Infectious Diseases

Infectious Diseases

SECOND EDITION

Sherwood L. Gorbach, MD
Professor of Community Health, Medicine, and Molecular Biology
Tufts University School of Medicine
Attending Physician, New England Medical Center and
St. Elizabeth's Hospital
Boston, Massachusetts

John G. Bartlett, MD
Stanhope Bayne Jones Professor of Medicine
The Johns Hopkins University School of Medicine
Chief, Division of Infectious Diseases
The Johns Hopkins Hospital
Baltimore, Maryland

Neil R. Blacklow, MD
Chairman, Department of Medicine
Richard M. Haidack Distinguished Professor of Medicine,
Molecular Genetics, and Microbiology
University of Massachusetts Medical School
Worcester, Massachusetts

W.B. SAUNDERS COMPANY
A Division of Harcourt Brace & Company
Philadelphia • London • Toronto • Montreal • Sydney • Tokyo

W.B. SAUNDERS COMPANY
A Division of Harcourt Brace & Company

The Curtis Center
Independence Square West
Philadelphia, Pennsylvania 19106

Library of Congress Cataloging-in-Publication Data

Infectious diseases / [edited by] Sherwood L. Gorbach, John G. Bartlett, Neil R. Blacklow.—2nd ed.

p. cm.

Includes bibliographical references and index.

ISBN 0–7216–6119–X

1. Communicable diseases. I. Gorbach, Sherwood L. II. Bartlett, John G. III. Blacklow, Neil R.

[DNLM: 1. Communicable Diseases. WC 100 I433 1998]

RC111.I5174 1998 616.9—dc20

DNLM/DLC 96–28575

INFECTIOUS DISEASES ISBN 0–7216–6119–X

Printed in the United States of America.

Last digit is the print number: 9 8 7 6 5 4 3 2 1

To Judy, Jean, and Margery
Who supported us in this, and in every other, endeavor;

To our students, house officers,
fellows, and colleagues
Who inspired us to learn and study,
and for whom we have written it down; and

To our patients
Who made it worth the while.

CONTRIBUTORS

MICHELLE J. ALFA, PhD
Associate Professor, Department of Medical Microbiology, University of Manitoba; Assistant Director, Microbiology, St. Boniface General Hospital, Winnipeg, Manitoba, Canada
Chancroid, Lymphogranuloma Venereum, and Granuloma Inguinale

BAN MISHU ALLOS, MD
Assistant Professor of Medicine and Preventive Medicine, Vanderbilt University School of Medicine, Nashville, Tennessee
Campylobacter Infections; *Campylobacter*

LARRY J. ANDERSON, MD
Chief, Respiratory and Enterovirus Branch, Centers for Disease Control and Prevention, Atlanta, Georgia
Poliovirus; Coxsackievirus, Echovirus, and Other Enteroviruses

VINCENT T. ANDRIOLE, MD
Professor of Medicine, Yale University School of Medicine; Attending Physician, Yale–New Haven Hospital, New Haven, Connecticut
Quinolones

ADRIANO ARGUEDAS, MD
Professor of Pediatrics, Universidad Autonoma de Ciencias Medicas; Attending Physician, Pediatric Infectious Diseases, Medicine 1 Department, National Children's Hospital, San Jose, Costa Rica
Mumps; Mumps Virus

DAVID M. ASHER, MD
Chief, Laboratory of Method Development, Center for Biologics Evaluation and Research, Food and Drug Administration, Rockville, Maryland
Slow Viral Infections of the Central Nervous System; Transmissible Spongiform Encephalopathies

ROBERT AUSTRIAN, MD, DSc (Hon)
John Herr Musser Professor and Chairman Emeritus, Department of Research Medicine, University of Pennsylvania School of Medicine; Visiting Physician, Hospital of the University of Pennsylvania, Philadelphia, Pennsylvania
Streptococcus pneumoniae

MICHAEL C. BACH, MD
Clinical Professor of Medicine, University of South Florida, Tampa; Hospital Epidemiologist, Infectious Disease Consultant, Manatee Memorial Hospital, Bradenton; Sarasota Memorial Hospital, Sarasota; Doctor's Hospital, Sarasota; and Columbia Blake Medical Center, Bradenton, Florida
Nocardia

ANN SULLIVAN BAKER, MD
Late Associate Professor of Medicine, Harvard Medical School; Physician, Infectious Disease Unit, Massachusetts General Hospital; Director, Infectious Diseases, Massachusetts Eye and Ear Infirmary, Boston, Massachusetts
Infections of Head and Neck Spaces and Salivary Glands; Infections of the Pharynx, Larynx, Epiglottis, Trachea, and Thyroid; Orbital Infections

JUAN C. BANDRES, MD, PhD
Research Assistant Professor, Departments of Medicine and Pathology, New York University; Staff Physician, Manhattan VA Medical Center, New York, New York
Approach to the Patient with Diarrhea

NEIL L. BARG, MD
Associate Professor, University of Michigan Medical School; Assistant Chief, Infectious Diseases, Department of Veterans Affairs Medical Center, Ann Arbor, Michigan
Infections Associated with Corticosteroids and Immunosuppressive Therapy

JOHN G. BARTLETT, MD
Stanhope Bayne Jones Professor of Medicine, The Johns Hopkins University School of Medicine; Chief, Division of Infectious Diseases, The Johns Hopkins Hospital, Baltimore, Maryland
Tables of Antimicrobial Agents; Approach to the Patient with Pneumonia; Bacterial Pneumonia; Bronchitis; Aspiration Pneumonia; Lung Abscess and Necrotizing Pneumonia; Empyema; *Clostridium difficile*–Associated Diarrhea and Colitis; Pyogenic Liver Abscess; Gastrointestinal Complications of Human Immunodeficiency Virus Infection; Human Immunodeficiency Virus Serology and Viral Burden; Antiretroviral Treatment; Glanders; Anaerobic Bacteria; Anaerobic Cocci; *Clostridium tetani;* Agents of Actinomycosis

MICHAEL BARZA, MD
Professor of Medicine, Tufts University School of Medicine; Associate Chief, Division of Geographic Medicine and Infectious Diseases, New England Medical Center, Boston, Massachusetts
Pharmacologic Principles; Infections of the Eye

ROBERT E. BAUGHN, PhD
Professor of Dermatology, Professor of Microbiology and Immunology, Baylor College of Medicine; Director, Syphilis Research Laboratory, Veterans Affairs Medical Center, Houston, Texas
Syphilis; Treponemes: Microbiology

JULES BAUM, MD
Research Professor of Ophthalmology, Tufts University School of Medicine, Boston, Massachusetts
Infections of the Eye

STEPHEN G. BAUM, MD
Professor of Medicine, Microbiology, and Immunology, Albert Einstein College of Medicine, Bronx; Chairman, Department of Medicine, Beth Israel Medical Center, New York, New York
Viral Pneumonia; Acute Viral Meningitis and Encephalitis

THEODORE M. BAYLESS, MD
Professor of Medicine, Department of Medicine, Division of Gastroenterology, The Johns Hopkins University School of Medicine; Clinical Director, Meyerhoff Digestive Disease–Inflammatory Bowel Disease Center, The Johns Hopkins Hospital, Baltimore, Maryland
Whipple's Disease

IRMGARD BEHLAU, MD
Research Fellow, Tufts University School of Medicine, Molecular Biology and Microbiology, Boston, Massachusetts
Infections of the Pharynx, Larynx, Epiglottis, Trachea, and Thyroid

JEFFREY D. BERNHARD, MD
Professor of Medicine, Director, Division of Dermatology, University of Massachusetts Medical School; Director, Division of Dermatology, University of Massachusetts Medical Center, Worcester, Massachusetts
Warts

DAVID I. BERNSTEIN, MD
Professor of Pediatrics, University of Cincinnati College of Medicine; Associate Director, Division of Infectious Diseases, Children's Hospital Medical Center, Cincinnati, Ohio
Measles; Rubeola (Measles) and Subacute Sclerosing Panencephalitis Virus

ALICE N. BESSMAN, MD
Emeritus Professor of Medicine, University of Southern California, Los Angeles; Former Chief, Ortho-Diabetes Service, Rancho Los Amigos Medical Center, Downey, California
Foot Infections in the Diabetic Patient and Infections Associated with Pressure Sores

NEIL R. BLACKLOW, MD
Chairman, Department of Medicine, Richard M. Haidack Distinguished Professor of Medicine, Molecular Genetics, and Microbiology, University of Massachusetts Medical School, Worcester, Massachusetts
Viral Gastroenteritis; Virus Classification; Caliciviruses and Astroviruses

CHARLES D. BLUESTONE, MD
Eberly Professor of Pediatric Otolaryngology, University of Pittsburgh School of Medicine; Director, Department of Pediatric Otolaryngology, Children's Hospital of Pittsburgh, Pittsburgh, Pennsylvania
Ear and Mastoid Infections

GERALD P. BODEY, MD
Emeritus Professor of Medicine, University of Texas M. D. Anderson Cancer Center; Professor of Internal Medicine and Pharmacology, University of Texas Health Science Center at Houston; Adjunct Professor of Microbiology and Immunology and Medicine, Baylor College of Medicine, Houston, Texas
Infections Associated with Malignancy

ROGER C. BONE, MD
Distinguished Professor of Medicine, Rush Medical College, Chicago, Illinois
Sepsis

JOHN W. BOSLEGO, MD
Director, Vaccine Infectious Diseases Clinical Research, Merck Research Laboratories, West Point, Pennsylvania
Neisseria gonorrhoeae; Neisseria meningitidis

EDWARD J. BOTTONE, PhD
Professor of Medicine, Professor of Microbiology, Professor of Pathology, Mount Sinai School of Medicine; Director for Consultative Microbiology, Division of Infectious Diseases, Department of Medicine, The Mount Sinai Hospital, New York, New York
Yersinia enterocolitica Infections; *Francisella tularensis, Pasteurella,* and *Yersinia pestis*

THOMAS G. BOYCE, MD
Medical Epidemiologist, Foodborne and Diarrheal Diseases Branch, Division of Bacterial and Mycotic Diseases, National Center for Infectious Diseases, Centers for Disease Control and Prevention, Atlanta, Georgia
Escherichia coli O157:H7 and Other Shiga Toxin–Producing *E. coli*

CLAIRE BROOME, MD
Deputy Director, Centers for Disease Control and Prevention, Atlanta, Georgia
Listeria monocytogenes

THOMAS BUTLER, MD
Professor of Internal Medicine, Texas Tech University Health Sciences Center; Attending Physician, University Medical Center, Lubbock, Texas
Relapsing Fever; *Borrelia* Species and *Spirillum minus*

FRANK M. CALIA, MD
Professor of Medicine, Vice-Dean and Senior Associate Dean for Academic Affairs, University of Maryland School of Medicine, Baltimore, Maryland
Clindamycin; Macrolide (and Azalide) Antibiotics: Erythromycin, Azithromycin, Clarithromycin, and Dirithromycin; Chloramphenicol

CARLOS CARRILLO, MD
Principal Professor of Microbiology, Universidad Peruana Cayetano Heredia; Director, Instituto Nacional de Salud, Lima, Peru
Brucella

KENNETH G. CASTRO, MD
Director, Division of Tuberculosis Elimination, National Center for HIV, STD, and TB Prevention, Centers for Disease Control and Prevention, Atlanta, Georgia
Antimycobacterial Drugs

MARSHA L. CHAFFINS, MD
Henry Ford Hospital, Detroit, Michigan
Cutaneous Infections in Human Immunodeficiency Virus Disease

RICHARD E. CHAISSON, MD
Associate Professor of Medicine, Epidemiology, and International Health, The Johns Hopkins University; Director, AIDS Service, The Johns Hopkins Hospital, Baltimore, Maryland
International Epidemiology of the Human Immunodeficiency Virus

SARAH H. CHEESEMAN, MD
Professor of Medicine, Pediatrics, and Molecular Genetics and Microbiology, Division of Infectious Diseases, University of Massachusetts Medical School, Worcester, Massachusetts
Cytomegalovirus Infections; Cytomegalovirus

JAMES E. CHILDS, ScD
Epidemiology Section Chief, Viral and Rickettsial Zoonoses Branch, Centers for Disease Control and Prevention, Atlanta, Georgia
Rabies; Rabies Virus

ANTHONY W. CHOW, MD, FRCPC, FACP
Professor of Medicine, Division of Infectious Diseases, Department of Medicine, and Director, MD/PhD Program, University of British Columbia; Attending Physician, Division of Infectious Diseases, Department of Medicine, Vancouver Hospital and Health Sciences Center, Vancouver, British Columbia, Canada
Infections of the Sinuses and Parameningeal Structures

CLAY J. COCKERELL, MD
Associate Professor of Dermatology and Pathology, Training Director, Division of Dermatopathology, University of Texas Southwestern Medical School, Dallas, Texas
Cutaneous Infections in Human Immunodeficiency Virus Disease

MITCHELL L. COHEN, MD
Director, Division of Bacterial and Mycotic Diseases, National Center for Infectious Diseases, Centers for Disease Control and Prevention, Atlanta, Georgia
Epidemiology of Community-Acquired Infections

ROBERT E. CONDON, MD
Ausman Foundation Professor of Surgery, Medical College of Wisconsin; Staff Surgeon, Froedtert Memorial Lutheran Hospital, Milwaukee, Wisconsin
Intraabdominal Infections; Appendicitis

DEBORAH COTTON, MD, MPH
Associate Professor of Medicine, Harvard Medical School; Associate Professor in the Department of Health Policy and Management, Harvard School of Public Health; Director of Clinical Epidemiology, Partners' AIDS Research Center, Massachusetts General Hospital, Boston, Massachusetts
Women with Acquired Immunodeficiency Syndrome

WILLIAM A. CRAIG, MD
Professor of Medicine, University of Wisconsin; Associate Chief of Staff for Education, Chief, Infectious Diseases, William S. Middleton Memorial VA Hospital, Madison, Wisconsin
Penicillins; Rifampin and Related Drugs

MARINELLA CARDELLO CUMMINGS, MS
Director, Sexually Transmitted Diseases Research Laboratory, State University of New York, Health Science Center, Brooklyn, New York
Mycoplasmas and Ureaplasmas

BURKE A. CUNHA, MD
Chief, Infectious Disease Division, Winthrop–University Hospital, Mineola, New York; Professor of Medicine, State University of New York School of Medicine, Stony Brook, New York
Clinical Approach to Fever; Fever of Unknown Origin

JOHN S. CZACHOR, MD
Associate Professor of Medicine, Wright State University School of Medicine; Infectious Disease Staff Physician, Miami Valley Medical Center, Dayton, Ohio
Trimethoprim-Sulfamethoxazole

JENNIFER S. DALY, MD
Associate Professor of Medicine, Division of Infectious Diseases, University of Massachusetts Medical School, Worcester, Massachusetts
Cat-Scratch Disease; *Bartonella* Species

RICHARD F. D'AMATO, PhD
Clinical Associate Professor, Laboratory Medicine, Albert Einstein College of Medicine, Bronx; Director, Clinical Microbiology, Co-Director, Infection Control and Environmental Health, Catholic Medical Center of Brooklyn and Queens, Jamaica, New York
Enterobacteriaceae

RAYMOND J. DATTWYLER, MD
Professor of Medicine, Division Chief, Allergy Department, and Director, Lyme Disease Center, State University of New York School of Medicine, Stony Brook; Attending Physician, Northport VA Medical Center, Northport, New York
Borrelia burgdorferi

LAWRENCE J. DAVIS, MD
Instructor in Clinical Medicine, Cornell University Medical College; Assistant Attending Physician, The New York Hospital–Cornell Medical Center, New York, New York
Cryptosporidium, Isospora, Cyclospora, Microsporidia, and *Dientamoeba*

GEORGE S. DEEPE, JR., MD
Professor of Medicine, University of Cincinnati College of Medicine, Cincinnati, Ohio
Skin Testing; *Blastomyces* and *Paracoccidioides: Blastomyces; Paracoccidioides*

E. PATCHEN DELLINGER, MD
Professor of Surgery, University of Washington School of Medicine; Chief, Division of General Surgery, Department of Surgery, University of Washington Medical Center, Seattle, Washington
Approach to the Patient with Postoperative Fever

STANLEY C. DERESINSKI, MD
Clinical Professor of Medicine, Stanford University, Stanford; Associate Chief, Division of Infectious Diseases, Santa Clara Valley Medical Center, San Jose; Medical Director, AIDS Health Services, Santa Clara County; Medical Director, AIDS Community Research Consortium, Redwood City, California
Coccidioides immitis

DICKSON D. DESPOMMIER, PhD
Professor of Public Health and Microbiology, Columbia University, New York, New York
Intestinal Nematodes; Tissue Nematodes

WILLIAM E. DISMUKES, MD
Professor and Vice Chairman, Department of Medicine, Director, Division of Infectious Diseases, University of Alabama at Birmingham, Birmingham, Alabama
Antifungal Drugs

GARY DOERN, PhD
Professor of Medicine, Molecular Genetics and Microbiology, and Pathology, University of Massachusetts Medical Center; Director, Clinical Microbiology Laboratories, Worcester, Massachusetts
Streptobacillus moniliformis; Calymmatobacterium granulomatis

J. STEPHEN DUMLER, MD
Associate Professor of Pathology, Director, Division of Medical Microbiology, and Associate Professor of Molecular Microbiology and Immunology, The Johns Hopkins University School of Medicine and Hygiene and Public Health; Director, Division of Medical Microbiology, Department of Pathology, The Johns Hopkins Hospital, Baltimore, Maryland
Rocky Mountain Spotted Fever; *Rickettsia rickettsii* (Rocky Mountain Spotted Fever)

HERBERT L. DuPONT, MD
Mary W. Kelsey Professor of Medicine, University of Texas Medical School; Chairman, Department of Medicine, St. Luke's Episcopal Hospital, Houston, Texas
Approach to the Patient with Diarrhea

WILLIAM A. DURBIN, JR., MD
Professor of Pediatrics and Medicine, Director, Division of Pediatric Infectious Diseases, University of Massachusetts Medical School, Worcester, Massachusetts
Bordetella

GEORGE M. ELIOPOULOS, MD
Associate Professor of Medicine, Harvard Medical School; Assistant Chairman, Department of Medicine, Deaconess Hospital, Boston, Massachusetts
Mechanisms of Bacterial Resistance to Antimicrobial Drugs

RICHARD T. ELLISON, III, MD
Professor of Medicine, University of Massachusetts Medical School; Clinical Director, Infectious Diseases, University of Massachusetts Medical Center, Worcester, Massachusetts
Infections Associated with Bone Marrow Transplantation

JERROLD J. ELLNER, MD
Professor of Medicine and Pathology, Case Western Reserve University; Physician, Acting Chairman, Department of Medicine, University Hospitals of Cleveland, Cleveland, Ohio
Tuberculosis; *Mycobacterium tuberculosis* and Other Mycobacteria

LAWRENCE J. ERON, MD
Infectious Diseases Consultant, Kanai Medical Clinic, Lihue, Hawaii
Human Papillomaviruses and Anogenital Disease

DAVID A. ESCHENBACH, MD
Professor, Chief, Division of Gynecology, Department of Obstetrics and Gynecology, University of Washington, Seattle, Washington
Vaginitis, Cervicitis, and Endometritis

JOSEPH J. ESPOSITO, PhD
Director, World Health Organization Collaborating Centre for Smallpox and Other Poxvirus Infections; Chief, Poxvirus Section, Centers for Disease Control and Prevention, Atlanta, Georgia
Smallpox

MAX ESSEX, DVM, PhD
Chairman, Department of Cancer Biology; Chairman, Harvard AIDS Institute; and Mary Woodard Lasker Professor of Health Sciences, Harvard School of Public Health, Boston, Massachusetts
Human Immunodeficiency Virus and Other Retroviruses

CHRISTOPHER H. FANTA, MD
Pulmonary Division, Brigham and Women's Hospital and Harvard Medical School, Boston, Massachusetts
Pneumonias in Immunocompromised Hosts

MICHAEL J. G. FARTHING, MD, FRCP
Professor of Gastroenterology, St. Bartholomew's Hospital Medical College; Professor of Gastroenterology and Honorary Consultant Physician, St. Bartholomew's and St. Mark's Hospitals, London, England
Giardia lamblia

DAVID S. FEINGOLD, MD
Professor of Dermatology and Medicine, Tufts University School of Medicine; Dermatologist-in-Chief, New England Medical Center, Boston, Massachusetts
Approach to the Patient with Skin or Soft Tissue Infection, Normal Cutaneous Flora and Infections They Cause; Staphylococcal and Streptococcal Skin or Soft Tissue Infections; Gram-Negative Bacillary Skin or Soft Tissue Infections; Cutaneous Abscesses and Ulcers

MAKONNEN FEKADU, DVM, PhD
Epidemiology Section, Viral and Rickettsial Zoonoses Branch, Centers for Disease Control and Prevention, Atlanta, Georgia
Rabies Virus

ROBERT FEKETY, MD
Professor Emeritus, Division of Infectious Diseases, Department of Medicine, University of Michigan Medical School, Ann Arbor, Michigan
Infections Associated with Corticosteroids and Immunosuppressive Therapy

SYDNEY M. FINEGOLD, MD
Professor of Medicine, Professor of Microbiology and Immunology, UCLA School of Medicine; Staff Physician, Infectious Diseases Section, VA Medical Center, West Los Angeles, Los Angeles, California
Anaerobic Gram-Negative Rods: *Bacteroides, Prevotella, Porphyromonas, Fusobacterium, Bilophila, Sutterella*

STACI A. FISCHER, MD
Assistant Professor of Medicine, Rush Medical College; Attending Physician, Section of Infectious Disease, Rush–Presbyterian–St. Luke's Medical Center, Chicago, Illinois
Brain Abscess

CONSTANTINE T. FRANTZIDES, MD, PhD
Associate Professor of Surgery, Medical College of Wisconsin, Milwaukee, Wisconsin
Diverticulitis

THOMAS R. GADACZ, MD
Professor of Surgery, Chair, Department of Surgery, Medical College of Georgia, Augusta, Georgia
Splenic Abscess

PIERCE GARDNER, MD, FACP
Professor of Medicine, Associate Dean for Academic Affairs, State University of New York at Stony Brook, Stony Brook, New York
Central Nervous System Shunt Infections

ROBERT P. GAYNES, MD
Chief, Nosocomial Infections Surveillance Activity Hospital Infections Program, Centers for Disease Control and Prevention, Atlanta, Georgia
Aminoglycosides

BRUCE G. GELLIN, MD, MPH
Medical Officer, Division of Microbiology and Infectious Diseases, National Institute of Allergy and Infectious Diseases, National Institutes of Health, Bethesda, Maryland
Reye's Syndrome

DAVID F. GIANSIRACUSA, MD
Professor of Medicine, Vice Chair, Department of Medicine, University of Massachusetts Medical School, Worcester, Massachusetts
Septic Arthritis

RONALD S. GIBBS, MD
Professor and Chair, Department of Obstetrics and Gynecology, University of Colorado School of Medicine, Denver, Colorado
Infections Associated with Pregnancy, Delivery, and Abortion

RICHARD GLECKMAN, MD
Professor of Medicine, Boston University School of Medicine; Director of Medicine and Residency Program Director, Carney Hospital, Boston, Massachusetts
Trimethoprim-Sulfamethoxazole

RICHARD H. GLEW, MD
Professor of Medicine, Molecular Genetics, and Microbiology, University of Massachusetts Medical School; Chairman, Chief Medical Officer, Department of Medicine, The Memorial Hospital, Worcester, Massachusetts
Vancomycin and Teicoplanin

W. PAUL GLEZEN, MD
Professor and Head, Preventive Medicine Section, Departments of Microbiology and Immunology and Pediatrics, Baylor College of Medicine; Senior Attending Pediatrician, Ben Taub General Hospital, Houston, Texas
The Common Cold

MARCIA B. GOLDBERG, MD
Assistant Professor, Department of Medicine, Division of Infectious Diseases, Albert Einstein College of Medicine, Bronx, New York
Salmonella Infections; *Salmonella*

DONALD A. GOLDMANN, MD
Professor of Pediatrics, Harvard Medical School; Hospital Epidemiologist, Director of Microbiology Laboratory, and Chief, Janeway Medical Service, Children's Hospital, Boston, Massachusetts
Epidemiology of Nosocomial Infections; Control of Nosocomial Infections

ANA M. GOMEZ, MD, PhD
Resident, Department of Pathology, University of Cincinnati School of Medicine, Cincinnati, Ohio
Blastomyces and *Paracoccidioides: Paracoccidioides*

SHERWOOD L. GORBACH, MD
Professor of Community Health, Medicine, and Molecular Biology, Tufts University School of Medicine; Attending Physician, New England Medical Center and St. Elizabeth's Hospital, Boston, Massachusetts
Side Effects of Antimicrobial Therapy; Traveler's Diarrhea; Gas Gangrene and Other Clostridial Skin and Soft Tissue Infections; Necrotizing Skin and Soft Tissue Infections; *Clostridium perfringens* and Other Clostridia

EDUARDO GOTUZZO, MD, FACP
Principal Professor of Medicine, Universidad Peruana Cayetano Heredia; Director, Instituto de Medicina Tropical "Alexander von Humboldt," and Chairman, Department of Transmissible Diseases, Hospital Nacional Cayetano Heredia, Lima, Peru
Brucella

JOHN R. GRAYBILL, MD
Professor and Chief, Division of Infectious Diseases, Department of Medicine, University of Texas Health Science Center; Staff Physician, Audie Murphy Memorial Veterans Administration Hospital, San Antonio, Texas
Cryptococcus neoformans

RONALD A. GREENFIELD, MD
Professor of Medicine, University of Oklahoma Health Sciences Center; Chief, Infectious Diseases Section, Department of Veterans Affairs Medical Center, Oklahoma City, Oklahoma
Sporothrix schenckii

MICHAEL H. GRIECO, MD
Professor of Clinical Medicine, Columbia University College of Physicians and Surgeons; Director, Department of Medicine, St. Luke's–Roosevelt Hospital Center, New York, New York
Approach to the Immunocompromised Patient

DIANE E. GRIFFIN, MD, PhD
Professor and Chair, Molecular Microbiology and Immunology, Professor, Medicine and Neurology, The Johns Hopkins University School of Hygiene and Public Health, The Johns Hopkins University School of Medicine, Baltimore, Maryland
Approach to the Patient with Infection of the Central Nervous System

PATRICIA M. GRIFFIN, MD
Chief, Foodborne Diseases Epidemiology Section, Centers for Disease Control and Prevention, Atlanta, Georgia
Escherichia coli O157:H7 and Other Shiga Toxin–Producing *E. coli*

JEFFREY K. GRIFFITHS, MD, MPHTM
Assistant Professor of Medicine and Comparative Medicine, Divisions of Geographic Medicine and Infectious Diseases, Tufts University Schools of Medicine and Veterinary Medicine; Staff Physician, Division of Infectious Diseases, St. Elizabeth's Medical Center of Boston, Boston, Massachusetts
Serum Therapy and Augmentation of the Host Response

CHARLES GROSE, MD
Professor of Pediatrics and Microbiology, The University of Iowa College of Medicine; Director of Infectious Diseases, Department of Pediatrics, The University of Iowa Hospital, Iowa City, Iowa
Varicella and Herpes Zoster; Varicella-Zoster Virus

ALEJANDRA C. GURTMAN, MD
Assistant Professor of Medicine, Mount Sinai School of Medicine; Attending Physician, Assistant Director, AIDS Center, The Mount Sinai Hospital, New York, New York
Miscellaneous Drugs; Phycomycetes

NEAL HALSEY, MD
Professor and Director, Division of Disease Control, Department of International Health, and Professor, Department of Pediatrics, The Johns Hopkins University, Baltimore, Maryland
Corynebacteria

SCOTT B. HALSTEAD, MD
Senior Scientist, Department of Molecular Microbiology and Immunology, School of Hygiene and Public Health, The Johns Hopkins University, Baltimore; Scientific Director, Infectious Diseases, Naval Medical Research and Development Command, National Naval Medical Center, Bethesda, Maryland
Dengue Viruses

DAVIDSON H. HAMER, MD
Assistant Professor of Medicine, Tufts University School of Medicine; Director, Traveler's Health Service, Associate Director, Infectious Diseases Center, New England Medical Center, Boston, Massachusetts
Intestinal Nematodes; Tissue Nematodes

MARGARET R. HAMMERSCHLAG, MD
Professor of Pediatrics and Medicine, State University of New York Health Science Center at Brooklyn; Co-Director, Division of Pediatric Infectious Diseases, University Hospital of Brooklyn, Kings County Hospital Center, Brooklyn, New York
Chlamydia Pneumonia

H. HUNTER HANDSFIELD, MD
Professor of Medicine, University of Washington School of Medicine; Director, Sexually Transmitted Disease Control Program, Seattle–King County Department of Public Health, Seattle, Washington
Approach to the Patient with Sexually Transmitted Disease

ALAN A. HARRIS, MD
Professor of Medicine and Preventive Medicine, Rush Medical College; Senior Assistant Chairman and Program Director, Department of Internal Medicine, and Hospital Epidemiologist, Rush–Presbyterian–St. Luke's Medical Center, Chicago, Illinois
Chronic Meningitis; Brain Abscess

CHARLES L. HATHEWAY, PhD
Chief, Botulism Laboratory, Centers for Disease Control and Prevention, National Center for Infectious Diseases, Division of Bacterial and Mycotic Diseases, Atlanta, Georgia
Clostridium botulinum

JAMES A. HELLINGER, MD
Research Physician, Community Research Initiative of New England, Brookline, Massachusetts
Human Immunodeficiency Virus and Other Retroviruses

H. FRANKLIN HERLONG, MD
Associate Professor of Medicine, The Johns Hopkins School of Medicine, Baltimore, Maryland
Approach to the Patient with Infection of the Liver

JOHN E. HERRMANN, PhD
Professor of Medicine, Molecular Genetics and Microbiology, Division of Infectious Diseases, University of Massachusetts Medical School, Worcester, Massachusetts
Rotaviruses and Other Reoviridae

DAVID W. HINES, MD
Section Head, Infectious Diseases, Rush/Westlake Hospital, Melrose Park; Assistant Professor, Rush Medical College, Chicago, Illinois
Sepsis

JAN V. HIRSCHMANN, MD
Professor of Medicine, University of Washington School of Medicine; Assistant Chief, Medical Service, Puget Sound VA Medical Center, Seattle, Washington
Antimicrobial Prophylaxis for Nonsurgical Infections; Approach to the Patient with Skin or Soft Tissue Infection; Normal Cutaneous Flora and Infections They Cause; Staphylococcal and Streptococcal Skin or Soft Tissue Infections; Gram-Negative Bacillary Skin or Soft Tissue Infections; Cutaneous Abscesses and Ulcers

CHARLES H. HOKE, JR., MD
Attending Physician, Infectious Diseases Service, Walter Reed Army Medical Center; Director, Division of Communicable Diseases and Immunology, Walter Reed Army Institute of Research, Washington, DC
Encephalitis Viruses Belonging to the Families Flaviviridae, Togaviridae, and Bunyaviridae

DAVE HOLLANDER, MD
Assistant Professor of Neurology, Tufts University School of Medicine; Associate Director, Neuromuscular Research Unit, New England Medical Center, Boston, Massachusetts
Infections of Muscle

JAMES W. C. HOLMES, MD, FACS
Professor of Clinical Surgery, Head, Section of Colo-Rectal Surgery, Tulane University School of Medicine, The Tulane University Hospital and Clinic, New Orleans, Louisiana
Peritonitis

PAUL D. HOLTOM, MD
Assistant Professor of Clinical Medicine and Orthopaedics, University of Southern California, Los Angeles, California
Coxiella burnetii (Q Fever)

EDWARD W. HOOK, MD
Professor of Medicine, University of Alabama at Birmingham; University of Alabama Hospital, Birmingham, Alabama
Gonorrhea

PHILIP C. HOPEWELL, MD
Professor of Medicine, University of California, San Francisco; Chief, Division of Pulmonary and Critical Care Medicine, San Francisco General Hospital Medical Center, San Francisco, California
Pulmonary Infections in Patients with Human Immunodeficiency Virus Infections

CYRUS C. HOPKINS, MD
Associate Professor of Medicine, Harvard Medical School; Hospital Epidemiologist, Clinical Chief, Infectious Diseases Unit, Massachusetts General Hospital, Boston, Massachusetts
Epidemiology of Nosocomial Infections; Control of Nosocomial Infections

C. ROBERT HORSBURGH, JR., MD
Professor of Medicine, Emory University School of Medicine; Director, Mycobacterial Center, Grady Memorial Hospital, Atlanta, Georgia
Antimycobacterial Drugs

MARSHALL S. HORWITZ, MD
Leo and Julie Forchheimer Professor and Chair, Microbiology and Immunology, Albert Einstein College of Medicine of Yeshiva University, Bronx, New York
Adenoviruses

WALTER T. HUGHES, MD
Arthur Ashe Chair in Pediatric AIDS Research and Professor of Pediatrics, University of Tennessee College of Medicine; Department of Infectious Diseases, St. Jude Children's Research Hospital, Memphis, Tennessee
Pneumocystis carinii Pneumonia; *Pneumocystis carinii*

NEWTON E. HYSLOP, JR., MD
Professor of Medicine, Tulane University School of Medicine; Chief, Infectious Disease Section, Co-Principal Investigator, Tulane-LSU AIDS Clinical Trials Unit, and Medical Director, HIV/AIDS/Tuberculosis In-Patient Unit at Charity Hospital, Tulane University Medical Center, New Orleans, Louisiana
Infectious Diseases of the Spinal Cord and Peripheral Nervous System

MICHAEL D. ISEMAN, MD
Professor of Medicine, Divisions of Pulmonary Sciences and Infectious Diseases, University of Colorado School of Medicine; Chief, Clinical Mycobacterial Disease Service, National Jewish Center for Immunology and Respiratory Medicine, Denver, Colorado
Nontuberculous Mycobacterial Infections

HENRY D. ISENBERG, PhD
Professor, Laboratory Medicine, Albert Einstein College of Medicine, Bronx; Chief, Microbiology, The Long Island Jewish Medical Center, The Long Island Campus for Albert Einstein College of Medicine, New Hyde Park, New York
Clinical Microbiology; *Enterobacteriaceae*

HILLEL K. JANAI, MD
General Pediatrics, Pediatric Infectious Diseases, Pediatric Pulmonary, Arroyo Grande Community Hospital, Arroyo Grande, California
Mumps; Mumps Virus

STEVEN A. JENISON, MD
Assistant Professor, University of New Mexico Health Sciences Center, Albuquerque, New Mexico
Hantaviruses

RICHARD T. JOHNSON, MD
Professor and Director of Neurology, Professor of Microbiology and Professor of Neuroscience, The Johns Hopkins University School of Medicine; Neurologist-in-Chief, The Johns Hopkins Hospital, Baltimore, Maryland
Human T-Cell Lymphotropic Virus Type I and Neurologic Diseases

WARREN D. JOHNSON, JR., MD
B. H. Kean Professor of Tropical Medicine, Chief, Division of International Medicine and Infectious Diseases, Cornell University Medical College; Attending Physician, The New York Hospital, New York, New York
Leishmania

KEITH A. JOINER, MD
Professor of Medicine, Epidemiology and Public Health, Cell Biology, Yale University School of Medicine, New Haven, Connecticut
Other Virulence Factors

RONALD C. JONES, MD
Chief of Surgery, Baylor University Medical Center, Dallas, Texas
Surgical Infections in Trauma

ADOLF W. KARCHMER, MD
Professor of Medicine, Harvard Medical School; Chief, Division of Infectious Diseases, Beth Israel Deaconess Medical Center, Boston, Massachusetts
Infections in a Prosthetic Device

DENNIS L. KASPER, MD
William Ellery Channing Professor of Medicine, Harvard Medical School; Director, Channing Laboratory, Co-Director, Division of Infectious Diseases, and Executive Vice Chairman, Department of Medicine, Brigham and Women's Hospital, Boston, Massachusetts
Group B *Streptococcus*

AMALIE M. KASS, MEd
Lecturer in The History of Medicine, Harvard Medical School, Boston, Massachusetts
A Perspective on the History of Infectious Diseases

EDWARD H. KASS, PhD, MD
Late William Ellery Channing Professor Emeritus, Harvard Medical School, Boston, Massachusetts
A Perspective on the History of Infectious Diseases

DONALD KAYE, MD
Klinghoffer Professor of Medicine and Executive Vice President for Health Affairs, Allegheny University of the Health Sciences, Philadelphia, Pennsylvania
Endocarditis

KENNETH M. KAYE, MD
Assistant Professor of Medicine, Harvard Medical School; Associate Physician, Brigham and Women's Hospital, Boston, Massachusetts
Epstein-Barr Virus Infection and Infectious Mononucleosis; Epstein-Barr Virus

PATRICK W. KELLEY, MD, DrPH
Adjunct Assistant Professor, Department of Preventive Medicine and Biostatistics, Uniformed Services University of the Health Sciences, Bethesda, Maryland; Director, Division of Preventive Medicine, Walter Reed Army Institute of Research, Washington, DC
Leptospirosis; *Leptospira*

CAROL A. KEMPER, MD
Clinical Assistant Professor of Medicine, Stanford University School of Medicine; Co-Medical Director, AIDS Health Services, Division of Infectious Diseases, Santa Clara Valley Medical Center, Stanford University, Stanford, California
Coccidioides immitis

MARK A. KEROACK, MD
Associate Professor of Medicine, University of Massachusetts Medical School; Chief, Infectious Disease Section, The Memorial Hospital, Worcester, Massachusetts
Vancomycin and Teicoplanin

GERALD T. KEUSCH, MD
Professor of Medicine, Tufts University School of Medicine; Chief, Division of Geographic Medicine and Infectious Diseases, New England Medical Center, Boston, Massachusetts
Shigellosis; *Shigella*

OLEN M. KEW, PhD
Chief, Molecular Virology Section, Centers for Disease Control and Prevention, Atlanta, Georgia
Poliovirus

ELLIOTT KIEFF, MD, PhD
Harriet Ryan Albee Professor of Medicine, Chairman, Committee on Virology, Harvard Medical School; Chief, Division of Infectious Diseases, Brigham and Women's Hospital, Boston, Massachusetts
Epstein-Barr Virus Infection and Infectious Mononucleosis; Epstein-Barr Virus

J. MICHAEL KILBY, MD
Assistant Professor of Medicine, University of Alabama at Birmingham; Medical Director, 1917 Clinic, Birmingham, Alabama
Antifungal Drugs

SEUNG H. KIM, MD
Chief, Pathology Branch, U.S. Army Institute of Surgical Research, Fort Sam Houston, San Antonio, Texas
Burns

CHARLES H. KING, MD
Associate Clinical Professor of Medicine, Case Western Reserve University; Physician, University Hospitals, Cleveland, Ohio
Schistosoma and Other Trematodes

KENNETH W. KIZER, MD, MPH
Adjunct Professor, University of Southern California, Los Angeles, California; Under Secretary for Health, U.S. Department of Veterans Affairs, Washington, DC
Animal Bites

ERNST KLAR, MD
Associate Professor of Surgery, University of Heidelberg, Heidelberg, Germany
Infection After Acute Pancreatitis

BRUCE S. KLEIN, MD
Associate Professor of Pediatrics, University of Wisconsin, Madison, Wisconsin
Blastomyces and *Paracoccidioides: Blastomyces*

JEROME O. KLEIN, MD
Professor of Pediatrics, Boston University School of Medicine; Director, Division of Pediatric Infectious Diseases, Maxwell Finland Laboratory for Infectious Diseases, Boston Medical Center, Boston, Massachusetts
Immunization of Children and Adults

MARK S. KLEMPNER, MD
Louisa C. Endicott Professor of Medicine, Professor of Microbiology and Molecular Biology, Tufts University School of Medicine; Associate Physician-in-Chief, Vice Chairman for Scientific Affairs, Department of Medicine, New England Medical Center, Boston, Massachusetts
Phagocytes: Normal and Abnormal Neutrophil Host Defenses

STEPHEN A. KLOTZ, MD
Professor of Medicine, University of Kansas School of Medicine, Kansas City, Kansas; Chief, Section of Infectious Diseases, Veterans Affairs Medical Center, Kansas City, Missouri
Anthrax; *Bacillus anthracis* and Other Aerobic Spore Formers

RAYMOND S. KOFF, MD
Professor of Medicine, University of Massachusetts Medical School, Worcester; Chairman, Department of Medicine, Columbia MetroWest Medical Center, Framingham and Natick, Massachusetts
Hepatitis B and Hepatitis D; Hepatitis C; Hepatitis E; Hepatitis B Virus and Hepatitis D Virus; Hepatitis C Virus; Hepatitis E Virus

OKSANA M. KORZENIOWSKI, MD
Professor of Medicine, Allegheny University; President, Medical/Dental Staff, Hospital Epidemiologist, Assistant Medical Director, and Medical Director, Quality Assurance, Allegheny University Hospital, East Falls, Philadelphia, Pennsylvania
Endocarditis

FREDERICK T. KOSTER, MD
Professor of Medicine, University of New Mexico Health Sciences Center, Albuquerque, New Mexico
Hantaviruses

CALVIN M. KUNIN, MD
Pomerene Professor of Internal Medicine, The Ohio State University; Attending Physician, The Ohio State University Hospital, Columbus, Ohio
Management of Urinary Catheters

JOHN R. LA MONTAGNE, PhD
Director, Division of Microbiology and Infectious Diseases, National Institute of Allergy and Infectious Diseases, National Institutes of Health, Bethesda, Maryland
Reye's Syndrome

TIMOTHY S. LEACH, MD, MPHTM
Assistant Professor of Medicine, University of New Jersey College of Medicine and Dentistry, Newark; Chief, Infection Control, Veterans Administration Medical Center, East Orange, New Jersey
Infectious Diseases of the Spinal Cord and Peripheral Nervous System

WILLIAM J. LEDGER, MD
Professor and Chairman, Department of Obstetrics and Gynecology, Cornell Medical College; Obstetrician-Gynecologist in Chief, New York–Presbyterian Hospital, New York, New York
Approach to the Patient with Infection of the Pelvis

JOHN M. LEEDOM, MD
Professor of Medicine, Chief, Division of Infectious Diseases, University of Southern California, Los Angeles, California
Coxiella burnetii (Q Fever)

THOMAS J. LEIPZIG, MD
Assistant Clinical Professor of Neurosurgery, Indiana University School of Medicine; Indianapolis Neurosurgical Group, Indianapolis, Indiana
Central Nervous System Shunt Infections

STANLEY M. LEMON, MD
Professor and Chairman, Department of Microbiology and Immunology, University of Texas Medical Branch, Galveston, Texas
Type A Viral Hepatitis; Hepatitis A Virus

STEPHEN A. LERNER, MD
Professor of Medicine, Vice Chief and Director of Research, Division of Infectious Diseases, Wayne State University School of Medicine, Detroit, Michigan
Aminoglycosides

DONALD Y. M. LEUNG, MD, PhD
Professor of Pediatrics, University of Colorado Health Sciences Center; Head of Division of Allergy-Immunology, National Jewish Medical and Research Center, Denver, Colorado
Kawasaki Syndrome

ROLAND A. LEVANDOWSKI, MD
Supervisory Medical Officer, Laboratory of Respiratory Viruses, Division of Viral Products, Center for Biologics Evaluation and Research, Bethesda, Maryland
Rhinoviruses

MYRON M. LEVINE, MD, DTPH
Professor, Department of Medicine and Department of Pediatrics, University of Maryland at Baltimore, Baltimore, Maryland
Specific and Nonspecific Treatment of Diarrhea

PAMELA A. LIPSETT, MD
Associate Professor of Surgery, Anesthesiology, and Critical Care Medicine, The Johns Hopkins University School of Medicine; Co-Director of the Surgical Intensive Care Unit, The Johns Hopkins Hospital, Baltimore, Maryland
Splenic Abscess

JEFFREY M. LISOWSKI, MD
Assistant Professor, Rush Medical College; Physician, Grant Hospital, Chicago, Illinois
Sepsis

NANCY Y. LIU, MD
Associate Professor of Clinical Medicine, Division of Rheumatology, University of Massachusetts Medical School, Worcester, Massachusetts
Septic Arthritis

DIANA N. J. LOCKWOOD, MD, MRCP
Senior Lecturer, Department of Infectious and Tropical Diseases, London School of Hygiene and Tropical Medicine; Consultant Leprologist, Hospital for Tropical Diseases, London, England
Leprosy; *Mycobacterium leprae*

WALTER J. LOESCHE, DMD, PhD
Professor, University of Michigan School of Dentistry; Professor of Microbiology, University of Michigan Medical School, Ann Arbor, Michigan
Dental Infections

DONALD B. LOURIA, MD
Professor and Chairman, Department of Preventive Medicine and Community Health, University of Medicine and Dentistry of New Jersey–New Jersey Medical School, Newark, New Jersey
Fungal Pneumonias

BENJAMIN J. LUFT, MD
Professor and Chair, Department of Medicine, State University of New York Health Science Center, Stony Brook, New York
Borrelia burgdorferi

KRISTINE L. MacDONALD, MD
Adjunct Associate Professor, University of Minnesota School of Public Health; Assistant State Epidemiologist, Minnesota Department of Health, Minneapolis, Minnesota
Toxic Shock Syndrome

JANINE R. MAENZA, MD
Assistant Professor of Medicine, The Johns Hopkins University School of Medicine, Baltimore, Maryland
Candida albicans and Related Species

JAMES H. MAGUIRE, MD
Associate Professor of Medicine, Harvard Medical School; Associate Professor in Tropical Public Health, Harvard School of Public Health; Clinical Director, Division of Infectious Disease, Brigham and Women's Hospital, Boston, Massachusetts
Trypanosoma

ADEL A. F. MAHMOUD, MD, PhD
Professor of Medicine, Chairman, Department of Medicine, Case Western Reserve University; Chairman of Medicine and Physician-in-Chief, Case Western Reserve University and University Hospitals, Cleveland, Ohio
Schistosoma and Other Trematodes

HARRY L. MALECH, MD
Deputy Chief, Laboratory of Host Defenses, National Institute of Allergy and Infectious Diseases, National Institutes of Health, Bethesda, Maryland
Phagocytes: Normal and Abnormal Neutrophil Host Defenses

LEONARD C. MARCUS, VMD, MD
Consultant in Tropical and Travel Medicine and Animal-Transmitted Diseases, Travelers' Health and Immunization Services, Newton, Massachusetts
Approach to the Patient with Zoonotic Infection

RICHARD B. MARKHAM, MD
Associate Professor of Molecular Microbiology and Immunology, The Johns Hopkins University School of Hygiene and Public Health, and Associate Professor, Department of Medicine, The Johns Hopkins University School of Medicine, Baltimore, Maryland
Cell-Mediated Immunity

MELVIN I. MARKS, MD
Professor and Vice-Chair, Department of Pediatrics, University of California, Irvine; Executive Director, Memorial Miller Children's Hospital and Health System, Long Beach, California
Mumps; Mumps Virus

J. JOSEPH MARR, MD
Executive Vice-President for Research and Development and Chief Scientific Officer, Immunologic Pharmaceutical Corporation, Waltham, Massachusetts
Amebic Liver Abscess

PHILIP D. MARSDEN, MD
Professor of Medicine, University of Brasilia, Brasilia, Brazil
Leishmania

HENRY MASUR, MD
Clinical Professor of Medicine, George Washington University School of Medicine, Washington, DC; Chief, Critical Care Medicine Department, Clinical Center, National Institutes of Health, Bethesda, Maryland
Approach to the Patient with Human Immunodeficiency Virus Infection: Clinical Features

GLENN E. MATHISEN, MD
Associate Clinical Professor of Medicine, University of California, Los Angeles; Chief, Infectious Disease Service, Olive View–UCLA Medical Center, Sycmar, California
Metronidazole and Other Nitroimidazoles

ZENE MATSUDA, MD, DSc
Research Associate, National Institute of Health of Japan, Tokyo, Japan
Human Immunodeficiency Virus and Other Retroviruses

KEITH P. W. J. McADAM, MA, FRCP
Director, Medical Research Council (UK) Laboratories, Fajara, Banjul, The Gambia
Leprosy; *Mycobacterium leprae*

JUSTIN C. McARTHUR, MBBS, MPH
Associate Professor of Neurology, The Johns Hopkins University School of Medicine; The Johns Hopkins Hospital, Baltimore, Maryland
Neurologic Complications of Human Immunodeficiency Virus Infections

WILLIAM M. McCORMACK, MD
Professor of Medicine and of Obstetrics and Gynecology, Director, Infectious Diseases Division, State University of New York Health Science Center, Brooklyn, New York
Mycoplasmas and Ureaplasmas

JOSEPH E. McDADE, PhD
Associate Director for Laboratory Science, National Center for Infectious Diseases, Centers for Disease Control and Prevention, Atlanta, Georgia
Ehrlichiosis, Q Fever, Typhus, Rickettsialpox, and Other Rickettsioses; *Rickettsia typhi* and *Rickettsia prowazekii; Rickettsia tsutsugamushi* and *Rickettsia akari*

JOHN E. McGOWAN, JR., MD
Professor of Pathology and Laboratory Medicine, Professor of Medicine (Infectious Diseases), Emory University Schools of Medicine and Public Health; Director, Clinical Microbiology, Grady Memorial Hospital, Atlanta, Georgia
Blood Stream Invasion

KELLY T. McKEE, JR., MD, MPH
Chief, Preventive Medicine Service, Womack Army Medical Center, Fort Bragg, North Carolina
Hemorrhagic Fever Viruses Belonging to the Families Arenaviridae, Filoviridae, and Bunyaviridae

RIMA McLEOD, MD
Jules and Doris Stein RPB Professor, Visual Sciences, Medicine, Pathology, and Immunology, The Pritzker School of Medicine of The University of Chicago; Attending Physician, Michael Reese Hospital and Medical Center, The University of Chicago Hospitals, Chicago, Illinois
Toxoplasmosis; *Toxoplasma gondii*

ALBERT T. McMANUS, PhD
Chief, Laboratory Division, U.S. Army Institute of Surgical Research, Fort Sam Houston, Texas
Burns

EDWIN M. MEARES, JR., MD
Professor of Urology, Emeritus, Department of Urology, Tufts University School of Medicine; Former Chairman, Department of Urology, New England Medical Center, Boston, Massachusetts
Urethritis, Prostatitis, Epididymitis, and Orchitis; Renal Abscess

H. CODY MEISSNER, MD
Associate Professor of Pediatrics, Tufts University School of Medicine; Chief, Division of Pediatric Infectious Disease, New England Medical Center, Boston, Massachusetts
Kawasaki Syndrome

WILLIAM G. MERZ, PhD
Associate Professor, Department of Pathology, Dermatology, Epidemiology, and Molecular Microbiology and Immunology, The Johns Hopkins University, Baltimore, Maryland
Candida albicans and Related Species

RICHARD D. MEYER, MD
Clinical Professor of Medicine, UCLA School of Medicine, Los Angeles; Staff, Northridge Hospital Medical Center, Northridge, California
Aspergillus Species

BURT R. MEYERS, MD
Professor of Medicine, The Mount Sinai School of Medicine; Director, Transplantation Infectious Diseases, The Mount Sinai Medical Center, New York, New York
Miscellaneous Drugs; Phycomycetes

MARCO K. MICHELSON, MD
Epidemiologist, Division of Parasitic Diseases, National Center for Infectious Diseases, Centers for Disease Control and Prevention, Atlanta, Georgia
Trichinosis

ROBERT C. MOELLERING, JR., MD, DSc (Hon)
Shields Warren-Mallinckrodt Professor of Medical Research, Harvard Medical School; Vice Chairman, Department of Medicine, Beth Israel Deaconess Medical Center, Boston, Massachusetts
Cephalosporins

BERNARD MOSS, MD, PhD
Chief, Laboratory of Viral Diseases, National Institute of Allergy and Infectious Diseases, National Institutes of Health, Bethesda, Maryland
Poxviruses

ROBERT R. MUDER, MD
Associate Professor of Medicine, University of Pittsburgh School of Medicine; Chief, Infection Control, VA Medical Center, Pittsburgh, Pennsylvania
Legionnaires' Disease

BRIGITTA U. MUELLER, MD
Assistant Professor of Pediatrics, Harvard Medical School; Assistant in Medicine, Children's Hospital, Boston, Massachusetts
Pediatric Human Immunodeficiency Virus Infection

MAURICE A. MUFSON, MD
Professor and Chair, Department of Medicine, Professor, Department of Microbiology, Marshall University School of Medicine; Active Staff, St. Mary's Hospital and Cabell Huntington Hospital; Medical Staff, Veterans Administration Medical Center, Huntington, West Virginia
Mycoplasma Pneumonia

THEODORE L. MUNSAT, MD
Professor of Pharmacology and Neurology, Tufts University School of Medicine; Director, Neuromuscular Research Unit, Tufts–New England Medical Center, Boston, Massachusetts
Infections of Muscle

BRIAN R. MURPHY, MD
Head, Respiratory Viruses Section, Laboratory of Infectious Diseases, National Institute of Allergy and Infectious Diseases, National Institutes of Health, Bethesda, Maryland
Parainfluenza Viruses

TIMOTHY F. MURPHY, MD
Professor of Medicine and Microbiology and Director, Division of Infectious Diseases, State University of New York at Buffalo, Buffalo, New York
Miscellaneous Gram-Negative Cocci: Other *Neisseria, Branhamella, Moraxella,* and *Kingella* Species; *Haemophilus*

BARBARA E. MURRAY, MD
Professor and Director, University of Texas Medical School at Houston, Division of Infectious Diseases, Houston, Texas
Enterococci

DANIEL M. MUSHER, MD
Professor of Medicine, Professor of Microbiology and Immunology, Chief of Infectious Diseases, Baylor College of Medicine; Chief, Infectious Disease Section, Veterans Affairs Medical Center, Houston, Texas
Syphilis; Treponemes: Microbiology

AVERY B. NATHENS, MD
Resident, Department of Surgery, University of Toronto, Toronto, Ontario, Canada
Intraabdominal Abscesses

GERARD J. NAU, MD, PhD
Clinical and Research Fellow, Harvard Medical School and Massachusetts General Hospital, Infectious Disease Unit, Boston; Visiting Scientist, The Whitehead Institute for Biomedical Research, Cambridge, Massachusetts
Infections of Head and Neck Spaces and Salivary Glands

JUDITH L. NERAD, MD
Assistant Professor of Medicine, Rush Medical College; Attending Physician, Cook County Hospital, Chicago, Illinois
Erysipelothrix rhusiopathiae; Miscellaneous Gram-Negative Bacilli: *Acinetobacter, Cardiobacterium, Actinobacillus, Chromobacterium, Capnocytophaga,* and Others

HAROLD C. NEU, MD
Professor of Medicine and Pharmacology, Columbia University College of Physicians and Surgeons; Hospital Epidemiologist, The Presbyterian Hospital in the City of New York, Columbia-Presbyterian Medical Center, New York, New York
Side Effects of Antimicrobial Therapy

KATHLEEN M. NEUZIL, MD
Assistant Professor of Medicine, Vanderbilt University School of Medicine; Assistant Chief, Medical Service, Department of Veterans Affairs Medical Center, Nashville, Tennessee
Human Herpesvirus 6 and Other Newly Recognized Human Herpesviruses

RONALD LEE NICHOLS, MD, FACS
William Henderson Professor of Surgery, Professor of Microbiology and Immunology, Tulane University School of Medicine; Attending Surgeon, The Tulane University Hospital and Clinic, New Orleans, Louisiana
Prophylaxis for Surgical Infections; Peritonitis; Surgical Wound Infection

RICHARD A. NITZBERG, MD
Assistant Clinical Professor of Surgery, Columbia University Medical School, New York, New York; Staff Vascular Surgeon, Overlook Hospital, Summit, New Jersey
Vascular Graft Infections

DONALD Z. NOAH, DVM, MPH
Epidemic Intelligence Service Officer, Viral and Rickettsial Zoonoses Branch, Centers for Disease Control and Prevention, Atlanta, Georgia
Rabies

JOHN NOBLE, MD
Professor of Medicine, Boston University School of Medicine; Chief, Section of General Internal Medicine, Boston Medical Center, Boston, Massachusetts
Smallpox

LISBETH NORDSTRÖM-LERNER, MD
Infection Control Coordinator, Holy Cross Hospital, Detroit, Michigan
Aminoglycosides

THOMAS F. O'DONNELL, JR., MD
Andrews Professor and Chairman, Department of Surgery, and Surgeon-in-Chief, Tufts University School of Medicine; New England Medical Center, Boston, Massachusetts
Vascular Graft Infections

PEARAY L. OGRA, MD
Professor of Pediatrics, University of Texas Medical Branch at Galveston; Chairman, Department of Pediatrics, Children's Hospital, Galveston, Texas
Respiratory Syncytial Virus

PATRICK I. OKOLO, III, MD
Post Doctoral Fellow in Gastroenterology and Hepatology, The Johns Hopkins University; Clinical Fellow, The Johns Hopkins Hospital, Baltimore, Maryland
Whipple's Disease

DAVID W. OLDACH, MD
Assistant Professor of Medicine, Division of Infectious Diseases, University of Maryland School of Medicine, Baltimore, Maryland
Clindamycin; Macrolide (and Azalide) Antibiotics: Erythromycin, Azithromycin, Clarithromycin, and Dirithromycin; Chloramphenicol

JAMES G. OLSON, PhD
Chief, Viral and Rickettsial Zoonoses Branch, Centers for Disease Control and Prevention, Atlanta, Georgia
Ehrlichiosis, Q Fever, Typhus, Rickettsialpox, and Other Rickettsioses; *Rickettsia typhi* and *Rickettsia prowazekii; Rickettsia tsutsugamushi* and *Rickettsia akari*

MICHAEL N. OXMAN
Professor of Medicine and Pathology, University of California, San Diego, School of Medicine; Physician, Infectious Diseases Section, Veterans Affairs Medical Center, San Diego, California
Genital Herpes; Herpes Simplex Viruses

MARK A. PALLANSCH, PhD
Chief, Enterovirus Section, Centers for Disease Control and Prevention, Atlanta, Georgia
Poliovirus; Coxsackievirus, Echovirus, and Other Enteroviruses

DARWIN PALMER, MD
Emeritus Professor, Department of Medicine, University of New Mexico School of Medicine, Albuquerque, New Mexico; Visiting Professor, Department of Medicine, University of Zimbabwe, Harare, Zimbabwe
Plague

JULIE PARSONNET, MD
Associate Professor of Medicine and of Health Research Policy, Stanford University School of Medicine, Stanford, California
Helicobacter

CHRISTOPHER C. PENN, MD
Private Clinician, Lawrence, Kansas
Anthrax; *Bacillus anthracis* and Other Aerobic Spore Formers

JAMES E. PENNINGTON, MD
Clinical Professor of Medicine, University of California, San Francisco; Vice President, Biological Clinical Research, Bayer Pharmaceutical Company, Berkeley, California
Pneumonias in Immunocompromised Hosts

DAVID C. PERLMAN, MD
Associate Professor of Medicine, Albert Einstein College of Medicine, Bronx; Director, AIDS Inpatient Unit, Beth Israel Medical Center, New York, New York
Viral Pneumonia

ROBERT PINNER, MD
Special Assistant for Surveillance, National Center for Infectious Diseases, Centers for Disease Control and Prevention, Atlanta, Georgia
Listeria monocytogenes

PHILIP A. PIZZO, MD
Thomas Morgan Rotch Professor and Chair, Department of Pediatrics, Harvard Medical School; Physician-in-Chief and Chair, Department of Medicine, Children's Hospital, Boston, Massachusetts
Pediatric Human Immunodeficiency Virus Infection

RICHARD PLATT, MD
Associate Professor of Medicine, Harvard Medical School; Hospital Epidemiologist, Brigham and Women's Hospital, Boston, Massachusetts
Epidemiology of Nosocomial Infections; Control of Nosocomial Infections

MATTHEW POLLACK, MD
Professor of Medicine, Uniformed Services University of the Health Sciences, F. Edward Hebert School of Medicine; Attending Physician, National Naval Medical Center, Bethesda, Maryland
Pseudomonas aeruginosa and Related Bacteria

DONALD M. PORETZ, MD
Clinical Professor of Medicine, Georgetown University School of Medicine, Washington, DC; Chief, Infectious Diseases, Fairfax Hospital, Falls Church, Virginia
Outpatient Parenteral Therapy

JOHN C. POTTAGE, JR., MD
Associate Professor, Rush Medical College; Associate Attending Physician, Rush–Presbyterian–St. Luke's Medical Center, Chicago, Illinois
Chronic Meningitis

BASIL A. PRUITT, JR., MD
Clinical Professor of Surgery, University of Texas Health Science Center at San Antonio; Editor, Journal of Trauma, San Antonio, Texas; Professor of Surgery, Uniformed Services University of the Health Sciences, Bethesda, Maryland
Burns

THOMAS C. QUINN, MD
Professor of Medicine, International Health, and Molecular Microbiology and Immunology, The Johns Hopkins University School of Medicine, Baltimore; Senior Investigator, National Institute of Allergy and Infectious Diseases, National Institutes of Health, Bethesda, Maryland
International Epidemiology of the Human Immunodeficiency Virus

GERALD V. QUINNAN, JR., MD
Professor of Preventive Medicine, Medicine, and Microbiology, Uniformed Services University of the Health Sciences, Bethesda, Maryland
Cytokines in the Treatment and Prevention of Infectious Diseases

RICHARD QUINTILIANI, MD
Professor of Medicine, University of Connecticut School of Medicine, Farmington; Director, Anti-Infective Research and Pharmacoeconomic Studies, Hartford Hospital, Hartford, Connecticut
Strategies for the Cost-Effective Use of Antibiotics

ALEXANDER RAKOWSKY, MD
Medical Officer, Division of Anti-Infective Drug Products, Food and Drug Administration, Rockville; Attending Staff, Pediatric Emergency Department, St. Agnes Hospital, Baltimore, Maryland
Rubella (German Measles); Rubella Virus

C. GEORGE RAY, MD
Professor and Chairman, Department of Pediatrics, St. Louis University School of Medicine; Pediatrician-in-Chief, Cardinal Glennon Children's Hospital, St. Louis, Missouri
Coronavirus

SHARON L. REED, MD, CTM
Associate Professor of Pathology and Medicine, Division of Infectious Diseases, University of California, San Diego, Medical School; Director, Microbiology and Virology Laboratories, UCSD Medical Center, San Diego, California
Entamoeba histolytica and Other Intestinal Amoebae

JACK S. REMINGTON, MD
Professor of Medicine, Stanford University; Professor of Medicine, Division of Infectious Diseases and Geographic Medicine, Stanford University School of Medicine, Stanford; Marcus A. Krupp MD Research Chair and Chairman, Department of Immunology and Infectious Diseases, Research Institute, Palo Alto Medical Foundation, Palo Alto, California
Toxoplasmosis

PETER D. REUMAN, MD, MPH
Associate Professor, Pediatric Immunology and Infectious Diseases, University of Florida College of Medicine, Gainesville, Florida
Rubeola (Measles) and Subacute Sclerosing Panencephalitis Virus

CRAIG ROBERTS, PhD
Lecturer, Strathclyde University, Glasgow, Scotland
Toxoplasma gondii

ALLAN ROSS RONALD, MD, FRCPC, FACP
Professor, Associate Dean of Research, University of Manitoba; Consultant, Infectious Diseases, St. Boniface General Hospital, Winnipeg, Manitoba, Canada
Chancroid, Lymphogranuloma Venereum, and Granuloma Inguinale

NOEL R. ROSE, MD, PhD
Professor of Pathology, and Professor of Molecular Microbiology and Immunology, The Johns Hopkins University; Attending Pathologist, Director of Immunology, The Johns Hopkins Hospital, Baltimore, Maryland
Immunodiagnosis

JILL R. ROSENTHAL, MD
Assistant Professor of Dermatology, Tufts University School of Medicine; Dermatologist and Director of Pediatric Dermatology, Department of Medical and Surgical Dermatology, New England Medical Center, Boston, Massachusetts
Fungal Infections of the Skin; Dematiaceous Fungi

KAREN F. ROTHMAN, MD
Assistant Professor, Department of Medicine and Pediatrics, University of Massachusetts Medical School, Worcester, Massachusetts
Warts

ORI D. ROTSTEIN, MD, FRCSC
Professor of Surgery, University of Toronto; Staff Surgeon, Toronto Hospital, Toronto, Ontario, Canada
Intraabdominal Abscesses

DONALD H. RUBIN, MD
Professor of Medicine, Microbiology and Immunology, Vanderbilt University School of Medicine; Associate Chief of Staff for Research and Development, Nashville Veterans Affairs Medical Center, Nashville, Tennessee
Human Herpesvirus 6 and Other Newly Recognized Human Herpesviruses

ROBERT H. RUBIN, MD
Gordon and Marjerie Osborne Chair of Health Sciences and Technology, Director, Harvard-MIT Center for Experimental Pharmacology and Therapeutics, Harvard-MIT Division of Health Sciences and Technology, Cambridge; Chief of Transplantation Infectious Disease, Massachusetts General Hospital, Boston, Massachusetts
Salmonella Infections; Infections in Organ Transplant Recipients; *Salmonella*

CHARLES E. RUPPRECHT, VMD, PhD
Rabies Section Chief, Viral and Rickettsial Zoonoses Branch, Centers for Disease Control and Prevention, Atlanta, Georgia
Rabies; Rabies Virus

DAVID A. SACK, MD
Professor, Department of International Health, and Head, Vaccine Testing Unit, The Johns Hopkins University; The Johns Hopkins Hospital, Baltimore, Maryland
Cholera and Related Illnesses Caused by *Vibrio* Species and *Aeromonas;* Vibrios

R. BRADLEY SACK, MD, ScD
Professor of International Health and Medicine, The Johns Hopkins University School of Hygiene and Public Health, Baltimore, Maryland
Escherichia coli Infections

MAJID SADIGH, MD
Associate Clinical Professor of Medicine, Associate Program Director/Primary Care Internal Medicine Residency Program, Yale University School of Medicine, New Haven; Attending Physician, St. Mary's Hospital, Waterbury, Connecticut
Central Nervous System Shunt Infections

SANDRA SALLUSTIO, MD, PhD
Emergency Medicine Resident, Department of Emergency Medicine, The Mount Sinai Medical Center, New York, New York
Salmonella

CHRISTINE C. SANDERS, PhD
Professor of Medical Microbiology and Director, Center for Research in Anti-Infectives and Biotechnology, Creighton University School of Medicine, Omaha, Nebraska
Other β-Lactam Antibiotics

JAY P. SANFORD, MD
Late Clinical Professor of Internal Medicine, University of Texas Southwestern Medical Center at Dallas, Dallas, Texas
Tularemia

FRANCISCO L. SAPICO, MD
Professor of Medicine, University of Southern California, Los Angeles; Chief of Infectious Diseases, Rancho Los Amigos Medical Center, Downey, California
Foot Infections in the Diabetic Patient and Infections Associated with Pressure Sores

STEPHEN J. SAVARINO, MD, MPH
Associate Professor of Pediatrics, Uniformed Services University of the Health Sciences, Bethesda, Maryland; Head, Applied Field Science Division, U.S. Naval Medical Research Unit No 3, Cairo, Egypt
Specific and Nonspecific Treatment of Diarrhea

DENNIS R. SCHABERG, MD
Professor and Chairman, Department of Medicine, University of Tennessee College of Medicine, Memphis, Tennessee
Staphylococci

JULIUS SCHACHTER, PhD
Professor of Laboratory Medicine, University of California, San Francisco, San Francisco, California; Director, World Health Organization Collaborating Center for Reference and Research on Chlamydia, World Health Organization, Geneva, Switzerland
Chlamydial Infections; *Chlamydia*

PETER M. SCHANTZ, MD, PhD
Epidemiologist, Division of Parasitic Diseases, National Center for Infectious Diseases, Centers for Disease Control and Prevention, Atlanta, Georgia
Trichinosis; Larva Migrans Syndromes Caused by *Toxocara* Species and Other Nematodes

MOSHE SCHEIN, MD, FCS (SA)
Associate Professor of Surgery, Cornell University Medical College, New York; Attending Surgeon, New York Methodist Hospital, Brooklyn, New York
Diverticulitis

GILBERT M. SCHIFF, MD
Professor of Medicine and Pediatrics, University of Cincinnati College of Medicine; Associate Chairman, Department of Pediatrics, and Director, Gamble Program for Clinical Studies, Infectious Diseases Division, Children's Hospital Medical Center, Cincinnati, Ohio
Measles; Rubeola (Measles) and Subacute Sclerosing Panencephalitis Virus

PATRICK M. SCHLIEVERT, PhD
Professor, Microbiology, University of Minnesota Medical School, Minneapolis, Minnesota
Toxic Shock Syndrome

ANNE SCHUCHAT, MD
Medical Epidemiologist, Division of Bacterial and Mycotic Diseases, National Center for Infectious Diseases, Centers for Disease Control and Prevention, Atlanta, Georgia
Listeria monocytogenes

E. NAN SCOTT, PhD
Associate Professor of Research Medicine, College of Medicine, University of Oklahoma Health Sciences Center; Microbiologist, VA Medical Center, Oklahoma City, Oklahoma
Sporothrix schenckii

DARRYL SEE, MD
Assistant Professor of Medicine, Department of Medicine, Division of Infectious Diseases, University of California, Irvine, Irvine, California
Pericarditis and Myocarditis

DEBORAH E. SENTOCHNIK, MD
Attending Staff, Infectious Diseases, Lahey Clinic Medical Center, Burlington, Massachusetts
Cephalosporins

JOHN L. SEVER, MD, PhD
Professor of Pediatrics, Obstetrics and Gynecology, Microbiology and Immunology, The George Washington University Medical Center and The Children's National Medical Center, Washington, DC
Rubella (German Measles); Rubella Virus

MARIA TERESA SEVILLE, MD
Infectious Disease Fellow, Loyola University, Stritch School of Medicine, Maywood, Illinois
Miscellaneous Gram-Negative Bacilli: *Acinetobacter, Cardiobacterium, Actinobacillus, Chromobacterium, Capnocytophaga,* and Others

KEERTI V. SHAH, PhD, MD
Professor, The Johns Hopkins University School of Hygiene and Public Health, Baltimore, Maryland
Human Papillomaviruses (Including Wart Viruses); Human Polyomavirus (Including the Agent Causing Progressive Multifocal Leukoencephalopathy)

JOHN N. SHEAGREN, MD
Professor of Medicine, Rush Medical College; Chairman, Department of Internal Medicine, Illinois Masonic Medical Center, Chicago, Illinois
Staphylococci

KALPANA D. SHERE, MD
Research Associate, Department of Medicine, Division of Infectious Diseases, Albert Einstein College of Medicine, Bronx, New York
Salmonella Infections

DAVID M. SHLAES, MD, PhD
Vice President, Infectious Disease Research, Wyeth Ayerst Research, Pearl River, New York
Miscellaneous Streptococci

JOHN W. SHORE, MD
Ophthalmic Consultant, Boston, Massachusetts
Orbital Infections

JONAS A. SHULMAN, MD
Executive Associate Dean and Professor of Medicine (Infectious Diseases), Emory University School of Medicine, Atlanta, Georgia
Blood Stream Invasion

PATRICIA M. SIMONE, MD
Acting Branch Chief, Field Services Branch, Division of Tuberculosis Elimination, National Center for HIV, STD, and TB Prevention, Centers for Disease Control and Prevention, Atlanta, Georgia
Antimycobacterial Drugs

CHARLES B. SMITH, MD
Associate Dean and Professor, Department of Medicine, University of Washington School of Medicine; Chief of Staff, VA Puget Sound Health Care System, Seattle, Washington
Influenza Viruses

JEFFREY W. SMITH, MS, MPH
Assistant Professor, Surgical Microbiology Research Laboratory, Tulane University School of Medicine, Department of Surgery, New Orleans, Louisiana
Peritonitis

DAVID R. SNYDMAN, MD
Professor of Pathology, Medicine, Microbiology and Molecular Biology, Tufts University School of Medicine; Director, Clinical Microbiology, and Attending Physician in Infectious Diseases, New England Medical Center, Boston, Massachusetts
Serum Therapy and Augmentation of the Host Response; Food Poisoning; *Erysipelothrix rhusiopathiae;* Miscellaneous Gram-Negative Bacilli: *Acinetobacter, Cardiobacterium, Actinobacillus, Chromobacterium, Capnocytophaga,* and Others

ROSEMARY SOAVE, MD
Associate Professor of Medicine and Public Health, Cornell University Medical College; Associate Attending Physician, The New York Hospital–Cornell Medical Center, New York, New York
Cryptosporidium, Isospora, Cyclospora, Microsporidia, and *Dientamoeba*

ANDREW SPIELMAN, ScD
Professor of Tropical Public Health, Department of Tropical Public Health, Harvard School of Public Health, Boston, Massachusetts
Arthropods

WALTER E. STAMM, MD
Professor of Medicine, Head, Division of Allergy and Infectious Diseases, University of Washington School of Medicine, Seattle, Washington
Approach to the Patient with Urinary Tract Infection

ANN E. STAPLETON, MD
Assistant Professor of Medicine, Division of Allergy and Infectious Diseases, University of Washington School of Medicine, Seattle, Washington
Approach to the Patient with Urinary Tract Infection

GENE H. STOLLERMAN, MD
Professor of Medicine and Public Health, Emeritus, Boston University, Boston, Massachusetts
Streptococcus pyogenes (Group A Streptococci)

DAVID R. STONE, MD
Assistant Professor, Tufts University School of Medicine; Attending Physician, Division of Geographic Medicine and Infectious Diseases, New England Medical Center, Department of Medicine, Lemuel Shattuck Hospital, Boston, Massachusetts
Approach to the Patient with Zoonotic Infection

JANET E. STOUT, PhD
Research Assistant Professor, Department of Medicine, University of Pittsburgh School of Medicine; Microbiologist, VA Medical Center, Pittsburgh, Pennsylvania
Legionella

STEPHEN E. STRAUS, MD
Chief, Laboratory of Clinical Investigation, National Institute of Allergy and Infectious Diseases, Bethesda, Maryland
Chronic Fatigue Syndrome

ALAN M. SUGAR, MD
Associate Professor of Medicine, Boston University School of Medicine; Assistant Visiting Physician, Boston Medical Center, Boston; Director, HIV/AIDS Program, Cape Cod Hospital, Hyannis, Massachusetts
Miscellaneous Fungi

MORTON SWARTZ, MD
Professor of Medicine, Harvard Medical School; Chief, Jackson Firm Department of Medicine, Massachusetts General Hospital, Boston, Massachusetts
Acute Bacterial Meningitis

RICHARD L. SWEET, MD
Professor and Chair, Department of Obstetrics, Gynecology and Reproductive Science, University of Pittsburgh; Chair, Department of Obstetrics and Gynecology, Magee-Women's Hospital, Pittsburgh, Pennsylvania
Pelvic Inflammatory Disease and Tuboovarian Abscess

DAVID L. SWERDLOW, MD
Assistant Chief, Foodborne Diseases Epidemiology Section, Foodborne and Diarrheal Diseases Branch, Division of Bacterial and Mycotic Diseases, National Center for Infectious Diseases, Centers for Disease Control and Prevention, Atlanta, Georgia
Escherichia coli 0157:H7 and Other Shiga Toxin–Producing *E. coli*

ELLA M. SWIERKOSZ, PhD
Associate Professor, Departments of Pathology and Pediatrics, St. Louis University School of Medicine; Director, Microbiology Laboratory, St. Louis University Hospital, St. Louis, Missouri
Coronavirus

GORDON L. TELFORD, MD
Professor of Surgery, Medical College of Wisconsin; Chief of General Surgery, Veterans Affairs Medical Center; Staff Surgeon, Froedtert Memorial Lutheran Hospital, Milwaukee, Wisconsin
Appendicitis

FRED C. TENOVER, PhD
Adjunct Professor of Epidemiology, Rollins School of Public Health, Emory University; Adjunct Professor of Laboratory Medicine and Pathology, Emory University School of Medicine; Chief, Nosocomial Pathogens Laboratory Branch, Hospital Infections Program, Centers for Disease Control and Prevention, Atlanta, Georgia
Molecular Techniques for the Detection and Identification of Infectious Agents

KENNETH S. THOMSON, PhD
Assistant Professor of Medical Microbiology and Immunology, Creighton University School of Medicine; Associate Director, Center for Research in Anti-Infectives and Biotechnology, Creighton University School of Medicine, Omaha, Nebraska
Other β-Lactam Antibiotics

GRACE M. THORNE, PhD
Assistant Professor of Pediatrics, Harvard Medical School; Research Associate, Infectious Diseases Division, Department of Medicine, and Research Director, General Clinical Research Center, Children's Hospital, Boston, Massachusetts
Toxins

MAUREEN R. TIERNEY, MD
Assistant Professor, Harvard Medical School, Boston; Medical Director, Spence Center for Women's Health, Cambridge, Massachusetts
Infections of the Pharynx, Larynx, Epiglottis, Trachea, and Thyroid

JEREMIAH TILLES, MD
Professor of Medicine, University of California, Irvine, School of Medicine, Irvine, California
Pericarditis and Myocarditis

NINA E. TOLKOFF-RUBIN, MD
Associate Professor of Medicine, Harvard Medical School; Chief of Hemodialysis and CAPD Units and Director of The End Stage Renal Disease Program, Massachusetts General Hospital, Boston, Massachusetts
Infections in Organ Transplant Recipients

LUCY S. TOMPKINS, MD, PhD
Professor, Medicine (Division of Infectious Diseases and Geographic Medicine) and Microbiology and Immunology, Stanford University; Clinical Chief, Infectious Diseases Services, Director, Clinical Microbiology/Virology Laboratory, and Director, Infection Prevention Program, Stanford Health Systems, Stanford, California
Molecular Epidemiology in Infectious Diseases

ZAHRA TOOSSI, MD
Associate Professor of Medicine, Case Western Reserve University; Physician, Veterans Administration Medical Center, Cleveland, Ohio
Tuberculosis; *Mycobacterium tuberculosis* and Other Mycobacteria

EDMUND C. TRAMONT, MD
Professor and Director, Medical Biotechnology Center, University of Maryland Biotechnology Center; Staff, University of Maryland Medical Systems, Baltimore, Maryland
Neisseria gonorrhoeae; Neisseria meningitidis

THEODORE F. TSAI, MD, MPH
Medical Officer, Centers for Disease Control, Fort Collins, Colorado
Yellow Fever Virus

WALTER W. TUNNESSEN, JR., MD
Senior Vice President, The American Board of Pediatrics, Chapel Hill, North Carolina
Erythema Infectiosum, Roseola, and Enteroviral Exanthems

SHAHE VARTIVARIAN
Private Clinician, Metropolitan Infectious Diseases Associates, Houston, Texas
Infections Associated with Malignancy

MITCHELL WACHTEL, MD
Pathologist, American Medical Laboratories, Chantilly, Virginia
Arthropods

FRANCIS A. WALDVOGEL, MD
Professor of Medicine and Chairman, Department of Internal Medicine, University Hospital, Geneva, Switzerland
Osteomyelitis

ANDREW L. WARSHAW, MD
Harold and Ellen Danser Professor of Surgery, Harvard Medical School; Chief of General Surgery, Massachusetts General Hospital, Boston, Massachusetts
Infection After Acute Pancreatitis

HAROLD J. WELCH, MD
Assistant Professor of Surgery, Tufts University School of Medicine, and Staff Vascular Surgeon, New England Medical Center, Boston, Massachusetts; Clinical Assistant Professor of Surgery, Uniformed Services University of the Health Sciences, Bethesda, Maryland
Vascular Graft Infections

ROBERT C. WELLIVER, MD
Professor of Pediatrics, State University of New York at Buffalo; Co-Director, Division of Infectious Diseases, Children's Hospital of Buffalo, Buffalo, New York
Respiratory Syncytial Virus

MICHAEL R. WESSELS, MD
Associate Professor of Medicine, Harvard Medical School; Associate Physician, Brigham and Women's Hospital; Physician, Beth Israel Deaconess Medical Center, Boston, Massachusetts
Group B *Streptococcus*

CHRISTOPHER T. WESTFALL, MD
Clinical Associate Professor, Uniformed Services University of the Health Sciences, Bethesda, Maryland
Orbital Infections

JOE WHEAT, MD
Professor of Medicine, Indiana University School of Medicine; Wishard Memorial Hospital; Chief, Infectious Diseases, Roudebush Veterans Hospital, Indianapolis, Indiana
Histoplasma

RICHARD J. WHITLEY, MD
Professor of Pediatrics, Microbiology, and Medicine, Loeb Eminent Scholar Chair in Pediatrics, University of Alabama at Birmingham, Birmingham, Alabama
Antiviral Therapy

DAVID N. WILLIAMS, MB, ChB, FRCP
Professor of Clinical Medicine, University of Minnesota Medical School; Vice-Chairman, Department of Internal Medicine, Hennepin County Medical Center, Minneapolis, Minnesota
Tetracyclines

RUSSELL A. WILLIAMS, MD
Professor of Surgery, University of California, Irvine, Irvine; Vice Chairman, Department of Surgery, and Director, Surgery Training Program, UCI Medical Center, Orange, California
Cholecystitis and Cholangitis

KAETHE WILLMS, MD
Professor, Department of Microbiology and Parasitology, School of Medicine, National University of Mexico, UNAM, Mexico City, Mexico
Cestodes (Tapeworms)

MARY E. WILSON, MD, FACP
Assistant Professor, Departments of Population and International Health and Epidemiology, Harvard School of Public Health; Assistant Clinical Professor, Harvard Medical School, Boston; Chief of Infectious Diseases and Director, Travel Resource Center, Mount Auburn Hospital, Cambridge, Massachusetts
Advice to Travelers

SAMUEL E. WILSON, MD
Professor of Surgery and Chair, Department of Surgery, University of California, Irvine, Medical Center, Orange, California
Cholecystitis and Cholangitis

JERRY A. WINKELSTEIN, MD
Professor of Pediatrics, The Johns Hopkins University School of Medicine; Director, Division of Immunology, Department of Pediatrics, The Johns Hopkins Hospital, Baltimore, Maryland
The Complement System

DIETMAR H. WITTMANN, MD, PhD
Professor of Surgery, Medical College of Wisconsin, Milwaukee, Wisconsin; Privat Dozent, Hamburg University Medical School, Hamburg, Germany
Intraabdominal Infections; Diverticulitis

MARTIN S. WOLFE, MD
Clinical Professor of Medicine, George Washington University Medical School; Clinical Associate Professor of Medicine, Georgetown University Medical School, Washington, DC
Antiparasitic Drugs

DAVID J. WYLER, MD
Professor of Medicine, Molecular Biology, and Microbiology, Tufts University School of Medicine, Boston; Physician, New England Medical Center, Boston; Attending Physician in Medicine and Consultant in Infectious Diseases, Martha's Vineyard Hospital, Oak Bluffs, Massachusetts
Plasmodium and *Babesia*

NEAL S. YOUNG, MD
Chief, Hematology Branch, National Heart, Lung, and Blood Institute, National Institutes of Health, Bethesda, Maryland
Human Parvovirus

RONALD J. ZABRANSKY
Private Clinician, Cleveland, Ohio
Miscellaneous Streptococci

JOHN A. ZAIA, MD
Director of Virology and Infectious Diseases, Department of Pediatrics, City of Hope National Medical Center, Duarte, California
Varicella and Herpes Zoster; Varicella-Zoster Virus

JONATHAN M. ZENILMAN, MD
Associate Professor of Medicine and Gynecology, The Johns Hopkins University School of Medicine; Attending Physician, The Johns Hopkins Hospital, Baltimore, Maryland
Gonorrhea; Prevention of Human Immunodeficiency Virus Transmission

STEPHEN H. ZINNER, MD
Professor and Interim Chairman, Department of Medicine, and Director, Division of Infectious Diseases, Brown University School of Medicine; Director, Division of Infectious Diseases, Rhode Island Hospital and Roger Williams Medical Center, Providence, Rhode Island
Treatment and Prevention of Infections in Immunocompromised Hosts

PREFACE

During the past half century, the frontiers of infection have undergone dramatic expansion. Our predecessors thought of infection as synonymous with contagion. The "fever doctor" treated the classic exanthems, typhoid fever, polio, and meningitis, each of which exacted a costly toll in premature death and disability.

A combination of public health measures, vaccines, and antimicrobial drugs has caused a merciful decline in the traditional contagious diseases. Even the freestanding infectious disease hospitals were eliminated as their census fell and the remnants of such units were absorbed into the modern hospital complex.

Yet these developments have not removed infection from the register of human afflictions. Insidious microbes still threaten the well-being of our patients, often in a different venue (acquired in the hospital instead of the community) or in the guise of a modern plague (AIDS). Ironically, advances in surgical techniques, such as insertion of prosthetic devices and organ transplantation, have virtually created a new field, postoperative infection. Contemporary diagnosis and treatment of infection are no longer the domain of the solitary physician. They now require a cooperative approach involving multiple specialties and utilizing a vast array of laboratory methods, imaging techniques, pharmacologic agents, and surgical intervention.

The field of infectious diseases has expanded at a rapid rate since the publication of the first edition of this book. As a result the second edition embodies many changes to keep pace with this escalating knowledge. Special emphasis has been added in both revised and newly written chapters on what are viewed by many authorities as the leading concerns in infectious diseases as we approach the new millennium: the advancing AIDS epidemic, emerging infections, and antimicrobial resistance in human pathogens. Besides dealing with these issues, the continuing chapters from the last edition have all been updated with new text and references that reflect the most recent scientific and clinical discoveries.

Among the topics of the new diagnostic and clinical chapters are the following: molecular diagnostics, probes, and polymerase chain reaction analysis; Kawasaki syndrome; Creutzfeldt-Jakob disease and kuru; diabetic foot ulcers and decubitus ulcers; toxic shock syndrome (including staphylococcal and streptococcal forms); and clinical approach to the patient with recurrent infection.

Chapters on emerging infections and recently discovered microorganisms are also added: *Escherichia coli* O157:H7, *Helicobacter pylori*, *Chlamydia pneumoniae*, *Bartonella*, and Microsporidia; and among the viruses, hepatitis viruses C, D, and E, herpesvirus 6, hantavirus, calicivirus, and astrovirus.

In the following areas the chapters have been expanded and/or have new authors: side effects of antimicrobial therapy; antimycobacterial drugs; advice to travelers; *Campylobacter*; *Yersinia*; cholera and related illnesses caused by *Vibrio* species and *Aeromonas*; surgical wound infections; skin and soft tissue infections; fungal infections of the skin; septic arthritis; slow virus infections of the central nervous system; infections associated with bone marrow transplantation; prevention of human immunodeficiency virus transmission; approach to the patient with a zoonotic infection; rabies; Rocky Mountain spotted fever; cat-scratch disease; *Entamoeba histolytica* and other intestinal amoebae; and intestinal and tissue nematodes.

We have attempted to select authors with recognized expertise in each subject. As a result, the list of contributors is a veritable "Who's Who" of contemporary authorities in medical and surgical infections. We are particularly proud of our section on surgical infections, which currently represent a significant portion of infection within the hospital, written by preeminent surgeons in their area of interest. The editors have read and critiqued every chapter. The authors themselves bear the responsibility for their chapters, but they have cooperated fully in meeting the requests of the editors for clarification and expansion.

The reader might note the liberal inclusion of tables and figures. The generous use of illustrative material is intended to highlight the seminal points of the chapter; in addition, we believe that illustrations render the text more accessible.

Our efforts were supported by an outstanding team at W. B. Saunders, particularly our editor, Richard Zorab, who serially encouraged, cajoled, empathized, stroked, and hammered—all with consummate skill and good grace. And we are grateful for the expert editing and quiet perseverance of Janice Gaillard and for the support of the production team, led by Linda R. Garber and Judith Gandy. In our offices, many hands have contributed to this effort, and we express our sincere thanks to Jane Patrick, Louise Kelly, Daphne Reilly, Suzanne Howatt, and Denise Guise.

Finally, a few thoughts on why we who work in this field are so committed to the enterprise of fighting infection. In all candor, most of us admit to the unqualified excitement of the quest, the perceptual challenge, the relentless pursuit of conquest over these microscopic agents of disease. Hans Zinsser captured in words the spirit of this calling in his classic book *Rats, Lice and History:*

> Infectious disease is one of the few genuine adventures left in the world . . . however secure and well-regulated life may become, bacteria, Protozoa, viruses, infected fleas, ticks, mosquitoes, and bedbugs will always lurk in the shadows ready to pounce when neglect, poverty, famine, or war lets down the defenses. And even in normal times they prey on the weak, the very young and the very old, living along with us, in mysterious obscurity waiting their opportunities. About the only genuine sporting proposition that remains unimpaired by the relentless domestication of a once free-living human species is the war against these ferocious little fellow creatures, which lurk in the dark corners and stalk us in the bodies of rats, mice, and all kinds of domestic animals; which fly and crawl with the insects, and waylay us in our food and drink and even in our love.

The challenge of infection is quite unlike any other in medicine, for it goes beyond the boundaries of humankind, requiring a mastery over the biology of the offending microorganism; its habitats; how it lives, feeds, and makes its way in a hostile world; its allies and vectors; its strengths; and most important, its vulnerabilities. Most fields of medicine encourage an anthropocentric image of the world. But an understanding of infectious diseases requires a vision beyond the human biosphere, which encompasses the ecosystem of microscopic creatures that share our environment.

Yet treating infection is more than an intellectual challenge; it is the added dimension of caring for its victims that is the driving spirit behind these endeavors. Whether in the laboratory, in the epidemiology office, or at the bedside, we all recognize that the focus of our efforts is the hapless patient suffering with an infectious disease. Fortunately, many infectious agents yield to the appropriate use of an antimicrobial drug or can be prevented by a vaccine or skillful application of public health measures. We do accept the reality that many microorganisms cannot be treated with current therapies or have established themselves in a host incapable of mustering a sufficient response in his own defense. And we also recognize, sadly, that many people still succumb to infectious diseases that are either treatable or readily preventable.

Ultimately, the practice of infectious diseases is the art of the possible. The editors and contributors have tried to set down what is known about infections in medicine and surgery in a way that conveys the excitement of the science and the satisfaction that follows the judicious application of appropriate diagnosis, therapy, and preventive measures.

SHERWOOD L. GORBACH
JOHN G. BARTLETT
NEIL R. BLACKLOW

CONTENTS

PART XII ▪ PARASITES 2393

PLATE 1

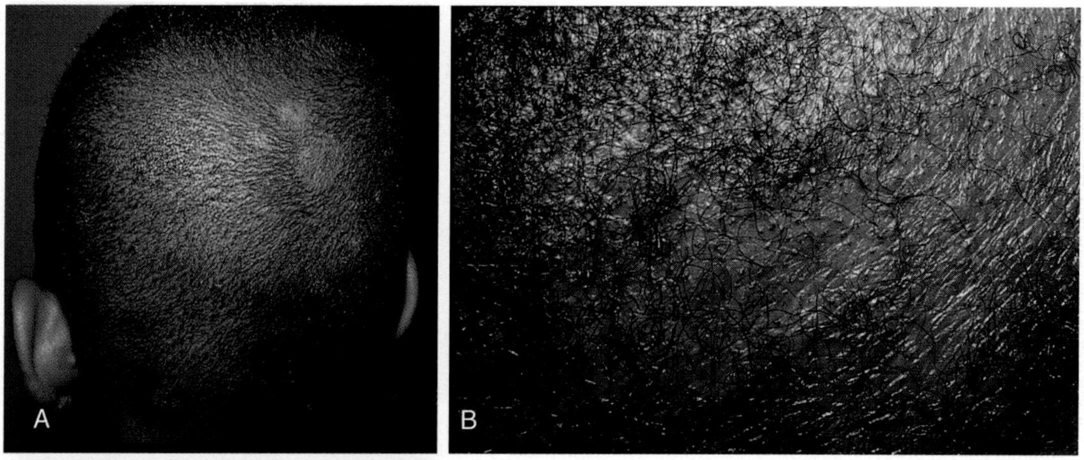

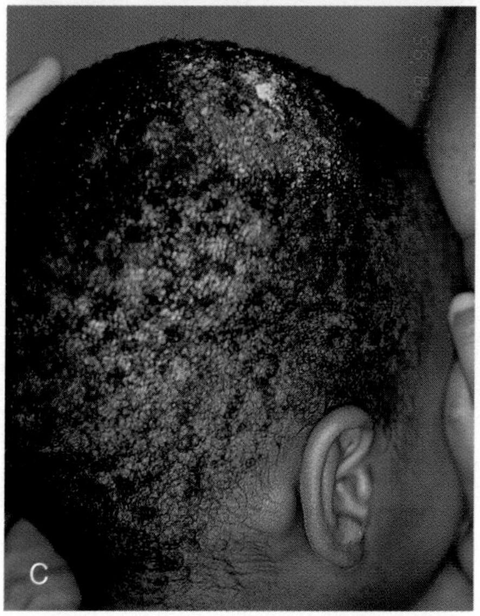

FIGURE 145–1 □ Tinea capitis. *A*, Multiple scaly alopecic plaques. *B*, Black-dot tinea capitis. *C*, Kerion with visibly enlarged post-auricular lymph node.

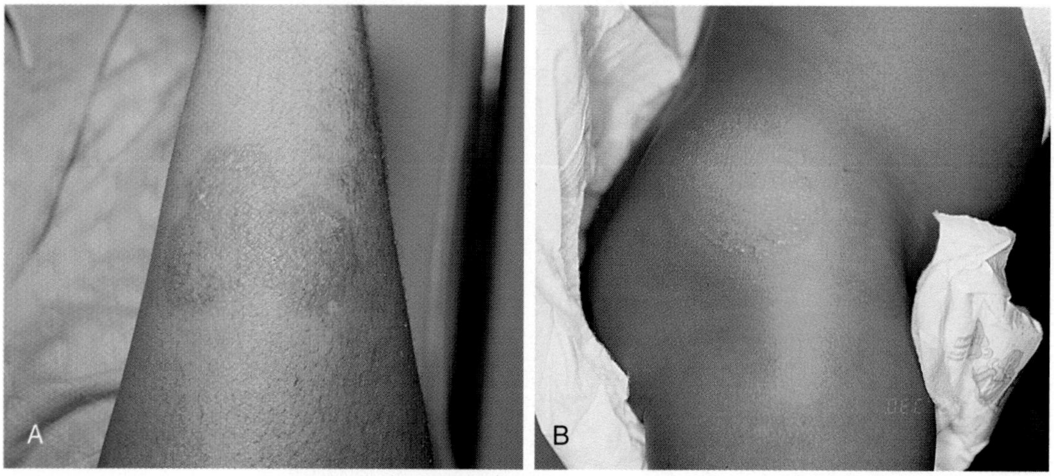

FIGURE 145–3 □ Tinea corporis. *A*, Coalescing scaly annular plaques on the forearm. *B*, Annular erythematous plaque on an infant's hip, occluded by the diaper.

PLATE 2

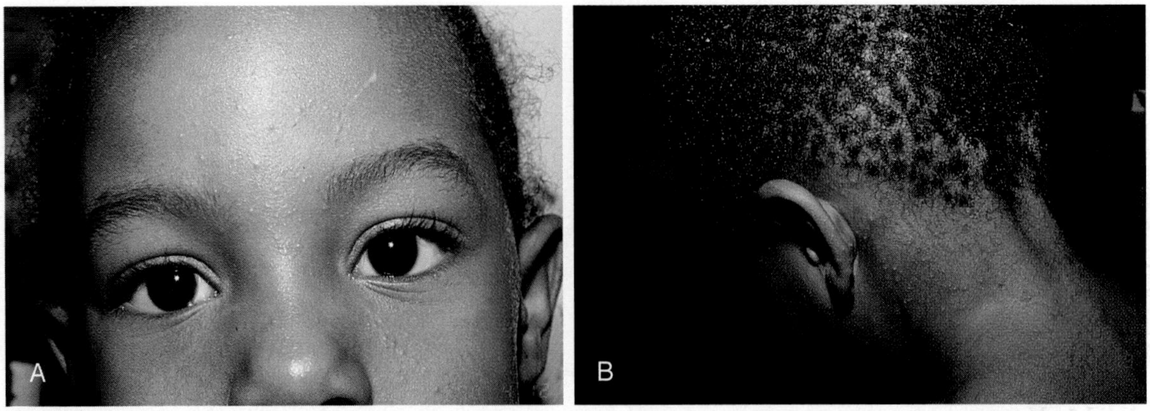

FIGURE 145–14 □ Id reaction. *A,* Fine papular eruption on the face in a 3-year-old girl with tinea capitis. *B,* Tinea capitis with fine papular id reaction on the neck.

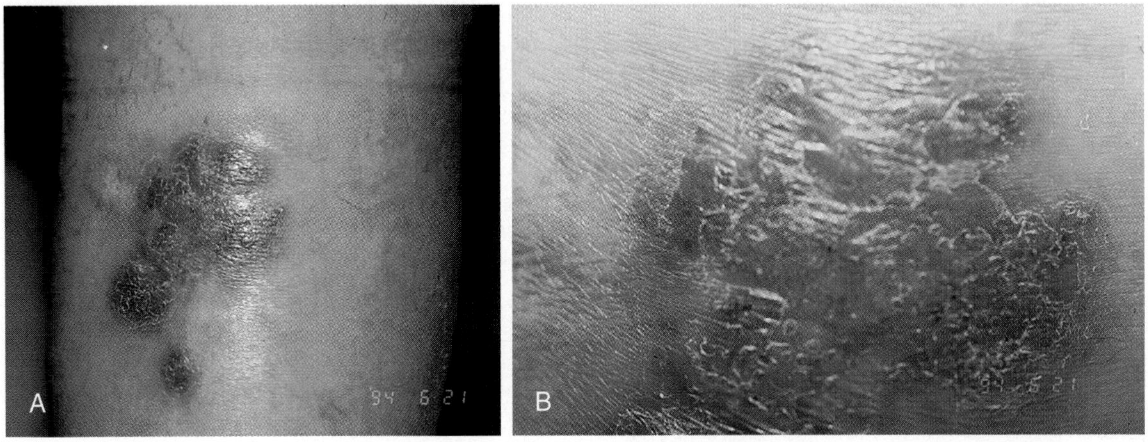

FIGURE 282–1 □ Chromoblastomycosis. *A,* Multiple plaques on the lower leg. *B,* Close-up of *A*. (*A* and *B* courtesy of Nellie Konnikov, MD, New England Medical Center, Boston, MA.)

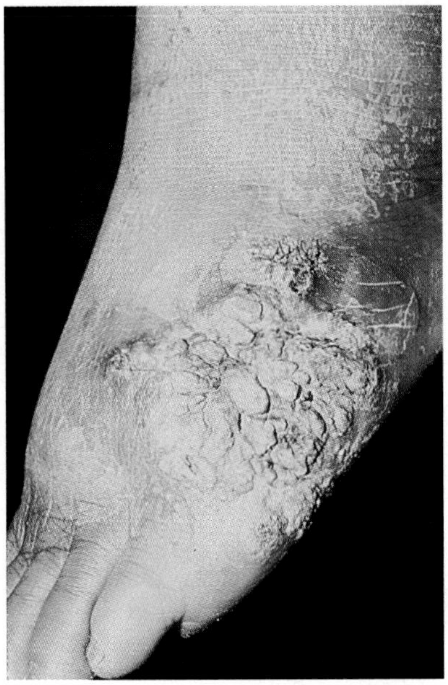

FIGURE 282–2 □ Chromoblastomycosis. Verrucous plaques on the lateral aspect of the foot.

PART I THE HISTORY OF INFECTIOUS DISEASES

1

A Perspective on the History of Infectious Diseases

Amalie M. Kass
*Edward H. Kass**

For most of recorded time, understanding of infectious diseases rested on theories that only recently have been replaced by the discoveries of science and the advances of technology. Until the development of bacteriology in the mid-19th century revealed the nature of infection and until vaccines, antisera, and antibiotics permitted some reliable modes of prevention and treatment, the understanding of infection in Western societies was based on theoretical and empirical doctrines and only a few preventive and therapeutic approaches had any validity. By the end of the 20th century, scientific investigation had increased the understanding of infectious diseases and produced a broad array of therapeutic agents.

The Classical Heritage

Greek philosophers and observers laid the foundation for medical theories and practices that persisted for two millennia. By recognizing that disease was not caused by evil spirits invading the body and by attempting to exclude magical incantations and potions, they made a quantum advance from the medical understandings of earlier cultures. For Hippocrates and his followers, disease was a process in nature that could be understood and treated by rational means. The Greeks believed nature to be composed of four basic elements: air, fire, water, and earth. Greek physicians taught that the human body was similarly composed of four constituent humors: blood, phlegm, black bile, and yellow bile. These were thought to arise in the heart, brain, spleen, and liver, respectively; for health to be maintained, all four were required to be in harmony. Fevers, poxes, pus, and other signs of infection represented the body's attempts to rid itself of damaging environmental factors that were upsetting the humoral balance.

The physician treated the individual, not a disease. Because all living things came from the earth, remedies were sought principally in plants. Fever, for example, was regarded as due to heating of the humors and required debilitating herbs to reduce the heat, followed by a restorative diet to strengthen the weakened body. Inasmuch as most patients survived, the efficacy of the treatments received general if not unanimous support.

The Greek physicians and those who followed them made important clinical observations and were particularly adept at recognizing symptoms and signs that indicated prognosis. Although historians delight in pointing to descriptions of specific diseases as found in the writings of seemingly prescient medical writers of antiquity and later periods, these references had little effect on practice because of the overwhelming influence of humoral doctrine. Similarly, mention of unseen organisms—such as seeds, germs, worms, and other animalcula that caused disease—permits interesting suggestions that classical or medieval scientists and physicians were foretelling infectious agents, but such allusions were purely speculative and had no scientific basis.

Theory and empiricism also lay behind the efforts of physicians and politicians to control the spread of disease. Personal and public cleanliness was obviously effective; the Jews and the Romans especially encouraged bathing, clean food, and pure water. The well off, who tended to be better bathed and fed, clearly seemed to have less disease than the relatively unwashed poor. However, in northern climates, bathing was less common, and the lessons from the exponents of cleanliness were often forgotten or ignored. Isolation of sick persons within a society and quarantines to protect a city or state from invasion by outsiders exposed to sickness were public health measures that could be used only by a government strong enough to enforce such regulations.

With the rapid spread of new religious doctrines during the post-Roman era, external causes of disease were once again viewed as visitations from a divine providence or from an underworld counterpart. The great plagues that afflicted Europe during and after the Middle Ages were often attributed to supernatural causes or to the influence of unwanted members of the population, leading to trials, expulsions, and executions. Historically, however, these epidemics correlated with the demise of feudalism, increased trade, greater movement of people, and growth of cities, with inevitable crowding, lack of sanitation, and strain on basic resources. The Crusades, warfare, and trade with distant lands brought, along with people and goods, hitherto unknown infections or provided a means whereby indigenous infections might be more readily spread.

Nevertheless, the basic humoralism that had been codified by Galen, the Greek physician who practiced in Rome during the second century of the Christian era, although modified and commented on by each succeeding generation, remained unchanged for almost 2000 years. Within the confines of this theoretical structure, treatment varied in emphasis rather than in intent. At one time, bleeding and purging might take priority; at another time, emetics and diaphoretics or stimulation of the nervous system would be in vogue, as one or another minor modification of the basic Hippocratic and Galenic doctrines assumed temporary ascendancy.

Chemical and Iatrochemical Discoveries

The first significant changes in doctrine occurred with the discoveries of postmedieval chemists, who incorporated minerals such as antimony and mercury into the pharmacopoeia; but again, benefits were more in the perception than in the demonstration. Infections remained life threatening, epidemics were common, and cures were often due as much to good fortune as to treatment, which was on occasion as harmful as the disease. Surgery—which was primarily devoted to repair of trauma, such as amputations, and to operations for

*Deceased.

the removal of kidney stones and cataracts—was especially dangerous. Mortality rates might reach 80% even for these limited surgical procedures, and pus was such a normal accompaniment that gradations of pus from "good and laudable" to "foul" were taught as prognostic signs.

Renaissance Medicine

The Renaissance brought more permanent questioning of traditional wisdom and hence of the teaching of ancient medical authorities. Universities were founded, and physicians who had university training acquired increased recognition for their learning. Anatomic studies, which were essential to the work of Renaissance painters and sculptors, received attention from physicians as well. The direct observations of Andreas Vesalius (1514–1564) at the autopsy table led to the correction of many of Galen's errors and laid the foundations of modern anatomy and surgery. His work also demonstrated the necessity for dissection, which in time would lead to investigation in pathologic anatomy and have a profound impact on the understanding of disease. Vesalius himself remained wedded to humoralism.

Renaissance anatomists also pointed to ways by which surgeons might operate to relieve the effects of trauma or adventitious growths, although always with the great risk of uncontrollable infection. Ambroise Paré (1510–1590), the barber-surgeon who served in the French army, where his skills were in great demand for soldiers wounded by newly invented gunpowder, made remarkable improvements in surgical treatment. Paré substituted the ligature for cautery and used clean, dry bandages and wine and honey, instead of boiling oil, to dress wounds. He too was acting empirically without understanding the reasons for his success.

In this same period, Girolamus Frascatorius (1484–1553) developed the first consistent concept of contagion, hypothesizing the existence of germs specific for different diseases, capable of multiplying in the body and of being spread either by direct contact or through objects that carried the infectious organisms. However, his contributions to the understanding of infectious diseases, significant because his guesses turned out to be correct, were based only on broad theorization and observation; there were no technical means to prove such theories.

The Enlightenment

New ways of thinking and new instruments continued to produce significant change. By the 17th century, profound challenges to religious, political, and cultural doctrines were accompanied by formal statements of scientific methods of experimentation and observation. The new mathematics, physics, and chemistry were often applied to physiologic observations and moved medicine closer to a scientific understanding of infection. Scientific academies and learned societies sprang up in the capitals of many European countries, while medical journals made their first appearance. The development of the microscope, starting with Anton van Leeuwenhoek (1632–1723), and improved fabrication of surgical and other scientific instruments were the result of technical skill and confidence that exploration of the unknown was possible. In turn, these intellectual and technical changes and the prosperity that an expanding market engendered fueled the growing sense that scientific exploration of disease was possible.

A brief flirtation with iatrophysics and the mechanistic explanation of disease as disturbance of solids (i.e., the atoms that were the essential bodily elements—an idea that had surfaced with some of the Greek physicians) seemed to challenge humoralism during the 17th century but did not prevail. Clinical observation and study of infectious diseases, especially by Thomas Sydenham (1624–1689), hinted at the notion of individual diseases with specific causes and remedies; like his contemporaries, however, Sydenham continued to believe in humors and to rely on bleeding, a practice that became more extensive than in earlier centuries. It was thought that fever, presumably a consequence of increased friction of blood flow, might be reduced by bleeding.

Thoughtful scientists and physicians were increasingly dissatisfied with humoral theory and sought alternative explanations of disease. By the mid-18th century, various classification systems were advanced, but they were not sufficiently convincing to replace basic humoralism. The importance of sanitation and cleanliness became more accepted and standards of living gradually improved, with a noticeable although dimly perceived effect on mortality patterns and population growth.

Jenner, Morgagni, and the French Pathologic Anatomists

One of the most important advances in public health was brought to Europe by observers who, taking their lead from folk practices in the Orient and Turkey, found that inoculation with material from the smallpox vesicle would protect against further attacks of the dreaded smallpox. Occasional fatalities followed such a procedure, and epidemics of smallpox were frequent enough that the inoculations were blamed. Edward Jenner (1749–1823), a practitioner trained as an apothecary (as were most practitioners of the time), was impressed with the common finding that milkmaids, renowned for their unscarred facial complexions, often had scars on their hands—scars produced by prior infection with cowpox, a common disorder of cows. Such women did not develop smallpox when there were outbreaks of the disease. Jenner's use of cowpox lymph as a means of protection against smallpox (Fig. 1–1) began a whole system of preven-

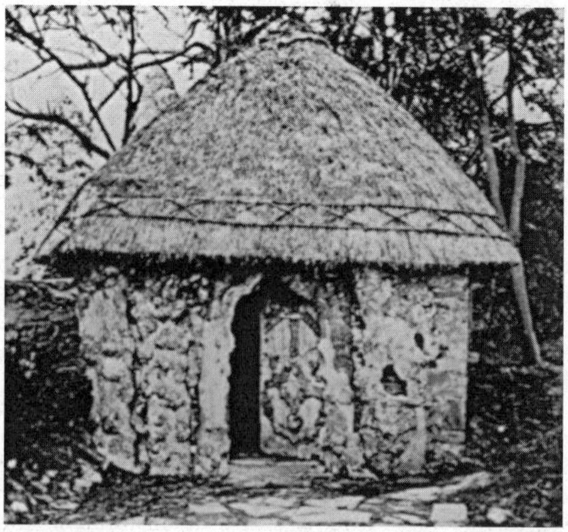

FIGURE 1–1 □ Hut in the garden of the vicarage in Gloucestershire where Jenner gave the first smallpox vaccinations. (Photograph by J. Eatough in publications of the Jenner Museum, Berkeley, Gloucestershire, UK.)

tive medicine based on vaccination (the word derived from the Latin root for cows).

Meanwhile, Giovanni Battista Morgagni (1682–1771) began his systematic observations at the autopsy table. His monumental treatise, based on the findings of some 700 dissections, correlated clinical symptoms and autopsy findings. By the beginning of the next century, numerous followers in France and England came to see pathologic anatomy as a key to understanding disease. They began to delineate specific disease syndromes, slowly coming to the realization that diseases might have specific causes as well as specific manifestations and might not represent solely attempts by the body to restore humoral balance. As chemical discoveries progressed, there was also a recognition that many manifestations of disease might be explained in chemical, as opposed to purely anatomic, changes in the body. Although these same pioneers continued to use bleeding, sweating, and purging as foundations for their treatments, they often espoused more "judicious" use of these methods and depended on their growing understanding of the natural history of disease to guide their therapy. A few drugs had become available, particularly cinchona, or Jesuit's bark, brought to Europe from the New World. Its value for certain remittent fevers led to its use for all fevers (for which it often proved ineffective) and thus to its being discarded as useless until later discoveries delineated its special role in the treatment of malaria. The only other drugs of the time that later turned out to have demonstrable value were opium, atropine, and digitalis.

Accompanying the newer ways of studying disease at autopsy, new ways of teaching medicine replaced the sterile didacticism of previous centuries. The growth of hospitals for treatment of the sick poor—as opposed to their earlier function as religious refuges—and of medical schools associated with hospitals established a locale for more systematic observation of illness and for the performance of autopsies. Hospital-trained physicians and surgeons began to acquire diagnostic and therapeutic skills and gradually to replace wound healers, bleeders, cuppers, leechers, and midwives, all of whom, trained by apprenticeship, had traditionally provided medical care to most of the population.

Nowhere was this bedside method as well employed as in France, which renounced traditional medical institutions along with the monarchy at the end of the 18th century. By the beginning of the 19th century, Paris had become the medical and scientific capital of Europe. Parisian hospitals were larger than those in other countries; autopsies were allowed by law (although still unlawful in Great Britain) and a group of medical greats dominated French thinking and teaching. Marie François Xavier Bichat (1771–1802) extended Morgagni's work, with careful dissections that led him to produce broad generalizations about the structure of diseased tissue. René Théophile Hyacinthe Laënnec (1781–1826), improvising a means by which he could tactfully examine an obese woman with heart disease, first employed the stethoscope, which was destined to become one of the most valuable tools of physical diagnosis. Laënnec correlated physical findings with pathologic anatomy in a variety of diseases of the heart, lungs, and liver. Pierre Charles Alexandre Louis (1787–1872) began the systematic analysis of disease, particularly of typhoid fever and pneumonia, which became a forerunner of quantitative bedside analysis. The influence of the Parisian school extended well beyond France. Students from England, Ireland, and the United States as well as other continental nations went there to study. Nonetheless, the persistence of humoral therapeutics is dramatically illustrated by the single fact that in 1833, France imported 42 million leeches.

Contagionism and Anticontagionism

Recurrent epidemics led contagionists and anticontagionists to debate the value and necessity of quarantines, lazarettos, and other sanitary measures to combat epidemics. Urbanization, industrialization, and growing trade made their arguments increasingly important to governmental officials, who paid close attention to the economic and social ramifications of a decision to close a port, exclude foreign traders, or undertake expensive public health measures. Without a satisfactory explanation regarding the agents of contagion, many denied the transmissibility of disease from person to person; rather, they insisted on environmental causes of disease, such as climate, bad air, and urban slums, or on moral culpability, such as the habits of the poor. Because quarantines were often unsuccessful and epidemics usually ended without stringent public health measures, it was not difficult to assume that the drastic bloodletting and purges prescribed by Benjamin Rush (1745–1813) in Philadelphia had brought an end to a yellow fever epidemic or that a change in weather had caused the cessation of outbreaks of cholera.

Throughout the 19th century, evidence accumulated regarding the validity of contagionism. British and Irish obstetricians had already shown that puerperal fever, which caused women to dread childbirth and to fear death after delivery, could be reduced if extreme cleanliness of attendants and bed linen was enforced and vaginal examinations were limited. In 1843 in Boston, Oliver Wendell Holmes (1809–1894) reviewed the pertinent literature and sided with those who suggested that puerperal fever was caused by contagious agents transmitted from infected persons to the parturient woman by the physician. Holmes outraged many obstetricians, whose sense of personal insult was abetted by the absence of scientific proof. Four years later in Vienna, Ignaz Semmelweis (1818–1865) deduced from a difference in mortality between one clinic staffed by midwives and another staffed by doctors and medical students that the latter attendants were carrying infection with them from autopsies or other patients. Semmelweis further recognized the similarity at autopsy between death from puerperal sepsis and that caused by wound infection and noted the efficacy of hand washing with chlorinated lime before attending parturient women. That Semmelweis was hounded out of Vienna is evidence that until the agent of infection was identified, most of the medical and scientific world was not yet ready to accept such a notion.

Interactive improvements in basic science and technology during the first part of the 19th century helped to clear the way for the germ theory, which would emerge in the following half-century. The development and use of the achromatic microscope by Joseph Lister (1786–1869, father of Lord Lister) and Thomas Hodgkin (1798–1866) in the late 1820s ended the problem of chromatic aberration and permitted more extensive use of the microscope than had heretofore been possible. The great discoveries in cell pathology and later discoveries in bacteriology were made possible partly by improved staining methods as well as by the technology that produced relatively inexpensive glass implements, piped gas, and other day-to-day usable technology.

A new kind of scientist was also emerging. Whereas research had previously been the hobby of practicing physicians and surgeons or of gifted amateurs, full-time employment of scientists in a laboratory or clinic attached to a university or scientific institute was becoming more common. This was especially true in France and Germany, which modernized the universities and gave governmental support to scientific research before other countries did so. In the second half of the 19th century, in consequence of the political turmoil in France, scientific and medical preeminence shifted to Germany, much as it would move to the United States in the second half of the 20th century.

Scientific Bacteriology

It was the genius of a Frenchman trained as a chemist that put to rest notions of spontaneous generation, firmly established the germ theory of disease, demonstrated the principle of immunity, and created the biologic basis for prevention and modern health practices. Bacteria had been observed under the microscope, especially in spoiled food, since the days of Leeuwenhoek, and by 1840 Jakob Henle (1809–1885) had revived the notion of microorganisms as the agents of disease. Casimir Davaine (1812–1882) and Pierre Rayer (1793–1867) discovered the anthrax bacillus in the blood of infected animals in 1850, and they succeeded in transferring the disease to other animals. Others had shown that fungi caused certain diseases of the skin and of silkworms. Many scientists—notably Virchow, Zenker, Obermeier, Klencke, and Villemin—made important but isolated discoveries without developing an accompanying theory.

Louis Pasteur (1822–1895) studied bacteria first because of their action in spoiling wine. He had already observed that tartaric acid formed crystals that were mirror images and thus discovered racemization. His experiments with beer and wine provided the proof that, contrary to the doctrine of many chemists including the reknowned Baron Justus von Liebig (1803–1873), microorganisms were the active agents of fermentation and that spontaneous generation was a myth. His demonstration that spoilage of wine could be prevented by the application of heat led in time to the pasteurization of many foods. Having benefited the French wine industry, Pasteur also applied his formidable talents to finding the causes of disease in silkworms and thereby rescued the silk industry. The close association of the fundamental discoveries of bacteriology with industrial problems has often been forgotten by succeeding generations.

After 20 years of fruitful research in the biology of microorganisms, in 1877 Pasteur began to investigate human and animal diseases (Fig. 1–2). He and his associates developed vaccines for anthrax, chicken cholera, and rabies. Despite the now obvious truth of Pasteur's work and its immense significance for medicine, in his lifetime he was continuously beset by critics and disbelievers—many from the medical profession, which resented him as an outsider.

Robert Koch (1843–1910), working in Germany, ranks as the second founder and major teacher of bacteriology. Koch trained in medicine and was a general practitioner in the early years of his career. He made great technical improvements in bacteriology, especially by using solid culture media and developing new methods of fixing and staining. In 1879 he studied the bacteria causing wound infection and destroyed the notion that the same pathogens might take on many different microscopic appearances, an idea that had been used by others to mask their own inability to obtain pure cultures. Koch's postulates, following those of Henle, laid down criteria for the identification of microbiologic pathogens. Koch also discovered the tubercle bacillus and cholera vibrio. His researches included investigations in Egypt, India, and South Africa. His claims for tuberculin as a treatment for tuberculosis proved to be unfounded, although tuberculin became an effective diagnostic aid.

With Pasteur and Koch training many gifted students, a spate of important discoveries followed. By the end of the 19th century, the infectious agents of amoebic and bacillary dysentery, gonorrhea, typhoid fever, leprosy, malaria, glanders, erysipelas, diphtheria, tetanus, pneumonia, epidemic meningitis, Malta fever (brucellosis), soft chancre, gas gangrene, plague, and botulism were identified. The existence of filterable viruses was hypothesized and proved, and many other infectious agents were identified during the first decades of the 20th century. The new discoveries extended to therapeutics. In 1889, Alexandre Yersin and Emile Roux showed that a toxin or toxins produced by the diphtheria bacillus circulated in the blood stream and accounted for the disease. Arthur Nicolaier made an analogous finding for tetanus, leading to the discovery of antitoxins against these toxins by Emil von Behring and Shibasaburo Kitasato and to the development of effective antitoxin therapy. Paul Ehrlich (1854–1915), having done important work on antibodies and immunity, proposed the concept of passive immunization as distinguished from active immunization produced by vaccination. He also began his search for antimicrobial drugs. Serum diagnosis began with the development in 1896 of Georges Widal's agglutination test for typhoid fever.

By the end of the 19th century, a coherent and scientifically proven explanation of the causes of many febrile diseases was firmly established. The long-debated question of the specificity of diseases had been laid to rest, and the belief in humors and in miasmas as causes of infection was largely dispelled.

The new thinking and new techniques spilled over into other medical areas. Holmes and Semmelweis had been vin-

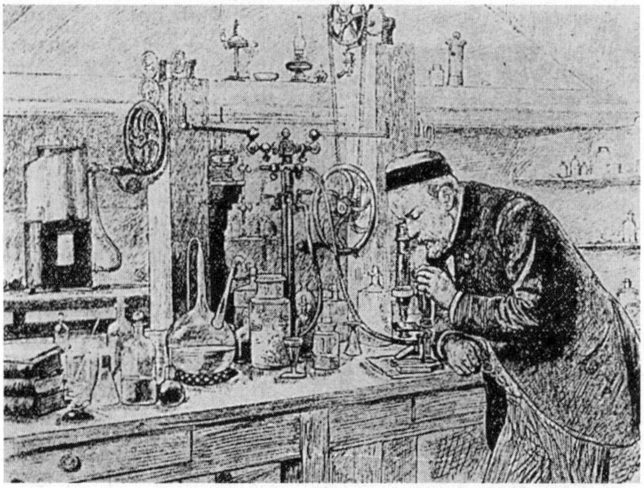

FIGURE 1–2 □ Pasteur in his laboratory. (Courtesy of the Countway Library of Medicine, Harvard Medical School, Cambridge, MA.)

dicated by the discovery of streptococci in pus by Theodor Billroth (1829–1894). In Glasgow, the surgeon Joseph Lister (1827–1912) applied Pasteur's lessons of bacterial infection to problems of sepsis in surgery and began to treat open fractures with carbolic acid to kill bacteria. When this proved successful in reducing the rate of infection of the wounds, he extended his "antiseptic" principle to all surgical procedures (Fig. 1–3). As in many areas of science, it took years before most surgeons accepted Lister's teaching. In the 1880s, Ernst von Bergmann (1836–1907) in Berlin developed the techniques of asepsis, in which instruments, operating areas, and hands of medical personnel were disinfected. Antisepsis and asepsis demolished the notion that pus was an inevitable and useful consequence of surgery.

The Sanitary Movement

Bacteriology also fueled the sanitary movement, especially in cities, where severe crowding and wretched housing, unpaved and unlit streets, limited running water, and inadequate waste disposal and sanitation were the norm for hundreds of thousands of inhabitants. John Snow (1813–1858) demonstrated in 1854 that cholera was more prevalent in London households receiving water from a lower part of the Thames than in households receiving water from a source farther up the river. Snow postulated but could not prove that a multiplying agent carried in the excreta of cholera victims via the water supply was causing the spread of the disease. Many sanitarians were already advocating improved water supply and sanitation without accepting the germ theory. After Koch's work revealed the etiology of cholera, public health officials concentrated on discovering the vectors of other food- and water-borne diseases and on improving disposal of sewage and providing clean supplies of water and food.

Arthropod-Borne Infections

The accomplishments of Theobald Smith (1859–1934), an American, in showing that cattle fever was transmitted by ticks, initiated the understanding of arthropod vectors. A series of discoveries by French, British, and Italian observers demonstrated that the plasmodia of malaria are transmitted by the female *Anopheles* mosquito. Control of yellow fever, also a mosquito-borne disease, enabled the United States to occupy Cuba after the Spanish-American War in 1898 and contributed to the successful construction of the Panama Canal a few years later. Public awareness of these accomplishments added to the demand for clean water, pure food, and a healthier environment and led to passage of legislation designed to protect the population from contagious diseases. Bacterial causes of diseases of plants, such as pear blight, were also receiving recognition.

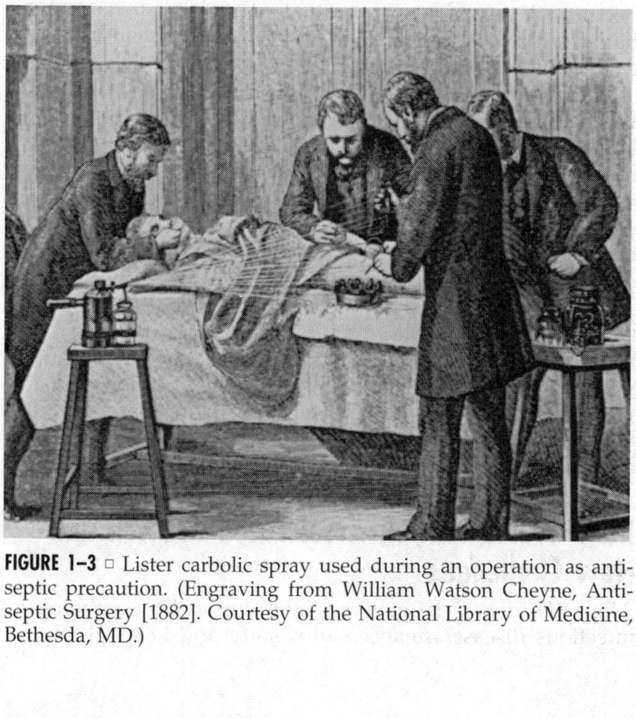

FIGURE 1–3 □ Lister carbolic spray used during an operation as antiseptic precaution. (Engraving from William Watson Cheyne, Antiseptic Surgery [1882]. Courtesy of the National Library of Medicine, Bethesda, MD.)

There was a natural tendency to assume that the decline in mortality and morbidity rates related to the major infectious diseases was the effect of immunization and specific therapy. In reality, however, much of the decline occurred before vaccines or serum therapy was available or widespread. The major reasons for the change were related to general socioeconomic improvement, with rising standards of living, improved nutrition, diminished crowding as family size decreased and housing became more abundant, and enforcement of sanitary regulations. With this improvement came increasing concern with infections that are not communicable but are due to autochthonous bacteria such as the gram-negative rods and staphylococci.

World War I

World War I gave a tremendous stimulus to the study of infectious diseases, especially those that were widespread among the armed forces, such as meningitis, diarrhea, trench fever, typhus, and gonorrhea. Scientific groups were appointed to investigate means of controlling these diseases. By the time the United States entered the war, Allied soldiers wounded in battle routinely received a prophylactic dose of tetanus antitoxin, with remarkably effective results. However, the influenza pandemic that swept the world in the years after the war, killing more than 20 million people worldwide and 500,000 in the United States alone, showed that much about infectious diseases remained unknown. The influenza virus had not been isolated and the cause of the pandemic was still uncertain. Various vaccines, many with severe side effects, were developed but had little success until more purified and more broadly effective products later became available.

Chemotherapy

The possibilities for chemotherapy had received much attention before World War I because of the work of Ehrlich and his associates in Germany. Drawing on the chemistry of staining, Ehrlich had developed the theory that a special chemical affinity exists between some chemicals and certain cells and that particular chemicals might be more lethal to the disease-causing microorganism than to the host. Ehrlich's dogged persistence in looking for the chemical compound that would specifically bind to and destroy pathogens such as *Treponema pallidum* led to the discovery of salvarsan (arsphenamine) and then to other organic arsenicals. The use of salvarsan and its derivatives not only reduced the dangers of syphilis but also provided another stimulus to the pharmaceutical industry.

Among the next major events in chemotherapeutics was the discovery in 1935 by Gerhardt Domagk, building on the German dye industry, that Prontosil, a dye prepared by diazotization of sulfanilamide, specifically cured infections due to β-hemolytic streptococci. Within a short time it was shown that the sulfanilamide portion of the dye accounted for the antibacterial activity. Derivatives of the basic molecule broadened the antibacterial spectrum to include a larger number of common bacterial pathogens. World War II stimulated the development of the sulfonamide drugs and a search for other antimicrobial agents, which led to renewed interest in penicillin. Penicillin had been discovered earlier by Alexander Fleming, but its potential was not explored because of its lability. As part of a systematic examination of potential candidates for further study, Howard Florey, Ernest Chain, Edward Abraham, and their associates established the value of penicillin and later of the cephalosporins. The cephalosporins, discovered by Giuseppe Brotzu in an isolate from a Sardinian sewage treatment pond, were developed in response to the growing resistance of many bacteria to sulfonamides and to penicillin.

The general concept of antibiosis, a term coined by Selman Waksman, went back more than half a century, to the time when it was first recognized that some molds had the ability to destroy bacteria. Soil microbiologists, among whom Waksman was an eminent leader, recognized that the complex ecology of the soil microflora depended in part on the capacity of some organisms to inhibit the multiplication of others. Some antibiotics were isolated and purified by Waksman, his former student René Dubos, and others, but toxicity limited their use. However, Waksman continued to search for effective and less toxic antibiotics in soil, and, with his students Elizabeth Bugie and Albert Schatz, he isolated streptomycin from a strain of *Streptomyces,* beginning a method of search that dominated the world of antibiotics for decades.

The initial discoveries of penicillin and streptomycin were made by academic investigators who used relatively few resources. The pharmaceutical industry responded rapidly to these discoveries and, within a remarkably short time, many additional and relatively inexpensive products became available (Fig. 1–4). When the search became more difficult and governmental requirements for approval more stringent, economic constraints drove up the price of newly discovered drugs.

As knowledge accumulated about the chemical structure and mechanisms of action of antimicrobial drugs, it became possible to alter the structure of the parent compound or of its active nucleus and to make large numbers of derivatives, some of which displayed greater activity, wider ranges of antimicrobial action, diminished susceptibility to the mechanisms that led to resistance by the microbes, or diminished toxicity. However, most discoveries of antimicrobial drugs were empirical. Only more recently has understanding of mechanisms led to the development of drugs, such as trimethoprim, that were specifically targeted against a vital mechanism within the microbes—a mechanism that was necessarily more susceptible to the drug in the microbe than in the host.

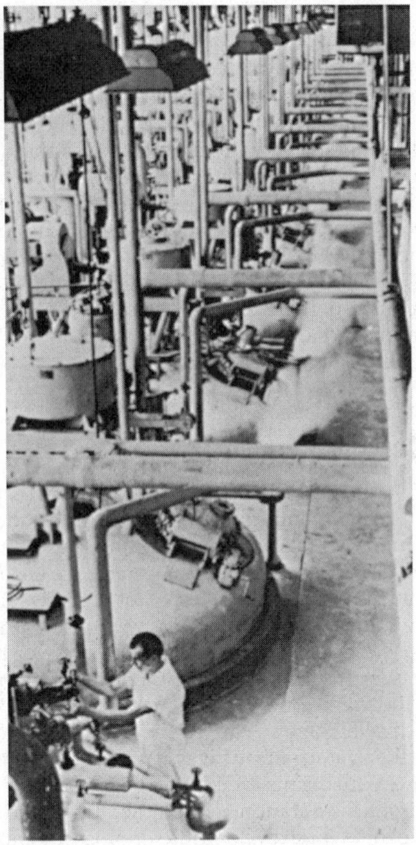

FIGURE 1–4 □ Industrial production of antibiotics. (Courtesy of United Press International. Reprinted by permission of The Bettmann Archive.)

Immunization

Interest never flagged in the promise of active immunization. The classic tetanus and diphtheria toxins were purified and thus became less likely to produce side effects when attenuated into toxoids. Infectious agents had to be isolated and grown, and their virulence attenuated, without destroying immunogenicity. Careful evaluation in a critical environment led to the sifting of conflicting claims, to the establishment of a growing number of active immunizing agents, and to a growing number of restrictions, constraints, and advice that produced an evolving and remarkably dynamic field, sparked by utility to the public health, potential profitability, and expanding scientific interest. The chemical capacity to isolate fragments of an antigen that could stimulate active immunity with a minimum of side effects, to enlarge the range of effectiveness of vaccines by conjugating them to protein carriers that might increase effectiveness, to combine vaccines with immunomodulating substances that might make vaccines more economical or more effective, and more recently to use cloning techniques to provide large supplies of vaccines that otherwise might be difficult to obtain (in hepatitis B, the agent was, until cloned, available only in the blood of previously infected individuals) all give testimony to the visions that illuminate the field.

There have been failures of doctrine and of procedure. When the doctrine, based on experiments in macaque monkeys, held that the poliomyelitis virus could enter the body only through nerve endings, as in the upper nasopharynx, many children were given compounds to destroy these nerve endings (and the accompanying sense of smell and much of taste) in what proved to be a futile attempt to halt the spread of poliomyelitis. The discovery in 1949 by John Enders, Thomas Weller, and Frederick Robbins that the poliovirus would multiply in cell cultures unrelated to nervous tissue provided a concept of the disease that was discontinuous with the prevailing wisdom; it led to the isolation of many viral agents and to effective vaccines. How many of these have the potential to eliminate certain diseases, as smallpox has been eliminated, remains to be determined.

Post–World War II: Accelerated Growth and New Challenges

After World War II, governmental support for research in infectious diseases financed university and hospital laboratories and facilitated the training of specialists in infectious diseases. National and then international organizations were created that further stimulated important work in the causes and treatment of infections. Publication, in many countries, of journals specifically for infectious diseases added to dissemination of new knowledge. International collaboration in the control and eradication of infectious diseases led to some major successes, most especially with worldwide elimination of smallpox.

Antimicrobial drugs made many surgical and other therapeutic procedures possible, procedures that otherwise would have been associated with prohibitive rates of infection. On the other hand, the increased number of immunocompromised patients has led to problems that require increasingly specialized information for their management. Nosocomial infections and drug-resistant strains of pathogens have produced additional clinical problems.

In the community, a more informed and demanding public, the desire for more effective preventive tactics, and more responsive governmental officials have not only broadened the demand for medical care but also increased the demand for services connected with infectious disease.

Many questions remain unanswered and many problems remain unsolved. Some well-known diseases—for example, malaria and schistosomiasis—continue to take a terrible toll in human suffering. The notion of "newly emerging infectious diseases" has begun to attract increased attention, as diseases hitherto unknown or unrecognized have appeared. Some, such as acquired immunodeficiency syndrome, have caused fear such as has not been seen since the days of the great plagues, whereas others, such as hantavirus pulmonary syndrome and the hemorrhagic fevers, raise serious problems of control. Diseases once thought to be under complete control have reawakened concern among public health officials. In the United States, for example, the emergence of multidrug-resistant strains has compounded the problems associated with tuberculosis, whereas in South America, cholera has once again become a serious threat. Finally, there remains the likelihood that diseases not now thought of as infectious may be caused by infectious agents. Identification of *Helicobacter pylori* as the cause of gastric ulcers is one example.

Acquisition of resistance to available drugs and inadequate understanding of the response of the host to infection are stimulating a search for new strategies. Less toxic, more effective vaccines will be based on genetic or biochemical manipulation of the chemical structure of their component antigens. Furthermore, medical personnel will need to work more closely than ever with social scientists and makers of public policy to better educate people throughout the world regarding the relationship of individual behavior to disease. The realization that the changes in ecosystems that accompany economic development schemes are major factors in the emergence of new diseases will also force closer ties between infectious disease researchers, epidemiologists, economists, and international agencies.

The ease with which people and goods now traverse the world and the intractable ties that bind all parts of our planet make it clear that laboratory research, clinical treatment, and control of infectious diseases will play increasingly important parts in the improvement of life for people throughout that world.

Acknowledgment

Richard Platt, MD, provided helpful suggestions and advice for the revision of this chapter.

Bibliography

- Ackerknecht EH: A Short History of Medicine, rev ed. Baltimore, Johns Hopkins University Press, 1982.
- Bynum WF, Nutton V (eds): Theories of Fever from Antiquity to the Enlightenment. London, Wellcome Institute for the History of Medicine, 1981.
- Dowling HF: Fighting Infection. Cambridge, MA, Harvard University Press, 1977.
- Duffy J: The Sanitarians. Urbana, IL, University of Illinois Press, 1990.
- Foster WD: A History of Medical Bacteriology and Immunology. London, William Heinemann, 1970.
- Kiple KF (ed): The Cambridge World History of Human Disease. New York, Cambridge University Press, 1993.
- Lyons AS, Petrucelli RJ: Medicine: An Illustrated History. New York, Harry N Abrams, 1987.
- Magner LN: A History of Medicine. New York, Marcel Dekker, 1992.
- Roizman B (ed): Infectious Diseases in an Age of Change. Washington, DC, National Academy Press, 1995.
- Rosenberg CE: Explaining Epidemics and Other Studies in the History of Medicine. New York, Cambridge University Press, 1992.
- Sigerist HE: Civilization and Disease. Chicago, University of Chicago Press, 1962.
- Silverstein AM: A History of Immunology. San Diego, CA, Academic Press, 1989.

HOW MICROORGANISMS CAUSE DISEASE

2

Toxins

Grace M. Thorne

Bacterial toxins were recognized approximately 100 years ago as the potent substances responsible for the effects of infectious diseases like diphtheria,[1] tetanus,[2] and botulism.[3] Roux and Yersin[4] were the first to use the term toxin in their description of the poisonous substance precipitated from a broth culture of diphtheria bacillus, and they rightly conjectured that the substance was a kind of enzyme. Nearly 80 years were to pass before Honjo[5, 6] and Gill[7] and coworkers demonstrated that nicotinamide adenine dinucleotide and elongation factor-2 were substrates in a reaction catalyzed by diphtheria toxin. Many toxins have subsequently been identified, and some confusion has arisen owing to the different terminology used as classification systems have evolved. Toxins have been named for the diseases they produce or the species name of the organism. Examples include cholera toxin (CT) produced by *Vibrio cholerae,* the causative agent of cholera; tetanus toxin (TeTx) produced by *Clostridium tetani,* the cause of tetanus; and Shiga toxin (STX) produced by *Shigella dysenteriae* (originally named Shiga's bacillus), a cause of bacillary dysentery or shigellosis. Toxins have been given simple letter designations, such as toxins A and B of *Clostridium difficile* and exotoxin A of *Pseudomonas aeruginosa.* Other toxins have been named for a physicochemical characteristic of the toxin preparations; the heat-labile toxins (LTs) and heat-stable toxins (STs) of *Escherichia coli* are good examples. Toxins have also been named for the cell types they affect; cytotoxins affect a variety of cell types (e.g., hepatotoxins), and neurotoxins refer to the specific organ affected. Once the mode of action is discovered, toxins are named for their enzyme activity, such as the α-toxin of *Clostridium perfringens,* which is known as a lecithinase, and the adenylate cyclase toxin of *Bordetella pertussis.*

In bacteriology, the term toxin is applied only to cell-associated endotoxin (lipopolysaccharide of the cell wall is described in Chapter 3) and to protein exotoxins, which are discussed in this chapter. Exotoxins are proteinaceous substances generally secreted from gram-positive or gram-negative bacteria and therefore can be isolated in the culture supernatant. Most important, exotoxins have a lethal effect on the host. The potent lethal nature of these proteins sets them apart from extracellular enzymes that may cause cell death and tissue damage but are not potent (i.e., median lethal dose greater than 1 mg/kg) and should not be considered toxins. Gill[8, 9] tabulated the lethal amounts of various toxins.

Exotoxins occur in many different sizes, ranging from 15 to 18 amino acids in length (*E. coli* ST) to 308 kDa (*C. difficile* toxin A), and molecular structures; however, a number of the important exotoxins conform to the A-B model described by Gill.[10] The so-called A-B toxins are composed of a binding B domain, component, or subunit(s) and an enzymatic A domain, component, or subunit(s) that is responsible for the toxic effect on the host cell.

There are also a large number of toxins that directly attack the cell membrane either by creating "channels," causing rearrangement of the membrane structure, or by digesting components of the membrane.

A few toxins affect intracellular reactions through transmembrane transducing systems. These toxins, like hormones, remain bound to the cell's exterior.

Some toxins are now known to function as superantigens because they are potent stimulators of T-cell proliferation. Toxicity is then mediated by subsequent release of cytokines like tumor necrosis factor, interleukin-1, interleukin-2, and interferon-γ.

Well-characterized examples of each type of toxin are discussed with emphasis on common themes in structure, molecular size, and shared DNA sequence motifs as well as molecular modes of action. The molecular technologies of the past 15 years have provided exciting discoveries of new toxins as well as identified families of toxins that share structural arrangements, receptor targets, and mechanisms of action.

The A-B Exotoxins

Toxins with some version of an A-B structure are shown in Figure 2–1. Each can bind by the B moiety to cell receptors and thereby concentrate toxin at the cell surface, and the B portion may even assist passage of the A portion across the membrane. Isolated A components exhibit "toxic" enzymatic activity in an in vitro broken cell system but are inactive against intact cells. Likewise, isolated B subunits usually have no toxic activity but can act to interfere with binding of intact toxin molecules. Only holotoxin can produce a toxic effect on intact eukaryotic cells or host. Although the A-B toxins differ in structure, receptor specificity, entry mechanism, and enzymatic reaction catalyzed, they are similar in that once bound, all trigger transfer of the A portion across the cell membrane into the cytosol.

Toxins with Adenosine Diphosphate–Ribosyltransferase Activity

A family of bacterial protein toxins exert their toxic effects through the nicotinamide adenine dinucleotide–dependent adenosine diphosphate (ADP) ribosylation of guanine nucleotide binding proteins of the adenylate cyclase complex in eukaryotic cell membranes. These toxins include CT, heat-labile enterotoxin (LT) produced by *E. coli,* and pertussis toxin (Table 2–1). One of the best understood toxins of this type is CT, which causes the voluminous dehydrating diarrhea characteristic of cholera. The crystal structures of CT and the approximately 80% homologous *E. coli* heat-labile enterotoxin are well defined.[11] Both CT and LT are synthesized as multisubunit toxins with A and B components. These toxins have their initial interaction with host cell membrane receptor G_{M1}, which is Gal-β1–3-Gal-NAc-β1-(NeuAc-

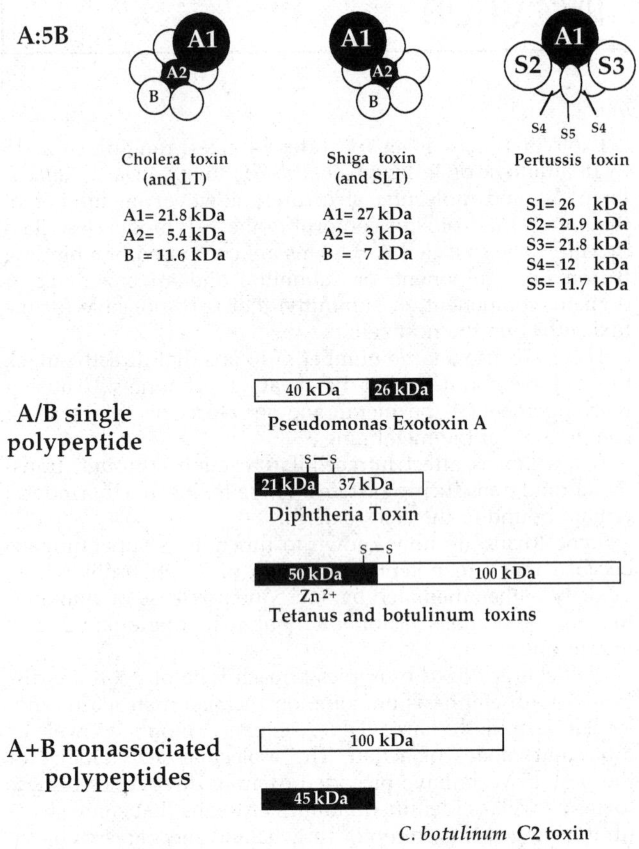

FIGURE 2–1 □ Representations of A-B toxins. (Structures are stylized and not drawn to scale.)

α2–3)→G1c ceramide. The pentameric B subunits appear to bind to the terminal galactose of the receptor. X-ray crystallography has shown the binding of the five subunits to be virtually identical.[12] The toxin A subunit is then nicked by proteolysis and reduced, yielding an A1 "enzyme" and an A2 "linker" polypeptide. The A1 and A2 peptides are still linked by a disulfide bond before internalization.[13] It is the A1 peptide that catalyzes the transfer of ADP ribose from nicotinamide adenine dinucleotide to subunits of the guanine nucleotide regulatory component G_s of the adenylate cyclase system.[14, 15] This modification leads to persistent activation of the cyclase and elevation of intracellular cyclic adenosine monophosphate (cAMP). The cAMP in turn activates a cAMP-dependent protein kinase, leading to phosphorylation alterations of ion transport and the development of diarrhea.

One area that is still unclear is the mode of entry of the toxin into the eukaryotic cell. Three possible scenarios have been proposed, which are reviewed by Kaper and colleagues.[16] The most likely explanation is that whole CT enters by endocytosis; the endosome travels through the cell with A1 peptide still associated with the endosomal membrane. Eventually A1 peptide ADP ribosylates G_s α-subunit located in the basolateral membrane. This theory is supported by studies reporting inhibition of CT by brefeldin A, which is known to interfere in vesicular transport in endosomal pathways of eukaryotic cells.[17, 18] These results support the requirement of an intact Golgi region for intracellular trafficking of the toxin and implicate endocytosis as the toxin's entry mechanism. Spangler[19] has written a detailed description of cellular factors that promote CT activity. The review by Kaper and coworkers[16] provides details of cholera enterotoxin as well as of other toxins (zonula occludens toxin [ZOT], Ace, ST, and new CT) produced by *V. cholerae* and their proposed mechanisms of action.

All the ADP ribosylating toxins listed in Table 2–1 modify nucleotide binding proteins. Elongation factor-2, the target of pertussis toxin and *P. aeruginosa* exotoxin A, is a guanosine triphosphate binding protein. Actin, the target of the clostridial C2 toxin, binds to adenosine triphosphate. The most recently described ADP-ribosyltransferase, the C3 toxin of *Clostridium botulinum,* targets Rho and Rac, which are small guanosine triphosphate binding proteins.[20] The role that C3 plays in disease is unclear at present.

Several different bacterial toxins with different enzymatic activities share the 1A:5B structural stoichiometry. These include the CT and *E. coli* LT family, pertussis toxin, and the STX and Shiga-like toxin (SLT) family (see Fig. 2–1). Crystallographic studies of two families of toxins (CT and LT, SLT-1 B subunit and STX) have revealed some structural similarities, which include conformation of the B subunits in a ring shape with a central pore (doughnut shape), similar length of the A2 subunit, and presence of an oligosaccharide binding fold within the B subunits of several of the toxins.[11, 21–25] Whereas these striking structural similarities have been observed, neither of the two families of toxins have significant similarities in amino acid sequences.

Shiga Toxin Family of Cytotoxins: RNA Glycosylases

STX is one of the most potent biologic substances known. Purified STX is cytotoxic, lethal, neurotoxic, and enterotoxic,[26] yet its role in human enteric disease has been unclear for many years. In the early 1980s, a rare serotype of diarrheogenic *E. coli* was shown to produce a Vero cell toxin.[27] Shortly thereafter, both immunologic and biochemical evidence linked STX and the newly named Shiga-like cytotoxins isolated from outbreak strains of *E. coli* O157:H7. The SLT-producing *E. coli* strains (particularly serotype O157:H7) are associated with the development of hemorrhagic colitis and hemolytic-uremic syndrome.[28] Infection with *S. dysenteriae* (which produces STX) is also known to lead to hemolytic-uremic syndrome. The role of SLT and STX in the development of these diseases has focused on the potential for damage of endothelial cells documented to be induced by SLT and endotoxin.[29] Sjogren and coworkers[30] have provided new evidence of the importance of SLT-1 (STX) in the pathogenicity of SLT-producing *E. coli.* This group compared isogenic strains of an enteroadherent rabbit diarrheal pathogen with and without SLT in a rabbit model of bacterial enteritis. They concluded that SLT-1 is an important virulence factor causing vascular changes consistent with endothelial damage. Such changes were similar to microvascular changes seen in humans with *E. coli* O157:H7 infection. The development of this animal model will assist in future studies of the STX family of toxins.

At the molecular level, cloning and genetic sequencing have shown STX and SLT-1 to be essentially identical; the SLT-2 family members are 55% homologous to STX.[31] The structural genes for two of the toxins, SLT-1 and SLT-2, are encoded on temperate bacteriophage, but the genes for STX are chromosomal, and other members of the SLT family (i.e., SLT-2c and SLT-2e) are not known to be on mobile genetic elements. Expression of STX and SLT-1 is repressed by iron, whereas production of the SLT-2 toxins is not.

These toxins have A and B subunits in a 1:5 ratio. The B subunit binds to globotriaosylceramide (P1) glycolipid on the surface of eukaryotic cells.[32] The A subunits of the STX toxin family are homologous to the A subunits of ricin, the plant toxin. This family of toxins acts directly on the ribosome. The *N*-glycosidase activity of the A subunit results in depurination of a specific adenine residue near the 3′ end of the 28S

TABLE 2–1 ■ Certain A-B Toxins with ADP-Ribosyltransferase Activity

TOXIN	SOURCE	MOLECULAR SUBUNITS	GENETIC CONTROL	ENZYME TARGET	TOXIN RECEPTOR	BIOLOGIC EFFECT
Cholera toxin	*Vibrio cholerae*	AB 5	Bacteriophage	G_s α-subunit of adenylate cyclase	G_{M1} ganglioside	Increase cAMP,* severe watery diarrhea
Heat-labile (LT) enterotoxin	*Escherichia coli*	AB 5	Plasmid	G_s α-subunit of adenylate cyclase	G_{M1} ganglioside; LT-2 binds several gangliosides	Increase cAMP, watery diarrhea
Pertussis toxin	*Bordetella pertussis*	AB 1–5	Chromosome	G_i, G_o, G_t subunits of adenylate cyclase	Different carbohydrate moieties	Increase cAMP, cellular effects
Diphtheria toxin	*Corynebacterium diphtheriae*	A/B	Bacteriophage	Elongation factor-2	Heparin-binding epidermal growth factor precursor	Inhibition of protein synthesis, necrosis
Pseudomonas exotoxin A	*Pseudomonas aeruginosa*	A/B	Chromosome	Elongation factor-2	α_2-Macroglobulin/low-density lipoprotein receptor	Inhibition of protein synthesis, necrosis
C2 toxin	*Clostridium botulinum*	A and B		Actin	Unknown	Cell death, loss of cell architecture
Iota toxin	*Clostridium perfringens*			Actin	Unknown	Loss of cell architecture
Iota-like toxin	*Clostridium spiroforme*			Actin	Unknown	Loss of cell architecture
C3 toxin	*Clostridium botulinum*	A/B	Bacteriophage	Rho and Rac proteins	Unknown	Cell death

*cAMP, Cyclic adenosine monophosphate.

ribosomal RNA and inactivation of the 60S ribosomal subunit, thus catalytically halting protein synthesis. The structure-function relationship of STX and SLTs is detailed in a review by Jackson and O'Brien.[33]

The Anthrax Toxin Complex: A Lethal Toxin and a Calmodulin-Dependent Adenylate Cyclase

Bacillus anthracis exotoxin has a tripartite structure composed of protective antigen (PA), edema factor (EF), and lethal factor (LF).[34] The individual protein components have no known biologic effect when they are administered alone; however, EF with PA injected into skin of test animals causes edema, and PA with LF injected into rats causes rapid death. Therefore, both EF and LF share the same cell receptor binding protein, PA. Once PA binds to a high-affinity cell receptor[35] and is proteolytically cleaved,[36] releasing a 20-kDa fragment, a site is exposed on the remaining cell-bound 63-kDa protein to which EF or LF can bind. Reaction of PA with EF or LF creates two separate toxins, edema toxin and lethal toxin; each conforms to the A-B model by possessing a cell receptor–binding B component and an enzymatically active A component responsible for toxicity. The complete toxins are internalized by receptor-mediated endocytosis.[37, 38] The entry of edema toxin by target cells leads to a rapid increase in cAMP levels, and edema toxin has been characterized as a calmodulin-dependent adenylate cyclase.[39–42] The exact mode of action of lethal toxin is less well known, but it is lethal for many species of experimental animals and is assumed to be the major virulence factor causing death in anthrax. No enzymatic activity has been associated with lethal factor, but a report suggests that it may be a metalloprotease.[43]

The plasmid pXO1 encodes all three components of the anthrax toxin. Presence of this plasmid along with a second plasmid, pXO2, which encodes the poly-D-glutamic acid capsule, is required for full pathogenicity of strains.[44–46]

Neurotoxins with Zinc-Binding Endopeptidase Activity

The most potent toxins known are the botulinal neurotoxins (BoNTs). Seven types (A to G) of BoNT are distinguished by their antigenic properties. The BoNTs are structurally and functionally related to TeTx and share conserved amino acid sequences. The structural genes for TeTx and BoNT type G are carried on plasmids; those of BoNT types C1 and D are located on bacteriophages. The genes for the remaining BoNTs are thought to reside in chromosomal locations.[47] Clostridia other than *C. botulinum* (i.e., *Clostridium butyricum* and *Clostridium baratii*) can produce BoNT, which suggests that genetic transfer between strains can occur.[48]

TeTx and the seven serotypes of BoNT are produced as single polypeptides that undergo proteolytic cleavage to generate toxins with two chains joined by a single disulfide bond. The heavy chain (100 kDa) is responsible for specific binding to neuronal cells; the light chain (50 kDa) blocks neurotransmitter release. The cell surface receptor recognized by the heavy chain has not been identified. Once bound, the two toxins produce different clinical signs. BoNT induces flaccid paralysis by inhibiting neurotransmitter release at the neuromuscular junction; TeTx is believed to travel by retrograde axonal transport to neurons in the spinal cord, where it blocks release of neurotransmitters, leading to the spasms characteristic of tetanus. It is only recently that these two toxins were found to share a common mechanism of action.

TeTx and BoNT are zinc endopeptidases.[49–52] The molecular targets of this group of neurotoxins have been identified. Synaptobrevin, a membrane protein of small synaptic vesicles, was the first target found and is proteolyzed by TeTx and BoNT types B, D, F, and G. Only TeTx and BoNT type B cleave the target at the same site. BoNT type C1 exclusively cleaves syntaxin, a presynaptic membrane protein. BoNT types A and E cleave SNAP-25, a synaptosome-associated protein, at different peptide bonds. The zinc-dependent protease activity is localized in the light chain of these toxins, and mutagenesis of the zinc-binding motif results in loss of activity. Whereas each toxin performs precise and different cleavage of these proteins, sequence analysis of the essential regions of the light chain has not provided any clues to their individual substrate specificities. However, future studies using these toxins that block neuron function should help increase understanding of interneural communication[53] as well as improve treatments for two important neuroparalytic diseases.

Other Clostridial Exotoxins

Strains of *C. botulinum* types C and D also produce a different cytotoxin termed C2, which is structurally, immunologically, and functionally distinct from BoNT. The C2 toxin is also known as a binary toxin because it is composed of two separate components: component 1, which ribosylates cellular actin, inhibiting its polymerization and therefore affecting the shape of target cells; and component 2, which binds to cell surface receptors. This toxin is now the prototype of a family of clostridial ADP ribosylating toxins that modify actin[54] (see Table 2–1).

Strains of *C. difficile* linked with antibiotic-associated diarrhea and pseudomembranous colitis have been found to produce both toxin A (enterotoxin) and toxin B (cytotoxin) (Table 2–2). Genes for both toxins have been cloned and sequenced, and the molecular masses of these two single-chain molecules have been estimated to be 308 kDa (toxin A) and 270 kDa (toxin B).[55] DNA repeat sequences found in toxin A are thought to play a role in attachment to eukaryotic target receptor.[56] Toxin A has been shown to elicit a hemorrhagic diarrheal response in rabbit ileal loops and to have a cytotoxic effect.[57] Toxin A, like another enterotoxin found in *V. cholerae* named ZOT,[58] also increases permeability of the small intestinal mucosa by affecting the structure of the intercellular tight junctions. There appears to be no amino acid sequence homology between these toxins.[59] Toxin B is a 1000-fold more potent cytotoxin than toxin A and is not enterotoxic in animals. There is still disagreement about the relative importance of each toxin in production of disease. Whereas inoculation with purified toxin A can reproduce the disease in animals, vaccination against both toxins is needed for complete protection in the hamster model.[60]

A specific receptor for toxin A has been identified as a trisaccharide present on rabbit red cells and on brush border membranes of hamster intestine.[61] The toxin A receptor appears to be linked to a guanine nucleotide regulatory protein. Rho proteins have been implicated as the cellular targets of *C. difficile* toxins A and B.[62, 63] The actual chemical modification is unclear but does not appear to be an ADP-ribosyltransferase. Pathogenic *C. difficile* apparently produce two large exotoxins with similar activities. Although one receptor is known for toxin A, the receptor for B and cellular effects toward Rho remain to be determined.

Membrane-Disrupting Toxins

A large class of exotoxins lyse eukaryotic cells by disrupting their membranes. Two types are described: one type has enzyme activity like phospholipase; exotoxins of the second type insert themselves in the membrane, forming a protein pore.

TABLE 2–2 ■ Properties of Bacterial Toxins

TOXIN	SOURCE	MOLECULAR SUBUNITS	GENETIC CONTROL	ENZYME ACTIVITY	TOXIN RECEPTOR	BIOLOGIC EFFECT
Shiga toxin	*Shigella dysenteriae*	AB 5	Chromosome	28S rRNA* glycosidase	P1	Inhibit protein synthesis, cell death, diarrhea
Shiga-like cytotoxins	*Escherichia coli*	AB 5	Bacteriophage, chromosome	28S rRNA glycosidase	P1	Inhibit protein synthesis, cell death, diarrhea
Adenylate cyclase toxin	*Bordetella* spp.	A/B	Chromosome	Adenylate cyclase	Unknown	Increase cAMP*
Anthrax toxin	*Bacillus anthracis*	Edema factor/ protective antigen	Plasmid	Adenylate cyclase	Unknown	Increase cAMP, edema
		Lethal factor/ protective antigen	Plasmid	Metalloprotease		Cell death, lethal
Tetanus toxin	*Clostridium tetani*	A/B	Plasmid	Zn^{2+} protease	Unknown	Spastic paralysis
Botulinal toxin (A–G)	*Clostridium botulinum, Clostridium butyricum, Clostridium baratii*	A/B	Chromosome, plasmid, bacteriophage	Zn^{2+} proteases	Unknown	Flaccid paralysis
Enterotoxin A	*Clostridium difficile*	A/B	Chromosome	Modify Rho	Trisaccharide	Enterotoxic, cytotoxic
Cytotoxin B	*Clostridium difficile*	A/B	Chromosome	Modify Rho	Unknown	Cytotoxic

*rRNA, Ribosomal RNA; cAMP, cyclic adenosine monophosphate.

Examples of toxins with enzyme activity include the α-toxin of *C. perfringens,* which is a phospholipase C; the β-toxin of *Staphylococcus aureus,* which is a sphingomyelinase C; and the β-toxin of *Clostridium novyi,* which is a lecithinase. The changes caused by these toxins that digest the membrane lipids are often sufficient to cause cell lysis.

The δ-toxin of *S. aureus* is a small peptide (26 amino acids) that forms an amphipathic helical rod long enough to span the lipid bilayer. Clusters of this toxin form hydrophilic pores and in high concentration can dissolve the membrane.[64]

The α-toxin, the major cytotoxin of *S. aureus,* also damages cells by generating pores in the plasma membrane. The protein is secreted as a single-chain 34-kDa protein.[65] The work of Jonas and coworkers[66] appears to show a new mode of cell destruction by this toxin in human T lymphocytes. At low concentrations, the toxin binds to as yet unidentified sites on the membrane and forms small pores that allow passage of monovalent ions but not calcium ions or adenosine triphosphate. The T cells were found to undergo internucleosomal DNA degradation characteristic of programmed cell death (apoptosis). The specific triggering of these events is still unclear. At higher concentrations, the toxin binds to specific sites and nonspecifically to the lipid membranes. The resulting formation of hexameric channels with diameters of 1 to 2 nm allows passage of monovalent and divalent ions and small macromolecules including adenosine triphosphate (molecular masses less than 1 to 2 kDa). Cells appear to die from massive influx of calcium ions and leakage of adenosine triphosphate.[67]

Molecular and genetic analysis of the β-toxin of *C. perfringens* has revealed sequence homology with the α-toxin and two other toxins of *S. aureus.*[68] The β-toxin of *C. perfringens* is known to play a major role in development of necrotic enteritis in humans (termed pigbel)[69, 70] and in animals. The purified toxin has been characterized for its biologic activity in animals, but its mode of action has not been identified. However, like the *S. aureus* α-toxin, the β-toxin can exist as monomeric and multimeric forms and may prove to be a pore-forming enteric toxin.

Streptolysin O is an oxygen-labile, thiol-activated pore former. This toxin binds to cholesterol, where it is thought to form pores after oligomerization.[71] Streptolysin S, an oxygen-stable hemolysin, is the principal agent of the beta hemolysis of many pyogenic streptococci.

Exotoxins That Act like Hormones

The heat-stable enterotoxins of *E. coli* are a heterogeneous group of small peptides that are plasmid encoded. Production of these toxins by enterotoxigenic *E. coli* is known to be responsible for worldwide cases of secretory diarrhea in humans and young animals.[72] There are two different ST types. ST-2 toxins cause disease primarily in piglets, and the mode of action has not been defined. The mechanism by which the ST-1 toxins cause diarrhea has been linked to activation of intestinal membrane-bound guanylate cyclase. The resulting elevation in cyclic guanosine monophosphate acts as an intracellular messenger causing the onset of diarrhea. Possibly two classes of ST-1 receptors have been described.[73, 74] A naturally occurring peptide, guanylin, isolated from rat jejunum, was found to activate guanylate cyclase.[75] The new peptide hormone was also found to be highly homologous in structure to ST-1. The intestinal peptide shares identical residues at eight positions within the 13–amino acid–long enterotoxin–receptor binding domain. Although the exact function of guanylin is still unclear, it does not cause a diarrheal response in test animals except at doses at least four orders of magnitude higher than those of ST-1.[76]

A new ST-related enterotoxin has been described in enteroaggregative *E. coli,* which are associated with persistent diarrhea in children.[77] The predicted amino acid sequence of this toxin suggests that it is the prototype for another subfamily of *E. coli* STs because it shares significant homology with the enterotoxic domain of ST-1 and with the hormone guanylin. Whereas bacteria have been known to produce hormone-like substances, no pathologic process had been associated with these compounds. ST-1 appears to be the first bacterial toxin to function as a hormone analog.

The Pyrogenic Toxin Family: Superantigens

The best characterized members of the pyrogenic toxin family include staphylococcal enterotoxins, the toxic shock syndrome toxin (TSST-1), and the streptococcal pyrogenic (erythrogenic) exotoxins. These toxins share some biologic activities: (1) pyrogenicity, (2) ability to enhance endotoxin shock in test animals, and (3) T-cell mitogenicity. These last two activities have led to distinction of these toxins as superantigens.[78] As such, the toxins function as potent T-cell mitogens, thereby causing immune interference. The toxins bind to class II major histocompatibility complex molecules on antigen-presenting cells. These toxins appear to stimulate T cells almost exclusively through the Vβ region of the T-cell receptor. At present, it is postulated that some or all of the pathologic effects of these toxins are caused by their ability to activate a large proportion of all T cells. The result of the T-cell stimulation by superantigens is massive cytokine release, which includes interleukin-2 and tumor necrosis factor. These two cytokines are known to cause shocklike symptoms when they are given to patients in high concentrations. Further interactions of superantigens with T cells are detailed in the reviews of Marrack and Kappler[79] and Schlievert.[80] These toxins are thought to play a causative role in several important diseases: toxic shock syndrome, toxic shock–like syndrome, streptococcal scarlet fever, staphylococcal food poisoning, and severe invasive disease due to group A streptococci described as the "flesh-eating" bacteria (Table 2–3). Studies providing evidence for the direct association of staphylococcal TSST-1, staphylococcal enterotoxins, and streptococcal pyrogenic exotoxins in these acute diseases, as well as their possible association with various chronic diseases, have been reviewed.[81] The human Vβ specificity of each of the toxins has also been elucidated. At present, it is not possible to predict the specificity of a superantigen for a particular Vβ element from its primary structure, although several toxins have amino acid sequences in common.

The staphylococcal enterotoxins include six serogroups designated by letters A through E and G; serogroup C has three subtypes. These protein toxins are all in the range of 25 to 30 kDa in size, and each has a single internal disulfide bond (cystine loop). Although these exotoxins continue to be called enterotoxins, they do not elicit the characteristic intestinal fluid accumulation of enterotoxins when they are inoculated into test animals, nor do they cause accumulation of cAMP or cyclic guanine monophosphate in enterocytes as described for CT or ST, respectively. The staphylococcal enterotoxins are presumed to function by affecting emetic receptors in the abdominal viscera that stimulate the emetic and diarrheal response. Just how these toxin superantigens may induce these symptoms is not easily explained. They may stimulate T cells or mast cells (or other cells) in the lining of the gut, causing a release of mediators that induce the diarrhea and vomiting.

The development of recombinant DNA technology allowed

TABLE 2–3 ■ Staphylococcal and Streptococcal Pyrogenic Toxin Superantigens and Their Associated Diseases

SOURCE	TOXIN*	GENETIC LOCATION	DISEASE ASSOCIATION
Staphylococcus aureus	SEA	Bacteriophage	Food poisoning, toxic shock syndrome (nonmenstrual toxic shock syndromes are associated with SEB and SEC)
	SEB	Plasmid, chromosome	
	SEC	Plasmid, chromosome	
	SED	Plasmid	
	SEE	Chromosome	
	TSST-1	Chromosome	Toxic shock syndrome (menstrual and nonmenstrual)
Streptococcus pyogenes group A	SPEA	Bacteriophage	Scarlet fever, toxic shock–like syndrome, invasive disease, erysipelas
	SPEC	Bacteriophage	
	SPEB	Chromosome	

*SE(A through E) are staphylococcal enterotoxins; SPE(A through C), streptococcal pyrogenic exotoxins; TSST-1, toxic shock syndrome toxin. Pyrogenic toxin superantigens have also been isolated from streptococcal groups B, C, F, and G and from viridans streptococci causing toxic shock–like syndrome.[80]

the genes of the enterotoxins of *S. aureus* and group A streptococcus to be identified, cloned, and sequenced. The history of detection of the genes involved in production of these toxins is reviewed by Lee and Schlievert.[82] As shown in Table 2–3, the genes for these toxins have been found on bacteriophages, plasmids, and genetically mobile elements with chromosomal locations. The amino acid sequences of many of the toxins listed have been deduced from the DNA encoding them. Staphylococcal enterotoxins A and E are more than 90% alike in amino acid sequence, as are members of the serogroup C. Comparison of all the staphylococcal enterotoxins and the streptococcal toxins has shown shared sequences that distinguish two groups within this family of toxins: staphylococcal enterotoxins A, E, and D and streptococcal pyrogenic exotoxin C in one group; and staphylococcal enterotoxins C1, C2, C3, and B and streptococcal pyrogenic exotoxin A in the second group.[83]

TSST-1 is serologically distinct from the staphylococcal enterotoxins and streptococcal pyrogenic exotoxins, does not contain the cystine loop of the staphylococcal enterotoxins, and cannot readily be aligned with the enterotoxin common sequences. The evolutionary relationship of TSST-1 is unclear; it may have descended from an earlier common ancestral gene.[82]

Streptococcal pyrogenic exotoxin B does not appear to be significantly associated with toxic shock–like syndrome. It shares minimal similarity with TSST-1 but has significantly high nucleotide sequence relatedness with a streptococcal proteinase precursor.[82]

The relationship of other toxins to this pyrogenic group is less clear. *S. aureus* can produce two other serologically distinct toxins, exfoliative toxins A and B, which cause scalded skin syndrome. These two toxins do share the Vβ restricted T-cell mitogenicity with the other pyrogenic toxins; however, they are not pyrogenic, nor do they synergize lethal endotoxic shock in test animals. The exfoliative toxins are similar in size to the enterotoxins, but no alignments are similar enough to predict any common modes of action. Substitution of serine 195 residue of exfoliatin A by a cysteine residue led to loss of biologic activity.[84] This result is consistent with the hypothesis that exfoliatin A could be a serine protease or lipase[85]; however, no enzyme activity has been detected with native toxin. While investigators hypothesize about the binding of exfoliatins to intracellular proteins such as profilaggrin and filaggrin[86] or GM4-like glycolipid[87] and histone-like proteins, the intracellular events brought about by these toxins are yet to be demonstrated.

Genetics of Toxin Production

Among the best studied examples of pathogenic diversity are the diarrheogenic *E. coli*. Most *E. coli* strains are nonpathogenic; however, certain strains have acquired different characteristic sets of virulence genes (e.g., adhesins, toxins, hemolysins) that enable them to colonize the intestinal tract and cause diarrhea.[88] The nature of the virulence genes determines the clinical and epidemiologic features of the diarrheal disease caused by a particular *E. coli* group.[89] Toxin production plays a key role in at least two of the three groups outlined in Table 2–4. The enterotoxigenic *E. coli*, which synthesize LT and/or ST, are responsible for worldwide occurrence of traveler's diarrhea, a watery diarrhea similar to that of cholera. A more recently recognized group termed enteroaggregative *E. coli* has been found to make a new ST-type toxin as well as a hemolysin. The relevance of this group

TABLE 2–4 ■ Toxins Produced by *Escherichia coli*

PATHOGENIC TYPE*	TOXINS†	ENTERIC INFECTIONS	COMMON RISK
Enterotoxigenic *E. coli*	LT-1	Traveler's diarrhea	Foreign travel
	LT-2	No role in human disease	
	ST-1	Traveler's diarrhea	Foreign travel
	ST-2	Diarrhea (usually swine pathogen)	
Enteroaggregative *E. coli*	EAST-1	Chronic, acute diarrhea (role of toxin?)	Unknown
Enterohemorrhagic *E. coli*	SLT-1	Diarrhea, hemorrhagic colitis	Raw ground beef
	SLT-2	Diarrhea, hemorrhagic colitis	Raw ground beef
	SLT-2	Disease in swine	

*Enteropathogenic *E. coli* (classic serotypes) and enteroinvasive *E. coli* do not produce toxins. SLT-producing *E. coli* strains are associated with the development of hemolytic-uremic syndrome.

†LT, Heat-labile toxin; ST, heat-stable toxin; EAST, enteroaggregative ST-like toxin; SLT, Shiga-like toxin.

is still under investigation. The SLT toxin family is produced by strains collectively termed enterohemorrhagic *E. coli.* These pathogens are capable of eliciting diarrhea and hemorrhagic colitis, and they are related to the development of hemolytic-uremic syndrome. In *E. coli,* the LT and ST genes are borne by plasmids; bacteriophages mediate SLT production.

The genetic regulation of exotoxin production demonstrates wide variation. Temperate bacteriophages encode the structural gene for diphtheria toxin, but its synthesis is inhibited by elevated iron and interaction with a factor of bacterial origin.[90] Three *Bordetella* species carry the pertussis toxin gene chromosomally, but it is expressed only in *B. pertussis* because of mutations in the promoter region of the toxin genes in both *B. parapertussis* and *B. bronchiseptica.*[91]

For full virulence, *V. cholerae* must produce CT and toxin-coregulated pili (TCP), which are surface, hairlike structures required for intestinal colonization. The structural genes for CT are known to be encoded by a filamentous bacteriophage, CTXΦ, related to the coliphage M13.[92] This is the first description of a filamentous phage's participating in lysogenic conversion of a bacterial pathogen. The TCP are the bacterial receptors for CTXΦ entry. Production of TCP and CT is coordinately regulated by the same virulence regulatory gene, *toxR*. Peterson and Mekalanos[93] have found 17 distinct genes that are controlled by *toxR*. The importance of *toxR* for development of infection and diarrhea was demonstrated by Herrington and coworkers,[94] who carried out human challenge studies with a classic *V. cholerae* O:1 strain in which the *toxR* gene was mutated. None of the volunteers was colonized or had diarrhea.

Understanding of the genetic expression of *C. perfringens* toxins has greatly expanded. Three regulatory genes have been identified that control the production of θ-toxin (perfringolysin O).[95] Two of the regulatory genes make up a two-component sensor-kinase system that also controls the production of other toxins. This regulatory system, as well, has been shown to affect virulence.[96] Such elaborate regulatory cascades allow the organism to quickly adapt to changing "environmental" external stimuli, whether in mammalian tissues or in the environment. The minireview by Mekalanos[97] provides an interesting discussion of the emerging themes that characterize virulence regulatory systems.

Studies of toxin operons have provided insight into the complexities of toxin assembly and secretion. Weiss and colleagues[98] have isolated mutants of *B. pertussis* that are defective in secretion of pertussis toxin. A region of the *B. pertussis* chromosome downstream from the structural gene for pertussis toxin was found to encode for eight proteins necessary for pertussis toxin transport. Seven of the predicted proteins show striking homology with the VirB proteins of *Agrobacterium tumefaciens,* which transport tumor-inducing DNA from *A. tumefaciens* into plant cells. These results appear to support a family of proteins involved in secretion of macromolecules from gram-negative bacteria.

Therapeutic Strategies: The Magic Bullets

Understanding the mode of action and structure-function relationships of certain of these potent toxins has provided unexpected and exciting new approaches to production of vaccines and therapeutic agents. Whereas the use of BoNT for treatment of painful muscle spasms has become an approved therapy,[99] a new generation of hybrid molecules is being created and tested experimentally for efficacy as vaccines[100, 101] and as treatment of infectious diseases including human immunodeficiency virus infection[102] as well as for cure of cancers,[103] leukemia,[104] and autoimmune diseases. As was pointed out by Strom and associates[105] in a review, the great German scientist Paul Ehrlich first suggested that fusion of cell-specific antibodies with the enzyme-active portion of a toxin could create magic bullets. Several immunotoxins have been developed, and new cytokine-toxin fusions are being genetically engineered and tested.[105] Monoclonal antibody–superantigen conjugates are also being examined for their abilities to eradicate tumors in an approach known as superantigen-directed T-cell killing.[106] Studies of bacterial and plant toxins have provided better understanding of how these lethal molecules trigger disease and show promise for exploitation of these same lethal mechanisms for potential cures.

References

1. Loeffler F: Untersuchungen über die Bedeutung der Mikroorganismen für die Entstehung der Diphtherie beim Menschen, bei der Taube und beim Kalbe. Mitt Reichsgesundheitsamt 2:421–499, 1884.
2. von Behring E, Kitasato S: Über das Zustandekommen der Diphtherie-Immunität und der Tetanus-Immunität bei Thieren. Dtsch Med Wochenschr 16:1113–1114, 1890.
3. van Ermengen E: De l' étiologie du botulisme. Compt Rend Soc Biol 49:155, 1897.
4. Roux E, Yersin A: Contribution à l'étude de la diphtérie. Ann Inst Pasteur (Paris) 2:629–661, 1888.
5. Honjo T, Nishizuka Y, Hayaishi O: Adenosine diphosphoribosylation of aminoacyl transferase II by diphtheria toxin. Cold Spring Harb Symp Quant Biol 34:603–610, 1969.
6. Honjo T, Nishizuka Y, Kato I, et al: Adenosine diphosphate ribosylation of aminoacyl transferase II and inhibition of protein synthesis by diphtheria toxin. J Biol Chem 246:4251–4260, 1971.
7. Gill DM, Pappenheimer AM Jr, Brown R, et al: Studies on the mode of action of diphtheria toxin VII. Toxin-stimulated hydrolysis of nicotinamide adenine dinucleotide in mammalian cell extracts. J Exp Med 129:1–21, 1969.
8. Gill DM: Bacterial toxins: A table of lethal amounts. Microbiol Rev 46:86–94, 1982.
9. Gill DM: Bacterial toxins: Lethal amounts. *In* Laskin AI, Lechevalier H (eds): CRC Handbook of Microbiology, Vol 8. Boca Raton, FL, CRC Press, 1987, pp 127–136.
10. Gill DM: Bacterial toxins: Description. *In* Laskin AI, Lechevalier H (eds): CRC Handbook of Microbiology, Vol 8. Boca Raton, FL, CRC Press, 1987, pp 3–18.
11. Sixma TK, Pronk SE, Kalk KH, et al: Crystal structure of a cholera toxin–related heat-labile enterotoxin from *E. coli.* Nature 351:371–377, 1991.
12. Sixma TK, Pronk SE, Kalk KH, et al: Lactose binding to heat-labile enterotoxin revealed by x-ray crystallography. Nature 355:561–564, 1992.
13. Gill DM, Rappaport RS: Origin of the enzymatically active A1 fragment of cholera toxin. J Infect Dis 139:674–680, 1979.
14. Cassel D, Pfeuffer T: Mechanism of cholera toxin action: Covalent modification of the guanyl nucleotide–binding protein of the adenylate cyclase system. Proc Natl Acad Sci USA 75:2669–2673, 1978.
15. Gill DM, Meren R: ADP-ribosylation of membrane proteins catalyzed by cholera toxin: Basis of the activation of adenylate cyclase. Proc Natl Acad Sci USA 75:3050–3054, 1978.
16. Kaper JB, Morris JG Jr, Levine MM: Cholera. Clin Microbiol Rev 8:48–86, 1995.
17. Lencer WI, Delp C, Neutra MR, Madara JL: Mechanism of cholera toxin action on a polarized human intestinal epithelial cell line: Role of vesicular traffic. J Cell Biol 117:1197–1209, 1992.
18. Orlandi PA, Curran PK, Fishman PH: Brefeldin A blocks the response of cultured cells to cholera toxin: Implications for intracellular trafficking in toxin action. J Biol Chem 268:12010–12016, 1993.
19. Spangler BD: Structure and function of cholera toxin and the related *Escherichia coli* heat-labile enterotoxin. Microbiol Rev 56:622–647, 1992.
20. Aktories K, Frevert J: ADP-ribosylation of a 21–24kDa eukaryo-

tic protein(s) by C3, a novel botulinum ADP-ribosyltransferase, is regulated by guanine nucleotide. Biochem J 247:363–368, 1987.

21. Fraser ME, Chernaia MM, Kozlov YV, James MNG: X-ray crystal structure of the holotoxin from *Shigella dysenteriae* at 2.5Å resolution. Nat Struct Biol 1:59–64, 1994.
22. Tamura M, Nogimori K, Murai S, et al: Subunit structure of islet-activating protein, pertussis toxin, in conformity with the A-B model. Biochemistry 21:5516–5522, 1982.
23. Ribi HO, Ludwig DS, Mercer KL, et al: Three-dimensional structure of cholera toxin penetrating a lipid membrane. Science 239:1272–1276, 1988.
24. Murzin AG: OB (oligonucleotide/oligosaccharide binding)-fold: Common structural and functional solution for non-homologous sequences. EMBO J 12:861–867, 1993.
25. Sixma TK, Aguirre A, Terwisscha van Scheltinga AC, et al: Heat-labile enterotoxin crystal forms with variable A/B5 orientation. Analysis of conformational flexibility. FEBS Lett 305:81–85, 1992.
26. Eiklid K, Olsnes S: Animal toxicity of *Shigella dysenteriae* cytotoxin: Evidence that the neurotoxic, enterotoxic, and cytotoxic activities are due to one toxin. J Immunol 130:380–384, 1983.
27. Konowalchuk J, Speirs JI, Stavric S: Vero response to a cytotoxin of *Escherichia coli*. Infect Immun 18:775–779, 1977.
28. Karmali MA, Petric M, Lim C, et al: The association between idiopathic hemolytic uremic syndrome and infection by verotoxin-producing *Escherichia coli*. J Infect Dis 151:775–782, 1985.
29. Kaye SA, Louise CB, Boyd B, et al: Shiga toxin–associated hemolytic uremic syndrome: Interleukin-1β enhancement of shiga toxin cytotoxicity toward human vascular endothelial cells in vitro. Infect Immun 61:3886–3891, 1993.
30. Sjogren R, Neill R, Rachmilewitz D, et al: Role of Shiga-like toxin 1 in bacterial enteritis: Comparison between isogenic *Escherichia coli* strains induced in rabbits. Gastroenterology 106:306–317, 1994.
31. Jackson MP, Neill RJ, O'Brien AD, et al: Nucleotide sequence analysis and comparison of the structural genes for Shiga-like toxin I and Shiga-like toxin II encoded by bacteriophages from *Escherichia coli* 933. FEMS Microbiol Lett 44:109–114, 1987.
32. Calderwood SB: Section II overview—Toxin structure-function, receptors, cell biology. *In* Karmali MA, Goglio AG (eds): Recent Advances in Verocytotoxin-Producing *Escherichia coli* Infections. Amsterdam, Elsevier Science Publishing, 1994, pp 119–122.
33. Jackson MP, O'Brien AD: Structure-function relationships of Shiga toxin and the Shiga-like toxins to bacterial enterotoxins and ribosome-inactivating proteins. *In* Karmali MA, Goglio AG (eds): Recent Advances in Verocytotoxin-Producing *Escherichia coli* Infections. Amsterdam, Elsevier Science Publishing, 1994, pp 123–130.
34. Leppla SH: Production and purification of anthrax toxin. Methods Enzymol 165:103–116, 1988.
35. Friedlander AM, Bhatnagar R, Leppla SH, et al: Characterization of macrophage sensitivity and resistance to anthrax lethal toxin. Infect Immun 61:245–252, 1993.
36. Klimpel DR, Molloy SS, Thomas G, Leppla SH: Anthrax toxin protective antigen is activated by a cell surface protease with sequence specificity and catalytic properties of furin. Proc Natl Acad Sci USA 89:10277–10281, 1992.
37. Friedlander AM: Macrophages are sensitive to anthrax lethal toxin through an acid-dependent process. J Biol Chem 261:7123–7126, 1986.
38. Gordan VM, Leppla SH, Hewlett EL: Inhibitors of receptor-mediated endocytosis block the entry of *Bacillus anthracis* adenylate cyclase toxin but not that of *Bordetella pertussis* adenylate cyclase toxin. Infect Immun 56:1066–1069, 1988.
39. Leppla SH: Anthrax toxin edema factor: A bacterial adenylate cyclase that increases cAMP concentrations in eukaryotic cells. Proc Natl Acad Sci USA 79:3162–3166, 1982.
40. Leppla SH: Purification and characterization of adenylyl cyclase from *Bacillus anthracis*. Methods Enzymol 195:153–168, 1991.
41. Tippetts MT, Robertson DL: Molecular cloning and expression of the *Bacillus anthracis* edema factor toxin gene: A calmodulin-dependent adenylate cyclase. J Bacteriol 170:2263–2266, 1988.
42. Munier H, Blanco FJ, Precheur B: Characterization of a synthetic calmodulin-binding peptide derived from *Bacillus anthracis* adenylate cyclase. J Biol Chem 268:1695–1701, 1993.
43. Klimpel KR, Arora N, Leppla SH: Anthrax toxin lethal factor contains a zinc metalloprotease consensus sequence which is required for lethal activity. Mol Microbiol 13:1093–1100, 1994.
44. Green BD, Battisti L, Koehler TM, et al: Demonstration of a capsule plasmid in *Bacillus anthracis*. Infect Immun 49:291–297, 1985.
45. Kaspar RL, Robertson DL: Purification and physical analysis of *Bacillus anthracis* plasmids pXO1 and pXO2. Biochem Biophys Res Commun 149:362–368, 1987.
46. Mikesell P, Ivins BE, Ristroph JD, Dreier TM: Evidence for plasmid-mediated toxin production in *Bacillus anthracis*. Infect Immun 39:371–376, 1983.
47. Niemann H: Molecular biology of clostridial neurotoxins. *In* Alouf JE, Freer J (eds): Sourcebook of Bacterial Toxins. New York, Academic Press, 1991, pp 299–344.
48. Hauser D, Gibert M, Marvaud JC, et al: Botulinal neurotoxin C1 complex genes, clostridial neurotoxin homology and genetic transfer in *Clostridium botulinum*. Toxicon 33:515–526, 1995.
49. Schiavo G, Benfenati F, Poulain B, et al: Tetanus and botulinum-B neurotoxins block neurotransmitter release by proteolytic cleavage of synaptobrevin. Nature 359:832–835, 1992.
50. Schiavo G, Poulain B, Rossetto O, et al: Tetanus toxin is a zinc protein and its inhibition of neurotransmitter release and protease activity depend on zinc. EMBO J 11:3577–3583, 1992.
51. Schiavo G, Rossetto O, Santucci A, et al: Botulinum neurotoxins are zinc proteins. J Biol Chem 267:23479–23483, 1992.
52. Blasi J, Chapman ER, Link E, et al: Botulinum neurotoxin A selectively cleaves the synaptic protein SNAP-25. Nature 365:160–163, 1993.
53. Niemann H, Blasi J, Jahn R: Clostridial neurotoxins: New tools for dissecting exocytosis. Trends Cell Biol 4:179–185, 1994.
54. Aktories K, Mohr C, Koch G: Clostridial actin-ADP-ribosylating toxins. Curr Top Microbiol Immunol 175:97–113, 1992.
55. von Eichel-Streiber C: Molecular biology of the *Clostridium difficile* toxins. *In* Sebald M (ed): Genetics and Molecular Biology of Anaerobic Bacteria. New York, Springer-Verlag, 1993, pp 264–289.
56. Dove DH, Wang SZ, Price SB, et al: Molecular characterization of the *Clostridium difficile* toxin A gene. Infect Immun 58:480–488, 1990.
57. Lyerly DM, Johnson JL, Wilkins TD: The toxins of *Clostridium difficile*. *In* Boriello SP (ed): Clinical and Molecular Aspects of Anaerobes. Petersfield, UK, Wrightson Biomedical Publishing, 1990, pp 137–145.
58. Fasano A, Baudry B, Pumplin DW, et al: *Vibrio cholerae* produces a second enterotoxin, which affects intestinal tight junctions. Proc Natl Acad Sci USA 88:5242–5246, 1991.
59. Hecht G, Pothoulakis C, LaMont JT, Madara JL: *Clostridium difficile* toxin A perturbs cytoskeletal structure and tight junction permeability of the cultured human intestinal epithelial monolayers. J Clin Invest 82:1516–1524, 1988.
60. Lyerly DM, Drivan HC, Wilkins TD: *Clostridium difficile:* Its disease and toxins. Clin Microbiol Rev 1:1–18, 1988.
61. Tucker KD, Wilkins TD: Toxin A of *Clostridium difficile* binds to the human carbohydrate antigens I, X, Y. Infect Immun 59:73–78, 1991.
62. Just I, Dritz G, Aktories D, et al: *Clostridium difficile* toxin B acts on the GTP binding protein Rho. J Biol Chem 269:10706–10712, 1994.
63. Dillon ST, Rubin EJ, Jakubovich M, et al: Involvement of Ras-related Rho proteins in the mechanisms of action of *Clostridium difficile* toxin A and toxin B. Infect Immun 63:1421–1426, 1995.
64. Freer JH, Birkbeck TH, Bhakoo M: Interaction of staphylococcal delta lysin with phospholipid monolayers and bilayers—a short review. *In* Alouf JE, Fehrenbach FJ, Jeljaszewicz J (eds): Bacterial Protein Toxins. New York, Academic Press, 1984, pp 181–189.
65. Tobkes N, Wallace BA, Bayley H: Secondary structure and assembly mechanism of an oligomeric channel protein. Biochemistry 24:1915–1920, 1985.
66. Jonas D, Walev I, Berger T, et al: Novel path to apoptosis: Small transmembrane pores created by staphylococcal alpha-toxin in T lymphocytes evoke internucleosomal DNA degradation. Infect Immun 62:1304–1312, 1994.
67. Bhakdi S, Tranum-Jensen J: Alpha-toxin of *Staphylococcus aureus*. Microbiol Rev 55:733–751, 1991.
68. Hunter SEC, Brown JE, Oyston PCF, et al: Molecular genetic analysis of beta-toxin of *Clostridium perfringens* reveals sequence

homology with alpha-toxin, gamma-toxin, and leudocidin of *Staphylococcus aureus.* Infect Immun 61:3958–3965, 1993.
69. Lawrence G, Walker PD: Pathogenesis of enteritis necroticans in Papua, New Guinea. Lancet 1:125–126, 1976.
70. Johnson S, Echeverria P, Taylor DN, et al: Enteritis necroticans among Khmer children at an evacuation site in Thailand. Lancet 2:496–500, 1987.
71. Bhakdi S, Tranum-Jensen J: Damage to mammalian cells by proteins that form transmembrane pores. Rev Physiol Biochem Pharmacol 107:147–223, 1987.
72. Sack RB: Human diarrheal disease caused by enterotoxigenic *Escherichia coli.* Annu Rev Microbiol 29:333–353, 1975.
73. Hughes M, Crane M, Hakki S, et al: Identification and characterization of a new family of high-affinity receptors for *Escherichia coli* heat-stable enterotoxin in rat intestinal membranes. Biochemistry 30:10738–10745, 1991.
74. Mann EA, Cohen MB, Giannella RA: Comparison of receptors for *Escherichia coli* heat-stable enterotoxin novel receptor present in IEC-6 cells. Am J Physiol 264:G172–G178, 1993.
75. Currie MG, Fok KF, Kato J, et al: Guanylin: An endogenous activator of intestinal guanylate cyclase. Proc Natl Acad Sci USA 89:947–951, 1992.
76. Carpick BW, Gariepy J: The *Escherichia coli* heat-stable enterotoxin is a long-lived superagonist of guanylin. Infect Immun 61:4710–4715, 1993.
77. Savarino SJ, Fasano A, Watson J, et al: Enteroaggregative *Escherichia coli* heat-stable enterotoxin 1 represents another subfamily of *E. coli* heat stable toxin. Proc Natl Acad Sci USA 90:3093–3097, 1993.
78. Bohach GA, Fast DJ, Nelson RD, Schlievert PM: Staphylococcal and streptococcal pyrogenic toxins involved in toxic shock syndrome and related illnesses. Crit Rev Microbiol 17:251–272, 1990.
79. Marrack P, Kappler J: The staphylococcal enterotoxins and their relatives. Science 248:705–711, 1990.
80. Schlievert PM: Role of superantigens in human disease. J Infect Dis 167:997–1002, 1993.
81. Kotb M: Bacterial pyrogenic exotoxins as superantigens. Clin Microbiol Rev 8:411–426, 1995.
82. Lee PK, Schlievert PM: Molecular genetics of pyrogenic exotoxin "superantigens" of group A streptococci and *Staphylococcus aureus.* Curr Top Microbiol Immunol 174:1–19, 1991.
83. Van den Bussche RA, Lyon JD, Bohach GA: Molecular evolution of the staphylococcal and streptococcal pyrogenic toxin gene family. Mol Phylogenet Evol 2:281–292, 1993.
84. Prevost G, Rifai S, Chaix ML, Piemont Y: Functional evidence that the Ser-195 residue of staphylococcal exfoliative toxin A is essential for biological activity. Infect Immun 59:3337–3339, 1991.
85. Dancer SJ, Garrat R, Saldanha J, et al: The epidermolytic toxins are serine proteases. FEBS Lett 268:129–132, 1990.
86. Smith TP, Bailey CJ: Epidermolytic toxin from *Staphylococcus aureus* binds to filaggrins. FEBS Microbiol Lett 194:309–312, 1986.
87. Tanabe T, Sato H, Ueda K, et al: Possible receptor for exfoliative toxins produced by *Staphylococcus hyicus* and *Staphylococcus aureus.* Infect Immun 63:1591–1594, 1995.
88. Whittam TS, Wolfe ML, Wachsmuth IK, et al: Clonal relationships among *Escherichia coli* strains that cause hemorrhagic colitis and infantile diarrhea. Infect Immun 61:1619–1629, 1993.
89. Levine MM: *Escherichia coli* that cause diarrhea: Enterotoxigenic, enteropathogenic, enteroinvasive, enterohemorrhagic, and enteroadherent. J Infect Dis 155:377–389, 1987.
90. Tao X, Murphy JR: Binding of the metalloregulatory protein DtxR to the diphtheria tox operator requires a divalent heavy metal ion and protects the palindromic sequence from DNase I digestion. J Biol Chem 267:21761–21764, 1992.
91. Arico B, Rappuoli R: *Bordetella parapertussis* and *Bordetella bronchiseptica* contain transcriptionally silent pertussis toxin genes. J Bacteriol 169:2847–2853, 1987.
92. Waldor MK, Mekalanos JJ: Lysogenic conversion by a filamentous phage encoding cholera toxin. Science 272:1910–1914, 1996.
93. Peterson KM, Mekalanos JJ: Characterization of the *Vibrio cholerae* ToxR regulon: Identification of novel genes involved in intestinal colonization. Infect Immun 56:2822–2829, 1988.
94. Herrington DA, Hall RH, Losonsky G, et al: Toxin, toxin-coregulated pili, and the toxR regulon are essential for *Vibrio cholerae* pathogenesis in humans. J Exp Med 168:1487–1492, 1988.
95. Rood JI, Lyristis M: Regulation of extracellular toxin production by *Clostridium perfringens.* Trends Microbiol 3:192–196, 1995.
96. Lyristis M, Bryant AE, Sloan J, et al: Identification and molecular analysis of a locus that regulates extracellular toxin production in *Clostridium perfringens.* Mol Microbiol 12:761–777, 1994.
97. Mekalanos JJ: Environmental signals controlling expression of virulence determinants in bacteria. J Bacteriol 174:1–7, 1992.
98. Weiss AA, Johnson FD, Burns DL: Molecular characterization of an operon required for pertussis toxin secretion. Proc Natl Acad Sci USA 90:2970–2974, 1993.
99. Schantz E, Johnson E: Properties and use of botulism toxin and other medicinal neurotoxins in medicine. Microbiol Rev 56:80–99, 1992.
100. Ryd M, Verma N, Lindbert AA: Induction of a humoral immune response to a Shiga toxin B subunit epitope expressed as chimeric LamB protein in a *Shigella flexneri* live vaccine strain. Microb Pathog 12:399–407, 1992.
101. Dale JB, Chiang EC: Intranasal immunization with recombinant group A streptococcal M protein fragment fused to a B subunit of *Escherichia coli* labile toxin protects mice against systemic challenge infections. J Infect Dis 171:1038–1041, 1995.
102. al-Jaufy AT, Haddad JE, King SR, et al: Cytotoxicity of a Shiga toxin A subunit–CD4 fusion protein to human immunodeficiency virus–infected cells. Infect Immun 62:956–960, 1994.
103. Siegall CB: Targeted toxins as anticancer agents. Cancer 74:1006–1012, 1994.
104. Kreitman RJ, Pastan I: Recombinant single-chain immunotoxins against T and B cell leukemias. Leukemia Lymphoma 13:1–10, 1994.
105. Strom TB, Anderson PL, Rubin-Kelley VE, et al: Immunotoxins and cytokine toxin fusion proteins. Ann N Y Acad Sci 636:233–250, 1991.
106. Kalland T, Dohlsten M, Lind P, et al: Monoclonal antibodies and superantigens: A novel therapeutic approach. Med Oncol Tumor Pharmacother 10:37–47, 1993.

3

Other Virulence Factors

Keith A. Joiner

Pathogenic microorganisms invade the host at specific sites, then evade host defenses. To cause disease, microbes must circumvent mucosal and cutaneous defenses, systemic humoral defenses, destruction by phagocytic cells, and killing via the cell-mediated immune system. The diseases that result from evasion may be almost solely a consequence of unchecked microbial replication, may result from toxic components produced by the microorganisms, or may be a byproduct of an ineffectual, diverted, or overblown immune response. Specific microbial constituents are implicated in these evasion processes. It is therefore instructive to consider illustrative virulence determinants[1] with suspected roles in attachment and invasion or in evasion of specific arms of the host defense system or with defined capacities to produce direct toxicity for the host. Although the last category has often assumed premier importance, a modern view of pathogenicity is consistent with the statement by Mims[2]: "Well-established infectious agents have . . . generally reached a state of balanced pathogenicity in the host, and cause the smallest amount of damage compatible with the need to enter, multiply, and be discharged from the body."

Attachment and Invasion

Interaction with Matrix Proteins

Bacteria often express specialized organelles for attachment—pili or fimbriae—which are discussed in Chapter 2.[3] Additional molecules that play specialized roles in attachment are defined. One prominent class of potential adhesion components consists of microbial molecules that bind to extracellular matrix proteins or basement membrane constituents.[4] Among the best characterized bacterial proteins active in these interactions are the fibronectin and collagen binding proteins of staphylococci and streptococci,[5–8] the mycobacterial fibronectin binding proteins, specific enterobacterial fimbrial types, and the polymeric surface proteins YadA of *Yersinia*[9] and the A protein of *Aeromonas.*[10] A variety of other bacteria, fungi, and protozoa are reported to bind fibronectin or other extracellular matrix proteins such as laminin, collagen, and vitronectin. Redundant and overlapping interactions are the rule rather than the exception. For example, *Staphylococcus aureus* binds to fibronectin,[11] laminin,[12] collagen,[7] and fibrinogen.[13] Binding is mediated by either protein-protein or protein-carbohydrate interactions. Among gram-positive organisms, the microbial receptor shares common motifs.[14]

It is often unclear whether binding of extracellular matrix proteins by microorganisms is a virulence trait or is an epiphenomenon. Mycobacteria provide a case in point. Binding of a *Mycobacterium leprae* cell wall protein to fibronectin potentiates bacterial entry into Schwann cells and epithelial cells.[15] In contrast, a secreted fibronectin binding protein of *Mycobacterium tuberculosis* (antigen 85) was identified as mycolyltransferase, a critical enzyme in cell wall synthesis. This suggests either that the protein is multifunctional or more likely that fibronectin binding is an epiphenomenon. Arguably, potentiation of cell entry by matrix protein binding is most important for organisms entering nonphagocytic cells lacking prototypic phagocytic receptors.

Interaction with Cell Surface Receptors

Microbial constituents may mimic the natural ligands for mammalian cell surface receptors, particularly those of the integrin and selectin families.[16, 17] Selected examples with bacteria, protozoa, and viruses illustrate the point. The best characterized interaction is with the invasin protein of *Yersinia pseudotuberculosis,* which binds directly to a variety of integrin receptors of the β_1 family, mediating bacterial uptake by target cells.[18, 19] Binding of *Bordetella pertussis* to phagocytic cells is promoted by the bacterial surface protein filamentous hemagglutinin, via the tripeptide amino acid sequence arginine-lysine–aspartic acid, known to be critical for fibronectin binding.[20] *Borrelia burgdorferi* bind integrin $\alpha_{IIb}\beta_3$ on human platelets.[21] Both the major surface protein (gp63) and the major surface glycolipid (lipophosphoglycan, or LPG) of *Leishmania mexicana* bind directly to different domains within the complement receptor CR3, a member of the β_2 integrin family, in macrophages.[22] Epstein-Barr virus enters cells by binding to another complement receptor, CR2, via the viral glycoprotein gp350/220, which has amino acid sequence homology with the natural complement ligand.[23] Adenovirus 2 encodes two proteins, the fiber protein and the penton base protein, which attach to integrin receptors (the latter to $\alpha_v\beta_3$ and $\alpha_v\beta_5$, which promote internalization but not attachment).[24]

Organisms may simultaneously recognize matrix proteins and cellular receptors. Infected erythrocytes containing *Plasmodium falciparum* trophozoites, in addition to binding to thrombospondin, another component of the extracellular matrix, bind to members of the immunoglobulin gene superfamily (intercellular adhesion molecule 1, vascular cell adhesion molecule) and the selectin family (endothelial leukocyte adhesion molecule) and to the differentiation antigen CD36. These interactions mediate attachment of the infected cells to vascular endothelium, sequestering the infected cells from clearance by the spleen.[25, 26]

Interactions Dependent on Carbohydrates or Pattern Recognition Molecules

Another class of adherence molecules consists of lectins produced by microorganisms that bind to carbohydrate residues on target cells or sites. Pili generally serve this function in bacteria. With *Mycoplasma* and influenza virus, specific microbial components bind to sialic acid on host cells. In *Entamoeba histolytica,* a galactose- or *N*-acetyl-D-galactosamine–inhibitable lectin mediates attachment of trophozoites to colonic mucins or mammalian target cells.[27–29] Organisms may bind to specialized cell surface glycoconjugates, such as glyosaminoglycans, as is the case with *Chlamydia.*[30] Conversely, carbohydrate-containing ligands on the organism may mediate attachment to tissues or surfaces. Microbes such as *Mycobacterium, Leishmania, Candida, Pneumocystis,* and specific strains of enterobacteria, containing mannose-rich components within the cell wall, bind to the mannose receptor in macrophages.[31–35] Finally, pattern recognition receptors, such as the macrophage scavenger receptor and CD14, bind gram-negative bacterial lipopolysaccharide (LPS), gram-positive bacterial lipoteichoic acid, and mycobacterial lipoarabinomannan,[36–38] providing broad-spectrum binding and clearance mechanisms for the host.

Summary

The net effect of the foregoing interactions is to target organisms to specific tissues or to specific sites on a cell and in some cases to facilitate microbial uptake. It is often impossible to isolate and identify the effects of a single ligand-receptor interaction, given the multitude of microbial cell surface components and host receptors as well as the multivalent nature of many receptor-ligand interactions. Redundant mechanisms for attachment are the rule. It is also generally difficult to determine whether the interaction of microbe and host cell only facilitates binding or potentiates cell entry. Experimental systems in which the effects of the microbial and host cell components can be studied in isolation, although difficult to devise, provide the best avenue to an accurate understanding of the interactions.

Evasion of Humoral Defenses

Whether localized to a specific tissue site, disseminated throughout the blood stream, or in transit to an intracellular locale, pathogenic microorganisms must evade humoral defenses. For most prokaryotes, the components of nearly impenetrable cell walls are intimately involved in evasion of the most important components of the humoral defense system, antibody and complement.

Gram-Negative Bacteria

The cell wall of gram-negative enteric bacteria is a trilamellar structure, consisting of an outer membrane, a thin peptidoglycan layer within the periplasmic space, and an inner membrane.[39] Often, there is a polysaccharide capsule external to the outer membrane along with pili (Fig. 3–1). The most

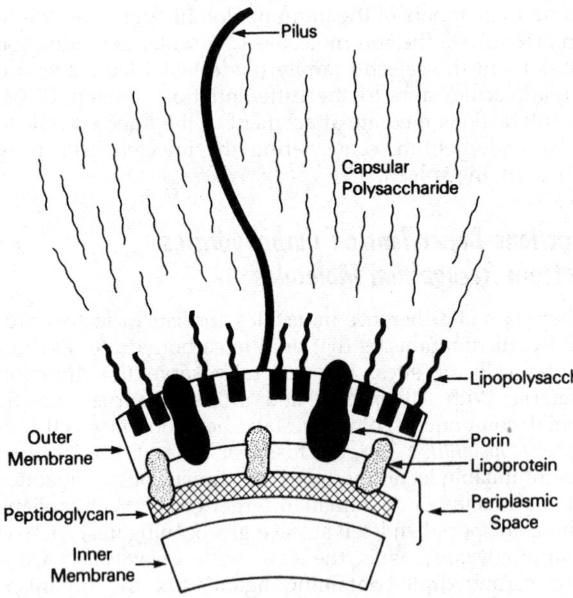

FIGURE 3–1 □ Diagram of the structure of the cell wall and the capsule of enteric gram-negative bacteria. The trilamellar cell wall is composed of an outer membrane, the peptidoglycan and periplasmic space, and the inner membrane. The two major components of the outer leaflet of the outer membrane are the LPS (containing O-polysaccharide) and outer membrane porin proteins. Lipoprotein anchors the outer membrane to the peptidoglycan. The polysaccharide capsule, which sits external to the outer membrane, is permeable to soluble molecules of large and small sizes but precludes interaction of phagocytic cells with components of the outer membrane or humoral ligands bound to outer membrane constituents. A single pilus is shown extending through the capsule.

prevalent component in the outer membrane is LPS, composed of three regions termed lipid A, core oligosaccharide, and O-polysaccharide (Fig. 3–2). Each portion of the LPS molecule has important interactions with the host immune system. Most important for the purposes of this section, LPS forms a confluent layer on the bacterial surface and serves as an impermeable physical barrier to attack by the humoral immune system. Direct lysis of organisms by the serum complement system is precluded by LPS, because lytic components of the cascade cannot gain access to the outer membrane bilayer or the inner membrane.[40] Although antibodies directed to determinants within the core oligosaccharide or to outer membrane proteins are generally present in normal human serum, these antibodies do not have access to core determinants in the native organism and cannot mediate direct opsonic functions or complement-dependent opsonic or lytic activities. In selected instances in which organisms produce shorter LPSs (termed lipooligosaccharides), such as with *Neisseria gonorrhoeae,* addition of sialic acid to lipooligosaccharide catalyzed by bacterial transsialidase blocks complement activation.[41] Hence, LPS can play a multifunctional role in serum resistance.

Outer membrane proteins of gram-negative bacteria, and particularly of nonenteric organisms, participate in evasion of the humoral immune system. Components from a family of related outer membrane proteins in *Salmonella* (Rck) and *Yersinia* (Ail) confer serum resistance independently of LPS.[42–45] At least in the case of the Rck protein, inefficient formation of the lytic C5b,6,7,8,9 complex of complement is the mechanism for serum resistance. With *Aeromonas*[10] and *Campylobacter fetus,*[46] confluent fibrillar protein arrays (termed S layers) coating the organism serve a barrier function, blocking antibody- and complement-dependent lytic and opsonic activity. Outer membrane proteins, such as protein III in *N. gonorrhoeae,* serve as targets for antibodies in normal serum that block the lytic activity of the complement cascade for the organism.[47]

Gram-Positive Bacteria

The cell wall of gram-positive organisms functions in evasion of the humoral immune system. The most striking feature of the gram-positive cell wall is the thick peptidoglycan.[48] The peptidoglycan is composed of covalently cross-linked, repeating subunits of *N*-acetylglucosamine and *N*-acetylmuramic acid, further cross-linked by peptide extensions. This rigid structure serves as a physical barrier, protecting the inner membrane from lytic attack by complement. Specific components also facilitate complement and antibody evasion. M protein from group A streptococci is one of the best studied and best understood virulence determinants in gram-positive bacteria.[49] Strains lacking M protein or in which the M protein has been deleted have decreased virulence. The molecule has conserved domains within the midportion of the α-helical coiled structure and has a polypeptide membrane anchor at the C-terminal of the molecule (see Fig. 3–2). Hypervariability occurs within the distal 20 to 25 residues of the N-terminal of the M protein, the only portion exposed to external macromolecules such as antibody and complement. Strains bearing M protein block complement activation, and in at least one M type the mechanism is known. M protein directly binds a negative complement regulatory molecule, factor H.[50, 51] In addition, the opsonic complement fragment C3b deposited on M protein–bearing strains is less capable of interacting with phagocyte C3 receptors than is C3b deposited on strains lacking M protein, possibly owing to steric hindrance of C3 bound to neighboring cells.[52]

Additional components unique to the gram-positive cell wall include the teichoic acids and the group-specific carbohydrates in streptococci. Lipoteichoic acid in group A streptococci is involved in attachment of the organism to fibronectin, as mentioned earlier, and also mediates binding of organisms to the macrophage scavenger receptor[36] and the pattern recognition receptor, CD14.[38] Teichoic acids are also implicated in complement activation by some but not all gram-positive bacteria. Protein A, a major component within the cell wall of pathogenic strains of *S. aureus,* directly binds immunoglobulin G (IgG). Protein A binds to the Fc portion of the immunoglobulin molecule and in so doing may either block or enhance IgG-mediated phagocytosis by interacting with Fc receptors on professional phagocytes. Analogous situations may exist with protein G from streptococci, which binds IgG, with the CR2- and CR3-like molecules produced by *Candida albicans,*[53, 54] and potentially even with the Fc receptor–like components produced by members of the herpesvirus family.

Protozoa and Helminths

Evasion of humoral defenses by protozoa and helminths is developmentally regulated; evasion mechanisms are generally manifest only in the life cycle stages that infect or reside within the vertebrate host. Infective vertebrate stages but not noninfective insect stages of *Trypanosoma cruzi* produce a complement regulatory molecule[55, 56] functionally analogous to human decay-accelerating factor, which limits complement activation and prevents lysis by the terminal portion of the complement cascade. Schistosomula of *Schistosoma mansoni* shed the complement-activating surface glycocalyx coat during transformation from the cercarial stage[57] and also acquire the complement regulatory molecule decay-accelerating factor from the vertebrate host,[58, 59] thus rendering the worms incapable of activating complement. Other surface compo-

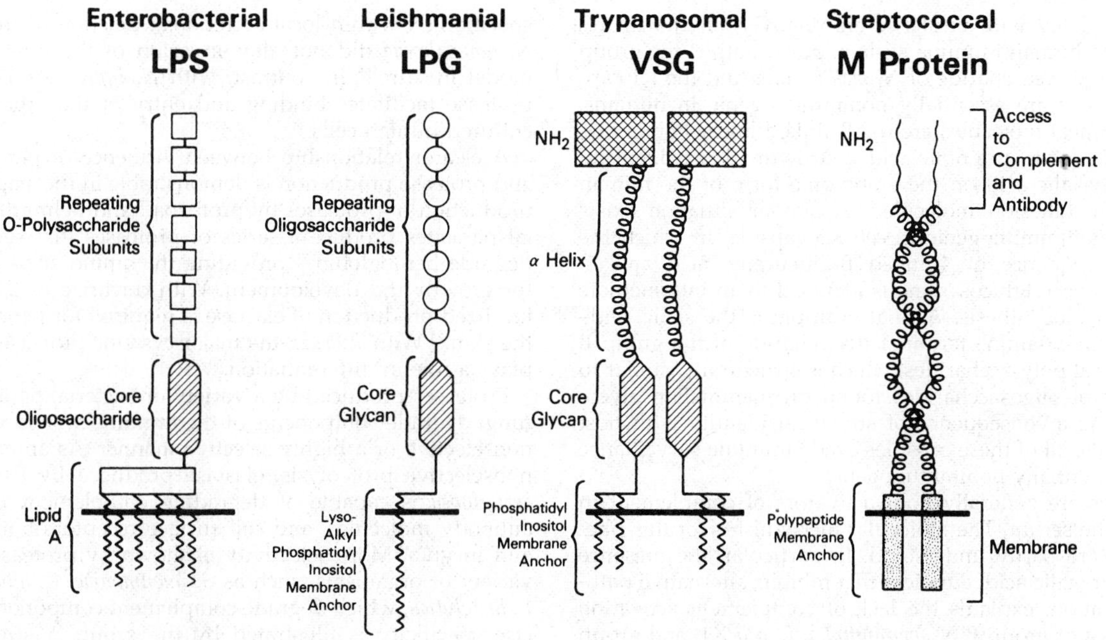

FIGURE 3–2 □ Structure of four microbial virulence determinants, which mediate evasion of humoral defenses. Common overall structural features are illustrated, along with the parts of each molecule that are exposed to external macromolecules, such as antibody and complement. Both enteric gram-negative bacterial LPS and leishmanial LPG contain variable numbers of repeating oligosaccharide subunits that are linked to a single core oligosaccharide or to a core glycan moiety, which is bound in turn to a lipid-containing membrane anchor. In LPS, the anchor is a portion of lipid A; whereas in LPG the anchor is a lyso-alkyl phosphatidylinositol. Trypanosomal variable surface glycoprotein (VSG) exists normally as a dimer, wherein each monomer is composed of a series of parallel α-helical polypeptide domains. For simplicity, only a single α-helix is shown for each monomer. The peptide component is linked to a core glycan moiety, which is bound to the membrane by a dimyristoyl phosphatidylinositol membrane anchor. Although the crystallographic structure of the α-helical portion of the molecule is known, the structure of the surface exposed portion, which is presumed to be in a β-sheet configuration, has not yet been solved. M protein consists of a dimer of α-helical chains in a coiled structure, with the N-terminal 20 to 25 residues in a random conformation. M protein is the only one of the constituents shown that has a polypeptide membrane anchor.

nents of the schistosomula may serve as the target for blocking antibodies capable of abrogating antibody-, complement-, and cell-dependent lytic activities against the helminth. The galactose-specific lectin of *E. histolytica,* described earlier for its role in cell attachment and target cytolysis, is a multifunctional protein that also blocks complement-mediated killing of the organism (and shares homology with the mammalian complement inhibitor CD59).[60] Some parasites bear confluent surface components analogous to bacterial LPS capable of preventing complement lysis in the absence of specific antibody. A confluent glycoprotein layer (variable surface glycoprotein; see Fig. 3–2) produced by infective stages but not noninfective procyclic stages of *Trypanosoma brucei*[61] limits complement activation on the trypomastigote surface. A confluent LPG (see Fig. 3–2) similar in overall structure to bacterial LPS is produced by infective stages of *Leishmania major* and sterically precludes complement lysis in a fashion exactly analogous to that with serum-resistant strains of *Salmonella* and *Escherichia coli.*

Antigenic Variation as a Mechanism for Evasion of Humoral Defense Mechanisms

T. brucei, N. gonorrhoeae, and *Borrelia* are the clearest examples of organisms in which major surface proteins or glycoproteins undergo spontaneous, rapid, and extensive antigenic variation. Additional organisms, including *Pneumocystis* and *Giardia,* also have an abundant family of genes encoding a major cell surface protein.[62, 63] A repertoire of different variable surface glycoprotein genes of *T. brucei,*[61] pilin genes of *N. gonorrhoeae,*[64] and variable major protein genes of *Borrelia*[65] are present. Only a single version of the protein is expressed at a given time, but expression of a new or altered copy of the gene occurs by a variety of processes, including transposition of silent copies of structural genes into a single expression site.[61] Antigenic variation in pili of *N. gonorrhoeae* can also result from transformation by DNA from autolysed gonococci. Although antigenic variation for these three organisms is not driven by the immune response, the result of rapid antigenic switching is evasion of the detrimental consequences of a developing antibody response against the critical surface or attachment component. In contrast, spontaneous antigenic variation on a longer time scale, driven in part by the immune response, occurs in the surface-exposed portions of many if not all microbial surface proteins that are potential or real targets for protective antibody. This concept is well illustrated by the perpetual changes in the hemagglutinin of influenza virus.

Evasion of Phagocytosis

Successful extracellular pathogens must evade phagocytosis and killing by both circulating and fixed phagocytic cells. The prototypic encapsulated bacteria, such as *Streptococcus pneumoniae, Klebsiella pneumoniae, S. aureus, Haemophilus influenzae,* and *Neisseria meningitidis,* are extracellular pathogens and grow in unrestrained fashion unless they are cleared by circulating and fixed phagocytic cells. As effective phagocytosis requires opsonization of the target particle, a common mechanism for preventing phagocytosis is prevention or blockade of opsonization by antibody or complement. The most common structure serving this function in bacteria is the polysaccharide capsule. Many bacterial capsular serotypes associated with virulence are relatively inert with regard to the human immune system. For example, the group B capsular polysaccharide of *N. meningitidis* and the K1 capsule of *E. coli* are essentially nonimmunogenic in humans. These identical molecules are α-2-8–linked linear homopolymers of *N*-acetylneuraminic acid, a structure that is identical to the polysialic acid on the embryonic form of the human neural cell adhesion molecule.[66] A similar situation exists with the nonimmunogenic *E. coli* K5 capsule, in which the repeating sequence of 4-linked β-glucuronic acid and 4-linked α-*N*-acetylglucosamine is identical to an intermediate in heparin biosynthesis. A final example is the sialic acid–galactose-glucosamine terminal trisaccharide of the group B streptococcal polysaccharides, which is structurally similar to a number of oligosaccharides found on mammalian glycoproteins. As a consequence of structural identity with host components, all of these capsules evade immune surveillance and are essentially nonimmunogenic.

Capsules are generally poor activators of complement in nonimmune serum. The molecular mechanisms for this phenomenon are partly understood. In particular, the presence of capsular sialic acid, a moiety that inhibits alternative pathway activation, explains the lack of complement activation by capsules of group B *N. meningitidis, E. coli* K1, and group B streptococci. Capsules are permeable to large protein molecules, permitting deposition of subcapsular antibody and complement components. For opsonization and phagocytosis of encapsulated organisms to occur, however, opsonic complement or antibody, or both, must be deposited on the capsular surface in a location accessible to phagocytic receptors on neutrophils, monocytes, and macrophages. In the absence of specific antibody, phagocytosis does not occur.[67]

Even more elaborate mechanisms for blocking phagocytosis have also been described. *Yersinia* secretes proteins that block phagocytosis by macrophages. These molecules are apparently inserted across the host cell plasma membrane and dephosphorylate host cell components involved in phagocytosis or disassemble actin filaments in the host cell.[68–70]

Dissemination and Evasion of Local Defenses

Proteases may function to facilitate initial invasion or subsequent spread of extracellular pathogens through normal tissues, to facilitate the normal process of development within or rupture out of cells, or to destroy or override components of the immune system. Only a limited number of enzymes produced by microorganisms, including proteinases, collagenases, lipases, and nucleases, are definitively associated with virulence. A few examples illustrate the point. Streptococci produce hyaluronidase, which liquefies hyaluronic acid and facilitates spreading; however, production of the enzyme by *Bacteroides* and *S. aureus* does not result in analogous dissection through tissue planes. Sialyltransferases in *T. cruzi*[71] and in *N. gonorrhoeae*[41, 72] play roles in transferring sialic acid from host cells to the microbial surface, either facilitating attachment or invasion or influencing susceptibility to complement killing or phagocytosis. In contrast, microbial production of neuraminidases is associated with but not definitively linked to virulence for a variety of organisms including *Bacteroides fragilis*. Pathogens that invade the respiratory mucosa, such as *H. influenzae* and *N. meningitidis*; occupy mucosal surfaces of the genitourinary tract, such as *N. gonorrhoeae*; or occupy the gastrointestinal tract, such as *B. fragilis* and *Giardia lamblia*, produce proteases specific for immunoglobulin A (IgA),[73] all of which are secreted by bacteria via a common mechanism.[74] Although the function of IgA protease would appear self-evident (i.e., destruction of specific IgA within local secretions), deletion of the gene in *N. gonorrhoeae* did not alter invasion of the organism in a model in vitro.[75] In contrast, with *H. influenzae* an IgA-like protease facilitates binding and entry of the organism into cultured human cells.[76]

A clearer relationship between virulence or pathogenicity and protease production is demonstrable in the stage-specific production of proteases by protozoa[77] and helminths. Malarial parasites produce a series of proteases that sequentially degrade hemoglobin,[78] providing the amino acids necessary for growth and development. With cercariae of *Schistosoma,* localized production of elastase is required for penetration of the skin.[79] With *T. cruzi,* the major cysteine protease (cruzain) plays a role in differentiation.[80, 81]

Proteases produced by a variety of bacteria, parasites, and fungi degrade components of the immune system in either a nonselective or a highly selective manner. As an example of nonselective proteolysis, elastase produced by *Pseudomonas aeruginosa* is capable of degrading complement molecules, antibody molecules, and cell surface receptors both in vitro and in vivo. More selectivity is shown by proteases from a variety of organisms, such as *S. pneumoniae, C. albicans,* and *E. histolytica,* which degrade complement component C3. Precise specificity is illustrated by the group A streptococcal protease, which specifically inactivates the complement chemotactic factor C5a.[82]

Figure 3–3 shows an overview of the mechanisms involved in microbial evasion of humoral defenses.

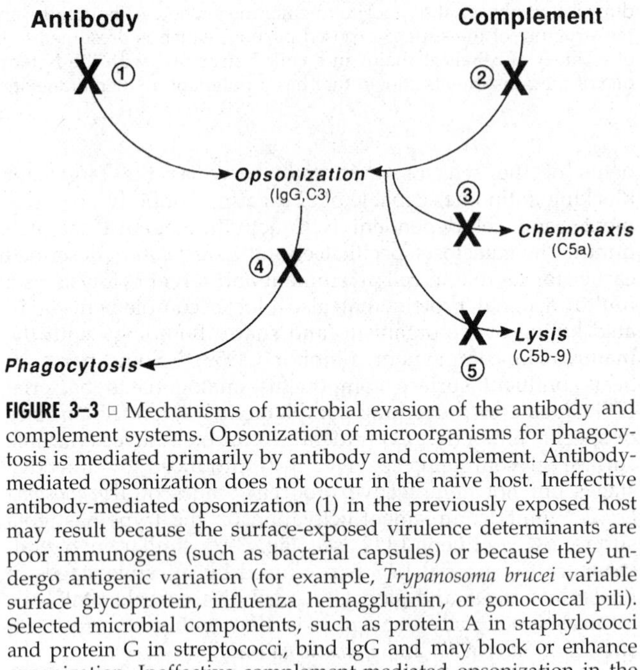

FIGURE 3–3 □ Mechanisms of microbial evasion of the antibody and complement systems. Opsonization of microorganisms for phagocytosis is mediated primarily by antibody and complement. Antibody-mediated opsonization does not occur in the naive host. Ineffective antibody-mediated opsonization (1) in the previously exposed host may result because the surface-exposed virulence determinants are poor immunogens (such as bacterial capsules) or because they undergo antigenic variation (for example, *Trypanosoma brucei* variable surface glycoprotein, influenza hemagglutinin, or gonococcal pili). Selected microbial components, such as protein A in staphylococci and protein G in streptococci, bind IgG and may block or enhance opsonization. Ineffective complement-mediated opsonization in the naive host generally results from blockade of alternative complement pathway activation (2) by microbial components, such as capsular sialic acid, streptococcal M protein, or the *Trypanosoma cruzi* C3 convertase inhibitor. Specific inactivation of the chemotactic component C5a (3) is mediated by group A streptococci. A block in phagocytosis of organisms exposed to antibody and complement (4) may occur because opsonic ligands are deposited below a polysaccharide capsule or because ligands or receptors or both are degraded by microbial proteases, such as elastase of *Pseudomonas aeruginosa.* Ineffective complement-mediated lysis (5) often occurs because surface components (enteric gram-negative LPS, gram-positive peptidoglycan, *Leishmania* LPG) sterically block access of the lytic C5b,6,7,8,9 complex to deeper, complement-susceptible sites on the microbial cell wall.

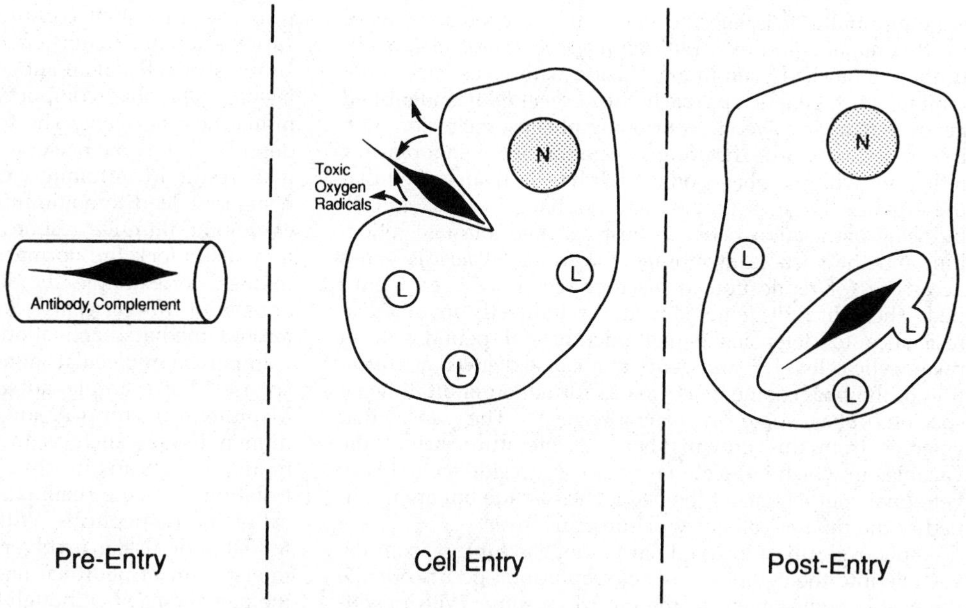

FIGURE 3–4 □ Intracellular pathogens must evade destruction before, during, and after cell entry. Specific examples of each process are described in the text. Evasion of the humoral defense system before cell entry *(left)* is illustrated in more detail in Figure 3–3. Organisms entering phagocytic cells *(center)* must circumvent killing by toxic oxygen metabolites. Once inside any cell *(right)*, pathogens must evade killing by nonoxidative processes, including lysosomal enzymes.

Evasion of Killing by Cells

Evasion During Cell Entry

Organisms that reside within cells must evade killing during the process of cell entry (Fig. 3–4). Although this may be a relatively simple task for entry into nonprofessional phagocytes, the task is more daunting for organisms entering neutrophils, monocytes, and macrophages. These professional phagocytes are capable, via NADPH oxidase, of producing a respiratory burst, with generation of toxic products of reduced oxygen (superoxide, hydrogen peroxide, singlet oxygen, hydroxyl radical) with potent antimicrobial activity. Conceptually, pathogens may evade the consequences of these products by entering cells without substantial generation of the burst or by producing products that block generation of the burst or inactivate products of the respiratory burst. Many intracellular pathogens that reside predominantly within macrophages, such as *Leishmania* species,[22] *Legionella pneumophila,*[83] and *M. tuberculosis, Mycobacterium avium,* and *M. leprae,*[84, 85] contain membrane components that direct the organism to enter the macrophage via receptors for complement component C3. These receptors, unlike those for the Fc portion of IgG, are not linked to triggering of the NADPH oxidase responsible for generating products of the respiratory burst. An alternative strategy is used by *Toxoplasma gondii,* which enters macrophages and nearly all nucleated cells by an active process that does not require the presence of any phagocytic receptors potentially involved in signal transduction or generation of a respiratory burst.[86] *L. pneumophila* produces a surface protein with homology to binding proteins for the immunosuppressive agent FK-506[87]; this protein facilitates microbial entry into macrophages via a route that does not result in killing.[88]

Several microbial molecules that block generation of the respiratory burst have been identified. Among the best studied is the abundant membrane component LPG of *Leishmania donovani,* which inhibits triggering of the NADPH oxidase.[89] LPG is a known inhibitor of protein kinase C, the central component in signal transduction leading to NADPH oxidase activation.

Most intracellular pathogens produce catalase or superoxide dismutase, or both, enzymes capable of specifically inactivating hydrogen peroxide and superoxide, respectively. Other microbial components containing large polysaccharide moieties, including the secreted phenolic glycolipid I of *M. leprae*[90] and the acid phosphatase and LPG of *L. donovani,* are nonspecific scavengers of products of the respiratory burst.[91]

Evasion of Killing Inside Cells

Three general strategies are adopted by intracellular organisms for evasion of nonoxidative killing inside cells. Intracellular organisms must evade killing by the acidic environment containing hydrolytic enzymes from lysosomes, organelles that are present in substantial quantities in nearly all cells. A selected group of intracellular pathogens reside within a vacuole that neither acidifies nor fuses with lysosomes (Table 3–1). On theoretical grounds it can be argued that the organisms must either produce an inhibitor of acidification and lysosomal fusion or actively form a compartment that does not contain signals for fusion with other intracellular compartments. Evidence for the latter concept exists for *T. gondii.*[92] The phagosome in which mycobacteria reside lacks the vacuolar proton adenosinetriphosphatase[93] and is blocked in maturation through the endocytic pathway.[94] Although sulfated glycolipids and ammonia produced by mycobacteria

TABLE 3–1 ■ Evasion of Nonoxidative Killing Inside Cells: The Role of Specialized Compartments

INHIBITION OF PHAGOSOME-LYSOSOME FUSION
Toxoplasma gondii
Legionella pneumophila
Chlamydia psittaci
Mycobacterium tuberculosis
RUPTURE OUT OF PHAGOSOME INTO CYTOPLASM
Trypanosoma cruzi
Shigella flexneri
Rickettsia spp.
Listeria monocytogenes
SURVIVAL AND REPLICATION WITHIN PHAGOLYSOSOME
Leishmania spp.
Salmonella typhimurium
Mycobacterium lepraemurium
Coxiella burnetii

were originally postulated to inhibit fusion events, evidence for this remains indirect. With *Histoplasma capsulatum,* acidification is blocked even though fusion with lysosomes is not inhibited.[95] A genetic approach with *Legionella* has identified genes that are involved in controlling phagosome fusion with lysosomes, as well as dictating association of the endoplasmic reticulum with the phagosome.[96–99] It has been suggested that these genes trigger a process of autophagy in the host cell, inducing association between host cell endoplasmic reticulum and the vacuole membrane.[100] Various *Salmonella* genes necessary for replication in macrophages have been identified. These include genes directly or indirectly involved in resistance to defensins (small microbicidal peptides from phagocytic cells)[101, 102] and genes that cause delayed acidification of the phagosome,[103] as well as formation of an unusual spacious phagosome in macrophages.[104] The sense that emerges from this growing body of literature is that the vacuoles in which intracellular pathogens reside are not conventional components of the endocytic cascade but are modified at the time of cell entry or subsequently.[105]

Another group of intracellular pathogens rupture from the vacuole into the cytoplasm, where replication occurs outside the hostile environment of the phagolysosome. With rickettsiae,[106] shigellae,[107] *Listeria monocytogenes,*[108] and *T. cruzi,*[109] the process of rupture has been associated with production by the organism of a hemolysin, whose activity may be triggered or facilitated by the acidic environment of the early endosomal compartment that forms immediately after microbial uptake into the cells. Interestingly, for *T. cruzi,* the process of cell entry involves recruitment of host cell lysosomes to the plasma membrane of the host cell[110] in a process that is calcium dependent and results from calcium transients induced by the parasite in the host cell.[111, 112]

Finally, some pathogens replicate within the apparently hostile environment of the phagolysosome. Major metabolic pathways in the intracellular form of *Coxiella burnetii*[113] and the intracellular amastigote form but not the extracellular promastigote form of *L. donovani*[114] have a pH optimum of 4.0 to 5.5, found in the phagolysosome. Emerging evidence suggests that these organisms actively induce fusion of phagosomes with lysosomes.[115] Nonetheless, the mechanism by which this group of pathogens evades destruction by lysosomal enzymes is unclear. The suggestion has been offered that LPSs, glycolipids, or LPGs that form a confluent surface coat are resistant to lysosomal hydrolases and thus provide an effective barrier to destruction within the phagolysosomal environment.

Proteins and Other Molecules That Alter Immune Responsiveness

There are three general mechanisms by which microbial components may ablate, divert, or subvert the host immune response. Microbial constituents may lead to immunologic suppression of immune effector cells or induction of immune suppressor cells, in an antigen-specific or antigen-nonspecific fashion. Microbial components may perfectly or imperfectly mimic host antigens. The former case leads to tolerance, as described for some bacterial capsular antigens; the latter case may result in autoimmune phenomena. Microbial components may lead to nonimmunologic destruction of cells critical for the immune response. Finally, microbial components may also block the normal activity of lymphokines and cytokines. For example, the dominant carbohydrate-containing antigen of *M. tuberculosis,* lipoarabinomannan, inhibits interferon-γ–mediated activation of macrophages.

Imperfect molecular mimicry results in autoimmune responses. For example, antigenic cross-reactivity between the M protein of group A streptococci and antigens in specific human tissues such as muscle (myosin),[116, 117] kidney, and brain provides an attractive explanation for the disease manifestations in acute rheumatic fever and acute poststreptococcal glomerulonephritis. With *T. cruzi,* autoantibodies specific for sites of tissue involvement, such as endocardium and interstitium of neuronal tissue, react with laminin and with the parasite itself, although the link between these antibodies and disease manifestations is not clear.

Some organisms may incapacitate or lyse effector cells by selective, immunologic means or by nonselective nonimmunologic mechanisms. The premier example of the selective depletion is the destruction of $CD4^+$ cells by human immunodeficiency virus. *E. histolytica* lyses granulocytes, lymphocytes, and macrophages in a contact-dependent fashion requiring the participation of the adherence lectin described earlier and the additional contribution of a pore-forming molecule and phospholipases produced by the ameba.[118]

Toxicity

Toxic components of microbial cell walls have been studied in large part in relation to septic shock and multiple organ failure[119] (Table 3–2). In this arena, endotoxin plays a central role. The biologic effects of LPS are legion. LPS interacts with the humoral defense system, causing disseminated intravascular coagulation by activation of the contact system and direct activation of factor XII, and causes antibody-independent complement activation with generation of the anaphylatoxins C3a and C5a.

Endotoxin has wide-ranging interactions with cells, inducing production by macrophages of prostaglandins, interferon-α, interleukin-1 (IL-1), and tumor necrosis factor and causing release from endothelial cells of IL-1, plasminogen activator inhibitor, and tissue factor.[120, 121] IL-1 and tumor necrosis factor in particular have a panoply of effects that are either beneficial or toxic, such as release of stress hormones, muscle degradation, development of fever, and cell activation. Per-

TABLE 3–2 ■ Biologic Properties of Selected Components from the Cell Wall of Gram-Negative and Gram-Positive Bacteria

BACTERIAL PRODUCT	STIMULATES PRODUCTION OF INTERLEUKIN-1	STIMULATES PRODUCTION OF TUMOR NECROSIS FACTOR	ACTIVATES COMPLEMENT	PRIMES PHAGOCYTIC CELLS	LETHAL ANIMALS
Gram-negative LPS	+	+	+	+	+
Gram-positive lipoteichoic acid*	+	+	±	−	−
Peptidoglycan*	+	+	+	−	+
Muramyl dipeptide	+	+	−	+	−
Pyrogenic exotoxins	+	+	−	+	+

*Higher concentrations than for LPS.

Modified from Danner RL, Suffredini AF, Natanson C, Parrillo JE: Microbial toxins: Role in the pathogenesis of septic shock and multiple organ failure. *In* Bihari DJ, Cerra FB (eds): Multiple Organ Failure. Fullerton, CA, Society of Critical Care Medicine, 1989, 151–191.

haps most important in relation to this last point, effector cell (neutrophil, monocyte/macrophage) inflammatory reactions, including endogenous mediator–induced release of toxic oxygen radicals,[122] lysosomal constituents, arachidonic acid metabolites, and platelet-activating factor, can be markedly augmented by prior exposure of cells to levels of endotoxin (<10 μg/mL) found circulating in patients with septicemia. This phenomenon, which has been termed endotoxin priming, is central to understanding the pathogenesis of septic shock, because LPS concentrations typically achieved in the blood stream and tissues of infected individuals "prime" cells for a markedly enhanced response to cytokines and chemotactic factors generated simultaneously during infection.

In almost all instances, the effects just described result from the lipid A moiety of LPS. The mechanism for LPS interaction with cells is largely defined, with a major role played by the serum LPS binding protein and the cell surface receptor CD14. The involvement of other cell surface receptors in the signal transduction process seems clear. The presence of specific fatty acid side chains, especially myristic acid in the acyloxyacyl position, correlates with biologic activity. The LPS molecule is largely resistant to the degradative effects of host cell enzymes. An important exception is neutrophil acyloxyacyl hydrolase, which detoxifies LPS by removing the critical myristic acid in the acyloxyacyl position.[123, 124]

Gram-positive organisms possess cellular components that also have toxic effects (see Table 3–2), although not generally at the doses or with the lethality seen with LPS. Recognition that peptidoglycan could induce the Shwartzman reaction, shock, and death led to the search for the smallest biologically active component in the structure capable of eliciting the same effects. Muramyl dipeptide or *N*-acetylmuramyl-L-alanyl-D-isoglutamine[125] has some but not all of the biologic activity of peptidoglycan, including the release from macrophages of tumor necrosis factor, IL-1, colony-stimulating factor, and interferon-α. Lipoteichoic acid also induces many of the effects seen with endotoxin, although again at much higher concentrations. It has now become evident that secreted exotoxins from streptococci and staphylococci, many of which are superantigens, are the most potent molecules at inducing cytokine release and toxicity for the host.[126, 127]

One newly recognized phenomenon is the ability of microbial components to induce programmed cell death, or apoptosis.[128] For example, the secreted hemolysin of *Shigella* induces apoptosis in macrophages, which can in turn induce IL-1 release. Staphylococcal α-toxin[129] also causes apoptosis, as does *E. histolytica.*

Finally, several interesting observations regarding cell biologic mechanisms for activity of bacterial toxins deserve note. Shiga toxin and other protein toxins that act on targets in the cytosol are transported after endocytosis by retrograde transport into the Golgi complex and endoplasmic reticulum, an effect that is apparently necessary for toxin action.[130] Several toxins, including cholera toxin, contain sequences at the C-terminal of the proteins that lead to their retention in the endoplasmic reticulum. Equally of interest, the mechanism of action of clostridial neurotoxins is now defined. These molecules act as proteases that specifically cleave protein components necessary for synaptic vesicle docking and fusion.[131]

Summary

Categorization of virulence factors is an increasingly complex task. As more microbial components are identified, cloned, synthesized, and specifically altered or deleted, the appreciation of the vast microbial repertoire of virulence determinants grows. Simultaneously, there is the recognition that many if not most virulence traits are redundant—organisms demonstrate multiple mechanisms for attachment, invasion, and evasion of host defenses. One consequence is the increasing need to define virulence factors expressed and operative in vivo.[132] This provides the best prospect for developing novel strategies of intervention aimed at blocking virulence traits.

References

1. Falkow S: Molecular Koch's postulates applied to microbial pathogenicity. Rev Infect Dis 10(Suppl 2):S274–S276, 1988.
2. Mims CA: The Pathogenesis of Infectious Disease. London, Academic Press, 1987.
3. Hultgren SJ, Abraham S, Caparon M, et al: Pilus and nonpilus bacterial adhesins: Assembly and function in cell recognition. Cell 73:887–901, 1993.
4. Westerlund B, Korhonen T: Bacterial proteins binding to the mammalian extracellular matrix. Mol Microbiol 9:687–694, 1993.
5. Valentin-Weigand P, Talay S, Kaufhold A, et al: The fibronectin binding domain of the Sfb protein adhesin of *Streptococcus pyogenes* occurs in many group A streptococci and does not cross-react with heart myosin. Microb Pathog 17:111–120, 1994.
6. Sela S, Aviv A, Tovi A, et al: Protein F: An adhesin of *Streptococcus pyogenes* binds fibronectin via two distinct domains. Mol Microbiol 10:1049–1055, 1993.
7. Foster T, McDevitt D: Surface-associated proteins of *Staphylococcus aureus:* Their possible roles in virulence. FEMS Microbiol Lett 118:199–205, 1994.
8. Frick I, Crossin K, Edelman G, Bjorck L: Protein H—a bacterial surface protein with affinity for both immunoglobulin and fibronectin type III domains. EMBO J 14:1674–1679, 1995.
9. Tamm A, Tarkkanen A, Korhonen T, et al: Hydrophobic domains affect the collagen-binding specificity and surface polymerization as well as the virulence potential of the YadA protein of *Yersinia enterocolitica.* Mol Microbiol 10:995–1011, 1993.
10. Kay WW, Trust TJ: Form and functions of the regular surface array (S-layer) of *Aeromonas salmonicida.* Experientia 15:412–414, 1991.
11. Proctor RA: The staphylococcal fibronectin receptor: Evidence for its importance in invasive infections. Rev Infect Dis 9(Suppl 4):S335–S340, 1987.
12. Lopes JD, dos Resi M, Bretani RR: Presence of laminin receptors in *Staphylococcus aureus.* Science 229:275–277, 1985.
13. Cheung AI, Projan SJ, Edelstein RE, Fischetti VA: Cloning, expression and nucleotide sequence of a *Staphlococcus aureus* gene *(fbpA)* encoding a fibrinogen binding protein. Infect Immun 63:1914–1920, 1995.
14. Joh H, House-Pompeo K, Patti J, et al: Fibronectin receptors from gram-positive bacteria: Comparison of active sites. Biochemistry 33:6086–6092, 1994.
15. Schorey J, Li Q, McCourt D, et al: A *Mycobacterium leprae* gene encoding a fibronectin binding protein is used for efficient invasion of epithelial cells and Schwann cells. Infect Immun 63:2652–2657, 1995.
16. Falkow S, Isberg RR, Portnoy DA: The interaction of bacteria with mammalian cells. Annu Rev Cell Biol 8:333–363, 1992.
17. Isberg RR, Tran Van Nhieu G: Binding and internalization of microorganisms by integrin receptors. Trends Microbiol 2:10–14, 1994.
18. Isberg RR, Leong JM: Multiple β_1 Chain integrins are receptors for invasin, a protein that promotes bacterial penetration into mammalian cells. Cell 60:861–871, 1990.
19. Leong JM, Morrissey PE, Marra A, Isberg RR: An aspartate residue of the *Yersinia pseudotuberculosis* invasin protein that is critical for integrin binding. EMBO J 14:422–431, 1995.
20. Relman D, Toumanen E, Falkow S, et al: Recognition of a bacterial adhesion by an integrin: Macrophage CR3 (alpha M beta 2, CD11b/CD18) binds to filamentous hemagglutinin of *Bordetella pertussis.* Cell 61:1375–1382, 1990.
21. Coburn J, Barthold SW, Leong JM: Diverse Lyme disease spirochetes bind integrin alpha IIb beta 3 on platelets. Infect Immun 62:5569–5567, 1994.
22. Russell DG, Talamas-Rohana P: *Leishmania* and the macrophage: A marriage of inconvenience. Immunol Today 10:328–333, 1989.

23. Nemerow GR, Houghten RA, Moore MD, Cooper NR: Identification of an epitope in the major envelope protein of Epstein-Barr virus that mediates viral binding to the B lymphocyte EBV receptor (CR2). Cell 56:369–377, 1989.
24. Wickham TJ, Mathias P, Cheresh DA, Nemerow GR: Integrins alpha v beta 3 and alpha v beta 5 promote adenovirus internalization but not virus attachment. Cell 73:309–319, 1993.
25. Chulay J, Ockenhouse H: Host receptors for malaria-infected erythrocytes. Am J Trop Med Hyg 43:6–14, 1990.
26. Crandall I, Sherman I: Cytoadherence and the *Plasmodium falciparum*–infected erythrocyte. Methods Cell Biol 45:193–210, 1994.
27. Mann BJ, Torian BE, Vedvick TS, Petri WAJ: Sequence of a cysteine-rich galactose-specific lectin of *Entamoeba histolytica.* Proc Natl Acad Sci USA 88:3248–3252, 1991.
28. Saffer LD, Petri WAJ: Role of the galactose lectin of *Entamoeba histolytica* in adherence-dependent killing of mammalian cells. Infect Immun 59:4681–4683, 1991.
29. Adler P, Wood SJ, Lee YC, et al: High affinity binding of the *Entamoeba histolytica* lectin to polyvalent *N*-acetylgalactosaminides. J Biol Chem 270:5164–5170, 1995.
30. Chen JC, Stephens RS: Trachoma and LGV biovars of *Chlamydia trachomatis* share the same glysoaminoglycan-dependent mechanism for infection of eukaryotic cells. Mol Microbiol 11:501–507, 1994.
31. Schlesinger L: Macrophage phagocytosis of virulent but not attenuated strains of *Mycobacterium tuberculosis* is mediated by mannose receptors in addition to complement receptors. J Immunol 150:2920–2930, 1993.
32. Schlesinger L, Hull S, Kaufman T: Binding of the terminal mannosyl units of lipoarabinomannan from a virulent strain of *Mycobacterium tuberculosis* to human macrophages. J Immunol 152:4070–4079, 1994.
33. Blackwell JM, Ezekowitz RAB, Roberts MB, et al: Macrophage complement and lectin-like receptors bind *Leishmania* in the absence of serum. J Exp Med 162:324–331, 1985.
34. Ezekowitz RA, Williams DJ, Koziel H, et al: Uptake of *Pneumocystis carinii* mediated by the macrophage mannose receptor. Nature 351:155–158, 1991.
35. Marodi L, Schreiber S, Anderson DC, et al: Enhancement of macrophage candidacidal activity by interferon-gamma. Increased phagocytosis, killing, and calcium signal mediated by a decreased number of mannose receptors. J Clin Invest 91:2596–2601, 1993.
36. Dunne DW, Resnick D, Greenberg J, et al: The type I macrophage scavenger receptor binds to gram positive bacteria and recognizes lipoteichoic acid. Proc Natl Acad Sci USA 91:1863–1867, 1994.
37. Hampton RT, Golenbock DT, Penman M, et al: Recognition and clearance of endotoxin by scavenger receptor. Nature 352:342–344, 1991.
38. Pugin J, Heumann ID, Tomasz A, et al: CD14 is a pattern recognition receptor. Immunity 1:509–516, 1994.
39. Inouye M: Bacterial Outer Membranes. New York, John Wiley & Sons, 1979.
40. Joiner KA: Complement evasion by bacteria and parasites. Annu Rev Microbiol 42:201–230, 1988.
41. van Putten JP: Phase variation of lipopolysaccharide directs interconversion of invasive and immuno-resistant phenotypes of *Neisseria gonorrhoeae.* EMBO J 12:4043–4051, 1993.
42. Heffernan E, Reed S, Hackett J, et al: Mechanism of resistance to complement-mediated killing of bacteria encoded by the *Salmonella typhimurium* virulence plasmid gene *rck.* J Clin Invest 90:953–964, 1992.
43. Heffernan E, Harwood J, Fierer J, Guiney D: The *Salmonella typhimurium* virulence plasmid complement resistance gene *rck* is homologous to a family of virulence-related outer membrane protein genes, including *pageC* and *ail.* J Bacteriol 174:84–91, 1992.
44. Heffernan E, Wu L, Louie J, et al: Specificity of the complement resistance and cell association phenotypes encoded by the outer membrane protein genes *rck* from *Salmonella typhimurim* and *ail* from *Yersinia enterocolitica.* Infect Immun 62:5183–5186, 1994.
45. Bliska J, Falkow S: Bacterial resistance to complement killing mediated by the Ail protein of *Yersinia enterocolitica.* Proc Natl Acad Sci USA 89:3561–3565, 1992.
46. Blaser M: Role of the S-layer proteins of *Campylobacter fetus* in serum-resistance and antigenic variation: A model of bacterial pathogenesis. Am J Med Sci 306:325–329, 1993.
47. Rice P, Vayo H, Tam M, Blake M: Immunoglobulin G antibodies directed against protein III block killing of serum-resistant *Neisseria gonorrhoeae* by immune serum. J Exp Med 164:1735–1748, 1986.
48. Tomasz A: Surface components of *Streptococcus pneumoniae.* Rev Infect Dis 3:190–211, 1981.
49. Fischetti V, Jones K, Hollingshead S, Scott J: Structure, function, and genetics of streptococcal M protein. Rev Infect Dis 10(Suppl 2):S356–S359, 1988.
50. Horstmann RD, Sieverstsen HJ, Knobloch J, Fischetti VA: Antiphagocytic activity of streptococcal M protein: Selective binding of complement control protein factor H. Proc Natl Acad Sci USA 85:1657–1661, 1988.
51. Fischetti VA, Horstmann RD, Pancholi V: Location of the complement factor H binding site on streptococcal M6 protein. Infect Immun 63:149–153, 1995.
52. Weis JJ, Law SK, Levine RP, Cleary PP: Mechanism of resistance to phagocytosis by group A streptococci: Failure of deposited complement opsonins to interact with cellular receptors. J Immunol 134:500–505, 1985.
53. Alaei S, Larcher C, Ebenbichler C, et al: Isolation and biochemical characterization of the iC3b receptor of *Candida albicans.* Infect Immun 61:1395–1399, 1993.
54. Franzke S, Calderone RA, Schaller K: Isolation of avirulent clones of *Candida albicans* with reduced ability to recognize the CR2 ligand C3d. Infect Immun 61:2662–2669, 1993.
55. Joiner KA, da Silva WD, Rimoldi MT, et al: Biochemical characterization of a factor produced by trypomastigotes of *Trypanosoma cruzi* which accelerates the decay of complement C3 convertases. J Biol Chem 263:11327–11335, 1988.
56. Tambourgi DV, Kipnis TL, da Silva WD, et al: A partial cDNA clone of trypomastigote decay-accelerating factor (T-DAF), a developmentally regulated complement inhibitor of *Trypanosoma cruzi,* has genetic and functional similarities to the human complement inhibitor DAF. Infect Immun 61:3656–3663, 1993.
57. Marikovsky M, Levi-Schaffer F, Arnon R, Fischelson Z: *Schistosoma mansoni:* Killing of transformed schistosomula by the alternative pathway of human complement. Exp Parasitol 61:86–94, 1986.
58. Walter EI, Ratnoff WD, Long KE, et al: Effect of glycoinositolphospholipid anchor lipid groups on functional properties of decay accelerating factor protein in cells. J Biol Chem 267:1245–1252, 1992.
59. Horta MF, Ramalho-Pinto FJ, Horta MF: Role of human decay-accelerating factor in the evasion of *Schistosoma mansoni* from the complement-mediated killing in vitro. J Exp Med 174:1399–1406, 1991.
60. Braga LL, Ninomiya H, McCoy JJ, et al: Inhibition of the complement membrane attack complex by the galactose specific adhesin of *Entamoeba histolytica.* J Clin Invest 90:1131–1137, 1992.
61. Donelson J: Unsolved mysteries of trypanosome antigenic variation. *In* Englund PT, Sher A (eds): The Biology of Parasitism. New York, Alan R Liss, 1988, pp 349–370.
62. Kovacs JA, Powell F, Edman JC, et al: Multiple genes encode the major surface glycoprotein of *Pneumocystis carinii.* J Biol Chem 268:6034–6040, 1993.
63. Mowatt MR, Nguyen BY, Conrad JT, et al: Size heterogeneity among antigenically related *Giardia lamblia* variant specific surface proteins is due to differences in tandem repeat copy number. Infect Immun 62:1213–1218, 1994.
64. Siefert H, So M: Genetic mechanisms of bacterial antigenic variation. Microbiol Rev 52:327–336, 1988.
65. Barbour AG: Antigenic variation of surface proteins of *Borrelia* species. Rev Infect Dis 10(Suppl 2):S399–S402, 1988.
66. Jann K, Jann B: Polysaccharide antigens of *Escherichia coli.* Rev Infect Dis 9(Suppl 5):S517–S526, 1987.
67. Brown E: Interaction of gram-positive organisms with complement. Curr Top Microbiol Immunol 121:159–187, 1985.
68. Forsberg A, Rosqvist R, Wolf-Watz H: Regulation and polarized transfer of the *Yersinia* outer proteins (Yops) involved in antiphagocytosis. Trends Microbiol 2:14–19, 1994.
69. Straley SC, Skrzypek E, Plano GV, Bliska JB: Yops of *Yersinia* spp. pathogenic for humans. Infect Immun 61:3105–3110, 1993.
70. Rosqvist R, Magnusson K-E, Wolf-Watz H: Target cell contact

triggers expression and polarized transfer of *Yersinia* YopE cytotoxin into mammalian cells. EMBO J 13:964–972, 1994.
71. Schenkman S, Jiang MS, Hart GW, Nussenzweig V: A novel cell surface trans-sialidase of *Trypanosoma cruzi* generates a stage-specific epitope required for invasion of mammalian cells. Cell 65:1117–1125, 1991.
72. Mandrell RE, Apicella MA: Lipo-oligosaccharides (LOS) of mucosal pathogens: Molecular mimicry and host-modification of LOS. Immunobiology 187:382–402, 1993.
73. Mulks M: Microbial IgA proteases. *In* Holder IA (ed): Bacterial Enzymes and Virulence. Boca Raton, FL, CRC Press, 1985, pp 81–100.
74. Klauser T, Pohlner J, Meyer TF: The secretion pathway of IgA protease-type proteins in gram-negative bacteria. Bioessays 15:799–805, 1993.
75. Koomey JM, Gill RE, Falkow S: Genetic and biochemical analysis of gonococcal IgA1 protease: Cloning in *Escherichia coli* and construction of mutants of gonococci that fail to produce the activity. Proc Natl Acad Sci USA 79:7881–7885, 1982.
76. St. Geme JW 3rd, de la Morena M, Falkow S: A *Haemophilus influenzae*-IgA protease-like protein promotes intimate interaction with human epithelial cells. Mol Microbiol 14:217–233, 1994.
77. McKerrow JH, Sun E, Rosenthal PJ, Bourvier J: The proteases and pathogenicity of parasitic protozoa. Annu Rev Microbiol 47:821–853, 1993.
78. Gluzman I, Francis S, Oksman A, et al: Order and specificity of the *Plasmodium falciparum* hemoglobin degradation pathway. J Clin Invest 93:1602–1608, 1994.
79. McKerrow JH: Parasite proteases. Exp Parasitol 68:111–115, 1989.
80. Meirelles MN, Juliano L, Carmona E, et al: Inhibitors of the major cysteinyl proteinase (gp57/51) impair host cell invasion and arrest the intracellular development of *Trypanosoma cruzi* in vitro. Mol Biochem Parasitol 52:175–184, 1992.
81. Harth G, Andrews N, Mills AA, et al: Peptide-fluoromethyl ketones arrest intracellular replication and intercellular transmission of *Trypanosoma cruzi.* Mol Biochem Parasitol 58:17–24, 1993.
82. Wexler C, Chenoweth D, Cleary P: Mechanism of action of the group A strepococcal C5a inactivator. Proc Natl Acad Sci USA 82:8144–8148, 1980.
83. Bellinger-Kawahara C, Horwitz MA: Complement component C3 fixes selectively to the major outer membrane protein (MOMP) of *Legionella pneumophila* and mediates phagocytosis of liposome-MOMP complexes by human monocytes. J Exp Med 172:1201–1210, 1990.
84. Schlesinger LS, Horwitz MA: Phagocytosis of leprosy bacilli is mediated by complement receptors CR1 and CR3 on human monocytes and complement component C3 in serum. J Clin Invest 85:1304–1314, 1990.
85. Schlesinger L, Bellinger-Kawahara C, Payne N, Horwitz M: Phagocytosis of *Mycobacterium tuberculosis* is mediated by human monocyte complement receptors and complement component C3. J Immunol 144:2771–2780, 1990.
86. Wilson CB, Tsai V, Remington JS: *Toxoplasma gondii:* Failure to trigger the oxidative burst by normal macrophages. J Exp Med 151:328–346, 1980.
87. Engleberg NC, Carter C, Weber DR, et al: DNA sequence of *mip*, a *Legionella pneumophila* gene associated with macrophage infectivity. Infect Immun 57:1263–1270, 1989.
88. Cianciotto NP, Eisenstein BI, Mody CH, et al: A *Legionella pneumophila* gene encoding a species specific surface protein potentiates initiation of intracellular infection. Infect Immun 57:1255–1262, 1989.
89. McNeely TB, Rosen G, Londner MV, Turco SJ: Inhibitory effects on protein kinase C activity by lipophosphoglycan fragments and glycosylphosphatidylinositol antigens of the protozoan parasite *Leishmania.* Biochem J 259:601–604, 1989.
90. Brennan P: Structure of mycobacteria: Recent developments in defining cell wall carbohydrates and proteins. Rev Infect Dis 11:S420–S430, 1989.
91. Chan J, Fujiwara T, Brennan PJ, et al: Microbial glycolipids: Possible virulence factors that scavenge oxygen radicals. Proc Natl Acad Sci USA 86:2453–2457, 1989.
92. Joiner KA, Fuhrman SA, Mietinnen H, et al: *Toxoplasma gondii:* Fusion competence of parasitophorous vacuoles in Fc receptor transfected fibroblasts. Science 249:641–646, 1990.
93. Sturgill-Koszycki S, Schlesinger PH, Chakraborty P, et al: Lack of acidification in *Mycobacterium* phagosomes produced by exclusion of the vesicular proton ATPase. Science 263:678–681, 1994.
94. Clemens DL, Horwitz MA: Characterization of the *Mycobacterium tuberculosis* phagosome and evidence that phagosome maturation is inhibited. J Exp Med 181:257–270, 1995.
95. Eissenberg L, Goldman W, Schlesinger P: *Histoplasma capsulatum* modulates the acidification of phagolysosomes. J Exp Med 177:1605–1611, 1993.
96. Berger KH, Isberg RR: Two distinct defects in intracellular growth complemented by a single genetic locus in *Legionella pneumophila.* Mol Microbiol 7:7–19, 1993.
97. Berger KH, Merriam JJ, Isberg RR: Altered intracellular targeting properties associated with mutations in the *Legionella pneumophila dotA* gene. Mol Microbiol 14:809–822, 1994.
98. Brand BC, Sadosky AB, Shuman HA: The *Legionella pneumophila* icm locus: A set of genes required for intracellular multiplication in human macrophages. Mol Microbiol 14:797–808, 1994.
99. Sadosky AB, Wiater LA, Shuman HA: Identification of *Legionella pneumophila* genes required for growth within and killing of human macrophages. Infect Immun 61:5361–5373, 1993.
100. Swanson MS, Isberg RR: Association of *Legionella pneumophila* with the macrophage endoplasmic reticulum. Infect Immun 63:3609–3620, 1995.
101. Fields PI, Groisman EA, Heffron F: A *Salmonella* locus that controls resistance to microbicidal proteins from phagocytic cells. Science 243:1059–1062, 1989.
102. Baumler A, Kusters J, Stojiljkovic I, Heffron F: *Salmonella typhimurium* loci involved in survival within macrophages. Infect Immun 62:1623–1630, 1994.
103. Alpuche-Aranda CM, Swanson JA, Loomis WP, Miller SI: *Salmonella typhimurium* activates virulence gene transcription within acidified macrophage phagosomes. Proc Natl Acad Sci USA 89:10079–10083, 1992.
104. Alpuche-Aranda CM, Racoosin EL, Swanson JA, Miller SI: *Salmonella* stimulate macrophage macropinocytosis and persist within spacious phagosomes. J Exp Med 179:601–608, 1994.
105. Small P, Ramakrishnan L, Falkow S: Remodeling schemes of intracellular pathogens. Science 263:637–639, 1994.
106. Winkler TS, Winkler HH: Penetration of cultured mouse fibroblasts (L cells) by *Rickettsia prowazekii.* Infect Immun 22:200–208, 1978.
107. Sansonetti PJ, Ryter A, Clerc P, et al: Multiplication of *Shigella flexneri* within HeLa cells: Lysis of the phagocytic vacuole and plasmid-mediated contact hemolysis. Infect Immun 51:461–469, 1986.
108. Portnoy DA, Jacks PS, Hinrichs DJ: Role of hemolysin for the intracellular growth of *Listeria monocytogenes.* J Exp Med 167:1459–1471, 1988.
109. Andrews NW, Whitlow MB: Secretion by *Trypanosoma cruzi* of a hemolysin active at low pH. Mol Biochem Parasitol 33:249–256, 1989.
110. Tardieux I, Webster P, Ravesloot J, et al: Lysosome recruitment and fusion are early events required for trypanosome invasion of mammalian cells. Cell 71:1117–1130, 1992.
111. Rodriguez A, Rioult MG, Ora A, Andrews NW: A trypanosome-soluble factor induces IP_3 formation, intracellular Ca^{2+} mobilization and microfilament rearrangement in host cells. J Cell Biol 129:1263–1273, 1995.
112. Burleigh BA, Andrews NW: A 120-kDa alkaline peptidase from *Trypanosoma cruzi* is involved in the generation of a novel $Ca2^{+}$-signaling factor for mammalian cells. J Biol Chem 270:5172–5180, 1995.
113. Hackstadt T, Williams J: Biochemical stratagem for obligate parasitism of eukaryotic cells by *Coxiella burnetii.* Proc Natl Acad Sci USA 78:3240–3244, 1981.
114. Mukkeda AJ, Meade JC, Glaser TA, Bonventre PF: Enhanced metabolism of *Leishmania donovani* amastigotes at acid pH: An adaptation for intracellular growth. Science 229:1099–1101, 1985.
115. Veras P, de Chastellier C, Moreau M: Fusion between large phagocytic vesicles: Targeting of yeast and other particulates to phagolysosomes that shelter the bacterium *Coxiella burnetii* or the protozoan *Leishmania amazonensis* in Chinese hamster ovary cells. J Cell Sci 107:3065–3076, 1994.

116. Dale JB, Beachey EH: Epitopes of streptococcal M protein shared with cardiac myosin. J Exp Med 162:583–591, 1985.
117. Cunningham MW, Antone SM, Gulizia JM, et al: Cytotoxic and viral neutralizing antibodies crossreact with streptococcal M protein, enteroviruses, and human cardiac myosin. Proc Natl Acad Sci USA 89:1320–1324, 1992.
118. Ravdin JI: *Entamoeba histolytica:* From adherence to enteropathy. J Infect Dis 159:420–429, 1989.
119. Danner RL, Suffredini AF, Natanson C, Parrillo JE: Microbial toxins: Role in the pathogenesis of septic shock and multiple organ failure. *In* Bihari DJ, Cerra FB (eds): Multiple Organ Failure. Fullerton, CA, Society of Critical Care Medicine, 1989, pp 151–191.
120. Watson RW, Redmond HP, Bouchier-Hayes D: Role of endotoxin in mononuclear phagocyte–mediated inflammatory responses. J Leukoc Biol 56:95–103, 1994.
121. Ulevitch RJ, Tobias PS: Recognition of endotoxin by cells leading to transmembrane signalling. Curr Opin Immunol 6:125–130, 1994.
122. Guthrie LA, McPhail LC, Henson PM, Johnson RB Jr: Priming of neutrophils for enhanced release of oxygen metabolites by bacterial lipopolysaccharide. J Exp Med 160:1656–1671, 1984.
123. Munford RS, Hall CL: Detoxification of bacterial lipopolysaccharides (endotoxins) by a human neutrophil enzyme. Science 234:203–205, 1986.
124. Munford RS, Hunter JP: Acyloxyacyl hydrolase, a leukocyte enyzme that deacylates bacterial lipopolysaccharides, has phospholipase, lysophospholipase, diacylglycerollipase, and acyltransferase activities in vitro. J Biol Chem 267:10116–10121, 1992.
125. Chedid L, Audibert F, Johnson AG: Biological properties of muramyl dipeptide, a synthetic glycopeptide analogous to bacterial immunoregulating agents. Prog Allergy 25:63–105, 1978.
126. Kapur V, Topouzis S, Majesky M, et al: A conserved *Streptococcus pyogenes* extracellular cysteine protease cleaves human fibronectin and degrades vitronectin. Microb Pathog 15:327–346, 1993.
127. Zumla A: Superantigens, T cell and microbes. Clin Infect Dis 15:313–320, 1992.
128. Chen Y, Zychlinsky A: Apoptosis induced by bacterial pathogens. Microb Pathog 17:203–212, 1994.
129. Jonas D, Walev I, Berger T: Novel path to apoptosis: Small transmembrane pores created by staphylococcal alpha-toxin in T lymphocytes evoke internucleosomal DNA degradation. Infect Immun 62:1304–1312, 1994.
130. Sandvig K, Garred O, Prydz K, et al: Retrograde transport of endocytosed Shiga toxin to the endoplasmic reticulum. Nature 358:510–511, 1992.
131. Huttner WB: Snappy exocytoxins. Nature 365:104–105, 1993.
132. Mahan MJ, Slauch JM, Mekalanos JJ: Selection of bacterial virulence genes that are specifically induced in host tissues. Science 259:686–688, 1993.

4

Molecular Epidemiology in Infectious Diseases

Lucy S. Tompkins

The term molecular epidemiology was first used to describe DNA-based methods to type, or fingerprint, strains of infectious microbes. During the past 15 years, many molecular methods have been adapted for use as typing schemes to assist the course of epidemiologic investigations. More recently, molecular techniques have been applied to detect infectious disease agents in clinical or environmental samples, providing greater sensitivity than was possible with conventional culture methods in the laboratory. Moreover, similar approaches have been taken to detect and identify microbes that are nonculturable. Therefore, molecular epidemiology now includes four applications of molecular techniques in infectious diseases: (1) to demonstrate relatedness between strains for epidemiologic investigations, (2) to facilitate diagnosis, (3) to identify the agents of syndromes whose causes are unknown, and (4) to identify genes involved in pathogenesis of infection and/or disease.

Epidemics of infectious diseases in the community or hospital usually occur as the result of transmission of a single strain (clone) to susceptible hosts. Thus, one would expect all case patients to be infected with identical isolates, whereas a group of control patients who were not epidemiologically linked to the outbreak would either be uninfected or be infected with different strains. The discovery of a single epidemic strain often suggests that patients were exposed to a common source or reservoir. Once this has been identified, measures are taken to eliminate the source, thereby preventing further cases. In contrast, an unusual increase in nosocomial infections caused by a particular species, for example, *Pseudomonas aeruginosa,* could also be caused by transmission of unrelated strains having different reservoirs and unique modes of transmission. The ability to discriminate among isolates of the same microbial species, therefore, offers an important tool to evaluate sources and modes of transmission and to solve the epidemiologic puzzle.

As noted by Jarvis,[1] although molecular techniques are powerful adjuncts to epidemiologic investigations, traditional clinical epidemiology must also accompany these studies. In practice, the clinical evaluation is usually done first, to guide subsequent studies that culture and type strains from suspected cases and reservoirs. Nonepidemiologically directed culture studies may lead to expensive exercises that are not helpful.[1] For instance, wide-scale culture-based studies of hospital personnel before risk factor analysis may not disclose carriers. The solution to an outbreak of wound infections caused by a strain of *Serratia marcescens* after cardiothoracic surgery was expedited by the concomitant use of molecular genotyping on suspected case and control strains and by classic case-control analysis to determine which hospital personnel were most closely linked to the cases. This study disclosed that a single nurse wearing artificial fingernails, who used a hand cream contaminated with the outbreak strain, was the carrier and transmitter of infection during surgery. Rapidly produced molecular fingerprints enabled the clinical epidemiologists to distinguish true cases (and the associated personnel) from pseudocases, focusing more refined investigations on the nurse who was highly associated with all the cases and few of the controls and her household exposure to the contaminated cream (Passaro D, et al, manuscript submitted).

In the case of bacterial strains, for which genotyping has been most widely applied, a single method may suffice to confirm relatedness of case strains and those obtained from suspected carriers or reservoirs. This is especially true in outbreaks occurring at a single institution, where the investigation is usually conducted for a relatively short time. Larger outbreaks in the community or nationwide may require several typing systems. Sometimes isolates are nontypeable with a single technique, whereas other methods may lack discriminatory power. There is currently no "gold standard" method for the comparison of new techniques. Therefore, investigators developing or applying new approaches are obligated to evaluate new schemes rigorously by testing them with a large battery of well-defined control strains and comparing results. Assessment of discriminatory power must be done by examining epidemiologically unrelated isolates.[2]

In practice, rapid methods, such as plasmid profile analysis or restriction digestion analysis, are usually employed first to obtain a "snapshot" of the situation and to organize clinical investigations. For instance, the study of an apparent outbreak of *Pseudomonas* pneumonia in a hospital intensive care unit should first determine whether the isolates are related (clonal) or not. If they are, subsequent studies should focus on likely reservoirs and proven modes of transmission, such as use of contaminated water in ventilation therapy humidifiers. If strains are shown to be unrelated by molecular analysis, this suggests that more nonspecific environmental factors, such as antibiotic usage or lapses in infection control practices, are responsible for the increase. If the initial method lacks discriminatory power, then other less rapid, more refined methods, such as pulsed-field gel electrophoresis (PFGE), should be tried.

Molecular Fingerprinting

Traditional methods of strain typing for bacteria, such as the antibiotic susceptibility profile, biochemical analysis of enzyme patterns or metabolic by-products, and identification of cell surface antigens with a panel of specific antibodies, depend on phenotypic characteristics. Conventional diagnostic laboratories frequently utilize antibiotic resistance patterns and biotyping, and these are often helpful, especially if the antibiotic resistance pattern is unusual or when the bacterial species is uncommon. However, other phenotyping methods are too complex and require special reagents, which routine laboratories do not utilize. In these instances, the strains may be referred to a reference laboratory for testing. As an example, *Escherichia coli* serotyping used to confirm verotoxin-encoding strains of enterohemorrhagic strains utilizes a large bank of specific antisera and is rarely performed in diagnostic laboratories. Because phenotypic characteristics reflect genes unique to a species or strain, phenotyping can be thought of as a simple type of genotyping. In many instances, the results of phenotyping correlate well with those of molecular fingerprinting. However, numerous examples have been noted in which phenotypic methods have low discriminatory power. Therefore, techniques that more directly examine DNA molecules or nucleotide base sequences provide a more sophisticated and accurate means of typing microbial strains.

Plasmids were the first molecules to be used to discriminate among bacterial strains.[3–7] A great majority of conventional bacterial pathogens contain plasmids that are circular, double-stranded molecules present in the cytoplasm. Plasmids encode genes that govern their own replication and transmissibility and also often contain antibiotic resistance genes or virulence determinants. For epidemiologic purposes, it is not necessary to determine which genes are contained on each plasmid. Rather, the technique of plasmid profile analysis depends primarily on separation of plasmid molecules by agarose gel electrophoresis, which separates each plasmid species on the basis of relative molecular weight, producing a unique profile. Small plasmid molecules move more quickly through the gel than large ones, creating bands at the position of each molecular species, which can be identified by staining the gel with ethidium bromide and examining the pattern under ultraviolet light. An example of plasmid profile analysis is shown in Figure 4–1. In this particular example,[8] the epidemic strain of *Staphylococcus epidermidis* causing prosthetic valve endocarditis contained several plasmids, ranging from 1.7 to 42 μDa in size. Not all plasmids were stably maintained in each patient's isolate, which produced a series of different fingerprints and widely var-

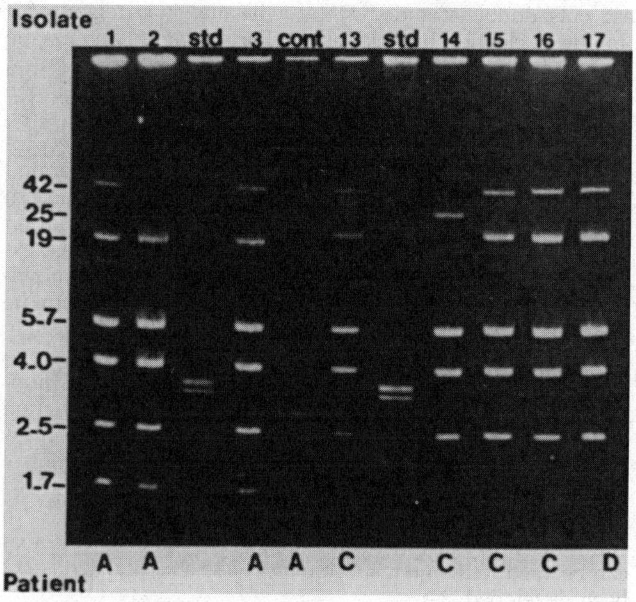

FIGURE 4–1 □ Agarose gel electrophoresis of plasmids extracted from several isolates of *Staphylococcus epidermidis,* which were collected from patients with hospital-acquired prosthetic valve endocarditis. Although some isolates lacked one or more plasmids, patients A, C, and D were found to be infected with a single strain of *S. epidermidis* in which plasmids were not stably maintained. One isolate (labeled "cont") was shown to be a skin contaminant. (From Mickelsen PA, Plorde JJ, Gordon KP, et al: Instability of antibiotic resistance in a strain of *Staphylococcus epidermidis* isolated from an outbreak of prosthetic valve endocarditis. J Infect Dis 152:50–58, 1985. University of Chicago, publisher.)

iable antibiotic susceptibility plasmids. Nonetheless, the "basic" fingerprint was identical among all clinical isolates, suggesting that a common strain and a common source were the cause of the outbreak. Subsequent clinical epidemiologic investigations confirmed this hypothesis, implicating the operating surgeon as the most likely carrier.

Plasmid profile analysis is rapid, requiring minimal equipment, and can be carried out in many routine diagnostic laboratories. It is an excellent initial method to employ for rapid assessment, and its utility has been confirmed by many studies. The method has proved to be more specific than serotyping for conducting investigations of salmonellosis.[9, 10] However, not all strains contain plasmids, and conversely, some pathogenic species such as *Salmonella* contain common plasmids encoding essential virulence determinants. Therefore, it would not be helpful to include the virulence plasmids in an analysis, because every pathogenic strain contains identical virulence plasmid molecules. Also, antibiotic usage may operate to induce selective pressure to maintain specific plasmid-containing resistance genes among a population of different strains. Moreover, well-documented examples have been cited in which the plasmid profile analysis failed to detect differences.[11]

Shortly after the initial application of plasmid profile analysis, second-generation molecular fingerprinting techniques were applied using the genomic DNA of microbial species based on the finding that each strain has unique chromosomal markers. The first of these methods is known as restriction endonuclease analysis (REA) or chromosomal digestion fingerprinting. Genomic fingerprinting encompasses an analysis of the entire DNA content of the microbe and can be applied to bacteria, viruses, fungi, and protozoa. The REA fingerprint is based on the unique distribution of specific endonuclease restriction sites along the chromosome; these sites constitute unique markers. Each restriction endonuclease cuts double-stranded DNA molecules in a region of a unique nucleotide base sequence. For example, the enzyme *Eco*RI recognizes GATTC, reading from the 5′ end to the 3′ end on each DNA strand. As shown in Figure 4–2, if the chromosome (which is circular) contained eight *Eco*RI sites, theoretically eight linear fragments of DNA would be produced by cleavage. These fragments can then be separated by agarose gel electrophoresis and visualized by ethidium bromide staining (see Fig. 4–2). All isolates of the same strain would produce identical REA patterns, as shown in the example (Fig. 4–3). Thus, one need not have any specific knowledge about the genes per se or their products to differentiate strains, and, therefore, the technique is applicable to virtually any infectious agent. One shortcoming of the method, however, is that extremely complex patterns composed of hundreds of bands are produced when conventional restriction endonucleases are used. These are difficult to compare unless each isolate is analyzed on the same gel or with control strains. Furthermore, the fingerprint patterns are often assessed visually, although sophisticated densitometry with computer analysis can be performed. A typing scheme that can be used to assign a specific type, like a serotype, has not been developed.

REA has proved to be extremely useful in conducting epidemiologic investigations[12–15] and has also been utilized to study the natural history of some persistent infections (with *Mycobacterium tuberculosis,* for example)[16] in which isolates with identical fingerprints can be isolated throughout the course of illness. This is because the chromosome of most microbes is stable and the random mutation rate is low. However, some bacterial species, including *Helicobacter,* undergo frequent nucleotide base changes, possibly through recombination with naturally transformed DNA, making it more difficult to define the term strain as applied to a collection of isolates. In this sense, *Helicobacter, Campylobacter,* and others seem to be "nonclonal," that is, natural infection occurs with a large number of different "strains," as compared with uropathogenic *E. coli,* for example, in which only a few of the more than 100 serotypes are capable of causing urinary tract infection.

There are now several new techniques, which are broadly classified as other types of restriction fragment length polymorphism (RFLP) analysis, to simplify genomic analysis. In Southern hybridization, the prototype RFLP technique, a limited number of restriction digestion fragments can be identified by their ability to hybridize with a single-stranded nucleic acid probe molecule encoding a complementary nucleotide base sequence. RFLP is the standard method used to examine allelic heterogeneity in human genetic studies, including the type used in forensic pathology. After washing away unhybridized, single-stranded probe DNA, the duplex molecules are then revealed by detecting the label used to tag the probe. The probe can be labeled with radioactivity such as phosphorus 32 (^{32}P), which is detected by autoradiography, or nonradiolabel markers can be employed (fluorescein, biotin, and so on). Because the probe will combine with only one or a few of the linear genomic fragments, the restriction profile is greatly simplified, and it is easy to compare differences among isolates.

Figure 4–4 demonstrates the differences between REA and RFLP fingerprints produced with a probe hybridizing to a single homologous sequence or a limited number of them, illustrating the ease of comparison of RFLP as compared with REA. Another example of the technique (Fig. 4–5) discloses similarities among isolates of *M. tuberculosis* cultured from different clinical specimens that were sequentially contaminated by material carried over from a true-positive clinical specimen in the diagnostic laboratory.[17] Because many bacterial species contain repetitive DNA sequences distributed

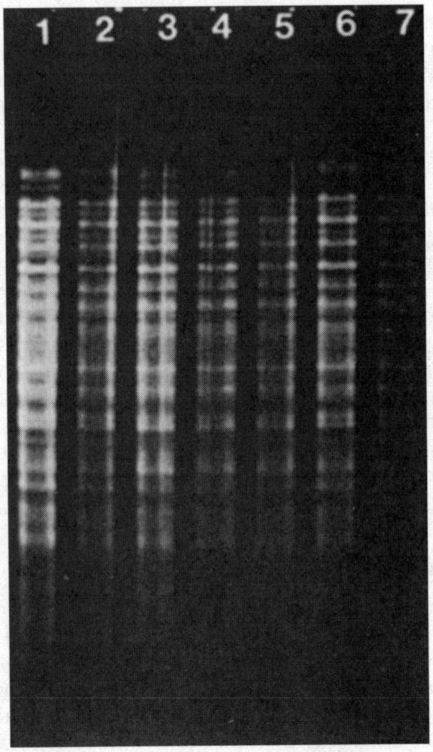

FIGURE 4–3 □ Agarose gel electrophoresis of restriction fragments produced by digestion with *Eco*RI from seven isolates of *Legionella pneumophila,* which were isolated from patients and from potable water in a hospital. An arrow indicates the location of an extra band that is seen in some isolates. All isolates share a common REA pattern and have identical electrophoretic typing types, which indicates that the isolates from patients and the isolates from water were derived from a common clonal ancestor. (From Tompkins LS, Troup NJ, Woods T, et al: Molecular epidemiology of *Legionella* species by restriction endonuclease and alloenzyme analysis. J Clin Microbiol 25:1875–1880, 1987.)

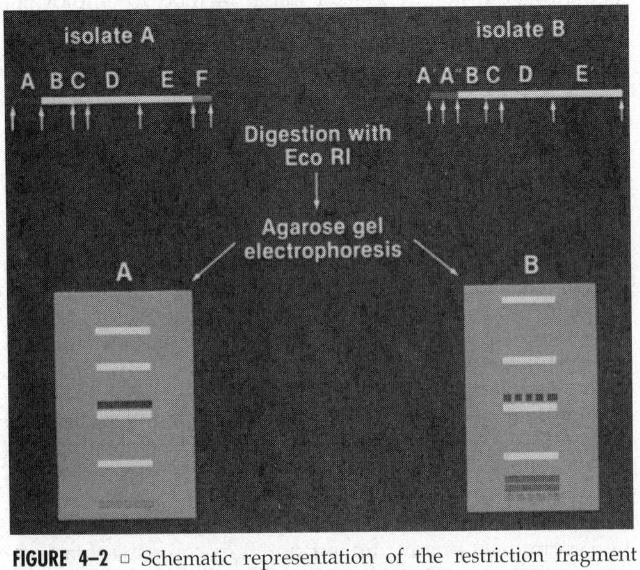

FIGURE 4–2 □ Schematic representation of the restriction fragment digestion patterns produced by cleavage with a single restriction endonuclease. The addition of a single restriction site (A′) and the deletion of another (between E and F) produces two unique REA patterns, which shows that isolates A and B are derived from different strains.

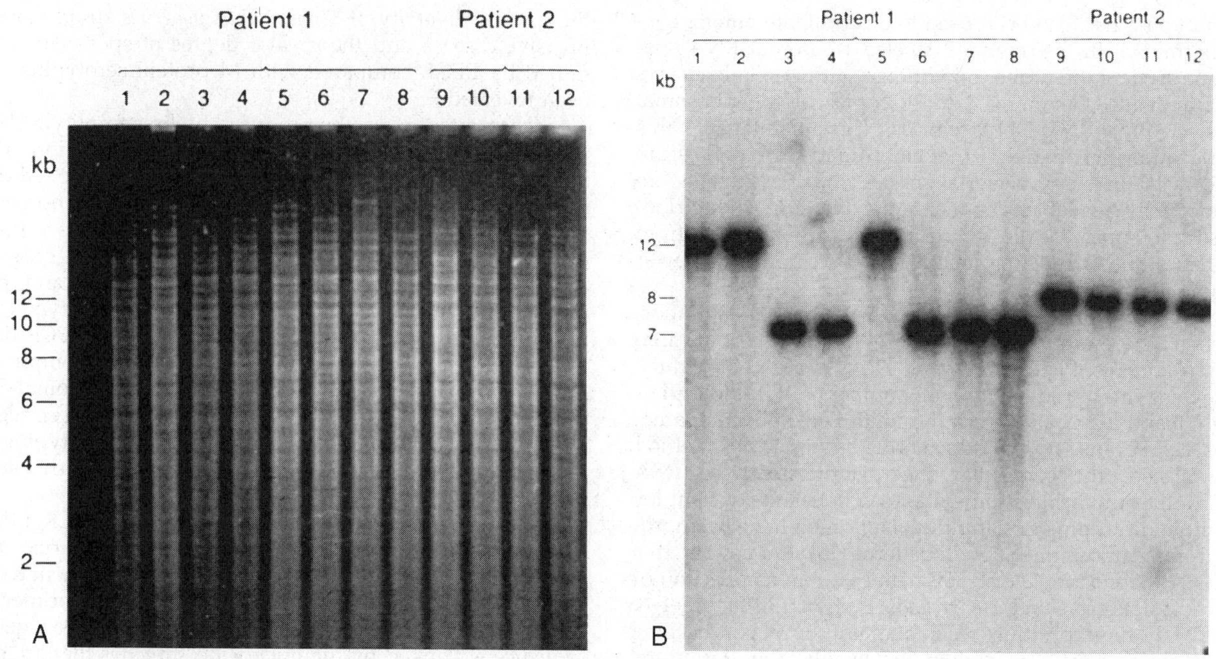

FIGURE 4–4 □ REA *(A)* and Southern hybridization fingerprinting *(B)* of whole-cell DNA extracted from isolates of *Pseudomonas aeruginosa* obtained from two patients with cystic fibrosis. *A,* The DNA was cleaved with the enzyme *Sma*I and subjected to agarose gel electrophoresis, generating a complex pattern with multiple bands. Isolates shown in lanes 1, 2, and 5 are identical. Isolates shown in lanes 3, 4, 6, 7, and 8 are virtually identical, thereby showing that these constitute a single strain that differs from the first strain, indicating that patient 1 was infected with two different strains during an 8-year period. Patient 2 was colonized with a different strain (lanes 9, 10, 11, and 12). *B,* The Southern hybridization fingerprint of genomic DNA cleaved with *Eco*RI and hybridized to a probe encoding a portion of the *Pseudomonas* exotoxin A gene plus upstream sequences. Clear-cut differences are readily noted. The different RFLP patterns are compatible with results of the REA analysis but are easier to distinguish. (*A* and *B* from Loutit JS, Tompkins LS: Restriction enzyme and Southern hybridization analyses of *Pseudomonas aeruginosa* strains from patients with cystic fibrosis. J Clin Microbiol 29:2897–2900, 1991.)

with the genome, it has been possible to type strains using the repetitive sequence as a probe in Southern hybridization. Although these are usually untranslated regions, their distribution in endonuclease restriction fragments serves as a strain marker.[18] Randomly distributed insertion sequences serve a similar function in mycobacterial genotyping.[19, 20] However, the limitation of the method for the epidemiology of infectious diseases lies in the fact that radiolabeled or fluorescent probes may be needed and the complexity of the method is greater. Thus, few diagnostic or reference laboratories rely on this, even though it has been successfully employed.

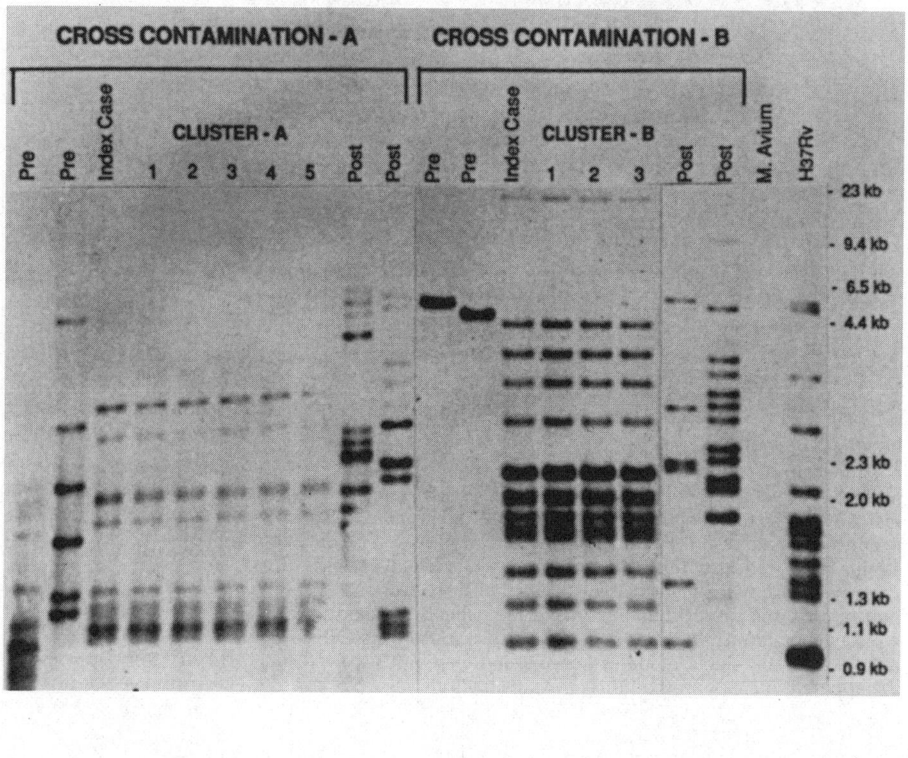

FIGURE 4–5 □ RFLP patterns of *M. tuberculosis* isolates obtained from sequential cultures processed in the diagnostic laboratory. Identical RFLP patterns indicate that cross-contamination occurred on two occasions (clusters A and B) in samples that were processed immediately after a true-positive specimen was sampled. Isolates following the index case have identical patterns. Molecular sizes are in kilobase pairs. (From Small PM, McClenny NB, Singh SP, et al: Molecular strain typing of *Mycobacterium tuberculosis* to confirm cross-contamination in the mycobacteriology laboratory and modification of procedures to minimize occurrence of false-positive cultures. J Clin Microbiol 31:1677–1682, 1993.)

Ribotyping has also been used to discriminate among bacterial strains.[21] In this method, labeled ribosomal RNA species are used as the probe to hybridize with genomic restriction fragments containing 2 to 10 copies of the ribosomal genes, creating RNA-DNA hybrids. The advantage of this fingerprinting technique is that ribosomal RNA probes are "universal" for every bacterial species and the reagents are commercially available. The major disadvantage is that ribotypes that appear to be identical may be produced from different strains, reflecting insufficient discriminatory power in some instances.

Compared with conventional REA and RFLP methods, which utilize endonucleases that cut the chromosome into many fragments, PFGE of genomic DNA treated with "rare" cutting enzymes produces a small number of high-molecular-weight bands that can easily be identified and compared. Moreover, because no hybridization is required, this method has replaced other molecular fingerprinting methods (REA and Southern hybridization) as a less expensive or complex and more discriminatory application. Criteria have been proposed for interpreting PFGE patterns to standardize this method.[21a] An example of PFGE patterns from a collection of clinical isolates of *Citrobacter freundii* is shown in Figure 4–6. The PFGE fingerprinting technique not only has become widely used in routine and public health laboratories for epidemiologic investigations but also has proved to be quite useful in tracing the evolution of pathogenicity. For example, the genetic diversity of *Streptococcus pyogenes* strains causing invasive disease and the greater degree of specificity determined by PFGE compared with M protein serotyping have been revealed.[22]

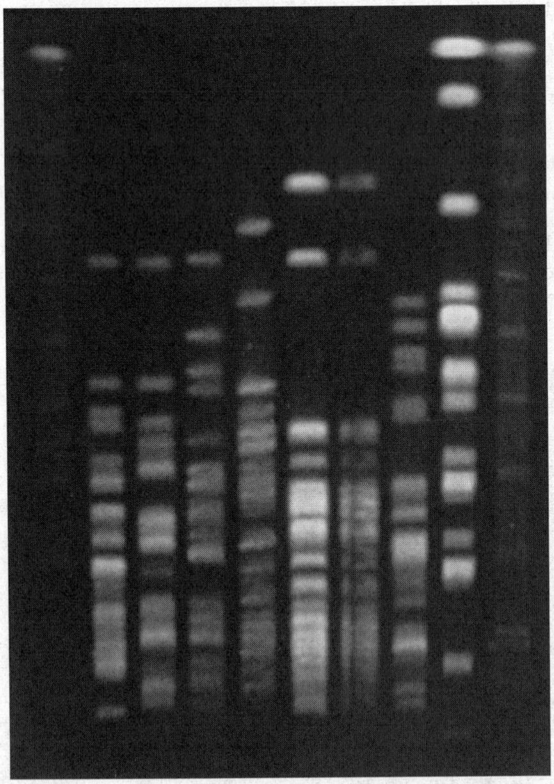

FIGURE 4–6 □ PFGE of a collection of *Citrobacter freundii* clinical isolates obtained during the course of an outbreak investigation. The genomic DNA was cleaved with a "rare" cutting enzyme and the fragments were separated by PFGE. The PFGE of DNA from each isolate produced a unique fingerprint (none are similar), even though the strains were collected during an apparent outbreak in a hospital. Further clinical assessment demonstrated that there were no epidemiologic risk factors in common among the patients. Therefore, the molecular fingerprint evidence supports the conclusion that a common source and single mode of transmission were not involved in the apparent increase in the *Citrobacter* infection rate.

Fingerprints can also be produced by first amplifying chromosomal sequences with polymerase chain reaction (PCR) amplification techniques with unique primers to create a large concentration of material to react with restriction endonucleases, essentially producing REA patterns. This variation on the technique may be especially useful when only tiny amounts of nucleic acid are present in the sample and, theoretically, the microorganism can be detected and typed in a noncultivable form. As an example of another PCR-based fingerprinting method, oligonucleotide primers complementary to conserved regions of the 16S and 23S ribosomal RNA genes can be used to amplify the intergenic spacer region, creating a variant on ribotyping called PCR ribotyping. As discussed later, a unique simplified band pattern can be produced from each bacterial species and strain.[23, 24]

Another variation, known as arbitrary primer PCR, utilizes a single short primer composed of a random series of 10 nucleotide bases, which can anneal to complementary sequences distributed along the chromosome.[25] The primer amplifies an unpredictable number of bands wherever a genetic sequence is flanked by the nucleotide stretches that are complementary to the arbitrary primer (Fig. 4–7). The number and size of fragments generated form the basis for the fingerprint pattern. The advantage of arbitrary primer PCR is that specific primer pairs are not needed and, theoretically, any random nucleotide primer sequence will work. However, in practice, not all arbitrary primers produce sufficient discrimination among strains, and the patterns may not always be reproducible.

The ultimate fingerprinting method with the highest degree of discriminatory power is, of course, DNA sequence analysis. This method requires a uniform population of DNA molecules, which are often cloned into a plasmid or phage vector; however, direct sequencing is now possible. A primer with a sequence complementary to the template DNA or to the junction of plasmid where it joins the cloned insert is hybridized to the template to start the polymerization of nucleotides into a complementary strand with DNA polymerase. All four nucleotides and a single dideoxynucleotide (ddGTP, ddATP, ddCTP, or ddTTP) are added to four tubes containing the template-primer hybrid. During the reaction, the polymerase incorporates nucleotides into the elongating chain. The dideoxynucleotide cannot be used in chain elongation. Thus, the chain is terminated wherever the dideoxynucleotide has been substituted. In manual DNA sequence analysis, electrophoresis of the four reactions on a gel followed by autoradiography reveals radiolabeled fragments aligned by size. Each band in each lane of the gel corresponds to the nucleotide in the DNA sequence at that position. Automated DNA sequencing machines utilize four different fluorescent tags to mark the primer. After chain elongation, each incorporated nucleotide fluoresces at a specific wavelength, corresponding to the dideoxynucleotide that stopped elongation. The sequence is then analyzed by computer and displayed, showing each nucleotide in a different color. This process has been clearly outlined by Rosenthal.[26]

Because manual DNA sequence analysis is tedious and slow, it has rarely been used for mere strain identification, but occasionally this is the only method to compare strains that will suffice. One example of the relevance of DNA sequence analysis to the solution to a serious epidemiologic problem has proved the occasional necessity for this technique, namely the analysis of human immunodeficiency virus isolates obtained from several patients of a known human immunodeficiency virus–positive dentist.[27] In this case, the

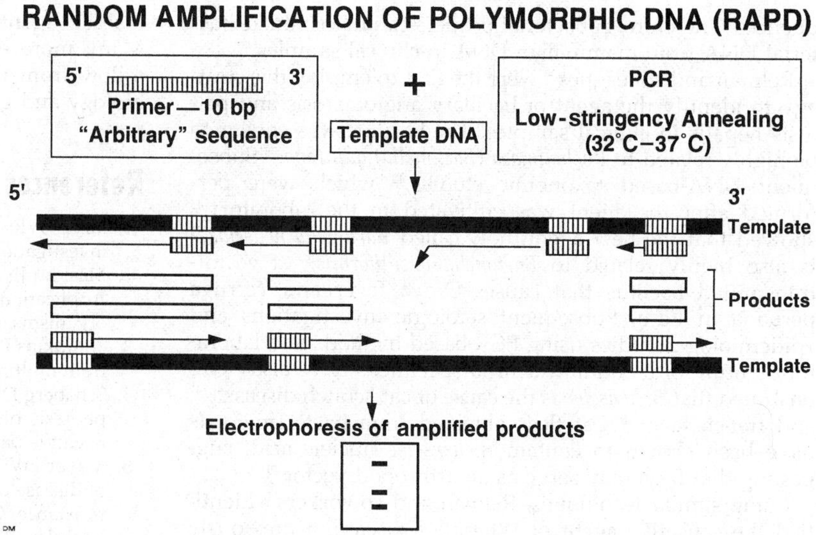

FIGURE 4–7 ▫ Schematic representation of PCR fingerprinting using an arbitrary primer. Under relatively low stringency, the short oligonucleotide composed of 10 to 11 random nucleotides can anneal to each strand of the genomic DNA (target). When two primers anneal to opposite strands at the appropriate interval, a double-stranded fragment (products) consisting of the intervening sequence is produced by polymerization. Primers that are not close enough together on opposite strands cannot amplify an intervening sequence, as indicated. This generates a unique fingerprint depending on the location of the complementary sites distributed through the genomic DNA. (Courtesy of Patricia Mickelsen, PhD, Division of Infectious Diseases, Stanford University Medical Center, Stanford, CA.)

discovery that the dentist's and patients' viral isolates were closely related by DNA sequence analysis strongly suggested that his viral strain had been transmitted in some fashion during dental procedures. In other instances, transmission of hepatitis B virus from patients and their contacts was documented by DNA sequence analysis of DNA amplified by PCR from the patients' sera.[28, 29] The speed and resolution provided by automated DNA sequencers now make DNA sequencing more widely applicable as a fingerprinting tool.

Identification of Infectious Microbes in Clinical or Environmental Samples

The infectious disease literature is replete with the description of syndromes thought to be infectious in nature but in which the agent had not been identified. These include cat-scratch disease, Whipple's disease, bacillary angiomatosis, sarcoidosis, Kawasaki disease, and many others. The application of PCR to clinical and environmental samples to detect infectious disease agents that have not yielded positive laboratory cultures has underscored the limitations of in vitro growth methods by detecting uncultivated microorganisms. For example, in environmental microbiology, the use of PCR to amplify all bacterial species from hostile environments, water, or soil has revealed the presence of numerous uncultured species.[30, 31] By extension to human infectious diseases, it is now clear that laboratory culture methods are most useful in detecting common pathogens, but these are clearly insensitive. Thus, the "plating efficiency" of a particular microorganism in a clinical specimen may be low, leading to a failure to detect small numbers of viable microorganisms. Similarly, the cultural or environmental incubation conditions may not allow growth of fastidious microbes.

The advent of molecular methods to amplify nucleic acid molecules enzymatically—in particular, through PCR amplification and other methods that can also detect and discriminate among foreign DNA sequences of infectious disease agents within samples containing eukaryotic cell nucleic acid sequences—has led to the detection of several new infectious disease agents and to the discovery of the pathogenesis of both old and new infectious disease syndromes. PCR has also been widely applied in more routine diagnostic microbiology. The basis of this revolutionary amplification method has opened a new chapter in infectious disease epidemiology. The method and its application have been reviewed extensively.[32, 33] Among the essential elements of conventional PCR to amplify a target sequence are specific oligonucleotide primers, complementary to regions on either side of the intervening target sequence. These are added to the sample containing the target sequence, which has been rendered into single strands to prime the polymerization reaction. This, in turn, incorporates nucleotides into complementary copies of each strand, creating a double-stranded copy of the original. The newly formed sequences are heated to produce single-stranded targets for a second round of amplification. After 30 or more rounds of amplification, the target sequence can be amplified 1 million–fold to produce sufficient DNA to clone and sequence the target or to detect it by conventional hybridization techniques.

In 1993, PCR amplification was exploited to quickly identify the cause of a mysterious pulmonary syndrome first seen in New Mexico.[34, 35] Once seroepidemiologic studies had suggested that this new, highly fatal syndrome was associated with a rise in antibodies to the Hantavirus family, specific primers were constructed to amplify the putative virus from clinical samples and later from suspected animals and their excreta. These studies and large-scale clinicoepidemiologic studies[36] demonstrated conclusively that a new species of *Hantavirus,* which is related to Hantaan virus, the agent of hemorrhagic fever with renal syndrome, caused the new pulmonary syndrome.[37] In addition to the application of molecular techniques to detect and identify the virus, other molecular fingerprinting methods have been utilized to type clinical strains from outbreaks and from suspected rodent reservoirs in many other locales in the United States.

Conventional PCR is based on the knowledge of the sequences flanking the target, which serve as a template for the oligonucleotide primers. How is it possible, then, to use PCR to detect unknown microorganisms that cannot be cultured in the laboratory? The first strategy used to determine the nature of an unculturable agent[38] utilized "universal" primers consisting of oligonucleotides complementary to highly conserved regions of the 16S ribosomal DNA genes from all eubacteria (now known as domain bacteria).[39] These 16S ribosomal genes from eubacteria contain regions that are identical within all genera and species interspersed with short stretches of unique oligonucleotide sequences.[40] Mammalian and other eukaryotic 16S ribosomal RNA has a similar secondary structure and also contains highly conserved sequences.[41] However, the eukaryotic ribosomal DNA sequences are different from the eubacterial conserved sequences. Therefore, eubacterial primers can discriminate bacterial DNA from mammalian DNA in clinical samples.

Relman and colleagues[38] were the first to employ this strategy to identify the agent of bacillary angiomatosis and peliosis hepatis in clinical samples. The bacillus was shown to be highly related to *Rochalimaea (Bartonella) quintana.*[38] Subsequent DNA-based taxonomic studies,[42] which were performed after the agent was cultivated in the laboratory,[43] showed that the new agent, now called *Bartonella henselae,*[44] is also highly related to *Bartonella bacilliformis,*[45] a vector-transmitted bacillus that causes Oroya fever and verruga peruana in Peru. Subsequent serologic investigations and epidemiologic studies using PCR-based methods and laboratory culture of blood and clinical specimens have also demonstrated that *B. henselae* is the cause of cat-scratch disease[46, 47] and trench fever.[48] Cat fleas obtained from bacteremic cats have been shown to contain *B. henselae* nucleic acid, suggesting that fleas may serve as an arthropod vector.[49]

Using similar techniques, Relman and coworkers[50] identified the causative agent of Whipple's disease, a previously unknown gram-positive bacterial species in the actinomycete group, named *Trophyrema whippellii,* whose environmental niche is soil and water samples in many geographic areas. Similarly, other investigators have detected new species of *Ehrlichia (E. chaffeensis)* as the agent of human ehrlichiosis.[51] Since 1992, a whole host of other bacteria, including many new *Helicobacter* species,[52] have been identified in clinical or environmental samples with this approach.

A somewhat different molecular method was used to discover the putative cause of Kaposi's sarcoma, a common tumor in patients with human immunodeficiency virus infection long thought to be initiated by an infectious disease agent. Chang and colleagues[53] first reported identification of herpesvirus-like DNA sequences in acquired immunodeficiency syndrome–associated Kaposi's sarcoma biopsy samples using the method of representational difference analysis to identify and characterize DNA sequences unique to Kaposi's sarcoma lesions, which were not found in adjacent normal skin from the same patient. The method[54] is performed by making simplified "representations" of genomic DNA extracted from diseased tissue and normal tissues obtained from the same individual, utilizing PCR amplification of short restriction fragments. Essentially, the genomic DNA from normal tissue was used to "subtract out" homologous DNA from the tumor tissue, providing a higher concentration of unique sequences presumably encoding the Kaposi's sarcoma agent. Ultimately only unique sequences found in the diseased tissue are preferentially amplified during PCR. Subsequent studies[55] have demonstrated that African Kaposi's sarcoma samples, including those that are not infected with human immunodeficiency virus, also contain the new herpesvirus-like virus, which has not been cultivated. Although a causal association between the new virus species and Kaposi's sarcoma has not been claimed, the molecular and epidemiologic evidence to indicate that this is the agent of this unique angiogenic tumor is mounting.

Summary

It is clear that the molecular methods developed during the recombinant DNA revolution and in the past few years have proved to be exquisitely sensitive techniques that permit the examination of many previously unknown facets of the epidemiology of infectious microorganisms. These methods are exceptionally useful for typing strains to pinpoint the modes of transmission and reservoirs of infection, to trace the natural evolution of pathogenic determinants in strains of infectious agents, and to discover new and old infectious disease agents and the clinical syndromes they produce. Many more exciting and important discoveries will surely follow from the development and application of molecular biology and genetics.

References

1. Jarvis WR: Usefulness of molecular epidemiology for outbreak investigations. Infect Control Hosp Epidemiol 15:500, 1994.
2. Maslow JN, Mulligan ME, Arbeit RD: Molecular epidemiology: Application of contemporary techniques to the typing of microorganisms. Clin Infect Dis 17:153, 1993.
3. Tompkins LS, Plorde JJ, Falkow S: Molecular analysis of R-factors from multiresistant nosocomial isolates. J Infect Dis 141:625, 1980.
4. Schaberg DR, Tompkins LS, Falkow S: Use of agarose gel electrophoresis of plasmid deoxyribonucleic acid to fingerprint gram-negative bacilli. J Clin Microbiol 13:1105, 1981.
5. Mayer LW: Use of plasmid profiles in epidemiologic surveillance of disease outbreaks and in tracing the transmission of antibiotic resistance. Clin Microbiol Rev 1:228, 1988.
6. Locksley RM, Cohen ML, Quinn TC, et al: Multiple antibiotic-resistant *Staphylococcus aureus:* Introduction, transmission, and evolution of nosocomial infection. Ann Intern Med 97:317, 1982.
7. Parisi JT, Hecht DW: Plasmid profiles in epidemiologic studies of infections by *Staphylococcus epidermidis.* J Infect Dis 141:637, 1980.
8. Mickelsen PA, Plorde JJ, Gordon KP, et al: Instability of antibiotic resistance in a strain of *Staphylococcus epidermidis* isolated from an outbreak of prosthetic valve endocarditis. J Infect Dis 152:50, 1985.
9. Holmberg SD, Wachsmuth IK, Hickman BG, Cohen ML: Comparison of plasmid profile analysis, phage typing, and antimicrobial susceptibility testing in characterizing *Salmonella typhimurium* isolates from outbreaks. J Clin Microbiol 19:100, 1984.
10. Wachsmuth K: Molecular epidemiology of bacterial infections: Examples of methodology and investigations of outbreaks. Rev Infect Dis 8:682, 1986.
11. Wachsmuth IK, Kiehlbach JA, Bopp CA, et al: The use of plasmid profiles and nucleic acid probes in epidemiologic investigations of food-borne, diarrheal diseases. Int J Food Microbiol 12:77, 1991.
12. Kaper JB, Bradford HB, Roberts NC, Falkow S: Molecular epidemiology of *Vibrio cholerae* in the U.S. Gulf Coast. J Clin Microbiol 16:129, 1982.
13. Tompkins LS, Troup NJ, Woods T, et al: Molecular epidemiology of *Legionella* species by restriction endonuclease and alloenzyme analysis. J Clin Microbiol 25:1875, 1987.
14. Loutit JS, Tompkins LS: Restriction enzyme and Southern hybridization analyses of *Pseudomonas aeruginosa* strains from patients with cystic fibrosis. J Clin Microbiol 29:2897, 1991.
15. Stout JE, Yu VL, Joly J, et al: Potable water as a cause of sporadic cases of community-acquired Legionnaires' disease. N Engl J Med 326:151, 1992.
16. Hermans PWM, Messadi F, Guebraxabher H, et al: Analysis of the population structure of *Mycobacterium tuberculosis* in Ethiopia, Tunisia, and the Netherlands: Usefulness of DNA typing for global tuberculosis epidemiology. J Infect Dis 171:1504, 1995.
17. Small PM, McClenny NB, Singh SP, et al: Molecular strain typing of *Mycobacterium tuberculosis* to confirm cross-contamination in the mycobacteriology laboratory and modification of procedures to minimize occurrence of false positive cultures. J Clin Microbiol 31:1677, 1993.
18. Versalovic J, Koeuth T, Lupski JR: Distribution of repetitive DNA sequences in eubacteria and application to fingerprinting of bacterial genomes. Nucleic Acids Res 19:6823, 1991.
19. Small PM, Hopewell PC, Singh SP, et al: The epidemiology of tuberculosis in San Francisco: A population-based study using conventional and molecular methods. N Engl J Med 330:1703, 1994.
20. Casper C, Singh SP, Rave S, et al: Transcontinental transmission of tuberculosis: A molecular epidemiological assessment. Am J Public Health 86:551, 1996.
21. Stull TL, LiPuma JJ, Edlind TD: A broad-spectrum probe for molecular epidemiology of bacteria: Ribosomal RNA. J Infect Dis 157:280, 1988.

21a. Tenover FC, Arbeit RD, Goering RV, et al: Interpreting chromo-

somal DNA restriction patterns produced by pulsed-field gel electrophoresis: Criteria for bacterial strain typing. J Clin Microbiol 33:2233, 1995.
22. Musser JM, Kapur V, Szeto J, et al: Genetic diversity and relationships among *Streptococcus pyogenes* strains expressing serotype M1 protein: Recent intercontinental spread of a subclone causing episodes of invasive disease. Infect Immun 63:994, 1995.
23. Kostman JR, Alden MB, Mair M, et al: A universal approach to bacterial molecular epidemiology by polymerase chain reaction ribotyping. J Infect Dis 171:204, 1995.
24. Kostman JR, Edlind TD, LiPuma JJ, Stull TL: Molecular epidemiology of *Pseudomonas cepacia* determined by polymerase chain reaction ribotyping. J Clin Microbiol 30:2084, 1992.
25. Welsh J, McClelland M: Fingerprinting genomes using PCR with arbitrary primers. Nucleic Acids Res 24:7213, 1990.
26. Rosenthal N: Molecular medicine: Fine structure of a gene–DNA sequencing. N Engl J Med 332:589, 1995.
27. Update: Transmission of HIV infection during an invasive dental procedure—Florida. MMWR Morb Mortal Wkly Rep 40:21, 1991.
28. Omata M, Ehata T, Yokosuka O, et al: Mutations in the precore region of hepatitis B virus DNA in patients with fulminant and severe hepatitis. N Engl J Med 324:1699, 1991.
29. Liang TJ, Hasegawa K, Rimon N, et al: A hepatitis B virus mutant associated with an epidemic of fulminant hepatitis. N Engl J Med 324:1705, 1991.
30. Liesack W, Stackebrandt K: Occurrence of novel groups of the domain bacteria as revealed by analysis of genetic material isolated from an Australian terrestrial environment. J Bacteriol 174:5072, 1992.
31. Ward DM, Weller R, Bateson MM: 16S rRNA sequences reveal numerous uncultured microorganisms in a natural community. Nature 345:63, 1990.
32. Saiki RK, Gelfand DH, Stoffel S, et al: Primer-directed enzymatic amplification of DNA with a thermostable DNA polymerase. Science 239:487, 1988.
33. Eisenstein BI: The polymerase chain reaction: A new method of using molecular genetics for medical diagnosis. N Engl J Med 322:178, 1990.
34. Outbreak of acute illness—Southwestern United States, 1993. MMWR Morb Mortal Wkly Rep 42:421, 1993.
35. Nichol ST, Spiropoulou CF, Morzunov S, et al: Genetic identification of a Hantavirus associated with an outbreak of acute respiratory illness. Science 262:914, 1993.
36. Duchin JS, Koster FT, Peters CJ, et al: Hantavirus pulmonary syndrome: A clinical description of 17 patients with a newly recognized disease. The Hantavirus Study Group. N Engl J Med 330:949, 1994.
37. Lee HW, Lee PW, Johnson KM: Isolation of the etiologic agent of Korean hemorrhagic fever. J Infect Dis 137:298, 1978.
38. Relman DA, Loutit JS, Schmidt TM, et al: The agent of bacillary angiomatosis. An approach to the identification of uncultured pathogens. N Engl J Med 323:1573, 1990.
39. Olsen GJ, Woese CR, Overbeek R: The winds of (evolutionary) change: Breathing new life into microbiology. J Bacteriol 176:1, 1994.
40. Woese CR: Bacterial evolution. Microbiol Rev 51:221, 1987.
41. Olsen GJ, Woese CR: Ribosomal RNA: A key to phylogeny. FASEB J 7:113, 1993.
42. Relman DA, Falkow S, LeBoit PE, et al: The organism causing bacillary angiomatosis, peliosis hepatis, and fever and bacteremia in immunocompromised patients (Letter). N Engl J Med 324:1514, 1991.
43. Slater LN, Welch DF, Hensel D, Coody DW: A newly recognized fastidious gram-negative pathogen as a cause of fever and bacteremia. N Engl J Med 323:1587, 1990.
44. Regnery RI, Anderson BE, Clarridge JE III, et al: Characterization of a novel *Rochalimaea* species, *R. henselae* sp. nov., isolated from blood of a febrile, human immunodeficiency virus–positive patient. J Clin Microbiol 30:265, 1992.
45. Relman DA, Lepp PW, Sadler KN, Schmidt TM: Phylogenetic relationships among the agent of bacillary angiomatosis, *Bartonella bacilliformis*, and other alpha-proteobacteria. Mol Microbiol 6:1801, 1992.
46. Dolan MJ, Wong MT, Regnery RL, et al: Syndrome of *Rochalimaea henselae* adenitis suggesting cat scratch disease. Ann Intern Med 118:331, 1993.
47. Regnery RI, Olson JG, Perkins BA, Bibb W: Serological response to *Rochalimaea henselae* antigen in suspected cat-scratch disease. Lancet 339:1443, 1992.
48. Lucey D, Dolan MJ, Moss CW, et al: Relapsing illness due to *Rochalimaea henselae* in immunocompetent hosts: Implication for therapy and new epidemiological associations. Clin Infect Dis 14:683, 1992.
49. Koehler JE, Glaser CA, Tappero JW: *Rochalimaea henselae* infection: A new zoonosis with the domestic cat as reservoir. JAMA 271:531, 1994.
50. Relman DA, Schmidt TM, MacDermott RP, Falkow S: Identification of the uncultured bacillus of Whipple's disease. N Engl J Med 327:293, 1992.
51. Anderson BE, Sumner JW, Dawson JE, et al: Detection of the etiologic agent of human ehrlichiosis by polymerase chain reaction. J Clin Microbiol 30:775, 1992.
52. Solnick J, O'Rourke J, Lee A, et al: An uncultured gastric spiral organism is a newly identified species of *Helicobacter* in humans. J Infect Dis 168:379, 1993.
53. Chang Y, Cesarman E, Pessin MS, et al: Identification of *Herpesvirus*-like DNA sequences in AIDS-associated Kaposi's sarcoma. Science 266:1865, 1994.
54. Lisitsyn N, Lisitsyn N, Wigler M: Cloning the differences between two complex genomes. Science 259:946, 1993.
55. Moore PS, Chang Y: Detection of *Herpesvirus*-like DNA sequences in Kaposi's sarcoma in patients with and those without HIV infection. N Engl J Med 332:1181, 1995.

HOST FACTORS

5

The Complement System

Jerry A. Winkelstein

Resistance to infection depends on the cooperative efforts of a number of different components of the immune system. One of these, the complement system, plays an important role in the defense against a wide variety of bacterial, viral, and fungal infections in both the nonimmune and immune host. This chapter summarizes current knowledge about the biochemistry and biology of the complement system, its significance in the host's defense against infection, and those clinical situations in which deficiencies of the complement system lead to an increased susceptibility to infection.

Biochemistry of Complement

The complement system is composed of a series of plasma proteins and cell membrane receptors that are important mediators of host defense and inflammation.[1] Most of the biologically significant effects of the complement system are mediated by the third component (C3) and the terminal components (C5-C9). To subserve their protective and inflammatory functions, however, C3 and C5-C9 must first be activated. At least two mechanisms exist by which they can be activated, the classical and alternative pathways (Fig. 5–1).

Activation of the classical pathway is usually initiated by antigen-antibody complexes.[2] Antibodies of the appropriate immunoglobulin class (IgG and IgM) and subclass (IgG1, IgG2, and IgG3) bind to antigen and in doing so create an immune complex that in turn binds and activates the first component of complement (C1). The first component of complement is a macromolecular complex composed of three biochemically distinct subcomponents, C1q, C1r, and C1s. The binding of C1q to the Fc portion of immunoglobulin leads to the activation of C1r, which in turn activates C1s. Activated C1s possesses serine esterase activity and is able to cleave the fourth component of complement (C4) into a high-molecular-weight fragment (C4b) and a low-molecular-weight fragment (C4a). The reaction continues with the activation of C2 by C1s. The cleavage of C2 results in the liberation of a small peptide (C2b). The larger fragment, C2a, then combines with C4b to form a bimolecular enzyme, $\overline{C4b,2a}$, which is responsible for activating C3 and assembling C5-C9 into the membrane attack complex.

Activation of the alternative pathway begins with the C3 molecule.[3] Native C3 contains an internal thiol ester. Under normal conditions, there is continuous low-grade hydrolysis of this thiol ester to create a molecule [termed $C3(H_2O)$] that can bind native factor B and allow its cleavage by factor D. Two cleavage products of factor B are generated, a larger product (Bb) and a smaller product (Ba). The association of the hydrolyzed C3 with Bb then creates a C3-cleaving enzyme [$C3(H_2O)$,Bb] termed the priming C3 convertase, which is responsible for the continuous, low-grade cleavage of C3 and, hence, the generation of nascent C3b. If the nascent C3b binds to a suitable surface, it forms a reversible complex with native factor B, which is then cleaved by factor D to create a highly efficient C3-cleaving enzyme ($\overline{C3b,Bb}$), termed the amplification C3 convertase. Properdin stabilizes the binding of Bb to C3b, thereby retarding its intrinsic decay.

Whether C3 is activated by the classical or alternative pathway, the C3 is cleaved, generating two fragments of unequal size, C3a and C3b. The smaller fragment, C3a, is released into the fluid phase, where it acts as an anaphylatoxin (see later). The larger fragment, C3b, binds to the surface of cells such as bacteria, where it is able to act as an opsonin (see later) or combine with either of the two C3-cleaving enzymes to create two new enzymes, the alternative pathway ($\overline{C3b_2,Bb}$) and classical pathway ($\overline{C4b,2a,3b}$) C5-cleaving enzymes.

Activation of C5 by either the alternative or the classical pathway C5-cleaving enzymes creates a smaller fragment, C5a, and a larger fragment, C5b. The smaller cleavage product, C5a, is released into the fluid phase, where it, like C3a, can act as an anaphylatoxin (see later). In addition, C5a possesses potent chemotactic activity (see later). If the C5b combines with native C6 while it is still attached to the C5-cleaving enzymes, it is stabilized and can initiate formation of the membrane attack complex, a multimolecular assembly of C5b, C6, C7, C8, and C9 that is capable of inserting into cell membranes and thereby expressing cytolytic activity.[4]

If the activation of the classical or alternative pathway were to proceed in an uncontrolled fashion, this would result in the generation of excessive amounts of the phlogistic fragments of complement, which in turn could cause widespread immunopathologic damage to the host. Fortunately, a number of mechanisms act to control the assembly and expression of both the classical and alternative pathway C3-cleaving enzymes. Each of these C3-cleaving enzymes is relatively labile and rapidly undergoes intrinsic decay under physiologic conditions. In addition, a number of control proteins inhibit the classical pathway (C1 esterase inhibitor, C4 binding protein, factor I, and decay-accelerating factor) and the alternative pathway (factor H, factor I). Thus, in the usual situation, the activation of C3 and C5-C9 proceeds in a controlled fashion and is limited to the immediate vicinity of the initiating substance (e.g., microbial surface or immune complex).

Activation of the classical pathway is usually initiated by antigen-antibody complexes and is therefore considered to be especially important in acquired immunity. However, some enveloped RNA viruses, some *Mycoplasma* species, and certain strains and species of both gram-negative and gram-positive bacteria can bind C1q directly and activate the classical pathway without a requirement for antibody. Activation of the alternative pathway does not usually require the participation of antibody; thus, it is generally viewed as an important mechanism of natural immunity. However, antibody can participate functionally in the activation of the alternative pathway by a variety of particles such as bacteria and virus-infected cells. Thus, under some circumstances, the classical pathway may function in "natural" immunity, and the alternative pathway may participate in "acquired" immunity.[5]

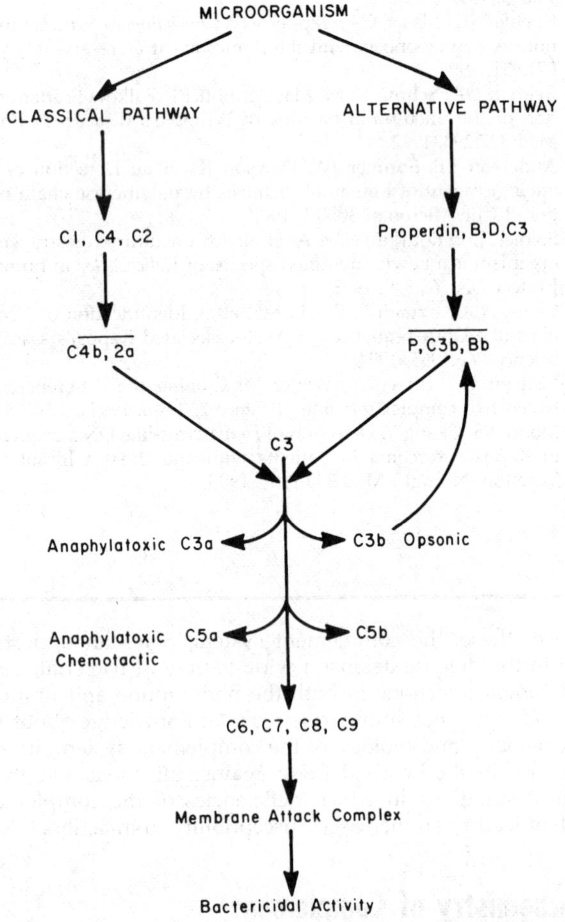

FIGURE 5–1 □ The complement system in humans. Microorganisms can activate C3 and the terminal components (C5-C9) by either the classical pathway or the alternative pathway. Activation of C3 and the terminal components generates a variety of biologically significant activities important in the host's defense against infection. (From Oski FA, De Angeles C, Feigen R, et al: Principles and Practice of Pediatrics. Philadelphia, JB Lippincott, 1990, p 837.)

Biologic Consequences of Complement Activation

Whether C3 and C5-C9 are activated by the classical or alternative pathway, they generate a wide variety of biologically significant activities that are important in the host's defense against infection.

The smaller cleavage products of C3 and C5, C3a and C5a, are potent anaphylatoxins.[6] They were originally identified through their ability to cause histamine release from basophils and mast cells, promote smooth muscle contraction, and increase vascular permeability. Additional functions of these peptides have been identified and include the ability to aggregate platelets and leukocytes, causing the production and release of arachidonic acid metabolites from them, and the ability to induce neutrophils to produce toxic oxygen metabolites and discharge their granular enzymes.[7]

In addition to its anaphylatoxic activities, C5a is a potent chemotactic factor.[8] Not only does it cause the directed movement of polymorphonuclear leukocytes and monocytes toward a focus of microbial invasion, but it also promotes the adherence of phagocytic cells to vascular endothelium, a necessary prerequisite to their exit from the intracellular compartment.

The larger cleavage product of C3, C3b, acts as a potent opsonin when it is fixed to the surface of a microorganism.[9] It appears that C3b subserves different opsonic functions, depending on the nature of the phagocytic cell and its state of activation.[10] In the case of neutrophils and nonactivated macrophages, C3b promotes attachment of the particle, whereas immunoglobulin G acts to favor ingestion. In the case of activated macrophages, C3b serves to aid in both attachment and ingestion.

The generation of efficient complement-mediated serum bactericidal activity requires the participation of the entire terminal complement sequence, C5b-C9.[11] Only gram-negative bacteria can be killed by complement. Although protoplasts of gram-positive organisms are susceptible to lysis by complement, intact gram-positive organisms are not, which suggests that their thick cell wall somehow interferes with the bactericidal action of C5-C9. The site of action of C5-C9 appears to be the outer lipid membrane of gram-negative organisms.

Role of Complement in Host Defense

A number of studies have established the biologic significance of the complement system in the host's defense against infection and have also provided valuable insight into the mechanisms by which the complement system exerts its protective effects. Studies in experimental animals have shown that the complement system plays an important role in resistance to a variety of bacteria, viruses, and fungi. For example, animals that have been pharmacologically depleted of C3 or are genetically deficient in C4, C3, or C5 are markedly more susceptible than normal animals to challenge with the pneumococcus,[12] *Staphylococcus,*[13] *Haemophilus influenzae,*[14] rabies virus,[15] Sindbis virus,[16] influenza A virus,[17] and *Candida,*[18] to mention just a few.

Other studies have addressed the mechanisms by which the complement system exerts its protective effect. For example, one such study has shown that C3b is responsible for a major portion of serum opsonic activity in vivo,[12] and another has shown that C5a plays a critical role in the initial migration of polymorphonuclear leukocytes to a focus of invading microorganisms.[19]

Finally, the complement system also appears to play an important defensive role in a number of different locations in the body. Not only is complement important in the clearance of microorganisms from the blood stream,[20] but it can also be shown to play an important role in local resistance to pneumonia,[21] meningitis,[14] and soft tissue infections.[13]

Primary Complement Deficiency Diseases

Although most of the genetically determined complement deficiencies are inherited as autosomal recessive disorders, one of them, properdin deficiency, is inherited as an X-linked recessive disorder (Table 5–1); another, C1 esterase inhibitor deficiency, is inherited as an autosomal dominant disorder. Most patients with genetically determined deficiencies of individual complement components present with an increased susceptibility to infection, rheumatic diseases, or angioedema.[22, 23] The kinds of infections seen in complement-deficient patients relate to the biologic functions of the missing component. Thus, patients with a deficiency of C3, or with a deficiency of a component in either of the two pathways necessary for the activation of C3, usually have an increased susceptibility to infections caused by bacteria for which C3b-dependent opsonization is an important host defense (e.g., *Streptococcus pneumoniae* and *H. influenzae*). In contrast, patients with deficiencies of C5-C9 have normal resistance to the pneumococcus and *H. influenzae* because C3b-mediated opsonization is intact, but they are unusually susceptible to infection with *Neisseria meningitidis* because they lack C5-C9–mediated serum bactericidal activity, an important host defense against this organism.

Complement deficiency diseases may be more common among patients with certain infectious diseases than was previously appreciated. For example, a number of studies have shown that approximately 5% to 15% of patients with systemic meningococcal infections have a genetically determined deficiency of a terminal component.[24–26] The prevalence of complement deficiencies appears to be particularly high in patients with infections caused by "uncommon" serogroups (such as X, Y, and W135),[27] in patients with meningococcemia caused by unencapsulated organisms,[28] in patients with a positive family history of systemic meningococcal

TABLE 5–1 ■ Genetically Determined Complement Deficiencies

DEFICIENCY	INHERITANCE	MAJOR CLINICAL MANIFESTATIONS
C1q	Autosomal recessive	Rheumatic disorders and systemic bacterial infections
C1r/C1s	Autosomal recessive	Rheumatic disorders
C4	Autosomal recessive	Rheumatic disorders and systemic bacterial infections
C2	Autosomal recessive	Rheumatic disorders and systemic bacterial infections
C3	Autosomal recessive	Systemic bacterial infections
C5	Autosomal recessive	Meningococcal sepsis and meningitis
C6	Autosomal recessive	Meningococcal sepsis and meningitis
C7	Autosomal recessive	Meningococcal sepsis and meningitis
C8	Autosomal recessive	Meningococcal sepsis and meningitis
C9	Autosomal recessive	Meningococcal sepsis and meningitis
Factor H	Autosomal recessive	Hemolytic-uremic syndrome
Factor I	Autosomal recessive	Systemic bacterial infections
Properdin	X-linked recessive	Meningococcal sepsis and meningitis

infections,[29] and in patients with recurrences.[26, 29] Although patients with complement deficiencies have an increased susceptibility to infection and are more likely to have recurrent infections, if their infections are recognized early, they can usually be treated successfully.

C1q Deficiency

There appear to be two distinct forms of C1q deficiency: one in which C1q cannot be detected by either functional or immunochemical analysis, and another in which immunochemical C1q is present but lacks functional activity.[22, 23, 30] The most common clinical presentation of either form of C1q deficiency has been a lupus-like syndrome. Some patients have also had an increased susceptibility to infection as manifested by bacterial sepsis or meningitis.

C1r/C1s Deficiency

Genetically determined deficiencies of C1r are characterized by a marked reduction of C1r (less than 1% of normal) and a moderate reduction of C1s (20% to 50% of normal).[22, 23, 30] The clinical presentation of C1r/C1s deficiency has included both a lupus-like illness and glomerulonephritis; to this date, an increased susceptibility to infection has not been prominent.

C4 Deficiency

Two loci within the major histocompatibility complex encode for C4, termed C4A and C4B. Patients with total C4 deficiency are homozygous for a double-null C4 haplotype and have severely depressed serum levels of both antigenic and functional C4 (less than 1%).[22, 23, 31] Patients with total C4 deficiency may present with an increased susceptibility to infection; however, the predominant clinical manifestation of C4 deficiency has been a systemic lupus erythematosus–like illness. Homozygous deficiencies of either C4A or C4B are relatively common among the general population, occurring in 1% and 3% of individuals, respectively.[31] Although the products of the two loci share some functional, structural, and antigenic characteristics that identify them as C4, they nevertheless differ slightly. For example, C4B possesses approximately four times the functional activity that C4A does. Studies have shown that homozygous C4B-deficient children have an increased susceptibility to bacteremia or meningitis, presumably because they have to rely on the less functional C4A isotype for the activation of C3 and C5-C9.[32]

C2 Deficiency

A deficiency of C2 is the most common of the inherited complement deficiencies.[33] The frequency of the gene for C2 deficiency has been estimated between 0.5% and 1%,[34] with homozygous deficient individuals occurring as frequently as 1 per 10,000.[33] The clinical manifestations of C2 deficiency have varied. Although some individuals are asymptomatic, most are clinically affected with an increased susceptibility to infection or rheumatic diseases, or both.[22, 23] For the most part, the infections have been blood-borne and systemic (e.g., sepsis, meningitis, arthritis, and osteomyelitis) and caused by encapsulated bacteria (e.g., pneumococcus, *H. influenzae*). A variety of rheumatic diseases have been seen in association with C2 deficiency. The most common of these has been a disorder that resembles systemic lupus erythematosus, but glomerulonephritis, dermatomyositis, anaphylactoid purpura, and vasculitis have also been seen.

C3 Deficiency

Patients with C3 deficiency generally have less than 1% of the normal amount of C3 in their serum.[22, 23, 35] Those serum activities directly dependent on C3, or indirectly dependent on C3 because of its role in the activation of C5-C9, are markedly reduced. Thus, serum opsonic, chemotactic, and bactericidal activities are either absent or markedly diminished in patients with C3 deficiency. The clinical manifestations of C3 deficiency have included an increased susceptibility to infection and rheumatic disorders.[22, 23, 35] Patients with C3 deficiency have had a variety of infections caused by encapsulated bacteria, including pneumonia, bacteremia, meningitis, and osteomyelitis. A number of patients have also presented with a clinical picture consistent with systemic lupus erythematosus or membranoproliferative glomerulonephritis.

C5 Deficiency

The sera of patients with C5 deficiency have markedly reduced levels of C5 and are therefore unable to generate normal chemotactic or bactericidal activity.[22, 23, 36] Like patients with deficiencies of the other terminal components, patients with C5 deficiency have usually presented with systemic meningococcal infections.

C6 Deficiency

The only abnormality relating to the complement system in C6-deficient patients is a marked deficiency of serum bactericidal activity.[22, 23, 37] The major clinical manifestation of C6 deficiency has been systemic neisserial infections. Whereas most patients have had meningococcal sepsis and meningitis, a few have had disseminated gonococcal infections.

C7 Deficiency

Only a few patients with C7 deficiency have been identified, and as expected, serum bactericidal activity has been markedly reduced in those patients in whom it has been tested.[22, 23, 38] A number of clinical presentations have been associated with C7 deficiency. As with the other deficiencies of terminal components, systemic meningococcal infections or disseminated gonococcal infections have predominated. Individual patients have also presented with a lupus-like syndrome, rheumatoid arthritis, and scleroderma.

C8 Deficiency

Native C8 is composed of three chains (α, β, and γ). The α-chain and γ-chain are covalently linked to form one subunit (C8 α-γ), which is joined by noncovalent bonds to the other subunit composed of the β-chain (C8 β). In one form of C8 deficiency, patients lack the C8 α-γ–subunit; in the other, the C8 β-subunit is deficient.[22, 23, 39] In either case, C8 activity is markedly reduced (less than 1% of normal). The only functional defect in C8-deficient sera is a marked reduction in bactericidal activity. The clinical presentation of C8 deficiency has consisted of systemic meningococcal infections, but systemic lupus erythematosus has also rarely been seen.

C9 Deficiency

Although genetically determined C9 deficiency is rare in the West, it is the most common complement deficiency in Japan.[22, 23, 40] Serum bactericidal activity can be generated by C5b-C8 without a requirement for C9, although the rate of killing is significantly reduced. Nevertheless, evidence suggests that patients with C9 deficiency, like patients with deficiencies of the other terminal components, have an increased susceptibility to meningococcal sepsis and meningitis.[41]

Factor I Deficiency

Patients with factor I deficiency have uncontrolled activation of C3 by the alternative pathway because, in the absence of factor I, there is no control imposed on the formation and expression of the alternative pathway C3 convertase.[42–44] Therefore, they have a secondary consumption of C3 resulting in markedly reduced levels of native C3 in the serum. As expected, those serum activities that depend on C3, either directly or indirectly, such as opsonic, chemotactic, and bactericidal activity, are reduced in patients with factor I deficiency. The most common clinical expression of factor I deficiency is an increased susceptibility to infection.[22, 23] As with primary C3 deficiency, the organisms most commonly responsible for these infections have been encapsulated bacteria, organisms for which C3 is an important opsonic ligand.

Factor H Deficiency

Factor H deficiency has only rarely been described.[22, 45] As with factor I deficiency, there is uncontrolled activation of the alternative pathway and, as a consequence, markedly reduced levels of C3. The clinical manifestations have included membranoproliferative glomerulonephritis and the hemolytic-uremic syndrome.

Properdin Deficiency

Properdin deficiency is inherited in an X-linked recessive pattern[22, 23] and exists in three different forms. In one form, properdin is undetectable in the serum of affected males.[46, 47] In a second form, serum properdin is reduced but detectable.[48] In a third form, properdin is present in normal amounts but lacks function.[49] To this date, the only clinical manifestation of properdin deficiency has been systemic meningococcal infections.

Secondary Complement Deficiencies

A number of clinical conditions exist in which the complement system is secondarily affected. In some of these, the secondary defect in complement function may be responsible, at least in part, for an increased susceptibility to infection.

The Newborn Infant

Newborn infants are unusually susceptible to a variety of infections. A number of defects in host defense have been identified in these infants, each of which has the potential to contribute to their increased susceptibility to infection.[50] Among these, defects in two complement-mediated functions, serum opsonizing and chemotactic activities, have been described.[51] The levels of most components of complement are mildly to moderately decreased in full-term infants, averaging between 50% and 80% of adult levels.[51] The levels in premature infants are more markedly reduced; in general, the more premature the infant, the more the given component is decreased relative to adult levels. Although the levels of individual components are only moderately reduced in newborns, it is likely that they contribute to the newborn's susceptibility to infection because nearly all components are reduced, and therefore the functional integrity of the complete cascade is impaired.[52]

Nephrotic Syndrome

Patients with the idiopathic nephrotic syndrome are remarkably susceptible to peritonitis and sepsis caused by the pneumococcus or *Escherichia coli*.[53] The infections occur most commonly when the patient is in relapse, losing large amounts of protein in the urine and accumulating significant amounts of extracellular fluid. Studies of such patients have shown that they have decreased serum opsonizing activity.[54] The defect appears to be related to a reduction in factor B levels because other complement components are normal and purified factor B corrects the defect.[54] Presumably, factor B is lost in the urine along with albumin.

Sickle Cell Disease

Patients with sickle cell disease have an increased susceptibility to bacterial sepsis and meningitis, particularly due to the pneumococcus.[55] In one study, the risk of acquiring pneumococcal meningitis for children with sickle cell disease was 300 to 500 times that for children without sickle cell disease.[56] Children with sickle cell disease have two immunologic defects that could contribute to their susceptibility to the pneumococcus: functional or anatomic asplenia[57] and decreased serum opsonizing activity.[58, 59] A number of studies have shown that the decrease in serum opsonizing activity in sickle cell disease is secondary to a functionally significant defect in the alternative pathway,[59–61] but the basis for that defect is unclear. It is likely that the decrease in complement-mediated serum opsonizing activity contributes to the increased susceptibility to infection seen in sickle cell disease because these patients have a higher risk for sepsis and meningitis than could be accounted for by splenectomy alone.

C3 Nephritic Factor

Some individuals develop significant and sustained hypocomplementemia that is due to an autoantibody aimed at the alternative pathway C3-cleaving enzyme $\overline{\text{C3b,Bb}}$.[62, 63] The autoantibody, termed C3 nephritic factor (C3NeF), apparently binds to the convertase and prolongs its half-life. This in turn leads to the persistent activation and consumption of C3 and results in markedly reduced levels of native C3. Nephritic factor was first identified in patients with glomerulonephritis[64] and partial lipodystrophy.[65] Subsequently, at least two patients with C3NeF have been identified who have had sepsis and meningitis presumably secondary to their marked decrease in serum C3 levels.[66, 67]

Burn Patients

Patients with burns typically have many problems with bacterial infections. In one series, more than 50% of deaths in burn-injured patients were related to sepsis.[68] A number of studies have shown that components of the complement system are reduced in burn patients in the days immediately after injury[69, 70]; apparently, the alternative pathway is affected to a greater degree than the classical pathway.[70] The decrease in function of the alternative pathway leads to decreased levels of serum opsonic and chemotactic activities,[71, 72] which in turn could contribute to the marked susceptibility to infection seen in these patients.

Laboratory Assessment of the Complement System

Genetically determined deficiencies of the classical activating pathway (C1, C4, and C2), of C3, and of the terminal components (C5, C6, C7, C8, and C9) can be detected by use of antibody-sensitized sheep erythrocytes in a total serum hemolytic complement (CH_{50}) assay. The lysis of sensitized erythrocytes can occur in the absence of C9, although it occurs at a lower rate and to a lesser extent than in the presence of C9. Therefore, a severe deficiency of any of the first eight components leads to a marked reduction in total hemolytic complement activity; a deficiency of C9 results in a CH_{50} that is one third to half the lower limit of normal.

Deficiencies of factor H, factor I, and properdin can be detected by a hemolytic assay that assesses lysis of rabbit erythrocytes, because rabbit erythrocytes are potent activators of the alternative pathway. Obviously, the serum of patients with deficiencies of C3 or C5-C9 will also be abnormal when it is tested in the rabbit erythrocyte assay, because the lysis of rabbit erythrocytes depends on these components as well as on components of the alternative activating pathway.

The identification of the specific component that is deficient usually rests on both functional and immunochemical tests. Functional assays are available for each of the individual components. They depend on reagents that lack the specific component in question but possess the other components of the hemolytic pathway in excess. Monospecific antibodies are also available for many of the individual components, allowing their detection by immunochemical techniques. In most cases, functional and immunochemical assessment of the specific component shows the deficiency. There are some exceptions, however. For example, one form of C1 inhibitor deficiency and one form of C1q deficiency are characterized by dysfunctional proteins that can be detected by immunochemical assays but are markedly reduced in functional activity.

References

1. Frank MM: The complement system in host defense and inflammation. Rev Infect Dis 1:483, 1979.
2. Porter RR, Reid KBM: The biochemistry of complement. Nature 275:699, 1978.
3. Fearon DT: Activation of the alternative complement pathway. Crit Rev Immunol 1:1, 1979.
4. Mayer MM, Michaels DW, Ramm LE, et al: Membrane damage by complement. Crit Rev Immunol 22:133, 1981.
5. Winkelstein JA: Complement and natural immunity. Clin Immunol Allergy 3:421, 1983.
6. Hugli TE: The structural basis for anaphylatoxin and chemotactic functions of C3a, C4a, and C5a. Crit Rev Immunol 22:321, 1981.
7. Vogt W: Anaphylatoxins: Possible roles in diseases. Complement 3:177, 1986.
8. Synderman R, Goetzl EJ: Molecular and cellular mechanisms of leukocyte chemotaxis. Science 213:830, 1981.
9. Hostetter MK, Gordon DL: Biochemistry of C3 and related thiolester proteins in infection and inflammation. Rev Infect Dis 9:97, 1987.
10. Griffin FM: Opsonizations, phagocytosis, and intracellular killing in the complement system. *In* Rother K, Till GO (eds): The Complement System. Berlin, Springer-Verlag, 1988, pp 395–418.
11. Joiner KA: Studies on the mechanism of bacterial resistance to complement-mediated killing and on the mechanisms of action of bactericidal antibody. Curr Top Microbiol Immunol 121:99, 1985.
12. Winkelstein JA, Smith MR, Shin HS: The role of C3 as an opsonin in the early stages of infection. Proc Soc Exp Biol Med 149:397, 1975.
13. Easmon CSF, Glynn AA: Comparison of subcutaneous and intraperitoneal staphylococcal infections in normal and complement-deficient mice. Infect Immunol 13:399, 1976.
14. Crosson FJ Jr, Winkelstein JA, Moxon ER: Participation of complement in the nonimmune host defense against experimental *Haemophilus influenzae* type b septicemia and meningitis. Infect Immun 14:882, 1976.
15. Miller A, Morse HC, Winkelstein JA, Nathanson N: The role of antibody in recovery from experimental rabies. J Immunol 121:321, 1978.
16. Hirsch RL, Griffin DE, Winkelstein JA: The effect of complement depletion on the course of Sindbis virus infection in mice. J Immunol 121:1276, 1978.
17. Hicks JT, Ennis FA, Kim E, Verbonitz M: The importance of an intact complement pathway in recovery from a primary viral infection: Influenza in decomplemented and C5-deficient mice. J Immunol 121:1437, 1978.
18. Gelfand JA, Hurley DL, Fauci AS, Frank MM: Role of complement in host defense against experimental candidiasis. J Infect Dis 138:9, 1978.
19. Snyderman R, Phillips JK, Merganhagen SE: Biological activity of complement in vivo. Role of C5 in the accumulation of polymorphonuclear leukocytes in inflammatory exudates. J Exp Med 134:1131, 1971.
20. Hosea SW, Brown EJ, Frank MM: The critical role of complement in experimental pneumococcal sepsis. J Infect Dis 142:903, 1980.
21. Bakker-Wondenberg IAJM, DeJong-Hoenderop JYT, Michel MF: Efficacy of antimicrobial therapy in experimental pneumococcal pneumonia: Effects of impaired phagocytosis. Infect Immun 25:366, 1979.
22. Ross SC, Densen P: Complement deficiency states and infections: Epidemiology, pathogenesis and consequences of neisserial and other infections in an immune deficiency. Medicine (Baltimore) 63:243, 1984.
23. Figueroa JE, Densen P: Infectious diseases associated with complement deficiencies. Clin Microbiol Rev 4:359, 1991.
24. Ellison RT, Kohler PH, Curd JG, et al: Prevalence of congenital or acquired complement deficiency in patients with sporadic meningococcal disease. N Engl J Med 308:913, 1983.
25. Leggiardro RJ, Winkelstein JA: Prevalence of complement deficiencies in children with systemic meningococcal infections. Pediatr Infect Dis 6:75, 1987.
26. Merino J, Rodriguez-Valverde V, Lamelas JA, et al: Prevalence of deficits of complement components in patients with recurrent meningococcal disease. J Infect Dis 148:331, 1983.
27. Fijen CAP, Kuijper EJ, Hannema AJ, et al: Complement deficiencies in patients over ten years old with meningococcal disease due to uncommon serogroups. Lancet 2:585, 1989.
28. Hummel DS, Mocca LF, Frasch CE, et al: Meningitis caused by an unencapsulated strain of *Neisseria meningitidis* in twin infants with C6 deficiency. J Infect Dis 155:815, 1987.
29. Nielsen HE, Koch C, Magnussen P, Lind I: Complement deficiencies in selected groups of patients with meningococcal disease. Scand J Infect Dis 21:389, 1989.
30. Loos M, Heinz HP: Hereditary and acquired complement deficiencies in animals and man: The first component. Prog Allergy 39:212, 1986.
31. Hauptmann G, Tappeiner G, Schifferli JA: Inherited deficiency of the fourth component of complement. Immunodeficiency Rev 1:3, 1988.
32. Rowe PC, McLean RH, Wood RA, et al: Association of homozygous C4B deficiency with bacterial meningitis. J Infect Dis 160:448, 1989.
33. Ruddy S: Hereditary and acquired complement deficiencies in animals and man: The second component. Prog Allergy 39:267, 1986.
34. Sullivan KE, Petri M, Schmeckpeper B, et al: The prevalence of a mutation that causes C2 deficiency in SLE. J Rheumatol 21:6, 1994.
35. Singer L, Colten HR, Wetsel RA: Complement C3 deficiency: Human, animal, and experimental models. Pathobiology 62:14, 1994.
36. McCarty GA, Snyderman R: Hereditary and acquired complement deficiencies in animals and man: The fifth component. Prog Allergy 39:272, 1986.
37. Rother V: Hereditary and acquired complement deficiencies in animals and man: The sixth component. Prog Allergy 39:283, 1986.

38. Zeitz HJ, Lint TF, Gewurz A, Gewurz H: Hereditary and acquired complement deficiencies in animals and man: The seventh component. Prog Allergy 39:289, 1986.
39. Tedesco F: Hereditary and acquired complement deficiencies in animals and man: The eighth component. Prog Allergy 39:295, 1986.
40. Lint TF, Gewurz H: Hereditary and acquired complement deficiencies in animals and man: The ninth component. Prog Allergy 39:307, 1986.
41. Nagata M, Hara T, Aoki T, et al: Inherited deficiency of the ninth component of complement: An increased risk of meningococcal meningitis. J Pediatr 114:260, 1989.
42. Abramson N, Alper CA, Lachmann PJ, et al: Deficiency of C3 inactivator in man. J Immunol 107:19, 1971.
43. Thompson RA, Lachmann PJ: A second case of human C3b inhibitor (KAF) deficiency. Clin Exp Immunol 27:23, 1977.
44. Barrett DJ, Boyle MDP: Restoration of complement function in vivo by plasma infusion in factor I deficiency. J Pediatr 104:76, 1984.
45. Thompson RA, Winterborn MH: Hypocomplementaemia due to a genetic deficiency of beta 1H globulin. Clin Exp Immunol 46:110, 1981.
46. Sjoholm AG, Braconier JH, Soderstrom C: Properdin deficiency in a family with fulminant meningococcal infections. Clin Exp Immunol 50:291, 1982.
47. Densen P, Weiler JM, Griffiss JM, Hoffmann LG: Familial properdin deficiency and fatal meningococcemia: Correction of the bactericidal defect by vaccination. N Engl J Med 316:922, 1987.
48. Sjoholm AG, Soderstrom C, Nilsonn LA: A second variant of properdin deficiency: The detection of properdin at low concentrations in affected males. Complement Inflamm 5:130, 1988.
49. Sjoholm AG, Kuijper EJ, Tijssen CC, et al: Dysfunctional properdin in a Dutch family with meningococcal disease. N Engl J Med 319:33, 1988.
50. Miller ME: Host defenses in the human neonate. Pediatr Clin North Am 24:413, 1977.
51. Johnston RB Jr, Altenburger KM, Atkinson AW Jr, Curry RH: Complement in the newborn infant. Pediatrics 64:S781, 1979.
52. Winkelstein JA, Kurlandsky LE, Swift AJ: Defective activation of the third component of complement in the sera of newborn infants. Pediatr Res 13:1093, 1979.
53. Churg J, Habib RR, White RHR: Pathology of the nephrotic syndrome in children: A report of the International Study of Kidney Disease in Children. Lancet 1:1299, 1970.
54. McLean RH, Forsgren A, Bjorksten B, et al: Decreased serum factor B concentration associated with decreased opsonization of *Escherichia coli* in the idiopathic nephrotic syndrome. Pediatr Res 11:910, 1977.
55. Barrett-Connor E: Bacterial infection and sickle cell anemia. Medicine (Baltimore) 50:97, 1971.
56. Robinson MG, Watson RJ: Pneumococcal meningitis in sickle cell anemia. N Engl J Med 274:1006, 1966.
57. Pearson HA, Spencer RP, Cornelius EA: Functional asplenia in sickle cell anemia. N Engl J Med 281:923, 1969.
58. Winkelstein JA, Drachman RH: Deficiency of pneumococcal serum opsonizing activity in sickle-cell disease. N Engl J Med 279:459, 1968.
59. Johnston RB Jr, Newman SL, Struth AG: An abnormality of the alternative pathway of complement activation in sickle cell disease. N Engl J Med 288:803, 1973.
60. Wilson WA, Thomas EJ, Sissons JEP: Complement activation in asymptomatic patients with sickle cell anemia. Clin Exp Immunol 36:130, 1979.
61. Koethe SM, Casper JT, Rodney GE: Alternative complement pathway activity in sera from patients with sickle cell disease. Clin Exp Immunol 23:56, 1976.
62. Daka MR, Fearon DT, Austen KF: C3 nephritic factor: Stabilization of fluid phase and cell bound alternative pathway convertase. J Immunol 116:1, 1976.
63. Davis AE III, Arnaout MA, Alper CA, Rosen FS: Transfer of C3 nephritic factor from mother to fetus: Is C3 nephritic factor IgG? N Engl J Med 297:144, 1977.
64. Spitzer RE, Vallota EH, Forrestal J, et al: Serum C3 lytic system in patients with glomerulonephritis. Science 164:436, 1969.
65. Sissons JGP, West RJ, Fallows J, et al: Complement abnormalities in lipodystrophy. N Engl J Med 294:461, 1976.
66. Edwards KM, Alford R, Gemurz H, Mold C: Recurrent bacterial infections associated with C3 nephritic factor and hypocomplementemia. N Engl J Med 308:1138, 1983.
67. Thompson RA, Yap PL, Brettle RB, et al: Meningococcal meningitis associated with persistent hypocomplementemia due to circulating nephritic factor. Clin Exp Immunol 52:153, 1983.
68. Sevitt S: A review of the complications of burns, their origin and importance for illness and death. J Trauma 19:358, 1979.
69. Bjornson AB, Altemeier WA, Bjornson HS: Complement, opsonins and the immune response to bacterial infection in burned patients. Ann Surg 191:323, 1980.
70. Gelfand JA, Donelan M, Burke JF: Preferential activation and depletion of the alternative pathway by burn injury. Ann Surg 198:58, 1983.
71. Bjornson AB, Alexander JW: Alterations of serum opsonins in patients with severe thermal injury. J Lab Clin Med 83:372, 1974.
72. Nathenson G, Miller ME, Myers KA, et al: Decreased opsonic and chemotactic activities in sera of postburn patients and partial opsonic restoration with properdin and properdin convertase. Clin Immunol Immunopathol 9:269, 1978.

6

Phagocytes: Normal and Abnormal Neutrophil Host Defenses

Mark S. Klempner
Harry L. Malech

Anatomy

The circulating polymorphonuclear neutrophil (PMN) is round, about 5 μm in diameter with a distinctive multilobed nucleus and many small granules[1, 2] (Fig. 6–1). In the process of exiting the circulation at sites of inflammation, the neutrophil demonstrates ameboid movement and pleomorphic changes in shape. The most distinctive morphologic feature of the mature neutrophil is the multilobed nucleus, typically appearing as two to four distinct lobes connected by thin strands of chromatin. This pattern appears late in myeloid differentiation. With stress or infection, immature neutrophils released from the marrow pool may have nuclei that lack distinct nuclear lobes, instead appearing bandlike, sometimes with a midpoint constriction. These immature neutrophils are often called bands because of the shape of the nucleus. The presence of increased numbers of band forms in the circulating blood (greater than 1% to 2% of the neutrophil count) is a useful indicator of increased flux of neutrophils from the marrow pool and may be the only indicator of infection or other inflammatory process when leukocytosis and fever are absent. Compared with fully mature neutrophils, bands may be less capable of performing functions essential to host defense against microorganisms.[3, 4]

Excessive segmentation of the neutrophil nucleus (five or more lobes) may be a manifestation of folate or vitamin B_{12} deficiency. The Pelger-Huët anomaly,[1] an infrequent codominant benign inherited trait, results in neutrophils with distinctive bilobed nuclei that must be distinguished from band

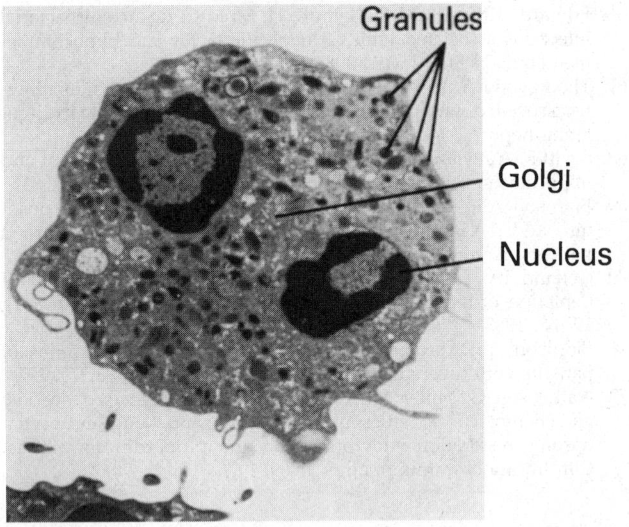

FIGURE 6–1 □ Electron micrograph of a human peripheral blood neutrophil. Two lobes of the segmented nucleus and many cytoplasmic granules are the most prominent features of this cell. Without specific staining for peroxidase, it is not possible to accurately distinguish the azurophil granules. However, the specific granules tend to be smaller and less electron dense than the azurophil granules. A portion of the Golgi membranes is evident as vesicular structures near the center of this cell. Just discernible is the grainy appearance of the cytoplasm, representing glycogen particles. (× 10,000.)

forms. The physiologic role for the multilobed nucleus of neutrophils is unknown, but it may allow greater deformation of neutrophils during migration into tissues to sites of inflammation.

Neutrophils contain many small granules at the limit of resolution by light microscopy. Classic descriptions of the granules of neutrophils define two types.[5] Azurophil (primary) granules are lysosome-like; contain acid hydrolases and many proteases; and are associated with a large number of cationic microbicidal proteins, such as defensins,[6] bactericidal/permeability increasing (BPI) protein,[7] azurocidin,[8] cathepsin G,[9] gp37,[10] and gp57.[11] They are peroxidase-positive, containing a large amount of myeloperoxidase (MPO),[12] and are produced mainly at the promyelocyte stage of neutrophil differentiation (Fig. 6–2). Specific (secondary) granules are produced primarily at the myelocyte-metamyelocyte stage of neutrophil differentiation and are three times more numerous than azurophil granules in the mature neutrophil. Specific granules contain lactoferrin,[13] a vitamin B_{12} binding protein,[14] a unique procollagenase,[15] and other distinctive components. The specific granule membrane appears to contain many integral membrane proteins also found in the plasma membrane, including formylpeptide chemotactic receptors,[16, 17] iC3b receptors,[18] the cytochrome *b*-558 component of the respiratory burst oxidase,[19] and adhesion receptors for a number of connective tissue elements (laminin).[20] Many stimuli cause degranulation of specific granules, a process that results in fusion of specific granule membranes with both the plasma membrane and the forming phagosome. Thus, specific granules appear to be an integral storage pool for a number of functionally important membrane proteins that are inserted into the plasma membrane or forming phagosome of the stimulated neutrophil. Additional exocytic vesicular storage compartments distinct from primary and secondary granules have been described. For example, a low-density vesicular compartment containing alkaline phosphatase[21] and a slowly sedimenting gelatinase-containing granule[22] have been reported. Under conditions of stimulation that do not lead to specific granule exocytosis as determined by lactoferrin secretion, plasma membrane–associated alkaline phosphatase increases, and both gelatinase[22, 23] and a mast cell histamine-releasing factor are released from neutrophils.[24]

The cytoplasm of unstimulated blood neutrophils contains large amounts of glycogen particles that are visible by electron microscopy. The predominant cellular energy source of neutrophils is anaerobic glycolysis, and stimulated neutrophils at sites of inflammation deplete these glycogen stores. Neutrophils contain few mitochondria. Neutrophils also contain relatively few ribosomes but are capable of limited protein synthesis. Protein synthesis by neutrophils may play a more important role in the inflammatory process than was formerly appreciated. For example, under some conditions, neutrophils synthesize interleukin-1, an important inflammatory mediator.[25] A prominent Golgi apparatus is present in neutrophils and may be important for recycling of membrane components and processing of newly synthesized proteins. A pair of centrioles with associated microtubule organizing centers are usually found near the Golgi apparatus.[26] In resting neutrophils, scant cytoskeletal elements are seen by electron microscopy, but in response to chemoattractants, there is an increase in cortical microfilaments containing F-actin and an increased number and length of microtubules extending radially from the microtubule organizing centers.[26] Microfilaments generate the contractile forces responsible for cell motility, including migration and phagocytosis.[27] Microtubules are important for maintaining a sterotypic polarized internal organization of cellular organelles during neutrophil migration[26] and possibly also play a role in movements of vesicular components.[28] Microtubules are not essential for neutrophil migration, including chemotaxis, or for phagocytosis and exocytosis, but they do influence the efficiency of migration during the chemotactic response.[29]

Granulopoiesis and Distribution

Myeloid precursors constitute the majority of cells in bone marrow. Neutrophil precursors are distributed in a reticular pattern; most immature forms are found near the bony spicules, and more mature forms are found nearest sinusoids. Neutrophils mature from myeloblasts to mature neutrophils in about 10 days.[30, 31] Morphologically mature neutrophils reside in the marrow pool for several additional days before release into the circulation. This marrow pool exceeds the number of neutrophils in the circulation by severalfold. Although interleukin-1, tumor necrosis factor, and perhaps other inflammatory response cytokines enhance release of both morphologically mature and immature marrow pool neutrophils, the mechanisms controlling release of neutrophils from the marrow in the normal uninfected host are unknown.[32, 33] Marrow pool neutrophils released to the circulation in response to endotoxin challenge differ in the expression of some surface markers compared with neutrophils released spontaneously in the normal host. These antigenically immature neutrophils and band forms that are released from the marrow in response to infection or stress appear to be functionally less capable than are mature neutrophils.[3, 4, 32, 33]

The normal adult bone marrow produces about 100 billion neutrophils daily. Whereas senescent neutrophils are probably cleared by the spleen, large numbers of neutrophils migrate into the alimentary tract, providing surveillance protection in the mouth and gut against bacteria breaching the mucosal barrier. Marrow production may be increased to 1 trillion neutrophils per day during serious infection. The normal half-life of circulating neutrophils is 6 to 10 hours and may be shortened to less than 1 hour in severe infection.[1, 30, 31] With ongoing infection, neutrophil precursors mature more rapidly, leading to cells with distinctive characteristics.

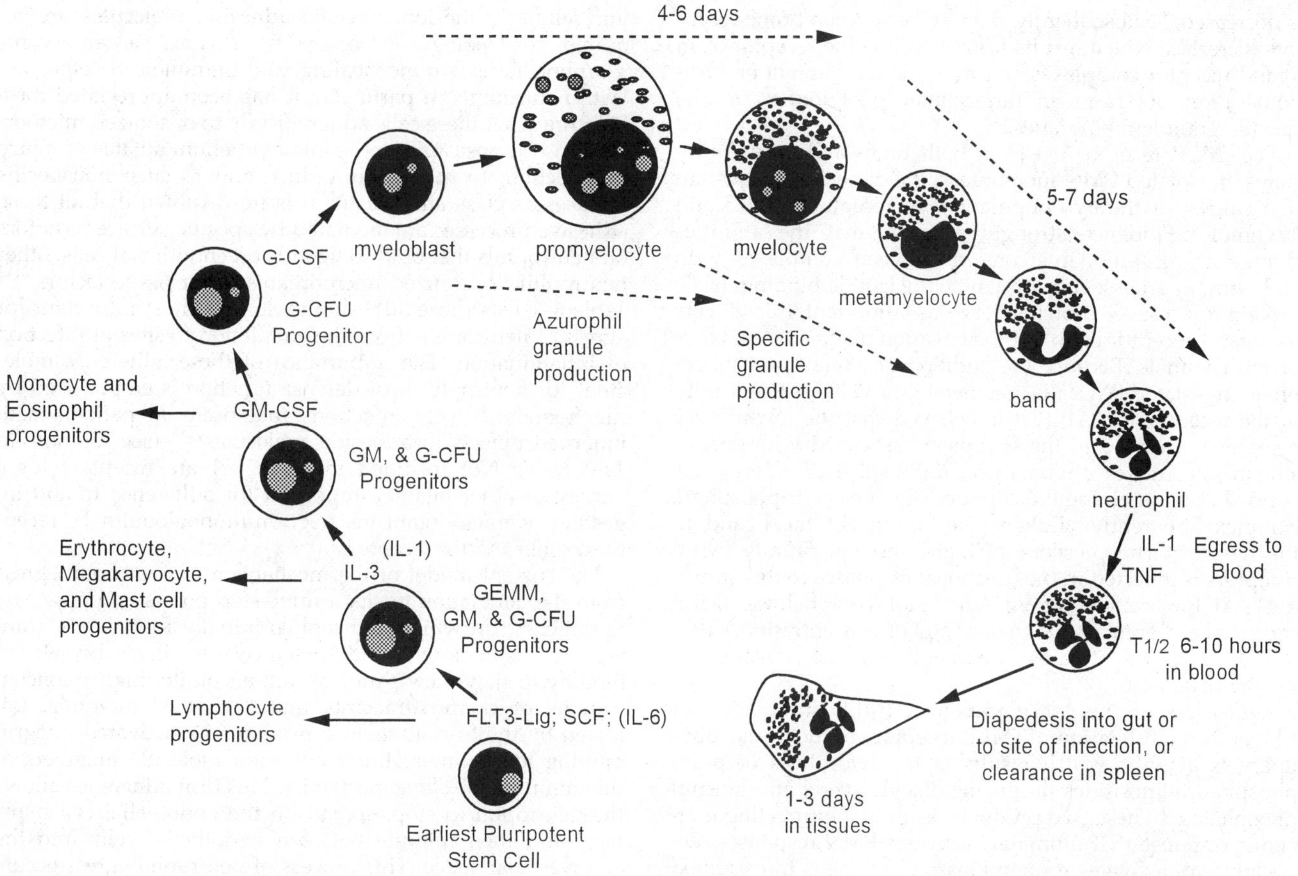

FIGURE 6–2 □ The production, differentiation, and distribution of neutrophils. FLT3 ligand, stem cell factor (SCF), and possibly interleukin-6 (IL-6), growth factors produced by marrow stroma cells, probably act synergistically to support proliferation of primitive pluripotent stem cells. Interleukin-3 (IL-3), possibly synergistically augmented by interleukin-1 (IL-1) and other later acting factors, enhances proliferation at a slightly later stage. Granulocyte-macrophage colony-stimulating factor (GM-CSF) appears to act only on monomyeloid precursors; granulocyte colony-stimulating factor (G-CSF) influences neutrophil precursors only. Both GM-CSF and G-CSF are also produced at sites of inflammation and can augment host defense functions of mature neutrophils. In addition, G-CSF appears to enhance the life span of mature neutrophils, possibly by delaying progression to apoptosis. G-CSF and GM-CSF have a proven role in the treatment of neutropenias or to enhance marrow recovery after transplantation or chemotherapy. Preliminary reports of several studies indicate that G-CSF and GM-CSF may also eventually find a place as useful therapeutic agents to enhance neutrophil host defense function in the setting of severe infections in the elderly or others with impaired host defense, even when neutropenia and compromised marrow function are not factors. By the myeloblast stage of neutrophil differentiation, cells under the influence of G-CSF enter the committed differentiation phase of development. Azurophil and specific granules are synthesized at the stages indicted by the arrows above the relevant labels. The overlap of two arrows indicates an overlap in the later stages of azurophil granule production and the earliest stage of specific granule production. When neutrophils are fully mature, they may remain in the marrow for a few days, but these cells are released early under the influence of IL-1 and tumor necrosis factor (TNF) and possibly other factors in the setting of infections. Neutrophil half-time in the blood is 6 to 10 hours, followed by egress from the blood to the gut or to sites of infection. Neutrophil senescence is an apoptotic process with clearing by the spleen from the blood or by macrophages at other tissue sites. GEMM, Granulocyte-erythrocyte-macrophage-megakaryocyte.

Toxic granulation can be seen, corresponding to the presence of an increased number of large primary granules. Döhle bodies consisting of retained ribosome-rich endoplasmic reticulum can also be seen.[1]

Activation of Neutrophils: Signal Transduction Pathways

PMNs circulate in a metabolically quiescent state. Their basal expression of membrane receptors for opsonins and chemotactic peptides, adherence glycoprotein molecules, or oxygen consumption is considerably less than the cells' capacity. However, when stimuli-like chemotactic factors, arachidonate metabolites, or complement cleavage fragments interact with specific membrane receptors, the neutrophil rapidly becomes activated. The cellular changes are so rapid and so profound that the neutrophil has served as one of the prototypic cells used to define the signal transduction pathways common to activation of many cell types.

Chemoattractants activate neutrophils through a sequence typical of many ligands that stimulate neutrophil function and that begin by binding to specific membrane receptors.[34] Whereas distinct receptors have been identified for the major chemoattractants, including the *N*-formylated peptides such as formyl-methionyl-leucyl-phenylalanine (fMLP)[34] and leukotrienes B_4[35] and C5a,[36] the most extensively characterized receptor is for the *N*-formylated peptides. Direct binding studies of the radiolabeled peptide [^{3}H]fMLP to intact neutrophils demonstrate approximately 50,000 receptor sites per cell.[37] The membrane receptor has been partially purified and appears to be a heavily glycosylated protein that is static neither in number nor in affinity for its ligand. After peptide-receptor interaction, the complex is internalized, leading to an interval during which the number of membrane receptors is decreased.[38] Subsequently, the number of membrane receptors increases, which results from recycling the receptor from ligand-receptor complexes and from the recruitment of additional receptors from an intracellular pool located in the specific granule membranes.[16, 17]

The fMLP receptor exists in both high- and low-affinity states. In isolated PMN membranes, the dissociation constant (K_d) values for the two populations of receptors are 0.5 and 20 nmol.[39] Evidence strongly suggests that the affinities change as receptors interconvert between complexes with and without an associated guanine nucleotide binding, or G, protein.[40] These G proteins serve as important transducers for ligand-receptor coupling to activation of effector enzymes or ion channels. Because the addition of guanosine triphosphate to isolated PMN plasma membranes lowers the affinity of the receptor for fMLP, it is believed that the low-affinity receptor is coupled to the G protein associated with guanosine triphosphate or guanosine diphosphate.[41] Energy expended in maintaining the G protein–guanosine triphosphate complex apparently weakens the binding of the ligand to the receptor. The presence of high- and low-affinity fMLP receptors is reflected in the functional responses to this stimulus.[16] At low concentrations (10^{-9} mol/L or below), fMLP serves as a chemotactic signal; at higher concentrations (10^{-6} mol/L or above), it causes degranulation and activates the respiratory burst.

Regardless of the concentration of fMLP, stimulation of PMNs through ligation of fMLP receptors induces phospholipase C activity, which results in the hydrolysis of polyphosphatidylinositides producing diacylglycerol and inositol phosphates.[42] These two products result in a bifurcating metabolic response that ultimately activates PMN responses. Diacylglycerol activates protein kinase C, which is translocated from the cytosol to the plasma membrane, where it phosphorylates proteins critical to the functional responses.[43] The inositol 1,4,5-trisphosphate that is formed by the action of phospholipase C leads to a rise in the cytosolic calcium concentration.[44] Calcium can be mobilized from intracellular stores, either granules or specialized organelles termed calciosomes, or from influx across the cell membrane.[45, 46] The amount of inositol 1,4,5-trisphosphate generated appears to be sufficient to release calcium from intracellular stores,[47] whereas conversion products of inositol 1,4,5-trisphosphate, such as 1,3,4,5-tetrakisphosphate, may signal calcium influx from the extracellular fluid. The regional rise in cytosolic calcium concentration has a major effect on the physical state of contractile proteins (see later), which results in the locomotion of the cell.

The metabolic events involved in signal transduction of PMNs are transient, lasting no more than a few minutes. Termination of the activation cascade has not been as well defined but may be regulated at several steps. Chemotactic peptide receptors can be internalized, or the ligand can be hydrolyzed at the cell surface. The rise in cytosolic cyclic adenosine monophosphate that follows stimulation of PMNs with fMLP also has an inhibitory action on PMN function, perhaps by inhibiting calcium influx across the plasma membrane.[48]

Adherence

Because neutrophils crawl by ameboid motion toward chemoattractants, one of the crucial steps in their exit from the intravascular space into specific tissue sites is their adherence to endothelial cells. During the past 15 years, the availability of monoclonal antibodies directed at a vast array of cell surface epitopes has led to the identification and classification of an equally vast array of cell surface molecules mediating cellular adhesion. Specific adhesion molecules are required for biologic processes as diverse as embryonic morphogenesis, wound healing, and immune cell responses. With neutrophils in particular, it has been appreciated for a long time that these cells adhere firmly to opsonized microorganisms, to postcapillary venule epithelium at sites of injury or infection, to other neutrophils, and to such nonspecific surfaces as glass and plastic. It is now known that all these adhesive processes are mediated by specific surface receptors on neutrophils that bind to ligands on endothelial cells, other neutrophils, opsonized microorganisms, or tissue factors.[49–51] Table 6–1 lists those adhesion molecules most important for egress of neutrophils from the circulation to sites of infection or inflammation. The importance of these adherence molecules for neutrophil host defense function is emphasized by the frequent, severe infections that occur in patients with inherited defects in adhesion molecules[49–51] (see footnote to Table 6–1). Not included in Table 6–1 are receptors for a variety of other ligands important for adherence to and ingestion of microorganisms (e.g., immunoglobulin Fc receptors or fibronectin receptors).

The current model of the mechanism of neutrophil egress from the circulation posits a three-step process proposed by Springer[50, 51] in which neutrophils initially form labile, transient interactions with endothelial cells mediated by selectin binding to sialyl Lewis mucins and encounter higher concentrations of chemoattractants that "activate" integrins, followed by the firm adherence provided by activated integrin binding to the intercellular adhesion molecule members of the immunoglobulin superfamily. This firm adherence allows the neutrophil to stop, spread on the endothelial cell's surface, and then migrate between endothelial cells into the extravascular space. This process of neutrophil egress occurs in the postcapillary venule.

To understand this process, it is useful to know about the properties of the four groups of surface molecules mediating this process. The selectin family of adhesion molecules has an N-terminal domain related to the calcium-dependent lectins that is extended from the cell surface by a variable number of repeating domains with homology to the epidermal growth factor repeat domain.[52, 53] L-selectin is present on neutrophils; P-selectin and E-selectin are found on endothelial cells. The ligand or counterreceptors to which selectins bind are sialyl mucins.[54] Whereas selectins are lectin-like molecules targeting the sialyl Lewis x or sialyl Lewis a carbohydrate moieties, there appears to be some selectivity for specific carbohydrate-rich mucins. For example, P-selectin has selectivity for the P-selectin glycoprotein ligand on the neutrophil surface.[55, 56] Selectin-mucin interactions tether the neutrophil to the activated endothelial cell surface, but shear forces of blood flow are capable of breaking these bonds. This results in a slowing of neutrophil passage through the venule as the neutrophil alternately sticks briefly to the endothelium and rolls along it.

This rolling with slowed passage through the venule allows more time for chemoattractant factors diffusing from sites of inflammation to interact with specific receptors and activate the neutrophil. This activation results in changes in an $\alpha_1\beta_2$ integrin family of neutrophil adhesion receptors. As indicated in Table 6–1, the three integrin molecules found on neutrophils are heterodimers in which the α-subunit is unique to each integrin (CD11a, CD11b, or CD11c) but the β-subunit is a 95-kDa glycopeptide (CD18) shared by all three integrins. Because these receptors were initially identified by their function, by their size, or by the monoclonal antibody used to identify them, different names in the literature actually refer to the same molecule as indicated in Table 6–1.[50, 51, 57] Thus, CD11b/CD18 or complement receptor type 3 (CR3) is the membrane receptor for the opsonic complement

TABLE 6–1 ■ Neutrophil Adhesion Molecules*

NEUTROPHIL RECEPTOR	LIGAND	FUNCTION
L-selectin	Sialyl Lewis sulfate-rich mucins	Labile leukocyte-endothelial adhesion mediating rolling
P-selectin glycoprotein ligand (PSGL-1)	P-selectin	Labile leukocyte-endothelial adhesion mediating rolling
Sialyl Lewis x mucins	E-selectin	Early firm leukocyte-endothelial adhesion mediating tethering
CD11a/CD18 (LFA-1)	ICAM-1 (CD54), ICAM-2 (CD102), ICAM-3	Firm but reversible leukocyte-endothelial and leukocyte-leukocyte adhesion
CD11b/CD18 (Mac-1, CR3)	ICAM-1 iC3b, fibrinogen, factor X	Firm but reversible leukocyte-endothelial and leukocyte-leukocyte adhesion; complement binding; phagocytosis
CD11c/CD18 (p150,95)	iC3b, fibrinogen	Complement binding; phagocytosis
ICAM-1	LFA-1, Mac-1	Homotypic reversible neutrophil aggregation

*Selectins are lectins mediating early events ("rolling") in neutrophil–endothelial cell interactions. L-selectin is shed from leukocytes during the detachment phase. The ligands are receptors for neutrophil surface adhesion molecules found on endothelial cells (P-selectin and E-selectin, ICAMs, sialyl Lewis), neutrophils (LFA-1, Mac-1), or opsonized microorganisms (iC3b) or at sites of inflammation. LFA-1, Mac-1, and p150,95 are $\alpha_1\beta_2$ integrins mediating firm cell-cell attachments. Enhanced adhesion and then later de-adhesion result from regulatable conformational changes in the integrin molecules. This mediates arrest of rolling with firm attachment to endothelium at a site of inflammation followed by transendothelial migration. ICAMs are members of the immunoglobulin superfamily. ICAM-1 is found on neutrophils and can interact with LFA-1 or MAC-1 on neutrophils to mediate homotypic adhesion (neutrophil aggregation), which serves to pile up a plug of neutrophils attached to endothelium in the postcapillary venule at sites of inflammation. Leukocyte adhesion deficiency type 1 (LAD-1) results from genetic defects in the CD18 gene leading to lack of leukocyte integrin (or in rare instances abnormal integrin function) and impaired transendothelial egress associated with recurrent infections. LAD-2, reported in only a few kindreds, may result from abnormalities of fucose metabolism leading to failure to produce the E-selectin and P-selectin ligands, resulting in clinical features similar to LAD-1. CR3, Complement receptor type 3; ICAM, intercellular adhesion molecule; LFA-1, lymphocyte function–associated antigen-1; Mac-1, heterodimer of the CD11/CD18 complex.

fragment iC3b and is a dimer of the 95-kDa common β-chain linked to an α-chain of 185 kDa; CD11a/CD18 or lymphocyte function–associated antigen-1 contains an α-chain of 190 kDa; and the α-chain of CD11c/CD18 or p150,95 is 150 kDa. The polypeptide α-chains are all coded on chromosome 16, the β-chain is coded on chromosome 21, and they are assembled into the heterodimer configuration before transport to the plasma membrane.[50, 51, 58]

The leukocyte integrins mediate adhesion by binding to specific ligands. In particular, a family of molecules known as intercellular adhesion molecules, which are related to the immunoglobulin superfamily, are important counterreceptors or ligands for the leukocyte integrins.[50, 51, 59–61] The specific targets for specific neutrophil integrins are indicated in Table 6–1. Localization of neutrophils at sites of inflammation depends on the dynamics of changes in neutrophil selectin and integrin molecules and endothelial cell adhesion receptors in response to activation by inflammatory cytokines, such as interleukin-1 or tumor necrosis factor, or by endotoxin (lipopolysaccharide).[50, 51, 59–62] It has been demonstrated that after exposure of neutrophils to chemotactic factors, new epitopes appear on leukocyte integrin molecules associated with increased adherence mediated by the integrins. Monoclonal antibodies directed at these neoepitopes inhibit adherence. This suggests that changes in conformation of integrin receptors probably play an important role in regulating adhesion.[63] This regulated integrin adhesion is reversible, allowing the neutrophil to firmly adhere to the endothelium and then to follow a chemotactic gradient through the endothelium into the extravascular space.

Migration

Unstimulated neutrophils in the circulation are round and without apparent polarity. Neutrophils stimulated by contact with adherent surfaces or on exposure to chemoattractants demonstrate ameboid movement. There is development of a polarized structure characterized by elongation of the cell and formation of an active pseudopodium. At sites of inflammation, neutrophils adhere to postcapillary endothelium, migrating between endothelial cells and through the basement membrane.[64] During migration, there is some secretion of degradative enzymes by neutrophils, possibly serving to facilitate migration through connective tissues.[65]

Several classes of chemotactic factors have been shown to bind to specific receptors at the neutrophil surface, enhancing motile responses of these cells. Formylmethionyl peptides are a potent class of human neutrophil chemoattractants produced in large amounts as a by-product of bacterial protein synthesis.[34] C5a and its metabolite C5a desArg are endogenous chemoattractants produced at sites of complement activation and are particularly important in mediating accumulation of neutrophils at sites of inflammation.[36] Another endogenous peptide neutrophil chemoattractant is interleukin-8,[66] originally called neutrophil-activating protein factor. Although initially reported as a monocyte secretory product, it is also produced by endothelial cells and perhaps other cell types in response to inflammatory mediators. Leukotriene B_4[35] and platelet-activating factor[67] are two lipid chemoattractants for neutrophils that are released at sites of inflammation or injury.

The motile process in neutrophils involves the formation and retraction of many types of cell surface protrusions, which must coordinate with the formation and severing of adhesive attachments of the neutrophil plasma membrane to other cells and to extracellular matrix elements. Cytoplasmic nonmuscle actin plays a central role in these events, generating motile forces in the neutrophil during migration or phagocytosis.[27] Neutrophils contain millimolar concentration of actin, much of which is monomeric in resting cells. On activation of neutrophils, there is a fourfold increase in the proportion of this actin incorporated into filaments. Much has been learned about a large number of other proteins interactive with actin to coordinate the proper configuration and timing of actin assembly and disassembly.

In the presence of adenosine triphosphate, purified monomeric actin spontaneously forms long filaments.[68] This is a polarized process, in which there is preferential addition of monomers to one end of the forming filament. Within the cytoplasm of living cells there is a family of proteins that bind actin monomers, inhibiting their incorporation into filaments. The prototype of this group is profilin.[69] There is evidence that membrane phosphatidylinositol phosphates dissociate actin monomer from profilin and increase availability of monomeric actin for spontaneous assembly into filaments.[70]

With purified actin, the elongation of actin filaments is energetically favored over the nucleation process required to begin the formation of a new filament. In cells are a number of proteins that either initiate nucleation or inhibit filament elongation by binding to what should be the rapidly elongating end of the actin filament. This favors the formation of many short filaments over fewer long filaments. Other proteins, such as gelsolin, are capable of severing actin filaments, also favoring an increased number of short filaments.[71] Calcium transients occurring during cell activation may enhance the severing activity of gelsolin and nucleating activity of other proteins, creating many short actin filaments.[69, 72] As calcium levels fall, the effect of increased phosphorylation of membrane phosphatidylinositols predominates, resulting in elongation of this increased number of short filaments.[27, 69–73] The mechanical stability of these filaments is further enhanced by actin cross-linking proteins. In leukocytes, the submembranous cortical actin networks tend to be orthogonal.[74] This may be a result of the action of actin binding protein (nonmuscle filamin), which both links actin filaments to membrane glycoproteins and promotes right-angle branching of these filaments.[75]

Phagocytosis

The process of internalizing particles by cells is termed phagocytosis and involves the attachment of the particle to the cell surface, which in turn triggers the extension of a pseudopod to enclose the particle in an endocytic vesicle or phagosome. Specific particle recognition and attachment to the PMN membrane are facilitated by PMN membrane receptors for the Fc portion of immunoglobulin G (IgG) and for cleavage fragments of the third complement component C3. At least three Fc-γ receptors (designated Fc-γ RI to RIII) have been identified; these differ in their molecular structure, affinity for IgG and its subclasses, expression on different cell types, and functional role in promoting particle internalization.

Fc-γ RI has the highest affinity for IgG with an association constant (K_a) of approximately 1 to 3 $\times$ 10^{-8} mol/L. This high-affinity Fc-γ receptor is a 72-kDa protein that is present on monocyte/macrophages but not on PMNs.[76, 77] Strong evidence points to a prominent role for this receptor in phagocytosis and antibody-dependent cellular cytotoxicity by monocyte/macrophages.[78] Fc-γ RII, which is expressed on neutrophil membranes, has a lower affinity for binding IgG, and the binding activity differs substantially according to the physical state of the IgG.[79] Monomeric IgG1 binds minimally to neutrophils, whereas multimeric IgG binds to the neutrophil Fc-γ RII with a high affinity.[80] This observation explains why circulating neutrophils, which are constantly bathed in serum IgG, do not have their Fc receptors occupied when they encounter an opsonized particle that presents multimers of IgG Fc to the neutrophil surface. In addition to Fc-γ RII, which has a broad electrophoretic mobility with an apparent molecular mass between 50 and 70 kDa, is Fc-γ RIII, with a molecular mass of 40 kDa.[81] This Fc receptor is widely distributed on leukocytes, including neutrophils, monocyte/macrophages, platelets, and B cells. Like Fc-γ RII, Fc-γ RIII exhibits a low binding avidity for monomeric IgG but a much higher affinity for IgG aggregates. Because of the molecular diversity of the Fc receptors and the presence of multiple receptors on the same cells, it has been difficult to assign specific function to the different receptor classes. However, Fc receptor expression is not uniform on all neutrophils and may play a role in the functional heterogeneity of both mature and immature cells.[82]

At least two neutrophil plasma membrane receptors for complement function as opsonin receptors and promote particle attachment to the neutrophil surface. Complement receptor type 1 (CR1) binds C3b but not uncleaved C3 and is a glycoprotein with four different allelic forms ranging in molecular mass from 160 to 250 kDa. Homozygotes express CR1 with a single molecular mass, whereas heterozygotes express two CR1 species. No disease has been linked to a specific CR1 phenotype. CR1 is expressed on both neutrophils and monocyte/macrophages, where it mediates attachment of particles coated with C3b.[83] It is also expressed on erythrocytes, lymphocytes, and glomerular podocytes, where its function is unknown. CR3, which is one of the leukocyte integrins, binds particles coated with iC3b, which is the cleavage fragment of C3b.[49] In addition, several microorganisms and particles· such as *Escherichia coli, Staphylococcus aureus, Histoplasma capsulatum,* and zymosan appear to bind directly to the phagocyte CR3 receptor in the absence of complement.[84, 85] At least in macrophages, the *E. coli* ligand that binds to CR3 is the lipid A portion of lipopolysaccharide or endotoxin. It remains unclear whether the CR3 receptor is the major lipopolysaccharide binding site on phagocytic cells that is coupled to the synthesis of cytokines such as interleukin-1 and tumor necrosis factor.

A major characteristic of CR1 and CR3 on phagocytic cells is their regulation by extracellular matrix proteins and soluble mediators. Both the binding affinity and the apparent numbers of CR1 and CR3 receptors are transiently increased when neutrophils are activated by spreading on surfaces coated with fibronectin, serum amyloid P component, or laminin as well as by soluble stimuli such as the tumor promoter phorbol myristate acetate.[18] The increased number of CR3 receptors appears to result from mobilization of an intracellular pool of receptors from specific granules to the plasma membrane, whereas the origin of additional CR1 is not known. Regulation of the binding affinity of CR3 for iC3b-coated particles may involve conversion of low-affinity receptors to higher affinity CR3 by phosphorylation, and this process may be important in the phagocytic capacity of neutrophils in the course of different diseases.[86]

Occupation of the Fc receptor appears to be linked to endosome formation and particle ingestion. Studies of intact macrophages, macrophage membranes, and isolated macrophage Fc receptor proteins reconstituted into lipid vesicles have demonstrated that the cross-linked Fc receptor functions as a monovalent cation channel.[87] Multimeric IgG binding to the Fc receptor leads to depolarization in the presence of either sodium or potassium ions, indicating that the channel is nonselective. Even cells that are not normally able to phagocytose particles, such as Chinese hamster ovary cells, will ingest some IgG-coated targets when they are transfected with and express Fc receptor.[88]

Once the opsonized particle is bound to the phagocyte plasma membrane by CR1, CR3, or Fc receptor, engulfment occurs by the localized extension of a pseudopod. The pseudopod progressively surrounds the particle as membrane receptors engage opsonin molecules on the surface in a process that has been analogized to "zippering up" the particle within the developing phagosome.[89] The ionic and biochemical events that propel the peripheral cytoplasm to surround the opsonized particle appear similar to those that propel the whole cell during chemotactic locomotion. Before and after complete closure of the extended pseudopod, cytoplasmic granule movement increases at the base of the phagosome, where the granule membranes of both specific and azurophil granules fuse with the phagosome to form the phagolysosome. The precise composition of the piece of plasma membrane that forms the endosome has a major influence on the fusion of the endosome with these intracellular organelles. It is within the phagolysosomal environment that the full microbicidal power of neutrophils and monocyte/macrophages is exerted on ingested microorganisms.

Microbicidal Mechanisms

Oxygen-Independent Killing

For convenience, the microbicidal components bathing the microorganism in the phagolysosome are divided into oxygen-independent and oxygen-dependent categories. The former refers to those factors that contribute to phagocyte killing of microorganisms in an anaerobic environment. Of the non–oxygen-dependent microbicidal factors of phagocytic cells, most attention has focused on granule-associated proteins, because fusion of granules with the phagosome to form the phagolysosome provides a mechanism for exposing the organism to these substances within a closed space.[90] Table 6–2 lists the granule-associated proteins of neutrophils and monocyte/macrophages and their location within the cell.

Several granule-associated proteins with microbicidal activity have been well characterized. BPI protein is a constituent of PMN azurophil granules that is lethal for many enteric gram-negative organisms but has no activity against gram-positive bacteria, fungi, or eukaryotic cells.[91] BPI protein appears to act by binding to and inserting into the outer membrane of gram-negative bacteria, where it destabilizes the membrane, leading to increased permeability.[92] Hydrolysis of bacterial phospholipids and changes in the synthesis of outer membrane proteins also occur early after BPI protein binding, although the exact nature of the bactericidal action of BPI protein remains to be defined.[93] The defensins are a family of polypeptide molecules containing 29 to 34 amino acids that are also localized in the azurophil granules of neutrophils.[94] In human PMNs, there are four different defensins designated human neutrophil protein-1, -2, -3, and -4. Similar cysteine-rich antimicrobial peptides have also been isolated from rabbit, rat, and guinea pig leukocytes as well as from Paneth cells in the mouse small intestine. The defensins exhibit broad antimicrobial activity against gram-positive and gram-negative bacteria, fungi, and certain enveloped viruses.[95] They are also cytotoxic for some human and murine cells. As with BPI protein, the mechanism of action of these polypeptides involves destabilization and permeabilization of the target membrane.[96] Other azurophil granule proteins with documented antimicrobial activities have been described.[8–11]

Lysozyme is a well-characterized, small (molecular mass of 14,500), highly cationic protein that cleaves the β-(1,4)-glycosidic linkage between *N*-acetylglucosamine and *N*-acetylmuramic acid present in the bacterial cell wall. Although this protein, which is present in both azurophil and specific granules of PMN, rapidly lyses some nonpathogenic grampositive bacteria (e.g., *Micrococcus lysodeikticus*), most organisms are resistant to the direct microbicidal action of lysozyme because the peptidoglycan is protected either by extensive cross-linking or by the outer membrane of gram-negative organisms. Lactoferrin, a constituent of the specific granules of PMNs, is an iron binding protein that exerts its antimicrobial effect by competing with bacteria for this essential growth factor. Lactoferrin may also play a role in granulopoiesis and in the adhesion of PMNs to endothelial cells and phagocytic particles. An acid pH in the phagolysosome contributes to the microbicidal activity of PMNs by directly inhibiting the growth of some bacteria and by promoting the activity of the peroxide-dependent killing mechanism and BPI protein. Within 15 minutes after particle ingestion, the pH in the developing phagosome progressively decreases to pH 4.0 to 6.5. Acidification is due to the action of proton pumps located in the lysosomal and plasma mem-

TABLE 6–2 ■ Contents of Human Neutrophil Granules

TYPE OF CONSTITUENT	AZUROPHIL (PRIMARY) GRANULE	SPECIFIC (SECONDARY) GRANULE	OTHER
Antimicrobial enzyme	Lysozyme Myeloperoxidase	Lysozyme	
Antimicrobial peptides and proteins	Bactericidal/permeability increasing protein Defensins Azurocidin	Lactoferrin	
Enzymes	Acid phosphatase β-Glucosaminidase α-Mannosidase Arylsulfatase α-Fucosidase Cathepsin G Cathepsin D Elastase Phospholipase A Histonase Deoxyribonuclease 5′-Nucleotidase Collagenase β-Glycerophosphatase β-Glucuronidase	Cytochrome *b* Collagenase	Acid phosphatase β-Glucosaminidase α-Mannosidase Cathepsin D β-Glucuronidase
Receptors		iC3b fMLP Laminin	Laminin
Other	Glycosaminoglycans Chondroitin sulfate Heparin sulfate	Flavoproteins Vitamin B_{12} binding protein	

branes as well as protons released during the respiratory burst.

Oxidative Killing

During phagocytosis or in response to high concentrations of chemoattractants, neutrophils are triggered to produce large amounts of superoxide that dismutates to hydrogen peroxide and other microbicidal oxidants.[97] This response has been called a respiratory burst because of the rapid consumption of oxygen associated with it (Fig. 6–3). When neutrophils, monocytes, or eosinophils are stimulated, a unique NADPH oxidase is activated. Activation of this oxidase requires assembly of an electron transport chain at the plasma membrane or the membrane of the forming phagosome. Activation of the NADPH oxidase requires the interaction of both membrane and cytoplasmic components.[98]

Figure 6–3 is a schematic representation of the components of the phagocytic cell NADPH oxidase. Early events in activation result in phosphorylation of a cationic cytoplasmic protein, p47phox (47-kDa phagocyte oxidase protein).[99] The phosphorylated p47phox together with p67phox[100] and Rac2, a Rho-related member of the Ras superfamily of guanosine triphosphates,[101–104] then translocate to the membrane of the forming phagosome.[105, 106] At the cell membrane, these cytoplasmic factors interact together[107, 108] and with a unique phagocyte flavocytochrome *b*-558[109–111] to form the active oxidase complex.[112, 113] Flavocytochrome *b*-558 is a heterodimer composed of two tightly associated subunits,[114, 115] p22phox[115] and a highly glycosylated[116] transmembrane large subunit gp91phox.[117–119] The gp91phox glycopeptide appears to have flavin and NADPH binding consensus sequences[110, 111] and together with the p22phox peptide coordinates the binding of two heme groups.[120] This flavin- and heme-containing flavocytochrome has an electron potential of −245 mV[109] and is the terminal electron donor to molecular oxygen, forming superoxide anion. Although much is now known about the fine structure of the NADPH oxidase components and the molecular basis of the protein-protein interactions leading to oxidase assembly, details of the three-dimensional structure of these proteins and the flow of electrons from NADPH to molecular oxygen remain to be determined. In addition, the

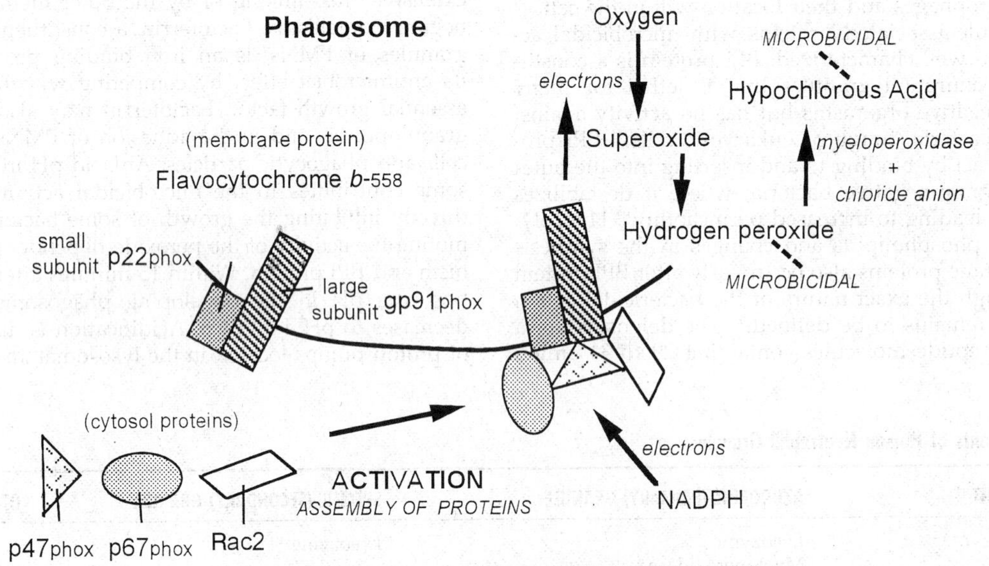

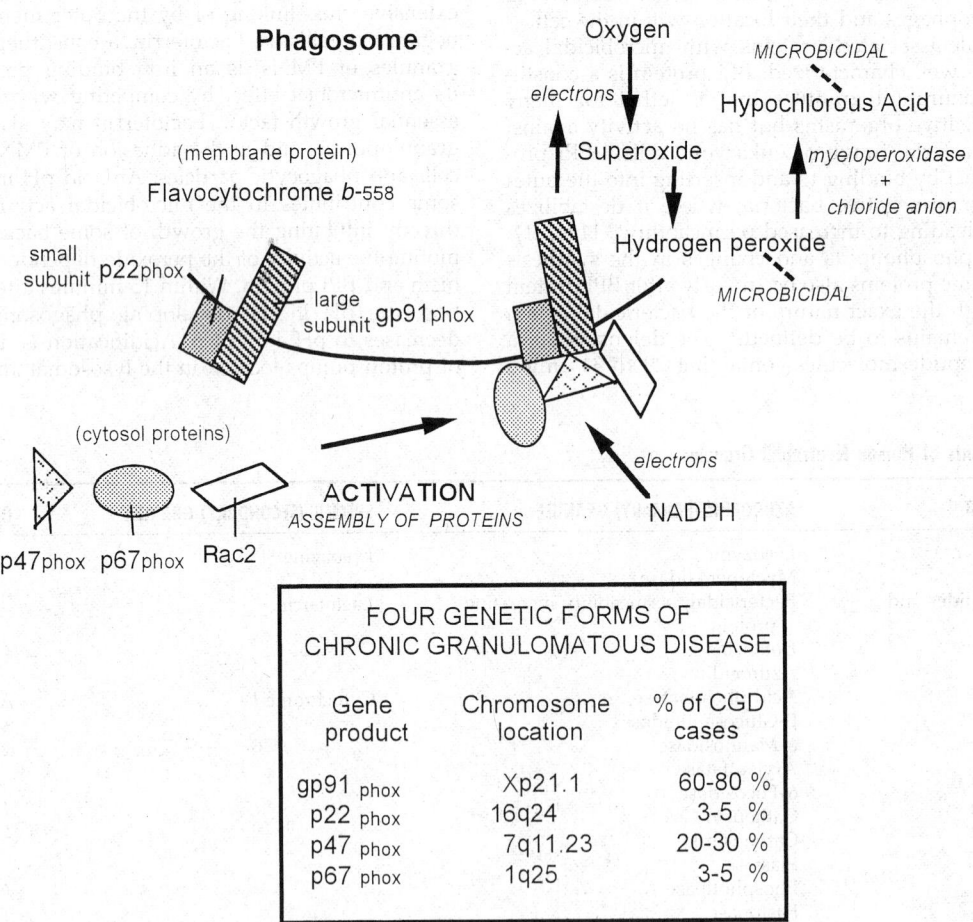

FOUR GENETIC FORMS OF CHRONIC GRANULOMATOUS DISEASE

Gene product	Chromosome location	% of CGD cases
gp91 phox	Xp21.1	60-80 %
p22 phox	16q24	3-5 %
p47 phox	7q11.23	20-30 %
p67 phox	1q25	3-5 %

FIGURE 6–3 ▫ Components of the phagocytic cell respiratory burst and the genetic lesions affecting these components in chronic granulomatous disease. The flavocytochrome *b*-558, consisting of a heterodimer of gp91phox and p22phox, is an integral membrane protein containing flavin, heme, and an NADPH binding site. The p47phox, p67phox, and Rac2 (a Ras-related guanosine triphosphatase) are cytoplasmic proteins in the resting cell. On activation, the p47phox is multiply phosphorylated and together with the other cytoplasmic factors translocates to the membrane of the forming phagosome; there they interact with the cytoplasmic domain of the flavocytochrome to form the enzymatically active NADPH oxidase. The cytoplasmic surface of the membrane lies beneath the line; above the line indicates the inside of the phagosome or the cell surface. After activation, electrons are transferred from NADPH to molecular oxygen to form superoxide. This breaks down into hydrogen peroxide, which together with chloride anion interacts with myeloperoxidase derived from azurophil granules fusing with the phagosome to form hypochlorous acid. The hydrogen peroxide and hypochlorous acid are the major oxidase-derived microbicidal substances. Chronic granulomatous disease results from mutations in the genes encoding any of the phox proteins. The chromosome location and frequency of genetic abnormalities are shown in the box.

terminal signal events that trigger assembly of these components appear to involve phospholipid mediators and kinases,[121, 122] and it is an active area of investigation.

The NADPH substrate for the oxidative burst is supplied by a sudden increase in anaerobic glucose metabolism through the hexose monophosphate shunt.[97] In mildly acidic conditions, superoxide rapidly reacts with water to form hydrogen peroxide. Superoxide dismutase, present in all cellular cytoplasm, further accelerates this reaction. Hydrogen peroxide is a more potent antimicrobial and cytocidal oxidant than is superoxide. Furthermore, in the presence of neutrophil MPO and halide (Cl^-, Br^-, I^-), the hydrogen peroxide reacts to form hypohalous acids, of which hypochlorous acid is the most abundant.[97, 98] Additional reactions may occur to produce free halogens and other reactive compounds. These halous oxidants are extremely potent antimicrobial substances. These oxidants not only damage microorganisms but also enhance the susceptibility of pathogens to some of the nonoxidative antimicrobial substances present in neutrophil granules, including proteases and other degradative enzymes. It is possible to speculate that the anaerobic environment within some abscesses deprives neutrophils of the oxygen necessary to produce this array of antimicrobial substances. Drainage of abscesses not only removes the bulk of organisms within the abscess but also achieves another important physiologic effect by enhancing neutrophil access to oxygen.

Some of the oxidants produced by neutrophils may also damage host tissues. In the presence of iron salts, hydrogen peroxide and superoxide can interact to form hydroxyl radical.[97] Whereas hydroxyl radical does have antimicrobial activity, it is particularly damaging to host tissues.[123–125] There is evidence that apolactoferrin present in large amounts in neutrophil specific granules may limit hydroxyl radical formation by sequestering iron. MPO may similarly limit formation of hydroxyl radical by shunting hydrogen peroxide into other reactions more appropriate to host defense.[126] Nonetheless, studies using hydroxyl radical scavengers in animals[123, 125, 126] indicate that sufficient hydroxyl radical is formed at sites of inflammation and neutrophil activation to have an impact on the pathophysiologic process of a number of conditions including adult respiratory distress syndrome, myocardial infarction, and autoimmune disorders.[127]

Neutropenia and Abnormal Neutrophil Function

Neutropenia

The peripheral blood neutrophil count normally ranges between 1500 and 8000/mm^3 but can be as low as 1000/mm^3.[128] Neutrophil counts in a normal individual are generally constant if that person is examined for a period of several years. A rule of thumb is that neutrophil counts lower than 1000/mm^3 are associated with some increased risk for infection; patients with counts below 500/mm^3 are at high risk for development of bacterial or fungal infection. The risk is further increased in patients with absolute neutrophil counts below 100/mm^3.[129, 130] This rule should be tempered by taking into account the clinical setting. A falling neutrophil count or a significant decrease over steady-state levels, together with a failure to increase counts in the setting of infection or other challenge to bone marrow reserve, requires investigation as to the cause of the neutropenia. Such neutropenia is also more likely to be associated with increased risk for infection than if the neutropenia has remained constant for many months or years and if there is some increased response to infections.[131, 132]

Some causes of inherited and acquired neutropenias are listed in Table 6–3. The most common neutropenias are iatrogenic, resulting from the widespread use of cytotoxic or immunosuppressive therapies for malignant neoplasm or control of autoimmune disorders. These drugs cause neutropenia because they are toxic to rapidly growing cells of the marrow. Cytotoxic chemotherapeutic agents fall into this category, but certain antibiotics such as chloramphenicol, trimethoprim-sulfamethoxazole (TMP-SMX), flucytosine, vidarabine, and the antiretroviral drug zidovudine may also cause neutropenia by inhibiting myeloid precursor proliferation. The marrow suppression is generally dose related and dependent on continued administration of the drug.

Drugs may also cause neutropenia by serving as immune haptens, resulting in sensitization of neutrophils or neutrophil precursors to immune-mediated destruction.[133] Drug-dependent immune neutropenia may appear as early as 7 days after exposure to a drug, but when there has been prior exposure, it may occur after only a few hours of exposure. Although almost any drug can cause this type of immune neutropenia, it is important to consider any of the commonly used antibiotics, particularly sulfa-containing compounds, penicillins, and cephalosporins.[134, 135] There may be associated fever or eosinophilia, but these signs are often not present. However, all medications, including common over-the-counter drugs, are possible causes of acute idiopathic neutropenia. Drug-induced immune neutropenia can be severe but usually requires only that the sensitizing drug be discontinued. Neutrophil counts usually begin to increase within 5 to 7 days and not longer than 10 days after the drug is stopped. Readministration of the sensitizing drug is usually associated with abrupt decreases in neutrophil counts. Diagnostic challenge with a suspect drug should not be done, because even short periods of neutropenia entail some risk for infection. Drugs can also be associated with aplastic anemia, affecting all formed blood elements, or with agranulocytosis; continued use may result in a prolonged neutropenia that may remit spontaneously but may be permanent. Some substances such as aromatic hydrocarbons, phenothiazines, and chloramphenicol have been specifically connected with idiosyncratic reactions resulting in prolonged or permanent neutropenia.[136, 137]

Other acquired forms of neutropenia are caused by an autoimmune disorder and may be associated with circulating antineutrophil antibodies.[138, 139] Acquired neutropenia is also associated with viral infections, including human immunodeficiency virus infection.[140, 141] Rarely, acquired neutropenia may manifest as a cyclic phenomenon occurring at intervals of several weeks.[142–144] Acquired cyclic neutropenia may be associated with an increase in natural killer–type large granulocytes and may be responsive to steroids.[142, 144, 145] Hereditary neutropenia may manifest in early childhood as a profound constant neutropenia or agranulocytosis.[146–152] Hereditary cyclic neutropenia is a rare autosomal dominant disorder characterized by a remarkably regular 3-week cycle.[142–144] A severe neutropenia of the newborn can result from maternal antibody response to neutrophil specific antigens on the child's neutrophils.[153, 154] This is a self-limited process, resolving as maternal antibodies are cleared.

Neutropenia may be associated with diseases in which there is splenomegaly with trapping and destruction of neutrophils (Felty syndrome, portal hypertension, or lysosomal storage diseases).[139] A transient neutropenia may be seen acutely in gram-negative bacteremia as circulating neutrophils abruptly marginate in response to circulating bacterial endotoxin.[33, 155] Severe infection in a premature infant or an elderly individual may occasionally be related to a more gradual decline in neutrophil counts to neutropenic levels when large numbers of circulating early neutrophil precursors are also seen. This may be evidence of bone marrow

TABLE 6–3 ■ Causes of Inherited and Acquired Neutropenias

NEUTROPENIAS	DESCRIPTION	REFERENCE
Immune		
Alloimmune neonatal neutropenia	Maternal-fetal neutrophil antigen incompatibility	153, 154
Primary autoimmune neutropenia	Antineutrophil antibodies	138, 139
Acquired cyclic neutropenia	Probably related to a benign clonal expansion of large granular lymphocytes	142–145
Aplastic anemia–agranulocytosis	Cause unknown, possibly drug related	136, 137
Drug-related autoimmune neutropenia	Drugs as haptens interacting with neutrophils	133–135
Secondary to other autoimmune disorders	Lupus erythematosus, Felty syndrome, rheumatoid arthritis	132, 139
Infection		
Epstein-Barr virus infection, hepatitis	Direct marrow suppression or immune phenomena	140
Human immunodeficiency virus infection		141
Marrow failure in neonates	Results from overwhelming infection	156
Acute endotoxinemia neutropenia (transient, not a true neutropenia)	Acute margination of neutrophils in postcapillary venules from bacteremia	30, 33, 155
Cytotoxic Drug Effects		
Therapy for cancer, immune disorders, or side effect of other drugs	Direct suppression of progenitors, iatrogenic and most common cause of neutropenia	130
Inherited Neutropenic Syndromes		
Familial benign neutropenia	Benign dominant inherited trait with marrow response to infection	152
Congenital agranulocytosis (Kostmann syndrome)	Abnormality at early myeloid development; responsive to granulocyte colony-stimulating factor	146, 167, 168
Inherited cyclic neutropenia	Abnormality of early progenitors; responsive to granulocyte colony-stimulating factor	142–144, 166
Abnormal marrow release syndromes (a feature of several rare disorders, e.g., lazy leukocyte syndrome, myelokathexis, WHIM syndrome)	Several different disorders with normal marrow production of neutrophils and failure of release; functional and morphologic abnormalities of neutrophils	147–149, 152
Reticular dysgenesis	Defective myeloid and lymphoid series	151
Shwachman syndrome	Myeloid dysgenesis, abnormal bone formation and abnormal pancreatic secretion	150

failure and, in the setting of severe infection in infants or the elderly, is a grave prognostic sign.[156]

In neutropenia, the inflammatory response is modified. The absence of neutrophil accumulation means that pus is not seen and the degree of swelling and redness is decreased. Fever and malaise are more reliable systemic signs of infection, and local signs may be limited to pain, warmth, and limitation of movement. Significant pulmonary infections may be evident despite only minor changes on chest radiographs. On physical examination, it is essential to look for gingivitis and aphthous ulcers, lymphadenitis, rectal abscess or fistula, splenomegaly, and liver tenderness. The skin should be carefully examined for early signs of cutaneous infection. In acute, severe neutropenia, the gastrointestinal and respiratory tracts are common sources of infection, although the site may be difficult to demonstrate. Blood cultures, urine cultures, and complete blood count as well as a chest radiograph should be obtained. Other studies should be dictated by history and physical findings. In cases of chronic neutropenia, laboratory studies should include a chest radiograph and possibly liver-spleen scan; complete blood count with differential; blood folate, vitamin B_{12}, and copper determinations; serum protein electrophoresis; immunoglobulin levels; and renal and liver function studies. When appropriate, a white cell count and differential should be done at least 3 days a week for an 8-week period to identify any cyclic pattern.[142] A bone marrow aspirate and biopsy for histologic examination and culture are an essential part of the work-up in chronic neutropenias, but they may be delayed in some cases of acute neutropenia when the cause is clear and recovery is likely.

For patients with chronic neutropenia, management of infection risk should be dictated by the medical history, although any infection, no matter how minor, should receive prompt attention. Patients whose neutrophil counts generally remain above 500/mm^3 or who show a significant marrow reserve in the setting of infection (or by steroid challenge) and whose history does not reveal major problems with recurrent infections should not receive prophylactic antibiotics and should not limit their activities.[138–142] Patients with constant or cyclic neutrophil counts below 500/mm^3 who show little marrow reserve response to infection are made susceptible, although a history of infections may differ significantly among individuals with similar degrees of chronic neutropenia. These patients may benefit from prophylactic antibiotics. Oral TMP (160 mg)–SMX (800 mg) twice daily is a commonly used regimen,[129] although concerns about its predisposing to fungal infection have been raised.[157] Others have suggested the use of oral quinolones such as norfloxacin or ciprofloxacin.[158, 159] In the setting of cytotoxic chemotherapy with severe persistent neutropenia, the proven effectiveness of TMP-SMX in preventing *Pneumocystis carinii* pneumonia may offer another incentive to use this form of antibacterial prophylaxis.[160] These patients should try to avoid heavy exposure to airborne soil, dust, or decaying organic matter to decrease the exposure to *Aspergillus* spores. Restriction of activities or social contacts probably makes little difference in infection risk. Good oral hygiene is essential. In addition to routine dental care, neutropenic patients can decrease gingivitis by using chlorhexidine mouthwash and brushing with hydrogen peroxide–sodium bicarbonate paste.

There is some evidence that in cytotoxic therapy–induced severe acute neutropenia, a simple reverse isolation regimen can be helpful in reducing infection during the neutropenic period.[161] This regimen consists of wearing a face mask and of careful hand washing by staff and visitors. More stringent isolation is probably unnecessary and serves only to impede contact of the patient with family and medical personnel. Prophylactic TMP-SMX or a quinolone (e.g., ciprofloxacin at 500 mg twice daily) is useful[129, 158, 159] as is the use of mouthwash and an oral nonabsorbable antifungal agent, such as nystatin, to reduce colonization with *Candida* species.

As noted previously, signs of inflammation are muted with severe neutropenia, such that fever or hypotension and occasionally pain at the site of infection may be the only signs of life-threatening infection. Slight infiltrates on chest radiography may be the only sign of severe pneumonia. Bacteremia without an obvious source of infection is common. When a site of infection can be determined, it is usually the mouth, sinuses, gastrointestinal tract, rectum, lungs, or skin. Bowel wall cellulitis and necrosis can present insidiously with fever and abdominal pain and is a surgical emergency.[162] Urinary tract infection occurs, but in the absence of instrumentation or anatomic abnormality, it is less common. With neutropenic individuals, it is essential in the presence of fever or other potential sign of infection, including hypotension in the absence of fever, that the patient be evaluated rapidly; that blood, sputum, urine, and other cultures be obtained; and that intravenous administration of broad-spectrum antibiotics be started promptly. The last measure markedly reduces mortality from infection.[163] Cultures and diagnostic studies must be performed expeditiously, and antibiotic therapy must take precedence over a more extensive evaluation.

Most of the principles of infection management have been determined from studies of patients receiving cytotoxic therapy in whom neutropenia is severe and little or no marrow reserve of neutrophils is present. In this setting, the major bacterial pathogens causing infection[129] are often those commonly colonizing the skin, oropharynx, and gastrointestinal tract. These include gram-negative organisms of the gastrointestinal tract, such as *E. coli* and *Klebsiella, Enterobacter, Proteus,* and *Salmonella* species; aerophilic organisms such as *Pseudomonas aeruginosa* and *Serratia* species; and *Haemophilus influenzae.* Common gram-positive pathogens include *S. aureus* (which in some institutions may include a high frequency of methicillin-resistant isolates), *Staphylococcus epidermidis, Streptococcus* and *Corynebacterium* species, and enterococci. Anaerobic species such as *Bacteroides, Clostridium, Fusobacterium,* and *Propionibacterium* must also be considered. Survey cultures before infection have not proved to be useful in predicting the infectious agent. Many studies have been done to demonstrate that a number of combination or single antibiotic choices appear to be similarly effective.[129]

It is important to cover a broad spectrum that is likely to provide bactericidal activity against the organisms listed. A combination of a broad-spectrum penicillin with activity against both *Pseudomonas* and *Klebsiella* (mezlocillin or piperacillin) with an aminoglycoside (gentamicin, tobramycin, or amikacin) is one such choice. Blood aminoglycoside levels should be obtained after 48 hours and then periodically to guide dose and schedule to achieve optimal bactericidal blood levels and minimize renal toxic effects. Imipenem-cilastatin or a broad-spectrum antipseudomonal third-generation cephalosporin (cefoperazone, ceftazidime) may be substituted for the broad-spectrum penicillin. Some studies have indicated that an extended-spectrum third-generation cephalosporin alone may be equally effective.[129, 164] These combinations are only moderately effective against *S. aureus* and are ineffective against *S. epidermidis* and methicillin-resistant *S. aureus.* It has been suggested that vancomycin be added to the regimen if these organisms are suspected or prevalent in a particular setting. In the hospital, organism prevalence and susceptibility patterns are important in choosing initial antibiotic coverage.

Changes in antibiotic should be dictated by culture results. In the absence of isolation of a specific organism and when fever persists for more than 4 or 5 days, one should consider adding an antibiotic (e.g., vancomycin) or changing antibiotics. There is strong agreement that if fever persists for 7 days, amphotericin B should be added because of the high risk for fungal infection with *Candida* or *Aspergillus* species.[129] For the same reason, the persistence of fever and infiltrate at chest radiography requires bronchoscopy and often open lung biopsy to rule out fungal infection. In the case of unexplained fever, antibiotics should be continued for 5 to 7 days or until the patient is afebrile; some have suggested, however, continuing antibiotics until resolution of the acute neutropenia regardless of the febrile response.[165] Granulocyte transfusions should not be used prophylactically in neutropenic patients, and controversy continues regarding any role for granulocyte transfusions in infected, severely neutropenic patients.[129, 166]

The identification and molecular cloning of a number of growth factors capable of enhancing production of neutrophils and other hematopoietic cells have resulted in the possibility of new therapies for both inherited and iatrogenic neutropenia.[167–172] Figure 6–2 illustrates the differentiation steps in production of neutrophils by bone marrow and the likely sites of action of some of the different factors affecting myeloid cell proliferation and differentiation. Most recently identified and cloned is a multipotent growth factor, which appears to act on early, self-regenerating pluripotent stem cells.[172–175] There is evidence to suggest that the multipotent growth factor may work in synergy with interleukin-6.[173, 175] Interleukin-3 acts to enhance replication of monomyeloid cell precursors at a slightly later stage of maturation[167, 170, 171, 176] and appears to work in synergy with granulocyte-macrophage colony-stimulating factor.[167, 168] Granulocyte colony-stimulating factor (G-CSF), acting at an even later stage, specifically enhances the production of neutrophils.[167, 169] Besides being growth factors, granulocyte-macrophage colony-stimulating factor and possibly also G-CSF are capable of enhancing the functional capacity of mature neutrophils.[177] G-CSF appears to have a profound effect on prolonging survival of neutrophils, probably by delaying the normal apoptotic process that limits the neutrophil life span.[178–180] Theoretically, this effect combined with the increase in neutrophil production associated with administration of G-CSF might augment host defense even in the nonneutropenic infected patient.[181] This has led to current research interest in the potential of G-CSF administration for treatment of severe infections in the nonneutropenic host. In a rabbit model of infection without neutropenia, G-CSF has been shown to enhance survival after bacterial challenge.[182] It is possible that current and future studies will define a role for G-CSF administration in patients without neutropenia but with severe life-threatening bacterial infection (e.g., the elderly with pneumonia or bacteremia).

Leukocyte Adhesion Deficiency

Defects in the gene for the common subunit of the leukocyte adhesion molecules CD11a/CD18 (lymphocyte function–associated antigen-1), CD11b/CD18 (macrophage-1 antigen, CR3), and CD11c/CD18 (p150,95) result in a spectrum of clinical manifestations collectively known as leukocyte adhesion deficiency (LAD), which are inherited in an autosomal recessive pattern.[183] This is a rare disorder with frequency of only a few per million or less. A few individuals have been identified with a similar spectrum of clinical features who have defects in fucose metabolism leading to a failure to produce the carbohydrate ligands required for selectin binding.[184, 185] To distinguish the two types of LAD genetic diseases, the more common (although still rare) inherited adhesion deficiency resulting from mutations in the CD18 gene is designated LAD-1; the selectin ligand defect currently reported in only a few individuals is designated LAD-2.

Most of the following discussion of diagnosis and treatment relates to experience with LAD-1, but many of the clinical features of LAD-2 and approaches to treatment would be similar. However, some features of LAD-2 are unique in that the patients reported have craniofacial dysmorphism, neurologic defects, and lack of the red blood cell H antigen, thus manifesting the Bombay (hh) erythrocyte phenotype. The patients have normal levels of CD11/CD18 integrins but appear to have a defect in glycosylation resulting in defective expression of sialyl Lewis x.[184, 185]

CD18 is encoded on chromosome 21q22.3 and is the site of mutations causing LAD-1. Primary defects in the genes encoding any of the CD11 α-subunit integrins have not been seen. However, proper translation and processing of the CD18 subunit are required for both stability and proper trafficking to cell membrane of any normally synthesized CD11 subunits. Inherited defects in production or structure of CD18 subunit result in instability of the associated CD11 subunits, leading to absent or deficient lymphocyte function–associated antigen, Mac-1 (heterodimer of the CD11/CD18 complex), and p150,95 at the cell surface.[186] A number of specific mutations have been identified that either impair messenger RNA (mRNA) production or alter or prevent posttranslational processing of CD18 to such a degree that detectable leukocyte integrins at the surface of neutrophils are scarce or absent. However, certain mutations lead to production of some functional CD18, leading to low levels (1% to 10%) of integrin molecules on the cell surface.[187–189]

The magnitude of the deficiency is reflected in the clinical spectrum of disease.[190] Completely absent expression of the leukocyte adhesion proteins by resting neutrophils results in the severe phenotype in which inflammatory cytokines do not increase their expression and activated T and B cells are also deficient.[191] By immunofluorescence flow cytometry (fluorescence-activated cell sorting [FACS] analysis), neutrophils from patients with a moderate phenotype express between 1% and 10% of the normal amount of CD11a/CD18, CD11b/CD18, and CD11c/CD18. Currently, an LAD-1 diagnosis is confirmed by demonstrating low or absent levels of these integrins on the surface of neutrophils or lymphocytes by FACS analysis. However, there is unpublished evidence of a CD18 point mutation leading to abnormal integrin function with normal levels of surface antigen associated with a mild LAD-1 phenotype.

The functional abnormalities of neutrophils from patients with LAD-1 are predictably based on the role these molecules play in normal neutrophil function.[192, 193] Cells adhere poorly to endothelial cells or protein-coated surfaces. Adherence-dependent functions, including chemotaxis and aggregation, are deficient in direct relationship to the severity of the integrin deficiency. Particles coated with iC3b, which normally adhere to the CR3 (CD11b/CD18) receptor, fail to bind to or induce phagocytosis or the respiratory burst of LAD-1 neutrophils. Whereas a variety of T- and B-lymphocyte abnormalities have been described in LAD-1, other lymphocyte-adhesive molecules that are expressed normally must be sufficient to account for the fact that LAD-1 patients do not appear to have a higher frequency of viral or protozoal infections.

Patients with severe LAD-1 experience recurrent, indolent bacterial infections primarily involving the skin, oral and genital mucosa, and respiratory and intestinal tracts.[194] Infections usually begin shortly after birth, often with an episode of omphalitis. One of the hallmarks of severe LAD-1 is delayed separation of the umbilical cord. Infections, especially of the skin, tend to become necrotic with progressively enlarging borders, slow healing, and development of dysplastic scars. The most frequently encountered bacteria are *S. aureus* and enteric gram-negative organisms. Like patients with severe neutropenia, patients with severe LAD-1 fail to form pus at sites of infection and are unusually susceptible to fungi such as *Candida* and *Aspergillus*. As with neutropenic patients, redness, heat, and swelling may be absent from an infected site, with only pain and fever indicating the presence and site of infection. Other than specific FACS analysis for integrin levels or specialized studies of neutrophil phagocytosis, aggregation, or spreading on glass or plastic surfaces, the only laboratory sign of severe LAD-1 is a persistent leukocytosis that may reach levels above 100,000 neutrophils per mm^3 during acute infection, although 30,000 to 60,000/mm^3 is more typical. When infection is not present, a persistent baseline neutrophil count above 12,000/mm^3 in a child or young adult with a history of recurrent or unusual infections should include LAD-1 in the differential diagnosis.

Expression of even a small amount of functional leukocyte integrin molecules results in a more moderate phenotype. Although these patients also experience recurrent infections, these infections are usually less frequent and less severe and may begin or be identified later in childhood. However, the spectrum of pathogens causing these problems is similar to that seen in the severe form of LAD-1. Recurrent episodes of sinusitis, otitis, and pneumonia as well as severe gingivitis, periodontitis, and poor dentition have been particularly frequent in these patients. Of particular note is that infections of the lower extremities may result in indolent enlarging and ulcerating lesions that require aggressive and prolonged antibiotics and débridement and may require skin grafting. These infections may become polymicrobial in type and include anaerobic organisms.

Treatment of LAD-1 depends on the severity of the deficiency of leukocyte integrin expression and its associated clinical phenotype. All patients are likely to benefit from prophylaxis with TMP-SMX.[194] This antibiotic has been successfully used as antibiotic prophylaxis in other pediatric populations with abnormal neutrophil function and is active against the most common organisms causing infections in these patients. Actuarial survival data for patients with moderate LAD-1 ($N = 24$) indicate that approximately 35% survive into the fourth decade. However, earlier recognition of these patients, institution of prophylactic antibiotics, and aggressive treatment of established infection should improve the overall outlook for those with the moderate phenotype. Patients with severe LAD-1 have a poor prognosis, with more than 75% mortality in the first decade. As a result, bone marrow transplantation has become the treatment of choice for these severe LAD-1 patients, and it should be considered early because of the otherwise high mortality of affected individuals in their first year.[195] Human leukocyte antigen partially mismatched bone marrow successfully engrafts in these patients, probably owing to their abnormal T-cell function, making bone marrow transplantation a particularly attractive treatment. Although gene replacement therapy is not yet possible, this disease is an ideal candidate because even low levels of expression of CD18 would probably provide clinical benefit. Demonstration of correction of LAD-1 in vitro in marrow progenitors or lymphocytes from human subjects is an important first step in demonstrating the feasibility of development of gene therapy for this inherited defect.[196–198]

Disorders of Neutrophil Motility

Recurrent bacterial infections, particularly those associated with gingivitis and aphthous ulcers of the mouth, may be caused by a defect in neutrophil motility.[199, 200] Neutrophil motility can be assessed with use of a number of types of micropore filter chemotactic chambers[199, 201–203] or by under-agarose migration methods.[204] In general, neutrophils are placed on one side of a porous filter or well of the agarose and buffer, or any of a number of chemotactic substances are placed on the other side. A normal donor should always be tested at the same time. Because chemotactic assays generally have a wide range of normal distribution,[205] repeated studies may be required to confirm a mild to moderate defect; only profound defects of 50% of normal or less are likely to be of clinical significance. It is useful to test both the cellular response of the patient to normal activated serum (C5a) and the ability of the patient's activated serum to induce a response in normal cells, because serum inhibitors of chemotaxis may be detected.

Although skin windows are sometimes used to assess in vivo neutrophil responses, there is such a broad range of normal that this study is best interpreted at a center where large numbers of patients and normal subjects have been tested previously. This study is done by abrading the skin and then taping a sterile glass coverslip to the surface, changing the glass several times in a 24-hour period, and assessing both the number of cells per area and the normal change from predominantly neutrophils at 6 to 8 hours to predominantly monocytes at 24 hours.[206]

Given the large number of proteins involved in cellular motility, it is likely that nonlethal inherited defects are possible in either actin or one of these actin binding proteins that would cause faulty phagocytic cell motility. Patients in whom phagocytic cell motility is impaired and actin assembly is abnormal have been described.[207, 208] The lazy leukocyte syndrome is probably another primary cellular disorder or group of disorders in motility.[149] The specific molecular defect responsible for these primary motility disorders has not yet been elucidated.

Mild to moderate impairment of neutrophil motility has been reported in the context of a number of physiologic states and disease processes. Neutrophils of neonates show impaired migration in comparison with neutrophils from older children.[209] Motility defects have been reported in association with a number of autoimmune disorders, diabetes, and other metabolic derangements.[199, 200] The mechanism by which these disorders produce abnormal motility is not understood, and except in cases of a profound defect, it is not clear whether the degree of impairment seen is of clinical significance. Patients with inherited neutrophil specific granule deficiency also have a defect in neutrophil chemotaxis in vitro and abnormal migration in vivo to skin windows. This possibly results from both the failure to release proinflammatory factors and the inability to achieve increase in certain surface receptors that normally accompanies degranulation.[206] Patients with hyperimmunoglobulinemia E recurrent infection syndrome, also called Job syndrome,[210, 211] have a variable defect in neutrophil chemotaxis. This disease was initially thought to involve a primary defect in chemotaxis, but this feature does not appear to be consistent even in the same patient over time. The primary defect may be a dysregulation of lymphocyte function that secondarily affects neutrophil motility. A profound defect in neutrophil chemotactic responses was reported in cancer patients receiving therapy with interleukin-2; this may account in part for the increased morbidity from bacterial infections associated with this therapy.[212] Neutrophil chemotactic responses may also be abnormal owing to the presence of serum factors that inhibit the generation of chemotactic factors or the response to such factors.[213] This can be seen in malignant neoplasm[214] or with trauma in which a cellular defect has also been described.[32, 215] Patients with LAD[183] or with Chédiak-Higashi syndrome (CHS)[216] also have significant abnormalities of neutrophil migration into tissues.

Abnormalities of Neutrophil Granule Formation and Content

Chédiak-Higashi Syndrome

One of the most profound defects in the formation of intracellular granules occurs in CHS, a rare autosomal recessive hereditary disorder.[216] The major morphologic abnormality in this disease is the fusion of intracellular granules with each other to form giant granules that are not uniformly distributed in the cytoplasm of the cell.[217] The formation of giant intracellular granules is not limited to leukocytes but is also seen in other granule-containing cells, including platelets, melanocytes, renal tubular cells, Schwann cells, thyroid follicle cells, and mast cells and pancreatic acinar cells in animal homologs of CHS.[218] The function of cells containing the giant granules is impaired, resulting in neutrophil and natural killer lymphocyte dysfunction, bleeding time prolongation, partial oculocutaneous albinism, mixed sensorimotor peripheral neuropathy, and nystagmus.[216, 219] Neutrophils from patients with CHS migrate slowly in response to chemotactic factors despite a normal or increased number of receptors. Opsonized bacteria (e.g., *S. aureus*) are ingested normally, but viable bacteria persist intracellularly, presumably owing to the deficiency of normal granules to fuse with the phagosome to form the phagolysosome.[220, 221] The respiratory burst of neutrophils in CHS is intact and often more exuberant than normal.

Patients with CHS experience recurrent bacterial infections, most frequently involving the skin and soft tissues and the upper and lower respiratory tracts.[216] Viral, fungal, and parasitic infections are not common in the early stage of CHS. Episodes of recurrent pyogenic infections usually begin in early childhood. Extensive scars from repeated drainage procedures of subcutaneous abscesses are usually present in older children. Three to six major infectious episodes per year are not uncommon. The inflammatory response at sites of such abscesses is usually less impressive than the extent of the infection. *S. aureus* and *H. influenzae* are the most common organisms isolated from pyogenic infections. *S. epidermidis* and enteric gram-negative rods are also seen. Many if not all patients who survive the recurrent infections develop a lymphoma-like accelerated phase of the syndrome characterized by hepatosplenomegaly, lymphadenopathy, and lymphocytic infiltration of multiple organs.

Complementation studies have shown that the genetic lesion in the beige mouse model of CHS is probably the same as in the human form of CHS.[222] With use of the beige mouse locus as a probe,[223] the human gene for CHS has been mapped to chromosome segment 1q42.1-q42.2.[224] From this information, it is anticipated that the gene for CHS will be cloned in the near future.

Because the fundamental abnormality in CHS is unknown, specific therapy is not available. One study of antibiotic prophylaxis with cloxacillin did not demonstrate prevention of recurrences of bacterial infections.[225] Success with other prophylactic antibiotics has not been reported. TMP-SMX would be a reasonable choice for prophylaxis because it has an appropriate spectrum of activity against the most common bacteria that cause infections in patients with CHS. Ascorbic acid has been reported to improve neutrophil function in some[226] but not all[227] patients. The rationale for this therapy is the beneficial effects of ascorbate on microtubule assembly, which has been reported to be abnormal in neutrophils from CHS patients.[228] However, it remains unclear whether the observed defects of microtubules are primary or secondary abnormalities of this disorder. Bone marrow transplantation has been successful in a limited number of individuals.[229] Long-term follow-up has not been reported.

Myeloperoxidase Deficiency

Deficiency of the enzyme MPO in the azurophil granules of neutrophils occurs with a prevalence of approximately 1 in 2000 individuals, making it the most common neutrophil abnormality by a large margin.[230] Automated white blood cell differentials that detect peroxidase in neutrophils by flow cytometry have enabled the widespread screening of individuals for peroxidase-negative granulocytes, providing accurate prevalence estimates.[231] Inherited and acquired types of MPO deficiency are recognized. The mode of inheritance of congenital MPO deficiency has not been precisely defined. Kindred studies have suggested an autosomal recessive pattern of inheritance with variable expression, possibly reflecting polygenic control of MPO production.[232] The structure, organization, and expression of the gene for MPO, which is located on the long arm of chromosome 17, have been characterized[233]; close coordination exists between MPO gene expression and genes that encode for other azurophil granule enzymes (e.g., human neutrophil elastase), but there is dissocation from the expression of genes for proteins, such as lactoferrin and gelatinase, that are constituents of the specific granules.[234, 235] There is strong evidence that hereditary MPO deficiency results from both pretranslational and posttranslational abnormalities.[236, 237] In some patients, the gene for MPO is apparently normal; however, there are only trace amounts of MPO mRNA and no proMPO or mature enzyme. Other patients with the same MPO-deficient phenotype express normal amounts of proMPO but no mature enzyme, suggesting that the defect is in the posttranslational processing of MPO.

Specific mutations have been identified for some individuals with MPO deficiency.[238, 239] Analysis of one of these mutations, a change at amino acid 569 from arginine to tryptophan, has been shown to specifically interfere with heme binding, leading to an unstable apoprotein that does not undergo the normal posttranslational process.[240] This is consistent with previous findings regarding lack of mature protein and trace amounts of larger sized preprocessed peptide in the mature neutrophils from a number of MPO-deficient individuals.[232]

Acquired MPO deficiency is most often associated with hematologic disorders, including acute and chronic myelogenous leukemias; myelodysplastic syndrome, refractory megaloblastic anemia, and aplastic anemia.[241, 242] The disappearance of the MPO phenotype occurs in patients with acute myelogenous leukemia in complete remission, and relapse may be presaged by the reappearance of MPO-deficient malignant cells before leukemic cells are seen in peripheral blood smears. As in most forms of hereditary MPO deficiency, mRNA for MPO may be detectable in leukemic cells that are cytochemically negative for MPO. This may be helpful in the classification of acute leukemias.[243]

Acquired MPO deficiency has also been reported in lead intoxication and ceroid lipofuscinosis and transiently during the neonatal period and pregnancy.[230]

The function of MPO-deficient neutrophils offers some clues to the minimal clinical manifestations of MPO deficiency.[244, 245] Phagocytosis, chemotaxis, and degranulation are normal, whereas the respiratory burst is often more sustained than in normal neutrophils. Microbicidal activity for bacteria is delayed but not absent. When the kinetics of bacterial killing are examined, MPO-deficient neutrophils are defective for the first 45 minutes but usually reach normal levels by 1 hour. In contrast, killing of *Candida albicans, Candida tropicalis, Candida stellatoidea,* and *Candida krusei* is absent. *Torulopsis glabrata, Candida parapsilosis* and *Candida pseudotropicalis* are killed normally by MPO-deficient neutrophils. These studies indicate the sensitivity of bacteria and some fungi to the MPO-independent microbicidal mechanisms of neutrophils and the complete dependence on the MPO–hydrogen peroxide–halide system for killing some clinically significant *Candida* species. Of the many with the MPO phenotype, only six patients with clinically significant recurrent and severe infections have been reported, four of whom suffered from disseminated candidiasis.[230, 246] Three of these four patients also had diabetes mellitus, which has been independently associated with abnormal neutrophil function in some patients with uncontrolled diabetes. The other two patients had MPO deficiency as one component of their abnormal neutrophil function, suggesting that MPO deficiency alone is not sufficient to cause recurrent bacterial or fungal infections. It is clear that the majority of patients with isolated MPO deficiency are clinically normal and do not require prophylactic antibiotics or further evaluation of their host defense systems.

Specific Granule Deficiency

Because the secondary or specific granules of neutrophils contain a mobilizable store of chemotactic factor receptors (fMLP), adhesion molecules and opsonin receptors (iC3b), and cytochrome *b*, which all modulate the function of neutrophils, it is not surprising that patients whose neutrophils either lack or are deficient in these granules experience recurrent bacterial infections. Both congenital and acquired forms of specific granule deficiency are recognized. Congenital specific granule deficiency appears to be inherited in an autosomal recessive pattern.[247] Neutrophils from neonates[248] and thermally injured patients[249, 250] are also deficient in specific granules, and the magnitude of the depletion of these granules correlates with the functional impairment.

Neutrophils that are deficient in specific granules display abnormal chemotaxis in vivo and in vitro, fail to up-regulate the number of chemotactic receptors after stimulation, have an impaired respiratory burst, and do not kill bacteria normally. Microscopic, protein, mRNA, and DNA studies of leukocytes from patients with the rare inherited form of specific granule deficiency suggest a more complex abnormality than simply a failure to produce specific granules. Not only are neutrophils missing specific granules, but eosinophils are also missing their normal complement of large, eosin-staining cytoplasmic granules, making them difficult to distinguish from neutrophils at the light microscopic level.[251] Neutrophils lack seven of the usual proteins found in specific granules including lactoferrin, vitamin B_{12} binding protein, neutrophil procollagenase, and others.[252, 253] Neutrophil marrow precursors are markedly deficient in the mRNA transcripts for these proteins.[252, 253] Neutrophils are also missing defensins and some other but not all proteins that are usually found in the azurophil granules.[254] For example, they have normal amounts of MPO. The morphologically abnormal eosinophils lack three of the eosinophil specific granule proteins, eosinophil-cationic protein, eosinophil-derived neurotoxin, and major basic protein.[251] Of note is that even though there is only a single gene for lactoferrin, these patients make normal amounts of lactoferrin in tears and nasal secretions but, as noted, fail to transcribe mRNA for lactoferrin in myeloid precursors.[252] When taken together, all of this information points to a genetic defect in some regulatory element involved in gene activation during myeloid differentiation. In contrast, neutrophils from patients with thermal injury appear to be deficient in specific granule contents by virtue of premature specific granule fusion with the plasma membrane, as indicated by their increased surface expression of specific granule membrane-associated proteins, such as p150,95 or the iC3b receptor.[255]

Patients with congenital specific granule deficiency experience recurrent bacterial infections that usually begin in early childhood. No particular predilection for certain bacterial pathogens has been noted. As with LAD patients, the inflammatory response at the infected site is often minimal and underestimates the severity of the infection. Cutaneous, sinopulmonary, and otic infections are the most common. Treatment is directed toward the specific pathogens, and therapy must usually be prolonged. No trials of antibiotic prophylaxis or experimental therapies have been reported. In patients with thermal injury–associated neutrophil specific granule deficiency, the other host defense abnormalities (impaired skin and respiratory barriers, complement deficiency) contribute to more profound infections, including sepsis and severe pneumonia.

Chronic Granulomatous Diseases of Childhood

Chronic granulomatous diseases (CGDs) are a group of four inherited disorders resulting from mutations in the genes encoding the subunits of the phagocyte NADPH oxidase[106, 256–260] (see Fig. 6–3). All forms of CGD have a common phenotype characterized by the failure of phagocytic cells to generate superoxide and the derivative microbicidal products hydrogen peroxide and hypochlorous acid. The establishment of a registry in the United States and ongoing demographic studies from Sweden[261] and Japan suggest a frequency of four to five living patients per million population. Current mortality is one death per year per 50 patients, which is a significant improvement from the high rate of early childhood mortality 20 years ago. There are currently more adult patients with CGDs. This is probably due to improvements in both diagnosis and treatments.[261–265]

The defect in oxidase activity in CGDs involves neutrophils, monocytes, eosinophils, and certain fixed tissue macrophages. The normal array of microbicidal oxidants is not produced, and these patients are susceptible to recurrent, often life-threatening infections. These patients also tend to form granulomata in all tissues, particularly in lungs, liver, and spleen. Formation of a large granuloma can occasionally obstruct the urinary or gastrointestinal tracts, and granulomatous colitis is also a complication seen in a significant subset of patients.[200, 266–270]

GENETICS

As noted before, there are four genetic forms of CGD, one X linked and the other three autosomal recessive, each resulting from a defect in a distinct component required for activation of the NADPH oxidase. For each genetic form of CGD, the defective or missing gene product,[99, 100, 118, 271, 272] chromosome location,[117, 118, 273–275] and frequency[271, 259–261] are indicated in Figure 6–3. The most common form of CGD is X linked, resulting from defects in the gene encoding the gp91phox large subunit of flavocytochrome *b*-558. Many types of distinct defects in this gene in a large number of affected kindreds have been documented, including deletions, inversions, and point mutations.[117, 256–260, 273] Depending on the X-linked kindred, gp91phox mRNA transcripts may be present or absent. No flavocytochrome is detectable in most individuals, but a nonfunctional flavocytochrome protein is made in some cases. A rare autosomal form of CGD resulting from defective gene encoding p22phox is phenotypically similar to the X-linked CGD in that no flavocytochrome *b*-558 is detectable in most cases, but a nonfunctional protein can be made with certain point mutations.[256, 259, 272] Of note is that with both forms of flavocytochrome *b*-558–negative CGD, neither flavocytochrome subunit peptide is immunologically detectable even though the gene defect involves the gene encoding only one of the two subunits.[272] This indicates that normal transcripts for both subunits are required for either translation or stability of the subunits. The second most common form of CGD affects the cytoplasmic p47phox.[256, 259, 271] With these patients, p47phox transcripts are present, but no p47phox protein is detectable in their phagocytes.[99] Although a number of mutations in this gene have been defined, more than 90% of the mutant alleles have a GT dinucleotide deletion at the start of the second exon. This mutation results in a frameshift leading to a shortened and unstable protein.[256, 259, 276, 277] The relatively high frequency of a specific mutation in a number of racial groups is unusual without some specific cause. A pseudogene highly homologous to the gene encoding p47phox and containing this mutation has been identified. It is likely that recombination of this pseudogene with the p47phox gene may account for the high frequency of this mutation.[278] Another rare genetic form of CGD is a result of mutations identified in the gene encoding the cytoplasmic p67phox protein. In this form of CGD, all patients studied to date have detectable mRNA but no p67phox protein.[100, 259, 271, 279–281] A 40-kDa protein (p40phox) with some homology to p47phox has been identified in neutrophils.[282] The role of this protein in NADPH oxidase function is not clear, but it appears to bind to p67phox and is reduced or absent in patients with the p67phox-deficient form of CGD.[283]

DIAGNOSIS

When CGD is suspected (see diagnostic indicators later), a screening assay should be performed.[200, 284] For more than 25 years, some variation of the nitroblue tetrazolium (NBT) dye reduction slide test has been the standard screening assay,[200, 203, 285] but fluorescence flow cytometric (FACS) assays have been developed that are rapid and more accurate.[286–288] Because many hospital laboratories at major medical centers have FACS equipment, and the assay is simple to perform, this has become the screening assay of choice. If a diagnosis of CGD is made by use of such screening assays, the results should be confirmed with a quantitative measurement of superoxide output by purified neutrophils using the ferricytochrome *c* reduction assay or a chemoluminescence assay.[200, 203] Such a quantitative assay is also useful for determining whether the defect in superoxide output is complete or partial because production of 1% or more superoxide relative to normal neutrophils can be associated with a less severe phenotype.

The principle behind the NBT assay is that when neutrophils produce superoxide, the yellow, soluble NBT is reduced to insoluble blue-black formazan, which precipitates on and within activated cells. Normal neutrophils produce a "positive" NBT test result, whereas CGD neutrophils are "negative." A normal control assay should always be done, and more than 95% of neutrophils in that control specimen should be positive. If not, then the test is invalid. It is also important that the assay be run for only 20 minutes before the reaction is terminated. Neutrophils from a few patients with X-linked CGD and many of the patients with the autosomal recessive, p47phox-deficient form of CGD may make trace amounts of superoxide. If the NBT assay is allowed to develop too long, formazan product accumulates in neutrophils from such patients, leading to a falsely "normal" phenotype. These principles (inclusion of a normal control specimen and proper timing of the reaction) also apply to the FACS assay, which measures the oxidation of dihydrorhodamine 123 by products of the phagocyte NADPH oxidase.[286, 287] Whereas the NBT test generally involves subjective scoring of formazan precipitate, the FACS assay involves machine-generated quantitative assessment of oxidase production on an individual cell basis.

The screening assay should be performed on both the affected individual and the mother because this may provide an early indication of the genotype. Female carriers of the X-linked form of CGD demonstrate phenotypic mosaicism of oxidase activity between individual neutrophils because of the normal embryonic process of lyonization, or inactivation of one of the two X chromosomes in different myeloid precursor cells.[285, 289] This mosaicism (a mixture of NBT-positive and NBT-negative neutrophils; or two distinct peaks of fluorescent-bright and fluorescent-negative neutrophils in the FACS assay[286, 287]) is pathognomonic of the X-linked CGD female carrier state. A female carrier can occasionally show extremes of lyonization in which 5% or less of neutrophils are normal or vice versa. The extreme CGD phenotype at the cellular level in these carriers is generally not associated with increased susceptibility to infection. However, X-linked CGD female carriers with less than 3% oxidase normal neutrophils can have infections characteristic of CGD and may be misdiagnosed as having an autosomal recessive form of CGD. The FACS assay is particularly sensitive at detecting neutrophils of the normal phenotype at a level even below 1%, thus revealing the X-linked carrier state in this setting. None of the assays is capable of reliably detecting the X-linked carrier state when lyonization has resulted in 95% or more of the neutrophils having the normal phenotype. Because of this, it is not possible to distinguish this situation from the significant number of cases of X-linked CGD that are a result of new mutations. This distinction has important implications for genetic counseling of the mother regarding the risk for CGD in children of any future pregnancies. Testing of the proband's maternal grandmother and the mother's sisters as well as the proband's siblings can sometimes clarify these issues. Although the etiology is unclear, there is an association of the female carrier state of X-linked CGD with discoid lupus erythematosus, which may hint at the genotype of the proband when it is present.[290, 291]

In specialized centers, protein electrophoretic immunoblot analysis of neutrophils for the presence of oxidase proteins together with cell-free assays of oxidase activation using cytosol and membrane fractions from neutrophils can be used to identify the genetic subtype of most patients with CGD.* Knowledge of the genetic subtype can be helpful for family genetic counseling and for guiding more detailed mutational analysis at the mRNA and genomic DNA level. However, detailed knowledge of the genotype or specific mutation responsible for the CGD currently does not alter the approach to the clinical care of the patient as outlined later. There is some evidence that as a group, patients with the p47phox autosomal recessive type of CGD, or patients with any type of CGD genotype in which more than 0.5% of the normal rate of superoxide production occurs, have a better prognosis.[257, 292] However, "mild" or "severe" infection history can characterize a particular CGD kindred regardless of other laboratory findings, and the clinical history of even siblings may vary considerably.

Advances in methods for mutational analysis and ease of sequencing together with a strong scientific interest in mapping critical functional domains of the oxidase proteins and identifying mutational "hot spots" have led to mutational analysis of hundreds of CGD patients worldwide.[259, 260] A portion of this information is contained in a database available through a World Wide Web site (http://www.helsinki.fi/science/signal/databases/x-cgdbase).[260] In addition to the scientific value, mutation analysis is important to patients and families for confirmation of CGD genotype and for prenatal diagnosis. Although gene therapy (see later discussion) is not yet developed as a working therapy for any disorder, it is an area of active investigation. If gene therapy is developed for treatment of CGD, it may be important to know the specific mutation responsible for the CGD. Mutation analysis for CGD is currently available only in a small number of research centers, requires considerable time and effort, and may not be successful in identifying all mutations. However, current advances in techniques for identifying mutations and in automation of sequence analysis may eventually make mutation analysis for CGD cheap, rapid, and accurate.

*References 99–101, 112, 256–260, 271–274.

Even without detailed mutation analysis, in a few X-linked kindreds including those involving substantial deletions, disease-related restriction fragment length polymorphisms (RFLPs) have been identified that may be informative for prenatal diagnosis.[117, 293] Normal allelic RFLPs flanking the gene encoding X-linked CGD have also been used for prenatal diagnosis.[294] However, for most X-linked CGD kindreds, prenatal RFLP analysis is not helpful and requires detailed sequence information about the specific mutation. Although a normal allelic RFLP has been documented in the gene encoding p67phox[295] and used for prenatal diagnosis,[296, 297] there are as yet no known disease-related RFLPs that can be used for prenatal diagnosis or carrier identification in any of the autosomal recessive forms of CGD.

CLINICAL MANIFESTATIONS

The clinical presentation of CGD can be varied.* Testing may be prompted by the knowledge that a sibling or other family member has CGD. A family history of unexplained deaths of infant or young boys may hint at X-linked CGD. However, the severity of the defect can be variable, and infections can be episodic. Particularly with the autosomal recessive forms of CGD, the average age at diagnosis is almost 10 years, considerably later than that seen with X-linked CGD. Increasingly, the medical community has become aware that the first severe infection in a CGD patient may not appear until the middle teen years or even far into adulthood.[263–265] This highlights the importance of screening for CGD in teenagers or adults with even one episode of a type of infection or with a pathogen suggestive of CGD. CGD should be part of the differential diagnosis in patients with unexplained pneumonia with *S. aureus*, *Aspergillus*, *Nocardia*, *Burkholderia* (formerly *Pseudomonas*) *cepacia*, or *Serratia*. These and other organisms that are catalase-positive are particularly pathogenic in CGD patients. Any child with a pneumonia that does not rapidly resolve with conventional therapy should have a CGD screening assay. Particularly pathognomonic of CGD is an osteomyelitis with *Serratia marcescens* or any type of infection with one of the organisms newly reclassified within the *Burkholderia* group (*B. cepacia, B. pseudomallei, or B. gladioli*).[296] It is particularly important to note that *Aspergillus* infection in CGD either may present as an indolent infection associated with a dense infiltrate or may present acutely with severe respiratory distress associated with a panlobular miliary or reticulonodular infiltrate. The latter presentation as a first severe infection in an older child or adult patient not previously known to have CGD may be misdiagnosed as hypersensitivity pneumonitis with potentially fatal consequences when *Aspergillus* is seen in sputum or bronchial lavage. CGD testing and recognition of the invasive nature of this *Aspergillus* infection are critical to institution of appropriate lifesaving therapy (see later). In addition to *Aspergillus*,

*References 200, 257, 261, 264, 265, 268, 298.

a large number of fungi have been demonstrated to cause infection in CGD patients.[299] *Paecilomyces* is of note as a CGD pathogen[300] because many microbiology diagnostic laboratories misclassify this organism as a *Penicillium* and thus report it as a contaminant or nonpathogenic species. Therefore, a pneumonia or soft tissue infection from which "*Penicillium*" is the only isolate also should prompt testing for CGD. Unexplained liver abscess is an indication for CGD testing. Needle biopsy of the liver often isolates no organism. CGD patients also have an increased susceptibility to *Mycobacterium tuberculosis*, and this infection in a child in populations in which this infection is uncommon is an indication for CGD testing. Chronic infections with cytomegalovirus can also be seen in a small subset of CGD patients, although such infection is not particularly diagnostic of CGD.

In some patients, problems with granuloma formation and other inflammatory manifestations of CGD may predominate over problems with infections.[298, 301–303] These patients may first present from early childhood through young adulthood with symptoms of partial gastric outlet obstruction or dysphagia resulting from obstructive granuloma of the pylorus or esophagus.[270, 301, 302] Granuloma of the bladder may present as deep pain associated with urination or as acute bladder outlet obstruction.[269, 303, 304] CGD patients may occasionally go unrecognized, carrying a diagnosis of inflammatory bowel disease with symptoms of abdominal pain and chronic diarrhea, with or without rectal fissures or abscesses, and with or without radiographic and histologic evidence of a granulomatous process in the small or large intestine.[305–307] If such patients should also have an infection of a type or with a pathogen suggestive of CGD, then CGD screening should be done. Inflammatory ocular problems, including a chorioretinitis, can be seen in a small subset of CGD patients. A few CGD patients may develop an arthritis resembling juvenile rheumatoid arthritis.[308]

MANAGEMENT: PROPHYLAXIS

Infection prophylaxis is an important element of the care of CGD patients. Particular attention to oral hygiene can control the gingivitis and aphthous ulcers that affect a subset of (but not all) patients. Use of chlorhexidine mouthwash and bicarbonate–hydrogen peroxide–based toothpaste for brushing can help. Prompt local care of cuts and minor skin infections with washing, hydrogen peroxide, and application of topical antibiotic are recommended. The activities and social interactions of children with CGD should not be limited. The only exception is that patients must avoid extremely dusty environments and should specifically not use power mowers, should not dig holes in the ground, and should carefully avoid sites of dispersion of decaying organic material such as spreading animal manure or garden mulch piles. They should also avoid construction sites and should not be near or participate in major renovations of old buildings. All of these activities are associated with high risk for fungal pneumonia, particularly the acute reticulonodular form. Daily prophylactic administration of oral TMP-SMX has been shown to significantly decrease the frequency of bacterial infections.[268, 309] Dicloxacillin or other oral antibiotic with antistaphylococcal activity can be used in sulfa-allergic individuals. The prophylactic daily administration of itraconazole is controversial in that no specific studies have been done to establish dosing or efficacy as prophylaxis, and mild chemical hepatitis can be seen in a small number of individuals with long-term administration. Nonetheless, in Europe and Japan and in some centers in the United States, itraconazole is used as fungal infection prophylaxis. It has been shown that prophylactic administration of subcutaneously injected recombinant interferon gamma results in a more than 70% reduction in infection risk in CGD patients, leading to regulatory approval of this treatment.[310] This protective effect is additive to the effect of prophylactic antibiotics and appears to be sustained for long periods.[264, 311–314] It is currently recommended that all CGD patients receive both prophylactic antibiotics and prophylactic interferon gamma. At the doses of interferon gamma recommended (50 $\mu g/m^2$ of body surface, 3 days a week), there are few side effects. Occasional fever, malaise, or headache can be handled with acetaminophen. These symptoms or neutropenia may rarely require dose reduction. The mechanism of protective effect is not understood but relates to partial amelioration of the defect in phagocyte oxidative burst in only a small subset of individuals.[315, 316] Of note is that a first manifestation of infection in a CGD patient receiving prophylactic interferon gamma may be the new appearance of fever associated with dosing of the interferon. This suggests that this fever results from a synergy between the exogenously administered interferon gamma and endogenous cytokines generated as a result of infection. Because interferon gamma administration requires chronic injections and is expensive, common questions are whether certain patients may benefit more than others and whether it could or should be used to treat infection rather than prophylactically. Unfortunately, no studies have been done to answer these two questions. A mouse model of the p47phox-deficient form of CGD has been developed in which the animals develop spontaneous infections similar to those of CGD patients.[317, 318] Preliminary studies with this animal model have confirmed that prophylactic interferon gamma can prolong survival. This model may allow determination of optimal dosing and whether exogenously administered interferon gamma may help treat established infections. The experience with bone marrow transplantation for CGD is discussed in more detail later.[319]

MANAGEMENT: TREATMENT OF INFECTIONS AND COMPLICATIONS

Despite these maneuvers, patients with CGD may get infections including those that are life threatening. The approach to diagnosis and management of infections in CGD patients follows many of the general principles applicable to patients with defects in host defense.[200, 266–268, 298] Early recognition of infection, diligent attempts to identify a pathogen, adequate doses of antibiotics, and relatively long courses of treatment ensure the best outcome. In addition, CGD patients have such extensive granuloma formation associated with infection that in a number of circumstances, partial or complete surgical extirpation of infected tissue is required to effect a cure.[320, 321] Infections tend to occur with the catalase-positive pathogens indicated in the previous discussion. Although the frequency of deep fungal infections has not increased, fungal infections now account for more than 50% of total infections seen in CGD patients.[309]

The most common infections are cellulitis and lymphadenitis. These often respond to local care and oral antibiotics, but lymphadenitis may require surgical treatment and intravenous antibiotics. Liver abscess and pneumonia are the most common deep organ infections, followed by infection of bone. Computed tomography (CT) of the chest is far more sensitive for early diagnosis of pneumonia in CGD patients than is chest radiography. Because early diagnosis may allow a shorter course of therapy or oral therapy for resolution, may require shorter hospitalization, and may catch an infection of the lung before spread to ribs or vertebrae, the early use of CT for diagnosis and follow-up is highly recommended. Because the only sign of liver abscess in a CGD patient may be intermittent fever or malaise, or liver abscess may silently complicate major infection elsewhere, CT of the liver is also highly recommended as part of an "infection work-up" in a CGD patient. For liver abscess, magnetic resonance imaging actually appears to be more sensitive than CT at picking up additional early lesions and should be performed before proceeding to surgical drainage, but it is often more convenient to obtain liver CT at the time of chest CT in the context of the initial search for the site of a suspected infection.

Infections in lung or liver may occasionally be accompanied by metastatic infection at other sites including bone, spleen, or brain. With *Nocardia* infections, it is particularly important to perform CT of the head and bone scans. It is therefore important to have a low threshold for embarking on a more extensive work-up even when a single site of infection is obvious. Bacteremia and meningitis are uncommon; bacteremia is most commonly seen with infection with *Burkholderia* species or other gram-negative organisms. Signs and symptoms of infection may occasionally be limited to malaise or pain. Fever may be absent or intermittent. With pneumonia, the presence of cough and shortness of breath are variable. Neutrophilia is not always present. An increase of the erythrocyte sedimentation rate from some previous baseline value can be a valuable indicator of infection and, when elevated, is a useful parameter to monitor during treatment. The erythrocyte sedimentation rate is a more reliable indicator of infection than is elevation of the white cell count.

Identification of a pathogen may often require biopsy for histologic examination and culture. Advances in interventional radiology have made it safe and convenient to perform needle biopsy under CT guidance of lung, liver, or other tissue. When histologic identification of a pathogen by cytopathologic examination with special stains is combined with results from microbiology, needle biopsy can identify a pathogen in more than 80% of cases, particularly if repeated biopsy is performed when no organism is found by a first biopsy. Whereas surgical drainage and débridement of liver abscess or major bone infection[320] continue to be critical for eradication of infection and shortening the time to cure, surgical intervention in pulmonary infections appears to be needed only when there is a large segment of devitalized lung or there is clear spread of infection to bone.[320, 321] Surgical drainage, débridement, or extirpation of nonviable tissue is essential in treatment of extensive infections of lung, liver, or bone. In cases of pneumonia, bronchoscopy is often done, but particularly with fungal infections, it often will not yield a credible pathogen. For this reason, needle biopsy is the preferred diagnostic procedure unless the lesion is not reachable by the transthoracic approach. Infection with more than one pathogen in CGD patients is not uncommon, particularly in cases of pneumonia. For example, mixed infection with *Aspergillus* species and *Nocardia* or *Burkholderia* species may be seen. Sometimes the second infection may become apparent because it is not covered in the specific treatment for the first identified pathogen.

As noted, pneumonia due to either *Burkholderia* species (particularly *B. cepacia*)[296, 297] or *Aspergillus* species is generally life threatening in CGD patients.[296, 297, 309, 322] With *B. cepacia*, patients often have high temperature with shortness of breath. In addition, the infection may progress rapidly in these patients. Furthermore, in many centers, this organism may be highly resistant to many first-line antibiotics. *Aspergillus* pneumonia usually presents with insidious onset, appearing as dense segmental or lobar infiltrates on the chest radiograph.[266, 323] Extension to ribs or vertebrae is a grave prognostic sign.[320, 321] Treatment with amphotericin B at doses of 1 to 1.5 mg/kg per day for 8 weeks or more is required. Segmental and occasionally lobar resection of devitalized tissue may be an essential component of the treatment.[321] Extension to bony structures always requires débridement. In some centers, daily granulocyte transfusions are used for the first 3 to 4 weeks of treatment of fungal pneumonia.[323–325] The amphotericin B therapy and granulocyte transfusions are spaced as far apart as possible to minimize adverse interactions. Transfused granulocytes should be ABO matched, should be obtained by centrifugation leukapheresis, and should not be irradiated because this adversely affects oxidase activity.[200] Other details regarding granulocyte transfusions are discussed in the section on neutropenia. There are no studies demonstrating efficacy of granulocyte transfusions in the treatment of CGD patients, but the transfused granulocytes do reach sites of infection,[324] and there is in vitro evidence of synergy of fungal killing by the combination of small numbers of normal neutrophils mixed with a larger number of CGD neutrophils.[326] As noted before, *Aspergillus* pneumonia in CGD patients may present as an acute febrile illness with shortness of breath associated with a miliary infiltrate on the chest radiograph affecting the entire field of both lungs. High-dose amphotericin B therapy with transient use of flucytosine to obtain some immediate antifungal effect is essential. In this setting, early compromise of oxygenation can be life threatening. Because this diffusion defect appears to be exacerbated by the exuberant granuloma formation characteristic of CGD, short-term use of steroids at an equivalent of 1 to 1.5 mg/kg of prednisone for 4 or 5 days may be lifesaving. Although theoretically this might also compromise host defense against the fungal infection, keeping the steroid dosing to less than a week and instituting aggressive antifungal therapy have led to cure of this type of infection in most cases. Amphotericin B therapy at 1.0 to 1.5 mg/kg per day for 6 weeks is typically effective for treatment of most fungal pneumonias in CGD. Prolonged follow-up therapy with oral itraconazole is recommended.

In about 20% of infections in CGD patients, no organism is isolated despite multiple biopsies and bronchoscopy and even surgical débridement. Empirical therapy for infection should begin with antibacterial therapy aimed at the most likely organisms in that setting. With pneumonias in CGD patients receiving TMP-SMX prophylaxis, *Staphylococcus* is rarely a pathogen and is easy to isolate when it is present. When no organism is isolated, empirical therapy with high-dose intravenous TMP-SMX plus ceftriaxone appears to be most successful. If infection progresses with this regimen, then ciprofloxacin or imipenem-cilastatin can be added. If 10 to 14 days of this approach suggest that the infection is progressing, then empirical antifungal therapy with amphotericin B must be begun after repeated biopsy. In certain settings, such as acute presentation with the reticulonodular, panlobular pattern, it is important to begin amphotericin B empirically early.

Obstructive granulomata of the gastrointestinal or urinary tract may result from infection or may occur in the absence of any apparent infectious process.[269, 270, 298, 301–307] Symptoms of gastrointestinal granuloma may include difficulty swallowing, early satiety, unexplained periodic vomiting, or just chronic indolent abdominal pain. The gastrointestinal granulomatous process may occasionally be indistinguishable from Crohn disease or ulcerative colitis, involving chronic diarrhea and abdominal pain, except that it is occurring in a CGD patient. Instrumentation and biopsy should be done with caution but may be helpful in diagnosis. Because CGD patients are particularly susceptible to *Clostridium difficile*, this pathogen must be excluded as a cause of the problem. Genitourinary tract granulomata may present as bladder discomfort or pain or as acute bladder outlet obstruction. In this setting, surgical correction of the process should be avoided, because trauma may exacerbate the process. For both the gastrointestinal and the genitourinary obstructive granulomatous processes, if no pathogen is identified, an empirical course of antibiotics is recommended, together with starting a course of steroids. There is probably only a slightly increased infection risk associated with steroid use, but patients should be monitored closely. A dose in the range of 0.5 to at most 1 mg/kg of prednisone daily for 2 weeks is recommended, followed by a taper because CGD obstructive granulomata are often responsive to steroids.[301, 302] The taper should aim at rapidly progressing to an alternate-day regimen, when no steroid is administered on one of the days. The taper can then be extended for several weeks. A patient may rarely need a repeated course or even require long-term alternate-day low doses to prevent repeated obstruction. Sometimes only extraordinarily low alternate-day dosing is required to prevent the problem. In the case of CGD-related colitis with chronic diarrhea, if *C. difficile* is ruled out, a prolonged empirical course of a combination of metronidazole and ciprofloxacin is recommended. This may be combined after a while with a course of steroids in the manner indicated before. In about two thirds of cases, this will control the colitis. For the others, this may remain a prolonged intractable problem, often of greater concern to the patient than infection. There is one report of the successful use of cyclosporine in this setting.[300]

FUTURE PROSPECTS FOR BONE MARROW TRANSPLANTATION AND GENE THERAPY

Bone marrow transplantation has been performed for CGD,[264, 319, 327–329] and successful engraftment can result in permanent cure of the disorder. Complications of the procedure have included failure of the graft, graft-versus-host disease, and fatal progression of infection present at the time of transplantation. Long-term follow-up data with regard to late complications are generally not available with respect to the "cured" patients. The availability of a human leukocyte antigen–identical matched donor is correlated with much better outcome, and transplantation should be a consideration for a CGD patient when such a donor is available. On balance, the risks of bone marrow transplantation when there is no fully human leukocyte antigen–identical donor appear to be greater than with conventional therapy. Advances in transplantation procedures may change this equation and make this approach a more general consideration for CGD patients.

As noted before, bone marrow transplantation can cure CGD, and the genes for all four genetic forms of CGD have been cloned. This has raised the theoretical possibility of developing gene therapy for CGD by targeting hematopoietic progenitor cells from CGD with the normal oxidase gene. Despite this promise of gene therapy for the future of medicine in general and CGD in particular, as of this writing, no gene therapy technique has been developed to a degree that unequivocal clinical benefit to any patient for any disease process has been demonstrated. A large number of studies have been reported in which virus or plasmid gene transfer vectors have been used to correct the CGD phenotype in tissue culture. The target cells have been cultured lines from CGD patients, cell lines engineered to have the CGD defect, and primary hematopoietic cells from CGD patients.[330–343] In addition, mouse models of both the X-linked form and the p47phox-deficient autosomal recessive form of CGD have been created and used for gene transfer studies.[318, 344–346] In the mouse model, prolonged but not permanent partial correction of the CGD phenotype with enhancement of resistance to infection has been demonstrated.[346] Engraftment in the mouse model did require radiation-based bone marrow conditioning. Preliminary results of a phase I human clinical trial of gene therapy for the p47phox-deficient form of CGD have been reported in abstract form.[347] This trial involved a single cycle of retrovirus-mediated gene transfer into autologous hematopoietic $CD34^+$ progenitor cells cultured short term ex vivo and then reinfused without any prior conditioning of the recipient to suppress bone marrow. After this infusion of gene-corrected autologous hematopoietic progenitors, small numbers of oxidase-positive granulocytes were detected in the peripheral blood at a level of 1 in 2000 to 1 in 30,000 granulocytes for up to 6 months. Although this is an encouraging demonstration of feasibility, it points out that considerable further development of gene therapy techniques is required before any clinical benefit from this technique can be expected.

References

1. Cline MJ: The White Cell. Cambridge, MA, Harvard University Press, 1975, pp 1–221.
2. Gallin JI, Goldstein IM, Snyderman R (eds): Inflammation: Basic Principles and Clinical Correlates. New York, Raven Press, 1988.
3. Altman AJ, Stossel TP: Functional immaturity of bone marrow bands and polymorphonuclear leucocytes. Br J Haematol 27:241, 1974.
4. Berkow RL, Dodson RW: Purification and functional evaluation of mature neutrophils from bone marrow. Blood 68:853, 1986.
5. Bainton DF, Ullyot JL, Farquhar MG: The development of neutrophilic polymorphonuclear leukocytes in human bone marrow. Origin and content of azurophil and specific granules. J Exp Med 134:907, 1971.
6. Ganz T, Selsted ME, Szklarek D, et al: Defensins: Natural peptide antibiotics of human neutrophils. J Clin Invest 76:1427, 1985.
7. Weiss J, Victor M, Elsbach P: Role of charge and hydrophobic interactions in the action of the bactericidal/permeability increasing protein of neutrophils on gram-negative bacteria. J Clin Invest 71:540, 1983.
8. Campanelli D, Detmers PA, Nathan CF, Gabay JE: Azurocidin and a homologous serine protease from neutrophils. Differential antimicrobial and proteolytic properties. J Clin Invest 85:904, 1990.
9. Shafer WM, Onunka VC, Martin LE: Antigonococcal activity of human neutrophil cathepsin G. Infect Immun 54:184, 1986.
10. Pohl J, Pereira HA, Martin NM, Spitznagel JK: Amino acid sequence of CAP37, a human neutrophil granule–derived antibacterial and monocyte-specific chemotactic glycoprotein structurally similar to neutrophil elastase. FEBS Lett 272:200, 1990.
11. Pereira HA, Spitznagel JK, Winton EF, et al: The ontogeny of a 57-Kd cationic antimicrobial protein of human polymorphonuclear leukocytes: Localization to a novel granule population. Blood 76:825, 1990.
12. Johnson KR, Nauseef WM, Care A, et al: Characterization of cDNA clones for human myeloperoxidase: Predicted amino acid sequence and evidence for multiple mRNA species. Nucleic Acids Res 15:2013, 1987.
13. Rado TA, Wei X, Benz EJ Jr: Isolation of lactoferrin cDNA from a human myeloid library and expression of mRNA during normal and leukemic myelopoiesis. Blood 70:989, 1987.
14. Johnston J, Bollekens J, Allen RH, Berliner N: Structure of the cDNA encoding transcobalamin I, a neutrophil granule protein. J Biol Chem 264:15754, 1989.
15. Hasty KA, Pourmotabbed TF, Goldberg GI, et al: Human neutrophil collagenase. A distinct gene product with homology to other matrix metalloproteinases. J Biol Chem 265:11421, 1990.
16. Sklar A, Jesaitis AJ, Painter RG: The neutrophil *N*-formyl peptide receptor: Dynamics of ligand-receptor interactions and their relationship to cellular responses. Contemp Top Immunobiol 14:29, 1984.
17. Fletcher MP, Gallin JI: Human neutrophils contain an intracellular pool of putative receptors for the chemoattractant *N*-formyl methionylleucylphenylalanine with a density of specific granules. J Cell Biol 95:444a, 1982.
18. Wright SD, Meyer BC: Phorbol esters cause sequential activation and deactivation of complement receptors on polymorphonuclear leukocytes. J Immunol 136:1759, 1986.
19. Jesaitis AJ, Buescher ES, Harrison D, et al: Ultrastructural local-

ization of cytochrome b in the membranes of resting and phagocytosing human granulocytes. J Clin Invest 85:821, 1990.
20. Yoon PS, Boxer LA, Mayo LA, et al: Human neutrophil laminin receptors: Activation-dependent receptor expression. J Immunol 138:259,1987.
21. Borregaard N, Miller LJ, Springer TA: Chemoattractant-regulated mobilization of a novel intracellular compartment in human neutrophils. Science 237:1204, 1987.
22. Petrequin PR, Todd RF, Devall LJ, et al: Association between gelatinase release and increased plasma membrane expression of the Mo-1 glycoprotein. Blood 69:605, 1987.
23. Deward B, Bretz U, Baggiolini M: Release of gelatinase from a novel secretory compartment of human neutrophils. J Clin Invest 70:518, 1982.
24. White MV, Kaplan AP, Haak-Frendscho M, Kaliner M: Neutrophils and mast cells. Comparison of neutrophil-derived histamine-releasing activity with other histamine-releasing factors. J Immunol 141:3575, 1988.
25. Marucha PT, Zeff RA, Kreutzer DL: Cytokine regulation of IL-1 beta gene expression in the human polymorphonuclear leukocyte. J Immunol 145:2932, 1990.
26. Malech HL, Root RK, Gallin JI: Structural analysis of human neutrophil migration: Centriole, microtubule and microfilament orientation and function during chemotaxis. J Cell Biol 75:666, 1977.
27. Stossel TP: From signal to pseudopod: How cells control cytoplasmic actin assembly. J Biol Chem 264:18261, 1989.
28. Rothwell SW, Nath JI, Wright DG: Interactions of cytoplasmic granules with microtubules in human neutrophils. J Cell Biol 108:2313, 1989.
29. Allan RB, Wilkinson PC: A visual analysis of chemotactic and chemokinetic locomotion of human neutrophil leukocytes. Exp Cell Res 111:191, 1978.
30. Malech HL: Phagocytic cells: Egress from marrow and diapedesis. *In* Gallin JI, Goldstein IM, Synderman R (eds): Inflammation: Basic Principles and Clinical Correlates. New York, Raven Press, 1988, pp 297–308.
31. Athens JW, Haab OP, Raab SO, et al: Leukokinetic studies. IV. The total blood, circulatory and marginal pools and the granulocyte turnover rate in normal subjects. J Clin Invest 40:989, 1961.
32. Krause PJ, Maderazo EG, Bannon P, et al: Neutrophil heterogeneity in patients with blunt trauma. J Lab Clin Med 112:208, 1988.
33. Brown CC, Malech HL, Gallin JI: Intravenous endotoxin recruits a distinct subset of human neutrophils, defined by monoclonal antibody 31D8, from bone marrow to peripheral circulation. Cell Immunol 123:294, 1989.
34. Snyderman R, Uhing RI: Chemoattractant stimulus-response coupling. *In* Gallin JI, Goldstein IM, Snyderman R (eds): Inflammation: Basic Principles and Clinical Correlates, ed 2. New York, Raven Press, 1992, pp 421–440.
35. Goldman DW, Gifford LA, Marotti T, et al: Molecular and cellular properties of human polymorphonuclear leukocyte receptors for leukotriene B_4. Fed Proc 46:200, 1987.
36. Chenowith EE, Hugli TE: Demonstration of specific C5a receptors on intact human polymorphonuclear leukocytes. Proc Natl Acad Sci USA 75:3943, 1978.
37. Williams LT, Snyderman R, Pike MC, Lefkowitz RJ: Specific receptor sites for chemotactic peptides on human polymorphonuclear leukocytes. Proc Natl Acad Sci USA 74:1204, 1977.
38. Niedel J, Kahane I, Cuatrecasas P: Receptor-mediated internalization of fluorescent chemotactic peptide by human neutrophils. Science 205:1412, 1979.
39. Koo C, Lefkowitz RJ, Snyderman R: The oligopeptide chemotactic factor receptor on human polymorphonuclear leukocyte membranes exists in two affinity states. Biochem Biophys Res Commun 106:442, 1982.
40. Snyderman R, Smith CD, Verghese MW: Model for leukocyte regulation by chemoattractant receptors: Role of a guanine nucleotide regulatory protein and polyphosphoinositide metabolism. J Leukoc Biol 40:785, 1986.
41. Koo C, Lefkowitz RJ, Snyderman R: Guanine nucleotides modulate the binding affinity of the oligopeptide chemoattractant receptor on human polymorphonuclear leukocytes. J Clin Invest 72:748, 1983.
42. Majerus PW, Connolly TM, Deckmyn H, et al: The metabolism of phosphoinositide-derived messenger molecules. Science 234:1519, 1986.
43. O'Flaherty JT, Schmitt JD, McCall CE, Wykle RL: Diacylglycerols enhance human neutrophil degranulation responses: Relevancy to a multiple mediator hypothesis of cell function. Biochem Biophys Res Commun 123:64, 1984.
44. Dougherty RW, Godfrey PP, Hoyle PC, et al: Secretagogue-induced phosphoinositide metabolism in human leucocytes. Biochem J 222:307, 1984.
45. Prentki M, Wollheim CG, Lew PD: Ca^{2+} homeostasis in permeabilized human neutrophils: Characterization of Ca^{2+}-sequestering pools and the action of inositol 1,4,5-triphosphate. J Biol Chem 259:13777, 1984.
46. Klempner MS: An adenosine triphosphate–dependent calcium uptake pump in human neutrophil lysosomes. J Clin Invest 76:303, 1985.
47. Bradford PG, Rubin RP: Quantitative changes in inositol 1,4,5-triphosphate in chemoattractant-stimulated neutrophils. J Biol Chem 261:15644, 1986.
48. Verghese MW, Fox K, McPhail LC, Snyderman R: Chemoattractant-elicited alterations of cAMP levels in human polymorphonuclear leukocytes require a Ca^{++}-dependent mechanism which is independent of transmembrane activation of adenylate cyclase. J Biol Chem 260:6769, 1985.
49. Albelda SM, Buck CA: Integrins and other cell adhesion molecules. FASEB J 4:2868, 1990.
50. Springer TA: Traffic signals for lymphocyte recirculation and leukocyte emigration: The multistep paradigm. Cell 76:301, 1994.
51. Springer TA: Traffic signals on endothelium for lymphocyte recirculation and leukocyte emigration. Annu Rev Physiol 57:827, 1995.
52. Rosen SD: Cell surface lectins in the immune system. Semin Immunol 5:237, 1993.
53. Bevilacqua MP: Endothelial-leukocyte adhesion molecules. Annu Rev Immunol 11:767, 1993.
54. Berg EL, Magnani J, Warnock RA, et al: Comparison of L-selectin and E-selectin ligand specificities: The L-selectin can bind the E-selectin ligands sialyl Le(x) and sialyl Le(a). Biochem Biophys Res Commun 184:1048, 1992.
55. Moore KL, Stults NL, Diaz S, et al: Identification of a specific glycoprotein ligand for P-selectin (CD62) on myeloid cells. J Cell Biol 118:445, 1992.
56. Sako D, Chang XJ, Barone KM, et al: Expression cloning of a functional glycoprotein ligand for P-selectin. Cell 75:1179, 1993.
57. Sanchez-Madrid F, Nagy JA, Robbins E, et al: A human leukocyte differentiation antigen family with distinct alpha-subunits and a common beta-subunit: The lymphocyte function–associated antigen (LFA-1), the C3bi complement receptor (OKM1/Mac-1), and the p150,95 molecule. J Exp Med 158:1785, 1983.
58. Marlin SD, Morton CC, Anderson DC, Springer TA: LFA-1 immunodeficiency disease: Definition of the genetic defect and chromosomal mapping of alpha and beta subunits by complementation in hybrid cells. J Exp Med 164:855, 1986.
59. Rothlein R, Dustin ML, Marlin SD, Springer TA: A human intercellular adhesion molecule (ICAM-1) distinct from LFA-1. J Immunol 137:1270, 1986.
60. Bevilacqua MP, Stengalin S, Gimbrone MA, Seed B: Endothelial leukocyte adhesion molecule 1, an inducible receptor for neutrophils related to complement regulatory proteins and lectins. Science 243:1160, 1989.
61. Johnson GI, Cook RG, McEver RP: Cloning of GMP-140, a granule membrane protein of platelets and endothelium: Sequence similarity to proteins involved in cell adhesion and inflammation. Cell 56:1033, 1989.
62. Dustin ML, Rothlein R, Bhan AK, et al: Induction by IL-1 and interferon-gamma: Tissue distribution, biochemistry and function of a natural adherence molecule (ICAM-1). J Immunol 137:245, 1986.
63. Diamond MS, Springer TA: A subpopulation of Mac-1 (CD11b/CD18) molecules mediates neutrophil adhesion to ICAM-1 and fibrinogen. J Cell Biol 120:545, 1993.
64. Marchesi VT, Florey HW: Electron micrographic observations on the emigration of leucocytes. Q J Exp Physiol 45:343, 1960.

65. Wright DG, Gallin JI: Secretory responses of human neutrophils: Exocytosis of specific (secondary) granules by human neutrophils during adherence in vitro and during exudation *in vivo*. J Immunol 123:285, 1979.
66. Peveri P, Walz A, Dewald B, Baggiolini M: A novel neutrophil-activating factor produced by human mononuclear phagocytes. J Exp Med 167:1547, 1988.
67. Goetzl EJ, Derian CK, Tauber AI, Valone FH: Novel effects of 1-*O*-hexadecyl-2-acyl-*sn*-glycero-3-phosphorylcholine mediators on human leukocyte function: Delineation of the specific roles of the acyl substituents. Biochem Biophys Res Commun 94:881, 1980.
68. Janmey PA, Hvidt S, Peetermans J, et al: Viscoelasticity of F-actin and F-actin/gelsolin complexes. Biochemistry 27:8218, 1988.
69. Lind SE, Janmey PA, Chaponnier C, et al: Reversible binding of actin to gelsolin and profilin in human platelet extracts. J Cell Biol 105:833, 1987.
70. Lassing I, Lindberg U: Specific interaction between phosphatidylinositol 4,5-bisphosphate and profilactin. Nature 314:472, 1985.
71. Hartwig JH, Chambers KA, Stossel TP: Association of gelsolin with actin filaments and cell membranes of macrophages and platelets. J Cell Biol 108:469, 1989.
72. Yin HL, Stossel TP: Purification and structural properties of gelsolin, a Ca^{2+}-activated regulatory protein of macrophages. J Cell Biol 255:9490, 1980.
73. Janmey PA, Ida K, Yin HL, Stossel TP: Polyphosphoinositide micelles and polyphosphoinositide-containing vesicles dissociate endogenous gelsolin-actin complex and promote actin assembly from the fast-growing end of actin filaments blocked by gelsolin. J Biol Chem 262:12228, 1987.
74. Hartwig JH, Shevlin PA: The architecture of actin filaments and the ultrastructural location of actin-binding protein in the periphery of lung macrophages. J Cell Biol 103:1007, 1986.
75. Gorlin JB, Yamin R, Egan S, et al: Human endothelial actin-binding protein (ABP-280, nonmuscle filamin): A molecular leaf spring. J Cell Biol 111:1089, 1990.
76. Anderson CL: Isolation of the receptor for IgG from a human monocyte cell line (U937) and from human peripheral blood monocytes. J Exp Med 156:1794, 1982.
77. Anderson CL, Spence JM, Edwards TS, Nusbacher J: Characterization of a polyvalent antibody directed against the IgG Fc receptor of human mononuclear phagocytes. J Immunol 134:465, 1985.
78. Shen L, Guyre PM, Anderson CL, Fanger MW: Heteroantibody-mediated cytotoxicity: Antibody to the high affinity Fc receptor for IgG mediates cytotoxicity by human monocytes that is enhanced by interferon-gamma and is not blocked by human IgG. J Immunol 137:3378, 1986.
79. Fleit HB, Wright SD, Unkeless JC: Human neutrophil Fc gamma receptor distribution and structure. Proc Natl Acad Sci USA 79:3275, 1982.
80. Kurlander RJ, Batker J: The binding of human immunoglobulin G1 monomer and small, covalently cross-linked polymers of immunoglobulin G1 to human peripheral blood monocytes and polymorphonuclear leukocytes. J Clin Invest 69:1, 1982.
81. Kulczycki A Jr: Human neutrophils and eosinophils have structurally distinct Fc receptors. J Immunol 133:849, 1984.
82. Klempner MS, Gallin JI: Separation and functional characterization of human neutrophil subpopulations. Blood 4:659, 1978.
83. Fearon DT: Identification of the membrane glycoprotein that is the C3b receptor of the human erythrocyte, polymorphonuclear leukocyte, B lymphocyte, and monocyte. J Exp Med 152:20, 1980.
84. Bullock WE, Wright SD: The role of adherence-promoting receptors, CR3, LFA-1, and p150,95 in binding of *Histoplasma capsulatum* by human macrophages. J Exp Med 165:195, 1987.
85. Wright SD, Jong MTC: Adhesion-promoting receptors on human macrophages recognize *E. coli* by binding to lipopolysaccharide. J Exp Med 164:1876, 1986.
86. Wright SD, Griffin FM Jr: Activation of phagocytic cells' C3 receptors for phagocytosis. J Leukoc Biol 38:327, 1985.
87. Young JD, Unkeless JC, Young TM, et al: Mouse macrophage Fc receptor for IgG gamma 2b/gamma 1 in artificial and plasma membrane vesicles functions as a ligand-dependent ionophore. Proc Natl Acad Sci USA 80:1636, 1983.
88. Joiner KA, Fuhrman SA, Miettinen HM, et al: *Toxoplasma gondii*: Fusion competence of parasitophorous vacuoles in Fc receptor–transfected fibroblasts. Science 249:641, 1990.
89. Griffin FM, Griffin JA, Leider JE, et al: Studies on the mechanism of phagocytosis. I. Requirements for circumferential attachment of particle bound ligands to specific receptors on the macrophage plasma membrane. J Exp Med 142:1263, 1975.
90. Spitznagel JK: Non-oxidative antimicrobial reactions of leukocytes. Contemp Top Immunobiol 14:283, 1984.
91. Weiss J, Elsbach P, Wolsson I, Odeberg H: Purification and characterization of a potent bactericidal and membrane-active protein from the granules of human polymorphonuclear leukocytes. J Biol Chem 235:2664, 1978.
92. Elsbach P, Weiss J: A reevaluation of the roles of the O_2-dependent and O_2-independent microbicidal systems of phagocytes. Rev Infect Dis 5:843, 1983.
93. Elsbach P, Weiss J: Oxygen-independent antimicrobial systems. *In* Gallin JI, Goldstein IM, Snyderman R (eds): Inflammation: Basic Principles and Clinical Correlates. New York, Raven Press, 1988, pp 445–470.
94. Ganz T, Selsted ME, Lehrer RI: Defensins. Eur J Haematol 44:1, 1990.
95. Ganz T, Selsted ME, Szklarek D, et al: Natural peptide antibiotics of human neutrophils. J Clin Invest 76:1427, 1985.
96. Lehrer RI, Barton A, Daher KA, et al: Interaction of human defensins with *E. coli*. Mechanism of bactericidal action. J Clin Invest 84:553, 1989.
97. Klebanoff SJ: Phagocytic cells: Products of oxygen metabolism. *In* Gallin JI, Goldstein IM, and Snyderman R (eds): Inflammation: Basic Principles and Clinical Correlates. New York, Raven Press, 1988, pp 297–308.
98. Segal AW: The electron transport chain of the microbicidal oxidase of phagocytic cells and its involvement in the molecular pathology of chronic granulomatous disease. J Clin Invest 83:1785, 1989.
99. Lomax KJ, Leto TL, Nunoi H, et al: Recombinant 47-kD cytosol factor restores NADPH oxidase in chronic granulomatous disease [published erratum in Science 246:987, 1989]. Science 245:409, 1989.
100. Leto TL, Lomax KJ, Volpp BD, et al: Cloning of a 67K neutrophil oxidase factor with similarity to a noncatalytic region of $p60^{c\text{-}src}$. Science 248:727, 1990.
101. Nunoi H, Rotrosen D, Gallin JI, Malech HL: Two forms of autosomal chronic granulomatous disease lack distinct neutrophil cytosol factors. Science 242:1298, 1988.
102. Abo A, Pick E, Hall A, et al: Activation of the NADPH oxidase involves the small GTP-binding protein p21rac1. Nature 353:668, 1991.
103. Knaus UG, Heyworth PG, Evans T, et al: Regulation of phagocyte oxygen radical production by the GTP-binding protein Rac2. Science 254:1512, 1991.
104. Kwong CH, Malech HL, Rotrosen D, Leto TL: Regulation of the human neutrophil NADPH oxidase by rho-related G-proteins. Biochemistry 32:5711, 1993.
105. Clark RA, Volpp BD, Leidal KG, Nauseef WM: Two cytosolic components of the human neutrophil respiratory burst oxidase translocate to the plasma membrane during cell activation. J Clin Invest 85:714, 1990.
106. Malech HL: Phagocyte oxidative mechanisms. Curr Opin Hematol 1993 1:123, 1993.
107. Diekmann D, Abo A, Johnston C, et al: Interaction of Rac with p67phox and regulation of phagocytic NADPH oxidase activity. Science 265:531, 1994.
108. de Mendez I, Adams AG, Sokolic RA, et al: Multiple SH3 domain interactions regulate NADPH oxidase assembly in whole cells. EMBO J 15:1221, 1996.
109. Cross AR, Jones OT, Harper AM, Segal AW: Oxidation-reduction properties of the cytochrome *b* found in the plasma-membrane fraction of human neutrophils: A possible oxidase in the respiratory burst. Biochem J 194:599, 1981.
110. Rotrosen D, Yeung CL, Leto, TL, et al: Cytochrome *b*558: The flavin-binding component of the phagocyte NADPH oxidase. Science 256:1459, 1992.
111. Abo A, Boyhan A, West I, et al: Reconstitution of neutrophil NADPH oxidase activity in the cell-free system by four components: p67-phox, p47-phox, p21rac1, and cytochrome *b*-245. J Biol Chem 267:16767, 1992.

112. Rotrosen D, Kleinberg ME, Nunoi H, et al: Evidence for a functional cytoplasmic domain of phagocyte oxidase cytochrome *b*558. J Biol Chem 265:8745, 1990.
113. Kleinberg ME, Malech HL, Rotrosen D: The phagocyte 47 kilodalton cytosolic oxidase protein is an early reactant in the activation of the respiratory burst. J Biol Chem 265:15577, 1990.
114. Harper AM, Dunne MJ, Segal AW: Purification of cytochrome *b*-245 from human neutrophils. Biochem J 219:519, 1984.
115. Parkos CA, Allen RA, Cochrane CG, Jesaitis AJ: The purified cytochrome b from human granulocyte plasma membrane is composed of two polypeptides with relative molecular weights of 91,000 and 22,000. J Clin Invest 80:732, 1987.
116. Kleinberg ME, Rotrosen D, Malech HL: Asparagine-linked glycosylation of cytochrome b_{558} large subunit varies in different human phagocytic cells. J Immunol 143:4152, 1989.
117. Royer-Pokora B, Kunkel LM, Monaco AP, et al: Cloning the gene for an inherited human disorder—chronic granulomatous disease—on the basis of its chromosome location. Nature 322:32, 1986.
118. Dinauer MC, Orkin SH, Brown R, et al: The glycoprotein encoded by the X-linked chronic granulomatous disease locus is a component of the neutrophil cytochrome *b* complex. Nature 327:717, 1987.
119. Teahan C, Rowe P, Parker P, et al: The X-linked chronic granulomatous disease gene codes for the beta-chain of cytochrome *b*-245. Nature 327:720, 1987.
120. Cross AR, Rae J, Curnutte JT: Cytochrome *b*-245 of the neutrophil superoxide-generating system contains two nonidentical hemes. Potentiometric studies of a mutant form of gp91phox. J Biol Chem 270:17075, 1995.
121. McPhail LC, Qualliotine-Mann D, Agwu DE, McCall CE: Phospholipases and activation of the NADPH oxidase. Eur J Haematol 51:294, 1993.
122. McPhail LC, Qualliotine-Mann D, Waite KA: Cell-free activation of neutrophil NADPH oxidase by a phosphatidic acid–regulated protein kinase. Proc Natl Acad Sci USA 92:7931, 1995.
123. Umeda T, Hara T, Hayashida M, Niijima T: Role of hydroxyl radical in neutrophil-mediated cytotoxicity. Cell Mol Biol 31:229, 1985.
124. Fox RB: Prevention of granulocyte-mediated oxidant lung injury in rats by a hydroxyl radical scavenger dimethyl thiourea. J Clin Invest 74:1456, 1984.
125. Hatherill JR, Till GO, Bruner LH, Ward PA: Thermal injury, intravascular hemolysis, and toxic oxygen products. J Clin Invest 78:629, 1986.
126. Britigan BE, Hassett DJ, Rosen GM, et al: Neutrophil degranulation inhibits potential hydroxyl-radical formation. Relative impact of myeloperoxidase and lactoferrin release on hydroxyl-radical production by iron-supplemented neutrophils assessed by spin-trapping techniques. Biochem J 264:447, 1989.
127. Malech HL, Gallin JI: Neutrophils in human diseases. N Engl J Med 317:687, 1987.
128. Zacharsk LKR, Elveback LR, Linman JW: Leukocyte counts in healthy adults. Am J Clin Pathol 56:148, 1971.
129. Hughes WT, Armstrong D, Bodey GP, et al: Guidelines for the use of antimicrobial agents in neutropenic patients with unexplained fever. J Infect Dis 161:381, 1990.
130. Bodey GP, Buckley M, Sathe YS, Freireich EJ: Quantitative relationships between circulating leukocytes and infections in patients with acute leukemia. Ann Intern Med 64:328, 1966.
131. Dale DC, Guerry D, Wewerka IV Jr, et al: Chronic neutropenia. Medicine (Baltimore) 58:128, 1979.
132. Russin SJ, Fillipo BH, Adler AG: Neutropenia in adults. What is its clinical significance? Postgrad Med 88:209, 1990.
133. Claas FHJ: Drug-induced immune granulocytopenia. Baillieres Clin Immunol Allergy 1:357, 1987.
134. Murphy MF, Riordan T, Minchinton RM, et al: Demonstration of an immune-mediated mechanism of penicillin-induced neutropenia and thrombocytopenia. Br J Haematol 55:155, 1983.
135. Murphy MF, Metcalfe P, Grint PCA, et al: Cephalosporin-induced immune neutropenia. Br J Haematol 59:9, 1985.
136. Gordon-Smith EC: Aplastic anaemia—Aetiology and clinical features. Baillieres Clin Haematol 2:1, 1989.
137. International Agranulocytosis and Aplastic Anemia Study: Risks of agranulocytosis and aplastic anemia: A first report of their relation to drug use with special reference to analgesics. JAMA 256:1749, 1986.
138. Lalezari P, Khorshidi M, Petrosova M: Autoimmune neutropenia of infancy. J Pediatr 109:764, 1986.
139. McCullough J, Clay ME, Thompson HW: Autoimmune granulocytopenia. Baillieres Clin Immunol Allergy 1:303, 1987.
140. Kurtzman G, Young N: Viruses and bone marrow failure. Baillieres Clin Haematol 2:51, 1989.
141. Murphy MF, Metcalfe P, Waters AH, et al: Incidence and mechanisms of neutropenia and thrombocytopenia in patients with human immunodeficiency virus infection. Br J Haematol 66:337, 1987.
142. Wright DG, Dale DC, Fauci AS, Wolff SM: Human cyclic neutropenia. Clinical review and long term follow-up of patients. Medicine (Baltimore) 60:1, 1981.
143. Dale DC, Hammond WP IV: Cyclic neutropenia: A clinical review. Blood Rev 2:178, 1988.
144. Lange RD, Jones JB: Cyclic neutropenia: Review of clinical manifestations and management. Am J Pediatr Hematol Oncol 3:363, 1987.
145. Loughran TP Jr, Hammond WP IV: Adult-onset cyclic neutropenia is a benign neoplasm associated with clonal proliferation of large granular lymphocytes. J Exp Med 164:2089, 1986.
146. Kostmann R: Infantile genetic agranulocytosis. A review with presentation of ten new cases. Acta Paediatr Scand 64:362, 1975.
147. O'Regan S, Newman AJ, Graham RC: Myelokathexis: Neutropenia with marrow hyperplasia. Am J Dis Child 131:655, 1977.
148. Wetzler M, Talpaz M, Kleinerman ES, et al: A new familial immunodeficiency disorder characterized by severe neutropenia, a defective marrow release mechanism, and hypogammaglobulinemia. Am J Med 89:663, 1990.
149. Miller ME, Oski FA, Harris MB: Lazy-leukocyte syndrome. Lancet 1:665, 1971.
150. Woods WG, Roloff JS, Lukens JN, Krivit W: The occurrence of leukemia in patients with the Shwachman syndrome. J Pediatr 99:425, 1981.
151. Roper M, Parmley RT, Crist WM, et al: Severe congenital leukopenia (reticular dysgenesis). Am J Dis Child 139:832, 1985.
152. Evans DIK: Congenital defects of the marrow stem cell. Baillieres Clin Haematol 2:163, 1989.
153. Lalezari P: Alloimmune neonatal neutropenia. Baillieres Clin Immunol Allergy 1:443, 1987.
154. Madyastha PR, Glassman AB: Neutrophil antigens and antibodies in the diagnosis of immune neutropenias. Ann Clin Lab Sci 19:146, 1989.
155. Wolff SM, Rubenstein M, Mulholland JH, Alling DW: Comparison of hematologic and febrile response to endotoxin in man. Blood 26:190, 1965.
156. Christensen RD, Rothstein G: Exhaustion of mature marrow neutrophils in neonates with sepsis. J Pediatr 96:316, 1980.
157. Pizzo P: Granulocytopenia and cancer chemotherapy. Past problems, current solutions, future challenges. Cancer 54(Suppl 1):2649, 1984.
158. Bow EJ, Rayner E, Louie TJ: Comparison of norfloxacin with cotrimazole for infectious prophylaxis in acute leukemia. Am J Med 84:847, 1988.
159. Dekker A, Rozenberg-Arska M, Verhoef J: Infection prophylaxis in acute leukemia: A comparison of ciprofloxacin with trimethoprim-sulfamethoxazole and colistin. Ann Intern Med 106:7, 1987.
160. Hughes WT, Kuhn S, Chaudhary S, et al: Successful chemoprophylaxis for *Pneumocystis carinii* pneumonitis. N Engl J Med 297:1419, 1977.
161. Nauseef WM, Maki DG: A study of the value of simple protective isolation in patients with granulocytopenia. N Engl J Med 304:448, 1981.
162. Glenn J, Funkhouser WK, Schneider PS: Acute illnesses necessitating urgent abdominal surgery in neutropenic cancer patients: Description of 14 cases and review of the literature. Surgery 105:778, 1989.
163. Young LS: Neutropenia: Antibiotic combinations for empiric therapy. Eur J Clin Microbiol Infect Dis 8:118, 1989.
164. Pizzo PA, Hathorn JW, Hiemenz J, et al: A randomized trial comparing ceftazidime alone with combination antibiotic therapy in cancer patients with fever and neutropenia. N Engl J Med 315:552, 1986.
165. Pizzo PA, Robichaud KJ, Gill FA, et al: Duration of empiric antibiotic therapy in granulocytopenic patients with cancer. Am J Med 67:194, 1979.

166. Alavi JB, Root RK, Djerassi I, et al: A randomized clinical trial of granulocyte transfusions for infection in acute leukemia. N Engl J Med 296:706, 1977.
167. Groopman JE, Molina J-M, Scadden DT: Hematopoietic growth factors. Biology and clinical applications. N Engl J Med 321:1449, 1989.
168. Mitsuyasu RT, Golde DW: Clinical role of granulocyte-macrophage colony stimulating factor. Hematol Oncol Clin North Am 3:411, 1989.
169. Gabrilove JL, Jakubowski A: Granulocyte colony-stimulating factor: Preclinical and clinical studies. Hematol Oncol Clin North Am 3:427, 1989.
170. Yang Y-C, Clark SC: Interleukin-3: Molecular biology and biologic activities. Hematol Oncol Clin North Am 3:441, 1989.
171. Garnick MB, O'Reilly RJ: Clinical promise of new hematopoietic growth factors: M-CSF, IL-3, IL-6. Hematol Oncol Clin North Am 3:495, 1989.
172. Witte ON: Steel locus defines new multipotent growth factor. Cell 63:5, 1990.
173. Zsebo KM, Wypych J, McNiece IK, et al: Identification, purification, and biological characterization of hematopoietic stem cell factor from buffalo rat liver–conditioned medium. Cell 63:195, 1990.
174. Martin FH, Suggs SV, Langley KE, et al: Primary structure and functional expression of rat and human stem cell factor DNAs. Cell 63:203, 1990.
175. Zsebo KM, Williams DA, Geissler EN, et al: Stem cell factor is encoded at the S1 locus of the mouse and is the ligand for the c-kit tyrosine kinase receptor. Cell 63:213, 1990.
176. Gillio AP, Gasparetto C, Laver J, et al: Effects of interleukin-3 on hematopoietic recovery after 5-fluorouracil or cyclophosphamide treatment of cynomolgus primates. J Clin Invest 85:1560, 1990.
177. Weisbart RH, Golde DW: Physiology of granulocyte and macrophage colony-stimulating factors in host defense. Hematol Oncol Clin North Am 3:401, 1989.
178. Adachi S, Kubota M, Lin YW, et al: In vivo administration of granulocyte colony stimulating factor promotes neutrophil survival in vitro. Eur J Haematol 53:129, 1994.
179. Liles WC, Dale DC, Klebanoff SJ: Glucocorticoids inhibit apoptosis of human neutrophils. Blood 86:3181, 1995.
180. Rex JH, Bhalla SC, Cohen DM, et al: Protection of human polymorphonuclear leukocyte function from the deleterious effects of isolation, irradiation, and storage by interferon-gamma and granulocyte-colony-stimulating factor. Transfusion 35:605, 1995.
181. Daifuku R, Andresen J, Morstyn G: Recombinant methionyl human granulocyte colony-stimulating factor for the prevention and treatment of non-neutropenic infectious diseases. J Antimicrob Chemother 32(Suppl A):91, 1993.
182. Smith WS, Sumnicht GE, Sharpe RW, et al: Granulocyte colony-stimulating factor versus placebo in addition to penicillin G in a randomized blinded study of gram-negative pneumonia sepsis: Analysis of survival and multisystem organ failure. Blood 86:1301, 1995.
183. Andersson DC, Springer TA: Leukocyte adhesion deficiency: An inherited defect in the Mac-1, LFA-1 and p150,95 glycoproteins. Annu Rev Med 38:175, 1987.
184. Etzioni A, Frydman M, Pollack S, et al: Recurrent severe infections caused by a novel leukocyte adhesion deficiency. N Engl J Med 327:1789, 1992.
185. von Adrian UH, Berger EM, Ramezani L, et al: In vivo behavior of neutrophils from two patients with distinct inherited leukocyte adhesion deficiency syndromes. J Clin Invest 91:2893, 1993.
186. Kishimoto TK, Hollander N, Roberts TM, et al: Heterogeneous mutations in the beta subunit common to the LFA-1, Mac-1 and p150,95 glycoproteins cause leukocyte adhesion deficiency. Cell 50:193, 1987.
187. Lopez-Rodriguez C, Nueda A, Grospierre B, et al: Characterization of two new CD18 alleles causing severe leukocyte adhesion deficiency. Eur J Immunol 23:2792, 1993.
188. Back AL, Kerkering M, Baker D, et al: A point mutation associated with leukocyte adhesion deficiency type 1 of moderate severity. Biochem Biophys Res Commun 193:912, 1993.
189. Wright AH, Douglass WA, Taylor GM, et al: Molecular characterization of leukocyte adhesion deficiency in six patients. Eur J Immunol 25:717, 1995.
190. Andersson DC, Schmalstieg FC, Finegold MJ, et al: The severe and moderate phenotypes of heritable Mac-l, LFA-1 deficiency: Their quantitative definition and relation to leukocyte dysfunction and clinical features. J Infect Dis 152:668, 1985.
191. Nunoi H, Yanabe Y, Higuchi S, et al: Severe hypoplasia of lymphoid tissues in Mo 1 deficiency. Hum Pathol 19:753, 1988.
192. Crowley CA, Curnutte JT, Rossin RE, et al: An inherited abnormality of neutrophil adhesion: Its genetic transmission and its association with mining protein. N Engl J Med 302: 1163, 1980.
193. Anderson DC, Schmalstieg FC, Arnaout MA, et al: Abnormalities of polymorphonuclear leukocyte associated with a heritable deficiency of high molecular weight surface glycoproteins (GP138): Common relationship to diminish cell adherence. J Clin Invest 74:536, 1984.
194. Fischer A, Lisowska-Grospierre B, Anderson DC, Springer TA: Leukocyte adhesion deficiency: Molecular basis and functional consequences. Immunodef Rev 1:39, 1988.
195. Fischer A, Blanche S, Veber F, et al: Correction of immune disorders by HLA-matched and mismatched bone marrow transplantation. *In* Gale RP (ed): Recent Advances in Bone Marrow Transplantation. New York, Alan R Liss, 1987, pp 911–918.
196. Wilson JM, Ping AJ, Krauss JC, et al: Correction of CD-18 deficient lymphocytes by retrovirus-mediated gene transfer. Science 248:1413, 1990.
197. Yorifugi T, Wilson, RW, Beaudet AL: Retroviral mediated expression of CD18 in normal and deficient human bone marrow progenitor cells. Hum Mol Genet 2:1443, 1993.
198. Wilson RW, Yorifugi T, Lorenzo I, et al: Expression of human CD18 in murine granulocytes and improved efficiency for infection of deficient human lymphoblasts. Hum Gene Ther 4:25, 1993.
199. Gallin JI, Quie PG (eds): Leukocyte Chemotaxis: Methods, Physiology and Clinical Implications. New York, Raven Press, 1979.
200. Gallin JI: Disorders of phagocytic cells. *In* Gallin JI, Goldstein IM, Snyderman R (eds): Inflammation: Basic Principles and Clinical Correlates, ed 2. New York, Raven Press, 1992, pp 859–874.
201. Gallin JI, Clark RA, Kimball HR: Granulocyte chemotaxis: An improved assay employing 51-Cr–labelled granulocytes. J Immunol 110:233, 1973.
202. Capsoni F, Minonzio F, Ongari AM, Zanussi C: A new simplified single-filter assay for 'in vitro' evaluation of chemotaxis of 51 Cr–labeled polymorphonuclear leukocytes. J Immunol Methods 120:125, 1989.
203. Metcalf JA, Gallin JI, Nauseef WM, Root RK: Laboratory Manual of Neutrophil Function. New York, Raven Press, 1986.
204. Nelson RD, Quie PG, Simmons RL: Chemotaxis under agarose: A new and simple method for measuring chemotaxis and spontaneous migration of human polymorphonuclear leukocytes and monocytes. J Immunol 115:1650, 1975.
205. Terpstra GK, Hoube LA: Directional cellular movement of cell populations: Its description by chemotactic assays. Agents Actions 26:224, 1989.
206. Gallin JI, Fletcher MP, Seligmann BE, et al: Human neutrophil-specific granule deficiency: A model to assess the role of neutrophil-specific granules in the evolution of the inflammatory response. Blood 59:1317, 1982.
207. Boxer LA, Hedley-Whyte ET, Stossel TP: Neutrophil actin dysfunction and abnormal neutrophil behavior. N Engl J Med 291:1093, 1974.
208. Southwick FS, Howard TH, Holbrook T, et al: The relationship between CR3 deficiency and neutrophil actin assembly. Blood 73:1973, 1989.
209. Hill HR: Biochemical, structural and functional abnormalities of polymorphonuclear leukocytes in the neonate. Pediatr Res 22:375, 1987.
210. Donabedian H, Gallin JI: The hyperimmunoglobulin E recurrent-infection (Job's) syndrome. A review of the NIH experience and the literature. Medicine (Baltimore) 62:195, 1983.
211. Leung DY, Geha RS: Clinical and immunologic aspects of the hyperimmunoglobulin E syndrome. Hematol Oncol Clin North Am 2:81, 1988.
212. Klempner MS, Noring R, Mier JW, Atkins MB: An acquired chemotactic defect in neutrophils from patients receiving interleukin-2 immunotherapy. N Engl J Med 322:959, 1990.
213. Moy JN, Nelson RD, Richards KL, Hostetter MK: Identification

of an IgA inhibitor of neutrophil chemotaxis and its membrane target for the metabolic burst. Immunology, 69:257, 1990.
214. Siegbahn A, Venge P, Nilsson K: Cellular origin of the chemokinetic inhibitor of polymorphonuclear leucocytes found in sera from patients with chronic lymphocytic leukaemia. Scand J Haematol 31:184, 1983.
215. Maderazo EG, Albano SD, Woronick CL, et al: Polymorphonuclear leukocyte migration abnormalities and their significance in seriously traumatized patients. Ann Surg 198:736, 1983.
216. Blume RS, Wolff SM: The Chédiak-Higashi syndrome: Studies in four patients and a review of the literature. Medicine (Baltimore) 51:247, 1972.
217. Rausch PG, Pryzwansky KB, Spitznagel JK: Immunochemical characterization of Chédiak-Higashi neutrophils. N Engl J Med 298:693, 1978.
218. Prieur DJ, Collier LL: Animal models of human diseases: Chédiak-Higashi syndrome. Am J Pathol 90:533, 1978.
219. Haliotis T, Roder J, Klein M, et al: Chédiak-Higashi gene in humans. I. Impairment of natural killer function. J Exp Med 151:1039, 1980.
220. Root RK, Rosenthal AS, Balestra DJ: Abnormal bactericidal, metabolic, and lysosomal functions of Chédiak-Higashi syndrome leukocytes. J Clin Invest 51:649, 1972.
221. Clark RA, Kimball HR: Defective granulocyte chemotaxis in the Chédiak-Higashi svndrome. J Clin Invest 50:2465, 1971.
222. Perou CM, Kaplan J: Complementation analysis of Chédiak-Higashi syndrome: The same gene may be responsible for the defect in all patients and species. Somat Cell Mol Genet 19:459, 1993.
223. Perou CM, Moore KJ, Nagle DL, et al: Identification of the murine beige gene by YAC complementation and positional cloning. Nat Genet 13:303, 1996.
224. Barrat FJ, Auloge L, Pastural E, et al: Genetic and physical mapping of the Chédiak-Higashi syndrome on chromosome 1q42-43. Am J Hum Genet 59:625, 1996.
225. Dale DC, Alling DW, Wolff SM: Cloxacillin prophylaxis in the Chédiak-Higashi syndrome. J Infect Dis 125:393, 1972.
226. Boxer LA, Wantanabe AM, Rister M, et al: Correction of leukocyte function in CHS by ascorbate. N Engl J Med 295:1041, 1976.
227. Gallin JI, Elin RJ, Hubert RT, et al: Efficacy of ascorbic acid in Chédiak-Higashi syndrome: Studies in humans and mice. Blood 53:226, 1979.
228. Pryzwandky KB, Schliwa M, Boxer LA: Microtubule organization of unstimulated and stimulated adherent human neutrophils in Chédiak-Higashi syndrome. Blood 66:1398, 1985.
229. Fischer A, Griscelli C, Friedrich W, et al: Bone marrow transplantation for immunodeficiencies and osteopetrosis. European survey, 1968–1985. Lancet 2:1080, 1986.
230. Nauseef WM: Myeloperoxidase deficiency. Hematol Oncol Clin North Am 2:135, 1988.
231. Parry MF, Root RK, Metcalf JA, et al: Myeloperoxidase deficiency: Prevalence and clinical significance. Ann Intern Med 95:483, 1981.
232. Nauseef WM, Root RK, Malech HL: Biochemical and immunologic analysis of hereditary myeloperoxidase deficiency. J Clin Invest 71:1297, 1983.
233. Johnson KR, Nauseef WM: Molecular biology of myeloperoxidase. *In* Everse J, Grisham M (eds): Peroxidases in Chemistry and Biology. Boca Raton, FL, CRC Press, 1990, pp 63–83.
234. Gouret P, duBois RM, Bernaudin JF, et al: Expression of the neutrophil elastase gene during human bone marrow cell differentiation. J Exp Med 169:833, 1989.
235. Rosmarin AG, Weil SC, Rosner GL, et al: Differential expression of CD11b/CD18 (Mol) and myeloperoxidase genes during myeloid differentiation. Blood 73:131, 1989.
236. Nauseef WM: Aberrant restriction endonuclease digests of DNA from subjects with hereditary myeloperoxidase deficiency. Blood 3:290, 1989.
237. Tobler A, Selsted ME, Miller CW, et al: Evidence of a pretranslational defect in hereditary and acquired myeloperoxidase deficiency. Blood 73:1980, 1989.
238. Nauseef WM, Brigham S, Cogley M: Hereditary myeloperoxidase deficiency due to a missense mutation of arginine 569 to tryptophan. J Biol Chem 269:1212, 1994.
239. Kizaki M, Miller CW, Selsted ME, Koeffler HP: Myeloperoxidase (MPO) gene mutation in hereditary MPO deficiency. Blood 83:1935, 1994.
240. Nauseef WM, Cogley M, McCormick S: Effect of the R569W missense mutation on the biosynthesis of myeloperoxidase. J Biol Chem 27:9546, 1996.
241. Davey FR, Erber WN, Gatter KC, Mason DY: Abnormal neutrophils in acute myeloid leukemia and myelodysplastic syndrome. Hum Pathol 19:454, 1988.
242. Bendix-Hansen K: Myeloperoxidase deficient polymorphonuclear leucocytes in leukaemia and allied disorders. Dan Med Bull 35:501, 1988.
243. Ferrari S, Tagliafico E, Ceccherelli G, et al: Expression of the myeloperoxidose gene in acute and chronic myeloid leukemias: Relationship to expression of cell cycle–related genes. Leukemia 3:423, 1989.
244. Cech P, Schneider P, Bachmann F: Partial myeloperoxidase deficiency. Acta Haematol 67:180, 1982.
245. Larrocha C, de Castro MF, Fontan G, et al: Hereditary myeloperoxidase deficiency: Study of 12 cases. Scand J Haematol 29:389, 1984.
246 Cech P, Papathanassiou A, Boreaux G, et al: Hereditary myeloperoxidase deficiency. Blood 53:403, 1979.
247. Gallin JI: Neutrophil specific granule deficiency. Annu Rev Med 36:263, 1985.
248. Falloon J, Gallin JI: Neutrophil granules in health and disease. J Allergy Clin Immunol 77:653, 1986.
249. Davis J, Dineen P, Gallin JI: Neutrophil degranulation and abnormal chemotaxis after thermal injury. J Immunol 124:1467, 1980.
250. Wolach B, Coates TD, Hugli TE, et al: Plasma lactoferrin reflects granulocyte activation via complement in burn patients. J Lab Clin Med 103:284, 1984.
251. Rosenberg HF, Gallin JI: Neutrophil-specific granule deficiency includes eosinophils. Blood 82:268, 1993.
252. Lomax KJ, Gallin JI, Rotrosen D, et al: Selective defect in myeloid cell lactoferrin gene expression in neutrophil specific granule deficiency. J Clin Invest 83:514, 1989.
253. Johnston JJ, Boxer LA, Berliner N: Correlation of messenger RNA levels with protein defects in specific granule deficiency. Blood 80:2088, 1992.
254. Ganz T, Metcalf JA, Gallin JI, Lehrer RI: Two genetic disorders that affect human neutrophils are associated with deficiencies of microbicidal and cytotoxic granule proteins (Abstr). Clin Res 35:424A, 1987.
255. Moore FD, Davis C, Roderick M, et al: Neutrophil activation in thermal injury as assessed by increased expression of complement receptors: N Engl J Med 314:948, 1986.
256. Roos D: The genetic basis of chronic granulomatous disease. Immunol Rev 138:121,1994.
257. Forehand JR, Johnston RB Jr: Chronic granulomatous disease: Newly defined molecular abnormalities explain disease variability and normal phagocyte physiology. Curr Opin Pediatr 6:668, 1994.
258. Segal AW: The NADPH oxidase and chronic granulomatous disease. Mol Med Today 2:129, 1996.
259. Roos D, de Boer M, Kuribayashi F, et al: Mutations in the X-linked and autosomal recessive forms of chronic granulomatous disease. Blood 87:1663, 1996.
260. Roos D, Curnutte JT, Hossle JP, et al: X-CGDbase: A database of X-CGD–causing mutations. Immunol Today 17:517, 1996.
261. Ahlin A, de Boer M, Roos D, et al: Prevalence, genetics and clinical presentation of chronic granulomatous disease in Sweden. Acta Paediatr 84:1386, 1995.
262. Finn A, Hadzic N, Morgan G, et al: Prognosis of chronic granulomatous disease. Arch Dis Child 65:942, 1990.
263. Schapiro BL, Newburger PE, Klempner MS, Dinauer MC: Chronic granulomatous disease presenting in a 69-year-old man. N Engl J Med 325:1786, 1991.
264. Weening RS, Leitz GJ, Seger RA: Recombinant human interferon-gamma in patients with chronic granulomatous disease—European follow up study. Eur J Pediatr 154:295, 1995.
265. Liese JG, Jendrossek V, Jansson A, et al: Chronic granulomatous disease in adults. Lancet 347:220, 1996.
266. Gallin JI, Malech HL: Update on chronic granulomatous diseases of childhood: Immunotherapy and potential for gene therapy. JAMA 263:1533, 1990.
267. Forrest CB, Forehand JR, Axtell RA, et al: Clinical features and current management of chronic granulomatous disease. Hematol Oncol Clin North Am 2:253, 1988.

268. Gallin JI: Recent advances in chronic granulomatous disease. Ann Intern Med 99:657, 1983.
269. Walther MM, Malech HL, Choyke P, et al: The urologic manifestations of chronic granulomatous disease. J Urol 147:1314, 1992.
270. Hiller H, Fisher D, Abrahamov A, Blinder G: Esophageal involvement in chronic granulomatous disease. Case report and review. Pediatr Radiol 25:308, 1995.
271. Clark RA, Malech HL, Gallin JI, et al: Genetic variants of chronic granulomatous disease: Prevalence of deficiencies of two discrete cytosolic components of the NADPH oxidase system. N Engl J Med 321:647, 1989.
272. Parkos CA, Dinauer MC, Jesaitis AJ, et al: Absence of both the 91kD and 22kD subunits of human neutrophil cytochrome *b* in two genetic forms of chronic granulomatous disease. Blood 73:1416, 1989.
273. Dinauer MC, Curnutte JT, Rosen H, Orkin SH: A missense mutation in the neutrophil cytochrome *b* heavy chain in cytochrome-positive X-linked chronic granulomatous disease. J Clin Invest 84:2012, 1989.
274. Dinauer MC, Pierce EA, Bruns GA, et al: Human neutrophil cytochrome *b* light chain (p22-phox). Gene structure, chromosomal location, and mutations in cytochrome-negative autosomal recessive chronic granulomatous disease. J Clin Invest 86:1729, 1990.
275. Francke U, Hsieh CL, Foellmer BE, et al: Genes for two autosomal recessive forms of chronic granulomatous disease assigned to 1q25 (*NCF2*) and 7q11.23 (*NCF1*). Am J Hum Genet 47:483, 1990.
276. Casimir CM, Bu-Ghanuim HN, Rodaway ARF, et al: Autosomal recessive chronic granulomatous disease caused by deletion at a dinucleotide repeat. Proc Natl Acad Sci USA 88:2753, 1991.
277. Iwata M, Nunoi H, Yamazaki H, et al: Homologous dinucleotide (GT or TG) deletion in Japanese patients with chronic granulomatous disease with p47-phox deficiency. Biochem Biophys Res Commun 199:1372, 1994.
278. Roesler J, Gorlach A, Rae J, et al: Recombination events between the normal p47-phox gene and a highly homologous pseudogene are the main cause of autosomal recessive chronic granulomatous disease (Abstr). Blood 86(Suppl 1):260a, 1995.
279. Nunoi H, Iwata M, Tatsuzawa S, et al: AG dinucleotide insertion in a patient with chronic granulomatous disease lacking cytosolic 67-kD protein. Blood 86:329, 1995.
280. Tanugi-Cholley LC, Issartel JP, Lunardi J, et al: A mutation located at the 5′ splice junction sequence of intron 3 in the p67phox gene causes the lack of p67phox mRNA in a patient with chronic granulomatous disease. Blood 85:242, 1995.
281. de Boer M, Hilarius-Stokman PM, Hossle JP, et al: Autosomal recessive chronic granulomatous disease with absence of the 67-kD cytosolic NADPH oxidase component: Identification of mutation and detection of carriers. Blood 83:531, 1994.
282. Wientjes FB, Hsuan JJ, Totty NF, Segal AW: p40phox, a third cytosolic component of the activation complex of the NADPH oxidase to contain src homology 3 domains. Biochem J 296:557, 1993.
283. Tsunawaki S, Mizunari H, Nagata M, et al: A novel cytosolic component, p40phox, of respiratory burst oxidase associates with p67phox and is absent in patients with chronic granulomatous disease who lack p67phox. Biochem Biophys Res Commun 199:1378, 1994.
284. Domachowske JB, Malech HL: Phagocytes. *In* Rich RR, Fleisher TA, Schwartz BD, et al (eds): Clinical Immunology: Principles and Practice. St. Louis, Mosby–Year Book, 1995, pp 392–407.
285. Buescher ES, Alling DW, Gallin JI: Use of an X-linked human neutrophil marker to estimate timing of lyonization and size of the dividing stem pool. J Clin Invest 76:1581, 1985.
286. Vowells SJ, Sekhsaria S, Malech HL, Fleisher TA: Flow cytometric analysis of the granulocyte respiratory burst: A comparison study of fluorescent probes. J Immunol Methods 178:89, 1995.
287. Vowells SJ, Fleisher TA, Sekhsaria S, et al: Genotype dependent variability in flow cytometric evaluation of NADPH oxidase function in patients with chronic granulomatous disease. J Pediatr 128:104, 1996.
288. Kenney RT, Malech HL, Epstein ND, et al: Characterization of the p67phox gene: Genomic organization and restriction fragment length polymorphism analysis for prenatal diagnosis in chronic granulomatous disease. Blood 82:3739, 1993.
289. Mills EL, Quie PG: Inheritance of chronic granulomatous disease. *In* Gallin JI, Fauci AS (eds): Advances in Host Defense Mechanisms, Vol 3, Chronic Granulomatous Disease. New York, Raven Press, 1983, pp 25–53.
290. Kragballe K, Borregaard N, Brandrup F, et al: Relation of monocyte and neutrophil oxidative metabolism to skin and oral lesions in carriers of chronic granulomatous disease. Clin Exp Immunol 43:390, 1981.
291. Brandrup F, Koch C, Petri M, et al: Discoid lupus erythematosus–like lesions and stomatitis in female carriers of X-linked chronic granulomatous disease. Br J Dermatol 104:495, 1981.
292. Weening RS, Adriaansz LH, Weemaes CMR, et al: Clinical differences in chronic granulomatous disease in patients with cytochrome *b*–negative or cytochrome *b*–positive neutrophils. J Pediatr 107:102, 1985.
293. Pelham A, O'Rielly M-A J, Malcolm S, et al: RFLP and deletion analysis for X-linked chronic granulomatous disease using the cDNA probe: Potential for improved prenatal diagnosis and carrier determination. Blood 76:820, 1990.
294. Lindlof M, Kere J, Ristola M, et al: Prenatal diagnosis of X-linked chronic granulomatous disease using restriction fragment length polymorphism analysis. Genomics 1:87, 1987.
295. Kenney RT, Leto TL: A *Hind*III polymorphism in the human *NCF2* gene. Nucleic Acids Res 18:7193, 1990.
296. Ross JP, Holland SM, Gill VJ, et al: Severe *Burkholderia* (*Pseudomonas*) *gladioli* infection in chronic granulomatous disease: Report of two successfully treated cases. Clin Infect Dis 21:1291, 1995.
297. Lacy DE, Spencer DA, Goldstein A, et al: Chronic granulomatous disease presenting in childhood with *Pseudomonas cepacia* septicaemia. J Infect 27:301, 1993.
298. Mouy R, Fischer A, Vilmer E, et al: Incidence, severity, and prevention of infections in chronic granulomatous disease. J Pediatr 114:555, 1989.
299. Kenney RT, Kwon-Chung KJ, Witebsky FG, et al: Invasive infection with *Sarcinosporon inkin* in a patient with chronic granulomatous disease. Am J Clin Pathol 94:344, 1990.
300. Cohen-Abbo A, Edwards KM: Multifocal osteomyelitis caused by *Paecilomyces varioti* in a patient with chronic granulomatous disease. Infection 23:55, 1995.
301. Chin TW, Stiehm ER, Falloon J, Gallin JI: Corticosteroids in treatment of obstructive lesions of chronic granulomatous disease. J Pediatr 111:349, 1987.
302. Quie PG, Belani KK: Corticosteroids for chronic granulomatous disease. J Pediatr 111:393, 1987.
303. Southwick FS, Van der Meer JW: Recurrent cystitis and bladder mass in two adults with chronic granulomatous disease. Ann Intern Med 109:118, 1988.
304. Casale AJ, Balcom AH, Wells RG, Chusid MJ: Bilateral complete ureteral obstruction and renal insufficiency, secondary to granulomatous disease. J Urol 142:812, 1989.
305. Stopyrowa J, Fyderek K, Sikorska B, et al: Chronic granulomatous disease of childhood: Gastric manifestation and response to salazosulfapyridine therapy. Eur J Pediatr 149:28, 1989.
306. Fisher JE, Khan AR, Heitlinger L, et al: Chronic granulomatous disease of childhood with acute ulcerative colitis: A unique association. Pediatr Pathol 7:91, 1987.
307. Rosh JR, Tang HB, Mayer L, et al: Treatment of intractable gastrointestinal manifestations of chronic granulomatous disease with cyclosporin. J Pediatr 126:143, 1995.
308. Lee BW, Yap HK: Polyarthritis resembling juvenile rheumatoid arthritis in a girl with chronic granulomatous disease. Arthritis Rheum 37:773, 1994.
309. Margolis DM, Melnick DA, Alling DW, Gallin JI: Trimethoprim-sulfamethoxazole prophylaxis in the management of chronic granulomatous disease. J Infect Dis 162:723, 1990.
310. The International Chronic Granulomatous Disease Cooperative Study Group: A phase III study establishing efficacy of recombinant human interferon gamma for infection prophylaxis in chronic granulomatous disease. N Engl J Med 324:509, 1991.
311. Gallin JI, Farber JM, Holland SM, Nutman TB: Interferon-gamma in the management of infectious diseases. Ann Intern Med 123:216, 1995.
312. Bemiller LS, Roberts DH, Starko KM, Curnutte JT: Safety and effectiveness of long-term interferon gamma therapy in patients with chronic granulomatous disease. Blood Cells Mol Dis 21:239, 1995.

313. Malech HL: Interferon gamma as infection prophylaxis in chronic granulomatous disease. *In* Baron S, Coppenhaver D, Dianzani F, et al (eds): Interferons: Principles and Medical Applications. Galveston, TX, University of Texas at Galveston, 1992, pp 563–573.
314. Malech HL: Cytokine therapy for chronic granulomatous disease: Gamma interferon. *In* Oppenheim JJ, Rossio JL, Gearing AJH (eds): Clinical Applications of Cytokines: Role in Pathogenesis, Diagnosis, and Therapy. New York, Oxford University Press, 1993, pp 75–78.
315. Sechler JMG, Malech HL, White CJ, Gallin JI: Recombinant human interferon-gamma reconstitutes defective phagocyte function in patients with chronic granulomatous disease of childhood. Proc Natl Acad Sci USA 85:4874, 1988.
316. Ezekowitz RAB, Dinauer MC, Jaffe HS, et al: Partial correction of the phagocyte defect in patients with X-linked chronic granulomatous disease by subcutaneous interferon gamma. N Engl J Med 319:146, 1988.
317. Jackson SH, Malech HL, Kozak CA, et al: Cloning and functional expression of the mouse homologue of p47phox. Immunogenetics 39:272, 1994.
318. Jackson SH, Gallin JI, Holland SM: The p47phox mouse knockout model of chronic granulomatous disease. J Exp Med 182:751, 1995.
319. Kamani N, August CS, Campbell DE, et al: Marrow transplantation in chronic granulomatous disease: An update with 6-year follow-up. J Pediatr 113:697, 1988.
320. Sponseller PD, Malech HL, McCarthy EF Jr, et al: Skeletal involvement in children who have chronic granulomatous disease. J Bone Joint Surg Am 73:37, 1991.
321. Pogrebniak HW, Gallin JI, Malech HL, et al: Surgical management of pulmonary infections in chronic granulomatous disease of childhood. Ann Thorac Surg 55:844, 1993.
322. O'Neil KM, Herman JH, Modlin JF, et al: *Pseudomonas cepacia*: An emerging pathogen in chronic granulomatous disease. J Pediatr 108:940, 1986.
323. Cohen MS, Isturiz RE, Malech HL, et al: Fungal infection in chronic granulomatous disease: The importance of the phagocyte in defense against fungi. Am J Med 71:59, 1981.
324. Buescher ES, Gallin JI: Leukocyte transfusions in chronic granulomatous disease. N Engl J Med 307:800, 1982.
325. Quie PG: The white cells: Use of granulocyte transfusions. Rev Infect Dis 9:189, 1987.
326. Rex JH, Bennett JE, Gallin JI, et al: Normal and deficient neutrophils can cooperate to damage *Aspergillus fumigatus* hyphae. J Infect Dis 162:523, 1990.
327. Rappaport JM, Newburger PE, Golblum RM, et al: Allogeneic bone marrow transplantation for chronic granulomatous disease. J Pediatr 101:952, 1982.
328. Di Bartolomeo P, Di Girolamo G, Angrilli F, et al: Reconstitution of normal neutrophil function in chronic granulomatous disease by bone marrow transplantation. Bone Marrow Transplant 4:695, 1989.
329. Hobbs JR, Monteil M, McCluskey DR, et al: Chronic granulomatous disease 100% corrected by displacement bone marrow transplantation from a volunteer unrelated donor. Eur J Pediatr 151:806, 1992.
330. Cobbs CS, Malech HL, Leto TL, et al: Retroviral expression of recombinant p47phox protein by EBV-transformed B lymphocytes from a patient with autosomal chronic granulomatous disease. Blood 79:1829, 1992.
331. Sekhsaria S, Gallin JI, Linton GF, et al: Peripheral blood progenitors as a target for genetic correction of p47phox-deficient chronic granulomatous disease. Proc Natl Acad Sci USA 90:7446, 1993.
332. Li F, Linton GF, Sekhsaria S, et al: CD34 positive peripheral blood progenitors as a target for genetic correction of the two flavocytochrome *b*558 defective forms of chronic granulomatous disease. Blood 84:53, 1994.
333. Sokolic RA, Sekhsaria S, Sugimoto Y, et al: A bicistronic retrovirus vector containing a picornavirus internal ribosome entry site allows for correction of X-linked CGD by selection for MDR1 expression. Blood 87:42, 1996.
334. Weil WM, Linton GF, Whiting-Theobald N, et al: Genetic correction of p67phox deficient chronic granulomatous disease using peripheral blood progenitor cells as a target for retrovirus mediated gene transfer. Blood (in press).
335. Porter CD, Parkar MH, Collins MK, et al: Efficient retroviral transduction of human bone marrow progenitor and long-term culture-initiating cells: Partial reconstitution of cells from patients with X-linked chronic granulomatous disease by gp91-phox expression. Blood 87:3722, 1996.
336. Thrasher AJ, Casimir CM, Kinnon C, et al: Gene transfer to primary chronic granulomatous disease monocytes. Lancet 346:92, 1995.
337. Zentilin L, Tafuro S, Grassi G, et al: Functional reconstitution of oxidase activity in X-linked chronic granulomatous disease by retrovirus-mediated gene transfer. Exp Cell Res 225:257, 1996.
338. Thrasher AJ, de Alwis M, Casimir CM, et al: Functional reconstitution of the NADPH-oxidase by adeno-associated virus gene transfer. Blood 86:761, 1995.
339. Kume A, Dinauer MC: Retrovirus-mediated reconstitution of respiratory burst activity in X-linked chronic granulomatous disease cells. Blood 84:3311, 1994.
340. Porter CD, Parkar MH, Verhoeven AJ, et al: p22-phox–deficient chronic granulomatous disease: Reconstitution by retrovirus-mediated expression and identification of a biosynthetic intermediate of gp91-phox. Blood 84:2767, 1994.
341. Maly FE, Schuerer-Maly CC, Quilliam L, et al: Restitution of superoxide generation in autosomal cytochrome-negative chronic granulomatous disease (A22(0) CGD)–derived B lymphocyte cell lines by transfection with p22phox cDNA. J Exp Med 178:2047, 1993.
342. Zhen L, King AA, Xiao Y, et al: Gene targeting of X chromosome–linked chronic granulomatous disease locus in a human myeloid leukemia cell line and rescue by expression of recombinant gp91phox. Proc Natl Acad Sci USA 90:9832, 1993.
343. Porter CD, Parkar MH, Levinsky RJ, X-linked chronic granulomatous disease: Correction of NADPH oxidase defect by retrovirus-mediated expression of gp91-phox. Blood 82:2196, 1993.
344. Pollock JD, Williams DA, Gifford MA, et al: Mouse model of X-linked chronic granulomatous disease, an inherited defect in phagocyte superoxide production. Nat Genet 9:202, 1995.
345. Ding C, Kume A, Bjorgvinsdottir H, et al: High-level reconstitution of respiratory burst activity in a human X-linked chronic granulomatous disease (X-CGD) cell line and correction of murine X-CGD bone marrow cells by retroviral-mediated gene transfer of human gp91phox. Blood 88:1834, 1996.
346. Mardiney M III, Jackson SH, Spratt SK, et al: Enhanced host defense after gene transfer in the murine p47phox-deficient model of chronic granulomatous disease. Blood 88(Suppl 1):487a, 1996.
347. Malech HL, Sekhsaria S, Whiting-Theobald N, et al: Prolonged detection of oxidase-positive neutrophils in the peripheral blood of five patients following a single cycle of gene therapy for chronic granulomatous disease. Blood 88(Suppl 1):486a, 1996.

7

Cell-Mediated Immunity

Richard B. Markham

Since the time of Pasteur, microbiologists and immunologists studying acquired resistance to microbial invasion have emphasized the role of humoral immunity in protecting against infection. Those, such as Metchnikoff and his heirs, who argued that phagocytic cells were the major element in antimicrobial immunity, would be supplanted by investigators who could show the remarkable increase in phagocytic efficiency achieved when microbes were opsonized before exposure to phagocytic cells. Not until the 1960s and 1970s, as the immunobiology of the T lymphocyte became better understood, did the significance of this cell for the development and control of all immune responses become appreciated. This understanding was greatly facilitated by the development of tissue culture systems in which cells could be maintained for long periods, by the realization that T cells were composed of functionally distinct and phenotypically distinguishable subsets, and by the appreciation of the requirement for histocompatibility between interacting immune cells. Nevertheless, the direct and dramatic protective effects achieved in animal models of infectious diseases by passive transfer of neutralizing or opsonizing antibody to nonimmune hosts continued to diminish the perceived importance of T cells in antimicrobial resistance.

In the late 1970s and 1980s, understanding of T-cell immunity finally achieved the sophistication that had been realized decades earlier with antibody responses. The discoveries of the T-cell receptor (TCR), of the mechanisms by which T cells recognize foreign antigens, and of the importance of secreted products of T cells and macrophages in the development of immune responses all provided the necessary foundation for understanding how T cells participate in antimicrobial immunity. The devastating consequences of the T-lymphocyte deficits associated with the acquired immunodeficiency syndrome—also a phenomenon of the 1980s—only underscored the critical role this cell plays in the development of the immune responses that prevent and control infection.

Cells Involved in Cell-Mediated Immunity

The cells of the immune system, in the aggregate, display a remarkable diversity of function. T lymphocytes can promote antibody formation, kill tumor cells or virus-infected cells, and generate delayed-type hypersensitivity, or alternatively they may suppress any or all of those immunologic activities. Although all of these functions are performed by T cells, each individual function is attributable to a distinct subset of T cells with more restricted capabilities. The discovery that each of the functionally distinct T-cell subsets carries a characteristic set of proteins on its surface has greatly facilitated the task of determining the role of the different immune cells.[1,2] The T lymphocyte, so named because of its obligatory migration through the thymus during its maturation, is the central cell in the development and expression of cell-mediated immunity. It bears a specific antigen receptor (called Ti) distinct from that of B cells,[3,4] and the TCR complex includes another protein, cluster of differentiation antigen 3 (CD3),[5,6] which also distinguishes T cells from other cells of the immune system. The broad class of T cells has been further subdivided into distinct functional subsets. Helper/inducer T cells facilitate the generation of immune responses by other T cells or B cells[7] and bear, in addition to CD3, the CD4 protein on their surface. Cytotoxic T cells lyse tumor or virus-infected cells and carry, in addition to CD3, the CD8 protein on their surface.[8]

Studies with cloned murine T-cell populations have indicated that helper/inducer $CD4^+$ T cells consist of two subsets, termed Th1 and Th2, that can be distinguished by the lymphokines they secrete.[9] Th1 cells secrete interleukin-2 (IL-2), interferon-γ (IFN-γ), and lymphotoxin but not interleukin-4 (IL-4), interleukin-5 (IL-5), or interleukin-10 (IL-10). Conversely, Th2 cells secrete IL-4, IL-5, and IL-10, but not IL-2, IFN-γ, or lymphotoxin. In addition, T lymphocytes can be functionally distinguished by their expression of surface proteins termed CD45RA, found on immunologically naive T cells, or CD45RO, found on T cells that have been exposed to antigens or mitogens.[10–12]

Although the association of specific surface proteins with specific functional activities is generally valid, studies with T-cell clones have demonstrated the potential existence of variants from this pattern, such as T cells with cytotoxic activity that bear the surface proteins characteristic of helper/inducer T cells.[13,14] The in vivo significance of these variant clones is controversial.

Five percent to 15% of lymphocytes in the peripheral blood are natural killer (NK) cells,[15] which, on exposure to IL-2, become lymphokine-activated killer cells.[16] These cells can lyse malignant or virus-infected target cells and are also capable of directly killing certain bacteria.[17] They are included in a group of cells that, because of their appearance, are referred to as large granular lymphocytes.[18] Although some of these cells may bear the T-cell marker CD3[19] or CD8,[20] they are identified in humans by the presence of two surface antigens, referred to as CD16 and CD56.[21,22] The CD16 surface marker is a receptor for the Fc region of immunoglobulin (Fc receptors),[23] and cells participating in antibody-dependent antimicrobial[24] or cytotoxic activity attach to and destroy antibody-coated targets via these receptors.

Antigen Recognition by T Cells

An essential distinction between T cells and B cells is the mechanism by which foreign antigens are recognized. Analysis of B-cell activation was facilitated by the fact that the antigen receptor on B cells, the immunoglobulin molecule, is also the secreted effector product of B cells and is present in large quantities in soluble form in the serum. Furthermore, an immunoglobulin molecule is capable of reacting directly and specifically with a foreign protein or microbial pathogen in its native state, permitting a conceptually straightforward analysis of how immunoglobulin protects against infectious diseases.

The process by which T cells recognize foreign antigens is remarkably more complex than that of B cells. T cells cannot bind crude antigens directly[25]; the TCR has no known direct effector function and is not secreted.

A key element in understanding antigen recognition and subsequent T-cell activation was the observation that T cells could recognize foreign antigens only when those antigens were presented to the T cell by other cells of the immune system. Furthermore, the antigen-presenting cells and the T cells being activated both had to possess the same set of major histocompatibility complex (MHC) proteins. The MHC genes encode the proteins that permit an individual to distinguish self from nonself and are therefore the primary antigens recognized when the immune system rejects tissue from an unrelated donor. Rosenthal and Shevach[26] reported in 1973 that T lymphocytes could not be activated in tissue culture by a foreign antigen unless macrophages of the same MHC haplotype as the T cells were also present. Katz and colleagues[27] demonstrated that helper T cells could help only B cells that shared their MHC proteins, and Zinkernagel and Dougherty[28] and Shearer and colleagues[29] proved that cytotoxic T cells could kill only histocompatible cellular targets.

The MHC products of both human and mouse have been divided into three major classes of molecules and two of these, termed class I and class II, are important in T-cell activation. Three class I loci have been identified: H-2K, H-2D, and H-2L in the mouse and human leukocyte antigen locus A (HLA-A), HLA-B, and HLA-C in humans.[30] Class II genes are encoded in the I-A and I-E regions of the mouse MHC and the HLA-D, -DR, -DQ, and -DP regions of the human MHC.[31] All of these loci are strikingly polymorphic in both human and mouse, the two most studied species. Class I antigens are the primary antigens recognized as foreign during tissue graft rejection and are also the antigens that must be shared between the classic cytotoxic T cell and its target for killing of the target cell to occur.[32] Similarly, helper T cells can be activated by and can "help" only cells that possess the same class II antigens as the helper cell.[27]

Class I antigens are found in varying amounts on virtually all mammalian cells.[33] The cellular distribution of class II antigens is more restricted, with expression primarily on activated macrophages,[34] dendritic cells,[34] and B cells.[35] Much smaller quantities of class II antigens are found on activated CD4+ T cells,[36] endothelial cells,[37] and epithelial cells.[38] Other cells may express these antigens under pathologic conditions.[39]

The importance of the class I and class II MHC molecules in T-cell immunity derives from the inability of T cells to be activated by a foreign antigen unless that antigen is physically associated with one of these molecules (Fig. 7–1). Only peptides, not complex proteins, are capable of associating with the MHC products,[40–42] which explains the inability of T cells to react to native proteins. The need for an accessory cell to activate T cells, as originally defined by Rosenthal and Shevach, results from a requirement for a cell that can take up complex proteins, process them into small peptides, and then attach those peptides to MHC proteins, which are subsequently expressed on the cell surface. Contact between the TCR of a specific T cell and the peptide-MHC complex is required for that T cell to be activated.

Not all peptides can bind to the class I or class II molecule of a given individual,[43] and which peptide binds depends on the structure of the class I or class II proteins produced by that individual. In some cases, none of the peptides that result from processing of a protein are capable of binding to MHC products of a specific individual, and that individual is then incapable of generating a T-cell response to those peptides or to the protein from which they were derived. On the other hand, T lymphocytes from two different individuals could appear to be activated by exposure of the immune system to the same complex protein, whereas in fact the T cells from the two individuals are reacting to processed peptides derived from different portions of that protein. This issue is particularly important for the development of vaccines that activate T lymphocytes: any successful vaccine must contain proteins that can be processed into peptides that bind to the wide variety of MHC proteins expressed by diverse human populations.

There are significant gaps in our understanding of the binding of proteins to the surface of cells that ultimately process those proteins into peptides for presentation to T cells. Proteins that have been opsonized by antibody or complement attach to macrophages via Fc or C3b receptors[44, 45]; the immunoglobulin molecule on the surface of B cells binds to the protein antigen for which it is specific, thereby enabling the B cell to ingest and process that protein, presenting its peptide degradation products to T cells.[35] For some viruses, specific cell receptors that permit the attachment of the virus have been identified.[46] However, most complex proteins that are taken up by phagocytic, antigen-presenting cells are unopsonized and what specific receptors, if any, are involved in their binding and uptake by antigen-presenting cells are undefined.

Once the foreign protein bound to the cell surface is ingested, it can be processed through at least two different pathways,[47] and which pathway the protein enters determines whether its peptide degradation product reappears on the cell surface in association with class I or class II MHC gene products.[14] The class of MHC gene product with which the peptide associates in turn determines whether the peptide stimulates CD4+ or CD8+ T cells. CD4+ T cells respond to antigens associated with class II MHC gene products and CD8+ T cells respond to antigens associated with class I MHC gene products. Because viruses are capable of infecting a broad range of cells, the nearly universal expression of class I antigens is critical for the control of virus infections by CD8+ cytotoxic T cells.

The two protein degradation pathways existing within antigen-presenting cells can be distinguished by the agents that inhibit their activity. Antigen processing that results in the association of peptides with class II antigens (leading to helper T-cell activation) can be blocked by agents that inhibit metabolic activity within lysosomes and endosomes.[40, 48] On the other hand, the processing of proteins into peptides that typically associate with class I MHC proceeds normally despite exposure of the antigen-presenting cells to agents that inhibit lysosomal metabolism.[48]

The discovery that peptides from ultraviolet light–inactivated influenza virus are presented in association with class II antigens, whereas peptides from live virus are presented in association with class I antigens,[14] provided a framework for understanding the differences in antigen processing. This observation suggested that endogenous synthesis of proteins within the cytoplasm of the antigen-presenting cell, as would occur with live virus infection of a cell, directed the proteins away from entry into lysosomes and favored their association with class I antigens. This association occurs as class I MHC proteins are synthesized in the endoplasmic reticulum (Lapham CK, et al, submitted), and the release of class I proteins from the endoplasmic reticulum requires their association with peptides.[49] Studies in which ultraviolet light–inactivated virions microinjected into the cytoplasm of antigen-presenting cells could generate class I–restricted cytotoxic T-cell responses indicate that presence in the cytoplasm alone is sufficient to promote association of antigen with class I MHC gene products.[50] The movement of

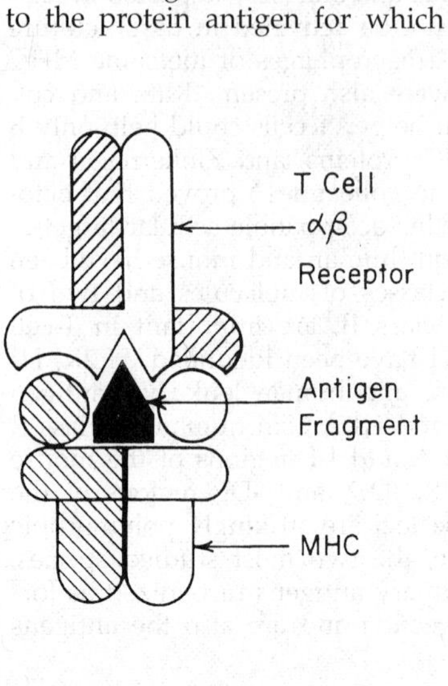

FIGURE 7–1 □ Interaction between a T-cell αβ receptor and an antigen-MHC ligand. (From Marrack P, Kappler J: The T-cell repertoire for antigen and MHC. Immunol Today 9:308–315, 1988.)

cytosolic peptides to the endoplasmic reticulum from the cytoplasm depends on the activity of two polymorphic transport proteins, termed TAP-1 and TAP-2, that are embedded in the membrane of the endoplasmic reticulum.[51–53] Both the polymorphism of the two TAP proteins and their variable expression in different cells[54] are possible sources of variation in immune responses among different individuals.

A nontraditional class I molecule, termed class Ib or, in the mouse, H-2M3, binds specifically to the N-terminal of peptides containing a terminal formylmethionine.[55–57] An N-terminal formylmethionine is frequently added as bacterial polypeptides are being synthesized. In contrast, this amino acid motif is rarely found in human cells. The presence of a conserved, nonpolymorphic region of the mammalian class I molecule that binds this bacterial peptide provides the infected host cell with a mechanism for presenting bacterial peptides to cytotoxic T cells, leading to the destruction of the infected cell. Such an H-2M3–dependent antigen presentation pathway has, in fact, been shown to be involved in protection against disease caused by *Listeria monocytogenes* in a mouse model system.[56, 57]

Although the macrophage may be the most important cell for presenting microbial antigens to T cells, any cell that expresses class I or II MHC gene products may present antigen to and activate the T cell capable of interacting with that MHC protein. From the structure of the TCR it is apparent that only a single receptor is involved in the binding of the MHC gene product–foreign peptide complex, so that interaction between the TCR and the MHC gene product is an integral part of the attachment of the TCR to a foreign peptide.

The inability of T cells to recognize peptides not associated with self-MHC is attributed to positive selection of self-MHC–restricted T cells within the thymus during T-cell differentiation. Studies with transgenic mice suggest that T cells with receptors capable of binding to self-MHC continue to mature within the thymus and ultimately populate the peripheral T-cell pools.[58] More than 90% of the T cells entering the thymus fail to mature and die there,[59] indicating that most T-cell precursors lack the receptors necessary for interacting with self-MHC in a manner that promotes their survival. Somewhat paradoxically, interactions between MHC-expressing thymic epithelial and maturing T lymphocytes are also believed to play a role in eliminating T cells reactive to self-antigens.[60] Elimination of such cells is essential to the prevention of autoimmune disease. Whether a cell is destined for preservation or destruction within the thymus may depend on the affinity of the interaction between the T cell and the thymic epithelial cell, with either too low or too high an affinity resulting in death of the T cell.

The T-Cell Receptor

Binding of the TCR to the foreign peptide–MHC complex, in combination with accessory signals provided by antigen-presenting cells, results in clonal expansion of the resting T cell bearing the receptor specific for that peptide–MHC gene product complex.[61, 62] The TCR is composed of two distinct molecular entities, a protein whose structure does not vary among T-cell clones, termed T3 or CD3, and a second set of proteins, the Ti molecule, consisting of heterologous α- and β-chains, each of which contains the variable regions that define a receptor with antigen specificity[63] (Fig. 7–2). Elegant studies by Yague and colleagues,[64] Dembic and colleagues,[65] and Saito and coworkers in Germain's laboratory[66] demonstrated that the αβ heterodimer complex is sufficient to recognize the MHC gene product–peptide complex. The Ti molecule has a small cytoplasmic domain (6 or 7 amino acids), whereas that of CD3 exceeds 40 amino acids, suggesting that binding of Ti may result in intracellular signaling via the associated CD3 molecule.[67, 68]

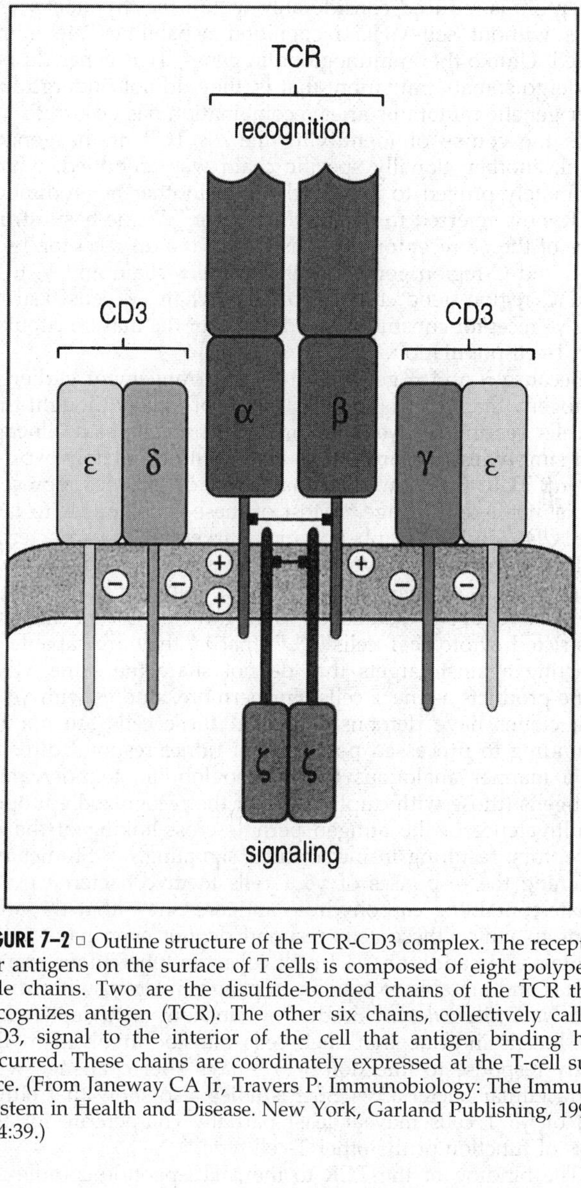

FIGURE 7–2 □ Outline structure of the TCR-CD3 complex. The receptor for antigens on the surface of T cells is composed of eight polypeptide chains. Two are the disulfide-bonded chains of the TCR that recognizes antigen (TCR). The other six chains, collectively called CD3, signal to the interior of the cell that antigen binding has occurred. These chains are coordinately expressed at the T-cell surface. (From Janeway CA Jr, Travers P: Immunobiology: The Immune System in Health and Disease. New York, Garland Publishing, 1996, p 4:39.)

As is the case for immunoglobulin, the diversity of the TCR derives from the fact that each of its two chains is encoded in three or four different gene segments and each of those segments is composed of a cluster of genes, each of which can code for the individual segment of the receptor protein.[61] The β-chain, for example, is composed of four different regions, the variable region (V), the diversity segment (D), the joining region (J), and the constant region (C). There are approximately 25 different V region genes for the β-chain, and only one of those genes is selected during rearrangement of the V, D, and J genes that ultimately encode a β-chain. Similarly, there are 100 V region genes capable of encoding the V region of a single human α-chain TCR. The different gene combinations that are generated as the V, D, and J region genes rearrange and combine to encode a single αβ-chain could theoretically produce approximately 10^{15} distinct TCRs.[69] Additional diversity is generated by the folding together of the α- and β-chains. Clearly, this degree of receptor variation would provide the ability to recognize an extremely large repertoire of foreign antigens. It should be remembered, however, that this large repertoire of potential receptors is reduced considerably within the thymus, where cells without self-MHC recognition capabilities are eliminated. Unlike the immunoglobulin genes, TCR genes do not undergo somatic mutation; that is, they do not undergo further genetic mutations after recombination has occurred.

In the course of identifying the αβ TCR at the genetic level, another clonally specific chain was identified, which ultimately proved to be one chain of another heterodimeric TCR, now referred to as the γδ receptor.[70, 71] The basic structure of the γδ receptor parallels that of the αβ receptor, with V, J, and C region gene clusters for the γ-chain and V, J, D, and C region gene clusters for the δ-chain. T cells bearing the γδ receptor constitute less than 5% of the mature circulating T-cell population.[72, 73]

Because γ and δ genes undergo rearrangement earlier in ontogeny than α and β genes,[74] it was originally thought that T cells bearing the γδ receptor were from the same lineage but simply less mature T cells that would ultimately express the αβ TCR. It is now clear that γδ-bearing T cells represent a distinct T-cell lineage.[74] Most of these cells appear to lack the CD4 and CD8 phenotypic markers that characterize helper/inducer and cytotoxic T-cell subsets, and they are referred to as double-negative T cells.[75] Lines of γδ-bearing T cells have been established that function as non–MHC-restricted cytotoxic T cells[71, 76, 77]; that is, they are capable of reacting against targets that do not share the same MHC gene products as the T cells. Furthermore, studies with γδ T-cell clones have demonstrated that these cells are not responding to processed peptides but rather respond directly, in a manner analogous to immunoglobulin, to polyvalent antigens (those with duplications of the recognized epitope). Multivalence of the antigen permits cross-linking of the γδ receptors, resulting in intracellular signaling.[78, 79] Studies examining the responses of γδ T cells to mycobacterial phosphate-containing carbohydrate antigens show that the antigens to which these cells respond do not even have to be proteins.[80] In addition, γδ T cells collect in tuberculous granulomas and are able to lyse macrophages infected with *Mycobacterium tuberculosis*.[81] Studies of knockout mice depleted of γδ T cells indicate that such cells may be involved in the early response to infection 3 to 5 days after challenge with intracellular bacteria.[82, 83] Such studies also show that either αβ or γδ T cells may at least partially compensate for the loss of function of the other T-cell type.[84, 85]

The binding of the TCR to the MHC-peptide complex is not sufficient to promote the T-cell proliferation associated with effective immune responses. Cytokines, such as interleukin-1 (IL-1) or IL-6, secreted by antigen-presenting cells during interactions with T cells markedly enhance the proliferation of the responding cells. Interactions between another set of cell surface proteins, CD28 on αβ T cells and B7 on antigen-presenting cells, such as B cells, dendritic cells, or macrophages, are also required[86] (Fig. 7–3). Almost all $CD4^+$ T cells carry the CD28 protein on their surface, as do 50% of $CD8^+$ T cells, and expression of this protein is up-regulated during T-cell stimulation. Interaction between CD28 and B7 stabilizes the message for various T-cell–derived cytokines, such as IL-2 and the resulting enhanced expression of these cytokines may account, at least in part, for the increased proliferation observed when CD28 binds to its B7 ligand on the antigen-presenting cell. CD28 activation also contributes to expansion of the responding T-cell population by inhibiting the programmed death of proliferating T cells, which typically occurs 4 to 5 days after cell stimulation.[87] CD28 is not found on γδ T cells. One other protein on the T-cell surface, gp39, has also been shown to be critical, through its interactions with a protein termed CD40 on antigen-presenting cells, to T-cell activation.[88] Other surface proteins on T cells and antigen-presenting cells serve to secure the binding of the T cell to the antigen-presenting cell but play less important roles in the intracellular processes associated with T-cell activation. Among these, the MHC class II–CD4 and the MHC class I–CD8 interactions determine the specificity of $CD4^+$ and $CD8^+$ T cells for antigens bound by the respective MHC molecules.

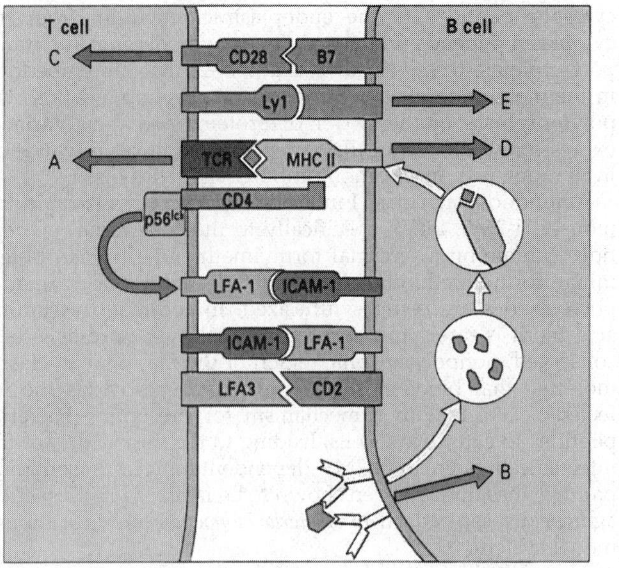

FIGURE 7–3 ▫ Multiple molecules are involved in the interactions between T cells and antigen-presenting or target cells. In this diagram the cell surface molecules involved in the interactions between antigen-presenting B cells and helper T cells are shown. The white arrows represent membrane immunoglobulin–directed delivery of antigen to an intracellular compartment where it is degraded and peptides can combine with MHC class II molecules. Other arrows show the discrete signal transduction events that have been established. A and B indicate the antigen-receptor signal transduction events involving tyrosine phosphorylation and phosphoinositide breakdown. The antigen receptors also regulate lymphocyte function–associated antigen-1 (LFA-1) affinity for intercellular adhesion molecule-1 (ICAM-1), possibly through the signal transduction events. In the T cell, CD28 also sends a unique signal to the T cell (C). In the B cell, class II MHC molecules and Lyb2 (CD72 in humans) appear to induce distinct signaling events (D and E). Not shown is the interaction between gp39 on T cells and CD40 on antigen-presenting cells. Also not demonstrated in this figure is the exchange of soluble interleukins and binding to the corresponding receptors on the other cell. (Adapted from DeFranco AL: Between B cells and T cells. Nature 351:603–604, 1991. Reprinted with permission from Nature. Copyright 1991 Macmillan Magazines Limited.)

The mechanism by which NK and lymphokine-activated killer cells recognize their targets in the absence of antibody is incompletely defined but does not involve the TCR. The critical interactions that influence NK cell activation are, in fact, negative influences. NK cells express on their surface either of two proteins, termed p58.1 and p58.2, that interact with class I MHC antigens on potential target cells.[89, 90] If an interaction between the p58 proteins and class I molecules occurs, the NK activity of the cell is negatively modulated or eliminated. Thus, cells that serve as targets for NK cells do not express class I antigens. The well-characterized targets of NK cells, tumor cells and virus-infected cells, are targets specifically because they fail to express class I antigens. Although the ability of certain viruses to down-regulate expression of class I could provide a mechanism of escape from class I–dependent cytotoxic T-cell activity, this same capability renders the virally infected cells susceptible to NK activity. Other cell surface structures have been implicated in the interaction between the NK cell and its target, including CD2, first identified as the sheep erythrocyte receptor on human T cells,[91] CD16,[92] and a protein termed NKR-P1A, which is found on both murine and human NK cells and is believed to provide an activating signal that stimulates killing of NK targets if the inhibitory class I MHC-p58 interaction does not occur.[52, 93–95] The effect of cellular interactions through these receptors appears to be secondary to that of the MHC class I–p58 receptor interactions.

Expression of the receptors and ligands involved in NK activity is not increased by specific immunization; any killer activity observed is, therefore, "natural" or preexisting in the nonimmune host. However, NK activity can be enhanced by specific lymphokines, such as the interferons, and by immunologic stimuli that promote release of those lymphokines.[96]

Intracellular Events Associated with T-Cell Activation

Binding of antigen to the TCR ultimately results in secretion of the biologically active proteins associated with an immune response. Secretion of those proteins is the end product of a complex series of biochemical events that link the TCR on the cell's membrane and the transcription factors that promote expression of lymphokine genes (Fig. 7–4). This movement of signals from cell surface to cell genome requires the conversion of biochemically inactive proteins in the cytoplasm to forms that interact with other cytoplasmic proteins, resulting in a cascade of reactions leading to lymphokine gene expression. The activation of these biochemically inert proteins results primarily from the phosphorylation of tyrosine sites, a process that is catalyzed by different tyrosine kinases.[97, 98] The pathways involved in this process have been reviewed in great detail[99] and are only summarized here.

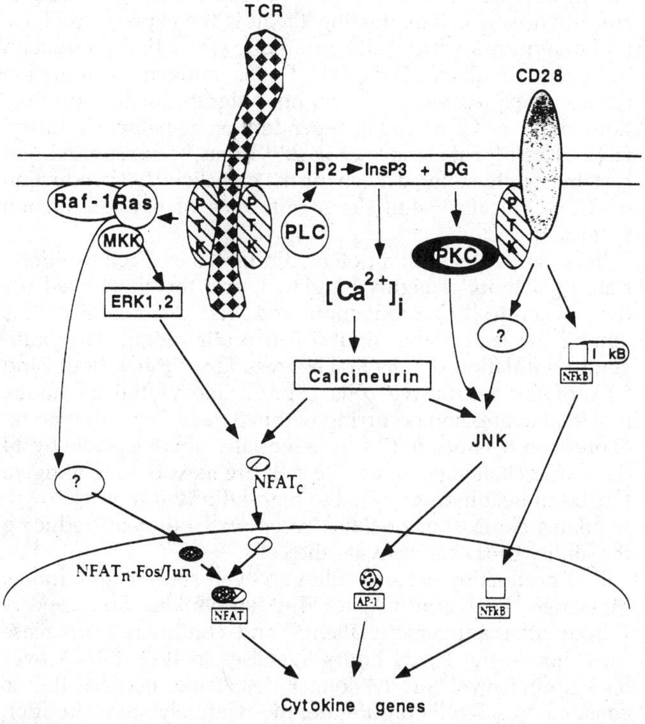

FIGURE 7–4 □ Pathways by which binding of the antigen receptor and other cell surface molecules result in T-cell activation. See text for an explanation of mechanisms of cytotoxic T cell killing. AP-1, Activator protein 1; ERK, extracellular signal–regulated kinase; JNK, Jun amino terminal kinase; MKK, mitogen-activated protein kinase kinase; NFAT, nuclear factor of activated T cells; NF-κB, nuclear factor κB; PKC, protein kinase C; PLC, phospholipase C; PTK, protein tyrosine kinase. (From Cantrell D: T cell antigen receptor signal transduction pathways. Annu Rev Immunol 14:266, 1996. Reproduced, with permission, from the Annual Review of Immunology, Volume 14, © 1996, by Annual Reviews Inc.)

The TCR complex can be perceived as composed of two functionally distinct regions. The variable portion, consisting of the polymorphic T-cell αβ receptor, recognizes antigen in the context of MHC proteins on antigen-presenting cells. The αβ-chains have a short cytoplasmic tail and therefore depend for their intracellular signaling on the invariant proteins to which they are noncovalently linked. These conserved proteins consist of the TCR ζ-chain and the γ-, δ-, and ε-chains of the CD3 antigen complex.[100] All of these invariant proteins have a long intracellular tail containing a critical series of amino acids characterized by the presence of two tyrosine residues.[101] This essential amino acid sequence or motif is referred to as the immunoglobulin receptor family tyrosine-based activation motif. The binding of cytoplasmic protein tyrosine kinases to this motif results in activation of the kinases,[102, 103] which can then phosphorylate tyrosine residues on other intracellular proteins. The kinases associated with binding of the TCR include $p59^{fyn}$, ZAP-70, and $p56^{lck}$.[104]

One target protein for the activity of these kinases is phospholipase C.[104] Phosphatidylinositol 4,5-bisphosphate is found in small quantities in mammalian cell membranes. Interaction of the TCR with antigen activates phospholipase C in the membrane, resulting in the hydrolysis of phosphatidylinositol 4,5-bisphosphate to diacylglycerol and inositol 1,4,5-trisphosphate. These hydrolysis products act as second messengers activating two distinct pathways.

Diacylglycerol increases the affinity of protein kinase C for calcium, which causes this enzyme to move from the cytosol to the cell membrane, where it catalyzes phosphorylation of different membrane proteins, including the Na^+-H^+ exchanger. This in turn leads to the increases in intracellular pH that are associated with cellular activation and proliferation. Inositol 1,4,5-trisphosphate releases calcium from intracellular stores such as the endoplasmic reticulum, which results in the activation of calcium-dependent protein kinases.

In addition to acting on phospholipase C, the tyrosine kinases that are activated by binding to the cytoplasmic domain of the TCR regulate the activation of a guanine nucleotide binding protein termed $p21^{ras}$. When guanine binds to $p21^{ras}$, it facilitates the binding of this kinase to a serine-threonine kinase termed Raf-1, thereby attracting Raf-1 to the cell membrane. At that site, Raf-1 initiates a cascade of mitogen-activated protein kinases, which include proteins termed extracellular signal–regulated kinases 1 and 2.[105] These two kinases in turn interact with the calcium signals generated through the phospholipase C pathway to activate the series of transcriptional activators, including nuclear factor of activated T cells, nuclear factor-κB, and activator protein 1, involved in the expression of cytokine genes. This process requires the activity of the tyrosine kinases that are activated as a result of binding of CD28 to its B7 ligand. The interaction of signals generated through the TCR and those generated through CD28 binding activate another mitogen-activated protein kinase, termed Jun amino-terminal kinase 1. The activation of this kinase is calcium dependent, requiring the activity of calcineurin, a calcium phosphatase that is essential for T-cell activation.[106] It appears to be critical for both the CD28 and TCR activation pathways.

As indicated earlier, interactions between gp39 on T cells and CD40 on antigen-presenting cells are also important for T-cell activation. However, the intracellular enzyme systems that are activated by these interactions have not yet been defined but are distinct from those associated with binding of the TCR and the binding of CD28 on T cells by the B7 ligand on antigen-presenting cells.

Most of the pathways elucidated to date have resulted from studies focusing on IL-2 production as the end product of T-cell activation. Clearly, IL-2 production is not the end point of immune activation for all cellular immune functions, and other pathways may be involved in the secretion of other lymphokines. Although the details of this pathway are now well described, the extent to which different intracellular biochemical interactions account for the lymphokine patterns associated with other subsets of T lymphocytes remains to be elucidated.

Cytokines

The ability of T lymphocytes to participate in antimicrobial resistance ultimately depends on the secretion of proteins that indirectly promote phagocytosis of bacteria or fungi, directly kill or inhibit the growth of microbial organisms, destroy virus-infected cells, or enhance the activity of other T cells or B cells that contribute to antimicrobial activity. Whereas the antimicrobial activity of the B lymphocyte is dependent on a single product (the antibody molecule), T cells and macrophages, viewed collectively, produce or are acted on by many different proteins, termed cytokines, that usually achieve effective concentrations only within short distances of the cells that produce them. Immunologically active proteins secreted by macrophages are termed monokines, and those produced by T cells are called lymphokines. It is likely that a given immunologic challenge results in the simultaneous secretion of many different cytokines, the cumulative effect of which might be difficult to predict. Furthermore, specific receptors have been defined for many of these cytokines and any biologic effect achieved by secretion of a given cytokine is determined as much by which cells are expressing cytokine receptors as by which cytokines are actually produced.

The ability to clone and express the cytokine genes has provided opportunities to explore in detail the functional capabilities of purified forms of these agents. Although this approach has been extremely useful for attributing specific activities to the different cytokines, in vivo effects depend on which particular "cocktail" of cytokines is produced after a specific immunologic challenge. It is not within the scope of this chapter to describe the functions of all known cytokines, but those with established functions relevant to antimicrobial immunity are briefly described.

Interleukin-1

Originally discovered as the "endogenous pyrogen" produced by white blood cells after endotoxin challenge,[107] IL-1 is now known to be a molecularly heterogeneous polypeptide produced by many different types of cells and possessing diverse biologic functions in addition to production of fever.[108] IL-1 is found in the extracellular environment of both mice and humans as two distinct proteins, referred to as IL-1α (pI 5) and IL-1β (pI 7.0), each of an approximate molecular mass of 17 kDa.[109, 110] In addition to its ability to induce fever, IL-1 promotes differentiation of T cells, thereby enhancing all of the other functions of which T cells are capable.

IL-1 activity in cell culture supernatant fluids is frequently assayed by measuring lymphocyte proliferation in the presence of the material being assayed.[111] Such proliferation actually results from the activity of IL-2, but IL-1 increases cellular proliferation by increasing both IL-2 production and expression of the receptor for IL-2 on T cells.[112] IL-1 also increases production of IFN-γ,[113] IL-4,[113] and colony-stimulating factor.[114] Osteoclasts exposed to IL-1 increase bone resorption,[113] and fibroblasts and monocytes increase prostaglandin production after IL-1 exposure.[113] These different activities of IL-1 provide some idea of the scope of its action, but they represent only a fraction of the many different functions that have been ascribed to it.

IL-1 induces its effect on cells by binding to specific receptors on the surface of IL-1–sensitive cells.[115] The IL-1 receptor binds both IL-1α and IL-1β, despite the structural differences between those two proteins.

As indicated, one of the more potent stimulators of IL-1 secretion is endotoxin or lipopolysaccharide from gram-negative bacteria.[108] The ability of a single cytokine, produced on exposure of the host to gram-negative bacteria, to stimulate T-cell differentiation and proliferation, to increase antibody production by B cells, to enhance macrophage chemotaxis, and to augment oxidative metabolism in neutrophils emphasizes the central role played by IL-1 in host defense against bacterial challenge.[108]

Interleukin-2

IL-2 is a 15-kDa polypeptide produced primarily by $CD4^+$ T cells that stimulates proliferation of T cells that have been activated by exposure to antigens or nonspecific stimuli.[116, 117] Binding of the TCR by a specific peptide-MHC protein, in the presence of accessory molecules such as IL-1, results in increased metabolic activity of the T cell, resulting in the expression of 55- and 75-kDa proteins on the cell surface that together act as a high-affinity receptor, termed Tac, for IL-2.[118] The 55- and 75-kDa proteins can individually form a low-affinity bond with IL-2.[119, 120] Because IL-2 acts nonspecifically on any cell expressing Tac, it is the expression of Tac that determines which cells proliferate when IL-2 production has been stimulated. For $CD8^+$ T cells, antigenic stimulation results in expression of Tac without significant IL-2 production. Thus, the $CD8^+$ cell is dependent on a "helper/inducer" $CD4^+$ T cell for its source of IL-2.[121] It has been reported that certain nonphysiologic mechanisms can elicit IL-2 production by $CD8^+$ T cells,[122] but the significance of that production is unclear.

Because IL-2 is such a potent stimulator of T-cell proliferation, its activity is highly regulated, and the short-lived nature of both IL-2 production and Tac expression[123–125] is among the factors that limit T-cell proliferation. After antigenic stimulation, T cells first express Tac within 6 hours and 50% of the responsive cells express Tac within 24 hours, maximal expression occurring within 3 days. From that point, expression declines until it is essentially nondetectable by 14 days after challenge, unless the cells are reexposed to antigen. Furthermore, binding of IL-2 to high-affinity receptors down-regulates expression of those receptors,[126] thereby reducing the ability of IL-2 to activate the cells.

IL-2 production occurs within an even shorter time frame. Messenger RNA (mRNA) for this lymphokine first appears 1 hour after antigenic challenge and continues to increase for 8 hours, but by 24 hours increases in IL-2 mRNA over background levels are no longer detectable. Because IL-2 is consumed as T cells proliferate, the relatively short duration of its production would appear to be a major factor limiting T-cell proliferation. Without additional IL-2, the proliferating T cells revert back to a resting state, in which they presumably serve as an expanded population of memory T cells capable of an accelerated response to secondary antigenic challenge.

In addition to stimulation of lymphocyte proliferation, IL-2 enhances the activity of NK cells, as measured by the range of tumor cells that can be lysed and by the degree of lysis of an individual tumor cell line that occurs when IL-2 is added both in vitro[127] and in vivo.[128] This activity of IL-2 has been exploited in clinical trials evaluating its efficacy as an antitumor agent.[129]

Interleukin-4

IL-4, also known as B-cell stimulatory factor 1, is a 20-kDa protein produced by certain classes of activated T cells and mast cells and is known to stimulate growth of T cells,[130] B cells, eosinophils, mast cells,[131] and macrophages.[132] It produces multiple effects on B cells, including increasing class II MHC expression in a calcium-independent fashion[133, 134]; antigen-induced class II expression requires calcium.[135] Once B cells are stimulated by antigen, B-cell proliferation is enhanced by the presence of IL-4, and certain antigens that fail to stimulate B-cell proliferation at all do so in the presence of IL-4.[136] IL-4 specifically stimulates secretion of both immunoglobulin (Ig) G1 and IgE in mice,[137, 138] and antibody to IL-4 reduces the concentration of IgE obtained in serum after stimulation with parasites that normally generate a large IgE response.[139] It thus appears that IL-4 functions as a major B-cell regulatory molecule, controlling both B-cell proliferation and the switch from IgM production to production of certain immunoglobulin isotypes.

Although IL-4 was first identified by its activity on B cells, it is now clear that IL-4 affects other hematopoietic cells as well. In the presence of IL-4, both CD4+ and CD8+ T cells stimulated with phorbol myristate acetate, an analog of diacylglycerol (see earlier), proliferate, whereas T cells stimulated with either agent alone show no proliferation.[140] This effect of IL-4 is totally independent of IL-2.[141] Macrophages exposed to IL-4 demonstrate increased cytotoxic activity and increased expression of class II MHC antigens.[142] IL-4 also acts synergistically with other lymphokines or cytokines to promote cell growth: IL-4 plus interleukin-3 (IL-3) promotes the growth of mast cell lines,[131] IL-4 plus granulocyte-macrophage colony-stimulating factor enables the establishment of granulocyte colonies in soft agar, and IL-4 plus erythropoietin promotes in vitro growth of erythrocyte precursors. Similarly, IL-4 enhances the growth of megakaryocyte precursors.[141]

Of particular importance is the role that IL-4 plays in the determination of whether immune responses to microbial pathogens are predominantly humoral or whether the cell-mediated limb of the immune response is activated.[143, 144] In some animal models of infection, IL-4 can divert a cellular immune response to a humoral response. Inbred mouse strains with predominant IL-4 responses to certain pathogens may be more susceptible to the effects of infection than their counterparts in which infection fails to elicit a predominant IL-4 response.

Interleukin-6

Interleukin-6 (IL-6) is a protein of approximately 23 kDa that was first defined as a macrophage product but is now known to be produced by many other types of cells, including T and B lymphocytes, endothelial cells, and fibroblasts.[145–148] IL-6 has multiple biologic effects, including the promotion of B-cell differentiation,[149] T-cell proliferation,[150, 151] and cytotoxic T-cell differentiation,[149] as well as the stimulation of growth of macrophage and granulocyte progenitors in vitro.[152] Its reported interferon-like antiviral activity has caused it to be termed interferon-β_2,[153] although the antiviral activity of this cytokine is controversial.[154] IL-6 is released by monocytes and macrophages under the same stimuli (e.g., exposure to endotoxin) that result in release of IL-1 and tumor necrosis factor (TNF), and each of these three cytokines interacts in a way that promotes the secretion and activity of the other. IL-6 is capable by itself, however, of inducing fever and production of acute-phase proteins, the latter effect attributable to a direct stimulatory activity of IL-6 on hepatocytes.[155]

Interferon

As one of the earliest described lymphokines, interferon was originally named for its ability to interfere with virus replication.[156] Subsequent analysis revealed that this activity is shared by three different classes of proteins produced by different types of cells.[157] Furthermore, the purification and cloning of these proteins have permitted analyses that indicate that, in addition to their antiviral activity, interferons have potent immunomodulatory functions.[158, 159]

The type I interferons include IFN-α and IFN-β, which are acid stable and produced by leukocytes and fibroblasts[160, 161] in response to viral challenge. An acid-labile form of IFN-α has also been described[162] that cross-reacts with antibodies to the acid-stable form but does not cross-react with IFN-γ, which is also acid labile.[163] IFN-γ, also called type II interferon or immune interferon, is produced by activated T lymphocytes.[164] IFN-α and IFN-β bind to the same receptor, but IFN-γ binds to a distinct receptor that has low affinity for the other types of interferon.[165] Interferons are produced in response to numerous different types of stimuli, including viruses, especially those producing double-stranded RNA,[166] certain bacteria,[96] and bacterial lipopolysaccharide.[167]

The antiviral activity of the interferons can be viewed as one manifestation of a broad range of modulatory effects, including marked inhibition of cell growth,[168] that these agents have on cellular functions. Antiviral activity has been most clearly demonstrated by the appearance of increased viral proliferation in animals that received antiinterferon antibodies before viral challenge.[169] Within cells, interferons induce the synthesis of proteins that have antiviral activity, the most frequently described being 2′,5′-oligo(A) synthetase,[170] a protein kinase,[171] and a protein termed Mx that, when generated in vivo, protects against infection with influenza virus.[172] These proteins inhibit viral protein synthesis and promote degradation of viral mRNA in cell-free systems, and they are presumed to act similarly within cells.[173]

In addition to the direct antiviral activity of all of the interferons, IFN-γ possesses a wide spectrum of antimicrobial activities that are achieved indirectly through its effects on the immune system. It up-regulates expression of both class I[174] and class II[175] MHC antigens on the surface of antigen-presenting cells, thereby facilitating the antigen-stimulated activation of helper/inducer and cytotoxic T cells. Similar up-regulation of Fc receptors for IgG by IFN-γ promotes ingestion by phagocytic cells of opsonized microorganisms.[176] The ability of macrophages to kill certain tumor cells lines or to kill intracellular bacteria is also markedly enhanced by exposure to IFN-γ.[177, 178] To varying degrees, all of the interferons enhance the ability of NK cells to destroy virus-infected targets.[96]

Tumor Necrosis Factor (Cachectin) and Lymphotoxin

TNF, also called cachectin, is a macrophage-secreted polymer of 17-kDa subunits[179] that was independently discovered by different investigators pursuing distinct biologic effects.[180, 181] TNF was identified by several groups as an activity found in the serum of mice treated with lipopolysaccharide[181] that caused hemorrhagic necrosis of implanted tumors and of certain tumor cell lines.[182] Rouzer and Cerami[183] identified cachectin as a serum product associated with the wasting syndrome of rabbits infected with *Trypanosoma brucei*.[183] The identity of these products with distinct activities was determined when amino acid sequencing studies revealed their homology.[184] This cytokine is referred to here as TNF.

Lymphotoxin was identified as a product of T lymphocytes stimulated by antigen or phytohemagglutinin that caused the destruction of fibroblasts and was therefore thought to be associated with the delayed-type hypersensitivity reaction.[185] Although it is structurally distinct from TNF, sharing only 30% amino acid homology,[186] lymphotoxin binds to the same receptor as TNF and therefore shares its biologic activities.[187] To distinguish these proteins, the macrophage product has been termed TNF-α and lymphotoxin, TNF-β. An additional level of complexity arises from the fact that T cells[188] as well as NK cells[189] may produce TNF-α, although in much lower concentrations than macrophages.

The activities of TNF, which generally apply to lymphotoxin as well, are to promote inflammation and destruction of tissue. It is the primary mediator of endotoxic shock, producing diverse effects on vascular endothelium.[190–192] It causes neutrophils to marginate[193] and promotes their ability to phagocytose foreign materials.[194] Enzyme systems and processes within the neutrophil that promote destruction of ingested material all demonstrate increased activity under the influence of TNF.[195] The activity of eosinophils against schistosomula is enhanced,[196] and the enhanced ability of TNF-stimulated macrophages to destroy ingested parasites or bacteria is also well documented.[197, 198]

With such potent inflammatory activity, TNF production and release must be tightly controlled.[199–202] This molecule is not stored in macrophages but must be newly synthesized each time its production and release are activated. When macrophages are stimulated with lipopolysaccharide, TNF mRNA levels increase by a factor of 50 to 100 and actual production of TNF increases by a factor of 10,000. On the other hand, TNF mRNA can be generated under certain conditions without any TNF production. Thus, control of production of this protein appears to occur primarily at the translational level by mechanisms not yet fully defined. Further control is maintained by the presence of unstable sequences within TNF mRNA, resulting in a short half-life for these molecules once they are generated. Glucocorticoid hormones have been demonstrated to interfere with TNF production at both the transcriptional and posttranscriptional levels.[199] Thus, whereas administration of corticosteroids to experimental animals before exposure to endotoxin ameliorates the effects of endotoxic shock, once shock has occurred, that is, once TNF has been synthesized and secreted, dexamethasone has little impact on the course of the clinical syndrome.[203]

TNF has multiple biologic effects in vitro, altering the activity of many different types of cells in tissue culture systems. Its ability to promote destruction of many, but not all, transformed cell lines is the origin of its name and led to early speculation that its primary function was to promote destruction of tumors in vivo. As has been indicated, its actual in vivo activity is more varied and quite dose dependent. When it is administered to animals in large boluses, the induced effect mimics endotoxic shock.[204] Continuous administration of lower doses results in the chronic wasting syndrome attributed to the effects of "cachectin" and is associated with suppression of both lipoprotein lipase activity and hepatic protein synthesis.[204–207] Manipulation of TNF levels to promote or restrict inflammatory responses may prove to be a useful therapeutic tool in the treatment of infectious diseases.

Granulocyte-Macrophage Colony-Stimulating Factor

Granulocyte-macrophage colony-stimulating factor is a protein of 14 to 35 kDa released by activated T cells and, to a lesser extent, macrophages, endothelial cells, and fibroblasts. It was first identified by its ability to promote in vitro growth of hematopoietic stem cells[208] but has subsequently been shown to stimulate enzymatic activity in mature macrophages, resulting in increased antimicrobial and antitumor activity.[209, 210] Clinical studies with recombinant granulocyte-macrophage colony-stimulating factor have demonstrated its ability in vivo to increase the number of circulating granulocytes in patients who have received bone marrow transplants[211] or chemotherapy.[212] These types of observations offer the promise of more extensive therapeutic use of this lymphokine.

Interleukin-12

Interleukin-12 (IL-12) is a 70-kDa heterodimeric cytokine produced predominantly by phagocytic cells in response to exposure to bacterial products. It consists of two covalently linked glycoproteins of 35 and 40 kDa. IL-12 secretion results in increased production of IFN-γ by both T cells and NK cells,[213, 214] and many of its biologic effects result from enhanced production of this lymphokine. Because IFN-γ is itself an important determinant of whether a microorganism elicits predominantly an antibody or a cell-mediated immune response, IL-12 becomes a critical factor in activating the cellular instead of the humoral limb of the immune response.[215–217] In addition to eliciting IFN-γ, IL-12 up-regulates production of TNF-α and granulocyte-macrophage colony-stimulating factor,[218] thereby further enhancing the early response to invading pathogens. This indirect antimicrobial activity of IL-12 is best understood in the context of different functions of Th1 and Th2 subsets of $CD4^+$ T cells.

T-Cell Subsets Distinguished by Lymphokine Secretion Patterns

Although the functions of the various lymphokines acting individually have been well defined, the effect of these lymphokines on immune responses to pathogens depends on which lymphokine responses are elicited by exposure to a given invading organism. The answer to this question has been greatly simplified by the realization that lymphokines are secreted in certain patterns and that secretion of certain lymphokines precludes the secretion of others. These patterns are attributable to the fact that different $CD4^+$ T-cell populations preferentially secrete different cocktails of lymphokines. Those secreting primarily IL-2 and IFN-γ are referred to as Th1 T cells and those secreting interleukins IL-4, IL-5, IL-6, and IL-10 are termed Th2 T cells.[219] The lymphokines secreted by Th1 T cells favor the induction of delayed-type hypersensitivity and cell-mediated immune responses. Those secreted by Th2 lymphocytes favor the development of IgG1 and IgE antibody responses. IFN-γ secretion by Th1 cells inhibits proliferation of Th2 clones but does not inhibit lymphokine secretion by those clones.[220, 221] However, IFN-γ can inhibit the effects that secreted IL-4, a Th2 product, can have on its target cells.[222–224] IL-10 from Th2 cells, in turn, can inhibit the production of IFN-γ by Th1 T cells. It does this by inhibiting the release from macrophages of cytokines that would normally enhance Th1 function.[225]

Whether exposure to a given microbial pathogen ultimately elicits a Th1 or a Th2 response depends on the activity of certain cytokines secreted by macrophages (IL-12) and T cells (IL-4). The most interesting studies of these effects have been in inbred mouse strains that differ in their response to parasitic or bacterial pathogens. It has been shown, for example, that mouse strains that produce IL-4 as part of a Th2 response to challenge with *Leishmania major* succumb to the infection, but those that respond with IL-12 production by macrophages and a predominant Th1 response develop only a localized, self-limited infection.[226] In contrast, Th1 responses exacerbate the arthritis and the proliferation of *Borrelia burgdorferi* in a mouse model of Lyme disease, and manipulation of the response to favor the activity of the Th2 cell population greatly ameliorates the symptoms and results in a reduction in the bacterial proliferation in affected joints.[227] The different effects of Th1 and Th2 cells in these two models systems may reflect the role of *L. major* as an intracellular pathogen, whereas *B. burgdorferi* establishes infection extracellularly. However, the properties that cause antigens to elicit primarily a Th1 or Th2 response are poorly defined, as is the genetic basis for the predominance of Th1 or Th2 responses in different inbred mouse strains.

Cells with Direct Antimicrobial Activity

Although the different lymphokines just discussed are likely to enhance nonspecifically both the elicitation and the execution of cell-mediated immune reactions to microbial infection, no specific antimicrobial activity can be directly attributed to these lymphokines, with the exception of the interferons. On the other hand, the direct antiviral activity of cytotoxic T cells and NK cells has been well described, and other studies have demonstrated a role for T cells in resistance to bacteria that normally reside in the extracellular environment.[228, 229]

Cytotoxic T Cells

Cell-mediated resistance to influenza virus provides a well-studied model of how cytotoxic T lymphocytes (CTLs) function and affords important insights into current concepts of antigen recognition by T cells. Serologic studies have indicated that the appearance of epidemics of influenza results from changes in two glycoproteins, neuraminidase and hemagglutinin, that extend outside the envelope of the virus. Populations without circulating antibodies to specific epitopes of these proteins are at risk for influenza.[230, 231] Antibody to the hemagglutinin prevents attachment of the virus to sialic acid residues on the cell surface, thereby interfering with infection of the cell. Studies in mice by Townsend and Skehel[232] demonstrated that CTLs were capable of reacting against influenza virus strains independent of hemagglutinin serotype and that the target of most CTL activity was not viral surface proteins but rather nucleoprotein, which, in the intact virion, is unexposed to the external environment. Furthermore, by deleting segments of the nucleoprotein gene from the virus, Townsend and colleagues[233] showed that different inbred mouse strains were responding to different segments of the nucleoprotein. These studies provided important indirect evidence that CTLs were not recognizing intact proteins and that an intracellular processing event, leading to expression of different segments of nucleoprotein on the surface of the infected cell, preceded recognition of that cell by CTLs. Because CTLs recognize only processed peptides, it is apparent that they would be effective in destroying only cells that are already infected by virus and could not prevent infection from occurring, as antibody might. Although antibody could prevent virus from spreading through the extracellular environment from one cell to the next, it could not inhibit ongoing viral replication in cells that were already infected. Antibody also could not interfere with direct cell-to-cell viral spread. This has been well demonstrated in models of herpes simplex virus infection of T-cell–deficient mice, in which the host mice are never able to eradicate the virus and eventually succumb to overwhelming infection.[234] Cellular and humoral immune mechanisms therefore act in a complementary manner to limit the spread of virus and to abort ongoing viral infection.

Two mechanisms have been described by which activated CTLs kill virus-infected cells (Fig. 7–5). Direct contact between the CTLs and their target is required and occurs at a membrane region of the CTL that is close to the cell's microtubule organizing center, centrioles, and Golgi apparatus.[235, 236] Model systems in which various esterases and proteases within the granules of CTLs destroy the target cell have been described. Particular emphasis has been placed on a complement-like CTL secretory product called perforin, which produces pores in the membrane of target cells.[237] This mechanism of cell lysis now appears to be the predominant one used by CTLs. The importance of perforin-mediated activity for CTL function has been most directly shown with knockout mice deficient in the perforin gene.[238]

Although the reduction in CTL activity observed in perforin-deficient mice clearly demonstrates the importance of this protein for normal CTL function, some residual CTL activity is observed in perforin-deficient mice. This activity results from the interaction of Fas ligand on T cells with Fas on target cells.[238–242] Fas, also called Apo-1, is a protein that may be expressed on the surface of potential CTL targets. Binding of Fas by its ligand on $CD8^+$ T cells results in death of the target cells, a death characterized by fragmentation of target cell DNA. This type of cell death, termed programmed cell death or apoptosis, is mediated by the activation of cellular endonucleases and is, therefore, quite distinct from the membrane disruption associated with perforin.[243] Fas ligand on the T cell is identical to membrane-bound TNF, and its expression is up-regulated by binding of the TCR on cytotoxic T cells.[244] Obviously, the killing of target cells through the Fas–Fas ligand pathway depends on the expression of Fas by the target cells. Macrophages and hepatocytes are among the cells that express Fas. Target cells lacking Fas, such as epithelial cells, can be killed only through perforin-dependent mechanisms.

The DNA disruption observed in Fas-mediated cell killing is also seen in perforin-mediated killing. However, in the case of perforin-mediated cell killing, the membrane disruption precedes the DNA fragmentation, whereas the opposite is true of Fas-mediated cell death. The DNA fragmentation observed in perforin-mediated cell killing probably results from entry of enzymes from the granules of the CTLs into the target cell through pores created by the activity of perforin.[245–247]

Natural Killer Cells

NK cells lyse their targets by the perforin-dependent pathway, although the membrane signals that stimulate the release of perforin are, as indicated, different for NK cells and CTLs. NK function exists normally in humans and requires no "immunization" to be elicited. In vitro studies have demonstrated that cell lines normally resistant to lysis by NK cells are lysed by NK cells if the target cell lines are infected with virus. This observation has been described for a number of different viruses, including the human immunodeficiency virus,[248] herpes simplex virus,[249] and varicella-zoster virus.[250] Mice treated in vivo with antibodies to NK cell surface markers are more susceptible to murine cytomegalovirus and hepatitis virus.[251] This observation in mice is supported by reports of an NK-deficient human patient who was subject to severe varicella and cytomegalovirus infections.[252]

In addition to their antiviral activity, NK cells have been shown to lyse directly the trypomastigote and epimastigote forms of *Trypanosoma cruzi*,[253] and mice infected with *Toxoplasma gondii* generate NK cells capable of killing that parasite in vitro.[254] High concentrations of NK cells can also inhibit the in vitro growth of *Cryptococcus neoformans*.[255]

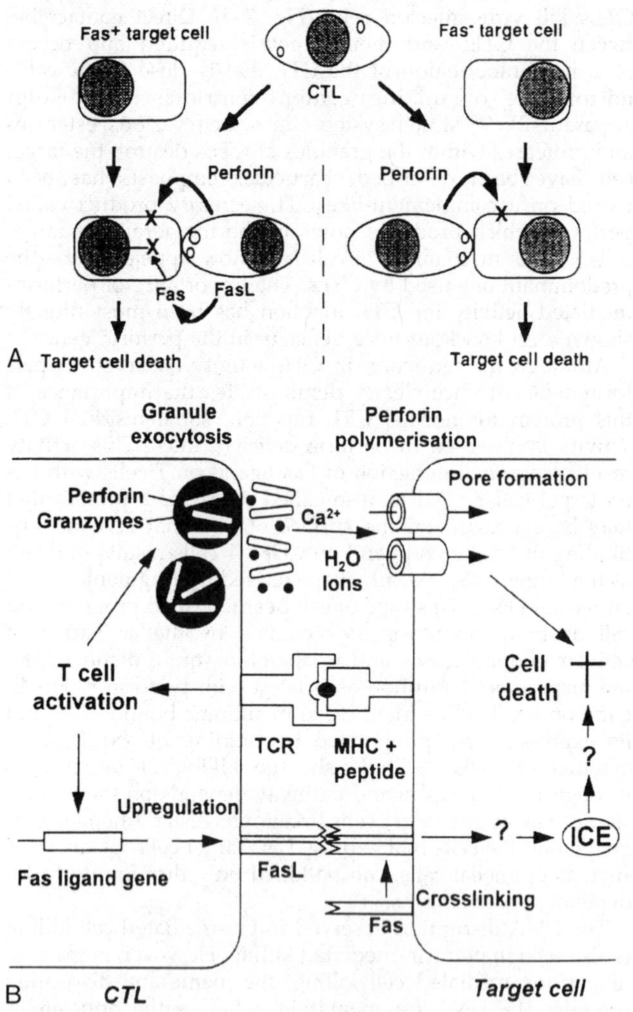

FIGURE 7–5 ▫ Schematic representation of the two pathways in T-cell–mediated cytotoxicity. *A*, The two pathways of cytotoxicity: Fas-negative target cells are lysed by the action of the perforin-dependent pathway. Fas-expressing target cells, however, are killed by the concomitant effect of the perforin- and the Fas-dependent pathways. *B*, Steps and molecules involved in the two pathways of T-cell–mediated cytotoxicity. For both pathways the engagement of the specific TCR complex and T-cell activation are primary events. The perforin-dependent granule exocytosis pathway *(top)* is then initiated by accumulation of cytoplasmic granules containing perforin and granzymes at the interface between effector T cell and target cell, followed by directed exocytosis of these granules on the target cell. The elevated free calcium ion concentration in the extracellular space compared with the granular compartment induces a conformational change of the perforin molecules, rendering them amphipathic and able to insert into the target cell membrane. There, 10 to 18 perforin molecules aggregate to form polyperforin pores, which make the target cell membrane permeable to water and small ions. This permeabilization eventually, together with effects of additional molecules such as granzymes entering through the polyperforin pore into the target cell cytoplasm, leads to death of the target cell. The Fas-dependent pathway *(bottom)* is initiated by up-regulation of Fas ligand (FasL) expression on the T cell. Binding and cross-linking of the Fas ligand molecule, which is probably present on the membrane in a trimeric form, with Fas molecules on the target cell lead to the induction of apoptosis. A death-inducing cytoplasmic domain on the Fas molecule triggers an apoptosis program that probably involves several interacting molecules, one of which may be IL-1β–converting enzyme (ICE) and/or a related protease. (From Kägi D, Ledermann B, Bürki K, et al: Molecular mechanisms of lymphocyte-mediated cytotoxicity and their role in immunological protection and pathogenesis in vivo. Annu Rev Immunol 14:210, 1996. Reproduced, with permission, from the Annual Review of Immunology, Volume 14, © 1996, by Annual Reviews Inc.)

T Cells with Activity Against Extracellular Bacteria

Two different laboratories, using either *Bacteroides fragilis*[228] or *Pseudomonas aeruginosa*,[229] have described murine model infection systems in which T cells protect against challenge with extracellular bacteria. In both systems the antibacterial activity has been attributed to soluble products of CD8+ T cells. In the *P. aeruginosa* model, secretion of the antibacterial factor results from binding of bacteria to Fc receptors on T cells that have previously been occupied by *P. aeruginosa*–specific antibody.[256] Thus, specific antibody on the T cell's Fc receptor acts as the antigen binding site for bacteria. The secreted factor has been shown to inhibit in vitro growth of bacteria in a direct but nonspecific manner.[257]

Immune Destruction of Intracellular Bacteria

The immune mechanisms by which bacteria, fungi, and parasites that survive and multiply within phagocytic cells can be destroyed have undergone reanalysis within the past several years. Early studies by Zinkernagel and colleagues[258] showed adoptive protection against infection with the intracellular pathogen *L. monocytogenes* to be class II restricted, indicating that cytotoxic mechanisms, which are predominantly class I restricted, were not involved. *Listeria* then became widely used in model systems for in vitro analysis of the basis for this protection.[259] Such in vitro studies with intracellular pathogens demonstrated that lymphokines produced by CD4+ T cells that were exposed to microbial antigens could activate macrophages to kill organisms that were not killed by macrophages that had not been exposed to immune T cells. This activation was nonspecific in that, once activated, the macrophages showed increased ability to destroy unrelated organisms or even tumor cells.[260] IFN-γ was subsequently identified as the primary T-cell product that activated macrophages to increased microbicidal activity.[177]

Although the term activated macrophage is readily understood on a functional level as related to whether a macrophage can destroy the organism residing within it, the biochemical basis for activation differs depending on the setting in which the activation occurs. This is best exemplified by the caseous necrosis that typically characterizes tuberculous lesions but is not observed in inflammatory lesions associated with other intracellular pathogens. This property of tuberculous lesions is attributable to products of the mycobacterial cell wall that stimulate increased production of TNF-α by the macrophage.[197, 261] Therefore, the inflammatory response to a given organism is influenced both by the T cells that organism stimulates and the biochemical pathways it triggers within the macrophage.

Studies have indicated that CD8+, as well as CD4+, T cells may be important in resistance to *Listeria*.[262, 263] Like CD4+ T cells, these cells can activate macrophages by secretion of IFN-γ.[264] Furthermore, Kaufmann and colleagues[265] have shown that cloned CD8+ T cells that are not MHC restricted are able to lyse infected macrophages in vitro and protect mice from in vivo challenge with these organisms. This non–MHC-restricted protection appears to be mediated through the interaction of T cells with bacterial proteins carrying the fMet-Leu-Phe signal sequence, which binds to the nonpolymorphic class Ib MHC gene products on antigen-presenting cells, as described earlier. As has been indicated, non–MHC-restricted T cells with γδ TCR have been shown to have similar activity against mycobacteria-infected macrophages.[81]

Conclusion

Although the explosive growth in our understanding of T-lymphocyte biology in the past decade has increased our knowledge of this cell's importance for host defense, it has also provided an appreciation of the variety and complexity of the responses that can be generated to different microbial pathogens. Analysis of Th1 and Th2 subsets and their associated lymphokine profiles has yielded a framework for understanding the different effects that T lymphocytes might produce in response to infection. In addition, the development of mouse strains deficient in certain immune capabilities has clarified the relative importance of different immune mechanisms of antimicrobial resistance. Armed with this new and rapidly increasing knowledge, the physician may be approaching the time when immunologic intervention is an important adjunct in the battle against increasingly antibiotic-resistant microbial pathogens.

References

1. Cantor H, Boyse EA: Functional subclasses of T lymphocytes bearing different Ly antigens. I. The generation of functionally distinct T-cell classes is a differentiative process independent of antigen. J Exp Med 141:1376, 1975.
2. Swain SL: Significance of Lyt phenotypes: Lyt2 antibodies block activities of T cells that recognize class I major histocompatibility complex antigens regardless of their function. Proc Natl Acad Sci USA 78:7101, 1981.
3. Allison J, McIntyre B, Bloch D: Tumor-specific antigen of murine T lymphoma defined with monoclonal antibody. J Immunol 129:2293, 1982.
4. Meuer D, Fitzgerald K, Hussey R, et al: 1983. Clonotypic structures involved in antigen-specific human T-cell function. Relationship to the T3 molecular complex. J Exp Med 157:705, 1983.
5. Weiss A, Imboden JB: 1987. Cell surface molecules and early events involved in T lymphocyte activation. Adv Immunol 41:1, 1987.
6. van Agthoven A, Terhorst C, Reinherz C, Schlossman SF: 1981. Characterization of T cell surface glycoproteins T1 and T3 present on all human peripheral T lymphocytes and functionally mature thymocytes. Eur J Immunol 11:18, 1981.
7. Cantor H, Shen FW, Boyse EA: Separation of helper T cells from suppressor T cells expressing different Ly components. II. Activation by antigen: After immunization, antigen-specific suppressor and helper activities are mediated by distinct T-cell subclasses. J Exp Med 143:1391, 1976.
8. Littman DR, Thomas Y, Maddon PJ, et al: The isolation and sequence of the gene encoding T8: A molecule defining functional classes of T lymphocytes. Cell 40:237, 1985.
9. Mosmann TR, Cherwinski H, Bond MW, et al: Two types of murine helper T cell clone. J Immunol 136:2348, 1986.
10. Clement LT, Yamashita N, Martin AM: The functionally distinct subpopulations of human CD4+ helper/inducer T lymphocytes defined by anti-CD45R antibodies derive sequentially from a differentiation pathway that is regulated by activation-dependent post-thymic differentiation. J Immunol 141:1464, 1988.
11. Serra HM, Krowka JF, Ledbetter JA, Pilarski LM: Loss of CD45R (Lp220) represents a post-thymic T cell differentiation event. J Immunol 140:1435, 1988.
12. Abbas AK, Williams ME, Burstein HJ, et al: Activation and functions of CD4+ T cell subsets. Immunol Rev 123:5, 1991.
13. Siliciano RF, Lawton T, Knall C, et al: Analysis of host-virus interaction in AIDS and with anti-gp120 T cell clones: Effect of HIV sequence variation and a mechanism for CD4+ cell depletion. Cell 54:561, 1988.
14. Morrison LA, Lukacher AE, Braciale VL, et al: Differences in antigen presentation to MHC class I– and class II–restricted influenza virus specific CTL clones. J Exp Med 163:903, 1986.
15. Lanier LL, Phillips JH, Hackett JH Jr, et al: Natural killer cells: Definition of a cell type rather than a function. J Immunol 137:2735, 1986.
16. Phillips JH, Lanier LL: Dissection of the lymphokine-activated killer phenomenon. J Exp Med 164:814, 1986.
17. Lopez C, Kirkpatrick D, Fitzgerald PA, et al: Studies of the cell lineage of the effector cells that spontaneously lyse HSV-1 infected fibroblasts (NK(HSV-1)). J Immunol 129:824, 1982.
18. Timonen T, Ortaldo JR, Herberman RB: Characteristics of human large granular lymphocytes and relationship to natural killer and K cells. J Exp Med 153:569, 1981.
19. Ortaldo JR, Herberman RB: Heterogeneity of natural killer cells. Annu Rev Immunol 2:359, 1984.
20. Perussia B, Fanning V, Trinchieri G: A human NK and K cell subset shares with cytotoxic T cell expression of the antigen recognized by OKT8. J Immunol 131:223, 1983.
21. Hercend T, Reinherz EL, Meuer S, et al: Phenotypic and functional heterogeneity of human cloned natural killer cell lines. Nature 301:158, 1983.
22. Lanier LL, Kipps TJ, Phillips JH: Functional properties of a unique subset of cytotoxic CD3+ T lymphocytes that express Fc receptors for IgG (CD1b/Leu-11 antigen). J Exp Med 162:2089, 1985.
23. Lanier LL, Le AM, Civin CI, et al: The relationship of CD16 (Leu-11) and Leu-19 (NKH-1) antigen expression on human peripheral blood NK cells and cytotoxic T lymphocytes. J Immunol 136:4480, 1986.
24. Shore SL, Melewicz FM, Gordon DS: The mononuclear cell in human blood which mediates antibody-dependent cellular cytotoxicity to virus-infected target cells. I. Identification of the population of effector cells. J Immunol 118:558, 1977.
25. Schwartz RH: T-lymphocyte recognition of antigen in association with gene products of the major histocompatibility complex. Annu Rev Immunol 3:237, 1985.
26. Rosenthal AS, Shevach EM: Function of macrophages in antigen recognition by guinea pig T lymphocytes. I. Requirement for histocompatible macrophages and lymphocytes. J Exp Med 138:1194, 1973.
27. Katz DH, Hamaoka T, Benacerraf B: Cell interactions between histocompatible T and B lymphocytes. Failure of physiologic cooperative interactions between T and B lymphocytes from allogeneic donor strains in humoral response to hapten-protein conjugates. J Exp Med 137:1405, 1973.
28. Zinkernagel RM, Doherty PC: Restriction of in vitro T cell–mediated cytotoxicity in lymphocytic choriomeningitis within a syngeneic or semiallogeneic system. Nature 248:701, 1974.
29. Shearer GM, Rhen TG, Garabrino CA: Cell mediated lympholysis of trinitrophenyl-modified autologous lymphocytes. Effector cell specificity to modified cell surface components controlled by the H-2K and H-2D serological regions of the murine major histocompatibility complex. J Exp Med 141:1348, 1975.
30. Srivastava R, Duceman BW, Biro PA, et al: Molecular organization of the class I genes of the human major histocompatibility complex. Immunol Rev 84:93, 1985.
31. Bell JI, Denny DW, McDevitt HO: Structure and polymorphism of murine and human class II major histocompatibility antigens. Immunol Rev 84:52, 1985.
32. Rouse BT, Norley S, Martin S: Antiviral cytotoxic T lymphocyte induction and vaccination. Rev Infect Dis 10:16, 1988.
33. Harris HW, Gill TJ III: Expression of class I transplantation antigens. Transplantation 42:109, 1986.
34. Brooks CF, Moore M: Differential MHC class II expression on human peripheral blood monocytes and dendritic cells. Immunology 63:303, 1988.
35. Krieger JI, Chestnut RW, Grey HM: Capacity of B cells to function as stimulators of a primary mixed leukocyte reaction. J Immunol 137:3117, 1986.
36. Kirkham BW, Pitzalis C, Kingsley GH, et al: Rheumatoid T lymphocyte MHC class II expression: In vitro stimulation produces normal MHC class II expression, independent of proliferation. J Rheumatol 16:270, 1989.
37. Manyak CL, Tse H, Fischer P, et al: Regulation of class II MHC molecules on human endothelial cells. Effects of IFN and dexamethasone. J Immunol 140:3817, 1988.
38. Dib SA, Vardi P, Bonner-Weir S, Eisenbarth GS: Selective localization of factor VIII antigenicity to islet endothelial cells and expression of class II antigens by normal human pancreatic ductal epithelium. Diabetes 37:482, 1988.
39. Ziegler-Heitbrock HW, Stachel D, Schlunk T, et al: Class II (DR) antigen expression on CD8+ lymphocyte subsets in acquired immune deficiency syndrome (AIDS). J Clin Immunol 8:473, 1988.
40. Allen PM: Antigen processing at the molecular level. Immunol Today 8:270, 1987.

41. Grey HM, Chestnut R: Antigen processing and presentation to T cells. Immunol Today 6:101, 1985.
42. Townsend ARM, Gotch FM, Davey J: Cytotoxic T lymphocytes recognize fragments of the influenza nucleoprotein. Cell 42:457, 1985.
43. Buus S, Sette A, Colon SM, et al: The relation between major histocompatibility complex (MHC) restriction and the capacity of Ia to bind immunogenic peptides. Science 235:1353, 1987.
44. Fearon DT, Wong WW: Complement ligand-receptor interactions that mediate biological responses. Annu Rev Immunol 1:243, 1983.
45. Morgan EL, Weigle WO: Biological activities residing in the Fc region of immunoglobulin. Adv Immunol 40:61, 1987.
46. Klatzman D, Champagne E, Chamaret S, et al: T-lymphocyte T4 molecule behaves as the receptor for human retrovirus LAV. Nature 312:767, 1984.
47. Germain RN: The ins and outs of antigen processing and presentation. Nature 322:687, 1986.
48. McCoy KL, Miller J, Jenkins M, et al: Diminished antigen processing by endosomal acidification mutant antigen-presenting cells. J Immunol 143:29, 1989.
49. Degen E, Cohendoyle MF, Williams DB: Efficient dissociation of the p88 chaperone from major histocompatibility complex class-1 molecules requires both β_2-microglobulin and peptide. J Exp Med 175:1653, 1992.
50. Yewdell JW, Bennin JR, Hosaka Y: Cells process exogenous proteins for recognition by cytotoxic T lymphocytes. Science 239:637, 1988.
51. Spies T, DeMars R: Restored expression of major histocompatibility class I molecules by gene transfer of a putative peptide transporter. Nature 351:323, 1991.
52. Spies T, Cerundolo V, Colonna M, et al: Presentation of viral antigen by MHC class I molecules is dependent on a putative peptide transporter heterodimer. Nature 355:644, 1992.
53. Powis SJ, Deverson EV, Bastin J, et al: Restoration of antigen presentation to the mutant cell line RMA-S by an MHC-linked transporter. Nature 354:528, 1991.
54. Powis SJ, Deverson EV, Coadwell WJ, et al: Effect of polymorphism of a MHC-linked transporter on the peptides assembled in a class-I molecule. Nature 357:211, 1992.
55. Lindahl KF, Hermel E, Loveland BE, Wang CR: Maternally transmitted antigen of mice: A model transplantation antigen. Annu Rev Immunol 9:351, 1991.
56. Pamer EG, Wang CR, Flaherty L, et al: H-2M3 presents a *Listeria monocytogenes* peptide to cytotoxic T lymphocytes. Cell 70:215, 1992.
57. Kurlander RJ, Shawar SM, Brown ML, Rich RR: Specialized role for murine class I-b MHC molecule in prokaryotic host defenses. Science 257:678, 1992.
58. Sha WC, Nelson CA, Newberry RD, et al: Positive and negative selection of an antigen receptor on T cells in transgenic mice. Nature 336:73, 1988.
59. Scollay R, Shortman K: Cell traffic in the adult thymus: Cell entry and exit, cell birth and death. *In* Watson JD, Marbrook J (eds): Recognition and Regulation in Cell-Mediated Immunity. New York, Marcel Dekker, 1985, p 3.
60. Kappler JW, Roehm N, Marrack P: T cell tolerance by clonal elimination in the thymus. Cell 49:273, 1987.
61. Davis MM, Bjorkman PJ: T-cell antigen receptor genes and T-cell recognition. Nature 334:395, 1988.
62. Schwartz RH: Immune response (Ir) genes of the murine major histocompatibility complex. Adv Immunol 38:31, 1986.
63. Saito H, Kranz DM, Takagaki Y, et al: Complete primary structure of a heterodimeric T-cell receptor deduced from cDNA sequences. Nature 309:757, 1984.
64. Yague J, White J, Coleclough C, et al: The T cell receptor: The alpha and beta chains define idiotype, and antigen and MHC specificity. Cell 42:81, 1985.
65. Dembic Z, Haas W, Weiss S, et al: Transfer of specificity by murine alpha and beta T-cell receptor genes. Nature 320:232, 1986.
66. Saito T, Weiss A, Miller J, et al: Specific antigen-Ia activation of transfected human T cells expressing murine Ti alpha beta-human T3 receptor complexes. Nature 325:125, 1987.
67. Clevers H, Alacron B, Wileman T, Terhorst C: The T cell receptor/CD3 complex: A dynamic protein ensemble. Annu Rev Immunol 6:629, 1988.
68. Weiss A, Imboden J, Terhorst C, Stobo J: The role of the T3/antigen receptor complex in T-cell activation. Annu Rev Immunol 4:593, 1986.
69. Elliott JF, Rock EP, Patten PA, et al: The adult T-cell receptor δ-chain is diverse and distinct from that of fetal thymocytes. Nature 331:627, 1988.
70. Brenner MB, McLean J, Dialynas DP, et al: Identification of a putative second T-cell receptor. Nature 322:145, 1986.
71. Bank I, DePinho RA, Brenner MB, et al: Functional T3 molecule associated with a novel heterodimer on the surface of immature human thymocytes. Nature 322:179, 1986.
72. Borst J, van Dongen JJM, Bolhuis RLH, et al: Distinct molecular forms of human T cell receptor γ-δ detected on viable T cells by a monoclonal antibody. J Exp Med 167:1625, 1988.
73. Lanier LL, Ruitenberg JJ, Phillips JH: Human $CD3^+$ T lymphocytes that express neither CD4 nor CD8 antigens. J Exp Med 164:339, 1986.
74. Pardoll DM, Fowlkes BJ, Bluestone JA, et al: Differential expression of two distinct T-cell receptors during thymocyte development. Nature 326:79, 1987.
75. Lew AM, Pardoll DM, Maloy WL, et al: Characterization of T cell receptor γ chain expression in a subset of murine thymocytes. Science 234:1401, 1986.
76. Moingeon P, Ythier A, Goubin G, et al: A unique T-cell receptor complex expressed on human fetal lymphocytes displaying natural-killer-like activity. Nature 323:638, 1986.
77. Moingeon P, Jitsukawa S, Faure F, et al: A γ-chain complex forms a functional receptor on cloned human lymphocytes with natural killer–like activity. Nature 325:723, 1987.
78. Lang F, Peyrat M, Constant P, et al: Early activation of human Vγ9Vδ2 T cell broad cytotoxicity and TNF production by nonpeptidic mycobacterial ligands. J Immunol 154:5986, 1995.
79. Morita CT, Beckman EM, Bukowski JF, et al: Direct presentation of nonpeptide prenyl pyrophosphate antigens to human γ-δ T cells. Immunity 3:495, 1995.
80. Schoel B, Sprenger S, Kaufmann SH: Phosphate is essential for stimulation of V-γ-9V-δ-2 T-lymphocytes by mycobacterial low-molecular-weight ligand. Eur J Immunol 24:1886, 1994.
81. Janis EM, Kaufmann SH, Schwartz RH, Pardoll DM: Activation of γ δ T cells in the primary immune response to *Mycobacterium tuberculosis*. Science 244:713, 1989.
82. Mombaerts P, Arnoldi J, Russ F, Kaufmann SHE: Different roles of alpha/beta and gamma/delta T cells in immunity against an intracellular bacterial pathogen. Nature 365:53, 1993.
83. Hiromatsu K, Yoshikai Y, Matsuzaki G, et al: A protective role of gamma/delta T cells in primary infection with *Listeria monocytogenes* in mice. J Exp Med 175:49, 1992.
84. Kaufmann SHE, Ladel CH: Role of T cell subsets in immunity against intracellular bacteria: Experimental infections of knock-out mice with *Listeria monocytogenes* and *Mycobacterium bovis* BCG. Immunobiology 191:509, 1994.
85. Fu XY, Roark CE, Kelly K, et al: Immune protection and control of inflammatory tissue necrosis by γ δ T cells. J Immunol 153:3115, 1994.
86. Lenschow DJ, Walunas TL, Bluestone JA: CD28/B7 system of T cell costimulation. Annu Rev Immunol 14:233, 1996.
87. Boise LH, Minn AJ, Noel PJ, et al: CD28 costimulation can promote T cell survival by enhancing the expression of Bcl-xL. Immunity 3:87, 1995.
88. Larsen CP, Elwood ET, Alexander DZ, et al: Long-term acceptance of skin and cardiac allografts after blocking CD40 and CD28 pathways. Nature 381:434, 1996.
89. Vitale M, Sivori S, Pende D, et al: The coexpression of two functionally independent p58 inhibitory receptors in human NK cell clones results in the inability to kill all normal allogeneic target cells. Proc Natl Acad Sci USA 92:3536, 1995.
90. Kaufman DS, Schoon RA, Leibson PJ: MHC class I expression on tumor targets inhibits natural killer cell–mediated cytotoxicity without interfering with target recognition. J Immunol 150:1429, 1993.
91. Siliciano RF, Pratt JC, Schmidt RE, et al: Activation of cytotoxic T lymphocyte and natural killer cell function through the T11 sheep erythrocyte binding protein. Nature 317:428, 1985.
92. Moretta A, Tambussi G, Ciccone E, et al: CD16 surface molecules regulate the cytolytic functions of $CD3\text{-}CD16^+$ human "natural killer" cells. Int J Cancer 44:727, 1989.

93. Giorda R, Trucco M: Mouse NKR-P1. A family of genes selectively coexpressed in adherent lymphokine-activated killer cells. J Immunol 147:1701, 1991.
94. Ryan JC, Niemi EC, Goldfien RD, et al: NKR-P1, an activating molecule on rat natural killer cells, stimulates phosphoinositide turnover and a rise in intracellular calcium. J Immunol 147:3244, 1991.
95. Lanier LL, Chang C, Phillips J: Human NKRP1A. A disulfide-linked homodimer of the C-type lectin superfamily expressed by a subset of NK and T lymphocytes. J Immunol 153:2417, 1994.
96. Djeu JY, Heinbaugh JA, Holden HT, Herberman RB: Augmentation of mouse natural killer cell activity by interferon and interferon inducers. J Immunol 122:175, 1979.
97. Samelson LE, Klausner RD: Tyrosine kinases and tyrosine-based activation motifs. J Biol Chem 267:24913, 1992.
98. Gauen LKT, Zhu YX, Letourneur F, et al: Interactions of $p59^{fyn}$ and ZAP-70 with T-cell receptor activation motifs; defining the nature of a signalling motif. Mol Cell Biol 14:3729, 1994.
99. Cantrell D: T cell antigen receptor signal transduction pathways. Annu Rev Immunol 14:259, 1996.
100. Weiss A: T cell antigen receptor signal transduction: A tale of tails and cytoplasmic protein-tyrosine kinases. Cell 73:209, 1993.
101. Cambier J: Conserved signaling motifs in antigen and Fc receptors. Semin Immunol 7, 1995.
102. Iwashima M, Irving BA, van Oers NSC, et al: Sequential interactions of the TCR with two distinct cytoplasmic tyrosine kinases. Science 263:1136, 1996.
103. Weil R, Cloutier JF, Fournel M, Veillette A: Regulation of ZAP70 by Src family tyrosine kinases in an antigen specific T cell line. J Biol Chem 270:2791, 1995.
104. Weiss A, Littman DR: Signal transduction by lymphocyte antigen receptors. Cell 76:263, 1994.
105. Cooper JA: Straight and narrow or tortuous and intersecting? Curr Biol 4:1118, 1994.
106. Clipstone NA, Crabtree GR: Identification of calcineurin as a key signaling enzyme in T-lymphocyte activation. Nature 357:695, 1992.
107. Wolff SM: Biological effects of bacterial endotoxins in man. J Infect Dis 128:S733, 1973.
108. Dinarello CA: Interleukin 1: Amino acid sequences, multiple biological activities and comparison with tumor necrosis factor (cachectin). Year Immunol 2:68, 1986.
109. LoMedico PT, Gubler U, Hellmann CP, et al: Cloning and expression of murine interleukin 1 cDNA in *Escherichia coli*. Nature 312:458, 1984.
110. Auron PE, Webb AC, Rosenwasser LJ, et al: Nucleotide sequence of human monocyte interleukin-1 precursor cDNA. Proc Natl Acad Sci USA 81:7907, 1984.
111. Gery I, Gershon RK, Waksman BH: Potentiation of the T lymphocyte response to mitogens. I. The responding cell. J Exp Med 136:128, 1972.
112. Mannel DN, Mizel SB, Diamanstein T, Falk W: Induction of interleukin 2 responsiveness in thymocytes by synergistic action of interleukin 1 and interleukin 2. J Immunol 134:3108, 1985.
113. Durum SK, Oppenheim JJ, Neta R: Immunophysiologic role of interleukin 1. *In* Oppenheim JJ, Shevach EM (eds): Textbook of Immunophysiology. New York, Oxford University Press, 1988, pp 210–225.
114. Kaushansky K, Lin N, Adamson JW: Interleukin 1 stimulates fibroblasts to synthesize granulocyte-macrophage and granulocyte colony-stimulating factors. J Clin Invest 81:92, 1988.
115. Dower SK, Kronheim SR, March CJ, et al: Detection and characterization of high-affinity plasma membrane receptors for human interleukin 1. J Exp Med 162:501, 1985.
116. Morgan DA, Ruscetti FW, Gallo R: Selective in vivo growth of T lymphocytes from normal human bone marrows. Science 193:1007, 1976.
117. Mier JW, Gallo RC: Purification and some characteristics of human T-cell growth factor from phytohemagglutinin stimulated lymphocyte conditioned media. Proc Natl Acad Sci USA 77:6134, 1980.
118. Leonard WJ, Depper JM, Robb RJ, et al: Characterization of the human receptor for T cell growth factor. Proc Natl Acad Sci USA 80:6957, 1983.
119. Robb RJ, Munck A, Smith KA: T-cell growth factors: Quantification, specificity, and biological relevance. J Exp Med 154:1455, 1981.
120. Depper JM, Leonard WJ, Kronke M, et al: Regulation of interleukin 2 receptor expression: Effects of phorbol diester, phospholipase C, and reexposure to lectin and antigen. J Immunol 133:3054, 1984.
121. Singer A, Munitz TI, Golding H, et al: Recognition requirements for the activation, differentiation and function of T-helper cells specific for class I MHC alloantigens. Immunol Rev 98:143, 1987.
122. Kaufmann Y, Berke G, Eshhar Z: Cytotoxic T lymphocyte hybridomas that mediate specific tumor cell lysis in vitro. Proc Natl Acad Sci USA 78:2502, 1981.
123. Leonard WJ, Kronke M, Peffer NJ, et al: Interleukin-2 receptor gene expression in normal human T lymphocytes. Proc Natl Acad Sci USA 82:6281, 1985.
124. Kronke M, Leonard WJ, Depper JM, et al: Sequential expression of genes involved in human T lymphocyte growth and differentiation. J Exp Med 161:1593, 1985.
125. Cantrell DA, Smith KA: Transient expression of interleukin 2 receptors. Consequences for T cell growth. J Exp Med 158:1895, 1983.
126. Smith KA, Cantrell DA: Interleukin 2 regulates its own receptors. Proc Natl Acad Sci USA 82:864, 1985.
127. West WH, Cannon GB, Kay H, et al: Natural cytotoxic reactivity of human lymphocytes against a myeloid cell line: Characterization of effector cells. J Immunol 118:355, 1977.
128. Grimm EA, Mazumber A, Zhang HZ, Rosenberg SA: Lymphokine-activated killer cell phenomenon: Lysis of natural killer–resistant fresh solid tumor cells by interleukin 2–activated autologous human peripheral blood lymphocytes. J Exp Med 155:1823, 1982.
129. Rosenberg SA, Lotze MT, Muul LM, et al: Observations on the systemic administration of autologous lymphokine-activated killer cells and recombinant interleukin-2 to patients with metastatic cancer. N Engl J Med 313:1485, 1985.
130. Hu-Li J, Shevach EM, Mizuguchi J, et al: B cell stimulatory factor-1 (interleukin 4) is a potent costimulant for normal resting T lymphocytes. J Exp Med 165:157, 1987.
131. Mosmann TR, Bond MW, Coffman RL, et al: T cell and mast cell lines respond to B cell stimulatory factor-1. Proc Natl Acad Sci USA 83:5654, 1986.
132. Zlotnick A, Daine B, Ransom J, Zipori D: Effects of recombinant B cell growth factor 1 on a macrophage cell line. J Leukoc Biol 40:314, 1986.
133. Smith CA, Rennick DM: Characterization of a murine lymphokine distinct from interleukin 2 and interleukin 3 (IL-3) possessing a T-cell growth factor activity and a mast-cell growth factor activity that synergizes with IL-3. Proc Natl Acad Sci USA 83:1857, 1986.
134. Rousset F, Malefijt FW, Slierendregt B, et al: Regulation of Fc receptor for IgE (CD23) and class II MHC antigen expression on Burkitt's lymphoma cell lines by human IL-4 and IFN-γ. J Immunol 140:2625, 1988.
135. Dennis GJ, Mizuguchi J, McMillan V, et al: Comparison of the calcium requirement for the induction and maintenance of B cell class II molecule expression and for B cell proliferation stimulated by mitogens and purified growth factors. J Immunol 138:4307, 1987.
136. Stein P, DuBois P, Greenblatt D, Howard M: Induction of antigen-specific proliferation in affinity-purified small B lymphocytes: Requirement for BSF-1 by type 2 but not type 1 thymus-independent antigens. J Immunol 136:2080, 1986.
137. Coffman RL, Carty J: A T cell activity that enhances polyclonal IgE production and its inhibition by interferon-γ. J Immunol 136:949, 1986.
138. Sideras P, Bergstedt-Lindqvist S, MacDonald HR, Severinson E: Secretion of IgG1 induction factor by T cell clones and hybridomas. Eur J Immunol 15:586, 1985.
139. Finkelman FD, Katona I, Urban JF Jr, et al: Suppression of in vivo polyclonal IgE responses by monoclonal antibody to the lymphokine B cell stimulatory factor-1. Proc Natl Acad Sci USA 83:9675, 1986.
140. Grabstein KH, Park LS, Morrisey PJ, et al: Regulation of murine T cell proliferation by B cell stimulatory factor-1. J Immunol 139:1148, 1987.

141. Paul WE, Ohara J: B-cell stimulatory factor/interleukin 4. Annu Rev Immunol 5:429, 1987.
142. Crawford RM, Finbloom DS, Ohara J, et al: B-cell stimulatory factor-1 (interleukin-4) activates macrophages for increased tumoricidal activity and expression of Ia antigens. J Immunol 139:135, 1987.
143. Sadick MD, Heinzzel FP, Holaday BJ, et al: Cure of murine leishmaniasis with anti–interleukin-4 monoclonal antibody. Evidence for a T cell–dependent, interferon γ–independent mechanism. J Exp Med 171:115, 1990.
144. Chatelain R, Varkila K, Coffman RL: IL-4 induces a Th2 response in *Leishmania major*–infected mice. J Immunol 148:1182, 1992.
145. Aarden L, Lansdorp P, Degroot E: A growth factor for B cell hybridomas produced by human monocytes. Lymphokines 10:175, 1985.
146. Kawano M, Hirano T, Matsuda T, et al: Autocrine generation and requirement of BSF-2/IL-6 for human multiple myelomas. Nature 332:83, 1988.
147. Zilberstein A, Ruggieri R, Korn JH, Revel M: Structure and expression of cDNA and genes for human interferon-β_2, a distinct species inducible by growth-stimulatory cytokines. EMBO J 5:2529, 1986.
148. Hirano T, Yaga T, Nakano N, et al: Purification to homogeneity and characterization of human B cell differentiation factor (BCDF or BSFp-2). Proc Natl Acad Sci USA 82:5490, 1985.
149. Takai Y, Wong GG, Clark SC, et al: B cell stimulatory factor-2 is involved in the differentiation of cytotoxic T lymphocytes. J Immunol 140:508, 1988.
150. Garman TD, Jacobs KA, Clark SC, Rautlet DH: B-cell–stimulatory factor 2 (β_2 interferon) functions as a second signal for interleukin 2 production by murine T cells. Proc Natl Acad Sci USA 84:7629, 1987.
151. Lotz M, Jirik F, Kabouridis P, et al: B cell stimulating factor 2/interleukin 6 is a costimulant for human thymocytes and T lymphocytes. J Exp Med 167:1253, 1988.
152. Michalevicz R, Revel M: Interferons regulate the in vitro differentiation of multilineage lympho-myeloid stem cells in hairy cell leukemia. Proc Natl Acad Sci USA 84:2307, 1987.
153. Weissenbach J, Chernajovsky Y, Zeevi M, et al: Two interferon mRNAs in human fibroblasts: In vitro translation and *Escherichia coli* cloning studies. Proc Natl Acad Sci USA 77:7152, 1980.
154. Content J, De Wit L, Pierard D, et al: Secretory proteins induced in human fibroblasts under conditions used for the production of interferon β. Proc Natl Acad Sci USA 79:2768, 1982.
155. Ritchie DG, Fuller GM: Hepatocyte-stimulating factor: A monocyte-derived acute-phase regulatory protein. Ann N Y Acad Sci 408:490, 1983.
156. Isaacs A, Lindemann J: Virus interference. I. The interferon. Proc Natl Acad Sci USA 147:258, 1957.
157. Pestka S, Langer JA, Zoon KC, Samuel CE: Interferons and their actions. Annu Rev Biochem 56:727, 1987.
158. Revel M, Chebath J: Interferon-activated genes. Trends Biochem Sci 11:166, 1986.
159. Moore RN, Larsen HS, Horohoo DW, Rouse BT: Endogenous regulation of macrophage proliferative expansion by colony stimulating factor–induced interferon. Science 223:178, 1984.
160. Havell EA, Yip YK, Vilcek J: Characteristics of human lymphoblastoid (Namalva) interferon. J Gen Virol 38:51, 1978.
161. Senussi OA, Cartwright T, Thompson P: Resolution of human fibroblast interferon into two distinct classes by thiol exchange chromatography. Arch Virol 62:323, 1979.
162. Pomerantz RJ, Hirsch MJ: Interferon and human immunodeficiency virus infection. *In* Interferon 9. London, Academic Press, 1987, p 113.
163. Falcoff E, Wietzerbin J, Stefanos S, et al: Properties of mouse immune T-interferon (type II). Ann N Y Acad Sci 350:145, 1980.
164. Kirchner H, Zawatzky R, Engler H, et al: Production of interferon in the murine mixed lymphocyte culture: II. Interferon production is a T cell–dependent function, independent of proliferation. Eur J Immunol 9:824, 1979.
165. Friedman RM: Interferons. *In* Oppenheim JJ, Shevach EM (eds): Textbook of Immunophysiology. New York, Oxford University Press, 1988, pp 194–209.
166. De Clerco E: Interferon inducers. Antibiot Chemother 27:251, 1980.
167. Wada M, Okamura H, Nagata K, et al: Cellular mechanisms in in vivo production of γ interferon induced by lipopolysaccharide in mice infected with *Mycobacterium bovis* BCG. J Interferon Res 5:431, 1985.
168. Gewert DR, Clemens MJ: Inhibition by interferon of thymidine uptake and deoxyribonucleic acid synthesis in human lymphoblastoid cells. Biochem Soc Trans 8:353, 1980.
169. Reis LFL, Le J, Hirano T: Antiviral action of tumor necrosis factor in human fibroblasts is not mediated by B cell stimulatory factor 2/IFN-β_2, and is inhibited by specific antibodies to IFN-β. J Immunol 140:1566, 1988.
170. Ball NA, White CN: Nuclease activation by double-stranded RNA and by 2′,5′-oligoadenylate in extracts of interferon-treated chick cells. Virology 93:348, 1979.
171. Epstein DA, Torrence PF, Friedman RM: Double-stranded RNA inhibits a phosphoprotein phosphatase present in interferon-treated cells. Proc Natl Acad Sci USA 350:621, 1980.
172. Horisberger MA, De Staritzky K: Expression and stability of the Mx protein in different tissues of mice, in response to interferon inducers or to influenza virus infection. J Interferon Res 9:583, 1989.
173. Whitaker-Dowling P, Younger JS: Antiviral effects of interferon in different virus-host cell systems. *In* Pfeffer LM (ed): Mechanisms of Interferon Actions. Boca Raton, FL, CRC Press, 1987, p 83.
174. Marley GM, Doyle LA, Ordonez JV, et al: Potentiation of interferon induction of class I major histocompatibility complex antigen expression by human tumor necrosis factor in small cell lung cancer cell lines. Cancer Res 49:6232, 1989.
175. Virelizier JL, Perez N, Arenzana-Seisdedos F, Devos R: Pure interferon γ enhances class II HLA antigens on human monocyte cell lines. Eur J Immunol 14:106, 1984.
176. Vogel SN, Finbloom DS, English KE, et al: Interferon-induced enhancement of macrophage Fc receptor expression: Beta interferon treatment of C3H/HeJ macrophages results in increased numbers and density of Fc receptors. J Immunol 130:1210, 1982.
177. Buchmeier NA, Schreiber RD: Requirement of endogenous interferon-γ production for resolution of *Listeria monocytogenes* infection. Proc Natl Acad Sci USA 82:7404, 1985.
178. Schultz RM, Chirigos MA: Similarities among factors that render macrophages tumoricidal in lymphokine and interferon preparations. Cancer Res 38:1003, 1978.
179. Smith RA, Baglioni C: The active form of tumor necrosis factor is a trimer. J Biol Chem 262:6951, 1987.
180. Cerami A, Ikeda Y, Le Trang N, et al: Weight loss associated with an endotoxin-induced mediator from peritoneal macrophages: The role of cachectin (tumor necrosis factor). Immunol Lett 11:173, 1985.
181. Carswell EA, Old LJ, Kassel RL, et al: An endotoxin-induced serum factor that causes necrosis of tumors. Proc Natl Acad Sci USA 72:3666, 1975.
182. Helson L, Green S, Carswell E, Old LJ: Effect of tumour necrosis factor on cultured human melanoma cells. Nature 258:731, 1975.
183. Rouzer CA, Cerami A: Hypertriglyceridemia associated with *Trypanosoma brucei brucei* infection in rabbits: Role of defective triglyceride removal. Mol Biochem Parasitol 2:31, 1980.
184. Beutler B, Greenwald D, Hulmes JD, et al: Identity of tumour necrosis factor and the macrophage-secreted factor cachectin. Nature 316:552, 1985.
185. Ruddle NH, Waksman BH: Cytotoxic effect of lymphocyte-antigen interaction in delayed hypersensitivity. Science 157:1060, 1967.
186. Pennica D, Nedwin GE, Hayflick JS, et al: Human tumour necrosis factor: Precursor structure, expression and homology to lymphotoxin. Nature 312:724, 1984.
187. Aggarwal B, Eessalu TE, Hass PI: Characterization of receptors for human tumour necrosis factor and their regulation by interferon γ. Nature 318:665, 1985.
188. Cuturi MC, Murphy M, Costa-Giomi MP, et al: Independent regulation of tumor necrosis factor and lymphotoxin production by human peripheral blood lymphocytes. J Exp Med 165:1581, 1987.
189. Ortaldo J, Ransom RM, Sayers TJ, Herbermann RB: Analysis of cytostatic/cytotoxic lymphokines: Relationship of natural killer cytotoxic factor to recombinant lymphotoxin, recombinant tu-

mor necrosis factor, and leukoregulin. J Immunol 137:2857, 1986.
190. Stern DM, Nawroth PP: Modulation of endothelial hemostatic properties by tumor necrosis factor. J Exp Med 163:740, 1986.
191. Nawroth P, Bank I, Handley D, et al: Tumor necrosis factor/cachectin interacts with endothelial cell receptors to induce release of interleukin 1. J Exp Med 163:1363, 1986.
192. Libby P, Ordovas JM, Auger KR, et al: Endotoxin and tumor necrosis factor induce interleukin-1 gene expression in adult human vascular endothelial cells. Am J Pathol 124:179, 1986.
193. Pohlman TH, Stanness KA, Beatty PG, et al: An endothelial cell surface factor(s) induced in vitro by lipopolysaccharide, interleukin 1, and tumor necrosis factor-α increases neutrophil adherence by CDw18-dependent mechanism. J Immunol 136:4548, 1986.
194. Shalaby MR, Aggarwal BB, Rinderknecht E, et al: Activation of human polymorphonuclear neutrophil functions by interferon-γ and tumor necrosis factors. J Immunol 135:2069, 1985.
195. Klebanoff SJ, Vadas MA, Harlan JM, et al: Stimulation of neutrophils by tumor necrosis factor. J Immunol 136:4220, 1986.
196. Silberstein DS, Dessein AJ: Tumor necrosis factor enhances eosinophil toxicity to *Schistosoma mansoni* larvae. Proc Natl Acad Sci USA 83:1055, 1986.
197. Bermudez LEM, Young LM: Tumor necrosis factor, alone or in combination with IL-2, but not IFN-γ, is associated with macrophage killing of *Mycobacterium avium* complex. J Immunol 140:3006, 1988.
198. Esparza I, Mannel D, Ruppel A, et al: Interferon-γ and lymphotoxin or tumor necrosis factor synergize to activate macrophages for tumoricidal and schistosomulicidal functions. Lymphokine Res 6:1715, 1987.
199. Beutler B, Krochin N, Milsark IW, et al: Control of cachectin (tumor necrosis factor) synthesis: Mechanisms of endotoxin resistance. Science 232:977, 1986.
200. Sariban E, Imamura K, Luebbers R, Kufe D: Transcriptional and posttranscriptional regulation of tumor necrosis factor gene expression in human monocytes. J Clin Invest 81:1506, 1988.
201. Collart MA, Berlin D, Vassalli JD, et al: Gamma interferon enhances macrophage transcription of the tumor necrosis factor/cachectin, interleukin 1, and urokinase genes, which are controlled by short-lived repressors. J Exp Med 164:2113, 1986.
202. Gifford GE, Lohmann-Matthes ML: Requirement for the continual presence of lipopolysaccharide for production of tumor necrosis factor by thioglycollate-induced peritoneal murine macrophages. Int J Cancer 38:135, 1986.
203. Veterans Administration Systemic Sepsis Cooperative Study Group: Effect of high dose glucocorticoid therapy on mortality in patients with clinical signs of systemic sepsis. N Engl J Med 317:659, 1987.
204. Bauss F, Droge W, Mannel DN: Tumor necrosis factor mediates endotoxic effects in mice. Infect Immun 55:1622, 1987.
205. Oliff A, Defeo-Jones D, Boyer M, et al: Tumors secreting human TNF/cachectin induce cachexia in mice. Cell 50:555, 1987.
206. Moldawer LL, Andersson C, Gelin J, Lundholm KG: Regulation of food intake and hepatic protein synthesis by recombinant-derived cytokines. Am J Physiol 254:G450, 1988.
207. Beutler B, Mahoney J, Le Trang N, et al: Purification of cachectin, a lipoprotein lipase–suppressing hormone secreted by endotoxin-induced RAW 264.7 cells. J Exp Med 161:984, 1985.
208. Metcalf D, Johnson GR, Burgess AW: Direct stimulation by purified GM-CSF of the proliferation of multipotential and erythroid precursor cells. Blood 55:138, 1980.
209. Grabstein KH, Urdal DL, Tushinski RJ, et al: Induction of macrophage tumoricidal activity by granulocyte-macrophage colony-stimulating factor. Science 232:506, 1986.
210. Weiser WY, van Neil A, Clark SC, et al: Recombinant human granulocyte/macrophage colony-stimulating factor activates intracellular killing of *Leishmania donovani* by human monocyte-derived macrophages. J Exp Med 166:1436, 1987.
211. Blazar BR, Widmer MB, Kersey JH, et al: Recombinant granulocyte/macrophage-colony stimulating factor in human and murine bone marrow transplantation. Behring Inst Mitt 83:170, 1988.
212. Gabrilove JL, Jakubowski A, Scher H, et al: Recombinant human granulocyte colony stimulating factors: Therapeutic application in the prevention of chemotherapy-induced neutropenia. Behring Inst Mitt 83:229, 1988.
213. Kobayaski M, Fitz L, Ryan M, et al: Identification and purification of natural killer cell stimulatory factor (NKSF), a cytokine with multiple biologic effects on human lymphocytes. J Exp Med 170:827, 1989.
214. Chan SH, Perussia B, Gupta JW, et al: Induction of IFN-gamma production by NK cell stimulatory factor (NKSF); characterization of the responder cells and synergy with other inducers. J Exp Med 173:869, 1991.
215. Manetti R, Parronchi P, Giudizi MG, et al: Natural killer cell stimulatory factor (interleukin 12 [IL-12]) induces T helper type 1 (Th1)–specific immune responses and inhibits the development of IL-4–producing Th cells. J Exp Med 177:1199, 1993.
216. Manetti R, Gerosa F, Giudizi MG, et al: Interleukin-12 induces stable priming for interferon-γ (IFN-γ) production during differentiation of human T helper (Th) cells and transient IFN-γ production in established Th2 cell clones. J Exp Med 179:1273, 1994.
217. Wu CY, Demeure C, Kiniwa M, et al: IL-12 induces the production of IFN-γ by neonatal human CD4 T cells. J Immunol 151:1938, 1993.
218. Kubin M, Kamoun M, Trinchieri G: Interleukin-12 synergizes with B7/CD28 interaction in inducing efficient proliferation and cytokine production of human T cells. J Exp Med 180:211, 1994.
219. Mosmann TR, Coffman RL: Th1 and Th2 cells: Different patterns of lymphokine secretion lead to different functional properties. Annu Rev Immunol 7:145, 1989.
220. Gajewski TF, Fitch FW: Anti-proliferative effect of IFN-γ in immune regulation. I. IFN-gamma inhibits the proliferation of Th2 but not Th1 murine HTL clones. J Immunol 140:4245, 1988
221. Fernandez-Botran R, Sanders VM, Mosmann TR, Vitetta ES: 1988. Lymphokine-mediated regulation of the proliferative response of clones of T helper 1 and T helper 2 cells. J Exp Med 168:543, 1988.
222. Gajewski TF, Goldwasser E, Fitch FW: Anti-proliferative effect of IFN-γ in immune regulation. II. IFN-γ inhibits the proliferation of murine bone marrow cells stimulated with IL-3, IL-4, or granulocyte-macrophage colony-stimulating factor. J Immunol 141:2635, 1988.
223. Coffman RL, Seymour B, Lebman DA, et al: The role of helper T cell products in mouse B cell differentiation and isotype regulation. Immunol Rev 102:5, 1988.
224. Boom WH, Liano D, Abbas AK: Heterogeneity of helper/inducer T lymphocytes. II. Effects of interleukin 4— and interleukin 2–producing T cell clones on resting B cells. J Exp Med 167:1350, 1988.
225. Fiorentino DF, Zlotnik A, Vieira P, et al: IL-10 acts on the antigen-presenting cell to inhibit cytokine production by Th1 cells. J Immunol 146:3444, 1991.
226. Locksley RM, Scott P: Helper T-cell subsets in mouse leishmaniasis: Induction, expansion and effector function. Immunol Today 12:A58, 1991.
227. Keane-Meyers S, Nickell SP: T cell subset modulation of immunity to *Borrelia burgdorferi* in mice. J Immunol 154:1770, 1995.
228. Onderdonk AB, Markham RB, Zeleznik DF, et al: Evidence for T cell–dependent immunity to *Bacteroides fragilis* in an intraabdominal abscess model. J Clin Invest 69:9, 1982.
229. Powderly WG, Pier GB, Markham RB: T lymphocyte–mediated protection against *Pseudomonas aeruginosa* infection in granulocytopenic mice. J Clin Invest 78:375, 1986.
230. Murphy BR, Kasel JA, Chanock RM: Association of serum anti-neuraminidase antibody with resistance to influenza in man. N Engl J Med 286:1329, 1972.
231. Douglas RG Jr, Markoff LJ, Murphy BR, et al: Live Victoria/75-ts-1(E) influenza A virus vaccines in adult volunteers. Role of hemagglutinin immunity in protection against illness and infection caused by influenza A virus. Infect Immun 26:274, 1979.
232. Townsend ARM, Skehel JJ: The influenza A virus nucleoprotein gene controls the induction of both subtype specific and cross reactive cytotoxic T cells. J Exp Med 160:552, 1984.
233. Townsend ARM, Rothbard J, Gotch FM, et al: The epitopes of

influenza nucleoprotein recognized by CTL can be defined with short synthetic peptides. Cell 44:959, 1986.
234. Shore SL, Feorino PM: Immunology of primary herpes virus infections in humans. *In* Nahmias AJ, Dowdle WR, Schinazi RF (eds): The Human Herpes Viruses. New York, Elsevier, 1981, p 267.
235. Geiger B, Rosen D, Berke G: Spatial relationships of microtubule-organizing centers and the contact area of cytotoxic T lymphocytes and target cells. J Cell Biol 95:137, 1982.
236. Bykovskaja SN, Rytenko AN, Rauschenbach MO, Mykovsky AF: Ultrastructural alteration of cytolytic T lymphocytes following their interaction with target cells. I. Hypertrophy and change of orientation of the Golgi apparatus. Cell Immunol 40:164, 1978.
237. Podack ER: Molecular mechanisms of cytolysis by complement and by cytolytic lymphocytes. J Cell Biochem 3:133, 1986.
238. Kägi D, Ledermann B, Bürki K, et al: Cytotoxicity mediated by T cells and natural killer cells is greatly impaired in perforin-deficient mice. Nature 369:31, 1994.
239. Kägi D, Vignaux F, Ledermann B, et al: Fas and perforin pathways as major mechanisms of T cell–mediated cytotoxicity. Science 265:528, 1994.
240. Walsh CM, Matloubian M, Liu C, et al: Immune functions in mice lacking the perforin gene. Proc Natl Acad Sci USA 91:10854, 1994.
241. Kojima H, Shinohara N, Hanaoka S, et al: Two distinct pathways of specific killing revealed by perforin mutant cytotoxic T lymphocytes. Immunity 1:357, 1994.
242. Lowin B, Hahne M, Mattmann C, Tschopp J: Cytolyic T-cell cytotoxicity is mediated through perforin and Fas lytic pathways. Nature 370:650, 1994.
243. Dhein J, Daniel PT, Traugh BC, et al: Induction of apoptosis by monoclonal antibody anti–APO-1 class switch variants is dependent on cross-linking of APO-1 cell surface antigens. J Immunol 149:3166, 1992.
244. Suda T, Takahaski T, Goldstein P, Nagata S: Molecular cloning and expression of the Fas ligand, a novel member of the tumor necrosis factor family. Cell 75:1169, 1993.
245. Shiver JW, Su L, Henkart PA: Cytotoxicity with target DNA breakdown by rat basophilic leukemia cells expressing both cytolysin and granzyme A. Cell 71:315, 1992.
246. Nakajima H, Henkart PA: Cytotoxic lymphocyte granzymes trigger a target cell internal disintegration pathway leading to cytolysis and DNA breakdown. J Immunol 152:1057, 1994.
247. Heusel JW, Wesselschmidt RL, Shresta S, et al: Cytotoxic lymphocytes require granzyme-B for the rapid induction of DNA fragmentation and apoptosis in allogenic target-cells. Cell 76:977, 1994.
248. Ruscetti FW, Mikovits JA, Kalyanaraman VS, et al: Analysis of effector mechanisms against HTLV-1 and HTLV-III/LAV infected lymphoid cells. J Immunol 136:3619, 1986.
249. Fitzgerald PA, Mendelsohn M, Lopez C: Human natural killer cells limit replication of herpes simplex virus type 1 in vitro. J Immunol 134:2666, 1985.
250. Hayward AR, Herberger M, Laszlo M: Cellular interactions in the lysis of varicella-zoster virus infected human fibroblasts. Clin Exp Immunol 63:141, 1986.
251. Bukowski JF, Woda BA, Habu S, et al: Natural killer cell depletion enhances virus synthesis and virus-induced hepatitis in vivo. J Immunol 131:1531, 1983.
252. Biron CA, Byrons KS, Sullivan JL: Susceptibility to viral infections in an individual with complete lack of natural killer cells. Nat Immun Cell Growth Regul 7:47, 1988.
253. Albright JW, Hatcher FM, Albright JF: Interaction between murine natural killer cells and trypanosomes of different species. Infect Immun 44:315, 1984.
254. Hauser WE, Tsai V: Acute toxoplasma infection of mice induces spleen NK cells that are cytotoxic for *T. gondii* in vitro. J Immunol 136:313, 1986.
255. Hidore MR, Murphy JW: Correlation of natural killer cell activity and clearance of *Cryptococcus neoformans* from mice after adoptive transfer of splenic nylon wool–nonadherent cells. Infect Immun 137:3624, 1986.
256. Markham RB, Pier GB, Schreiber JR: The role of cytophilic IgG3 antibody in T cell–mediated resistance to infection with the extracellular bacterium, *Pseudomonas aeruginosa.* J Immunol 146:316, 1991.
257. Markham RB, Goellner J, Pier GB: In vitro T cell killing of *Pseudomonas aeruginosa.* I. Evidence that a lymphokine mediates killing. J Immunol 133:962, 1984.
258. Zinkernagel RM, Althage A, Alder B, et al: H-2 restriction of cell-mediated immunity to an intracellular bacterium: Effector T cells are specific for *Listeria* antigen in association with H-2I region–coded self-markers. J Exp Med 145:1353, 1977.
259. Beller DI, Kiely JM, Unanue ER: Regulation of macrophage populations. I. Preferential induction of Ia-rich peritoneal exudates by immunologic stimuli. J Immunol 124:1426, 1980.
260. Ruco LP, Meltzer MS: Macrophage activation for tumor cytotoxicity: Induction of tumoricidal macrophages by PPD in BCG-immunized mice. Cell Immunol 32:203, 1977.
261. Moreno C, Taverne J, Mehlert A, et al: Lipoarabinomannan from *Mycobacterium tuberculosis* induces the production of tumour necrosis factor from human and murine macrophages. Clin Exp Immunol 76:240, 1989.
262. Kaufmann SHE: Possible role of helper and cytolytic T lymphocytes in antibacterial defense: Conclusions based on a murine model of listeriosis. Rev Infect Dis 9:S650, 1987.
263. Kaufmann SH: Which T cells are relevant to resistance against *Listeria monocytogenes* infection? Adv Exp Med Biol 239:135, 1988.
264. Pawelec G, Schaudt K, Rehbein A, Busch FW: Differential secretion of tumor necrosis factor-alpha and granulocyte/macrophage colony-stimulating factors but not interferon-gamma from $CD4^+$ compared to $CD8^+$ human T cell clones. Eur J Immunol 19:197, 1989.
265. Kaufmann SH, Rodewald HR, Hug E, De Libero G: Cloned *Listeria monocytogenes* specific non–MHC-restricted Lyt-2^+ T cells with cytolytic and protective activity. J Immunol 140:3173, 1988.

8

Clinical Approach to Fever

Burke A. Cunha

If a physician is skilled enough to induce fever, it would be useless to search for another remedy against disease.

RUFUS OF EPHESUS

Historical Aspects

Fever has evolutionary significance as a primal host defense mechanism. The ancients recognized fever as a beneficial sign in infection. Hippocrates believed and wrote that during infection, "fever intervening is favorable." Rufus of Ephesus also considered fever vital and even advocated fever therapy. The concept of fever therapy, that is, the deliberate induction of fever by an infectious agent (malaria was given to cause fever and cure syphilis), was awarded the Nobel Prize in Medicine in 1927. Thomas Sydenham wrote that "fever is nature's engine which she brings into the field to remove her enemy." The German physician Carl von Liebermeister studied fever extensively in the 1800s and also appreciated the benefits of fever in infection. However, salicylates became popular at the turn of the century, and physicians noticed that patients felt better with salicylates and assumed the effect was due to lowering of temperature. Since then, physicians have tried to eliminate fevers in a variety of ways, depriving the host of the benefits of fever.[1]

General Concepts

Thermoregulation

The average temperature of individuals varies considerably (approximately 1°F) from what is called normal (e.g., 98°F). Temperature normally increases with exercise, eating, hot weather, and ovulation. Daily temperature varies in each individual (e.g., diurnal tap rhythm, which peaks in late afternoon and evenings and is at its lowest in the early morning). An increase in temperature above normal for an individual is called fever. Fever is caused by an increase in heat production mediated by the preoptic nucleus of the anterior hypothalamus. The hypothalamus may be viewed conceptually as a thermostat. When the hypothalamus thermostat is reset to normal, temperatures fall when heat production is terminated, and vasodilation and sweating restore the body to normal temperature levels. Epithelial cells and mononuclear cells (but not polymorphonuclear leukocytes or lymphocytes), when contacted by microscopic or antigenic stimuli, elaborate chemical mediators (e.g., cytokines) that reach the hypothalamus through the circulation. The most important cytokines in the febrile response are interleukin-1, tumor necrosis factor, and interleukin-6. Although much is known about the role of cytokines and thermoregulation, this has contributed little to our understanding of the febrile response.[2]

Benefits of Fever

Fever exerts a profound influence on all measurable host defense mechanisms. Increased temperature optimizes chemotaxis, complement activity, and phagocytosis. No discernible adverse effects on the immune system are attributable to lowered temperature. Elevated temperatures also have a direct inhibitory effect on many microorganisms. The effect of high temperature on various microorganisms is substantial (e.g., gonococci are lysed, gram-negative bacillary replication is inhibited, viral replication is slowed, syphilitic spirochetes are destroyed). Fever also indirectly augments host defenses by increasing lysosomal lysis and decreasing serum iron concentration. The entire acute-phase response is initiated and mediated by fever. Furthermore, the activity of many antibiotics is enhanced by fever.[1]

Fever is the clinical expression of an inadequate initial response to an infectious challenge. In the battle between the microbes and the host, fever is the main manifestation of the mobilization of the host's defenses in the life or death struggle against microbial attack.

Clinical Aspects

Fever and Acute-Phase Reactions

The febrile response is accompanied by a variety of signs and symptoms that are associated with fever. Headache, arthralgias, or myalgias may occur with fever, and mild confusion or delirium is common in the elderly. Fever, being a manifestation of the inflammatory response to tissue injury, is accompanied by a variety of nonspecific acute-phase reactions. In addition to fever, there may be leukocytosis or leukopenia, thrombocytosis or thrombocytopenia, a decrease in serum cations (iron, copper, and zinc), and many changes in serum proteins. Increases in C-reactive protein and erythrocyte sedimentation rate occur frequently along with modest increases of serum fibrinogen, haptoglobin, ceruloplasmin, α_1-antitrypsin, and the C3 component of complement. Serum albumin concentration decreases as an acute-phase response. Thyroxine and glucocorticoid levels are also nonspecifically increased. Proteinuria, but not hematuria, frequently accompanies acute febrile infectious diseases.[3, 4]

Fever Blisters

Fever blisters are perioral herpes simplex virus reactivation. Fever alone does not result in fever blisters. The common recurrent perioral vesicular lesions of herpes simplex virus are not associated with fever. Fever blisters are associated with pneumococcal meningitis, meningococcal meningitis, and malaria.[3, 4]

Fever and Chills

Rigors (i.e., true chills) often precede or accompany fever. True rigors (e.g., involuntary teeth-chattering chills) must be differentiated from the sensation of chilliness. Rigors, increasing muscle contraction that generates heat, have the effect of increasing core temperature. Rigors are commonly associated with bacterial infections and are not characteristic of viral (except viral influenza), chlamydial, or fungal infections.[3, 5, 6]

Chills are characteristic of relatively few infectious diseases: bacteremia, cholangitis, abscesses, viral influenza, pyelonephritis, bacterial pneumonias (especially pneumococcal), typhoid fever, typhus, arthropod-borne viral infections, and plague. Single chills occur with viral influenza, pneumococcal pneumonia, leptospirosis, typhoid, typhus, and transient or sustained bacteremias. Recurrent chills are associated with persistent bacteremias, abscesses, septic thrombophlebitis, cholangitis, rat-bite fever, and brucellosis. Noninfectious diseases may have recurrent chills with fever (e.g., renal cell carcinoma, lymphomas, and overzealous antipyretic therapy).[3, 5, 6]

Duration of Fever

Most acute infectious diseases have fever at some point during the course of the illness. Fever with most acute infections usually resolves within 2 weeks, with or without treatment. Superficial and chronic infections have little or no febrile component. Neutropenic and elderly patients frequently have an absent or blunted febrile response. In contrast, high fevers develop rapidly in children, even with mild infections.[3, 5] The inability to mount a fever is a sign of poor prognosis, but a decrease in temperature in a febrile patient signals that the host is responding to the infection.[6–9]

Clinical Approach

Fever usually indicates an inflammatory, infectious, or neoplastic disorder. The absence of fever does not rule out any of these conditions, but the abruptness of the onset of illness, the appearance of the patient, the fever's magnitude and pattern, and the associated clinical and laboratory findings usually provide sufficient information for assessment of the probable cause of the fever. Diseases behave biologically in a predictable manner even though the clinical presentation may be varied. The pattern of organ involvement and detached analysis of the key characteristic aspects of the fever determine the differential diagnosis of the cause of the fever.

For diagnostic purposes, fevers may be viewed as acute, subacute, or chronic, with or without localizing signs. Fevers with localizing signs present few difficulties in diagnosis, but febrile illnesses without localizing signs are a diagnostic challenge. In patients with fever only, careful analysis of the fever pattern may be the only way to arrive at a presumptive diagnosis. The most helpful localizing signs are hepatic or splenic enlargement, regular or generalized lymphadenopathy, and cutaneous findings (e.g., rash). Clinically, fever should be viewed as an important sign and as an essential host defense mechanism.[6, 7, 10]

Fever in the Ambulatory Setting

Most ambulatory patients with noncritical infectious diseases have self-limited illnesses and become afebrile in 1 to 2 weeks. High temperatures (≥102°F) in ambulatory patients are usually due to community-acquired pneumonia, pyelonephritis, intraabdominal or pelvic abscesses, pharyngitis, pelvic inflammatory disease, septic arthritis, acute osteomyelitis, and intravenous (IV) line infections from home IV fluid therapy. Skin infections, urethritis, cystitis, prostatitis, subacute bacterial endocarditis, chlamydial infections, common respiratory viral infections (excluding viral influenza), viral hepatitis, and infectious diarrhea (excluding enteric fevers) usually present with temperatures of 102°F or lower. Many infections are not associated with much fever, such as sexually transmitted diseases (excluding disseminated gonococcal disease), lymphogranuloma venereum, human immunodeficiency virus infection, Lyme disease, superficial or chronic skin infections, chronic or recurrent pharyngitis, and chronic osteomyelitis.[6, 9]

Fever in Hospitalized Patients

Fever in hospitalized patients may be due to many infectious and noninfectious diseases. Fever patterns help to eliminate diagnostic possibilities as often as they provide diagnostically meaningful information. Medical diagnosis usually depends on assessing the significance of multiple clinical variables that combine to form a clinical syndrome. The syndromic approach permits the clinician to rapidly arrive at a working diagnosis on which to base further tests and empirical therapy. The main clinical problem in practice is to differentiate infectious from noninfectious diseases (e.g., noninfectious pulmonary infiltrates from pneumonia). Once this diagnosis is narrowed to an organ system, specific diagnostic tests can determine the definitive diagnosis[7–10] (Table 8–1).

Fever and Recent Foreign Travel

Visitors or host country nationals returning from Latin America, Asia, or Africa with acute febrile illness or rash

TABLE 8–1 ■ Differential Diagnosis of Fever in Hospitalized Patients Based on Temperature

TEMPERATURE ≤102°F	TEMPERATURE ≥102°F
Acute cholecystitis	Cholangitis
Acute myocardial infarction	Pericarditis
Simple phlebitis	Suppurative thrombophlebitis
Pulmonary emboli or infarction	Septic pulmonary emboli
Acute pancreatitis	Pancreatic abscess, infected pseudocyst
Viral hepatitis (hepatitis viruses A, B, C, and others)	Nonhepatitis viral liver disease (Epstein-Barr virus, leptospirosis, drug fever)
Uncomplicated wound infections	Severe or complicated wound infections (invasive group A streptococcus, *Vibrio vulnificus*)
	Abscess deep to wound
Gastrointestinal tract bleeding	Bowel infarction
Catheter-associated bacteriuria (cystitis)	Pyelonephritis

Adapted from Cunha BA: Clinical implications of fever. Postgrad Med 85:188–200, 1989.

TABLE 8–2 ■ Fever and Recent Foreign Travel

	INCUBATION PERIOD		
	2 Weeks	2–3 Weeks	>3 Weeks
COMMON			
Malaria		•	•
Pulmonary tuberculosis			•
Viral hepatitis (hepatitis viruses A, B, C, and others)			•
Typhoid fever		•	
Diarrhea	•		
Toxigenic *Escherichia coli* infection			
Cholera			
Amebic dysentery			
Shigella dysentery			
Campylobacteriosis			
Giardiasis			
Yersinia infection			
Cryptosporidiosis			
Cyclospora infection			
UNCOMMON			
Human immunodeficiency virus infection			•
Typhus	•		
Viral hemorrhagic fevers		•	
Asian		•	
African		•	
Latin American		•	
Leptospirosis		•	
Brucellosis		•	
Arboviral infections (dengue fever)	•		
Visceral leishmaniasis			•
Trypanosomiasis		•	

present a specific problem. Returning travelers usually have common rather than exotic rare infections. Patients should be approached syndromically (e.g., acute diarrheal illness, pulmonary symptoms–pneumonia, jaundice), or an acute undifferentiated febrile illness may be diagnosed. The conditions associated with traveler's diarrhea are well known. Lung findings point to a typical or atypical pneumonia or tuberculosis. Fever (temperature of ≤102°F) and jaundice point to viral hepatitis. Typhoid fever and malaria are then left as common diagnostic considerations, and arboviral and zoonotic infections are uncommon[4, 9, 11–18] (Table 8–2).

Fever Patterns

Fever patterns are of most help in diagnosing febrile illnesses without localizing signs and are of limited usefulness in

TABLE 8–3 ■ Diagnostic Significance of Extreme Hyperpyrexia and Hypothermia

EXTREME PYREXIA (≥106°F)	HYPOTHERMIA (≤97°F)
Central fevers (neoplastic, trauma, or infection)	Elderly age
	Cold exposure
Drug fever	Hypothyroidism
Heat stroke	Overwhelming infection
Human immunodeficiency virus infection	Sepsis in chronic renal failure
	Overzealous treatment with antipyretics
Malignant hyperthermia	
Malignant neuroleptic syndrome	

Adapted from Cunha BA: Clinical implications of fever. Postgrad Med 85:188–200, 1989.

nosocomial fevers. The classic fever patterns retain their usefulness and validity in many areas of the world where traditional infectious diseases are common and still important.

Intermittent fevers are temperature elevations that return to normal at least once during most days. Sustained or continuing fevers do not vary more than a few degrees per day. Remittent fevers do not return to normal each day. Relapsing fevers are recurrent for a period of days or weeks and may have any underlying fever pattern (e.g., intermittent, continuous, remittent). Biphasic illnesses are not truly recurrent and occur only once. Relapsing fevers should be differentiated from febrile diseases likely to relapse.[3, 5, 6]

Magnitude of Fever

Although temperature elevation does not correlate with disease severity, the height of the temperature elevation has important diagnostic significance at temperature extremes (e.g., hyperpyrexia or hypothermia). Temperatures above 106°F are not due to infectious diseases, and a noninfectious cause should be the focus of the diagnostic approach (Table 8–3). Hypothermia or subnormal temperature, if associated with bacteremia, is a sign of poor prognosis. Slight hypothermia may be a normal variant in the elderly or not infrequently is due to overzealous antipyretic measures.[7, 8]

Most temperature elevations are encountered clinically between the extremes of hyperpyrexia and hypothermia. Temperatures between 98°F and 102°F may be related to an infection but are usually due to noninfectious conditions common in hospitalized patients, especially in critical care units. For diagnostic purposes, it is clinically useful to divide fevers into those capable of temperature elevations to 102°F or higher and those that nearly always remain below 102°F. The differential diagnosis of most commonly encountered causes of fever in the hospital and intensive care unit may be approached efficiently by applying this principle.[6, 9]

Frequency of Fever

Fever spikes may be classified for diagnostic purposes as occurring once (quotidian) or more (double-quotidian) daily, every third day (tertian), or every fourth day (quartan). Fevers may also be described as intermittent, continuous or sustained, and remittent. Relapsing fevers recur at various intervals after the initial febrile episode. In a hospitalized patient with temperatures of 102°F or lower for 1 to 2 weeks, a single fever spike to 103°F that returns to normal without treatment by the next day is probably not due to a systemic infectious disease. Single fever spikes are never due to infection and are commonly due to the transfusion of blood or blood products or to manipulation of a colonized or infected mucosal surface.

The most specific fever pattern is the double-quotidian, because only a few diseases are associated with two fever spikes a day (e.g., adult Still disease, right-sided gonococcal endocarditis, visceral leishmaniasis [kala-azar]). A double-quotidian fever is an important clue to the diagnosis of adult Still disease, because there are no other physical or laboratory findings to establish the diagnosis.

Most infectious diseases have no specific fever pattern. The classic fever curves are of limited diagnostic usefulness in hospitalized patients, because most nosocomial fevers are not due to classic infectious diseases. The most important fever patterns are presented in Table 8–4.

Duration of Fever

The majority of acute infectious diseases improve or worsen within 2 weeks. Not uncommonly, many infectious diseases cause persistent fever after clinical improvement that may last 2 to 4 weeks. The diagnosis of the cause of such fevers is usually straightforward, but the cause of some remains obscure. These are best termed prolonged fevers to avoid confusing them with bona fide fevers of unknown origin. Fevers of unknown origin, by definition, must have temperatures of 101°F or above for at least 3 weeks and remain undiagnosed after a week of inpatient or outpatient work-up (see Chapter 189).

Recurring Fevers

Relapsing fevers may be due to a variety of infectious and noninfectious diseases. Multisystem disease characterized by exacerbation or remission may mimic infectious relapsing fever. Most temperature elevations occur at night as an exaggeration of our normal diurnal temperature variation, but the reversal of diurnal pattern occurs with a few infectious diseases.

A biphasic fever is characterized by two fever spikes during the illness, usually during the course of 1 week or more (e.g., African hemorrhagic fever). This is in contrast to relapsing fevers, which are recurrent and not necessarily biphasic[3, 5, 6] (Table 8–5).

Pulse-Temperature Relationships

The relationship of the pulse to the temperature is often more useful than the fever pattern. If the pulse is elevated out of proportion to the temperature, the relationship is termed relative tachycardia. Relative tachycardia is associated with noninfectious conditions and toxin-mediated infections (e.g., gas gangrene). When the pulse is not elevated proportionately to the temperature elevation, a pulse-temperature deficit exists (e.g., relative bradycardia). The finding of relative bradycardia has important diagnostic significance. For example, if a hospitalized patient presents with fevers and relative bradycardia, the differential diagnosis is limited to Legionnaires' disease or drug fever (Fig. 8–1). If the findings on chest x-ray examination are normal, the work-up should be focused toward drug fever. Drug fever is usually accompanied by relative bradycardia; associated findings include negative blood culture results (excluding contaminants), slightly elevated serum transaminase activities, elevated erythrocyte sedimentation rate, and presence of eosinophils in the peripheral smear (eosinophilia is uncommon). Relative bradycardia is an early clue to malaria or typhoid fever in a traveler without localized findings[7–9] (Table 8–6).

High fever in patients looking inappropriately well suggests drug or factitious fever. Both drug fever and factitious fever are associated with relative bradycardia.

Fever Defervescence Patterns

Viral illnesses have a slow defervescence usually during a period of a week. Temperatures of febrile, noninfectious diseases do not decrease without specific therapy. Steroids and antipyretics decrease temperatures nonspecifically, and this needs to be taken into account in assessing therapeutic responses. Clinicians may be misled into thinking that an antibiotic is being effective as evidenced by a decrease in temperature only to learn later that the patient was concomitantly receiving an antipyretic medication. For this and other reasons, fevers should not be eliminated without reason.[1, 6, 7]

Bacterial infections usually manifest a prompt drop in temperature with appropriate treatment. However, infections respond at different rates, and this may be useful clinically. For example, enterococcal subacute bacterial endocarditis defervesces slowly for a week, in contrast to viridans streptococcal

TABLE 8–4 ■ Diagnostic Significance of Fever Patterns

FEVER PATTERN	USUAL CAUSES
Single fever spike	Manipulation of a colonized or infected mucosal surface Transfusion of blood or blood products Infusion-related sepsis (contaminated infusate) Temperature error Not a systemic infectious disease
Double-quotidian fevers	Adult Still disease (adult-juvenile rheumatoid arthritis) Visceral leishmaniasis Miliary tuberculosis Mixed malarial infections Right-sided gonococcal endocarditis
Tertian fevers	Malaria *(Plasmodium vivax)*
Quartan fevers	Malaria *(Plasmodium malariae)*
Intermittent fevers	Gram-negative or gram-positive sepsis Abscesses (renal, abdominal, pelvic) Acute bacterial endocarditis Kawasaki disease Malaria Miliary tuberculosis Peritonitis Toxic shock syndrome Antipyretics
Remittent fevers	Viral upper respiratory tract infections *Plasmodium falciparum* malaria Acute rheumatic fever *Legionella* infection *Mycoplasma* infection Tuberculosis Subacute bacterial endocarditis (viridans streptococci)
Continuous or sustained fevers	Central fevers Roseola infantum (human herpesvirus 6) Brucellosis Kawasaki disease Psittacosis Rocky Mountain spotted fever Scarlet fever Enterococcal subacute bacterial endocarditis (tularemia) Typhoid fever Drug fever
Biphasic (camelback) fevers	Colorado tick fever Dengue fever Leptospirosis Brucellosis Lymphocytic choriomeningitis Yellow fever Poliomyelitis Smallpox Rat-bite fever *(Spirillum minus)* Chikungunya fever Rift Valley fever African hemorrhagic fevers (Marburg, Ebola, Lassa) Echovirus infection (echovirus 9)
Relapsing fevers	Relapsing fever *(Borrelia recurrentis)* Yellow fever Smallpox Ascending (intermittent) cholangitis Brucellosis Dengue Chronic meningococcemia Malaria Rat-bite fever *(Streptobacillus moniliformis)*

Adapted from Cunha BA: Infectious diseases. *In* Samiy AH, Bardoness J, Douglas RG (eds): Textbook of Diagnostic Medicine. Philadelphia, Lea & Febiger; 1987, pp 131–166.

subacute bacterial endocarditis. Similarly, temperature from *Haemophilus influenzae* or *Klebsiella* pneumonia comes down more slowly than if the patient had pneumococcal pneumonia. Pneumococcal or *H. influenzae* meningitis, in contrast, has a slower rate of temperature decrease than does meningococcal meningitis. Even the febrile response to antibiotic therapy may vary, as is the case with pneumococcal pneumonia, which has three patterns of defervescence. The usual pattern of proven pneumonia is rapidly decreasing temperature during the first 24 to 36 hours of antibiotic therapy. The second pattern is a more gradual decrease during 3 to 4 days, usually seen in compromised hosts (e.g., alcoholic patients). Last, after initial defervescence, a small group of patients will have another temperature spike on day 3 or 4.[6]

After an initial response to antimicrobial therapy, patients usually continue with low-grade or no fever until discharge. Reappearance of fever during treatment suggests an infectious complication (septic emboli in a patient with subacute bacterial endocarditis). The reappearance of fever after an initial response is virtually never due to resistant organisms, but it may be due to superinfection. The diagnostic approach should be directed accordingly, and antibiotic therapy should not be changed because of the possibility of resistant organisms. Immunocompromised hosts, in general, respond more slowly to antibiotic therapy than do normal hosts.[7, 8]

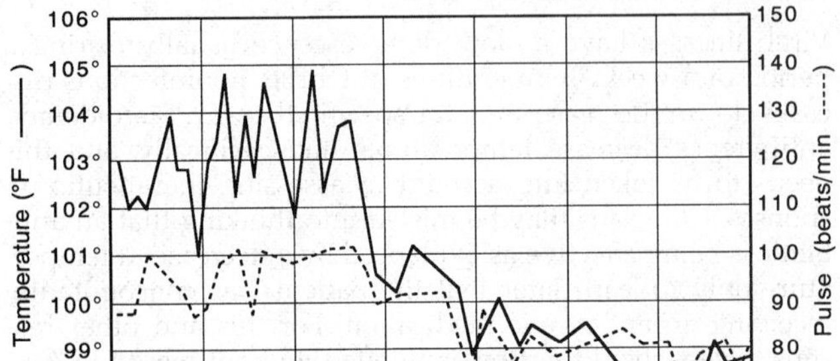

FIGURE 8–1 □ The temperature chart shows relative bradycardia in a patient with Legionnaires' disease.

Fever Without Localizing Signs

Fever can be approached from a diagnostic perspective as presenting with or without localizing signs. Infectious diseases presenting as acute febrile illnesses without localizing signs are the most difficult diagnostic problem (e.g., typhoid fever, malaria, ehrlichiosis, roseola infantum, typhoidal tularemia, Epstein-Barr virus mononucleosis, miliary tuberculosis). The preeruptive stages of Rocky Mountain spotted fever,

TABLE 8–5 ■ Fevers Likely to Relapse

INFECTIOUS CAUSES	
Relapsing fever *(Borrelia recurrentis)*	Colorado tick fever
Trench fever *(Bartonella quintana)*	Dengue fever
Q fever	Leptospirosis
Typhoid fever	Brucellosis
Campylobacter fetus infection	Bartonellosis (Oroya fever)
Syphilis	Acute rheumatic fever
Tuberculosis	Rat-bite fever *(Spirillum minus)*
Histoplasmosis	Visceral leishmaniasis
Coccidioidomycosis	Lyme disease
Blastomycosis	Malaria
Melioidosis *(Pseudomonas pseudomallei)*	Babesiosis
Lymphocytic choriomeningitis	Noninfluenzal respiratory viral infections
Dengue fever	Epstein-Barr virus mononucleosis
Yellow fever	Cytomegalovirus mononucleosis
Chronic meningococcemia	
NONINFECTIOUS CAUSES	
Behçet disease	Fever, adenopathy, pharyngitis, aphthous ulcers (FAPA) syndrome
Crohn disease	Systemic lupus erythematosus
Weber-Christian disease (panniculitis)	Hyperimmunoglobulinemia D syndrome
Leukocytoclastic angiitis	
Sweet syndrome	
Familial Mediterranean fever	

viral hepatitis, and the childhood exanthems are further examples. If no localizing signs are present, analysis of temperature and fever pattern is of clinical importance and may provide the only clue to guide further testing or suggest the diagnosis.[7–10]

Fever with Localizing Signs

Fever and Rash

The approach to the acutely ill patient with rash and fever is to evaluate the location and character of the rash and the severity of the illness. Many subacute and chronic rashes are associated with temperature elevations, but the clinical challenge is to rapidly and accurately diagnose acutely ill patients with exanthems. Rash distribution may be viewed as primarily central or peripheral. If the rash involves the palms and soles, the diagnostic possibilities are narrowed considerably[11–18] (Table 8–7).

In addition to the location of the rash, its nature (i.e., predominantly petechial-hemorrhagic or maculopapular) is important. Associated clinical and laboratory findings then permit approaching both types of rash in acutely ill febrile patients (Table 8–8). Miscellaneous cutaneous findings may provide diagnostic clues. For example, it may be difficult to distinguish acute malaria from typhoid fever early in the illness, but rose spots appearing late in the first week point to typhoid fever. Typhoid fever usually causes few truncal rose spots, but the paratypical enteric fevers and *Shigella sonnei* infection may be associated with many rose spots, so that even the number of rose spots has diagnostic value. Similarly, fever blisters are an important finding in patients with meningitis. Meningococcal and pneumococcal pneumonitis are associated with fever blisters, but herpes simplex meningoencephalitis is not. In herpes simplex meningoencephalitis, the fever blister precedes but does not usually appear simultaneously with the meningoencephalitis (Table 8–9). Rash and fever usually occur together, but in some illnesses, the fever abates when the rash appears (e.g., roseola infantum due to human herpesvirus 6).[11–13]

TABLE 8–6 ■ Diagnostic Significance of Temperature-Pulse Relationships

RELATIVE BRADYCARDIA*	RELATIVE TACHYCARDIA
Dengue fever	Anemia
Drug fever	Clostridial sepsis
Typhus	Diphtheria
Legionnaires' disease	Hyperthyroidism
Leptospirosis	Pulmonary emboli
Lymphomas	Supraventricular arrhythmias
Malaria	
Psittacosis	
Typhoid fever	
Yellow fever	
Central fevers	
African hemorrhagic fevers (Marburg, Ebola, Lassa)	
Factitious fever	

*In immunocompetent adults (not receiving β-blockers) with temperature ≥102°F. (To determine whether relative bradycardia is present, take the temperature in °F, subtract 1 from the ones digit, multiply that number by 10, and add 100. For example, if the temperature is 104°F, $3 \times 10 \rightarrow 30 + 100 = 130$. Therefore, the appropriate pulse response for a temperature of 104°F is a pulse rate of 130 per minute.)

Adapted from Cunha BA: Clinical implications of fever. Postgrad Med 85:188–200, 1989.

Fever and Jaundice

Jaundice may be considered a localizing sign in a febrile patient. Relatively few infectious diseases present with jaundice and fever. Many infectious and noninfectious diseases cause hyperbilirubinemia but not jaundice. Bacteremias, not uncommonly, are accompanied by elevated bilirubin levels, but clinical jaundice is less common. Aside from disease primarily affecting the liver, several systemic infections may result in jaundice with fever[7, 10] (Table 8–10).

Fever and Erythema Nodosum or Erythema Multiforme

Erythema nodosum or erythema multiforme in a patient with or without fever can be a clue to an underlying condition. Diagnostic accuracy is enhanced if multiple variables (e.g., diagnostic findings) are combined to increase diagnostic specificity. If a patient with sore throat, diarrhea, and an ill-defined pulmonary infiltrate has erythema multiforme, the

TABLE 8–7 ■ Fever and Rash Involving the Palms and Soles

Acute or subacute bacterial endocarditis	Orf
Scarlet fever	*Capnocytophaga canimorsus* infection (DF-2 bacillus)
Toxic shock syndrome	Measles
Kawasaki disease	Gonococcemia
Ehrlichiosis (rare)	Meningococcemia
Rocky Mountain spotted fever	Milker's nodule
Erythema multiforme	Drug fever
Secondary syphilis	Atypical measles
Smallpox	Enterovirus infection (echovirus 9)
Chickenpox	Rat-bite fever *(Streptobacillus moniliformis)*
Overwhelming staphylococcal or pneumococcal sepsis	Epstein-Barr virus mononucleosis
Hand-foot-and-mouth disease	
Dengue fever	
Rubella	

Adapted from Cunha BA: Infectious diseases. *In* Samiy AH, Bardoness J, Douglas RG (eds): Textbook of Diagnostic Medicine. Philadelphia, Lea & Febiger, 1987, pp 131–166.

TABLE 8–8 ■ Differential Diagnosis of Petechial-Hemorrhagic Rashes in the Acutely Ill Patient

DISEASE	PRIMARY DISTRIBUTION OF RASH		APPEARANCE OF RASH AFTER FEVER	ASSOCIATED FEATURES*
	Central	Peripheral		
Acute meningococcemia	+	+	1–2 h	Bilateral conjunctivitis Irregular lesions and distribution Late winter and early spring Severe headache Herpes labialis (if meningitis) History of mild recent upper respiratory tract infection
Disseminated intravascular coagulation	+	+	Variable	Source tumor or infection Thrombocytopenia Microangiopathic hemolytic anemia Bleeding from venipuncture sites Renal insufficiency
Overwhelming staphylococcal sepsis	−	+	Variable	Usually obvious staphylococcal focus or staphylococcal acute bacterial endocarditis Distal extremity hemorrhagic nodules or infarcts (asymmetric)
Overwhelming pneumococcal sepsis	−	+	1–2 d	Asplenic patients (trauma, staging procedures for lymphoma, sickle cell anemia)
Typhus	+	−	3–6 d	Begins in axilla Severe headache, dry cough Relative bradycardia Gangrene of nose, earlobes, scrotum, vulva, fingers, toes Occasional splenomegaly
Rocky Mountain spotted fever	−	+	2–3 d	Late spring and early fall Begins on wrists and ankles Severe headache, splenomegaly Periorbital and peripheral edema No lung involvement Positive OX-2, OX-19 serologic test results Leukopenia, thrombocytopenia
Dengue fever	+	−	3–4 d	Appropriate travel history Begins in thorax and axilla Biphasic fever curve Severe headache, severe myalgias "Palpable pinpoint petechiae" Relative bradycardia Leukopenia
Toxic shock syndrome	+	+	1–2 d	Persistent hypotension despite fluid replacement Conjunctivitis Tampon user, surgical wound, menses Liver or kidney dysfunction Maculopapular rash Periorbital, facial, and extremity edema Sore throat and vagina (oral-vaginal erythema) Watery diarrhea Nausea and vomiting Headache and myalgias
Enterovirus infections (echoviruses 4, 9, 11; coxsackieviruses A9, B3)	+	−	5–7 d	Rash may have maculopapular component Sore throat and diarrhea Aseptic meningitis; may resemble early meningococcemia
African hemorrhagic fevers (Marburg virus, Ebola virus)	+	−	1–2 d	Rash scarlatiniform-maculopapular before becoming petechial-purpuric Conjunctival suffusion Severe headache Dry cough and sore throat Nausea, vomiting, diarrhea Leukopenia, thrombocytopenia ↑ LFTs Biphasic fever pattern
Capnocytophaga canimorsus infection (DF-2 bacillus)	−	+	Variable	Common in splenectomized patients Associated with lymphomas, steroids Usually history of dog exposure or bite Acute renal failure Hypotension or shock Thrombocytopenia Purpura, eschar, and gangrene may develop Buffy coat positive for DF-2 organisms

TABLE 8–8 ■ Differential Diagnosis of Petechial-Hemorrhagic Rashes in the Acutely Ill Patient *(Continued)*

DISEASE	PRIMARY DISTRIBUTION OF RASH: Central	PRIMARY DISTRIBUTION OF RASH: Peripheral	APPEARANCE OF RASH AFTER FEVER	ASSOCIATED FEATURES*
Scarlet fever	+	−	1–2 d	Nausea and vomiting Circumoral pallor Strawberry tongue Pastia lines on arms "Sandpaper skin" Pseudoappendicitis (right rectus syndrome) Abdominal pain Eosinophilia Palatal petechiae
Measles	+	−	2–3 d	Toxic appearance Deep red, purple, or brown rash begins on face Cough Conjunctivitis Pneumonia (giant cell) Encephalitis Pseudoappendicitis Koplik spots Desquamation late
Rubella	+	−	1–7 d	Postcervical-suboccipital adenopathy Palatal petechiae (Forschheimer spots) No upper respiratory tract infection Face to feet in 3 d Conjunctivitis
Atypical measles	−	+	2–3 d	History of "killed" measles vaccine (1963–1967) Begins on extremities, may be vesicular, urticarial, or petechial Always pneumonia, pulmonary infiltrate ↑ ESR ↑ Rheumatoid factors Eosinophilia
Kawasaki disease	+	−	Variable	Conjunctivitis Edema of hands and feet Erythema of tongue and mouth Erythema multiforme–like lesions Thrombocytosis Nonspecific electrocardiographic changes <5 y of age Sustained, high fever <1 wk Negative streptococcal throat cultures
Drug fever	+	−	Variable	Negative blood cultures Looks "relatively well" unless coexistent infection ↑ LFTs, ↑ ESR Relative bradycardia
Spotted fevers	+	−	5–7 d	Rash maculopapular, may become petechial Severe headache Ankle and wrist rash spreads to trunk Palms and soles rash
Leptospirosis	+	−	4–5 d	Morbilliform or scarlatiniform rash Biphasic fever Conjunctival suffusion ↑ LFTs, ↑ bilirubin Leukocytosis Jaundice (Weil disease) Rose spots (rarely)
Epstein-Barr virus mononucleosis	+	−	Variable	Bilateral upper lid edema (Hoagland sign) Bilateral posterior cervical adenopathy Exudative or nonexudative pharyngitis Palatal petechiae ↑ LFTs, ↑ ESR ~30% group A streptococcal, pharyngeal colonization *(not infection)*

*ESR, Erythrocyte sedimentation rate; LFTs, liver function tests.

Adapted from Cunha BA: Infectious diseases. *In* Samiy AH, Bardoness J, Douglas RG (eds): Textbook of Diagnostic Medicine. Philadelphia, Lea & Febiger, 1987, pp 131–166.

TABLE 8–9 ■ Fever and Miscellaneous Skin Findings

ROSE SPOTS	**HEMORRHAGIC BULLAE**
Salmonella enteric fever (few spots)	Leukemias
Non–*Salmonella typhi* enteric fevers (many spots)	*Capnocytophaga canimorus* (DF-2 bacillus)
Pseudomonas aeruginosa	Gas gangrene
Shigella sonnei	*Vibrio vulnificus*
Leptospirosis	Necrotizing fasciitis
	Aeromonas hydrophila
HORDER SPOTS	Invasive group A streptococci
Psittacosis	Anthrax
ESCHARS	**SPLINTER HEMORRHAGES**
All rickettsial infections (except Q fever and rickettsialpox)	Severe anemia
Capnocytophaga canimorus (DF-2 bacillus)	Trauma
	Acute or subacute bacterial endocarditis
ECTHYMA GANGRENOSUM	Postpericardiotomy (Dressler syndrome)
Pseudomonas aeruginosa	Systemic lupus erythematosus
Aeromonas hydrophila	
Serratia marcescens	
ANNULAR LESIONS	**FEVER BLISTERS**
Erythema migrans (Lyme disease)	Pneumococcal meningitis
Erythema marginatum	Meningococcal meningitis
Tinea	Nontyphoidal salmonella
Erythema multiforme	Malaria
Kawasaki disease	**CELLULITIS-LIKE LESIONS**
Yaws, pinta	Leukocytoclastic angiitis
	Sweet syndrome
	Systemic lupus erythematosus
	Cutaneous lymphomas

diagnosis of *Mycoplasma* infection can confidently be made. Erythema nodosum has historically been due to systemic mycoses and tuberculosis and associated with sarcoidosis, streptococcal infection, and inflammatory bowel disease[9, 10] (Tables 8–11 and 8–12).

Fever and Hepatosplenomegaly

An enlarged liver or spleen is an important diagnostic finding. Relatively few infectious diseases cause isolated enlargement of the liver or spleen, and the diseases are not the same for the liver and spleen. This information can be used to diagnostic advantage in a febrile patient. Similarly, enlargement of both the liver and spleen (hepatosplenomegaly) has its own differential diagnosis[9, 10] (Table 8–13).

Fever and Lymphadenopathy

Lymph node enlargement may be regional or general. Local lymph node enlargement suggests a regional or local cause

TABLE 8–10 ■ Fever and Jaundice

Malaria	Hepatic abscesses (pyogenic, amebic)
Typhoid fever (rare)	Epstein-Barr virus mononucleosis
Ascending cholangitis	Leptospirosis (Weil disease)
Yersinia infection	Yellow fever
Viral hepatitis (hepatitis viruses A, B, C, and others)	Dengue fever
Biliary ascariasis	Hepatic *Pneumocystis carinii* pneumonia
Portal pyemia (pylephlebitis)	Toxic shock syndrome
Overwhelming gram-positive or gram-negative sepsis	Relapsing fever *(Borrelia recurrentis)*
Babesiosis	
Human immunodeficiency virus infection *(Cryptosporidium)*	

TABLE 8–11 ■ Differential Diagnosis of Erythema Multiforme

INFECTIOUS CAUSES	
Herpes simplex virus	*Mycoplasma pneumoniae*
Epstein-Barr virus	*Francisella tularensis*
Vaccinia virus	*Yersinia*
Enterovirus	*Vibrio parahaemolyticus*
Adenovirus (7)	*Mycobacterium tuberculosis*
Hepatitis B virus	*Treponema pallidum*
Influenza A virus	*Histoplasma capsulatum*
Coxsackievirus (B5, B16)	*Coccidioides immitis*
NONINFECTIOUS CAUSES	
Neoplasms (leukemia, lymphoma, leiomyoma, pelvic tumor)	
Systemic lupus erythematosus	
Radiation therapy	
Inflammatory bowel disease (regional enteritis, ulcerative colitis)	
Sarcoidosis	
Pregnancy	
Sunlight	
Immunization (diphtheria-pertussis, poliomyelitis, typhoid, measles vaccine)	
Drugs (especially sulfonamides, phenylbutazone, penicillin, phenytoin)	

for enlargement. However, enlargement in certain regional lymph node groups may suggest a systemic illness (e.g., preauricular nodes in tularemia, postoccipital nodes in rubella, postcervical nodes in Epstein-Barr virus mononucleosis). Some diseases may present with either local or general node enlargement (e.g., Epstein-Barr virus mononucleosis).

Generalized adenopathy usually signifies a systemic disorder that may be infectious or noninfectious. Adenopathy alone or with liver or spleen enlargement provides additional diagnostic information[6, 9, 10] (Table 8–14).

Treatment of Fever

Fever is a key diagnostic sign and should not be diminished or eliminated without good cause. A fever spike should initiate a search for the cause of the temperature elevation rather than elicit a therapeutic response. Because fever optimizes all known host defense mechanisms, fever should not be treated unless it poses a threat to the patient. Conditions in which fever should elevate temperature to 102°F and above include severe cardiopulmonary disease, recent cardiac surgery, extreme hyperpyrexia (106°F and above), and high fe-

TABLE 8–12 ■ Differential Diagnosis of Erythema Nodosum

INFECTIOUS CAUSES	
Streptococci (β-hemolytic)	*Yersinia*
Mycobacteria	*Campylobacter jejuni*
Lymphogranuloma venereum	*Salmonella*
Coccidioidomycosis	Cat-scratch disease
Blastomycosis	Tularemia
Histoplasmosis	Hepatitis C
Coxsackievirus (B5)	Epstein-Barr virus mononucleosis
Psittacosis	Tuberculosis
NONINFECTIOUS CAUSES	
Ulcerative colitis	Sarcoidosis
Crohn disease	Leukemia
Systemic lupus erythematosus	Lymphomas
Sulfonamides	Pregnancy
Bromides	Behçet disease
Barbiturates	Oral contraceptives

vers in children. Extreme hyperpyrexia (106°F and above) may result in central nervous system damage, and temperature should be decreased to approximately 102°F. Patients with recent coronary bypass surgery or severe cardiopulmonary disease should not be allowed to have temperatures much above 102°F to avoid myocardial infarction for increased tissue oxygen demands.

Children, but not adults, may experience febrile seizures with high fevers, and temperature should be lowered to remain at 102°F or below. Most patients in good health tolerate high temperature fairly well, but some individuals complain of feeling ill with low-grade fevers. If the diagnosis is secure in such patients, it is not unreasonable to treat with antipyretics. If it is necessary to decrease body temperature for the reasons stated, it should be done slowly and not be continued until the patient is afebrile. The temperature should be lowered gradually by antipyretics, sponging, or hypothermia blanket to approximately 102°F. In contrast, high fevers in children should be brought down rapidly because temperatures increase so rapidly in children and because of the concern for febrile seizures.

Lowering elevated temperatures in adults should be done gradually, unless the fever is life threatening, to avoid inducing shaking chills and myalgias. Fever should remain untreated, if possible, to permit assessment of the response to antimicrobial therapy. The febrile course of an illness may help to differentiate bacterial from viral infection or infection from noninfection. Fever not only is needed as a host response but often is the only way to monitor many infectious diseases. Antipyretics may also have a direct deleterious effect on the host. There is no rationale for treating fever excluding the exceptions mentioned. Blunting or eliminating the febrile response may deprive the patient of an essential host defense mechanism, fever.[1, 19, 20]

TABLE 8–13 ■ Fever and Hepatomegaly, Splenomegaly, and Hepatosplenomegaly

ORGAN INVOLVEMENT	USUAL CAUSES
Hepatomegaly	Amebic liver abscess
	Brucellosis
	Chagas disease
	Clonorchiasis
	Echinococcosis
	Fascioliasis
	Histoplasmosis
	Malaria
	Viral hepatitis
	Opisthorchiasis
	Schistosomiasis
	Toxocariasis
	Typhoid fever
	Visceral leishmaniasis
	Bartonellosis
	Hydatid cyst disease
Splenomegaly*	Typhus
	Chagas disease
	Malaria
	Subacute bacterial endocarditis
	Schistosomiasis
	Typhoid fever
	Brucellosis
	Histoplasmosis
	Myelofibrosis
	Systemic lupus erythematosus
	Visceral leishmaniasis
	Leukemia
	Lymphoma
	Tuberculosis
	Epstein-Barr virus mononucleosis
Hepatosplenomegaly	Typhoid fever
	Tularemia
	Brucellosis
	South American trypanosomiasis
	Hypernephroma
	Histoplasmosis
	Visceral larva migrans *(Toxocara)*
	Visceral leishmaniasis
	Schistosomiasis
	Relapsing fever
	Epstein-Barr virus mononucleosis
	Cytomegalovirus mononucleosis
	Psittacosis
	Malaria
	Syphilis
	Typhus
	Rocky Mountain spotted fever
	Tuberculosis
	Babesiosis

*Extremely large spleen: chronic myelogenous leukemia, myelofibrosis, malaria, visceral leishmaniasis, lymphoma.

TABLE 8–14 ■ Differential Diagnosis of Lymphadenopathy

REGIONAL ADENOPATHY	GENERALIZED ADENOPATHY
Any local infection	Brucellosis
Tularemia (ulceroglandular)	Leptospirosis
Syphilis (primary)	Miliary tuberculosis
Tuberculosis (typical or atypical)	Histoplasmosis
Sporotrichosis	Epstein-Barr virus mononucleosis
Herpes simplex virus infection	Cytomegalovirus mononucleosis
Cat-scratch disease	Dengue fever
Scrub typhus	Syphilis
Lymphogranuloma venereum	Toxoplasmosis
Rat-bite fever *(Spirillum minus)*	Rubella
Metastatic carcinoma	Waldenström macroglobulinemia
Lymphomas	Lymphomas
Bubonic plague	Human immunodeficiency virus infection
Kawasaki disease	Serum sickness
Toxoplasmosis	Pseudolymphomas
Epstein-Barr virus mononucleosis	Hyperthyroidism
	Systemic lupus erythematosus
	Rheumatoid arthritis
	Sarcoidosis
	Viral hepatitis
	Myeloid metaplasia
	Immunoblastic lymphadenopathy

References

1. Kluger MJ (ed): Fever. Its Biology, Evolution, and Function. Princeton, NJ, Princeton University Press, 1979.
2. Dinarello CA, Cannon JG, Wolff SM: New concepts on the pathogenesis of fever. Rev Infect Dis 10:168–189, 1988.
3. Isaac B, Kernbaum S, Burke M (eds): Unexplained Fever. Boca Raton, FL, CRC Press, 1991.
4. Strickland GT (ed): Hunter's Tropical Medicine, ed 7. Philadelphia, WB Saunders, 1991.
5. Mackowiak PA (ed): Fever. Basic Mechanisms and Management. New York, Raven Press, 1991.
6. Cluff LE, Johnson JE (eds): Clinical Concepts of Infectious Diseases, ed 3. Boston, Williams & Wilkins, 1982, pp 61–74.

7. Cunha BA: Clinical implications of fever. Postgrad Med 85:188–200, 1989.
8. Cunha BA: Infectious diseases. *In* Samiy AH, Bardoness J, Douglas RG (eds): Textbook of Diagnostic Medicine. Philadelphia, Lea & Febiger, 1987, pp 131–166.
9. Cunha BA (ed): Fever. Infect Dis Clin North Am 10:33–222, 1996.
10. Schlossberg D, Shulman JA (eds): Differential Diagnosis of Infectious Disease. Baltimore, Williams & Wilkins, 1996.
11. Canizares O, Harman RRM (eds): Clinical Tropical Dermatology, ed 2. Boston, Blackwell Scientific Publications, 1992.
12. Corey L, Kirby P: Rash and fever. *In* Braunwald E, Isselbacher KJ, Petersdorf RG, et al (eds): Harrison's Principles of Internal Medicine, ed 11. New York, McGraw-Hill, 1987, pp 240–244.
13. Fitzpatrick TB, Johnson RA: Differential diagnosis of rashes in the acutely ill febrile patient and in life-threatening diseases. *In* Jeffers JD, Scott E, White J (eds): Dermatology in General Medicine. Textbook and Atlas, ed 3. New York, McGraw-Hill, 1987, pp 21–22.
14. Manson-Bahr PEC, Bell DR (eds): Manson's Tropical Diseases, ed 19. London, Baillière Tindall, 1987.
15. Oblinger MJ, Sande MA: Fever and Rash. *In* Stein JH (ed): Internal Medicine. Boston, Little, Brown, 1983, pp 1173–1178.
16. Pankey GA (ed): Dermatologic manifestations of infectious diseases. Infect Dis Clin North Am 8:677–688, 1994.
17. Lawson JH (ed): A Synopsis of Fevers and Their Treatment, ed 12. London, Lloyd-Luke, 1977.
18. Warren KS, Mahmoud AAR (eds): Tropical and Geographical Medicine, ed 2. New York, McGraw-Hill Information Services, 1990.
19. Esposito AL: Aspirin impairs antibacterial mechanisms in experimental pneumococcal pneumonia. Am Rev Respir Dis 130:857–862, 1984.
20. Shann F: Antipyretics in severe sepsis. Lancet 1:338–339, 1995.

9

Cytokines in the Treatment and Prevention of Infectious Diseases

Gerald V. Quinnan, Jr.

Cytokines are secreted soluble proteins that affect the proliferation or differentiation of specific cell types through processes that involve binding to specific cell surface receptors.[1] The number of cytokines recognized and knowledge of the nature of their actions are continuously increasing, adding progressively to our understanding of infectious diseases and new options for treatment and prevention. The cytokines that are currently applicable to the management of infectious diseases are substances that either affect leukocyte function or are involved in hematopoiesis. In the near future applications are likely to be developed for other cytokines by virtue of their effects on infectious disease manifestations or conditions that predispose to infections. This chapter reviews information pertinent to understanding the actions and use of the cytokines of current clinical relevance, the interleukins (ILs), the interferons (IFNs), and the hematopoietic growth factors.

The binding of cytokines to their cell surface receptors leads to induction of cytokine effects through the process of signal transduction.[2] The receptors for cytokines are proteins or protein complexes that are induced as a result of cytokine binding to interact with other cytosolic or membrane-bound proteins, such that protein phosphorylation or dephosphorylation events occur.[3] Such events activate functions of proteins, initiating a series of events that lead to the activation of expression of a particular gene or genes via the effects of DNA binding proteins, eventually resulting in the change in cell growth or differentiation that is the specific phenotypic effect of the cytokine.[4] There is some sharing of components of receptor signal transduction pathways by different cytokines. Cytokine receptors are typically composed of subunits, some of which are subunits of other cytokine receptors, and distinct cytokine-receptor binding events may result in phosphorylation of the same cytosolic proteins or induction of the same DNA binding proteins.[4, 5] Nevertheless, cytokines mediate specific effects by virtue of the variable expression of specific receptors on different cell types or other distinguishing biochemical characteristics of the responding cells.

The action of any cytokine on a particular cell changes the state of differentiation of that cell and may change the responsiveness of the cell to other cytokines. As a result of such effects, multiple cytokines often affect one type of cell and may act additively, synergistically, sequentially, or interdependently. They may act in either an autocrine (affecting the cell that produces them) or a paracrine (affecting nearby cells) manner, and one cytokine may induce or suppress the production of another. These complex interactions are sometimes referred to as the cytokine cascade, although the specific sequence of interactions that affect one cell type is probably different from the sequence of those that affect another cell type, even though some of the same cytokines may be involved.

Cytokine effects are important in disease pathogenesis. The genomes of some organisms encode protein homologs of mammalian cytokines, on which they may be dependent for growth or disease manifestations.[6, 7] Alternatively, they may depend on host cytokines for their own growth, may utilize cytokine receptors for their own attachment to target cells, or may modulate cytokine production or receptor expression in the host.[8–10] Many, perhaps all, of the components of signal transduction pathways are the products of protooncogenes; that is, they are products of normal genes that can be associated with oncogenesis through mutation or change in expression or function. Not surprisingly, therefore, the intracellular processes activated by cytokines are being increasingly implicated in the mechanisms of oncogenesis, including viral oncogenesis,[11, 12] and much of the clinical research that has been conducted regarding cytokines has been oriented toward oncology. These extensive interactions between cytokines and infectious agents will undoubtedly result in many new approaches to treatment and prevention of infectious diseases in the years to come.

Interleukins

The ILs are cytokines that transmit signals between cells of the different leukocyte lineages. At the time of this writing, 13 ILs are listed on Medline by the National Library of Medicine, as described in Table 9-1, and publications have appeared describing others. Many of the ILs have descriptive names reflecting functions that were discovered in advance of molecular cloning of their encoding genes or demonstration that a source and target of the cytokine were both of

TABLE 9–1 ■ Sources and Effects of Interleukins

NUMBER	SYNONYM	SOURCES	EFFECTS
1	Lymphocyte-activating factor[13–15]	Monocytes, macrophages, neutrophils	Inflammatory response induction, T-cell activation
2	T-cell growth factor[16–18]	Th1 helper T cells	T- and B-cell proliferation, reduced immunoglobulin production, induction of IL-4 production
3	Multipotential colony-stimulating factor[19–21]	Activated lymphocytes and macrophages, granulocytes	Erythroid, megakaryocytic, and multipotential stem cell proliferation
4	B-cell growth factor[22–24]	Th2 helper T cells	Differentiation of Th2 cells, B-cell proliferation, suppression of proinflammatory cytokine production, chemotaxis of monocytes and neutrophils
5	B-cell growth factor II[22–26]	Th2 helper T cells	B-cell and eosinophil proliferation
6	B-cell differentiation factor 2[27]	Monocytes, T cells, others	Acute-phase response induction, B- and T-cell growth
7	Lymphopoietin 1[28, 29]	Stromal cells	Proliferation of thymocyte stem cells and pre-B and pre-T cells
8	Neutrophil, monocyte-derived chemotactic factor[30–33]	Monocytes and neutrophils	Neutrophil and T-cell chemotaxis
9	P40 T-cell growth factor[34–37]	T cells	T-cell and erythroid precursor proliferation
10	Cytokine synthesis inhibitory factor[38–40]	Th2 helper T cells, macrophages, B cells, keratinocytes	Suppressed IL-2 and IFN-γ production, proliferation of megakaryocytes, mast cells, and multilineage colonies
11	Adipogenesis inhibitory factor[41, 42]	Stromal cells	Modulation of antigen-specific immunoglobulin production, proliferation of pre-B and macrophage cells
12	Natural killer cell stimulatory factor[43]	Monocytes and macrophages	Lymphokine secretion by Th1 cells, cytotoxic T-cell and natural killer cell cytotoxicity
13	None[13, 44]	Th2 helper T cells	Reduced macrophage production of proinflammatory cytokines, suppression of $CD8^+$ T-cell responses

leukocyte lineage. In fact, some of the substances have many names that are not listed in Table 9–1. The utility of descriptive names is limited because all of the ILs have a variety of effects depending on the type of cell affected and its state of activation or differentiation. The recognized effects of the ILs include the induction of proliferation of both precursors and mature cells of all leukocyte lineages, as well as some other hematopoietic cell types, modulation of mononuclear cell chemotaxis, and modulation of the production of other cytokines or the responsiveness of cells to other cytokines.

A number of important relationships among the ILs have emerged, some of which are summarized in Table 9–2. One particularly significant set of relationships is based on the recognition that helper T cells can be divided into different subsets on the basis of the cytokines they produce. One subset, designated Th1, produces IL-2 and IFN-γ, and the other, Th2, produces IL-4, IL-5, IL-10, and IL-13.[45–48] Th0 cells

TABLE 9–2 ■ Examples of Significant Functional Relationships Among Cytokines

FUNCTIONAL GROUP	CYTOKINES
Helper T-cell subset specific	
Th1 produced	IL-2, IFN-γ
Th2 produced	IL-4, IL-5, IL-10, IL-13
Proinflammatory	IL-1β, tumor necrosis factor-α, IL-6
Antiinflammatory	IL-4, IL-10, transforming growth factor-β, IL-13
Eosinophilogenic	IL-3, IL-5, granulocyte-macrophage colony-stimulating factor
IL-4 gene family	IL-3, IL-4, IL-5, granulocyte-macrophage colony-stimulating factor

can produce all of these lymphokines and are driven to mature into Th1 or Th2 cells by IL-12 and IL-4, respectively. These Th1 and Th2 subsets cross-regulate each other. As examples, IL-2 induces production of IL-4 and subsequent differentiation of Th2 cells,[16] and IL-4 can block production of IL-2 and IFN-γ and induce apoptosis of Th1 cells.[49] The cytokines produced by these two subsets generally have reciprocal effects. The Th1 cytokines promote cell-mediated immune responses, including production of cytokines by and chemotaxis of monocytes and cytotoxic lymphocyte responses, but suppress immunoglobulin production by B cells. Conversely, Th2 cytokines suppress macrophage and T-cell responses and enhance immunoglobulin production. Unique patterns of regulation of Th1 and Th2 responses characterize the pathogenesis of certain infectious diseases, such as acquired immunodeficiency syndrome (AIDS), those caused by mycobacterial infections, and many parasitic diseases.[50–52] Better understanding of these regulatory phenomena may lead to new approaches to therapy. In addition, regulation of Th1 and Th2 induction has become an important focus of adjuvant research.[53] The demonstration that production of IL-6 at a mucosal surface can markedly enhance immunoglobulin A production exemplifies the potential to induce selectively the type of immune response most likely to be of value against any particular infection.[54]

The macrophage-deactivating effects of Th2 cytokines are shared in part by transforming growth factor-β and are the basis for their being grouped with the antiinflammatory cytokines. The proinflammatory cytokines include IL-1β, tumor necrosis factor-α, and IL-6.[55] The proinflammatory cytokines induce the acute-phase response, B-cell differentiation, and antibacterial macrophage activities. The signal transduction that follows binding of these proinflammatory cytokines to their receptors results in induction of high levels of a common nuclear binding protein that enhances the expression of genes involved in the acute-phase response, such as IL-8, granulocyte colony-stimulating factor (G-CSF), IL-1, and immunoglobulin genes.[4]

Certain of the ILs are hematopoietic growth factors, including IL-3, IL-4, IL-5, IL-7, IL-9, IL-10, and IL-11 (see Table 9–1 for references). The induction of eosinophilia involves the proliferative effects of IL-5 and granulocyte-macrophage colony-stimulating factor (GM-CSF), as well as promoting effects of IL-3.[56] Because of these effects, these three cytokines are referred to as eosinophilogenic cytokines. Their effects are significant in diseases characterized by eosinophilia, particularly a number of parasitic diseases. The relationship between these factors is further evident in the finding that IL-4, IL-5, GM-CSF, and IL-3 are in a single gene family clustered in a region of a single chromosome.[14] Such a gene clustering implies an ancestral relationship between them, which is not surprising in view of their related functions. It is likely that other related cytokines will be found to be ordered in families and that the complex interactions between the various cytokines will come to be viewed as the interplay between proteins in a limited number of families, with substantial redundancy in receptor subunits, signal transduction pathways, and DNA-binding, gene-activating proteins used within each family and possibly among them.

Interleukin-2

The only IL licensed by the U.S. Food and Drug Administration at this time is IL-2. It is indicated for use in the treatment of metastatic renal cell carcinoma. Potential usefulness as therapy for infectious diseases is anticipated, because of its role in cell-mediated immune responses, such as cytotoxic T-cell and natural killer cell responses, that are important in many viral infections.[57, 58] Interest in its potential use in AIDS was evoked when studies demonstrated that exposure of lymphocytes from infected patients to IL-2 in vitro resulted in differentiation of cytomegalovirus-specific cytotoxic T-cell precursors into mature effector cells and that the blood of these patients contained activity that inhibited IL-2 production.[59, 60] Initial clinical studies of continuous infusion of IL-2 in patients with human immunodeficiency virus (HIV) infection were disappointing, however, because no effect on cytotoxic cell activity was observed and an initial increase in $CD4^+$ cell numbers was followed by a progressive decline.[61, 62] The cause of the decline was unknown, but it may have been due in part to induction of increased HIV replication. Subsequently, it has been learned that there is a progressive decline in Th1 cell function during the course of HIV infection, with a switch to Th2 predominance possibly being the factor that finally results in progression of the infection to AIDS.[63] Kovacs and colleagues[64] have reported that sustained increases in $CD4^+$ cell numbers could be induced in some patients early but not late in the course of HIV infection by intermittent infusion of IL-2. There were no sustained increases in HIV replication in patients who responded positively to treatment but there were in those in the late stages of infection. These results raise intriguing possible explanations for the observed effects of IL-2, particularly when considered in light of evidence that Th2, but not Th1, cells support replication of HIV.[65] It is possible that by treating with IL-2 intermittently, the secondary Th2-inducing effects of IL-2 can be avoided, allowing enhanced cell-mediated immunity but limiting the differentiation of helper T cells into Th2 cells, the target cells for HIV replication. The results of this clinical trial do not establish the efficacy of IL-2 for treatment of HIV infection but do justify the conduct of a controlled efficacy trial.

IL-2 has significant toxicity, particularly when used in the high doses recommended for treatment of renal cell carcinoma.[66]

Other Interleukins

A number of additional ILs have been introduced into phase I clinical trials, mostly for attempted treatment of malignancies. The capacity of IL-3 to induce proliferation of multipotential stem cells has evoked interest in its possible use for stimulating bone marrow in individuals with deficient production. It has been used in conjunction with GM-CSF in patients with myelodysplastic syndrome and after bone marrow transplantation to enhance hematopoiesis, with the possibility that the combination might reduce infectious complications associated with these conditions.[67, 68] A fusion protein consisting of parts of IL-3 and GM-CSF, named PIXY321, has been produced by recombinant DNA techniques and is also in clinical trials.[69]

Interferons

IFNs were the first cytokines introduced into clinical trials. The three main types of IFN are designated α, β, and γ. IFN-α and IFN-β are produced primarily by leukocytes and fibroblasts, respectively, in response to viral infection or other biochemical stimuli. IFN-γ is produced by T lymphocytes, primarily in response to immune stimulation.[47] They share the properties of interference with virus growth in cell culture (the reason for their names), potent immunomodulatory effects, and antiproliferative effects against tumor cells and normal cells.[58] They are, however, molecularly distinct.

Interferon-α

There are more than 17 different molecular species of IFN-α.[70] Each is the product of a specific gene and has its own unique profile of biologic activities. Among the three forms currently licensed in the United States, IFN alfa-2a (Roferon-A) and IFN alfa-2b (Intron A) are the products of single genes and are produced by recombinant DNA technology; IFN alfa-n3 (Alferon) is purified from supernatant fluids of cultured human leukocytes and is a mixture of 15 different molecular species.

INTERFERON ALFA-2A

IFN alfa-2a is indicated for use in treatment of hairy cell leukemia and AIDS-related Kaposi's sarcoma. Although neither of these is an infectious disease in the classic sense, hairy cell leukemia may be caused by human T-cell lymphotropic virus type II, and Kaposi's sarcoma has been associated with a previously unrecognized herpesvirus.[71, 72] Furthermore, an important manifestation of hairy cell leukemia is predisposition to infections, and Kaposi's sarcoma appears in the context of the immunodeficiency caused by HIV. The clinical responses obtained in these diseases are summarized in Table 9–3.

The response rates indicated for hairy cell leukemia are based on a grading system used to evaluate residual disease in the bone marrow.[73] Many patients with less than complete response benefit from treatment. There are significant reductions in the rate of secondary infections and requirements for red blood cell and platelet transfusion and improvement in average performance status. A patient should be treated for at least 6 months before being classified as a nonresponder. The optimum duration of treatment for responders has not been established. The recommended treatment regimen is 3 million international units (IU) subcutaneously or intramus-

TABLE 9–3 ■ Interferons Approved for Treatment or Prevention of Infectious Diseases by the U.S. Food and Drug Administration

INTERFERON	INDICATION FOR USE	RESPONSES
IFN alfa-2a	Hairy cell leukemia	Complete or partial response, 61%
		Minimal response or stable, 39%
	AIDS-associated Kaposi's sarcoma	Complete or partial response, 28%–45%
IFN alfa-2b	Hairy cell leukemia	Complete, partial, or minimal response, 90%
	AIDS-associated Kaposi's sarcoma	Complete or partial response, 35%–71%
	Condyloma acuminatum	Complete or partial response, 84%
	Chronic hepatitis C	Alanine aminotransferase response, 54%; histologic response, 69%
	Chronic hepatitis B	Alanine aminotransferase and virologic responses, 39%–54%
IFN alfa-n3	Condyloma acuminatum	Complete response, 54%
IFN gamma-1b	Chronic granulomatous disease	Reduction in serious infections, 67%

cularly daily for 16 to 24 weeks for response induction, then three times weekly for maintenance therapy. Doses may be held constant or reduced as needed because of toxic effects.

The beneficial effects of IFN alfa-2a in treatment of Kaposi's sarcoma are the result of shrinkage of tumor size and consist of palliation of the cosmetically disfiguring or physically disabling effects of the tumors.[74] IFN treatment of the malignancy is not curative and does not stop the progression of HIV infection. The benefit is most significant in patients with less severely impaired immunity. Patients with prior opportunistic infections or $CD4^+$ cell counts less than 200/mm^3 of peripheral blood respond rarely. Treatment is eventually discontinued for all patients, mostly as a result of adverse effects or lack of response. The decision regarding when to treat a particular patient should be based on a clinical judgment regarding the status of the Kaposi's sarcoma in comparison with the expected adverse effects and the knowledge that the duration of therapy is likely to be limited and the likelihood of response is greater early in infection. The recommended treatment is 36 million IU daily for 10 to 12 weeks for induction and three times a week for maintenance. Frequent dose adjustments are needed for toxicity.

The adverse effects of all forms of IFN alfa are similar and are described later. Serum neutralizing activity against IFN alfa-2a develops in about 25% of patients who undergo treatment for hairy cell leukemia. The clinical significance of this neutralizing activity is uncertain.[73, 74]

INTERFERON ALFA-2B

Hairy Cell Leukemia and Kaposi's Sarcoma. Interferon alfa-2b is also indicated for use in the treatment of hairy cell leukemia and AIDS-associated Kaposi's sarcoma.[75, 76] The response rates in these two diseases are similar to those observed after treatment with IFN alfa-2a. The recommended treatment for hairy cell leukemia is 2 million IU subcutaneously or intramuscularly three times a week and for Kaposi's sarcoma is 30 million IU three times a week, with dosage adjustment as needed. Serum neutralizing activity was not detected in patients treated for these diseases.

Condyloma Acuminatum. Intralesional treatment with IFN alfa-2b ordinarily involves a 3-week course, but responses continue to be observed for up to 8 weeks after the start of treatment (5 weeks after completion of treatment).[77, 78] The complete response rate after a single 3-week course of treatment has been 31% to 43% of treated lesions and after two courses 57% to 85%. Significant partial responses occur in many additional patients, for whom IFN may serve as useful presurgical therapy. Among completely responding patients 81% remained lesion free 16 weeks after initiation of treatment. The recommended treatment regimen is 1 million IU per lesion three times a week for 3 weeks, with treatment of up to five lesions at one time.

Chronic Hepatitis C. The benefits of treatment of chronic hepatitis C are difficult to evaluate because of the fluctuating nature of the disease and because the fibrotic and cirrhotic changes that are often present at biopsy may not resolve even if the progression of the disease is completely arrested. Nevertheless, treatment with IFN alfa-2b has value for a significant proportion of patients with this disease. In three different studies the average rate of normalization of alanine aminotransferase (ALT) activity was 54%[79, 80] (see also manufacturer's product package insert). Improvements in abnormal hepatic histology were observed in 61% to 69% of patients, depending on the type of scoring system used. During 6 months of posttreatment follow-up, 51% of ALT responses were maintained and new responses were observed in 83% of patients with relapses who were retreated. The diagnosis of hepatitis C should be confirmed by liver biopsy before treatment. The recommended treatment regimen is 3 million IU three times a week for 16 weeks if no ALT response is observed and for 26 weeks if an ALT response is observed.

Autoimmune disorders associated with hepatitis C virus infections have been evaluated during IFN treatment. In two studies improvements were demonstrated in the clinical manifestations of hepatitis C virus–associated mixed cryoglobulinemia.[81, 82] In another study of 14 patients with chronic hepatitis C virus infection and antineutrophil antibodies, 12 patients became antineutrophil autoantibody negative within 5 months of initiation of treatment.[83] In contrast, in a study of six patients with chronic hepatitis C virus infection and liver or kidney microsomal antibody type 1, three patients experienced a significant increase in ALT levels soon after beginning IFN alfa treatment.[84]

Clearance of detectable hepatitis C virus RNA from plasma or liver biopsy tissue occurs in about 50% of patients with chronic infection treated with IFN alfa, but relapse occurs in half of those responders.[85, 86]

Chronic Hepatitis B. The safety and effectiveness of IFN alfa-2b for treatment of chronic hepatitis B was demonstrated in three clinical trials.[87–89] Adult patients with documented chronic hepatitis B virus (HBV) infection of greater than 6 months' duration and positive hepatitis B e antigen and HBV DNA serum markers of HBV replication were studied. Virologic responses, consisting of elimination of the serum markers of HBV replication, were observed in 39% to 54% of patients; normalization of ALT levels, in 42% to 50% (including 87% of virologic responders); and improvements in liver histopathology, in 85% of responders in one study. Responses were durable and were associated with loss of serum hepatitis B surface antigen positivity in some patients, with the proportion converting to negative possibly increasing with increasing duration of response. The recommended treatment

TABLE 9–4 ■ Approximate Rates of Adverse Effects of Treatment with Interferon Alfa

	INTENDED WEEKLY IFN DOSAGE (IU × 10⁶)				
ADVERSE EFFECT*	≤5	5–15	30–35	90	≥245
Influenza-like illness	+ + +	+ + + +	+ + + +	+ + + +	+ + + +
Gastrointestinal	+	+ +	+ + +	+ + +	+ + +
Neuropsychiatric	±	+	+	+	+ +
Respiratory	−	±	±	±	+ +
Leukopenia	+	+ +	+ + +	+ + +	+ + +
Transaminasemia†	−	+	NA‡	+	+ + +

*Approximate rates corresponding to symbols: −, not reported; ±, occurring in <5% of recipients; +, in 5% to <15%; + +, in 15% to <30%; + + +, in 30% to <50%; + + + +, in ≥50%.
†Rates of transaminasemia in patients treated for chronic hepatitis are not included.
‡NA, Not available.

is 30 to 35 million IU/wk given either as 5 million IU daily or 10 million IU three times a week for 16 weeks. The safety and effectiveness of IFN alfa-2b in patients with combined HBV and hepatitis D virus infections were not evaluated in these studies, and treatment is not recommended for these patients.

INTERFERON ALFA-N3

This product is purified from the supernatant medium of cultured pooled leukocytes from human sources and treated in various ways that inactivate viruses that might be present in human leukocytes. Before the advent of recombinant DNA technology, IFN manufactured in similar ways was the principal source of material for use in clinical trials. IFN alfa-n3 is indicated for use in treatment of condyloma acuminatum. In a clinical trial of 156 patients, most of whom had relapses after or had disease refractory to treatment with other modalities, the rate of complete resolution of all warts was 54% and that of individually treated warts was 73%.[90] Treatment was continued for up to 8 weeks, and about half of the responses that did occur did so during the 3 months after treatment. Recurrence followed in about 24% of responders. The recommended treatment is 250,000 IU (0.05 mL) injected into the base of each wart twice weekly for up to 8 weeks, unless resolution occurs sooner. The maximum dose recommended for any one treatment session is 2.5 million IU.

OTHER CLINICAL TRIALS OF INTERFERON ALFA

There have been clinical trials of IFN alfa for treatment or prevention of a wide variety of diseases, of which a few infectious diseases are mentioned briefly here: various manifestations of papillomavirus infections, chronic hepatitis D, and HIV infection. Forms of IFN alfa not currently licensed in the United States have been shown to be active when administered systemically to children with papillomatosis of the middle and lower respiratory tract.[91, 92] Despite observations that some patients responded to treatment, it is not clear that the benefit is of sufficient magnitude and duration in those who respond to merit its routine use in all children with this condition. Positive effects of IFN alfa treatment on cervical, vaginal, and vulvar intraepithelial neoplasia have been reported.[93–95]

IFN alfa has been found to suppress chronic hepatitis D virus infections, but relapses occur soon after treatment. The mean time to relapse in one study after 1 year of treatment was 3.8 months.[96] Hepatitis D virus superinfection was observed in a patient being treated with IFN alfa for chronic hepatitis B.[97] On the basis of induction of long-term remission in three of five patients with recent onset of progressive hepatitis D infection, Marzano and colleagues[98] recommended treatment of patients early in the course of disease. Additional controlled study of larger populations of patients may establish the role of IFN alfa, if any, in this condition.

Despite the activity of IFN alfa against HIV in vitro, clinical trials of systemic IFN alfa alone or in combination with zidovudine for treatment of Kaposi's sarcoma have not demonstrated an effect of IFN treatment on the progression of AIDS.[99, 100] In view of that experience, initial reports of dramatic effectiveness of low-dose oral IFN in AIDS were surprising.[101, 102] Two subsequent randomized, placebo-controlled trials of low-dose oral IFN alfa have not confirmed the earlier positive reports.[103, 104]

ADVERSE EFFECTS OF INTERFERON ALFA

The adverse effects of the different forms of IFN alfa are similar. The available data are derived mostly from clinical trials in adults, and none of the IFN alfa currently licensed in the United States is labeled as indicated for use in children. The frequency and severity of adverse reactions vary with respect to dosage and the disease being treated. The most common side effects are influenza-like symptoms. About 30% of patients who receive IFN alfa-n3, at 250,000 IU per lesion twice weekly, and most patients who receive doses higher than that of any IFN alfa experience these symptoms, as summarized in Table 9–4. The severity of the reaction also tends to increase as the dose is increased. These symptoms include fever, headache, myalgias, arthralgias, and malaise. Gastrointestinal symptoms, including nausea, diarrhea, and others, occur at all dose levels, with the frequency and severity increasing at higher doses. Neuropsychiatric symptoms, including depression, anxiety, and others, are infrequent except at doses of 35 million IU/d or greater. Respiratory symptoms, including cough, dyspnea, and others, are also infrequent except at the highest dose levels. A variety of other adverse effects have been reported. The most common laboratory abnormalities are leukopenia and hepatic enzyme elevation, which vary according to dose, and possibly the disease being treated.

The adverse effects of IFN alfa therapy can be managed in a variety of ways. For serious or severe adverse effects, it is often necessary to withhold doses and/or to reduce subsequent dosages, generally by 50%. Such adverse effects occur most frequently, but not exclusively, during treatment with the higher doses used (e.g., >100 million IU/wk). Less severe adverse effects can often be ameliorated to a satisfactory degree by the judicious use of antipyretics or analgesics and by administration of doses at bedtime. During therapy with low or moderate dosage regimens (e.g., <100 million IU/wk), patients may become tolerant to the adverse effects; at the highest doses used adverse effects eventually necessitate discontinuation of treatment for many or all patients.

Interferon Beta

IFN beta-1b (Betaseron) is licensed in the United States for use for treatment of relapsing, remitting multiple sclerosis to reduce the frequency of relapses.[105, 106] It is produced by recombinant DNA technology. The mechanism of action of IFN beta-1b in this disease is unknown. Relapse of multiple sclerosis is highly associated with the occurrence of recent respiratory infection, and the beneficial effect may involve prevention of respiratory infections in these patients.[107] The adverse effects of IFN beta are similar to those of IFN alfa.

Interferon-γ

IFN-γ is produced primarily by T lymphocytes and has a variety of effects, many of which are mediated through macrophage activation. The IFN gamma licensed in the United States, IFN gamma-1b (Actimmune), is made by recombinant DNA technology. It is indicated for use in reducing the frequency and severity of serious infections associated with chronic granulomatous disease. This is a group of X-linked and autosomal recessive inherited disorders characterized by increased rates of serious pyogenic infections resulting from defective phagocyte superoxide production and function.[108] IFN gamma partially corrects the phagocytic defects in vitro.[108] After a phase I study demonstrated that administration of IFN gamma-1b in vivo also improved phagocyte function, a randomized, placebo-controlled study was conducted.[109, 110] The IFN treatment group experienced highly significant improvements in the time to first serious infection, the number of people who developed serious infections, and the number of serious infections developed. A serious infection was defined as one requiring hospitalization and parenteral antibiotics. The recommended treatment regimen is 50 $\mu g/m^2$ per dose (approximately 1.5 million U/m^2) subcutaneously three times a week (1.5 μg/kg per dose for children with a body surface area ≤ 0.5 m^2). As with other IFNs, dosages should be reduced or withheld should severe reactions occur. The adverse reactions attributable to IFN gamma-1b are similar to those seen with equivalent dosages of other IFNs, with influenza-like reactions occurring in the majority of individuals.

Promising results have been obtained using IFN gamma-1b for other purposes, as well. It has been used in chronic granulomatous disease as an adjunct to antibiotics for treatment of established infections with *Aspergillus* and *Pseudallescheria boydii*.[111, 112] A pilot study of IFN gamma-1b treatment of six patients with congenital osteopetrosis was conducted because of the known defect in leukocyte superoxide formation in that condition.[113] Enhancement of bone resorption and improvement in bone marrow production and leukocyte function were noted. A controlled trial of treatment of this condition has not been reported.

Treatment with IFN gamma has not been reported to be beneficial for patients with AIDS.[114]

Hematopoietic Growth Factors

The three hematopoietic growth factors licensed for use in the United States for treatment or prevention of infectious diseases are erythropoietin, GM-CSF, and G-CSF (Table 9–5). All three are produced by recombinant DNA technology.

Erythropoietin

The proper name for the licensed recombinant erythropoietin is epoietin alfa. It is sold under the trade names Epogen and Procrit. It was first licensed for the treatment of anemia and reduction of the need for blood transfusion for patients with chronic renal failure.[115, 116] Subsequently, it was approved for use in cancer patients receiving chemotherapy and in conjunction with zidovudine for treatment of HIV infection. It is indicated for elevation or maintenance of the red blood cell level and to decrease the need for transfusions of these HIV-infected patients. Its utility was demonstrated in placebo-controlled studies involving anemic, HIV-infected patients who were being treated with zidovudine. The benefit was limited to the subgroup (which constituted 84% of the total population studied) who had serum erythropoietin levels of 500 IU/mL or less.[117–119] Among patients who were transfusion dependent at baseline, 43% of epoietin alfa recipients and 18% of placebo recipients became transfusion independent. Furthermore, it was possible to maintain hematocrits in the normal range in the absence of reduction of the zidovudine dose at a significantly higher rate in the epoietin alfa recipients. The study was not designed to determine whether the epoietin alfa actually increased the efficacy of zidovudine. The recommended starting dose of epoietin alfa as an adjunct to zidovudine therapy is 100 U/kg intravenously or subcutaneously three times a week for 8 weeks. The dose can be adjusted subsequently, with monitoring of the hematocrit, if an unsatisfactory response is obtained initially. If the hematocrit exceeds 40%, the dose should be adjusted downward. Patients can be maintained with an established effective dose, with adjustments for changing circumstances as needed. The adverse experiences observed in the epoietin alfa–treated patients were similar to those observed in the placebo recipients. There is concern that treatment may contribute to severe hypertension in patients with chronic renal failure, and it is advised in general that treatment not be initiated for patients with uncontrolled hypertension. Allergic reactions have been observed.

Granulocyte Colony-Stimulating Factor

The proper name of the G-CSF licensed in the United States is filgrastim (Neupogen). It is normally produced in the body by a variety of cell types and acts selectively to enhance the proliferation of granulocyte precursors in the bone marrow.[120] It is indicated to decrease the incidence of infection, as manifest by febrile neutropenia, in patients with nonmyeloid malignancies who are receiving myelosuppressive anticancer drugs associated with a significant incidence of severe neutropenia with fever. In a randomized, placebo-controlled

TABLE 9–5 ■ Cytokine Growth Factors Approved by the U.S. Food and Drug Administration for Treatment or Prevention of Infectious Diseases

GROWTH FACTOR	INDICATION	RESPONSE
Erythropoietin (epoietin alfa)	In conjunction with zidovudine for HIV infection	43% transfusion independent
G-CSF (filgrastim)	Reduction of infection after chemotherapy for malignancy	47% reduction in febrile neutropenia
GM-CSF (sargramostim)	Myeloid reconstitution after autologous bone marrow transplantation	Duration of infection, neutropenia, and hospitalization reduced
	Bone marrow engraftment failure or delay	Survival extended almost threefold

study of patients being treated for small-cell lung cancer, there was a statistically significant reduction in the number of patients experiencing febrile neutropenia from 76% in the placebo group to 40% in the treatment group.[121] There were also reductions in the requirements for hospitalization and antibiotic use and in the duration of severe neutropenia. Increases in neutrophil counts have been observed in other, smaller studies of patients with different malignancies and chemotherapy regimens. The recommended dose of filgrastim is 5 μg/kg per day intravenously or subcutaneously, beginning at least 24 hours after the initiation of chemotherapy and continued daily for up to 2 weeks or until the postsuppression absolute neutrophil count exceeds 10,000/mm^3. Treatment with filgrastim causes bone pain, which is dose related and usually responsive to nonnarcotic analgesics. It has also been associated with a capillary leak syndrome.[122]

Filgrastim has been studied for treatment of neutropenia in many circumstances, including treatment after a variety of types of chemotherapy for malignancy,[123] cyclic neutropenia,[124, 125] chronic severe neutropenia,[126, 127] severe neutropenia of the newborn,[128, 129] and neutropenia occurring as an idiosyncratic reaction to drug therapy.[130, 131] It has also been used to mobilize peripheral blood stem cells so that they can be harvested for later use in autologous transfusion.[132, 133]

Granulocyte-Macrophage Colony-Stimulating Factor

Recombinant human GM-CSF (Leukine), the proper name of which is sargramostim, induces the growth and differentiation of myelomonocytic precursor cells in the bone marrow.[134] It is indicated for use in myeloid reconstitution after autologous bone marrow transplantation and in bone marrow transplantation failure or engraftment delay. The randomized, placebo-controlled clinical trials in autologous bone marrow transplantation demonstrated efficacy in patients who received transplants for non-Hodgkin's lymphoma and acute lymphocytic leukemia.[135] Treatment with sargramostim significantly reduced the number of days with absolute neutrophil counts below 500/mm^3 and below 1000/mm^3 and the mean durations of hospitalization, infection, and antibacterial therapy. Survival was not affected by treatment, leaving the role of sargramostim in this condition somewhat controversial.[136]

The clinical trial of sargramostim in bone marrow transplantation failure or engraftment delay was historically controlled. Treatment improved the mean survival of patients who had autologous marrow transplants from 161 days to 474 days and of patients who had allogeneic marrow transplants from 35 days to 97 days, compared with historical control subjects (manufacturer's product package insert).

The adverse events observed after sargramostim administration in the concurrently controlled trials were not more frequent than after placebo. The adverse effects that are considered attributable to sargramostim include bone pain, a capillary leak syndrome, and renal and hepatic dysfunction. It is necessary to monitor white cell counts and platelet counts during therapy to avoid excessive leukocytosis or thrombocytosis. Progression of underlying malignancy during therapy is a reason to discontinue treatment.

For myeloid reconstitution after autologous bone marrow transplantation, treatment is begun 2 to 4 hours after marrow infusion and is administered in doses of 250 μg/m^2 per day as a 2-hour intravenous infusion for 21 days. For treatment of failure of engraftment or engraftment delay the treatment course is 14 days, and treatment may be repeated after 7-day rest periods for second and third courses, if needed. Dosages can be reduced or withheld, as needed for management of adverse reactions.

References

1. Fauci AS: Immunomodulators in clinical medicine. Ann Intern Med 106:421, 1987.
2. Taniguchi T: Cytokine signaling through nonreceptor protein tyrosine kinases. Science 286:251, 1995.
3. Pazin MJ, Williams LT: Triggering signaling cascades by receptor tyrosine kinases. Trends Biochem Sci 17:374, 1992.
4. Akira S, Kishimoto T: IL-6 and NF-IL6 in acute-phase response and viral infection. Immunol Rev 127:25, 1992.
5. Leonard WJ, Noguchi M, Russell SM, et al: The molecular basis of X-linked severe combined immunodeficiency: The role of the interleukin-2 receptor gamma chain as a common gamma chain, gamma c. Immunol Rev 138:61, 1994.
6. Pickup DJ: Poxviral modifiers of cytokine responses to infection. Infect Agents Dis 3:116, 1994.
7. Opgenorth A, Nation N, Graham K, et al: Transforming growth factor alpha, Shope fibroma growth factor, and vaccinia growth factor can replace myxoma growth factor in the induction of myxomatosis in rabbits. Virology 192:701, 1993.
8. Todd B, Pope JH, Georghiou P: Interleukin-2 enhances production in 24 hours of infectious human immunodeficiency virus type 1 in vitro by naturally infected mononuclear cells from seropositive donors. Arch Virol 121:227, 1991.
9. Pace J, Hayman MJ, Galan E: Signal transduction and invasion of epithelial cells by *S. typhimurium*. Cell 72:505, 1993.
10. Verheijden GF, Moolenaar WH, Ploegh HL: Retention of epidermal growth factor receptors in the endoplasmic reticulum of adenovirus-infected cells. Biochem J 282:115, 1992.
11. McGlennen RC, Ostrow RS, Carson LF, et al: Expression of cytokine receptors and markers of differentiation in human papillomavirus-infected cervical tissues. Am J Obstet Gynecol 165:696, 1991.
12. Kuivinen E, Hoffman BL, Hoffman PA, et al: Structurally related class I and class II receptor protein tyrosine kinases are down-regulated by the same E3 protein coded for by human group C adenoviruses. J Cell Biol 120:1271, 1993.
13. Dinarello CA: Interleukin-1. Adv Pharmacol 25:21, 1994.
14. Boulay JL, Paul WE: The interleukin-4 family of lymphokines. Curr Opin Immunol 4:294, 1992.
15. Dinarello CA: The proinflammatory cytokines interleukin-1 and tumor necrosis factor and treatment of the septic shock syndrome. J Infect Dis 163:1177, 1991.
16. Le Gros G, Ben-Sasson SZ, Seder R, et al: Generation of interleukin 4 (IL-4)–producing cells in vivo and in vitro: IL-2 and IL-4 are required for in vitro generation of IL-4–producing cells. J Exp Med 172:921, 1990.
17. Mier JW, Gallo RC: Purification and some characteristics of human T-cell growth factor from phytohemagglutinin-stimulated lymphocyte–conditioned media. Proc Natl Acad Sci USA 77:6134, 1980.
18. Gottlieb DJ, Prentice HG, Heslop HE, et al: IL-2 infusion abrogates humoral immune responses in humans. Clin Exp Immunol 87:493, 1992.
19. Baines P, Truran L, Bailey-Wood R, et al: Haemopoietic colony-forming cells from peripheral blood stem cell harvests: Cytokine requirements and lineage potential. Br J Haematol 88:472, 1994.
20. Elmslie RE, Dow SW, Ogilvie GK: Interleukins: Biological properties and therapeutic potential. J Vet Intern Med 5:283, 1991.
21. Chen YZ, Gu XF, Caen JP, et al: Interleukin-3 is an autocrine growth factor of human megakaryoblasts, the DAMI and MEG-01 cells. Br J Haematol 88:481, 1994.
22. Rocken M, Urban J, Shevach EM: Antigen-specific activation, tolerization, and reactivation of the interleukin 4 pathway in vivo. J Exp Med 179:1885, 1994.
23. Miossec P: Interleukin-4 and interleukin-10 as antagonists of interferon-gamma. J Interferon Res 14:285, 1994.
24. Wang P, Wu P, Anthes JC, et al: Interleukin-10 inhibits interleukin-8 production in human neutrophils. Blood 83:2678, 1994.
25. Limaye AP, Abrams JS, Silver JE: Regulation of parasite-induced eosinophilia: Selectively increased interleukin 5 production in helminth-infected patients. J Exp Med 172:399, 1990.

26. Mahanty S, Nutman TB: The biology of interleukin-5 and its receptor. Cancer Invest 11:624, 1993.
27. Ruef C, Budde K, Lacy J, et al: Interleukin 6 is an autocrine growth factor for mesangial cells. Kidney Int 38:249, 1990.
28. Schmitt C, Ktorza S, Sarun S, et al: CD34-expressing human thymocyte precursors proliferate in response to interleukin-7 but have lost myeloid differentiation potential. Blood 82:3675, 1993.
29. Dokter WH, Sierdsema SJ, Esselink MT, et al: Interleukin-4 mRNA and protein activated human T cells are enhanced by interleukin-7. Exp Hematol 22:74, 1994.
30. Zachariae CO: Chemotactic cytokines and inflammation. Biological properties of the lymphocyte and monocyte chemotactic factors ELCF, MCAF and IL-8. Acta Derm Venereol Suppl (Stockh) 181:1, 1993.
31. Kimata H, Lindley I: Interleukin-8 differentially modulates interleukin-4– and interleukin-2–induced human B cell growth. Eur J Immunol 24:3237, 1994.
32. Wertheim WA, Kunkel SL, Standiford TJ, et al: Regulation of neutrophil-derived IL-8: The role of prostaglandin E_2, dexamethasone, and IL-4. J Immunol 151:2166, 1993.
33. Cassatella MA, Meda L, Bonora S, et al: Interleukin-10 (IL-10) inhibits the release of proinflammatory cytokines from human polymorphonuclear leukocytes. Evidence for an autocrine role of tumor necrosis factor and IL-1 beta in mediating the production of IL-8 triggered by lipopolysaccharide. J Exp Med 178:2207, 1993.
34. Schmitt E, Germann T, Goedert S, et al: IL-9 production of naive $CD4^+$ T cells depends on IL-2, is synergistically enhanced by a combination of TGF-beta and IL-4, and is inhibited by IFN-gamma. J Immunol 153:3989, 1994.
35. Lehrnbecher T, Poot M, Orscheschek K: Interleukin 7 as interleukin 9 drives phytohemagglutinin-activated T cells through several cell cycles: No synergism between interleukin 7, interleukin 9 and interleukin 4. Cytokine 6:279, 1994.
36. Lemoli RM, Fortuna A, Fogli M, et al: Stem cell factor (*c-kit* ligand) enhances the interleukin-9 dependent proliferation of human $CD34^+$ and $CD34^+CD33^-DR^-$ cells. Exp Hematol 22:919, 1994.
37. Houssiau FA, Renauld JC, Stevens M: Human T cell lines and clones respond to IL-9. J Immunol 150:2634, 1993.
38. Del Prete G, De Carli M, Almerigogna F, et al: Human IL-10 is produced by both type 1 helper (Th1) and type 2 helper (Th2) T cell clones and inhibits their antigen proliferation and cytokine production. J Immunol 150:353, 1993.
39. Schlaak JF, Schmitt E, Huls C, et al: A sensitive and specific bioassay for the detection of human interleukin-10. J Immunol Methods 168:49, 1994.
40. Rennick D, Hunte B, Dang W: Interleukin-10 promotes the growth of megakaryocyte, mast cell, and multilineage colonies: Analysis with committed progenitors and $Thy1loSca1^+$ stem cells. Exp Hematol 22:136, 1994.
41. Suen Y, Chang M, Lee SM, et al: Regulation of interleukin-11 protein and mRNA expression in neonatal and adult fibroblasts and endothelial cells. Blood 84:4125, 1994.
42. Lee BL, Cumano A, Iscove NN, et al: Stromal cell independent growth of bipotent B cell–macrophage precursors from murine fetal liver. Int Immunol 6:401, 1994.
43. Chehimi J, Trinchieri G: Interleukin-12: A bridge between innate resistance and adaptive immunity with a role in infection and acquired immunodeficiency. J Clin Immunol 14:149, 1994.
44. Magazin M, Guillemot JC, Vita N, et al: Interleukin-13 is a monocyte chemoattractant. Eur Cytokine Netw 5:397, 1994.
45. Mosmann TR, Cherwinski H, Bond MW, et al: Two types of murine helper T cell clone. I. Definition according to profiles of lymphokine activities and secreted proteins. J Immunol 136:2348, 1986.
46. Romagnani S: Type 1 T helper and type 2 T helper cells: Functions, regulation and role in protection and disease. Int J Clin Lab Res 21:152, 1991.
47. Stout RD, Bottomly K: Antigen specific activation of effector macrophages of IFN-gamma producing (TH1) T cell clones. Failure of IL-4–producing (TH2) T cell clones to activate effector function in macrophages. J Immunol 142:760, 1989.
48. Mosmann TR, Schumacher JH, Fiorentino DF, et al: Isolation of monoclonal antibodies specific for IL-4, IL-5, IL-6, and a new Th2-specific cytokine (IL-10), cytokine synthesis inhibitory factor, by using a solid phase radioimmunoadsorbent assay. J Immunol 145:2938, 1990.
49. D'Andrea A, Ma X, Aste-Amezaga M, et al: Stimulatory and inhibitory effects of interleukin (IL)-4 and IL-13 on the production of cytokines by human peripheral blood mononuclear cells: Priming for IL-12 and tumor necrosis factor alpha production. J Exp Med 181:537, 1995.
50. Berman MA, Zaldivar F Jr, Imfeld KL, et al: HIV-1 infection of macrophages promotes long-term survival and sustained release of interleukins 1 alpha and 6. AIDS Res Hum Retroviruses 10:529, 1994.
51. Modlin RL, Nutman TB: Type 2 cytokines and negative immune regulation in human infections. Curr Opin Immunol 5:511, 1993.
52. Urban JF Jr, Katona IM, Paul WE, et al: Interleukin-4 is important in protective immunity to a gastrointestinal nematode infection in mice. Proc Natl Acad Sci USA 88:5513, 1991.
53. Golding B, Zaitseva M, Golding H: The potential for recruiting immune responses toward type 1 or type 2 T cell help. Am J Trop Med Hyg 50(Suppl):33, 1994.
54. Ramsay AJ, Husband AJ, Ramshaw IA, et al: The role of interleukin-6 in mucosal IgA antibody responses in vivo. Science 264:561, 1994.
55. Yano S, Sone S, Nishioka Y, et al: Differential effects of anti-inflammatory cytokines (IL-4, IL-10 and IL-13) on tumoricidal and chemotactic properties of human monocytes induced by monocyte chemotactic and activating factor. J Leukoc Biol 57:303, 1995.
56. Yano A, Yasukawa M, Yanagisawa K, et al: Adult T cell leukemia associated with eosinophilia: Analysis of eosinophil-stimulating factors produced by leukemic cells. Acta Haematol 88:207, 1992.
57. Quinnan GV Jr, Kirmani N, Rook AH, et al: Cytotoxic T cells in cytomegalovirus infection: HLA-restricted T-lymphocyte and non–T-lymphocyte cytotoxic responses correlate with recovery from cytomegalovirus infection in bone-marrow-transplant recipients. N Engl J Med 307:7, 1982.
58. Wittek AE, Quinnan GV: Immunology of viral infections. *In* Belshe RB (ed): Textbook of Human Virology, ed 2. St. Louis, Mosby–Year Book, 1991, p 116.
59. Rook AH, Masur H, Lane HC, et al: Interleukin-2 enhances the depressed natural killer and cytomegalovirus-specific cytotoxic activities of lymphocytes from patients with the acquired immune deficiency syndrome. J Clin Invest 72:398, 1983.
60. Siegal JP, Djeu JY, Stocks NI, et al: Sera from patients with the acquired immunodeficiency syndrome inhibit production of interleukin-2 by normal lymphocytes. J Clin Invest 75:1957, 1985.
61. Lane HC, Siegal JP, Rook AH, et al: Use of interleukin-2 in patients with acquired immunodeficiency syndrome. J Biol Response Modifiers 3:512, 1984.
62. Scwartz DH, Skowron G, Merigan TC: Safety and effects of interleukin-2 plus zidovudine in asymptomatic individuals infected with human immunodeficiency virus. J Acquir Immune Defic Syndr 4:11, 1991.
63. Clerici M, Sarin A, Coffman RL, et al: Type 1/type 2 cytokine modulation of T-cell programmed cell death as a model for human immunodeficiency virus pathogenesis. Proc Natl Acad Sci USA 91:11811, 1994.
64. Kovacs JA, Baseler M, Dewar RJ, et al: Increases in CD4 lymphocytes with intermittent courses of interleukin-2 in patients with human immunodeficiency virus infection. N Engl J Med 332:567, 1995.
65. Maggi E, Mazzetti M, Ravina A, et al: Ability of HIV to promote a TH1 to TH0 shift and to replicate preferentially in TH2 and TH0 cells. Science 265:244, 1994.
66. Siegal JP, Puri RK: Interleukin-2 toxicity. J Clin Oncol 9:694, 1991.
67. Maurer AB, Ganser A, Buhl R, et al: Restoration of impaired cytokine secretion from monocytes of patients with myelodysplastic syndromes after in vivo treatment with GM-CSF or IL-3. Leukemia 7:1728, 1993.
68. Fleischman RA: Southwestern Internal Medicine Conference: Clinical use of hematopoietic growth factors. Am J Med Sci 305:248, 1993.
69. Vadhan-Raj S: PIXY321 (GM-CSF/IL-3 fusion protein): Biology and early clinical development. Stem Cells (Dayt) 12:253, 1994.

70. Baron S, Tyring SK, Fleischman WR Jr, et al: The interferons: Mechanisms of action and clinical applications. JAMA 266: 1375, 1991.
71. Kalyanaraman VS, Sarngadharan MG, Robert-Guroff M, et al: A new subtype of human T cell leukemia virus (HTLV-II) associated with a T-cell variant of hairy cell leukemia. Science 218:571, 1982.
72. Moore PS, Chang Y: Detection of herpesvirus-like DNA sequences in Kaposi's sarcoma in patients with and those without HIV infection. N Engl J Med 332:1181, 1995.
73. Golomb HM, Jacobs A, Fefer A, et al: Alpha-2 interferon therapy of hairy-cell leukemia: A multicenter study of 64 patients. J Clin Oncol 4:900, 1986.
74. Real FX, Oettegen HF, Krown SE: Kaposi's sarcoma and the acquired immunodeficiency syndrome: Treatment with high and low doses of recombinant leukocyte A interferon. J Clin Oncol 4:544, 1986.
75. Golomb HM, Fefer A, Golde DW, et al: Sequential evaluation of alpha-2b-interferon treatment in 128 patients with hairy cell leukemia. Semin Oncol 14(Suppl 2):13, 1987.
76. Mitsuyasu RT: Interferon alpha in the treatment of AIDS-related Kaposi's sarcoma. Br J Haematol 79(Suppl 1):69, 1991.
77. Reichman RC, Oakes D, Bonnez W, et al: Treatment of condyloma acuminatum with three different interferon-alpha preparations administered parenterally: A double-blind, placebo-controlled trial. J Infect Dis 162:1270, 1990.
78. Vance JC, Bart BJ, Hansen RC, et al: Intralesional recombinant alpha-2 interferon for the treatment of patients with condyloma acuminatum of verruca plantaris. Arch Dermatol 122:272, 1986.
79. Weiland O, Schvarcz R, Wejstal R, et al: Interferon alpha-2b treatment of chronic posttransfusion non-A, non-B hepatitis: Interim results of a randomized controlled open study. Scand J Infect Dis 21:127, 1989.
80. Hoofnagle JH, Di Bisceglie AM, Shindo M: Antiviral therapy of hepatitis C—Present and future. J Hepatol 17(Suppl 3):S130, 1993.
81. Durand JM, Cretel E, Kaplanski G, et al: Long-term results of therapy with interferon alpha for cryoglobulinemia associated with hepatitis C virus infection. Clin Rheumatol 13:123, 1994.
82. Ferri C, Zignego AL, Longombardo G: Effect of alpha-interferon on hepatitis C virus chronic infection in mixed cryglobulinemia patients. Infection 21:93, 1993.
83. Warny M, Brenard R, Cornu C, et al: Anti-neutrophil antibodies in chronic hepatitis and the effect of alpha-interferon therapy. J Hepatol 17:294, 1993.
84. Muratori L, Lenzi M, Cataleta M, et al: Interferon therapy in liver/kidney microsomal antibody type 1–positive patients with chronic hepatitis C. J Hepatol 21:199, 1994.
85. Qian C, Camps J, Muluenda MD, et al: Replication of hepatitis C virus in peripheral blood mononuclear cells. Effect of alpha-interferon therapy. J Hepatol 16:380, 1992.
86. Lau JY, Mizokami M, Ohno T, et al: Discrepancy between biochemical and virological responses to interferon-alpha in chronic hepatitis C. Lancet 342:1208, 1993.
87. Perillo RP, Schiff ER, Davis GL, et al: A randomized, controlled trial of interferon alfa-2b alone and after prednisone withdrawal for the treatment of chronic hepatitis B. The Hepatitis Interventional Therapy Group. N Engl J Med 323:295, 1990.
88. Hoofnagle JH, Peters M, Mullen KD, et al: Randomized, controlled trial of recombinant human alpha-interferon in patients with chronic hepatitis B. Gastroenterology 95:1318, 1988.
89. Korenman J, Baker B, Waggoner J, et al: Long-term remission of chronic hepatitis B after alpha-interferon therapy. Ann Intern Med 114:629, 1991.
90. Friedman-Kien AE, Eron LJ, Conant M, et al: Natural interferon alfa for treatment of condylomata acuminata. JAMA 259:533, 1988.
91. Sessions RB, Dichtel WJ, Goepfert H: Treatment of recurrent respiratory papillomatosis with interferon. Ear Nose Throat J 63:488, 1984.
92. Lusk RP, McCabe BF, Mixon JH: Three-year experience of treating recurrent respiratory papilloma with interferon. Ann Otol Rhinol Laryngol 96:158, 1987.
93. Yliskoski M, Cantell K, Syrjanen K, et al: Topical treatment with human leukocyte interferon of HPV 16 infections associated with cervical and vaginal intraepithelial neoplasias. Gynecol Oncol 36:353, 1990.
94. Dunham AM, McCartney JC, McCance DJ, et al: Effect of perilesional injection of alpha-interferon on cervical intraepithelial neoplasia and associated human papillomavirus infection. J R Soc Med 83:490, 1990.
95. Spirtos NM, Smith LH, Teng NN: Prospective randomized trial of topical alpha-interferon (alpha-interferon gels) for the treatment of vulvar intraepithelial neoplasia III. Gynecol Oncol 37:34, 1990.
96. Hadziyannis SJ: Use of alpha-interferon in the treatment of chronic delta hepatitis. J Hepatol 13(Suppl 1):S21, 1991.
97. Craxi A, Di Marco V, Bruno R, et al: Hepatitis delta superinfection during alpha-interferon treatment for hepatitis B. Ital J Gastroenterol 24:19, 1992.
98. Marzano A, Ottrobelli A, Spezia C, et al: Treatment of early chronic delta hepatitis with lymphoblastoid alpha interferon: A pilot study. Ital J Gastroenterol 24:119, 1992.
99. Lane HC, Feinberg J, Davey V, et al: Anti-retroviral effects of interferon-alpha in AIDS-associated Kaposi's sarcoma. Lancet 2:1218, 1988.
100. Krown SE, Gold JW, Niedzweicki D, et al: Interferon-alpha with zidovudine: Safety, tolerance, and clinical and virologic effects in patients with Kaposi sarcoma associated with the acquired immunodeficiency syndrome (AIDS). Ann Intern Med 112:812, 1990.
101. Obel AO, Koech DK: Outcome of intervention with or without low dose oral interferon alpha in thirty-two HIV-1 seropositive patients in a referral hospital. East Afr Med J 67(7 Suppl 2):SS71, 1990.
102. Koech DK, Obel AO: Efficacy of Kemron (low dose oral natural human interferon alpha) in the management of HIV-1 infection and acquired immune deficiency syndrome (AIDS). East Afr Med J 67(7 Suppl 2):SS64, 1990.
103. Hulton MR, Levin DL, Freedman LS: Randomized, placebo-controlled, double-blind study of low-dose oral interferon-alpha in HIV-1 antibody positive patients. J Acquir Immune Defic Syndr 5:1084, 1992.
104. Kaiser G, Jaeger H, Birkman J, et al: Low-dose oral natural human interferon-alpha in 29 patients with HIV-1 infection: A double-blind, randomized, placebo-controlled trial. AIDS 6:563, 1992.
105. The IFNB Multiple Sclerosis Study Group: Interferon beta-1b is effective in relapsing-remitting multiple sclerosis. I. Clinical results of a multicenter, randomized, double-blind, placebo-controlled trial. Neurology 43:655, 1993.
106. Paty DW, Li DK: Interferon beta-1b is effective in relapsing-remitting multiple sclerosis. II. MRI analysis results of a multicenter, randomized, double-blind, placebo-controlled trial. Neurology 43:662, 1993.
107. Panitch HS: Influence of infection on exacerbations of multiple sclerosis. Ann Neurol 36(Suppl):S25, 1994.
108. Rex JH, Bennett JE, Gallin JI, et al: In vivo interferon-gamma therapy augments the in vitro ability of chronic granulomatous disease neutrophils to damage *Aspergillus* hyphae. J Infect Dis 163:849, 1991.
109. Gallin JI, Sechler JM, Malech HL: Reconstitution of defective phagocyte function in chronic granulomatous disease of childhood with recombinant human interferon-gamma. Trans Assoc Am Physicians 101:12, 1988.
110. The International Chronic Granulomatous Disease Cooperative Study Group: A controlled trial of interferon gamma to prevent infection in chronic granulomatous disease. N Engl J Med 324:509, 1991.
111. Bernhisel-Broadbent J, Camargo EE, Jaffe HS, et al: Recombinant human interferon-gamma as adjunct therapy for *Aspergillus* infection in a patient with chronic granulomatous disease. J Infect Dis 163:908, 1991.
112. Phillips P, Forbes JC, Speert DP: Disseminated infection with *Pseudallescheria boydii* in a patient with chronic granulomatous disease: Response to gamma-interferon plus antifungal chemotherapy. Pediatr Infect Dis J 10:536, 1991.
113. Key LL Jr, Ries WL, Rodriguiz RM, et al: Recombinant human interferon gamma therapy for osteopetrosis. J Pediatr 121:119, 1992.
114. Mitsuyasu RT: Use of recombinant interferons and hematopoietic growth factors in patients infected with human immunodeficiency virus. Rev Infect Dis 13:979, 1991.

115. Eschbach JW, Adamson JW, Cooperative Multicenter r-HuEpo Trial Group: Correction of the anemia of hemodialysis (HD) patients with recombinant human erythropoietin (r-HuEPO): Results of a multicenter study. Kidney Int 33:189, 1988.
116. Lim VS, DeGowin RL, Zavala D, et al: Recombinant human erythropoietin treatment in pre-dialysis patients: A double-blind placebo-controlled trial. Ann Intern Med 110:108, 1989.
117. Henry DH, Beall GN, Benson CA, et al: Recombinant human erythropoietin in the treatment of anemia associated with human immunodeficiency virus (HIV) infection and zidovudine therapy. Ann Intern Med 117:739, 1993.
118. Phair JP, Abels RI, McNeill MV, et al: Recombinant human erythropoietin treatment: Investigational new drug protocol for the anemia of the acquired immunodeficiency syndrome. Overall results. Arch Intern Med 153:2669, 1993.
119. Revicki DA, Brown RE, Henry DH, et al: Recombinant human erythropoietin and health-related quality of life of AIDS patients with anemia. J Acquir Immune Defic Syndr 7:474, 1994.
120. Zsebo KM, Cohen AM, Murdock DC, et al: Recombinant human granulocyte colony-stimulating factor: Molecular and biological characterization. Immunobiology 172:175, 1986.
121. Crawford J, Ozer H, Stoller R, et al: Reduction by granulocyte colony-stimulating factor of fever and neutropenia induced by chemotherapy in patients with small-cell lung cancer. N Engl J Med 325:164, 1991.
122. Oeda E, Shinohara K, Kamei S, et al: Capillary leak syndrome likely the result of granulocyte colony-stimulating factor after high-dose chemotherapy. Intern Med 33:115, 1994.
123. Bronchud MH: Recombinant human granulocyte colony-stimulating factor in the management of cancer patients: Five years on. Oncology 51:189, 1994.
124. Marcolongo R, Zambello R, Trentin L, et al: Childhood onset cyclic neutropenia: G-CSF therapy restores neutrophil count but does not influence superoxide anion and cytokine release by neutrophils. Br J Haematol 89:277, 1995.
125. Boxer LA, Hutchinson R, Emerson S: Recombinant human granulocyte-colony-stimulating factor in the treatment of patients with neutropenia. Clin Immunol Immunopathol 62:S39, 1992.
126. Jones EA, Bolyard AA, Dale DC: Quality of life of patients with severe chronic neutropenia receiving long-term treatment with granulocyte colony-stimulating factor. JAMA 270:1132, 1993.
127. Welte K, Zeidler C, Reiter A, et al: Effects of granulocyte colony-stimulating factor in children with severe neutropenia. Acta Haematol Pol 25(Suppl 1):155, 1994.
128. Makhlouf RA, Doron MW, Bose CL, et al: Administration of granulocyte colony-stimulating factor to neutropenic low birth weight infants of mothers with preeclampsia. J Pediatr 126:454, 1995.
129. La Gamma EF, Alpan O, Kocherlakota P: Effect of granulocyte colony-stimulating factor on preeclampsia-associated neonatal neutropenia. J Pediatr 126:457, 1995.
130. Weide R, Koppler H, Heymanns J, et al: Successful treatment of clozapine induced agranulocytosis with granulocyte-colony stimulating factor (G-CSF). Br J Haematol 80:557, 1992.
131. Means RT Jr, Sandidge DR, Rankin KM, et al: Treatment of phenothiazine-induced agranulocytosis with recombinant granulocyte colony-stimulating factor. Am J Hematol 41:296, 1992.
132. Fukuda M, Kojima S, Matsumoto K, et al: Autotransplantation of peripheral blood stem cells mobilized by chemotherapy and recombinant human granulocyte colony-stimulating factor in childhood neuroblastoma and non-Hodgkin's lymphoma. Br J Haematol 80:327, 1992.
133. Schwartzberg LS, Birch R, Hazelton B, et al: Peripheral blood stem cell mobilization by chemotherapy with and without recombinant human granulocyte colony-stimulating factor. J Hematother 1:317, 1992.
134. Metcalf D: The molecular biology and functions of the granulocyte-macrophage colony-stimulating factors. Blood 67:257, 1986.
135. Nemunaitis J, Rabinowe SN, Singer JW, et al: Recombinant human granulocyte-macrophage colony-stimulating factor after autologous bone marrow transplantation for lymphoid malignancy: Pooled results of a randomized, double-blind, placebo controlled trial. N Engl J Med 324:1773, 1991.
136. Nemunaitis J, Singer JW, Buckner CD, et al: Long-term follow-up of patients who received recombinant human granulocyte-macrophage colony stimulating factor after autologous bone marrow transplantation for lymphoid malignancy. Bone Marrow Transplant 7:49, 1991.

EPIDEMIOLOGY

10

Epidemiology of Community-Acquired Infections

Mitchell L. Cohen

Epidemiology involves the study of almost any aspect of an infectious disease and the populations it affects. Such studies might include defining the occurrence of the disease, its clinical manifestations and management, characteristics of the affected population, the mechanisms of transmission, and the characteristics of the causative organism. The clinical aspects, microbiology, diagnostics, and management of specific diseases are discussed in other chapters. The purpose of this chapter is to examine the application of general concepts of epidemiology to community-acquired infections.

The Epidemiologic Method and Its Limitations

Epidemiology defines the who, what, when, where, how, and why of infectious diseases. The *who* is the populations at risk for infection. The *what* is the scope and impact of infections. The *when* is the temporal trends. The *where* is the geographic location of disease. The *how* defines the reservoirs of disease and the mechanisms of transmission. The *why* addresses the issue of risk factors, or the reasons disease affects some persons but not others.

Descriptive and Analytic Epidemiology

The two most commonly used methods for studying infectious diseases are descriptive and analytic epidemiology.[1] Descriptive epidemiology involves the collection and analysis of all data that describe the disease in the population. Analysis of these data frequently leads to the development of hypotheses. Analytic epidemiology typically involves the testing of hypotheses—the comparison of characteristics among persons who are ill and those who are well. This approach frequently leads to the identification of associations with or risk factors for disease.

There are important limitations to both epidemiologic approaches. One of the important limitations in descriptive epidemiology is underreporting or underascertainment of cases of a specific disease. For many diseases, calculated incidences are underestimates, because many variables affect reporting. For example, for a case of an illness such as salmonellosis to be reported, a culture must be referred to the state health laboratory for serotyping. For many cases of salmonellosis, physicians are not consulted, or cultures are not obtained or sent for serotyping. From outbreak investigations it has been estimated that only 1 in 10 to 1 in 100 salmonellosis cases are reported.[2] Thus, reported incidences[3] of 18 per 100,000 may be only a fraction of an estimated actual incidence of 18 per 1000.

Analytic epidemiology is limited by several additional factors. Associations demonstrated by epidemiologic studies do not necessarily ensure causation. A statistically significant association simply implies that the likelihood of the association occurring by chance alone is small. Inferring causation requires statistical and logical epidemiologic associations,[4] but proving it often requires results from animal studies to fulfill Koch's postulates. Analytic studies may be affected by confounding and by a variety of biases. Confounding is a spurious identification of a risk factor because it is associated with a true causative factor, such as age and smoking. In addition, bias can be introduced unsuspectedly during the collection or analysis of data.[5] Comparison groups different in some systematic fashion may indicate a selection bias. Differences in how or what data are collected for different groups result in ascertainment bias. Sound epidemiologic studies attempt to minimize such bias by appropriate design and analysis of findings.

Endemic and Epidemic Disease

Epidemiologic methods may be used to study either endemic or epidemic disease. Illness occurs as sporadic or isolated cases or as parts of recognized outbreaks or epidemics. The term endemic is typically used for cases of an illness that are not associated and that occur at an expected frequency. Several studies, however, have demonstrated that the distinction between the endemic or sporadic disease and epidemic illness can be somewhat artificial. Riley and coworkers[6] investigated both endemic and epidemic *Salmonella newport* infections in the northeastern United States in 1982. Using plasmid profile analysis to subtype the *S. newport* isolate, the investigators demonstrated that the same organism was causing what was interpreted as cases of an epidemic and of sporadic or endemic disease. The organism was transmitted by the same vehicle, precooked roast beef. Because the individual endemic cases had not been investigated, they were assumed to be endemic and to be transmitted by various vehicles. In fact, detailed analysis of the *S. newport* isolates over time suggested that the relatively constant occurrence of this serotype was, in fact, the result of successive introduction and transmission of different strains, some of which produced recognized epidemics. Thus, endemic disease was simply a summation of miniepidemics caused by discrete clones.

An epidemic can be defined as an occurrence of disease at a rate greater than expected. Increased frequency of disease may not indicate a true increase but may be related to changes in recognition (i.e., better diagnosis or an increase in reporting). An increased incidence of disease, however, usually indicates changes in exposure, in the population at risk, or in the characteristics of the organism (e.g., antigens or pathogenicity). In practice, an increase in disease frequency often suggests increased exposure, and thus an opportunity for intervention and prevention.

Much epidemiologic information is gathered by investigating epidemics, or outbreaks of disease. The investigation of an outbreak requires an orderly approach of data collection, hypothesis generation and testing, and intervention.[7] Outbreaks frequently provide sufficiently large numbers of ill persons to allow statistical analyses to determine risk factors for infection, mechanisms of transmission, and reservoirs of the agent organism.

Such investigations can also lead to the identification of new pathogens. The investigations of bloody diarrhea outbreaks in Oregon and Michigan in 1982 led to the identification of *Escherichia coli* O157:H7 as a cause of hemorrhagic colitis.[8] In this instance, the presence of the same serotype in a number of ill persons suggested that the organism might be a pathogen despite the fact that it lacked any recognized toxin or other pathogenic characteristic.

Case Definition

For many epidemiologic studies or epidemic investigations it is necessary for the epidemiologist to develop a case definition. This definition may be based solely on the results of a laboratory test, such as a blood culture, or may depend principally on the presence of certain clinical manifestations, such as the signs and symptoms of toxic shock syndrome. The development of a case definition is an important step that can profoundly affect the outcome of the analysis. For example, a strict clinical case definition may limit the recognized spectrum of disease, whereas a loose clinical case definition may be likely to include persons whose illness may have an entirely different cause.

In a sense, an epidemiologist can manipulate a case definition to achieve desired degrees of sensitivity and specificity. In case-control studies, a specific definition is often desirable, because including too many persons as cases who do not have the illness under study would reduce the likelihood of demonstrating associations between cases and risk factors. As with diagnostic tests in clinical medicine, it would be desirable in epidemiology to have a case definition that was 100% sensitive and 100% specific—a situation that is not realistic.

Different case definitions can identify different populations of cases. A vaccine efficacy study that uses sputum cultures could misidentify pneumococci as the cause of a certain number of pneumonia cases, because patients are commonly colonized with *Streptococcus pneumoniae*. Thus, this less specific case definition might falsely lower the values for vaccine efficacy by allowing inclusion of cases caused by other organisms. On the other hand, a study that uses a more specific case definition that requires isolation of the pneumococci from blood excludes the nonbacteremic cases of pneumococcal pneumonia and examines only vaccine efficacy for preventing the more severe, invasive disease. The impact of different case definitions may partially explain conflicting values for pneumococcal vaccine efficacy obtained in two studies.[9, 10]

Epidemiology and the Laboratory

Epidemiologic studies have been much assisted by laboratory advances, particularly in molecular biology.[11, 12] In the past, many epidemiologic investigations were stymied by the inability to distinguish between strains of common microorganisms and thus more accurately define a case. When *Salmonella typhimurium* infection, which accounts for 25% of all *Salmonella* serotypes, occurred in the community, the epidemiologist was unable to distinguish between strains unless they were carrying unusual antibiotic-resistant markers. Thus, epidemiologic studies might be unable to show associations, because studying all *S. typhimurium* isolates included different strains transmitted by different vehicles (a classification error). With the advent of plasmid profile analysis, ribotyping, enzyme typing, and DNA probes, subtyping has become possible and practical.[13, 14] These methods, which allowed a greater degree of subtyping, have made possible many important epidemiologic studies.

Epidemiologic Concepts

Incidence

Epidemiology attempts to quantify the frequency of disease. Knowing the number of cases of disease and the number of persons in the population, one can calculate the incidence of an infectious disease. For the purposes of this chapter, an *incidence rate* is defined as the number of times an infection is noted in an observed population during the defined period divided by the number of persons observed in that time.[15] For most infectious diseases, the incidence is reported as an annual rate. For a few infectious diseases that cause a chronic illness, it may be more appropriate to refer to the *prevalence* of disease, the proportion of the population ill in a defined time period.[15] Because most infectious diseases have a short duration, however, the frequency of the illness is usually given as an annual rate. The incidence of the disease can be determined by a variety of methods. Most commonly, an illness is declared reportable by state law and a formal surveillance system is established. Programs at state and federal levels conduct surveillance for these diseases and tabulate the reported cases. A crude annual incidence can be calculated by dividing the number of reported cases by the size of the population.

The incidence of a disease can provide important information. Observed over time, changes in incidence can identify an emerging problem or the effectiveness of prevention or control measures. Comparing incidences can assist public health officials in allocating resources or the clinician in considering the most likely causes of a particular syndrome. Comparing the incidence of disease in different populations can provide clues to how the disease is being transmitted or indicate the presence of specific susceptibilities in the population.

Study Populations

Infectious disease epidemiology studies the occurrence and characteristics of specific infections in defined populations. A population may be defined by a specific geographic location, host characteristic, or exposure—all residents of a county or state, participants in a church supper, children in a daycare center, or patients in an intensive care unit. In different populations the same infection may have different epidemiologic characteristics, such as incidence, clinical manifestations, and mechanisms of transmission. Some infections are grouped by somewhat arbitrary criteria that make epidemiologic sense, for example, nosocomial and community-acquired infections. The hospital is a relatively discrete ecosystem: it has self-contained populations and epidemics and often unique pathogens, reservoirs, and mechanisms of transmission. The community, on the other hand, is a more diverse ecosystem without clear physical boundaries that involves many different pathogens and many populations. Individual populations frequently interact, and ample opportunities often exist for transmission of infectious agents. For example, instances are well-documented in which organisms are transmitted into the hospital from the community and vice versa. An investigation of multidrug-resistant *Salmonella* species in Brazil demonstrated that the apparently community-acquired infections were occurring among infants who were colonized during the hospitalization after their birth but had no symptoms until after discharge.[16] A number of investigations have demonstrated the introduction of drug-resistant *Salmonella* species into hospitals from persons who acquired infections after eating contaminated foods in the community.[17] The interactions between the hospital and the community are only a small part of the complex interactions that occur between populations in the community.

Temporal Characteristics

The incidence of many infectious diseases varies over time. A *secular trend* is a change in the incidence of disease over an extended period. Diseases that are transmitted by the fecal-oral route, such as typhoid, have decreased with improvements in sanitation, water treatment, and sewage disposal. On the other hand, the occurrence of diseases such as nontyphoid salmonellosis has increased as a result of changes in food production and distribution (Fig. 10–1). A *periodic trend* is a change in the secular trend that tends to recur at consistent intervals. Before the widespread use of vaccine, measles demonstrated a periodic trend in the United States, with peaks every 2 years. Most periodic trends have been attributed to either changes in the organism or changes in population immunity. A *seasonal trend* is a consistent pattern in the annual occurrence of a disease. Meningococcal meningitis has a clear late winter–early spring peak[18] (Fig. 10–2). Many of the bacterial enteric pathogens, such as *Salmonella, Shigella,* and *Campylobacter,* have a seasonal peak in summer to fall. Another enteric pathogen, rotavirus, has a winter peak in the United States. The explanation for the presence of a seasonal trend is usually not known but is frequently the subject of speculation. The greater occurrence of salmonellosis in the summer has been attributed to factors such as inadequate refrigeration during times when refrigeration is most critical. The sharp year-end peak observed for certain serotypes has been attributed to poor food handling in association with holiday dinners at which turkey is served.

Geographic Characteristics

Disease may occur with different frequencies in different geographic areas, as does Rocky Mountain spotted fever, for example (Fig. 10–3). Differences in the occurrence of spotted

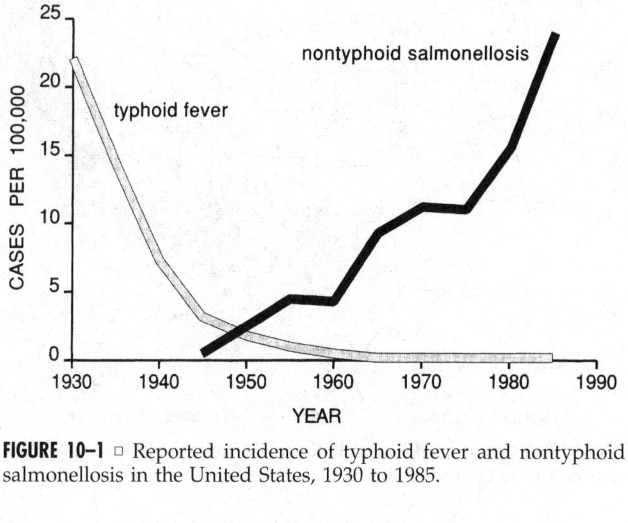

FIGURE 10–1 □ Reported incidence of typhoid fever and nontyphoid salmonellosis in the United States, 1930 to 1985.

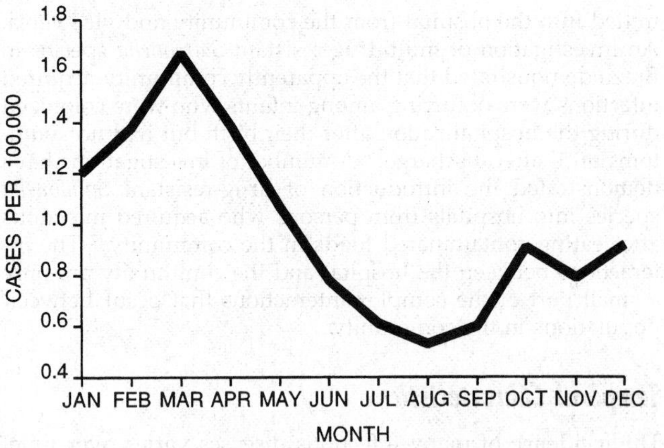

FIGURE 10–2 ▫ Distribution of meningococcal disease, by month, 1982 to 1984. (Adapted from Harrison LH, Broome CV: The epidemiology of meningococcal meningitis in the U.S. civilian population. *In* Vedros NA [ed]: Evolution of Meningococcal Disease. Boca Raton, FL, CRC Press, 1987, pp 27–45.)

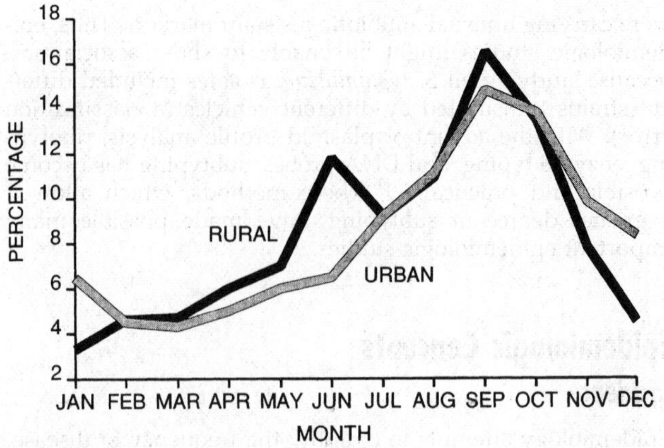

FIGURE 10–4 ▫ Distribution of *S. newport* isolates from urban and rural counties in the United States, by month, 1968 to 1982.

fever correlates with the distribution of its vectors.[19] Other diseases may reflect differences in the demographic characteristics of the population, varying exposures, or differences in reporting. One specific *Salmonella* serotype, *S. newport*, peaks in the spring in rural areas and in the summer in both rural and urban areas (Fig. 10–4). The explanation for the additional spring peak in rural areas is unknown, but it may be related to close contact with infected animals. The summer peak in both rural and urban areas is likely due to foodborne infections.

Reservoirs and Routes of Transmission

Public health officials attempt to devise appropriate intervention strategies by using both descriptive and analytic epidemiology to identify reservoirs for infectious agents and define the routes and mechanisms of transmission. For an organism to perpetuate itself, it must have an ecologic niche, or reservoir, where it can replicate either in the environment or in animal or human populations. These reservoirs can vary from the environment (*Legionella* in cooling towers or hot-water systems), to animals (*Salmonella* in food animals), to human populations (the agents of tuberculosis, smallpox, measles, or typhoid). Some organisms may be sustained in several reservoirs (*Giardia* or influenza virus).

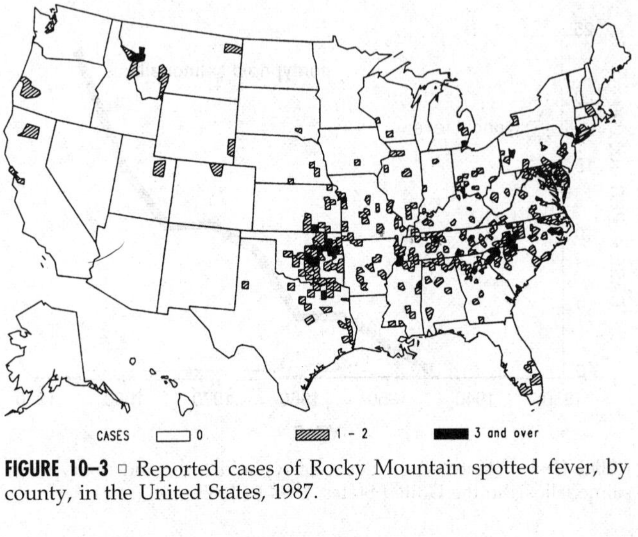

FIGURE 10–3 ▫ Reported cases of Rocky Mountain spotted fever, by county, in the United States, 1987.

To be a successful pathogen the organism must be transmitted from the reservoir to a susceptible host in sufficient numbers and in a site where it can persist and replicate. The precise route of transmission is determined by characteristics of both organism and host. In a healthy adult, salmonellae are transmitted primarily in food, because infection requires relatively large numbers of organisms. In the more susceptible neonates, salmonellosis can be caused by the fewer organisms transmitted person to person by fecal-oral contact. On the other hand, shigellae, which require only a small dose for infection, are readily transmitted to both children and adults by person-to-person fecal-oral contact.

The routes of transmission can be straightforward: *Legionella* may be transmitted in aerosol from a contaminated cooling tower or in shower water from a contaminated water heating system. Hepatitis B virus and human immunodeficiency virus (HIV) may be transmitted by blood transfusion, parenteral drug abuse, or sexual contact with infected persons. Alternatively, the routes of transmission can be extremely convoluted. In one *Salmonella heidelberg* outbreak, the organism was transmitted from ill calves to a farmer's pregnant daughter, who subsequently transmitted the organism to her newborn infant. The organism was then transmitted in the hospital nursery from the infected newborn to two other infants, probably by direct contact with the hands of nurses.[20]

Risk Factors

One of the purposes of analytic epidemiology is to identify the risk factors associated with disease. This is typically accomplished by case-control or cohort analysis that attempts to identify different frequencies of characteristics or exposures in ill (cases) and well (controls) persons. Risk factors are typically characteristics of the ill person, such as age, sex, race, socioeconomic status, area of residence, or exposures such as foods, smoking, medications, illicit drug use, travel history, daycare attendance, or sexual activity. In perhaps the first example of analytic epidemiology, John Snow examined the occurrence of cholera in 1853 in two areas of London, which differed only in the source of their water. He was able to demonstrate that the death rate from cholera was 10 times higher in the houses supplied by a company whose source of water was in a more sewage-contaminated area of the Thames River.[21] Some factors, such as breast-feeding or immunization, may be associated with decreased risk of disease and be protective. An epidemiologic investigation of a typhoid outbreak might demonstrate an association between eating a certain food and disease as well as an association between having received typhoid vaccine and remaining well. Determining the risk factors that are associated with disease can lead to identification not only of the exposures and the vehicles or route of transmission, but also of susceptibilities present in cases, which can allow targeting of specific control strategies to that portion of the population.

Prevention and Control

The ultimate goal of epidemiology is control and prevention. Prevention strategies operate in three general areas: (1) interruption or prevention of transmission, (2) prevention of infection, and (3) prevention of disease. The tools to implement these strategies include physical or chemical methods, immunology, and education.

A wide variety of physical and chemical interventions are available. Most attempt to prevent transmission of pathogenic microorganisms. The simple measure of adequate cooking can block the transmission of a variety of food-borne pathogens. Pasteurization of milk has led to the elimination of milk-borne outbreaks of streptococcal disease and typhoid. Filtration and chlorination of water provide barriers to the water-borne transmission of various enteric bacteria and parasites. Heating or disinfecting implicated water supplies can prevent the transmission of *Legionella*. The most time-honored methods of prevention are providing physical barriers to transmission such as use of quarantine, surgical masks, gloves, condoms, or protective environments. Chemotherapy can also be used to prevent transmission. Antimicrobial treatment of a typhoid carrier or a patient with tuberculosis eliminates human reservoirs for infection. In addition, chemotherapy can prevent infection of exposed persons as well as disease in those already infected (e.g., prophylaxis of tuberculosis, *Haemophilus influenzae* type b infection, or meningococcal disease).

Immunologic tools such as vaccination can also reduce transmission by reducing the number of infected individuals. Immunologic methods, however, are more often used to prevent infection (oral polio vaccine) or to prevent an infected person from developing disease (inactivated polio vaccine). Immunization is one of the most effective control measures. The elimination of susceptible persons from a population not only leads to the reduction of transmission but also to the real (smallpox) or potential (measles, poliomyelitis) elimination of diseases that are restricted to a human reservoir.

A final and important tool of prevention is education. Education has impact in all areas of prevention. Epidemiologists have long appreciated the importance of behavior in the occurrence of disease, whether it be smoking, sexual activity, or food handling. As evidenced by current efforts in encouraging safe sex, education is playing a renewed and increasingly important role in the prevention and control of infectious diseases. Behaviors that pose a risk of infectious disease, such as unprotected sexual activity, are targets of educational efforts aimed at interrupting transmission. Frequently, education becomes an important prevention strategy for a disease that cannot be effectively treated or controlled through immunization (e.g., HIV infection).

The clinician plays an important role in the prevention of disease by ensuring appropriate immunization, treatment, prophylaxis, and education of patients and by recognizing and reporting public health problems. Unfortunately, preventive measures are not maximally utilized. Low rates of immunization for many adult populations at high risk for certain vaccine-preventable diseases[22] and insufficient educational efforts in the prevention of disease indicate a need for more intensive prevention activities.

TABLE 10–1 ■ Estimated Impact of Infectious Diseases in the United States, by Pathogen Group

PATHOGEN GROUP	DEATHS	INCIDENCE
Viral	17,000	207,329,000
Bacterial	68,200	36,026,000
Parasitic	1,800	26,620,000
Fungal	1,200	18,027,000

Adapted from Bennett JV, Holmberg SD, Rogers MF, Solomon SL: Infectious and parasitic diseases. *In* Amler RW, Dull HB (eds): Closing the Gap. The Burden of Unnecessary Illness. New York, Oxford University Press, 1987, pp 102–114.

Frequency and Impact of Infectious Disease in the United States

Few data are available that estimate the impact of infectious diseases or the relative importance of various syndromes or microbial infections. Even for illnesses for which national surveillance systems exist, it may be misleading to compare the incidences of diseases reported in different surveillance systems, because different variables, many of which often are not defined, can affect reporting. For example, by using isolates reported to the Centers for Disease Control and Prevention (CDC), the 1986 incidence of salmonellosis and campylobacteriosis was 18 and 4 per 100,000, respectively[23]; however, a population-based study conducted in a large health maintenance organization in Seattle, Washington, between May 1985 and April 1986 defined rates for salmonellosis and campylobacteriosis of 21 and 50 per 100,000, respectively.[24] Data from many of the surveillance systems are best used for following trends or changes in the descriptive epidemiology of a specific pathogen.

In 1984, a Carter Center report attempted to quantify the impact of various infectious diseases.[25] The authors estimated that infectious diseases accounted for more than 740 million cases and 190,000 deaths each year in the United States. The cost of infectious diseases exceeded $17 billion and resulted in 1 billion disability days. Each year, infectious diseases accounted for more than 2 million of the 12 million (18%) years of life lost before age 65 years. Using a different source of data (a survey of experts from the CDC), the authors estimated the impact of the four major pathogen groups (Table 10–1). The most common infectious syndromes and their relative impact are shown in Table 10–2. The figures in Table 10–2 are not mutually exclusive but provide a framework for defining the most common community-acquired infections.

Another source for estimating the impact of infectious dis-

TABLE 10–2 ■ Estimated Impact of Selected Infections in the United States

TYPE OF INFECTION	DEATHS (× 1000)	INCIDENCE (× 1000)
Cutaneous	11.8	53,534
Enteric	10.8	25,227
Meningitis	3.5	229
Pneumonia, lower respiratory tract	52.0	29,321
Sexually transmitted	8.2	16,234
Upper respiratory tract	3.3	160,590

Adapted from Bennett JV, Holmberg SD, Rogers MF, Solomon SL: Infectious and parasitic diseases. *In* Amler RW, Dull HB (eds): Closing the Gap. The Burden of Unnecessary Illness. New York, Oxford University Press, 1987, pp 102–114.

eases is the National Health Interview Survey conducted by the National Center for Health Statistics.[26] This survey examined the occurrence of acute conditions that either required medical attention or restricted activity for persons in randomly sampled households in the United States. These findings indicate that, for 1987, the incidence of infectious diseases is at least 111 acute conditions per 100 persons per year. More than half the acute conditions resulted in the ill person's seeking medical attention. Based on these survey results, the most common conditions leading to a visit to a physician were, in decreasing order, influenza, common cold, otitis media, upper respiratory tract infection, unspecified viral infection, acute bronchitis, unspecified intestinal virus, and pneumonia.

Trends in Community-Acquired Infections

The 20th century has witnessed several technologic and societal changes that have had major impact on infectious diseases. With increasing development, better nutrition, increasing emphasis on personal hygiene, better sewage disposal, and provision of safe drinking water, a number of diseases have become less frequent. Immunization has led to the eradication of smallpox and the control of several childhood diseases. Antimicrobial chemotherapy has reduced mortality rates for a number of diseases, such as typhoid fever, meningitis, and endocarditis, and reduced the incidence of complications of other infections.

Technology has provided ways to identify previously unrecognized pathogens and to more rapidly diagnose infectious diseases. Technologic advances have enabled the identification of previously unrecognized causative agents of diarrheal disease such as *Campylobacter* or *E. coli* O157:H7 as well as Legionnaires' disease, toxic shock syndrome, and acquired immunodeficiency syndrome. Rapid diagnostic tests for a variety of microorganisms using polyclonal antisera, monoclonal antibodies, DNA probes, or the polymerase chain reaction (PCR) are currently in use in several clinical laboratories. It is likely that over-the-counter diagnostic tests will become available for common illnesses such as streptococcal pharyngitis. Such diagnostic advances are likely to have an important impact on the epidemiology of infectious diseases.

On the other hand, societal and technologic changes have also resulted in the emergence of new diseases and altered the epidemiologic character of old infections. In October 1992, the Institute of Medicine published a report titled *Emerging Infections: Microbial Threats to Health in the United States.*[27] This report defined emerging diseases as "ones whose incidence had increased within the past two decades, or whose incidence threatens to increase in the near future." The factors that were influencing the emergence of infectious diseases were placed into six categories (Table 10–3). Each of these factors is having a significant impact.[28] Technologic advances that enable the rapid distribution of large amounts of contaminated food to wide geographic areas have converted food-borne outbreaks from events involving dozens at church suppers to interstate or international outbreaks involving hundreds of thousands of people. In 1985, a multistate outbreak of *S. typhimurium* infection caused by contaminated pasteurized milk affected an estimated 200,000 persons in the midwestern United States.[29] In 1984, a food-borne outbreak aboard multiple planes of a British airline disseminated cases of *Salmonella enteritidis* infection over at least four continents.[30] Advances in transportation itself are changing the geographic distribution of diseases. The febrile patient in a U.S. emergency department can be a tourist returning from an African vacation with a case of malaria or trypanosomiasis. Immigration to the United States in the 1970s and 1980s after natural disasters or political change has increased the incidence of diseases such as leprosy and drug-resistant tuberculosis and provided patients infected with a variety of exotic parasitic diseases.

TABLE 10–3 ■ Factors Influencing the Emergence of Infectious Diseases

Changes in human demographics and behavior
Changes in technology and industry
Economic development and land use
International travel and commerce
Microbial adaption and change
Breakdown of public health measures

Technologic and social changes not only have affected the occurrence of established pathogens but also have been associated with the emergence of new agents. Technologic advances, such as air conditioning, cooling towers, and hot-water systems, have provided reservoirs and mechanisms for transmission of *Legionella.* Certain superabsorbent menstrual tampons with specific chemical compositions were associated with toxic shock syndrome.

Social changes can have similar impact on the epidemiology of community-acquired infections. The sexual revolution of the 1960s and 1970s provided opportunity for sexually transmitted diseases such as HIV infection. The return of mothers to the workplace has prompted a tremendous increase in the use of daycare. An article estimated that in the United States, by 1990, more than 6 million children younger than age 6 years will have received full- or part-time daycare.[31] This analysis of published articles suggested that diarrheal diseases, hepatitis A, meningitis, and otitis media are transmitted at increased rates in daycare settings. Daycare is an apparent risk factor for the acquisition of certain community-acquired infections for family members and daycare staff as well as for attending children. Daycare is also playing an important role in the emergence of antimicrobial resistance of *S. pneumoniae.*[32]

The emergence of antimicrobial resistance is a trend of particular concern.[33–35] Strains of *Mycobacterium tuberculosis* and enterococci had become essentially untreatable with existing antibiotics by the early 1990s. Strains of other organisms including *Staphylococcus aureus* and *S. pneumoniae* were susceptible to only one or two antimicrobial agents. The emergence of resistance was related to both the selective pressures of antimicrobial use and factors increasing the transmission of drug-resistant organisms.

Changes in the age distribution of the population also affect the epidemiology of community-acquired infections. As the population ages, the age-specific incidence of certain diseases may remain the same but the overall incidence may change. Childhood diseases may become less frequent as infections in elderly persons increase.

New pathogens have gained prominence as a result of HIV infections and medical manipulations that have increased the population of immunocompromised patients. These patients are susceptible to a variety of bacterial, viral, fungal, and parasitic organisms that seldom cause illness in the immunocompetent person. Although many of these infections are nosocomial, several can be community acquired, particularly by patients infected with HIV. In addition, patients with HIV infection have 100 to 200 times greater risk of developing infections that are not traditionally thought to be opportunistic, such as tuberculosis and pneumococcal pneumonia.[36, 37] An increase in the incidence of *Shigella* bacteremia in men aged 25 to 49 years suggests that HIV infections will affect the epidemiologic characteristics of many infectious diseases[38] (Fig. 10–5). With estimates of 650,000 to 900,000[39] HIV-

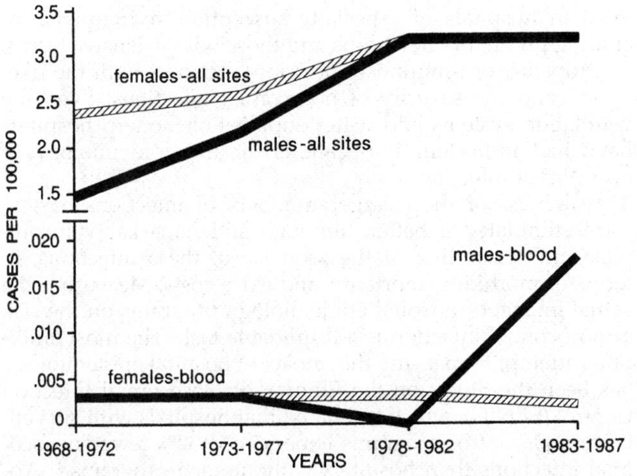

FIGURE 10–5 □ Reported *Shigella* isolates in the United States from men and women aged 25 to 49 years, by culture site, 1968 to 1987.

infected persons in the United States, thousands of additional cases of infections with opportunistic and nonopportunistic pathogens will occur in the next decade.

The impact of technology and social change on infectious diseases is not new. In the Middle Ages, advances in agriculture, overpopulation, and urbanization were some of the factors in the emergence and transmission of the Black Death.[40] With the current rate of technologic and societal change, we should anticipate continued changes in the epidemiology of established community-acquired infections and the emergence of new pathogens as important causes of morbidity and mortality.

References

1. Evans AS: Epidemiological concepts. *In* Evans AS, Feldman HA (eds): Bacterial Infections of Humans. New York, Plenum Publishing, 1982, pp 3–4.
2. Cohen M, Tauxe RV: Drug-resistant *Salmonella* in the United States: An epidemiologic perspective. Science 234:964, 1986.
3. Hargrett-Bean NT, Pavia AT, Tauxe RV: *Salmonella* isolates from humans in the United States, 1984–1986. MMWR CDC Surveill Summ 37:25, 1988.
4. Rothman KJ: Modern Epidemiology. Boston, Little, Brown, 1986, pp 7–21.
5. Sackett DL: Bias in analytic research. J Chronic Dis 32:51–63, 1979.
6. Riley LW, DiFerdinando GT Jr, DeMelfi TM, et al: Evaluation of isolated cases of salmonellosis by plasmid profile analysis: Introduction and transmission of a bacterial clone by precooked roast beef. J Infect Dis 148:12, 1983.
7. Gregg MB: The principles of an epidemic field investigation. *In* Holland WW, Detels R, Knox G (eds): Oxford Textbook of Public Health. Oxford, Oxford University Press, 1985, p 284.
8. Riley LW, Remis RS, Helgerson SD, et al: Hemorrhagic colitis associated with a rare *Escherichia coli* serotype. N Engl J Med 308:681, 1983.
9. Simberkoff MS, Cross AP, Al-Ibrahim M, et al: Efficacy of pneumococcal vaccine in high-risk patients: Results of a Veterans Administration cooperative study. N Engl J Med 315:1318, 1986.
10. Bolan G, Broome CV, Facklam RR, et al: Pneumococcal vaccine efficacy in selected populations in the United States. Ann Intern Med 104:1, 1986.
11. Mayer LW: Use of plasmid profiles in epidemiologic surveillance of disease outbreaks and in tracing the transmission of antibiotic resistance. Clin Microbiol Rev 1:228, 1988.
12. Wachsmuth K: Molecular epidemiology of bacterial infections: Examples of methodology and of investigations of outbreaks. Rev Infect Dis 8:682, 1986.
13. Tompkins LS, Troup N, Labigne-Roussel A, et al: Cloned, random chromosomal sequences as probes to identify *Salmonella* species. J Infect Dis 154:156, 1986.
14. Holmberg SD, Wachsmuth IK, Hickman-Brenner FW, et al: Comparison of plasmid profile analysis, phage typing, and antimicrobial susceptibility testing in characterizing *Salmonella typhimurium* isolates from outbreaks. J Clin Microbiol 19:100, 1984.
15. MacMahon B, Pugh TF: Epidemiology: Principles and Methods. Boston, Little, Brown, 1970.
16. Riley LW, Ceballos BSO, Trabulsi LR, et al: The significance of hospitals as reservoirs for endemic multiresistant *Salmonella typhimurium* causing infection in urban Brazilian children. J Infect Dis 150:236, 1984.
17. Holmberg SD, Osterholm MT, Senger KA, et al: Drug-resistant *Salmonella* from animals fed antimicrobials. N Engl J Med 311:617, 1984.
18. Harrison LH, Broome CV: The epidemiology of meningococcal meningitis in the U.S. civilian population. *In* Vedros NA (ed): Evolution of Meningococcal Disease. Boca Raton, FL, CRC Press, 1987, pp 27–45.
19. Centers for Disease Control: Summary of notifiable diseases, United States, 1987. MMWR Morb Mortal Wkly Rep 36:48, 1988.
20. Lyons RW, Samples CL, Desilva NN, et al: An epidemic of resistant *Salmonella* in a nursery: Animal to human spread. JAMA 243:546, 1980.
21. Fox JP, Hall CE, Elveback LR: Epidemiology: Man and Disease. London, Macmillan, 1970, pp 24–26.
22. Williams WW, Hickson MA, Kane MA, et al: Immunization policies and vaccine coverage among adults. Ann Intern Med 108:616, 1988.
23. Tauxe RV, Hargrett-Bean N, Patton CM, Wachsmuth IK: *Campylobacter* isolates in the United States, 1982–1986. MMWR CDC Surveill Summ 37:1, 1988.
24. MacDonald KL, O'Leary MJ, Cohen ML, et al: *Escherichia coli* O157:H7, an emerging gastrointestinal pathogen. JAMA 259:3567, 1988.
25. Bennett JV, Holmberg SD, Rogers MF, Solomon SL: Infectious and parasitic diseases. *In* Amler RW, Dull HB (eds): Closing the Gap. The Burden of Unnecessary Illness. New York, Oxford University Press, 1987, pp 102–114.
26. National Center for Health Statistics: Current estimates from the National Health Interview Survey. Vital Health Stat 10(166):1, 1988.
27. Institute of Medicine: Emerging Infections: Microbial Threats to Health in the United States. Washington DC, National Academy Press, 1992.
28. Cohen ML: Infectious diseases: New and forgotten risks. Health Environ Digest 7:1, 1993.
29. Ryan CA, Nickels MK, Hargrett-Bean NT, et al: Massive outbreak of antimicrobial-resistant salmonellosis traced to pasteurized milk. JAMA 258:3269, 1987.
30. Tauxe RV, Tormey MP, Mascola L, et al: Salmonellosis outbreak on trans-Atlantic flights: Foodborne illness on aircraft: 1947–1984. Am J Epidemiol 125:150, 1987.
31. Haskins R, Kotch J: Day care and illness: Evidence, costs, and public policy. Pediatrics 77:951, 1986.
32. Reichler MR, Allphin AA, Breeman RF, et al: The spread of multiply resistant *Streptococcus pneumoniae* at a day care center in Ohio. J Infect Dis 166:1346, 1992.
33. Cohen ML: Epidemiology of drug resistance: Implications for a post-antimicrobial era. Science 257:1050, 1992.
34. Cohen ML: Antimicrobial resistance: Prognosis for public health. Trends Microbiol 2:422, 1994.
35. Hofmann J, Cetron MS, Farley M, et al: The prevalence of drug-resistant *Streptococcus pneumoniae* in Atlanta. N Engl J Med 333:481, 1995.
36. Redd SC, Rutherford GW, Sande MA, et al: The role of human immunodeficiency virus infection in pneumococcal bacteremia in San Francisco residents. J Infect Dis 162:1012, 1990.
37. Castro KG: Tuberculosis as an opportunistic disease in persons infected with human immunodeficiency virus. Clin Infect Dis 21:566, 1995.
38. Angulo FJ, Swerdlow DL: Bacterial enteric infections in persons infected with human immunodeficiency virus. Clin Infect Dis 21:584, 1995.
39. Karon JM, Rosenberg PS, McQuillan G, et al: Prevalence of HIV infection in the United States. JAMA 276:126, 1996.
40. Gottfried RS: The Black Death: Natural and Human Disaster in Medieval Europe. New York, The Free Press, 1983.

11

Epidemiology of Nosocomial Infections

Richard Platt
Donald A. Goldmann
Cyrus C. Hopkins

Infections acquired in the hospital are a major problem because of their frequency, severity, and cost. About 5% of patients admitted to acute care hospitals in the United States acquire a new infection, resulting in approximately 2 million nosocomial infections each year. Approximately 39% of these infections involve the urinary tract, 17% are surgical wound infections, 18% are pneumonias, and 7% are bacteremias.[1] These figures are extrapolations, and they reflect the pooled risks of a heterogeneous group of individuals and institutions. No matter what the specific numbers of infections are, nosocomial infections cause substantial morbidity and excess mortality. They also prolong hospitalizations and increase the costs of medical care. Estimates of morbidity, mortality, and costs vary, but most estimates place the average cost of a nosocomial infection at more than $1000 in 1990 dollars.[2–6] Thus, the aggregate annual cost easily exceeds $2 billion. In addition, many estimates indicate at least a doubling of the odds of death.[4, 7–18]

Hospital epidemiology, in its usual sense, is the application of epidemiologic methods to hospital-acquired, or nosocomial, infections. There is ample reason to believe that similar epidemiologic methods can contribute to other areas of hospital administration and quality assurance.[19–21] In this chapter, however, we confine our attention to the original meaning of the term and largely discuss the application of hospital epidemiology to infections in acute care institutions. Many of the same principles also apply in chronic care hospitals and nursing homes.

The central aim of hospital epidemiology is to prevent the acquisition of nosocomial infection. Many of the principles required to accomplish this purpose have been appreciated for decades, long before a formal discipline of hospital epidemiology evolved. However, five factors have played an important role in the development of formal, structured infection control programs. These are (1) an increased awareness of the number and importance of nosocomial infections; (2) an actual increase in certain nosocomial infections, many of which are consequences of advances in medical care; (3) a desire to control the direct costs of nosocomial infections; (4) regulatory requirements; and (5) an increasing involvement of infection control personnel in policy development and educational activities for health care workers and patients.

Formal surveillance can identify previously unappreciated nosocomial infections. Nosocomial infections also result directly or indirectly from technologic advances in medical care. Many of the most important innovations of the past century have created opportunities for infection. Examples include surgery, transfusion therapy and blood banking, mechanical ventilation, intravascular therapy, and urinary catheter drainage, all of which have been responsible for many serious nosocomial infections. In addition, the prolonged survival in hospitals of especially susceptible individuals, including premature newborns and those with extensive burns, neutropenia, or immunosuppression, increases both the likelihood and the severity of nosocomial infections. Even the ventilation systems and water supplies of modern hospitals have had important implications for the epidemiology of nosocomial infections.

Awareness of these larger numbers of infections has, in turn, stimulated a better, although still remarkably incomplete, understanding of the sequelae of these infections, in terms of morbidity, mortality, and extra costs. Measuring the actual impact of hospital epidemiology programs on the risk of nosocomial infection is a formidable task. The most ambitious attempt to measure the impact of hospital epidemiology has been the Study on the Efficacy of Nosocomial Infection Control (SENIC), which estimated that hospitals with surveillance and control programs experienced 32% fewer nosocomial infections than hospitals without such programs.[22] Application of these results to a single teaching hospital with 700+ beds indicated that current infection control practices yielded approximately $2.4 million in avoided charges in 1985.[23] The ability to decrease unnecessary expense by practical infection control measures should provide a motivation for continued support for such measures.

A corollary development has been heightened concern about infections transmitted to hospital workers. Hepatitis B, hepatitis C, tuberculosis, human immunodeficiency virus (HIV) infection, and influenza are examples of serious threats to health care workers. In addition, infectious agents such as cytomegalovirus that are rarely transmitted in hospitals cause great anxiety. The assessment of the actual risks and the formulation of policies for containment of such infections usually fall largely within the domain of hospital infection control programs.

Finally, the need for hospitals to maintain infection control programs as a requirement for accreditation has established such programs as fixtures in modern U.S. hospitals.[24]

This chapter focuses on methods for identifying nosocomial infections; on the occurrence and consequences of these infections; and on the principal etiologic agents, reservoirs, and modes of transmission. Chapter 42 discusses the application of these findings to infection control.

Identification of Infections

It would be extremely useful to have broadly applicable information on the occurrence of nosocomial infections in a variety of settings. Such data would be immediately useful to individual institutions as an initial way to determine whether their infection experience is "acceptable." This information will become especially important if hospitals are required to make public their experience with nosocomial infections or if this becomes a basis for accreditation or reimbursement.

Definitions of Infection

As in any epidemiologic endeavor, one needs to apply meaningful definitions of infections; to identify and count the infections accurately; and to classify them appropriately with respect to important risk factors, such as neutropenia, intubation, obesity, and diabetes. None of these requirements is straightforward and free from controversy. A variety of definitions have been proposed. The widely accepted definitions promulgated by the Centers for Disease Control and Prevention (CDC) are a useful starting point, given their widespread use.[25–27]

However, review of these criteria (Table 11–1) raises several

TABLE 11–1 ■ Selected CDC Surveillance Definitions of Nosocomial Infections

SURGICAL SITE INFECTION

A. *Superficial incisional infection* must occur at the incision site within 30 d after surgery AND involve only skin, subcutaneous tissue, or muscle located above the fascial layer

AND any of the following:

1. Purulent drainage from the incision or drain located above the fascial layer

or

2. Organism isolated from aseptically obtained culture of fluid from wound closed primarily

or

3. Pain or tenderness or localized swelling or redness or heat and the surgeon deliberately opens wound, unless wound is culture-negative

or

4. Surgeon's or attending physician's diagnosis of infection

The following are not classified as superficial surgical site infections: stitch abscess, infection at an episiotomy or circumcision site, infected burn wound, and infections that extend into the fascial and muscle layers.

B. *Deep incisional surgical site infection* must occur at the operative site within 30 d after surgery if no implant is left in place or within 1 y if implant is in place AND infection involves tissues or spaces at or beneath the fascial layer

AND any of the following:

1. Purulent drainage from the deep incision but not from the organ/space component of the surgical site

or

2. Wound spontaneously dehisces or is deliberately opened by surgeon when patient has fever (>38°C) and/or localized pain or tenderness, unless wound is culture-negative

or

3. An abscess or other evidence of infection seen on direct examination, during surgery, or by histopathologic or radiologic examination

or

4. Surgeon's diagnosis of deep incisional infection

C. *Organ/space surgical site infection* involves any part of the anatomy other than the incision that was opened or manipulated during the operative procedure. It must occur within the time periods noted for deep surgical site infection. It must meet at least one of these criteria:

1. Purulent drainage from a drain that is placed through a stab wound into the organ/space

or

2. An abscess or other evidence of infection involving the organ/space seen on direct examination, during surgery, or by histopathologic or radiologic examination

or

3. Surgeon's or attending physician's diagnosis of organ/space infection

Specific organs or spaces that can be affected include: arterial or venous infection, breast abscess or mastitis, disk space, ear (mastoid), endometritis, endocarditis, eye (other than conjunctivitis), gastrointestinal tract, intraabdominal, joint or bursa, mediastinitis, meningitis or ventriculitis, myocarditis or pericarditis, oral cavity, osteomyelitis, other infections of the lower respiratory tract, other infections of the genitourinary tract, other male or female reproductive tract, sinusitis, spinal abscess without meningitis, upper respiratory tract or pharyngitis, vaginal cuff

URINARY TRACT INFECTION (bacteriuria in adults only)

A. *Symptomatic urinary tract infection*

1. Fever (>38°C) or urgency or frequency or dysuria or suprapubic tenderness AND urine culture with >100,000 colonies/mL with no more than two species of organism

or

2. Two of the preceding symptoms

AND any of the following

a. Dipstick test positive for leukocyte esterase and/or nitrate

or

b. Pyuria ($\geq$10 white cells per mm^3 or $\geq$3 white cells per high-power field of unspun urine)

or

c. Organism seen on Gram stain of unspun urine

or

d. Two urine cultures with repeated isolation of the same uropathogen with $\geq$100 colonies/mL in nonvoided specimens

or

e. Urine culture with $\leq$100,000 colonies/mL of a single uropathogen in a patient being treated with appropriate antimicrobial therapy

or

f. A physician's diagnosis

or

g. A physician institutes appropriate antimicrobial therapy

B. *Asymptomatic bacteriuria*

1. An indwelling catheter is present within 7 d before urine is cultured AND patient has no symptoms (see above) AND patient has a urine culture with $\geq$100,000 colonies/mL with no more than two species of organisms

or

2. No indwelling urinary catheter has been present within 7 d before the first of two urine cultures with $\geq$100,000 colonies/mL, of the same organism, and the patient has no symptoms

PNEUMONIA (adults only)

A. Rales or dullness to percussion on physical examination of chest

AND any one of the following:

1. New onset of purulent sputum or change in character of sputum

or

2. Organism isolated from blood culture

or

3. Isolation of pathogen from specimen obtained by transtracheal aspirate, bronchial brushing, or biopsy

or

B. Chest radiographic examination shows new or progressive infiltrate, consolidation, cavitation, or pleural effusion AND any one of the following

1. One of the additional criteria noted above

or

2. Isolation of virus or detection of viral antigen in respiratory secretions

or

3. Diagnostic single antibody titer (immunoglobulin M) or fourfold increase in paired serum samples (immunoglobulin G) for pathogen

or

4. Histopathologic evidence of pneumonia

LABORATORY-CONFIRMED BLOOD STREAM INFECTION (adults only)

A. Recognized pathogen isolated from blood culture AND pathogen is not related to infection at another site

or

B. There is fever (>38°C), chills, or hypotension

AND one of the following is present:

1. A common skin contaminant is isolated from two blood cultures drawn on separate occasions AND the organism is not related to infection at another site

or

2. A common skin contaminant is isolated from a blood culture from a patient with an intravascular access device, AND the physician institutes appropriate antimicrobial therapy

or

3. There is a positive antigen test on blood AND the organism is not related to infection at another site.

Data from references 25 and 27.

questions. For example, even the apparently straightforward finding of "purulence" in sputum or wound drainage can have a broad range of interpretations, especially when used by individuals of different backgrounds, including nurses, surgeons, laboratory technologists, and patients. In addition, the physician's diagnosis of infection recorded in the chart is sufficient to establish the diagnosis. This allows the possibility of false-positive diagnoses (especially for conditions such as urinary tract infection) and biased ascertainment, because some physicians are more likely to make the diagnosis of infection and to note it than others. False-negative diagnoses are also a potential problem, because the likelihood of obtaining cultures and of documentation must vary widely. The problems of establishing the diagnosis of nosocomial pneumonia have engendered considerable discussion, as pneumonia often occurs in the context of ventilatory support that is associated with pulmonary infiltrates.[28–32]

Even the time of onset of some infections is unclear, because colonization with a pathogen can be present on admission to the hospital but symptoms of clinical disease appear much later. *Clostridium difficile* enterocolitis, for example, can occur weeks after admission. Initial acquisition of the organism could have occurred either as cross-infection within the hospital or at some time before admission.

Ascertainment of Infection

METHODOLOGICAL ISSUES

The range of surveillance methods is broad, extending from self-reporting by patients and physicians to universal, prospective surveillance by trained personnel.[33–37] Virtually all widely used surveillance systems depend on review of the medical record, which is labor intensive. The accuracy of such systems depends on the completeness of the medical record and the submission of cultures when infection is suspected. Additional surveillance methods include review of microbiology laboratory results and reports of chest radiography before they are returned to the medical records, review of nurses' records, interviews with the nursing staff, and interviews with and examinations of patients.[38] In general, the more intensive the surveillance, the larger the number of infections identified but at a correspondingly greater cost. For example, review of nursing records, interviews with clinical staff, and examination of patients increase the yield but may place an unacceptable burden on the infection control program's resources.

Striking a balance between exhaustive efforts to capture nearly every infection and targeted surveillance aimed at detecting the most important problems remains a difficult and controversial problem. For example, there is legitimate debate about the merits of identifying and reporting superficial postoperative wound infections. Although they rarely cause substantial morbidity, they may serve as indicators for more serious events that occur so infrequently they are difficult to study. Similar considerations apply for asymptomatic nosocomial urinary tract infections.

Several methods have been proposed to allow more efficient utilization of reviewer time, including review of laboratory data as a primary source to target patients for intensive review or to identify important colonization, for example, by methicillin-resistant *Staphylococcus aureus*, before infection occurs. Additional methods include prescreening of the nursing records and intensive care unit checklists.[39] Especially interesting research endeavors at present focus on methods for using automated data systems to identify patients who are likely to have nosocomial infections.[40–42] These systems draw on data from the microbiology laboratory, the pharmacy, the radiology department, the operating room, coded medical record diagnoses, and admission diagnoses to identify patients with characteristics that suggest infection. Skilled personnel can then direct their efforts preferentially at assessing these patients.[43–45]

A substantial proportion of infections become manifest after discharge from the hospital. This phenomenon will become increasingly important as the duration of hospitalization decreases and as more and more surgery is performed on an outpatient basis. Although hospitals are required to identify such infections to maintain their accreditation, there is little agreement on the methods that should be used.[46] Unless the infections prompt readmission to the original institution, conventional surveillance methods detect only a minority of infections. A number of methods have been tried in an effort to increase the yield, including physical examination of the patient by surveillance personnel and physicians' or patients' responses to telephoned queries or to mailed questionnaires, but one assessment suggests that both their sensitivity and their specificity limit their value.[47, 48] Automated claims data, pharmacy dispensing data, and other administrative data sets may become useful resources for surveillance.

DATA SOURCES FOR NOSOCOMIAL INFECTION RATES

There are several useful, reasonably broad-based data sets. The most complete and best described data set is that of SENIC, conducted by the CDC, which involved 339,000 patients in 338 hospitals, representing a wide range of size and complexity of services and patients.[49] These patients were hospitalized during 1970 and 1975 to 1976. SENIC involved review of a representative selection of medical records by specially trained reviewers who used detailed algorithms for identifying infections.[50] There was extensive validation of the reliability of record abstraction[51] and of the sensitivity of record abstraction compared with a physician's review,[52] as well as of a variety of other features. Several caveats apply in interpreting this information. The most important include use of attending physicians' stated diagnosis of infection as one criterion for diagnosing infection and highly variable test ordering and data recording practices. In addition, SENIC data do not apply to new conditions that have emerged as medical practice has evolved during the past 15 years.

The CDC also sponsors the National Nosocomial Infection Survey (NNIS), which obtains information submitted to it by participating hospitals across the United States.[26] This information is published periodically in *Morbidity and Mortality Weekly Reports* (available by subscription and on the Internet at http://www.cdc.gov/epo/mmwr/mmwr.html) and elsewhere and provides an assessment of contemporary infection experience.[1, 53–61] Although this information is a major resource, it is important to realize that the participating hospitals are a nonrandom sample, that the surveillance definitions have changed with time, and that the information the hospitals provide has not been extensively validated. Moreover, although NNIS has proposed methods for adjusting for differences in case mix and severity of illness (see later), these are not completely efficient, which limits the usefulness of NNIS data for comparisons that would be of interest.

Additional sources of information obtained in a uniform way from more than one institution include the South Florida Hospital Consortium for Infection Control,[62] the Israeli Study of Surgical Infections,[35] and hospitals in Rhode Island[63, 64] and New Jersey, where a broad-based surveillance system for antimicrobial-resistant pathogens has been instituted.[65] There are also many useful reports of the infection experience within a small number of institutions. These include a landmark report of postoperative wound infections after more than 60,000 procedures[36] and analyses of specific types of infections including those associated with selected surgical procedures,[66] bacteremias,[8, 67–71] pneumonias,[72–77] and urinary tract infections.[78–80] There are also useful reports of infections in intensive care units[81–93] and among immunocompromised patients,[94] those with intravascular catheters,[64] and newborns.[17, 61, 95–98] In addition, many clinical trials provide useful information.

Risk Factors and Sequelae of Nosocomial Infection

Interpretation of information on the numbers of nosocomial infections depends critically on an understanding of the population being evaluated. Some factors have such a strong influence on the risk of infection that an admirably low infection rate in one population is unacceptably high in another.

One approach to dealing with this problem is to adjust for severity of illness. Several systems have been proposed to adjust for severity,[99–105] and a number of investigators have created ad hoc systems to accomplish this purpose.[106–108] Although the formal severity scoring systems are promising and have received considerable use in research settings, they have not been widely incorporated into nosocomial infection practice. One reason for this is that several scoring systems depend on information that must be obtained by labor-intensive review of the medical records.

DISCOVERY OF RISK FACTORS

The discovery of risk factors has been a major focus of research efforts. This has been made possible by the development of data sets of appropriate size and reliability and also by the application of analytic methods noted in the following. There are several reasons for wanting to identify risk factors and quantify their contribution to the overall burden of infections. The most important is to identify potentially alterable factors to guide preventive measures. It is also useful to identify and estimate the contribution of nonalterable risk factors, such as underlying disease, to facilitate informed decisions about risks and benefits of various interventions.

Detailed information on risk factors is rarely obtained in a general surveillance effort because this information is difficult to obtain from standard review of the medical record. More detailed information, such as duration of procedures, dates of insertion and removal of catheters or intravascular cannulas, the presence of drains, and metabolic or physiologic parameters that are needed to construct severity of illness scales, may be time-consuming to obtain or unavailable altogether unless it is collected prospectively. Studies involving detailed surveillance of specific procedures or services have often been able to obtain much more specific information concerning factors that may have predisposed the patient to develop infection. Risk factors for specific types of infections are noted in the following.

ASSESSMENT OF SEQUELAE

Identifying the nature and magnitude of consequences of nosocomial infections is a second major focus of hospital epidemiology research. The consequences of interest include excess morbidity and mortality, as well as increased utilization of resources. The problems of confounding (see later) are especially relevant here, because patients who acquire infection are almost always inherently sicker and receive more intensive and invasive medical care than patients who do not.

IMPACT OF CONFOUNDING AND EFFECT MODIFICATION ON IDENTIFICATION OF RISK FACTORS AND CONSEQUENCES OF NOSOCOMIAL INFECTION

Interpretation of the significance of risk factors and sequelae of nosocomial infections requires appreciation of two major issues, confounding and effect modification.

Confounding. Confounding is the distortion of a relationship between two factors by their separate and independent association with a third factor. Confounding can affect identification of risk factors and consequences of infection, as characteristics that are neither risk factors nor consequences may appear to be one or the other because they are associated both with acquisition of infection and with genuine risk factors or consequences. For instance, if one hospital performs a large proportion of "clean" procedures, such as orthopedic implantations, and another performs a large proportion of "contaminated" procedures, such as colectomies, the second hospital's overall infection rate is almost certain to be higher. The difference between hospitals is misleading, however, because it is explained by the difference in the mix of procedures, not by the quality of care that the hospitals deliver. In this example, procedure type is a confounder of the relationship between hospital and infection rate because it is itself a predictor of infection and is also associated with the putative risk factor (procedure) and the outcome (infection).

Effect Modification. Effect modification is a separate phenomenon that bears on identification of risk factors and consequences. Effect modifiers are factors that influence the risk in some circumstances, but not others. For example, intestinal colonization by *C. difficile* is a risk factor for pseudomembranous colitis, but the risk is principally restricted to individuals who are treated with antibiotics that allow overgrowth of the organism.[109]

Compensating for Confounding and Effect Modification. Three approaches have been used to compensate for these distortions. One can match infected patients to uninfected ones, matching on potential risk factors that are not the subject of immediate investigation. In the preceding example, in which the relation between hospital and infection was evaluated, one would match on procedure type. Matching imposes important constraints, including the requirement for careful selection of comparison subjects, the inability to study factors used in matching, and the possibility that overmatching can hide an important difference between the groups being compared. It is usually necessary to preserve the matched groups through the analyses. Techniques that do not require explicit matching during selection of subjects are stratification and a variety of multivariate methods. Discussion of these methods is beyond the scope of this chapter.

Some investigators have also attempted to deal with confounding of outcomes by having knowledgeable observers review cases individually and determine which of the outcomes is attributable to infection.[3] This approach is intuitively appealing and, in essence, uses expert knowledge to perform informal adjustment for confounding and effect modification. However, it has important drawbacks, including the reliance on sufficient information about the patients being available to the reviewers, the existence of a sufficiently detailed understanding of the mechanisms by which infection causes adverse outcomes, and the potential differences within and between reviewers.

Epidemiology of Specific Types of Nosocomial Infections

Surgical Wounds

OCCURRENCE

The reported rates of postoperative wound infection depend critically on both the definition of infection and the intensity and duration of surveillance. The latter point is especially important in light of the decreases in duration of hospitalization and the increases in the proportion of procedures performed on an ambulatory basis. The duration of follow-up required depends in part on the type of procedure. As an example, wound infections involving orthopedic prostheses can occur many months after implantation.

Among infections detected during hospitalization, the overall risk is 1.2% for infections detected by the combination of surveillance procedures used by the hospitals participating in the NNIS,[1] 4.1% for infections noted on detailed medical record review performed after discharge by specially trained reviewers,[110] and 4.7% when prospective surveillance with telephone follow-up is added.[36]

ETIOLOGIC AGENTS

The principal etiologic agents vary with the hospital's flora and the procedure, particularly with the anatomic site involved. *S. aureus* remains a leading pathogen in clean surgery, but coagulase-negative staphylococci are increasingly important pathogens in surgical site infections complicating operations involving implantation of foreign bodies and devices. Aerobic and anaerobic gram-negative bacilli are the predominant pathogens in infections after abdominal and pelvic procedures. Although enterococci are less virulent than these other microorganisms, the emergence of strains resistant to penicillins, aminoglycosides, and glycopeptides makes treatment especially difficult.

RISK FACTORS

The risk of infection depends on many risk factors. Procedure type is among the most important. One of the best known classification systems creates four categories of procedures,[111] assigned on the basis of wound contamination. The classes are clean, clean-contaminated, contaminated, and infected. This scoring system allows separation of procedures into classes whose risks of infection are 2.9% for clean procedures, 3.9% for clean-contaminated procedures, 8.5% for procedures at a contaminated site, and 12.6% for procedures that involve an infected site.[110]

A more sophisticated system developed by the CDC takes into account characteristics of the host as well as the procedure, thereby allowing a more accurate estimate of the underlying risk of postoperative surgical site infection.[110, 112] This scoring system assigns one point each for the following risk factors: Anesthesiology Society of America score of 3 or more, contaminated or dirty surgery, and procedure length greater than the 75th percentile for similar procedures in the NNIS data set. Although this risk stratification system reduces the risk of making misleading comparisons (e.g., between hospitals) because of differences in underlying severity of illness or case mix, it is still does not account for much of the variability in infection risk. For instance, the risk can vary by nearly an order of magnitude among clean procedures for low-risk individuals, from less than 1% for orthopedic surgery to 5% to 10% for breast surgery. In addition, this scoring system shares the feature of many such systems in that it depends on the availability and accuracy of the clinical information recorded in medical records. In many hospitals, substantial effort is required to collect these data on a routine basis for all procedures (uninfected as well as infected); in addition, the accuracy of the classification is not known. Finally, risk factors such as duration of surgery are almost certainly approximations of the actual factors that increase risk.

Additional risk factors include recent prior surgery at the same site,[113] operator's experience,[114] infection at another anatomic site, shaving the operative site on the day before surgery, obesity, and diabetes. The role of operative drains is not clear, as there are both observational studies and randomized studies that support a role for drains[115, 116] and others that find no contribution.[117–119] Environmental factors, such as ultraviolet light[120, 121] or ultraclean air,[122, 123] and special tightly woven barrier clothing for personnel have also been shown to be effective in certain circumstances, but a number of issues complicate the interpretation of these studies.

For many procedures, the use (or lack of use) of appropriately timed perioperative antibiotic prophylaxis is a major, modifiable, risk factor.[124, 125] This issue is discussed in detail in Chapter 42.

SEQUELAE

Estimates of the extra length of hospitalization vary from 5 to 24 days.[2, 3, 126–128]

Urinary Tract Infections

OCCURRENCE

Urinary tract infections are the most common nosocomial infections, accounting for 39% of the total. The majority of these infections are asymptomatic and can be detected only by quantitative urine culture.

ETIOLOGIC AGENTS

The principal etiologic agents are enteric gram-negative rods, enterococci, and *Pseudomonas aeruginosa*.[129]

RISK FACTORS

The majority of nosocomial urinary tract infections result from instrumentation of the urinary tract, most often by indwelling catheter drainage systems. Other forms of instrumentation, such as cystoscopy, and procedures such as nephrostomy placement or creation of an ileal bladder also put the patient at high risk. Among catheterized patients, the most important risk factor is the duration of catheterization.[78–80] Overall, the incremental risk of infection is 1% to 5% for each day the catheter remains in place. Other risk factors include female sex, impaired renal function, diabetes, absence of a urinometer, colonization of the catheter drainage bag, and catheterization for purposes other than drainage during surgery or measurement of urine output. Use of systemic antibiotics appears to decrease the risk of infections for catheters that stay in place for a small number of days but to increase the risk if the catheter is in place for more than 6 days. Moreover, the risk of infection with antibiotic-resistant organisms is increased. The use of catheters with a seal on the junction between the catheter and the collection system also decreased the risk of infection for patients who did not receive systemic antibiotics, presumably because disconnection of the junction allowed contamination of the drainage system.[80, 130]

SEQUELAE

The difficulties of distinguishing between consequences of infection and the bad outcomes associated with increased susceptibility to infection are especially prominent here, as prolonged catheterization is a major risk factor and is also plausibly related to the severity of the underlying illness. A study that adjusted for severity of underlying illness identified a 2.8-fold excess mortality during hospitalization associated with nosocomial urinary tract infections occurring during acute care hospitalizations.[9] Randomization to a sealed-junction catheter drainage system resulted in a reduction in deaths that was commensurate with the reduction in infections. The putative mechanism for this excess mortality is occult bacteremia; however, this explanation is speculative. Several studies have assessed the effect of nosocomial urinary tract infection on length of stay and total cost of hospital care. Although the findings vary widely, every study has identified both increased length of hospitalization and cost. The increased durations ranged from 0.6[131] to 7.6 days.[127] The estimates of excess cost ranged from $88[3] to $558[6]; these costs are conservative estimates as they were derived in the mid-1970s. All of these studies attempted to control for confounders.

Pneumonia

OCCURRENCE

Nosocomial pneumonia was reported during 0.6% of hospitalizations.[1, 49, 132–135] The risk among patients undergoing mechanical ventilation has been reported to be as high as 27%.[136]

ETIOLOGIC AGENTS

Most studies that have attempted to define the etiologic agents of nosocomial pneumonia have relied on cultures of expectorated sputum samples or endotracheal sputum aspirates. The pathogens recovered in such studies vary from hospital to hospital, with gram-negative bacilli predominating.[1, 137] Studies using a protected specimen brush and bronchoalveolar lavage have stressed the potential importance of gram-positive cocci and *Haemophilus influenzae*.[32] Viruses are also important causes of nosocomial pneumonia[138]; improved understanding of the epidemiology of these infections should emerge as viral diagnostic techniques become more readily available. Immunosuppressed patients are also at risk for a variety of special pathogens, including fungi, such as *Aspergillus*, and *Legionella*.

RISK FACTORS

Risk factors include mechanical ventilation, aspiration, depressed level of consciousness, underlying chronic lung disease, thoracic or abdominal surgery, antimicrobial exposure, and age greater than 70 years.[7, 73–75, 139] The use of agents that decrease gastric acidity as prophylaxis against stress ulcers in ventilated patients may further increase the risk, presumably by allowing a greater role for microbial growth in a gastric reservoir.[82, 140, 141] Because manipulation of gastric pH is an alterable risk factor, it is important to clarify the contribution of increased pH and to determine the impact of such control. Contamination of respiratory equipment, discussed later, is also a well-recognized risk factor.

SEQUELAE

The overall risk of dying with nosocomial pneumonia is reported to range from 30% to more than 50%.[7, 72, 73] After adjustment for confounders, one study identified an excess risk of death[7] but another did not.[72] There are several possible explanations for the absence of significant excess mortality in the latter study, among them the relatively limited power of that analysis. The risk of death is higher for patients with bilateral pneumonia, respiratory failure, age greater than 60 years, increased severity of the underlying disease, or neoplastic disease.[7, 72] The duration of hospitalization until onset of pneumonia is also associated with mortality.[72] Nosocomial pneumonia has been reported to increase the duration of hospitalization by 7 days.[2, 72]

Bacteremia

OCCURRENCE

The overall risk of bacteremia is 0.3% of hospital discharges,[49] and bacteremia accounts for 5% to 7% of nosocomial infections.[1, 49, 71] Although it is usually straightforward to identify patients with positive blood culture results, it is important to realize that the indications for obtaining these cultures may vary widely. A potential bias is also introduced by clinicians in attempts to distinguish "contaminants" from truly positive cultures.[142] It is not clear how often bacteremia is asymptomatic and whether asymptomatic bacteremia, if it occurs, is associated with substantial morbidity.

ETIOLOGIC AGENTS

The most common etiologic agents are coagulase-negative staphylococci, *S. aureus*, *Escherichia coli*, *P. aeruginosa*, and enterococci.[1, 67, 68, 143] Fungi, including several *Candida* species such as *Candida torulopsis*, *Candida fusarium*, and *Candida trichosporum*, have become considerably more common during the past 10 years.[144] This is a result, in part, of the use of broad-spectrum antibiotics for susceptible hosts, especially those with profound immunosuppression.

RISK FACTORS

The major sources of nosocomial bacteremia are intravascular catheters and the nosocomial infections already described.[1, 67, 68, 145–147] Short peripheral catheters are quite low in risk, particularly if they are removed within a few days. Percutaneous central venous catheters, especially catheters used for hemodialysis, involve the highest risk. The risk of infection is greater for internal jugular catheters than for subclavian catheters, although the latter are associated with a higher risk of noninfectious complications. Tunneled, cuffed catheters, such as Hickman or Broviac catheters, are associated with lower rates of infection than are nontunneled catheters, and totally implanted catheter systems are even less likely to become infected. In general, rates of infection are higher with multiple-lumen than with single-lumen catheters. For the first week or two of central catheterization the skin is the principal source of microorganisms contaminating and infecting the catheter. Contamination of the hub of the catheter may become more important after that.

SEQUELAE

For all nosocomial bacteremias, the crude risk of death is approximately 40%, ranging from 2% for infections among obstetric-gynecologic patients to 60% for transplant recipients.[8, 67, 148] A case-control evaluation indicated that bacteremia increased the risk of death in hospital 14-fold.[4] The excess duration of hospitalization has been estimated to range from 14 to 32 days.[2]

Ecology and Transmission

Acquisition of a nosocomial infection is often the end of a complex sequence of events, including spread of an organism

TABLE 11–2 ■ The Invasive Device as Conduit of Infection: A Comparison of Sources of Contamination

SITE OF NOSOCOMIAL INFECTION	INVASIVE DEVICE	INFECTED SITE	SOURCE OF ORGANISMS Extraluminal*	SOURCE OF ORGANISMS Intraluminal
Urinary tract	Bladder catheter	Bladder, kidney	Perineal flora	Catheter lumen, from catheter junction, and drainage bag
Lower respiratory tract	Endotracheal tube	Trachea, lung	Pharynx or skin around tracheostomy tubing	Ventilator reservoir and tubing
Intravascular	Intravascular cannula	Blood vessel	Skin	Intravascular fluids, tubing connections, or catheter hubs
Surgical wound	Drains and wicks	Subcutaneous tissues	Skin	Lumen of drains

*Organisms may arise from the flora at that site or others that gain access to it.

to an individual patient and invasion of a susceptible site. Organisms may reach the patient by several routes (see later). Access to a site is often provided by invasive devices, including intravascular catheters, endotracheal tubes, urinary drainage catheters, and surgical drains. Such devices provide a route of access, by breaching local host defenses; an indwelling foreign body that hampers systemic host defenses; and a reservoir for survival and multiplication of the organisms. The characteristics of some devices favor persistence of specific organisms, and each organism tends to spread by characteristic routes, as illustrated by Tables 11–2 and 11–3.

Reservoirs of Pathogens

PATIENTS

Patients are often either colonized or infected with organisms that are disseminated by the hands of health care workers, as well as other means noted in the following. Their flora changes quickly during hospitalization to favor organisms that are found less frequently in the community. These organisms tend to be more resistant to antibiotics and therefore more difficult to treat.[149, 150] The extensive contact that patients have with health care workers and the high concentration of organisms that may be present in wound drainage, bladder catheter drainage bags, and stool allow them to be efficient disseminators of this flora. Examples of organisms for which both patients and health care workers may be the reservoir include *S. aureus*, *Staphylococcus epidermidis*, enteric gram-negative bacilli, enterococci, and a wide array of viruses, including hepatitis B virus, rotavirus, and respiratory syncytial virus.

HEALTH CARE WORKERS

One must distinguish between health care workers' common role in carrying organisms that persist transiently on the skin of their hands and their much less frequent role as carriers and disseminators of nosocomial pathogens. Among the best known examples of infections for which health care workers have been identified as reservoirs are nasal carriage of *S. aureus* and pharyngeal, rectal, and vaginal carriage of group A streptococci.[151–154] A finding of penicillin- and gentamicin-resistant enterococci was attributed to a health care worker with heavy colonization of stool and hands. Outbreaks of infection with gram-negative bacilli have rarely been linked to carriers on the hospital staff. However, chronic

TABLE 11–3 ■ Relative Roles of Selected Sources and Modes of Transmission for Selected Pathogens

PRINCIPAL MODE OF TRANSMISSION AND INFECTION OR AGENT	RESERVOIR OR SOURCE Human	RESERVOIR OR SOURCE Dry Environment	RESERVOIR OR SOURCE Moist Environment
Contact*			
Influenza (also airborne)	+ + +		
Respiratory syncytial virus	+ + +	+ + (fomites)	
Staphylococcus aureus (rare airborne)	+ + +	+ (fomites)	
Escherichia coli	+ +		
Enterobacter	+		+ (intravenous fluids)
Salmonella	+ + +		
Pseudomonas aeruginosa (also common source)	+		+ + (intensive care unit fluids)
Stenotrophomonas maltophilia (also common source)			+ + + (intensive care unit fluids)
Clostridium difficile	+ + +	+ + (fomites)	
Airborne			
Measles	+ + +		
Varicella (also contact)	+ + +		
Legionella			+ + (hot-water supply, ventilator cooling towers)
Tuberculosis	+ + +		
Aspergillus		+ + (ventilating systems, construction sites, dusty and/or moist environments)	
Blood-borne			
Hepatitis B virus	+ + +		
Human immunodeficiency virus	+ + +		

*Contact transmission includes transmission via large respiratory droplets that travel only a few feet.

colonization of the hands with gram-negative pathogens has been documented and represents a potential source of transmission to patients. Rarely, colonized individuals are especially efficient disseminators of these organisms, apparently by virtue of shedding colonized skin scales or generating aerosols. Certain conditions, such as symptomatic upper respiratory tract infection or rash, appear to increase the likelihood of transmitting pathogens.

VENTILATING SYSTEMS

Contamination of the air is an uncommon source of nosocomial infection in U.S. hospitals. It is possible for the air to become contaminated from external sources, for example, with fungal spores liberated during construction that occurs near the hospital.[155] Recirculated air can also become contaminated by environmental organisms such as *Aspergillus*, which can colonize the insulation that lines ventilation ducts or air filters. Potential pathogens, such as *Legionella*, can also colonize central humidifiers and then be disseminated through the air. Contamination of ventilating systems need not be a hospital-wide problem. For instance, problems have occurred in systems intended to protect immunocompromised patients from the outside environment by supplying air to single rooms.[156]

WATER

The water supplies in U.S. hospitals are rarely the source of enteric pathogens. They can serve as reservoirs for some organisms in special circumstances, however. Water supplies, especially hot-water systems, and environmental cooling systems can be colonized by *Legionella*.[157–161] Ventilator reservoirs, respiratory cascades, and room humidifiers can also become colonized, especially by *Pseudomonas* species and other "water-loving" species.[162–165] Other moist areas, including faucets (especially with aerators), shower heads, sinks and sink drains, and flower vases, can become colonized with gram-negative bacilli.[166–169] The importance of these other moist areas in propagating infections is clear for *Legionella* but not for many other potential pathogens, because they are usually colonized but have only rarely been recognized to cause problems. The role of hospital water supplies as sources of atypical mycobacterial infection among individuals with acquired immunodeficiency syndrome is being investigated.

OTHER ENVIRONMENTAL SOURCES

In general, environmental surfaces such as floors and walls are not hazardous to the patient. However, gram-positive pathogens, such as methicillin-resistant *S. aureus* and vancomycin-resistant *Enterococcus*, can survive for long periods and may represent a source of contamination of the hands of caregivers. *C. difficile* may also persist and disseminate in this fashion. Some viruses, especially respiratory syncytial virus, persist on environmental surfaces, and caregivers who touch these surfaces may transmit these organisms. If the caregivers are susceptible, they may infect themselves. These pathogens are usually a hazard only insofar as they come in direct contact with the patient or with the hands of health care workers. Floors, walls, and remote surfaces are unlikely to present a problem unless they accumulate dust that can harbor organisms.[170]

MEDICAL DEVICES

Medical devices can be reservoirs for infecting organisms.[171–173] Some devices are contaminated during use and others during manufacture. The array of organisms that can contaminate such devices is quite large, ranging from atypical mycobacteria colonizing prosthetic heart valves[174] to the Creutzfeldt-Jakob agent contaminating implantable electrodes.[175] Most problems attributed to contaminated devices occur when the devices remain moist, especially during intended disinfection procedures that are inadequate.

SOLUTIONS

There is considerable tropism of specific agents for particular kinds of fluids. For example, nutrient-poor fluids such as dextrose solutions have been colonized by bacteria that can fix atmospheric nitrogen.[176] Lipid-containing solutions, either alone or in combination with other nutrients, support the growth of many types of organisms but have been especially associated with infections caused by *Malassezia*[177, 178] and *S. epidermidis*.[179] Even disinfectants can be colonized. Especially well-known examples include the ready colonization of benzalkonium chloride and iodophors by *Burkholderia* (formerly *Pseudomonas*) *cepacia*.[180–182]

Modes of Spread

CONTACT

Contact is probably the most common mode of spread of nosocomial infection. Typically, health care workers' hands transmit organisms acquired from patients (sometimes referred to as indirect contact) (see earlier) or their own flora (direct contact). Such transmission is involved in transfer of common skin flora, such as staphylococci, but can also serve in transfer of gram-negative bacilli, *C. difficile*, and respiratory or gastrointestinal viruses. Such transmission can often be interrupted by hand washing or by the use of gloves.

Hand-to-skin contact is not required to effect contact transmission of disease. Transmission of infection by large respiratory droplets that travel only a few feet is usually regarded as a special case of contact transmission. Bacterial pathogens including *Bordetella pertussis, Neisseria meningitidis*, and group A streptococci are transmitted by this route, as are viral respiratory pathogens such as adenovirus and parainfluenza virus.

FECAL-ORAL

Fecal-oral transmission of infection requires that the reservoir of the organism be the intestinal tract and that colonization or infection occur via inoculation of the mouth. In the hospital, this cycle rarely transmits the usual enteric infections, such as salmonellosis or shigellosis. However, it does play a major role in transmitting organisms that colonize the gut, such as *Enterobacter, Serratia*, and *Pseudomonas*, as well as *E. coli, C. difficile*, and rotavirus. In this setting, the fecal-oral route depends on contamination of the hands of health care workers, who then carry the organism to open wounds, urinary catheter systems, respiratory equipment, and the mouths of other patients. Deposition of organisms on fomites can expand the range of distribution between individuals. Rarely, organisms may colonize the gastrointestinal tracts of employees, who then disseminate them.

VECTOR-BORNE

Vector-borne transmission, in the usual sense of arthropod vectors, is rarely a problem in the well-built modern hospital, although it is often productive for us to view the health care worker as a potential vector of hospital flora.

AIRBORNE

Airborne spread of infection from other patients should be distinguished from airborne spread from environmental sources.[183] When patients and personnel are the source of airborne infection, microorganisms are disseminated via droplet nuclei, which are only a few micrometers in diameter, remain suspended in air for long periods, and evade normal upper respiratory defense mechanisms. Diseases spread by droplet nuclei or a combination of large and small droplets include measles, chickenpox, and *Mycobacterium tuberculosis* infection, which should therefore be managed in a private room, preferably at negative pressure with respect to the corridor and with frequent exchanges of air. Fungal spores originating in the environment are also efficiently transmitted by the airborne route and sophisticated air-handling and filtration systems are required to eliminate these. Both small droplets and spores are small enough that they remain airborne for extended periods and can travel long distances. In addition, their small size enables them to evade the normal upper respiratory defense mechanisms. Larger respiratory droplets were discussed earlier as a special case of contact spread.

BLOOD-BORNE

Blood-borne transmission of infection was the major means of dissemination of hepatitis B virus infection before the widespread use of screening and volunteer donors. For a brief period, it was a growing mechanism for transmission of HIV infection. Blood can also be a principal means of transmitting cytomegalovirus infection. This can be a life-threatening problem for certain immunosuppressed patients and is also a problem for individuals who receive multiple transfusions. Current blood-screening procedures have greatly reduced the threat of hepatitis B and C and HIV infection by this route. Screening for cytomegalovirus can greatly reduce the blood-borne transmission of this virus to immunosuppressed patients and neonates. Blood transfusion also occasionally transmits malaria, trypanosomiasis, and bacterial infections. Blood components can also transmit infection, as in the case of intravenous globulin transmitting hepatitis C. Blood-borne transmission of infections to health care workers is also a problem and is discussed later.

Means of Entry

Indwelling medical devices provide nosocomial pathogens with direct access to normally sterile sites, particularly the lungs, urinary tract, and blood stream. In addition, surgical drains predispose to postoperative infection. In all of these cases, organisms colonizing the skin or a mucosal surface are either dragged in when a device is inserted, migrate along the external surface of the device, or enter through an internal, fluid-lined channel. Each body surface is, or can be, colonized with its own flora, and each such catheter is often connected to a larger reservoir that can serve as a source of growth and multiplication of a different set of organisms. A summary is given in Table 11–2.

The Agent

The reservoirs and routes of transmission of some representative examples of important nosocomial pathogens are listed in Table 11–3.

BACTERIA

S. aureus remains the major cause of surgical wound and intravenous catheter entry site infections.[184] People are the most common source of *S. aureus*, although it can also be found in the environment. In most cases, the human host carries the pathogen only transiently on the hands, but contaminated hands are by far the main problem in transmission of *S. aureus* in the hospital. Although persistent colonization of hospital staff occurs frequently (up to 50% in some studies), such colonization is rarely the source of nosocomial infection. When individuals are colonized, the major reservoir is the anterior nares. The pathogen is also found on skin, especially of the lower face, and hands. The perineum and anus are also occasionally colonized. Health care workers with dermatitis or active staphylococcal infections are more likely to disseminate staphylococci or skin squames and to be a source of outbreaks of infection.

Evaluation of clusters of staphylococcal wound infections should focus first on identification of individuals involved in the care of infected patients and then on reviewing their practices rather than on a search for a colonized individual or an environmental source. Failure to use standard barrier precautions for care of wounds or to perform standard hand washing appears to cause the largest number of nosocomial staphylococcal infections. If epidemiologic evidence points to a specific carrier of staphylococci on the hospital staff, genotyping and or phage typing of isolates from the caregiver and patients should be performed. Although organisms can be isolated from the environment or equipment, these are less likely to provide the source than is either another patient or an infected or colonized employee. Coagulase-negative staphylococci, especially *S. epidermidis*, are ubiquitous environmental and skin-colonizing organisms. They rarely invade, except when they cause infections related to indwelling foreign bodies (from prostheses to intravascular cannulas). Application of plasmid fingerprinting or endonuclease restriction enzyme mapping indicates that cross-infection plays an important role in introducing strains to patients.[185]

Enterococci, which are part of the normal intestinal flora, have become much more common pathogens during the past several years, especially as causes of nosocomial bacteremia.[186] This phenomenon may be a consequence in part of heavy selection pressure exerted by the use of broad-spectrum antimicrobials, such as cephalosporins, that have relatively less activity against enterococci. Separately, the increasing use of vancomycin may play a role in the emergence of vancomycin-resistant enterococci, discussed later.

Group A streptococcal infections are almost always the result of close contact with a colonized human. In community settings, the organism is transmitted principally by large respiratory droplets and causes pharyngitis. In hospitals, the principal risk is wound infection, which follows transmission from pharyngeal, anal, and vaginal sites. The likelihood that a colonized health care worker is involved in transmission of nosocomial group A streptococcal infection is high enough that even a single case should prompt a search for additional cases and potential carriers.

There are two major groups of gram-negative bacillary pathogens. Enterics, such as *E. coli*, are most likely to originate from a human source (urine or feces). Other nonenteric and water-loving organisms, such as *Stenotrophomonas* (formerly *Xanthomonas*) *maltophilia* or *Aeromonas hydrophila*, can often be traced to a water source, such as contaminated medical equipment.

The enteric gram-negative bacilli, including organisms such as *E. coli*, *Proteus*, and *Klebsiella*, are normal inhabitants of the human gastrointestinal tract, from which they colonize the perineum and the introitus, thereby gaining access to the urinary tract. They are also among the early colonizers of the pharynx of the hospitalized patient and hence cause a large proportion of lower respiratory tract infections.

As noted earlier, some strains of the genus *Enterobacter* are able to live and grow in nitrogen-poor fluids, for example, in 5% dextrose in water. Accordingly, these organisms can play a disproportionate role in outbreaks of contaminated intravascular fluid systems. Conversely, this provides a clue to the source of such infection when they cause bacteremia without an identifiable source.

Nonenteric gram-negative organisms, especially *P. aeruginosa* and *Acinetobacter,* may be found among normal flora but less often and in smaller numbers than the enterics. Under appropriate selection pressure by antibiotics, these organisms can proliferate and be an endogenous source of infection.[187–189] Transient carriage on hands of health care workers can provide access to patients, resulting in cross-infection and clusters of infection. Such clusters have been well described for patients with indwelling bladder catheters. As noted earlier, nonenteric gram-negative bacilli can survive and proliferate in virtually any moist environment, solution, or medication. Failure to disinfect medical devices properly or to ensure the sterility of solutions and medication can lead to common-source outbreaks of infection.

Anaerobes are rarely documented as causes of nosocomial infections. However, it is not clear whether this is a function of biology or of technique or failure to culture. Outbreaks of infection with *C. difficile* have, however, been identified,[190–192] and the ability of these organisms to form hardy spores may make them more likely to persist in the environment.[193] They can presumably be transmitted either on the hands of employees or on fomites touched by patients' or employees' hands.

Antibiotic-resistant bacteria have become increasingly serious problems in many hospitals.[194–198] Methicillin-resistant *S. aureus* is widespread, prompting major dislocations in care, as hospitals attempt to control transmission.[199, 200] The increased prevalence of methicillin-resistant organisms, including coagulase-negative staphylococci, has also been a major factor in the increased use of vancomycin. This use of vancomycin, in turn, is probably responsible in part for the emergence of vancomycin-resistant *Enterococcus* as a serious pathogen.[186, 201] The potential for vancomycin resistance to transfer across species to the much more pathogenic *S. aureus* is a serious concern, because the combination of methicillin and vancomycin resistance would be essentially untreatable with currently available antimicrobials that are approved for use against this organism.

MYCOBACTERIUM TUBERCULOSIS AND FUNGI

Tuberculosis, transmitted by the airborne route, has its principal reservoir in infected patients. It is occasionally transmitted by health care workers. On rare occasions, contaminated endoscopes have been implicated in the transmission of tuberculosis.[202] The emergence of multidrug-resistant tuberculosis and the demonstration that it has caused nosocomial transmission[203] have prompted a major reworking of hospital infection control practices. These are addressed in Chapter 42.

Aspergillus, a pathogen for immunosuppressed hosts, is widespread, thriving on moisture and decaying organic matter. The principal issues in environmental control are related to the need to prevent a large burden of organisms from accumulating, and from being circulated in the hospital.[32, 139, 204–206] This often requires attention to construction activities and ventilating equipment.[155, 207–209]

Candida albicans and other *Candida* species have become important nosocomial pathogens.[10, 210–212] *Candida* commonly colonizes the gastrointestinal tract and has, like *S. epidermidis,* has been considered an endogenous infection. *Candida* blood stream infections have been reported to be associated with parenteral nutrition.[213] Techniques that distinguish among different strains indicate that cross-infection is also an important problem.[214]

VIRUSES

Patients and health care workers are usually the source of nosocomial viral infections. Viral infections are commonly transferred between patients and employees but are often unrecognized, partly because the lesser symptoms are not as well documented and also because viral cultures are obtained less frequently. Greater availability of viral cultures and other diagnostic tests should increase the recognition of these infections.

Respiratory viruses, especially respiratory syncytial virus and rhinovirus, may be among the most common nosocomial infectious agents. These infections appear to be transmitted by direct contact,[138] although there is also evidence for respiratory spread of rhinovirus.[215] Adenovirus, which is also transmitted by direct contact, can cause life-threatening infections among immunosuppressed patients, and specific serotypes have also caused explosive epidemics of conjunctivitis among patients or health care workers who are exposed to contaminated equipment, such as tonometers and the oculars of microscopes. In pediatrics, some viral infections represent particular problems. Transmission of respiratory syncytial virus from other infected children on the hands of health care workers is a major mode of transmission.[216] Contaminated fomites may also play a role. Respiratory syncytial virus can also cause symptomatic infections in adult personnel, who may in turn serve as an important reservoir for infection in pediatric patients.

Common childhood respiratory diseases, such as measles and chickenpox, may also provide airborne hazards to other susceptible patients and staff on the same floor. Airborne isolation is required for these infections. Influenza virus, a respiratory tract pathogen, is spread principally by large droplets but can also be transmitted by droplet nuclei.

Enteric viruses, like rotavirus, are also common causes of nosocomial infection.[217–219] Hepatitis A virus and enteroviruses have not been recognized as major pathogens outside nurseries, probably because shedding of virus diminishes by the time symptoms prompt hospitalization.

Health Care Workers

Health care workers are at risk both of acquiring infections from patients and of transmitting their own illnesses to patients. These issues require considerable effort by infection control and occupational health service staffs. The epidemiology of infections in health care workers can be described in the same terms as those used for patients, although the emphasis and priorities differ. The same modes of spread operate: close person-to-person contacts may result in acquisition of organisms, as in the acquisition of nasal carriage with *S. aureus.* Most infections, including respiratory infections, infectious diarrhea, and soft tissue infections (such as boils, paronychia, and whitlows), are not routinely identified, however, unless looked for during a specific epidemiologic survey.

A few exposures have been studied well enough to allow a specific estimate of risk: tuberculin conversion among employees involved in general care of patients in the United States occurs at about 1% per year, slightly above what is expected in the population as a whole. Occupationally acquired tuberculosis has become an important concern, especially in light of the emergence of drug resistance.[220] This has led to major changes in control procedures, which are discussed in Chapter 42.

Needlestick injuries involving transfer of blood from a hepatitis B–positive source result in a 15% to 20% seroconversion rate in susceptible individuals.[221] Similar exposure to HIV-infected blood involves a risk less than 0.5%,[222, 223] and exposure to hepatitis C involves a risk of approximately 3%.[224]

Some infections pose essentially no risk to employees. The risk of acquisition of cytomegalovirus infection is not measurably greater for heavily exposed health care workers than for other individuals. Even pregnant employees can reasonably be expected to care for patients with cytomegalovirus infection, provided routine barrier precautions are used. HIV is transmitted infrequently when barrier techniques that are part of universal precautions can be applied. These precautions should also reduce the risk of transmission of hepatitis B, although vaccination remains a principal preventive measure.

Some diseases in employees present sufficient risk to patients to require their exclusion from the workplace or evaluation by trained personnel to make a more specific diagnosis. Infections that require such attention include those spread by respiratory droplets, such as pertussis and streptococcal infections of the throat; those spread by direct contact with lesions, such as adenoviral conjunctivitis; those spread by draining wounds; those spread by contact with diarrheal stools; and some diseases transmitted by an airborne or droplet contact route, such as measles, rubella, chickenpox, and tuberculosis. In influenza epidemic situations, it may also be practical to immunize, to identify cases of influenza infection, and to exclude infected personnel. Control measures are described in Chapter 42.

References

1. Horan TC, White JW, Jarvis WR, et al: Nosocomial infection surveillance, 1984. MMWR CDC Surveill Summ 35:17SS–29SS, 1986.
2. Haley RW, Schaberg DR, Von Allmen SD, McGowan JE Jr: Estimating the extra charges and prolongation of hospitalization due to nosocomial infections: A comparison of methods. J Infect Dis 141:248–257, 1980.
3. Haley RW, Schaberg DR, Crossley KB, et al: Extra charges and prolongation of stay attributable to nosocomial infections: A prospective interhospital comparison. Am J Med 70:51–58, 1981.
4. Spengler RF, Greenough WB: Hospital costs and mortality attributed to nosocomial bacteremias. JAMA 240:2455–2458, 1978.
5. Davies TW, Cottingham J: The cost of hospital infection in orthopaedic patients. J Infect 11:329–338, 1989.
6. Givens CD, Wenzel RP: Catheter-associated urinary tract infections in surgical patients: A controlled study on the excess morbidity and costs. J Urol 124:646–648, 1980.
7. Celis R, Torres A, Gatell JM, et al: Nosocomial pneumonia. A multivariate analysis of risk and prognosis. Chest 93:318–324, 1988.
8. Weinstein MP, Murphy JR, Reller LB, Lichtenstein KA: The clinical significance of positive blood cultures: A comprehensive analysis of 500 episodes of bacteremia and fungemia in adults. II. Clinical observations, with special reference to factors influencing prognosis. Rev Infect Dis 5:54–70, 1983.
9. Platt R, Polk BF, Murdock B, Rosner B: Mortality associated with nosocomial urinary-tract infection. N Engl J Med 307:637–642, 1982.
10. Wey SB, Mori M, Pfaller MA, et al: Hospital-acquired candidemia. The attributable mortality and excess length of stay. Arch Intern Med 148:2642–2645, 1988.
11. Miller PJ, Wenzel RP: Etiologic organisms as independent predictors of death and morbidity associated with bloodstream infections. J Infect Dis 156:471–477, 1987.
12. Bryan CS, Reynolds KL, Brown JJ: Mortality associated with enterococcal bacteremia. Surg Gynecol Obstet 160:557–561, 1985.
13. Martin MA, Pfaller MA, Wenzel RP: Coagulase-negative staphylococcal bacteremia. Mortality and hospital stay. Ann Intern Med 110:9–16, 1989.
14. Wenzel RP: The mortality of hospital-acquired bloodstream infections: Need for a new vital statistic? Int J Epidemiol 17:225–227, 1988.
15. Rose R, Hunting KJ, Townsend TR, Wenzel RP: Morbidity/mortality and economics of hospital-acquired blood stream infections: A controlled study. South Med J 70:1267–1269, 1977.
16. Gross PA, Van Antwerpen C: Nosocomial infections and hospital deaths. A case-control study. Am J Med 75:658–662, 1983.
17. Goldmann DA, Freeman J, Durbin WA: Nosocomial infection and death in a neonatal intensive care unit. J Infect Dis 147:635–641, 1983.
18. Gross PA, Neu HC, Aswapokee P, et al: Deaths from nosocomial infections: Experience in a university hospital and a community hospital. Am J Med 68:219–223, 1980.
19. Crede W, Hierholzer WJ Jr: Linking hospital epidemiology and quality assurance: Seasoned concepts in a new role. Infect Control 9:42–44, 1988.
20. Wenzel RP: Expanding roles of hospital epidemiology: Quality assurance. Infect Control Hosp Epidemiol 10:255–256, 1989.
21. Wenzel RP: Quality assessment. An emerging component of hospital epidemiology. Diagn Microbiol Infect Dis 13:197–204, 1990.
22. Haley RW, Culver DH, White JW, et al: The efficacy of infection surveillance and control programs in preventing nosocomial infections in US hospitals. Am J Epidemiol 121:182–205, 1985.
23. Follow CDC guidelines for protection from AIDS. Mich Nurse 60:3, 1987.
24. Joint Commission on Accreditation of Hospitals: Accreditation Manual for Hospitals. Chicago, Joint Commission on Accreditation of Hospitals, 1989.
25. Garner JS, Jarvis WR, Emori TG, et al: CDC definitions for nosocomial infections, 1988. Am J Infect Control 16:128–140, 1988.
26. Emori TG, Culver DH, Horan TC, et al: National nosocomial infections surveillance system (NNIS): Description of surveillance methods. Am J Infect Control 19:19–35, 1991.
27. Horan TC, Gaynes RP, Martone WJ, et al: CDC definitions of nosocomial surgical site infections, 1992: A modification of CDC definitions of surgical wound infections. Infect Control Hosp Epidemiol 13:606–608, 1992.
28. Wunderink RG, Mayhall CG, Gibert C: Methodology for clinical investigation of ventilator-associated pneumonia. Epidemiology and therapeutic intervention. Chest 102:580S–588S, 1992.
29. Baselski VS, el-Torky M, Coalson JJ, Griffin JP: The standardization of criteria for processing and interpreting laboratory specimens in patients with suspected ventilator-associated pneumonia. Chest 102:571S–579S, 1992.
30. Bonten MJ, Gaillard CA, Wouters EF, et al: Problems in diagnosing nosocomial pneumonia in mechanically ventilated patients: A review. Crit Care Med 22:1683–1691, 1994.
31. Cook DJ, Brun-Buisson C, Guyatt GH, Sibbald WJ: Evaluation of new diagnostic technologies: Bronchoalveolar lavage and the diagnosis of ventilator-associated pneumonia. Crit Care Med 22:1314–1322, 1994.
32. Tablan OC, Anderson LJ, Arden NH, et al: Guideline for prevention of nosocomial pneumonia. The Hospital Infection Control Practices Advisory Committee, Centers for Disease Control and Prevention. Infect Control Hosp Epidemiol 15:587–627, 1994.
33. Abrutyn E, Talbot GH: Surveillance strategies: A primer. Infect Control 8:459–464, 1987.
34. Garvey JM, Buffenmyer C, Rycheck RR, et al: Surveillance for postoperative infections in outpatient gynecologic surgery. Infect Control 7:54–58, 1986.
35. Simchen E, Wax Y, Pevsner B, et al: The Israeli study of surgical infections (ISSI): I. Methods for developing a standardized surveillance system for a multicenter study of surgical infections. Infect Control 9:232–240, 1988.
36. Cruse PJE, Foord R: The epidemiology of wound infection. A 10-year prospective study of 62,939 wounds. Surg Clin North Am 60:27–40, 1980.
37. Birnbaum D: Nosocomial infection surveillance programs. Infect Control 8:474–479, 1987.
38. Wenzel RP, Osterman CA, Hunting KJ, Gwaltney JM: Hospital-

acquired infections. I. Surveillance in a university hospital. Am J Epidemiol 103:251–260, 1976.
39. Milliken J, Tait GA, Ford-Jones EL, et al: Nosocomial infections in a pediatric intensive care unit. Crit Care Med 16:233–237, 1988.
40. Burke JP, Classen DC, Pestotnik SL, et al: The HELP system and its application to infection control. J Hosp Infect 18(Suppl A):424–431, 1991.
41. Classen DC, Burke JP, Pestotnik SL, et al: Surveillance for quality assessment: IV. Surveillance using a hospital information system. Infect Control Hosp Epidemiol 12:239–244, 1991.
42. Evans RS, Burke JP, Classen DC, et al: Computerized identification of patients at high risk for hospital-acquired infection. Am J Infect Control 20:4–10, 1992.
43. Thornsberry C: Methicillin-resistant staphylococci. Clin Lab Med 9:255–267, 1989.
44. Wenzel RP, Streed SA: Surveillance and use of computers in hospital infection control. J Hosp Infect 13:217–229, 1989.
45. Yokoe DS, Platt R: Surveillance for surgical site infections: The uses of antibiotic exposure. Infect Control Hosp Epidemiol 15:717–723, 1994.
46. Holtz TH, Wenzel RP: Postdischarge surveillance for nosocomial wound infection: A brief review and commentary. Am J Infect Control 20:206–213, 1992.
47. Sands K, Vineyard G, Platt R: Surgical site infections occurring after hospital discharge. J Infect Dis 173:963–970, 1996.
48. Manian FA, Meyer L: Comparison of patient telephone survey with traditional surveillance and monthly physician questionnaires in monitoring surgical wound infections. Infect Control Hosp Epidemiol 14:216–218, 1993.
49. Haley RW, Culver DH, White JW, et al: The nationwide nosocomial infection rate. A new need for vital statistics. Am J Epidemiol 121:159–167, 1985.
50. Haley RW, Quade D, Freeman HE, Bennett JV: The SENIC Project. Study on the efficacy of nosocomial infection control (SENIC Project). Summary of study design. Am J Epidemiol 111:472–485, 1980.
51. Whaley FS, Quade D, Haley RW: Effects of method error on the power of a statistical test. Implications of imperfect sensitivity and specificity in retrospective chart review. Am J Epidemiol 111:534–542, 1980.
52. Haley RW, Schaberg DR, McClish DK, et al: The accuracy of retrospective chart review in measuring nosocomial infection rates. Results of validation studies in pilot hospitals. Am J Epidemiol 111:516–533, 1980.
53. Centers for Disease Control: National Nosocomial Infections Study Report, 1977 (6 Month Summaries). Atlanta, Centers for Disease Control, 1979.
54. Centers for Disease Control: National Nosocomial Infections Study Report, Annual Summary 1978. Atlanta, Centers for Disease Control, 1981.
55. Centers for Disease Control: National Nosocomial Infections Study Report, Annual Summary 1979. Atlanta, Centers for Disease Control, 1982.
56. Centers for Disease Control: Nosocomial infection surveillance, 1980–1982. MMWR CDC Surveill Summ 32:1SS–16SS, 1983.
57. Centers for Disease Control: Nosocomial infection surveillance, 1983. MMWR CDC Surveill Summ 33:9SS–22SS, 1984.
58. Nosocomial infection rates for interhospital comparison: Limitations and possible solutions. A report from the National Nosocomial Infections Surveillance (NNIS) System. Infect Control Hosp Epidemiol 12:609–621, 1991.
59. Horan TC, Culver DH, Gaynes RP, et al: Nosocomial infections in surgical patients in the United States, January 1986–June 1992. National Nosocomial Infections Surveillance (NNIS) System. Infect Control Hosp Epidemiol 14:73–80, 1993.
60. Consensus paper on the surveillance of surgical wound infections. The Society for Hospital Epidemiology of America; The Association for Practitioners in Infection Control; The Centers for Disease Control; The Surgical Infection Society. Infect Control Hosp Epidemiol 13:599–605, 1992.
61. Gaynes RP, Martone WJ, Culver DH, et al: Comparison of rates of nosocomial infections in neonatal intensive care units in the United States. National Nosocomial Infections Surveillance System. Am J Med 91:192S–196S, 1991.
62. Ehrenkranz NJ: South Florida Hospital Consortium for Infection Control: Structure and function. Am J Infect Control 15:36–41, 1987.
63. Tager IB, Ginsberg MB, Simchen E, et al: Rationale and methods for a statewide, prospective surveillance system for the identification and prevention of nosocomial infections. Rev Infect Dis 3:683–693, 1981.
64. Tager IB, Ginsberg MB, Ellis SE, et al: An epidemiologic study of the risks associated with peripheral intravenous catheters. Am J Epidemiol 118:839–851, 1983.
65. Paul SM, Finelli L, Crane GL, Spitalny KC: A statewide surveillance system for antimicrobial-resistant bacteria: New Jersey [see comments]. Infect Control Hosp Epidemiol 16:385–390, 1995.
66. Nagachinta T, Stephens M, Reitz B, Polk BF: Risk factors for surgical-wound infection following cardiac surgery. J Infect Dis 156:967–973, 1987.
67. Brenner ER, Bryan CS: Nosocomial bacteremia in perspective: A community-wide study. Infect Control 2:219–226, 1981.
68. Weinstein MP, Reller LB, Murphy JR, Lichtenstein KA: The clinical significance of positive blood cultures: A comprehensive analysis of 500 episodes of bacteremia and fungemia in adults. I. Laboratory and epidemiologic observations. Rev Infect Dis 5:35–53, 1983.
69. Spengler RF, Greenough WB 3d, Stolley PD: A descriptive study of nosocomial bacteremias at The Johns Hopkins Hospital, 1968–1974. Johns Hopkins Med J 142:77–84, 1978.
70. Bryan CS, Reynolds KL, Derrick CW: Patterns of bacteremia in pediatrics practice: Factors affecting mortality rates. Pediatr Infect Dis 3:312–316, 1984.
71. Maki DG: Nosocomial bacteremia. An epidemiologic overview. Am J Med 70:719–732, 1981.
72. Leu HS, Kaiser DL, Mori M, et al: Hospital-acquired pneumonia. Attributable mortality and morbidity. Am J Epidemiol 129:1258–1267, 1989.
73. Graybill JR, Marshall LW, Charache P, et al: Nosocomial pneumonia. A continuing major problem. Am Rev Respir Dis 108:1130–1140, 1973.
74. Garibaldi RA: Postoperative pneumonia and urinary-tract infection: Epidemiology and prevention. J Hosp Infect 11:265–272, 1988.
75. Garibaldi RA, Britt MR, Coleman ML, et al: Risk factors for postoperative pneumonia. Am J Med 70:677–680, 1981.
76. Gross PA: Epidemiology of hospital-acquired pneumonia. Semin Respir Infect 2:2–7, 1987.
77. Sinclair DG, Evans TW: Nosocomial pneumonia in the intensive care unit. Br J Hosp Med 51:177–180, 1994.
78. Garibaldi RA, Burke JP, Dickman ML, Smith CB: Factors predisposing to bacteriuria during indwelling urethral catheterization. N Engl J Med 291:215–219, 1974.
79. Shapiro M, Simchen E, Izraeli S, Sacks TG: A multivariate analysis of risk factors for acquiring bacteriuria in patients with indwelling urinary catheters for longer than 24 hours. Infect Control 5:525–532, 1984.
80. Platt R, Polk BF, Murdock B, Rosner B: Risk factors for nosocomial urinary tract infection. Am J Epidemiol 124:977–985, 1986.
81. Pingleton SK: Enteral nutrition as a risk factor for nosocomial pneumonia. Eur J Clin Microbiol Infect Dis 8:51–55, 1989.
82. Tryba M: Risk of acute stress bleeding and nosocomial pneumonia in ventilated intensive care unit patients: Sucralfate versus antacids. Am J Med 83:117–124, 1987.
83. Rountree PM, Beard MA: Sources of infection in an intensive care unit. Med J Aust 1:577–582, 1968.
84. Peacock JE, Marsik FJ, Wenzel RP: Methicillin-resistant *Staphylococcus aureus*: Introduction and spread within a hospital. Ann Intern Med 93:526–532, 1980.
85. Donowitz LG, Wenzel RP, Hoyt JW: High risk of hospital-acquired infection in the ICU patient. Crit Care Med 10:355–357, 1982.
86. Wenzel RP, Thompson RL, Landry SM, et al: Hospital-acquired infections in intensive care unit patients: An overview with emphasis on epidemics. Infect Control 4:371–375, 1983.
87. Fagon JY, Novara A, Stephan F, et al: Mortality attributable to nosocomial infections in the ICU. Infect Control Hosp Epidemiol 15:428–434, 1994.
88. Trilla A: Epidemiology of nosocomial infections in adult intensive care units. Intensive Care Med 20(Suppl 3):S1–S4, 1994.

89. Chernoff AE, Snydman DR: Viral infections in the intensive care unit. New Horiz 1:279–301, 1993.
90. Kim YS, Pons VG: Infections in the neurosurgical intensive care unit. Neurosurg Clin North Am 5:741–754, 1994.
91. Vincent JL, Bihari DJ, Suter PM, et al: The prevalence of nosocomial infection in intensive care units in Europe. Results of the European Prevalence of Infection in Intensive Care (EPIC) Study. EPIC International Advisory Committee. JAMA 274:639–644, 1995.
92. Emmerson AM: The epidemiology of infections in intensive care units. Intensive Care Med 16(Suppl 3):S197–S200, 1990.
93. Emmerson AM, Enstone JE, Kelsey MC: The Second National Prevalence Survey of infection in hospitals: Methodology. J Hosp Infect 30:7–29, 1995.
94. Rubin RH, Wolfson JS, Cosimi AB, Tolkoff RNE: Infection in the renal transplant recipient. Am J Med 70:405–411, 1981.
95. Goldmann DA, Leclair J, Macone A: Bacterial colonization of neonates admitted to an intensive care environment. J Pediatr 93:288–293, 1978.
96. Townsend TR, Wenzel RP: Nosocomial bloodstream infections in a newborn intensive care unit: A case-matched control study of morbidity, mortality and risk. Am J Epidemiol 114:73–80, 1981.
97. Haley RW, Bregman DA: The role of understaffing and overcrowding in recurrent outbreaks of staphylococcal infection in a neonatal special-care unit. J Infect Dis 145:875–885, 1982.
98. Donowitz LG, Haley CE, Gregory WW, Wenzel RP: Neonatal intensive care unit bacteremia: Emergence of gram-positive bacteria as major pathogens. Am J Infect Control 15:141–147, 1987.
99. Gross PA, Beyt BE, Decker MD, et al: Description of case-mix adjusters by the Severity of Illness Working Group of the Society of Hospital Epidemiologists of America (SHEA). Infect Control Hosp Epidemiol 9:309–316, 1988.
100. Horn SD: Measuring severity of illness: Comparison across institutions. Am J Public Health 73:25–31, 1983.
101. Barriere SL, Lowry SF: An overview of mortality risk prediction in sepsis [see comments]. Crit Care Med 23:376–393, 1995.
102. Richardson DK, Gray JE, McCormick MC, et al: Score for Neonatal Acute Physiology: A physiologic severity index for neonatal intensive care. Pediatrics 91:617–623, 1993.
103. Gray JE, Richardson DK, McCormick MC, et al: Neonatal therapeutic intervention scoring system: A therapy-based severity-of-illness index. Pediatrics 90:561–567, 1992.
104. Haley RW: Nosocomial infections in surgical patients: Developing valid measures of intrinsic patient risk. Am J Med 91:145S–151S, 1991.
105. Gray JE, Richardson DK, McCormick MC, Goldmann DA: Coagulase-negative staphylococcal bacteremia among very low birth weight infants: Relation to admission illness severity, resource use, and outcome. Pediatrics 95:225–230, 1995.
106. McCabe WR, Jackson GG: Gram-negative bacteremia. I. Etiology and ecology. Arch Intern Med 110:847–855, 1962.
107. Britt MR, Schleupner CJ, Matsumiya S: Severity of underlying disease as a predictor of nosocomial infection. Utility in the control of nosocomial infection. JAMA 239:1047–1051, 1978.
108. Gross PA, DeMauro PJ, Van Antwerpen C, et al: Number of comorbidities as a predictor of nosocomial infection acquisition. Infect Control Hosp Epidemiol 9:497–500, 1988.
109. McFarland LV, Mulligan ME, Kwok RY, Stamm WE: Nosocomial acquisition of *Clostridium difficile* infection. N Engl J Med 320:204–210, 1989.
110. Haley RW, Culver DH, Morgan WM, et al: Identifying patients at high risk of surgical wound infection. A simple multivariate index of patient susceptibility and wound contamination. Am J Epidemiol 121:206–215, 1985.
111. CDC Guidelines for the Prevention and Control of Nosocomial Infections. Guidelines for prevention of surgical wound infections, 1985. Am J Infect Control 14:71–82, 1986.
112. Culver DH, Horan TC, Gaynes RP, et al: Surgical wound infection rates by wound class, operative procedure, and patient risk index. National Nosocomial Infections Surveillance System. Am J Med 91:152S–157S, 1991.
113. Beatty JD, Robinson GV, Zaia JA, et al: A prospective analysis of nosocomial wound infection after mastectomy. Arch Surg 118:1421–1424, 1983.
114. Miller PJ, Searcy MA, Kaiser DL, Wenzel RP: The relationship between surgeon experience and endometritis after cesarean section. Surg Gynecol Obstet 165:535–539, 1987.
115. Simchen E, Wax Y, Pevsner B: The Israeli study of surgical infections (ISSI): II. Initial comparisons among hospitals with special focus on hernia operations. Infect Control 9:241–249, 1988.
116. Loong RL, Rogers MS, Chang AM: A controlled trial on wound drainage in caesarean section. Aust N Z J Obstet Gynaecol 28:266–269, 1988.
117. Garibaldi RA, Cushing D, Lerer T: Risk factors for postoperative infection. Am J Med 91:158S–163S, 1991.
118. Shaffer D, Benotti PN, Bothe A Jr, et al: A prospective, randomized trial of abdominal wound drainage in gastric bypass surgery. Ann Surg 206:134–137, 1987.
119. Lubowski D, Hunt DR: Abdominal wound drainage—A prospective, randomized trial. Med J Aust 146:133–135, 1987.
120. Bagshawe KD, Blowers R, Lidwell OM: Isolating patients in hospital to control infection. Part III—Design and construction of isolation accommodation. Br Med J 2:744–748, 1978.
121. Levenson SM, Trexler PC, van der Waaij D: Nosocomial infection: Prevention by special clean-air, ultraviolet light, and barrier (isolator) techniques. Curr Probl Surg 23:453–558, 1986.
122. Lidwell OM, Towers AG: Protection from microbial contamination in a room ventilated by a uni-directional air flow. J Hyg (Lond) 67:95–106, 1969.
123. Lidwell OM, Towers AG: Unidirectional ("laminar") flow ventilation system for patient isolation. Lancet 1:347–350, 1972.
124. Dellinger EP, Gross PA, Barrett TL, et al: Quality standard for antimicrobial prophylaxis in surgical procedures. The Infectious Diseases Society of America. Infect Control Hosp Epidemiol 15:182–188, 1994.
125. Classen DC, Evans RS, Pestotnik SL, et al: The timing of prophylactic administration of antibiotics and the risk of surgical-wound infection [see comments]. N Engl J Med 326:281–286, 1992.
126. Freeman J, Rosner BA, McGowan JE: Adverse effects of nosocomial infection. J Infect Dis 140:732–740, 1979.
127. Freeman J, McGowan JE: Methodologic issues in hospital epidemiology. III. Investigating the modifying effects of time and severity of underlying illness on estimates of cost of nosocomial infection. Rev Infect Dis 6:285–300, 1984.
128. Pinner RW, Haley RW, Blumenstein BA, et al: High cost nosocomial infections. Infect Control 3:143–149, 1982.
129. Horan TC, White JW, Jarvis WR, et al: Nosocomial infection surveillance, 1984. MMWR CDC Surveill Summ 35:17SS–29SS, 1986.
130. Platt R, Polk BF, Murdock B, Rosner B: Reduction of mortality associated with nosocomial urinary tract infection. Lancet 1:893–897, 1983.
131. Scheckler WE: Hospital costs of nosocomial infections: A prospective three-month study in a community hospital. Infect Control 1:150–152, 1980.
132. Craven DE, Steger KA, Barat LM, Duncan RA: Nosocomial pneumonia: Epidemiology and infection control. Intensive Care Med 18(Suppl 1):S3–S9, 1992.
133. George DL: Epidemiology of nosocomial ventilator-associated pneumonia. Infect Control Hosp Epidemiol 14:163–169, 1993.
134. Inglis TJ: Pulmonary infection in intensive care units. Br J Anaesth 65:94–106, 1990.
135. Niederman MS: Nosocomial pneumonia in the elderly patient. Chronic care facility and hospital considerations. Clin Chest Med 14:479–490, 1993.
136. Jimenez P, Torres A, Rodriguez-Roisin R, et al: Incidence and etiology of pneumonia acquired during mechanical ventilation. Crit Care Med 17:882–885, 1989.
137. McHenry MC, Alfidi RJ, Deodhar SD, et al: Hospital-acquired pneumonia. Med Clin North Am 58:565–580, 1974.
138. Anderson LJ, Patriarca PA, Hierholzer JC, Noble GR: Viral respiratory illnesses. Med Clin North Am 67:1009–1030, 1983.
139. Rhame FS, Streifel AJ, Kersey JH, McGlave PB: Extrinsic risk factors for pneumonia in the patient at high risk of infection. Am J Med 76:42–52, 1984.
140. Craven DE, Daschner FD: Nosocomial pneumonia in the intubated patient: Role of gastric colonization. Eur J Clin Microbiol Infect Dis 8:40–50, 1989.
141. Driks MR, Craven DE, Celli BR, et al: Nosocomial pneumonia

in intubated patients given sucralfate as compared with antacids or histamine type 2 blockers. The role of gastric colonization. N Engl J Med 317:1376–1382, 1987.
142. Freeman J, Platt R, Sidebottom DG, et al: Coagulase-negative staphylococcal bacteremia in the changing neonatal intensive care unit population. Is there an epidemic? JAMA 258:2548–2552, 1987.
143. McGowan JE: Changing etiology of nosocomial bacteremia and fungemia and other hospital-acquired infections. Rev Infect Dis 73:S357–S370, 1985.
144. Pfaller M, Wenzel R: Impact of the changing epidemiology of fungal infections in the 1990s. Eur J Clin Microbiol Infect Dis 11:287–291, 1992.
145. Ehrenkranz NJ, Eckert DG, Phillips PM: Sporadic bacteremia complicating central venous catheter use in a community hospital: A model to predict frequency and aid in decision-making for initiation of investigation. Am J Infect Control 17:69–76, 1989.
146. McGowan JE, Parrott PL, Duty VP: Nosocomial bacteremia. Potential for prevention of procedure-related cases. JAMA 237:2727–2729, 1977.
147. Moro ML, Vigano EF, Cozzi Lepri A: Risk factors for central venous catheter–related infections in surgical and intensive care units. The Central Venous Catheter–Related Infections Study Group [published erratum in Infect Control Hosp Epidemiol 15:508–509, 1994]. Infect Control Hosp Epidemiol 15:253–264, 1994.
148. Jamulitrat S, Meknavin U, Thongpiyapoom S: Factors affecting mortality outcome and risk of developing nosocomial bloodstream infection. Infect Control Hosp Epidemiol 15:163–170, 1994.
149. Rosenthal S, Tager IB: Prevalence of gram-negative rods in the normal pharyngeal flora. Ann Intern Med 83:355–357, 1975.
150. Axelrod P, Talbot GH: Risk factors for acquisition of gentamicin-resistant enterococci. A multivariate analysis. Arch Intern Med 149:1397–1401, 1989.
151. Schaffner W, Lefkowitz LB, Goodman JS, Koenig MG: Hospital outbreak of infections with group a streptococci traced to an asymptomatic anal carrier. N Engl J Med 280:1224–1225, 1969.
152. Berkelman RL, Martin D, Graham DR, et al: Streptococcal wound infections caused by a vaginal carrier. JAMA 247:2680–2682, 1982.
153. Ogden E, Amstey MS: Puerperal infection due to group A beta hemolytic streptococcus. Obstet Gynecol 52:53–55, 1978.
154. Berg U, Bygdeman S, Henningsson A, et al: An outbreak of group A streptococcal infection in a maternity unit. J Hosp Infect 3:333–339, 1982.
155. Sarubbi FA, Kopf HB, Wilson MB, et al: Increased recovery of *Aspergillus flavus* from respiratory specimens during hospital construction. Am Rev Respir Dis 125:33–38, 1982.
156. Hopkins CC, Weber DJ, Rubin RH: Invasive aspergillus infection: Possible non-ward common source within the hospital environment. J Hosp Infect 13:19–25, 1989.
157. Parry MF, Stampleman L, Hutchinson JH, et al: Waterborne *Legionella bozemanii* and nosocomial pneumonia in immunosuppressed patients. Ann Intern Med 103:205–210, 1985.
158. England AC, Fraser DW: Sporadic and epidemic nosocomial legionellosis in the United States. Epidemiologic features. Am J Med 70:707–711, 1981.
159. Cohen ML, Broome CV, Paris AL, et al: Fatal nosocomial Legionnaires' disease: Clinical and epidemiologic characteristics. Ann Intern Med 90:611–613, 1979.
160. Haley CE, Cohen ML, Halter J, Meyer RD: Nosocomial Legionnaires' disease: A continuing common-source epidemic at Wadsworth Medical Center. Ann Intern Med 90:583–586, 1979.
161. Stout J, Yu VL, Vickers RM, Shonnard J: Potable water supply as the hospital reservoir for Pittsburgh pneumonia agent. Lancet 1:471–472, 1982.
162. Kaiser AB: Humidifiers and pseudomonas infections. N Engl J Med 283:708, 1970.
163. Hewitt WL, Sanford JP: Workshop on hospital-associated infections. J Infect Dis 130:680–686, 1974.
164. McNeil MM, Solomon SL, Anderson RL, et al: Nosocomial *Pseudomonas pickettii* colonization associated with a contaminated respiratory therapy solution in a special care nursery. J Clin Microbiol 22:903–907, 1985.
165. Goldmann DA, Klinger JD: *Pseudomonas cepacia:* Biology, mechanisms of virulence, epidemiology. J Pediatr 108:806–812, 1986.
166. Levin MH, Olson B, Nathan C, et al: *Pseudomonas* in the sinks in an intensive care unit: Relation to patients. J Clin Pathol 37:424–427, 1984.
167. Berkelman RL, Godley J, Weber JA, et al: *Pseudomonas cepacia* peritonitis associated with contamination of automatic peritoneal dialysis machines. Ann Intern Med 96:456–458, 1982.
168. Martone WJ, Osterman CA, Fisher KA, Wenzel RP: *Pseudomonas cepacia:* Implications and control of epidemic nosocomial colonization. Rev Infect Dis 3:708–715, 1981.
169. Martone WJ, Tablan OC, Jarvis WR: The epidemiology of nosocomial epidemic *Pseudomonas cepacia* infections. Eur J Epidemiol 3:222–232, 1987.
170. Anderson RL, Mackel DC, Stoler BS, Mallison GF: Carpeting in hospitals: An epidemiological evaluation. J Clin Microbiol 15:408–415, 1982.
171. Stamm WE, Colella JJ, Anderson RL, Dixon RE: Indwelling arterial catheters as a source of nosocomial bacteremia. An outbreak caused by *Flavobacterium* species. N Engl J Med 292:1099–1102, 1975.
172. Weinstein RA, Emori TG, Anderson RL, Stamm WE: Pressure transducers as a source of bacteremia after open heart surgery. Report of an outbreak and guidelines for prevention. Chest 69:338–344, 1976.
173. Nosocomial infection and pseudoinfection from contaminated endoscopes and bronchoscopes—Wisconsin and Missouri. MMWR Morb Mortal Wkly Rep 40:675–678, 1991.
174. Wallace RJ Jr, Musser JM, Hull SI, et al: Diversity and sources of rapidly growing mycobacteria associated with infections following cardiac surgery. J Infect Dis 159:708–716, 1989.
175. Jarvis WR: Precautions for Creutzfeldt-Jakob disease. Infect Control 3:238–239, 1982.
176. Goldmann DA, Dixon RE, Fulkerson CC, et al: The role of nationwide nosocomial infection surveillance in detecting epidemic bacteremia due to contaminated intravenous fluids. Am J Epidemiol 108:207–213, 1978.
177. Richet HM, McNeil MM, Edwards MC, Jarvis WR: Cluster of *Malassezia furfur* pulmonary infections in infants in a neonatal intensive-care unit. J Clin Microbiol 27:1197–1200, 1989.
178. Powell DA, Hayes J, Durrell DE, et al: *Malassezia furfur* skin colonization of infants hospitalized in intensive care units. J Pediatr 111:217–220, 1987.
179. Jarvis WR, Highsmith AK, Allen JR, Haley RW: Polymicrobial bacteremia associated with lipid emulsion in a neonatal intensive care unit. Pediatr Infect Dis 2:203–208, 1983.
180. Frank MJ, Schaffner W: Contaminated aqueous benzalkonium chloride. An unnecessary hospital infection hazard. JAMA 236:2418–2419, 1976.
181. Kaslow RA, Mackel DC, Mallison GF: Nosocomial pseudobacteremia. Positive blood cultures due to contaminated benzalkonium antiseptic. JAMA 236:2407–2409, 1976.
182. Craven DE, Moody B, Connolly MG, et al: Pseudobacteremia caused by povidone-iodine solution contaminated with *Pseudomonas cepacia.* N Engl J Med 305:621–623, 1981.
183. Eickhoff TC: Airborne nosocomial infection: A contemporary perspective. Infect Control Hosp Epidemiol 15:663–672, 1994.
184. Grosserode MH, Wenzel RP: The continuing importance of staphylococci as major hospital pathogens. J Hosp Infect 19(Suppl B):3–17, 1991.
185. Archer GL, Mayhall CG: Comparison of epidemiological markers used in the investigation of an outbreak of methicillin-resistant *Staphylococcus aureus* infections. J Clin Microbiol 18:395–399, 1983.
186. Moellering RC Jr: Emergence of *Enterococcus* as a significant pathogen. Clin Infect Dis 14:1173–1176, 1992.
187. Weinstein RA, Nathan C, Gruensfelder R, Kabins SA: Endemic aminoglycoside resistance in gram-negative bacilli: Epidemiology and mechanisms. J Infect Dis 141:338–345, 1980.
188. Olson B, Weinstein RA, Nathan C, et al: Epidemiology of endemic *Pseudomonas aeruginosa:* Why infection control efforts have failed. J Infect Dis 150:808–816, 1984.
189. Flynn DM, Weinstein RA, Nathan C, et al: Patients' endogenous flora as the source of "nosocomial" *Enterobacter* in cardiac surgery. J Infect Dis 156:363–368, 1987.
190. Samore MH: Epidemiology of nosocomial *Clostridium difficile* infection. Compr Ther 19:151–156, 1993.

191. Nath SK, Thornley JH, Kelly M, et al: A sustained outbreak of *Clostridium difficile* in a general hospital: Persistence of a toxigenic clone in four units [see comments]. Infect Control Hosp Epidemiol 15:382–389, 1994.
192. Olson MM, Shanholtzer CJ, Lee JT Jr, Gerding DN: Ten years of prospective *Clostridium difficile*–associated disease surveillance and treatment at the Minneapolis VA Medical Center, 1982–1991 [see comments]. Infect Control Hosp Epidemiol 15:371–381, 1994.
193. Fraser DW: Bacteria newly recognized as nosocomial pathogens. Am J Med 70:432–438, 1981.
194. Tomasz A: Multiple-antibiotic-resistant pathogenic bacteria. A report on the Rockefeller University Workshop [see comments]. N Engl J Med 330:1247–1251, 1994.
195. Morris JG Jr, Shay DK, Hebden JN, et al: Enterococci resistant to multiple antimicrobial agents, including vancomycin. Establishment of endemicity in a university medical center. Ann Intern Med 123:250–259, 1995.
196. Recommendations for preventing the spread of vancomycin resistance. Hospital Infection Control Practices Advisory Committee (HICPAC). Infect Control Hosp Epidemiol 16:105–113, 1995.
197. Schaberg DR, Culver DH, Gaynes RP: Major trends in the microbial etiology of nosocomial infection. Am J Med 91:72S–75S, 1991.
198. McGowan JE Jr: Do intensive hospital antibiotic control programs prevent the spread of antibiotic resistance? Infect Control Hosp Epidemiol 15:478–483, 1994.
199. Boyce JM: Methicillin-resistant *Staphylococcus aureus* in hospitals and long-term care facilities: Microbiology, epidemiology, and preventive measures. Infect Control Hosp Epidemiol 13:725–737, 1992.
200. Boyce JM, Jackson MM, Pugliese G, et al: Methicillin-resistant *Staphylococcus aureus* (MRSA): A briefing for acute care hospitals and nursing facilities. The AHA Technical Panel on Infections Within Hospitals [see comments]. Infect Control Hosp Epidemiol 15:105–115, 1994.
201. Nosocomial enterococci resistant to vancomycin—United States, 1989–1993. MMWR Morb Mortal Wkly Rep 42:597–599, 1993.
202. Wheeler PW, Lancaster D, Kaiser AB: Bronchopulmonary cross-colonization and infection related to mycobacterial contamination of suction valves of bronchoscopes. J Infect Dis 159:954–958, 1989.
203. Nosocomial transmission of multidrug-resistant tuberculosis among HIV-infected persons—Florida and New York, 1988–1991. MMWR Morb Mortal Wkly Rep 40:585–591, 1991.
204. Herman LG: Aspergillus in patient care areas. Ann N Y Acad Sci 353:140–146, 1980.
205. Rose HD, Hirsch SR: Filtering hospital air decreases *Aspergillus* spore counts. Am Rev Respir Dis 119:511–513, 1979.
206. Fanti F, Conti S, Campani L, et al: Studies on the epidemiology of *Aspergillus fumigatus* infections in a university hospital. Eur J Epidemiol 5:8–14, 1989.
207. Arnow PM, Andersen RL, Mainous PD, Smith EJ: Pulmonary aspergillosis during hospital renovation. Am Rev Respir Dis 118:49–53, 1978.
208. Lentino JR, Rosenkranz MA, Michaels JA, et al: Nosocomial aspergillosis: A retrospective review of airborne disease secondary to road construction and contaminated air conditioners. Am J Epidemiol 116:430–437, 1982.
209. Iwen PC, Davis JC, Reed EC, et al: Airborne fungal spore monitoring in a protective environment during hospital construction, and correlation with an outbreak of invasive aspergillosis. Infect Control Hosp Epidemiol 15:303–306, 1994.
210. Harvey RL, Myers JP: Nosocomial fungemia in a large community teaching hospital. Arch Intern Med 147:2117–2120, 1987.
211. Butler KM, Baker CM: *Candida:* An increasingly important pathogen in the nursery. Pediatr Clin North Am 35:543–563, 1988.
212. Burnie JP, Odds FC, Lee W, et al: Outbreak of systemic *Candida albicans* in intensive care unit caused by cross infection. Br Med J 290:746–748, 1985.
213. Moro ML, Maffei C, Manso E, et al: Nosocomial outbreak of systemic candidosis associated with parenteral nutrition. Infect Control Hosp Epidemiol 11:27–35, 1990.
214. Matthews R, Burnie J: Assessment of DNA fingerprinting for rapid identification of outbreaks of systemic candidiasis. Br Med J 298:354–357, 1989.
215. Dick EC, Jennings LC, Mink KA, et al: Aerosol transmission of rhinovirus colds. J Infect Dis 156:442–448, 1987.
216. Leclair JM, Freeman J, Sullivan BF, et al: Prevention of nosocomial respiratory syncytial virus infections through compliance with glove and gown isolation precautions. N Engl J Med 317:329–334, 1987.
217. Vial PA, Kotloff KL, Losonsky GA: Molecular epidemiology of rotavirus infection in a room for convalescing newborns. J Infect Dis 157:668–673, 1988.
218. Cone R, Mohan K, Thouless M, Corey L: Nosocomial transmission of rotavirus infection. Pediatr Infect Dis 7:103–109, 1988.
219. Cubitt WD, Holzel H: An outbreak of rotavirus infection in a long-stay ward of a geriatric hospital. J Clin Pathol 33:306–308, 1980.
220. Menzies D, Fanning A, Yuan L, Fitzgerald M: Tuberculosis among health care workers. N Engl J Med 332:92–98, 1995.
221. Grady GF, Lee VA: Hepatitis B immune globulin—Prevention of hepatitis from accidental exposure among medical personnel. N Engl J Med 293:1067–1070, 1975.
222. Gerberding JL: Management of occupational exposures to blood-borne viruses. N Engl J Med 332:444–451, 1995.
223. Henderson DK: Risks for exposures to and infection with HIV among health care providers in the emergency department. Emerg Med Clin North Am 13:199–211, 1995.
224. Lanphear BP, Linnemann CC Jr, Cannon CG, et al: Hepatitis C virus infection in healthcare workers: Risk of exposure and infection [see comments]. Infect Control Hosp Epidemiol 15:745–750, 1994.

12

Clinical Microbiology

Henry D. Isenberg

The microbiologic diagnosis of infectious diseases is based on (1) direct examination of specimens by microscopic, immunologic, or genetic techniques; (2) isolation of microorganisms from various body fluids or sites and the response of pertinent isolates to antimicrobic drugs to guide therapy; and (3) specific antibody responses to the pathogen. Serologic diagnosis is the subject of another chapter. This chapter focuses on approaches to direct examination and culture.

Specimen Collection and Processing

General Principles

Proper specimen collection is the key element in the microbiologic diagnosis of infectious disease. The major challenge in collecting specimens is to avoid contamination of the specimen with microorganisms that are indigenous to the skin and mucous membranes (Table 12–1). General approaches to the problem of contamination include disinfecting the body surface before aspiration or biopsy, bypassing the area with indigenous microbiota, using selective culture techniques, and performing quantitative cultures. Disinfection of the skin is reasonably successful, provided that the skin is exposed to the disinfectant for at least 30 seconds. Disinfection of mucous membranes is far less successful; for example, contamination of specimens obtained through the surface of the oral cavity or the vagina is frequently unavoidable. Aspiration, such as transtracheal or suprapubic, is a method used to bypass an area that is heavily colonized by indigenous microbiota. Specimens for the culture of mycobacteria are decontaminated and then inoculated onto media containing antimicrobial agents, which minimizes contamination of cultures by other bacteria. Such selective techniques are also used for the culture of fungi, viruses, chlamydiae, and mycoplasmas. Quantitation is often used to differentiate between indigenous microbiota and pathogens. Quantitation has formed the basis for diagnosis of urinary tract infection for many years; it has been applied to bronchoalveolar lavage specimens and protected brushes for the diagnosis of bacterial pneumonia and to efforts to distinguish colonizing from infecting microorganisms in wounds, surgical or traumatic, and in burns.

Swabs, especially cotton swabs, are the favorite device used for the collection and transport of specimens for microbiologic analysis. Unfortunately, the amount of specimen provided in a swab is usually insufficient for culture, let alone culture and smear preparation. Cotton contains substances injurious to some microorganisms. Small samples are not released readily from the swab, which interferes with accurate evaluations of specimens. Commercially available porous plastic cotton substitutes have improved the utility of swabs; they are capable of releasing all of the specimen while protecting against desiccation, and they are not detrimental to any constituents of the population in the specimen. The use of swabs should be restricted to lesions of the skin and mucous membranes. Swabs are no substitute for the aspiration of fluid or pus from a body site. A variety of transport vials for accumulated body fluids or pus are available commercially that preserve anaerobic and aerobic bacteria for an adequate time until they can be analyzed in the microbiology laboratory. Material should be aspirated into a syringe and injected into the vial for transport to the laboratory. If the amount of fluid or pus in a lesion is limited, the lesion may be irrigated with a small amount of bacteriostat-free saline or, preferably, lactated Ringer solution.

Specimens obtained by invasive procedures must be collected carefully, because it is unlikely that the procedure will be repeated if the specimen is unsatisfactory or insufficient for complete microbiologic examination. All invasive procedures must be performed with constant attention to universal precautions, which must at all times extend to the proper conditions of transport containers and requisitions. Microbiology laboratory staff cannot be expected to handle grossly contaminated containers, lids, and especially syringes with needles attached. The surgeon obtaining tissue at operation should take a large enough block to provide material for both histologic and microbiologic examinations. Ideally, the block of tissue is divided at the operating table and a portion submitted for each type of examination. If a single large lesion or abscess is present, several portions of the lesion or abscess wall should be obtained for microbiologic examination. If, on the other hand, there are multiple smaller lesions or abscesses, the surgeon should obtain specimens from more than one of them. Because the number of microorganisms diminishes with the duration of infection, the more chronic the infection, the larger the portion of a lesion that should be obtained.

Despite all efforts, the laboratory may still have difficulty establishing the pathogen of an infectious disease. Technical difficulties may preclude obtaining specimens that are representative of the disease process, or it may simply be impossible to obtain a specimen that is not contaminated with indigenous microbiota. Specimens, although appropriate, may be taken after the initiation of antimicrobial therapy. In patients who have received antimicrobial agents, in alcoholic individuals, and in various populations of patients whose immune function is compromised, indigenous bacteria may be replaced by gram-negative bacilli belonging to Enterobacteriaceae and Pseudomonadaceae, further clouding the distinction between indigenous and pathogenic microorganisms of the skin and mucous membranes. Laboratories establish procedures to detect the most likely pathogens by site of origin of the specimen and so may not seek to detect a rare pathogen in the absence of a clinical impression and history. Related to all of the foregoing, laboratories are seldom if ever aware of the suspected diagnosis because the information is not provided on the requisition form. Misunderstandings between clinician and microbiologist are the result more often of poor communication than of laboratory negligence. Finally, with the exception of those instances in which the identity of the pathogen can be established on the basis of direct specimen examination, diagnosis depends on growth of the microorganism, which may take 1 day to 8 weeks, depending on the microorganism. Results, for example, of mycobacterial cultures, may therefore be reported long after a patient's discharge from the hospital.

TABLE 12–1 ■ Bacteria Commonly Found on Healthy Human Body Surfaces*

BACTERIA	SKIN	CONJUNCTIVA	UPPER RESPIRATORY TRACT	MOUTH	LOWER INTESTINE	GENITOURINARY TRACT External Genitalia	Anterior Urethra	Vagina
Aerobic and Facultatively Anaerobic								
Staphylococci	+	+	+	+	±	+	++	+
Streptococci								
Viridans	±	±	+	++	+	+	±	+
Group A			±	±				
Group D			±	+	+	+	+	+
Streptococcus pneumoniae		±	+	+				
Neisseriae		±	±	+			+	±
Corynebacteria	+	+	+	+	+	+	+	+
Haemophili		±	+	+				
Enterobacteriaceae			±	±	++	+	+	±
Anaerobic								
Clostridia				±	++		±	±
Propionibacteria	++		+	±	±		±	
Actinomycetes			+	+	±			
Lactobacilli				+	+		±	++
Bifidobacteria				+	++			++
Bacteroides			+	++	++	+	+	+
Fusobacteria			+	++	+	+	+	±
Cocci								
Gram-positive	+		+	++	++	+	±	+
Gram-negative			+	++	+		±	+

*±, Irregular; +, common; ++, prominent.
From Washington JA II: Medical bacteriology. *In* Henry JB (ed): Clinical Diagnosis and Management by Laboratory Methods, ed 18. Philadelphia, WB Saunders, 1991, pp 1025–1073.

The extent of microbiologic services provided varies considerably from one laboratory to the next. Most clinical microbiology laboratories provide a full range of services in bacteriology, but their services in mycology, mycobacteriology, virology, and parasitology are variable. For example, many laboratories provide acid-fast smears and cultures for mycobacteria but refer positive cultures to a reference facility for identification and susceptibility testing. Many laboratories provide services for the isolation of fungi and identification of yeast, but filamentous fungi that grow in cultures may be sent to a reference laboratory for identification. These different services are recognized by national laboratory inspection and accreditation agencies so that proficiency testing programs can be graded accordingly.

All clinical laboratories must provide medical and nursing personnel with instructions on proper specimen collection and transport[1] (Table 12–2). Microbiologists, moreover, need to participate actively in in-service educational programs for nurses, because it is they who are frequently responsible for specimen collection and transport. Interns, residents, and medical students also require attention. Most have not been exposed to the rigorous demands for asepsis, the variety of collection kits, and the need for rapid delivery to the laboratory to preserve the microbiologic integrity of each specimen. Educational efforts by microbiologists should alleviate this steadily increasing problem. This participation is particularly important for operating room personnel, who often assist surgeons with specimen collection. Another group of particular importance is intensive care unit personnel, who are frequently responsible for obtaining blood specimens from intravascular lines and other specimens from critically ill patients. Special attention must also be devoted to nurses caring for hematology-oncology patients, who are at high risk for infection and from whom specimens are frequently obtained by nurses. The microbiologist is responsible for selecting the most appropriate specimen collection and transport devices and for ensuring that they are distributed to areas where they are needed. For example, operating room personnel need to have sterile anaerobic transport vials available, so operating rooms must have a supply at all times. There are also occasions on which the microbiologist must provide for preparation of smears and inoculation of cultures at the bedside. A prime example is for a corneal or intraocular infection from which the amount of specimen collected is so minute that it would be lost in any transport system. Ophthalmologists, either in the outpatient department or in the operating room, must be trained in the methods for preparation of smears and inoculation of cultures. Although transport media may ensure the viability of some microorganisms for 24 hours, viability of certain microorganisms during storage and transport is limited and measures must be taken to ensure prompt delivery to the laboratory. If such transport is not possible, consideration must be given to providing special storage conditions that will allow the organism to recover when the specimen is finally received at the laboratory. There are now a variety of commercially available devices that contain fixative to preserve parasites in fecal specimens for detection by staining in the laboratory. Specimens for *Chlamydia* culture may be placed into a special transport medium; if transport is delayed, it can be frozen so that the organism may be cultured on arrival in the laboratory. Such specialized transport systems have been devised for a variety of microorganisms.

Specific Guidelines

SEPTICEMIA

The prompt detection of septicemia is one of the most important functions of the microbiology laboratory. Certain principles are important to bear in mind in this process. First, with the notable exception of intravascular infections such as

TABLE 12–2 ■ Specimen Collection and Transport for Bacteriology

SPECIMEN	COLLECTION AND TRANSPORT	COMMENTS
Blood	Adults 1. 10 mL into each of two 100-mL vacuum bottles (may include one bottle with SeptiChek attachment) *or* 2. 5 mL into each of two 50-mL vacuum bottles + 10 mL into Isolator *or* 3. 10 mL into one 100-mL vacuum bottle + 10 mL into Isolator *or* 4. 10 mL into each of two BACTEC high-volume resin bottles Infants 1. 1–3 mL into each of two 50- or 100-mL vacuum bottles *or* 2. 0.5–1.5 mL into pediatric Isolator + any remaining blood into 50- or 100-mL vacuum bottle	A minimum of two and a maximum of four cultures per septic episode are recommended.
Intravascular catheter	Remove catheter aseptically, clip one (from 2- to 3-inch catheter) or two (from 8- to 24-inch catheter) 2-inch segments, and transfer into swab transport device (e.g., Culturette)	Catheter segments should be cultured semiquantitatively.
Exudate (transudate, drainage, ulcer)	Swab or sterile, screw-capped tube	Such specimens are rarely suitable for anaerobic culture.
Eye	See text of source book for table	
Feces	Freshly passed specimen in sealed container or rectal swab	Transport medium is recommended if delay is anticipated.
Fluids		
Cerebrospinal	Sterile, screw-capped tube to be delivered to the laboratory immediately	Refrigeration may be harmful to *Neisseria* or *Haemophilus.*
Peritoneal (including dialysate)	Inoculate 10 mL into Isolator or into blood culture bottles	Direct inoculation of blood culture systems has increased yield of bacteria from patients with spontaneous peritonitis and continuous ambulatory peritoneal dialysis–associated peritonitis.
Pleural	Inoculate a portion of the specimen into an anaerobic transport system	Pleural or empyema fluid is a major source of anaerobic bacteria causing pleuropulmonary infection.
Genitourinary system		
For *Neisseria gonorrhoeae*	Send swab moistened with Stuart or Amies transport medium directly to the laboratory (4 h maximal transport time) or directly inoculate modified Thayer-Martin medium in Transgrow or JEMBEC device	Women Cervix: Moisten speculum with water before inserting into vagina; insert swab into cervical canal. Anal swab: Insert swab approximately 2 cm and move from side to side to sample crypts. Urethra or vagina: Cultures indicated when cervical not possible. Men Urethra: Swab may be used when a discharge is present; otherwise, a sterile bacteriologic loop is inserted to obtain scrapings for smear and culture. Anal canal: As for women.
Cervix, vagina for other bacteria	Swab	Specimens from these sites are not suitable for anaerobic culture.
Urine		
Midstream Catheter	Collect in sterile screw-capped container, which must be transported to the laboratory within 2 h unless refrigerated.	
Suprapubic aspirate	Inject portion of aspirate into an anaerobic transport tube or vial	This is the only type of urine specimen that is acceptable for anaerobic culture.
Abscess, traumatic or postoperative wound	Aspirate pus with syringe and needle and transport to laboratory by injecting aspirate into an anaerobic transport vial or taking the syringe directly to the laboratory	A swab provides too little material for Gram-stained smear or aerobic and anaerobic cultures. If the amount of pus is limited, one may inject the area with 0.5–1.0 mL bacteriostat-free lactated Ringer, and aspirate material.

Table continued on following page

TABLE 12–2 ■ Specimen Collection and Transport for Bacteriology *(Continued)*

SPECIMEN	COLLECTION AND TRANSPORT	COMMENTS
Respiratory tract		
For *Bordetella pertussis*	Use flexible wire calcium-tipped swab or soft rubber catheter to obtain nasopharyngeal specimen	Cough plate is not recommended.
Throat	Swab posterior pharynx, tonsils, any areas of purulence or ulceration; dry swab acceptable if cultured within 2 h; otherwise, moisten swab with Stuart or Amies transport medium	Avoid contamination with oral secretions. Ordinarily, testing for group A streptococci is sufficient. The laboratory must be notified in case of suspected diphtheria, pertussis, or gonococcal infection.
Sputum	Obtain specimen by expectorating a deep cough in a sterile, screw-capped jar	Specimens should be screened cytologically and another specimen requested when >25 squamous epithelial cells are observed per low-power field.
Transtracheal aspirate	Collect aspirate in a Lukens trap or inject into an anerobic transport vial	Such specimens are suitable for anaerobic culture.
Protected brush	The brush is severed from the inner cannula and transported to the laboratory in 1 mL of bacteriostat-free lactated Ringer solution	Quantitative culture of the vortexed lactated Ringer solution helps differentiate upper from lower respiratory tract bacterial origin.
Bronchoalveolar lavage	Obtain at least 40 mL for complete microbiologic examination	Cytocentrifuge smears should be made for Gram and other appropriate stains. Quantitative culture will help to differentiate upper from lower respiratory tract bacterial origin.
Tissue	Sterile, screw-capped container	A sufficient amount of tissue must be obtained for both histopathologic and microbiologic examinations.

From Washington JA II: Medical microbiology. *In* Henry JB (ed): Clinical Diagnosis and Management by Laboratory Methods, ed 18. Philadelphia, WB Saunders, 1991, pp 1025–1073.

endocarditis, most bacteremias are intermittent. For this reason, a single blood culture is rarely if ever indicated. Two separate blood cultures are necessary, and usually sufficient, to rule out or establish the diagnosis of bacteremia; however, three or four may be necessary to rule out bacteremia when the probability of bacteremia is high and either the anticipated pathogen is also a common contaminant (as in prosthetic valve endocarditis) or the patient received prior antimicrobial therapy for suspected endocarditis.[1, 2]

The second important principle for detection of septicemia is that the volume of blood per culture is the single most important determinant of yield. The difference in yield between cultures of 10 and 20 mL of blood is often as great as 40%. The incremental yield is smaller (about 10% to 15%) for cultures of 30 mL of blood versus 20 mL. Regardless of the blood culture system used in the laboratory, the microbiologist should design the system to accommodate 20 mL of blood per culture from adults. The volume of blood per culture is often of concern to nursing personnel and physicians in intensive care units and in hematology-oncology units, where patients are frequently subjected to phlebotomy; however, this concern needs to be tempered by the higher probability of yield with a 20-mL specimen than with 10 mL or even less and the consequently greater likelihood of appropriate antimicrobial therapy being given.

Blood is better collected by peripheral venipuncture than from an intravascular line, because manipulation of a line increases the likelihood of contamination of the line and of the specimen. Cultures of blood taken from intravascular lines have significantly greater yields of coagulase-negative staphylococci, the significance of which is frequently difficult to assess unless these organisms are isolated concurrently from a peripheral venipuncture sample. Some investigators have advocated concurrent quantitative culture of blood obtained from an intravascular line and by venipuncture to assist in the diagnosis of intravascular line–related bacteremia.[2] Others, however, have not noted line-related bacteremia to be consistently associated with larger numbers of bacteria per milliliter in blood taken from the intravascular line than in blood taken from a peripheral vein.[2] Currently, quantitation of organisms in blood is most practically done with a lysis-centrifugation blood culture system.

The third important point regarding blood cultures entails the use of sterile technique to obtain and handle them. Disinfection of the skin can be performed with a variety of agents, including iodine, iodophor, chlorhexidine, and even 70% alcohol. The disinfectant should remain in contact with the skin surface for at least 30 seconds before venipuncture. The vein should be palpated after skin preparation only with a sterile-gloved finger. The rubber diaphragms of blood culture bottles or devices must be similarly disinfected before blood is injected into them. Although experimental data suggest that the optimal time for blood collection for culture is before the onset of fever and chills, the usual practice is to obtain the first blood culture specimen as soon as possible after the onset of these signs. Subsequent blood culture specimens should be collected at intervals of 1 to 2 hours to enhance the probability of detecting intermittent bacteremia.

It is routine practice in laboratories today to use blood culture systems that allow the recovery of aerobic and anaerobic bacteria as well as *Candida* species. For this purpose, it is necessary to inoculate blood into two separate devices, which are usually two separate bottles but may be a bottle and a lysis-centrifugation tube or another combination. At the moment, there is no single-bottle system or single-device system that satisfactorily detects organisms that cause bacteremia and candidemia. The device that comes closest to meeting this goal is the lysis-centrifugation tube, but it has reduced capability for detecting anaerobic bacteria and so should rarely be used alone.

Blood cultures from infants and small children are a problem, because the volume of blood that can be obtained is limited. The question often arises whether a 0.5- to 1.0-mL sample should be inoculated into an aerobic or anaerobic blood culture bottle. This dilemma may be eased by the use of a pediatric lysis-centrifugation tube, which allows the user to distribute the lysed blood onto as many media as are needed for aerobic and anaerobic culture.

Mycobacteremia due to *Mycobacterium avium* complex (and, to a lesser extent, *Mycobacterium tuberculosis*) has been noted with increasing frequency since the advent of the acquired immunodeficiency syndrome (AIDS). There are two approaches to the detection of mycobacteremia: (1) lysis-centrifugation with culture of the lysed sediment on mycobacterial isolation media; and (2) direct inoculation of blood into mycobacterial liquid medium containing carbon 14–radiolabeled substrates, metabolism of which by mycobacteria results in the evolution of radioactive carbon dioxide.

Although *Candida* species are usually detected reasonably well in the aerobic bottle of blood culture systems, optimal detection of yeast and filamentous fungi requires the use of the lysis-centrifugation tube and culture of the lysed sediment on suitable fungus isolation media incubated at 25°C to 30°C for up to 6 weeks. For the most part, blood culture for viruses is restricted to the isolation of cytomegalovirus from buffy coat preparations of blood of organ transplant recipients.

Leptospira organisms can be isolated only from cultures of blood taken during the first few days of illness. Requests for blood cultures for leptospires should be screened by the laboratory director to ascertain the duration of illness. Cultures of urine may be indicated during the first 2 to 3 weeks of illness but are unproductive thereafter. When leptospirosis is suspected, it is probably most important to obtain acute- and convalescent-phase sera for antibody testing.[1]

When malaria is suspected, the optimal time for blood collection is midway between febrile paroxysms; the least optimal time is during or immediately after febrile paroxysms, when species differentiation is most difficult because the red blood cells have ruptured and freed the parasites. *Wuchereria* and *Brugia* have a nocturnal periodicity, so the microfilariae are most likely to be found in smears of blood collected between 10:00 PM and 8:00 AM. In contrast, *Loa loa* has diurnal periodicity, so the optimal time for preparation of blood smears is around noon. Whereas anticoagulated blood is satisfactory for the preparation of smears for detection of microfilariae, anticoagulants may distort red blood cell morphologic features. Smears for malaria diagnosis (both thin and thick smears are necessary) should be prepared from a finger stick. The thin film is prepared as for hematologic examination. For the thick film, a drop of blood is applied to the slide and spread with the corner of another glass slide in a circular motion to form a film approximately the size of a dime. The film should be thin enough that newsprint can be read through it. If too thick, the film will simply peel off the slide during the staining procedure. The purpose of the thick film is to allow more rapid screening of blood for the presence of parasites, whereas the purpose of the thin film is to provide the cellular detail required for identification of the malarial parasite.[3]

CENTRAL NERVOUS SYSTEM INFECTIONS

Central nervous system infections are caused by a variety of bacteria, mycobacteria, fungi, viruses, and some parasites; the likelihood that a given agent is responsible varies with the patient's age and immune status, the season, and other variables. Neonatal meningitis, for example, is most frequently associated with *Streptococcus agalactiae* or *Escherichia coli;* meningitis in children aged 4 months to 4 years immunized against *Haemophilus influenzae* is now most likely due to *Neisseria meningitidis* or *Streptococcus pneumoniae.* In nonimmunized infants and children, *H. influenzae* serogroup b remains the major scourge. The type of agent suspected may also be suggested by various cerebrospinal fluid (CSF) parameters, including glucose and protein levels, or by the differential white cell counts.

Culturing provides the definitive diagnosis of bacterial, mycobacterial, and fungal meningitis. The isolation of viruses from CSF is highly variable, depending on the particular virus involved. For example, mumps virus is readily isolated from CSF, whereas herpes simplex virus seldom is. Enteroviruses are isolated with moderate frequency from CSF but are more frequently isolated from the throat or stool specimens (Table 12–3). Brain biopsy specimens provide the definitive diagnosis of herpes simplex encephalitis. In many instances of viral central nervous system infections, the diagnosis is based on serologic testing (see Table 12–3). A major impediment to the detection in CSF of various microorganisms, and particularly mycobacteria and viruses, is the small volume of

TABLE 12–3 ■ Appropriate Tests for Laboratory Diagnosis of Viral Agents of Central Nervous System Infections

AGENT IN VIRUS ISOLATION	POSITIVE YIELDS* FROM SOURCE: Throat	Stool	CSF	Urine	Other
Enteroviruses	+ + +	+ + + +	+ +	−	Autopsy tissue
Mumps virus	+ + + +	−	+ + +	+	−
Herpes simplex virus					
Type 1	−	−	±	−	Brain biopsy (+ + + +)
Type 2	±	−	+ +	±	Genital or rectal swabs (+ + +)
Arboviruses†	−	−	+ +	−	Blood (+), autopsy tissue (+ +)

AGENT IN SERODIAGNOSIS	SEROLOGIC TESTS OF GREATEST USEFULNESS (PAIRED SERA)
Echovirus	Neutralization
Coxsackievirus	Neutralization
Poliovirus	Neutralization, complement fixation
Mumps virus	Complement fixation, hemagglutination inhibition
Herpes simplex virus	Compliment fixation, neutralization, indirect immunofluorescence, passive hemagglutination
Arboviruses	Hemagglutination inhibition or complement fixation

*Indicates relative frequency of positive yield in culture attempts. CSF, Cerebrospinal fluid.

†Because it is frequently difficult to isolate these agents from the disease in question, it is emphasized that serologic tests are particularly important to ensure a diagnosis.

From Ray CG, et al: Cumitech 14: Laboratory Diagnosis of Central Nervous System Infections. Washington, DC, American Society for Microbiology, 1982.

fluid frequently sent for microbiologic examination. At least 1 mL of fluid should be obtained for each of these examinations.

A presumptive diagnosis of bacterial meningitis may frequently be made on the basis of direct examination of the specimen. The Gram-stained smear is positive, on average, in 80% of cases of *H. influenzae* meningitis and in a somewhat smaller portion of cases of *N. meningitidis* or *S. pneumoniae* meningitis. The accuracy of the Gram-stained smear depends to a large extent on the skill and experience of the microscopist. A variety of commercial products have become available that allow detection of antigens of *H. influenzae, N. meningitidis, S. pneumoniae,* and *S. agalactiae.* The sensitivity of these immunochemical tests is approximately the same as that of the Gram-stained smear, because the sensitivity of each varies directly with the amount of microbial polysaccharide in the CSF. The sensitivity, therefore, varies according to whether the Gram-stained smear is positive or negative. In some previously treated patients, the immunochemical test results may be positive in the face of a negative culture. Overall, when CSF culture is negative and the immunologic test result is positive, more often than not bacterial meningitis is present.[4] False-positive immunochemical results are more likely to occur when the tests are performed with concentrated urine specimens. Immunologic tests for bacterial pathogens in CSF are, for the most part, vastly overused in laboratories and may have limited clinical utility, because it appears that culture is considered to provide the definitive result in most cases. In other words, immunologic testing of CSF is unlikely to modify empirical antimicrobial therapy. In sharp contrast, the latex agglutination test for cryptococcal antigen is a highly sensitive and specific test for the diagnosis of *Cryptococcus neoformans* meningitis and should, therefore, replace the traditional India ink preparation, which has less than 50% sensitivity.

Material aspirated from a brain abscess should be handled in such a way as to ensure recovery of both aerobic and anaerobic bacteria and should be transported to the laboratory either in the syringe used for the aspiration or in an anaerobic transport vial.

Microscopic examination of CSF is much facilitated by the use of cytocentrifuge techniques. Bacterial cultures are frequently propagated with material concentrated by either centrifugation or filtration. The concentrate is then used for inoculation of bacteriologic media. Concentrates obtained by centrifugation are also used for the culture of mycobacteria and fungi. Viral cultures involve the inoculation of a variety of cell lines. For more specific details on media and cell lines to be inoculated, the reader should consult the *Clinical Microbiology Procedures Handbook.*[1]

UPPER RESPIRATORY TRACT INFECTIONS (Table 12–4)

The definitive approach to identifying the agent of sinusitis or otitis media is direct aspiration of the sites rather than nasopharyngeal culture. Because the microbiology of acute sinusitis and acute otitis media is predictable and amenable to empirical therapy, sinus aspiration is generally limited to cases of more chronic disease, in which a greater variety of aerobic, facultatively anaerobic, and anaerobic bacteria as well as fungi may be involved. In such instances, therefore, it is important to submit a specimen in a container suitable for both aerobic and anaerobic bacterial culture.

The most common agents of sore throat are viruses and group A streptococci. Rare ones are *Neisseria gonorrhoeae, Corynebacterium diphtheriae,* and *Bordetella pertussis.* Streptococci belonging to Lancefield groups C and G may cause pharyngitis, particularly in epidemic situations, but they are not generally known to be associated with nonsuppurative sequelae. In practice, it is sufficient to examine throat swabs for the presence or absence of group A streptococci unless one of the other known causes of pharyngitis is specifically to be sought. The rate of positivity of cultures and the degree of positivity of cultures for group A streptococci may be related to the vigor with which the throat is swabbed, including the posterior pharynx, areas of purulence in the tonsillar areas, and any other obvious areas of inflammation and exudation. Because there is considerable variation in this practice by physicians and other allied health personnel who obtain throat swabs, it is often impossible for the laboratory to assign any greater significance to a culture that yields many colonies of group A streptococci than to one that yields a few colonies. Moreover, studies in children and in adults have demonstrated that seroconversion (antistreptolysin O and anti-DNase B) occurs as frequently in patients with weakly positive throat cultures for group A streptococci as in patients with strongly positive throat cultures.[5,6] These observations are of some relevance to the use of rapid antigen tests for the detection of group A streptococci, because the sensitivity of such tests is directly related to the number of colonies present in a culture of a specimen taken at the same time. Therefore, it has been recommended by an American Heart Association Council on Cardiovascular Disease in the Young that negative rapid test results be confirmed with a culture, because sparse growth of group A streptococci does not necessarily reflect the carrier state and may indicate acute infection.[7]

A dry swab is suitable for the isolation of group A streptococci if cultures are inoculated within 2 hours of specimen collection. If longer storage and transport time is anticipated, swabs should be placed into a transport medium, such as Stuart or Amies or one of the numerous variations thereof. The swabs of Culturette EZ II (Becton Dickinson Microbiology Systems) consist of polymers that are porous and permit microorganisms to survive for at least 24 hours without the addition of transport media. Because two swabs are provided and can be used simultaneously, cultures and smears or antigen detection can be performed. Many such swab transport systems are commercially available today, and they are also satisfactory for throat swabs for viruses.

LOWER RESPIRATORY TRACT INFECTIONS

Lower respiratory tract infections are caused by a variety of bacteria, mycobacteria, fungi, viruses, some parasites, *Chlamydia trachomatis, Chlamydia pneumoniae,* and *Mycoplasma pneumoniae.* What is the most likely agent varies according to the patient's age, occupation, travel history, and immune status and the season. Diagnostic approaches also vary according to the suspected agent and the patient's underlying disease, history, and clinical condition. Procedures can be broadly classified as noninvasive or invasive.[8]

The major noninvasive approach to the diagnosis of lower respiratory tract infection is the collection of expectorated sputum. What laboratories actually receive is more often saliva than sputum, and it is important for all specimens labeled as sputum to be screened before bacterial culture to ascertain whether they are predominantly sputum or predominantly saliva. Screening is easily accomplished by preparing a Gram-stained smear of the sample submitted and examining the smear under low-power (×100) magnification (Fig. 12–1). To assess the acceptability of a routine sputum specimen for culture, 10 to 20 low-power microscopic fields should be screened. The following conditions make such specimens acceptable for culture analysis: neutrophils, 1 to 9 per field, epithelial cells, none or few (less than 9 per field); neutrophils, 10 to 25 per field, epithelial cells, less than 25 per field. Specimens that do not meet these criteria should

TABLE 12–4 ■ Microorganisms Encountered in Respiratory Tract Specimens

ORGANISM	FREQUENCY OF ISOLATION*	DISEASE INVOLVEMENT†
Absidia spp.	C	2
Acinetobacter spp.	B	2
Actinomyces spp.	A	2
Adenovirus	B	3
Aerococcus viridans	B	1
Agrobacterium tumefaciens	C	2
Arachnia propionica	B	1
Arcanobacterium haemolyticum	B	3
Ascaris lumbricoides larvae	C	3
Aspergillus spp.	B	2
Bacillus anthracis	C	3
Bacillus spp.	B	1
Bacteroides spp.	A	2
Bifidobacterium spp.	B	1
Bipolaris spp.	C	2
Blastomyces dermatitidis	C	3
Bordetella pertussis	B	3
Borrelia spp.	B	1
Branhamella (Moraxella) catarrhalis	B	2
Brucella spp.	C	3
Campylobacter rectus (formerly *Wolinella recta*)	B	1
Campylobacter spp.	B	1
Candida spp.	B	2
Capnocytophaga spp.	B	2
Cardiobacterium hominis	B	1
Chlamydia spp.	B	3
Clostridium spp.	B	2
Coccidioides immitis	B	3
Coronavirus	B	2
Corynebacterium diphtheriae (toxigenic)	C	3
Corynebacterium spp.	B	1
Coxiella burnetii	C	3
Cryptococcus neoformans	C	3
Cryptosporidium spp.	C	3
Cytomegalovirus	B	2
Echinococcus spp. protoscolices or hooklets	C	3
Eikenella corrodens	B	2
Entamoeba gingivalis	B	1
Entamoeba histolytica trophozoites	C	3
Enterobacteriaceae	B	2
Enterococcus spp.	C	1
Enterovirus	B	2
Epstein-Barr virus	C	2
Flavobacterium spp.	C	2
Fonsecaea spp.	C	2
Francisella tularensis	C	3
Fusobacterium spp.	A	2
Gamella spp	B	1
Haemophilus spp.	A	2
Herpes simplex virus	B	3
Histoplasma capsulatum	B	3
Human immunodeficiency virus	C	3
Influenza viruses	B	3
Kingella spp.	C	2
Lactobacillus spp.	B	1
Legionella spp.	B	2
Leptotrichia buccalis	B	1
Measles virus	B	3
Micrococcus spp.	A	1
Moraxella spp.	B	1
Mucor spp.	C	2
Mumps virus	B	3
Mycobacterium spp.	B	2
Mycobacterium tuberculosis group	B	3
Necator americanus	C	3
Neisseria gonorrhoeae	C	3
Neisseria meningitidis	B	2
Neisseria spp.	A	1
Nocardia spp.	B	3
Papillomaviruses	C	2
Paracoccidioides brasiliensis	C	3
Paragonimus spp. ova	C	3
Parainfluenza viruses	B	2
Pasteurella spp.	C	2
Penicillium spp.	C	1
Peptostreptococcus spp.	A	2
Pneumocystis carinii	B	2
Porphyromonas spp.	A	2
Prevotella spp.	A	2
Pseudallescheria boydii	C	2
Respiratory syncytial virus	B	3
Rhinoviruses	B	2
Rhizomucor spp.	C	2
Rhizopus spp.	C	2
Rhodococcus spp.	C	2
Rothia dentocariosa	B	1
Rubella virus	B	3
Sarcinosporon inkin	B	2
Selenomonas spp.	C	1
Sporothrix schenckii	C	3
Staphylococcus spp.	A	2
Stenotrophomonas (formerly *Xanthomonas*) *maltophilia*	B	2
Stomatococcus mucilaginosus	B	1
Streptococcus pneumoniae	B	2
Streptococcus pyogenes	B	2
Streptococcus spp.	A	2
Strongyloides stercoralis larvae	C	3
Treponema spp.	B	2
Trichomonas tenax	B	1
Varicella-zoster virus	B	3
Veillonella spp.	B	1
Vibrio spp.	B	1

*A, Commonly encountered in clinical specimens; B, occasionally encountered in clinical specimens; C, rarely encountered in clinical specimens.

†1, When present, it is rarely if ever involved in disease production; 2, when present, it is occasionally involved in disease production; 3, when present, it is commonly involved in disease production.

From Isenberg HD, D'Amato RF: Indigenous and pathogenic microorganisms of humans. *In* Murray PR, Baron EJ, Pfaller MA, et al (eds): Manual of Clinical Microbiology, ed 6. Washington, DC, ASM Press, 1994, pp 5–18.

not be analyzed further, and the ordering clinician should be advised to submit another specimen. When sputum is obtained from a truly neutropenic patient, the presence of ciliated epithelial cells can serve as an indicator of the lower respiratory tract origin of the specimen.[9] Acceptable smears may be examined by oil immersion (×1000) and the preponderance of any characteristic morphologic type of bacteria (e.g., pneumococcus-like, *Neisseria*-like, *Staphylococcus*-like, enterobacillus-like) reported. The presence of *Haemophilus*-like or *Neisseria*-like bacteria in the Gram-stained smear should prompt the laboratory to include a chocolate agar medium for the isolation of *Haemophilus* or *N. meningitidis* and to examine the culture carefully for *Branhamella (Moraxella) catarrhalis.* Because *Haemophilus* and *Neisseria* species are often present in the indigenous microbiota of the oropharynx, isolation of these organisms and *Branhamella* is indicated

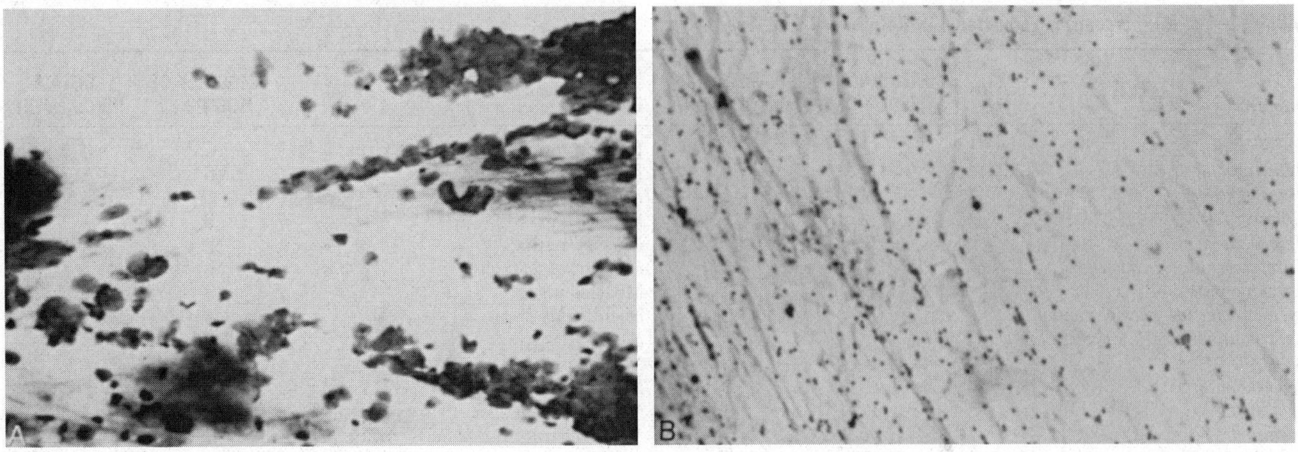

FIGURE 12–1 □ Smears of representative sputum specimens (Gram stain, × 100). *A,* Unacceptable specimen displaying numerous squamous epithelial cells and rare polymorphonuclear leukocytes. *B,* Acceptable specimen displaying numerous polymorphonuclear leukocytes, occasional alveolar macrophages, and rare squamous epithelial cells. (From Murray PR, Washington JA II: Microscopic and bacteriologic analysis of expectorated sputum. Mayo Clin Proc 50:339–344, 1975.)

only when organisms resembling these genera are predominant in the Gram-stained smear of sputum.

Throat swabs are suitable for the isolation of *C. trachomatis* from infants with pneumonitis, *M. pneumoniae,* and a variety of respiratory viruses, including influenza virus, parainfluenza virus, and adenovirus. The optimal specimen for respiratory syncytial virus is obtained by nasal washings rather than with a throat swab. The presence of respiratory syncytial virus can be detected rapidly and accurately by immunofluorescence or immunoassay of the specimen. As noted before, the isolation of respiratory viruses can be made from swabs in Stuart or Amies transport medium as well as from viral transport media. Swabs taken for the culture of *C. trachomatis,* on the other hand, must be placed into a sucrose-phosphate medium and, if not cultured shortly thereafter, frozen at −70°C. Sucrose-phosphate transport medium is also recommended for swabs taken for culture of *M. pneumoniae.*

For the diagnosis of mycobacterial disease, it is recommended that a single, freshly expectorated sputum specimen be collected on each of three consecutive days. Pooled sputum specimens are not acceptable because of heavy bacterial overgrowth. In patients with suspected mycobacterial or fungal infection who do not have a productive cough, it is useful to induce sputum production by having the patient inhale a hypertonic sodium chloride aerosol. There is no established role for the utility of induced sputum for the diagnosis of bacterial pneumonia. Induced sputum is also useful for the diagnosis of *Pneumocystis carinii* pneumonia, both in patients with AIDS and in other immunocompromised patients.[8, 9]

The second major category of specimens from the lower respiratory tract represents those obtained by invasive techniques. The primary techniques in use today are based on fiberoptic bronchoscopy with bronchoalveolar lavage or a protected catheter brush.[9] Bronchoalveolar lavage is performed by instilling 40 to 50 mL of saline solution into the affected lobe and then aspirating as much of the instilled fluid as possible for a specimen for examination. This process is repeated four or five times, so the total volume of instilled saline is about 240 or 250 mL. The aspirated lavage fluid is examined microscopically for cellular content and stained for the presence of bacteria, mycobacteria, fungi, and *P. carinii.* Microscopic examination should be performed with smears prepared by cytocentrifugation. The fluid is cultured quantitatively for the presence of bacteria and is then concentrated for culture of mycobacteria, fungi, and viruses. An alternative approach for the diagnosis of bacterial pneumonia in seriously ill patients is to use the protected catheter brush by which a double-lumen, distally occluded catheter is passed through the bronchoscope into an area of purulence. The inner cannula is then advanced to dislodge the distally occluded plug at the area to be sampled. The inner brush is then used to obtain the material and is withdrawn into the inner cannula, which in turn is withdrawn through the outer cannula and removed. After the external surface of the inner cannula is disinfected, the brush is advanced and the bristles are severed with sterile scissors into 1 mL of sterile lactated Ringer solution for transport to the laboratory. After the mixing of the contents on a mechanical stirrer, quantitative bacterial cultures are made of the lactated Ringer solution for the detection of aerobic and anaerobic bacteria. A colony count of at least 10,000 colony-forming units (CFU)/mL is usually indicative of the species causing infection. Contaminating microorganisms are usually present in smaller numbers. Both procedures have been used for the diagnosis of bacterial pneumonia in intubated, intensive care unit patients and have been found to provide complementary results. In immunosuppressed patients, it may also be useful to perform transbronchial biopsy for histologic examination and complete microbiologic analysis.

Other invasive procedures include thoracocentesis, transtracheal aspiration, and transthoracic needle aspiration. Thoracocentesis may be useful in the diagnosis of *H. influenzae* pneumonia in children and in the diagnosis of anaerobic pleuropulmonary disease in adults. In general, transtracheal aspiration should be performed only by experienced operators and only when a bacterial pathogen is suspected or is to be ruled out, the severity of the illness justifies the risk of the procedure, alternative specimens obtained by less invasive methods provide inconclusive results, and laboratory resources are available for prompt processing of specimens.[9] Moreover, there should be no contraindications to the procedure. One limitation to the procedure appears to be in the diagnosis of pneumonia in patients who have received antimicrobial therapy. Transthoracic needle aspiration is carried out principally for the diagnosis of malignant neoplasms and has had relatively limited use, except in children, for the diagnosis of pneumonia.

Open lung biopsy is used primarily for the diagnosis of pneumonia in immunosuppressed patients and for instances when a diagnosis has not been established by the procedures described before. With the advent of induced sputum examination for *P. carinii* and bronchoalveolar lavage with transbronchial biopsy, the need for open lung biopsy has diminished. Nonetheless, when the procedure is performed, it is essential that a protocol be established for both histologic and microbiologic examination of the specimen. A freshly cut surface of the specimen is used to make impression smears for Gram and Gomori methenamine silver stains and for direct immunofluorescence stains for *Legionella.* The specimen is homogenized, and the homogenate is used for a potassium hydroxide and, preferably, calcofluor wet preparation and for cultures for bacteria, *Legionella,* mycobacteria, fungi, and viruses. Sections of the lung should be stained for bacteria, mycobacteria, and fungi.

URINARY TRACT INFECTIONS (Table 12–5)

Urinary tract infections may arise from various sites along the genitourinary tract. For the purpose of diagnosis of urinary tract infection in the laboratory, a variety of specimens may be submitted, depending on the suspected site of infection or suspected agent, but the majority are clean-voided midstream urine samples. Proper instruction of patients or of allied health personnel in correct antiseptic procedure for collection of urine from female patients is important to minimize contamination by introital and periurethral flora. Because the urethra is normally colonized by a diverse aerobic and anaerobic bacteria, it is customary to discard the first ounce or so of voided urine and to collect a midstream sample for culture.[2, 10]

The goal of urethral catheterization is usually therapeutic, and it is not performed solely for the purpose of obtaining a urine specimen for culture. In such instances, specimens may be collected immediately after catheterization or from chronic indwelling urethral catheters. Another procedure for obtaining urine specimens performed less frequently is suprapubic aspiration. This procedure is useful for collecting specimens from infants and small children, when results of clean-voided midstream specimens are inconclusive, and when bacteriuria due to anaerobic or other fastidious bacteria is suspected. The possibility of infection due to fastidious microorganisms is suggested by a positive Gram stain examination and failure to propagate the organism on routine culture of urine. Anaerobic bacteriuria does occur rarely and can be accurately documented only by examination of urine obtained by suprapubic aspiration. *Gardnerella vaginalis,* for example, is not infrequently isolated from midstream clean-catch specimens from women, but the role of this organism in bacteriuria can be accurately determined only by suprapubic aspiration. In another example, a small number of yeast organisms may be isolated repeatedly from midstream specimens; however, the role of yeast in causing bacteriuria can be established definitively only by isolating them from suprapubically aspirated urine. Less frequently, urine specimens

TABLE 12–5 ■ Microorganisms Encountered in Genitourinary Tract Specimens

ORGANISM	FREQUENCY OF ISOLATION*	DISEASE INVOLVEMENT†	ORGANISM	FREQUENCY OF ISOLATION*	DISEASE INVOLVEMENT†
Acinetobacter spp.	B	2	*Histoplasma capsulatum*	C	3
Actinomyces spp.	B	2	Human immunodeficiency virus	B	3
Adenoviruses	B	1	*Lactobacillus* spp.	A	1
Alcaligenes spp.	C	2	*Leptospira interrogans*	C	3
Aspergillus spp.	C	1	*Listeria* spp.	C	2
Bacillus spp.	C	1	*Mobiluncus* spp.	B	2
Bacteroides spp.	A	2	Molluscum contagiosum virus	C	3
Bifidobacterium spp.	C	1	*Moraxella* spp.	B	1
Bilophila wadsworthia	C	2	Mumps virus	C	3
Blastomyces dermatitidis	C	3	*Mycobacterium* spp.	B	2
Branhamella (Moraxella) catarrhalis	B	1	*Mycoplasma hominis*	B	2
Brugia malayi	C	3	*Neisseria gonorrhoeae*	B	3
Calymmatobacterium granulomatis	C	3	*Neisseria meningitidis*	C	3
Campylobacter spp.	C	2	*Neisseria* spp.	B	1
Candida spp.	B	2	Papillomaviruses	C	3
Chlamydia spp.	B	2	*Penicillium* spp.	C	1
Clostridium spp.	A	2	*Peptostreptococcus* spp.	B	1
Corynebacterium spp.	B	2	*Porphyromonas* spp.	A	2
Cryptococcus spp.	C	2	*Prevotella* spp.	A	2
Cytomegalovirus	B	2	*Propionibacterium* spp.	B	1
Dioctophyma renale	C	3	*Pseudomonas* spp.	B	2
Entamoeba histolytica	C	3	*Rhodotorula* spp.	C	1
Enterobacteriaceae	A	2	*Saccharomyces* spp.	C	1
Enterobius vermicularis	B	2	*Schistosoma haematobium*	C	3
Enterococcus spp.	B	2	*Staphylococcus* spp.	A	2
Flavobacterium spp.	C	2	*Streptococcus* spp.	B	2
Fusobacterium spp.	B	1	*Torulopsis glabrata*	B	2
Gardnerella vaginalis	B	2	*Treponema pallidum*	B	3
Geotrichum candidum	C	1	*Trichomonas vaginalis*	B	3
Haemophilus ducreyi	B	3	*Ureaplasma urealyticum*	B	1
Hepatitis A and B viruses	B	2	*Wuchereria bancrofti*	C	3
Herpes simplex virus	B	3	Zygomycetes	C	1

*A, Commonly encountered in clinical specimens; B, occasionally encountered in clinical specimens; C, rarely encountered in clinical specimens.

†1, When present, it is rarely if ever involved in disease production; 2, when present, it is occasionally involved in disease production; 3, when present, it is commonly involved in disease production.

From Isenberg HD, D'Amato RF: Indigenous and pathogenic microoganisms of humans. *In* Murray PR, Baron EJ, Pfaller MA, et al (eds): Manual of Clinical Microbiology, ed 6. Washington, DC, ASM Press, 1994, pp 5–18.

are submitted for the purpose of localizing infections to the bladder or to a kidney. Because an accurate determination is based on relative differences in the numbers of bacteria in specimens from different sites, localization studies require careful quantitation of each sample.

When urine specimens are to be cultured for mycobacteria and fungi, freshly voided specimens, rather than pooled specimens, should be collected.

Urine is generally obtained for culture when there is a problem in differentiating among urinary tract infection, vaginitis, and sexually transmitted disease; when bacteriuria is suspected in infants, children, male patients, and elderly patients; when pyelonephritis is suspected; when there are recurrent infections, particularly when short-course therapy fails; when covert bacteriuria is suspected in a pregnant woman; when there is a symptomatic catheter- or instrument-associated nosocomial infection; and before urinary tract instrumentation. Urine culture is generally not indicated for young, otherwise healthy women with uncomplicated urinary tract infections or for asymptomatic patients with chronic, indwelling urethral catheters.[11]

Urine should ordinarily be cultured within 2 hours of collection, or it should be refrigerated until culture can be performed. Urine is an excellent culture medium, so a small and probably insignificant number of bacteria can rapidly proliferate if the specimen is stored at room temperature longer than 2 hours. Commercially available urine transport devices may be useful for follow-up of outpatients, as long as the devices are returned to the laboratory within 24 hours of urine collection. With a variety of "miniculture" devices, a small agar surface on a slide or paddle is dipped into a voided urine specimen; the device is returned to a laboratory, where the specimen is incubated. Such devices are useful for screening purposes, but the small size of the agar surface makes isolation, identification, and susceptibility testing of bacteria difficult.

A variety of rapid detection methods for bacteriuria have been devised,[12] among them Gram-stained smears, enzyme methods for detection of leukocyte esterase and nitrite, filtration methods, bioluminescence, and photometry. A variety of methods for urine microscopy for bacteriuria have been used.[13] Observation by a trained microscopist of at least two bacteria in each of several oil-immersion fields ($\times 1000$) examined has at least a 95% correlation with bacteriuria of at least 10^5 CFU/mL. The sensitivity of the leukocyte esterase-nitrite dipstick is only about 85% for the detection of the same level of bacteriuria. The leukocyte esterase-nitrite dipstick, although increasingly popular, should be used with caution, especially in evaluating patients with diminished cellular responses or patients infected with microorganisms that do not reduce nitrate. Whereas it is useful in clinics frequented by patients from the community, the use of the dipstick for patients in tertiary facilities should be approached with caution. The sensitivity of filtration methods and of bioluminescence is also approximately 95%; each method can be carried out in 2 minutes or less per specimen, in contrast to photometric methods, which require anywhere from 1 to 12 hours. The negative predictive value for all of these tests is at least 95% when the criterion for bacteriuria is 10^5 CFU/mL. If it is 10^4 CFU/mL, only Gram stain and bioluminescence have negative predictive values of at least 95%. Therefore, it may be feasible and practical for urine specimens to be screened as a prerequisite for culture, depending on the criterion being used to define bacteriuria and depending on test volume, prevalence of bacteriuria, and cost. In the typical hospital laboratory, the prevalence of bacteriuria, even at a level of 10^4 CFU/mL, is only approximately 10% of samples received, so a test with a high negative predictive value may be a useful, quick screen. Although culture is seldom if ever indicated for acute dysuric syndrome in young women, bacteriuria as low as 100 CFU/mL may be significant in this particular population; if cultures are requested, special techniques must be used.

The concept of significant bacteriuria and the criterion of 100,000 or more CFU/ml is a useful, but not absolute, criterion that has stood well the test of time. . . . There have been efforts on the part of some workers to lower the criterion for significant bacteriuria in women with the urethritis syndrome. This is a special group. . . . In my view, it would be most unfortunate if findings in this group are projected to other individuals. It would be far better to single them out for special attention by the . . . laboratory.[14]

This statement by Kunin is reassuring to many microbiologists, because urine specimens usually constitute the single largest type of specimen received in their laboratories and because the requisitions accompanying the specimens rarely contain any diagnostic information that would permit special studies to be carried out in those instances in which lower levels of bacteriuria are considered significant.

Cultures of urine from patients who have long-term indwelling urethral catheters are complicated by a number of factors. In a study by Warren and coworkers[15] of 605 consecutive weekly urine specimens from 20 such patients, 98% contained bacteria in high concentrations and 77% were polymicrobial (mean, 2.6 species per weekly specimen). Moreover, in a study by Tenney and Warren,[16] significantly larger numbers of bacteria and more species per specimen were found with long-term indwelling catheterization than with a replacement catheter. *Proteus mirabilis, Morganella morganii, Providencia* species, *Pseudomonas aeruginosa,* and other gram-negative bacilli as well as enterococci were significantly more common in specimens from patients catheterized long term than from those whose catheter had been replaced. Thus, although cultures of urine from indwelling catheters provide a sensitive method for detection of organisms causing urosepsis in bacteremia, cultures of such specimens are highly nonspecific.[16] For this reason, it is common practice in many laboratories to limit identification of isolates from urine of patients who have indwelling catheters long term to specimens that contain no more than two species in concentrations of at least 10^5 CFU/mL and to report the presence of larger numbers of species at high concentrations as "mixed" and suggest a repeated specimen. Most clinical laboratories desist from analyzing catheter-obtained cultures unless there is a clinical need.[10]

GASTROENTERITIS (Table 12–6)

The list of microorganisms that cause diarrheal diseases has increased considerably in the last decade. To the traditional enteric bacterial pathogens—*Salmonella* and *Shigella*—have been added *Campylobacter jejuni, Plesiomonas shigelloides,* the *Aeromonas hydrophila* group (?), *Clostridium difficile, E. coli* (enterotoxigenic, enteroinvasive, enteropathogenic, enterohemorrhagic, and enteroadherent), a variety of *Vibrio* species in addition to *Vibrio cholerae,* and a variety of species of *Yersinia* in addition to *Yersinia enterocolitica. Giardia lamblia* and *Entamoeba histolytica* remain the parasitic pathogens of major concern in diarrheal disease; however, the importance of *Cryptosporidium* species, microsporidia, and *Cyclospora* in causing diarrhea in both immunosuppressed and immunocompetent patients has been appreciated only since the advent of AIDS. The list of viruses that have been associated with diarrhea includes not only rotaviruses and Norwalk or Norwalk-like viruses but also enteric adenoviruses, caliciviruses, astroviruses, and coronaviruses. Other microorganisms have been shown to infect the gastrointestinal tract of AIDS patients. These include *N. gonorrhoeae, C. trachomatis, M.*

TABLE 12–6 ■ Microorganisms Encountered in Gastrointestinal Tract Specimens*

ORGANISM	FREQUENCY OF ISOLATION†	DISEASE INVOLVEMENT‡
Absidia spp.	C	1
Acidaminococcus fermentans	C	1
Acinetobacter spp.	B	1
Adenoviruses	B	2
Aeromonas spp.	B	2
Alcaligenes spp.	B	2
Anaerobiospirillum succiniciproducens	C	2
Ancylostoma duodenale	B	3
Angiostrongylus costaricensis	C	3
Anisakis spp. larvae	C	3
Ascaris lumbricoides	B	3
Astroviruses	C	2
Bacillus spp.	B	2
Bacteroides spp.	A	2
Balantidium coli	C	3
Bifidobacterium spp.	B	1
Blastocystis hominis	B	2
Caliciviruses	C	2
Campylobacter spp.	B	3
Candida spp.	B	2
Capillaria spp.	C	3
Chilomastix mesnili	B	1
Clonorchis sinensis	C	3
Clostridium spp.	A	2
Coronaviruses	C	2
Corynebacterium spp.	B	1
Cryptosporidium spp.	C	3
Dicrocoelium dendriticum ova	C	1
Dientamoeba fragilis	B	2
Diphyllobothrium latum	B	3
Dipylidium caninum	C	3
Endolimax nana	B	1
Entamoeba coli	B	1
Entamoeba hartmanni	B	1
Entamoeba histolytica	B	3
Enterobacteriaceae	A	2
Enterobius vermicularis	B	3
Enterococcus spp.	A	2
Enteromonas hominis	C	1
Enteroviruses	A	1
Eubacterium spp.	A	1
Fasciola hepatica	C	3
Fasciolopsis buski	C	3
Fusobacterium spp.	A	2
Gastrodiscoides hominis	C	3
Geotrichum candidum	C	1
Giardia lamblia	B	3
Helicobacter pylori	B	3
Heterophyes heterophyes	C	3
Histoplasma capsulatum	C	3
Hymenolepis spp.	C	3
Iodamoeba butschlii	B	1
Isospora belli	C	2
Lactobacillus spp.	B	1
Metagonimus yokogawai	C	3
Microsporidian genera (several)	C	3
Mucor spp.	C	2
Mycobacterium spp.	B	2
Mycoplasma spp.	C	1
Necator americanus	B	3
Neisseria gonorrhoeae	C	3
Neisseria spp.	B	1
Norwalk and Norwalk-like viruses	B	3
Opisthorchis viverrini	C	3
Paracoccidioides brasiliensis	C	3
Paragonimus spp.	C	3
Pediococcus spp.	C	1
Peptostreptococcus spp.	B	2
Plesiomonas shigelloides	C	2
Pseudomonas spp.	B	2
Retortamonas intestinalis	C	1
Rhizomucor spp.	C	1
Rhizopus spp.	C	1
Rhodotorula spp.	C	1
Rotavirus	B	3
Ruminococcus bromii	C	1
Saccharomyces spp.	B	1
Sapporo agent	B	2
Sarcocystis spp.	C	2
Schistosoma spp.	B	3
Selenomonas spp.	B	1
Staphylococcus spp.	B	2
Streptococcus spp.	B	2
Strongyloides stercoralis	B	3
Succinimonas spp.	B	1
Succinivibrio spp.	B	1
Taenia spp.	C	3
Trichinella spiralis larvae	C	3
Trichomonas hominis	B	1
Trichosporon beigelii	C	1
Trichostrongylus spp.	C	2
Trichuris trichiura	B	2
Veillonella spp.	B	2
Vibrio spp.	B	2

*Diseases other than gastroenteritis may be caused by organisms listed. Several species of the genera listed may be found; not all of the species are involved in disease processes.

†A, Commonly encountered in clinical specimens; B, occasionally encountered in clinical specimens; C, rarely encountered in clinical specimens.

‡1, When present, it is rarely if ever involved in disease production; 2, when present, it is occasionally involved in disease production; 3, when present, it is commonly involved in disease production.

From Isenberg HD, D'Amato RF: Indigenous and pathogenic microorganisms of humans. *In* Murray PR, Baron EJ, Pfaller MA, et al (eds): Manual of Clinical Microbiology, ed 6. Washington, DC, ASM Press, 1994, pp 5–18.

avium complex, *Treponema pallidum, Isospora belli,* cytomegalovirus, and herpes simplex virus. Of this lengthy list of enteric pathogens, only the various pathogenic categories of *E. coli* and the viruses other than rotaviruses cannot be readily detected by clinical laboratories today. The inability of *E. coli* O157:H7 to ferment sorbitol provides a ready means for the microbiologist to screen for this bacterium with the use of sorbitol-MacConkey agar. However, other verotoxin-producing *E. coli* strains will not be detected in this fashion.

Direct microscopic examination of fecal material is required for the diagnosis of parasitic infections. The accurate detection of parasites requires examination of more than one stool specimen; a minimum of three specimens, collected on separate days, should be examined. When parasitic infection is suspected but the patient does not have diarrhea, it may be helpful to prescribe a saline purgative, such as magnesium sulfate (Epsom salts) or buffered sodium phosphate (Fleet Phospho-Soda) to be taken on arising in the morning, followed by breakfast, and then collection of the specimen at home or in an outpatient setting. Stool specimens for ova and parasites should be collected in commercially available two-vial transport systems—one vial containing 10% formalin, the other polyvinyl alcohol—that preserve the morphologic character and number of the parasites and ova. The polyvinyl alcohol specimens of especially diarrheal stools should be smeared for staining with trichrome stain for protozoa, with acid-fast stain for cryptosporidia and *Cyclospora*, and with modified trichrome stain for the demonstration of microsporidia (*Nosema, Encephalitozoon, Enterocytozoon, Pleistophora,* and *Microsporidia* species).[3] Ova and larvae can be discerned by direct or centrifuged aliquots of the formalin-fixed submission.[3] When giardiasis is suspected and at least three separately collected stool specimen examinations are negative, it may be necessary to obtain duodenal material by aspiration or an enteric string technique.

Direct microscopic examination of fecal specimens is also useful in differentiating between inflammatory processes due to organisms such as *Shigella, Campylobacter,* and enteroinvasive *E. coli* and noninflammatory processes, such as those associated with *V. cholerae,* enterotoxigenic *E. coli,* and viral agents. Although some have advocated limiting stool culture to specimens that contain leukocytes, the presence of leukocytes is variable with *Salmonella, Yersinia,* and *Aeromonas* infections. In addition, limiting the type of specimen that should be cultured on the basis of consistency of the specimen or the presence or absence of leukocytes may preclude detection of carrier states of *Salmonella* and *Yersinia,* although the clinical significance of the carrier state of *Y. enterocolitica* remains under discussion. Laboratory procedures should include routine culture of stool for *Salmonella, Shigella,* and *Campylobacter* organisms submitted in an appropriately buffered, commercially available stool preservative (e.g., buffered glycerol with indicator), along with a history of travel and food consumption when unusual pathogens are suspected.[1] Whether specimens should be routinely cultured for *Yersinia* remains a subject of debate, because the frequency of yersiniosis varies widely around the United States and may vary widely in any particular geographic region. Laboratory procedures in coastal areas and for patients with a history of diarrhea after ingestion of shellfish should include cultures for vibrios. The role of the *A. hydrophila* group in diarrheal disease remains controversial, so the decision to culture for this organism is often based on local prejudice. If laboratory procedures include a selective medium for the isolation of *Yersinia,* it is likely that organisms belonging to the *A. hydrophila* group will also be isolated. Routine stool cultures for *Salmonella, Shigella,* and *Campylobacter* species are among the most time-consuming and expensive procedures carried out in the microbiology laboratory. They include inoculation of a variety of differential and selective media and, in most laboratories, inoculation of enrichment broths, which are then subcultured onto differential and selective media after overnight incubation. Although shigellae are not usually isolated after culture in an enrichment broth, salmonellae often are. It is customary for lactose-negative colonies on enteric differential and selective media to be screened with a limited number of biochemical tests to rule out *Salmonella* or *Shigella,* after which the laboratory proceeds with definitive identification of those isolates for which the biochemical test screen results are compatible with these organisms. Thus, the entire process of ruling out the presence of *Salmonella* or *Shigella* may require 4 or 5 days. Unless examination of stool specimens for vibrios is part of the routine procedure of the laboratory, it is necessary for the examination to be specifically requested when the diagnosis of vibriosis is suspected, because a selective medium is also necessary for this purpose.

The laboratory diagnosis of *C. difficile* diarrhea is also controversial. Culture for the organism is the most sensitive but also the least specific approach, because nontoxigenic *C. difficile* may be present in stool from asymptomatic, healthy persons. The tissue culture assay for *C. difficile* toxin is the most specific test but is probably less sensitive than culture. The culture technique is time-consuming, slow, and nonspecific. The cytotoxic assay requires the use of tissue cultures that are not available in laboratories that do not also perform viral isolation. Enzyme immunoassays that correspond well with tissue culture results are now available commercially and can be employed readily in most clinical laboratories. The latex agglutination assay does not detect either of the two significant toxins of *C. difficile.*

Rotaviruses and enteric adenoviruses can be detected by enzyme immunoassay or, in the case of rotaviruses, by latex agglutination. The sensitivity of latex agglutination for rotaviruses appears to be somewhat less than that of enzyme immunoassay, but latex agglutination appears to be as sensitive as enzyme immunoassay when the test is applied to specimens collected within the first day or two of illness. Sensitivity of latex agglutination appears to diminish on subsequent days.

SEXUALLY TRANSMITTED DISEASES (See Table 12–5)

The focus of sexually transmitted diseases has expanded substantially from gonorrhea and syphilis to include infections by *C. trachomatis,* herpes simplex virus, *Trichomonas vaginalis, Ureaplasma urealyticum,* scabies, and a variety of other infections with extragenital manifestations such as those associated with AIDS. The major activity in this area in microbiology laboratories, however, remains diagnosis of gonorrhea, syphilis, and infections due to *C. trachomatis,* herpes simplex virus, and *T. vaginalis.*

Specimens from the genital tract include urethral, cervical, and anorectal swabs. In some cases, it may also be appropriate to obtain a pharyngeal swab.

Culture for *N. gonorrhoeae* remains the standard against which other diagnostic methods are compared. For specimens from normally sterile sites, culture on chocolate agar medium incubated in an atmosphere of enriched carbon dioxide is satisfactory; however, specimens from the urethra and cervix that are heavily colonized with indigenous microorganisms should be inoculated onto Thayer-Martin medium or one of its variations. To facilitate direct inoculation of specimens onto media without delay, Thayer-Martin medium is available either in a bottle containing carbon dioxide (Transgrow) or in a rectangular plate (JEMBEC). After inoculation into the plate, a tablet of sodium bicarbonate is placed into the device and the entire system is placed into a sealable plastic bag. The humidity from the medium activates the sodium bicarbonate to produce carbon dioxide during incubation. Both Transgrow and JEMBEC facilitate the transport of cultures to a laboratory for examination; however, if a transport delay is anticipated, each system requires overnight incubation before transport. If a delay of 6 hours or less between specimen collection and culture is anticipated, the use of a swab in a transport medium such as Stuart or Amies is satisfactory.

Presumptive identification of isolated colonies may be based on results of Gram stain and the oxidase reaction. Definitive identification of *N. gonorrhoeae* can be made with carbohydrate utilization tests or by immunofluorescence.

The Gram-stained smear remains the most accurate rapid method for detecting *N. gonorrhoeae* in urethral specimens from symptomatic men. The sensitivity and specificity of this test are 95% and 95%, respectively, in contrast with those of the Gram-stained smear of urethral specimens from asymptomatic men (approximately 60% and 95%, respectively).[17] The sensitivity and specificity of the Gram-stained smear of cervical material from symptomatic women are 40% to 70% and 95%, respectively.[17]

A more recent approach to the diagnosis of gonorrhea is with genetic probes using nucleic hybridization. A nonisotopic, RNA-directed DNA probe based on liquid-phase hybridization (GenProbe PACE) has been found to be highly sensitive and highly specific compared with culture for the detection of *N. gonorrhoeae* in a population at high risk.[18] The test provides results within 2 hours. Microbiologists will require a specimen for culture as well, because positive test results must be followed with susceptibility studies.

The definitive diagnosis of *C. trachomatis* genitourinary tract infections is made by cell culture techniques superseded in most clinical microbiology laboratories by direct methods described later. Urethral specimens should be collected with a small cotton-tipped, aluminum-shafted swab; endocervical specimens should be collected with a cotton- or Dacron-tipped, aluminum- or plastic-shafted swab. To collect urethral specimens, the swab should be inserted 3 to 5 cm into the urethra and withdrawn. To collect endocervical specimens, the cervix should first be cleaned to remove excess discharge; the swab used to collect the specimen is placed within the endocervical canal and rubbed vigorously against its wall. An important point is to obtain as much cellular material as possible to enhance the chances for recovery of the organism from culture or antigen detection testing. Although the use of a cytobrush has provided specimens that contain significantly more of elementary bodies than do specimens collected with a swab or with a cytologic scraper, there does not appear to be a significant increase in the number of patients with positive immunofluorescence or enzyme immunoassay test results from cytobrush specimens than from swab specimens.[19, 20]

Specimens should be placed into a sucrose-phosphate medium for transport to the laboratory. Specimens in the transport medium may be stored under refrigeration for up to 72 hours before being inoculated into cell cultures, but specimens that require a longer period of storage should be frozen at −70°C immediately after collection.[21] Specimens are inoculated by low-speed centrifugation onto cycloheximide-treated McCoy cells in a monolayer on coverslips in 1-dram vials[21] or, alternatively, onto monolayers in microdilution plate wells. The latter technique facilitates the processing of a large number of specimens but appears to demand more stringent technique[21] to achieve results comparable to those of the shell vial technique. Because published reports often fail to describe these technical variables, it is difficult to assess the accuracy of a culture method and, therefore, also difficult to assess the sensitivity and specificity of nonculture methods. The presence of *C. trachomatis* in the cell monolayers is detected by immunofluorescent staining with genus-reactive monoclonal antibody.

Because cell culture techniques are not usually available in laboratories that do not perform diagnostic virology, nonculture methods have become popular. Two methods in wide use today are the direct immunofluorescent test and the enzyme immunoassay test (Chlamydiazyme).[22] Fluorescent-labeled monoclonal antibodies are available from several commercial sources. The results of numerous published evaluations of both methods have been reviewed by Stamm,[20, 23] who pointed out that any analysis of published data needs to take into account variations in specimen collection, culture technique, study populations, laboratory equipment, and expertise of laboratory workers. In his review of 15 published studies of the use of the direct immunofluorescent test, he found that test sensitivity in a population of symptomatic men averaged 92% (range, 90% to 100%) and specificity 97% (range, 72% to 99%). The advantages of direct immunofluorescence[20, 22] include the ability to assess the quality of the specimen on the basis of its cell content and a short turnaround time; its disadvantages include the need for a fluorescence microscope, expertise in immunofluorescence microscopy, and inefficiency when more than a few specimens must be examined at one time. The advantages of the enzyme immunoassay method include greater technical simplicity, easy examination of multiple specimens, objective results, and economy in batch processing of specimens; its disadvantages include a 4-hour turnaround time, and it is economical only when multiple specimens are processed in batches. DNA probes for *C. trachomatis* have been developed and are available commercially[20, 22] even in conjunction with molecular probes for gonococcus. They are highly sensitive and specific. The advantages and disadvantages of DNA probes may be similar to those of the enzyme immunoassay. Implementation of any of these techniques in the laboratory must be preceded by a careful analysis of advantages and disadvantages and cost.

Because the diagnosis of syphilis is usually made serologically (see Chapter 113), the discussion in this chapter is limited to darkfield examination for the diagnosis of primary syphilis. The examiner obtaining specimens from a chancre should wear surgical gloves to prevent transmission of infection. The lesion should be abraded with a dry gauze sponge until it bleeds. The excess blood is blotted with a gauze sponge, and a coverslip is applied to the serous exudate. It may be necessary to apply pressure to the base of the chancre to increase the amount of serous exudate for examination. The coverslip is inverted onto a glass microscope slide, and the edge is sealed with Vaspar or lanolin to prevent evaporation of the specimen, which should be examined as soon as possible with a darkfield microscope at a magnification of ×450. Diagnosis is based on observation of motile spirochetes. The person performing darkfield examinations for *T. pallidum* must be experienced with this procedure; the untrained observer may confuse various artifacts.[24]

Isolation of herpes simplex virus in tissue culture remains the standard against which nonculture methods are compared. Isolation of the virus is optimal when material is obtained from intact vesicles by needle aspiration or on a Dacron- or cotton-tipped swab after unroofing the vesicle. Isolation rates are lower when crusted lesions are sampled. Swabs should be placed into a transport medium, such as Stuart, Amies, or viral transport medium. Swab extracts are inoculated into cell culture monolayer, which in a period of anywhere from 24 to 96 hours demonstrates a typical cytopathic effect if the virus is present. The virus may be detected more rapidly when inoculation includes low-speed centrifugation of the specimen onto a monolayer of cells on a coverslip in a 1-dram vial. After approximately 15 hours' incubation, the coverslip is stained with a fluorescent-labeled monoclonal antibody and examined by immunofluorescence microscopy. The sensitivity of this procedure is equivalent to that of conventional cell culture techniques. A disadvantage of both methods is the requirement for cell cultures. The major nonculture methods are direct immunofluorescence and enzyme immunoassay. The sensitivity of direct immunofluorescence with monoclonal antibody is 85% to 90%. As with culture, the rate of viral detection is diminished with progression of the lesion. Similar levels of sensitivity have been reported with immunoperoxidase staining and with enzyme immunoassay.[25–28]

The laboratory diagnosis of vaginitis and vaginosis remains a problem. Perhaps least problematic is the detection of *T. vaginalis,* which is almost always made by direct microscopic examination of vaginal secretions, although some investigators have found that conventional wet mount examination is insensitive relative to culture.[3] Microscopic detection of the organism appears to be improved by the use of direct immunofluorescence with monoclonal antibodies. The diagnosis of vaginal candidiasis is complicated by the fact that vaginal cultures of as many as 25% of healthy, asymptomatic women yield *Candida* organisms. Laboratory diagnosis of *Candida* vaginitis is usually made by direct microscopic examination revealing budding yeasts and pseudohyphae. Compared with culture, however, direct microscopic examination has only approximately 75% sensitivity.[29] The etiology of nonspecific vaginitis or bacterial vaginosis is as yet incompletely resolved. Initially considered to be associated with *G. vaginalis,* the entity is currently thought to involve infection with a variety of *Bacteroides* species, *Peptostreptococcus* species, and anaerobic curved rods including *Mobiluncus* species, with a concurrent decrease in lactobacilli.[30, 31] *G. vaginalis* is frequently present in cases with bacterial vaginosis, but the organism may also be isolated from 20% to 50% of vaginal material from healthy, asymptomatic women. Because of the complexity of microbiology and, therefore, the isolation techniques required, diagnosis is often made on the basis of the character of the discharge, a vaginal pH above 4.5, a positive test response for amines, and the presence of clue cells.[32] Krohn and colleagues[31] studied the vaginal flora of patients with bacterial vaginosis diagnosed by clinical signs, gas-liquid chromatography, and Gram-stained vaginal smears to assess the predictive value of each method. *G. vaginalis, Bacteroides* species, *Peptostreptococcus* species, *U. urealyticum,* and *Mycoplasma hominis* were more common in women who had bacterial vaginosis than in women who did not. *Mobiluncus* species was recovered from less than 50% of the women with vaginosis. The character of the discharge, amine odor, clue cells, and pH of at least 4.7 were less frequently present in the pregnant women studied by Krohn and coworkers[31] than in previous studies of nonpregnant women.[32] Improved sensitivity was observed with a Gram-stained smear demonstrating fewer than five *Lactobacillus* species morphotypes per oil-immersion field and five or more *G. vaginalis* morphotypes together with five or more other morphotypes, including curved gram-variable rods or fusiforms in each oil-immersion field. In conclusion, direct microscopic examination for the presence of *T. vaginalis,* budding yeast with pseudohyphae, reduced numbers of lactobacilli morphotypes with increased numbers of other gram-negative and gram-variable bacteria, and presence of clue cells can provide rapid diagnostic information. It may, however, have only moderate sensitivity relative to culture and, in the case of bacterial vaginosis, gas-liquid chromatography, or a combination of any three of the following four test results: vaginal pH at least 4.7, the presence of clue cells, amine odor, and homogeneous character of the discharge. For *Candida* vaginitis, culture is highly sensitive but lacks specificity; for bacterial vaginosis, it is expensive, time-consuming, and probably impractical for routine laboratory purposes.

MUSCULOSKELETAL INFECTIONS (Table 12–7)

Musculoskeletal infections are most frequently due to aerobic, facultatively anaerobic, and anaerobic bacteria and less frequently to mycobacteria or fungi. Microorganisms can be recovered in the majority of instances from a previously undrained and unopened wound abscess, provided that the specimen is properly collected and transported to the laboratory. Open wounds, ulcers, and sinus tracks are usually contaminated with cutaneous, mucosal, or environmental organisms. Generally speaking, a swab specimen provides the laboratory with too small a sample of material for adequate examination, so a generous quantity of material should be aspirated through a sterile needle into a syringe. Then, the contents are injected into an anaerobic transport vial for transport to the laboratory. Anaerobic transport media, available commercially, allow the recovery of facultatively or obligately aerobic bacteria with impunity. In many laboratories, swab specimens are unacceptable for anaerobic cultures. Sinus tracts frequently originate in bone secondary to chronic osteomyelitis, but the predictive value of culture of swabs taken at the orifice of a sinus track is poor compared with that of operative specimens.[33] Uncontaminated material is difficult to obtain from diabetic foot infections, but every effort must be made to avoid contamination from ulcers or other open lesions when culture material is obtained from bullae, abscesses, necrotic soft tissues, or bone.[34, 35]

The microbiology of musculoskeletal infections has changed somewhat through the years, from a predominance of staphylococci, streptococci, pneumococci, and clostridia to an increasing frequency of gram-negative bacilli. This shift has been apparent in postoperative wound infection, chronic osteomyelitis, and trauma wounds.[36] However, the past 2 to 3 years have seen the reemergence of gram-positive bacteria in this setting; many of these organisms display resistance to commonly used antimicrobial agents. Practical anaerobic bacteriology methods have increasingly enabled laboratories to recognize musculoskeletal infections associated with anaerobic gram-negative bacilli and anaerobic cocci.[37]

Quantitative bacteriology of wound biopsy specimens has been found useful in the management of patients with acute open wounds, those for whom delayed wound closure is contemplated, and those who receive skin grafts.[38] Numerous studies have shown a correlation between the presence of more than 10^5 CFU/g of tissue at the time of wound closure and the development of wound sepsis.[39–41] Important requirements of quantitative microbiology of wounds are cleansing and débridement of the wound before biopsy and biopsy of a tissue sample of about 1 cm^3. If the wound is large, multiple specimens should be obtained. The tissue is carefully weighed in a preweighed, sterile vessel and homogenized for preparation of an immediate quantitative Gram-stained smear and for culture[38, 41] (Fig. 12–2). For the Gram-stained smear, 0.4 mL of the undiluted homogenate is transferred to a clean glass microscope slide and spread over an area not

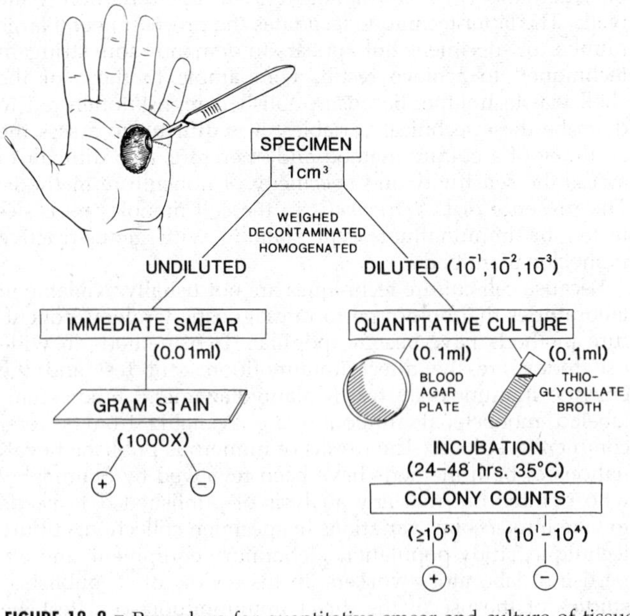

FIGURE 12–2 □ Procedure for quantitative smear and culture of tissue from traumatically acquired wounds after cleansing and débridement. (From Cooney WP III, Fitzgerald RH Jr, Dobyns JH, Washington JA II: Quantitative wound cultures in upper extremity trauma. J Trauma 22:112–117, 1982.)

TABLE 12–7 ■ Microorganisms Encountered in Skin, Wound, and Burn Specimens

ORGANISM	FREQUENCY OF ISOLATION*	DISEASE INVOLVEMENT†
Absidia spp.	A	1
Acinetobacter spp.	B	2
Actinomadura madurae	C	2
Actinomyces spp.	B	2
Aeromonas spp.	B	2
Agrobacterium tumefaciens	C	2
Ancylostoma spp.	C	3
Arcanobacterium haemolyticum	C	2
Aspergillus spp.	B	1
Bacillus anthracis	C	3
Bacillus spp.	B	1
Bacteroides spp.	B	2
Bartonella bacilliformis	C	3
Basidiobolus ranarum	C	2
Bifidobacterium spp.	B	2
Bipolaris spp.	C	2
Blastomyces dermatitidis	B	3
Brugia spp.	C	3
Candida spp.	A	2
Cephalosporium spp.	B	2
Cladosporium carrionii	C	2
Clostridium spp.	B	2
Coccidioides immitis	B	3
Conidiobolus coronatus	C	2
Corynebacterium diphtheriae	C	3
Corynebacterium spp.	B	2
Cryptococcus neoformans	C	3
Cryptococcus spp.	C	1
Dematiaceous fungi	B	2
Dirofilaria spp.	C	3
Dracunculus medinensis	C	3
Ehrlichia spp.	C	3
Entamoeba histolytica	C	3
trophozoites		2
Enterobacteriaceae	B	2
Enterococcus spp.	B	3
Epidermophyton floccosum	B	3
Erysipelothrix spp.	C	2
Eubacterium spp.	B	2
Exophilia (Wangiella) dermatitidis	C	2
Flavobacterium spp.	B	2
Fonsecaea spp.	C	2
Fusarium spp.	B	2
Fusobacterium spp.	B	2
Geotrichum candidum	B	1
Herpes simplex virus	A	3
Histoplasma capsulatum	B	3
Leishmania spp.	C	3
Leptospira spp.	C	3
Listeria spp.	C	2
Loboa loboi	C	2
Madurella spp.	C	2
Malassezia spp.	B	2
Monsonella streptocerca	C	3
Micrococcus spp.	A	1
Microsporum spp.	B	3
Moraxella spp.	B	2
Mucor spp.	A	1
Mycobacterium spp.	B	2
Neisseria spp.	B	2
Neotestudina rosatii	C	2
Nocardia spp.	C	2
Oerskovia spp.	C	2
Onchocerca volvulus	C	3
Papillomaviruses	B	3
Paracoccidioides brasiliensis	C	3
Pasteurella spp.	C	2
Penicillium spp.	B	1
Peptostreptococcus spp.	B	2
Plesiomonas shigelloides	C	2
Poxviruses	B	3
Propionibacterium spp.	A	2
Pseudallescheria boydii	C	2
Pseudomonas spp.	B	2
Rhinocladiella aquaspersa	C	2
Rhizomucor spp.	B	1
Rhizopus spp.	B	1
Rhodococcus spp.	C	2
Rhodotorula spp.	B	1
Rickettsia spp.	B	3
Sarcinosporon inkin	B	2
Scopulariopsis brevicaulis	B	2
Spirillum minus	C	3
Sporothrix schenckii	B	2
Staphylococcus spp.	A	2
Stenotrophomonas (formerly *Xanthomonas*) *maltophilia*	B	2
Streptobacillus moniliformis	C	2
Streptococcus spp.	B	2
Streptomyces somaliensis	C	2
Strongyloides spp.	C	3
Taenia solium cysticerci	C	3
Treponema spp.	B	3
Trichophyton spp.	B	3
Varicella-zoster virus	B	3
Veillonella spp.	B	2
Vibrio spp.	C	2

*A, Commonly encountered in clinical specimens; B, occasionally encountered in clinical specimens; C, rarely encountered in clinical specimens.
†1, When present, it is rarely if ever involved in disease production; 2, when present, it is occasionally involved in disease production; 3, when present, it is commonly involved in disease production.
From Isenberg HD, D'Amato RF: Indigenous and pathogenic microorganisms of humans. *In* Murray PR, Baron EJ, Pfaller MA, et al (eds): Manual of Clinical Microbiology, ed 6. Washington, DC, ASM Press, 1994, pp 5–18.

exceeding 15 mm in diameter. Drying is expedited by placing the slide in a 75°C oven for 15 minutes before Gram staining. The entire smear is examined under oil immersion (×1000); the presence of any organism in any of the fields examined constitutes a positive smear, which correlates with the presence of at least 10^5 CFU/g of tissue.

NORMALLY STERILE BODY FLUIDS[42]

The processing of CSF and thoracocentesis fluid has already been discussed; this section deals only with peritoneal, pericardial, and synovial fluids. Formerly, small aliquots of peritoneal fluid or dialysate were cultured for bacteria and fungi in a routine manner. More recently, centrifugation or filtration concentrates of larger volumes of fluid have been used. Increasing attention has been given to processing peritoneal fluid with the advent of continuous ambulatory peritoneal dialysis. Methods used for microbiologic analysis of continuous ambulatory peritoneal dialysis effluent have been reviewed by von Graevenitz,[43] who found four principal reasons for negative cultures in the presence of at least 100 leukocytes per mm³ effluent: (1) inadequate quantity of fluid examined, (2) use of insufficient media, (3) antimicrobial agents in the peritoneal cavity, and (4) phagocytosis of microorganisms in stored effluent. From his review of the literature, von Graevenitz[43] came to the following conclusions. (1) Yield from broth enrichment was not superior to that from primary agar cultures, although the optimal dilution factor in broth remains undefined. (2) The use of various isolation media with incubation for up to 7 days contributed to the detection of bacteria, mycobacteria, nocardiae, and fungi. (3) Storage of effluent at 4°C for up to 12 hours did not appear to diminish the yield, but surprisingly, neither did storage at room temperature for up to 5 days as long as no antibiotics were present in the effluent. (4) Patients receiving antimicrobial therapy had lower yields from cultures than did those not taking antimicrobial agents. (5) Measures that neutralize antibiotic or phagocytic activity by use of sodium polyanetholesulfonate, Triton X, antimicrobial removal resins, washing of sediment, physical or chemical disruption of phagocytes by sonication, freezing, thawing, or sodium deoxycholate significantly increase yield. (6) Filtration methods carry the risk of filter clogging and contamination. (7) Pour-plate cultures do not increase yield. (8) Lysis-centrifugation methods may be superior to plating of centrifugates in detection of polymicrobial infection and in the speed with which microorganisms can be identified and undergo susceptibility tests.

Although von Graevenitz[43] did not think that data were available to determine the minimal volume that would be sufficient for culture, he and his colleagues[44] found that the yield from centrifuged sediment of 50 mL of dialysate was equivalent to that from 1000 mL of dialysate. Ludlam and colleagues[45] compared direct quantitative cultures without leukocyte lysis with quantitative culture after leukocyte lysis by a proteolytic enzyme and found that culture of the sediment of 50 mL of effluent after lysis provided the best rate of recovery, but they thought that the procedure was technically demanding. Although the value of a Gram-stained smear of the centrifuged sediment has been variable, Ludlam and colleagues[45] found the Gram-stained smear to be positive in about a third of cases. In a comparison of direct inoculation of 10 mL of dialysate into a lysis-centrifugation tube (Isolator), direct inoculation of 5 mL of dialysate into each of two BACTEC blood culture bottles, and centrifugation of 50 mL of dialysate with culture of the sediment, Woods and Washington[46] found that the number of pathogens recovered was greatest by lysis-centrifugation, followed by the BACTEC blood culture method, and finally by centrifugation. Although differences among methods were not statistically significant in this study, culture of 10 mL of effluent by lysis-centrifugation or by the BACTEC system was superior to culture of the centrifuged sediment of 50 mL of effluent. It would appear, therefore, that the culture of 10 mL of effluent in a blood culture system would be a more practical approach to the diagnosis of peritonitis than culture-centrifuged or filtered sediment. Lysis of phagocytes does appear to be helpful and can be accomplished by a variety of techniques summarized by von Graevenitz,[43] including lysis-centrifugation. The Gram-stained smear, if positive, can help direct initial antimicrobial therapy.

The etiology of purulent pericarditis is diverse—aerobic and anaerobic gram-positive and gram-negative bacteria, *Nocardia,* mycobacteria, and fungi—and specimens must be cultured appropriately for this range of pathogenic microorganisms. Similar procedures must be used with synovial fluid, and particular attention must be given to choosing procedures for the isolation of *N. gonorrhoeae* and *H. influenzae.* Anyone who considers using heparinized syringes to collect pericardial or synovial fluid must remember that all commercially available heparin products contain preservatives that could interfere with microbial recovery.

Methods for Detecting Microbes

Microscopy

Microscopic examination of specimens often provides the most rapid means for detecting microorganisms, but it must be understood that the sensitivity of microscopy may be different from that of culture. Simultaneous submission of smears with specimens for cultural analysis should be practiced whenever feasible. For example, the observation of at least two bacteria per oil-immersion field (×1000) in a urine specimen indicates the presence of at least 10^5 CFU/mL. The sensitivity of the Gram-stained smear in this instance is approximately 95%. On the other hand, the sensitivity of the Gram-stained smear of sputum for the diagnosis of pneumococcal pneumonia is only about 50% if a preponderance of lancet-shaped gram-positive diplococci is the criterion for positivity. Obviously, a less strict criterion increases the sensitivity of the Gram-stained smear, but at the expense of specificity. The sensitivity of a Gram-stained smear of CSF from children with meningitis is approximately 75%, whereas that of a Gram-stained smear of peritoneal or ascites fluid in patients with peritonitis is ordinarily about 30% but may be as high as 50%. Urine is not ordinarily concentrated by centrifugation for purposes of microscopic examination for bacteria, whereas other body fluids, including CSF, are. Concentration of normally sterile body fluids, as well as of bronchoalveolar lavage fluid, for purposes of microscopic examination is enhanced by the use of cytocentrifugation.[47, 48] In many clinical laboratories, the sensitivity of acid-fast smears of sputum for tubercle bacilli is approximately 50%, although it varies according to the extent of disease.[49]

The traditional method for detecting *C. neoformans* in CSF has been the microscopic examination of an India ink wet mount preparation, but because the sensitivity of this approach is less than 50%, the latex agglutination test for cryptococcal antigen is now recommended instead. This test requires careful control for the presence of rheumatoid factor, which may cause a false-positive reaction that may be inactivated by a proteolytic enzyme. A potassium hydroxide wet mount preparation may be used to examine sputum and other specimens for *Blastomyces dermatitidis, Coccidioides immitis,* and certain other fungi; potassium hydroxide–calcofluor will enhance detection still further.[50]

Immunofluorescence microscopy, latex agglutination, enzyme immunoassay, and genetic probes are being used with increasing frequency to detect a variety of microorganisms. Specific applications of such techniques have been described in the section on specimen collection, transport, and processing. The decision to use any one of these methods is complex. In rare instances, these approaches represent the only means of detecting the microorganism (e.g., human papillomavirus, hepatitis viruses). In other instances, these approaches increase the speed of detection of microorganisms with fastidious growth requirements. Each of the rapid methods (except those for microorganisms that cannot be detected in culture) requires careful clinical evaluation in comparison with culture. In all instances, careful analysis of the sensitivity, specificity, positive and negative predictive values, and costs of false-negative and false-positive results must be made, taking into account the prevalence of the disease in the population under study. One must be careful to differentiate between a screening test and a confirmatory test. A screening test should have high sensitivity, but it may have low specificity provided that a confirmatory test is available. If no confirmatory test is available, a screening test must be highly sensitive *and* specific. A confirmatory test should generally be highly specific; its sensitivity may vary according to whether a screening test is available. The risk of a false-negative result must be assessed in terms of the impact of missed diagnosis or delayed initiation of therapy and the impact of a false-positive result in terms of the risks of inappropriate therapy and of missing another diagnosis. Other considerations are spectrum bias, the failure to consider the heterogeneity of the diseased and nondiseased populations in assessing test performance; the availability and use of adequate reference standards; the appropriateness of the selection of a specific cutoff point for immunoassays; referral bias, bias that may be introduced when an initially nonreactive or equivocally reactive specimen is retested with a different assay or when equivocal or positive specimens are retested with another assay; sample size; and the level of expertise of those who perform the test.[51]

Reference standards are not always as "golden" as they are thought to be. There is continuing debate about the use of nonselective versus selective media, atmosphere and duration of incubation, and adequacy of the swab procedure for throat cultures for group A streptococci. For *C. difficile,* culture is regarded as highly sensitive but highly nonspecific and the cytotoxin assay as somewhat insensitive but highly specific. Multiple variables, including specimen collection and processing and the culture procedure, affect the sensitivity of culture for *C. trachomatis.* New technologies are often evaluated in laboratories where the evaluating investigators and technologists are expert in the diagnosis of a specific infection. Bias may be introduced by virtue of the expertise or by virtue of the investigators' interest in the product, and their results may not reflect how the product will perform in routine clinical or office laboratory settings or even in the home setting. Assuming that all of the factors involved in a test's evaluation have been studied adequately and that the data indicate that a particular new technology performs satisfactorily, other decisions remain to be made. The first is whether a new immunoassay or genetic probe can be used as a substitute for culture. Are the statistical parameters such that the results of any of these tests are equal to those of culture? If not, the potential value of the probe or immunoassay as a screening test must be carefully assessed. This assessment must take into account not only the added cost of the screening test but any potential value to the patient in terms of initiation of appropriate therapy or to the hospital in terms of reducing length of stay. Although the screening test may increase the cost of detecting a microorganism in the laboratory, a positive result may provide a specific diagnosis and allow initiation of appropriate therapy sooner than would otherwise be the case and could reduce the length of stay in the hospital. In analyzing laboratory costs, it is important to realize that most immunoassay and probe kits are designed to handle 10 or 20 tests concurrently; therefore, maximal cost-effectiveness is achieved only when batches of 10 or 20 tests are processed at a time. Testing a single sample or just a few samples at a time becomes expensive, especially when standard controls must be used to calibrate each run and reagents have a limited shelf life. Thus, for example, the more cost-effective test for single-sample analysis for *C. trachomatis* and *Legionella pneumophila* is immunofluorescence microscopy, whereas immunoassay or a genetic probe is more cost-effective when batches of approximately 20 tests can be processed at one time. Respiratory syncytial virus infection is a situation in which speedy diagnosis accelerates initiation of therapy and may obviate hospitalization and the attendant risk of transmission of infection to other patients; in this case, the higher cost of immunofluorescence (versus culture) may be clinically and epidemiologically justifiable. A rapid method employing immunostaining is now commercially available. A final problem arises when the sensitivity level of a screening test is so low relative to culture that physicians have no confidence in the results and opt to administer therapy on an empirical basis. This phenomenon has been observed with currently available antigen detection tests for group A streptococci in throat swabs, which, although highly specific, may be only 50% sensitive. Experience with these tests demonstrates that although appropriate treatment increases in frequency for children with positive test results, so does the likelihood of inappropriate therapy for children who do not have group A streptococcal pharyngitis, because therapy is administered on the basis of clinical judgment rather than a negative test result.

Genetic probes have been developed experimentally for the detection of plasmid-mediated β-lactamases and plasmid-mediated aminoglycoside-modifying enzymes. Such tests could, therefore, be used to detect the specific resistance mechanisms of microorganisms in clinical specimens. Certain problems are associated with this approach. First, genotypic resistance may not reflect phenotypic resistance. Second, resistance may be due to other mechanisms, such as chromosomal β-lactamases, alterations in penicillin binding proteins, or alterations or deletions of outer membrane proteins (porins). Third, direct specimen testing may reveal a resistance mechanism in the indigenous microbiota but not in the pathogen, so the result will be false-positive.

Microbial Identification

Microorganisms are identified in cultures by a variety of methods, which are described in detail in standard clinical microbiology textbooks.[1] Many bacteria and yeasts are identified by commercially available kits and devices, some of which are semiautomated or automated and combine identification with antimicrobial susceptibility testing in a single process. The major responsibility of the clinical microbiologist is to design procedures that allow isolation of the most likely pathogens by source or site and that limit identification of isolates to those that are clinically important. The microbiologist must make every effort to differentiate among indigenous microbiota, contaminating microorganisms, and pathogenic microorganisms. Reporting the indigenous microorganisms, particularly with their antimicrobial susceptibility, implies that such microorganisms are clinically important and often leads to inappropriate use of antimicrobial agents. For example, only a limited number of bacterial species are proved to be associated with pharyngitis, and *H. influenzae, Staphylococcus aureus,* viridans streptococci, Enterobacteriaceae, and *Neisseria* species other than *N. gonorrhoeae* are not among them. If any or all of these components of the indigenous microbiota of the pharynx are reported, they may be misinterpreted as being clinically significant, and inappropriate therapy may be instituted. To cite another example, the agents of vaginitis are a relatively limited number of bacteria, fungi, and parasites. Although *S. aureus* is unusual in vaginal material except in association with the toxic shock syndrome, other microorganisms such as Enterobacteriaceae are not known to cause vaginitis or cervicitis, and reporting such species may, again, lead to inappropriate therapy. The identification and susceptibility testing of indigenous microorganisms are also terribly time-consuming and use time that might better be devoted to the performance of clinically relevant tests and procedures. The implementation of suitable blood culture systems that can handle inocula of 20 mL of blood is often cited as an excessive expense for the laboratory; however, those same laboratories often spend more money in time identifying indigenous microorganisms and providing useless antimicrobial susceptibility data along with the identification. The microbiologist must set priorities according to the severity of disease and the importance of microbial identification and susceptibility testing of a pathogen in reducing the morbidity or the mortality from an infection. This goal cannot be achieved unless pertinent information about the clinical impression and history is provided by the clinician requesting analysis. There are few more important functions of the microbiology laboratory than optimal detection of the microbial pathogens of septicemia or meningitis and few less important functions than identifying indigenous microbes.

Tests of Antimicrobial Activity

Antimicrobial Susceptibility Testing

INDICATIONS FOR TESTING AND SELECTION OF ANTIMICROBIALS

Antimicrobial susceptibility tests are performed when the susceptibility of a pathogen to commonly employed antimicrobial agents cannot be predicted. Such organisms include staphylococci, the Enterobacteriaceae, *Pseudomonas* species, *Acinetobacter* species, *H. influenzae, S. pneumoniae, Enterococcus* species, and *N. gonorrhoeae. Streptococcus pyogenes* has predictable susceptibility to penicillin, so it does not need to be tested for susceptibility unless a patient is allergic to penicillins and requires alternative therapy such as macrolides or tetracyclines, to which resistance may occur. Susceptibility of anaerobic bacteria to ampicillin-sulbactam, ticarcillin-clavulanate, imipenem, chloramphenicol, and metronidazole is sufficiently predictable that susceptibility testing of the Bacteroidaceae to these antimicrobials is not ordinarily indicated. Standardized procedures have been established by the National Committee for Clinical Laboratory Standards for disk diffusion testing and dilution testing of bacteria that grow under aerobic conditions and for dilution testing of anaerobic bacteria.[52–54] The E-test (AB Biodisc North America, Piscataway, NJ) is now available as a means to determine susceptibility of aerobic and anaerobic microorganisms. These strips are especially useful for anaerobic minimal inhibitory concentrations and for rapid determination of penicillin-tolerant or penicillin-resistant pneumococci.[55]

Susceptibility testing should be limited to bacteria of presumed clinical importance, and the laboratory should minimize testing of indigenous microorganisms whenever possible. Regardless of what method is used for susceptibility testing, it must be understood that the term susceptible implies that an infection due to the isolated microorganism may be treated appropriately with the recommended dosage of antimicrobial to which the organism is susceptible unless it is otherwise contraindicated. The term resistant indicates that the microorganism isolated is not inhibited by safely achievable concentrations of the antimicrobial agent administered at the recommended dosage or that the organism possesses or is likely to possess resistance mechanisms and that therapy with the antimicrobial agent tested is unlikely to be effective. Clearly, antimicrobial activity in vivo depends on multiple factors besides whether the organism is susceptible in vitro—absorption characteristics, volume of distribution, and pharmacokinetics of the antimicrobial; its route of excretion; impairment of renal or hepatic function; extent of its protein binding; degree of postantibiotic effect; administration in combination with another antimicrobial; and the presence of any serious, underlying diseases in the patient, including immunosuppression. In some instances, organisms are reported to be moderately susceptible to a particular antimicrobial agent. Such a report implies that the organism is inhibited by concentrations of the drug (usually a β-lactam) that may be obtainable either by maximal doses or by concentration of the drug in a body site (such as the urinary tract). "Intermediate" is a "buffer zone" that should prevent small, uncontrolled technical factors from causing major errors in interpretation, and it is usually applied to antimicrobial agents with a narrow toxic/therapeutic ratio (e.g., aminoglycosides) that cannot be administered in doses higher than those recommended without serious risk of toxicity. However, most clinical microbiology reports indicate that the organism is susceptible, intermediate, or resistant to a given agent. Clinicians must understand the grading of the microbial response practiced in a specific microbiology laboratory. Changes in interpretation of susceptibility occur with some frequency, advocated to accommodate the laboratory results to clinical experience.

The selection of antimicrobial agents for testing in the laboratory is a complex matter.[56] In principle, the agents to be tested should be selected from those in the hospital formulary. Thus, it is important for the microbiologist to work in coordination with the formulary committee. Unfortunately, the antimicrobials in different hospitals' formularies differ so much that it is often difficult for the microbiologist using a commercially available kit or device for susceptibility testing to obtain complete concordance between what is in the formulary and what is in the kit or device. In some instances, equivalence of activity among agents in a particular category of antimicrobials is so great that the activity of one can be used to predict the activity of others. For example, susceptibility of staphylococci to oxacillin indicates susceptibility to methicillin, nafcillin, and other penicillinase-resistant penicillins. Susceptibility to cephalothin also indicates susceptibility to other first-generation parenteral and oral cephalosporins. Susceptibility of Enterobacteriaceae to cefotaxime also indicates susceptibility to ceftizoxime and ceftriaxone. Conversely, staphylococcal resistance to oxacillin indicates resistance to other penicillinase-resistant penicillins as well as to cephalosporins, imipenem, ampicillin-sulbactam, and ticarcillin-clavulanate. Because some isolates of oxacillin-resistant staphylococci may appear to be susceptible to some cephalosporins in vitro, the laboratory should report such isolates as being resistant not only to oxacillin but also to the other β-lactam antibiotics that have been listed. Cross-resistance or cross-susceptibility among aminoglycosides is not always predictable; the aminoglycoside-modifying enzymes may be specific to one particular agent, although a gram-negative bacillus that is resistant to amikacin is usually resistant to all other aminoglycosides.

Laboratories may elect to selectively report the activity in vitro of certain antimicrobial agents. For example, if a gram-negative bacillus is susceptible to cefazolin or cephalothin, the laboratory may report this result and not report its susceptibility to second- or third-generation cephalosporins, which are no more effective but certainly more expensive. Likewise, if a gram-negative bacillus is susceptible to gentamicin, the laboratory may elect not to report the susceptibilities of the gram-negative bacillus to tobramycin, amikacin, or netilmicin. Such selective reporting becomes unmanageable when microorganisms of differing susceptibilities are propagated in mixed culture. A guideline for selecting antimicrobial agents to be tested against various categories of bacteria that grow aerobically is presented in Table 12–8.

For clinically significant isolates of *H. influenzae,* the first and simplest test to be performed is one for β-lactamase. β-Lactamase–negative isolates should be tested for their susceptibility to ampicillin because ampicillin resistance due to chromosome mutation cannot be detected with a test for β-lactamase. Therapy with ampicillin or amoxicillin may proceed if the β-lactamase test result is negative and the isolate is susceptible to ampicillin. If the isolate does produce β-lactamase or is resistant to ampicillin, further susceptibility testing may or may not be indicated. β-Lactamase–producing isolates of *H. influenzae* are uniformly susceptible to amoxicillin-clavulanate, ampicillin-sulbactam, and ticarcillin-clavulanate, and ampicillin-resistant isolates are uniformly suscepti-

TABLE 12–8 ■ Guidelines for Selection of Antibacterial Agents for Susceptibility Testing*

ANTIMICROBIAL AGENT	STAPHYLOCOCCI	ENTEROCOCCI	NONENTEROCOCCAL STREPTOCOCCI	PSEUDOMONADS	ENTEROBACTERIACEAE
Amikacin				P	P
Ampicillin	S	P			P
Ampicillin-sulbactam (or amoxicillin-	S				S
clavulanate)					S
Azlocillin (or mezlocillin or piperacillin				P	
or ticarcillin)					
Aztreonam				S	S
Cefamandole (or cefonicid or					S
cefuroxime)					
Cefotaxime (or cefoperazone or					P
ceftazidime or ceftizoxime or					
ceftriaxone or moxalactam)				P	
Cefoxitin (or cefotetan)					S
Ceftazidime (or cefoperazone)					
Cephalothin	P†		P		P‡
Chloramphenicol	S			S	S
Ciprofloxacin	S			S	S
Clindamycin	P		P		
Erythromycin	P	U	P		
Gentamicin (or tobramycin)	S	S		P	P
Imipenem				S	S
Mezlocillin (or piperacillin or ticarcillin)					P
Netilmicin				S	S
Oxacillin (or methicillin or nafcillin)	P†				
Penicillin G	P		P		
Tetracycline	S				S, U
Ticarcillin-clavulanate					S
Trimethoprim-sulfamethoxazole	S			S§	P
Vancomycin	P	S			
Cinoxacin (or nalidixic acid)					U
Nitrofurantoin	U	U	U		U
Norfloxacin	U	U	U	U	U
Trimethoprim	U				U

*P, Primary agents to be tested routinely; S, secondary agents to be tested under special circumstances such as in institutions harboring endemic or epidemic resistance to one or more of the primary agents, for treatment of patients who are allergic to a primary agent, or as an epidemiologic aid; U, urinary tract–specific agent to be tested against urinary isolates only.

†Oxacillin (or methicillin or nafcillin)–resistant staphylococci should be considered resistant to cephalosporins, penicillins (including combinations with β-lactamase inhibitors), and imipenem.

‡Gentamicin should be tested at a concentration of 500 or 2000 g/mL to detect highly resistant strains that are not synergistically affected by the combination of a penicillin and gentamicin.

§Applies only to species other than *Pseudomonas aeruginosa*.

ble to third-generation cephalosporins. Confirmed resistance of *H. influenzae* has not yet been reported for third-generation cephalosporins. Chloramphenicol-resistant isolates of *H. influenzae* remain rare in the United States; however, if therapy with chloramphenicol is contemplated, resistance may be determined by the disk diffusion method or most rapidly by a test for chloramphenicol acetyltransferase, the enzyme responsible for inactivating chloramphenicol. Testing of amoxicillin-clavulanate, cefaclor, and trimethoprim-sulfamethoxazole should be limited to isolates of *Haemophilus* from localized, non–life-threatening diseases. Cefuroxime, to which *Haemophilus* susceptibility is unpredictable, poses a unique problem: susceptibility to the parenteral form is defined by a minimal inhibitory concentration of not more than 8 μg/mL, whereas susceptibility to the oral form is not more than 4 μg/mL. Thus, the laboratory must issue its susceptibility report according to the site or source of origin of the isolate.

Of particular concern today is the increasing frequency of antimicrobial resistance of gonococci. Resistance is mediated either by plasmids or by chromosome mutations. Plasmids mediate resistance to the penicillins and tetracyclines; chromosome mutations mediate resistance to β-lactams, tetracyclines, erythromycin, and spectinomycin. Although gene probes have been developed for the detection of plasmids that mediate penicillin resistance, none is yet commercially available, so the detection of penicillinase-producing *N. gonorrhoeae* requires testing isolated colonies with a rapid β-lactamase test. On the other hand, the detection of chromosomally mediated resistance to penicillins requires either disk diffusion or dilution testing of isolated colonies. At this time, clinical laboratories should include β-lactamase testing on a routine basis and may wish to test isolates from treatment failures for their susceptibility to penicillin by the disk diffusion or a dilution method. If the prevalence of chromosomally mediated penicillin resistance in the community is known to be on the order of at least 3% to 5%, susceptibility testing of β-lactamase–negative isolates should be added. Because tetracyclines are no longer recommended primarily for treatment of gonococcal infection, susceptibility testing of isolates to tetracyclines is probably not usually necessary. Susceptibility testing should be performed by either the disk diffusion method or an agar dilution method using GC agar base according to methods described by the National Committee for Clinical Laboratory Standards.[52, 53] Resistance to spectinomycin remains rare in the United States, and resistance to third-generation cephalosporins such as ceftriaxone may be emerging and require laboratory documentation of susceptibility.[57]

Anaerobic bacteria may be tested to determine patterns of

susceptibility in medical centers in the United States; to monitor the emergence of resistance over time in medical centers; and to assist in the antimicrobial management of patients with central nervous system infections, endocarditis, osteomyelitis, joint infections, prosthetic device infections, vascular graft infections, and refractory or recurrent bacteremia.[54] Susceptibility tests of isolates of *M. tuberculosis* are usually performed routinely for the primary drugs used for chemotherapy—isoniazid, streptomycin, rifampin, and ethambutol. In some instances, susceptibility testing may be reserved for isolates from patients with life-threatening disease or at high risk for having resistant strains, but when selective testing is used, isolates should be stored in case the need arises in the future to determine their susceptibility. Although the reference method for susceptibility testing of mycobacteria is usually considered to be the proportion method, it is not practical for routine clinical laboratory use. An alternative method for testing *M. tuberculosis* is the radiometric method. Rapidly growing mycobacteria may be tested by a microdilution or a disk diffusion method. The radiometric method is being adapted to provide accurate results with some *Mycobacterium* species that are slower growing than *M. tuberculosis,* but it is important to ensure that data validating this procedure are available for a specific species-antimicrobial combination before the combination is tested in the clinical laboratory.

Antifungal susceptibility testing is not standardized. Difficulties have arisen in correlating results in vitro with efficacy in vivo. The activity of antifungal agents is both inoculum and medium dependent, and much work needs to be done to establish the various test parameters necessary to produce results that are reproducible in vitro and also clinically meaningful.

Antiviral susceptibility testing is assuming some increasing importance with the finding of acyclovir- and ganciclovir-resistant isolates of herpes simplex virus and cytomegalovirus. Antiviral susceptibility testing remains technically complex, however, and will therefore continue to be performed in research laboratories in the foreseeable future.

SUSCEPTIBILITY TEST VARIABLES

Variations in inoculum size remain the major cause of day-to-day variations in susceptibility test results. Because an increasing number of clinical laboratories have implemented microdilution testing for routine purposes, it is essential that procedures be used that ensure an inoculum of approximately 5×10^5 CFU/mL.[53] In no case should the manufacturer's directions be totally relied on to achieve this level of inoculum; each laboratory must perform the steps necessary to enumerate organisms in the inoculum that they use. Failure to achieve the recommended inoculum of 5×10^5 CFU/mL will lead to false susceptible results with penicillinase-producing staphylococci, oxacillin-resistant staphylococci, and β-lactamase–producing gram-negative bacilli. Currently, the frequency of non–penicillinase-producing staphylococci is sufficiently small that any *Staphylococcus* species for which the minimal inhibitory concentration of penicillin is 0.12 μg/mL or less requires confirmation with a β-lactamase test. A minimal inhibitory concentration for penicillin of 0.12 μg/mL or less for a β-lactamase–producing staphylococcus almost invariably results from an inadequate inoculum size. Another clue to the inadequacy of inoculum can be obtained by reviewing the results of ampicillin activity against *Enterobacter cloacae.* If more than 5% of strains are susceptible, it is likely that the inoculum used in the laboratory was too small.[56]

Another variable that affects the activity of antimicrobial agents against certain organism groups is the cation content of the medium. The activity of aminoglycosides in vitro against *P. aeruginosa* is inversely proportional to the amount of calcium and magnesium in the test medium. Because the Mueller-Hinton broth medium used in laboratories today may be deficient in cation, adjustment of the medium to contain calcium at 20 to 25 mg/L and magnesium at 10 to 12.5 mg/L is recommended.[52] Mueller-Hinton medium must be supplemented with growth requirements for susceptibility testing of *H. influenzae.* Susceptibility testing of gonococci should be performed with GC agar base.[52, 53] For reference purposes, susceptibility of anaerobic bacteria should be tested by the agar dilution technique, using either Wilkins-Chalgren agar or *Brucella* agar; however, because agar dilution is not practical for routine laboratory purposes, a broth microdilution or E test procedures are recommended.[54, 55] Criteria for disk diffusion testing of rapidly growing aerobic bacteria must not be extrapolated to disk diffusion testing of anaerobic bacteria. Instead, the E test with appropriate controls should be used.

Bactericidal Testing

There are several categories of bactericidal test parameters: the minimal bactericidal or lethal concentration, the serum bactericidal titer (Schlichter test), and the time-kill curve. Although each is useful in the investigation of a new antimicrobial agent, their clinical value remains limited owing to problems of technique and considerable difficulty of interpretation. The minimal bactericidal concentration is determined by introducing a specified inoculum of a microorganism into a series of test tubes or wells in a microdilution plate containing serially diluted concentrations of an antimicrobial agent and then incubating them overnight. After 16 or 18 hours of incubation, those tubes or wells that show no visible growth are subcultured onto antibiotic-free medium, which is incubated overnight. The minimal bactericidal concentration is the lowest concentration of antimicrobial that kills at least 99.9% of the initial inoculum. Hypothetically, the minimal bactericidal concentration is the same as or within one or two dilutions of the minimal inhibitory concentration when bactericidal activity has taken place. If the minimal bactericidal concentration exceeds the minimal inhibitory concentration by a factor of 32 or more, the organism is considered to be tolerant. Although tolerant viridans streptococci and pneumococci have been identified on the basis of autolytic defects, the clinical significance of such strains is incompletely understood. A considerable volume of information has been published on tolerant strains of *S. aureus;* nevertheless, variables such as the growth phase of the inoculum, the survival of organisms on the inside wall of the test tube above the meniscus, and the subculture volume can determine whether a strain of *S. aureus* is shown to be tolerant. In other words, the outcome of the test can be affected by how the test is performed. Such variables render the clinical literature that purports to show that "tolerant" staphylococci are associated with more frequent complications or require more protracted therapy virtually impossible to interpret.

Similar test variability, plus lack of consensus on the optimal time for specimen collection and the maximal titer associated with treatment success or failure, makes the clinical literature on the value of the serum bactericidal test difficult to interpret. In most published studies, the number of patients with low serum bactericidal titers is too small for statistical analysis. Obviously, it would be unethical to limit the antibiotic dose to perform the critical experiment needed to assess the true clinical value of the serum bactericidal titer.

The time-kill curve is a research tool that assesses how much of the original inoculum was killed and measures the rate of killing. Because tolerance, particularly of staphylococci, is most accurately demonstrated by a slow rate of killing, it is recommended that a foreshortened time-kill study be used to determine tolerance in staphylococci.[58, 59] Time-kill curves have also been used to study the interaction between combinations of antimicrobial agents and, more specifically, to determine whether the interaction is synergistic, antagonistic, or indifferent. For example, it can be demonstrated that a combination of penicillin plus gentamicin produces statistically significantly greater killing of enterococci than either one alone. This interaction is of considerable importance clinically, because serious enterococcal infections, particularly endocarditis, require such combinations for cure. A more practical approach to the determination of whether synergy will occur between penicillin and either streptomycin or gentamicin can be obtained by determining whether an enterococcus is inhibited by either 2000 μg/mL of streptomycin or 500 μg/mL of gentamicin. Inhibition of the enterococcus by either of these concentrations of aminoglycosides is predictive of a synergistic interaction between that aminoglycoside and penicillin, whereas failure of inhibition is predictive of lack of synergy between that aminoglycoside and penicillin. In this particular case, the clinical laboratory can easily provide results that are analogous to those of a time-kill curve. No simple alternative to the time-kill curve is available for other species of microorganisms.[60–62]

Antibiotic Assay

The concentration of an antimicrobial agent that is achieved in the serum depends not only on the dose administered but also on the route of administration, the formulation or form, the patient's compliance and body weight, the extracellular fluid volume, the extent of protein binding of the antimicrobial agent, the agent's elimination or excretion rate, the disease state, the interaction of the antimicrobial with other drugs being administered, the timing of blood sampling for assay, and the analytic method. Patients for whom antimicrobial assays are usually indicated include those who are receiving prolonged (more than 5 days) antimicrobial therapy, those who do not respond to antimicrobial therapy, those who develop signs or symptoms of ototoxicity or nephrotoxicity while receiving antimicrobial therapy, those with impaired or rapidly changing renal function, those undergoing dialysis, elderly persons, those with cystic fibrosis or burns, those who are obese or have expanded extracellular fluid volume, those who may not comply with prescribed antimicrobial therapy, those with infections at sites where penetration of an antimicrobial may be uncertain or variable (e.g., CSF), those with malabsorption syndromes who are receiving oral antimicrobials, and those with normal renal function (to ensure that peak concentrations are in the recommended therapeutic range and that trough concentrations are not excessive).

In practice, antibiotic assays are most often performed to determine concentrations of antimicrobials that have a narrow toxic/therapeutic ratio, such as the aminoglycosides and vancomycin. Chloramphenicol is another such drug, but the expanded-spectrum cephalosporins have largely replaced it, and relatively few assays for chloramphenicol are performed today. The usual doses, therapeutic ranges, and concentrations associated with potential toxicity of antimicrobials with narrow toxic/therapeutic ratios are listed in Table 12–9.

Assays of antimicrobials with large toxic/therapeutic ratios (e.g., β-lactams) are rarely indicated unless the route of administration or presence of an underlying disease may cause serum levels to differ markedly from the usual range and the infection is in a fluid where penetration is variable or uncertain.

To assay for peak levels, blood should be collected 30 minutes after an intravenous dose, 60 minutes after an intramuscular dose, or 60 to 120 minutes after an oral dose; however, trough levels are more sensitive indicators of decreased clearance and accumulation of drug. If assays cannot be performed immediately, it is recommended that serum specimens be frozen at −70°C or that a β-lactamase be added to prevent inactivation of aminoglycosides by β-lactam antibiotics.

Today, immunoassays are usually performed to determine serum concentrations of aminoglycosides and vancomycin. Such assays are quick, simple, sensitive, and specific. Assays for other antimicrobial agents are generally performed by microbiologic assay or, if the equipment and expertise are available, high-performance liquid chromatography.

This cursory account of clinical microbiology represents an

TABLE 12–9 ■ Factors That Affect Monitoring of Selected Antimicrobials

ANTIMICROBIAL AGENT	USUAL DOSE	DOSAGE INTERVAL (h)	MAXIMAL DOSE (24 h)	NORMAL SERUM HALF-LIFE (h)	MAJOR ROUTE OF ELIMINATION	REMOVED BY DIALYSIS		THERAPEUTIC RANGE (μg/mL)		RECOMMENDED BASIS FOR DOSAGE ADJUSTMENT*
						Hemodialysis	Peritoneal Dialysis	Peak	Trough	
Amikacin	5–7.5 mg/kg	8–12	15 mg/kg	2–3	Renal	Yes	Yes	20–25	5–10	P, T
Gentamicin	1.7 mg/kg	8	5 mg/kg	2–3	Renal	Yes	Yes	4–8	1–2	P, T
Kanamycin	5–7.5 mg/kg	8–12	15 mg/kg	2–3	Renal	Yes	Yes	20–25	5–10	P, T
Netilmicin	2–2.5 mg/kg	8	7.5 mg/kg	2–3	Renal	Yes	Yes	6–10	0.5–2	P, T
Streptomycin	0.5–1 g	8–12	2 g	2–3	Renal	Yes	—	5–20	<5	P, T
Tobramycin	1.7 mg/kg	8	5 mg/kg	2–3	Renal	Yes	Yes	4–8	1–2	P, T
Chloramphenicol	0.5–1 g	6	4 g	4†	Hepatic/renal	Yes	No	15–25	8–10	T
Flucytosine	37.5 mg/kg	6	150 mg/kg	4	Renal	Yes	Yes	100	50	T
TMP-SMX‡										
TMP	5 mg/kg	6	20 mg/kg	11	Renal	Yes	—	≥5	—	P
SMX	25 mg/kg	6	100 mg/kg	13	Renal	Yes	—	≥100	—	P
Vancomycin	0.5–1 g	8–12	2 g	6	Renal	No	Yes	20–40	5–10	T

*P, Peak level; T, trough level. These recommendations are valid when dose interval is no greater than twice the usual. Blood for peak levels should be drawn 30 min after completion of an IV infusion, 1 h after an intramuscular dose, and 1 to 2 h after an oral dose.

†Half-life in children younger than 4 wk can be much prolonged. Half-life is affected only slightly in renal failure but can be greatly prolonged with liver disease.

‡Maximal dosages of trimethoprim-sulfamethoxazole (TMP-SMX) apply to treatment of *Pneumocystis carinii* infection. Serum half-life is shortened in adolescents and children. Measurement of either TMP or SMX alone is sufficient for dosage adjustment.

From Anhalt JP, Wilkowske CJ, Washington JA II: Manual of Antimicrobial Agents, ed 11. Philadelphia, BC Decker, 1989. Reprinted by permission of Mayo Foundation.

effort to present the essential role this discipline plays in the diagnosis of infectious disease. The paramount message of this chapter is the need for constant dialogue between clinicians and microbiologists to provide pertinent information as rapidly and accurately as possible at a time when the financial resources available for all of health care are diminishing and justification for analyses is demanded, often by individuals with little appreciation of the reasons for the performance of examinations. Simultaneously, a variety of heretofore rare or unknown microorganisms are intruding into the intimate biosphere of patients in medical facilities and even in the community, complicating the decision process of clinical microbiologists still further. Usually exaggerated coverage by poorly informed television and printed media commentators of emerging or reemerging pathogens succeeds in creating confusion if not fear among the public, increasing the demand for clinical and laboratory demonstrations of such microorganisms. Only cooperation between the clinician and the laboratorian can maintain the perspective that reassures the public of our awareness of and efforts to control these microorganisms.

References

1. Isenberg HD (ed): Clinical Microbiology Procedures Handbook. Washington, DC, American Society for Microbiology, 1992.
2. Baron EJ, Peterswon LR, Finegold SM: Bailey & Scott's Diagnostic Microbiology, ed 9. St. Louis, CV Mosby, 1994.
3. Garcia LS, Bruckner DA: Diagnostic Medical Parasitology, ed 2. Washington, DC, American Society for Microbiology, 1993.
4. Wilson CB, Smith AL: Rapid tests for the diagnosis of bacterial meningitis. Clin Top Infect Dis 134:56, 1986.
5. Gerber MA, Randolph MF, Chanatry J, et al: Antigen detection tests for streptococcal pharyngitis: Evaluation of sensitivity with respect to true infections. J Pediatr 108:654, 1986.
6. Komaroff A, Pas TM, Aronson MD, et al: The prediction of streptococcal pharyngitis in adults. J Gen Intern Med 1:1, 1986.
7. Dajani AS, Bisno AL, Chung KJ, et al: Prevention of acute rheumatic fever: A statement for health professionals by the Committee on Rheumatic Fever, Endocarditis and Kawasaki Disease of the Council on Cardiovascular Disease in the Young, the American Heart Association. Pediatr Infect Dis J 8:263, 1989.
8. Isenberg HD, Fritsche TR, Lancz G, et al: Lower respiratory tract specimens. *In* Howanitz JH, Howanitz PJ (eds): Laboratory Medicine: Test Selection and Interpretation. New York, Churchill Livingstone, 1991, pp 655–674.
9. Bartlett JG, Ryan KJ, Smith TF, Wilson WR: Laboratory diagnosis of lower respiratory tract infections. *In* Washington JA (ed): Cumitech 7A. Washington, DC, American Society for Microbiology, 1987, pp 1–18.
10. Pezzlo M: Urine culture procedure. *In* Isenberg HD (ed): Clinical Microbiology Procedures Handbook. Washington, DC, American Society for Microbiology, 1992, pp 1.17.1–1.17.15.
11. Mobley HLT, Warren JW: Urinary Tract Infections: Molecular Pathogenesis and Clinical Management. Washington, DC, American Society for Microbiology, 1995.
12. Pezzlo M: Detection of urinary tract infections by rapid methods. Clin Microbiol Rev 1:268, 1988.
13. Jenkins RD, Fenn JP, Matsen JM: Review of urine microscopy for bacteriuria. JAMA 255:3397, 1986.
14. Kunin C: Detection, Prevention and Management of Urinary Tract Infections, ed 4. Philadelphia, Lea & Febiger, 1987, p 60.
15. Warren JW, Tenney JH, Hoopes JM, et al: Prospective microbiologic study of bacteriuria in patients with chronic indwelling urethral catheters. J Infect Dis 146:719, 1982.
16. Tenney JH, Warren JW: Bacteriuria in women with long-term catheters: Comparison of indwelling and replacement catheters. J Infect Dis 157:199, 1988.
17. Dallabetta G, Hook EW: Gonococcal infections. Infect Dis Clin North Am 1:25, 1987.
18. Granato PA, Roefaro Franz MA: Evaluation of a prototype DNA probe test for the noncultural diagnosis of gonorrhea. J Clin Microbiol 27:632, 1989.
19. Boyle JF: Laboratory diagnosis of chlamydial infections: Introduction. *In* Isenberg HD (ed): Clinical Microbiology Procedures Handbook. Washington, DC, American Society for Microbiology, 1992.
20. Schracter J, Stamm WE: *Chlamydia*. *In* Murray PR, Baron EJ, Pfaller MA, et al (eds): Manual of Clinical Microbiology, ed 6. Washington, DC, ASM Press, 1994, pp 669–677.
21. Peterson E: Isolation of *Chlamydia* spp in cell culture. *In* Isenberg HD (ed): Clinical Microbiology Procedures Handbook. Washington, DC, American Society for Microbiology, 1992.
22. Boyle JF, Clarke LM: Direct assays for the laboratory diagnosis of chlamydial infections. *In* Isenberg HD (ed): Clinical Microbiology Procedures Handbook. Washington, DC, American Society for Microbiology, 1992.
23. Stamm WE: Diagnosis of *Chlamydia trachomatis* genitourinary infections. Ann Intern Med 108:710, 1988.
24. Norris JN, Larsen SA: Treponema and other host-associated spirochetes. *In* Murray PR, Baron EJ, Pfaller MA, et al (eds): Manual of Clinical Microbiology, ed 6. Washington, DC, ASM Press, 1994, pp 636–651.
25. Clarke LM: Laboratory diagnosis of viral and rickettsial infections: Introduction. *In* Isenberg HD (ed): Clinical Microbiology Procedures Handbook. Washington, DC, American Society for Microbiology, 1992, pp 8.1.1–8.1.6.
26. Clarke LM, McPhee JM, Cummings RV: Isolation of viruses in conventional tube culture: Selection and inoculation of cell cultures. *In* Isenberg HD (ed): Clinical Microbiology Procedures Handbook. Washington, DC, American Society for Microbiology, 1992, pp 8.5.1–8.5.13.
27. Wold AD: Shell vial assay for the rapid detection of viral infections. *In* Isenberg HD (ed): Clinical Microbiology Procedures Handbook. Washington, DC, American Society for Microbiology, 1992, pp 8.6.1–8.6.10.
28. Keller EW: Detection and identification of viruses by immunofluoresecense. *In* Isenberg HD (ed): Clinical Microbiology Procedures Handbook. Washington, DC, American Society for Microbiology, 1992, pp 8.9.1–8.9.10.
29. Fredricsson B, Frisk Å, Hagström B, et al: Vaginal mycoses: Aspects on diagnosis and their treatment with econazole nitrate. Curr Ther Res 27:309, 1980.
30. Holst E, Wathne B, Hovelius B, Mårdh P-A: Bacterial vaginosis: Microbiological and clinical findings. Eur J Clin Microbiol 6:536, 1987.
31. Krohn MA, Hillier SL, Eschenbach DA: Comparison of methods for diagnosing bacterial vaginosis among pregnant women. J Clin Microbiol 27:1266, 1989.
32. Amsel R, Totten PA, Spiegel CA, et al: Nonspecific vaginitis: Diagnostic criteria and microbial and epidemiologic associations. Am J Med 74:14, 1983.
33. Mackowiak PA, Jones SR, Smith JW: Diagnostic value of sinustract cultures in chronic osteomyelitis. JAMA 239:2772, 1978.
34. Wheat J, Allen SD, Henry M, et al: Diabetic foot infections: Bacteriologic analysis. Arch Intern Med 146:1935, 1986.
35. Bamberger DM, Daus GP, Gerding DM: Osteomyelitis in the feet of diabetic patients: Long-term results, prognostic factors, and the role of antimicrobial and surgical therapy. Am J Med 83:653, 1987.
36. Washington JA II: The microbiology of musculoskeletal infection. Orthop Clin North Am 6:115, 1975.
37. Summanen P, Baron EJ, Citron DM, et al: Wadsworth Anaerobic Bacteriology Manual, ed 5. Belmont, CA, Star Publishing, 1993.
38. Strain B: Quantitative bacteriology: Tissues and aspirates. *In* Isenberg HD (ed): Clinical Microbiology Procedures Handbook. Washington, DC, American Society for Microbiology, 1992, pp 1.16a.1–1.16a.4.
39. Raahav D, Friis-Møller A, Bjerre-Jepsen K, Thiis-Knudsen J: The infective dose aerobic and anaerobic bacteria in postoperative wound sepsis. Arch Surg 121:924, 1986.
40. Marshall KA, Edgerton MT, Rodeheaver GT, et al: Quantitative microbiology: Its application to hand injuries. Am J Surg 131:730, 1976.
41. Cooney WP III, Fitzgerald RH Jr, Dobyns JH, Washington JA II: Quantitative wound cultures in upper extremity trauma. J Trauma 22:112, 1982.
42. Isenberg HD, D'Amato RF: Indigenous and pathogenic microorganisms of humans. *In* Murray PR, Baron EJ, Pfaller MA, et al

(eds): Manual of Clinical Microbiology, ed 6. Washington, DC, ASM Press, 1994, pp 5–18.
43. von Graevenitz A: Is there an optimal methodology for the microbiological analysis of effluent in CAPD peritonitis? Zentralbl Bakteriol Mikrobiol Hyg A 267:331, 1988.
44. Hächler H, Vogt K, Binswanger U, von Graevenitz A: Centrifugation of 50 ml of peritoneal fluid is sufficient for microbiological examination in continuous ambulatory peritoneal dialysis (CAPD) patients with peritonitis. Infection 14:102, 1986.
45. Ludlam HA, Price TNC, Berry HA, Phillips I: Laboratory diagnosis of peritonitis in patients on continuous ambulatory peritoneal dialysis. J Clin Microbiol 26:1757, 1988.
46. Woods GS, Washington JA II: Comparison of methods for processing dialysate in suspected continuous ambulatory peritoneal dialysis–associated peritonitis. Diagn Microbiol Infect Dis 7:155, 1987.
47. Shanholtzer CJ, Schaper PJ, Peterson LR: Concentrated Gram stains prepared with a Cytospin centrifuge. J Clin Microbiol 16:1052, 1982.
48. Gill VJ, Nelson NA, Stock F, Evans G: Optimal use of the cytocentrifuge for recovery and diagnosis of *Pneumocystis carinii* in bronchoalveolar lavage and sputum specimens. J Clin Microbiol 26:1641, 1988.
49. Kim TC, Lackman RS, Heatwole KN, Rochester D: Acid-fast bacilli in sputum smears of patients with pulmonary tuberculosis: Prevalence and significance of negative smears pretreatment and positive smears posttreatment. Am Rev Respir Dis 129:264, 1984.
50. Pasareh L, Schell WA: Potassium hydroxide–calcofluor white procedure. *In* Isenberg HD (ed): Clinical Microbiology Procedures Handbook. Washington, DC, American Society for Microbiology, 1992, pp 6.4.1–6.4.2.
51. Washington JA: Evaluation of new in vitro diagnostic test procedures in clinical microbiology. Infect Control Hosp Epidemiol 10:77, 1989.
52. National Committee for Clinical Laboratory Standards: Performance Standard for Antimicrobial Disk Susceptibility Tests, ed 5. Villanova, PA, NCCLS, 1990. NCCLS document M2-A4.
53. National Committee for Clinical Laboratory Standards: Methods for Dilution Antimicrobial Susceptibility Tests for Bacteria That Grow Aerobically, ed 3. Villanova, PA, NCCLS, 1990. NCCLS document M7-A2.
54. National Committee for Clinical Laboratory Standards: Methods for Antimicrobial Susceptibility Testing of Anaerobic Bacteria, ed 2. Villanova, PA, NCCLS, 1989. NCCLS publication M11-T2.
55. Novak SM: E-test susceptibility testing. *In* Isenberg HD (ed): Clinical Microbiology Procedures Handbook. Washington, DC, American Society for Microbiology, 1992, pp 5.2a.1–5.2a.17.
56. Hindler J, Barriere SL: Selecting antimicrobial agents for testing and reporting. *In* Isenberg HD (ed): Clinical Microbiology Procedures Handbook. Washington, DC, American Society for Microbiology, 1992, pp 5.24.1–5.24.14.
57. Jorgensen JH, Sahm DF: Antimicrobic susceptibility testing: General considerations. *In* Murray PR, Baron EJ, Pfaller MA, et al (eds): Manual of Clinical Microbiology, ed 6. Washington, DC, ASM Press, 1994, pp 1277–1280.
58. Handwerger S, Tomasz A: Antibiotic tolerance among clinical isolates of bacteria. Rev Infect Dis 7:368, 1985.
59. Sherris JC: Problems in in vitro determination of antibiotic tolerance in clinical isolates. Antimicrob Agents Chemother 30:633, 1986.
60. Knapp C, Moody JA: Tests to assess bactericidal activity. *In* Isenberg HD (ed): Clinical Microbiology Procedures Handbook. Washington, DC, American Society for Microbiology, 1992, pp 5.16.1–5.16.33.
61. Griffin J: Serum inhibitory and bactericidal filters. *In* Isenberg HD (ed): Clinical Microbiology Procedures Handbook. Washington, DC, American Society for Microbiology, 1992, pp 5.17.1–5.17.18.
62. Moody JH: Synergism testing: Broth microdilution checker board and broth macrodilution methods. *In* Isenberg HD (ed): Clinical Microbiology Procedures Handbook. Washington, DC, American Society for Microbiology, 1992, pp 5.18.1–5.18.28.

13

Immunodiagnosis

Noel R. Rose

Since the remarkable specificity of antigen-antibody reactions was recognized at the end of the 19th century, a number of diagnostic tests based on immunologic specificity have been developed. We employ the term immunodiagnosis as more appropriate than the older term serodiagnosis, because some of the most important procedures measure cell-mediated rather than humoral immunity. Immunodiagnosis implies evaluation of total immune response rather than simply the study of the antibody products of the immune response found in the serum. Two different approaches to the application of immunologic methods should be distinguished: (1) a known antigen is employed to detect an immune response in patients' serum; (2) an antibody of defined specificity serves as reagent for the identification of the corresponding pathogen. Both of these principal applications of immunologic methods are discussed in this chapter.

Measurement of the Immune Response

Under favorable circumstances, the etiologic diagnosis of infectious disease is based on the isolation and identification of the causative agent. Frequently, we seek indirect evidence of infection by demonstrating an antibody response in the serum of a patient or by performing a skin test on the patient. For such a test for an infectious disease, it is necessary to make a reasonable speculation about the causative agent, based on either clinical or epidemiologic findings. The appropriate antigen or antigens can then be used as a reagent for measuring antibodies in serum or for eliciting skin test reactions.

Because of their outstanding sensitivity and specificity, antigen-antibody reactions lend themselves to diagnostic applications. In an immunochemical sense, *sensitivity* refers to the ability of an immunologic reagent to detect small amounts of antigen, whereas *specificity* describes the selective reaction between antigen and its corresponding antibody. The great sensitivity of antibody-mediated reactions allows the detection of minuscule amounts of antibody, which is often useful for demonstrating a response early in the course of disease or a long time after an infection. The specificity of antibody reactions permits precise delineation of the antigen responsible for the immune response. It must be remembered, however, that a given antigen can be represented on a number of different microorganisms. Although the antigen-antibody reaction itself is specific, the identification of the antibody may sometimes be ambiguous.

The terms sensitivity and specificity are defined somewhat differently in a clinical or statistical context. Sensitivity is defined as the proportion of subjects with the disease who have a positive test for the disease. Specificity is the proportion of subjects without the disease who have a negative test. Equally important in evaluating a test is its *predictive value.* Positive predictive value is the probability of disease in a patient with a positive test result. Negative predictive value is the probability of not having the disease if the test result is negative or normal. The predictive value, therefore, is determined by the sensitivity and specificity of the test and the prevalence of disease in the population being studied.

In evaluating antibody-mediated reactions, the terms false-negative and false-positive are often employed. *False-negative* refers to the fact that antibody may not always be present in diagnostic quantities in cases of the disease. A false-negative result may represent a problem in sampling (for example, the serum specimen may have been taken too early in the course of infection) or a defect in the patient's immune response. The antigen preparation itself may not be appropriate for the individual case, because different patients recognize different antigenic determinants. False-negative results, therefore, limit the sensitivity of serologic methods.

A distinction is sometimes made between biologic false-positive and technical false-positive reactions. Technical false-positive results accrue from faults in the test procedure itself; for example, ill patients sometimes produce acute-phase reactants, such as C-reactive protein, that mimic in some respects the antigen-antibody reactions. Rheumatoid factors representing antibody to the immunoglobulin molecule may invalidate serologic tests. In fact, high levels of globulins themselves may result in a nonspecific interaction between a patient's serum and antigen. Biologic false-positive results, on the other hand, are not really false but reflect the fact that the same antigenic determinant may appear on a number of different pathogens. False-positive results, then, may compromise the specificity of serologic diagnosis.

Because the predictive value of a test depends on prevalence, it varies with the population to which it is applied. For example, even with a very specific test, positive results applied to a disease of low prevalence are more likely to be false-positives. Conversely, negative results, even with a very sensitive test, are likely to be false-negatives when applied to a disease of higher prevalence. Thus, the interpretation of an immunodiagnostic test depends on the setting.

The first immunodiagnostic procedure based on the demonstration of an antibody response in patients' serum was described by Widal in 1896, when he showed that the serum of patients suffering from typhoid fever agglutinated typhoid bacilli. His test, which is still a cornerstone of the diagnosis of typhoid fever, depends on the fact that typhoid bacilli are antigenically homogeneous. Were there many different antigenic types of typhoid bacilli, it would be impractical to demonstrate antibody by such a test. Usually it is not feasible to perform a Widal-type test for other salmonelloses, because there are many different antigenic varieties of *Salmonella.* Unless there is information to suggest which species of *Salmonella* is likely involved in a particular case, all 1500 serotypes would have to be tested. Sometimes an organism isolated from patients in an outbreak, or even from an individual patient, can be used as antigen in a Widal-type test for *Salmonella* infection. Another problem is that gram-negative bacilli share many somatic and flagellar antigens. Because so many antigens are shared among related or even unrelated microorganisms, normal persons have a low level of antibody to most pathogens. Therefore, antibody-based diagnosis generally depends on demonstrating a rise in antibody titer during the course of the disease. A comparison of titers of "acute" and "convalescent" serum specimens taken at least 2 weeks apart is a most important criterion for establishing the diagnosis. A fourfold increase in titer is usually indicative of current infection. If only a single sample is available, a high titer of antibody—well beyond the range found in normal persons—is required.

In addition to antigen specificity, the class of an antibody provides important clinical information. Immunoglobulin M (IgM) antibodies generally appear 7 to 10 days after infection and reach a peak after 2 or 3 weeks. The titer then drops, and immunoglobulin G (IgG) antibodies follow, which may persist in the patient's serum for long periods. IgM antibody, therefore, generally represents recent infection, whereas IgG antibody may reflect infection in the past. IgG antibody is capable of crossing the placenta from mother to fetus, but IgM antibody is not. The presence of IgG antibody in cord serum, therefore, may be a reflection of antibody in the maternal serum. IgM antibody in the serum of a newborn is taken as evidence of antibody production by the infant.

There are other instances when the class of antibody is important; for example, the presence of immunoglobulin A (IgA) antibody in infections involving mucosal surfaces indicates a local response. IgA antibody in fecal specimens is sometimes useful in documenting intestinal infections such as cholera or poliomyelitis.

There are instances when the absence of antibody in the face of infection must be interpreted with caution. Infants, for example, are usually unable to produce antibody against carbohydrate antigens such as bacterial capsules. Patients receiving immunosuppressive drugs may also fail to produce antibody to a variety of antigenic stimuli. In fact, the absence of antibody to common antigens and the failure to produce antibody after appropriate stimuli are important for the diagnosis of immunodeficiency disease.

Immunodeficient patients often fail to produce antibodies when given a powerful antigenic stimulus, such as tetanus toxoid or pneumococcus polysaccharide. They may even lack the "natural" blood group antibodies, anti-A and anti-B. Infection with human immunodeficiency virus leads to a decrease in $CD4^+$ T cells, which serve as helpers for antibody formation. Patients with acquired immunodeficiency syndrome often produce relatively weak IgM antibodies and fail to produce IgG antibodies on stimulation, because $CD4^+$ T cells are needed for isotype class switching.

In addition to using antibody, it is possible to use skin test reactions for the indirect diagnosis of infectious disease. Two types of skin tests can be employed. In the case of diseases such as diphtheria and scarlet fever, the symptoms are due to a discrete exotoxin. A toxin neutralization skin test can be performed. Microorganisms that are primarily intracellular in their habitat often induce cell-mediated responses. They can be measured by means of the delayed hypersensitivity skin test.

Identification of Microorganisms

Defined antisera are widely used in medical microbiology for the identification of microorganisms. Labeled antisera may be applied directly to specimens from the patient, including body fluids and tissue. Such methods are often of great value because they can provide an immediate diagnosis.

Another application of antibody reagents is the identification of microorganisms in culture. The identification of viral isolates, for example, frequently depends on the ability of an antiserum to neutralize some discernible effect of the cultured virus. An additional use of defined antibodies is in grouping and typing of microorganisms. Identification of the serotypes of *Salmonella* is possible only by the application of a panel of defined serologic reagents.

There has been a great effort to apply molecular methodology rather than antibody probes to the identification of microorganisms directly in specimens from patients. Molecular testing can be divided into two approaches: the use of DNA probes to detect directly a specific target sequence or nucleic acid amplification to detect specific target DNA or RNA. The direct use of DNA probes is now widely accepted as a rapid approach to identifying certain specific pathogens in tissues or cultures. Amplification techniques are more sensitive but subject to false-positives caused by contamination.

Antibody Response

Neutralization

From a theoretical point of view, the antibodies most relevant to infectious diseases are those that neutralize the pathogenic effects of the microorganism. In the case of toxigenic diseases, such as tetanus, diphtheria, and *Clostridium difficile* gastroenteritis, direct tests of toxin neutralization are feasible in specially equipped laboratories. It has proved to be simpler and less expensive, however, to measure the toxin immunochemically, using one of the immunoassays to be discussed subsequently. In the past, mouse protection tests were the standard procedure for identifying type-specific antibodies to pneumococci, but this method has also been largely replaced by simpler immunochemical procedures in vitro. Viruses that produce obvious cytopathic effects in tissue culture, such as those of measles and mumps, lend themselves to neutralization tests, which are both sensitive and specific. They require, however, that stocks of living virus be available in the laboratory. Rather than by cytopathic effects, some viruses can be detected by their ability to produce hemagglutination. Hemagglutination inhibition reactions are used for measurement of antibodies to influenza virus, adenovirus, and rubella virus. *Mycoplasma* infection produces measurable metabolic changes in infected cells, so that metabolic inhibition tests can be performed for this group of organisms.

Neutralization tests can also be performed with major bacterial products that produce biologic effects. The β-hemolytic streptococcus is remarkable for the number of biologically active secretions it produces. Antibodies to streptolysin O, to DNase B, streptokinase, and hyaluronidase are conveniently measured in the diagnostic laboratory and are useful as evidence of current or recent streptococcal infection. Their greatest application is in the diagnosis of sequelae of streptococcal infection, such as glomerulonephritis and rheumatic fever.

Another approach is to measure the direct effect of antibody on the living microorganism. The original demonstration of antibody-directed, complement-mediated bacteriolysis was carried out by Pfeiffer using *Vibrio cholerae,* and this method is still used occasionally in specialized laboratories. Complement-mediated lysis of *Neisseria meningitidis* is sometimes a useful procedure, not only for demonstrating the presence of antibody but also for determining the integrity of the complement system in a patient's serum. Persons with deficiency in the later components of the complement cascade are inordinately susceptible to meningococcal infections. Opsonization followed by phagocytosis is mediated by antibody to the microbial surface and is a useful technique for measuring protective antibody to *Brucella.*

Agglutination

Agglutination occurs when antibody molecules combine with particulate antigens. The most commonly used particulate antigens are whole bacterial cells and red blood cells. The ready availability of standardized suspensions of killed bacteria enables the clinical laboratory to make an indirect diagnosis of an infectious disease even when the pathogen cannot be isolated from the patient. A rising titer of antibody during the progression and resolution of the illness is an indication of infection with that organism.

The so-called febrile agglutination test uses a panel of possible pathogens to identify the microorganism against which there is the most marked immunologic response. The panel is made up of organisms that are appropriate for the patient's symptoms and correspond with local epidemiologic findings. A typical panel may be composed of suspensions of *Salmonella typhi* (both H and O antigen suspensions are usually included), other *Salmonella* species prevalent in the particular community, *Brucella, Yersinia pestis,* and *Francisella tularensis.* In addition, *Proteus vulgaris* suspensions are included because of their cross-reaction with certain rickettsiae, as represented by the Weil-Felix reaction to be described later. Similar agglutination reactions are sometimes performed with suspensions of *Bordetella pertusis, V. cholerae, Listeria monocytogenes,* and *Leptospira icterohaemorrhagiae* if there is clinical evidence of infection by one of these organisms.

The interpretation of the results of these diagnostic agglutination tests requires considerable knowledge and experience. Several points must be kept in mind:

1. Microorganisms, particularly gram-negative bacilli, share many antigens, so the presence of even a high titer of antibody is not necessarily indicative of infection by that particular species.
2. A test result usually does not become positive until 2 or 3 weeks after infection. Therefore, a negative result early in disease does not exclude the diagnosis.
3. Antibodies may persist long after infection has subsided or may be produced by previous vaccination. A high titer of antibody, therefore, is not always indicative of current infection.

The interpretation of agglutination tests, therefore, depends much on the clinical situation and past history of the patient.

Some of the most useful agglutination tests depend on the presence of shared antigens. Members of the typhus spotted fever and scrub typhus groups of *Rickettsia* share some antigens with certain strains of *Proteus,* providing the basis for the Weil-Felix reaction referred to before. Patients with *Mycoplasma* pneumonia generally produce high titers of cold hemagglutinins that act on normal human erythrocytes, and patients with infectious mononucleosis produce heterophil antibodies to sheep and ox erythrocytes.

Precipitation

When a soluble antigen comes in contact with its corresponding antibody in solution, antigen-antibody complexes result, which may become insoluble. Precipitation is highly dependent on the proportions of antibody and antigen, as well as the temperature, salt concentration, and pH of the solution. Therefore, precipitation reactions must be carried out under carefully controlled conditions. In particular, it must be remembered that precipitation can be inhibited by an excess of antigen, so a range of antigen concentrations must be tested. In addition, precipitation is relatively insensitive as a measure of antibody, although it may be quite sensitive as far as testing antigen is concerned.

Originally, precipitin reactions were carried out in fluid media. Under these conditions, however, it is not possible to distinguish different antigen-antibody combinations that occur simultaneously in the same tube. Therefore, precipitin reactions are now usually carried out in gelified media. An advantage of precipitation in agar, in addition to separating individual reactions, is that it is possible to relate an unknown antigen-antibody reaction with a known one. One can definitively identify antibodies to pathogenic fungi, such as *Blastomyces, Coccidioides,* and *Aspergillus,* and parasites, such as *Entamoeba, Trypanosoma, Trichinella,* and *Echinococcus,* by reactions of identity in agar. In addition, antibodies to important constituents of microorganisms, such as staphylococcal teichoic acid, can be precisely identified by precipitation in gel, because the patient's serum forms a single precipitin line of identity with the positive control serum and purified teichoic acid.

Counterimmunoelectrophoresis makes use of endosmotic flow to concentrate antigen and antibody at an interface. During electrophoresis, the slow-moving immunoglobulins migrate toward the cathode while most antigens move in a concentrated front toward the anode. By appropriate arrangement of wells, antigen and antibody can thus be made to collide, forming a precipitate between the two wells. The precipitation lines develop rapidly, usually giving maximum intensity within 30 to 90 minutes, depending on the strength of the reagents. This technique provides a sensitive measure of antigens of mycotic pathogens such as *Cryptococcus* and can be applied to cerebrospinal fluid. Bacterial antigens from *N. meningitides, Haemophilus influenzae* type b, and *Streptococcus pneumoniae* can also be demonstrated in cerebrospinal fluid by counterimmunoelectrophoresis.

Methodologically, flocculation tests resemble precipitin reactions. The Venereal Disease Research Laboratory (VDRL) test for syphilis contains as antigen cardiolipin fortified with cholesterol and lecithin. The test measures both IgG and IgM antibodies formed by the host in response to release of cardiolipin from damaged host cells during syphilitic infection as well as to the lipid of the treponeme itself. Antibody acts on this lipidic suspension to produce visible floccules, which can be seen either macroscopically or microscopically. Because of its sensitivity, the VDRL test is widely used as an exclusionary screening test. With cerebrospinal fluid, it is valuable in the diagnosis of neurosyphilis. For large-scale screening programs, the highly sensitive rapid plasma reagin test is widely used, but it is usually combined with a less sensitive confirmatory test.

Conditioned, Indirect, or Passive Agglutination

The greater sensitivity and convenience of agglutination testing rather than of precipitin reactions have encouraged the development of methods to convert precipitation to agglutination. This is done by attaching the soluble antigen to an inert particle. The most widely used carrier is the red blood cell, but latex, bentonite, and even collodion particles have been used. The red blood cells may be used in their native state or fixed. Fixation not only increases the life span of the red blood cell but sometimes removes native cell surface antigens to which the patient might have antibodies. Alternatively, when fresh red blood cells can be employed, complement-mediated lysis with consequent release of hemoglobulin can be used as an indication of antigen-antibody interaction at the red blood cell surface.

The first requirement in developing a passive hemagglutination reaction is to coat the red blood cell. Some substances adhere to red blood cells spontaneously, but most require chemical coupling, which may be effected by treating the cells with tannic acid or chromic chloride or by covalently bonding the antigen with bisdiazotized benzene or some similar linker. Sometimes carbohydrates and lipopolysaccharides bind directly to red blood cells without chemical linkage. The coated cells must then be washed thoroughly to remove any soluble antigen and added to dilutions of serum. Antibody titers are determined exactly by agglutination.

Among the antigens that are often used in passive hemagglutination tests are pneumococcus and *Meningococcus* polysaccharides and capsular antigens of *Y. pestis* and *H. influenzae* type b. Protein antigens, such as diphtheria and tetanus toxins and the Vi antigen of the typhoid bacillus, lend themselves to passive hemagglutination. Antibodies to *Treponema pallidum* can be detected by using a microhemagglutination assay. Latex particles have proved useful carriers for a number of microbial antigens, including those of *Histoplasma, Cryptococcus,* and other systemic fungi and *Entamoeba histolytica* and other parasitic protozoa.

A related method that has been exploited extensively is coagglutination. It employs selected strains of staphylococci that express protein A on their surface. This surface protein binds the Fc portion of an antibody molecule. Such antibody-coated staphylococcal organisms readily take up the corresponding antigen and provide an appropriate coated particle for agglutination reactions. The method has proved to be a useful adjunct for the diagnosis of gonorrhea.

Complement Fixation

The complement fixation reaction is valuable if the antigen is not present in a readily accessible or purified form. It represents a highly sensitive technique for measuring low concentrations of antibody. Because each antibody molecule may trigger the activation of hundreds of complement molecules, a considerable amplification of the antigen-antibody reaction can be achieved.

The test is performed in two stages. In the first, antigen-antibody mixtures are incubated with a measured amount of complement; in the second stage, a suspension of sheep red blood cells sensitized with rabbit antibody to sheep red blood cells is added as an indicator system to detect free or unfixed complement after the original antigen-antibody reaction. Complement can be measured most accurately by determining the quantity necessary to lyse 50% of a standard suspension of antibody-coated red blood cells. The test then can be quantitated by measuring the amount of complement actually consumed. Alternatively, the dilution of serum able to give 50% fixation of a standard quantity of complement with a previously determined optimal dilution of antigen can be determined.

The complement fixation test is rather intricate, because it depends on the standardization of a number of reagents; however, the indicator system is the same for all tests used. The only difference is in the antigen employed. Therefore, once the complement fixation method has been established in a laboratory, it is readily applicable to a number of different tests. A major drawback of complement fixation is that certain human sera are anticomplementary, that is, they inactivate complement directly. Anticomplementarity may be due to the presence of circulating antigen-antibody complexes, to elevated levels of immunoglobulin, or to unknown factors in the serum. In any case, it invalidates the complement fixation test.

Historically, the greatest application of complement fixation has been for serologic diagnosis of syphilis. The antigen employed in the test is cardiolipin, which was originally obtained as an alcohol extract of beef heart. Complement fixation is particularly appropriate as a test for syphilis because the sensitivity and specificity are readily adjusted. For screening purposes it is often necessary to have a highly sensitive test, that is, one that detects all patients suffering from the disease. Such tests inevitably have a high proportion of false-positive results. For diagnosis, on the other hand, a more specific test may be advantageous to determine only the active cases of syphilis. It is important that both the immunologist and the clinician agree on the optimal sensitivity/specificity ratio of the test in particular circumstances.

The list of other pathogens to which the complement fixation method has been applied is lengthy. It includes bacteria such as *Bordetella, Listeria, Neisseria,* and *Nocardia;* fungi such as *Aspergillus, Blastomyces, Coccidioides,* and *Histoplasma; Chlamydia; Rickettsia;* and viruses, including herpes simplex virus, cytomegalovirus, respiratory syncytial virus, adenovirus, and influenza virus.

Immunofluorescence and Immunoenzyme Procedures

Antigen-antibody reactions can be visualized directly by labeling either antigen or antibody with an appropriate marker. Possible markers are fluorochromes, enzymes, and electron-opaque substances. In the diagnostic immunology laboratory, fluorescein isothiocyanate is the most commonly used reagent. Fluorochromes absorb radiation (e.g., ultraviolet light) and emit visible light. Immunofluorescence techniques, therefore, require a special microscope capable of admitting ultraviolet light. As a method for demonstrating antibodies, immunofluorescence is highly versatile. Indirect immunofluorescence is performed by adding a patient's serum to a slide containing the appropriate microorganism. The microorganism might be obtained from a pure culture, a tissue culture, or a tissue section. After the serum is incubated with this substrate, the slide is washed and a fluorescein-labeled antiglobulin reagent is added. The slide is washed again, mounted, and studied under an ultraviolet microscope. If antibodies are present in the serum, the microorganism will be seen to fluoresce brightly.

Immunofluorescence is widely used for organisms that cannot be grown in pure culture. *T. pallidum* has yet to be cultured; however, the organism can be grown in the rabbit testis and films prepared on slides for an indirect immunofluorescence reaction, referred to as the fluorescent treponemal antigen test. A further refinement of the test is necessary because many human sera contain antibodies to treponemes, presumably induced by the common spirochetal inhabitants of the mouth. Therefore, the fluorescent treponemal antibody absorption test has been developed. In this procedure, the patient's serum is first absorbed with a suspension of nonpathogenic treponemes and then tested by the fluorescent antibody method. Because the method is rather complex and expensive, it is reserved for confirmatory testing when the clinical signs or history disagree with the rapid plasma reagin, VDRL, or other nontreponemal test results.

The indirect fluorescent antibody test has proved to be equally useful for the serologic diagnosis of many viral infections, such as infectious mononucleosis. The viral capsid antigen is present in cultured cells harboring Epstein-Barr virus. Smears of these cells are prepared, along with controls of uninfected cell lines; they are treated with the patient's serum and the reaction is developed with a fluorescein-labeled antiglobulin. The results are read under the fluorescence microscope. By using a class-specific antiglobulin, the isotype of the patient's antibody can be determined. The same procedure can be used for other Epstein-Barr virus antigens, such as Epstein-Barr nuclear antigen, which is localized in the cell nucleus.

Fluorescent methods have proved to be useful for many other pathogens that are most readily grown in tissue culture, such as *Chlamydia* and *Rickettsia*.

Radioimmunoassay and Enzyme Immunoassay

Immunoassays are performed by measuring direct binding of antibody to antigen. In the simplest test, a radiolabeled antigen is added to bind the antibody. The test can be carried out either in fluid medium or on a solid surface. In fluid, the antigen-antibody complex must be separated from free antibody, usually by addition of ammonium sulfate or antiglobulin. The radioactivity of the precipitate is then measured. A solid-phase test is carried out by attaching the antigen to a glass or plastic surface. In some cases, the attachment requires first putting down a layer of antibody and then adding the appropriate antigen. The patient's serum is then added, followed by the labeled antiglobulin. After washing, the reaction is quantitated by the amount of radioactivity attached to the surface. Because this method is highly sensitive as well as quantitative, it has been widely adopted in the diagnostic immunology laboratory. Radioimmunoassays are, for example, the most common method for measuring antibodies to the hepatitis viruses.

For immunodiagnostic purposes, enzyme immunoassays offer a number of important advantages. The enzyme-linked reagents have a long half-life, are free from the legal limitations surrounding radioisotopes, and are adaptable to single tests or to large-scale automation. Enzyme immunoassays can be divided into two major groups: homogeneous assays, in which the enzyme activity is altered during the immune reaction, and heterogeneous assays, in which the enzyme activity of the labeled reagent is not affected by precipitation in the immune reaction. In heterogeneous assays, there must be an additional step to separate the bound from the unreacted labeled reagent. Although homogeneous assays are simpler in principle, the enzyme-linked immunosorbent assay is most widely used in immunodiagnosis. In principle, it can be used for the measurement of antibody to virtually any infectious agent. A particular attraction of the method is that the same conjugate can be used in any application. Class-specific, enzyme-labeled antiglobulins permit recognition of the immunoglobulin class, if such information is desired. Anticomplement antibodies may provide a useful alternative if complement is added to the antigen-antibody combination. The procedure calls for coating the wells of plastic microplates with the relevant antigen, adding the patient's serum in one or more dilutions, washing, and adding enzyme-labeled antihuman immunoglobulin conjugate. After further incubation, the enzyme substrate is added and incubated, and the degradation of a chromogenic substrate is measured by means of color intensity. The reaction can be stopped at a selected point in time, or kinetic measurements can be made of substrate breakdown. In this manner, a relationship can be calculated between the enzymatic activity and the amount of antibody in the serum.

The basic method can be modified in a number of ways. If the antigen is not present in reasonably purified form, the wells can be coated with specific antibody, either polyclonal or monoclonal antibody, followed by addition of crude antigen. These tests are referred to as capture assays. The test is then carried out in the usual manner. Enzyme-labeled staphylococcal protein A can be used instead of the antiglobulin reagent. This method is effective only to detect antibody classes IgG1, IgG2, and IgG4, which react with protein A. In the sandwich method, the well is coated with antigen and then the sample of serum to be tested is added, followed by enzyme-labeled antigen and substrate. It is obvious that the versatility of the method enzyme-linked immunosorbent assay accounts for its broad applications in immunodiagnosis.

A number of fluorescent immunoassays have been widely adopted by clinical laboratories. These procedures are rapid and sensitive and lend themselves to automation. The fluorescent labels used are generally the same as in immunofluorescence, and the test procedures resemble enzyme immunoassays. Homogeneous assays are feasible when the antigen-antibody reaction leads to quenching of the fluorescence. As an example, such an assay was introduced for the serologic diagnosis of syphilis. Fluorescein-labeled liposomes containing cardiolipin antigen are added to a patient's serum. The antibody-antigen interaction sterically inhibits the reaction of the fluorescein-labeled cardiolipin with antifluorescein antibody. When reacted with fluorescein, the antifluorescein antibody will quench the fluorescence. The anticardiolipin antibody level correlates with the degree of fluorescence emitted.

WESTERN IMMUNOBLOT

A specialized application of enzyme immunoassays valuable for crude antigens is the Western immunoblot. A complex antigen mixture is first separated by electrophoresis in detergent-containing gel and then transferred to a nitrocellular membrane. The membrane is covered with the patient's serum, washed, and exposed to labeled antiglobulin reagent. The reactions, seen as colored bands, are localized according to the approximate molecular weight of the particular components. This method is widely used for confirmation of human immunodeficiency virus infection.

Skin Tests

Toxin Neutralization

The exotoxins of organisms such as *Corynebacterium diphtheriae* are potent antigens and regularly evoke neutralizing antibodies, which are protective against the disease in humans. The measurement of this immune response during the course of disease in an individual patient plays little role in diagnosis or management; however, information about the immune status of populations is valuable for epidemiologic studies. Antitoxin levels can be estimated by use of hemagglutination tests with toxin-coated red blood cells, but sometimes it is necessary to determine the levels of antibodies that actually neutralized the toxin. These studies employ the Schick test for estimating diphtheria antitoxin levels. The Schick test is capable of dividing a population into susceptible and nonsusceptible groups based on their response to a standard dose of diphtheria toxin. Persons who are Schick-positive possess a serum antitoxin level of more than 0.01 antitoxin units (AU) per milliliter, whereas most persons who are Schick-negative possess levels of less than 0.01 AU/mL. The test is performed by intracutaneous injection of an appropriate dilution of diphtheria toxin into the flexor surface of the arm and the same amount of heat-inactivated toxin in the other arm. This inactivated control serves to detect allergic reactions to the medium. The control is important because most toxin preparations used in the Schick test are not highly purified. This control material may give rise to an immediate wheal and flare reaction or to a delayed erythematous response that can be mistaken for a positive Schick test.

In nonimmune persons, the toxin produces an area of redness in about 18 hours, which grows in size and intensity in 3 to 5 days. A central area of necrosis may develop. With adequate levels of circulating antitoxin and no sensitivity to other corynebacterial antigens, no reaction will be seen at the site of either injection.

Delayed Hypersensitivity

Delayed hypersensitivity skin tests are a cost-effective way to evaluate cellular immunity in patients with infectious diseases. Demonstration of cutaneous hypersensitivity reduces the need for costly studies of cellular immunity in vitro. Demonstration of the cellular response complements measurement of humoral immunity. The information may be useful diagnostically, especially in chronic intracellular infections produced by bacteria, viruses, and fungi. A positive skin test may also be useful in prognosis, because patients with delayed hypersensitivity sometimes have a better outlook than patients who lack such responses. Finally, tests of cell-mediated immunity are an important part of the evaluation of possible immunodeficiency.

The presence of hypersensitivity reactions accompanying an infection was first demonstrated in Robert Koch's description of local induration and swelling after subcutaneous reaction of tuberculin. The value of tuberculin tests for diagnosis was recognized by von Pirquet and Schick in 1903, using percutaneous skin tests, and Mantoux in 1910, using intradermal injections of tuberculin. The Mantoux test remains the standard method for clinical applications of delayed hypersensitivity assessment in infectious diseases.

It is critical to recognize the different types of cutaneous reactions that may follow injection of a microbial product into the skin. Immediate hypersensitivity reactions appear in the form of a wheal and erythema within a few minutes of the injection. They result from the interaction of cell-fixed antibodies, usually IgE, with the injected antigen. The Jones-Mote reaction begins within 2 to 4 hours of antigen challenge and reaches a maximum intensity in 24 to 72 hours. It is characterized by a basophil-rich cell infiltrate and is usually accompanied by the production of circulating IgG antibodies. The Arthus reaction, manifested by local erythema and edema and sometimes even necrosis, can occur 18 to 24 hours after challenge. This reaction is caused by the interaction of circulating complement-fixing antibodies (IgG or IgM) with locally deposited antigen. Delayed hypersensitivity reactions are usually maximal 48 to 72 hours after injection. Perivascular infiltrates of small and large lymphocytes develop by 4 to 6 hours, followed by a diffuse infiltrate composed of lymphocytes, monocytes, and basophils. Most of the infiltrating cells bear the phenotypic markers of helper T lymphocytes. The induration of delayed hypersensitivity is believed to be due to the production of cytokines by these invading lymphocytes.

The application and reading of delayed hypersensitivity skin tests require considerable skill and experience. It is necessary first to ensure that the antigen is delivered intracutaneously. Next, the reaction must be evaluated carefully 48 and 72 hours after administration. A positive reaction is denoted by the presence of induration, defined as palpable thickening of the skin, and is independent of erythema and swelling.

The appearance of delayed hypersensitivity is dependent on prior contact with the microorganism. The interpretation of the test, therefore, depends on particular circumstances. A positive tuberculin test result in a child, for example, is probably indicative of infection. On the other hand, the absence of skin reaction to common microorganisms in adults can be used as evidence of immunodeficiency. Such deficiency may be general or antigen specific. General tests are usually performed by applying a panel of common microbial antigens, including streptococcal streptokinase, *Trichophyton, Candida,* and tetanus toxoid.

The tuberculin test is the classic method of detecting infection with *Mycobacterium tuberculosis.* The original tuberculin, old tuberculin, is made by cultivating a virulent strain of *M. tuberculosis* on liquid medium for several months, at which time the medium containing numerous bacterial products is filtered, sterilized, and concentrated. In 1934, Seibert developed the purified protein derivative as a way of isolating the principal antigen. For clinical purposes, the intradermal Mantoux test is indicated. The tine tests, in which the prongs of the tine are covered with dried tuberculin, are more feasible for extensive epidemiologic studies. The indications for a tuberculin test are suspected tuberculosis, evaluation of contacts, and exclusion of tuberculosis. The specificity of the test is sufficiently high that a positive result provides compelling evidence of past or present mycobacterial infection; however, because of extensive sharing of antigenic determinants within the genus, there is cross-reaction among the various mycobacteria. For instance, a patient infected with *Mycobacterium intracellulare* is more likely to develop a reaction to purified protein derivative. A positive reaction is also found in persons vaccinated with bacille Calmette-Guerin. False-negative reactions may be attributable to technical errors. More substantive causes of negative reactions are transient anergy associated with viral exanthemata (such as measles) and treatment with immunosuppressive drugs, particularly corticosteroids. Patients with early tuberculosis who are tested before the development of delayed hypersensitivity have a negative reaction. On the other hand, patients with extensive pulmonary or miliary tuberculosis are sometimes specifically anergic, and this represents a sign of poor prognosis.

Delayed hypersensitivity skin tests are available for a number of other infectious diseases—histoplasmosis, coccidioidomycosis, candidiasis, nocardiosis, and leprosy, among others. In general, their application and interpretation are similar to those for the tuberculin test; however, the test reagents are often poorly standardized. Some skin test reagents, such as that for histoplasma, may elicit production of antibodies. Blood samples for serologic tests, therefore, should be taken before the skin test reagent is applied.

Skin test reagents are difficult to apply in infants and older persons with atrophic skin. Additional contraindications may prevent the use of skin tests. In these instances, tests in vitro of cell-mediated immunity can be used. There are two major analogs in vitro of delayed hypersensitivity, lymphocyte transformation and production of lymphokines such as interleukin-2. These tests are normally performed on peripheral blood lymphocytes, but lymph node and pleural fluid cells can sometimes be used. The validation of these tests depends on their correlation with skin tests in large-scale studies.

In some diseases, protective immunity seems to depend mainly on cytotoxic T cells. Tests in vitro of T-cell-mediated destruction of virus-infected target cells have been introduced for human immunodeficiency virus infection.

Identification of Microorganisms by Immunologic Methods

Direct Applications

At times it is advantageous to demonstrate the organism or antigenic products of the organism directly in clinical specimens. This approach does not require waiting for an antibody response; these tests are effective even in immunocompromised individuals. The diagnosis of pneumococcal pneumonia, for example, can be made rapidly by demonstrating *S. pneumoniae* in sputum by means of the quellung capsular swelling test. The organism also releases copious amounts of polysaccharide that can be demonstrated in body fluids. Sputum samples can be tested for capsular antigens with pools of type-specific antisera using counterimmunoelectrophoresis or coagglutination. Serum is not as reliable a specimen as sputum for detection of pneumococcal antigen in pneumonia patients, although antigenemia is present in 20% to 40% of cases. Moreover, the detection of circulating antigen is a sign of poor prognosis. Urine does not yield as high an antigen positivity rate as sputum in cases of pneumococcal pneumonia; however, pneumococcal antigen can be detected by counterimmunoelectrophoresis in the cerebrospinal fluid of some patients with pneumococcal meningitis. A great advantage of these tests for antigen in cerebrospinal fluid is that an etiologic diagnosis can be made immediately without waiting for the results of culture.

Because meningitis can be considered a medical emergency, speed is important in the diagnosis. Therefore, latex reagents are available for the demonstration in cerebrospinal fluid of antigen from a number of different pathogens, including *S. pneumoniae, Streptococcus pyogenes, H. influenzae, Cryptococcus neoformans, Candida albicans,* and *N. meningitidis* as well as group B streptococci.

An alternative approach for etiologic diagnosis is to demonstrate the pathogen directly in the affected tissues. Biopsy and autopsy specimens are generally used for this purpose. If specific antisera are available, immunofluorescence and immunoperoxidase can often be applied successfully. For example, fluorescein-labeled antibodies can be used to demonstrate *T. pallidum* in tissue samples, replacing the more demanding darkfield method. DNA or RNA probes for particular organisms have been produced, which can be applied to tissue sections, using radioautography to develop the localized reaction. The polymerase chain reaction greatly amplifies the microbial nucleic acid and increases the sensitivity of the method considerably. The great sensitivity of the method requires special attention to technical details, because even trace contamination of specimens can produce false-positive reactions.

Because of their speed and cost-effectiveness, antigen detection methods are being used more often in clinical laboratories as specific antisera become available. They are also applicable in previously treated patients when there is trouble isolating the pathogen in culture. Sometimes, in fact, they are the only means of identifying the agent of infection. The methods are, however, limited by the cross-reactions known to occur among microorganisms. Moreover, antigen detection methods do not permit assessment of antibiotic susceptibility. They are, therefore, likely to remain auxiliary techniques for the foreseeable future.

Identification of Microorganisms in Culture

Because of their specificity, antibodies are ideal reagents for identification of microorganisms. The wide availability of monoclonal antibodies has greatly increased the specificity of immunologic methods of species identification. Many of the techniques described earlier in this chapter can be applied to antigen identification, including agglutination of bacterial cells, precipitation of microbial products, and neutralization of toxins or infectious virus. Immunofluorescent methods are widely used, as are enzyme immunoassays and radioimmunoassays. All of these methods depend on the specificity and potency of the antibody reagents. In the past, this goal required purification of the respective antigens before immunization and removal of unwanted antibodies by specific absorption. These steps are unnecessary if carefully selected monoclonal antibodies are employed.

In addition to species identification, specific antibodies can be used for grouping and typing isolated microorganisms. The many serotypes of *Salmonella* are defined primarily by means of their antigenic specificity. The grouping of streptococci and the typing of pneumococci and of *H. influenzae* all depend on the availability of appropriate antisera. The information obtained is sometimes of clinical value but more often is needed for epidemiologic studies. Grouping and typing, therefore, are generally carried out in specialized central or reference laboratories.

Summary

This chapter describes the application of immunologic methods to the diagnosis of infectious diseases. The major method of immunodiagnosis depends on the demonstration of a rising titer of circulating antibodies to the particular pathogen in the serum of the patient. The method is of great value because serum is generally readily available and the tests are technically straightforward. Its usefulness is limited, however, by the fact that antibodies require time to appear in the blood stream and may remain for a considerable period after infection. Moreover, related organisms may induce production of cross-reactive antibodies. In a few diseases, the presence of cell-mediated immunity to an organism has more diagnostic value than the presence of circulating antibody. In these cases, delayed hypersensitivity skin tests or their correlates in vitro are employed. Finally, immunologic means and molecular hybridization can be used to aid in the identification of infectious microorganisms. Monoclonal and selected polyclonal antibodies and DNA and RNA probes can detect microorganisms in specimens from patients. The polymerase chain reaction greatly amplifies microbial nucleic acid and offers an extraordinarily sensitive technique for identifying pathogens directly in specimens. The tests may be carried out directly on body fluids or tissues from the patient, providing a relatively rapid means of identification. Antibody reagents are also used in the laboratory to assist in identification of cultured pathogens.

Bibliography

- Murray PR, Baron EJ, Pfaller MA, et al (eds): Manual of Clinical Microbiology, ed 6. Washington, DC, American Society for Microbiology, 1995.
- Rose NR, et al (eds): Manual of Clinical Laboratory Immunology, ed 5. Washington, DC, American Society for Microbiology (in press).

14

Molecular Techniques for the Detection and Identification of Infectious Agents

Fred C. Tenover

Today, the emphasis in clinical microbiology is on rapid diagnostic techniques that will reduce the time required to identify the presence of pathogenic microorganisms in clinical samples. Rapid techniques can be divided into three major categories; microscopic methods, immunologic methods, and molecular methods. Whereas each has a role to play in the laboratory diagnosis of infectious diseases, nucleic acid–based methods have the greatest potential for increasing the sensitivity of detecting infectious agents directly in clinical samples while maintaining high specificity. Molecular techniques also have the broadest diagnostic applications, including the ability to detect and identify infectious agents that cannot be cultured in vitro.[1] Although the major strength of molecular methods is for organism identification, molecular techniques can also be adapted for strain typing and for detection of antimicrobial resistance genes to guide therapy early in the course of disease. Although many of the newer nucleic acid amplification methods appear complex, they are based on simple DNA-to-DNA or DNA-to-RNA hybridization reactions. In this chapter, the basic principles of nucleic acid hybridization and amplification are presented along with examples of how these molecular methods are applied to the diagnosis of infectious diseases.

Types of Molecular Methods

The two major formats of molecular diagnostic testing are hybridization assays using nucleic acid probes and nucleic acid amplification assays. The underlying premise of molecular diagnostic technologies is that each organism contains, within its genetic complement, sequences of either DNA or RNA that are absolutely unique to that species. The goal of the technology is to indicate the presence or absence of those unique sequences in clinical samples in lieu of culturing the organism in vitro. The hybridization assay is the simplest molecular test, which involves (1) denaturing the target nucleic acid in the sample to single strands, usually by exposure to sodium hydroxide; (2) adding the probe (which can be either DNA or RNA) to the reaction mixture and allowing it to bind to its complementary target sequences, forming a stable double-stranded molecule; and (3) detecting the new double-stranded molecules. Most probes tend to be short molecules (50 bases in length or less) so that hybridization times require less than an hour to complete, and the detection system usually employs chemoluminescent substrates that are chemically coupled to the probes (Fig. 14–1). Most diagnostic DNA probe assays are homogeneous, that is, hybridization and detection of reaction products take place in a single tube, which simplifies assay conditions. The specificity of the assay is a function of the sequences chosen for the probe and the stringency of the reaction, which in turn is a function of the temperature, salt concentration, and pH of the assay. Each of these parameters must be optimized to prevent binding of the probe to nontarget sequences.

DNA probes were introduced by Moseley and coworkers[2] in 1980 as a means of detecting enterotoxigenic *Escherichia coli* present in stool samples. Stool samples were spotted onto filter papers resting on MacConkey agar plates and incubated overnight. After incubation, the filters were removed, and the colonies present on the filters were examined for the presence of enterotoxin genes by use of radioactively labeled DNA probes. The technique was highly sensitive and specific compared with the "gold standard," which was a cell culture assay. This procedure made use of a biologic amplification step, that is, the growth of organisms on agar plates, to increase the amount of target present before DNA probe testing. Amplification was the key to achieving high assay sensitivity.

Molecular diagnostic tests of the second broad class employ biochemical amplification steps instead of biologic amplification. In some techniques, this occurs before hybridization analysis; in others, it is in lieu of hybridization analysis.[3, 4] Amplification methods include increasing the quantity of target nucleic acid sequences, amplifying probe sequences after hybridization occurs, and amplifying the signal produced after hybridization. All of the biochemical amplification techniques incorporate hybridization reactions in some phase of the reaction. The primary advantages of biochemical amplification over biologic amplification are sensitivity and speed. A millionfold amplification of target is achievable with some methods in little more than 1 hour.

Applications of DNA Probes

DNA probe assays can be used to identify organisms already available in pure culture (culture confirmation) or to identify

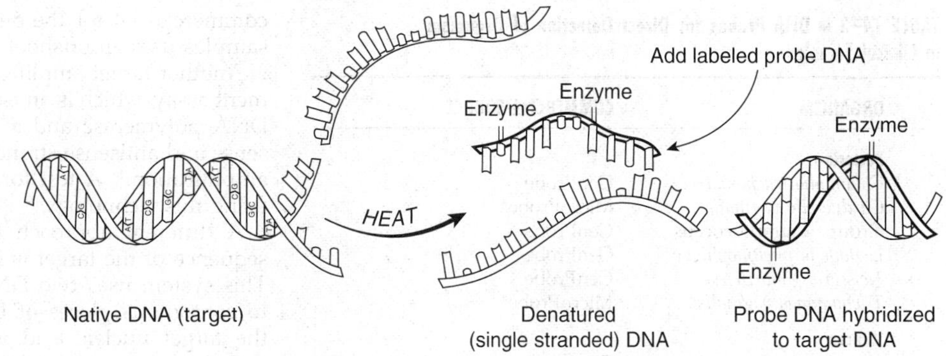

FIGURE 14–1 □ DNA probes.

organisms directly in clinical samples, including organisms fixed in tissue sections.[5] In culture confirmation assays, unique sequences of DNA or RNA are used to identify organisms in place of a set of biochemical or immunologic reactions. For slow-growing or fastidious organisms, this can result in significant time savings over conventional methods. Ribosomal RNA sequences are typical targets of DNA probes. Identification of mycobacteria growing either on agar or in the BACTEC* liquid growth system is the most common application of DNA probes for culture confirmation.[6, 7] The combination of the BACTEC system plus DNA probes often identifies *Mycobacterium tuberculosis* in an average of 2 weeks or less from the time of specimen collection. Sputum samples showing large numbers of organisms per high-power field can often be identified as containing *M. tuberculosis* in less than a week. However, DNA probes are not sensitive enough to detect mycobacteria directly in clinical samples. DNA probes for other bacterial species are listed in Table 14–1. Some microbiologists have used commercial probes, such as those for enterococci or *Staphylococcus aureus*, to identify organisms growing directly in blood culture vials[8]; however, this application is not approved by the U.S. Food and Drug Administration and requires independent laboratory validation before use. DNA probes can also be used to identify a number of yeasts and dimorphic molds (Table 14–2). Probes are particularly effective in identifying molds in the early stages of hyphal growth before diagnostic fruiting structures are apparent.[9, 10]

PROBES FOR DIRECT DETECTION OF INFECTIOUS AGENTS IN CLINICAL SAMPLES

The most common use of probes is for detecting organisms directly in clinical samples, particularly the agents of sexually transmitted diseases. Commercial DNA probes are used widely in the United States and Europe to detect *Neisseria gonorrhoeae* and *Chlamydia trachomatis* in urethral and endocervical specimens.[11, 12] In fact, both tests can be performed on material obtained with a single swab. Organisms need not be viable to be detected by this test. In contrast to direct fluorescent antibody–based tests, however, the quality of the specimen cannot be assessed to determine that collection was satisfactory before the DNA probe is used. These tests, on occasion, produce indeterminate values that require retesting to ensure accuracy.

Other commercial probe tests that have been cleared for use by the U.S. Food and Drug Administration are shown in Table 14–3. The tests for *Trichomonas vaginalis* and *Gardnerella vaginalis* are approved but no longer commercially available.

*Trade names are used for identification purposes only and do not imply endorsement by the U.S. Public Health Service or the U.S. Department of Health and Human Services.

Applications of Nucleic Acid Amplification Tests

At present, the polymerase chain reaction (PCR) is the most widely used amplification technology for detection and identification of infectious agents.[3, 13] An extensive list of the research applications of this technology has been reported,[3] although new applications for infectious diseases are continually being introduced in the literature. However, alternative amplification technologies, including other target amplification strategies (such as the strand displacement assay; the transcription amplification system and its sister technologies, the self-sustaining sequence replication reaction and nucleic acid sequence–based amplification), are beginning to show promise as both sensitive and specific methods for identifying infectious agents.[3, 4] Probe amplification systems, including the ligase chain reaction and signal amplification systems, such as branched DNA, will soon be competitive technologies.[3] Examples of potential commercial applications of these technologies are listed in Table 14–4.

BRIEF REVIEW OF AMPLIFICATION METHODS

PCR assays require a source of target nucleic acid, small DNA primers that are complementary to sequences at the 5′ and 3′ ends of the region of DNA to be amplified, an enzyme to synthesize DNA (i.e., the polymerase), and an instrument to modulate reaction temperatures during the various cycles. PCR usually consists of a three-step cycle of (1) denaturing

TABLE 14–1 ■ Culture Confirmation Assays for Bacterial Pathogens

ORGANISM	COMMERCIAL SOURCE
Haemophilus influenzae	GenProbe
Mycobacterium tuberculosis complex	GenProbe
Mycobacterium avium	GenProbe
Mycobacterium avium complex	GenProbe
Mycobacterium intracellulare	GenProbe
Mycobacterium gordonae	GenProbe
Neisseria gonorrhoeae	GenProbe
Streptococcus pneumoniae	GenProbe
Enterococci	GenProbe
Group B streptococci	GenProbe
Thermophilic campylobacters*	GenProbe

*Includes *Campylobacter jejuni, Campylobacter coli,* and *Campylobacter lari.*

TABLE 14–2 ■ Culture Confirmation Assays for Fungal Pathogens

ORGANISM	COMMERCIAL SOURCE
Candida albicans	GenProbe
Coccidioides immitis	GenProbe
Cryptococcus neoformans	GenProbe
Histoplasma capsulatum	GenProbe

TABLE 14–3 ■ DNA Probes for Direct Detection of Organism in Clinical Samples

ORGANISM	COMMERCIAL SOURCE
Bacteria	
Chlamydia trachomatis	GenProbe
Gardnerella vaginalis	MicroProbe*
Group A streptococcus	GenProbe
Legionella pneumophila	GenProbe
Neisseria gonorrhoeae	GenProbe
Trichomonas vaginalis	MicroProbe*
Viruses	
Human papillomavirus	Digene

*Approved but not marketed.

the DNA present in a sample; (2) allowing the single-stranded DNA primers to bind (anneal) to the denatured DNA; and (3) duplicating the target material between the primers by using DNA polymerase, which results in two double-stranded copies of the target DNA (Fig. 14–2). The cycle is initiated again with the denaturation of the newly created double-stranded DNA. The second cycle yields four copies of the target DNA; additional cycles increase the amount of target DNA exponentially. Thirty cycles yield approximately a millionfold amplification of the original target sequence. PCR can be adapted to the amplification of RNA targets by incorporating a reverse transcription step before the first amplification cycle. A single enzyme is now available that is capable of both reverse transcription and polymerization steps.

The major drawback to PCR is the potential for contamination of samples by previously amplified material that strays into a clinical sample during specimen preparation. Such DNA may serve as a template for amplification, producing a false-positive result. Chemical approaches to prevent carryover contamination have been developed to help alleviate this problem.[14] The opposite problem, the presence of substances inhibitory to the PCR reaction, is also encountered in samples such as whole blood and stool. Controls to indicate the presence of inhibitors in samples should be incorporated into the assay format. A commercial kit is now available for detection of *C. trachomatis* using PCR.[15]

The transcription amplification system, which is a different target amplification method, is a two-step process that begins with production of a double-stranded DNA molecule from target RNA. In the second step, RNA copies are then produced from the DNA strands in an exponential manner.[16] A commercial kit for the detection of *M. tuberculosis* in clinical samples uses an offshoot of this system.[17]

Another target amplification system is the strand displacement assay, which is an isothermal process that uses a unique DNA polymerase and a complement of four probes to the sense and antisense strands of nucleic acid to effect sequence amplification.[18] A test for *M. tuberculosis* has been described using this technology.[19]

A different approach to amplification, if the nucleotide sequence of the target is known, is the ligase chain reaction. This system uses two DNA probes that are complementary to contiguous pieces of DNA on the target nucleic acid. If the target nucleic acid is present in the sample, the two probes are joined by DNA ligase, and the newly ligated probe is replicated enzymatically in a continuous reaction.[20] One such application of the ligase chain reaction is for detection of *C. trachomatis*.[21]

Branched DNA is a true signal amplification system in which a DNA probe first captures a target molecule, and the DNA complex is then bound to a second DNA backbone on a solid support. A third DNA probe containing numerous reporter moieties is then allowed to bind to the complex, which dramatically increases the signal initiated by the binding of the first probe to the target. Either DNA or RNA sequences can be targeted in this method. One application of branched DNA technology has been to follow the viral load of hepatitis C virus during interferon therapy.[22]

Finally, the use of nucleic acid sequencing techniques for identification of microorganisms and detection of mutations associated with drug resistance is gaining acceptance in the clinical laboratory. New technologies, such as automated sequence analysis of PCR products using high-density oligonucleotide arrays on silicone chips, are proving both rapid and highly accurate. Clinical applications of sequencing techniques are already beginning to have an impact on infectious disease management.[23]

Detection of Antimicrobial Resistance Genes

The goal of using molecular methods to identify bacteria directly in clinical samples is to speed identification and improve sensitivity, obviating the need for culture. However, by eliminating culture, the laboratory also eliminates its ability to perform antimicrobial susceptibility testing. Although this is not an issue for *C. trachomatis*, it is an important issue for drug-resistant *N. gonorrhoeae* and especially for *M. tuberculosis*, for which multidrug resistance has been described.[24] Particularly for amplification-based methods, the loss of susceptibility results to guide therapy could be a major deficit. One approach to this problem is to use PCR,

TABLE 14–4 ■ Current and Proposed Commercial Target, Probe, and Signal Amplification Assays

ORGANISM	METHOD	COMMERCIAL SOURCE
Bacteria		
Chlamydia trachomatis	Polymerase chain reaction	Roche
	Ligase chain reaction*	Abbot
Mycobacterium tuberculosis	Polymerase chain reaction	Roche
	Amplified *M. tuberculosis**	GenProbe
	Strand displacement assay	Becton Dickinson
Viruses		
Human immunodeficiency virus	Polymerase chain reaction	Roche
	Branched DNA	Chiron
Hepatitis C virus	Branched DNA	Chiron

*Clearance received from the U.S. Food and Drug Administration.

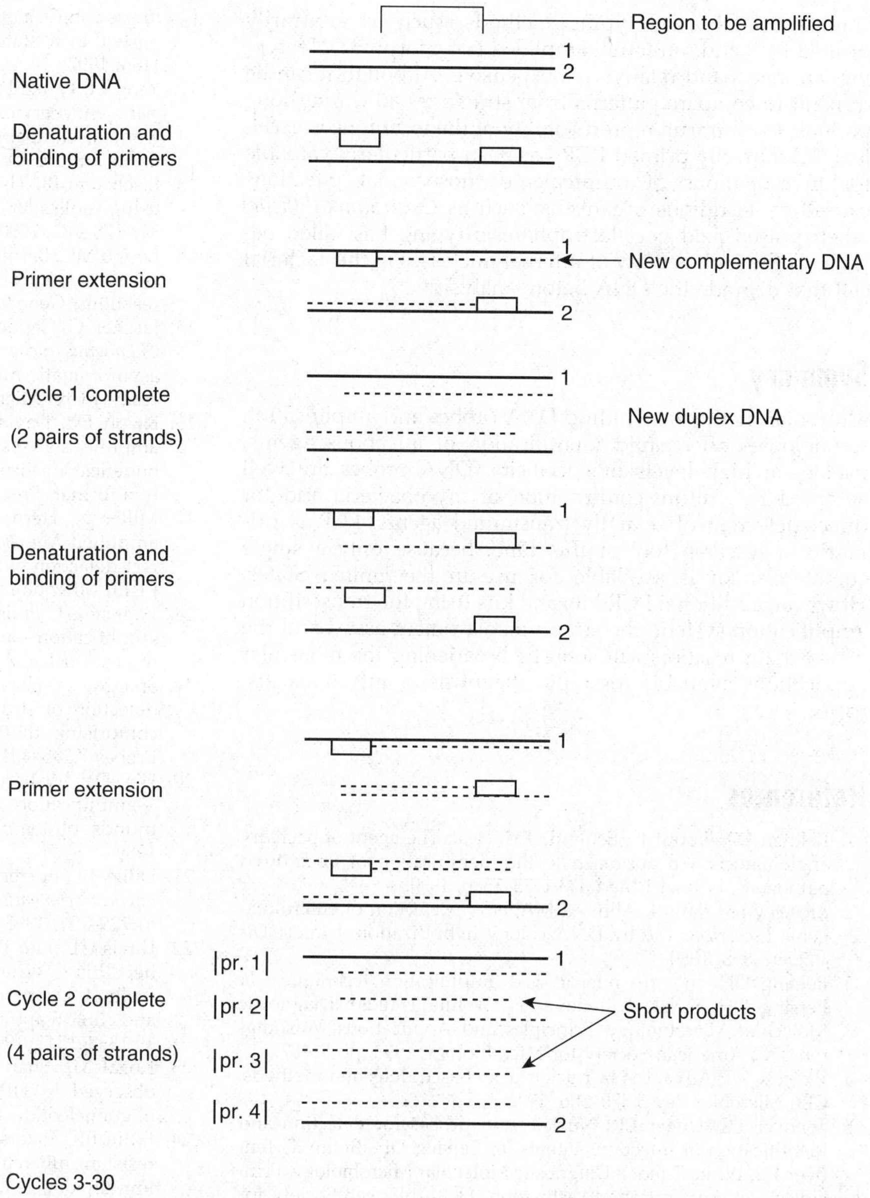

FIGURE 14–2 ▫ Polymerase chain reaction. (From Tenover FC: Molecular methods for the clinical microbiology laboratory. *In* Balows A, Hausler WJ Jr, Herrmann KL, et al [eds]: Manual of Clinical Microbiology, ed 5. Washington, DC, American Society for Microbiology, 1991, pp 119–127.)

or other amplification methods, to detect key resistance determinants in the organism directly in the clinical sample. More than 30 PCR assays targeting resistance genes have been described to date,[25] and the utility of such an approach for detecting mutations associated with rifampin resistance in *M. tuberculosis*[26] and ampicillin resistance in *H. influenzae* directly in cerebrospinal fluid[27] has been demonstrated. Additional organism–resistance gene combinations are currently undergoing evaluation.

Strain-Typing Techniques

Strain typing is becoming more commonplace in many microbiology laboratories, and molecular methods have replaced the more traditional typing procedures, such as serotyping, phage typing, and antibiogram typing. Whereas these tests still have some utility, molecular methods are more discriminatory, more reproducible, and in many cases easier to apply in a clinical laboratory. Three have proved to be particularly useful: plasmid fingerprinting, pulsed-field gel electrophoresis, and arbitrarily primed PCR.[28]

Plasmid fingerprinting was the first molecular typing method to be applied to outbreaks of both nosocomial and community-acquired infections. It uses the size and number of extrachromosomal elements as a means of strain identification. This technique, especially coupled with restriction endonuclease digestion, is a cost-effective typing method. Unfortunately, not all pathogens carry extrachromosomal DNA, which limits its utility.

Pulsed-field gel electrophoresis is a more universal strain-typing procedure that has been used successfully to type more than 50 different species of bacteria.[29] It uses a novel electrophoresis system to separate the large pieces of chromosomal DNA produced by restriction enzymes that cleave at infrequent intervals. This technique is less variable than plasmid fingerprinting but more discriminating than other genotypic typing methods, such as ribotyping or multilocus enzyme electrophoresis. Although start-up costs are relatively high because of the requirement for specialized equipment, the ability to type both bacteria and yeast makes it a key tool for epidemiologic studies of outbreaks of disease. Criteria for interpretation of the fragment patterns produced during pulsed-field gel electrophoresis have been proposed.[29]

Finally, PCR-based typing methods, such as arbitrarily primed PCR and randomly amplified polymorphic DNA typing, are rapid and relatively inexpensive. Although it can be difficult to compare patterns from strains tested during long periods, the intrarun reproducibility of the technique is excellent.[30] Arbitrarily primed PCR has been particularly valuable for investigations of outbreaks of nosocomial infections caused by fastidious organisms, such as *Clostridium difficile*, when pulsed-field gel electrophoresis typing has failed because of the high activity of internal nucleases in the bacterial cell that degrade the DNA before analysis.

Summary

Molecular methods including DNA probes and amplification technologies offer rapid identification of infectious agents, usually at high levels of specificity. DNA probes are well accepted for culture confirmation of mycobacteria and for direct detection of sexually transmitted agents. PCR is primarily a research tool at this time, because only a single commercial kit is available for use in the United States. However, additional PCR kits and kits using the transcription amplification system, the strand displacement assay, and the ligase chain reaction will soon be broadening the molecular applications available for rapid diagnosis of infectious diseases.

References

1. Relman DA, Loutit JS, Schmidt TM, et al: The agent of bacillary angiomatosis: An approach to the identification of uncultured pathogens. N Engl J Med 323:1573–1580, 1990.
2. Moseley SM, Huq I, Alim ARMA, et al: Detection of enterotoxigenic *Escherichia coli* by DNA colony hybridization. J Infect Dis 142:892–898, 1980.
3. Persing DH: In vitro nucleic acid amplification techniques. *In* Persing DH, Smith T, Tenover FC, White T (eds): Diagnostic Molecular Microbiology. Principles and Applications. Washington, DC, American Society for Microbiology, 1993, pp 51–87.
4. Wolcott MJ: Advances in nucleic acid–based detection methods. Clin Microbiol Rev 5:370–386, 1992.
5. Tenover FC, Unger ER: Nucleic acid probes for detection and identification of infectious agents. *In* Persing DH, Smith T, Tenover FC, White T (eds): Diagnostic Molecular Microbiology. Principles and Applications. Washington, DC, American Society for Microbiology, 1993, pp 3–25.
6. Ellner PD, Kiehn TE, Cammarata R, Hosmer M: Rapid detection and identification of pathogenic *Mycobacterium* by combining radiometric and nucleic acid probe methods. J Clin Microbiol 26:1349–1352, 1988.
7. Evans KD, Nakasone AS, Sutherland PA, et al: Identification of *Mycobacterium tuberculosis* and *Mycobacterium avium–M. intracellulare* directly from primary BACTEC cultures by using acridinium-ester–labeled DNA probes. J Clin Microbiol 30:2427–2431, 1992.
8. Davis TE, Fuller DD: Direct identification of bacterial isolates in blood cultures by using a DNA probe. J Clin Microbiol 29:2193–2196, 1991.
9. Sandin RL, Isada CM, Hall GS, et al: Aberrant *Histoplasma capsulatum* confirmation of identity by a chemiluminescence-labeled DNA probe. Diagn Microbiol Infect Dis 17:235–238, 1993.
10. Stockman L, Clark KA, Hunt JM, Roberts GD: Evaluation of commercially available acridinium ester–labeled chemiluminescent DNA probes for culture identification of *Blastomyces dermatitidis, Coccidioides immitis, Cryptococcus neoformans*, and *Histoplasma capsulatum*. J Clin Microbiol 31:845–850, 1993.
11. Limberger RJ, Biega R, Evancoe A, et al: Evaluation of culture and the Gen-Probe PACE-2 assay for detection of *Neisseria gonorrhoeae* and *Chlamydia trachomatis* in endocervical specimens transported to a state health laboratory. J Clin Microbiol 30:1162–1166, 1992.
12. Yang LI, Panke ES, Leist PA, et al: Detection of *Chlamydia trachomatis* endocervical infection in asymptomatic and symptomatic women; comparison of deoxyribonucleic acid probe test with tissue culture. Obstet Gynecol 165:1444–1453, 1991.
13. Eisenstein BI: The polymerase chain reaction: A new method of using molecular genetics for medical diagnosis. N Engl J Med 322:178–183, 1990.
14. Longo MC, Bernionger MS, Hartley JL: Use of uracil DNA glycosylase to control carryover contamination in polymerase chain reactions. Gene 93:125–128, 1990.
15. Jaschek G, Gaydos CA, Welsh LE, Quinn TC: Direct detection of *Chlamydia trachomatis* in urine specimens from symptomatic and asymptomatic men by using a rapid polymerase chain reaction assay. J Clin Microbiol 31:1209–1212, 1993.
16. Kwoh DY, Davis GR, Whitfield KM, et al: Transcription-based amplification system, and detection of amplified human immunodeficiency virus type 1 with a bead-based sandwich hybridization format. Proc Natl Acad Sci USA 86:1173–1177, 1989.
17. Miller N, Hernandez SG, Cleary TJ: Evaluation of Gen-Probe amplified *Mycobacterium tuberculosis* direct test and PCR for direct detection of *Mycobacterium tuberculosis* in clinical specimens. J Clin Microbiol 32:393–397, 1994.
18. Walker GT, Fraiser MS, Schram JL, et al: Strand displacement amplification—an isothermal, in vitro DNA amplification technique. Nucleic Acids Res 20:1691–1696, 1992.
19. Spargo CA, Haaland PD, Jurgensen SR, et al: Chemiluminescent detection of strand displacement amplified DNA from species comprising the *Mycobacterium tuberculosis* complex. Mol Cell Probes 7:395–404, 1993.
20. Wu DY, Wallace B: The ligase amplification reaction (LAR)—amplification of specific DNA sequences using sequential rounds of template-dependent ligations. Genomics 4:560–569, 1989.
21. Dillie BJ, Butzen CC, Birkenmeyer LG: Amplification of *Chlamydia trachomatis* DNA by ligase chain reaction. J Clin Microbiol 31:729–731, 1993.
22. Davis GL, Lau JY-N, Urdea MS, et al: Quantitative detection of hepatitis C virus RNA with a solid phase signal amplification method: Definition of optimal conditions for specimen collection and clinical application in interferon-treated patients. Hepatology 19:1337–1341, 1994.
23. Kozal MJ, Shah N, Shwen N, et al: Extensive polymorphisms observed in HIV-1 clade B protease gene using high-density oligonucleotide arrays. Nat Med 2:753–759, 1996.
24. Edlin BR, Tokars JI, Grieco MH, et al: An outbreak of multidrug resistant tuberculosis among hospitalized patients with acquired immunodeficiency syndrome. N Engl J Med 326:1514–1521, 1992.
25. Tenover FC, Popovic T, and Olsvik Ø: Genetic methods for detecting antibacterial resistance genes. *In* Murray PR, Baron EJ, Pfaller MA, et al (eds): Manual of Clinical Microbiology, ed 6. Washington, DC, ASM Press, 1995, pp 1368–1378.
26. Telenti A, Imboden P, Marchesi F, et al: Direct, automated detection of rifampin-resistant *Mycobacterium tuberculosis* by polymerase chain reaction and single-strand confirmation polymorphism analysis. Antimicrob Agents Chemother 37:2054–2058, 1993.
27. Tenover FC, Huang MB, Rasheed JK, Persing DH: Development of PCR assays to detect ampicillin resistance genes in cerebrospinal fluid samples containing *Haemophilus influenzae*. J Clin Microbiol 32:2729–2737, 1994.
28. Arbeit RD: Laboratory procedures for the epidemiologic analysis of microorganisms. *In* Murray PR, Baron EJ, Pfaller MA, et al (eds): Manual of Clinical Microbiology, ed 6. Washington, DC, ASM Press, 1995, pp 190–208.
29. Tenover FC, Arbeit RD, Goering RV, et al: Interpreting chromosomal DNA restriction patterns produced by pulsed-field gel electrophoresis: Criteria for bacterial strain typing. J Clin Microbiol 33:2233–2239, 1995.
30. van Belkum A: DNA fingerprinting of medically important microorganisms by PCR. Clin Microbiol Rev 7:174–184, 1994.

15

Skin Testing

George S. Deepe, Jr.

History

Skin testing originated in 1890, when Robert Koch described the inflammatory response induced by tubercle bacilli that were injected into the skin of *Mycobacterium tuberculosis*–infected guinea pigs.[1] In the following year, he discovered that injected culture medium from growing tubercle bacilli also evoked an inflammatory response. The active constituent was called old tuberculin.[2] Because this material, when injected into infected guinea pigs, appeared to inhibit growth of *M. tuberculosis*, Koch advocated its use as specific therapy for tuberculosis. Extensive clinical trials, however, failed to demonstrate efficacy of old tuberculin; nevertheless, it was quite evident that the substance was useful as a skin test reagent to detect exposure to *M. tuberculosis*. Widespread application of skin testing in clinical medicine became possible after the introduction of two techniques, intracutaneous and contact testing, by Mantoux[3] and von Pirquet,[4] respectively. Indeed, von Pirquet[5] was the first to recognize the cutaneous tuberculin reaction as an allergic phenomenon, and he also termed the lack of tuberculin reactivity in children with active measles anergy.

That cutaneous reactivity was mediated by specific cells was demonstrated by Landsteiner and Chase,[6] who successfully transferred contact sensitivity to naive animals using peritoneal exudate cells from sensitized ones. Shortly thereafter, Chase[7] transferred tuberculin reactivity to naive animals and similar studies were performed in humans.[8] Since that time, skin testing has provided a powerful and simple technique for detecting past or recent infection with certain pathogenic microbes (Table 15–1), for assessing the integrity of cellular immune responses, and for evaluating immediate hypersensitivity to antibiotics. In general, however, skin testing with antigens prepared from pathogenic microbes is not useful as a diagnostic procedure because it does not distinguish active *disease* from remote sensitization.

Morphology and Histology

The delayed cutaneous hypersensitivity response should be considered a dynamic process involving the ingress and egress of immunocompetent cells. Much of what is known about the morphologic features of cutaneous reactivity to protein antigens is derived from studies of tuberculin hypersensitivity. Presumably, the response to other antigens is similar, if not identical. In humans, the earliest macroscopic finding is erythema, which is evident by 12 hours after intradermal challenge. Induration develops within 24 hours and peaks by 48 to 72 hours. Histologically, the erythema results from vasodilatation that is induced by various cytokines, principally vasoactive amines; induration is accompanied by a vigorous influx of mononuclear cells, into the perivascular areas initially and then into the dermis and subcutaneous tissues.[9–11] Only a few scattered polymorphonuclear leukocytes are evident. Immunohistologic studies have demonstrated that both $CD4^+$ and $CD8^+$ T cells are present in lesions, at ratios of 2:1 to 5:1.[11, 12] A sizable proportion of T cells contain surface markers that suggest an activated state (i.e., anti–interleukin 2 receptor, CD71, CD38).[13]

Within 12 hours of challenge, the number of Langerhans cells in the epidermis increases. Subsequently, these cells are observed in the dermis, suggesting that they emigrate from the area of inflammation to distant organs. Because Langerhans cells can function as antigen-presenting cells, it is possible that they also transport antigen during migration.[11]

A second type of response to foreign antigen was discovered by Jones and Mote,[14, 15] who tested subjects with filter-sterilized peritoneal fluid from rabbits injected intraperitoneally with hemolytic streptococci. The cutaneous reaction followed the kinetics of hypersensitivity to other antigens, but macroscopically there was a softened induration with a large area of erythema. Studies of experimental animals using a variety of antigens have shown that, in contrast to the cells present in tuberculin responses, basophils are a prominent cell population in the Jones-Mote reaction.[16]

Immunology of Cutaneous Reactivity

The skin test stands as one of the major manifestations of the cell-mediated immune system. Although it is a relatively simple test to perform, expression of a positive skin response requires a complex series of cellular interactions culminating in induration (Fig. 15–1). Studies of experimental models of infection have indicated that with few exceptions the principal T-cell subset involved in elaborating cutaneous reactivity

TABLE 15–1 ■ Skin Tests That Are Useful in Human Infectious Diseases

INFECTIOUS DISEASE	MICROBE	SKIN TEST REAGENT	SOURCE OF REAGENT
Coccidioidomycosis	*Coccidioides immitis*	Coccidioidin	Culture filtrate of mycelial-phase organisms
		Spherulin	Autolysate of spherules
Histoplasmosis	*Histoplasma capsulatum*	Histoplasmin	Culture filtrate from mycelial-phase organisms
Leishmaniasis	*Leishmania braziliensis* *Leishmania mexicana* *Leishmania donovani* *Leishmania major* *Leishmania tropica*	Leishmanin	Phenol-treated promastigotes suspended in saline at concentration of 1–2 × 10⁶ per mL
Leprosy	*Mycobacterium leprae*	Lepromin	Extract of organisms obtained from armadillo liver or from nodules of patients with lepromatous leprosy (bacilli suspended at 1.6 × 10⁸ per mL)
		Dharmendra antigen	Formalin and ether extract of *M. leprae*
Paracoccidioidomycosis	*Paracoccidioides brasiliensis*	Paracoccidioidin	Culture filtrate from mycelial-phase organisms
Tuberculosis	*Mycobacterium tuberculosis*	Purified protein derivative	Purified culture filtrate of *M. tuberculosis*

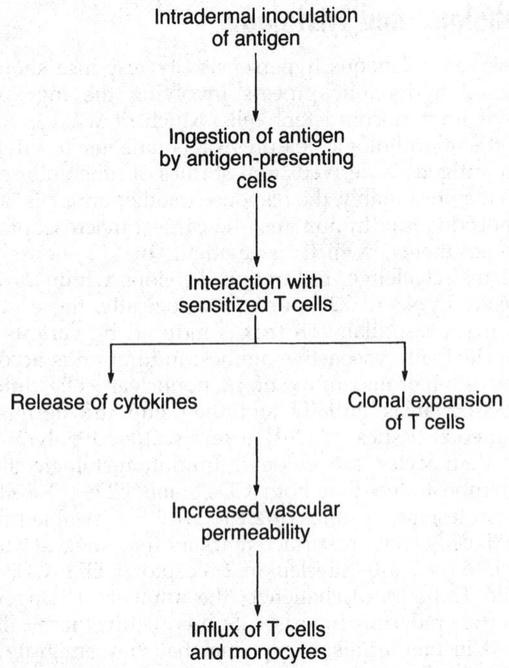

FIGURE 15–1 □ Schema for cellular events that lead to a positive skin test result. After intradermal inoculation of antigen, the antigen is ingested by antigen-presenting cells and immunogenic peptides become bound to class II major histocompatibility complex molecules. Antigen-specific T cells ($CD4^+$) recognize the bimolecular complex and become activated. Consequently, there is proliferation of T cells as well as release of cytokines. Vascular permeability is increased, and T cells and monocytes begin to infiltrate into the inflamed area.

is the $CD4^+$ T cell.[17–19] Those exceptions are viral infections. Cells that mediate delayed-type hypersensitivity (DTH) responses have been referred to as T_{DTH}. The presence of DTH often correlates with the capacity of T cells to exert a protective immune response; thus, it was generally believed that these two cell subsets were one and the same. However, evidence exists that T_{DTH} cells and T cells that mediate protection are distinct functional subpopulations.[18, 20, 21] The capacity to propagate cloned T cells offered a way to assess whether a monoclonal population of cells could both express DTH and provide protection, but these studies have been hampered by the finding that cloned T cells are unable to traffic normally in hosts.[17, 22, 23]

The biochemical, molecular, and cellular events that lead to expression of DTH are currently under intense investigation. After intradermal inoculation of antigen, it is ingested by accessory cells that include macrophages, dendritic cells, and Langerhans cells. With few exceptions, $CD4^+$ T cells recognize native antigen that has been degraded or "processed" into immunogenic peptides that become associated with class II major histocompatibility complex molecules.[24–27] Within accessory cells, native antigen is denatured by proteolytic enzymes and is then transported in conjunction with major histocompatibility complex molecules to the surface. The α/β receptor on T cells engages this bimolecular complex.[28–30] In turn, T cells become activated to release a number of cytokines, including interleukins-2, -3, and -4, interferon-γ, and colony-stimulating factors, and to undergo clonal proliferation. Subsequently, large numbers of monocytes and T cells are found in the area of inflammation.

Evidence indicates that $CD4^+$ T cells can be separated into two functionally distinct subsets, termed Th1 and Th2 cells. The division is based on the profile of cytokines secreted by each subset. Thus, Th1 cells produce interleukin-2 and interferon-γ, whereas Th2 cells release interleukins-4, -5, and -10.[31, 32] Both subsets elaborate tumor necrosis factor-β and colony-stimulating factors. Th1 cells have been identified as the cells that mediate DTH reactivity.[31, 32]

Anergy signifies the failure to mount a response to an antigen.[5] Although this obviously happens in nonsensitized persons, there are numerous ways, at the cellular and molecular levels, to explain unresponsiveness in previously sensitized subjects (Table 15–2). In infectious disease states, the highest prevalence of anergy is among persons with progressive disseminated infections, but nonresponsiveness may be found in those with limited infections[33–36] (Table 15–3). Moreover, experimental models of infection have suggested a direct correlation between the presence of anergy and the burden of microorganisms or microbial antigens.[37–40] The significance of this has yet to be explained.

Pharmacologic Modulation of Skin Test Reactivity

Human studies concerning the modification of skin test reactivity by pharmacologic agents are sparse. Corticosteroids, when given at dosages greater than 15 mg/d for 3 weeks, inhibit expression of tuberculin hypersensitivity in humans.[41, 42] The mechanism of the inhibition has not been defined precisely, but it is presumably alterations in number of T cells and in biologic function. Short-term administration of large doses of methylprednisolone, on the other hand, does not render a subject anergic.[43]

Prostaglandins have been shown to be inhibitors of immune responses in vitro.[44] A single study has demonstrated that indomethacin, which irreversibly blocks prostaglandin synthesis, has improved skin test responses in two patients with common variable immunodeficiency.[45] In normal subjects, however, indomethacin did not alter intradermal skin test responses.[46]

In experimental animals, the effects of various immunomodulators on DTH responses have been examined. Only a few are listed here. Amphotericin B can enhance contact sensitivity in mice, probably by inhibiting suppressor cell activity.[47] Cyclophosphamide can also enhance DTH responses by the same mechanism.[48] Other immunodepressants such as 6-mercaptopurine can cause depression of DTH,[49] but in humans it may be difficult to separate the effects of the drug and those of the underlying disease.

Skin Tests for Specific Infectious Diseases

Mycobacterial Infections

Tuberculosis. Two to four weeks after infection with *M. tuberculosis*, most immunocompetent persons mount a posi-

TABLE 15–2 ■ Putative Cellular and Molecular Causes of Anergy in Infectious Diseases

Activation of suppressor T cells or suppressor macrophages
Production of suppressor factors
Defects in antigen presentation
Lack of antigen-reactive T cells
Clonal deletion
Human immunodeficiency virus–mediated destruction
Pharmacologic modulation
Iatrogenic or idiopathic cytopenia
Defective cytokine production
Viral infections other than human immunodeficiency virus (e.g., measles)

TABLE 15–3 ■ Skin Test Anergy in Infectious Diseases

MICROBE	INFECTIOUS DISEASE STATE	ANERGY TO SPECIFIC ANTIGEN* (%)
Coccidioides immitis	Acute pulmonary coccidioidomycosis	<10
	Chronic pulmonary coccidioidomycosis	30–75
	Disseminated coccidioidomycosis	30–70
Histoplasma capsulatum	Acute pulmonary histoplasmosis	<10
	Chronic pulmonary histoplasmosis	10–30
	Disseminated histoplasmosis	45–70
Leishmania tropica	Cutaneous leishmaniasis	<10
Leishmania major	Cutaneous leishmaniasis	<10
Leishmania mexicana	Cutaneous leishmaniasis	<10
Leishmania braziliensis	Cutaneous leishmaniasis	<10
Leishmania braziliensis	Mucocutaneous leishmaniasis	<10
Leishmania aethiopica	Diffuse cutaneous leishmaniasis	>90
Leishmania mexicana	Diffuse cutaneous leishmaniasis	>90
Leishmania donovani	Visceral leishmaniasis	>90
Mycobacterium leprae	Tuberculoid leprosy	<20
	Borderline leprosy	40–100
	Lepromatous leprosy	>80
Mycobacterium tuberculosis	Pulmonary tuberculosis	10–20
	Disseminated tuberculosis	50–70
Paracoccidioides brasiliensis	Asymptomatic paracoccidioidomycosis	<10
	Progressive pulmonary paracoccidioidomycosis	30–55
	Disseminated paracoccidioidomycosis	>70

*Compiled from references 33–36, 50–62, 71, 83, 88, 93, 99, 112–122.

tive skin test response to intermediate-strength (5 tuberculin units [TU]) purified protein derivative. This response mirrors the healing process exerted by cell-mediated immune mechanisms in vivo. Among persons with active pulmonary tuberculosis, up to 20% may manifest either antigen-specific anergy or a more generalized lack of reactivity to a battery of recall antigens.[50–52] In disseminated tuberculosis, the incidence of anergy approaches 50% to 70%, especially in miliary disease and meningitis.[53–60] Furthermore, the responsiveness to tuberculin may be diminished by immunosuppressive therapy or by certain underlying diseases such as chronic renal failure, hematologic disorders, and immunodeficiency syndromes.[61–66] In normal hosts, cutaneous sensitivity usually recovers after weeks to months of antituberculous therapy. The cause of the immunoregulatory disturbance in those without known preexisting immunologic defects is incompletely understood. Studies in vitro have implicated circulating monocytes as mediators of antigen-specific suppression in anergic subjects who had pulmonary tuberculosis.[67] Removal of these cells from peripheral mononuclear blood cells enhances responsiveness in vitro of T cells to tuberculin.

For clinical diagnosis and epidemiologic studies, the tuberculin skin test with 5 TU of purified protein derivative remains an important tool. Certain problems with this test are acknowledged. Because *M. tuberculosis* shares antigens with numerous nontuberculous mycobacteria, cross-reactivity may lead to a false-positive skin test result. Moreover, persons vaccinated with bacille Calmette-Guérin may also show a positive tuberculin reaction. Another difficulty in construing the significance of a positive skin test result arises with the so-called booster phenomenon. If reactivity to tuberculin in infected persons has waned over time, skin testing may produce either a small reaction or no reaction. Rechallenge, however, may prompt an amnestic response with an increase in the size of the tuberculin reaction.[68] This problem is most often observed in situations of repeated testing in short periods and may lead to the false impression of conversion. The booster phenomenon may be overcome by retesting those with a response less than 10 mm within a week.[69]

Exactly how long a skin test result remains positive is not known. In general, it appears that tuberculin sensitivity is lifelong.[70] As the population of many countries ages, the possibility of waning reactivity may become a significant clinical problem in elderly persons. Lack of hypersensitivity may be misinterpreted as indicating that tuberculosis cannot be the cause of a patient's illness.

Leprosy. Both the clinical manifestations and the immunologic features of leprosy are spectral. Patients with the limited forms of infection, tuberculoid and borderline tuberculoid leprosy, exhibit a skin test response to lepromin, a heat-killed suspension of bacilli prepared from infected armadillos or skin nodules of patients with lepromatous disease. At 48 to 72 hours after challenge, an area of induration becomes apparent (the Fernandez reaction). Subsequently, the response progresses to nodule formation and possibly ulceration (the Mitsuda reaction) during the 3 to 4 weeks after injection. Also, it is important to emphasize that many normal persons who have not been exposed to *Mycobacterium leprae* may manifest a reaction to lepromin. In contrast, untreated patients with borderline disease or lepromatous leprosy do not mount a response to lepromin; moreover, the anergy is frequently generalized.[71] Responses to nonspecific antigens may be regained after antibiotic therapy in lepromatous patients, but unlike the situation in tuberculosis, the specific response to lepromin often remains negative.[71]

The cutaneous reactivity to purified protein derivative of patients with untreated and treated lepromatous leprosy has been examined in detail. Fifty-eight percent of patients with lepromatous leprosy responded, and the percentage was higher in those treated longer than 18 months.[72] The reaction was characterized by early onset of induration, which was maximal at 4 days and was observed for up to 21 days. T cells and circulating monocytes constituted the majority of cells in positive responders, and $CD4^+$ T cells were predominant. One interesting feature was the destruction of macrophages containing leprosy bacilli in areas of skin testing. This is reminiscent of Koch's original observation that skin testing with tuberculin reduced the number of tubercle bacilli in skin of *M. tuberculosis*–infected guinea pigs.

Several reasons have been proposed to explain anergy in

lepromatous leprosy, among them the existence of suppressor cells,[73, 74] defective production of cytokines,[75, 76] impaired expression of interleukin-2 receptors,[77] and the presence of serum factors that depress cell-mediated immunity.[78]

Fungal Diseases

Useful skin test reagents are available for *Candida, Histoplasma, Coccidioides,* and *Paracoccidioides.* Blastomycin, which has been employed to detect blastomycosis, is not an adequate preparation. It should be emphasized that, in contrast to the tuberculin test in immunocompetent hosts, the definition of a positive skin reaction in fungal diseases is a 5-mm area of induration, not 10 mm.[79]

Approximately 50% to 90% of normal persons respond to *Candida* antigens as a result of colonization by this ubiquitous organism.[80–82] Because such a large percentage of individuals demonstrate a positive response to the *Candida* antigen skin test, it is included in a battery of recall antigens to test for immunocompetence in an individual. This skin test preparation is not useful in the detection of infection with *Candida* species.

It is presumed that between 90% and 100% of those who have convalesced from acute pulmonary histoplasmosis, coccidioidomycosis, or paracoccidioidomycosis manifest a positive skin reaction to the respective antigen.[34, 83] Cross-reactivity has been observed between histoplasmin and coccidioidin and between paracoccidioidin and histoplasmin. The time required for conversion to a positive skin test appears to be approximately 4 weeks.[84, 85] The persistence of a positive skin response to these fungal antigens in immunocompetent persons apparently is lifelong, although several studies have suggested that it may be short-lived. Waning reactivity has been reported in persons residing in endemic areas.[86–88] It has been argued that reversion of coccidioidin reactivity to negative suggests susceptibility to reactivation of infection.[88]

In disseminated forms of histoplasmosis, coccidioidomycosis, and paracoccidioidomycosis, the percentage of positive responders drops to 30% to 50%.[33, 34, 83, 89] Anergy in histoplasmosis or coccidioidomycosis may have important prognostic value and may indicate progression of infection beyond the pulmonary system. Also, the failure to detect a positive skin reaction in an ill patient may be misconstrued as an indication that the person is not infected with fungus. This incorrect assumption could lead to marked delay in diagnosis and treatment. Experimental evidence suggests that anergy in these diseases may be caused in part by suppressor cells[37, 90, 91] or deficient cytokine production.[92]

Leishmaniasis

The vast majority of persons with cutaneous or mucocutaneous leishmaniasis manifest skin test positivity to specific antigen.[93, 94] As with many other intracellular pathogens, skin test reactivity is usually evident 4 to 6 weeks after primary infection and appears to persist indefinitely. A positive skin response may provide indirect evidence of active infection but only in conjunction with the appropriate clinical findings. False-positive reactions may be seen in those exposed to nonpathogenic *Leishmania* species.

On the other hand, skin test responses to specific antigens are absent in a large proportion of persons with diffuse cutaneous leishmaniasis or visceral leishmaniasis.[95–99] After treatment, most patients mount a skin response to antigen. One study of humans with diffuse cutaneous leishmaniasis has demonstrated that anergy is associated with a circulating population of adherent suppressor cells.[35] Addition of indomethacin restored reactivity in vitro to *Leishmania* antigens by peripheral blood cells from infected patients.[35] There are, however, no data to suggest that treatment with this pharmacological agent in vivo restores cellular immune responses of such patients.

Studies of both humans and experimental animals infected with *Leishmania donovani* have described several mechanisms to account for the loss of DTH associated with visceral leishmaniasis—impaired production of interleukins-1 and -2,[100, 101] generation of suppressor T cells and suppressor macrophages,[102, 103] and suppression of macrophage expression of class I and class II major histocompatibility complex molecules.[104]

Prognostic Value of Skin Testing in Human Immunodeficiency Virus Infection

Human immunodeficiency virus infection is associated with a progressive loss of $CD4^+$ T cells. Therefore, it can be anticipated that skin test responses may become negative at some point in infection. Individuals with a $CD4^+$ T-cell count below 400 cells per mm^3 exhibit a lower incidence of skin test positivity to one or more of a battery of recall antigens than those with greater than 400 cells per mm^3 (67% versus 94%). Moreover, the lack of cutaneous reactivity on presentation was predictive of the development of acquired immunodeficiency syndrome. Thus, skin tests may be useful as a predictor of progression to acquired immunodeficiency syndrome.[105]

Skin Testing to Detect Antibiotic Hypersensitivity

Skin testing to assess antibiotic allergy is used to measure immediate (immunoglobulin E–mediated) hypersensitivity but not DTH reactions (cell-mediated immune mechanism). Among reactions to antibiotics, penicillin allergy has been studied most thoroughly, and it is the one antibiotic for which standard skin tests exist. Penicillin G forms antigenic determinants categorized as major and minor. The major determinant is benzylpenicilloyl, and some of the minor determinants are benzyl-D-penicilloate and benzyl-D-penicilloic acid.[106] Testing with the major determinants detects many but not all patients at risk for anaphylaxis. The minor determinants, however, appear to be responsible for most of the severe immediate reactions to penicillin.[107] Unfortunately, there is no adequate preparation of minor determinants. Some have used aged penicillin G, but studies have shown that this is not a reliable preparation for minor determinants.[108]

The prevalence of a positive skin test is related to the time that has elapsed between clinical reaction and application of the skin test.[108] A positive skin test is highly indicative of immediate hypersensitivity, and a negative skin test strongly suggests that no allergy exists.[109] Approximately 1% to 2% of individuals who are skin test–negative for penicillin react to systemic administration of this antibiotic.[108–111] In such cases, the symptoms are usually mild and develop several days after initiation of therapy; none of the reactions has been life threatening. Skin testing is, therefore, exceptionally safe, and only mild reactions have been noted in studies of several thousand subjects.[109] The utility of testing with other antibiotics remains to be determined because of a lack of uniform preparations for skin testing.

References

1. Koch R: Weitere Mitteilung über ein Heilmittel gegen Tuberkulose. Dtsch Med Wochenschr 16:1029, 1890.

2. Koch R: Weitere Mitteilung über das Tuberkulin. Dtsch Med Wochenschr 17:1189, 1891.
3. Mantoux C: L'intradermal réaction à la tuberculine et son interprétation clinique. Presse Med 18:10, 1910.
4. von Pirquet C: Quantitative experiments with cutaneous tuberculin reaction. J Pharmacol Exp Ther 1:151, 1909.
5. von Pirquet C: Das Verhalten der kutanen Tuberkulinreaktion während der Masern. Dtsch Med Wochenschr 34:1297, 1908.
6. Landsteiner K, Chase MW: Experiments on transfer of cutaneous sensitivity to simple compounds. Proc Soc Exp Biol Med 49:688, 1942.
7. Chase MW: The cellular transfer of cutaneous hypersensitivity to tuberculin. Proc Soc Exp Biol Med 59:134, 1945.
8. Lawrence HS: The cellular transfer of cutaneous hypersensitivity to tuberculin in man. Proc Soc Exp Biol Med 71:516, 1949.
9. Bosnan C, Feldman JD: Composition, morphology, and source of cells in delayed skin reactions. Am J Pathol 58:201, 1970.
10. Dvorak HF, Mihm MC Jr, Dvorak AC, et al: Morphology of delayed-type hypersensitivity reactions in man. I. Quantitative description of the inflammatory response. Lab Invest 31:111, 1974.
11. Poulter LW, Seymour GJ, Duke O, et al: Immunohistological analysis of delayed-type hypersensitivity in man. Cell Immunol 74:358, 1982.
12. Platt JL, Grant BW, Eddy AA, et al: Immune cell populations in cutaneous delayed-type hypersensitivity. J Exp Med 158:1227, 1983.
13. Fullmer MA, Shen JY, Modlin RL, et al: Immunohistological evidence of lymphokine production and lymphocyte activation antigens in tuberculin reactions. Clin Exp Immunol 67:383, 1987.
14. Jones TD, Mote JR: The phases of foreign protein sensitization in human beings. N Engl J Med 210:120, 1934.
15. Mote JR, Jones TD: The development of foreign protein sensitization in human beings. J Immunol 30:149, 1936.
16. Richerson HB, Dvorak HF, Leskowitz S: Cutaneous basophil hypersensitivity. I. A new look at the Jones-Mote reaction, general characteristics. J Exp Med 132:546, 1970.
17. Deepe GS Jr: Protective immunity in murine histoplasmosis: Functional comparison of adoptively transferred T-cell clones and splenic T cells. Infect Immun 56:2350, 1988.
18. Hussein S, Curtis J, Akuffo H, et al: Dissociation between delayed-type hypersensitivity and resistance to pathogenic mycobacteria demonstrated by T-cell clones. Infect Immun 55:564, 1987.
19. Czuprynski CJ, Brown JF, Young KM, et al: Administration of purified anti-L3T4 monoclonal antibody impairs the resistance of mice to *Listeria monocytogenes* infection. Infect Immun 57:100, 1989.
20. Murphy JW: Effects of first-order *Cryptococcus*-specific T suppressor cells on induction of cells responsible for delayed-type hypersensitivity. Infect Immun 48:439, 1985.
21. Orme IM: Induction of nonspecific acquired resistance and delayed-type hypersensitivity, but not specific acquired resistance in mice inoculated with killed mycobacterial vaccines. Infect Immun 56:3310, 1988.
22. Dailey MO, Fathman CG, Butcher EC, et al: Abnormal migration of T-lymphocyte clones. J Immunol 128:2134, 1982.
23. Dailey MO, Gallatin WM, Weissman IL: The in vivo behavior of T-cell clones: Altered migration due to loss of the lymphocyte homing receptor. J Mol Cell Immunol 2:27, 1985.
24. Ziegler HK, Unanue ER: Identification of a macrophage antigen-processing event required for I region–restricted antigen presentation to T lymphocytes. J Immunol 127:1869, 1981.
25. Unanue ER: Antigen presenting function of the macrophage. Annu Rev Immunol 2:395, 1984.
26. Allen PM, Beller DI, Braun J, et al: The handling of *Listeria monocytogenes* by macrophages: The search for an immunogenic molecule in antigen presentation. J Immunol 132:323, 1984.
27. Babbitt BP, Allen PM, Matseuda G, et al: Binding of immunogenic peptides to Ia histocompatibility molecules. Nature 316:359, 1985.
28. Unanue ER, Allen PM: The basis for the immunoregulatory role of macrophages and other accessory cells. Science 236:551, 1987.
29. Marrack P, Kappler J: The antigen-specific, major histocompatibility complex–restricted receptor on T cells. Adv Immunol 38:1, 1986.
30. Marrack P, Kappler J: The T-cell receptor. Science 238:1073, 1987.
31. Sher A, Coffman RL: Regulation of immunity to parasites by T cells and T-cell derived cytokines. Annu Rev Immunol 10:385, 1992.
32. Fitch FW, McKisic MD, Lancki DW, et al: Differential regulation of murine T lymphocyte subsets. Annu Rev Immunol 11:29, 1993.
33. Furculow MF: Comparison of treated and untreated severe histoplasmosis. JAMA 183:823, 1963.
34. Drutz DJ, Catanzaro A: Coccidioidomycosis. Am Rev Respir Dis 117:559, 1978.
35. Petersen EA, Neva FA, Oster CN, et al: Specific inhibition of lymphocyte-proliferation by adherent suppressor cells in diffuse cutaneous leishmaniasis. N Engl J Med 306:387, 1982.
36. Turk JL, Bryceson ADM: Immunological phenomena in leprosy and related diseases. Adv Immunol 13:209, 1971.
37. Nickerson DA, Havens RA, Bullock WE: Immunoregulation in disseminated histoplasmosis. Cell Immunol 60:287, 1981.
38. Cox RA, Kennell W: Suppression of T-lymphocyte response by *Coccidioides immitis* antigen. Infect Immun 56:1424, 1988.
39. Murphy JW, Moorhead JW: Regulation of cell-mediated immunity in cryptococcosis. I. Induction of speciic afferent suppressor cells by cryptococcal antigen. J Immunol 128:276, 1982.
40. Fahey JR, Herman R: Relationship between delayed hypersensitivity response and acquired cell-mediated immunity in C57BL/6J mice infected with *Leishmania donovani*. Infect Immun 49:447, 1985.
41. Bovornkitti S, Kangsadal P, Sathirapat P, et al: Reversion and reconversion rate of tuberculin skin reactions in correlation with the use of prednisone. Dis Chest 38:51, 1960.
42. Schatz M, Patterson R, Kloner R: The prevalence of tuberculin positive skin tests in a steroid-treated asthmatic population. Ann Intern Med 84:261, 1976.
43. Fan PT, Yu DTY, Clements PJ, et al: Effects of corticosteroids on the human immune response: Comparison of one and three daily 1 gm intravenous pulses of methylprednisolone. J Lab Clin Med 91:625, 1978.
44. Goodwin JS, Webb DR: Regulation of the immune response by prostaglandins. Clin Immunol Immunopathol 15:106, 1980.
45. Goodwin JS, Bankhurst AD, Murphy SA, et al: Partial reversal of the cellular immune defect in common variable immunodeficiency with indomethacin. J Clin Lab Immunol 1:197, 1978.
46. Goodwin JS, Selinger DS, Messner RP, et al: Effect of indomethacin in vivo on humoral and cellular immunity in humans. Infect Immun 19:430, 1978.
47. Shirley SF, Little JR: Immunopotentiating effects of amphotericin B. I. Enhanced contact sensitivity in mice. J Immunol 123:2878, 1979.
48. Askenase PW, Hayden BJ, Gershon RK: Augmentation of delayed-type hypersensitivity by doses of cyclophosphamide which do not affect antibody responses. J Exp Med 141:697, 1975.
49. Phillips SM, Zweiman B: Mechanisms of the suppression of delayed hypersensitivity in the guinea pig by 6-mercaptopurine. J Exp Med 137:149, 1973.
50. McMurray DN, Echeverri A: Cell-mediated immunity in anergic patients with pulmonary tuberculosis. Am Rev Respir Dis 118:827, 1978.
51. Nash D, Douglass JE: Anergy in active pulmonary tuberculosis. A comparison between positive and negative reactors and an evaluation of 5 TU and 250 TU skin test doses. Chest 77:1, 1980.
52. Daniel TM, Oxtoby MJ, Pinto EM, et al: The immune spectrum in patients with pulmonary tuberculosis. Am Rev Respir Dis 123:556, 1981.
53. Proudfoot AT, Akhtar AJ, Douglas AC, et al: Miliary tuberculosis in adults. Br Med J 2:273, 1969.
54. Munt PW: Miliary tuberculosis in the chemotherapy era: With a clinical review in 69 American adults. Medicine 51:139, 1971.
55. Sahn SA, Neff TA: Miliary tuberculosis. Am J Med 56:495, 1974.
56. Grieco MH, Chmel H: Acute disseminated tuberculosis as a diagnostic problem. A clinical study based on twenty-eight cases. Am Rev Respir Dis 109:554, 1974.
57. Barrett-Connor E: Tuberculous meningitis in adults. South Med J 60:1061, 1969.
58. Haas EJ, Madhavan T, Quinn EL: Tuberculous meningitis in an urban general hospital. Arch Intern Med 137:1518, 1977.

59. Klein NC, Damsker B, Hirschman SZ: Mycobacterial meningitis. Retrospective analysis from 1970 to 1983. Am J Med 79:29, 1985.
60. Ogawa SK, Smith MA, Brennessel DJ, et al: Tuberculous meningitis in an urban medical center. Medicine (Baltimore) 66:317, 1987.
61. Andrew OT, Schoenfeld PY, Hopewell PC: Tuberculosis in patients with end-stage renal disease. Am J Med 68:59, 1980.
62. Rutsky EA, Rostand SG: Mycobacteriosis in patients with chronic renal failure. Arch Intern Med 140:57, 1980.
63. Navari RM, Sullivan KM, Springmeyer SC, et al: Mycobacterial infection in marrow transplant patients. Transplantation 36:509, 1983.
64. Kaplan MH, Armstrong D, Rosen P: Tuberculosis complicating neoplastic disease. A review of 201 cases. Cancer 33:850, 1974.
65. Pitchenik AE, Cole C, Russell BW, et al: Tuberculosis, atypical mycobacteriosis, and the acquired immunodeficiency syndrome among Haitian and non-Haitian patients in south Florida. Ann Intern Med 101:641, 1984.
66. Centers for Disease Control: Tuberculosis and human immunodeficiency virus infection: Recommendations of the Advisory Committee for the Elimination of Tuberculosis (ACET). MMWR Morb Mortal Wkly Rep 38:236, 1989.
67. Ellner JJ: Suppressor adherent cells in human tuberculosis. J Immunol 121:2573, 1978.
68. Narain R, Nair SS, Rao GR, et al: Enhancing of tuberculin allergy by previous tuberculin testing. Bull WHO 34:623, 1966.
69. Thompson NJ, Glassroth JL, Snider DE Jr, et al: The booster phenomenon in serial tuberculin skin testing. Am Rev Respir Dis 119:587, 1979.
70. Stead WW, To T: The significance of tuberculin skin testing in elderly persons. Ann Intern Med 107:837, 1987.
71. Bullock WE: Studies on immune mechanisms in leprosy. I. Depression of delayed allergic response to skin test antigens. N Engl J Med 278:298, 1968.
72. Kaplan G, Laal S, Sheftel G, et al: The nature and kinetics of a delayed immune response to purified protein derivative of tuberculin in the skin of lepromatous leprosy patients. J Exp Med 168:1811, 1988.
73. Mehra V, Mason LH, Rothman W, et al: Delineation of a human T-cell subset responsible for lepromin-induced suppression in leprosy patients. J Immunol 125:1183, 1980.
74. Modlin RL, Kato H, Mehra V, et al: Genetically restricted suppressor T-cell clones derived from lepromatous leprosy lesions. Nature 322:459, 1986.
75. Watson S, Bullock W, Nelson K, et al: Interleukin 1 production by peripheral blood mononuclear cells from leprosy patients. Infect Immun 45:787, 1984.
76. Haregewoin A, Godal T, Mustafa AS, et al: T cell–conditioned media reverse T-cell unresponsiveness in lepromatous leprosy. Nature 303:342, 1983.
77. Mohagheghpour N, Gelber RH, Larrick JW, et al: Defective cell-mediated immunity in leprosy: Failure of T cells from lepromatous leprosy patients to respond to *Mycobacterium leprae* is associated with defective expression of interleukin 2 receptors and is not reconstituted by interleukin 2. J Immunol 135:1443, 1985.
78. Bullock WE, Fasal P: Studies of immune mechanisms in leprosy. III. The role of cellular and humoral factors in impairment of the in vitro immune response. J Immunol 106:888, 1971.
79. Sarosi GA, Catanzaro A, Daniel TM, et al: Clinical usefulness of skin testing in histoplasmosis, coccidioidomycosis, and blastomycosis. Am Rev Respir Dis 138:1081, 1988.
80. Hassett AM, Woods RJ, Temperly IJ, et al: Cell-mediated immunity to recall antigens in vivo and in vitro. Irish J Med Sci 146:167, 1977.
81. Ferguson AC, Kershar HE, Collin WK, et al: Correlation of cutaneous hypersensitivity with lymphocyte response to *Candida albicans*. Am J Clin Pathol 68:499, 1977.
82. Shannon DC, Johnson G, Rosen F, et al: Cellular activity to *Candida albicans* antigen. N Engl J Med 275:690, 1966.
83. Schwarz J: Histoplasmosis. New York, Praeger, 1981.
84. Loosli CG, Grayston JT, Alexander ER, et al: Epidemiological studies of pulmonary histoplasmosis in a farm family. Am J Hyg 55:392, 1952.
85. Murray JF, Lurie HI, Kaye J, et al: Benign pulmonary histoplasmosis (cave disease) in South Africa. S Afr Med J 31:245, 1957.
86. Zeidberg LD, Dillon A, Gass RS: Some factors in the epidemiology of histoplasmin sensitivity in Williamson County, Tennessee. Am J Public Health 41:80, 1951.
87. Pappagianis D: Epidemiological aspects of respiratory mycotic infections. Bacteriol Rev 31:25, 1967.
88. Sievers ML: Disseminated coccidioidomycosis among southwestern American Indians. Am Rev Respir Dis 109:602, 1974.
89. Catanzaro A, Spitler LE, Moser KM: Cellular immune response in coccidioidomycosis. Cell Immunol 15:360, 1975.
90. Catanzaro A: Suppressor cells in coccidioidomycosis. Cell Immunol 64:235, 1981.
91. Stobo JD, Paul S, Van Scoy RE, et al: Suppressor thymus-derived lymphocytes in fungal infection. J Clin Invest 57:319, 1976.
92. Watson SR, Schmitt SK, Hendricks DE, et al: Immunoregulation in disseminated murine histoplasmosis: Disturbances in the production of interleukins 1 and 2. J Immunol 135:3487, 1985.
93. Carvalho EM, Johnson WD, Barreto E, et al: Cell mediated immunity in American cutaneous and mucosal leishmaniasis. J Immunol 135:4144, 1985.
94. Jones TC, Johnson WD Jr, Barretto AC, et al: Epidemiology of American cutaneous leishmaniasis due to *Leishmania braziliensis braziliensis*. J Infect Dis 156:73, 1987.
95. Bryceson ADM: Diffuse cutaneous leishmaniasis in Ethiopia. III. Immunological studies. Trans R Soc Trop Med Hyg 64:380, 1970.
96. Convit J, Pinardi ME, Rondon A: Diffuse cutaneous leishmaniasis. A disease due to an immunological defect. Trans R Soc Trop Med Hyg 66:603, 1972.
97. Rezai HR, Ardekalai SM, Amirhakimi G, et al: Immunological features of kala-azar. Am J Trop Med Hyg 27:1079, 1978.
98. Carvalho EM, Teixeira RS, Johnson WD: Cell mediated immunity in American visceral leishmaniasis: Reversible immunosuppression during acute infection. Infect Immun 33:498, 1981.
99. Ho M, Koech DK, Iha DW, et al: Immunosuppression in Kenyan visceral leishmaniasis. Clin Exp Immunol 51:207, 1983.
100. Crawford GD, Wyler DJ, Dinarello CA: Parasite-monocyte interactions in human leishmaniasis: Production of interleukin 1 in vitro. J Infect Dis 152:315, 1985.
101. Reiner N, Finke JH: Interleukin 2 deficiency in murine *Leishmaniasis donovani* and its relationship to depressed spleen cell responses to phytohemagglutinin. J Immunol 131:1487, 1983.
102. Nickol AD, Bonventre PF: Visceral Leishmaniasis in congenic mice of susceptible and resistant phenotypes: T lymphocyte–mediated immunosuppression. Infect Immun 50:169, 1984.
103. Murray HW, Carriero SM, Donelly DM: Presence of a macrophage-mediated suppressor cell mechanism during cell-mediated immune response in experimental visceral leishmaniasis. Infect Immun 54:487, 1986.
104. Reiner NE, Ng W, McMaster WR: Parasite–accessory cell interactions in murine leishmaniasis. II. *Leishmania donovani* suppresses macrophage expression of class I and class II major histocompatibility complex products. J Immunol 138:1926, 1987.
105. Blatt SP, Hendrix CW, Butzin CA, et al: Delayed-type hypersensitivity skin testing predicts progression to AIDS in HIV-infected patients. Ann Intern Med 119:177, 1994.
106. Ressler C, Mendelson LM: Skin test for diagnosis of penicillin allergy—Current status. Ann Allergy 59:167, 1987.
107. Levine RB, Redmond AP, Fellner MJ, et al: Penicillin allergy and the heterogeneous immune response to benzylpenicillin. J Clin Invest 45:1895, 1966.
108. Ressler C, Neag PM, Mendelson LM: A liquid chromatographic study of stability of the minor determinants of penicillin allergy. A stable minor determinant mixture skin test preparation. J Pharm Sci 74:448, 1985.
109. Sullivan TJ, Wedner HJ, Shatz GS, et al: Skin testing to detect penicillin allergy. J Allerg Clin Immunol 68:171, 1981.
110. Green GR, Rosenblum AH, Sweet LC: Evaluation of penicillin hypersensitivity: Value of clinical history and skin testing with penicilloyl-polylysine and penicillin G. J Allergy Clin Immunol 60:339, 1977.
111. Sogn DD, Evans R 3d, Shepherd GM, et al: Results of the National Institute of Allergy and Infectious Diseases Collaborative Clinical Trial to test the predictive value of skin testing with major and minor penicillin derivatives in hospitalized patients. Arch Intern Med 152:1025, 1992.
112. Smith CE, Whiting EG, Baker EE, et al: The use of coccidioidin. Am Rev Tuberc 57:330, 1955.
113. Smith CE, Beard RR, Saito MT: Pathogenesis of coccidioidomy-

cosis with special reference to pulmonary cavitation. Ann Intern Med 29:623, 1948.
114. Winn WA: A long term study of 300 patients with cavitary-abscess lesions of the lung of coccidioidal origin. An analytical study with special reference to treatment. Dis Chest 54:268, 1968.
115. Hyde L: Coccidioidal pulmonary cavitation. Dis Chest 54:273, 1968.
116. Wiant JR, Smith JW: Coccidioidin skin reactivity in pulmonary coccidioidomycosis. Chest 63:100, 1973.
117. Myrvang V, Godal T, Ridley DS, et al: Immune responsiveness to *Mycobacterium leprae* and other mycobacterial antigens throughout the clinical and histopathological spectrum of leprosy. Clin Exp Immunol 14:541, 1973.
118. Nath I, Curtiss J, Sharma AK, et al: Circulating T-cell numbers and their mitogenic potential in leprosy—Correlation with mycobacterial load. Clin Exp Immunol 29:363, 1977.
119. Restrepo A: Immune response to *Paracoccidioides brasiliensis* in human and animal hosts. Curr Top Med Mycol 2:239, 1988.
120. Mussatti C, Rezkallah-Iwasso MT, Mendes E, et al: In vivo and in vitro evaluation of cell-mediated immunity in patients with paracoccidioidomycosis. Cell Immunol 24:365, 1978.
121. Mota NGS, Rezkallah-Iwasso MT, Peracoli MT, et al: Correlation between cell-mediated immunity and clinical forms of paracoccidioidomycosis. Trans R Soc Trop Med Hyg 79:765, 1985.
122. Mok WY, Fava-Netto C: Paracoccidioidin and histoplasmin sensitivity in Coari (state of Amazonas), Brazil. Am J Trop Med Hyg 27:808, 1978.

PRINCIPLES OF TREATMENT

16

Pharmacologic Principles

Michael Barza

The physician must have a basic understanding of pharmacologic principles to use antimicrobial agents in the safest and most effective way. My purpose in this chapter is to outline the most important of these principles from the point of view of a clinical consultant in infectious diseases.

For most antimicrobial agents, the bulk of the pharmacokinetic information available deals with the concentrations of the drugs in plasma or serum. Data on the concentrations of drugs in peripheral sites are more scarce; furthermore, when the concentrations of drugs are monitored during treatment, it is generally serum concentrations that are studied, even when the primary focus of infection is extravascular, because serum is more accessible than other body fluids. Fortunately, measurements of concentrations in serum may provide a good guide to concentrations in peripheral sites, provided that a few basic principles are borne in mind. Accordingly, this chapter begins with a consideration of the determinants of the concentration profile in serum and goes on to discuss the relation between the concentrations in serum and in peripheral sites. Data regarding the intracellular penetration of drugs are also reviewed.

Antibiotic Concentrations in Serum

Serum Concentrations and Time for Equilibration

After a rapid intravenous injection (bolus injection) of an antibiotic, the concentration of drug in the serum promptly reaches a peak and then begins to decline (Fig. 16–1). The first portion of the decline, the α-phase, is steep as a result of mixing of the bolus with the blood and distribution to rapidly equilibrating compartments. In the second portion, the β-phase (or elimination phase), the decline is mainly the result of drug elimination. The β-phase is used to determine the serum half-life ($t_{1/2}$) of the drug. For most drugs, diffusion between the tissues and the plasma occurs quickly enough that the serum half-life in the β-phase not only is the time in which the serum concentration drops by half but also approximates the time in which the total amount of drug in the body is reduced by half. The serum half-life is related to the elimination rate as

$$t_{1/2} = 0.693/K \qquad (1)$$

where K is the elimination rate constant. If $t_{1/2}$ is expressed in hours, then the units of K are hour^{-1}.

If a drug is administered at regular intervals without a loading dose, there will be a steady rise in the peak and trough concentrations in the serum until an equilibrium is reached, at which time the rate of drug elimination is equal to the rate of administration (Fig. 16–2). The number of doses (N) required for the peak serum concentration to reach 95% of the equilibrium concentration can be determined by dividing the serum half-life by the dosing interval (t_i) and multiplying by 4.32. The time required for the peak concentrations to reach 95% of the equilibrium value (by definition, $N \times t_i$) can be calculated by multiplying the half-life of the drug by 4.32.[1] For example, if gentamicin has a serum half-life of 8 hours in a patient with renal impairment and is administered at a fixed dosage every 24 hours, the number of doses required for the peak serum concentration to reach 95% of the equilibrium value is $4.32 \times 8/24$, or 1.44 dose, and the time to reach 95% of the equilibrium value is 34.6 hours.

Equilibrium can be achieved quickly if a loading dose is given initially (Fig. 16–2*A*). In general, a loading dose is about 1.5 to 2 times larger than the maintenance dose. With drugs that have a short serum half-life in relation to the dosing interval (e.g., most penicillins and cephalosporins), there is little or no accumulation between doses and there is no need for a loading dose; however, with agents that have a longer half-life and a relatively narrow therapeutic index (such as the aminoglycosides), it is common practice to administer a loading dose to patients with serious infections to achieve equilibrium concentrations quickly.

If a drug is given by continuous infusion (Fig. 16–2*B*) rather than by rapid intravenous injection, again the serum concentration rises slowly until equilibrium is reached. As with intermittent infusions, the time required to achieve 95% of the equilibrium concentration is the product of 4.32 and the half-life of the drug. Thus, the time required to achieve equilibrium is independent of whether the drug is given by intermittent or continuous infusion. As with intermittent dosing, equilibrium can be achieved much more quickly if a loading dose is given.

The analysis of serum concentration curves is more complicated when drugs are administered by the oral or intramuscular route than when they are given by the intravenous route because drug elimination and absorption occur simultaneously. The elimination half-life cannot be reliably determined until drug absorption is complete. Nevertheless, the

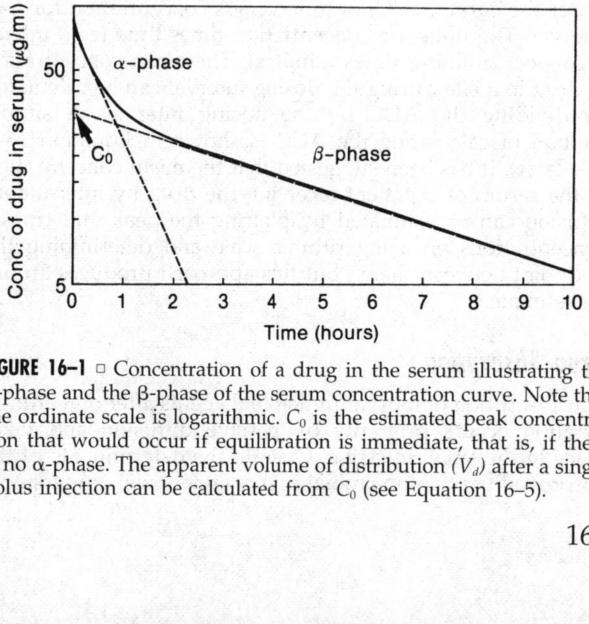

FIGURE 16–1 ▫ Concentration of a drug in the serum illustrating the α-phase and the β-phase of the serum concentration curve. Note that the ordinate scale is logarithmic. C_0 is the estimated peak concentration that would occur if equilibration is immediate, that is, if there is no α-phase. The apparent volume of distribution (V_d) after a single bolus injection can be calculated from C_0 (see Equation 16–5).

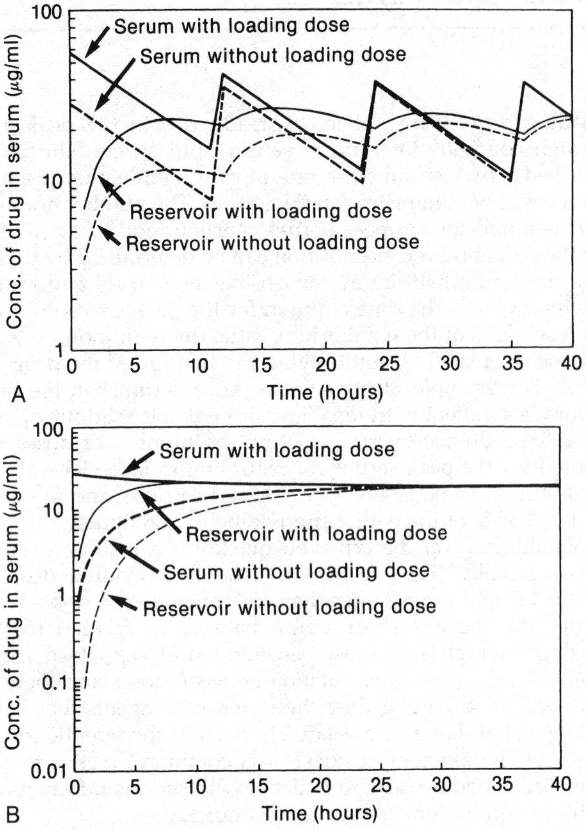

FIGURE 16–2 □ Concentrations of vancomycin in the serum and in a large reservoir (e.g., peritoneal fluid) during administration by intermittent infusion *(A)* or during continuous infusion *(B)* with or without a loading dose. The dosage is 1 g every 12 hours, and the half-life is 6 hours. The initial dose (loading dose) is 1.5 g. Whether the drug is given by intermittent or continuous infusion, about 4 half-lives of the drug are required for the peak serum concentration to reach 95% of the equilibrium peak concentration in the absence of a loading dose. Equilibration is markedly hastened by the administration of a loading dose.

underlying pharmacologic principles are the same for all routes.

The Area Under the Curve

A convenient way to take into account the changes in concentration in a given site over time is to calculate the area under the curve (AUC) of time versus concentration for that interval. The units are concentration times time (e.g., micrograms per milliliter times minutes). The mean concentration of drug in a site during the dosing interval can be calculated by dividing the AUC by the dosing interval. A simple method of calculating the AUC is shown in Equation 16–4 (see later). It has been suggested that the mean concentration in the serum of a patient receiving the drug by intermittent infusion can be estimated by plotting the peak and trough concentrations on a logarithmic scale and determining the midpoint between them,[2] but this approach produces an underestimate.[3]

Drug Absorption

The absorption of most antimicrobial agents after oral administration occurs primarily by passive diffusion and takes place in the small intestine. Overall, the determinants of the absorbability of antimicrobial agents are not well understood. Lipid solubility appears to be important for the oral absorption of penicillins in relatively acidic conditions but perhaps not at more neutral pH values.[4] Among cephalosporins, the possession of an arylglycine side chain favors oral absorption. Despite these general observations, it is difficult to predict from the structure of a compound how well it will be absorbed by mouth, and the final determination rests on the results of clinical studies.

Some penicillins and cephalosporins have been formulated as prodrugs to facilitate absorption when they are taken by the oral route. Many prodrugs are esters of the parent compound, the ester being split off by enzymes in the intestinal mucosa or in the plasma to release the free drug into the serum.

The absorption of many antimicrobial agents is affected when they are ingested with food. The effect of food on most penicillins is to delay absorption but not to reduce the total amount absorbed; other drugs, such as several cephalosporins, show reduced absorption when they are taken with food.[5] For still other compounds, food has no effect or even enhances absorption. There have been some variations in the results from study to study.[5]

The coadministration of nonabsorbable antacids or histamine H_2-receptor blockers may diminish the absorption of some antimicrobial agents by at least two mechanisms, reduction of gastric acidity and, in the case of antacids, chelation. For example, the absorption of ketoconazole requires an acid environment and is sharply diminished in patients with diminished gastric acidity. Tetracyclines are chelated by the divalent cations present in antacids and dairy products. The coadministration of antacids or zinc markedly reduces the oral absorption of fluoroquinolones.

Appreciable quantities of antibiotics may be absorbed from sites of topical application, as in lavage of joints or the peritoneum and irrigation of tissues. In the case of drugs such as the aminoglycosides, systemic toxic effects may occur, especially in patients with unsuspected renal impairment. Most such applications are unnecessary if a well-chosen antimicrobial agent is given by conventional routes. Indeed, the U.S. Food and Drug Administration has advised against using solutions containing neomycin for irrigation of wounds, joints, or body cavities (except the urinary bladder) because these treatments carry an appreciable risk of toxic effects without conferring a clear benefit.

Drug Elimination

There are three major routes of drug elimination. A fourth route, back-diffusion across the colonic epithelium, is important for only a few antibiotics.

Kidneys. The principal route of elimination of many antimicrobial agents, including the penicillins, cephalosporins, aminoglycosides, and vancomycin, is by the kidneys. Renal elimination may occur either by glomerular filtration or tubular secretion. Glomerular filtration is a passive diffusional process. For drugs that are bound to serum proteins, only the unbound fraction is eliminated by glomerular filtration. The rate of elimination of free drug by glomerular filtration is roughly proportional to the rate of clearance of creatinine, but not precisely proportional because a small proportion of the creatinine is secreted into the urine. In contrast to glomerular filtration, tubular secretion is an active transport process that is not affected by serum protein binding. Tubular secretion is a more efficient excretory process than is glomerular filtration; hence, drugs that are eliminated by tubular secretion have shorter serum half-lives than those that are eliminated by glomerular filtration alone. Probenecid inhibits the active transport pump for penicillins and many cephalosporins and prolongs the half-life of these agents.

Liver and Gallbladder. The hepatobiliary system is a dominant route of elimination for a few commonly used antimicrobial agents, notably cefoperazone, of which about 60% of an intravenous dose is eliminated in the bile, and ceftriaxone, of which about 40% is eliminated in the bile.

There are several consequences of a high degree of biliary elimination of an antibiotic. First, little dose adjustment is necessary for patients with renal impairment. Second, depending on the antibacterial spectrum of the drug, there may be major alterations in the fecal flora and a tendency of the drug to produce diarrhea. By contrast, if biliary elimination is slight, alterations in the fecal flora will be minimal even if the drug has a broad spectrum; this is the case with imipenem. Although it might be speculated that there should be a direct relation between the extent of alterations in the fecal flora and the degree of colonization by resistant strains, this has not been shown experimentally.[6] Most antimicrobial agents are excreted in appreciable concentrations in the bile if the biliary tract is unobstructed but are undetectable in the bile when there is high-grade biliary obstruction. An exception is cefoperazone, which achieves appreciable concentrations even with complete biliary obstruction.

Severe hepatobiliary disease is likely to alter the clearance rate for drugs that are eliminated mainly by hepatobiliary mechanisms. However, in contrast to the usefulness of the serum creatinine value for estimating the effect of renal failure on the half-life of drugs eliminated primarily by glomerular filtration, no simple clinical laboratory test is available to allow the physician to estimate changes in hepatic clearance and to make precise dosage adjustments in patients with hepatobiliary disease; as a consequence, the adjustments are generally crude.

Metabolism. Metabolism is an important means of elimination for a number of antimicrobial agents, including many penicillins and cephalosporins, clindamycin, chloramphenicol, macrolides, metronidazole, rifampin, sulfonamides, isoniazid, and some tetracyclines. Metabolism generally occurs in the liver and results in a loss of antibacterial activity. In most instances, the metabolites are more polar—and thus more water soluble—than the parent compound, so they are more readily eliminated in urine or bile than the parent compound is. The rate of acetylation of isoniazid is genetically determined; subjects can be classified as rapid acetylators or slow acetylators. Dosages of drugs that are extensively metabolized do not have to be adjusted for patients with renal failure unless the metabolites have an adverse effect.

Back-Diffusion. A fourth means of eliminating drugs from the circulation is by back-diffusion across the colonic epithelium and elimination in the feces. Although this is not an important route for most drugs, minocycline and ciprofloxacin are eliminated to some degree by this route.

RENAL FAILURE

Drugs that are eliminated primarily by renal mechanisms accumulate in patients whose renal function is impaired. In general, the total daily dose must be reduced to about the same extent as renal function is reduced. The calculation is easiest for drugs that are eliminated mainly by glomerular filtration. For example, in a patient with stable renal impairment and a serum creatinine concentration (Cr_S) of 5.0 mg/dL, it may be inferred that the rate of glomerular filtration is about 20% of normal and that the total daily dose should be reduced by 80%. A more precise way of assessing renal function in men is to estimate the creatinine clearance rate as follows[7]:

$$\text{Creatinine clearance (mL/min)} = \frac{(140 - \text{age})(\text{weight})}{Cr_S\,(\text{mg/dL}) \times 72} \qquad (2)$$

where age is expressed in years and weight in kilograms. For women, the factor in the divisor is 85 rather than 72.

The daily dose may be reduced to compensate for the effects of renal failure by prolonging the interval between doses, by reducing the dose given at each administration, or by combining these approaches. The choice of whether to modify the dose or the dosing interval is a difficult one that touches on many controversial issues in antimicrobial chemotherapy. The issue has been debated extensively with respect to the aminoglycosides. On the one hand, giving the usual dose at longer intervals (Fig. 16–3) results in widely fluctuating serum concentrations; the trough concentrations may be below the inhibitory threshold for the infecting microorganisms in vitro. On the other hand, decreasing the dose but maintaining the usual dosing interval produces higher trough concentrations. Some investigators believe that high trough concentrations are an important risk factor for the nephrotoxic effects of aminoglycosides, whereas others suggest that high trough concentrations are simply an early manifestation of renal impairment from infection or other conditions rather than a cause of renal impairment. As a practical matter, in using aminoglycosides to treat patients with serious infections, I have generally opted to decrease the dose rather than change the dosing interval to ensure maximal antibacterial effect, despite the possibly higher risk for nephrotoxic effects. For severely neutropenic patients, it may be more crucial to avoid subinhibitory concentrations with β-lactam antibiotics than with aminoglycosides because the postantibiotic effect on gram-negative species is appreciable with aminoglycosides but not with β-lactam antibiotics.[8]

REMOVAL OF DRUGS BY DIALYSIS

Peritoneal dialysis removes little of most antimicrobial agents that accumulate in renal failure, but hemodialysis removes substantial amounts. This is not because the peritoneum is poorly permeable to antibiotics; on the contrary, drugs instilled into the peritoneal cavity are rapidly absorbed into the systemic circulation. In fact, a convenient means of maintaining serum concentrations at a specific level is to add the drug to the dialysis fluid at the desired concentration. The apparent paradox whereby equilibrium between peritoneal fluid and the systemic circulation appears to occur more rapidly when drugs are placed in the peritoneal fluid than

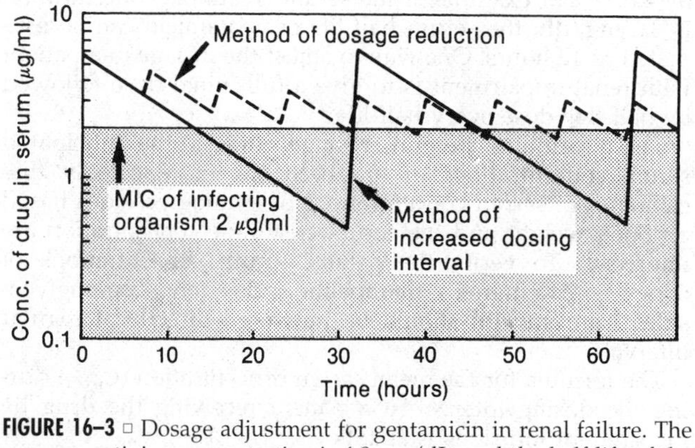

FIGURE 16–3 □ Dosage adjustment for gentamicin in renal failure. The serum creatinine concentration is 4.0 mg/dL, and the half-life of the drug is 8.5 hours. The method of increasing the dosing interval, shown here as the administration of 80 mg every 32 hours, results in low trough concentrations, which could be below the minimal inhibitory concentration (MIC) of the infecting organism for prolonged periods. The dosage reduction method, shown here as the administration of 20 mg every 8 hours, results in higher trough concentrations, which some believe could predispose to nephrotoxic effects.

when they are placed in the systemic circulation may be explained by the fact that the peritoneal surface area is larger in relation to the peritoneal cavity than it is in relation to the total systemic circulation (see later).

Sample Estimations of Serum Concentrations

Before the distribution of antibiotics to extravascular sites is considered, it may be useful to give some examples of calculations that allow clinicians to estimate peak and trough concentrations of antimicrobial agents using the information available from standard textbooks of pharmacology.

INTERMITTENT ADMINISTRATION

The *increase* in peak serum concentration from a dose of drug is equal to the intravenous dose (expressed in milligrams) divided by the apparent volume of distribution (V_d, expressed in liters). Values for V_d may be obtained from the literature. The concept of apparent V_d is discussed later.

For a drug such as gentamicin, which is negligibly protein bound, a typical loading dose might be 2.25 mg/kg, which is about 1.5 times the maintenance dose of 1.5 mg/kg, given every 8 hours. For a 70-kg patient with a calculated V_d of 18 L, the dose of about 160 mg would produce a peak serum concentration of 8.9 μg/mL. If a once-daily dosing schedule is used instead, as is becoming a common approach, the loading dose could be omitted. The daily dose of 4.5 mg/kg would produce a peak serum concentration of 17.5 μg/mL.

The calculation of peak concentration applies to free drug in the serum. For an agent that is appreciably bound to serum protein, the total serum concentration (free plus bound drug) could be calculated by dividing the concentration of free drug by the fraction that is free. For example, if a drug is 70% protein bound and the concentration of free drug in the serum is 10 μg/mL, the total concentration can be estimated to be 33 μg/mL (10/0.3).

Once the peak serum concentration is known, values at intervals after the peak can be estimated on the assumption that the concentration will fall by half every half-life. In patients with stable renal impairment, the serum half-life of an aminoglycoside (hours) can be estimated roughly by multiplying the steady-state serum creatinine concentration by 4.0.[9, 10] For example, if the serum creatinine concentration is 3.0 mg/dL, the serum half-life of gentamicin can be estimated as 12 hours. One way to adjust the dosage in a patient with renal impairment is to give a full initial dose followed by half this dose every half-life.

These formulas are only a rough guide to the anticipated serum concentrations. It has been shown repeatedly that estimates of serum concentrations of aminoglycosides based on body weight and the serum creatinine concentration are imprecise. To verify the results, serum concentrations of drugs with a narrow therapeutic index (e.g., aminoglycosides, vancomycin) should be measured directly at regular intervals.

The formula for the mean serum concentration (C_{mean}) during the dosing interval in a patient receiving the drug by intermittent infusions is as follows:

$$C_{mean} = \frac{\text{dose}}{V_d \times t_i \times K} = \frac{\text{dose} \times t_{1/2}}{V_d \times t_i \times 0.693} \quad (3)$$

where V_d is the volume of distribution, t_i is the dosing interval, K is the elimination rate constant, and $t_{1/2}$ is the serum half-life of the drug. Because $t_i \times C_{mean}$ is the AUC during the dosing interval, or AUC_i, it can be calculated as follows:

$$AUC_i = \frac{\text{dose} \times t_{1/2}}{V_d \times 0.693} \quad (4)$$

CONTINUOUS INFUSION

The steady-state serum concentration (C_S) of free drug during continuous infusion can be calculated by varying Equation 16–3 so that dose/t_i is replaced by I, the infusion rate:

$$C_S = \frac{I}{V_d \times K} = \frac{I \times t_{1/2}}{V_d \times 0.693} \quad (5)$$

Suppose that carbenicillin is being given at a rate of 1000 mg/h, that V_d (from the literature) is estimated to be 14 L, and that the serum half-life is estimated to be 1 hour. Then C_S is 1000 mg/h divided by (14 × 0.693), or 103 mg/L (μg/mL). Assuming that the drug is 50% bound to serum protein, the total serum concentration is 206 mg/L.

Distribution to Peripheral Sites

Major Influences on Distribution

There are three major determinants of the distribution of drugs between the plasma (central compartment) and extravascular sites (peripheral compartment). The first is the nature of the capillary bed. In most tissues and organs, the capillary bed is fenestrated by small pores that permit the ready diffusion of substances with molecular masses up to about 1000 daltons. This encompasses most antimicrobial agents. A few sites in the body, which may be termed specialized sites, possess unfenestrated capillaries. Because drugs must pass through the endothelial cells of the capillaries to reach the extravascular space in these specialized sites, the rate of diffusion is determined by the degree of lipid solubility of the drug.

The most clinically important specialized sites are the central nervous system, the retina, and the prostate gland. Drugs that are weakly lipid soluble, such as the β-lactams, aminoglycosides, some tetracyclines, and vancomycin, penetrate poorly into the brain and cerebrospinal fluid (CSF), the vitreous humor, and the secretions of the prostate gland. Weakly lipid soluble drugs also penetrate poorly into most cells, an important consideration in the concept of V_d. Drugs that are more lipid soluble, such as metronidazole, rifampin, chloramphenicol, trimethoprim, doxycycline, and minocycline, penetrate more readily into these specialized sites and into cells.

A second major determinant of the distribution of drugs into the periphery is the degree of serum protein binding of the drug. Protein binding is a reversible process; however, at any moment, only the proportion of drug that is unbound (free drug) is available for diffusion across capillaries. Only free drug is antibacterially active. The major binding protein for most drugs is albumin. Accordingly, the extent of binding is greatest in the plasma. Nevertheless, there may be an appreciable degree of protein binding in extravascular sites. For example, in cellulitis, there may be extensive leakage of serum albumin into the extravascular compartment.

Active transport pumps are a third major determinant of distribution for certain agents. The best studied of these pumps act on organic anions and are located in the choroid plexus of the brain and the retina of the eye; the pumps transport β-lactam drugs out of the central nervous system and the vitreous humor. They are competitively inhibited by probenecid. Similar pumps in the cells of the proximal tubule of the kidney and in the biliary ducts are responsible for secretion of drugs into the urine and bile.

Estimating Concentration in Extravascular Sites

NONSPECIALIZED SITES

It is much easier to envision the relation between drug concentrations in serum and extravascular sites in a state of equilibrium than in nonequilibrium situations. At equilibrium, the average concentration of free drug in nonspecialized extravascular sites is equal to that in the serum during the dosing interval. This assumes that no drug is destroyed in the site. If there is local destruction of the drug, as might occur in an abscess because of bacterial enzymes, the equilibrium concentration in the extravascular site will be lower than that in the serum.

The rapidity with which equilibrium is reached and the shape of the concentration curve in peripheral sites are related to the ratio of surface area to volume in the site,[11, 12] as described later. Examples of results for sites with large and small ratios of surface area to volume in a patient receiving antibiotic by intermittent intravenous injection are shown in Figure 16–4. Estimating the time required to reach the equilibrium concentration in the extravascular compartment is difficult because it requires knowledge of the permeability coefficient, *P*, for the site; *P* may vary strikingly from site to site.[12]

Interstitial Fluid Model (see Fig. 16–4*A*). In the thin layer of interstitial fluid that surrounds capillaries, the ratio of surface area to volume is great (i.e., diffusion distances are short). There is a large area for exchange of drug between serum and site compared with the volume into which the drug must be distributed. Equilibration occurs promptly, and the concentration of drug in the interstitial fluid follows closely the concentration of free drug in the plasma.

Large Fluid Collections (see Fig. 16–4*B*). In collections such as pleural or ascitic fluid, in which the ratio of surface area to volume is low and the diffusional distances are great, equilibration with serum occurs slowly, and the concentration of drug in the center of the collection fluctuates much less than in the serum. The mean concentration of free drug in the extravascular site at equilibrium can be easily inferred because it is equal to that in the serum. The serum value can be estimated by use of Equation 16–3 if the drug is being given by intermittent infusion and by use of Equation 16–5 if the drug is being given by continuous infusion. For sites with intermediate ratios of surface area to volume, the curves lie between those shown in Figure 16–4*A* and *B*.

Diffusion into abscesses may occur somewhat less readily than into interstitial fluid; however, the difficulty of sterilizing abscesses by chemotherapy probably is related not to impediments to drug penetration but to the large bacterial inoculum (inoculum effect), the degradation of drug by bacterial enzymes, and the adverse effect of the milieu (including the low pH) on the activity of the drug. Bacteria that are dividing slowly (e.g., in an abscess) are much less susceptible than rapidly dividing bacteria to a variety of antimicrobial agents, including not only drugs that act on the cell wall but those that act on DNA and on protein synthesis as well.

SPECIALIZED SITES

For specialized tissues with unfenestrated capillaries, primarily the brain, CSF, and vitreous humor, the situation is more complicated (see Fig. 16–4C). These sites behave like large reservoirs, not only because of their low ratios of surface area to volume but because of the slowness of diffusion through the unfenestrated capillaries, especially for drugs that are not lipid soluble. Nevertheless, in the absence of drug destruction, the mean concentrations of drugs in these sites would be expected eventually to be equal to those in the plasma, were it not for the active transport pumps, principally those for β-lactam drugs. Although the transport

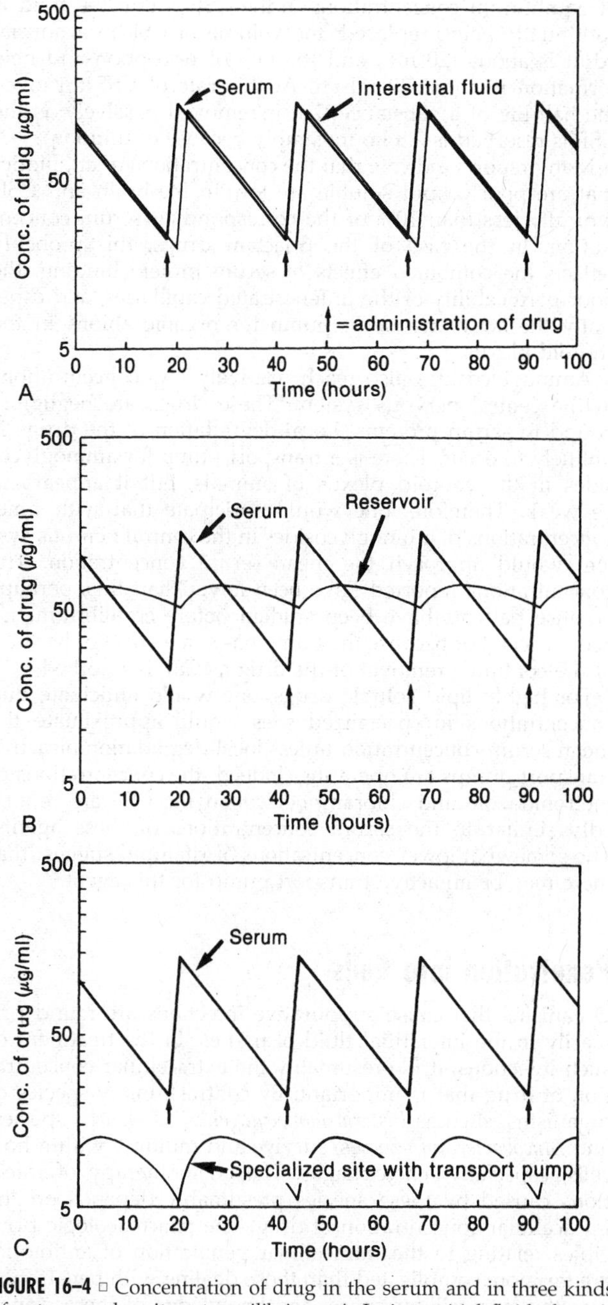

FIGURE 16–4 □ Concentration of drug in the serum and in three kinds of extravascular sites at equilibrium. *A*, In interstitial fluid, there is ready transport between the vascular and extravascular sites, and concentrations in the extravascular site closely mimic those in the serum. *B*, In a large reservoir, such as pleural fluid, equilibration between serum and the site occurs slowly, as shown in Figure 16–2. At equilibrium, the mean concentration in the large reservoir is equal to that in the serum, but the fluctuations in concentration are much less in the large reservoir than in the serum. *C*, In a specialized site, such as CSF, there is a barrier to drug transport because the capillaries are nonfenestrated. The combination of a penetration barrier and active transport (e.g., of a β-lactam drug) results in concentrations that are much lower in the extravascular site than in the serum, even at equilibrium.

pumps are relatively inefficient, their effect is exaggerated by the diffusional barriers. In evaluating clinical reports of the concentrations of antibiotics in these sites, it should be borne in mind that equilibrium may not have been achieved even after prolonged periods of drug administration.

One other factor that may militate against the achievement

of equilibrium concentrations in the CSF is that the fluid is continually being replaced; the volume of CSF in a normal adult is about 120 mL, and the rate of resorption and new formation is about 30 mL/h. At this rate of CSF turnover, the half-life of a substance that is removed passively as the CSF is resorbed is 2.8 hours simply because of dilution.

Many reports indicate that the concentrations of antibiotics that are poorly lipid soluble are low in the brain and CSF, typically less than 10% of the corresponding serum concentration. In the case of the β-lactam drugs, this probably reflects the combined effects of serum protein binding, the poor permeability of the unfenestrated capillaries, and especially the active transport pump for organic anions in the choroid plexus.

Aminoglycosides also reach relatively low concentrations in the central nervous system. These drugs are negligibly bound to serum proteins. Local degradation of the drugs is unlikely to occur. There is a transport pump for aminoglycosides in the choroid plexus of animals, but it appears to be weak. Therefore, one would anticipate that with time, concentrations of aminoglycosides in the central nervous system would approach the mean serum concentration. The concentrations reported have been lower than this, perhaps because patients have been studied before equilibrium has been reached or because the pump has some effect or because of the continual removal of the drug as CSF is resorbed.

For highly lipid soluble drugs, one would anticipate that concentrations in specialized sites would approximate the mean serum concentration unless local degradation or active transport pumps are operating. Indeed, the concentrations of metronidazole and chloramphenicol in the CSF are reportedly similar to the serum concentrations of these agents. The somewhat lower concentrations of rifampin suggest that there may be an active transport pump for this agent.[13]

Penetration into Cells

Organisms that cause suppurative infections are found primarily in the interstitial fluid of tissues. In the treatment of such infections, it is presumably the extracellular concentration of drug that is important. By contrast, many species of organisms, such as *Listeria monocytogenes*, *Salmonella* species, and *Mycobacterium* species, survive and multiply within host cells, especially macrophages. The chemotherapy of infections caused by these species presumably depends on the intracellular concentration of drug. The pharmacologic principles relating to the intracellular penetration of antibiotics are far more complicated than those dealing with penetration into the extracellular space, and knowledge of these principles is rudimentary.

A significant issue in studying the intracellular penetration of antibiotics relates to the subcellular distribution of the drug. Many studies report the "average" intracellular concentration of drug, but for most agents, it is unlikely that intracellular concentrations are homogeneous. For example, many drugs that are accumulated intracellularly, such as lincosamides, macrolides, and aminoglycosides, are weak bases and are found primarily in the acidic lysosomes. Paradoxically, in this location, their antibacterial activity may be diminished. In some instances, the intracellular microorganism is found in a subcellular location different from that in which the antibiotic is accumulated. This appears to be the case with azithromycin and *Toxoplasma gondii*.[14] Nevertheless, the drug has some activity against the parasite. To further complicate the issue, drug penetration may vary depending on the type of cell under study. Although many issues concerning the intracellular penetration and activity of drugs remain unclear, there is evidence to suggest that the most effective drugs for the treatment of infection by intracellular pathogens are those that are well accumulated within cells.

Table 16–1 summarizes the pharmacologic and pharmacodynamic properties of selected antibiotics as derived from extensive reviews.[15–17] The experiments have been done in a variety of cell types, polymorphonuclear leukocytes, macrophages, fibroblasts, and HeLa cells, with somewhat different results in the various cell types. For most drugs, entry is mainly by simple diffusion, and distribution is in accord with pH partition. There is some suggestion of active transport of clindamycin and the macrolides. In general, the β-lactam drugs penetrate poorly into cells, even after prolonged exposure. Aminoglycosides are accumulated slowly to concentrations exceeding those in the extracellular fluid by twofold to fourfold. Clindamycin (but not lincomycin) and the macrolides, especially clarithromycin and azithromycin, reach much higher concentrations in cells than in the extracellular fluid; much of the accumulated drug is within lysosomes, where activity may not be optimal. The fluoroquinolones show moderate accumulation within cells, to about twofold to eightfold the extracellular concentration. Efflux from cells appears to be rapid for all agents except the aminoglycosides and azithromycin. This observation probably accounts for the finding of low levels of aminoglycosides in urine long after the end of treatment and for the efficacy of azithromycin in brief treatment courses, such as the single-dose treatment of chlamydial urethritis and cervicitis.

Intracellular drug not only may exert an effect against intracellular pathogens but could be slowly released into the interstitial fluid. In this manner, the intracellular space could serve as a "reservoir" or depot, leading to more sustained drug concentrations in interstitial fluid between doses. This may be the case with azithromycin. It has also been suggested that antibiotic-laden neutrophils could carry antibiotic to sites of infection with beneficial effects, but this is unclear.

Additional Considerations

As discussed, drugs that are weakly lipid soluble penetrate most types of cells poorly. For these agents, most of the drug in tissues lies in the interstitial fluid. Calculations based on the assumption that the total amount of drug detected in a sample of tissue is distributed evenly throughout cells and the interstitial fluid will lead to a marked underestimate of the interstitial fluid concentration.

The methods of homogenizing and assaying tissues may have a major impact on the results. For example, a number of studies purport to show that different cephalosporins penetrate bone to different degrees. In fact, these variations probably relate to differences in the methods used to extract the drug from the bone. Careful studies indicate that the concentrations of cephalosporins in the interstitial fluid of normal and osteomyelitic bone are similar to those in the serum.[18, 19]

There is still controversy about both theoretical and experimental aspects of drug penetration into the prostate gland. The capillary bed of the organ is unfenestrated, so drugs that are poorly lipid soluble penetrate with difficulty. The barrier appears to be maintained in all but the most acute states of inflammation. The unique pharmacologic feature of the prostate gland relates to the issue of pH partition, or ion trapping. The prostatic secretions of the dog have a pH of only 6.4. Most β-lactam drugs are anions, which are less intensely ionized, and therefore are more lipid soluble, in the acidic secretions of the prostate gland than in the serum. Accordingly, they diffuse more readily out of the prostate gland than into it. At equilibrium, concentrations in the prostate are lower than in the serum. In contrast, weak bases such as the aminoglycosides and erythromycin exhibit the

TABLE 16–1 ■ Intracellular Accumulation and Activity of Selected Antibiotics

AGENT	DRUG CONCENTRATION*	MECHANISM OF CELLULAR DRUG UPTAKE	LOCALIZATION IN CELL	KINETICS OF INFLUX AND EFFLUX	ACTIVITY IN CELLS
β-Lactams	Intracellular/extracellular ratio of ≤0.7 in PMNs,† macrophages, fibroblasts, and HeLa cells, even after prolonged incubation	Diffusion and pH partition	Free in cytoplasm	Rapid influx and efflux (half-life, 20–30 min)	Variable, from no activity (especially in PMNs) to some activity (especially in macrophages and monocytes); some activity evident by best methods
Aminoglycosides	Slow intracellular accumulation to 2–4 times extracellular level after 72 h of incubation	Endocytosis and diffusion	50% in lysosomes, 50% in cytoplasm	Slow	Less activity than at same concentration extracellularly; possible reduction of activity as pH falls with phagosome-lysosome fusion; better activity in macrophages than in PMNs
Rifampin	Intracellular level 2–3 times extracellular level	Diffusion	In cytoplasm	Rapid	Activity in cells equal to activity in cell-free medium
Lincosamides	Intracellular versus extracellular level: clindamycin, 10- to 50-fold in PMNs and macrophages: lincomycin, ratio of ≤2	Diffusion and pH partition; clindamycin may use energy-requiring nucleoside transport system	50% in lysosomes, 50% in cytoplasm	Rapid	Despite high intracellular concentrations of clindamycin, intracellular no greater than extracellular activity
Macrolides	Intracellular versus extracellular level: erythromycin, 10- to 30-fold in PMNs and alveolar macrophages, lower in cultured human and HeLa cells; intracellular levels higher for newer macrolides	Diffusion and pH partition; active transport different from nucleoside transport of clindamycin	50% in lysosomes, 50% in cytoplasm	Rapid influx and efflux (half-life, 15–20 min) of all except azithromycin	Erythromycin potent against obligate intracellular organisms such as *Legionella*; no effect on *Staphylococcus aureus* in PMNs
Fluoroquinolones	Intracellular level 2–8 times extracellular level in macrophages and fibroblasts	Not known	In cytoplasm or loosely associated with organelles	Rapid	Active against *S. aureus* in PMNs

*Average concentration in whole cells.
†Polymorphonuclear leukocytes.
From Barza M: Tissue-directed antibiotic therapy: Antibiotic dynamics in cells and tissue. Challenges to antibiotic activity in tissue. Clin Infect Dis 19:910–915, 1994. © by The University of Chicago.

reverse phenomenon; they are trapped in the prostate gland. However, the mean pH of prostatic secretions from normal men is 7.28 and from men with bacterial prostatitis is 8.32, values that are strikingly different from those in the prostate gland of dogs. The alkaline pH in patients with chronic prostatitis should favor the accumulation of weak acids such as penicillins, cephalosporins, sulfonamides, and rifampin. It is difficult to test the validity of these hypotheses clinically. Studies of the concentration of drugs in human prostatic secretions are complicated by the fact that contamination of ejaculate by even minute amounts of urine produces spurious results because most drugs are excreted in high concentrations in the urine.

The Apparent Volume of Distribution

Drugs that are highly lipid soluble penetrate readily into most tissues and fluids of the body and are said to have a large V_d. By contrast, drugs that are weakly lipid soluble tend to be restricted to the extracellular fluid, which composes about 20% to 30% of the body weight. For a given dose, the serum concentration of a highly lipid soluble agent would be much lower than that of a weakly lipid soluble agent because the highly lipid soluble agent is distributed into a much larger volume. The V_d of a hydrophilic drug is much increased in a patient with a large "third space" (e.g., with abundant ascites). V_d values for a number of drugs are available from standard textbooks of pharmacology. In addition, the V_d can be estimated during continuous infusion by use of Equation 16–5 and during intermittent infusion by use of Equation 16–3. An even simpler way of estimating the V_d after a single rapid injection of a drug is to project the β-phase curve to time zero (see Fig. 16–1). This value is the peak concentration after correcting for the α-phase. The dose divided by this concentration is the V_d.

Measurements of the V_d provide only a gross idea of the peripheral distribution of a drug. Peculiarities of a drug sometimes lead to spuriously low serum concentrations and, therefore, spuriously high V_d values, even if tissue penetration is not unusually good. For example, the apparent V_d of nafcillin is larger and the serum concentrations are lower than would be expected from the degree of lipid solubility or of penetration into peripheral sites because nafcillin is taken up extensively by the liver. Amphotericin B is not well distributed to the periphery, but its serum concentrations are low, resulting in a large estimated V_d because the drug binds to cholesterol-containing membranes of cells. Thus, the V_d should be considered only as a rough guide to the actual penetration of drugs into cells and specialized sites.

Clinical Relevance of Antibiotic Concentrations in Vivo

The antimicrobial effect of a drug in vivo cannot be fully predicted by simple extrapolation from its pharmacokinetic behavior and its effects in vitro. This fact is not surprising. Aside from the important effects of host defenses, which are difficult to simulate in vitro, there are likely to be marked differences between the situations in vitro and in vivo in inoculum size and rate of growth of microbial cells, as well as in pH and other aspects of the microenvironment, all of which may have a marked influence on the antibacterial efficacy of the drug.

For most infections, it is not necessary to maintain drug concentrations in the serum at an inhibitory level throughout the treatment period to have a good result. There are several explanations for this finding. One is that the antibacterial effect of the drug may persist up to several hours after the substance is no longer detectable in the environment; the duration of this "postantibiotic effect" depends on the particular species of bacterium and the drug.[8] Another explanation is that drug concentrations in extravascular sites may fluctuate much less than in serum (see Fig. 16–4). A third reason is the protective effect of host defenses.

Many studies have attempted to relate the bactericidal titer of antibiotics in the serum to the outcome of infections.[20] A few have shown a significant correlation between the serum bactericidal titer and cure of the infection[21–23]; others have shown little correlation, again indicating the difficulties in extrapolating from the situation in vitro to that in vivo. It is to be hoped that increased knowledge of the interaction between drugs and microbes in vitro and in vivo and greater sophistication in the application of computer models may render such extrapolations more useful. In the last analysis, the determination of the value of an antibiotic in the treatment of clinical infectious diseases must rest on carefully conducted trials in humans.

References

1. Tallarida RJ, Murray RB: Manual of Pharmacologic Calculations. New York, Springer-Verlag, 1981, pp 46–47.
2. Peterson LR, Gerding DN: Prediction of cefazolin penetration into high- and low-protein–containing fluid: New method for performing simultaneous studies. Antimicrob Agents Chemother 14:533, 1978.
3. Gonda I: On predictions of free antibiotic (cefazolin) concentrations in extravascular fluids from "logarithmic mean serum concentrations." J Antimicrob Chemother 9:53, 1982.
4. Tsuji A, Miyamoto E, Kubo O, Yamana T: GI absorption of β-lactam antibiotics III. Kinetic evidence for in situ absorption of ionized species of monobasic penicillins and cefazolin from the rat small intestine and structure-absorption rate relationships. J Pharm Sci 68:812, 1979.
5. Welling PG, Tse FLS: The influence of food on the absorption of antimicrobial agents. J Antimicrob Chemother 9:7, 1982.
6. Barza M, Giuliano M, Jacobus NV, Gorbach SL: Effect of broad-spectrum antibiotics on "colonization resistance" of intestinal microflora of humans. Antimicrob Agents Chemother 31:723, 1987.
7. Cockcroft DW, Gault MH: Prediction of creatinine clearance from serum creatinine. Nephron 16:31, 1976.
8. Vogelman B, Gudmundsson S, Turnidge J, et al: In vivo postantibiotic effect in a thigh infection in neutropenic mice. J Infect Dis 157:287, 1988.
9. Cutler RE, Gyselynck AM, Fleet WP, et al: Correlation of serum creatinine concentration and gentamicin half-life. JAMA 219:1037, 1972.
10. McHenry MC, Tavan TL, Gifford RW Jr: Gentamicin dosages for renal insufficiency. Ann Intern Med 74:192, 1971.
11. Van Etta L, Peterson LR, Fasching CE, Gerding DN: Effect of the ratio of surface area to volume on the penetration of antibiotics into extravascular spaces in an in vitro model. J Infect Dis 146:423, 1982.
12. Barza M, Cuchural G: General principles of antibiotic tissue penetration. J Antimicrob Chemother 15(Suppl A):59, 1985.
13. Thea D, Barza M: Use of antibacterial agents in infections of the central nervous system. Infect Dis Clin North Am 3:553, 1989.
14. Schwab JC, Cao Y, Slowik MR, Joiner KA: Localization of azithromycin in *Toxoplasma gondii*–infected cells. Antimicrob Agents Chemother 38:1620, 1994.
15. Barza M: Challenges to antibiotic activity in tissue. Clin Infect Dis 19:910, 1994.
16. Tulkens PM: Intracellular distribution and activity of antibiotics. Eur J Clin Microbiol Infect Dis 10:100, 1991.
17. van den Broek PJ: Antimicrobial drugs, microorganisms, and phagocytes. Rev Infect Dis 11:213, 1989.
18. Lunke RJ, Fitzgerald RH Jr, Washington JA II: Pharmacokinetics of cefamandole in osseous tissue. Antimicrob Agents Chemother 19:851, 1981.
19. Daly RC, Fitzgerald RH Jr, Washington JA II: Penetration of cefazolin into normal and osteomyelitic canine cortical bone. Antimicrob Agents Chemother 22:461, 1982.
20. Wolfson JS, Swartz MN: Serum bactericidal activity as a monitor of antibiotic therapy. N Engl J Med 312:968, 1985.
21. Sculler JP, Klastersky J: Significance of serum bactericidal activity in gram-negative bacillary bacteremia in patients with and without granulocytopenia. Am J Med 76:429, 1984.
22. Weinstein MP, Stratton CW, Ackley A, et al: Multicenter collaborative evaluation of a standardized serum bactericidal test as a prognostic indicator in infective endocarditis. Am J Med 78:262, 1985.
23. Weinstein MP, Stratton CW, Hawley HB, et al: Multicenter collaborative evaluation of a standardized serum bactericidal test as a predictor of therapeutic efficacy in acute and chronic osteomyelitis. Am J Med 83:218, 1987.

ANTIMICROBIAL DRUGS

17

Penicillins

William A. Craig

Although Fleming isolated penicillin from *Penicillium notatum* in 1928,[1] it took another decade for this discovery to achieve clinical utility. Investigators at Oxford University, including Florey, Chain, and Abraham, systematically studied the physical, chemical, and structural characteristics of penicillin. They solved its stability problems, determined its structure, and isolated sufficient quantities of the drug to begin clinical testing in 1941.[2,3] Trials in Great Britain and the United States demonstrated dramatic benefits.[4,5] Production improvements brought about by deep fermentation procedures, use of cornsteep liquor, and a new strain, *Penicillium chrysogenum,* led to widespread availability of the drug by the end of the 1940s.[6,7]

Chemistry

The basic structure of the penicillins is a nucleus with fused β-lactam and thiazolidine rings and a side chain group (Fig. 17–1). The penicillin nucleus, 6-aminopenicillanic acid, can be obtained from *P. chrysogenum* in a medium devoid of precursors for a side chain or after removal of the side chain by enzymatic treatment with an amidase.[8] The biosynthesis of penicillins represents a combination of two amino acids, cysteine and valine.[9] The presence of an intact β-lactam ring is essential for activity. Because a free carboxyl group is also required for activity, most penicillins are available as salts. Carboxyl ester formulations require hydrolysis by nonspecific esterases in serum and tissues for in vivo activity.

The side chain provides diversity in the physicochemical and biologic characteristics of the penicillins.[10] Different side chains occur naturally (e.g., penicillins F and G), by addition of precursors to the fermentation medium (e.g., penicillin V), or by chemical attachment of specific structures to 6-aminopenicillanic acid. The last-named method has led to the development of many clinically useful semisynthetic penicillins.

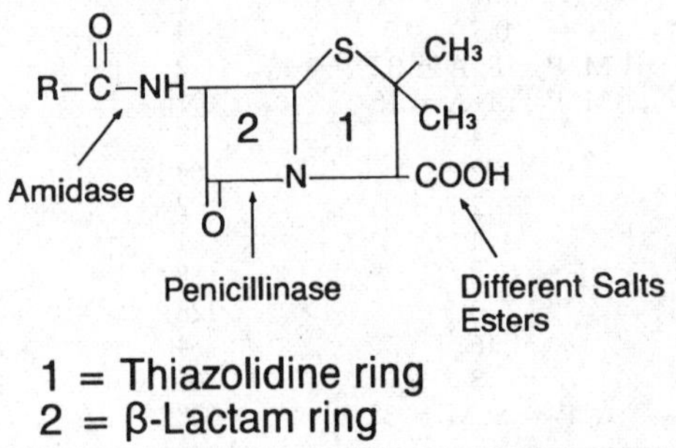

FIGURE 17–1 ▫ Basic structure of penicillins and sites of β-lactamase inactivation, amidase removal of side chains in synthesis of semisynthetic analogs, and salt and ester formulations.

Mechanism of Action

Penicillins inhibit bacterial growth by interfering with the synthesis of the cell wall. The first two steps in cell wall synthesis (i.e., formation of an acetylmuramyl pentapeptide followed by alternating linkage to acetylglucosamine to form peptidoglycan chains) are unaffected by penicillin. It is the final step in this process, in which strands of peptidoglycan are cross-linked by peptide side chains, that is inhibited by penicillin.[11] This transpeptidation reaction occurs at the surface of the cell membrane. Penicillins, because of their structural similarity to the terminal D-alanine-D-alanine of the pentapeptide, bind covalently to the active site of the transpeptidase enzyme.[12]

Although acylation of the transpeptidase enzyme is of major importance for the inhibitory effects of penicillin on bacterial growth, there are additional targets or proteins at the cell membrane that bind penicillins.[13–15] These membrane components, with molecular weights from 35,000 to 120,000, are called penicillin binding proteins (PBPs). They are numbered by convention in the order of decreasing molecular weight. PBPs with similar molecular weights are differentiated by letters. Gram-negative bacilli typically contain 7 to 10 PBPs; gram-positive and gram-negative cocci have 3 to 5 PBPs. In addition, some proteins are found in small amounts, whereas others are abundant. In *Escherichia coli,* PBPs 2 and 5 account for about 1% and 65%, respectively, of the binding of penicillin G to these proteins.[16]

Some of the PBPs correspond to known enzymes (i.e., transpeptidases and carboxypeptidases) involved in cell wall synthesis. Others have not yet been identified. Binding to some PBPs is associated with bacterial cell death, whereas attachment to others changes bacterial morphologic characteristics. With *E. coli,* binding to the PBP 1 complex correlates with the lethal activity of penicillin. Preferential binding to PBP 2 is associated with loss of rod shape and formation of large ovoid cells. High affinity for PBP 3 results in filament formation without septa.[15–17]

Although penicillins are bactericidal drugs, the mechanisms by which they kill bacteria vary for different species. For pneumococci and *E. coli,* killing is caused by lysis resulting from deregulation of the autolytic enzyme system (i.e., peptidoglycan hydrolases).[18,19] Penicillin appears to trigger autolysis by causing the loss of normally present inhibitors (e.g., lipoteichoic acid) of peptidoglycan hydrolases.[20] Penicillins may also directly enhance autolytic activity.[21] For staphylococci, autolytic activity actually decreases during exposure to penicillin.[22] Lysis of these organisms is apparently due to punching of a few minute holes into the cell wall, caused by the lytic activity of vesicular structures called murosomes.[23,24] Under normal circumstances, murosomes initiate the separation of bacteria into daughter cells. For *Streptococcus pyogenes,* killing is not due to lysis.[25] It results, instead, from a penicillin-induced hydrolysis of cellular RNA.[26]

In general, the rate of killing of bacteria by penicillins exhibits minimal dependence on the concentration of drug.[27] Maximal killing rates are usually observed at concentrations of four times the minimal inhibitory concentration. Although penicillins induce persistent suppression of bacterial growth (i.e., postantibiotic effect) of several hours' duration with gram-positive cocci, extremely short or no postantibiotic ef-

TABLE 17–1 ■ Activity of Penicillins Against Aerobic Cocci, *Haemophilus influenzae*, and Gram-Positive Bacilli

	MEAN MINIMAL INHIBITORY CONCENTRATION (mg/L)*								
ORGANISM	Penicillin G	Penicillin V	Methicillin	Nafcillin, Oxacillin, Cloxacillin, Dicloxacillin	Ampicillin, Amoxicillin	Carbenicillin, Ticarcillin	Azlocillin, Mezlocillin, Piperacillin	Amdinocillin	Temocillin
Staphylococcus aureus	0.02 (>32)	0.02 (>32)	1 (2)	0.2 (0.4)	0.1 (>32)	1 (16)	1 (16)	2 (>128)	>128
Staphylococcus epidermidis	0.02 (>32)	0.02 (>32)	2 (2)	0.2 (0.4)	0.1 (>32)	2 (16)	0.2 (16)	4 (>128)	>128
Streptococcus pyogenes	0.005	0.01	0.2	0.02	0.01	0.2	0.02	2	128
Streptococcus agalactiae	0.05	0.05	2	0.1	0.2	1	0.2	2	>128
Streptococcus pneumoniae	0.01	0.02	0.1	0.05	0.02	0.4	0.02	2	>128
Penicillin intermediate	0.5	—	—	2	0.5; amox = 0.2	8	1	—	—
Penicillin resistant	2	—	—	8	2; amox = 1	64	4	—	—
Viridans group streptococci	0.05	0.05	1	0.2	0.05	0.4	0.2	4	>128
Enterococcus faecalis	2	4	>32	16	1	32	1	>128	>128
Neisseria gonorrhoeae	0.05 (>32)	0.2 (>32)	0.4 (1)	1 (2)	0.05 (>32)	0.1 (8)	0.05 (2)	0.1 (>32)	0.5 (1)
Neisseria meningitidis	0.05	0.2	0.5	4	0.05	0.05	0.01	1	—
Moraxella catarrhalis	0.1 (2)	—	—	—	0.01 (2)	0.1 (4)	0.1 (0.5)	—	—
Haemophilus influenzae	0.4 (>16)	4	2	16	0.4 (>16)	0.4 (4)	0.1 (0.5)	16	0.5 (0.5)
Listeria monocytogenes	0.4	—	>4	4	0.2	2	1	—	—
Corynebacterium diphtheriae	0.1	—	—	0.1	0.2	0.2	0.5	—	—

*Mean minimal inhibitory concentration for β-lactamase–positive strains is given in parentheses.
Data from references 30–45.

fects are observed for these drugs with gram-negative bacilli.[28, 29]

Spectrum of Activity

The penicillins are active against a wide variety of aerobic and anaerobic bacteria[30–51] (Tables 17–1 to 17–3). Because the peptidoglycan cell wall of gram-negative bacteria lies within a lipid membrane, a penicillin must pass this outer barrier before reaching the site of action. Thus, penicillins are more active against gram-positive bacteria than against gram-negative bacteria. However, the presence of different side chains on the penicillin nucleus has significantly altered the spectrum of activity of some derivatives. This also provides a method for classification of the different penicillins. The *natural penicillins* (penicillin G and V) are highly active against streptococci, penicillinase-negative staphylococci, meningococci, anaerobic cocci, *Clostridium perfringens,* and spirochetes. However, penicillin G is 5 to 10 times more active than penicillin V against *Haemophilus influenzae* and gram-negative cocci. The *penicillinase-resistant penicillins* (methicillin, nafcillin, oxacillin, cloxacillin, and dicloxacillin) are active against most penicillinase-producing staphylococci. However, they are less potent than other penicillins against other organisms.

The extended-spectrum penicillins consist of three groups of drugs. The aminopenicillins (ampicillin and amoxicillin) have enhanced activity against *E. coli, Proteus mirabilis,* salmonellae, shigellae, *H. influenzae,* and enterococci. The carboxypenicillins (carbenicillin and ticarcillin) are active against *Pseudomonas aeruginosa* and *Proteus vulgaris* as well as *Providencia, Morganella,* and *Enterobacter* species. However, they are significantly less potent than ampicillin against streptococci and enterococci. The ureidopenicillins (mezlocillin, azlocillin, and piperacillin) combine characteristics of both of the other two groups of extended-spectrum penicillins. Some of these drugs are also active against most *Klebsiella* species.

Resistance

The primary mechanism for resistance to the penicillins is enzymatic hydrolysis of the β-lactam ring by β-lactamases.[52]

TABLE 17–2 ■ Activity of Penicillins Against Enterobacteriaceae and *Pseudomonas*

	MEAN MINIMAL INHIBITORY CONCENTRATION (mg/L)					
ORGANISM*	Penicillin G	Ampicillin, Amoxicillin	Carbenicillin (C), Ticarcillin (T)	Azlocillin (A), Mezlocillin (M), Piperacillin (P)	Amdinocillin	Temocillin
Escherichia coli	64	4	4	8	1	4
Proteus mirabilis	32	4	2	0.5	4	1
Klebsiella pneumoniae	>128	>128	>128	M, P = 8; A = 32	2	2
Enterobacter sp.	>128	128	8	M, P = 4; A = 16	2	2
Citrobacter sp.	>128	32	8	4	2	4
Serratia sp.	>128	>128	128	32	64	16
Salmonella sp.	8	2; amox = 1	4	2	2	4
Shigella sp.	16	2; amox = 4	2	4	1	2
Morganella sp.	>128	128	16	8	8	2
Providencia sp.	>128	>128	16	8	128	1
Proteus vulgaris	>128	64	8	16	64	2
Acinetobacter sp.	>128	32	16	8	64	>128
Pseudomonas aeruginosa	>128	>128	T = 32; C = 64	A, P = 8; M = 32	>128	>128

*Strains resistant to penicillins are frequently observed; 90% minimal inhibitory concentrations are listed for ampicillin, amoxicillin, ticarcillin, and piperacillin in Table 17–5.
Data from references 44–48.

TABLE 17–3 ■ Activity of Penicillins Against Anaerobic Bacteria

	MINIMAL INHIBITORY CONCENTRATION (MEAN/90%) (mg/L)					
ORGANISM	Penicillin G	Oxacillin	Amoxicillin, Ampicillin	Carbenicillin, Ticarcillin	Azlocillin, Mezlocillin, Piperacillin	Temocillin
Clostridium perfringens	0.1/0.5	0.5/1	0.1/0.5	0.5/2	0.5/2	>128
Eubacterium sp.	0.5/2	2/16	0.2/1	2/16	2/16	—
Peptococcus sp.	0.1/0.5	0.5/4	0.1/0.5	0.1/1	0.1/0.5	128/>128
Peptostreptococcus sp.	0.1/1	0.4/8	0.2/1	0.5/4	0.5/2	16/>128
Propionibacterium sp.	0.1/0.5	0.5/1	0.1/0.5	0.2/1	0.2/1	—
Bacteroides fragilis	16/64	>128	16/64	32/128	32/128	32/64
Prevotella sp.	0.2/8	32	0.2/8	0.5/4	0.5/4	16/64
Fusobacterium sp.	0.1/2	>128	0.1/8	0.5/4	0.1/4	8/64
Veillonella sp.	0.2/1	8/32	0.2/1	2/8	4/32	—

Data from references 44, 45, and 49–51.

Most penicillins are susceptible to inactivation by the penicillinase elaborated by most hospital strains and about 80% of community isolates of *Staphylococcus aureus.* β-Lactamase production in gram-positive cocci is plasmid mediated and inducible. When exposed to penicillins, such organisms secrete large amounts of enzyme into the surrounding environment to destroy all available drug. The development of penicillins with bulky side chains resulted in drugs that were more resistant to inactivation by these β-lactamases. However, some strains of *S. aureus* produce excessive amounts of the enzyme and can exhibit borderline susceptibility or resistance to the penicillinase-resistant penicillins.[53]

In gram-negative bacilli, β-lactamases are located in the periplasmic space between the outer and inner cell membranes. Penicillin molecules that pass the outer membrane could come in contact with a β-lactamase before reaching the site of action. Although all gram-negative bacteria appear to contain β-lactamase, the type and amount can vary markedly.[52] They can be chromosome or plasmid mediated, constitutive or inducible, and active against only certain classes of β-lactam drugs or against a broad spectrum of such drugs. The ability of penicillins to inhibit the growth of gram-negative bacilli is dependent on the rate of influx across the outer membrane being greater than the rate of hydrolysis by β-lactamases.[54] Alterations in the penicillin side chain that governs gram-negative activity generally enhance penetration across the outer membrane rather than reduce the rate of hydrolysis.[55] Temocillin, the 6-α-methoxy derivative of ticarcillin, is an exception in that it is highly stable to most β-lactamases.[56]

The spread of plasmid-mediated β-lactamases such as TEM-1 among Enterobacteriaceae and to *H. influenzae* and *Neisseria gonorrhoeae* has greatly altered susceptibility to the penicillins.[57, 58] Penicillins are also inactivated by the newer extended-spectrum β-lactamases. Plasmid-mediated staphylococcal penicillinase has also apparently spread to *Enterococcus faecalis.*[59] Selection of stable derepressed clones producing a chromosome-mediated β-lactamase has increased resistance to penicillins in *P. aeruginosa* and *Enterobacter* species.[60] The ureidopenicillins appear to be more susceptible than the carboxypenicillins to overprotection of pseudomonal β-lactamase.[61]

Another mechanism of increasing importance for resistance to penicillins involves alteration of the target site. This form of resistance accounts for penicillin resistance in pneumococci; methicillin resistance in staphylococci; and non–β-lactamase resistance to penicillins in *Neisseria* species, *H. influenzae,* and some gram-negative bacilli.[62–66] PBPs with reduced affinity for penicillin result from amino acid substitutions and insertions in PBPs. For example, penicillin-resistant isolates of *Streptococcus pneumoniae* have shown up to 38 amino acid substitutions in the sequence of PBP 2b.[67] In *S. pneumoniae* and *Neisseria* species, altered PBPs can apparently result from replacement of part of the gene coding for PBP with corresponding genes from related species. For example, the DNA sequences of the gene coding for PBP of penicillin-resistant *S. pneumoniae* exhibit striking similarities with those from viridans streptococci.[68] Likewise, the gene coding for PBP 2 in penicillin-resistant isolates of *Neisseria meningitidis* and *N. gonorrhoeae* contains part of the gene coding for PBP 2 from *Neisseria flavescens.*[69] The chromosomal gene (i.e., *mec* determinant) that encodes the low-affinity PBP 2a in methicillin-resistant staphylococci may be a fusion product of a regulatory region of the staphylococcal penicillinase gene and a gene coding for PBP of *E. coli.*[70]

Altered permeability of the outer membrane of gram-negative bacilli provides another mechanism for resistance to the penicillins. Mutants with reduced or altered porin channels show 2- to 16-fold higher minimal inhibitory concentrations to the broad-spectrum penicillins.[71, 72] However, in most resistant clinical isolates, decreased permeability has occurred jointly with altered PBPs or inducible β-lactamases.[73, 74]

Resistance to the bactericidal effects of penicillins is known as tolerance.[75] This phenomenon is considered present when the minimal bactericidal concentration is significantly greater (usually more than 16-fold) than the minimal inhibitory concentration.[76] It is observed primarily with staphylococci, streptococci, enterococci, and *Listeria monocytogenes.*[76, 77] Organisms exhibiting tolerance appear to have reduced or altered autolytic activity with exposure to penicillin. Infections with tolerant bacteria may be associated with a reduced or slower response to penicillin therapy.[76, 78]

Pharmacokinetic Properties

Changes in the penicillin side chain alter pharmacokinetic properties as well as the spectrum of activity[79–96] (Table 17–4). Penicillin G, methicillin, the carboxypenicillins, and the ureidopenicillins are unstable in the acidic milieu of the stomach (i.e., half-life less than 30 minutes at pH 2) and are largely restricted to parenteral administration. Penicillin V, the isoxazolyl penicillins, the aminopenicillins, and the indanyl ester formulation of carbenicillin are acid stable with half-lives of 2 to 6 hours at pH 2; all are available for use as oral preparations. The acid stability of nafcillin is intermediate. Penicillins not inactivated by gastric acid are generally well absorbed and exhibit peak serum levels in 1 to 2 hours. Among the aminopenicillins, ampicillin exhibits only 30% to 60% absorption; amoxicillin and the carboxyl ester formulations of ampi-

TABLE 17–4 ■ Pharmacokinetic Characteristics of the Penicillins

DRUG	ACID STABLE	PROTEIN BINDING (%)	PEAK SERUM LEVEL (mg/L) Oral Dose (500 mg)	PEAK SERUM LEVEL (mg/L) Intravenous Infusion (1 g)	ROUTE OF EXCRETION	HALF-LIFE (h) Normal	HALF-LIFE (h) Creatinine Clearance < 10 mL/min
Penicillin G	No	60	2	60*	Renal	0.5	5
Penicillin V	Yes	78	5	—	Renal	0.5	4
Methicillin	No	37	—	100	Renal	0.5	4
Nafcillin	Slight	89	4	160	Renal + hepatic	0.5	1
Oxacillin	Yes	93	6	200	Renal + hepatic	0.4	1
Cloxacillin	Yes	94	12	200	Renal + hepatic	0.4	1
Dicloxacillin	Yes	97	15	—	Renal + hepatic	0.7	1.5
Ampicillin	Yes	18	3.5	100	Renal	1.0	10
Amoxicillin	Yes	17	8	100	Renal	0.9	10
Bacampicillin	Yes	—	10	—	Renal	See ampicillin	
Carbenicillin	No	47	5†	170	Renal	1.1	15
Ticarcillin	No	45	—	170	Renal	1.2	15
Azlocillin	No	40	—	220	Renal + hepatic	1.0	5
Mezlocillin	No	35	—	200	Renal + hepatic	1.0	4
Piperacillin	No	50	—	200	Renal + hepatic	1.0	4
Temocillin	No	83	—	200	Renal	4	18
Clavulanate	Yes	Low	3‡	5*	Renal	0.8	10
Sulbactam	No	Low	18‡	100	Renal	1	10
Tazobactam	No	Low	—	26*	Renal	1	7

*Based on a dose of 1 million units for penicillin G; 100 mg intravenously for clavulanate; and 375 mg intravenously for tazobactam.
†Administered as indanyl ester, which is stable to acid.
‡Based on a dose of 125 mg orally for clavulanate and a dose of 590 mg for sulbactam administered as sultamicillin.
Data from references 79–96.

cillin are almost completely absorbed. Food delays absorption and reduces peak levels of most penicillins. Amoxicillin is affected less by food than ampicillin is.[88] The ampicillin esters show enhanced absorption when they are taken with food.

Absorption from intramuscular injection sites is also generally rapid, with peak serum levels occurring within 1 hour. Procaine and benzathine salts of penicillin G are relatively insoluble preparations that are absorbed slowly from intramuscular injection sites. The water solubility of procaine and benzathine penicillin G is 4- and 60-fold less, respectively, than is observed with sodium and potassium salts of the drug.[80] Intramuscular administration of these formulations results in lower but more sustained blood levels than those that result from penicillin G.

Distribution of the penicillins within the body is governed by the lipid solubility of the drug and the extent of protein binding. Although penicillins bind almost exclusively to albumin, the extent of binding can vary from 20% to 97%.[81] Because only unbound drug can pass through capillary pores into interstitial fluid or across cell membranes into intracellular fluid, avidly bound penicillins tend to exhibit high serum concentrations and low tissue concentrations.[97] Likewise, fetal serum and amniotic fluid concentrations of the penicillins tend to correlate with the unbound drug level in maternal serum, rather than the total drug level.[98]

In general, the penicillins are largely confined to the extracellular compartment. Nafcillin and the isoxazolyl penicillins have the highest lipid solubility and the best potential for passage across cell membranes into intracellular fluid.[99] However, these are the same penicillins that have the highest degree of protein binding (89% to 97%). Drug penetration ex vivo into human erythrocytes is higher for nafcillin and isoxazolyl penicillins than for ampicillin and penicillin G.[100] However, the presence of albumin markedly reduces penetration of the highly bound drugs.

Concentrations of unbound drug in various tissues and inflammatory fluids are close to those in serum.[81, 101] In the absence of infection, concentrations in cerebrospinal fluid (CSF) are less than 3% of the value in serum. The presence of an active transport system that transports penicillins from CSF back to serum contributes to the low drug levels in CSF.[102] Infection results in higher, therapeutic levels in CSF, because inflammation enhances penetration and interferes with efflux by active transport.[103] Probenecid also blocks active transport and elevates penicillin concentrations in CSF.[104] Drug concentrations in human milk, aqueous humor, saliva, tears, respiratory secretions, and prostatic fluid are also lower than those in serum and further reflect the low penetration of penicillins across cell membranes.[98, 101]

Penicillins are eliminated primarily by the kidney; the major mechanism for renal excretion is tubular secretion. This active transport process is largely unaffected by protein binding and results in rapid excretion of the penicillins, with half-lives ranging from 30 to 80 minutes, and high urinary concentrations. Maximal tubular excretion rates can vary for different penicillins (e.g., 5.5 and 1.0 g/h for penicillin G and cloxacillin, respectively).[105] Probenecid inhibits this organic acid transport system and prolongs the half-life of penicillins. A daily dose of 2 g gives maximal inhibition of tubular secretion of penicillin G.[106] Because tubule function is not fully developed until a month or two of life, renal excretion of penicillins in newborns is markedly slower than in older children, which necessitates dosage modification.

Temocillin differs from the other penicillins in that it is eliminated almost entirely by glomerular filtration. Because the rate of elimination by filtration is slowed by protein binding, the half-life of temocillin, which is 83% bound, is prolonged to 4 hours.[107] It has also been shown that the rapid elimination of penicillin G is followed after several hours by a slow elimination phase with a half-life of about 3 hours[82] (Fig. 17–2). As a result, 1 million units of intravenous penicillin G will provide serum concentrations above the minimal inhibitory concentration for many streptococci for more than 9 hours. Other penicillins may have a similar slow elimination phase. However, it would be of therapeutic importance only for susceptible organisms.

Penicillins are not extensively metabolized.[108] However,

breakdown products, such as penicilloic and penicillanic acids, are produced, which can contribute to the development of hypersensitivity. Penicillins are excreted into bile, but only nafcillin, the isoxazolyl penicillins, and the ureidopenicillins exhibit significant elimination (25% to 40%) by this route. Bile levels are 2 to 10 times higher than serum concentrations for penicillin G and the aminopenicillins and 20 to 40 times higher than simultaneous serum levels for nafcillin and the ureidopenicillins.[101]

The maximal daily dosages of many penicillins need to be reduced in renal impairment.[96] However, significant modification of the ureidopenicillins and the penicillinase-resistant penicillins is required only with creatinine clearances less than 10 mL/min. Although longer half-lives of certain penicillins have been observed in patients with liver disease, the extent of impaired elimination does not require dosage modification unless there is concomitant renal disease.[109]

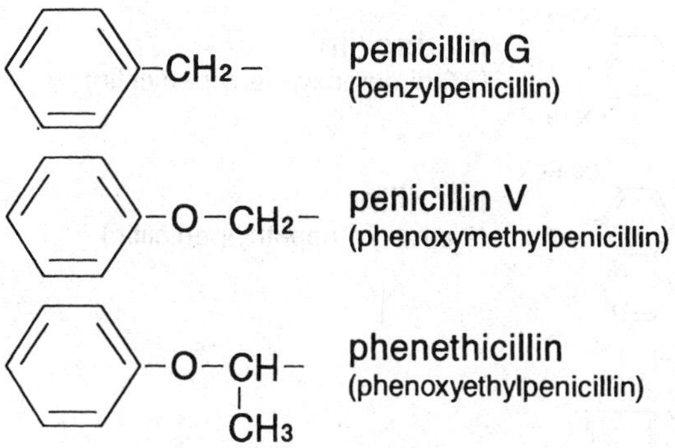

FIGURE 17–3 ▫ Structure of side chains for natural and related penicillins.

Clinical Use of Specific Agents

Natural Penicillins (Fig. 17–3)

Penicillin G. Benzylpenicillin, or penicillin G, is still a major drug for the treatment of streptococcal infections. Although *S. pneumoniae* organisms resistant to penicillin have been found in various parts of the world, decreased efficacy of penicillin G has been observed primarily in meningitis.[110] In pneumococcal pneumonia, there appears to be no difference with high-dose penicillin therapy in the mortality rates of patients infected by susceptible or resistant strains.[111] Penicillin G is highly effective in treatment of *S. pyogenes* infections. It is the major agent for viridans streptococcal endocarditis. The drug is also useful for prophylaxis of bacterial endocarditis and to prevent recurrences of rheumatic fever.

Because nearly all *N. meningitidis* strains are still susceptible, penicillin G remains the drug of choice for meningococcal infections. However, the drug is ineffective in eliminating the meningococcal carrier state. Penicillin G is no longer the drug of choice for *N. gonorrhoeae* infections because a significant number of resistant strains have emerged. Treponemal infections, including all stages of syphilis, are best treated with penicillin G. Although penicillin G is beneficial in late Lyme disease, ceftriaxone may be a more effective agent.[112] Penicillin G also reduces morbidity in severe leptospirosis.[113]

Penicillin G is still the recommended drug for actinomycosis, anthrax, rat-bite fever (due to *Streptobacillus moniliformis* or *Spirillum minus*), erysipeloid, fusospirochetal infections, gas gangrene, and periodontal infections.[114] Although penicillin G in moderately high concentrations is effective in many anaerobic infections of the lung, clindamycin appears to be more effective in cases of lung abscess.[115]

Because penicillin G is acid labile, it is generally given by intravenous injection in doses of 0.5 to 1 million units (equivalent to 300 to 600 mg) every 6 hours for many streptococcal infections. However, 12 million to 20 million units (7.2 to 12 g) per day is required for meningitis, endocarditis, and severe infections and for pneumonia caused by resistant strains. Procaine penicillin G, 600,000 units intramuscularly every 12 hours, is as effective as 20 million units of intravenous penicillin G for pneumococcal pneumonia caused by penicillin-susceptible strains.[116] In areas where penicillin resistance is not a problem, treatment for gonorrhea is a dose of 4.8 million units of procaine penicillin G, divided between two sites, injected after a 1-g oral dose of probenecid. Benzathine penicillin G (1.2 to 2.4 million units) provides low serum levels for 3 to 4 weeks. It is indicated for treatment of syphilis, group A β-hemolytic streptococcal pharyngitis, and skin infections and for prevention of streptococcal infections in patients with previous rheumatic fever. Both repository forms produce CSF levels that are too low and variable to be recommended for neurosyphilis, especially in patients infected with human immunodeficiency virus.[117]

Penicillin V. The phenoxymethyl penicillin is stable in gastric acid and is thus suitable for oral dosing. It can substitute for penicillin G for mild to moderate streptococcal infections of the upper respiratory tract, skin, and soft tissues. Daily dosages of 0.5 to 2 g for adults and 25 to 50 mg/kg for children should be given in two to four divided doses. Once-daily dosing for streptococcal pharyngitis results in an unacceptable failure rate.[118] Although penicillin V is effective in early Lyme disease, it may not be as effective as tetracycline in preventing late complications.[119] Phenethicillin, the phenoxyethyl derivative of penicillin G, has pharmacologic properties similar to those of penicillin V but is not available in the United States.

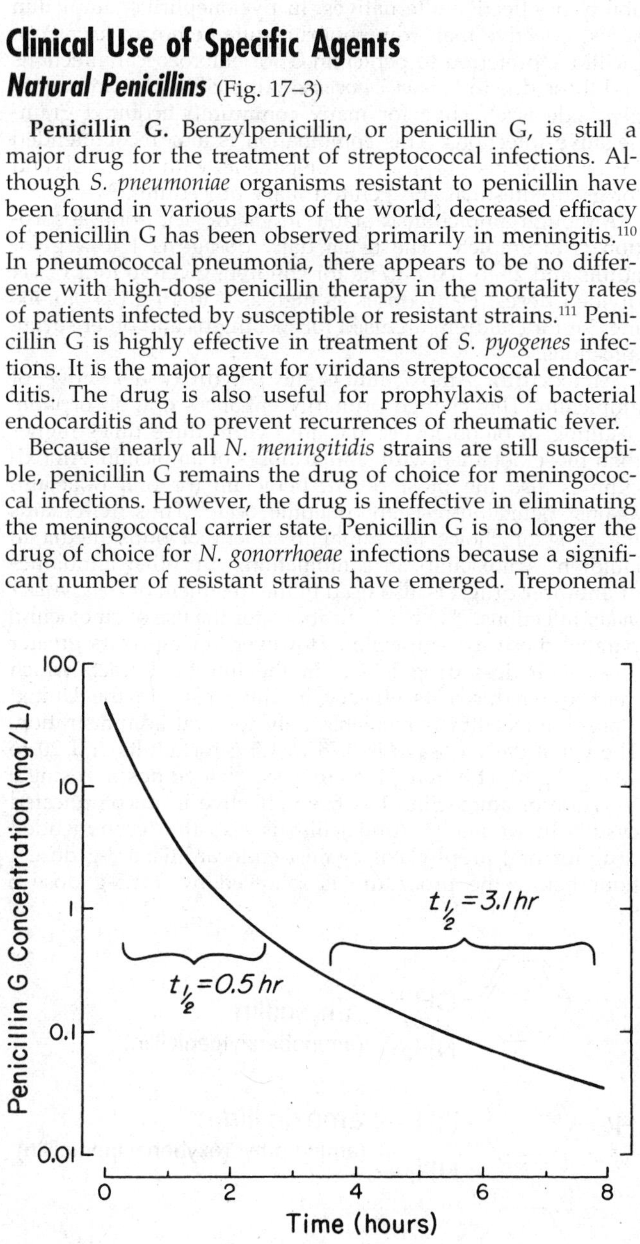

FIGURE 17–2 ▫ Mean serum concentrations for penicillin G in eight normal subjects. (Data from Ebert SC, Leggett J, Vogelman B, et al: Evidence for a slow elimination phase for penicillin G. J Infect Dis 158:200, 1988.)

Penicillinase-Resistant Penicillins (Fig. 17–4)

Methicillin. Methicillin was the first available penicillin that was resistant to the penicillinase of staphylococci. Despite the increasing occurrence of methicillin-resistant strains

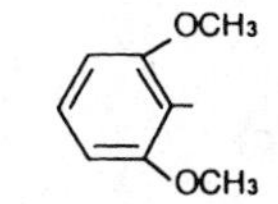

methicillin
(2,6-dimethoxyphenylpenicillin)

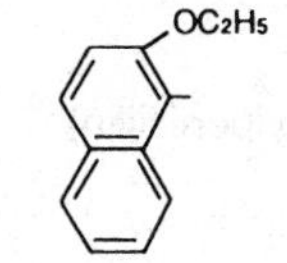

nafcillin
(2-ethoxy-1-naphthylpenicillin)

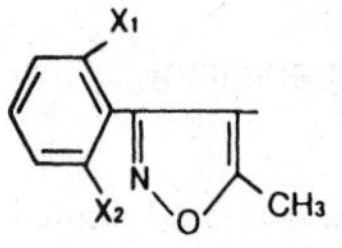

X_1=H	X_2=H	oxacillin (3-phenyl-5-methyl-4-isoxazolylpenicillin)
X_1=Cl	X_2=H	cloxacillin (2-chlorophenyl derivative)
X_1=Cl	X_2=Cl	dicloxacillin (2,6-dichlorophenyl derivative)
X_1=Cl	X_2=F	flucloxacillin (2-chloro-6-fluorophenyl derivative)

FIGURE 17–4 □ Structure of side chains for penicillinase-resistant penicillins.

(which are resistant to all penicillins), this drug and the other penicillinase-resistant penicillins remain the drugs of choice for most *S. aureus* infections. However, the high prevalence of methicillin resistance in coagulase-negative staphylococci has reduced the use of these drugs for these organisms.[120] Because methicillin is rapidly destroyed by gastric acid, the drug is available only for parenteral administration. The usual daily dosage is 4 to 12 g for adults and 100 to 300 mg/kg for children, given in four to six divided doses.

Nafcillin. Nafcillin is about 10 times more potent than methicillin against staphylococci and streptococci. It is, however, more highly protein bound than methicillin. When both binding and intrinsic antimicrobial activity are taken into consideration, the biologic activities of both drugs in serum are similar.[121] Although the indications and dosage regimens for this drug are the same as those for methicillin, nafcillin may be the preferred agent for staphylococcal central nervous system infections because of enhanced CSF penetration.[122] Nafcillin may also be associated with a lower frequency of adverse reactions than methicillin.[123] The drug's high biliary excretion rate eliminates the need for dosage modification in renal impairment. Because nafcillin is not completely stable to acid, its absorption is erratic and results in variable serum levels.

Isoxazolyl Penicillins. These drugs are stable to gastric acid. Thus, they are used for oral therapy for less severe staphylococcal infections. Osteomyelitis and septic arthritis, in both children and adults, have been effectively treated with oral therapy.[124, 125] As with nafcillin, the avid protein binding of these drugs is compensated for by their high intrinsic activity. Cloxacillin and dicloxacillin yield higher total and unbound serum concentrations than does oxacillin.[86] Flucloxacillin, which is not available in the United States, exhibits the best oral absorption. The usual oral daily dosage for these drugs is 1 to 4 g for adults and 50 to 100 mg/kg for children, given in four divided doses. Parenteral oxacillin is available, which can be used at dosages similar to those of nafcillin and methicillin in place of nafcillin and methicillin. Parenteral cloxacillin, which is also not available in the United States, has been shown to reduce perioperative infections after craniotomy.[126] All of the isoxazolyl penicillins have extensive hepatic elimination and do not require modification with renal impairment.

Aminopenicillins (Fig. 17–5)

Ampicillin. Aminobenzylpenicillin or ampicillin provides effective therapy for many upper respiratory tract infections and exacerbations of chronic bronchitis due to *S. pneumoniae, Bronhamella (Moraxella) catarrhalis,* and *H. influenzae.* However, the relatively high frequency of β-lactamase–positive strains of *H. influenzae* and *M. catarrhalis* in many locations has reduced empirical use of ampicillin in more severe infections. Its use for meningitis in children, *Salmonella* and *Shigella* infections, and urinary tract infections has also been curtailed by the appearance of resistant strains and the availability of effective alternatives. In pyelonephritis, ampicillin is less effective than trimethoprim-sulfamethoxazole.[127] Ampicillin is preferred to penicillin G for enterococcal infections and those due to *L. monocytogenes.* Ampicillin plus an aminoglycoside is effective for many community-acquired gram-negative infections. This combination is also recommended for endocarditis prophylaxis for patients with high risk and for gastrointestinal and genitourinary procedures.[128]

Although ampicillin is stable in gastric acid, oral absorption is incomplete. The usual daily dosage is 1 to 4 g for adults and 25 to 100 mg/kg for children, given in four or six divided doses. Daily doses as high as 8 to 16 g (200 to 400 mg/kg for children) are used for meningitis and other severe infections.

Amoxicillin. Amoxicillin is the *p*-hydroxy derivative of ampicillin. This change primarily enhances oral absorption, resulting in blood levels that are two to three times higher than those obtained with similar doses of ampicillin. Amoxicillin is also the most potent penicillin (or oral β-lactam) against penicillin-resistant pneumococci.[36] Thus, it remains the drug of choice for initial treatment of otitis media in children. Amoxicillin, in combination with other antibiotics or antiulcer drugs, is also used in the treatment of *Helicobacter pylori* infections.[129] Other indications for the use of amoxicillin parallel those for ampicillin. However, owing to its greater absorption, less drug is left in the intestinal tract, which markedly reduces its efficacy in shigellosis. In the United States, amoxicillin is available only for oral administration. The usual daily dosage is 0.75 to 1.5 g for adults and 20 to 40 mg/kg for children, given in three divided doses. A single 3-g dose of amoxicillin has been effective in uncomplicated cystitis in women.[130] Amoxicillin is also the recommended drug for oral prophylaxis against endocarditis; a 3-g dose 1 hour before the procedure is followed by a 1.5-g dose 6

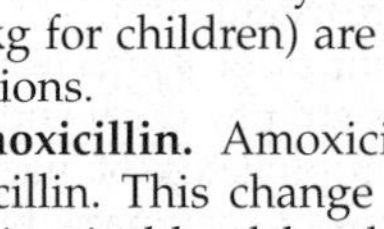

ampicillin
(aminobenzylpenicillin)

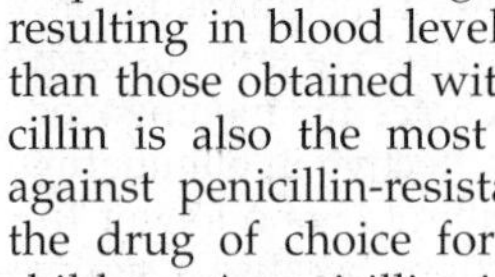

amoxicillin
(amino-p-hydroxybenzylpenicillin)

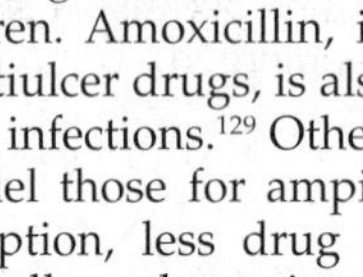

cyclacillin
(aminocyclohexylpenicillin)

FIGURE 17–5 □ Structure of side chains for aminopenicillins.

hours later.[128] Cyclacillin, another well-absorbed analog of ampicillin, is no longer available in the United States.

Ampicillin Esters. Bacampicillin, pivampicillin, and talampicillin are 1-carboxyl esters of ampicillin. They are inactive until hydrolyzed to ampicillin by esterase enzymes present in the gastrointestinal epithelium and in serum.[131] These ester formulations result in almost complete absorption of ampicillin. Only bacampicillin is available in the United States. It produces peak blood levels of ampicillin that are even slightly higher than those of amoxicillin.[89] The indications for use are the same as for amoxicillin. The usual daily dosage is 0.8 to 1.6 g (equivalent to 0.56 to 1.12 g of ampicillin) for adults and 12.5 to 25 mg/kg for children, given in two divided doses.

Carboxypenicillins (Fig. 17–6)

Carbenicillin. Carbenicillin is the carboxybenzyl derivative of penicillin. Although the main indications for its use are infections caused by *P. aeruginosa*, carbenicillin is active against other ampicillin-resistant gram-negative bacilli, such as *P. vulgaris,* as well as *Enterobacter, Morganella,* and *Providencia* species.[132] A daily intravenous dose of 30 to 40 g (400 to 600 mg/kg for children) is required for systemic pseudomonal infections. Because carbenicillin is a disodium salt, each gram contains 4.7 mEq of sodium; large doses can precipitate congestive heart failure as well as induce hypokalemia and inhibit platelet function. Parenteral carbenicillin is no longer available in the United States. Indanyl carbenicillin is an α-carboxyl ester of carbenicillin that is resistant to acid inactivation.[133] This oral formulation is useful only for urinary tract infections, especially those due to *P. aeruginosa.* The daily dose is 1.5 to 3.0 g, given in four divided doses.

Ticarcillin. Ticarcillin has replaced carbenicillin in the treatment of serious pseudomonal infections because it has similar pharmacologic properties but is twofold to fourfold more active against *P. aeruginosa.*[134] This reduces the recommended daily dose to 4 g for urinary tract infections and 200 to 300 mg/kg (about 15 to 21 g) for systemic infections, given in four to six divided doses. The lower dose of ticarcillin also reduces the frequency of adverse reactions observed with carbenicillin.[135]

Ureidopenicillins (Fig. 17–7)

Mezlocillin. The antimicrobial spectrum of mezlocillin combines the activities of ampicillin and ticarcillin. The drug is also active against many isolates of *Klebsiella.* Its pharmacologic properties are similar to those of the carboxypenicillins except that about a third of the drug is eliminated by biliary excretion. Thus, dosage modification is required only with severe renal impairment. The drug is used for the treatment of serious gram-negative infections, including those due to

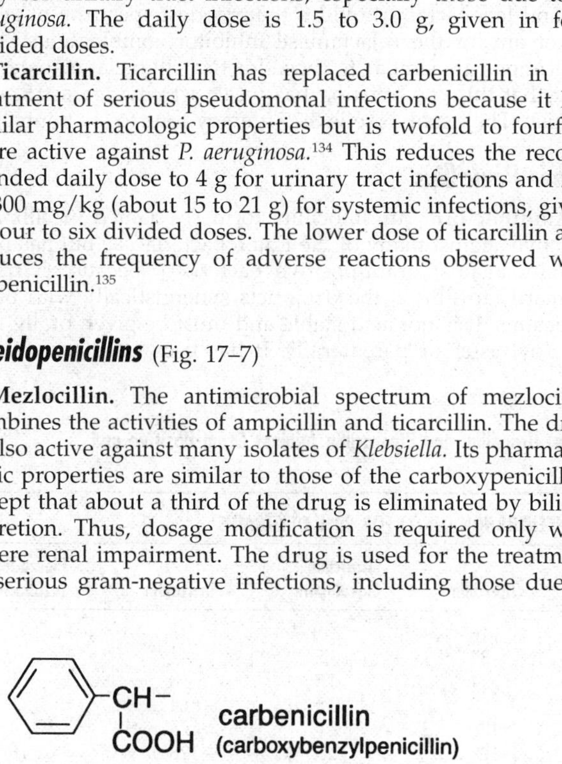

FIGURE 17–6 ▫ Structure of side chains for carboxypenicillins.

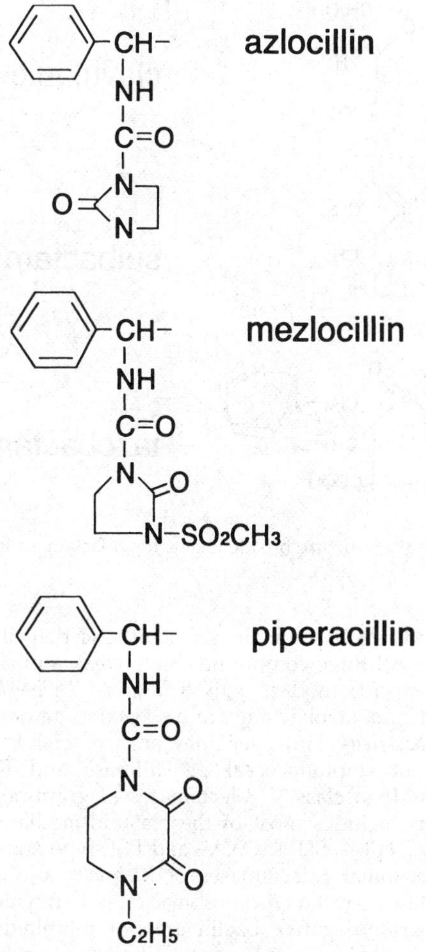

FIGURE 17–7 ▫ Structure of side chains for ureidopenicillins.

P. aeruginosa.[136] Its high biliary excretion may enhance efficacy in the treatment of biliary tract infections.[137] Its clearance with increasing concentrations is nonlinear because of saturation of biliary excretion.[138] This allows less frequent dosing than with the carboxypenicillins (i.e., every 6 hours rather than every 4 hours). The usual daily dose is 4 to 8 g for urinary tract infections and 12 to 18 g (200 to 300 mg/kg) for systemic infections. Because the drug is a derivative of ampicillin, it is a monosodium salt and less likely to result in the adverse reactions associated with the carboxypenicillins.

Azlocillin. Azlocillin is similar in pharmacologic action and antimicrobial spectrum to mezlocillin, except that it is twofold to fourfold more active against *P. aeruginosa* but relatively inactive against *Klebsiella* species.[139] Dosage regimens are similar to those for mezlocillin. It is no longer available in the United States.

Piperacillin. Piperacillin is also about fourfold more active than mezlocillin against *P. aeruginosa,* but unlike azlocillin, it maintains its activity against *Klebsiella* species.[140] Its pharmacologic properties, indications for use, and usual dosage regimens are similar to those for mezlocillin.[141]

β-Lactamase Inhibitors (Fig. 17–8)

Clavulanic acid, the first β-lactamase inhibitor, is produced by *Streptomyces clavuligerus.*[142] Its structure differs from penicillin in that it has no side chain on the β-lactam ring, has an oxygen atom in place of the sulfur atom, and contains a hydroxyethylidene substitution on the oxazolidine ring. Sul-

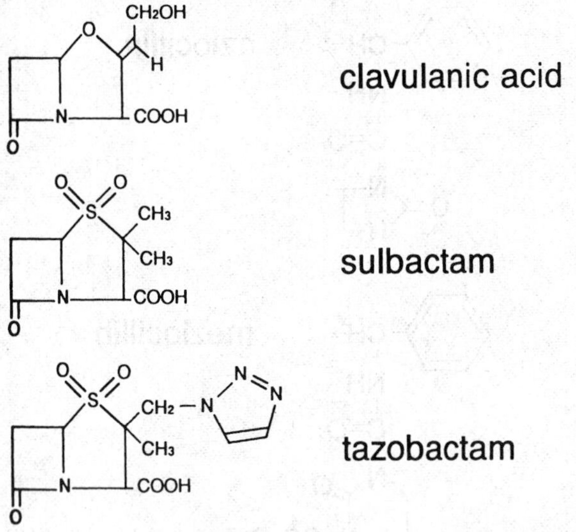

FIGURE 17–8 □ Structure of side chains for β-lactamase inhibitors.

bactam and tazobactam are semisynthetic penicillanic acid sulfones.[143] All three compounds have weak antibacterial activity except for modest activity against *Neisseria* species. Sulbactam and tazobactam are also active against *Acinetobacter calcoaceticus.* However, they are irreversible "suicide" inhibitors of staphylococcal penicillinase and Richmond-Sykes class II to class V β-lactamases of gram-negative bacilli.[144] This includes most of the plasmid-mediated β-lactamases (e.g., TEM-, SHV-, OXA-, and PSE-type enzymes) and the chromosomal β-lactamases of *Klebsiella* and *Bacteroides* species. However, the chromosomal class I enzymes present in many gram-negative bacilli are not inhibited by these drugs. Nevertheless, a β-lactamase inhibitor combined with amoxicillin, ampicillin, ticarcillin, and piperacillin enhances their activity against β-lactamase–producing strains of staphylococci, gonococci, *H. influenzae, M. catarrhalis, Bacteroides* and *Klebsiella* species, and *E. coli*[145–151] (Table 17–5). The activity against other gram-negative bacilli is largely unaffected by these β-lactamase inhibitors.

The pharmacokinetic profile of clavulanic acid is similar to that of amoxicillin.[94] In contrast, sulbactam and tazobactam are poorly absorbed orally. With intravenous administration, the pharmacologic action of sulbactam and tazobactam is similar to that of ampicillin.[95, 152] All three β-lactamase inhibitors are eliminated predominantly by the kidney with a half-life of about 1 hour, have low protein binding, and distribute primarily to extracellular fluid.

Amoxicillin-Clavulanate. Only the oral formulation of amoxicillin-clavulanate is available in the United States. It has been especially useful for otitis media, sinusitis, and lower respiratory tract infections due to β-lactamase–producing *H. influenzae* and *M. catarrhalis.*[153] It is effective in staphylococcal and streptococcal skin infections and is the recommended agent for infections after animal and human bites.[154] The usual daily dose is 0.75 to 1.5 g of amoxicillin plus 0.375 g of clavulanate, given in three divided doses. Administration of more than 0.375 g of clavulanate per day is associated with a high frequency of diarrhea.

Ampicillin-Sulbactam. Only the parenteral fixed 2:1 ratio of ampicillin-sulbactam is currently available in the United States. Its indications are similar to those for amoxicillin-clavulanate but include intraabdominal and gynecologic infections and more severe skin and soft tissue infections.[155] The usual dose is 6 to 12 g/d (4 to 8 g of ampicillin), divided into four doses.

Ticarcillin-Clavulanate. A fixed 30:1 ratio of ticarcillin-clavulanate is available for intravenous administration. Its broad spectrum of activity has resulted in successful treatment of nosocomial pneumonia, intraabdominal infections, and severe skin and soft tissue infections.[156] This combination is also active against many *Stenotrophomonas* (formerly *Xanthomonas*) *maltophilia* strains.[157] A dose of 3.1 g is given four to six times daily.

Piperacillin-Tazobactam. A fixed 8:1 mixture of piperacillin and tazobactam provides the broadest spectrum of activity of any of the β-lactamase inhibitor combinations.[158] Its indications are similar to those for ticarcillin-clavulanate, except that this combination has weak activity against *S. maltophilia.* The usual dose is 3.75 g every four to six hours.

Other Penicillins

Amdinocillin. Amdinocillin, formerly named mecillinam, is active against many of the Enterobacteriaceae but has poor activity against gram-positive bacteria.[159] Because it binds primarily to PBP 2, the drug acts synergistically with other β-lactams. It is not acid stable and must be given orally as a pivaloyl ester or parenterally. It has been used for urinary

TABLE 17–5 ■ Effect of β-Lactamase Inhibitors on Activity of Amoxicillin, Ampicillin, Ticarcillin, and Piperacillin Against Gram-Positive and Gram-Negative Bacteria

	MINIMAL INHIBITORY CONCENTRATION (mg/L) FOR 90% OF STRAINS						
ORGANISM	Amoxicillin, Ampicillin	Amoxicillin-Clavulanate	Ampicillin-Sulbactam	Ticarcillin	Ticarcillin-Clavulanate	Piperacillin	Piperacillin-Tazobactam
Staphylococcus aureus	>128	0.5	2	16	2	32	2
Neisseria gonorrhoeae	128	1	1	32	0.5	—	—
Moraxella catarrhalis	16	0.2	0.25	4	0.5	8	1
Haemophilus influenzae	64	2	1	8	0.5	64	1
Bacteroides fragilis	128	2	2	>128	2	>128	4
Escherichia coli	>128	32	16	>128	32	>128	16
Proteus mirabilis	4	0.5	1	8	1	32	2
Proteus vulgaris	>128	8	16	32	1	32	2
Klebsiella pneumoniae	>128	8	16	>128	8	>128	16
Enterobacter sp.	>128	>128	16	128	128	>128	128
Serratia sp.	>128	>128	>128	128	64	>128	32
Acinetobacter sp.	64	64	4	32	32	64	16
Pseudomonas aeruginosa	>128	>128	>128	64	64	64	64

Data from references 145–151.

tract infections, but it is not currently available in the United States.[160]

Temocillin. This 6-α-methoxy derivative of ticarcillin is resistant to inactivation by β-lactamases. It is active against most of the Enterobacteriaceae but has poor activity against gram-positive bacteria and *P. aeruginosa*.[161] Because of its long half-life, it is administered twice daily. Although it has been effective in severe gram-negative infections, it is not available in the United States.[162]

Adverse Reactions

Hypersensitivity reactions are the most common adverse effects associated with penicillin therapy. They are mediated by antibodies, whose production is induced by penicillin degradation products bound to protein (i.e., haptens). The penicilloyl derivative, which results from the opening of the β-lactam ring, accounts for the largest amount of protein-bound degradation products and is known as the major determinant of penicillin allergy.[163] Additional metabolites (e.g., penicilloate and penilloate derivatives) are present in smaller amounts and are called the minor determinants. Virtually everyone makes antibodies after exposure to penicillins, but these are primarily of the immunoglobulin M and immunoglobulin G classes. However, the rarer immunoglobulin E antibodies are associated with immediate hypersensitivity reactions. Anaphylaxis is seen in 0.004% to 0.015% of cases; urticaria occurs in 1% to 5%.[164] Both determinants can mediate each reaction. However, minor determinants are associated more with anaphylaxis; the major determinant is involved more with urticarial reactions.

Immunoglobulin M and immunoglobulin G antibodies may be involved in nonurticarial skin reactions. Morbilliform rashes occur in 5% to 9% of individuals receiving ampicillin but in only 2% to 3% of those receiving penicillin G.[165–167] The occurrence of ampicillin rashes is also enhanced by Epstein-Barr virus and cytomegalovirus infections and by concomitant use of allopurinol.[168] Although erythema multiforme and exfoliative dermatitis are rare reactions to penicillin, these β-lactams are the most common known cause of Stevens-Johnson syndrome.[169] Serum sickness is an uncommon adverse effect of penicillins and results from deposition of immune complexes in tissue. Drug fever may have a similar mechanism.

Cytotoxic reactions from immunoglobulin G and immunoglobulin M antibodies can account for hematologic side effects observed with the penicillins. Coombs-positive hemolytic anemia usually results from antipenicillin antibodies reacting with drug already bound to red blood cell membranes.[170] Complement is not activated, and intravascular hemolysis rarely occurs. Instead, these cells are removed extravascularly and destroyed by the reticuloendothelial system. Similar mechanisms may cause the more commonly observed neutropenia, which appears to be enhanced by high-dose therapy.[171, 172] Although platelet dysfunction can also result from large doses, especially those of carbenicillin and ticarcillin, clinical bleeding is uncommon. By binding to platelet membranes, penicillins impair the interaction of agonists with receptors on the platelet surface.[173, 174]

The interstitial nephritis seen with penicillins is basically a cytotoxic hypersensitivity reaction. Penicilloyl metabolites initially bind to kidney tissue. Antipenicillin antibodies then react with the penicillin and complement is activated, resulting in cellular damage.[175] Tubule basement membrane can be released in the process, and antibodies to this antigen may contribute to the kidney damage.[176] Cell-mediated toxicity may also play a role in this adverse reaction.[177] Although this complication has been reported with most penicillins, it is apparently most commonly observed with methicillin, prolonged therapy, and daily doses greater than 6 g.[123]

High doses of penicillins, especially the carboxypenicillins, can produce fluid overload because of their sodium content. Hypokalemia results because large amounts of these drugs in the distal tubule act as nonreabsorbable anions, creating a favorable gradient for excessive excretion of potassium.[178, 179]

Myoclonic jerks, hyperreflexia, seizures, and coma have been associated with intrathecal instillations of various penicillins and with high-dose intravenous therapy, primarily in patients with renal impairment.[180] Decreased protein binding and inhibition of active transport from the CSF occur in uremia and may contribute to enhanced toxicity in patients with renal impairment.[181, 182]

Gastrointestinal reactions, including enterocolitis due to *Clostridium difficile*, can occur with all penicillins. Diarrhea has been most common with oral ampicillin and combinations with β-lactamase inhibitors. Hepatotoxicity is uncommon and observed primarily with oxacillin and carbenicillin.[183, 184] The frequency of oxacillin hepatotoxicity appears to be increased in patients infected with human immunodeficiency virus.[185]

Drug interactions with penicillins are uncommon. Nafcillin has resulted in a few cases of warfarin resistance and subtherapeutic cyclosporine levels.[186, 187] Penicillins, especially the carboxypenicillins and ureidopenicillins, can inactivate gentamicin and tobramycin.[188] This inactivation is insignificant in patients with normal renal function. With renal impairment, concomitant administration of a penicillin can shorten aminoglycoside half-lives, necessitating more frequent dosing.[189]

References

1. Fleming A: On antibacterial action of cultures on *Penicillium*, with special reference to their use in isolation of *B. influenzae*. Br J Exp Pathol 10:226, 1929.
2. Chain E, Florey HW, Gardner AD, et al: Penicillin as chemotherapeutic agent. Lancet 2:226, 1940.
3. Abraham EP, Chain E, Fletcher CM, et al: Further observations on penicillin. Lancet 2:177, 1941.
4. Florey ME, Florey HW: General and local administration of penicillin. Lancet 1:387, 1943.
5. Keefer CS, Blake FG, Marshall EK Jr, et al: Penicillin in the treatment of respiratory infections; a report of 500 cases; statement by committee on chemotherapeutic and other agents. JAMA 122:1217, 1943.
6. Raper KB, Alexander DF, Coghill RD: Penicillin; natural variation and penicillin production in *Penicillium notatum* and allied species. J Bacteriol 48:639, 1944.
7. Moyer AJ, Coghill RD: Penicillin; production of penicillin in surface cultures. J Bacteriol 51:57, 1946.
8. Batchelor FR, Doyle FP, Naylor JHC, et al: Synthesis of penicillin: 6-Aminopenicillanic acid in penicillin fermentations. Nature 183:257, 1959.
9. Queener SW: Molecular biology of penicillin and cephalosporin biosynthesis. Antimicrob Agents Chemother 34:943, 1990.
10. Hou JP, Poole JW: β-Lactam antibiotics; their physicochemical properties and biological activities in relation to structure. J Pharm Sci 60:503, 1971.
11. Wise EM Jr, Park JT: Penicillin: Its basic site of action as an inhibitor of a peptide cross-linking reaction in cell wall mucopeptide synthesis. Proc Natl Acad Sci USA 54:75, 1965.
12. Tipper DJ, Strominger JL: Mechanism of action of penicillins: A proposal based on their structural similarity to acyl-D-alanyl-D-alanine. Proc Natl Acad Sci USA 54:1133, 1965.
13. Tomasz A: Penicillin-binding proteins in bacteria. Ann Intern Med 96:502, 1982.
14. Waxman DJ, Strominger JL: Penicillin binding proteins and the mechanism of action of beta-lactam antibiotics. Annu Rev Biochem 52:825, 1983.
15. Spratt BG: Distinct penicillin-binding proteins involved in the

division, elongation and shape of *Escherichia coli* K12. Proc Natl Acad Sci USA 72:2999, 1975.
16. Tomasz A: From penicillin-binding proteins to the lysis and death of bacteria: A 1979 view. Rev Infect Dis 1:434, 1979.
17. Suzuki H, Nishimura Y, Hirota Y: On the process of cellular division in *Escherichia coli:* A series of mutants of *E. coli* altered in the penicillin-binding proteins. Proc Natl Acad Sci USA 75:664, 1978.
18. Tomasz A, Waks S: Mechanism of action of penicillin: Triggering of the pneumococcal autolytic enzyme by inhibitors of cell wall synthesis. Proc Natl Acad Sci USA 72:4162, 1975.
19. Kitano K, Tomasz A: *Escherichia coli* mutants tolerant to beta-lactam antibiotics. J Bacteriol 140:955, 1979.
20. Höltje JV, Tomasz A: Lipoteichoic acid: A specific inhibitor of autolysin activity in pneumococcus. Proc Natl Acad Sci USA 72:1690, 1975.
21. Fontana R, Satta G, Romanzi CA: Penicillins activate autolysins extracted from both *Escherichia coli* and *Klebsiella pneumoniae* envelopes. Antimicrob Agents Chemother 12:745, 1977.
22. Reinicke B, Blümel P, Labischinski H, et al: Neither an enhancement of autolytic wall degradation nor an inhibition of the incorporation of cell wall material are pre-requisites for penicillin-induced bacteriolysis in staphylococci. Arch Microbiol 141:309, 1985.
23. Giesbrecht P, Labischinski H, Wecke J: A special morphogenetic wall defect and the subsequent activity of "murosomes" as the very reason for penicillin-induced bacteriolysis in staphylococci. Arch Microbiol 141:315, 1985.
24. Maidhof H, Johannsen L, Labischinski H, et al: Onset of penicillin-induced bacteriolysis in staphylococci is cell cycle dependent. J Bacteriol 171:2252, 1989.
25. McDowell TD, Lemanski CL: Absence of autolytic activity (peptidoglycan nicking) in penicillin-induced nonlytic death in a group A streptococcus. J Bacteriol 170:1783, 1988.
26. McDowell TD, Reed KE: Mechanism of penicillin killing in the absence of bacterial lysis. Antimicrob Agents Chemother 33:1680, 1989.
27. Vogelman B, Craig WA: Kinetics of antimicrobial activity. J Pediatr 108:835, 1986.
28. Bundtzen RW, Gerber AU, Cohn DL, et al: Postantibiotic suppression of bacterial growth. Rev Infect Dis 3:28, 1981.
29. Craig WA, Vogelman B: The postantibiotic effect. Ann Intern Med 106:900, 1987.
30. Sabath LD, Garner C, Wilcox C, et al: Susceptibility of *Staphylococcus aureus* and *Staphylococcus epidermidis* to 65 antibiotics. Antimicrob Agents Chemother 9:962, 1976.
31. Finland M, Garner C, Wilcox C, et al: Susceptibility of beta-hemolytic streptococci to 65 antibacterial agents. Antimicrob Agents Chemother 9:11, 1976.
32. Baker CN, Thornsberry C, Facklam RR: Synergism, killing kinetics, and antimicrobial susceptibility of group A and B streptococci. Antimicrob Agents Chemother 19:716, 1981.
33. Persson KM-S, Forsgren A: Antimicrobial susceptibility of group B streptococci. Eur J Clin Microbiol 5:165, 1986.
34. Finland M, Garner C, Wilcox C, et al: Susceptibility of pneumococci and *Haemophilus influenzae* to antibacterial agents. Antimicrob Agents Chemother 9:274, 1976.
35. Linares J, Alonso T, Perez JL, et al: Decreased susceptibility of penicillin-resistant pneumococci to twenty-four β-lactam antibiotics. J Antimicrob Chemother 30:279, 1992.
36. Spangleer SK, Jacobs MR, Appelbaum PC: In vitro susceptibilities of 185 penicillin-susceptible and -resistant pneumococci to WY-49605 (SUN/SY 5555), a new oral penem, compared with those to penicillin G, amoxicillin, amoxicillin-clavulanate, cefixime, cefaclor, cefpodoxime, cefuroxime, and cefdinir. Antimicrob Agents Chemother 38:2902, 1994.
37. Pankuch GA, Jacobs MR, Appelbaum PC: Susceptibilities of 200 penicillin-susceptible and -resistant pneumococci to piperacillin, piperacillin-tazobactam, ticarcillin, ticarcillin-clavulanate, ampicillin, ampicillin-sulbactam, ceftazidime, and ceftriaxone. Antimicrob Agents Chemother 38:2905, 1994.
38. Cooksey RC, Swenson JM: In vitro antimicrobial inhibition patterns of nutritionally variant streptococci. Antimicrob Agents Chemother 16:514, 1979.
39. Toala P, McDonald A, Wilson C, et al: Susceptibility of group D streptococci (enterococcus) to 21 antibiotics in vitro, with special reference to species differences. Am J Med Sci 258:416, 1969.
40. Pérez JL, Riera L, Valls F, et al: A comparison of the in-vitro activity of seventeen antibiotics against *Streptococcus faecalis.* J Antimicrob Chemother 20:357, 1987.
41. Hall WH, Schierl EA, Maccani JE: Comparative susceptibility of penicillinase-positive and -negative *Neisseria gonorrhoeae* to 30 antibiotics. Antimicrob Agents Chemother 15:562, 1979.
42. Trallero EP, Arenzana JMG, Ayestaran I, et al: Comparative activity in vitro of 16 antimicrobial agents against penicillin-susceptible meningococci and meningococci with diminished susceptibility to penicillin. Antimicrob Agents Chemother 33:1622, 1989.
43. Doern GV, Tubert TA: In vitro activities of 39 antimicrobial agents for *Branhamella catarrhalis* and comparison of results with different quantitative susceptibility test methods. Antimicrob Agents Chemother 32:259, 1988.
44. Phillips I, King A, Shannon K, et al: Temocillin (BRL 17421): In-vitro antibacterial activity and susceptibility to β-lactamases. J Antimicrob Chemother 10:271, 1982.
45. Wiedemann B, Atkinson BA: Susceptibility to antibiotics: Species incidence and trends. *In* Lorian V (ed): Antibiotics in Laboratory Medicine, ed 3. Baltimore, Williams & Wilkins, 1991, pp 962–1208.
46. Neu HC: Structure-activity relationships of new β-lactam compounds and in vitro activity against common bacteria. Rev Infect Dis 5(Suppl 2):S319, 1983.
47. Parry MF, Folta D: The in vitro activity of mezlocillin against community hospital isolates in comparison to other penicillins and cephalosporins. J Antimicrob Chemother 11(Suppl C):97, 1983.
48. Verbist L: Comparison of the activities of the new ureidopenicillins piperacillin, mezlocillin, azlocillin, and Bay k 4999 against gram-negative organisms. Antimicrob Agents Chemother 16:115, 1979.
49. Sutter VL, Finegold SM: Susceptibility of anaerobic bacteria to 23 antimicrobial agents. Antimicrob Agents Chemother 10:736, 1976.
50. Appelbaum PC, Chatterton SA: Susceptibility of anaerobic bacteria to ten antimicrobial agents. Antimicrob Agents Chemother 14:371, 1978.
51. Gill VJ, MacLowry JD: Antibiotic susceptibilities of commonly encountered anaerobic bacteria. *In* Seligson D (ed): Handbook Series in Clinical Laboratory Science. Section E. Clinical Microbiology, Vol II. Cleveland, OH, CRC Press, 1977, pp 281–292.
52. Livermore DM: β-Lactamases in laboratory and clinical resistance. Clin Microbiol Rev 8:557, 1995.
53. McDougal LK, Thornsberry C: The role of β-lactamase in staphylococcal resistance to penicillinase-resistant penicillins and cephalosporins. J Clin Microbiol 23:832, 1986.
54. Nikaido H: Outer membrane barrier as a mechanism of antimicrobial resistance. Antimicrob Agents Chemother 33:1831, 1989.
55. Nikaido H: Role of permeability barriers in resistance to β-lactam antibiotics. Pharmacol Ther 27:197, 1985.
56. Jules K, Neu HC: Antibacterial activity and β-lactamase stability of temocillin. Antimicrob Agents Chemother 22:453, 1982.
57. Medeiros AA, O'Brien TF: Ampicillin-resistant *Haemophilus influenzae* type B possessing a TEM-type beta-lactamase but little permeability barrier to ampicillin. Lancet 1:716, 1975.
58. Elwell LP, Roberts M, Mayer LW, et al: Plasmid-mediated β-lactamase production in *Neisseria gonorrhoeae.* Antimicrob Agents Chemother 11:528, 1977.
59. Murray BE, Mederski-Samoraj B, Foster SK, et al: In-vitro studies of plasmid-mediated penicillinase from *Streptococcus faecalis* suggest a staphylococcal origin. J Clin Invest 77:289, 1986.
60. Sanders CC, Sanders WE Jr: Type 1 beta-lactamases of gram-negative bacteria: Interactions with beta-lactam antibiotics. J Infect Dis 154:792, 1986.
61. Livermore DM, Yang Y-J: β-Lactamase lability and inducer power of newer β-lactam antibiotics in relation to their activity against β-lactamase–inducibility mutants of *Pseudomonas aeruginosa.* J Infect Dis 155:755, 1987.
62. Malouin F, Bryan LE: Modification of penicillin-binding proteins as mechanisms of β-lactam resistance. Antimicrob Agents Chemother 30:1, 1986.
63. Chambers HF: Methicillin-resistant staphylococci. Clin Microbiol Rev 1:173, 1988.
64. Jabes D, Nachman S, Tomasz A: Penicillin-binding protein fami-

lies: Evidence for the clonal nature of penicillin resistance in clinical isolates of pneumococci. J Infect Dis 159:16, 1989.
65. Mendelman PM, Campos J, Chaffin DO, et al: Relative penicillin G resistance in *Neisseria meningitidis* and reduced affinity of penicillin-binding protein 3. Antimicrob Agents Chemother 32:706, 1988.
66. Mendelman PM, Chaffin DO, Kalaitzoglou G: Penicillin-binding proteins and ampicillin resistance in *Haemophilus influenzae.* J Antimicrob Chemother 25:525, 1990.
67. Smith AM, Klugman KP: Alterations in penicillin-binding protein 2B from penicillin-resistant wild-type strains of *Streptococcus pneumoniae.* Antimicrob Agents Chemother 39:859, 1995.
68. Coffey TJ, Dowson CG, Daniels M, et al: Genetics and molecular biology of β-lactam–resistant pneumococci. Microb Drug Resist 1:29, 1995.
69. Spratt BG, Zhang Q-Y, Jones DM, et al: Recruitment of a penicillin-binding protein gene from *Neisseria flavescens* during the emergence of penicillin resistance in *Neisseria meningitidis.* Proc Natl Acad Sci USA 86:8988, 1989.
70. Song MD, Wachi M, Doi M, et al: Evolution of an inducible penicillin-target protein in methicillin-resistant *Staphylococcus aureus* by gene fusion. FEBS Lett 221:167, 1987.
71. Harder KJ, Nikaido H, Matsuhashi M: Mutants of *Escherichia coli* that are resistant to certain beta-lactam compounds lack the *ompF* porin. Antimicrob Agents Chemother 20:549, 1981.
72. Jaffé A, Chabbert YA, Derlot E: Selection and characterization of β-lactam–resistant *Escherichia coli* K-12 mutants. Antimicrob Agents Chemother 23:623, 1983.
73. Hancock RE, Woodruff WA: Roles of porin and β-lactamase in β-lactam resistance in *Pseudomonas aeruginosa.* Rev Infect Dis 10:770, 1988.
74. Mirelman D, Nuchamowitz Y, Rubenstein E: Insensitivity of peptidoglycan biosynthetic reactions to beta-lactam antibiotics in a clinical isolate of *Pseudomonas aeruginosa.* Antimicrob Agents Chemother 19:687, 1981.
75. Tomasz A, Albino A, Zanati E: Multiple antibiotic resistance in a bacterium with suppressed autolytic system. Nature 227:138, 1970.
76. Handwerger S, Tomasz A: Antibiotic tolerance among clinical isolates of bacteria. Rev Infect Dis 7:368, 1985.
77. Sabath LD, Wheeler N, Laverdiere M, et al: A new type of penicillin resistance of *Staphylococcus aureus.* Lancet 1:443, 1977.
78. Rajashekaraiah KR, Rice T, Rao VS, et al: Clinical significance of tolerant strains of *Staphylococcus aureus* in patients with endocarditis. Ann Intern Med 93:796, 1980.
79. McCarthy CG, Finland M: Absorption and excretion of four penicillins: Penicillin G, penicillin V, phenethicillin and phenylmercaptomethyl penicillin. N Engl J Med 263:315, 1960.
80. Bergan TB: Penicillins. Antibiot Chemother 25:1, 1978.
81. Craig WA, Suh B: Protein binding and the antimicrobial effects: Methods for the determination of protein binding. *In* Lorian V (ed): Antibiotics in Laboratory Medicine, ed 3. Baltimore, Williams & Wilkins, 1991, pp 367–402.
82. Ebert SC, Leggett J, Vogelman B, et al: Evidence for a slow elimination phase for penicillin G. J Infect Dis 158:200, 1988.
83. Bryan CS, Stone WJ: "Comparable massive" penicillin G therapy in renal failure. Ann Intern Med 82:189, 1975.
84. Bulger RJ, Lindholm DD, Murry JS, et al: Effect of uremia on methicillin and oxacillin blood levels: Excretion and inactivation in renal failure and hemodialysis. JAMA 187:319, 1964.
85. Nauta EH, Mattie H: Dicloxacillin and cloxacillin pharmacokinetics in healthy and hemodialysis patients. Clin Pharmacol Ther 20:98, 1976.
86. Kunin CM: Clinical pharmacology of the new penicillins. I. The importance of serum protein binding in determining antimicrobial activity and concentration in serum. Clin Pharmacol Ther 7:166, 1966.
87. Spyker DA, Ruglowski RJ, Vann RL, et al: Pharmacokinetics of amoxicillin: Dose dependence after intravenous, oral and intramuscular administration. Antimicrob Agents Chemother 11:132, 1977.
88. Welling PG, Huang H, Koch PA, et al: Bioavailability of ampicillin and amoxicillin in fasted and nonfasted subjects. J Pharm Sci 66:549, 1977.
89. Craig WA: Pharmacokinetics of bacampicillin tablets in adults. Bull N Y Acad Med 59:457, 1983.
90. Libke RD, Clarke JT, Ralph ED, et al: Ticarcillin vs carbenicillin: Clinical pharmacokinetics. Clin Pharmacol Ther 17:441, 1975.
91. Bergan T: Overview of acylureidopenicillin pharmacokinetics. Scand J Infect Dis Suppl 29:33, 1981.
92. Neu HC, Srinivasan S, Francke EL, et al: Pharmacokinetics of amdinocillin and pivamdinocillin in normal volunteers. Am J Med 75(Suppl 2A):60, 1983.
93. Boelaert J, Daneels R, Schurgers M, et al: The pharmacokinetics of temocillin in patients with normal and impaired renal function. J Antimicrob Chemother 11:349, 1983.
94. Adam D, De Visser I, Koeppe P: Pharmacokinetics of amoxicillin and clavulanic acid administered alone and in combination. Antimicrob Agents Chemother 22:353, 1982.
95. Johnson CA, Halstenson CE, Kelloway JS, et al: Single-dose pharmacokinetics of piperacillin and tazobactam in patients with renal disease. Clin Pharmacol Ther 51:32, 1992.
96. Gilbert DN, Bennett WM: Use of antimicrobial agents in renal failure. Infect Dis Clin North Am 3:517, 1989.
97. Wise R, Gillet AP, Cadge B, et al: Influence of protein binding on the tissue levels of 6 β-lactams. J Infect Dis 142:77, 1980.
98. Nau H: Clinical pharmacokinetics in pregnancy and perinatology. Dev Pharmacol Ther 10:174, 1987.
99. Craig WA, Welling PG: Protein binding of antimicrobials: Clinical, pharmacokinetic and therapeutic implications. Clin Pharmacokinet 2:252, 1977.
100. Kornguth ML, Kunin CM: Uptake of antibiotics by human erythrocytes. J Infect Dis 133:175, 1976.
101. Gerding DN, Peterson LR, Hughes CE, et al: Extravascular antimicrobial distribution and the respective blood concentrations in humans. *In* Lorian V (ed): Antibiotics in Laboratory Medicine, ed 3. Baltimore, Williams & Wilkins, 1991, pp 880–961.
102. Dixon RL, Owens ES, Rall DP: Evidence of active transport of benzyl-^{14}C-penicillin from cerebrospinal fluid to blood. J Pharm Sci 58:1106, 1969.
103. Spector R, Lorenzo AV: Inhibition of penicillin transport from the cerebrospinal fluid after intracisternal inoculation of bacteria. J Clin Invest 54:316, 1974.
104. Dacey RG, Sande MA: Effect of probenecid on cerebrospinal fluid concentration of penicillin and cephalosporin derivatives. Antimicrob Agents Chemother 6:437, 1974.
105. Bins JW, Mattie H: Saturation of the tubular excretion of β-lactam antibiotics. Br J Clin Pharmacol 25:41, 1988.
106. Overbosch D, Van Gulpen C, Hermans J, et al: The effect of probenecid on the renal tubular excretion of benzylpenicillin. Br J Clin Pharmacol 25:51, 1988.
107. Overbosch D, Van Gulpen C, Mattie H: Renal clearance of temocillin in volunteers. Drugs (Suppl 5):128, 1985.
108. Cole M, Kenig MD, Hewitt VA: Metabolism of penicillins to penicilloic acids and 6-aminopenicillanic acid in man and its significance in assessing penicillin absorption. Antimicrob Agents Chemother 3:463, 1973.
109. Turnidge JD, Craig WA: β-Lactam pharmacology in liver disease. J Antimicrob Chemother 11:499, 1990.
110. Klugman KP: Pneumococcal resistance to antibiotics. Clin Microbiol Rev 3:171, 1990.
111. Pallares R, Linares J, Vadillo M, et al: Resistance to penicillin and cephalosporin and mortality from severe pneumococcal pneumonia in Barcelona, Spain. N Engl J Med 333:474, 1995.
112. Dattwyler RJ, Halperin JJ, Volkman DJ, Luft BJ: Treatment of late Lyme borreliosis—Randomised comparison of ceftriaxone and penicillin. Lancet 1:1191, 1988.
113. Watt G, Padre LP, Tuazon ML, et al: Placebo-controlled trial of intravenous penicillin for severe and late leptospirosis. Lancet 1:433, 1988.
114. MacGowan A: When is penicillin monotherapy the antibiotic treatment of choice? J Antimicrob Chemother 29:239, 1992.
115. Levison ME, Mangura CT, Lorber B, et al: Clindamycin compared with penicillin for the treatment of anaerobic lung abscess. Ann Intern Med 98:466, 1983.
116. Brewin A, Arango L, Hadley WK, et al: High-dose penicillin therapy and pneumococcal pneumonia. JAMA 230:409, 1974.
117. Musher DM, Hamill RJ, Baughn RE: Effect of human immunodeficiency virus (HIV) infection on the course of syphilis and on the response to treatment. Ann Intern Med 113:872, 1990.
118. Gerber MA, Randolph MF, DeMeo K, et al: Failure of once-

daily penicillin V therapy for streptococcal pharyngitis. Am J Dis Child 143:153, 1989.
119. Steere AC, Hutchinson GJ, Rahn DW, et al: Treatment of the early manifestations of Lyme disease. Ann Intern Med 99:22, 1983.
120. Thornsberry C: The development of antimicrobial resistance in staphylococci. J Antimicrob Chemother 21(Suppl C):9, 1988.
121. Craig WA, Ebert SC: Protein binding and its significance in antibacterial therapy. Infect Dis Clin North Am 3:407, 1989.
122. Kane JG, Parker RH, Jordan GW, et al: Nafcillin concentration in cerebrospinal fluid during treatment of staphylococcal infections. Ann Intern Med 87:309, 1977.
123. Kancir LM, Tuazon CU, Cardella TA, et al: Adverse reactions to methicillin and nafcillin during treatment of serious *Staphylococcus aureus* infections. Arch Intern Med 138:909, 1978.
124. Tetzlaff TR, McCracken GH, Nelson JD: Oral antibiotic therapy for skeletal infections of children. II. Therapy of osteomyelitis and suppurative arthritis. J Pediatr 92:485, 1978.
125. Black J, Hunt TL, Godley PJ, et al: Oral antimicrobial therapy for adults with osteomyelitis or septic arthritis. J Infect Dis 155:968, 1987.
126. Van Ek B, Dijkmans BAC, Van Dulken H, et al: Antibiotic prophylaxis in craniotomy: A prospective double-blind placebo-controlled study. Scand J Infect Dis 20:633, 1988.
127. Stamm WE, McKevitt M, Counts GW: Acute renal infection in women: Treatment with trimethoprim-sulfamethoxazole or ampicillin for two or six weeks. A randomized trial. Ann Intern Med 106:341, 1987.
128. Prevention of bacterial endocarditis. Med Lett 31:112, 1989.
129. Bayerdorffer E, Miehlke S, Mannes G, et al: Double-blind trial of omeprazole and amoxicillin to cure *Helicobacter pylori* infection in patients with duodenal ulcers. Gastroenterology 108:1412, 1995.
130. Philbrick JT, Bracikowski JP: Single-dose antibiotic treatment for uncomplicated urinary tract infections. Arch Intern Med 145:1672, 1985.
131. Swahn A: Gastrointestinal absorption and metabolism of two 35S-labelled ampicillin esters. Eur J Clin Pharmacol 9:299, 1976.
132. Neu HC, Swarz H: Carbenicillin: Clinical and laboratory experience with a parenterally administered penicillin for treatment of *Pseudomonas* infections. Ann Intern Med 71:903, 1969.
133. Butler K, English AR, Briggs B, et al: Indanyl carbenicillin: Chemistry and laboratory studies with a new semisynthetic penicillin. J Infect Dis 127:S97, 1973.
134. Fuchs PC, Thornsberry C, Barry AL, et al: Ticarcillin: A collaborative in vitro comparison with carbenicillin against 9,000 clinical bacterial isolates. Am J Med Sci 274:255, 1977.
135. Parry MF, Neu HC: A comparative study of ticarcillin plus tobramycin versus carbenicillin plus gentamicin for the treatment of serious infections due to gram-negative bacilli. Am J Med 64:961, 1978.
136. Pancoast SJ, Jahre JA, Neu HC: Mezlocillin in the therapy of serious infections. Am J Med 67:747, 1979.
137. Gerecht WB, Henry NK, Hoffman WW, et al: Prospective randomized comparison of mezlocillin therapy alone with combined ampicillin and gentamicin therapy for patients with cholangitis. Arch Intern Med 149:1279, 1989.
138. Bergan T: Pharmacokinetics of mezlocillin in healthy volunteers. Antimicrob Agents Chemother 14:801, 1978.
139. Parry MF: The in-vitro activity of azlocillin: A community hospital study of 1900 clinical isolates. J Antimicrob Chemother 11(Suppl B):15, 1983.
140. Holmes B, Richard DM, Brodgen RN, et al: Piperacillin: A review of antibacterial activity, pharmacokinetic properties, and their therapeutic use. Drugs 28:375, 1984.
141. Winston DJ, Murphy W, Young LS, et al: Piperacillin therapy for serious bacterial infections. Am J Med 69:255, 1980.
142. Reading C, Cole M: Clavulanic acid: A beta-lactamase–inhibiting beta-lactam from *Streptomyces clavuligerus*. Antimicrob Agents Chemother 11:852, 1977.
143. Aronoff SC, Jacobs MR, Johenning S, Yamabe S: Comparative activities of the β-lactamase inhibitors YTR 830, sodium clavulanate, and sulbactam combined with amoxicillin or ampicillin. Antimicrob Agents Chemother 26:580, 1984.
144. Bush K: β-Lactamase inhibitors from laboratory to clinic. Clin Microbiol Rev 1:109, 1988.
145. Fuchs PC, Barry AL, Thornsberry C, et al: In vitro evaluation of Augmentin by both microdilution and disk diffusion susceptibility testing: Regression analysis, tentative interpretive criteria, and quality control limits. Antimicrob Agents Chemother 24:31, 1983.
146. Jones RN: In vitro evaluations of aminopenicillin/β-lactamase inhibitor combinations. Drugs 35(Suppl 7):17, 1988.
147. Barry AL, Ayers LW, Gavan TL, et al: In vitro activity of ticarcillin plus clavulanic acid against bacteria isolated in three centers. Eur J Clin Microbiol 3:203, 1984.
148. Fuchs PC, Barry AL, Thornsberry C, et al: In vitro activity of ticarcillin plus clavulanic acid against 632 clinical isolates. Antimicrob Agents Chemother 25:392, 1984.
149. Barry AL, Pfaller MA, Fuchs PC, et al: In vitro activities of 12 orally administered antimicrobial agents against four species of bacterial respiratory pathogens from U.S. medical centers in 1992 and 1993. Antimicrob Agents Chemother 38:2419, 1994.
150. Kuck NA, Jacobus NV, Petersen PJ, et al: Comparative in vitro and in vivo activities of piperacillin combined with the β-lactamase inhibitors tazobactam, clavulanic acid, and sulbactam. Antimicrob Agents Chemother 33:1964, 1989.
151. Murray P, Cantrell HF, Lankford RB, et al: Multicenter evaluation of the in vitro activity of piperacillin-tazobactam compared with eleven selected β-lactam antibiotics and ciprofloxacin against more than 42,000 aerobic gram-positive and gram-negative bacteria. Diagn Microbiol Infect Dis 19:111, 1994.
152. Noguchi JK, Gill MA: Sulbactam: A β-lactamase inhibitor. Clin Pharmacokinet 7:37, 1988.
153. Todd PA, Benfield P: Amoxicillin/clavulanic acid. An update of its antibacterial activity, pharmacokinetic properties and therapeutic use. Drugs 39:264, 1990.
154. Goldstein EJC, Reihardt JF, Murray PM, et al: Outpatient therapy of bite wounds: Demographic data, bacteriology, and a prospective, randomized trial of amoxicillin/clavulanic acid versus penicillin I dicloxacillin. Int J Dermatol 26:123, 1987.
155. Lees L, Milson JA, Knirsch AK, et al: Sulbactam plus ampicillin: Interim review of efficacy and safety for therapeutic and prophylactic use. Rev Infect Dis 8(Suppl 5):S644, 1986.
156. Meylan PR, Calandra T, Casey PA, et al: Clinical experience with timentin in severe hospital infections. J Antimicrob Chemother 17(Suppl C):127, 1986.
157. Khardori N, Elting L, Wong E, et al: Nosocomial infections due to *Xanthomonas maltophilia (Pseudomonas maltophilia)* in patients with cancer. Rev Infect Dis 12:997, 1990.
158. Bryson HM, Brogden RN: Piperacillin/tazobactam. A review of its antibacterial activity, pharmacokinetic properties and therapeutic potential. Drugs 47:506, 1994.
159. Neu HC: Penicillin-binding proteins and role of amdinocillin in causing bacterial cell death. Am J Med 75(Suppl 2A):9, 1983.
160. Cox CE: Parenteral amdinocillin for treatment of complicated urinary tract infections. Am J Med 75(Suppl 2A):82, 1983.
161. Verbist L: In vitro activity of temocillin (BRL 17421), a novel beta-lactamase–stable penicillin. Antimicrob Agents Chemother 22:157, 1982.
162. Lindsay G, Beattie AD, Taylor EW: Temocillin in the treatment of serious gram-negative infections. Drugs 29(Suppl 5):191, 1985.
163. Saxon A, Beall GN, Rohr AS, et al: Immediate hypersensitivity reactions to beta-lactam antibiotics. Ann Intern Med 107:204, 1987.
164. Idsoe O, Guthe T, Wilcox RR, et al: Nature and extent of penicillin side reactions, with particular reference to fatalities from anaphylactic shock. Bull World Health Organ 38:159, 1968.
165. Shapiro S, Siskin V, Slone D, et al: Drug rash with ampicillin and other penicillins. Lancet 2:69, 1969.
166. Arndt KA, Jick H: Rates of cutaneous reactions to drugs. A report from the Boston Collaborative Drug Surveillance Program. JAMA 235:918, 1976.
167. Ressler C, Mendelson LM: Skin test for diagnosis of penicillin allergy—current status. Ann Allergy 59:167, 1987.
168. Kerns DL, Shira JE, Go S, et al: Ampicillin rash in children. Relationship to penicillin allergy and infectious mononucleosis. Am J Dis Child 125:187, 1973.
169. Huff JC: Erythema multiforme. Dermatol Clin 3:141, 1985.
170. Kerr RO, Cardamone J, Dalmasso AP, et al: Two mechanisms of erythrocyte destruction in penicillin-induced hemolytic anemia. N Engl J Med 287:1322, 1972.

171. Olaison L, Alestig K: A prospective study of neutropenia induced by high doses of β-lactam antibiotics. J Antimicrob Chemother 25:449, 1990.
172. Markowitz SM, Rothkopf M, Holden FD, et al: Nafcillin-induced agranulocytosis. JAMA 232:1150, 1975.
173. Shattil SJ, Bennett JS, McDonough M, et al: Carbenicillin and penicillin G inhibit platelet function in vitro by impairing the interaction of agonists with the platelet surface. J Clin Invest 71:619, 1980.
174. Burroughs SF, Johnson GJ: β-Lactam antibiotic–induced platelet dysfunction: Evidence for irreversible inhibition of platelet activation in vitro and in vivo after prolonged exposure to penicillin. Blood 75:1473, 1990.
175. Baldwin DS, Levine BB, McCluskey RT, et al: Renal failure and interstitial nephritis due to penicillin and methicillin. N Engl J Med 279:1245, 1968.
176. Border WA, Lehman DH, Egan JD, et al: Antitubular basement-membrane antibodies in methicillin-associated interstitial nephritis. N Engl J Med 291:381, 1974.
177. Colvin RB, Burton JR, Hyslop NE Jr, et al: Penicillin-associated interstitial nephritis. Ann Intern Med 81:404, 1974.
178. Brunner FP, Frick PG: Hypokalaemia, metabolic alkalosis and hypernatraemia due to "massive" sodium penicillin therapy. Br Med J 4:550, 1968.
179. Klastersky J, Vanderkelen B, Daneau D, et al: Carbenicillin and hypokalemia. Ann Intern Med 78:774, 1973.
180. Manian FA, Stone WJ, Alford RH: Adverse antibiotic effects associated with renal insufficiency. Rev Infect Dis 12:236, 1990.
181. Craig WA, Evenson MA, Sarver KP, et al: Correction of protein binding defect in uremic sera by charcoal treatment. J Lab Clin Med 87:637, 1976.
182. Spector R, Snodgrass SR: The effect of uremia on penicillin flux between blood and cerebrospinal fluid. J Lab Clin Med 87:749, 1976.
183. Wilson FM, Belamavic J, Lauter CB, et al: Anicteric carbenicillin hepatitis. Eight episodes in four patients. JAMA 232:818, 1967.
184. Onorato JM, Axelrod JM: Hepatitis from intravenous high-dose oxacillin therapy. Ann Intern Med 89:497, 1978.
185. Saliba B: Oxacillin hepatotoxicity in HIV-infected patients. Ann Intern Med 120:1048, 1994.
186. Heilker GM, Fowler JW, Self TH: Possible nafcillin-warfarin interaction. Arch Intern Med 154:822, 1994.
187. Vermis S, Maddux MS, Pollak R, et al: Subtherapeutic cyclosporin concentrations during nafcillin therapy. Transplantation 43:913, 1987.
188. Wallace SM, Chan L-Y: In vitro interaction of aminoglycosides with β-lactam penicillins. Antimicrob Agents Chemother 28:274, 1985.
189. Riff LJ, Jackson GG: Laboratory and clinical conditions for gentamicin inactivation by carbenicillin. Arch Intern Med 130:887, 1972.

18

Cephalosporins

Robert C. Moellering, Jr.
Deborah E. Sentochnik

Historical Background

The discovery of penicillin by Alexander Fleming in 1928 and its subsequent characterization a decade later by Howard Florey, Ernst Chain, Norman Heatley, E. P. Abraham, and others at Oxford University set the stage for the first clinical use of penicillin in the early 1940s. The success of this venture led numerous other investigators to search for antibiotic-producing microorganisms. The first microbial producer of a cephalosporin, *Cephalosporium acremonium* (now also known as *Acremonium chrysogenum*), was isolated from a sewage outlet in the harbor at Cagliari, Sardinia, by Giuseppi Brotzu, a professor of bacteriology at the University of Cagliari.[1] Brotzu suspected that the occasional clearing of the waters surrounding the sewage outfall might be related to the presence of antibiotic-producing microorganisms, the search for which led to isolation of the initial strain of *C. acremonium.* Brotzu was able to make crude filtrates from his original isolate, which he utilized to treat a variety of infections. He injected the material directly into boils and other skin infections with moderate success and even administered the filtrates intramuscularly and intravenously to Sardinian patients suffering from typhoid fever and brucellosis.[2] Although the patients receiving these filtrates had severe febrile reactions, Brotzu thought that the material was instrumental in their recovery from the infections. This is ironic, because none of the early cephalosporins exhibited any useful clinical activity against either typhoid fever or brucellosis!

Brotzu was unable to carry out further studies on his antibiotic-producing microorganisms, and he was unable to interest the Italian pharmaceutical industry in his findings. So, in 1948, he sent a culture of his *C. acremonium* to Sir Howard Florey at Oxford. Initial studies there showed that Brotzu's microorganism produced a substance (named cephalosporin P) that had activity only against gram-positive bacteria. It seemed unlikely, however, that this compound could have accounted for the clinical activity noted by Brotzu. Further studies revealed that in the aqueous phase that remained after extraction of cephalosporin P there remained another compound, initially called cephalosporin N. This compound was active against gram-negative bacilli (especially *Salmonella* species) and undoubtedly was the substance that was responsible for the original clinical activity reported by Brotzu. Subsequent studies, however, showed that this compound was actually a penicillin, not a cephalosporin, and it was renamed penicillin N and proved to be identical to another antibiotic isolated in the United States called synnematin B. In 1953 a third antibiotic was isolated from *C. acremonium.* This compound, named cephalosporin C, was only about 1/10 as active against *Salmonella typhi* and staphylococci as penicillin N; however, unlike penicillin N, which was readily destroyed by penicillinase-producing strains of staphylococci and *Bacillus cereus,* cephalosporin C was noted to be active against microorganisms that produced these enzymes. Interest in this compound was heightened when it was noted to be relatively nontoxic and was effective in treating various infections in animal models.[2]

Chemistry and Nomenclature

Cephalosporin C was subsequently shown to be quite similar to penicillin N in that it had a D-α-aminoadipyl side chain attached to a β-lactam ring. However, in the case of cephalosporin C, the β-lactam ring was fused to a six-membered dihydrothiazine (cephem) ring rather than the five-membered thiazolidine (penam) ring found in penicillin N (Figs. 18–1 and 18–2). This initial observation showed that the presence of a cephem ring, as opposed to a thiazolidine ring, conferred relative resistance to certain β-lactamases, including those produced by *Staphylococcus aureus* and *B. cereus.* Although cephalosporin C was used to treat a few urinary tract infections in children, it was not active enough for serious clinical development. The discovery that the nucleus of penicillin (6-aminopenicillanic acid) could be pro-

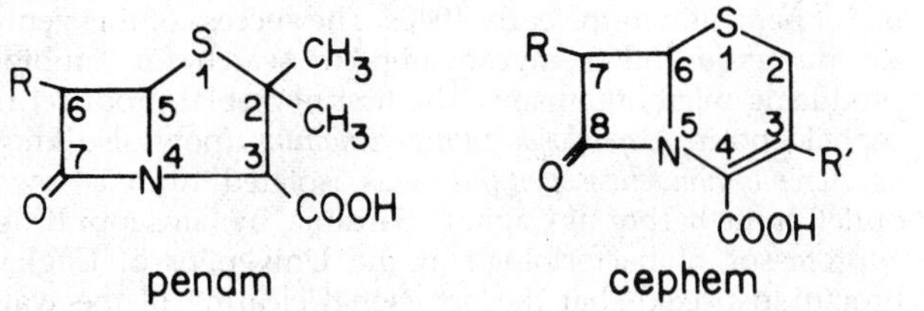

FIGURE 18–1 □ Nuclear structure of the penicillins (penam nucleus) and cephalosporins (cephem nucleus).

duced in pure crystalline form in 1958 led to the discovery of a variety of new semisynthetic penicillins produced by chemically adding side chains at the 6 position of 6-aminopenicillanic acid.[3] The subsequent production of 7-aminocephalosporanic acid set the stage for the development of a number of new and potentially clinically useful cephalosporins. Unlike the penicillins, chemical modification can be made at both the 7 and the 3 positions of the cephalosporin molecule. The initial cephalosporins produced for clinical use (cephalothin, cephaloridine, and, several years later, cefazolin) all exhibited good activity against gram-positive organisms (with the exception of enterococci and methicillin-resistant staphylococci), and they also showed activity against certain gram-negative bacilli, including *Escherichia coli, Proteus mirabilis,* and *Klebsiella pneumoniae,* as well as *Salmonella* and *Shigella* (see Fig. 18–2). Unfortunately, although these compounds were active in vitro against *Salmonella,* they were not effective for the treatment of systemic salmonellosis. Although the cephalosporins are relatively stable to the staphylococcal β-lactamases, there are a broad variety of other β-lactamases, particularly those produced by gram-negative bacilli, that are capable of destroying these compounds. The presence of a methoxy group at the 7 position markedly enhances the stability of cephalosporins to a broad variety of gram-negative cephalosporinases, especially those produced by *Bacteroides* species. Cefoxitin was the first compound with a 7-methoxy group to be developed for clinical use (Fig. 18–3). Technically, cefoxitin is not a true cephalosporin but a cephamycin, having been initially derived from a strain of *Streptomyces lactamdurams.*[4] Despite this technicality, most authors have considered cefoxitin and other cephamycins to be cephalosporins, and these compounds are considered along with the true cephalosporins in this chapter. In general, cephalosporins containing a 7α-methoxy group (such as cefoxitin, cefmetazole, cefotetan, and moxalactam) (Fig. 18–4; see Fig. 18–3) exhibit enhanced activity against β-lactamase–producing strains of *Bacteroides fragilis,* but this advantage is, to a degree, offset by a moderate loss of intrinsic activity against gram-positive organisms, including *S. aureus.*[5] Various substitutions at both the 3 and the 7 positions of the cephalosporin molecule have produced enhanced activity against gram-negative bacilli. One such substitution is the methylthiotetrazole (MTT) moiety that is present at the 3 position in compounds such as cefamandole, cefotetan, cefoperazone, moxalactam, and cefmetazole. As a result, each of these compounds exhibits enhanced activity against a broad range of gram-negative bacilli. Unfortunately, however, the MTT group is also associated with the disulfiram-like reactions and prolongation of prothrombin time that can accompany the use of cephalosporins containing this moiety.[5] Another modification that has resulted in enhanced activity against gram-negative bacteria is the incorporation of an aminothiazolyl group in the acyl side chain at the 7 position of various cephalosporins.[6] It is also possible to add a methoxy group directly to the oxime residue that abuts the aminothiazolyl portion of the side chain at the 7 position. The resultant aminothiazolylmethoxy group confers enhanced resistance to β-lactamase without the loss of activity against gram-positive organisms seen when the methoxy group is, instead, attached directly to the β-lactam ring at the 7 position.[7] It appears that the presence of an aminothiazolyl group enhances the ability of the resulting cephalosporins to penetrate through the outer cell envelope of gram-negative bacilli and may enhance the affinity of these

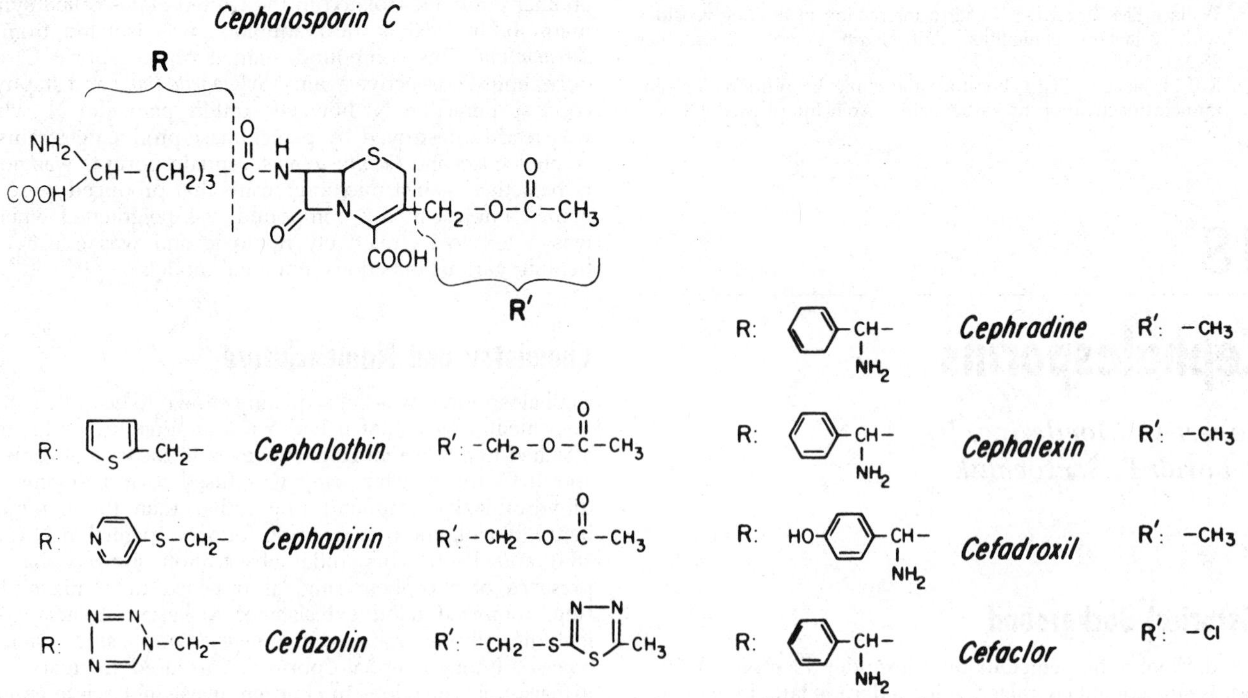

FIGURE 18–2 □ Structural formulae of cephalosporin C and the first-generation cephalosporins. (From Calderwood SB, Moellering RC Jr: Principles of anti-infective therapy. *In* Stein JH [ed]: Internal Medicine, ed 3. Boston, Little, Brown, 1990, pp 1202–1218.)

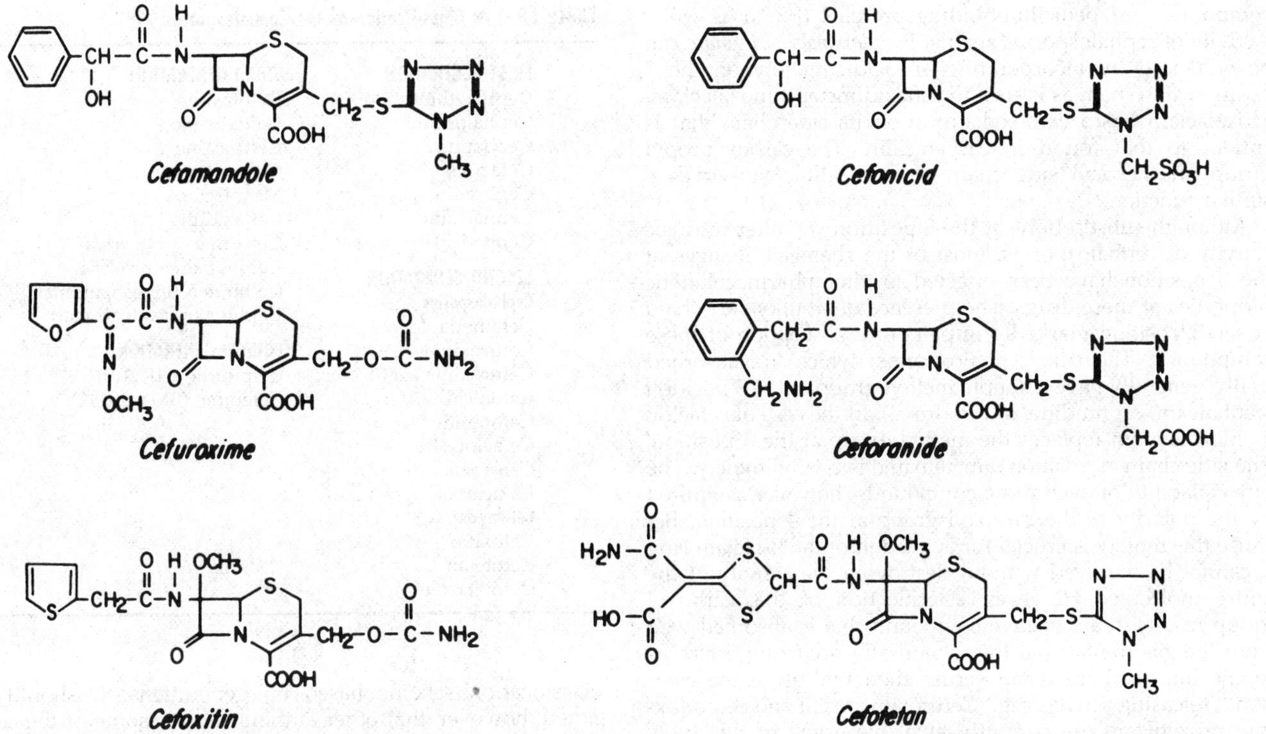

FIGURE 18–3 □ Structural formulae of the parenteral second-generation cephalosporins. (From Calderwood SB, Moellering RC Jr: Principles of anti-infective therapy. *In* Stein JH [ed]: Internal Medicine, ed 3. Boston, Little, Brown, 1990, pp 1202–1218.)

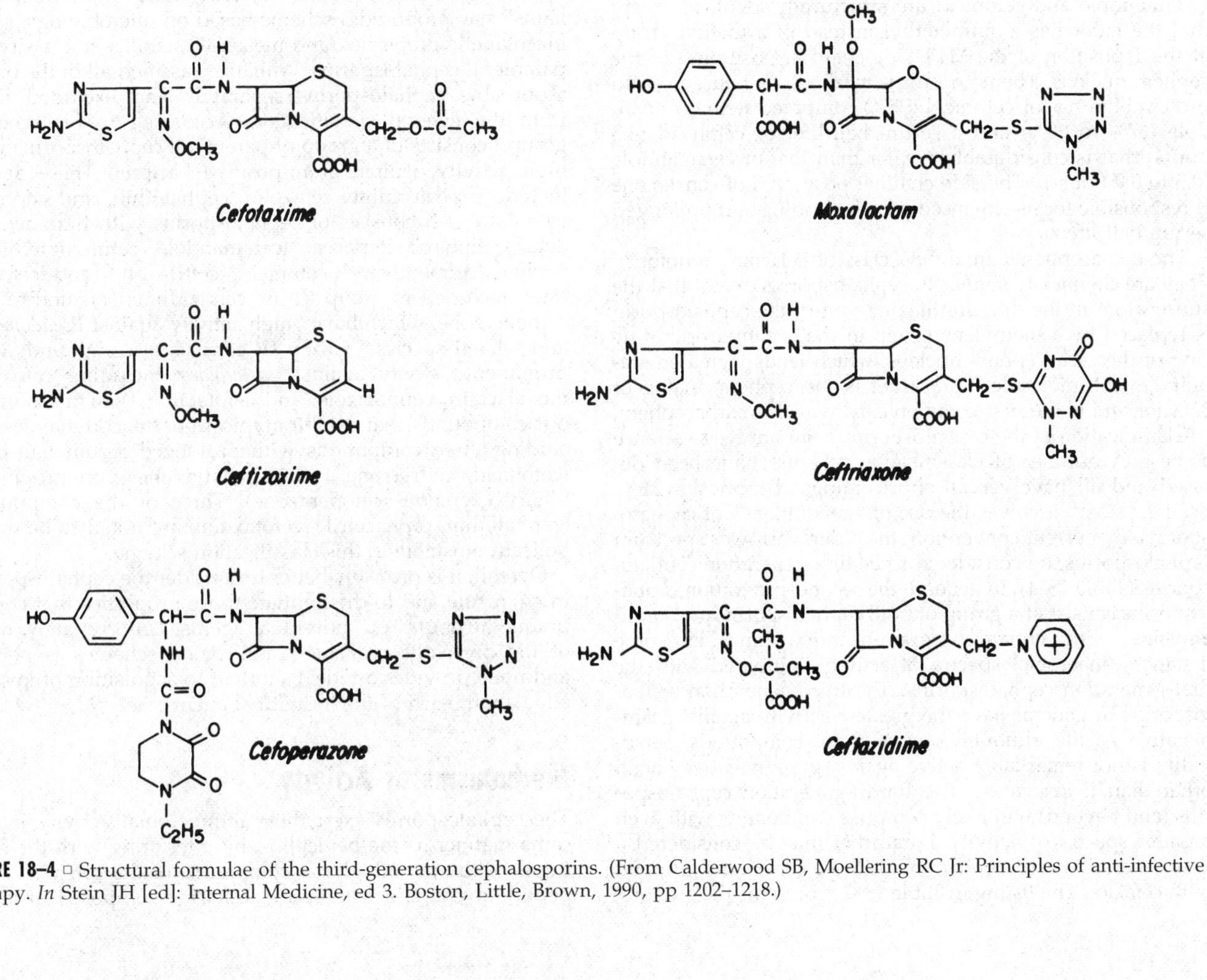

FIGURE 18–4 □ Structural formulae of the third-generation cephalosporins. (From Calderwood SB, Moellering RC Jr: Principles of anti-infective therapy. *In* Stein JH [ed]: Internal Medicine, ed 3. Boston, Little, Brown, 1990, pp 1202–1218.)

compounds for penicillin-binding proteins (PBPs) as well.[5] Activity of cephalosporins against *Pseudomonas aeruginosa* can be enhanced by incorporating an acidic moiety on the 7 position side chain as is seen in ceftazidime and moxalactam. Moxalactam has a carboxyl group on its side chain that is similar to that found in carbenicillin. The carboxypropyl group on the acyl side chain of ceftazidime subserves a similar function.[5]

Although substitutions at the 3 position can alter intrinsic activity of cephalosporins, most of the chemical changes at the 3 position have been effected to alter pharmacokinetic properties of these drugs. The presence of a bulky side chain at the 3 position markedly impairs oral absorption of these compounds. The true cephalosporins, which are absorbed orally, generally have a simple methyl group at the 3 position (cephalexin, cephradine, or cefadroxil). In the case of cefaclor, a chlorine atom replaces the methyl group at the 3 position. The side chain at position 3 in cefixime is a vinyl moiety. The bioavailability of even these compounds, however, is limited by the polarity of the carboxyl group at the 4 position. Because this moiety is crucial for activation of the β-lactam ring it cannot be removed without destroying the activity of the entire molecule.[5] However, esterification of this carboxyl group results in an inactive compound that is absorbed well from the gastrointestinal tract. Naturally occurring esterases in the intestinal tract and serum then hydrolyze the ester bond, releasing active drug.[5] Cefuroxime axetil and cefpodoxime proxetil are the currently available esters of this type. Cefetamet pivoxil remains an investigational agent in the United States.[8]

Finally, alterations in the side chain at the 3 position of the cephalosporin molecule can also have a striking influence on protein binding and renal excretion of these compounds. Cefamandole and cefonicid are structurally identical except that the latter has a sulfomethyl instead of a methyl group at the 1 position of the MTT side chain at position 3 of the cephem nucleus. The net result is markedly enhanced serum protein binding for cefonicid (98%) compared with cefamandole (67% to 80%) and a serum half-life for cefonicid (4.5 hours) that is considerably greater than that of cefamandole (0.5 to 0.9 hours).[5] The side chain at position 3 of ceftriaxone is responsible for its enhanced protein binding and prolonged serum half-life as well.

The carbacephems are a new class of β-lactam antibiotic.[9] They are chemically similar to cephalosporins except that the sulfur atom in the dihydrothiazine ring of the cephalosporin is replaced by a methylene group in the tetrahydropyridine ring of the carbacephem nucleus, which lends increased stability to the molecule. Loracarbef is the cephem analog of cefaclor and is the first commercially available carbacephem.

Classification of the cephalosporins is an imprecise science at best. A number of classification schemes have been devised and all have certain shortcomings. The most widely used "system" involves the use of "generations" of cephalosporins. By current convention, the older, narrower spectrum cephalosporins are considered to be first-generation cephalosporins (Table 18–1). In general, the second-generation cephalosporins consist of a group of both cephalosporins and cephamycins with enhanced gram-negative (and in some instances anaerobic) spectra of activity compared with the first-generation cephalosporins. The third-generation cephalosporins in general have the greatest activity against gram-negative bacilli, although one of these compounds, cefsulodin, is not remarkably active against gram-negative bacilli other than *P. aeruginosa.* The fourth-generation cephalosporins (and beyond) will likely comprise compounds with even broader spectra of activity. Loracarbef may be considered a first-generation carbacephem but is more commonly grouped with cefaclor. The listing in Table 18–1 represents the authors' classification scheme based on generations. It should be noted, however, that other authors classify some of the compounds differently. For instance, cefaclor is sometimes called a first-generation cephalosporin, whereas cefotetan, cefmetazole, and cefixime have occasionally been classified as third-generation cephalosporins.

TABLE 18–1 ■ Classification of the Cephalosporins

FIRST GENERATION	**THIRD GENERATION**
Cephalothin	Cefotaxime
Cephaloridine	Ceftizoxime
Cephapirin	Ceftriaxone
Cefazolin	Cefoperazone
Cephradine	Moxalactam
Cephalexin	Ceftazidime
Cephadroxil	Cefixime
	Cefpodoxime proxetil
SECOND GENERATION	Ceftibuten (investigational)
Cephalosporins	Cefdinir (investigational)
Cefamandole	
Cefuroxime	**FOURTH GENERATION**
Cefuroxime axetil	Cefpirome (HR 810)
Cefonicid	Cefepime (BMY 28142)
Ceforanide	
Cefaclor	
Cefprozil	
Loracarbef	
Cefamycins	
Cefoxitin	
Cefotetan	
Cefmetazole	

In an effort to avoid using the term generation in relationship to cephalosporins (because it is clearly imprecise), Williams[10] has proposed a scheme based on microbiology, pharmacokinetic properties, and metabolic stability to classify the parenteral cephalosporins. Williams classified all of the orally absorbable cephalosporins separately and excluded them from the general classification. According to his schema, group I consists of a group of parenteral cephalosporins with high activity against gram-positive bacteria. These agents include cephaloridine, cefazolin, cephalothin, and cephacetrile. Group II consists of cephalosporins with high activity against Enterobacteriaceae (cefamandole, cefuroxime, ceftizoxime, cefmenoxime, cefonicid, ceftriaxone, and cefotaxime). Included in group III are ceftazidime, cefsulodin, and cefoperazone, which have "high activity against *Pseudomonas* and related species." Group IV consists of compounds with prominent activity against *Bacteroides,* including cefoxitin, moxalactam, cefmetazole, and cefotetan.[10] Williams pointed out compounds that exhibit atypical pharmacodynamics, including three compounds with prolonged serum half-lives (cefonicid, ceftriaxone, cefotetan) and one with prominent biliary excretion (cefoperazone). Three of the compounds (cephalothin, cephacetrile, cefotaxime) are noted to be metabolically unstable in this classification scheme.

Overall, it is probably better to consider the cephalosporins in aggregate and to differentiate those properties that confer unique attributes on individual agents. Unfortunately, none of the presently available classification schemes is perfect and none provides an ideal shortcut to acquisition of knowledge about each of the individual agents.

Mechanisms of Activity

The cephalosporins exert their antimicrobial activity in the same manner as the penicillins, by interfering with the synthesis of the peptidoglycan component of the cell wall. The peptidoglycan is a heteropolysaccharide composed of alternating *N*-acetylglucosamine and *N*-acetylmuramic acid residues that are cross-linked by oligopeptide bridges, thus forming a lattice structure. After being formed in the cytoplasm and transported to the outer surface of the cell membrane, the new sugar residues are inserted into the existing cross-linked structure through the action of trans-, carboxy-, and endopeptidases. The highly stressed amide group of the β-lactam ring in β-lactam antibiotics is conformationally similar to the D-alanyl-D-alanine bond of the peptidoglycan pentapeptides, thereby causing the peptidases to "mistake" the drug for their natural substrate.[11] Once bound to this site, the enzymes lose their catalytic activity. Such enzymes have become known as PBPs.

The precise makeup and number of PBPs in a cell vary among species. These enzymes differ in their affinity for various β-lactams and in the effect that their lack of appropriate participation in cell wall synthesis has on the cell. Inactivation of some PBPs affects cell wall growth; of others, cell morphology. Precisely how the inhibition of PBPs results in an antibacterial effect is not yet clear.[12] There may be more than one mechanism, even in one organism, depending on which PBP is bound to the β-lactam.

Mechanisms of Resistance

Resistance to β-lactam antimicrobials, including cephalosporins,[13] can occur by three mechanisms, which have a dynamic relationship: (1) alterations in target PBPs, (2) enzymatic destruction of the antibiotic, and (3) inability of the drug to reach its binding site in the cell. Resistance can occur intrinsically or as a result of selection of resistant subclones or mutants during exposure to cephalosporins.[14] Target PBPs can be modified to have decreased affinity for a β-lactam antibiotic.[15, 16] Functional replacement of a sensitive PBP by one that is less sensitive to the antibiotic has also been documented.[17]

To reach its target PBP, a cephalosporin must penetrate an organism's cell envelope. This is done relatively easily in the case of gram-positive organisms, as the peptidoglycan structure that makes up the cell wall routinely allows the passage of cephalosporin-sized particles. Gram-negative organisms possess a more formidable barrier, a complex structure composed of polysaccharides, lipids, and proteins. Materials penetrate this outer cell envelope through water-filled channels, or porins, produced by various outer membrane proteins.[18] Passage by a cephalosporin depends on channel size, charge, and hydrophilic properties. There appear to be other pathways across the cell envelope, but they remain to be elucidated.[19]

β-Lactamases[20] are enzymes produced by bacteria that can destroy β-lactams by hydrolyzing the bond between the carbon and nitrogen atom of the β-lactam ring. Their effectiveness in doing so depends on a combination of enzyme location and quantity, as well as target affinity. Gram-positive bacteria release large amounts of β-lactamases directly into their extracellular space. Growth of susceptible cells in an environment containing cephalosporins depends on their collective ability to decrease the amount of active drug present to tolerable levels. In gram-negative bacilli, β-lactamases are found in the periplasmic space and are not released "nonspecifically" into the surrounding environment. The ability of gram-negative bacilli to grow in the presence of a cephalosporin is thus a function of the individual cell. Several classification schemes for the β-lactamases exist based on characteristics such as amino acid sequences, molecular weight, or isoelectric point and are discussed further in Chapter 31. Genetic information for coding of the enzymes can be carried chromosomally, or on transposons on plasmids, with production being inducible or constitutive.[21, 22] Of note is that in addition to the plasmid-mediated β-lactamases that have a broad spectrum of activity, a number of more cephalosporin-specific enzymes have been discovered. They have been found in some gram-negative bacteria and are active against the third-generation cephalosporins, and aztreonam in particular.[23–25]

TABLE 18–2 ■ Pharmacokinetics of Parenteral Cephalosporins

AGENT	HALF-LIFE (HOURS)	STANDARD DOSE (GRAMS)	USUAL DOSE INTERVAL (HOURS)
Cephalothin	0.6	1–2	4
Cefazolin	1.9	0.5–1.5	8
Cephapirin	0.6	1–2	4
Cephradine	0.8	0.5–2	4–6
Cefamandole	0.7	1–2	4–6
Cefuroxime	1.2	0.75–3	6–8
Cefonicid	4.4	1–2	24
Cefoxitin	0.8	1–2	6–8
Cefotetan	3.5	1–2	12
Cefmetazole	1.1	2	6–12
Cefotaxime	1.0	1–2	6
Ceftizoxime	1.7	1–2	6–12
Ceftriaxone	6.4	1–2	12–24
Ceftazidime	2.0	1–3	8
Cefoperazone	2.1	1–3	8
Moxalactam	2.3	1–3	8

Pharmacokinetics

The pharmacokinetics of the cephalosporins[26–28] are summarized in Tables 18–2 and 18–3. Ceftriaxone is noteworthy for its prolonged half-life, which allows once- or twice-daily dosing.[29] Cefotaxime is special in that 20% to 40% is excreted as desacetyl cefotaxime, which may be synergistic with the parent compound in antibacterial activity against certain organisms.[30] The primary mode of excretion for the cephalosporins is renal, with the exception of cefoperazone,[31] which has a major degree of hepatic excretion. Ceftriaxone also has some hepatic secretion (about 40%) in humans. Dosing adjustments for the cephalosporins in renal failure are outlined in Table 18–4. Although tissue penetration by the cephalosporins is, in general, excellent, only the third-generation agents and cefuroxime reach clinically useful levels in the cerebrospinal fluid.[32]

Spectrum of Antimicrobial Activity

The cephalosporins are broad-spectrum agents.[33] As a rule, gram-positive activity diminishes while gram-negative activ-

TABLE 18–3 ■ Pharmacokinetics of Oral Cephalosporins

AGENT	HALF-LIFE (HOURS)	STANDARD DOSE (GRAMS)	USUAL DOSE INTERVAL (HOURS)
Cephradine	0.8	0.5–1	6
Cephalexin	0.9	0.25–0.5	6
Cefadroxil	1.5	1	12
Cefaclor	0.6	0.25–0.5	8
Cefprozil	1.2	0.25–0.5	12–24
Loracarbef	1.1	0.2–0.4	12
Cefuroxime axetil	1.3	0.125–0.5	12
Cefixime	3	0.2–0.4	12–24
Cefpodoxime proxetil	2.2	0.2–0.4	12

TABLE 18–4 ■ Suggested Dosage of Cephalosporins in Patients in Renal Failure

	MAXIMUM DOSAGE (GRAMS/DOSING INTERVAL [HOURS])			REMOVED BY	
AGENT	GFR* of >50	GFR of 10–50 mL/min	GFR of 10 mL/min	Hemodialysis	Peritoneal Dialysis
Cephalothin	2/4	2/6	1/8	X	X
Cefazolin	1.5/8	1/12	1/24	X	
Cephapirin	2/6	2/6	1/8	X	
Cephradine	0.5/6	0.25/6	0.25/12	X	X
Cefadroxil	0.5/12	0.5/24	0.5/36	X	
Cephalexin	0.5/6	0.25/8	0.25/12	X	
Cefuroxime	1.5/6	1.5/8	0.75/24	X	X
Cefamandole	2/6	2/8	1/8	X	
Cefonicid	2/24	1/24	1/72		
Cefoxitin	2/6	2/8	1/12	X	
Cefotetan	2/12	2/24	1/24	X	?
Cefaclor	0.5/8	0.25/8	0.25/8	X	X
Cefotaxime	2/6	2/8	2/12	X	
Ceftizoxime	2/6	1/12	0.5/12	X	
Cefoperazone	3/8	3/8	3/8	X	
Ceftazidime	2/8	2/12	1/24	X	X
Ceftriaxone	2/12	2/12	2/12		
Moxalactam	3/8	2/8	1/8	X	

*GFR, Glomerular filtration rate.

ity improves as one progresses from first- to third-generation agents. Anaerobic coverage is best by the second-generation agents, specifically the cefamycins, and moxalactam. None of the cephalosporins is active against enterococci, *Listeria monocytogenes*, or methicillin-resistant *S. aureus*. Disk-diffusion susceptibility tests may sometimes provide misleading results against methicillin-resistant *S. aureus*, but all such *S. aureus* should be considered cross-resistant to all cephalosporins.[34] Ceftazidime has the most substantial anti–*P. aeruginosa* activity, but neither this nor any of the other agents is particularly active against other *Pseudomonas* species.

The first-generation agents have excellent activity against gram-positive organisms such as methicillin-susceptible staphylococci and penicillin-susceptible streptococci. They have good activity against the large majority of community-acquired *E. coli*, *K. pneumoniae*, and *P. mirabilis*, but other gram-negative organisms should be considered resistant until proved otherwise. Although most mouth anaerobes, especially those usually considered penicillin susceptible, are susceptible to these agents, *B. fragilis* is not. All the first-generation agents, both oral[35, 36] and parenteral,[37–40] have essentially the same antibacterial activity with a few minor exceptions. Although cephalothin has slightly better gram-positive coverage and cefazolin slightly better gram-negative activity than the remaining drugs in the group, this is not clinically significant.

Cefuroxime[41, 42] compares favorably with the first-generation cephalosporins for streptococcal coverage but is slightly less active against staphylococci. It has enhanced gram-negative coverage, for in addition to being active against *E. coli*, *K. pneumoniae*, and *P. mirabilis*, it has good activity against *Haemophilus influenzae*, including β-lactamase producers. Cefuroxime is active against about 30% more of the Enterobacteriaceae, including *Klebsiella oxytoca*, *Morganella morganii*, and *Citrobacter* species, than are the first-generation cephalosporins. Activity is not good against *Proteus vulgaris* or *Providencia* and *Serratia* species. The drug is fairly active in vitro against gastrointestinal pathogens such as *Yersinia*, *Salmonella*, and *Shigella*. Cefuroxime is also quite active against many isolates of *Neisseria* species. Anaerobic coverage is similar to that of the first-generation agents.[43] The spectrum of activity of cefamandole is similar to that of cefuroxime, except that it is more active in vitro against coagulase-negative staphylococci and it is not as resistant as cefuroxime to certain gram-negative β-lactamases, including the plasmid-mediated (TEM) β-lactamase found in ampicillin-resistant *H. influenzae*. Cefuroxime axetil[44] is an oral preparation of cefuroxime with more gram-negative coverage than that offered by the older second-generation oral agent cefaclor.[45] The spectrum of activity of cefaclor is identical to that of the first-generation cephalosporins except that it also has good activity against *H. influenzae*, including some β-lactamase–producing strains. Loracarbef[46] has essentially the same coverage, although with further enhanced activity against *Bronhamella (Moraxella) catarrhalis* and *H. influenzae*, including β-lactamase–producing strains. The spectrum of activity of cefprozil is also similar to that of cefaclor but with gram-negative coverage approaching that of cefuroxime.

The cephamycins cefoxitin,[49] cefotetan,[50, 51] and cefmetazole[52] are noteworthy for their anaerobic coverage. However, they are inferior to metronidazole and chloramphenicol in their coverage of *B. fragilis*,[53, 54] generally being active against about 80% of isolates. Compared with cefoxitin, cefotetan and cefmetazole have slightly inferior coverage of non–*B. fragilis* in the group *B. fragilis*, with marginally more coverage of anaerobic gram-negative bacilli. These differences appear to be of little clinical consequence. Compared with cefuroxime, cefoxitin and cefmetazole have less gram-positive and gram-negative coverage overall, with only moderate activity against *H. influenzae*. Although the gram-positive coverage of cefotetan is similar, its gram-negative coverage approaches that of the third-generation cephalosporins. The cephamycins have good (although not outstanding) activity against *Neisseria gonorrhoeae*. Cefonicid[55] is slightly more active against gonococcal organisms but has less gram-positive coverage than cefuroxime and about equivalent gram-negative activity. Its anaerobic activity is comparable to that of the first-generation drugs.

All of the third-generation agents[56–62] have excellent activity in vitro against gram-negative organisms. More than 90% of the Enterobacteriaceae are susceptible to the third-generation cephalosporins. Nonfermentors such as *Acinetobacter* and *Pseudomonas* species are less susceptible. Of note, resistance has been seen to develop during therapy of *Serratia marcescens*, *Citrobacter freundii*, *Enterobacter cloacae*, and *P. aeruginosa* and is due to the selection of mutants that are derepressed for the production of chromosomally mediated type I cephalosporinases, which can destroy the third-generation cephalosporins.[13] Ceftazidime[63–65] has the greatest activity against *P. aeruginosa*. All the drugs, particularly ceftriaxone,[66] are extremely active against *N. gonorrhoeae* (including penicillinase producers). The gram-positive coverage is slightly inferior to that of the second-generation agents, ceftazidime and moxalactam being by far the least active in the group. Overall, anaerobic coverage is approximately the same as that of the first-generation agents, except for moxalactam, which is roughly as active as cefoxitin and cefotetan against *B. fragilis* and other anaerobes. It is not clear whether the in vitro activity of ceftizoxime against anaerobes reported in some studies is of any clinical significance.[67]

Cefepime[68–70] is a new parenteral cephalosporin with such a broad range of coverage that, although it is generally classified with the third-generation agents, some would consider it a "fourth-generation" cephalosporin. Cefepime is active against *Streptococcus pneumoniae*, *Streptococcus pyogenes*, *H. influenzae*, *Neisseria* spp., and the Enterobacteriaceae. Compared with ceftazidime, cefepime has less antipseudomonal activity (50% of *P. aeruginosa* organisms are inhibited by 8 μg/mL[69]) but substantially more against *S. aureus*. Cefpirome and cefpiramide are investigational third-generation cephalosporins with antipseudomonal activity.

A spate of oral preparations marketed as third-generation cephalosporins has been released, with more on the horizon.[71] Cefixime[72, 73] has excellent activity against *S. pneumoniae, S. pyogenes, H. influenzae, Neisseria* spp., and many of the Enterobacteriaceae but poor antistaphylococcal coverage. The spectrum of cefpodoxime axetil[74] is similar, with the addition of moderate antistaphylococcal coverage. Ceftibuten,[75, 76] which is likely to be released soon, is highly active against the Enterobacteriaceae, *H. influenzae, Neisseria* spp., and *M. catarrhalis*. It has only moderate activity against streptococci and relatively poor activity against *S. aureus*. Cefdinir[77] and cefetamet pivoxil,[78, 79] which are widely used in Europe, remain investigational in the United States. Gram-positive coverage of cefdinir is similar to that of cefpodoxime. The activity against Enterobacteriaceae is moderately less than that provided by cefixime. Cefetamet pivoxil is highly potent against the Enterobacteriaceae, *M. catarrhalis,* and *H. influenzae,* including β-lactamase producers. It has moderate coverage for *S. pneumoniae* and *S. pyogenes* but no appreciable activity against α-hemolytic streptococci or against staphylococci.

Clinical Applications

The dazzling array of oral and parenteral cephalosporins can be made comprehensible if physicians become familiar with the outstanding general features of several of the more useful agents and apply some of the basic tenets of proper antibiotic use. Empirical therapy should be aimed at the most likely responsible organisms, which depends on whether an infection is community acquired or nosocomial, the site of the infection, and specific host factors, such as immune status. Antimicrobial therapy should be as narrowly focused as possible, particularly when bacteriologic data become available. Although a cephalosporin is rarely a drug of first choice for an established infection, these antibiotics are important, especially for initial coverage, because of their low toxicity and broad activity spectra. They may be tolerated well by patients allergic to penicillins provided the allergy is not of the immediate or anaphylactic type. In addition, aminoglycoside therapy can sometimes be avoided by substituting these agents for aminoglycosides in established infections and using them to replace β-lactam–aminoglycoside combinations for initial empirical coverage in some settings. Limitations of this class of antibiotics include lack of activity against enterococci, methicillin-resistant staphylococci, and *Listeria*; poor penetration into cerebrospinal fluid by older agents; and undependable activity against *P. aeruginosa* except by ceftazidime.

In general, first-generation agents are reasonable choices for predominantly gram-positive infections, especially community-acquired pneumonia or skin and soft tissue infections, if one is trying to avoid using a penicillin. The first-generation agents are the mainstay of surgical prophylaxis. The second-generation agents can be thought of in two groups: the cephamycins, which are effective for community-acquired mixed aerobic and anaerobic infections of mild to moderate severity; and cefuroxime, with excellent activity against *H. influenzae*–related illnesses such as pneumonia and various head and neck infections. The importance of the third-generation agents lies in their coverage for gram-negative organisms, including many multiresistant Enterobacteriaceae. Because of their excellent penetration into the cerebrospinal fluid, these drugs (except cefoperazone) are agents of choice for gram-negative meningitis. They may need to be combined with other antibiotics to treat infections with a heavy gram-positive or anaerobic component. Ceftazidime is outstanding in its activity against *P. aeruginosa.*

First-Generation Cephalosporins

The first-generation parenteral cephalosporins,[80] cephalothin,[2, 81] cephapirin, cephradine, and cefazolin,[82] are essentially interchangeable in most clinical situations. The longer half-life of cefazolin has made it the most widely used agent in this category.[83] These antibiotics are rational choices for infections due to gram-positive organisms such as staphylococci and nonenterococcal streptococci when one would like to avoid administration of penicillin for community-acquired pneumonia or skin and soft tissue infections.[84] Of note, staphylococcal endocarditis is one of the rare situations in which cephalothin may be preferable to the slightly less β-lactamase–stable cefazolin.[85] The gram-negative coverage of the first-generation cephalosporins might allow one to use them for complicated community-acquired urinary tract infections, but to be certain of good coverage of most Enterobacteriaceae, one should either combine these agents with an aminoglycoside[86] or avoid them altogether. If a second- or third-generation cephalosporin is empirically chosen in such a situation and susceptibility testing reveals that a first-generation agent has good activity, it is appropriate to switch to the less costly and narrower spectrum drug. The first-generation agents have a unique role in surgical prophylaxis and remain the standard for cardiac, thoracic, orthopedic, vascular, and most abdominal and obstetric surgery.[87–89] Cefazolin and its relatives should not be used when *Pseudomonas* species, enterococci, *H. influenzae,* or nonstreptococcal anaerobes are of primary concern. In addition, these drugs are useless in central nervous system infection, because they do not penetrate even into inflamed meninges. These drugs have little role as single agents in treating nosocomial infections of any kind (except those caused by *S. aureus*), owing to their limited gram-negative coverage, but they may be combined with aminoglycosides for initial coverage in this setting.

Cephalexin, cephradine, and cefadroxil are the so-called first-generation oral cephalosporins.[80] They are equivalent in clinical use, including applications for urinary tract and soft tissue infections. Although cefadroxil is promoted for once- or twice-daily dosing, it remains extremely expensive and without advantages other than serum half-life over the other two drugs in the group.

Second-Generation Cephalosporins

The extended anaerobic spectrum of the cephamycins renders them especially useful as single-agent therapy of mild to moderately severe community-acquired mixed aerobic and anaerobic infections[57]: intraabdominal infections such as mild complications of diverticulitis; pelvic infections (cefoxitin is part of the Centers for Disease Control and Prevention recommendations[90] for in-hospital therapy of pelvic inflammatory disease); aspiration pneumonia; and certain skin and soft tissue infections such as infected diabetic feet and sacral decubiti, where multidrug-resistant gram-negative organisms are not of utmost concern. Although most experience in these areas has been with cefoxitin, the smaller clinical trials done to date with cefotetan and cefmetazole suggest that the equivalent efficacy and the less frequent dosing of the newer agent are attractive for cost containment.[50, 91, 92] The clinical significance, if any, of the slightly inferior coverage of *Bacteroides* other than *B. fragilis* by cefotetan and cefmetazole compared with cefoxitin remains to be shown. These drugs should not be employed empirically if *B. fragilis* is thought to be a significant component of an infection in a life-threatening situation. They are not appropriate for empirical therapy of nosocomial infections, including intraabdominal ones, as gram-negative coverage in these situations is not predictable. These agents are also inappropriate for infections that are caused primarily by gram-positive organisms. They are gaining popularity as prophylactic agents in colorectal surgery, especially when oral agents cannot be used.[6, 93]

Cefuroxime and cefamandole have roughly comparable spectra of activity, but cefuroxime[94] has assumed the role of cefamandole in many clinical situations because of its longer half-life and lack of an MTT side chain. Cefuroxime occupies a special niche in the treatment of infections such as certain pneumonias, epiglottitis, and complicated sinusitis, where β-lactamase–producing *H. influenzae* is the major potential pathogen but staphylococci and nonenterococcal streptococci are also of concern. Bacteremias, urinary tract infections, and soft tissue infections due to susceptible organisms can also be treated with this agent. Its initially promising role in the therapy of meningitis has largely been usurped by the third-generation agents. The same is true of empirical therapy of nosocomial infections or life-threatening gram-negative bacteremia, owing to the broader scope of gram-negative coverage provided by the third-generation cephalosporins. The potential advantage of cefamandole for therapy and prevention of staphylococcal infections (including those due to coagulase-negative staphylococci) remains to be determined, although both cefuroxime and cefamandole may be slightly more effective than cefazolin in preventing postoperative staphylococcal infections.[88]

Although cefonicid has been available for clinical use for a number of years, its precise clinical role remains to be defined. It has been shown to be effective in a variety of situations,[95, 96] but there is concern that once-daily dosing, which was the original selling point, produces trough levels inadequate for treating serious infections such as endocarditis and bacteremias. Even when shown to be effective, it is unclear whether it offers any cost or efficacy benefits over other currently available cephalosporins. There is some interest in using one-time dosing of the drug for prolonged surgical procedures.

The second-generation oral agents, including loracarbef, may be useful in a wide range of community-acquired infections of mild to moderate severity. Potential indications include sinusitis, bronchitis, skin and soft tissue infections, otitis media, and urinary tract infections. However, these agents are expensive and often provide a broader range of coverage than what is indicated. Cefuroxime axetil has been shown to have efficacy for the treatment of early Lyme disease.[97]

Third-Generation Cephalosporins

The third-generation cephalosporins are important in clinical medicine owing to their general characteristics of broad antibacterial, especially gram-negative, activity and their penetration into the cerebrospinal fluid. Particular agents in the group are outstanding because of their antipseudomonal activity (ceftazidime) or their long half-life (ceftriaxone).

Cefotaxime[98–101] and ceftizoxime[102] can be considered equivalent in terms of clinical use. They are especially useful for treating gram-negative nosocomial infections such as pneumonia, complicated urinary tract infections, osteomyelitis, and wound infections. For life-threatening infections, it is prudent to add an aminoglycoside until the infecting organism(s) and susceptibilities are known, to ensure coverage of organisms such as *Citrobacter, Enterobacter,* and *Serratia.* Better agents are available for treatment of primarily gram-positive or anaerobic infections. These relative gaps in coverage must be provided for by the use of additional drugs if resistant gram-positive or anaerobic bacteria are playing a significant role in an infection where cefotaxime or ceftizoxime is thought to be required for gram-negative coverage, as in hospital-acquired intravascular catheter–related bacteremia or intraabdominal infection. These drugs are rarely necessary for community-acquired infections but may be reasonable empirical therapy for a severe illness, especially if *Klebsiella* might be responsible, until bacteriologic data are available. Cefotaxime may have a role in the treatment of neurologic manifestations of Lyme disease.[103]

Ceftriaxone can be categorized in the same way as the previous two agents for excellent coverage of many multidrug-resistant gram-negative organisms, with the same general indications.[104] There are several settings in which the newer agent has a unique role. For example, ceftriaxone is effective therapy for typhoid fever[105] as well as for focal *Salmonella* infection.[106] Intramuscular ceftriaxone, which is gaining popularity in the treatment of various sexually transmitted diseases, is now the agent recommended by the Centers for Disease Control and Prevention for therapy of gonococcal disease in areas with significant numbers of penicillinase-producing organisms[107, 108]; it is effective for both pharyngeal and anorectal disease.[109] Gonococcal ophthalmia neonatorum is likewise successfully treated with the drug.[110] It also appears to be effective therapy for chancroid.[111] Ceftriaxone has gained prominence for the treatment of refractory acute Lyme disease, including meningitis, as well as for late neurologic complications.[103, 112] As the focus on home antibiotic therapy increases, so does the interest in using ceftriaxone in this setting, owing to its infrequent dosing and effectiveness as either an intravascular or an intramuscular agent.[113, 114] Twice-daily dosing is still preferred by many physicians for serious infections such as meningitis and endocarditis, but once-daily dosing is effective even in these settings.[114–116]

The empirical use of ceftriaxone or cefotaxime is recommended for community-acquired meningitis (typically caused by *N. meningitides, S. pneumoniae,* or *H. influenzae*) in children and in adults older than 50 years.[117] Ceftizoxime may also be effective in this setting, but it has less activity than the other two agents against pneumococci, especially those resistant to penicillin.[118] These agents can be useful in the treatment of meningitis due to gram-negative organisms; only ceftazidime is reliable in the treatment of cases caused by *P. aeruginosa.*[119] There have been reports of ceftriaxone failures in the treatment of meningitis due to *S. pneumoniae* with relative and especially high-level resistance to penicillin.[120] Recommendations, pending results of susceptibility testing, suggest preferential therapy with vancomycin in suspected cases of pneumococcal meningitis in areas where intermediate or high-level penicillin resistance has been identified.[121] None of the cephalosporins has a role in treatment of *L. monocytogenes* meningitis.

Ceftazidime is similar to the agents already discussed in general effectiveness for gram-negative infections,[122] but it is the only cephalosporin that can be employed routinely in the therapy of *P. aeruginosa*–related infection and should be reserved for situations in which this organism is likely to be implicated. Many studies have examined the role of ceftazidime, alone or in combination with an aminoglycoside, as empirical therapy for febrile neutropenic patients.[123–125] Although controversy exists, it seems most prudent to use the combination in this setting as well as in treating most serious *P. aeruginosa* infections in normal hosts. Special clinical situations in which ceftazidime can be considered the treatment of choice for *Pseudomonas* infections include *P. aeruginosa* meningitis[126, 127] and cystic fibrosis pulmonary infections.[128, 129]

It might also be acceptable to use ceftazidime alone for therapy of infections of the urinary tract or skin and soft tissue due to *P. aeruginosa.* Ceftazidime can be uniquely useful in treatment of other *Pseudomonas* infections, such as melioidosis (*P. pseudomallei*).[106]

Cefoperazone, released before ceftazidime, was originally hoped to be an effective anti-*Pseudomonas* agent; however, minimal concentrations inhibiting 90% of the isolates of *P. aeruginosa* are often in the 16 to 32 μg/mL range for cefoperazone. The drug has no clear-cut indications. Its moderately prolonged serum half-life allows twice-daily dosing for non–life-threatening infections. Its biliary route of excretion has made it favored by some surgeons as prophylaxis in right upper quadrant surgery, but this practice has not been examined in controlled trials. It does not require dose adjustment for patients with impaired renal function.

Even as the third-generation cephalosporins are proving to be of great clinical importance, their precise clinical roles are still being defined. Some of the evolving issues that need to be evaluated systematically include the problems of superinfection with enterococci[130, 131] and highly resistant gram-negative organisms as well as the likelihood of resistance developing during therapy.[14] Such resistance has been documented, especially in *Citrobacter* species and *Enterobacter* species and in *Acinetobacter,* but the true incidence and clinical significance remain to be elucidated. A report of a nosocomial outbreak of infections due to *Klebsiella* spp. resistant to third-generation cephalosporins[23] is sobering. Whether addition of an aminoglycoside is warranted, or even effective, in trying to prevent the emergence of resistance is not known, but aminoglycosides are widely used for this purpose at present. The prudent use of the broad-spectrum late-generation cephalosporins and stringent adherence to infection control measures appear to be the best available methods for containing emergence and nosocomial spread of organisms resistant to these agents.[132]

The precise role of the third-generation oral cephalosporins in the outpatient armamentarium remains to be defined. As is true of the second-generation agents, these oral cephalosporins are expensive and may cover a broader range of organisms than is appropriate in the treatment of a specific outpatient infection. Although many of these agents are touted as providing the answer for children with multiple episodes of otitis media, for example, a review of this topic did not stress the use of these agents.[132] They may have a place in the early conversion to oral antibiotics from intravenous therapy with second- or third-generation cephalosporins.[133]

Toxicity

Local Reactions

The cephalosporins are quite safe: grave adverse effects are rare. As with any intravenous agent, the potential for phlebitis[134] exists. Prevalence rates from different studies vary from 1% to 5%, with no agent being more irritating than others. Cefoxitin and cephalothin are poorly tolerated when administered via the intramuscular route unless accompanied by a local anesthetic.

Hypersensitivity Reactions

Immediate hypersensitivity reactions to the cephalosporins rarely occur.[135, 136] More common but still infrequent are drug fever, eosinophilia, angioedema, and rash. The true incidence of these manifestations is not known, but a rash, the most common reaction, has been estimated to occur in 1% to 3% of patients.[33, 137]

The extent to which cross-allergy between the penicillins and cephalosporins exists has long been debated, and although various degrees of cross-reactivity have been demonstrated in the laboratory, the question has been more difficult to address in the clinical setting.[135, 138] It has often been stated that persons with a history of penicillin allergy are more likely to have an allergic response to a cephalosporin,[139] but Smith[140] found that persons with a history of allergy to penicillin are three times more likely to react even to unrelated drugs. Results from penicillin skin tests have not proved reliable in predicting reactions to cephalosporins.[141, 142] The true incidence of cross-reactivity probably lies in the range of 3% to 7%.[136] Among the cephalosporins, the first-generation agents demonstrate the most cross-reactivity with penicillin.[143] The incidence of anaphylaxis due to cephalosporins in penicillin-allergic patients is not known, but because there appears to be some cross-reactivity and there have been cases of anaphylaxis due to cephalosporins,[144] it is recommended that persons who have a history of immunoglobulin E–mediated hypersensitivity reaction (anaphylaxis, angioedema, urticaria) to a penicillin not receive a cephalosporin.[33] The utility of skin tests for cephalosporin sensitivity is too limited to warrant their recommendation.[145]

Serum sickness–like reactions can result from the tissue deposition of β-lactam specific immunoglobulin G or immunoglobulin M antibodies and circulating β-lactam antigens.[145] Although this occurs rarely with cephalosporin use overall, cefaclor use in children has been associated with serum sickness 15 times more frequently than has ampicillin.[146] There are reports of serum sickness–like reactions associated with cefprozil use.[147]

Hepatic and Gastrointestinal Disturbances

Elevated transaminase values have been reported in conjunction with use of almost all the cephalosporins, occurring at a frequency of 1% to 7%,[144] but whether this is due to the antibiotic or to the underlying condition the antibiotic is treating is unclear.[148] Profound hepatic injury has been reported but is quite rare.[149]

The reported frequency of nonspecific antibiotic-associated diarrhea varies greatly among various studies but likely occurs about 5% of the time. Pseudomembranous colitis has been reported in patients receiving cephalosporins but does not occur disproportionately after cephalosporin therapy as compared with other antibiotic therapy.[150] It has been suggested that cefoperazone and ceftriaxone are more commonly associated with diarrhea because biliary excretion may favor suppression of normal intestinal flora, but similar rates have been seen with other cephalosporins and are influenced by the patient's age, renal function, and underlying condition.[151]

Ceftriaxone has been associated with formation of biliary sludge detectable by ultrasound examination. This is typically asymptomatic, but symptoms of cholecystitis can occur. Sludge formation (pseudolithiasis) is most common in children, patients receiving ceftriaxone at more than 2 g/d, and those with biliary stasis.[152, 153] Under these circumstances, ceftriaxone is excreted in high concentrations into the bile and forms an insoluble calcium salt, which can precipitate out of solution.[154] Although this sludge can be expected to resolve spontaneously after a variable time, cholelithiasis can occur rarely.[152]

Neurotoxicity

Although seizures have been associated with several of the cephalosporins, they have occurred generally in the setting of excessive doses.[155, 156] The neurotoxicity of these agents is quite low, and they have been used safely intraventricularly.[155]

Disulfiram-Like Reactions

Disulfiram-like reactions have occurred with the ingestion of alcohol several hours after administration of cephalosporins with 3-methylthiotetrazole side chains[157, 158] such as are found on molecules of moxalactam, cefoperazone, cefotetan, cefonicid, and cefamandole. This is likely due to an accumulation of acetaldehyde, which is the result of the ability of the MTT metabolite to inhibit aldehyde dehydrogenase. This enzyme normally metabolizes the ethanol breakdown product acetaldehyde to water and carbon dioxide.[155]

Nephrotoxicity

One of the older cephalosporins,[33] cephaloridine, became renowned for its dose-dependent nephrotoxicity[159] and is no longer in clinical use. Cephalothin has, on rare occasion, been associated with renal failure, probably due to tubular injury.[160] Although ceftazidime may cause a decrease in glomerular filtration rate, tubule function is affected to only a small degree[161] and clinical problems are not apparent.[162] Overall, the potential for nephrotoxicity by currently available agents is extremely low.[163] Interstitial nephritis can be seen as part of a hypersensitivity reaction to cephalosporins.[148]

Hematologic Toxicity

Although development of a positive reaction to the Coombs test is thought to be relatively frequent (3%) in patients receiving cephalosporins,[164] most reports and reviews[164–166] focus on the older drugs. The actual incidence with use of the more recently developed members of the group is unclear. The incidence of hemolytic anemia is extremely low, even in patients with a positive Coombs reaction, and is most often due to an immune complex–mediated process.[167, 168] Neutropenia is an unusual (1%) complication that reverses rapidly with cessation of therapy and typically occurs only after several weeks of treatment. Eosinophilia or thrombocytosis is frequently seen (5%), but these conditions are most likely results of the underlying infection. Isolated cases of immune-mediated platelet dysfunction have been reported for several cephalosporins.

The cephalosporins can affect hemostasis. Moxalactam has an adverse effect on both platelet aggregation and prothrombin levels, which produced significant bleeding frequently enough that the drug is no longer in widespread clinical use.[169, 170] The other cephalosporins are not known to affect platelet aggregation. Hypoprothrombinemia with the use of many antibiotics, including cephalosporins, has been thought to arise from depletion of vitamin K–processing intestinal flora.[171] There is compelling evidence that those cephalosporins with an MTT side chain induce hypoprothrombinemia by inhibiting vitamin K metabolism and carboxylation of glutamic acid.[172, 173] Estimates of the prevalence of hypoprothrombinemia due to these agents range from 4% to 68%[173, 174] with the highest frequencies accompanying moxalactam use. The precise incidence of bleeding due to cephalosporins has been difficult to assess, as multiple confounding factors appear to be involved. Among agents currently in use, clinically apparent bleeding has been reported with cefoperazone[175] and cefotetan[176] and is more likely to occur in the setting of renal failure and debilitation. A single subcutaneous injection of vitamin K reverses hypoprothrombinemia, usually in a matter of hours unless the cephalosporin has an MTT side chain, in which case the prothrombin time may take 24 to 36 hours to normalize.[174] If bleeding is present, fresh-frozen plasma may be necessary. Prophylactic use of once- or twice-weekly parenteral doses of 10 mg of vitamin K has been suggested for use in settings where hypoprothrombinemia is more likely to occur, as in renal failure, malnutrition, intraabdominal infection, or recent gastrointestinal surgery, at least when cefotetan or cefoperazone is used. Although bleeding is theoretically possible with the use of cefonicid, given its MTT side chain, it has not yet been reported.

References

1. Abraham EP: Cephalosporins 1945–1986. *In* Williams JD (ed): The Cephalosporin Antibiotics. Auckland, New Zealand, Adis Press, 1987, pp 1–14.
2. Abraham EP, Loder PB: Cephalosporin C. *In* Flynn EH (ed): Cephalosporins and Penicillins: Chemistry and Biology. New York, Academic Press, 1972, pp 2–26.
3. Rolinson GN: The influence of 6-aminopenicillanic acid on antibiotic development. J Antimicrob Chemother 22:5, 1988.
4. Oniski HR, Daoust DR, Zimmerman SB, et al: Cefoxitin, a semisynthetic cephamycin antibiotic: Resistance to β-lactamase inactivation. Antimicrob Agents Chemother 5:38, 1974.
5. Allan JD, Eliopoulos GM, Moellering RC Jr: Antibiotics: Future directions by understanding structure-function relationships. *In* Root RK, Trunkey DD, Sande MA (eds): Contemporary Issues in Infectious Diseases, Vol 6. New York, Churchill Livingstone, 1987, pp 263–284.
6. Dunn GL: Ceftizoxime and other third generation cephalosporins: Structure-activity relationships. J Antimicrob Chemother 10(Suppl C):1, 1982.
7. Neu HC: Relation of structural properties of β-lactam antibiotics to antibacterial activity. Am J Med 79:2, 1985.
8. Fassbender M, Lode H, Schaberg T, et al: Pharmacokinetics of new cephalosporins, including a new carbacephem. Clin Infect Dis 16:646, 1993.
9. Cooper RD: The carbacephems: A new β-lactam antibiotic class. Am J Med 92:25, 1992.
10. Williams JD: Classification of cephalosporins. *In* Williams JD (ed): The Cephalosporin Antibiotics. Auckland, New Zealand, Adis Press, 1987, pp 15–22.
11. Yocum RR, Rasmussin JR, Strominger SL: The mechanism of action of penicillin: Penicillin activates the active site of *Bacillus stearothermophilus* D-alanine carboxypeptidase. J Biol Chem 255:3977, 1980.
12. Tomasz A: Penicillin-binding proteins in bacteria. Ann Intern Med 96:502, 1982.
13. Jacoby GA, Archer GL: New mechanisms of bacterial resistance to antimicrobial agents. N Engl J Med 324:601, 1991.
14. Sanders CC, Sanders WE Jr: Microbial resistance to newer generation β-lactam antibiotics: Clinical and laboratory implications. J Infect Dis 151:399, 1985.
15. Fontano R, Grossato A, Rossi L, et al: Transition from resistance to hypersusceptibility to β-lactam antibiotics associated with loss of a low-affinity penicillin-binding protein in a *Streptococcus faecium* mutant highly resistant to penicillin. Antimicrob Agents Chemother 28:678, 1985.
16. Hartman BJ, Tomasz A: Low-affinity penicillin-binding protein associated with β-lactam resistance in *Staphylococcus aureus*. J Bacteriol 158:513, 1984.
17. Handwerger S, Tomasz A: Alterations in the penicillin-binding proteins of clinical and laboratory isolates of *Streptococcus pneumoniae* with low levels of penicillin resistance. J Infect Dis 153:83, 1986.
18. Gutmann L, Williamson R, Collatz E: The possible role of porins in antibiotic resistance. Ann Intern Med 101:554, 1984.
19. Mitsuyama J, Hiruma R, Jagamuchi A, et al: Identification of porins in outer membrane of *Proteus, Morganella* and *Providencia* spp. and their role in outer membrane permeation of β-lactams. Antimicrob Agents Chemother 31:379, 1987.
20. Sanders CC: Beta-lactamases of gram-negative bacteria: New challenges for new drugs. Clin Infect Dis 14:1089, 1992.
21. Sanders WE, Sanders CC: Inducible β-lactamases: Clinical and

epidemiologic implications for use of newer cephalosporins. Rev Infect Dis 10:830, 1988.
22. Cullmann W, Opferkuch W, Stieglitz M, et al: Influence of spontaneous and inducible β-lactamase production in the antimicrobial activity of recently developed β-lactam compounds. Chemotherapy 30:175, 1984.
23. Medeiros AA: Nosocomial outbreaks of multiresistant bacteria: Extended-spectrum beta-lactamases have arrived in North America. Ann Intern Med 119:428, 1993.
24. Jacoby GA, Medeiros AA: More extended-spectrum β-lactamases. Antimicrob Agents Chemother 35:1697, 1991.
25. Sanders CC: New beta-lactams: New problems for the internist. Ann Intern Med 115:650, 1991.
26. Donowitz GR, Mandell GL: Beta-lactam antibiotics. N Engl J Med 313:490, 1988.
27. Brogard JM, Conte F: Pharmacokinetics of the new cephalosporins. Antimicrob Agents Chemother 21:592, 1982.
28. Bergan T: Pharmacokinetic properties of the cephalosporins. *In* Williams JD (ed): The Cephalosporin Antibiotics. Auckland, New Zealand, Adis Press, 1987, pp 89–104.
29. Patel IH, Kaplan SA: Pharmacokinetic profile of ceftriaxone in man. Am J Med 77(Suppl 4G):17, 1984.
30. Chin NX, Neu HC: Cefotaxime and desacetyl cefotaxime: An example of advantageous antimicrobial metabolism. Diagn Microbiol Infect Dis 2:215, 1984.
31. Kemmerich B, Lode H, Borner K, et al: Biliary excretion and pharmacokinetics of cefoperazone in humans. J Antimicrob Chemother 12:27, 1983.
32. Cherubin CE, Eng RH, Norrby R, et al: Penetration of newer cephalosporins into cerebrospinal fluid. Rev Infect Dis 11:526, 1989.
33. Gustaferro CA, Steckelberg JM: Cephalosporin antimicrobial agents and related compounds. Mayo Clin Proc 66:1064, 1991.
34. Basker MJ, Edmonson RA, Sutherland R: Comparative stabilities of penicillins and cephalosporins to staphylococcal β-lactamase and activities against *Staphylococcus aureus.* J Antimicrob Chemother 6:333, 1980.
35. Hartstein AI, Patrick KE, Jones SR, et al: Comparison of pharmacologic and antimicrobial properties of cephadroxil and cephalexin. Antimicrob Agents Chemother 12:93, 1977.
36. Silver MS, Counts GW, Zeleznik D, et al: Comparison of in vitro antibacterial activity of three oral cephalosporins: Cefaclor, cephalexin and cephradine. Antimicrob Agents Chemother 12:591, 1977.
37. Renzini G, Ravagnan G, Oliva B: In vitro and in vivo microbiological evaluation of cephapirin, a new antibiotic. Chemotherapy 21:289, 1975.
38. Bergeron MG, Brusch JL, Barza M, et al: Bactericidal activity and pharmacology of cefazolin. Antimicrob Agents Chemother 4:396, 1973.
39. Phair JP, Carlton J, Tan JS: Comparison of cefazolin, a new cephalosporin antibiotic, with cephalothin. Antimicrob Agents Chemother 2:329, 1972.
40. Turck M, Anderson KN, Smith RH, et al: Laboratory and clinical evaluation of a new antibiotic: Cephalothin. Ann Intern Med 63:199, 1965.
41. Neu HC, Fu KP: Cefuroxime, a β-lactamase–resistant cephalosporin with a broad spectrum of gram-positive and -negative activity. Antimicrob Agents Chemother 13:657, 1978.
42. O'Callaghan CH, Sykes RB, Griffiths A, et al: Cefuroxime, a new cephalosporin antibiotic: Activity in vitro. Antimicrob Agents Chemother 9:511, 1976.
43. Rolfe D, Finegold SM: Comparative in vitro activity of new β-lactam antibiotics against anaerobic bacteria. Antimicrob Agents Chemother 20:600, 1981.
44. Ginsburg CM: Pharmacokinetics and bactericidal activity of cefuroxime axetil. Antimicrob Agents Chemother 28:504, 1985.
45. Medical Letter: Two new oral cephalosporins. Med Lett Drugs Ther 31:85, 1979.
46. Brogden RN, McTavish D: Loracarbef: A review of its antimicrobial activity, pharmacokinetic properties and therapeutic efficacy. Drugs 45:716, 1993.
47. Wiseman LR, Benfield P: Cefprozil: A review of its antibacterial activity, pharmacokinetic properties and therapeutic potential. Drugs 45:295, 1993.
48. Thornsberry C: Review of the in vitro antibacterial activity of cefprozil, a new cephalosporin. Clin Infect Dis 1:95, 1992.
49. Birnbaum J, Stapley EO, Miller AK, et al: Cefoxitin, a semisynthetic cephamycin: A microbiologic overview. J Antimicrob Chemother 4:15, 1978.
50. Ward A, Richards DM: Cefotetan: A review. Drugs 30:382, 1985.
51. Ayres LW, Jones RN, Barry AL, et al: Cefotetan, a new cephamycin. Antimicrob Agents Chemother 22:859, 1982.
52. Jones RN: Review of the in-vitro spectrum and characteristics of cefmetazole. J Antimicrob Chemother 12(Suppl D):1, 1989.
53. Goldstein EJC, Citron DM: Annual incidence, epidemiology and comparative in vitro susceptibilities to cefoxitin, cefotetan, cefmetazole and ceftizoxime of recent community-acquired isolates of the *Bacteroides fragilis* group. J Antimicrob Chemother 26:2361, 1988.
54. Back VT, Roy I, Thadepalli H: Susceptibility of anaerobic bacteria to cefoxitin and related compounds. Antimicrob Agents Chemother 11:912, 1977.
55. Actor P: In vitro experience with cefonicid. Rev Infect Dis 64:S783, 1984.
56. Neu HC: Pathophysiologic basis for the use of third-generation cephalosporins. Am J Med 88(Suppl 4A):35, 1990.
57. Goldberg DM: The cephalosporins. Med Clin North Am 71:1113, 1987.
58. Thornsberry C: Review of in vitro activity of third-generation cephalosporins and other newer β-lactam antibiotics against clinically important bacteria. Am J Med 79:14, 1985.
59. Carmine AA, Brogden RN, Heel RC, et al: Cefotaxime: A review of its antibacterial activity, pharmacological properties and therapeutic use. Drugs 25:223, 1983.
60. Fass RJ: Comparative in vitro activities of third-generation cephalosporins. Arch Intern Med 143:1743, 1983.
61. Jones RN, Thornsberry C: Cefotaxime: A review of in vitro antimicrobial properties and spectrum of activity. Rev Infect Dis 4(Suppl):5300, 1982.
62. Fu KP, Neu HC: Antibacterial activity of ceftizoxime, a β-lactamase stable cephalosporin. Antimicrob Agents Chemother 17:583, 1980.
63. Neu HC, Labthavikul P: Antibacterial activity and β-lactamase stability of ceftazidime. Antimicrob Agents Chemother 21:11, 1982.
64. Gozzard DJ, Geddes AM, Farrell ID, et al: Ceftazidime—A new extended-spectrum cephalosporin. Lancet 1:1152, 1982.
65. Brogden RN, Carmine A, Heel RC, et al: Cefoperazone: A review of its in vitro antimicrobial activity, pharmacological properties and therapeutic efficacy. Drugs 22:423, 1981.
66. Cleeland R, Squires E: Antimicrobial activity of ceftriaxone: A review. Am J Med 77:3, 1984.
67. Johnson CC: Susceptibility of anaerobic bacteria to beta-lactam antibiotics in the United States. Clin Infect Dis 16(Suppl 4):S371, 1993.
68. Barradell LB, Bryson HM: Cefepime: A review of its antibacterial activity, pharmacokinetic properties and therapeutic use. Drugs 47:471, 1994.
69. Grassi GG, Grassi C: Cefepime: An overview of activity in vitro and in vivo. J Antimicrob Chemother 32(Suppl B):87, 1993.
70. Sanders CC: Cefepime: The next generation? Clin Infect Dis 15:369, 1993.
71. Neu HC: Oral beta-lactam antibiotics from 1960–1993. Infect Dis Clin Pract 6:394, 1993.
72. Bluestone CD: Review of cefixime in the treatment of otitis media in infants and children. Pediatr Infect Dis J 12:75, 1993.
73. Leggett NJ, Caravaggio C, Rybak MJ: Cefixime. DICP 24:489, 1990.
74. Chocas EC, Paap CM, Godley PJ: Cefpodoxime proxetil: A new, broad-spectrum oral cephalosporin. Ann Pharmacother 27:1369, 1993.
75. Wiseman LR, Balfour JA: Ceftibuten. A review of its antibacterial activity, pharmacokinetic properties and clinical efficacy. Drugs 47:784, 1994.
76. Bragman SG, Casewell MW: The in-vitro activity of ceftibuten against 475 clinical isolates of gram-negative bacilli. J Antimicrob Chemother 25:221, 1990.
77. Sultan T, Baltch AL, Smith RF, Ritz W: In vitro activity of cefdinir (FK482) and ten other antibiotics against gram-positive and gram-negative bacteria isolated from adult and pediatric patients. Chemotherapy 40:80, 1994.
78. Schito GC, Pesce A, Debbia EA: Stability in the presence of

widespread beta-lactamases. A prerequisite for the antibacterial activity of beta-lactam drugs. Drugs 47(Suppl 3):1, 1994.
79. Bryson HM, Brogden RN. Cefetamet pivoxil. A review of its antibacterial activity, pharmacokinetic properties and therapeutic use. Drugs 45:589, 1993.
80. Moellering RC Jr, Swartz MN: The newer cephalosporins. N Engl J Med 294:24, 1976.
81. Van Scoy RE, Wilkowske CJ: Prophylactic use of anti-microbial agents in adult patients. Mayo Clin Proc 67:288, 1992.
82. Perkins RL, Saslaw S: Experiences with cephalothin. Ann Intern Med 64:13, 1966.
83. Quintiliani R, Nightingale CH: Cefazolin. Ann Intern Med 89:650, 1978.
84. Neu HC: The place of cephalosporins in antibacterial treatment of infectious diseases. J Antimicrob Chemother 6(Suppl A):1, 1980.
85. Quinn EL, Pohlod D, Madhavan T, et al: Clinical experience with cefazolin and other cephalosporins in bacterial endocarditis. J Infect Dis 128(Suppl):S386, 1983.
86. Giamerellou H: Aminoglycoside plus β-lactams against gram-negative organisms: Evaluation of in vitro synergy and chemical interactions. Am J Med 80(Suppl B):126, 1986.
87. Sanford JP, Sande MA, Gilbert DN: Guide to Antimicrobial Therapy, ed 26. Dallas, TX, Antimicrobial Therapy, 1996, p 106.
88. Kaiser AB: Antimicrobial prophylaxis in surgery. N Engl J Med 315:1129, 1986.
89. Di Piro JT, Bowden TA Jr, Hooks VH III: Prophylactic parenteral cephalosporins in surgery. JAMA 252:3277, 1984.
90. Centers for Disease Control and Prevention: 1993 sexually transmitted diseases treatment guidelines. MMWR Morbid Mortal Wkly Rep 42(RR-14):1, 1993.
91. Poindexter AN III, Sweet R, Ritter M: Cefotetan in the treatment of obstetric and gynecologic infections. Am J Obstet Gynecol 154:946, 1986.
92. Griffith DL, Novak E, Greenwald CA, et al: Clinical experience with cefmetazole sodium in the United States. J Antimicrob Chemother 23(Suppl D):21, 1989.
93. Gorbach SL: The role of cephalosporins in surgical prophylaxis. J Antimicrob Chemother 23(Suppl D):61, 1989.
94. Jones RN, Thornsberry C: In vitro antimicrobial activity, physical characteristics and other microbiology features of cefuroxime: A new study and review. *In* Moellering RC Jr (ed): The Clinical Significance of the Newer β-Lactam Antibiotics: Focus on Cefuroxime. Auckland, New Zealand, Adis Press, 1983, pp 30–45.
95. Kaye D: An overview: Evaluation of cefonicid in infections of the urinary tract, lower respiratory tract, and skin and soft tissue. Rev Infect Dis 6(Suppl 11):S835, 1984.
96. Jacob CS, Layne P: Cefonicid: An overview of clinical studies in the United States. Rev Infect Dis 6(Suppl 4):S791, 1984.
97. Luger SW, Paparone P, Wormser GP, et al: Comparison of cefuroxime axetil and doxycycline in treatment of patients with early Lyme disease associated with erythema migrans. Antimicrob Agents Chemother 39:661, 1995.
98. Smith CR, Ambinder R, Lipsky JJ, et al: Cefotaxime compared with nafcillin plus tobramycin for serious bacterial infections: A randomized, double-blind trial. Ann Intern Med 101:469, 1984.
99. Karakusis PH, Feczko JM, Goodman LJ, et al: Clinical efficacy of cefotaxime in serious infections. Antimicrob Agents Chemother 21:119, 1982.
100. Francke EL, Neu HC: Use of cefotaxime, a β-lactamase stable cephalosporin in therapy of serious infection, including those due to multiresistant organisms. Am J Med 71:435, 1981.
101. Young JPW, Hussan JM, Bruch K, et al: The evaluation of efficacy and safety of cefotaxime: A review of 2500 cases. J Antimicrob Chemother 6(Suppl A):293, 1980.
102. Scully BE, Neu HC: The use of ceftizoxime in the treatment of critically ill patients infected with multiply antibiotic resistant bacteria. J Antimicrob Chemother 10:141, 1982.
103. Halperin JJ: Neuroborreliosis. Am J Med 98(Suppl 4A):53S, 1995.
104. Steele RW: Ceftriaxone therapy of meningitis and serious infections. Am J Med 79(Suppl 2A):52, 1985.
105. Islam A, Butler T, Nath SK, et al: Randomized treatment of patients with typhoid fever using ceftriaxone or chloramphenicol. J Infect Dis 158:742, 1988.
106. Finch RG: Third-generation cephalosporins in the treatment of rare infections. Am J Med 88(Suppl 4A):25S, 1990.
107. Le Saux N, Ronald AR: Role of ceftriaxone in sexually transmitted diseases. Rev Infect Dis 11:299, 1989.
108. Judson FN: Management of antibiotic-resistant *Neisseria gonorrhoeae*. Ann Intern Med 110:5, 1989.
109. Judson FN, Ehret JM, Handsfield HH: Comparative study of ceftriaxone and spectinomycin for treatment of pharyngeal and anorectal gonorrhea. JAMA 253:1417, 1985.
110. Laga M, Naamara W, Brunham RC, et al: Single-dose therapy of gonococcal ophthalmia neonatorum with ceftriaxone. N Engl J Med 315:1382, 1986.
111. Taylor DN, Pitarangsi C, Escheverria P, et al: Comparative study of ceftriaxone and trimethoprim-sulfamethoxazole for treatment of chanchroid in Thailand. J Infect Dis 152:1002, 1985.
112. Dattwyler RJ, Halperin JJ, Volkman DJ, Luft BJ: Treatment of late Lyme borreliosis—randomised comparison of ceftriaxone and penicillin. Lancet 1:1191, 1988.
113. Baumgartner JD, Glauser MP: Single daily dose treatment of severe refractory infections with ceftriaxone: Cost savings and possible outpatient treatment. Arch Intern Med 143:1868, 1983.
114. Francioli PB: Ceftriaxone and outpatient treatment of infective endocarditis. Infect Dis Clin 7:97, 1993.
115. Cabellos C, Viladrich PF, Verdaguer R, et al: A single daily dose of ceftriaxone for bacterial meningitis in adults. Clin Infect Dis 20:1164, 1995.
116. Francioli P, Etienne J, Hoigne R, et al: Treatment of streptococcal endocarditis with a single daily dose of ceftriaxone sodium for four weeks. JAMA 267:264, 1992.
117. Tunkel AR, Wispelway B, Scheld WM: Bacterial meningitis: Recent advances in pathophysiology and treatment. Ann Intern Med 112:610, 1990.
118. Overturf AD, Cable DC, Farthal DN, et al: Treatment of bacterial meningitis with ceftizoxime. Antimicrob Agents Chemother 25:258, 1984.
119. Norrby SR: Role of cephalosporins in the treatment of bacterial meningitis in adults. Overview with special emphasis on ceftazidime. Am J Med 79(Suppl 2A):56, 1985.
120. John CC: Treatment failure with use of a third-generation cephalosporin for penicillin-resistant pneumococcal meningitis: Case report and review. Clin Infect Dis 18:188, 1994.
121. Austrian R: Confronting drug-resistant pneumococci. Ann Intern Med 121:807, 1994.
122. Scully BE, Neu HC: Clinical efficacy of ceftazidime: Treatment of serious infection due to multiresistant *Pseudomonas* and other gram-negative bacteria. Arch Intern Med 144:5, 1984.
123. Bodey GP: Empirical antibiotic therapy for fever in neutropenic patients. Clin Infect Dis 17(Suppl 2):S378, 1993.
124. Hughes WT, Armstrong D, Bodey GP, et al: Guidelines for the use of antimicrobial agents in neutropenic patients with unexplained fever. J Infect Dis 161:381, 1990.
125. EORTC International Antimicrobial Therapy Cooperative Group: Ceftazidime combined with a short or long course of amikacin for empirical therapy of gram-negative bacteremia in cancer patients with granulocytopenia. N Engl J Med 317:1692, 1987.
126. Fong IW, Tomkins B: Review of *Pseudomonas aeruginosa* meningitis with special emphasis on treatment with ceftazidime. Rev Infect Dis 7:604, 1985.
127. Hudson SJ, Ingham HR: Ceftazidime for *Pseudomonas* meningitis (Letter). Lancet 1:464, 1985.
128. Blumer JL, Stern RC, Klinger JD, et al: Ceftazidime therapy in patients with cystic fibrosis and multiply drug-resistant *Pseudomonas.* Am J Med 79(Suppl 2A):37, 1985.
129. Gold R, Overmeyer A, Knie B, et al: Controlled trial of ceftazidime vs. ticarcillin and tobramycin in the treatment of acute respiratory exacerbations in patients with cystic fibrosis. Pediatr Infect Dis 4:172, 1985.
130. Pallares R, Pujol M, Pena C, et al: Cephalosporins as risk factor for nosocomial *Enterococcus faecalis* bacteremia. Arch Intern Med 153:1581, 1993.
131. Moellering RC Jr: Enterococcal infections in patients treated with moxalactam. Rev Infect Dis 4(Suppl):S708, 1982.
132. Berman S: Otitis media in children. N Engl J Med 332:1560, 1995.
133. Ramirez JA, Srinath L, Ahkee S, et al: Early switch from intravenous to oral cephalosporins in the treatment of hospitalized patients with community-acquired pneumonia. Arch Intern Med 155:1273, 1995.

134. Berger S, Ennst EC, Barza M: Comparative incidence of phlebitis due to buffered cephalothin, cephapirin, and cefamandole. Antimicrob Agents Chemother 9:575, 1976.
135. Lin RY: A perspective on penicillin allergy. Arch Intern Med 152:930, 1992.
136. Saxon A, Beall GN, Rohr AS, et al: Immediate hypersensitivity reactions to β-lactam antibiotics. Ann Intern Med 107:204, 1987.
137. Young EJ, Fainstein V, Mosher DM: Drug-induced fever: Cases seen in evaluation of unexplained fever in a general hospital population. Rev Infect Dis 4:69, 1982.
138. Blanca M, Fernandez J, Miranda A, et al: Cross-reactivity between penicillins and cephalosporins: Clinical and immunologic studies. J Allergy Clin Immunol 83:381, 1989.
139. Petz LD: Immunologic nonreactivity between penicillins and cephalosporins: A review. J Infect Dis 137:S74, 1978.
140. Smith JW, Johnson JE, Cluff LE: Studies on the epidemiology of adverse drug reactions. N Engl J Med 274:998, 1966.
141. Wendel GD Jr, Stark BJ, Jamison RB, et al: Penicillin allergy and desensitization in serious infections during pregnancy. N Engl J Med 312:1229, 1985.
142. Solley GO, Gleich GJ, Van Dellen RG: Penicillin allergy: Clinical experience with a battery of skin test reagents. J Allergy Clin Immunol 69:238, 1982.
143. Sullivan TJ: Drug allergy. *In* Middleton E, Reed C, Ellis E, et al (eds): Allergy: Principles and Practice. St. Louis: CV Mosby, 1989, pp 1523–1534.
144. Norrby SR: Side effects of cephalosporins. *In* Williams JD (ed): The Cephalosporin Antibiotics. Auckland, New Zealand, Adis Press, 1987, pp 105–120.
145. Weiss ME: Evaluation and treatment of patients with prior reactions to β-lactam antibiotics. Clin Top Infect Dis 13:131, 1993.
146. Heckbert SR, Stryker WS, Coltin KL, et al: Serum sickness in children after antibiotic exposure. Am J Epidemiol 132:336, 1990.
147. Lowery N, Kearns GL, Young RA, et al: Serum sickness–like reactions associated with cefprozil therapy. J Pediatr 125:325, 1994.
148. Norrby SR: Problems in evaluation of adverse reactions to β-lactam antibiotics. Rev Infect Dis 8(Suppl 3):S358, 1986.
149. Ammann R, Neftel K, Hardmeier TH, et al: Cephalosporin-induced cholestatic jaundice. Lancet 2:336, 1982.
150. Kelly CP, Pothoulakis C, LaMont JT: *Clostridium difficile* colitis. N Engl J Med 330:257, 1994.
151. Trollfors B, Alestig K, Norrby R: Cecal and gastrointestinal reactions to intravenously administered cefoxitin and cefuroxime. J Infect Dis 11:315, 1979.
152. Lopez AJ, O'Keefe P, Morrissey M, et al: Ceftriaxone-induced cholelithiasis. Ann Intern Med 115:712, 1991.
153. Heim-Duthoy KL, Caperton EM, Pollack R, et al: Apparent biliary pseudolithiasis during ceftriaxone therapy. Antimicrob Agents Chemother 34:1146, 1990.
154. Park HZ, Lee SP, Schy AL: Ceftriaxone-associated gallbladder sludge: Identification of calcium-ceftriaxone salt as a major component of gallbladder precipitate. Gastroenterology 100:1665, 1991.
155. Klion AD, Kallsen J, Cowl CT, et al: Ceftazidime-related nonconvulsive status epilepticus. Arch Intern Med 154:586, 1994.
156. Fekety FR: Safety of parenteral third-generation cephalosporins. Am J Med 88(Suppl 4A):38S, 1990.
157. Elenbaas RM, Ryan JL, Robinson WA, et al: On the disulfiram-like activity of moxalactam. Clin Pharmacol Ther 32:347, 1982.
158. Buening MK, Wold JS, Israel KS, et al: Disulfiram-like reactions to β-lactams. JAMA 245:2027, 1981.
159. Tune BM, Fravert D: Mechanisms of cephalosporin nephrotoxicity: A comparison of cephaloridine and cephaloglycin. Kidney Int 18:591, 1980.
160. Barza M: Nephrotoxicity of cephalosporins: An overview. J Infect Dis 137(Suppl):S60, 1978.
161. Alestig K, Trollfors B, Andersson R, et al: Ceftazidime and renal function. J Antimicrob Chemother 13:177, 1984.
162. Meyers BR: Comparative toxicities of third-generation cephalosporins. Am J Med 79(Suppl 7A):96, 1985.
163. Zhanel AA: Cephalosporin-induced nephrotoxicity: Does it exist? DICP 24:262, 1990.
164. Bang NA, Kammer RB: Hematologic complications associated with β-lactam antibiotics. Rev Infect Dis 5(Suppl):S380, 1983.
165. Spath P, Garratty A, Petz LD: Studies on the immune response to penicillin and cephalothin in humans: II. Immunohematologic reactions to cephalothin administration. J Immunol 107: 860, 1971.
166. Kuwahara S, Miney L, Nishata M: Immunogenicity of cefazolin. Antimicrob Agents Chemother 1:374, 1971.
167. Chenoweth CE, Judd WJ, Steiner EA, et al: Cefotetan-induced immune hemolytic anemia. Clin Infect Dis 15:863, 1992.
168. Garratty G, Postoway N, Schwellenbach J, et al: A fatal case of ceftriaxone-induced hemolytic anemia associated with intravascular immune hemolysis. Transfusion 31:176, 1991.
169. Pakter RL, Russel TR, Mielke H, et al: Coagulopathy associated with the use of moxalactam. JAMA 248:1100, 1982.
170. Nichols RL, Wikler MA, McDevitt JT, et al: Coagulopathy associated with extended-spectrum cephalosporins in patients with serious infections. Antimicrob Agents Chemother 31:281, 1987.
171. Conly JM, Ramotark S, Chubb H: Hypoprothrombinemia in febrile, neutropenic patients with cancer association with antimicrobial suppression of intestinal flora. J Infect Dis 150:202, 1984.
172. Lipsky JJ: Antibiotic associated hypoprothrombinemia. J Antimicrob Chemother 21:281, 1988.
173. Shevchuk YM, Conly JM: Antibiotic-associated hypoprothrombinemia. A review of prospective studies, 1966–1988. Rev Infect Dis 12:1109, 1990.
174. Sattler FR, Weitekamp MR, Ballard JO: Potential for bleeding with the new β-lactam antibiotics. Ann Intern Med 105:924, 1986.
175. Sattler FR, Colao DJ, Caputo GM, et al: Cefoperazone for empiric therapy in patients with impaired renal function. Am J Med 81:229, 1986.
176. Conjura A, Bell W, Lipsky JJ: Cefotetan and hypoprothrombinemia. Ann Intern Med 108:643, 1988.

19

Other β-Lactam Antibiotics

Christine C. Sanders
Kenneth S. Thomson

The β-lactam antibiotics are a large family of diverse compounds each of which contains a four-membered β-lactam ring (Fig. 19–1). There are three major groups within this family. They differ from each other in the general nature of the substituent adjacent to the β-lactam ring.[1] The first group contains compounds with a five-membered ring fused to the β-lactam ring (see Fig. 19–1). Included in this group are the penicillins, which are penams with a sulfur atom located at position 1. Other penams include mecillinam (amdinocillin) and the β-lactamase inhibitors sulbactam and tazobactam. The introduction of a double bond between C-2 and C-3 creates a penem for which there are currently no compounds available clinically. However, several penems are currently under investigation. Substitution of an oxygen at position 1 creates the clavams and clavems, which are oxapenams and oxapenems, respectively. The β-lactamase inhibitor clavulanic acid is a clavam. Substitution of a carbon at position 1 creates the carbapenams and carbapenems, the latter of which include the thienamycins such as imipenem. Similar structural variations are possible within the second major group of β-lactam antibiotics, which have a six-membered ring fused to the β-lactam ring (see Fig. 19–1). The cephalo-

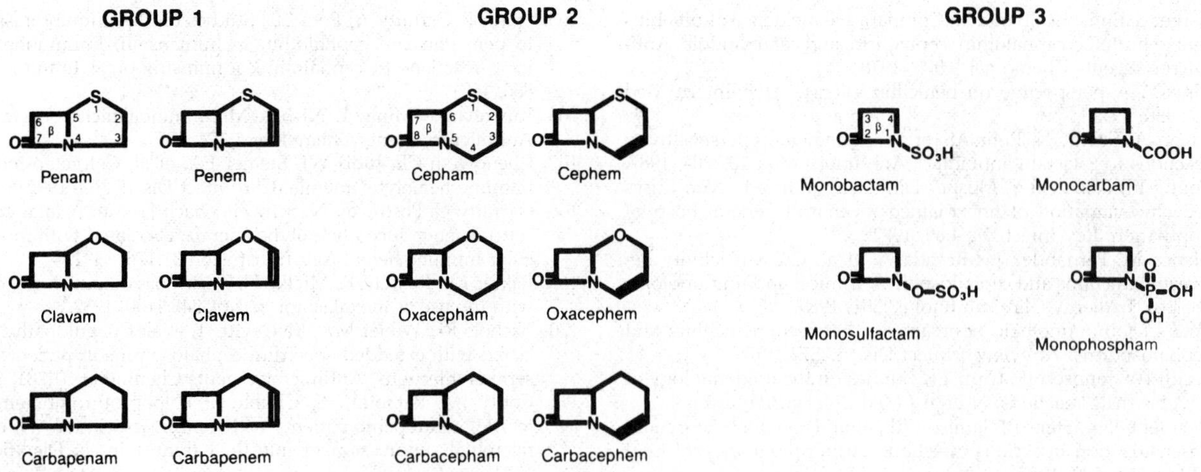

FIGURE 19–1 □ Major structures within the β-lactam family.

sporins and cephamycins are the best known cephem antibiotics. Moxalactam is the only oxacephem approved for clinical use to date. Loracarbef is the only carbacephem approved for clinical use to date. Numerous other compounds within this second group are under investigation. The third group of β-lactam antibiotics contains the monocyclic compounds (see Fig. 19–1). This group includes the monobactams such as aztreonam and numerous related investigative compounds.

This chapter covers β-lactam antibiotics not dealt with elsewhere in this text: the carbapenems, the carbacephems, and the monocyclic β-lactam antibiotics. These groups each contain one compound that is currently available for clinical use, and ongoing research promises new compounds within these groups in the near future.

Monocyclic β-Lactam Antibiotics

Structure-Activity Relationships

Among the monocyclic β-lactam antibiotics, the monobactams have been studied the most intensively.[2–4] These monocyclic, bacterially produced β-lactam antibiotics were discovered as naturally occurring compounds in gram-negative bacteria. They had only weak antibacterial activity, but intensive studies of structure-activity relationships led to the development of the synthetic monobactams, which have good antibacterial activity and stability to β-lactamases.[2–4] Aztreonam, the only parenteral monobactam currently available for clinical use, has the same side chain as ceftazidime and a 4-α-methyl group. Its activity is confined to gram-negative bacteria including *Pseudomonas aeruginosa*.[5] It is not active against gram-positive bacteria or obligate anaerobes, but neither is it susceptible to inactivation by most β-lactamases produced by gram-negative bacteria.[5, 6] Monobactams with simple arylacetyl side chains are active primarily against gram-positive bacteria (Fig. 19–2). α-Methoxylation at C-3 renders such compounds resistant to hydrolysis by staphylococcal penicillinase.[3]

The overall structure of the monocyclic β-lactam antibiotics has also been modified to improve activity against *P. aeruginosa* and to provide good oral bioavailability.[2] SQ 83360 is an investigative monocarbam derivative with a hydroxypyridone function added to the side chain at N-1 (see Fig. 19–2). In tests with *P. aeruginosa*, this modification has enhanced the in vitro and in vivo activity of the compound 3- to 62-fold over that of aztreonam.[2] Unlike penicillin derivatives, phenylglycylmonobactams are poorly active, owing in part to their chemical instability.[3] Thus, development of an orally absorbable monocyclic β-lactam required synthesis of 4-disubstituted monosulfactams such as tigemonam (see Fig. 19–2). This investigative monocyclic β-lactam is similar to aztreonam in its antibacterial spectrum except that it is not active against *P. aeruginosa*.[7]

Aztreonam

ACTIVITY RESISTANCE

Aztreonam is the only monocyclic β-lactam antibiotic currently available for clinical use. It is a synthetic parenteral monobactam with clinically useful activity only against gram-negative bacteria.[5, 8, 9] Like other β-lactam antibiotics, it is bactericidal and interferes with cell wall biosynthesis. It binds primarily to penicillin binding protein (PBP) 3.[8] Among gram-negative bacteria, it is active in vitro against most Enterobacteriaceae, *Aeromonas* species, *Neisseria gonorrhoeae*, *Haemophilus influenzae*, and *P. aeruginosa*, but its efficacy in treatment of infections with some of these organisms has not been documented to date.[5, 8, 9] It is not active in vitro against gram-positive bacteria, obligate anaerobes, and various nonfermentative gram-negative bacteria such as *Acinetobacter* species, *Alcaligenes denitrificans*, and *Achromobacter, Moraxella*, and *Flavobacterium* species.[8] Although it is not readily hydrolyzed by the most prevalent plasmid-mediated β-lactamases,[5, 8, 9] certain enzymes are responsible for resistance to aztreonam. These include (1) the chromosomal β-lactamases found in some strains of *Klebsiella oxytoca*, (2) high levels of chromosomal AmpC β-lactamases found in mutants of various Enterobacteriaceae and *P. aeruginosa*, (3) extended-spectrum β-lactamases that are new derivatives of the TEM and SHV plasmid-mediated β-lactamases and are produced by various Enterobacteriaceae, and (4) plasmid-mediated derivatives of AmpC β-lactamases found in *Klebsiella pneumoniae* and *Escherichia coli*.[5, 8, 10–13] Laboratory mutants less susceptible to aztreonam via nonenzymatic mechanisms have also been described.[14–16] Most of these have been shown to be less permeable to the drug.

PHARMACOKINETICS

Therapeutic levels of aztreonam can be achieved via either intravenous or intramuscular injection but not via oral administration.[8, 9] The time to peak serum levels after an intramuscular dose is 1 hour, and the half-life in serum averages 1.7 hours after parenteral administration. Levels in

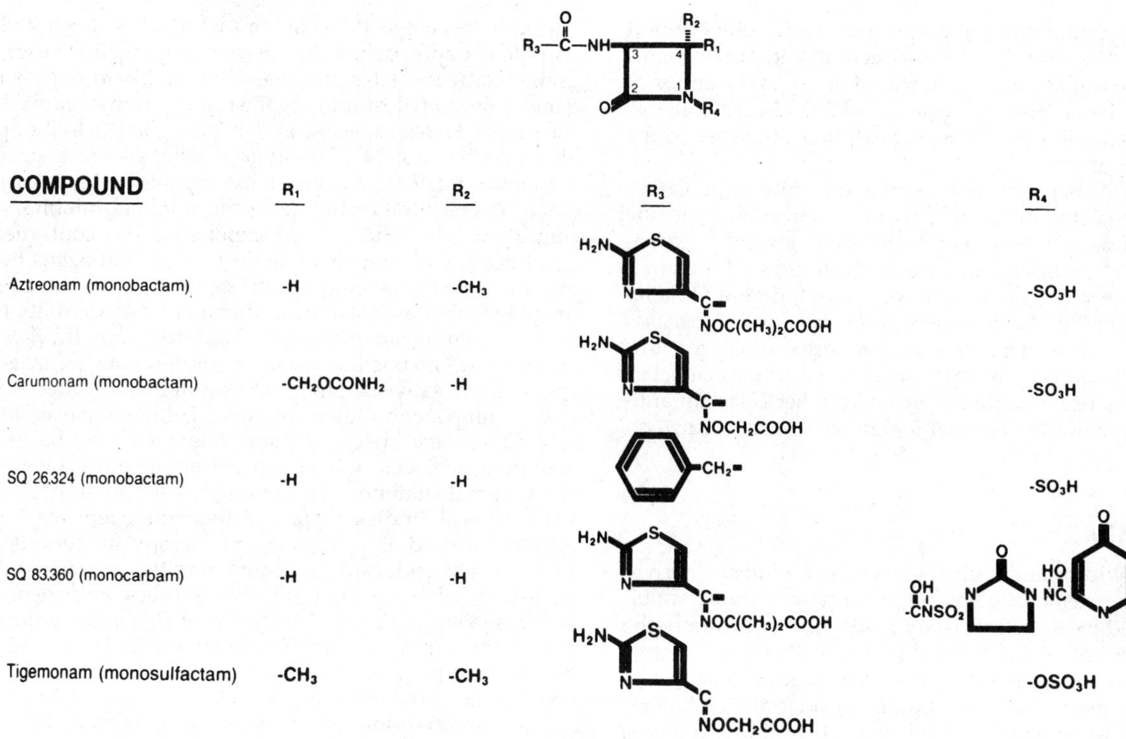

FIGURE 19–2 □ Monocyclic β-lactam antibiotics.

the cerebrospinal fluid are significantly lower than those in serum, even in the presence of meningeal inflammation,[8, 17] and efficacy in meningitis has yet to be investigated thoroughly. Aztreonam is metabolized to a limited extent, and the major metabolite is the biologically inactive open ring structure.[8] Two thirds of a dose is excreted unchanged in urine, and only 1% is excreted unchanged in feces. Twenty-six percent of a dose is excreted as inactive metabolites, half in urine and half in feces.[8, 9] Aztreonam is excreted equally by active tubular secretion and glomerular filtration in the kidneys, and probenecid and furosemide do not significantly increase serum levels of the drug. Aztreonam doses must be adjusted in patients with compromised renal function, and the drug is effectively removed by both hemodialysis and peritoneal dialysis.[8, 9] To date there is no evidence for pharmacologic interactions with other antibiotics that might be used in combination with aztreonam.[18]

ADVERSE REACTIONS

The safety profile of aztreonam seems to be similar to that of most other β-lactam antibiotics.[19, 20] The most commonly encountered side effects include local reaction at the infusion site (1.7%), rash (1.8%), nausea and vomiting (0.6%), and diarrhea (0.8%). Pseudomembranous colitis has been reported in patients receiving aztreonam, although its occurrence is quite low.[19] Superinfections, when they occur, are often due to gram-positive bacteria, especially the enterococci.[8, 21] Cross-allergenicity between aztreonam and other β-lactam antibiotics is quite low.[8, 22] Thus, aztreonam may be a valuable therapeutic agent for patients with known allergy to penicillin or other β-lactam antibiotics.

CLINICAL USE

Clinical trials have shown aztreonam to be effective in the treatment of a variety of infections with gram-negative bacteria. These include both complicated and uncomplicated urinary tract infections, lower respiratory tract infections, septicemia, skin and skin structure infections, intraabdominal infections, and gynecologic infections including endometritis and pelvic cellulitis.[8, 9, 23] Because of its relatively narrow spectrum, aztreonam is not recommended for empirical therapy in clinical settings that might involve gram-positive bacteria or obligate anaerobes; however, because of its low cross-allergenicity with other β-lactam antibiotics, it is a useful therapeutic alternative for patients allergic to penicillins or cephalosporins. Although not approved for use in children or neonates, aztreonam may ultimately prove useful in certain pediatric settings.[24] These include treatment of pyelonephritis, use for patients allergic to penicillins or cephalosporins (especially those with cystic fibrosis), and use for patients who cannot tolerate the disruption of the gastrointestinal tract flora that broader spectrum β-lactam antibiotics produce.

Carbapenems

Structure-Activity Relationships

The thienamycins, the first carbapenems to be discovered, are naturally occurring antibiotics produced by *Streptomyces cattleya*.[25] Now this family has grown to include compounds produced by diverse microorganisms as well as synthetic antibiotics.[26] The nucleus of the carbapenems resembles that of a penicillin except that a carbon atom has been substituted for the sulfur atom at position 1 in the five-membered ring and there is a double bond in that ring (see Fig. 19–1). The carbapenems are highly active in vitro against most aerobic and anaerobic bacteria, including many that are resistant to other β-lactam antibiotics.[27] At C-6, the carbapenems possess an alkyl or substituted alkyl group. Carbapenems that have a side chain in the trans conformation at C-6 are resistant to hydrolysis by most β-lactamases.[25, 28] This conformation is different from that of other β-lactams, which have an acylamino substituent in the cis position as the side chain at C-6 or C-7. The anti-*Pseudomonas* activity of carbapenems appears to be due to the attachment of an exocyclic sulfur at C-2[25, 28] (Fig. 19–3). The side chain at C-2 is also responsible for susceptibility to hydrolysis by dipeptidases located in the brush border of the kidney.[28]

Inhibition of β-lactamase activity is a feature of all carbapenems that is due either to enzyme inactivation or to the formation of long-lived enzyme-drug complexes.[29, 30] Carbapenems are also strong inducers of Bush group 1 enzymes and various chromosomal metalloenzymes found in *Stenotrophomonas* (formerly *Xanthomonas*) *maltophilia* and *Aeromonas hydrophila*.[31, 32] The structural feature responsible for this strong inducer potency is unknown; however, this characteristic precludes use of carbapenems with other β-lactam antibiotics because of the potential for antagonism to occur.

Imipenem

ACTIVITY RESISTANCE

Imipenem (*N*-formimidoylthienamycin) is a synthetic derivative of thienamycin, a potent but chemically unstable antibiotic produced by *S. cattleya* (see Fig. 19–3). It is currently the only carbapenem available for clinical use. It is highly active in vitro against gram-positive and gram-negative bacteria as well as obligate anaerobes.[25–31] Like other β-lactam antibiotics, imipenem is bactericidal and inhibits cell wall biosynthesis; however, unlike other β-lactam antibiotics, its major lethal targets in most bacteria are PBP 1 and PBP 2.[26, 27, 30] The potency of imipenem in vitro against gram-negative bacteria has been attributed to resistance to hydrolysis by β-lactamases, the relatively small number of lethal targets in the cell, and good penetration through the outer membrane. Good penetration into gram-negative bacteria has been attributed to its small size and the zwitterionic nature of the molecule.[26, 28] In *P. aeruginosa*, penetration appears to be further enhanced by a selective porin that permits entry of imipenem.[33]

Imipenem has the broadest antibacterial spectrum of any currently available β-lactam. Initial studies suggested that its potency approached that of penicillin against susceptible gram-positive isolates and was comparable to that of third-generation cephalosporins against most gram-negative bacteria except *Proteus* species, and it had good activity against all anaerobes except *Clostridium difficile* and rare strains of *Bacteroides fragilis*.[31] Against most organisms it was bactericidal at concentrations close to the minimal inhibitory concentration.[27, 31, 34] Subsequent experience has confirmed the good activity of imipenem against many pathogens but has also identified gaps in its spectrum, emerging resistance, and organisms that are tolerant to therapeutic concentrations.[34–40] Among gram-positive bacteria, *Corynebacterium* JK, *Enterococcus faecium*, methicillin-resistant *Staphylococcus aureus*, and coagulase-negative staphylococci should be regarded as resistant to imipenem. Other enterococci, *Listeria monocytogenes*, and *Clostridium* species exhibit tolerance (i.e., bactericidal activity is achieved only at concentrations much higher than the minimal inhibitory concentrations for these organisms). Early clinical studies suggested that imipenem may not be effective if used as a single-agent therapy for serious infections such as endocarditis and meningitis caused by tolerant bacteria.[36, 37, 40, 41] For gram-negative aerobes, imipenem is not active against *S. (X.) maltophilia*, most *Burkholderia* (formerly *Pseudomonas*) *cepacia*, many flavobacteria, an increasing number of strains of *P. aeruginosa*, and rare strains of *Proteus* species and *Serratia marcescens*.[38, 39]

Three mechanisms of resistance to imipenem have been documented to date: altered target, drug hydrolysis, and decreased penetration of imipenem across the outer membrane of gram-negative bacteria. In gram-positive bacteria, altered PBPs are responsible for imipenem resistance as well as tolerance in strains of staphylococci, pneumococci, and enterococci.[29, 42] Resistance mechanisms have not been elucidated in *Corynebacterium* JK, *L. monocytogenes*, or *Clostridium* species. Resistance has emerged during therapy of infections caused by enterococci and methicillin-resistant staphylococci.[37, 39] Imipenem-hydrolyzing enzymes have been reported in some infrequently isolated gram-negative pathogens.[30, 34] and in a variety of common gram-negative pathogens.[13, 30, 34, 43–47] *S. (X.) maltophilia, A. hydrophila, Flavobacterium odoratum, Legionella gormanii*, and rare strains of *B. fragilis, P. aeruginosa*, and *S. marcescens* produce metallo-β-lactamases that hydrolyze imipenem and require zinc as a cofactor.[13] In a study of seven hospitals in the midland of Japan, 19% of strains of *S. marcescens* recovered from patients were resistant to imipenem, and those with high-level resistance produced a metallo-β-lactamase.[48] Thus, strains producing these enzymes, although once rare, may be on the increase. In addition to these metallo-β-lactamases, other enzymes capable of hydrolyzing imipenem have been reported.[13, 49, 50] These have been found in rare strains of *Enterobacter cloacae* and *S. marcescens*. Resistance attributed to diminished permeability has emerged during imipenem therapy of infections caused by *P. aeruginosa, Proteus* species, *E. cloacae*, and *S. marcescens*.[27, 29, 39, 45, 51, 52] In *E. cloacae*, diminished permeability combined with production of high levels of AmpC β-lactamase is required for resistance to imipenem, whereas in most *P. aeruginosa* strains diminished permeability alone can produce resistance.[47] In *P. aeruginosa*, imipenem resistance emerges more frequently than it does in other organisms and is associated with loss of the D2 (Opr) porin in the outer membrane.[51, 53] Because this porin is specific for diffusion of certain basic amino acids and small peptides containing them, resistance emerges solely to the carbapenems—the only β-lactams that use this porin pathway.[54]

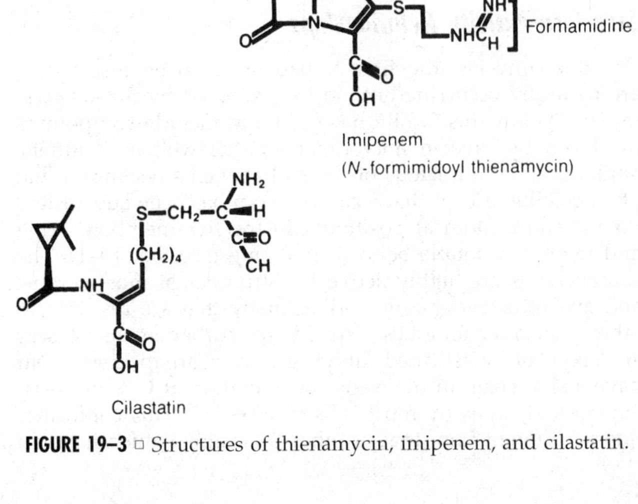

FIGURE 19–3 □ Structures of thienamycin, imipenem, and cilastatin.

PHARMACOKINETICS

Imipenem is not absorbed orally. After intravenous administration, it is readily hydrolyzed by the mammalian renal dipeptidase, dehydropeptidase I (DHP-I), located on the luminal surface of proximal tubular cells.[54] This postexcretory metabolism is a unique phenomenon that does not occur with other major groups of β-lactam antibiotics. Degradation caused by DHP-I results in loss of antibacterial activity in the urine and the formation of a product that in animals exhibits nephrotoxicity similar to that of cephaloridine.[54] This problem has been overcome by coadministering imipenem in a 1:1 ratio with the DHP inhibitor cilastatin[27, 34] (Fig. 19–4; see Fig. 19–3).

In patients with normal renal function, imipenem and cilastatin when administered intravenously have similar kinetic parameters, both having serum half-lives of about 1 hour.[27] In such patients, 50% of an administered dose of imipenem is eliminated by glomerular filtration, 25% by active renal tubule secretion, and 25% by nonrenal mechanisms.[27] The concurrent administration of probenecid blocks tubule secretion of imipenem and extends its half-life. In neonates, the elderly, and patients with diminished renal function, the half-lives of both imipenem and cilastatin are increased. Cilastatin, which is much less subject to extrarenal metabolism, tends to accumulate if therapeutic levels of imipenem are maintained and renal function is severely impaired.[30, 55] In complete renal failure the serum half-life is 3.5 to 4 hours for imipenem and 16 hours for cilastatin. Hemodialysis substantially removes imipenem and cilastatin.[27] Intravenous imipenem is well distributed in most tissues and fluids; only 20% binds to plasma proteins. Cerebrospinal fluid levels of imipenem are significantly lower than serum levels, even in the presence of inflamed meninges.[27, 56]

ADVERSE REACTIONS

The major adverse effects of intravenous imipenem-cilastatin are gastrointestinal, such as nausea (2.0%), diarrhea (1.8%), and vomiting (1.5%); allergic reactions (2.7%); phlebitis or erythema at the infusion site (3.1%); transiently elevated liver function tests (1.0%); and seizures (0.4%). Seizures usually occur in elderly persons or in patients with underlying abnormalities of the central nervous system.[26, 57–59] Other associated predisposing factors include renal impairment and chronic alcoholism.[26, 45, 56, 58] Anticonvulsant therapy and dosage adjustment or withdrawal of antibiotics are required if seizures occur.[27, 45, 58] Dosage adjustment is also required for patients with diminished renal function (creatinine clearance rate ≤ 70 mL/min) to avoid induction of seizures.[60] Colonization and superinfection—particularly by fungi and imipenem-resistant pseudomonads—occur in 16% or less of patients receiving imipenem-cilastatin. Pseudomembranous

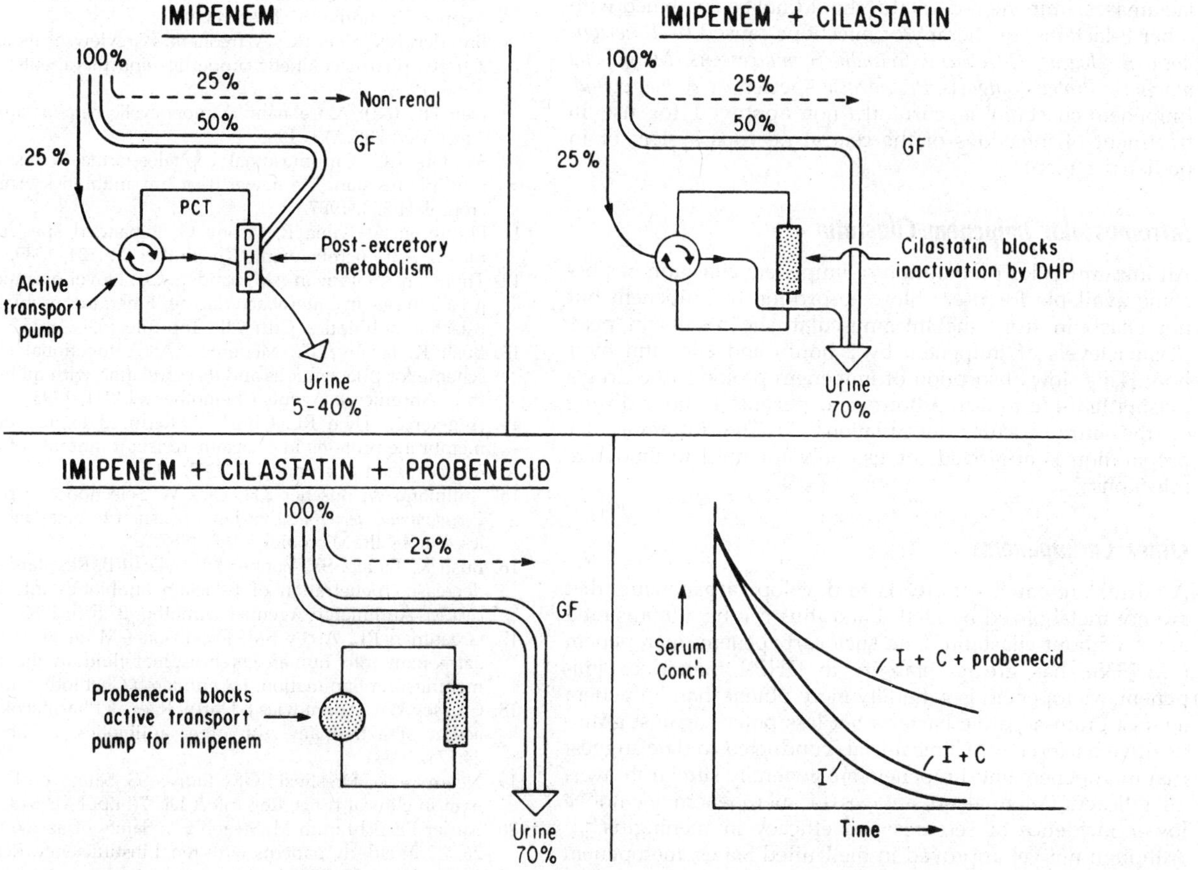

FIGURE 19–4 □ Imipenem administered by itself *(upper left)* has a serum half-life of about 1 hour. About 25% is eliminated by nonrenal mechanisms, 50% by glomerular filtration (GF), and 25% by active tubular secretion; however, both filtered and secreted drug is metabolized by the dehydropeptidase (DHP) enzyme on the brush border of the proximal convoluted tubular (PCT) cell, so that only 5% to 40% reaches the urine. Coadministration of cilastatin *(upper right)* inhibits the DHP enzyme and allows most renally eliminated imipenem to reach the urine. For reasons that are not clear, cilastatin (C) slightly increases serum levels of imipenem (I) without changing its serum half-life *(bottom right)*. Addition of probenecid *(bottom left)* blocks the active transport pump for imipenem by diverting all renal elimination to glomerular filtration. Impairment of active tubule secretion by probenecid prolongs the serum half-life of imipenem *(bottom right)*. (From Barza M: Imipenem: First of a new class of beta-lactam antibiotics. Ann Intern Med 103:552–560, 1985.)

colitis has also been reported (0.1%). There is no evidence of renal impairment or bleeding related to therapy with imipenem-cilastatin.[27, 45, 56, 57, 59] Imipenem is contraindicated for patients with a history of β-lactam allergy. The 2.7% incidence of allergy was observed in trials that excluded patients with serious β-lactam allergy and may therefore underestimate the true incidence of allergic reactions to imipenem-cilastatin.[27]

CLINICAL USE

In general, intravenous imipenem-cilastatin should be regarded as a reserve antibiotic for the treatment of hospital-acquired infections caused by multiantibiotic-resistant bacteria and complicated polymicrobial infections caused by mixtures of aerobic and anaerobic bacteria. Clinical trials have demonstrated imipenem-cilastatin efficacy in a range of infections of lower respiratory tract, abdomen, female reproductive tract, bones and joints, skin, and soft tissues and in bacteremia. It is relatively expensive and should not be used when cheaper or narrower spectrum antibiotics would suffice. Indiscriminate use escalates costs and promotes the emergence of resistant bacteria.[27, 45, 56]

Imipenem-cilastatin should not be used for therapy of infections caused by methicillin-resistant staphylococci or as monotherapy for serious *Pseudomonas* or *Enterococcus* infections. Because of its ability to induce certain chromosomal β-lactamases, imipenem-cilastatin should not be combined with other β-lactams for therapy of infections caused by *P. aeruginosa, E. cloacae, Citrobacter freundii, S. marcescens, Morganella morganii, Proteus vulgaris, Providencia* species, or *A. hydrophila*. Imipenem-cilastatin is currently not approved for use in treatment of infections of the central nervous system or in pediatric patients.

Intramuscular Imipenem-Cilastatin

An intramuscular preparation of imipenem-cilastatin has become available for use.[61] Slow absorption of imipenem but not cilastatin from the intramuscular site results in peak plasma levels of imipenem by 2 hours and cilastatin by 1 hour. This slow absorption of imipenem prolongs the drug's plasma half-life to 2 to 3 hours and permits 12-hour dosing of the intramuscular formulation.[62, 63] The intramuscular preparation is approved for use only for mild to moderate infections.[61]

Other Carbapenems

A current research priority is to develop carbapenems that are not metabolized by DHP-I and thus can be administered alone without cilastatin. One such carbapenem, meropenem (SM-7338), has greater stability to DHP-I than does imipenem. Meropenem is generally more potent than imipenem against gram-negative bacteria but less potent against gram-positive bacteria.[64, 65] Clinical trials conducted to date suggest that meropenem and imipenem are generally similar in overall efficacy. Potential advantages of meropenem include a lower incidence of seizures and efficacy in meningitis.[64–72] Although not yet approved in the United States, meropenem is undergoing review by the U. S. Food and Drug Administration.

Carbacephems

Loracarbef is the only carbacephem currently available for clinical use. It is chemically identical to cefaclor, an oral cephalosporin, except for the presence of a carbon atom at position 1 instead of a sulfur atom (see Fig. 19–1, group 2). Loracarbef and cefaclor are similar in antimicrobial spectrum, clinical efficacy, and toxicity profiles.[73–78] Like cefaclor, it is readily hydrolyzed by most β-lactamases encountered in clinical isolates of gram-negative bacteria and thus would not be a first-line agent for infections with such organisms.[73, 76, 78] As a new synthetic agent, loracarbef is an expensive alternative to older, less expensive but equally efficacious agents.[79]

References

1. Brown AG: β-Lactam nomenclature. J Antimicrob Chemother 10:365, 1982.
2. Sykes RB, Koster WH, Bonner DP: The new monobactams: Chemistry and biology. J Clin Pharmacol 28:113, 1988.
3. Cimarusti CM, Sykes RB: Monocyclic β-lactam antibiotics. Med Res Rev 4:1, 1984.
4. Cimarusti CM, Sykes RB: Monobactams. *In* Grayson M, Eckroth D(eds): Encyclopedia of Chemical Technology, ed 3, Suppl Vol. New York, John Wiley & Sons, 1984, pp 131–144.
5. Sykes RB, Bonner DP: Discovery and development of the monobactams. Rev Infect Dis 7(Suppl 4):S579, 1985.
6. Imada A, Kondo M, Okonogi K, et al: In vitro and in vivo antibacterial activities of carumonam (AMA-1080), a new N-sulfonated monocyclic β-lactam antibiotic. Antimicrob Agents Chemother 27:821, 1985.
7. Tanaka SK, Schwind Summerill RA, Minassian BF, et al: In vitro evaluation of tigemonam, a novel oral monobactam. Antimicrob Agents Chemother 31:219, 1987.
8. Brogden RN, Heel RC: Aztreonam. A review of its antibacterial activity, pharmacokinetic properties and therapeutic use. Drugs 31:96, 1986.
9. Neu HC (ed): Aztreonam: A monocyclic beta-lactam antibiotic. Am J Med 78(2A):1, 1985.
10. Sanders CC: Chromosomal cephalosporinases responsible for multiple resistance to newer β-lactam antibiotics. Annu Rev Microbiol 41:573, 1987.
11. Philippon A, Labia R, Jacoby G: Expanded spectrum β-lactamases. Antimicrob Agents Chemother 33:1131, 1989.
12. Thomson KS, Prevan AM, Sanders CC: Novel plasmid-mediated β-lactamases in Enterobacteriaceae: Emerging problems for new β-lactam antibiotics. Curr Clin Top Infect Dis 16:151, 1996.
13. Bush K, Jacoby GA, Mederos AA: A functional classification scheme for β-lactamases and its correlation with molecular structure. Antimicrob Agents Chemother 39:1211, 1995.
14. Aggeler R, Then RL, Ghosh R: Reduced expression of outer-membrane proteins in β-lactam–resistant mutants of *Enterobacter cloacae*. J Gen Microbiol 133:3383, 1987.
15. Cullmann W, Büscher KH, Dick W: Selection and properties of *Pseudomonas aeruginosa* variants resistant to beta-lactam antibiotics. Eur J Clin Microbiol 6:467, 1987.
16. Bush K, Tanaka SK, Bonner DP, Sykes RB: Resistance caused by decreased penetration of β-lactam antibiotics into *Enterobacter cloacae*. Antimicrob Agents Chemother 27:555, 1985.
17. Greenman RL, Arcey SM, Dickinson GM, et al: Penetration of aztreonam into human cerebrospinal fluid in the presence of meningeal inflammation. J Antimicrob Chemother 15:637, 1985.
18. Creasey WA, Adamovics J, Dhruv R, et al: Pharmacokinetic interaction of aztreonam with other antibiotics. J Clin Pharmacol 24:174, 1984.
19. Newman TJ, Dreslinski GR, Tadros SS: Safety profile of aztreonam in clinical trials. Rev Infect Dis 7(Suppl 4):S648, 1985.
20. Sattler FF, Schramm M, Swabb EA: Safety of aztreonam and SQ 26,922 in elderly patients with renal insufficiency. Rev Infect Dis 7(Suppl 4):S622, 1985.
21. Chandrasekar PH, Smith BR, LeFrock JL, Carr B: Enterococcal superinfection and colonization with aztreonam therapy. Antimicrob Agents Chemother 26:280, 1984.
22. Adkinson NF Jr, Saxon A, Spence MR, Swabb EA: Cross-allergenicity and immunogenicity of aztreonam. Rev Infect Dis 7(Suppl 4):S613, 1985.
23. Acar JF, Neu HC (eds): Gram-negative aerobic bacterial infections: A focus on directed therapy, with special reference to aztreonam. Rev Infect Dis 7(Suppl 4), 1985.

24. Aronoff SC (ed): Aztreonam: New developments in the treatment of gram-negative infection in children. Pediatr Infect Dis J 8(Suppl 4):S99, 1989.
25. Kahan FM, Kropp H, Sundelof JG, Birnbaum J: Thienamycin: Development of imipenem-cilastatin. J Antimicrob Chemother 12(Suppl D):1, 1983.
26. Wise R: In vitro and pharmacokinetic properties of the carbapenems. Antimicrob Agents Chemother 30:343, 1986.
27. Barza M: Imipenem: First of a new class of beta-lactam antibiotics. Ann Intern Med 103:552, 1985.
28. Neu HC: β-Lactam antibiotics: Structural relationships affecting in vitro activity and pharmacologic properties. Rev Infect Dis 8(Suppl 3):S237, 1986.
29. Neu HC: Carbapenems: Special properties contributing to their activity. Am J Med 78(Suppl 6A):33, 1985.
30. Norrby SR: Imipenem/cilastatin. *In* Peterson PK, Verhoef J (eds): The Antimicrobial Agents Annual 3. Amsterdam, Elsevier, 1988, pp 151–157.
31. Braveny I: In vitro activity of imipenem—A review. Eur J Clin Microbiol 3:456, 1984.
32. Sanders CC, Sanders WE Jr, Thomson KS, Iaconis JP: Meropenem: Activity against resistant gram-negative bacteria and interactions with β-lactamases. J Antimicrob Chemother 24(Suppl A):187, 1989.
33. Studemeister AE, Quinn JP: Selective imipenem resistance in *Pseudomonas aeruginosa* associated with diminished outer membrane permeability. Antimicrob Agents Chemother 32:1267, 1988.
34. Birnbaum J, Kahan FM, Kropp H: Carbapenems, a new class of beta-lactam antibiotics. Discovery and development of imipenem/cilastatin. Am J Med 78(Suppl 6A):3, 1985.
35. Berry AJ, Johnston JL, Archer GL: Imipenem therapy of experimental *Staphylococcus epidermidis* endocarditis. Antimicrob Agents Chemother 29:784, 1986.
36. Chandrasekar PH, Levine DP, Price S, Rybak MJ: Comparative efficacies of imipenem-cilastatin and vancomycin in experimental aortic valve endocarditis due to methicillin resistant *Staphylococcus aureus*. J Antimicrob Chemother 21:461, 1988.
37. Chambers HF: Methicillin-resistant staphylococci. Clin Microbiol Rev 1:173, 1988.
38. Kropp H, Gerckens L, Sundelof JG, Kahan FM: Antibacterial activity of imipenem: The first thienamycin antibiotic. Rev Infect Dis 7(Suppl 3):S389, 1985.
39. Neu HC: New antibiotics: Areas of appropriate use. J Infect Dis 155:403, 1987.
40. Auckenthaler R, Wilson WR, Wright AJ, et al: Lack of in vivo and in vitro bactericidal activity of *N*-formimidoyl thienamycin against enterococci. Antimicrob Agents Chemother 22:448, 1982.
41. Lipman B, Neu HC: Imipenem: A new carbapenem antibiotic. Med Clin North Am 72:567, 1988.
42. Carsenti-Etesse H, Durant J, DeSalvador F, et al: In vitro development of resistance of *Streptococcus pneumoniae* to β-lactam antibiotics. Microb Drug Resist 1:85, 1995.
43. Mitsuhashi S: Resistance to β-lactam antibiotics in bacteria. *In* Ishigami J (ed): Recent Advances in Chemotherapy. Tokyo, University of Tokyo Press, 1985.
44. Iaconis J, Sanders CC: Purification and characterization of inducible β-lactamases in *Aeromonas* spp. Antimicrob Agents Chemother 34:44, 1990.
45. Fujii T, Sato K, Miyata K, et al: Biochemical properties of β-lactamase produced by *Legionella gormanii*. Antimicrob Agents Chemother 23:925, 1986.
46. Watanabe M, Iyobe S, Inoue M, Mitsuhashi S: Transferable imipenem resistance in *Pseudomonas aeruginosa*. Antimicrob Agents Chemother 35:147, 1991.
47. Livermore D: Carbapenemases. J Antimicrob Chemother 29:609, 1992.
48. Ito H, Arakawa Y, Ohsuka S, et al: Plasmid-mediated dissemination of the metallo-β-lactamase gene *bla*IMP among clinically isolated strains of *Serratia marcescens*. Antimicrob Agents Chemother 39:824, 1995.
49. Naas T, Livermore D, Nordmann P: Characterization of an LysR family protein, Sme R from *Serratia marcescens* S6, its effect on expression of the carbapenem-hydrolyzing β-lactamase Sme-1, and comparison of this regulator with other β-lactamase regulators. Antimicrob Agents Chemother 39:629, 1995.
50. Nordmann P, Mariotte S, Naas T, et al: Biochemical properties of a carbapenem-hydrolyzing β-lactamase from *Enterobacter cloacae* and clonings of the gene into *Escherichia coli*. Antimicrob Agents Chemother 37:939, 1993.
51. Quinn JP, Studemeister AE, DiVincenzo CA, Lerner SA: Resistance to imipenem in *Pseudomonas aeruginosa*: Clinical experience and biochemical mechanisms. Rev Infect Dis 10:892, 1988.
52. Winston DJ, McGrattan MA, Busuttil RW. Imipenem therapy of *Pseudomonas aeruginosa* and other serious bacterial infections. Antimicrob Agents Chemother 26:673, 1984.
53. Trias J, Nikaido H: Outer membrane D2 catalyzes facilitated diffusion of carbapenems and penems through the outer membrane of *Pseudomonas aeruginosa*. Antimicrob Agents Chemother 34:52, 1990.
54. Norrby SR. Imipenem/cilastatin. *In* Peterson PK, Verhoef J (eds): The Antimicrobial Agents Annual 2. Amsterdam, Elsevier, 1987, pp 144–152.
55. Bégué PC, Baron S, Challier P, et al: Pharmacokinetic and clinical evaluation of imipenem/cilastatin in children and neonates. Scand J Infect Dis Suppl 52:40, 1987.
56. Canadian Infectious Disease Society Committee on Antimicrobial Agents: Imipenem: A new carbapenem. Can Med Assoc J 139:505, 1988.
57. Calandra GB, Ricci FM, Wang C, Brown KR: The efficacy results and safety profile of imipenem/cilastatin from the clinical research trials. J Clin Pharmacol 28:120, 1988.
58. Calandra G, Lydick E, Carrigan J, et al: Factors predisposing to seizures in seriously ill infected patients receiving antibiotics: Experience with imipenem/cilastatin. Am J Med 84:911, 1988.
59. Primaxin® I.V. (imipenem-cilastatin sodium for injection) package insert. West Point, PA, Merck and Co. 1994.
60. Pestonik SL, Classen DC, Evans RS, et al: Prospective surveillance of imipenem/cilastatin use and associated seizures using a hospital information system. Ann Pharmacother 27:497, 1993.
61. Primaxin® I.M. (imipenem-cilastatin sodium for suspension). *In* Physicians' Desk Reference, ed 50. Montvale, NJ, Medical Economics, 1996, p 1727.
62. Kahan FM, Rogers JD: Imipenem/cilastatin: Evolution of the sustained-release intramuscular formulation. Chemotherapy 37(Suppl 2):21, 1991.
63. Onishi A, Otawa M, Hara K: A clinical phase I study on intramuscular imipenem/cilastatin sodium. Jpn J Antibiot 44:860, 1991.
64. Pryka RD, Haig GM: Meropenem, a new carbapenem antimicrobial. Ann Pharmacother 28:1045, 1994.
65. Edwards JR, Turner PJ, Wannop C, et al: In vitro antibacterial activity of SM-7338, a carbapenem antibiotic with stability to dehydropeptidase I. Antimicrob Agents Chemother 33:215, 1989.
66. Rizzato L, Montemurro L, Fanti D, et al: Meropenem versus imipenem: Relationship between microbiological parameters and clinical outcome in lower respiratory tract infections. Curr Ther Res 54:731, 1993.
67. Chmelik V, Gutvirth J: Meropenem treatment of post-traumatic meningitis due to *Pseudomonas aeruginosa*. J Antimicrob Chemother 32:922, 1993.
68. Livingstone D, Gill MJ, Wise R: Mechanisms of resistance to the carbapenems. J Antimicrob Chemother 35:1, 1995.
69. Masuda N, Ohya S: Cross-resistance to meropenem, cephems, and quinolones in *Pseudomonas aeruginosa*. Antimicrob Agents Chemother 36:1847, 1992.
70. Donnelly JP, Horrevorts A, Sauerwein R, de Pauw BE: High dose meropenem in meningitis due to *Pseudomonas aeruginosa*. Lancet 339:1117, 1992.
71. Klugman KP, Dagan R, Meropenem Meningitis Study Group: Randomized comparison of meropenem with cefotaxime for treatment of bacterial meningitis. Antimicrob Agents Chemother 39:1140, 1995.
72. Brismar B, Malmborg AS, Tunevall G, et al: Meropenem versus imipenem/cilastatin in the treatment of intra-abdominal infections. J Antimicrob Chemother 35:139, 1995.
73. Howard AJ, Dunkin KT: Comparative in-vitro activity of a new carbapenem, LY163892. J Antimicrob Chemother 22:445, 1988.
74. Jones RN, Barry AL: Antimicrobial activity of LY163892, an orally administered 1-carbacephem. J Antimicrob Chemother 22:315, 1988.
75. Jones RN, Barry AL: Beta-lactamase hydrolysis and inhibition studies of the new 1-carbacephem LY163892. Eur J Clin Microbiol 6:570, 1987.

76. Pelosi E, Fontana R: In vitro activity and β-lactamase stability of LY163892. Eur J Clin Microbiol 7:549, 1988.
77. Knapp CC, Washington JA II: In vitro activities of LY163892, cefaclor and cefuroxime. Antimicrob Agents Chemother 32:131, 1988.
78. Cao C, Chin NX, Neu HC: In-vitro activity and β-lactamase stability of LY163892. J Antimicrob Chemother 22:155, 1988.
79. Loracarbef. Med Lett Drugs Ther 34:87, 1992.

20

Aminoglycosides

Stephen A. Lerner
Robert P. Gaynes
Lisbeth Nordström-Lerner

The aminoglycoside antibiotics have been a bulwark for treatment of gram-negative bacillary infections for more than 30 years. Their rapid, predictable bactericidal activity has cast them as lead players, especially in blood stream infections. Their potential for synergistic activity with β-lactams and the relative infrequency of permanent aminoglycoside resistance emerging in bacteria during therapy have made these agents ideal for combating the multidrug-resistant organisms, such as *Pseudomonas* and *Enterobacter*, that are often found in nosocomial infections. Although aminoglycosides have the potential for nephro- and ototoxicity, their utility has been enhanced by dosage management based on monitoring of serum levels and renal function. Moreover, allergic reactions and other adverse effects are rare. Thus, despite the advent of new β-lactams and fluoroquinolones, the aminoglycosides continue to serve as important antibacterial agents for serious infections.

History

The first systematic examination of soil microorganisms for antibacterial activity yielded the isolation of the first aminoglycoside antibiotic, streptomycin, from *Streptomyces griseus*.[1] The activity of streptomycin against aerobic gram-negative bacilli was soon compromised by the emergence of resistance. However, the revolutionary use of streptomycin for the treatment of tuberculosis[2] was generally preserved by the advent of combination drug therapy, which reduced the emergence of resistance in *Mycobacterium tuberculosis*. With clinical use, ototoxicity, an important limiting side effect of the aminoglycosides, soon became evident.[2–6] Dihydrostreptomycin (produced by catalytic reduction of streptomycin or naturally by *Streptomyces humidus*) was developed in an attempt to reduce the primarily vestibular toxicity of the drug,[7] but this analog was so severely toxic to the auditory system that it had to be dropped from clinical use.[8–12] With the introduction of effective but less toxic antitubercular agents, streptomycin is used today as a second-line agent for tuberculosis and in the therapy of specific infections such as tularemia, plague, brucellosis, and systemic enterococcal infections. Neomycin, isolated from *Streptomyces fradiae*, was developed to overcome the problem of streptomycin resistance,[13] but it proved to be too ototoxic and nephrotoxic for systemic use[14–18] and has since been restricted to topical application.[19] Paromomycin was first described in 1959[20]; it is used principally as an antiparasitic agent.

A broader spectrum of activity against aerobic gram-negative bacilli was achieved by the isolation of kanamycin from *Streptomyces kanamyceticus* in the 1950s.[21] The broadened antibacterial spectrum of gentamicin, isolated from *Micromonospora purpurea*,[22] including *Pseudomonas aeruginosa* and many kanamycin-resistant strains of Enterobacteriaceae, eventually ushered in the modern era of aminoglycoside therapy. The subsequent development of tobramycin, amikacin, and netilmicin as well as other aminoglycosides that are not used in the United States, such as sisomicin,[23, 24] dibekacin,[25] and isepamicin,[26] was directed toward improved activity against gram-negative bacilli and reduction of nephro- and ototoxicity. The suffix -micin reflects an origin from *Micromonospora* (gentamicin, sisomicin) or a semisynthetic derivative (netilmicin, isepamicin) of one of these, rather than an origin from *Streptomyces* (-mycin).

The research and development of new aminoglycosides have been curtailed, in part by the introduction of potent extended-spectrum β-lactam and fluoroquinolone antibiotics that lack the liability of nephro- and ototoxicity.[27] Nonetheless, the continued activity of aminoglycosides against nosocomial pathogens that are increasingly resistant to other classes of antibiotics, their use in synergistic combination with β-lactams, the relative ease of blood level monitoring and dosage adjustment, and their decreasing cost as they go off patent ensure their place in the antibiotic armamentarium in selected but important niches.

Chemistry

All aminoglycosides consist of a central six-membered aminocyclitol ring linked to two or more amino sugar residues by glycosidic bonds (Fig. 20–1). The aminocyclitol of streptomycin is streptidine, whereas that of all other available aminoglycosides is 2-deoxystreptamine. Spectinomycin (Fig. 20–2), isolated from *Streptomyces spectabilis*, is also an aminocyclitol, but it lacks amino sugars and glycosidic bonds. Although it thus is not strictly speaking an aminoglycoside and its action differs somewhat from that of these compounds, it is generally considered with the aminoglycosides.

The 2-deoxystreptamine aminoglycosides are further classified by their amino sugars. Those in the neomycin family (neomycins and paromomycin) have two aminohexoses and one pentose. Those in the kanamycin family (kanamycins, tobramycin, and amikacin) and the gentamicin family (gentamicin, sisomicin, and netilmicin) have two aminohexoses attached to the 2-deoxystreptamine. The 3-aminohexose in the C ring is kanosamine for the kanamycin family and garosamine for the gentamicin family. Neomycin consists of roughly equal proportions of neomycins B and C; kanamycin is principally kanamycin A, with less than 5% kanamycin B; and commercial gentamicin is the gentamicin C complex, which includes roughly equal proportions of gentamicins C_1, C_{1a}, and C_2. Tobramycin is 3′-deoxykanamycin B; dibekacin is 3′,4′-dideoxykanamycin B. Amikacin is derived from kanamycin A by acylation of the 1-amino group by 2-hydroxy-4-aminobutyric acid. Netilmicin is derived from sisomicin by ethylation of the 1-amino group of sisomicin.

Aminoglycosides are highly polar, water-soluble polycations and are generally stable to heat and to pH change within the range 5 to 8.[28] They interact with penicillins, apparently by nucleophilic opening of the β-lactam ring, resulting in acylation of an amino group of the aminoglycoside to form an inactive amide.[29, 30] Amikacin and netilmicin

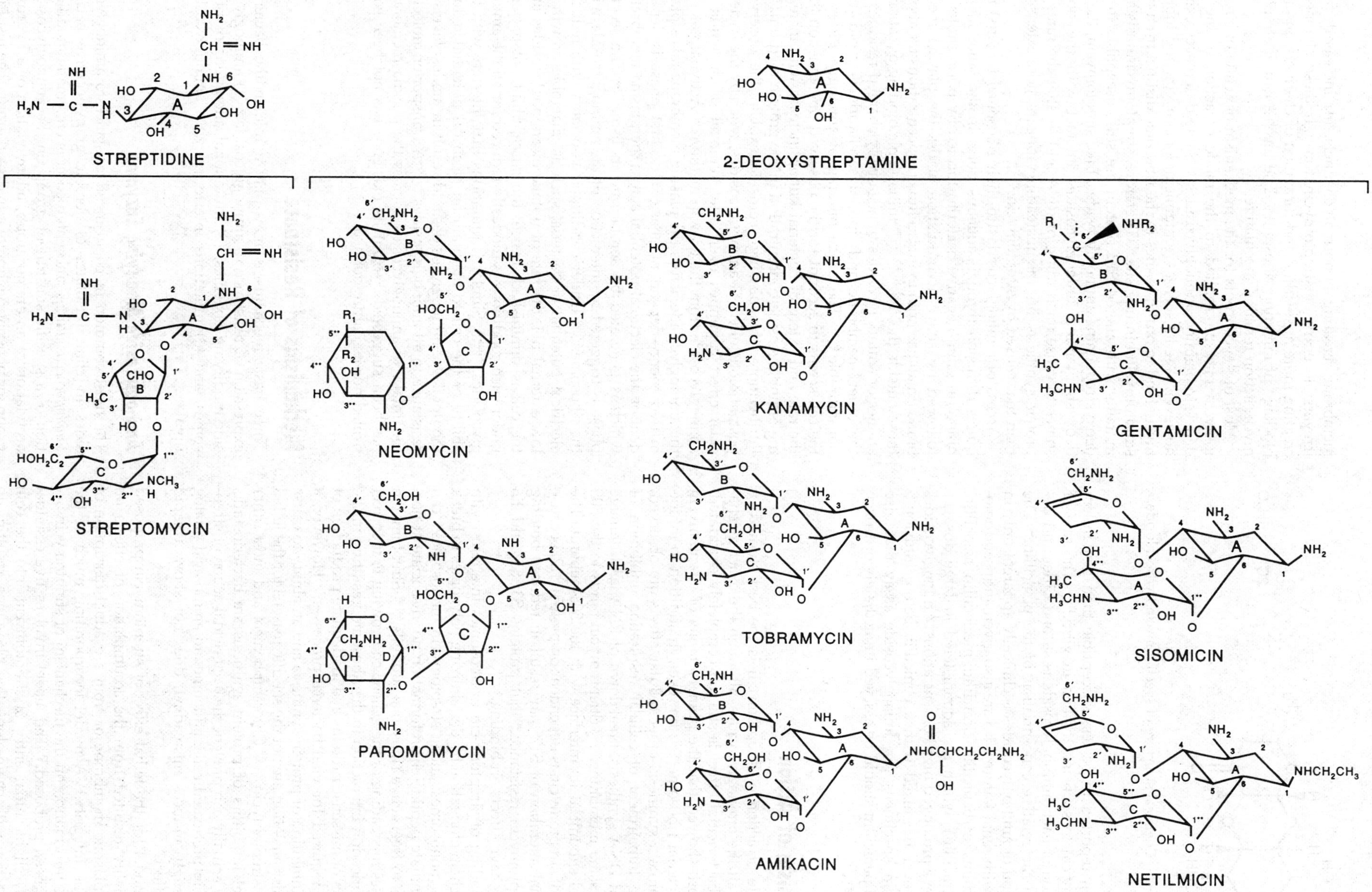

FIGURE 20–1 □ Chemical structures of the aminoglycosides. Neomycin contains approximately equal amounts of neomycin B (R_1 = H; R_2 = CH_2NH_2) and C (R_1 = CH_2NH_2; R_2 = H). Kanamycin is principally kanamycin A (structure shown). Gentamicin is gentamicin C complex, with approximately equal amounts of gentamicin C_1 (R_1 = R_2 = CH_3), C_{1a} (R_1 = R_2 = H), and C_2 (R_1 = CH_3; R_2 = H).

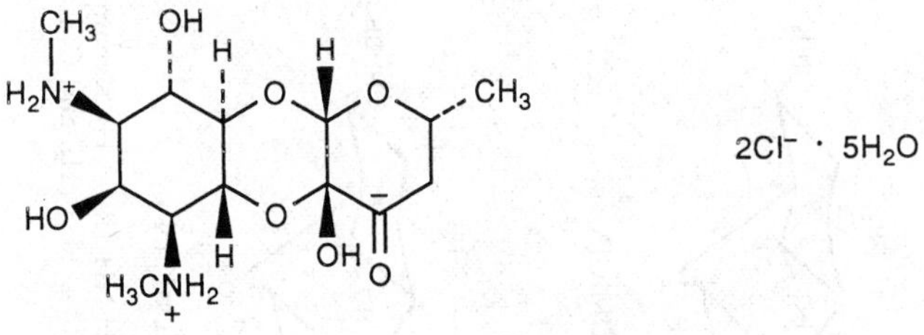

FIGURE 20–2 ▫ Chemical structure of spectinomycin hydrochloride.

have been reported to be less susceptible than gentamicin or tobramycin to such inactivation in vitro.[31–33] The rate of inactivation of each aminoglycoside is second order and depends on the relative concentration of the penicillin.[34] The inactivation of aminoglycosides is clinically apparent only in patients with renal failure who are also given antipseudomonal penicillins (carbenicillin, ticarcillin, mezlocillin, azlocillin, and piperacillin), which are administered in large dosages and achieve prolonged high concentrations. Aminoglycosides should never be mixed with a penicillin before infusion,[35] and serum specimens for aminoglycoside assay that also contain a penicillin should be assayed immediately or frozen until assay.[32]

Mechanism of Action

The mode of action of streptomycin is the best studied of those of all the aminoglycosides, although the exact mechanism of bactericidal effect is still not completely elucidated. Early work showed that the primary target of streptomycin is the bacterial ribosome[36, 37]; however, in addition to inhibition of protein synthesis other cellular effects are observed, including impairment of cellular respiration, inhibition of RNA and DNA synthesis, breakdown of RNA, and damage to the plasma membrane.[38, 39] Streptomycin binds to the 30S ribosomal subunit at its interface with the 50S subunit. The binding of streptomycin is dependent on protein S12, because mutational alteration of S12 may result in reduced binding and streptomycin resistance,[40] but proteins S3, S5, and L6 may also have effects on binding.[41–43]

The binding of streptomycin to ribosomes interferes with peptide chain elongation by destabilizing polysomes to break down to monosomes; such "streptomycin monosomes" can neither initiate peptide chain formation nor dissociate at normal rates to free, active ribosomal subunits.[44–47] Streptomycin also causes misreading of the genetic code owing to incorrect codon-anticodon interaction in the ribosome, resulting in the formation of missense proteins and inadequate production of proteins required for vital bacterial processes.[48] However, a general inhibition of protein synthesis and an ability to cause codon mistranslation are not the specific reasons for the lethal effect of streptomycin.[49, 50] Chloramphenicol and most other ribosomal inhibitors of protein synthesis are bacteriostatic, and they actually can prevent the bactericidal action of streptomycin in pretreated cells; ethionine, an amino acid analog that strongly induces misreading, does not show a rapid killing effect.[51–53]

One model for the lethal effect of streptomycin proposed that lethality resulted from the accumulation of effects on the cytoplasmic membrane or from a gradual disruption of membrane integrity.[49] A model incorporating much of the available information on the mechanism of streptomycin action has been proposed.[53] The model involves five essential steps: (1) slight initial entry of streptomycin into the cell; (2) interaction with chain-elongating ribosomes, resulting in misreading; (3) incorporation of false proteins into the cell membrane, creating abnormal channels; (4) increased and irreversible entry of streptomycin through these channels, creating more misreading and formation of channels; and (5) blockage of initiating ribosomes. The mechanism of streptomycin action remains speculative.

Most of the concepts for the mechanism of action of streptomycin may be applied to the mode of action of the 2-deoxystreptamine aminoglycosides.[54] Some differences exist, however. Agents such as gentamicin, kanamycin, and tobramycin bind to multiple sites in the ribosome distinct from the streptomycin binding site.[55] Therefore, streptomycin-resistant mutants with altered S12 protein are still susceptible to 2-deoxystreptamine aminoglycosides. Like streptomycin, the 2-deoxystreptamine aminoglycosides interact with the ribosomes to cause misreading of RNA and to alter the rates of protein synthesis, but the misreading appears more extensive than that caused by streptomycin.[55]

Access of aminoglycosides to their ribosomal target(s) requires diffusion through aqueous pores in the outer membrane (in gram-negative bacteria) formed by porin proteins, followed by active accumulation across the plasma membrane (in all bacteria) to intracellular concentrations far above those outside the cell.[49, 50, 56–59] Initial ionic binding of cationic amines of aminoglycosides to negatively charged residues of the outer membrane and lipopolysaccharide is rapid and nonsaturable.[60–63] The initial binding of aminoglycosides to the cell seems to account for the observed phenomenon that the rate and extent of bacterial killing increase with increasing aminoglycoside concentration in the growth medium.[64–66] Furthermore, this binding seems to explain the observed postantibiotic effect of aminoglycosides, whereby the bactericidal effect continues even after removal or depletion of aminoglycoside from the growth medium.[67] Active uptake of the aminoglycoside across the plasma membrane takes place in two energy-dependent phases. The first phase is dependent on the electrical potential across the plasma membrane, which is generated by aerobic metabolism.[49, 68] The second phase is triggered by interaction of the aminoglycoside with the ribosome.[49, 59] Under conditions associated with reduced electrical potential of bacteria, such as anaerobic growth or low external pH, the rate of uptake of aminoglycosides into the cell is diminished; hence, the susceptibility of bacteria under such conditions is modestly reduced for all the aminoglycosides.[49, 68–71] Similarly, mutations that interfere with the ability of the cell to maintain an electrical potential reduce the uptake of aminoglycosides and result in modest levels of resistance to all aminoglycosides.[49, 68] A transporter molecule for uptake of aminoglycosides across the plasma membrane has been suggested,[72, 73] but its existence has not been confirmed nor its nature defined.

Mechanisms of Resistance

Three basic mechanisms may play a role in the bacterial expression of resistance to aminoglycosides: (1) aminoglycoside-modifying enzymes, (2) mutational alterations of ribosomes, and (3) mutations interfering with aminoglycoside uptake.

Aminoglycoside-Modifying Enzymes

The most common mechanism of resistance to aminoglycosides in clinical isolates of aerobic gram-negative bacilli, *Staphylococcus aureus*, and enterococci is enzymatic modification of a specific substituent group on the aminoglycoside: acetylation of an amino group, adenylylation of a hydroxyl group, or phosphorylation of a hydroxyl group. The resulting modified aminoglycoside binds poorly to the ribosomes, and the accelerated second energy-dependent phase of aminoglycoside uptake does not occur.[74] The level of resistance to substrate aminoglycosides conferred by modifying enzymes is relatively high, as little unmodified aminoglycoside reaches the ribosomes.[73] The location of these enzymes in the cell has been investigated. Dickie and coworkers[74] concluded that an aminoglycoside-modifying enzyme was loosely associated with the outer aspect of the cytoplasmic membrane. On the other hand, evidence suggests that at least one aminoglycoside-modifying enzyme resides in the cytosol or is loosely associated with the inner leaflet of the plasma membrane.[75] Further evidence against a periplasmic location includes the demonstration that preformed modified aminoglycoside placed outside the plasma membrane is not taken into the cell, even though an aminoglycoside modified by intact cells ends up within the cell.[76] Thus, these enzymes may in some cases inactivate an aminoglycoside substrate as it enters the cytoplasm[75] or perhaps during its transport across the plasma membrane.[73]

A diverse array of aminoglycoside-modifying enzymes and the frequent clustering of their genes on plasmids account for the variety of patterns of cross-resistance to the aminoglycosides seen in different strains.[73] Enzymes that attack different substituent sites may, of course, have different substrate specificities.[77] Even families of isoenzymes that carry out the same modification of the same substituent at the same site on a variety of aminoglycosides may have different specificities across the spectrum of substrates.[78] In some cases, demonstration of activity against an aminoglycoside substrate in vitro may not be reflected as resistance to the aminoglycoside in vivo. This results from the fact that the Michaelis constant K_m of the substrate is so high (i.e., the affinity of the enzyme for the substrate is so poor) that there is little enzymatic modification at the concentrations encountered in the cell.[79–81]

There are several clinical implications of the observation that the majority of aminoglycoside resistance in clinical isolates is determined by enzymatic modification. Whereas the emergence of β-lactamase–mediated resistance to β-lactams occurs readily by derepression of enzyme synthesis[82, 83] or by mutational alteration of substrate specificity,[84, 85] the appearance of new enzyme-mediated aminoglycoside resistance in a strain as a result of mutation is rare. Thus, the aminoglycoside resistance pattern within a strain is generally stable. On the other hand, the location of the genes for most aminoglycoside-modifying enzymes on plasmids[86, 87] allows ready transfer of enzyme-mediated resistance between strains of a species and even from species to species. Thus, introduction of a plasmid R factor into a hospital environment can dramatically change aminoglycoside resistance patterns within its nosocomial strains.[88, 89] The demonstration of genes for aminoglycoside-modifying enzymes on transposons has increased the complexity of assortment of resistance to aminoglycosides and other antibiotics within strains.[89] Thus, it is important to monitor aminoglycoside resistance patterns in the nosocomial pathogens periodically within each hospital as a guide to initiation of therapy.

In an attempt to circumvent enzymatic resistance to aminoglycosides, semisynthetic aminoglycosides such as amikacin have been developed; the formation of amikacin by substitution of kanamycin A at its 1-*N* site reduces the efficiency of enzymatic modification of the resulting amikacin at most of its target substituents.[90] Thus, in the past, resistance to amikacin was conferred only by 6′-acetyltransferase and 4′-adenylyltransferase activities.[71, 90, 91] However, new 3′-phosphotransferase activity has been found to modify amikacin efficiently and thus to confer high-level resistance to it.[92–94] Fortunately, amikacin resistance is relatively rare in the United States. Isepamicin has been developed because of its effectiveness against amikacin-resistant strains that have aminoglycoside acetyltransferase 6′-I, which is relatively common in Japan.[95]

Alterations in Ribosomal Aminoglycoside Binding Sites

Streptomycin-resistant mutants of *Escherichia coli* that arise in the laboratory have ribosomes that fail to bind radiolabeled dihydrostreptomycin.[40] This type of resistance has been found to occur in clinical isolates of *Neisseria gonorrhoeae*[96] and enterococci.[97] Although mutational changes in ribosomal binding proteins may account for some resistance to streptomycin, this mechanism has been relatively unimportant for resistance to 2-deoxystreptamine aminoglycosides in clinical settings.[71] However, one investigation revealed infection and colonization in a neonatal intensive care unit with a strain of *E. coli* that was multiply resistant to aminoglycosides, apparently from mutational alteration of ribosomes.[98] Such resistance, fortunately, is rare.

Mutations Interfering with Aminoglycoside Uptake

In contrast to the occurrence of β-lactam resistance,[99] the emergence of resistance to aminoglycosides during therapy is considered unusual.[100] Emergence of aminoglycoside-resistant mutants with decreased uptake of aminoglycosides has been observed, however, in aerobic gram-negative bacilli and staphylococci.[73] As a rule, the level of resistance is less than that related to aminoglycoside-modifying enzymes, and there is complete cross-resistance to all aminoglycosides.[73]

In many cases, the resistant isolates are small-colony variants produced by mutations affecting the membrane electrical potential and various components of the electron transport chain.[56, 59, 69, 73] Some of these resistant isolates retain their virulence.[101–103] In other cases the small-colony variants can be less virulent, but such variants can persist during therapy and then revert to the original virulent phenotype after cessation of therapy, causing relapse.[104] Combination therapy with a β-lactam may circumvent this problem.[73]

In some cases, especially with *P. aeruginosa*, decreased aminoglycoside uptake is not associated with altered membrane electrical potential or electron transport or with abnormal aerobic growth.[73] Such permeability mutants may have an alteration in the outer membrane[105] or the lipopolysaccharide,[106] and in some cases the responsible alterations have not been demonstrated.[107]

Although chromosomal mutations reducing the uptake of aminoglycosides normally cause only low-level resistance, dramatic resistance to an aminoglycoside may arise in the laboratory from such mutations in cells containing a modifying enzyme with inefficient activity against the aminoglycoside that by itself is not sufficient to confer resistance to it.[81] Such synergistic resistance resulting from inefficient enzymatic modification and reduced uptake has not yet been reported in clinical isolates.

A transient resistance to aminoglycosides develops after the early, concentration-dependent phase of rapid killing after exposure of bacteria to an aminoglycoside.[108] This period of refractoriness to the bactericidal effect of aminoglycosides lasts for several hours and is maximal during recovery of growth after the postantibiotic effect. It depends on the temporary cessation of energy-dependent uptake of aminoglycosides into the bacteria, and it seems to be an adaptive response rather than a result of selection of unstable mutants.

Epidemiology of Aminoglycoside Resistance

Several hospitals have reported their experience with aminoglycoside-resistant organisms.[71, 109–118] The following organisms account for 93% to 100% of the aminoglycoside-resistant clinical isolates in these reports: *P. aeruginosa, Stenotrophomonas* (formerly *Xanthomonas*) *maltophilia, Burkholderia* (formerly *Pseudomonas*) *cepacia*, other *Pseudomonas* sp., *Serratia marcescens, Klebsiella* sp., *Enterobacter* sp., *E. coli, Proteus-Providencia-Morganella* sp., *Haemophilus* sp., and *Acinetobacter calcoaceticus* var. *anitratus* and var. *lwoffi*. High-level resistance to aminoglycosides may also be an important problem in enterococci[119–124] and *S. aureus*.[125, 126]

In general, activity of aminoglycosides has held up well over the years. A report of antimicrobial resistance rates among almost 34,000 isolates of aerobic gram-negative bacilli from patients in 396 intensive care units across the United States revealed rates of susceptibility to gentamicin, tobramycin, and amikacin each greater than 90% for *E. coli, Klebsiella pneumoniae*, and *Enterobacter* spp. For *P. aeruginosa*, the rates were 93% and 89%, respectively, for tobramycin and amikacin but only 65% for gentamicin.[127]

Aminoglycoside resistance patterns differ from region to region and among hospitals. These patterns are usually the result of variations in the prevalence of various aminoglycoside-modifying enzymes, which generally confer high-level resistance; however, isolates may also have generalized low-level resistance to aminoglycosides, which is indicative of reduced uptake.[95] Strikingly different resistance patterns to aminoglycosides have been seen among isolates from Japan, Taiwan, and Korea; Chile; and the United States.[95] Of the aminoglycoside-resistant strains from East Asia, 88% showed some type of 6′-acetylating activity that conferred resistance to the aminoglycosides most widely used there—dibekacin, kanamycin, and amikacin. Among the isolates from Chile, almost 94% had 3-acetylating activity, but those isolates appeared to be from a single hospital outbreak. In the United States, where gentamicin is the most widely used aminoglycoside and gentamicin resistance was seen in 92% of isolates that were resistant to at least one aminoglycoside, resistant isolates were equally likely to have 2″-adenylylating, 6′-acetylating, or 3-acetylating activity.

In addition to variation of resistance mechanisms among geographic regions, it has been suggested by one study that aminoglycoside-resistant isolates of *P. aeruginosa* have a greater frequency of nonenzymatically mediated (presumably because of reduced uptake) resistance than is found in isolates of Enterobacteriaceae, in which resistance was mediated predominantly by modifying enzymes.[128] Other studies have confirmed this finding.[107, 117, 118] Aminoglycoside resistance in *P. aeruginosa* often appeared in mutants after aminoglycoside therapy in patients who had prior carriage of susceptible strains of the same serotype, usually from wound or sputum specimens.[128] Environmental contamination or patient-to-patient spread seemed an unlikely explanation for the appearance of such resistance, so it is not surprising that barrier precautions were less effective in controlling the appearance of aminoglycoside-resistant *P. aeruginosa* than aminoglycoside-resistant Enterobacteriaceae.[128, 129]

Strategies for the control of endemic and epidemic aminoglycoside resistance have been reviewed elsewhere.[130] Traditional control measures include improved aseptic techniques and hand washing, isolation or cohorting of infected or colonized patients, and elimination of any significant environmental reservoirs such as urinary catheters, if possible. Limitation of aminoglycoside use, especially where resistant *P. aeruginosa* has been a problem, may be helpful. Barrier-type "antibiotic resistance precautions" have been used aggressively with considerable success in limiting transmission of most aminoglycoside-resistant Enterobacteriaceae.[128, 131]

Spectrum of Antimicrobial Activity

The principal antibacterial activity of aminoglycosides in vitro is directed against a broad spectrum of aerobic and facultative gram-negative bacilli, including *Pseudomonas, Acinetobacter*, and some other nosocomial nonfermenters.[71, 132–135] Susceptibility is assessed by determination of the minimal inhibitory concentration (MIC)[136] or by other methods, such as disk testing,[137] which can be related to the MIC. Susceptibility is defined as MIC within the range of concentrations that are clinically achievable in blood. The concentration of divalent cations, such as calcium and magnesium, in the medium may have a profound antagonistic effect on the in vitro activity of aminoglycosides, especially against *P. aeruginosa*,[138, 139] presumably by competition for binding sites on the outer membrane or lipopolysaccharide.[63] Supplementation of Mueller-Hinton broth medium with physiologic concentrations of calcium (50 mg/L) and magnesium (25 mg/L) has been adopted as standard for the testing of aminoglycoside susceptibility.[136, 140] Cation supplementation has a greater effect on the MIC of netilmicin for *P. aeruginosa* than is seen with other aminoglycosides.[139] Nonetheless, the clinical efficacy of netilmicin against this organism seemed to correlate better with susceptibility determined with lower or no cation supplementation of broth or with disk testing.[139, 141] Therefore, it has been suggested that testing of *P. aeruginosa* for netilmicin susceptibility be carried out either with disk testing[142] or with lower cation supplementation of broth.[139]

Neither streptomycin nor kanamycin has activity against *P. aeruginosa*. The development of widespread resistance of Enterobacteriaceae to streptomycin and, in hospitals, even to kanamycin has precluded the use of streptomycin and severely curtailed the use of kanamycin against these organisms. Against Enterobacteriaceae, gentamicin, tobramycin, amikacin, and netilmicin are generally equivalently active, although gentamicin is often more potent than tobramycin against isolates of *S. marcescens*.[143] All four aminoglycosides are active against *P. aeruginosa*, although tobramycin is generally more potent than gentamicin.[144] Amikacin is less potent on a molar basis than are the other commonly used aminoglycosides,[145] but the higher serum levels allowable by its lower molar toxicity compensate for this and produce equivalent activity against susceptible strains. There is no evidence that minor differences in potency among aminoglycosides to which a strain is susceptible are reflected in differences in clinical efficacy.

Although there is little intrinsic resistance to aminoglycosides among aerobic and facultative gram-negative bacilli, acquired resistance may reduce the effectiveness of these agents, especially among isolates in major medical centers, where published studies are generally carried out. Because of the aminoglycoside-modifying enzymes that are prevalent in the United States, cross-resistance to gentamicin and tobramycin is common in most hospitals, although some gentamicin-resistant *P. aeruginosa* strains are susceptible to tobramycin. Because it is a poor substrate for many enzymes that modify gentamicin and tobramycin, amikacin has activity against strains that are resistant because of such enzymes; it is thus especially useful where such strains are prevalent. Netilmicin may also be useful against many gentamicin- and tobramycin-resistant strains. Thus, in general, the rank order of aminoglycosides against which there is resistance is gentamicin tobramycin netilmicin amikacin. Nonetheless, because the patterns of resistance may vary among strains, all aerobic gram-negative isolates must be tested individually for susceptibility to the aminoglycosides of interest. As aminoglycoside resistance usually occurs in endemic and epidemic strains within a hospital,[129] depending principally on the content of aminoglycoside-modifying enzymes, it is important for hospitals to maintain updated tabulations of antibiotic susceptibility profiles for their isolates as a guide to initial therapy as well as an indication for epidemiologic measures to contain new resistant strains that may appear occasionally.

Against gram-positive organisms, aminoglycosides have the greatest activity for staphylococci.[71, 146] Aminoglycosides are not used as single agents for staphylococcal infections because of the availability of less toxic agents of more certain clinical efficacy. However, gentamicin may be administered in a regimen with a penicillin or vancomycin for synergistic activity (see the section on synergistic activity). Enterococci and streptococci are resistant to aminoglycosides, although an aminoglycoside (generally gentamicin, occasionally streptomycin) is often administered with a penicillin or vancomycin for synergistic treatment of systemic enterococcal infections and, rarely, for streptococcal infections (see the section on synergistic activity). High-level resistance (MIC 2000 μg/mL) of the aminoglycoside is correlated with enterococcal resistance to synergistic activity, so enterococcal isolates are tested for susceptibility at this concentration as a screen for synergism.[147] *Listeria monocytogenes* is generally susceptible to aminoglycosides, and because of in vitro synergistic activity with ampicillin against this organism, gentamicin is often used with ampicillin for listerial infections.

Aminoglycosides are generally active against *Haemophilus* and *Legionella* species, but they are not used clinically for such infections. Aminoglycosides are also active against *Neisseria* species, but only the aminocyclitol spectinomycin is used for gonococcal infections.

Streptomycin has major activity for *M. tuberculosis*, but kanamycin and amikacin are also clinically active.[148] Amikacin also has clinically useful activity against some atypical mycobacteria.[149, 150]

Aminoglycosides are inactive against anaerobes, including *Bacteroides*, because they lack respiratory quinones and an electron transport chain, and the active uptake that is necessary for activity does not take place under anaerobic growth conditions.[73] Viruses, rickettsiae, and fungi are not affected by aminoglycosides.

Paromomycin has activity against various parasites: *Entamoeba histolytica* and various tapeworms, including *Taenia saginata, Taenia solium, Dipylidium caninum, Diphyllobothrium latum*, and *Hymenolepis nana*.

Synergistic Activity

The demonstration of synergistic activity in vitro[151, 152] between aminoglycosides and antibiotics that interfere with cell wall biosynthesis, such as β-lactams and vancomycin, and the utility of such activity in the treatment of infections in animal model systems[151, 153–155] and in humans[156] have broadened the useful spectrum of activity of the aminoglycosides. The classic example of such synergistic activity is in enterococci, against which combinations of sublethal concentrations of an aminoglycoside and an agent that interferes with cell wall biosynthesis produce a lethal effect.[157] Gentamicin is the most reliably active aminoglycoside, although streptomycin may be utilized if the strain is inhibited by a concentration of 2000 μg/mL.[158] Synergistic effects between an aminoglycoside and a penicillin may also be observed with some strains of viridans streptococci.[159] For enterococci and streptococci, the aminoglycoside may not be bactericidal at clinically achievable concentrations, but combined therapy with synergistic activity is critical for treatment of enterococcal endocarditis,[156, 160, 161] and it may reduce the duration of successful treatment of viridans streptococcal endocarditis.[162] Even though staphylococci and various gram-negative pathogens may be susceptible to the aminoglycoside alone, the use of synergistic combinations may permit reduction of the dose (and presumably toxicity) of the aminoglycoside and/or enhance the overall effectiveness of therapy. The early demonstration that the mechanism of synergism in *E. coli* is enhancement by the β-lactam of the uptake of sublethal concentrations of the aminoglycoside has been confirmed in enterococci,[159, 163] *S. aureus*,[164] and *P. aeruginosa*.[165] In addition to the effects of synergistic activity, the use of an aminoglycoside and a β-lactam may prevent or forestall the regrowth of mutant subpopulations that are resistant to one of the drugs.[151, 166, 167]

Virtually all enterococci fail to be inhibited by clinically achievable concentrations of aminoglycosides, yet synergistic therapy with ampicillin or vancomycin renders most strains treatable.[168] High-level resistance to an aminoglycoside (MIC 500 μg/mL) in an enterococcal strain, resulting from an aminoglycoside-modifying enzyme[169] or, in the case of streptomycin, possibly an altered ribosomal binding site,[97, 170] is generally correlated with a failure of synergism between the aminoglycoside and ampicillin or vancomycin.[168] The aminoglycosides of choice for enterococcal infections are gentamicin and streptomycin. Both agents should be tested against enterococcal isolates, because high-level resistance to one does not necessarily predict resistance to the other.[168, 169] Other aminoglycosides are not useful against *Enterococcus faecium*. Amikacin may be used for an *Enterococcus faecalis* infection if susceptibility to high-level kanamycin is demonstrated; susceptibility to high-level amikacin may falsely indicate synergistic activity.[169]

Pharmacokinetics

The aminoglycosides are sufficiently similar in their pharmacokinetics to be considered as a class.[171–180]

Absorption. Aminoglycosides must be administered parenterally to achieve therapeutic concentrations reliably. For systemic therapy, they are generally infused intravenously, or they may be injected intramuscularly. They are well tolerated by either route. Peak serum levels achieved between 30 and 90 minutes after intramuscular injection are similar to those at 30 minutes after a 30-minute intravenous infusion. Poor perfusion, as in shock, retards absorption from intramuscular sites. Aminoglycosides are poorly absorbed from the gastrointestinal tract after either oral or rectal administration; oral aminoglycosides are quantitatively passed in the feces without alteration.[181] Repeated oral administration of large doses of aminoglycosides, such as of neomycin for alteration of intestinal flora in patients with hepatic encephalopathy, may result in detectable systemic concentrations.[182–192] Rectal and colostomy irrigations could also lead to absorption and accumulation.[193] Such systemic accumulation is exacerbated by reduced excretion in patients with renal impairment. Because of its greater toxic potential, the risk of toxicity with gastrointestinal administration of neomycin is greater than for other aminoglycosides. Similarly, although absorption of aminoglycosides through intact skin is minimal, topical application to large denuded areas, such as burns, ulcers, or wounds, can result in significant accumulation, especially in the presence of reduced excretion related to renal failure.[194–198] Instillation of aminoglycosides into body cavities with large serosal surfaces, such as pleural or peritoneal spaces, may result in rapid absorption by diffusion that is dependent on concentration.[192, 199–202] The risk of toxicity resulting from topical application or irrigation of aminoglycosides is enhanced by the use of neomycin or the presence of renal failure. Detectable, but low, concentrations of aminoglycosides are found in serum after aerosolized or endotracheal administration.[203–205] This may contribute to systemic accumulation, especially in patients with renal failure who are also receiving systemic aminoglycoside therapy.[206]

Distribution. The volume of distribution of aminoglycosides is similar to the extracellular fluid compartment.[180, 207–209] Binding to serum proteins is less than 10% and does not affect their distribution freely into interstitial fluid.[210–212] The α-phase of aminoglycoside pharmacokinetics after intravenous infusion represents the initial rapid decline in aminoglycoside concentration in serum as the drug distributes from the vascular space into its volume of distribution. After this distribution, the serum level is similar to the peak level attained after intramuscular injection.

There is little penetration across membranes into cells, with the exception of the proximal tubule cells of the renal cortex, where they are actively accumulated.[213–215] Because virtually all of each aminoglycoside is filtered through the glomerulus and excreted unchanged in the urine, the peak concentrations achieved in urine may reach 100 times those in serum.[216, 217] In contrast to the situation in the kidney and urine, aminoglycosides enter prostatic fluid poorly.[218] Aminoglycosides penetrate well into most body fluids and spaces, achieving concentrations close to those in serum in synovial fluid, pleural and pericardial spaces, and peritoneal cavity, especially in the presence of inflammation.[219–222] Concentrations of aminoglycosides in bile may approach 30% of those in serum, but they may be reduced in the presence of biliary obstruction.[223, 224] Penetration of systemically administered aminoglycosides into bronchial secretions is poor.[225] For this reason, some have administered aminoglycosides endotracheally as well as parenterally for gram-negative bacillary pneumonia.[226, 227]

The pharmacology of antibiotics, including aminoglycosides, in the eye of the rabbit and of humans has been reviewed.[228] Modest concentrations of aminoglycosides penetrate from the blood into the cornea and aqueous humor, and somewhat higher concentrations are reached in the presence of inflammation. However, more reliable levels are achieved in the cornea and aqueous humor by topical application and subconjunctival injection, respectively. Penetration of aminoglycosides into the vitreous humor after systemic administration or subconjunctival injection is poor, even with inflammation. For this reason, direct intravitreal injection is recommended for the treatment of bacterial endophthalmitis.

The blood-brain barrier of the nonfenestrated capillaries of the central nervous system and the blood–cerebrospinal (CSF) barrier imposed by the specialized epithelium of the choroid plexus[229] result in poor penetration of the highly polar aminoglycosides into the CSF, even in the presence of meningitis, and into the brain and brain abscess.[230] Despite the high concentrations of aminoglycosides in lumbar CSF after intrathecal injection, they are much lower in ventricular CSF because of the caudal flow of CSF from the ventricle.[231, 232] It is thus preferable to administer aminoglycosides intraventricularly as well as parenterally for meningitis. With a CSF volume of approximately 160 mL in the adult, after intraventricular injection of 5 mg of an aminoglycoside, a peak concentration of about 30 μg/mL is expected and is in the range of concentrations found in ventricular and lumbar CSF after distribution.[219] In the neonate, CSF levels resulting from parenteral administration are higher than in the adult.[233] In fact, a prospective, controlled study of the treatment of gram-negative bacillary meningitis in neonates showed no therapeutic advantage of the addition of intraventricular aminoglycoside to systemic therapy over systemic therapy alone.[232]

Elimination. Aminoglycosides are excreted unchanged and virtually completely by the kidneys. They are filtered by the glomerulus, and a small fraction is actively absorbed into proximal tubular cells,[234] as implied by the finding that the renal clearance of aminoglycosides is somewhat less than the simultaneous creatinine clearance.[235] The β (excretory) phase of aminoglycoside pharmacokinetics, which follows the α (distributive) phase, represents renal excretion and thus is correlated with the glomerular filtration rate. Therefore, impairment of renal function leads to a prolonged half-life of aminoglycosides in serum and requires alteration of dosage. A prolonged, slow terminal (γ) phase of excretion probably represents eventual release of drug from the proximal tubule cells into the urine. Whereas the β-phase half-life of aminoglycoside excretion is 1.5 to 3.5 hours,[236, 237] that of the γ-phase is 30 to 700 hours.[238] As the total amount of drug in this deep compartment is relatively small, it has little effect on clinical dosing.

Determination of Dosage Regimen

The goal of aminoglycoside dosing is to adjust the dose and interdose interval to achieve serum levels sufficiently high to be considered therapeutic[239–242] and to avoid excessive drug exposure, which is thought to increase the risk of toxicity.[243–247] The aim is the achievement of peak (drawn about 30 minutes after a 30- to 60-minute infusion or about 1 hour after an intramuscular injection) and trough (drawn within 30 minutes of the next dose) serum levels within generally accepted ranges: for gentamicin, tobramycin, and netilmicin, peak levels of 4 to 10 μg/mL and trough levels less than 2 μg/mL; for amikacin, peak levels of 15 to 32 μg/mL and trough levels less than 10 μg/mL. The levels (and doses) of amikacin are generally three to four times higher than those of gentamicin, tobramycin, and netilmicin, to compensate for the lower antibacterial activity of amikacin on a molar basis. Fortunately, these higher levels of amikacin are not correlated with an increased risk of toxicity. These ranges of desired serum levels are not absolute but rather general guides for monitoring and adjustment of dosage. Clearly, they may be adjusted upward when warranted, such as for an infection caused by a relatively resistant organism or a serious infection at a site to which aminoglycosides penetrate relatively poorly. Of course, use of an aminoglycoside in such situations may be avoided, if possible. Similarly, the range can be adjusted downward if the aminoglycoside is an adjunct to combination therapy or if the infection is localized in the urine, where aminoglycosides are concentrated.

Because several doses may be required before a steady state is reached (four to five drug half-lives), in clinical situations that require rapid attainment of optimal peak serum levels, an initial loading dose is often administered. This is also employed for patients with renal failure whose subsequent doses will be delayed. The peak serum level after a loading dose is determined by the dose divided by the volume of distribution, regardless of renal function. The volume of distribution is estimated to be approximately 0.25 L/kg.[248] Thus, appropriate loading doses for patients with a usual volume of distribution are as follows: 2 mg/kg for gentamicin, tobramycin, and netilmicin; and 7.5 mg/kg for amikacin.

Subsequent maintenance dosing is affected by renal function as well as by volume of distribution. To adjust for reduced renal clearance, one can reduce the individual dose and/or widen the interdose interval. Although the peak and trough levels obviously are interrelated, adjustment of the dose principally affects the peak level and adjustment of the interdose interval principally affects the trough level. Thus, both types of dosage adjustment are generally employed. Various nomograms are used to assist with dosing, a common example being that of Sarubbi and Hull.[249] Although such nomograms are useful for initial therapy, dosing should be verified by actually checking serum levels and making further dosage adjustments accordingly, as the underlying assumptions of uniform volume of distribution and excellent correlation of aminoglycoside clearance with calculated creatinine clearance may not be valid for all patients.[250] Individualized pharmacokinetic dosing, using multiple serum levels and pharmacokinetic analysis, is the most precise method for achieving desired serum levels and is preferred when available. Examples of this approach are the method of Sawchuck and Zaske and colleagues[251–254] and the Bayesian feedback method.[248] Pharmacists may be helpful in implementing such methods. When pharmacokinetically based dosing is not available, dosage regimens should be individualized by trial and error, according to peak and trough serum levels and estimates of renal function. There are no firm guidelines for such monitoring. The serum creatinine level is usually monitored one to three times a week, as long as it seems stable, and more often if renal function is changing. Generally, peak and trough serum levels are checked within about 24 to 48 hours after initiation of therapy, and dosage is adjusted as needed. Once the peak and trough serum levels are in the desired ranges, trough levels are rechecked once or twice a week, because a rising trough level is a sensitive indicator of declining renal function. If the volume of distribution does not change, the peak levels are a constant increment above the trough levels for a given dose. Of course, serum levels should be rechecked within a day or two after any dosage adjustment or in situations of changing renal function or volume of distribution.

Special Situations with Altered Aminoglycoside Pharmacokinetics

The neonate, especially the premature infant, has a large volume of distribution and slower renal clearance than do older children and adults.[255–257] Elderly patients have loss of renal function that may not be reflected simply in the serum creatinine values. Estimates of creatinine clearance, such as that of Cockroft and Gault,[258] take into account age, weight, and sex as well as serum creatinine value. Patients who are cachectic and bedridden may have a serum creatinine value that underestimates impairment of renal function. Cachectic patients, with little fat, may also have a higher proportion of body weight as extracellular fluid. Conversely, obese patients may have a smaller than average volume of distribution on a weight basis,[259–261] so ideal body weight may be better estimated according to height and bone structure. Conditions such as ascites or congestive heart failure increase the volume of distribution, and dosage may have to be adjusted accordingly. Furthermore, these third spaces may fluctuate during therapy, so levels may have to be monitored more frequently. The clearance of aminoglycosides in patients with extensive burns may be increased, owing to increased rate of glomerular filtration and also possibly to oozing of extracellular fluid.[251, 262, 263] As a result, the dosage may have to be increased according to serum levels. Cystic fibrosis patients have a higher glomerular filtration rate and thus clear aminoglycosides more rapidly. Higher dosages of aminoglycosides are required to maintain adequate serum levels, especially considering that the organisms associated with this disease (such as *P. aeruginosa*) are relatively resitant to antibiotics and that there is poor penetration of aminoglycosides into respiratory secretions.[264, 265] It has been reported that febrile patients have increased glomerular filtration rates and therefore require larger doses of aminoglycosides,[266] but that observation has not been widely confirmed. One study reported that febrile neutropenic patients with hematologic malignancy have a larger volume of distribution and rate of clearance for aminoglycosides than do matched control patients, but there was no correlation with fever or leukocyte count.[267] On the other hand, another study failed to find any differences in pharmacokinetics of gentamicin between febrile neutropenic and matched control patients.[268] The inactivation of aminoglycosides by penicillins (see the section on chemistry) has little clinical impact on aminoglycoside pharmacokinetics in patients with normal renal function[269] for the following reasons. The rate of inactivation slows considerably as the concentration of β-lactam drops as a result of rapid excretion and also is slowed in the presence of plasma proteins; and the rate of inactivation of aminoglycoside even at peak serum concentrations of penicillin and aminoglycoside is significantly slower than the rate of normal renal clearance. In the presence of renal failure, however, higher concentrations of aminoglycoside and penicillin interact over longer periods, and the resulting rate of aminoglycoside inactivation is relatively fast compared with the rate of renal clearance. The consequent shortening of half-life of the free, active aminoglycoside may be clinically significant, and dosage should be adjusted according to serum levels.[270–272]

Dialysis

In the anuric patient the half-life of aminoglycosides is increased to 40 to 50 hours.[162, 273–278] Hemodialysis reduces the serum aminoglycoside level by 50% in about 6 to 8 hours.[172, 275, 279, 280] Generally, one half of a loading dose is administered after hemodialysis to replace what has been removed. Actual serum levels should be verified because of poor predictability. Removal of aminoglycosides by peritoneal dialysis may be efficient but is less reliable.[172, 281] For patients without peritonitis, a loading dose is given, and subsequent doses are administered when the serum level drops sufficiently. For patients with peritonitis, after a parenteral loading dose the aminoglycoside may be added to the dialysis fluid at a therapeutic concentration (e.g., 4 to 5 μg/mL for gentamicin, tobramycin, and netilmicin, and 15 to 20 μg/mL for amikacin) and instilled in the peritoneal cavity for local therapy and maintenance of serum levels.

Once-Daily Dosing

The conventional divided daily dosing of aminoglycosides was originally established on toxicologic and therapeutic premises that were preliminary and mainly hypothetic. Subsequently, attention has been given to the attractive possibility of administering the entire daily dose in a single infusion every 24 hours, even in patients with normal renal function.[282–284] Microbiologic considerations suggest that the resulting high peaking serum levels may enhance efficacy. Aminoglycosides, unlike the β-lactams, kill bacteria in a concentration-dependent manner; that is, the higher the concentration, the more rapid the killing and the greater its extent.[285, 286] In fact, clinical studies support a correlation between higher peak serum concentrations of aminoglycosides,[240, 241, 287] or ratio of peak serum levels to MIC for the infecting organism,[242] an efficacy. One might anticipate a therapeutic disadvantage from the long interdose interval, especially in the period when the serum level falls below the MIC. However, such a potential disadvantage may be mitigated by the observed postantibiotic effect with aminoglycosides, in contrast to β-lactams; the bacterial growth continues to be inhibited for a period after the aminoglycoside concentration falls below the MIC both in vitro[288–290] and in vivo.[291, 292] Also, higher aminoglycoside concentrations, which would be expected with once-daily dosing, produce a longer postantibiotic effect.[286] Thus, the postantibiotic effect may prolong killing and inhibition through much of the longer interdose interval produced by once-daily dosing, especially in the presence of adjunctive β-lactam activity or adequate neutrophils. A longer interdose interval might even be advantageous in permitting bacteria to recover their aminoglycoside susceptibility after the refractory period that is maximal during recovery of growth after the postantibiotic effect (see the section on mechanisms of resistance). In animal models of infection, once-daily dosing has been shown to be at least as effective as conventional divided dosing, either with adjunctive β-lactam treatment or in the presence of adequate neutrophils.[286, 292–295]

In animal model systems of nephrotoxicity, the daily administration of aminoglycoside in several divided doses was associated with greater accumulation of drug in the renal cortex and with more nephrotoxicity than was seen in animals receiving the same total dose once a day.[286, 295–298] Continuous infusion of aminoglycoside produced even greater renal accumulation of drug and/or nephrotoxicity, compared with those effects after administration of the entire daily dose in a single treatment.[295, 299, 300] A similar influence of aminoglycoside dosing regimen on renal cortical accumulation of drug has been reported in humans.[301]

Experiments on aminoglycoside ototoxicity in animals have shown less cochlear damage with the total dose given once daily than with multiple divided doses.[302, 303] In similar experiments, however, once-daily amikacin was only minimally and inconsistently less cochleotoxic than the daily administration of the same total amount in three divided doses[304]; another study showed that varying the dosing regimen of kanamycin did not affect the incidence or severity of cochlear toxicity.[305] As with many studies of ototoxicity in animals, renal function was not monitored, so it is possible that the results reflect prior nephrotoxicity causing drug accumulation and potentiating ototoxicity. In animal studies of aminoglycoside uptake into the organ of Corti in the inner ear, the uptake was dose dependent, with rapid saturation kinetics as in the proximal tubule cell of the kidney.[306, 307] Thus, it was postulated that the shorter exposure of tissues to drug with larger but less frequent doses should be associated with less ototoxicity. Indeed, administration of an aminoglycoside by continuous infusion (the ultimate limit of frequent dosing) produced even greater accumulation of the drug in the organ of Corti than was seen when the same total dose was administered in less frequent intermittent doses.[308, 309]

Despite the obvious advantages of cost and convenience and the theoretical and experimental evidence suggesting benefits with once-daily dosing of aminoglycosides, relatively few patients have been studied with such regimens. In no study has once-daily dosing been associated with inferior efficacy or with greater nephrotoxicity or ototoxicity than conventional regimens.[300, 310–318] Although most of the studies comparing once-daily dosing with conventional multiple daily dosing have been relatively small and not all have been appropriately randomized and "blinded," a metaanalysis of the available published clinical studies attempted to overcome some of the difficulties by combining the data from the various trials.[319] This analysis led to the conclusion that once-daily administration of aminoglycoside regimens results in a small but significant improvement in clinical efficacy over that seen with multiple daily administration but that both modes of administration result in similar rates of bacteriologic eradication and drug toxicity. Thus, one can state cautiously that patients with normal and stable renal function can be treated safely and efficaciously for short periods with once-daily administration.

Toxicity

The principal adverse effects of aminoglycosides are nephrotoxicity and ototoxicity. Despite problems with these reactions, other side effects are exceedingly rare. Fortunately, hypersensitivity reactions are rare, allowing the implantation of bone cement and orthopedic beads containing aminoglycosides without fear of allergic reactions. Furthermore, aminoglycosides do not provoke inflammation, which allows their use in orthopedic implants and permits intramuscular injection, intravenous infusion without phlebitis, and instillation in body cavities (e.g., peritoneal and pleural spaces) and CSF. They are not hepatotoxic or phototoxic, nor do they depress bone marrow or derange coagulation. Neuromuscular blockade is a potentially serious, but rare, problem.

Neuromuscular Blockade

The presence of sufficiently high concentrations of an aminoglycoside at neuromuscular junctions can produce blockade, leading to flaccid paralysis and respiratory arrest. Internalization of calcium into the presynaptic region of the axon is inhibited, ultimately preventing release of acetylcholine, and there is blockade of the postsynaptic receptor for acetylcholine.[320] This effect is the cause of acute fatality in experimentally treated animals. Fortunately, it is rare in humans, being seen virtually exclusively in special situations. It would generally require rapid bolus intravenous infusion or rapid absorption from a highly concentrated solution instilled in the peritoneal or pleural space to achieve a sufficiently high concentration at the neuromuscular junction for paralysis. Susceptibility to neuromuscular blockade is enhanced by neuromuscular blocking agents used with anesthesia, excess magnesium, hypocalcemia, botulism, or myasthenia gravis.[320–326] Intravenous aminoglycosides should be infused during 20 to 60 minutes, special care being taken in the presence of potentiating conditions. Established neuromuscular blockade can usually be reversed by the prompt administration of calcium gluconate; response to cholinesterase inhibitors, such as neostigmine, has been variable.[327]

Nephrotoxicity

All aminoglycosides are associated with the development of nephrotoxicity. The clinical manifestation of this toxicity is generally nonoliguric acute renal failure, but virtually all patients receiving aminoglycosides show evidence of early subclinical renal tubular damage,[328] with release in the urine of tubular brush border and lysosomal enzymes,[329–333] tubular casts,[334] and β_2-microglobulin.[330, 331, 335, 336] In practice, these early manifestations are too sensitive and nonspecific to be used as indicators for the development of nephrotoxicity.[337, 338] Therefore, nephrotoxicity is usually assessed as reduction of glomerular filtration rate, reflected in a rise of the serum creatinine value or decline in creatinine clearance. Such determinations are more convenient and more clinically relevant than the sensitive early indicators. A rise of the serum creatinine value may be detected as early as several days after initiation of aminoglycoside treatment, but the risk of toxicity rises with duration of treatment,[247] so the toxicity often is not detected until after 7 to 10 days or more. The degree of decline in creatinine clearance is generally mild, especially if serum levels and renal function are monitored and the dosing is adjusted to avoid excessive accumulation. In rare cases, renal damage may be severe.[339] Renal compromise is almost always completely reversible after cessation of therapy,[283, 338, 340] as the proximal tubule cells regenerate. In animals, tubule cells may regenerate even during therapy, and newly regenerated cells are less sensitive to aminoglycoside damage.[341, 342] This may underlie the finding that renal function of patients with nephrotoxicity may improve even during continued therapy.[343] There may be early polyuria, but there is usually no change in urine volume associated with toxicity.[340, 344] Oliguria may occur rarely with severe toxicity.

The incidence of aminoglycoside nephrotoxicity in published reports of prospective clinical trials varies from 0% to

50%[345] but is generally in the range of 5% to 15%. There are several reasons for the wide variation in reported incidence. First, the defining criteria for toxicity have not been standardized. Various studies have utilized a criterion of a fixed rise in the serum creatinine value, such as 0.5 mg/dL[343]; a two-tiered rise (0.5 mg/dL for baseline less than 3.0 mg/dL and 1.0 mg/dL for baseline 3.0 mg/dL or higher)[346]; a fixed percentage rise, such as 50%[334] or 100% (equivalent to a 50% decline of the calculated creatinine clearance)[244]; or a combination of fixed and percentage rises.[347] It was shown that application of different criteria for nephrotoxicity could significantly affect the observed incidence in the same study.[347] Populations of patients and treatment course vary among studies, and this also contributes to the variability in the reported incidence of nephrotoxicity. Risk factors associated with development of nephrotoxicity have been analyzed in an attempt to identify characteristics of patients and their aminoglycoside treatment courses that might alert the physician to an increased risk,[244, 247] although the applicability of this approach has been questioned and debated.[348–351] Risk factors have included older age, shock, the presence of liver disease, female sex, and duration of therapy. The association of liver disease and nephrotoxicity has been supported by experimental results[352] and by a retrospective clinical analysis.[353] Drugs with their own potential for nephrotoxicity, such as amphotericin B, cisplatin, and cyclosporine, may enhance the renal toxicity of aminoglycosides when they are administered concomitantly. Furthermore, vancomycin, which has little demonstrable nephrotoxicity of its own, has been shown to enhance the nephrotoxicity of aminoglycosides in animals[354] and in humans,[355–357] although other studies have failed to show this effect.[358, 359]

The desire to develop an aminoglycoside with reduced toxic potential has led to numerous comparative clinical studies. With respect to efficacy, there is no evidence of benefit from the use of one aminoglycoside over another with equivalent activity in vitro.[360] Comparative studies in animal models and examination of in vitro attributes have suggested differences in nephrotoxic potential among aminoglycosides.[307, 361] Nonetheless, it is difficult to demonstrate any clinically significant differences in nephrotoxic activity in humans among various members of this class.[345, 360] Although amikacin may be less toxic on a molar basis, it is used clinically and tested for toxicity with doses and serum levels three to four times those for gentamicin and tobramycin to produce comparable antibacterial activity. Neomycin may be more nephrotoxic than other aminoglycosides, and streptomycin may be less toxic.[362] However, these drugs have not been subjected to careful scrutiny by prospective, comparative testing with current standards for assessment of toxicity.

Elements of the mechanisms of aminoglycoside nephrotoxicity have been elucidated in animal models.[307, 344, 363, 364] After filtration of aminoglycosides through the glomerulus, a small fraction is actively accumulated by proximal tubule cells, with initial binding to phospholipids of the brush border membrane, such as phosphatidylinositol, and subsequent internalization by pinocytosis. This uptake into proximal tubule cells produces concentrations of 1 to 2 mg per gram of tissue in the renal cortex and represents the deep compartment from which the third phase of excretion has a prolonged half-life. The pinocytotic vesicles formed by uptake fuse with lysosomes, where phospholipids accumulate into osmiophilic, lamellar structures, called myeloid bodies, probably as a result of inhibition of lysosomal phospholipases by the aminoglycosides. Binding of aminoglycosides to the basolateral membranes of proximal tubule cells may also be important for the inhibition of membrane-bound sodium-potassium adenosinetriphosphatase. Mitochondria become altered structurally and functionally, perhaps as a result of the observed overwhelming phospholipidosis and rupture of lysosomes with release of their contents. Necrosis of tubule cells and shedding of debris into the tubular lumen ensue. The mechanism of the consequent decline in glomerular filtration has not been established, although various hypotheses have been proposed.[320, 365–369] After cessation of aminoglycoside exposure, and sometimes even before, regeneration of tubule cells begins and usually proceeds to completion. This is followed by restoration of tubular function and generally complete recovery of baseline glomerular filtration. The observation[370] that the concomitant administration of polyaspartic acid prevents the pathophysiologic effects of gentamicin nephrotoxicity in the rat model is of great interest, especially because it has no effect on the antibacterial activity of the drug. Because polyaspartic acid enhances the uptake of gentamicin into tubule cells, the nature of its protective effect remains to be determined. The applicability of such protective therapy in humans requires exploration.

Ototoxicity

All aminoglycosides are associated with the risk of development of ototoxicity. However, severe symptomatic ototoxicity is now rare, in part because of careful monitoring of renal function and serum levels, with appropriate dosage adjustment. It has been stated that different aminoglycosides cause toxicity predominantly for one or the other modality of inner-ear function,[327] but certainly auditory (cochlear) and vestibular toxicity can occur with any aminoglycoside.[345, 347, 371, 372] Clinical symptoms of auditory toxicity may appear as hearing loss or tinnitus, but patients sometimes report merely a feeling of fullness in the ear. Symptoms of severe vestibular toxicity may appear as nausea, vomiting, vertigo, nystagmus, and/or difficulty with gait, especially in the dark or on uneven ground. Some patients report difficulty in fixating visually on objects, especially when the head is moving, such as reading signs or recognizing faces while walking; others report simply a vague feeling of queasiness. Reports of dizziness are common in hospitalized patients but may represent other causes, such as postural hypotension when getting up from the bed.

An individual may sustain cochlear and/or vestibular damage,[347, 372] and ototoxicity may affect one or both inner ears.[347, 372] The ototoxic effect may progress after cessation of aminoglycoside therapy, and symptoms may not appear until after the end of the treatment.[372] Because the target cells of ototoxicity, the cochlear and vestibular hair cells, do not regenerate once they have died, severe ototoxicity is generally irreversible.[306, 372] However, reversibility can be demonstrated in some cases, which are usually mild or even subclinical.[306, 347, 372, 373]

Subclinical loss of auditory or vestibular function can sometimes be detected before symptoms.[347, 372, 374] The earliest toxic effects on the auditory system reduce sound perception at the higher frequencies, and lower frequencies may be affected progressively over time.[372, 374] Thus, an appreciable loss at higher frequencies may take place before the patient notices more obvious loss of speech perception (at lower frequencies up to 2 to 3 kHz); diminished appreciation of music and other subtle functions requiring acute perception at higher frequencies might even go unnoticed. Similarly, considerable vestibular deficit might arise before the perception of any related symptoms.[372] In some cases, the effects are truly mild. However, patients given aminoglycosides are generally quite ill and often restricted to bed. Therefore, even with greater vestibular deficit, symptoms may not be provoked or noticed. Because vestibular deficit may be compensated by proprioceptive and visual cues, especially in the young, even ambulatory patients with vestibular toxicity may be unaware of symptoms. It can be argued that auditory toxicity that compromises speech perception can be more damaging than vestibular toxicity. However, vestibular toxicity that profoundly affects ambulation can certainly alter one's life. Fortunately, symptomatic auditory or vestibular toxicity is rare.

Cochlear toxicity is generally assessed by pure tone audiometric testing of air and bone conduction at doubling frequencies from 0.5 to 8.0 kHz.[372, 375] Testing at 3.0 and 6.0 kHz is also often included.[376] Although it is optimal to conduct the test in a soundproof room, audiometry may be carried out satisfactorily at the bedside,[372, 375] even though some patients may not be sufficiently alert to cooperate. Ambient noise is usually in the range of frequencies below 2.0 kHz, which is less important for detecting early ototoxicity.[375] The presence of loud, higher pitched noise, such as hissing from a respirator, may interfere with bedside testing.

Although criteria for defining auditory toxicity have not been standardized, an increase in threshold of at least 15 dB from baseline (within 72 hours after initiation of therapy)[376] in either ear is considered meaningful.[374] To reduce the incidence of false-positive results,[377] such a change at two or more frequencies in the same ear is generally required.[374]

Because the earliest effects of aminoglycosides are noted at higher frequencies, audiometric testing at frequencies above the 8.0-kHz limit of conventional audiometers may increase sensitivity so that ototoxic changes are detected earlier, before they might affect lower frequencies and cause symptoms.[372, 374] Although there are technical problems with high-frequency audiometric testing and neither the methodology nor the criteria for evaluation have been well standardized,[372, 375] such testing has been employed in the assessment of aminoglycoside toxicity.[313, 378, 379]

The testing of vestibular function is more arduous than audiometry and generally requires transportation to the audiology suite. Furthermore, the testing methodology for evaluation of vestibular toxicity is less well established. Therefore, relatively few patients have been evaluated objectively for vestibular toxicity in clinical studies of aminoglycosides.[345, 372] Vestibular stimulation is usually accomplished by bithermal caloric irrigation with water or air, and responses are recorded on an electronystagmogram.[372, 376, 380] A decrease of 50% from baseline in the maximal speed of the slow component of nystagmus in either ear is generally accepted as evidence of vestibular toxicity.[372, 376, 380]

Since 1973,[381] various prospective studies of aminoglycoside treatment have examined the incidence of and risk factors for ototoxicity for the different aminoglycosides, using objective testing and defined criteria for toxicity, when possible. The incidences of cochlear toxicity have ranged from 9% to 43% and of vestibular toxicity from 0% to 19%.[382] The reasons for such a spread include (1) variations in definitions of toxicity, (2) variations in populations of patients, (3) general lack of control arms without aminoglycoside treatment, and (4) variations in aminoglycosides used and treatment courses. Surveys of the literature have estimated an overall incidence of cochlear toxicity of about 5% to 10%[345, 382]; for vestibular toxicity the incidence is similar[371] or somewhat less.[345] Analysis of comparative studies that have examined the relative cochlear or vestibular toxic potential reveals generally comparable ototoxicity among gentamicin, tobramycin, and amikacin, but netilmicin appears to be associated with lower rates of audiovestibular toxicity.[345, 360, 382] Even when netilmicin is associated with a comparable incidence of ototoxicity, it has often been given at higher doses than gentamicin or tobramycin. It has been estimated that clinically detectable (symptomatic) ototoxicity occurs in less than 0.5% of patients treated with gentamicin, tobramycin, or amikacin.[320]

Clinical studies have examined the association of various risk factors with the development of ototoxicity in patients monitored for renal function and serum levels. Utilizing stepwise discriminant analysis, Moore and coworkers[245] found ototoxicity associated with duration of therapy (or total aminoglycoside dose), bacteremia, higher serum urea nitrogen/creatinine ratio (as an indication of hypovolemia), higher fever, and the presence of liver dysfunction. Other studies have found an association with age[383]; elevation of mean trough serum levels (suggesting impairment of renal excretion) and the development of nephrotoxicity[247]; and elevated trough levels, nephrotoxicity, duration of therapy, and treatment with furosemide.[246] Although ethacrynic acid use, even in single doses, is apparently associated with increased risk of aminoglycoside ototoxicity,[384, 385] other studies have failed to implicate furosemide use as a risk factor.[386] Although vancomycin enhanced the ototoxicity of gentamicin in an animal model,[387] vancomycin use has not been implicated as a risk factor for the development of aminoglycoside ototoxicity in humans. Because cisplatin produces cochlear (rarely vestibular) and renal toxicity similar to that of the aminoglycosides,[372] it may be considered to increase the risk of aminoglycoside ototoxicity. Studies of patients treated with larger than usual doses of gentamicin or tobramycin for extended courses revealed an increased incidence of ototoxicity.[243, 343] This finding and an association in other studies of ototoxicity with higher trough levels[381, 388, 389] confirm the impression that the area under the serum concentration–time curve may be related to the risk of ototoxicity, perhaps by fostering penetration of aminoglycoside into the deep compartment of the inner ear. Renal impairment can lead to higher trough levels and accumulation of drug, increasing the risk of ototoxicity if dosage is not adjusted appropriately.

Patients treated with aminoglycosides do not generally undergo routine testing of inner-ear function. Audiometric or vestibular function testing may be undertaken to confirm a possible symptom of cochleotoxic or vestibulotoxic change, although interpretation without a baseline test may be difficult. Patients who are at greater risk for ototoxicity, especially with long duration of therapy, higher dosage to achieve higher levels, or marked renal impairment, should be alerted to the possibility of ototoxic symptoms. Such patients may be considered for periodic (every 1 to 2 weeks) audiometry, if the clinical condition permits. Some may also be able to tolerate periodic electronystagmography, although the testing is more arduous and not well standardized.

Histopathologic studies of aminoglycoside ototoxicity in animals have revealed that the principal targets are the sensory hair cells of the organ of Corti and of the vestibular epithelia.[390, 391] In the cochlea, the order of sensitivity is the first through third rows of outer hair cells and then the row of inner hair cells, and from cells in the basal turn (corresponding to perception of the highest frequencies) to those in the apical turn. The degeneration of the vestibular sensory cells also follows a regular pattern.[392] Histopathologic reports of ototoxicity in humans are few, but the findings of cochlear hair cell loss parallel those in animals.[393–396] One histopathologic study of two cases with ototoxicity has reported preservation of hair cells but reduction in cochlear ganglion cells.[397]

Current concepts of the mechanism of aminoglycoside ototoxicity at the cellular and molecular levels have been formulated principally by Schacht and coworkers.[306, 398–400] As aminoglycosides pass from the blood stream to the target hair cells of the cochlea, they enter the perilymph. Their rate of entry is slow, and their rate of elimination from the perilymph is also quite slow. There is no active accumulation in perilymph, because the maximal level in the perilymph is not higher than that in serum. One might expect that the high concentrations achieved in the CSF by intraventricular injection, as for gram-negative bacillary meningitis, would diffuse via the cochlear aqueduct into the perilymph, resulting in higher, potentially toxic concentrations. However, at autopsy a patient treated with both intraventricular and intravenous tobramycin had a low level of tobramycin in the perilymph, as is found in patients treated with intravenous aminoglycoside alone.[401] Therefore, in this case there seemed to be no significant penetration of aminoglycoside from the CSF into the perilymph. Kinetics studies of aminoglycoside in various tissues of the rat have shown rapid uptake, early saturation, and increasingly lengthy half-lives of elimination from deeper compartments in inner ear tissue with prolonged exposure.[306] The only other tissue to show similar results was the renal cortex, although there the saturation concentration was much higher. In all other tissues, entry was slower and nonsaturable. Ototoxicity was correlated with later penetration into deeper compartments of inner-ear tissue. Biochemical studies of the molecular basis of toxicity, suggest a multistep mechanism.[398–400] Initially the drug binds electrostatically to the plasma membrane of hair cells, producing acute, reversible electrophysiologic effects. The binding and acute effects are antagonized by divalent cations, such as calcium. The drug is then taken into the cell by an energy-dependent process. Inside the cell, aminoglycosides bind to phosphatidylinositol bisphosphate, inhibiting its hydrolysis and thus preventing its physiologic function as a second messenger. Aminoglycosides may interfere with other important reactions regulated by polyphosphoinositides, and their competition with divalent cations or polyamines may further compromise the cell. The binding to phosphatidylinositol bisphosphate may be the critical step in toxicity, because physicochemical studies have shown exceptional binding of various aminoglycosides to that compound; the resulting disturbance in membrane structure is correlated with the rank order of ototoxic potential among aminoglycosides in animal models.[402] Furthermore, the presence of polyphosphoinositides and active metabolism of these compounds appear to be characteristic principally of inner ear and kidney tissue. This similarity and the presence of an active cellular uptake mechanism for aminoglycosides may explain the tissue specificity for the aminoglycosides.

Review of Drugs

For general use against aerobic gram-negative bacillary infections, four of the currently available aminoglycosides are considered: gentamicin, tobramycin, amikacin, and netilmicin. The choice among these is usually dictated by in vitro susceptibility and by cost. Each of these drugs is discussed briefly, and the other aminoglycosides and their specialized applications are reviewed.

Gentamicin. As the first of the modern aminoglycosides, with effective activity against *P. aeruginosa* and many kanamycin-resistant strains of Enterobacteriaceae, gentamicin displaced kanamycin as the preferred drug for aerobic gram-negative bacillary infections. Its extremely low cost has made it the workhorse aminoglycoside in hospitals where the incidence of gentamicin resistance is relatively low. Besides its cost, gentamicin has no clear advantage over other aminoglycosides against gram-negative bacilli, although it is generally preferred over tobramycin for *S. marcescens* because of its greater activity in vitro. Tobramycin is generally preferred in *P. aeruginosa* infection, because it is usually more active against gentamicin-susceptible strains and may even have activity against some gentamicin-resistant strains. In hospitals where gentamicin resistance is prevalent, amikacin is generally preferred for empirical therapy. Gentamicin is most often the optimal aminoglycoside for synergistic use with a penicillin against enterococci, streptococci, or staphylococci, although occasional strains of gentamicin-resistant enterococci are subject to the synergistic activity of streptomycin. Gentamicin is also preferred (alternative, streptomycin) for prophylaxis of endocarditis with penicillin G, ampicillin, or vancomycin. A preservative-free preparation is available for central nervous system and ocular administration.

Tobramycin. Tobramycin is generally comparable to gentamicin, except that it is usually considered preferable for tobramycin-susceptible strains of *P. aeruginosa*, but less active against *S. marcescens*. Some trials have suggested that tobramycin may be less nephrotoxic than gentamicin,[345, 360] but such a difference has not been clearly determined. Although some hospitals prefer to use tobramycin for this reason, cost analysis of a possible difference in nephrotoxicity suggests that gentamicin may still be cost-effective over tobramycin for general use.[403] A preservative-free preparation is available for central nervous system and ocular administration.

Amikacin. Although cross-resistance between gentamicin and tobramycin is common in Enterobacteriaceae and *P. aeruginosa*, in most hospitals such resistant strains remain susceptible to amikacin. Thus, amikacin should be used for infections caused by gram-negative bacilli known to be resistant to gentamicin and tobramycin and for empirical therapy for nosocomial infections caused by these organisms in hospitals where resistance to gentamicin and tobramycin is common. The use of amikacin as the principal aminoglycoside for empirical therapy of gram-negative bacillary infections in the absence of a high prevalence of strains resistant to both gentamicin and tobramycin is controversial. It is commonly believed that restriction of amikacin usage reduces the selective pressure for emergence of amikacin resistance or the proliferation of amikacin-resistant strains. Nonetheless, use of amikacin as the primary aminoglycoside has not been associated with marked increases of amikacin-resistant isolates, and the incidence of gentamicin and tobramycin resistance has dropped.[404, 405] On the other hand, although emergence of new resistance to amikacin is not common, primary use of this agent may be associated with the appearance of new amikacin resistance that does not confer resistance to gentamicin and tobramycin.[406–408] The relatively high cost of amikacin is also a consideration against the general replacement of gentamicin and tobramycin. Amikacin may be useful for the treatment of mycobacterial infections, such as those caused by *M. tuberculosis, Mycobacterium fortuitum*, and *Mycobacterium avium-intracellulare*. A preservative-free preparation is available for central nervous system and ocular administration.

Netilmicin. Netilmicin is active against some, but not all, strains of gram-negative bacilli that are resistant to gentamicin and tobramycin. Thus, it may provide a less expensive alternative to amikacin for the treatment of infections caused by gentamicin-, tobramycin-resistant strains that are netilmicin susceptible. Although netilmicin appears to be effective for the treatment of *P. aeruginosa* infections, some concern exists about its use against this organism, because of its inferior activity in cation-supplemented media in vitro (see the section on spectrum of antimicrobial activity). One study showed that netilmicin was effective as a single agent for the treatment of *P. aeruginosa* infections.[409] However, another study suggesting greater efficacy of amikacin than netilmicin as a single agent for *P. aeruginosa* infections[410] has kept alive concern about the use of netilmicin against *P. aeruginosa*. The usual practice of including an antipseudomonal β-lactam with an aminoglycoside in the treatment regimen for *P. aeruginosa* infections may overcome and obscure any inferiority of netilmicin. Because of evidence suggesting a lower ototoxic potential of netilmicin compared with other modern aminoglycosides (see the section on toxicity), netilmicin may be considered for use in situations in which the risk of ototoxicity is increased or in which its appearance would be especially devastating. Some hospitals have chosen netilmicin as their first-line aminoglycoside, despite its cost, because of its lower potential for ototoxicity.

Kanamycin. Because of its inactivity against *P. aeruginosa* and the frequency of resistance to kanamycin among Enterobacteriaceae, parenteral kanamycin has been largely replaced by gentamicin and the other modern aminoglycosides, although it still may be used as an alternative to streptomycin in tuberculosis treatment.

Streptomycin. Streptomycin is used as a second-line agent for the treatment of tuberculosis, as when the isolate is resistant to isoniazid and rifampin or when parenteral therapy is desirable. It may also be used in place of gentamicin with a penicillin or with vancomycin for the treatment of serious enterococcal or streptococcal infections (e.g., endocarditis); for enterococci, susceptibility to synergism with streptomycin should be demonstrated (see the section on spectrum of antimicrobial activity and synergistic activity). Streptomycin is preferred for treatment of tularemia and plague and is often used (with a tetracycline) for severe brucellosis.

Neomycin. Neomycin may be administered orally with erythromycin base as prophylaxis for elective colorectal surgery. Oral neomycin also may be used as an adjunct in the treatment of hepatic coma. Because of possible systemic accumulation, oral neomycin should be used with great caution in patients with renal impairment. Concern about absorption should also limit the use of this agent as a peritoneal or pleural irrigant. Neomycin may be used topically with other agents in otic drops for external otitis and in ophthalmic drops or ointment for superficial bacterial infections of the eye. For limited primary pyodermas, it may be used topically alone or in combination with other agents. Neomycin may produce hypersensitivity, especially in the patient with contact dermatitis or chronic dermatosis. Cross-sensitization may restrict the use of other aminoglycosides. (Hypersensitivity may be seen with other aminoglycosides, but they are rarely used on the skin.) Topical application of an aminoglycoside, such as neomycin, to the middle ear or the round window membrane in experimental animals readily produces ototoxicity. Although the use of neomycin otic drops has not been clearly shown to be associated with ototoxicity in humans, this possibility should be considered for patients with perforated tympanic membranes or tympanostomy tubes.

Paromomycin. Paromomycin may be used in combination with iodoquinol as an alternative in the treatment of mild to moderately severe intestinal amebiasis. It may also be used as an alternative to niclosamide for the treatment of tapeworm infections.

Spectinomycin. Although spectinomycin as an aminocyclitol is often classified with the aminoglycosides, it differs from them in a number of ways. Structurally it lacks an amino sugar and has no glycosidic bond (see the section on chemistry). Although its target site appears to be on the 30S ribosomal subunit, it does not cause misreading of messenger RNA.[400] Spectinomycin is active against the vast majority of *N. gonorrhoeae* strains, including penicillinase-producing and chromosomally mediated penicillin-resistant strains. Although its activity against susceptible strains of enteric bacilli is bacteriostatic, its activity against gonococci is bactericidal.[411, 412] In contrast to the inactivity of the aminoglycosides against *Bacteroides fragilis*, this organism may be susceptible to achievable concentrations of spectinomycin, although many strains are resistant.[413] Spectinomycin is inactive against *Chlamydia trachomatis* and *Treponema pallidum* but does inhibit some isolates of *Ureaplasma urealyticum*.[411] *Gardnerella vaginalis* is generally susceptible to spectinomycin.[414]

Spectinomycin is well absorbed after intramuscular injection and is well tolerated. Mean peak serum levels 1 hour after intramuscular injection of 2 g are about 100 μg/mL. Plasma protein binding is minimal, and unchanged drug is completely excreted in the urine with a half-life in serum of about 1 hour.[413] Unlike the aminoglycosides, spectinomycin has not been shown to cause renal or inner-ear toxicity, although it has not been tested extensively in long treatment courses in human subjects.

The clinical use of spectinomycin is limited to the treatment of gonococcal infections.[413] The agent is highly effective for anogenital gonorrhea as a single 2-g intramuscular injection and for disseminated gonococcal infection by intravenous administration.[320] It is not reliably effective for the treatment of pharyngeal gonorrhea or anorectal gonococcal infections in men or for *C. trachomatis* infections coexisting with gonorrhea.[327] Spectinomycin is used as an alternative to ceftriaxone and other third-generation cephalosporins in the treatment of susceptible types of gonococcal infection caused by known or suspected penicillin-resistant strains of gonococci. Because spectinomycin does not cure incubating syphilis, follow-up serologic tests for syphilis must be carried out.

Clinical Uses

The principal uses of aminoglycosides are for the treatment of aerobic gram-negative bacillary infections and in synergistic combinations for the treatment of gram-positive coccal infections. For treatment of other organisms, see the previous section on review of drugs. For gram-negative bacilli, aminoglycosides are used especially for empirical therapy in situations in which the likelihood of resistance to other agents is high, as in nosocomial infections, and also when predictable, rapid bactericidal activity is critical, as in bacteremias. The attributes of aminoglycosides that make them highly suitable for such use include rapid bactericidal action, with increased rates of killing at higher concentrations, and a relatively predictable susceptibility pattern among nosocomial isolates in a given hospital, with fewer problems of emerging resistance than with other agents. Although aminoglycosides may be used as monotherapy in the treatment of urinary tract infections, they are generally administered with other agents for infections elsewhere. Because aminoglycosides are frequently used for initial, empirical therapy, other agents may be used to broaden the effective activity of the treatment regimen to include gram-positive cocci and anaerobes and/or to provide synergistically enhanced activity with aminoglycosides against gram-positive cocci and gram-negative bacilli in serious infections and in compromised patients. With the advent of potent broad-spectrum β-lactams and fluoroquinolones, some clinical studies have suggested that monotherapy with these agents may be as effective in some settings as combination therapy with aminoglycosides and β-lactams. Therefore, once the patient's condition has stabilized and the clinical situation and the microbial etiology have been clarified after the first few days of combination therapy including an aminoglycoside, the physician may consider whether the initial regimen may be safely replaced by a less toxic one.

The clinical utility of aminoglycosides depends on the pathogen, the site of infection, and the nature of the infected host.

P. aeruginosa may be only moderately susceptible to aminoglycosides and β-lactams and may develop resistance to either of these classes of drugs during therapy.[415, 416] Therefore, a combination of an aminoglycoside and a β-lactam is generally used for the treatment of *P. aeruginosa* infections. In some situations, the combination can be shown to be superior to monotherapy with an antipseudomonal β-lactam.[417, 418] The same rationale is often applied to the treatment of other susceptible nosocomial pathogens, including Enterobacteriaceae such as *Enterobacter, S. marcescens, Morganella,* and *Citrobacter* and nonfermenters such as *Acinetobacter.* Systemic enterococcal infections as a rule are treated with the combination of gentamicin with ampicillin or vancomycin.[419, 420] Similarly, gentamicin or streptomycin may be added to penicillin G for viridans streptococcal endocarditis,[420–422] and gentamicin may be added to an antistaphylococcal penicillin or vancomycin for *S. aureus* endocarditis or for the first 2 weeks of treatment with a course of vancomycin and rifampin for coagulase-negative staphylococcal prosthetic valve endocarditis.[423]

Septicemia. For the reasons stated earlier, septicemia (i.e., suspected gram-negative bacteremia with a clinical septic picture) is generally treated presumptively with an aminoglycoside at a dosage to achieve high serum levels in combination with a broad-spectrum β-lactam, especially when the infection is nosocomial. If an underlying site of infection is strongly suspected or documented, the β-lactam may be selected to target particular types of pathogens. In neonates, gentamicin is generally used with ampicillin for initial therapy of group B streptococcal infections.[424]

Urinary Tract Infections. Because of the high concentrations of aminoglycosides in urine and their persistence in renal tissue, they are favorable for the treatment of urinary tract infections. Aminoglycosides may be used alone for community-acquired gram-negative bacillary infection, although ampicillin should be added for enterococcal infection. When an aminoglycoside is used alone at low dosage, one must remember that low pH and high solute concentrations in the urine may be unfavorable for its activity.[425, 426] Usually the high concentration of the aminoglycoside in urine provides adequate antibacterial activity, but in case of a suboptimal response, one might consider alkalinization and dilution of the urine. For nosocomial infections, a β-lactam is generally administered with the aminoglycoside. The selection of a particular aminoglycoside and a β-lactam depends in large part on the suspected pathogens and their susceptibility profiles. Because of poor penetration into the prostate, aminoglycosides normally are not recommended for the treatment of prostatic infections, although they have been used for multidrug-resistant organisms. The availability of fluoroquinolones, which penetrate well into the prostate,[427] makes the use of aminoglycosides unnecessary for the treatment of prostatic infections.

Endocarditis. Gentamicin (or streptomycin) plus ampicillin (or penicillin G) or vancomycin is virtually obligatory in the treatment of enterococcal endocarditis,[419, 420] unless high-level resistance to the aminoglycoside is present (see the section on synergistic activity). Gentamicin is also used initially with vancomycin and rifampin for the treatment of coagulase-negative staphylococcal prosthetic valve endocarditis.[423] In some cases of *S. aureus* endocarditis, gentamicin with an antistaphylococcal penicillin may be useful. Combination therapy may not improve results for *S. aureus* endocarditis in intravenous drug abusers,[428] but it may allow a shorter course of therapy.[429] In nonaddicts with *S. aureus* endocarditis, gentamicin may be used for the first few days of therapy with a penicillin, because a controlled trial showed more rapid clearing of bacteremia in the patients receiving combination therapy, even though continued combination therapy had no effect on mortality.[430] For the rare case of endocarditis caused by *P. aeruginosa* or other gram-negative rod, the synergistic action of an aminoglycoside and a β-lactam may be advantageous.[431–433]

Respiratory Tract Infections. Because of their relatively poor penetration into respiratory tract secretions and their relatively poor activity at the low pH that is prevalent there, aminoglycosides do not generally play a role in the treatment of pneumonia. Furthermore, most community-acquired pneumonias are caused by organisms for which aminoglycoside therapy is not optimal. However, the use of an aminoglycoside with an appropriate β-lactam may be critical for the treatment of nosocomial gram-negative rod pneumonia,[434, 435] especially if bacteremia is suspected. Use of such combinations of agents with antipseudomonal activity may be important for acute exacerbations of respiratory infections in cystic fibrosis patients, as the resident tracheobronchial flora becomes more resistant to various agents, including the aminoglycosides.[436–438] The use of endotracheal plus parenteral aminoglycoside has been investigated for the treatment of gram-negative bacterial pneumonia.[227] Bacterial clearing was improved with the endotracheal therapy, but there was no significant improvement in clinical efficacy.

Intraabdominal Infections. For the treatment of intraabdominal infection, drainage of abscesses naturally is of prime importance. For antibiotic treatment of peritoneal infections, gentamicin has been utilized with antianaerobic agents,[439] such as clindamycin, metronidazole, or a β-lactam such as cefoxitin, cefotetan, or imipenem. The availability of these β-lactams with potent activity against both anaerobes such as *B. fragilis* and a broad spectrum of aerobic gram-negative bacilli has raised the possibility of monotherapy for intraabdominal infections. For example, a report indicates that imipenem may be superior to the conventional combination of clindamycin and an aminoglycoside for the treatment of intraabdominal infections.[440] For the management of biliary infections such as cholangitis or infectious complications of acute cholecystitis, relief of obstruction and drainage are most important, but associated antibiotic therapy may include an aminoglycoside, as in the regimens for peritonitis. As discussed in the section on pharmacokinetics, aminoglycosides penetrate poorly into obstructed bile but may be useful once obstruction is relieved. For peritonitis associated with peritoneal dialysis, aminoglycosides have been used effectively by intraperitoneal lavage.[441]

Similarly, aminoglycosides have been used effectively as standard therapy with an antianaerobic agent for the treatment of pelvic infections in the female,[442] but such infections may be treated solely with a β-lactam having sufficient activity against anaerobes as well as aerobes.

Meningitis. Newer β-lactam antibiotics that have great potency against gram-negative bacilli and produce therapeutic concentrations in CSF, such as cefuroxime and third-generation cephalosporins, have largely replaced the aminoglycosides in the treatment of meningitis caused by Enterobacteriaceae. However, aminoglycosides may be indicated in combination therapy for the treatment of meningitis caused by gram-negative bacilli such as *P. aeruginosa* and *Enterobacter,* which are unlikely to be cleared by a parenteral β-lactam alone.[230] The poor penetration of aminoglycosides into CSF, even with inflammation, mandates their direct instillation into the CSF for the treatment of gram-negative bacillary meningitis. The intraventricular route through an Ommaya reservoir is more reliable for delivering adequate concentrations of drug throughout the CSF than is the intrathecal route.[232, 443] Because the penetration of aminoglycosides into CSF is much better in neonates than in older children and adults, parenteral therapy with an aminoglycoside is adequate for gram-negative bacillary meningitis in the neonate; in a multicenter study, additional intraventricular therapy appeared to confer no advantage, and the death rate was higher in the dual-route treatment group.[233] For direct administration into the CSF, gentamicin, tobramycin, and amikacin are available in preservative-free preparations.

Ocular Infections. Aminoglycosides play an important role in the treatment of ocular infections suspected or known to involve gram-negative bacilli.[228] They are applied topically in drops for the treatment of corneal infections, and they are administered by direct intravitreal injection for the treatment of endophthalmitis.

Bone and Joint Infections. Aminoglycosides may be indicated, usually in combination with a suitable β-lactam, for the treatment of acute or chronic osteomyelitis caused by gram-negative bacilli, especially *P. aeruginosa*. Chronic infections require aggressive débridement of necrotic tissue; despite extended courses of antibiotic therapy, they may relapse or fail to improve. Long-term follow-up therapy with an oral quinolone after an initial 3- to 6-week course of parenteral therapy with an aminoglycoside plus a β-lactam may improve the ultimate results, but long-term studies are needed.

High local concentrations of aminoglycosides can be delivered for prophylaxis or therapy of osteomyelitis by diffusion from polymethyl methacrylate impregnated with gentamicin or tobramycin.[444–453] Aminoglycosides are well suited to this method of delivery, because they are fairly inert in tissue, rarely produce hypersensitivity reactions, are physically stable to the heat generated by exothermic polymerization of the methyl methacrylate, and do not adversely affect the physical properties of the cement. Furthermore, although aminoglycoside concentrations in wound drainage fluid are high and the drug may continue to be released for weeks to months, serum levels are low and neither nephrotoxicity nor ototoxicity has been reported with the use of this material. Gentamicin-impregnated polymethyl methacrylate cement has been used successfully for prophylaxis in total hip arthroplasty and for treatment of infected sites by reimplantation of a new prosthesis with gentamicin cement. Aminoglycoside-impregnated polymethyl methacrylate in the form of beads can be implanted temporarily for one to several weeks in débrided sites for the treatment of chronic osteomyelitis. Therapeutic results are best with staphylococci but less favorable with gram-negative bacilli, including *Pseudomonas*, and with enterococci. Adjunctive parenteral therapy may be administered as well.

Gram-negative bacillary septic arthritis may be treated with a suitable β-lactam, but combined therapy with an aminoglycoside may be considered for infection with *P. aeruginosa* or other relatively resistant organism.

The Febrile Neutropenic Patient. Although aminoglycosides by themselves are not as effective in the neutropenic patient as in those with adequate neutrophils,[454] in various combinations with antipseudomonal β-lactams they have provided standard empirical regimens for the treatment of febrile neutropenic patients.[455–457] The presumed advantages of this combination therapy include potential synergistic activity against gram-negative bacilli, such as *P. aeruginosa*, and possible reduction of emergence of resistance to the β-lactam. Nonetheless, clinical study regimens with two β-lactam drugs and monotherapy with a single β-lactam have demonstrated comparable efficacy in this setting without the risk of aminoglycoside toxicity.[458, 459] Such avoidance of an aminoglycoside may be desirable for patients receiving another toxic agent, such as cisplatin, cyclosporine, or amphotericin B. However, inclusion of an aminoglycoside in a combination regimen may be warranted by the prevalence in these patients of *P. aeruginosa* and other nosocomial gram-negative bacilli that develop β-lactam resistance.

Future Uses

With the availability of potent, broad-spectrum β-lactams and fluoroquinolones that have in vitro activity and clinical efficacy against most organisms in the aminoglycoside spectrum, the use of aminoglycosides for general first-line therapy is likely to decline. They will continue to be used against organisms for which synergistic activity is advantageous, such as enterococci and *P. aeruginosa*, and for *Pseudomonas, Enterobacter,* and *Serratia* in hospitals where emergence of β-lactam resistance in these organisms has been a problem. They may also continue to be used in initial, empirical therapy when the susceptibility of infecting pathogens to other agents is uncertain. Persistence of aminoglycoside effectiveness in the presence of resistance to alternative agents may ultimately lead us back to broader reliance on this class of drugs.

References

1. Schatz A, Bugie E, Waksman SA: Streptomycin, a substance exhibiting antibiotic activity against gram-positive and gram-negative bacteria. Proc Soc Exp Biol Med 55:66, 1944.
2. Hinshaw HC, Feldman WH: Streptomycin in the treatment of clinical tuberculosis: A preliminary report. Proc Mayo Clin 20:313, 1945.
3. Farrington RF, Hull-Smith H, Bunn PA, McDermott W: Streptomycin toxicity: Reactions to highly purified drug on long-continued administration to human subjects. JAMA 134:678, 1947.
4. Chase JS: Toxic effects of streptomycin on eighth nerve. Am Rev Tuberc 56:418, 1947.
5. Barr B, Floberg LE, Hamberger CA, Köck HJ: Otological aspects of streptomycin therapy. Acta Otolaryngol Suppl (Stockh) 75:5, 1949.
6. Waksman SA: Streptomycin: Nature and Practical Applications. Baltimore, Williams & Wilkins, 1949.
7. Edison AD, Frost BM, Graessle OE, et al: An experimental evaluation of dihydrostreptomycin. Am Rev Tuberc 58:487, 1948.
8. Glorig A: The effect of dihydrostreptomycin hydrochloride and sulphate on the auditory mechanism. Ann Otol 60:327, 1951.
9. Liden G: Loss of hearing following treatment with dihydrostreptomycin or streptomycin. Acta Otolaryngol 43:551, 1954.
10. Cohen SS, Johnson L, Lichtenstein MR, Lynch WJ: A comparative study of streptomycin and dihydrostreptomycin in pulmonary tuberculosis. Am Rev Tuberc 68:229, 1953.
11. Mahady SCF, Armstrong FL, Beck F: A comparative study of streptomycin and dihydrostreptomycin in pulmonary tuberculosis. Am Rev Tuberc 68:238, 1953.
12. Shambaugh GE, Derlacki EL, Harrison WH, et al: Dihydrostreptomycin deafness. JAMA 170:1657, 1959.
13. Waksman SA, Lechevalier HA: Neomycin: A new antibiotic active against streptomycin-resistant bacteria, including tuberculous organisms. Science 109:305, 1949.
14. Carr DT, Pfuetze KH, Brown HA, et al: Neomycin in clinical tuberculosis. Am Rev Tuberc 63:427, 1951.
15. Waisbren BA, Spink WW: A clinical appraisal of neomycin. Ann Intern Med 33:1099, 1950.
16. Ballantyne J: Iatrogenic deafness. J Laryngol Otol 84:967, 1970.
17. Greenwood GJ: Neomycin ototoxicity. Arch Otolaryngol 69:340, 1959.
18. De Beauklaer MM, Travis LB, Dodge WF, Guerral FA: Deafness and acute tubular necrosis following parenteral administration of neomycin. Am J Dis Child 121:250, 1971.
19. De Oliveira JAA: Audiovestibular Toxicity of Drugs, Vols I and II. Boca Raton, FL, CRC Press, 1989.
20. Haskell TH, French JL, Bartz QR: Paromomycin. J Am Chem Soc 81:3480, 1959.
21. Umezawa H, Ueda M, Maeda K, et al: Production and isolation of a new antibiotic, kanamycin. J Antibiot 10:181, 1957.
22. Weinstein MJ, Luedemann GM, Oden EM, Wagman GH: Gentamicin: A new broad-spectrum antibiotic complex. Antimicrob Agents Chemother 1963:1, 1964.
23. Shadomy S, Jutz C, Wagner G: In vitro studies with sisomicin, gentamicin and tobramycin. Infection 4(Suppl):S305, 1976.
24. Sanders CC, Sanders WE, Goering RV: In vitro studies with SCH21420 and SCH22591: Activity in comparison with six other aminoglycosides and synergy with penicillin against enterococci. Antimicrob Agents Chemother 14:178, 1978.
25. Paradelis AG, Douboyas J, Stathopoulos G, et al: In vitro comparison of kanamycin, kanendomycin, gentamicin, amikacin,

sisomicin, and dibekacin against 200 strains of *Pseudomonas aeruginosa*. Antimicrob Agents Chemother 14:514, 1978.
26. Nagabushan TL, Cooper AB, Tsai H, et al: The syntheses and biological properties of 1-*N*-(*S*-4-amino-2-hydroxybutyryl)-gentamicin B and 1-*N*(*S*-3-amino-2-hydroxyproprionyl)-gentamicin B. J Antibiot 31:687, 1978.
27. Price KE: Aminoglycoside research 1975–1985: Prospects for development of improved agents. Antimicrob Agents Chemother 29:543, 1986.
28. Windholz M, Budavari SF, Otterbein ES (eds): The Merck Index, ed 10. Rahway, NJ, Merck, 1983.
29. Waitz JA, Drube CG, Moss EL Jr, et al: Biological aspects of the interaction between gentamicin and carbenicillin. J Antibiot 25:219, 1972.
30. Josephs HB, Lerner SA: The inactivation of gentamicin and tobramycin by carbenicillin requires an intact β-lactam ring. Presented at the 13th International Congress of Chemotherapy; Vienna, Austr SE8.4/1-8; 1983.
31. Holt HA, Broughall JM, McCarthy M, Reeves DS: Interactions between aminoglycoside antibiotics and carbenicillin or ticarcillin. Infection 4:107, 1976.
32. Pickering LK, Rutherford I: Effect of concentration and time upon inactivation of tobramycin, gentamicin, netilmicin, and amikacin by azlocillin, carbenicillin, mecillinam, mezlocillin, and piperacillin. J Pharmacol Exp Ther 217:345, 1981.
33. Glew RH, Pavuk RA: Stability of gentamicin, tobramycin, and amikacin in combination with four β-lactam antibiotics. Antimicrob Agents Chemother 24:474, 1983.
34. Wallace SM, Chan L-Y: In vitro interaction of aminoglycosides with β-lactam penicillins. Antimicrob Agents Chemother 28:274, 1985.
35. McLaughlin JE, Reeves DS: Clinical and laboratory evidence for inactivation of gentamicin and carbenicillin. Lancet 1:261, 1971.
36. Spotts CR, Stanier RY: Mechanism of streptomycin action on bacteria: A unitary hypothesis. Nature 192:663, 1961.
37. Weisblum B, Davies J: Antibiotic inhibitors of the bacterial ribosome. Bacteriol Rev 32:493, 1968.
38. Dubin DT, Hancock R, Davis BD: The sequence of some effects of streptomycin in *Escherichia coli*. Biochim Biophys Acta 74:476, 1963.
39. Arnad N, Davis BD, Armitage AK: Damage by streptomycin to the cell membrane of *Escherichia coli*. Nature 185:23, 1960.
40. Ozaki M, Mizuchima S, Nomura M: Identification and functional characterization of the protein controlled by the streptomycin-resistant locus in *E. coli*. Nature 222:333, 1969.
41. Schreiner G, Nierhaus KH: Protein involved in the binding of dihydrostreptomycin to ribosomes of *Escherichia coli*. J Mol Biol 81:71, 1973.
42. Kühberger R, Piepersberg W, Petzet A, et al: Alteration of ribosomal protein L6 in gentamicin-resistant strains of *Escherichia coli*. Effects on fidelity of protein synthesis. Biochemistry 18:187, 1979.
43. Hummel H, Piepersberg W, Böck A: 30S subunit mutations relieving restriction of ribosomal misreading caused by L6 mutations. Mol Gen Genet 179:147, 1980.
44. Modolell J, Davis BD: Mechanism of inhibition of ribosomes by streptomycin. Nature 224:345, 1969.
45. Modolell J, Davis BD: Breakdown by streptomycin of initiation complexes formed on the ribosomes of *Escherichia coli*. Proc Natl Acad Sci USA 67:1148, 1970.
46. Wallace BJ, Davis BD: Cyclic blockade of initiation sites by streptomycin-damaged ribosomes in *Escherichia coli*: An explanation for dominance of sensitivity. J Mol Biol 75:377, 1973.
47. Wallace BJ, Tai P-C, Davis BD: Effect of streptomycin on the response of *Escherichia coli* ribosomes to the dissociation factor. J Mol Biol 75:391, 1973.
48. Davies J, Gorini L, Davis BD: Misreading of RNA codewords induced by aminoglycoside antibiotics. Mol Pharmacol 1:93, 1965.
49. Bryan LE, Kwan S: Roles of ribosomal binding, membrane potential, and electron transport in bacterial uptake of streptomycin and gentamicin. Antimicrob Agents Chemother 23:835, 1983.
50. Hancock REW: Aminoglycoside uptake and mode of action with special reference to streptomycin and gentamicin. II. Effects of aminoglycosides on cells. J Antimicrob Chemother 8:429, 1981.
51. Pine MJ: Comparative physiological effects of incorporated amino acid analogs in *Escherichia coli*. Antimicrob Agents Chemother 13:676, 1978.
52. Matsunaga K, Hiroshi Y, Nishimura T, Tanaka N: Inhibition of DNA replication by aminoglycoside antibiotics. Antimicrob Agents Chemother 30:468, 1986.
53. Davis BD, Chen L, Tai PC: Misread protein creates membrane channels: An essential step in the bactericidal action of aminoglycosides. Proc Natl Acad Sci USA 83:6164, 1986.
54. Davies J: Aminoglycoside-aminocyclitol antibiotics and their modifying enzymes. *In* Lorian V (ed): Antibiotics in Laboratory Medicine. Baltimore, Williams & Wilkins, 1980, pp 474–489.
55. Cabanas MJ, Vazquez D, Modolell J: Dual interference of hygromycin B with ribosomal translocation with aminoacyl tRNA recognition. Eur J Biochem 87:21, 1978.
56. Hancock REW: Aminoglycoside uptake and mode of action with special reference to streptomycin and gentamicin. I. J Antimicrob Chemother 8:249, 1981.
57. Hancock REW, Raffle VJ, Nicas TI: Involvement of the outer membrane in gentamicin and streptomycin uptake and killing in *Pseudomonas aeruginosa*. Antimicrob Agents Chemother 19:777, 1981.
58. Bryan LE, van den Elzen HM: Effects of membrane-energy mutations and cations on streptomycin and gentamicin accumulation by bacteria: A model for entry of streptomycin and gentamicin in susceptible and resistant bacteria. Antimicrob Agents Chemother 12:163, 1977.
59. Ahmad MH, Rechenmacher A, Böck A: Interaction between aminoglycoside uptake and ribosomal resistant mutations. Antimicrob Agents Chemother 18:798, 1980.
60. Peterson AA, Hancock REW, McGroarty EJ: Binding of polycationic antibiotics and polyamines to lipopolysaccharides of *Pseudomonas aeruginosa*. J Bacteriol 164:1256, 1985.
61. Moore RA, Bates NC, Hancock REW: Interaction of polycationic antibiotics with *Pseudomonas aeruginosa* lipopolysaccharide and lipid A studied by using dansyl-polymyxin. Antimicrob Agents Chemother 29:496, 1986.
62. Rocque WJ, Fesik SW, Haug A, McGroarty EJ: Polycation binding to isolated lipopolysaccharide from antibiotic-hypersusceptible mutant strains of *Escherichia coli*. Antimicrob Agents Chemother 32:308, 1988.
63. Jackson GG, Lolans VT, Daikos GL: The inductive role of ionic binding in the bactericidal and postexposure effects of aminoglycoside antibiotics with implications for dosing. J Infect Dis 162:408, 1990.
64. Vogelman BS, Craig WA: Postantibiotic effects. J Antimicrob Chemother 15:37, 1985.
65. Vogelman B, Craig WA: Kinetics of antimicrobial activity. J Pediatr 108:835, 1986.
66. Kapusnik JE, Hackbarth CJ, Chambers HF, et al: Single, large, daily dosing versus intermittent dosing of tobramycin for treating experimental pseudomonas pneumonia. J Infect Dis 158:7, 1988.
67. Bundtzen RW, Gerber AU, Cohn DL, Craig WA: Postantibiotic suppression of bacterial growth. Rev Infect Dis 3:28, 1981.
68. Damper PD, Epstein W: Role of the membrane potential in bacterial resistance to aminoglycoside antibiotics. Antimicrob Agents Chemother 20:803, 1981.
69. Bryan LE, Kwan S: Mechanisms of aminoglycoside resistance of anaerobic bacteria and facultative bacteria grown anaerobically. J Antimicrob Chemother 8(Suppl D):1, 1981.
70. Mates SM, Patel L, Kaback HR, et al: Membrane potential in anaerobically growing *Staphylococcus aureus* and its relationship to gentamicin uptake. Antimicrob Agents Chemother 23:526, 1983.
71. Moellering RC Jr: In vitro antibacterial activity of the aminoglycoside antibiotics. Rev Infect Dis 5(Suppl):S212, 1983.
72. Höltje JV: Streptomycin uptake via an inducible polyamine transport system in *Escherichia coli*. Eur J Biochem 86:345, 1978.
73. Bryan LE: Aminoglycoside resistance. *In* Bryan LE (ed): Antimicrobial Drug Resistance. Orlando, FL, Academic Press, 1984.
74. Dickie P, Bryan LE, Pickard MA: Effect of enzymatic adenylation on dihydrostreptomycin accumulation in *Escherichia coli* carrying an R-factor: Model explaining aminoglycoside resistance by inactivating mechanisms. Antimicrob Agents Chemother 14:569, 1978.

75. Perlin MH, Lerner SA: Localization of an amikacin 3′-phosphotransferase in *Escherichia coli*. J Bacteriol 147:320, 1981.
76. Garcia-Riestra C, Perlin MH, Lerner SA: Lack of accumulation of exogenous adenylyl dihydrostreptomycin by whole cells or spheroplasts of *Escherichia coli*. Antimicrob Agents Chemother 27:114, 1985.
77. Davies J: Resistance to aminoglycosides: Mechanisms and frequency. Rev Infect Dis 5(Suppl 2):S261, 1983.
78. Trieu-Cuot P, Courvalin P: Evolution and transfer of aminoglycoside resistance genes under natural conditions. J Antimicrob Chemother 18(Suppl C): 93, 1986.
79. Vastola AP, Altschaefl J, Harford S: 5-*epi*-Sisomicin and 5-*epi*-gentamicin B: Substrates for aminoglycoside-modifying enzymes that retain activity against aminoglycoside-resistant bacteria. Antimicrob Agents Chemother 13:41, 1980.
80. DeHertogh DA, Lerner SA: Correlation of aminoglycoside resistance with the K_ms and V_{max}/K_m ratios of enzymatic modification of aminoglycosides by 2″-*O*-nucleotidyltransferase. Antimicrob Agents Chemother 27:670, 1985.
81. Perlin MH, Lerner SA: High-level amikacin resistance in *Escherichia coli* due to phosphorylation and impaired aminoglycoside uptake. Antimicrob Agents Chemother 27:216, 1986.
82. Lodge JM, Piddock LJV: The control of class I β-lactamase expression in Enterobacteriaceae and *Pseudomonas aeruginosa*. J Antimicrob Chemother 28:167, 1991.
83. Collatz E, Labia R, Gutmann L: Molecular evolution of ubiquitous β-lactamases towards extended-spectrum enzymes active against new β-lactam antibiotics. Mol Microbiol 4:1615, 1990.
84. Jacoby GA, Medeiros AA: More extended spectrum β-lactamases. Antimicrob Agents Chemother 35:1697, 1991.
85. Sanders CC: Chromosomal cephalosporinases responsible for multiple resistance to newer β-lactam antibiotics. Annu Rev Microbiol 41:573, 1987.
86. Davies J, Kagen SA: What is the mechanism of plasmid-determined resistance to aminoglycoside antibiotics? *In* Drew J, Hagemauer G (eds): R-Factors. Their Properties and Possible Control. New York, Springer-Verlag, 1978, p 207.
87. Young FE, Mayer L: Genetic determinants of microbial resistance to antibiotics. Rev Infect Dis 1:55, 1979.
88. O'Brien TF, Ross, OG, Guyman MA, et al: Dissemination of an antibiotic resistance plasmid in hospital patient flora. Antimicrob Agents Chemother 17:537, 1980.
89. Schaberg DR, Rubens CE, Alford RH, et al: Evolution of antimicrobial resistance and nosocomial infection: Lessons learned from the Vanderbilt experience. Am J Med 70:445, 1981.
90. Siegenthaler WE, Bonetti A, Lüthy R: Aminoglycoside antibiotics in infectious diseases: An overview. Am J Med 80(Suppl 6B):2, 1986.
91. Price KE, DeFuria MD, Pursiano TA: Amikacin, an aminoglycoside with marked activity against antibiotic-resistant clinical isolates. J Infect Dis 134(Suppl):S249, 1976.
92. Torres C, Lerner DL, Perlin MH, et al: Purification and characterization of a new aminoglycoside phosphotransferase (3′) with a low K_m for amikacin (Abstr 718). Presented at the 26th Interscience Conference on Antimicrobial Agents and Chemotherapy, 1986.
93. Lambert T, Gerbaud G, Courvalin P: Transferable amikacin resistance in *Acinetobacter* spp. due to a new type of 3′-aminoglycoside phosphotransferase. Antimicrob Agents Chemother 32:15, 1988.
94. Gaynes RP, Groisman E, Nelson E, et al: Isolation, characterization, and cloning of a plasmid-borne gene encoding a phosphotransferase that confers high-level amikacin resistance in enteric bacilli. Antimicrob Agents Chemother 32:1379, 1988.
95. Shimizu K, Kumada T, Hsieh W-C, et al: Comparison of aminoglycoside resistance patterns in Japan, Formosa, Korea, Chile, and the United States. Antimicrob Agents Chemother 28:282, 1985.
96. Maness MJ, Foster GC, Sparling PF: Ribosomal resistance to streptomycin and spectinomycin in *Neisseria gonorrhoeae*. J Bacteriol 120:1293, 1974.
97. Eliopoulous GM, Farber BF, Murray BE, et al: Ribosomal resistance of clinical enterococcal isolates to streptomycin. Antimicrob Agents Chemother 25:398, 1984.
98. Gaynes RP, Simpson D, Reeves S, et al: Colonization and infection of neonates with multiply resistant *Escherichia coli*. Infect Control 5:519, 1984.
99. Sanders CC, Sanders WE Jr: Emergence of resistance during therapy with the newer β-lactam antibiotics: Role of inducible beta-lactamases and implications for the future. Rev Infect Dis 5:639, 1983.
100. Sugarman B, Pesanti E: Treatment failures secondary to in vivo development of drug resistance by microorganisms. Rev Infect Dis 2:153, 1980.
101. Musher DN, Baughn RE, Templeton GB, Minuth JN: Emergence of variant forms of *Staphylococcus aureus* after exposure to gentamicin and infectivity of the variants in experimental animals. J Infect Dis 136:360, 1977.
102. Musher DN, Baughn RE, Merrell GL: Selection of small-colony variants of Enterobacteriaceae by in vitro exposure to aminoglycosides: Pathogenicity for experimental animals. J Infect Dis 140:209, 1979.
103. Funada H, Hattori K, Kosaki N: Catalase-negative *Escherichia coli* isolated from blood. J Clin Microbiol 7:474, 1978.
104. Rusthoven JJ, Davies TA, Lerner SA: Clinical isolation and characterization of aminoglycoside-resistant small colony variants of *Enterobacter aerogenes*. Am J Med 67:702, 1979.
105. Nicas TI, Hancock REW: Outer membrane protein H1 of *Pseudomonas aeruginosa*: Involvement in adaptive and mutational resistance to ethylenediaminetetraacetate, polymyxin B, and gentamicin. J Bacteriol 143:872, 1980.
106. Bryan LE, O'Hara K, Wong S: Lipopolysaccharide changes in impermeability-type aminoglycoside resistance in *Pseudomonas aeruginosa*. Antimicrob Agents Chemother 26:250, 1984.
107. Maloney J, Rimland D, Stephens DS, et al: Analysis of amikacin-resistant *Pseudomonas aeruginosa* developing in patients receiving amikacin. Arch Intern Med 149:630, 1989.
108. Daikos GL, Jackson GG, Lolans VT, Livermore DM: Adaptive resistance to aminoglycoside antibiotics from first-exposure down-regulation. J Infect Dis 162:414, 1990.
109. Moellering RC, Wennersten C, Kunz LJ, Portras JW: Resistance to gentamicin, tobramycin and amikacin among clinical isolates of bacteria. Am J Med 62:873, 1977.
110. Jauregui L, Cushing RD, Lerner AM: Gentamicin/amikacin resistant gram-negative bacilli at Detroit General Hospital. Am J Med 62:882, 1977.
111. Kauffman CA, Ramundo NC, Williams SG, et al: Surveillance of gentamicin-resistant gram-negative bacilli in a general hospital. Antimicrob Agents Chemother 13:918, 1978.
112. Snelling CFT, Ronald AR, Cates CY, Forsythe WC: Resistance of gram-negative bacilli. J Infect Dis 124(Suppl):S264, 1971.
113. Guerrant RL, Strausbaugh LJ, Wenzel RP, et al: Nosocomial bloodstream infection caused by gentamicin-resistant gram-negative bacilli. Am J Med 62:894, 1977.
114. Korzeniowski OM, Hook EW: Aminocyclitols: Aminoglycosides and spectinomycin: *In* Mandell GL, Douglas RG, Bennett JE (eds): Principles and Practice of Infectious Diseases. New York, Wiley, 1979, pp 249–272.
115. Acar JF, Goldstein FW, Menard R, Beriot JP: Strategies in aminoglycoside use and impact upon resistance. Am J Med 80(Suppl 6B):82, 1986.
116. Van Landuyt HW, Boelaert J, Glibert B, et al: Surveillance of aminoglycoside resistance. European data. Am J Med 80(Suppl 6B):76, 1986.
117. Legakis NJ, Velonaki A, Velonakis EM, Lyberopoulou T: Survey of aminoglycoside resistance patterns. Chemioterapia 5:185, 1986.
118. Young EJ, Sewell CM, Koza MA, Clarridge JE: Antibiotic resistance patterns during aminoglycoside restriction. Am J Med 290:223, 1985.
119. Calderwood SA, Wennersten C, Moellering RC Jr, et al: Resistance to six aminoglycosidic aminocyclitol antibiotics among enterococci: Prevalence, evolution, and relationship to synergism with penicillin. Antimicrob Agents Chemother 12:401, 1977.
120. Mederski-Samoraj BD, Murray BE: High-level resistance to gentamicin in clinical isolates of enterococci. J Infect Dis 147:751, 1983.
121. Zervos MJ, Dembinski S, Mikesell T, Schaberg DR: High-level resistance to gentamicin in *Streptococcus faecalis*: Risk factors and evidence for exogenous acquisition of infection. J Infect Dis 153:1075, 1986.
122. Zervos MJ, Kauffman CA, Therasse PM, et al: Nosocomial infec-

tion by gentamicin-resistant *Streptococcus faecalis*: An epidemiologic study. Ann Intern Med 106:687, 1987.
123. Gordon S, Svenson J, Facklam R, et al: (Abstr 790). Presented at the 29th Interscience Conference on Antimicrobial Agents and Chemotherapy, 1989.
124. Patterson JE, Zervos MJ: High-level gentamicin resistance in *Enterococcus*: Microbiology, genetic basis, and epidemiology. Rev Infect Dis 12:644, 1990.
125. Archer GL, Johnston JL: Self-transmissible plasmids in staphylococci that encode resistance to aminoglycosides. Antimicrob Agents Chemother 24:70, 1983.
126. Schaberg DR, Power G, Betzold J, Forbes BA: Conjugative R-plasmids in antimicrobial resistance of *Staphylococcus aureus* causing nosocomial infections. J Infect Dis 152:43, 1985.
127. Itokazu GS, Quinn JP, Bell-Dixon C, et al: Antimicrobial resistances rates among aerobic gram-negative bacilli recovered from patients in intensive care units: Evaluation of a national post-marketing surveillance program. Clin Infect Dis 23:779, 1996.
128. Weinstein RA, Nathan C, Gruensfelder R, Kabins SA: Endemic aminoglycoside resistance in gram-negative bacilli. J Infect Dis 141:338, 1980.
129. Alford RH, Hall A: Epidemiology of infections caused by gentamicin-resistant Enterobacteriaceae and *Pseudomonas aeruginosa* over 15 years at the Nashville Veterans Administration Medical Center. Rev Infect Dis 9:1079 1987.
130. Weinstein RA, Kabins SA: Strategies for prevention and control of multiply drug-resistant nosocomial infection. Am J Med 70:449, 1981.
131. Gaynes RP, Weinstein RA, Smith J, et al: Control of aminoglycoside resistance by barrier precautions. Infect Control 4:221, 1983.
132. Breidis DJ, Robson HG: Comparative activity of netilmicin, gentamicin, amikacin, and tobramycin against *Pseudomonas aeruginosa* and Enterobacteriaceae. Antimicrob Agents Chemother 10:592, 1976.
133. Fu KP, Neu HC: In vitro study of netilmicin compared with other aminoglycosides. Antimicrob Agents Chemother 10:526, 1976.
134. Kabins SA, Nathan C, Cohen S: In vitro comparison of netilmicin, a semisynthetic derivative of sisomicin, and four other aminoglycoside antibiotics. Antimicrob Agents Chemother 10:139, 1976.
135. Dhawan V, Marso E, Martin WJ, et al: In vitro studies with netilmicin compared with amikacin, gentamicin, and tobramycin. Antimicrob Agents Chemother 11:64, 1977.
136. National Committee for Clinical Laboratory Standards: Approved standard M7-A: Methods for dilution antimicrobial susceptibility tests for bacteria that grow aerobically. Villanova, PA, National Committee for Clinical Laboratory Standards, 1985.
137. National Committee for Clinical Laboratory Standards: Approved standard M2-A3: Performance standards for antimicrobic disk susceptibility tests. Villanova, PA, National Committee for Clinical Laboratory Standards, 1984.
138. Reller LB, Schoenknecht FD, Kenny MA, Sherris JC: Antibiotic susceptibility testing of *Pseudomonas aeruginosa*: Selection of a control strain and criteria for magnesium and calcium content in media. J Infect Dis 130:454, 1974.
139. Barry AL, Miller GH, Thornsberry C, et al: Influence of cation supplements on activity of netilmicin against *Pseudomonas aeruginosa* in vitro and in vivo. Antimicrob Agents Chemother 31:1514, 1987.
140. Jones RN, Barry AL, Gawan TL, Washington JA II: Susceptibility tests: Microdilution and macrodilution, broth procedures. *In* Lennette EH, Balows A, Hausler WA Jr, Shadomy HJ (eds): Manual of Clinical Microbiology, ed 4. Washington, DC, American Society for Microbiology, 1985, p 972.
141. Greenberg RN, Hansbrough JN, Lorber RR, Miller GH: Netilmicin sulfate as single-agent therapy for *Pseudomonas* infections. South Med J 82:715, 1989.
142. Barry AL, Miller GH, Hare RS, et al: Modification of interpretive breakpoints for netilmicin disk susceptibility tests with *Pseudomonas aeruginosa*. J Clin Microbiol 19:311, 1984.
143. Juvin ME, Drugeon HB, Caillon J, Pirault JL: Comparaison de l'activité bactéricide de trois aminosides: Gentamicine, tobramycin, amikacine. Pathol Biol 35:461, 1987.
144. Sanders CC, Sanders WE, Goering RV: In vitro studies with SCH21420 and SCH22591: Activity in comparison with six other aminoglycosides and synergy with penicillin against enterococci. Antimicrob Agents Chemother 14:178, 1978.
145. Yu PKW, Washington JA II: Comparative in vitro activity of three aminoglycoside antibiotics: BB-K8, kanamycin, and gentamicin. Antimicrob Agents Chemother 4:133, 1973.
146. Young LS, Hewitt WL: Activity of five aminoglycoside antibiotics in vitro against gram-negative bacilli and *Staphylococcus aureus*. Antimicrob Agents Chemother 4:617, 1973.
147. Sahm DF, Torres C: Effects of medium and inoculum variations on screening for high-level aminoglycoside resistance in *Enterococcus faecalis*. J Clin Microbiol 26:250, 1988.
148. Garcia Rodriguez JA, Martin Luengo F, Saenz Gonzalez MC: Activity of amikacin against *Mycobacterium tuberculosis*. J Antimicrob Chemother 4:293, 1978.
149. Dalovisio JR, Pankey GA: In vitro susceptibility of *Mycobacterium fortuitum* and *Mycobacterium chelonei* to amikacin. J Infect Dis 137:318, 1978.
150. Chiu J, Nussbaum J, Bozzette S, et al: California Collaborative Treatment Group: Treatment of disseminated *Mycobacterium avium* complex infection in AIDS with amikacin, ethambutol, rifampin, and ciprofloxacin. Ann Intern Med 113:358, 1990.
151. Allan JD, Moellering RC Jr: Management of infections caused by gram-negative bacilli: The role of antimicrobial combinations. Rev Infect Dis 7(Suppl 4):S559, 1985.
152. Holm SE: Interaction between β-lactam and other antibiotics. Rev Infect Dis 8(Suppl 3):S305, 1986.
153. Hook EW, Roberts RB, Sande MA: Antimicrobial therapy of experimental enterococcal endocarditis. Antimicrob Agents Chemother 8:564, 1975.
154. Johnson DE, Thompson B, Calia FM: Comparative activities of piperacillin, ceftazidime, and amikacin, alone and in all possible combinations, against experimental *Pseudomonas aeruginosa* infections in neutropenic rats. Antimicrob Agents Chemother 28:735, 1985.
155. Gordin FM, Rusnak MG, Sande MA: Evaluation of combination chemotherapy in a lightly anesthetized animal model of *Pseudomonas* pneumonia. Antimicrob Agents Chemother 31:398, 1987.
156. Mandell GL, Kaye D, Levison ME, Hook EW: Enterococcal endocarditis: An analysis of 38 patients observed at the New York Hospital Cornell Medical Center. Arch Intern Med 125:258, 1970.
157. Moellering RC Jr, Wennersten C, Weinberg AN: Studies on antibiotic synergism against enterococci. I. Bacteriologic studies. J Lab Clin Med 77:821, 1971.
158. Moellering RC Jr, Korzeniowski OM, Sande MA, Wennersten CB: Species-specific resistance to antimicrobial synergism in *Streptococcus faecium* and *Streptococcus faecalis*. J Infect Dis 140:203, 1979.
159. Miller MH, El-Sokkary MA, Feinstein SA, Lowy FD: Penicillin-induced effects on streptomycin uptake and early bactericidal activity differ in viridans group and enterococcal streptococci. Antimicrob Agents Chemother 30:763, 1986.
160. Geraci JE, Martin WJ: Antibiotic therapy of bacterial endocarditis. VII. Subacute enterococcal endocarditis: Clinical, pathologic, and therapeutic consideration of 33 cases. Circulation 10:173, 1954.
161. Dowling HF: Present status of therapy with combinations of antibiotics. Am J Med 39:796, 1965.
162. Tan JS, Terhume CA Jr, Kaplan S, Hamberger M: Successful two-week treatment schedule for penicillin-susceptible *Streptococcus viridans* endocarditis. Lancet 2:1340, 1971.
163. Moellering RC Jr, Weinberg AN: Studies on antibiotic synergism against enterococci. II. Effect of various antibiotics on the uptake of C^{14}-labeled streptomycin by enterococci. J Clin Invest 50:2580, 1971.
164. Zenilman JM, Miller MH, Mandel LJ: In vitro studies simultaneously examining effect of oxacillin on uptake of radiolabeled streptomycin and on associated bacterial lethality in *Staphylococcus aureus*. Antimicrob Agents Chemother 30:877, 1986.
165. Miller MH, Feinstein SA, Chow RT: Early effects of β-lactams on aminoglycoside uptake, bactericidal rates, and turbidimetrically measured growth inhibition in *Pseudomonas aeruginosa*. Antimicrob Agents Chemother 31:108, 1987.
166. Eliopoulos GM, Moellering RC Jr: Antibiotic synergism and antimicrobial combinations in clinical infections. Rev Infect Dis 4:282, 1982.

167. Gerber AU, Vastola AP, Brandel J, Craig WA: Selection of aminoglycoside-resistant variants of *Pseudomonas aeruginosa* in an in vivo model. J Infect Dis 146:691, 1982.
168. Herman DJ, Gerding DN: Antimicrobial resistance among enterococci. Antimicrob Agents Chemother 35:1, 1991.
169. Herman DJ, Gerding DN: Screening and treatment of infections caused by resistant enterococci. Antimicrob Agents Chemother 35:215, 1991.
170. Zimmerman RA, Moellering RC Jr, Weinberg AN: Mechanism of resistance to antibiotic synergism in enterococci. J Bacteriol 105:873, 1971.
171. Clarke JT, Libke RD, Regamey C, Kirby WM: Comparative pharmacokinetics of amikacin and kanamycin. Clin Pharmacol Ther 15:610, 1974.
172. Jaffe G, Meyers BR, Hirschman SZ: Pharmacokinetics of tobramycin in patients with stable renal impairment, patients undergoing peritoneal dialysis, and patients on chronic hemodialysis. Antimicrob Agents Chemother 5:611, 1974.
173. Jahre JA, Fu KP, Neu HC: Kinetics of netilmicin and gentamicin. Clin Pharmacol Ther 23:591, 1978.
174. Kahlmeter G, Hallberg T, Kamme C: Gentamicin and tobramycin in patients with various infections: Concentrations in serum and urinary excretion. J Antimicrob Chemother 4(Suppl A):37, 1978.
175. Meyers BR, Hirschman SZ, Warmser G, et al: Pharmacokinetic study of netilmicin. Antimicrob Agents Chemother 12:122, 1977.
176. Regamey C, Gordon RC, Kirby WM: Comparative pharmacokinetics of tobramycin and gentamicin. Clin Pharmacol Ther 14:296, 1973.
177. Riff LJ, Mareschi G: Netilmicin and gentamicin: Comparative pharmacology in humans. Antimicrob Agents Chemother 11:609, 1977.
178. Schentag JJ, Jusko WJ: Renal clearance and tissue accumulation of gentamicin. Clin Pharmacol Ther 22:364, 1977.
179. Schentag JJ, Lasezkay G, Cumbo TJ, et al: Accumulation pharmacokinetics of tobramycin. Antimicrob Agents Chemother 13:649, 1978.
180. Walker JM, Wise R, Michard M: The pharmacokinetics of amikacin and gentamicin in volunteers: A comparison of individual differences. J Antimicrob Chemother 5:95, 1979.
181. Kunin CM: Absorption, distribution, excretion and fate of kanamycin. Ann N Y Acad Sci 132:811, 1966.
182. Kunin CM, Chalmers TC, Leevy CM: Absorption of orally administered neomycin and kanamycin. N Engl J Med 262:380, 1960.
183. Breen KJ, Bryant RE, Levinson JD, Schenker S: Neomycin absorption in man. Ann Intern Med 76:211, 1972.
184. Last PM, Sherlock S: Systemic absorption of orally administered neomycin in liver disease. N Engl J Med 262:385, 1960.
185. Berk DP, Chalmers T: Deafness complicating antibiotic therapy of hepatic encephalopathy. Ann Intern Med 73:393, 1970.
186. Greenberg JH, Momay H: Audiotoxicity and nephrotoxicity due to orally administered neomycin. JAMA 194:827, 1965.
187. Halpern EB, Heller MW: Ototoxicity of orally administered neomycin. Arch Otolaryngol 73:675, 1961.
188. Gibson WS: Deafness due to orally administered neomycin. Arch Otolaryngol 86:163, 1967.
189. Ruben RJ, Daly JF: Neomycin ototoxicity and nephrotoxicity. Laryngoscope 78:734, 1968.
190. Kalbian VV: Deafness following oral use of neomycin. South Med J 65:499, 1972.
191. Ward KM, Rounthwaite FJ: Neomycin ototoxicity. Ann Otol 87:211, 1978.
192. Masur H, Whelton PK, Whelton A: Neomycin toxicity revisited. Arch Surg 111:822, 1976.
193. Fields RL: Neomycin ototoxicity. Arch Otolaryngol 79:67, 1964.
194. Fuller A: Ototoxicity of neomycin aerosol. Lancet 1:1026, 1960.
195. Stewart IF: The ototoxic effects of some antibiotics. Can Otolaryngol Soc 20:202, 1966.
196. Kelley DR, Nilo ER, Berggreu RB: Deafness after topical neomycin wound irrigation. N Engl J Med 280:1338, 1969.
197. Bamford MFM, Jones LF: Deafness and biochemical imbalance after burns treatment with topical antibiotics in young children. Arch Dis Child 53:326, 1978.
198. Manuel MA, Kurtz I, Saiphoo CS, Nedzelski JM: Nephrotoxicity and ototoxicity following irrigation of wounds with neomycin. Can J Surg 22:274, 1979.
199. Helm WH: Ototoxicity of neomycin aerosol. Lancet 1:1294, 1960.
200. Myerson M, Knight HF, Gambarcini AJ: Intrapleural neomycin causing ototoxicity. Ann Thorac Surg 9:483, 1970.
201. Weinstein AJ, McHenry MC, Gavan TL: Systemic absorption of neomycin irrigating solution. JAMA 238:152, 1977.
202. DePaepe M, Lameire N, Belpaire F, et al: Peritoneal pharmacokinetics of gentamicin in man. Clin Nephrol 19:107, 1983.
203. Odio W, Van Laer E, Klastersky J: Concentrations of gentamicin in bronchial secretions after intramuscular and endotracheal administration. J Clin Pharmacol 15:518, 1975.
204. Gough PA, Schuddekopf-Jordan N: A review of the therapeutic efficacy of aerosolized and endotracheally instilled antibiotics. Pharmacotherapy 2:367, 1982.
205. Stout SA, Derendorf H: Local treatment of respiratory infections with antibiotics. Drug Intell Clin Pharm 21:322, 1987.
206. Lake KB, Van Dyke JJ, Rumsfeld JA: Combined topical pulmonary and systemic gentamicin: The question of safety. Chest 68:62, 1975.
207. Hall WH, Gerding DN, Schierl EA: Penetration of tobramycin into infected intravascular fluids and its therapeutic effectiveness. J Infect Dis 135:957, 1977.
208. Leroy A, Humburt G, Oksenhendler G, Fillastre JP: Pharmacokinetics of aminoglycosides in subjects with normal and impaired renal function. Antibiot Chemother 25:163, 1978.
209. Edwards DJ, Mangione A, Cumbo TJ, Schentag JJ: Predicted tissue accumulation of netilmicin in patients. Antimicrob Agents Chemother 20:714, 1981.
210. Gordon RC, Regamey C, Kirby WM: Serum protein binding of the aminoglycoside antibiotics. Antimicrob Agents Chemother 2:214, 1972.
211. Chisholm GD, Waterworth PM, Calnan JS, et al: Concentration of antibacterial agents in interstitial tissue fluid. Br Med J 1:569, 1973.
212. Barza M, Scheife RT: Antimicrobial spectrum, pharmacology, and therapeutic use of antibiotics. J Maine Med Assoc 68:194, 1977.
213. Collier VU, Lietman PS, Mitch WE: Evidence for luminal uptake of gentamicin in perfused rat kidney. J Pharmacol Exp Ther 210:247, 1979.
214. Silverblatt FJ, Kuehn C: Autoradiography of gentamicin uptake by the rat proximal tubular cell. Kidney Int 15:335, 1979.
215. Bennett WM: Mechanisms of aminoglycoside nephrotoxicity. Clin Exp Pharmacol Physiol 16:1, 1989.
216. Wood MJ, Farrell W: Comparison of urinary excretion of tobramycin and gentamicin in adults. J Infect Dis 134(Suppl):S133, 1976.
217. Jackson GG: Present status of aminoglycoside antibiotics and their safe effective use. Clin Ther 1:200, 1977.
218. Alftan O, Renkonen OV, Sironen A: Concentration of gentamicin in serum, urine and urogenital tissue in man. Acta Pathol Microbiol Scand [B] 81(Suppl 241):92, 1973.
219. Chow A, Hecht R, Witners R: Gentamicin and carbenicillin penetration into the septic joint. N Engl J Med 285:178, 1971.
220. Dee TH, Kozin F: Gentamicin and tobramycin penetration into synovial fluid. Antimicrob Agents Chemother 12:548, 1977.
221. Chisholm GD, Waterworth PM, Calnan JS, et al: Concentration of antibacterial agents in interstitial tissue fluid. Br Med J 1:569, 1973.
222. Scherrer JJ, Kearns GL, Jackson JW: Tobramycin penetration into pericardial fluid. Am J Hosp Pharm 38:1039, 1981.
223. Mendelson J, Portnoy J, Sigman H: Pharmacology of gentamicin in the biliary tract of humans. Antimicrob Agents Chemother 4:538, 1973.
224. Pitt HA, Roberts RB, Johnson WD Jr: Gentamicin levels in the human biliary tract. J Infect Dis 127:299, 1973.
225. Odio W, Van Laer E, Klastersky J: Concentrations of gentamicin in bronchial secretions after intramuscular and endotracheal administration. J Clin Pharmacol 15:518, 1975.
226. Klastersky J, Geuning C, Mouawad E, Daneau D: Endotracheal gentamicin in bronchial infections in patients with tracheostomy. Chest 61:117, 1972.
227. Brown RB, Kruse JA, Counts GW, et al: Double-blind study of endotracheal tobramycin in the treatment of gram-negative bacterial pneumonia. Antimicrob Agents Chemother 34:269, 1990.
228. Barza M: Antibacterial agents in the treatment of ocular infections. Infect Dis Clin North Am 3:533, 1989.

229. Rall DP, Stabenau JR, Zubrod CG: Distribution of drugs between blood and cerebrospinal fluid: General methodology and effect of pH gradients. J Pharmacol Exp Ther 125:185, 1959.
230. Thea D, Barza M: Use of antibacterial agents in infections of the central nervous system. Infect Dis Clin North Am 3:553, 1989.
231. Moellering RC Jr, Fisher EG: Relationship of intraventricular gentamicin levels to cure of meningitis. J Pediatr 81:532, 1972.
232. Kaiser AB, McGee ZA: Aminoglycoside therapy of gram-negative bacillary meningitis. N Engl J Med 293:1215, 1975.
233. McCracken GH Jr, Mize S, Threlkeld N: Intraventricular gentamicin therapy in gram-negative bacillary meningitis of infancy. Lancet 1:787, 1980.
234. Silverblatt FJ, Kuehn C: Autoradiography of gentamicin uptake by the rat proximal tubular cell. Kidney Int 15:335, 1979.
235. Barza M, Scheife RT: Antimicrobial spectrum, pharmacology, and therapeutic use of antibiotics. J Maine Med Assoc 68:194, 1977.
236. Gyselynck A-M, Forrey A, Cutler R: Pharmacokinetics of gentamicin: Distribution and plasma and renal clearance. J Infect Dis 124(Suppl):S70, 1971.
237. Plantier J, Forrey AW, O'Neill MA, et al: Pharmacokinetics of amikacin in patients with normal or impaired renal function: Radioenzymatic acetylation assay. J Infect Dis 134(Suppl):S323, 1976.
238. Schentag JJ, Jusko WJ: Renal clearance and tissue accumulation of gentamicin. Clin Pharmacol Ther 22:364, 1977.
239. Anderson ET, Young LS, Hewitt WL: Simultaneous antibiotic levels in "breakthrough" gram-negative rod bacteremia. Am J Med 61:493, 1976.
240. Moore RD, Smith CR, Lietman PS: The association of aminoglycoside plasma levels with mortality in patients with gram-negative bacteremia. J Infect Dis 149:443, 1984.
241. Moore RD, Smith CR, Lietman PS: Association of aminoglycoside plasma levels with therapeutic outcome in gram-negative pneumonia. Am J Med 77:657, 1984.
242. Moore RD, Lietman PS, Smith CR: Clinical response to aminoglycoside therapy: Importance of the ratio of peak concentration to minimal inhibitory concentration. J Infect Dis 155:93, 1987.
243. Tablan OC, Reyes MP, Rintelmann WF, Lerner AM: Renal and auditory toxicity of high-dose, prolonged therapy with gentamicin and tobramycin in pseudomonas endocarditis. J Infect Dis 149:257, 1984.
244. Moore RD, Smith CR, Lipsky JJ, et al: Risk factors for nephrotoxicity in patients treated with aminoglycosides. Ann Intern Med 100:352, 1984.
245. Moore RD, Smith CR, Lietman PS: Risk factors for the development of auditory toxicity in patients receiving aminoglycosides. J Infect Dis 149:23, 1984.
246. Lerner SA, Matz GJ, Schmitt BA: Prospective, randomized, blinded assessment of nephro- and ototoxicity in patients treated with gentamicin, netilmicin, and tobramycin (Abstr 488). Presented at the 24th Interscience Conference on Antimicrobial Agents and Chemotherapy, 1984.
247. Sawyers CL, Moore RD, Lerner SA, Smith CR: A model for predicting nephrotoxicity in patients treated with aminoglycosides. J Infect Dis 153:1062, 1986.
248. Burton ME, Brater DC, Chen PS, et al: A Bayesian feedback method of aminoglycoside dosing. Clin Pharmacol Ther 37:349, 1985.
249. Sarubbi FA Jr, Hull JH: Amikacin serum concentrations: Prediction of levels and dosage guidelines. Ann Intern Med 89:612, 1978.
250. Zaske DE, Cipolle RJ, Strate RJ: Gentamicin dosage requirements: Wide interpatient variations in 242 surgery patients with normal renal function. Surgery 87:164, 1980.
251. Sawchuck RJ, Zaske DE: Pharmacokinetics of dosing regimens which utilize intravenous infusions: Gentamicin in burn patients. J Pharmacokinet Biopharm 4:183, 1976.
252. Sawchuck RJ, Zaske DE, Cipolle RJ, et al: Kinetic model for gentamicin dosing with use of individual patient parameters. Clin Pharmacol Ther 21:362, 1977.
253. Cipolle RJ, Seifert RD, Zaske DE, Strate RG: Systematically individualizing tobramycin dosage regimens. J Clin Pharmacol 20:570, 1980.
254. Zaske DE: Aminoglycosides: Counterpoint discussion. *In* Evans WE, Schentag JJ, Jusko WJ (eds): Applied Pharmacokinetics: Principles of Therapeutic Drug Monitoring. San Francisco, Applied Therapeutics, 1980, p 210.
255. Howard JB, McCracken GH, Trujillo H, et al: Amikacin in newborn infants: Comparative pharmacology with kanamycin and clinical efficacy in 45 neonates with bacterial diseases. Antimicrob Agents Chemother 10:205, 1976.
256. Haughey DB, Hilligoss DM, Grassi A, et al: Two compartment gentamicin pharmacokinetics in premature neonates: A comparison to adults with decreased glomerular filtration rate. J Pediatr 96:325, 1980.
257. McCracken G: Aminoglycoside toxicity in infants and children. Am J Med 80(Suppl 6B):172, 1986.
258. Cockroft DW, Gault MH: Prediction of creatinine clearance from serum creatinine. Nephron 16:31, 1976.
259. Schwartz SN, Pazin GJ, Lyon JA, et al: A controlled investigation of the pharmacokinetics of gentamicin and tobramycin in obese patients. J Infect Dis 138:499, 1978.
260. Blovin RA, Mann HJ, Griffen WO Jr, et al: Tobramycin pharmacokinetics in morbidly obese patients. Clin Pharmacol Ther 26:508, 1979.
261. Hallynck TH, Soep HH, Thomas JA, et al: Lean body mass and amikacin dosage. J Antimicrob Chemother 6:286, 1980.
262. Zaske DE, Sawchuck RJ, Strate RG: The necessity of increased doses of amikacin in burn patients. Surgery 84:603, 1978.
263. Loirat P, Rohan J, Baillet A, et al: Increased glomerular filtration rate in patients with major burns and its effect on the pharmacokinetics of tobramycin. N Engl J Med 299:915, 1978.
264. Marks MI, Prentice R, Swarson R, et al: Carbenicillin and gentamicin: Pharmacologic studies in patients with cystic fibrosis and *Pseudomonas* pulmonary infections. J Pediatr 79:822, 1971.
265. McCrae WM, Raeburn JA, Hanson EJ: Tobramycin therapy of infections due to *Pseudomonas aeruginosa* in patients with cystic fibrosis: Effect of dosage and concentration of antibiotic in sputum. J Infect Dis 134(Suppl):S191, 1976.
266. Pennington JE, Dale DC, Reynolds HY, et al: Gentamicin sulfate pharmacokinetics: Lower levels of gentamicin in blood during fever. J Infect Dis 132:270, 1975.
267. Zeitany RG, El Saghir NS, Santhosh-Kuvan CR, Sigmon MA: Increased aminoglycoside dosage requirements in hematologic malignancy. Antimicrob Agents Chemother 34:702, 1990.
268. Bianco TM, Dwyer PN, Bertino JS Jr: Gentamicin pharmacokinetics, nephrotoxicity, and prediction of mortality in febrile neutropenic patients. Antimicrob Agents Chemother 33:1890, 1989.
269. Wallace SM, Chan L-Y: In vitro interaction of aminoglycosides with β-lactam penicillins. Antimicrob Agents Chemother 28:274, 1985.
270. Ervin TR, Bullock WE, Nuttall CE: Inactivation of gentamicin by penicillins in patients with renal failure. Antimicrob Agents Chemother 9:1004, 1976.
271. Blair DC, Duggan DO, Schroeder ET: Inactivation of amikacin and gentamicin by carbenicillin in patients with end-stage renal failure. Antimicrob Agents Chemother 22:376, 1982.
272. Thompson MIB, Russo MC, Saxon BJ, et al: Gentamicin inactivation by piperacillin or carbenicillin in patients with end-stage renal disease. Antimicrob Agents Chemother 21:268, 1982.
273. Giusti DL, Hayton WL: Dosage regimen adjustments in renal impairment. Drug Intell Clin Pharm 7:382, 1973.
274. Lockwood WR, Bower JD: Tobramycin concentrations in the serum of normal and anephric patients. Antimicrob Agents Chemother 3:125, 1973.
275. Madhavan T, Yaremchuk K, Levin N, et al: Effect of renal failure and dialysis on the serum concentration of the aminoglycoside amikacin. Antimicrob Agents Chemother 10:464, 1976.
276. McHenry MC, Wagner JG, Hall PM, et al: Pharmacokinetics of amikacin patients with impaired renal function. J Infect Dis 134(Suppl):S343, 1976.
277. Pijick J, Hallynck T, Soep H, et al: Pharmacokinetics of amikacin in patients with renal insufficiency: Relationship of half-life to creatinine clearance. J Infect Dis 134(Suppl):S331, 1976.
278. Leroy A, Humbert G, Oksenhendler G, Fillastre JP: Pharmacokinetics of aminoglycosides in subjects with normal and impaired renal function. Antibiot Chemother 25:163, 1978.
279. Pechere JC, Dugal R: Pharmacokinetics of intravenously administered tobramycin in normal volunteers and in renally impaired and hemodialyzed patients. J Infect Dis 134(Suppl):S118, 1976.

280. Regeur L, Colding H, Jensen H, et al: Pharmacokinetics of amikacin during hemodialysis and peritoneal dialysis. Antimicrob Agents Chemother 11:214, 1977.
281. Atkins RC, Mion C, Despaux E, et al: Peritoneal transfer of kanamycin and its use in peritoneal dialysis. Kidney Int 3:391, 1973.
282. Jackson GG: Chairman's summary: The impact of novel dosing regimens on the safety and efficacy of aminoglycosides. J Drug Dev 1(Suppl 3):155, 1988.
283. Gilbert DN, Bennett WM: Use of antimicrobial agents in renal failure. Infect Dis Clin North Am 3:517, 1989.
284. Nordström L, Lerner SA: Single daily dose therapy with aminoglycosides. J Hosp Infect 18(Suppl A):117, 1991.
285. Vogelman B, Craig WA: Kinetics of antimicrobial activity. J Pediatr 108:835, 1986.
286. Kapusnik JE, Hackbarth CJ, Chambers HF, et al: Single, large, daily dosing versus intermittent dosing of tobramycin for treating experimental pseudomonas pneumonia. J Infect Dis 158:7, 1988.
287. Noone P, Parsons TM, Pattison JR, et al: Experience in monitoring gentamicin therapy during treatment of serious gram-negative sepsis. Br Med J 1:477, 1974.
288. Bundtzen RW, Gerber AU, Cohn DL, Craig WA: Postantibiotic suppression of bacterial growth. Rev Infect Dis 3:28, 1981.
289. Craig WA, Gundmundsson S: The postantibiotic effect. *In* Lorian V (ed): Antibiotics in Laboratory Medicine, ed 2. Baltimore, Williams & Wilkins, 1984, pp 515–536.
290. Vogelman BS, Craig WA: Postantibiotic effects. J Antimicrob Chemother 15:37, 1985.
291. Gerber AU, Faller-Segessenmann C: In vivo assessment of in vitro killing patterns of *Pseudomonas aeruginosa*. J Antimicrob Chemother 15(Suppl A):201, 1985.
292. Vogelman B, Gundmundsson S, Turnidge J, et al: In vivo postantibiotic effect in a thigh infection in neutropenic mice. J Infect Dis 157:287, 1988.
293. Gerber AU, Craig WA, Brugger HP, et al: Impact of dosing intervals on activity of gentamicin and ticarcillin against *Pseudomonas aeruginosa* in granulocytopenic mice. J Infect Dis 147:910, 1983.
294. Herscovici L, Grise G, Thauvin C, et al: Efficacy and safety of once daily versus intermittent dosing of tobramycin in rabbits with acute pyelonephritis. Scand J Infect Dis 20:205, 1988.
295. Wood CA, Norton DR, Kohlhepp SJ, et al: The influence of tobramycin dosage regimens on nephrotoxicity, ototoxicity and antibacterial efficacy in a rat model of subcutaneous abscess. J Infect Dis 158:13, 1988.
296. Frame PT, Phair JP, Watanakunakorn C, Bannister TWP: Pharmacologic factors associated with gentamicin nephrotoxicity in rabbits. J Infect Dis 135:952, 1977.
297. Bennett WM, Plamp CE, Gilbert DN, et al: The influence of dosage regimen on experimental gentamicin nephrotoxicity: Dissociation of peak serum levels from renal failure. J Infect Dis 140:576, 1979.
298. Olier B, Viotte G, Morin JP, Fillastre JP: Influence of dosage regimen on experimental tobramycin nephrotoxicity. Chemotherapy 29:385, 1983.
299. Reiner NE, Bloxham DD, Thompson WL: Nephrotoxicity of gentamicin and tobramycin given once daily or continuously in dogs. J Antimicrob Chemother 4:85, 1978.
300. Powell SH, Thompson WL, Luthe MA, et al: Once-daily vs continuous aminoglycoside dosing: Efficacy and toxicity in animal and clinical studies of gentamicin, netilmicin, and tobramycin. J Infect Dis 147:918, 1983.
301. Verpooten GA, Giuliano RA, Verbist L, et al: Once daily dosing decreases renal accumulation of gentamicin and netilmicin. Clin Pharmacol Ther 45:22, 1989.
302. Brummett RE: Ototoxicity of aminoglycoside antibiotics in animal models. *In* Fillastre J-P (ed): Nephrotoxicity and Ototoxicity of Drugs. Rouen, France, INSERM, 1982, p 359.
303. Pechere JC, Bernard PA: Gentamicin ototoxicity can be avoided if a new therapeutic regimen is used (Abstr 484). Presented at the 24th Interscience Conference on Antimicrobial Agents and Chemotherapy, 1984.
304. Bamonte F, Dionisotti S, Gamba M, et al: Relation of dosing regimen to aminoglycoside ototoxicity: Evaluation of auditory damage in the guinea pig. Chemotherapy 36:41, 1990.
305. Davis RR, Brummett RE, Bendrick TW, Himes DL: Dissociation of maximum concentration of kanamycin in plasma and perilymph from ototoxic effect. J Antimicrob Chemother 14:291, 1984.
306. Tran Ba Huy P, Bernard P, Schacht J: Kinetics of gentamicin uptake and release in the rat: Comparison of inner ear tissues and fluid with other organs. J Clin Invest 77:1492, 1986.
307. Tulkens PM: Nephrotoxicity of aminoglycoside antibiotics. Toxicol Lett 46:107, 1989.
308. Tran Ba Huy P: Aminoglycoside ototoxicity: Influence of dosage regimen on drug uptake, correlation between membrane binding and clinical features. J Drug Dev 1(Suppl 3):93, 1988.
309. Tran Ba Huy P, Deffrennes D: Aminoglycoside ototoxicity: Influence of dosage regimen on drug uptake and correlation between membrane binding and some clinical features. Acta Otolaryngol 105:511, 1988.
310. Fan ST, Lau WY, Teoh-Chan CH, et al: Once daily administration of netilmicin compared with thrice daily, both in combination with metronidazole, in gangrenous and perforated appendicitis. J Antimicrob Chemother 22:69, 1988.
311. Maller R, Isaksson B, Nilsson L, Sören L: A study of amikacin given once versus twice daily in serious infections. J Antimicrob Chemother 22:75, 1988.
312. Muijsken MA, Vreede RW, Haverkorn MJ, et al: New approach in antimicrobial therapy: An open, randomized study of efficacy and safety of once-daily versus conventional dosing of netilmicin in combination therapy in patients with severe infections. *In* Vreede R (ed): Infections by Gram-Negative Bacilli: Humoral Defense of the Host and Antimicrobial Therapy. Utrecht, Netherlands, 1988, p 143.
313. Tulkens PM, Clerckx-Braun F, Donnez J, et al: Safety and efficacy of aminoglycosides once-a-day: Experimental data and randomized, controlled evaluation in patients suffering from pelvic inflammatory disease. J Drug Dev 1(Suppl 3):71, 1988.
314. Hollender LF, Bahnini J, DeManzini N, et al: A multicentric study of netilmicin once daily versus thrice daily in patients with appendicitis and other intra-abdominal infections. J Antimicrob Chemother 23:773, 1989.
315. Mauracher EH, Lau WY, Kartowisastro H, et al: Comparison of once-daily and thrice-daily netilmicin regimens in serious infections: A multicenter study in six Asian countries. Clin Ther 11:604, 1989.
316. Sturm AW: Netilmicin in the treatment of gram-negative bacteremia: Single daily versus multiple daily dosage. J Infect Dis 159:931, 1989.
317. Nordström L, Ringberg H, Cronberg S, et al: Does administration of an aminoglycoside in a single daily dose affect its efficacy and toxicity? J Antimicrob Chemother 25:159, 1990.
318. ter Braak EW, de Vries PJ, Bouter KP, et al: Once-daily dosing regimen for aminoglycoside plus beta-lactam combination therapy of serious bacterial infections: Comparative trial with netilmicin plus ceftriaxone. Am J Med 89:58, 1990.
319. Munckhof WJ, Grayson ML, Turnidge JD: A meta-analysis of studies on the safety and efficacy of aminoglycosides given either once daily or as divided doses. J Antimicrob Chemother 37:645, 1996.
320. Lietman PS: Aminoglycosides and spectinomycin: Aminocyclitols. *In* Mandell GL, Douglas RG Jr, Bennett JE (eds): Principles and Practice of Infectious Diseases, ed 3. New York, Churchill Livingstone, 1990, pp 269–284.
321. Chinyanga HM, Stoyka WW: The effect of colymycin M, gentamycin and kanamycin on depression of neuromuscular transmission induced by pancuronium bromide. Can Anaesth Soc J 21:569, 1974.
322. L'Hommedieu CS, Huber PA, Rasch DK: Potentiation of magnesium-induced neuromuscular weakness by gentamicin. Crit Care Med 11:55, 1983.
323. L'Hommedieu C, Stough R, Brown L, et al: Potentiation of neuromuscular weakness in infant botulism by aminoglycosides. J Pediatr 95:1065, 1979.
324. Hokkanen E: The aggravating effect of some antibiotics on the neuromuscular blockade in myasthenia gravis. Acta Neurol Scand 40:346, 1964.
325. Sanders DB, Kim YI, Howard JF, et al: Intercostal muscle biopsy studies in myasthenia gravis: Clinical correlations and the direct effects of drugs and myasthenic serum. Ann N Y Acad Sci 377:544, 1981.

326. Pittinger CB, Adamson R: Antibiotic blockade of neuromuscular function. Annu Rev Pharmacol 12:169, 1972.
327. American Medical Association Department of Drugs, Division of Drugs and Technology: Aminoglycosides. Miscellaneous antibacterial agents. *In* Drug Evaluations, ed 6. Chicago, American Medical Association, 1986, p 1425.
328. Schentag JJ: Aminoglycoside pharmacokinetics as a guide to therapy and toxicology. *In* Whelton A, Neu HC (eds): The Aminoglycosides: Microbiology, Clinical Use and Toxicology. New York, Marcel Dekker, 1982, pp 143–167.
329. Patel V, Luft FC, Yum MN, et al: Enzymuria in gentamicin induced kidney damage. Antimicrob Agents Chemother 7:364, 1975.
330. Gibey R, Dupond JL, Alber D, et al: Predictive value of urinary *N*-acetyl-beta-d-glucosaminidase (NAG), alanine aminopeptidase (AAP), and beta-2-microglobulin in evaluating nephrotoxicity of gentamicin. Clin Chim Acta 116:25, 1981.
331. Sethi K, Diamond LH: Aminoglycoside nephrotoxicity and its predictability. Nephron 27:265, 1981.
332. Davey PG, Geddes AM: Study of alanine aminopeptidase excretion as a test of gentamicin nephrotoxicity. J Antimicrob Chemother 11:455, 1983.
333. Mondorf AW, Heynold FT, Scherberich JE, et al: Assessment of the nephrotoxic potential of ceftazidime and a ceftazidime/tobramycin combination in volunteers. Infection 11(Suppl 1):557, 1983.
334. Schentag JJ, Gengo FM, Plaut ME, et al: Urinary casts as an indicator of renal tubular damage in patients receiving aminoglycosides. Antimicrob Agents Chemother 16:468, 1979.
335. Schentag JJ, Plaut ME: Patterns of beta-2 microglobulin excretion by patients treated with aminoglycosides. Kidney Int 17:654, 1980.
336. Trollfors B, Alestig K, Krantz I, Norrby R: Quantitative nephrotoxicity of gentamicin in nontoxic doses. J Infect Dis 3:306, 1980.
337. Zaske DE: Aminoglycosides: *In* Evans WE, Schentag JJ, Jusko WJ (eds): Applied Pharmacokinetics. Spokane, WA, Applied Therapeutics, 1986, p 331.
338. Garrison MW, Zaske DE, Rotschafer JC: Aminoglycosides: Another perspective. DICP 24:267, 1990.
339. Lietman PS, Smith CR: Aminoglycoside nephrotoxicity in humans. J Infect Dis 5(Suppl 2):S284, 1983.
340. Tulkens PM: Nephrotoxicity of aminoglycoside antibiotics. Toxicol Lett 46:107, 1989.
341. Luft FC, Rankin LI, Sloan RS, Yum MN: Recovery from aminoglycoside nephrotoxicity with continued drug administration. Antimicrob Agents Chemother 14:284, 1978.
342. Elliott WC, Houghton DC, Gilbert DN, et al: Gentamicin nephrotoxicity: I. Degree and permanence of acquired insensitivity. J Lab Clin Med 100:501, 1982.
343. Rybak MJ, Boike SC, Levine DP, Erickson SR: Clinical use and toxicity of high-dose tobramycin in patients with pseudomonal endocarditis. J Antimicrob Chemother 17:115, 1986.
344. Appel GB: Aminoglycoside nephrotoxicity. Am J Med 88(Suppl 3C):16S, 1990.
345. Kahlmeter G, Dahlager JI: Aminoglycoside toxicity–A review of clinical studies published between 1975 and 1982. J Antimicrob Chemother 13(Suppl A):9, 1984.
346. Smith CR, Lipsky JJ, Laskin OL, et al: Double-blind comparison of the nephrotoxicity and auditory toxicity of gentamicin and tobramycin. N Engl J Med 302:1106, 1980.
347. Lerner SA, Schmitt BA, Seligsohn R, Matz GJ: Comparative study of ototoxicity and nephrotoxicity in patients randomly assigned to treatment with amikacin or gentamicin. Am J Med 80(Suppl 6B):98, 1986.
348. Lam YW, Arana CJ, Shikuma LR, Rotschafer JC: The clinical utility of a published nomogram to predict aminoglycoside nephrotoxicity. JAMA 256:639, 1986.
349. Moore RD, Smith CR, Lietman PS: Predicting aminoglycoside nephrotoxicity (Letter). JAMA 256:864, 1986.
350. Rotschafer JC, Shikuma L, Lam F: Reply (Letter). JAMA 256:865, 1986.
351. Garrison MW, Rotschafer JC: Clinical assessment of a published model to predict aminoglycoside-induced nephrotoxicity. Ther Drug Monit 11:171, 1989.
352. Moore RD, Smith CR, Lietman PS: Increased risk of renal dysfunction due to interaction of liver disease and aminoglycosides. Am J Med 80:1093, 1986.
353. Desai TK, Tsang T-K: Aminoglycoside nephrotoxicity in obstruction jaundice. Am J Med 85:47, 1988.
354. Wood CA, Kohlhepp SJ, Kohnen PW, et al: Vancomycin enhancement of experimental tobramycin nephrotoxicity. Antimicrob Agents Chemother 30:20, 1986.
355. Farber BF, Moellering RC Jr: Retrospective study of the toxicity of preparations of vancomycin from 1974 to 1981. Antimicrob Agents Chemother 23:138, 1983.
356. Rybak MJ, Frankowski JJ, Edwards DJ, Albrecht LM: Alanine aminopeptidase and β_2-microglobulin excretion in patients receiving vancomycin and gentamicin. Antimicrob Agents Chemother 31:1461, 1987.
357. Rybak MJ, Albrecht LM, Boike SC, Chandrasekar PH: Nephrotoxicity of vancomycin, alone and with an aminoglycoside. J Antimicrob Chemother 25:679, 1990.
358. Mellor JA, Kingdom J, Cafferkey M, Keane CT: Vancomycin toxicity: A prospective study. J Antimicrob Chemother 15:773, 1985.
359. Sorrell TC, Collignon PJ: A prospective study of adverse reactions associated with vancomycin therapy. J Antimicrob Chemother 16:235, 1985.
360. Buring JE, Evans DA, Mayreut SL, et al: Randomized trials of aminoglycoside antibiotics: Quantitative overview. Rev Infect Dis 10:951, 1988.
361. Williams PD, Bennett DB, Gleason CR, Hottendorf GH: Correlation between renal membrane binding and nephrotoxicity of aminoglycosides. Antimicrob Agents Chemother 31:570, 1987.
362. Appel GB, Neu HC: The nephrotoxicity of antimicrobial agents. N Engl J Med 296:663, 722, 784, 1977.
363. Tulkens PM: Experimental studies on nephrotoxicity of aminoglycosides at low doses. Am J Med 80(Suppl 6B):105, 1986.
364. Bennett WM: Mechanisms of aminoglycoside nephrotoxicity. Clin Exp Pharmacol Physiol 16:1, 1989.
365. Baylis C, Rennke HR, Brenner BM: Mechanisms of the defect in glomerular ultrafiltration associated with gentamicin administration. Kidney Int 12:344, 1977.
366. Appel GB, Siegel NJ, Appel AS, Hayslett JP: Studies on the mechanism of nonoliguric experimental acute renal failure. Yale J Biol Med 54:273, 1981.
367. Appel GB: Aminoglycoside nephrotoxicity: Physiologic studies of the sites of nephron damage. *In* Whelton A, Neu HC (eds): The Aminoglycosides. New York, Marcel Dekker, 1982, pp 269–282.
368. Humes HD, Weinberg JM, Krauss TC: Clinical and pathophysiological aspects of aminoglycoside nephrotoxicity. Am J Kidney 2:5, 1982.
369. Neugarten J, Aynedjian HS, Bank N: The role of tubular obstruction in acute renal failure due to gentamicin. Kidney Int 24:330, 1983.
370. Gilbert DN, Wood CA, Kohlhepp SJ, et al: Polyaspartic acid prevents experimental aminoglycoside nephrotoxicity. J Infect Dis 159:945, 1989.
371. Matz GJ, Lerner SA: Prospective studies of aminoglycoside ototoxicity in adults. *In* Lerner SA, Matz GJ, Hawkins JE Jr (eds): Aminoglycoside Ototoxicity. Boston, Little, Brown, 1981, p 327.
372. DeOliveira JAA: Audiovestibular Toxicity of Drugs, Vols I and II. Boca Raton, FL, CRC Press, 1989.
373. Black FO, Peterka RJ, Elardo SM: Vestibular reflex changes following aminoglycoside induced ototoxicity. Laryngoscope 97:582, 1987.
374. Brummett RE, Fox KE: Aminoglycoside-induced hearing loss in humans. Antimicrob Agents Chemother 33:797, 1989.
375. Thompson PL, Northern JL: Audiometric monitoring of patients treated with ototoxic drugs. *In* Lerner SA, Matz GJ, Hawkins JE Jr (eds): Aminoglycoside Ototoxicity. Boston, Little, Brown, 1981, pp 237–245.
376. Mowry HJ, Roeder JW, Matz GJ, Lerner SA: Auditory and vestibular assessment of patients receiving aminoglycosides. *In* Lerner SA, Matz GJ, Hawkins JE Jr (eds): Aminoglycoside Ototoxicity. Boston, Little Brown, 1981, pp 249–254.
377. Meyerhoff WL, Maale GE, Yellin W, Roland PS: Audiologic threshold monitoring of patients receiving ototoxic drugs: A preliminary report. Ann Otol Rhinol Laryngol 98:950, 1989.
378. Jacobson EJ, Downs MP, Fletcher JL: Clinical findings in high-frequency thresholds during known ototoxic drug usage. J Aud Res 9:379, 1969.
379. McRorie TI, Bosso J, Randolph L: Aminoglycoside ototoxicity

in cystic fibrosis: Evaluation by high-frequency audiometry. Am J Dis Child 143:1328, 1989.
380. Roeder JW, Mowry HJ, Matz GJ, Lerner SA: Serial vestibular testing in normal subjects. *In* Lerner SA, Matz GJ, Hawkins JE Jr (eds): Aminoglycoside Ototoxicity. Boston, Little, Brown, 1981, pp 309–319.
381. Nordström L, Banck G, Belfrage S, et al: Prospective study of the ototoxicity of gentamicin. Acta Pathol Microbiol Scand [B] 81(Suppl 241):58, 1973.
382. Govaerts PJ, Claes J, Van De Heyning PH, et al: Aminoglycoside-induced ototoxicity. Toxicol Lett 52:227, 1990.
383. Gatell JM, Ferran F, Araujo V, et al: Univariate and multivariate analyses of risk factors predisposing to auditory toxicity in patients receiving aminoglycosides. Antimicrob Agents Chemother 31:1383, 1987.
384. Mathog RH, Klein WJ Jr: Ototoxicity of ethacrynic acid and aminoglycoside antibiotics in uremia. N Engl J Med 280:1223, 1969.
385. Brummett RE, Brown RT, Himes DL: Quantitative relationships of the ototoxic interaction of kanamycin and ethacrynic acid. Arch Otolaryngol 105:240, 1979.
386. Smith CR, Lietman PS: Effect of furosemide on aminoglycoside-induced nephrotoxicity and auditory toxicity in humans. Antimicrob Agents Chemother 23:133, 1983.
387. Brummett RE, Fox KE, Jacobs F, et al: Augmented gentamicin ototoxicity induced by vancomycin in guinea pigs. Arch Otolaryngol Head Neck Surg 116:61, 1990.
388. Line DH, Poole GW, Waterworth PM: Serum streptomycin levels and dizziness. Tubercle 51:76, 1970.
389. Black RE, Lau WK, Weinstein RJ, et al: Ototoxicity of amikacin. Antimicrob Agents Chemother 9:956, 1976.
390. Hawkins JE Jr, Johnsson L-G: Histopathology of cochlear and vestibular ototoxicity in laboratory animals. *In* Lerner SA, Matz GJ, Hawkins JE Jr (eds): Aminoglycoside Ototoxicity. Boston, Little, Brown, 1981, pp 175–195.
391. Wersäll J: Structural damage to the organ of Corti and the vestibular epithelia caused by aminoglycoside antibiotics in the guinea pig. *In* Lerner SA, Matz GJ, Hawkins JE Jr (eds): Aminoglycoside Ototoxicity. Boston, Little, Brown, 1981, pp 197–214.
392. Lindemann HH: Regional differences in sensitivity of the vestibular sensory epithelia to ototoxic antibiotics. Acta Otolaryngol 67:177, 1969.
393. Johnsson L-G, Hawkins JE Jr, Kingsley TC, et al: Aminoglycoside-induced inner ear pathology in man, as seen by microdissection. *In* Lerner SA, Matz GJ, Hawkins JE Jr (eds): Aminoglycoside Ototoxicity. Boston, Little, Brown, 1981, pp 389–408.
394. Nadol JB Jr: Histopathology of human aminoglycoside ototoxcoside ototoxicity. *In* Lerner SA, Matz GJ, Hawkins JE Jr (eds): Aminoglycoside Ototoxicity. Boston, Little, Brown, 1981, p 409.
395. Backus RM, De Groot JCMJ, Tange RA, Huizing EH: Pathological findings in the human auditory system following longstanding gentamicin ototoxicity. Arch Otorhinolaryngol 344:69, 1987.
396. Huizing EH, De Groot JCMJ: Human cochlea pathology in aminoglycoside ototoxicity—A review. Acta Otolaryngol Suppl (Stockh) 436:117, 1987.
397. Hinojosa R, Lerner SA: Cochlear neural degeneration without hair cell loss in two patients with aminoglycoside ototoxicity. J Infect Dis 156:449, 1987.
398. Schacht J: Molecular mechanisms of drug-induced hearing loss. Hear Res 22:297, 1986.
399. Williams SE, Zenner H-P, Schacht J: Three molecular steps of aminoglycoside ototoxicity demonstrated in outer hair cells. Hear Res 30:11, 1987.
400. Henley CM III, Schacht J: Pharmacokinetics of aminoglycoside antibiotics in blood, inner-ear fluids and tissues and their relationship to ototoxicity. Audiology 27:137, 1988.
401. Lerner SA, Seligsohn R, Bhattacharya I, et al: Aminoglycoside levels in the inner ear perilymph of man. *In* Fillastre J-P (ed): Nephrotoxicity and Ototoxicity of Drugs. Rouen, France, INSERM, 1982, p 387.
402. Wang BM, Weiner ND, Takada A, Schacht J: Characterization of aminoglycoside-lipid interactions and development of a refined model for ototoxicity testing. Biochem Pharmacol 33:3257, 1984.
403. Holloway JJ, Smith CR, Moore RD, et al: Comparative cost effectiveness of gentamicin and tobramycin. Ann Intern Med 101:764, 1984.
404. Betts RF, Valenti WM, Chapman SW: Five-year surveillance of aminoglycoside usage in a university hospital. Ann Intern Med 100:219, 1984.
405. Gerding DN, Larson TA: Aminoglycoside resistance in gram-negative bacilli during increased amikacin use. Am J Med 19(Suppl 1A):1, 1985.
406. Torres C, Lerner DL, Perlin MH, et al: Purification and characterization of a new aminoglycoside phosphotransferase (3′) with a low K_m for amikacin (Abstr 718). Presented at the 26th Interscience Conference on Antimicrobial Agents and Chemotherapy, 1986.
407. Gaynes RP, Groisman E, Nelson E, et al: Isolation, characterization, and cloning of a plasmid-borne gene encoding a phosphotransferase that confers high-level amikacin resistance in enteric bacilli. Antimicrob Agents Chemother 32:1379, 1988.
408. Green P, Lerner SA, Gaynes R: Transfer of a plasmid containing an amikacin resistance gene encoding a novel phosphotransferase [APH(3′)] from a clinical isolate of *Serratia marcescens* (Abstr A4). Presented at the 29th Interscience Conference on Antimicrobial Agents and Chemotheraphy. Washington, DC, American Society for Microbiology, 1989.
409. Greenberg RN, Hansbrough JN, Lorber RR, Miller GH: Netilmicin sulfate as single-agent therapy for *Pseudomonas* infections. South Med J 82:715, 1989.
410. Noone M, Pomeroy L, Sage R, Noone P: Prospective study of amikacin versus netilmicin in the treatment of severe infection in hospitalized patients. Am J Med 86:809, 1989.
411. McCormack WM, Finland M: Spectinomycin. Ann Intern Med 84:712, 1976.
412. Ward ME: The bactericidal action of spectinomycin on *Neisseria gonorrhoeae*. J Antimicrob Chemother 3:323, 1977.
413. Holloway WJ: Spectinomycin. Med Clin North Am 66:169, 1982.
414. Virtanen S: Sensitivity of *Haemophilus vaginalis (Corynebacterium vaginale)* to oleandomycin and spectinomycin. Pathol Microbiol 42:36, 1975.
415. Bryan LE: Aminoglycoside resistance. *In* Bryan LE (ed): Antimicrobial Drug Resistance. Orlando, FL, Academic Press, 1984, pp 241–277.
416. Sanders CC, Sanders WE Jr: Emergence of resistance during therapy with the newer β-lactam antibiotics: Role of inducible β-lactamases and implications for the future. Rev Infect Dis 5:639, 1983.
417. Gordin FM, Rusnak MG, Sande MA: Evaluation of combination chemotherapy in a highly anesthetized animal model of *Pseudomonas* pneumonia. Antimicrob Agents Chemother 31:398, 1987.
418. Hilf M, Yu VL, Sharp J, et al: Antibiotic therapy for *Pseudomonas aeruginosa* bacteremia: Outcome correlations in a prospective study of 200 patients. Am J Med 87:540, 1989.
419. Serra P, Brandimarte C, Martino P, et al: Synergistic treatment of enterococcal endocarditis. Arch Intern Med 137:1562, 1977.
420. Bisno AL, Dismukes WE, Durack DT, et al: Antimicrobial treatment of infective endocarditis due to viridans streptococci, enterococci, and staphylococci. JAMA 261:1471, 1989.
421. Wilson WR, Geraci JE: Treatment of streptococcal infective endocarditis. Am J Med 78(Suppl 6B):128, 1985.
422. Scheld WM: Therapy of streptococcal endocarditis: Correlation of animal model and clinical studies. J Antimicrob Chemother 20(Suppl A):71, 1987.
423. Karchmer AW, Archer GL, Dismukes WE: *Staphylococcus epidermidis* causing prosthetic valve endocarditis: Microbiologic and clinical observations as guides to therapy. Ann Intern Med 98:447, 1983.
424. Edwards MS, Baker CJ: *Streptococcus agalactiae* (group B *Streptococcus*). *In* Mandell GL, Douglas RG Jr, Bennett JE (eds): Principles and Practice of Infectious Diseases, ed 3. New York, Churchill Livingstone, 1990, pp 1554–1563.
425. Sabath LD, Gerstein DA, Leaf CD, Finland M: Increasing the usefulness of antibiotics: Treatment of infections caused by gram-negative bacilli. Clin Pharm Ther 11:161, 1970.
426. Minuth JN, Musher DM, Thorsteinsson SB: Inhibition of the antibacterial activity of gentamicin by urine. J Infect Dis 133:14, 1976.
427. Norrby SR: Treatment of urinary tract infections with quinolone antimicrobial agents. *In* Wolfson JS, Hooper DC (eds): Quinolone Antimicrobial Agents. Washington, DC, American Society for Microbiology, 1989, pp 107–123.

428. Abrams B, Sklaver A, Hoffman T, et al: Single or combination therapy of staphylococcal endocarditis in intravenous drug abusers. Ann Intern Med 90:789, 1979.
429. Chambers HF, Miller RT, Newman MD: Right-sided *Staphylococcus aureus* endocarditis in intravenous drug abusers: Two week combination therapy. Ann Intern Med 109:619, 1988.
430. Korzeniowski OM, Sande MA, The National Collaborative Endocarditis Study Group: Combination antimicrobial therapy for *Staphylococcus aureus* endocarditis in patients addicted to parenteral drugs and in nonaddicts. Ann Intern Med 97:496, 1982.
431. Reyes MP, Brown WJ, Lerner AM: Treatment of patients with *Pseudomonas* endocarditis with high dose aminoglycoside and carbenicillin therapy. Medicine (Baltimore) 57:57, 1978.
432. Crane LR, Levine DP, Zervos MJ, et al: Bacteremia in narcotic addicts at the Detroit Medical Center: I. Microbiology, epidemiology, risk factors and empiric therapy. Rev Infect Dis 8:364, 1986.
433. Levine DP, Crane LR, Zervos MJ: Bacteremia in narcotic addicts at the Detroit Medical Center: II. Infectious endocarditis: A prospective comparative study. Rev Infect Dis 8:374, 1986.
434. Donowitz GR, Mandell GL: Empiric therapy for pneumonia. Rev Infect Dis 5(Suppl 1):40, 1983.
435. Lynch JP III: Pathogenesis and treatment of nosocomial pneumonia. Intern Med Certif 3:21, 1989.
436. Penketh A, Pitt T, Roberts D, et al: The relationship of phenotype changes in *Pseudomonas aeruginosa* to the clinical conditions of patients with cystic fibrosis. Am Rev Respir Dis 127:605, 1983.
437. Pier GB: Pulmonary disease associated with *Pseudomonas aeruginosa* in cystic fibrosis: Current status of the host-bacterium interaction. J Infect Dis 151:575, 1985.
438. Smith AL, Redding G, Doershuk C, et al: Sputum changes associated with therapy for endobronchial exacerbation in cystic fibrosis. J Pediatr 112:547, 1988.
439. Nichols RL: Management of intra-abdominal sepsis. Am J Med 80(Suppl 6B):195, 1986.
440. Solomkin JS, Dellinger EP, Christou NV, Busuttil RW: Results of a multicenter trial comparing imipenem/cilastatin to tobramycin/clindamycin for intra-abdominal infections. Ann Surg 212:581, 1990.
441. de Paepe M, Belpaire F, Bogaert M, et al: Gentamicin for treatment of peritonitis in continuous ambulatory peritoneal dialysis (Letter). Lancet 2:424, 1981.
442. Ledger W: Aminoglycosides in gynecologic infections. Am J Med 80(Suppl 6B):216, 1986.
443. Wirt TC, McGee ZA, Oldfield EH, Meacham WF: Intraventricular administration of amikacin for complicated meningitis and ventriculitis. J Neurosurg 50:95, 1979.
444. Carlsson AS, Josefsson G, Lindberg L: Revision with gentamicin-impregnated cement for deep infections in total hip arthroplasties. J Bone Joint Surg Am 60:1059, 1978.
445. Josefsson G, Lindberg L, Wiklander B: Systemic antibiotics and gentamicin-containing bone cement in the prophylaxis of postoperative infections in total hip arthroplasty. Clin Orthop Relat Res 159:194, 1981.
446. Veesci V, Barquet A: Treatment of chronic osteomyelitis by necrectomy and gentamicin-PMMA beads. Clin Orthop Relat Res 159:201, 1981.
447. Soto-Hall R, Saenz L, Tavernetti R, et al: Tobramycin in bone cement: An in-depth analysis of wound, serum, and urine concentrations in patients undergoing total hip revision arthroplasty. Clin Orthop Relat Res 175:60, 1983.
448. Buchholz HW, Elson RA, Heinert K: Antibiotic-loaded acrylic cement: Current concepts. Clin Orthop Relat Res 190:96, 1984.
449. Wahlig H, Dingeldein E, Buchholz HW, et al: Pharmacokinetic study of gentamicin-loaded cement in total hip replacements: Comparative effects of varying dosage. J Bone Joint Surg Br 66:175, 1984.
450. Salvati EA, Callaghan JJ, Brause BD, et al: Reimplantation in infection: Elution of gentamicin from cement and beads. Clin Orthop Relat Res 207:83, 1986.
451. Walenkamp GHIM, Vree TB, Van Rens TJG: Gentamicin-PMMA beads: Pharmacokinetic and nephrotoxicological study. Clin Orthop Relat Res 205:171, 1986.
452. Scott DM, Rotschafer JC, Behrens F: Use of vancomycin and tobramycin polymethylmethacrylate impregnated beads in the management of chronic osteomyelitis. DICP 22:480, 1988.
453. Bunetel L, Segui A, Cormier M, et al: Release of gentamicin from acrylic bone cement. Clin Pharmacokinet 17:291, 1989.
454. Feld R, Valdivieso M, Bodey GP, et al: A comparative trial of sisomicin therapy by intermittent versus continuous infusion. Am J Med Sci 274:179, 1977.
455. DeJongh CA, Joshi JH, Newman KA, et al: Antibiotic synergism and response in gram-negative bacteremia in granulocytopenic cancer patients. Am J Med 80:96, 1986.
456. Young LS: Empirical antimicrobial therapy in the neutropenic host. N Engl J Med 315:580, 1986.
457. Klastersky J, Zinner SH, Calandra T, et al and EORTC Antimicrobial Therapy Cooperative Group: Empiric antimicrobial therapy for febrile granulocytopenic cancer patients: Lessons from four EORTC trials. Eur J Clin Oncol 24(Suppl 1):S35, 1988.
458. Hughes WT, Armstrong D, Bodey GP, et al: Guidelines for the use of antimicrobial agents in neutropenic patients with unexplained fever. J Infect Dis 151:381, 1990.
459. Deresinski S, De Pauw BE, Feld R: Empirical treatment of gram-negative bacteremia in granulocytopenic patients with leukemia (Abstr 251). Presented at the 30th Interscience Conference on Antimicrobial Agents and Chemotherapy, 1990.

21

Tetracyclines

David N. Williams

The tetracycline antibiotics were the first broad-spectrum antibiotics and were initially effective against a wide range of microorganisms. Tetracyclines are now less generally used, in large part because of the development of antimicrobial resistance and the appearance of newer and more effective chemotherapeutic agents. For the most part, tetracyclines are used outside the hospital, where they account for up to 39% of antibiotic prescriptions in the United Kingdom.[1] In the United States, data on the use of antimicrobial agents in the outpatient setting are not readily available.[2] A study by the National Center for Health Statistics of the antimicrobial drug prescribing practices of office-based physicians from 1980 to 1992 found that although there was no trend in the rate of prescriptions for tetracyclines during the decade, they ranked third (behind amoxicillin and erythromycin) among generic antimicrobial drugs in 1992.[2]

Classification

Tetracyclines can be divided into three groups, based on pharmacologic characteristics: (1) short-acting compounds—chlortetracycline, oxytetracycline, and tetracycline; (2) an intermediate group, consisting of demeclocycline and methacycline; and (3) long-acting compounds—doxycycline and minocycline. Novel analogs, the glycylcyclines, show promise in vitro against organisms with characterized tetracycline resistance determinants, including methicillin-resistant *Staphylococcus aureus* and *Enterococcus faecium*.[3]

Structure

The basic structure consists of a hydroxynaphthacene nucleus containing, as the name implies, four fused benzene rings.

Substitution on the rings accounts for the number and diversity of tetracyclines. Chlortetracycline and oxytetracycline were the first to be discovered, as a result of an intensive screening of soil organisms for antimicrobial properties. Chlortetracycline was isolated from *Streptomyces aureofaciens* in 1947 and oxytetracycline from *Streptomyces rimosus* in 1950. The parent compound, tetracycline, was produced by the catalytic dehalogenation of chlortetracycline in 1953. Doxycycline and minocycline are semisynthetic derivatives discovered in 1966 and 1972, respectively.

Mechanisms of Action

Tetracyclines are bacteriostatic drugs and act on the bacterial ribosome. Penetration of the bacterial cell wall by tetracycline probably occurs as a result of both passive diffusion and active transport. Once the drug is within the bacterial cell, inhibition of protein synthesis occurs by binding to a specific domain on the 30S ribosomal subunit, so as to block the binding of aminoacyl–transfer RNA to the acceptor site on the messenger RNA ribosome complex. This prevents the addition of new amino acids to the growing peptide chain.[4]

Spectrum of Activity

Tetracycline is the most representative congener, and sensitivities for all tetracyclines are determined by using the standard 30-μg tetracycline antimicrobial disk. Differences in antimicrobial activities between the congeners do exist, with doxycycline and minocycline being the most active. Although minocycline is more active against *S. aureus* and *Nocardia asteroides* and doxycycline is more active against *Bacteroides fragilis,* the clinical relevance of these differences is debatable. Tetracyclines retain activity against community isolates of aerobic gram-negative organisms, such as *Escherichia coli* and *Klebsiella,* but isolates of *Pseudomonas aeruginosa* and *Proteus mirabilis* are generally resistant. Tetracyclines retain activity against a wide variety of microorganisms, including the three *Chlamydia* species (*C. trachomatis, C. pneumoniae,* and *C. psittaci*), *Mycoplasma* spp., rickettsiae, *Ehrlichia* spp., and spirochetal organisms. The utility of tetracyclines against these organisms has increasingly important clinical implications. They are also active to some degree against other organisms, including mycobacterial, fungal, and protozoal organisms[5–14] (Table 21–1).

Increasing microbial resistance has led to a decline in the utility of tetracyclines. Resistance was initially noted with strains of *S. aureus,* but later resistance was seen in *Streptococcus pneumoniae* and β-hemolytic streptococci. Resistance has been increasingly found in isolates of *Haemophilus influenzae* and *Neisseria gonorrhoeae,* but the precise incidence of resistance varies from place to place. Resistance to tetracyclines is primarily genetically mediated. The genes usually reside in plasmids and/or transposons and are transferrable. There are two major mechanisms of resistance: (1) an active efflux mechanism (mediated by resistant proteins inserted into the bacterial cytoplasmic membrane), which results in a reduction of the intracellular accumulation of tetracycline, and (2) ribosomal protection (in which a cytoplasmic protein interacts with the ribosome, reducing its sensitivity to tetracycline). For a detailed review, the reader is referred to Chopra and coworkers.[4] There has also been concern of late regarding the use of tetracyclines in animal husbandry as a food additive for growth promotion and prophylaxis, particularly as it relates to resistance in gram-negative organisms.[15]

TABLE 21–1 ■ Susceptibility of Selected Microorganisms to Tetracycline, Minocycline, and Doxycycline

	MIC_{90} (μg/mL)* OF		
ORGANISM	**Tetracycline**	**Minocycline**	**Doxycycline**
Gram-Positive Bacteria			
Staphylococcus aureus	100.00	3.1–6.3	25.00
Streptococcus pyogenes	3.10	0.80	0.80
Streptococcus pneumoniae	0.80	0.20	0.20
Gram-Negative Bacteria			
Neisseria gonorrhoeae	1.60	1.60	1.60
Haemophilus influenzae	6.30	3.10	3.10
Brucella species	2.00	2.00	1.00
Pasturella multocida	0.40	0.40	0.40
Anaerobes			
Bacteroides fragilis	32.00	8.00	8.00
Clostridium perfringens	64.00	32.00	8.00
Other			
Mycoplasma pneumoniae	1.60	1.60	1.60
Legionella pneumophila		4.00	4.00
Chlamydia trachomatis	0.12	0.06	
Nocardia asteroides	32.00	4.00	32.00
Mycobacterium marinum	20.00	10.00	10.00

*MIC_{90}, Antimicrobial concentration required to inhibit 90% of isolates. Organisms should be considered susceptible if the MIC values are 4 μg/mL or less.

From Williams DN: Tetracyclines. *In* Peterson PK, Verhoef J (eds): The Antimicrobial Agents Annual 3. New York, Elsevier Science Publishers, 1988, pp 218–228.

Clinical Pharmacology

Ten tetracyclines are currently in clinical use, although not all are available in all countries. This discussion focuses on tetracycline (as a standard or parent drug), doxycycline, and minocycline. Tetracycline has a half-life of 10 hours, compared with 15 hours for minocycline and 18 hours for doxycycline. Tetracycline is traditionally given four times a day; doxycycline and minocycline are usually given on a once- and twice-daily basis, respectively. The reported degree of protein binding varies, depending on the methods used: tetracycline is about 60% protein bound, whereas doxycycline and minocycline are 80% to 90% protein bound.

After oral administration, drug absorption occurs in the stomach and proximal small intestine. The degree of absorption varies from 60% to 80% for tetracycline and reaches almost 100% for doxycycline and minocycline. Tetracycline absorption is impaired with the concomitant ingestion of milk, antacids, or food, although this is thought to be less of a problem with doxycycline, as it binds less avidly to calcium and magnesium ions. After oral administration of 500 mg of tetracycline, peak serum levels of about 3 to 4 μg/mL occur at approximately 1 to 3 hours, falling to about 2 μg/mL at 8 hours. Peak serum levels of about 2.5 μg/mL (after about 2 hours) occur after a 200-mg dose of oral doxycycline or minocycline. The peak serum level after a 200-mg intravenous dose of doxycycline or minocycline is approximately 4 μg/mL. Doxycycline is the best tolerated and thus most favored intravenous formulation but should be given slowly, over about 60 minutes, to reduce the likelihood of local thrombophlebitis. Intramuscular administration of tetracycline, doxycycline, and minocycline should be avoided because of local irritation and severe pain.

After oral absorption of tetracycline, there is an active enterohepatic circulation, resulting in biliary levels that are at least 5- to 10-fold higher than the corresponding serum levels. Minocycline and doxycycline are lipophilic and are thus more diffusible, resulting in penetration into the brain, eye, and prostate. Minocycline appears to be the most diffusible of the tetracyclines. It is able to penetrate respiratory secretions, hence its former role in the treatment of the meningococcal carrier state. Tetracyclines also penetrate the sebum and are excreted in perspiration, properties that attest to the usefulness of these drugs in the treatment of acne. The ability of tetracyclines to cross the placental barrier may lead to problems with dental and bone growth in the unborn child because of the avidity with which they bind to calcium.

The degree to which tetracyclines are excreted in the urine and feces varies. Urinary excretion depends on the glomerular filtration rate, and urinary recovery rates vary from 60% for tetracycline to 35% for doxycycline to 10% for minocycline.[16] Note that the antimicrobial activity of tetracyclines is enhanced in an acid environment. Tetracyclines should be avoided in renal insufficiency. Doxycycline is the exception, because in renal failure it diffuses into the intestinal lumen, where it becomes chelated, and the chelated doxycycline cannot be reabsorbed.[17]

Toxicity

The use of tetracyclines may result in a number of adverse effects. True hypersensitivity is rare. Occasionally rashes and even anaphylaxis can occur. During the treatment of spirochetal infections, a Jarisch-Herxheimer reaction can occur. Photosensitivity was classically described with demeclocycline. Photosensitivity now appears to be a toxic rather than an allergic reaction, presumably related to drug accumulation in the skin. It occurs infrequently with doxycycline (a potential concern because of its use in malaria prophylaxis) and minocycline. Minocycline, however, has been associated with increased skin pigmentation.

Tetracycline is a notorious cause of unwanted dental staining. This reaction is most likely to occur between the fourth and sixth months of intrauterine life, but the threat of interference with dental and bone growth persists through to the age of 8 years. Most authorities urge avoidance of tetracycline until the age of 12 years. Dental staining seems to be dose dependent and to some degree drug dependent. It is least likely to occur with doxycycline, presumably because of less avid chelation. Thus, in pediatric practice, when a tetracycline is deemed appropriate (for example, for Rocky Mountain spotted fever or other rickettsial or spirochetal infections), doxycycline would be the drug of choice. Repeated courses of any tetracycline should be avoided in childhood.

Tetracyclines can cause diarrhea. Diarrhea is more likely with the less well absorbed congeners. Tetracyclines are quite acidic in solution and have caused esophageal irritation and ulceration, particularly in elderly patients with preexisting gastroesophageal disease. For that reason, patients should be encouraged to take tetracycline (and especially doxycycline) with liberal amounts of fluid and at least an hour or so before retiring. Hepatotoxicity, manifested histologically as microvesicular fatty change, has been described. This was classically described in pregnant women with preexisting renal insufficiency receiving more than 2 g/d of intravenous tetracycline. A case-control study[18] using Medicaid billing data on patients hospitalized with acute liver disease found an adjusted odds ratio for acute hepatitis for tetracycline of 3.6. There have been case reports of acute liver failure associated with minocycline.[19]

Renal insufficiency may occur as a result of tetracycline-induced reduction of protein synthesis, resulting in increased azotemia from amino acid catabolism. Demeclocycline can cause renal tubular damage. The Fanconi syndrome of renal tubular acidosis was associated with the use of outdated tetracycline that degraded to the epianhydro form. This is no longer seen. One report noted that minocycline could induce a lupus-like syndrome,[20] whereas others have linked minocycline with hypersensitivity pneumonitis.[21] Dizziness, vertigo, and ataxia are seen exclusively with minocycline, and these side effects seem to occur primarily in women.[22] Vestibular symptoms appear to be related to concentration of the drug in the lipid-laden cells of the vestibular apparatus.

Of the drug interactions, reduced absorption of all tetracyclines due to the interaction with divalent metals (calcium, magnesium, and aluminum) is well known, hence the admonishment to avoid taking tetracyclines with milk, antacids, and iron preparations. Tetracyclines chelate divalent metals, and the resulting compound cannot be absorbed. A number of drugs, particularly the antiepileptic drugs carbamazepine, diphenylhydantoin, and barbiturates, induce the hepatic metabolism of tetracyclines, thus shortening their serum half-lives.

Clinical Indications

Tetracyclines are no longer used as initial single-drug therapy for unknown acute infections. They should also be avoided in children younger than the age of 12 years, in pregnant women, and in patients with liver or kidney disease. Their use today is restricted to specific situations, some of which are discussed here (Table 21–2).

Acne

In the National Ambulatory Medical Care Survey[2] of oral antimicrobial drug prescribing by office-based physicians, acne was the most frequently reported complaint associated with the use of tetracyclines. If the inflammatory response is severe enough to warrant systemic antibiotic therapy, many authorities believe that tetracylines are the drugs of choice, based on effectiveness, toxicity, and cost.

Spirochetal Infections

Tetracycline is the drug of choice in adults for the treatment of the primary stage of Lyme disease (erythema migrans). Tetracycline in a dose of 250 mg four times a day (qid) for 10 days has been shown to both reduce the duration of the rash and prevent the important sequelae of arthritis, meningitis, and carditis. However, longer courses of up to 30 days may be necessary based on the severity of disease (e.g., disseminated lesions) and clinical response. Doxycycline at 100 mg twice daily (bid) has largely replaced tetracycline, based on convenience and the increased likelihood for compliance.[23] Oral antibiotics, such as doxycycline at a dose of 100 mg bid for 30 days, are recommended for patients with Lyme arthritis who do not have concomitant neurologic involvement.[24] In the event of failure to respond, a 2- to 4-week course of intravenous ceftriaxone is recommended, along with careful follow-up for consideration of other therapeutic modalities.

Tetracycline has also been used in the treatment of relapsing fever *(Borrelia recurrentis)* and as an alternative drug in the treatment of first, second, and early latent stages of syphilis. In those circumstances, doxycycline at 100 mg bid for 2 weeks is recommended. Note that for neurosyphilis, congenital syphilis, or syphilis in pregnancy, penicillin desensitization is recommended.[25] Doxycycline is also effective in the treatment and prophylaxis of leptospirosis.[26]

Genital Infections

C. trachomatis is an important pathogen in a number of genital infections, including urethritis, pelvic inflammatory dis-

TABLE 21–2 ■ Some Uses of Tetracyclines

PROPHYLAXIS

Malaria (doxycycline); leptospirosis (doxycycline); cholera

THERAPY

Single Drug	Combination
Bacterial	***Bacterial***
Chancroid Granuloma inguinale Cholera Bartonellosis Lyme disease Relapsing fever *Legionella* infection *Pasturella multocida* infection *Actinomyces israelii* infection *Vibrio parahaemolyticus* infection *Vibrio vulnifiscus* infection	Resistant *Staphylococcus aureus* infection (minocycline and rifampin) Plague (with streptomycin) Melioidosis (with chloramphenicol) Brucellosis (with streptomycin or doxycycline with rifampin) Tularemia (with streptomycin) *Helicobacter pylori* infection (with metronidazole, bismuth subsalicylate, and a histamine H_2-blocker)
Other Microorganisms	**Other Microorganisms**

Genital *Mycoplasma* infection
Ureaplasma urealyticum infection
Rickettsial infections
  Endemic typhus
  Rocky Mountain spotted fever
  Tick fever
  Trench fever
  Scrub typhus
Coxiella burnetti infection
Ehrlichia chaffeensis infection
Human granulocytic ehrlichiosis (*Ehrlichia phagocytophila, Ehrlichia equi*)
Chlamydia trachomatis infection
Chlamydia psittaci infection
Chlamydia pneumoniae (TWAR)
Mycobacterium marinum infection (minocycline)
Nocardiosis
	Mycobacterium fortuitum and *M. chelonae* infection (doxycycline with amikacin)
	Mycobacterium leprae infection (minocycline and various combinations)
	Amebiasis
	Malaria

Syndromes	
Acne vulgaris, acne rosacea Malabsorption syndromes (Whipple's disease; sprue and blind loop syndromes) Chronic bronchitis Uncomplicated urinary tract infection; dysuria-frequency syndrome Prostatitis; epididymitis Pelvic inflammatory disease Periodontal disease (minocycline) ?Acute aphthous ulcers (topical tetracycline)	

NONINFECTIOUS USES

Rheumatoid arthritis (minocycline)
Pleurodesis (minocycline and doxycycline)

ease, and epididymitis. Because of the known sequelae of chlamydial infections, which include infertility and ectopic pregnancy, oral tetracycline at 500 mg qid or (increasingly) doxycycline at 100 mg bid for 14 days is invariably included as part of any therapeutic regimen for pelvic inflammatory disease.[25] Patients with uncomplicated urethritis, epididymitis, or proctitis should be treated with doxycycline at 100 mg bid for 7 days pending culture results. Doxycycline is now prescribed in conjunction with another drug (usually a cephalosporin) for *N. gonorrhoeae.* Note that doxycycline alone cannot be recommended as the therapy for gonococcal infection because of increasing drug resistance. Azithromycin in a single 1-g dose has been shown to be as effective as doxycycline at 100 mg bid for 7 days for uncomplicated chlamydial infection.[25] Lymphogranuloma venereum caused by serovars L1, L2, or L3 of *C. trachomatis* is a rare disease in the United States. Doxycycline at 100 mg bid for 21 days is the recommended therapy.

Urinary Tract Infections

The utility of tetracyclines in urinary tract infections has diminished during the past decade; however, the dysuria-frequency syndrome, which presents clinically rather insidiously with pyuria and a negative urine culture, is often due to *C. trachomatis,* thus prompting consideration of tetracycline therapy. Although in acute prostatitis virtually all antibiotics penetrate the inflamed prostate, the treatment of chronic prostatitis is a formidable challenge. Some work has emphasized the etiologic role of *C. trachomatis,* and pharmacologic data demonstrate that doxycycline is one of the few drugs that penetrates the noninflamed prostate.[27]

Respiratory Infections

Tetracyclines are also less widely used today in the treatment of various respiratory problems. They are sometimes used in the treatment of acute exacerbations of chronic bronchitis, although the role of antibiotics in this setting remains controversial. However, patients with atypical pneumonia—when *Mycoplasma pneumoniae, Legionella pneumophila, C. pneumoniae, C. psittaci, Coxiella burnetti,* and *Francisella tularensis* are all etiologic possibilities—should be considered for tetracycline therapy, either alone or in combination. Note that the in vitro activity of doxycycline against *L. pneumophila* is inferior to that of the macrolides.[28]

Malaria Prophylaxis

Doxycycline is used as a causal prophylactic agent against *Plasmodium falciparum.* The need to take doxycycline daily raises concerns about compliance, thus limiting its use to travelers for whom mefloquine is contraindicated and those traveling to areas where mefloquine-resistant strains of *P. falciparum* have been documented (e.g., eastern Thailand, Thailand-Myanmar border, and Cambodia).[29] Doxycycline should be taken at a dose of 100 mg/d starting a day before and continuing during and for 4 weeks after leaving a malarious area. Doxycycline in combination with quinine can be used to treat chloroquine-resistant *P. falciparum.*

Other Infections

Tetracyclines retain an important role in the treatment of a diverse list of organisms either alone or in combination with other drugs (see Table 21–2). The tetracyclines have long been used in the treatment of various rickettsial infections, including Rocky Mountain spotted fever. More recently they have been used in the treatment of infections due to *Ehrlichia chaffeensis* and human granulocytic ehrlichiosis.[30, 31] Ehrlichiosis causes a rickettsia-like infection, characterized by fever, myalgias, pancytopenia, and a history of tick bites. In human granulocytic ehrlichiosis, morulae in the cytoplasm of neutrophils can usually be detected on examination of a blood smear. In both ehrlichiosis and rickettsial infection, prompt initiation of doxycycline therapy is indicated if infection is suspected so as to avoid potentially significant mortality and morbidity.

Tetracycline, usually in combination with chloramphenicol or trimethoprim-sulfamethoxazole, remains an important drug in the treatment of melioidosis (due to *Pseudomonas pseudomallei*). In 1986, the World Health Organization recommended a 6-week course of doxycycline combined with rifampin as the treatment of choice in brucellosis. A randomized double-blind study compared 45 days of the combination of doxycycline and rifampin with doxycycline and streptomycin for the treatment of brucellosis due to *Brucella melitensis*. Overall, the doxycycline-rifampin combination was less effective in preventing relapses (14.4%) than the doxycycline-streptomycin combination (5.9%).[32] However, if the treatment failures in patients with spondylitis were excluded, the results of therapy for both groups were similar.

In the treatment of *Mycobacterium fortuitum* and *Mycobacterium chelonae* infections, doxycycline plus amikacin is a useful combination, whereas minocycline alone for 8 to 16 weeks is appropriate initial therapy for *Mycobacterium marinum* infection. Studies have shown bactericidal activity of minocycline, either alone or in combination with clarithromycin, against *Mycobacterium leprae* in lepromatous leprosy.[33] Minocycline shows promise as a component in the multidrug treatment of this disease.

A double-blind placebo-controlled trial showed that minocycline (200 mg/d) was safe and effective for patients with mild to moderate rheumatoid arthritis.[34] It should be emphasized that the benefit was modest but was statistically significant for joint swelling and joint tenderness and for several laboratory parameters. The mechanism of action is unclear.

References

1. Hamilton-Miller JMT: Use and abuse of antibiotics. Br J Clin Pharmacol 18:469–474, 1984.
2. McCaig LF, Hughes JM: Trends in antimicrobial drug prescribing among office-based physicians in the United States. JAMA 273:214–219, 1995.
3. Testa RT, Petersen PJ, Jacobus NV, et al: In vitro and in vivo antibacterial activities of the glycylcyclines, a new class of semisynthetic tetracyclines. Antimicrob Agents Chemother 37:2270–2277, 1993.
4. Chopra I, Hawkey PM, Hinton M: Tetracyclines, molecular and clinical aspects. J Antimicrob Chemother 29:245–277, 1992.
5. Neu HC: A symposium on the tetracyclines: A major appraisal. Bull N Y Acad Med 54:141–155, 1978.
6. Steigbigel NH, Reed CW, Finland M: Susceptibility of common pathogenic bacteria to seven tetracycline antibiotics in vitro. Am J Med Sci 255:179–195, 1968.
7. Hall WH, Opfer BJ: Influence of inoculum size on comparative susceptibilities of penicillinase-positive and -negative *Neisseria gonorrhoeae* to 31 antimicrobial agents. Antimicrob Agents Chemother 26:192–195, 1984.
8. Farrell ID, Hinchliffe PM, Robinson L: Sensitivity of *Brucella* spp to tetracycline and its analogues. J Clin Pathol 29:1097–1100, 1976.
9. Rosenthal SL, Freundlich LF: In vitro antibiotic sensitivity of *Pasturella multocida*. Health Lab Sci 13:246–249, 1976.
10. Sutter VL, Finegold SM: Susceptibility of anaerobic bacteria to 23 antimicrobial agents. Antimicrob Agents Chemother 10:736–752, 1976.
11. Edelstein PH, Meyer RD: Susceptibility of *Legionella pneumophila* to 20 antimicrobial agents. Antimicrob Agents Chemother 18:403–408, 1980.
12. Oriel JD, Ridgway GL: Comparison of tetracycline and minocycline in the treatment of nongonococcal urethritis. Br J Vener Dis 59:245–248, 1983.
13. Gutmann L, Goldstein FW, Kitzis MD, et al: Susceptibility of *Nocardia asteroides* to 46 antibiotics, including 22 β-lactams. Antimicrob Agents Chemother 23:248–251, 1983.
14. Sanders WJ, Wolinsky E: In vitro susceptibility of *Mycobacterium marinum* to eight antimicrobial agents. Antimicrob Agents Chemother 18:529–531, 1980.
15. Holmberg SD, Osterholm MT, Senger KA, Cohen ML: Drug-resistant *Salmonella* from animals fed antimicrobials. N Engl J Med 3111:617–622, 1984.
16. Fabre J, Milek E, Kalfopoulos P: The kinetics of tetracycline in man. Excretion, penetration in normal inflammatory tissues, behavior in renal insufficiency and hemodialysis. Schweiz Med Wochenschr 101:625–633, 1971.
17. Whelton A, Schach von Wittenau M, Twomey TM, et al: Doxycycline pharmacokinetics in the absence of renal function. Kidney Int 5:365–371, 1974.
18. Carson JL, Strom BL, Duff A, et al: Acute liver disease associated with erythromycins, sulfonamides, and tetracyclines. Ann Intern Med 119:576–583, 1993.
19. Min DI, Burke PA, Lewis WD, Jenkins RL: Acute hepatic failure associated with oral minocycline: A case report. Pharmacotherapy 12:68–71, 1992.
20. Byrne PAC, Williams BD, Pritchard MH: Minocycline-related lupus. Br J Rheumatol 33:674–676, 1994.
21. Guillon J, Joly P, Autran B, et al: Minocycline-induced cell-mediated hypersensitivity pneumonitis. Ann Intern Med 117:476–481, 1992.
22. Williams DN, Laughlin LW, Lee Y: Minocycline: Possible vestibular side effects. Lancet 2:744–746, 1974.
23. Massarotti EM, Rahn DW, Messner RP, et al: Treatment of early Lyme disease. Am J Med 92:396–403, 1992.
24. Steere AC, Levin RC, Molloy PJ, et al: Treatment of lyme arthritis. Arthritis Rheum 37:878–888, 1994.
25. Centers for Disease Control and Prevention: 1993 sexually transmitted diseases treatment guidelines (Abstr). MMWR Morb Mortal Wkly Rep 42(RR-14):1–102, 1993.
26. McLain JBL, Ballou WP, Harrison SM, Steinweg DL: Doxycycline therapy for leptospirosis. Ann Intern Med 100:696–698, 1984.
27. Ristuccia AM, Cunha BA: Current concepts in antimicrobial therapy of prostatitis. Urology 20:338–345, 1982.
28. Reda C, Quaresima T, Pastoris MC: In-vitro activity of six intracellular antibiotics against *Legionella pneumophila* strains of human and environmental origin. J Antimicrob Chemother 33:757–764, 1994.
29. Wyler DJ: Malaria chemoprophylaxis for the traveler. N Engl J Med 329:31–37, 1993.
30. Fishbein DB, Dawson JE, Robinson LE: Human ehrlichiosis in the United States, 1985 to 1990. Ann Intern Med 120:736–743, 1994.
31. Bakken JS, Dumler S, Chen S, et al: Human granulocytic ehrlichiosis in the upper midwest United States. JAMA 272:212–218, 1994.
32. Ariza J, Gudiol F, Pallares R, et al: Treatment of human brucellosis with doxycycline plus rifampin or doxycycline plus streptomycin. Ann Intern Med 117:25–30, 1992.
33. Ji B, Jamet P, Perani EG, et al: Powerful bactericidal activities of clarithromycin and minocycline against *Mycobacterium leprae* in lepromatous leprosy. J Infect Dis 168:188–190, 1993.
34. Tilley BC, Alarcon GS, Heyse SP, et al: Minocycline in rheumatoid arthritis. A 48-week, double-blind, placebo-controlled trial. MIAA Trial Group. Ann Intern Med 122:81–89, 1995.

22

Clindamycin

David W. Oldach
Frank M. Calia

Two lincosamide antimicrobials, lincomycin and clindamycin, are currently available in the United States. The former drug is of historical interest only, having been replaced by its derivative, clindamycin. Lincomycin was isolated in 1962 by Mason and coworkers[1] from a soil actinomycete, *Streptomyces lincolnensis,* found near Lincoln, Nebraska; hence its name. The drug was modified by Magerlein[2] in 1966 to the 7-deoxy, 7-chloro derivative clindamycin. This chemical modification resulted in improved gastrointestinal absorption, increased activity against aerobic gram-positive cocci, and a broader spectrum of activity against anaerobic organisms and the protozoa *Toxoplasma* and *Plasmodium.*[3–17] Because lincomycin has no therapeutic advantages and some disadvantages, it has been replaced by the more versatile derivative clindamycin.

Structure

Clindamycin is composed of the amino acid *trans*-L-4*n*-propylhygrinic acid, which is attached to a sulfur-containing derivative of an octose (Fig. 22–1).

Mechanisms of Action

The lincosamides inhibit bacterial protein synthesis. Their major target is the site of peptide bond formation (the peptidyl transferase loop) in the 23S ribosomal RNA of the 50S ribosomal subunit.[18, 19] Lincomycin and clindamycin have equivalent affinities for their shared ribosomal target site, suggesting that the increased activity of clindamycin for gram-negative bacteria is due to more effective penetration of the bacterial membranes.[19] The lincosamides interact with ribosomes free of nascent peptides, and either interfere with the subsequent ribosomal binding of aminoacyl transfer RNAs or induce their dissociation.[20–24] Clindamycin is considered a bacteriostatic drug because it inhibits protein synthesis; however, it may be bactericidal in some circumstances.[25, 26] Because chloramphenicol, the macrolides, and the lincosamides bind at nearby or overlapping sites, each may interfere with the effect of the other.

The drug has been found to potentiate opsonization and phagocytosis of bacteria at subinhibitory concentrations.[27] Complement is consumed in the process.[28] By inhibiting bacterial protein synthesis, clindamycin may alter the bacterial cell surface, facilitating phagocytosis and enhancing intracellular killing of the organism.[29, 30]

In culture, the drug inhibits the production of the *Staphylococcus aureus* toxin associated with the toxic shock syndrome[31] and of the B toxin of *Clostridium perfringens.*[32] In experimental models, clindamycin prevents the development of glycocalyx biofilms by *S. aureus.*[33] By enveloping themselves in this fibrous exopolysacchride, bacteria are protected from host defenses and the action of antibiotics.[34–38] Theoretically, by inhibiting biofilm production, the drug renders the organisms more vulnerable.

Clindamycin may also have a significant immune-modulating role through its effects on eukaryotic protein synthesis. In cell culture, clindamycin demonstrated dose-dependent suppression of lipopolysaccharide-induced tumor necrosis factor-β production by human monocytes.[32]

Spectrum of Activity

The antimicrobial spectrum of clindamycin includes aerobic gram-positive cocci, gram-positive and gram-negative anaerobes, and certain protozoa[3, 7–17, 39–44] (Table 22–1). Aerobic gram-negative bacilli, including the Enterobacteriaceae and *Pseudomonas* species, are resistant as a rule.[3, 7, 40] Certain gram-negative organisms such as *Haemophilus influenzae, Neisseria meningitidis, Neisseria gonorrhoeae,* and *Campylobacter fetus* are moderately sensitive.[3, 7, 8, 43, 45] The drug is active at clinically achievable concentrations against *Streptococcus pyogenes, Streptococcus pneumoniae, Streptococcus viridans,* and *Streptococcus bovis.*[3, 7, 8, 40–42] *Enterococcus faecalis* and *Enterococcus faecium,* however, are usually resistant.[41] Approximately 80% to 90% of *S. aureus* strains are sensitive to clindamycin.[3, 7, 8, 46, 47] Although the drug is usually active against *S. aureus* and *Staphylococcus epidermidis,* sufficient resistance exists in these two species to necessitate sensitivity studies before initiation of therapy for serious infection.[7, 46–50] Some strains of erythromycin-resistant staphylococci are sensitive to clindamycin, whereas others are cross-resistant.[3, 7, 8, 51] During clindamycin treatment of infections due to erythromycin-resistant, clindamycin-sensitive strains of staphylococci, clindamycin resistance (dissociated cross-resistance) may emerge.[48, 52, 53] Most methicillin-resistant strains of *S. aureus* are resistant to clindamycin.[54] Clindamycin is bactericidal for *S. aureus, S. pyogenes,* and *S. pneumoniae.*[3, 7–9, 25] Most strains of *Corynebacterium*

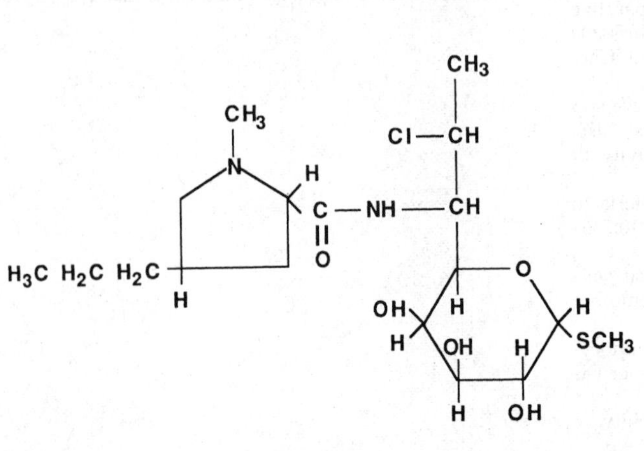

FIGURE 22–1 □ Chemical structure of clindamycin.

TABLE 22–1 ■ In Vitro Susceptibility of Selected Organisms to Clindamycin and Percentage of Sensitive Isolates*

ORGANISM	MINIMAL INHIBITORY CONCENTRATION (μg/mL) Median	Range	% OF SENSITIVE ISOLATES
Staphylococcus aureus†	0.1	0.05–1.5	80–90
Staphylococcus epidermidis†	0.1	0.1–1.5	50–90
Streptococcus pyogenes	0.04	0.02–0.1	Majority
Streptococcus pneumoniae†	0.01	0.002–0.05	Changing rapidly
Streptococcus viridans	0.02	0.005–0.05	Majority
Enterococcus faecalis, E. faecium	100	12.5≥100	<10–20
Corynebacterium diphtheriae	0.2		Majority
Neisseria gonorrhoeae	3.1	0.01–6.3	N/A
Neisseria meningitidis	12.5	6.3–25	N/A
Haemophilus influenzae	12.5	1.6–25	N/A
Clostridium difficile	4	0.06>128	<10
Clostridium perfringens	0.12–1.0	0.06–8.0	80–100
Clostridium spp. (other)	1.0–4.0	0.06≥128.0	70–90
Nocardia asteroides	64	0.75–400	<10
Bacteroides fragilis group	0.25–1.0	0.125≥256	80–100
Bacteroides thetaiotaomicron	1.0–8.0	0.5–128	44–88
Prevotella/Porphyromonas spp.	0.06–4.0	0.06≥128	93–100
Fusobacterium spp.†	0.06–16	0.06≥128	97–100
Peptococcus spp.	0.25	0.06≥128	78–100
Mobiluncus spp.	0.25–1.0	0.5	100
Gardnerella vaginalis	0.5	<0.12–1.0	100
Propionibacterium spp.	0.03	0.03	100
Mycoplasma pneumoniae	3.1	1.6–3.1	N/A
Chlamydia trachomatis	1	0.25–2.0	N/A

*See references 3, 7–12, 39–44, 63, 64, 261–266. N/A, Not available.
†Some strains are markedly more resistant.

diphtheriae are also sensitive.[43, 55] Although the drug is active in vitro against some *Nocardia asteroides* isolates, clinical efficacy data are insufficient to recommend its use in *Nocardia* infections.[56]

A major clinical role for the drug has been defined by its consistent activity for anaerobic organisms, especially the clinically important *Bacteroides fragilis* group.[10–12, 57–61] Although most species and strains are sensitive, clindamycin resistance may be significant in some of the *Bacteroides* subspecies, particularly *Bacteroides thetaiotaomicron* and *Bacteroides vulgatus.* A survey of 1229 strains of the *B. fragilis* group from eight hospitals in the United States reported in 1988 indicated that the prevalence of clindamycin resistance in all species was 6.4% (*B. thetaiotaomicron,* 9.7%; *B. vulgatus,* 14.8%; *Bacteroides distasonis,* 5.8%; *B. fragilis,* 4.9%; and *Bacteroides ovatus,* 6.5%).[62] Chloramphenicol and metronidazole were found to be the most active non–β-lactams; clindamycin was noted to have good activity. A gradual increase in resistance to clindamycin has been noted during the past decade, in one center rising from a 2.5% rate of resistance to 8% *(B. fragilis),* whereas rates for non-*fragilis* species ranged between 7% and 22%.[63, 64] The drug is bactericidal for some strains of *B. fragilis* and is bacteriostatic for others.[26] Clindamycin is usually active against anaerobic streptococci, *Peptococcus, Veillonella, Prevotella melaninogenica* (formerly *Bacteroides melaninogenicus*), *C. perfringens, Actinomyces* spp. (including *Actinomyces israelii*), *Clostridium tetani,* and *Fusobacterium.*[57–61, 65–67] Approximately 33% of *Fusobacterium varium* organisms, 10% of peptococci, and 10% to 20% of non–*C. perfringens* clostridia are resistant.[11, 12, 50, 68] *Clostridium ramosum,* which is frequently recovered from intraabdominal and pelvic infections, and *Clostridium difficile* are often resistant.[60, 67, 69, 70] Because of its overall activity against anaerobes, the drug has found a useful niche in the treatment of pelvic, abdominal, and pulmonary infections by this group of organisms. Clindamycin has in vitro and in vivo activity against *Chlamydia trachomatis* and has been a cornerstone in regimens for the treatment of pelvic inflammatory disease.[71–74] The drug also has activity against anaerobic vaginal flora and *Gardnerella vaginalis,* and it has been effective for the treatment of bacterial vaginosis.[75, 76]

Clindamycin is active against chloroquine-sensitive and -resistant strains of *Plasmodium falciparum.*[16, 17, 77–81] *Plasmodium vivax* is also sensitive, but the extraerythrocytic phase is resistant. The drug is also active against *Toxoplasma gondii* and *Pneumocystis carinii.*[13–15, 82–89] Unlike erythromycin, an antibiotic it closely resembles, clindamycin is ineffective against *Mycoplasma pneumoniae* and *Treponema pallidum.*[3, 90–92]

Mechanisms of Resistance

Clindamycin resistance can develop during therapy. This has been documented for strains of *S. aureus, S. epidermidis, S. pyogenes, S. pneumoniae, H. influenzae, C. diphtheriae,* and *Propionibacterium acnes.*[53, 93–99] Resistance has also developed in certain anaerobes, including *Eubacterium, F. varium, Peptococcus,* and *B. fragilis.*[11, 57–59, 63, 64, 68, 100] Exposing subcultures of *S. aureus* daily to clindamycin leads to slow incremental emergence of resistance.[40] This phenomenon may be the product of chromosomal mutations or plasmid transfer.[93, 100–102]

Clindamycin resistance is caused by changes in the ribosomal binding site, which overlaps that of the macrolide antibiotics.[103] Resistance in staphylococci, *C. diphtheriae,* and *Bacteroides* species has been attributed to methylation of the 23S ribosomal RNA of the 50S ribosome subunit, preventing attachment of antimicrobials.[48, 98] Expression of the methylase responsible for this alteration can be constitutive (resulting in the full macrolide-lincosamide-streptogramin resistance phenotype) or inducible. The greater potency of erythromycin as an inducer of expression of this gene can result in the in vitro erythromycin-resistant, clindamycin-sensitive phenotype (dissociated cross-resistance),[48, 52, 53] probably accounting for the development of resistance to clindamycin in vivo during therapy. Inducible clindamycin resistance has been demonstrated in both gram-positive and gram-negative anaerobic species.[103–106]

Plasmids have been found that code for clindamycin resistance and are transferable within the genus *Bacteroides*.[102] Clindamycin resistance has also been shown to be transferable in a strain of *C. perfringens*.[102] The transfer of clindamycin and tetracycline resistance from one strain of *B. fragilis* to another has been demonstrated in an experimental abscess model.[104] Resistance transference has also been shown to occur in the intestinal tracts of humans and animals.[106, 107] These observations suggest that in polymicrobial infections, resistance may be transferred between strains and species of varying antibiotic susceptibility.[108]

Enzymatic inactivation of clindamycin is rare and probably not clinically important. *Streptomyces coelicolor* phosphorylates clindamycin, producing a derivative that cannot be hydrolyzed to active drug.[109]

Clinical Pharmacology

Clindamycin is available in two oral formulations and one parenteral preparation. The hydrochloride salt tastes bitter and comes in capsules. The water-soluble palmitate ester, which does not have the bitter taste of the hydrochloride, is used in the oral suspension. Clindamycin phosphate is the water-soluble ester of clindamycin and phosphoric acid used for parenteral administration. The palmitate and phosphate esters are inactive and must be hydrolyzed in vivo to be biologically active.[110, 111] Approximately 90% of the oral formulations are absorbed from the gastrointestinal tract.[3, 4, 112, 113] Absorption of the hydrochloride is rapid, producing peak serum levels in 45 minutes.[4, 5] Slightly higher levels are produced by the palmitate[114] (Table 22–2).

Gastrointestinal absorption is delayed in elderly persons.[115] Although food delays absorption, total absorption is not decreased.[3–6] After oral administration, patients with gastrointestinal diseases have higher serum levels of drug than do normal control subjects.[109] Serum concentrations are higher with renal failure.[116] A trivial amount of the drug is absorbed dermally after topical application.[117, 118] The phosphate ester causes little pain on intramuscular injection and is absorbed well, reaching a serum peak level in 1 hour in children and 3 hours in adults.[110, 119, 120] Intravenously administered drug produces a serum peak at the end of infusion.[120–122] Clindamycin achieves high concentrations in many tissues but does not cross the blood-brain barrier, precluding its use in meningitis.[123, 124] The drug reaches therapeutic levels in the iris, choroid, retina, adenoids, and tonsils.[124, 125] The concentrations in saliva and sputum are close to those in serum.[110, 126, 127] The level of drug in the atrial appendage is 250% of that in serum.[128] Excellent levels are found in dental alveolar serum.[129] The bone-tissue concentration is approximately one third that of serum.[129–133] Therapeutic concentrations are easily reached in synovial, pleural, and peritoneal fluids.[120, 124, 133–135] Clindamycin crosses the placenta and enters the fetus, but teratogenic effects have not been described in animals.[136] (Safety has not been fully established in pregnant women.) The concentration in the human appendix, with or without inflammation, is 1.5 times the level in serum.[137] The drug reaches therapeutic concentrations in the uterus, fallopian tubes, surgical wound tissue, and decubitus ulcers.[138–140] High concentrations are found in abscesses produced experimentally.[141] Like erythromycin, clindamycin is actively transported into macrophages and polymorphonuclear leukocytes.[142, 143] The concentrations in neutrophils and pulmonary macrophages are, respectively, 9 to 33 times and 50 times the concentrations in serum. These intracellular concentrations may be therapeutically important. From 60% to 95% of the drug is protein bound and its half-life varies from 2 to 2.5 hours.[5, 39, 110, 144, 145] In adults, 6% to 10% of the administered dose is excreted in the urine,[113, 115, 120] and twice as much is excreted by infants and children.[119]

Clindamycin and its metabolites are mainly eliminated in the bile, where high concentrations are achieved in the absence of biliary tract obstruction.[4, 94, 110] Most of the drug is metabolized in the liver to the biologically active *N*-dimethyl derivative and sulfoxide.[4, 146] These metabolites are found in bile and urine but not in serum.[110] The serum half-life is prolonged to 8 to 12 hours in the presence of active liver disease, and the dose should be adjusted accordingly for patients with moderate to severe liver dysfunction.[94, 143, 147, 148] The percentage excreted by the kidneys is increased with liver disease and markedly decreased with renal failure.[94, 145, 149] No dosage adjustment is usually required for renal dysfunction, because most of the drug is eliminated by the liver, but some suggest that the dosage be reduced in the face of severe renal failure.[116, 149–151] When both renal and liver disease are present, the dosage should be reduced significantly and serum clindamycin levels should be monitored.[94] Clindamycin is not removed by peritoneal dialysis or hemodialysis.[145, 149, 150, 152, 153] Levels in the bile are two to five times those in serum and peak in 2 hours.[110] With biliary obstruction, the amount of drug in the bile is negligible even though it is elevated in liver tissue.[154, 155] Because clindamycin and its metabolites are eliminated in the bile, high concentrations are found in the stool even after parenteral administration.[110] The drug's suppression of anaerobic flora in the gut leads to one of its major complications, antibiotic-associated colitis.[156] The sulfoxide metabolite is less active than the parent compound, whereas the *N*-dimethyl derivative is four times more active and accounts for the high biologic activity in the bile.[4] This route of excretion is responsible for the considerable biologic activity found in feces after parenteral administration, which persists in the intestine for long periods.[110, 157] In animals, there is an enterohepatic circulation of clindamycin

TABLE 22–2 ■ Serum Concentration of Clindamycin in Adults*

PREPARATION	DOSE (mg)	ROUTE	TIME (h)	PEAK CONCENTRATION (μg/mL)
Clindamycin hydrochloride	150	PO	0.75	2.55 ± 0.92†
	300	PO	1	3.6
Clindamycin palmitate	150	PO	0.75	3.8
Clindamycin phosphate	300	IM	3	5
Clindamycin phosphate	300	IM	End of infusion	2.6–26
Clindamycin phosphate	600	IV	End of infusion	6.0–30

*See references 3–6, 62, 89–92, 95–101. PO, Oral; IM, intramuscular; IV, intravenous.
†With renal failure 3.39 ± 0.68 μg/mL.

and its *N*-dimethyl metabolite.[109] Antimicrobial activity persists in the stool for 5 days after a 48-hour course of parenteral drug and causes a major reduction of numbers of susceptible bacteria in the colon.[158] This alteration of gut flora may last up to 14 days after the drug is discontinued. The presence of *N*-dimethyl clindamycin in the urine for days after a single dose suggests slow tissue release of the antibiotic.

Toxicity and Adverse Effects

Hypersensitivity reactions—including morbilliform rashes, urticaria, erythema multiforme (Stevens-Johnsons syndrome), drug fever, eosinophilia, and anaphylactoid reactions—have been attributed to clindamycin.[159] Exanthems may develop in as many as 10% of patients.[160] Contact dermatitis with burning, itching, and peeling may occur with topical use.[161] Local irritation at the intramuscular injection site and phlebitis at the site of intravenous infusion are also possible. Hypotension, electrocardiographic changes, and cardiovascular collapse have been described after bolus administration of lincomycin.[159] Infusion during 10 to 60 minutes precludes this complication. By inhibiting neuromuscular transmission, clindamycin has been associated with neuromuscular blockade.[162, 163] The drug can also potentiate the action of neuromuscular blocking agents.[164, 165] Hematopoietic effects, including neutropenia, agranulocytosis, and thrombocytopenia, have been reported but are rare.[159] Clindamycin has been associated with elevations of serum transminase levels (aspartate transaminase, alanine transaminase) without other liver function abnormalities.[120, 166] Most of these represent false-positive elevations due to drug interference with the colorimetric measurement.[3] True hepatotoxicity with hepatocellular damage and jaundice has been reported; in one case it was attributed to the vanishing bile duct syndrome.[167, 168] The drug has been given to patients with liver disease without further deterioration of liver function.[148] Patients may complain of a bitter metallic taste during parenteral administration of the drug.[120, 122, 168]

The most significant adverse effect, however, is on the gastrointestinal tract.[169–176] Diarrhea may represent a trivial annoyance or a life-threatening antibiotic-associated colitis. Approximately 2% to 30% (average 8%) of patients develop diarrhea while taking clindamycin. The vast majority suffer from simple diarrhea, and perhaps less than 10% of persons with loose stools develop colitis. Antibiotic-associated diarrhea is self-limited and abates when the drug is discontinued.[176, 177] These complications are not unique to clindamycin and are encountered with the cephalosporins, the penicillins, and other antimicrobials as well as immunosuppressive and antitumor drugs.[178] The actual attack rate of antibiotic-associated colitis per 1000 doses has been estimated to be 1.5 for cephalosporin, 1.9 for clindamycin, and 2.1 for ampicillin.[179] The incidence of significant colitis associated with clindamycin treatment ranges from 0.1% to 10%.[169, 180] Antibiotic-associated colitis should be viewed as a superinfection of the bowel with *C. difficile,* which is commonly found in the hospital environment.[181] Restriction of clindamycin usage may curtail nosocomial epidemics of *C. difficile*–associated diarrhea.[182] Antibiotic-associated diarrhea and colitis caused by *C. difficile* are discussed in Chapter 79.

Drug Interactions

Clindamycin may potentiate the action of neuromuscular blocking drugs, including pancuronium and *d*-tubocurarine chloride.[163–165] In solution, clindamycin phosphate is physically incompatible with ampicillin, aminophylline, barbiturates, calcium gluconate, magnesium sulfate, and phenytoin sodium. Clindamycin is highly protein bound in vivo and may induce drug toxicities through displacement of bound fractions of other medications.[183]

The interactions of clindamycin with other antimicrobials have been well studied. Synergy between clindamycin and gentamicin has been reported for *Escherichia coli, Proteus mirabilis,* and *Pseudomonas aeruginosa.*[159, 184] In one study, the combination was synergistic for half of the strains of Enterobacteriaceae and *Pseudomonas* tested.[185] Others have found antagonism between clindamycin and gentamicin or amikacin for some strains of *E. coli* and of *Klebsiella.*[186] Clindamycin and an aminoglycoside may be synergistic for *Streptococcus sanguis, Streptococcus salivarius,* and *S. aureus,* but antagonism has been noted for many strains of *Streptococcus mutans.*[187–189] The combination of clindamycin and trimethoprim-sulfamethoxazole has an additive effect for *S. aureus, S. pyogenes, E. coli, Klebsiella* and *Enterobacter* species, and *H. influenzae.*[43, 190]

Preparations

Clindamycin is available as the hydrochloride salt in 75-, 150-, and 300-mg capsules; the palmitate hydrochloride, a water-soluble salt of the ester in flavored granules for reconstitution in suspension (75 mg/5 mL); and the phosphate ester (150 mg/mL) for intramuscular and intravenous use. Clindamycin phosphate is also prepared as a topical solution and topical gel (10 mg/mL) for external use in the treatment of acne vulgaris.

Daily Dosing Recommendations

Peak serum levels depend on formulation, dose, and route (see Table 22–2). Levels that follow administration of the hydrochloride and the palmitate are comparable; parenteral drug produces higher levels. Serum concentrations of clindamycin required to inhibit sensitive organisms are clinically achievable (see Table 22–1). The recommended oral dosage for children is 8 to 16 mg/kg per day in three or four equal doses; for severe infections, it is 16 to 20 mg/kg per day in three or four doses. For adults, the recommended oral dosage is 150 to 300 mg every 6 hours; for more severe infections, it is 300 to 450 mg every 6 hours. The dosage of parenteral drug recommended for neonates is 15 to 20 mg/kg per day in three or four doses; for children older than 1 month, 15 to 25 mg/kg per day in three or four doses; and for more serious infections, 25 to 40 mg/kg per day in three or four doses. For adults, the recommended dosage of clindamycin phosphate is 600 to 1200 mg/d in three or four equal doses. For more severe infections, especially when *B. fragilis, Peptococcus,* or *C. perfringens* is suspected, the adult dosage is 1200 to 2700 mg/d in three or four doses. In one institution, a systematic change in intravenous clindamycin dosing schedules from four times a day (600 mg four times daily) to three times a day (600 mg three times daily) was not associated with adverse outcomes.[191]

Assay

The half-life of clindamycin is prolonged in patients with active liver disease and to a small extent in those with renal failure.[94, 116, 147–151] When both are present, dose reduction is indicated. Measurements of serum drug levels are rarely required, and assays are not widely available. A bioassay has been described that is capable of measuring clindamycin in the presence of aminoglycoside.[192] High-pressure liquid chromatography has also been used to measure clindamycin and the phosphate and palmitate esters.[193]

Clinical Indications

Clindamycin should be used in situations that capitalize on its unique antimicrobial spectrum and pharmacokinetics. Serious gram-positive coccal infections, especially of bone and synovium, occurring in penicillin-allergic patients, and infections in the abdomen, pelvis, and lung involving anaerobes, particularly *B. fragilis,* are obvious examples (Table 22–3). Fear of antibiotic-associated colitis has led many clinicians to substitute other antimicrobials in situations in which in the past clindamycin would have been used. The drug remains a relatively safe antibiotic if patients are monitored closely.

Clindamycin is quite useful in treating infections caused by polymicrobial flora including anaerobes: intraabdominal sepsis, pelvic infections in women, diabetic foot ulcers, decubitus ulcers, and certain respiratory tract infections.[59, 109, 194–204] Experimentally, the drug prevented intraabdominal abscess formation in an animal model.[194, 195] Clindamycin is not as pH sensitive as the macrolides and aminoglycosides, and it enters polymorphonuclear cells.[141–143] For these reasons, it may be more active within abscesses.

Clindamycin has a proven role in the treatment of intraabdominal sepsis. As these infections are generally due to perforation of the gastrointestinal tract, the antibiotic regimen selected must have activity against both anaerobes and gram-negative aerobes. In the past, clindamycin, metronidazole, and chloramphenicol have been used in combination with aminoglycoside or β-lactam antibiotics to achieve this goal.

TABLE 22–3 ■ Clinical Uses of Clindamycin

Mixed anaerobic and aerobic infections
Intraabdominal,* e.g., ruptured or gangrenous appendix, diverticulitis, penetrating trauma, perforated ulcer, intestinal fistula, ischemic bowel, hepatic and pancreatic abscess
Pelvic,* e.g., ovarian abscess, chronic salpingitis, septic abortion, endometritis, posthysterectomy vaginal cuff infections, Bartholin gland abscess
Pulmonary, e.g., aspiration pneumonia, necrotizing pneumonia, empyema, putrid lung abscess
Odontogenic†
Upper respiratory tract,* e.g., chronic sinusitis, chronic otitis
Diabetic foot ulcers*
Decubitus ulcers*
Soft tissue,† e.g., clostridial infections, necrotizing fasciitis, synergistic gangrene
Gram-positive infections
Group A streptococcus pharyngeal carriers
Recurrent tonsillitis
Staphylococcal infections
Corynebacterium diphtheriae carrier state
Acne vulgaris (topical)
Osteomyelitis
Staphylococcal
Anaerobic
Toxoplasma
Chorioretinitis
Encephalitis
Malaria
Plasmodium falciparum (chloroquine sensitive and resistant)
Pneumocystis carinii pneumonia
Treatment

*Plus an aminoglycoside or aztreonam.
†Gram-negative aerobic coverage may be necessary.

In fact, in the past 20 years, the combination of clindamycin plus an aminoglycoside or broad-spectrum β-lactam has been a "gold standard" against which alternative regimens have been compared.[73, 74, 196, 201, 203, 205–212] However, an increasing prevalence of clindamycin-resistant *B. fragilis* as well as of non–*fragilis Bacteroides* isolates has been reported.[63, 64, 208] Antimicrobial susceptibility of aerobic and anaerobic isolates from abdominal and pulmonary infections has been statistically correlated with clinical outcomes, emphasizing the need for complete antimicrobial sensitivity data.[213, 214] Alternative drugs recommended for intraabdominal infection include cefotan, cefoxitin, cefmetazole, ticarcillin-clavulanate, ampicillin-sulbactam, piperacillin-tazobactam, and imipenem-cilastatin. Although clindamycin-containing regimens are clearly effective for life-threatening aerobic sepsis, alternative regimens incorporating metronidazole (particularly if clindamycin resistance is a local problem) or imipenem-cilastatin should be considered.[208]

Infections of the female genital tract—ovarian abscess, chronic salpingitis, endometritis, septic abortion, posthysterectomy vaginal cuff infection, and Bartholin gland abscess—typically contain mixed flora.[73, 74, 199, 212] Clindamycin-aminoglycoside and clindamycin–β-lactam combinations in conjunction with appropriate surgical intervention have been shown repeatedly to decrease morbidity and mortality.[74, 198, 199, 215–217] For the treatment of pelvic inflammatory disease, the Centers for Disease Control and Prevention has recommended that antibiotic therapy target *N. gonorrhoeae, C. trachomatis,* and common genital tract flora such as *E. coli, Prevotella* species, *Bacteroides* species, and anaerobic streptococci.[218] The three regimens currently recommended by the Centers for Disease Control and Prevention (cefoxitin-doxycycline, clindamycin-gentamicin, cefotetan-doxycycline) were demonstrated to be comparable in efficacy and safety.[73] Clindamycin is active against *C. trachomatis,* although minimum inhibitory concentrations tend to be higher than those of tetracycline and erythromycin.[71, 219] Despite this, clindamycin has proven efficacy in the treatment of *C. trachomatis* infections.[72, 73] Topical and systemic clindamycin therapy has been found to be effective in the treatment of bacterial vaginosis.[75, 76]

Clindamycin is effective therapy for pulmonary infections involving anaerobes, including aspiration pneumonia, necrotizing pneumonia, empyema, and putrid lung abscesses.[210, 220–222] Anaerobic bacteria have become major pathogens in the etiology of empyema, with a mean of two or three isolates per pleural fluid specimen.[223] Commonpathogens include *Fusobacterium nucleatum, Prevotella* spp. (including former *B. melaninogenicus*), *Peptostreptococcus,* and *B. fragilis.*[223] β-Lactamase production is found in up to 35% of isolates, explaining the superiority of clindamycin to penicillin in controlled trials for these infections.[224, 225] However, the increasing prevalence of clindamycin resistance among *Bacteroides* species is of concern, and some now advocate the combination of penicillin plus clindamycin or alternative treatment regimens such as β-lactam–β-lactamase inhibitors, imipenem, or penicillin plus metronidazole.[223]

Pyogenic oral-facial infections may arise from a dental source and cause suppurative complications including maxillary sinusitis, mediastinitis, retropharyngeal abscess, infection of the floor of the mouth (Ludwig angina), cavernous sinus thrombosis, pleuropulmonary abscess, and hematogenously disseminated abscesses of brain, liver, kidneys, and bone.[226–229] Anaerobes play a major role in such infections. Penicillin-resistant organisms, including *Prevotella* and *Bacteroides* species, are frequently isolated. Clindamycin is effective therapy in this setting, with the same caveat regarding resistance described earlier, as well as the need for coverage of aerobic gram-negative bacilli in some cases.

Diabetic foot ulcers and decubitus ulcers are common infections that contain anaerobes and aerobic gram-positive and gram-negative flora.[230–235] Clindamycin combined with ciprofloxacin, an aminoglycoside, aztreonam, or a β-lactam antibiotic provides appropriate antibacterial activity.[140, 234, 236] Clindamycin may have an important therapeutic role in the treatment of mixed soft tissue infections such as necrotizing fasciitis and *C. perfringens* infections. In an animal model, clindamycin was superior to penicillin and metronidazole for group A streptococcal cellulitis and *C. perfringens* gas gangrene, perhaps because of its rapid effect on bacterial toxin production.[32, 237–238] However, it should be stressed that some *C. perfringens* isolates are clindamycin resistant, and in this context, the drug should be used in combination therapy until sensitivities are known. In addition, clindamycin's minimum inhibitory concentrations for *C. perfringens* isolates are variable, and higher than usual doses of the drug should be used.[57, 67] Clindamycin is not indicated for the treatment of brain abscess or other central nervous system infection involving mixed flora because of its inability to penetrate the blood-brain barrier.[123, 124]

Chronic pharyngeal carriage of β-hemolytic streptococci that fails to respond to penicillin has been treated successfully with clindamycin; in one trial, a 10-day course of oral clindamycin was demonstrated to be superior to intramuscular benzathine penicillin plus oral rifampin for treatment of chronic carriers.[239, 240] Carriers of group A streptococci harbor organisms in the pharynx, including *S. aureus, Bacteroides,* and *Prevotella* species, which produce sufficient β-lactamase to inactivate penicillin.[241] Clindamycin, by eliminating the carrier state, can terminate recurrent tonsillitis.[242] The drug is as effective as erythromycin and benzathine penicillin in eliminating the carrier state of *C. diphtheriae.*[243] Clindamycin may be used as an alternative to the penicillin in the treatment of staphylococcal infections other than endocarditis, for which it is not recommended.[53, 244] The sensitivity of the organism must be established before severe infections are treated. Clindamycin has been recommended as an appropriate alternative agent for endocarditis prophylaxis for patients with penicillin allergy and erythromycin intolerance.[245, 246]

Therapeutic concentrations of the drug are found in bone, especially in the presence of inflammation.[247–249] This antibiotic has proven value in the treatment of staphylococcal and anaerobic osteomyelitis.[235, 247–251] Several unique features of the drug may help explain its success against osteomyelitis caused by these organisms. Clindamycin is bactericidal against *S. aureus* and many strains of *Bacteroides,* an important virtue in the treatment of osteomyelitis.[3, 25, 26] Both of these species elaborate a glycocalyx, which in experimental models plays a major role in the adherence of bacteria to bone as well as in protection from phagocytosis, antibodies, and the effect of antibiotics.[33–38] Clindamycin interferes with the production of this glycocalyx.[33, 252] Because therapeutic levels are achievable by oral administration, the prolonged treatment course required by these infections is feasible on an outpatient basis.[253]

Topical clindamycin is superior to tetracycline in the treatment of acne vulgaris.[254] Oral clindamycin is effective therapy for severe pustular acne.[255]

The combination of intravenous clindamycin plus oral pyrimethamine has been demonstrated to have equivalent or superior efficacy in the treatment of *Toxoplasma* encephalitis in patients with acquired immunodeficiency syndrome when compared with pyrimethamine plus sulfadiazine.[84, 85] Toxicities with this regimen are comparable in frequency, although gastrointestinal manifestations are more common with pyrimethamine-clindamycin, whereas bone marrow suppression occurs more often with pyrimethamine-sulfadiazine.[84, 85, 256–258] Although the drug does not usually cross the blood-brain barrier, in the presence of inflammation there is sufficient penetration; however, higher daily dosages are recommended. Because of high relapse rates after initial therapy, maintenance therapy for this infection is required; during 60 weeks of follow-up in one study, pyrimethamine-sulfadiazine was demonstrated to be superior to pyrimethamine-clindamycin.[259] Clindamycin is not appropriate for primary prophylaxis because of a high toxicity rate.[260] Ocular toxoplasmosis has been treated successfully with oral clindamycin.[261] Subconjunctival and retrobulbar injections of the drug have also been used for *Toxoplasma* chorioretinitis.[14] Retrobulbar injections may cause diplopia and papillitis.[14]

Clindamycin in combination with primaquine has been shown to be safe and effective (compared with trimethoprim-sulfamethoxazole) in the treatment of mild to moderately severe *P. carinii* pneumonia in patients with acquired immunodeficiency syndrome.[86, 87] In addition, this regimen has proved effective as salvage therapy for patients unable to tolerate primary therapy with trimethoprim-sulfamethoxazole or pentamidine.[261] Rash and methemoglobinemia were frequent side effects of the combination of clindamycin and primaquine. Clindamycin does not have a role in *P. carinii* pneumonia prophylaxis because of its gastrointestinal side effects.

Clindamycin has been used alone and in combination with quinine to treat chloroquine-sensitive and chloroquine-resistant falciparum malaria.[77–81] In addition, clindamycin with oral quinine has been recommended for the treatment of *Babesia* infections.[262]

References

1. Mason KJ, Dietz A, Deboer C: Lincomycin, a new antibiotic. I. Discovery and biologic properties. Antimicrob Agents Chemother 1962:555, 1963.
2. Magerlein BJ, Birkenmeyer RD, Kagan F: Clinical modification of lincomycin. Antimicrob Agents Chemother 1966:727, 1967.
3. McGehee RF Jr, Smith CB, Wilcox C, Finland M: Comparative studies of antibacterial activity in vitro and absorption and excretion of lincomycin and clinimycin. Am J Med Sci 256:279, 1968.
4. Wagner JG, Novak E, Patel NC, et al: Absorption, excretion and half-life of clinimycin in normal adult males. Am J Med Sci 256:25, 1968.
5. DeHaan RM, Metzler CM, Schellenberg D, et al: Pharmacokinetic studies of clindamycin hydrochloride in human. Int J Clin Pharmacol Ther Toxicol 6:105, 1972.
6. DeHaan RM, Vanden Bosch WD, Metzler CM, et al: Clindamycin serum concentrations after administration of clindamycin palmitate with food. J Clin Pharmacol 12:205, 1972.
7. Garrison DW, DeHaan RM, Lawson JB: Comparison in vitro antibacterial activities of 7-chloro-7-deoxylincomycin, lincomycin and erythromycin. Antimicrob Agents Chemother 1967: 397, 1968.
8. Phillips I, Fernandes R, Warren C: In vitro comparison of erythromycin, lincomycin, and clindamycin. Br Med J 2:89, 1970.
9. Garrod LP, Lambert HP, O'Grady F: Antibiotic and Chemotherapy, ed 5. Edinburgh, Churchill Livingstone, 1981, p 183.
10. Tally FP, Cuchural GJ, Jacobus NV, et al: Susceptibility of the *Bacteroides fragilis* group in the United States in 1981. Antimicrob Agents Chemother 23:536, 1983.
11. Sutter VL: In vitro susceptibility of anaerobes: Comparison of clindamycin and other antimicrobial agents. J Infect Dis 135(Suppl):S7, 1977.
12. Bartlett JG: Anti-anaerobic antibacterial agents. Lancet 2:478, 1982.
13. Araujo FG, Remington JS: Effect of clindamycin on acute and chronic toxoplasmosis in mice. Antimicrob Agents Chemother 5:647, 1974.
14. Tate GW Jr, Martin RG: Clindamycin in the treatment of human ocular toxoplasmosis. Can J Ophthalmol 12:188, 1977.

15. Tabbara KF, O'Connor GR: Treatment of ocular toxoplasmosis with clindamycin and sulfadiazine. Ophthalmology 87:129, 1980.
16. Miller LH, Glew RH, Wyler DJ, et al: Evaluation of clindamycin in combination with quinine against multidrug-resistant strains of *Plasmodium falciparum*. Am J Trop Med Hyg 23:565, 1974.
17. Lewis C: Antiplasmodial activity of 7-halogenated lincomycins. J Parasitol 54:169, 1968.
18. Chang FN, Weisblum B: The specificity of lincomycin binding to ribosomes. Biochemistry 6:836, 1967.
19. Douthwaite S: Interaction of the antibiotics clindamycin and lincomycin with *E. coli* 23S ribosomal RNA. Nucleic Acids Res 20:4717, 1992.
20. Contreras A, Vasquez D: Cooperative and antagonistic interactions of peptidyl-tRNA and antibiotics with bacterial ribosomes. Eur J Biochem 74:539, 1977.
21. Chang FN: Lincomycin. *In* Hahn FE (ed): Antibiotics V-1. New York, Springer-Verlag, 1979, p 127.
22. Cundliffe E: Antibiotics and polyribosomes. II. Some effects of lincomycin, spiramycin and streptogramin A in vivo. Biochemistry 8:2063, 1969.
23. Reusser F: Effect of lincomycin and clindamycin on peptide chain initiation. Antimicrob Agents Chemother 7:32, 1975.
24. Menninger JR, Coleman RA: Lincosamide antibiotics stimulate dissociation of peptidyl-tRNA from ribosomes. Antimicrob Agents Chemother 37:2027, 1993.
25. Sande MA, Johnson ML: Antimicrobial therapy of experimental endocarditis caused by *Staphylococcus aureus*. J Infect Dis 131:367, 1975.
26. Nastro LJ, Finegold SM: Bactericidal activity of five antimicrobial agents against *Bacteroides fragilis*. J Infect Dis 126:104, 1972.
27. Gemmell CG, Peterson PK, Schmeling D, et al: Potentiation of opsonization and phagocytosis of *Streptococcus pyogenes* following growth in the presence of clindamycin. J Clin Invest 67:1249, 1981.
28. Milatovic D, Braveny I, Verhoef J: Clindamycin enhances opsonization of *Staphylococcus aureus*. Antimicrob Agents Chemother 24:413, 1983.
29. Kempner MS: Interactions of polymorphonuclear leukocytes with anaerobic bacteria. Rev Infect Dis 6:540, 1984.
30. Proctor RA, Olbrantz PJ, Mosher DF: Subinhibitory concentrations of antibiotics alter fibronectin binding to *Staphylococcus aureus*. Antimicrob Agents Chemother 24:823, 1983.
31. Schlievert PM, Kelly JA: Clindamycin-induced suppression of toxic shock syndrome–associated exotoxin production. J Infect Dis 149:471, 1984.
32. Stevens DL, Bryant AE, Hackett SP: Antibiotic effects on bacterial viability, toxin production, and host response. Clin Infect Dis 20(Suppl 2):S154, 1995.
33. Mayberry-Carson KJ, Tober-Meyer B, Lambe DW Jr, et al: An electron microscopic study of the effect of clindamycin therapy on bacterial adherence and glycocalyx formation in experimental *Staphylococcus aureus* osteomyelitis. Microbios 43:189, 1986.
34. Speers DJ, Sydney MLN: Ultrastructure studies of adherence of *Staphylococcus aureus* in experimental acute hematogenous osteomyelitis. Infect Immun 49:443, 1985.
35. Gristina AG, Costerton JW: Bacterial adherence and the glycocalyx and their role in musculoskeletal infection. Orthop Clin North Am 15:517, 1984.
36. Mayberry-Carson KJ, Tober-Meyer B, Smith JK, et al: Bacterial adherence and glycocalyx formation in osteomyelitis experimentally induced with *Staphylococcus aureus*. Infect Immun 43:825, 1984.
37. Gristina AG, Oga M, Webb LY, et al: Adherent bacterial colonization in the pathogenesis of osteomyelitis. Science 228:990, 1985.
38. Lambe DW Jr, Mayberry-Carson KJ, Ferguson KP: Morphological stabilization of the glycocalyces of 23 strains of five *Bacteroides* species using specific antisera. Can J Microbiol 30:809, 1984.
39. Leigh DA: Antibacterial activity and pharmacokinetics of clindamycin. J Antimicrob Chemother 7(Suppl A):3, 1981.
40. Meyers BR, Kaplan K, Weistein L: Microbiological and pharmacological behavior of 7-chlorolincomycin. Appl Microbiol 17:653, 1969.
41. Karchmer AW, Moellering RC Jr, Watson BK: Susceptibility of various serogroups of streptococci to clindamycin and lincomycin. Antimicrob Agents Chemother 7:164, 1975.
42. Hatch LA: An in vitro survey of sensitivity of clindamycin in a hospital laboratory. Can J Public Health 60:41, 1969.
43. Marks MI: In vitro activity of clindamycin and other antimicrobials against gram-positive bacteria and *Hemophilus influenzae*. Can Med Assoc J 112:170, 1975.
44. Harrison HR, Riggins RM, Alexander ER, et al: In vitro activity of clindamycin against strains of *Chlamydia trachomatis*, *Mycoplasma hominis* and *Ureaplasma urealyticum* isolated from pregnant women. Am J Obstet Gynecol 149:477, 1985.
45. Chow AW, Patten V, Bednorz D: Susceptibility of *Campylobacter fetus* to twenty-two antimicrobial agents. Antimicrob Agents Chemother 13:416, 1978.
46. Reeves DS, Holt HA, Phillips I, et al: Activity of clindamycin against *Staphylococcus aureus* and *Staphylococcus epidermidis* from four UK centers. J Antimicrob Chemother 27:469, 1991.
47. Lemmen S, Kropec A, Engels I, et al: MIC and serum bactericidal activity of clindamycin against methicillin-resistant and -sensitive staphylococci. Infection 21:407, 1993.
48. McGehee RF, Barrett FF, Finland M: Resistance of *Staphylococcus aureus* to lincomycin, clindamycin and erythromycin. Antimicrob Agents Chemother 1968:392, 1969.
49. Nunnery AW, Riley HD: Clinical and laboratory studies of lincomycin in children. Antimicrob Agents Chemother 1964:142, 1965.
50. Barrett FF, McGehee RF Jr, Finland M: Methicillin-resistant *Staphylococcus aureus* at Boston City Hospital. N Engl J Med 279:441, 1968.
51. Desmyter J, Reybrouck G: Lincomycin sensitivity of erythromycin-resistant staphylococci. Chemotherapia 9:183, 1964.
52. Duncan IBR: Development of lincomycin resistance by staphylococci. Antimicrob Agents Chemother 1967:723, 1968.
53. Watanakunakorn C: Clindamycin therapy of *Staphylococcus aureus* endocarditis. Clinical relapse and development of resistance to clindamycin, lincomycin and erythromycin. Am J Med 60:419, 1976.
54. Maple PA, Hamilton-Miller JM, Brumfitt W: World-wide antibiotic resistance in methicillin-resistant *Staphylococcus aureus*. Lancet 1:537, 1989.
55. Zamiri I, McEntegart MG: The sensitivity of diphtheria bacilli to eight antibiotics. J Clin Pathol 25:716, 1972.
56. Black WA, McNellis DA: Susceptibility of *Nocardia* species to modern antimicrobial agents. Antimicrob Agents Chemother 1970:346, 1971.
57. Martin WJ, Garner M, Washington JA II: In vitro antimicrobial susceptibility of anaerobic bacteria isolated from clinical specimens. Antimicrob Agents Chemother 1:148, 1972.
58. Bach VT, Thadepalli H: Susceptibility of anaerobic bacteria in vitro to 23 antimicrobial agents. Chemotherapy 26:344, 1980.
59. Chow AW, Montgomerie JZ, Guze LB: Parenteral clindamycin therapy for severe anaerobic infections. Arch Intern Med 134:78, 1974.
60. Staneck JL, Washington JA II: Antimicrobial susceptibilities of anaerobic bacteria: Recent clinical isolates. Antimicrob Agents Chemother 6:311, 1974.
61. Sutter VL, Finegold SM: In vitro susceptibility of anaerobic bacteria to 23 antimicrobial agents. Antimicrob Agents Chemother 10:736, 1976.
62. Cuchural GJ Jr, Tally FP, Jacobus NV, et al: Susceptibility of the *Bacteroides fragilis* group in the United States: Analysis by site of isolation. Antimicrob Agents Chemother 32:717, 1988.
63. Appleman MD, Heseltine PNR, Cherubin CE: Epidemiology, antimicrobial susceptibility, pathogenicity, and significance of *Bacteroides fragilis* group organisms isolated at Los Angeles County–University of Southern California Medical Center. Rev Infect Dis 13:12, 1991.
64. Aldridge KE, Gelfand M, Reller LB, et al: A five year multicenter study of the susceptibility of the *Bacteroides fragilis* group isolates to cephalosporins, cephamins, penicillins, clindamycin, and metronidazole in the United States. Diagn Microbiol Infect Dis 18:235, 1994.
65. Pien FD, Thompson RL, Martin WJ: Clinical and bacteriologic studies of anaerobic gram-positive cocci. Mayo Clin Proc 47:251, 1972.
66. Holmberg K, Nord CE, Dornbusch K: Antimicrobial in vitro susceptibility of *Actinomyces israelii* and *Arachnia propionica*. Scand J Infect Dis 9:40, 1977.

67. Wilkins TD, Thiel T: Resistance of some species of *Clostridium* to clindamycin. Antimicrob Agents Chemother 3:136, 1973.
68. Bartlett JG, Sutter VL, Finegold SM: Treatment of anaerobic infections with lincomycin and clindamycin. N Engl J Med 287:1006, 1972.
69. Tally FP, Armfield AY, Dowell VR Jr, et al: Susceptibility of *Clostridium ramosum* to antimicrobial agents. Antimicrob Agents Chemother 5:589, 1974.
70. Dornbusch K, Nord CE, Dahlback A: Antibiotic susceptibility of *Clostridium* species isolated from human infections. Scand J Infect Dis 7:127, 1975.
71. Harrison HR, Riggin RM, Alexander ER, et al: In vitro activity of clindamycin against strains of *Chlamydia trachomatis, Mycoplasma hominis,* and *Ureaplasma urealyticum* isolated from pregnant women. Am J Obstet Gynecol 149:477, 1984.
72. Alger LS, Lovchik JC: Comparative efficacy of clindamycin versus erythromycin in eradication of antenatal *Chlamydia trachomatis.* Am J Obstet Gynecol 165:375, 1991.
73. Hemsell DL, Little BB, Faro S, et al: Comparison of three regimens recommended by the Centers for Disease Control and Prevention for the treatment of women hospitalized with acute pelvic inflammatory disease. Clin Infect Dis 19:70, 1994.
74. Dodson MG: Antibiotic regimens for treating acute pelvic inflammatory disease. An evaluation. J Reprod Med 39:285, 1994.
75. Schlicht JR: Treatment of bacterial vaginosis. Ann Pharmacother 28:483, 1994.
76. Sweet RL: New approaches for the treatment of bacterial vaginosis. Am J Obstet Gynecol 169:479, 1993.
77. Hall AP, Doberstyn ED, Nanakorn A, et al: *Falciparum malaria* semiresistant to clindamycin. Br Med J 2:12, 1975.
78. Metzger W, Mordmuller B, Graninger W, et al: High efficacy of short-term quinine-antibiotic combinations for treating adult malaria patients in an area in which malaria is hyperendemic. Antimicrob Agents Chemother 39:245, 1995.
79. Kremsner PG, Winkler S, Brandts C, et al: Curing of chloroquine-resistant malaria with clindamycin. Am J Trop Med Hyg 49:650, 1993.
80. Kremsner PG, Winkler S, Brandts C, et al: Clindamycin in combination with chloroquine or quinine is an effective therapy for uncomplicated *Plasmodium falciparum* malaria in children from Gabon. J Infect Dis 169:467, 1994.
81. Kremsner PG, Radloff P, Metzer W, et al: Quinine plus clindamycin improves chemotherapy of severe malaria in children. Antimicrob Agents Chemother 39:1603, 1995.
82. Fichera MP, Bhopale MK, Roos D: In vitro assays elucidate peculiar kinetics of clindamycin action against *Toxoplasma gondii.* Antimicrob Agents Chemother 39:1530, 1995.
83. Blais J, Tardif C, Chamberland S: Effect of clindamycin on intracellular replication, protein synthesis, and infectivity of *Toxoplasma gondii.* Antimicrob Agents Chemother 37:2571, 1993.
84. Dannemann B, McCutchan A, Israelski D, et al: Treatment of toxoplasma encephalitis in patients with AIDS. A randomized trial comparing pyrimethamine plus clindamycin to pyrimethamine plus sulfadiazine. Ann Intern Med 116:33, 1992.
85. Luft B, Hafner R, Korzun AH, et al: Toxoplasmic encephalitis in patients with the acquired immunodeficiency syndrome. N Engl J Med 329:995, 1993.
86. Toma E, Fournier S, Dumont M, et al: Clindamycin/primaquine versus trimethoprim-sulfamethoxazole as primary therapy for *Pneumocystis carinii* pneumonia in AIDS: A randomized, double-blind pilot trial. Clin Infect Dis 17:178, 1993.
87. Black JR, Feinberg J, Murphy RL, et al: Clindamycin and primaquine therapy for mild-to-moderate episodes of *Pneumocystic carinii* pneumonia in patients with AIDS. AIDS Clinical Trials Group 044. Clin Infect Dis 18:905, 1994.
88. Queener SF, Bartlett MS, Richardson JP, et al: Activity of clindamycin with primaquine against *Pneumocystic carinii* in vitro and in vivo. Antimicrob Agents Chemother 32:807, 1988.
89. Kovacs JA, Masur H: *Pneumocystis carinii* pneumonia. Therapy and prophylaxis. J Infect Dis 158:254, 1988.
90. Axelrod J, Myers BR, Hirschman SZ: 7-Chloro-lincomycin therapy of pulmonary infections due to *Mycoplasma pneumoniae.* Antimicrob Agents Chemother 2:499, 1972.
91. Smilak JD, Burgin WW Jr, Moore WL Jr, et al: *Mycoplasma pneumoniae* pneumonia and clindamycin therapy. Failure to demonstrate efficacy. JAMA 228:729, 1974.
92. Brause BD, Borges JS, Roberts RB: Relative efficacy of clindamycin, erythromycin and penicillin in treatment of *Treponema pallidum* in skin syphilomas of rabbits. J Infect Dis 134:93, 1976.
93. Semel JD, Trenholme GM, Levin S: Gentamicin and clindamycin-resistant *Staphylococcus aureus.* Am J Med Sci 280:4, 1980.
94. Williams DN, Crossley K, Hoffman C, et al: Parenteral clindamycin phosphate: Pharmacology with normal and abnormal liver function and effect on nasal staphylocci. Antimicrob Agents Chemother 7:153, 1975.
95. Drapkin MS, Karchmer AW, Moellering RC Jr: Bacteremia infections due to clindamycin-resistant streptococci. JAMA 236:263, 1976.
96. Champion LAA, Wald ER, Luddy RE, et al: *Streptococcus pneumoniae* resistant to erythromycin and clindamycin. J Pediatr 92:505, 1978.
97. Newell AC: Clinical trial of a new antibiotic. Med J Aust 2:321, 1970.
98. Coyle MB, Minshew BH, Bland JA, et al: Erythromycin and clindamycin resistant *Corynebacterium diphtheriae* from skin lesions. Antimicrob Agents Chemother 16:525, 1979.
99. Crawford WW, Crawford IP, Stoughton RB, et al: Laboratory induction and clinical occurrence of combined clindamycin and erythromycin resistance in *Corynebacterium acnes.* J Invest Dermatol 72:187, 1979.
100. Salaki JS, Black R, Tally FP, et al: *Bacteroides fragilis* resistant to the administration of clindamycin. Am J Med 60:426, 1976.
101. Tally FP, Snydman DR, Gorbach SL, et al: Plasmid-mediated transferable resistance to clindamycin and erythromycin in *Bacteroides fragilis.* J Infect Dis 139:83, 1979.
102. Tally FP, Cuchural GJ Jr, Malamy MH: Mechanisms of resistance and resistance transfer in anaerobic bacteria: Factors influencing antimicrobial resistance. Rev Infect Dis 6(Suppl 1):260, 1984.
103. Lai CJ, Weisblum B, Fahnestock SR, et al: Alteration of 23S ribosomal RNA and erythromycin-induced resistance to lincomycin and spiramycin in *Staphylococcus aureus.* J Mol Biol 74:67, 1973.
104. Reig M, Moreno A, Baquero F: Resistance of *Peptostreptococcus* species to macrolides and lincosamides: Inducible and constitutive phenotypes. Antimicrob Agents Chemother 36:662, 1992.
105. Butler EB, Joiner KA, Malmy M, et al: Transfer of tetracycline or clindamycin resistance among strains of *Bacteroides fragilis* in experimental abscesses. J Infect Dis 150:20, 1984.
106. Reig M, Fernandez MC, Ballesta JPG, et al: Inducible expression of ribosomal clindamycin resistance in *Bacteroides vulgatus.* Antimicrob Agents Chemother 36:639, 1992.
107. Guinee PAM: Resistance transfer to the resident intestinal *Escherichia coli* of rats. J Bacteriol 102:291, 1970.
108. Smith HW: Transfer of antibiotic resistance from animal and human strains of *Escherichia coli* to resident *E. coli* in the alimentary tract of man. Lancet 1:1174, 1969.
109. Sugarman B, Pesanti E: Treatment failures secondary to in vivo development of drug resistance by microorganisms. Rev Infect Dis 2:153, 1980.
110. DeHaan RM, Metzler CM, Schnellenberg D: Pharmacokinetic studies of clindamycin phosphate. J Clin Pharmacol 13:190, 1973.
111. Forist AA, DeHaan RM, Metzler CM: Clindamycin bioavailability from clindamycin-2 palmitate and clindamycin-2 hexadecylcarbonate in man. J Pharmacokinet Biopharmacol 1:89, 1973.
112. DeHaan RM, Schellenberg D: Clindamycin palmitate flavored granules. Multidose tolerance, absorption, and urinary excretion study in healthy children. J Clin Pharmacol 12:74, 1972.
113. Sun FF, His RSP: Metabolism of clindamycin: I. Absorption and excretion of clindamycin in rat and dog. J Pharm Sci 62:1265, 1973.
114. Stillerman M, Isenberg HD, Facklam RR: Streptococcal pharyngitis therapy: Comparison of clindamycin palmitate and potassium phenoxymethyl penicillin. Antimicrob Agents Chemother 4:514, 1973.
115. Cambell IW, Hossack DJN, Munro JF: Absorption and urinary excretion of clindamycin palmitate in the elderly. Curr Med Res Opin 1:369, 1973.
116. Joshi A, Stein R: Altered serum clearance of intravenously administered clindamycin phosphate in patients with uremia. J Clin Pharmacol 14:140, 1974.
117. Algra RJ, Rosen T, Waisman M: Topical clindamycin in acne vulgaris. Safety and stability. Arch Dermatol 113:1380, 1977.

118. Vordon DA: Systemic absorption of topical clindamycin (Letter). Arch Dermatol 114:798, 1978.
119. Kauffman RE, Shoeman DW, Wan SH, et al: Absorption and excretion of clindamycin-2-phosphate in children after intramuscular injection. Clin Pharmacol Ther 13:704, 1972.
120. Fass RJ, Saslaw S: Clindamycin: Clinical and laboratory induction of parenteral therapy. Am J Med Sci 263:369, 1972.
121. Rodriguez W, Ross S, Khan W, et al: Clindamycin in the treatment of osteomyelitis in children. A report of 29 cases. Am J Dis Child 131:1088, 1977.
122. Hugo H, Dornbusch K, Sterner G: Studies on the clinical efficacy, serum levels and side effects of clindamycin phosphate administered intravenously. Scand J Infect Dis 9:221, 1977.
123. Picardi JL, Lewis HP, Tan JS, et al: Clindamycin concentrations in the central nervous system in primates before and after head trauma. J Neurosurg 43:717, 1975.
124. Panzer JD, Brown DC, Epstein WL, et al: Clindamycin levels in various body tissue and fluids. J Clin Pharmacol 12:259, 1972.
125. Tabbara KF, O'Connor GR: Ocular tissue absorption of clindamycin phosphate. Arch Ophthalmol 93:1180, 1975.
126. Stephen KW, McCrossan J, MacKenzie D, et al: Factors determining the passage of drugs from blood into saliva. Br J Clin Pharmacol 9:51, 1980.
127. Raeburn JA, Devine JD: Clindamycin levels in sputum in a patient with purulent chest disease due to cystic fibrosis. Postgrad Med J 47:366, 1971.
128. Mandal AK, Thadepalli H, Bach VT, et al: Antibiotic concentration in the human right atrial appendage. Curr Ther Res 28:504, 1980.
129. Bystedt H, Dahlback A, Nord CE: Concentration of azidocillin, erythromycin, doxycycline and clindamycin in dental alveolar serum after single oral dose. Int J Oral Surg 6:65, 1977.
130. Nicholas P, Meyers PB, Levy RN, et al: Concentration of clindamycin in human bone. Antimicrob Agents Chemother 8:220, 1975.
131. Smilack JD, Flittie WH, Williams TW Jr: Bone concentrations of antimicrobial agents after parenteral administration. Antimicrob Agents Chemother 9:169, 1976.
132. Dornbusch K, Carlsom A, Hugo H, et al: Antibacterial activity of clindamycin and lincomycin in human bone. J Antimicrob Chemother 3:153, 1977.
133. Baird P, Sullivan M, Hughes S, et al: Penetration into bone and tissues of clindamycin phosphate. Postgrad Med J 54:65, 1978.
134. Plott MA, Roth H: Penetration of clindamycin into synovial fluid. Clin Pharmacol Ther 11:577, 1970.
135. Gerding DN, Hall WH, Schierl EA: Antibiotic concentrations in ascitic fluid of patients with ascites and bacterial peritonitis. Ann Intern Med 86:708, 1977.
136. Philipson A, Sabath LD, Charles D: Transplacental passage of erythromycin and clindamycin. N Engl J Med 288:1219, 1973.
137. Berger SA, Barza M, Leslie SW, et al: Penetration of clindamycin into the human appendix. Arch Surg 113:1094, 1978.
138. Elder MG, Bywater MJ, Reeves DS: Pelvic tissue and serum concentrations of various antibiotics given as preoperative medication. Br J Obstet Gynecol 84:886, 1977.
139. Bagley DH, MacLowry J, Beazley RM, et al: Antibiotic concentration in human wound fluid after intravenous administration. Ann Surg 188:202, 1978.
140. Borger SA, Barza M, Haher J, et al: Penetration of clindamycin into decubitus ulcers. Antimicrob Agents Chemother 14:498, 1978.
141. Joiner KA, Lowe BR, Dzink JL, et al: Antibiotic levels in infected and sterile abscesses in mice. J Infect Dis 143:487, 1981.
142. Johnson JD, Hand WL, Francis JB, et al: Antibiotic uptake by alveolar macrophages. J Lab Clin Med 95:429, 1980.
143. Prokesch RC, Hand WL: Antibiotic entry into human polymorphonuclear leukocytes. Antimicrob Agents Chemother 23:373, 1982.
144. Gordon RC, Regamey C, Kirby WMM, et al: Serum protein binding of erythromycin, lincomycin and clindamycin. J Pharm Sci 62:1074, 1973.
145. Bennett WM, Muther RS, Parker RA, et al: Drug therapy in renal failure: Dosing guidelines for adults. Part I. Antimicrobial agents, analgesics. Ann Intern Med 93:62, 1980.
146. Brodasky TF, Argoudelis AD, Eble TE: The characterization and thin-layer chromatographic quantitation of the human metabolite of 7-deoxy-7(*S*)chlorolincomycin (U-21,251 F). J Antibiot 21:327, 1968.
147. Avant GR, Schenker S, Alford RH, et al: The effect of cirrhosis on the disposition and elimination of clindamycin. Am J Dig Dis 20:223, 1975.
148. Hinthron DR, Baker LH, Romig DA, et al: Use of clindamycin in patients with liver disease. Antimicrob Agents Chemother 9:498, 1976.
149. Peddie BA, Dann E, Bailey RR: The effect of impairment of renal function and dialysis on the serum and urine levels of clindamycin. Aust N Z J Med 5:198, 1975.
150. Eastwood JB, Gower PE: A study of the pharmacokinetics of clindamycin in normal subjects and patients with chronic renal failure. Postgrad Med J 50:710, 1974.
151. Van Scoy RE, Wilson WR: Antimicrobial agents in patients with renal insufficiency. Mayo Clin Proc 52:704, 1977.
152. Malacoff RF, Finkelstein FO, Andriole VT: Effect of peritoneal dialysis on serum levels of tobramycin and clindamycin. Antimicrob Agents Chemother 8:574, 1975.
153. Golper TA: Drugs and peritoneal dialysis. Dialysis Transplant 8:41, 1979.
154. Brown RB, Martyak SN, Barza M, et al: Penetration of clindamycin phosphate into the abnormal human biliary tract. Ann Intern Med 84:168, 1976.
155. Sales JEL, Sutcliffe M, O'Grady F: Excretion of clindamycin in the bile of patients with biliary tract disease. Chemotherapy 19:11, 1973.
156. Silva J, Fekety R: Clostridia and antimicrobial enterocolitis. Annu Rev Med 32:327, 1981.
157. McCall CE, Steigbigel NH, Finland M: Lincomycin: Activity in vitro and absorption and excretion in normal young men. Am J Med Sci 254:144, 1967.
158. Kager L, Liljequist L, Malmborg AS, et al: Effect of clindamycin prophylaxis on the colonic microflora in patients undergoing colorectal surgery. Antimicrob Agents Chemother 20:736, 1981.
159. Dhawan VK, Thadepalli H: Clindamycin: A review of fifteen years of experience. Rev Infect Dis 4:1133, 1982.
160. Geddes AM, Bridgewater FAJ, Williams DN, et al: Clinical and bacteriologic studies with clindamycin. Br Med J 2:703, 1970.
161. Thompsen RJ, Stranieri A, Knutson D, et al: Topical clindamycin treatment of acne. Clinical, surface lipid composition and quantitative surface microscopy response. Arch Dermatol 1116:1031, 1980.
162. Fiekers JF, Marshall IG, Parsons RL: Clindamycin and lincomycin alter miniature endplate current decay. Nature 281:680, 1979.
163. Pittinger C, Adamson R: Antibiotic blockage of neuromuscular function. Annu Rev Pharmacol 12:169, 1972.
164. Fogdall RP, Miller RD: Prolongation of a pancuronium-induced neuromuscular blockage by clindamycin. Anesthesiology 41:407, 1974.
165. Becker LD, Miller RD: Clindamycin enhances a nondepolarizing neuromuscular blockade. Anesthesiology 45:84, 1976.
166. Geddes AM, Dwyer N St J, Ball AP, et al: Clindamycin in bone and joint infection. J Antimicrob Chemother 3:501, 1977.
167. Elmore M, Rissing JP, Rink L, et al: Clindamycin-associated hepatotoxicity. Am J Med 57:627, 1974.
168. Altraif F, Lilly L, Wanless IR, Heathcote J: Cholestatic liver disease with ductopenia (vanishing bile duct syndrome) after administration of clindamycin and trimethoprim-sulfamethoxazole. Am J Gastroenterol 89:1230, 1994.
169. Tedesco FJ, Barton RW, Alpers DH: Clindamycin-associated colitis: A prospective study. Ann Intern Med 81:429, 1974.
170. Swartzberg JE, Maresca RM, Remington JS: Gastrointestinal side effects associated with clindamycin. Arch Intern Med 136:876, 1976.
171. Condon RE, Anderson MJ: Diarrhea and colitis in clindamycin-treated surgical patients. Arch Surg 113:794, 1978.
172. Friedman GD, Gerard MJ, Ury HK: Clindamycin and diarrhea. JAMA 236:2498, 1976.
173. Swartzberg JE, Maresca RM, Remington JS: Clinical study of gastrointestinal complications associated with clindamycin therapy. J Infect Dis 135(Suppl):S99, 1977.
174. Gurwith MJ, Rabin HR, Love K, and the Cooperative Antibiotic Diarrhea Study Group: Diarrhea associated with clindamycin and ampicillin therapy: Preliminary results of a cooperative study. J Infect Dis 135(Suppl):S104, 1977.

175. Lusk RH, Fekety FR Jr, Silva J Jr, et al: Gastrointestinal side effects of clindamycin and ampicillin therapy. J Infect Dis 135(Suppl):S120, 1977.
176. Neu HC, Prince A, Neu CO, et al: Incidence of diarrhea and colitis associated with clindamycin therapy. J Infect Dis 135(Suppl):S120, 1977.
177. Brause BD, Romankiewick JA, Gotz V, et al: Comparative study of diarrhea associated with clindamycin and ampicillin therapy. Am J Gastroenterol 73:244, 1980.
178. Bartlett JG: Infections of the large intestine. Curr Opin Infect Dis 2:90, 1989.
179. Pierce PF Jr, Wilson R, Silva J Jr, et al: Antibiotic-associated pseudomembranous colitis: An epidemiologic investigation of a cluster of cases. J Infect Dis 145:269, 1982.
180. Ramirez-Ronda CH: Incidence of clindamycin-associated colitis (Letter). Ann Intern Med 81:860, 1974.
181. McFarland LV, Mulligan ME, Kwok MS, et al: Nosocomial acquisition of *Clostridium difficile* infections. N Engl J Med 320:204, 1989.
182. Pear SM, Williamson TH, Bettink K, et al: Decrease in nosocomial *Clostridium difficile*–associated diarrhea by restricting clindamycin use. Ann Intern Med 120:272, 1994.
183. Kishore K, Raina A, Misra V, et al: Acute verapamil toxicity in a patient with chronic toxicity: Possible interaction with ceftriaxone and clindamycin. Ann Pharmacother 27:877, 1993.
184. Leng B, Meyer BP, Hirschman SZ, et al: Susceptibilities of gram-negative bacteria to combinations of antimicrobial agents in vitro. Antimicrob Agents Chemother 8:164, 1975.
185. Fass RJ, Rotilie CA, Prior RB: Interaction of clindamycin and gentamicin in vitro. Antimicrob Agents Chemother 6:582, 1974.
186. Zinner SH, Provonchee RB, Elias K, et al: Effect of clindamycin on the in vitro activity of amikacin and gentamicin against gram-negative bacilli. Antimicrob Agents Chemother 9:661, 1976.
187. Watanakunakorn C, Glotzbecker C: Enhancement of the effects of antistaphylococcal antibiotics by aminoglycosides. Antimicrob Agents Chemother 6:802, 1974.
188. Duperval R, Bill NJ, Geraci JE, et al: Bactericidal activity of combinations of penicillin or clindamycin with gentamicin or streptomycin against species of viridans streptococci. Antimicrob Agents Chemother 8:673, 1975.
189. Snyder RJ, Wilkowske CJ, Washington JA III: Bactericidal activity of combinations of gentamicin with penicillin or clindamycin against *Streptococcus mutans.* Antimicrob Agents Chemother 7:333, 1975.
190. Brumfitt W, Miller H, Grey D: Antibacterial activity of combinations of clindamycin and antifolate agents (Letter). Microbios 4:95, 1977.
191. Yellin AE, Berne TV, Heseltine PNR, et al: Prospective randomized study of two different doses of clindamycin admixed with gentamicin in the management of perforated appendicitis. Am Surg 59:248, 1993.
192. Ervin FR, Bullock WE Jr: Simple assay for clindamycin in the presence of aminoglycosides. Antimicrob Agents Chemother 6:831, 1974.
193. Brown LW: High-pressure liquid chromotographic assays for clindamycin, clindamycin phosphate, and clindamycin palmitate. J Pharm Sci 67:1254, 1978.
194. Weinstein WM, Onderdonk AB, Bartlett JG, et al: Antimicrobial therapy of experimental intraabdominal sepsis. J Infect Dis 132:282, 1975.
195. Louie TJ, Onderdonk AB, Gorbach SL, et al: Therapy for experimental intraabdominal sepsis: Comparison of four cephalosporins with clindamycin plus gentamicin. J Infect Dis 135(Suppl):S18, 1977.
196. Fass RJ, Ruiz DE, Garner WG, et al: Clindamycin and gentamicin for aerobic and anaerobic sepsis. Arch Intern Med 137:28, 1977.
197. Gorbach SL, Thadepalli H: Clindamycin in pure and mixed anaerobic infections. Arch Intern Med 134:87, 1974.
198. Chow AW, Ota JK, Guze LB: Clindamycin plus gentamicin as expectant therapy for presumed mixed infections. Can Med Assoc J 115:1225, 1976.
199. Leigh PA, Simmons K, Williams S: The treatment of abdominal and gynecological infections with parenteral clindamycin phosphate. J Antimicrob Chemother 3:493, 1977.
200. Nichols RL: Intraabdominal sepsis: Characterization and treatment. J Infect Dis 135(Suppl):S54, 1977.
201. Fass RJ: Treatment of mixed bacterial infections with clindamycin and gentamicin. J Infect Dis 135(Suppl):S74, 1977.
202. Thadepalli H, Gorbach SL, Broido PW, et al: Abdominal trauma, anaerobes and antibiotics. Surg Gynecol Obstet 137:270, 1973.
203. Berne TV, Yellin AW, Appleman MD, et al: Antibiotic management of surgically treated gangrenous or perforated appendicitis. Comparison of gentamicin and clindamycin versus cefamandole versus cefaperazone. Am J Surg 144:8, 1982.
204. Kislak JW: The susceptibility of *Bacteroides fragilis* to 24 antibiotics. J Infect Dis 125:295, 1972.
205. Pitkin D, Sheikh W, Wilson S, et al: Comparison of the activity of meropenem with that of other agents in the treatment of intraabdominal, obstetric/gynecological, and skin and soft tissue infections. Clin Infect Dis 20(Suppl 2):S372, 1995.
206. deGroot AGW, Hustinx PA, Lampe AS, et al: Comparison of imipenem/cilastatin with the combination of aztreonam and clindamycin in the treatment of intraabdominal infections. J Antimicrob Chemother 32:491, 1993.
207. Dougherty SH, Sirinek KR, Schauer PR, et al: Ticarcillin/clavulanate compared with clindamycin/gentamicin (with or without ampicillin) for the treatment of intraabdominal infections in pediatric and adult patients. Am Surg 61:297, 1995.
208. McClean KL, Sheehan GJ, Harding GKM: Intraabdominal infections: A review. Clin Infect Dis 19:100, 1994.
209. Smith JA, Skidmore AG, Forward AD, et al: Prospective, randomized, double-blind comparison of metronidazole and tobramycin with clindamycin and tobramycin in the treatment of intraabdominal sepsis. Ann Surg 192:213, 1980.
210. Levinson ME, Santoro J, Bran JL, et al: In vitro activity and clinical efficacy of clindmycin in the treatment of infections due to anaerobic bacteria. J Infect Dis 135(Suppl):S49, 1977.
211. Sheehan G, Harding G: Intraperitoneal infections. *In* Finegold SM, George WL (eds): Anaerobic Infections in Human. San Diego, CA, Academic Press, 1989, pp 349–384.
212. Harding GKM, Buckwold FJ, Ronald AR, et al: Prospective, randomized comparative study of clindamycin, chloramphenicol, and ticarcillin each in combination with gentamicin in therapy for intraabdominal and female genital tract sepsis. J Infect Dis 142:384, 1980.
213. Wilson SE, Hopkins JA: Clinical correlates of anaerobic bacteriology in peritonitis. Clin Infect Dis 20(Suppl 2):S251, 1995.
214. Hopkins JA, Lee JCH, Wilson SE: Susceptibility of intraabdominal isolates at operation. A predictor of post-operative infection. Ann Surg 59:791, 1993.
215. Swenson RM, Michaelson TC, Daly MJ, et al: Clindamycin in infections of the female genital tract. Obstet Gynecol 44:699, 1974.
216. Ledger WJ, Kriewall TJ, Sweet RL, et al: The use of parenteral clindamycin in the treatment of obstetric-gynecologic patients with severe infection. A comparison of clindamycin-kanamycin combination with penicillin-kanamycin. Obstet Gynecol 43:490, 1974.
217. DiZerega G, Yonekura L, Roy S, et al: A comparison of clindamycin-gentamicin and penicillin-gentamicin in the treatment of post–cesarean section endomyometritis. Am J Obstet Gynecol 134:238, 1979.
218. Centers for Disease Control: Sexually transmitted diseases treatment guidelines. MMWR Morb Mortal Wkly Rep 38:25, 1989.
219. Stamm WE, Holmes KK: *Chlamydia trachomatis* infections of the adult. *In* Holmes KK, Mardh P-A, Sparling PF, et al (eds): Sexually Transmitted Diseases. New York, McGraw-Hill, 1984, pp 258–270.
220. Bartlett JG, Gorbach SL: Treatment of aspiration pneumonia and primary lung abscess. JAMA 234:935, 1975.
221. Brook I: Clindamycin in treatment of aspiration pneumonia in children. Antimicrob Agents Chemother 15:342, 1979.
222. Sen P, Tecson F, Kapila R, et al: Clindamycin in the oral treatment of putative anaerobic pneumonias. Arch Intern Med 134:73, 1974.
223. Civen R, Somer HJ, Marina M, et al: A retrospective review of cases of anaerobic empyema and update of bacteriology. Clin Infect Dis 20(Suppl 2):S224, 1995.
224. Levinson ME, Magura CT, Lorber B, et al: Clindamycin compared with penicillin for the treatment of anaerobic lung abscess. Ann Intern Med 98:466, 1983.

225. Bartlett JG, Gorbach SL: Penicillin or clindamycin for primary lung abscess? An editorial. Ann Intern Med 98:546, 1983.
226. Chow AW, Roser SM, Brady FA: Orofacial odontogenic infections. Ann Intern Med 88:392, 1978.
227. Murray DR, Rosenblatt JE: Penicillin resistance and penicillinase production in clinical isolates of *Bacteroides melaninogenicus*. Antimicrob Agents Chemother 11:605, 1977.
228. Kannangara DW, Thadepalli H, McQuirter JL: Bacteriology and treatment of dental infections. Oral Surg 50:103, 1980.
229. Brook I: Bacteriologic features of chronic sinusitis in children. JAMA 246:967, 1981.
230. Louie TJ, Bartlett JG, Tally FP, et al: Aerobic and anaerobic bacteria in diabetic foot ulcers. Ann Intern Med 85:461, 1976.
231. Sapico FL, Canawati HA, Witte JL, et al: Quantitative aerobic and anaerobic bacteriology of infected diabetic feet. J Clin Microbiol 12:413, 1980.
232. Galpin JW, Chow AW, Bayer AS, et al: Sepsis associated with decubitus ulcers. Am J Med 61:346, 1976.
233. Peromet M, Labbe M, Yourassowsky, et al: Anaerobic bacteria isolated from decubitus ulcers. Infection 1:205, 1978.
234. Chow AW, Galpin JE, Guze LB: Clindamycin for treatment of sepsis caused by decubitus ulcers. J Infect Dis 135(Suppl):S65, 1977.
235. Gerding D: Foot infections in diabetic patients: The role of anaerobes. Clin Infect Dis 20(Suppl 2):S283, 1995.
236. Simons WJ, Lee TJ: Aztreonam in the treatment of bone and joint infections caused by gram-negative bacilli. Rev Infect Dis 7(Suppl 4):S783, 1985.
237. Stevens DL, Gibbons AE, Bergstrom R, Winn V: The Eagle effect revisited: Efficacy of clindamycin, erythromycin, and penicillin in the treatment of streptococcal myositis. J Infect Dis 158:23, 1988.
238. Stevens DL, Laine BM, Mitten JE: Comparison of single and combination antimicrobial agents for prevention of experimental gas gangrene caused by *Clostridium perfringens*. Antimicrob Agents Chemother 31:312, 1987.
239. Brook I, Leyva F: The treatment of the carrier state of group A β-hemolytic streptococci with clindamycin. Chemotherapy 27:360, 1981.
240. Tanz RR, Poncher JR, Corydon KE, et al: Clindamycin treatment of chronic pharyngeal carriage of group A streptococci. J Pediatr 119:123, 1991.
241. Brook I, Yocum P, Friedman EM: Aerobic and anaerobic bacteria in tonsils of children with recurrent tonsillitis. Ann Otol Rhinol Laryngol 90:261, 1981.
242. Brook I, Hirokawa S: Treatment of patients with a history of recurrent tonsillitis due to group A β-hemolytic streptococci. Clin Pediatr 24:331, 1985.
243. McCloskey RV, Green MJ, Eller J, et al: Treatment of diphtheria carriers: Benzathine penicillin, erythromycin and clindamycin. Ann Intern Med 81:788, 1974.
244. Tuazon CU, Sheagren JN: Relapse of staphylococcal endocarditis after clindamycin therapy. Am J Med Sci 269:145, 1975.
245. Dajani AS, Bisno AL, Chung KJ, et al: Prevention of bacterial endocarditis: Recommendations by the American Heart Association. JAMA 264:2919, 1990.
246. Endocarditis working party of the British Society for Antimicrobial Chemotherapy. Antibiotic prophylaxis of infective endocarditis. Lancet 335:88, 1990.
247. Wharton MR, Beddon FH: Clindamycin for acute osteomyelitis in children. Postgrad Med J 51:166, 1975.
248. Feigin RD, Pickering LK, Anderson D, et al: Clindamycin treatment of osteomyelitis and septic arthritis in children. Pediatrics 55:213, 1975.
249. Smilak JD, Flittie WH, Williams TW Jr: Bone concentration of antimicrobial agents after parenteral administration. Antimicrob Agents Chemother 9:169, 1976.
250. Klainer AS, Urba WJ, Katz-Pollock H: Anaerobic osteomyelitis: A serious sequela of diabetes. Infect Med 3:34, 1986.
251. Templeton WC III, Wawrukiewicz A, Melo JC, et al: Anaerobic osteomyelitis of long bones. Rev Infect Dis 5:692, 1983.
252. Norden CW: Lessons learned from animal models of osteomyelitis. Rev Infect Dis 10:103, 1988.
253. Norden CW, Shinners E, Niederriter K: Clindamycin treatment of experimental chronic osteomyelitis due to *Staphylococcus aureus*. J Infect Dis 153:956, 1986.
254. Stoughton RB, Cornell RC, Gange RW, et al: Double-blind comparison of topical 1 percent clindamycin phosphate (Cleocin T) and oral tetracycline 500 mg/day in the treatment of acne vulgaris. Cutis 26:424, 1980.
255. Basler RSW: Clindamycin for tetracycline-resistant acne. Cutis 25:527, 1980.
256. Dannemann BR, Israelski DM, Remington JS: Treatment of toxoplasmic encephalitis with intravenous clindamycin. Arch Intern Med 148:2477, 1988.
257. Rolston KVI, Hoy J: Role of clindamycin in the treatment of central nervous system toxoplasmosis. Am J Med 83:551, 1987.
258. Tuazon CU: Toxoplasmosis in AIDS patients. J Antimicrob Chemother 23(Suppl A):77, 1989.
259. Duerden BI: Role of the reference laboratory in susceptibility testing of anaerobes and a survey of isolates referred from laboratories in England and Wales during 1993–1994. Clin Infect Dis 20(Suppl 2):S180, 1995.
260. Summanen PA, Jousimies-Somer H, Manby S, et al: *Bilophila wadsworthia* isolates from clinical specimens. Clin Infect Dis 20(Suppl 2):S210, 1995.
261. Civen H, Jousimies-Somer H, Marina M, et al: A retrospective review of cases of anaerobic empyema and update of bacteriology. Clin Infect Dis 20(Suppl 2):S224, 1995.
262. Hecht DW, Lederer L, Osmolski JR, et al: Susceptibility results for the *Bacteroides fragilis* group: Comparison of the broth microdilution and agar dilution methods. Clin Infect Dis 20(Suppl 2):S342, 1995.
263. Citron DM, Goldstein EJC, Kenner MA, et al: Activity of ampicillin/sulbactam, ticarcillin/clavulanate, clarithromycin and eleven other antimicrobial agents against anaerobic bacteria isolated from infections in children. Clin Infect Dis 20(Suppl 2):S356, 1995.
264. Pitkin D, Sheikh W, Wilson S, et al: Comparison of the activity of meropenem with that of other antimicrobial agents in the treatment of intraabdominal, obstetric/gynecologic, and skin and soft tissue infections. Clin Infect Dis 20(Suppl 2):S372, 1995.
265. Hecht DW, Osmolski JR, O'Keefe JP: Variation in the susceptibility of *Bacteroides fragilis* group isolates from six Chicago hospitals. Clin Infect Dis 16(Suppl 4):S357, 1993.
266. Sheikh W, Pitkin DA, Nadler H: Antibacterial activity of meropenem and selected comparative agents against anaerobic bacteria at seven North American centers. Clin Infect Dis 16(Suppl 4):S361, 1993.

23

Macrolide (and Azalide) Antibiotics: Erythromycin, Azithromycin, Clarithromycin, and Dirithromycin

Frank M. Calia
David W. Oldach

Erythromycin was isolated in 1952 from the actinomycete *Streptomyces erythraeus*, a soil organism found in the Philippines.[1] The spectrum of activity of this drug encompasses gram-positive cocci and bacilli, *Legionella*, *Mycoplasma*, *Chla-*

mydia, and some gram-negative organisms including *Bordetella pertussis, Haemophilus ducreyi, Campylobacter jejuni*, and *Branhamella (Moraxella) catarrhalis*.[2] A long-standing record of safety and effectiveness has sustained erythromycin's clinical usefulness, although it can no longer be relied on to treat serious staphylococcal and gonococcal infections.[3, 4] The limited activity of erythromycin for treatment of many gram-negative infections (in particular with *Haemophilus influenzae*), its acid lability, and the desire for improved pharmacokinetics led to a successful search for semisynthetic derivative compounds. Three such agents, azithromycin, clarithromycin, and dirithromycin, are now approved for use in the United States. Azithromycin, an azalide antibiotic, differs from erythromycin by insertion of a methyl-substituted nitrogen in the lactone ring, generating a 15-membered macrolide (or azalide).[5] This change broadens activity against gram-negative organisms (and other selected pathogens), diminishes acid lability, and results in striking changes in pharmacokinetics (most notably, accumulation of high drug levels intracellularly and in tissues). Clarithromycin, which like erythromycin has a 14-membered lactone ring, has substitution of an *O*-methyl group at position 6 of the ring, with resultant acid stability and improved antimicrobial and pharmacokinetic properties (most notably, excellent activity against *Mycobacterium* species).[6] In addition, the primary metabolite of clarithromycin (14-hydroxyclarithromycin) has significant antimicrobial activity. Dirithromycin is a semisynthetic macrolide antibiotic derived through the condensation of erythromycylamine and an aliphatic aldehyde.[7] It is rapidly hydrolyzed in vivo, generating the active drug erythromycylamine. Its antimicrobial spectrum is similar to that of erythromycin, but it offers the potential advantage of once-daily dosing because of an extended half-life. Clinical experience with dirithromycin, the most recently approved (in the United States) of the macrolide antibiotics, is limited at present; until greater experience has accumulated in appropriate clinical trials, the older agents would be preferred for serious infection.[8]

It is of interest to note that other macrolide products of the Actinomycetales (e.g., cyclosporine, tacrolimus, and rapamycin), which have been developed to exploit their immunosuppressive properties, demonstrate varying degrees of antifungal and antibacterial activity as well.

Structure

Erythromycin is one of the 14-membered macrolides, consisting of a macrocyclic lactone ring attached to two sugar moieties. Clarithromycin differs only in the substitution of an *O*-methyl group at position 6 of the lactone ring. The major metabolite of clarithromycin, 14-hydroxyclarithromycin, has significant antimicrobial activity. Azithromycin has a methyl-substituted nitrogen inserted in the ring, generating a 15-membered ring structure. Dirithromycin is the condensation product of an erythromycin derivative, erythromycylamine, and an aliphatic aldehyde. Erythromycylamine, the active agent, is readily released in vivo and in vitro through hydrolysis (Fig. 23–1).

Mechanism of Action

Erythromycin binds reversibly to a single high-affinity site on the 50S subunit of the 70S bacterial ribosome.[9, 10] This site is located in the peptidyl–transfer RNA binding region of the 50S ribosome subunit; binding of the antibiotic is thought to prevent translocation of peptidyl–transfer RNA.[11, 12] Azithromycin and clarithromycin have a similar mechanism of action. In contrast, chloramphenicol, which also binds the 50S subunit of the 70S bacterial ribosome, blocks the peptidyltransferase reaction of protein synthesis. In some bacterial systems, erythromycin (and presumptively azithromycin and clarithromycin) interferes with ribosomal binding of chloramphenicol, lincomycin, clindamycin, and other macrolide antimicrobials.[13, 14] Erythromycin does not bind to mammalian 80S ribosomes, which explains much of its lack of toxicity in humans.[15] In cell-free systems, erythromycin, like chloramphenicol, can inhibit protein synthesis in ribosomes derived from mammalian mitochondria.[16]

As members of the group of drugs that inhibit bacterial protein synthesis, the macrolide antibiotics are considered bacteriostatic antimicrobials. In fact, each of these drugs may be bactericidal, depending on the species of organism, inoculum size, growth phase, and drug concentration tested.[6, 17, 18]

Erythromycin, azithromycin, and clarithromycin have all been demonstrated to inhibit bacterial growth of typical respiratory tract pathogens for 2 to 8 hours after exposure to the antibiotic (postantibiotic effect).[19, 20] The postantibiotic effects of azithromycin and clarithromycin are extended in the presence of concentrations of the drugs lower than the minimal inhibitory concentration from the observed 2 to 8 hours for common respiratory pathogens to 6 to 20 hours.[20] This property may account, in part, for the successful use of these drugs at long dosing intervals, during which prolonged periods of low serum antibiotic concentration are observed. More significantly, erythromycin, erythromycylamine, azithromycin, and clarithromycin accumulate to high levels within cells, with prolonged intracellular half-lives. This enhances their activity against organisms that proliferate intracellularly. The mechanism of cellular accumulation and concentration is believed to be passive diffusion, with trapping through ribosomal binding and within cell lysosomes.

Spectrum of Activity

Erythromycin is active against many gram-positive and some gram-negative bacteria (Table 23–1). The drug is inactive against Enterobacteriaceae and *Pseudomonas* species, except in an alkaline environment.[2, 21] These gram-negative bacteria are resistant because of the inability of erythromycin to enter the cell; organisms rendered cell wall deficient are susceptible.[22, 23] Erythromycin is a weak base and becomes less ionized as the pH rises; in a nonionized state, the drug can pass through the cell wall of gram-negative enteric bacteria.[17, 21] Thus, the pH of the growth medium has a profound effect on in vitro bacterial susceptibility patterns.

Erythromycin is active in vitro against many strains of *Staphylococcus aureus* and streptococcal species, including groups A and B streptococci, *Streptococcus pneumoniae*, and *Streptococcus viridans*.[2, 24, 25] However, increasing resistance among these species has been noted[26]; for instance, erythromycin resistance is common among *Streptococcus pyogenes* isolates in Japan and Europe.[27, 28] Among 78 *S. pyogenes* isolates obtained in Korea, the values for the minimal inhibitory concentration for 90% of strains (MIC-90) for erythromycin and azithromycin were each greater than 128 μg/mL.[29] In a report of patients with invasive pneumococcal disease in Atlanta, Georgia, 15% of isolates were resistant to erythromycin and clarithromycin.[30] In the Georgia study, among isolates with resistance to penicillin or ceftriaxone, more than 40% were also resistant to erythromycin. Thus, although erythromycin has been a drug of choice for the treatment of streptococcal pharyngitis or community-acquired pneumonia, such decisions now must be made in the context of the ongoing pandemic of antibiotic resistance. Less than 50% of strains of enterococci are sensitive.[31] Other sensitive gram-positive

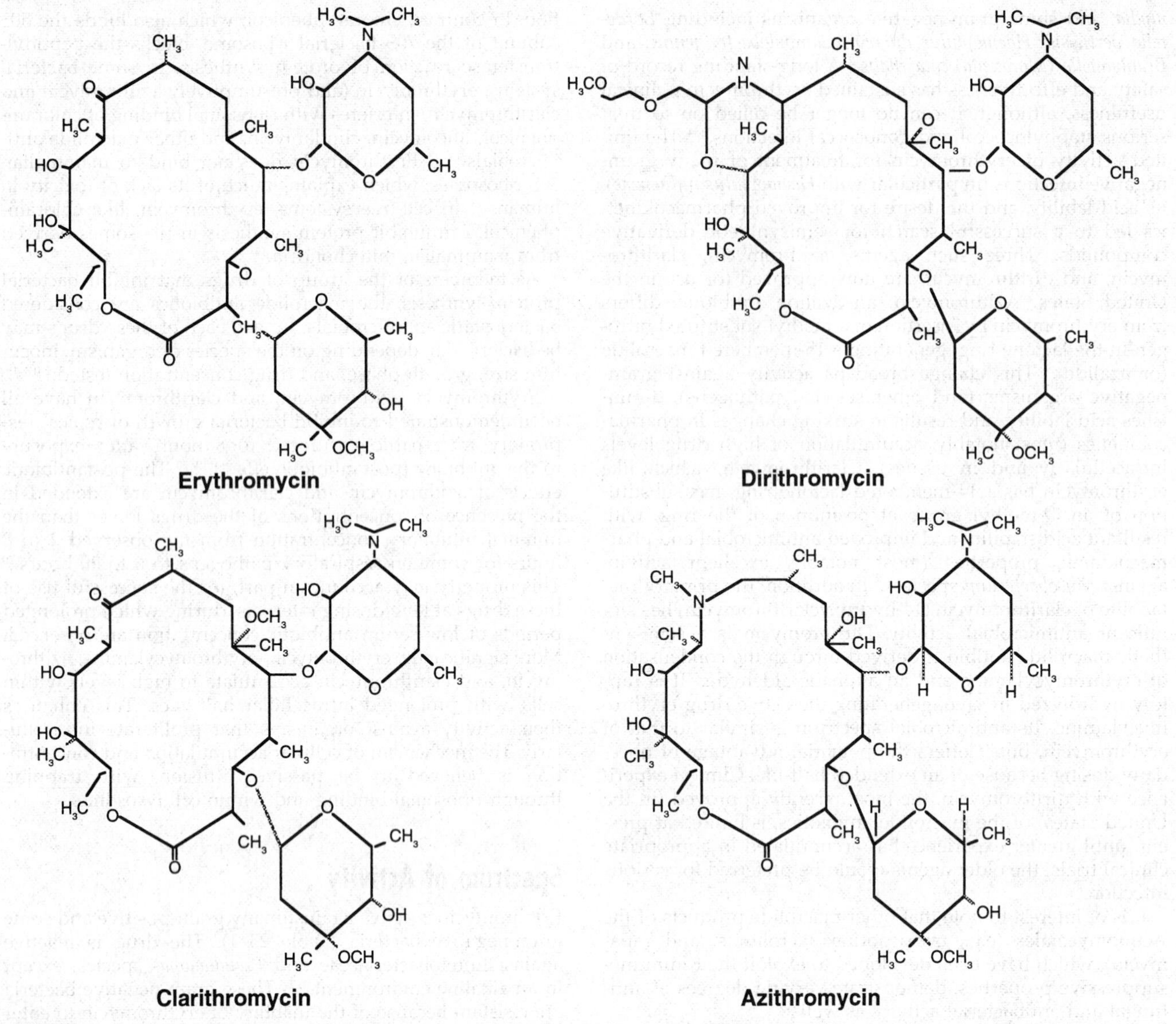

FIGURE 23–1 ▫ Chemical structures of erythromycin, dirithromycin, clarithromycin (14-membered lactone ring macrolide antibiotics), and azithromycin (15-membered ring azalide antibiotic).

bacteria include *Actinomyces israelii*, *Bacillus anthracis*, *Listeria monocytogenes*, *Corynebacterium diphtheriae*, *Clostridium perfringens*, *Clostridium tetani*, and *Erysipelothrix rhusiopathiae*.[2] Some strains of *C. perfringens* are only moderately sensitive.[32] Susceptible gram-negative organisms include *Neisseria meningitidis*, *Neisseria gonorrhoeae*, *B. catarrhalis*, *B. pertussis*, *Legionella* species, *H. ducreyi*, *Campylobacter fetus*, and *C. jejuni*.[2] The drug is active against *H. influenzae*, although strain sensitivity is variable.[33, 34] *Treponema pallidum*, *Borrelia burgdorferi*, *Bartonella* species, *Chlamydia trachomatis*, *Mycoplasma pneumoniae*, and some *Ureaplasma urealyticum* isolates are also sensitive.[2, 6, 18, 35–37] Erythromycin is active against many strains of *Bacteroides*, but the sensitivity of strains of *Bacteroides fragilis* varies widely and is quite pH dependent.[38, 39]

The active agent in dirithromycin, erythromycylamine, does not differ significantly from erythromycin in antimicrobial activity.[7]

Azithromycin and clarithromycin have microbiologic activities similar to those of erythromycin, with some important differences. Azithromycin is less active than erythromycin, based on minimal inhibitory concentration values, against gram-positive organisms. Gram-positive organisms with resistance to erythromycin are also resistant to azithromycin and clarithromycin,[5, 40] and thus the statements made earlier regarding increasing antimicrobial resistance apply to these newer macrolides as well. Azithromycin is much more active than erythromycin against a number of pathogens in vitro, including *Haemophilus* species, *B. pertussis*, *B. catarrhalis*, *N. gonorrheae*, *N. meningitidis*, and *Campylobacter* species.[18] *Actinobacillus actinomycetemcomitans*, *Bartonella* species, *Brucella melitensis*, *Gardnerella vaginalis*, *Helicobacter pylori*, and *Mobiluncus* species are sensitive. *Yersinia enterocolitica* isolates are usually sensitive, although *Yersinia pestis* isolates are not.[41] Azithromycin has comparable activity against *Chlamydia* species and *M. pneumoniae* and appears to be more active than erythromycin against *Mycoplasma hominis* and *U. urealyticum*.[42, 43] Azithromycin has significant activity against *Toxoplasma gondii* and *B. burgdorferi*.[44, 45, 46] The drug has activity against both doxycycline-sensitive and -resistant strains of *Rickettsia tsutsugamushi*,[47] as well as *Plasmodium* species and *Babesia microti*.[48, 49]

Clarithromycin, in conjunction with its primary metabolite, 14-hydroxyclarithromycin, has a broad range of activity similar to that of azithromycin and erythromycin. In vitro, the drug is comparable or superior to erythromycin (and generally superior to azithromycin) in its activity against gram-positive organisms.[6] Clarithromycin is the most active of the currently approved macrolide antibiotics against *H. pylori*, *Mycobacterium chelonae* (subspecies *chelonae* and *abscessus*), *Mycobacterium fortuitum*, *Mycobacterium avium* complex (MAC), and *Mycobacterium leprae*.[50–55] Clarithromycin is, in general, less active than azithromycin against gram-negative bacteria but retains clinical efficacy in the treatment of infections caused by *H. influenzae* because of the activity of 14-hydroxyclarithromycin.[56–58] The drug is active in vitro against *B. catarrhalis*, *Legionella pneumophila*, *M. pneumoniae*, *Chlamydia pneumoniae*, *C. trachomatis*, and *B. burgdorferi*.[56, 58–67] Like azithromycin, clarithromycin suppresses *T. gondii* tachyzoite replication.[68–71]

Mechanisms of Resistance

Several mechanisms may result in bacterial resistance to the macrolide antibiotics, including impermeability of the bacterial cell wall,[17] active efflux pumping of the antibiotic,[72] target site alteration,[73, 74] and drug inactivation.[75]

The cell envelopes of the Enterobacteriaceae and *Pseudomonas* species are relatively impermeable to macrolides.[17] However, the protoplast of these organisms, formed by stripping

TABLE 23–1 ▪ Mean Minimal Inhibitory Concentrations of Selected Pathogens to Macrolide Antibiotics*

	MINIMAL INHIBITORY CONCENTRATION (μg/mL)			
PATHOGEN	**Erythromycin**	**Dirithromycin**	**Azithromycin**	**Clarithromycin**
Bacteroides spp. (including *B. fragilis*)	>12	≥32	>8	2
Bartonella spp. (*B. quintana, B. henselae*)	0.06–0.25	—	0.006–0.03	0.006–0.015
Bordetella parapertussis	0.25	—	0.13	0.25
Bordetella pertussis	0.03	0.03	0.03	0.03
Borrelia burgdorferi	0.03–0.06	—	0.015	0.015
Branhamella catarrhalis	0.13–0.5	0.25	<0.25–0.50	<0.25
Brucella melitensis	—	—	0.6	—
Campylobacter jejuni	1.0–2.0	1.0	0.24–0.5	2–4
Chlamydia pneumoniae	<0.125	0.25–2.5	0.25	<0.03
Chlamydia trachomatis	0.064–>1.0	0.25–2.5	0.12	—
Clostridium spp.	>5.1	0	>3.7	1.5
C. perfringens	1.0–1.56	—	0.25–0.78	—
C. difficile	1.0–1.56	8.0	2.0–6.25	1.0
Corynebacterium spp.	>46	—	88	4
Eikenella corrodens	4	—	2.0–4.0	—
Escherichia coli	>64	—	4	—
Fusobacterium spp.	16	—	4	—
Haemophilus ducreyi	0.03	—	<0.01	0.01
Haemophilus influenzae	4.0–8.0	8.0	0.5–2.0	4–16
Haemophilus parainfluenzae	4.0	16.0	2.0	8.0
Helicobacter pylori	0.22	—	<0.25	0.03
Legionella spp.	0.06–0.5	1.0	0.25–2.0	0.25
Listeria monocytogenes	0.25	4.0	0.5	0.13
Mycobacterium avium complex (MAC)	16–>64	—	32–64	1.0–8.0
Mycobacterium chelonae subspecies *abscessus*	>8.0	—	8	0.50
Mycobacterium chelonae subspecies *chelonae*	8	—	2	0.25
Mycoplasma hominis	—	>128	4.0–32.0	—
Mycoplasma pneumoniae	—	0.02	0.002–0.01	—
Neisseria gonorrhoeae	2.0	2.0	0.25	0.25
Pasteurella spp.	1.56	—	0.1–2.0	—
Peptostreptococcus spp.	>8	2.3	2.3	2.6
Propionibacterium acnes	0.03	—	0.03	0.03
Salmonella enteritidis	128	—	4.0–8.0	—
Staphylococcus aureus	0.41–1.76	—	—	—
Erythromycin sensitive	0.41–1.76	—	0.8–1.6	0.06
Erythromycin resistant	>61	>64	>64	>59
Staphylococcus epidermidis				
Erythromycin sensitive or nonselected isolates	<0.05	—	<0.27	0.06
Erythromycin resistant	>4	—	>4	—
Streptococcus pneumoniae	<0.25	0.25	<0.25	<0.25
Streptococcus pyogenes	<0.25	0.25	0.1–0.5	<0.25
Streptococcus spp. (groups B, C, E)	0.06	0.25	0.13	0.06
Streptococcus spp.	—	>64		
(group D, including enterococci)	>50	>64	>50	>50
Streptococcus viridans	1.24	—	<2.0	0.03
Ureaplasma urealyticum	0.25–4.0	4.0	0.064–2.0	—
Yersinia enterocolitica	>50	—	3.12	—
Yersinia pestis	—	—	32	—

*Data from references 5–7, 18, 25–67, 301–316. The — indicates not available.

off the cell wall, is sensitive to erythromycin.[23] Raising the pH of the environment also increases permeability and susceptibility of these bacteria to the drug.[21] Energy-dependent efflux of 14- and 15-membered macrolides is another mechanism of resistance and may be plasmid associated.[72] Efflux pumps with broad ligand specificity that confer resistance to multiple antibiotics may be induced by single agents.[76]

Chromosomal mutation may produce a one-step high-level resistance. Mutations causing alteration of a single amino acid in the 50S ribosomal protein can decrease the binding affinity for erythromycin (and often other macrolide and lincosamide antimicrobials), rendering organisms resistant.[77] This mechanism of resistance has been described in some strains of *Escherichia coli, S. pyogenes, Campylobacter* species, and *S. aureus*. Resistance caused by chromosomal mutation is usually unstable and occurs at a low frequency.[78]

Posttranscriptional modification of the 23S ribosomal RNA by an adenine-specific *N*-methyltransferase is a common mechanism of resistance. The class of genes coding for this methylase has been named *erm* (erythromycin ribosome methylation), and approximately 30 such genes from diverse sources have been described.[73] The *erm* genes have been identified in multiple gram-positive bacteria, including *Staphylococcus, Lactobacillus,* and *Bacillus*, as well as enterococcal, streptococcal, and enterobacterial species and some anaerobes (e.g., *Bacteroides, Clostridium*). Multiple *erm* genes have been isolated from *Streptomyces* species, the source organisms of most macrolide antibiotics.[73] Resistance to erythromycin related to 23S ribosomal RNA modification confers resistance to other macrolides (clarithromycin, azithromycin), clindamycin, and the streptogramin antibiotics, thus the term MLS resistance (macrolides, lincosamides, streptogramins). The *erm* genes are frequently plasmid associated. Expression may be constitutive (the entire bacterial population is resistant) or inducible by subinhibitory levels of drug.[73, 79] The latter mechanism probably accounts for what Garrod[80] described as the phenomenon of dissociated resistance found in some strains of staphylococci. When grown in large concentrations of erythromycin, only a small portion of the population of organisms was resistant. When grown in a subinhibitory concentration of drug, however, almost the entire population was resistant to erythromycin, other macrolides, and the lincosamides. These organisms appeared to be sensitive to these antibiotics when grown in the absence of erythromycin.

Certain strains of *E. coli* and gram-positive organisms inactivate macrolides enzymatically.[75] A gene for an inducible macrolide 2′-phosphotransferase of *E. coli* that inactivates 14-membered macrolide ring antibiotics (erythromycin, clarithromycin) has been characterized.[81, 82] Macrolides can be inactivated by glycosylation.[83] Some bacterial strains inactivate erythromycin with a plasmid-encoded esterase that cleaves the lactone ring (*ereA* and *ereB* genes).[84, 84a, 85]

Up to 50% of *S. aureus* isolates in hospitals are erythromycin resistant because of the selective pressure of drug use. Resistant staphylococci are more common in large teaching hospitals.[2] Emergence of staphylococcal resistance to erythromycin during therapy has been repeatedly observed, and for this reason the macrolides cannot be considered first-line therapy for serious staphylococcal infections.[17, 86, 87] In areas of the world where erythromycin is commonly used, strains of resistant *S. pyogenes* and pneumococci are increasingly common.[27, 28, 29, 30, 88, 89] In the United States, group A streptococcal resistance has been found to vary from 5% in Oklahoma to 0.5% in Tennessee,[90, 91] and the prevalence of resistant strains can be expected to increase with time.

The newer macrolide antibiotics face the same challenge of antimicrobial resistance. Organisms with acquired resistance to erythromycin, in particular through the acquisition of *erm* (the MLS phenotype) and *ere* genes, are generally resistant to azithromycin and clarithromycin.[5, 72] When used as monotherapy, azithromycin was associated with the development of resistance in four of six *H. pylori* infections treated.[92] Similarly, increases in the drug concentration required to inhibit *H. influenzae* isolates obtained from patients with chronic bronchitis during therapy have been observed.[93] Resistance to azithromycin or clarithromycin develops rapidly when these drugs are used as monotherapy in the treatment of MAC infections.[94, 95] In vitro, the rate of acquisition of resistance to clarithromycin by *M. avium* (when the selection pressure was clarithromycin alone) was comparable to that found for *Mycobacterium tuberculosis* with rifampin, suggesting a single-step mutation mechanism.[96] Although the development of resistance is believed to be related to a point mutation in 23S ribosomal RNA, the precise locus has not been identified.[96]

Pharmacology

All of the macrolide antibiotics undergo enterohepatic circulation; after oral administration of drug, significant serum levels accumulate only after saturation of first-pass metabolism and biliary excretion has occurred. This fact complicates calculations of oral bioavailability.[97] As a class, these antibiotics are characterized by the ability to achieve higher tissue concentrations than plasma concentrations and the persistence of tissue concentrations. Rapid and significant intracellular accumulation of each of the antibiotics described in this chapter has been demonstrated. The drugs vary somewhat in the degree to which they can accumulate both intracellularly and within tissues; however, the clinical significance of these differences remains unclear.[97]

Erythromycin

Erythromycin is slightly water soluble and has a pK_a of 8.8. The bitter-tasting base is the biologically active form of the drug, and its activity increases as the pH rises from 5.5 to 8.5.[86] A major problem in erythromycin pharmacokinetics is its rapid inactivation by gastric acid and variable absorption after oral administration. Serum levels are higher if the drug is taken on an empty stomach.[98] To prevent degradation by gastric acid and to improve absorption, the pharmaceutical industry has prepared acid-resistant enteric coatings that protect the compound in the stomach and dissolve in the duodenum.[99] Another strategy has been to alter the chemical structure of the base to improve absorption by forming a salt (the stearate), an ester (the ethylsuccinate), or the estolate (the lauryl sulfate salt of the propionyl ester). The salt and esters are more acid resistant, form a stable suspension in water, and are tasteless. Pediatric liquid suspensions depend on these characteristics. The stearate dissolves in the duodenum, releasing the base, which is subsequently absorbed in the upper small intestine.[99] Absorption of the stearate form of erythromycin is improved when it is taken with a meal.[100] The two ester derivatives are absorbed intact and must be partially hydrolyzed to the biologically active base in the blood.[101, 102] Although the ester and estolate are less affected by gastric acid and food in the stomach than the base or salt, higher plasma levels are produced when they are taken in the fasting state.[103]

The absorption of base is variable and produces peak serum concentrations within 4 hours of ingestion[98–101, 104–108] (Table 23–2). The stearate and ethylsuccinate are more evenly absorbed, producing peak serum levels after 3 and 2 hours, respectively. Approximately 45% of the ethylsuccinate reaches the serum as inactive ester and 55% as active base.[101, 103] The estolate is absorbed from the intestine as the propionate

TABLE 23–2 ■ Serum Concentrations of Macrolide Antibiotics*

PREPARATION	DOSE (mg)	ROUTE	HOURS AFTER DOSE	PEAK SERUM CONCENTRATION RANGE (μg/mL) (AT STEADY STATE)	TERMINAL HALF-LIFE (h)†
Erythromycin					
Base	250	PO	4	0.3–1.7	—
	500	PO	4	0.3–1.9	—
Stearate	250	PO	2–3	0.2–1.3	—
	500	PO	3	0.4–1.8	1.2–2.0
Ethylsuccinate	400	PO	0.5–2.5	0.6	—
Estolate	250	PO	2–4	1.2	—
	500	PO	2–4	3.0	—
Gluceptate	250	IV	1	2.6–3.5	—
	1000	IV	1	9.9	—
Lactobionate	500	IV	1	9.9	—
Clarithromycin	250	PO	3	2.0	3–4
14-Hydroxyclarithromycin	—	—	3	0.7	5–7
Azithromycin	500	PO	3.2	.24–0.4	68
Dirithromycin (erythromycylamine)	500	PO	4.1	0.48	45

*Data from references 5–7, 18, 98–110, 133–139. PO, Oral; IV, intravenous.
†Terminal half-life, at the end of a 5- to 14-d course of therapy.

ester. More estolate is absorbed from the gut within 2 hours of ingestion than with the other erythromycin compounds. Although serum levels of total drug are higher, only 23% to 35% of the total is active base.[101] Consequently, enteric-coated base tablets taken in the fasting state produce as high a plasma level of active erythromycin as estolate capsules.[106]

The characteristics of erythromycin preparation absorption have practical implications. For instance, erythromycin is recommended as appropriate antimicrobial prophylaxis to prevent endocarditis in patients with penicillin allergy who are undergoing dental procedures. The current guidelines from the American Heart Association recommend erythromycin ethylsuccinate (800 mg) or erythromycin stearate (1 g), given orally 2 hours before a procedure is performed, followed by a second dose of antibiotic 6 hours later.[109] Use of enteric-coated erythromycin as a substitute would be inappropriate in this context, given the all-or-none effect of pH on drug release from the preparation.[110] Peak serum levels are not achieved for 4 to 5 hours, and 2 hours after ingestion the antibiotic may be undetectable in serum.[111]

Intravenous preparations of erythromycin include the gluceptate and lactobionate. Peak concentrations are achieved within an hour and are higher than levels produced by comparable doses of oral preparations.[107] Intramuscular erythromycin is painful, is irregularly absorbed, and causes sterile abscesses. This route of administration is not recommended.

Erythromycin is distributed throughout the body water.[108] Protein binding of active drug varies between 40% and 90% (average 70%).[104, 112] The drug passes readily into ascites and pleural fluid, reaching concentrations approximately 50% of that in serum.[113] Levels in prostatic fluid and semen are about one third those in blood.[113] After a delay, erythromycin diffuses into middle-ear fluid in concentrations therapeutic for group A streptococci and pneumococci but not for *H. influenzae*.[114] The drug also passes into sinus fluid after a lag period similar to that observed with middle-ear fluid.[115, 116] Erythromycin achieves higher levels that are sustained longer in pulmonary tissues and secretions than do comparable doses of ampicillin and amoxicillin.[117, 118] Intravenous administration of erythromycin produces drug concentrations in sputum three to four times higher than those produced by oral administration.[117] High concentrations of drug are also found in tonsillar and adenoidal tissue.[119] Erythromycin does not readily cross the meninges and blood-brain barrier; consequently, therapeutic levels are not achieved in cerebrospinal fluid or brain.[113] This antimicrobial should not be used to treat infections of the central nervous system. The drug is not recommended for septic arthritis because of inadequate penetration into synovial fluid.[120] Orally administered base produces sufficient concentrations in stool to suppress most anaerobic bacteria.[113] For this reason, erythromycin combined with an oral aminoglycoside is commonly administered preoperatively to patients undergoing elective colorectal surgery to reduce bowel flora.

Erythromycin is concentrated in the liver and may be partially inactivated by demethylation.[121] Most of the drug is excreted unaltered in the bile, so high levels are found in the stool.[122, 123] Concentrations of drug in the bile are reduced in patients with obstructive biliary disease.[123] Approximately 2.5% of an oral dose and 15% of an intravenous dose of erythromycin are excreted unchanged in the urine.[98] The serum half-life of the drug is normally 1.5 hours but increases to 4 to 6 hours in anuric patients.[107, 108] Peritoneal dialysis and hemodialysis do not significantly reduce serum levels.[124] The antibiotic remains longer in tissue than in serum, a characteristic shared by all of the macrolide antibiotics.[6, 18, 97, 125, 126] Because the major site of elimination is the liver, changes in dosing are not recommended for most patients with renal failure[124]; ototoxicity has been reported, however, in elderly patients with renal failure.[127] A reduction in dose is recommended for patients with some degree of liver disease and renal failure. Erythromycin is found in maternal milk, and the drug crosses the placenta to the fetus.[128] In more than four decades of use, there have been no reported cases of teratogenic effects.[2]

Erythromycin is concentrated in neutrophils and macrophages by a process that requires energy.[129, 130] Concentrations in alveolar macrophages and neutrophils are 9 to 23 times and 10 to 13 times greater, respectively, than extracellular fluid concentrations.[130–132] The clinical implications of these high intracellular concentrations of drug are not established, although in the case of *Legionella* species they are suggestive.[132] These intracellular pathogens respond to erythromycin but not to other antimicrobials that demonstrate activity in vitro but do not enter the cell.

Azithromycin

Azithromycin is available in multiple formulations, described later, for oral dosing. After oral dosing, the drug is rapidly absorbed and distributed widely throughout the body. Ingestion with food decreases drug bioavailability (peak concentrations drop by 50%, area-under-curve concentrations by 43%). Accordingly, the drug should be taken 1 hour before or 2 hours after meals. Approximately 37% of a single 500-mg dose is bioavailable. Aluminum- and magnesium-containing antacids reduce peak serum levels; their use with the antimicrobial should be avoided. The drug is 50% protein bound at concentrations of 0.02 to 0.05 μg/mL, and as concentrations rise, the protein-bound fraction diminishes rapidly (at 1.0 μg/mL, 7% protein bound).[18, 133–141]

Drug concentrations in tissues are higher than those in serum, and elimination is more gradual. Tissue concentrations after a single dose of 500 mg of azithromycin ranged from 1 to 10 μg/mL in gastric, muscle, fat, bone, prostate, lung, kidney, and tonsil tissues. Elimination half-life from tissues after a single dose was estimated to be 56 to 76 hours.[133–141] Concentrations of azithromycin in serum, sputum, bronchial mucosa, and alveolar macrophages were measured in patients undergoing bronchoscopy, after a single 500-mg dose of drug. Within 96 hours after the dose, the drug was concentrated in macrophages, bronchial mucosa, and sputum at concentration ratios (relative to serum levels) of 52:1 to 1150:1.[142] Azithromycin concentrations in monocytes and neutrophils exceed plasma levels by 400- to 1200-fold, respectively, after multiple doses.[143] Accumulation of azithromycin in phagocytes does not affect their function.[144] Such extraordinary levels of drug in cells and tissues allow 5-day, once-daily therapy for conditions such as community-acquired pneumonia and bronchitis.

In children 7 months to 5 years old treated with azithromycin for otitis media, once-daily dosing with azithromycin at 5 mg/kg (after a single 10 mg/kg dose on the first day of therapy) led to steady-state serum levels by the fifth dose (serum trough concentration before the final dose, 51 ng/mL, and at 24 hours after the final dose, 47 ng/mL).[138]

Azithromycin and metabolites are excreted primarily in feces; approximately 75% of excreted drug-related material is unchanged. Less than 6% of an oral dose of azithromycin is excreted in the urinary tract within 1 week of consumption.[135]

Clarithromycin

Clarithromycin is available in tablet form and in granules for oral suspension. The drug is rapidly absorbed from the gastrointestinal tract but undergoes substantial first-pass metabolism, reducing bioavailability to approximately 50% after a single 250-mg dose. Peak clarithromycin plasma concentrations after a single dose of 250 or 500 mg of drug were achieved in 3 hours (0.62 to 0.84 μg/mL and 1.77 to 1.89 μg/mL, respectively).[6] Clarithromycin undergoes rapid biotransformation to the active metabolite 14-hydroxyclarithromycin (peak concentrations of 3.1 to 4.9 μg/mL and 6.1 to 6.9 μg/mL were measured after single doses of 250 and 500 mg, respectively).[6] Steady-state peak serum concentrations of the drug are achieved after four to six doses and are approximately 1 μg/mL (250 mg twice a day [bid]) and 2 to 3 μg/mL (500 mg bid). The drug is 42% to 70% protein bound at these concentrations.[143, 145–6] Unlike the effects with erythromycin base and azithromycin, coadministration of food does not appreciably alter clarithromycin pharmacokinetic parameters.[6, 146]

As with the other macrolide antibiotics, clarithromycin and its metabolites have exceptional tissue penetration and accumulation within cells.[143, 144, 147] Concentrations of the drug within alveolar cells were 1700-fold greater than those in plasma (17 versus 0.01 μg/mL) 48 hours after the fifth and final dose of a dosing regimen of 500 mg each 12 hours; at that time point, lung epithelial lining fluid concentrations were 23.4 μg/mL.[144] As with azithromycin, no data are available regarding cerebrospinal fluid concentrations of the drug.

Approximately 50% of administered doses of clarithromycin are excreted by the kidneys, in the form of clarithromycin or its 14-hydroxy metabolite. The elimination half-life of the drug is approximately 3 to 4 hours when it is given as 250 mg every 12 hours, increasing to 7 to 8 hours when it is given as 500 mg every 12 hours.[142–147] In the setting of significant liver disease, there is diminished generation of the 14-hydroxy metabolite. In the setting of severe renal impairment, dosage adjustment is required.

Unlike erythromycin, which has an unsurpassed safety record for use in pregnant patients (pregnancy category B), and azithromycin, which is probably safe (pregnancy category B), clarithromycin has demonstrated teratogenic effects in animal studies (pregnancy category C). The drug should be used for pregnant women only in clinical circumstances in which no alternative therapy is appropriate.

Dirithromycin

Dirithromycin is rapidly hydrolyzed to a primary metabolite after absorption. The active agent, erythromycylamine, reaches peak serum concentrations in 4 to 5 hours after a single dose. Unlike absorption of azithromycin and clarithromycin, absorption of dirithromycin is increased when it is taken with food. Serum concentrations are lower than those achieved by other macrolides, but high tissue concentrations accumulate. The drug is excreted primarily in the bile and feces, with an elimination half-life of 30 to 44 hours, allowing use of single daily doses. After single dosing with oral dirithromycin, 62% to 81% of the drug (primarily as erythromycylamine) is excreted in feces; less than 3.0% is recovered from urine. Erythromycylamine is not cleared by hemodialysis.[7, 126]

Toxicity and Adverse Effects

Erythromycin has a deserved reputation as a safe, nontoxic antimicrobial. The most frequent side effects of oral therapy are abdominal cramps, nausea, vomiting, and mild diarrhea.[113] Gastrointestinal upset is dose related and may be ameliorated by decreasing the dose. Approximately 45% of children treated with erythromycin ethylsuccinate and 14% given erythromycin estolate developed sufficiently severe gastrointestinal symptoms to stop taking the drug.[119] Cases of hypertrophic pyloric stenosis have been attributed to erythromycin estolate.[148] A prospective comparison of patients' tolerance of enteric-coated versus non–enteric-coated oral erythromycin preparations demonstrated dose-related gastrointestinal side effects for each but no significant difference between the two formulations.[149] The gastrointestinal effects of erythromycin are attributed to the drug's ability to mimic the effects of the gastrointestinal polypeptide hormone motilin (it is not clear whether the drug binds motilin receptors or induces endogenous motilin secretion).[150, 151] These otherwise undesired effects have been exploited clinically in the treatment of diabetic gastroparesis.[152, 153]

Gastrointestinal intolerance was the primary adverse effect reported on the basis of pooled data from 1676 pediatric patients receiving clarithromycin suspension in phase II and phase III trials.[154] Overall, 15.5% of patients reported gastrointestinal side effects; most common were diarrhea (6.6%), vomiting (6.3%), abdominal pain (2.5%), and nausea (1.0%). The rates of these observed side effects were similar to those seen with comparative drugs. Similar observations were made for adult patients receiving clarithromycin.[6, 155] Among approximately 4000 patients assessed who had received azithromycin, the incidence of adverse events was 12%; as with clarithromycin, these were predominantly gastrointestinal in nature.[156] These side effects rarely resulted in discontinuation of the drug and occurred less frequently than among those patients treated with erythromycin.

Cholestatic jaundice accompanied by fever, abdominal pain, eosinophilia, hyperbilirubinemia, and elevated transaminase values has been associated with erythromycin estolate.[157] This uncommon complication, which may be accompanied by rash and leukocytosis, occurs 10 to 20 days after initiation of therapy; the majority of cases are attributed to erythromycin estolate, although similar disease has been reported with erythromycin base and the salt (stearate) and ester (ethylsuccinate) preparations.[158–162] Cholestatic liver disease has an incidence of less than 1 in 1000 treated patients and is more common in adults, especially pregnant women, than children.[160, 163, 164] Jaundice is reversible in days to weeks after discontinuation of the medication, and chronic liver disease or death has not been described.[156] Histologically, cholestatic hepatitis consists of biliary stasis, periportal infiltration by inflammatory cells, and some hepatocellular damage to the point of cellular necrosis.[156] Rechallenge of patients with erythromycin estolate–induced hepatitis has resulted in recurrent disease with a shorter incubation period, suggesting a hypersensitivity reaction as the cause of this syndrome, although direct hepatocyte toxicity of erythromycin propionate has been described.[157, 165] Interference of the estolate with colorimetric determinations of transaminase levels may result in artifactual elevations[166]; this phenomenon should not be confused with drug-associated cholestasis. Because the estolate has no therapeutic advantage, it should not be given to adults, although it is probably safe for children and is better tolerated than the ethylsuccinate preparation.

Elevated transaminase levels (<1% to 5%) are observed in patients receiving clarithromycin,[6, 167] although significant hepatic injury is uncommon. The U.S. Food and Drug Administration has records of nine cases of hepatic failure associated with clarithromycin, although in most of those episodes drug interactions (particularly with acetaminophen) possibly contributed (Moldina N, personal communication, 1996). Rates of transaminase elevation of 1% to 2% among patients treated with azithromycin have been reported.[18]

Many reports of erythromycin-associated ototoxicity, including tinnitus, deafness, high-frequency hearing loss, and vertigo, have been described.[168] The ototoxicity of erythromycin was assessed prospectively with serum drug concentrations and audiograms in patients with pneumonia by Swanson and associates.[169] Twenty-one percent of patients receiving erythromycin at 4 g/d developed varying degrees of hearing impairment; the majority of symptomatic patients (four of five) were older than 60 years of age. Patients receiving erythromycin at less than 4 g/d in this study did not develop ototoxicity. In all patients, ototoxicity was reversible, requiring 6 to 14 days for return to normal.[169] In rare cases, erythromycin-associated ototoxicity can be irreversible. Reversible ototoxicity has been reported with azithromycin, occurring in approximately 14% of a cohort of patients receiving long-term azithromycin in combination with ethambutol and clofazimine for *M. avium* infection.[170] Similar ototoxicity has not been described with clarithromycin or dirithromycin, but the possibility of such an effect should be anticipated for any patient receiving macrolide antibiotic therapy, particularly for patients receiving high doses of drug for extended periods.

Although macrolide antibiotics reduce anaerobic and aerobic flora of the gut, antibiotic-associated colitis has rarely been associated with these antibiotics.[171] Superinfection of the vagina or gut with *Candida* species does occur. Allergic reactions—fever, rashes, eosinophilia—are uncommon for this class of antibiotics.[2, 18, 172, 173] Pancreatitis is an extremely uncommon complication of erythromycin therapy, but the related macrolide roxithromycin was removed from U.S. development during phase II trials because of severe episodes of pancreatitis. Significant episodes of pancreatitis attributed to azithromycin and clarithromycin have been reported to the U.S. Food and Drug Administration, although this is an uncommon event (Moldina N, personal communication, 1996).

Intravenous infusions of erythromycin lactobionate frequently produce side effects. Local pain at the infusion site and a feeling of lightheadedness are common, especially in young adults.[107, 174] The development of thrombophlebitis during intravenous administration can be prevented by diluting the drug and slowing the infusion rate.

Drug Interactions

Members of the cytochrome P-450 isozyme family are important in the metabolic clearance of numerous medications and are inducible by a wide variety of drugs. Macrolide antibiotics have varying effects on cytochrome P-450, the significant concern being formation of stable drug-enzyme complexes, resulting in competitive inhibition of metabolism of other medications.[175] This inhibition may occur even in the setting of increased cytochrome P-450 enzyme levels induced by the binding of macrolide antibiotics. Drugs metabolized by the cytochrome P-450 system, which may be significantly affected by the coadministration of macrolide antibiotics, include carbamazepine, valproate, ergotamine, glucocorticoids, theophylline, oral contraceptives, warfarin, clozapine, benzodiazepines, terfenadine, cisapride, cyclosporine, and tacrolimus.[141, 176] Simultaneous use of any of the macrolide antibiotics with these drugs (and others metabolized by the cytochrome P-450 system) should be done with attention to the potential for adverse interactions. In addition, macrolide antibiotics may improve absorption of digoxin to the point of toxicity in some patients by suppressing gut flora that normally degrades some of the drug before it is absorbed.[176, 177]

Among the macrolide antibiotics reviewed in this chapter, erythromycin and clarithromycin have been unequivocally demonstrated to form complexes with cytochrome P-450, with resultant inhibition or inactivation of the enzyme.[178] Dirithromycin and erythromycylamine were not shown to bind cytochrome P-450 and thus may not share the same potential for adverse drug interactions as erythromycin.[179] This premise awaits clinical validation. Azithromycin does interact with the cytochrome P-450 system; however, significant drug interactions with warfarin, terfenadine, and theophylline have not been observed clinically.[141, 180] Theophylline toxicity has been observed when erythromycin was administered concurrently.[181, 182] Erythromycin may elevate levels of warfarin, causing excessive hypoprothrombinemia.[183, 184] Elevation of cyclosporine and tacrolimus blood levels, in some cases with associated nephrotoxicity, has been attributed to impaired cytochrome P-450 metabolism of the drug in the setting of coadministration of erythromycin and clarithromycin.[185–187] We have observed a similar effect with azithromycin; accordingly, we routinely reduce the cyclosporine or tacrolimus dosage by 30% to 50% at the time of initiation of therapy with macrolide antibiotics and follow drug levels closely. Erythromycin and clarithromycin (and presumptively all of the macrolides) should not be taken concomitantly with cisapride. Serious cardiac arrhythmias including ventricular tachycardia, ventricular fibrillation, polymorphic ventricular tachycardia (torsades de pointes), and QT prolongation have been reported in this setting.[188] QT prolongation and associated arrhythmias occurring as a complication of erythromycin administration alone have been reported in 11 patients.[189] Coadministration of clarithromycin and carbamazepine led to significant increases in carbamazepine levels (exceeding toxic thresholds), despite lowering of the dosage by 30% to 40%. Coadministration should be avoided and, if it is considered necessary, the carbamazepine dosage should be decreased by 30% to 50% and levels monitored.[190] Clinically significant interaction of erythromycin and carbamazepine, resulting in hepatorenal syndrome, has been reported.[191] Adverse interactions with clozapine and benzodiazepines have been described. When given to patients with acquired immunodeficiency syndrome (AIDS) receiving long-term zidovudine therapy, clarithromycin may result in more rapid absorption of the drug, but in one investigation it appeared to have no significant effect on overall zidovudine bioavailability, based on mean area-under-curve levels of the drug before and after clarithromycin administration.[192] Prior studies had suggested that clarithromycin led to a significant decrease in zidovudine absorption[193]; these conflicting results have not been reconciled.

Erythromycin may cause false elevations of urinary catecholamines and 17-hydroxycorticosteroids and false reductions of urinary estriol levels as measured by colorimetric techniques.[98, 194]

Intravenous preparations of erythromycin are incompatible with certain other drugs, including vitamin B complex, vitamin C, chloramphenicol, cephalothin, colistin, heparin, tetracyclines, and phenytoin.

The interaction of erythromycin and other antimicrobials has been well studied. The combination of erythromycin and penicillin has demonstrated synergy against some strains of *S. aureus*.[195] Erythromycin inhibits the biosynthesis of penicillinase by these organisms and protects the penicillin from being inactivated by the enzyme; this phenomenon may occur in the presence of subinhibitory concentrations of erythromycin.[196, 197] In other instances, subinhibitory concentrations of the drug actually induce an increase in the production of penicillinase. Antagonism between erythromycin and ampicillin, cefamandole, or gentamicin has been demonstrated in some strains of *S. aureus* and *H. influenzae*.[198] Erythromycin and ampicillin may have a synergistic or additive effect on *Nocardia asteroides*.[199] Rifampin or penicillin and erythromycin may have antagonistic effects on *Listeria*,[200, 201] yet erythromycin and rifampin may have synergistic bactericidal effects on some strains of *S. aureus*.[202] The combination of erythromycin and sulfonamide has a synergistic effect on β-lactamase–producing and other strains of *H. influenzae*.[203] This may have important therapeutic implications for the treatment of otitis media.

Available Preparations

Erythromycin is available in several oral and parenteral preparations, as described here (Table 23–3). Erythromycin base comes prepared as enteric-coated tablets, enteric-coated pellets in capsules, and film-coated tablets. The stearate or salt is available in film-coated tablets; the ethylsuccinate or ester in chewable tablets, tablets, and liquid; and the lauryl sulfate salt of the proprionyl ester or estolate in capsules, liquid, and tablets. Enteric and film coatings are used to protect the drug from the effects of gastric acid. Two water-soluble erythromycin salts, erythromycin gluceptate and erythromycin lactobionate, are available for intravenous use. The drug should not be given intramuscularly. Topical solutions and ointments of 1.5%, 2%, and 3% erythromycin base are used to treat acne vulgaris. Ophthalmic ointments of 0.5% are also available for the treatment of bacterial conjunctivitis and prophylaxis against neonatal chlamydial and gonococcal ophthalmic infections.

TABLE 23–3 ■ Preparations of Erythromycin

Oral
Base
Enteric-coated tablets
Enteric-coated pellets in capsules
Film-coated tablets
Stearate (salt)
Film-coated tablets
Ethylsuccinate (ester)
Chewable, liquids, tablets
Lauryl sulfate salt of the propionyl ester (estolate)
Capsules, liquids, tablets
Intravenous
Erythromycin gluceptate
Erythromycin lactobionate
Topical solutions and ointments
Ophthalmic ointments

Dirithromycin is available as 250-mg enteric-coated tablets; no intravenous or oral suspension formulations are available.

Azithromycin is available in gelatin capsules containing 250 mg of the active ingredient azithromycin dihydrate; in tablets containing 600 mg of the active agent; in granules for oral suspension for pediatric use; and in 1000-mg single-dose packets containing granules for oral suspension. The formulation for flavored pediatric oral suspension results in drug concentrations of 100 or 200 mg/5 mL. No intravenous formulation of azithromycin is available.

Clarithromycin is available as film-coated tablets and granules for oral suspension. Film-coated tablets contain 250 or 500 mg of clarithromycin. Clarithromycin granules when resuspended result in drug concentrations of 125 or 250 mg per 5 mL in flavored preparations for pediatric use. No intravenous formulation of clarithromycin is available.

Dosing Recommendations

Peak serum levels of erythromycin base depend on formulation, dose, and route (see Table 23–2). Available oral formulations yield comparable serum concentrations of active drug. The serum levels of erythromycin required to inhibit sensitive organisms are listed in Table 23–1 and are clinically attainable. The recommended dose of drug for most indications varies between 250 and 500 mg four times daily. For moderate to severe infections, including those caused by *Legionella* species, the recommended dose of intravenous erythromycin is 4 g/d.

The recommended dose of dirithromycin for treatment of respiratory tract and skin and soft tissue infections is 500 mg, given once a day for 7 days.[8, 126]

The recommended dose of azithromycin for treatment of respiratory tract and skin and soft tissue infections in adults is 500 mg, given on day 1 of therapy, followed by 250 mg given once a day on days 2 through 5 of therapy. For treatment of otitis media in children, dosage is administered at 10 mg/kg of body weight on day 1, followed by 5 mg/kg for the next 4 days. For treatment of pharyngitis or tonsillitis in children aged 2 years and older, the recommended dose is 12 mg/kg, given once each day for 5 days. Azithromycin prophylaxis at a dose of 1200 mg given once a week is effective for prevention of *M. avium* infection in AIDS patients.[18, 204–207] Single-dose therapy with 1000 mg of azithromycin is effective for genital *Chlamydia* infections.

The recommended dose of clarithromycin for treatment of

respiratory tract and skin and soft tissue infections in adults is 250 to 500 mg bid given for 7 to 14 days. For prophylaxis against MAC infections in adults, 500 mg bid is recommended, whereas for therapy for established infection, multidrug regimens including clarithromycin at 500 to 1000 mg bid are recommended[204–206]; for children, the dosage is calculated as 7.5 mg/kg bid.[6, 204]

Assay

The most common dose-related toxicities of erythromycin are various gastrointestinal symptoms.[113] Reducing the dose or temporarily interrupting therapy ameliorates these complaints. In the presence of renal failure or hepatic dysfunction in elderly patients, reducing the dose seems prudent and may avoid the hearing loss they often experience.[168] Serum assays for all of the macrolide antibiotics are rarely indicated and when performed are used as a research tool.

Clinical Indications

Overview

The macrolide antibiotics reviewed in this chapter have proved safe and efficacious. Erythromycin is the drug of choice for certain infections and in other instances may be an effective alternative to penicillin G or the tetracyclines. Such a substitution may be dictated by allergy, intolerance, contraindications, or cost. It has also found a niche as a prophylactic drug. Erythromycylamine, the active moiety in the prodrug dirithromycin, in comparison with erythromycin, has a similar spectrum of activity and markedly prolonged half-life, allowing once-daily dosing. Although fewer data have accumulated concerning the clinical efficacy and toxicity of dirithromycin, the drug appears to be equivalent to erythromycin, with greater ease of administration. Unless specifically noted, discussion of the clinical indications for dirithromycin therapy is covered here within the broader topic of erythromycin. Azithromycin and clarithromycin induce less gastrointestinal intolerance than erythromycin, a significant improvement. Azithromycin and clarithromycin have longer half-lives, allowing once-daily (azithromycin) or twice-daily (clarithromycin) dosing, another significant improvement. The long tissue half-life of azithromycin allows a 5-day course of therapy for some indications, in comparison with 7 to 14 days for other agents. These improvements in pharmacokinetics and patients' tolerance must be balanced against the greater costs of these agents in comparison with erythromycin. Azithromycin differs significantly from erythromycin and clarithromycin in having enhanced activity against gram-negative organisms, in particular *H. influenzae.* Azithromycin has proven efficacy for treatment of *C. trachomatis* infections. Conversely, erythromycin and clarithromycin have, in general, 2- to 10-fold lower minimal inhibitory concentrations for susceptible gram-positive organisms (e.g., *S. pneumoniae, S. aureus, S. pyogenes*) than azithromycin. Clarithromycin is unique in having lower minimal inhibitory concentrations, as noted, for gram-positive organisms (compared with azithromycin) and exceptional activity against mycobacteria, in particular, MAC members. In addition, the major metabolite of clarithromycin, 14-hydroxyclarithromycin, is active against *H. influenzae.* Numerous "novel" indications that are under study for azithromycin and/or clarithromycin (treatment or prophylaxis of infections with *M. leprae,* MAC, *H. pylori, Cryptosporidium parvum, Bartonella henselae, T. gondii,* and others) are presented in the following.

Respiratory Tract Infections

Respiratory infections caused by susceptible organisms are effectively treated with macrolide antibiotics. Erythromycin is considered the drug of choice for infection with *L. pneumophila* and other *Legionella* species.[208–210] No data are available proving equivalent efficacy of dirithromycin in the treatment of confirmed *L. pneumophila* pneumonia, and intravenous therapy would most often be indicated in this circumstance. Azithromycin and clarithromycin do not have U.S. Food and Drug Administration approval for the treatment of confirmed *L. pneumophila* infection; however, the minimal inhibitory concentrations for these drugs are similar or superior to those of erythromycin (clarithromycin shows increased activity). Clarithromycin was demonstrated to be effective in the treatment of *Legionella* pneumonia in an open-label study of Pakistani patients with moderate to severe disease,[211] and in treatment trials for community-acquired pneumonia both azithromycin and clarithromycin have demonstrated efficacy in suspected cases of *Legionella* pneumonia of mild to moderate severity.[212–218] Erythromycin is considered the drug of choice for *Mycoplasma* infections, although tetracycline is an effective alternative.[219] Azithromycin and clarithromycin have demonstrated similar excellent activity against *M. pneumoniae* both in vitro and in the treatment of atypical pneumonias with documentation of *Mycoplasma* infection.[60, 214] The macrolide antibiotics reduce the duration of respiratory symptoms and fever and hasten resolution of pulmonary infiltrates but have not been demonstrated to eliminate the organism from the nasopharynx.[220] Erythromycin, azithromycin, and clarithromycin all have good activity against *C. pneumoniae*[221, 222] and have demonstrated clinical efficacy in the treatment of pneumonia caused by this agent.[214, 215, 217, 218] Erythromycin is effective therapy for the treatment of *Chlamydia psittaci* and *Coxiella burnetii* infection[223, 224]; clinical experience with azithromycin or clarithromycin in treatment of disease caused by these pathogens is not available, but both should be effective agents on the basis of in vitro susceptibility data. Thus, each of these antibiotics is a rational choice for treatment of the agents associated with atypical pneumonia when oral therapy is indicated.

The macrolide antibiotics have efficacy against the most common bacterial pathogens isolated in cases of community-acquired pneumonia and bronchitis (e.g., *S. pneumoniae, M. catarrhalis, S. pyogenes, H. influenzae*) and are acceptable agents for the treatment of these infections when of mild to moderate severity.[8, 204] Erythromycin may be used to treat acute bronchitis and acute exacerbations of chronic bronchitis.[225] Despite the variable sensitivity of *H. influenzae* to this antibiotic, erythromycin has been shown to decrease symptom severity and duration in treated patients.[225] The antibiotic may also be used as chronic suppressive therapy in patients with chronic obstructive pulmonary disease to prevent recurrences of respiratory infections.[172] Clarithromycin has also been demonstrated to be effective in the treatment of *H. influenzae* infection associated with bronchitis or pneumonia. In comparative trials with ampicillin, erythromycin, cefixime, cefaclor, and cefuroxime, clarithromycin achieved comparable bacteriologic eradication rates and clinical responses in the treatment of lower respiratory tract infection. However, it should be noted that in these studies, bacterial eradication rates for *H. influenzae* were diminished (64% to 100%) in comparison with *S. pneumoniae* and *M. catarrhalis.*[155, 217, 218, 226] For treatment of adult patients with purulent bronchitis, a 5-day course of clarithromycin was demonstrated to be as effective as 10 days of therapy.[216] Azithromycin has similar efficacy in the treatment of pneumonia and bronchitis and has been demonstrated in clinical trials to be comparable or superior to amoxicillin, amoxicillin-clavulanate, erythromycin, and cefaclor.[18] In one study of hospitalized patients with exacerbations of chronic bronchitis attributed to *H. influenzae*, failure to eradicate the pathogen despite high sputum concentrations of the antibiotic was associated with diminished clinical cure rates and the emergence of antibiotic resistance among isolates.[93]

Otitis Media and Pharyngitis

The most common agents of otitis media are *S. pneumoniae*, *H. influenzae*, group A streptococci, and *M. pneumoniae*. Erythromycin has been compared with ampicillin, amoxicillin, erythromycin with sulfonamide, and triple sulfonamides alone in the treatment of this infection. Patients with purulent otitis treated with erythromycin had a higher cure rate than those treated with sulfonamides alone.[227] The erythromycin-sulfonamide combination was found to be superior to erythromycin alone and as effective as ampicillin or amoxicillin.[228, 229] In vitro the combination is more active against *H. influenzae* than the macrolide alone.[230] These data support the recommendation that erythromycin be used in combination with sulfonamides for treating acute otitis media in children. In randomized treatment trials, clarithromycin was found to have safety and efficacy equivalent to those of amoxicillin,[231, 232] amoxicillin-clavulanate,[233, 234] and cefaclor[235] in the treatment of pediatric patients with acute otitis media. Similarly, azithromycin has been found to have efficacy comparable to that of amoxicillin-clavulanate, with a lower incidence of side effects, in the treatment of pediatric acute otitis media.[236]

The pathogens responsible for purulent sinusitis are similar to those recovered from patients with otitis media. Although amoxicillin is considered by many to be the drug of choice, erythromycin can be used for penicillin-allergic patients. Sinusitis caused by *H. influenzae* may respond more slowly to erythromycin.[237] Clarithromycin and azithromycin have demonstrated efficacy in the treatment of sinusitis,[238–242] although less expensive alternatives such as trimethoprim-sulfamethoxazole or amoxicillin should be considered. In addition, clarithromycin was less effective than amoxicillin and ampicillin in the treatment of sinusitis caused by *H. influenzae*.[240, 241]

Streptococcal pharyngitis responds to erythromycin treatment, and the drug is as effective as the penicillins in preventing acute rheumatic fever.[17, 243] Clarithromycin was demonstrated to be equivalent to penicillin VK in the treatment of streptococcal pharyngitis among children, with superior bacterial eradication rates (92% versus 81%).[244] The presence of β-lactamase–producing organisms in the oral pharynx probably accounts for the superior eradication rates observed with the macrolide antibiotics compared with penicillin VK. Azithromycin was demonstrated to be equivalent to penicillin V in the treatment of streptococcal pharyngitis in adults[245] and equivalent to erythromycin in children.[246] Thus, the macrolide antibiotics are reasonable alternatives for the treatment of pharyngitis in penicillin-allergic patients, although increasing reports of erythromycin resistance among group A β-hemolytic streptococcal isolates must be considered.

Administered early in the course of pertussis, erythromycin reduces the contagiousness of this infection but does not shorten the duration of clinical illness.[247, 248] The drug is effective prophylaxis for nonimmunized children who have been exposed to whooping cough.[247] On the basis of in vitro sensitivity data, azithromycin and clarithromycin should have comparable efficacy. Although antibiotics do not alter the course of infection by lysogenic *C. diphtheriae*, erythromycin effectively eliminated the acute and chronic carrier state in more than 90% of adults.[249]

Skin and Soft Tissue Infections

Skin infections with *S. pyogenes*, including cellulitis, erysipelas, impetigo, and lymphangitis, have been treated successfully with erythromycin.[98, 250] The cure rate approaches that achieved with penicillin G. Treatment failure suggests a mixed infection with erythromycin-resistant strains of *S. aureus*.[2] Penicillinase-resistant penicillins (if not contraindicated), cephalosporins, or vancomycin may be required in this situation or, for impetigo, topical mupirocin.[251] Clarithromycin and azithromycin have demonstrated efficacy equivalent to that of erythromycin, cefadroxil, and cephalexin in the treatment of skin and skin structure infections.[252, 253] Erythromycin is safe, inexpensive therapy for chronic acne vulgaris.[254] Erythrasma, a superficial skin infection caused by *Corynebacterium minutissimum*, responded dramatically to this drug.[255] In penicillin-allergic patients, *C. tetani* was eliminated from contaminated wounds by erythromycin.[2, 120]

Gastrointestinal Tract Infections

Erythromycin has consistent activity against *C. jejuni* and has been demonstrated to reduce the duration of positive stool cultures and to moderate symptoms of gastroenteritis related to this pathogen.[256, 257] Fluorinated quinolones are active against this organism and are preferred therapy.[258, 259] Azithromycin and clarithromycin have significant activity against *H. pylori* and have each been successful in the eradication of infection when used in triple therapy (bismuth, tetracycline or amoxicillin, and clarithromycin or azithromycin) or dual therapy (omeprazole plus clarithromycin or azithromycin).[260–262] However, clarithromycin is preferred. Monotherapy of *Helicobacter* infection with clarithromycin was associated with the development of resistance in 21% of subjects and thus combination regimens must be used.[263] Azithromycin has excellent in vitro activity against other enteric bacteria (*Shigella* spp., *Salmonella* spp., *Campylobacter* spp.)[264]; however, a preliminary report suggested that the drug may not be adequate therapy for the treatment of typhoid fever.[265]

Sexually Transmitted Diseases

Azithromycin, in a single 1-g dose, has become a mainstay in the treatment of uncomplicated genital tract infection with *C. trachomatis* because of high efficacy, ease of administration, and assurance of compliance.[266, 267] Single-dose azithromycin had efficacy comparable to that of a 7-day course of doxycycline or single-dose ceftriaxone in the treatment of uncomplicated *N. gonorrhoeae* infection.[268, 269] However, the Centers for Disease Control and Prevention has not recommended routine use of azithromycin for the treatment of gonorrhea, because of the high frequency of adverse reactions observed in clinical trials and the high cost of the drug compared with alternative regimens.[270] Erythromycin is recommended for treatment of *U. urealyticum*, *Chlamydia* infections including lymphogranuloma venereum, and chancroid[36, 251, 267, 271–273]; for each of these pathogens, azithromycin has demonstrated equivalent or superior efficacy.[268, 274–276] Erythromycin may be used to treat early syphilis in immunocompetent patients with penicillin allergy, but treatment failures have been observed when the drug has been used to treat primary syphilis infection in pregnant women.[277] Azithromycin has in vitro activity against *T. pallidum*, and in a pilot study a 10-day course of the drug was effective in the treatment of primary or secondary syphilis.[278] However, the effectiveness of single-dose azithromycin for the eradication of incubating syphilis is unknown, and the drug is not recommended by the Centers for Disease Control and Prevention for treatment of syphilis at this time.[279] Azithromycin was demonstrated to be comparable to penicillin V for the treatment of early Lyme borreliosis.[280] Topical erythromycin (0.5% ointment) is effective in preventing neonatal gonococcal conjunctivitis.[271, 281]

Mycobacterial Infections

Therapy of MAC infection in AIDS patients has been dramatically enhanced by the development of clarithromycin and azithromycin. When used as monotherapy for MAC disease, clarithromycin (500 mg bid) was associated with reduction or clearance of bacteremia and reduced fever and constitutional symptoms; however, recurrence of bacteremia with clarithromycin-resistant strains occurred frequently.[95] Similarly, azithromycin has been demonstrated to reduce bacteremia and relieve symptoms in AIDS patients (with rapid development of resistance).[282] A consensus committee convened by the U.S. Public Health Service has recommended that therapy for disseminated MAC infection in patients with human immunodeficiency virus infection consist of clarithromycin or azithromycin in combination with one or more additional agents (in particular, ethambutol and/or clofazimine).[283] Although such combination therapy is required for effective treatment, it is also associated with an increased frequency of drug toxicity.[206, 284] Azithromycin and clarithromycin have also been demonstrated to be highly effective agents for the prevention of MAC disease in AIDS patients. Prophylaxis with clarithromycin was compared with placebo in AIDS patients with CD4$^+$ T cell counts of less than 100/mm^3, and a significant reduction in the incidence of MAC bacteremia, constitutional symptoms, and mortality was observed.[205] In patients with human immunodeficiency virus infection and CD4$^+$ T cell counts of less than 100/mm^3 randomized to receive prophylactic clarithromycin (500 mg bid), rifabutin (450 mg/d), or combination therapy, MAC disease or bacteremia occurred in 9%, 15%, and 7%, respectively, during a median follow-up of 336 days.[285] A once-weekly dose of 1200 mg of azithromycin was demonstrated to reduce the occurrence of MAC bacteremia from 23.3% (placebo) to 8.2% (azithromycin) during 400 days of follow-up.[286] Combination of once-weekly azithromycin (1200 mg) with daily rifabutin was demonstrated to be superior to azithromycin or rifabutin alone.[207]

Clarithromycin has been used effectively in the treatment of other mycobacterial infections. In vitro sensitivity data and preliminary clinical experience suggest that the drug is highly effective for the treatment of infection with disseminated *M. chelonae*.[287] Case reports suggest that the drug is effective in the treatment of *Mycobacterium marinum* infection.[287, 288] Short-course clarithromycin monotherapy was associated with significant clinical improvement in patients with lepromatous leprosy, suggesting that the agent is bactericidal for *M. leprae* and should have a significant role in the treatment of this disease.[289] In addition, clarithromycin may be of benefit in the treatment of multidrug-resistant *M. tuberculosis* infections.[290]

Other Uses in Patients with Human Immunodeficiency Virus Infection

The newer macrolides have proved useful or promising in the treatment of other infectious diseases associated with the human immunodeficiency virus epidemic. In animal models, combination therapy with clarithromycin and sulfonamides was associated with improved clearance of *Pneumocystis carinii* infection,[291] and case reports suggest that the drug may have a role in salvage therapy for AIDS patients with *P. carinii* pneumonia.[292] Clarithromycin in combination with minocycline has been used as effective salvage and/or maintenance treatment for cerebral toxoplasmosis in AIDS patients,[293, 294] and azithromycin has shown promise in combination with pyrimethamine for treatment of acute disease.[295] Erythromycin and azithromycin have been used successfully in the treatment of AIDS-related bacillary angiomatosis (*Bartonella henselae* infection).[296–298] Azithromycin and clarithromycin may have a role in the treatment of AIDS-associated cryptosporidiosis, although currently available data are limited to case reports. Although these data are promising, determination of the definitive role for the macrolides in the treatment of each of the foregoing infections awaits further clinical evaluation.

Potential Role in Treatment of Malaria

Finally, a role for azithromycin in the treatment and prophylaxis of malaria appears plausible. The drug was demonstrated to have schizonticidal activity against rodent and human plasmodia in vivo[48] and in pilot studies demonstrated promise as a prophylactic agent against chloroquine-resistant *Plasmodium falciparum*.[299]

References

1. McGuire JM, Bunch RL, Anderson RC, et al: "Ilotycin" a new antibiotic. Antibiot Chemother 2:281, 1952.
2. Washington JA II, Wilson WR: Erythromycin: A microbial and clinical perspective after 30 years of clinical use (1). Mayo Clin Proc 60:189, 1985.
3. Thomson EF, Rountree PM, Freeman BM: Observations on the sensitivity to erythromycin of *Staphylococcus aureus*. *In* Antibiotics Annual 1955–1956. New York, Medical Encyclopedia, 1957, pp 63–72.
4. Brown ST, Pederson AHB, Holmes KK: Comparison of erythromycin base and estolate in gonococcal urethritis. JAMA 238:1371, 1977.
5. Retsema J, Girard A, Schelkly W, et al: Spectrum and mode of action of azithromycin (P-62,993), a new 15-membered ring macrolide with improved potency against gram-negative organisms. Antimicrob Agents Chemother 31:1939, 1987.
6. Peters DH, Clissold SP: Clarithromycin: A review of its antimicrobial activity, pharmacokinetic properties, and therapeutic potential. Drugs 44:117, 1992.
7. Brogden R, Peters D: Dirithromycin. A review of its antimicrobial activity, pharmacokinetic properties, and therapeutic efficacy. Drugs 48:599, 1994.
8. Dirithromycin. Med Lett 37:109, 1995.
9. Pestka S: Binding of ^{14}C-erythromycin to *Escherichia coli* ribosomes. Antimicrob Agents Chemother 6:474, 1974.
10. Oleinick NL, Corcoran JW: Two types of binding of erythromycin to ribosomes from antibiotic-sensitive and -resistant *Bacillus subtilis* 168. J Biol Chem 244:727, 1969.
11. Pestka S: Antibiotics as probes of ribosome structure: Binding of chloramphenicol and erythromycin to polyribosomes; effects of other antibiotics. Antimicrob Agents Chemother 5:255, 1974.
12. Otaka T, Kaji A: Release of (oligo) peptidyl-tRNA from ribosomes by erythromycin. Proc Natl Acad Sci USA 72:2649, 1975.
13. Oleinick NL, Wilhelm JM, Corcoran JW: Nonidentity of the site of action of erythromycin A and chloramphenicol on *Bacillus subtilis* ribosomes. Biochim Biophys Acta 155:290, 1968.
14. Chang FN, Weisblum B: The specificity of lincomycin binding to ribosomes. Biochemistry 6:836, 1967.
15. Mao JCH, Putterman M, Wiegand RG: Biochemical basis of the selective toxicity of erythromycin. Biochem Pharmacol 19:391, 1970.
16. Ibrahim NG, Beattie DS: Protein synthesis on ribosomes isolated from rat liver mitochondria: Sensitivity to erythromycin. FEBS Lett 36:102, 1973.
17. Haight TH, Finland M: Observations on mode of action of erythromycin. Proc Soc Exp Biol Med 81:188, 1952.
18. Peters DH, Friedel HA, McTavish D: Azithromycin. A review of its antimicrobial activity, pharmacokinetic properties and clinical efficacy. Drugs 44:750, 1992.
19. Gerber AU, Craig WA: Growth kinetics of respiratory pathogens

after short exposures to ampicillin and erythromycin in vitro. J Antimicrob Chemother 8(Suppl C):81, 1981.
20. Odenholt-Tornqvist I, Lowdin E, Cars O: Postantibiotic effects and postantibiotic sub-MIC effects of roxithromycin, clarithromycin and azithromycin on respiratory tract pathogens. Antimicrob Agents Chemother 39:221, 1995.
21. Sabath LD, Gerstein PA, Loder PB, et al: Excretion of erythromycin and its enhanced activity in urine against gram-negative bacilli with alkalinization. J Lab Clin Med 72:916, 1968.
22. Mao JCH, Putterman M: Accumulation in gram-positive and gram-negative bacteria as a mechanism of resistance to erythromycin. J Bacteriol 95:1111, 1968.
23. Taybeneck U: Susceptibility of *Proteus mirabilis* and its stable L-forms to erythromycin and other macrolides. Nature 196:195, 1962.
24. Barrett FF, Casey JI, Wilcox C, et al: Bacteriophage types and antibiotic susceptibility of *Staphylococcus aureus*: Boston City Hospital. Arch Intern Med 125:867, 1970.
25. Finland M: Changing patterns of susceptibility of common bacterial pathogens to antimicrobial agents. Ann Intern Med 76:1009, 1972.
26. Sorbello AF: Group A streptococcal resistance to clindamycin and erythromycin. JAMA 262:1329, 1989.
27. Seppala H, Nissinen A, Jarvinen H, et al: Resistance to erythromycin in group A streptococci. N Engl J Med 326:292, 1992.
28. Maruyama S, Yoshioka H, Fujita K, et al: Sensitivity of group A streptococci to antibiotics. Am J Dis Child 133:1143, 1979.
29. Hsueh PR, Chen HM, Huang AH, Wu JJ: Decreased activity of erythromycin against *Streptococcus pyogenes* in Taiwan. Antimicrob Agents Chemother 39:2239, 1992.
30. Hofmann J, Cetron MS, Farley MM, et al: The prevalence of drug-resistant *Streptococcus pneumoniae* in Atlanta. N Engl J Med 333:481, 1995.
31. Toala P, McDonald A, Wilcox C, et al: Susceptibility of group D streptococcus (enterococcus) to 21 antibiotics in vitro, with special reference to species differences. Am J Med Sci 258:416, 1969.
32. Martin WJ, Gardner M, Washington JA II: In vitro antimicrobial susceptibility of anaerobic bacteria isolated from clinical specimens. Antimicrob Agents Chemother 1:148, 1972.
33. Emerson BB, Smith AL, Harding AL, et al: *Haemophilus influenzae* type b susceptibility to 17 antibiotics. J Pediatr 86:617, 1975.
34. Finland M, Garner C, Wilcox C, et al: Susceptibility of pneumococci and *Haemophilus influenzae* to antibacterial agents. Antimicrob Agents Chemother 9:274, 1976.
35. Centers for Disease Control: Sexually transmitted disease treatment guidelines. MMWR Morbid Mortal Wkly Rep 334(Suppl):755, 1985.
36. Spaepen MS, Kundsin RB: Simple, direct broth-disk method for antibiotic susceptibility testing of *Ureaplasma urealyticum.* Antimicrob Agents Chemother 11:267, 1977.
37. Maurin M, Gasquet S, Ducco C, Raoult D: MICs of 28 antibiotic compounds for 14 *Bartonella* (formerly *Rochalimaea*) isolates. Antimicrob Agents Chemother 39:2387, 1995.
38. Tally FP, Cuchural GJ, Jacobus NV, et al: Susceptibility of the *Bacteroides* group in the United States in 1981. Antimicrob Agents Chemother 23:536, 1983.
39. Ingham HR, Selkon JB, Codd AA, et al: The effect of carbon dioxide on the sensitivity of *Bacteroides fragilis* to certain antibiotics in vitro. J Clin Pathol 23:254, 1970.
40. Neu HC: The development of macrolides: Clarithromycin in perspective. J Antimicrob Chemother 27(Suppl A):1, 1992.
41. Smith MD, Vinh DX, Hoa NTT, et al: In vitro antimicrobial susceptibilities of strains of *Yersinia pestis.* Antimicrob Agents Chemother 39:2153, 1995.
42. Renaudin H, Bebear C: Comparative in vitro activity of azithromycin, clarithromycin, erythromycin, and lomeloxacin against *Mycoplasma pneumoniae, Mycoplasma hominis* and *Ureaplasma urealyticum.* Eur J Clin Microbiol Infect Dis 9:838, 1990.
43. Rylander M, Hallander HO: In vitro comparison of the activity of doxycycline, tetracycline, erythromycin, and a new macrolide, CP 62993, against *Mycoplasma pneumoniae, Mycoplasma hominis,* and *Ureaplasma urealyticum.* Scand J Infect Dis Suppl 53:12, 1988.
44. Preac-Mursic V, Wilske B, Schierz G, et al: Comparative antimicrobial activity of the new macrolides against *Borrelia burgdorferi.* Eur J Clin Microbiol Infect Dis 8:651, 1989.
45. Stamm LV, Parrish EA: In vitro activity of azithromycin and CP-63,956 against *Treponema pallidum.* J Antimicrob Chemother 25(Suppl A):11, 1990.
46. Derouin F, Caroff B, Chau F, et al: Synergistic activity of clarithromycin and minocycline in an animal model of acute experimental toxoplasmosis. Antimicrob Agents Chemother 36:2852, 1992.
47. Strickman D, Sheer T, Salata K, et al: In vitro effectiveness of azithromycin against doxycycline-resistant and -susceptible strains of *Rickettsia tsutsugamushi*, etiologic agent of scrub typhus. Antimicrob Agents Chemother 39:2406, 1995.
48. Andersen SL, Ager A, McGreevy P, et al: Activity of azithromycin as a blood schizonticide against rodent and human plasmodia in vivo. Am J Trop Med Hyg 52:159, 1995.
49. Weiss LM, Wittner M, Wasserman S, et al: Efficacy of azithromycin for treating *Babesia microti* infection in the hamster model. J Infect Dis 168:1289, 1993.
50. Eliopoulos GN, Reiszner F, Ferraro MJ, Moellering RC: Comparative in vitro activity of A-56268 (TE-031), a new macrolide antibiotic. J Antimicrob Chemother 21:671, 1988.
51. Hardy D, Hensey D, Beyer J, et al: Comparative in vitro activities of new 14-, 15-, and 16-membered macrolides. Antimicrob Agents Chemother 32:1710, 1988.
52. Fernandes P, Bailer R, Swanson R, et al: In vitro and in vivo evaluation of A-5628, a new macrolide. Antimicrob Agents Chemother 30:865, 1986.
53. Naik S, Ruck R: In vitro activities of several new macrolide antibiotics against *Mycobacterium avium* complex. Antimicrob Agents Chemother 33:591, 1989.
54. Gornyski E, Gutman S, Allen W: Comparative antimycobacterial activities of difloxacin, emafloxacin, enoxacin, peloxacin, reference fluoroquinolones, and a new macrolide, clarithromycin. Antimicrob Agents Chemother 33:5591, 1989.
55. Brown B, Wallace R, Onyi G, et al: Activities of four macrolides, including clarithromycin, against *Mycobacterium fortuitum, Mycobacterium chelonae,* and *M. chelonae–like organisms. Antimicrob Agents Chemother 36:180, 1992.*
56. Barry AL, Jones RN, Thornsberry C: In vitro activities of azithromycin (CP 63,993), clarithromycin (A-56268; TE-031), erythromycin, roxitromycin, and clindamycin. Antimicrob Agents Chemother 32:752, 1988.
57. Barry AL, Jurgensen JH, Hardy DJ: Reproducibility of disc susceptibility tests with *Haemophilus influenzae.* J Antimicrob Chemother 27:295, 1991.
58. Olsson-Liljequist B, Hoffman BM: In vitro activity of clarithromycin combined with its 14-hydroxy metabolite A-62671 against *H. influenzae.* J Antimicrob Chemother 27(Suppl A):11, 1991.
59. Benson C, Segreti J, Kessler H, et al: Comparative in vitro activity of A-56268 (TE-031) against gram-positive and gram-negative bacteria and *Chlamydia trachomatis.* Eur J Clin Microbiol Infect Dis 6:173, 1987.
60. Cassell GH, Drnec J, Waites KB, et al: Efficacy of clarithromycin against *Mycoplasma pneumoniae.* J Antimicrob Chemother 27(Suppl A):47, 1991.
61. Edelstein PM, Meyer RD: Susceptibility of *Legionella pneumophila* to twenty antimicrobial agents. Antimcrob Agents Chemother 18:403, 1980.
62. Hammerschlag MR, Qumei KK, Roblin PM: In vitro activities of azithromycin, clarithromycin, L-ofloxacin, and other antibiotics against *Chlamydia pneumoniae.* Antimicrob Agents Chemother 36:1573, 1992.
63. Kuo C, Wang S, Grayston T: Antimicrobial activity of several antibiotics and a sulfonamide against *Chlamydia trachomatis* organisms in cell culture. Antimicrob Agents Chemother 12:80, 1977.
64. McNulty CA, Dent JC: Susceptibility of clinical isolates of *Campylobacter pylori* to twenty-one antimicrobial agents. Eur J Clin Microbiol Infect Dis 7:566, 1988.
65. Metchock B: In-vitro activity of azithromycin compared with other macrolides and oral antibiotics against *Salmonella typhi.* J Antimicrob Chemother 25(Suppl A):29, 1990.
66. Benson CA, Segreti J, Kessler H, et al: Comparative in vitro activity of A-56268 (TE-031), a new macrolide, compared with that of erythromycin and clindamycin against selected gram-positive and gram-negative organisms. Antimicrob Agents Chemother 31:328, 1987.

67. Ridgway GL, Mumtaz G, Fenelon L: The in vitro activity of clarithromycin and other macrolides in the type strain of *Chlamydia pneumoniae.* J Antimicrob Chemother 27(Suppl A):43, 1991.
68. Araujo F, Prokocimer P, Lin T, et al: Activity of clarithromycin alone or in combination with other drugs for treatment of murine toxoplasmosis. Antimicrob Agents Chemother 36:2454, 1992.
69. Araujo FG, Shepard RM, Remington JS: In vivo activity of the macrolide antibiotics azithromycin, roxithromycin and spiramycin against *Toxoplasma gondii.* Eur J Clin Microbiol Infect Dis 10:519, 1991.
70. Chang HR, Rudareanu FC, Pechere JC: Activity of A-56268 (TE-031), a new macrolide, against *Toxoplasma gondii* in mice. J Antimicrob Chemother 22:359, 1988.
71. Chang H, Pechere J: In vitro effects of four macrolides on *Toxoplasma gondii.* Antimicrob Agents Chemother 32:524, 1988.
72. Goldman RC, Capobianco JO: Role of an energy-dependent efflux pump in plasmid pNE24-mediated resistance to 14- and 15-membered macrolides in *Staphylococcus epidermidis.* Antimicrob Agents Chemother 34:1973, 1990.
73. Weisblum B: Erythromycin resistance by ribosome modification. Antimicrob Agents Chemother 39:577, 1995.
74. Lai CJ, Weisblum B: Altered methylation of ribosomal RNA in an erythromycin-resistant strain of *Staphylococcus aureus.* Proc Natl Acad Sci USA 68:856, 1971.
75. Barthelemy P, Autissier D, Gerbaud G, et al: Enzymic hydrolysis of erythromycin by a strain of *Escherichia coli.* J Antibiot (Tokyo) 37:1692, 1984.
76. Charvalos E, Tselentis Y, Hamzehpour MM, et al: Evidence for an efflux pump in multidrug-resistant *Campylobacter jejuni.* Antimicrob Agents Chemother 39:2019, 1995.
77. Oleinick NL: The erythromycins. *In* Corcoran JW, Hahn FE (eds): Mechanisms of Action of Antimicrobial and Antitumor Agents. New York, Springer-Verlag, 1975, p 396.
78. Lacey RW: Lack of evidence for mutation to erythromycin resistance in clinical strains of *Staphylococcus aureus.* J Clin Pathol 30:602, 1977.
79. Weisblum B: Inducible erythromycin resistance in bacteria. Br Med Bull 40:47, 1984.
80. Garrod LP: The erythromycin group of antibiotics. Br Med J 2:57, 1957.
81. O'Hara K, Kanda T, Ohmiya K, et al: Purification and characterization of macrolide 2′-phosphotransferase from a strain of *Escherichia coli* that is highly resistant to erythromycin. Antimicrob Agents Chemother 33:1354, 1989.
82. Noguchi N, Emura A, Matsuyama H, et al: Nucleotide sequence and characterization of erythromycin resistance determinant that encodes macrolide 2′-phosphotransferase I in *Escherichia coli.* Antimicrob Agents Chemother 39:2359, 1995.
83. Jenkins G, Cundliffe E: Cloning and characterization of two genes from *Streptomyces lividans* that confer inducible resistance to lincomycin and macrolide antibiotics. Gene 108:55, 1991.
84. Arthur M, Andremont A, Courvalin P: Distribution of erythromyxin esterase and rRNA methylase genes in members of the family Enterobacteriaceae highly resistant to erythromycin. Antimicrob Agents Chemother 31:404, 1987.
84a. Leclerq R, Courvalin P: Intrinsic and unusual resistance to macrolide, lincosamide, and streptogramin antibiotics in bacteria. Antimicrob Agents Chemother 35:1273, 1991.
85. O'Brien TF, Acar JF, Medeiros AA, et al: International comparison of prevalence of resistance to antibiotics. JAMA 239:1518, 1978.
86. Haight TH, Finland M: The antibacterial action of erythromycin. Proc Soc Exp Biol Med 81:175, 1952.
87. Haight TH, Finland M: Resistance of bacteria to erythromycin. Proc Soc Exp Biol Med 81:183, 1952.
88. Dixon JMS, Lipinski AE: Pneumococci resistant to erythromycin. Can Med Assoc J 119:1044, 1978.
89. Linares J, Garau J, Dominquez C, et al: Antibiotic resistance and serotypes of *Streptococcus pneumoniae* from patients with community-acquired pneumococcal disease. Antimicrob Agents Chemother 23:545, 1983.
90. Istre GR, Welch DF, Marks MI, et al: Susceptibility of group A β-hemolytic *Streptococcus* isolates to penicillin and erythromycin. Antimicrob Agents Chemother 20:244, 1981.
91. Saroglou G, Bisno AL: Susceptibility of skin and throat strains of group A streptococci to rosamicin and erythromycin. Antimicrob Agents Chemother 13:701, 1978.
92. Glupczynski Y, Burette A: Failure of azithromycin to eradicate *Campylobacter pylori* from the stomach because of acquired resistance during treatment. Am J Gastroenterol 85:98, 1990.
93. Davies BI, Maesen FPV, Gubbelmans R: Azithromycin (CP-62,993) in acute exacerbations of chronic bronchitis; an open clinical, microbiological and pharmacokinetic study. J Antimicrob Chemother 23:743, 1989.
94. Young LS, Wiviott L, Wu M, et al: Azithromycin for treatment of *Mycobacterium avium-intracellulare* complex infection in patients with AIDS. Lancet 338:1107, 1991.
95. Chaisson RE, Benson CA, Dube MP, et al: Clarithromycin therapy for bacteremic *Mycobacterium avium* complex disease in patients with AIDS. A randomized double-blind dose-ranging study in patients with AIDS. Ann Intern Med 121:905, 1994.
96. Doucet-Populaire F, Truffot-Pernot C, Grosset J, Jarlier V: Acquired resistance in *Mycobacterium avium* complex strains isolated from AIDS patients and beige mice during treatment with clarithromycin. J Antimicrob Chemother 36:129, 1995.
97. Williams JD, Sefton AM: Comparison of macrolide antibiotics. J Antimicrob Chemother 31(Suppl C):11, 1993.
98. Nicholas P: Erythromycin: Clinical review 1. Clinical pharmacology. N Y State J Med 77:2088, 1977.
99. Fraser DG: Selection of an oral erythromycin product. Am J Hosp Pharm 37:1199, 1980.
100. Malmborg AS: Effect of food on absorption of erythromycin. A study of two derivatives, the stearate and the base. J Antimicrob Chemother 5:591, 1979.
101. Bechtol LD, Stephens VC, Pugh CT, et al: Erythromycin esters—Comparative in vivo hydrolysis and bioavailability. Curr Ther Res 20:610, 1976.
102. Tardrew PC, Mao JCH, Kenney D: Antibacterial activity of 2′-esters of erythromycin. Appl Microbiol 18:159, 1969.
103. Thompson PJ, Burgess KR, Marlin GE: Influence of food on absorption of erythromycin ethylsuccinate. Antimicrob Agents Chemother 18:829, 1980.
104. Welling PG: The esters of erythromycin. J Antimicrob Chemother 5:633, 1979.
105. McCracken GH, Ginsburg CM: Pharmacologic evaluation of orally administered antibiotics in infants and children. Pediatrics 62:738, 1978.
106. DiSanto AR, Tserng KY, Chodos DJ, et al: Comparative bioavailability evaluation of erythromycin base and its salts and esters. I. Erythromycin estolate capsules versus enteric-coated erythomycin base tablets. J Clin Pharmacol 20:437, 1980.
107. Austin KL, Mather LE, Philpot CR, et al: Intersubject and dose-related variability after intravenous administration of erythromycin. Br J Clin Pharmacol 10:273, 1980.
108. Houin G, Tillement JP, Lhoste F, et al: Erythromycin pharmacokinetics in man. J Int Med Res 8(Suppl):9, 1980.
109. Dajani AS, Bisno AL, Chung KJ, et al: Prevention of bacterial endocarditis: Recommendations by the American Heart Association. JAMA 264:2919, 1990.
110. Chun A, Seitz JA: Pharmacokinetics and biological availability of erythromycin. Infection 5(Suppl 1):S14, 1977.
111. Schlicht JR: Letter to the editor reply. Ann Pharmacother 26:716, 1992.
112. Prandota J, Tillement JP, d'Athis P, et al: Binding of erythromycin base to human plasma proteins. J Int Med Res 8(Suppl 2):1, 1980.
113. Griffith RS, Black HR: Erythromycin. Med Clin North Am 54:1199, 1970.
114. Bass JW, Steele RW, Wiebe RA, et al: Erythromycin concentrations in middle ear exudates. Pediatrics 48:417, 1971.
115. Axelsson A, Brorson JE: The concentration of antibiotics in sinus secretions. Ampicillin, cephradine and erythromycin estolate. Ann Otol Rhinol Laryngol 83:232, 1974.
116. Paavolainen M, Kohonen A, Palva T, et al: Penetration of erythromycin stearate into maxillary sinus mucosa and secretions in chronic maxillary sinusitis. Acta Otolaryngol (Stockh) 84:292, 1977.
117. Wollmer P, Rhodes CG, Pike VW, et al: Measurement of pulmonary erythromycin concentrations in patients with lobar pneumonia by means of positron tomography. Lancet 2:1361, 1982.

118. Brun Y, Forey F, Gamondes JP, et al: Levels of erythromycin in pulmonary tissue and bronchial mucus compared to those of amoxicillin. J Antimicrob Chemother 8:459, 1981.
119. Ginsburg CM, McCracken GH, Culbertson MC: Concentrations of erythromycin in serum and tonsils. Comparisons of the estolate and ethylsuccinate suspensions. J Pediatr 89:1011, 1976.
120. Rapp GF, Griffith RS, Hebble WM: The permeability of traumatically inflamed synovial membrane to commonly used antibiotics. J Bone Joint Surg Am 48:1534, 1966.
121. Mao JCH, Tardrew PL: Demethylation of erythromycins by rabbit tissue in vitro. Biochem Pharmacol 14:1049, 1965.
122. Hammond JH, Griffith RS: Factors affecting the absorption and biliary excretion of erythromycin and two of its derivatives in humans. Clin Pharmacol Ther 2:308, 1961.
123. Chelvan P, Hamilton-Miller JMT, Brumfitt W: Biliary excretion of erythromycin after parenteral administration. Br J Clin Pharmacol 8:233, 1979.
124. Bennett WM, Muther RS, Parker RA, et al: Drug therapy in renal failure: Dosing guidelines for adults. Part I: Antimicrobial agents, analgesics. Ann Intern Med 93:62, 1980.
125. Martin JR, Johnson P, Miller MF: Uptake, accumulation, and egress of erythromycin by tissue culture cells of human origin. Antimicrob Agents Chemother 27:314, 1985.
126. Sides GD, Cerimele BJ, Black HR, et al: Pharmacokinetics of dirithromycin. J Antimicrob Chemother 31(Suppl C):65, 1993.
127. Mery JP, Kanfer A: Ototoxicity of erythromycin in patients with renal insufficiency. N Engl J Med 301:944, 1979.
128. Philipson A, Sabath LD, Charles D: Transplacental passage of erythromycin and clindamycin. N Engl J Med 288:1219, 1973.
129. Johnson JD, Hand WL, Francis JB, et al: Antibiotic uptake by alveolar macrophages. J Lab Clin Med 95:429, 1980.
130. Prokesch RC, Hand WL: Antibiotic entry into human polymorphonuclear leukocytes. Antimicrob Agents Chemother 21:373, 1982.
131. Hand WL, Corwin RW, Steinberg TH, et al: Uptake of antibiotics by human alveolar macrophages. Am Rev Respir Dis 129:933, 1984.
132. Miller MF, Martin JR, Johnson P, et al: Erythromycin uptake and accumulation by human polymorphonuclear leukocytes and efficacy of erythromycin in killing ingested *Legionella pneumophila*. J Infect Dis 119:714, 1984.
133. Lalak NJ, Morris DL: Azithromycin clinical pharmacokinetics. Clin Pharmacokinet 25:370, 1993.
134. Bahal N, Nahata M: The new macrolide antibiotics: Azithromycin, clarithromycin, dirithromycin, and roxithromycin. Ann Pharmacother 26:46, 1992.
135. Foulds G, Shepard RM, Johnson RB: The pharmacokinetics of azithromycin in human serum and tissues. J Antimicrob Chemother 25(Suppl A):73, 1990.
136. Glaude RP, Bright GM, Isaacson RF, et al: In vitro and in vivo uptake of azithromycin (CP-62,993) by phagocytic cells: Possible mechanism of delivery and release at sites of infection. Antimicrob Agents Chemother 33:277, 1989.
137. Glaude RP, Snider ME: Intracellular accumulation of azithromycin by cultured human fibroblasts. Antimicrob Agents Chemother 34:1056, 1990.
138. Nahata MC, Koranyi KI, Gadgil SD, et al: Pharmacokinetics of azithromycin in pediatric patients after oral administration of multiple doses of suspension. Antimicrob Agents Chemother 37:314, 1993.
139. Piscitelli SC, Danziger LH, Rodvold KA: Clarithromycin and azithromycin: New macrolide antibiotics. Clin Pharm 11:137, 1992.
140. Zithromax product information, manufacturer's package insert. Parsippany, NJ, Pfizer, 1995.
141. Lode HC: The pharmacokinetics of azithromycin and their clinical significance. Eur J Clin Microbiol Infect Dis 10:807, 1991.
142. Baldwin DR, Ashby JP, Andrews JM, et al: Pulmonary disposition of azithromycin following a single 500 mg oral dose. Thorax 45:324, 1990.
143. Honeybourne D, Kees F, Andrews JM, et al: The levels of clarithromycin and its 14-hydroxy metabolite in the lung. Eur Respir J 7:1275, 1994.
144. Conte JR Jr, Golden JA, Duncan S, et al: Intrapulmonary pharmacokinetics of clarithromycin and of erythromycin. Antimicrob Agents Chemother 39:334, 1995.
145. Chu S, Wilson D, Guay D: Clarithromycin pharmacokinetics in healthy young and elderly volunteers. J Clin Pharmacol 32:1045, 1992.
146. Chu S, Park B, Locke C, et al: Drug-food interaction potential of clarithromycin, a new macrolide antimicrobial. J Clin Pharmacol 32:32, 1992.
147. Fraschini F, Scaglione F, Pintucci G, et al: The diffusion of clarithromycin and roxithromycin into nasal mucosa, tonsil and lung in humans. J Antimicrob Chemother 27(Suppl A):61, 1991.
148. Filippo JA: Infantile hypertrophic pyloric stenosis related to ingestions of erythromycin estolate. A report of five cases. J Pediatr Surg 11:177, 1976.
149. Ellsworth AJ, Christensen DB, Volpone-McMahon MT: Prospective comparison of patient tolerance to enteric-coated vs. nonenteric-coated erythromycin. J Fam Pract 31:265, 1990.
150. Itoh Z, Suzuki T, Nakaya M, et al: Gastrointestinal motor-stimulating activity of macrolide antibiotics and analysis of their side effects on the canine gut. Antimicrob Agents Chemother 26:863, 1984.
151. Tomomasa T, Kurooume T, Arai H, et al: Erythromycin induces migrating motor complex in human gastrointestinal tract. Dig Dis Sci 31:157, 1986.
152. Erbas T, Varoglu E, Erbas B, et al: Comparison of metoclopramide and erythromycin in the treatment of diabetic gastroparesis. Diabetes Care 16:1511, 1993.
153. Janssens J, Peeters TL, Vantrappen G, et al: Improvement of gastric emptying in diabetic gastroparesis by erythromycin. N Engl J Med 322:1028, 1990.
154. Craft JC, Siepman N: Overview of the safety profile of clarithromycin suspension in pediatric patients. Pediatr Infect Dis J 12:S142, 1993.
155. Guay DRP, Patterson DR, Siepman N, Craft JC: Overview of the tolerability profile of clarithromycin in preclinical and clinical trials. Drug Saf 8:350, 1993.
156. Hopkins S: Clinical toleration and safety of azithromycin. Am J Med 91(Suppl A):75, 1991.
157. Braun P: Hepatotoxicity of erythromycin. J Infect Dis 119:300, 1969.
158. Sullivan D, Csuka ME, Blanchard B: Erythromycin ethylsuccinate hepatotoxicity. JAMA 243:1074, 1980.
159. Viteri AL, Greene JR, Dyck WP: Erythromycin ethylsuccinate–induced cholestasis. Gastroenterology 76:1007, 1979.
160. Carson JL, Strom BL, Duff A, et al: Acute liver disease associated with erythromycins, sulfonamides, and tetracyclines. Ann Intern Med 119:576, 1993.
161. Derby LE, Jick H, Henry DA, Dean AD: Erythromycin-associated cholestatic hepatitis. Med J Aust 158:600, 1993.
162. Shirin H, Schapiro JM, Arber N, et al: Erythromycin base–induced rash and liver function disturbances. Ann Pharmacother 26:1522, 1992.
163. McCormack WM, George H, Donner A, et al: Hepatotoxicity of erythromycin estolate during pregnancy. Antimicrob Agents Chemother 12:630, 1977.
164. Inman WHN, Rawson NSB: Erythromycin estolate and jaundice. Br Med J 286:1954, 1983.
165. Dujoune CA, Shoeman D, Bianchine J, et al: Experimental bases for the different hepatotoxicity of erythromycin preparations in man. J Lab Clin Med 70:832, 1972.
166. Sabath LD, Gerstein DA, Finland M: Serum glutamic oxalactic transaminase: False elevation during administration of erythromycin. N Engl J Med 279:1137, 1968.
167. Barradell LB, Plosker GL, McTavish D: Clarithromycin. A review of its pharmacological properties and therpaeutic use in *Mycobacterium avium-intracellulare* complex infection in patients with acquired immune deficiency syndrome. Drugs 46:289, 1993.
168. Brummett RE: Ototoxic liability of erythromycin and analogues. Otolaryngol Clin North Am 26:811, 1993.
169. Swanson DJ, Sung RJ, Fine MJ, et al: Erythromycin ototoxicity: Prospective assessment with serum concentrations and audiograms in a study of patients with pneumonia. Am J Med 92:61, 1992.
170. Wallace RM, Miller LK, Nguyen M, Shields AR: Ototoxicity with azithromycin. Lancet 343:241, 1994.
171. Gantz NM, Zawacki JK, Dickerson WJ, et al: Pseudomembranous colitis associated with erythromycin. Ann Intern Med 91:866, 1979.

172. Washington JA II, Wilson WR: Erythromycin: A microbial and clinical perspective after 30 years of clinical use (second of two parts). Mayo Clin Proc 60:271, 1985.
173. Sides GD, Conforti PM: Safety profile of dirithromycin. J Antimicrob Chemother 31(Suppl C):175, 1993.
174. Putzi R, Blaser J, Luthy R, et al: Side effects due to the intravenous infusion of erythromycin lactobionate. Infection 11:161, 1983.
175. Larrey D, Tinel M, Pessayre D: Formation of inactive cytochrome P_{450} Fe(II)-metabolite complexes with several erythromycin derivatives but not with josamycin and midecamycin in rats. Biochem Pharmacol 39:1487, 1983.
176. Lunden TM: Pharmacokinetic interactions of the macrolide antibiotics. Clin Pharmacokinet 10:63, 1985.
177. Dobkin JF, Saha JR, Butler VP, et al: Digoxin-inactivating bacteria: Identification in human gut flora. Science 220:325, 1983.
178. Periti P, Mazzei T, Mini E, Novelli A: Pharmacokinetic drug interactions of macrolides. Clin Pharmacother 23:106, 1992.
179. Lindstrom TD, Hanssen BR, Wrighton SA: Cytochrome P-450 complex formation by dirithromycin and other macrolides in rat and human livers. Antimicrob Agents Chemother 37:265, 1993.
180. Honig PK, Wortham DC, Zamani K, Cantilena LR: Comparison of the effect of the macrolide antibiotics erythromycin, clarithromycin and azithromycin on terfenadine steady-state pharmacokinetics and electrocardiographic parameters. Drug Invest 7:148, 1994.
181. LaForce CF, Szefler SJ, Miller MF, et al: Inhibition of methylprednisolone elimination in the presence of erythromycin therapy. J Allergy Clin Immunol 72:34, 1983.
182. Reisz G, Pingleton SK, Melethil S, et al: The effect of erythromycin on theophylline pharmacokinetics in chronic bronchitis. Am Rev Respir Dis 127:581, 1983.
183. Schwartz JI, Bachmann K: Erythromycin-warfarin interaction. Arch Intern Med 144:2094, 1984.
184. Sato RI, Gray DR, Brown SE: Warfarin interactions with erythromycin. Arch Intern Med 144:2413, 1984.
185. Ferrari SL, Goffin E, Mourad M, et al: The interaction between clarithromycin and cyclosporine in kidney transplant recipients. Transplantation 58:725, 1994.
186. Ptachinski RJ, Carpentier BJ, Burckart GJ, et al: Effect of erythromycin on cyclosporine levels. N Engl J Med 313:1416, 1985.
187. Shaeffer MS, Collier D, Sorrell MF: Interaction between FK506 and erythromycin. Ann Pharmacother 28:280, 1994.
188. Cisapride. *In* Physicians' Desk Reference, ed 49. Montvale, NJ, Medical Economics Data Production, 1995, p 1191.
189. Brandriss MW, Richardson WS, Barold SS: Erythromycin-induced QT prolongation and polymorphic ventricular tachycardia (torsades de pointes): Case report and review. Clin Infect Dis 18:995, 1994.
190. O'Connor NK, Fris J: Clarithromycin-carbamazepine interaction in a clinical setting. J Am Board Fam Pract 7:489, 1994.
191. Viani F, Claris-Appiani AC, Rossi LN, et al: Severe hepatorenal failure in a child receiving carbamazepine and erythromycin. Eur J Pediatr 151:715, 1992.
192. Vance E, Watson-Bitar M, Gustavson L, Kazanjian P: Pharmacokinetics of clarithromycin and zidovudine in patients with AIDS. Antimicrob Agents Chemother 39:1355, 1995.
193. Petty B, Polis M, Haneiwick S, et al: Pharmacokinetic assessment of clarithromycin plus zidovudine in HIV patients (Abstr). Presented at the 32nd Interscience Conference on Antimicrobial Agents and Chemotherapy; October 1992; Anaheim, CA.
194. Gallagher JC, Ismail MA, Aladjem S: Reduced urinary estriol levels with erythromycin therapy. Obstet Gynecol 56:381, 1980.
195. Herrell WE, Balows A, Becker J: Erythromycin: A new approach to the problem of antibiotic-resistant staphylococci. Antibiot Med Clin Ther 7:637, 1960.
196. Allen NE, Epp JK: Mechanism of penicillin-erythromycin synergy on antibiotic-resistant *Staphylococcus aureus.* Antimicrob Agents Chemother 13:849, 1978.
197. Michel J, Ferne M, Borinski R, et al: Effects of subminimal inhibitory concentrations of chloramphenicol, erythromycin, and penicillin on group A streptococci. Eur J Clin Microbiol 1:375, 1982.
198. Cohn JR, Jungkind DL, Baker JS: In vitro antagonism by erythromycin of the bactericidal action of antimicrobial agents against common respiratory pathogens. Antimicrob Agents Chemother 18:872, 1980.
199. Finland M, Bach MC, Garner C, et al: Synergistic action of ampicillin and erythromycin against *Nocardia asteroides*: Effect of time of incubation. Antimicrob Agents Chemother 5:344, 1974.
200. Tuazon CU, Shamsuddin D, Miller H: Antibiotic susceptibility and synergy of clinical isolates of *Listeria monocytogenes.* Antimicrob Agents Chemother 21:525, 1982.
201. Penn RL, Ward TT, Steigbigel RT: Effects of erythromycin in combination with penicillin, ampicillin or gentamicin on the growth of *Listeria monocytogenes.* Antimicrob Agents Chemother 22:289, 1982.
202. Peard MC, Fleck DG, Garrod LP, et al: Combined rifampicin and erythromycin for bacterial endocarditis. Br Med J 4:410, 1970.
203. Marks MI: In vitro activity of clindamycin and other antimicrobials against gram-positive bacteria and *Haemophilus influenzae.* Can Med Assoc J 112:170, 1975.
204. Clarithromycin and azithromycin. Med Lett Drugs Ther 34:45, 1992.
205. Pierce M, Crampton S, Henry D, et al: A randomized trial of clarithromycin as prophylaxis against disseminated *Mycobacterium avium* complex infection in patients with advanced acquired immunodeficiency syndrome. N Engl J Med 335:384, 1996.
206. Shafran SD, Singer J, Zarowny DP, et al: A comparison of two regimens for the treatment of *Mycobacterium avium* complex bacteremia in AIDS: Rifabutin, ethambutol and clarithromycin versus rifampin, ethambutol, clofazimine, and ciprofloxacin. N Engl J Med 335:337, 1996.
207. Havilir DV, Dube MP, Sattler FR, et al: Prophylaxis against disseminated *Mycobacterium avium* complex with weekly azithromycin, daily rifabutin, or both. N Engl J Med 335:392, 1996.
208. Swartz MN: Clinical aspects of legionnaire's disease. Ann Intern Med 90:492, 1979.
209. Gump DW, Frank RO, Winn WC Jr, et al: Legionnaire's disease in patients with associated serious disease. Ann Intern Med 90:538, 1979.
210. Wing EJ, Schafer FJ, Pasculle AW: Successful treatment of *Legionella micdadei* (Pittsburg pneumonia agent) pneumonia with erythromycin. Am J Med 71:836, 1981.
211. Hamedani P, Ali J, Hafeez S, et al: The safety and efficacy of clarithromycin in patients with *Legionella* pneumonia. Chest 1991:1503, 1991.
212. Dark D: Multicenter evaluation of azithromycin and cefaclor in acute lower respiratory tract infections. Am J Med 91(Suppl 3A):31, 1991.
213. Kinasewitz G, Wood RG: Azithromycin versus cefaclor in the treatment of acute bacterial pneumonia. Eur J Clin Microbiol Infect Dis 10:872, 1991.
214. Schonwald S, Gunjaca M, Kolacny L, et al: Comparison of azithromycin and erythromycin in the treatment of atypical pneumonias. J Antimicrob Chemother 25(Suppl A):123, 1990.
215. Schonwald S. Skerk V, Petricevic I, et al: Comparison of three-day and five-day courses of azithromycin in the treatment of atypical pneumonia. Eur J Clin Microbiol Infect Dis 10:877, 1991.
216. Adam D: Clarithromycin in the treatment of respiratory tract infections. Infection 21: 265, 1993.
217. Anderson G, Esmonde TS, Coles S, et al: A comparative safety and efficacy study of clarithromycin and erythromycin stearate in community-acquired pneumonia. J Antimicrob Chemother 27(Suppl A):117, 1991.
218. Chien SM, Pichotta P, Siepmann N, et al: Treatment of community-acquired pneumonia. A multicenter, double-blind, randomized study comparing clarithromycin with erythromycin. Chest 103:697, 1993.
219. Rasch JR, Mogabgab WJ: Therapeutic effect of erythromycin on *Mycoplasma pneumoniae* pneumonia. Antimicrob Agents Chemother 5:693, 1965.
220. Smith CB, Friedewald WT, Chanock RM: Shedding of *Mycoplasma pneumoniae* after tetracycline and erythromycin. N Engl J Med 276:1172, 1967.
221. Chirwin K, Roblin PM, Hammerschlag MR: In vitro susceptibilities of *Chlamydia pneumoniae* (*Chlamydia* sp. strain TWAR). Antimicrob Agents Chemother 33:1634, 1989.
222. Welsh LA, Gaydos CA, Quinn TC: In-vitro evaluation of activities of azithromycin, erythromycin and tetracycline against *Chlamydia trachomatis* and *Chlamydia pneumoniae.* Antimicrob Agents Chemother 36:291, 1992.

223. Covelli HD, Husky DL, Dolphin RE: Psittacosis: Clinical presentations and therapeutic observations. West J Med 132:242, 1980.
224. D'Angelo LJ, Hetherington R: Q fever treated with erythromycin. Br Med J 2:305, 1979.
225. Fraschini F, Avallon R, Copponi V, et al: Bactericidal action of an average dose of erythromycin in the bronchi. Curr Med Res Opin 6:111, 1979.
226. Bachand R: Comparative study of clarithromycin and ampicillin in the treatment of patients with acute bacterial exacerbations of chronic bronchitis. J Antimicrob Chemother 27(Suppl A):90, 1991.
227. Lenoski EF, Wingert WA, Wehrle PF: Drug trials in acute otitis media. Curr Ther Res 10:631, 1968.
228. Sell SH, Wilson DA, Stamm JM, et al: Treatment of otitis media caused by *Haemophilus influenzae*: Evaluation of three antimicrobial regimens. South Med J 171:1143, 1978.
229. Howard JE, Nelson JD, Clahsen J, et al: Otitis media of infancy and early childhood: A double-blind study of four treatment regimens. Am J Dis Child 130:965, 1976.
230. Sell SHW: In vitro sensitivity studies of *Haemophilus influenzae* typeable and nontypeable strains. Pediatrics 39:214, 1967.
231. Coles SJ, Addlestone MB, Kamdar MK, Macklin JL: A comparative study of clarithromycin and amoxycillin suspensions in the treatment of pediatric patients with acute otitis media. Infection 21:272, 1993.
232. Pukander JS, Jero JP, Kaprio EA, Sorri MJ: Clarithromycin vs. amoxicillin suspensions in the treatment of pediatric patients with acute otitis media. Pediatr Infect Dis J 12:S1181, 1993.
233. Aspin MM, Hoberman A, McCarty J, et al: Comparative study of the safety and efficacy of clarithromycin and amoxicillin-clavulanate in the treatment of acute otitis media in children. J Pediatr 125:136, 1994.
234. McCarty JM, Phillips A, Wiisanen R: Comparative safety and efficacy of clarithromycin and amoxicillin/clavulanate in the treatment of acute otitis media in children. Pediatr Infect Dis J 12:S122, 1993.
235. Gooch WM, Gan VN, Corder WT, et al: Clarithromycin and cefaclor suspensions in the treatment of acute otitis media in children. Pediatr Infect Dis J 12:S128, 1993.
236. McLinn S: Double blind and open label studies of azithromycin in the management of acute otitis media in children: A review. Pediatr Infect Dis J 14:S62, 1995.
237. Kalm O, Kamme C, Bergstrom B, et al: Erythromycin stearate in acute maxillary sinusitis. Scand J Infect Dis 7:209, 1975.
238. Dubois J, Saint-Pierre C, Tremblay C: Efficacy of clarithromycin vs. amoxicillin/clavulanate in the treatment of acute maxillary sinusitis. Ear Nose Throat J 72:804, 1993.
239. Calhoun KH, Hokanson JA: Multicenter comparison of clarithromycin and amoxicillin in the treatment of acute maxillary sinusitis. Arch Fam Med 2:837, 1993.
240. Bachand RT Jr: Comparative study of clarithromycin and ampicillin in the treatment of patients with acute bacterial exacerbations of chronic bronchitis. J Antimicrob Chemother 27(Suppl A):91, 1991.
241. Karma P, Pukander J, Penttila M, et al: The comparative efficacy and safety of clarithromycin and amoxycillin in the treatment of outpatients with acute maxillary sinusitis. J Antimicrob Chemother 27(Suppl A):83, 1990.
242. Casiano R: Azithromycin and amoxicillin in the treatment of acute maxillary sinusitis. Am J Med 91(Suppl 3A):27, 1991.
243. Ginsburg CM, McCracken GH, Crow SD, et al: Erythromycin therapy for group A streptococcal pharyngitis. Results of a comparative study of the estolate and ethylsuccinate formulations. Am J Dis Child 138:536, 1984.
244. Still JG, Hubbard WC, Poole JM, et al: Comparison of clarithromycin and penicillin VK suspensions in the treatment of children with streptococcal pharyngitis and review of currently available alternative antibiotic therapies. Pediatr Infect Dis J 12:S134, 1993.
245. Hooton TM: A comparison of azithromycin and penicillin V for the treatment of streptococcal pharyngitis. Am J Med 91(Suppl 3A):23S, 1991.
246. Weippl G: Multicentre comparison of azithromycin versus erythromycin in the treatment of paediatric pharyngitis or tonsillitis caused by group A streptococci. J Antimicrob Chemother 31(Suppl E):95, 1993.
247. Lambert H: Antimicrobial drugs in the treatment and prevention of pertussis. J Antimicrob Chemother 5:329, 1979.
248. Bass JW, Klenk EL, Klotheimer CC, et al: Antimicrobial treatment of pertussis. J Pediatr 75:768, 1969.
249. Miller LW, Bickham S, Jones WL, et al: Diphtheria carriers and the effect of erythromycin therapy. Antimicrob Agents Chemother 6:166, 1974.
250. McKendrick MW: Erythromycin revisited. J Antimicrob Chemother 5:432, 1979.
251. Dagan R, Bar-David Y: Double-blind study comparing erythromycin and mupirocin for treatment of impetigo in children: Implications of a high prevalence of erythromycin-resistant *Staphylococcus aureus* strains. Antimicrob Agents Chemother 36:287, 1992.
252. Hebert AA, Still JG, Reuman PD: Comparative safety and efficacy of clarithromycin and cefadroxil suspensions in the treatment of mild to moderate skin and skin structure infections in children. Pediatr Infect Dis J 12:S112, 1993.
253. Kiani R: Double blind, double-dummy comparison of azithromycin and cephalexin in the treatment of skin and skin structure infections. Eur J Clin Microbiol Infect Dis 10:880, 1991.
254. Rivkin L, Rapaport M: Clinical evaluation of a new erythromycin solution for acne vulgaris. Cutis 25:552, 1980.
255. Sarkany I, Tarplin D, Blank H: The etiology and treatment of erythrasma. J Invest Dermatol 37:283, 1961.
256. Wang WL, Reller LB, Blaser MJ: Comparison of antimicrobial susceptibility patterns of *Campylobacter jejuni* and *Campylobacter coli*. Antimicrob Agents Chemother 26:351, 1984.
257. Mandal BK, Ellis ME, Dunbar EM, et al: Double-blind placebo controlled trial of erythromycin in the treatment of clinical *Campylobacter* infection. J Antimicrob Chemother 13:619, 1984.
258. DuPont HL, Ericsson CD, Robinson A, et al: Current problems in antimicrobial therapy for bacterial enteric infection. Am J Med 82(Suppl 4A):324, 1987.
259. Pichler HET, Diridl G, Stickler K, et al: Clinical efficacy of ciprofloxacin compared with placebo in bacterial diarrhea. Am J Med 82(Suppl 4A):329, 1987.
260. Al-Assi MT, Genta RM, Karttunen TJ, et al: Azithromycin triple therapy for *Helicobacter pylori* infection: Azithromycin, tetracycline, and bismuth. Am J Gastroenterol 90:403, 1995.
261. Al-Assi MT, Ramirez FC, Lew GM, et al: Clarithromycin, tetracycline, and bismuth: A new non-metronidazole therapy for *Helicobacter pylori* infection. Am J Gastroenterol 89:1203, 1994.
262. Labenz J, Stolte M, Domian C, et al: High-dose omeprazole plus amoxicillin or clarithromycin cures *Helicobacter pylori* infection in duodenal ulcer disease. Digestion 56:14, 1995.
263. Peterson WL, Graham DY, Marshall B, et al: Clarithromycin as monotherapy for eradication of *Helicobacter pylori:* A randomized double-blind trial. Am J Gastroenterol 88:1860, 1993.
264. Gordillo ME, Singh KV, Murray BE: In vitro activity of azithromycin against bacterial enteric pathogens. Antimicrob Agents Chemother 37:1203, 1993.
265. Wallace MR, Yousif AA, Habib NF, Tribble DR: Azithromycin and typhoid. Lancet 343:1498, 1993.
266. Martin DH, Mroczkowski TF, Dalu ZA, et al: A controlled trial of a single dose of azithromycin for the treatment of chlamydial urethritis and cervicitis. N Engl J Med 327:921, 1992.
267. Weber JT, Johnson RE: New treatments for *Chlamydia trachomatis* genital infection. Clin Infect Dis 20(Suppl 1):566, 1995.
268. Steingrimsson O, Olafsson J, Thorarinsson H, et al: Azithromycin in the treatment of sexually transmitted disease. J Antimicrob Chemother 25(Suppl A):109, 1990.
269. Handsfield HH, Dalv ZA, Martin DA, et al: Multicenter trial of single-dose azithromycin vs ceftriaxone in the treatment of uncomplicated gonorrhea. Sex Transm Dis 21:107, 1994.
270. Moran JS, Levine WC: Drugs of choice for uncomplicated gonococcal infections. Clin Infect Dis 20(Suppl 1):547, 1995.
271. Schachter J: Chlamydia infections. Part III. N Engl J Med 298:540, 1978.
272. Bilgeri YR, Ballard RC, Duncan MD, et al: Antimicrobial susceptibility of 103 strains of *Haemophilus ducreyi* isolated in Johannesburg. Antimicrob Agents Chemother 22:686, 1982.
273. Schulte JM, Schmid GP: Recommendations for treatment of chancroid, 1993. Clin Infect Dis 20(Suppl 1):539, 1995.
274. Bush MR, Rosa C: Azithromycin and erythromycin in the treatment of cervical chlamydial infection during pregnancy. Obstet Gynecol 84:61, 1994.

275. Tyndall MW, Agoki E, Plummer FA, et al: Single dose azithromycin for the treatment of chancroid: A randomized comparison with erythromycin. Sex Transm Dis 21:231, 1994.
276. Steingrimsson O, Olafsson JH, Thorarinsson H, et al: Single dose azithromycin treatment of gonorrhea and infections caused by *C. trachomatis* and *U. urealyticum* in men. Sex Transm Dis 21:43, 1994.
277. Tramont E: *Treponema pallidum* (syphilis). *In* Mandell GL, Bennett JE, Dolin R (eds): Principles and Practice of Infectious Diseases, ed 4. New York, Churchill Livingstone, 1995, pp 1794–1808.
278. Verdon MS, Handsfield HH, Johnson RB: Pilot study of azithromycin for the treatment of primary and secondary syphilis. Clin Infect Dis 19:486, 1994.
279. Rolfs RT: Treatment of syphilis, 1993. Clin Infect Dis 20(Suppl 1):523, 1995.
280. Weber K, Wilske B, Preac-Mursic V, Thurmayr R: Azithromycin versus penicillin V for the treatment of early Lyme borreliosis. Infection 21:367, 1993.
281. Rothenberg R: Ophthalmia neonatorum due to *Neisseria gonorrhoeae*; prevention and treatment. Sex Transm Dis 6(Suppl):187, 1979.
282. Young LS, Wiviott L, Wu M, et al: Azithromycin for treatment of *Mycobacterium avium-intracellulare* complex infection in patients with AIDS. Lancet 338:1107, 1991.
283. Masur H, US Public Health Service Task Force on Prophylaxis and Therapy for *Mycobacterium avium* complex: Recommendations on the prophylaxis and therapy for disseminated *Mycobacterium avium* complex disease in patients infected with the human immunodeficiency virus. N Engl J Med 329:898, 1993.
284. Goldberger M, Masur H: Clarithromycin therapy for *Mycobacterium avium* complex disease in patients with AIDS: Potential and problems. Ann Intern Med 121:974, 1994.
285. Benson CA, Cohn DL, Williams P, et al: A phase III prospective, randomized, double-blind study of the safety and efficacy of clarithromycin vs. rifabutin vs. clarithromycin plus rifabutin for prevention of *Mycobacterium avium* complex disease in HIV and patients with CD4 counts less than 100 cells/microliter (Abstr 205). Abstracts of the Third National Conference on Retroviruses and Opportunistic Infections; January 28–February 1, 1996; Washington, DC.
286. Oldfield EC, Dickinson G, Chung R, et al: Once weekly azithromycin for the prevention of *Mycobacterium avium* complex infection in AIDS patients (Abstr 203). Abstracts of the Third National Conference on Retroviruses and Opportunistic Infections; January 28–February 1, 1996; Washington, DC.
287. Wallace RJ, Tanner D, Brennan PJ, Brown BA: Clinical trial of clarithromycin for cutaneous (disseminated) infection due to *Mycobacterium chelonae*. Ann Intern Med 119:482, 1993.
288. Laing RBS, Wynn RF, Leen CLS: New antimicrobials against *Mycobacterium marinum* infection. Br J Dermatol 131:914, 1994.
289. Chan GP, Garcia-Ignacio BYY, Chavez VE, et al: Clinical trial of clarithromycin for lepromatous leprosy. Antimicrob Agents Chemother 38:515, 1994.
290. Cavalieri SJ, Biehle JR, Sanders WE: Synergistic activities of clarithromycin and antituberculous drugs against multidrug-resistant *Mycobacterium tuberculosis*. Antimicrob Agents Chemother 39:1542, 1995.
291. Alder J, Mitten M, Shipkowitz N, et al: Treatment of experimental *Pneumocystis carinii* infection by combination of clarithromycin and sulphamethoxazole. J Antimicrob Chemother 33:253, 1994.
292. Price DA, Hollings NP, Janes SM, et al: Clinical response to the addition of clarithromycin in *Pneumocystis carinii* pneumonia refractory to high dose co-trimoxazole. J Antimicrob Chemother 34:303, 1994.
293. Rabaud C, Amiel C, Maignan M, et al: Clarithromycin plus minocycline as a treatment for cerebral toxoplasmosis in HIV-infected patients (Abstr). Presented at the Third Conference on Retroviruses and Opportunistic Infections; January 28–February 1, 1996; Washington, DC.
294. Lacassin F, Schaffo D, Perronne C, et al: Clarithromycin-minocycline combination as salvage therapy for toxoplasmosis in patients infected with human immunodeficiency virus. Antimicrob Agents Chemother 39:276, 1995.
295. Saba J, Morlat P, Raffi F, et al: Pyrimethamine plus azithromycin for treatment of acute toxoplasmic encephalitis in patients with AIDS. Eur J Clin Microbiol Infect Dis 12:853, 1993.
296. Guerra LG, Neira CJ, Boman D, et al: Rapid response of AIDS-related bacillary angiomatosis to azithromycin. Clin Infect Dis 17:264, 1993.
297. Koehler JE, LeBoit PE, Egbert BM, Berger TG: Cutaneous vascular lesions and disseminated cat-scratch disease in patients with the acquired immunodeficiency syndrome (AIDS) and AIDS-related complex. Ann Intern Med 109:449, 1988.
298. Slater LN, Welch DF, Min KW: *Rochalimaea henselae* causes bacillary angiomatosis and peliosis hepatitis. Arch Intern Med 152:602, 1992.
299. Kuschner RA, Heppner DG, Andersen SL, et al: Azithromycin prophylaxis against a chloroquine-resistant strain of *Plasmodium falciparum*. Lancet 343:1396, 1994.
300. Barry AL, Fuchs PC: In vitro activities of a streptogramin (RP59500), three macrolides, and an azalide against four respiratory tract pathogens. Antimicrob Agents Chemother 39:238, 1995.
301. Fattorini L, Li B, Piersimoni C, et al: In vitro and ex vivo activities of antimicrobial agents used in combination with clarithromycin, with or without amikacin, against *Mycobacterium avium*. Antimicrob Agents Chemother 39:680, 1995.
302. Goldstein EJC, Citron DM: Comparative susceptibilities of 173 aerobic and anaerobic bite wound isolates to sparfloxacin, temafloxacin, clarithromycin, and older agents. Antimicrob Agents Chemother 37:1150, 1993.
303. Goldstein EJC, Nesbit CA, Citron DM: Comparative in vitro activities of azithromycin, Bay y 3118, levofloxacin, sparfloxacin, and 11 other oral antimicrobial agents against 194 aerobic and anaerobic bite wound isolates. Antimicrob Agents Chemother 39:1097, 1995.
304. Gomez-Garces JL, Cogollos R, Alos JI: Susceptibilities of fluoroquinolone-resistant strains of *Campylobacter jejuni* to 11 oral antimicrobial agents. Antimicrob Agents Chemother 39:542, 1995.
305. Inderlied C: In vitro and in vivo activity of azithromycin against the *Mycobacterium avium* complex. J Infect Dis 159:994, 1989.
306. Rastogi N, Labrousse V: Extracellular and intracellular activities of clarithromycin used alone and in association with ethambutol and rifampin against *Mycobacterium avium* complex. Antimicrob Agents Chemother 35:462, 1991.
307. Dangor Y, Miller SD, Exposto F da L, et al: Antimicrobial susceptibilities of southern African isolates of *Haemophilus ducreyi*. Antimicrob Agents Chemother 32:1458, 1988.
308. Dautzenberg B, Truffot C, Legris S, et al: Activity of clarithromycin against *Mycobacterium avium* infection in patients with the acquired immune deficiency syndrome. Am Rev Respir Dis 144:564, 1991.
309. Johnson R, Kodner C, Russell M, et al: In vitro and in vivo susceptibility of *Borrelia burgdorferi* to azithromycin. Antimicrob Agents Chemother 32:755, 1990.
310. Maskell JP, Sefton AM, Williams JD: Comparative in vitro activity of azithromycin and erythromycin against gram positive cocci, *H. influenzae*, and anaerobes. J Antimicrob Chemother 25(Suppl A):19, 1990.
311. Scieux C, Bianchi A, Cappey B, et al: In vitro activity of azithromycin against *C. trachomatis*. J Antimicrob Chemother 25(Suppl A):7, 1990.
312. Slaney L, Chubb H, Ronald A, Brunham R: In vitro activity of azithromycin, erythromycin, ciprofloxacin, and norfloxacin against *Neisseria gonorrhoeae, H. ducreyi*, and *Chlamydia trachomatis*. J Antimicrob Chemother 25(Suppl A):1, 1990.
313. Vanhoof R, Gordts B, Dierickx R, et al: Bacteriostatic and bactericidal activities of 24 antimicrobial agents against *Campylobacter fetus* subsp *jejuni*. Antimicrob Agents Chemother 18:118, 1980.
314. Yajko D, Nassos P, Sanders C: Comparison of the intracellular activities of clarithromycin and erythromycin against *Mycobacterium avium* complex strains in J774 cells and in alveolar macrophages from human immunodeficiency virus type 1–infected individuals. Antimicrob Agents Chemother 36:1163, 1992.
315. Williams JD: Spectrum of activity of azithromycin. Eur J Clin Microbiol Infect Dis 10:813, 1991.

24

Vancomycin and Teicoplanin

Richard H. Glew
Mark A. Keroack

Vancomycin, a narrow-spectrum glycopeptide antibiotic directed primarily against gram-positive bacteria, was discovered in 1956 from an actinomycete, *Streptomyces* (currently *Amycolatopsis*) *orientalis,* isolated from a soil sample from Borneo.[1] Among the active fermentation by-products of this organism was a compound initially referred to as 05865 and subsequently given the generic name vancomycin (from the word vanquish). Vancomycin was introduced clinically in 1958, 2 years before methicillin, and enjoyed widespread use in the treatment of infections caused by penicillin-resistant gram-positive bacteria, particularly *Staphylococcus aureus.*[2] After the introduction of the bactericidal antistaphylococcal penicillins and cephalosporins, vancomycin was generally relegated to the role of alternative therapy in patients allergic to β-lactam antibiotics, largely because of the perception that vancomycin was more toxic. In more recent years, vancomycin use has increased dramatically; one academic medical center noted a 20-fold increase in use in the decade of the 1980s.[3] Much of the use has been directed at known or suspected oxacillin-resistant strains of *S. aureus* and, in association with vascular catheters and other indwelling medical devices, coagulase-negative staphylococci.

Advances in the manufacturing process have produced purer clinical preparations of vancomycin, and it has been suggested that many of the systemic and local reactions noted in the early years may have been due to impurities in the more primitive formulations.[1, 4–6] The rarity of ototoxicity and nephrotoxicity in new formulations of vancomycin together with the availability of several dosing nomograms has reduced concerns about adverse effects and led to a reexamination of the need for assiduous monitoring of serum concentrations of the drug.[7–12]

For years, vancomycin maintained consistent bactericidal activity against nearly all gram-positive organisms. However, the 1990s have witnessed the epidemic spread of vancomycin-resistant organisms, particularly among enterococci.[13–19] Strategies to treat and contain these organisms are problematic and continue to evolve.[20–23]

Chemistry

Vancomycin is a complex glycopeptide (Fig. 24–1) with the chemical formula $C_{66}H_{75}Cl_2N_9O_{24}$ and a molecular weight of 1449, much larger than any of the penicillins, cephalosporins, macrolides, tetracyclines, or aminoglycosides.[6, 24] Other glycopeptide antibiotics include actinoidin, ristocetin, and teicoplanin. Vancomycin hydrochloride is most soluble at pH 3 to 5; solubility decreases rapidly with increasing pH, reaching a minimum of about 15 mg/mL at pH 7.[25] In distilled water or 0.9% sodium chloride solution, vancomycin has a pH of approximately 4; solutions of vancomycin hydrochloride are stable for 14 days at room temperature.[26, 27] Vancomycin is unstable in alkaline solutions and forms insoluble salts in solution with certain chemical compounds; thus, vancomycin must not be mixed with drugs or diluents with which it is incompatible, such as sodium bicarbonate, heparin, certain penicillins and sulfonamides, chloramphenicol, corticosteroids, aminophylline, vitamin preparations, warfarin, and barbiturates.[26, 28–30] Vancomycin for human administration is provided as a hydrochloride salt and is usually reconstituted with sterile water and then diluted with 0.9% sodium chloride or 5% dextrose.

Microbiology

Mode of Antimicrobial Action

The principal mode of bactericidal action of vancomycin is to inhibit bacterial cell wall synthesis in dividing organisms. During the second stage of cell wall synthesis, vancomycin prevents polymerization of UDP-*N*-acetylmuramyl pentapeptide and *N*-acetylglucosamine into peptidoglycan[31] by virtue of tight binding of D-alanyl-D-alanine at the free carboxyl end of the cross-linking pentapeptide to the cleft in the chlorine-bearing face of vancomycin,[24] thereby sterically preventing binding of the peptide to the enzyme peptidoglycan synthetase. Because penicillins and cephalosporins inhibit the subsequent cross-linkage of the pentapeptide side chains of peptidoglycan, it is not surprising that there is no cross-resistance between vancomycin and the β-lactams. The large molecular size of vancomycin prevents it from crossing the outer cell membrane of gram-negative bacteria, thus restricting its activity to gram-positive species.

Antimicrobial Spectrum

Vancomycin is highly active and bactericidal against most species of gram-positive cocci and bacilli.[32, 33] Virtually all strains of *S. aureus,* including those that are methicillin resistant, are susceptible to vancomycin in low concentrations, with minimal inhibitory concentrations (MICs) lower than 5 mg/L. Vancomycin susceptibility is noted with most of the non-*aureus Staphylococcus* species, including *S. epidermidis, S.*

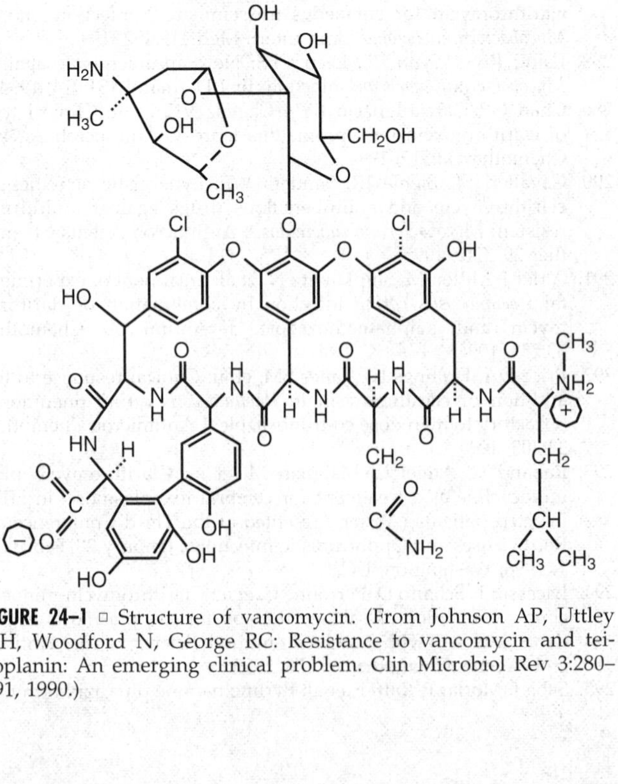

FIGURE 24–1 □ Structure of vancomycin. (From Johnson AP, Uttley AH, Woodford N, George RC: Resistance to vancomycin and teicoplanin: An emerging clinical problem. Clin Microbiol Rev 3:280–291, 1990.)

saprophyticus, S. haemolyticus, S. hominis, and *S. warneri,* as well as with unspeciated coagulase-negative staphylococci.[34]

All strains of *Streptococcus pneumoniae,* including penicillin-resistant isolates, have been susceptible to vancomycin.[35, 36] Vancomycin is bactericidal for all strains of *Streptococcus pyogenes* (group A streptococci), group C and group G streptococci, viridans streptococci, and *Streptococcus bovis.* Vancomycin is usually not bactericidal even for susceptible strains of enterococci at concentrations that can be achieved safely in humans; minimal bactericidal concentrations (MBCs) are usually more than 32 times higher than MICs.[37] Occasional isolates of group B streptococci (*Streptococcus agalactiae*) appear resistant to vancomycin, although most isolates exhibit MICs lower than 4.0 mg/L. In addition, vancomycin may have relatively high MBCs for occasional strains of viridans streptococci, *S. bovis,* and group B streptococci.[32, 37–39] Most strains of *Listeria monocytogenes* are inhibited by clinically achievable levels of vancomycin, but MBCs are much higher than MICs and generally exceed achievable serum levels.[33, 40] All strains of diphtheroids (nondiphtheria *Corynebacterium* species including *Corynebacterium jeikeium* and *Corynebacterium* D2) appear to be susceptible to modest concentrations (MICs lower than 1 mg/L) of vancomycin.[41–44] Some strains of *Lactobacillus* species are resistant to vancomycin.[19, 45, 46]

Among anaerobes, vancomycin is active against most clostridial isolates, including *Clostridium perfringens* and *Clostridium difficile*; most isolates are inhibited by less than 1 mg/L.[47, 48] On the other hand, no more than half of *Actinomyces* species appear susceptible to vancomycin.[49] Microaerophilic and anaerobic streptococci are usually susceptible, whereas *Bacteroides* species and other gram-negative anaerobes are not.

Vancomycin exhibits no significant activity against most gram-negative bacteria, including the Enterobacteriaceae and Pseudomonadaceae as well as *Legionella* species.[26] Although successful treatment with vancomycin of cases of meningitis caused by *Flavobacterium meningosepticum* has been reported, all strains of this gram-negative bacillus demonstrate resistance to vancomycin in vitro.[50, 51] Rickettsiae, chlamydiae, and mycobacteria are resistant as well.[26] Some strains of *Neisseria* appear susceptible in vitro,[52] but the clinical significance of these findings is unknown.

Resistance

Vancomycin enjoyed consistent activity against virtually all gram-positive species for the first 30 years of its clinical use, but subsequent years have witnessed a dramatic increase in the prevalence of vancomycin-resistant enterococci (VRE).[13–16, 53–57] Among the members of the National Nosocomial Infection Survey, hospitals reporting any isolates of VRE rose from 0.3% to 7.9% of facilities from 1989 to 1993, with larger, university-affiliated hospitals and intensive care unit settings reporting a disproportionate number of cases.[20] Clinical infection with VRE is associated with prolonged length of hospital stay, prior antibiotic use, and renal failure requiring hemodialysis or peritoneal dialysis.[54–56]

The majority of VRE isolates from U.S. hospitals (67% in one series) bear the VanA phenotype.[15, 16] This is characterized by high-level resistance to vancomycin (MIC, 64 μg/mL or higher) and teicoplanin (MIC, 16 to 128 μg/mL or higher). The *vanA* is a 9-gene complex that alters the usual target of vancomycin, the terminal D-alanyl-D-alanine of the muramyl pentapeptide, substituting instead D-alanyl-D-lactate.[58, 59] It is located on a transposable genetic element, transposon 1546, which may be plasmid associated. VanA has been observed in *Enterococcus faecium, Enterococcus faecalis,* and *Enterococcus avium.* The VanB phenotype usually displays lower level vancomycin resistance (MIC, 16 to 1024 μg/mL), with preservation of teicoplanin susceptibility (MIC, 2 μg/mL or lower), and is seen in both *E. faecium* and *E. faecalis.*[16, 57] The VanC pattern, isolated from *E. gallinarum,* has low-level resistance to vancomycin (MIC, 4 to 16 μg/mL) with teicoplanin susceptibility. VanC-like phenotypes have also been observed in *Enterococcus casseliflavus* and *Enterococcus raffinosus.*[16] The low-level resistance that characterizes the VanB and VanC isolates may be missed by some short-incubation automated susceptibility systems.[60] There have been reports of enterococci that have evolved from the VanB phenotype to actually require the presence of vancomycin for growth.[61, 62]

No clear consensus has emerged regarding the therapy for VanA isolates, many of which are β-lactam resistant as well as glycopeptide resistant; suggestions have included use of β-lactam–aminoglycoside combinations,[21, 22, 63] chloramphenicol,[64] and experimental macrolides (e.g., quinupristin-dalfopristin[65]). VRE with low-level resistance have been treated with teicoplanin, although acquired resistance to this agent has been observed in some cases.[63, 66]

The Centers for Disease Control and Prevention has issued guidelines to prevent the epidemic spread of VRE.[20] The guidelines detail educational efforts, isolation procedures, laboratory screening methods, and survey techniques to detect asymptomatic colonization. In an attempt to limit the impact of VRE, medical facilities are advised to (1) establish methods for screening for VRE,[67] (2) use barrier methods (gowns, gloves) to prevent transmission from known cases,[20, 68] and (3) curtail the use of vancomycin when reasonable therapeutic alternatives exist or when cultures fail to document β-lactam–resistant gram-positive infection.

Other gram-positive species have manifested vancomycin resistance, including less frequently encountered genera such as *Leuconostoc, Pediococcus,* group G streptococci, *Lactobacillus,* and *Erysipelothrix.*[19, 69–72] Strains of coagulase-negative staphylococcus, including *S. epidermidis* and *S. haemolyticus,* have been found to demonstrate vancomycin resistance, often in an incremental fashion after drug exposure.[72–74] So far, none of these organisms has shown the potential for rapid epidemic spread noted for VRE.

Antibiotic Combinations

Evaluation in vitro of the interaction between various antibiotic combinations may produce conflicting results, probably owing to differences in testing methods (checkerboard titrations versus time-kill curves), end points (bacteriostatic versus bactericidal), size and growth phase of the starting inoculum, and sampling times. Results must be interpreted with caution in the absence of data in vivo. Vancomycin and gentamicin are synergistic against most sensitive strains of enterococci, viridans streptococci, *S. bovis,* methicillin-sensitive and methicillin-resistant *S. aureus,* and one third to one half of strains of *S. epidermidis.*[6, 75–78] The combination of vancomycin plus rifampin has generally produced less favorable and often conflicting results. Against *S. epidermidis,* the combination of vancomycin plus rifampin is commonly synergistic and rarely demonstrates antagonism[78, 79]; however, vancomycin-rifampin synergism has been demonstrated against only one fifth to one third of *S. aureus* isolates,[80–82] and antagonism is noted frequently.[83–85] Furthermore, clinical experience with the combination of vancomycin plus rifampin in the treatment of serious *S. aureus* infections has been inconsistent.[86] The combination of vancomycin plus rifampin is not synergistic and is occasionally antagonistic against enterococci.[77] In summary, the most predictable situations for obtaining synergism with vancomycin combinations are (1) vancomycin plus gentamicin against enterococci, *S. bovis,* and viridans streptococci; (2) vancomycin plus gentamicin against methicillin-sensitive and methicillin-resistant *S. aureus*; and

(3) vancomycin plus rifampin against non-*aureus* staphylococci.

Pharmacokinetics

Absorption

Vancomycin absorption from the gastrointestinal tract is ordinarily minimal, although occasional reports have documented therapeutic (and, rarely, potentially toxic) serum concentrations during administration of oral or intracolonic vancomycin to patients with pseudomembranous colitis and marked renal impairment.[87–89] Intramuscular injection of vancomycin produces severe pain and tissue necrosis, and only the intravenous (IV) route is employed. To minimize phlebitis and infusion-related reactions, it is recommended that the IV dose be reconstituted in 100 to 250 mL of dextrose or normal saline solution and infused at a rate not exceeding 1 g/h.[90]

Distribution

The distribution of vancomycin after IV administration appears to be a biphasic process and most closely fits a three-compartment, open pharmacokinetic model.[91, 92] The distribution half-life, about 8 minutes, is followed by an intermediate half-life of 30 to 90 minutes, then an elimination half-life that is long and highly variable, ranging from 3 to 13 hours (average, 6 hours) in persons with normal renal function.[91–95]

Peak serum levels of vancomycin after IV infusion are proportional to the administered dose. Serum levels of vancomycin measured 2 hours after single-dose IV infusion are 2 to 10 mg/L after a dose of 500 mg, 25 mg/L after 1 g, and 45 mg/L after 2 g.[92]

With multiple-dose administration, penetration of vancomycin is good (more than 75% of serum levels) into ascitic, pericardial, and synovial fluids and moderately good (more than 50% of serum levels) into pleural fluid; therapeutic concentrations (more than 2.5 mg/L) are obtained in all these fluids after IV administration of one or more doses.[90, 96] Penetration of vancomycin from serum into peritoneal dialysis fluid is highly variable and unpredictable.[97]

Penetration of vancomycin into the cerebrospinal fluid (CSF) is variable in general and poor in patients with uninflamed meninges,[90] but it appears to be fair to moderately good (1% to 37% of serum levels) in patients with inflamed meninges; many patients with meningitis are likely to have therapeutic CSF concentrations with IV therapy alone.[90, 92] In one case series of pneumococcal meningitis, an initial response to vancomycin was seen in all 11 patients, but subsequent clinical failure occurred in 4 patients on days 4 to 8 associated with falling levels of vancomycin in the CSF.[98] In cases of meningitis associated with neurosurgical devices, coagulase-negative staphylococci and corynebacteria are encountered commonly.[99] Intrathecal or intraventricular administration of vancomycin is frequently employed in these cases; however, the CSF levels achieved are variable, and therapeutic drug levels in the CSF should be monitored.[100, 101]

Vancomycin is not concentrated in bile. Although biliary levels are about 30% to 50% of serum levels[90, 96] and may be therapeutic in vitro against streptococci (including enterococci), the drug should not be considered first-line treatment for gram-positive biliary tract infection. Like many other antibiotics, vancomycin does not penetrate well into ocular tissues.[102]

Animal studies have demonstrated good penetration and high tissue levels of vancomycin in kidney, liver, and spleen.[103] Limited data for humans indicate tissue levels higher than serum levels in heart, aorta, kidney, liver, and lung.[104] Penetration of vancomycin into abscess fluid is good; pus exhibits levels about equal to those in serum.[104] Penetration of vancomycin into bone is variable and is generally modest; higher concentrations are achieved in medullary bone than in cortical bone. About 3 hours after infusion of a single IV dose of 15 mg/kg vancomycin into normal subjects, Graziani and associates[105] noted cancellous bone levels of vancomycin of less than 2 μg/g in most patients; the mean bone/serum ratio was 13% for cancellous bone and 7% for cortical bone. In patients with osteomyelitis, vancomycin therapy resulted in cancellous bone concentrations of 3.6 μg/g (21% of serum level) in one patient; cortical bone levels were 3.5 and 8.5 μg/g (21% to 38% of serum levels) in two specimens and were undetectable in three.[105] Penetration into uninfected sternal bone was 30% to 70% of serum levels in another study with mean osseous concentrations of 9.3 μg/g.[106]

Elimination

Vancomycin is excreted almost entirely by the kidneys, primarily by glomerular filtration, and there is no evidence of tubular secretion or reabsorption.[90] There is a linear relationship between vancomycin clearance (C_{vanc}) and creatinine clearance (C_{cr}).[8, 91] The ratio of C_{vanc} to C_{cr} is about 70% in all patients, and the difference between the two clearance rates is explained by the approximately 55% binding of vancomycin to serum proteins.[91]

Administration and Dosing

In adults with normal renal function, dosing of vancomycin is simple: administration of 30 mg/kg per day (i.e., 2 g/d to the average adult) in two to four divided doses results in trough and peak serum levels in the desired therapeutic range. Traditional therapeutic drug monitoring requires (1) that a trough serum value be obtained just before (and not more than 1 hour before) a dose, with a target of 5 to 10 mg/L for patients receiving vancomycin at 12-hour intervals and 10 to 15 mg/L for 6-hour dosing intervals, and (2) that a peak serum level be measured 1 to 2 hours after completion of an IV infusion; the desired range is 25 to 40 mg/L, depending on the infecting organism and the site and severity of infection.[90, 92, 94] Some authors have argued that vancomycin dosing without determination of therapeutic drug levels should be adopted into common practice.[11, 12] This is based on the lack of clear data linking drug concentrations to clinical efficacy and the relative rarity of ototoxic and nephrotoxic effects caused by modern preparations of vancomycin when it is used alone. However, we continue to advocate therapeutic drug monitoring in critically ill patients, those with altered renal function or diminished renal perfusion, those receiving concomitant nephrotoxins (especially aminoglycosides), and those undergoing prolonged therapy.

Because the kidney is the only significant route of excretion of vancomycin, the dosage must be reduced for patients with impaired renal function. To avoid potentially toxic serum levels of vancomycin, C_{cr} can be used to determine the appropriate dosing schedule for these patients. C_{cr} can be estimated with reasonable accuracy[107] using the patient's age, sex, weight, and serum creatinine value:

$$C_{cr} = \frac{(140 - \text{age}) \times (1.00\ [\text{males}];\ 0.85\ [\text{females}]) \times \text{wt}}{72 \times \text{serum creatinine}}$$

where C_{cr} is in milliliters per minute, weight is in kilograms, and the serum creatinine value is in milligrams per deciliter. This formula is especially important for elderly patients, in whom the serum creatinine value often overestimates C_{cr}.

Several dosing methods have been proposed to sustain appropriate serum vancomycin concentrations in patients with varying degrees of renal insufficiency.[8, 108–110] Most methods employ a dose-variable principle for modifying maintenance dosing. Moellering and coworkers[8] produced a nomogram that establishes the total daily dose of vancomycin required to achieve a steady-state serum vancomycin concentration of 15 mg/L by use of a graph or calculated from the following formula:

$$\text{Dose (mg/kg/24 h)} = 15.4 \times C_{cr}$$

where C_{cr} is measured or calculated in milliliters per minute per kilogram. This method commonly results in trough serum levels within the range of 5 to 10 mg/L and peak serum levels from 25 to 30 mg/L.

This nomogram is awkward to use for patients with severe renal insufficiency, in which case it is more convenient to administer a maintenance dose infrequently rather than smaller doses on a daily basis.[110] In fact, it is possible to administer vancomycin to anephric patients at 15 mg/kg once weekly.[111] Matzke and coworkers[9] recommended a fixed-dose variable-interval method beginning with a loading dose of 25 mg/kg followed by a maintenance dose of 19 mg/kg administered at dosing intervals derived from a graph or calculated according to the following formula:

$$\text{Dosing interval (h)} = 12 \times \frac{86}{0.689C_{cr}\,(\text{mL/min}) + 3.66}$$

This formula is designed to provide a dose that attains trough and peak serum vancomycin concentrations of 7.5 and 30 mg/L, respectively.

Results of studies designed to evaluate the comparative predictability and reliability of various nomograms have been inconclusive.[94, 112, 113] Regardless of the dosing nomogram employed, serum vancomycin concentrations together with serum creatinine concentrations should be monitored at least once weekly for patients with renal insufficiency, because there is substantial interpatient variation in vancomycin clearance.

The oral administration of vancomycin produces negligible serum and tissue concentrations and is used exclusively for the treatment of *C. difficile* colitis.[114, 115]

Dialysis

Vancomycin is commonly used to treat gram-positive infections in hemodialysis patients; traditionally, a dosage of 1 g/wk has been employed. The use of high-flux dialyzer membranes has been associated with an abrupt drop in vancomycin concentration (by up to 40%) after treatment, followed by a reequilibration of serum with tissue levels of the drug.[116, 117] The net effect was a reduction by 16% of serum levels with each treatment or removal of one third of the dose in a typical week with three dialysis treatments.[116]

Vancomycin is commonly used in the treatment of peritonitis associated with continuous ambulatory peritoneal dialysis (CAPD).[118, 119] IV administration of vancomycin to CAPD patients results in intraperitoneal (IP) levels that are 20% to 25% of serum levels or about 1 to 5 mg/L.[120, 121] IP dosing of vancomycin is therapeutically equivalent to IV administration and is complicated by fewer side effects.[121–123] Both intermittent (30 mg/kg per week) and continuous (15 mg/kg initially, followed by 30 mg/L dialysate) IP dosing regimens produce therapeutic serum levels and are effective clinically.[121, 122] Reports of chemical peritonitis after IP administration of a particular formulation of vancomycin have not been common in more recent years.[124]

Vancomycin's pharmacokinetics can be affected by patient-related factors other than renal function. As with aminoglycosides, the half-life of vancomycin appears to be shorter and the dose requirements higher in burn patients.[125] Obese patients exhibit a relatively large volume of distribution for vancomycin, which indicates that vancomycin dosage should be calculated on total body weight rather than lean body weight (as with aminoglycosides).[126] Vancomycin clearance appears to be delayed in patients with liver impairment.[127]

Pediatric Dosing

Schaad and associates[7] recommended that dosing of vancomycin for children be based on age: for neonates younger than 1 week, 15 mg/kg every 12 hours; for neonates 8 to 30 days, 15 mg/kg every 8 hours; and for older infants and children, 10 mg/kg every 6 hours. Considerably higher doses were required to achieve therapeutic concentrations of vancomycin among a group of pediatric cancer patients.[128] In this group, accelerated drug clearance was predictable from elevated creatinine clearance.

James and coworkers[129] offered recommendations for administering vancomycin to preterm infants on the basis of postconceptional age and using lower total doses than those recommended by Schaad: for premature infants of gestational age younger than 27 weeks, 27 mg/kg every 36 hours; for gestational age 27 to 30 weeks, 24 mg/kg every 24 hours; for gestational age 31 to 36 weeks, 18 mg/kg every 12 hours; and for gestational age older than 37 weeks, 22.5 mg/kg every 12 hours. Longer drug half-lives requiring lower dosages among critically ill neonates who had low urine output or who required dopamine were noted by Seay and colleagues.[130]

Adverse Effects

Clinical experience with purified formulations of vancomycin suggests that it is a relatively safe antibiotic.[4, 5, 11, 12, 131]

INFUSION-RELATED REACTIONS

The most frequent adverse reactions associated with vancomycin therapy are those related to IV administration. The red man syndrome is an infusion rate–dependent, nonimmunologic reaction to vancomycin related to histamine release.[132–135] It consists of pruritus and erythematous flushing of the head, face, neck, and upper torso, often with hypotension (occasionally profound and dangerous); these effects usually subside within minutes when the infusion is terminated. This reaction occurred in 35% to 90% of volunteers receiving 1000 mg of vancomycin during 1 hour and in up to 10% of patients receiving 500 mg during 1 hour.[4, 132–134] In patients manifesting the reaction, its effects can be minimized by infusing 500 mg in 1 hour or 1000 mg in 2 hours.[134] Pretreatment with antihistamines also reduces the likelihood of the reaction and facilitates the dosing of 1000 mg in 1 hour.[135, 136] Concomitant administration of narcotics may potentiate the red man syndrome.[137] In rare instances, the reaction has been observed after oral administration of the drug.[138] Although early preparations of vancomycin were associated with high rates of chemical thrombophlebitis (about 50% of patients), the frequency with modern formulations has been in the range of 5% to 13%.[90, 139]

ALLERGIC REACTIONS

Hypersensitivity reactions, including skin eruptions (typically an erythematous, maculopapular rash and less often urticaria) as well as medication-associated fevers, have been noted in about 1% to 8% of patients receiving vancomycin.[131, 140] One case of a systemic lupus erythematosus–like vasculitis syndrome has been reported.[141]

HEMATOPOIETIC COMPLICATIONS

Adverse hematopoietic reactions associated with vancomycin therapy appear to be uncommon.[131] Thrombocytopenia has been reported rarely.[142] Eosinophilia occurs sporadically. Vancomycin-associated neutropenia has been reported occasionally, usually about 2 to 3 weeks into therapy, and appears to be unrelated to vancomycin serum levels.[131, 143, 144] An immune mechanism is probably involved, because some of these patients exhibit concomitant fever or rash. Periodic monitoring of the neutrophil count is recommended in patients receiving IV vancomycin therapy, particularly when it is administered for longer than 2 weeks.

OTOTOXICITY

Impairment of auditory function caused by vancomycin therapy is extremely uncommon; most cases have been reported in patients who are receiving other ototoxic medications (particularly aminoglycosides) concurrently.[11, 145, 146] Sorrell and Collignon[140] evaluated 54 patients prospectively, 11 with serial audiograms; 1 patient (also receiving gentamicin) was noted to have unilateral mild hearing impairment. Vancomycin does not appear to produce ototoxic effects in experimental animals.[145, 147]

NEPHROTOXICITY

Studies suggest that nephrotoxic effects associated with vancomycin occur occasionally and are most common in certain clinical settings: (1) elderly patients; (2) concomitant administration of an aminoglycoside; (3) prolonged therapy; (4) elevated serum vancomycin concentrations; (5) high-grade bacteremia; and (6) acute cardiovascular insufficiency. Farber and Moellering[131] noted nephrotoxic reactions in 35% of patients receiving vancomycin plus an aminoglycoside and in only 5% of patients receiving vancomycin alone. Sorrell and Collignon[140] reported nephrotoxic reactions in 14% of patients who received vancomycin plus an aminoglycoside and in no patients who received vancomycin alone. In a study of older patients, Downs and associates[148] reported nephrotoxic reactions in 27% of patients who had received recent or concurrent aminoglycoside therapy; of elderly individuals who received vancomycin alone, 7% had a nephrotoxic reaction, a rate that was not significantly different from the frequency noted in age-matched patients being treated with nonnephrotoxic antibiotics. Vancomycin may augment the nephrotoxic effects of aminoglycosides,[131, 149] but this effect has not been observed consistently.[12, 148]

Clinical Applications

Staphylococcus aureus

Vancomycin is the treatment of choice in β-lactam–intolerant patients who have serious infections due to *S. aureus*, including bacteremia, endocarditis, skin and soft tissue infections, pneumonia, and septic arthritis.[4, 150, 151] The relatively low rate of sterilization of blood cultures by vancomycin in cases of *S. aureus* endocarditis has led some investigators to suggest that the drug is inferior to traditional β-lactams for this indication and should be used with caution for serious *S. aureus* infections in nonallergic individuals solely for convenience of dosing.[152, 153] Vancomycin is indicated for the treatment of staphylococcal osteomyelitis in patients allergic to penicillins, although the variable and modest penetration of vancomycin into bone[104, 105] suggests that first-generation cephalosporins and clindamycin probably are superior. Vancomycin is the drug of choice for the treatment of methicillin-resistant *S. aureus* infections.[139, 154, 155]

Coagulase-Negative Staphylococci

Vancomycin is the mainstay of therapy for infections due to the coagulase-negative staphylococci.[156] Indeed, the most common setting for vancomycin use is the empirical or directed therapy of infection caused by these organisms involving indwelling medical devices, including bacteremia associated with vascular catheters, prosthetic valve endocarditis, vascular graft infections, prosthetic joint infections, and central nervous system shunt infections.[3, 99, 156–160] In general, the device must be removed to achieve cure of most staphylococcal infections associated with a foreign body.[161, 162] This is probably due to the ability of coagulase-negative staphylococci to form biofilms, which impair the killing power of vancomycin in vitro.[163] However, vancomycin therapy without removal of the device is often successful in CAPD-associated peritonitis and in postoperative endophthalmitis in recipients of intraocular lens implants.[118, 164] Occasionally, vancomycin is curative as well in prosthetic valve endocarditis, bacteremia associated with tunneled central venous (Hickman or Broviac) catheters, and meningitis due to CSF shunts.[158–162, 165, 166] Combination therapy (vancomycin plus rifampin or gentamicin) is often employed in prosthetic valve endocarditis due to non-*aureus* staphylococci.[158]

Streptococci

Vancomycin is an effective antibiotic for treatment of serious infections caused by streptococci in patients allergic to β-lactam antibiotics and can be used successfully to treat endocarditis due to viridans streptococci or *S. bovis*.[151, 167] Vancomycin is an alternative for penicillin-allergic patients with serious infections due to enterococci but must be used in combination with an aminoglycoside (gentamicin) for endocarditis.[151, 167] Vancomycin is the drug of choice for pneumococci highly resistant to penicillin (MIC above 2.0 μg/mL), but late failures in cases of meningitis have been observed.[35, 36, 98]

Diphtheroids

Vancomycin is the antibiotic of choice for treatment of infections due to diphtheroids, a group of nonsporulating, nondiphtheria corynebacteria that have emerged as important pathogens in patients with underlying malignant disease and neutropenia or with indwelling prosthetic devices.[168, 169]

Other Clinical Settings

Orally administered vancomycin in doses as low as 125 mg four times daily is as effective as metronidazole for treating antibiotic-associated colitis.[114, 115] IV administration of vancomycin produces low fecal concentrations of drug, probably owing to minimal biliary excretion, and is not effective in the treatment or prevention of antibiotic-associated colitis.[170] Vancomycin has often been part of antibiotic therapy for fever in the neutropenic host. However, Rubin and coworkers[171] found that outcomes for patients were not affected adversely by omitting vancomycin from the treatment regimen until β-lactam–resistant gram-positive infection had been documented by culture. The empirical use of vancomycin should be considered when febrile neutropenic patients show clinical signs of gram-positive infection (e.g., inflammation near vascular catheters) or in those treated prophylactically with fluoroquinolones, in whom fever indicates gram-positive infection more frequently.[172]

The agents of bacterial peritonitis in patients receiving CAPD are commonly gram-positive organisms, particularly *S. aureus* and non-*aureus* staphylococci, against which vancomycin is highly effective. Although continuous IP administration of vancomycin at a concentration of 25 to 50 mg/L in the dialysate (often with an initial IV loading dose) has been the most common mode of treatment, studies suggest that intermittent IP administration can be employed for CAPD-associated peritonitis. Studies have demonstrated that once-weekly IP administration of vancomycin (30 mg/kg in 2 L of dialysate with 6-hour dwell time) results in prolonged, effective peritoneal concentrations of vancomycin,[121] and two IP doses (30 mg/kg in 2 L 1 week apart) can be as effective and safe as continuous IP vancomycin therapy in managing CAPD-associated peritonitis.[122]

Vancomycin has been used successfully to treat bacterial meningitis and central nervous system shunt infections caused by susceptible organisms, especially coagulase-negative staphylococci.[159, 166] The shunt is typically removed completely, with a ventriculostomy device used for drainage and intrathecal drug administration. However, acceptable cure rates have been achieved by some investigators with exteriorization of the distal end of the shunt alone. The usual intrathecal doses of vancomycin range from 5 to 10 mg in infants to 10 to 20 mg in children and adults.[101] Vancomycin has also been used in the treatment of nonneurosurgical meningitis due to susceptible organisms in patients with severe (anaphylactic) penicillin allergy, or in patients infected with penicillin-resistant pneumococci, but experience with this therapy is limited.[35, 36, 98, 173]

Vancomycin can be employed for surgical prophylaxis in procedures involving implantation of a prosthesis in β-lactam–allergic patients. It is also the drug of choice for endocarditis prophylaxis in β-lactam–allergic individuals.[174]

Teicoplanin

Teicoplanin (formerly known as teichomycin A_2) is a newer glycopeptide antibiotic similar to vancomycin but with novel structural and pharmacologic properties.[175] Derived from fermentation products of *Actinoplanes teichomyceticus*,[176] teicoplanin differs chemically from vancomycin in that its carbohydrate moieties are D-glycosamine and D-mannose instead of D-glucose and vancosamine, and two dihydroxyphenyglycines are present instead of aspartic acid and *N*-methylleucine; it is distinct from all other glycopeptides in having an acyl substituent, which is a fatty acid.[177] It is larger than vancomycin, with a molecular weight of about 2000. As with vancomycin, its mechanism of action is the inhibition of polymerization of peptidoglycan by interacting with the D-alanyl-D-alanine terminus of the muramyl pentapeptide, which fits into a cleft inside the antibiotic molecule.[175] Owing to the presence of the fatty acid moiety, teicoplanin is far more lipophilic than vancomycin, which probably accounts for its greater tissue and cellular penetration.[175, 177] Teicoplanin exhibits a much higher degree of protein binding than does vancomycin (about 90% versus 55%), and it is likely that this feature and strong tissue binding explain its delayed clearance and much longer half-life (33 to 48 hours, compared with about 6 hours for vancomycin).[178, 179] The acidic charge provided teicoplanin by its phenolic groups and terminal carboxyl and amino groups renders it soluble as a sodium salt at physiologic pH, which probably accounts for the favorable tolerability and absorption obtained with intramuscular injection.[175, 177]

Teicoplanin has excellent activity against gram-positive organisms. It is about as active as vancomycin against staphylococci but generally four to eight times more active against streptococci and clostridia.[179–182] Like vancomycin, teicoplanin is bactericidal against growing cells; the MBC is typically no more than two to four times the MIC for most organisms.[175, 181] Although teicoplanin has greater inhibitory activity than vancomycin against enterococci, each is only bacteriostatic; the MBC is usually above achievable serum concentrations and more than 32 times the MIC.[182] Teicoplanin and vancomycin exhibit similar bactericidal synergism in combination with gentamicin against sensitive strains of enterococci. Teicoplanin is active against vancomycin-resistant enterococci bearing the VanB phenotype, but the in vivo development of teicoplanin resistance has been observed.[16, 57, 66] It has no activity against VanA isolates, nor does it demonstrate synergistic killing with β-lactams against these isolates.[63] Like vancomycin, teicoplanin is bacteriostatic for *L. monocytogenes*.[182]

Because of its long terminal half-life, teicoplanin can be administered much less frequently than vancomycin. Many early studies indicated clinical success with teicoplanin administered in a loading dose of about 6 mg/kg (about 400 to 600 mg) followed by a maintenance regimen of 2 to 3 mg/kg (about 200 mg) once daily.[183–185] However, subsequent studies with serious staphylococcal infections suggested that more aggressive loading therapy is needed to obtain adequate serum levels rapidly.[186, 187] A high loading dose, or administration of two or three initial maintenance doses at 12-hour intervals after the loading dose, may be necessary to establish adequate serum levels promptly (trough concentration of 5 to 10 mg/L and peak serum levels of 25 to 30 mg/L) in seriously ill patients. Bibler and associates[185] recommended that teicoplanin treatment of patients with gram-positive bacteremia should begin with three IV doses of 6 to 7 mg/kg at 12-hour intervals followed by single daily doses of the same amount. However, Fortún and colleagues[188] noted breakthrough bacteremia at doses of 7 mg/kg per day in cases of *S. aureus* endocarditis, suggesting that the optimal dosage of teicoplanin for this disease remains to be defined.

At doses of 6 mg/kg per day, teicoplanin was as effective as and less toxic than vancomycin for treatment of gram-positive infections in neutropenic hosts.[189, 190] The drug has also been employed in the treatment of infections caused by sensitive strains of enterococci, although its role in serious infection and endocarditis remains uncertain.[191] Teicoplanin has been used in oral form to treat *C. difficile* colitis.[192]

Teicoplanin appears to be less toxic than vancomycin. Intramuscular injection is tolerated well except for mild pain at the injection site and results in excellent absorption (90% bioavailability).[175, 180] Phlebitis is uncommon with IV administration of teicoplanin,[185] and infusion-related red man syndrome does not seem to occur.[180, 184] Occasional allergic reactions (rash, eosinophilia) have been noted with teicoplanin. Transient elevations and liver chemistries have been noted to occur occasionally. Renal and otic toxic effects appear to be extremely uncommon.[175, 183–185]

References

1. Griffith RS: Introduction to vancomycin. Rev Infect Dis 3:S200, 1981.
2. Geraci JE, Heilman FR, Wellman WE, Ross GT: Some laboratory and clinical experiences with a new antibiotic, vancomycin. Proc Staff Meet Mayo Clin 31:564, 1956.
3. Ena J, Dick RW, Jones RN, Wenzel RP: The epidemiology of

intravenous vancomycin usage in a university hospital: A 10-year study. JAMA 269:598, 1993.
4. Cook FV, Farrar WE Jr: Vancomycin revisited. Ann Intern Med 88:813, 1978.
5. Levine JF: Vancomycin: A review. Med Clin North Am 71:1135, 1987.
6. Cooper GL, Given DB: Vancomycin: A Comprehensive Review of 30 Years of Clinical Experience. Indianapolis, IN, Park Row Publishers, 1986.
7. Schaad UB, Nelson JD, McCracken GH Jr: Pharmacology and efficacy of vancomycin for staphylococcal infections in children. Rev Infect Dis 3:S282, 1981.
8. Moellering RC Jr, Krogstad DJ, Greenblatt DJ: Vancomycin therapy in patients with impaired renal function: A nomogram for dosage. Ann Intern Med 94:343, 1981.
9. Matzke GR, McGory RW, Halstenson CE, Keane WF: Pharmacokinetics of vancomycin in patients with various degrees of renal function. Antimicrob Agents Chemother 25:433, 1984.
10. Cutler NR, Narang PK, Lesko LJ, et al: Vancomycin disposition: The importance of age. Clin Pharmacol Ther 36:803, 1984.
11. Freeman CD, Quintiliani R, Nightingale CH: Vancomycin therapeutic drug monitoring: Is it necessary? Ann Pharmacother 27:594, 1993.
12. Cantú TG, Yamanaka-Yuen NA, Lietman PS: Serum vancomycin concentrations: Reappraisal of their clinical value. Clin Infect Dis 18:533, 1994.
13. Leclercq R, Derlot E, Duval J, Courvalin P: Plasmid-mediated resistance to vancomycin and teicoplanin in *Enterococcus faecium.* N Engl J Med 319:157, 1988.
14. Shlaes DM, Bouvet A, Devine C, et al: Inducible, transferable resistance to vancomycin in *Enterococcus faecalis* A256. Antimicrob Agents Chemother 33:198, 1989.
15. Leclercq R, Derlot E, Weber M, et al: Transferable vancomycin and teicoplanin resistance in *Enterococcus faecium.* Antimicrob Agents Chemother 33:10, 1989.
16. Clark NC, Cooksey RC, Hill BC, et al: Characterization of glycopeptide-resistant enterococci from U.S. hospitals. Antimicrob Agents Chemother 37:2311, 1993.
17. Handwerger S, Raucher B, Altarac D, et al: Nosocomial outbreak due to *Enterococcus faecium* highly resistant to vancomycin, penicillin, and gentamicin. Clin Infect Dis 16:750, 1993.
18. Livornese LL, Dias SD, Samel C, et al: Hospital-acquired infection with vancomycin-resistant *Enterococcus faecium* transmitted by electronic thermometers. Ann Intern Med 117:112, 1992.
19. Johnson AP, Uttley AH, Woodford N, George RC: Resistance to vancomycin and teicoplanin: An emerging clinical problem. Clin Microbiol Rev 3:280, 1990.
20. Centers for Disease Control and Prevention: Preventing the spread of vancomycin resistance—A report from the Hospital Infection Control Practices Advisory Committee prepared by the Subcommittee on Prevention and Control of Antimicrobial-resistant Microorganisms in Hospitals. Fed Regist 59:25758, 1994.
21. Caron F, Pestel M, Kitzis MD, et al: Comparison of different β-lactam-glycopeptide-gentamicin combinations for an experimental endocarditis caused by a highly β-lactam–resistant and highly glycopeptide-resistant isolates of *Enterococcus faecium.* J Infect Dis 171:106, 1995.
22. Green M, Binczewski B, Pasculle AW, et al: Constitutively vancomycin-resistant *Enterococcus faecium* resistant to synergistic β-lactam combinations. Antimicrob Agents Chemother 37:1238, 1993.
23. Murray BE: Editorial response: What can we do about vancomycin-resistant enterococci? Clin Infect Dis 20:1134, 1995.
24. Sheldrick GM, Jones PG, Kennard O, et al: Structure of vancomycin and its complex with acetyl-D-alanyl-D-alanine. Nature 271:223, 1978.
25. Pfeiffer RR: Structural features of vancomycin. Rev Infect Dis 3:S205, 1981.
26. Cheung RPF, DiPiro JT: Vancomycin: An update. Pharmacotherapy 6:153, 1986.
27. Mann JM, Coleman DL, Boylan JC: Stability of parenteral solutions of sodium cephalothin, cephaloridine, potassium penicillin G (buffered) and vancomycin HCl. Am J Hosp Pharm 28:760, 1971.
28. Barg NL, Supena RB, Fekety R: Persistent staphylococcal bacteremia in an intravenous drug abuser. Antimicrob Agents Chemother 29:209, 1986.
29. Misgen R: Compatibilities and incompatibilities of some intravenous admixtures. Am J Hosp Pharm 22:92, 1965.
30. Grant HR: Compatibilities of intravenous admixtures. Hosp Pharm 15:67, 1962.
31. Perkins HR, Nieto M: The chemical basis for the action of the vancomycin group of antibiotics. Ann N Y Acad Sci 235:348, 1974.
32. Watanakunakorn C: Mode of action and in vitro activity of vancomycin. J Antimicrob Chemother 14(Suppl):7, 1984.
33. Watanakunakorn C: The antibacterial action of vancomycin. Rev Infect Dis 3:S210, 1981.
34. Kloos WE, Bannerman TL: Update on clinical significance of coagulase-negative staphylococci. Clin Microbiol Rev 7:117, 1994.
35. Jacobs MR: Treatment and diagnosis of infections caused by drug-resistant *Streptococcus pneumoniae.* Clin Infect Dis 15:119, 1992.
36. Friedland IR, McCracken GH Jr: Management of infections caused by antibiotic-resistant *Streptococcus pneumoniae.* N Engl J Med 331:377, 1994.
37. Krogstad DJ, Parquette AR: Defective killing of enterococci: A common property of antimicrobial agents acting on the cell wall. Antimicrob Agents Chemother 17:965, 1980.
38. Stratton CW, Liu C, Ratner HB, Weeks LS: Bactericidal activity of daptomycin (LY 146032) compared with those of ciprofloxacin, vancomycin and ampicillin against enterococci as determined by kill-kinetic studies. Antimicrob Agents Chemother 31:1014, 1987.
39. Kim MJ, Weiser M, Gottschall S, Randall EL: Identification of *Streptococcus faecalis* and *Streptococcus faecium* and susceptibility studies with newly developed antimicrobial agents. J Clin Microbiol 25:787, 1987.
40. Tuazon CU, Shamsuddin D, Miller H: Antibiotic susceptibility and synergy of clinical isolates of *Listeria monocytogenes.* Antimicrob Agents Chemother 21:525, 1982.
41. Jadeja L, Fainstein V, LeBlanc B, Bodey GP: Comparative in vitro activities of teichomycin and other antibiotics against JK diphtheroids. Antimicrob Agents Chemother 24:145, 1983.
42. Riley PS, Hollis DG, Utter GB, et al: Characterization and identification of 95 diphtheroid (group JK) cultures isolated from clinical specimens. J Clin Microbiol 9:418, 1979.
43. Gill VJ, Manning C, Lamson M, et al: Antibiotic-resistant group JK bacteria in hospitals. J Clin Microbiol 13:472, 1981.
44. Santamaria M, Ponte C, Wilhelmi I, Soriano F: Antimicrobial susceptibility of *Corynebacterium* group D2. Antimicrob Agents Chemother 28:845, 1985.
45. Bayer AS, Chow AW, Betts D, Guze B: Lactobacillemia: Report of nine cases. Am J Med 4:808, 1978.
46. Holliman RE, Bone GP: Vancomycin resistance of clinical isolates of lactobacilli. J Infect 16:279, 1988.
47. Sapico FL, Kwok Y-Y, Sutter VI, Finegold SM: Standardized antimicrobial disc susceptibility testing of anaerobic bacteria. In vitro susceptibility of *Clostridium perfringens* to nine antibiotics. Antimicrob Agents Chemother 2:320, 1972.
48. George WL, Sutter VL, Finegold SM: Toxigenicity and antimicrobial susceptibility of *Clostridium difficile,* a cause of antimicrobial agent–associated colitis. Curr Microbiol 1:55, 1978.
49. Lerner PI: Susceptibility of pathogenic actinomycetes to antimicrobial compounds. Antimicrob Agents Chemother 5:302, 1974.
50. Aber RC, Wennersten C, Moellering RC Jr: Antimicrobial susceptibility of flavobacteria. Antimicrob Agents Chemother 14:483, 1978.
51. Altman G, Bogokovsky G: In vitro testing of *Flavobacterium meningosepticum* to antimicrobial agents. J Med Microbiol 4:296, 1971.
52. Jaffe HW, Lewis JS, Wiesner PJ: Vancomycin-sensitive *Neisseria gonorrhoeae.* J Infect Dis 144:198, 1981.
53. Uttley AH, Collins CH, Naidoo J, George RC: Vancomycin-resistant enterococci (Letter). Lancet 1:57, 1988.
54. Edmond MB, Ober JF, Weinbaum DL, et al: Vancomycin-resistant *Enterococcus faecium* bacteremia: Risk factors for infection. Clin Infect Dis 20:1126, 1995.
55. Herman DJ, Gerding DN: Minireview: Antimicrobial resistance among enterococci. Antimicrob Agents Chemother 35:1, 1991.

56. Courvalin P: Minireview: Resistance of enterococci to glycopeptides. Antimicrob Agents Chemother 34:2291, 1990.
57. Quintiliani R Jr, Evers S, Courvalin P: The *vanB* gene confers various levels of self-transferable resistance to vancomycin in enterococci. J Infect Dis 167:1220, 1993.
58. Walsh CT: Vancomycin resistance: Decoding the molecular logic. Science 261:308, 1993.
59. Fan C, Moews PC, Walsh CT, Knox JR: Vancomycin resistance: Structure of D-alanine:D-alanine ligase at 2.3 Å resolution. Science 266:439, 1994.
60. Tenover FC, Tokars J, Swenson J, et al: Ability of clinical laboratories to detect antimicrobial agent–resistant enterococci. J Clin Microbiol 31:1695, 1993.
61. Fraimow HS, Jungkind DL, Lander DW, et al: Urinary tract infection with an *Enterococcus faecalis* isolate that requires vancomycin for growth. Ann Intern Med 121:22, 1994.
62. Green M, Shlaes JH, Barbadora K, Shlaes DM: Bacteremia due to vancomycin-dependent *Enterococcus faecium*. Clin Infect Dis 20:712, 1995.
63. Hayden MK, Koenig GI, Trenholme GM: Bactericidal activities of antibiotics against vancomycin-resistant *Enterococcus faecium* blood isolates and synergistic activities of combinations. Antimicrob Agents Chemother 38:1225, 1994.
64. Norris AH, Reilly JP, Edelstein PH, et al: Chloramphenicol for the treatment of vancomycin-resistant enterococcal infections. Clin Infect Dis 20:1137, 1995.
65. Lynn WA, Clutterbuck E, Want S, et al: Treatment of CAPD-peritonitis due to glycopeptide-resistant *Enterococcus faecium* with quinupristin/dalfopristin. Lancet 344:1025, 1994.
66. Hayden MK, Trenholme GM, Schultz JE, Sahm DF: In vivo development of teicoplanin resistance in a VanB *Enterococcus faecium* isolate. J Infect Dis 167:1224, 1993.
67. Edberg SC, Hardalo CJ, Kontnick C, Campbell S: Rapid detection of vancomycin-resistant enterococci. J Clin Microbiol 32:2182, 1994.
68. Boyce JM, Opal SM, Chow JW, et al: Outbreak of multidrug-resistant *Enterococcus faecium* with transferable *vanB* class vancomycin resistance. J Clin Microbiol 32:1148, 1994.
69. Rubin LG, Vellozzi E, Shapiro J, Isenberg HD: Infection with vancomycin-resistant "streptococci" due to *Leuconostoc* species. J Infect Dis 157:216, 1988.
70. Swenson JM, Facklam RR, Thornsberry C: Antimicrobial susceptibility of vancomycin-resistant *Leuconostoc, Pediococcus,* and *Lactobacillus* species. Antimicrob Agents Chemother 34:543, 1990.
71. Noble JT, Tyburski MB, Berman M: Antimicrobial tolerance in group G streptococci. Lancet 2:982, 1980.
72. Ruoff KL, Kuritzkes DR, Wolfson JS, Ferraro MJ: Vancomycin-resistant gram-positive bacteria isolated from human sources. J Clin Microbiol 26:2064, 1988.
73. Schwalbe RS, Stapleton JT, Gilligan PH: Emergence of vancomycin resistance in coagulase-negative staphylococci. N Engl J Med 316:927, 1987.
74. Archer GL, Climo MW: Minireview: Antimicrobial susceptibility of coagulase-negative staphylococci. Antimicrob Agents Chemother 38:2231, 1994.
75. Mandell GL, Lindsey E, Hook EW: Synergism of vancomycin and streptomycin for enterococci. Am J Med Sci 259:346, 1970.
76. Harwick HB, Kalmanson GM, Guze LB: In vitro activity of ampicillin or vancomycin combined with gentamicin or streptomycin against enterococci. Antimicrob Agents Chemother 4:383, 1973.
77. Watanakunakorn C, Tisone JC: Synergism between vancomycin and gentamicin or tobramycin for methicillin-susceptible and methicillin-resistant *Staphylococcus aureus* strains. Antimicrob Agents Chemother 22:903, 1982.
78. Ein ME, Smith NJ, Aruffo JF, et al: Susceptibility and synergy studies of methicillin-resistant *Staphylococcus epidermidis*. Antimicrob Agents Chemother 16:655, 1979.
79. Lowy F, Wexler MA, Steigbigel NH: Therapy of methicillin-resistant *Staphylococcus epidermidis* experimental endocarditis. J Lab Clin Med 100:94, 1982.
80. Tuazon CU, Lin MYC, Sheagren JN: In vitro activity of rifampin alone and in combination with nafcillin and vancomycin against pathogenic strains of *Staphylococcus aureus*. Antimicrob Agents Chemother 13:759, 1978.
81. Tuazon CU, Miller H: Comparative in vitro activities of teichomycin and vancomycin alone and in combination with rifampin and aminoglycosides against staphylococci and enterococci. Antimicrob Agents Chemother 25:411, 1984.
82. Bayer AS, Morrison JO: Disparity between time-kill and checkerboard methods for determination of in vitro bactericidal interactions of vancomycin plus rifampin versus methicillin-susceptible and -resistant *Staphylococcus aureus*. Antimicrob Agents Chemother 26:220, 1984.
83. Zinner SH, Lagast H, Klastersky J: Antistaphylococcal activity of rifampin with other antibiotics. J Infect Dis 144:365, 1981.
84. Watanakunakorn C, Guerriero JC: Interaction between vancomycin and rifampin against *Staphylococcus aureus*. Antimicrob Agents Chemother 19:1089, 1981.
85. Hackbarth CJ, Chambers HF: Methicillin-resistant staphylococci: Genetics and mechanisms of resistance. Antimicrob Agents Chemother 33:991, 1989.
86. Levine DP, Cushing RD, Ji J, Brown WJ: Community-acquired methicillin-resistant *Staphylococcus aureus* endocarditis in the Detroit Medical Center. Ann Intern Med 97:330, 1982.
87. Bryan CS, White WL: Safety of oral vancomycin in functionally anephric patients. Antimicrob Agents Chemother 14:634, 1978.
88. Spitzer PG, Eliopoulos GM: Systemic absorption of enteral vancomycin in a patient with pseudomembranous colitis. Ann Intern Med 100:533, 1984.
89. Pasic M, Carrel T, Opravil M, et al: Systemic absorption after local intracolonic vancomycin in pseudomembranous colitis. Lancet 342:443, 1993.
90. Matzke GR, Zhanel GG, Guay DRP: Clinical pharmacokinetics of vancomycin. Clin Pharmacol 11:257, 1986.
91. Krogstad DJ, Moellering RC Jr, Greenblatt DJ: Single-dose kinetics of intravenous vancomycin. J Clin Pharmacol 20:197, 1980.
92. Moellering RC Jr: Pharmacokinetics of vancomycin. J Antimicrob Chemother 14:43, 1984.
93. Cunha BA, Quintiliani R, Deglin JM, et al: Pharmacokinetics of vancomycin in anuria. Rev Infect Dis 3:S269, 1981.
94. Healy DP, Polk RE, Garson ML, et al: Comparison of steady-state pharmacokinetics of two dosage regimens of vancomycin in normal volunteers. Antimicrob Agents Chemother 31:393, 1987.
95. Rotschafer JC, Crossley K, Zaske DE, et al: Pharmacokinetics of vancomycin: Observations in 28 patients and dosage recommendations. Antimicrob Agents Chemother 22:391, 1982.
96. Geraci JE, Heilman FR, Nichols DR, et al: Some laboratory and clinical experiences with a new antibiotic, vancomycin. Antibiot Ann 1956–1957:90, 1957.
97. Glew RH, Pavuk RA, Hennick K: Vancomycin pharmacokinetics and toxicity. Presented at the 13th International Congress of Chemotherapy; August 28–September 2, 1983; Vienna, Austria.
98. Viladrich PF, Gudiol F, Linares J, et al: Evaluation of vancomycin for therapy of adult pneumococcal meningitis. Antimicrob Agents Chemother 35:2467, 1991.
99. Shoenbaum SC, Gardner P, Shillito J: Infections of cerebrospinal fluid shunts: Epidemiology, clinical manifestations and therapy. J Infect Dis 131:543, 1975.
100. Krontz DP, Strausbaugh LJ: Effect of meningitis and probenecid on the penetration of vancomycin into cerebrospinal fluid in rabbits. Antimicrob Agents Chemother 18:882, 1980.
101. Luer MS, Hatton J: Vancomycin administration into the cerebrospinal fluid: A review. Ann Pharmacother 27:912, 1995.
102. MacIlwaine WA, Sande MA, Mandell GL: Penetration of antistaphylococcal antibiotics into the human eye. Am J Ophthalmol 77:589, 1974.
103. Engineer MS, Ho DW, Bodey GP: Comparison of vancomycin disposition in rats with normal and abnormal renal functions. Antimicrob Agents Chemother 20:718, 1981.
104. Torres JR, Sanders CV, Lewis AC: Vancomycin concentration in human tissues: Preliminary report. J Antimicrob Chemother 5:475, 1979.
105. Graziani AL, Lawson LA, Gibson GA, et al: Vancomycin concentrations in infected and noninfected human bone. Antimicrob Agents Chemother 32:1320, 1988.
106. Massias L, Dubois C, deLentdecker P, et al: Penetration of vancomycin in uninfected sternal bone. Antimicrob Agents Chemother 36:2539, 1992.
107. Cockcroft DW, Gault MH: Prediction of creatinine clearance from serum creatinine. Nephron 16:31, 1976.

108. Nielsen HE, Hansen HE, Korsager B, Skov PE: Renal excretion of vancomycin in kidney disease. Acta Med Scand 197:261, 1975.
109. Leonard AE, Boro MS: Vancomycin pharmacokinetics in middle-aged and elderly men. Am J Hosp Pharm 51:798, 1994.
110. Rodvold KA, Blum RA, Fischer JH, et al: Vancomycin pharmacokinetics in patients with various degrees of renal function. Antimicrob Agents Chemother 32:848, 1988.
111. Eykyn S, Phillips I, Evans J: Vancomycin for staphylococcal shunt site infections in patients on regular hemodialysis. Br Med J 3:80, 1970.
112. Rybak MJ, Boike SC: Monitoring vancomycin therapy. Drug Intell Clin Pharm 20:757, 1986.
113. Musa DM, Pauly DJ: Evaluation of a new vancomycin dosing method. Pharmacotherapy 7:69, 1987.
114. Teasley DG, Gerding DN, Olson MM, et al: Prospective randomised trial of metronidazole versus vancomycin for *Clostridium difficile*–associated diarrhoea and colitis. Lancet 2:1043, 1983.
115. Fekety R, Silva J, Kaufman C, et al: Treatment of antibiotic-associated *Clostridium difficile* colitis with oral vancomycin: Comparison of two dosage regimens. Am J Med 86:15, 1989.
116. Böhler J, Reetze-Bonorden P, Keller E, et al: Rebound of plasma vancomycin levels after haemodialysis with highly permeable membranes. Eur J Clin Pharmacol 42: 635, 1992.
117. Quale JM, O'Halloran JJ, DeVincenzo N, Barth RH: Removal of vancomycin by high-flux hemodialysis membranes. Antimicrob Agents Chemother 36:1424, 1992.
118. Keane WF, Everett ED, Fine RN, et al: Continuous ambulatory peritoneal dialysis (CAPD) peritonitis treatment recommendations: 1989 update. Perit Dial Int 9:247, 1989.
119. Peterson PK, Matzke G, Keane WF: Current concepts in the management of peritonitis in patients undergoing continuous ambulatory peritoneal dialysis. Rev Infect Dis 9:604, 1987.
120. Blevins RD, Halstenson CE, Salem NG, Matzke GR: Pharmacokinetics of vancomycin in patients undergoing continuous ambulatory peritoneal dialysis. Antimicrob Agents Chemother 25:603, 1984.
121. Morse GD, Farolino DF, Apicella MA, Walsh JW: Comparative study of intraperitoneal and intravenous vancomycin pharmacokinetics during continuous ambulatory peritoneal dialysis. Antimicrob Agents Chemother 31:173, 1987.
122. Boyce NW, Wood C, Thompson NM, et al: Intraperitoneal (IP) vancomycin therapy for CAPD peritonitis—A prospective, randomized comparison of intermittent versus continuous therapy. Am J Kidney Dis 4:304, 1988.
123. Bailie GR, Morton R, Ganguli L, et al: Intravenous or intraperitoneal vancomycin for the treatment of continuous ambulatory peritoneal dialysis–associated gram-positive peritonitis? Nephron 46:316, 1987.
124. Freiman JP, Graham DJ, Reed TG, McGoodwin EB: Chemical peritonitis following the intraperitoneal administration of vancomycin. Perit Dial Int 12:57, 1992.
125. Garrelts JC, Peterie JD: Altered vancomycin dose vs. serum concentration relationship in burn patients. Clin Pharmacol Ther 44:9, 1988.
126. Blouin RA, Bauer LA, Miller DD, et al: Vancomycin pharmacokinetics in normal and morbidly obese subjects. Antimicrob Agents Chemother 21:575, 1982.
127. Brown N, Ho DHW, Fong K-LL, et al: Effects of hepatic function on vancomycin clinical pharmacology. Antimicrob Agents Chemother 23:603, 1983.
128. Chang D, Liem L, Malogolowkin M: A prospective study of vancomycin pharmacokinetics and dosage requirements in pediatric cancer patients. Pediatr Infect Dis 13:969, 1994.
129. James A, Koren G, Milliken J, et al: Vancomycin pharmacokinetics and dose recommendations for preterm infants. Antimicrob Agents Chemother 31:52, 1987.
130. Seay RE, Brundage RC, Jensen PD, et al: Population pharmacokinetics of vancomycin in neonates. Clin Pharmacol Ther 56:169, 1994.
131. Farber BF, Moellering RC Jr: Retrospective study of the toxicity of preparations of vancomycin from 1974 to 1981. Antimicrob Agents Chemother 23:138, 1983.
132. Polk RE, Healy DP, Schwartz LB, et al: Vancomycin and the red-man syndrome: Pharmacodynamics of histamine release. J Infect Dis 157:502, 1988.
133. Newfield P, Roizen MF: Hazards of rapid administration of vancomycin. Ann Intern Med 91:581, 1979.
134. Healy DP, Sahai JV, Fuller SH, Polk RE: Vancomycin-induced histamine release and "red man syndrome": Comparison of 1- and 2-hour infusions. Antimicrob Agents Chemother 34:550, 1990.
135. Wallace MR, Mascola JR, Oldfield EC: Red man syndrome: Incidence, etiology, and prophylaxis. J Infect Dis 164:1180, 1991.
136. Sahai J, Healy DP, Garris R, et al: Influence of antihistamine pretreatment on vancomycin-induced red man syndrome. J Infect Dis 160:876, 1989.
137. Wong JT, Ripple RE, MacLean JA, et al: Vancomycin hypersensitivity: Synergism with narcotics and "desensitization" by a rapid continuous intravenous protocol. J Allergy Clin Immunol 94:189, 1994.
138. Bergeron L, Boucher FD: Possible red-man syndrome associated with systemic absorption of oral vancomycin in a child with normal renal function. Ann Pharmacother 28:581, 1994.
139. Wilhelm MP: Vancomycin. Mayo Clin Proc 66:1165, 1991.
140. Sorrell TC, Collignon PJ: A prospective study of adverse reactions associated with vancomycin therapy. J Antimicrob Chemother 16:235, 1985.
141. Markman M, Lim HW, Bluestein HG: Vancomycin-induced vasculitis. South Med J 79:382, 1986.
142. Zenon GJ, Cadle RM, Hamill RJ: Vancomycin-induced thrombocytopenia. Arch Intern Med 151:995, 1991.
143. Kesarwala HH, Rahill WJ, Amaram N: Vancomycin-induced neutropenia (Letter). Lancet 1:1423, 1981.
144. Farwell AP, Kendall LG Jr, Vakil RD, Glew RH: Delayed appearance of vancomycin-induced neutropenia in a patient with chronic renal failure. South Med J 77:664, 1984.
145. Brummet RE, Fox KE: Vancomycin- and erythromycin-induced hearing loss in humans. Antimicrob Agents Chemother 33:791, 1989.
146. Bailie GR, Neal D: Vancomycin ototoxicity and nephrotoxicity. A review. Med Toxicol 3:376, 1988.
147. Wold JS, Turnipseed SA: Toxicology of vancomycin in laboratory animals. Rev Infect Dis 3:S224, 1981.
148. Downs NJ, Niehart RE, Dolezal JM, Hodges GR: Mild nephrotoxicity associated with vancomycin use. Arch Intern Med 149:1777, 1989.
149. Rybak MJ, Albrecht LM, Boike SC, Chandrasekar PH: Nephrotoxicity of vancomycin, alone and with an aminoglycoside. J Antimicrob Chemother 25:679, 1990.
150. Kirby WMM: Vancomycin therapy in severe staphylococcal infections. Rev Infect Dis 3:S236, 1981.
151. Geraci JE, Wilson WR: Vancomycin therapy for infective endocarditis. Rev Infect Dis 3:S250, 1981.
152. Levine DP, Fromm BS, Reddy BR: Slow response to vancomycin or vancomycin plus rifampin in methicillin-resistant *Staphylococcus aureus* endocarditis. Ann Intern Med 115:674, 1991.
153. Small PM, Chambers HF: Vancomycin for *Staphylococcus aureus* endocarditis in intravenous drug users. Antimicrob Agents Chemother 34:1227, 1990.
154. Myers JP, Linnemann CC Jr: Bacteremia due to methicillin-resistant *Staphylococcus aureus.* J Infect Dis 145:532, 1982.
155. Cafferkey MT, Hone R, Keane CT: Antimicrobial chemotherapy of septicemia due to methicillin-resistant *Staphylococcus aureus.* Antimicrob Agents Chemother 28:819, 1985.
156. Lowy FD, Hammer SM: *Staphylococcus epidermidis* infections. Ann Intern Med 99:834, 1983.
157. Wade JC, Schimpff SC, Newman KA, Wiernik PH: *Staphylococcus epidermidis:* An increasing cause of infection in patients with granulocytopenia. Ann Intern Med 97:503, 1982.
158. Karchmer AW, Archer GL, Dismukes WE: *Staphylococcus epidermidis* causing prosthetic valve endocarditis: Microbiology and clinical observation as guides to therapy. Ann Intern Med 98:447, 1983.
159. Swayne R, Rampling A, Newsom SWB: Intraventricular vancomycin for treatment of shunt-associated ventriculitis. J Antimicrob Chemother 19:249, 1987.
160. Inman RD, Gallegos KV, Brause BD, et al: Clinical and microbial features of prosthetic joint infection. Am J Med 77:47, 1984.
161. Dickinson GM, Bisno AL: Infections associated with indwelling devices: Concepts of pathogenesis; infections associated with intravascular devices. Antimicrob Agents Chemother 33:597, 1989.
162. Dickinson GM, Bisno AL: Infections associated with indwelling

devices: Infections related to extravascular devices. Antimicrob Agents Chemother 33:602, 1989.
163. Evans RC, Holmes CJ: Effect of vancomycin hydrochloride on *Staphylococcus epidermidis* biofilm associated with silicone elastomer. Antimicrob Agents Chemother 31:889, 1987.
164. Weber DJ, Hoffman KL, Thoft RA, Baker AS: Endophthalmitis following intraocular lens implantation: Report of 30 cases and review of the literature. Rev Infect Dis 8:12, 1986.
165. Press OW, Ramsey PG, Larson EB, et al: Hickman catheter infections in patients with malignancies. Medicine (Baltimore) 63:189, 1984.
166. McLaurin RL, Frame PT: Treatment of infections of cerebrospinal fluid shunts. Rev Infect Dis 9:595, 1987.
167. Bisno AL, Dismukes WE, Durack DT, et al: Antimicrobial treatment of infective endocarditis due to viridans streptococci, enterococci, and staphylococci. JAMA 261:1471, 1989.
168. Lipsky BA, Goldberger AC, Tompkins LS, Plourde JJ: Infections caused by nondiphtheria corynebacteria. Rev Infect Dis 4:1220, 1982.
169. Riebel W, Frantz N, Adelstein D, Spagnuolo PJ: *Corynebacterium* JK: A cause of nosocomial device-related infection. Rev Infect Dis 8:42, 1986.
170. Oliva SL, Guglielmo BJ, Jacobs R, Pons VG: Failure of intravenous vancomycin and intravenous metronidazole to prevent or treat antibiotic-associated pseudomembranous colitis. J Infect Dis 159:1154, 1989.
171. Rubin M, Hathorn JW, Marshall D, et al: Gram-positive infections and the use of vancomycin in 550 episodes of fever and neutropenia. Ann Intern Med 108:30, 1988.
172. Bow EJ, Loewen R, Vaughan D: Reduced requirement for antibiotic therapy targeting gram-negative organisms in febrile, neutropenic patients with cancer who are receiving antibacterial chemoprophylaxis with oral quinolones. Clin Infect Dis 20:907, 1995.
173. Gump DW: Vancomycin for treatment of bacterial meningitis. Rev Infect Dis 3:S289, 1981.
174. Dajani AS, Bisno AL, Chung KJ, et al: Prevention of bacterial endocarditis: Recommendations by the American Heart Association. JAMA 264:2919, 1990.
175. Brogden RN, Peters DH: Teicoplanin: A reappraisal of its antimicrobial activity, pharmacokinetic properties and therapeutic efficacy. Drugs 47:823, 1994.
176. Somma S, Gastaldo L, Corti A: Teichoplanin, a new antibiotic from *Actinoplanes teichomyceticus* nov. sp. Antimicrob Agents Chemother 26:917, 1984.
177. Parenti F: Structure and mechanism of action of teichoplanin. J Hosp Infect 7(Suppl):79, 1986.
178. Parenti F: Glycopeptide antibiotics. J Clin Pharmacol 28:136, 1988.
179. Lagast H, Dodion P, Klastersky J: Comparison of pharmacokinetics and bactericidal activity of teichoplanin and vancomycin. J Antimicrob Chemother 18:513, 1986.
180. Verbist L, Tjandramaga B, Hendrickx B, et al: In vitro activity and human pharmacokinetics of teichoplanin. Antimicrob Agents Chemother 26:881, 1984.
181. Williams AH, Gruneberg RN: Teichoplanin. J Antimicrob Chemother 14:441, 1984.
182. Pallanza R, Berti M, Goldstein BP, et al: Teichoplanin: In vitro and in vivo evaluation and comparison to other antibiotics. J Antimicrob Chemother 11:419, 1983.
183. Drabu YJ, Walsh B, Blakemore PH, Mehtar S: Teichoplanin in infections caused by methicillin-resistant staphylococci. J Antimicrob Chemother 21(Suppl):89, 1987.
184. Stille W, Sietzen W, Dieterich H-A, Fell JJ: Clinical efficacy and safety of teichoplanin. J Antimicrob Chemother 21(Suppl):69, 1988.
185. Bibler MR, Frame PT, Hagler DN, et al: Clinical evaluation of efficacy, pharmacokinetics, and safety of teichoplanin for serious gram-positive infections. Antimicrob Agents Chemother 31:207, 1987.
186. Calain P, Krause K-H, Vaudaux P, et al: Early termination of a prospective, randomized trial comparing teichoplanin and flucloxacillin for treating severe staphylococcal infections. J Infect Dis 155:187, 1987.
187. Galanakis N, Giamarellou H, Vlachogiannis N, et al: Poor efficacy of teicoplanin in treatment of deep-seated staphylococcal infections. Eur J Clin Microbiol Infect Dis 7:130, 1988.
188. Fortún J, Pérez-Molina JA, Anón MT, et al: Right-sided endocarditis caused by *Staphylococcus aureus* in drug abusers. Antimicrob Agents Chemother 39:525, 1995.
189. Rolston KVI, Nguyen H, Amos G, et al: A randomized double-blind trial of vancomycin versus teicoplanin for the treatment of gram-positive bacteremia in patients with cancer. J Infect Dis 169:350, 1994.
190. Menichetti F, Martino P, Bucaneve G, et al: Effects of teicoplanin and those of vancomycin in initial empirical antibiotic regimen for febrile, neutropenic patients with hematologic malignancies. Antimicrob Agents Chemother 38:2041, 1994.
191. Schmit JL: Efficacy of teicoplanin for enterococcal infections: 63 cases and review. Clin Infect Dis 15:302, 1992.
192. de Lalla F, Privitera G, Rinaldi E, et al: Treatment of *Clostridium difficile*–associated disease with teicoplanin. Antimicrob Agents Chemother 33:1125, 1989.

25

Trimethoprim-Sulfamethoxazole

Richard Gleckman
John S. Czachor

Trimethoprim-sulfamethoxazole (TMP-SMX) is a fixed-dose combination chemotherapeutic agent that became available in the United States in oral form in 1973. The parenteral preparation was released in 1981. The drug is marketed in the United States under the trade names Bactrim and Septra and is known in numerous countries as co-trimoxazole. Although it possesses a fixed dose ratio of one part TMP to five parts SMX, the relative amount of each drug varies with the preparation. Standard-dose oral tablets have 80 mg of TMP and 400 mg of SMX; double-strength tablets contain twice those amounts. The liquid form has 40 mg of TMP and 200 mg of SMX per 5 mL (1 teaspoon). Each 5-mL vial of parenteral TMP-SMX for infusion contains 80 mg of TMP and 400 mg of SMX.

Mechanism of Action

The two components of this drug provide sequential inhibition of enzyme systems involved in bacterial synthesis of tetrahydrofolic acid and thereby disrupt nucleic acid synthesis. Bacterial nucleic acid synthesis is selectively attacked by this agent because bacteria, in contrast to humans, cannot use exogenous folate to metabolize proteins. Sulfonamides inhibit synthesis of dihydrofolic acid, an intermediate step in the formation of tetrahydrofolic acid. TMP, in turn, binds avidly to bacterial dihydrofolate reductase in preference to human dihydrofolate reductase, thereby preventing the formation of the active metabolite tetrahydrofolic acid[1] (Fig. 25–1). On occasion, the combination of TMP and SMX provides inhibitory or even synergistic activity for bacteria, even when the action of the individual components is not inhibitory. Thymidine synthesis seems to be the critical point of activity for TMP-SMX.

Bacteria develop resistance to TMP-SMX less frequently

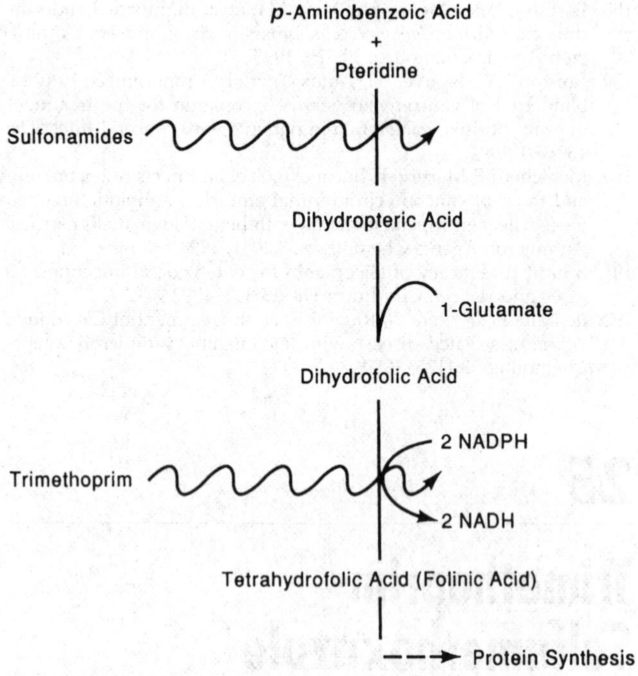

FIGURE 25–1 □ Competitive blockade of folinic acid by TMP-SMX.

than to either component. However, there has been an increase in the incidence of TMP resistance, superimposed on a background of considerable sulfonamide resistance.[2] Daycare centers, long-term care facilities, and intensive care units are reservoirs for TMP-SMX–resistant organisms.[3, 4] Susceptibility to TMP generally is more critical to the agent's effectiveness, as on occasion synergy is demonstrated despite sulfonamide resistance. TMP resistance can be mediated by several mechanisms: overproduction of dihydrofolate reductase by the bacteria; deletion of the thymidine requirement in protein synthesis; or impermeability to TMP. The most important mechanism of resistance is plasmid mediated and results in diminished affinity for TMP to dihydrofolate reductase.[5]

Pharmacokinetics

For most susceptible bacteria, maximal synergistic inhibition occurs at a serum ratio for TMP-SMX of 1:20. By preparing the drugs in a fixed 1:5 ratio, peak serum concentrations of TMP and SMX of approximately 1:20 are achieved by administration of the oral and parenteral compounds. Absorption, distribution, metabolism, and excretion of both compounds follow first-order kinetics.

Oral Administration

Both TMP and SMX are absorbed well from the gastrointestinal tract, even by patients with enteritis. The absorption of SMX and TMP after ingestion of the combination compound is comparable to that measured when the individual components are administered independently. Peak serum levels average approximately 1.75 μg/mL for TMP and 37.5 μg/mL for SMX after a single double-strength tablet is ingested by patients with normal renal function. The peak serum levels of TMP and SMX occur at 1 and 4 hours, respectively. One half to two thirds of both drugs is bound to plasma proteins.

Parenteral Administration

After intravenous infusion, peak concentrations of TMP and SMX are more predictable and occur more rapidly—in approximately 1 to 1.5 hours. After administration of two vials of TMP-SMX, the serum concentration of TMP is 3.5 μg/mL and that of SMX is 47.3 μg/mL. Although comparative distribution properties of intravenous and oral TMP-SMX have not been reported, it appears that cerebrospinal fluid (CSF) concentrations of TMP are enhanced by intravenous administration.[6]

Penetration of TMP and SMX into tissues and body fluids is not identical, often resulting in a therapeutic ratio that deviates from the presumed ideal serum ratio of 1:20. Although ratios of TMP to SMX in tissues and fluids range from 1:1 to 1:40, synergistic bacterial killing has been documented.[7] Less than 30% of TMP and SMX is metabolized, primarily via hepatic mechanisms. Approximately half of each drug's dose is excreted in the urine; however, nearly all the TMP is excreted in an active, nonmetabolized form, whereas only 20% of SMX is excreted intact.[8]

Tissue concentrations of SMX are generally less than the corresponding serum or plasma concentrations. The concurrent tissue concentrations for TMP often exceed those of SMX. In fact, TMP concentrations in saliva, breast milk, uninflamed prostatic tissue, seminal fluid, inflamed lung tissue, and bile often exceed those measured in the serum. Penetration of TMP-SMX into CSF is variable; concentration ranges of TMP vary from 20% to 60% of the levels obtained in the serum and those of SMX from 12% to 50%.

In patients with normal renal function, the half-life of TMP is 22 hours and that of SMX, 9 hours. The usual adult parenteral dosage is 2 to 3 vials every 8 hours administered intravenously; the typical oral dose is one single- or double-strength tablet every 12 hours. Dosage of TMP-SMX in children is based on the severity of the infectious process and on body weight: the usual oral dose is 8 mg/kg per day for TMP and 40 mg/kg per day for SMX given at 12-hour intervals; daily parenteral doses are based on 10 mg/kg for TMP and 50 mg/kg for SMX divided in three doses. The dose of TMP-SMX must be adjusted for patients with renal insufficiency, particularly when the creatinine clearance rate approaches 30 mL/min. For both oral and parenteral use, a single loading dose of TMP-SMX is given as if no renal impairment existed, followed by one half to one third of the usual amount administered at the same dose interval for the duration of therapy.

Hemodialysis effectively removes the metabolically unaltered and active forms of both TMP and SMX, but crystalluria can result, because the metabolized SMX derivatives are not removed by this process and the metabolized components can be deposited in the kidneys.[8, 9] Serum drug concentrations should be monitored in patients undergoing dialysis to help adjust the dosage. After a loading dose, follow-up doses (one half or one third of the original dose) are administered every 24 to 48 hours to patients undergoing dialysis.

The pharmacokinetics of TMP-SMX is not altered in patients with acquired immunodeficiency syndrome (AIDS), and no dosage adjustment is necessary when oral medication replaces the intravenous preparation.[10]

Adverse Reactions

Untoward reactions are associated with the administration of TMP-SMX in 6% to 8% of patients who do not have AIDS.[11, 12] Nearly half of the adverse reactions occur within 72 hours after oral administration.[13] Although toxicity can be life threatening, it is almost always reversible by stopping use of the drug (Table 25–1). The more common untoward reactions include gastrointestinal distress and cutaneous events, such as morbilliform rash and pruritus. Life-threatening side effects include hematologic abnormalities and severe skin reac-

TABLE 25–1 ■ Adverse Effects of Trimethoprim-Sulfamethoxazole

Anaphylaxis
Serum sickness
Cutaneous reactions
Morbilliform rash
Stevens-Johnson syndrome (exfoliative dermatitis)
Erythema multiforme
Toxic epidermal necrolysis
Photosensitivity rash
Hematologic reactions
Leukopenia
Thrombocytopenia
Agranulocytosis
Hemolytic anemia
Bone marrow suppression
Gastrointestinal reactions
Nausea
Vomiting
Diarrhea
Hepatotoxicity
Glossitis
Stomatitis
Pancreatitis
Altered taste
Pseudomembranous colitis
Neurologic reactions
Headache
Confusion
Peripheral neuropathy
Aseptic meningitis
Tremor
Acute psychosis
Fever
Nephrotoxicity
Phlebitis
Vasculitis
Pruritus (not associated with rash)
Hyperkalemia

tions, such as exfoliative dermatitis and toxic epidermal necrolysis.

Patients who are allergic to either component should not be given TMP-SMX. The hematologic reactions attributed to TMP-SMX are identical to those of sulfonamides, but it may not be the sulfonamides themselves that are responsible for the hypersensitivity reactions commonly ascribed to them. Preliminary evidence suggests that patients who are "slow acetylators" may be more prone to idiosyncratic adverse reactions from sulfonamides. Theoretically, slow acetylation shunts more drug into other metabolic pathways, specifically oxidative processes that produce toxic metabolites. Thus, metabolites of sulfa compounds, rather than the sulfonamide itself, are the agents incriminated in hypersensitivity and allergic reactions.[13, 14] By testing peripheral blood lymphocytes with sulfonamide hydroxylamine compounds, it may be possible to gauge the nature of the adverse reaction in advance, without endangering the patient.[14] Acetylator phenotype is also a risk factor that predisposes patients infected with human immunodeficiency virus (HIV) to hypersensitivity events.[15] A CD4/CD8 ratio higher than 0.10 and treatment for less than 14 days are independently predictive of drug-induced hypersensitivity for HIV-infected patients.

TMP-SMX should not be prescribed to patients who have a folic acid deficiency state or glucose-6-phosphate dehydrogenase deficiency or those who are pregnant. Teratogenicity is a potential risk. Long-term use of TMP-SMX has been associated with evidence of altered folate metabolism.[16] Coadministration of folinic acid may reduce or prevent the antifolate activity of TMP-SMX without interfering with its antimicrobial activity.[17]

Several adverse effects of TMP-SMX have unique associations. Thrombocytopenia seems to be more frequent in elderly patients receiving thiazide diuretic therapy.[18] A higher incidence of reversible neutropenia can be demonstrated in children receiving TMP-SMX parenterally.[19] Crystalluria with resultant renal insufficiency can occur in hypoalbuminemic patients.[20]

Parenteral administration of TMP-SMX has resulted in the development of reversible hyperkalemia.[21–23] The compound appears to resemble the drug amiloride, an agent that impedes renal potassium secretion.

Although not an untoward reaction, fluid overload due to the dilution requirements of parenterally administered TMP-SMX can present a challenge. The manufacturers recommend that 125 mL of 5% dextrose solution be used for each vial of TMP-SMX (80 mg of TMP, 400 mg of SMX). On occasion, 12 to 16 vials per day are required to treat life-threatening infections. Patients whose fluids are restricted or who have congestive heart failure or precarious fluid-electrolyte balance may be unable to tolerate the extra fluid, which can amount to 2 L/d. The amount of additional fluid can be limited by diluting each ampule with only 75 mL of 5% dextrose solution as long as the mixture is administered within 2 hours.

TMP-SMX has the potential to interact with additional prescribed medications, including procainamide and cyclosporine. The anticoagulant effect of warfarin is enhanced when this drug is administered with TMP-SMX.[24] Serum levels of phenytoin can become elevated because TMP-SMX inhibits its metabolic clearance, and this can result in toxic side effects. Moreover, TMP-SMX can potentiate the hypoglycemic effects of oral sulfonylurea compounds.[25] When TMP-SMX is coadministered with methotrexate, enhanced bone marrow suppression can result.

Antimicrobial Spectrum

Many gram-positive and gram-negative bacteria are susceptible to TMP-SMX.[26] It is important to realize, however, that this compound possesses minimal if any anaerobic inhibitory activity. Synergy for bacterial inhibition is demonstrated even when microorganisms are resistant to SMX and moderately resistant to TMP. A maximal synergistic action occurs when microbes are susceptible to both drugs.

Many gram-positive aerobic cocci are inhibited by TMP-SMX in vitro. Among the organisms that are susceptible to TMP-SMX are some strains of *Staphylococcus aureus*, including some methicillin-resistant variants; *Staphylococcus saprophyticus*; some group A β-hemolytic streptococci; *Streptococcus agalactiae*; and most but not all *Streptococcus pneumoniae*.[26] *Enterococcus faecalis* is often resistant to TMP-SMX, and resistance can develop during therapy. *Corynebacterium diphtheriae* is inhibited by TMP-SMX in vitro.

Many gram-negative cocci are susceptible to TMP-SMX. It usually inhibits *Neisseria meningitidis*, some but not all strains of *Neisseria gonorrhoeae*, and *Branhamella (Moraxella) catarrhalis*. Gram-negative aerobic bacilli are often susceptible to its inhibitory activity. *Escherichia coli*, many *Klebsiella* spp., *Citrobacter (C. diversus* and *C. freundii)*, *Enterobacter* spp. (including *E. cloacae*, *E. aerogenes*, and *E. agglomerans*), some *Salmonella* and some *Shigella* spp., most strains of *Haemophilus influenzae* (including some ampicillin-resistant strains), some strains of *Haemophilus ducreyi*, *Morganella morganii*, *Proteus (P. vulgaris* and *P. mirabilis)*, and some *Serratia* spp. are susceptible to TMP-SMX. Other commonly susceptible gram-negative bacilli include *Acinetobacter* spp., *Providencia rettgeri* and *Providencia stuartii*, and *Aeromonas*, *Brucella*, and *Yersinia* spp. *Xanthomonas maltophilia*, formerly *Pseudomonas maltophilia*, is inhibited in vitro by TMP-SMX, and this compound has emerged as one of the preferred treatments for patients infected with this organism. *Pseudomonas aeruginosa* is invariably resistant to TMP-SMX, but the compound has shown inhibitory activity for other *Pseudomonas* species, such as *Pseudomonas cepacia*.

TMP-SMX has also inhibitory activity directed at a variety of additional organisms, including *Nocardia asteroides, Pneumocystis carinii*, some strains of *Chlamydia trachomatis, Listeria monocytogenes*, some nontuberculous *Mycobacterium* species (including *M. marinum, M. kansasii*, and *M. scrofulaceum*), *Isospora belli*, and *Pseudomonas pseudomallei*.

Therapeutic Uses

Genitourinary Tract Infections

TMP-SMX is effective therapy for acute, symptomatic urinary tract infections—namely, urethritis, cystitis, and pyelonephritis—caused by susceptible bacteria. Single-dose therapy (two double-strength tablets) has been an acceptable treatment for young women with acute, uncomplicated cystitis, but this treatment course remains less effective than the traditional 10-day course of therapy.[27] A 3-day course of therapy is appropriate for most young women with acute bacterial cystitis.[28] TMP-SMX has an established track record in treating women with acute symptomatic, nonobstructive, community-acquired pyelonephritis,[29] and it has been used successfully when administered for 6 weeks to treat men with invasive infection of the urinary tract.[30] The availability of an intravenous preparation provides an additional dimension for patients who require hospitalization. The efficacy of long-term prophylaxis with TMP-SMX to prevent recurrent cystitis among young women has been consistently confirmed.[31–34] Half of a single-strength tablet per day or one single-strength tablet every other day is effective.

Therapy with TMP-SMX has been used successfully to treat acute and chronic bacterial prostatitis. The parenteral form of this agent is a useful adjunct to surgery for prostatic abscess caused by susceptible bacteria.

Previously, TMP-SMX was an appropriate therapeutic choice for some patients with chancroid, a sexually transmitted infection caused by *H. ducreyi*. However, the emergence of resistant strains is being reported throughout the world, and TMP-SMX is no longer the preferred therapy.

Respiratory Tract Infections

TMP-SMX has demonstrated efficacy in the treatment of patients with community-acquired otitis media and sinusitis[35] as well as acute exacerbation of chronic bronchitis and pneumonia. The compound provides some distinct advantages for therapy of these infections: it is an inexpensive drug that inhibits the growth of most strains of *S. pneumoniae, B. catarrhalis*, and most strains (both ampicillin susceptible and resistant) of *H. influenzae*; it can be administered orally or parenterally, and it often represents a therapeutic alternative for the patient who is allergic to penicillin.

Nosocomial pneumonias caused by susceptible strains of facultative aerobic gram-negative bacilli have also been treated successfully with TMP-SMX as exclusive therapy or as one component of a combination regimen.

Intestinal Infections

TMP-SMX is one of the preferred drugs for infectious diarrhea when the patient requires an antimicrobial agent in addition to fluid replacement and correction of electrolyte imbalance. It has a role in the therapy of enterocolitis caused by susceptible strains of *Shigella*, enterotoxigenic *E. coli, Aeromonas hydrophila*,[36] *Plesiomonas shigelloides*,[37, 38] *Cyclospora*,[39] and *I. belli*.[40–42]

Selected patients with *Salmonella* enterocolitis—namely, those with an aneurysm, a lymphoproliferative disease, a prosthesis, an organ transplant, or AIDS,[43, 44] who are at enhanced risk of morbidity and mortality if bacteremia develops—are potential candidates for TMP-SMX treatment. This compound is one of a number of agents that could be offered to these patients as well as to patients with extraintestinal disease caused by *Salmonella* spp. and *Yersinia enterocolitica*.

TMP-SMX is one option for the prevention of traveler's diarrhea for those patients (with selective associated disorders) who plan to enter the interior of Mexico.[45] The increased resistance of bacterial enteropathogens has reduced the current role of TMP-SMX as therapy for traveler's dysentery.

Prophylaxis with TMP-SMX is efficacious, safe, and cost-effective for prevention of spontaneous bacterial peritonitis in patients with cirrhosis.[46]

Infections in Neutropenic Hosts

The majority of infections in neutropenic patients arise from endogenous microbial flora. When gastrointestinal epithelial surfaces are damaged by the disease process or chemotherapy, infections often result. Patients with hematologic or lymphoreticular malignancies are at particular risk, especially during induction therapy. If transmigration of pathogens is prevented, the incidence of infectious complications may be reduced. In some studies, TMP-SMX has been employed successfully as prophylaxis, presumably because of its selective decontamination of gut flora.[47, 48] Although enterococci, resistant gram-negative aerobic bacilli, anaerobes, and fungi are not inhibited, a reduction in the number of infections caused by susceptible gram-negative bacteria has been noted. The prophylactic use of TMP-SMX in leukopenic patients has, however, on occasion, been associated with the emergence of infections caused by fungi and resistant gram-negative bacilli. The usual prophylactic dose is one double-strength tablet twice daily until the neutropenia resolves.

TMP-SMX has also proved to be an effective component of empirical antibiotic therapy for febrile neutropenic patients.[46, 49] This compound penetrates throughout the body, is relatively free of toxic effects, and inhibits many bacteria that are often responsible for infections in these patients. This agent may be particularly useful in penicillin-allergic, febrile, granulocytic patients, especially when combined with an aminoglycoside to treat susceptible aerobic gram-negative bacillary infections.

Miscellaneous Indications

TMP-SMX has proved to be effective therapy for meningitis caused by susceptible strains of *S. pneumoniae, N. meningitidis, H. influenzae*, and *L. monocytogenes*[50]; thus, it represents an alternative treatment for patients who are allergic to penicillin. It can be considered appropriate therapy for patients with gram-negative meningitis caused by a susceptible strain, especially when the patient cannot tolerate third-generation cephalosporins. This drug has also emerged as one of the preferred treatments for respiratory or central nervous system infection caused by *N. asteroides*.[51] Combined with polymyxin B or an aminoglycoside, it has been used successfully to treat endocarditis caused by *P. cepacia* and *X. maltophilia*.[52] Limited data indicate that when vancomycin therapy is precluded, TMP-SMX could represent an option for the treatment of selected patients with infection caused by methicillin-resistant *S. aureus*.[53] When added to the standard cyclosphosphamide-corticosteroid treatment, or, alternatively, administered as the exclusive therapy, TMP-SMX appears to be useful in the therapy of Wegener granulomatosis.[54–57]

Pneumocystis carinii *Infections*

The efficacy of TMP-SMX in the prophylaxis and treatment of *P. carinii* pneumonia (PCP) was established before the AIDS epidemic.[58–62] Daily prophylaxis with low-dose TMP-SMX or thrice-weekly administration of the compound are both accepted strategies to prevent the development of PCP in immunosuppressed persons, particularly those with organ transplants, systemic necrotizing vasculitis, and malignancies. This drug is the preferred treatment for the primary and secondary prevention of PCP in the patient with AIDS and is the therapy of choice for the patient with established PCP.[63–66] However, HIV-infected recipients of TMP-SMX often experience untoward events.[67] Adverse events usually do not develop in the first week of treatment. Anemia, neutropenia, and azotemia increase with increasing TMP plasma concentrations, whereas other untoward events (gastrointestinal adverse reactions, rash, fever, and liver function abnormalities) are independent of plasma concentration of TMP or SMX.[68] When adverse reactions develop, consideration should be given to discontinuing therapy, with the possibility of rechallenge or desensitization in the future.[69–72] Guidelines for desensitization have been published.[73, 74] Decisions regarding discontinuation and subsequent reintroduction will be predicated on the nature of the untoward event, the urgency of treatment, and the availability of alternative therapies. Unfortunately, however, the extent of initial TMP-SMX–induced toxicity may not correlate with the severity of reactions associated with readministration of the drug, and, in fact, patients who have previously manifested intolerance to TMP-SMX are at risk of developing life-endangering anaphylactoid reactions ("re-challenge" reactions) when this medication is readministered.[74]

The untoward effects of TMP-SMX for patients with AIDS are often identical to those for other persons (see Table 25–1), but HIV-infected patients appear to be unusually predisposed to develop fever, maculopapular eruptions, gastrointestinal symptoms, peripheral blood cytopenias, and, rarely, tremors.[75] The bone marrow–suppressive effect of TMP-SMX is of particular concern in patients with AIDS, because the disease itself, neoplasms, and opportunistic infections can invade the bone marrow; moreover, the drugs often prescribed to these patients, such as zidovudine and ganciclovir, have the potential to cause neutropenia and thrombocytopenia. An acute hypotensive event, resembling septic shock, has occurred in HIV-infected patients prescribed TMP-SMX.[76]

TMP-SMX has caused both hepatocellular and cholestatic liver injury. Intrahepatic cholestasis produced by this medication can be severe and may persist for years after the drug is discontinued.

The daily dose of TMP-SMX traditionally used to treat PCP in immunocompromised hosts is 15 to 20 mg/kg for TMP and 100 mg/kg for SMX. When untoward reactions occur during treatment, a reduced daily dose of 10 to 12 mg/kg for TMP has proved to be as effective as the usual dose and to cause fewer adverse reactions. The administration of corticosteroid to the AIDS patient with PCP appears to reduce the incidence of adverse skin reactions attributed to TMP-SMX.[77] The coadministration of folinic acid and TMP-SMX, designed to reduce the number of TMP-SMX–induced side effects, has, in fact, been reported to result in the recovery of fewer patients treated for PCP.[78]

Miscellaneous Infections Associated with HIV Infection

TMP-SMX is appropriate therapy for patients with infectious diarrhea associated with *I. belli* and *Cyclospora* and invasive disease caused by susceptible strains of *Salmonella*.[79–82] Limited studies also indicate a role for TMP-SMX for the prophylaxis and treatment of *Toxoplasma gondii* encephalitis.[83, 84] It has been observed that HIV-infected patients who receive prophylactic TMP-SMX to prevent PCP appear to be at reduced risk for toxoplasmic encephalitis, bacterial pneumonias, and infectious diarrhea caused by *I. belli* and *Salmonella* spp.[67, 84]

References

1. Burchall JJ, Hitchings GH: Inhibitor-binding analysis of dihydrofolate reductases from various species. Mol Pharmacol 1:126, 1965.
2. Huovinen P, Sundström L, Swedberg G, et al: Trimethoprim and sulfonamide resistance. Antimicrob Agents Chemother 39:279, 1995.
3. Wingard E, Shlaes JH, Mortimer EA, et al: Colonization and cross-colonization of nursing home patients with trimethoprim-resistant gram-negative bacilli. Clin Infect Dis 16:75, 1993.
4. Fornasini M, Reves RR, Murray BE, et al: Trimethoprim-resistant *Escherichia coli* in households of children attending day care centers. J Infect Dis 166:326, 1994.
5. Cockerill FR III, Edson RS: Trimethoprim-sulfamethoxazole. Mayo Clin Proc 62:921, 1987.
6. Svedhem A, Iwarson S: Cerebrospinal fluid concentrations of trimethoprim during oral and parenteral treatment. J Antimicrob Chemother 5:717, 1979.
7. Hansen I: The combination trimethoprim-sulfamethoxazole. Antibiot Chemother 25:217, 1978.
8. Rubin RH, Swartz MN: Trimethoprim-sulfamethoxazole. N Engl J Med 303:426, 1980.
9. Craig WA, Kunin CM: Trimethoprim-sulfamethoxazole. Pharmacodynamic effects of urinary pH and impaired renal function: Studies in humans. Ann Intern Med 78:491, 1973.
10. Chin TWF, Vandenbroucke A, Fong IW: Pharmacokinetics of trimethoprim-sulfamethoxazole in critically ill and non–critically ill AIDS patients. Antimicrob Agents Chemother 39:28, 1995.
11. Jick H: Adverse reactions to trimethoprim-sulfamethoxazole in hospitalized patients. Rev Infect Dis 4:426, 1982.
12. Lawson DH, Jick H: Adverse reactions to co-trimoxazole in hospitalized medical patients. Am J Med Sci 275:53, 1978.
13. Shear NH, Speilberg SP, Grant DM, et al: Differences in metabolism of sulfonamides predisposing to idiosyncratic toxicity. Ann Intern Med 105:179, 1986.
14. Rieder MJ, Vetrecht J, Shear NH, et al: Diagnosis of sulfonamide hypersensitivity reactions by in vitro "rechallenge" with hydroxylamine metabolites. Ann Intern Med 110:286, 1989.
15. Carr A, Gross AS, Hoskins JM et al: Acetylation phenotype and cutaneous hypersensitivity to trimethroprim-sulphamethoxazole in HIV-infected patients. AIDS 8:333, 1994.
16. Kahn SB, Fein SA, Brodsky I: Effect of trimethoprim on folate metabolism in man. Clin Pharmacol Ther 9:550, 1968.
17. Gleckman R, Alvarez S, Joubert DW: Drug therapy reviews: Trimethoprim-sulfamethoxazole. Am J Hosp Pharm 36:893, 1979.
18. Frisch JM: Clinical experience with adverse reactions to trimethoprim-sulfamethoxazole. J Infect Dis 128(Suppl):607, 1973.
19. Ardati KO, Thirumoorthi MC, Oajani AS: Intravenous trimethoprim-sulfamethoxazole in the treatment of serious infection in children. J Pediatr 95:801, 1979.
20. Buchanan N: Sulphamethoxazole, hypoalbuminaemia, crystalluria, and renal failure. Br Med J 2:172, 1978.
21. Greenberg S, Reiser IN, Chou SY, et al: Trimethoprim-sulfamethoxazole induces reversible hyperkalemia. Ann Intern Med 119:291, 1993.
22. Choi MJ, Fernandez PC, Patnaik A, et al: Trimethoprim-induced hyperkalemia in a patient with AIDS. N Engl J Med 328:703, 1993.

23. Velázquez H, Perazella MA, Wright FS, et al: Renal mechanism of trimethoprim-induced hyperkalemia. Ann Intern Med 119:296, 1993.
24. O'Reilly RA: Stereoselective interaction of trimethoprim-sulfamethoxazole with the separated enantiomorphs of racemic warfarin in man. N Engl J Med 302:33, 1980.
25. Lawson DH, Paice BJ: Adverse reactions to trimethoprim-sulfamethoxazole. Rev Infect Dis 4:429, 1982.
26. Bushby SRM: Trimethoprim-sulfamethoxazole: In vitro microbiological aspects. J Infect Dis 128(Suppl):442, 1973.
27. Fihn SD, Johnson C, Roberts PL, et al: Trimethoprim-sulfamethoxazole for acute dysuria in women: A single-dose or 10-day course. Ann Intern Med 108:350, 1988.
28. Hooton JM, Winter C, Tiu F, et al: Randomized comparative trial and cost analysis of 3-day antimicrobial regimens for treatment of acute cystitis in women. JAMA 273:41, 1995.
29. Stamm WE, McKevitt M, Counts GW: Acute renal infection in women: Treatment with trimethoprim-sulfamethoxazole or ampicillin for 2 or 6 weeks. A randomized trial. Ann Intern Med 106:341, 1987.
30. Gleckman R, Crowley M, Natsios GA: Treatment of recurrent invasive urinary tract infections of men. N Engl J Med 301:878, 1979.
31. Harding GKM, Ronald AR: A controlled study of antimicrobial prophylaxis of recurrent urinary tract infection in women. N Engl J Med 291:597, 1974.
32. Harding GKM, Buckwold FJ, Marrie TJ, et al: Prophylaxis of recurrent urinary tract infection in female patients. Efficacy of low-dose, thrice-weekly therapy with trimethoprim-sulfamethoxazole. JAMA 242:1975, 1979.
33. Stamm WE, Counts GW, Wagner KF, et al: Antimicrobial prophylaxis of recurrent urinary tract infections: A double-blind, placebo-controlled trial. Ann Intern Med 92:770, 1980.
34. Nicolle LE, Harding GKM, Thomson M, et al: Efficacy of five years of continuous, low-dose trimethoprim-sulfamethoxazole prophylaxis for urinary tract infection. J Infect Dis 158:1239, 1988.
35. Williams JW Jr, Holleman DR Jr, Samsa GP, et al: Randomized controlled trial of 3 vs 10 days of trimethoprim/sulfamethoxazole for acute maxillary sinusitis. JAMA 273:1015, 1995.
36. Holmberg SD, Schell WL, Fanning GR, et al: *Aeromonas* intestinal infections in the United States. Ann Intern Med 105:683, 1986.
37. Brenden RA, Miller MA, Janda SM: Clinical disease spectrum and pathogenic factors associated with *Plesiomonas shigelloides* infections in humans. Rev Infect Dis 10:303, 1988.
38. Holmberg SD, Wachsmuth K, Hickman-Brenner FN, et al: *Plesiomonas* enteric infection in the United States. Ann Intern Med 105:690, 1986.
39. Hoge CH, Shlim DR, Ghimire M, et al: Placebo-controlled trial of co-trimoxazole for *Cyclospora* infections among travellers and foreign residents in Nepal. Lancet 345:691, 1995.
40. DeHovitz JA: Management of *Isospora belli* infections in AIDS patients. Infect Med 5:437, 1988.
41. Weiss LM, Perlman DC, Sherman J, et al: *Isospora belli* infection: Treatment with pyrimethamine. Ann Intern Med 109:474, 1988.
42. Pape J, Verdier R-I, Johnson W Jr: Treatment and prophylaxis of *Isospora belli* infection in patients with the acquired immunodeficiency syndrome. N Engl J Med 320:1044, 1990.
43. Celum CL, Chaisson RI, Rutherford GW, et al: Incidence of salmonellosis in patients with AIDS. J Infect Dis 156:998, 1987.
44. Jacobs JL, Gold JW, Murray HW, et al: *Salmonella* infections in patients with the acquired immunodeficiency syndrome. Ann Intern Med 102:186, 1985.
45. Dupont HL, Ericsson CD: Prevention and treatment of traveler's diarrhea. N Engl J Med 328:1821, 1993.
46. Singh N, Gayowski T, Yu VL, et al: Trimethoprim-sulfamethoxazole for the prevention of spontaneous bacterial peritonitis in cirrhosis: A randomized trial. Ann Intern Med 122:595, 1995.
47. EORTC International Antimicrobial Therapy Project Group: Trimethoprim-sulfamethoxazole in the prevention of infection in neutropenic patients. J Infect Dis 150:372, 1984.
48. DePauw BE, Novakova IRO, Ubachs E, et al: Co-trimoxazole in patients with haemotologic malignancies: A review of 10 years' clinical experience. Curr Med Res Opin 11:64, 1988.
49. Stuart RK, Braine HG, Lietman PS, et al: Carbenicillin-trimethoprim-sulfamethoxazole versus carbenicillin-gentimicin as empiric antibiotic therapy of infection in granulocytopenic patients. Am J Med 68:876, 1980.
50. Spitzer PG, Hammer SM, Karchmer AVV: Treatment of *Listeria monocytogenes* infection with trimethoprim-sulfamethoxazole: Case report and review of the literature. Rev Infect Dis 8:427, 1986.
51. Smego RA, Moeller MB, Gallis HA: Trimethoprim-sulfamethoxazole therapy for *Nocardia* infections. Arch Intern Med 143:711, 1983.
52. Street AC, Durack DT: Experience with trimethoprim-sulfamethoxazole in treatment of infective endocarditis. Rev Infect Dis 10:915, 1988.
53. Markowitz N, Quinn EL, Saravolatz LD: Trimethoprim-sulfamethoxazole compared with vancomycin for the treatment of *Staphylococcus aureus* infection. Ann Intern Med 117:390, 1992.
54. DeRemee RA, McDonald TJ, Weiland LH: Wegener's granulomatosis: Observations on treatment with antimicrobial agents. Mayo Clin Proc 60:27, 1985.
55. West BC, Todd JR, King JW: Wegener's granulomatosis and trimethoprim-sulfamethoxazole: Complete remission after a twenty-year course. Ann Intern Med 106:840, 1987.
56. Spiera H, Lawson W, Weinrauch H: Wegener's granulomatosis treated with sulfamethoxazole-trimethoprim. Report of a case. Arch Intern Med 148:2065, 1988.
57. Israel HL: Sulfamethoxazole-trimethoprim therapy for Wegener's granulomatosis. Arch Intern Med 148:2293, 1988.
58. Hughes WT, Rivera GK, Schell MJ, et al: Successful intermittent chemoprophylaxis for *Pneumocystis carinii* pneumonia. N Engl J Med 316:1627, 1987.
59. Hughes WT: Five-year *Pneumocystis* pneumonitis-free survival in an oncology center. J Infect Dis 150:305, 1984.
60. Hughes WT, NcNobb PC, Malcres TD, et al: Efficacy of trimethoprim and sulfamethoxazole in the prevention and treatment of *Pneumocystis carinii* pneumonitis. J Infect Dis 128:607, 1973.
61. Hughes WT, Feldman S, Chaudhary SC, et al: Comparison of pentamidine isethionate and trimethoprim-sulfamethoxazole in the treatment of *Pneumocystis carinii* pneumonia. J Pediatr 92:285, 1978.
62. Siegel SE, Wolff LJ, Baehner RL, Hammond D: Treatment of *Pneumocystis carinii* pneumonitis. A comparative trial of sulfamethoxazole-tremethoprim v pentamidine in pediatric patients with cancer: Report from the Children's Cancer Study Group. Am J Dis Child 138:1051, 1984.
63. Wharton JM, Coleman DL, Wofsy CB, et al: Trimethoprim-sulfamethoxazole or pentamidine for *Pneumocystis carinii* pneumonia in the acquired immunodeficiency syndrome. A prospective randomized trial. Ann Intern Med 105:37, 1986.
64. Sattler FR, Cowan R, Nielsen DM, et al: Trimethoprim-sulfamethoxazole compared with pentamidine for treatment of *Pneumocystis carinii* pneumonia in the acquired immunodeficiency syndrome: A prospective, noncrossover study. Ann Intern Med 109:280, 1988.
65. Montgomery AB, Feigal DW Jr, Sattler F, et al: Pentamidine aerosol versus trimethoprim-sulfamethoxazole for *Pneumocystis carinii* in acquired immune deficiency syndrome. Am J Respir Crit Care Med 151:1068, 1995.
66. Gallant JE, Moore RD, Chaisson RE. Prophylaxis for opportunistic infections in patients with HIV infection. Ann Intern Med 120:932, 1994.
67. Jung AC, Paauw DS. Management of adverse reactions to trimethoprim-sulfamethoxazole in human immunodeficiency virus–infected patients. Arch Intern Med 154:2402, 1994.
68. Hughes WT, LaFon SW, Scott JD, et al: Adverse events associated with trimethoprim-sulfamethoxazole and atovaquone during the treatment of AIDS-related *Pneumocystis carinii* pneumonia. J Infect Dis 171:1295, 1995.
69. Shafer RW, Seitzman PA, Tapper ML: Successful prophylaxis of *Pneumocystis carinii* pneumonia with trimethoprim-sulfamethoxazole in AIDS patients with previous allergic reactions. J Acquir Immune Defic Syndr 2:389, 1989.
70. Carr A, Penny R, Cooper DA. Efficacy and safety of rechallenge with low-dose trimethoprim-sulphamethoxazole in previously hypersensitive HIV-infected patients. AIDS 7:65, 1993.
71. Hardy WD, Feinberg J, Finkelstein DM, et al: A controlled trial of trimethoprim-sulfamethoxazole or aerosolized pentamidine for secondary prophylaxis of *Pneumocystis carinii* pneumonia in patients with the acquired immunodeficiency syndrome. N Engl J Med 327:1842, 1992.

72. Bozzette SA, Finkelstein DM, Spector SA, et al: A randomized trial of three antipneumocystis agents in patients with advanced human immunodeficiency virus infection. N Engl J Med 332:693, 1995.
73. Absar N, Daneshuar H, Beall G: Desensitization to trimethoprim-sulfamethoxazole in HIV-infected patients. J Allergy Clin Immunol 93:1001, 1994.
74. Gluckstein D, Ruskin J: Rapid oral desensitization to trimethoprim-sulfamethoxazole (TMP-SMZ): Use in prophylaxis for *Pneumocystis carinii* pneumonia in patients with AIDS who were previously intolerant to TMP-SMZ. Clin Infect Dis 20:849, 1995.
75. Borucki MJ, Matzke DS, Pollard RB: Tremor induced by trimethoprim-sulfamethoxazole in patients with the acquired immunodeficiency syndrome (AIDS). Ann Intern Med 109:77, 1988.
76. Nguyen BY, Landucci DI, Cunnion RE, et al: A case of hyperdynamic shock caused by trimethoprim-sulfamethoxazole in which no tumor necrosis factor or features of anaphylaxis were detected. Clin Infect Dis 17:885, 1993.
77. Caumes E, Roudier C, Rogeaux O, et al: Effect of corticosteroids on the incidence of adverse cutaneous reactions to trimethoprim-sulfamethoxazole during treatment of AIDS-associated *Pneumocystis carinii* pneumonia. Clin Infect Dis 18:319, 1994.
78. Safrin S, Lee BL, Sande MA: Adjunctive folinic acid with trimethoprim-sulfamethoxazole for *Pneumocystis carinii* pneumonia in AIDS patients is associated with an increased risk of therapeutic failure and death. J Infect Dis 170:912, 1994.
79. Wurtz R: *Cyclospora*: A newly identified intestinal pathogen of humans. Clin Infect Dis 18:620, 1994.
80. Pape JW, Verdier RI, Boncy M, et al: *Cyclospora* infection in adults infected with HIV: Clinical manifestations, treatment, and prophylaxis. Ann Intern Med 121:654, 1994.
81. Pape JW, Verdier R, Johnson WD, et al: Treatment and prophylaxis of *Isospora belli* infection. N Engl J Med 320:1044, 1989.
82. Gruenewald R, Blum S, Chan J: Relationship between human immunodeficiency virus infection and salmonellosis in 20- to 59-year-old residents of New York City. Clin Infect Dis 18:358, 1994.
83. Canessa A, Del Bono V, DeLeo P, et al: Cotrimoxazole therapy for *Toxoplasma gondii* encephalitis in AIDS patients. Eur J Clin Microbiol Infect Dis 11:125, 1992.
84. Podzamczer D, Salazar A, Jimenez J, et al: Intermittent trimethoprim-sulfamethoxazole compared with dapsone-pyrimethamine for the simultaneous primary prophylaxis of *Pneumocystis* pneumonia and toxoplasmosis in patients infected with HIV. Ann Intern Med 122:755, 1995.

26

Quinolones

Vincent T. Andriole

The history of the newer quinolone antibacterial agents began with the introduction of nalidixic acid in 1962.[1] Oxolinic acid and cinoxacin were introduced in the 1970s. Shortly thereafter the insertion of a fluorine at the 6 position and a piperazine at the 7 position in the basic nucleus was observed to enhance and broaden the antibacterial activity of these agents. This procedure led to the discovery of newer quinolones with antibacterial activities 1000 times those of nalidixic acid.[2]

The clinical importance of the newer quinolones derives from their broad antibacterial spectrum, unique mechanism of action, good absorption from the gastrointestinal tract after oral administration, excellent tissue distribution, and low incidence of adverse reactions.[3]

Chemistry and Classification

The quinolone antibacterial agents are all structurally similar compounds. They can be divided into four general groups—naphthyridines, cinnolines, pyridopyrimidines, and quinolines (Fig. 26–1). A common skeleton, 4-oxo-1,4-dihydroquinolone (4-quinolone), is produced by adding an oxygen molecule at the 4 position in the basic nucleus.[2] The naphthyridines (nalidixic acid, enoxacin, tosufloxacin, and trovafloxacin), with an additional nitrogen in the 8 position, are 8-aza-4-quinolones. The cinnolines (cinoxacin), with an additional nitrogen in the 2 position, are 2-aza-4-quinolones. The pyridopyrimidines (pipemidic and piromidic acids), with additional nitrogens in the 6 and 8 positions, are 6,8-diaza-4-quinolones (Fig. 26–2). All of the other highly active agents (Fig. 26–3) are classified as 4-quinolones.[2, 3] Numerous additional compounds have been synthesized and are undergoing development.[3]

The 1,8-naphthyridine derivatives include nalidixic acid (1-ethyl-7-methyl-1,8-naphthyridin-4-one-3-carboxylic acid), enoxacin [1-ethyl-6-fluoro-1,4-dihydro-4-oxo-7-(1-piperazinyl)-1,8-naphthyridine-3-carboxylic acid], tosufloxacin [7-(3-amino-1-pyrrolidinyl)-1-(2,4-difluorophenyl)-6-fluoro-1,4-dihydro-4-oxo-1,8-naphthyridine-3-carboxylic acid], and trovafloxacin [7-(1*a*,5*a*,6*a*)-6-amino-3-azabicyclo[3.1.0]hex-3-yl)-6-fluoro-1-(2,4-difluorophenyl)-1,4-dihydro-4-oxo-1,8-naphthyridine-3-carboxylic acid]. Cinoxacin (1-ethyl-1,4-dihydro-4-oxo[1,3]dioxolo[4,5-g]cinnoline-3-carboxylic acid) is the only cinnoline derivative.[4] The quinoline derivatives include oxolinic acid (5-ethyl-5,8-dihydro-8-oxo-1,3-dioxolo[4,5-*g*]quinoline-7-carboxylic acid),[5–7] norfloxacin [1-ethyl-6-fluoro-1,4 dihydro-4-oxo-7-(1-piperazinyl)-3-quinolinecarboxylic acid],[8, 9] ciprofloxacin [1-cyclopropyl-6-fluoro-1,4-dihydro-4-oxo-7-(1-piperazinyl)-3-quinolinecarboxylic acid hydrochloride,[10] ofloxacin [9-fluoro-2,3-dihydro-3-methyl-10-(4-methyl-1-piperazinyl)-7-oxo-7*H*-pyrido[1,2,3-*de*]-1,4-benzoxazine-6-carboxylic acid], fleroxacin [6,8-difluoro-1-(2-fluoroethyl)-1,4-dihydro-7-(4-methyl-1-piperazinyl)-4-oxo-3-quinolinecarboxylic acid], lomefloxacin [1-ethyl-6,8-difluoro-1,4-dihydro-7-(3-methyl-1-piperazinyl)-4-oxo-3-quinolinecarboxylic acid], pefloxacin [1-ethyl-6-fluoro-1,4-dihydro-7-(4-methyl-1-piperazinyl)-4-oxo-3-quinolinecarboxylic acid],[3] sparfloxacin [5-amino-1-cyclopropyl-7-(*cis*-3,5-dimethyl-1-piperazinyl)-6,8-difluoro-1,4-dihydro-4-oxo-3-quinolinecarboxylic acid],[11, 12] clinafloxacin [7-(3-amino-1-pyrrolidinyl)-8-chloro-1-cyclopropyl-6-fluoro-1,4-dihydro-4-oxo-3-quinolinecarboxylic acid],[13] and levofloxacin [(−)-(*S*)-9-fluoro-2,3-dihydro-3-methyl-10-(4-methyl-1-piperazinyl)-7-oxo-7*H*-pyrido[1,2,3,-*de*] [1,4] benzoxazine-6-carboxylic acid].[3, 11–14] Many other newer quinolone compounds are being developed.[3, 12]

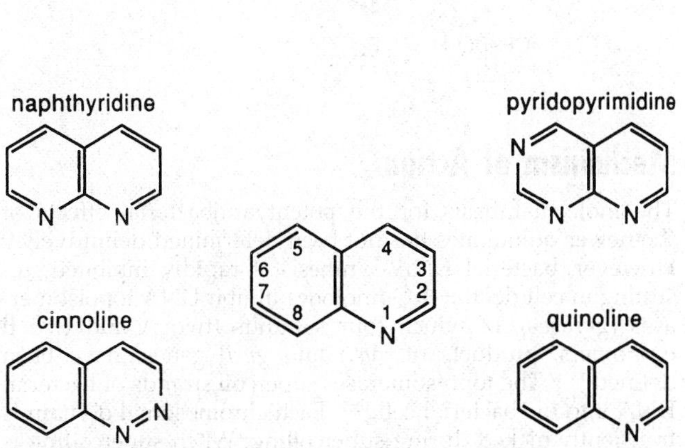

FIGURE 26–1 ▫ Chemical structure of the four general groups of the 4-quinolones and the system of ring numbering.

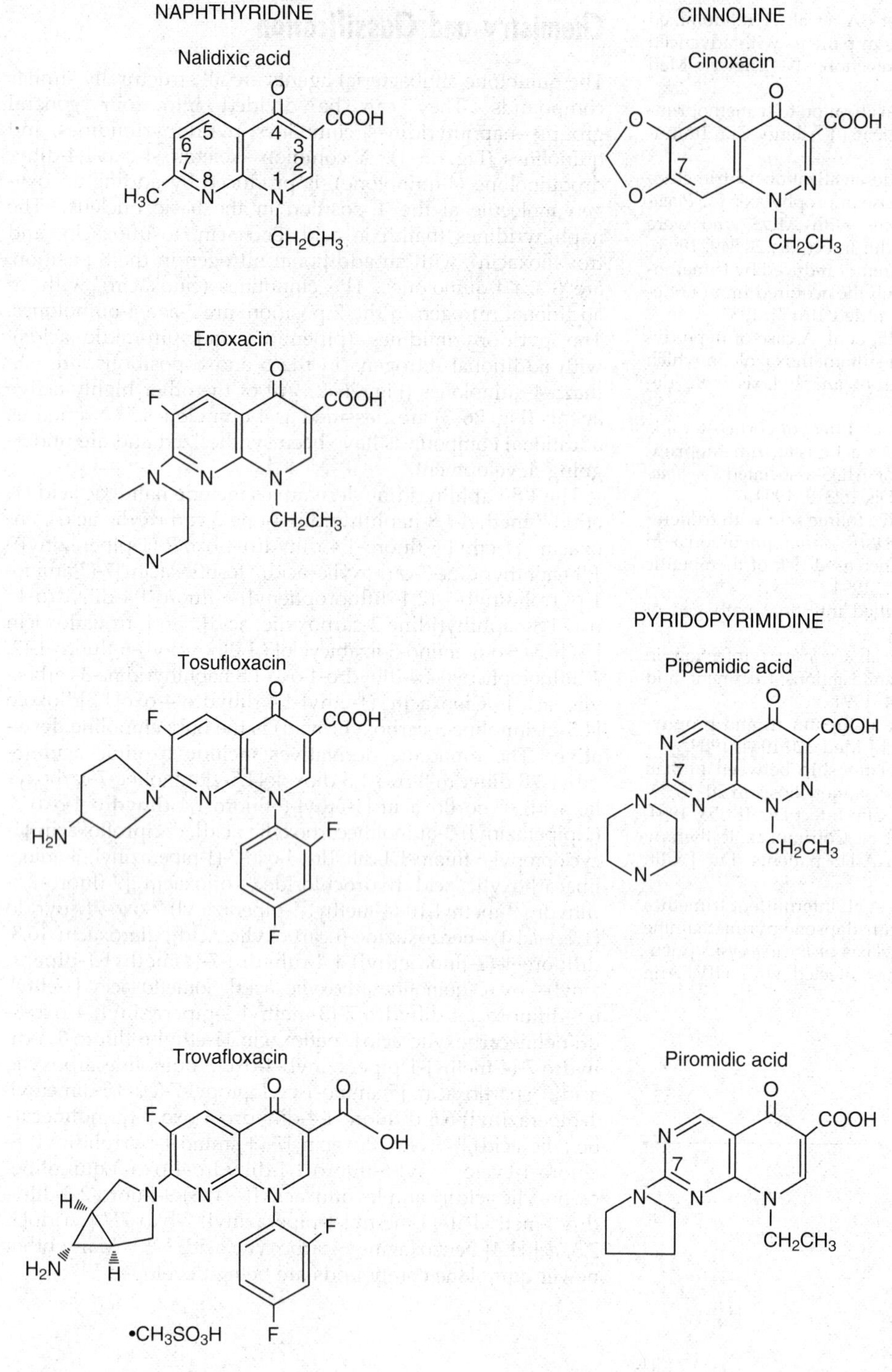

FIGURE 26–2 □ Structures of naphthyridine, cinnoline, and pyridopyrimidine derivatives.

Mechanism of Action

The molecular basis for the potent antibacterial effects of the newer quinolones has not been determined definitively.[15] However, bacterial DNA synthesis is rapidly inhibited, resulting in cell death.[2, 15] Quinolones inhibit DNA topoisomerases (gyrases), of which four subunits (two A and two B monomers, products of *gyrA* and *gyrB* genes) have been defined.[16, 17] The topoisomerases supercoil strands of bacterial DNA into the bacterial cell.[18, 19] Each chromosomal domain is transiently nicked during supercoiling. When supercoiling is completed, an enzyme seals the nicked DNA. The enzyme, identified by Gellert and coworkers[20] and termed DNA gyrase or topoisomerase II (nicking-closing enzyme), nicks double-stranded chromosomal DNA, introduces supercoils, and seals the nicked DNA.[2, 3, 20–22] The A subunits are thought to introduce the nicks, the B subunits to supercoil, and then the A subunits to seal the nick they produced initially.[2, 22] Quinolones bind to the DNA–DNA gyrase complex.[23] Quinolones also inhibit topoisomerase IV, the specific role of which has not yet been defined.[24] The bacterial activity of the 4-quinolones is reduced significantly if RNA or protein synthesis is inhibited.[25] Although all 4-quinolones are bactericidal, these drugs have a single most bactericidal concentration and in greater or lesser concentrations kill fewer bacteria.[2, 26] This paradoxical effect of decreased killing at higher concentrations is most likely the result of dose-dependent inhibition of RNA synthesis.[2, 26] Also, some quinolones may kill by more than one mechanism.[27] Other non-antibacterial quinolone compounds, particularly those with acetyl substituents on the C-7 piperazine ring, have potent activity against eukaryotic topoisomerase II and may prove useful as antitumor agents.[28]

Antimicrobial Activity

Table 26–1 presents an overview of the antimicrobial activity of selected 4-quinolones in vitro. The newer quinolones are quite active against enteric gram-negative aerobic bacteria and against other aerobic gram-negative organisms including gram-negative cocci, that is, *Branhamella (Moraxella) catarrhalis*

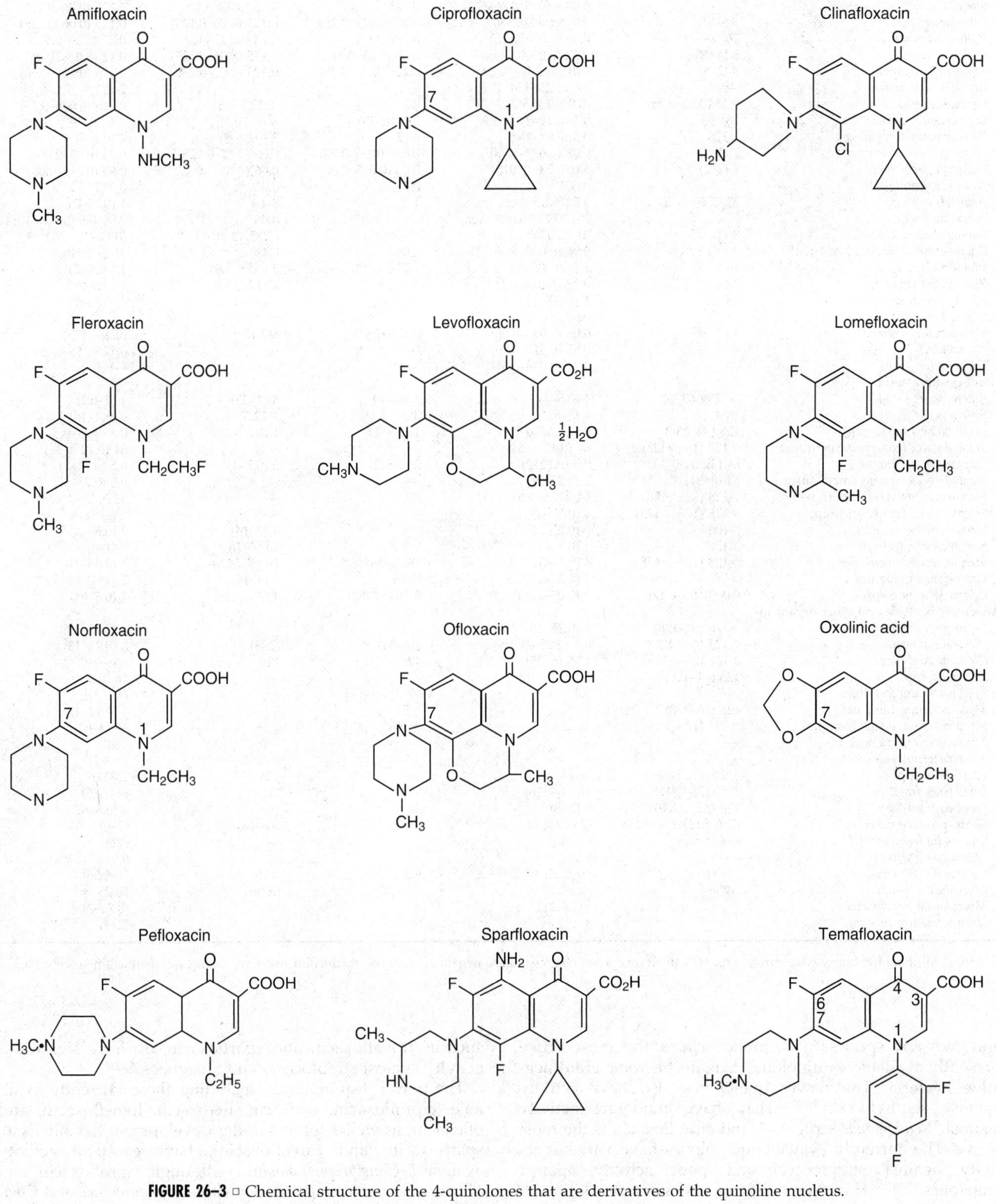

FIGURE 26–3 □ Chemical structure of the 4-quinolones that are derivatives of the quinoline nucleus.

TABLE 26–1 ■ In Vitro Antimicrobial Activity of Selected 4-Quinolones*

	MIC$_{90}$ (RANGE) (μg/mL)				
ORGANISM	**Nalidixic Acid**	**Ciprofloxacin**	**Enoxacin**	**Norfloxacin**	**Ofloxacin**
Gram-negative aerobes					
Escherichia coli	8 (4–128)	0.03 (0.015–0.06)	0.5 (0.25–1)	0.125 (0.06–0.5)	0.125 (0.06–0.25)
Klebsiella pneumoniae	8 (1–128)	0.125 (0.06–0.25)	0.5	0.25 (0.125–1)	0.25 (0.03–0.25)
Enterobacter spp.	32 (4–128)	0.125 (0.03–0.5)	0.5 (0.25–4)	0.5 (0.125–2)	0.5 (0.125–1)
Citrobacter spp.	8 (4–>100)	0.03 (0.03–0.06)	0.5	0.25 (0.125–0.5)	0.5 (0.03–2)
Serratia marcescens	>128 (16–>256)	0.25 (0.06–0.5)	2 (0.5–4)	1 (0.5–8)	1 (0.25–2)
Shigella spp.	4	0.03 (0.015–0.06)	0.125	0.06 (0.03–0.125)	0.125 (0.06–0.125)
Salmonella spp.	8 (4–8)	0.015 (≤0.015–0.03)	0.25 (0.125–0.25)	0.125 (0.06–0.125)	0.125 (0.06–0.125)
Proteus mirabilis	16 (4–32)	0.06 (0.03–0.125)	0.5 (0.25–1)	0.25 (0.125–0.5)	0.25 (0.25–0.5)
Proteus vulgaris	8 (4–16)	0.12 (0.03–0.25)	0.25 (0.25–0.5)	0.125 (0.06–0.125)	0.12 (0.03–1)
Morganella morganii	8 (2–8)	0.015 (0.015–0.03)	0.125 (0.03–0.25)	0.125 (0.03–0.25)	0.125 (0.125–0.25)
Brucella melitensis	—	0.5 (0.25–0.5)	—	—	2
Legionella spp.	0.25 (0.12–0.25)	(0.03–0.125)	0.2	(0.125–0.5)	0.015 (0.008–0.15)
Pseudomonas cepacia	16	0.5 (0.12–2)	25 (16–25)	8 (8–50)	3.1 (3–32)
Pseudomonas aeruginosa	≥128	0.5 (0.25–1)	4 (2–8)	2 (0.06–8)	4 (0.5–4)
Haemophilus influenzae	1 (1–2)	0.03 (0.007–0.06)	0.125 (0.06–0.25)	0.06 (0.03–0.125)	0.03 (0.03–0.06)
Neisseria gonorrhoeae	1 (1–2)	≤0.015 (≤0.015)	0.03 (0.015–0.06)	0.06 (0. 015–0.125)	0.03 (0.015–0.06)
Neisseria meningitidis	2	0.004	0.06	0.03	0.015
Acinetobacter spp.	32–256	0.5 (0.015–1)	1–2	8–64	1 (0.12–2)
Aeromonas spp.	0.5	≤0.008 (≤0.008–0.05)	—	0.06	0.03–0.5 (0.003–10)
Campylobacter jejuni	8	(0.12–0.78)	(1–32)	(0.25–2)	(0.12–2)
Branhamella (Moraxella) catarrhalis	2	0.06 (0.007–0.06)	0.06	0.4	(0.06–0.50)
Providencia rettgeri	16	1 (≤0.008–2)	1 (0.5–6.25)	2 (0.25–3.1)	1 (0.25–2)
Providencia stuartii	32	0.25 (≤0.008–1)	1–2	2 (≤0.25–2)	1 (0.6–4)
Stenotrophomonas (formerly *Xanthomonas) maltophilia*	16	4 (1–4)	8 (3–16)	4 (4–>64)	4 (0.5–4)
Yersinia enterocolitica	4 (1–8)	0.06 (0.015–0.06)	0.12–0.25	≤0.12	(0.06–0.25)
Hafnia alvei	—	0.03 (0.015–0.06)	—	—	0.12 (0.15–0.25)
Helicobacter pylori	—	0.31 (0.039–0.31)	—	—	—
Gram-positive aerobes					
Enterococcus faecalis	>128 (>128)	4 (0.5–4)	8 (8–16)	8 (4–32)	4 (2–6.2)
Enterococcus faecium	>64	4 (2–8)	32	≥12.5	6.2 (2–16)
Staphylococci (coag neg)	128 (32–256)	0.5 (0.06–0.5)	1 (0.5–1)	1 (0.25–2)	0.5 (0.25–0.5)
Staphylococci (coag neg/meth res)	>128 (16–>128)	64 (0.12–>64)	—	—	64 (0.12–>64)
Staphylococcus aureus	64 (32–128)	0.5 (0.12–2)	2 (0.5–2)	2 (0.5–4)	0.5 (0.12–1)
Staphylococcus aureus (meth susc)	64 (8–64)	1 (0.25–2)	—	—	0.5 (0.25–32)
Staphylococcus aureus (meth res)	>128 (32–>128)	64 (0.25–>64)	—	—	32 (0.25–>128)
Streptococcus (*viridans* group)	>128 (128–>128)	4 (0.12–8)	—	—	4 (1–8)
Streptococcus pyogenes	>100	1 (0.25–2)	>8	4 (2–16)	2 (0.05–4)
Streptococcus agalactiae	>128	2 (0.5–4)	>8	16 (4–16)	2 (1–4)
Streptococcus pneumoniae	>128 (128–>128)	4 (0.5–4)	16 (8–16)	16 (4–>16)	4 (0.05–4)
Listeria monocytogenes	>64	2 (0.5–4)	8–16	8 (4–16)	2 (1–4)
Corynebacterium spp.	0.06 (0.03–0.12)	1 (0.05–128)	8 (4–>128)	4 (4–>128)	1 (0.5–64)
Anaerobic bacteria and other organisms					
Peptostreptococcus spp.	>128 (64–128)	4 (0.25–16)	—	—	8 (0.25–32)
Clostridium spp.	>128 (4–>128)	0.5 (0.25–2)	(16–32)	(2–8)	8 (0.25–16)
Clostridium difficile	>128 (64–>128)	12.5 (8–25)	128	128	8 (8–16)
Prevotella spp.	128 (64–128)	16 (0.25–16)	—	—	16 (0.5–16)
Mycobacterium fortuitum	—	0.3	—	2	(1–3.1)
Mycobacterium tuberculosis	128 (16–128)	1	>5	8	1 (0.12–4)
Mycobacterium avium complex	>256 (128–>256)	16	>256	≥16	32 (4–64)
Mycobacterium chelonae	—	8	—	>16	>20
Mycobacterium kansasii	—	1	≥5	8	(1–3.1)
Bacteriodes spp.	512	16 (4–>16)	16	128	(2–32)
Bacteroides fragilis	128 (128–>128)	16 (4–>16)	32	>128	(2–12.5)
Fusobacterium spp.	128 (32–>128)	8 (2–8)	32	16	4 (0.5–8)
Gram-positive cocci	(256–512)	(2–6.25)	(2–8)	(16–64)	(2–8)
Chlamydia pneumoniae	(>64)	(1–2)	—	—	0.25
Chlamydia psittaci	—	1	—	—	0.5
Chlamydia trachomatis	(>64)	(1–1.56)	6.3	≥16	(1–1.56)
Mycoplasma hominis	>256	(0.5–2)	8	(8–16)	(1–2)
Mycoplasma pneumoniae	—	(0.78–2)	8	12	(0.78–2)
Ureaplasma urealyticum	—	4	—	—	(2–4)

*MIC$_{90}$, Minimal inhibitory concentration for 90% of strains; coag neg, coagulase negative; meth res, methicillin resistant; meth susc, methicillin susceptible.

and *Neisseria* species.[29–32] Ciprofloxacin is the most active presently available 4-quinolone[29–32] against aerobic gram-negative bacteria. The newer quinolones also have activity against staphylococci.[29–32] They have moderate activity against *Pseudomonas aeruginosa*, and ciprofloxacin is the most active. The currently available quinolones have variable activity against streptococci and poor activity against anaerobes.[29–31, 33] However, a few agents under development, such as trovafloxacin and sparfloxacin, do have significant activity against streptococci and anaerobes.[33, 34]

The newer 4-quinolones, including those currently available (ciprofloxacin, enoxacin, fleroxacin, lomefloxacin, and ofloxacin) as well as others under development (levofloxacin, sparfloxacin, and trovafloxacin), have excellent activity against *Legionella pneumophila.* Although ciprofloxacin and ofloxacin are active against *Mycoplasma pneumoniae* and *Chla-*

TABLE 26–1 ■ In Vitro Antimicrobial Activity of Selected 4-Quinolones* *Continued*

MIC$_{90}$ (RANGE) (μg/mL) *CONTINUED*						
Pefloxacin	**Lomefloxacin**	**Fleroxacin**	**Sparfloxacin**	**Trovafloxacin**	**Clinafloxacin**	**Levofloxacin**
0.125 (0.125–0.25)	0.2 (0.06–1.0)	0.1 (0.03–2)	0.03 (≤0.015–0.12)	0.06 (≤0.008–0.12)	≤0.03 (≤0.03–0.06)	0.10
0.5	1 (0.2–6.25)	0.5 (0.12–6.25)	0.012 (≤0.008–0.25)	0.05 (0.05–1)	0.13 (≤0.03–0.13)	0.25
0.5 (0.25–1)	0.5 (≤0.25–1)	(0.12–0.25)	0.06–.25 (0.015–1)	0.05	0.13 (≤0.03–0.25)	(0.18–0.39)
0.5	0.5 (0.12–25)	0.12 (≤0.06–25)	0.06–0.5 (≤0.015–1)	0.1 (0.06–0.25)	—	(0.03–0.78)
1 (0.25–2)	2 (0.25–25)	0.5 (0.25–25)	1 (0.25–1)	0.5 (0.05–2)	—	3.13
0.125	(0.06–0.25)	≤0.125	0.06 (0.015–0.12)	0.06 (0.03–0.12)	—	—
0.125 (0.06–0.25)	0.25	(≤0.12–0.25)	0.06 (0.015–0.12)	0.05	≤0.03 (≤0.03)	0.12
0.5 (0.25–1)	0.5–1	0.5 (≤0.12–0.5)	0.5 (0.06–0.5)	(0.2–2)	≤0.03 (≤0.03)	0.19
0.25	0.5 (0.25–1)	0.12 (≤0.12–0.25)	0.5 (0.12–1)	0.5	—	0.20
0.25 (0.25–0.5)	0.25 (0.25–12.5)	0.12 (<0.06–12.5)	0.25 (≤0.015–0.5)	0.25	≤0.03 (≤0.03)	0.12
—	—	—	0.25	—	0.06 (0.03–0.06)	—
—	≤0.06	≤0.06	≤0.06	—	—	(0.05–0.12)
4 (2–8)	4 (4–>50)	2 (2–>50)	(1–8)	3 (0.5–32)	0.25 (≤0.03–0.25)	5.12
—	16	4 (4–16)	1 (0.12–2)	.25	0.25 (≤0.03–0.12)	3.13
0.06 (0.03–0.06)	(≤0.06–0.12)	(≤0.06–1)	≤0.015 (≤0.015–0.03)	0.03 (0.03–0.12)	≤0.03 (≤0.03)	0.02
0.06 (0.03–0.06)	0.12	0.2	≤0.015 (≤0.015–0.03)	0.25 (≤0.001–0.25)	—	0.02
0.03	(≤0.06–0.42)	(0.03–0.25)	≤0.06	0.008 (0.004–0.015)	—	—
(1–8)	4	0.5–4 (0.5–32)	0.25 (0.015–0.5)	8	—	—
0.03	0.12	0.12–0.25 (0.12–1)	0.12 (≤0.015–0.25)	0.03	—	—
0.5	(0.125–1)	0.5	(0.1–0.12)	—	—	—
0.25	(≤0.1–1)	(0.25–2)	(0.01–0.12)	0.03 (0.007–0.03)	(≤0.03)	0.10
0.5	4 (1.6–6.2)	0.5 (0.12–1)	0.5 (0.12–1)	0.5	—	—
4	1 (1–4)	1 (0.5–2)	2 (0.12–8)	2	—	0.39
4.0	8 (8–25)	3 (3–25)	0.5 (0.03–1)	2 (0.2–2)	—	3.13
	(≤0.06–0.25)	(≤0.06–2)	0.06 (≤0.015–0.25)	(0.03–0.05)	≤0.03 (≤0.03)	
0.25						—
—	—	—	0.25 (0.015–0.25)	0.06 (0.008–0.06)	—	—
—	—	—	(0.25–4)	0.25 (0.031–0.25)	—	—
4–8	8 (4–16)	8 (8–>16)	0.5 (0.25–0.5)	2	0.25 (0.01–1)	1.56
—	8	8	1 (0.5–1)	2	0.5 (0.015–0.5)	3.13
0.5 (0.25–1)	1 (0.5–1)	1 (0.25–8)	0.125 (0.03–8)	1–4 (0.015–16)	0.03 (≤0.007–0.25)	0.78
—	—	4 (0.5–64)	4 (0.06–>16)	4 (0.015–16)	—	2.12
0.5 (0.25–1)	1 (0.5–2)	1 (0.25–1)	0.06 (0.03–2)	—	0.03 (≤0.007–0.125)	—
—	—	32 (0.2–64)	0.25 (0.03–0.25)	0.06 (0.015–4)	—	0.39
—	—	64 (32–64)	0.25 (0.03–1)	2 (0.015–8)	—	0.78
—	—	—	0.25 (0.03–0.5)	0.25 (0.015–0.25)	0.06 ((0.06–0.13)	(≤0.007–0.06)
8 (8–16)	8 (4–12.5)	8 (4–12.5)	0.5 (0.12–0.5)	0.12	(≤0.03–0.06)	1.56
32	16 (8–32)	8 (≥8)	0.5 (0.12–0.5)	0.25	(≤0.06–0.13)	2 (0.5–2)
12 (8–16)	8 (2–16)	8 (8–25)	0.5 (0.064–0.5)	0.25 (0.064–0.5)	0.06 (≤0.008–0.06)	1.56
6–8	(6.2–8)	8 (4–>16)	2 (0.12–2)	0.25 (0.12–0.25)	—	—
8 (8–>128)	>12.5	2 (1–32)	0.25 (0.25–64)	(0.03–>32)	—	—
—	—	—	4 (0.25–4)	1 (0.06–2)	0.5 (0.015–0.5)	5.56
(1–8)	(2–16)	(2–32)	0.25 (0.015–2)	(<0.06–4)	0.12 (0.06–0.12)	0.78
64	≥32	(16–32)	6.25	4 (0.5–4)	0.5 (0.03–1)	6.25
—	—	—	(8–16)	2 (0.06–4)	—	8.0
2	—	≤0.05	1.56	—	—	2.78
8	4	≤0.05	0.2	32 (2–64)	—	0.32
>64	—	16	12.5	64 (4–64)	—	16.50
>64	—	>32	(6.25–>100)	—	—	—
4	—	≥0.5	—	—	—	2.39
—	(8–32)	(2–64)	2	0.5 (0.5–2)	—	5.12
16	(8–64)	≥16	2 (1–2)	0.5 (0.12–4)	—	4.0
32	16	16	2	2 (0.12–2)	—	—
16	(4–25)	(8–12.5)	—	—	—	—
—	4	2	(0.01–0.25)	0.12	—	0.5
—	—	—	0.03	—	—	—
—	(2–3.1)	(1.5–6.3)	(0.05–0.063)	0.06	—	—
4	2	2	≤0.06 (0.01–0.06)	—	—	—
4	(4–8)	4	(0.1–0.25)	—	—	0.50
—	—	—	0.5	—	—	2.0

mydia pneumoniae, newer quinolones under development (levofloxacin, sparfloxacin, and trovafloxacin) are more active. The 4-quinolones are also active against *Chlamydia trachomatis, Mycoplasma hominis,* and *Ureaplasma urealyticum.*[35, 36]

The 4-quinolones have variable activity against *Mycobacterium* species. In general, they are not so active against *Mycobacterium avium-intracellulare,* whereas some newer 4-quinolones are active against *Mycobacterium tuberculosis, Mycobacterium kansasii,* and *Mycobacterium fortuitum* but have less activity against *Mycobacterium chelonae.*[37, 38] Sparfloxacin and ofloxacin have activity against *Mycobacterium leprae* and have also shown efficacy in patients with lepromatous leprosy.[39, 40]

Combinations of other classes of antimicrobial agents with the 4-quinolones generally show an additive or indifferent effect, occasionally show a synergistic effect but only in a few strains, and rarely show antagonism.[41, 42] The bactericidal activity of 4-quinolones is reduced, however, during the postantibiotic effect by rifampin.[43]

Mechanisms of Bacterial Resistance

The selection in vitro of both gram-positive and gram-negative variants with reduced susceptibility to the quinolones has occurred after serial exposure of bacteria to subinhibitory drug concentrations.[29] The resulting strains may exhibit cross-resistance to other quinolones. The mechanism of resistance usually involves either (1) mutations in the gene coding for DNA gyrase so that there is reduced quinolone affinity for the A or B subunit or (2) mutations that alter the outer membrane porins, which have been described in *Esherichia coli* and *P. aeruginosa*.[15, 29, 44–56] Relative resistance to antibiotics that are not related to the quinolones has been observed when reduced susceptibility to the quinolones is caused by reduced outer membrane porin P activity.[29, 52, 56, 57]

Although the exact mechanism for the development of bacterial resistance to the quinolones has not been determined, high-level resistance to the quinolones occurs most commonly when serine in the 83 position of subunit A is replaced by tryptophan or leucine, as has been observed in *Staphylococcus aureus*. These and other alterations in amino acids have also resulted in quinolone resistance in *E. coli*.[15, 49–51, 55]

Because quinolones interfere with DNA gyrase activity, which is necessary for plasmid replication, quinolones were expected to promote loss of plasmids and to inhibit transfer of R factor–mediated resistance[52, 53, 58]; however, although plasmid-mediated resistance may be possible, it has not yet been observed in clinical isolates.[29, 59, 60]

Pharmacology

The currently available quinolones as well as others under development are well absorbed from the gastrointestinal tract after oral administration and have excellent bioavailability. Most of the quinolones are excreted by the kidney into the urine, although some are metabolized in the liver.[61–64]

The pharmacokinetic properties of some of the newer quinolones are summarized in Table 26–2. An intravenous preparation is also available for ciprofloxacin, fleroxacin, ofloxacin, and pefloxacin. In general, the newer quinolones exhibit linear pharmacokinetics. Peak serum concentrations occur 1 to 3 hours after oral administration. Food and histamine H_2 blockers (ranitidine) delay absorption so that serum peaks appear later and are moderately lower.[61] Absorption is also reduced by concurrent administration of magnesium hydroxide or aluminum hydroxide antacids and by other drugs that decrease peristalsis or delay gastric emptying time.[61] The newer quinolones are not extensively bound to serum proteins. Their long serum half-life allows twice-daily or once-daily dosing. The newer quinolones are metabolized in the kidneys and liver. Renal elimination is by glomerular filtration and active tubular secretion, which is blocked by probenecid (except for fleroxacin). The antibacterial activity of the quinolones is reduced at lower urinary pH values (pH 5.5 to 6.0 versus pH 7.4).[3] Pefloxacin and nalidixic acid undergo extensive hepatic metabolism, followed by enoxacin and, to a lesser degree, norfloxacin, ciprofloxacin, and fleroxacin. Lomefloxacin and ofloxacin undergo the least hepatic metabolism. Biliary concentrations of ciprofloxacin, enoxacin, ofloxacin, and pefloxacin are two to eight times serum concentrations.[61]

Quinolones provide good tissue distribution, with excellent interstitial fluid levels, entry into phagocytic cells, and high urinary concentrations after oral administration.[61–64] Quinolones, except for nalidixic acid,[65] accumulate in the prostate gland, and concentrations in prostatic tissue, prostatic fluid, and seminal fluid are higher than those in plasma.[61–64, 66, 67] Ciprofloxacin, ofloxacin, nalidixic acid, and pefloxacin are excreted into breast milk of lactating women.[68] The tissue penetration of some of the newer quinolones is summarized in Table 26–3.

Dosage Adjustments for Renal or Hepatic Insufficiency

For patients whose creatinine clearance rate is below 50 mL/min, dosage adjustments of ofloxacin, fleroxacin, and lomefloxacin are suggested because these drugs are excreted largely unchanged in the urine and undergo minimal hepatic metabolism.[69] The suggested adjustment for ofloxacin is a standard dose and for fleroxacin and lomefloxacin is an initial standard dose followed by one half a standard dose at 24-hour intervals for patients with creatinine clearance rates of 10 to 50 mL/min; the suggested adjustment for ofloxacin, fleroxacin, and lomefloxacin is one half the standard dose every 24 hours for patients with creatinine clearance rates less than 10 mL/min.[61, 69, 70] Dosage adjustments for cinoxacin, ciprofloxacin, enoxacin, and norfloxacin may be necessary for patients with moderate renal insufficiency but only when the creatinine clearance rate is substantially depressed, that is, less than 30 mL/min, when maintenance doses can be given at 18- to 24-hour intervals.[61, 69, 71] Dosage adjustments are not required for pefloxacin and nalidixic acid. Hemodialysis has a minimal effect on the clearance of the newer quinolones

TABLE 26–2 ■ Pharmacokinetic Properties of Selected Newer Quinolones

QUINOLONE	DOSE (mg)	PEAK SERUM CONCENTRATION (mg/L)	HALF-LIFE (h)	PROTEIN BINDING (%)	BIOAVAILABILITY (%)	VOLUME OF DISTRIBUTION (L)	URINARY EXCRETION Unchanged (%)	URINARY EXCRETION Metabolites (%)
Ciprofloxacin	500	2–3	3–4.5	35	85	250	30–60	10
Enoxacin	400	2–3	4–6	43	90	190	50–55	15
Fleroxacin	400	4–6	10	23	96	100	60–70	10
Levofloxacin	500	5.7	7.6	—	—	102	—	—
Lomefloxacin	400	3	8	14–25	>95	190	70	10
Norfloxacin	400	1.5	3–4.5	15	80	225	20–40	20
Ofloxacin	400	3.5–5	5–6	8–30	85–95	100	70–90	5–10
Pefloxacin	400	4–5	10–11	25	90	110	5–15	55
Sparfloxacin	400	1.2–1.6	15.2–20.6	45	>60	322	<15	25
Trovafloxacin	100–300	1.4–4.3	7.1–9.6	70	60–85	90–110	8.8	—

TABLE 26–3 ■ Penetration of Selected Quinolones into Body Fluids and Tissues*

FLUID OR TISSUE	CIPROFLOXACIN	NORFLOXACIN	OFLOXACIN	ENOXACIN	PEFLOXACIN	FLEROXACIN	SPARFLOXACIN	TROVAFLOXACIN
Blister fluid	++++	++++	++++	++++	+++	++++	++++	+++
Saliva	++	++	+++	+++	+++	+++	+++	–
Bronchial secretions	++	–	+++	++++	++++	–	++++	–
Pleural fluid	+++	–	–	–	–	–	+++	–
Nasal secretions	+++	+++	++++	++++	+++	++++	++++	–
Tears	++	++	+++	++	+++	+++	+++	–
Sweat	+	+	++	++	++	++	+++	–
Cerebrospinal fluid	+	–	++	–	+++	–	++	++
Prostatic fluid	+++	++	++++	++	–	++	–	–
Ejaculate	+++++	–	++++	++++	–	++++	–	–
Vaginal secretions	–	–	–	–	–	–	+++++	–
Lung	++++	–	++++	+++++	++++	++++	+++++	+++++
Kidney	+++++	+++++	+++++	++++	–	–	–	–
Bone	++++	–	++	++	++	++++	–	–
Skin	++++	–	–	++++	–	–	–	–
Muscle	++++	–	–	++++	–	–	–	–
Fat	++++	–	–	+++	–	++	–	–

* +, Area under the curve (AUC) ratios or concentration ratios <0.1; ++, AUC ratios or concentration ratios 0.1–0.5; +++, AUC ratios or concentration ratios 0.5–1; ++++, AUC ratios or concentration ratios 1–4; +++++, AUC ratios or concentration ratios >4.

Adapted from Sorgel F, Jaehde U, Naber K, Stephan U: Pharmacokinetic disposition of quinolones in human body fluids and tissues. Clin Pharmacokinet 16(Suppl 1):5, 1989.

(i.e., ciprofloxacin, enoxacin, fleroxacin, lomefloxacin, norfloxacin, and ofloxacin) and a slightly higher effect on the clearance of pefloxacin.[69, 70, 71] Peritoneal dialysis has no substantial effect on the clearance of ciprofloxacin, fleroxacin, and ofloxacin.[70, 71] Nevertheless, a maintenance dose for ciprofloxacin is recommended after hemodialysis or peritoneal dialysis and for fleroxacin but only after hemodialysis. Dosage recommendations based on renal function are summarized in Table 26–4.

For patients with hepatic disease without concomitant renal insufficiency, no dosage adjustment is needed for ciprofloxacin, fleroxacin, lomefloxacin, norfloxacin, or ofloxacin. However, the dosage of pefloxacin and possibly of enoxacin may have to be adjusted in patients with hepatic disease.[61, 69, 72] Also, norfloxacin and ciprofloxacin may accumulate but only in patients with severe hepatic failure.[61]

Toxicity and Adverse Reactions

Toxicities with the earlier newer quinolones were low. Compared with other commonly used antimicrobial agents, the fluoroquinolones can be considered relatively safe.[3, 30, 73, 74] Gastrointestinal disturbances (anorexia, nausea, diarrhea, vomiting, dyspepsia, and abdominal discomfort) are the adverse reactions reported most frequently (2% to 11%). Central nervous system (CNS) reactions (1% to 7%) may occur in the form of headache, dizziness, tiredness, vertigo, syncope, restlessness, insomnia, tinnitus, and sensory changes.[3, 30, 73, 74] Severe neurotoxic reactions are rare (<0.5%) and include psychotic reactions, hallucinations, depression, and grand mal seizures, which are reversible with cessation of therapy. Thus, the quinolones should be used with caution in patients with known or suspected CNS disorders (e.g., epilepsy) or other conditions that predispose to seizures. These direct CNS effects correlate roughly with quinolone binding at the γ-aminobutyric acid (GABA) type A receptors in the brain, blocking GABA and leading to CNS stimulation.[74] Hypersensitivity reactions are also rare (0.4% to 2%) and include erythema, pruritus, urticaria, and rash. Equally rare are episodes of hypotension, tachycardia, nephrotoxic reactions (crystalluria) with elevated serum creatinine levels, thrombocytopenia, leukopenia, and anemia. Transient elevations in liver enzyme values have been observed rarely.[3, 30, 73]

Moderate to severe phototoxicity, manifested by an exaggerated sunburn reaction, has been observed in patients who are exposed to direct sunlight while receiving some members of the quinolone class of drugs, especially lomefloxacin, pefloxacin, and fleroxacin. Quinolones that accumulate in high concentrations in skin have a higher risk of producing phototoxicity.[74]

Quinolone-associated arthropathy is a potential adverse reaction in humans, because quinolones have been shown to cause arthropathy (cartilage erosions and effusions) in immature weight-bearing joints of animals. Although there is limited experience with the use of quinolones in children, to date there is little evidence of quinolone-induced arthropathy in humans.[73–75] Nevertheless, quinolones are not recommended for routine use in children and have not yet been approved for pediatric use in the United States.

Some quinolones (ciprofloxacin, ofloxacin, nalidixic acid, and pefloxacin) are excreted into breast milk, and quinolones, in general, should not be given to nursing mothers.[30, 68] Quinolones should also be avoided during pregnancy because their safety has not been established.

Oral nalidixic acid, oxolinic acid, and cinoxacin are usually tolerated well, although a number of adverse reactions have been reported. Gastrointestinal side effects include nausea, vomiting, diarrhea, and abdominal pain. Dermatologic reactions include pruritus, nonspecific rashes, urticaria associated with eosinophilia, and edema of the extremities. Nalidixic acid also produces photosensitivity reactions (sunburn or rarely a bullous eruption) on skin surfaces exposed to sunlight.[76] Ophthalmic side effects include blurred vision, diplopia, photophobia, abnormal accommodation, and changes in color perception, all of which disappear with cessation of therapy. CNS reactions include headaches, drowsiness, asthenia, giddiness, vertigo, syncope, restlessness, insomnia, tinnitus, and sensory changes.[77] Nalidixic acid has also been associated with grand mal seizures and acute reversible toxic psychosis,[77] as well as pseudotumor cerebri with intracranial hypertension, papilledema, and bulging of fontanelles in infants and young children,[78–80] which reverses after cessation of therapy. Rarely, abnormal results of liver function tests and renal function values and reduced hematocrit, hemoglobin, and leukocyte counts have been observed. Nalidixic acid has been associated, rarely, with cholestatic jaundice and with hemolytic anemia that is sometimes associated with glucose-6-phosphate dehydrogenase–deficient red blood cells.[81] Administration of nalidixic acid, oxolinic acid, and cinoxacin to prepubertal children and pregnant women is not recommended.

The newer fluoroquinolones, norfloxacin, ciprofloxacin, ofloxacin, enoxacin, lomefloxacin, fleroxacin, and pefloxacin, have similar side effects, which, however, are relatively infrequent, and these agents are considered relatively safe.[73] Gas-

TABLE 26–4 ■ Dosage Guide for Adult Patients Based on Renal Function

	DOSES FOR CREATININE CLEARANCE OF (mL/min)				
DRUG	>80	80–50	50–10	<10	DOSE AFTER DIALYSIS
Cinoxacin	250 mg q 6 h 500 mg q 12 h	250 mg q 8 h	250 mg q 12 h	250 mg q 24 h	None
Ciprofloxacin	250–500 mg q 12 h	250–500 mg q 12 h	250–500 mg q 18 h	250–500 mg q 24 h	250–500 mg hemodialysis + peritoneal
Enoxacin	200–400 mg q 12 h	200–400 mg q 12 h	100–200 mg q 12 h	100–200 mg q 24 h	None
Fleroxacin	400 mg q 24 h	400 mg q 24 h	200 mg q 24 h*	200 mg q 24 h*	400 mg hemodialysis, none peritoneal
Lomefloxacin	400 mg q 24 h	400 mg q 24 h	200 mg q 24 h*	200 mg q 24 h*	None
Nalidixic acid	0.5–1.0 g q 6 h	0.5–1.0 g q 6 h	0.5–1.0 g q 6 h	0.5–1.0 g q 6 h	—
Norfloxacin	400 mg q 12 h	400 mg q 12 h	400 mg q 24 h	400 mg q 24 h	None
Ofloxacin	200–400 mg q 12 h	200–400 mg q 12 h	200–400 mg q 24 h	100–200 mg q 24 h	None
Pefloxacin	400 mg q 12 h	400 mg q 12 h	400 mg q 12 h	400 mg q 12 h	None

*Daily maintenance dose after initial 400-mg loading dose.

trointestinal side effects are the most frequent (2% to 11% of patients) and include nausea, vomiting, dyspepsia, epigastric or abdominal pain, anorexia, diarrhea, flatulence, and dry mouth.[73] Antibiotic-associated colitis has been seen but rarely.[82]

CNS side effects, the next most common, occur in 1% to 7% of patients. Mild reactions include headache, dizziness, fatigue, insomnia, faintness, agitation, listlessness, restlessness, abnormal vision, and bad dreams. Severe reactions (<0.5%) include hallucinations, depression, psychotic reactions, and grand mal convulsions. The side effects occur after only a few days of treatment and disappear when therapy is discontinued.[73, 82]

Skin and allergic reactions, the next most common side effects (0.6% to 2.4% of patients), include erythema, urticaria, rash, pruritus, and photosensitivity reactions on skin surfaces exposed to sunlight.[73, 82] Rarely, hypotension, tachycardia, nephrotoxicity, thrombocytopenia, leukopenia, anemia, and transient elevations in liver enzyme values have been observed.[73, 82]

Drug Interactions

The quinolones are known to interact with a variety of other compounds. Specifically, bioavailability of some quinolones is reduced after oral administration with alkaline earth and transition metal cations because quinolones form chelates with several polyvalent cations such as calcium, magnesium, iron, and aluminum.[61, 74, 83, 84] Therefore, administration of quinolones with antacids containing calcium, aluminum, or magnesium; with sucralfate; with divalent or trivalent cations, such as iron; or with multivitamins containing zinc may substantially interfere with the absorption of the quinolones, resulting in low systemic levels, so simultaneous oral administration should be avoided. These agents should not be taken within the 2-hour period before or after quinolone administration. Even then, there is sufficient variability between patients to warrant avoidance of these compounds during oral quinolone therapy. Also, the absorption of some quinolones may be affected minimally by food.

Two other frequently referenced quinolone drug interactions are those with either theophylline or caffeine and those with certain nonsteroidal antiinflammatory drugs (NSAIDs), such as fenbufen or its metabolite biphenylacetic acid.[30, 74, 85–89] These are important interactions because they may result in significant CNS toxicity. Data have shown that some quinolones strongly inhibit the hepatic cytochrome P-450 enzymes that metabolize theophylline and caffeine, thereby reducing their clearance and leading to their accumulation and toxicity.[74, 90, 91] These studies have shown a structure–side effect profile for theophylline interactions that is controlled primarily by the R_7 side chain, somewhat by the R_1 substituent, and to a lesser extent by X_8[74, 90, 91] and not by the oxo metabolites of the side chains as was suggested previously.[86, 92] The highest interactions occur for small nonbulky R_7 substituents, whereas bulkier R_7 side chains diminish the interaction. Also, a nitrogen in the X_8 position (naphthyridines, see Fig. 26–2) is the least preferred, although a bulky R_7 substituent can compensate for a nitrogen at X_8.[74] These data explain prior observations that enoxacin (a naphthyridine compound) has the greatest effect on theophylline metabolism, that is, significant increases in theophylline plasma concentrations (111%) with reduced clearance.[83, 86, 87] In contrast, theophylline plasma concentrations are increased by ciprofloxacin (23%), ofloxacin (12%), and minimally by norfloxacin, fleroxacin, and lomefloxacin.[85–87] Pefloxacin reduces theophylline clearance by 30%.[85] Theophylline doses should probably be halved for patients receiving enoxacin, and theophylline serum levels should be monitored for patients receiving enoxacin or ciprofloxacin. No routine reduction in theophylline dose is recommended for patients receiving norfloxacin, ofloxacin, fleroxacin, or lomefloxacin. Caffeine clearance is interfered with by the newer quinolones. Enoxacin increases the plasma concentration of caffeine by 41% and reduces the clearance by 78%. Ciprofloxacin increases the half-life of caffeine only modestly (15%) and ofloxacin and lomefloxacin do so only minimally.[88, 89]

The quinolones may interact to varying degrees with other drugs, including warfarin, H_2-receptor antagonists, cyclosporine, rifampin, and NSAIDs. Concomitant administration of an NSAID with a quinolone may increase the risk of CNS stimulation and convulsive seizures. Quinolones at high concentrations inhibit GABA receptor binding, which leads to CNS stimulation, but the inhibitory concentrations are not therapeutically relevant unless these quinolones are combined with certain NSAIDs, which potentiate quinolone GABA receptor binding by 100- to 3000-fold. This brings the inhibitory concentration into the therapeutic range. Again, the R_7 group has the greatest influence on the NSAID-potentiated CNS effects of the quinolones. However, the real clinical importance of the effects of NSAIDs and quinolones remains to be determined because of the low incidence of NSAID-induced CNS effects.[74, 93]

Disturbances of blood glucose, including symptomatic hyper- and hypoglycemia, have been reported, usually in diabetic patients receiving concomitant treatment with an oral hypoglycemia agent or insulin. For these patients, careful monitoring of blood glucose is recommended, and the quinolone should be discontinued if a hypoglycemic reaction occurs. Nalidixic acid–glucuronide conjugates may produce a false-positive reaction for urine glucose when tested with Benedict solution but not with glucose oxidase strips. Nitrofurantoin interferes with the therapeutic action of nalidixic acid.

Clinical Applications

Certain infectious diseases are amenable to oral therapy, including infections of the respiratory tract, especially those that are chronic; urinary tract infections, except urosepsis; bone and joint infections; skin and soft tissue infections; certain gastrointestinal infections; some sexually transmitted diseases; and some pelvic infections. Also, prophylaxis can be given orally, particularly for immunocompromised patients. Adequate evidence of efficacy with the newer quinolones, particularly ciprofloxacin and ofloxacin, has been demonstrated by clinical investigation in most of these infectious diseases.[3, 30] Enoxacin, fleroxacin, and lomefloxacin have been efficacious in some of these infections; norfloxacin, in urinary tract infections and some sexually transmitted diseases; and cinoxacin and nalidixic acid, in urinary tract infections only. The availability of intravenous preparations of ciprofloxacin, fleroxacin, ofloxacin, and pefloxacin has broadened the use of quinolones for these and other types of infections.

Urinary Tract Infections

Nalidixic acid, cinoxacin, norfloxacin, ciprofloxacin, ofloxacin, enoxacin, fleroxacin, lomefloxacin, and pefloxacin have established roles in treating urinary tract infections. Nalidixic acid (adults, 1 g four times daily for 1 to 2 weeks, thereafter, if needed, 0.5 g; children, 55 mg/kg per day in four divided doses for 1 to 2 weeks, thereafter, if needed, 33 mg/kg) and cinoxacin (adults, 250 mg four times daily or 500 mg twice daily for 1 to 2 weeks; not recommended for children) have been used in acute and recurrent uncomplicated urinary infections with susceptible organisms. Nalidixic acid has also been used as long-term therapy for frequent recurrent bacteriuria, but cure rates have not been optimal and resistance commonly emerges during treatment.[3, 30] Rapid emergence of resistant organisms during short- and long-term treatment with cinoxacin has not been observed.[94, 95]

The newer quinolones are as effective as other well-established agents for treating uncomplicated urinary infections.[3, 30, 67] Single doses of norfloxacin (800 mg), ciprofloxacin (100 or 250 mg), fleroxacin (400 mg), and ofloxacin (200 mg) are highly effective for simple cystitis caused by Enterobacteriaceae in women but may be less effective against *Staphylococcus saprophyticus*.[3, 67, 96–99] Excellent bacterial cure rates have also been achieved in uncomplicated urinary infections with norfloxacin, ciprofloxacin, ofloxacin, fleroxacin, lomefloxacin, or enoxacin given for 3 to 10 days.[3, 67, 96–102]

Excellent cure rates have been observed when norfloxacin, ciprofloxacin, ofloxacin, fleroxacin, lomefloxacin, and enoxacin were given for 5 to 14 days to patients with nosocomial or complicated urinary infections.[3, 96, 103, 104]

Ciprofloxacin (1000 mg/d), ofloxacin (300 to 600 mg/d), pefloxacin (800 mg/d), and norfloxacin (800 mg/d), given to patients with either acute or chronic prostatitis for 28 (range 5 to 84) days, cured 63% to 92% of patients.[3, 67, 105–108]

Respiratory Tract Infections

The quinolones have excellent in vitro activity (except for *Streptococcus pneumoniae* and other streptococcal species) against the respiratory tract pathogens responsible for community-acquired pneumonia, including the agents responsible for atypical pneumonia, such as *L. pneumophila, M. pneumoniae,* and *C. pneumoniae* (see Table 26–1). The quinolones are also effective against the majority of organisms responsible for acute bacterial exacerbations of chronic bronchitis and for nosocomial respiratory tract infections (see Table 26–1). Most patients with purulent bronchitis, acute exacerbations of chronic bronchitis, or pneumonia treated for 10 (range 7 to 15) days with ciprofloxacin, ofloxacin, enoxacin, fleroxacin, lomefloxacin, or pefloxacin experienced clinical cure or improvement (76% to 95%) and bacterial cure (68% to 96%).[3, 109–116] Bacterial persistence, relapse, or treatment failure occurred in 49% of *P. aeruginosa* infections, in 39% of *S. pneumoniae* infections, and in 33% of *S. aureus* infections.[3, 109]

Ciprofloxacin and ofloxacin have been used successfully to treat patients with community-acquired pneumonias caused by *M. catarrhalis, Haemophilus influenzae, M. pneumoniae, Legionella,* and *C. pneumoniae*.[3, 109, 116] Although some patients with pneumococcal pneumonia have been cured with intravenous ciprofloxacin or ofloxacin, treatment failures have occurred.[3, 109] Therefore, physicians are reluctant to use the currently available quinolones to treat either community-acquired or aspiration pneumonia because of their reduced activity against *S. pneumoniae* and against the microaerophilic and anaerobic bacteria associated with aspiration pneumonia. However, intravenous ciprofloxacin, ofloxacin, pefloxacin, and fleroxacin have been used successfully in hospital-acquired pneumonia caused by aerobic gram-negative bacteria, although the bacteriologic eradication rate for *P. aeruginosa* is lower.[3, 109, 117–119] Exacerbations of acute pulmonary infections in patients with cystic fibrosis who have *P. aeruginosa* in their sputum have responded to ciprofloxacin (750 mg twice daily orally) or ofloxacin (400 mg twice daily orally), although resistant organisms may emerge.[3, 120, 121] Malignant external otitis caused by *P. aeruginosa* may also respond to ciprofloxacin therapy (750 mg twice daily orally) given for 1 to 6 months.[122]

Although the newer quinolones may be useful in specific cases of chronic sinusitis caused by susceptible aerobic gram-negative bacteria, they should not be used for acute sinusitis or acute otitis media because of the possible presence of pneumococci.

Gastrointestinal Infections

The bacterial pathogens that cause diarrheal disease, including toxigenic *E. coli, Salmonella, Shigella, Campylobacter,* and *Vibrio* species, are highly susceptible to the newer quinolones. These agents also provide high drug concentrations in the lumen of the gut and the mucosa, which contribute to eradication of these pathogens from the intestine within 48 hours of initiation of therapy.[123] Ciprofloxacin, 500 mg twice daily, and norfloxacin, 400 mg twice daily, for 3 to 5 days or a single oral 400-mg dose of fleroxacin cures more than 90% of cases of acute bacterial diarrhea and acute traveler's diarrhea, and these are comparable to trimethoprim-sulfamethoxazole.[3, 123–125] Single-dose fleroxacin was as effective as 2 or 3 days of therapy in patients with cholera, shigellosis, and *Vibrio parahaemolyticus* infections.[125] Single-dose therapy with 800 mg of norfloxacin[126] or 1 g of ciprofloxacin[127] was also effective in treating shigellosis except for patients infected with *Shigella dysenteriae* type 1.[127] Quinolones are not routinely recommended as prophylaxis against acute traveler's diarrhea because the disease responds promptly to treatment when symptoms develop and because resistance may develop more rapidly with indiscriminate use of the newer quinolones. However, prophylaxis is recommended for patients with impaired health, and daily doses of 400 mg of norfloxacin, 500 mg of ciprofloxacin, 300 mg of ofloxacin, or 400 mg of fleroxacin have been highly effective in preventing traveler's diarrhea.[127]

Patients with typhoid fever have responded to ciprofloxacin, 500 mg twice daily, or fleroxacin, 400 mg daily, for 7 days or to ofloxacin, 200 mg twice daily, with greater than 90% cure rates.[3, 128–131] Also, ciprofloxacin, 500 to 750 mg twice daily for 4 weeks, eliminated the chronic *Salmonella* carrier state in 86% of patients followed up for 10 to 12 months.[3]

Although the newer quinolones inhibit *Helicobacter pylori,* these agents have not been effective in the treatment of *H. pylori*–associated gastritis and treatment has resulted in quinolone resistance.[132–134] Ciprofloxacin may have some value in *Clostridium difficile* enterocolitis.[135] Relapses have been reported in patients with *Brucella* infections who have been treated with quinolones.[136]

Skin and Soft Tissue Infections

Oral therapy with ciprofloxacin, ofloxacin, enoxacin, and fleroxacin effectively treats a variety of bacterial skin and skin structure infections in patients with cellulitis, subcutaneous abscesses, and wound infections and infected ulcers in patients with diabetes.[3, 137–143] Most patients received oral ciprofloxacin (750 mg twice daily for 10 to 14 days), ofloxacin (400 mg twice daily), or fleroxacin (400 mg daily) and clinical cure or improvement was observed in 80% to 90%. Bacterial cure rates were lower for gram-positive infections than for gram-negative aerobic infections. Quinolone therapy failed in 25% of anaerobic infections and to a lesser extent in infections caused by *S. aureus,* streptococci, and *P. aeruginosa.* Ciprofloxacin, 750 mg orally twice daily for 7 to 28 days, eradicated colonization with methicillin-resistant *S. aureus* (MRSA) in 50% to 79% of evaluable patients.[144, 145] When rifampin was combined with ciprofloxacin, the eradication rate was 100% when the isolates were susceptible to both agents, and these patients remained free of MRSA for at least 1 month.[144] Although ciprofloxacin may eradicate MRSA colonies or cure MRSA infection, resistant strains have rapidly emerged.[3, 146, 147]

Osteomyelitis

The newer oral quinolones have been effective as monotherapy for osteomyelitis, particularly when it is caused by gram-negative aerobic organisms.[3, 148–151] Most patients with acute or chronic osteomyelitis, either in native bone or complicating a foreign body, have been treated with ciprofloxacin, ofloxacin, fleroxacin, or pefloxacin for 6 to 8 weeks (range 4 days to 6 months). Clinical cure or improvement occurred in approximately 80% of patients treated with ciprofloxacin with adequate follow-up of at least 6 months to more than 1 year. Treatment failures occurred in 15% to 20%, and a few patients developed recurrent infection. Resistant strains developed in some patients, principally those with *P. aeruginosa* infections.[148–151] Ciprofloxacin, ofloxacin, and fleroxacin have had modest success in a small number of patients with septic arthritis.

Sexually Transmitted Diseases

The newer quinolones are extremely active in vitro against *Neisseria gonorrhoeae*, including penicillinase-producing strains, and against *Haemophilus ducreyi*.[3, 29] *C. trachomatis* isolates are most susceptible to ciprofloxacin, ofloxacin, sparfloxacin, and trovafloxacin but are resistant to enoxacin and norfloxacin[152] (see Table 26–1). Although *Gardnerella vaginalis* and *U. urealyticum* are relatively resistant to these agents, ciprofloxacin is active against the latter about 50% of the time.[3, 153] Thus, quinolones have been used to treat a variety of sexually transmitted diseases but are not effective against *Treponema pallidum*.

Gonococcal Infections

Single oral doses of 250 mg of ciprofloxacin, 400 mg of enoxacin, 400 mg of pefloxacin, 400 mg of ofloxacin, 400 mg of fleroxacin, 200 mg of sparfloxacin, or 800 mg of norfloxacin cured 95% to 100% of uncomplicated gonococcal infections in both men and women, including infections with penicillinase-producing *N. gonorrhoeae*. Thus, 100 mg of ciprofloxacin, the lowest effective oral single dose of the newer quinolones, has cured almost 100% of patients with urethral as well as rectal gonorrhea and is probably effective for pharyngeal gonococcal infections. There is little experience with the quinolones in the treatment of disseminated gonococcal infections.

Chlamydia Urethritis and Postgonococcal and Nongonococcal Urethritis

None of the current quinolones is effective as single-dose therapy for *C. trachomatis* urethritis, nor do they prevent postgonococcal urethritis when used as single-dose therapy for gonococcal infections. Although ciprofloxacin at 750 mg orally twice daily for 4 days eradicated *C. trachomatis* in 60% of coinfected patients and reduced the incidence of postgonococcal urethritis from 35% to 12.8%, the response rates with 7 days of therapy with ciprofloxacin or norfloxacin were not optimal.[154] Ofloxacin (300 mg twice daily) for 7 days was as effective as doxycycline in patients with nongonococcal urethritis or *C. trachomatis* cervicitis.[154–156] The quinolones are less effective than doxycycline or azithromycin for nongonococcal urethritis regardless of the presence or absence of *Chlamydia* or *Ureaplasma* infection.[157]

Chancroid

Patients with chancroid (*H. ducreyi*) infections have responded successfully to a single 500-mg oral dose of ciprofloxacin (95% cure rate); however, 500 mg of ciprofloxacin twice daily for 3 days cured 100% of patients with chancroid.[158] Fleroxacin, at a single dose of 400 mg in human immunodeficiency virus–negative men or at 400 mg daily for 5 days in human immunodeficiency virus–positive men, cured more than 90% of these patients with chancroid.[159]

Other Infections

IMMUNOCOMPROMISED HOST

Ciprofloxacin (500 mg twice daily), norfloxacin (400 mg twice or three times daily), ofloxacin (300 mg twice daily), and pefloxacin (400 mg twice daily) given orally have been used successfully for prophylaxis in granulocytopenic patients. The incidence of bacteremia and colonization with gram-negative bacilli and the amount and duration of antibiotic therapy directed against gram-negative bacilli were significantly reduced in febrile neutropenic patients,[3, 160, 161] which was most effectively accomplished with ciprofloxacin.[160] The emergence of quinolone-resistant gram-negative organisms has been observed in neutropenic cancer patients who received quinolone prophylaxis.[160–162] Limited clinical experience with intravenous ciprofloxacin, ofloxacin, and pefloxacin in the treatment of severe infections in immunocompromised patients suggests a potential role for these agents when used in combination with other agents, such as aminoglycosides.[163] Monotherapy with the quinolones for febrile neutropenic patients is not recommended.[3]

CENTRAL NERVOUS SYSTEM INFECTIONS

Ciprofloxacin, ofloxacin, and pefloxacin penetrate the cerebrospinal fluid and brain tissue.[3, 164–166] Clinical experience with the quinolones as therapeutic agents for CNS bacterial infections is limited.[166, 167] These agents should be reserved for special cases caused by multiantibiotic-resistant aerobic gram-negative bacteria. In nasopharyngeal carriers of *Meningococcus*, oral ciprofloxacin, 500 mg twice daily for 5 days, 250 mg twice daily for 2 days, or at a 750-mg single dose (15 mg/kg single dose for 2- to 18-year-old patients) eradicated the organism in more than 90% of patients.[168–171]

Ciprofloxacin and ofloxacin have been used with some success, in combination with other drugs, to treat multidrug-resistant pulmonary tuberculosis (ciprofloxacin and ofloxacin) and *M. avium-intracellulare* bacteremia in patients with acquired immunodeficiency syndrome (ciprofloxacin).[172–174] In general, the current quinolones are, at best, second-line agents to be used in combination for treating mycobacterial disease, except for *M. leprae*. Sparfloxacin, pefloxacin, and ofloxacin have shown efficacy in patients with lepromatous leprosy.[39, 40]

Ciprofloxacin (intravenously for 1 week and then orally for 3 weeks) plus oral rifampin (4 weeks) cured 10 patients who were intravenous drug abusers with right-sided *S. aureus* endocarditis who completed 4 weeks of therapy.[175] Nineteen patients with Mediterranean spotted fever caused by *Rickettsia conorii* were cured with oral ciprofloxacin (500 mg twice daily) for 2 days,[176] and five patients with cat-scratch disease experienced rapid improvement when treated with oral ciprofloxacin at 500 mg twice daily.[177]

References

1. Lesher GY, Froelich EJ, Gruett MD, et al: 1,8-Naphthyridine derivatives. A new class of chemotherapeutic agents. J Med Pharm Chem 5:1063, 1962.
2. Smith JT, Lewin CS: Chemistry and mechanisms of action of the

quinolone antibacterials. *In* Andriole VT (ed): The Quinolones. London, Academic Press, 1988, pp 23–81.
3. Andriole VT: Clinical overview of the newer 4-quinolone antibacterial agents. *In* Andriole VT (ed): The Quinolones. London, Academic Press, 1988, pp 155–200.
4. Wick WE, Preston DS, White WA, et al: Compound 64716, a new synthetic antibacterial agent. Antimicrob Agents Chemother 4:415, 1973.
5. Turner FJ, Ringel SM, Martin JF, et al: Oxolinic acid, a new synthetic antimicrobial agent. I. In vitro and in vivo activity. Antimicrob Agents Chemother 7:475, 1967.
6. Ringel SM, Turner FJ, Lindo FL, et al: Oxolinic acid, a new synthetic antimicrobial agent. II. Bactericidal rate and resistance development. Antimicrob Agents Chemother 7:480, 1967.
7. Ringel SM, Turner FJ, Roemer S, et al: Oxolinic acid, a new synthetic antimicrobial agent. III. Concentrations in serum, urine, and renal tissue. Antimicrob Agents Chemother 7:486, 1967.
8. Ito A, Hirai K, Inoue M, et al: In vitro antibacterial activity of Am 715, a new nalidixic acid analog. Antimicrob Agents Chemother 17:103, 1980.
9. Downs J, Andriole VT, Ryan JL: In vitro activity of MK-0366 against clinical urinary pathogens including gentamicin-resistant *Pseudomonas aeruginosa.* Antimicrob Agents Chemother 21:670, 1982.
10. Wise R, Andrew JM, Edwards LJ: In vitro activity of Bay 09867, a new quinolone derivative, compared with those of other antimicrobial agents. Antimicrob Agents Chemother 23:559, 1983.
11. Chin NX, Gu JW, Yu KW, et al: In vitro activity of sparfloxacin. Antimicrob Agents Chemother 35:567, 1991.
12. Andriole VT: The future of the quinolones. Drugs 45(3):1, 1993.
13. Norrby SR, Jonsson M: Comparative in vitro activity of PD 127,391, a new fluorinated 4-quinolone derivative. Antimicrob Agents Chemother 32:1278, 1988.
14. Tanaka M, Kurata T, Fujisawa C, et al: Mechanistic study of inhibition of levofloxacin absorption by aluminum hydroxide. Antimicrob Agents Chemother 37:2173, 1993.
15. Cullen ME, Wyke AW, Kuroda R, et al: Cloning and characterization of a DNA gyrase A gene from *Escherichia coli* that confers clinical resistance to 4-quinolones. Antimicrob Agents Chemother 33:886, 1989.
16. Higgins NP, Peebles CL, Sugino A, et al: Purification of subunits of *Escherichia coli,* DNA gyrase and reconstitution of enzymic activity. Proc Natl Acad Sci USA 75:1773, 1978.
17. Pedrini A: Nalidixic acid. *In* Hahn FE (ed): Antibiotics, Vol 5. Berlin, Springer-Verlag, 1979.
18. Wang JC: Interactions between DNAs and enzymes. The effect of superhelical turns. J Mol Biol 87:797, 1974.
19. Wang JC: DNA topoisomerases. Annu Rev Biochem 54:665, 1985.
20. Gellert M, Mizuuchi K, O'Dea MH, et al: DNA gyrase. Proc Natl Acad Sci USA 73:3872, 1976.
21. Sugino A, Peebles CL, Krenzer KN, Cozzarelli NR: Mechanism of action of nalidixic acid: Purification of *Escherichia coli nalA* gene product and its relationship to DNA gyrase and a novel nicking-closing enzyme. Proc Natl Acad Sci USA 74:4767, 1977.
22. Gellert M, Mizuuchi K, O'Dea MH, et al: Nalidixic acid resistance. A second genetic character involved in DNA gyrase activity. Proc Natl Acad Sci USA 74:4772, 1977.
23. Shen LL, Kohlbrenner WE, Weigl D, et al: Mechanism of quinolone inhibition of DNA gyrase. Appearance of unique norfloxacin binding sites in enzyme-DNA complexes. J Biol Chem 264:2973, 1989.
24. Hoshino K, Kitamura A, Morrissey I, et al: Comparison of inhibition of *Escherichia coli* topoisomerase IV by quinolones with DNA gyrase inhibition. Antimicrob Agents Chemother 38:2623, 1994.
25. Smith JT: Awakening the slumbering potential of the 4-quinolone antibacterials. Pharm J 233:299, 1984.
26. Crumplin GC, Smith JT: Nalidixic acid: An antibacterial paradox. Antimicrob Agents Chemother 8:251, 1975.
27. Lewin CS, Morrissey I, Smith JT: The mode of action of quinolones. The paradox in activity of low and high concentrations and activity in the anaerobic environment. Eur J Clin Microbiol Infect Dis 10:240, 1991.
28. Gootz TD, McGuirk PR, Moynihan MS, et al: Placement of alkyl substituents on the C-7 piperazine ring of fluoroquinolones: Dramatic differential effects on mammalian topoisomerase II and DNA gyrase. Antimicrob Agents Chemother 38:130, 1994.
29. Phillips I, King A, Shannon K: In vitro properties of the quinolones. *In* Andriole VT (ed): The Quinolones. London, Academic Press, 1988, pp 83–118.
30. Andriole VT: Quinolones. Encycl Hum Biol 6:399, 1991.
31. Eliopoulos GM, Eliopoulos CT: Activity in vitro of the quinolones. *In* Hooper DC, Wolfson JS (eds): Quinolone Antimicrobial Agents, ed 2. Washington, DC, American Society for Microbiology, 1993, pp 161–194.
32. Garcia-Rodriguez JA, Garcia Sanchez JE, Trujillano I, et al: Susceptibilities of *Brucella melitensis* isolates to clinafloxacin and four other new fluoroquinolones. Antimicrob Agents Chemother 39:1194, 1995.
33. Piddock LJV: New quinolones and gram-positive bacteria. Antimicrob Agents Chemother 38:163, 1994.
34. Neu HC, Chin NX: In vitro activity of the new fluoroquinolone CP-99,219. Antimicrob Agents Chemother 38:2515, 1994.
35. Heessen FWA, Myutjens HL: In vitro activities of ciprofloxacin, norfloxacin, pipemidic acid, cinoxacin, and nalidixic acid against *Chlamydia trachomatis.* Antimicrob Agents Chemother 25:123, 1984.
36. Kenny GE, Hooton TM, Roberts MC, et al: Susceptibilities of genital mycoplasmas to the newer quinolones as determined by the agar dilution method. Antimicrob Agents Chemother 33:103, 1989.
37. Leyson DC, Haemers A, Pattyn SR: Mycobacteria and the new quinolones. Antimicrob Agents Chemother 33:1, 1989.
38. Tomioka H, Saito H, Sato K: Comparative antimycobacterial activities of the newly synthesized quinolone AM-1155, sparfloxacin, and ofloxacin. Antimicrob Agents Chemother 37:1259, 1993.
39. Chan GP, Garcia-Ignacio BY, Chavez VE, et al: Clinical trial of sparfloxacin for lepromatous leprosy. Antimicrob Agents Chemother 38:61, 1994.
40. Ji B, Perani EG, Petinom C, et al: Clinical trial of ofloxacin alone and in combination with dapsone plus clofazimine for treatment of lepromatous leprosy. Antimicrob Agents Chemother 38:662, 1994.
41. Neu HC: Synergy and antagonism of combinations with quinolones. Eur J Clin Microbiol Infect Dis 10:255, 1991.
42. Neu HC: Quinolone antimicrobial agents. Annu Rev Med 41:465, 1992.
43. Meng X, Nightingale CH, Sweeney KR, et al: Loss of bactericidal activities of quinolones during the post-antibiotic effect induced by rifampicin. J Antimicrob Chemother 33:721, 1994.
44. Hirai K, Aoyama H, Suzue S, et al: Isolation and characterization of norfloxacin-resistant mutants of *Escherichia coli* K-12. Antimicrob Agents Chemother 30:248, 1986.
45. Hirai K, Suzue S, Irikura T, et al: Mutations producing resistance to norfloxacin in *Pseudomonas aeruginosa.* Antimicrob Agents Chemother 31:582, 1987.
46. Chapman JS, Bertasso A, Georgopapadakou NH: Fleroxacin resistance in *Escherichia coli.* Antimicrob Agents Chemother 33:239, 1989.
47. Nakamura S, Nakamura M, Kojima T, et al: *gyrA* and *gyrB* mutations in quinolone-resistant strains of *Escherichia coli.* Antimicrob Agents Chemother 33:254, 1989.
48. Legakis NJ, Tzouvelekis LS, Makris A, et al: Outer membrane alterations in multiresistant mutants of *Pseudomonas aeruginosa* selected by ciprofloxacin. Antimicrob Agents Chemother 33:124, 1989.
49. Reece RJ, Maxwell A: DNA gyrase: Structure and function. Crit Rev Biochem Mol Biol 26:335, 1991.
50. Willmott CJR, Maxwell A: A single point mutation in the DNA gyrase A protein greatly reduces binding of fluoroquinolones to the gyrase-DNA complex. Antimicrob Agents Chemother 37:126, 1993.
51. Sreedharan S, Oram M, Jensen B, et al: DNA gyrase *gyrA* mutations in ciprofloxacin-resistant strains of *Staphylococcus aureus*: Close similarity with quinolone resistance mutations in *Escherichia coli.* J Bacteriol 172:7260, 1990.
52. Cohen SP, McMurry LM, Levy SB: *marA* locus causes decreased expression of OmpF porin in multiple-antibiotic-resistant (Mar) mutant of *Escherichia coli.* J Bacteriol 170:6416, 1988.

53. Okazaki T, Hirai K: Cloning and nucleotide sequence of the *Pseudomonas aeruginosa nfxB* gene, conferring resistance to new quinolones. FEMS Microbiol Lett 97:197, 1992.
54. Takiff HE, Salazar L, Guerrero C, et al: Cloning and nucleotide sequence of *Mycobacterium tuberculosis gyrA* and *gyrB* genes and detection of quinolone resistance mutations. Antimicrob Agents Chemother 38:773, 1994.
55. Vila J, Ruiz J, Goni P, et al: Mutation in the *gyrA* gene of quinolone-resistant clinical isolates of *Acinetobacter baumannii.* Antimicrob Agents Chemother 39:1201, 1995.
56. Piddock LJV, Panchal S, Norte V: Comparison of the mechanism of action and resistance of two new fluoroquinolones, rufloxacin and MF961 with those of ofloxacin and fleroxacin in gram-negative and gram-positive bacteria. J Antimicrob Chemother 31:855, 1993.
57. Sanders CC, Sanders WE Jr, Goering RV, Werner V: Selection of multiple antibiotic resistance by quinolones, β-lactams, and aminoglycosides with special reference to cross-resistance between unrelated drug classes. Antimicrob Agents Chemother 26:797, 1984.
58. Hirai K, Irikura T, Iyobe S, et al: Inhibition of conjugal transfer of R plasmids by norfloxacin in *Pseudomonas aeruginosa.* Chemotherapy 32:471, 1984.
59. Crumplin GC: Plasmid-mediated resistance to nalidixic acid and new 4-quinolones? Lancet 2:854, 1987.
60. Munshi MH, Sack DA, Haider K, et al: Plasmid-mediated resistance to nalidixic acid in *Shigella dysenteriae* type I. Lancet 2:419, 1987.
61. Bergan T: Pharmacokinetics of fluorinated quinolones. *In* Andriole VT (ed): The Quinolones. London, Academic Press, 1988, pp 119–154.
62. Sorgel F, Jaehde U, Naber K, Stephan U: Pharmacokinetic disposition of quinolones in human body fluids and tissues. Clin Pharmacokinet 16(Suppl 1):5, 1989.
63. Lode H, Hoffken G, Boeckk M, et al: Quinolone pharmacokinetics and metabolism. J Antimicrob Chemother 26(Suppl B):41, 1990.
64. Sorgel F, Kinzig M: Pharmacokinetics of gyrase inhibitors, Part 1: Basic chemistry and gastrointestinal disposition. Am J Med 94(Suppl 3A):44, 1993.
65. Stamey TA, Meares EM, Winningham DG: Chronic bacterial prostatitis and the diffusion of drugs into prostatic fluid. J Urol 103:187, 1970.
66. Burt RAP, Morgan T, Payne JP, et al: Cinoxacin concentrations in plasma, urine and prostatic tissue after oral administration in man. Br J Urol 49:147, 1977.
67. Andriole VT: Use of quinolones in treatment of prostatitis and lower urinary tract infections. Eur J Clin Microbiol Infect Dis 10:342, 1991.
68. Giamarellou H, Kilokythas E, Petrikkos G, et al: Pharmacokinetics of three newer quinolones in pregnant and lactating women. Am J Med 87(Suppl 5A):49, 1989.
69. Lode H, Hoffken G, Olschewski P, et al: Pharmacokinetics of ofloxacin after parenteral and oral administration. Antimicrob Agents Chemother 31:1338, 1987.
70. Weidekamm E: Pharmacokinetics of fleroxacin in renal impairment. Am J Med 94(Suppl 3A):70, 1993.
71. Fillastre JP, Leroy A, Moulin B, et al: Pharmacokinetics of quinolones in renal insufficiency. J Antimicrob Chemother 26(Suppl B):51, 1990.
72. Montay G, Gaillot J: Pharmacokinetics of fluoroquinolones in hepatic failure. J Antimicrob Chemother 26(Suppl B):61, 1990.
73. Stahlmann R, Lode H: Safety overview: Toxicity, adverse effects and drug interactions. *In* Andriole VT (ed): The Quinolones. London, Academic Press, 1988, 201–233.
74. Domagala JM: Structure-activity and structure–side-effect relationships for the quinolone antibacterials. J Antimicrob Chemother 33:685, 1994.
75. Adam D: Use of quinolones in pediatric patients. Rev Infect Dis 11(Suppl 5):1113, 1989.
76. Zelickson AS: Phototoxic reaction with nalidixic acid. JAMA 190:556, 1964.
77. Cahal DA: Reactions to nalidixic acid. Br Med J 2:590, 1965.
78. Boreus LO, Sundstrom B: Intracranial hypertension in a child during treatment with nalidixic acid. Br Med J 2:744, 1967.
79. Cohen DN: Intracranial hypertension and papilledema associated with nalidixic acid therapy. Am J Ophthalmol 76:680, 1973.
80. Rao KG: Pseudotumor cerebri associated with nalidixic acid. Urology 4:204, 1974.
81. Belton EM, Jones RV: Haemolytic anaemia due to nalidixic acid. Lancet 2:691, 1965.
82. Adam D, Syndrassy K, Christ W, et al: Arbeitsgemeinschaft "Arzneimittelsicherheit" der Paul Ehrlich Gesellschaft fur Chemotherapie. Vertraglichkeit der Gyrase Hemmer. Muench Med Wochenschr 129:45, 1987.
83. Radandt JM, Marchbanks CR, Dudley MN: Interactions of fluoroquinolones with other drugs: Mechanisms, variability, clinical significance, and management. Clin Infect Dis 14:272, 1992.
84. Polk RE, Healy DP, Sahai J, et al: Effect of ferrous sulfate and multivitamins with zinc on absorption of ciprofloxacin in normal volunteers. Antimicrob Agents Chemother 33:1141, 1989.
85. Robson RA: The effects of quinolone on xanthine pharmacokinetics. Am J Med 92(Suppl 4A):22, 1992.
86. Wijnands WJA, Vree TB, van Herwaarden CLA: The influence of quinolone derivatives on theophylline clearance. Br J Clin Pharmacol 22:677, 1986.
87. Gregoire SL, Grasela TH Jr, Freer JP, et al: Inhibition of theophylline clearance by coadministered ofloxacin without alteration of theophylline effects. Antimicrob Agents Chemother 31:375, 1987.
88. Staib AH, Harder S, Mieke S, et al: Gyrase inhibitors impair caffeine elimination in man. Methods Find Exp Clin Pharmacol 9:193, 1987.
89. Stille W, Harder S, Mieke S, et al: Decrease of caffeine elimination in man during co-administration of 4 quinolones. J Antimicrob Chemother 20:729, 1987.
90. Fuhr U, Anders EM, Mahr G, et al: Inhibitory potency of quinolone antibacterial agents against cytochrome P450IA2 activity in vivo and in vitro. Antimicrob Agents Chemother 36:942, 1992.
91. Fuhr U, Strobl G, Manaut F, et al: Quinolone antibacterial agents: Relationship between structure and in vitro inhibition of human cytochrome P-450 isoform CYP1A2. Mol Pharmacol 43:191, 1993.
92. Hasegawa T, Nadai M, Kuzuya T, et al: The possible mechanism of interaction between xanthines and quinolones. J Pharm Pharmacol 42:767, 1990.
93. Janknegt R: Drug interactions with quinolones. J Antimicrob Chemother 26(Suppl D):7, 1990.
94. Landes RR: Long term low-dose cinoxacin therapy for the prevention of recurrent urinary tract infections. J Urol 123:47, 1980.
95. Schaeffer AJ, Jones JM, Flynn SS: Prophylactic efficacy of cinoxacin in recurrent urinary tract infections: Biologic effect on the vaginal and fecal flora. J Urol 127:1118, 1982.
96. Malinverni R, Glauser MP: Comparative studies of fluoroquinolones in the treatment of urinary tract infections. Rev Infect Dis 10(Suppl):153, 1988.
97. Iravani A: Multicenter study of single-dose and multiple-dose fleroxacin versus ciprofloxacin in the treatment of uncomplicated urinary tract infections. Am J Med 94(Suppl 3A):89, 1993.
98. Pfau A, Sacks TG: Single dose quinolone treatment in acute uncomplicated urinary tract infection in women. J Urol 149:532, 1993.
99. Saginur R, Nicolle LE: Single dose compared with 3-day norfloxacin treatment of uncomplicated urinary tract infection in women. Arch Intern Med 152:1233, 1992.
100. Nicolle LE, DuBois J, Martel AY, et al: Treatment of acute uncomplicated urinary tract infections with 3 days of lomefloxacin compared with treatment with 3 days of norfloxacin. Antimicrob Agents Chemother 37:574, 1993.
101. Andrade-Villanueva J, Flores-Gaxiola A, Lopez-Guillen P, et al: Comparison of the safety and efficacy of lomefloxacin and trimethoprim/sulfamethoxazole in the treatment of uncomplicated urinary tract infections: Results from a multicenter study. Am J Med 92(Suppl 4A):71, 1992.
102. Iravani A: Efficacy of lomefloxacin as compared to norfloxacin in the treatment of uncomplicated urinary tract infections in adults. Am J Med 92(Suppl 4A):75, 1992.
103. Pittman W, Moon JO, Hamrick LC, et al: Randomized double-blind trial of high- and low-dose fleroxacin versus norfloxacin for complicated urinary tract infection. Am J Med 94(Suppl 3A):101, 1993.
104. Cox CE: A comparison of the safety and efficacy of lomefloxacin and ciprofloxacin in the treatment of complicated or recurrent urinary tract infections. Am J Med 92(Suppl 4A):82, 1992.

105. Bologna M, Vaggi L, Flammini D, et al: Norfloxacin in prostatitis; correlation between HPLC tissue concentrations and clinical results. Drugs Exp Clin Res 11:95, 1985.
106. Suzuki K, Tamai H, Naide Y, et al: Laboratory and clinical study of ofloxacin in the treatment of bacterial prostatitis. Hinyokika Kiyo 30:1505, 1984.
107. Weidner W, Schiefer HG, Dalhoff A: Treatment of chronic bacterial prostatitis with ciprofloxacin. Am J Med 82(Suppl):280, 1987.
108. Remy G, Rouger C, Chavanet P, et al: Use of ofloxacin for prostatitis. Rev Infect Dis 10(Suppl):173, 1988.
109. Thys JP, Jacobs F, Byl B: Role of quinolones in the treatment of bronchopulmonary infections, particularly pneumococcal and community-acquired pneumonia. Eur J Clin Microbiol Infect Dis 10:304, 1991.
110. Kemper P, Kohler D: A double-blind study of two dosage regimens of lomefloxacin in bacteriologically proven exacerbations of chronic bronchitis of gram-negative etiology. Am J Med 92(Suppl 4A):98, 1992.
111. Grassi C, Albera C, Pozzi E: Lomefloxacin versus amoxicillin in the treatment of acute exacerbations of chronic bronchitis: An Italian multicenter study. Am J Med 92(Suppl 4A):103, 1992.
112. Gotfried MH, Ellison WT: Safety and efficacy of lomefloxacin versus cefaclor in the treatment of acute exacerbations of chronic bronchitis. Am J Med 92(Suppl 4A):108, 1992.
113. Chodosh S: Efficacy of fleroxacin versus amoxicillin in acute exacerbations of chronic bronchitis. Am J Med 94(Suppl 3A):131, 1993.
114. Ulmer W: Fleroxacin versus amoxicillin in the treatment of acute exacerbation of chronic bronchitis. Am J Med 94(Suppl 3A):136, 1993.
115. Andriole VT: The use of quinolones in respiratory tract infections: Summary. Proceedings of the 17th International Congress of Chemotherapy, Berlin, Germany, 1991. Infection 19(Suppl 7):391, 1991.
116. Lipsky BA, Tack KJ, Kuo C, et al: Ofloxacin treatment of *Chlamydia pneumoniae* (strain TWAR) lower respiratory tract infections. Am J Med 89:722, 1990.
117. Peloquin CA, Cumbo TJ, Nix DE, et al: Evaluation of intravenous ciprofloxacin in patients with nosocomial lower respiratory tract infections. Impact of plasma concentrations, organism, minimum inhibitory concentration, and clinical condition on bacterial eradication. Arch Intern Med 149:2269, 1989.
118. Gentry LO, Rodriguez-Gomez G, Kohler RB, et al: Parenteral followed by oral ofloxacin for nosocomial pneumonia and community-acquired pneumonia requiring hospitalization. Am Rev Respir Dis 145:31, 1992.
119. Farkas SA: Intravenous fleroxacin versus ceftazidime in the treatment of acute nonpneumococcal lower respiratory tract infections. Am J Med 94(Suppl 3A):142, 1993.
120. Bosso JA, Black PG, Matsen JM: Ciprofloxacin versus tobramycin plus azlocillin in pulmonary exacerbations in adult patients with cystic fibrosis. Am J Med 82(Suppl):180, 1987.
121. Scully BE, Nakatomi M, Ores C, et al: Ciprofloxacin therapy in cystic fibrosis. Am J Med 82(Suppl):196, 1987.
122. Giamarellou H: Use of quinolones in malignant otitis externa. Quinolone Bull 10:19, 1993.
123. DuPont HL, Ericsson CD: Prevention and treatment of traveler's diarrhea. N Engl J Med 328:1821, 1993.
124. Steffen R, Jori R, DuPont HL, et al: Efficacy and toxicity of fleroxacin in the treatment of traveler's diarrhea. Am J Med 94(Suppl 3A):182, 1993.
125. Butler T, Lolekha S, Rasidi C, et al: Treatment of acute bacterial diarrhea: A multicenter international trial comparing placebo with fleroxacin given as a single dose or once daily for three days. Am J Med 94(Suppl 3A):187, 1993.
126. Gotuzzo E, Oberhelman RA, Maguina C, et al: Comparison of single-dose treatment with norfloxacin and standard 5-day treatment with trimethoprim-sulfamethoxazole for acute shigellosis in adults. Antimicrob Agents Chemother 33:1101, 1989.
127. Bennish ML, Salam MA, Khan WA, et al: Treatment of shigellosis. III. Comparison of one- and two-dose ciprofloxacin with standard 5-day treatment. A randomized, blinded trial. Ann Intern Med 117:7278, 1992.
128. Uwaydah AK, Al Soub H, Matar I: Randomized prospective study comparing two dosage regimens of ciprofloxacin for treatment of typhoid fever. J Antimicrob Chemother 30:707, 1992.
129. Wang F, Gu X-J, Zhang M-F, et al: Treatment of typhoid fever with ofloxacin. J Antimicrob Chemother 23:785, 1989.
130. Arnold K, Hong CS, Nelwan R, et al: Randomized comparative study of fleroxacin and chloramphenicol in typhoid fever. Am J Med 94(Suppl 3A):195, 1993.
131. Gotuzzo E, Guerra JG, Benavente L, et al: Use of norfloxacin to treat chronic typhoid carriers. J Infect Dis 157:1221, 1988.
132. Simor AE, Ferro S, Low DE: Comparative in vitro activities of six new fluoroquinolones and other oral antimicrobial agents against *Campylobacter pylori*. Antimicrob Agents Chemother 33:108, 1989.
133. Glupczynski Y, Labbe M, Burette A, et al: Treatment failure of ofloxacin in *Campylobacter pylori* infection. Lancet 2:1096, 1987.
134. Mertens JCC, Dekker W, Ligtvoet EEJ, et al: Treatment failure of norfloxacin against *Campylobacter pylori* and chronic gastritis in patients with nonulcerative dyspepsia. Antimicrob Agents Chemother 33:245, 1989.
135. Lettau LA: Oral fluoroquinolone therapy in *Clostridium difficile* enterocolitis. JAMA 260:2216, 1988.
136. Lang R, Rubinstein E: Quinolones for the treatment of brucellosis. J Antimicrob Chemother 29:1063, 1992.
137. Valainis GT, Pankey GA, Katner HP: Ciprofloxacin in the treatment of bacterial skin infections. Am J Med 82(Suppl):230, 1987.
138. Self PL, Zeluff BA, Sollo D, et al: Use of ciprofloxacin in the treatment of serious skin and skin structure infections. Am J Med 82(Suppl):239, 1987.
139. Gentry LO: Review of quinolones in treatment of infections of the skin and skin structure. J Antimicrob Chemother 28(Suppl C):97, 1991.
140. Smith JW, Nichols RL: Comparison of oral fleroxacin with oral amoxicillin/clavulanate for treatment of skin and soft tissue infections. Am J Med 94(Suppl 3A):150, 1993.
141. Powers RD: Open trial of oral fleroxacin versus amoxicillin/clavulanate in the treatment of infections of skin and soft tissue. Am J Med 94(Suppl 3A):155, 1993.
142. Tassler H: Comparative efficacy and safety of oral fleroxacin and amoxicillin/clavulanate potassium in skin and soft tissue infections. Am J Med 94(Suppl 3A):159, 1993.
143. Parish IC, Jungkind DL: Systemic antimicrobial therapy for skin and skin structure infections: Comparison of fleroxacin and ceftazidime. Am J Med 94(Suppl 3A):166, 1993.
144. Mulligan ME, Ruane PJ, Johnston L, et al: Ciprofloxacin for eradication of methicillin-resistant *Staphylococcus aureus* colonization. Am J Med 82(Suppl):215, 1987.
145. Smith SM, Eng RHK, Tecson-Tumang F: Ciprofloxacin therapy for methicillin-resistant *Staphylococcus aureus* infections or colonizations. Antimicrob Agents Chemother 33:181, 1989.
146. Piercy EA, Barbaro D, Luby JP, et al: Ciprofloxacin for methicillin-resistant *Staphylococcus aureus* infections. Antimicrob Agents Chemother 33:128, 1989.
147. Trucksis M, Hooper DC, Wolfson JS: Emerging resistance to fluoroquinolones in staphylococci: An alert. Ann Intern Med 114:424, 1991.
148. Andriole VT: Treatment of osteomyelitis with quinolones. Quinolone Bull 3:15, 1987.
149. Gentry LO: Oral antimicrobial therapy for osteomyelitis (Editorial). Ann Intern Med 114:986, 1991.
150. Green SL: Efficacy of oral fleroxacin in bone and joint infections. Am J Med 94(Suppl 3A):174, 1993.
151. Putz PA: A pilot study of oral fleroxacin given once daily in patients with bone and joint infections. Am J Med 94(Suppl 3A):177, 1993.
152. Hartinger A, Hartmut B, Korting HC: In vitro activity of ciprofloxacin and ofloxacin against clinical isolates of *Chlamydia trachomatis*. Rev Infect Dis 10(Suppl):151, 1988.
153. Krausse R, Ulmann U: In vitro-Aktivitat von Enoxazin, Ciprofloxacin und Tetracyclin gegenüber *Mycoplasma hominis* und *Ureaplasma urealyticum*. Z Antimikrob Antineoplast Chemother 2:83, 1984.
154. Fong IW: Treatment of chlamydial urethritis with ofloxacin or ciprofloxacin. Quinolone Bull 2:10, 1986.
155. Hooton TM, Batteiger BE, Judson FN, et al: Ofloxacin versus doxycycline for treatment of cervical infection with *Chlamydia trachomatis*. Antimicrob Agents Chemother 36:1144, 1992.
156. Kitchen VS, Donegan C, Ward H, et al: Comparison of ofloxacin with doxycycline in the treatment of non-gonococcal urethritis

and cervical chlamydial infection. J Antimicrob Chemother 26(Suppl D):99, 1990.
157. Stamm WE, Hicks CB, Martin DH, et al: Azithromycin for empirical treatment of the nongonococcal urethritis syndrome in men. A randomized double-blind study. JAMA 274:545, 1995.
158. Naamara W, Plummer FA, Greenblatt RM, et al: Treatment of chancroid with ciprofloxacin. Am J Med 82(Suppl):317, 1987.
159. Tyndall MW, Plourde PJ, Agoki E, et al: Fleroxacin in the treatment of chancroid: An open study in men seropositive or seronegative for the human immunodeficiency virus type I. Am J Med 94(Suppl 3A):85, 1993.
160. D'Antonio D, Piccolomini R, Iacone A, et al: Comparison of ciprofloxacin, ofloxacin and pefloxacin for the prevention of the bacterial infection in neutropenic patients with haematological malignancies. J Antimicrob Chemother 33:837, 1994.
161. Bow EJ, Loewen R, Vaughan D: Reduced requirement for antibiotic therapy targeting gram-negative organisms in febrile, neutropenic patients with cancer who are receiving antibacterial chemoprophylaxis with oral quinolones. Clin Infect Dis 20:907, 1995.
162. Kern WV, Andriof E, Oethinger M, et al: Emergence of fluoroquinolone-resistant *Escherichia coli* at a cancer center. Antimicrob Agents Chemother 38:681, 1994.
163. Chan CC, Oppenheim BA, Anderson H, et al: Randomized trial comparing ciprofloxacin plus netilmicin versus piperacillin plus netilmicin for empiric treatment of fever in neutropenic patients. Antimicrob Agents Chemother 33:87, 1989.
164. Wolff M, Regnier B, Daldoss C, et al: Penetration of pefloxacin into cerebrospinal fluid of patients with meningitis. Antimicrob Agents Chemother 26:289, 1984.
165. Pioget JC, Wolff M, Singlas E, et al: Diffusion of ofloxacin into cerebrospinal fluid of patients with purulent meningitis or ventriculitis. Antimicrob Agents Chemother 33:933, 1989.
166. Segev S, Barzilai A, Rosen N, et al: Pefloxacin treatment of meningitis caused by gram-negative bacteria. Arch Intern Med 149:1314, 1989.
167. Schonwald S, Beus I, Lisic M, et al: Brief report: Ciprofloxacin in the treatment of gram-negative bacillary meningitis. Am J Med 87(Suppl 5A):248, 1989.
168. Renkonen OV, Sivonen A, Visakorpi R: Effect of ciprofloxacin on carrier rate of *Neisseria meningitidis* in army recruits in Finland. Antimicrob Agents Chemother 31:962, 1987.
169. Pugsley MP, Dworzack DL, Horowitz EA, et al: Efficacy of ciprofloxacin in the treatment of nasopharyngeal carriers of *Neisseria meningitidis*. J Infect Dis 156:211, 1987.
170. Dworzack DL, Sanders CC, Horowitz EA, et al: Evaluation of single-dose ciprofloxacin in the eradication of *Neisseria meningitidis* from nasopharyngeal carriers. Antimicrob Agents Chemother 21:1740, 1988.
171. Cuevas LE, Kazembe P, Mughogho GK, et al: Eradication of nasopharyngeal carriage of *Neisseria meningitidis* in children and adults in rural Africa: A comparison of ciprofloxacin and rifampicin. J Infect Dis 171:728, 1995.
172. Yew WW, Kwan SY, Ma WK, et al: In vitro activity of ofloxacin against *Mycobacterium tuberculosis* and its clinical efficacy in multiply resistant pulmonary tuberculosis. J Antimicrob Chemother 26:227, 1990.
173. de Lalla F, Maserati R, Scarpellini P, et al: Clarithromycin-ciprofloxacin-amikacin for therapy of *Mycobacterium avium–Mycobacterium intracellulare* bacteremia in patients with AIDS. Antimicrob Agents Chemother 36:1567, 1992.
174. Kemper CA, Meng T-C, Nussbaum J, et al: Treatment of *Mycobacterium avium* complex bacteremia in AIDS with a four-drug oral regimen. Ann Intern Med 116:466, 1992.
175. Dworkin RJ, Sande MA, Lee BL, et al: Treatment of right-sided *Staphylococcus aureus* endocarditis in intravenous drug abusers with ciprofloxacin and rifampicin. Lancet 2:1071, 1989.
176. Gudiol F, Pallares R, Carratala J, et al: Randomized double-blind evaluation of ciprofloxacin and doxycycline for Mediterranean spotted fever. Antimicrob Agents Chemother 33:987, 1989.
177. Holley HP: Successful treatment of cat-scratch disease with ciprofloxacin. JAMA 265:1563, 1991.

27

Chloramphenicol

Frank M. Calia
David W. Oldach

After the discovery and manufacture of penicillin in the 1940s, soil organisms were actively screened for antimicrobial production. Chloramphenicol was isolated from the organism *Streptomyces venezuelae*, which was discovered in a field near Caracas, Venezuela.[1,2] Released in 1949 under the name Chloromycetin, the drug proved to be efficacious in the treatment of infections caused by gram-positive and gram-negative bacteria, including anaerobes and ricksettsiae. For several decades, chloramphenicol was the only antimicrobial available that was consistently active against *Salmonella* species, including *Salmonella typhi*.[3] The recognition of life-threatening toxic effects (i.e., gray syndrome in premature and newborn infants and aplastic anemia) caused clinicians to restrict the use of this drug.[4,5] The emergence of ampicillin-resistant strains of *Haemophilus influenzae* and the recognition of the importance of penicillin-resistant strains of *Bacteroides* led to a renewed interest in chloramphenicol.[6,7] Less toxic antimicrobials have since replaced the drug in many instances. Because of its potential toxicity, although rare, chloramphenicol should be used only for seriously ill patients in well-defined clinical situations.

Structure

Chloramphenicol has a simple structure and is now mass-produced by chemical synthesis.[8] The drug is composed of a *p*-nitrobenzene ring attached to a propanediol moiety with a dichloracetamide side chain (Fig. 27–1). The antimicrobial activity depends on the integrity of the propanediol moiety and dichloracetamide side chain. The aromatic ring and the acyl side chain may be substituted without loss of bacteriostasis.[9,10]

In addition to chloramphenicol base, two esters of the drug are commercially available, chloramphenicol succinate and chloramphenicol palmitate.[11,12] The esters must be hydrolyzed to chloramphenicol to be biologically active.

Mechanism of Action

Chloramphenicol inhibits protein synthesis in bacteria. Nucleic acid synthesis is not affected.[13] The drug binds only to

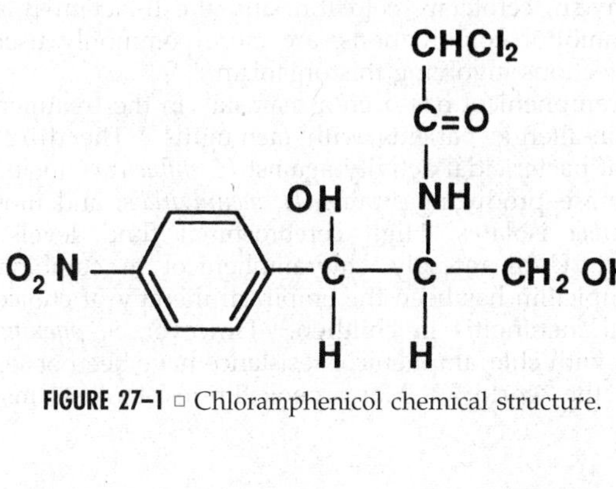

FIGURE 27–1 □ Chloramphenicol chemical structure.

the 70S ribosome, where high-affinity reversible binding occurs at a particular site on the 50S subunit. This interaction of drug with ribosome is responsible for protein synthesis inhibition, which causes bacteriostasis of sensitive organisms.[14] Because most protein synthesis in mammals occurs on 80S ribosomes, protein synthesis inhibition does not occur in host cells. Mammalian mitochondria are an important exception.[15, 16] These cellular organelles may have been primitive infecting organisms that gradually evolved into obligatory endosymbionts. Chloramphenicol-induced inhibition of mitochondrial protein synthesis accounts for some of the significant toxicity encountered with this agent.

Chloramphenicol acts by blocking the addition of new amino acids to a growing protein chain by inhibiting peptide bond formation.[17] Specifically, chloramphenicol inhibits the binding of the amino acid–containing end of transfer RNA to the 50S binding site.[18] By interfering with the attachment of aminoacyl-transfer RNA, the amino acid substrate is unavailable to peptidyl transferase. This prevents the formation of the peptide bond.[19]

Chloramphenicol is bactericidal for some organisms, including *Streptococcus pneumoniae, H. influenzae*, and *Neisseria meningitidis*.[20, 21] The killing mechanism has not been elucidated.

Spectrum of Activity

Chloramphenicol is the prototype of the broad-spectrum antimicrobial. The drug demonstrates activity against bacteria, ricksettsiae, ehrlichiae, chlamydiae, and spirochetes.[22–24] Sensitive organisms are susceptible to serum levels that are easily achieved clinically. The drug is active against most aerobic and anaerobic gram-positive bacteria, with the exception of *Nocardia* species, group D streptococci, and methicillin-resistant *Staphylococcus aureus*.[25] Many of the Enterobacteriaceae, especially *Escherichia coli* and *Proteus mirabilis*, are quite sensitive to chloramphenicol, whereas *Klebsiella, Enterobacter, Serratia*, and indole-positive *Proteus* species have varying sensitivities.[26] *Pseudomonas* species, with the exception of *Pseudomonas pseudomallei*, and *Acinetobacter* species are almost always resistant.[27] Other gram-negative organisms—*N. meningitidis, Neisseria gonorrhoeae, H. influenzae* (β-lactamase–positive and β-lactamase–negative strains), *Vibrio cholerae, Brucella* species, *Bordetella pertussis, P. pseudomallei*, and *Salmonella* species including *S. typhi*—are usually sensitive, with exceptions as noted in the following.[24, 28, 29] Chloramphenicol is active in vitro against most anaerobes, including *Bacteroides fragilis*.[30]

Other antimicrobials have replaced chloramphenicol in our armamentarium because of the potential for toxicity. β-Lactam antibiotics are highly effective against most gram-positive organisms, and second- and third-generation cephalosporins are active against most of the Enterobacteriaceae and many *Pseudomonas* species. Although *B. fragilis* is susceptible to chloramphenicol, other drugs, including metronidazole, clindamycin, cefotetan, cefoxitin, and the β-lactam–β-lactamase inhibitor combinations, are more commonly used to treat infections involving this organism.[31, 32]

Chloramphenicol has been a mainstay in the treatment of penicillin-allergic patients with meningitis.[33] The drug has excellent bactericidal activity against *H. influenzae*, including β-lactamase–producing strains, *N. meningitidis*, and most *S. pneumoniae* isolates. High cerebrospinal fluid levels are achieved. Until recently, chloramphenicol in combination with ampicillin has been the empirical therapy of choice for bacterial meningitis in children.[34] However, *S. pneumoniae* isolates with chloramphenicol resistance have been observed around the world.[35–39] Many penicillin-resistant strains are also resistant to chloramphenicol, with elevated minimal inhibitory concentrations of chloramphenicol. In addition, intermediate resistance to chloramphenicol has been described in penicillin-resistant isolates; minimal inhibitory concentrations suggest chloramphenicol sensitivity (4 μg/mL or less), whereas minimal bactericidal concentrations (8 μg/mL or greater) demonstrate relative resistance.[38, 39] Failure of chloramphenicol therapy for penicillin-resistant pneumococcal meningitis in this setting has been attributed to inadequate bactericidal activity in cerebrospinal fluid.[37–39] It is not known whether higher doses of chloramphenicol can overcome this intermediate resistance pattern. In addition, in vitro antagonism between chloramphenicol and β-lactam antibiotics has been observed repeatedly,[39, 40] although the clinical significance of this effect remains uncertain. Strains of *H. influenzae* have been isolated that are resistant to both chloramphenicol and ampicillin.[41] The third-generation cephalosporins have supplanted chloramphenicol use for the treatment of bacterial meningitis[42, 43] when these drugs are accessible and affordable.

Salmonella species, including *S. typhi*, with resistance to chloramphenicol have been isolated in the United States.[44–51] *S. typhi* strains resistant to all of the traditional first-line agents (chloramphenicol, ampicillin, trimethoprim-sulfamethoxazole) are now endemic throughout the Indian subcontinent, the Middle East, South Africa, and Southeast Asia.[50–53] For this reason, many now consider ciprofloxacin (and newer quinolones) to be alternative first-line agents for the treatment of typhoid fever.[53, 54] Shortened courses of ceftriaxone (3 to 7 days) have been shown to be as effective as 14 days of chloramphenicol therapy for *S. typhi* infection,[55, 56] although clinical relapse can occur with these regimens.

Shigella isolates resistant to multiple antibiotics, including chloramphenicol, are common in developing countries.[45] These strains have become prevalent because of the common practice of selling antimicrobials over-the-counter in these countries. Increasing resistance to ampicillin and trimethoprim-sulfamethoxazole, drugs of choice for shigellosis, has been reported for *Shigella dysenteriae* isolates in Africa and Asia.[45] Chloramphenicol's role in the treatment of this disease is limited; newer fluorinated quinolones, however, are effective substitutes.[57, 58]

Chloramphenicol is active against the majority of clinically important ricksettsiae, ehrlichiae, chlamydiae, spirochetes, and mycoplasmas; however, other less toxic therapeutic alternatives, such as the tetracyclines or erythromycin, are often recommended.[59–62]

Mechanisms of Resistance

Five mechanisms of resistance to chloramphenicol have been described: drug inactivation through acetylation or nitroreduction, alteration of bacterial ribosomal binding proteins, alteration of chloramphenicol transport across the bacterial cell wall, and active efflux pumping of the drug. The most significant of these mechanisms is the plasmid-mediated production of chloramphenicol acetyltransferase.[63] The R factors carrying this gene may confer simultaneous resistance to multiple antibiotics.[45, 51] Outbreaks of chloramphenicol-resistant typhoid fever and shigella dysentery have been associated with these plasmids.[50, 64, 65] A report from California traced an outbreak of plasmid-mediated chloramphenicol-resistant *Salmonella enteritidis* serotype *newport* infections in humans to contaminated hamburger prepared from cattle raised on a dairy farm where chloramphenicol use was common.[66] Thus, a direct link between antibiotic use, selection of resistance phenotypes, and human disease was established.

Chloramphenicol use in animals raised for food production has never been legal in the United States.

Chloramphenicol can be rapidly inactivated in vitro by some strains of *Bacteroides* and *Clostridium* through nitroreduction.[67] Altered binding of chloramphenicol to the 50S ribosomal subunit of *Bacillus subtilis* has been described.[68] Altered cell wall permeability to chloramphenicol has been described in *E. coli, Pseudomonas aeruginosa, Serratia,* and *H. influenzae*.[69–71] Transposon-mediated resistance genes encoded on bacterial plasmids have been identified in *Pseudomonas*. Presence of the transposon was associated with the loss of an outer membrane protein, with subsequent diminished chloramphenicol uptake.[72] A chromosomally mediated resistance gene, associated with loss of an outer membrane protein, has been identified in *H. influenzae* isolates.[73] An efflux mechanism has been proposed to further explain the intrinsic resistance of *P. aeruginosa* to chloramphenicol.[74]

Pharmacology

Serum concentrations of chloramphenicol are determined by dose, route of administration, and product form. Chloramphenicol is well absorbed from the gastrointestinal tract after oral administration and produces peak serum levels within 1 to 2 hours.[75] The drug is only slightly water soluble and is bitter to taste. Consequently, the oral suspension used in children is the more soluble tasteless palmitate ester. The intravenous formulation is a 3-monosuccinate ester. Because the esters are not microbiologically active, they must be hydrolyzed in the gastrointestinal tract by pancreatic lipase or in the body by the liver, kidneys, and lungs to the active chloramphenicol base.[11, 76] Hydrolysis is variable, and serum levels of active drug after palmitate administration are usually less than levels achieved after comparable doses of the base drug.[77] Chloramphenicol succinate is rapidly cleared from the plasma during intravenous administration.[78] The renal clearance of prodrug is 27% in adults and 41% in children.[79] Approximately 70% of intravenously administered succinate ester undergoes hydrolysis to the active base. As a result, serum levels produced by intravenous dosing are approximately 70% of those achieved after a similar oral dose of nonester.[80] Chloramphenicol palmitate produces lower levels than chloramphenicol base but higher levels than intravenous chloramphenicol succinate.[79] Hydrolysis is less complete after intramuscular injection of the succinate because of delayed absorption of the ester from the injection site.[81] Serum levels of active drug after an intramuscular dose are approximately one half to two thirds of a comparable intravenous dose. Studies of patients with typhoid fever and Rocky Mountain spotted fever have demonstrated delayed therapeutic responses and an increased frequency of relapse after intramuscular therapy compared with oral or intravenous treatment.[82] The use of intramuscular chloramphenicol is therefore not recommended.

Chloramphenicol in ophthalmic ointments and solutions is absorbed into the aqueous humor, producing bacteriostatic concentrations of the drug.[83] Subconjunctival injections do not produce adequate levels in the aqueous humor.[84] In the face of panophthalmitis due to susceptible organisms, systemic therapy is required. Topical drug should not be used to treat bacterial conjunctivitis.[85]

Chloramphenicol gains access into most body fluids, including cerebrospinal, pleural, pericardial, peritoneal, and joint fluids.[12, 86, 87] Forty percent to 65% of the plasma concentration is achieved in cerebrospinal fluid in the presence or absence of inflamed meninges.[12, 88, 89] The drug is lipophilic, and concentrations in brain tissue may be as high as nine times that of serum.[90] Only small concentrations of active drug are found in the bile.[91]

The drug is conjugated in the liver to glucuronate. Chloramphenicol glucuronide is microbiologically inactive and nontoxic.[91] When given concurrently, phenobarbital may increase the rate of conjugation of chloramphenicol, resulting in a significant decrease in the serum level of active drug.[92] The glucuronide is excreted by renal tubular secretion; only 5% to 10% of the drug is excreted in the active form by glomerular filtration.[91] Probenecid increases serum concentrations of inactive glucuronide but does not affect levels of active drug. Although chloramphenicol concentrations in the urine are sufficient to treat urinary tract infections in patients with normal renal function, urinary concentrations are inadequate in patients with renal failure.[93] Because the glucuronide is nontoxic, little dosage modification is required for decreased renal function. A reduction in glomerular filtration rate has little effect on plasma drug clearance.[94] There is no need for dosage change in patients undergoing dialysis; hemodialysis and peritoneal dialysis do not affect the serum half-life.[95]

Patients with significant parenchymal liver disease metabolize chloramphenicol at a lower rate. Increased levels of active chloramphenicol have been reported in patients with hepatic insufficiency, and bone marrow depression may ensue.[96] The dose should be reduced in such patients, and the course of therapy should be as brief as possible.

The hydrolysis of chloramphenicol succinate in children is variable, especially during the neonatal period.[97] Newborns have a deficiency of the glucuronide-conjugating mechanism as well as a reduced glomerular filtration rate.[88] The low rate of conjugation and reduction in renal clearance produces higher levels of drug per dose than in older infants. Reduced dosing and careful monitoring of serum levels of drug are required in this age group.[97] The drug crosses the placenta and is also found in breast milk. Caution is advised in treating pregnant or lactating women.[98]

In adults with normal liver function, chloramphenicol has a half-life of 3 to 4 hours and is 25% to 50% protein bound.[94, 99] Recommended doses usually produce serum concentrations of 5 to 25 μg/mL. Susceptible bacteria are defined as organisms inhibited by a concentration of 16 μg/mL or less.[100, 101]

Chloramphenicol interferes with the metabolism of phenytoin, tolbutamide, cyclosporine, and warfarin.[102–105] Similar interference probably occurs with tacrolimus (FK-506) as well. When these drugs are administered with chloramphenicol, their doses may have to be reduced and levels monitored. Because phenobarbital may increase or decrease the rate of metabolism of chloramphenicol, serum chloramphenicol levels should be assayed when these drugs are given concurrently.[92]

Toxicity and Adverse Reactions

Gray Syndrome

A symptom complex of vomiting, abdominal distention, lethargy, cyanosis, hypotension, irregular respirations, hypothermia, and death has been described in full-term neonates and premature infants treated with chloramphenicol.[5, 106] The syndrome is due to an accumulation of unaltered drug caused by a reduced ability to conjugate and excrete chloramphenicol in this age group.[97] Mitochondrial inner membrane enzyme activity is affected, including protein synthesis and oxidative phosphorylation.[107, 108] At moderately elevated concentrations, chloramphenicol inhibits the cytochrome system; at concentrations greater than 100 μg/mL, it interferes with electron transport in the NADPH oxidase portion of the mitochondrial respiratory chain.[109, 110] Organs with a high rate of oxygen consumption, such as the heart, liver, kidneys, and skeletal muscle, are particularly susceptible to the toxic effects of chloramphenicol.

Gray syndrome begins typically 3 to 4 days after the initiation of therapy. Concentrations of serum chloramphenicol are usually greater than 75 μg/mL.[5] An early finding is unexplained metabolic acidosis, caused by the inhibition of oxidation and production of lactic acid.[111] The acidosis does not respond to bicarbonate therapy, and cardiovascular collapse ensues in 6 to 12 hours. Generalized hypoperfusion causes the peculiar pallor and cyanosis that result in the characteristic gray color of the skin. Tissue hypoperfusion leads to further accumulation of lactic acid. As the drug accumulates, hepatocyte metabolism is inhibited and the rate of conjugation is slowed. Serum concentrations climb still higher, perpetuating the vicious circle.

This syndrome is reversible if the drug is terminated immediately after the onset of symptoms. Approximately 40% of affected infants die within 2 to 3 days. Exchange transfusions and charcoal-column hemoperfusion have been used successfully.[112, 113] Although most cases occur in infants younger than 30 days, the syndrome has been described in children 25 months of age and older who have elevated serum levels of drug and in adults who have accidentally ingested excessive quantities of chloramphenicol.[114, 115]

Hematologic Toxicity

Chloramphenicol may affect the hematopoietic system in several ways. Two potentially life-threatening toxic effects involving the bone marrow are well described.[4, 67, 101, 116, 117]

A dose-related, reversible depression of the marrow is a direct toxic effect. Chloramphenicol inhibits mammalian mitochondrial enzymes at serum concentrations of 10 μg/mL or higher, including the enzyme ferrochelatase, which catalyzes the final step in heme synthesis.[15, 116, 118] A reduction of serum iron use and incorporation into red blood cell precursors results from this inhibition.[119] The earliest sign of toxicity is reticulocytopenia, which occurs after 5 to 7 days of drug therapy.[120] Reticulocytopenia may also be caused by the underlying infection. Serum iron concentrations increase because of underuse and may double within 6 to 10 days. At chloramphenicol serum concentrations of 30 μg/mL or greater, the bone marrow develops morphologic changes.[120] Mitochondria are fragmented and the mitochondrial matrix is condensed, producing vacuolization in erythroid and myeloid precursors.[121] Vacuolization of precursors in the marrow is not specific for chloramphenicol intoxication; similar changes have been described in alcoholism, Di Guglielmo syndrome, phenylketonuria, and riboflavin deficiency.[122]

Bone marrow depression may cause anemia, granulocytopenia, and thrombocytopenia.[120] Thrombocytopenia develops late in the course of treatment, on day 16 or later. Patients deficient in folic acid and vitamin B_{12} do not respond to replacement therapy if they are given chloramphenicol concurrently.[123] Factors commonly associated with marrow depression are doses in excess of 4 g/d, liver disease, and serum concentrations in excess of 25 μg/mL.[96, 120] Marrow depression is reversible with discontinuation of the antibiotic. Failure to recognize this complication in time may result in terminal infection or hemorrhage.

The second type of bone marrow toxicity, thought to be idiosyncratic, is usually fatal.[4] Data suggest that chloramphenicol produces this irreversible aplastic anemia in 1 in 25,000 to 45,000 patients exposed to the drug.[124] An frequency as rare as 1 in 200,000 has also been reported.[125] Approximately 26% of all cases of aplastic anemia are attributed to chloramphenicol.[126] A slight predominance in female patients is noted. The majority of cases occur 3 to 12 weeks after chloramphenicol therapy is initiated, although aplasia may develop months and even years after therapy.[101, 124, 125, 127] This reaction is not dose related; indeed, numerous cases of aplastic anemia or pancytopenia occurring after the administration of chloramphenicol eyedrops have been reported.[128] The exact mechanism producing aplasia is not clearly defined. Concordance in identical twins suggests a genetic predisposition.[125, 129] Initially, idiosyncratic aplastic anemia was described only after oral administration.[130] For this reason, toxic bacterial degradation products of chloramphenicol absorbed from the gut were the suspected cause. This view is supported by the observation that bacterial degradation products of the drug have been shown to cause damage to human bone marrow cells and lymphocytes in culture.[131, 132] Subsequently, however, aplasia has been reported in patients treated with parenteral drug only.[133] Two additional patients have developed aplastic anemia after receiving parenteral chloramphenicol in conjunction with cimetidine.[134] Cimetidine is also known to have a suppressive effect on the bone marrow. Although aplasia may be more common after oral therapy, parenteral drug remains a risk.[135] Thiamphenicol, a chloramphenicol analog available in Europe and Japan but not in the United States, has been associated with reversible bone marrow depression but not with idiosyncratic aplastic anemia.[136] Because this drug has a methylsulfone group replacing the nitro group on the aromatic ring, the nitrobenzene moiety of chloramphenicol is suspected to be the inducer of aplastic anemia.[116]

Most cases of aplasia occur after chloramphenicol therapy has been completed, although this complication occasionally occurs during antibiotic administration. Accordingly, it makes sense to perform complete blood counts at least twice weekly for all patients receiving this antibiotic. The development of leukopenia, anemia, or thrombocytopenia would signal a need to discontinue the drug immediately. Although monitoring blood cell counts may not be a reliable way to predict most cases of aplastic anemia, dose-related marrow depression can be identified early in this way.[137] Treatment of aplasia has been unsatisfactory, although bone marrow transplantation is now recommended. Before the use of transplantation, all patients were dead within 18 months of the diagnosis.[101, 138]

Some patients with bone marrow hypoplasia attributed to chloramphenicol have subsequently developed acute myeloblastic leukemia.[139] Chloramphenicol is widely prescribed in China for infectious diseases in children. In Shanghai, children who received more than 10 days of chloramphenicol were found to have a greater risk for development of acute nonlymphocytic and acute lymphocytic leukemia than were control subjects. Acute nonlymphocytic leukemia developed more frequently than acute lymphocytic leukemia.[140] Although the methods of the Shanghai study have been criticized, chloramphenicol and several metabolites have been demonstrated to induce chromosomal aberrations and DNA strand breakage in cultured rat and human cell lines.[132, 141, 142] The drug is classified as a probable carcinogen by the International Agency for Research on Cancer.[143]

Chloramphenicol may induce acute hemolysis in patients with the Mediterranean form of glucose-6-phosphate dehydrogenase deficiency. Hemolysis has not been reported in black persons, who have the milder A type of this deficiency.[144]

Optic Neuritis

Optic nerve injury has been reported in patients with cystic fibrosis and others receiving prolonged courses of chloramphenicol.[145, 146] Reversible decreases in vision, central scotoma, and alterations in red-green color discrimination have been noted, but permanent changes have also been described.[147] Other neurologic syndromes including ophthalmoplegia, peripheral neuropathy, acute encephalopathy, depression, and headache have also been observed.[148]

Other Types of Reactions

Hypersensitivity reactions associated with chloramphenicol are uncommon but include drug fever and various dermatologic reactions.[149, 150] Jarisch-Herxheimer reactions have been reported in patients with relapsing fever, brucellosis, typhoid fever, and syphilis who were treated with chloramphenicol. Gastrointestinal complaints such as nausea, vomiting, and diarrhea have been noted, and glossitis has been produced by high doses of the drug.[150] Chloramphenicol has been demonstrated to suppress the primary immune response and cell-mediated immunity in animal models. The clinical significance of this immunosuppression is not known.[151, 152]

Drug Interactions

Chloramphenicol inhibits the hepatic drug-metabolizing microsomal enzymes, the cytochrome P-450 complex.[153] This inhibition is irreversible, and new enzymes must be synthesized.[154] The drug prolongs the half-life of warfarin, phenytoin, cyclosporine, and the oral hypoglycemic agents tolbutamide and chlorpropamide by this mechanism.[103–105, 154] Prothrombin times, phenytoin levels, cyclosporine levels, and blood glucose levels should be monitored when these drugs are given concurrently with chloramphenicol. Similar caution with tacrolimus (FK-506) is warranted. Because phenytoin and phenobarbital induce hepatic microsomal enzymes, including glucuronyl transferase, either or both of these drugs may decrease the serum half-life of chloramphenicol.[155] Acetaminophen has been reported to block hepatic uptake of chloramphenicol and prolong clearance of the drug.[156] The occurrence of aplasia in patients receiving concurrent chloramphenicol and cimetidine or acetazolamide may indicate additional important drug interactions.[128, 134]

Available Preparations

Preparations of chloramphenicol are listed in Table 27–1. Chloramphenicol capsules are no longer manufactured or marketed in the United States (since April 1995) but can be obtained from international pharmacies if required. Similarly, the oral suspension form of chloramphenicol (chloramphenicol palmitate) is not available in the United States. Questions regarding drug availability should be directed to the manufacturer (Parke-Davis, Morris Plains, New Jersey).

TABLE 27–1 ■ Preparations of Chloramphenicol

Oral	
Chloramphenicol capsules*	250 mg 500 mg
Chloramphenicol palmitate suspension*	150 mg/5 mL
Intravenous	
Chloramphenicol sodium succinate	1 g/vial
Ophthalmic	
Chloramphenicol ophthalmic solution	25 mg/vial
Chloramphenicol ophthalmic cream	1%
Otic	
Chloramphenicol otic solution	5 mg/mL

*Not available in the United States (see text).

TABLE 27–2 ■ Dosing of Chloramphenicol

AGE	DOSE	COMMENTS
Newborn younger than 2 wk and premature infants	25 mg/kg/d in 6-h intervals	Assay of serum levels mandatory
Infants 2–4 wk old	25 mg/kg q 12 h	
Older children and adults	50 mg/kg/d in 6-h intervals	
Older children and adults with meningitis	100 mg/kg/d in 6-h intervals	

Dosing Recommendations

Because oral chloramphenicol is well absorbed from the gastrointestinal tract and the intravenous ester formulation must be hydrolyzed in the body, oral and parenteral dosing recommendations are similar.[79, 80] Most susceptible organisms are inhibited by concentrations of chloramphenicol ranging between 5 and 20 μg/mL (below 16 μg/mL).[100, 101] The schedules listed in Table 27–2 produce serum levels within this range for most of the treatment period.

Assay

Bone marrow depression in children and adults and the gray syndrome in newborns and premature infants are dose related.[5, 120] Serum levels of chloramphenicol should be monitored in newborns, premature infants, patients with liver disease, and those receiving drugs that interfere with the metabolism of the antibiotic.[96, 97, 153] Serum concentrations should range between 10 and 25 μg/mL. Bone marrow depression occurs at concentrations greater than 25 μg/mL.[120]

Early chemical assays did not distinguish among prodrug, active drug, and conjugate.[157] Currently available methods include microbiologic and radioenzymatic assays and high-performance liquid chromatography. Although specific, bioassays are not sensitive. They require an appropriate test organism and may be confounded when other antibiotics are given simultaneously.[158, 159] Radioenzymatic assays using chloramphenicol acetyltransferase are rapid and specific but require expensive equipment.[160, 161] High-performance liquid chromatography has all the advantages of the radioenzymatic assay and can distinguish among prodrug, active drug, and conjugate.[162, 163]

Clinical Indications

Although rare, major chloramphenicol intoxication is life threatening. Accordingly, the clinical indications for this otherwise valuable drug are narrow and well defined.

Chloramphenicol is the first choice for treatment of rickettsial or ehrlichial infections in pregnancy or in the setting of tetracycline allergy.[3, 164] At present, the American Academy of Pediatrics recommends that Rocky Mountain spotted fever in children younger than 9 years be treated with chloramphenicol[165] to avoid tooth discoloration. However, this recommendation has been moderated by the observation that tooth discoloration did not occur in one study of children younger than 5 years who received repeated short courses (6 days) of tetracycline.[166] In addition, the risk of tooth discoloration may be lower still when doxycycline is used because of its lower calcium-binding avidity.[167] Thus, some pediatricians avoid chloramphenicol use, even in children younger than 9 years.[168] Chloramphenicol is, however, highly effective in both parenteral and oral forms when it is used to treat Rocky Mountain spotted fever and typhus. For nonpregnant patients older than 8 years in the absence of allergy, tetracycline or doxycycline should be considered the drug of first choice for treatment of Rocky Mountain spotted fever.[169] In a retrospective review of 237 cases of human ehrlichiosis, patients not receiving a chloramphenicol- or tetracycline-containing antibiotic regimen were more likely to have prolonged fever, require hospitalization, and have an increased mortality rate.[170]

As described before, chloramphenicol has been considered the drug of choice by many for severe *Salmonella* infections, particularly typhoid fever.[3, 28] For this reason, chloramphenicol remains a "gold standard" with which alternative therapeutic agents are compared.[171] However, the prevalence of chloramphenicol resistance is increasing throughout Asia, Africa, and the Middle East, and higher mortality rates have been observed in patients with drug-resistant *S. typhi* infections.[171–174] Thus, although chloramphenicol still has a significant role in the treatment of typhoid in developing countries, because of both cost and overall efficacy[175] it can no longer be considered the drug of choice for patients with severe disease (particularly in endemic areas with multidrug resistance). Alternative agents (for *S. typhi* strains resistant to ampicillin, trimethoprim-sulfamethoxazole, and chloramphenicol) include ciprofloxacin,[53, 54] ofloxacin,[176] and ceftriaxone.[55, 56] Drug therapy should be restricted to patients with systemic disease and is not indicated in the treatment of uncomplicated gastroenteritis. The carrier state responds to fluorinated quinolones.[54, 177, 178]

Chloramphenicol remains an important drug in the treatment of central nervous system infections. The drug is able to cross the blood-brain barrier and penetrate brain tissue because of its lipophilicity.[89, 90] Chloramphenicol is an effective alternative to the penicillins and cephalosporins in treating older children and adults with meningitis who have a severe penicillin allergy; it is bactericidal for sensitive isolates of *S. pneumoniae, N. meningitidis,* and *H. influenzae*.[21, 33, 179] Third-generation cephalosporins, particularly cefotaxime and ceftriaxone, have replaced penicillin-chloramphenicol or ampicillin-chloramphenicol combinations as empirical therapy of bacterial meningitis in nonallergic patients.[42] Chloramphenicol is not reliably effective in the treatment of gram-negative bacillary meningitis, perhaps because the drug is only bacteriostatic for this group of organisms.[21] The drug is also not useful in the treatment of neonatal meningitis, from which the most common organisms recovered are group B streptococci, gram-negative bacilli, and *Listeria*; chloramphenicol is bacteriostatic for this group of organisms as well.[79] Because of its activity against anaerobic organisms and favorable kinetics, chloramphenicol in combination with large doses of aqueous penicillin G has remained a mainstay in the treatment of pyogenic brain abscesses.[90, 180] High-dose penicillin and third-generation cephalosporins plus metronidazole are alternative therapies for brain abscess, which may result in more rapid sterilization of abscess fluid.[181–183]

Chloramphenicol is useful in treating penicillin-allergic patients with epiglottitis, septic arthritis, and osteomyelitis due to *H. influenzae*.[184] Chloramphenicol has been used in the treatment of nosocomial infections due to vancomycin-resistant *Enterococcus faecium*.[185] Optimal therapy for these infections has not been defined.

Several uncommon diseases may require the use of chloramphenicol. Melioidosis, a disease most commonly encountered in Southeast Asia and Australia, is treated with chloramphenicol in combination with tetracycline and an aminoglycoside. The use of cetazidime-containing regimens in the treatment of this disease, however, has been associated with lower mortality and relapse rates.[186, 187] Brucellosis may be treated with chloramphenicol or a tetracycline as an alternative.[188] Chloramphenicol is bacteriostatic for *Francisella tularensis* and *Yersinia pestis* but in extraordinary circumstances could be expected to treat clinical disease due to these pathogens effectively.[189–191]

Although chloramphenicol was once considered an option in treating abdominal and pelvic anaerobic infections because of the role of *B. fragilis*, a number of alternative drugs that are now available have rendered the use of chloramphenicol unnecessary in this situation.[31, 32]

References

1. Ehrlich J, Bartz QR, Smith RM, et al: Chloromycetin, a new antibiotic from a soil actinomycete. Science 106:417, 1947.
2. Ehrlich J, Gottlieb D, Burkholder RR, et al: *Streptomyces venezuelae*: N. sp., the source of chloromycetin. J Bacteriol 56:467, 1948.
3. Kucers A: Current position of chloramphenicol chemotherapy. J Antimicrob Chemother 6:1, 1980.
4. Rich ML, Ritterhof RJ, Hoffman RJ: A fatal case of aplastic anemia following chloramphenicol (Chloromycetin) therapy. Ann Intern Med 33:1459, 1950.
5. Burns LE, Hodgman JE, Cass AB: Fatal circulatory collapse in premature infants receiving chloramphenicol. N Engl J Med 261:1318, 1959.
6. Cole FS, Daum RS, Teller L, et al: Effect of ampicillin and chloramphenicol alone and in combination on ampicillin: Susceptible and resistant *Haemophilus influenzae* type B. Antimicrob Agents Chemother 15:415, 1979.
7. Chow AW, Guze LB: Bacteroidaceae bacteremia: Clinical experience with 112 patients. Medicine (Baltimore) 53:93, 1974.
8. Malik VS: Chloramphenicol. Adv Appl Microbiol 15:297, 1972.
9. Hahn FE, Gund P: A structured model of chloramphenicol receptor site. *In* Drews J, Hahn FE (eds): Drug Receptor Interactions in Antimicrobial Chemotherapy. New York, Springer-Verlag, 1975, pp 245–266.
10. Pongs O: Chloramphenicol. *In* Hahn FE (ed): Antibiotics, Vol 1. New York, Springer-Verlag, 1979, pp 26–42.
11. Glazko AJ, Edgerton WH, Dill WA, et al: Chloromycetin palmitate: A synthetic ester of chloromycetin. Antibiot Chemother 2:234, 1952.
12. McCrumb FR Jr, Snyder MJ, Hicken WJ: The use of chloramphenicol acid succinate in the treatment of acute infections. *In* Antibiotics Annual 1957–1958. New York, Medical Encyclopedia, 1958, pp 837–841.
13. Wisseman CL, Smadel JE, Hahn FE, et al: Mode of action of chloramphenicol. 1. Action of chloramphenicol on assimilation of ammonia and on synthesis of proteins and nucleic acids in *Escherichia coli*. J Bacteriol 67:662, 1954.
14. Vazquez D: Uptake and binding of chloramphenicol by sensitive and resistant organisms. Nature 203:257, 1964.
15. Martelo OJ, Manyan DR, Smith US, et al: Chloramphenicol and bone marrow mitochondria. J Lab Clin Med 74:927, 1969.
16. Freeman KB: Inhibition of mitochondrial and bacterial protein synthesis by chloramphenicol. Can J Biochem 48:479, 1970.
17. Pestka S: Inhibitors of ribosome functions. Annu Rev Microbiol 25:487, 1971.
18. Pestka S: Studies on the formation of transfer ribonucleic acid–ribosome complexes. XI. Antibiotic effects on phenylalanyl-oligonucleotide binding to ribosomes. Proc Natl Acad Sci USA 64:709, 1969.
19. Vazquez D, Barbacid M, Fernandez-Munoz R: Antibiotic action on the ribosomal peptidyl transferase center. *In* Drews J, Hahn FE (eds): Drug Receptor Interactions in Antimicrobial Chemotherapy. New York, Springer-Verlag, 1975, pp 193–216.
20. Wehrle PF, Mathies AW, Leedom JM, et al: Bacterial meningitis. Ann N Y Acad Sci 145:488, 1967.

21. Rahal JJ Jr, Simberkoff MS: Bactericidal and bacteriostatic action of chloramphenicol against meningeal pathogens. Antimicrob Agents Chemother 16:13, 1979.
22. Dajani AS, Kauffman RE: The renaissance of chloramphenicol. Pediatr Clin North Am 28:195, 1981.
23. Feder HM Jr, Osier C, Maderazo EG: Chloramphenicol: A review of its use in clinical practice. Rev Infect Dis 3:479, 1981.
24. Barry AL, Thornsberry C: Susceptibility testing: Appendix 2. *In* Lennette EH (ed): Manual of Clinical Microbiology, ed 3. Washington, DC, American Society for Microbiology, 1980, pp 498–499.
25. Finland M: Changing patterns of susceptibility of common bacterial pathogens to antimicrobial agents. Ann Intern Med 76:1009, 1972.
26. Finland M, Garner C, Wilcox C, et al: Susceptibility of "Enterobacteria" to aminoglycoside antibiotics: Comparisons with tetracyclines, polymyxins, chloramphenicol and spectinomycin. J Infect Dis 134(Suppl):S57, 1976.
27. Eickhoff TC, Bennett JV, Hayes PS, et al: *Pseudomonas pseudomallei* susceptibility to chemotherapeutic agents. J Infect Dis 121:95, 1970.
28. Robertson RP, Wahab MFA, Rasch FO: Evaluation of chloramphenicol and ampicillin in *Salmonella* enteric fever. N Engl J Med 278:171, 1968.
29. Rubinstein E, Shamberg B: In vitro activity of cinoxacin, ampicillin, and chloramphenicol against *Shigella* and non-typhoid *Salmonella*. Antimicrob Agents Chemother 11:577, 1977.
30. Finegold SM: Therapy for infections due to anaerobic bacteria: An overview. J Infect Dis 135(Suppl):S25, 1977.
31. Harding GKM, Buckwald FJ, Ronald AR, et al: Prospective, randomized comparative study of clindamycin, chloramphenicol, and ticarcillin, each and in combination with gentamicin, in therapy for intraabdominal and female genital tract sepsis. J Infect Dis 142:384, 1980.
32. Cuchural GJ Jr, Tally FP, Jacobus NV, et al: Susceptibility of the *Bacteroides fragilis* group in the United States: Analysis by site of infection. Antimicrob Agents Chemother 32:717, 1988.
33. Westenfeld GO, Paterson PY: Life-threatening infections: Choice of alternate drugs when penicillin cannot be given. JAMA 210:845, 1969.
34. Klein JO, Feigin RD, McCracken GH: Report of the task force on diagnosis and management of meningitis. Pediatrics 78(Suppl):959, 1986.
35. Klugman KP: Pneumococcal resistance to antibiotics. Clin Microbiol Rev 3:171, 1990.
36. Lee HJ, Park JY, Jang SH, et al: High incidence of resistance to multiple antimicrobials in clinical isolates of *Streptococcus pneumoniae* from a University Hospital in Korea. Clin Infect Dis 20:826, 1995.
37. Ridgway EJ, Allen KD, Neal TJ, et al: Penicillin-resistant pneumococcal meningitis (Letter). Lancet 339:931, 1992.
38. Friedland IR, Shelton S, McCracken GH: Chloramphenicol in penicillin-resistant pneumococcal meningitis (Letter). Lancet 342:240, 1993.
39. Friedland IR, Klugman KP: Failure of chloramphenicol therapy in penicillin-resistant pneumococcal meningitis. Lancet 339:405, 1992.
40. Wallace JF, Smith RH, Arcia M, et al: Studies on the pathogenesis of meningitis: Antagonism between penicillin and chloramphenicol in experimental pneumococcal meningitis. J Clin Lab Med 70:408, 1967.
41. Kenny JF, Isburg CD, Michaels RH: Meningitis due to *Haemophilus influenzae* type b resistant to both ampicillin and chloramphenicol. Pediatrics 66:14, 1980.
42. McCracken GH Jr, Nelson JD, Kaplan SL, et al: Consensus report: Antimicrobial therapy for bacterial meningitis in infants and children. Pediatr Infect Dis J 6:501, 1987.
43. Strandberg DA, Jorgensen JH, Drutz DJ: Activities of newer beta-lactam antibiotics against ampicillin, chloramphenicol, or multiply-resistant *Haemophilus influenzae*. Diagn Microbiol Infect Dis 2:333, 1984.
44. Cohen ML, Tauxe RV: Drug-resistant *Salmonella* in the United States: An epidemiologic perspective. Science 234:964, 1986.
45. Murray BE: Resistance of *Shigella, Salmonella* and other selected enteric pathogens to antimicrobial agents. Rev Infect Dis 8(Suppl):S172, 1986.
46. MacDonald KL, Cohen ML, Hargrett-Bean NT, et al: Changes in antimicrobial resistance of *Salmonella* isolated from humans in the United States. JAMA 258:1496, 1987.
47. Baine WB, Farmer JJ, Gangarosa EJ, et al: Typhoidal fever in the United States associated with the 1972–1973 epidemic in Mexico. J Infect Dis 135:649, 1977.
48. Ryder RW, Blake PA: Typhoid fever in the United States, 1975 and 1976. J Infect Dis 139:124, 1979.
49. Tacket CO, Dominguez LB, Fisher HJ, et al: An outbreak of multiple-drug-resistant *Salmonella* enteritis from raw milk. JAMA 253:2057, 1985.
50. Smith SH, Palumbo PE, Edelson PJ: *Salmonella* strains resistant to multiple antibiotics: Therapeutic implications. Pediatr Infect Dis 3:455, 1984.
51. Goldstein FW, Chumpitaz JC, Guevara JM, et al: Plasmid-mediated resistance to multiple antibiotics in *Salmonella typhi*. J Infect Dis 153:261, 1986.
52. Coovadia YM, Gathiram V, Bhamjee A, et al: An outbreak of multiresistant *Salmonella typhi* in South Africa. Q J Med 82:91, 1992.
53. Mourad AS, Metwally M, Nor El Deen A, et al: Multiple-drug-resistant *Salmonella typhi* (Letter). Clin Infect Dis 17:135, 1993.
54. DuPont HL: Quinolones in *Salmonella typhi* infection. Drugs 45(Suppl 3):119, 1993.
55. Lasserre R, Sangalang RP, Santiago L: Three-day treatment of typhoid fever with two different doses of ceftriaxone, compared to a 14-day therapy with chloramphenicol: A randomized trial. J Antimicrob Chemother 28:765, 1991.
56. Islam A, Butler T, Kabir I, et al: Treatment of typhoid fever with ceftriaxone for 5 days or chloramphenicol for 14 days: A randomized clinical trial. Antimicrob Agents Chemother 37:8, 1993.
57. DuPont HL, Corrado ML, Sabbaj J: Use of norfloxacin in the treatment of acute diarrheal disease. Am J Med 82(Suppl):79, 1987.
58. DuPont HL, Ericsson CD, Robinson A, et al: Current problems in antimicrobial therapy for bacterial enteric infections. Am J Med 82(Suppl):325, 1987.
59. Harrel GT: Treatment of Rocky Mountain spotted fever with antibiotics. Ann N Y Acad Sci 55:1027, 1952.
60. McLean IW Jr, Schwab JH, Hillegas AB, et al: Susceptibility of microorganisms to chloramphenicol (Chloromycetin). J Clin Invest 28:953, 1949.
61. Romansky MJ, Olansky S, Taggart SR, et al: The antitreponemal effect of oral chloromycetin in 23 cases of early syphilis in man: A preliminary report. Science 110:639, 1949.
62. Denny FW, Clyde WA Jr, Glezen WP: *Mycoplasma pneumoniae* disease: Clinical spectrum, pathophysiology, epidemiology and control. J Infect Dis 123:74, 1971.
63. Benveniste R, Davies J: Mechanisms of antibiotic resistance in bacteria. Annu Rev Biochem 42:471, 1973.
64. Datta N, Richards H, Datta C: *Salmonella typhi* in vivo acquires resistance to both chloramphenicol and co-trimoxazole. Lancet 1:1181, 1981.
65. Cherubin CE, Neu HC, Rahal JJ, et al: Emergence of resistance to chloramphenicol in *Salmonella*. J Infect Dis 135:807, 1977.
66. Spika JS, Waterman SH, Soo Hoo GW, et al: Chloramphenicol resistant *Salmonella newport* traced through hamburger to dairy farms. N Engl J Med 316:565, 1987.
67. Yunis A: Chloramphenicol: Relation of structure to activity and toxicity. Annu Rev Pharmacol Toxicol 28:83, 1988.
68. Osawa S, Takata R, Tanaka K, et al: Chloramphenicol resistant mutants of *Bacillus subtilis*. Mol Gen Genet 127:163, 1973.
69. Gaffney DF, Cundliffe E, Foster TJ: Chloramphenicol resistance that does not involve chloramphenicol acetyltransferase encoded by plasmids from gram negative bacteria. J Gen Microbiol 125:113, 1981.
70. Irvin JE, Ingram JM: Chloramphenicol-resistant variants of *Pseudomonas aeruginosa* defective in amino acid transport. Can J Biochem 58:1165, 1980.
71. Traub WH, Fukushima PI: Nonspecific resistance of *Serratia marcescens* against antimicrobial drugs. Chemotherapy 25:196, 1979.
72. Burns JL, Rubens CE, Mendelman PM, et al: Cloning and expression in *Escherichia coli* of a gene encoding nonenzymatic chloramphenicol resistance from *Pseudomonas aeruginosa*. Antimicrob Agents Chemother 29:445, 1986.

73. Burns JL, Mendelman PM, Levy J, et al: A permeability barrier as a mechanism of chloramphenicol resistance in *Haemophilus influenzae*. Antimicrob Agents Chemother 27:46, 1985.
74. Li XZ, Livermans DM, Nikaido H: Role of efflux pump(s) in intrinsic resistance of *Pseudomonas aeruginosa*: Resistance to tetracycline, chloramphenicol, and norfloxacin. Antimicrob Agents Chemother 38:1732, 1994.
75. Bartelloni PJ, Calia FM, Minchew BH, et al: Absorption and excretion of two chloramphenicol products in humans after oral administration. Am J Med Sci 258:203, 1969.
76. Kaufman RE, Miceli JN, Strebel L, et al: Pharmacokinetics of chloramphenicol and chloramphenicol succinate in infants and children. J Pediatr 98:315, 1981.
77. Sack CM, Koup JR, Smith AL: Chloramphenicol pharmacokinetics in infants and young children. Pediatrics 66:579, 1980.
78. Pickering LK, Hoecker JL, Kramer WG, et al: Clinical pharmacology of two chloramphenicol preparations in children: Sodium succinate (IV) and palmitate (oral) esters. J Pediatr 96:757, 1980.
79. Smith AL, Weber A: Pharmacology of chloramphenicol. Pediatr Clin North Am 30:209, 1983.
80. Glazko AJ, Dill AW, Kinkel JR, et al: Absorption and excretion of parenteral doses of chloramphenicol sodium succinate in comparison with peroral doses of chloramphenicol. Clin Pharmacol Ther 21:104, 1977.
81. Shah PN, D'Souza J, Dathani KK: Absorption of chloramphenicol by various routes of administration. Indian J Med Res 65:549, 1977.
82. DuPont HL, Hornick RB, Weiss RB, et al: Evaluation of chloramphenicol acid succinate therapy of induced typhoid fever and Rocky Mountain spotted fever. N Engl J Med 282:53, 1970.
83. George FJ, Hanna C: Ocular penetration of chloramphenicol. Arch Ophthalmol 93:184, 1977.
84. McPherson SD Jr, Presley GD, Crawford JR: Aqueous humor assays of subconjunctival antibiotics. Am J Ophthalmol 66:430, 1968.
85. Jarudi N: Comparison of antibiotic therapy in presumptive bacterial conjunctivitis. Am J Ophthalmol 79:790, 1975.
86. Bennett WM, Singer I, Golper T, et al: Guidelines for drug therapy in renal failure. Ann Intern Med 86:754, 1977.
87. Rapp GF, Griffith RS, Hebble WM: The permeability of traumatically inflamed synovial membrane to commonly used antibiotics. J Bone Joint Surg Am 48:1534, 1966.
88. Friedman CA, Lovejoy FC, Smith AL: Chloramphenicol disposition in infants and children. J Pediatr 95:1071, 1979.
89. Rensimer ER, Pickering LK, Ericsson C, et al: Sequential CSF concentration of chloramphenicol after administration of oral chloramphenicol palmitate. Lancet 1:165, 1981.
90. Kramer PW, Griffith RS, Campbell RL: Antibiotic penetration of the brain. J Neurosurg 31:295, 1969.
91. Glazko AJ, Wolf LM, Dill WA, et al: Biochemical studies on chloramphenicol (Chloromycetin). J Pharmacol Exp Ther 96:445, 1949.
92. Bloxham RA, Durbin GM, Johnson T, et al: Chloramphenicol and phenobarbitone: A drug interaction. Arch Dis Child 54:76, 1979.
93. Lindberg AA, Nilsson LH, Bucht H, et al: Concentrations of chloramphenicol in the urine and blood in relation to renal function. Br Med J 2:724, 1966.
94. Kunin CM, Glazko AJ, Finland M: Persistence of antibiotics in blood of patients with acute renal failure. II. Chloramphenicol and its metabolism products in the blood of patients with severe renal disease or hepatic cirrhosis. J Clin Invest 38:1498, 1959.
95. Kunin CM: A guide to use of antibiotics in patients with renal disease. Ann Intern Med 67:151, 1967.
96. Suhrland LG, Weisberger AS: Chloramphenicol toxicity in liver and renal disease. Arch Intern Med 112:161, 1963.
97. Weiss CF, Glazko AJ, Weston JK: Chloramphenicol in the newborn infant: A physiologic explanation of its toxicity when given in excessive doses. N Engl J Med 262:787, 1960.
98. Havelka J, Hejzlar M, Popov V, et al: Excretion of chloramphenicol in human milk. Chemotherapy 13:204, 1968.
99. Grafnetterova J, Grafnetter D, Schuck O, et al: The effect of endogenous compounds isolated from sera of uremic patients on chloramphenicol binding to proteins. Biochem Pharmacol 28:2923, 1979.
100. Ericsson HM, Sherris JC: Antibiotic sensitivity testing. Report of an international collaborative study. Acta Pathol Microbiol Scand Sect B 217(Suppl 217):1, 1971.
101. National Committee for Clinical Laboratory Standards: Methods for Antimicrobial Susceptibility Testing of Anaerobic Bacteria, ed 2, approved standard. Villanova, PA, National Committee for Clinical Laboratory Standards, 1990. NCCLS publication M11-A2.
102. Christiansen LK, Skovsted L: Inhibition of drug metabolism by chloramphenicol. Lancet 2:1397, 1969.
103. Adams HR, Isaacson EL, Masters BS: Inhibition of hepatic microsomal enzymes by chloramphenicol. J Pharmacol Exp Ther 203:388, 1977.
104. Serino F, Grevel J, Napoli KL, et al: Oxygen radical formation by the cytochrome P450 system as a cellular mechanism for cyclosporine toxicity. Transplant Proc 26:2916, 1994.
105. Steinfort CL, McConachy KA: Cyclosporin-chloramphenicol drug interaction in a heart-lung transplant recipient (Letter). Med J Aust 161:455, 1994.
106. Sutherland JM: Fatal cardiovascular collapse of infants receiving large amount of chloramphenicol. Am J Dis Child 97:761, 1959.
107. Abou-Khalil S, Abou-Khalil WH, Yunis AA: Differential effects of chloramphenicol and its nitrosoanalogue on protein synthesis and oxidative phosphorylation in rat liver mitochondria. Biochem Pharmacol 29:2605, 1980.
108. Hallman M: Oxygen uptake in neonatal rats: A developmental study with particular reference to the effects of chloramphenicol. Pediatr Res 7:923, 1973.
109. Freeman KB, Halder D: The inhibition of mammalian mitochondrial NADPH oxidation by chloramphenicol and its isomer and analogues. Can J Biochem 46:1003, 1968.
110. Freeman KB: Effects of chloramphenicol and its isomers and analogues on the mitochondrial respiratory chain. Can J Biochem 48:469, 1970.
111. Evans LS, Kleiman MB: Acidosis as a presenting feature of chloramphenicol toxicity. J Pediatr 108:475, 1986.
112. Kessler DL, Smith AL, Woodrum DE: Chloramphenicol toxicity in a neonate treated with exchange transfusion. J Pediatr 96:140, 1980.
113. Mauer SM, Chavers BM, Kjellstrand CM: Treatment of an infant with severe chloramphenicol intoxication using charcoal column hemoperfusion. J Pediatr 96:136, 1980.
114. Craft AW, Brocklebank JT, Hey EN, et al: The "grey toddler" chloramphenicol toxicity. Arch Dis Child 49:235, 1974.
115. Thompson WL, Anderson SE Jr, Lipsky JJ, et al: Overdoses of chloramphenicol (Letter). JAMA 243:149, 1975.
116. Yunis AA: Chloramphenicol toxicity: 25 years of research (Review). Am J Med 87:44N, 1989.
117. Holt D, Harvey D, Harvey R: Chloramphenicol toxicity. Adverse Drug React Toxicol Rev 12:93, 1993.
118. Mangan DR, Arimura GK, Yunis AA: Chloramphenicol-induced erythroid suppression and bone marrow ferrochelatase in dogs. J Lab Clin Med 79:137, 1972.
119. Rubin D, Weisberger AS, Botti RE, et al: Changes in iron metabolism in early chloramphenicol toxicity. J Clin Invest 37:1286, 1958.
120. Scott JL, Finegold SM, Belkin GA, et al: A controlled double blind study of the hematologic toxicity of chloramphenicol. N Engl J Med 272:1137, 1965.
121. Yunis AA, Smith US, Restrepo A: Reversible bone marrow suppression from chloramphenicol: A consequence of mitochondrial injury. Arch Intern Med 126:272, 1970.
122. Meissner HC, Smith AL: The current status of chloramphenicol. Pediatrics 64:3348, 1979.
123. Saidi P, Wallerstein RO, Aggeler PM: Effect of chloramphenicol on erythropoiesis. J Lab Clin Med 57:247, 1961.
124. Wallerstein RO, Condit PK, Kasper CK, et al: Statewide study of chloramphenicol therapy and fatal aplastic anemia. JAMA 208:2045, 1969.
125. Best WK: Chloramphenicol-associated blood dyscrasias. JAMA 201:181, 1967.
126. Alter BP, Potter NU, Li FP: Classification and etiology of the aplastic anemias. Clin Haematol 7:431, 1978.
127. Clarke WTW: Fatal aplastic anemia and chloramphenicol. Can Med Assoc J 97:815, 1967.
128. Frannfelder FT, Morgan RL, Yunis AA: Blood dyscrasias and

topical chloramphenicol (Letter). Am J Ophthalmol 115:812, 1992.
129. Nagao T, Mauer AM: Concordance for drug induced aplastic anemia in identical twins. N Engl J Med 281:7, 1969.
130. Holt R: The bacterial degradation of chloramphenicol. Lancet 1:1259, 1967.
131. Jiminez JJ, Arimura GK, Abou-Khalil WH, et al: Chloramphenicol-induced bone marrow injury: Possible role of bacterial metabolites of chloramphenicol. Blood 70:1180, 1987.
132. Frayssinet CL, Robba NA, Barnat S, et al: Cytotoxicity and DNA damaging potency of chloramphenicol and six metabolites: A new evaluation in human lymphocytes and Raji cells. Mutat Res 320:207, 1994.
133. Fink TJ, Gump DW: Chloramphenicol: An inpatient study of use and abuse. J Infect Dis 138:690, 1978.
134. West BC, DeVault GA Jr, Clement JC, et al: Aplastic anemia associated with parenteral chloramphenicol: Review of 10 cases, including the second case of possible increased risk with cimetidine. Rev Infect Dis 10:1048, 1988.
135. Plaut ME, Best WR: Aplastic anemia after parenteral chloramphenicol: Warning reviewed (Letter). N Engl J Med 306:1486, 1982.
136. Keiser C, Buchegger U: Hematologic side effects of chloramphenicol and thiamphenicol. Helv Med Acta 37:265, 1973.
137. Daum RS, Cohen DL, Smith AL: Fatal aplastic anemia following apparent dose-related chloramphenicol toxicity. J Pediatr 94:403, 1979.
138. Pillow PR, Epstein RB, Buckner CD: Treatment of bone marrow failure by isogenic marrow infusion. N Engl J Med 275:94, 1966.
139. Adamson RH, Seiber SM: Clinically induced leukemia in humans. Environ Health Res 39:93, 1981.
140. Shu XO, Gao YT, Linet MS, et al: Chloramphenicol use and childhood leukaemia in Shanghai. Lancet 2:934, 1987.
141. Serana I, Caretto S, Rainaldi G, et al: Induction of chromosomal aberrations and sister-chromatid exchanges by chloramphenicol. Mutat Res 248:145, 1991.
142. Martelli A, Mattioli F, Pastorino G, et al: Genotoxicity testing of chloramphenicol in rodent and human cells. Mutat Res 260:65, 1991.
143. International Agency for Research on Cancer: Monograph on the Evaluation of Carcinogenic Risks to Humans, Vol 50. Lyon, France, International Agency for Research on Cancer, pp 169–173.
144. McCaffrey RP, Halsted CH, Wahab MFA, et al: Chloramphenicol-induced hemolysis in Caucasian glucose-6-phosphate dehydrogenase deficiency. Ann Intern Med 74:722, 1971.
145. Wallenstein L, Snyder J: Neurotoxic reactions to chloromycetin. Ann Intern Med 36:1526, 1952.
146. Huang NN, Harley RD, Promadhattavedi V, et al: Visual disturbances in cystic fibrosis following chloramphenicol administration. J Pediatr 68:32, 1966.
147. Cocke JG, Brown RE, Geppert LJ: Optic neuritis with prolonged use of chloramphenicol. J Pediatr 68:27, 1981.
148. Levine PH, Regelson W, Holland JF: Chloramphenicol associated encephalopathy. Clin Pharmacol Ther 11:194, 1970.
149. Smadel JE: Chloramphenicol (Chloromycetin) in the treatment of infectious diseases. Am J Med 7:671, 1949.
150. Woodward TE, Wisseman CL Jr: Chloromycetin (chloramphenicol). New York, Medical Encyclopedia, 1958, pp 24–28.
151. Weisberger AS, Daniel TM: Suppression of antibody synthesis by chloramphenicol analogs. Proc Soc Exp Biol Med 131:570, 1969.
152. DaMert GJ, Sohle PG: Effect of chloramphenicol on in vitro function of lymphocytes. J Infect Dis 139:220, 1979.
153. Halpert J: Further studies of the suicide inactivation of purified rat liver cytochrome P-450 by chloramphenicol. Mol Pharmacol 21:166, 1982.
154. Koup J, Gibaldi M, McNamara P, et al: Interaction of chloramphenicol with phenytoin and phenobarbital. Clin Pharmacol Ther 24:571, 1978.
155. Krasinski K, Kusmiez H, Nelson JD: Pharmacologic interactions among chloramphenicol, phenytoin and phenobarbital. Pediatr Infect Dis 1:232, 1982.
156. Buchanan M, Moodley GP: Interaction between chloramphenicol and paracetamol. Br Med J 2:307, 1979.
157. Mason EO Jr, Kaplan SL, Baker CJ, et al: Modification of the colorimetric assay for chloramphenicol in the presence of bilirubin. Antimicrob Agents Chemother 15:544, 1979.
158. Bannatyne RM, Cheung R: Chloramphenicol bioassay. Antimicrob Agents Chemother 16:43, 1979.
159. Jorgenson JH, Alexander GA: Rapid bioassay for chloramphenicol in the presence of other antibiotics. Am J Clin Pathol 4:472, 1981.
160. Smith AL, Smith DH: Improved enzymatic assay of chloramphenicol. Clin Chem 24:1452, 1978.
161. Robison LR, Seligsohn R, Lerner SA: Simplified radioenzymatic assay for chloramphenicol. Antimicrob Agents Chemother 13:25, 1978.
162. Koup JR, Brodsky B, Lau A, et al: High performance liquid chromatographic assay of chloramphenicol in serum. Antimicrob Agents Chemother 14:439, 1978.
163. Velagapudi R, Smith RV, Ludden TM, et al: Simultaneous determination of chloramphenicol and chloramphenicol succinate in plasma using high-performance liquid chromatography. J Chromatogr 228:423, 1982.
164. Kelsey DS: Rocky Mountain spotted fever. Pediatr Clin North Am 26:369, 1979.
165. American Academy of Pediatrics: Rocky Mountain spotted fever. *In* Peter G (ed): 1994 Red Book: Report of the Committee on Infectious Diseases, ed 23. Elk Grove, IL, American Academy of Pediatrics, 1994.
166. Grossman ER, Walchek A, Freedman H, et al: Tetracyclines and permanent teeth: The relation between dose and tooth color. Pediatrics 47:567, 1971.
167. Forti G, Benincari C: Doxycycline and the teeth (Letter). Lancet 1:78, 1969.
168. Abramson JS, Givner LB: Should tetracycline be contraindicated for therapy of presumed Rocky Mountain spotted fever in children less than 9 years of age? Pediatrics 86:123, 1990.
169. Walker D: Rocky Mountain spotted fever: A seasonal alert. Clin Infect Dis 20:1111, 1995.
170. Fishbein DB, Dawson JE, Robinson LE: Human ehrlichiosis in the United States, 1985 to 1990. Ann Intern Med 120:736, 1994.
171. Gupta A: Multidrug resistant typhoid fever in children: Epidemiology and therapeutic approach. Pediatr Infect Dis J 13:134, 1994.
172. Sharma KB, Bhat MB, Pasricha A, et al: Multiple antibiotic resistance among salmonellae in India. J Antimicrob Chemother 5:15, 1979.
173. Mandal BK: *Salmonella typhi* and other salmonellas. Gut 35:726, 1994.
174. Bhutta ZA, Naqui SA, Razzaq RA, et al: Multi-drug resistant typhoid in children: Presentation and clinical features. Rev Infect Dis 13:832, 1991.
175. Chakravorty B, Jain N, Gupta B, et al: Chloramphenicol resistant enteric fever. J Indian Med Assoc 91:10, 1993.
176. Khan MA, Hayat Z, Sadick A: Ofloxacin in the treatment of typhoid fever resistant to chloramphenicol and amoxicillin. Clin Ther 16:815, 1994.
177. Gotuzzo E, Guerra JG, Benavente L: Use of norfloxacin to treat chronic typhoid carriers. J Infect Dis 157:1221, 1988.
178. Ferreccio C, Morris JG Jr, Valdivieso C, et al: Efficacy of ciprofloxacin in the treatment of chronic typhoid carriers. J Infect Dis 157:1235, 1988.
179. Hornick RB, Gallager LR, Ronald AR, et al: Chloramphenicol treatment of pyogenic meningitis. Bull Sch Med Univ Maryland 51:43, 1966.
180. Brewer NS, MacCarty CS, Wellman WE: Brain abscess: A review of recent experience. Ann Intern Med 82:571, 1975.
181. Overturf GD: Pyogenic bacterial infections of the CNS. Neurol Clin 4:69, 1986.
182. Chun CH, Johnson JD, Hofstetter M, et al: Brain abscess: A study of 45 consecutive cases. Medicine (Baltimore) 65:415, 1986.
183. Sjolin J, Lilja A, Eriksson N, et al: Treatment of brain abscess with cefotaxime and metronidazole: Prospective study on 15 consecutive patients. Clin Infect Dis 17:857, 1993.
184. Dajani AS, Asmar BI, Thirumoorthi MC: Systemic *Haemophilus influenzae* disease: An overview. J Pediatr 94:355, 1979.
185. Norris AH, Reilly JP, Edelstein PA, et al: Chloramphenicol for the treatment of vancomycin-resistant enterococcal infections. Clin Infect Dis 20:1137, 1995.
186. Sookpranee M, Boonma P, Susaengut W, et al: Multicenter pro-

spective randomized trial comparing ceftazidime plus co-trimoxazole with chloramphenicol plus doxycycline and co-trimoxazole for treatment of severe melioidosis. Antimicrob Agents Chemother 36:158, 1992.
187. Chaowagul W, Suputtamongkol I, Dance DA, et al: Relapse in melioidosis: Incidence and risk factors. J Infect Dis 168:1181, 1993.
188. Rizzo-Naudi J, Griseti-Soler N, Canado W: Human brucellosis: An evaluation of antibiotics in the treatment of brucellosis. Postgrad Med J 13:520, 1967.
189. McCrumb FR, Mercier S, Robic G, et al: Chloramphenicol and Terramycin in the treatment of pneumonic plague. Am J Med 14:284, 1953.
190. McCrumb FR, Snyder MJ, Woodward TE: Studies on human infection with *Pasteurella tularensis*: Comparison of streptomycin and chloramphenicol in the prophylaxis of clinical disease. Trans Assoc Am Physicians 70:74, 1957.
191. Meyer KF, Quan SF, McCrumb FR, et al: Effective treatment of plague. Ann N Y Acad Sci 55:1228, 1952.

28

Metronidazole and Other Nitroimidazoles

Glenn E. Mathisen

Metronidazole

Metronidazole, an antimicrobial agent that has excellent activity against strict anaerobic bacteria and certain parasites, has become an important agent in the treatment of a wide variety of anaerobic infections. Its excellent penetration into all tissues (including the central nervous system) and bactericidal activity against strict anaerobes have made it especially useful for treatment of certain deep-seated infections, such as brain abscess and anaerobic osteomyelitis. Although questions about the mutagenicity of the drug have been raised, increasing experience suggests that it is a safe, well-tolerated drug that has few major side effects when used properly.

Mode of Action

The mode of action of metronidazole can be thought of as involving four successive steps[1]: (1) entry of the drug into the bacterial cell, (2) reductive activation, (3) toxic effect of the reduced intermediate product(s), and (4) release of inactive end products. Reductive activation occurs when the nitro group of the drug (which acts as a preferential electron acceptor) is reduced by low-redox-potential electron transport proteins. This reduces the intracellular concentration of unchanged drug and produces a gradient that promotes further entry of the unchanged drug into the cell. Short-lived intermediate compounds or free radicals are believed to damage the cell through interaction with DNA or other macromolecular compounds. The cytotoxic intermediate compounds decompose into nontoxic and inactive end products, including acetamide and 2-hydroxyethyl oxamic acid.

Metronidazole acts as a potent bactericidal agent; organisms are typically killed at the same concentration as or within a twofold dilution of that required for inhibition.[2] The metabolic products of metronidazole include a hydroxy derivative that also has significant anaerobic activity.[3] Other breakdown products (e.g., acid derivative) may have considerably less activity or may not be taken up by the target organism.[1]

Spectrum of Activity and Resistance

The activity of metronidazole against 793 strains of anaerobic and microaerophilic bacteria is summarized in Table 28–1.[3] Note the excellent activity of metronidazole against strict anaerobic organisms such as *Bacteroides fragilis*—virtually all the organisms were inhibited by 16 μg/mL or less, the breakpoint for the drug. Despite widespread use of metronidazole, susceptibility surveys suggest that *B. fragilis* and related organisms remain almost uniformly susceptible to metronidazole.[4, 5] Metronidazole is much less active against gram-positive non–spore-forming anaerobes; only 25% of *Actinomyces* and *Arachnia* strains are susceptible to metronidazole at achievable levels. *Propionibacterium acnes* is often resistant, with some strains requiring greater than 100 μg/mL for inhibition.[6, 7] In vitro studies have also indicated the drug's poor activity against facultative anaerobes and microaerophilic streptococci—organisms that are frequently found in mixed aerobic-anaerobic infections. In these infections, metronidazole alone is inadequate and antimicrobial agents active against microaerophilic streptococci (e.g., penicillin G) and gram-negative facultative anaerobes should also be administered.

Metronidazole also has activity against a variety of other organisms such as *Treponema pallidum*, oral spirochetes, *Campylobacter fetus*, *Helicobacter pylori*, and *Gardnerella vaginalis*. It is rare to see resistance to metronidazole among strict anaerobic bacteria; however, it does occur and can lead to a clinical relapse of infection.[8, 9] Resistance has been noted among isolated strains of *B. fragilis*, *Bacteroides distasonis*, *Prevotella melaninogenica* (formerly *Bacteroides melaninogenicus*), and *Bacteroides bivius*. The mechanism of this resistance is unclear; however, Tally and colleagues[10] studied a resistant strain of *B. fragilis* and found both slower cellular uptake and decreased intracellular reduction of the drug. Resistance of *Trichomonas vaginalis* to metronidazole is well recognized and may occasionally lead to treatment failure; the mechanism of this resistance is unknown but it can usually be overcome with higher doses of metronidazole.[11–14] Unfortunately, plasmid-transferable resistance to metronidazole has been described; this could lead to relatively rapid widespread development of resistance in the future, although it does not seem to be a clinical problem at the present time.

Pharmacology

Metronidazole is almost completely absorbed after oral administration. Serum levels are similar after equivalent oral and intravenous doses. The drug is generally given in an intravenous loading dose of 15 mg/kg followed by a maintenance dose of 7.5 mg/kg every 6 hours. This results in peak and trough steady-state plasma levels averaging 25 and 18 μg/mL; serum half-life is approximately 8 hours, so dosage at longer intervals is certainly feasible. Although total absorption of the drug is not affected by administration with food, peak serum levels are markedly delayed. Metronidazole is well absorbed via the rectal route, with peak levels occurring approximately 3 hours after administration. Metronidazole is absorbed after vaginal administration, although peak levels (mean 1.2 μg/mL) and bioavailability (20%) are lower than after administration via the oral or intravenous route.[15, 16] Metronidazole readily crosses the placenta; intrave-

TABLE 28–1 ■ Activity of Metronidazole Against Anaerobic and Microaerophilic Bacteria

BACTERIA	NUMBER OF STRAINS	CUMULATIVE PERCENTAGE SUSCEPTIBLE TO INDICATED CONCENTRATION (μg/mL) 4	8	16	32
*Bacteroides fragilis**	161	90	99	100	—
Prevotella melaninogenica†	60	98	100	—	—
Other *Bacteroides* and *Selenomonas* spp.	154	95	98	100	—
Fusobacterium sp.	65	100	—	—	—
Anaerobic gram-negative cocci	24	92	96	100	—
Anaerobic gram-positive cocci	124	98	—	—	—
Clostridium perfringens	18	94	100	—	—
Other *Clostridium* spp.	73	97	99	—	100
Gram-positive nonsporulating bacilli	87	57	60	62	66
Capnocytophaga spp.	27	52	70	93	—

*Includes all species of the *B. fragilis* group.
†Includes *P. melaninogenica* (formerly *Bacteroides melaninogenicus*) and *Porphyromonas asaccharolytica* (formerly *Bacteroides asaccharolyticus*).
From Sutter VL: *In* In vitro susceptibility of anaerobic and microaerophilic bacteria to metronidazole and its hydroxy metabolite. Finegold SM, George WL, Rolfe RD (eds): Proceedings of the First United States Metronidazole Conference, Tarpon Springs, FL, February 1982. New York, Biomedical Information, 1982, p 61.

nous administration to pregnant women produces equivalent fetal serum levels.[17]

Metronidazole has excellent penetration at almost all sites and has been shown to achieve therapeutic levels in the following tissues and fluids: alveolar bone, amniotic fluid, unobstructed biliary tract, cerebrospinal fluid and brain abscess contents, cord blood, pleural empyema fluid, hepatic abscesses, middle-ear discharge, middle-ear mucosa, breast milk, pelvic tissues, saliva, seminal fluid, and vaginal secretions. Penetration into aqueous humor results in levels one half to one third of serum levels.[18] Metronidazole has little protein binding, and its volume of distribution is approximately 80% of body weight.

Metronidazole is metabolized in the liver with the formation of five major metabolic products: the hydroxy derivative, an acid metabolite, acetylmetronidazole, metronidazole glucuronide, and the glucuronide conjugate of hydroxymetronidazole. Metronidazole and its metabolites are eliminated primarily in the urine (60% to 80%); 6% to 15% is excreted in the feces.

In patients with severe renal failure, the hydroxy metabolite of metronidazole accumulates; this is not generally a problem, and dose adjustment is not required unless there is concomitant hepatic failure. Metronidazole is rapidly eliminated during hemodialysis, which reduces the elimination half-life of the drug to 2.6 hours. The drug is also eliminated during peritoneal dialysis, and dose reduction is generally not recommended during chronic ambulatory peritoneal dialysis.[19] Serum clearance of metronidazole is delayed in patients with impaired hepatic function. Although data are limited, a dose reduction of 50% has been recommended in patients with severe hepatic dysfunction regardless of the presence of renal failure.[20, 21]

Administration and Dosage

Current recommended dosing schedules for metronidazole are shown in Table 28–2. Intravenous administration is recommended for seriously ill patients, although the excellent serum levels after oral administration allow this route to be used as conditions warrant. The manufacturer recommends intravenous administration during a 1-hour period, although a number of investigators have administered the drug in as little as 20 minutes without any apparent adverse effects.

After reconstitution, metronidazole hydrochloride should be diluted with intravenous fluid to a concentration not exceeding 8 μg/mL and should be neutralized to a pH of 6.0 to 7.0 with sodium bicarbonate before administration. The drug is also available from the manufacturer in a premixed, ready-to-use isotonic solution that does not require dilution or buffering before infusion.

The recommended duration of therapy in various situations is noted in Table 28–2. For serious infections, 2 to 4 weeks of therapy is recommended; certain patients may require more prolonged therapy depending on the clinical situation and the physician's judgment.

TABLE 28–2 ■ Major Indications for Metronidazole: Administration and Dosage*

INDICATION	ROUTE OF ADMINISTRATION	DOSAGE
Susceptible anaerobic infections	IV	Loading dose of 15 mg/kg, then 7.5 mg/kg q 6 h
	PO	1–2 g/d in 2–4 doses q 6–12 h
Nonspecific vaginitis	PO	500 mg bid for 7 d
	Intravaginally	5 g 0.75% metronidazole gel bid for 5 d
Trichomonas vaginitis	PO	250 mg tid for 7 d or 500 mg bid for 5 d or 2 g in a single dose
Amebiasis (intestinal or extraintestinal)	IV or PO	750 mg tid for 10 d
Giardiasis	PO	250 mg bid or tid for 5–7 d or 2 g/d for 3 d
Pseudomembranous enterocolitis	PO	500 mg q 6–12 h for 7–10 d
	IV†	500 mg q 6–8 h

*IV, Intravenous; PO, oral; bid, twice daily; tid, three times daily.
†For use in patients unable to take oral therapy. The optimal drug and dose in this situation have not been determined. See references 30, 31, and 63.

Dosage adjustment for patients with severe hepatic dysfunction was discussed in a previous section.

Adverse Reactions

Metronidazole is well tolerated, and major adverse reactions are uncommon when the drug is used properly. Table 28–3 lists the most common major and minor adverse reactions. The most serious adverse reactions involve the central nervous system and include seizures, cerebellar ataxia, and peripheral neuropathy. These reactions are rare and generally occur in patients who are receiving high doses of the drug for a prolonged period. Caution should be exercised when the drug is administered to patients with a history of seizures or neurologic problems; administration of the drug should be discontinued immediately if any of these toxic effects develop. Gastrointestinal side effects include nausea, anorexia, and epigastric distress; diarrhea and vomiting are less common. Although metronidazole is used to treat pseudomembranous colitis, it has rarely been reported to cause pseudomembranous colitis. This possibility should be considered in patients who develop diarrhea while receiving the drug. In addition to these side effects, other reactions such as stomatitis, dry mouth, furring of the tongue, glossitis, headache, fever, dizziness, pneumonitis, syncope, aseptic meningitis, and oral or vaginal candidiasis may be seen.

Concerns have been raised about the potential mutagenicity of the drug on the basis of tests in the Ames *Salmonella* mutant system and the evidence of possible carcinogenicity of metronidazole in some animal models.[22] It is believed that antibacterial activity and mutagenic activity are related to nitroreduction of the drug. The fact that little nitroreduction takes place in eukaryotic cells suggests that mutagenicity is less likely to occur in humans. Indeed, when metronidazole was studied for mutagenic potential in eukaryotic test systems, no evidence of mutagenicity could be detected.[23, 24] Results of animal carcinogenicity studies are confusing. Although prolonged administration of metronidazole has resulted in increased tumor rates in some animal models, other studies have been negative or even suggested that metronidazole reduced the effect of some carcinogens.[25, 26] Long-term follow-up of a cohort of 771 women who received metronidazole therapy for the treatment of vaginal trichomoniasis during the 1960s has not shown an increased incidence of malignancy.[27] On the other hand, a report raised the possibility of carcinogenicity in patients with Crohn disease who received prolonged therapy.[28] These cases remain anecdotal, and great caution should be exercised in attributing carcinogenicity to metronidazole in this situation. Metronidazole appears safe when used in standard doses for limited periods (weeks); patients should not be given more prolonged therapy unless absolutely necessary.

Metronidazole crosses the placental barrier, and concerns have been raised about possible teratogenicity. However, a study of pregnant women who had received metronidazole during pregnancy uncovered no evidence of an increased incidence of birth defects or adverse events in infants born after the exposure.[29] Animal studies[30] and one anecdotal human case[31] have suggested the possibility of teratogenicity, but it is difficult to extrapolate from these few data. A meta-analysis reviewed 32 published studies referring to the use of metronidazole in pregnancy; no excess of teratogenicity was demonstrated in the 7 evaluable studies (1336 patients).[32] Although use of metronidazole appears to be safe during the later part of pregnancy, it should be restricted to situations in which it is clearly needed. Metronidazole should probably not be given during the first trimester unless clearly necessary.

TABLE 28–3 ■ Adverse Effects Related to Metronidazole Therapy

MAJOR ADVERSE REACTIONS (RARE)
Seizures, encephalopathy
Cerebellar dysfunction, ataxia
Peripheral neuropathy
Disulfiram reaction with alcohol
Potentiation of effects of warfarin
Pseudomembranous colitis
Pancreatitis
Aseptic meningitis
Hepatotoxicity
MINOR ADVERSE REACTIONS
Minor gastrointestinal disturbances
Reversible neutropenia
Metallic taste
Dark or red-brown urine
Maculopapular rash, urticaria
Urethral, vaginal burning
Gynecomastia

Clinical Use

ANAEROBIC INFECTIONS

Metronidazole is used for treatment of a wide variety of anaerobic infections. An important caveat is that the microbial flora of anaerobic infections is frequently mixed and often includes microaerophilic streptococci and other organisms resistant to metronidazole (e.g., anaerobic non–spore-forming gram-positive rods). In these situations, the addition of penicillin G or ampicillin (erythromycin for the penicillin-allergic patient) is necessary for optimal antimicrobial coverage. The presence of facultative anaerobic gram-negative rods would also require an additional drug for adequate coverage. These considerations help to explain the suboptimal response described when metronidazole alone is used in the treatment of anaerobic pleuropulmonary infection.[33]

Metronidazole's excellent tissue penetration and bactericidal activity make it a useful agent for deep-seated infections that are difficult to treat such as anaerobic central nervous system infections (e.g., brain abscess), endocarditis caused by susceptible anaerobes, and anaerobic infection in the immunocompromised host. For example, metronidazole (in combination with penicillin) has become the agent of choice for anaerobic brain abscess and is probably one factor that has enhanced survival of these patients. Metronidazole has been found to be useful in the treatment of a number of other anaerobic infections including bacteremia, infections of bones and joints, soft tissue infections, oral and dental infections, intravaginal infections, and head and neck infections. Metronidazole is useful for therapy of nonspecific vaginitis, a condition in which various anaerobes (and *G. vaginalis*) may play a role.[34–36] Its use in the treatment of bacterial vaginosis during the later stages of pregnancy appears to be helpful in preventing preterm birth in some patients.[37, 38] Metronidazole's role in the therapy of pseudomembranous colitis has already been mentioned; several studies suggest that metronidazole may even be effective as parenteral therapy when oral agents cannot be taken because of ileus or toxic megacolon.[39, 40] In the treatment of tetanus, a clinical study suggests that metronidazole may be more effective than procaine penicillin.[41]

PARASITIC INFECTIONS

Metronidazole is quite useful in the therapy of a number of parasitic infections with single-cell parasites such as *Ent-*

amoeba histolytica, Giardia lamblia, and T. vaginalis. Metronidazole is the treatment of choice for amebic liver abscess and invasive intestinal amebiasis; data even suggest that it effectively eradicates cysts in the asymptomatic intestinal carrier. Vaginitis caused by *T. vaginalis* can be successfully treated with any one of a number of regimens utilizing metronidazole (see Table 28–2). Treatment failures resulting from resistant strains have been described but can generally be overcome with higher doses or the use of other drugs such as clindamycin.[11–13, 42] Metronidazole is quite useful in the therapy of giardiasis, although occasional treatment failures may require alternative therapy. *Blastocystis hominis* may cause intestinal infection with diarrhea, which can be treated with metronidazole.[43] Although metronidazole may have some value in therapy for cutaneous leishmaniasis, it appears to be less effective than other agents.[44]

Other Therapeutic Uses

Metronidazole has been shown to be helpful in the treatment of a number of syndromes believed to be related to overgrowth of intestinal bacterial flora. These conditions include the complications of jejunoileal bypass for obesity[45] and dysfunction of the continent ileostomy[46]; it can also be used to prevent intrahepatic cholestasis associated with total parenteral nutrition.[47] Although use in Crohn disease is controversial, some studies have suggested that metronidazole may have a beneficial effect in this condition. It appears to be able to lessen the diarrhea and may be effective for other complications such as perianal fistula, erythema nodosum, and metastatic skin lesions.[48, 49] Unfortunately, prolonged therapy is necessary in this situation, and the frequent occurrence of peripheral neuropathy[50] and concerns about potential carcinogenicity[28] may limit its usefulness.

Several studies have shown metronidazole to be an effective prophylactic agent (alone or in combination with other antimicrobials) in patients undergoing elective colon surgery, gynecologic surgery, and emergency appendectomy. Although metronidazole may be useful in these situations, it should be kept in mind that true intraabdominal infection requires additional agents. Some studies showed metronidazole to be less effective than other agents in both appendectomy for nonperforated appendicitis and hysterectomy.[51, 52]

Tinidazole

Tinidazole is a nitroimidazole compound that is similar to metronidazole in its mechanism of action, antimicrobial spectrum, and toxicity. Although there is far less clinical experience with tinidazole, its longer half-life suggests that it may have some advantages in certain clinical situations. Oral absorption of the drug is almost complete, and serum levels are comparable to those seen after intravenous administration; after the standard oral dose of 2 g, serum levels between 40 and 60 μg/mL are reached.[53] The prolonged serum half-life (12.5 hours) allows therapeutic levels (10 μg/mL) to be present 24 hours after oral administration.

Because of the drug's pharmacokinetics, single-dose regimens are effective for treatment of trichomoniasis in both men and women.[54–56] Several studies have shown that single-dose tinidazole is as effective as (or more effective than) various single- and multiple-dose regimens of metronidazole in the treatment of giardiasis.[57–59] Tinidazole is also active against *E. histolytica*; relatively short courses (3 days) of therapy appear to be as effective as longer courses of metronidazole in the therapy of intestinal amebiasis,[60] although one study has shown more prolonged cyst excretion with tinidazole. Tinidazole appears to be as effective as metronidazole in the treatment of amebic liver abscess, although treatment may occasionally fail if other adjunctive measures (i.e., needle aspiration and drainage) are not used for more seriously ill patients.

The single-dose regimens of tinidazole offer definite advantages in clinical situations in which cost and compliance are an issue. Although it would be reasonable to assume that tinidazole would be as effective as metronidazole in the therapy of serious intraabdominal infection, there are relatively few clinical data at this time.

Other Nitroimidazole Compounds

Several other agents are closely related to metronidazole; however, some are investigational and far fewer data are available concerning their clinical use. Nimorazole is comparable to metronidazole and tinidazole in the treatment of giardiasis and trichomoniasis[59, 61]; however, it appears to be far less active against obligately anaerobic gram-negative bacilli.[62] Ornidazole is similar to tinidazole and metronidazole and has been used successfully to treat a variety of bacterial and parasitic infections; one potential drawback is its increased incidence of side effects. Few data are available on two other agents—carnidazole and secnidazole; however, both have proved effective in the single-dose treatment of vaginal trichomoniasis.[63, 64]

References

1. Müller M: Mode of action of metronidazole on anaerobic bacteria and protozoa. Surgery 93:165, 1983.
2. Nastro LJ, Finegold SM: Bacterial activity of five antimicrobial agents against *Bacteroides fragilis*. J Infect Dis 136:104, 1972.
3. Sutter VL: In vitro susceptibility of anaerobic and microaerophilic bacteria to metronidazole and its hydroxy metabolite. *In* Finegold SM, George WL, Rolfe RD (eds): Proceedings of the First United States Metronidazole Conference, Tarpon Springs, FL, February 1982. New York, Biomedical Information, 1982, p 61.
4. Turgeon P, Turgeon V, Gourdeau M, et al: Longitudinal study of susceptibilities of species of the *Bacteroides fragilis* group to five antimicrobial agents in three medical centers. Antimicrob Agents Chemother 38:2276, 1994.
5. Aldridge KE, Gelfand M, Reller LB, et al: A five-year multicenter study of the susceptibility of the *Bacteroides fragilis* group isolates to cephalosporins, cephamins, penicillins, clindamycin, and metronidazole in the United States. Diagn Microbiol Infect Dis 18:235, 1994.
6. Wust J: Susceptibility of anaerobic bacteria to metronidazole, ornidazole, and tinidazole and routine susceptibility testing by standardized methods. Antimicrob Agents Chemother 11:631, 1977.
7. Rosenblatt JE, Edson RS: Metronidazole. Mayo Clin Proc 58:154, 1983.
8. Ingham HR, Eaton S, Venables CW, et al: *Bacteroides fragilis* resistant to metronidazole after long-term therapy. Lancet 1:214, 1978.
9. Sprott MS, Ingham HR, Hickman JE, et al: Metronidazole-resistant anaerobes. Lancet 1:1220, 1983.
10. Tally FP, Snydman DR, Shimell MJ, et al: Mechanisms of antimicrobial resistance of *Bacteroides fragilis*. *In* Phillips I, Collier J (eds): Metronidazole: Proceedings of the Second International Symposium on Anaerobic Infections, Geneva, April 1979. New York, Grune & Stratton, 1979, p 19.
11. Robertson DHH, Heyworth R, Harrison C, Lumsden WHR: Treatment failure in *Trichomonas vaginalis* infections in females. I. Concentrations of metronidazole in plasma and vaginal content during normal and high dosage. J Antimicrob Chemother 21:373, 1988.
12. Lumsden WHR, Harrison C, Robertson DHH: Treatment failure in *Trichomonas vaginalis* infections in females. II. In-vitro estimation of the sensitivity of the organism to metronidazole. J Antimicrob Chemother 21:555, 1988.

13. Müller M, Lossick JG, Gorrell TE: In vitro susceptibility of *Trichomonas vaginalis* to metronidazole and treatment outcome in vaginal trichomoniasis. Sex Transm Dis 15:17, 1988.
14. Ahmed-Jushuf IH, Murray AE, McKeown J: Managing trichomonal vaginitis refractory to conventional treatment with metronidazole. Genitourin Med 64:25, 1988.
15. Fredricsson B, Hagstrom B, Nord C-E, et al: Systemic concentrations of metronidazole and its main metabolites after intravenous, oral and vaginal administration. Gynecol Obstet Invest 24:200, 1987.
16. Cunningham E, Kraus DM, Brubaker L, Fischer JH: Pharmacokinetics of intravaginal metronidazole gel. J Clin Pharmacol 34:1060, 1994.
17. Visser AA, Hundt HKL: The pharmacokinetics of a single intravenous dose of metronidazole in pregnant patients. J Antimicrob Chemother 13:279, 1984.
18. Mattila J, Nerdrum K, Rouhiainen H, et al: Penetration of metronidazole and tinidazole into the aqueous humor in man. Chemotherapy 29:188, 1983.
19. Guay DR, Meatherall RC, Baxter H, et al: Pharmacokinetics of metronidazole in patients undergoing continuous ambulatory peritoneal dialysis. Antimicrob Agents Chemother 25:306, 1984.
20. Lau AH, Evans R. Chang C-W, et al: Pharmacokinetics of metronidazole in patients with alcoholic liver disease. Antimicrob Agents Chemother 31:1662, 1987.
21. Loft S, Sonne J, Dossing M, et al: Metronidazole pharmacokinetics in patients with hepatic encephalopathy. Scand J Gastroenterol 22:117, 1987.
22. Dobias L, Cerna M, Rossner P, Sram R: Genotoxicity and carcinogenicity of metronidazole. Mutat Res 317:177, 1994.
23. Lambert B, Lindblad A, Lindsten H, et al: Genotoxic effects of metronidazole in human lymphocytes in vitro and in vivo. *In* Phillips I, Collier J (eds): Metronidazole: Proceedings of the Second International Symposium on Anaerobic Infections, Geneva, April 1979. New York, Grune & Stratton, 1979, p 229.
24. Hartley-Asp AB: Chromosomal studies on human lymphocytes exposed to metronidazole in vivo and in vitro. *In* Phillips I, Collier J (eds): Metronidazole: Proceedings of the Second International Symposium on Anaerobic Infections, Geneva, April 1979. New York, Grune & Stratton, 1979, p 237.
25. Finegold SM: Metronidazole. Ann Intern Med 93:585, 1980.
26. Rainey JB, Maeda M, Williams C et al: The carcinogenic effect of intrarectal deoxycholate in rats is reduced by oral metronidazole. Br J Cancer 49:631, 1984.
27. Beard CM, Noller KL, O'Fallon WM, et al: Cancer after exposure to metronidazole. Mayo Clin Proc 63:147, 1988.
28. Krause JR, Ayuyang HQ, Ellis LD: Occurrence of three cases of carcinoma in individuals with Crohn's disease treated with metronidazole. Am J Gastroenterol 80:978, 1985.
29. Robbie MO, Sweet RL: Metronidazole use in obstetrics and gynecology: A review. Am J Obstet Gynecol 145:865, 1983.
30. Garry VF, Nelson RL: Host-mediated transformation: Metronidazole. Mutat Res 190:289, 1987.
31. Cantu JM, Garcia-Cruz D: Midline facial defect as a teratogenic effect of metronidazole. Birth Defects 18:85, 1982.
32. Burtin P, Taddio A, Ariburnu O, et al: Safety of metronidazole in pregnancy: A meta-analysis. Am J Obstet Gynecol 172:525, 1995.
33. Sanders CV, Hanna BJ, Lewis AC, et al: The use of metronidazole in the treatment of anaerobic pleuropulmonary infections *In* Phillips I, Collier J (eds): Metronidazole: Proceedings of the Second International Symposium on Anaerobic Infections, Geneva, April 1979. New York, Grune & Stratton, 1979, p 83.
34. Swedberg J, Steiner JD, Deiss F, et al: Comparison of single-dose vs one-week course of metronidazole for symptomatic bacterial vaginosis. JAMA 254:1046, 1985.
35. Livengood CH 3rd, McGregor JA, Soper DE, et al: Bacterial vaginosis: Efficacy and safety of intravaginal metronidazole treatment. Am J Obstet Gynecol 170:759, 1994.
36. Mikamo H, Izumi K, Ito K, et al: Study on treatment of bacterial vaginosis with oral administration of metronidazole or cefdinir. Chemotherapy 40:362, 1994.
37. McDonald HM, O'Loughlin JA, Vigneswaran R, et al: Bacterial vaginosis in pregnancy and efficacy of short-course oral metronidazole treatment: A randomized controlled trial. Obstet Gynecol 84:343, 1994.
38. Morales WJ, Schorr S, Albritton J: Effect of metronidazole in patients with preterm birth in preceding pregnancy and bacterial vaginosis: A placebo-controlled, double-blind study. Am J Obstet Gynecol 171:345, 1994.
39. Kleinfeld DI, Sharpe RJ, Donta ST: Parenteral therapy for antibiotic-associated pseudomembranous colitis. J Infect Dis 157:389, 1988.
40. Bolton RP, Culshaw MA: Faecal metronidazole concentrations during oral and intravenous therapy for antibiotic associated colitis due to *Clostridium difficile*. Gut 27:1169, 1986.
41. Ahmadsyah I, Salim A: Treatment of tetanus: An open study to compare the efficacy of procaine penicillin and metronidazole. Br Med J (Clin Res) 291:648, 1985.
42. Tepper RS, Ives TJ, Kebede M: Recurrent bacterial vaginosis unresponsive to metronidazole: Successful treatment with oral clindamycin. J Am Board Fam Pract 7:431, 1994.
43. Guirges SY, Al-Waili NS: *Blastocystis hominis:* Evidence for human pathogenicity and effectiveness of metronidazole therapy. Clin Exp Pharmacol Physiol 14:333, 1987.
44. Chong H: Oriental sore: A look at trends in and approaches to the treatment of leishmaniasis. Int J Dermatol 25:615, 1986.
45. Drenick E: Extraintestinal complications of jejunoileal bypass for obesity. *In* Finegold SM, George WL, Rolfe RD (eds): Proceedings of the First United States Metronidazole Conference, Tarpon Springs, FL, February 1982. New York, Biomedical Information, 1982, p 371.
46. Kelly DG, Phillips SF, Kelly KA, et al: Dysfunction of the continent ileostomy: Clinical features and bacteriology. Gut 24:193, 1983.
47. Capron J-P, Herve M-A, Gineston J-L, et al: Metronidazole in prevention of cholestasis associated with total parenteral nutrition. Lancet 1:446, 1983.
48. Gilat T: Metronidazole in Crohn's disease (Editorial). Gastroenterology 83:702, 1982.
49. Duhra P, Paul CJ: Metastatic Crohn's disease responding to metronidazole. Br J Dermatol 119:87, 1988.
50. Duffy LF, Daum F, Fisher SE, et al: Peripheral neuropathy in Crohn's disease patients treated with metronidazole. Gastroenterology 88:681, 1985.
51. Vinceletto J, Finkelstein F, Aoki FY, et al: Double-blind trial of perioperative intravenous metronidazole prophylaxis for abdominal and vaginal hysterectomy. Surgery 93:185, 1983.
52. Keiser TA, MacKenzie RL, Feld R, et al: Prophylactic metronidazole in appendectomy: A double-blind controlled trial. Surgery 93:201, 1983.
53. Wood BA, Faulkner JK, Monro AM: The pharmacokinetics, metabolism and tissue distribution of tinidazole. J Antimicrob Chemother 10(Suppl):43, 1982.
54. Wallin J, Forsgren A: Tinidazole: A new preparation for *T. vaginalis* infections. II. Clinical evaluation of treatment with a single oral dose. Br J Vener Dis 50:148, 1974.
55. Jones R, Enders P: An evaluation of tinidazole as single-dose therapy for the treatment of *Trichomonas vaginalis*. Med J Aust 2:679, 1977.
56. Hillstrom L, Pettersson L, Palsson E: Comparison of ornidazole and tinidazole in single-dose treatment of trichomoniasis in women. Br J Vener Dis 53:193, 1977.
57. Farid Z, El-Masry NA, Miner WF, Hassan A: Tinidazole in treatment of giardiasis (Letter). Lancet 2:721, 1974.
58. Pettersson T: Single-dose tinidazole therapy for giardiasis. Br Med J 1:395, 1975.
59. Levi GC, De Avila CA, Neto VA: Efficacy of various drugs for treatment of giardiasis: A comparative study. Am J Trop Med Hyg 26:564, 1977.
60. Swami B, Lavakusulu D, Sitha Devi C: Tinidazole and metronidazole in the treatment of intestinal amoebiasis. Curr Med Res Opin 5:152, 1977.
61. Willcox RR: How suitable are available pharmaceuticals for the treatment of sexually transmitted diseases? I. Conditions presenting as genital discharges. Br J Vener Dis 53:314, 1977.
62. Reynolds AV, Hamilton-Miller JMT, Brumfitt W: A comparison of the in vitro activity of metronidazole, tinidazole, and nimorazole against gram-negative anaerobic bacilli. J Clin Pathol 28:775, 1975.
63. Notowicz A, Stolz E, DeKoning GAJ: First experiences with single-dose treatment of vaginal trichomoniasis with carnidazole (R25831). Br J Vener Dis 53:129, 1977.

64. Symonds J: Secnidazole: A nitroimidazole with a prolonged serum half-life. J Antimicrob Chemother 5:484, 1979.

Bibliography

- Finegold SM: Metronidazole. Ann Intern Med 93:585, 1980.
- Finegold SM, George WL (eds): Anaerobic Infections in Humans. San Diego, CA, Academic Press, 1989.
- Finegold SM, George WL, Rolfe RD (eds): Proceedings of the First United States Metronidazole Conference, Tarpon Springs, FL, February 1982. New York, Biomedical Information, 1982.
- Finegold SM, McFadzean JA, Roe FJC (eds): Metronidazole: Proceedings of the International Metronidazole Conference, Montreal, 1 May 1976. Princeton, NJ, Excerpta Medica, 1977.
- "Flagyl" (Metronidazole) in Anaerobic Infections. Essex, England, May & Baker, 1979.
- Kucers A, Bennett NM, Kemp RJ (eds): Metronidazole. *In* The Use of Antibiotics. Philadelphia, JB Lippincott, 1987, pp 1290–1329.
- Phillips I, Collier J (eds): Metronidazole: Proceedings of the Second International Symposium on Anaerobic Infections, Geneva, April 1979. New York, Grune & Stratton, 1979.
- Proceedings of the North American Metronidazole Symposium on Anaerobic Infections, Scottsdale, AZ. Surgery 93:123, 1983.
- Rosenblatt JE, Edson RS: Metronidazole. Mayo Clin Proc 62:1013, 1987.
- Stanz MH, Bradley WE: Metronidazole (Flagyl IV, Searle). Drug Intell Clin Pharm 15:838, 1981.

29

Rifampin and Related Drugs

William A. Craig

The rifamycin antibiotics were first isolated in 1957 as fermentation products from *Streptomyces mediterranei*.[1] Rifamycin SV and rifamide were the first clinically released semisynthetic compounds, but both were poorly absorbed when taken by mouth. Rifampin (also called rifampicin) was discovered in 1965 and found to be the most active derivative after oral administration.[2] More recent semisynthetic derivatives with increased activity against mycobacteria include rifabutin (Ansamycin), rifapentine, rifaximin, and the benzoxazinorifamycins.[3–6]

Chemistry

The rifamycins consist of a naphthalenic ring that is spanned by a long aliphatic loop or "ansa" (Fig. 29–1). Changes primarily in the 3 and 4 positions of the naphthalenic ring have led to the different semisynthetic derivatives. Alterations in the aliphatic loop result in loss of activity.[6] They are lipid-soluble compounds, display their best aqueous solubility at acidic pH, and behave like zwitterions in solution.

Mechanism of Action

The rifamycins inhibit DNA-dependent RNA polymerase by binding to the β-subunit of the enzyme in susceptible micro-

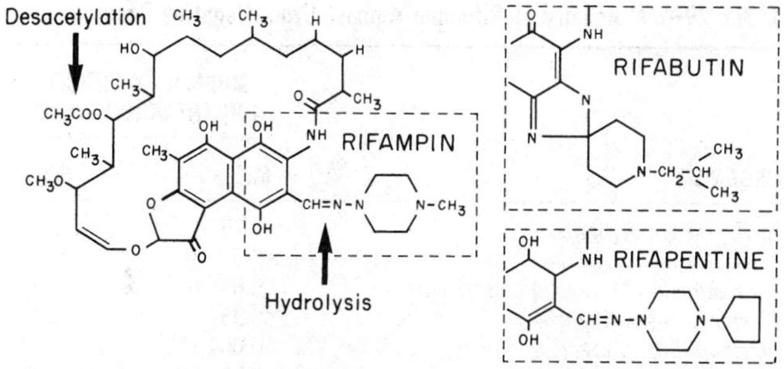

FIGURE 29–1 ▫ Structure of rifamycins.

organisms.[7] This interferes with protein synthesis by preventing chain initiation but not elongation. Inhibition of mammalian enzymes requires concentrations more than 1000 times greater than those active against bacterial enzymes.[8] The drugs are bactericidal. Intermittent exposure to rifampin results in some of the longest durations of persistent suppression of bacterial growth (i.e., postantibiotic effect) observed with any antimicrobial.[9]

Spectrum of Activity

Rifampin is active against a large variety of aerobic and anaerobic bacteria[10–23] (Tables 29–1 to 29–3). Among the gram-positive bacteria (see Table 29–1), rifampin is most active against staphylococci. Minimal inhibitory concentrations for methicillin-resistant strains are similar to those for methicillin-susceptible staphylococci.[10] Except for *Enterococcus faecalis*, most gram-positive bacteria have minimal inhibitory concentrations of 1.0 mg/L or less. Against *Clostridium difficile*, rifampin is as active as metronidazole and vancomycin.[13]

With gram-negative bacteria (see Table 29–2), rifampin exhibits excellent activity against *Neisseria gonorrhoeae, Neisseria meningitidis, Branhamella (Moraxella) catarrhalis, Haemophilus influenzae*, and *Haemophilus ducreyi*. It is one of the most active antimicrobials against all of the *Legionella* species.[15] Most strains of *Brucella* are also susceptible to rifampin.[20] Although Enterobacteriaceae and *Pseudomonas* species have minimal inhibitory concentrations for rifampin that are greater than 2 mg/L, the RNA polymerase enzymes from these organisms

TABLE 29–1 ▪ Activity of Rifampin Against Gram-Positive Bacteria

	MINIMAL INHIBITORY CONCENTRATION (mg/L)	
ORGANISM	MIC_{50}	MIC_{90}
Staphylococcus aureus	0.015	0.015
Staphylococcus epidermidis	0.015	0.015
Streptococcus pyogenes	0.12	0.12
Streptococcus agalactiae	1.0	1.0
Streptococcus pneumoniae	0.12	4.0
Viridans group streptococci	0.06	0.12
Enterococcus faecalis	4.0	16.0
JK diphtheroids	0.05	0.05
Listeria monocytogenes	≤0.12	0.25
Clostridium difficile	≤0.2	≤0.2
Clostridium perfringens	≤0.1	≤0.1
Eubacterium spp.	≤0.1	0.4
Peptococcus spp.	0.2	1.6
Peptostreptococcus spp.	≤0.1	1.6
Propionibacterium acnes	≤0.1	≤0.1

Data from references 10–14.

TABLE 29–2 ■ Activity of Rifampin Against Gram-Negative Bacteria

ORGANISM	MINIMAL INHIBITORY CONCENTRATION (mg/L) MIC50	MIC90
Neisseria gonorrhoeae	0.25	0.5
Neisseria meningitidis	≤0.03	0.12
Branhamella (Moraxella) catarrhalis	0.03	0.03
Haemophilus influenzae	0.25	0.5
Haemophilus ducreyi	0.004	0.03
Legionella pneumophila	0.03	0.03
Brucella spp.	2.5	4.0
Rochalimaea spp.	≤0.125	≤0.125
Escherichia coli	8	16
Klebsiella pneumoniae	32	32
Proteus mirabilis	4	8
Enterobacter spp.	32	64
Citrobacter spp.	32	32
Serratia marcescens	64	64
Providencia spp.	8	32
Acinetobacter spp.	8	8
Pseudomonas aeruginosa	32	64
Bacteroides fragilis	0.4	0.8
Prevotella spp.	≤0.1	0.2
Fusobacterium spp.	0.2	1.6
Veillonella spp.	1.6	1.6

Data from references 14–23.

are only slightly less sensitive to the drug than those from staphylococci. Despite its apparent difficulty 1n penetrating the outer membrane of aerobic gram-negative bacilli, rifampin has demonstrated in vitro synergy with aminoglycoside and β-lactam antibiotics against *Pseudomonas aeruginosa*.[22, 23]

The rifamycins vary markedly in their activity against different mycobacteria[24–28] (see Table 29–3). Rifampin is active against *Mycobacterium tuberculosis*, *Mycobacterium kansasii*, and *Mycobacterium marinum*; intermediate against *Mycobacterium avium-intracellulare*; and inactive against *Mycobacterium fortuitum* and *Mycobacterium chelonae*. *Mycobacterium leprae* is also susceptible to rifampin.[26]

Chlamydia trachomatis (including lymphogranuloma venereum strains), *Chlamydia psittaci*, and *Coxiella burnetii* are also quite susceptible to rifampin.[27, 28] The drug even exhibits activity against all erythrocytic forms of *Plasmodium vivax*[29] and against several fungi in the presence of other drugs such as amphotericin B.[30]

TABLE 29–3 ■ Activity of Rifampin and Rifabutin Against *Mycobacterium* Species

ORGANISM	Rifampin MIC50	Rifampin MIC90	Rifabutin MIC50	Rifabutin MIC90
M. tuberculosis	0.3	0.6	0.06	0.06
M. avium-intracellulare	5.0	20	0.5	2.0
M. kansasii	0.6	2.5	≤0.5	≤0.5
M. marinum	1.25	2.5	≤0.5	≤0.5
M. fortuitum	>20	>20	>2.0	>2.0
M. chelonae	>20	>20	>2.0	>2.0

MINIMAL INHIBITORY CONCENTRATION (mg/L)

Based on agar minimal inhibitory concentration data from references 24, 25, and 104.

Resistance

The rapid emergence of resistant bacteria has been a common problem for monotherapy with the rifamycins. Susceptible bacteria develop resistance to these drugs by insertion, deletion, or point mutations in the gene encoding the β-subunit of the RNA polymerase enzyme (*rpoB* gene).[31] These mutations, which result in extra, missing, or substituted amino acids in the enzyme, can occur at various sites in the *rpoB* gene and at frequencies ranging from 1 per 10^6 to 1 per 10^9 bacteria.[31, 32]

Except for prophylaxis, the rifamycins should not be used alone. In combination with rifampin, a variety of antituberculous drugs are effective in preventing the emergence of resistant tubercle bacilli. Primary resistance of *M. tuberculosis* to rifampin occurs in about 3.5% of newly diagnosed patients in the United States.[33] With staphylococci, β-lactam antibiotics appear to be more effective than vancomycin in preventing the emergence of rifampin-resistant organisms with combined use.[34, 35]

Pharmacokinetic Properties

Rifampin is rapidly and virtually completely absorbed after oral dosing, resulting in serum concentrations similar to those after intravenous administration[36, 37] (Fig. 29–2). The drug is cleared from the circulation primarily by hepatic metabolism and biliary excretion; its half-life is 2 to 5 hours. Because the excretory capacity of the liver for rifampin tends to saturate at doses of 300 to 450 mg, larger amounts result in a disproportionate increase in maximal serum levels and area under the curve.[36] Peak serum concentrations after ingestion of 600 mg or 10 mg/kg can vary from 4 to 32 mg/L but usually fall in the range of 7 to 15 mg/L.[36–39] About 80% of the drug is bound to serum proteins.

Rifampin and other rifamycins are metabolized in the liver by desacetylation to a less active metabolite[37] (see Fig. 29–1). The desacetyl derivative accounts for most of the drug in bile. Hydrolysis of rifampin to the inactive 3-formylrifampin apparently occurs only in the urine. Because rifampin is a potent inducer of hepatic microsomal enzymes (cytochrome

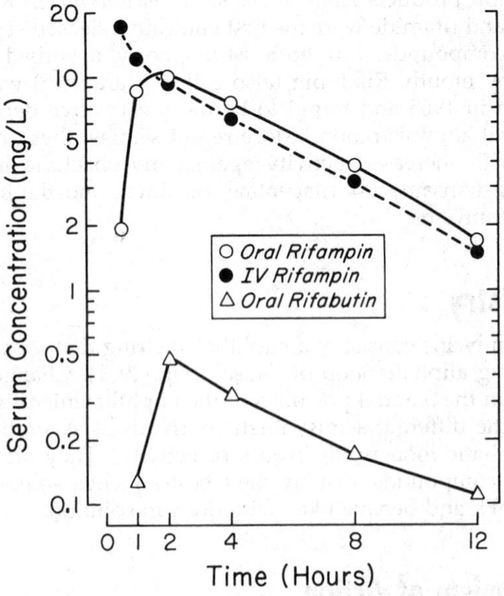

FIGURE 29–2 □ Serum concentrations of rifampin after oral and intravenous (IV) administration of 600 mg and of rifabutin after oral dosing of 600 mg. (Data from references 36, 37, 106, and 113.)

P-450 mixed-function oxidase system), it stimulates its own metabolism. Repeated administration increases clearance of the drug and decreases peak serum concentrations and area under the curve about 30% to 40%. Because only 6% to 25% of rifampin is excreted in the urine, dosage modification is not required in patients with renal impairment. Although use of rifampin in patients with liver disease is not recommended except in case of necessity, hepatic dysfunction only doubles the drug's half-life.[40] The pharmacokinetics of rifampin in children and in elderly patients is similar to that in adults.[41, 42]

The high lipid solubility of rifampin results in tissue concentrations similar to those observed in serum.[37] Therapeutic concentrations are obtained in saliva, tears, sputum, and pancreatic juice; bone; cardiac valve tissue; and pleural, ascitic, blister, and tubercle cavitary fluids.[37–39, 43] Rifampin levels up to 0.8 mg/L are observed in cerebrospinal fluid of normal individuals after a 600-mg oral dose.[44] Intravenous infusions of 20 mg/kg in children and 600 mg in adults with uninflamed meninges produces cerebrospinal fluid concentrations of 0.1 to 3.0 mg/L.[45, 46] Higher concentrations up to 2.4 mg/L are observed in patients with meningitis.[44, 47] Oral doses of 600 mg produce concentrations of 0.2 to 1.3 mg/L in the aqueous humor.[48] The drug also readily enters phagocytic cells and is capable of killing intracellular bacteria and sterilizing abscesses.[49, 50]

Rifampin is available for both oral and intravenous administration. The intravenous preparation should not be administered by the intramuscular or subcutaneous route. The recommended dosage is 600 mg in adults and 10 to 20 mg/kg, not to exceed 600 mg, in children. A 1% suspension can be prepared by adding the powder from four 300-mg capsules to 120 mL of syrup.[51]

Clinical Usage

Mycobacterial Infections

Since its introduction into clinical medicine in 1968, rifampin has joined isoniazid as one of the cornerstones in the chemotherapy of tuberculosis. As with other drugs, monotherapy with rifampin is associated with a high failure rate owing to the emergence of resistant organisms[52]; however, drug combinations including rifampin have produced cure rates after 6 to 9 months of therapy equivalent to those obtained with 18 months of therapy with regimens lacking rifampin.[53, 54] Currently recommended regimens include 6 months of treatment with a combination of rifampin at 10 to 20 mg/kg per day (maximum, 600 mg), isoniazid at 300 mg/d, and pyrazinamide at 15 to 30 mg/kg per day (maximum, 2 g) during the first 8 weeks of therapy.[55] In areas where the primary resistance rate is greater than 4%, ethambutol or streptomycin is added to the regimen until susceptibility results are known. Two- and three-drug fixed combinations of rifampin, isoniazid, and pyrazinamide are available to enhance compliance and prevent drug resistance.[56] Rifampin is recommended for prophylactic therapy of contacts exposed to isoniazid-resistant organisms[55]; however, the efficacy of rifampin prophylaxis is not well documented. Rifampin, in combination with other drugs, is also useful in the treatment of infections due to *M. kansasii, M. marinum, Mycobacterium xenopi*, and *M. avium-intracellulare*.[57–62]

Rifampin is currently the major drug for the treatment of leprosy. Once-monthly therapy with rifampin is highly bactericidal against *M. leprae* but is used in combination with dapsone to prevent the emergence of resistant strains.[63]

Prophylaxis

Rifampin can eradicate a variety of organisms from the nasopharynx of carriers and is therefore useful in the prophylaxis of infection. For prophylaxis of close contacts of patients with severe meningococcal infections, a single daily dose of 10 mg/kg or 600 mg for 2 or 4 days has reduced the carriage of *N. meningitidis* by 75% to 95%.[64–66]

The drug is also effective in eradicating carriage of *H. influenzae* type b. A single daily dose of rifampin at 20 mg/kg (maximum, 600 mg) for 2 or 4 days reduces carriage of *H. influenzae* in more than 90% of children.[67] This has likewise been shown to reduce the frequency of secondary infections. Prophylaxis is recommended for household contacts when there are children younger than 4 years. Rifampin prophylaxis for contacts in daycare centers is also recommended by the Centers for Disease Control and Prevention.[68]

A 4-day course of rifampin, 10 mg/kg twice daily, plus benzathine penicillin G is highly effective in eradicating carriage of *Streptococcus pyogenes*,[69] but such therapy is rarely indicated.

Although a 5- to 10-day course of rifampin can reduce the carriage of *Staphylococcus aureus* by 73% to 95%,[70–72] there are no published studies on its efficacy in reducing the frequency of recurrent skin infections. However, 5-day courses of rifampin repeated every 3 months reduce the frequency of shunt infections in patients undergoing hemodialysis[72] and decrease the episodes of catheter site infection and peritonitis in patients undergoing peritoneal dialysis.[73] Rifampin, in combination with trimethoprim or minocycline, has good efficacy in eradicating the nasal carriage of methicillin-resistant *S. aureus* in hospitalized patients.[74, 75] However, these regimens have had less success in eliminating the organism from extranasal sites.

Staphylococcal Infections

The absence of adequate controlled clinical trials makes the use of rifampin in the treatment of staphylococcal infections a controversial topic. The addition of rifampin to standard therapy has resulted in some dramatic responses in patients with endocarditis due to *S. aureus*.[76, 77] However, one of the concerns with the use of rifampin in serious staphylococcal infections is the reported antagonism by rifampin of the killing of staphylococci by β-lactam drugs and vancomycin.[78] Animal studies, on the other hand, usually demonstrate similar or enhanced activity of drug combinations containing rifampin.[79] Although an unblinded, prospective clinical trial suggested that the addition of rifampin to oxacillin improved clinical outcome in patients with serious staphylococcal infections,[80] a subsequent double-blind, placebo-controlled trial by the same investigators showed no major benefit.[81] In general, the addition of rifampin is recommended for cases of staphylococcal infection associated with myocardial and metastatic abscesses. Rifampin has been combined with ciprofloxacin or ofloxacin to provide an entirely oral regimen for the treatment of right-sided *S. aureus* endocarditis in intravenous drug abusers.[82]

Rifampin, in combination with vancomycin and gentamicin, is recommended for the treatment of prosthetic valve endocarditis due to *Staphylococcus epidermidis*. In the only prospective trial, the three-drug regimen was as effective as the combination of rifampin and vancomycin but resulted in a lower frequency of rifampin resistance during therapy.[83]

Osteomyelitis is another infection caused by *S. aureus* in which the use of rifampin has been studied. In animal models, the best efficacy is observed with regimens containing rifampin.[84] The only controlled clinical trial in patients with chronic staphylococcal osteomyelitis demonstrated a trend toward better response (80% versus 50%) with the nafcillin plus rifampin regimen than with nafcillin alone,[85] although the small number of patients in the study made it impossible to demonstrate statistical significance. Rifampin combinations have also been useful in the treatment of orthopedic implant-related infections caused by gram-positive cocci.[86]

Brucella *Infections*

Rifampin appears to have an increasing role in the treatment of brucellosis. Treatment for 45 days with doxycycline plus rifampin exhibits a clinical response similar to that seen with tetracycline plus streptomycin.[87] Rifampin has also been successful in the treatment of *Brucella* endocarditis.[88]

Other Infections

Despite limited clinical experience, a combination of rifampin, vancomycin, and a third-generation cephalosporin has been recommended by some physicians for meningitis caused by penicillin-resistant pneumococci.[89] Although rifampin has been added when *Legionella* infection responded poorly to erythromycin, no clinical trials have demonstrated enhanced activity of combined therapy. The addition of rifampin to ticarcillin plus tobramycin resulted in a dramatic improvement in a few cases of infection due to *P. aeruginosa* that were failing to respond to combination therapy.[90] In a prospective, randomized trial, the addition of rifampin to combination therapy of an antipseudomonal penicillin and aminoglycoside significantly increased the frequency of bacteriologic cure, but this did not reduce mortality.[91] Last, rifampin has also demonstrated clinical efficacy in a few cases of cutaneous leishmaniasis, pulmonary actinomycosis, relapsing *C. difficile*–associated diarrhea, and meningitis due to *Flavobacterium meningosepticum*.[92]

Side Effects

The most common side effect observed with rifampin is an orange-red discoloration of the urine. Permanent staining of soft contact lenses can also occur during rifampin therapy. Two- to 4-day courses of rifampin for prophylaxis are associated with a variety of mild, reversible side effects, such as abdominal pain or diarrhea (11%), nausea and vomiting (5% to 13%), headache or visual change (4% to 10%), dizziness or drowsiness (2% to 8%), and pruritus or rash (2% to 8%).[93]

Important side effects with more prolonged therapy include hepatitis, interstitial nephritis, influenza-like syndrome, thrombocytopenia, anemia, and leukopenia.[94–96] Although elevated liver enzyme activities are observed in about 5% to 10% of patients, hepatitis occurs in only 0.15% to 0.43% of patients treated with rifampin alone.[94] The frequency of hepatitis rises to 2.5% in patients receiving multiple-drug therapy for tuberculosis; however, most studies suggest that rifampin does not enhance the hepatotoxicity of isoniazid.

Interstitial nephritis is a rare complication of rifampin and occurs primarily with intermittent dosing. Renal failure due to massive hemolysis, glomerulonephritis, and the tubular precipitation of light chain proteins produced by rifampin have also been reported.[94, 97]

An influenza-like syndrome, with fever, chills, malaise, and headache, has also been associated with intermittent dosing of rifampin. It rarely occurs with daily dosing and is most common with intermittent dosing less than twice weekly and with doses greater than 900 mg.[94] It most likely represents an immunologic reaction due to the formation of rifampin-antibody complexes. Most hematologic toxic effects also appear to be immunologic reactions related to rifampin-induced antibodies. In healthy subjects, rifampin did not produce any detectable effect on immunoglobulin levels, antigen responsiveness, and skin test reactivity.[98]

Because the rifamycins are potent stimulators of the hepatic microsomal enzymes, especially cytochrome P-450IIIA4, their use may enhance the metabolism of other drugs cleared by these enzymes. Rifampin has been shown to increase the rate of elimination of a large number of drugs[99–103] (Table 29–4). This can result in decreased efficacy of concomitant drug therapy with rifampin therapy or in concomitant drug toxicity after rifampin is stopped. The complications resulting from rifampin therapy have been unwanted pregnancies in patients taking oral contraceptives, relapse of asthma and Addison disease in patients receiving glucocorticoid therapy, relapse of arrhythmia in patients taking quinidine or verapamil, exacerbation of diabetes in individuals receiving oral hypoglycemic agents, acute rejection in transplant recipients taking cyclosporine, and relapse of hypothyroidism in patients receiving thyroxine replacement. Rifampin can also reduce the concentrations of clarithromycin, doxycycline, fluconazole, itraconazole, and zidovudine, which may have therapeutic consequences.[100–103]

Because the rifamycins are lipid soluble, they readily penetrate the placenta. Large doses of rifampin can produce teratogenic effects in rodents. Although similar effects have not been observed in humans, rifampin should be given to pregnant women only to treat active cases of tuberculosis.[55]

Rifabutin

Rifabutin is a semisynthetic derivative of rifamycin S that is about 10 times more active than rifampin against *M. tuberculosis* and *M. avium-intracellulare*[104–106] (see Table 29–3). The drug is currently used for the treatment and prevention of *M. avium-intracellulare* infections. Clinical trials in patients with acquired immunodeficiency syndrome with $CD4^+$ cell counts less than 200/mm^3 demonstrated that 300 mg of rifabutin daily reduces the acquisition of *M. avium-intracellulare* bacteremia by about 50%.[107] The Centers for Disease Control and Prevention now recommends rifabutin prophylaxis in patients infected with human immunodeficiency virus with $CD4^+$ cell counts less than 100/mm^3.[108] Rifabutin has also been used in the treatment of *M. avium-intracellulare* infections in patients with acquired immunodeficiency syndrome with variable results.[109–112]

The pharmacologic properties of rifabutin differ somewhat from those of rifampin. Although the drug is rapidly absorbed, oral bioavailability is only 12% to 20%.[113] In addition, the drug has a larger volume of distribution than rifampin does. As a result, the serum concentrations of rifabutin are markedly less than those of rifampin (see Fig. 29–2). With oral doses of 300 to 600 mg, peak serum concentrations of rifabutin have ranged from 0.3 to 0.9 mg/L.[113–115] Approximately 70% of the drug is bound to serum proteins. Tissue levels of rifabutin are two to eight times higher than serum concentrations.[116] The concentrations of rifabutin in cerebrospinal fluid are 30% to 70% of those in serum.[116] The drug is

TABLE 29–4 ■ Drugs That Exhibit Increased Hepatic Clearance with Concomitant Rifampin Therapy

Barbiturates	Estrogens	Quinidine
Chloramphenicol	Fluconazole	Sulfasalazine
Cimetidine	Glucocorticoids	Sulfonylureas
Clarithromycin	Glyburide	Theophylline
Clofibrate	Itraconazole	Thyroxine
Cyclosporine	Ketoconazole	Verapamil
Dapsone	Metoprolol	Warfarin
Digitoxin	Methadone	Zidovudine
Digoxin	Phenytoin	
Doxycycline	Propranolol	

eliminated from the circulation like rifampin, with only 10% recovered in the urine.

The side effects with rifabutin therapy differ from those observed with rifampin. Uveitis and an arthralgia-arthritis syndrome have been the major toxic effects observed with long-term prophylaxis with rifabutin.[117, 118] The drug also appears to induce the hepatic microsomal enzymes to a lesser degree than rifampin does.[119] Thus, concomitant use of rifabutin results in smaller decreases in serum concentrations of clarithromycin and zidovudine than those observed with rifampin.[103, 120] Rifabutin may be the preferred rifamycin to combine with clarithromycin for treating *M. avium-intracellulare* infection; however, clarithromycin can slow the elimination of rifabutin and increase the frequency of rifabutin-associated side effects.[121]

Other Rifamycins

Rifapentine is two to three times more active than rifampin against *M. avium-intracellulare* and *M. tuberculosis*.[4, 122] Rifapentine exhibits good oral bioavailability and results in mean peak serum concentrations of 8 to 15 mg/L after ingestion of 600 mg or a dose of 8 mg/kg.[123, 124] The drug has a longer serum half-life (14 to 20 hours) than is observed with rifampin and rifabutin. The extensive hepatic metabolism, high biliary excretion, low renal elimination, and wide tissue distribution of the drug are similar to those of rifampin. The results of clinical trials with rifapentine are not yet available.

The more recently developed benzoxazinorifamycin KRM-1648 is 16 to 64 times more potent than rifampin against most mycobacteria.[5, 125] It is even active against many rifampin-resistant strains of *M. avium-intracellulare*.

Rifaximin is a poorly absorbed rifamycin derivative that is used primarily to reduce bacterial numbers within the gastrointestinal tract.[126] In initial clinical trials, it has demonstrated efficacy in hepatic encephalopathy, acute diverticulitis, and surgical prophylaxis.

References

1. Sensi P: History of the development of rifampin. Rev Infect Dis 5(Suppl 3):S402, 1983.
2. Maggi N, Pasqualucci CR, Ballotta R, Sensi P: Rifampicin: A new orally active rifamycin. Chemotherapy 11:285, 1966.
3. Della Bruna C, Schioppacassi G, Ungheri D, et al: LM 427, a new spiropiperidylrifamycin: In vitro and in vivo studies. J Antibiot (Tokyo) 36:1502, 1983.
4. Arioli V, Berti M, Carniti G, et al: Antibacterial activity of DL 473, a new semisynthetic rifamycin derivative. J Antibiot (Tokyo) 34:1026, 1981.
5. Saito H, Tomioka H, Emori M, et al: In vitro antimycobacterial activities of newly synthesized benzoxazinorifamycins. Antimicrob Agents Chemother 35:542, 1991.
6. Wehrli W, Staehelin M: The rifamycins—Relation of chemical structure and action on RNA polymerase. Biochim Biophys Acta 182:24, 1969.
7. Hartman G, Honikel KO, Knüsel F: The specific inhibition of the DNA-directed RNA synthesis by rifamycin. Biochim Biophys Acta 145:843, 1967.
8. Buss WC, Morgan R, Guttmann J, et al: Rifampicin inhibition of protein synthesis in mammalian cells. Science 200:432, 1978.
9. Bundtzen RW, Gerber AU, Cohn DL, et al: Postantibiotic suppression of bacterial growth. Rev Infect Dis 3:28, 1981.
10. Pohlod DJ, Saravolatz LD, Somerville MM: In-vitro susceptibility of gram-positive cocci to LY146032 teicoplanin, sodium fusidate, vancomycin, and rifampicin. J Antimicrob Chemother 20:197, 1987.
11. Pérez JL, Riera L, Valls F, et al: A comparison of the in-vitro activity of seventeen antibiotics against *Streptococcus faecalis*. J Antimicrob Chemother 20:357, 1987.
12. Jadeja L, Fainstein V, LeBlanc B, et al: Comparative in vitro activities of teichomycin and other antibiotics against JK diphtheroids. Antimicrob Agents Chemother 24:145, 1983.
13. Fekety R, Silva J, Toshniwal R, et al: Antibiotic-associated colitis: Effects of antibiotics on *Clostridium difficile* and the disease in hamsters. Rev Infect Dis 1:386, 1979.
14. Martin WJ, Gardner M, Washington JA II: In vitro antimicrobial susceptibility of anaerobic bacteria isolated from clinical specimens. Antimicrob Agents Chemother 2:148, 1972.
15. Thornsberry C, Hill BC, Swenson JM, et al: Rifampin: Spectrum of antibacterial activity. Rev Infect Dis 5(Suppl 3):S412, 1983.
16. Doern GV, Jorgensen JH, Thornsberry C, et al: National collaborative study of the prevalence of antimicrobial resistance among clinical isolates of *Haemophilus influenzae*. Antimicrob Agents Chemother 32:180, 1988.
17. Doern GV, Tubert TA: In vitro activities of 39 antimicrobial agents for *Branhamella catarrhalis* and comparison of results with different quantitative susceptibility test methods. Antimicrob Agents Chemother 32:259, 1988.
18. Dangor Y, Miller SD, Exposto FDL, et al: Antimicrobial susceptibilities of southern African isolates of *Haemophilus ducreyi*. Antimicrob Agents Chemother 32:1458, 1988.
19. Trallero EP, Arenzana JMG, Ayestaran I, et al: Comparative activity in vitro of 16 antimicrobial agents against penicillin-susceptible meningococci and meningococci with diminished susceptibility to penicillin. Antimicrob Agents Chemother 33:1622, 1989.
20. Rubinstein E, Lang R, Shasha B, et al: In vitro susceptibility of *Brucella melitensis* to antibiotics. Antimicrob Agents Chemother 35:1925, 1991.
21. Maurin M, Raoult D: Antimicrobial susceptibility of *Rochalimaea quintana, Rochalimaea vinsonii*, and the newly recognized *Rochalimaea henselae*. J Antimicrob Chemother 32:587, 1993.
22. Zuravleff JJ, Yu VL, Yee RB: Ticarcillin-tobramycin-rifampin: In vitro synergy of the triplet combination against *Pseudomonas aeruginosa*. J Lab Clin Med 101:896, 1983.
23. Valdes JM, Baltch AL, Smith RP, et al: The effect of rifampicin on the in-vitro activity of cefpirome or ceftazidime in combination with aminoglycosides against *Pseudomonas aeruginosa*. J Antimicrob Chemother 25:575, 1990.
24. Lorian V, Finland M: In vivo effect of rifampin on mycobacteria. Appl Microbiol 17:202, 1969.
25. Rynearson TK, Shronts JS, Wolinsky E: Rifampin: In vitro effect on atypical mycobacteria. Am Rev Respir Dis 104:272, 1971.
26. Rees RJW: Rifampicin: The investigation of a bactericidal antileprosy drug. Lepr Rev 46(Suppl 1):121, 1975.
27. Schachter J: Rifampin in chlamydial infections. Rev Infect Dis 5(Suppl 3):S562, 1983.
28. Yeaman MR, Mitscher LA, Baca OG: In vitro susceptibility of *Coxiella burnetti* to antibiotics including several quinolones. Antimicrob Agents Chemother 31:1079, 1987.
29. Pukrittayakamee S, Viravan C, Charoenlarp P, et al: Antimalarial effects of rifampin in *Plasmodium vivax* malaria. Antimicrob Agents Chemother 38:511, 1994.
30. Medoff G: Antifungal action of rifampin. Rev Infect Dis 5(Suppl 3):S614, 1983.
31. Wehrli W: Rifampin: Mechanisms of action and resistance. Rev Infect Dis 5(Suppl 3):S407, 1983.
32. Mendelman PM, Roberts MC, Smith AL: Mutation frequency of *Haemophilus influenzae* to rifampin resistance. Antimicrob Agents Chemother 22:531, 1982.
33. Bloch AB, Cauthen GM, Onorato IM, et al: Nationwide survey of drug-resistant tuberculosis in the United States. JAMA 271:665, 1994.
34. Simon GL, Smith RH, Sande MA: Emergence of rifampin-resistant strains of *Staphylococcus aureus* during combination therapy with vancomycin and rifampin: A report of two cases. Rev Infect Dis 5(Suppl 3):S507, 1983.
35. Eng RHK, Smith SM, Buccini FJ, et al: Differences in ability of cell-wall antibiotics to suppress emergence of rifampicin resistance in *Staphylococcus aureus*. J Antimicrob Chemother 15:201, 1985.
36. Acocella G: Clinical pharmacokinetics of rifampicin. Clin Pharmacokinet 3:108, 1978.
37. Kenny MT, Strates B: Metabolism and pharmacokinetics of the antibiotic rifampin. Drug Metab Rev 12:159, 1981.

38. Archer GL, Armstrong BC, Kline BJ: Rifampin blood and tissue levels in patients undergoing cardiac valve surgery. Antimicrob Agents Chemother 21:800, 1982.
39. Pederzoli P, Falconi M, Guaglianone O, et al: Rifampicin concentrations in pancreatic juice. J Antimicrob Chemother 16:129, 1985.
40. Acocella G, Bonollo L, Garimoldi M, et al: Kinetics of rifampicin and isoniazid administered alone and in combination to normal subjects and patients with liver disease. Gut 13:47, 1972.
41. Koup JR, Williams-Warren J, Weber A, et al: Pharmacokinetics of rifampin in children. I. Multiple dose intravenous infusion. Ther Drug Monit 8:11, 1986.
42. Advenier C, Gobert C, Houin G, et al: Pharmacokinetic studies of rifampicin in the elderly. Ther Drug Monit 5:61, 1983.
43. Solberg CO, Halstensen A, Digranes A, et al: Penetration of antibiotics into human leukocytes and dermal suction blisters. Rev Infect Dis 5(Suppl 3):S468, 1983.
44. Bobrowitz ID: Levels of rifampin in cerebrospinal fluid. Chest 63:648, 1973.
45. Nahata MC, Fan-Havard P, Barson WJ, et al: Pharmacokinetics, cerebrospinal fluid concentration, and safety of intravenous rifampin in pediatric patients undergoing shunt placements. Eur J Clin Pharmacol 38:515, 1990.
46. Nau R, Prange HW, Menck S, et al: Penetration of rifampicin into the cerebrospinal fluid of adults with uninflamed meninges. J Antimicrob Chemother 29:719, 1992.
47. D'Oliveira JJG: Cerebrospinal fluid concentrations of rifampin in meningeal tuberculosis. Am Rev Respir Dis 106:432, 1972.
48. Outman WR, Levitz RE, Hill DA, et al: Intraocular penetration of rifampin in humans. Antimicrob Agents Chemother 36:1575, 1992.
49. Hand WL, King-Thompson NL: Contrasts between phagocyte antibiotic uptake and subsequent intracellular bactericidal activity. Antimicrob Agents Chemother 29:135, 1986.
50. Mandell GL, Vest TK: Killing of intraleukocytic *Staphylococcus aureus* by rifampin: In vitro and in vivo studies. Rev Infect Dis 5(Suppl 3):S463, 1983.
51. Krukenberg CC, Mischler PG, Massad EN, et al: Stability of 1% rifampin suspensions prepared in five syrups. Am J Hosp Pharm 43:2225, 1986.
52. Baronti A, Lukinovich N: A pilot trial of rifampicin in tuberculosis. Tubercle 49:180, 1968.
53. British Thoracic and Tuberculosis Association: Short-course chemotherapy in pulmonary tuberculosis. A controlled trial by the British Thoracic and Tuberculosis Association. Lancet 2:1102, 1976.
54. British Thoracic Association: A controlled trial of six months chemotherapy in pulmonary tuberculosis. Second report: Results during the 24 months after the end of chemotherapy. Am Rev Respir Dis 126:460, 1982.
55. American Thoracic Society: Treatment of tuberculosis and tuberculosis infection in adults and children. Am J Respir Crit Care Med 149:1359, 1994.
56. Moulding T, Dutt AK, Reichman LB: Fixed-dose combination of antituberculous medications to prevent drug resistance. Ann Intern Med 122:951, 1995.
57. Ahn CH, Lowell JR, Ahn SS, et al: Chemotherapy for pulmonary disease due to *Mycobacterium kansasii*: Efficacies of some individual drugs. Rev Infect Dis 3:1028, 1981.
58. Donta ST, Smith PW, Levitz RE, et al: Therapy of *Mycobacterium marinum* infections. Arch Intern Med 146:902, 1986.
59. Bogaerts Y, Elinck W, van Renterghem D, et al: Pulmonary disease due to *Mycobacterium xenopi*: Report of two cases. Eur J Respir Dis 63:298, 1982.
60. Kemper CA, Meng TC, Nussbaum J, et al: Treatment of *Mycobacterium avium* complex bacteremia in AIDS with a four-drug oral regimen. Rifampin, ethambutol, clofazimine, and ciprofloxacin. Ann Intern Med 116:466, 1992.
61. Chiu J, Nussbaum J, Bozzette S, et al: Treatment of disseminated *Mycobacterium avium* complex infection in AIDS with amikacin, ethambutol, rifampin, and ciprofloxacin. Ann Intern Med 113:358, 1990.
62. Jacobson MA, Yajko D, Northfelt D, et al: Randomized, placebo-controlled trial of rifampin, ethambutol, and ciprofloxacin for AIDS patients with disseminated *Mycobacterium avium* complex infection. Ann Intern Med 168:112, 1993.
63. Ellard GA: Chemotherapy of leprosy. Br Med Bull 44:775, 1988.
64. Beam WE Jr, Newberg NR, Devine LF, et al: The effect of rifampin on the nasopharyngeal carriage of *Neisseria meningitidis* in a military population. J Infect Dis 124:39, 1971.
65. Schwartz B, Al-Tobaiqi A, Al-Ruwais A, et al: Comparative efficacy of ceftriaxone and rifampin in eradicating pharyngeal carriage of group A *Neisseria meningitidis*. Lancet 1:1239, 1988.
66. Nicolle LE, Postl B, Kotelewetz E, et al: Chemoprophylaxis for *Neisseria meningitidis* in an isolated arctic community. J Infect Dis 145:103, 1982.
67. Green M, Li KI, Wald ER, et al: Duration of rifampin chemoprophylaxis for contacts of patients infected with *Haemophilus influenzae* type B. Antimicrob Agents Chemother 36:545, 1992.
68. Update: Prevention of *Hemophilus influenzae* type b disease. MMWR 35:170, 1986.
69. Tanz RR, Shulman ST, Barthel MJ, et al: Penicillin plus rifampin eradicates pharyngeal carriage of group A streptococci. J Pediatr 106:876, 1985.
70. Wheat LJ, Kohler RB, White AL, et al: Effect of rifampin on nasal carriage of coagulase-positive staphylococci. J Infect Dis 144:177, 1981.
71. McAnally TP, Lewis MR, Brown DR: Effect of rifampin and bacitracin on nasal carriage of *Staphylococcus aureus*. Antimicrob Agents Chemother 25:422, 1984.
72. Yu VL, Goetz A, Wagener M, et al: *Staphylococcus aureus* nasal carriage and infection in patients on hemodialysis. Efficacy of antibiotic prophylaxis. N Engl J Med 315:91, 1986.
73. Zimmerman SW, Ahrens E, Johnson CA, et al: Randomized, controlled trial of prophylactic rifampin for peritoneal dialysis catheter-related infections and peritonitis. Kidney Int 37:335, 1990.
74. Roccaforte JS, Bittner MJ, Stumpf LA, Preheim LC: Attempts to eradicate methicillin-resistant *Staphylococcus aureus* colonization with the use of trimethoprim-sulfamethoxazole, rifampin, and bacitracin. Am J Infect Control 16:141, 1988.
75. Darouiche R, Wright C, Hamill R, et al: Eradication of colonization by methicillin-resistant *Staphylococcus aureus* by using oral minocycline-rifampin and topical mupirocin. Antimicrob Agents Chemother 35:1612, 1991.
76. Acar JF, Goldstein FW, Duval J: Use of rifampin for the treatment of serious staphylococcal and gram-negative bacillary infections. Rev Infect Dis 5(Suppl 3):502, 1983.
77. Faville RJ, Zaske DE, Kaplan EL, et al: *Staphylococcus aureus* endocarditis: Combined therapy with vancomycin and rifampin. JAMA 240:1963, 1978.
78. Watanakunakorn C, Tisone JC: Antagonism between nafcillin or oxacillin and rifampin against *Staphylococcus aureus*. Antimicrob Agents Chemother 22:920, 1982.
79. Zak O, Scheld WM, Sande MA: Rifampin in experimental endocarditis due to *Staphylococcus aureus* in rabbits. J Infect Dis 5(Suppl 3):S481, 1983.
80. Van Der Auwera P, Meunier-Carpentier F, Klatersky J: Clinical study of combination therapy with oxacillin and rifampin for staphylococcal infections. Rev Infect Dis 5(Suppl 3):S515, 1983.
81. Van der Auwera P, Klastersky J, Thys JP, et al: Double-blind, placebo-controlled study of oxacillin combined with rifampin in the treatment of staphylococcal infections. Antimicrob Agents Chemother 28:467, 1985.
82. Dworkin RJ, Lee BL, Sande MA, et al: Treatment of right-sided *Staphylococcus aureus* endocarditis in intravenous drug users with ciprofloxacin and rifampicin. Lancet 2:1071, 1989.
83. Karchmer AW, Archer GA: Methicillin-resistant *Staphylococcus epidermidis* (SE) prosthetic valve (PV) endocarditis (E): A therapeutic trial. *In* Program and Abstracts of the 24th Interscience Conference on Antimicrobial Agents and Chemotherapy; October 8–10, 1984. Abstract 476.
84. Norden CW: Experimental chronic staphylococcal osteomyelitis in rabbits: Treatment with rifampin alone and in combination with other antimicrobial agents. Rev Infect Dis 5(Suppl 3):S491, 1983.
85. Norden CW, Bryant R, Palmer D, et al: Chronic osteomyelitis caused by *Staphylococcus aureus*: Controlled clinical trial of nafcillin therapy and nafcillin-rifampin therapy. South Med J 79:947, 1986.
86. Widmer AF, Gaechter A, Ochsner PE, et al: Antimicrobial treatment of orthopedic implant-related infections with rifampin combinations. Clin Infect Dis 14:1251, 1992.

87. Ariza J, Gudiol F, Pallares R, et al: Treatment of human brucellosis with doxycycline plus rifampin or doxycycline plus streptomycin. A randomized, double-blind study. Ann Intern Med 117:25, 1992.
88. Jacobs F, Abramowicz D, Vereerstraeten P, et al: *Brucella* endocarditis: The role of combined medical and surgical treatment. Rev Infect Dis 12:740, 1990.
89. Catalan MJ, Fernandez JM, Varquez A, et al: Failure of cefotaxime in the treatment of meningitis due to relatively resistant *Streptococcus pneumoniae*. Clin Infect Dis 18:766, 1994.
90. Yu VL, Zuravleff JJ, Peacock JE, et al: Addition of rifampin to carboxypenicillin-aminoglycoside combination for the treatment of *Pseudomonas aeruginosa* infection: Clinical experience with four patients. Antimicrob Agents Chemother 26:575, 1984.
91. Korvick JA, Peacock JE Jr, Muder RR, et al: Addition of rifampin to combination antibiotic therapy for *Pseudomonas aeruginosa* bacteremia: Prospective trial using the Zelen protocol. Antimicrob Agents Chemother 36:620, 1992.
92. Morris AB, Brown RB, Sands M: Use of rifampin in nonstaphylococcal, nonmycobacterial disease. Antimicrob Agents Chemother 37:1, 1993.
93. Band JD, Fraser DW: Adverse effects of two rifampicin dosage regimens for the prevention of meningococcal infection. Lancet 1:101, 1984.
94. Girlin DJ: Adverse reactions to rifampicin in antituberculosis regimens. J Antimicrob Chemother 3:115, 1977.
95. Van Assendelft AHW: Leucopenia in rifampicin chemotherapy. J Antimicrob Chemother 16:407, 1985.
96. Grosset J, Leventis S: Adverse effects of rifampin. Rev Infect Dis 5(Suppl 3):S440, 1983.
97. Soffer O, Nassar VH, Campbell WG Jr: Light chain cast nephropathy and acute renal failure associated with rifampin therapy. Am J Med 82:1052, 1987.
98. Humber DP, Nsanzumuhire H, Aluoch HA, et al: Controlled double-blind study of the effect of rifampin on humoral and cellular immune responses in patients with pulmonary tuberculosis and in tuberculosis contacts. Am Rev Respir Dis 122:425, 1980.
99. Baciewicz AM, Self TH, Bekemeyer WB: Update on rifampin drug interactions. Arch Intern Med 147:565, 1987.
100. Venkatesan K: Pharmacokinetic drug interactions with rifampicin. Clin Pharmacokinet 22:47, 1992.
101. Burger DM, Meenhorst PL, Koks CHW, et al: Pharmacokinetic interaction between rifampin and zidovudine. Antimicrob Agents Chemother 37:1426, 1993.
102. Colmenero JD, Fernandez-Gallardo LC, Agundez JAG, et al: Possible implications of doxycycline-rifampin interaction for treatment of brucellosis. Antimicrob Agents Chemother 38:2798, 1994.
103. Wallace RJ Jr, Brown BA, Griffith DE, et al: Reduced serum levels of clarithromycin in patients treated with multidrug regimens including rifampin or rifabutin for *Mycobacterium avium–M. intracellulare* infection. J Infect Dis 171:747, 1995.
104. Heifets LB, Iseman MD: Determination of in vitro susceptibility of mycobacteria to Ansamycin. Am Rev Respir Dis 132:710, 1985.
105. Heifets LB, Lindholm-Levy PJ, Iseman MD: Rifabutine: Minimal inhibitory and bactericidal concentrations for *Mycobacterium tuberculosis*. Am Rev Respir Dis 137:719, 1988.
106. Heifets LB, Iseman MD, Lindholm-Levy PJ, et al: Determination of Ansamycin MICs for *Mycobacterium avium* complex in liquid medium by radiometric and conventional methods. Antimicrob Agents Chemother 28:570, 1985.
107. Nightingale SD, Cameron DW, Gordin FM, et al: Two controlled trials of rifabutin prophylaxis against *Mycobacterium avium* complex infection in AIDS. N Engl J Med 329:828, 1993.
108. U.S. Public Health Service Task Force on Prophylaxis and Therapy for *Mycobacterium avium* complex: Recommendations on prophylaxis and therapy for disseminated *Mycobacterium avium* complex for adults and adolescents infected with human immunodeficiency virus. MMWR Morbid Mortal Wkly Rep 42(RR-9):14, 1993.
109. Masur H, Tuazon C, Gill V, et al: Effect of combined clofazimine and Ansamycin therapy on *Mycobacterium avium–Mycobacterium intracellulare* bacteremia in patients with AIDS. J Infect Dis 155:127, 1987.
110. Agins BD, Berman DS, Spicehandler D, et al: Effect of combined therapy with Ansamycin, clofazimine, ethambutol, and isoniazid for *Mycobacterium avium* infection in patients with AIDS. J Infect Dis 159:784, 1989.
111. Hoy J, Mijch A, Sandland M, et al: Quadruple-drug therapy for *Mycobacterium avium-intracellulare* bacteremia in AIDS patients. J Infect Dis 161:801, 1990.
112. Sullam PM, Gordin FM, Wynne BA, et al: Efficacy of rifabutin in the treatment of disseminated infection due to *Mycobacterium avium* complex. Clin Infect Dis 19:84, 1994.
113. Skinner MH, Hsieh M, Torseth J, et al: Pharmacokinetics of rifabutin. Antimicrob Agents Chemother 33:1237, 1989.
114. Narang PK, Lewis RC, Bianchine JR: Rifabutin absorption in humans: Relative bioavailability and food effect. Clin Pharmacol Ther 52:335, 1992.
115. Battaglia R, Pianezzola E, Salgarollo G, et al: Absorption, disposition and preliminary metabolic pathway of ^{14}C-rifabutin in animals and man. J Antimicrob Chemother 26:813, 1990.
116. Brogden RN, Fitton A: Rifabutin. A review of its antimicrobial activity, pharmacokinetic properties and therapeutic efficacy. Drugs 47:983, 1994.
117. Havlir D, Torriani F, Dube M: Uveitis associated with rifabutin prophylaxis. Ann Intern Med 121:510, 1994.
118. Siegel FP, Eilbott D, Burger H, et al: Dose-limiting toxicity of rifabutin in AIDS-related complex: Syndrome of arthralgia/arthritis. AIDS 4:433, 1990.
119. Perucca E, Grimaldi R, Frigo GM, et al: Comparative effects of rifabutin and rifampicin on hepatic microsomal enzyme activity in normal subjects. Eur J Clin Pharmacol 34:595, 1988.
120. Gallicano K, Sahai J, Swick L, et al: Effect of rifabutin on the pharmacokinetics of zidovudine in patients infected with human immunodeficiency virus. Clin Infect Dis 21:1008, 1995.
121. Griffith DE, Brown BA, Girard WM, et al: Adverse events associated with high-dose rifabutin in macrolide-containing regimens for the treatment of *Mycobacterium avium* complex lung disease. Clin Infect Dis 21:594, 1995.
122. Cynamon MH: Comparative in vitro activities of MDL 473, rifampin, and Ansamycin against *Mycobacterium intracellulare*. Antimicrob Agents Chemother 28:440, 1985.
123. Birmingham AT, Coleman AJ, Orme MLE, et al: Antibacterial activity in serum and urine following oral administration in man of DL473 (a cyclopentyl derivative of rifampicin). Br J Clin Pharmacol 6:445, 1978.
124. Buniva G, Sassella D, Frigo GM: Pharmacokinetics of rifapentine in man. *In* Spitzy KH, Karrer K (eds): Proceedings of the 13th International Congress of Chemotherapy. Vienna, Egermann Druckerei, 1983, pp 111/29–33.
125. Luna-Herrera J, Reddy MV, Gangadharam PRJ: In vitro activity of the benzoxazinorifamycin KRM-1648 against drug-susceptible and multidrug-resistant tubercle bacilli. Antimicrob Agents Chemother 39:440, 1995.
126. Gillis JC, Brogden RN: Rifaximin. A review of its antibacterial activity, pharmacokinetic properties and therapeutic potential in conditions mediated by gastrointestinal bacteria. Drugs 49:467, 1995.

30

Miscellaneous Drugs

Burt R. Meyers
Alejandra C. Gurtman

Polymyxin B/Colistin

The polymyxins are a group of polypeptide antibiotics isolated from a soil bacillus *(Bacillus polymyxa)*; a number of these compounds (A, B, C, D, E) are isolated from different strains of the bacillus. Colistin, produced by *Bacillus colistinus*, was originally thought to be different but was soon found to be identical to polymyxin E. All of these drugs have molecular weights of approximately 1000. Of the five polymyxins, only two are currently in clinical use, polymyxins B and E (colistin).

Mode of Action and Antibiotic Activity

All the polymyxins act on bacterial membranes, interacting with phospholipids; their lipophobic groups disrupt the membranes, changing their permeability. Polymyxins are cationic detergents and attach to anionic binding sites in the cell membrane. Antibiotic sensitivity of these compounds is probably related to the phospholipid content of the cell wall. Damage to this structure breaks the osmotic barrier and leads to a leaking of intracellular materials and perhaps allows entry of other agents. Toxic effects due to this binding have been postulated.[1] Binding to phospholipids may explain some of the biologic activity of polymyxin B, which has been found to block the biologic effect of endotoxin lipopolysaccharide (LPS). Polymyxin B inhibits pyrogenicity from LPS[2] and LPS-induced interleukin-1 release by monocytes.[3] It also inhibits the endotoxin effect of decreasing natural killer cell activity in burn patients.[4] Mortality in experimentally induced endotoxemia in animals was reduced. Polymyxin B also protected against gram-negative septicemia.[5–8] It was demonstrated in an *Escherichia coli* sepsis rabbit model that polymyxin B moderated acidosis and decreased hypotension compared with control subjects, whereas corticosteroids and antibodies to LPS failed.[9] Polymyxin B also prevents LPS release of tumor necrosis factor-α from alveolar macrophages.[10] Further studies have shown that incubation of polymyxin B with LPS inhibits the tumoricidal action of these macrophages.[11] Polymyxin B decreases endotoxin concentrations in experimental animals with meningitis due to *E. coli* after treatment with antibiotics.[12]

Antibacterial Activity

Both polymyxin B and colistin are active against gram-negative organisms, including *E. coli, Klebsiella* spp., *Enterobacter* spp., *Salmonella* spp., *Shigella* spp., and *Pseudomonas aeruginosa*. In vitro, polymyxin B is more active than colistin against *P. aeruginosa*.[13–15] Minimal inhibitory concentrations (MICs) vary between 0.02 and 2.0 μg/mL; the MICs for *P. aeruginosa* are somewhat higher. Species of *Pseudomonas* other than *P. aeruginosa* (i.e., *P. cepacia, P. maltophilia*, and so forth) are usually resistant. These agents have less activity against *Serratia marcescens* and are inactive against *Proteus* spp. Other sensitive gram-negative bacteria include *Haemophilus influenzae, Bordetella pertussis, Neisseria meningitidis, Neisseria gonorrhoeae, Brucella* spp., and cholera strains excluding *Vibrio cholerae* (biotype *eltor*). Although some strains of *Bacteroides* spp. and *Fusobacterium* spp. are sensitive, *Bacteroides fragilis* is resistant. All gram-positive organisms are resistant. Bacterial resistance of previously sensitive organisms is not commonly acquired. There is cross-resistance between polymyxin B and colistin for all strains.[16] Resistance is most likely due to decreased permeability across the outer membrane.[17] In vitro synergy has been demonstrated with sulfa compounds for resistant strains of *P. aeruginosa, Proteus* spp., and *S. marcescens*. Synergy with trimethoprim and polymyxin B has been demonstrated in vitro for *Serratia* spp. Combinations of sulfamethoxazole, trimethoprim, and colistin have also demonstrated synergy.[18, 19] In vitro polymyxin B may affect the cell membranes of certain fungi, increasing permeability to tetracycline with inhibition of the growth.[20] Other studies have shown polymyxin B to enhance amphotericin B activity against *Coccidioides immitis*.[21] Synergy with bacitracin and miconazole and polymyxin B against *Staphylococcus aureus* and *Staphylococcus epidermidis* suggests that entry of these agents occurs because of membrane perturbation.[22] Colistin has activity against strains of *Mycobacterium* including *M. tuberculosis, M. intracellulare, M. xenopi*, and *M. fortuitum*.[15, 23]

The antibacterial effect of the polymyxins can be prevented by the divalent cations magnesium and calcium and by ethylenediaminetetraacetic acid[24]; they stabilize membranes, preventing polymyxin B from competitively displacing these ions on negatively charged phosphate groups on membrane lipids. This may be clinically significant because physiologic concentrations of calcium affect polymyxin, suggesting less activity in vivo than could be predicted by susceptibility in vitro.[25] Polymyxin B exerts an antiinsulin effect[26]; it is a protein kinase C inhibitor, and this has the effect on glucose metabolism of decreasing glucose-stimulated insulin secretion.[27–29]

Pharmacokinetics

Polymyxin B and colistin are not absorbed when given orally. After intramuscular injection of polymyxin B, peak serum levels of 2 to 8 μg/mL are observed. The half-life ($t_{1/2}$) in serum is 6 hours.[30, 31] Serum levels decline slowly during 8 to 12 hours. Accumulation has been reported in patients given 2.5 mg/kg per day, with peak levels reported 7 days later of 15 μg/mL. When colistin methane sulfonate (polymyxin E) is given intramuscularly at a dose of 2.5 mg/kg to adults, peak serum levels of 5 to 7 μg/mL occur between 1 and 2 hours; the $t_{1/2}$ is 1.6 to 2.7 hours. Drug accumulation was found, with peak levels of 12 μg/mL. When given intravenously by bolus and then by slow infusion, serum levels of 5 to 6 μg/mL are maintained.[32] Excretion of polymyxin B is mainly renal via glomerular filtration, although only a small amount of polymyxin B is recovered in the first 12 hours; 60% of the injected dose of polymyxin B sulfate can be found in the urine for a period of days. Urinary concentration varies between 20 and 100 μg/mL after parenteral therapy. Colistin is excreted more rapidly by the kidney, with 40% excretion in the first 8 hours; a high fluid intake decreases urinary concentrations to 20 μg/mL[33] from the usual level of 200 μg/mL. In the presence of renal insufficiency, the $t_{1/2}$ is 48 to 72 hours.[30, 34] Polymyxins are not found in the biliary tract and do not enter the cerebrospinal fluid even in the presence of inflammation.

Others have found a shorter $t_{1/2}$.[35] In animals, the drug is distributed to liver, kidney, brain, heart, muscle, and lung[1] and persists up to 72 hours after a single injection. Protein binding is low with both of these compounds. The exact method of inactivation is not known.

Administration and Dosage

Both agents can be given by the intramuscular and intravenous routes. The usual dose of polymyxin is 15,000 to 25,000 units/kg per day (1.5 to 2.5 mg/kg per day) (1 mg polymyxin B = 10,000 units). The intramuscular dose of polymyxin B is 2.5 to 5 mg/kg per day every 4 or 6 hours. In patients with normal renal function, the usual intravenous dosage of polymyxin is 50 mg/500 mL infused during 8 hours (not to exceed 25,000 units/kg per day). The same dose can be added to 100 mL and infused during 30 minutes; rapid intravenous injection should be avoided. For colistimethate, the intramuscular and intravenous dosage is 2.5 to 5.0 mg/kg per day in two to four divided doses; the higher dosage is reserved for severe infections. Because both these agents accumulate in renal failure, the doses should be modified.[31, 35–39] Regimens include giving the standard dose 150 mg polymyxin B or 120 mg colistin at adjusted intervals according to renal function.[37] Colistin at 2 to 3 mg/kg may be given after each session of hemodialysis.[40]

Polymyxin B can be administered intrathecally. The usual dosage for adults is 5 to 10 mg given daily for 3 days and then on alternate days. Treatment is continued for at least 3 days after the cerebrospinal fluid is sterile, usually more than 2 weeks. The dosage in children younger than 2 years of age is 2.0 mg daily for 3 or 4 days, then 2.5 mg every other day. This drug should be delivered in sterile saline (not procaine) to obviate toxic effects. Polymyxin B can be given orally in doses of 100 to 200 mg, three or four times daily. A dose of 800 mg daily has been used for intestinal decontamination in patients with leukemia or to prevent infection in the intensive care unit.[41] Colistin sulfate can be administered orally at a dosage of 5 to 15 mg/kg per day in three equally divided doses, but the oral preparation is no longer available in the United States.

Adverse Effects

Nephrotoxicity is commonly seen with polymyxin B and, less frequently, with colistin; this may be because methane sulfonate is used and believed to be less toxic than the sulfate derivative used in polymyxin E. Toxicity is manifested by proteinuria, hematuria, and casts. Renal dysfunction is manifested by an elevated serum creatinine level. Nephrotoxicity is usually noted in the first few days of therapy but may be found after the drug is stopped. In one study, nephrotoxicity occurred in 20% of patients[42]; oliguric renal failure and tubular necrosis were reported, although usually at higher dosages. These agents are poorly dialyzed during hemodialysis; colistin is only partially cleared by peritoneal dialysis.[43] Great caution is necessary when these drugs are used in the presence of renal dysfunction. Serum levels reach high concentrations and may further increase nephrotoxicity. Administration with cephalothin increases toxicity.

Numbness, paresthesias (often perioral), peripheral neuropathy, slurred speech, dyphasia, and ataxia have been noted, usually in the first 4 days. More serious events, including psychosis, convulsions, coma, and ataxia, may occur. Facial flushing and dizziness are more commonly seen in those with renal insufficiency.

Neuromuscular blockade manifested as respiratory paralysis may occur, even after the first dose of either drug; it is more common in renal failure with high serum concentrations. Restlessness and dyspnea may be the first signs. In most cases, other factors—including anesthesia, sedation, hypoxia, and hypocalcemia—are noted. The neuromuscular blockade is different than that seen with aminoglycosides, which can be reversed by neostigmine. However, with polymyxin B, a noncompetitive blockade occurs that is not reversible by drugs. Treatment requires support of respiratory function usually for 24 hours until the drug has dissipated. Because aminoglycosides may interfere with nerve conduction, they should not usually be administered concomitantly.

After oral administration, nausea, vomiting, and diarrhea often occur. The polymyxins are not absorbed through denuded skin, and side effects are rarely noted with topical administration. Hypersensitivities such as rash and pruritus are found infrequently.

Clinical Applications

Polymyxin B and colistin should be considered only as second-line drugs in the treatment of gram-negative infections. Experimental *P. aeruginosa* infection in animals revealed that other agents such as gentamicin and tobramycin were more effective and less toxic than colistin and polymyxin B.[44] Polymyxin B and colistin have been used in the past to treat infections caused by *P. aeruginosa*, including bacteremia, pneumonia, burns, meningitis, and urinary tract infections.[14, 43] In the early 1960s, *Pseudomonas* septicemia was treated with polymyxin.[45] Other infections treated included *Pseudomonas* meningitis, in which the agents were used parenterally and intrathecally, and infected burns, in which the agents were used both parenterally and topically. Polymyxin B has been used parenterally in the treatment of pulmonary infections with some success and was effective in six of seven patients with septicemia.[43] It has also been aerosolized and given prophylactically into the respiratory tract for critically ill patients in an attempt to prevent pneumonia due to *P. aeruginosa;* in this study, however, patients developed pneumonia with polymyxin B–resistant organisms (i.e., *P. maltophilia* and *P. cepacia*).[46] Investigators have attempted to prevent colonization and subsequent respiratory tract infections with local antimicrobial prophylaxis. This prophylaxis consisted of polymyxin B administered orally, either alone or in combination with gentamicin, parenteral cefotaxime, nalidixic acid, and neomycin. Colistin has been substituted for polymyxin B with these agents.[47–49] Intestinal decontamination has been used to control nosocomial infections with multidrug-resistant gram-negative bacilli.[50] When polymyxin B and gentamicin were administered as a paste to the nose or oral pharynx and orally in patients in an intensive care unit, there were decreased colonization of the oral pharynx and trachea and decreased cases of pneumonia compared with control patients.[51] Emergence of bacterial resistance was studied in a surgical intensive care unit in patients receiving parenteral cefotaxime and oral polymyxin during a 30-month period. There was an 8% increase in strains of *Proteus* and *Morganella* spp.; 10% of the patients were colonized with cefotaxime-resistant strains, which were eliminated with the nonabsorbable oral therapy.[52]

In one study, 600 mg daily of polymyxin B orally or intravenously suppressed intestinal microflora but was associated in half the volunteers with severe gastrointestinal side effects.[53] Polymyxin B and colistin have been used orally as prophylaxis of infection of leukopenic patients. These agents have been combined with neomycin, gentamicin, trimethoprim-sulfamethoxazole, ofloxacin, and nalidixic acid[54–60]; in some cases, however, candidal overgrowth was seen when amphotericin B was not included. When used alone, the dose of polymyxin for decontamination was 800 mg daily.[41] Polymyxin B is moderately inactivated by food and feces.[48, 50] In combination with tobramycin, inactivation of polymyxin was reduced; the dose could be decreased to 400 mg daily to prevent infection in trauma patients.

In a prospective but nonblinded or controlled study using polymixin B lozenges at 2 mg, tobramycin at 1.8 mg, and amphotericin B at 10 mg four times daily to patients undergoing radiation for head and neck cancer, the incidence of mucositis was decreased compared with historical control subjects. Colonization by gram-negative bacilli was decreased, and no oral fungal infections occurred.[61] Polymyxin B may offer an alternative for the treatment of infections due to gram-negative bacilli that are resistant to commonly used antibiotics; ceftazidime-resistant *Klebsiella pneumoniae, Enterobacter* spp., and *P. aeruginosa* infections have been treated successfully. It has been combined with rifampin to treat resistant *S. marcescens* infection and with trimethoprim-sulfamethoxazole to treat infections with *P. cepacia* and *S. marcescens*. Urinary tract infections caused by *P. aeruginosa* have been treated with these agents; colistin may be a better choice of therapy because higher urinary concentrations are more rapidly obtained than with polymyxin B.

In patients with central nervous system infections, polymyxin B may have a role in the treatment of multidrug-resistant gram-negative bacilli, including *P. aeruginosa*; because levels are not obtained after systemic administration, intrathecal therapy is required. A patient has been treated successfully with colistin and piperacillin.[62]

Colistin has been combined with trimethoprim-sulfamethoxazole for the prevention of infection in patients with acute nonlymphocytic leukemia. The authors concluded that combination therapy was better than trimethoprim-sulfamethoxazole alone.[60] In another study, polymyxin was included in a regimen of oral nonabsorbable antibiotics used to prevent infection in cirrhotic patients with gastrointestinal hemorrhage; infections with enteric bacteria occurred less frequently in patients given this prophylaxis.[63] It has also been suggested that polymyxin B be studied as adjuvant therapy for severe gram-negative infection.[9] Although it has been demonstrated that serum endotoxin levels are increased in patients with obstructive jaundice, polymyxin B had no effect on endotoxemia and outcome after operation to relieve jaundice.[64] Others have recommended that this agent be used as preoperative bowel decontamination to prevent infection after orthotopic liver transplantation.[65]

Polymyxin B sulfate has been prepared for topical and ophthalmic use, usually in combination with other compounds such as neomycin and bacitracin. These preparations include creams, ointments, drops, and sprays. When these drugs are used topically, bacterial resistance and allergic reactions are uncommon. Absorption through denuded burn surfaces and mucous membranes is poor; thus, infections of the external ear canal, skin, eyes, and mucous membranes are often treated with these agents. Corneal ulcers caused by *P. aeruginosa* have been treated both topically and with subconjunctival injection of polymyxin B; the drug has been used topically in the eye to treat *Acanthamoeba* sp. infections associated with contact lens wear.[66]

Colistin sulfate (Coly-Mycin) has been used to treat diarrheal infections in infants and children caused by susceptible strains of enteropathogenic *E. coli*; the usual dosage is 5 to 15 mg/kg per day in three divided doses. Others believe that these agents are of no clinical efficacy for treating gastroenteritis caused by gram-negative bacilli.[67, 68]

Future Use of Polymyxin

The association of circulating endotoxin with the development of adult respiratory distress syndrome has been demonstrated.[69] Polymyxin B obviates the effects of endotoxin, as demonstrated in multiple models, by blocking the effect of cytokines that are liberated from cellular elements. Its role in these clinical situations (e.g., adult respiratory distress syndrome, septic shock) mandates clinical testing.

Polymyxin E paste (2%) can be combined with tobramycin and applied to the buccal mucosa and oral cavity in intensive care units as prophylaxis for nosocomial pneumonia.[70] No infections occurred in 27 patients who were studied this way.

Methenamine

Methenamine was discovered in 1894. It is a cyclic hydrocarbon condensation product of ammonia and formaldehyde with properties of a monoacidic base; it is soluble in water and forms a weak basic solution at a pH of 8.0 to 8.5. It is available in three different forms: alone as a pure base or in combination with mandelic acid or hippuric acid.

Mode of Action

In acidic urine, methenamine is hydrolyzed to formaldehyde and ammonia by the following reaction: $N_4(CH_2)_6 + 6H_2O + 4H^+ = 4NH_4^+ + 6HCHO$. Because the release of formaldehyde occurs only in an acidic medium, the antimicrobial activity of methenamine is related to the urinary pH.

Antibacterial Activity

Methenamine is active against all gram-negative and gram-positive bacteria, even fungi, except for urea-splitting organisms such as *Proteus* spp.[71] Bacterial resistance to formaldehyde does not develop, and no cross-resistance with any other antibiotic has been reported.[72]

Pharmacokinetics

After oral ingestion, methenamine is well absorbed and circulates unchanged. About 10% to 30% is hydrolyzed by gastric fluid. After a single (1-g) dose, approximately 82% of methenamine is recovered in urine in 24 hours, and 90% is recovered during continuous administration. The peak serum level is 35 μg/mL at 1 hour; 20% of methenamine is converted to formaldehyde in the urine. Concentrations of formaldehyde of 10 to 15 μg/mL have bacteriostatic activity; concentrations greater than 28 μg/mL are bactericidal.[73] A urinary pH less than 6.0 is necessary to achieve the bactericidal effect; the addition of hippurate or mandelic acid ensures the acidity of the urine. The mean half-life is 4.3 hours.[74]

Renal clearance of methenamine approximates creatinine clearance; caution is required in patients with renal insufficiency.[75] Methenamine is widely distributed throughout the body fluids (e.g., cerebrospinal fluid, aqueous humor, and pericardial and synovial fluids).

Dosage

For adults the oral dose is 1 g every 6 hours for methenamine mandelate and 1 g every 12 hours for the hippurate form. In children, half the adult dose is recommended.

Adverse Effects

This drug is well tolerated; gastrointestinal disturbances such as nausea, vomiting, and diarrhea have occasionally been reported.[76] Skin reactions, bladder irritation, and inflammation accompanied by dysuria, hematuria, and proteinuria may occur.[77] It has been associated with bilateral anterior uveitis.[78] Methenamine should not be administered in conjunction with sulfonamides, which may precipitate when formaldehyde is released.[79] It is contraindicated in patients with gout, because urate crystals may precipitate in urine.[80]

Clinical Applications

Methenamine is indicated only for treatment of lower urinary tract infections, and even this is controversial.[81, 82] It is effective as preoperative prophylaxis in bacteriuric patients undergoing transurethral prostatic resection,[83] cystoscopy, and vaginal surgery.[84] Use with urinary acidifying agents in combination (e.g., hemiacidrin) is recommended. In patients receiving methenamine, bacteriuria is reduced in those requiring intermittent catheterization[85, 86]; however, relapses or reinfections in patients with spinal cord injuries who have neurogenic bladders have been reported.[87]

Methenamine is not more effective than trimethoprim alone; its failure may be due to the drug's inability to alter the periurethral flora.[88] A potential use for methenamine is in the treatment of calcium stone disease because renal secretion of oxalate is decreased.[89] Further clinical trials are necessary to confirm this activity.

Fusidic Acid

Fusidic acid, available since 1962, was isolated from the fungus *Fusidium coccineum*; it has a steroid-like structure and is related chemically to cephalosporin P. It is poorly soluble in water and thus is prepared as a sodium salt for oral administration and as a diethanolamine salt for intravenous administration. It is a weak acid (pH 5.7) that is largely ionized at the pH values of the blood.[90]

Mode of Action

Fusidic acid inhibits bacterial protein synthesis by interacting with the ribosome and interfering with the polypeptide chain elongation. It inhibits the elongation factor G and guanosine diphosphate, decreasing guanosine triphosphate hydrolysis. This inhibition leads to less protein A on the surface of gram-positive bacteria (*S. aureus*), increasing susceptibility to phagocytosis.[91]

Antibacterial Activity

Fusidic acid is highly effective against staphylococci, including penicillin-sensitive *S. aureus*, β-lactamase–producing strains, methicillin-resistant strains,[92, 93] and *S. epidermidis*.[94] The MIC for *S. aureus* ranges between 0.063 and 1.0 mg/L (median, 0.125 mg/L); the minimal bactericidal concentration ranges between 0.25 and 16 mg/dL (median, 8 mg/dL).[95] Synergy with rifampin and dicloxacillin has been demonstrated[96] and antagonism between fusidic acid and rifampin reported.[97] Other gram-positive bacteria, such as streptococci, are much less susceptible to fusidic acid, with MIC values of 8.6 μg/mL for *S. pneumoniae*, 6.8 μg/mL for *Streptococcus pyogenes*, and 1.6 μg/mL for *Streptococcus viridans*; in vitro synergism with gentamicin against enterococcus has been demonstrated.[98] Gram-positive anaerobes such as *Clostridium tetani* (MIC of 0.016 μg/mL) and *Clostridium perfringens* are sensitive. The MIC of fusidic acid for *B. fragilis* is 0.25 to 4.0 μg/mL.[99] All gram-negative bacilli are resistant, but some gram-negative cocci (i.e., *N. meningitidis* and *N. gonorrhoeae*) with MIC values of 0.56 and 0.66 μg/mL, respectively,[100] are susceptible. Other sensitive organisms include *Nocardia asteroides* (MIC of 2.5 mg/mL)[101] and *M. tuberculosis* (MIC of 1.0 μg/mL).

Pharmacokinetics

After oral dosing of 500 mg of fusidic acid, the peak serum level of 20 mg/mL was achieved in 2 hours, although the variation for the rate of absorption is variable among subjects. The $t_{1/2}$ is 5 to 6 hours[90]; some accumulation may occur when the drug is administered every 8 hours. After 96 hours of therapy, a plasma concentration between 21 and 71 μg/mL was obtained. With the oral suspension, a faster peak but lower mean peak concentration is observed than with the tablets.[90] After intravenous administration, an initial high level of 20 mg/L is noted (mean, 44 μg/mL) after a 2-hour infusion.[102]

Excretion

Fusidic acid is metabolized in the liver and probably undergoes enterohepatic circulation. At least seven different metabolites have been found in bile,[103] some of them with microbiologic activity. About 2% of fusidic acid is found in the feces, probably due to biliary excretion, as well as a small quantity of nonabsorbed drug. Small amounts of fusidic acid are renally excreted, and less than 1% of the drug can be recovered from the urine.[104] Fusidic acid is not renally excreted, so patients with renal failure or undergoing hemodialysis do not need dose adjustments.[105] The drug should be avoided in patients with hepatic failure, because it competes with bilirubin for albumin binding sites.

Distribution

Fusidic acid is strongly protein bound (99%)[106]; it is well distributed throughout the body, with good diffusion into different cell types including lymphocytes, macrophages, and fibroblasts.[107] Fusidic acid penetrates the synovial fluid of inflamed joints with levels that approach those of plasma. In bone, concentrations that exceed the MIC for most strains of *S. aureus* have been observed. Some of these levels may exceed the MIC by a factor of 100.[108] Heart tissue levels are one third those of plasma, and the drug penetrates better into atrial appendages than do cephalosporins. It is not affected by cardiopulmonary bypass.[109] Fusidic acid enters purulent collections, prostatic fluid, and aqueous humor. Cerebrospinal fluid concentrations are quite low, although in cerebral abscesses levels approach the serum concentrations.[110] Fusidic acid passes through the placenta and can be detected in fetal tissue.

The usual oral dose for adults is 500 mg given three times daily, but the dose can be doubled in severe infections. A suspension of 250 mg of fusidic acid hemihydrate per 5 mL is available but has less bioavailability than the enteric-coated tablets with 250 mg of fusidic acid. For children younger than 1 year of age the recommended dose is 50 mg/kg per day. The intravenous preparation contains, per vial, 580 mg of diethanolamine salt, equivalent to 500 mg of fusidic acid. The dose is diluted in saline and should be infused during 6 hours. The dosage for adults is 580 mg diethanolamine fusidate three times daily; it is 10 mg/kg for children. A 2% ointment for topical administration is available.

Adverse Effects

After oral administration, nausea, vomiting, and diarrhea may occur. Ingestion of food decreases dyspepsia without affecting blood levels. After intravenous administration, severe local pain may occur, as well as venospasm and thrombophlebitis[111] resulting from an irritant effect on the vein wall. This effect can be minimized with slow infusions in a large peripheral vein. Because fusidic acid is highly protein bound, it competes with bilirubin for albumin binding sites, reversibly increasing free bilirubin concentrations.[112] Fusidic acid should be used cautiously in patients with liver impairment, especially in neonates, because of the potential for brain damage.[106] Neutropenia and rashes have rarely been reported.[113]

Clinical Applications

Fusidic acid in its oral, parenteral, and topical forms has been used to treat staphylococcal infections of skin and soft tissue (e.g., abscesses, furunculosis, and infected burns). It is an alternative therapy to penicillinase-resistant penicillins and cephalosporins for osteomyelitis, septic arthritis, endocarditis, sepsis, and pneumonia when *S. aureus* is isolated or suspected.[114] Children with cystic fibrosis have been treated for *S. aureus* infections.[115] Because of the development of drug resistance, fusidic acid is not recommended as monotherapy but should be given with other antistaphylococcal agents (e.g., β-lactamase–resistant penicillins or cephalosporins).[96] Fusidic acid has been added to bone cement for prophylaxis of infections before hip replacement. Fusidic acid has been used to treat nasal carriers of methicillin-resistant *S. aureus*[116]; pseudomembranous colitis due to *Clostridium difficile* may benefit from fusidic acid therapy.[117] It appears to be a weak bactericidal antileprosy agent, which may have a role in the multidrug treatment of leprosy.[118] A case of successfully treated legionellosis has been reported.[119] Fusidic acid is active in vitro against many methicillin-resistant *S. aureus* strains, so it should be considered for use with other agents such as vancomycin, rifampin, and possibly ciprofloxacin in refractory cases.[93] There are few reports in the literature suggesting that fusidic acid may be a promising candidate for prophylaxis in neurosurgery.[120, 121] Fusidic acid is excreted into the bile and discharged into the small intestine where the colonization with *Giardia* organisms is maximal; thus, a potential use in combination with metronidazole can be considered in refractory cases of giardiasis.[122] It has also been used as self-administration prophylaxis before cataract surgery with significant reduction of *S. aureus* and *S. epidermidis* infection and attainment of sterile eyes.[123] Finally, because fusidic acid penetrates lymphocytes and macrophages, an attempt was made to treat patients with human immunodeficiency virus infection; no response of p24 antigen or increase in $CD4^+$ cells was detected.[124]

Nitrofurantoin

Nitrofurantoin has been available since 1953 and is one of the nitrofuran compounds, which consist of a primary nitro group joined to a heterocycle ring. It is poorly soluble in water and is available in crystalline and macrocrystalline forms.

Mode of Action

The precise mechanism of action is unknown; it is probably due to inhibition of bacterial enzymes and may also interfere with DNA. Drug activity is increased in acidic urine.

Antibacterial Activity

Nitrofurantoin is active against most gram-negative bacteria that cause urinary tract infection. *E. coli* strains are sensitive, with an MIC of 16 μg/mL; other gram-negative bacilli with an MIC of 32 μg/mL or less are considered susceptible to the drug. *Enterobacter* spp. and *Klebsiella* spp. are less susceptible, with MIC values usually greater than 100 μg/mL, whereas *Proteus* spp. and *P. aeruginosa* are almost always resistant, with MIC values greater than 200 μg/mL.[125]

Nitrofurantoin is also active against gram-positive bacteria that sometimes produce urinary tract infections, such as *Enterococcus, S. aureus, S. epidermidis,* and *Staphylococcus saprophiticus*. The MIC values for gram-positive cocci are lower: 4 μg/mL for *S. aureus* and 25 μg/mL for *Enterococcus*.

Other microorganisms, such as *S. pyogenes, S. pneumoniae, Corynebacterium* spp., *Salmonella* spp., *Shigella* spp., and *B. fragilis*, are sensitive in vitro. Organisms usually do not develop resistance to nitrofurantoin, but cross-resistance with aminoglycosides with *E. coli* has been reported.[126]

Pharmacokinetics

The standard crystalline form is more rapidly absorbed than the macrocrystalline form. Nitrofurantoin has an extremely short half-life ($t_{1/2}$ = 20 minutes).[127] Serum levels are low, with peak concentrations in plasma near 0.72 mg/L detected after 2 hours.[128]

Excretion

About one third of the dose appears in urine as active drug, with urine levels of 50 to 250 μg/mL. Recovery from the urine is related to creatinine clearance. The drug tends, however, to accumulate in patients with abnormal renal function.[129] Nitrofurantoin also penetrates the interstitial tissue of the renal medulla.[130] Some drug is excreted into the bile; it is inactivated in all body tissues, but hepatic degradation may be the most significant.

Administration

Nitrofurantoin is available for oral use but not for intravenous administration in the United States. Sustained-release nitrofurantoin in the form of microcapsules may decrease the severity of side effects.[131, 132] Oral dosage for adults is 50 to 100 mg every 6 hours.

Adverse Effects

Adverse reactions to nitrofurantoin are quite common, varying from mild, reversible effects to severe reactions with long-term sequelae. The most common side effects include gastrointestinal reactions (e.g., nausea and vomiting), usually dose related. These reactions tend to occur during the first week of therapy and are more frequent in women. The macrocrystalline form, which is more slowly absorbed, has fewer gastrointestinal side effects.[133, 134] Diarrhea, abdominal pain, and gastrointestinal bleeding are rare complications.[127]

Three different types of hepatic toxicity may occur: (1) acute hepatocellular damage; (2) cholestatic jaundice, more common in elderly patients and sometimes associated with rash and eosinophilia[135]; and (3) chronic active hepatitis with severe necroinflammatory disease associated with hypergammaglobulinemia and high titers of antinuclear antibodies, usually seen in women.[136] There is a possible association between particular human leukocyte antigen (HLA) molecules and immunoallergic hepatitis; HLA-DRG and HLA-DRS have been linked to nitrofurantoin-associated hepatitis.[137] Discontinuation of the drug often results in clinical and laboratory improvement. However, in one report, a patient required orthotopic liver transplantation after chronic therapy with low-dose nitrofurantoin.[138] Pancreatitis and parotitis have been reported, sometimes associated with fever and increased serum amylase level[139, 140]; thyroid inflammation has also been noted.

PULMONARY REACTIONS

Nitrofurantoin can produce different types of adverse pulmonary effects. The first type is acute bronchitis, asthma, and pneumonitis[141]; these usually occur 5 to 10 days after therapy is initiated. Cough, dyspnea, and fever with or without infiltrates on the chest radiograph may be observed; eosinophilia has been seen. This reaction is believed to be allergic and usually resolves with discontinuation of the drug. The two other types of pulmonary effect are subacute pneumonitis and chronic lung involvement with interstitial fibrosis producing chronic cough and dyspnea.[142, 143] The chronic form is more common in women; hypergammaglobulinemia and antinuclear antibodies may be found. Pathologic examination reveals interstitial inflammation and fibrosis. It is believed that nitrofurantoin generates toxic oxygen radicals that produce this lung injury. Indirect damage resulting from nitrofurantoin may have the ability to recruit neutrophils to the lung tissue[144] and produce an inflammatory response. Clinical and radiographic resolution of this severe side effect is unpredictable.

HEMATOLOGIC REACTIONS

There are different types of blood dyscrasia: acute hemolytic anemia in patients with glucose-6-phosphate dehydrogenase deficiency and red cell enzyme deficiencies such as enolase and glutathione peroxidase deficiencies.[145, 146]

Megaloblastic anemia, probably due to folic acid deficiency; leukopenia[147]; thrombocytopenia; agranulocytosis; and aplastic anemia have been described.[127]

NEUROLOGIC REACTIONS

Polyneuropathy with a stocking-glove distribution is one of the most severe side effects. It is seen more frequently in patients with renal insufficiency. Although the clinical presentation is variable, sensory loss, pain, and motor weakness occur. Nitrofurantoin has also been associated with retrobulbar neuritis,[148] seventh cranial nerve palsy,[149] and pseudotumor cerebrii.[150] The mechanism is believed to be related to a direct toxic effect of the drug.

HYPERSENSITIVITY REACTIONS

Eosinophilia, rashes, and drug fever have been reported, as has drug-induced lupus erythematosus.[151]

Clinical Applications

Today the only indication for nitrofurantoin is the treatment of urinary tract infections involving the upper and lower genitourinary tract. It has also been used for prostatitis, in prophylaxis of recurrent urinary tract infection, and in prevention of bacteriuria after prostatectomy.[152] Suppressive therapy with nitrofurantoin has the advantage that resistance does not usually occur.

Bacitracin

Bacitracin was isolated in 1943 from a strain of *Bacillus subtilis*, today known as *Bacillus licheniformis*. It is a polypeptide composed of peptide-linked amino acids containing a thiazolidine ring and is highly soluble in water. The commercial product is a mixture of several bacitracins. The activity of bacitracin is expressed in a unit that represents 26 μg of a standard preparation.

Mode of Action

Bacitracin acts at stage 2 in cell wall synthesis, inhibiting conversion of phospholipid pyrophosphate to phospholipid, which is an essential reaction for the regeneration of the lipid carrier involved in cell wall synthesis.[153]

Antibacterial Activity

Bacitracin is active against gram-positive cocci and bacilli, particularly *S. aureus* and *S. pyogenes*; groups C and G are less susceptible, whereas group B strains are resistant. *Neisseria* spp., *H. influenzae, Treponema pallidum, Actinomyces* spp., and *Fusobacterium* spp. are also sensitive. Gram-negative bacilli are usually resistant.[154] The development of resistance to bacitracin is uncommon in patients treated with this compound.

Pharmacokinetics

After oral administration of 25,000 or 50,000 units of intramuscular bacitracin, the serum concentration varied between 0.006 and 1.0 unit/mL at 2 hours.[155, 156] Bacitracin penetrates pleural and ascitic fluid well; extremely small concentrations can be detected in cerebrospinal fluid. Most of the drug is inactivated, and 30% can be found in a 24-hour urine sample in the active form.[156]

Adverse Effects

When used parenterally, bacitracin is highly nephrotoxic, producing dose-related renal tubular damage.[153] When bacitracin is used as a topical preparation, skin irritation and allergic reactions are unusual.[157] Anaphylaxis after intraoperative irrigation in patients previously sensitized[158] or after topical therapy when the drug can penetrate the systemic circulation through ulcerated skin or open cancellous bone has been reported.[159]

Clinical Applications

Bacitracin is available in a variety of different topical forms as creams, ointments, sprays, powders, and irrigating solutions for treatment of staphylococcal infections of the skin and soft tissue, including furunculosis, impetigo, pyoderma, and abscesses.[154] It has also been used for intraoperative irrigation in neurosurgery and orthopedic surgery, which has decreased the incidence of postoperative wound infection.[160, 161] Bacitracin alone or a bacitracin-zinc combination has been used to treat patients infected with *Giardia lamblia*. Cure rates were higher than 86%.[162] Colonization with methicillin-resistant *S. aureus* may be treated with a combination of bacitracin, rifampin, and trimethoprim-sulfamethoxazole. This causes short-term eradication of the microorganism, although relapse or reinfection may be seen.[163, 164] Bacitracin appears to be as effective as vancomycin in the treatment of pseudomembranous colitis due to *C. difficile*.[155] Oral bacitracin may be an effective alternative to oral vancomycin for the eradication of vancomycin-resistant *Enterococcus faecium* from the enteric tract.[165]

References

1. Kunin CM, Bugg A: Binding of polymyxin antibratus to tissue: The major determinant of distribution and persistence in the body. J Infect Dis 124:394, 1971.
2. Warner SJ, Mitchell D, Savage N, McClain E: Dose-dependent reduction of lipopolysaccharide pyrogenicity by polymyxin B. Biochem Pharmacol 34:3995, 1985.
3. Cavaillon JM, Haeffner-Cavaillon N: Polymyxin-B inhibition of LPS-induced interleukin-1 secretion by human monocytes is dependent upon the LPS origin. Mol Immunol 23:965, 1986.
4. Bender BS, Winchurch RA, Thupari JN, et al: Depressed natural killer cell function in thermally injured adults: Successful in vivo and in vitro immunomodulation and the role of endotoxin. Clin Exp Immunol 71:120–125, 1988.
5. Rifkind D: Prevention by polymyxin B of endotoxin lethality in mice. J Bacteriol 93:1463, 1966.
6. From AHL, Fong JSC, Good RA: Polymyxin B sulfate modification of bacterial endotoxin: Effects on the development of endotoxin shock in dogs. Infect Immun 23:660, 1979.
7. Hughes B, Madan BR, Parratt JR: Polymyxin B sulphate protects cats against the haemodynamic and metabolic effects of *E. coli* endotoxin. Br J Pharmacol 74:701, 1981.
8. Craig WA, Turner JH, Kunin CM: Prevention of generalized Shwartzman reaction and endotoxin lethality by polymyxin B localized in tissues. Infect Immun 10:287, 1974.
9. Flynn PM, Shenep JL, Stokes DC, et al: Polymyxin B moderates acidosis and hypotension in established, experimental gram-negative septicemia. J Infect Dis 156:706, 1987.
10. Stokes DC, Shenep JL, Fishman M, et al: Polymyxin B prevents lipopolysaccharide-induced release of tumor necrosis factors from alveolar macrophages. J Infect Dis 160:52, 1989.
11. Cameron DJ, Churchill MH: Cytotoxicity of human macrophages for tumor cells: Enhancement mycobacterial lipopolysaccarides (LPS). J Immunol 124:708, 1980.

12. Tauber MG, Shibl AM, Hackbarth CJ, et al: Antibiotic therapy, endotoxin concentration in cerebrospinal fluid, and brain edema in experimental *Escherichia coli* meningitis in rabbits. J Infect Dis 156:456, 1987.
13. Duncan IB: Susceptibility of 1500 isolates of *Pseudomonas aeruginosa* to gentamicin, carbenicillin, colistin and polymyxin B. Antimicrob Agents Chemother 5:9, 1974.
14. Nord NM, Hoeprich PD: Polymyxin B and colistin. N Engl J Med 270:1030, 1965.
15. Rastogi N, Potar MC, David HL: Antimycobacterial spectrum of colistin (polymixin E). Ann Inst Pasteur Microbiol 137A:45, 1986.
16. Moore RA, Hancock RE: Involvement of outer membrane of *Pseudomonas cepacia* in aminoglycoside and polymyxin resistance. Antimicrob Agents Chemother 30:923, 1986.
17. Peterson AA, Fesik SW, McGroarty EJ: Decreased binding of antibiotics to lipopolysaccharides from polymyxin-resistant strains of *Escherichia coli* and *Salmonella typhimurium*. Antimicrob Agents Chemother 31:230, 1987.
18. Nord C-E, Wadstrom T, Wretlind B: Synergistic effect of combinations of sulfamethoxazole, trimethoprim, and colistin against *Pseudomonas maltophilia* and *Pseudomonas cepacia*. Antimicrob Agents Chemother 6:521, 1974.
19. Rosenblatt JE, Stewart PR: Combined activity of sulfamethoxazole, trimethoprim, and polymyxin B against gram-negative bacilli. Antimicrob Agents Chemother 6:84, 1974.
20. Schwartz SN, Medoff G, Kobayashi GS, et al: Antifungal properties of polymyxin B and its potentiation of tetracycline as an antifungal agent. Antimicrob Agents Chemother 2:36, 1972.
21. Collins MS, Pappagagionis D: Inhibition of *Coccidiodes immitis* in vitro and enhancement of amphotericin B by polymyxin B. Antimicrob Agents Chemother 7:781, 1975.
22. Cornelissen F, Van de Bossche H: Synergism of the antimicrobial agents miconazole, bacitracin and polymyxin B. Chemotherapy 29:419, 1983.
23. Rastogi N, Henrotte JG, David HL: Colistin (polymyxin E)–induced cell leakage in *Mycobacterium aurum*. Zentralbl Bakteriol Mikrobiol Hyg (A) 263:548, 1987.
24. Nicas TI, Hancock RE: Alteration of susceptibility to EDTA, polymyxin B and gentamicin in *Pseudomonas aeruginosa* by divalent cation regulation of outer membrane protein H1. J Gen Microbiol 129:509, 1983.
25. Davis SD, Ianetta A, Wedgwood RJ: Activity of colistin against *Pseudomonas aeruginosa*: Inhibition by calcium. J Infect Dis 124:610, 1971.
26. Gremeaux T, Tanti JF, Van Obberghen E, et al: Polymyxin B selectively inhibits insulin effects on transport in isolated muscle. Am J Physiol 252:E248, 1987.
27. Strutchfield J, Jones PM, Howell SL: The effects of polymyxin B, a protein kinase C inhibitor, on insulin secretion from intact and permeabilized islets of Langerhans. Biochem Biophys Res Commun 136:1001, 1986.
28. Henriksen EJ, Sleeper MD, Zierath JR, Holloszy JO: Polymyxin B inhibits stimulation of glucose transport in muscle by hypoxia or contractions. Am J Physiol 256:E662, 1989.
29. Amir S, Sasson S, Kaiser N, et al: Polymyxin B is an inhibitor of insulin-induced hypoglycemia in the whole animal model: Studies on the mode of inhibitory action. J Biol Chem 262:6663, 1987.
30. Kunin CM: A guide to the use of antibiotics in patients with renal disease. Ann Intern Med 67:151, 1967.
31. Fekety R: Polymyxin. *In* Mandell G, Douglas RC, Bennett JE (eds): Principles and Practices of Infectious Diseases, ed 2. New York, John Wiley & Sons, 1985, p 235.
32. Cox CE, Harrison LH: Intravenous sodium colistimethate therapy of urinary-tract infections: Pharmacological and bacteriological studies. Antimicrob Agents Chemother 10:296, 1970.
33. McMillar M, Price TML, MacLaren DM, et al: *Pseudomonas pyocyanea* infection treated with colistin methane sulphonate. Lancet 2:737, 1962.
34. Kunin CM: More on antimicrobials in renal failure. Ann Intern Med 69:397, 1968.
35. Goodwin NJ, Fredman EA: The effects of renal compartment, peritoneal dialysis and hemodialysis on serum colistimethate levels. Ann Intern Med 68:984, 1968.
36. Appel GB, Neu HC: The nephrotoxicity of antimicrobial agents. N Engl J Med 296:663, 1977.
37. Bennett WM, Muther RS, Parker RA, et al: Drug therapy in renal failure: Dosing guidelines for adults. Part 1. Antimicrobial agents. Ann Intern Med 93:62, 1980.
38. Froman J, Gross L, Curatala S: Serum and urine levels following parenteral administration of sodium colistimethate to normal individuals. J Urol 103:210, 1970.
39. MacKay D, Kaye D: Serum concentrations of colistin in patients with normal and impaired renal function. N Engl J Med 270:394, 1964.
40. Curtis JR, Eastwood JB: Colistimethate sodium administration during hemodialysis and peritoneal dialysis. Br Med J 1:484, 1968.
41. Slejjfer DTh, Mulder NH, deVries-Hospens HG, et al: Infection prevention in granulocytopenic patients by selective decontamination of the digestive tract. Eur J Cancer 16:859, 1980.
42. Koch-Weser J, Sidel VW, Federman EB, et al: Adverse effects of sodium colistimethate: Manifestations and specific reaction rates during 317 courses of therapy. Ann Intern Med 72:857, 1970.
43. Fekety Jr FR, Norman PS, Cluff LE: The treatment of gram-negative bacillary infections with colistin. Ann Intern Med 57:214, 1962.
44. Pedersen MF, Pederson JF, Madsen PO: A clinical and experimental comparative study of sodium colistimethate and polymyxin B sulfate. Invest Urol 9:234, 1971.
45. Murdock J MCC: The treatment of severe *Pseudomonas pyocyanea* infections with colistin. *In* Proceedings of the Third International Congress of Chemotherapy; 1964; Stuttgart, Germany; p 319.
46. Feeley TW, DuMoulin GC, Hedley-Whyte J, et al: Aerosol polymyxin and pneumonia in seriously ill patients. N Engl J Med 193:471, 1975.
47. Klastersky J, Hensgens C, Noterman J, et al: Endotracheal antibiotics for the prevention of tracheo-bronchial infections in tracheotomized unconscious patients: A comparative study of gentamicin and aminosidin-polymyxin B combination. Chest 68:302, 1975.
48. Ledingham IM, Alcock SR, Eastaway AT, et al: Triple regimen of selective decontamination of the digestive tract, systemic cefotaxime, and microbiological surveillance for prevention of acquired infection in intensive care. Lancet 1:785, 1988.
49. Johanson WG Jr, Seidenfeld JJ, de los Santos R, et al: Prevention of nosocomial pneumonia using topical and parenteral antimicrobial agents. Am Rev Respir Dis 137:265, 1988.
50. Hazenberg MP, Pennock-Schroder AM, van de Merwe JP: Reversible binding of polymyxin B and neomycin to the solid part of faeces. J Antimicrob Chemother 17:333, 1986.
51. Unertl K, Ruckdeschel G, Selbmann HK, et al: Prevention of colonization and respiratory infections in long-term ventilated patients by local antimicrobial prophylaxis. Intensive Care Med 13:106, 1987.
52. VanSaene HK, Stontenbeck CP, Zandstra DF: Cefotaxime combined with selective decontamination in intensive care unit patients: Virtual absence of emergence of resistance. Drugs 35:29, 1988.
53. Van Saene JJ, van Saene HK, Tarko-Smit NJ, Beukeveld GJ: Enterobacteriaceae suppression by three different oral doses of polymyxin E in human volunteers. Epidemiol Infect 100:407, 1988.
54. Clasener HAL, Yollaard EJ, van Saene HKF: Long-term prophylaxis of infection by selective decontamination in leukopenia and in mechanical ventilation. Rev Infect Dis 9:295, 1987.
55. de Vries-Hospers H, Sleijfer DT, Mulder NH, et al: Bacteriological aspects of selective decontamination of the digestive tract as a method of infection prevention in granulocytopenic patients. Antimicrob Agents Chemother 19:813, 1981.
56. Storring RA, Jameson B, McElwain TJ, Wiltshaw E: Oral nonabsorbed antibiotics prevent infection in acute non-lymphoblastic leukaemia. Lancet 2:837, 1977.
57. Dekker AW, Rozenberg-Arska M, Verhoef J: Infection prophylaxis in acute leukemia: A comparison of ciprofloxacin with trimethoprim-sulfamethoxazole and colistin. Ann Intern Med 106:7, 1987.
58. Manan P, Kibbler CC, Noone P: Activity of ciprofloxacin and colistin against *Pseudomonas aeruginosa* isolates from neutropenic patients: A possible approach to prophylaxis (letter). J Antimicrob Chemother 22:953, 1988.

59. Kurrle E, DeKiler AW, Gaus W, et al: Prevention of infection in acute leukemia: A prospective randomized study of two different drug regimens for antimicrobial prophylaxis. Infection 14:226, 1986.
60. Rosenberg-Arska M, Dekker AW, Berhoef J: Colistin and trimethoprim-sulfamethoxazole for the prevention of infection in patients with acute non-lymphocytic leukaemia: Disease in emergence of resistant bacteria. Infection 11:167, 1983.
61. Spijkervet FKL, van Saene HKF, van Saene JJM, et al: Effect of selective elimination of the oral flora on mucositis in irradiated head and neck cancer patients. J Surg Oncol 46:167, 1991.
62. Karpuch J, Schiffer J, Boldur I, et al: Purulent meningitis due to *Pseudomonas aeruginosa* successfully treated with colistin and piperacillin. J Infect 11:272, 1985.
63. Rimola A, Bory F, Teres J, et al: Oral non-absorbable antibiotics to prevent infection in cirrhotics with gastrointestinal hemorrhage. Hepatology 5:463, 1985.
64. Ingoldby CJ, McPherson GA, Blumgart LH: Endotoxemia in human obstructive jaundice: Effect of polymyxin B. Am J Surg 147:766, 1984.
65. Wiesner RH, Hermans P, Rakela J, et al: Selective bowel decontamination to prevent gram-negative bacterial and fungal infection following orthotopic liver transplantation. Transplant Proc 19:2420, 1987.
66. Moore MB, McCulley JP: Acanthamobea keratitis associated with contact lenses: Six consecutive cases of successful management. Br J Ophthalmol 73:271, 1989.
67. Marsden HB, Hyde WA: Colistin methane sulphonate in childhood infections. Lancet 2:144, 1962.
68. Gotoff SP, Lepper MH: Treatment of *Salmonella* carriers with colistin sulfate. Am J Med Sci 249:399, 1965.
69. Parsons P, Worthen GS, Moore EE, et al: The association of circulating endotoxin with the development of the adult respiratory distress syndrome. Am Rev Respir Dis 140:294, 1989.
70. vanUffenen R, Rommes JH, vanSawne HK: Preventing lower airway colonization and infection in mechanically ventilated patients. Crit Care Med 15:99, 1987.
71. Kucers A: Fusidate sodium. *In* Kucers A, Bennett NM (eds): The Use of Antibiotics, ed 4. London, William Heinemann Medical Books, 1987, pp 808–818.
72. Scudi JV, Duca CJ: Some antibacterial properties of Mandelamine (methenamine mandelate). J Urol 61:459, 1949.
73. Pearman JW, Peterson GJ, Nash JB: The antimicrobial activity of urine of paraplegic patients receiving methenamine mandelate. Invest Urol 16:91, 1978.
74. Klinge E, Mannisto P, Mantyla R, et al: Pharmacokinetics of methenamine in healthy volunteers. J Antimicrob Chemother 9:209, 1982.
75. Bennett WM, Singer I, Coggins CM: A practical guide to drug usage in adult patients with impaired renal function. JAMA 214:1468, 1970.
76. Gleckman R, Alvarez S, Joubert DW, et al: Drug therapy reviews: Methenamine mandelate and methenamine hippurate. Am J Hosp Pharm 36:1509, 1979.
77. Elo J, Sarna S, Ahava K, et al: Methenamine hippurate in urinary tract infections in children: Prophylaxis, treatment and side effects. J Antimicrob Chemother 4:355, 1978.
78. Kolker RJ: Medication-induced bilateral anterior uveitis. Arch Ophthalmol 109:1343, 1991.
79. Lipton JH: Incompatibility between sulfamethizole and methenamine mandelate. N Engl J Med 268:92, 1963.
80. U.S. Public Health Service Cooperative Study: Prevention of recurrent bacteriuria with continuous chemotherapy. Ann Intern Med 69:655, 1968.
81. Cronberg S, Welin CD, Henriksson L, et al: Prevention of recurrent acute cystitis by methenamine hippurate: Double blind controlled crossover long term study. Br Med J (Clin Res) 294:1507, 1987.
82. Vainrub B, Musher DM: Lack of effect of methenamine in suppression of, or prophylaxis against, chronic urinary infection. Antimicrob Agents Chemother 12:625, 1977.
83. Olsen JM, Friss-Moller A, Jensen SK, et al: Cefotaxime for prevention of infectious complications in bacteriuric men undergoing transurethral prostatic resection: A controlled comparison with methenamine. Scand J Urol Nephrol 17:299, 1983.
84. Tyreman NO, Andersson PO, Kroon L, et al: Urinary tract infection after vaginal surgery: Effect of prophylactic treatment with methenamine hippurate. Acta Obstet Gynecol Scand 65:731, 1986.
85. Kevorkian CG, Merritt JL, Ilstrup DM: Methenamine mandelate with acidification: An effective urinary antiseptic in patients with neurogenic bladder. Mayo Clin Proc 59:523, 1984.
86. Krebs M, Halvorsen RB, Fishman IJ, et al: Prevention of urinary tract infection during intermittent catheterization. J Urol 131:82, 1984.
87. Kuhlemeier KV, Stover SL, Lloyd LK: Prophylactic antibacterial therapy for preventing urinary tract infections in spinal cord injury patients. J Urol 134:514, 1985.
88. Brumfitt W, Hamilton-Miller JMT, Gargan RA, et al: Long-term prophylaxis of urinary infections in women: Comparative trial of trimethoprim, methenamine hippurate and topical povidone-iodine. J Urol 130:1110, 1983.
89. Fellstrom B, Butz M, Bo G, et al: The effects of methenamine-hippurate upon urinary risk factors for renal stone formation. Scand J Urol Nephrol 19:125, 1985.
90. Reeves DS: The pharmacokinetics of fusidic acid. J Antimicrob Chemother 20:467, 1987.
91. Kucers A: Methenamine mandelate and methenamine hippurate. *In* Kucers A, Bennett NM (eds): The Use of Antibiotics, ed 4. London, William Heinemann Medical Books, 1987, pp 1344–1348.
92. Moorhouse EC, Mulvihill TE, Jones L, et al: The in vitro activity of some antimicrobial agents against methicillin-resistant *Staphylococcus aureus*. J Antimicrob Chemother 15:291, 1985.
93. Foldes M, Munro R, Sorell TC, et al: In vitro effects of vancomycin, rifampicin, and fusidic acid, alone and in combination against methicillin-resistant *Staphylococcus aureus*. J Antimicrob Chemother 77:21, 1983.
94. Yu VL, Zuravleff JJ, Bornholm J, et al: In vitro synergy testing of triple antibiotic combination against *Staphylococcus epidermidis* isolates from patients with endocarditis. J Antimicrob Chemother 14:359, 1984.
95. McDonald M, Hurse A, Sim KN: Methicillin-resistant *Staphylococcus aureus* bacteremia. Med J Aust 2:191, 1981.
96. Jensen K, Lassen HC: Combined treatment with antibacterial chemotherapeutical agents in staphylococcal infections. Q J Med 38:91, 1969.
97. Zinner SH, Lagast H, Klastersky J: Antistaphylococcal activity of rifampicin with other antibiotics. J Infect Dis 144:365, 1981.
98. Traub WH, Spohr M, Bauer D: *Streptococcus faecalis*: In vitro susceptibility to antimicrobial drugs, single and combined, with and without defibrinated human blood. Chemotherapy 32:270, 1986.
99. Stirling J, Goodwin S: Susceptibility of *Bacteroides fragilis* to fusidic acid. J Antimicrob Chemother 3:522, 1977.
100. Miles RS, Moyes A: Comparison of susceptibility of *Neisseria meningitidis* to sodium sulphadiazine and sodium fusidate in vitro. J Clin Pathol 31:355, 1978.
101. Black WA, McNellis DA: Comparative in vitro sensitivity of *Nocardia* species to fusidic acid and sulphonamides. J Med Microbiol 4:293, 1971.
102. Copperman IJ: The prolonged use of intravenous fusidic acid in severe staphylococcal infection. Br J Clin Pract 26:83, 1972.
103. Godtfredsen WO, Vangedal S: On the metabolism of fusidic acid in man. Acta Chem Scand 20:1599, 1966.
104. Wise R, Pippard M, Mitchard M: The disposition of sodium fusidate in man. Br J Clin Pharmacol 4:615, 1977.
105. Hobby JA: Fucidin in patients on hemodialysis. J Clin Pathol 23:484, 1970.
106. Brodersen R: Fusidic acid binding to serum albumin and interaction with binding of bilirubin. Acta Paediatr Scand 74:874, 1985.
107. Brown KN, Percival A: Penetration of antimicrobials into tissue culture cells and leukocytes. Scand J Infect Dis Suppl 14:251, 1978.
108. Sattar MA, Barrett SP, Cawley ID: Concentrations of some antibiotics in synovial fluid after oral administration, with special reference to antistaphylococcal activity. Ann Rheum Dis 42:67, 1983.
109. Bergeron MG, Desaulniers D, Lessard C, et al: Concentrations of fusidic acid, cloxacillin and cefamandole in sera and atrial appendages of patients undergoing cardiac surgery. Antimicrob Agents Chemother 27:928, 1985.

110. Louvois J, Gortvai P, Hurley R: Antibiotic treatment of abscess of the central nervous system. Br Med J 2:985, 1977.
111. Iwarson S, Fasth S, Olaison L, et al: Adverse reactions to intravenous administration of fusidic acid. Scand J Infect Dis 13:65, 1981.
112. Humble MW, Eykyn S, Phillips I: Staphylococcal bacteraemia, fusidic acid, and jaundice. Br Med J 280:1495, 1980.
113. Evans DI: Granulocytopenia due to fusidic acid (letter). Lancet 2:851, 1988.
114. Anderson JD: Fusidic acid: New opportunities with an old antibiotic. Can Med Assoc J 122:765, 1980.
115. Kraemer R: Sputum penetration of fusidic acid in patients with cystic fibrosis. Eur J Pediatr 138:172, 1982.
116. Guenthner SH, Wenzel RP: In vitro activities of teichomycin, fusidic acid, flucloxacillin, fosfomycin and vancomycin against methicillin-resistant *Staphyloccus aureus*. Antimicrob Agents Chemother 26:268, 1984.
117. Cronberg S, Castor B, Thoren A: Fusidic acid for the treatment of antibiotic-associated colitis induced by *Clostridium difficile*. Infections 12:276, 1984.
118. Franzblau SG, Chan GP, Garcia-Ignacio BG, et al: Clinical trial of fusidic acid for lepromatous leprosy. Antimicrob Agents Chemother 38:1651, 1994.
119. Friis-Moller A, Rechnitzer C, Nielsen L, et al: Treatment of *Legionella* lung abscess in a renal transplant recipient with erythromycin and fusidic acid (letter). Eur J Clin Microbiol 4:513, 1985.
120. Mindermann T, Zimmerli W, Gratzl O: Randomized placebo-controlled trial of single-dose antibiotic prophylaxis with fusidic acid in neurosurgery. Acta Neurochir 121:9, 1993.
121. Mindermann T, Zimmerli W, Rajacic Z, Gratzl O: Penetration of fusidic acid into human brain tissue and cerobrospinal fluid. Acta Neurochir 121:12, 1993.
122. Farthing MJ, Inge MG: Antigiardial activity of the bile salt-like antibiotic sodium fusidate. J Antimicrob Chemother 17:165, 1986.
123. Gray TB, Keenan JI, Clemett RS, Allardyce RA: Fusidic acid prophylaxis before cataract surgery: Patient self-administration. Austr N Z J Ophthalmol 21:99, 1993.
124. Youle MS, Hawkins DA, Lawrence AG, et al: Clinical, immunological, and virological effects of sodium fusidate in patients with AIDS or AIDS-related complex (ARC): An open study. J Acquir Immune Defic Syndr 2:59, 1989.
125. Kucers A: Nitrofurans. *In* Kucers A, Bennett NM (eds): The Use of Antibiotics, ed 4. London, William Heinemann Medical Books, 1987, pp 1276–1289.
126. Obaseiki-Ebor EE: Cross resistance to nitrofurans of aminoglycoside-aminocyclitol resistant strains of *Escherichia coli*. J Antimicrob Chemother 11:485, 1983.
127. D'Arcy PF: Nitrofurantoin. Drug Intell Clin Pharmacol 19:540, 1985.
128. Mannisto PT, Lammingsivu U: Nitrofurantoin is highly bound to plasma protein. J Antimicrob Chemother 9:327, 1982.
129. Sachs J, Geer T, Noell P, et al: Effect of renal function on urinary recovery of orally administered nitrofurantoin. N Engl J Med 278:1032, 1968.
130. Currie GA, Little PJ, McDonald SJ: The localization of cephaloridine and nitrofurantoin in the kidney. Nephron 3:282, 1966.
131. Spencer RC, Moseley DJ, Greensmith MJ: Nitrofurantoin modified release versus trimethoprim or co-trimoxazole in the treatment of uncomplicated urinary tract infection in general practice. J Antimicrob Chemother 33(Suppl A):121,1994.
132. Ertan G, Karasulu E, Abou-nada M, et al: Sustained-release dosage form of nitrofurantoin. Part 2. In vivo urinary excretion in man. J Microencaps 11:1 37, 1994.
133. Hailey FJ, Glascock HW Jr: Gastrointestinal tolerance to a new form of nitrofurantoin: A collaborative study. Curr Ther Res 9:600, 1967.
134. Kalowski S, Radford N, Kincaid-Smith P: Crystalline and macrocrystalline nitrofurantoin in the treatment of urinary tract infection. N Engl J Med 290:385, 1974.
135. Ernaelsteen D, Williams R: Jaundice due to nitrofurantoin. Gastroenterology 41:590, 1961.
136. Black M, Rabin L, Schatz N: Nitrofurantoin-induced chronic active hepatitis. Ann Intern Med 92:62, 1980.
137. Berson A, Freneaux E, Larrey D, et al: Possible role of HLA in hepatotoxicity. An exploratory study in 71 patients with drug-induced idiosyncratic hepatitis. J Hepatol 20:336, 1994.
138. Hebert MF, Roberts JP: Endstage liver disease associated with nitrofurantoin requiring liver transplantation. Ann Pharmacother 27:1193, 1993.
139. Nelis GF: Nitrofurantoin-induced pancreatitis: Report of a case. Gastroenterology 84:1032, 1983.
140. Christophe JL: Pancreatitis induced by nitrofurantoin. Gut 35:712, 1994.
141. Pineura RF, Hartnett JS: Acute pulmonary reaction to nitrofurantoin. Thorax 29:599, 1974.
142. Sovijari AR, Lemola M, Stenius B, et al: Nitrofurantoin induced acute subacute and chronic pulmonary reactions. Scand J Respir Dis 58:41, 1977.
143. Holmberg L, Boman G, Bottiger LE, et al: Adverse reactions to nitrofurantoin: Analysis of 921 reports. Am J Med 69:733, 1980.
144. Martin WJ: Nitrofurantoin: Potential direct and indirect mechanisms of lung injury. Chest 83:51S, 1983.
145. Stefanin M: Chronic hemolytic anemia associated with erythrocyte deficiency exacerbated by ingestion of nitrofurantoin. Am J Clin Pathol 58:408, 1972.
146. Steinberg M, Brauer MJ, Necheles TF: Acute hemolytic anemia associated with erythrocyte glutathione-peroxidase deficiency. Arch Intern Med 125:302, 1970.
147. Levy S, Meyers BR, Mellin H: Reversible granulocytopenia in a patient with polycythemia vera taking nitrofurantoin. J Mt Sinai Hosp 36:26, 1969.
148. Hakamies L: Die Nitrofurantoin-Polyneuropathie. Schweiz Med Wochenschr 100:2212, 1970.
149. Thomson RG, James OF: Seventh-nerve palsy and hepatitis associated with nitrofurantoin. Hum Toxicol 5:387, 1986.
150. Korzets A, Rathaus M, Chen B, et al: Pseudotumor cerebrii and nitrofurantoin (Letter). Drug Intell Clin Pharmacol 22:345, 1988.
151. Chapman JA: An unusual nitrofurantoin-induced drug reaction. Ann Allergy 56:16, 1986.
152. Weiss J, Wein A, Jacobs J, et al: Use of nitrofurantoin macrocrystals after transurethral prostatectomy. J Urol 130:479, 1983.
153. Harshberger SE (ed): Medical Pharmacology. St. Louis, CV Mosby, 1984, p 605.
154. Kucers A: Bacitracin and gramicidin. *In* Kucers A, Bennett NM (eds): The Use of Antibiotics, ed 4. London, William Heinemann Medical Books, 1987, pp 751–753.
155. Dudley MN, McLaughlin JC, Carrington G, et al: Oral bacitracin vs vancomycin therapy for *Clostridium difficile*–induced diarrhea. Arch Intern Med 146:1101, 1986.
156. Zintel HA, Ma RA, Nicholas AC, et al: The absorption, distribution, excretion and toxicity of bacitracin in man. Am J Med Sci 218:439, 1949.
157. Fischer AA: Adverse reactions to bacitracin, polymyxin and gentamicin sulfate. Cutis 32:510, 1983.
158. Netland PA, Baumgartner JE, Andrews BT: Intraoperative anaphylaxis after irrigation with bacitracin: Case report. Neurosurgery 21:927, 1987.
159. Schechter JF, Wilkinson RD, DelCarpia J: Anaphylaxis following the use of bacitracin ointment. Arch Dermatol 120:909, 1984.
160. Benjamin JB, Volz RG: Efficacy of a topical antibiotic irrigant in decreasing or eliminating bacterial contamination in surgical wounds. Clin Orthop 184:114, 1984.
161. Cannon SC, Graham MD, Bojrab DI, et al: Use of bacitracin for neurotologic surgery. Laryngoscope 98:1050, 1988.
162. Andrews BJ, Panitescu D, Jipa GH, et al: Chemotherapy for giardiasis: Randomized clinical trial of acitracin, bacitracin zinc, and a combination of bacitracin zinc with neomycin. Am J Trop Med Hyg 52:318, 1995.
163. Roccaforte JS, Bitner MJ, Stumpf CA, et al: Attempts to eradicate methicillin-resistant *Staphylococcus aureus* colonization with the use of trimethoprim-sulfamethoxazole, rifampin, and bacitracin. Am J Infect Control 16:141, 1988.
164. Yu VL, Goetz A, Wagener M, et al: *Staphyloccus aureus* nasal carriage and infection in patients on hemodialysis. N Engl J Med 315:91, 1986.
165. O'Donovan CA, Fan-Havard P, Tecson-Tumang FT, et al: Enteric eradication of vancomycin-resistant *Enterococcus faecium* with oral bacitracin. Diagn Microbiol Infect Dis 18:105, 1994.

31

Mechanisms of Bacterial Resistance to Antimicrobial Drugs

George M. Eliopoulos

In response to the ongoing evolution of bacterial resistance traits, an impressive variety of antimicrobial compounds have been developed and introduced into clinical practice over the last several decades. Nevertheless, the continued emergence of increasingly resistant bacteria challenges both the ingenuity of medicinal chemists who seek to develop more effective agents and the skill of clinicians who wish to apply available antimicrobials to the best effect. To this end, a general understanding of microbial resistance mechanisms will assist the clinician in identifying situations in which standard laboratory methods may not reveal the full potential of drug resistance, in anticipating circumstances that favor the emergence of resistant strains during therapy, and in assessing the likelihood that alternative antimicrobials would prove useful against resistant bacterial isolates.

Requirements for Antimicrobial Activity and General Mechanisms of Resistance

To understand bacterial resistance mechanisms, it is useful first to consider the properties of an antibiotic required for efficacy. Simply stated, the antibiotic must be able to (1) penetrate to the site of its normal molecular target in adequate amounts; (2) encounter target molecules capable of interacting with the drug in such a manner as to initiate the desired antimicrobial effect; and (3) escape inactivation by intracellular or extracellular bacterial enzymes. Bacterial resistance mechanisms have evolved that can impede antibiotic efficacy at any of these steps (Fig. 31–1). First, because the principal targets of most antibiotics lie deep to the external surface of bacteria, any barrier to penetration of the drug through the bacterial cell wall can reduce activity. In some cases, intracellular accumulation of the antibiotic is reduced by efflux pumps, which actually remove drug that has already entered the cell. Second, the natural molecular targets may be altered in a way that reduces effective interaction with the antibiotic yet does not interfere with important physiologic functions. Bacteria may also use alternative biochemical pathways, insensitive to drug action, that bypass the functions of the primary target. Finally, inactivating or modifying enzymes may act on the antimicrobial agent, rendering it ineffective. Frequently, interactions between two or more of these mechanisms may result in levels of resistance substantially greater than any one mechanism alone would achieve. These mechanisms of resistance are examined in detail as they relate to antimicrobial compounds in common use (Table 31–1).

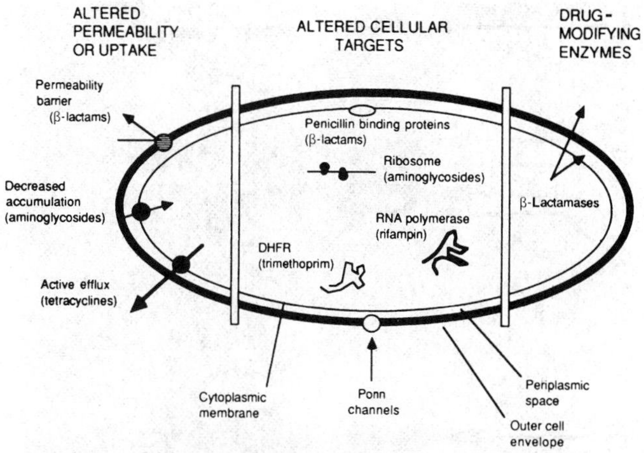

FIGURE 31–1 □ General mechanisms of bacterial resistance to antimicrobials. Examples are given of resistance mechanisms against representative antimicrobials (in parentheses) that may be encountered in gram-negative bacilli.

Resistance Due to Altered Target Molecules

β-*Lactam Antibiotics*

The primary targets of β-lactam antibiotics are penicillin binding proteins (PBPs) associated with the bacterial cytoplasmic membrane (Fig. 31–2). The number (generally four to eight) and molecular sizes of PBPs vary with individual species.[1, 2] Several PBPs have been associated with enzymatic activities (e.g., transpeptidase or carboxypeptidase) involved in cell wall synthesis and remodeling. Individual β-lactams display differential binding to specific PBPs, and such binding may result in predictable morphologic changes in the bacteria. Binding by β-lactams to essential PBP targets results in inhibition of cell growth and may culminate in cell death and lysis.[2, 3] Alterations of PBP targets have been implicated

TABLE 31–1 ■ Antimicrobial Compounds and Their Resistance Mechanisms

DRUG CLASS	RESISTANCE MECHANISM
β-Lactams	Altered penicillin binding proteins Reduced permeability β-Lactamases
Aminoglycosides	Decreased ribosomal binding Reduced permeability or uptake Modification of enzymes
Macrolide-lincosamide	Decreased ribosomal binding Reduced permeability Modification of enzymes Active efflux pump
Chloramphenicol	Decreased ribosomal binding Reduced permeability Chloramphenicol acetyltransferase Active efflux pump
Tetracyclines	Target (ribosome) resistance Active efflux pump Drug detoxification
Quinolones	Target (DNA gyrase) resistance Reduced permeability Active efflux pump
Rifampin	Reduced RNA polymerase binding Modification of drug
Inhibitors of folate synthesis	Dihydropteroate synthase or dihydrofolate reductase target resistance Reduced permeability

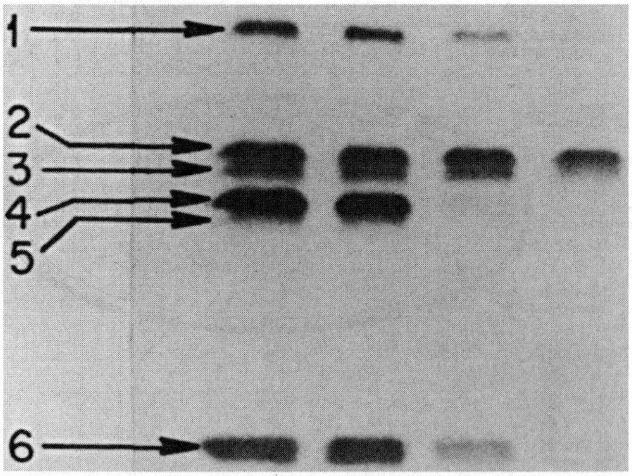

FIGURE 31–2 □ Penicillin binding proteins of a strain of *Enterococcus faecium* (numbered top to bottom) as separated by polyacrylamide gel electrophoresis and visualized fluorographically after binding to [^{3}H]benzyl penicillin. The penicillin was added at concentrations (right to left, beginning in far right lane) ranging from 0.06 to 32 μg/mL. (Reproduced in part from Eliopoulos GM, Wennersten C, Moellering RC Jr: Resistance to β-lactam antibiotics in *Streptococcus faecium*. Antimicrob Agents Chemother 22:295–301, 1982.)

in resistance to β-lactam antibiotics in a number of important pathogens.

Resistance or relative resistance to penicillin among pneumococci is an important problem in the United States and elsewhere.[4–8] In 1980 it was shown that stepwise transformation of DNA from a penicillin-resistant South African strain of *Streptococcus pneumoniae* (penicillin minimal inhibitory concentration of 6.2 μg/mL) into a susceptible recipient pneumococcus (penicillin minimal inhibitory concentration of 0.06 μg/mL) resulted in a series of organisms with incremental increases in penicillin resistance associated with changes in PBP patterns to progressively resemble those of the donor strain.[9] Multiple changes in PBPs, including changes in electrophoretic patterns and reduced binding of penicillin, have now been described in penicillin-resistant pneumococci.[2] Genes mediating production of reduced-affinity PBPs may have been acquired from other bacterial species by recombinational events.[10] Reduced-affinity PBPs have also been implicated in relative resistance to third-generation cephalosporins in this species.[11]

Methicillin resistance in *Staphylococcus aureus* has been attributed to the presence of a PBP, termed PBP 2′ or PBP 2a, with markedly reduced binding affinities for β-lactams.[12, 13] Synthesis of this PBP is inducible in the presence of β-lactams.[14–16] It is believed that in the presence of β-lactams at concentrations fully saturating—hence inactivating—other PBPs, PBP 2a retains critical synthetic functions necessary for cell survival. The structural gene for PBP 2a, *mecA,* is necessary but not sufficient to produce homogeneous high-level resistance to antistaphylococcal penicillins; the nature of additional factors contributing to resistance continues to be elucidated.[17–20] The *mecA* gene and low-affinity PBP 2a it specifies account also for the high rate of methicillin resistance encountered among nosocomial isolates of coagulase-negative staphylococci.[21–24]

Low-affinity PBP target molecules result in resistance to β-lactams among enterococci.[25, 26] Markedly reduced affinity of PBP 5 accounts for particularly high levels of resistance to penicillin encountered in *Enterococcus faecium,* with minimal inhibitory concentrations sometimes reaching 500 μg/mL.[25–29] Analysis of the amino acid sequence of an enterococcal low-affinity PBP showed considerable similarity with the sequence of PBP 2a.[30] β-Lactam resistance in various gram-negative bacteria, including *Neisseria gonorrhoeae, Neisseria meningitidis, Haemophilus influenzae,* and *Pseudomonas aeruginosa,* has been related to altered PBP targets.[2, 31–35] The precise role of target site modifications in resistance to β-lactams is more difficult to assess in gram-negative bacteria because β-lactamases are so common and there may be coexisting permeability barriers.

Glycopeptide Antibiotics

Vancomycin-resistant enterococci have emerged as a major clinical problem.[36] The normal molecular target of this antibiotic is the D-alanine-D-alanine dipeptide terminal of UDP-*N*-acetylmuramyl pentapeptide peptidoglycan precursors. In strains representative of the most common resistance phenotypes (class A and class B), an altered peptidoglycan target terminating in the D-alanine-D-lactate depsipeptide demonstrates substantially reduced binding affinity for vancomycin.[37] A 10,851 base pair transposon has been described that contains several genes that contribute to glycopeptide resistance in enterococci.[38]

Aminoglycosides

Mutations affecting the binding of aminoglycosides to ribosomal targets have been reported, mostly pertaining to streptomycin.[39] For example, mutation in the *rpsL* gene results in alteration of a protein (S12) that controls binding of streptomycin to the 30S ribosomal subunit.[39, 40] Other mutations affecting a 16S ribosomal RNA gene confer resistance to streptomycin in some bacteria.[41, 42] Ribosomal resistance to streptomycin has been documented in clinical isolates of various species including *N. gonorrhoeae,*[43] *S. aureus,*[44] *P. aeruginosa,*[45] *Enterococcus faecalis,*[46] and *Mycobacterium tuberculosis.*[41, 42, 47] Ribosomal resistance to deoxystreptamine aminoglycosides (e.g., kanamycin) has been described[48, 49] but is probably uncommon among clinical isolates; ribosomal resistance to gentamicin has been described[50] but has not been reported in clinical isolates.[51, 52]

Macrolide-Lincosamide Antibiotics

Although barriers to penetration account for the intrinsic resistance of Enterobacteriaceae to erythromycin,[53] resistance in gram-positive organisms usually occurs at the 50S ribosomal subunit target. Target resistance commonly involves not only macrolides (erythromycin) but also antibiotics of the lincosamide (clindamycin, lincomycin) and streptogramin B classes and is thus referred to as MLS resistance. The MLS resistance genes are commonly plasmid mediated and often found on transposons, which facilitate exchange of genetic material between plasmid and chromosomal DNA.[52, 54] Numerous erythromycin (target) resistance genes have been described in a broad range of bacterial species.[55, 56] These resistance genes mediate production of methylase enzymes, which methylate adenine residues on 23S ribosomal RNA, thus rendering the ribosome resistant to the antibiotics.[55, 57] Resistance may be inducible or constitutive. Bacteria with inducible resistance often demonstrate dissociated resistance, appearing to be resistant to erythromycin (a good inducer) but susceptible to clindamycin; once resistance is induced, cells generally demonstrate resistance to other members of the MLS_B class.[58] The mechanism by which exposure to erythromycin results in methylase induction is complex and termed translational attenuation. In short, in the absence of erythromycin, the relevant messenger RNA is sequestered in a form not available for translation. Association of erythromycin with the ribosome complex induces a conformational change that yields a translationally active form of messenger RNA.[58] Inducible resistance to erythromycin and streptogramins without resistance to clindamycin[59] (which may be due to efflux mechanisms in some isolates[24]) as well as ribosomal resistance to lincosamides alone[60] has been observed.

MLS-resistant gram-positive cocci have been encountered commonly in some parts of the world. In the mid-1970s, approximately 50% of group A streptococci isolated in Japan were macrolide resistant.[57] Erythromycin resistance was seen in approximately 50% of pneumococci recovered in Hungary in the late 1980s[8] and is now being encountered among many penicillin-resistant pneumococci in the United States and abroad.[4–6, 61] Macrolide resistance is widespread among current isolates of coagulase-negative staphylococci, with the majority of isolates expressing constitutive MLS resistance.[24, 59]

Chloramphenicol

Resistance to chloramphenicol because of decreased binding of drug to bacterial 50S ribosomal subunits has been reported in laboratory mutants, but target site resistance does not appear to be common among clinical isolates.[62]

Tetracyclines

Resistance to tetracycline at the level of ribosomal protein synthesis has been described in streptococci that have acquired the *tet*(M) gene.[63] The presence of this gene product in some fashion protects ribosomal protein synthesis from inhibition by tetracyclines.[64] The amino acid sequence of the Tet(M) protein resembles that of elongation factors which associate with the ribosome during protein synthesis, which may be relevant to its mode of action, but the exact mechanism by which resistance occurs in the presence of *tet*(M) is as yet unknown.[64] The *tet*(M) gene has been found in various gram-positive and gram-negative bacteria and confers resistance to tetracycline in *Ureaplasma urealyticum* and *Mycoplasma hominis* as well.[65–67]

Quinolones

The principal target of quinolone antimicrobials is the enzyme DNA gyrase (bacterial topoisomerase II).[68] Mutations in genes coding for DNA gyrase confer resistance to inhibition by quinolones.[68] In gram-negative organisms, permeability barriers may contribute to levels of resistance seen; in *S. aureus*, inhibitory activities of various quinolones on partially purified gyrase parallel growth-inhibitory activities of the drugs.[69, 70] With the introduction of fluoroquinolones into hospital environments, resistance in *S. aureus*, especially among methicillin-resistant strains, has emerged in a large proportion of isolates.[71–73] This often reflects clonal spread of a limited number of strains.

Rifampin

Antimicrobial activity of rifampin requires binding of the drug to the β-subunit of RNA polymerase. Single-step mutations resulting in single amino acid substitutions occur with moderate frequency (approximately 10^{-8} in *Escherichia coli*). Resulting polymerases vary in degree of sensitivity to rifampin and in levels of resistance conferred.[74]

Folate Pathway Inhibitors

Target alterations can confer resistance to sulfonamides and trimethoprim. In this case, resistance typically results from acquisition of drug-resistant enzymes rather than from mutations affecting chromosomal enzymes. Two distinct types of low-affinity dihydropteroate synthase mediating sulfonamide resistance have been described in gram-negative organisms. Genetic determinants for these occur on transposons and plasmids with a broad host range, which permits efficient dissemination among bacteria.[75]

Several dihydrofolate reductases with reduced sensitivity to inhibition by trimethoprim have been described, genes for which can also be acquired via resistance plasmids and transposons.[76–78] In some species (e.g., *Bacteroides* spp., *Clostridium* spp., *Neisseria* spp., *Branhamella* spp., and *Nocardia* spp.), intrinsic insensitivity of the native dihydrofolate reductase to trimethoprim contributes to drug resistance.[76] Trimethoprim resistance due to overproduction of structurally altered chromosomal enzyme has been described in laboratory mutants and some clinical isolates.[76, 79, 80] Mutational loss of thymidylate synthase activity, with the resulting requirement for exogenous thymine or thymidine, can uncommonly result in trimethoprim resistance.[80]

Resistance Due to Permeability Barriers or Diminished Drug Uptake or Accumulation

β-Lactams

Studies with *E. coli* demonstrate that water-filled transmembrane pores created by outer membrane proteins (especially those designated OmpF and OmpC) serve as a major route by which β-lactams, and cephalosporins in particular, traverse the lipid-rich outer membrane of gram-negative bacteria.[81] The rate of antibiotic penetration through these porin protein channels depends on the physical characteristics of each drug.[82] There is evidence that penicillins may also penetrate the cell envelope directly through the lipid bilayer. Laboratory mutants of Enterobacteriaceae selected for β-lactam resistance may demonstrate diminished amounts of OmpF or other putative porin proteins. Such permeability mutants often demonstrate small increases in resistance to other antibiotics as well; higher levels of resistance to other antimicrobials such as aminoglycosides, chloramphenicol, tetracyclines, trimethoprim, or quinolones probably reflect pleiotropic mutations rather than porin deficiency alone.[82–85] The activity of imipenem is often preserved against porin-deficient mutants, probably because its compact zwitterionic structure permits rapid penetration, it is inherently β-lactamase stable, and the limited number of primary PBP 2 targets (approximately 20 per bacterium) require that only a few drug molecules penetrate for initiation of antibacterial effect.[86] This example illustrates the fact that because defects in cell permeability retard but do not prevent penetration of β-lactams, significant increases in resistance typically require the interplay of additional resistance mechanisms such as periplasmic β-lactamases or target alterations.[87] Diminished permeability through the outer membrane also contributes to intrinsic and acquired β-lactam resistance in *P. aeruginosa*.[82, 88, 89] For example, imipenem resistance emerges relatively commonly when this antibiotic is used alone to treat *P. aeruginosa* infections.[90] Impaired penetration of the carbapenem is associated with loss of specific outer membrane proteins.[82, 91, 92] In *P. aeruginosa*, imipenem penetration appears to occur through a specific channel consisting of trimers of a protein termed OprD, which is selective for small zwitterionic compounds.[93] Evidence has been suggested that active efflux mechanisms may also contribute to resistance to some β-lactam antibiotics in this species.[94]

Aminoglycosides

Factors impeding penetration of aminoglycosides to their ribosomal target sites are complex and not yet completely understood. Resistance to multiple aminoglycosides has been associated with loss or reduction of outer membrane proteins in Enterobacteriaceae[95] or even with the appearance of new outer membrane proteins in *P. aeruginosa*.[96] In the latter species, alterations in surface lipopolysaccharide composition may affect intracellular uptake of aminoglycosides,[97] but only a few strains have been studied thoroughly. Amikacin-resistant strains of *P. aeruginosa* arising during treatment with this aminoglycoside demonstrate impaired intracellular uptake of the drug.[98] Studies with "small colony variant" strains of aminoglycoside-resistant *P. aeruginosa* recovered from experimental animals failing to respond to therapy with these agents reveal defective aminoglycoside uptake. In these slow-growing, unstable mutants, uptake is negligible, like that seen in normal cells poisoned with cyanide.[99] Such strains generate inadequate transmembrane electrical potentials compared with normal isolates of *P. aeruginosa*. Generation of transmembrane electrical gradients also appears to be important for the uptake of aminoglycosides in *S. aureus*,[100] with aminoglycoside-resistant small colony variants of this species also showing defective uptake of the antibiotic.[101] One strain of *E. faecalis* has been described that displayed a specific transport defect for gentamicin (but not tobramycin), resulting in failure of penicillin-gentamicin synergism.[102]

Macrolides

Intrinsic low-level resistance to erythromycin in Enterobacteriaceae can be attributed to limited drug permeability. Enhanced penetration of nonionized drugs at alkaline pH is reflected by greater antimicrobial activity under these conditions.[53, 54] Selective resistance to erythromycin (without resistance to lincosamides or streptogramins) reported in an isolate of *Staphylococcus epidermidis* was initially believed to be due to reduced drug uptake in the absence of evidence of drug inactivation or altered ribosomal binding.[103] However, subsequent studies revealed that a plasmid contained in that strain was associated with both erythromycin resistance and an adenosine triphosphate–dependent efflux system specific to 14- and 15-membered macrolide antibiotics.[104, 105] Thus, resistance in this strain was related to active removal of the macrolide from cell cytoplasm rather than to any intrinsic barriers to penetration of the drug.

Chloramphenicol

Reduced intracellular penetration of chloramphenicol has been described in several bacterial species, sometimes associated with loss of specific outer membrane proteins or altered lipopolysaccharide patterns.[62, 106, 107] Efflux systems for removal of chloramphenicol from the cell have been demonstrated in both gram-positive and gram-negative bacteria.[64, 108, 109] In contrast to the adenosine triphosphate–dependent pump described for macrolides, these efflux systems are energized by the electrochemical proton gradient across the bacterial cell membrane.

Tetracyclines

Although mutations affecting outer membrane (porin) proteins or surface lipopolysaccharides of gram-negative bacteria have been associated with reduced activities of hydrophilic (tetracycline) or lipophilic (minocycline) tetracycline analogs, respectively, efflux systems are now thought to be more important than permeability barriers in determining ultimate levels of intracellular accumulation of tetracyclines within the bacterial cytoplasm.[110, 111] Tetracycline efflux systems, which derive energy from proton-motive force, may be either intrinsic (chromosomal) or plasmid mediated.[104] Acquisition of a tetracycline resistance gene results in the inducible synthesis of a transmembrane protein (Tet), which pumps cation-complexed drug out of the cell cytoplasm, resulting in markedly increased levels of resistance to the drug.[104, 112]

Quinolones

Mutations resulting in decreased outer membrane permeability can reduce the susceptibility of gram-negative bacteria to quinolones. Mutant strains of Enterobacteriaceae selected for resistance to one or more of the fluoroquinolones have demonstrated decreased expression of major outer membrane proteins (e.g., OmpF) and diminished susceptibility to structurally unrelated compounds including tetracycline, aminoglycosides, and chloramphenicol.[68, 83, 85, 113] Cellular lipopolysaccharide composition in Enterobacteriaceae may affect penetration of hydrophobic quinolones such as nalidixic acid.[114] Spontaneous mutants conferring resistance to fluoroquinolones alone or cross-resistance to quinolones, β-lactams, and other antimicrobials have also been reported for *P. aeruginosa*, associated with decreases or even increases in quantities of various outer membrane proteins.[115–119]

Energy-dependent efflux systems affecting fluoroquinolones have now been described in a variety of organisms including Enterobacteriaceae, *P. aeruginosa*, and *S. aureus*.[64, 104, 109, 120] When studied in *Bacillus subtilis*, expression of the NorA membrane protein of *S. aureus* (analogous to the Tet transporter protein) conferred resistance not only to fluoroquinolones but also to unrelated compounds such as chloramphenicol, puromycin, and ethidium bromide but not to tetracycline.[121]

Folate Pathway Inhibitors

Permeability barriers to trimethoprim occur intrinsically in *P. aeruginosa* and, when acquired in Enterobacteriaceae, are associated with diminished levels of putative porin proteins and pleiotropic resistance to drugs of other antimicrobial classes.[76, 84, 95] Intrinsic or acquired resistance to sulfonamides in gram-negative organisms may also result from decreased intracellular penetration.[122]

Resistance to Multiple Antibiotics

In some cases, mutations affecting a single genetic locus may result in changes in susceptibility to several unrelated antimicrobials. One such locus, termed *mar* (multiple antibiotic resistance), appears to control expression of resistance to multiple antibiotics including chloramphenicol, tetracycline, fluoroquinolones, and β-lactams.[123] With such mutations, evidence of both increased efflux and decreased drug penetration (reduced OmpF) can be observed.[124] When *E. coli mar* mutants selected on exposure to low concentrations of chloramphenicol or tetracycline were subsequently exposed to norfloxacin, substantially higher frequencies of resistance to norfloxacin were observed ($\sim 10^{-7}$) as compared with exposure of the initial wild-type isolate to the fluoroquinolone, in which case resistant mutants were rarely observed ($<10^{-9}$).[125] Existence of such phenomena, involving simultaneous activation of multiple resistance determinants and resulting in cross-resistance to unrelated classes of antimicrobials, illustrates the enormous complexity of antibiotic resistance mechanisms in gram-negative bacteria.

Resistance Due to Inactivation of Antimicrobials

β-Lactam Antibiotics

Inactivation of β-lactams by enzymatic hydrolysis of the β-lactam ring is the most common and best understood mecha-

TABLE 31–2 ■ Classification of β-Lactamases

ENZYME CLASS	CHARACTERISTICS	EXAMPLES
Group 1	Cephalosporinases not inhibited by clavulanic acid	Chromosomal enzymes of *P. aeruginosa, Enterobacter cloacae*
Groups 2a–2e	Penicillinase and/or cephalosporinases inhibited by clavulanic acid	Plasmid-mediated TEM type; staphylococcal; *Klebsiella* chromosomal enzyme
Group 3	Metalloenzymes	Imipenem-hydrolyzing enzyme of *Xanthomonas maltophilia*
Group 4	Penicillinases not inhibited by clavulanic acid	Chromosomal enzyme of *P. cepacia*

Data from references 126–129.

nism of resistance to this class of drugs. Dozens of enzymes from various bacteria, differing in substrate profiles, potential for inhibition, and physical characteristics, have been described. Several classification schemes have been proposed, the most recent and comprehensive of which was developed by Bush.[126–129] This method divides β-lactamases into four major groups based largely on preferred antibiotic substrates and inhibition profiles (Table 31–2).

GRAM-POSITIVE BACTERIA

β-Lactamase–mediated resistance to penicillins among gram-positive cocci is exemplified by the exoenzymes of *S. aureus.* These enzymes and those of coagulase-negative staphylococci are less active against cephalosporins and antistaphylococcal penicillins than they are against penicillin G, and they are inhibited by β-lactamase inhibitors such as clavulanic acid, sulbactam, and tazobactam. Some isolates of *S. aureus* demonstrate modestly reduced susceptibility to antistaphylococcal penicillins, activities of which are restored when combined with β-lactamase inhibitors.[130] Such strains, termed borderline oxacillin resistant, have been noted to be hyperproducers of β-lactamase.

Penicillinase-producing enterococci were first described in 1983.[131] Molecular studies suggest that genetic determinants of this enzyme arose in staphylococci.[132] Although these enterococci are still exceedingly uncommon, sporadic isolates of β-lactamase–producing enterococci have been encountered on several continents, and two large outbreaks of infection or colonization have been described in U.S. hospitals.[133] β-Lactamases have been described in various gram-positive bacilli, but such strains are relatively uncommon human pathogens.

GRAM-NEGATIVE BACTERIA

Numerous β-lactamases have been described in gram-negative organisms, including plasmid-mediated and chromosomally determined enzymes. The former are important because of their potential for dissemination, whereas the latter have contributed to β-lactam resistance among troublesome nosocomial pathogens such as *P. aeruginosa* and *Enterobacter* spp.

Plasmid-Mediated β-Lactamases. Plasmid-mediated penicillin-hydrolyzing enzymes of the type designated TEM have long been recognized as a common cause of resistance to ampicillin among various gram-negative bacteria, including *E. coli, H. influenzae,* and *N. gonorrhoeae.* The development of β-lactamase–stable second- and third-generation cephalosporins initially offered predictably active alternatives against strains bearing common plasmid-mediated enzymes[134] (Table 31–3). However, as discussed later, plasmid-mediated β-lactamases now occur that can inactivate these newer agents.

Inducible, Chromosomally Mediated Enzymes. In most clinical isolates of *P. aeruginosa, Enterobacter cloacae,* and several other species of gram-negative bacilli, chromosomally mediated β-lactamases (primarily cephalosporins) are produced at extremely low levels unless organisms are exposed to β-lactams. Frequently referred to as inducible enzymes, these β-lactamases are under control of a complex system of genetic regulation.[135, 136] Exposure to β-lactams can result in reversible augmentation of enzyme production and resistance to a broad range of β-lactam antibiotics. Alternatively, selection of spontaneous stably derepressed mutant hyperproducers of β-lactamase can occur[86] (Table 31–4). At the extremely low substrate concentrations calculated to exist in the periplasmic space of organisms with intact permeability barriers, these β-lactamases can effectively hydrolyze even "stable" third-generation cephalosporins.[137] The emergence of resistance to third-generation cephalosporins among gram-negative species with inducible chromosomal β-lactamases is a significant clinical problem, occurring in up to 30% of treatment courses and leading to primary treatment failure or relapse in a significant proportion of these.[138] In a multicenter study of *Enterobacter* spp. bacteremias, resistance emerged in 6 of 31 (19%) cases treated with a third-generation cephalosporin but in only 1 of 89 and none of 50 patients receiving an aminoglycoside or another β-lactam, respectively.[139] Sanders[140] has cautioned that organisms of this type should not be considered truly susceptible to the third-generation cephalosporins, regardless of routine susceptibility test results.

Additional Problems with β-Lactamases. Within the past few years, several new β-lactamases have been recognized

TABLE 31–3 ■ Activity of β-Lactams Against Derivatives of *Pseudomonas aeruginosa* Strain PU21 Expressing Specific Plasmid-Mediated β-Lactamases*

	MINIMAL INHIBITORY CONCENTRATION (g/mL) OF				
β-LACTAMASE	TIC	PIP	CPZ	CAZ	IMI
None	32	16	16	2	4
TEM-1	128	128	128	4	4
TEM-2	128	128	128	2	8
OXA-2	128	128	128	8	8
OXA-3	128	128	128	16	8
PSE-1	128	128	64	2	8
PSE-2	128	128	128	2	8

*TIC, Ticarcillin; PIP, piperacillin; CPZ, cefoperazone; CAZ, ceftazidime; IMI, imipenem.

Data from Allan JD, Eliopoulos GM, Ferraro MJ, et al: Comparative in vitro activities of cefpiramide and apalcillin individually and in combination. Antimicrob Agents Chemother 27:782, 1985.

TABLE 31–4 ■ Antimicrobial Susceptibility of a Laboratory Mutant Strain of *Pseudomonas aeruginosa* with Stable Overproduction of Chromosomal β-Lactamase Compared with the Normally Inducible Parent Strain from Which It Was Derived

ANTIMICROBIAL	MINIMAL INHIBITORY CONCENTRATION (μg/mL) Parent	Mutant
Piperacillin	4	64
Cefotaxime	16	128
Ceftazidime	2	32
Imipenem	4	4
Gentamicin	2	2
Ciprofloxacin	0.25	0.25

that have created or threaten to create additional therapeutic difficulties.

Extended-Spectrum β-Lactamases. Beginning in the early 1980s, several plasmid-mediated β-lactamases were recognized that conferred resistance to third-generation cephalosporins.[141] For the most part, these enzymes belong to the TEM or SHV families, with minor alterations in amino acid sequences accounting for marked changes in substrate specificity.[142, 143] Currently, more than two dozen such enzymes have been identified. Genes mediating their production tend to occur on large plasmids also encoding additional resistance determinants.[144] Several outbreaks of infection and/or colonization with such organisms have occurred in the United States and abroad. In one French hospital, five distinct plasmid-mediated extended-spectrum β-lactamases were identified in *Klebsiella pneumoniae* over a short period.[145] In the United States, the frequency of ceftazidime-resistant *K. pneumoniae* increased slightly from 1987 to 1991, although in one center frequencies of resistant organisms increased from 1% to 40% in this time period.[146]

Resistance to β-Lactamase Inhibitors. In the late 1980s, several isolates of *E. coli* were encountered that produced TEM-1 β-lactamase (which should have been susceptible to inhibition by β-lactamase inhibitors) but that were resistant to amoxicillin-clavulanate combinations. These isolates were found to produce the enzyme at levels up to 30-fold greater than those of typical enzyme-producing strains, mediated by genes localized on small, multicopy plasmids.[147] Later, strains of *E. coli* were identified that produced a TEM-related enzyme that was relatively insensitive to inhibition by β-lactamase inhibitors.[148] Two of these genes have been sequenced, and the corresponding enzymes have been designated TEM-30 and TEM-31.[149]

Plasmid-Mediated "Chromosomal" β-Lactamases. An extremely broad spectrum enzyme that was plasmid mediated and insensitive to inhibition by the standard β-lactamase inhibitors was identified in *K. pneumoniae* and designated MIR-1.[150] Partial sequencing of the responsible gene demonstrated approximately 90% identity to the chromosomal *(ampC)* cephalosporinase of *E. cloacae.* Sequencing of another plasmid-mediated, noninhibitable enzyme from *E. coli* (BIL-1) revealed 94% homology at the amino acid sequence level with the chromosomal *ampC* cephalosporinase of *Citrobacter freundii.*[151] These two cases illustrate the potential for introduction of chromosomal resistance genes into plasmids, increasing the possibility of subsequent dissemination.

Carbapenemases. Chromosomal β-lactamases of *P. aeruginosa* and possibly *Enterobacter* spp. contribute only to a slight degree to carbapenem resistance. In contrast, zinc metalloenzymes found in *Stenotrophomonas* (formerly *Xanthomonas*) *maltophilia* and *Aeromonas* spp. contribute substantially to resistance.[152] Chromosomal carbapenem-hydrolyzing enzymes have been encountered in rare isolates of *Serratia marcescens* and *E. cloacae.*[153, 154] These enzymes shared considerable amino acid sequence identity and appeared to be of the serine (as opposed to metalloenzyme) active site type. Carbapenem-hydrolyzing metalloenzymes resembling those of *Aeromonas, Bacillus cereus,* and *Bacteroides fragilis* have been found in *S. marcescens.*[155] Initially thought to be chromosomal, such enzymes were subsequently demonstrated on plasmids from *S. marcescens* isolated in Japan.[156] Imipenem-hydrolyzing β-lactamase, resistant to inhibition by currently available inhibitors, was encountered in *P. aeruginosa* on a plasmid with multiple antibiotic resistance genes (gentamicin, sulfonamides).[157]

Aminoglycosides

Enzymatic modification of aminoglycosides is achieved by acetylation of vulnerable amino groups or by adenylylation or phosphorylation of hydroxyl groups on these compounds.[158] Differences in susceptibilities of various aminoglycosides to modifying enzymes depend on the presence or absence of such vulnerable groups and whether these are accessible to the enzyme in three-dimensional conformation. Genetic elements mediating production of aminoglycoside-modifying enzymes are usually plasmid mediated but may exist on the bacterial chromosome as well. Several genes are associated with transposons.[159–161] Enzymes are produced constitutively, although multiplication of gene copy number, with increased levels of resistance, has been reported.[51]

A large number of distinct modifying enzymes have been described.[162–164] For example, at least nine genes have been identified to date yielding enzymes that acetylate 2-deoxystreptamine aminoglycosides at the 6′ position alone.[165] Production of an aminoglycoside-modifying enzyme does not necessarily render bacteria resistant to a modifiable drug. For example, *E. coli* producing 2″-adenylyltransferase and *S. aureus* producing 3′-phosphotransferase may remain susceptible in vitro to netilmicin and amikacin, respectively, despite the ability to demonstrate modification of the aminoglycoside in each case.[164, 166] Susceptibility appears to depend on a balance of opposing forces: the efficiency of drug inactivation versus the effectiveness of inhibitory or bactericidal drug activity. Other bacterial cell factors, such as the level of permeability, can markedly affect phenotypic expression of plasmid-mediated aminoglycoside resistance determinants.[167] In enterococci, the presence of aminoglycoside-modifying enzymes may confer resistance to penicillin-aminoglycoside bacterial synergism even when levels of enzyme activity are not sufficient to raise minimal inhibitory concentrations above those for strains lacking enzyme activity.[168]

Several aminoglycoside-modifying enzymes may be present simultaneously within a single organism. For example, among recent isolates of *E. faecium,* it would not be uncommon to encounter high-level streptomycin resistance based on nucleotidyltransferase, chromosomal 6′-acetyltransferase inherent to the species,[165] plasmid (transposon)-mediated resistance to gentamicin, and other deoxystreptamine aminoglycosides based on the bifunctional 6′-acetyltransferase-2″-phosphotransferase enzyme[169] and additional kanamycin- and amikacin-modifying activity due to a 3′-phosphotransferase.

It may not always be possible to deduce susceptibility to aminoglycoside-modifying enzymes based on the presence or absence of groups vulnerable to modification. In one example, overproduction of a 3′-phosphotransferase in *E. coli* led to low-level tobramycin resistance despite the absence of a vulnerable 3′-hydroxyl group on tobramycin.[170] It was postulated that resistance resulted from sequestration of the aminoglycoside due to formation of a heat-labile complex between the enzyme and aminoglycoside.

MLS Antimicrobials

Inactivation of MLS class antimicrobials has been reported in both gram-positive and gram-negative organisms.[54] Erythromycin esterases, which hydrolyze the antibiotic lactone ring, have been encountered among clinical isolates of *E. coli, K. pneumoniae,* and *Enterobacter agglomerans.* Genetic determinants of these enzymes are plasmid-borne. Presence of the enzymes confers levels of resistance that are substantially higher than can be attributed to the intrinsic low-level resistance to erythromycin among Enterobacteriaceae.[51, 171, 172] Erythromycin esterase genes may coexist with ribosome modification (ribosomal RNA methylase) genes in enteric bacteria.[173] A macrolide 2′-phosphotransferase has also been detected in *E. coli.*[174] Staphylococcal lincosamide-modifying enzymes (4-lincosamide-*O*-nucleotidyltransferases) have been described that fully inactivate lincomycin but confer only relative resistance to clindamycin. The latter is manifested only by high minimal bactericidal concentrations or decreased inhibitory activity when tested against high bacterial inocula.[175] Genetic elements mediating enzymes that inactivate streptogramin A and B drugs have been encountered in gram-positive bacteria.[173, 176]

Chloramphenicol

Drug inactivation is the major mechanism of resistance to chloramphenicol among gram-positive organisms. Chloramphenicol acetyltransferase production is plasmid mediated and inducible in *S. aureus.*[62] Similar enzymes are found in enterococci, pneumococci and other streptococci, clostridia, and *Bacillus* spp. In gram-negative organisms, chloramphenicol acetyltransferase genes are often plasmid-borne and located on transposable elements. Studies in enterococci have shown that acetylation occurs at the 3-hydroxyl position. Nonenzymatic transfer of the acetyl group to the 1 position follows, and the resulting 1-acetyl-chloramphenicol is subject to repeated acetylation at the 3 position.[177] Fluorinated chloramphenicol analogs, which resist enzymatic inactivation, have been synthesized but not further developed because of the limited practical utility of such compounds.[178]

Tetracycline and Rifampin

A *B. fragilis* transposon has been encountered that mediates tetracycline resistance both by promoting active drug efflux and by drug detoxification.[179] The exact nature of the chemical modification inactivating the drug is unknown but has been proposed to be accelerated autooxidation of the compound.[180] Minocycline, doxycycline, and other tetracycline analogs are subject to the detoxification pathway described. The clinical significance of such resistance mechanisms, if any, is unknown.[181]

Modification of rifampin to yield inactive compounds has been reported in *Nocardia* spp. and several *Mycobacterium* isolates.[182]

Antimicrobial Cross-resistance

Because several members of any one antimicrobial class often share common targets, routes of access to these target sites, and sometimes similar susceptibilities to inactivating enzymes, it is not surprising that bacteria often demonstrate extensive cross-resistance to several agents of a class. In some situations, cross-resistance may not be apparent by routine susceptibility testing. An example is methicillin-resistant staphylococci, with which standard tests may fail to detect subpopulations resistant to cephalosporins.[183] In other cases, resistance to one antimicrobial agent may signal decreased susceptibility but not absolute resistance to other members of the class. For example, compared with strains that are fully susceptible to nalidixic acid, nalidixic acid–resistant Enterobacteriaceae tend to display higher minimal inhibitory concentrations against several of the newer fluoroquinolones. Nevertheless, most isolates of the latter group remain susceptible to clinically achievable concentrations of the more potent, newer antimicrobials.[184]

Cross-resistance also occurs between antibiotics representing different classes. In gram-negative bacteria, permeability mutants with altered outer membrane (porin) proteins sometimes demonstrate resistance to diverse agents such as quinolones, trimethoprim, and chloramphenicol.[185] As already discussed, mutations affecting certain genetic loci may result in altered levels of resistance to several unrelated antimicrobials, apparently resulting from both activation of efflux systems and down-regulation of permeability channels.[123, 124]

Simultaneous resistance to two or more drug classes can also follow acquisition of multiantibiotic-resistant plasmids or of a single plasmid specifying resistance to multiple drug classes. Genes encoding β-lactamases and aminoglycoside-modifying enzymes may coexist on plasmids[141] or even on single transposons—a phenomenon that expands the potential host range of transmissible resistance elements.[186, 187] As exemplified by *M. tuberculosis,* multiple drug resistance in individual isolates can result from the accumulation of chromosomal mutations, each affecting a specific antibiotic resistance gene.[42] Multiple drug resistance can also occur through a combination of chromosomal mutational events and acquisition of exogenous resistance genes as seen in penicillin-resistant pneumococci, some isolates of which also demonstrate resistance to trimethoprim-sulfamethoxazole, chloramphenicol, and tetracycline.[4] As a result, selective pressure based on extensive use of one antimicrobial may promote continued resistance to drugs of other classes, even if use of those is restricted.

Strategies to Reduce Antimicrobial Resistance

Antibiotic Combinations

The use of two or more antimicrobials in combination to prevent bacterial resistance (with subsequent clinical treatment failure) is exemplified by multidrug regimens for the treatment of tuberculosis. Such combinations have proved highly effective, even though resistance to individual components of the regimens develops rapidly when they are used as single agents.[188, 189] The success of this approach rests on the mathematic improbability that mutational resistance to two or more drugs would develop simultaneously in a single bacterial colony.

Rifampin is a drug with excellent activity against a variety of bacterial pathogens but to which resistance develops rapidly. Rifampin has been employed in combination with other agents against nonmycobacterial infections. For example, rifampin-vancomycin combinations have proved effective in the treatment of prosthetic valve endocarditis due to coagulase-negative staphylococci.[190] It is now clear, however, that coadministration of a second antimicrobial may not completely prevent the development of rifampin resistance. This incomplete protection may result from differential penetration of the antibiotics deeply into tissues or into phagocytic cells that harbor viable bacteria.[168]

Antibiotic combinations, particularly β-lactams plus aminoglycosides, have been widely used in the treatment of serious gram-negative bacillary infections, at least in part in an attempt to minimize the development of resistance to either component.[168] This approach is supported by animal studies and some but not all clinical trials.[191] The value of adding an aminoglycoside (with its attendant cost and toxicities) to a highly potent β-lactam may be difficult to demonstrate unequivocally in most clinical situations. Still, many clinicians strongly favor use of such combinations in treating serious gram-negative infections, especially in neutropenic or otherwise immunocompromised patients and particularly when infection is due to *P. aeruginosa*.[168]

The strategy of using antimicrobial combinations to delay the emergence of resistance to individual agents is predicated on the assumption that resistance to one agent occurs with a probability independent of resistance to the other. As discussed in the preceding section, this is often *not* the case. Acquisition of resistance to two or more drugs simultaneously can arise in a number of ways, further limiting the usefulness of this strategy.

Minimization of Selective Pressure

Although for the individual patient appropriately aggressive use of antibiotic therapy targeted at a specific pathogen is likely to reduce the risk of microbial drug resistance, there is substantial evidence that extensive antibiotic use promotes the selection, propagation, and maintenance of drug-resistant microorganisms, especially in the hospital environment.[192–195] Particularly striking in this regard has been the experience with the liberal use of topical aminoglycoside (gentamicin) in burn units, which has resulted in outbreaks of colonization with gentamicin-resistant strains of *P. aeruginosa*.[196] In this and other examples, restricted use of the antimicrobial has dramatically decreased isolation rates of resistant microorganisms.[192, 194, 196] It is important to note, however, that the recognition of a serious institutional problem with antibiotic-resistant pathogens, leading to severe restrictions on the use of antimicrobials, is also likely to enhance awareness of and compliance with other infection control measures. The appropriate use of measures such as barrier precautions has been demonstrated to be effective in decreasing colonization of patients with nosocomial pathogens[197] and would contribute substantially to any beneficial effect of antibiotic restriction alone.

Given that the use of antibiotics for surgical prophylaxis accounts for a significant fraction of total antibiotic use in many hospitals, prophylactic regimens should adhere to accepted standards relating to antimicrobial spectrum (i.e., avoiding regimens with overly broad spectrums) and duration of administration.[198]

References

1. Eliopoulos GM, Wennersten C, Moellering RC Jr: Resistance to β-lactam antibiotics in *Streptococcus faecium*. Antimicrob Agents Chemother 22:295, 1982.
2. Georgopapadakou NH: Penicillin-binding proteins and bacterial resistance to β-lactams. Antimicrob Agents Chemother 37:2045, 1993.
3. Malouin F, Bryan LE: Modification of penicillin-binding proteins as mechanisms of β-lactam resistance. Antimicrob Agents Chemother 30:1, 1986.
4. Haglund LA, Istre GR, Pickett DA, et al: Invasive pneumococcal disease in central Oklahoma: Emergence of high-level penicillin resistance and multiple antibiotic resistance. J Infect Dis 168:1532, 1993.
5. Centers for Disease Control and Prevention: Drug-resistant *Streptococcus pneumoniae*—Kentucky and Tennessee, 1993. MMWR Morbid Mortal Wkly Rep 43:23, 1994.
6. Soares S, Kristinsson KG, Musser JM, et al: Evidence for the introduction of a multiresistant clone of serotype 6B *Streptococcus pneumoniae* from Spain to Iceland in the late 1980s. J Infect Dis 168:158, 1993.
7. Muñoz R, Coffey TJ, Daniels M, et al: Intercontinental spread of a multiresistant clone of serotype 23F *Streptococcus pneumoniae.* J Infect Dis 164:302, 1991.
8. Marton A, Gulyas M, Muñoz R, et al: Extremely high incidence of antibiotic resistance in clinical isolates of *Streptococcus pneumoniae* in Hungary. J Infect Dis 163:542, 1991.
9. Zighelboim S, Tomasz A: Penicillin-binding proteins of multiply antibiotic-resistant South African strains of *Streptococcus pneumoniae*. Antimicrob Agents Chemother 17:434, 1980.
10. Spratt BG: Resistance to antibiotics mediated by target alterations. Science 264:388, 1994.
11. Figueiredo AMS, Connor JD, Severin A, et al: A pneumococcal clinical isolate with high-level resistance to cefotaxime and ceftriaxone. Antimicrob Agents Chemother 36:886, 1992.
12. Hartman BJ, Tomasz A: Low-affinity penicillin-binding protein associated with β-lactam resistance in *Staphylococcus aureus*. J Bacteriol 158:513, 1984.
13. Chambers HF, Sachdeva M: Binding of β-lactam antibiotics to penicillin-binding proteins in methicillin-resistant *Staphylococcus aureus*. J Infect Dis 161:1170, 1990.
14. Ubukata K, Yamashita N, Konno M: Occurrence of a β-lactam-inducible penicillin-binding protein in methicillin-resistant staphylococci. Antimicrob Agents Chemother 27:851, 1985.
15. Chambers HF, Hartman BJ, Tomasz A: Increased amounts of a novel penicillin-binding protein in a strain of methicillin-resistant *Staphylococcus aureus* exposed to nafcillin. J Clin Invest 76:325, 1985.
16. Hackbarth CJ, Chambers HF: *blaI* and *blaR1* regulate β-lactamase and PBP 2a production in methicillin-resistant *Staphylococcus aureus*. Antimicrob Agents Chemother 37:1144, 1993.
17. Murakami K, Tomasz A: Involvement of multiple genetic determinants in high-level methicillin resistance in *Staphylococcus aureus*. J Bacteriol 171:874, 1989.
18. Hackbarth CJ, Miick C, Chambers HF: Altered production of penicillin-binding protein 2a can affect phenotypic expression of methicillin-resistance in *Staphylococcus aureus*. Antimicrob Agents Chemother 38:2568, 1994.
19. Gustafson J, Strässle A, Hächler H, et al: The *femC* locus of *Staphylococcus aureus* required for methicillin resistance includes the glutamine synthetase operon. J Bacteriol 176:1460, 1994.
20. Maki H, Yamaguchi T, Murakami K: Cloning and characterization of a gene affecting the methicillin resistance level and the autolysis rate in *Staphylococcus aureus*. J Bacteriol 176:4993, 1994.
21. Trees DL, Iandolo JJ: Identification of a *Staphylococcus aureus* transposon (Tn*4291*) that carries the methicillin resistance gene(s). J Bacteriol 170:149, 1988.
22. Chambers HF: Coagulase-negative staphylococci resistant to β-lactam antibiotics in vivo produce penicillin-binding protein 2A. Antimicrob Agents Chemother 31:1919, 1987.
23. Tesch W, Strässle A. Berger-Bachi B, et al: Cloning and expression of methicillin resistance from *Staphylococcus epidermidis* in *Staphylococcus carnosus*. Antimicrob Agents Chemother 32:1494, 1988.
24. Archer GL, Climo MW: Antimicrobial susceptibility of coagulase-negative staphylococci. Antimicrob Agents Chemother 38:2231, 1994.
25. Fontana R, Cerini R, Longoni P, et al: Identification of a streptococcal penicillin-binding protein that reacts very slowly with penicillin. J Bacteriol 155:1343, 1983.
26. Williamson R, LeBouguenec C, Gutmann L, et al: One or two low affinity penicillin-binding proteins may be responsible for the range of susceptibility of *Enterococcus faecium* to benzylpenicillin. J Gen Microbiol 131:1933, 1985.
27. Grayson ML, Eliopoulos GM, Wennersten CB, et al: Increasing resistance to β-lactam antibiotics among clinical isolates of *Enterococcus faecium:* A 22-year review of one institution. Antimicrob Agents Chemother 35:2180, 1991.
28. Klare I, Rodloff AC, Wagner J, et al: Overproduction of a penicillin-binding protein is not the only mechanism of penicillin resistance in *Enterococcus faecium*. Antimicrob Agents Chemother 36:783, 1992.
29. Fontana R, Aldegheri M. Ligozzi M, et al: Overproduction of a

low-affinity penicillin-binding protein and high-level ampicillin resistance in *Enterococcus faecium.* Antimicrob Agents Chemother 38:1980, 1994.
30. Piras G, El Kharroubi A, van Beeumen J, et al: Characterization of an *Enterococcus hirae* penicillin-binding protein 3 with low penicillin affinity. J Bacteriol 172:6856, 1990.
31. Godfrey AJ, Bryan LE, Rabin HR: β-Lactam-resistant *Pseudomonas aeruginosa* with modified penicillin-binding proteins emerging during cystic fibrosis treatment. Antimicrob Agents Chemother 19:705, 1981.
32. Dougherty TJ: Involvement of a change in penicillin target and peptidoglycan structure in low-level resistance to β-lactam antibiotics in *Neisseria gonorrhoeae.* Antimicrob Agents Chemother 28:90, 1985.
33. Mendelman PM, Chaffin DO, Stull TL, et al: Characterization of non-β-lactamase-mediated ampicillin resistance in *Haemophilus influenzae.* Antimicrob Agents Chemother 26:235, 1984.
34. Parr TR Jr, Bryan LE: Mechanisms of resistance of an ampicillin-resistant, β-lactamase-negative clinical isolate of *Haemophilus influenzae* type b to β-lactam antibiotics. Antimicrob Agents Chemother 25:747, 1984.
35. Spratt BG, Cromie KD: Penicillin-binding proteins of gram-negative bacteria. Rev Infect Dis 10:699, 1988.
36. Centers for Disease Control and Prevention: Nosocomial enterococci resistant to vancomycin—United States, 1989–1993. MMWR Morb Mortal Wkly Rep 42:597, 1993.
37. Arthur M, Courvalin P: Genetics and mechanisms of glycopeptide resistance in enterococci. Antimicrob Agents Chemother 37:1563, 1993.
38. Arthur M, Molinas C, Depardieu F, et al: Characterization of Tn*1546,* a Tn3-related transposon conferring glycopeptide resistance by synthesis of depsipeptide peptidoglycan precursors in *Enterococcus faecium* BM 4147. J Bacteriol 175:117, 1993.
39. Hancock REW: Aminoglycoside uptake and mode of action with special reference to streptomycin and gentamicin. J Antimicrob Chemother 8:249, 1981.
40. Bryan LE: General mechanisms of resistance to antibiotics. J Antimicrob Chemother 22(Suppl A):1, 1988.
41. Honoré N, Cole ST: Streptomycin resistance in mycobacteria. Antimicrob Agents Chemother 38:238, 1994.
42. Morris S, Han Bai G, Suffys P, et al: Molecular mechanisms of multiple drug resistance in clinical isolates of *Mycobacterium tuberculosis.* J Infect Dis 171:954, 1995.
43. Maness MJ, Foster GC, Sparling PF: Ribosomal resistance to streptomycin and spectinomycin in *Neisseria gonorrhoeae.* J Bacteriol 120:1293, 1974.
44. Lacey RW, Chopra I: Evidence for mutation to streptomycin resistance in clinical strains of *Staphylococcus aureus.* J Gen Microbiol 73:175, 1972.
45. Tseng JT, Bryan LE, Van den Elzen HM: Mechanisms and spectrum of streptomycin resistance in a natural population of *Pseudomonas aeruginosa.* Antimicrob Agents Chemother 2:136, 1972.
46. Eliopoulos GM, Farber, BF, Murray B, et al: Ribosomal resistance of clinical enterococcal isolates to streptomycin. Antimicrob Agents Chemother 25:398, 1984.
47. Shaila MS, Gopinathan KP, Ramakrishnan T: Protein synthesis in *Mycobacterium tuberculosis* H37Rv and the effect of streptomycin in streptomycin-susceptible and -resistant strains. Antimicrob Agents Chemother 4:205, 1973.
48. Yamada T, Nagata A, Ono Y, et al: Alteration of ribosomes and RNA polymerase in drug-resistant clinical isolates of *Mycobacterium tuberculosis.* Antimicrob Agents Chemother 27:921, 1985.
49. Ahmad MH, Rechenmacher A, Bock A: Interaction between aminoglycoside uptake and ribosomal resistance mutations. Antimicrob Agents Chemother 18:798, 1980.
50. Holmes DJ, Cundliffe E: Analysis of a ribosomal RNA methylase gene from *Streptomyces tenebrarius* which confers resistance to gentamicin. Mol Gen Genet 229:229, 1991.
51. Bryan LE: Aminoglycoside resistance. *In* Bryan LE (ed): Antimicrobial Drug Resistance. Orlando, FL, Academic Press, 1984, pp 241–277.
52. Jacoby GA, Archer GL: New mechanisms of bacterial resistance to antimicrobial agents. N Engl J Med 324:601, 1991.
53. Arthur M, Andremont A, Courvalin, P: Distribution of erythromycin esterase and rRNA methylase genes in members of the family *Enterobacteriaceae* highly resistant to erythromycin. Antimicrob Agents Chemother 31:404, 1987.
54. Auckenthaler RW, Zwahlen A, Waldvogel FA: Macrolides. *In* Peterson PK, Verhoef J (eds): Antimicrobial Agents Annual 1. Amsterdam, Elsevier Science Publishing, 1986, pp 115–126.
55. Weisblum B.: Erythromycin resistance by ribosomal modification. Antimicrob Agents Chemother 39:577, 1995.
56. Weisblum B: Inducible resistance to macrolides, lincosamides and streptogramin type B antibiotics: The resistance phenotype, its biological diversity, and structural elements that regulate expression—A review. J Antimicrob Chemother 16(Suppl A):63, 1985.
57. Mitsuhashi S, Inoue M: Resistance to macrolides and lincomycins. *In* Bryan LE (ed): Antimicrobial Drug Resistance. Orlando, FL, Academic Press, 1984, pp 279–291.
58. Weisblum B: Insights into erythromycin action from studies of its activity as inducer of resistance. Antimicrob Agents Chemother 39:797, 1995.
59. Jenssen WD, Thakker-Varia S, Dubin DT, et al: Prevalence of macrolides-lincosamides-streptogramin B resistance and *erm* gene classes among clinical strains of staphylococci and streptococci. Antimicrob Agents Chemother 31:883, 1987.
60. Quiros LM, Fidalgo S, Mendez FJ, et al: Novel mechanisms of resistance to lincosamides in *Staphylococcus* and *Arthrobacter* spp. Antimicrob Agents Chemother 32:420, 1988.
61. Lee H-J, Park J-Y, Jang S-H, et al. High incidence of resistance to multiple antimicrobials in clinical isolates of *Streptococcus pneumoniae* from a university hospital in Korea. Clin Infect Dis 20:826, 1995.
62. Smith AL, Burns JL: Resistance to chloramphenicol and fusidic acid. *In* Bryan LE (ed): Antimicrobial Drug Resistance. Orlando, FL, Academic Press, 1984, p 293.
63. Burdett V: Streptococcal tetracycline resistance mediated at the level of protein synthesis. J Bacteriol 165:564, 1986.
64. Coleman K, Athalye M, Clancey A, et al: Bacterial resistance mechanisms as therapeutic targets. J Antimicrob Chemother 33:1091, 1994.
65. Morse SA, Johnson SR, Biddle JW, et al: High-level tetracycline resistance in *Neisseria gonorrhoeae* is result of acquisition of streptococcal *tetM* determinant. Antimicrob Agents Chemother 30:664, 1986.
66. Knapp JS, Johnson SR, Zenilman JM, et al: High-level tetracycline resistance resulting from TetM in strains of *Neisseria* spp., *Kingella denitrificans,* and *Eikenella corrodens.* Antimicrob Agents Chemother 32:765, 1988.
67. Brown JT, Roberts MC: Cloning and characterization of *tetM* gene from a *Ureaplasma urealyticum* strain. Antimicrob Agents Chemother 31:1852, 1987.
68. Hooper DC and Wolfson JS: Mechanisms of quinolone action and bacterial killing. *In* Hooper DC and Wolfson JS (eds): Quinolone Antimicrobial Agents, ed 2. Washington, DC, American Society for Microbiology, 1993, p 53.
69. Eliopoulos GM, Eliopoulos, CT: Quinolone antimicrobial agents: Activity in vitro. *In* Wolfson JS, Hooper DC (eds): Quinolone Antimicrobial Agents. Washington, DC, American Society for Microbiology, 1989, p 35.
70. Takahata M, Nishino T: DNA gyrase of *Staphylococcus aureus* and inhibitory effect of quinolones on its activity. Antimicrob Agents Chemother 32:1192, 1988.
71. Isaacs RD, Kunke PJ, Cohen RL, et al: Ciprofloxacin resistance in epidemic methicillin-resistant *Staphylococcus aureus.* Lancet 2:843, 1988.
72. Shalit I, Berger SA, Gorea A, et al: Widespread quinolone resistance among methicillin-resistant *Staphylococcus aureus* isolates in a general hospital. Antimicrob Agents Chemother 33:593, 1989.
73. Blumberg HM, Rimland D, Carroll DJ, et al: Rapid development of ciprofloxacin resistance in methicillin-susceptible and -resistant *Staphylococcus aureus.* J Infect Dis 163:1279, 1991.
74. Wehrli W: Rifampin: Mechanisms of action and resistance. Rev Infect Dis 5(Suppl 3):S407, 1983.
75. Radstrom P, Swedberg G: RSF1010 and a conjugative plasmid contain *sulII,* one of two known genes for plasmid-borne sulfonamide resistance dihydropteroate synthase. Antimicrob Agents Chemother 32:1684, 1988.
76. Huovinen P, Sundström L, Swedberg G, et al: Trimethoprim and sulfonamide resistance. Antimicrob Agents Chemother 39:279, 1995.

77. Galetto DW, Johnston JL, Archer GL: Molecular epidemiology of trimethoprim resistance among coagulase-negative staphylococci. Antimicrob Agents Chemother 31:1683, 1987.
78. Wylie BA, Amyes SGB, Young HK, et al: Identification of a novel plasmid-encoded dihydrofolate reductase mediating high-level resistance to trimethoprim. J Antimicrob Chemother 33:429, 1988.
79. DeGroot R, Campos J, Moseley SL, et al: Molecular cloning and mechanisms of trimethoprim resistance in *Haemophilus influenzae.* Antimicrob Agents Chemother 32:477, 1988.
80. Hamilton-Miller JMT: Resistance to antibacterial agents acting on antifolate metabolism. *In* Bryan LE (ed): Antimicrobial Drug Resistance. Orlando, FL, Academic Press, 1984, p 173.
81. Yoshimura F, Nikaido H: Diffusion of β-lactam antibiotics through the porin channels of *Escherichia coli* K-12. Antimicrob Agents Chemother 27:84, 1985.
82. Nikaido H: Outer membrane barrier as a mechanism of antibiotic resistance. Antimicrob Agents Chemother 33:1831, 1989.
83. Sanders CC, Sanders WE Jr, Goering RV, et al: Selection of multiple antibiotic resistance by quinolones, β-lactams, and aminoglycosides with special reference to cross-resistance between unrelated drug classes. Antimicrob Agents Chemother 26:797, 1984.
84. Gutmann L, Billot-Klein D, Williamson R, et al: Mutation of *Salmonella paratyphi* A conferring cross-resistance to several groups of antibiotics by decreased permeability and loss of invasiveness. Antimicrob Agents Chemother 32:195, 1988.
85. Hooper DC, Wolfson JS, Souza KS, et al: Genetic and biochemical characterization of norfloxacin resistance in *Escherichia coli.* Antimicrob Agents Chemother 29:639, 1986.
86. Sanders CC, Sanders WE Jr: Type I beta-lactamase of gram-negative bacteria: Interactions with beta-lactam antibiotics. J Infect Dis 154:792, 1986.
87. Hancock REW: Role of porins in outer membrane permeability. J Bacteriol 169:929, 1987.
88. Hancock REW, Woodruff WA: Roles of porin and β-lactamase in β-lactam resistance of *Pseudomonas aeruginosa.* Rev Infect Dis 10:770, 1988.
89. Godfrey AJ, Bryan LE: Penetration of β-lactams through *Pseudomonas aeruginosa* porin channels. Antimicrob Agents Chemother 31:1216, 1987.
90. Quinn JP, Studemeister AE, DiVincenzo CA, et al: Resistance to imipenem in *Pseudomonas aeruginosa:* Clinical experience and biochemical mechanisms. Rev Infect Dis 10:892, 1988.
91. Lynch MJ, Drusano GL, Mobley HTL: Emergence of resistance to imipenem in *Pseudomonas aeruginosa.* Antimicrob Agents Chemother 31:1892, 1987.
92. Buscher K, Cullman W, Dick W, et al: Imipenem resistance in *Pseudomonas aeruginosa* resulting from diminished expression of an outer membrane protein. Antimicrob Agents Chemother 31:703, 1987.
93. Livingstone D, Gill MJ, Wise R: Mechanisms of resistance to carbapenems. J Antimicrob Chemother 35:1, 1995.
94. Li X-Z, Ma D, Livermore DM, Nikaido H: Role of efflux pump(s) in intrinsic resistance of *Pseudomonas aeruginosa:* Active efflux as a contributing factor to β-lactam resistance. Antimicrob Agents Chemother 38:1742, 1994.
95. Collatz E, Gutmann L: Bacterial porins as mediators of antibiotic susceptibility. *In* Peterson PK, Verhoef J (eds): Antimicrobial Agents Annual 2. Amsterdam, Elsevier Science Publishing, 1987, p 442.
96. Norris SA, Sciortino CV: Monoclonal antibody to an aminoglycoside-resistance factor from *Pseudomonas aeruginosa.* J Infect Dis 158:1324, 1988.
97. Bryan LE, O'Hara K, Wong S: Lipopolysaccharide changes in impermeability-type aminoglycoside resistance in *Pseudomonas aeruginosa.* Antimicrob Agents Chemother 26:250, 1984.
98. Maloney J, Rimland D, Stephens DS, et al: Analysis of amikacin-resistant *Pseudomonas aeruginosa* developing in patients receiving amikacin. Arch Intern Med 149:630, 1989.
99. Parr TR Jr, Bayer AS: Mechanisms of aminoglycoside resistance in variants of *Pseudomonas aeruginosa* isolated during treatment of experimental endocarditis in rabbits. J Infect Dis 158:1003, 1988.
100. Mates SM, Patel L, Kaback HR, et al: Membrane potential in anaerobically growing *Staphylococcus aureus* and its relationship to gentamicin uptake. Antimicrob Agents Chemother 23:526, 1983.
101. Miller MH, Edberg SC, Mandel LJ, et al: Gentamicin uptake in wild-type and aminoglycoside-resistant small-colony mutants of *Staphylococcus aureus.* Antimicrob Agents Chemother 18:722, 1980.
102. Moellering RC Jr, Murray BE, Schoenbaum SC, et al: A novel mechanism of resistance to penicillin-gentamicin synergism in *Streptococcus faecalis.* J Infect Dis 141:81, 1980.
103. Lampson BC, von David W, Parisi JT: Novel mechanisms for plasmid-mediated erythromycin resistance to pNE24 from *Staphylococcus epidermidis.* Antimicrob Agents Chemother 30: 653, 1986.
104. Levy SB: Active efflux mechanisms for antimicrobial resistance. Antimicrob Agents Chemother 36:695, 1992.
105. Goldman RC, Capobianco JO: Role of an energy-dependent efflux pump in plasmid pNE24-mediated resistance to 14- and 15-membered macrolides in *Staphylococcus epidermidis.* Antimicrob Agents Chemother 34:1973, 1990.
106. Burns JL, Rubens CE, Mendelman PM, et al: Cloning and expression in *Escherichia coli* of a gene encoding nonenzymatic chloramphenicol resistance from *Pseudomonas aeruginosa.* Antimicrob Agents Chemother 29:445, 1986.
107. Burns JL, Hedin LA, Lien DM: Chloramphenicol resistance in *Pseudomonas cepacia* because of decreased permeability. Antimicrob Agents Chemother 33:131, 1989.
108. McMurry LM, George AM, Levy SB: Active efflux of chloramphenicol in susceptible *Escherichia coli* strains and in multiple-antibiotic-resistant (Mar) mutants. Antimicrob Agents Chemother 38:542, 1994.
109. Li X-Z, Livermore DM, Nikaido H: Role of efflux pump(s) in intrinsic resistance of *Pseudomonas aeruginosa:* Resistance to tetracycline, chloramphenicol, and norfloxacin. Antimicrob Agents Chemother 38:1732, 1994.
110. Levy SB: Resistance to the tetracyclines. *In* Bryan LE (ed): Antimicrobial Drug Resistance. Orlando, FL, Academic Press, 1984, p 191.
111. McMurray L, Petrucci RE Jr, Levy SB: Active efflux of tetracycline encoded by four genetically different tetracycline resistance determinants in *Escherichia coli.* Proc Natl Acad Sci USA 77:3974, 1980.
112. Thanassi DG, Suh GSB, Nikaido H: Role of outer membrane barrier in efflux-mediated tetracycline resistance of *Escherichia coli.* J Bacteriol 177:998, 1995.
113. Diver J: The mode of action of the 4-quinolones: An update. Quinolone Bull 4:25, 1988.
114. Hirai K, Aoyama H, Irikura T, et al: Differences in susceptibility to quinolones of outer membrane mutants of *Salmonella typhimurium* and *Escherichia coli.* Antimicrob Agents Chemother 29:535, 1986.
115. Robillard NJ, Scarpa AL: Genetic and physiological characterization of ciprofloxacin resistance in *Pseudomonas aeruginosa* PAO. Antimicrob Agents Chemother 32:535, 1988.
116. Daikos GI, Lolans VT, Jackson GG: Alterations in outer membrane proteins of *Pseudomonas aeruginosa* associated with selective resistance to quinolones. Antimicrob Agents Chemother 32:785, 1988.
117. Hirai K, Suzue S, Irikura T, et al: Mutations producing resistance to norfloxacin in *Pseudomonas aeruginosa.* Antimicrob Agents Chemother 31:582, 1987.
118. Masuda N, Sakagawa E, Ohya S: Outer membrane proteins responsible for multiple drug resistance in *Pseudomonas aeruginosa.* Antimicrob Agents Chemother 39:645, 1995.
119. Zhanel GG, Karlowsky JA, Saunders MH, et al: Development of multiple-antibiotic-resistant (Mar) mutants of *Pseudomonas aeruginosa* after serial exposure to fluoroquinolones. Antimicrob Agents Chemother 39:489, 1995.
120. Cohen SP, Hooper DC, Wolfson JS, et al: Endogenous active efflux of norfloxacin in susceptible *Escherichia coli.* Antimicrob Agents Chemother 32:1187, 1988.
121. Neyfakh AA, Borsch CM, Kaatz GW: Fluoroquinolone resistance protein NorA of *Staphylococcus aureus* is a multidrug efflux transporter. Antimicrob Agents Chemother 37:128, 1993.
122. Then RL: Mechanisms of resistance to trimethoprim, the sulfonamides, and trimethoprim-sulfamethoxazole. Rev Infect Dis 4:261, 1982.

123. Cohen SP, Yan W, Levy SB: A multidrug resistance regulatory chromosomal locus is widespread among enteric bacteria. J Infect Dis 168:484, 1993.
124. Ariza RR, Li Z, Ringstad N, et al: Activation of multiple antibiotic resistance and binding of stress-inducible promoters by *Escherichia coli* Rob protein. J Bacteriol 177:1655, 1995.
125. Cohen SP, McMurry LM, Hooper DC, et al: Cross-resistance to fluoroquinolones in multiple-antibiotic resistant (Mar) *Escherichia coli* selected by tetracycline or chloramphenicol: Decreased drug accumulation associated with membrane changes in addition to OmpF reduction. Antimicrob Agents Chemother 33:1318, 1989.
126. Bush K: Characterization of β-lactamases. Antimicrob Agents Chemother 33:259, 1989.
127. Bush K: Classification of β-lactamases: Groups 1, 2a, 2b and 2b′. Antimicrob Agents Chemother 33:264, 1989.
128. Bush K: Classification of β-lactamases: Groups 2c, 2d, 2e, 3 and 4. Antimicrob Agents Chemother 33:271, 1989.
129. Bush K: Recent developments in β-lactamase research and their implications for the future. Rev Infect Dis 10:681, 1988.
130. McDougal LK, Thornsberry C: The role of β-lactamase in staphylococcal resistance to penicillinase-resistant penicillin and cephalosporin. J Clin Microbiol 23:832, 1986.
131. Murray BE, Mederski-Samoraj B: Transferable β-lactamase: A new mechanism for in vitro penicillin resistance in *Streptococcus faecalis*. J Clin Invest 72:1168, 1983.
132. Murray BE, Mederski-Samoraj B, Foster SK, et al: In vitro studies of plasmid-mediated penicillinase from *Streptococcus faecalis* suggest a staphylococcal origin. J Clin Invest 77:289, 1986.
133. Eliopoulos GM: Increasing problems in the therapy of enterococcal infections. Eur J Clin Microbiol Infect Dis 12:409, 1993.
134. Allan JD, Eliopoulos GM, Ferraro MJ, et al: Comparative in vitro activities of cefpiramide and apalcillin individually and in combination. Antimicrob Agents Chemother 27:782, 1985.
135. Lindberg F, Lindquist S, Normark S: Genetic basis of induction and overproduction of chromosomal class I β-lactamase in nonfastidious gram-negative bacilli. Rev Infect Dis 10:782, 1988.
136. Korfmann G, Wiedemann B: Genetic control of β-lactamase production in *Enterobacter cloacae*. Rev Infect Dis 10:793, 1988.
137. Vu H, Nikaido H: Role of beta-lactam hydrolysis in the mechanism of resistance of a beta-lactamase-constitutive *Enterobacter cloacae* strain to expanded spectrum beta-lactams. Antimicrob Agents Chemother 27:393, 1985.
138. Sanders WE Jr, Sanders CC: Inducible β-lactamases: Clinical and epidemiological implications for use of newer cephalosporins. Rev Infect Dis 10:830, 1988.
139. Chow JW, Fine MJ, Shales DM, Quinn JP, et al: *Enterobacter* bacteremia: Clinical features and emergence of antibiotic resistance during therapy. Ann Intern Med 115:585, 1991.
140. Sanders CC: New β-lactams: New problems for the internist. Ann Intern Med 115:650, 1991.
141. Sirot J, Chanal C, Petit A, et al: *Klebsiella pneumoniae* and other Enterobacteriaceae producing novel plasmid-mediated β-lactamases markedly active against third-generation cephalosporins. Epidemiologic studies. Rev Infect Dis 10:850, 1988.
142. Philippon A, Labia R, Jacoby G: Extended-spectrum β-lactamases. Antimicrob Agents Chemother 33:1131, 1989.
143. Du Bois SK, Marriott MS, Amyes SGB: TEM- and SHV-derived extended-spectrum β-lactamases: Relationship between selection, structure and function. J Antimicrob Chemother 35:7, 1995.
144. Jacoby GA, Medeiros AA: More extended-spectrum β-lactamases. Antimicrob Agents Chemother 35:1697, 1991.
145. Chanal CM, Sirot DL, Petit A, et al: Multiplicity of TEM-derived β-lactamases from *Klebsiella pneumoniae* strains isolated at the same hospital and relationships between the responsible plasmids. Antimicrob Agents Chemother 33:1915, 1989.
146. Burwen DR, Banerjee SN, Gaynes RP, et al: Ceftazidime resistance among selected nosocomial gram-negative bacilli in the United States. J Infect Dis 170:1622, 1994.
147. Martinez JL, Vincente MF, Delgado-Iribarren A, et al: Small plasmids are involved in amoxicillin-clavulanate resistance in *Escherichia coli*. Antimicrob Agents Chemother 33:595, 1989.
148. Vedel G, Belaaouaj A, Gilly L, et al: Clinical isolates of *Escherichia coli* producing TRI β-lactamases: Novel TEM-enzymes conferring resistance to β-lactamase inhibitors. J Antimicrob Chemother 30:449, 1992.
149. Zhou XY, Bordon F, Sirot D, et al: Emergence of clinical isolates of *Escherichia coli* producing TEM-1 derivatives or an OXA-1 β-lactamase conferring resistance to β-lactamase inhibitors. Antimicrob Agents Chemother 38:1085, 1994.
150. Papanicolaou GA, Medeiros AA, Jacoby GA: Novel plasmid-mediated β-lactamase (MIR-1) conferring resistance to oxyimino- and α-hydroxy-β-lactams in clinical isolates of *Klebsiella pneumoniae*. Antimicrob Agents Chemother 34:2200, 1990.
151. Fosberry AP, Payne DJ, Lawlor EJ, et al: Cloning and sequence analysis of bla_{BIL-1}, a plasmid-mediated class C β-lactamase gene in *Escherichia coli* BS. Antimicrob Agents Chemother 38:1182, 1994.
152. Livingstone D, Gill MJ, Wise R: Mechanisms of resistance to the carbapenems. J Antimicrob Chemother 35:1, 1955.
153. Naas T, Vandel L, Sougakoff W, et al: Cloning and sequence analysis of the gene for a carbapenem-hydrolyzing class A β-lactamase, Sme-1, from *Serratia marcescens* S6. Antimicrob Agents Chemother 38:1262, 1994.
154. Nordmann P, Mariotte S, Naas T, et al: Biochemical properties of a carbapenem-hydrolyzing β-lactamase from *Enterobacter cloacae* and cloning of the gene into *Escherichia coli*. Antimicrob Agents Chemother 37:939, 1993.
155. Osano E, Arakawa Y, Wacharotayankun R, et al: Molecular characterization of an enterobacterial metallo β-lactamase found in a clinical isolate of *Serratia marcescens* that shows imipenem resistance. Antimicrob Agents Chemother 38:71, 1994.
156. Ito H, Arakawa Y, Ohsuka S, et al: Plasmid-mediated dissemination of the metallo-β-lactamase gene bla_{IMP} among clinically isolated strains of *Serratia marcescens*. Antimicrob Agents Chemother 39:824, 1995.
157. Watanabe M, Iyobe S, Inoue M, et al: Transferable imipenem resistance in *Pseudomonas aeruginosa*. Antimicrob Agents Chemother 35:147, 1991.
158. Eliopoulos GM, Moellering RC Jr: A critical comparison of the newer aminoglycosidic aminocyclitol antibiotics. *In* Remington JS, Swartz MN (eds): Current Clinical Topics in Infectious Diseases, Vol 4. New York, McGraw-Hill, 1983, p 378.
159. Storrs MJ, Courvalin P, Foster TJ: Genetic analysis of gentamicin resistance in methicillin- and gentamicin-resistant strains of *Staphylococcus aureus* isolated in Dublin hospitals. Antimicrob Agents Chemother 32:1174, 1988.
160. Tomalsky ME, Chamorro RM, Crosa JH, et al: Transposon-mediated amikacin resistance in *Klebsiella pneumoniae*. Antimicrob Agents Chemother 32:1416, 1988.
161. Hodel-Christian SL, Murray BE: Characterization of the gentamicin resistance transposon Tn*5281* from *Enterococcus faecalis* and comparison to staphylococcal transposons Tn*4001* and Tn*4031*. Antimicrob Agents Chemother 35:1147, 1991.
162. Mitsuhashi S, Kawabe H: Aminoglycoside antibiotic resistance in bacteria. *In* Whelton A, Neu HC (eds): The Aminoglycosides: Microbiology, Clinical Use and Toxicology. New York, Marcel Dekker, 1982, p 97.
163. Carlier C, Courvalin P: Resistance of streptococci to aminoglycoside-aminocyclitol antibiotics. *In* Schlessinger D (ed): Microbiology: 1982. Washington, DC, American Society for Microbiology, 1982, p 162.
164. Shannon K, Phillips I: Mechanisms of resistance to aminoglycosides in clinical isolates. J Antimicrob Chemother 9:91, 1982.
165. Costa Y, Galimand M, Leclercq R, et al: Characterization of the chromosomal *acc(6′)-Ii* gene specific for *Enterococcus faecium*. Antimicrob Agents Chemother 37:1896, 1993.
166. Bongaerts GPA, Molendijk L: Relation between aminoglycoside 2″-*O*-nucleotidyl transferase activity and aminoglycoside resistance. Antimicrob Agents Chemother 25:234, 1984.
167. Perlin MH, Lerner SA: High-level amikacin resistance in *Escherichia coli* due to phosphorylation and impaired aminoglycoside uptake. Antimicrob Agents Chemother 29:216, 1986.
168. Eliopoulos GM, Eliopoulos CT: Antibiotic combinations: Should they be tested? Clin Microbiol Rev 1:139, 1988.
169. Ferretti JJ, Gilmore KS, Courvalin P: Nucleotide sequence analysis of the gene specifying bifunctional 6′-aminoglycoside acetyltransferase 2″-aminoglycoside phosphotransferase enzyme in *Streptococcus faecalis* and identification and cloning of gene regions specifying the two activities. J Bacteriol 167:631, 1986.
170. Menard R, Molinas C, Arthur M, et al: Overproduction of 3′-aminoglycoside phosphotransferase type I confers resistance to

tobramycin in *Escherichia coli.* Antimicrob Agents Chemother 37:78, 1993.
171. Courvalin P, Ounissi H, Arthur M: Multiplicity of macrolide-lincosamide-streptogramin antibiotic resistance determinants. J Antimicrob Chemother 16(Suppl A):91, 1985.
172. Andremont A, Gerbaud G, Courvalin P: Plasmid-mediated high-level resistance to erythromycin in *Escherichia coli.* Antimicrob Agents Chemother 29:515, 1986.
173. Leclercq R, Courvalin P: Intrinsic and unusual resistance to macrolide, lincosamide, and streptogramin antibiotics in bacteria. Antimicrob Agents Chemother 35:1273, 1991.
174. O'Hara K, Kanda T, Ohmiya K, et al: Purification and characterization of macrolide 2′-phosphotransferase from a strain of *Escherichia coli* that is highly resistant to erythromycin. Antimicrob Agents Chemother 33:1354, 1989.
175. Leclercq R, Brisson-Noel A, Duval J, et al: Phenotypic expression and genetic heterogeneity of lincosamide inactivations in *Staphylococcus* spp. Antimicrob Agents Chemother 31:1887, 1987.
176. Rende-Fournier R, Leclercq R, Galimand M, et al: Identification of the *satA* gene encoding a streptogramin A acetyltransferase in *Enterococcus faecium* BM4145. Antimicrob Agents Chemother 37:2119, 1993.
177. Nakagawa Y, Nitahara Y, Miyamura S: Kinetic studies on enzymatic acetylation of chloramphenicol in *Streptococcus faecalis.* Antimicrob Agents Chemother 16:719, 1979.
178. Neu HC, Fu KP: In vitro activity of chloramphenicol and thiamphenicol analogs. Antimicrob Agents Chemother 18:311, 1980.
179. Park BH, Levy SB: The cryptic tetracycline resistance determinants on Tn*4400* mediates tetracycline degradation as well as tetracycline efflux. Antimicrob Agents Chemother 32:1797, 1988.
180. Speer BS, Salyers AA: Novel aerobic tetracycline resistance gene that chemically modifies tetracycline. J Bacteriol 171:148, 1989.
181. Speer BS, Shoemaker NB, Salyers AA: Bacterial resistance to tetracycline: Mechanisms, transfers, and clinical significance. Clin Microbiol Rev 5:387, 1992.
182. Dabbs ER, Yazawa K, Mikami Y, et al: Ribosylation by mycobacterial strains as a new mechanism of rifampin inactivation. Antimicrob Agents Chemother 39:1007, 1995.
183. Archer GL: Antimicrobial susceptibility and selection of resistance among *Staphylococcus epidermidis* isolates recovered from patients with infections of indwelling foreign devices. Antimicrob Agents Chemother 14:353, 1978.
184. Thabaut A, Durosoir J-L: Comparative in vitro antibacterial activity of pefloxacin (1589RB), nalidixic acid, pipemidic acid and flumequin. Drugs Exp Clin Res 9:229, 1983.
185. Gutmann L, Williamson R, Moreau N, et al: Cross-resistance to nalidixic acid, trimethoprim, and chloramphenicol associated with alterations in outer membrane proteins of *Klebsiella, Enterobacter,* and *Serratia.* J Infect Dis 151:501, 1985.
186. Martin C, Gomez-Lus R, Ortiz JM, et al: Structure and mobility of an ampicillin and gentamicin resistance determinant. Antimicrob Agents Chemother 31:1266, 1987.
187. Jacoby GA: Resistance plasmids of *Pseudomonas aeruginosa. In* Bryan LE (ed): Antimicrobial Drug Resistance. Orlando, FL, Academic Press, 1984, p 497.
188. Tuberculosis Chemotherapy Trials Committee of the Medical Research Council: The treatment of pulmonary tuberculosis with isoniazid. Br Med J 2:735, 1952.
189. Cohn ML, Middlebrook G, Russell WF Jr: Combined drug treatment of tuberculosis. I. Prevention of emergence of mutant populations of tubercle bacilli resistant to both streptomycin and isoniazid. J Clin Invest 38:1349, 1959.
190. Karchmer AW, Archer GL, Dismukes WE Jr: Rifampin treatment of prosthetic valve endocarditis due to *Staphylococcus epidermidis.* Am J Med 75(Suppl 2A):90, 1983.
191. Eliopoulos GM, Moellering RC Jr: Antimicrobial combinations. *In* Lorian V (ed): Antibiotics in Laboratory Medicine, ed 3. Baltimore, Williams & Wilkins, 1991, p 432.
192. Spitzer PG, Eliopoulos GM: Antibiotic resistance in the intensive care unit and mechanisms of spread. *In* Farber BF (ed): Infection Control in Intensive Care. New York, Churchill Livingstone, 1987, p 189.
193. O'Brien TF, Acar JF: Antibiotic resistance worldwide. *In* Peterson PK, Verhoef J (eds): Antimicrobial Agents Annual 2. Amsterdam, Elsevier Science Publishing, 1987, p 457.
194. Rice LB, Willey SH, Papanicolaou GA, et al: Outbreak of ceftazidime resistance caused by extended-spectrum β-lactamases at a Massachusetts chronic care facility. Antimicrob Agents Chemother 34:2193, 1990.
195. Murray BE: Can antibiotic resistance be controlled? N Engl J Med 330:1229, 1994.
196. Shulman JA, Terry PM, Hough CE: Colonization with gentamicin-resistant *Pseudomonas aeruginosa,* pyocin type 5, in a burn unit. J Infect Dis 124(Suppl):S18, 1971.
197. Klein BS, Perloff WH, Maki DG: Reduction of nosocomial infection during pediatric intensive care by protective isolation. N Engl J Med 320:1714, 1989.
198. Anonymous. Antimicrobial prophylaxis in surgery. Med Lett Drugs Ther 34:5, 1992.

32

Antiviral Therapy

Richard J. Whitley

Compared with the remarkable progress made in the treatment of bacterial infections in the past four decades, advances in the chemotherapy of viral diseases have been slower. In the United States, only a few antiviral agents of proven value are available for a limited number of clinical indications. Unique problems are associated with the development of antiviral agents. First, viruses are obligate intracellular parasites that utilize many biochemical pathways of the infected host cell. Historically, clinically useful antiviral activity has been difficult to achieve without also adversely affecting normal host cell metabolism, causing toxic effects in uninfected cells. Second, early diagnosis of viral infection is crucial for effective antiviral therapy because, by the time symptoms appear, several cycles of viral multiplication have usually occurred and replication is waning. Precise diagnosis is difficult for many viral infections because of the lack of specificity of many viral syndromes, for example, coryza and cough for rhinovirus infection or the encephalopathy associated with herpes simplex encephalitis. As a consequence, effective antiviral therapy is dependent on rapid, sensitive, specific, and practical means of diagnosing viral diseases. Nevertheless, there are some viral infections, such as herpes zoster or genital herpes, for which a clinical diagnosis is relatively routine. Third, because many of the disease syndromes caused by viruses are common, relatively benign, and self-limiting, the therapeutic index, or ratio of efficacy to toxicity, must be extremely high for therapy to be acceptable. Obviously, there are exceptions to this observation, as encountered with herpes simplex encephalitis or cytomegalovirus (CMV) retinitis. Fortunately, research in molecular biology is helping solve two of these problems. Enzymes unique to viral replication have been identified and, therefore, clearly distinguish between virus and host cell functions. Unique events in viral replication serve as ideal targets for antiviral agents; examples include the thymidine kinase (TK) of herpes simplex virus (HSV) and reverse transcriptase of human immunodeficiency virus (HIV). Second, several early, sensitive, and specific diagnostic methods for viral illnesses have been made possible by recombinant DNA technology, such as methods using monoclonal antibodies, DNA hybridization, and the polymerase chain reaction.

As with all infectious diseases, the effectiveness of therapy often depends on host defenses, and this principle is of paramount importance when discussing antiviral agents. Immunocompromised patients are at increased risk for the development of symptomatic herpesvirus infections and deserve special note. All herpesviruses become latent, and reactivation results in an extremely high incidence of both infection and disease. In renal transplant recipients, for example, 40% to 70% reactivate latent HSV infections; 80% to 100% reactivate CMV infections; and 5% to 35% reactivate varicella-zoster virus (VZV) infections within 1 year, as summarized.[1, 2] Not only is the incidence of reactivation high but also these infections are often more severe in the immunocompromised population, for example, varicella in children with leukemia, mucocutaneous HSV infections in organ transplant recipients, and CMV infections in bone marrow transplant recipients and patients with acquired immunodeficiency syndrome (AIDS).

Whereas most of this chapter addresses specific drugs, antiviral therapy includes both supportive measures and other therapeutic modalities often not considered as drug therapy, such as immunoglobulin therapy. Similarly, the use of interferons (IFNs) deserves mention, as well. After a consideration of the "nondrug" therapies, the subsequent discussion focuses on antiviral drugs for herpesvirus and respiratory virus infections.

Nonspecific Management of Viral Infections

Supportive Care

Because chemotherapeutic approaches are limited, symptomatic and supportive treatments, including bed rest, hydration, and analgesics, remain the management modalities for many viral diseases, particularly acute upper respiratory infections. Although nonspecific, these approaches are important. Data obtained with animal models help elucidate this principle. Severe, repetitive, and exhausting exercise in mice infected with coxsackievirus B3 prolongs infection and results in a delay in the appearance of both circulating IFN and type-specific serum neutralizing antibodies. Virologically, there is a marked increase in the quantity of virus detected in the myocardium, which is associated with higher mortality.[3]

Immunoglobulin Therapy

Efficacy has been established for prophylactic immunoglobulin administration for several viral infections. Although it has been suggested, the use of immunoglobulin therapy of established disease has not been proved unequivocally beneficial for any viral infection. This approach has been tried for the treatment of echovirus meningoencephalitis associated with agammaglobulinemia, chronic Epstein-Barr virus infection in adolescents and adults, and respiratory syncytial virus (RSV) disease[4] in hospitalized children. Currently, another active area of research is the use of CMV hyperimmune globulin for prevention and treatment of infection in bone marrow transplant patients.[5–8] Benefit has been shown for the administration of intravenous immunoglobulin and CMV hyperimmune globulin when combined with ganciclovir in the treatment of CMV pneumonia in bone marrow transplant recipients. Survival increased to 52% to 79%.[9, 10] This survival rate is significantly better than that of historical control subjects treated with either agent alone. Studies of RSV monoclonal antibodies for disease prevention and therapy are in progress, as noted.

Therapy of Herpesvirus Infections

Acyclovir and Valacyclovir

Acyclovir is the most widely prescribed and clinically effective antiviral drug available to date. Valacyclovir, the L-valine ester oral prodrug of acyclovir, was developed to improve the oral bioavailability of acyclovir.

CHEMISTRY, MECHANISM OF ACTION, AND ANTIVIRAL ACTIVITY

Acyclovir, 9-[2-(hydroxyethoxy)methyl]guanine, a synthetic acyclic purine nucleoside analog, is a selective inhibitor of replication of HSV types 1 and 2 and VZV.[11, 12] Acyclovir is converted by virus-encoded TK to its monophosphate derivative, an event that does not occur to any significant extent in uninfected cells.[13] Subsequent di- and triphosphorylation is catalyzed by cellular enzymes, resulting in acyclovir triphosphate concentrations 40 to 100 times higher in HSV-infected than in uninfected cells. Acyclovir triphosphate inhibits viral DNA synthesis by competing with deoxyguanosine triphosphate as a substrate for viral DNA polymerase.[14] Because acyclovir triphosphate lacks the 3′-hydroxyl group required for DNA chain elongation, viral DNA synthesis is terminated. Viral DNA polymerase is tightly associated with the terminated DNA chain and is functionally inactivated.[15] Also, the viral polymerase has greater affinity for acyclovir triphosphate than does cellular DNA polymerase, resulting in little incorporation of acyclovir into cellular DNA. In vitro, acyclovir is most active against HSV-1 (average median effective concentration = 0.04 μg/mL), HSV-2 (0.10 μg/mL), and VZV (0.50 μg/mL).[16] Epstein-Barr virus requires higher acyclovir concentrations for inhibition and CMV, which lacks a virus-specific TK, is resistant.

Valacyclovir is cleaved by valine hydrolase to acyclovir, which is then metabolized in infected cells to the active triphosphate of acyclovir. Because it is metabolized to acyclovir, it has the same in vitro spectrum of activity.

ABSORPTION, DISTRIBUTION, AND ELIMINATION

Acyclovir is available in topical, oral, and intravenous preparations. The topical preparation is 5% acyclovir in a polyethylene glycol ointment base. Oral formulations include a 200-mg capsule, an 800-mg tablet, and a suspension (200 mg per 5 mL). Absorption of acyclovir after oral administration is slow and incomplete, with oral bioavailability of about 15% to 30%.[17] After multidose oral administration of 200 or 800 mg of acyclovir, the mean steady-state peak levels are about 0.57 and 1.57 μg/mL, respectively.[18] Much higher plasma acyclovir levels can be achieved with intravenous administration. Steady-state peak acyclovir concentrations after intravenous doses of 5 or 10 mg/kg every 8 hours are about 9.9 and 20.0 μg/mL, respectively. Acyclovir penetrates most body tissues well, including the brain. The terminal plasma half-life is 2 to 3 hours in adults with normal renal function. Acyclovir is minimally metabolized and about 85% is excreted unchanged in the urine via renal tubular secretion and glomerular filtration. Acyclovir dosage adjustment is required for patients with impaired renal function. In patients with creatinine clearance (C_{cr}) greater than 50 mL/min, 100% of the recommended intravenous dose is given at 8-hour intervals. For a C_{cr} of 25 to 50 or 10 to 25 mL/min, the dosing interval is extended to 12 or 24 hours, respectively. If the C_{cr} is less than 10 mL/min, the standard intravenous dose is reduced by 50% and is given every 24 hours. Recommendations for use in renal impairment appear in Table 32–1. For patients with severe renal failure (C_{cr} < 10 mL/min), the dose of oral acyclovir should be reduced to 200 mg (for HSV)

TABLE 32–1 ■ Dosage Adjustment for Intravenous Acyclovir in Patients with Impaired Renal Function

CREATININE CLEARANCE (mL/min/1.73 m²)	% OF STANDARD DOSE	DOSING INTERVAL (h)
>50	100	8
25–50	100	12
10–25	100	24
0–10*	50	24

*Administered after hemodialysis.

or 800 mg (for VZV) every 12 hours. Acyclovir is readily removed by hemodialysis but not by peritoneal dialysis.

Valacyclovir is available only as a tablet formulation. It is metabolized nearly completely to acyclovir within minutes after absorption. Notably, plasma levels of acyclovir that are achieved after 2 g of valacyclovir given by mouth three times a day (tid) approximate those achieved with 5 mg/kg administered every 8 hours intravenously. Dosage adjustments are not required unless the C_{cr} is less than 25 mL/min, at which time the dosing frequency is decreased to twice daily (bid).

CLINICAL INDICATIONS

Herpes Simplex Virus Infections

Genital Herpes. Initial genital HSV infection can be treated with topical, oral, or intravenous acyclovir. Topical application of acyclovir reduces the duration of virus shedding and the time to complete lesion crusting but is less effective than oral or intravenous therapy.[19, 20] Intravenous acyclovir is the most effective treatment for first-episode genital herpes and results in a significant reduction in the median duration of virus shedding, pain, and time to complete healing (8 versus 14 days).[21, 22] Because intravenous acyclovir therapy usually requires hospitalization, it should be reserved for patients with systemic complications. Oral therapy (200 mg five times daily) is nearly as effective as intravenous acyclovir for initial genital herpes[23, 24] and has become the standard treatment. Neither intravenous nor oral acyclovir treatment of acute HSV infection alters the frequency of subsequent recurrences.[22, 24]

Recurrent genital herpes is less severe and resolves more rapidly than primary infection, offering a shorter time interval for successful antiviral chemotherapy. Topically applied acyclovir reduces the duration of virus shedding but has no significant effect on the clinical symptoms.[25, 26] Orally administered acyclovir shortens the duration of virus shedding and time to healing (6 versus 7 days) when initiated early (within 24 hours of onset), but the duration of pain and itching and the time to subsequent recurrence are not affected.[27, 28] Nevertheless, some physicians recommend episodic therapy of recurrences at a dosage of 200 mg five times daily or 400 mg tid.

Oral acyclovir is dramatically effective for suppression of frequently recurring genital herpes.[29–31] Daily administration of acyclovir reduced the frequency of recurrences by up to 80% and 25% to 30% of patients had no further recurrences while taking acyclovir.[30, 32] Successful suppression for as long as 3 years has been reported with no evidence of significant adverse effects.[32] Titration of acyclovir (400 mg bid or 200 mg two to five times daily) may be required to establish the minimal acyclovir dose that is most effective and economic. Acyclovir treatment should be interrupted at 12-month intervals to reassess the need for continued suppression.[33] Emergence of acyclovir-resistant HSV appears to be an infrequent occurrence in immunologically normal individuals,[34] although it has been documented.[35] Asymptomatic virus shedding can continue despite clinically effective acyclovir suppression, resulting in the possibility of person-to-person transmission.[36]

Valacyclovir has been studied for the treatment of recurrent genital herpes at a dosages of 1 g tid. Therapeutic benefit is equivalent to that of acyclovir administered at 200 mg tid or five times daily.[37]

Herpes Labialis. Topical therapy with 5% acyclovir for HSV-1 orolabial infections produced no clinical benefit,[38] probably because of poor penetration of drug to the site of viral replication. Orally administered acyclovir at a dose of 200 mg five times daily for 5 days reduced the time to loss of crust by approximately 1 day (7 versus 8 days) but did not alter the duration of pain or time to complete healing.[39] If the dose was increased to 400 mg five times daily for 5 days, treatment started during prodrome or erythema stages reduced the mean duration of pain by 36% and time to loss of crust by 27%.[40] Thus, oral acyclovir has modest clinical benefit only if initiated early after recurrence and it cannot be recommended for routine therapy of herpes labialis.

Short-term prophylactic acyclovir may benefit some patients with recurrent herpes labialis who anticipate high-risk activity (e.g., intense exposure to sunlight).[41] Intermittent acyclovir administration does not alter the frequency of subsequent recurrences.

Mucocutaneous Herpes Simplex Virus Infections in Immunocompromised Patients. HSV infections of the lip, mouth, skin, perianal area, or genitals may be more severe in immunocompromised patients than in normal hosts. Lesions tend to be more invasive, slower to heal, and associated with prolonged virus shedding. Clinical benefit from intravenous acyclovir is well documented.[42] Acyclovir recipients had a significantly shorter duration of virus shedding and accelerated lesion healing.[43] Oral acyclovir therapy is also effective for these conditions.[44] It is the treatment of choice for this entity.

Acyclovir prophylaxis of HSV infections is of significant clinical value in severely immunocompromised patients, especially those undergoing induction chemotherapy or organ transplantation. Administration of intravenous or oral acyclovir reduced the incidence of symptomatic HSV infection from about 7% to 5% to 20%.[45, 46] A sequential regimen of intravenous acyclovir followed by oral acyclovir for 3 to 6 months can virtually eliminate symptomatic HSV infections in transplant recipients. Various oral dosing regimens, ranging from 200 mg tid to 800 mg bid, have been used successfully. Among bone marrow transplant recipients, acyclovir-resistant HSV isolates have been identified more frequently after therapeutic acyclovir administration than during prophylaxis.[47–49] Acyclovir has become a therapeutic mainstay for physicians in treating and suppressing herpesvirus infections in immunocompromised patients.

Herpes Simplex Encephalitis. Herpes simplex encephalitis is associated with significant morbidity and mortality in spite of antiviral therapy.[50, 51] Acyclovir therapy at 10 mg/kg every 8 hours for 10 to 14 days reduced mortality at 3 months to 19%, compared with approximately 50% among vidarabine recipients.[50] Furthermore, 38% of acyclovir recipients returned to normal function. These data stress the need for improved therapeutic regimens for herpes simplex encephalitis.

Neonatal Herpes Simplex Virus Infections. Newborns with HSV infections can be classified as having disease: (1) localized to skin, eye, and mouth; (2) of the central nervous system (CNS); or (3) disseminated (multiorgan). Acyclovir was shown to be as effective as (but not superior to) vidarabine treatment.[52] No infant with disease localized to the skin, eye, or mouth died, whereas 18% and 55% of infants with CNS or disseminated infection, respectively, died. Among infants with HSV localized to the skin, eye, and mouth, 90% and 98% of vidarabine and acyclovir recipients, respectively, were developing normally 2 years after infection. Among infants who survived encephalitis, 50% of vidarabine and 43% of acyclovir recipients were developing normally. Among survivors of disseminated infection, 62% of vidarabine and 57% of acyclovir recipients were developing normally. Thus, in contrast to the therapy of herpes simplex encephalitis in older patients, there were no significant differences in either morbidity or mortality between acyclovir and vidarabine treatments. Clearance of virus from infants who received acyclovir was slower than from immunocompromised adults, implying a requirement for host defense. To improve outcome, therapy must prevent progression of infection to the CNS or disseminated disease. The safety and ease of administration of acyclovir prompt its recommendation as the treatment of choice for neonatal HSV infections. The currently recommended intravenous dose is 10 mg/kg every 8 hours. Long-term oral suppressive therapy may be of value but warrants careful evaluation.[53]

Other Herpes Simplex Virus Infections. Case reports have described the successful use of acyclovir in the treatment of other HSV infections such as hepatitis, pulmonary infections, herpetic esophagitis, proctitis, eczema herpeticum, erythema multiforme, and herpetic whitlow. Topical acyclovir for HSV ocular infections is effective but probably not superior to trifluorothymidine.[54]

Varicella-Zoster Virus Infections

Varicella. Oral acyclovir therapy in normal children and adolescents with chickenpox shortened the duration of new lesion formation by about 1 day, reduced total lesion count, and improved constitutional symptoms.[55, 56] In a group of adolescents and adults with chickenpox, oral acyclovir therapy initiated within 24 hours of the appearance of the rash reduced the total number of lesions and time to total crusting from about 8 to 7 days.[57, 58] Therapy of older patients with chickenpox (who may have more severe manifestations) appears indicated, but treatment of younger children must be decided on a case-by-case basis. In uncontrolled studies, intravenous acyclovir may improve the outcome of varicella pneumonia in adults, including pregnant women.[59]

Acyclovir therapy of chickenpox in immunocompromised children substantially reduces morbidity and mortality. In placebo-controlled trials, treatment with intravenous acyclovir improved the outcome, as evidenced by a reduction of VZV pneumonitis from 45% to less than 5%.[60, 61] The treatment of choice is intravenous acyclovir at a dosage of 500 mg/m^3 every 8 hours for 7 to 10 days; oral acyclovir therapy is not indicated for immunocompromised children with chickenpox.

Herpes Zoster. Intravenous acyclovir therapy of herpes zoster in the normal host produced some acceleration of cutaneous healing but had no consistent beneficial effects on acute neuritis or postherpetic neuralgia.[62, 63] Oral acyclovir administration (800 mg five times a day) resulted in accelerated cutaneous healing and reduction of the severity of acute neuritis.[64, 65] In placebo-controlled trials, acyclovir therapy accelerated cessation of new vesicle formation from 7.4 to 6.2 days and time to crusting from 10.1 to 8.4 days.[64] Clinical benefits of therapy were most evident when drug administration was initiated within 48 hours of disease onset. Oral acyclovir treatment of herpes zoster ophthalmicus reduced the incidence of serious ocular complications such as keratitis and uveitis.[66] If therapy can be initiated within 48 hours of the onset of rash, oral acyclovir (800 mg five times per day) is one of two choices for immunocompetent patients with localized herpes zoster, especially those with trigeminal nerve involvement. Of note, metaanalysis of the acyclovir placebo-controlled data indicated statistically significant benefit for reduction of postherpetic neuralgia.[66a]

Valacyclovir has been extensively evaluated for the treatment of herpes zoster in the immunocompetent host at 1 g tid for 7 days or longer. These studies indicated that valacyclovir is superior to acyclovir for the reduction of persistent pain associated with shingles. Treatment with valacyclovir is recommended for the normal host suffering from shingles[67] and was approved by the U.S. Food and Drug Administration.

The increased frequency of significant morbidity in immunocompromised patients with herpes zoster highlights the need for effective antiviral chemotherapy. Intravenous acyclovir significantly reduced the frequency of cutaneous dissemination and visceral complications of herpes zoster in immunocompromised adults.[68, 69] Acyclovir has become the standard therapy at a dose of 10 mg/kg or 500 mg/m^2 every 8 hours for 7 to 10 days. No data exist to document the efficacy of oral acyclovir therapy in immunocompromised patients with herpes zoster, although oral acyclovir is frequently prescribed.

RESISTANCE

Resistance of HSV to acyclovir can develop through mutations in the viral gene encoding TK via generation of TK-deficient mutants or the selection of mutants possessing a TK that is unable to phosphorylate acyclovir.[70, 71] Clinical isolates resistant to acyclovir are almost uniformly deficient in TK, although DNA polymerase mutants have been recovered from HSV-infected patients.[72, 73] Drug resistance was considered rare, and resistant isolates were thought to be less pathogenic[47] until a series of acyclovir-resistant HSV isolates from patients with AIDS were characterized.[74] These resistant mutants were deficient in TK but remained sensitive to vidarabine and foscarnet, drugs that do not require viral TK for activation.[75, 76] Acyclovir-resistant HSV isolates have been identified as the cause of pneumonia,[77] encephalitis,[78] esophagitis,[72] and mucocutaneous infections,[79, 80] all occurring in immunocompromised patients. Acyclovir-resistant mutants have been described in the normal host.[35, 73] Acyclovir-resistant isolates of VZV have been identified much less frequently than acyclovir-resistant HSV but have been recovered from marrow transplant recipients and AIDS patients.[81, 82] The acyclovir-resistant VZV isolates all had altered or absent TK function but remained susceptible to vidarabine and foscarnet.[83]

Valacyclovir, because it is metabolized to acyclovir, should have the same sensitivity patterns as the parent compound.

ADVERSE EFFECTS

Acyclovir and valacyclovir therapies are associated with few adverse effects. Renal dysfunction induced by acyclovir has been reported but appears to be relatively uncommon and is usually reversible.[84, 85] Creatinine elevations have been noted in patients given large doses of acyclovir by rapid intravenous infusion and have been attributed to crystallization of drug in the renal tubules and collecting ducts, resulting in a transient nephropathy.[86] The risk of nephrotoxicity can be minimized by administering acyclovir by slow infusion during 1 hour and ensuring adequate hydration. Neither oral acyclovir nor valacyclovir therapy has been associated with renal dysfunction. A few reports have linked intravenous acyclovir use with CNS disturbances including agitation, hallucinations, disorientation, tremors, and myoclonus.[87, 88]

An Acyclovir in Pregnancy Registry has gathered data on prenatal acyclovir exposures. Although no significant risk to the mother or fetus has been documented, the total number of monitored pregnancies remains too small to detect any low-frequency events.[89] Because acyclovir crosses the placenta and can concentrate in amniotic fluid, there is concern about the potential for fetal nephrotoxicity, although none has been observed.[90]

CONCLUSIONS ON ACYCLOVIR AND VALACYCLOVIR

The synthesis of acyclovir was a true milestone in the development of selective and specific inhibitors of viral replication. A large number of carefully conducted clinical trials have clearly established acyclovir as the drug of choice for a wide range of infections caused by HSV and VZV. Because of the enhanced plasma concentrations of acyclovir that are achieved after valacyclovir administration, the latter drug is likely to be the treatment of choice for shingles and, perhaps, genital herpes. The appearance of isolates resistant to acyclovir underscores the necessity for continued development of new agents with alternative mechanisms of action.

Foscarnet

CHEMISTRY, MECHANISM OF ACTION, AND ANTIVIRAL ACTIVITY

Foscarnet, a pyrophosphate analog of phosphonoacetic acid, has potent in vitro and in vivo activity against herpesviruses. Unacceptable toxicity was demonstrated with phosphonoacetic acid (deposition in bone), but foscarnet is less toxic. These drugs inhibit the DNA polymerase of all human herpesviruses by blocking the pyrophosphate binding site, thus inhibiting the formation of the 3′-5′ phosphodiester bond between primer and substrate and preventing chain elongation. Unlike acyclovir, which requires activation by a virus-specific TK, foscarnet acts directly on the virus DNA polymerase. TK-deficient, acyclovir-resistant herpesviruses remain sensitive to foscarnet. Foscarnet has been used successfully to treat severe mucocutaneous HSV infections caused by acyclovir-resistant HSV-2.[91] It also inhibits influenza A RNA-dependent RNA polymerase and the reverse transcriptase of several other animal and human retroviruses, including HIV.

ABSORPTION, DISTRIBUTION, AND ELIMINATION

The oral bioavailability of foscarnet is extremely poor; thus, administration is by the intravenous route. An intravenous infusion of 60 mg/kg every 8 hours results in peak and trough plasma concentrations of approximately 450 to 575 and 80 to 150 μM, respectively. The cerebrospinal fluid concentration of foscarnet is approximately two thirds of the plasma level.

Renal excretion is the primary route of clearance of foscarnet, with more than 80% of the dose appearing in the urine. Bone sequestration also occurs, resulting in complex plasma elimination.

CLINICAL INDICATIONS

Foscarnet is licensed for the treatment of CMV retinitis in individuals with HIV infection as well HSV and VZV isolates that are resistant to acyclovir or penciclovir in immunocompromised hosts. Administration of foscarnet at 60 mg/kg every 8 hours for 14 to 21 days followed by maintenance therapy at 90 to 120 mg/kg per day was associated with stabilization of retinal disease in approximately 90% of patients.[92] However, as is with the case with ganciclovir therapy of CMV retinitis, relapse occurs.[93]

The clinical trial group studies of ocular complications of AIDS[94] demonstrated improved overall survival in HIV-infected patients with CMV retinitis who received foscarnet[94] compared with ganciclovir recipients. However, there was no difference between drugs in the overall stabilization or persistence of therapeutic value for CMV retinitis. Studies of the Ocular Complication of AIDS has terminated a clinical trial utilizing a combination of foscarnet and ganciclovir because of enhanced and significant clinical benefit in prevention of relapse of disease. The basis of prolonged survival in foscarnet recipients is unknown but may be related to the drug's anti-HIV activity.

Mucocutaneous infections caused by HSV and those caused by VZV in immunocompromised hosts can be treated with foscarnet at dosages lower than that for the management of CMV retinitis. Foscarnet dosages of 40 mg/kg administered every 8 hours for 7 days or longer resulted in cessation of virus shedding and healing of lesions in the majority of patients.[76] However, as one might imagine, relapses occur that may or may not be amenable to acyclovir therapy.

RESISTANCE

Isolates of HSV, CMV, and VZV have all been demonstrated to develop resistance to foscarnet both in the laboratory and in the clinical setting.[95, 96] Isolates of HSV that are resistant to foscarnet have median effective concentrations higher than 100 μg/mL. These isolates are all DNA polymerase mutants.

ADVERSE EFFECTS

Although foscarnet has significant activity in the management of herpesvirus infections, toxicity is a major problem with its administration. Significant nephrotoxicity, including acute tubular necrosis and interstitial nephritis, is associated with its administration and has resulted in limited clinical use of the compound. In addition, metabolic aberrations of calcium, magnesium, phosphate, and other electrolytes have been associated with foscarnet administration and, therefore, warrant careful monitoring. Symptomatic hypocalcemia is the most common metabolic abnormality. Seizures, secondary to hypocalcemia, have been associated with foscarnet therapy but usually in patients with an underlying CNS disease. Drug interactions have been encountered with nephrotoxic agents, pentamidine, and zidovudine. Increases in serum creatinine level develop in one half of patients who receive this medication but are usually reversible after cessation. Other CNS side effects include headache (25% of patients), tremor, irritability, and hallucinations.

CONCLUSIONS ON FOSCARNET

Clearly, foscarnet has a role in the physician's armamentarium for the management of CMV infections in high-risk populations of patients, particularly patients with AIDS who suffer from CMV retinitis. The utilization of this compound requires vigilance for potential untoward affects.

Ganciclovir

CHEMISTRY, MECHANISM OF ACTION, AND ANTIVIRAL ACTIVITY

CMV infections are a major cause of morbidity and mortality in immunocompromised patients. CMV retinitis occurs in 15% to 46% of patients with AIDS.[97] Infection rates in organ transplant recipients average 50% to 60% and higher.[98–102] CMV pneumonia can occur at a frequency as high as 17% in bone marrow transplant recipients and has an associated mortality as high as 85%, even with therapy.[103, 104] In 1982, four laboratories independently reported the activity of ganciclovir against CMV.[105–109] Ganciclovir, 9-[1,3-dihydroxy-2-propoxy)methyl]guanine (Cytovene), has enhanced in vitro activity against all herpesviruses compared with acyclovir, including 8 to 20 times greater antiviral activity against CMV.[106, 107] Although potential toxicity prevents the use of ganciclovir for relatively benign CMV diseases, the absence of any other therapeutic agents for CMV infection allows ganciclovir to be an important therapeutic agent for life- and sight-threatening diseases. As with acyclovir, the activity of ganciclovir in herpesvirus-infected cells depends on phosphorylation by virus-induced TK. Also as with acyclovir, ganciclovir monophosphate is further converted to its di- and triphosphate derivatives by cellular kinases. In cells infected by HSV-1 or HSV-2, ganciclovir triphosphate competitively inhibits the incorporation of guanosine triphosphate into viral DNA. Ganciclovir triphosphate is incorporated at internal and terminal sites of viral DNA and inhibits DNA synthesis. The mode of action of ganciclovir against CMV is mediated by a protein kinase, UL-97, that efficiently promotes the obligatory initial phosphorylation of ganciclovir to its monophosphate.[107, 110–113]

ABSORPTION, DISTRIBUTION, AND ELIMINATION

The oral bioavailability of ganciclovir is poor, approximately 5% to 7%.[114, 115] Peak and trough plasma levels are approximately 1 and 0.5 μg/mL, respectively, after administration of 1 g every 6 hours. Intravenous administration of a standard dose of 5 mg/kg results in peak and trough plasma concentrations of 8 to 11 and 0.5 to 1.2 μg/mL, respectively. Concentrations of ganciclovir in critical biologic fluids, including the aqueous humor and cerebrospinal fluid, tend to be less than those in the plasma. The plasma elimination half-life is 2 to 4 hours for individuals with normal renal function. The kidney is the major route of clearance of the drug, and therefore impaired renal function requires adjustment of dosage.

CLINICAL INDICATIONS

Human Immunodeficiency Virus–Infected Patients. In the absence of therapy, CMV retinitis in patients with AIDS is progressive and eventually causes blindness. Ganciclovir has been administered to large number of AIDS patients with CMV retinitis. Most patients (78%) experienced either improvement or stabilization of their retinitis as shown by fundoscopic examinations compared with only 2 of 20 historical controls.[116] Induction therapy is usually at a dosage of 5.0 mg/kg bid given intravenously for 10 to 14 days. Maintenance therapy is essential. Median time to relapse for patients receiving no maintenance therapy averages 47 days. Maintenance therapy at 25 to 35 mg/kg per week significantly lengthened the median time to relapse to 105 days.[117, 118] Virtually every patient treated experienced either a cessation or reduction of plasma viremia.[118] Cultures of urine and blood usually became negative after 7 to 10 days of treatment.[118] Visual acuity usually stabilizes at pretreatment levels but rarely improves dramatically. Relapse occurs quickly in the absence of maintenance therapy, but usually occurs, eventually, even in patients receiving maintenance therapy. The optimal dosing schedule for maintenance therapy is unknown, but doses of 5 mg/kg for 5 to 7 d/wk are currently recommended. The significance of bone marrow toxicity must be taken into consideration as well, because 30% to 40% of patients in these studies developed neutropenia.[117, 119]

Similar reports of benefit have appeared with the use of ganciclovir for the treatment of other CMV infections in AIDS patients, particularly those involving the gastrointestinal tract, as 85% of patients showed improvement or stabilization of disease.[120] Although benefit has been reported in the treatment of CMV pneumonia in AIDS patients, evaluation of therapies for CMV infection in the lungs (i.e., pneumonia) of these patients is particularly difficult because of the high incidence of concurrent lung infections and the high incidence of positive CMV cultures in the absence of disease. It must also be borne in mind that most CMV infections in AIDS patients recur after discontinuation of therapy.

During the past several years, oral administration of ganciclovir for the treatment for CMV retinitis in patients with AIDS as well as the prevention of CMV end organ disease in the same population has been studied. The utilization of ganciclovir at a dosage of 1 g three to six times daily after intravenous induction therapy provides a sustained period before the next episode of reactivated retinitis at intervals similar to, albeit smaller (but not significantly) than, those required when drug is given intravenously. These data are predicated on retinal photographs defining evidence of disease progression.[121]

Similarly, for HIV-infected individuals with $CD4^+$ cell counts less than 200/mm^3 a placebo-controlled prophylactic study demonstrated that end organ disease was significantly delayed in patients who received ganciclovir. Both of these observations have led to a recommendation of licensure by the U.S. Food and Drug Administration.

Organ Transplant Recipients. Therapy of opportunistic CMV infections in organ transplant recipients is complicated by the fact that decreasing immunosuppressants is usually impossible, hence elimination of CMV infection is rare if not impossible. Nonetheless, CMV infections are extremely common and the cause of significant morbidity and mortality in these populations of patients. The lung is among the most common sites of serious CMV disease for which therapy has been reported to be beneficial.[122, 123] Adverse effects were common; neutropenia and thrombocytopenia developed in 38% and 25% respectively, and CNS toxicity was noted in 25% of patients. Benefit from ganciclovir in treating CMV pneumonia in organ transplant patients is therefore suggested. Nonetheless, treatment of CMV pneumonia with ganciclovir has become standard as it has for other life- or sight-threatening CMV infections.

Bone Marrow Transplant Patients. CMV infections in bone marrow transplant recipients are more frequently devastating than in any other population of patients. CMV pneumonia can occur in as many as 17% of these patients and, if untreated, has a mortality as high as 85%.[124] Disease prevalence varies greatly from one transplant center to another. One trial demonstrated an excellent virologic response, with all CMV-infected patients becoming culture-negative by the fourth day of therapy, and respiratory secretions from 9 of the 10 patients becoming negative at a median of 8 days; however, only 1 of 10 patients survived.[124] Subsequent reports have suggested some benefit, including survival of 8 of 21 patients (38%) with documented CMV pneumonia.[125] An additional two patients responded to ganciclovir; one of these patients had a relapse with fatal CMV pneumonia 60 days after induction therapy, and the other died of disseminated aspergillosis on day 78. No CMV disease was demonstrated in the latter patient at autopsy. Ganciclovir combined with intravenous immunoglobulin adds benefit in the treatment of bone marrow transplant recipients with CMV pneumonia.[9, 10]

Ganciclovir has been administered in anticipation of CMV disease to bone marrow transplant recipients. Several clinical trials utilizing different designs (e.g., initiation of ganciclovir after engraftment versus initiation at the time of demonstration of infection by bronchial alveolar lavage but in the absence of clinical symptoms) have established the effectiveness of ganciclovir in preventing CMV pneumonia and reducing mortality during the period of treatment.[126–128] The utilization of ganciclovir under these circumstances is gaining enhanced support among transplant physicians; however, long-term survival benefit (>120 days) is not apparent.

RESISTANCE

A laboratory strain of CMV resistant to ganciclovir was demonstrated by Biron and colleagues.[129] Clinical resistance to CMV was reported by Erice and coworkers[130] for three patients who had ganciclovir-resistant virus, each with persistent CMV viremia and a deteriorating clinical course. With the prolonged ganciclovir treatment that many AIDS patients and other immunocompromised patients receive, resistance to this drug may soon become an important problem. Ganciclovir resistance should continue to attract our attention. With progressive CMV retinitis disease, switching to foscarnet therapy seems appropriate.

Two mechanisms of resistance to ganciclovir have been documented. First, the alteration of a protein kinase gene, identified as *UL97*, reduces the intracellular phosphorylation of ganciclovir, thereby rendering it inactive. The second mechanism of resistance is that of point mutations in the viral DNA polymerase gene.[131, 132] Resistance is associated with decreased sensitivity by a factor of up to 20.

ADVERSE EFFECTS

The most important side effects of ganciclovir, on the basis of animal studies and clinical trials, are the development of dose-limiting neutropenia and thrombocytopenia.[116] Neutropenia occurs in approximately 24% to 38% of all patients, most commonly in AIDS patients. The neutropenia is usually reversible with adjustment of the dosage of ganciclovir, including withholding treatment. Nevertheless, some patients have had irreversible leukopenia. Agents with significant myelotoxicity, such as antimetabolites or alkylating agents, cannot be used concomitantly with ganciclovir. Zidovudine (Retrovir, azidothymidine) is also contraindicated for patients receiving ganciclovir, which results in difficult management decisions for many patients with AIDS. Thrombocytopenia occurs in 6% to 19% of patients. Numerous other side effects possibly related to ganciclovir, such as nausea, vomiting, dizziness, and headache, are usually not of clinical significance.

Ganciclovir also has significant gonadal toxicity in animal models, most notably as a potent inhibitor of spermatogenesis.[116] It causes an increased incidence of tumors in the preputial gland of male mice, a finding of unknown significance. As an agent affecting DNA synthesis, ganciclovir has carcinogenic potential.[116]

CONCLUSIONS ON GANCICLOVIR

Ganciclovir has been the most widely tested drug for the treatment of CMV infections. There is support for clinical use for patients with AIDS who have CMV retinitis and gastrointestinal infection. Benefit is suggested but has been less dramatic for CMV pneumonia in immunocompromised hosts, but ganciclovir therapy has, nonetheless, become standard treatment.

Idoxuridine and Trifluorothymidine

CHEMISTRY, MECHANISM OF ACTION, AND ANTIVIRAL ACTIVITY

Idoxuridine (5-iodo-2′-deoxyuridine) and trifluorothymidine (trifluridine, Viroptic) are analogs of thymidine. When administered systemically, these nucleosides are phosphorylated by both viral and cellular TK to active triphosphorate derivatives that inhibit both viral and cellular DNA synthesis. The result is antiviral activity but also sufficient host cytotoxicity to prevent the systemic use of these drugs. The toxicity of idoxuridine was confirmed when it was administered parenterally for herpes simplex encephalitis in the early 1970s.[133] However, the toxicity of these compounds is not significant when they are applied topically to the eye in the treatment of HSV keratitis. Idoxuridine is, in fact, the first antiherpes drug with biologic activity.[134, 135] Both idoxuridine and trifluorothymidine are effective and licensed for treatment of HSV keratitis.

ABSORPTION, DISTRIBUTION, AND ELIMINATION

Topically applied idoxuridine or trifluorothymidine penetrates cells of the cornea. Low levels of drugs can be detected in the aqueous humor. Systemic concentrations of drug in the plasma are not detected after topical therapy of ocular disease.

CLINICAL INDICATIONS

Trifluorothymidine is the most efficacious of these compounds.[136] These agents are not of proven value in the treatment of stromal keratitis or uveitis, although trifluridine is more likely to penetrate the cornea and, ultimately, may prove to be beneficial for these conditions. Some forms of stromal keratitis and uveitis are thought to be caused by immune mechanisms and, thus, would not respond to antiviral drugs.[134] This suggested pathogenesis serves as the rationale for the use of topical corticosteroids in the treatment of these conditions.

RESISTANCE

Little effort has been directed to evaluating HSV isolates obtained from the eye, in large part because of the difficulty in accomplishing this task. As a consequence, clinical resistance to idoxuridine has not attracted attention from the biomedical community.

ADVERSE EFFECTS

The ophthalmic preparation of idoxuridine and trifluridine causes local irritation, photophobia, edema of the eyelids and cornea, punctual occlusion, and superficial punctate keratopathy.[136]

Penciclovir and Famciclovir

CHEMISTRY, MECHANISM OF ACTION, AND ANTIVIRAL ACTIVITY

A new member of the guanine nucleoside family of drugs is famciclovir (Famvir), the prodrug of penciclovir, which is approved worldwide. Penciclovir does not have significant oral bioavailability (less than 5%). However, famciclovir provides excellent oral bioavailability (approximately 77%) and appears to have a good therapeutic index for the therapy of both HSV and VZV infections.[137] Famciclovir is the diacetyl ester of 6-deoxypenciclovir. When administered orally, it is rapidly converted to penciclovir. The spectrum of activity of penciclovir and, therefore, famciclovir against human herpesviruses is similar to that of acyclovir.[138] Penciclovir is phosphorylated more efficiently than acyclovir in HSV- and VZV-infected cells. Host cell kinases phosphorylate both penciclovir and acyclovir to a small but comparable extent. The preferential metabolism in HSV- and VZV-infected cells is the major determinant of its antiviral activity. Penciclovir triphosphate has, on the average, a 10-fold longer intracellular half-life than acyclovir triphosphate in HSV-1–, HSV-2–, and VZV-infected cells after drug removal. Penciclovir triphosphate is formed at concentrations sufficient to be an effective inhibitor of viral DNA polymerase, albeit at a lower inhibition constant (K_i) than that of acyclovir triphosphate. Both compounds have good activity against HSV-1, HSV-2, and VZV. The activity of penciclovir in vitro, like that of acyclovir, depends on both the host cell and the assay (plaque reduction, virus yield, and viral DNA inhibition). The mean penciclovir median effective concentrations ± standard deviation for HSV-1 in MRC-5, human embryo lung (HEL), WISH, and WI38 cells are 0.4 ± 0.2, 0.6 ± 0.4, 0.2 ± 0.2, and 1.8 ± 0.8 μg/mL, respectively. These inhibitory concentrations are comparable to the inhibitory concentration of acyclovir. For HSV-2, similar levels of activity in the identical cell lines are 1.8 ± 0.6, 2.4 ± 2.5, 0.8 ± 0.1, and 0.3 ± 0.2 μg/mL, respectively. These assays utilize a plaque reduction procedure. In virus yield reduction assays, inhibition of VZV replication in MRC-5 cells is between 3.0 and 5.1 μg/mL, values virtually identical to those of acyclovir. Penciclovir, like acyclovir, is relatively inactive against CMV and Epstein-Barr virus. Penciclovir is also active against hepatitis B virus.

Activity against a variety of acyclovir-resistant strains has been examined. TK-negative strains are resistant to both penciclovir and acyclovir. The majority of acyclovir-resistant HSV and VZV clinical isolates are also cross-resistant to penciclovir; however, a few acyclovir-resistant strains have shown sensitivity to penciclovir. Foscarnet-resistant HSV isolates are susceptible to both penciclovir and acyclovir.

Cytotoxicity assays of uninfected cells, as assessed by thymidine incorporation, indicated median inhibitory concentrations (micrograms per milliliter) for both penciclovir and acyclovir in excess of the value of 100 μg/mL for most cell lines. Such values contribute to the conclusion that there is a high in vitro therapeutic index.

ABSORPTION, DISTRIBUTION, AND ELIMINATION

Conversion of famciclovir to penciclovir occurs at two levels. The major metabolic route of famciclovir is deacetylation of one ester group as the prodrug crosses the duodenal barrier of the gastrointestinal tract. The drug is transported to the liver via the portal vein, where the remaining ester group is removed and oxidation occurs at the sixth position of the side chain, resulting in penciclovir, the active drug. In humans, famciclovir is absorbed rapidly and extensively after oral administration. The first metabolite that appears in the plasma is almost entirely the deacetylated compound with little or no parent drug detected. Thus, the major metabolite, ultimately, of famciclovir is penciclovir. Maximal plasma concentrations of penciclovir indicate oral bioavailability of approximately 77% of famciclovir. Pharmacokinetic parameters for penciclovir are linear for famciclovir oral dose ranges of 125 to 750 mg. Penciclovir is eliminated rapidly and almost unchanged by active tubular secretion and glomerular filtration by the kidneys.[137] The elimination half-life in healthy subjects is approximately 2 hours. Food appears to slow the rate of conversion of famciclovir to penciclovir but has no effect on the ultimate extent of availability of penciclovir.[139] Dosages selected for human investigation include 125, 250, 500, and 750 mg per dose administered two or three times per day.

CLINICAL INDICATIONS

Herpes Zoster. In studies of shingles in individuals of all ages, more than 1200 patients have been evaluated in studies utilizing either placebo-controlled designs or administration of acyclovir as a control.[140, 141] Initial trials of famciclovir (250, 500, or 750 mg tid) indicated that it was equivalent to the standard acyclovir treatment of herpes zoster for cutaneous healing and, in a subgroup analysis, accelerated resolution of pain (zoster-associated pain).[140] A placebo-controlled study of famciclovir at a dosage of 500 or 250 mg tid indicated acceleration of cutaneous healing and a two- to threefold reduction of time to resolution of postherpetic neuralgia, the latter being most evident in patients older than 50 years. The interpretation of these studies has been questioned because of definitions and subgroup analyses, but the apparent finding of accelerated resolution of postherpetic neuralgia is important and warrants clarification. Future studies, clearly, will demonstrate the extent of this benefit.[142]

Genital Herpes Simplex Virus Infection. Studies of patients with recurrent genital HSV infection (with either intravenous penciclovir or oral famciclovir therapy) have indicated beneficial effects in acceleration of all aspects of improvement (e.g., pain, virus shedding, duration). For recurrent genital HSV infection, after intravenous penciclovir therapy, statistically significant benefit can be demonstrated for virtually all end points that reflect healing. Such end points include loss of lesions, pain, shorter duration of time for total healing, and decreased duration of viral excretion. Famciclovir given twice daily (125, 250, or 500 mg bid for 5 days) was found to be effective in the treatment of recurrent genital herpes. Studies of famciclovir therapy of primary genital HSV infection are in progress. Similarly, studies of the impact of famciclovir therapy on recurring HSV infections of immunocompromised hosts or effectiveness in suppressive therapy, particularly asymptomatic excretion of virus, remain to be completed.[143]

RESISTANCE

HSV and VZV isolates resistant to penciclovir have been identified in the laboratory. These isolates have similar patterns of resistance, as one might imagine, compared with acyclovir. Namely, resistance variance can be attributed to alterations or deficiencies of TK and DNA polymerase. The occurrence of clinically resistant mutants has not been identified. Acyclovir-resistant viruses share resistance, for the most part, with penciclovir.

ADVERSE EFFECTS

Therapy with oral famciclovir is well tolerated, being associated only with headache, diarrhea, and nausea, common findings with other orally bioavailable antiviral agents.[144] Preclinical studies of famciclovir found that chronic administration was tumorigenic (murine mammary tumors) and caused testicular toxicity in other rodents.[145] The implications of these findings for humans are unknown. Famciclovir also interacts with digoxin, resulting in increased plasma concentrations of this medication.[146]

CONCLUSIONS ON FAMCICLOVIR AND PENCICLOVIR

Famciclovir has significant activity in the treatment of herpes zoster in the elderly. The ease of administration three times daily compared with acyclovir (five times daily) provides a distinct advantage for famciclovir. Direct comparisons between valacyclovir and famciclovir are required to establish the choice between these medications.

Sorivudine

CHEMISTRY, MECHANISM OF ACTION, AND ANTIVIRAL ACTIVITY

Sorivudine (bromovinyl arabinosyluracil) is a nucleoside analog that was synthesized by Machida and colleagues.[147, 148]

Sorivudine has undergone field trial evaluation for the treatment of herpes zoster in Japanese volunteers and was licensed for the treatment of this disease in 1994 in that country. The compound is currently under evaluation in the United States, Canada, Europe, and Australia for the treatment of VZV infections in both normal and immunocompromised hosts.

Sorivudine is a pyrimidine nucleoside analog that has in vitro inhibitory activity against VZV at concentrations of 0.0001 to 0.004 μg/mL. These concentrations are more than 1000-fold lower than that required for the inhibition of VZV replication by acyclovir. Sorivudine is also an effective inhibitor of HSV-1 replication, with inhibitory concentrations ranging from 0.03 to 0.1 μg/mL. These concentrations are similar to those for acyclovir. Of note, sorivudine is inactive against HSV-2 and CMV.[149]

The uptake and phosphorylation of sorivudine have been studied in HSV-infected cells. Concentrations of drug and metabolites up to 40- to 190-fold higher can be detected in cells infected by HSV compared with mock infected cells. TK-deficient HSV isolates did not result in enhanced uptake of sorivudine. Not surprisingly, there was a significant 10-fold quantitative difference in the triphosphate derivatives of sorivudine with HSV-1 and HSV-2, implying the basis for the difference in sensitivity of these viruses.[150] K_i values were evaluated to determine the binding affinity of sorivudine to the virus-induced enzymes. Sorivudine has a high affinity for HSV-1–induced TK but virtually no affinity for HSV-2–induced TK human cytosol or mitochondrial induced TK. For example, the average K_i values were 0.94 μM for HSV-1 and 54.7 μM for HSV-2 but were greater than 100 μM for human kinases.[151] Initial phosphorylation is mediated by viral TK, and further metabolism to the diphosphate derivative is dependent on viral thymidylate kinase activity. Sorivudine triphosphate is a competitive inhibitor of viral DNA replication. Sorivudine triphosphate is not incorporated into viral DNA, as occurs with acyclovir triphosphate.[152] TK-negative VZV isolates are resistant to inhibition in the presence of sorivudine at varying concentrations.

ABSORPTION, DISTRIBUTION, AND ELIMINATION

Sorivudine is well absorbed when administered orally. Dose range studies have utilized sorivudine at 10, 20, 40, 80, and 100 mg given once a day for 14 days. The peak plasma level is achieved approximately 3 to 4 hours after administration. At dosages as low as 10 mg/d, a plasma level of 0.5 μg/mL is attained. At the highest dose evaluated, 100 mg, the peak plasma level was 5.0 μg/mL. The dosage evaluated in U.S. studies of sorivudine is 40 mg once daily. Mean peak and trough plasma concentrations for this dosage are 1.8 and 0.2 μg/mL, respectively. The plasma elimination half-life averages 5 to 7 hours. Plasma concentrations of sorivudine even at dosages as low as 10 mg once daily exceed by a factor of 10 the median effective dose for VZV.[149] The overall oral bioavailability of sorivudine is estimated to be in excess of 90%. Most drug is recovered unchanged in the urine, and less than 5% is excreted as the metabolite of sorivudine, namely bromovinyl uridine.

CLINICAL INDICATIONS

Three controlled clinical trials have been performed in the Western world that have evaluated sorivudine for the treatment of VZV infection. Additional studies are in progress. The studies that have been completed include a placebo-controlled study of chickenpox in Navy recruits and two acyclovir-controlled studies of localized zoster in individuals who have HIV infection.[153–155] None of these studies has yet appeared in the peer-reviewed literature. In the treatment of chickenpox, sorivudine accelerated the cessation of lesion formation and time to pustulation and healing when therapy was instituted within 72 hours after the onset of disease.

The European, Canadian, and Australian study of herpes zoster in HIV-infected individuals was terminated early because of evidence of accelerated cessation of lesion formation in sorivudine recipients.[155] The overall acceleration of cessation of lesion formation was approximately 1 day. The U.S. study of localized herpes zoster in HIV-infected individuals is currently under analysis.

RESISTANCE

Sorivudine-resistant VZV isolates have not been identified in the clinical arena. Serial laboratory passage will demonstrate that alteration of VZV TK will lead to resistance to sorivudine.

ADVERSE EFFECTS

During the pharmacokinetic studies of healthy volunteers, tolerance was acceptable. The most frequent complaints were nausea and vomiting, diarrhea, and headache. Elevated hepatic enzyme values were noted in a low percentage of patients.

In preclinical animal toxicology studies, a single-dose median lethal dose could not be achieved with the highest oral and intravenous doses tested. Further acceleration of the dosage administration regimen was limited because of the solubility of the compound. In animal toxicology studies conducted for 1, 3, and 6 months, the compound was well tolerated. Sorivudine was not teratogenic in rats. Mutagenicity studies with the Ames test, chromosome aberration test, and human lymphocyte sister chromatid exchange test were negative. At the highest doses tested (higher than anticipated for human administration), there was an increase in the incidence of hepatic and testicular neoplasms in rodents. The implication of these findings for human investigations is unknown.

CONCLUSIONS ON SORIVUDINE

Sorivudine is a unique nucleoside analog with significantly enhanced in vitro activity and oral bioavailability. Early indications from controlled studies indicate that sorivudine is superior to acyclovir for the treatment of localized zoster in individuals with HIV infection and chickenpox in adults. On the basis of experience in Japan, coadministration of sorivudine with 5-fluorouracil is contraindicated. Sorivudine inhibits dipyrimadole dehydrogenase, required for the metabolism of 5-fluorouracil. As a consequence, toxic levels of 5-fluorouracil accumulate in the plasma and have led to the deaths of nearly 30 patients in Japan.

Vidarabine

After the initial in vitro studies of de Rudder and colleagues[156] of the antiviral activity of vidarabine (Vira-A, adenine arabinoside, 9-β-D-arabinofuranosyladenine) against HSV, Miller and associates[157] demonstrated that other DNA viruses, particularly VZV and CMV, were sensitive to this compound in vitro as summarized.[50] Vidarabine is a purine nucleoside analog that is phosphorylated intracellularly to its mono-, di-, and triphosphate derivatives. The triphosphate derivative competitively inhibits DNA-dependent DNA polymerases of some DNA viruses approximately 40 times more than those of host cells. In addition, vidarabine is incorporated into terminal positions of both cellular and viral

DNA and thus inhibits elongation. Viral DNA synthesis is blocked at lower doses of drug than is host cell DNA synthesis, resulting in a relatively selective antiviral effect. However, large doses of vidarabine are cytotoxic to dividing host cells.

The benefit demonstrated in initial placebo-controlled clinical trials of this drug was a major impetus for the development of antiviral therapies. However, because of poor solubility and some toxicity, vidarabine was quickly replaced by acyclovir in the physician's armamentarium. Today, it is no longer available as an intravenous formulation. Vidarabine should be recognized historically as the first drug licensed for systemic use in the treatment of a viral infection.

Therapy of Respiratory Virus Infections

Background

It is difficult to overestimate the impact of respiratory viral illnesses on human health. Almost 90% of the population experience one of these illnesses each year, resulting in a staggering number of days lost from work and school and of visits to physicians, as well as in significant potential for serious morbidity and even death.[158] Nonetheless, because these conditions in most populations of patients are self-limited and rarely fatal, the requirements for new drugs are stringent: an extreme degree of safety, moderate to high effectiveness, ease of administration, and low cost.[158] Accordingly, only two such antiviral agents are approved for use in the United States, each with fairly limited indications. Because of the number of developmental programs identifying new antiviral agents for treatment of respiratory viruses, it seems likely that an expanded armamentarium will be forthcoming.

Amantadine and Rimantadine

CHEMISTRY, MECHANISM OF ACTION, AND ANTIVIRAL ACTIVITY

Amantadine was identified as effective against influenza A viruses and was soon shown to be effective against all type A variants.[159–162] Amantadine was first reported to be effective for the prophylaxis of influenza A more than two decades ago, being approved for this indication in the United States in 1966, as reviewed.[163] For a variety of reasons it was slow to achieve widespread use. Amantadine has a narrow spectrum of activity. At concentrations achievable in humans it is useful only against influenza A.[160] Influenza A viruses differ in their susceptibility to amantadine, and the drug may have different actions depending on the concentration and virus strain. Early studies indicated that amantadine acted by preventing the penetration or uncoating of influenza A viruses. Rimantadine is the α-methyl derivative of amantadine (α-methyl-1-adamantanemethylamine hydrochloride).

Rimantadine is 5- to 10-fold more active than amantadine and has the same spectrum of activity, mechanism of action, and clinical indications.[163] Rimantadine is somewhat more effective than amantadine against type A viruses at the same concentration.[164] Rimantadine is used extensively in the former Soviet Union and has been widely tested in the United States.[164, 165] The mechanism of action of these drugs involves the influenza A virus M2 protein, a membrane protein that is the ion channel for this virus. By interfering with the function of the M2 protein, amantadine and rimantadine inhibit the acid-mediated association of the matrix protein from the ribonuclear protein complex within endosomes. This event occurs early in the viral replication cycle. The consequences are the potentiation of acidic pH–induced conformational changes in the hemagglutinin during its intracellular transport.[166]

ABSORPTION, DISTRIBUTION, AND ELIMINATION

There are differences between rimantadine and amantadine.[158, 165] Absorption of rimantadine is delayed compared with that of amantadine, and equivalent doses of rimantadine produce lower plasma levels than amantadine, presumably because of a larger volume of distribution.[165, 167] The lower plasma levels may explain the lower incidence of side effects at similar doses. The side effects of rimantadine are similar to but less than those of amantadine and include gastrointestinal and CNS effects.[164, 168, 169] Rimantadine has similar CNS side effects even though, unlike amantadine, this drug does not affect CNS catecholamine release and is not effective in the treatment of Parkinson disease. The efficacy of rimantadine in both the prophylaxis and the treatment of influenza A is similar to that of amantadine.[168] Both amantadine and rimantadine are well absorbed after oral administration.

Amantadine is excreted in the urine by glomerular filtration and probably tubular secretion. It is not metabolized. The plasma elimination half-life is approximately 12 to 18 hours in individuals with normal renal function. However, the elimination half-life increases in elderly patients with impaired C_{cr}. Rimantadine is extensively metabolized after oral administration, having an elimination half-life that averages 24 to 36 hours. Approximately 15% of the dose is excreted unchanged in the urine.

CLINICAL INDICATIONS

As antiviral agents, amantadine and rimantadine are licensed for both chemoprophylaxis and treatment of influenza A. Because of a lower incidence of side effects associated with rimantadine compared with amantadine, it is used preferentially. Rimantadine can be given to any nonimmunized member of the general population who wishes to avoid influenza A, but prophylaxis is especially recommended for control of presumed influenza outbreaks in institutions housing high-risk persons. High-risk individuals include adults and children with chronic disorders of the cardiovascular or pulmonary system requiring regular follow-up or hospitalization during the preceding year, as well as residents of nursing homes and other chronic care facilities housing patients of any age with chronic medical conditions. In these instances, drug should be administered to all residents of the institution, whether or not they received an influenza vaccination the previous fall. To reduce the spread of virus and to minimize disruption of patients' care, it is also recommended that prophylaxis be offered to nonvaccinated staff who care for high-risk residents in chronic care institutions or hospitals experiencing a presumed influenza A outbreak. Rimantadine prophylaxis is also recommended in the following situations:

1. As an adjunct to late immunization of high-risk individuals. Rimantadine does not interfere with antibody response to the vaccine.
2. For persons who have not been immunized and who care for high-risk persons in home settings, both to reduce the spread of virus and to allow persons to maintain care for high-risk persons in the home setting.
3. For immunodeficient persons, who may be expected to have a poor antibody response to vaccine.
4. For persons for whom influenza vaccine is contraindicated, such as those hypersensitive to egg protein.[168]

There is general agreement that the efficacy of amantadine and rimantadine when used prophylactically for influenza A averages 70% to 80% (range, 0% to 100%), approximately the same as with influenza vaccines.[158] In general, efficacy is about 66% for infections and about 75% for infection-related illnesses.[158] Effectiveness has been demonstrated for prevention of both experimental (i.e., artificial challenge) and naturally occurring infections for all three major subtypes of influenza A virus.

These drugs are also presumed to be effective for the treatment of influenza A. All studies showed a beneficial effect on the signs and symptoms of acute influenza, as well as a significant reduction in quantity of virus in respiratory secretions at some time during the course of infection. Because of the short duration of disease, therapy must be administered within 48 hours of symptom onset to show benefit. Aerosol administration of amantadine and rimantadine has been reported, but this route of administration needs further testing.[161]

RESISTANCE

Rimantadine-resistant strains of influenza virus have been isolated from children treated for 5 days. There have been subsequent reports of rimantadine-resistant strains being transmitted from person to person and producing clinical influenza.[170, 171] The development of such resistance lends further support to the importance of vaccination in appropriate populations of patients.

Development of resistance of influenza A viruses is mediated by single nucleotide changes in RNA segment 7 that result in amino acid substitutions in the transmembrane of the M2 protein.[172, 173] Obviously, amantadine and rimantadine share cross-resistance.

ADVERSE EFFECTS

Amantadine is reported to cause side effects in 5% to 10% of healthy young adults taking the standard adult dose of 200 mg/d.[158, 174] These side effects are usually mild and cease soon after amantadine is discontinued, although they often disappear with continued use of the drug as well.[169] CNS side effects—5% to 33% of patients—are most common and include difficulty in thinking, confusion, lightheadedness, hallucinations, anxiety, and insomnia. Activities requiring mental alertness (e.g., driving) should be avoided until it is reasonable to assume that these symptoms will not occur. More severe adverse effects, such as mental depression and psychosis, are usually associated with doses exceeding 200 mg/d. About 5% of patients complain of nausea, vomiting, or anorexia. Older individuals are more likely to experience side effects. Rimantadine appears better tolerated.[164, 165]

Patients with renal disease should receive doses based on their C_{cr} values (Table 32–2). Doses for older people and children are usually lower, as well. Persons with an active seizure disorder may be at increased risk for seizures when amantadine is given at standard doses.

Side effects associated with rimantadine administration are significantly less than those encountered with amantadine, particularly those of the CNS. Rimantadine has been associated with exacerbations of underlying seizure disorders.

TABLE 32–2 ■ Dosage Adjustment for Oral Amantadine in Patients with Impaired Renal Function

CREATININE CLEARANCE (mL/min/1.73 m²)	SUGGESTED ORAL MAINTENANCE REGIMEN AFTER 200 mg (100 mg bid) ON THE FIRST DAY
≥80	100 mg bid
60–80	100 mg bid alternating with 100 mg daily
40–60	100 mg daily
30–40	200 mg (100 mg bid) twice weekly
20–30	100 mg three times each week
10–20	200 mg (100 mg bid) alternating with 100 mg every 7 d
<10	100 mg every 7 d

CONCLUSIONS ON AMANTADINE AND RIMANTADINE

Amantadine and rimantadine are efficacious for the prevention and treatment of influenza A. Because of the high incidence of adverse effects associated with amantadine administration, rimantadine has replaced this compound for the most part.

Ribavirin

CHEMISTRY, MECHANISM OF ACTION, AND ANTIVIRAL ACTIVITY

Ribavirin was synthesized in 1972 and shown shortly thereafter to exert antiviral effects against a variety of RNA- and DNA-containing viruses.[175–177] Ribavirin has been evaluated most as a therapy for respiratory virus infections, but its broad spectrum of activity has resulted in clinical trials for a number of viral infections.

Ribavirin is a nucleoside analog whose mechanisms of action are poorly understood and probably not the same for all viruses; however, its ability to alter nucleotide pools and the packaging of messenger RNA (mRNA) appears important.[175–178] This process is not totally virus specific, but there is a certain selectivity in that infected cells produce more mRNA than noninfected cells. A major action is the inhibition by ribavirin-5′-monophosphate of inosine-monophosphate dehydrogenase, an enzyme essential for DNA synthesis. This inhibition may have direct effects on the intracellular level of guanosine monophosphate; other nucleotide levels may be altered, but the mechanisms are at present unknown. Also, the 5′-triphosphate of ribavirin inhibits the formation of the 5′-guanylation capping on the mRNA of vaccinia and Venezuelan equine encephalitis viruses. In addition, the triphosphate is a potent inhibitor of viral mRNA (guanine-7) methyltransferase of vaccinia virus. The capacity of viral mRNA to support protein synthesis is markedly reduced by ribavirin. Of note, high concentrations of ribavirin also inhibit cellular protein synthesis. It has been suggested that ribavirin may inhibit RNA-dependent RNA polymerase of influenza A virus.[158]

ABSORPTION, DISTRIBUTION, AND ELIMINATION

Ribavirin can be administered orally (bioavailability of approximately 40% to 45%) or intravenously.[179] Aerosol administration has become standard for the treatment of RSV infections in children. Oral doses of 600 and 1200 mg result in peak plasma concentrations of 1.3 and 2.5 μg/mL, respectively. Intravenous dosages of 500 and 1000 mg result in 17 and 24 μg/mL plasma concentrations, respectively. Aerosol administration of ribavirin results in plasma levels that are a function of the duration of exposure. Whereas respiratory secretions contain milligram quantities of drug, only microgram quantities (0.5 to 3.5 μg/mL) can be detected in the plasma.

The kidney is the major route of clearance of drug, accounting for approximately 40%. Hepatic metabolism also contributes to the clearance of ribavirin. Notably, ribavirin triphosphate concentrates in erythrocytes and persists for a month or longer. The persistence of ribavirin in erythrocytes probably contributes to its hematopoietic toxicity.

CLINICAL INDICATIONS

Ribavirin is licensed for the treatment of carefully selected, hospitalized infants and young children with severe lower respiratory tract infections caused by RSV. The vast majority of infants and children with RSV infection have disease that is mild and self-limited and are not candidates for ribavirin. Use of aerosolized ribavirin for adults and children with RSV infections reduced the severity of illness and virus shedding.[180–183] In a double-blind, placebo-controlled trial, this form was evaluated in RSV lower respiratory tract disease in 26 infants, including those with underlying cardiopulmonary disease. Treated infants improved significantly faster as measured by illness severity score, arterial blood gas values, and amount of virus shed from nasal washes. In addition, a generally good outcome was observed in 27 nonrandomized, severely ill infants with congenital heart disease who were treated with a ribavirin aerosol. Notably, as many as one third of infants with congenital heart disease may die from RSV infection. No adverse effects were observed in any of the infants studied and no ribavirin-resistant RSV strains were isolated despite prolonged treatment of some infants.[182] Aerosol therapy with ribavirin appears to have the advantage of producing high pulmonary drug levels with little systemic absorption. In patients receiving 8 or more hours of continuous therapy, the mean peak level in tracheal secretions may be 100 times greater than the minimal inhibitory concentration preventing RSV replication in vitro. Furthermore, repeated courses eliminated simultaneous infection with both parainfluenza virus and RSV in an infant with severe combined immunodeficiency syndrome.[184] Ribavirin therapy has also been shown to decrease the duration of ventilatory support and oxygen supplementation.[185] The use of ribavirin for the treatment of RSV infections is controversial,[186] but it is indicated for the treatment of infants at high risk for severe illness and complications of RSV infection, including infants with severe respiratory compromise and underlying conditions such as bronchopulmonary dysplasia or cyanotic congenital heart disease. Treatment is also recommended for infants with severe combined immunodeficiency who develop parainfluenza virus infection of the lower respiratory tract.

Ribavirin has been reported to be effective by other (i.e., nonaerosol) routes in several other viral infections, including measles, genital herpes infections, and herpes zoster.[187–190] When given intravenously or orally, it has been reported to reduce mortality significantly in patients with Lassa fever.[191] Of perhaps greater interest for Eastern countries, ribavirin was demonstrated to be useful for epidemic hemorrhagic fever.[192]

Of interest, ribavirin is being administered intravenously to patients with presumed *Hantavirus* pulmonary syndrome. At this time, there is no evidence that therapy is efficacious.[193]

RESISTANCE

Emergence of viruses resistant to ribavirin has not been documented.

ADVERSE EFFECTS

No adverse effect has been clearly attributable to aerosol therapy with ribavirin, although reports of adverse effects during or after therapy of infants with RSV have included bronchospasm, changes in pulmonary function tests, pneumothorax in ventilated patients, apnea, cardiac arrest, hypotension, and concomitant digitalis toxicity. Changes in pulmonary function tests after ribavirin therapy in adults with chronic obstructive pulmonary disease have been noted as well, but one study reported no change in respiratory symptoms even though small changes in preliminary function tests were demonstrated.[194]

Precipitation of drug within the ventilatory apparatus of patients receiving mechanical ventilation can be a serious problem but is not a contraindication for its use. When proper precautions are taken, such as frequent changes in ventilator tubing, safe delivery of ribavirin to ventilated patients can be accomplished. Reticulocytosis, rash, and conjunctivitis have been associated with the use of ribavirin aerosol. When the drug was given orally or intravenously, transient elevations of serum bilirubin values and occurrence of mild anemia were reported. Although there are no pertinent human data, ribavirin has been found to be teratogenic and mutagenic in nearly all species in which it has been tested. This drug is, therefore, contraindicated for women who are or may become pregnant during exposure to the drug.

Some concern has been expressed about the risk to persons in the room with infants being treated with ribavirin aerosol, particularly women of childbearing age. Although this risk seems to be minimal with limited exposure, awareness and caution on the part of personnel are warranted, and continued evaluation is important.[195, 196] Furthermore, the use of a drug salvage hood is considered mandatory.

CONCLUSIONS ON RIBAVIRIN

Ribavirin has significant broad-spectrum antiviral activity. Its use in the management of RSV infection of high-risk children has been questioned of late; nevertheless, it is the only therapeutic agent currently available. In the absence of toxicity-related complications of treatment, it will remain available until additional medications are developed. Its use for other infections (e.g., measles, *Hantavirus* pulmonary syndrome, hepatitis A) warrants further investigation.

Miscellaneous Therapeutics

Interferons

CHEMISTRY, MECHANISM OF ACTION, AND ANTIVIRAL ACTIVITY

IFNs are glycoprotein cytokines (intracellular messengers) with a complex array of immunomodulating, antineoplastic, and antiviral properties. The name interferon was derived from landmark experiments by Isaacs and Lindemann in 1957 demonstrating the existence of a biological substance that interfered with viral replication in infected cells. IFNs are currently classified as α, β, or γ; natural sources of these classes, in general, are leukocytes, fibroblasts, and lymphocytes, respectively. Each type of IFN can now be produced via recombinant DNA technology. The complexity of the response to IFN, including the variability of dose response, duration of therapy, and combination with other treatments, creates enormous challenges to determining appropriate clinical scenarios in which IFN might be a worthwhile therapeutic agent.

Binding of IFN to the intact cell membrane is the first step in establishing an antiviral effect.[197] IFN binds to specific cell surface receptors; IFN-γ appears to have a different receptor from either IFN-α or IFN-β, which may explain the purported synergistic antiviral and antitumor effects sometimes observed when IFN-γ is given with either of the other two IFN species.

A prevalent view of IFN action is that, after binding, there is synthesis of new cellular RNAs and proteins, which mediate the antiviral effect. Chromosome 21 is required for this antiviral state in humans no matter which species of IFN is employed. At least three of the newly synthesized proteins in IFN-treated cells appear to be associated with the development of an antiviral state: 2′,5′-oligoadenylate synthetase, a protein kinase, and an endonuclease. The antiviral state is not fully expressed until these primed cells are infected with virus. In addition to their antiviral effect, IFNs have a number of other biologic activities, both useful and potentially deleterious, including inhibition of cell proliferation and enhancement of the cytotoxic activities of lymphocytes, the expression of cell surface antigens, and the phagocytic and tumoricidal activities of macrophages. These properties may play an important role in the in vivo antiviral and antitumor effects of the IFNs.[197, 198]

ABSORPTION, DISTRIBUTION, AND ELIMINATION

IFN must be administered intramuscularly or subcutaneously (including into a lesion, such as a wart). Plasma levels are dose dependent, peaking 4 to 8 hours after intramuscular administration and returning to baseline between 18 and 36 hours. There appears to be some variability in absorption in the three classes of IFN and in resultant plasma levels. Leukocyte and IFN-α appear to have an elimination half-life of 2 to 4 hours. IFN is inactivated by various organs of the body in as yet undefined method.

CLINICAL INDICATIONS

Although IFN is promising as a therapeutic agent for a number of viral infections, the only licensed use of IFN as an antiviral is its intralesional administration in the treatment of condyloma acuminatum, or genital wart, which is caused by human papillomaviruses. IFN alfa is licensed; it is the focus for further discussions. Among the many viral infections in which IFN has been tested, treatments of condyloma acuminatum, chronic hepatitis B and C, and recurrent respiratory papillomatosis have been most clinically useful.

Condyloma Acuminatum. Several large controlled trials have demonstrated the clinical benefit of IFN alfa therapy of condyloma acuminatum that was refractory to cytodestructive therapies. Eron and colleagues[199] compared patients with up to three external warts treated intralesionally with 1.0×10^6 IU of recombinant IFN alfa and placebo-treated patients. Significant benefit in the treatment group was demonstrated by complete clearing of treated lesions (36% versus 17% of placebo recipients), as well as by reduction in mean wart area (40% reduction versus 46% increase). In other well-controlled studies, either a similar (46%) or higher (62%) rate of clearance was reported. Notably, clearing responses of placebo recipients averaged 21% to 22%.[200, 201] When IFN is administered parenterally, the outcome is poorer.[202]

Although IFN has proven benefit in the treatment of condyloma acuminatum, much research remains to be done to examine the effects of different routes of administration, prolonged therapy, repeated courses of treatment, and combination of IFN with other therapeutic modalities (i.e., cryotherapy with liquid nitrogen, carbon dioxide destruction, and podophyllin or laser treatment).

Respiratory Papillomatosis. Recurrent respiratory papillomatosis is a disease in which squamous papillomas recur relentlessly within the larynx and trachea of both children and young adults. Standard management consists of careful microendoscopic excision, usually with a carbon dioxide laser. There have been numerous case reports and uncontrolled studies supporting benefit from the use of IFN as an adjunct to surgical treatment. Results of placebo-controlled trials have suggested benefit.[203, 204]

Hepatitis. The inhibitory effect of human leukocyte IFN alfa on hepatitis B virus replication was first reported by Greenberg and associates.[205] Levels of hepatitis B DNA polymerase, a marker of replication, were reduced on five separate occasions in three patients with chronic hepatitis who were treated with 6×10^3 to 16×10^4 IU/kg. Treatment with IFN alfa in chronic hepatitis B was subsequently investigated in several large, randomized, controlled trials.

Alexander and colleagues[206, 207] randomly assigned a group of males seropositive for hepatitis B e antigen and with DNA polymerase in the serum to receive IFN or no treatment. Interim analysis of the first 46 patients found 6 in the IFN group but no patient in the control group with simultaneous loss of both serum hepatitis B e antigen and HBV DNA polymerase. Similar data have been reviewed.[208, 209] Although this study and others are encouraging, the response rate has been low, namely 30% to 40%. A third phase of hepatitis B therapy with IFN involves its combinations with other agents, including a corticosteroid pulse. However, a large multicenter trial comparing patients randomly assigned to receive one or two doses of IFN alfa versus prednisolone followed by IFN alfa or no treatment failed to prove added benefit over IFN alone.[210] Alternative monotherapy and combination therapies are being investigated including famiciclovir alone and with IFN and lamivudine alone and with IFN.

The activity of IFN in the treatment of hepatitis C has been extensively evaluated.[211] IFN dosages have ranged from 1×10^6 subcutaneously three times weekly for 1 to 18 months. Only 2.6% of the placebo control subjects had normalized serum alanine aminotransferase values. In contrast, treatment led to serum alanine aminotransferase normalization in 33% to 45% of patients. Unfortunately 50% to 80% of patients had relapses. IFN alfa therapy induced remission, but relapse is common, as reviewed.[212]

Respiratory Infections. It has been reported that nasal spray or drops of IFN alfa provide prophylaxis against the common cold, if caused by rhinovirus infection, as evidenced by reduced severity of illness, frequency of illness, and virus shedding in both experimentally challenged subjects and patients naturally infected with rhinoviruses.[213–215] For example, in a series of trials reported by Tyrrell,[216] 1 of 62 patients treated prophylactically with IFN developed a cold after rhinovirus challenge compared with 28 of 72 placebo control subjects. In other studies, IFN alfa self-administered for 7 days by healthy individuals exposed to a family member with coldlike findings reduced the symptoms of respiratory illness in recipients by 39% to 41%.[217, 218] This beneficial effect was limited to rhinovirus infections. When rhinoviral colds alone were considered, IFN prevented illness in 78% to 79% of patients or shortened the course of colds by 76% fewer symptom days.

RESISTANCE

Resistance to administered IFN has not been documented, although neutralizing antibodies to recombinant IFNs have been reported. The clinical importance of the latter observation is unknown.

ADVERSE EFFECTS

Side effects are frequent with IFN administration and are usually dose limiting. Influenza-like symptoms—fever, chills, headache, and malaise—commonly occur, but these symptoms usually become less severe with repeated treatments. At doses used in the treatment of condyloma acuminatum, these side effects rarely cause termination of treatment. For local treatment (intralesional administration), pain at the injection site does not differ significantly from that experienced by placebo-treated patients and is short-lived. Leukopenia is the most common hematologic abnormality, occurring in up to 26% of patients treated for condyloma.[197] Leukopenia is usually modest, not clinically relevant, and reversible on discontinuation of therapy. Increased alanine aminotransferase levels may also occur, as well as nausea, vomiting, and diarrhea.

At higher doses of IFN, neurotoxicity is encountered, as manifested by personality changes, confusion, loss of attention, disorientation, and paranoid ideation. Early studies with IFN-γ show side effects similar to those with α and β IFNs but with the addition of dose-limiting hypotension and a marked increase in triglyceride levels.

It should also be recognized that amino acid sequences and differences in expression systems of IFN that are produced by recombinant DNA technology may lead to the development of neutralizing antibodies. The biologic significance of these antibodies is unknown.

CONCLUSIONS ON INTERFERONS

IFNs do have a role in the treatment of viral and other diseases. At present, they remain one of the mainstays in the treatment of genital warts and hepatitis B and C. Probably, over time, IFNs will be utilized with other antiviral drugs, particularly nucleoside analogs, in the management of both of these infections.

Future Prospects

Advances in molecular virology continue to identify and define at a molecular level the sites of viral replication that may be vulnerable to attack without harm to the host cell.[219] Further characterization of the viral DNA polymerase, required for viral replication but not utilized by the host cell, is thus a major research focus. In addition, classes of compounds, many of them nucleoside analogs, are being systematically evaluated to identify more efficacious and less toxic antivirals. A description of some of the most promising drugs follows.

Cidofovir. (*S*)-1-(3-Hydroxy-2-phosphonylmethoxypropyl) cytosine (HPMPC). Cidofovir, a novel acyclic phosphorate nucleoside analog, has been used to treat cases of acyclovir- and foscarnet-resistant HSV infection as well as CMV retinitis. Betaherpesviruses are particularly susceptible to the drug. The drug has a mechanism of action similar to those of the other nucleoside analog but employs cellular kinases to produce the active triphosphate form of the drug. Activated HPMPC has higher affinity for viral DNA polymerase and therefore selectively inhibits viral replication.[220] The drug is less potent than acyclovir in vitro; however, in vivo HPMPC persists in cells for prolonged periods, increasing drug activity.[221] In addition, HPMPC produces active metabolites with long half-lives (17 to 48 hours), permitting once-weekly dosing.[222] Unfortunately, HPMPC concentrates in kidney cells 100 time greater than in other tissues and produces severe proximal convoluted tubule nephrotoxicity when administered systemically.[220] Attempts to limit the drug's nephrotoxicity include coadministration of probenecid with intravenous hydration, synthesis of cyclic congener prodrugs of HPMPC, and use of topical formulations.[220] Cyclic HPMPC is a prodrug of HPMPC that undergoes intracellular conversion to HPMPC. In vitro systems demonstrated that cyclic HPMPC has activity comparable to that of HPMPC. In mice infected with HSV-2 and treated for 2 weeks, cyclic HPMPC was as potent as the parent drug but produced 1⁄13 the amount of nephrotoxicity.[223] HPMPC had limited and variable oral bioavailability (2% to 26%) when tested in rats and, therefore, is administered intravenously.[224]

Cidofovir is currently in phase II and phase III testing for treatment of CMV retinitis (Jaffee, H. personal communications) in HIV infections and in phase I and phase II trials as a topical treatment for acyclovir-resistant HSV infections. Probenecid has been added to intravenously administered HPMPC to prevent significant nephrotoxicity. Two of five patients with HIV and asymptomatic CMV infection treated with HPMPC (3.0 mg/kg) experienced increased creatinine levels after 6 to 14 doses.[223] Patients receiving higher doses (10 mg/kg) experienced nephrotoxicity after two doses. One case report documented systemic treatment of an acyclovir-resistant HSV infection; however, the drug was discontinued because of decreased renal function in this patient.[220]

Topical HPMPC (0.2%) is as effective as trifluridine (1%) in reducing HSV-1 shedding and healing time in rabbits with dendritic keratitis.[225] Other investigators have examined the role of topical HPMPC in treatment and prevention of HSV-2 infections in mice and guinea pigs. Animals infected with HSV-2 were treated 6 to 24 hours after infection with topical acyclovir (5%) or HPMPC (0.5% to 5%) three times a day. HPMPC-treated animals had reduced virus shedding and decreased lesion development compared with acyclovir recipients.[226] The 5% topical solution of HPMPC proved significantly toxic to guinea pigs. Lower concentrations (0.3%, 0.5%, and 1%) of HPMPC were more effective than 5% acyclovir. Moreover, these concentrations did not produce the same toxicity as 5% HPMPC.

Cyclobutyl Compounds. Cyclobutyl compounds represent a new group of carbocyclic nucleoside analog that provide broad-spectrum antiviral protection in experimental and animal studies. Moreover, these agents have in vitro activity against resistant strains of HIV, HSV-1, CMV, HSV-2, VZV, and HIV-1. The nucleoside analogs terminate DNA chain elongation. Broad-spectrum antivirals would benefit patients with multiple viral infections, namely HIV-infected persons with herpesvirus infections. Lobucavir is a member of the cyclobutyl class of drugs that has been tested in placebo-controlled phase II trials for patients infected with HIV and CMV. The drug exhibited linear kinetics at low doses, had good bioavailability (40%), and had a half-life of 2 hours. The drug was tolerated as well as placebo.[227] Only 1 of the 27 patients who completed the study excreted CMV at the outset of the study; therefore, data are not available on the effect of lobucavir on CMV shedding.

Newer Approaches. Antiviral medications can inhibit viral infection at any step in the infection process. Targets for antiviral development include herpesvirus attachment, entry, uncoating, protein synthesis or modification, replication, assembly, and egress. Many of the newer experimental agents target essential processes unique to virus replication and, therefore, potentially have high selectivity. Medications that augment the immune response constitute another pathway for combating herpesvirus infections. Recombinant cytokines, monoclonal antibodies, vaccines, and IFN inducers complement current antiviral agents and produce synergistic activity with acyclovir in vitro against some herpesviruses.[228] Most of these newer antiviral agents and immunotherapeutics are in preclinical trials and are presented with descriptions of viral pathogenesis and theoretical mechanisms of actions.

Studies of WIN 51711, a compound with activity against many rhinoviruses and enteroviruses, were the first to describe how a successful antiviral drug interacts with a virion at the atomic level.[229] This compound is one of a class of compounds that resemble arildone, a drug known to inhibit uncoating of poliovirus.[230] X-ray diffraction studies of WIN 51711 bound to rhinovirus 14 showed that the compound adheres tightly to a hydropic pocket formed by VP1, one of the structural proteins of rhinovirus 14.[229] These hydrophobic pockets were found in the VP1 proteins of poliovirus and

TABLE 32–3 ■ Indications for the Use of Available Antiviral Agents

INDICATION	ANTIVIRAL AGENT	ROUTE*	DOSE	COMMENTS
RSV infection (infants)	Ribavirin	Aerosol	Diluted in sterile water to a concentration of 20 mg/mL, then delivered via aerosol for 12–18 h/d for 3–7 d	Use only for infants at high risk.
Life- or sight-threatening infections in immunocompromised hosts caused by CMV	Ganciclovir	IV	5.0 mg/kg q 12 h for 14 d	Maintenance therapy of 5.0 mg/kg/d recommended for AIDS patients. Leukopenia is a frequent complication; in bone marrow transplant patients with CMV pneumonia, CMV immune globulin may be a useful adjunct.
Condyloma acuminatum	Interferon alfa	Intralesional	1.0 million units injected into the base of each lesion, up to three times per week for 3 wk	Influenza-like symptoms may occur with administrations.
Influenza A	Amantadine/rimantadine	PO	Adults: 100–200 mg/d for 5–7 d; children ≤9 y: 4.4–8.8 mg/kg/d for 5–7 d not to exceed 150 mg/d	Normal persons >65 y of age should receive 100 mg/d.
Prophylaxis against influenza A	Amantadine/rimantadine	PO	Adults: 100–200 mg/d; children ≤9 y: 4.4–8.8 mg/kg/d (not to exceed 150 mg/d)	Continued for the duration of the epidemic or for 2 wk in conjunction with influenza vaccination (until vaccine-induced immunity develops); normal persons >65 y of age should receive 100 mg/d.
HSV encephalitis	Acyclovir	IV	10 mg/kg (1-h infusion) 8 h for 10–14 d	Morbidity and mortality are significantly lower in patients treated with acyclovir than with vidarabine.
Neonatal herpes	Vidarabine	IV	30 mg/kg/d (continuous infusion during 12 h) for 10 d	Efficacy of vidarabine is established; vidarabine and acyclovir show equal efficacy.
	or			
	Acyclovir	IV	10 mg/kg (1-h infusion) q 8 h for 14–21 d	
Mucocutaneous HSV infection in immunocompromised hosts	Acyclovir	IV	5 mg/kg (1-h infusion) q 8 h for 7–10 d	Choice of topical, PO, or IV preparation depends on clinical severity and setting; topical acyclovir is appropriate only when it can be applied to all lesions; it does not affect untreated lesions or systemic symptoms.
	or			
	Acyclovir	PO		
	or			
	Acyclovir	Topical	5% ointment; four to six applications a day for 7 d or until healed	Least desirable.
Prophylaxis against mucocutaneous HSV during intense immunosuppression	Acyclovir	PO	200 mg three or four times a day	Oral therapy is most convenient; lesions recur when therapy stops.
	or			
	Acyclovir	IV	250 mg/m² q 8 h or 5 mg/kg q 12 h (1-h infusion)	Lesions recur when therapy stops.
Treatment of initial genital HSV infections	Acyclovir	PO	200 mg five times a day for 10 days	Drug of choice in most clinical settings; treatment has no effect on subsequent recurrence rates.
	or			
	Acyclovir	IV	5 mg/kg (1-h infusion) q 8 h for 5–7 d	For patients requiring hospitalization or with neurologic or other visceral complications.
Recurrent genital herpes	Acyclovir	PO	200 mg five times a day for 5 d	No effect on subsequent recurrence rates; efficacy is greater if used early in attack.
Prophylaxis against frequently recurring genital herpes	Acyclovir	PO	200 mg three to five times a day	Occasional "breakthrough" attacks and/or asymptomatic virus shedding during treatment; reevaluation every 6 mo is recommended.

TABLE 32–3 ■ Indications for the Use of Available Antiviral Agents *Continued*

INDICATION	ANTIVIRAL AGENT	ROUTE*	DOSE	COMMENTS
Treatment of HSV keratitis	Trifluridine	Topical	One drop of 0.1% ophthalmic solution q 2 h while awake (up 9 drops/d)	3% acyclovir ointment (ophthalmic) is equal or superior to idoxuridine, vidarabine, and trifluridine for treatment of HSV keratitis but is not available in the United States.
	or Vidarabine	Topical	One-half-inch ribbon of 3% ophthalmic ointment five times a day	
	or Idoxuridine	Topical	One-half-inch ribbon of 0.5% ophthalmic ointment five times a day	
Chickenpox in immunocompromised hosts	Acyclovir	IV	500 mg/m² (1-h infusion) q 8 h for 7 d	In the absence of comparative data, acyclovir is preferred because of its ease of administration and lower toxicity.
	or Vidarabine	IV	10 mg/kg/d (continuous infusion over 12 h) for 5 d	
Treatment of severe localized or disseminated herpes zoster in immunocompromised hosts	Acyclovir	IV	500 mg/m² or 5–10 mg/kg (1-h infusion) q 8 h for 5–7 d	Comparative trials in severe localized and disseminated herpes zoster are under way; pending results, acyclovir is preferred because of its ease of administration and lower toxicity.
	or Vidarabine	IV	10 mg/kg/d (continuous infusion over 12 h) for 5–7 d	

*IV, Intravenous; PO, oral.

meningovirus and may be common to all picornaviruses. Compounds like WIN 51711 may lock into the conformation of the VP1 so that the virus cannot disassemble.[230]

Conclusion

Although relatively few antiviral drugs are licensed for use at this time, there is significant interest in the development of antiviral compounds. Table 32–3 summarizes the use of currently available antivirals for indications other than therapy of HIV infections. Systematic approaches have revealed a number of promising new drugs that are in various stages of evaluation. A better understanding of the molecular biology of virus replication and pathogenesis should elucidate drugs with enhanced virus-specific activity.

Acknowledgments

Work that was performed and reported by the author was supported by contracts NO1-AI-15113, NO1-AI-62554, and NO1-AI-12667 from the Antiviral Research Branch of the National Institute of Allergy and Infectious Diseases, a grant from the Division of Research Resources (RR-032) from the National Institutes of Health, and a grant from the state of Alabama.

References

1. Whitley RJ: Herpes simplex virus. *In* Fields BN, Knipe DM, Howley PM, et al (eds): Fields Virology. Philadelphia, Lippincott-Raven Publishers, 1996, pp 2297–2342.
2. Levin MJ: Impact of herpesvirus infections in the future. J Med Virol 1(Suppl 1):158–164, 1993.
3. Lerner AM: An overview of virus infections. *In* Petersdorf RC, Adams RD, Braunwald E, et al (eds): Harrison's Principles of Internal Medicine, ed 10. New York, McGraw-Hill, 1983, pp 1091–1098.
4. Groothuis JR, Simoes EA, Levin MJ, et al: Prophylactic administration of respiratory syncytial virus immune globulin to high-risk infants and young children. The respiratory syncytial immune globulin study group. N Engl J Med 329:1524–1530, 1993.
5. Winston DJ, Ho WG, Lin CH, et al: Intravenous immune globulin for prevention of cytomegalovirus infection and interstitial pneumonia after bone marrow transplantation. Ann Intern Med 106:12–18, 1987.
6. Meyers JD, Leszczynski J, Zaia JA, et al: Prevention of cytomegalovirus infection by cytomegalovirus immune globulin after marrow transplantation. Ann Intern Med 98:442–446, 1983.
7. O'Reilly RJ, Reich L, Gold J: A randomized trial of intravenous hyper-immune globulin for the prevention of cytomegalovirus infections following marrow transplantation: Preliminary results. Transplant Proc 15:1405–1413, 1983.
8. Bowden RA, Sayers M, Flournoy N, et al: Cytomegalovirus immune globulin and seronegative blood products to prevent primary cytomegalovirus infection after marrow transplantation. N Engl J Med 314:1006–1110, 1986.
9. Emanuel D, Cunningham I, Jules-Elysee K, et al: Cytomegalovirus pneumonia after bone marrow transplantation successfully treated with the combination of ganciclovir and high-dose intravenous immune globulin. Ann Intern Med 109:777–782, 1988.
10. Reed EC, Raleigh BA, Dandliker PS, et al: Treatment of cytomegalovirus pneumonia with ganciclovir and intravenous cytomegalovirus immunoglobulin in patients with bone marrow transplants. Ann Intern Med 109:783–788, 1988.
11. Elion GB, Furman PA, Fyfe JA, et al: Selectivity of action of

an antiherpetic agent, 9-(2-hydroxyethoxymethyl) guanine. Proc Natl Acad Sci USA 74:5716–5720, 1977.
12. Schaeffer HJ, Beauchamp L, de Miranda P, et al: 9-(2-Hydroxyethoxymethyl) guanine activity against viruses of the herpes group. Nature 272:583–585, 1978.
13. Fyfe JA, Keller PM, Furman PA, et al: Thymidine kinase from herpes simplex virus phosphorylates the new antiviral compound, 9-(2-hydroxyethoxymethyl)guanine. J Biol Chem 253:8721–8727, 1978.
14. Derse D, Chang Y-C, Furman PA, et al: Inhibition of purified human and herpes simplex virus–induced DNA polymerase by 9-(2-hydroxyethoxy methyl) guanine [acyclovir] triphosphate: Effect on primer-template function. J Biol Chem 256:11447–11451, 1981.
15. Furman PA, St. Clair MH, Spector T: Acyclovir triphosphate is a suicide inactivator of the herpes simplex virus DNA polymerase. J Biol Chem 259:9575–9579, 1984.
16. Collins P, Bauer DJ: The activity in vitro against herpes virus of 9-(2-hydroxyethoxymethyl)guanine (acycloguanosine), a new antiviral agent. J Antimicrob Chemother 5:432–436, 1979.
17. deMiranda P, Blum MR: Pharmacokinetics of acyclovir after intravenous and oral administration. J Antimicrob Chemother 12:29–37, 1983.
18. Laskin OL: Acyclovir: Pharmacology and clinical experience. Arch Intern Med 144:1241–1246, 1984.
19. Corey L, Nahmias AJ, Guinan ME, et al: A trial of topical acyclovir in genital herpes simplex virus infections. N Engl J Med 306:1313–1319, 1982.
20. Corey L, Benedetti J, Critchlow C, et al: Treatment of primary first episode genital herpes simplex virus infections with acyclovir: Results of topical, intravenous, and oral therapy. J Antimicrob Chemother 12:79–88, 1983.
21. Corey L, Fife KH, Benedetti JK, et al: Intravenous acyclovir for the treatment of primary genital herpes. Ann Intern Med 98:914–921, 1983.
22. Peacock JE, Kaplowitz LG, Sparling PF, et al: Intravenous acyclovir therapy of first episodes of genital herpes: A multicenter double-blind, placebo-controlled trial. Am J Med 85:301–306, 1988.
23. Bryson YJ, Dillon M, Lovett M, et al: Treatment of first episodes of genital herpes simplex virus infection with oral acyclovir: A randomized double-blind controlled trial in normal subjects. N Engl J Med 308:916–921, 1983.
24. Mertz GJ, Critchlow CW, Benedetti J, et al: Double-blind placebo-controlled trial of oral acyclovir in first-episode genital herpes simplex virus infection. JAMA 252:1147–1151, 1984.
25. Reichman RC, Badger GJ, Guinan ME: Topically administered acyclovir in the treatment of recurrent herpes simplex genitalis: A controlled trial. J Infect Dis 147:336–340, 1983.
26. Luby JP, Gnann JW Jr, Alexander WJ, et al: A collaborative study of patient-initiated treatment of recurrent genital herpes with topical acyclovir or placebo. J Infect Dis 150:1–6, 1984.
27. Reichman RC, Badger GJ, Mertz GJ, et al: Treatment of recurrent genital herpes simplex infection with oral acyclovir. Controlled trial. JAMA 251:2103–2107, 1984.
28. Nilsen AE, Aasen T, Halsos AM, et al: Efficacy of oral acyclovir in the treatment of initial and recurrent genital herpes. Lancet 2:571–573, 1982.
29. Douglas JM, Critchlow C, Benedetti J, et al: Double-blind study of oral acyclovir for suppression of recurrences of genital herpes simplex virus infection. N Engl J Med 310:1551–1556, 1984.
30. Mertz GJ, Jones CC, Mills J, et al: Long-term acyclovir suppression of frequently recurring genital herpes simplex virus infection. JAMA 260:201–206, 1988.
31. Straus SE, Takiff HE, Seidlin M, et al: Suppression of frequently recurring genital herpes: Placebo-controlled double-blind trial of oral acyclovir. N Engl J Med 310:1545–1550, 1984.
32. Kaplowitz LG, Baker D, Gelb L, et al: Prolonged continuous acyclovir treatment of normal adults with frequently recurring genital herpes simplex virus infections. JAMA 265:747–751, 1991.
33. Straus SE, Croen KD, Sawyer MH, et al: Acyclovir suppression of frequently recurring genital herpes. Efficacy and diminishing need during successive years of treatment. JAMA 260:2227–2230, 1988.
34. Nusinoff-Lehrman S, Douglas JM, Corey L, et al: Recurrent genital herpes and suppressive oral acyclovir therapy. Ann Intern Med 104:786–790, 1986.
35. Kost RG, Hill EL, Tigges M, et al: Brief support: Recurrent acyclovir resistant genital herpes in an immunocompetent host. N Engl J Med 329:1777–1781, 1993.
36. Straus SE, Seidin M, Takiff HE, et al: Effect of oral acyclovir treatment on symptomatic and asymptomatic shedding in recurrent genital herpes. Sex Transm Dis 16:107–113, 1989.
37. Safrin S: Valtrex (valaciclovir) (VACV) for the treatment of recurrent genital herpes. Presented at the Eighth International Conference on Antiviral Research; April 23–28, 1995; Santa Fe, NM.
38. Spruance SL, Schnipper LE, Overall JC, et al: Treatment of herpes simplex labialis with topical acyclovir in polyethylene glycol. J Infect Dis 146:85–90, 1982.
39. Raborn GW, McGaw WT, Grace M, et al: Oral acyclovir and herpes labialis: A randomized, double-blind, placebo-controlled study. J Am Dent Assoc 115:38–42, 1987.
40. Spruance SL, Stewart JCB, Rowe NH, et al: Treatment of recurrent herpes simplex labialis with oral acyclovir. J Infect Dis 161:185–190, 1990.
41. Spruance SL, Hamill ML, Hoge WS, et al: Acyclovir prevents reactivation of herpes simplex labialis in skiers. JAMA 260:1597–1599, 1988.
42. Wade JC, Newton B, McLaren C, et al: Intravenous acyclovir to treat mucocutaneous herpes simplex virus infection after marrow transplantation: Double-blind trial. Ann Intern Med 96:265–269, 1982.
43. Meyers JD, Wade JC, Mitchell CD, et al: Multicenter collaborative trial of intravenous acyclovir for treatment of mucocutaneous herpes simplex virus infection in immunocompromised host. Am J Med 73:229–235, 1982.
44. Shepp DH, Newton BA, Dandliker PS, et al: Oral acyclovir therapy for mucocutaneous herpes simplex virus infections in immunocompromised marrow transplant recipients. Ann Intern Med 102:783–785, 1985.
45. Saral R, Burns WH, Laskin OL, et al: Acyclovir prophylaxis of herpes simplex virus infections: A randomized, double-blind, controlled trial in bone-marrow-transplant recipients. N Engl J Med 305:63–67, 1981.
46. Wade JC, Newton B, Flournoy N: Acyclovir for prevention of herpes simplex virus reactivation after marrow transplantation. Ann Intern Med 100:823–828, 1984.
47. Wade JC, McLaren C, Meyers JD: Frequency and significance of acyclovir-resistant herpes simplex virus isolated from marrow transplant patients receiving multiple courses of treatment with acyclovir. J Infect Dis 148:1077–1082, 1983.
48. Kimberlin DW: Research initiatives in studies of antiviral resistance and consensus points and recommendations. Antiviral Res 26:439–452, 1995.
49. Whitley RJ, Darby G: Antiviral therapy: Present approaches, clinical needs, and drug development strategies. Rev Contemp Pharmacother 7:91–107, 1996.
50. Whitley RJ, Alford CA Jr, Hirsch MS, et al: Vidarabine versus acyclovir therapy in herpes simplex encephalitis. N Engl J Med 314:144–149, 1986.
51. Skoldenberg B, Forsgren M, Alestig K, et al: Acyclovir versus vidarabine in herpes simplex encephalitis. Randomised multicentre study in consecutive Swedish patients. Lancet 2:707–711, 1984.
52. Whitley RJ, Arvin A, Prober C, et al: A controlled trial comparing vidarabine with acyclovir in neonatal herpes simplex virus infection. N Engl J Med 324:444–449, 1991.
53. Guttman LT, Wilfert CM, Eppes S: Herpes simplex virus encephalitis in children: Analysis of cerebrospinal fluid and progressive neurodevelopmental deterioration. J Infect Dis 154:415–421, 1986.
54. Hovding G: A comparison between acyclovir and trifluorothymidine ophthalmic ointment in the treatment of epithelial dendritic keratitis: A double-blind, randomized parallel group trial. Acta Ophthalmol 67:51–54, 1989.
55. Balfour HH, Kelly JM, Suarez CS, et al: Acyclovir treatment of varicella in otherwise healthy children. J Pediatr 116:633–639, 1990.
56. Dunkle LM, Arvin AM, Whitley RJ, et al: A controlled trial of acyclovir for chickenpox in normal children. N Engl J Med 325:1539–1544, 1991.

57. Balfour HH Jr, Rotbart HA, Feldman S, et al: Acyclovir treatment of varicella in otherwise healthy adolescents. J Pediatr 120:627–633, 1992.
58. Feder BM: Treatment of adult chickenpox with oral acyclovir. Arch Intern Med 150:2061–2065, 1990.
59. Haake DA, Zakowski PC, Haake DC, et al: Early treatment with acyclovir for varicella pneumonia in otherwise healthy adults: Retrospective controlled study and review. Rev Infect Dis 12:788–798, 1990.
60. Prober CG, Kirk LE, Keeney RE: Acyclovir therapy of chickenpox in immunosuppressed children—A collaborative study. J Pediatr 101:622–625, 1982.
61. Nyerges G, Meszner Z, Gyarmati E, et al: Acyclovir prevents dissemination of varicella in immunocompromised children. J Infect Dis 157:309–313, 1988.
62. Bean B, Braun C, Balfour HH Jr: Acyclovir therapy for acute herpes zoster. Lancet 2:118–121, 1982.
63. McGill J, MacDonad DR, Fall C, et al: Intravenous acyclovir in acute herpes zoster infection. J Infect Dis 6:157–161, 1983.
64. Wood MJ, Ogan PH, McKendrick MW, et al: Efficacy of oral acyclovir treatment of acute herpes zoster. Am J Med 85:79–83, 1988.
65. Morton P, Thomson AN: Oral acyclovir in the treatment of herpes zoster in general practice. N Z Med J 102:93–95, 1989.
66. Cobo LM, Foulks GN, Liesegang T: Oral acyclovir in the treatment of acute herpes zoster ophthalmicus. Ophthalmology 93:763–770, 1986.
66a. Wood MJ, Kay R, Dworkin RH, et al: Oral acyclovir accelerates pain resolution in herpes zoster: A meta-analysis of placebo-controlled trials. Clin Infect Dis 22:341–347, 1996.
67. Beutner KR, Friedman DJ, Forszpaniak C, et al: Valaciclovir compared with acyclovir for improved therapy for herpes zoster in immunocompetent adults. Antimicrob Agents Chemother 39:1547–1553, 1995.
68. Balfour HH, Bean B, Laskin O, et al: Acyclovir halts progression of herpes zoster in immunocompromised patients. N Engl J Med 308:1448–1453, 1983.
69. Shepp D, Dandliker PS, Meyers JD: Treatment of varicella-zoster virus in severely immunocompromised patients: A randomized comparison of acyclovir and vidarabine. N Engl J Med 314:208–212, 1987.
70. Crumpacker CS, Schnipper LE, Marlowe SI, et al: Resistance to antiviral drugs of herpes simplex virus isolated from a patient treated with acyclovir. N Engl J Med 305:343–346, 1982.
71. Kimberlin DW, Coen DM, Biron KK, et al: Molecular mechanisms of antiviral resistance. Antiviral Res 26:369–401, 1995.
72. Sacks SL, Wanklin RJ, Reece DE, et al: Progressive esophagitis from acyclovir-resistant herpes simplex. Clinical roles for DNA polymerase mutants and viral heterogeneity. Ann Intern Med 111:893–899, 1989.
73. Kimberlin DW, Kern ER, Sidwellm RW, et al: Models of antiviral resistance. Antiviral Res 26:415–422, 1995.
74. Erlich KS, Mills J, Chatis P, et al: Acyclovir-resistant herpes simplex virus infections in patients with the acquired immunodeficiency syndrome. N Engl J Med 320:293–296, 1989.
75. Safrin S, Crumpacker C, Chatis P, et al: A controlled trial comparing foscarnet with vidarabine for acyclovir-resistant mucocutaneous herpes simplex in the acquired immunodeficiency syndrome. N Engl J Med 325:551–555, 1991.
76. Erlich KS, Jacobson MA, Koehler JE: Foscarnet therapy for severe acyclovir-resistant herpes simplex virus type-2 infections in patients with the acquired immunodeficiency syndrome (AIDS). Ann Intern Med 110:710–713, 1989.
77. Ljungman P, Ellis MN, Hackman RC, et al: Acyclovir-resistant herpes simplex virus causing pneumonia after marrow transplantation. J Infect Dis 162:244–248, 1990.
78. Gateley A, Gander RM, Jonson PC, et al: Herpes simplex virus type 2 meningoencephalitis resistant to acyclovir in a patient with AIDS. J Infect Dis 161:711–715, 1990.
79. Englund JA, Zimmerman ME, Swierkosz EU, et al: Herpes simplex virus resistant to acyclovir. A study in a tertiary care center. Ann Intern Med 112:416–422, 1990.
80. Marks GL, Nolen PE, Erlich KS, et al: Mucocutaneous dissemination of acyclovir-resistant herpes simplex virus in a patient with AIDS. Rev Infect Dis 11:474–476, 1989.
81. Pahwa S, Biron K, Lim W, et al: Continuous varicella-zoster infection associated with acyclovir resistance in a child with AIDS. JAMA 260:2879–2882, 1988.
82. Jacobson MA, Berger TC, Fikrig S, et al: Acyclovir-resistant varicella zoster virus infection after chronic oral acyclovir in patients with the acquired immunodeficiency syndrome (AIDS). Ann Intern Med 112:187–191, 1990.
83. Safrin S, Berger TG, Gilson I: Foscarnet therapy in five patients with AIDS and acyclovir-resistant varicella zoster virus infection. Ann Intern Med 115:19–21, 1991.
84. Speigal DM, Lau K: Acute renal failure and coma secondary to acyclovir therapy. JAMA 155:1882–1883, 1986.
85. Bianchetti MG, Roduit C, Oetliker OH: Acyclovir induced renal failure: Course and risk factors. Pediatr Nephrol 5:238–239, 1991.
86. Brigden D, Rosling AE, Woods NC: Renal function after acyclovir intravenous injection. Am J Med 73:182–185, 1982.
87. Wade KC, Meyers JD: Neurologic symptoms associated with parenteral acyclovir treatment after bone marrow transplantation. Ann Intern Med 98:921–925, 1983.
88. Cohen SMZ, Minkove JA, Zebley JW 3d, Mulholland JH: Severe but reversible neurotoxicity from acyclovir (Letter). Ann Intern Med 100:920, 1984.
89. Andrews EB, Tilson HH, Hurin BA, Cordero JF: Acyclovir in Pregnancy Registry. An observational epidemiological approach. Am J Med 85(Suppl 2A):123–128, 1988.
90. Frenkel LM, Brown ZA, Bryson YJ, et al: Pharmacokinetics of acyclovir in the term human pregnancy and neonate. Am J Obstet Gynecol 164:569–576, 1991.
91. Chatis PA, Miller CH, Schrager LE, et al: Successful treatment with foscarnet of an acyclovir-resistant mucocutaneous infection with herpes simplex virus in a patient with acquired immunodeficiency syndrome. N Engl J Med 320:297–300, 1989.
92. Palestine AG, Polis MA, DeSmet MD, et al: A randomized controlled trial of foscarnet in the treatment of cytomegalovirus retinitis in patients with AIDS. Ann Intern Med 115:665–673, 1991.
93. Jacobson MA, Drew WL, Feinberg J, et al: Foscarnet therapy for ganciclovir-resistant cytomegalovirus retinitis in patients with AIDS. J Infect Dis 163:1348–1351, 1991.
94. Mortality in patients with the acquired immunodeficiency syndrome treated with either foscarnet or ganciclovir for cytomegalovirus retinitis. Studies of Ocular Complications of AIDS Research Group. In collaboration with the AIDS Clinical Trials Group. N Engl J Med 326:213–220, 1992.
95. Birch CJ, Tachedjian G, Doherty RR, et al: Altered sensitivity to antiviral drugs of herpes simplex virus isolates from a patient with the acquired immunodeficiency syndrome. J Infect Dis 162:731–734, 1990.
96. Safrin S, Kemmerly S, Plotkin B, et al: Foscarnet-resistant herpes simplex virus infection in patients with AIDS. J Infect Dis 169:193–196, 1994.
97. Palestine AG. Clinical aspects of cytomegalovirus retinitis. Rev Infect Dis 10(Suppl 3):S515–S521, 1988.
98. Ho M: Human cytomegalovirus infections in immunocompromised patients. *In* Greenough WB, Merigan TC (eds): Cytomegalovirus: Biology and Infection. New York, Plenum Medical Publishing, 1982, pp 171–204.
99. Gorensek MJ, Stewart RW, Keys TF, et al: A multivariate analysis of the risk of cytomegalovirus infection in heart transplant recipients. J Infect Dis 157:515–522, 1988.
100. Zaia JA, Kovacs A, Forman SJ: Human cytomegalovirus-associated pneumonitis: Pathogenesis, prevention, and treatment. Transplant Proc 19:125–131, 1987.
101. Frank I, Friedman HM: Progress in the treatment of cytomegalovirus pneumonia. Ann Intern Med 109:769–770, 1988.
102. Meyers JE, Flournoy N, Thomas ED: Risk factors for cytomegalovirus infection after human marrow transplantation. J Infect Dis 153:478–488, 1986.
103. Meyers JD: Cytomegalovirus infection following marrow transplantation: Risk, treatment and prevention. *In* Plotkin SA, Michelson S, Pagano JS, Rapp F (eds): CMV Pathogenesis and Prevention of Human Infection. New York, Alan R Liss, 1984, pp 101–117.
104. Meyers JD: Management of cytomegalovirus infection. Am J Med 85:102–106, 1988.
105. Verheyden JPH: Evaluation of therapy for cytomegalovirus infection. Rev Infect Dis 10:477–485, 1988.

106. Matthews T, Boehme R: Antiviral activity and mechanism of action of ganciclovir. Rev Infect Dis 10:490–494, 1988.
107. Mar E-C, Cheng YC, Huang ES: Effect of 9-(1,3 dihydroxy-2-propoxymethyl) guanine on human cytomegalovirus replication in vitro. Antimicrob Agents Chemother 24:518–521, 1983.
108. Martin JC, Dvorak CA, Smee DE, et al: 9-[(1,3-Dihydroxy-2-propoxy)methyl]guanine: A new potent and selective antiherpes agent. J Med Chem 26:759–761, 1983.
109. Tocci MJ, Livelli T, Perry HC, et al: Effects of the nucleoside analogue 2′-nor-2′-deoxyguanosine on cytomegalovirus replication. Antimicrob Agents Chemother 25:247–252, 1984.
110. Frank KB, Chiou JF, Cheng YC: Interaction of herpes simplex virus–induced DNA polymerase with 9-(1,3-dihydroxy-2-propoxymethyl) guanine triphosphate. J Biol Chem 259:1566–1569, 1984.
111. Biron KK, Stanat SC, Sorrell JB, et al: Metabolic ativation of the nucleoside analog 9-[(2-hydroxy-1-(hydroxymethyl)ethyoxy]-methyl)guanine in human diploid fibroblasts infected with human cytomegalovirus. Proc Natl Acad Sci USA 82:2473–2477, 1985.
112. Biron KK, Stenbuck PJ, Sorrell JB: Inhibition of the DNA polymerases of varicella-zoster virus and human cytomegalovirus by the nucleoside analogs ACV and BW795U (Abstr). J Cell Biochem 8B:207, 1984.
113. Smee DF, Bochme R, Chernow M, et al: Intracellular metabolism and enzymatic phosphorylation of 9-(1,3-dihydroxy-2-propoxymethyl) guanine and acyclovir in herpes simplex virus–infected and uninfected cells. Biochem Pharmacol 34:1049–1056, 1985.
114. Jacobson MA, De Miranda P, Cederberg DM, et al: Human pharmacokinetics and tolerance of oral ganciclovir. Antimicrob Agents Chemother 31:1251–1254, 1987.
115. Fletcher C, Sawchuk R, Chinnock B, et al: Human pharmacokinetics of the antiviral drug DHPG. Clin Pharmacol Ther 1:281–286, 1986.
116. Buhles WC Jr, Mastre BJ, Tinker AJ, et al: Ganciclovir treatment of life- or sight-threatening cytomegalovirus infection: Experience in 314 immunocompromised patients. Rev Infect Dis 10:495–504, 1988.
117. Holland GN, Sidikaro Y, Kreiger AE, et al: Treatment of cytomegalovirus retinopathy with ganciclovir. Ophthalmology 94:815–823, 1987.
118. Mills J, Jacobson MA, O'Donnell JJ, et al: Treatment of cytomegalovirus retinitis in patients with AIDS. Rev Infect Dis 10:522–526, 1988.
119. Burns WH, Saral R, Santos GW, et al: Isolation and characterisation of resistant herpes simplex virus after acyclovir therapy. Lancet 1:421–423, 1982.
120. Dieterich DT, Chachoua A, Lafleur F, et al: Ganciclovir treatment of gastrointestinal infections caused by cytomegalovirus in patients with AIDS. Rev Infect Dis 10:532–537, 1988.
121. Hayes K, Danks DM, Gibas H: Cytomegalovirus in human milk. N Engl J Med 287:177–178, 1972.
122. Sydman DR: Ganciclovir therapy for cytomegalovirus disease associated with renal transplants. Rev Infect Dis 10:554–560, 1988.
123. Keay S, Petersen E, Icenogle T, et al: Ganciclovir treatment of serious cytomegalovirus infection in heart and heart-lung transplant recipients. Rev Infect Dis 10:563–572, 1988.
124. Shepp DH, Dandliker PS, de Miranda P, et al: Activity of 9-[2-hydroxy-1-(hydroxymethyl)ethoxymethyl]guanine in the treatment of cytomegalovirus pneumonis. Ann Intern Med 103:368–373, 1985.
125. Crumpacker C, Marlowe S, Zhang JL, et al: Treatment of cytomegalovirus pneumonia. Rev Infect Dis 10(Suppl 3):S538–S546, 1988.
126. Schmidt GM, Horak DA, Niland JC, et al: A randomized, controlled trial of prophylactic ganciclovir for cytomegalovirus pulmonary infection in recipients of allogeneic bone marrow transplants. N Engl J Med 324:1005–1011, 1991.
127. Goodrich JM, Mori M, Gleaves CA, et al: Early treatment with ganciclovir to prevent cytomegalovirus disease after allogeneic bone marrow transplantation. N Engl. J Med 325:1601–1607, 1991.
128. Winston DJ, Ho WG, Bartoni K, et al: Ganciclovir prophylaxis of cytomegalovirus infection and disease in bone marrow transplant recipients. Results of a placebo-controlled, double-blind trial. Ann Intern Med 118:179–184, 1993.
129. Biron KK, Fyfe JA, Stanat SC, et al: A human cytomegalovirus mutant resistant to the nucleoside analog 9-([2-hydroxy-1-(hydroxymethyl)ethoxy]methyl)guanine (BW B759U) induces reduced levels of BW B759U triphosphate. Proc Natl Acad Sci USA 83:8769–8773, 1986.
130. Erice A, Chou S, Biron KK, et al: Progressive disease due to ganciclovir-resistant cytomegalovirus in immunocompromised patients. N Engl J Med 320:289–293, 1989.
131. Stanat SC, Reardon JE, Erice A, et al: Ganciclovir-resistant cytomegalovirus clinical isolates: Mode of resistance to ganciclovir. Antimicrob Agents Chemother 35:2191–2197, 1991.
132. Littler E, Stuart AD, Chee MS: Human cytomegalovirus UL97 open reading frame encodes a protein that phosphorylates the antiviral nucleoside analogue ganciclovir. Nature 358:160–162, 1992.
133. Boston Interhospital Virus Study Group and the NIAID Sponsored Cooperative Antiviral Clinical Study: Failure of high dose 5-deoxyuridine in the therapy of herpes simplex virus encephalitis: Evidence of unacceptable toxicity. N Engl J Med 292:600–603, 1975.
134. Prussoff WM, Bakkle YS, Sekely A: Cellular and antiviral effects of halogenated deoxyribonucleosides. Ann N Y Acad Sci 130:135–150, 1965.
135. Kaufman HE, Martola EL, Dohlman CH: The use of 5-iodo-2′-deoxyuridine in the treatment of herpes simplex keratitis. Arch Ophthalmol 68:235–239, 1962.
136. Pavan-Langston DR: Major ocular viral diseases. *In* Galasso G, Whitley RJ, Merigan T (eds): Antiviral Agents and Viral Diseases of Man. New York, Raven Press, 1990, pp 183–233.
137. Fowles SE, Pue MA, Pierce D, et al: Pharmacokinetics of penciclovir in healthy elderly subjects following a single oral administration of 750 mg famciclovir. Br J Clin Pharmacol 34(Suppl 1):450P, 1992.
138. Sutton D, Kern ER: Activity of famciclovir and penciclovir in HSV-infected animals: A review. Antiviral Chem Chemother 4(Suppl 1):37–46, 1993.
139. The International Valaciclovir HSV Study Group, Smiley L, Burroughs Wellcome Co: Valaciclovir and acyclovir for the treatment of recurrent genital herpes simplex virus infections. Presented at the 33rd Interscience Conference of Antimicrobial Agents and Chemotherapy; October 17–20, 1993; New Orleans, LA.
140. de Greef H, Famciclovir Herpes Zoster Clinical Study Group: Famciclovir, a new oral antiherpes drug: Results of the first controlled clinical study demonstrating its efficacy and safety in the treatment of uncomplicated herpes zoster in immunocompetent patients. Int J Antimicrob Chemother 4:241–246, 1994.
141. Tyring S, Barbarash RA, Nahlik JE, et al: Famciclovir for the treatment of acute herpes zoster. Effects on acute disease and postherpetic neuralgia: A randomized, double-blind, placebo-controlled trial. Ann Intern Med 123:89–96, 1995.
142. Whitley RJ: Famciclovir for herpes zoster. *In* Medical Letter Handbook of Antimicrobial Therapy. New Rochelle, NY, The Medical Letter, 1994, p 67.
143. Mertz GJ, Loveless MO, Kraus SJ, et al: Famciclovir for suppression of recurrent genital herpes. Presented at the 34th Interscience Conference on Antimicrobial Agents and Chemotherapy; October 4–7, 1994; Orlando, FL.
144. Saltzman R, Jurewicz R, Boon R: The safety of famciclovir in patients with herpes zoster and genital herpes. Antimicrob Agents Chemother 38:2454–2457, 1994.
145. Famvir (famciclovir) package insert. King of Prussia, PA, SmithKline Beecham Pharmaceuticals, 1994.
146. Daniels S, Schentag JJ: Drug interaction studies and safety of famciclovir in healthy volunteers: A review. Antiviral Chem Chemother 4(Suppl 1):57–64, 1993.
147. Machida H, Sakata S, Kuninaka A, Yoshino H: Antiherpesviral and anticellular effects of 1-β-D-arabinofuranosyl-*E*-5-(2-halogenovinyl) uracils. Antimicrob Agents Chemother 20:47–52, 1981.
148. Machida H, Sakata S: In vitro and in vivo antiviral activity of 1-β-D-arabinofuranosyl-*E*-5-(2-bromovinyl)uracil (BV-araU) and related compounds. Antiviral Res 4:135–141, 1984.
149. Machida H: Comparison of susceptibilities of varicella-zoster virus and herpes simplex virus to nucleoside analogs. Antimicrob Agents Chemother 29:524–526, 1986.
150. Suzutani T, Machida H, Sakuma T, Azuma M: Effects of various

nucleosides on antiviral activity and metabolism of 1-β-D-arabinofuranosyl-*E*-5-(2-bromovinyl)uracil against herpes simplex virus types 1 and 2. Antimicrob Agents Chemother 32:1547–1551, 1988.
151. Cheng YC, Dutschman G, Fox JJ, et al: Differential activity of potential antiviral nucleoside analogs on herpes simplex virus–induced and human cellular thymidine kinases. Antimicrob Agents Chemother 20:420–423, 1981.
152. Yokota T, Kono K, Mori S, et al: Mechanism of selective inhibition of varicella-zoster virus replication by 1-β-D-arabinofuranosyl-*E*-5-(2-bromovinyl) uracil. A report from Yamasa Shoyu Co, Japan. Antiviral Res 4:245–257, 1988.
153. Whitley RJ, Weiss H, Gnann J, et al: Sorivudine (BV-araU) versus acyclovir for herpes zoster in HIV-infected patients: Results of a multi-center controlled trial. J Invest Med 43:A114, 1995.
154. Wallace MR, Sawyer MH, Chamberlin CJ, et al: BV-araU for the treatment of adult varicella. Presented at the Second International Conference on Varicella Zoster Virus Infections; 1994; Paris, France.
155. DeHertog D. Sorivudine (BV-araU) versus acyclovir for herpes zoster in HIV-infected patients: Results of a multi-center controlled trial. Presented at the 34th Interscience Conference on Antimicrobial Agents and Chemotherapy; October 4–7, 1994; Orlando, FL.
156. Rudder J de, Andreeff F, Privat de Garilhe M: Action inhibitrice de la 9-D-xylofuranosyl-adenine sur la multiplication du virus de l'herpès en culture cellulaire. C R Hebd Seances Sci Ser D 264:677–680, 1967.
157. Miller FA, Dixon GJ, Ehrlich J, et al: Antiviral activity of 9-β-D-arabinofuranosyladenine (ara-A). I. Cell culture studies. Antimicrob Agents Chemother 8:136–147, 1968.
158. Couch R: Respiratory diseases. *In* Galasso G, Whitley R, Merigan T (eds): Antiviral Agents and Viral Diseases of Man. New York, Raven Press, 1990, pp 327–273.
159. Davies WL, Grunert RR, Haff RF, et al: Antiviral activity of 1-adamantanamine (amantadine). Science 144:862–863, 1964.
160. Hoffman CE: Amantadine HCI and related compounds. *In* Carter WA (ed): Selective Inhibitors of Viral Functions. Cleveland, OH, CRC Press, 1973, pp 199–211.
161. Sears SD, Clements ML: Protective efficacy of low-dose amantadine in adults challenged with wild-type influenza A virus. Antimicrob Agents Chemother 31:1470–1473, 1987.
162. Douglas RGJ: Drug therapy: Prophylaxis and treatment of influenza. N Engl J Med 322:443–450, 1990.
163. Reines ED, Gross PA: Antiviral agents. Med Clin North Am 72:691–721, 1988.
164. Dolin R, Reichman RC, Madone HP, et al: A controlled trial of amantadine and rimantadine in the prophylaxis of influenza A infection. N Engl J Med 307:580–584, 1982.
165. Tominack RL, Hayden FG: Rimantadine hydrochloride and amantadine hydrochloride use in influenza A virus infections. Infect Dis Clin North Am 1:459–478, 1987.
166. Hayden FG: Amantadine and rimantadine resistance in influenza A viruses. Curr Opin Infect Dis 7:674–677, 1994.
167. Jackson GG, Rubenis ME, Levandowski RA: Viral respiratory disease. Curr Ther Intern Med 2:765–770, 1987.
168. Centers for Disease Control: Prevention and control of influenza. Ann Intern Med 107:521–525, 1987.
169. Mostow SR: Prevention, management, and control of influenza. Am J Med 82:35–40, 1987.
170. Belshe RB, Burk B, Newman F: Resistance of influenza A virus to amantadine and rimantadine: Results of one decade of surveillance. J Infect Dis 159:430–435, 1989.
171. Belshe RB, Smith MH, Hall CB, et al: Genetic basis of resistance to rimantadine emerging during treatment of influenza virus infection. J Virol 62:1508–1512, 1988.
172. Hay AJ: The action of adamantanamines against influenza A viruses: Inhibition of the M2 ion channel protein. Semin Virol 3:21–30, 1992.
173. Hayden FG, Belshe RB, Clover RD, et al: Emergence and apparent transmission of rimantadine-resistant influenza A virus in families. N Engl J Med 321:696–702, 1989.
174. Hayden FG, Gwaltney JM Jr, Van de Castle RL, et al: Comparative toxicity of amantadine hydrochloride and rimantadine hydrochloride in healthy adults. Antimicrob Agents Chemother 19:226–233, 1981.
175. Sidwell RW, Huffman JH, Khare GP, et al: Broad-spectrum antiviral activity of virazole: 1-β-D-Ribofuranosyl-1,2,4-triazole-3-carboxamide. Science 177:705–706, 1972.
176. Huffman JH, Sidwell RW, Khare GP, et al: In vitro effect of 1-beta-D-ribofuranosyl-1,2,4-triaxole-3-carboxamide (virazole, ICN 1229) on deoxyribonucleic acid and ribonucletic acid viruses. Antimicrob Agents Chemother 3:235–241, 1973.
177. Wray SK, Gilbert BE, Noall MW, et al: Mode of action of ribavirin: Effect of nucleotide pool alterations on influenza virus ribonucleoprotein synthesis. Antiviral Res 5:29–37, 1985.
178. Eriksson B, Helgstrand E, Johansson NG, et al: Inhibition of influenza virus ribonucleic acid polymerase by ribavirin triphosphate. Antimicrob Agents Chemother 11:946–951, 1977.
179. Laskin OL, Longstreth JA, Hart CC, et al: Ribavirin disposition in high-risk patients for acquired immunodeficiency syndrome. Clin Pharmacol Ther 41:546–555, 1987.
180. Hall CB, McBride JT, Walsh EE, et al: Aerosolized ribavirin treatment of infants with respiratory syncytial viral infection: Randomized double-blind study. N Engl J Med 308:1443–1447, 1983.
181. Hall CB, Walsh EE, Hruska JF, et al: Ribavirin treatment of experimental respiratory syncytial viral infection: Controlled double-blind study in young adults. JAMA 249:2666–2670, 1983.
182. Hall CB, McBride JT, Gala CL, et al: Ribavirin treatment of respiratory syncytial virus infection in infants with underlying cardiopulmonary disease. JAMA 254:3047–3051, 1985.
183. Carmack MA, Prober CG: Respiratory syncytial virus and ribavirin: Quo vadis? Infect Agents Dis 1:99–107, 1992.
184. McIntosh K, Kurachek SC, Cairns LM, et al: Treatment of respiratory viral infection in immunodeficient infant with ribavirin aerosol. Am J Dis Child 138:305–308, 1984.
185. Smith DW, Frankel LR, Mathers LH, et al: A controlled trial of aerosolized ribavirin in infants receiving mechanical ventilation for severe respiratory syncytial virus infection. N Engl J Med 325:24–29, 1991.
186. Wald ER, Dashefasky B, Green M: In re ribavirin: Case of premature adjudication. J Pediatr 112:154–158, 1988.
187. Fernandez H: Summary of clinical trials—Herpes genitalis and measles. *In* Smith RA, Kirkpatrick W (eds): Ribavirin: A Broad Spectrum Antiviral Agent. New York, Academic Press, 1980, pp 215–230.
188. Uylangco CV, Beroy GJ, Santiago LT, et al: Double-blind placebo-controlled evaluation of ribavirin in treatment of acute measles. Clin Ther 3:389–396, 1981.
189. Bierman SM, Kirkpatrick W, Fernandex H: Clinical efficacy of ribavirin in treatment of genital herpes simplex virus infection. Chemotherapy 27:139–145, 1981.
190. Minkoff DL: Clinical use of ribavirin and treatment of herpes zoster in otherwise normal adults. *In* Smith RA, Kirkpatrick W (eds): Ribavirin: A Broad Spectrum Antiviral Agent. New York, Academic Press, 1980, pp 185–199.
191. McCormick JB, King IJ, Webb PA, et al: Lassa fever: Effective therapy with ribavirin. N Engl J Med 314:20–26, 1986.
192. Huggins JW: Prospects for treatment of viral ribavirin, a broad spectrum of antiviral drug. Rev Infect Dis 11(Suppl):S750–S761, 1989.
193. Chapman LE, Khabbaz RF: Etiology and epidemiology of the Four Corners hantavirus outbreak. Infect Agents Dis 3:234–244, 1994.
194. Liss HP, Bernstien J: Ribavirin aerosol in the elderly. Chest 93:1239–1240, 1988.
195. Rodriguez WJ, Dang Bui RH, Conner JD, et al: Environmental exposure of primary care personnel to ribavirin aerosol when supervising treatment of infants with respiratory syncytial virus infections. Antimicrob Agents Chemother 31:1143–1146, 1987.
196. Centers for Disease Control: Assessing exposures of health-care personnel to aerosols of ribavirin—California. JAMA 260:1844–1845, 1988.
197. Nokta MA, Reichman RC, Pollard RB: Pathogenesis of viral infections. *In* Galasso GJ, Whitley RJ, Merigan TC (eds): Antiviral Agents and Viral Diseases of Man. New York, Raven Press, 1989, pp 49–85.
198. Ho M: Interferon for the treatment of infections. Annu Rev Med 38:51–59, 1987.
199. Eron LJ, Judson F, Tucker S, et al: Interferon therapy for condylomata acuminata. N Engl J Med 315:1059–1064, 1986.

200. Friedman-Kien A, Eron LJ, Conant M, et al: Natural interferon alpha for treatment of condylomata acuminata. JAMA 259:533–538, 1988.
201. Reichman RC, Oakes D, Bonnez W, et al: Treatment of condyloma acuminatum with three different interferons administered intralesionally: A multicentered, placebo-controlled trial. Ann Intern Med 108:675–679, 1988.
202. Reichman RC, Oakes D, Bonnez W, et al: Treatment of condyloma acuminatum with three different alpha interferon preparations administered parenterally: A double-blind, placebo-controlled trial. J Infect Dis 162:248–258, 1990.
203. Haglund S, Jundquist P, Cantell K, et al: Interferon therapy in juvenile laryngeal papillomatosis. Arch Otolaryngol 107:327–332, 1981.
204. Goepfert H, Gutterman J, Dichtel W, et al: Leukocyte interferon in patients with juvenile papillomatosis. Ann Otol Rhinol Laryngol 91:431–436, 1982.
205. Greenberg HB, Pollard RB, Lutwick LI, et al: Effect of human leukocyte interferon on hepatitis B virus infection in patients with chronic active hepatitis. N Engl J Med 295:517–522, 1976.
206. Alexander GJM, Brahm J, Fagan EA: Loss of HBsAg with interferon therapy in chronic hepatitis B virus infection. Lancet 1:66–68, 1987.
207. Alexander GJM, Williams R: Natural history and therapy of chronic hepatitis in humans: A critical review of the state of the art. Am J Med 85:143–146, 1988.
208. Hoofnagle JH, Di Bisceglie AM: Antiviral therapy of viral hepatitis. *In* Galasso GJ, Whitley RJ, Merigan TC (eds): Antiviral Agents and Viral Diseases of Man. New York, Raven Press, 1989, pp 415–459.
209. Hoofnagle JH: Antiviral treatment of chronic type B hepatitis. Ann Intern Med 107:414–415, 1987.
210. Perrillo RP, Schiff ER, Davis GL, et al: A randomized, controlled trial of interferon alfa-2b alone and after prednisone withdrawal for the treatment of chronic hepatitis B. N Engl J Med 323:295–301, 1990.
211. Davis GL, Balart LA, Schiff ER, et al: Treatment of chronic hepatitis C with recombinant interferon alfa: A multicenter randomized, controlled trial. N Engl J Med 321:1501–1506, 1989.
212. Davis GL, Lim H: Current status of interferon therapy for chronic hepatitis C: A hepatologist's perspective. Infect Agents Dis 2:150–154, 1993.
213. Samo TC, Greenberg SB, Couch RB, et al: Efficacy and tolerance of intranasally applied recombinant leukocyte A interferon in normal volunteers. J Infect Dis 148:535–542, 1983.
214. Herzog C, Just M, Berger R, et al: Intranasal interferon for contact prophylaxis against common cold in families (Letter). Lancet 2:962, 1983.
215. Farr BM, Gwaltney JM Jr, Adams KF, et al: Intranasal interferon alpha 2 for prevention of natural rhinovirus colds. Antimicrob Agents Chemother 26:1–34, 1984.
216. Tyrrell DA: Interferons and their clinical value. Rev Infect Dis 9:243–249, 1987.
217. Douglas RM, Moore BW, Miles HB, et al: Prophylactic efficacy of intranasal alpha$_2$-interferon against rhinovirus infections in family setting. N Engl J Med 314:65–70, 1986.
218. Hayden FG, Albrecht JK, Kaiser DL, et al: Prevention of natural colds by contact prophylaxis with intranasal alpha-interferon. N Engl J Med 314:71–75, 1986.
219. Crumpacker CS 2d: Molecular targets for antiviral therapy. N Engl J Med 321:163–171, 1989.
220. Lalezari JP, Drew WL, Glutzer E, et al: Treatment with intravenous (*S*)-1-[3-hydroxy-2-(phosphonylmethoxy)propyl]-cytosine of acyclovir-resistant mucocutaneous infection with herpes simplex virus in a patient with AIDS. J Infect Dis 170:570–572, 1994.
221. Bronson JJ, Ferrara LM, Hitchcock MJ, et al: (*S*)-1-(3-Hydroxy-2-(phosphonylmethoxy)propyl)cytosine (HPMPC): A potent antiherpesvirus agent. Adv Exp Med Biol 278:277–283, 1990.
222. Yang H, Datema R: Prolonged and potent therapeutic and prophylactic effects of (*S*)-1-[(3-hydroxy-2-phosphonylmethoxy)-propyl] cytosine against herpes simplex virus type 2 infections in mice. Antimicrob Agents Chemother 35:1596–1600, 1991.
223. Bischofberger N, Hitchcock MJ, Chen MS, et al: 1-[((*S*)-2-Hydroxy-2-oxo-1,4,2-dioxaphosphorinan-5-yl) methyl] cytosine, an intracellular prodrug for (*S*)-1-(3-hydroxy-2-phosphonylmethoxypropyl) cytosine with improved therapeutic index in vivo. Antimicrob Agents Chemother 38:2387–2391, 1994.
224. Lee WA, Shaw J-P, Bidgood A, et al: Tissue distribution and bioavailability of cyclic HPMPC, an intracellular prodrug of HPMPC. Presented at the Eighth International Conference on Antiviral Research; April 23–28, 1995; Santa Fe, NM.
225. Gordon YJ, Romanowski EG, Araullo-Cruz T: HPMPC, a broad-spectrum topical antiviral gent, inhibits herpes simplex virus type 1 replication and promotes healing of dendritic keratitis in the New Zealand rabbit ocular model. Cornea 13:516–520, 1994.
226. Bravo FJ, Stanberry LR, Kier AB, et al: Evaluation of HPMPC therapy for primary and recurrent genital herpes in mice and guinea pigs. Antiviral Res 21:59–72, 1993.
227. Petty BG, Wachsman M, Jordan MC, et al: Sequential ascending multiple-dose safety and pharmacokinetic study of oral lobucavir (BMS-180194) in asymptomatic volunteers seropositive for HIV and CMV. Presented at the Eighth International Conference on Antiviral Research; April 23–28, 1995; Sante Fe, NM.
228. O'Brien WJ, Coe EC, Taylor JL: Nucleoside metabolism in herpes simplex virus–infected cells following treatment with interferon and acyclovir, a possible mechanism of synergistic antiviral activity. Antimicrob Agents Chemother 34:1178–1182, 1990.
229. Smith TJ, Kremer MJ, Lou M, et al: The site of attachment in human rhinovirus 14 for antiviral agents that inhibit uncoating. Science 233:1286–1293, 1986.
230. Otto MJ, Fox MF, Fancher MJ, et al: In vitro activity of WIN 51711, a new broad-spectrum antipicornavirus drug. Antimicrob Agents Chemother 27:883–886, 1985.

33

Antifungal Drugs

J. Michael Kilby
William E. Dismukes

The systemic mycoses are among the most difficult infectious diseases to treat. Long-term therapy for weeks to months is often necessary, as is close monitoring of the patient for potentially serious side effects of the antifungal agents. Amphotericin B, flucytosine, miconazole, ketoconazole, fluconazole, and itraconazole are the drugs currently available for the therapy of systemic fungal diseases. Although there is growing evidence that the azole compounds (which have minimal toxicity and can be given orally) are appropriate alternatives in many clinical situations, the fungicidal agent amphotericin B, available since 1957, is the traditional drug of choice for severe systemic infections caused by common fungal pathogens such as *Aspergillus* species, *Blastomyces dermatitidis*, *Candida* species, *Coccidioides immitis*, *Cryptococcus neoformans*, and *Histoplasma capsulatum*. The currently available drugs are discussed in detail here; the activity spectrum of each drug is summarized in Table 33–1. Investigational agents are described briefly.

Amphotericin B

Amphotericin B, a polyene macrolide antibiotic similar to nystatin, is a bacterial by-product of *Streptomyces nodosus*.[1] The name amphotericin B is derived from the ability of the drug to act as both an acid and a base. The drug is unstable at high or low pH and must be formulated in a neutral suspension of 5% dextrose in water (D5W). Amphotericin B,

TABLE 33–1 ■ Spectrum of Activity of Antifungal Agents Against Systemic Fungal Pathogens Based on Results of Tests in Vitro or in Vivo in Animals

PATHOGEN	AMPHOTERICIN B	FLUCYTOSINE	MICONAZOLE	KETOCONAZOLE	FLUCONAZOLE	ITRACONAZOLE
Aspergillus species	+	+	+			+
Blastomyces dermatitidis	+			+	+	+
Candida albicans	+	+	+	+	+	+
Agents of chromomycosis		+		+		+
Cryptococcus neoformans	+	+	+	+	+	+
Coccidioides immitis	+		+	+	+	+
Histoplasma capsulatum	+		+	+	+	+
Agents of mucormycosis	+					
Paracoccidioides brasiliensis	+		+	+	+	+
Pseudoallescheria boydii			+	+		
Sporothrix schenckii	+		+	+	+	+

which is complexed with desoxycholate, a bile salt, to improve its solubility in water, is marketed in 50-mg vials for intravenous use. Topical preparations are also available.

Amphotericin B has a lipophilic structure and binds to cholesterol in mammalian cell membranes and more avidly to ergosterol in fungal cytoplasmic membranes, resulting in a disruption of membrane integrity with subsequent leakage of intracellular contents and, ultimately, cell death.[2] Fungi may rarely become resistant to amphotericin B and other polyene agents by decreasing membrane ergosterol or by altering the binding characteristics of ergosterol to amphotericin B.[3] In addition, fungi may develop resistance to amphotericin B after being exposed to the antifungal azole compounds. Of potential clinical importance is the observation that outcome in immunocompromised hosts may be worse among patients with infections caused by yeasts that are more resistant to amphotericin B.[4–6] Several studies have suggested that the effectiveness of amphotericin B may be due in part to favorable immunomodulatory effects such as increased macrophage activation.[2, 7] Some of the enhanced fungicidal activity of monocytes and macrophages in the presence of amphotericin B may be attributable to accumulation of the drug within these cells rather than to immunomodulation.[8]

Absorption of amphotericin B after oral administration is minimal; therefore, intravenous dosing for treatment of systemic mycoses is required.[9] Peak serum concentrations are approximately 0.5 to 2.0 μg/mL after a 50-mg dose. Once the colloidal suspension has been administered, the desoxycholate salt separates from the amphotericin B complex, with the free drug being highly bound (90% to 95%) by plasma proteins. Amphotericin B is distributed principally into the liver (14% to 41%), lungs (1% to 6%), and kidneys (0.3% to 2%) and to a lesser extent into pleural, peritoneal, and joint fluids and aqueous humor. Distribution into the central nervous system, vitreous humor, and amniotic fluid is minimal. Because of slow release from tissue stores, the drug can be detected in the serum for 7 to 8 weeks after treatment ceases.

Amphotericin B has previously been the mainstay of systemic antifungal therapy[1] (Table 33–2). It remains the drug of choice for patients with progressive, life-threatening fungal disease such as invasive aspergillosis or mucormycosis. Although amphotericin B, alone or in combination, is effective therapy for candidemia and other forms of disseminated candidiasis, azole compounds may provide comparable efficacy with less toxicity in nonneutropenic hosts with uncomplicated candidemia.[10] Although there is limited experience supporting the effectiveness of fluconazole for hepatosplenic candidiasis,[11, 12] amphotericin B is often chosen for life-threatening candidal syndromes including meningitis, endocarditis, and hepatosplenic disease.[13, 14] The combination of amphotericin B and flucytosine is recommended for patients with cryptococcal meningitis,[15, 16] but fluconazole may be a reasonable alternative for patients infected with human immunodeficiency virus (HIV) who present with less severe manifestations of cryptococcal meningitis.[17] The azole compounds provide effective alternative therapy for patients with mild to moderately severe blastomycosis, coccidioidomycosis, and histoplasmosis,[18–23] but amphotericin B should be administered to all patients with serious, life-threatening forms of these diseases.

Amphotericin B is also the antifungal agent of choice for empirical therapy in a persistently febrile, granulocytopenic host.[24, 25] The role of amphotericin B for antifungal prophylaxis, in contrast to empirical therapy, in immunocompromised hosts is less clear. Patients undergoing bone marrow transplantation have less fungal colonization[26] and fewer invasive *Aspergillus* infections[27] when given prophylactic low-dose amphotericin B, but the overall risk/benefit ratio of this intervention is not known. If prophylaxis against fungal infection in the setting of bone marrow transplantation is used, fluconazole may be the preferred agent,[28] although the azole agent has less activity than amphotericin B against several fungal pathogens of emerging importance, such as *Aspergillus* species, *Candida glabrata,* and *Candida krusei.*

Therapy should be initiated with a test dose of 1.0 mg amphotericin B in 50 to 100 mL of D5W infused during 20 to

TABLE 33–2 ■ Therapy for Selected Systemic Mycoses

DISEASE	RECOMMENDED THERAPY	ALTERNATIVES
Aspergillosis	Amphotericin B (± flucytosine or rifampin)	Itraconazole
Blastomycosis	Amphotericin B or itraconazole	Ketoconazole ? Fluconazole
Candidiasis (invasive or disseminated)	Amphotericin B (± flucytosine) or fluconazole	? Itraconazole
Chromomycosis	Flucytosine ± amphotericin B	Ketoconazole Itraconazole
Coccidioidomycosis	Fluconazole or amphotericin B	Ketoconazole Itraconazole
Cryptococcosis	Amphotericin B (± flucytosine) or fluconazole	? Itraconazole
Histoplasmosis	Itraconazole or amphotericin B	Ketoconazole ? Fluconazole
Mucormycosis	Amphotericin B	None
Paracoccidioidomycosis	Ketoconazole or itraconazole	Amphotericin B Sulfonamide
Sporotrichosis (extracutaneous)	Itraconazole	Amphotericin B ? Fluconazole

30 minutes, and the patient's vital signs should be monitored closely over this period. Dosage may then be increased rapidly, or more slowly in increments.[2] For patients with neutropenia or rapidly progressing infection (e.g., invasive aspergillosis), a dose of 0.25 to 0.5 mg/kg should be given after the test dose. The daily dose may then be rapidly escalated to 0.75 to 1.0 mg/kg administered during a period of 2 to 6 hours, depending on the patient's tolerance. For patients who have significant side effects with the test dose, poor cardiopulmonary function, or more indolent fungal disease, amphotericin B may be administered in a slower, more cautious approach. For example, after the test dose, therapy may be initiated with a dose of 0.25 to 0.3 mg/kg per day, followed by a gradual increase in the daily dose by 5 to 10 mg until a dose of 0.4 to 0.6 mg/kg per day is reached. In the majority of patients, rapid infusions of amphotericin B (during 1 or 2 hours) are generally well tolerated,[29] although more initial adverse signs and symptoms—including rigors, tachycardia, nausea, and vomiting—were reported in patients given a 45-minute infusion compared with those given the standard 4-hour infusion.[30] Because amphotericin B is degraded in situ and only small amounts are excreted as unchanged drug in the urine and feces, downward dosage adjustments are not necessary for patients with preexisting renal or hepatic impairment. Patients receiving hemodialysis or peritoneal dialysis require no additional dose of amphotericin B after dialysis, owing to the extensive plasma protein binding and the wide volume of distribution of the drug. Routine measurement of amphotericin B concentrations in body fluids is not indicated.[1]

The significance of asymptomatic candiduria and the optimal therapy for various syndromes associated with funguria are unknown.[31] Amphotericin B may be administered locally to patients with candidal urinary tract infection by continuous or intermittent bladder irrigation. Continuous irrigation is carried out by infusing a solution of 50 μg/mL through a triple-lumen urinary catheter or suprapubic tube for 2 to 5 days. Amphotericin B has also been infused directly into the renal pelvis or ureter via nephrostomy tube. Intermittent irrigation is carried out by instilling 10 to 30 mg of amphotericin B in 250 to 400 mL of D5W via urinary catheter and cross-clamping the catheter for as long as possible; this dose is given one to four times daily for several days.

Amphotericin B is associated with a variety of major and minor adverse effects that often affect its use (Table 33–3). Anaphylaxis-type reactions manifested as hypotension, arrhythmias, and even cardiac arrest are rare but have occurred during initial exposure to the drug; hence, the need to give a test dose. Infusion of amphotericin B is frequently accompanied by headache, nausea, chills, and fever, which in general tend to subside or decrease after several days to several weeks of therapy. Premedication with oral aspirin, acetaminophen, indomethacin, or diphenhydramine has been used to minimize these infusion-related reactions. If these measures are ineffective, intravenous hydrocortisone or meperidine may be given before the infusion or added to the infusion solution in a further attempt to control the constitutional symptoms. Thrombophlebitis, which is associated with intravenous infusion of amphotericin B, may be minimized by administering heparin concomitantly (500 to 1000 units), prolonging the period of infusion, and frequently changing infusion sites. One study suggests that empirical pretreatment regimens may not provide any additional benefit over observation without premedication.[32] Instead, pretreatment regimens may be designed for subsequent doses based on an individual's adverse experience with initial amphotericin B doses.

The kidneys and bone marrow are the targets of the major toxic effects of amphotericin B. Some degree of nephrotoxicity occurs in most patients, often in the form of azotemia, decreased urinary concentrating ability, and hypokalemia to the degree that many patients require potassium supplementation. Clinically significant renal tubular acidosis and hypomagnesemia may develop. Renal damage is in part dose related and is reversible up to a total dose of 2.0 to 5.0 g.[33] The daily dose of amphotericin B should be decreased or the drug temporarily discontinued when a patient's creatinine level rises above 3.0 mg/dL. The use of an alternate-day dosing regimen reduces nephrotoxicity only if the total cumulative dose is reduced. Efforts to prevent renal toxicity involve primarily the avoidance of other nephrotoxic agents and diuretics and the maintenance of an adequate intravascular volume. Renal toxicity can be reversed and may be prevented with adequate sodium loading and maintenance of sodium intake, which interfere with tubuloglomerular feedback.[34] A mild to moderate normocytic, normochromic anemia secondary to decreased production of erythropoietin occurs in most patients who receive more than 2 to 3 weeks of amphotericin B therapy, and it is usually reversible on discontinuation of drug. Neutropenia and thrombocytopenia are rare adverse effects. Arachnoiditis and myelopathy are potential complications of intrathecal infusion. An acute, fatal deterioration in pulmonary function has been reported when amphotericin B and granulocyte infusions have been administered concomitantly, but the data to support this association are conflicting.[35, 36]

Flucytosine

Flucytosine (5-fluorocytosine) is an orally administered antifungal agent used principally in combination with amphotericin B for the treatment of cryptococcal meningitis and disseminated or invasive forms of candidiasis.[2] The fungistatic effects of this fluorine analog of cytosine result from its antimetabolite properties. After uptake by fungi, flucytosine is converted by intracellular deamination to fluorouracil, which is incorporated into fungal RNA and inhibits protein synthesis. Flucytosine is also converted to fluorodeoxyuridine monophosphate, which interferes with DNA synthesis by inhibiting thymidylate synthetase.

Flucytosine is available in 250- and 500-mg capsules. Approximately 90% of an orally administered dose is absorbed.[9] Minimal plasma protein binding and tissue accumulation result in a short half-life of 3 to 5 hours. Flucytosine concentrations in the cerebrospinal, peritoneal, and synovial fluids and in bronchial secretions are approximately 75% of simultaneous plasma concentrations regardless of the presence of inflammation. About 90% of a dose is excreted unchanged in the urine; consequently the urine concentration may be up to 100 times that in plasma.

For patients with normal renal function, the recommended dosage of flucytosine is 75 to 150 mg/kg per day at 6-hour intervals. As shown in Table 33–4, the daily dose must be adjusted for patients with renal dysfunction.[37] Patients receiving hemodialysis require an additional 37.5 mg/kg dose after dialysis. In addition, plasma levels of flucytosine should be monitored to maintain peak concentration between 50 and 100 μg/mL, as myelosuppression and other toxicities correlate with higher plasma levels of the drug.

Flucytosine is indicated for patients with cryptococcosis, invasive forms of candidiasis, and chromomycosis (see Table 33–2). The development of drug resistance is more common in patients treated with flucytosine alone. Combination therapy with flucytosine and amphotericin B is aimed at achieving a synergistic effect and preventing the emergence of drug-resistant fungi. Although combination therapy has been associated with conflicting results in a few patients with

TABLE 33–3 ■ Adverse Effects of Currently Available Systemic Antifungal Agents

TYPE OR LOCATION OF EFFECT	AMPHOTERICIN B	FLUCYTOSINE	KETOCONAZOLE	MICONAZOLE	FLUCONAZOLE	ITRACONAZOLE
Acute, life threatening	Hypotension, anaphylaxis, cardiac arrhythmias			Hypotension, anaphylaxis, cardiac arrhythmias		
Gastrointestinal tract	Anorexia, nausea, vomiting	Abdominal pain, diarrhea, nausea, vomiting	Abdominal pain, anorexia, nausea, vomiting	Nausea, vomiting	Anorexia, nausea, vomiting	Anorexia, nausea, vomiting
Skin		Rash	Pruritus ± rash	Pruritus ± rash	Rash	Rash
Kidney	Azotemia, renal tubular acidosis, hypokalemia, hypomagnesemia					
Liver		Hepatitis	Hepatitis		Hepatitis	Hepatitis
Bone marrow	Anemia	Anemia (less common), leukopenia, thrombocytopenia		Anemia, leukopenia, thrombocytosis, thrombocytopenia		
Endocrine			Decreased libido, impotence, oligospermia, gynecomastia, menstrual irregularities			
Other	Headache, fever, chills, phlebitis, weight loss	Confusion, headache	Photophobia, somnolence, headache	Fever, phlebitis, psychosis, hyperlipidemia, hyponatremia	Alopecia	Hypokalemia, pedal edema, hypertension

TABLE 33–4 ■ Flucytosine Dosing in Patients with Renal Failure

CREATININE CLEARANCE RATE (mL/min)	DOSAGE (mg/kg/d)
>50	100–150
26–50	75
13–25	37
≤12	Adjusted to keep 2-h peak level at 50–100 μg/mL
Hemodialysis patients	37.5 mg/kg after dialysis

Adapted and reprinted by permission of the publisher from Toxicity of amphotericin B plus flucytosine in 194 patients with cryptococcal meningitis, by Stamm AM, Diasio RB, Dismukes WE, et al, American Journal of Medicine, 83:236–242, 1987. Copyright 1987 by Excerpta Medica Inc.

Aspergillus infections, it is frequently used for more severe cases of cryptococcal meningitis,[15, 16] including patients who have acquired immunodeficiency syndrome (AIDS), and for those with serious, life-threatening candidal syndromes such as meningitis, endocarditis, and hepatosplenic disease.[13, 14]

As shown in Table 33–3, the toxicity of flucytosine is directed principally against the gastrointestinal tract, liver, and bone marrow. For the most part, these adverse effects are dose related and can be prevented or minimized by maintaining plasma levels below 100 μg/mL. In addition, the metabolite fluorouracil may exert a toxic effect. Data are conflicting about the risk of flucytosine toxicity in patients receiving combination amphotericin B and flucytosine therapy, for which safety evaluations are confounded by amphotericin B–induced renal dysfunction.[37] Close monitoring of hepatic, renal, and hematopoietic function is essential. If a patient develops abdominal pain, nausea, vomiting, or diarrhea, flucytosine should be withdrawn or the dose reduced until these symptoms subside or improve. Approximately 5% of patients develop asymptomatic elevations in hepatocellular enzymes. Clinically significant hepatitis is rare, but deaths have been attributed to flucytosine-induced hepatic disease. About 10% to 15% of patients develop leukopenia, thrombocytopenia, or both; anemia is much less common. In one study, most patients with AIDS were able to tolerate flucytosine at a dose of 100 mg/kg per day.[37a] Although flucytosine-induced blood dyscrasias are usually reversible on discontinuation of drug, fatal bone marrow suppression has been reported.

The Azoles

Since the introduction of ketoconazole in 1981, the azole compounds have been increasingly utilized as less toxic alternatives to amphotericin B and flucytosine for the treatment of superficial and systemic fungal infections.[38] The azole compounds exert fungistatic activity by inhibiting synthesis of ergosterol, an integral component of the cell membrane, via selective interaction with cytochrome P-450–dependent 14-α-demethylase, thus rendering the cytoplasmic membrane more permeable. The result is leakage of intracellular contents. Fungicidal activity, likely secondary to direct membrane damage, may occur at higher concentrations. The imidazoles (miconazole and ketoconazole) contain two nitrogen atoms in the five-membered azole ring; the triazoles (fluconazole and itraconazole) contain three. The triazoles have a more selective affinity for fungal as compared with mammalian cytochrome P-450 enzymes, resulting in fewer potential adverse effects of the triazoles compared with the imidazoles.

Ketoconazole

Ketoconazole is an orally and topically administered imidazole compound that has a broad spectrum of activity. However, the improved pharmacologic characteristics and better tolerability of the newer azole compounds have made these agents superior alternatives in many clinical situations.[38] As shown in Table 33–5, ketoconazole is highly protein bound. Although the drug is distributed fairly extensively to most tissues and body fluids, cerebrospinal fluid levels are low.[39, 40] The drug is metabolized in the liver and excreted principally as inactive drug in the bile. Less than 5% of active drug is eliminated by the kidneys.

Oral ketoconazole, available as a 200-mg tablet, is absorbed fairly well: peak plasma concentrations 1 to 4 hours after a 200-mg dose are 1.5 to 3.0 μg/mL. Controversy exists as to whether food interferes with or enhances absorption.[41] An increase in the dosage results in a nearly linear increase in corresponding plasma levels; however, there is marked patient-to-patient variation. Because ketoconazole is weakly dibasic, absorption depends on gastric acidity. Thus, plasma concentration may be diminished due to poor oral absorption, especially in patients with achlorhydria; in those taking antacids, histamine H_2-receptor antagonists, or anticholinergic agents; and in elderly patients with decreased gastric acidity. Some patients with AIDS have a gastropathy that decreases gastric acid production,[42] and therefore ketoconazole may not be effective in these patients. Absorption may be improved in achlorhydric patients with 240 mL of Coca-Cola or other beverage with a pH lower than 3.0.[43] Important interactions of ketoconazole with other drugs concomitantly administered have been documented (Table 33–6). For example, ketoconazole may enhance the effects of oral anticoagulants and sulfonylureas; decrease the clearance of cyclosporine, theophylline, and chlordiazepoxide; and variably interact with phenytoin, rifampin, and isoniazid.[38] Life-threatening arrhythmias due to prolongation of the QT interval can occur when ketoconazole and selected antihistamines (terfenadine, astemizole, or loratadine) are given concurrently; therefore, coadministration should be avoided.[44]

Ketoconazole can be used to treat mucosal and cutaneous infections caused by *Candida* species and the dermatophytoses caused by *Epidermophyton, Trichosporon,* and *Microsporum* species.[45] Although ketoconazole is an effective therapy for many forms of the systemic mycoses (see Table 33–2), one of the triazoles—fluconazole or itraconazole—is often preferred because of lesser toxicity and in some cases greater efficacy. Ketoconazole may be chosen when a cheaper

TABLE 33–5 ■ Pharmacologic Properties of Selected Antifungal Azole Drugs

PROPERTY	KETOCONAZOLE	ITRACONAZOLE	FLUCONAZOLE
Molecular weight	531	706	305
Water solubility	Poor	Poor	Good
Protein binding (%)	99	>99	11
Relative oral bioavailability (%)	75	>70	>80
Urinary excretion of active drug (%)	<5	<1	80
Terminal elimination half-life (h)	7–10	24–42	22–31
Cerebrospinal fluid/plasma concentration (%)	<10	<1	>70

Adapted from Como JA, Dismukes WE: Oral azole drugs as systemic antifungal therapy [see comments]. N Engl J Med, 1994, 330, 263–272. Copyright 1994. Massachuesetts Medical Society. All rights reserved.

TABLE 33–6 ■ Drug Interactions Involving Azole Antifungal Drugs

EFFECT OF INTERACTION	KETOCONAZOLE	FLUCONAZOLE	ITRACONAZOLE
Decreased absorption of azole	Antacids H_2-receptor antagonists Sucralfate		Antacids H_2-receptor antagonists
Decreased plasma concentration of azole due to metabolism	Rifampin Phenytoin Isoniazid	Rifampin	Rifampin Phenytoin
Increased plasma concentration of coadministered drug	Warfarin Sulfonylureas Cyclosporine Phenytoin Corticosteroids Theophylline Chlordiazepoxide Midazolam Astemizole Terfenadine Loratadine Cisapride	Warfarin Sulfonylureas Cyclosporine Phenytoin Zidovudine Theophylline Rifabutin	Warfarin Sulfonylureas Cyclosporine Phenytoin Midazolam Astemizole Terfenadine Loratadine Digoxin

alternative agent is necessary for patients with indolent, non–life-threatening infections requiring prolonged treatment such as recurrent mucosal candidiasis, coccidioidomycosis, paracoccidioidomycosis, blastomycosis, chromomycosis, penicilliosis, or pseudoallescheriasis.[18, 21, 46–51] In general, the dose of ketoconazole should be 400 mg/d initially and then 200 mg/d as chronic maintenance therapy. For patients who demonstrate no response after 4 to 6 weeks, the dosage should be increased by 200-mg increments at monthly intervals up to a total dose of 800 mg/d or other appropriate antifungal therapy should be substituted. Doses of 1200 mg/d or more are associated with unacceptable toxicity.[21, 40]

As Table 33–3 shows, the most common adverse effects attributed to ketoconazole therapy are dose-dependent anorexia, vomiting, and abdominal pain, which rarely necessitate discontinuation of drug provided the dosage is less than 600 to 800 mg/d.[18] These gastrointestinal side effects may be ameliorated or prevented by administering the drug with a meal. Asymptomatic elevation of serum transaminase levels is seen in 2% to 10% of patients, but symptomatic hepatotoxicity is seen in only 1 in 10,000 to 15,000 patients. Rash, pruritus, and headache are occasional side effects. At dosages in excess of 400 mg/d, ketoconazole may interfere with steroidogenesis, resulting in endocrine abnormalities.[52] Suppression of testosterone synthesis may cause gynecomastia, oligospermia, loss of libido, impotence, and menstrual irregularities. Clinically significant adrenal insufficiency secondary to ketoconazole suppression of corticosteroid synthesis is rare and usually reversible.[53, 54]

Miconazole

Miconazole, structurally similar to clotrimazole and ketoconazole, is used mostly for the topical treatment of mucocutaneous fungal infections. A colloidal suspension for intravenous infusion is available as a 20-mL ampule (10 mg/mL) for treatment of systemic mycoses, but currently the drug is rarely used because of safer alternatives. There is no oral formulation. Adverse effects are frequent during treatment with intravenous miconazole, and life-threatening complications—including anaphylaxis, hypotension, cardiac arrhythmias, and respiratory arrest—have been reported (see Table 33–3).

Fluconazole

Fluconazole, approved in 1990, differs pharmacologically from ketoconazole and itraconazole (see Table 33–5) in that it is highly water soluble, penetrates cerebrospinal fluid well (cerebrospinal fluid/plasma ratio greater than 70%), has a longer half-life (about 30 hours), is only weakly protein bound (approximately 11%), is evenly distributed throughout body fluids and tissues, and is excreted in the urine as active drug (80%).[38, 55, 56] To achieve steady-state concentrations more rapidly, a loading dose should be used at the start of treatment. Fluconazole is currently the only azole available in both oral (tablet and suspension) and intravenous formulations.

As with other antifungal azoles, drug interactions must be considered (see Table 33–6). Current data suggest no interaction with histamine H_2-receptor antagonists; some potentiation of the effects of oral anticoagulants and sulfonylureas; and elevation of plasma levels of cyclosporine, phenytoin, and theophylline.[38, 55, 57] Rifampin decreases serum concentrations of fluconazole; conversely, fluconazole therapy may increase levels (and therefore toxicity) of the closely related compound rifabutin.[58, 59] There is also evidence that fluconazole alters the pharmacokinetic disposition of zidovudine, and patients receiving this combination should be monitored carefully for adverse reactions.[60]

Fluconazole has activity against a broad range of fungal pathogens and is useful in diverse clinical settings (see Table 33–1).[38, 55] Fluconazole is effective therapy for dermatomycoses and mucocutaneous forms of candidiasis. A single 150-mg oral dose produces a high cure rate in uncomplicated vaginal candidiasis.[61] In daily doses of 50 to 400 mg, fluconazole appears to be more effective than ketoconazole or clotrimazole troches for oral and esophageal candidiasis in patients with immunocompromising conditions. All HIV-infected patients given fluconazole at 100 mg/d for oral candidiasis in one study had clinical resolution, compared with only 65% of those treated with clotrimazole troches, and the fluconazole-treated group had more prolonged clinical responses after therapy.[62] Fluconazole at 100 to 200 mg/d resulted in endoscopic cure of *Candida* esophagitis in 91% of patients with AIDS, compared with only 52% of cases treated with 200 to 400 mg/d of ketoconazole.[46] A study involving 37 cancer patients with oropharyngeal candidiasis demonstrated comparable responses to fluconazole at 100 mg/d and ketoconazole at 400 mg/d, but the patients treated with ketoconazole had earlier relapses.[63]

In addition, fluconazole is comparable to oral formulations of amphotericin B as prophylaxis against oropharyngeal and systemic fungal infections in neutropenic patients.[64, 65] However, there are conflicting data about the usefulness of prophylaxis with fluconazole in asymptomatic at-risk individuals (including neutropenic cancer patients, bone marrow transplant recipients, and patients with AIDS).[28, 66–68] Antifungal prophylaxis in these settings is not routinely recommended as increased survival and cost-effectiveness have not been proved. Azole-resistant fungal isolates, including *C. krusei* and *C. glabrata,* have become more common under the selective pressure of routine fluconazole prophylaxis in some clinical settings.[69–71] Although the interpretation of fungal susceptibility testing is not as well standardized as that for bacterial pathogens, it is clear that both microbiologic and clinical resistance to fluconazole occurs, particularly in HIV-infected patients treated with fluconazole for mucocutaneous candidiasis.[72, 73]

One study demonstrated that fluconazole was as effective as amphotericin B for the treatment of candidemia in nonneutropenic patients. The patients in this trial were not immunodeficient and the majority of *Candida* infections were catheter related. There was substantially less toxicity associated with fluconazole compared with amphotericin B.[10]

Although amphotericin B is considered to be standard therapy for hepatosplenic candidiasis, a limited number of patients with this entity have been successfully treated with fluconazole.[11, 12] A randomized multicenter comparison of fluconazole (200 to 400 mg/d) and amphotericin B (at least 0.3 mg/kg per day) with or without flucytosine as primary treatment of cryptococcal meningitis in AIDS demonstrated that fluconazole is also an effective, less toxic alternative for this disease.[17] Among 194 evaluable patients, the rates of favorable response (including quiescent disease) were similar for the two groups (fluconazole, 60%; amphotericin B, 64%). The mortality rates also were similar. However, more early deaths occurred in fluconazole-treated patients, and conversion of cerebrospinal fluid cultures from positive to negative was slower in these patients. Results of a smaller randomized trial (20 evaluable patients) in a similar population showed superiority of combination amphotericin B and flucytosine over fluconazole.[74] These collective data do not settle the issue as to the optimal primary therapy of cryptococcal meningitis in AIDS, but fluconazole appears to be an effective alternative to amphotericin B, especially in patients with less serious disease (e.g., normal mental status at the time of presentation). Some data suggest that an effective approach is to initiate therapy with amphotericin B and flucytosine followed by consolidation of acute therapy with fluconazole.[37a] Investigations involving novel approaches for primary therapy of cryptococcosis are ongoing and include an oral combination of fluconazole and flucytosine[75] and higher daily doses (800 mg/d) of fluconazole.[76] All AIDS patients with cryptococcal meningitis who survive the initial illness require some form of lifetime maintenance therapy.[77] Results of a prospective multicenter trial conducted by the National Institute of Allergy and Infectious Diseases Mycoses Study Group and the AIDS Clinical Trials Group indicate that fluconazole (200 mg/d) is more effective as maintenance therapy than is amphotericin B (1.0 mg/kg per week).[78] The failure rate in the fluconazole treatment group was 9%, compared with 33% in the amphotericin B group.

Oral azole drugs have replaced amphotericin B for the management of most non–life-threatening *C. immitis* infections.[21–23] Fluconazole is also effective therapy for coccidioidal meningitis and provides a welcome alternative to previous regimens involving prolonged intrathecal amphotericin B.[20] Higher doses of fluconazole appear to be necessary for a successful outcome in treating other endemic mycoses, including blastomycosis, histoplasmosis, and sporotrichosis.[38]

Fluconazole is well tolerated in dosages up to 400 mg/d. The most common adverse effects are nausea, vomiting, and rash (see Table 33–3). Asymptomatic elevations in hepatocellular enzyme levels occasionally occur; severe and even fatal hepatotoxicity has also been reported.[79] Otherwise, major toxicity has been minimal. There has been no evidence of suppression of steroidogenesis in animals or humans.[80] Alopecia has been associated with fluconazole and is usually reversible on discontinuation of the drug. The etiology of this potentially endocrinologic effect is not understood.[81]

Itraconazole

Itraconazole is an orally administered antifungal triazole that was approved for treatment of both superficial and systemic mycoses in 1992. When taken with meals, itraconazole has a bioavailability greater than 70%, is more than 99% protein bound after oral administration, and has a half-life in humans of more than 24 hours[38] (see Table 33–5). Concentrations of itraconazole in the lungs, kidneys, and epidermis are five times greater than simultaneous plasma concentrations; however, penetration into cerebrospinal fluid is less than 10% of the plasma concentration, regardless of the degree of meningeal inflammation. Less than 1% of active drug is excreted into the urine. No dose adjustment is required for patients with renal or hepatic dysfunction.

The interactions between itraconazole and other drugs represent a drawback to its clinical use in patients with complicated medical problems (see Table 33–6). Like that of ketoconazole, the absorption of itraconazole can be affected by drugs that alter gastric acidity. In addition, several other important itraconazole-drug interactions have been reported that may necessitate close monitoring of drug levels (phenytoin, cyclosporine) or avoidance altogether (terfenadine, astemizole, midazolam).[38]

Itraconazole is considered the drug of choice for several dimorphic fungal infections. It is recommended for the treatment of most patients with chronic indolent blastomycosis.[19] Although life-threatening histoplasmosis should be treated with amphotericin B, itraconazole is indicated for most patients with or without AIDS who have less severe *Histoplasma* infections.[19] In one study, 85% of patients with AIDS-associated mild to moderately severe disseminated histoplasmosis responded to itraconazole at 600 mg/d for 3 days, followed by 400 mg/d.[82] In addition, itraconazole, 200 to 400 mg/d, is the preferred agent in preventing relapse of disseminated histoplasmosis in patients with AIDS.[83] Itraconazole is the drug of choice in treating most patients with lymphocutaneous or osteoarticular forms of sporotrichosis.[84, 85] Open-label noncomparative clinical trials in humans indicate that itraconazole is effective therapy for dermatophytic infections including onychomycosis[86] as well as coccidioidomycosis,[22, 87] paracoccidioidomycosis,[88] chromomycosis,[88] and infections due to *Penicillium marneffei*[50] when administered in daily doses of 50 to 600 mg for at least 3 to 6 months.

Itraconazole is more active against *Aspergillus* species than are the other azoles. Open-label noncomparative trials involving patients with invasive aspergillosis suggest that itraconazole is sometimes effective for this devastating infection and is associated with less toxicity than is amphotericin B.[89, 90] Itraconazole is a reasonable alternative for patients who cannot take fluconazole as "consolidation" therapy after a 2-week induction phase consisting of amphotericin B with flucytosine.[37a] Preliminary studies indicate that itraconazole is also effective in the treatment of oropharyngeal and vaginal candidiasis, but results of large trials comparing the drug with the other azoles are not currently available.

To date, no serious adverse effects have been associated with itraconazole, including suppression of steroidogenesis (see Table 33–3). Minor side effects include nausea and vomiting, rash, anorexia, flatulence, headache, transient elevation of hepatocellular enzyme levels, and hypokalemia with or without pedal edema and increased blood pressure. No explanation for the latter effects has been determined.[38]

Investigational Antifungal Agents

Novel Forms and Routes of Administration of Amphotericin B

There are several promising investigational approaches to diminishing the toxicities of conventional intravenous amphotericin B administration. Intracavitary amphotericin B instillation for treatment of aspergilloma has been explored, as have aerosolized and intranasal formulations of amphotericin B for prophylaxis of pulmonary infections.

Lipid formulations of amphotericin B have been developed to permit larger doses of free drug to be given with a higher therapeutic index. Amphotericin B has been incorporated into unilamellar liposomes (AmBisome), a colloidal dispersion (ABCD, Amphocil, or Amphotec), and nonliposomal lipid complexes (ABLC or Abelcet). Other studies have investigated the emulsion of amphotericin B in common lipid parenteral nutrition solution (Intralipid).[91] Animal studies indicate that both the liposomal vesicles and the lipid complex are taken up rapidly by the reticuloendothelial system, including lymph nodes, liver, lungs, spleen, and kidneys. The tropism of these lipid preparations of amphotericin B for the reticuloendothelial system may be responsible for the enhanced efficacy. Amphotericin B is transferred efficiently from the vehicle to fungal cells primarily in monomeric form rather than in aggregated forms, which may explain its decreased adverse effects on leukocyte activity and other host tissues.[92] Lipid formulations have variable activity in vitro.[93] Although limited clinical studies carried out with lipid formulations of amphotericin B have yielded encouraging results,[94–96] the exact role of these awaits the outcome of large clinical trials comparing commercially standardized preparations of these investigational agents with conventional amphotericin B.

Other Drugs

New formulations of oral suspension and intravenous itraconazole are in development. Other investigational triazole compounds with an improved spectrum of antifungal activity, especially against *Aspergillus* species, are currently undergoing evaluation. Terbinafine, an allylamine compound that inhibits squalene epoxidase, resulting in ergosterol deficiency, has been used in the United States as a topical therapy for superficial dermatophyte infections. Oral terbinafine, available in Europe, has the potential to become an alternative therapy for onychomycosis as well as selected systemic fungal infections such as sporotrichosis and blastomycosis.

Compounds with novel modes of action involving the fungal cell wall rather than the fungal cell membrane are also in various stages of development. Because eukaryotic cells lack a cell wall, cell wall–active compounds theoretically will have more targeted activity and limited toxic effects on mammalian host cells compared with cell membrane–active antifungal agents. Investigational cell wall–active drugs include (1) the nikkomycins, inhibitors of chitin synthase; (2) echinocandins, pneumocandins, and other glucan synthase inhibitors; and (3) pradimicins and benanomicins, which interfere with the fungal cell wall by calcium-dependent binding to mannoproteins.

In addition, the manipulation of cytokines and other immunomodulatory approaches to antifungal therapy are actively being explored. Particularly intriguing are recombinant human gene products such as interferon-γ and colony-stimulating factors (including granulocyte and granulocyte-macrophage colony-stimulating factors), which are already used in specific clinical settings to aid in the prevention or treatment of bacterial infections. Preliminary studies suggest that interferon-γ and the colony-stimulating factor cytokines may also potentiate immune responses against systemic mycoses. Other immunomodulatory approaches to prophylaxis and adjunctive therapy under investigation include the use of interleukins (interleukin-12 and others) and monoclonal antibodies directed against specific fungal pathogens.

References

1. Gallis HA, Drew RH, Pickard WW: Amphotericin B: 30 years of clinical experience. Rev Infect Dis 12:308, 1990.
2. Medoff G, Kobayashi GS: Strategies in the treatment of systemic fungal infections. N Engl J Med 302:145, 1980.
3. Dick JD, Merz WG, Saral R: Incidence of polyene-resistant yeasts recovered from clinical specimens. Antimicrob Agents Chemother 18:158, 1980.
4. Dick JD, Rosengar BR, Merz WG, et al: Fatal disseminated candidiasis due to amphotericin B-resistant *Candida guilliermondii.* Ann Intern Med 102:67, 1985.
5. Powderly WG, Kobayashi GS, Herzig GP, et al: Amphotericin B–resistant yeast infection in severely immunocompromised patients. Am J Med 84:826, 1988.
6. Conly J, Rennie R, Johnson J, et al: Disseminated candidiasis due to amphotericin B–resistant *Candida albicans.* J Infect Dis 165:761, 1992.
7. Wilson E, Thorson L, Speert DP: Enhancement of macrophage superoxide anion production by amphotericin B. Antimicrob Agents Chemother 35:796, 1991.
8. Martin E, Stuben A, Gorz A, et al: Novel aspect of amphotericin B action: Accumulation in human monocytes potentiates killing of phagocytosed *Candida albicans.* Antimicrob Agents Chemother 38:13, 1994.
9. Daneshmend TK, Warnock DW: Clinical pharmacokinetics of systemic antifungal drugs. Clin Pharmacokinet 8:17, 1983.
10. Rex JH, Bennett JE, Sugar AM, et al: A randomized trial comparing fluconazole with amphotericin B for the treatment of candidemia in patients without neutropenia. N Engl J Med 331:1325, 1994.
11. Kauffman CA, Bradley SF, Ross SC, Weber DR: Hepatosplenic candidiasis: Successful treatment with fluconazole. Am J Med 91:137, 1991.
12. Anaissie E, Bodey GP, Kantargian H, et al: Fluconazole therapy for chronic disseminated candidiasis in patients with leukemia and prior amphotericin B therapy. Am J Med 91:142, 1991.
13. Smego RA Jr, Perfect JR, Durack DT: Combined therapy with amphotericin B and 5-fluorocytosine for *Candida* meningitis. Rev Infect Dis 6:791, 1984.
14. Thaler M, Pastakia B, Shawker TH, et al: Hepatic candidiasis in cancer patients: The evolving picture of the syndrome. Ann Intern Med 108:88, 1988.
15. Bennett JE, Dismukes WE, Duma RG, et al: A comparison of amphotericin B alone and combined with flucytosine in the treatment of cryptococcal meningitis. N Engl J Med 301:126, 1979.
16. Dismukes WE, Cloud G, Gallis HA, et al: Treatment of cryptococcal meningitis with combination amphotericin B and flucytosine for four as compared to six weeks. N Engl J Med 317:334, 1987.
17. Saag MS, Powderly WG, Cloud GA, et al: Comparison of amphotericin B with fluconazole in the treatment of acute AIDS-associated cryptococcal meningitis. The NIAID Mycoses Study Group and the AIDS Clinical Trials Group. N Engl J Med 326:83, 1992.
18. Dismukes WE, Cloud G, Bowles C, et al: Treatment of blastomycosis and histoplasmosis with ketoconazole. Results of a prospective randomized clinical trial. Ann Intern Med 103:861, 1985.
19. Dismukes WE, Bradsher RW Jr, Cloud GC, et al: Itraconazole therapy for blastomycosis and histoplasmosis: NIAID Mycoses Study Group. Am J Med 93:489, 1992.
20. Galgiani JN, Catanzaro A, Cloud GA, et al: Fluconazole therapy for coccidioidal meningitis. Ann Intern Med 119:28, 1993.
21. Galgiani JN, Stevens DA, Graybill JR, et al: Ketoconazole therapy of progressive coccidioidomycosis: Comparison of 400 and 800

mg doses and observations at higher doses. Am J Med 84:603, 1988.
22. Graybill JR, Stevens DA, Galgiani JN, et al: Itraconazole treatment of coccidioidomycosis. Am J Med 89:282, 1990.
23. Catanzaro A, Galgiani JN, Levine BE, et al: Fluconazole in the treatment of chronic pulmonary and nonmeningeal disseminated coccidioidomycosis. NIAID Mycoses Study Group. Am J Med 98:249, 1995.
24. Pizzo PA, Robichaud KJ, Gill FA, et al: Empiric antibiotic and antifungal therapy for cancer patients with prolonged fever and granulocytopenia. Am J Med 72:101, 1982.
25. EORTC International Antimicrobial Therapy Cooperative Group: Empiric antifungal therapy in febrile granulocytopenic patients. Am J Med 86:668, 1989.
26. Perfect JR, Klotman ME, Gilbert CC, et al: Prophylactic intravenous amphotericin B in neutropenic autologous bone marrow transplant recipients. J Infect Dis 165:891, 1992.
27. Rousey SR, Russler S, Gottlieb M, Ash RC: Low-dose amphotericin B prophylaxis against invasive *Aspergillus* infections in allogeneic marrow transplantation. Am J Med 91:484, 1991.
28. Goodman JL, Winston DJ, Greenfield RA, et al: A controlled trial of fluconazole to prevent fungal infections in patients undergoing bone marrow transplantation. N Engl J Med 326:845, 1992.
29. Cruz JM, Peacock JE Jr, Loomer L, et al: Rapid intravenous infusion of amphotericin B: A pilot study. Am J Med 93:123, 1992.
30. Ellis ME, al-Hokail AA, Clink HM, et al: Double-blind randomized study of the effect of infusion rates on toxicity of amphotericin B. Antimicrob Agents Chemother 36:172, 1992.
31. Sanford JP: The enigma of candiduria: Evolution of bladder irrigation with amphotericin B for management—From anecdote to dogma and a lesson from Machiavelli. Clin Infect Dis 16:145, 1993.
32. Goodwin SD, Clearly JD, Walawander CA, et al: Pretreatment regimens for adverse events related to infusion of amphotericin B. Clin Infect Dis 20:755, 1995.
33. Fisher MA, Talbot GH, Maislin G, et al: Risk factors for amphotericin B–associated nephrotoxicity. Am J Med 87:547, 1989.
34. Branch RA: Prevention of amphotericin B–induced renal impairment: Review on the use of sodium supplementation. Arch Intern Med 148:2389, 1988.
35. Wright DG, Robichaud KJ, Pizzo PA, et al: Lethal pulmonary reaction associated with the combined use of amphotericin B and leukocyte transfusions. N Engl J Med 304:1185, 1981.
36. Dana BW, Durie BGM, White RF, et al: Concomitant administration of granulocyte transfusions and amphotericin B in neutropenic patients: Absence of significant pulmonary toxicity. Blood 57:91, 1981.
37. Stamm AM, Diasio RB, Dismukes WE, et al: Toxicity of amphotericin B plus flucytosine in 194 patients with cryptococcal meningitis. Am J Med 83:236, 1987.
37a. Van Der Horst C, Saag M, Cloud G, et al: Randomized double blind comparison of amphotericin B plus flucytosine to amphotericin B alone followed by a comparison of fluconazole to itraconazole in the treatment of acute cryptococcal meningitis in patients with AIDS (Abstr). *In* Program of the 35th Interscience Conference on Antimicrobial Agents and Chemotherapy; 1995; San Francisco.
38. Como JA, Dismukes WE: Oral azole drugs as systemic antifungal therapy. N Engl J Med 330:263, 1994.
39. Daneshmend TK, Warnock DW, Turner A, et al: Pharmacokinetics of ketoconazole in normal subjects. J Antimicrob Chemother 8:299, 1981.
40. Craven PC, Graybill JR, Jorgensen JH, et al: High-dose ketoconazole for treatment of fungal infections of the central nervous system. Ann Intern Med 98:160, 1983.
41. Lelawongs P, Barone JA, Colaizzi JL, et al: Effect of food and gastric acidity on absorption of orally administered ketoconazole. Clin Pharm 7:228, 1988.
42. Lake-Bakaar G, Tom W, Lake-Bakaar D, et al: Gastropathy and ketoconazole malabsorption in the acquired immunodeficiency syndrome (AIDS). Ann Intern Med 109:471, 1988.
43. Chin TWF, Loeb M, Fong IW: Effects of an acidic beverage (Coca-Cola) on absorption of ketoconazole. Antimicrob Agents Chemother 39:1671, 1995.
44. Honig PK, Wortham DC, Zamani K, et al: Terfenadine-ketoconazole interaction: Pharmacokinetic and electrocardiographic consequences. JAMA 269:1513, 1993.
45. Cox FW, Stiller RL, South DA, et al: Oral ketoconazole for dermatophyte infections. J Am Acad Dermatol 6:455, 1982.
46. Laine L, Dretler RH, Conteas CN, et al: Fluconazole compared with ketoconazole for the treatment of *Candida* esophagitis in AIDS: A randomized trial. Ann Intern Med 117:655, 1992.
47. Negroni R, Robles AM, Arechavala A, et al: Ketoconazole in the treatment of paracoccidioidomycosis and histoplasmosis. Rev Infect Dis 2:643, 1980.
48. Dismukes WE, Stamm AM, Graybill JR: Treatment of systemic mycosis with ketoconazole: Emphasis on toxicity and clinical response in 52 patients. Ann Intern Med 98:13, 1983.
49. Galgiani JN, Stevens DA, Graybill JR, et al: *Pseudoallescheria boydii* infections treated with ketoconazole. Chest 86:219, 1984.
50. Suppartpinyo K, Nelson KE, Merz WG, et al: Response to antifungal therapy by human immunodeficiency virus-infected patients with disseminated *Penicillium marneffei* infections and in vitro susceptibilities of isolates from clinical specimens. Antimicrob Agents Chemother 37:2407, 1993.
51. Horsburgh CR, Kirkpatrick CH: Long-term therapy of chronic mucocutaneous candidiasis with ketoconazole: Experience with twenty-one patients. Am J Med 74:23, 1983.
52. Sonino N: The use of ketoconazole as an inhibitor of steroid production. N Engl J Med 317:812, 1987.
53. Pont A, Graybill JR, Craven PC, et al: High-dose ketoconazole therapy and adrenal and testicular function in humans. Arch Intern Med 144:2140, 1984.
54. Britton H, Shehab Z, Lightner E, et al: Adrenal response in children receiving high doses of ketoconazole for systemic coccidioidomycosis. J Pediatr 112:488, 1988.
55. Grant SM, Clissold SP: Fluconazole: A review of its pharmacodynamic and pharmacokinetic properties, and therapeutic potential in superficial and systemic mycoses. Drugs 39:877, 1990.
56. Tucker RM, Williams PL, Arathoon EG, et al: Pharmacokinetics of fluconazole in cerebrospinal fluid and serum in human coccidioidal meningitis. Antimicrob Agents Chemother 32:369, 1988.
57. Lazar JD, Wilner KD: Drug interactions with fluconazole. Rev Infect Dis 12(Suppl 3):S327, 1990.
58. Fuller JD, Stanfield LED, Craven EC: Rifabutin prophylaxis and uveitis. N Engl J Med 330:1315, 1994.
59. Narang PK, Tapnell CB, Schoenfelder JR, et al: Fluconazole and enhanced effect of rifabutin prophylaxis. N Engl J Med 330:1316, 1994.
60. Sahai J, Gallicano K, Pakuts A, Cameron DW: Effect of fluconazole on zidovudine pharmacokinetics in patients infected with human immunodeficiency virus. J Infect Dis 169:1103, 1994.
61. Kinghorn GR: Vulvovaginal candidiasis. J Antimicrob Chemother 28(Suppl A):59, 1991.
62. Koletar SL, Russell JA, Fass RJ, et al: Comparison of oral fluconazole and clotrimazole troches as treatment for oral candidiasis in AIDS. Lancet 1:746, 1989.
63. Meunier F, Aoun M, Gerard M: Therapy for oropharyngeal candidiasis in the immunocompromised host: A randomized double-blind study of fluconazole vs. ketoconazole. Rev Infect Dis 12(Suppl 3):S364, 1990.
64. Samonis G, Rolston K, Karl C: Prophylaxis of oropharyngeal candidiasis with fluconazole. Rev Infect Dis 12(Suppl 3):S369, 1990.
65. Menichetti F, Del Favero A, Martino P, et al: Preventing fungal infection in neutropenic patients with acute leukemia: Fluconazole compared with oral amphotericin B. The GIMEMA Infection Program. Ann Intern Med 120:913, 1994.
66. Winston DJ, Chandrasekar PH, Lazarus HM, et al: Fluconazole prophylaxis of fungal infections in patients with acute leukemia: Results of a randomized placebo-controlled, double-blind, multicenter trial. Ann Intern Med 118:495, 1993.
67. Powderly WG, Finkelstein DM, Feinberg J, et al: A randomized trial comparing fluconazole with clotrimazole troches for the prevention of fungal infections in patients with advanced human immunodeficiency virus infection. N Engl J Med 332:700, 1995.
68. Stevens DA, Greene SI, Lang OS: Thrush can be prevented in patients with AIDS and AIDS-related complex. A randomized, double-blind, placebo-controlled study of 100 mg oral fluconazole daily. Arch Intern Med 151:2458, 1991.
69. McQuillen DP, Zangman BS, Meunier F, Levitz SM: Invasive infections due to *Candida krusei*: Report of ten cases of fungemia that include three cases of endophthalmitis. Clin Infect Dis 14:472, 1992.

70. Wingard JR, Merz WG, Rinaldi MG, et al: Association of *Torulopsis glabrata* infections with fluconazole prophylaxis in neutropenic bone marrow transplant patients. Antimicrob Agents Chemother 37:1847, 1993.
71. Wingard JR, Merz WG, Rinaldi MG: Increase in *Candida krusei* infection among patients with bone marrow transplantation and neutropenia treated prophylactically with fluconazole. N Engl J Med 325:1274, 1991.
72. Cameron ML, Schell WA, Bruch S, et al: Correlation of in vitro fluconazole resistance of *Candida* isolates in relation to therapy and symptoms of individuals seropositive for human immunodeficiency virus type 1. Antimicrob Agents Chemother 37:2449, 1993.
73. Rex JH, Rinaldi MG, Pfaller MA: Resistance of *Candida* species to fluconazole. Antimicrob Agents Chemother 39:1, 1995.
74. Larsen RA, Leal MA, Chan LS: Fluconazole compared to amphotericin B plus flucytosine for the treatment of cryptococcal meningitis: A prospective study. Ann Intern Med 113:183, 1990.
75. Larsen RA, Bozzette SA, Jones BE, et al: Fluconazole combined with flucytosine for treatment of cryptococcal meningitis in patients with AIDS. Clin Infect Dis 19:741, 1994.
76. Haubrich RH, Haghighat D, Bozzette SA, et al: High-dose fluconazole for treatment of cryptococcal disease in patients with human immunodeficiency virus infection. The California Collaborative Treatment Group. J Infect Dis 170:238, 1994.
77. Bozzette SA, Larsen RA, Chiu J, et al: A placebo-controlled trial of maintenance therapy with fluconazole after treatment of cryptococcal meningitis in the acquired immunodeficiency syndrome. California Collaborative Treatment Group. N Engl J Med 324:580, 1991.
78. Powderly WG, Saag MS, Cloud GA, et al: A controlled trial of fluconazole or amphotericin B to prevent relapse of cryptococcal meningitis in patients with the acquired immunodeficiency syndrome. The NIAID AIDS Clinical Trials Group and Mycoses Study Group. N Engl J Med 326:793, 1992.
79. Jacobson MA, Hanks DK, Ferrell LD: Fatal hepatic necrosis due to fluconazole. Am J Med 96:188, 1994.
80. Hanger DP, Jerons S, Shaw JTB: Fluconazole and testosterone: in vivo and in vitro studies. Antimicrob Agents Chemother 32:646, 1988.
81. Pappas PG, Kauffman CA, Perfect J, et al: Alopecia associated with fluconazole therapy. Ann Intern Med 123:354, 1995.
82. Wheat J, Hafner R, Korzun A, et al: Itraconazole treatment of disseminated histoplasmosis in patients with the acquired immunodeficiency syndrome. Am J Med 98:336, 1995.
83. Wheat J, Hafner R, Wulfsohn M, et al: Prevention of relapse of histoplasmosis with itraconazole in patients with the acquired immunodeficiency syndrome. The NIAID Clinical Trials and Mycoses Study Group Collaborators. Ann Intern Med 118:610, 1993.
84. Sharkey-Mathis PK, Kauffman CA, Graybill JR, et al: Treatment of sporotrichosis with itraconazole. NIAID Mycoses Study Group. Am J Med 95:279, 1993.
85. Restreppo A, Robledo J, Gomez I, et al: Itraconazole therapy in lymphangitic and cutaneous sporotrichosis. Arch Dermatol 122:413, 1986.
86. Piepponen T, Blomqvist K, Brandt H, et al: Efficacy and safety of itraconazole in the long-term treatment of onychomycosis. J Antimicrob Chemother 29:195, 1992.
87. Diaz M, Puente R, de Hoyas LA, and Cruz S: Itraconazole in the treatment of coccidioidomycosis. Chest 100:682, 1991.
88. Cauwenbergh G, De Doncker P, Stoops K, et al: Itraconazole in the treatment of human mycoses: Review of three years of clinical experience. Rev Infect Dis 9(Suppl 1):S146, 1987.
89. Denning DW, Lee JY, Hostetler JS, et al: NIAID Mycoses Study Group Multicenter Trial of oral itraconazole therapy for invasive aspergillosis. Am J Med 97:135, 1994.
90. Dupont B: Itraconazole therapy in aspergillosis: Study in 49 patients. J Am Acad Dermatol 23:607, 1990.
91. Caillot D, Casasnovas O, Solary E, et al: Efficacy and tolerance of an amphotericin B lipid (Intralipid) emulsion in the treatment of candidaemia in neutropenic patients. J Antimicrob Chemother 31:161, 1993.
92. Brajtburg J, Elberg S, Kobayashi GS, Bolard J: Amphotericin B incorporated into egg lecithin-bile salt mixed micelles: Molecular and cellular aspects relevant to therapeutic efficacy in experimental mycoses. Antimicrob Agents Chemother 38:300, 1994.
93. Hanson LH, Stevens DA: Comparison of antifungal activity of amphotericin B deoxycholate suspension with that of amphotericin B cholesteryl sulfate colloidal dispersion. Antimicrob Agents Chemother 36:486, 1992.
94. Lopez-Berestein G, Bodey GP, Fainstein V, et al: Treatment of systemic fungal infections with liposomal amphotericin B. Arch Intern Med 149:2533, 1989.
95. Coker RJ, Viviani M, Gazzard BG, et al: Treatment of cryptococcosis with liposomal amphotericin B (AmBisome) in 23 patients with AIDS. AIDS 7:829, 1993.
96. Ringden O, Meunier F, Tollemar J, et al: Efficacy of amphotericin B encapsulated in liposomes (AmBisome) in the treatment of invasive fungal infections in immunocompromised patients. J Antimicrob Chemother 28(Suppl B):73, 1991.

34

Antimycobacterial Drugs

Patricia M. Simone
C. Robert Horsburgh, Jr.
Kenneth G. Castro

There are currently 58 accepted species of mycobacteria.[1] However, not all are pathogenic to humans; most are saprophytic and have been isolated from soil and water.[2] Bacteria in the *Mycobacterium tuberculosis* complex are the most common cause of disease affecting the pulmonary, lymphatic, meningeal, osteoarticular, and renal systems. In addition, they can cause disseminated disease. Nontuberculous mycobacteria have been described as causative of pulmonary disease, lymphadenitis, cutaneous ulcers, and disseminated disease.[3] This chapter provides an overview of the available therapeutic agents for human disease caused by the various mycobacteria.

Tuberculosis

Treatment of Active Disease

Tuberculosis is an ancient and deadly disease. In the 1800s, remedies such as bloodletting and cupping were replaced by regimens of bed rest and fresh air in sanatoria in the mountains or by the sea.[4] Effective treatment for tuberculosis became possible with the discovery of streptomycin in the 1940s. It was soon discovered, however, that the initial response to streptomycin therapy was quickly followed by a clinical deterioration as streptomycin resistance developed.[5, 6] Further investigation revealed that the development of resistance could be prevented by the use of two or more drugs in combination,[7–9] and standard regimens consisting of more than one drug (e.g., streptomycin, isoniazid, and *p*-aminosalicylic acid) given for 18 to 24 months were adopted.[10, 11] These early regimens were effective but frequently caused adverse reactions. The introduction of rifampin in the 1970s revolutionized antituberculosis treatment, and highly effective regimens of only 6 months in duration (short-course chemotherapy) have become the standard of care.[12] These regimens have consisted of an initial multidrug regimen or bactericidal phase (e.g., isoniazid, rifampin, and pyrazinamide with or without streptomycin or ethambutol) for the first 2 months, followed by a continuation or sterilizing phase with isoniazid and rifampin for a minimum of an additional 4 months. As tuberculosis patients were moved out of sanatoria, the problem of nonadherence of patients leading to treatment failure and multidrug resistance emerged. Finally, fully supervised therapy became feasible with the introduction of intermittent therapy during the continuation phase.[13]

GENERAL PRINCIPLES OF ANTITUBERCULOSIS THERAPY

Drugs used in currently recommended antituberculosis treatment regimens are selected on the basis of three important properties: (1) the early bactericidal activity, (2) the sterilizing activity, and (3) the ability to prevent the emergence of drug resistance[14] (Table 34–1). The early bactericidal activity is defined as the ability of the drug to decrease the number of bacilli in the sputum during the initial period of therapy.[15, 16] The sterilizing activity is defined as the drug's ability to kill semidormant bacilli in an acid environment or other semidormant bacteria. Drugs with potent sterilizing activity have enabled the duration of therapy to be reduced to the currently recommended short-course (i.e., 6-month) regimens. The ability to prevent the emergence of drug resistance is measured by the prevention of treatment failure due to drug resistance during therapy. Of the available antituberculosis drugs, isoniazid is the most bactericidal. Both isoniazid and rifampin are effective in preventing the emergence of drug resistance, but rifampin has more potent sterilizing activity than isoniazid.[17, 18] Compared with isoniazid and rifampin, ethambutol has intermediate bactericidal activity when relatively high dosage is used for intermittent therapy, moderate ability to prevent resistance, and intermediate sterilizing ability. Pyrazinamide is poor at preventing the emergence of drug resistance but has potent sterilizing activity.

PRACTICAL APPLICATION OF ANTITUBERCULOSIS THERAPY

The highest priority for tuberculosis prevention and control is promptly identifying patients who have active disease and ensuring that they complete an appropriate regimen of antituberculosis therapy. The main goals of tuberculosis treatment are to (1) provide the safest, most effective therapy in the shortest time to cure illness and prevent death from the disease and (2) ensure that patients adhere to the prescribed regimen to prevent failure, relapse, further transmission, and development of drug resistance.

TABLE 34–1 ■ Relative Activities of Antituberculosis Medications*

EARLY BACTERICIDAL ACTIVITY		PREVENTING DRUG	STERILIZING	
In Vitro	In Vivo	RESISTANCE	ACTIVITY	ACTIVITY
INH	INH	INH	RIF	High
RIF		RIF	PZA	
SM				
	EMB	SM	INH	
EMB	RIF			
PZA		EMB	SM	
	SM	THA	EMB	
	PZA			
THA	THA			
PAS	PAS	PZA	THA	Low

*EMB, Ethambutol; INH, isoniazid; PAS, *p*-aminosalicylic acid; PZA, pyrazinamide; RIF, rifampin; SM, streptomycin; THA, ethionamide.

To prevent the emergence of resistance, regimens must include two or more drugs to which the *M. tuberculosis* isolate has demonstrated in vitro susceptibility. However, the susceptibility pattern of the isolate is usually not known when the initial regimen is being chosen, and an inadequate regimen may result when primary resistance is not initially suspected. Therefore, an initial regimen consisting of four drugs (isoniazid, rifampin, pyrazinamide, and either ethambutol or streptomycin) is recommended.[19] When there is little possibility of drug resistance (i.e., there is less than 4% primary resistance to isoniazid in the community and the patient has had no previous treatment with antituberculosis medications, is not from a country with a high prevalence of drug resistance, and has no known exposure to a drug-resistant case), initial regimens containing only three drugs (isoniazid, rifampin, and pyrazinamide) may be adequate. However, in facilities experiencing outbreaks of multidrug-resistant tuberculosis, a five- or six-drug regimen may be more appropriate as initial therapy. Drug susceptibility tests should be obtained on all initial *M. tuberculosis* isolates obtained from patients with active tuberculosis. The results should be used to guide clinical decisions for individual patients and should be reported to the local health department for monitoring of drug resistance trends.

Nonadherence to therapy has been recognized as a major cause of treatment failure, relapse, and emergence of drug resistance.[20] Ensuring adherence is key to completing treatment successfully, and the most effective method of ensuring adherence is supervised or directly observed therapy.[21, 22] In directly observed therapy, a health care provider or other designated person observes the patient swallow each dose of antituberculosis medications. Directly observed therapy has been shown to be cost-effective when intermittent regimens are used[23] and to result in significant reductions in the rates of primary and acquired drug resistance and relapse when it is universally administered.[24] Clinicians caring for patients who have tuberculosis should be aware of the directly observed therapy services available through their local health department's tuberculosis control program.

Patients who are receiving antituberculosis therapy must be monitored for evidence of clinical and bacteriologic response. If there is a poor or suboptimal response to therapy, the patient should be evaluated for causes of treatment failure (e.g., nonadherence, drug resistance, or rarely malabsorption[25]). A single drug should never be added to a failing regimen. This may have the same effect as treating active tuberculosis with a single drug, which predictably leads to the emergence of drug resistance.[26]

CURRENTLY RECOMMENDED DRUG REGIMENS

The duration of therapy for tuberculosis depends on the drugs used, the drug susceptibility test results, and the patient's response to therapy. Because isoniazid resistance has been documented in nearly 10% of patients with tuberculosis nationwide,[27] efforts must be implemented to prevent the development of multidrug resistance. Therefore, most patients should be treated initially with a regimen containing isoniazid, rifampin, and pyrazinamide plus either ethambutol or streptomycin (Table 34–2). Pyrazinamide and ethambutol or streptomycin should be maintained in the initial regimen until susceptibility to isoniazid and rifampin is demonstrated, with pyrazinamide given for at least 2 months. If the isolate is susceptible to isoniazid and rifampin, or in situations when there is little possibility of drug resistance (i.e., less than 4% primary drug resistance to isoniazid in the community and the patient has had no previous treatment with antituberculosis medications, is not from a country with a high prevalence of drug resistance, and has no known

TABLE 34–2 ■ Regimen Options for Treatment of Tuberculosis*

OPTION	INDICATION	TOTAL DURATION (wk)	INITIAL PHASE	
			Drugs	Interval and Duration
1	Pulmonary and extrapulmonary tuberculosis in adults and children	24	INH RIF PZA EMB or SM	Daily for 8 wk
2	Pulmonary and extrapulmonary tuberculosis in adults and children	24	INH RIF PZA EMB or SM	Daily for 2 wk, and then 2 times/wk† for 6 wk
3	Pulmonary and extrapulmonary tuberculosis in adults and children	24	INH RIF PZA EMB or SM	3 times/wk† for 6 mo‡
4	Smear- and culture-negative pulmonary tuberculosis in adults	16	INH RIF PZA EMB or SM	Follow option 1, 2, or 3 for 8 wk
5	Pulmonary and extrapulmonary tuberculosis in adults and children when PZA is contraindicated	36	INH RIF EMB or SM	Daily for 4–8 wk

*Note: For all patients, if susceptibility results show resistance to any of the first-line drugs or if the patient remains symptomatic or smear- or culture-positive after 3 mo, consult a tuberculosis medical expert. Avoid streptomycin for pregnant women because of the risk for ototoxic injury to the fetus. INH, Isoniazid; RIF, rifampin; PZA, pyrazinamide; EMB, ethambutol; SM, streptomycin.

†Directly observed therapy should be used with all regimens administered two or three times weekly.

‡For infants and children with miliary tuberculosis, bone and joint tuberculosis, or tubercular meningitis, treatment should last at least 12 mo. For adults with these forms of extrapulmonary tuberculosis, response to therapy should be monitored closely. If response is slow or suboptimal, treatment may be prolonged as judged on a case-by-case basis.

exposure to drug-resistant tuberculosis), the initial 2-month regimen can be limited to isoniazid, rifampin, and pyrazinamide.[28] After the initial 2-month treatment phase is complete and susceptibility to isoniazid and rifampin has been demonstrated, these two drugs are continued for an additional 4 months (continuation phase of treatment). Several 6-month regimens have been demonstrated to be highly effective[12, 29–31] (Table 34–3). When treatment is directly observed, intermittent therapy may be used. Treatment should be extended for a total of 9 months for patients who cannot, or should not, take pyrazinamide.

Persons infected with human immunodeficiency virus (HIV) should receive a minimum of 6 months of antituberculosis therapy. HIV-infected patients with tuberculosis have been reported to respond adequately to antituberculosis therapy.[32, 33] However, in HIV-infected patients, it is critically important to monitor the clinical and bacteriologic response. If the response is slow or otherwise suboptimal, the patient should be reevaluated, and therapy should be prolonged.[28]

In general, these same regimens are also effective for the treatment of extrapulmonary tuberculosis. However, children who have miliary tuberculosis, osteoarticular tuberculosis, or tubercular meningitis should receive at least 12 months of therapy.[28]

The preferred treatment for pregnant or lactating women who have tuberculosis is isoniazid and rifampin for a minimum of 9 months.[34, 35] Ethambutol should be included initially unless resistance is unlikely. Streptomycin should be avoided during pregnancy because it interferes with fetal ear development and may cause congenital deafness. Pyrazinamide is not recommended for use during pregnancy in the United States because of inadequate data on its potential teratogenicity.

Shorter treatment is also effective for adults who are diagnosed with smear- and culture-negative pulmonary tuberculosis. Four months of isoniazid and rifampin, preferably with pyrazinamide for the first 2 months, has been demonstrated to be effective.[36, 37] Ethambutol should also be included unless drug resistance is unlikely.

For persons with tuberculosis whose isolates are resistant only to isoniazid, 6-month regimens containing isoniazid, rifampin, pyrazinamide, and either ethambutol or streptomycin have been shown to be effective.[38] When isolated isoniazid resistance is documented after a four-drug regimen has been initiated, the isoniazid should be discontinued and the other drugs continued for the entire 6 months.[28] Persons who cannot tolerate isoniazid or who have isoniazid-resistant tuberculosis can be treated with rifampin, pyrazinamide, and ethambutol for 2 months followed by rifampin and ethambutol for an additional 7 months. If pyrazinamide is not used initially, a minimum of 12 months of rifampin and ethambutol is an effective treatment alternative.[39, 40]

The treatment of tuberculosis resistant to both isoniazid and rifampin, often called multidrug-resistant tuberculosis, is not standardized and is often unsuccessful.[41] The key to successful treatment has been shown to be associated with prompt diagnosis and rapid initiation of at least two drugs to which the *M. tuberculosis* isolate is susceptible in vitro.[42–44] In general, the medications used to treat multidrug-resistant tuberculosis are less potent and more toxic and require much longer administration (18 to 24 months) than standard antituberculosis therapy. Therapy for multidrug-resistant tuberculosis should ideally consist of at least four drugs to which the isolate has documented in vitro susceptibility.[45] It is preferable that the regimen consist of "new" medications (ones that the patient has not received before), including one injectable medication. Ensuring adherence through the use of directly observed therapy and other adherence-promoting measures[46] is essential. Surgical resection of affected lung tissue has been used as an adjunct to medical therapy in

TABLE 34–3 ■ Regimen Options for Treatment of Tuberculosis

	CONTINUATION PHASE		
OPTION	Drugs*	Interval and Duration	COMMENTS
1	INH RIF	Daily or 2 or 3 times/wk† for 16 wk‡	EMB or SM should be continued until susceptibility to INH and RIF is demonstrated. In areas where primary INH resistance < 4%, EMB or SM may not be necessary for patients with no individual risk factors for drug resistance.
2	INH RIF	2 times/wk† for 16 wk‡	Regimen should be directly observed. After the initial phase, continue EMB or SM until susceptibility to INH and RIF is demonstrated, unless drug resistance is unlikely.
3	—	—	Regimen should be directly observed. Continue all four drugs for 6 mo. There is some evidence that SM may be discontinued after 4 mo if the isolate is susceptible to all drugs. This regimen has been shown to be effective for INH-resistant tuberculosis.
4	INH RIF PZA EMB or SM	Daily or 2 or 3 times/wk† for 8 wk	Continue all four drugs for 4 mo. If drug resistance is unlikely (primary INH resistance < 4% and patient has no individual risk factors for drug resistance), EMB or SM may not be necessary and PZA may be discontinued after 2 mo.
5	INH RIF	Daily or 2 times/wk† for 28–32 wk‡	EMB or SM should be continued until susceptibility to INH and RIF is demonstrated. In areas where primary INH resistance < 4%, EMB or SM may not be necessary for patients with no individual risk factors for drug resistance.

*INH, Isoniazid; RIF, rifampin; PZA, pyrazinamide; EMB, ethambutol; SM, streptomycin.

†Directly observed therapy should be used with all regimens administered two or three times weekly.

‡For infants and children with miliary tuberculosis, bone and joint tuberculosis, or tubercular meningitis, treatment should last at least 12 mo. For adults with these forms of extrapulmonary tuberculosis, response to therapy should be monitored closely. If response is slow or suboptimal, treatment may be prolonged as judged on a case-by-case basis.

selected cases of multidrug-resistant tuberculosis, with improved outcome.[47, 48]

Preventive Therapy

The main purpose of chemoprophylaxis is to prevent latent *M. tuberculosis* infection from progressing to active disease. In addition, preventive therapy is sometimes used to prevent infection in persons who have been exposed to patients with active pulmonary or laryngeal tuberculosis but who are not yet infected with *M. tuberculosis* (primary prophylaxis). The most common medication used for preventive therapy is isoniazid. Several large randomized placebo-controlled clinical trials of isoniazid preventive therapy have demonstrated that isoniazid is effective in preventing the progression of latent infection to active disease; however, the effectiveness is strongly dependent on the patient's adherence.[49–51]

CANDIDATES FOR PREVENTIVE THERAPY

By definition, persons with latent *M. tuberculosis* infection have no evidence of active disease. In the United States, infected persons are identified by the Mantoux tuberculin skin test with 5 units of purified protein derivative. Individuals with a true-positive tuberculin skin test reaction have a significant lifetime risk for development of active tuberculosis. However, this risk is variable, and the benefit of preventive therapy must always be weighed against the risk of adverse drug reactions. The most serious adverse reaction associated with isoniazid preventive therapy is drug-induced hepatitis.[52] Asymptomatic increases in hepatic enzyme activities are common, but occasionally serious and even fatal hepatitis may occur. Because the risk for hepatitis is associated with advancing age, recommendations for the use of preventive therapy are based on the age of the infected person and the risk for development of active tuberculosis (Table 34–4). Those who have the highest risk for the development of active disease are given the highest priority for preventive therapy and should be treated regardless of age. These include persons who have HIV infection, persons who have documented recent tuberculin skin test result conversions, and persons who are close contacts of a person with

TABLE 34–4 ■ Candidates for Preventive Therapy

HIGH-PRIORITY CANDIDATES FOR PREVENTIVE THERAPY

Persons with a positive skin test reaction in the following high-risk groups, regardless of age:
- Persons known to have or suspected of having human immunodeficiency virus infection (≥5 mm)
- Close contacts of a person with infectious tuberculosis (≥5 mm)
- Recent tuberculin skin test converters (≥10 mm increase if younger than 35 y; ≥15 mm increase if 35 y of age or older)
- Persons who have a chest radiograph suggestive of previous tuberculosis and who have received inadequate treatment (≥5 mm)
- Persons who inject drugs (≥10 mm)
- Persons with certain medical conditions* (≥10 mm)

Persons with a positive skin test reaction who are younger than 35 y and in the following groups:
- Foreign-born persons from areas where tuberculosis is common (≥10 mm)
- Medically underserved, low-income populations (≥10 mm)
- Children younger than 4 y (≥10 mm)
- Locally identified high-prevalence groups (e.g., migrant farm workers) (≥10 mm)

LOW-PRIORITY CANDIDATES FOR PREVENTIVE THERAPY

Persons younger than 35 y with no known risk factors for tuberculosis (≥15 mm)

*For example, diabetes mellitus, silicosis, low body weight (10% or more below the ideal), cancer of the head and neck, hematologic and reticuloendothelial diseases, end-stage renal disease, intestinal bypass or gastrectomy, chronic malabsorption syndrome, prolonged corticosteroid therapy, and other immunosuppressive therapy.

infectious tuberculosis. For other risk groups, persons with a positive tuberculin skin test reaction who are younger than 35 years are recommended for preventive therapy. Because anergic HIV-infected persons have been shown to have a high risk for active tuberculosis in selected settings, preventive therapy should also be considered for close contacts who are HIV infected and anergic.[53–55]

RECOMMENDED PREVENTIVE THERAPY REGIMENS

Most commonly, isoniazid is used alone for preventive therapy in a single daily dose of 300 mg in adults and 10 to 15 mg/kg in children (300-mg maximal dose). Every effort should be made to ensure that patients adhere to therapy for at least 6 months (Table 34–5). Children should receive at least 9 months of preventive therapy, and HIV-infected persons should receive at least 12 months. Isoniazid may be given twice weekly to high-risk infected persons in institutions and facilities where preventive therapy can be directly observed by a staff member, although data on the efficacy of twice-weekly preventive therapy are limited.

Persons who have a positive tuberculin skin test reaction and either silicosis or radiographic evidence of previous tuberculosis may be given preventive therapy with either (1) 12 months of isoniazid or (2) 4 months of isoniazid and rifampin, preferably with pyrazinamide for the first 2 months. Ethambutol should be included in the 4-month regimen unless drug resistance is unlikely.[28]

For close contacts of infectious patients who have isoniazid-resistant tuberculosis, preventive therapy with rifampin is recommended, in part on the basis of studies of rifampin preventive therapy in a mouse model.[56] It should be given in standard therapeutic doses for 6 months for adults and 9 months for children. For those likely to be infected with isoniazid- and rifampin-resistant tuberculosis, observation without preventive therapy has usually been recommended because other drugs have not been evaluated for their efficacy as preventive agents. However, for persons likely to be infected with multidrug-resistant tuberculosis who have a high risk for the development of active tuberculosis (e.g., HIV-infected persons), alternative forms of preventive therapy have been recommended.[57] Any such regimen should include at least two drugs to which the infecting organism has documented in vitro susceptibility. Potential regimens include ethambutol and pyrazinamide or pyrazinamide and a quinolone (ofloxacin or ciprofloxacin) given daily for at least 6 months in standard therapeutic doses. These patients should be monitored closely for the occurrence of side effects and for development of active tuberculosis.[58]

Antituberculosis Drugs

These drugs have been divided into first-line and second-line drugs on the basis of their antibacterial activity, relative safety, and studied efficacy. First-line drugs are considered most effective and have fewer side effects than second-line drugs. Unlike first-line drugs, second-line drugs have not been studied for use in intermittent regimens. Second-line drugs are reserved for cases of drug resistance or drug intolerance.

First-Line Drugs (Tables 34–6 and 34–7)

ISONIAZID

Isoniazid is highly active against *M. tuberculosis* and is the cornerstone of tuberculosis therapy. It inhibits mycolic acid synthesis, but the exact mechanism of action is unknown. It is active against both intracellular and extracellular organisms, primarily against those bacteria that are actively dividing. Isoniazid is primarily administered by the oral route and is

TABLE 34–5 ■ Regimen Options for Preventive Therapy for Tuberculosis in Adults and Children

INDICATION	MINIMAL DURATION (mo)	DRUG*	INTERVAL	CONDITIONS
Adult	6	INH	Daily or twice weekly†	HIV-negative Normal chest radiograph
Child	9	INH	Daily or twice weekly†	HIV-negative Normal chest radiograph
Adult with silicosis or radiographic evidence of old, healed tuberculosis	4	INH RIF (PZA for 2 mo) (EMB unless resistance unlikely)	Daily	Active disease ruled out
	12	INH	Daily	
HIV-infected child or adult	12	INH	Daily	Active disease ruled out
Adult Source case has INH-resistant tuberculosis	6	RIF	Daily	INH resistance of source case documented or likely
Child Source case has INH-resistant tuberculosis	9	RIF	Daily	INH resistance of source case documented or likely
Source case has multidrug-resistant tuberculosis	6	Two drugs to which the infecting organism is susceptible (e.g., PZA and EMB or PZA and a quinolone)	Daily	Contact at high risk for the development of active disease Multidrug resistance of source case documented or likely Active disease ruled out

*INH, Isoniazid; RIF, rifampin; PZA, pyrazinamide; EMB, ethambutol; HIV, human immunodeficiency virus. Note: Dosage recommendations for preventive therapy are the same as those for the treatment of tuberculosis.

†Preventive therapy regimens given intermittently should be dirtectly observed.

TABLE 34–6 ■ First-Line Antituberculosis Drugs: Dosages

		DOSE (mg/kg)*					
		Daily		2 Times/Week†		3 Times/Week†	
DRUG	ROUTE	*Children*	*Adults*	*Children*	*Adults*	*Children*	*Adults*
Isoniazid	Oral	10–20 (300 mg)	5 (300 mg)	20–40 (900 mg)	15 (900 mg)	20–40 (900 mg)	15 (900 mg)
Rifampin	Oral	10–20 (600 mg)	10 (600 mg)	10–20 (600 mg)	10 (600 mg)	10–20 (600 mg)	10 (600 mg)
Pyrazinamide	Oral	15–30 (2 g)	15–30 (2 g)	50–70 (4 g)	50–70 (4 g)	50–70 (3 g)	50–70 (3 g)
Ethambutol	Oral	15–25	15–25	50	50	25–30	25–30
Streptomycin	IM or IV	20–40 (1 g)	15 (1 g)	25–30 (1.5 g)	25–30 (1.5 g)	25–30 (1.5 g)	25–30 (1.5 g)

*Maximal dose is given in parentheses. Doses are for children younger than 12 y. Adjust weight-based dosages as weight changes. IM, Intramuscular; IV, intravenous.

†All regimens administered two or three times a week should be used with directly observed therapy.

well absorbed from the gastrointestinal tract. Its bioavailability may be reduced by antacids and high-carbohydrate foods. Peak blood concentrations of 3 to 7 μg/mL are achieved 1 to 2 hours after oral administration of the daily dose. A preparation for intravenous or intramuscular administration is available.

Hepatotoxic effects associated with isoniazid administration may be manifested as asymptomatic elevation of the hepatic enzyme activities, overt hepatitis requiring cessation of therapy, severe hepatitis followed by liver transplantation,[59] or fatal hepatitis.[60] The risk for hepatitis is approximately 1%, but the risk is increased in older age groups and in persons who consume alcohol. Isoniazid may also cause neurotoxic effects by interfering with pyridoxine metabolism. Peripheral neuropathy is the most common manifestation and occurs most frequently in persons who may be mildly pyridoxine deficient, such as pregnant women, alcohol abusers, and malnourished patients. Peripheral neuropathy can be prevented by as little as 6 mg of pyridoxine (vitamin B_6) a day.[61] Antinuclear antibodies develop in about 20% of patients receiving prolonged isoniazid therapy,[62] although few develop overt systemic lupus erythematosus.[63] Hypersensi-

TABLE 34–7 ■ First-Line Antituberculosis Drugs: Adverse Reactions

DRUG	ADVERSE REACTIONS	MONITORING	COMMENTS
Isoniazid	Hepatic enzyme elevation Hepatitis Peripheral neuropathy Mild effects on central nervous system Drug interactions	Baseline measurements of hepatic enzymes for adults Repeat measurements If baseline results are abnormal If patient is at high risk for adverse reactions If patient has symptoms of adverse reactions	Hepatitis risk increases with age and alcohol consumption Pyridoxine can prevent peripheral neuropathy
Rifampin	Gastrointestinal upset Drug interactions Hepatitis Bleeding problems Influenza-like symptoms Rash	Baseline measurements for adults Complete blood count and platelets Hepatic enzymes Repeat measurements If baseline results are abnormal If patient has symptoms of adverse reactions	Significant interactions with Methadone Birth control pills Many other drugs Colors body fluids orange May permanently discolor soft contact lenses
Pyrazinamide	Hepatitis Rash Gastrointestinal upset Joint aches Hyperuricemia Gout (rare)	Baseline measurements for adults Uric acid Hepatic enzymes Repeat measurements If baseline results are abnormal If patient has symptoms of adverse reactions	Treat hyperuricemia only if patient has symptoms
Ethambutol	Optic neuritis	Baseline and monthly tests Visual acuity Color vision	Not recommended for children too young to be monitored for changes in vision unless tuberculosis is drug resistant
Streptomycin	Ototoxicity (hearing loss or vestibular dysfunction) Renal toxicity	Baseline and repeated tests as needed Hearing Kidney function	Avoid or reduce dose in adults older than 60 y

tivity reactions, pancreatitis, gynecomastia, arthralgias, and arthritis have been reported rarely in association with isoniazid administration. Isoniazid may produce a monoamine oxidase inhibitor–like effect when foods such as cheese or red wine are ingested[64] or histidine reactions after ingestion of certain types of fish.[65] Isoniazid inhibits the metabolism of some anticonvulsant medications[66, 67] and may reduce ketoconazole serum levels.

RIFAMPIN

Rifampin has a marked bactericidal effect on intracellular and extracellular *M. tuberculosis,* including a unique effect against semidormant organisms. It inhibits DNA-dependent RNA polymerase, blocking RNA transcription. In addition, rifampin has a potent sterilizing activity. By inclusion of rifampin in tuberculosis therapy, short-course chemotherapy became possible. The drug is well absorbed from the gastrointestinal tract, although concomitant food intake may interfere with absorption.[68] Peak blood concentrations of 7 to 10 μg/mL are achieved 2 to 4 hours after oral administration of a 600-mg dose. An intravenous preparation is also available.

Rifampin is relatively nontoxic. It causes a harmless reddish or orange discoloration of the urine and other body fluids. Patients should be warned about this and about the possibility that contact lenses may become permanently discolored. The most common adverse reaction is gastrointestinal upset such as anorexia, nausea, and abdominal discomfort. Hepatitis occurs less frequently with rifampin than with isoniazid, although there are some reports of an increased risk for hepatitis when the two medications are given concurrently.[69] Some adverse reactions occur more frequently with intermittent rather than daily administration of rifampin. Thrombocytopenia, influenza-like syndromes, and renal failure have been reported with intermittent administration. As a potent inhibitor of hepatic cytochrome P-450 oxidative enzymes, rifampin accelerates the metabolism of many drugs, including anticoagulants, antiarrhythmics, anticonvulsants, glucocorticoids, cyclosporine, methadone, theophylline, ketoconazole, oral hypoglycemic agents, estrogens, and oral contraceptives.[70]

ETHAMBUTOL

Ethambutol appears to inhibit incorporation of mycolic acids into the cell wall and is effective only against actively growing bacteria. It is used as part of an initial four-drug regimen as a supplement to isoniazid and rifampin when primary resistance is suspected or in combination with other drugs when either isoniazid or rifampin or both cannot be used because of documented drug resistance or drug intolerance. Peak serum concentrations of 2 to 5 μg/mL are achieved 2 to 4 hours after the administration of a dose of 15 mg/kg. Ethambutol is administered by the oral route at a daily adult and pediatric dosage of 15 to 25 mg/kg. In general, the higher dose is used in retreatment cases and is lowered to 15 mg/kg per day after the first 2 months. The main adverse reaction associated with ethambutol administration is optic neuritis. Signs and symptoms include blurry vision, central scotomata, and color blindness. These are usually completely reversible if the drug is stopped promptly. The ocular injury appears to be dose related, occurring in about 5% of persons who receive 25 mg/kg per day for more than 2 months but only rarely in those getting 15 mg/kg per day. In general, ethambutol should not be given to children who are too young to be monitored for visual toxic effects. Other side effects include hypersensitivity reactions, elevated uric acid levels, and rarely peripheral neuropathy. The dosage should be reduced in renal failure.[71]

PYRAZINAMIDE

Pyrazinamide is a bactericidal drug in acid environments, and its potent sterilizing activity has resulted in effective 6-month regimens.[72] There is rapid absorption from the gastrointestinal tract after oral administration. Peak plasma concentrations of 33 to 65 μg/mL at 1 to 2 hours after an oral administration of 1.5 g have been reported. Hepatotoxic effects were fairly common when pyrazinamide was first used, but the risk is low at the currently recommended dosages. It may also produce elevated uric acid levels, occasionally associated with arthralgias and rarely with acute gout. Hypersensitivity reactions and gastrointestinal upset may occur.

STREPTOMYCIN

Streptomycin is an aminoglycoside antibiotic and was the first drug discovered for the treatment of tuberculosis. Streptomycin interferes with bacterial protein synthesis and is bactericidal against *M. tuberculosis.* It is most active in an alkaline environment and is usually given by intramuscular injection but may also be given intravenously. The mean plasma half-life of parenteral streptomycin is 2.4 to 2.7 hours in adults 40 years or younger, but it can be as long as 7 to 9 hours in newborn and elderly persons. The drug is cleared by the kidney and accumulates in the presence of renal insufficiency. The most important adverse effects of streptomycin are ototoxic and nephrotoxic, and both occur more frequently in older patients. Vestibular disturbances are more common than auditory damage. The risk for ototoxic effects is related to the total dose and the peak serum levels. Concomitant administration of other ototoxic drugs increases the risk. Nephrotoxic effects occur less frequently with streptomycin than with kanamycin and capreomycin. Hypersensitivity reactions, neuromuscular blockade, and hematologic effects have been reported. The dose should be reduced in persons with impaired renal function, and the drug should be avoided in pregnancy because it may produce auditory damage in the fetus.

FIXED-DOSE COMBINATIONS

Because drug resistance may develop in patients self-administering therapy who take only one drug when more than one is prescribed, the more widespread use of fixed-dose combination tablets containing more than one antituberculosis drug has been recommended.[73, 74] In the United States, combinations of isoniazid plus rifampin (Rifamate) and isoniazid plus rifampin and pyrazinamide (Rifater) are available. Two tablets of Rifamate provide the conventional dose of 300 mg of isoniazid and 600 mg of rifampin. Rifater, on the other hand, has 50 mg of isoniazid, 120 mg of rifampin, and 300 mg of pyrazinamide. The recommended dosage is five tablets a day for persons weighing less than 55 kg and six tablets a day for those weighing 55 kg or more. The six-tablet dosage provides a 720-mg dose of rifampin (which exceeds the maximal dose usually recommended) to compensate for the lower bioavailability of rifampin when it is given in the combination form. Although the use of fixed-dose combination tablets eliminates the possibility of monotherapy, these formulations are more expensive than the individual drugs purchased separately, and there is the possibility of underdosing if the patient does not take all of the prescribed tablets at once. Fixed-dose combination tablets are unnecessary when directly observed therapy is used.

Second-Line Drugs (Table 34–8)

CYCLOSERINE

Cycloserine was discovered in the 1950s and was mainly used because of drug resistance or drug intolerance. In sus-

TABLE 34–8 ■ Second-Line Antituberculosis Drugs

DRUG*	DAILY DOSE† {Maximal Dose} (Usual Dose)	ADVERSE REACTIONS	MONITORING	COMMENTS
Cycloserine	15–20 mg/kg PO in divided doses {1 g} (250–500 mg bid)	Psychosis Convulsions Depression Headaches Rash Drug interactions	Assess mental status Measure serum drug levels	Start with low dosage and increase as tolerated Pyridoxine may decrease central nervous system effects
Ethionamide	15–20 mg/kg PO in divided doses {1 g} (250–500 mg bid)	Gastrointestinal upset Hepatotoxicity Hypersensitivity Metallic taste Bloating	Measure hepatic enzyme levels	Start with low dosage and increase as tolerated May cause hypothyroid condition, especially if used with *p*-aminosalicylic acid
p-Aminosalicylic acid	150 mg/kg PO in divided doses {12 g} (4 g tid)	Gastrointestinal upset Hypersensitivity Hepatotoxicity Sodium load	Measure hepatic enzyme levels Assess volume status	Start with low dosage and increase as tolerated Monitor cardiac patients for sodium load
Capreomycin	15–30 mg/kg IM or IV qd {1 g}	Toxicity Auditory Vestibular Renal	Assess Vestibular function Hearing function Measure Blood urea nitrogen Creatinine level	After bacteriologic conversion, dosage may be reduced to 2 or 3 times/wk
Kanamycin and amikacin	15–30 mg/kg IM or IV qd {1 g}	Toxicity Auditory Vestibular Renal	Assess Vestibular function Hearing function Measure Blood urea nitrogen Creatinine level	After bacteriologic conversion, dosage may be reduced to 2 or 3 times/wk
Ciprofloxacin	750–1500 mg/d PO (750 mg bid)	Gastrointestinal upset Dizziness Hypersensitivity Drug interactions Headaches Restlessness	Drug interactions	Not approved by U.S. Food and Drug Administration for tuberculosis treatment Should not be used in children Avoid Antacids Iron Zinc Sucralfate
Ofloxacin	600–800 mg/d PO (400 mg bid)	Gastrointestinal upset Dizziness Hypersensitivity Drug interactions Headaches Restlessness	Drug interactions	Not approved by U.S. Food and Drug Administration for tuberculosis treatment Should not be used in children Avoid Antacids Iron Zinc Sucralfate

*Use these drugs only in consultation with a clinician experienced in the management of drug-resistant tuberculosis. Adjust weight-based dosages as weight changes. PO, Oral; IM, intramuscular; IV, intravenous; bid, twice daily; tid, three times daily; qd, every day.
†Doses for children are the same as those for adults.

ceptible bacteria, it interferes with cell wall synthesis; depending on serum concentrations, it may exert bactericidal or bacteriostatic activity against *M. tuberculosis.* Cycloserine is readily absorbed from the gastrointestinal tract after the administration of 250 mg twice daily. Peak serum levels are 25 to 30 μg/mL at 4 to 8 hours; the drug is excreted mainly by the kidneys.

Cycloserine frequently causes neurologic or psychiatric disturbances, ranging from headache and drowsiness to convulsions or psychosis. Peripheral neuritis has also been described. These effects appear to be dose related and exacerbated in renal insufficiency, but they generally disappear when the medication is discontinued. Concomitant use of pyridoxine and monitoring of serum levels may help prevent most serious reactions. The dosage should be adjusted for renal impairment.

ETHIONAMIDE

Ethionamide is a derivative of isonicotinic acid. It is an oral medication that may be given in single or divided doses. Its mechanism of action against *M. tuberculosis* is not known; it appears to interfere with peptide synthesis. Depending on the serum concentration, ethionamide may exert either bacteriostatic or bactericidal activity. Peak serum concentrations of 9 μg/mL are reached between 1.8 and 3.0 hours after a single dose of 1 g.

Because of its toxicity, ethionamide is usually reserved for retreatment or treatment of multidrug-resistant tuberculosis. It frequently causes nausea, vomiting, anorexia, and abdominal pain. Gradually increasing to a full dose or administering the drug with meals or at bedtime, or with an antiemetic, may improve tolerance. Hypersensitivity reactions, hepatitis, and various forms of neurotoxic effects may occur. Rarely, ethionamide administration has been associated with endocrinologic disturbances, such as hypothyroidism, menstrual irregularities, impotence, and gynecomastia.

p-AMINOSALICYLIC ACID

In the past, *p*-aminosalicylic acid was a standard first-line drug, but now it is reserved for use in the treatment of multidrug-resistant tuberculosis. Its exact mechanism of action is unknown, although it is thought to interfere with formation of folic acid. It is available in oral formulation, which is readily absorbed from the gastrointestinal tract and undergoes hepatic metabolism, and it is excreted in urine. Peak serum levels of 7 to 8 μg/mL are achieved 1 to 2 hours after ingestion of a 4-g dose. *p*-Aminosalicylic acid is now available in a granular formulation.[75]

The most commonly reported side effect with use of *p*-aminosalicylic acid is gastrointestinal irritation. Hypersensitivity reactions may occur in 5% to 10% of patients. Other reported adverse effects include Löffler syndrome, hepatitis (thought to result from a hypersensitivity reaction), thyroid dysfunction, crystalluria, hemolytic anemia, and a mononucleosis-like syndrome.

CAPREOMYCIN

Capreomycin has been described as a polypeptide antibiotic with four microbiologically active components. It approaches streptomycin in its therapeutic effect against susceptible *M. tuberculosis* isolates and can be administered only parenterally because of its lack of absorption from the gastrointestinal tract. In adults, peak serum levels of 30 μg/mL occur 1 to 2 hours after the intramuscular administration of 1 g.

The most common reaction described with capreomycin is a nephrotoxic effect manifested by decreased creatinine clearance. Renal function should be closely monitored. Renal function usually returns to normal after the drug is discontinued. Capreomycin may also cause auditory and vestibular toxic effects; audiometry should be performed during therapy. Other side effects include neuromuscular blockade after a large intravenous dose (enhanced by anesthesia; antagonized by neostigmine), eosinophilia, leukocytosis, leukopenia, and rarely thrombocytopenia. Capreomycin's safety for use in pregnancy or lactation has not been established.

KANAMYCIN AND AMIKACIN

Kanamycin and amikacin are aminoglycoside antibiotics active against *M. tuberculosis*. There is complete cross-resistance between kanamycin and amikacin, and cross-resistance may also occur with capreomycin. These agents are available in parenteral form for intramuscular or intravenous use. Side effects and precautions are similar to those related to the use of capreomycin. The most commonly reported toxic effects are auditory, renal, and vestibular. Therefore, patients taking these drugs should have audiometry, vestibular function testing, and monitoring of renal function.

QUINOLONES

The fluoroquinolones (ciprofloxacin and ofloxacin) are DNA gyrase (DNA topoisomerase II) inhibitors that have significant in vitro activity against *M. tuberculosis*. They are not licensed for the treatment of tuberculosis and controlled trials demonstrating their effectiveness are lacking, but they have been used extensively in recent years for treatment of multidrug-resistant tuberculosis. Acquisition of drug resistance has already been reported.[76] Peak serum concentrations of about 4.0 μg/mL are achieved after a 750-mg dose of ciprofloxacin and a 400-mg dose of ofloxacin. The minimal inhibitory concentration is about 1 μg/mL for both drugs. Quinolones are relatively nontoxic[77]; hypersensitivity reactions and gastrointestinal complaints are reported most commonly. They should not be used in children or during pregnancy because of arthropathies reported in animal studies. Concomitant use of quinolones may prolong the half-life of theophylline. In addition, ferrous sulfate and antacids may interfere with quinolone absorption.

Nontuberculous Mycobacteria: Regimens by Causative Organism

Mycobacterium avium *Complex*

The *M. avium* complex (MAC) comprises organisms of more than 40 serotypes. These organisms are broadly divided into two groups, *M. avium* and *M. intracellulare*. These groups differ in their in vitro susceptibility to antimycobacterial agents; however, such differences do not appear to be clinically meaningful, and the two groups can be considered together.

Disseminated MAC Disease. Disseminated disease due to MAC was uncommon before the acquired immunodeficiency syndrome (AIDS) epidemic, but it is now seen in about one quarter of patients with AIDS, making it nearly as common as tuberculosis in the United States and the most common bacterial infection of AIDS patients.[78] Early studies showed poor response to therapy, but the introduction of the azalide-macrolide antibiotics has resulted in suppression of bacteremia and substantial clinical improvement in patients with this disease. Studies of monotherapy with clarithromycin[79] or azithromycin[80] have demonstrated rapid reduction of bacteremia and clinical improvement. Clarithromycin use resulted in elimination of bacteremia in half of the patients by 8 weeks of therapy.[79] However, monotherapy with either agent leads to rapid development of resistance; thus, these drugs should never be given without another antimycobacterial agent. Moreover, resistance to clarithromycin and azithromycin is reciprocal, so that the two should not be used together, nor should one be substituted for the other when resistance is suspected.

A consensus committee of experts has suggested that at least one and possibly two other antimycobacterial agents be used in conjunction with an azalide-macrolide drug in treating disseminated MAC disease.[81] The optimal second drug is not known, but most experts prefer ethambutol because it appears effective as a single agent against MAC,[82] can be taken orally, and is well tolerated. Rifampin and rifabutin both show synergy with ethambutol against MAC in vitro[83, 84] and would be appropriate third agents. Addition of rifabutin to a suboptimal regimen demonstrated benefit in one clinical trial.[85] Clofazimine also shows in vitro activity against MAC and is concentrated in macrophages, where MAC persists; however, the prolonged time to tissue saturation with the usual oral dosing of this agent raises concerns that it may not provide benefit for a number of months after initiation of therapy and may fail to prevent macrolide resistance.[86–88] Fluoroquinolones also show in vitro activity, but this is marginal.[89, 90] Maximal oral doses of ciprofloxacin or ofloxacin are not well tolerated by patients with AIDS,[77, 91] but intravenous administration of higher doses may have a role in treating some patients. Amikacin also has activity against MAC in vitro, but a study showed no effect of addition of amikacin to a regimen for disseminated MAC.[92] However, that regimen may have already been optimal, thus obscuring potential usefulness of amikacin against MAC. In our clinic, we reserve amikacin for therapy of patients who do not respond to standard oral regimens or who relapse after initial response to such regimens. Comparative trials of treatment of disseminated MAC with multidrug regimens containing azalide-macrolide antibiotics are in progress, but no results are yet available.

The usefulness of antimicrobial susceptibility testing of MAC isolates is unproved, and such tests should not be routinely obtained. The only such tests with generally agreed on cutoffs are those for azithromycin and clarithromycin.[81] Because nearly all MAC isolates from patients who have not received prior therapy with these agents are susceptible to both agents, initial testing has little value. However, when patients do not respond clinically or microbiologically (after 4 to 6 weeks of therapy) or appear to relapse (usually after 12 weeks of therapy), susceptibility testing is indicated. Such testing, if it reveals resistance, allows discontinuation of expensive and potentially toxic medications. A report suggested that the level of resistance in initial MAC isolates was increasing, but no information was available on whether the patients had received prior therapy[93]; further evaluation of this worrisome possibility is needed.

Patients should be assessed at least biweekly for resolution of symptoms and suppression of bacteremia. Whereas quantitative blood cultures are generally not used outside of the research setting, a qualitative blood culture should be performed after 12 weeks of therapy; a positive blood culture at such time suggests treatment failure. Symptoms, particularly fevers and night sweats, should abate with successful therapy. Weight loss and anemia may not resolve,[94] despite sterilization of the blood, and may require specific supportive measures. Patients who initially respond may later have return of their symptoms, and such patients should have blood cultures repeated; positive blood cultures are an indication for alteration of the antimycobacterial regimen. As noted before, susceptibility testing should be performed for the azalide-macrolide antibiotics. Resistance to other agents has not been seen with prolonged therapy (unpublished observations) and may be related to the lesser potency of these agents against MAC. Although serum drug levels have been reported to be low in patients with AIDS and MAC,[91, 95] these low levels were not associated with a less successful clinical outcome, and monitoring serum drug levels is not recommended.[91]

If resistance to azalide-macrolide antibiotics occurs or patients are unable to tolerate either of these agents, a four-drug oral regimen not containing these agents (rifampin, ethambutol, clofazimine, and ciprofloxacin) has been shown to be useful in two studies[91, 96] and should be employed. As noted, intravenous agents, such as amikacin, may also be used. If this route is taken, we favor a 1-month course of daily amikacin with careful monitoring of drug levels; others have advocated less intensive courses of longer duration, but the efficacy and toxicity of such therapy have not been evaluated.

Treatment of disseminated MAC in patients with AIDS must be continued for the life of the patient. Treatment is generally suppressive rather than curative, and relapse after discontinuation of therapy can be expected.

MAC Pulmonary Disease. MAC pulmonary disease in the HIV-uninfected host was the most common form of MAC disease before AIDS. It currently accounts for roughly 3000 cases annually in the United States.[97] Treatment of this disease has also been improved by the advent of the azalide-macrolide drugs, and most experts recommend two- or three-drug oral regimens at doses similar to those used for disseminated disease.[98, 99] The optimal duration of therapy has not been established, but 12 months appears adequate in most cases. Some authors have reported good results with initial azalide-macrolide monotherapy,[100] followed by combination therapy, but we do not favor this approach because of the potential lengthening of duration of therapy and the risk for development of resistance in patients with a high burden of organisms.

Patients who have resistance or intolerance to azalide-macrolide drugs will have a more difficult course. We prefer to use the four-drug oral regimen, as outlined before, for treatment of disseminated disease without azalide-macrolide drugs, but many elderly patients cannot tolerate this regimen. Other authors have recommended isoniazid, rifampin, and ethambutol for 18 to 24 months with streptomycin added for the initial 3 to 6 months.[3, 101]

The utility of in vitro susceptibility testing of isolates in designing therapeutic regimens for pulmonary MAC disease is also limited; some studies have shown correlation between the results of such tests and clinical outcome, whereas others have not.[102–105] As with disseminated disease, initial testing is probably not warranted. Patients who do not respond or who appear to relapse while they are receiving an azalide-macrolide–containing regimen should have their isolate tested against azalide-macrolide drugs. The benefit of testing against other agents is less clear.

MAC Lymphadenitis. Isolated MAC lymphadenitis is largely a disease of children; more than 60% of cases occur in children younger than 3 years. The preponderance of cases are cervical nodes, usually a single node but less often multiple contiguous nodes. It is estimated that 500 cases a year occur in the United States.[97] Therapy has been largely surgical; excision of the node is the treatment of choice.[106] However, a report of cure with clarithromycin-ethambutol therapy in a case in which excision was not possible suggests that antimycobacterial therapy may be an alternative to surgery.[107]

MAC Prophylaxis. For persons at high risk for MAC disease, antibiotic prophylaxis has also been shown to be of value. In patients with AIDS and $CD4^+$ cell counts less than $75/mm^3$, rifabutin 300 mg orally per day reduced the frequency of MAC bacteremia by 50%.[108] Clarithromycin prophylaxis (500 mg orally twice per day) provides significant protection against MAC bacteremia in patients with advanced AIDS,[109] as does azithromycin (1200 mg once weekly).[110] These regimens appear to be of roughly equal effectiveness, with the slightly greater protection afforded by clarithromycin or azithromycin balanced by the risk for development of drug-resistant disease if prophylaxis fails[109]; such drug-resistant disease in breakthroughs was not seen with rifabutin prophylaxis.[108] The use of azithromycin plus rifabutin may provide even greater protection.[110] Other groups at high risk for MAC disease, such as persons with hairy cell leukemia, may also benefit from prophylactic therapy, but no studies have been reported.

Mycobacterium kansasii

M. kansasii causes disseminated disease in persons with AIDS and pulmonary disease in persons with or without HIV infection. All presentations are relatively uncommon, and data on therapeutic regimens are sparse. Early studies of therapy for *M. kansasii* pulmonary disease showed equivalent response rates with drug regimens of isoniazid, rifampin, and ethambutol or isoniazid, rifampin, and streptomycin.[111] Rifampin is an essential part of any treatment regimen for *M. kansasii*[112]; therapy should be continued for 18 months.

There is no clear role for in vitro susceptibility testing in selecting initial therapeutic regimens; isolates are routinely resistant to isoniazid at the doses tested, despite the usefulness of this drug in therapy. It is thought that the isolates are susceptible at levels slightly higher than those tested.[3] However, in patients who have had previous treatment with rifampin, resistance to this drug may have arisen, and susceptibility testing should be performed. One study has reported success with treatment of rifampin-resistant *M. kansasii* disease using regimens selected on the basis of in vitro susceptibility.[113] The reported exquisite susceptibility of *M. kansasii* to clarithromycin suggests a role for this drug in treatment of disease due to *M. kansasii*,[114] but no clinical experience has been reported.

Therapy for disseminated disease should follow the same principles. Case series of disseminated disease in patients with AIDS have reported limited success with regimens containing isoniazid, rifampin, ethambutol, and trimethoprim-sulfamethoxazole in some cases.[115, 116] Clarithromycin may also be a useful addition in these patients.

Mycobacterium fortuitum *biovar* fortuitum

M. fortuitum biovar *fortuitum* has been reported largely as a cause of skin and soft tissue disease, although disseminated disease, pulmonary infection, endocarditis, and keratitis have been reported.[117] Most isolates are susceptible to sulfamethoxazole, ciprofloxacin, cefoxitin, imipenem, and amikacin but not clarithromycin.[118, 119] Initial therapy should include two of these agents; subsequent modifications should be made on the basis of in vitro susceptibility testing, which is a reliable predictor of therapeutic outcome.[120] Therapy for uncomplicated skin lesions may require only 3 months. Invasive disease in the HIV-uninfected host should receive 3 to 6 months of therapy; disseminated disease in the HIV-infected host should continue for the life of the patient.

Mycobacterium fortuitum *biovar* peregrinum

M. fortuitum biovar *peregrinum* is an uncommon cause of skin and soft tissue infections. Invasive disease has not been reported.[117] Most isolates are susceptible to sulfamethoxazole, cefoxitin, amikacin, clarithromycin, and azithromycin.[118, 119] Initial therapy should include two of these agents; subsequent modifications should be made on the basis of in vitro susceptibility testing, which is a reliable predictor of therapeutic outcome.[120]

Mycobacterium fortuitum *Third Biovar*

This organism is also an uncommon cause of skin and soft tissue infections. Invasive disease has not been reported.[117] Most isolates are susceptible to sulfamethoxazole, cefoxitin, and amikacin but not clarithromycin or azithromycin.[118, 119] Initial therapy should include two of these agents; subsequent modifications should be made on the basis of in vitro susceptibility testing, which is a reliable predictor of therapeutic outcome.[120]

Mycobacterium chelonae

M. chelonae (formerly *M. chelonei* subsp. *chelonae*) has been reported as a cause of skin and soft tissue infection. Disseminated disease and keratitis have been seen but are rare.[117] Isolates are routinely susceptible to clarithromycin, azithromycin, and amikacin.[118] Clarithromycin appears to be the therapy of choice for this infection.[121] However, resistance may develop with monotherapy.[122] Invasive infection may require combination chemotherapy based on in vitro susceptibility testing.[120] Therapy for uncomplicated skin lesions may require only 3 months. Invasive disease in the HIV-uninfected host should receive 3 to 6 months of therapy; disseminated disease in the HIV-infected host should continue for the life of the patient.

Mycobacterium abscessus

M. abscessus (formerly *M. chelonae* subsp. *abscessus*) has been reported to cause pulmonary disease, skin and soft tissue infections, and disseminated disease.[117] Most isolates are susceptible to cefoxitin, amikacin, clarithromycin, and azithromycin.[118, 119] Initial therapy should include an azalide-macrolide antibiotic and one other agent[123]; subsequent modifications should be made on the basis of in vitro susceptibility testing, which is a reliable predictor of therapeutic outcome.[120]

Mycobacterium chelonae–*like Organisms*

These organisms have been reported as causes of wound infection and catheter-related sepsis and rarely as pathogens in patients with AIDS.[124] They are quite susceptible to most antibiotics, including amikacin, imipenem, cefoxitin, ciprofloxacin, and ofloxacin.[118] Initial therapy should include two of these agents; subsequent modifications should be made on the basis of in vitro susceptibility testing, which is a reliable predictor of therapeutic outcome.[120]

Mycobacterium marinum

M. marinum causes skin and soft tissue infections in nonimmunocompromised persons. Occasional cases of invasive arthritis and disseminated disease have been reported. In vitro susceptibilities are variable, and a relationship between such results and responses to therapy has not been demonstrated.[125–127] Most patients are treated with at least two of the following: rifampin, ethambutol, doxycycline, minocycline, or co-trimoxazole. In vitro studies suggest that clarithromycin may also be effective,[128] and cures have been reported with clarithromycin plus ethambutol.[129] Surgical removal of involved lymph nodes has improved outcomes in some series. Therapy is continued for a minimum of 3 months.[3]

Mycobacterium ulcerans

M. ulcerans causes necrotic skin ulcers, largely in Africa, Australia, and New Guinea. The mycobacteria secrete a potent cytotoxin that is responsible for the tissue damage. Antimycobacterial agents are not effective,[130, 131] presumably because they are not given until the toxin has been secreted; penetration to the site of infection may also be impaired by the extensive necrosis. Surgical excision of early lesions and skin grafting for extensive lesions are recommended.[131]

Mycobacterium leprae

Hansen's disease, or leprosy, affects more than 5 million persons worldwide but is uncommon in the United States.[132, 133] Dapsone, rifampin, clofazimine, and ethionamide are useful agents. Multidrug regimens are usually used, both to prevent emergence of drug resistance and to eliminate persistent organisms. However, a study showed that long-term outcomes of dapsone monotherapy were also satisfactory as long as dapsone-resistant organisms were not present.[134]

For paucibacillary leprosy, dapsone, 1 to 2 mg/kg, is given daily and rifampin 10 mg/kg monthly, both for a 6-month period. For multibacillary forms, daily dapsone, monthly rifampin, and clofazimine (at 300 mg monthly plus 50 mg daily) are given for 2 years.[135] Directly observed therapy of the monthly doses is strongly recommended. In vitro susceptibility testing is not available. Animal studies suggest that minocycline, ofloxacin, and clarithromycin may also be useful in treatment of leprosy.[136, 137]

Mycobacterium haemophilum

M. haemophilum is an infrequent cause of skin lesions; nearly all cases occur in immunocompromised patients, and dissemination can occur in the HIV-infected host.[138–140] In vitro susceptibility testing suggests that most isolates are susceptible to clarithromycin, ciprofloxacin, cycloserine, and rifabutin[140]; use of these agents for therapy appeared to be associated with an improved clinical outcome, but only 13 patients were described. Others have recommended a regimen of amikacin, ciprofloxacin, and rifampin.[141] The optimal duration of therapy and the role of in vitro susceptibility testing in guiding management are unknown.

Mycobacterium xenopi

M. xenopi is a cause of pulmonary disease in both immunologically normal and immunosuppressed hosts; disseminated disease in patients with AIDS has also been reported.[142, 143] The organism is routinely susceptible to isoniazid and streptomycin, but it is intermediate to rifampin and resistant to ethambutol[144]; in vitro synergy between rifampin and streptomycin has been reported,[145] but the relevance of this finding to clinical response is unclear. The optimal therapeutic regimen has not been defined, and response of pulmonary disease to therapy is variable[144, 146]; a consensus panel has recommended initiation of therapy with isoniazid, rifampin, and ethambutol, possibly with an initial period of streptomycin.[3] Therapy should be continued for 18 months. Those failing to respond to medical therapy may benefit from surgical resection.[147] Disseminated disease in AIDS has also shown a variable response to therapy.

Mycobacterium szulgai

M. szulgai is a rare cause of pulmonary disease; cutaneous infection and olecranon bursitis have also been reported.[148] Isolates of *M. szulgai* are usually susceptible to isoniazid, streptomycin, and rifampin; susceptibility to ethambutol is variable.[148] A report also showed susceptibility to clarithromycin.[128] Therapy with three of these drugs is recommended[3, 148]; at least 12 months of treatment would appear prudent.

Mycobacterium malmoense

M. malmoense is similar in clinical presentation to MAC; it causes pulmonary disease in normal hosts, cervical lymphadenitis in children, and disseminated disease in patients with AIDS.[149–151] It is common in Europe but rare in the United States. Most authors recommend 18 to 24 months of therapy with isoniazid, rifampin, and ethambutol, with an initial period of streptomycin for pulmonary or disseminated disease.[3, 152] The value of in vitro susceptibility testing as a guide to selection of drugs is unknown. Clarithromycin has not been clinically evaluated but may prove useful.

Mycobacterium genavense

M. genavense is biochemically and genetically related to *M. simiae* but produces a clinical picture more similar to that of MAC, with disseminated disease in AIDS patients the dominant clinical presentation.[153, 154] Susceptibility studies are limited by the failure of growth on solid media; limited experience suggests that three-drug regimens containing clarithromycin (such as those recommended for MAC) are effective.[155]

Mycobacterium simiae

M. simiae is a rare cause of pulmonary disease and also a rare cause of disseminated disease in patients with AIDS.[156–159] Most isolates are resistant to the majority of antimycobacterial agents, including clarithromycin,[128] and therapeutic results are poor.[156] An expert panel has recommended initiating therapy with isoniazid, rifampin, ethambutol, and streptomycin and adjusting the regimen on the basis of results of in vitro susceptibility tests.[3]

Mycobacterium scrofulaceum

M. scrofulaceum was a common cause of cervical lymphadenitis in children in the United States until the 1970s, but it is rare today[106]; it is also infrequently seen as a cause of pulmonary disease[160] and as disseminated disease in AIDS.[161] Treatment of isolated lymphadenitis should continue to be surgical. *M. scrofulaceum* is susceptible in vitro to clarithromycin,[128] and multidrug regimens containing clarithromycin have been advocated. Susceptibility to ethambutol and rifampin is variable, but these drugs might be useful additional drugs for initial therapy until susceptibility results are available. Duration of therapy is unknown, but treatment should be lifelong in patients with AIDS.

Mycobacterium celatum

This newly described pathogen is closely related to MAC and *M. xenopi*. The clinical spectrum includes pneumonia and disseminated disease in patients with AIDS.[162, 163] A report indicated that isolates may be susceptible to clarithromycin, azithromycin, amikacin, ciprofloxacin, ofloxacin, clofazimine, rifampin, and rifabutin.[162] We recommend a therapeutic strategy similar to that for MAC.

Mycobacterium smegmatis

M. smegmatis is rarely reported to cause skin and soft tissue infection, especially after inoculation.[164] Isolates are usually susceptible to amikacin, imipenem, ethambutol, ciprofloxacin, doxycycline, and sulfamethoxazole. Results of in vitro susceptibility testing are recommended as a guide to therapy, and clinical outcomes are, on the whole, favorable.[165] Superficial infection may be cured by excision without antibiotics.[166]

Mycobacterium gordonae

M. gordonae is a common saprophyte and almost never a pathogen; only a handful of well-documented cases of human infection have been reported.[167] Susceptibility in vitro to ethambutol, clarithromycin, rifampin, and amikacin has been reported.[128, 167] Few isolates have been tested against quinolones or trimethoprim-sulfamethoxazole. Results of treatment are mixed; the paucity of cases precludes conclusions about therapy.

Specific Antimycobacterial Drugs for Nontuberculous Mycobacteria (Table 34–9)

Azithromycin

Azithromycin is a macrolide antibiotic with a 15-membered macrolide ring known as an azalide. It inhibits bacterial protein synthesis by binding to the 50S ribosomal subunit; this is thought to be the mechanism of action in mycobacteria as well. Azithromycin is active in vitro against MAC and other nontuberculous mycobacteria, but it is not active against *M. tuberculosis.* The drug is well absorbed orally and is concentrated in tissues, where levels 10 to 100 times higher than serum levels may be achieved.[168, 169] The half-life is nearly 5 days, so that dosing may be at intervals greater than daily, although daily dosing is usually used for convenience. The drug is metabolized and excreted in the liver; it should be used with caution in persons with hepatic impairment. As with other macrolides, gastrointestinal disturbance can occur, although azithromycin appears to have less gastrointestinal toxicity than either erythromycin or clarithromycin. This toxicity is dose related and may be circumvented by dividing doses. Diarrhea and nausea, as well as frank abdominal pain, are seen. Rashes and other evidence of hypersensitivity are rare. More worrisome is hearing loss, which has been reported in patients receiving therapy for MAC with high doses of the drug.[170] Although this is reversible if the drug is discontinued early, continuation may result in permanent hearing loss. Little is known about interactions with rifamycins or antiretroviral agents. When the drug is given with rifabutin, uveitis appears to be rare, in contrast with the experience when clarithromycin is given with rifabutin.

Cefoxitin

Cefoxitin is a β-lactam antibiotic that interferes with cell wall synthesis of gram-negative and gram-positive bacteria; its mode of action against mycobacteria is unknown but may be similar. Cefoxitin is active against all biovars of *M. fortuitum, M. abscessus,* and *M. chelonae*–like mycobacteria, and it is used primarily for invasive infections with these organisms. Because the drug is poorly absorbed orally, it must be given by the intramuscular or intravenous route; the intravenous route is preferred. The half-life in the serum is 1 hour; 85% of the drug is excreted in the urine, so dose adjustment should be made when it is used in patients with altered renal function. High doses are recommended for treating mycobacterial infections with cefoxitin (12 g/d).[119] Toxic effects include rash, fever, eosinophilia, and mild leukopenia and elevations in liver function tests. All are uncommon (less than 3%).

Clarithromycin

Clarithromycin is a macrolide antibiotic that is closely related to erythromycin. It inhibits bacterial protein synthesis by binding to the 50S ribosomal subunit; this is thought to be the mechanism of action in mycobacteria as well. Clarithromycin is active in vitro against MAC and other nontuberculous mycobacteria, but it is not active against *M. tuberculosis.* The drug is well absorbed orally and is concentrated in tissues, where levels two to six times higher than in serum may be achieved.[171] The half-life is 2.6 to 4.4 hours; this has led to twice-daily dosing, although the slow growth rate of mycobacteria would undoubtedly allow daily dosing; however, gastrointestinal intolerance of the correspondingly larger single dose has effectively limited this strategy.[79] The drug is metabolized and excreted in the liver, but 30% is also excreted in the urine, and dose adjustment is needed in persons with impaired renal function. As with other macrolides, gastrointestinal disturbance can occur, but clarithromycin has substantially less gastrointestinal toxicity than erythromycin. This toxicity is dose related; persons unable to tolerate 500 mg twice daily (the highest recommended dose) may successfully tolerate 250 mg four times a day or may require dose reduction to 250 mg orally twice per day. Moreover, those who do not tolerate clarithromycin may tolerate azithromycin. Diarrhea and nausea as well as abdominal pain or dyspepsia are the most common manifestations, occurring in 11% of patients. Rashes and other evidence of hypersensitivity are rare. Hearing loss appears to be less common than with azithromycin. As with other macrolides, hepatic injury may occur with use of clarithromycin.[172] There is a bidirectional interaction between clarithromycin and rifa-

TABLE 34–9 ■ Agents Used in the Treatment of Nontuberculous Mycobacteria

DRUG	ROUTE*	PEDIATRIC DOSAGE	ADULT DOSAGE	FREQUENCY
Amikacin	IV	15 mg/kg	15 mg/kg	Once daily
Azithromycin	PO	7.5 mg/kg	500 mg	Once daily
Cefoxitin	IV	30 mg/kg	2 g	q 4 h
Ciprofloxacin	PO	NR†	750 mg	Twice daily
Clarithromycin	PO	7.5 mg/kg	500 mg	Twice daily
Clofazimine	PO	1–2 mg/kg	100 mg‡	Once daily
Co-trimoxazole	PO	4 mg/kg trimethoprim plus 20 mg/kg sulfamethoxazole	160 mg trimethoprim + 800 mg sulfamethoxazole	Twice daily
Dapsone	PO	1–2 mg/kg	100 mg	Once daily
Doxycycline	PO	1–2 mg/kg§	100 mg	Twice daily
Ethambutol	PO	15–25 mg/kg	15–25 mg/kg	Once daily
Imipenem	IV	15 mg/kg	1 g	q 6 h
Minocycline	PO	1–2 mg/kg§	100 mg	Twice daily
Ofloxacin	PO	NR	400 mg	Twice daily
Rifabutin	PO	10 mg/kg	300 mg	Once daily
Rifampin	PO	20 mg/kg	600 mg	Once daily
Sulfisoxazole	PO	30 mg/kg	2 g	Four times daily

*PO, Oral; IV, intravenous.
†NR, Not recommended.
‡50 mg for leprosy.
§Not recommended for children younger than 8 y.

butin, with increased levels of rifabutin and decreased levels of clarithromycin when the drugs are taken concurrently.[173–175] This interaction may be responsible for the occurrence of uveitis when clarithromycin is used in conjunction with 600 mg/d of rifabutin.[176] Uveitis appears uncommon, however, if the rifabutin dose does not exceed the recommended dose of 300 mg/d. This uveitis resolves when rifabutin doses are lowered or the drug is discontinued.

Clofazimine

Clofazimine is a riminophenazine dye that binds to DNA, but its mechanism of antimycobacterial action is unknown. It has activity against MAC and *M. leprae* and is primarily used in treatment of infections with these organisms. Clofazimine has variable absorption but is effective when given orally. It is extremely fat soluble, with a large volume of distribution; consequently, the drug is not detectable in the serum for up to 3 months after initiation of oral therapy, and the half-life is 70 days.[86, 87] It is excreted in the stool, with less than 1% of drug found in the urine. Toxicity is minimal; an orange-bronze discoloration of the skin is the most common effect in light-skinned individuals. This pigmentation gradually resolves if the drug is discontinued. Dry skin and scaling can also be bothersome to the patient. Gastrointestinal disturbances, including nausea, vomiting, and diarrhea, are uncommon when doses of 100 mg daily are employed but become more frequent as higher doses are used.

Dapsone

Dapsone is a long-acting sulfa compound that is effective against *M. leprae,* for which it is the primary antimycobacterial agent. Its mechanism of action is presumed to be inhibition of mycobacterial synthesis of folic acid, by analogy with its activity in other bacteria. The drug is well absorbed orally and has a mean plasma half-life of 28 hours. Excretion occurs in the stool after hepatic metabolism, and enterohepatic circulation leads to prolongation of the presence of the drug in the body. The major toxic effect is hemolytic anemia occurring in persons with glucose-6-phosphate dehydrogenase deficiency, and patients should be screened for this defect before beginning dapsone therapy. Rare individuals will have a hypersensitivity syndrome consisting of fever, jaundice, anemia, and exfoliative dermatitis; this syndrome resolves with discontinuation of the drug.

Sulfisoxazole

Sulfisoxazole is a sulfa drug with activity against all biovars of *M. fortuitum.* Its mechanism of antimycobacterial action is presumed to be inhibition of bacterial synthesis of folic acid, by analogy with its activity in other bacteria. The drug is absorbed well from the gastrointestinal tract and can be given orally. The half-life is 5 to 6 hours, and more than 95% of the drug is excreted in the urine; thus, dose adjustment must be made for patients with impaired renal function. Toxic effects include rash, fever, photosensitization, anemia, and (rarely) Stevens-Johnson syndrome.

Co-trimoxazole

Co-trimoxazole is a fixed combination of sulfamethoxazole and trimethoprim. The combination has activity against *M. marinum,* and this is the only mycobacterial species for which it is used. Its mechanism of antimycobacterial action is presumed to be inhibition of bacterial synthesis of folic acid, by analogy with its activity in other bacteria. The drug is absorbed well from the gastrointestinal tract and can be given orally. The half-life of the sulfa portion is 10 to 12 hours, and most of the drug is excreted in the urine; thus, dose adjustment must be made for patients with impaired renal function. The half-life of the trimethoprim moiety is 9 to 11 hours, and it is also excreted in the urine. Toxic effects include rash, fever, photosensitization, anemia, leukopenia, and (rarely) Stevens-Johnson syndrome.

Imipenem

Imipenem is a β-lactam antibiotic that is given with cilastatin to counter enzymatic breakdown of imipenem in the kidney. Imipenem acts by binding to penicillin binding proteins of many bacteria; the antimycobacterial activity is also thought to result from such binding. The drug is active against *M. fortuitum* biovar *fortuitum* and *M. chelonae*–like organisms. It is an alternative agent for treatment of invasive infections with these organisms. Imipenem is given intravenously and has a half-life of 1 hour. Seventy percent of the drug is excreted in the urine; thus, dose reduction is required in persons with impaired renal function. Toxic effects include rash and fever, nausea, and vomiting. Diarrhea and local thrombophlebitis at the site of infusion are also seen. Seizures have also been reported but are uncommon.

Doxycycline

Doxycycline is a long-acting tetracycline analog that is active against *M. marinum* and is used in treatment of infection with this organism. Tetracyclines inhibit protein synthesis by interfering with attachment of RNA to the ribosome, primarily at the 30S ribosomal subunit; presumably its activity against *M. marinum* involves such a mechanism. Doxycycline is well absorbed from the gut and is given orally. The serum half-life is 18 hours, and somewhat less than half of the drug appears in the urine. Dose adjustment in renal failure is not required. Toxic effects include nausea and photosensitivity, but these are uncommon.

Minocycline

Minocycline is a long-acting tetracycline analog that is active against *M. leprae* and *M. marinum* and is used as an alternative therapy in treatment of infections with these organisms. Tetracyclines inhibit protein synthesis by interfering with attachment of RNA to the ribosome, primarily at the 30S ribosomal subunit; presumably its activity against mycobacteria involves such a mechanism. Minocycline is well absorbed from the gut and is given orally. The serum half-life is 16 hours, and less than 10% of the drug appears in the urine. Dose adjustment in renal failure is therefore not required. Toxic effects include nausea and photosensitivity, but these are uncommon. Vertigo and ataxia may result from this agent and limit its use in some patients.

Rifabutin

Rifabutin is a rifamycin related to rifampin; its antimycobacterial effect is thought to be mediated by binding to DNA-dependent RNA polymerase. It is more active in vitro against mycobacteria than is rifampin, but this increased activity is balanced by lower achievable serum levels. Tissue concentrations may be higher, but the clinical importance of this is unknown. Peak serum levels of 0.4 μg/mL are achieved 2 hours after the 300-mg oral dose; the half-life is approximately 2 days. Excretion is primarily biliary. Rifabutin appears to be a less potent inducer of hepatic metabolism by the cytochrome P-450 pathway than is rifampin, but such enzyme induction is still substantial. Rifabutin, 300 mg/d orally, is effective in prophylaxis of MAC infection in patients with AIDS and a $CD4^+$ cell count less than 75/mm^3. The same dose is also commonly included in multidrug regimens for treatment of disseminated MAC infection in patients with AIDS. The contribution of rifabutin to the success of such regimens is theoretically likely but as yet unproved. Like rifampin, rifabutin causes a red-orange discoloration of the urine that is disturbing but harmless. Rash, gastrointestinal disturbance, hepatitis, and uveitis are possible but rare at the recommended dose. All side effects, and particularly uveitis, are more frequent when the drug is coadministered with clarithromycin, possibly because of a drug interaction between these two agents.[173–176]

Amikacin

Amikacin is an aminoglycoside antibiotic that interferes with bacterial protein synthesis, although the exact mechanism of its action in mycobacteria has not been elucidated. Amikacin is active against MAC, *M. fortuitum* (all biovars), *M. chelonae*-like organisms, *M. abscessus,* and *M. haemophilum.* However, its use is generally restricted to invasive infections with isolates that are not susceptible to oral agents. Amikacin is not absorbed from the gastrointestinal tract and is generally given intravenously, although intramuscular injections can also be given. The serum half-life is 8 hours; because of the slow growth of mycobacteria, once-daily dosing is sufficient. The drug is excreted by the kidney, and doses must be adjusted in patients with impaired renal function. Monitoring of serum drug levels is recommended. Amikacin has considerable ototoxicity and nephrotoxicity. Ototoxic injury can be either cochlear or vestibular, and the risk increases with the duration of therapy. This poses a particular problem in treatment of mycobacterial infections, for which months to years of treatment are often desirable. In practice, amikacin is given for only a brief period of 1 to 3 months; treatment for more than 3 months with full-dose amikacin almost guarantees ototoxic effects. Hearing loss is reversible if the drug is stopped promptly, but onset can be insidious and disability permanent. Nephrotoxic effects are more easily monitored but likewise common. Biweekly serum creatinine determinations and weekly amikacin levels should be obtained while the patient is receiving therapy; doses must be adjusted if renal function impairment occurs.

References

1. Good RC, Mastro TD: The modern mycobacteriology laboratory: How it can help the clinician. Clin Chest Med 10:315–322, 1989.
2. Wolinsky E, Rynearson TK: Mycobacteria in soil and their relation to disease-associated strains. Am Rev Respir Dis 97:1032–1037, 1968.
3. Wallace RJ Jr, O'Brien R, Glassroth J, et al: Diagnosis and treatment of disease caused by nontuberculous mycobacteria. Am Rev Respir Dis 142:940–953, 1990.
4. Ayvazian LF: History of tuberculosis. *In* Reichman LB, Herschfield ES (eds): Tuberculosis: A Comprehensive International Approach. New York, Marcel Dekker, 1993, pp 1–20.
5. Medical Research Council: A Medical Research Council Investigation. Streptomycin treatment of pulmonary tuberculosis. Br Med J 2:769–782, 1948.
6. Hinshaw HC, Feldman WH, Pfuetze KH: Treatment of tuberculosis with streptomycin. A summary of observation in one hundred cases. JAMA 13:778–782, 1946.
7. Medical Research Council: A Medical Research Council Investigation. Treatment of pulmonary tuberculosis with streptomycin and para-aminosalicylic acid. Br Med J 2:1073–1085, 1950.
8. Medical Research Council: The treatment of pulmonary tuberculosis with isoniazid, an interim report to the Medical Research Council by their Tuberculosis Chemotherapy Trials Committee. Br Med J 2:735–746, 1953.
9. Medical Research Council: Various combinations of isoniazid with streptomycin or with PAS in the treatment of pulmonary tuberculosis. Seventh report to the Medical Research Council by their Tuberculosis Chemotherapy Trials Committee. Br Med J 1:434–445, 1955.
10. Crofton J: Drug treatment of tuberculosis. Standard chemotherapy. Br Med J 2:370–373, 1960.
11. Medical Research Council–Tuberculosis Chemotherapy Trials Committee: Long-term chemotherapy in the treatment of chronic pulmonary tuberculosis with cavitation. Tubercle 43:201–267, 1962.
12. Combs DL, O'Brien RJ, Geiter LJ: USPHS short-course chemotherapy trial 21: Effectiveness, toxicity, and acceptability. The report of final results. Ann Intern Med 112:397–406, 1990.
13. Fox W: General considerations in intermittent drug therapy of pulmonary tuberculosis. Postgrad Med 47:729–736, 1971.
14. Mitchison DA: Basic mechanisms of chemotherapy. Chest 6(Suppl):771–781, 1979.
15. Jindani A, Aber VR, Edwards EA, Mitchison DA: The early bactericidal activity of drugs in patients with pulmonary tuberculosis. Am Rev Respir Dis 121:939–949, 1980.
16. Dickinson JM, Aber VR, Mitchison DA: Bactericidal activity of streptomycin, isoniazid, rifampin, ethambutol and pyrazinamide alone and in combination against *Mycobacterium tuberculosis.* Am Rev Respir Dis 116:627–635, 1977.
17. Grosset J: The sterilizing value of rifampicin and pyrazinamide in experimental short-course chemotherapy. Tubercle 59:287–297, 1978.
18. Mitchison DA: The action of antituberculosis drugs in short-course chemotherapy. Tubercle 66:219–226, 1985.
19. Centers for Disease Control: Initial therapy for tuberculosis in the era of multidrug resistance. MMWR Morbid Mortal Wkly Rep 42(RR-7):1–8, 1993.
20. Fox W: The problem of self-administration of drugs, with particular reference to pulmonary tuberculosis. Tubercle 39:269–274, 1958.
21. McDonald RJ, Memon AM, Reichman LB: Successful supervised ambulatory management of tuberculosis treatment failures. Ann Intern Med 96:297–302, 1982.
22. Sbarbaro JA: All patients should receive directly observed therapy in tuberculosis. Am Rev Respir Dis 138:1075–1076, 1988.
23. Iseman MD, Cohn DL, Sbarbaro JA: Directly observed treatment of tuberculosis—We can't afford not to try it. N Engl J Med 328:576–578, 1993.
24. Weis SE, Slocum PC, Blais FX, et al: The effect of directly observed therapy on the rates of drug resistance and relapse in tuberculosis. N Engl J Med 330:1179–1184, 1994.
25. Patel KB, Belmonte R, Crowe HM: Drug malabsorption and resistant tuberculosis in HIV-infected patients. N Engl J Med 332:336–337, 1995.
26. Mahmoudi A, Iseman MD: Pitfalls in the care of patients with tuberculosis. JAMA 270:65–68, 1993.
27. Bloch AB, Cauthen GM, Onorato IM, et al: Nationwide survey of drug-resistant tuberculosis in the United States. JAMA 271:665–671, 1994.
28. American Thoracic Society: Treatment of tuberculosis and tuberculosis infection in adults and children. Am J Respir Crit Care Med 149:1359–1374, 1994.
29. Cohn DL, Catlin BJ, Peterson KL, et al: A 62-dose 6-month therapy for pulmonary and extrapulmonary TB. A twice-weekly, directly observed, and cost-effective regimen. Ann Intern Med 112:407–415, 1990.
30. Hong Kong Chest Service/British Medical Research Council: Controlled trial of 4 three-times-weekly regimens and a daily regimen given for 6 months for pulmonary TB. Second report: The results up to 24 months. Tubercle 63:89–98, 1982.
31. Hong Kong Chest Service/British Medical Research Council: Five-year follow-up of a controlled trial of five 6-month regimens of chemotherapy for pulmonary tuberculosis. Am Rev Respir Dis 136:1339–1342, 1987.
32. Small PM, Schechter GF, Goodman PC, et al: Treatment of tuberculosis in patients with advanced human immunodeficiency virus infection. N Engl J Med 324:289–294, 1991.
33. Perriens JH, St Louis ME, Mukadi YB, et al: Pulmonary tubercu-

losis in HIV-infected patients in Zaire: A controlled trial of treatment for either 6 or 12 months. N Engl J Med 332:779–784, 1995.
34. Snider DE Jr: Should women taking antituberculosis drugs breast-feed? Arch Intern Med 144:589–590, 1984.
35. Snider DE Jr, Layde PM, Johnson MW, Lyle MA: Treatment of tuberculosis during pregnancy. Am Rev Respir Dis 122:65–79, 1980.
36. Dutt AK, Moers D, Stead WW: Smear- and culture-negative pulmonary tuberculosis: Four-month short-course chemotherapy. Am Rev Respir Dis 139:867–870, 1989.
37. Hong Kong Chest Service/Tuberculosis Research Centre, Madras/British Medical Research Council: A controlled trial of 3-month, 4-month, and 6-month regimens of chemotherapy for sputum-smear–negative pulmonary tuberculosis. Results at 5 years. Am Rev Respir Dis 139:871–876, 1989.
38. Mitchison DA, Nunn AJ: Influence of initial drug resistance on the response to short-course chemotherapy of pulmonary tuberculosis. Am Rev Respir Dis 133:423–430, 1986.
39. Babu Swai O, Aluoch JA, Githui WA, et al: Controlled clinical trial of a regimen of two durations for the treatment of isoniazid resistant pulmonary tuberculosis. Tubercle 69:5–14, 1988.
40. Zierski M: Prospects of retreatment of chronic resistant pulmonary tuberculosis patients: A critical review. Lung 154:91–102, 1977.
41. Goble M, Iseman MD, Madsen LA, et al: Treatment of 171 patients with pulmonary tuberculosis resistant to isoniazid and rifampin. N Engl J Med 328:527–532, 1993.
42. Salomon N, Perlman DC, Friedmann P, et al: Predictors and outcome of multidrug-resistant tuberculosis. Clin Infect Dis 21:1245–1252, 1995.
43. Telzak EE, Sepkowitz K, Alpert P, et al: Multidrug-resistant tuberculosis in patients without HIV infection. N Engl J Med 333:907–911, 1995.
44. Turett GS, Telzak EE, Torian LV, et al: Improved outcomes for patients with multidrug-resistant tuberculosis. Clin Infect Dis 21:1238–1244, 1995.
45. Iseman MD: Treatment of multidrug-resistant tuberculosis. N Engl J Med 329:784–791, 1993.
46. Centers for Disease Control and Prevention: Improving Patient Adherence to Tuberculosis Treatment. Atlanta, U.S. Department of Health and Human Services, Public Health Service, CDC, 1994.
47. Iseman MD, Madsen L, Goble M, Pomerantz M: Surgical intervention in the treatment of pulmonary disease caused by drug-resistant *M. tuberculosis*. Am Rev Respir Dis 141:623–625, 1990.
48. Treasure RL, Seaworth BJ: Current role of surgery in *Mycobacterium tuberculosis*. Ann Thorac Surg 59:1405–1409, 1995.
49. Ferebee SH: Controlled chemoprophylaxis trial in tuberculosis: A general review. Adv Tuberc Res 17:28–106, 1969.
50. Hsu KH: Thirty years after isoniazid: Its impact on tuberculosis in children and adolescents. JAMA 251:1283–1285, 1984.
51. International Union Against Tuberculosis Committee on Prophylaxis: Efficacy of various durations of isoniazid preventive therapy for tuberculosis: Five years of follow-up in the IUAT trial. Bull World Health Organ 60:555–564, 1982.
52. Kopanoff DE, Snider DE Jr, Caras GJ: Isoniazid-related hepatitis: A U.S. Public Health Service cooperative surveillance study. Am Rev Respir Dis 117:991–1001, 1978.
53. Selwyn PA, Sckell BM, Alcabes P, et al: High risk of active tuberculosis in HIV-infected drug users with cutaneous anergy. JAMA 268:504–509, 1992.
54. Moreno S, Baraia-Etxaburu J, Bouza E, et al: Risk for developing tuberculosis among anergic patients infected with HIV. Ann Intern Med 119:194–198, 1993.
55. Pape JW, Simone SJ, Ho JL, et al: Effect of isoniazid prophylaxis on incidence of active tuberculosis and progression of HIV infection. Lancet 342:268–272, 1993.
56. Lecoeur HF, Truffot-Pernot C, Grosset JH: Experimental short-course preventive therapy of tuberculosis with rifampin and pyrazinamide. Am Rev Respir Dis 140:1189–1193, 1989.
57. Centers for Disease Control: Management of persons exposed to multidrug-resistant tuberculosis. MMWR Morbid Mortal Wkly Rep 41:61–71, 1992.
58. Horn DL, Hewlett D, Alfalla C: Limited tolerance of ofloxacin and pyrazinamide prophylaxis against tuberculosis (Letter). N Engl J Med 330:1241, 1994.
59. Centers for Disease Control and Prevention: Severe isoniazid-associated hepatitis—New York, 1991–1993. MMWR Morbid Mortal Wkly Rep 42:545–547, 1993.
60. Moulding TS, Redeker AG, Kanel GC: Twenty isoniazid-associated deaths in one state. Am Rev Respir Dis 140:700–705, 1989.
61. Snider DE: Pyridoxine supplementation during isoniazid therapy. Tubercle 61:191–196, 1980.
62. Rothfield NF, Bierer MF, Garfield JW: Isoniazid induction of antinuclear antibodies. Ann Intern Med 88:650–652, 1978.
63. Alarcon-Segovia D, Fishbein E, Betancourt VM: Antibodies to nucleoprotein in tuberculous patients receiving isoniazid. Clin Exp Immunol 5:429–437, 1969.
64. Smith CK, Durack DT: Isoniazid and reaction to cheese. Ann Intern Med 88:520–521, 1978.
65. Uragoda CG: Histamine poisoning in tuberculous patients after ingestion of tuna fish. Am Rev Respir Dis 121:157–159, 1980.
66. Block SH: Carbamazepine-isoniazid interaction. Pediatrics 69:494, 1982.
67. Kutt H, Brennan R, Dehejia H, Verebely K: Diphenylhydantoin intoxication. A complication of isoniazid therapy. Am Rev Respir Dis 101:377–384, 1970.
68. Zent C, Smith P: Study of the effect of concomitant food on the bioavailability of rifampicin, isoniazid, and pyrazinamide. Tubercle 76:109–113, 1995.
69. Steele MA, Burk RF, Des Prez RM: Toxic hepatitis with isoniazid and rifampin. Chest 99:465–471, 1991.
70. Borcherding SM, Baciewicz AM, Self TH: Update on rifampin drug interactions II. Arch Intern Med 152:711–716, 1992.
71. Varughese A, Brater DC, Benet LZ, Lee CS: Ethambutol kinetics in patients with impaired renal function. Am Rev Respir Dis 134:34–38, 1986.
72. Steele MA, Des Prez RM: The role of pyrazinamide in tuberculosis chemotherapy. Chest 94:842–844, 1988.
73. Drugs for tuberculosis. Med Lett 37:67–70, 1995.
74. Moulding T, Dutt AK, Reichman LB: Fixed-dose combinations of antituberculous medications to prevent drug resistance. Ann Intern Med 122:951–954, 1995.
75. Ridzon R, Lloyd J, Geiter L, et al: Comparison of adverse reactions of para-aminosalicylate granules to tablets (Abstr M7). *In* Abstracts of the 34th Interscience Conference on Antimicrobial Agents and Chemotherapy. Washington, DC, American Society for Microbiology, 1994, p 197.
76. Sullivan EA, Kreiswirth BN, Palumbo L, et al: Emergence of fluoroquinolone-resistant tuberculosis in New York City. Lancet 345:1148–1150, 1995.
77. Berning SL, Madsen L, Iseman MD, Peloquin CA: Long-term safety of ofloxacin and ciprofloxacin in the treatment of mycobacterial infections. Am J Respir Crit Care Med 151:2006–2009, 1995.
78. Horsburgh CR: *Mycobacterium avium* complex infection in the acquired immunodeficiency syndrome. N Engl J Med 324:1332–1338, 1991.
79. Chaisson RE, Benson CA, Dube MP, et al: Clarithromycin therapy for bacteremic *Mycobacterium avium* complex disease. Ann Intern Med 121:905–911, 1994.
80. Young LS, Wiviott L, Wu M, et al: Azithromycin for treatment of *Mycobacterium avium-intracellulare* complex infection in patients with AIDS. Lancet 338:1107–1109, 1991.
81. Masur H, PHS Task Force: Recommendations on prophylaxis and therapy for disseminated *Mycobacterium avium* complex disease in patients infected with the human immunodeficiency virus. N Engl J Med 329:898–904, 1993.
82. Kemper CA, Havlir D, Haghighat D, et al: The individual microbiologic effect of three antimycobacterial agents, clofazimine, ethambutol, and rifampin, on *Mycobacterium avium* complex bacteremia in patients with AIDS. J Infect Dis 170:157–164, 1994.
83. Yajko DM, Kirhara J, Sanders C, et al: Antimicrobial synergism against *Mycobacterium avium* complex strains isolated from patients with acquired immune deficiency syndrome. Antimicrob Agents Chemother 32:1392–1395, 1988.
84. Heifets LB, Iseman MD, Lindholm-Levy PJ: Combinations of rifampin or rifabutine plus ethambutol against *Mycobacterium avium* complex. Bactericidal synergistic, and bacteriostatic additive or synergistic effects. Am Rev Respir Dis 137:711–715, 1988.
85. Sullam PM, Gordin FM, Wynne BA, et al: Efficacy of rifabutin

in the treatment of disseminated infection due to *Mycobacterium avium* complex. Clin Infect Dis 19:84–86, 1994.
86. Yawalkar SJ, Vischer W: Lamprene (clofazimine) in leprosy. Lepr Rev 50:135–144, 1979.
87. Levy L: Pharmacologic studies of clofazimine. Am J Trop Med Hyg 23:1097–1109, 1974.
88. May T, Brel F, Beuscart C: A French randomized open trial of combination therapy for MAC bacteremia (Abstr 1202). *In* Abstracts of the 35th Interscience Conference on Antimicrobial Agents and Chemotherapy. Washington, DC, American Society for Microbiology, 1995, p 241.
89. Heifets LB, Lindholm-Levy PJ: Bacteriostatic and bactericidal activity of ciprofloxacin and floxacin against *Mycobacterium tuberculosis* and *Mycobacterium avium* complex. Tubercle 68:267–276, 1987.
90. Young LS, Berlin OGW, Inderlied CD: Activity of ciprofloxacin and other fluorinated quinolones against mycobacteria. Am J Med 82(SA):23–26, 1987.
91. Gordon SM, Horsburgh CR, Peloquin CA, et al: Low serum levels of oral antimycobacterial agents in patients with disseminated *Mycobacterium avium* complex disease. J Infect Dis 168:1559–1562, 1993.
92. Parenti D, Ellner J, Hafner R, et al: A phase II/III trial of rifampin, ciprofloxacin, clofazimine, ethambutol, ± amikacin in the treatment of disseminated *Mycobacterium avium* infection in HIV-infected individuals. *In* Abstracts of the Second National Conference on Human Retroviruses. Washington, DC, American Society for Microbiology, 1995, p 56.
93. Gordin FA, Heifets LB, Wynne BA, et al: *Mycobacterium avium* complex (MAC) resistance identified to antimycobacterial drugs used in an ongoing MAC treatment study in AIDS. *In* Abstracts of the Second National Conference of Human Retroviruses. Washington, DC, American Society for Microbiology, 1995, p 171.
94. Burman W, Rietmeijer C, Reves R: Treatment of disseminated *Mycobacterium avium* complex with clarithromycin decreases transfusional requirements. *In* Abstracts of the Second National Conference on Human Retroviruses. Washington, DC, American Society for Microbiology, 1995, p 56.
95. Wallace RJ, Brown BA, Griffith DE, et al: Reduced serum levels of clarithromycin in patients on multidrug regimens including rifampin or rifabutin for treatment of *Mycobacterium avium-intracellulare*. *In* Abstracts of the 34th Interscience Conference on Antimicrobial Agents and Chemotherapy. Washington, DC, American Society for Microbiology, 1994, p 246.
96. Kemper KA, Meng T-C, Nussbaum J, et al: Treatment of *Mycobacterium avium* complex bacteremia in AIDS with a four-drug oral regimen. Ann Intern Med 116:466–472, 1992.
97. O'Brien RJ, Geiter LJ, Snider DE: The epidemiology of nontuberculous mycobacterial diseases in the United States. Results from a national survey. Am Rev Respir Dis 135:1007–1014, 1987.
98. Dautzenberg B, Piperno D, Diot P, et al: Clarithromycin in the treatment of *Mycobacterium avium* lung infections in patients without AIDS. Chest 107:1035–1040, 1995.
99. Griffith DE, Wallace RJ, Brown BA, et al: Azithromycin monotherapy for HIV^- patients with *Mycobacterium avium intracellulare* complex lung disease. Am J Respir Crit Care Med 151:A477, 1995.
100. Wallace RJ, Brown BA, Griffith DE: Drug intolerance to high-dose clarithromycin among elderly patients. Diagn Microbiol Infect Dis 16:215–221, 1993.
101. Iseman MD, Corpe RF, O'Brien RJ, et al: Disease due to *Mycobacterium avium-intracellulare*. Chest 87:139S–149S, 1985.
102. Ahn CH, Ahn SS, Anderson RA, et al: A four-drug regimen for initial treatment of cavitary disease caused by *Mycobacterium avium* complex. Am Rev Respir Dis 134:436–441, 1986.
103. Etzkorn ET, Aldarondo S, McCallister CK, et al: Medical therapy of *Mycobacterium avium-intracellulare* pulmonary disease. Am Rev Respir Dis 134:442–445, 1986.
104. Horsburgh CR, Mason UG III, Heifets L, et al: Response to therapy of pulmonary *Mycobacterium avium-intracellulare* infection correlates with the results of in vitro susceptibility testing. Am Rev Respir Dis 135:418–421, 1987.
105. Rosenzweig DR: Pulmonary mycobacterial infections due to *Mycobacterium intracellulare-avium* complex. Clinical features and course in 100 consecutive cases. Chest 76:115–119, 1979.
106. Wolinsky E: Mycobacterial lymphadenitis in children: A prospective study of 105 nontuberculous cases with long-term follow-up. Clin Infect Dis 10:954–963, 1995.
107. Green PA, von Reyn CF, Smith RP: *Mycobacterium avium* complex parotid lymphadenitis: Successful therapy with clarithromycin and ethambutol. Pediatr Infect Dis J 12:615–616, 1993.
108. Nightingale SD, Cameron DW, Gordin FM, et al: Two controlled trials of rifabutin prophylaxis against *Mycobacterium avium* complex infection in AIDS. N Engl J Med 329:828–833, 1993.
109. Pierce M, Crampton S, Henry D, et al: A randomized trial of clarithromycin as prophylaxis against disseminated *Mycobacterium avium* complex infection in patients with advanced acquired immunodeficiency syndrome. N Engl J Med 335:384–391, 1996.
110. Havlir DV, Dube MP, Sattler FR, et al: Prophylaxis against disseminated *Mycobacterium avium* complex with weekly azithromycin, daily rifabutin, or both. N Engl J Med 335:392–398, 1996.
111. Ahn CH, Hurst GA: The treatment of disease due to *Mycobacterium kansasii*. Semin Respir Med 2:228–232, 1981.
112. Lillo M, Orengo S, Cernoch P, et al: Pulmonary and disseminated infection due to *Mycobacterium kansasii*: A decade of experience. Rev Infect Dis 12:760–767, 1990.
113. Wallace RJ, Dunbar D, Brown BA, et al: Rifampin-resistant *Mycobacterium kansasii*. Clin Infect Dis 18:736–743, 1994.
114. Biehle J, Cavalieri SJ: In vitro susceptibility of *Mycobacterium kansasii* to clarithromycin. Antimicrob Agents Chemother 36:2039–2041, 1992.
115. Levine B, Chaisson RE: *Mycobacterium kansasii*: A cause of treatable pulmonary disease associated with advanced human immunodeficiency virus (HIV) infection. Ann Intern Med 114:861–868, 1991.
116. Carpenter JL, Parks JM: *Mycobacterium kansasii* infections in patients positive for human immunodeficiency virus. Rev Infect Dis 13:789–796, 1991.
117. Wallace RJ, Swenson JM, Silcox VA, et al: Spectrum of disease due to rapidly growing mycobacteria. Rev Infect Dis 5:657–679, 1983.
118. Brown BA, Wallace RJ Jr, Onyi GO, et al: Activities of four macrolides, including clarithromycin, against *Mycobacterium fortuitum, Mycobacterium chelonae,* and *M. chelonae*-like organisms. Antimicrob Agents Chemother 36:180–184, 1992.
119. Wallace RJ Jr: The clinical presentation, diagnosis, and therapy of cutaneous and pulmonary infections due to the rapidly growing mycobacteria, *M. fortuitum* and *M. chelonae*. Clin Chest Med 10:419–429, 1989.
120. Wallace RJ, Swenson JM, Silcox VA, Bullen MG: Treatment of nonpulmonary infections due to *Mycobacterium fortuitum* and *Mycobacterium chelonei* on the basis of in vitro susceptibilities. J Infect Dis 151:500–513, 1985.
121. Wallace RJ Jr, Tanner D, Brennan PJ, Brown BA: Clinical trial of clarithromycin for cutaneous (disseminated) infection due to *Mycobacterium chelonae*. Ann Intern Med 119:482–486, 1993.
122. Tebas P, Sultan F, Wallace RJ Jr, Fraser V: Rapid development of resistance to clarithromycin following monotherapy for disseminated *Mycobacterium chelonae* infection in a heart transplant patient. Clin Infect Dis 20:443–444, 1995.
123. Mushatt DM, Witzig RS: Successful treatment of *Mycobacterium abscessus* infections with multidrug regimens containing clarithromycin (Letter). Clin Infect Dis 20:1441–1442, 1995.
124. Wallace RJ, Silcox VA, Tsukamura M, et al: Clinical significance, biochemical features, and susceptibility patterns of sporadic isolates of the *Mycobacterium chelonae*–like organism. J Clin Microbiol 31:3231–3239, 1993.
125. Iredell J, Whitby M, Blacklock Z: *Mycobacterium marinum* infection: Epidemiology and presentation in Queensland 1971–1990. Med J Aust 157:596–598, 1992.
126. Donta ST, Smith PW, Levitz RE, et al: Therapy of *Mycobacterium marinum* infections. Arch Intern Med 146:902–904, 1986.
127. Kullavanijaya P, Sirimachan S, Bhuddhavudhikrai P: *Mycobacterium marinum* cutaneous infections acquired from occupations and hobbies. Int J Dermatol 32:504–507, 1993.
128. Brown BA, Wallace RJ, Onyi GO: Activities of clarithromycin against eight slowly growing species of nontuberculous mycobacteria, determined by using a broth microdilution MIC system. Antimicrob Agents Chemother 36:1987–1990, 1992.

129. Bonnet E, Debat-Zoguereh D, Petit N, et al: Clarithromycin: A potent agent against infections due to *Mycobacterium marinum.* Clin Infect Dis 18:664–666, 1994.
130. Revil WDL, Pike MC, Morrow RH, Ateng J: A controlled trial of the treatment of *Mycobacterium ulcerans* infection with clofazimine. Lancet 2:873–877, 1973.
131. Hayman J: *Mycobacterium ulcerans* infection (Letter). Lancet 337:124, 1991.
132. Noordeen SK, Lopez Bravo L, Sundaresan TK: Estimated number of leprosy cases in the world. Bull World Health Organ 70:7–10, 1992.
133. Mastro TD, Redd SC, Breiman RF: Imported leprosy in the United States, 1978 through 1988: An epidemic without secondary transmission. Am J Public Health 82:1127–1130, 1992.
134. Dietrich M, Gaus W, Kern P, et al: An international randomized study with long-term follow-up of single versus combination chemotherapy of multibacillary leprosy. Antimicrob Agents Chemother 38:2249–2257, 1994.
135. World Health Organization: Chemotherapy of leprosy for control programmes. World Health Organ Tech Rep Series 675, 1982.
136. Gelber RH: Hansen's disease. West J Med 158:583–590, 1993.
137. Miller RA: Hansen's disease—A time for cautious optimism. West J Med 158:631–633, 1993.
138. Dever LL, Martin JW, Seaworth B, et al: Varied presentations and responses to treatment of infections caused by *Mycobacterium haemophilum* in patients with AIDS. Clin Infect Dis 14:1195–1200, 1992.
139. Rogers PL, Walker RE, Lane HC, et al: Disseminated *Mycobacterium haemophilum* infection in two patients with the acquired immunodeficiency syndrome. Am J Med 84:640–642, 1988.
140. Straus WL, Ostroff SM, Jernigan DB, et al: Clinical and epidemiologic characteristics of *Mycobacterium haemophilum,* an emerging pathogen in immunocompromised patients. Ann Intern Med 120:118–125, 1994.
141. Kiehn TE, White M, Pursell KJ, et al: A cluster of four cases of *Mycobacterium haemophilum* infection. Eur J Clin Microbiol Infect Dis 12:114–118, 1993.
142. Eng RH, Forrester C, Smith SM, et al: *Mycobacterium xenopi* infection in a patient with acquired immunodeficiency syndrome. Chest 86:145–147, 1984.
143. Tecson-Tumang FT, Bright JL: *Mycobacterium xenopi* and the acquired immunodeficiency syndrome. Ann Intern Med 100:461–462, 1984.
144. Costrini AM, Mahler DA, Gross WM, et al: Clinical and roentgenographic features of nosocomial pulmonary disease due to *Mycobacterium xenopi.* Am Rev Respir Dis 123:104–109, 1981.
145. Banks J, Jenkins PA: Combined versus single antituberculosis drugs on the in vitro sensitivity patterns of non-tuberculous mycobacteria. Thorax 42:838–842, 1987.
146. Banks J, Hunter AM, Campbell IA, et al: Pulmonary infection with *Mycobacterium xenopi*: Review of treatment and response. Thorax 39:376–382, 1984.
147. Parrot RG, Grosset JH: Post-surgical outcome of 57 patients with *Mycobacterium xenopi* pulmonary infection. Tubercle 69:47–55, 1988.
148. Maloney JM, Gregg CR, Stephens DS, et al: Infections caused by *Mycobacterium szulgai* in humans. Rev Infect Dis 9:1120–1126, 1987.
149. Henriques B, Hoffner SE, Petrini B, et al: Infection with *Mycobacterium malmoense* in Sweden: Report of 221 cases. Clin Infect Dis 18:595–600, 1994.
150. Chocarro A, Gonzalez Lopez A, Breznes MF, et al: Disseminated infection due to *Mycobacterium malmoense* in a patient infected with human immunodeficiency virus. Clin Infect Dis 19:203–204, 1994.
151. Claydon EJ, Coker RJ, Harris JRW: *Mycobacterium malmoense* infection in HIV positive patients. J Infect 23:191–194, 1991.
152. Zaugg M, Salfinger M, Opravil M, et al: Extrapulmonary and disseminated infections due to *Mycobacterium malmoense*: Case report and review. Clin Infect Dis 16:540–549, 1993.
153. Bottger EC, Teske A, Kirschner P, et al: Disseminated "*Mycobacterium genavense*" infection in patients with AIDS. Lancet 340:76–80, 1992.
154. Pechère M, Opravil M, Wald A, et al: Clinical and epidemiologic features of infection with *Mycobacterium genavense.* Arch Intern Med 155:400–404, 1995.
155. Bessesen MT, Shlay J, Stone-Venohr B, et al: Disseminated *Mycobacterium genavense* infection: Clinical and microbiological features and response to therapy. AIDS 7:1357–1361, 1993.
156. Bell RC, Higuchi JH, Donovan WN, et al: *Mycobacterium simiae.* Clinical features and follow-up of twenty four patients. Am Rev Respir Dis 127:35–38, 1983.
157. Huminer D, Dux S, Samra Z, et al: *Mycobacterium simiae* infection in Israeli patients with AIDS. Clin Infect Dis 17:508–509, 1993.
158. Torres RA, Nord J, Feldman R, et al: Disseminated mixed *Mycobacterium simiae–Mycobacterium avium* complex infection in acquired immunodeficiency syndrome. J Infect Dis 164:432–433, 1991.
159. Levy-Frebault V, Pangon B, Bure A, et al: *Mycobacterium simiae* and *Mycobacterium avium–M. intracellulare* mixed infection in acquired immune deficiency syndrome. J Clin Microbiol 25:154–157, 1987.
160. Wolinsky E: Nontuberculous mycobacteria and associated diseases. Am Rev Respir Dis 119:107–159, 1979.
161. Sanders JW, Walsh A, Snider RL, Sahn EE: Disseminated *Mycobacterium scrofulaceum* infection: A potentially treatable complication of AIDS. Clin Infect Dis 20:549, 1995.
162. Tortoli E, Piersimoni C, Bacosi D: Isolation of the newly described species *Mycobacterium celatum* from AIDS patients. J Clin Microbiol 33:137–140, 1995.
163. Butler WR, O'Connor SP, Yakrus MA: *Mycobacterium celatum* sp. nov. Int J Syst Bacteriol 43:539–548, 1993.
164. Wallace RJ, Nash DR, Tsukamura M, et al: Human disease due to *Mycobacterium smegmatis.* J Infect Dis 158:52–59, 1988.
165. Newton JA, Weiss PJ, Bowler WA, et al: Soft-tissue infection due to *Mycobacterium smegmatis*: Report of two cases. Clin Infect Dis 16:531–533, 1993.
166. Plaus WJ, Hermann G: The surgical management of superficial infections caused by atypical mycobacteria. Surgery 110:99–103, 1991.
167. Weinberger M, Berg SL, Feuerstein IM, et al: Disseminated infection with *Mycobacterium gordonae*: Report of a case and critical review of the literature. Clin Infect Dis 14:1229–1239, 1992.
168. Foulds G, Shepard RM, Johnson RB: The pharmacokinetics of azithromycin in human serum and tissues. J Antimicrob Chemother 25:S73–S82, 1990.
169. Gladue RP, Bright GM, Isaacson RE, et al: In vitro and in vivo uptake of azithromycin by phagocytic cells: Possible mechanism of delivery and release at sites of infection. Antimicrob Agents Chemother 33:277–282, 1989.
170. Wallace MR, Miller LK, Nguyen M, et al: Ototoxicity with azithromycin (Letter). Lancet 343:241, 1994.
171. Barradell LB, Plosker GL, McTavish D: Clarithromycin: A review of its pharmacological properties and therapeutic use in *Mycobacterium avium-intracellulare* complex infection in patients with acquired immune deficiency syndrome. Drugs 46:289–312, 1993.
172. Brown BA, Wallace RJ, Griffith DE, et al: Clarithromycin-induced hepatotoxicity. Clin Infect Dis 20:1073–1074, 1995.
173. DATRI 001 Study Group: Clarithromycin plus rifabutin for MAC prophylaxis: Evidence for a drug interaction (Abstr 291). Abstracts of the First National Conference on Human Retroviruses. Washington DC, American Society for Microbiology, 1993, p 106.
174. DATRI 001 Study Group: Coadministration of clarithromycin alters the concentration-time profile of rifabutin (Abstr A2). *In* Abstracts of the 34th Interscience Conference on Antimicrobial Agents and Chemotherapy. Washington, DC, American Society for Microbiology, 1994, p 3.
175. Wallace RJ, Brown BA, Griffith DE, et al: Reduced serum levels of clarithromycin in patients on multidrug regimens including rifampin or rifabutin for treatment of *Mycobacterium avium-intracellulare* (Abstr M59). *In* Abstracts of the 34th Interscience Conference on Antimicrobial Agents and Chemotherapy. Washington, DC, American Society for Microbiology, 1994, p 246.
176. Shafran SD, Deschênes J, Miller M, et al: Uveitis and pseudojaundice during a regimen of clarithromycin, rifabutin, and ethambutol. N Engl J Med 438–439, 1994.

35

Antiparasitic Drugs

Martin S. Wolfe

Antiparasitic drugs are used in the treatment of protozoa, helminths, and parasitic arthropods. The drugs described in this chapter are for the most part those approved and available in the United States. Some of these available drugs are considered investigational for certain purposes in the United States.* Particular unavailable drugs may be obtained from the Centers for Disease Control and Prevention.†

The safety during pregnancy of many of the drugs listed has not been determined with certainty, and they are often contraindicated unless the benefit is thought to outweigh their potential hazard to the fetus.

For each drug, listed generically in alphabetic order, the following information is generally provided: brand name; major indications; mechanism of action when known; side effects, contraindications, and significant drug interactions; and doses for adults and children. Table 35–1 summarizes the drug's availability (brand name, manufacturer, formulation) and doses for adults and children for various parasites.

Albendazole (Albenza). Albendazole is a benzimidazole broad-spectrum anthelmintic. Studies outside the United States have shown a single 400-mg adult dose to be effective and well tolerated for treatment of ascariasis, hookworm infections, enterobiasis, and most cases of trichuriasis.[1] The same dose repeated for 3 consecutive days was effective against strongyloidiasis, cestodiasis, heavy trichuriasis,[1] and cutaneous larva migrans.[1a] In these doses, albendazole appeared to be nearly devoid of significant side effects. Safety has not been established in pregnancy or in children younger than 2 years. Albendazole has been used in hydatid disease. Indications included inoperable lesions, disseminated disease, and prophylaxis before surgery. A large proportion of cysts were affected beneficially by a treatment regimen of 800 mg/d for three 28-day cycles with 14 days' rest between cycles.[2] The frequency of clinical side effects was low. Albendazole has also been used against cerebral cysticercosis. In a comparative evaluation versus praziquantel for this condition, both appeared to be effective at the doses used (15 mg/kg per day for 30 days with albendazole); albendazole showed a slightly better overall response.[3] Albendazole has also been found to be an effective therapy for gnathostomiasis in Thailand.[4] Preliminary data suggest that albendazole has good clinical and antiparasitic efficacy in treating the intestinal microsporidian *Septata intestinalis* in patients with the acquired immunodeficiency syndrome (AIDS), but is less effective in treating another intestinal microsporidian, *Enterocytozoon bieneusi*.[5] In June 1996, albendazole was approved by the U.S. Food and Drug Administration (FDA) for treatment of *Echinococcus granulosis* infection and parenchymal neurocysticercosis caused by *Taenia solium*.

Amphotericin B (Fungizone).* Amphotericin B is an antifungal antibiotic used for amebic meningoencephalitis caused by *Naegleria* species[6] and as an alternative treatment for American mucocutaneous leishmaniasis[7] (see also Chapter 288). It is poorly absorbed from the gastrointestinal tract and for these infections is given intravenously (IV). A large number and variety of side effects have been described. Amphotericin B is considered an investigational drug for both these indications.

γ-Benzene Hexachloride (Kwell). γ-Benzene hexachloride (also known as lindane) is used to treat scabies and lice.[8] It is available as a cream, lotion, and shampoo. Eczematous eruptions due to sensitization may occur. It must be used with caution in infants and young children. With excessive or prolonged application, absorption through the skin can cause convulsions and rarely death in children; use of larger doses than recommended should be avoided.[8] Before it is applied, the patient should take a hot soapy bath or shower. For scabies and body lice, a thin layer of lotion or cream is applied over the entire skin surface from the neck down, left on for 24 hours, and then thoroughly washed off. A second application 1 week later may be useful in killing hatching progeny. For head and pubic lice, 1 ounce of shampoo is vigorously rubbed into the hair for at least 4 minutes, and the hair is then rinsed thoroughly. A second application is seldom required. Resistance to scabies may have developed in some endemic areas.

Benznidazole (Rochagan).* Benznidazole is a nitroimidazole drug available in South America for the treatment of the acute phase of *Trypanosoma cruzi* infection (Chagas disease). The efficacy of this drug in chronic Chagas disease has not been established.

It has been shown in only limited use to be effective in reducing the severity and duration of the acute phase. It remains controversial whether benznidazole is curative.[9] Side effects include gastrointestinal symptoms, headache, weight loss, and polyneuritis. The regimen used in adults is 5 to 7 mg/kg by mouth daily for 30 to 120 days.

Bithionol (Bitin).† Bithionol is used in the treatment of *Fasciola hepatica*[10] and *Paragonimus westermani* infections.[11] It is manufactured in Japan. The anthelmintic effect of oral bithionol is poorly understood. Side effects include photosensitivity, skin reactions, urticaria, and gastrointestinal disturbances. For treatment of fascioliasis and paragonimiasis, the dose for both adults and children is 30 to 40 mg/kg on alternate days for 10 to 15 doses. Maximal dosage is 2 g/d.

Chloroquine Phosphate (Aralen). Chloroquine is a 4-aminoquinoline used primarily for the suppression and treatment of susceptible strains of malaria. In the United States, chloroquine is marketed only as oral Aralen phosphate in 500-mg salt tablets (equal to 300 mg of base). In Europe and Africa, chloroquine sulfate is marketed as Nivaquine in tablet, liquid, and injectable forms. A chloroquine hydrochloride salt, Aralen hydrochloride, is a parenteral solution for intramuscular (IM) use (each milliliter contains 50 mg of the salt, equal to 40 mg of base), which can be substituted for the oral phosphate salt when severe nausea or vomiting is present, when oral absorption is in question, or when an infection is particularly severe. Most experts do not recommend IM administration of chloroquine into young children. If it is used in young children, great caution must be exercised, and oral administration should be substituted as soon as is practicable. Chloroquine's action is on the asexual erythrocytic forms of malaria parasites, but it does not affect the liver stages of plasmodia and therefore will not prevent relapses of malaria caused by species that have a liver stage in their life cycle. Chloroquine is almost completely absorbed from the

Text continued on page 383

*These investigational drugs, and some others described that are not at present available in the United States and are also considered investigational, are marked with a single asterisk in the text and in Table 35–1.

†Unavailable drugs that may be obtained from the CDC Drug Service, Centers for Disease Control and Prevention, Atlanta, GA 30333 (telephone 404–639–3356) are marked with a dagger in the text and in Table 35–1.

TABLE 35–1 ■ Drug Treatment of Parasitic Infections*

PARASITE AND DISEASE	DRUG	ADULT DOSAGE	PEDIATRIC DOSAGE	PROPRIETARY NAME, FORM (MANUFACTURER)
Intestinal Protozoa				
Entamoeba histolytica				
Amebic dysentery	***Drug of choice***			
	Metronidazole followed by	750 mg tid × 10 d	50 mg/kg/d in 3 doses × 10 d	Flagyl tablets, IV (Searle)
	Paromomycin	500 mg tid × 7 d	30 mg/kg/d in 3 doses × 7 d	Humatin tablets (Searle)
	or			
	Iodoquinol	650 mg tid × 20 d	40 mg/kg/d in 3 doses × 20 d	Yodoxin tablets (Searle)
	or			
	Diloxanide furoate†	500 mg tid × 10 d	20 mg/kg/d in 3 doses × 10 d	Furamide† tablets (Boots, England)
	Alternatives			
	Tinidazole‡ followed by paromomycin, iodoquinol, or diloxanide furoate† as for amebic dysentery	600 mg bid × 5–10 d	50 mg/kg/d (max 2 g) in 1 dose for 5–10 d	Fasigyn‡ tablets (Pfizer)
Moderately severe nondysenteric amebiasis	***Drug of choice***			
	Metronidazole	500 mg tid × 10 d	35 mg/kg/d in 3 doses × 10 d	
	Alternatives			
	Tinidazole‡ followed by paromomycin, iodoquinol, or diloxanide furoate† as for amebic dysentery	600 mg bid × 5 d	50 mg/kg/d (max 2 g) in 1 dose × 5 d	
Mildly symptomatic nondysenteric amebiasis	***Drug of choice***			
	Paromomycin	500 mg tid × 7 d	30 mg/kg/d in 3 doses × 7 d	
	Alternative			
	Diloxanide furoate†	500 mg tid × 10 d	20 mg/kg/d in 3 doses × 10 d	
Asymptomatic cyst-passing state	Paromomycin	500 mg tid × 7 d	30 mg/kg/d in 3 doses × 7 d	
	or			
	Iodoquinol	650 mg tid × 20 d	40 mg/kg/d in 3 doses × 20 d	
	or			
	Diloxanide furoate†	500 mg tid × 10 d	20 mg/kg/d in 3 doses × 10 d	
Amebic liver abscess	***Drug of choice***			
	Metronidazole followed by paromomycin, iodoquinolol, or diloxanide furoate† as for amebic dysentery	750 mg tid × 10 d	50 mg/kg/d in 3 doses × 10 d	
	Alternative			
	Tinidazole (alone)‡ followed by paromomycin, iodoquinol, or diloxanide furoate† as for amebic dysentery	800 mg tid × 5 d	50 mg/kg/d (max 2 g) in 1 dose × 3 d	
Giardia lamblia	Metronidazole‡	250 mg tid × 7 d	5 mg/kg tid × 7 d	
	or			
	Furazolidone	100 mg (tablet) qid × 7–10 d	1.25 mg/kg (suspension) qid × 7–10 d	Furoxone tablets and suspension (Roberts)
	or			
	Tinidazole‡	One 2-g dose	One 50 mg/kg dose	Fasigyn‡ tablets (Pfizer)
Dientamoeba fragilis	Paromomycin	500 mg tid × 7 d	30 mg/kg/d in 3 doses × 7 d	Humatin capsules (Parke-Davis)
	or			
	Iodoquinol	650 mg tid × 20 d	40 mg/kg/d in 3 doses × 20 d	Yodoxin tablets (Glenwood)
	or			
	Tetracycline‡	500 mg qid × 10 d	Not recommended for children younger than 8 y	

TABLE 35–1 ■ Drug Treatment of Parasitic Infections* *Continued*

PARASITE AND DISEASE	DRUG	ADULT DOSAGE	PEDIATRIC DOSAGE	PROPRIETARY NAME, FORM (MANUFACTURER)
Intestinal Protozoan *Continued*				
Balantidium coli	Iodoquinol‡ or Tetracycline‡	As for *D. fragilis*	As for *D. fragilis*	
Isospora belli	Trimethoprim-sulfamethoxazole (TMP-SMX)	TMP 160 mg + SMX 800 mg qid × 10 d, then bid × 3 wk	—	Bactrim tablets (Roche) Septra tablets (Burroughs Wellcome)
Cryptosporidium sp.	Paromomycin	500–750 mg qid	—	Humatin capsules (Parke-Davis)
Other Protozoan Infections				
Naegleria sp. (primary amebic meningoencephalitis)	Amphotericin B‡	1 mg/kg/d IV, for indefinite period	As for adults	Fungizone* injection (Apothecon)
Leishmania braziliensis, L. mexicana (American cutaneous and mucocutaneous leishmaniasis)	***Drug of choice*** Stibogluconate sodium†	20 mg/kg/d IV or IM × 28 d (may be repeated or continued until there is a response)	As for adults	Pentostam† injection (Glaxo-Wellcome, England)
	Alternative Amphotericin B‡	0.25–1 mg/kg by slow infusion daily or every 2 d for up to 8 wk	As for adults	
Leishmania donovani (kala-azar, visceral leishmaniasis)	***Drug of choice*** Stibogluconate sodium†	20 mg/kg/d IM or IV × 28 d (may be repeated)	As for adults	
	Alternative Pentamidine isethionate	2–4 mg/kg/d IM for up to 15 doses (may be repeated)	As for adults	Pentam 300 injection (Fujisawa)
Leishmania tropica, L. major (oriental sore, cutaneous leishmaniasis)	***Drug of choice*** Stibogluconate sodium†	20 mg/kg/d IM or IV × 20 d (may be repeated)	As for adults	
Pneumocystis carinii (pneumonia)	***Drug of choice*** Trimethoprim-sulfamethoxazole (TMP-SMX)	TMP 15 mg/kg/d + SMX 75 mg/kg/d PO or IV in 4 doses × 14–21 d	As for adults	Bactrim tablets (Roche) Septra tablets (Burroughs Wellcome)
	Alternative Pentamidine isethionate	3–4 mg/kg/d IM × 14–21 d	As for adults	
Toxoplasma gondii (toxoplasmosis)	***Drug of choice*** Pyrimethamine plus	25–100 mg/d × 3–4 wk	2 mg/kg/d × 3 d, then 1 mg/kg/d (max 25 mg/d) × 4 wk	Daraprim tablets (Burroughs Wellcome)
	Sulfadiazine	1–1.5 g/d × 3–4 wk	100–200 mg/kg/d × 3–4 wk	
	Alternative Spiramycin‡	3–4 g/d × 3–4 wk	50–100 mg/kg/d × 3–4 wk	Rovamycine‡ tablets (Rhône-Poulenc, Rorer)
Trichomonas vaginalis (trichomonas)	***Drug of choice*** Metronidazole	2 g once or 250 mg tid PO × 7 d	15 mg/kg/d PO in 3 doses × 7 d	Flagyl tablets (Searle)

Table continued on following page

TABLE 35–1 ■ Drug Treatment of Parasitic Infections* *Continued*

PARASITE AND DISEASE	DRUG	ADULT DOSAGE	PEDIATRIC DOSAGE	PROPRIETARY NAME, FORM (MANUFACTURER)
Other Protozoan Infections *Continued*				
Trypanosoma cruzi (South American trypanosomiasis, Chagas disease)	***Drug of choice***			
	Nifurtimox†	8–10 mg/kg/d PO in 4 doses × 120 d	Age 1–10 y: 15–20 mg/kg/d in 4 doses qod Age 11–16 y: 12.5–15 mg/kg/d in 4 doses qod	Lampit† tablets (Bayer, Germany)
	Alternative			
	Benznidazole‡	5–7 mg/kg × 30–120 d	—	Rochagan‡ tablets (Roche, Brazil)
Trypanosoma brucei gambiense, T. brucei rhodesiense (African trypanosomiasis, sleeping sickness) Hemolymphatic stage	***Drug of choice***			
	Suramin†	100–200 mg (test dose) IV, then 1 g IV on days 1, 3, 7, 14, and 21	20 mg/kg on days 1, 3, 7, 14, and 21, after a test dose	Germanin† injection (Bayer, Germany)
	Alternative			
	Pentamidine isethionate	4 mg/kg/d IM × 10 d	4 mg/kg/d IM × 10 d	Pentam 300 injection (Fujisawa)
Late disease with central nervous system involvement	***Drug of choice***			
	Melarsoprol†	2–3.6 mg/kg/d IV × 3 d; after 1 wk, 3.6 mg/kg/d IV × 3 d; repeat again after 10–21 d	18–25 mg/kg total over 1 mo: initial dose, 0.36 mg/kg IV, increasing gradually to max 3.6 mg/kg at intervals of 1–5 d for total of 9 or 10 doses	Arsobal† injection (Rhône-Poulenc, Rorer, France)
T. b. gambiense (both stages) (variable effectiveness with *T. b. rhodesiense*)	Eflornithine	100 mg/kg q 6 h IV for 14 d	—	Ornidyl (Merrell Dow)
Malaria Treatment Regimens				
Plasmodium falciparum acquired where chloroquine resistance does not occur and *P. malariae*	Chloroquine phosphate or	600 mg base PO stat, then 300 mg after 6 h, then 300 mg/d for 2 d (total 1500 mg base)	10 mg/kg base PO stat, 5 mg/kg after 6 h, then 5 mg/kg for 2 d	Aralen tablets (Sanofi Winthrop)
	Chloroquine hydrochloride	If patient is vomiting, give 200 mg IM every 6 h until oral ingestion is possible (max 800 mg/d)	IM chloroquine not recommended	Aralen hydrochloride injection (Sanofi Winthrop)
P. falciparum acquired in areas with chloroquine-resistant strains	Quinine sulfate (salt) plus	650 mg PO tid × 3 d	25 mg/kg/d in 3 doses × 3 d	Quinine sulfate capsules (various manufacturers)
	Pyrimethamine-sulfadoxine	One 3-tablet dose on last day of quinine	As for malaria prophylaxis	Fansidar tablets (Roche)
	Alternatives			
	For chloroquine resistance or where resistance occurs to pyrimethamine-sulfadoxine:			
	Quinine sulfate (salt) plus	650 mg PO tid × 3 d	25 mg/kg/d in 3 doses × 3 d	
	Tetracycline or	250 mg qid × 7 d	5 mg/kg qid × 7 d	Tetracycline tablets (various manufacturers)
	Mefloquine alone or	One 1250-mg dose PO	Children weighing <45 kg: one 25-mg/kg dose; ≥45 kg: as for adults	Lariam tablets (Roche)
	Halofantrine alone	500 mg q 6 h × 3 doses; repeat in 1 wk	8 mg/kg q 6 h × 3 doses (<40 kg); repeat in 1 wk	Halfan tablets (SmithKline Beecham)

TABLE 35–1 ■ Drug Treatment of Parasitic Infections* *Continued*

PARASITE AND DISEASE	DRUG	ADULT DOSAGE	PEDIATRIC DOSAGE	PROPRIETARY NAME, FORM (MANUFACTURER)
Malaria Treatment Regimens *Continued*				
P. falciparum (severe or complicated infection)	Quinine dihydrochloride (salt IV) or	20 mg/kg loading dose over 4 h, followed by 10 mg/kg over 2 to 8 h; repeat every 8 h until oral treatment can be started (max 1800 mg/d)	Same as for adults	Quinine dihydrochloride
	Quinidine gluconate (IV) followed by either quinidine or quinine orally (for total of 3 d) plus	See quinidine in text	See quinidine in text	Quinidine gluconate injection (Lilly)
	Tetracycline	250 mg qid × 7 d	5 mg/kg qid × 7 d	
Plasmodium vivax and *P. ovale*	Chloroquine phosphate followed by	As for nonresistant *P. falciparum* and *P. malariae*	As for nonresistant *P. falciparum* and *P. malariae*	
	Primaquine phosphate	15 mg base/d × 14 d	0.3 mg base/kg/d × 14 d	Primaquine tablets (Sanofi Winthrop)
Malaria Prophylaxis				
In areas with chloroquine-sensitive strains	Chloroquine phosphate	300 mg base/wk (500 mg salt) continue for 4 wk after leaving malarial area	5 mg base/kg/wk	Aralen and generic tablets
In areas with chloroquine-resistant strains	Mefloquine	250 mg once weekly and for 4 wk after leaving malarial area	Children weighing <15 kg: ¼ tablet/wk 15–19 kg: ¼ tablet/wk 20–30 kg: ½ tablet/wk 31–45 kg: ¾ tablet/wk >45 kg: 1 tablet/wk	
	Alternatives Doxycycline	100 mg/d during exposure and 4 wk thereafter	Contraindicated for children younger than 8 y After age 8 y: 2 mg/kg/d (max 100 mg/d)	Vibramycin tablets (Pfizer)
	Chloroquine phosphate plus	As for sensitive strains	As for sensitive strains	
	Proguanil‡ plus	200 mg/d during exposure and 4 wk thereafter	Children weighing 4–9 kg: 25 mg/d 10–14 kg: 50 mg/d 15–29 kg: 100 mg/d 30–50 kg: 150 mg/d >50 kg: 200 mg/d	Paludrine* tablets (ICI, England)
	Pyrimethamine-sulfadoxine	Carry one self-treatment dose (3 tablets)	Children weighing 5–10 kg: ½ tablet 11–20 kg: 1 tablet 21–30 kg: 1½ tablets 31–45 kg: 2 tablets >45 kg: 3 tablets	Fansidar tablets (Roche)
Against later relapses	Primaquine phosphate	15 mg base/d × 14 d	0.3 mg base/kg/d × 14 d	Primaquine tablets (Sanofi Winthrop)
Intestinal Helminths ***Nematoda*** *Ascaris lumbricoides*	***Drug of choice*** Mebendazole	100 mg bid × 3 d	For children aged >2 y, as for adults	Vermox tablets (Janssen)
	Alternative Pyrantel pamoate	One 11 mg/kg dose (max 1 g)	As for adults (max 1 g)	Reese's Pinworm Medicine (over-the-counter)
Trichuris trichiura	Mebendazole	As for *A. lumbricoides*	As for *A. lumbricoides*	

Table continued on following page

TABLE 35–1 ■ Drug Treatment of Parasitic Infections* *Continued*

PARASITE AND DISEASE	DRUG	ADULT DOSAGE	PEDIATRIC DOSAGE	PROPRIETARY NAME, FORM (MANUFACTURER)
Intestinal Helminths Nematoda *Continued*				
Necator americanus, Ancylostoma duodenale (hookworm)	***Drug of choice*** Mebendazole	As for *A. lumbricoides*	As for *A. lumbricoides*	
	Alternative Pyrantel pamoate‡	11 mg/kg (max 1 g) × 3 d	As for adults (max 1 g)	
Enterobius vermicularis	***Drug of choice*** Mebendazole	One 100-mg dose; repeat in 2 wk	As for adults	
	Alternative Pyrantel pamoate	One 11 mg/kg dose; repeat in 2 wk	As for adults	
Strongyloides stercoralis	***Drug of choice*** Thiabendazole	25 mg/kg bid × 2 d (max 3 g/d)	As for adults	Mintezol suspension (Merck)
	Alternative Ivermectin‡	200 μg/kg daily for 2 d	As for adults	Mectizan‡ (Merck)
Trichostrongylus sp.	Thiabendazole‡	As for *S. stercoralis*	As for *S. stercoralis*	
	or Pyrantel pamoate‡	As for *A. lumbricoides*	As for *A. lumbricoides*	
	or Mebendazole‡	As for *A. lumbricoides*	As for *A. lumbricoides*	
Cestoda				
Taenia saginata, Taenia solium, Diphyllobothrium latum, Dipylidium caninum	***Drug of choice*** Praziquantel‡	5–10 mg/kg once	As for adults	Biltricide‡ tablets (Miles)
Hymenolepis nana and *H. diminuta*	***Drug of choice*** Praziquantel‡	One 25 mg/kg dose	As for adults	
Cerebral cysticercosis cellulosae	Praziquantel‡	50 mg/kg/d in 3 doses × 15 d	As for adults	
	or Albendazole‡	15 mg/kg/d in 2 doses for 8–30 d	As for adults	Albenza (SmithKline Beecham)
Echinococcus granulosus	Albendazole or Mebendazole	As per text and prescribing information	As per prescribing information	
Trematoda				
Schistosoma mansoni	***Drug of choice*** Praziquantel	40 mg/kg/d in 2 doses for 1 d	As for adults	Biltricide tablets (Miles)
	Alternative Oxamniquine	Caribbean and S. American strains: one 15 mg/kg dose African strains: 40–60 mg/kg/d over 2–3 d	As for adults	Vansil tablets (Pfizer)
Schistosoma japonicum	Praziquantel	60 mg/kg/d in 3 doses × 1 d	As for adults	
Schistosoma mekongi	Praziquantel	As for *S. japonicum*	As for *S. japonicum*	
Schistosoma intercalatum	Praziquantel	As for *S. mansoni*	As for *S. mansoni*	
Schistosoma haematobium	Praziquantel	40 mg/kg/d in 2 doses for 1 d	As for adults	
Fasciolopsis buski	Praziquantel‡	25 mg/kg tid × 1 d	As for adults	Biltricide‡ tablets (Miles)
Heterophyes heterophyes	Praziquantel‡	25 mg/kg tid × 1 d	As for adults	
Metagonimus yokogawai	Praziquantel‡	25 mg/kg tid × 1 d	As for adults	
Liver and Lung Flukes				
Paragonimus westermani	Praziquantel‡	25 mg/kg tid × 2 d	As for adults	
Opisthorchis viverrini, Clonorchis sinensis	Praziquantel‡	25 mg/kg tid × 1 d	As for adults	
Fasciola hepatica	Bithionol†	30–40 mg/kg on alternate days × 10–15 doses (max 2 g/d)	As for adults	Bitin† capsule (Tanabe, Japan)

TABLE 35–1 ■ Drug Treatment of Parasitic Infections* *Continued*

PARASITE AND DISEASE	DRUG	ADULT DOSAGE	PEDIATRIC DOSAGE	PROPRIETARY NAME, FORM (MANUFACTURER)
Other Helminths				
Filarioidea				
Wuchereria bancrofti *Brugia malayi* *Loa loa* *Mansonella ozzardi* and *M. perstans*	Diethylcarbamazine	Day 1, 50 mg PO Day 2, 50 mg tid Day 3, 100 mg tid Days 4–28, 2 mg/kg tid	Day 1, 25–50 mg Day 2, 25–50 mg tid Day 3, 50–100 mg tid Days 4–28, 2 mg/kg tid	Hetrazan tablets (Lederle)
Tropical pulmonary eosinophilia	Diethylcarbamazine	2 mg/kg tid × 21 d	As for adults	
Onchocerca volvulus	Ivermectin‡	150 μg/kg PO once; repeat at approximately 1-y intervals	As for adults	Mectizan‡ tablets (Merck)
Miscellaneous Helminths				
Cutaneous larva migrans	Thiabendazole	25 mg/kg bid PO or topically (max 3 g/d) × 2–5 d	As for adults	Mintezol suspension (Merck)
Visceral larva migrans	Diethylcarbamazine‡ or	2 mg/kg tid × 7–10 d	As for adults	
	Mebendazole‡	100–200 mg bid × 5 d	As for adults	
Parasitic Arthropoda				
Pediculus humanus, P. humanus capitis, Phthirus pubis, Sarcoptes scabiei (scabies)	Lindane	One topical dose	One topical dose	Kwell lotion, shampoo (Reed & Carnrick)
	or Permethrin			
	Head lice	1% rinse, single application	As for adults	Nix Creme Rinse (Glaxo-Wellcome)
	Scabies	5% cream, single application	As for adults	Elimite Cream (Herbert)

*IM, Intramuscular; IV, intravenous; PO, oral; bid, twice daily; qid, four times a day; qod, every other day; tid, three times a day; max, maximum.
†In the United States, this drug is available from the CDC Drug Service, Centers for Disease Control and Prevention, Atlanta, GA 30333, telephone 404–639–3356; after office hours 404–639–2888.
‡Considered an investigational drug for this purpose in the United States.

gastrointestinal tract, is deposited in the tissues in considerable amounts, and is excreted slowly. Frequent side effects with suppressive use include gastrointestinal upset, headache, dizziness, and blurred vision. Less common side effects include rash, pruritus, partial alopecia, myopathy, and central nervous system (CNS) stimulation. Irreversible retinal damage, seen when chloroquine is used in large daily doses for prolonged periods for collagen diseases, is virtually unheard of in the usual doses recommended for malaria suppression and treatment.[12, 13] Chloroquine should not be given to patients with psoriasis or porphyria or in the presence of retinal changes of any cause. Chloroquine is considered safe in recommended doses for infants and pregnant women at risk for malaria.[14] Strains of *Plasmodium falciparum* in many malarious areas have developed resistance to chloroquine, and an additional or alternative drug should be used in areas of known chloroquine resistance for both suppression and treatment of malaria with these strains.[15] In more recent years, chloroquine-resistant *Plasmodium vivax* malaria has been documented in Indonesia, Papua New Guinea, and Myanmar.[16] For malaria suppression in adults, 300 mg of base is taken weekly, beginning 1 week before entering a malarious area and continuing while in the malarious area and for 4 weeks after leaving. For infants and children, a weekly dose of 5 mg/kg base is given, not to exceed the adult dose regardless of weight. For oral treatment of chloroquine-sensitive *P. falciparum* infection as well as the other three species of malaria, adults receive 600 mg of base initially, followed by 300 mg 6 hours later, and 300 mg 24 and 48 hours thereafter. For children, 10 mg/kg base is given initially, followed by 5 mg/kg in 6 hours, and 5 mg/kg 24 and 48 hours thereafter. When Aralen hydrochloride is used to treat acute malaria, adults should receive an initial IM dose of 200 mg of base, repeated every 6 hours until oral chloroquine can be taken. The total parenteral dosage in the first 24 hours should not exceed 800 mg of base.

Diethylcarbamazine Citrate (Hetrazan). Diethylcarbamazine is a piperazine derivative used to treat filariasis[17] and experimentally for visceral larva migrans. Although licensed, it is not presently available commercially in the United States and must be obtained from the manufacturer (Lederle). Abroad it is available as Banocide and Notezine. Diethylcarbamazine is readily absorbed from the gastrointestinal tract and kills microfilariae of most species of filariae found in humans. There is presumptive evidence that it kills adult worms of *Wuchereria bancrofti* and *Brugia malayi*. Repeated courses are often necessary to kill *Loa loa* and *Mansonella perstans* adult worms. It has relatively little action on adult *Onchocerca volvulus* worms. Diethylcarbamazine has no effect on *Mansonella ozzardi*.[18] A 50- to 100-mg dose of diethylcarbamazine is used as a provocative test for onchocerciasis (the Mazzotti reaction),[19] and a 200-mg dose has been used to increase the number of circulating microfilariae of *W. bancrofti* for diagnosis.[20] Common side effects include headache, dizziness, nausea, and fever. Rapid destruction of microfilariae in the initial days of treatment may cause allergic reactions, including exacerbation of rash and pruritus in onchocerciasis and lymphadenopathy and nodular swellings along the course of lymphatics in bancroftian and malayan filariasis.[21] In patients with heavy *L. loa* infections, encephalopathy has occurred.[22] To attempt to decrease these early allergic reactions, particularly in onchocerciasis with ocular involvement, the initial daily dose of diethylcarbamazine should be small and the dose should be increased gradually to the maximal daily recommended dose. An initial 50-mg dose is gradually increased until a maximum of 2 mg/kg three times daily (tid) is reached; this dose is given for a total of 28 days. For blood-borne filariasis, 2 mg/kg three times a day for 28 days is given to both adults and children. For tropical pulmonary eosinophilia, the same dose is given for 21 days. Antihistamines or corticosteroids may be required to control allergic reactions to diethylcarbamazine, particularly in onchocerciasis and bancroftian filariasis.[21] Diethylcarbamazine has also been used to treat visceral larva migrans, with mixed reports of effectiveness.

Diloxanide Furoate (Furamide).† Diloxanide furoate is used in the treatment of amebiasis. Its mode of action is unknown. It is poorly absorbed and is most effective in the asymptomatic cyst-passing state and in mild noninvasive amebiasis.[23] The most frequently observed side effect is excessive flatulence; mild gastrointestinal side effects occasionally occur. For asymptomatic and mildly symptomatic intestinal amebiasis in adults, it is used alone in a dose of 500 mg tid for 10 days. Children receive 20 mg/kg per day in three divided doses for 10 days. The same dose can be used in follow-up luminal treatment of invasive amebiasis. In the United States, diloxanide furoate is available only from the CDC Drug Service.

Eflornithine (Ornidyl). Eflornithine is highly effective in both CNS and non-CNS infections with *Trypanosoma brucei gambiense*. Eflornithine is much less effective against *Trypanosoma brucei rhodesiense*.[7] Side effects, including diarrhea, anemia, and hair loss, are common but tolerable and reversible. The usual treatment regimen is 100 mg/kg every 6 hours infused IV in 1 hour for 14 days, followed by 300 mg/kg per day for 3 to 4 weeks. Eflornithine is approved in the United States for this indication but is not marketed and must be obtained from the manufacturer (Merrell Dow).[24]

Furazolidone (Furoxone). Furazolidone is a nitrofuran derivative used in the treatment of giardiasis.[25] It is marketed in tablets and as a liquid. The liquid form is particularly useful in treating infants and young children because it is the only available liquid antigiardiasis drug produced in the United States. Furazolidone can produce a disulfiram-type reaction when it is taken with alcohol, and it is also a monoamine oxidase inhibitor. Occasional hypersensitivity reactions may occur, including hypotension, urticaria, fever, and arthralgia, as may nausea, vomiting, and headache. Furazolidone may cause mild hemolysis in glucose-6-phosphate dehydrogenase–deficient persons. Metabolic degradation products may give a brown color to the urine. The dosage for adults is 100 mg four times daily (qid) for 7 to 10 days. Children should receive 6 mg/kg per day in four divided doses for 7 to 10 days, but the drug should not be given to infants younger than 1 month.

Halofantrine (Halfan). Halofantrine is used in the treatment of chloroquine-resistant *P. falciparum* (CRPF) malaria. In some areas of mefloquine-resistant *P. falciparum*, there is also cross-resistance to halofantrine. Halofantrine is not recommended for malaria chemoprophylaxis. The drug is available in 500-mg tablets, and although it is approved in the United States, it is not being marketed. The adult treatment dosage is 500 mg every 6 hours for three doses in a 1-day course. Children's dosage is 8 mg/kg every 6 hours for three doses. The manufacturer recommends that a second full course be taken by nonimmune individuals 1 week after completion of the first course. Side effects have included abdominal pain, diarrhea, and nausea. The drug is contraindicated in pregnancy and during breast-feeding.[15, 26] Halofantrine has been found to cause dose-related lengthening of the PR and QT_c intervals.[27] It should not be taken 1 hour before to 3 hours after meals and should not be used for patients with known cardiac conduction defects. Cardiac monitoring is recommended.

Iodoquinol (Yodoxin). Iodoquinol is a halogenated oxyquinoline used in the treatment of amebiasis, *Dientamoeba fragilis* infection, and *Balantidium coli* infection.[28] It was formerly produced as Diodoquin, but this brand has been removed from the U.S. market. Iodoquinol acts against amoebae primarily in the intestinal lumen and by itself is ineffective against invasive amebiasis. Because so little of the drug is absorbed, it has relatively little toxicity. It rarely causes abdominal pain, diarrhea, or rash. It is contraindicated in persons with iodine intolerance. In doses recommended for intestinal protozoa, iodoquinol has not been shown to cause the optic atrophy occasionally seen with long-term administration to children in large doses for acrodermatitis enteropathica and nonspecific diarrhea. In the treatment of asymptomatic intestinal amebiasis by itself, or used as a follow-up luminal drug, the dosage for adults is 650 mg tid for 20 days. Children receive 40 mg/kg per day in three doses for 20 days. Similar doses have been used for *D. fragilis* and *B. coli* infections.

Ivermectin (Mectizan).† Ivermectin is now the drug of choice for the treatment of onchocerciasis.[29] It has also been used as a wide-spectrum antihelmintic in humans against intestinal helminths, including strongyloidiasis, and against blood-stage filariasis.[29] In onchocerciasis, ivermectin acts against microfilariae by paralyzing them and allowing them to be removed by the reticuloendothelial system. Intrauterine microfilariae are damaged and degenerate and are reduced in number. The drug has no effect against adult worms, and treatment must be repeated with buildup of microfilariae at approximately yearly intervals for the duration of the adult worms' lives (approximately 10 to 15 years). Side effects with the required single oral dose have generally been mild and include fever, pruritus, and rash. The dose for onchocerciasis for both adults and children is 150 μg/kg, once orally (PO), with repeated doses at approximately yearly intervals. A randomized trial comparing ivermectin and thiabendazole for treatment of chronic infection with *Strongyloides stercoralis* showed that ivermectin in a course of 200 μg/kg daily for 2 days had equal efficacy and was better tolerated.[30]

Mebendazole (Vermox). Mebendazole is a synthetic benzimidazole, a broad-spectrum anthelmintic used in the treatment of trichuriasis,[31] ascariasis,[31] enterobiasis,[32] and hookworm disease.[32] Mebendazole is also used in treating hydatid cysts when surgery is contraindicated or cysts rupture spontaneously during surgery; this is an experimental indication in the United States.[33] It acts by blocking glucose uptake by the susceptible helminths and is poorly absorbed from the gastrointestinal tract. Mebendazole is well tolerated and only rarely causes abdominal pain, nausea, and diarrhea. It is contraindicated in pregnant women and in children before age 2 years. For trichuriasis, ascariasis, and hookworm infections, both adults and children receive 100 mg twice daily (bid) for 3 days. For enterobiasis, a single 100-mg tablet is taken and the dose repeated 2 weeks later. Mebendazole has also been experimentally used, along with steroids, in the treatment of severe trichinosis.[34]

Mefloquine (Lariam). Mefloquine is used in the chemoprophylaxis and treatment of multidrug-resistant *P. falciparum* and *P. vivax* malaria.[35, 36] Mefloquine appears to act by blocking the invasion of malarial sporozoites into red blood cells. Side effects include vomiting and dizziness. Cases of CNS toxic effects have been seen after treatment doses and much less frequently with prophylactic use.[36-38] Mefloquine should not be used for self-treatment because of these side effects. Because mefloquine has occasionally been associated with cardiac problems, it should not be used by persons with cardiac conduction abnormalities. Ordinarily, mefloquine should not be given concurrently with quinine or quinidine; if these drugs are to be used in the initial treatment of severe malaria, mefloquine administration should be deferred until at least 12 hours after the last dose. Mefloquine is not recommended in persons with a history of epilepsy or psychiatric disorder. A review of mefloquine use in pregnancy suggests that it is not associated with adverse effects and it can be considered for use in women who are pregnant or likely to become so when exposure to CRPF is unavoidable.[39] For curative treatment of malaria, the total dose of mefloquine for adults and children weighing more than 45 kg is 1250 mg administered as a single dose. Alternatively, it can be given as 750 mg followed 6 to 8 hours later by 500 mg. A lower total dose of 750 to 1000 mg is sufficient for semiimmune patients living in malarious areas. Children who weigh less than 45 kg (regardless of immunity status) receive 25 mg/kg in a single dose. For chemoprophylaxis, adults and children who weigh more than 45 kg receive 250 mg once weekly while exposed to malaria and for 4 weeks afterward. Doses for children weighing less than 45 kg are given in Table 35–1. *P. falciparum* strains resistant to mefloquine are reported.[35]

Melarsoprol (Arsobal).† Melarsoprol is an organic compound of arsenic. It is the drug of choice for late-stage *T. brucei rhodesiense* infection with CNS involvement.[40] It is manufactured in France in a clear sterile solution. After IV administration, a small but therapeutically significant amount of the drug penetrates the cerebrospinal fluid and has a lethal effect on trypanosomes infecting the CNS. During administration, care must be taken to prevent leakage into the tissues. Side effects are common during treatment—encephalopathy, myocardial damage, albuminuria, hypertension, Jarisch-Herxheimer–type reaction, vomiting, and peripheral neuropathy.[40] Because of its toxicity, melarsoprol should not be used for early, untreated hemolymphatic trypanosomiasis. For adults, 2 to 3.6 mg/kg per day IV is given for three doses; this course is repeated after 1 week and again after 10 to 21 days. Children should receive 18 to 25 mg/kg total dose during 1 month; an initial dose of 0.36 mg/kg IV is given, increasing gradually to a maximum of 3.6 mg/kg at intervals of 1 to 5 days for a total of 9 or 10 doses.

Metronidazole (Flagyl). Metronidazole is a nitroimidazole compound used in the treatment of vaginal trichomoniasis, amebiasis, and giardiasis.[41] It is trichomonacidal and giardicidal; it is amebicidal at both intestinal and extraintestinal sites. It is absorbed well and is more effective for symptomatic or invasive amebiasis than for the asymptomatic cyst-passing state.[42] Common side effects are nausea, headache, and a metallic taste. Dizziness, vomiting, abdominal cramps, and diarrhea are less common. *Candida* overgrowth may occur. Dark urine may develop from a metabolite of the drug. Metronidazole should not be used with alcohol because it can give a disulfiram-like reaction. Metronidazole has caused lung tumors in mice but not in hamsters and is mutagenic to some bacteria. The risk to humans of carcinogenicity and mutagenicity is considered to be low, if not negligible.[43] Metronidazole is the drug of choice for *Trichomonas vaginalis* in a standard dose of 250 mg tid for 7 days. An alternative is a single 2-g dose, which has been found to have comparable efficacy and side effects.[44] For symptomatic nondysenteric intestinal amebiasis, adults should receive 500 mg tid and children 50 mg/kg per day in three divided doses for 10 days. For acute amebic dysentery and amebic liver abscess, adults should receive 750 mg tid and children 50 mg/kg per day in three divided doses, both for 10 days. Metronidazole is available as an IV preparation for use in severe infections.[45] When used for amebiasis, metronidazole should always be followed by a luminal active drug. Metronidazole has never been approved by the FDA for treatment of giardiasis, but it is regularly used for this infection. Dosage is 250 mg tid for adults and 5 mg/kg tid for children, both for 7 days.

Nifurtimox (Lampit).† Nifurtimox is used in the treatment of *T. cruzi* infection (Chagas disease).[9] It has been useful in the treatment of the acute phase of infection, but there is no evidence that it alters the development of the established lesions of chronic Chagas disease. Side effects can be severe and may include nervousness (and rarely hallucinations and convulsions), weight loss, and peripheral neuritis. It is tolerated better by younger than older patients and is not recommended during pregnancy. The adult dose is 8 to 10 mg/kg per day PO in four divided doses for 120 days. Children's doses are given in Table 35–1.

Oxamniquine (Vansil). Oxamniquine is an alternative to praziquantel in the treatment of *Schistosoma mansoni* infection.[46] Rare side effects include dizziness, drowsiness, neuropsychiatric disturbances, and gastrointestinal symptoms. For South American and Caribbean strains of *S. mansoni*, a single 15 mg/kg oral dose is effective. Some experts recommend 40 to 60 mg/kg over 2 to 3 days in all of Africa.[47]

Paromomycin (Humatin). Paromomycin is a broad-spectrum, poorly absorbed antibiotic used in the treatment of amebiasis[48] and *D. fragilis* infection. It should be given with caution to persons with ulcerative lesions of the bowel, to avoid renal toxic effects through inadvertent absorption. Because it is poorly absorbed, it is most effective for asymptomatic and mildly symptomatic intestinal amebiasis and should not be used by itself to treat invasive amebiasis. It can also be used as a follow-up luminal active drug for invasive amebiasis. The adult dose for amebiasis and *D. fragilis* infection is 500 mg bid for 7 days; children should receive 30 mg/kg per day in three divided doses, also for 7 days. IV paromomycin has been found to be effective against visceral and cutaneous leishmaniasis and in a topical formulation against Old World cutaneous leishmaniasis.[49] Oral paromomycin treatment has resulted in improvement of both clinical and parasitologic parameters in cryptosporidiosis in AIDS.[50]

Pentamidine Isethionate (Pentam 300). Pentamidine isethionate is an aromatic diamidine used as an alternative treatment of early Gambian sleeping sickness without CNS involvement, leishmaniasis, and *Pneumocystis carinii* pneumonia.[51] The mode of action of the diamidines is not completely understood, but they may act by interfering with nuclear metabolism. Side effects can include hypotension, ventricular arrhythmias, vomiting, blood dyscrasias, renal damage, and pain or sterile abscess at the injection site. Both hypoglycemia and hyperglycemia may occur. Pentamidine should be used with caution in patients with hypertension, diabetes, malnutrition, or hepatic or renal disease. Experience with Rhodesian sleeping sickness is more limited, and because of the associated early CNS involvement, pentamidine is not usually recommended.[51] There is potential confusion about the dose of pentamidine and its salts. In the United States and England, it is supplied as the isethionate salt in vials of 300 mg, and the doses given are in terms of this salt. In some other countries, the methane sulfonate salt is used, and the formulation and dose are different.[52] It should be freshly prepared by dissolving the powder in sterile distilled water, not saline solution. The dose for African trypanosomiasis for both adults and children is 4 mg/kg per day IM for 10 days. Pentamidine is an alternative treatment for leishmaniasis[7]; the dose is 2 to 4 mg/kg per day IM for up to 15 days. Formerly, pentamidine, in a dose of 3 to 4 mg/kg per day

IM for 14 to 21 days, was the only available treatment for *P. carinii* pneumonia for both adults and children. However, trimethoprim-sulfamethoxazole is at least as effective and less toxic and is presently considered the drug of choice for initial therapy.[53] Pentamidine is recommended for persons who have a severe allergy to a sulfonamide or are unable to tolerate or fail to respond to trimethoprim-sulfamethoxazole. Aerosolized pentamidine has been found effective for primary and secondary prophylaxis of *P. carinii* pneumonia.[53]

Permethrin. Permethrin is a synthetic pyrethroid used as an aerosol clothing spray for protection against mosquitoes and ticks. A 1% permethrin product (Nix Creme Rinse) is used for treatment of head lice,[54] and a 5% product (Elimite Cream) is used against scabies infestation,[55] both in single-dose treatments. Itching and burning may occur as side effects. No systemic reactions have been reported.

Praziquantel (Biltricide). Praziquantel is the drug of choice for most fluke infections, including schistosomiasis.[56, 57] In the United States, praziquantel is an investigational drug for the treatment of intestinal tapeworms and cysticercosis.[58] Side effects are mild and include dizziness and drowsiness. The only specific contraindication is ocular cysticercosis, because destruction of parasites in the eye may cause serious damage. For *S. mansoni, Schistosoma hematobium* and *Schistosoma intercalatum*, the dose for adults and children is 40 mg/kg per day in two doses for 1 day. For *Schistosoma japonicum* and *Schistosoma mekongi*, the dose for adults and children is 60 mg/kg per day in three doses for 1 day. For *P. westermani*, 25 mg/kg tid is given for 2 days. The same regimen for 1 day is given for *Clonorchis sinensis, Opisthorchis* species, *Fasciolopsis buski, Heterophyes heterophyes*, and *Metagonimus yokogawai. F. hepatica* infections do not respond well to praziquantel.[59] For the tapeworms, *D. latum, T. saginata, T. solium*, and *D. caninum*, 5 to 10 mg/kg in a single dose has been effective. For *H. nana*, 25 mg/kg in a single dose is effective. Praziquantel is replacing surgery as a treatment of choice for neurocysticercosis.[3, 60, 61] The regimen currently used is 50 mg/kg per day in three divided doses for 15 days. To decrease cerebral edema from dying parasites, corticosteroids should be administered concurrently, beginning 2 days before and continued during the 15-day course of praziquantel.[61]

Primaquine Phosphate. Primaquine phosphate is an 8-aminoquinoline used to prevent relapses and to provide radical cure of *P. vivax* and *Plasmodium ovale* malaria by acting on hypnozoites of these species in the liver. It also has a gametocidal effect against malaria parasites.[62] It is marketed as primaquine phosphate in 26.3-mg salt (15-mg base) tablets. Minor side effects include nausea, abdominal discomfort, and headache. Acute hemolytic anemia occurs in persons with glucose-6-phosphate dehydrogenase deficiency.[63] Primaquine should not be given to patients who are simultaneously receiving other potentially hemolytic drugs, agents capable of depressing the myeloid elements of the bone marrow.[63] Primaquine is contraindicated in pregnancy. For radical cure of acute *P. vivax* or *P. ovale* malaria to prevent relapses, adults receive 15 mg of base daily for 14 days, after completing initial schizonticidal therapy, usually with chloroquine. Children receive 0.3 mg/kg base daily for 14 days in broken up tablets because there is no liquid preparation and the tablets do not go into solution. Primaquine is also recommended to prevent relapses after travelers with prolonged exposure leave malarious areas where *P. vivax* or *P. ovale* occurs. This is best taken after completing the 4-week terminal doses of the chemosuppressive drug or drugs. A daily dose of 30 mg of base for 14 days may be required for adults exposed to so-called Chesson-strain *P. vivax* malaria in parts of the Southwest Pacific and Southeast and South Asia.[64] Primaquine alone has been found to be effective prophylaxis against falciparum malaria in studies in Kenya.[65] Primaquine plus clindamycin is used as an alternative treatment for *Pneumocystis* pneumonia in patients who have failed to respond to or are intolerant of standard therapy.[66]

Proguanil Hydrochloride (Paludrine).* Proguanil hydrochloride is used only for the chemoprophylaxis of malaria and has been found to be particularly useful in Africa.[67, 68] It acts by slowly arresting the development of maturing schizonts and is effective against the primary tissue phase of *P. falciparum*. It also renders gametocytes incapable of developing in the mosquito. It is rapidly absorbed, is readily excreted, does not accumulate in the body when given in therapeutic doses, and must be taken daily. Proguanil is not licensed for use in the United States, but it is widely available in Europe and Africa. It is tolerated well but can cause gastrointestinal side effects and occasionally mouth ulcers. It can be used as an alternative drug in persons intolerant of chloroquine in areas where *P. falciparum* is sensitive to chloroquine. In areas of CRPF malaria, proguanil is given daily and chloroquine weekly. The adult dosage is 200 mg daily during exposure and for 4 weeks afterward. Children's doses are given in Table 35–1.

Pyrantel Pamoate (Antiminth Oral Suspension). Pyrantel pamoate is a broad-spectrum anthelmintic used in the treatment of ascariasis and enterobiasis.[69, 70] It is effective against hookworms but is considered an investigational drug for this purpose in the United States.[69] It has also been used against *Trichostrongylus* species, with varying results in different parts of the world.[70] The anthelmintic activity is probably due to its neuromuscular blocking property. Pyrantel pamoate is tolerated well and only rarely causes gastrointestinal disturbances, headaches, dizziness, and rash. For treatment of ascariasis, enterobiasis, and trichostrongyliasis, both adults and children receive 11 mg/kg (maximum, 1 g) in a single dose. For enterobiasis, the dose is repeated after 2 weeks. For hookworms, the same single oral dose is given for 3 consecutive days. Pyrantel pamoate is available as an over-the-counter preparation (Reese's Pinworm Medicine).

Pyrimethamine (Daraprim). Pyrimethamine is an aminopyrimidine derivative formerly used alone for the suppression of susceptible strains of malaria[71] and for treatment of toxoplasmosis.[72] Pyrimethamine, 25 mg, combined with 500 mg sulfadoxine (a long-acting sulfonamide) is marketed as Fansidar and used for treatment of susceptible strains of chloroquine-resistant *P. falciparum*.[73] Pyrimethamine, 12.5 mg, is also combined with dapsone, 100 mg, as Maloprim, an antimalarial manufactured in England.[73, 74] Pyrimethamine is a folic acid antagonist, and its therapeutic action is based on the differential requirement between host and parasite for nucleic acid precursors involved in growth. This activity is highly selective against plasmodia and *Toxoplasma gondii*. In the recommended dosage of 25 mg weekly used for malaria suppression, side effects are uncommon. Excessive or prolonged doses required for toxoplasmosis may produce a macrocytic anemia because of interference with folic acid metabolism, and it is advisable to administer 10 mg of folinic acid per day in this situation.[72] There is widespread resistance by malaria parasites to pyrimethamine. Although it is available in the United States, it is probably the least effective antimalarial and is seldom recommended by itself.[71] Fansidar is no longer recommended for chemoprophylaxis of CRPF malaria because of the high risk of death from Stevens-Johnson syndrome. A single three-tablet adult dose of Fansidar can be used for self-treatment of a febrile illness thought to be CRPF malaria when medical care is not immediately available.[73] Children's emergency treatment doses are given in Table 35–1. *P. falciparum* is also resistant to Fansidar in many malarious areas. Fansidar is contraindicated for persons allergic to sulfonamides, in pregnancy at term, and for infants younger than 2 months. Maloprim is not approved in the United

States, and there is concern about the risk for toxic effects to bone marrow and resistance to CRPF malaria.[75] For treatment of toxoplasmosis in adults, 25 to 100 mg/d of pyrimethamine along with 1 to 1.5 g of sulfadiazine qid is taken for 3 to 4 weeks. For children, 2 mg/kg per day (maximum, 25 mg/d) of pyrimethamine along with 100 to 200 mg/kg per day of sulfadiazine is also taken for 3 to 4 weeks. In immunocompromised persons, including those with AIDS, with CNS toxoplasmosis, therapy with high doses of pyrimethamine and sulfonamides or clindamycin is recommended for prolonged periods.

Quinidine Gluconate. Quinidine gluconate, an isomer of quinine, is used for IV treatment of severe *P. falciparum* malaria where there is quinine resistance (in Thailand) or where IV quinine is not available (in the United States).[76] Adults and children receive an initial loading dose of 10 mg/kg salt (6.2 mg/kg base) administered in an hour, followed by a continuous infusion of 0.02 mg/kg salt (0.0125 mg/kg base) per minute.[76, 77] With both regimens, oral quinidine sulfate or quinine was substituted when patients could swallow and retain oral medications. Quinidine treatment should be continued for 72 hours total. During IV quinidine use, infusion speed must be carefully monitored, and the blood pressure and electrocardiogram should be monitored closely for evidence of toxic reactions.

Quinine. Quinine is an alkaloid extracted from the bark of the cinchona tree used for the treatment of CRPF malaria and of severe *P. falciparum* malaria.[78] It is available as oral quinine sulfate in 650-mg and 325-mg tablets and as quinine dihydrochloride for IV use. The IV preparation is not available in the United States. Quinine's primary action is schizonticidal, and no lethal effect is exerted on sporozoites or preerythrocytic tissue forms. Usual therapeutic doses of quinine frequently cause some degree of cinchonism (tinnitus, headache, nausea, abdominal pain, blurred vision, and altered auditory acuity), but these symptoms are usually not severe enough to require cessation of treatment. Blood dyscrasias rarely occur, as may urticaria, asthma, drug fever, and hypoglycemia. IV administration of quinine dihydrochloride may lead to arrhythmias, hypotension, and acute circulatory failure. It must be given slowly in dilute solutions with constant monitoring of the pulse and blood pressure, and oral quinine sulfate should be substituted when possible. For oral treatment of CRPF malaria in adults, quinine sulfate, 650 mg tid, is given for 3 days, followed by either tetracycline, 250 mg qid, for 7 days or three tablets of pyrimethamine-sulfadoxine (Fansidar). To children, 25 mg/kg per day is given in three divided doses for 3 days, followed by Fansidar in reduced doses. For IV treatment of severe *P. falciparum* malaria in adults, quinine dihydrochloride is administered as a 20 mg/kg loading dose in 4 hours, followed by 10 mg/kg in 2 to 8 hours, repeated every 8 hours until oral quinine therapy can be started.[77, 78] For children, the same dose as for adults is used (maximum, 1800 mg/d for children and adults). Fansidar, a tetracycline, or clindamycin should then be given to ensure total cure.

Spiramycin (Rovamycine).* Spiramycin is used as an alternative treatment for toxoplasmosis and has also proved safe in pregnant women with this condition.[79] Gastrointestinal symptoms and allergic reactions have occurred. For toxoplasmosis, 3 to 4 g/d is given and in pregnancy is continued until delivery. The FDA has not approved spiramycin for routine use, and it is not commercially available in the United States.

Stibogluconate Sodium; Sodium Antimony Gluconate (Pentostam).† Pentostam is a solution containing 30% to 34% pentavalent antimony. It is the drug of choice for visceral, cutaneous, and mucocutaneous leishmaniasis.[7, 80, 81] A related antimony drug, meglumine antimonate (Glucantime*) is manufactured in France but is not available in the United States.[80, 81] The mechanism of action of these pentavalent antimony compounds is unknown. Drug reactions, as a rule, are not severe, owing in part to rapid excretion of the drugs. Side effects can include gastrointestinal symptoms, muscle pain and joint stiffness, bradycardia and electrocardiographic changes, and rash. This drug should be used cautiously in those patients who have received antimony therapy within 2 months; should be withheld from those who manifest toxic reactions to the drug; and is best not given to patients with heart, liver, or kidney disease. For visceral and mucocutaneous leishmaniasis, the dose for both adults and children is 20 mg/kg per day IM or IV for 28 days. For cutaneous leishmaniasis, the standard treatment is 20 mg/kg per day for 20 days for adults and children. This is usually given IV but can be given IM.[81] Some types of visceral, cutaneous, and mucocutaneous leishmaniasis are more difficult to treat and may require higher doses, more prolonged treatment, or alternative drugs.[49]

Suramin (Germanin).† Suramin is a synthetic urea compound and the drug of choice for therapy of early blood-stage Rhodesian *(T. brucei rhodesiense)* and Gambian *(T. brucei gambiense)* trypanosomiasis.[40] Suramin is also used to kill adult worms in onchocerciasis.[82] The exact mechanism of action is uncertain, although it is known to inhibit numerous enzyme systems. Suramin clears the blood of trypanosomes, and a full course cures nearly all early cases. It does not cross the blood-brain barrier and does not cure the infection if CNS invasion has occurred. Suramin can cause a variety of side effects, including vomiting, pruritus, urticaria, fever, paresthesias, and hyperesthesia of the palms and soles. A moderate degree of albuminuria is usual, but if casts appear, indicating more severe kidney damage, treatment should be discontinued. It should not be used when renal or hepatic disease is present. Idiosyncrasy may lead to circulatory collapse, and deaths have occurred from immediate hypersensitivity. The drug powder must be mixed into a 10% solution with 5 mL of distilled water immediately before use, and this should not be stored for more than 0.5 hour. A 100- to 200-mg IV dose to test for sensitivity should be given initially. In trypanosomiasis, 1 g is then given slowly IV on days 1, 3, 7, 14, and 21. Children receive 20 mg/kg on the same schedule. A second course of treatment should not be given earlier than 3 months after the first course. For treatment of onchocerciasis, after initial treatment with diethylcarbamazine and a 100-mg test dose, 1 g IV for adults and 20 mg/kg IV for children are given once weekly for 5 weeks. Because suramin can be toxic to patients with mild cases of onchocerciasis without ocular involvement typically seen in areas where the disease is not endemic, suramin is rarely indicated. Ivermectin has replaced suramin for most onchocerciasis infections.

Tetracycline Hydrochloride. Tetracycline is an antibiotic used in the treatment of certain intestinal protozoa, including *D. fragilis* and *B. coli*.[28] Tetracycline is also used after quinine or quinidine, in treatment of CRPF malaria.[15] A long-acting form of tetracycline, doxycycline, can be used for chemoprophylaxis against multidrug-resistant *P. falciparum* malaria.[83] Tetracyclines have a relatively slow-acting schizonticidal effect against *P. falciparum* and cannot be relied on alone to treat acute attacks in nonimmune persons. (See Chapter 21 for a discussion of the side effects of tetracycline hydrochloride.) Its use could be justified in young children with severe, potentially life-threatening CRPF malaria, for whom the benefit clearly outweighs the risk of tooth staining. However, clindamycin could be substituted for treatment of young children and pregnant women. A dose of 500 mg qid for 10 days has been used for *D. fragilis* and *B. coli* infections in adults. For treatment of CRPF malaria, tetracycline, 250 mg qid for 7 days, is given after quinine or quinidine. For chemoprophylaxis of multidrug-resistant *P. falciparum* malaria, 100 mg of doxycycline daily is taken during exposure and for 4 weeks thereafter. Photosensitivity is a potential hazard with doxycycline.

Thiabendazole (Mintezol). Thiabendazole is a broad-spectrum benzimidazole anthelmintic used in treatment of strongyloidiasis,[84] trichostrongyliasis,[85] and cutaneous larva migrans.[86] It has been used experimentally against *Capillaria* species,[85] *Dracunculus medinensis*,[87] and *Trichinella spiralis* infections.[88] Thiabendazole is thought to act on parasites by interfering with microtubule aggregation and through inhibition of the enzyme fumarate reductase. It also has antiinflammatory properties, which may explain its usefulness in dracunculiasis and trichinosis. The most frequently encountered side effects are nausea, vomiting, headache, and dizziness, which occur more in adults than in children. Rare side effects include liver damage, hypotension, angioneurotic edema, and Stevens-Johnson syndrome. Because CNS side effects may occur, activities requiring mental alertness should be avoided, and it should be used with caution in patients with liver disease. The drug should be taken after meals. For strongyloidiasis and trichostrongyliasis, the dose for both adults and children is 25 mg/kg bid (maximum, 3 g/d) for 2 days. For disseminated strongyloidiasis, treatment should be continued for at least 5 days. For cutaneous larva migrans, similar oral doses are taken for 2 days. Alternatively, thiabendazole suspension may be applied topically to lesions.[86] Thiabendazole, 25 mg/kg bid for 5 days, has been used in trichinosis, but its effect on larvae in muscle is thought to be more antiinflammatory than lethal,[88] and it is less effective than mebendazole.

Tinidazole (Fasigyn).* Tinidazole is a nitroimidazole used outside the United States for giardiasis, amebiasis, and vaginal trichomoniasis.[89] In comparative trials with the related nitroimidazole metronidazole, tinidazole has been as effective in shorter, better tolerated courses.[90] About 10% of patients experience mild gastrointestinal side effects and headache. For giardiasis, adults are given a single 2-g oral dose, and children receive a single 50-mg/kg dose (maximum 2 g/d). Symptomatic intestinal amebiasis has been treated with 600 mg bid for 5 to 10 days for adults. Single daily doses of 2 g have been used for 2 to 6 days. For amebic liver abscess, the more successful regimens have been 800 mg tid for 5 days or a single daily dose of 2 g for 3 days. Children's doses are given in Table 35–1. As with metronidazole in treating amebiasis, tinidazole should always be followed with a luminal amebicide to decrease the possibility of relapse. For vaginal trichomoniasis, a single 2-g dose is given.

Trimethoprim-Sulfamethoxazole (Bactrim, Septra). Trimethoprim-sulfamethoxazole is a synthetic antibacterial combination used in treatment of *P. carinii*,[53] *Isospora belli* infections,[91] and *Cyclospora* infection.[92] Available evidence suggests that trimethoprim is relatively nontoxic to humans. Reactions to sulfamethoxazole are similar to those caused by other short- and medium-acting sulfonamides. For *P. carinii* infection, the dose for both children and adults is trimethoprim 15 mg/kg per day and sulfamethoxazole 75 mg/kg per day, PO or IV, in four divided doses for 14 to 21 days. AIDS patients should be treated for 21 days, and they may have exaggerated reactions to the drug—fever, rash, granulocytopenia, and bone marrow depression.[53] This drug is also used for prophylaxis of *P. carinii* infection.[53] For *I. belli* infection in adults, trimethoprim, 160 mg, and sulfamethoxazole, 800 mg, are given qid for 10 days and then bid for 3 weeks. The high rate of recurrence suggests that an initial shorter 1- to 2-week course followed by an indefinite period of daily doses prophylactically may be a better approach. For *Cyclospora* infection in adults, trimethoprim, 160 mg, plus sulfamethoxazole, 800 mg bid, is given for 7 days. Children receive trimethoprim, 5 mg/kg, plus sulfamethoxazole, 25 mg/kg bid, for 7 days. (See Chapter 25 for a more detailed discussion of this agent.)

References

1. Rossignol JF, Maisonneuve H: Albendazole: Placebo-controlled study in 870 patients with intestinal helminths. Trans R Soc Trop Med Hyg 77:707, 1983.

1a. Jones SK, Reynolds NJ, Oliewicki S, et al: Oral albendazole for treatment of cutaneous larva migrans. Br J Dermatol 122:99, 1990.

2. Horton RJ: Chemotherapy of *Echinococcus* infection in man with albendazole. Trans R Soc Trop Med Hyg 83:97, 1989.
3. Cruz M, Cruz I, Horton J: Albendazole versus praziquantel in the treatment of cerebral cysticercosis: Clinical evaluation. Trans R Soc Trop Med Hyg 85:244, 1991.
4. Kraivichian P, Kulkumthorn M, Yingyourd P, et al: Albendazole for the treatment of human gnathostomiasis. Trans R Soc Trop Med Hyg 86:418, 1992.
5. Molina JM, Oksenhendler E, Beauvais B, et al: Disseminated microsporidiosis due to *Septata intestinalis* in patients with AIDS: Clinical features and response to albendazole therapy. J Infect Dis 171:245, 1995.
6. Duma R: Disease caused by free-living amebae. Infect Dis Newslett 8:25, 1989.
7. Jernigan JA, Pearson RD: Chemotherapy of leishmaniasis, Chagas' disease and African trypanosomiasis. Curr Opin Infect Dis 6:794, 1993.
8. Kwell and other drugs for treatment of lice and scabies. Med Lett Drugs Ther 19:18, 1977.
9. Marr JJ, Docampo R: Chemotherapy for Chagas' disease: A perspective of current therapy and considerations for future research. Rev Infect Dis 8:884, 1986.
10. Farag HF, Salem A, El-Hifni SA, et al: Bithionol (Bitin) treatment in established fascioliasis in Egyptians. J Trop Med Hyg 91:240, 1988.
11. Singh TS, Mutum SS, Razaque MA: Pulmonary paragonimiasis: Clinical features, diagnosis and treatment of 39 cases in Manipur. Trans R Soc Trop Med Hyg 80:967, 1986.
12. Appleton B, Wolfe MS, Mishtowt GI: Chloroquine as a malarial suppressive: Absence of visual effects. Milit Med 138:225, 1973.
13. Lange WR, Frankenfield DL, Moriarty-Sheehan M, et al: No evidence for chloroquine-associated retinopathy among missionaries on long-term malaria chemoprophylaxis. Am J Trop Med Hyg 51:392, 1994.
14. Wolfe MS, Cordero JF: Safety of chloroquine in chemosuppresion of malaria during pregnancy. Br Med J 290:1496, 1985.
15. Kain KC: Chemotherapy and prevention of drug-resistant malaria. Wilderness Environ Med 6:307, 1995.
16. Marlar-Than, Myat-Phone-Kyaw, Aye-Yu-Soe, et al: Development of resistance to chloroquine by *Plasmodium vivax* in Myanmar. Trans R Soc Trop Med Hyg 89:307, 1995.
17. Mackenzie CD, Kron MA: Diethylcarbamazine: A review of its action in onchocerciasis, lymphatic filariasis, and inflammation. Trop Dis Bull 82:R1, 1985.
18. Weller PF, Simon HB, Parkhurst BH, et al: Tourism-acquired *Mansonella ozzardi* microfilaremia in a regular blood donor. JAMA 240:858, 1978.
19. Keystone JS, Davies D: Single-blind Mazzotti test for onchocerciasis. Lancet 339:678, 1992.
20. Sullivan TJ, Hembree SC: Enhancement of the density of circulating microfilariae with diethylcarbamazine. Trans R Soc Trop Med Hyg 64:787, 1970.
21. Ottesen EA: Description, mechanisms, and control of reactions to treatment in the human filariases. Ciba Found Symp 127:265, 1987.
22. Van Bogaert L, Dubois A, Janssens PG, et al: Encephalitis in *Loa loa* filariasis. J Neurol Neurosurg Psychiatry 18:103, 1955.
23. Wolfe MS: Nondysenteric intestinal amebiasis: Treatment with diloxanide furoate. JAMA 224:1601, 1973.
24. Milord F, Pepin J, Loko L, et al: Efficacy and toxicity of eflornithine for treatment of *Trypanosoma brucei gambiense* sleeping sickness. Lancet 340:652, 1992.
25. Murphy TV, Nelson JD: Five versus ten days' therapy with furazolidone for giardiasis. Am J Dis Child 137:267, 1983.

26. Bryson HM, Goa KL: Halofantrine. A review of its antimalarial activity, pharmacokinetic properties and therapeutic potential. Drugs 43:236, 1992.
27. Castot A, Rapoport P, LeCoz P: Prolonged QT interval with halofantrine. Lancet 341:1541, 1993.
28. Wolfe MS: The treatment of intestinal protozoan infections. Med Clin North Am 66:707, 1982.
29. Campbell WC: Ivermectin as an antiparasitic agent for use in humans. Annu Rev Microbiol 45:445, 1991.
30. Gann PH, Neva FA, Gam AA: A randomized trial of single- and two-dose ivermectin versus thiabendazole for treatment of strongyloidiasis. J Infect Dis 169:1076, 1994.
31. Wolfe MS, Wershing JM: Mebendazole: Treatment of trichuriasis and ascariasis in Bahamian children. JAMA 230:1408, 1974.
32. Keystone JS, Murdock JK: Mebendazole. Ann Intern Med 91:582, 1979.
33. Kammerer WS, Schantz PM: Echinococcal disease. Infect Dis Clin North Am 7:605, 1993.
34. Levin ML: Treatment of trichinosis with mebendazole. Am J Trop Med Hyg 32:980, 1983.
35. Palmer KJ, Holliday SM, Brogden RN: Mefloquine. A review of its antimalarial activity, pharmacokinetic properties, and therapeutic effect. Drugs 45:430, 1993.
36. White NJ: Mefloquine in the prophylaxis and treatment of falciparum malaria. Br Med J 308:286, 1994.
37. Hennequin C, Bouree P, Bazin N, et al: Severe psychiatric side effects observed during prophylaxis and treatment with mefloquine. Arch Intern Med 154:2360, 1994.
38. Barrett PJ, Emmins PD, Clark PD, et al: Comparison of adverse events associated with use of mefloquine and combination of chloroquine and proquanil as antimalarial prophylaxis: Postal and telephone survey of travellers. BMJ 313:525, 1996.
39. Centers for Disease Control and Prevention: Health Information for International Travel, 1995. Washington, DC, U.S. Government Printing Office, 1995. HHS publication (CDC) 95-8280.
40. Apted FIC: Present status of chemotherapy and chemoprophylaxis of human trypanosomiasis in the Eastern hemisphere. Pharmacol Ther 11:391, 1980.
41. Rosenblatt JE, Edson RS: Metronidazole. Mayo Clin Proc 62:1013, 1987.
42. Spillman R, Ayala S, DeSanchez CE: Double-blind test of metronidazole and tinidazole in the treatment of asymptomatic *Entamoeba histolytica* and *Entamoeba hartmanni* carriers. Am J Trop Med Hyg 25:549, 1976.
43. Goldman P: Metronidazole: Proven benefits and potential risks. Johns Hopkins Med J 147:1, 1980.
44. Hager WD, Brown ST, Kraus SJ, et al: Metronidazole for vaginal trichomoniasis: Seven day vs single dose regimens. JAMA 244:1219, 1980.
45. Wolfe MS: Amebiasis. *In* Strickland GT (ed): Hunter's Tropical Medicine, ed 7. Philadelphia, WB Saunders, 1991, pp 563–564.
46. Foster R: A review of clinical experience with oxamniquine. Trans R Soc Trop Med Hyg 81:55, 1987.
47. Shekhar KC: Schistosomiasis drug therapy and treatment considerations. Drugs 42:379, 1991.
48. Sullam PM, Slutkin G, Gottlieb AB, et al: Paromomycin therapy of endemic amebiasis in homosexual men. Sex Transm Dis 13:151, 1986.
49. Cook GC: Leishmaniasis: Some recent developments in chemotherapy. J Antimicrob Chemother 31:327, 1993.
50. White CA, Chappell CL, Hayat CS, et al: Paromomycin for cryptosporidiosis in AIDS: A prospective double-blind trial. J Infect Dis 170:419, 1994.
51. Sands M, Kron MA, Brown RB: Pentamidine: A review. Rev Infect Dis 7:625, 1985.
52. Arnott MA, Hay J, Croft SL: Pentamidine: Which salt? Lancet 1:1057, 1988.
53. Masur H: Prevention and treatment of *Pneumocystis* pneumonia. N Engl J Med 327:1853, 1992.
54. Permethrin for head lice. Med Lett Drugs Ther 28:89, 1986.
55. Permethrin for scabies. Med Lett Drugs Ther 32:21, 1990.
56. Pearson RD, Guerrant RC: Praziquantel: A major advance in anthelminthic therapy. Ann Intern Med 99:195, 1983.
57. King CH, Mahmoud AAF: Drugs five years later: Praziquantel. Ann Intern Med 110:290, 1989.
58. Groll E: Praziquantel for cestode infections in man. Acta Trop 37:293, 1980.
59. Farid Z, Trabolsi B, Boctor F, et al: Unsuccessful use of praziquantel to treat acute fascioliasis in children. J Infect Dis 154:920, 1986.
60. Vasconcelos D, Cruz-Segura H, Mateos-Gomez H, et al: Selective indications for the use of praziquantel in the treatment of brain cysticercosis. J Neurol Neurosurg Psychiatry 50:383, 1987.
61. Rikus van Dellen J, McKeown CP: Praziquantel in active cerebral cysticercosis. Neurosurgery 22:92, 1988.
62. Grewal RS: Pharmacology of 8-amino-quinolines. Bull World Health Organ 59:397, 1981.
63. Clyde DF: Clnical problems associated with the use of primaquine as a tissue schizonticidal and gametocytocidal drug. Bull World Health Organ 59:391, 1981.
64. Jelinek T, Nothdurft HD, Von Sonnenburg E, et al: Long-term efficacy of primaquine in the treatment of vivax malaria in nonimmune travelers. Am J Trop Med Hyg 52:322, 1995.
65. Weiss WR, Oloo AJ, Johnson A, et al: Daily primaquine is effective prophylaxis against falciparum malaria in Kenya: Comparison with mefloquine, doxycycline, and chloroquine plus proguanil. J Infect Dis 171:1569, 1995.
66. Ruf B, Pohle HD: Clindamycin/primaquine for *Pneumocystis carinii* pneumonia. Lancet 2:626, 1989.
67. Fogh S, Schapira A, Bygbjerg IC, et al: Malaria prophylaxis in travelers to East Africa: A comparative prospective study of chloroquine plus proguanil with chloroquine plus sulfadoxine-pyrimethamine. Br Med J 296:820, 1988.
68. Gozal D, Hengy C, Fodat G: Prolonged malaria prophylaxis with chloroquine and proguanil (chloroguanide) in a nonimmune resident population of an endemic area with a high prevalence of chloroquine resistance. Antimicrob Agents Chemother 35:373, 1991.
69. Seah SKK: Pyrantel pamoate in treatment of helminthiasis in a nonendemic area. Southeast Asian J Trop Med Public Health 4:534, 1973.
70. Farahmandian I, Sahba GH, Arfaa F, et al: A comparative evaluation of the therapeutic effect of pyrantel pamoate and bephenium hydroxynaphthoate on *Ancylostoma duodenale* and other intestinal helminths. J Trop Med Hyg 75:205, 1972.
71. Bruce-Chwatt L (ed): Essential Malariology, ed 2. London, Heinemann, 1985, pp 226–227.
72. McCabe RE, Remington JS: The diagnosis and treatment of toxoplasmosis. Eur J Clin Microbiol 2:95, 1983.
73. Brown GV: Chemoprophylaxis of malaria. Med J Austr 159:187, 1993.
74. Cook IF: Inadequate prophylaxis of malaria with dapsone-pyrimethamine. Med J Aust 142:340, 1985.
75. Bruce-Chwatt LJ, Hutchinson DBA: Maloprim and agranulocytosis. Lancet 2:1487, 1983.
76. Centers for Disease Control and Prevention: Treatment with quinidine gluconate of persons with severe *Plasmodium falciparum* malaria: Discontinuation of parenteral quinine from CDC Drug Service. MMWR Morbid Mortal Wkly Rep 40(RR-4):21, 1991.
77. White NJ: The treatment of malaria. N Engl J Med 335:800, 1996.
78. Severe and Complicated Malaria, ed 2. World Health Organization Malaria Action Programme. Trans R Soc Trop Med Hyg 84(Suppl 2):1, 1990.
79. Desmonts G, Couvseur J: Congenital toxoplasmosis: A prospective study of 378 pregnancies. N Engl J Med 290:1110, 1974.
80. Berman JD: Chemotherapy for leishmaniasis: Biochemical mechanisms, clinical efficacy, and future strategies. Rev Infect Dis 10:560, 1988.
81. Herwaldt BL, Berman JD: Recommendations for treating leishmaniasis with sodium stibogluconate (Pentostam) and review of pertinent clinical studies. Am J Trop Med Hyg 46:296, 1992.
82. Hawking F: Suramin: With special reference to onchocerciasis. Adv Pharmacol Chemother 15:289, 1978.
83. Pang LW, Limsomwong N, Singharaj P: Prophylactic treatment of vivax and falciparum malaria with low dose doxycycline. J Infect Dis 158:1124, 1988.
84. Grove DI: Treatment of strongyloidiasis with thiabendazole: An analysis of toxicity and effectiveness. Trans R Soc Trop Med Hyg 76:114, 1982.
85. Campbell WC, Cuckler AC: Thiabendazole in the treatment and control of parasitic infections in man. Tex Rep Biol Med 27 (Suppl 2):665, 1969.
86. Davies HD, Sakuls P, Keystone JS: Creeping eruption. A review of clinical presentation and management of 60 cases presenting to a tropical disease unit. Arch Dermatol 129:558, 1993.

87. Kale OO, Elemile T, Enahoro F: Controlled comparative trial of thiabendazole and metronidazole in the treatment of dracontiasis. Ann Trop Med Parasitol 77:151, 1983.
88. Campbell WC, Blair LS: Chemotherapy of *Trichinella spiralis* infections (a review). Exp Parasitol 35:304, 1974.
89. Sawyer PF, Brogden RN, Pinder RM, et al: Tinidazole: A review of its antiprotozoal activity and therapeutic efficacy. Drugs 11:423, 1976.
90. Bassily S, Farid Z, El-Masry A, et al: Treatment of intestinal *E. histolytica* and *G. lamblia* with metronidazole, tinidazole, and ornidazole: A comparative study. J Trop Med Hyg 90:9, 1987.
91. Pape JW, Verdier R-I, Johnson WD: Treatment and prophylaxis of *Isospora belli* infection in patients with the acquired immunodeficiency syndrome. N Engl J Med 320:1044, 1989.
92. Hoge CW, Shlim DR, Ghimire M, et al: Placebo-controlled trial of co-trimoxazole for cyclospora infections among travellers and foreign residents in Nepal. Lancet 345:691, 1995.

36

Serum Therapy and Augmentation of the Host Response

Jeffrey K. Griffiths
David R. Snydman

Overview and History

Products of serum can treat, ameliorate, and prevent many infectious diseases, including many of major public health importance. These preparations are used in therapy when the patient is unable to mount an early or adequate humoral response to a pathogen or its toxins. Most beneficial properties of serum lie in the immunoglobulin fraction, which has been used for many decades in the prevention of infectious diseases. Serum therapy has a unique place in medicine, as the administration of serum and its products predated the antibiotic era.

Intravenous immunoglobulin (IVIG) has proved beneficial in a number of specific circumstances, such as the replacement of immunoglobulin in the permanently or transiently deficient host. Those with congenital agammaglobulinemia or immunoglobulin G (IgG) subclass deficiency with recurrent infections fit into this group. Another major role for immunoglobulin is in the administration of specific antibody for a specific infection. This is especially useful if no specific drug therapy exists, such as with rabies exposure or parvovirus infection. An evolving role for IVIG is in the combination therapy of viral infections, such as cytomegalovirus (CMV) pneumonia after transplantation, with concurrent high-titer hyperimmune antibody and antiviral drugs.

An area of active research is the use of IVIG and similar products in sepsis, which remains a major final pathway in many infections. Mortality in sepsis has remained high despite the use of antibiotics and intensive resuscitation methods. Monoclonal antibody therapy for sepsis has been intensively pursued, with the aim of augmenting the host's immune response in a direction that decreases mortality. Conceptually, monoclonal antibody therapy is most similar to hyperimmune globulin therapy for a specific infection, with a mediator of sepsis as the target rather than a specific pathogen. The targets for these antibodies have been either the bacterial initiators of the sepsis syndrome, such as endotoxin, or the cytokine cascade mediators that mediate the sepsis syndrome. Thus, the potential benefit for exogenous administration of cytokine mediators is large.

The modern era of serum therapy began with three of Robert Koch's students.[1] Emil Behring and Shibasaburo Kitasato developed a sheep antiserum to diphtheria toxin, which was given in 1891 to a girl dying of diphtheria, who recovered within hours and survived.[2] Paul Ehrlich produced and used horse antisera to tetanus toxin in 1897.[3] In the 1920s and 1930s, Maxwell Finland and colleagues demonstrated that early, specific treatment with animal immune sera was efficacious in conditions such as pneumococcal pneumonia.[4, 5] Serum preparations derived from human placentas[6] were shown to prevent and treat measles in 1935.[7] Cohn and colleagues[8] fractionated serum using cold ethanol and produced fractions highly enriched in γ-globulins. It was used in World War II to prevent hepatitis A and measles.[9] This preparation was used by Bruton[10] to treat a child with recurrent sepsis and agammaglobulinemia in 1951, beginning the era of replacement therapy for the immunodeficient host.

From this collective experience, central observations about immunotherapy (first enunciated in Finland) were made. These included the realization that immunotherapy reduces the mortality and morbidity related to infection, as long as early and specific diagnosis of the infection was made and early administration of immunoglobulins was accomplished. At that time, toxicity was common with animal preparations, such as horse hyperimmune sera to *Streptococcus pneumoniae*. These principles have meaning today. Current clinical trials with agents such as murine anti–tumor necrosis factor (TNF) monoclonal antibodies in the treatment of human sepsis strongly suggest that early recognition of the sepsis syndrome is crucial to successful action, and it is of interest that animal and not human monoclonal antibodies are being tested.

Intravenous (IV) use of early gamma globulin preparations was limited because of the risk of cardiovascular collapse and death. Intramuscular (IM) or subcutaneous injections were used, although these methods were limited by volumes that could be given, pain at the site of injection, and abscess formation. Moreover, in immunoglobulin A (IgA)–deficient patients, antiallotypic IgA antibody reactions limited the use of gamma globulin, which contains IgA. Plasma infusions were used by some, but many difficulties (hepatitis transmission, large volumes needed) remained.[11] IVIG administration was reinvestigated in the 1960s, and reactions were found to be related to protein aggregates and complement activation.[12] Technology developed in the late 1970s and 1980s to prevent complement activation by aggregates has rendered current human IV preparations relatively free of these problems and resulted in a rebirth of the use of IVIG.

We review the inherent characteristics and pharmacology of immune globulins (IGs), their potential side effects, and their uses in normal and immunodeficient hosts and address a number of miscellaneous states in which IGs may be salubrious.

Immune Globulin Characteristics: Preparation, Pharmacology, and Side Effects

IG is a preparation of human IGs pooled from blood donors or plasmapheresis patients. Unselected immune serum globulin contains antibodies to various viruses and microorganisms as reflected in the plasma pool of the population sampled. IG that has not been denatured has been shown to exhibit good opsonic activity against a large number of gram-negative and gram-positive bacterial species. In addition, antibody to a wide variety of viral and fungal organisms can be found.

Incremental advances have led to preparations that are safe for IV use (Table 36–1). This goal has been attained by a variety of means, including chemical treatment, pepsin digestion, diethylaminoethyl (DEAE) column chromatography, acidification, ultracentrifugation, and ultrafiltration.[13, 14] Ideally, immunoglobulin for IV use should be composed of the native molecules (IgG subclasses) in proportion to that found in serum, with full biologic properties, a pharmacokinetic profile similar to that seen with other gamma globulins, and no impurities. Theoretically, minimal alteration of the immunoglobulin molecule should protect maximal biologic activity. Because 1 in 600 people are IgA deficient,[15] immunoglobulin preparations should have minimal IgA to reduce the risk of antiallotypic allergic reactions. Some currently available gamma globulin is nearly pure monomeric IgG, with little or no IgA and without complement-activating properties. However, variations exist in chemical properties, antibody titers to specific pathogens, IgA, and IgG subclasses[14, 16–19] in commercial products.

Virus inactivation steps, such as a solvent-detergent step, need not alter the function of IVIG, as measured by in vitro assays of Fc functional activity.[20] A variety of steps, such as ethanol fractionation, polyethylene glycol (PEG) precipitation, solvent-detergent treatment, and pasteurization, have been tested against a variety of viral pathogens, such as human immunodeficiency virus (HIV), hepatitis C virus (HCV), mumps virus, vaccinia virus, chikungunya virus, vesicular stomatitis virus, Sindbis virus, and echovirus. In some circumstances, multiple steps are required to inactivate infectious virus particles.[21] For example, Louie and colleagues[22] have shown that coupling the cold ethanol Cohn-Oncley process with formulation at pH 4.25 caused a 10,000-fold decrease in bovine viral diarrhea virus intentionally added to the plasma pool and complete inactivation of 1000 chimpanzee infectious doses per milliliter of HCV.

When IG is given intravenously to IgG-deficient individuals, peak serum levels are proportional to the doses adminis-

TABLE 36–1 ■ Characteristics of Commercially Available Intravenous Immunoglobulin*

		IgG SUBCLASSES AS A PERCENTAGE OF TOTAL IgG				
PRODUCT	METHOD OF PREPARATION	IgG1	IgG2	IgG3	IgG4	IgA (μg/mL)
IVIG preparations						
Gammagard S/D (Baxter/Hyland); also marketed as Polygam S/D (American Red Cross/Hyland)	Cohn fractionation, DEAE-Sephadex adsorption and ultrafiltration, and detergent treatment; stabilization with 2% glucose, 0.22% glycine, 0.2% PEG, 0.3% albumin	72.1	22	5.5	0.4	<3.7 (<10)
Gammar-P IV (Armour)	Cohn fractionation, filtration, pasteurization (60°C for 10 h), sterile filtration; stabilized with albumin and sucrose	69	23	6	2	25
Gamimune N, 5% (Miles Biologics)	Cohn fractionation–effluent III ultrafiltration, followed by formulation at pH 4.5 in 10% maltose	58.7	29.3	6.3	5.1	270
Gamimune N, 10% (Miles Biologics)	Cohn fractionation–effluent III ultrafiltration, followed by formulation at pH 4.5 in 0.16–0.24 M glycine	71.1	22.2	5.3	1.4	113
Iveegam (Immuno AG)	Cohn fractionation, immobilized trypsin treatment, followed by PEG fractionation; stabilized in 5% glucose	60–70 (64.1)	30–40 (29.4)	0 (4.0)	2 (1.5)	<100 (<10)
Sandoglobulin	Cohn fractionation, pepsin treatment at pH 4; stabilization in 5% sucrose	60.5	30.2	6.6	2.6	720
Venoglobulin-I	Cohn fractionation, followed by PEG fractionation and DEAE-Sephadex treatment; stabilized with 2% mannitol and 1% albumin	60.9	29.4	5.3	4.4	20–24
Venoglobulin-S	Cohn fractionation, followed by PEG fractionation and DEAE-Sephadex treatment, treatment with tri-*n*-butyl phosphate (TNBP) and polysorbate 80, and stabilization with 5% sorbitol	65.7–67.2	23.7–25.3	5.7–5.9	3.0–3.4	11–14
Reference IgG (World Health Organization)		60.0	29.4	6.5	4.1	
CMV hyperimmune globulin (CMVIg; CytoGam) (Massachusetts State Biological Laboratories; MedImmune)	Cohn fractionation, ultrafiltration, stabilization with sucrose and albumin, 0.22-μm filter filtration, solvent detergent	65–66	27–28	5.2	1.7–1.8	30–200
Respiratory syncytial virus hyperimmune globulin (RSVIg; (RespiGam) (Massachusetts State Biological Laboratories and MedImmune)	Cohn fractionation, ultrafiltration, stabilization with sucrose and albumin, 0.22-μm filter filtration, solvent detergent	65–66	27–28	5.2	1.7–1.8	30–200

*Data are from manufacturers and published comparisons (published values are in parentheses). As preparations change, the reader is urged to review the specific manufacturer's package insert information before use. The most biologically relevant characteristics of IG preparations may be the specific neutralizing titers to specific pathogens, not the distribution of IgG subclasses.

tered. A doses of 200 mg/kg leads to an increase of about 100 mg/dL and a dose of 1 g/kg to an increase of about 500 mg/dL. Serum IgG levels peak and fall rapidly, but 3 to 7 days after infusion the levels stabilize at 35% to 50% of the peak serum level.[23–25] Thereafter, serum IgG levels fall slowly in an exponential fashion, reaching baseline levels in 3 to 4 weeks. This has been interpreted as meaning that IgG redistributes from the vascular compartment into the extravascular space, accounting for the rapid fall, and is then eliminated at a slower pace from all compartments in a terminal elimination phase. Other reasons for a rapid initial fall include elimination of denatured IgG, immune complex formation, high catabolic states, steroid administration before transplant surgery, and binding of target antigens. When given IM, immune serum globulin results in an increment in peak serum levels of IgG that is about half that of IVIG and also has a half-life of 21 to 28 days. Greater increases of serum levels occur with IV than with IM administration when identical amounts of globulin are given.

Elimination of administered IgG is rapid in protein-losing states, such as after burning.[26, 27] Some but not all premature neonates eliminate IgG quickly.[25] In bone marrow transplant recipients, the half-life of immune serum globulin, as measured by CMV antibody determination, may be as short as hours.[28] Half-lives between 6 and 15 days have been observed for CMV hyperimmune globulin in other transplant settings.[29] After liver or kidney transplantation, the CMV antibody half-life is approximately 7 to 8 days during the first 2 months and increases to 16 to 18 days in the third month.[30] It is thought that infection with a specific agent leads to depletion of specific antibody, accounting for the shortened half-life noted during CMV and pneumococcal infections.[31]

It is believed that the mechanism of action of exogenous IG is the same as that of endogenously produced antibody, and it has been reviewed by Schiff[31] and others.[32] Immunoglobulins are discussed comprehensively in Chapter 5. The specific activity of a lot of IVIG against a certain pathogen appears to be most related to the donor pool and not to the method of manufacture. It has been suggested that clinicians may wish in the future to select IVIG on the basis of pathogen-specific antibody,[33] which may vary from lot to lot. Alas, this information is rarely available in the clinical setting. Current U.S. Food and Drug Administration (FDA) regulations specify that IGs have a minimal titer only against diphtheria, poliomyelitis, measles, and hepatitis B.

High-dose IVIG (600 mg/kg per month) does not appear to substantially improve phagocytic function (phagocytosis, intracellular bactericidal activity, chemotaxis, superoxide production) over that seen with lower dose IVIG (200 mg/kg per month).[34] Meissner and colleagues[35] have discussed the functional properties of IVIG, with particular attention to its use in Kawasaki syndrome and respiratory syncytial virus (RSV) prophylaxis.

Our understanding of the effects of IVIG on the immune system is incomplete. Aukrust and coworkers[36] have documented striking changes in plasma cytokine and interleukin (IL)–1 receptor antagonist levels after the administration of 400 mg/kg IVIG to 12 individuals with primary agammaglobulinemia. These included rapid rises in IL-6, IL-8, and TNF-α, which are proinflammatory. Subsequently, there were prolonged elevations in soluble TNF receptors and in IL-1 receptor antagonist, suggestive of a counterregulatory response. These compounds regulate the inflammatory response, and thus these findings may be relevant to the effects of IVIG in immunologically mediated disorders.

Serious side effects of IVIG are rare.[19] More common, minor side effects of IVIG, such as mild fever, mild headache, chills, fatigue, and diarrhea, are reported in about one third to one half of all IVIG recipients. Immediate severe reactions related to intact IgG appear to be vanishingly rare. IVIG should be administered cautiously to individuals with high levels of serum IgG, to decrease the risk of hyperviscosity syndromes, or to those with immune complex disease. It has been suggested that IVIG, given to raise platelet counts in patients with idiopathic thrombocytopenic purpura, could lead to thrombosis in individuals with severe atherosclerosis; the evidence for this is slight. Fears that high-dose IVIG, by blocking reticuloendothelial system clearance, could lead to decreased opsonization of bacterial or fungal pathogens also do not appear substantiated. As alluded to earlier, a reaction after IVIG administration in IgA-deficient individuals may occur, although it is unusual, and IVIG preparations with little IgA can be chosen for use in this circumstance. Aseptic meningitis, secondary to high-dose IVIG (2 g/kg) for the treatment of various immune-related neuromuscular diseases, has been reported to be more common in those with a history of migraine.[37] It can rarely occur after use of IVIG at normal doses.[38] Acute renal failure has been described as a rare complication of IVIG, with no evidence to date of immune complex–mediated, or inflammatory, renal disease.[39] This complication varies from asymptomatic decreases in glomerular filtration rates to anuric renal failure, usually with rapid recovery of function after cessation of therapy. As with any other manufactured product given intravenously, there is a risk of contamination or of infusion of infected material. It appears that IVIG is not supportive of bacterial growth but does support the growth of yeast at 25°C or 37°C in vitro.[40]

A major theoretical concern has been the potential transmission of blood-borne pathogens, such as HIV, hepatitis B virus, and HCV.[41] Before the advent of blood product screening for HIV, there were reports of false-positive HIV antibody test results after the administration of IVIG, representing passive transfer of antibody in the immunoglobulin. It has been demonstrated that HIV is inactivated by the Cohn-Oncley fractionation method for preparing IVIG, with an estimated[42, 43] reduction in HIV titer during IVIG manufacture on the order of 10^{15}. The use of screening for HIV antibody in blood donors and the use of the Cohn-Oncley procedure render the risk of HIV transmission essentially zero.

However, hepatitis C transmission has been documented in patients with primary hypogammaglobulinemia after treatment with IG.[44] Several commercial and experimental lots of IVIG from one manufacturer have been found to contain HCV RNA by polymerase chain reaction detection. Ethanol, which is used in the manufacture of IVIG by the Cohn-Oncley process, does not appear to affect HCV RNA at concentrations up to 25%.[45] This finding may help explain why HCV, unlike some other viruses such as HIV, may be found in some commercial preparations.

Paradoxically, lots of IVIG that lack antibody to HCV may be more likely to transmit HCV than lots with anti-HCV antibody. Yu and coworkers[46] have reported the detection of infectious HCV RNA in lots of IVIG manufactured by Baxter Healthcare, which withdrew its IVIG preparation Gammagard in February 1994 because of reports of HCV transmission. Of lots of plasma that had been screened and found negative for anti-HCV antibody, 20 of 24 were positive for HCV RNA by polymerase chain reaction assays. It has been suggested that this finding indicates that the presence of anti-HCV antibody in the IVIG plasma pools may assist in partitioning the infectious virus during the manufacturing process. Others have concluded on the basis of HCV RNA polymerase chain reaction testing that the reason for the Gammagard-associated HCV infections was probably the use of HCV-contaminated plasma and the lack of a potent HCV-inactivating step during production.[47] Consistent with this line of reasoning was the finding that chimpanzees that received unprocessed plasma from a pool of 2887 HCV-seronegative donors contracted HCV, but chimpanzees that received IVIG processed from the same plasma pool did not contract HCV. These studies suggest that withholding plasma that is HCV-seropositive does not render a plasma pool noninfectious and that the safety of IVIG manufactured from such pools is not compromised by withholding the seropositive units. Previous experience with hepatitis B suggests that antibody to hepatitis B surface antigen may assist in inactivating or precipitating the hepatitis B particle during manufacture.[48, 49] Thus, screening of donors may decrease the viral burden in plasma pools used for IVIG manufacture but may exclude antibody useful in inactivating infectious viruses.

Between 1983 and 1994, there were at least 17 reports of transmission of non-A, non-B hepatitis or transaminitis connected with the use of six different IVIG preparations. The latter were produced without including a validated virus inactivation method during manufacture. Key elements of safe IVIG production and safety from viral transmission must include minimization of virus contamination in the source plasma, good manufacturing practices, and the use of a rigorous virus inactivation procedure.[50] As a result of the outbreaks of hepatitis C, the FDA now requires evidence of HCV inactivation with a virus inactivation step, typically use of a solvent detergent or acidic pH, or evidence that no HCV RNA can be detected by the polymerase chain reaction.

Commercial lots of IVIG contain detectable levels of antibody to pathogens such as hepatitis B virus and CMV, and these passively transferred antibodies may confound the interpretation of laboratory studies.[51]

Cost

The cost of IG preparations varies widely, from only a dollar or so per milliliter of IG for IM administration to thousands of dollars for a monthly course of IVIG. Lifelong dependence on IVIG replacement is expensive. In the Boston region in January 1996, wholesale hospital pharmacy costs for 1 g of IVIG varied between $24 for volume customers to double that price on the spot market (St. Elizabeth's Medical Center Department of Pharmacy). Thus, the current cost of IVIG alone, at a dose of 400 mg/kg per month for a 70-kg individual, approaches $8640 wholesale per year. For the uninsured individual or small facility that has to pay these costs, the price might be double. To this sum must be added the costs of medical supervision and IVIG administration.

Home IV therapy has been touted as an inexpensive alternative to in-hospital therapy, as the cost of hospitalization is eliminated. Among 13 companies surveyed in New Jersey, the highest priced company charged approximately four times as much as the lowest priced company, and many agencies offered IVIG therapy at moderate costs. Thus, comparative pricing may significantly reduce the cost to the patient or health care system.[52] Hyperimmune preparations are usually far more potent than unselected preparations and may be less costly overall than larger amounts of less potent preparations. In addition, use of prophylactic CMV hyperimmune globulin after transplantation appears to be cost-effective.[53]

Prophylaxis and Treatment in the Normal Host

The normal host has relatively little need for immune serum globulin or IVIG, and there is little indication for its use. For example, IM immune serum globulin does not appear to reduce the frequency of otitis media in children with normal levels of IgG and recurrent episodes of otitis media.[54] There is no indication for serum product use in normal hosts without exposure to a specific pathogen. It was found decades ago that IM immune serum globulin prevented clinical illness caused by a number of specific pathogens such as diphtheria, tetanus, and measles in closed populations (such as army recruits or asylum residents) during an epidemic with the same pathogen. Indeed, this concept of specific exposure prophylaxis has led to the development of hyperimmune globulin preparations.

Use of Unselected Intramuscular Immune Serum Globulin

Traditionally, unselected IM immune serum globulin has been used for hepatitis A prophylaxis[55] as outlined in Table 36–2. Despite the availability of hepatitis A vaccine, IM globulin remains an attractive option for prophylaxis after exposure to hepatitis A because of its rapidity of action, low cost, and wide availability. Similarly, immune serum globulin can prevent or ameliorate measles in the normal host. Unselected IG may also be used when hyperimmune globulin preparations are not available for exposures to tetanus or hepatitis B, although hyperimmune globulin is preferable. Given the current requirement to screen plasma donors for the absence of antibody to hepatitis C, there is probably no longer any role for immune serum globulin after hepatitis C exposure.

Use of Hyperimmune Globulins

Hyperimmune globulins derived from donor pools of individuals immunized to, or selected for, specific pathogens with high titer to the pathogen or its toxin have been useful (see Table 36–2). The rationale for the production of hyperimmune globulins is to ensure lot-to-lot consistency of antibody titers with enriched preparations that may have some in vitro consistency as well. The incremental antibody titers of these hyperimmune preparations can be large. For example, unselected immune serum globulin has an anti–hepatitis B titer of 1:100, whereas the hepatitis B IG has an anti–hepatitis B surface antigen titer of 1:100,000.[56] For varicella-zoster and tetanus immune globulins, the hyperimmune antibody titers are approximately four- to eightfold higher than in the unselected preparations. Specific indications exist for the use of these hyperimmune globulin preparations for normal and immunodeficient hosts at risk of acquiring certain diseases[57, 58] (see Table 36–2). Diseases included in this category are hepatitis B, measles, rabies, varicella, vaccinia, tetanus, CMV infection, and pertussis. An RSV hyperimmune preparation has also been licensed for use in neonates and those with cardiopulmonary disorders[59] and is discussed later in this chapter.

Animal preparations of hyperimmune globulins are available in the developing world and the developed world for the treatment of some infectious diseases, such as rabies, diphtheria, botulism, and tetanus.[60] Being efficacious, they are preferable to no treatment at all, but they have more side effects. Equine antibody preparations are available in the United States from the Centers for Disease Control and Prevention (CDC; telephone 401-639-3670, 24 hours a day) against types A, B, and E botulism, diphtheria, tetanus, Western equine encephalitis, and vaccinia.

There is no intellectual reason why hyperimmune serum has to be limited to a single antigen or pathogen. For example, immunization and subsequent plasmapheresis of volunteers against a number of bacterial polysaccharide antigens (*S. pneumoniae*, *Haemophilus influenzae*, and *Neisseria meningitidis*) have been used to manufacture a polyvalent hyperimmune globulin termed bacterial polysaccharide IG. In studies of Apache infants, a group at high risk of developing *H. influenzae* type b and pneumococcal infections, protection

TABLE 36–2 ■ Indications for Unselected Immune Globulins and Hyperimmune Globulins in the Prevention of Specific Infectious Diseases

INFECTION	INDICATION	GLOBULIN PREPARATION AND DOSE
Botulism	Treatment and prevention of botulism in ingestor of botulinus toxin	Trivalent (types A, B, and E) specific equine antibody; call CDC (404-639-3670). Does not reverse toxin already bound to nerve endings but neutralizes circulating unbound toxin. Serum sickness seen in ~10% of treated patients.
Cytomegalovirus infection	Prophylaxis and treatment of CMV in CMV-seronegative kidney transplant recipients of CMV-seropositive donors	See package insert; hyperimmune anti-CMV IVIG is given IV.
Diphtheria	Respiratory diphtheria—probably no role in cutaneous diphtheria	Call CDC at 404-639-3670.*
Hepatitis A	Postexposure prophylaxis: family contacts; sexual contacts; institutional or daycare center outbreaks	Unselected IG; 0.02 mL/kg, up to 2 mL total for defined exposures. Administration more than 2 wk after exposure is not likely to be beneficial.
	Preexposure prophylaxis in travelers	0.06 mL/kg up to 5 mL for long-term travel, with repeated doses at intervals of 4–6 mo. Hepatitis A vaccine may replace IG in most preexposure situations. IG use does not replace avoidance behaviors, such as careful selection of safe food and water.
Hepatitis B	Percutaneous or mucosal exposure	Hepatitis B IG (HBIG); hyperimmune preparation; 0.06 mL/kg. Vaccinate with hepatitis B vaccine if repeated exposure (e.g., health care worker) is likely.*
	Newborns of hepatitis B surface antigen–positive mothers	HBIG, 0.5 mL at birth, and vaccinate with hepatitis B vaccine.
	Sexual contacts of persons with acute or chronic hepatitis B	HBIG, 0.06 mL/kg, and vaccinate with hepatitis B vaccine.*
Measles	Nonimmune contacts of acute cases exposed fewer than 6 d previously	Unselected IG 0.25 mL/kg up to 15 mL for normal hosts, 0.5 mL/kg up to 15 mL for immunocompromised persons.
Rabies	Exposure to rabid or potentially rabid animals, such as a bite injury, salivary contact, or aerosol	Hyperimmune rabies immune globulin, HRIG, 20 IU/kg IM, with half given in the region of the exposure.
Respiratory syncytial virus (RSV) infection	Prophylaxis of RSV infection in children with bronchopulmonary dysplasia or prematurity	Hyperimmune, monthly administration to susceptible children and neonates during the RSV transmission season.
Tetanus	Contaminated wound injury *and* either an uncertain tetanus toxoid vaccination history or a history of less than three doses of tetanus toxoid	Tetanus (hyper)immune globulin (TIG); 250 units IM if prior tetanus immunization history is unknown or if less than three doses of tetanus toxoid have been administered and if the wound is contaminated, for example, by feces, saliva, or dirt, or is a puncture wound, or is the result of a crush, burn, frostbite, or missile injury.*
Vaccinia	Severe reaction to vaccinia vaccination	Hyperimmune preparation, available from CDC (404-639-3670).
Varicella-zoster	*Substantial* exposure by immunosuppressed or newborn contacts, such as household contacts of the index case; close indoor contact lasting more than 1 h; sharing the same hospital room with an infected person; prolonged face-to-face contact with an infected person, such as occurs with nurses and physicians	Hyperimmune preparation; varicella-zoster IG (VZIG); 125 units/10 kg up to a maximum of 625 units. Higher doses in immunosuppressed adults may be necessary (insufficient data available). Fractional doses are not recommended (e.g., given in aliquots of 125 units). Pregnant women and infants born to mothers in whom varicella develops within 5 d or before 48 h after delivery should also receive VZIG. VZIG does not prevent infection but ameliorates the disease.*

*If hyperimmune preparations are not available and administration of VZIG, TIG, HBIG, or equine antidiphtheria globulins is indicated, unselected IG or IVIG may be given although the efficacy of unselected preparations is probably less than that of hyperimmune globulins. HIBG should be given at a dose of 0.06 mL/kg in this circumstance.

against serious *H. influenzae* type b or pneumococcal disease could be demonstrated after prophylaxis with bacterial polysaccharide IG.[61]

Augmentation of the Normal Response: Gram-Negative Bacterial Sepsis

There is intense interest in the use of IVIG or other similar products in gram-negative sepsis, which continues to result in high mortality despite aggressive use of antimicrobial agents and intravascular volume expanders.[62] Many studies have investigated the relative contributions of bacterial products (e.g., endotoxin) and host mediators (e.g., cytokines) in the sepsis syndrome, with the hope that antibody binding of these products will increase survival during sepsis.[63] Immune plasma from volunteers immunized with the J-5 *Escherichia coli* mutant prevented death in patients with gram-negative sepsis[64] and reduced infectious complications (but not overall mortality) in high-risk surgical patients.[65] Results of subsequent studies using plasma and IV gamma globulin were not as favorable,[66, 67] whereas somewhat more positive results were found with the use of a human or murine monoclonal IgM antiendotoxin antibody in a subset of patients with the sepsis syndrome caused by gram-negative organisms.[68, 69] These differences may be explained by the relatively low capacity of unselected IgG, and the relatively high capacity of hyperimmune or monoclonal IgM, to bind endotoxin and thus possibly to prevent shock related to endotoxin release. Nonetheless, overall, the treatment of sepsis with unselected IVIG or with antibody to endotoxin components has not proved statistically beneficial.[70, 71] Sepsis can be caused by organisms without endotoxin such as *Staphylococcus aureus*; moreover, once endotoxin has initiated the cytokine cascade that leads to the sepsis syndrome, antiendotoxin antibody therapy may be too late. Efforts have focused on the cytokine mediators of sepsis, which come into play after endotoxin release and which are the final common mediators of sepsis no matter what the etiology.[72, 73] TNF-α, IL-1β, IL-6, and IL-8 are consistently found elevated during sepsis.[74, 75] IL-1 receptor antagonist therapy seemed to have benefit in early trials and probably resulted in fewer deaths in a subsegment of patients but not overall.[76, 77] Current trials are investigating compounds such as anti-TNF murine monoclonal antibodies administered within hours of the onset of sepsis. Discussion of these mediators can be found in Chapter 9.

Prophylaxis and Treatment of the Deficient Host

Replacement Therapy of the Congenitally Deficient Host (Table 36–3)

Bruton's original description[10] of agammaglobulinemia and recurrent sepsis, controlled by IM gamma globulin, was of a child with X-linked hypogammaglobulinemia. Given the obvious benefit of IM IG, no controlled trial comparing IG with placebo was ever conducted, but few doubt the lifesaving consequences of IG in this situation. Subsequent randomized trials have demonstrated the superiority of IVIG over the IM product in the treatment of congenital hypogammaglobulinemia. High-dose IV therapy (i.e., 200 to 500 mg/kg per month) has been shown to be associated with fewer infections and decreased use of antibiotics compared with lower doses.[78] Other primary humoral deficiency states warrant IVIG prophylaxis. These include transient hypogammaglobulinemia of infancy, especially if accompanied by symptomatic infections; common variable immunodeficiency, especially if IgG levels fall below 250 mg/dL; X-linked hyper-IgM syndrome; and selective deficiency of IgG subclasses.[79, 80] Although total IgG may not be decreased in the last condition, replacement therapy is indicated.[81] Selective immunoglobulin deficiencies are being recognized as part of other syndromes, such as congenital heart disease and Down syndrome,[82–84] and replacement therapy may become part of standard management in these diseases. IgA deficiency is regarded as a contraindication to IVIG treatment, given the possibility of anti-IgA–mediated anaphylaxis, although some individuals with IgA and IgG subclass deficiency may benefit from IVIG.[85]

Another set of indications for the use of IVIG includes combined immunodeficiencies, in which abnormal T-lymphocyte function is associated with antibody production defects. Thus, individuals with ataxia-telangiectasia, Wiskott-Aldrich syndrome, hyper-IgE syndrome, or DiGeorge syndrome benefit from IVIG. Individuals with X-linked lymphoproliferative syndromes or Chédiak-Higashi disease may also reasonably receive IVIG.[86, 87]

TABLE 36–3 ■ Recommended and Probably or Possibly Beneficial (Investigational) Uses of Intravenous Immunoglobulin in the Augmentation of the Host Response

PRIMARY IMMUNODEFICIENCY SYNDROMES

Recommended use
- Agammaglobulinemia
- Ataxia-telangiectasia
- Common variable immunodeficiency
- DiGeorge syndrome
- Selective antibody deficiency (e.g., subclass deficiency) with a history of recurrent infections
- Severe combined immunodeficiency
- Short-limbed dwarfism
- Wiskott-Aldrich syndrome
- X-linked lymphoproliferative syndrome
- X-linked hyper-IgM syndrome
- X-linked agammaglobulinemia

Possible use*
- Congenital heart disease
- Down syndrome

ACQUIRED IMMUNODEFICIENCY SYNDROMES

Recommended
- Transplantation

Possible use*
- Neonatal sepsis
- After surgery or trauma
- Protein-losing nephropathy if total serum IgG < 600 mg/dL
- HIV-seropositive children
- Chronic lymphocytic leukemia†
- Multiple myeloma†

Recommended
- Hemorrhagic virus infections (immune plasma) such as Lassa fever or Argentinian hemorrhagic fever
- Kawasaki disease (mucocutaneous lymph node syndrome)
- Parovirus B19 infection
- RSV infection prevention in children and neonates with either bronchopulmonary dysplasia or prematurity

Possible use*
- Enteric infections with agents such as *Clostridium difficile* or *Cryptosporidium* using hyperimmune preparations
- Hepatitis C after exposure
- Prevention of necrotizing enterocolitis in premature neonates
- Toxic shock syndrome

*As yet unproved. Routine use of IVIG is *not* recommended at this time.
†May not be cost-effective; selection of patients is urged.

Replacement Therapy and Prophylaxis of the Transiently Deficient Host (see Table 36–3)

NEONATAL SEPSIS

Premature neonates are deficient in antibody and are at great risk of serious infection. Most maternal antibody crosses the placenta only after 34 weeks of gestation, and IgG2 subclass molecules are poorly transferred, as are IgM and IgA. Moreover, premature neonates have decreased complement and fibronectin levels, impaired phagocyte function, low levels of cytokine production, and small marrow reserves of neutrophils.[88–91] Although the indications for the use of IVIG in neonatal sepsis are still unclear, both fresh-frozen plasma and IVIG are becoming widely used for prophylaxis against, and treatment for, neonatal infections.

A large multicenter placebo-controlled double-blind study of 587 infants weighing 500 to 1750 g at birth revealed that IVIG at 500 mg/kg given periodically led to a significant decrease (approximately 30%) in the risk of a first nosocomial infection and, in infants with an infection, a decrease in the mean number of hospital days (from 101 to 80 days).[92] Another study of 753 neonates who were randomized to receive either IVIG at 500 mg/kg with high opsonic activity to group B streptococci or albumin found that survival during the first 7 days was higher in septic infants receiving IVIG, but by 8 weeks of age no significant difference in mortality was present.[93] A comparison of granulocyte transfusions versus 1000 mg/kg per day for the first 3 days of sepsis in neutropenic premature neonates showed higher survival in the group given granulocytes, but the dose of IVIG was so high that Fc receptor blockade may have occurred in the IVIG treatment group.[94]

Although some studies have suggested that prophylactic IVIG is useful in the prevention of infections in neonatal intensive care units, especially in the developing world, others have failed to show any efficacy, including those in the developing world.[95] One potential explanation for this contradictory set of data is the rise in infections caused by nosocomial (and otherwise unusual) pathogens such as *Staphylococcus epidermidis* in neonatal intensive care units. Many lots of IVIG derived from normal population pools may lack antibody to these unusual pathogens and thus not be able to offer any protection to the neonate.[96]

A single dose of IVIG soon after birth does not appear to decrease the risk of infection in the subsequent several months. In a large multicenter, randomized, double-blind, controlled trial,[97] 753 premature (gestational age 34 weeks or less) neonates with birth weights of 500 to 2000 g were randomly selected to receive a single IV infusion (10 mL/kg) of either IVIG (500 mg/kg) or albumin (5 mg/kg) within 12 hours of birth and were observed for 8 weeks for infection. This single infusion of IVIG did not result in a diminution of late-onset sepsis or infection in these neonates.

In the United States, group B *Streptococcus* and gram-negative enteric bacilli such as *E. coli* are the major cause of death resulting from sepsis in premature neonates.[98] Low maternal antibody levels to group B streptococci correlated with neonatal susceptibility to group B streptococcal infections.[99] Group B streptococcal immune or hyperimmune serum can be lifesaving to human neonates or animal models[100–104] if given early in infection. Studies from Europe and the Middle East have shown fewer deaths in IVIG-treated neonates.[105–109] However, it has been speculated that extremely high dose IVIG (2 g/kg) may impair host defenses[110] via blockade of the reticuloendothelial system, and extremely high doses of IVIG given with antibiotics to animals infected with group B streptococci increased mortality in one study.[111] Thus, the dose of IVIG must not be excessive, or it may adversely the patient. In addition, problems with the study designs and differences in pathogens leave it unclear whether all premature neonates should be treated with IVIG.[86–88, 112, 113]

Viral infections are also of major importance in neonates. In one study, prophylaxis for viral infection with IVIG in premature neonates (500 mg/kg in the first week of life, 7 days later, and then every 14 days for a maximum of five doses) did not prevent or alter CMV or adenovirus disease.[114] In contrast, CMV hyperimmune globulin (CMVIG) given to prevent CMV disease in multiply transfused premature neonates showed a trend toward benefit with fewer clinical CMV syndromes (14% versus 4%, $P = .18$), fewer ventilator days, and shorter hospital stay compared with neonates given albumin.[115] A conclusive answer to the benefit of CMVIG in premature neonates requires a larger cohort of infants.

Several recurrent elements are worth noting. First, the neonates at risk are deficient in defenses and at higher risk of sepsis than older children or adults. Second, hyperimmune or enriched preparations of IVIG appeared to be more efficacious than unselected IVIG in a number of studies, and experimental data strongly suggest that high titers of antibody to the pathogens involved in neonatal sepsis are desirable. Third, local factors such as the incidence of sepsis overall and the identity of the pathogens (common or nosocomial) may strongly affect any benefit of IVIG. Last, any benefit of extremely high-dose IVIG may be masked by its effects on the function of the immune system. In sum, the efficacy of unselected IG as general prophylaxis for bacterial sepsis in neonates is unproved, but the trend of studies is toward benefit. Which subgroups of neonates benefit, how to select IVIG on the basis of titers to specific pathogens, and the cost-effectiveness of this approach remain unresolved.

In the future it may prove true that specific hyperimmune serum products are more beneficial than unselected preparations for neonatal sepsis. An ideal IVIG preparation for the prevention of severe infections in neonates should perhaps be prepared from a population-based IVIG plasma pool supplemented by hyperimmune antibodies to specific pathogens, such as the common pathogens group B *Streptococcus* and *E. coli*, and nosocomial pathogens such as *S. epidermidis* and *Pseudomonas aeruginosa*.

ADULT SEPSIS

The role of IVIG in sepsis in adults has not been as intensively studied as that in neonates, perhaps because most adults are at much lower risk of sepsis and do not have the immunologic deficiencies of neonates outlined in the previous section. In addition, adults with sepsis are a far more heterogeneous population than neonates, and studies of prophylaxis are far harder to conduct in this group. Several trials have shown benefit of IVIG in preventing intensive care–related severe infections, yet a number of other studies have shown no benefit of the administration of hyperimmune antibodies directed against components of the sepsis cascade, such as endotoxin.[116] It appears that most commercial and academic interest in the prevention or treatment of sepsis in adults is focused on mediators of sepsis, such as endotoxin or cytokine mediators.

BURNS

In thermal burns, the major cause of death is sepsis resulting from opportunistic bacteria, such as *P. aeruginosa*.[117] Serum immunoglobulin levels fall rapidly after burns, and the size of the decrement is related to the size of the burn.[118] IG enriched in antibody to *P. aeruginosa* was protective when burned mice were inoculated with *Pseudomonas*.[119] Studies with IM IG in burn patients have produced contradictory results.[120, 121] One study found an antipseudomonal polyvalent vaccine or IM hyperimmune IG, in conjunction with antimicrobials, to be superior than antimicrobials alone for preventing death of burned patients.[122] However, a prospective, randomized, double-blind placebo-controlled study of IVIG (500 mg/kg) given twice weekly to 50 seriously burned patients found no difference in outcome[123]; similarly, a trial of IVIG at 500 mg/kg for 1 week versus albumin showed no difference in mortality.[124] Further studies are needed before IG can be recommended for burn patients.

MAJOR SURGERY AND TRAUMA

Surgery results in a temporary immunodeficiency state, called by some the postsurgery or posttraumatic immunodeficiency syndrome. This syndrome is characterized by elevations in serum acute-phase reactants, IL-2 receptors, and neopterin, concurrent with declines in serum immunoglobulins, complement components, circulating T cells, and natural killer cells.[125] The use of IVIG has been investigated in this syndrome both to replace antibody and to modulate the inflammatory changes.[126] In a multicenter double-blind study of 329 patients comparing placebo, IVIG, and IVIG high in antibody to endotoxin, a subset of patients who had undergone major surgical procedures appeared to have benefited from standard IVIG but not the hyperimmune preparation.[127] In another study of patients with gastrointestinal cancer, 159 patients were given either 15 g of IVIG on days 1 and 5 after surgery or placebo. Patients who had undergone colon surgery but not others appeared to have benefited from IVIG, although there was a trend toward benefit in the group overall.[128] These studies point out the need to conduct large randomized studies to evaluate any potential benefit of IVIG therapy and to identify subgroups in whom efforts should be concentrated.

CHRONIC LYMPHOCYTIC LEUKEMIA, MULTIPLE MYELOMA, AND CHEMOTHERAPY

Much of the γ-globulin produced by people with chronic lymphocytic leukemia (CLL), multiple myeloma (MM), or Waldenström macroglobulinemia is nonfunctional, and infection becomes increasingly common as the disease progresses.[129, 130] IVIG is known to reduce the number of bacterial infections in B-cell CLL, in which hypogammaglobulinemia is common. IVIG, 400 mg/kg given every 3 weeks, decreased by half the number of bacterial infections in people with CLL.[131, 132] In an attempt to determine the amount of IVIG needed to prevent infectious complications, Jurlander and colleagues[133] in Denmark gave 15 patients with CLL 10 g of IVIG every 3 weeks, which stabilized serum immunoglobulin levels just above the lower limit of normal after 11 doses. The number of hospitalizations and febrile episodes during therapy fell by 69% and 51%, respectively, compared with the pretherapy period. Similarly, Gamm and coworkers[134] found that doses of IVIG as low as 250 mg/kg per 4 weeks decreased the rate of infection in CLL. In a cautionary note, one study of patients with CLL has suggested that IVIG replacement is not cost-effective, as its benefits do not lead to reduced mortality despite reductions in infections.[135]

The benefit of IG in MM has been less clear. One early study with IM IG showed no benefit[136]; in contrast, evidence has been reported from a prospective, crossover study that higher doses of IVIG are beneficial.[137] IVIG does appear to decrease the incidence of severe bacterial infections in people with stable-phase MM. A double-blind, randomized, placebo-controlled multicenter study has shown a major impact of IVIG on infections in those with plateau-phase MM.[138] Eighty-two patients with stable plateau-phase MM received IVIG at 400 mg/kg per month or placebo during 1 year. Concurrent chemotherapy was not altered, and no one received prophylactic antibiotics. There were major decreases in the incidence of pneumonia or sepsis and the overall incidence of infections in the group given IVIG. This protective effect was most marked in patients with a poor (less than twofold increase) response to pneumococcal vaccine (Pneumovax), suggesting that a subpopulation of those with MM and altered humoral immunity can be identified and treated with IVIG. On the basis of this information, prophylactic IVIG is likely to be beneficial for patients with advanced CLL or MM, although more information is needed. There is no evidence that standard IG reduces the incidence of infection during chemotherapy,[139] and its use is not advocated.

NEPHROSIS AND PROTEIN-LOSING ENTEROPATHIES

Infection has long been recognized as a complication of the nephrotic syndrome. People with these conditions are frequently hypogammaglobulinemic and individuals may benefit from IG therapy,[140] but few controlled studies have been conducted from which to generalize. Among 86 consecutive adults with nephrotic syndrome and no diabetes, the relative risk of infection in individuals with a serum IgG level below 600 mg/dL was 6.74 times higher than in individuals with a serum IgG concentration above 600 mg/dL.[141] This risk of infection was independent of the increased risk (5.31-fold) seen in those with creatinine values above 2.0 mg/dL. When IVIG was administered prospectively to patients with serum IgG levels below 600 mg/dL to raise it above that level, the rate of infection was reduced to that seen in those whose unmanipulated serum level was higher than 600 mg/dL. We believe that further studies in this area are warranted given these encouraging results.

Prophylaxis and Treatment in Transplantation

The major risk of death in transplantation is from infection related to immunosuppression. The most common and significant infection is that with CMV.[142] CMV infection is associated with graft rejection, superinfections with both bacterial and fungal pathogens, serious morbidity, and death. Antirejection therapy, especially with OKT3 antibody or antilymphocyte serum, may increase the likelihood of infectious complications.[143] In those who undergo bone marrow transplantation, an additional risk is graft-versus-host disease. High doses of IVIG or CMVIG attenuate the severity of CMV disease and appear to significantly improve survival in kidney and bone marrow transplantation.[144, 145] The benefit of IG therapy is most marked in CMV-seronegative kidney transplant recipients whose donors are seropositive.

In a series of prospective studies of CMV-seronegative recipients of kidney transplants from seropositive donors, using CMVIG given within 72 hours of transplantation and then at 2, 4, 6, 8, 12, and 16 weeks, highly significant reductions in CMV-associated syndromes (from 60% in control subjects to 31% in CMVIG recipients) were seen, as well as decreases of about 50% in graft loss and overall death. Fungal and parasitic superinfections were markedly reduced in CMVIG recipients, with an overall reduction in incidence from 20% to 4%. It appears that CMV-induced immunosuppression, which when combined with transplantation provides the milieu for opportunistic fungal and protozoan infections, may be prevented by CMVIG. This appears true despite the fact that CMVIG does not appear to significantly alter infection rates in transplant recipients.[146–148] Allograft rejection is often linked to CMV infection, and reducing the rate of symptomatic CMV disease with CMVIG may protect the allograft from damage. Furthermore, prophylaxis with CMVIG appears to be cost-effective.[149]

In a review of clinical uses for IVIG during marrow transplantation,[144] Berkman and colleagues pooled the results of six controlled trials of prophylactic IgG for CMV infections in bone marrow transplantation[149–154] and concluded that prophylactic IgG decreases the incidence of CMV infection proceeding to interstitial pneumonia and of acute graft-versus-host disease. A study of IVIG in bone marrow transplantation patients showed, in patients who received IVIG, a marked diminution in interstitial pneumonia; a decreased relative risk of gram-negative sepsis and local infections; and, in patients 20 years of age or older, a reduction in the incidence of acute graft-versus-host disease and a decrease in deaths in some human leukocyte antigen–identical subgroups.[155] Several intravenous IGs have licensed indications for prevention of graft-versus-host disease.

Unlike the data for IVIG in prophylaxis, there is no evidence that CMVIG or unselected IVIG alone is useful in the therapy of CMV pneumonia in bone marrow transplantation. Ten of 14 bone marrow recipients with biopsy-proven CMV pneumonia who received CMVIG as treatment died.[156] CMV pneumonia in bone marrow transplantation, usually a lethal complication, has been treated successfully with a combination of IVIG and ganciclovir,[157, 158] neither of which, alone, provides any clear therapeutic benefit. Schmidt and colleagues[159] have shown in a randomized, controlled trial in which asymptomatic CMV-seropositive bone marrow transplant recipients who had positive culture results for CMV (as shown by bronchoalveolar lavage at day 35 after transplantation) and received prophylactic ganciclovir in addition to high-dose IVIG died less frequently (5 of 20, 25%) than control subjects who received IVIG alone (14 of 20, 70%, $P = .01$). Culture-negative marrow recipients who received IVIG alone had a 22% incidence of CMV pneumonia, similar to the 25% in those who had positive culture results and received dual prophylaxis. On the basis of these data, probably all individuals undergoing bone marrow transplantation should receive high-dose IVIG primarily to prevent graft-versus-host disease but also for the secondary benefits of action against CMV disease. A subset of CMV-seropositive patients benefit from additional ganciclovir prophylaxis.

In heart transplant recipients, CMV hyperimmune IG may reduce the severity of CMV disease.[160] Confirmatory studies are needed before IG use can be generally advocated in heart or heart-lung transplantation.

Two studies examining IVIG use in liver transplant recipients suggested trends in reduction of CMV disease.[161, 162] In a randomized, double-blind, placebo-controlled trial of CMVIG in liver transplantation, globulin reduced the rate of CMV disease from 31% in the placebo group to 19% in the treated group, although, as might be expected, the infection rate was similar (61% and 57%).[163] A retrospective analysis of 39 primary orthotopic liver transplants revealed no symptomatic CMV disease or deaths after prophylaxis with CMVIG and ganciclovir. In this study, ganciclovir alone was reported to be ineffective as CMV prophylaxis[164]; in a study of ganciclovir or acyclovir intravenous prophylaxis, ganciclovir alone reduced the CMV disease rate to 9%, but the effect was limited to CMV-seropositive recipients.[165] Studies of combination ganciclovir and CMVIG prophylaxis in liver transplant recipients are in progress.

Acquired Immunodeficiency Syndrome and Intravenous Immune Globulin

Polyclonal hypergammaglobulinemia is common in HIV disease, and it is associated with a decreased response to neoantigens and immunizations. The data on the role of IVIG in individuals with HIV infection are confusing. It is helpful to remember that some trials have been done with unselected IVIG administration and others with hyperimmune anti-HIV plasma and to think of them separately.

Children with congenital HIV infection appear to have more profound humoral deficits than do adults with HIV, presumably because adults have a pool of memory cells that predates the HIV infection.[166] Recurrent bacterial infection is a major problem in this group of children.[167] A number of studies, some of which had crossover designs (none of which were prospective and randomized), have shown major benefits of IVIG therapy in pediatric HIV infection, with decreased episodes of infection, resolution of intractable diarrhea, and fewer hospital days.[168–172]

Spector and colleagues[173] conducted a controlled trial of IVIG in children receiving azidothymidine for advanced HIV infection. They found a beneficial effect in children between the ages of 3 months and 12 years who received IVIG at 400 mg/kg every 28 days, compared with children who received a 0.1% albumin control solution. This decrease in the rate of infection of about 40% was most evident in children who were not receiving trimethoprim-sulfamethoxazole (TMP-SMX) prophylaxis for *Pneumocystis carinii* pneumonia. Paradoxically, the children who were receiving TMP-SMX prophylaxis and received IVIG had a higher rate of bacterial infection than did the control subgroup that was receiving TMP-SMX. In contrast, Mofenson and coworkers[174] found that IVIG was an effective prophylactic agent against bacterial infections in children. In an open-label study conducted as a follow-up to their randomized placebo-controlled study, they found that in the children who crossed over from placebo to IVIG, the rate of serious and of minor bacterial infections was significantly lower after the change. This decreased rate of infection was observed independently of the use of TMP-SMX. In contrast, in the group that had received IVIG during the first trial, there was no significant change in the rate of infection when IVIG was continued. We believe that there is a role for IVIG in children with the acquired immunodeficiency syndrome (AIDS) but that the exact indications are not yet understood and that prophylaxis with TMP-SMX probably independently diminishes the benefit of IVIG.

Lambert and Stiehm[175] have reviewed the protective role of passive immunity in the prevention of maternal-fetal HIV transmission. There is no current indication for the use of IVIG during the pregnancy of HIV-seropositive women, except perhaps for thrombocytopenia.[176]

The data for adults are also confusing and contradictory. For example, a group of investigators in Dusseldorf published a small study on the effects of IVIG in AIDS in 35 patients, stratified as placebo, low-dose therapy, and high-dose therapy, and found no beneficial effects after 1 year of IVIG therapy.[177] In contrast to these data, Kiehl and colleagues[178] in Germany have published preliminary data from their randomized outpatient trial of IVIG in adults with advanced HIV and AIDS suggesting that IVIG reduces the number of episodes of fever and diarrhea and the duration of hospitalization, as well as decreasing mortality related to infection.

In contrast, there is evidence that plasma with anti-HIV antibody is able to decrease AIDS-related complications in HIV-seropositive recipients. Vittecoq and coworkers[179] randomized 86 symptomatic HIV-seropositive individuals to receive plasma rich in anti–HIV-1 antibody or standard seronegative plasma. Each patient received 300 mL every 14 days over a 1-year period and every 28 days thereafter, in addition to antivirals and conventional prophylaxis. Donor serum was obtained from individuals with high titers of anti-p24 antibody, a negative p24 antigen serum assay, and a $CD4^+$ lymphocyte subset count of 400 cells per mm^3 or greater. Plasma was heat inactivated before use. The appearance of the first AIDS-defining event was delayed, and found only about one third as frequently, in recipients of the plasma containing anti-p24 antibody; moreover, the total number of deaths and of AIDS-defining events was significantly decreased by 38%. In a similarly designed study, 220 AIDS patients received a placebo or 250 or 500 mL of high-titer anti-HIV plasma in a 12-month double-blind study.[180] Positive effects were found only in the group who received 500 mL with $CD4^+$ lymphocyte counts between 50 and 200 cells per mm^3. In the group receiving 500 mL of plasma, both reduced deaths and a rise in $CD4^+$ lymphocyte counts were found.

Yap[181] has summarized the current indications for IVIG for AIDS patients as the prevention or treatment of respiratory and other infections in children with AIDS, potentially infections in adults, idiopathic thrombocytopenic purpura, severe parvovirus B19 infection or measles, or autoimmune disorders in which IVIG is helpful. What subgroups of people with AIDS will benefit from IVIG is still unresolved. A common problem in HIV infection is thrombocytopenia. As in HIV-seronegative people, high-dose IVIG may produce a rise in platelet counts. It is unclear how long the benefit of IVIG lasts in this situation.[182–184]

Interferon and Granulocyte Colony-Stimulating Factor Therapy

Modulation of the immune response to the benefit of the host can also be effected by the use of specific cytokines, such as interferon (IFN)–α. IFN-α is made principally by lymphocytes and mononuclear phagocytes and interferes with viral replication. IFNs have been extensively investigated for the treatment of chronic hepatitis B and C, as well as for upper respiratory tract virus infections, herpesvirus syndromes, and papillomavirus infections.[185, 186] In individuals with chronic hepatitis B, daily treatment with 5 million units of IFN, with or without prednisone pretreatment (given to enhance antiviral efficacy), led to remission in more than one third of patients.[187] Use of this regimen or of IFN alfa therapy at a dose of 10 million units three times weekly for 16 to 24 weeks induced a long-term remission with loss of HBV DNA and hepatitis B e antigen in 25% to 40% of patients, with about half of the responders losing all hepatitis B surface antigen and presumably becoming cured.[188, 189] People with low viral serum DNA levels and high initial aminotransferase levels responded best to treatment, whereas those with cirrhosis, male sex, high DNA levels, chronic persistent hepatitis, immunosuppressive therapy, HIV infection, or low initial aminotransferase levels were least likely to benefit.[190, 191] Chronic non-A, non-B hepatitis, caused principally by HCV, can also be treated with subcutaneous IFN alfa. Approximately half of those receiving at least 2 million units three times weekly for 24 to 36 weeks showed significant reductions in serum aminotransferase levels and improvement on liver biopsy specimens in three studies.[192–194] Relapse was common after stopping treatment, but those who were retreated appeared to respond once again. In a reported trial, continuance of IFN alfa therapy at a dose of 3 million units given three times a week for 18 months produced better histologic findings and serum aminotransferase values than regimens using lower doses or shorter treatment periods.[195] Thus, in chronic hepatitis, a cause of much morbidity and mortality, a subset of patients benefits from IFN alfa therapy. Excitement about this modality of treatment must be balanced by an appreciation of its costs, the need for selection of patients, and the inconvenience.

Papillomavirus infections are common, have malignant potential, and often recur no matter what the therapy.[196] IFN has been studied as an adjunct to other therapies and appears to have a role in the treatment of anogenital, laryngeal, and plantar warts.[197–201] It has also been studied in the treatment of cervical intraepithelial neoplasia associated with papillomavirus infection, and intralesional therapy appears to be more helpful than IFN topical gels.[202, 203] Overall it appears to have a role in increasing the success of surgical removal,[204] but the cost of IFN suggests that its use should be reserved for recalcitrant or anatomically problematic warts.[205, 206]

Chronic granulomatous disease is a rare, heterogeneous group of disorders in which NADPH oxidase deficiencies lead to a defect in the oxidative burst of monocytes and neutrophils used to kill bacteria.[207] Clinical trials of recombinant IFN-γ, using prophylactic subcutaneous treatment three times weekly, in patients with chronic granulomatous disease have shown approximately 70% reductions in infections and have led to its widespread use in this circumstance.[208–210] IFN-γ is synthesized principally by T and natural killer cells and has antiviral, antitumor, and macrophage-enhancing effects. Interestingly, IFN-γ does not appear to reconstitute the oxidative burst function directly and may work via other mechanisms.[211]

Leishmaniasis, caused by species of *Leishmania*, has emerged as a disease that is profoundly modulated by the immune system.[212] Both macrophages stimulated by IFN-γ and *Leishmania*-specific $CD4^+$ T cells are able to kill parasite amastigotes.[213, 214] IFN-γ has been studied as an adjunct to pentavalent antimony treatment, and it appears to be effective in the treatment of diffuse cutaneous leishmaniasis,[215] as well as antimony-resistant mucosal disease.[216] Prospective studies to determine the role for IFN-γ appear warranted.

Prophylactic human leukocyte IFN also appears to decrease the incidence of CMV-related syndromes in recipients of kidney transplants[217] but not when used as acute treatment[218] in a variety of other transplant settings. Although IFNs have appeared to be helpful in the treatment of herpes simplex virus infections, drug therapy with acyclovir is better tolerated and less expensive.

Prophylactic intranasal interferon alfa-2 protects against rhinovirus infections, but not other respiratory pathogens such as influenza virus A or B or coronavirus, in the household contacts of family members with respiratory infections.[219, 220] Nasal bleeding and other local symptoms were common in these studies. IFN is not cost-effective in rhinovirus prophylaxis, and its side effect profile is limiting, given the benign nature of most rhinovirus infections.

Granulocyte colony-stimulating factor (filgrastim) has been shown to increase peripheral blood granulocyte counts during chemotherapy for transitional cell cancer of the urothelium.[221] In so doing it decreased days of neutropenia and reduced the number of days during which antimicrobials were used because of fever and neutropenia. Similar findings were obtained for patients with small-cell lung cancer undergoing chemotherapy.[222] Granulocyte colony-stimulating factor stimulates the proliferation, differentiation commitment, and functional abilities of neutrophil progenitors.[223, 224] Its use is primarily in the prevention of neutropenic fever and infection during cancer chemotherapy. This augmentation of the host immune system is likely to be more widely used in other situations in which neutropenia is common, such as cyclic or congenital neutropenia, although little nonanectodal information is available.

Whereas cytokine therapy may help the immune response to malignancies, it may detract from host defenses against infections. Nosocomial infection associated with treatment with IL-2 is problematic[225] and appears to be associated with a defect in neutrophil chemotaxis that can be overcome by the use of steroids.[226]

Miscellaneous Conditions and Indications for Therapy

A number of other specific circumstances exist that clearly do, or may, benefit from IG, IVIG, or hyperimmune IVIG therapy. These include Kawasaki disease; the toxic shock syndrome; infections with parvovirus B19, RSV, and the hemorrhagic fever viruses; some enteric infections; and malaria (Table 36–4).

IVIG has been used in an uncontrolled fashion for a variety of reasons and in many cases has not proved helpful in the long run. In addition, for these FDA-unapproved, or "off-label," uses it is unclear what dose of IVIG should be used, if it should be used at all. Finally, the cost and difficulty of conducting placebo-controlled, randomized trials of IVIG for

TABLE 36–4 ■ What Criteria Seem to Predict Whether a Globulin Preparation Will Be Effective in the Treatment or Prevention of a Specific Disease?

- High levels of intact neutralizing antibody to the pathogen in the globulin preparation. Hyperimmune preparations are manufactured so as to increase the titers of the specific antibody desired.
- The infection is directly mediated by a toxin or viral particle, such as rabies or diphtheria. More complex pathogens, such as bacteria, fungi, and protozoa, have been less amenable to treatment with globulins, perhaps because the pathogenic process is complex and has multiple actions on the host or because evasion of the immune response is practiced by the pathogen.
- Early recognition of the disease process.
- Early administration of the globulin product.

rare or fatal conditions may mean that conducting these trials is difficult or practically impossible. We believe that caution is indicated in the use of IVIG in these circumstances.[227]

Kawasaki Disease (Mucocutaneous Lymph Node Syndrome)

It is controversial whether there is an infectious agent in the mucocutaneous lymph node syndrome, or Kawasaki disease, but it is clear that IVIG is helpful in treatment of the disease. The current treatment of choice in Kawasaki disease is IVIG and aspirin.[228, 229] IVIG at a dose of 400 mg/kg per day for 5 days in conjunction with aspirin prevented more coronary artery lesions than did a lower dose of 100 or 200 mg/kg per day for the same period, and it has been noted that alkylated IVIG was less effective than native unaltered IVIG.[230] Trials have shown that single-treatment, high-dose IVIG is also efficacious.[231–233] Some authors have pointed out that a delay in treatment during the presentation of Kawasaki disease often leads to high incidence of coronary lesions, and given the safety of IVIG, have recommended the early use of IVIG when a child presents with a syndrome consistent with early Kawasaki disease.[234, 235] Recurrence of Kawasaki disease does not appear to be related to the use of IVIG during the primary episode.[236] The mechanisms of action of IVIG in Kawasaki disease have been reviewed.[35]

Toxic Shock Syndrome

Toxic shock syndrome, a syndrome mediated by a toxin that can be produced by either *S. aureus* or group A *Streptococcus*, can be prevented in experimental rabbit models using monoclonal antibodies to the toxin.[237] Killing the invading bacteria with antimicrobials does not eliminate the toxic shock toxin, but the use of appropriately selected antibodies may. There is increasing evidence that the toxic shock syndrome is the result of superantigenic stimulation by the toxin, which is thought to bind to the major histocompatibility complex class II receptors of monocytes and macrophages outside the classic antigen groove. This toxin-receptor complex is then recognized nonspecifically by a broad variety of T lymphocytes, leading to nonspecific and disordered systemic release of IL-1, TNF, and INF-γ.[238] Experimental evidence supports the notion that IVIG inhibits superantigenic stimulation by staphylococcal toxins.[239, 240] Ogawa and colleagues[241] have reported the use of IVIG during the toxic shock syndrome after staphylococcal pneumonia. No randomized trial of IVIG in toxic shock syndrome has been reported, although on experimental and intellectual grounds IVIG would appear to be an attractive candidate for treatment.

Parvovirus B19 Infection

Parvovirus B19, the ubiquitous causative agent of fifth disease (erythema infectiosum), can also cause persistent anemia in children with sickle cell disease (aplastic crisis), individuals with aplastic anemia, or individuals with immunosuppression such as those with AIDS or malignancies. In addition, parvovirus B19 appears to be a rare cause of fetal hydrops. Usually, development of specific antibody to the virus leads to termination of the infection. IVIG has been reported to be curative in all of these circumstances, as resolution of the infection appears to be due to a neutralizing antibody response.[242–246] There is no other known treatment besides IVIG for serious parvovirus B19 infection. Kurtzman and colleagues[244] have described a young man with aplastic anemia of 10 years' duration related to persistent parvovirus B19 infection. He had no IgG specific for a viral capsid protein and had high levels of immunoglobulin M. He was cured of the infection with IVIG that contained parvovirus-neutralizing IgG. In addition, it appears that superficially unrelated symptoms or syndromes may also resolve with IVIG. For example, Nigro and coworkers[247] have reported the successful use of IVIG in hypogammaglobulinemic infant with anemia and neurologic disorders. Finkel and colleagues[248] have reported that three patients with a systemic necrotizing vasculitis and chronic parvovirus B19 infection had resolution of both the chronic infection and the vasculitis with IVIG after corticosteroids and cyclophosphamide failed to control the vasculitis.

Respiratory Syncytial Virus Infection

The FDA approved the licensure of hyperimmune anti-RSV IVIG in January 1996 (RespiGam, manufactured by the Massachusetts State Biological Laboratories) to prevent RSV disease in neonates and children younger than 24 months with bronchopulmonary dysplasia or a history of prematurity. RSV has been shown to be a major cause of death and morbidity in children with bronchopulmonary dysplasia, congenital heart disease, and immunodeficiency such as in AIDS or cancer.[249–251] Adults undergoing bone marrow transplantation are also at risk of death resulting from RSV.[252] Attempts to prevent RSV disease with vaccines in the 1960s resulted in an immunogenic product that paradoxically exacerbated naturally acquired disease in vaccinated children. Epidemiologic studies in the 1970s found that infants with serum anti-RSV titers higher than 1:200 were at significantly less risk of bronchiolitis and pneumonia than children with lower antibody levels.[253] Clinical trials with unselected IVIG and hyperimmune anti-RSV IVIG were conducted. Despite encouraging early results, unselected IVIG was not shown to be efficacious in reducing RSV morbidity and mortality in a series of trials, principally because commercial lots of IVIG did not contain sufficient amounts of RSV-neutralizing antibody and could not achieve a 1:400 target titer after infusion.[254–256] Siber and colleagues[257] at the Massachusetts State Biological Laboratories then selected lots of IVIG for high anti-RSV activity by microneutralization techniques. This product was used in a randomized prospective trial in which RespiGam was given at a dose of 750 mg/kg monthly during three RSV transmission seasons to 274 infants and children at high risk of RSV disease because of chronic pulmonary disease (principally bronchopulmonary dysplasia), congenital heart disease, or premature birth (35 weeks of gestation or less). RespiGam reduced the frequency of RSV lower respiratory tract infection by 62%, and hospitalization was decreased by 57%; moreover, the need for the number of intensive care unit hospitalizations was nearly eliminated with a 97% decrease, and mechanical ventilation was completely eliminated.[258] These benefits were not seen with a lower dose of 150 mg/kg. Efficacy in other groups, such as older children with congenital heart disease or cystic fibrosis, has not been established.

Enteric Infections

This chapter has focused on the use of parenteral IGs and cytokines, but gut mucosal immunity is increasingly recognized for its central role in host immunity. It is estimated that 70% to 80% of the IG-producing cells in humans are located in the intestinal mucosa, and the majority of antibodies produced daily are excreted into the gut.[259] Many studies have shown the protective effects of breast milk.[260] Eibl and colleagues[261, 262] administered an oral IG preparation enriched in IgA to low-birth-weight neonates and found that it significantly decreased the incidence of necrotizing enterocolitis.

This study was not "blinded" and had no control treatment group, yet none of 88 neonates given the supplement developed necrotizing enterocolitis but 6 of 91 control infants given standard feedings did develop it ($P = .0143$). It is likely that orally administered IG will be investigated for enteric diseases caused by enteric viruses,[263] bacteria,[264] and protozoa[265] in high-risk or immunodeficient populations. Trials investigating hyperimmune antitoxin globulin preparations given enterically for refractory *Clostridium difficile* colitis are under way. *Cryptosporidium parvum*, which causes cholera-like watery diarrhea in immunocompromised people with cancer or AIDS, has occasionally been controlled if not cured after the administration of bovine hyperimmune anti-*Cryptosporidium* colostrum.[266–268]

Hemorrhagic Fever and Other Hemorrhagic Virus Infections

Lassa virus and other viruses such as Bolivian and Argentinian hemorrhagic fever viruses are arenaviruses transmitted from peridomestic rodents. Survival after Lassa fever is directly dependent on the development of neutralizing antibody.[269] Infections with Lassa virus have been treated with immune plasma as well as ribavirin.[270–272] It appears that either agent is efficacious if given within the first week of illness, and the agents are especially effective if given together. This finding is analogous to the finding that CMVIG and ganciclovir are more effective given together than alone in the treatment of CMV pneumonia after bone marrow transplantation. In view of the prohibitive cost of antiviral agents in the developing world, hyperimmune plasma pools may be the most reasonable way to treat symptomatic disease, especially if plasma can be screened for HIV and other blood-borne infectious agents.

Argentinian hemorrhagic fever is caused by Junin virus, which is closely related to Machupo virus, the causative agent of Bolivian hemorrhagic fever. In the 1960s, empirical therapy with convalescent plasma was found to be therapeutic during Argentinian hemorrhagic fever, and in a controlled trial of Argentinian hemorrhagic fever plasma mortality was reduced from 16% to 1% compared with the placebo group.[273] Death usually occurs only in those given plasma after 8 days of illness or those given plasma with inadequate levels of neutralizing antibody.[274] Other hemorrhagic fever viruses, such as *Nairovirus*, which causes Crimean-Congo hemorrhagic fever, and *Hantavirus*, are global in distribution. They may be candidates for hyperimmune preparations. In a nosocomial outbreak of Crimean-Congo hemorrhagic fever in South Africa, six high-risk contacts who became infected received immune plasma and survived, whereas both the index case and a nosocomially infected physician never demonstrated any neutralizing antibody production and died.[275]

The thread that binds these diverse viral illnesses together would appear to be the ability of neutralizing antibody to prevent death. It can be argued that small lots of hyperimmune plasma should be available to public health authorities should outbreaks of these disease occur.[276]

Malaria

Malaria is rapidly becoming resistant to drug therapy, and in some regions such as the Myanmar (Burma)–Thailand border region, *Plasmodium falciparum* resistance to mefloquine and other agents has been documented.[277] An antimalarial IVIG preparation made from plasma donated in a malaria hyperendemic region of the Ivory Coast in Africa was administered to eight Thai patients with falciparum malaria. Asexual parasitemia was reduced by a mean of 728-fold, as fast as or faster than with drugs, and the effect was consistent in all eight patients.[278] This study demonstrated that protective antibody is not geographically limited and, although not curative, it is quite beneficial. As therapeutic options become more limited for the treatment of malaria, it is possible that a low-volume hyperimmune antimalaria preparation of IVIG may have a treatment role in selected circumstances. We are anecdotally aware of clinicians in Africa treating cerebral malaria in children with chloroquine-resistant falciparum malaria with plasma, but to our knowledge no prospective trials have been conducted.

References

1. Rousell RH, Pennington JE: An historical overview of immunoglobulin therapy. *In* Yap PL (ed): Clinical Applications of Intravenous Immunoglobulin Therapy. Edinburgh, Churchill Livingstone, 1992, pp 1–15.
2. Behring E: Zur Behandlung der Dipththerie mit Diptherie Heilserum. Dtsch Med Wochenschr 19:543, 1893.
3. Ehrlich P: Die Wertbemessung des Diphtherieheilserums und deren theoretische Grundlagen. Klin Jahrb 6:299, 1897.
4. Finland M: The serum treatment of lobar pneumonia. N Engl J Med 202:1244, 1930.
5. Finland M: Adequate dosage in the specific serum treatment of pneumococcus type I pneumonia. Am J Med Sci 192:849, 1936.
6. McKhann CF, Chu FT: Antibodies in placental extracts. J Infect Dis 52:268, 1933.
7. McKhann CF, Greene AA, Coady H: Factors influencing the effectiveness of placental extract in the prevention and modification of measles. J Pediatr 6:603, 1935.
8. Cohn EJ, Oncley JL, Strong LE, et al: Chemical, clinical and immunological studies on the products of human plasma fractionation. I. The characterization of protein fractions of human plasma. J Clin Invest 23:417, 1944.
9. Ordman CW, Jenning CG, Janeway CA: Chemical, clinical, and immunological studies on the products of human plasma fractionation. XII. The use of concentrated normal human serum gammaglobulin (human immune serum globulin) in the prevention and attenuation of measles. J Clin Invest 23:541, 1944.
10. Bruton OC: Agammaglobulinemia. Pediatrics 9:722, 1952.
11. Dwyer JM: Thirty years of supplying the missing link. Am J Med 73(Suppl 3A):46, 1984.
12. Barandun S, Kistler P, Jeunet F, Isliker H: Intravenous administration of human gammaglobulin. Vox Sang 7:157, 1962.
13. Lundblad JL, Londeree N: The effect of processing methods on intravenous immune globulin preparation. J Hosp Infect 12(Suppl D):3, 1988.
14. McIver J, Grady GF: Immunoglobulin preparations. *In* Churchill WH, Kurtz SR (eds): Transfusion Medicine. Boston, Blackwell Scientific Publications, 1988, pp 189–209.
15. Burks AW, Steele RW: Selective IgA deficiency. Ann Allergy 57:3, 1986.
16. Apfelzeig R, Piskiewicz D, Hooper JA: Immunoglobulin A concentrations in commercial immune globulins. J Clin Immunol 7:46, 1987.
17. Lewis RB, Matzke DS, Albrecht TB, Pollard RB: Assessment of the presence of cytomegalovirus-neutralizing antibody by a plaque-reduction assay. Rev Infect Dis 8(Suppl 4):S434, 1986.
18. Lundblad JL, Mitra G, Sternberg MM, Schroeder DD: Comparative studies of impurities in intravenous immunoglobulin preparations. Rev Infect Dis 8(Suppl 4):S382, 1986.
19. Yap PL, Williams PE: The safety of IVIG preparations. *In* Yap PL (ed): Clinical Applications of Intravenous Immunoglobulin Therapy. Edinburgh, Churchill Livingstone, 1992, pp 43–62.
20. Yang YH, Ngo C, Yeh IN, Uemura Y: Antibody Fc functional activity of intravenous immunoglobulin preparations treated with solvent-detergent for virus inactivation. Vox Sang 67:337, 1994.
21. Uemura Y, Yang YH, Heldebrant CM, et al: Inactivation and elimination of viruses during preparation of human intravenous immunoglobulin. Vox Sang 67:246, 1994.
22. Louie RE, Galloway CJ, Dumas ML, et al: Inactivation of hepatitis C virus in low pH intravenous immunoglobulin. Biologicals 22:13, 1994.

23. Schiff RI: Half-life and clearance of pH 6.8 and pH 4.25 immunoglobulin G intravenous preparations in patients with primary disorders of humoral immunity. Rev Infect Dis 8(Suppl 4):S449, 1986.
24. Pirofsky B: Safety and toxicity of a new serum immunoglobulin G intravenous preparation, IGIV pH 4.25. Rev Infect Dis 8(Suppl 4):S457, 1986.
25. Weisman LE, Fischer GW, Hemming VG, Peck CC: Pharmacokinetics of intravenous immunoglobulin (Sandoglobulin) in neonates. Pediatr Infect Dis 5(Suppl 3):S185, 1986.
26. Arturson G, Hogman CF, Johansson SGO, Killander J: Changes in immunoglobulin levels in severely burned patients. Lancet 1:546, 1969.
27. Munster AM, Hoagland HC, Pruitt BA Jr: The effect of thermal injury on serum immunoglobulins. Ann Surg 172:965, 1970.
28. Hagenbeek A, Brummelhuis HGJ, Donkers A, et al: Rapid clearance of cytomegalovirus-specific IgG after repeated intravenous infusions of human immunoglobulin into allogeneic bone marrow transplant recipients. J Infect Dis 155:897, 1987.
29. Snydman DR, McIver J, Leszczynski J, et al: A pilot trial of a novel cytomegalovirus immune globulin in renal transplant recipients. Transplantation 38:553, 1984.
30. Snydman DR: Prevention of cytomegalovirus-associated diseases with immunoglobulin. Transplant Proc 23(Suppl 1):131, 1991.
31. Schiff RI: Intravenous gammaglobulin: Pharmacology, clinical uses and mechanisms of action. Pediatr Allergy Immunol 5:63, 1994.
32. Ballow M: Mechanisms of action of intravenous immune serum globulin therapy. Pediatr Infect Dis J 13:806, 1994.
33. Weisman LE, Cruess DF, Fischer GW: Opsonic activity of commercially available standard intravenous immunoglobulin preparations. Pediatr Infect Dis J 13:1122, 1994.
34. Van T, Sussman G, Pruzanski W: Impact of intravenous infusion of low and high doses of gamma globulins (IVIG) on phagocytic functions in adults with primary humoral immunodeficiency. Inflammation 18:419, 1994.
35. Meissner HC, Schlievert PM, Leung DY: Mechanisms of immunoglobulin action: Observations on Kawasaki syndrome and RSV prophylaxis. Immunol Rev 139:109, 1994.
36. Aukrust P, Froland SS, Liabakk NB, et al: Release of cytokines, soluble cytokine receptors, and interleukin-1 receptor antagonist after intravenous immunoglobulin administration in vivo. Blood 84:2136, 1994.
37. Sekul EA, Cupler EJ, Dalakas MC: Aseptic meningitis associated with high-dose intravenous immunoglobulin therapy: Frequency and risk factors. Ann Intern Med 121:259, 1994.
38. De Vlieghere FC, Peetermans WE, Vermylen J: Aseptic granulocytic meningitis following treatment with intravenous immunoglobulin. Clin Infect Dis 18:1008, 1994.
39. Cantu TG, Hoehn-Saric EW, Burgess KM, et al: Acute renal failure associated with immunoglobulin therapy. Am J Kidney Dis 25:228, 1995.
40. Pfeiffer RW, Siegel J, Ayers LW: Assessment of microbial growth in intravenous immune globulin preparations. Am J Hosp Pharm 51:1676, 1994.
41. Schiff RI: Transmission of viral infections through intravenous immune globulin (Editorial). N Engl J Med 331:1649, 1994.
42. Mitra G, Wong MF, Mozen MM, et al: Elimination of infectious retroviruses during preparation of immunoglobulins. Transfusion 26:394, 1986.
43. Wells MA, Wittek AE, Epstein JS, et al: Inactivation and partition of human T-cell lymphotrophic virus, type III, during ethanol fractionation of plasma. Transfusion 26:210, 1986.
44. Bjoro K, Froland SS, Yun Z, et al: Hepatitis C infection in patients with primary hypogammaglobulinemia after treatment with contaminated immune globulin. N Engl J Med 331:1607, 1994.
45. Yu MY, Mason BL, Tankersley DL: Detection and characterization of hepatitis C virus RNA in immune globulins. Transfusion 34:596, 1994.
46. Yu MW, Mason BL, Guo ZP, et al: Hepatitis C transmission associated with intravenous immunoglobulins (Letter). Lancet 345:1173, 1995.
47. Nübling CM, Willkommen H, Löwer J: Hepatitis C transmission associated with intravenous immunoglobulins (Letter). Lancet 345:1174, 1995.
48. Tabor E, Gerety RJ: Transmission of hepatitis B by immune serum globulin. Lancet 2:1293, 1979.
49. Tabor E, Aronson DL, Gerety RJ: Removal of hepatitis B virus infectivity from factor IX complex by hepatitis B immune globulin. Experiments in chimpanzees. Lancet 2:69, 1980.
50. Hellstern P: Clinical experience with the viral safety of immunoglobulins. Blood Coagul Fibrinol 5(Suppl 3):S31, 1994.
51. Karna P, Murray DL, Valduss D, et al: Passive transfer of hepatitis antibodies during intravenous administration of immune globulin. J Pediatr 125:463, 1995.
52. Bielory L, Long GC: Home health care costs: intravenous immunoglobulin home infusion therapy. Ann Allergy Asthma Immunol 74:265, 1995.
53. Tsevat J, Snydman DR, Pauker SG, et al: Which renal transplant patients should receive cytomegalovirus immune globulin? A cost-effectiveness analysis. Transplantation 52:259, 1991.
54. Jorgensen F, Andersson B, Hanson LA, et al: Gamma-globulin treatment of recurrent acute otitis media in children. Pediatr Infect Dis J 9:389, 1990.
55. Committee on Infectious Diseases, American Academy of Pediatrics: The Report of the Committee on Infectious Diseases, ed 21 (Red Book). Elk Grove Village, IL, American Academy of Pediatrics, 1988.
56. Centers for Disease Control: Recommendations of the Immunization Practices Advisory Committee (ACIP): Recommendations for prevention against viral hepatitis. MMWR Morbid Mortal Wkly Rep 34:313, 329, 1985.
57. ACP Task Force on Adult Immunization and Infectious Diseases Society of America: Guide for Adult Immunizations, ed 2. Philadelphia, American College of Physicians, 1990.
58. Gershon AA, Steinberg S, Brunnell PA: Zoster immune globulin: A further assessment. N Engl J Med 290:243, 1974.
59. Respiratory syncytial virus hyperimmune globulin (RespiGam) package insert. Jamaica Plain, MA, Massachusetts State Biological Laboratories and MedImmune.
60. Wilde H, Chutivongse S: Equine rabies immune globulin: A product with an undeserved poor reputation. Am J Trop Med Hyg 42:175, 1990.
61. Santosham M, Reid R, Ambrosino DM, et al: Prevention of Haemophilus influenzae type b infections in high-risk infants treated with bacterial polysaccharide immune globulin. N Engl J Med 317:923, 1987.
62. Cohen J. Intravenous immunoglobulin (IVIG) for gram-negative infection—A critical review. J Hosp Infect 12(Suppl D):47, 1988.
63. Natanson C, Hoffman WD, Suffredini AF, et al: Selected treatment strategies for septic shock based on proposed mechanisms of pathogenesis. Ann Intern Med 120:771, 1994.
64. Ziegler EJ, McCutchan JA, Fierer J, et al: Treatment of gram-negative bacteremia and shock with human antiserum to a mutant UDP-GAL epimerase deficient mutant Escherichia coli. N Engl J Med 307:1225, 1982.
65. Baumgartner JD, Gauser MP, McCutcheon JA, et al: Prevention of gram-negative shock and death in surgical patients by antibody to endotoxin core glycolipid. Lancet 2:59, 1985.
66. Greisman SE, Johnston CA. Failure of antisera to J5 and R595 rough mutants to reduce endotoxemic lethality. J Infect Dis 157:54, 1988.
67. Ziegler EJ. Protective antibody to endotoxin core: The emperor's new clothes? J Infect Dis 158:286, 1988.
68. Ziegler EJ, Fisher CJ Jr, Sprung CL, et al: The HA-1A Sepsis Study Group. Treatment of gram-negative bacteremia and septic shock with HA-1A human monoclonal antibody against endotoxin: A randomized, double-blind placebo-controlled trial. N Engl J Med 324:429, 1991.
69. Greenman R, Schein R, Martin M, et al: A controlled clinical trial of E5 murine monoclonal IgM antibody to endotoxin in the treatment of gram-negative sepsis. JAMA 266:1097, 1991.
70. McCloskey RV, Straube RC, Sanders C, et al: Treatment of septic shock with human monoclonal antibody HA-1A. Ann Intern Med 121:1, 1994.
71. Cross AS: Antiendotoxin antibodies: A dead end? (Editorial). Ann Intern Med 121:58–59, 1994.
72. Dinarello CA, Gelfand JA, Wolff SM: Anticytokine strategies in the treatment of the systemic inflammatory syndrome. JAMA 269:1829, 1993.
73. Parillo JE: Pathogenic mechanisms of septic shock. N Engl J Med 328:1471, 1993.

74. Christman JW, Holden EP, Balckwell TS: Strategies for blocking the systemic effects of cytokines in the sepsis syndrome. Crit Care Med 23:955, 1995.
75. Goldie AS, Fearon KCH, Ross JA, et al: Natural cytokine antagonists and endogenous antiendotoxin core antibodies in sepsis syndrome. The Sepsis Intervention Group. JAMA 274:172, 1995.
76. Fisher CJ Jr, Slotman GJ, Opal SM, et al: Initial evaluation of human recombinant interleukin-1 receptor antagonist in the treatment of sepsis syndrome: A randomized, open-label, placebo-controlled multicenter trial. Crit Care Med 22:12, 1994.
77. Fisher CJ Jr, Dhainault JF, Pribble JP, et al: Recombinant human interleukin 1 receptor antagonist in the treatment of patients with sepsis syndrome. Results of a randomized, double-blind, placebo-controlled trial. Phase III rhIL-1ra Sepsis Study Group. JAMA 27:1836, 1994.
78. Roifman CM, Levison H, Gelfand EW: High-dose versus low-dose intravenous immunoglobulin in hypogammaglobulinaemia and chronic lung disease. Lancet 1:1075, 1987.
79. Rosen FS, Cooper MD, Wedgwood RJP: The primary immunodeficiencies (1). N Engl J Med 311:235, 1984.
80. Rosen FS, Cooper MD, Wedgwood RJ: The primary immunodeficiencies (2). N Engl J Med 311:300, 1984.
81. Beard LJ, Ferrante A: Aspects of immunoglobulin replacement therapy. Pediatr Infect Dis J 9(Suppl 8):S54, 1990.
82. Radford DJ, Thong YH: The association between immunodeficiency and congenital heart disease: A review. Pediatr Cardiol 9:103, 1988.
83. Loh RKS, Harth SC, Thong YH, Ferrante A: Immunoglobulin G subclass deficiency and predisposition to infection in Down's syndrome. Pediatr Infect Dis J 9:547, 1990.
84. Thong YH: Clinical value of IgG subclass investigations in pediatric practice. Pediatr Infect Dis J 9:S36, 1990.
85. Björkander J, Bengtsson U, Oxelius V, Hanson LÅ: Symptoms in patients with lowered levels of IgG subclasses, with or without IgA deficiency, and effects of immunoglobulin prophylaxis. Monogr Allergy 20:157, 1986.
86. Schiff RI: Intravenous gammaglobulin: Pharmacology, clinical uses and mechanisms of action. Pediatr Allergy Immunol 5:63, 1994.
87. Schiff RI: Intravenous gammaglobulin, 2: Pharmacology, clinical uses and mechanisms of action. Pediatr Allergy Immunol 5:127, 1994.
88. Gonzalez LA, Hill HR: The current status of intravenous gammaglobulin use in neonates. Pediatr Infect Dis J 8:315, 1989.
89. Edwards MS: Complement in neonatal infections: An overview. Pediatr Infect Dis 5(Suppl 3):S168, 1986.
90. Wilson CB, Lewis DB: Basis and implications of selectively diminished cytokine production in neonatal susceptibility to infection. Rev Infect Dis 12(Suppl 4):S410, 1990.
91. Berger M: Complement deficiency and neutrophil dysfunction as risk factors for bacterial infection in newborns and the role of granulocyte transfusion in therapy. Rev Infect Dis 12(Suppl 4):401, 1990.
92. Baker CJ, Melish ME, Hall RT, et al: Intravenous immune globulin for the prevention of nosocomial infection in low-birth-weight neonates. N Engl J Med 327:213, 1992.
93. Weisman LE, Stoll BJ, Kueser TJ, et al: Intravenous immune globulin therapy for early-onset sepsis in premature neonates. J Pediatr 121:434, 1992.
94. Cairo MS, Worcester CC, Rucker RW, et al: Randomized trial of granulocyte transfusions versus intravenous immune globulin therapy for neonatal neutropenia and sepsis. J Pediatr 120:281, 1992.
95. Paul V: Immunoglobulin prophylaxis does not prevent nosocomial infections in very low birth weight neonates. Natl Med J India 8:24, 1995.
96. Fischer GW: Use of intravenous immune globulin in newborn infants. Clin Exp Immunol 97(Suppl 1):73, 1994.
97. Weisman LE, Stoll BJ, Kueser TJ, et al: Intravenous immune globulin prophylaxis of late-onset sepsis in premature neonates. J Pediatr 125:922, 1994.
98. Ferrieri P: Neonatal susceptibility and immunity to major bacterial pathogens. Rev Infect Dis 12(Suppl 4):394, 1990.
99. Baker CJ, Kasper DL: Correlation of maternal antibody deficiency with susceptibility to neonatal group B infections. N Engl J Med 294:753–756, 1976.
100. Shigeoka AO, Hall RT, Hill HR: Blood transfusion in group B streptococcal sepsis. Lancet 1:636, 1978.
101. Gloser H, Bachmayer H, Helm A: Intravenous immunoglobulin with high activity against group B streptococci. Pediatr Infect Dis 5(Suppl 3):S176, 1986.
102. Hill HR, Shigeoka AO, Pincus S, Christensen RD: Intravenous IgG in combination with other modalities in the treatment of neonatal infection. Pediatr Infect Dis 5(Suppl 3):S180, 1986.
103. Christensen KK, Christensen P: Intravenous gamma-globulin in the treatment of neonatal sepsis with special reference to group B streptococci and pharmacokinetics. Pediatr Infect Dis 5(Suppl 3):S189, 1986.
104. Harper TE, Christensen RD, Rothstein G, Hill HR: Effect of intravenous immunoglobulin G on neutrophil kinetics during experimental group B streptococcal infection in neonatal rats. Rev Infect Dis 8(Suppl 4):S401, 1986.
105. Haque KN, Zaidi MH, Haque SK, et al: Intravenous immunoglobulin for prevention of sepsis in preterm and low birth weight infants. Pediatr Infect Dis 5:622, 1986.
106. Chirico G, Rondini G, Plebani A, et al: Intravenous gammaglobulin therapy for prophylaxis of infection in high-risk neonates. J Pediatr 110:437, 1987.
107. Sidiropoulos D, Boehme U, von Muralt G: Immunoglobulin supplementation in the management of neonatal sepsis. Schweiz Med Wochenschr 111:1649, 1981.
108. Haque KN, Zaidi MH, Bahakim H: IgM-enriched intravenous immunoglobulin therapy in neonatal sepsis. Am J Dis Child 142:1293, 1988.
109. Haque KN, Zaidi MH, Hasan B: IgM-enriched intravenous immunoglobulin therapy in neonatal sepsis. Am J Dis Child 142:1293, 1988.
110. Siegal G, Byrne W, Cross A, Finbloom D: High dose intravenous immunoglobulin may impair host defenses (Abstr). Clin Res 33:419A, 1985.
111. Kim KS: High-dose intravenous immune globulin impairs antibacterial activity of antibiotics. J Allergy Clin Immunol 84:579, 1989.
112. Noya FJD, Baker CJ: Intravenously administered immune globulin for premature infants: A time to wait (Editorial). J Pediatr 115:969, 1989.
113. Kliegman RM, Clapp DW, Berger M: Targeted immunoglobulin therapy for the prevention of neonatal infections. Rev Infect Dis 12(Suppl 4):443, 1990.
114. Piedra PA, Kasel JA, Norton HJ, et al: Evaluation of an intravenous immunoglobulin preparation for the prevention of viral infection among hospitalized low birth weight infants. Pediatr Infect Dis J 9:470, 1990.
115. Snydman DR, Werner BG, Meissner HC, et al: Use of cytomegalovirus immunoglobulin in multiply transfused, premature neonates. Pediatr Infect Dis J 14:34, 1995.
116. Commeta A, Baumgartner JD, Glauser MP: Polyclonal intravenous immune globulin for prevention and treatment of infections in critically ill patients. Clin Exp Immunol 97(Suppl 1):69, 1994.
117. Pruitt BA, McManus AT: Opportunistic infections in severely burned patients. Am J Med 76(Suppl 3A):146, 1984.
118. Liljedahl S-O, Olhagen B, Plantin L-O, Birke G: Studies on burns. VII. The problem of infection, with special reference to gammaglobulin. Acta Chir Scand [Suppl] 309:3, 1963.
119. Collins MS, Roby RE: Protective activity of an intravenous immune globulin (human) enriched in antibody against lipopolysaccharide antigens of *Pseudomonas aeruginosa*. Am J Med 76(Suppl 3A):168, 1984.
120. Stone HH, Graber CD, Martin JD Jr, Kolb L: Evaluation of gamma globulin for prophylaxis against burn sepsis. Surgery 58:810, 1965.
121. Wesley J, Fisher A, Fisher MW: Immunization against *Pseudomonas* in infection after thermal injury. J Infect Dis 130(Nov Suppl):S152, 1974.
122. Jones RJ, Roe EA, Gupta JL: Controlled trial of *Pseudomonas* immunoglobulin and vaccine in burn patients. Lancet 2:1263, 1980.
123. Waymack JP, Jenkins ME, Alexander JW, et al: A prospective trail of prophylactic intravenous immune globulin for the prevention of infections in severely burned patients. Burns 15:71, 1989.

124. Munster AM, Moran KT, Thupari J, et al: Prophylactic intravenous immunoglobulin replacement in high-risk burn patients. J Burn Care Rehabil 8:376, 1987.
125. Grob P, Holch M, Fierz W, et al: Immunodeficiency after major trauma and selective surgery. Pediatr Infect Dis J 7:S37, 1988.
126. Zanetti G, Glauser MP, Baumgartner J-D: Use of immunoglobulins in prevention and treatment of infection in critically ill patients: Review and critique. Rev Infect Dis 13:985, 1991.
127. Cometta A, Baumgartner J-D, Lee ML, et al: Prophylactic intravenous administration of standard immune globulin as compared with core-lipopolysaccharide immune globulin in patients at high risk of postsurgical infection. N Engl J Med 327:234, 1992.
128. Gipponi M, Canova G, Bonalumi U, et al: Immunoprophylaxis in "septic risk" patients undergoing surgery for gastrointestinal cancer. Results of a randomized, multicenter clinical trial. Int Surg 78:63, 1993.
129. Broder S, Humphrey R, Durm M, et al: Impaired synthesis of polyclonal (non-paraprotein) immunoglobulins by circulating lymphocytes from patients with multiple myeloma. N Engl J Med 293:887, 1975.
130. Besa EC: Recent advances in the treatment of chronic lymphocytic leukemia: Defining the role of intravenous gammaglobulin. Semin Hematol 29:14, 1992.
131. Cooperative Group for the Study of Immunoglobulin in Chronic Lymphocytic Leukemia: Intravenous immunoglobulin for the prevention of infection in chronic lymphocytic leukemia. A randomized, controlled clinical trial. N Engl J Med 319:902, 1988.
132. Griffiths H, Brennan V, Lea J, et al: Crossover study of immunoglobulin replacement therapy in patients with low-grade B-cell tumors. Blood 73:366, 1989.
133. Jurlander J, Geisler CH, Hansen MM: Treatment of hypogammaglobulinaemia in chronic lymphocytic leukaemia by low-dose intravenous gammaglobulin. Eur J Haematol 53:114, 1994.
134. Gamm H, Huber C, Chapel H, et al: Intravenous immune globulin in chronic lymphocytic leukaemia. Clin Exp Immunol 97(Suppl 1):17, 1994.
135. Weeks JC, Tierney MR, Weinstein MC: Cost effectiveness of prophylactic intravenous immune globulin in chronic lymphocytic leukemia. N Engl J Med 325:81, 1991.
136. Salmon SE, Samal BA, Hayes DM, et al: Role of gammaglobulin for immunoprophylaxis in multiple myeloma. N Engl J Med 277:1336, 1967.
137. Schedel I: Application of immunoglobulin preparations in multiple myeloma. *In* Morrell A, Nydegger UE (eds): Clinical Uses of Intravenous Immunoglobulins. London, Academic Press, 1986, pp 123–132.
138. Chapel HM, Lee M, Hargreaves R, et al: Randomised trial of intravenous immunoglobulin as prophylaxis against infection in plateau-phase multiple myeloma. The UK Group for Immunoglobulin Replacement Therapy in Multiple Myeloma. Lancet 343:1059, 1994.
139. Rubin M, Gress J, Marshall D, et al: Prophylaxis of infectious complications in neutropenic cancer patients with intravenous immunoglobulin (Abstr). Presented at the 28th Interscience Conference on Antimicrobial Agents and Chemotherapy; October 7, 1988; Los Angeles.
140. Wilfert CM, Katz SL: Etiology of bacterial sepsis in nephrotic children, 1963–1967. Pediatrics 42:840, 1968.
141. Ogi M, Yokoyama H, Tomosugi N, et al: Risk factors for infection and immunoglobulin replacement therapy in adult nephrotic syndrome. Am J Kidney Dis 24:427, 1994.
142. Emmanuel D: Treatment of cytomegalovirus disease. Semin Hematol 27:22–27, 1990.
143. Snydman DR: Prevention of cytomegalovirus disease with intravenous immune globulin. Transplant Proc 23(Suppl 1):20, 1991.
144. Berkman SA, Lee ML, Gale RP: Clinical uses of intravenous immunoglobulins. Ann Intern Med 112:278, 1990.
145. Champlin RE, Ho WG, Winston DJ: Acute graft-vs.-host disease and interstitial pneumonitis interrelated problems following allogeneic bone marrow transplantation: Effects of intravenous immune globulin and other interventions. J Hosp Infect 12(Suppl D):29, 1988.
146. Snydman DR, Werner BG, Heinze-Lacey B, et al: Use of cytomegalovirus immune globulin to prevent cytomegalovirus disease in renal-transplant recipients. N Engl J Med 317:1049, 1987.
147. Snydman DR, Werner BG, Tilney NL, et al: A final analysis of primary cytomegalovirus disease prevention in renal transplant recipients with a cytomegalovirus immune globulin: Comparison of randomized and open-label trials. Transplant Proc 23:1357, 1991.
148. Werner BG, Snydman DR, Freeman R, et al: Cytomegalovirus immune globulin for the prevention of primary CMV disease in renal transplant patients: Analysis of usage under treatment IND status. Transplant Proc 25:1442, 1993.
149. Winston DJ, Pollard RB, Ho WG, et al: Cytomegalovirus immune plasma in bone marrow transplant recipients. Ann Intern Med 97:11, 1982.
150. Meyers JD, Leszczynski J, Zaia JA, et al: Prevention of cytomegalovirus infection by cytomegalovirus immune globulin after marrow transplantation. Ann Intern Med 98:442, 1983.
151. Condie RM, O'Reilly RJ: Prevention of cytomegalovirus infection by prophylaxis with an intravenous hyperimmune, native, unmodified cytomegalovirus globulin. Am J Med 76:134, 1984.
152. Bowden RA, Sayers M, Flournoy N, et al: Cytomegalovirus immune globulin and seronegative blood products to prevent primary cytomegalovirus infection after marrow transplantation. N Engl J Med 314:1006, 1986.
153. Kubanek B, Ernst P, Ostendorff P, et al: Preliminary data of controlled trial of hyperimmune globulin in the prevention of cytomegalovirus in bone marrow transplant recipients. Transplant Proc 117:468, 1985.
154. Winston DJ, Ho WG, Lin TH, et al: Intravenous immune globulin for prevention of cytomegalovirus infection and interstitial pneumonia after bone marrow transplantation. Ann Intern Med 106:12, 1987.
155. Sullivan KM, Kopecky KJ, Jocom J, et al: Immunomodulatory and antimicrobial efficacy of intravenous immunoglobulin in bone marrow transplantation. N Engl J Med 323:705, 1990.
156. Reed EC, Bowden RA, Dandliker PS, et al: Efficacy of cytomegalovirus immunoglobulin in marrow transplant recipients with cytomegalovirus pneumonia. J Infect Dis 156:641, 1987.
157. Emmanuel D, Cunningham I, Jules-Elysee K, et al: Cytomegalovirus pneumonia after bone marrow transplantation successfully treated with the combination of ganciclovir and high-dose intravenous immune globulin. Ann Intern Med 109:777, 1988.
158. Reed EC, Bowden RA, Dandliker PS, et al: Treatment of cytomegalovirus pneumonia with ganciclovir and intravenous cytomegalovirus immunoglobulin in patients with bone marrow transplants. Ann Intern Med 109:783, 1988.
159. Schmidt GM, Horak DA, Niland JC, et al: A randomized, controlled trial of prophylactic ganciclovir for cytomegalovirus pulmonary infection in recipients of allogeneic bone marrow transplants. N Engl J Med 324:1005, 1991.
160. Schafers HJ, Wahlers T, Jurmann M, et al: Hyperimmunoglobulin for cytomegalovirus prophylaxis following heart transplantation. J Hosp Infect 12(Suppl D):61, 1988.
161. Saliba F, Arulnaden JL, Gugenheim J, et al: CMV hyperimmune globulin prophylaxis after liver transplantation: A prospective randomized controlled study. Transplant Proc 21:2260, 1989.
162. Dussaix E, Wood C: Cytomegalovirus infection in pediatric liver recipients. Transplantation 48:272, 1989.
163. Snydman DR, Werner BG, Dougherty NN, et al: Cytomegalovirus immune globulin prophylaxis in liver transplantation. A randomized, double-blind, placebo-controlled trial. Ann Intern Med 119:984, 1993.
164. Prian GW, Koep LJ: Elimination of cytomegalovirus disease in liver transplant patients treated prophylactically with combination cytomegalovirus hyperimmune globulin and ganciclovir. Transplant Proc 26(Suppl 1):54, 1994.
165. Winston DJ, Wirin D, Shaked A, Busuttil RW: Randomised comparison of ganciclovir and high-dose acyclovir for long-term cytomegalovirus prophylaxis in liver-transplant recipients. Lancet 346:69, 1995.
166. Bernstein LJ, Ochs HD, Wedgwood RJ, Rubinstein A: Defective humoral immunity in pediatric acquired immune deficiency syndrome. J Pediatr 107:352, 1985.
167. Krasinski K, Borkowsky W, Bonk S, et al: Bacterial infections in human immunodeficiency virus-infected children. Pediatr Infect Dis J 7:323, 1988.
168. Calvelli TA, Rubinstein A: Intravenous gammaglobulin in infant acquired immunodeficiency syndrome. Pediatr Infect Dis 5(Suppl 3):S207, 1986.

169. Oleske JM, Connor EM, Bobila R, et al: The use of IVIG in children with AIDS. Vox Sang 52:172, 1987.
170. Schaad UB, Gianella-Borradori A, Perret B, et al: Intravenous immune globulin in symptomatic pediatric human immunodeficiency virus infection. Eur J Pediatr 147:300, 1988.
171. Williams PE, Hague RA, Yap PL, et al: Treatment of human immunodeficiency virus antibody positive children with intravenous immunoglobulin. J Hosp Infect 12(Suppl D):67, 1988.
172. Hague RA, Yap PL, Mok JYQ, et al: Intravenous immunoglobulin in HIV infection: Evidence for the efficacy of treatment. Arch Dis Child 64:1146, 1989.
173. Spector SA, Gelber RD, McGrath N, et al: A controlled trial of intravenous immune globulin for the prevention of serious bacterial infections in children receiving zidovudine for advanced human immunodeficiency virus infection. N Engl J Med 331:1181, 1994.
174. Mofenson LM, Moye J Jr, Korelitz J, et al: Crossover of placebo patients to intravenous immunoglobulin confirms efficacy for prophylaxis of bacterial infections and reduction of hospitalization in human immunodeficiency virus–infected children. The National Institute of Child Health and Human Development Intravenous Immunoglobulin Clinical Trial Study Group. Pediatr Infect Dis J 13:477, 1994.
175. Lambert JS, Stiehm ER: Passive immunity in the prevention of maternal-fetal transmission of human immunodeficiency virus infection. Ann N Y Acad Sci 693:186, 1993.
176. Mandelbrot L, Schlienger I, Bongain A, et al: Thrombocytopenia in pregnant women infected with human immunodeficiency virus: Maternal and neonatal outcome. Am J Obstet Gynecol 171:252, 1994.
177. Jablonowski H, Sander O, Willers R, et al: The use of intravenous immunoglobulins in symptomatic HIV infection. Results of a randomized study. Clin Invest 72:220, 1994.
178. Kiehl M, Stoll R, Domschke W: Intravenose Immunoglobulinsubstitution bei Patienten mit ARC and AIDS (WR3-6). Immun Infekt 22:53, 1994.
179. Vittecoq D, Chevret S, Morand-Joubert L, et al: Passive immunotherapy in AIDS: A double-blind randomized study based on transfusions of plasma rich in anti–human immunodeficiency virus 1 antibodies vs. transfusions of seronegative plasma. Proc Natl Acad Sci USA 92:1195, 1995.
180. Levy J, Youvan T, Lee ML: Passive hyperimmune plasma therapy in the treatment of acquired immunodeficiency syndrome: Results of a 12-month multicenter double-blind controlled trial. The Passive Hyperimmune Therapy Study Group. Blood 84:2130, 1994.
181. Yap PL: Does intravenous immune globulin have a role in HIV-infected patients? Clin Exp Immunol 97(Suppl 1):59, 1994.
182. Pollak AN, Janinis J, Green D: Successful intravenous immune globulin therapy for human immunodeficiency virus–associated thrombocytopenia. Arch Intern Med 148:695, 1988.
183. Buseel JB, Haimi JS: Isolated thrombocytopenia in patients infected with HIV: Treatment with intravenous gammaglobulin. Am J Hematol 28:79, 1988.
184. Bierling P, Bettaieb A, Oksenhendler E: Human immunodeficiency virus–related immune thrombocytopenia. Semin Thromb Hemost 21:68, 1995.
185. Cantell K: Development of antiviral therapy with alpha interferons: Promises, false hopes and accomplishments. Ann Med 27:23, 1995.
186. Terrault N, Feinman SV: Interferons for viral hepatitis. Transfus Med Rev 9:29, 1995.
187. Perrillo RP, Schiff ER, Davis GL, et al: A randomized, controlled trial of interferon alfa-2b alone and after prednisone withdrawal for the treatment of chronic hepatitis B. N Engl J Med 323:295, 1990.
188. Alexander GJM, Fagan EA, Daniels HM, et al: Loss of HbsAg with interferon therapy in chronic hepatitis B virus infection. Lancet 2:66, 1988.
189. Hoofnagle JH: Therapy of acute and chronic viral hepatitis. Adv Intern Med 39:241, 1994.
190. Brook MG, McDonald JA, Karayiannis P, et al: Randomised controlled trial of interferon alfa 2a (Roferon-A) for the treatment of chronic hepatitis B virus (HBV) infection: Factors that influence response. Gut 30:1116, 1989.
191. Wong DKH, Cheung AM, O'Rourke K, et al: Effect of alpha-interferon treatment in patients with hepatitis B antigen–positive chronic hepatitis B. Ann Intern Med 119:312, 1993.
192. Davis GL, Balart LA, Schiff ER, et al: Treatment of chronic hepatitis C with recombinant interferon alfa. A multicenter randomized, controlled trial. N Engl J Med 321:1501, 1989.
193. Di Bisceglie AM, Martin P, Kassianides C, et al: Recombinant interferon alfa therapy for chronic hepatitis C. N Engl J Med 321:1506, 1989.
194. Schvarcz R, Weiland O, Wejstal R, et al: A randomized controlled open study of interferon alpha-2b treatment of chronic non-A, non-B posttransfusion hepatitis: No correlation of outcome to presence of hepatitis C virus antibodies. Scand J Infect Dis 21:617, 1989.
195. Poynard T, Bedossa P, Chevallier M, et al: A comparison of three interferon alfa-2b regimens for the long-term treatment of chronic non-A, non-B hepatitis. N Engl J Med 332:1457, 1995.
196. Stone KM: Human papillomavirus infection and genital warts: Update on epidemiology and treatment. Clin Infect Dis 20(Suppl 1):S91, 1995.
197. Vance JC, Bart BJ, Hansen RC, et al: Intralesional recombinant alpha-2 interferon for the treatment of patients with condyloma acuminatum or verruca plantaris. Arch Dermatol 122:272, 1986.
198. Eron LJ, Judson F, Tucker S, et al: Interferon therapy for condylomata acuminata. N Engl J Med 315:1059, 1986.
199. Reichman RC, Oakes D, Bonnez W, et al: Treatment of condyloma acuminatum with three different interferons administered intralesionally: A double blind, placebo-controlled trial. Ann Intern Med 108:675, 1988.
200. Friedman-Kien A, Eron LJ, Conant M, et al: Natural interferon alfa for treatment of condylomata acuminata. JAMA 259:533, 1988.
201. Leventhal BG, Kashima HK, Mounts P, et al: Long-term response of recurrent respiratory papillomatosis to treatment with lymphoblastoid interferon alfa-n1. N Engl J Med 325:613, 1991.
202. Penna C, Fallani MG, Gordigiani R, et al: Intralesional beta-interferon treatment of cervical intraepithelial neoplasia associated with human papillomavirus infection. Tumori 80:146, 1994.
203. Schneider A, Grubert T, Kirchmayr R, et al: Efficacy trail of topically administered interferon gamma-1 gel in comparison to laser treatment in cervical intraepithelial neoplasia. Arch Gynecol Obstet 256:75, 1995.
204. Fleshner PR, Freilich MI: Adjuvant interferon for anal condyloma. A prospective, randomized trial. Dis Colon Rectum 37:1255, 1994.
205. Ling MR: Therapy of genital human papillomavirus infections. Part I: Indications for and justification of therapy. Int J Dermatol 31:682, 1992.
206. Ling MR: Therapy of genital human papillomavirus infections. Part II: Methods of treatment. Int J Dermatol 31:769, 1992.
207. Thrasher AJ, Keep NH, Wientjes F, Segal AW: Chronic granulomatous disease. Biochim Biophys Acta 1227:1, 1994.
208. Gallin JI, Malech HL, Weening JT, et al: A controlled trial of interferon gamma to prevent infection in chronic granulomatous disease. International Chronic Granulomatous Disease Cooperative Study. N Engl J Med 324:509, 1991.
209. Fisher A, Segal AW, Seger R, Weening RS: The management of chronic granulomatous disease. Eur J Pediatr 152:896, 1993.
210. Weening RS, Leitz GJ, Seger RA: Recombinant human interferon-gamma in patients with chronic granulomatous disease—European follow up study. Eur J Pediatr 154:295–8, 1995.
211. Curnutte JT: Conventional versus interferon-gamma therapy in chronic granulomatous disease. J Infect Dis 167(Suppl 1):S8, 1993.
212. Pearson RD, Sousa AQ: Clinical spectrum of leishmaniasis. Clin Infect Dis 22:1, 1996.
213. Sypek JP, Wyler DJ: Antileishmanial defense in macrophages triggered by tumor necrosis factor expressed on CD4+ T lymphocyte plasma membrane. J Exp Med 174:755, 1991.
214. Murray HW, Rubin BY, Rothermel CD: Killing of intracellular *Leishmania donovani* by lymphokine-stimulated human mononuclear phagocytes. Evidence that interferon-gamma is the activating cytokine. J Clin Invest 72:1506, 1983.
215. Badaro R, Johnson WD Jr: The role of interferon-gamma in the treatment of visceral and diffuse cutaneous leishmaniasis. J Infect Dis 167(Suppl 1):S13, 1993.

216. Botasso O, Cabrine J, Falcoff R: Successful treatment of antimony-resistant American mucocutaneous leishmaniasis. Arch Dermatol 128:996, 1992.
217. Cheeseman SH, Rubin RH, Stewart JA, et al: Controlled clinical trial of prophylactic human-leukocyte interferon in renal transplantation. N Engl J Med 300:1345, 1979.
218. Verheyden JPH: Evolution of therapy for cytomegalovirus infection. Rev Infect Dis 10(Suppl 3):S477, 1988.
219. Douglas RM, Moore BW, Miles HB, et al: Prophylactic efficacy of intranasal alpha-2-interferon against rhinovirus infections in the family setting. N Engl J Med 314:65, 1986.
220. Hayden FG, Albrecht JK, Kaiser DL, Gwaltney JM Jr: Prevention of natural colds by contact prophylaxis with intranasal alpha-2-interferon. N Engl J Med 314:71, 1986.
221. Gabrilove JL, Jakubowski A, Scher H, et al: Effect of granulocyte colony-stimulating factor on neutropenia and associated morbidity due to chemotherapy for transitional-cell carcinoma of the urothelium. N Engl J Med 318:1414, 1988.
222. Crawford J, Ozer H, Stoller R, et al: Reduction by granulocyte colony-stimulating factor of fever and neutropenia induced by chemotherapy in patients with small-cell lung cancer. N Engl J Med 325:164, 1991.
223. Lieschke GJ, Burgess AW: Granulocyte colony-stimulating factor and granulocyte-macrophage colony-stimulating factor (1). N Engl J Med 327:28, 1992.
224. Lieschke GJ, Burgess AW: Granulocyte colony-stimulating factor and granulocyte-macrophage colony-stimulating factor (2). N Engl J Med 327:99, 1992.
225. Snydman DR, Sullivan B, Gill M, et al: Nosocomial sepsis associated with interleukin-2. Ann Intern Med 112:102, 1990.
226. Klempner MS, Noring R, Mier JW, Atkins MB: An acquired chemotactic defect in neutrophils from patients receiving interleukin-2 immunotherapy. N Engl J Med 332:959, 1990.
227. Ratko TA, Burnett DA, Foulke GE, et al: Consensus statement. Recommendations for off-label use of intravenously administered immunoglobulin preparations. JAMA 273:1865, 1995.
228. Plotkin SA, Daum RS, Giebink GS, et al: Intravenous γ-globulin use in children with acute Kawasaki disease. Pediatrics 82:122, 1988.
229. Rowley AH, Schulman ST: What is the status of intravenous gamma-globulin for Kawasaki syndrome in the United States and Canada? Pediatr Infect Dis J 7:463, 1988.
230. Onouchi Z, Yanagisawa M, Hirayama T, et al: Optimal dosage and differences in therapeutic efficacy of IGIV in Kawasaki disease. Acta Paediatr Jpn 37:40, 1995.
231. Engle MA, Fatica NS, Bussel JB, et al: Clinical trial of single-dose intravenous gamma globulin in acute Kawasaki disease. Am J Dis Child 143:1300, 1989.
232. Barron KS, Murphy DJ, Silverman ED, et al: Treatment of Kawasaki syndrome: A comparison of two dosage regimens of intravenously administered immune globulin. J Pediatr 117:638, 1990.
233. Newburger JW, Takahashi M, Beiser AS, et al: A single intravenous infusion of gamma globulin as compared with four infusions in the treatment of acute Kawasaki syndrome. N Engl J Med 324:1633, 1991.
234. Joffe A, Kabani A, Jadavji T: Atypical and complicated Kawasaki disease in infants. Do we need criteria? West J Med 162:322, 1995.
235. Rosenfeld EA, Corydon KE, Shulman ST: Kawasaki disease in infants less than one year of age. J Pediatr 126:524, 1995.
236. Nakamura Y, Hirose K, Yanagawa H, et al: Incidence rate of recurrent Kawasaki disease in Japan. Acta Paediatr 83:1061, 1994.
237. Best GK, Scott DF, Kling JM, et al: Protection of rabbits in an infection model of toxic shock syndrome (TSS) by a TSS toxin-1–specific monoclonal antibody. Infect Immun 56:998, 1988.
238. Zumla A: Superantigens, T cells, and microbes. Clin Infect Dis 15:313, 1992.
239. Takei S, Arora YK, Walker SM: Intravenous immunoglobulin contains specific antibodies inhibitory to activation of T cells by staphylococcal toxin superantigens. J Clin Invest 91:602, 1993.
240. Dwyer JM: Manipulating the immune system with immune globulin. N Engl J Med 326:107, 1992.
241. Ogawa M, Ueda S, Anzai N, et al: Toxic shock syndrome after staphylococcal pneumonia treated with intravenous immunoglobulin (Letter). Vox Sang 68:59, 1995.
242. Pattison JR, Jones SE, Hodgson J, et al: Parvovirus infections and hypoplastic crisis in sickle-cell anaemia. Lancet 1:664, 1981.
243. Serjeant GR, Topley JM, Mason K, et al: Outbreak of aplastic crises in sickle cell anaemia associated with parvovirus-like agent. Lancet 2:595, 1981.
244. Kurtzman GJ, Frickhofen N, Kimball J, et al: Pure red cell aplasia of ten years' duration due to B19 parvovirus infection and its cure with immunoglobulin therapy. N Engl J Med 321:519, 1989.
245. Frickhofen N, Abkowitz JL, Safford M, et al: Persistent B19 parvovirus infection in patients infected with human immunodeficiency virus-1: A treatable cause of anemia in AIDS. Ann Intern Med 113:926, 1990.
246. Gloning KP, Schramm T, Bruisis E, et al: Successful intrauterine treatment of fetal hydrops caused by parvovirus B19 infection. Behring Inst Mitt 85:79, 1990.
247. Nigro G, D'Eufemia P, Zerbini M, et al: Parvovirus B19 infection in a hypogammaglobulinemic infant with neurologic disorders and anemia: Successful immunoglobulin therapy. Pediatr Infect Dis J 13:1019, 1994.
248. Finkel TH, Torok TJ, Ferguson PJ, et al: Chronic parvovirus B19 infection and systemic necrotising vasculitis: Opportunistic infection or aetiological agent? Lancet 343:1255, 1994.
249. Groothuis JR, Gutierrez KM, Lauer BA: Respiratory syncytial virus infections in children with bronchopulmonary dysplasia. Pediatrics 82:199, 1988.
250. MacDonald NE, Hall CB, Suffin SC, et al: Respiratory syncytial viral infection in infants with congenital heart disease. N Engl J Med 307:397, 1982.
251. Hall CB, Powell KR, MacDonald NE, et al: Respiratory syncytial virus infection in children with compromised immune function. N Engl J Med 315:77, 1986.
252. Hertz MI, Englund JA, Snover D, et al: Respiratory syncytial virus–induced acute lung injury in adult patients with bone marrow transplants: A clinical approach and review of the literature. Medicine (Baltimore) 68:269, 1989.
253. Parrot RH, Kim HW, Arrobio JOP, et al: Epidemiology of respiratory syncytial virus in Washington DC. II. Infection and disease with respect to age, immunologic status, race, and sex. Am J Epidemiol 98:289, 1973.
254. Hemming VG, Rodriguez W, Kim HW, et al: Intravenous immunoglobulin treatment of respiratory syncytial virus infections in infants and young children. Antimicrob Agents Chemother 31:1882, 1987.
255. Groothuis JR, Levin MJ, Rodriguez W, et al: Use of intravenous gamma globulin to passively immunize high-risk children against respiratory syncytial virus: Safety and pharmacokinetics. Antimicrob Agents Chemother 35:1469, 1991.
256. Meissner HC, Fulton DR, Groothuis JR, et al: Controlled trial to evaluate protection of high risk infants against respiratory syncytial virus disease by using standard intravenous immune globulin. Antimicrob Agents Chemother 37:1655, 1993.
257. Siber GR, Leszczynski J, Pena-Cruz V, et al: Protective antibody of a human respiratory syncytial virus immune globulin prepared from donors screened by microneutralization assay. J Infect Dis 165:456, 1992.
258. Groothuis JR, Simoes EAF, Levin ML, et al: Prophylactic administration of respiratory syncytial virus immune globulin to high-risk infants and young children. N Engl J Med 329:1524, 1993.
259. Brandtzaeg P: Overview of the mucosal immune system. Curr Top Microbiol Immunol 146:13, 1989.
260. Welsh JK, May JT: Anti-infective properties of breast milk. J Pediatr 94:1, 1979.
261. Eibl MM, Wolf HM, Furnkranz H, Rosenkranz A: Prevention of necrotizing enterocolitis in low-birth-weight infants by IgA-IgM. N Engl J Med 319:1, 1988.
262. Eibl MM, Wolf HM, Furnkranz H, Rosenkranz A: Prophylaxis of necrotizing enterocolitis by oral IgA-IgG: Review of a clinical study in low birth weight infants and discussion of the pathogenic role of infection. J Clin Immunol 10(Nov Suppl):S72, 1990.
263. Yolken RH, Maldonado Y, Kinney J, Vonderfecht S: Epidemiology and potential methods for prevention of neonatal intestinal viral infections. Rev Infect Dis 12(Suppl 4):421, 1990.
264. Tacket CO, Losonsky G, Link H, et al: Protection by milk immunoglobulin concentrate against oral challenge with enterotoxigenic *Escherichia coli*. N Engl J Med 318:1240, 1988.

265. Tzipori S, Roberton D, Chapman C: Remission of diarrhoea due to cryptosporidiosis in an immunodeficient child treated with hyperimmune bovine colostrum. Br Med J 293:1276, 1986.
266. Tzipori S, Robertson D, Cooper DA, et al: Chronic cryptosporidial diarrhoea and hyperimmune cow colostrum. Lancet 2:344, 1987.
267. Ungar BLP, Ward DJ, Fayer RF, et al: Cessation of *Cryptosporidium*-associated diarrhea in an acquired immunodeficiency patient after treatment with hyperimmune bovine colostrum. Gastroenterology 98:486, 1990.
268. Fries L, Hillman K, Crabb J, et al: Clinical and microbiological effects of bovine anti-*Cryptosporidium* immunoglobulin (BACI) on cryptosporidial diarrhea in AIDS (Abstr). Presented at the 34th Interscience Conference on Antimicrobial Agents and Chemotherapy; October 7, 1994; Orlando, FL.
269. Jahrling PB, Peters CJ: Passive antibody therapy of Lassa fever in cynomolgus monkeys: Importance of neutralizing antibody and Lassa virus strain. Infect Immun 44:528, 1984.
270. Leifer E, Gocke DJ, Bourne H: Lassa fever, a new virus disease of man from West Africa. II. Report of a laboratory-acquired infection treated with plasma from a person recently recovered from the disease. Am J Trop Med Hyg 19:677, 1970.
271. Jahring PB, Frame JD, Rhoderick JB, Monson MH: Endemic Lassa fever in Liberia. IV. Selection of optimally effective plasma for treatment by passive immunization. Trans R Soc Trop Med Hyg 79:380, 1985.
272. McCormick JB, King IB, Webb PA, et al: Lassa fever: Effective therapy with ribavirin. N Engl J Med 314:20, 1986.
273. Maiztegui JI, Fernandez N, Damilano A: Efficacy of immune plasma in treatment of Argentine haemorrhagic fever and association between treatment and a late neurological syndrome. Lancet 2:1216, 1979.
274. Enria DA, Briggiler AM, Fernandez NJ, et al: Importance of dose of neutralising antibodies in treatment of Argentine haemorrhagic fever with immune plasma. Lancet 2:255, 1984.
275. van de Wal BW, Joubert JR, van Eeden PJ, King JB: A nosocomial outbreak of Crimean-Congo haemorrhagic fever at Tygerberg Hospital. S Afr Med J 68:729, 1985.
276. Griffiths JK, Snydman DR. The use of intravenous immunoglobulin in viral infections. *In* Yap PL (ed): Clinical Applications of Intravenous Immunoglobulin Therapy. Edinburgh, Churchill Livingstone, 1992, pp 167–202.
277. Centers for Disease Control and Prevention: Health Information for International Travel 1995. US Department of Health and Human Services, Public Health Service, National Center for Infectious Diseases. Washington, DC, US Government Printing Office; 1995. HHS publication (CDC) 95–8280.
278. Sabchareon A, Burnouf T, Ouattara D, et al: Parasitologic and clinical human response to immunoglobulin administration in falciparum malaria. Am J Trop Med Hyg 45:297, 1991.

37

Side Effects of Antimicrobial Therapy

Sherwood L. Gorbach
Harold C. Neu

Virtually any antimicrobial agent can produce side effects, which vary from mild to life threatening (Table 37–1). Adverse effects of antimicrobial agents vary greatly depending on the genetic background of the patient and are often influenced by renal and hepatic function. Dose, duration of therapy, and concurrent use of other therapy affect both the frequency and the intensity of adverse effects. In some situations the precise mechanism of the adverse effect is known, whereas in others the biochemical events are not fully established. Antimicrobial agents can also alter the normal flora of the body and cause adverse effects as a result of overgrowth of organisms or selection of normally saprophytic organisms that produce disease in compromised patients. A listing of common side effects of oral antimicrobial drugs, based on selected articles in the literature,[1–31] is presented in Table 37–2.

Hypersensitivity-Allergic Reactions

Every antimicrobial agent has been associated with hypersensitivity reactions. The antigenic potential of agents varies, but many provoke reactions due either to immunoglobulin combination or to sensitization of lymphocytes. Penicillins, perhaps because they are the most widely used agents, have been associated with the most hypersensitivity reactions.[32–36] Penicillin G is present in nature, and traces found in food products may act as sensitizing molecules in persons who have not received penicillin therapeutically. Penicillins, primarily penicillin G, and derivatives such as penicilloic acid, penicillanic acid, and other breakdown products of its metabolism can combine with human proteins.[32] The minor breakdown products benzylpenicilloate and penicillin itself are the most important components that produce the anaphylactic reactions observed in 0.004% to 0.04% of persons who receive a penicillin,[37] with deaths estimated to occur in 1 or 2 of 100,000 treated patients.[35, 37] Data on anaphylaxis with cephalosporins have been collected by various pharmaceutical companies during clinical trials. For example, among 8236 patients given cefaclor, 0.1% had urticaria, and there were no instances of anaphylaxis.[35] The major determinants, penicilloyl components, can be combined with lysine to make a penicilloyl-polylysine combination (Pre-Pen), which can be used as a skin test for penicillin allergy. Persons who do not demonstrate a skin reaction (immediate wheal and flare reaction) to the penicilloyl-polylysine combination have less than a 5% chance of having either an immediate (2 to 30 minutes) anaphylactic (wheezing, laryngeal or generalized edema) or an accelerated (1 to 72 hours) urticarial reaction.[32] In a large cooperative study, patients with or without a history of penicillin allergy were skin tested with the major and minor determinants and then treated with penicillin. The study confirmed the excellent positive and negative predictive values of the skin tests regardless of the history of allergy. Only 1.2% of history-positive, skin test–negative patients had a reaction. When patients with both a positive history and positive skin tests received incremental doses of penicillin, 22% (2 of 9) had a reaction.[38]

Skin tests with penicilloyl-polylysine and minor determinants do not predict skin reactions to penicillins such as rash. It is possible that these reactions are in part immunoglobulin M antibody mediated. In some patients, continued administration of penicillins elicits production of blocking immunoglobulin G antibodies and the rash abates. However, this cannot be predicted, and fulminant exfoliative reactions do occasionally develop. In general, ampicillin produces rashes twice as frequently as other penicillins, approximately 7% versus 3%.[39] The mechanism of the reaction is not established but appears to be related to polymers of the ampicillin because it can be reduced by ultrapurification of ampicillin during production. Whether rash is truly less frequent with amoxicillin than with ampicillin has not been established. Many patients who have acute Epstein-Barr virus infection

TABLE 37–1 ■ Adverse Reactions to Antimicrobial Agents*

REACTION	COMMON FOR	INFREQUENT FOR
Hypersensitivity-allergic		
Anaphylaxis	Penicillin G	Cephalosporins, imipenem
Fever		All agents
SLE-like reactions	Isoniazid	Griseofulvin, nitrofurantoin
Cutaneous reactions	Sulfonamides, penicillins	All agents
Histamine reactions	Vancomycin	
Phototoxicity	Tetracyclines	Quinolones, chloroquine, primaquine, griseofulvin
Hematopoietic		
Pancytopenia	Choramphenicol	
Neutropenia	Sulfonamides, trimethoprim, pyrimethamine, zoduvidine	Penicillins, cephalosporins, dapsone
Hemolytic anemia (G6PD associated)	Sulfonamides, nitrofurans, chloramphenicol, sulfones, nalidixic acid, primaquine	
Immune hemolysis	Penicillins, cephalosporins, isoniazid, rifampin	
Sideroblastic anemia	Isoniazid	
Thrombocytopenia	Sulfonamides, penicillins, cephalosporins, rifampin, trimethoprim, pyrimethamine	
Platelet dysfunction	Carbenicillin, ticarcillin, moxalactam	Extended-spectrum penicillins
Hypoprothrombinemia	Moxalactam, cefoperazone, cefamandole	Cefotetan, ceftriaxone, cefmetazole
Gastrointestinal		
Nausea, emesis, abdominal pain	Erythromycin	Oral penicillins, quinolones, metronidazole, nystatin, tetracyclines, TMP-SMX, ketoconazole
Diarrhea	Ampicillin-sulbactam, amoxicillin-clavulanate, cefixime, cefoperazone, ceftriaxone, clindamycin	Any agent
Pseudomonas enterocolitis (*Clostridium difficile*)	Any agent, more commonly ampicillin, TMP-SMX, cefoxitin, clindamycin	
Malabsorption	Neomycin	Other aminoglycosides
Hepatic		
Transaminase level increase	Penicillins, particularly oxacillin, aztreonam	
Cholestatic jaundice	Oleandomycin, erythromycin estolate, nitrofurans, sulfonamides	
Hepatitis	Isoniazid, nitrofurantoin	Rifampin, sulfonamides, ketoconazole
Pulmonary		
Histamine release	Polymyxin by aerosol	
Interstitial infiltrates	Nitrofurantoin	
Cardiovascular		
Arrhythmias	Amphotericin B, miconazole, penicillin G	
Hypotension	Pentamidine, emetine	
Metabolic		
Hypokalemia	Carbenicillin, amphotericin B	
Hypogonadal effects	Ketoconazole	
Hyperglycemia	Nalidixic acid	
Pancreatitis	Pentamidine, nitrofurantoin, TMP-SMX	
Diabetes	Pentamidine	
Hypomagnesemia	Amphotericin B, aminoglycosides	
Renal		
Hypersensitivity nephritis	Sulfonamides	
Interstitial nephritis	All β-lactams	
Tubular toxicity	Aminoglycosides, polymyxins	
Distal tubular acidosis	Amphotericin B, tetracyclines	
Crystal deposition	Fluoroquinolones, acyclovir	
Neurologic		
Peripheral neuropathy	Nitrofurans, metronidazole, polymyxins, griseofulvin, cycloserine, isoniazid	Tetracyclines
Muscular blockade	Polymyxins, aminoglycosides, capreomycin	Clindamycin, lincomycin
Central nervous excitation	Fluoroquinolones	
Seizures	Penicillin, imipenem, cycloserine	Amantadine, isoniazid, metronidazole, fluoroquinolones, thiabendazole
Ophthalmic		
Blindness	Ethambutol	Isoniazid, chloramphenicol, quinolones, chloroquine
Ototoxicity		
Deafness	Aminoglycosides, vancomycin	Erythromycin
Vestibulotoxicity	Aminoglycosides, minocycline	

*SLE, Systemic lupus erythematosus; G6PD, glucose-6-phosphate dehydrogenase; TMP-SMX, trimethoprim-sulfamethoxazole.

(infectious mononucleosis) will develop a skin reaction when they receive ampicillin. Such persons can subsequently receive a penicillin without reaction. Allergic reactions to the quinolone antibiotics are rare; transient rash is seen in less than 1% of treated patients and anaphylactic reactions are extremely rare.[40, 41]

Serum sickness–type reactions were reported in the past to penicillins, but they have been noted infrequently in the past two decades. A reaction of fever, edema, and arthralgia has followed use of the oral cephalosporin cefaclor, at a reported incidence of 0.02% to 0.5%, which is higher compared with amoxicillin or trimethoprim-sulfamethoxazole.[42, 43] Vasculitis-

TABLE 37–2 ■ Reported Percent Frequency of Selected Side Effects After Oral Administration of Antibacterial Drugs*

DRUG	REFERENCE NO.	NO. OF PATIENTS	PERCENTAGE WITH Nausea	Vomiting	Diarrhea	Rash	Therapy Stopped	Other Side Effects
Cephalosporins								
Cephalexin	1	116	4.0	10	6.0	1.0	NP	
	2	305	2.3	0.7	1.3	1.0	1.3	
	3	NP	—	No quantitative data			—	
Cefaclor	2	245	4.5	0.4	5.7	0.4	—	"Serum sickness" 0.02%–0.5%[21, 22]
	4	129	NP	NP	3.0	2.0	—	
	5	435	1.0	1.0	2.0	1.0	—	
	6	374	2.4	0.5	3.7	1.3	—	
	3	NP	NP	NP	1.0	1.5	2.4	
Cefuroxime axetil	6	84	5.0	1.0	8.0	0	—	
	3	NP	2.4	2.0	3.5	0.6	—	
Cefixime	4	134	NP	NP	16	3.0	—	
	3	NP	7	NP	16	<2	3.8	
Cefprozil	7	2,383	2.3	0.7	1.2	0.7	2.0	
	3	NP	3.5	1.0	2.9	0.9	2.0	
Cefpodoxime proxetil	8	762	1.0	NP	4	NP	2.0	
	9	3,650	—	2	—	NP	NP	
	10	1,468	1.0	0.2	4.6	0.5	2.3	
Loracarbef	11	4,506	1.9	1.4	4.1	1.2	1.5	
Ceftibuten	Investigator brochure	1,870	1.0	2.0	4.0	<1	—	
Penicillins								
Penicillin V	2	630	3.3	1.3	3.7	0.6	2.5	
	5	199	0	0	5.0	0	—	
	7	918	NP	NP	NP	1.2–3.0	—	
	3	NP	NP	NP	NP	2.5–4.2	—	
Ampicillin	7	1,775	NP	NP	NP	5.2	—	
	12	2,998	NP	NP	—	5.2	—	
Amoxicillin	2	574	1.7	0.5	4.5	1.6	1.9	
	7	1,225	NP	NP	NP	3.9–6.4	—	
Amoxicillin-clavulanate	2	129	NP	1.6	8.5	0.8	—	
	4	267	NP	2.0	22	1.0	1.0	
	6	110	5	2	18	4.0	—	
	8	306	NP	9.2	24	NP	—	
	3	NP	3	1	9	3	2–3	
Lincosamides								
Clindamycin	13	NP	NP	NP	Up to 20	NP	NP	CDT antibiotic-associated diarrhea in 0.01%–18% of treated patients[16,17]
	3	NP	NP	NP	NP	NP	NP	
	14	52	NP	NP	31	21	31	
Macrolides								
Erythromycin base	15	128	2.0	3.0	2.0	0	NP	Rare idiosyncratic hepatitis
	13	147	NP	NP	NP	NP	0.4–0.6	
Enteric coated	2	441	5.5	2.9	5.3	0.6	4.9	
	16	112	—	27	—	0	19	
	17	21	—	52	—	0	14	
	3	Multiple preparations. No data—general comments only						
Azithromycin	2	3,995	2.6	0.8	3.6	0.2	0.7	
	18	229	2.6	NP	5.2	NP	NP	
	3	NP	3.0	<1	5.0	<1	0.7	
Clarithromycin	19	3,768	3.8	NP	3.0	NP	NP	
	3	NP	3.0	NP	3.0	0	4	
Fluoroquinolines								
Ciprofloxacin	20	4,287	—	2.3	1.5	0.8	1.2	Symptoms referable to CNS (i.e., headache, agitation, dizziness, sleep disturbance in 1%–4%)[29]
	3	2,799	5.2	2.0	2.3	1.1	3.5	
Ofloxacin		3,184	—	5.4	—	NP	—	In high dose, headache, tremor, disorientation[30]
		15,641	—	0.9	0.4	0.3	1.5	
	3	NP	3.0	1.3	1.0	NP	4.0	
Lomefloxacin	3	2,869	3.7	<1	1.4	1.0	2.6	
Temafloxacin	3	2,602	5.6	1.1	2.8	1.5	4.1	
TMP-SMX	7	1,066	—	—	—	—	2.4–4.7	
	23	47	—	18	—	2	2	
	24	47	11	NP	0	6	11	
	25	196	8.2	—	0	5	4	
	26	180	—	4	—	2	3.9	
	27	129	—	7	—	7	NP	
	28	216	9.3	NP	NP	NP	5.1	
	3	—	—	—	No quantitative data		—	

*NP, Not provided; CNS, central nervous system; CDT, *Clostridium difficile* toxin; TMP-SMX, trimethoprim-sulfamethoxazole.
From Gilbert DN: Aspects of the safety profile of oral antibacterial agents. Infect Dis Clin Pract 4(Suppl 2):S103–S112, 1995.

type reactions and purpuric reactions of the Henoch-Schönlein type have occurred principally with penicillins, cephalosporins, and sulfonamides but have been reported for every type of antimicrobial agent.

The prevalence of cephalosporin cross-reactions of an anaphylactic or accelerated type in penicillin-allergic patients is less than 5%[32]; nonetheless, cephalosporins should not be administered to a patient who has had anaphylaxis to penicillin unless a skin test has been performed. A number of studies have demonstrated that patients who are allergic to penicillins as demonstrated by positive skin tests can receive aztreonam, a monobactam, without allergic reaction.[44, 45] Carbapenems, such as imipenem, produce anaphylaxis and rash in penicillin-allergic patients.[44] Because β-lactamase inhibitors such as clavulanate and sulbactam are always combined with penicillins, it is unclear how frequently these compounds by themselves would produce allergic reactions.

Fever as a result of antimicrobial therapy has been reported for every class of antimicrobial agent and for all antiparasitic agents as well. It is important to realize that fever may be the sole manifestation of allergic reaction and that an allergic person may never develop rash or eosinophilia.

Isoniazid, griseofulvin, and nitrofurantoins produce a systemic lupus erythematosus–type reaction and positive results on antinuclear antibody tests.[46] Patients have fever, joint symptoms, and rash similar to what occurs in systemic lupus erythematosus.

Cutaneous Reactions

Cutaneous reactions to drugs can vary from a minor erythematous maculopapular eruption to exfoliative dermatitis. Fixed drug eruptions, urticaria, and photodermatitis are possible drug reactions. The most common causes of reactions are β-lactams, particularly penicillins, as already noted, and the sulfonamides. Indeed, 5% to 8% of patients receiving a sulfonamide may develop a skin reaction. The most serious skin reactions have occurred with long-acting sulfonamides[47] such as sulfadoxine, the sulfonamide component of Fansidar, which has been associated with Stevens-Johnson syndrome.[48] Skin reactions have occurred with tetracyclines, clindamycin (lincomycin), antituberculosis drugs such as isoniazid, ethambutol, rifampin, pyrazinamide, quinolones such as nalidixic acid, ciprofloxacin, norfloxacin, enoxacin, and metronidazole. Skin eruptions are infrequent for chloramphenicol, macrolides such as erythromycin, and aminoglycosides. Trimethoprim-sulfamethoxazole causes rash in about 10% of immunocompetent patients and in about 50% of patients with human immunodeficiency virus infection.[49, 50] Some human immunodeficiency virus–positive patients with rash can continue to receive the drug, albeit at a reduced dose.

A cutaneous eruption of erythema after rapid infusion of vancomycin, so-called red neck syndrome, is due to release of histamine.[51, 52] This can be aborted by administering antihistamine agents. Other agents probably cause such a reaction occasionally.

Phototoxicity (erythema associated with ultraviolet light exposure) is most often associated with use of tetracyclines, particularly the chloro derivatives such as chlortetracycline and dimethylchlortetracycline.[53] Antimalarials such as chloroquine and primaquine also produce photosensitization, as does griseofulvin.[54] Photosensitivity and photoonycholysis (subungual hemorrhages) have been reported to occur during or a few days after treatment with any of the quinolone antibiotics. The most frequently implicated drugs in photosensitivity reactions are lomefloxacin, pefloxacin, fleroxacin, and ofloxacin, whereas norfloxacin and ciprofloxacin are less often involved.[40, 41, 55] Photosensitization can cause severe sunburn reactions and even bullous eruptions in areas exposed to sun. Ichthyosis and excess pigmentation of the skin have occurred with use of clofazimine.

Hematopoietic Reactions

The most serious hematopoietic drug reactions are pancytopenia and aplastic anemia. The drug most often associated with these reactions is chloramphenicol, for which an incidence of 1 in 40,000 or 1 in 60,000 is suggested.[56] Toxicity has followed oral, intramuscular, and intravenous administration and ophthalmic instillation. There appear to be two types of marrow reactions to chloramphenicol. The more common type occurs in most persons who receive chloramphenicol in doses that cause prolonged serum levels greater than 25 μg/mL. Cytochrome oxidase and ferrochelatase activities are affected, resulting in a breakdown of oxidative phosphorylation.[57] Anemia and thrombocytopenia gradually develop. The bone marrow cells show maturational arrest with vacuolization of the cytoplasm of erythroid cells. The reticulocyte count falls, and there is an increase in serum iron level. These marrow changes and peripheral blood changes revert to normal if chloramphenicol is withdrawn. The second type of marrow depression is the rare form of aplastic anemia that appears to be genetically controlled, because it occurs in identical twins, and may be related to metabolic products of chloramphenicol. Chloramphenicol can be removed from the body by exchange transfusion or charcoal hemoperfusion.[58, 59] This reaction is neither dose related nor reversible. It has been suggested that thiamphenicol, in which the *p*-nitro group on the benzene ring has been replaced by a methylsulfonyl group and so is not metabolized, will not cause aplastic anemia, but this is not established. Isoniazid produces a sideroblastic anemia in a few patients.

Leukopenia has been reported with most antimicrobial agents. Several mechanisms probably are involved. In some cases white blood cells may be destroyed in the spleen because they are bound to the compounds. In other situations high concentrations may alter the ability of granulocyte colony-stimulating factor to cause white blood cell production. In the case of penicillins and cephalosporins, the latter form of toxicity seems to occur most often when β-lactam agents are taken in large doses for prolonged periods. Leukopenia has been noted most for oxacillin, nafcillin, and piperacillin of the penicillins, but it can occur with all agents, even oral cephalosporins such as cephalexin and the newer β-lactam agents aztreonam and imipenem.[34, 60–64]

Sulfonamides, trimethoprim, pyrimethamine, and sulfones such as dapsone can produce leukopenia by interfering with folate metabolism.[65] At high concentrations they have affinity for mammalian dihydrofolate reductase. Zidovudine (AZT) produces leukopenia by a similar mechanism, interfering with synthesis of white blood cells.[66] Sulfonamides produce the pseudo–Pelger-Huët anomaly of white blood cells. Other agents that have been associated with leukopenia, albeit infrequently, are acyclovir and amantadine. Leukopenia and even pancytopenia have followed when the flucytosine dose was not adjusted to the patient's renal function. This occurs most often when it is administered with amphotericin B. The mechanism is conversion of the flucytosine by intestinal bacteria to 5-fluorouracil, which is the actual marrow depressant.[67]

Hemolytic anemia occurs in persons with glucose-6-phosphate dehydrogenase deficiency who receive sulfonamides, sulfones, nitrofurans, furazolidone, chloramphenicol, nalidixic acid, or 8-aminoquinolines such as primaquine.[68] Immune hemolysis has developed during use of penicillins, cephalosporins, isoniazid, and rifampin and was seen with *p*-aminosalicylic acid when it was used. It has also (rarely) been reported for erythromycin. Although amphotericin can cause red blood cell membrane hemolysis, the anemia associated with this drug appears to be due to inhibition of erythropoietin rather than a direct suppressive effect on the bone marrow.[69] Some agents such as cephalosporins produce false-positive results on the Coombs test, but actual hemolysis is rarely due to cephalosporins.[70, 71] The anemia that occurs with trimethoprim, pyrimethamine, and other folate antagonists is due to the effect on dihydrofolate reductase and is megaloblastic.

Thrombocytopenia can result from a number of different mechanisms. In the case of sulfonamides, cephalosporins, penicillins, and rifampin, it appears to be the result of immune reactions of the drugs with platelets that are destroyed in the spleen.[72] Folate antagonists such as trimethoprim and pyrimethamine produce thrombocytopenia by their effect on dihydrofolate reductase.[65] Prolonged bleeding time due to platelet dysfunction has occurred with the semisynthetic anti-*Pseudomonas* penicillins and with the oxacephem moxalactam.[73–76] The agents interfere with normal adenosine diphosphate aggregation of platelets by binding to the adenosine diphosphate receptor site. This effect is both agent adenosine diphosphate and dose related.[34, 71] It was most frequent with carbenicillin, followed by ticarcillin, piperacillin, azlocillin, and mezlocillin, in that order. It develops within 48 to 72 hours after administration of the drugs. At the doses of ticarcillin, ticarcillin-clavulanate, azlocillin, piperacillin, and mezlocillin currently used (12 to 24 g/d) actual bleeding is infrequent, although bleeding time is prolonged and platelet aggregation is impaired in assays in vitro. This adverse effect is worse in persons with abnormal platelet function such as those in renal failure, who already have a clotting problem.[77]

Synthesis of prothrombin can be affected by various antimicrobial agents. It has been studied best for the cephalosporins.[78] Agents that contain a methylthiotetrazole group at the C-3 position of the dihydrothiazine ring have, in plasma and liver, dimers of the methylthiotetrazole group. These compounds are thought to interfere with vitamin K synthesis by altering γ-carboxylation of glutamic acid.[79] Moxalactam used at doses greater than 4 g/d frequently prolongs prothrombin time. Cefoperazone, cefotetan, cefmetazole, and cefamandole all possess the side chain and can prolong prothrombin time, although they do so infrequently if renal and hepatic function is normal. Once-weekly administration of vitamin K corrects the defect, and vitamin K should be administered to malnourished patients who are to be treated with these drugs.

A multisystem disease, with greatest impact on the hematopoietic system, was associated with the new quinolone temofloxacin, forcing its withdrawal from market; the reactions included hemolytic anemia, thrombocytopenia, and disseminated intravascular coagulation, along with acute renal failure and hepatic dysfunction.[31, 40] These reactions occurred in 1 in 10,000 treated cases, for reasons unknown, and thus were not detected in prerelease investigational trials.

Gastrointestinal Toxicity

Gastrointestinal complaints have been reported for all antimicrobial agents whether they are administered by the oral or parenteral route. Several agents are associated with a particularly high incidence of nausea, abdominal pain, and emesis. Erythromycin preparations cause severe abdominal pain and nausea in adults, whereas children seem to tolerate the compounds without major distress.[80] The dose of antimicrobial seems to influence the frequency of gastrointestinal reactions. The incidence of nausea or abdominal discomfort ranges from 1% to 5% of patients and is more often noted with the oral antistaphylococcal compounds than with penicillin V.[81] Most oral cephalosporins are tolerated well, although nausea occurs with newer compounds such as cefixime at doses higher than 400 mg/d.[82] Orally administered aminoglycosides and polymyxin produce a sensation of nausea in many patients at the doses used for intestinal decontamination. Metronidazole, ketoconazole, methenamine, nystatin, rifampin, tetracyclines, trimethoprim, and trimethoprim-sulfamethoxazole all produce nausea. Rapid infusion of imipenem is frequently associated with nausea and emesis.[83]

Diarrhea has been reported to occur with virtually all antimicrobial agents. Several mechanisms are apparently involved. The most important form is that due to toxins produced by *Clostridium difficile,* which accounts for 15% to 30% of all cases of antibiotic-associated diarrhea.[84, 85] In studies from Sweden, *C. difficile* caused 18% of 4793 cases of diarrhea with antibiotics. Based on drug sales, the relative risk of developing *C. difficile* diarrhea for lincosamides (clindamycin and lincomycin) was 70; for cephalosporins, 40; for penicillinase-stable penicillins, 8; and for amoxicillin, 1.[86] *C. difficile* diarrhea is uncommon with erythromycin, metronidazole, ureidopenicillins, and tetracyclines and is extremely rare with quinolones, vancomycin, and aminoglycosides. Antibiotic-associated diarrhea may progress to fulminant pseudomembranous colitis. In contrast to this serious form of disease, many agents cause frequent loose stools. This occurs commonly with the β-lactamase inhibitor–β-lactam combination drugs amoxicillin-clavulanate and sulbactam-ampicillin.[87, 88] Diarrhea occurs with oral cephalosporins less frequently but is found after use of cefixime and other third-generation oral cephalosporins. Cefoperazone, of the parenteral cephalosporin agents, and ceftriaxone have caused diarrhea more often than other cephalosporins have.[89, 90] In most of these situations, alteration of gastrointestinal flora is the explanation, particularly for agents that are poorly absorbed or are largely excreted in bile.

Nonabsorbable aminoglycosides, particularly neomycin (because of the large dose used), produce malabsorption of fat, protein, carbohydrates, and certain drugs such as digoxin.[91, 92] Oral neomycin causes villus shortening, round-cell infiltration of the upper small bowel, and crypt-cell damage; it also binds to bile salts, causing them to be excreted in the feces.

Hepatic Toxicity

A number of different hepatic toxic reactions have followed use of antimicrobial agents. Penicillins have produced increases in hepatic aminotransferase activity.[34] Usually the levels of aspartate aminotransferase and alanine aminotransferase are less than twice normal. This has been seen most often with oxacillin and carbenicillin and when large doses were used.[93, 94] Similar reactions have followed the use of cephalosporins, aztreonam, and quite infrequently imipenem-cilastatin. Infrequently, β-lactams produce true hepatocellular and cholestatic liver damage.

Cholestatic jaundice has followed the use of erythromycin estolate, principally in adults, oleandomycin, tetracyclines, oxacillin, nitrofurans, and sulfonamides.[95–98] The hepatic toxicity of erythromycin appears to be related to the propionyl ester linkage at the C′2 position.[96] Erythromycin-induced jaundice usually starts 10 to 12 days after treatment but may appear within 1 or 2 days. Fever and rash often occur. Tetracyclines are not given to pregnant women; such use was formerly associated in the mother with extensive hepatic damage with fatty changes. The total daily dose of intravenous tetracycline should not exceed 1 g.

Isoniazid produces hepatocellular toxicity in varying numbers of patients depending on age.[99, 100] True serious hepatic reactions are uncommon in children even though 10% to 15% have some abnormality of aminotransferase activity. Risk of hepatitis before age 20 years is less than 0.03%, whereas that for persons older than 35 years is approximately 1%. Toxicity—apparently more common in "rapid acetylators"—is related to metabolic products. Studies that suggest that toxicity occurs more often in patients with underlying liver disease are probably not valid owing to inadequate statistical analysis of data. It is possible to anticipate toxic reactions by monthly monitoring of hepatic enzyme levels.[101] Rifampin itself has little potential for hepatic toxicity, but it appears to increase the likelihood of isoniazid toxicity. Other antituberculosis agents such as pyrazinamide, ethionamide, and the obsolete *p*-aminosalicylic acid have produced fulminant liver damage.

Sulfonamides may produce both hepatocellular and cholestatic liver damage. No particular sulfonamide has been more associated with severe liver injury, but the long-acting agents can remain in the body for a month. Among the antifungal drugs, ketoconazole has produced fulminant hepatic necrosis in a small number of patients, more frequently women.[102, 103] Amphotericin B can also cause increases in transaminase values, but rarely above twice normal, and it is questionable whether amphotericin B truly is hepatotoxic.

Nitrofurantoin has been the cause of chronic active hepatitis, focal nodular hyperplasia of the liver, and active hepatitis.[104] This has rarely been fatal. Thiabendazole administered for longer periods than the usual 2 days produces cholestatic hepatitis that can persist for weeks. Acyclovir and ribavirin occasionally cause elevation of bilirubin values.

Pulmonary Toxicity

Pulmonary reactions to antimicrobial agents are unusual. Aerosol administration of polymyxins can provoke histamine release and bronchospasm. In general, aerosol administration of aminoglycosides or penicillins does not cause bronchial reactions. Aerosol pentamidine is associated with cough and occasionally bronchospasm but generally it is tolerated well. Aerosol use of amphotericin B causes bronchospasm due to the desoxycholate used to solubilize the agent.

Nitrofurantoins produce two forms of pulmonary toxicity. The acute form consists of chills, fever, cough, and dyspnea, which begin within 2 to 10 days after the drug is started.[105, 106] There is eosinophilia, and pulmonary infiltrates are demonstrated by radiography. The reaction stops if the drug is withdrawn. A more chronic form of pulmonary disease has followed prolonged use of the agent.[107] Dyspnea and cough develop gradually. There are interstitial infiltrates at the lung bases, and pulmonary function tests show a restrictive lung pattern. Lung function does not completely return to normal when the agent is withdrawn.

An uncommon pulmonary reaction has occurred in neutropenic patients receiving amphotericin B at the time of infusion if they also receive a transfusion of white blood cells.[108] Pulmonary infiltrates develop due to the localization of white blood cells in the lungs.

Cardiovascular Toxicity

Cardiovascular toxic events are rarely due to antimicrobial agents. Rapid injection of large doses of a potassium salt of penicillin can cause cardiac arrhythmia. Arrhythmias have occurred infrequently with use of intravenous amphotericin B, particularly in patients with impaired renal function.[109] The mechanism is thought to be hyperkalemia. Miconazole has produced hypotension and arrhythmias. Pentamidine, emetine, stibogluconate, melarsoprol, all antiparasitic agents, have been associated with hypotension, arrhythmia, and shock, whereas quinine has been associated with conduction defects.[54, 110]

Metabolic Effects

A number of different metabolic effects can be associated with antimicrobial agents. Some could be considered renal toxic reactions, but the disorder is actually of electrolytes. Large doses of penicillins such as carbenicillin, a disodium salt that contains sodium at approximately 5 mEq/g, can produce sodium overload at doses of 24 to 40 g/d.[93] Ticarcillin is also a disodium salt, but it is rarely given in doses greater than 18 g/d. Azlocillin, mezlocillin, piperacillin, and penicillin G all contain sodium at less than 2 mEq/g.

Large doses of penicillins deliver so great a load of nonreabsorbable anion to the distal tubule that hydrogen ion exchange is altered and hypokalemia develops.[34] Loss of cations such as magnesium can be associated with administration of amphotericin B or aminoglycosides. Demethylchlortetracycline produces nephrogenic diabetes insipidus, and in years past outdated tetracycline that had formed epianhydro derivatives produced the Fanconi syndrome. Amphotericin B has also infrequently produced reversible diabetes insipidus.

Ketoconazole interferes with adrenal function and alters normal testosterone synthesis. Hyperglycemia had been reported to occur with nalidixic acid but not with the newer quinolones such as ciprofloxacin, norfloxacin, and ofloxacin. Hypoglycemia followed by diabetes mellitus occurs with pentamidine.[42] Pancreatitis has been seen with nitrofurantoins, pentamidine, and with trimethoprim-sulfamethoxazole and other sulfonamides.

Renal Toxicity

The kidney is, unfortunately, particularly vulnerable to the adverse effects of antimicrobial agents because so many are removed from the body by the kidney and it is exposed to much higher concentrations of drugs than are many other organs.[111] Damage to the kidney can be to the glomeruli or the proximal, distal, or collecting tubules.

Hypersensitivity glomerular damage has followed use of penicillins but is relatively rare compared with interstitial nephritis. Methicillin is the prototype penicillin that causes interstitial nephritis, although it has been seen with virtually all the penicillins and a number of cephalosporins.[112] Clinically, the reaction is a syndrome of fever, eosinophilia, and rash, which usually accompany the renal reaction. Urinalysis reveals white blood cells, casts, proteinuria, eosinophiluria, and microscopic hematuria. Urine output is initially normal, although serum creatinine and blood urea nitrogen values increase. Renal biopsy shows patchy tubular damage with interstitial edema, lymphocytes, eosinophils, monocytes, and plasma cells. Glomeruli are normal. The mechanism of the reaction is not established. When the drugs are withdrawn, renal function returns to normal. Whether the reaction will recur every time a penicillin is administered is not known. If a reaction has occurred with penicillins it can also occur with cephalosporins.

Rifampin has produced interstitial nephritis, and interstitial nephritis has rarely been reported to occur with minocycline with the new quinolones such as ciprofloxacin.[113]

Cephalosporins currently in general use rarely produce nephrotoxicity. Cephaloridine, no longer available in the United States, produced damage by accumulating in high concentrations in the proximal tubule cells.[114] Polymyxins bind to ligands in proximal tubule cells and damage cell membranes, producing loss of normal tubule function.

The nephrotoxicity of aminoglycosides has been investigated exhaustively. Aminoglycosides vary in toxicity from rarely nephrotoxic streptomycin to highly nephrotoxic neomycin. Tobramycin and netilmicin may be comparably nephrotoxic, and less so than amikacin, gentamicin, and sisomicin, in that order. Aminoglycosides are transported across the luminal brush border of the proximal renal tubule.[114] The positively charged aminoglycoside binds to negatively charged phosphatidylinositol. Pinocytosis of the aminoglycoside into vesicles occurs, with subsequent fusion with lysosomes. Aminoglycosides cause accumulation within lysosomes of multilaminar structures called myeloid bodies. The aminoglycosides inhibit lysosomal phospholipases, which may affect prostaglandin synthesis and reduce glomerular filtration due to alteration of normal vasodilator prostaglandin–vasoconstrictor angiotensin II interaction.[115]

Clinically about 5% to 25% of patients receiving aminoglycosides exhibit some reduction in glomerular filtration.[116] The initial signs are increased excretion of renal tubule enzyme and increased excretion of β_2-microglobulin. Initially, there is nonoliguric renal dysfunction with polyuria while the serum creatinine value increases and creatinine clearance rate slows. A few patients progress into renal failure, but the renal function of most is restored when the agents are withdrawn, and only a small fraction of patients require dialysis.

Amphotericin B can cause both vasoconstriction (hence decreased renal blood flow) and direct toxic reactions in proximal and distal tubules.[117] Tubule intracellular calcium deposits develop with extended use. Distal tubular acidosis develops with cells hyperpermeable to hydrogen ions and loss of potassium. Creatinine clearance rate declines with polyuria, acidosis, and hypokalemia. Most persons who are treated with amphotericin B develop some degree of nephrotoxicity. Renal function usually returns to normal after the drug is withdrawn, but calcium deposits in the tubules may persist.

Nephrotoxicity of amphotericin B can be lessened by hydration and administration of a sodium load before infusion of the amphotericin B.[114, 118] Mannitol infusions do not reduce nephrotoxicity.

Obstructive nephropathy secondary to crystallization of antimicrobial agents had occurred with sulfonamides when sulfadiazine was first used, owing to its relative insolubility. This has occurred in the era of acquired immunodeficiency syndrome, as large doses of sulfadiazine are used to treat toxoplasmosis. Other sulfonamides are much more soluble at a urinary pH of 5, and tubule deposits rarely form when sulfisoxazole or sulfamethoxazole is used. Sulfonamides can produce allergic vasculitis of the kidney. Trimethoprim does not appear to be nephrotoxic, but it alters renal handling of creatinine with a resulting rise in the serum creatinine value.[119] Quinolones such as norfloxacin and ciprofloxacin at an alkaline pH can form crystals producing renal damage in animals, but this does not appear to occur in humans at the doses used.[120] Acyclovir forms crystals when renal function is depressed, resulting in further damage to renal function but rarely renal failure.[121] Tetracyclines, with the exception of doxycycline, can also cause renal function to deteriorate and should not be given to patients whose renal function is impaired. It is not clear whether vancomycin truly causes nephrotoxicity or only aggravates the toxicity of other agents that often are administered with it, such as aminoglycosides or cisplatin.

Neurotoxicity

Central and peripheral nervous system toxicity has occurred with antimicrobial drug use. Peripheral neuropathy has developed with use of metronidazole,[122] nitrofurans,[105] polymyxins,[123] griseofulvin, cycloserine, and rarely tetracyclines. Polymyxins, aminoglycosides, capreomycin, clindamycin, lincomycin, and quinolones produce reversible neuromuscular blockade resembling myasthenia gravis. The toxicity is dose related and most likely to occur with polymyxins, owing to blockage at the myoneural end plate.[124] Aminoglycosides compete with acetylcholine for receptor sites, so the end plate is not depolarized.[125] The aminoglycoside inhibits internalization of calcium into the presynaptic region of the axon, preventing the ultimate release of acetylcholine. Neuromuscular paralysis caused by aminoglycosides is increased by curare-like drugs, botulinum toxin, and myasthenia gravis. Calcium salts reverse the aminoglycoside effects. The effect of polymyxins is also reversed by calcium infusion but not by neostigmine. The fluorinated quinolones can cause various central nervous system disorders, including dizziness, restlessness, confusion, depression, anxiety, euphoria, sleep disorders, catatonia, tremors, and in some cases convulsions.[40, 41] The overall incidence of nervous system reactions is reported as 1% to 5%.

Isoniazid produces peripheral neuropathy by interfering with pyridoxine cofactor. It occurs most frequently in persons who are slow acetylators of the drug. It can be prevented but not reversed by pyridoxine.[126]

Central nervous system toxicity varies from headache, nervousness, excitement, dizziness, agitation, insomnia, lethargy, paranoia, depression, psychosis, and vertigo to frank seizures. Virtually every antimicrobial agent has been reported to cause headache, nervousness, or insomnia. The true incidence of such reactions is not clear, because similar reactions occur with placebos.

Seizures are an important adverse effect and clearly follow use of penicillins, imipenem, cycloserine, amantadine, isoniazid, metronidazole, piperazine, quinolones, and thiabendazole.[127] Penicillin-related seizures usually are of the myoclonic type and occur principally in patients in renal failure whose dosage is not adjusted. They occur even with highly protein bound drugs such as oxacillin in this situation. Penicillin and imipenem have a high affinity for neuronal tissue. Imipenem seems to have a higher potential to cause seizures than other β-lactam antibiotics, reported in 3% (0.9% drug related) of treated patients.[128, 129] Renal insufficiency and underlying seizure disorder are associated with imipenem seizures.[130] A new carbapenem, meropenem, has a much lower seizure risk, recorded as 0.05% in nearly 4000 treated patients.[131]

Seizures are rare with quinolones but appear to be more common with compounds that are naphthyridine derivatives such as nalidixic acid and enoxacin.[120] Seizures have occurred when enoxacin has been used concomitantly with a nonsteroidal antiinflammatory agent.

Ophthalmic Toxicity

Direct ophthalmic toxicity is infrequent with antimicrobial drugs. Sudden loss of vision has been associated with amantadine.[132] It is reversible. Ethambutol produces an optic neuritis that progresses to blindness if the drug is not withdrawn.[133] Vision returns virtually to normal after the drug is withdrawn but this may take up to 8 months. Toxicity is dose related and cannot be anticipated by eye examination. Sudden alteration of visual acuity measured by the Snellen chart or of red-green discrimination should suggest that toxicity is developing and the drug should be stopped. Ophthal-

TABLE 37–3 ■ Selected Drug-Drug Interactions Involving an Oral Antibacterial Agent

ANTIBACTERIAL AGENT (A)	OTHER DRUG (B)	EFFECT	SIGNIFICANCE/CERTAINTY
Erythromycin (includes azithromycin and clarithromycin)	Carbamazepine	↑ Levels* of B	Avoid combination
	Corticosteroids	↑ Effects* of B	Awareness
	Digoxin	↑ Levels* of B	Awareness
	Theophylline	↑ Levels* of B	Dosage adjustment
	Terfenadine or astemizole	↑ Levels* of B	Avoid risk of serious cardiovascular adverse drug reactions
Fluoroquinolones			
All agents	Cimetidine	↑ Levels* of A	Awareness
	Multivalent cations (i.e., aluminum, chromium, iron, magnesium, zinc)	↓ Absorption of A	Awareness
Ciprofloxacin	Theophylline	↑ Levels* of B	Dosage adjustment
	Caffeine	↑ Levels* of B	Awareness
	Oral anticoagulants	↑ Prothrombin time	Monitor prothrombin time
Ofloxacin	Oral anticoagulants	↑ Prothrombin time	Monitor prothrombin time
Tetracyclines (includes doxycycline)	Multivalent cations i.e., aluminum, bismuth, iron, magnesium, and others)	↓ Absorption of A	Awareness
	Digoxin	↑ Levels* of B	Awareness
	Phenytoin	↓ Serum half-life of A	Awareness
TMP-SMX†	Phenytoin	↑ Levels* of B	Dosage adjustment
	Oral anticoagulants	↑ Prothrombin time	Monitor prothrombin time
	Sulfonylureas	↑ Effects of B	Monitor blood glucose

*Serum levels.
†TMP-SMX, Trimethoprim-sulfamethoxazole.
From Gilbert DN: Aspects of the safety profile of oral antibacterial agents. Infect Dis Clin Pract 4(Suppl 2):S103–S112, 1995.

mic toxicity is unusual at a dose of 15 mg/kg per day, provided renal function is not depressed. Rarely, optic neuritis develops with chronic use of isoniazid or chloramphenicol. Antimalarials such as chloroquine can produce irreversible retinal injury, particularly if total dose exceeds 100 g. Loss of vision due to a local reaction in the eye has followed killing of parasites in onchocerciasis by demethylcarbazine or ivermectin.

Ototoxicity

Deafness or vestibular dysfunction can be caused by antimicrobial agents. Aminoglycosides are the agents most often associated with deafness.[134] Neomycin is the most ototoxic agent, followed by kanamycin, amikacin, tobramycin, gentamicin, and netilmicin.[135] Deafness results from damage to outer hair cells of the organ of Corti. The outer hair cells are involved with hearing higher tones, which are destroyed, particularly at the basal turn. Cells do not regenerate, and hearing loss is permanent in those parts of the hearing range that have been destroyed by the aminoglycosides. Damage to outer cochlear-turn otic hair cells is increased by sound and by administering aminoglycosides with other ototoxic agents such as vancomycin, diuretics such as ethacrynic acid, and furosemide. High doses of erythromycin also produce temporary deafness, but hearing characteristically returns to normal. Capreomycin also causes deafness. Vancomycin causes hearing loss, particularly in the presence of renal failure and when it is administered with aminoglycosides.[136] The incidence of ototoxicity due to teicoplanin is not established, but teicoplanin appears to be much less ototoxic than vancomycin.

Because the hearing loss caused by antimicrobial agents is initially outside the range of the human voice it may not be detected. Tinnitus and a feeling of fullness in the ears can precede hearing loss, but hearing loss can occur without these symptoms. Generally, if aminoglycoside blood levels are kept within the accepted range, auditory toxicity does not occur. Hearing loss can be bilateral or unilateral and is cumulative with repeated aminoglycoside courses.

Vestibulotoxicity occurs with aminoglycosides and with minocycline.[137] Streptomycin, gentamicin, and sisomicin have a greater propensity to produce vestibular damage than auditory damage, but any aminoglycoside can produce vestibular defects in the presence of decreased renal function.[135] The exact frequency of the damage is unknown but is estimated to be between 5% and 15%. Vestibular damage is primarily to type I hair cells at the peak of the ampullar cristae. Cellular damage may be related to perilymph and endolymph concentrations that alter adenosine triphosphatase activity, with resulting distortion of ion gradients. Vestibular dysfunction is manifested by nausea, vertigo, dizziness, and unsteady gait. Unilateral or bilateral damage can occur. Minocycline causes temporary vestibulotoxicity that is dose related, is more common in females, and is reversible.[138] The mechanism of the vestibular effect is not known.

Drug Interactions

Many antimicrobial agents can cause important drug-drug interactions (Table 37–3). During their extensive clinical trial programs, the fluoroquinolones were found to be associated with many drug interactions.[41] Such interactions can occur with antimicrobial agents or with other compounds administered to treat noninfectious illness. Antimicrobial agents may affect the cytochrome P-450 microsomal enzyme production in the liver, altering the metabolism of certain agents. Competition for excretory pathways in the liver or kidney may result in accumulation of the antimicrobial agent or of another drug. Competition for binding sites on albumin or tissue may make available a larger than usual amount of a drug. Illustrations of clinically important drug interactions between antimicrobial agents and other drugs are presented in Table 37–3.[31]

References

1. Leigh DA, Faiers MC, Brumfitt W: Laboratory and clinical studies with cephalexin. Postgrad Med J 45(Suppl):69, 1970.

2. Hopkins S: Clinical toleration and safety of azithromycin. Am J Med 91(Suppl):40S, 1991.
3. Physicians' Desk Reference, ed 49. Montvale, NJ, Medical Economics Data Production, 1995.
4. Stutman HR, Argueadas AG: Comparison of cefprozil with other antibiotic regimens in the treatment of children with acute otitis media. Clin Infect Dis 14(Suppl):204S, 1992.
5. McCarty JM, Renteria A: Treatment of pharyngitis and tonsillitis with cefprozil: Review of three multicenter trials. Clin Infect Dis 14(Suppl):224S, 1992.
6. Pelletier LL: Review of the experience with cefprozil for the treatment of lower respiratory tract infections. Clin Infect Dis 14(Suppl):238S, 1992.
7. Bigby M, Jick S, Jick H, Arndt K: Drug-induced cutaneous reactions. JAMA 256:3358, 1986.
8. Cox CE, Graveline JF, Luongo JM: Review of clinical experience in the United States with cefpodoxime proxetil in adults with uncomplicated urinary tract infections. Drugs 42(Suppl):41S, 1991.
9. Kumazawa J: Summary of clinical experience with cefpodoxime proxetil in adults in Japan. Drugs 42(Suppl):1S, 1991.
10. Safron C: Cefpodoxime proxetil: Dosage, efficacy and tolerance in adults suffering from respiratory tract infections. J Antimicrob Chemother 26(Suppl):93S, 1990.
11. Therasse D: The safety profile of loracarbef: Clinical trials in respiratory, skin and urinary tract infections. Am J Med 92(Suppl):20S, 1992.
12. Arndt KA, Jick H: Rates of cutaneous reactions to drugs. JAMA 235:918, 1976.
13. Sogn DD, Evans R, Shepherd GM, et al: Results of the National Institute of Allergy and Infectious Diseases collaborative clinical trial to test the predicted value of skin testing with major and minor penicillin derivatives in hospitalized adults. Arch Intern Med 152:1025, 1992.
14. Petz LD: Immunologic cross-reactivity between penicillin and cephalosporins: A review. J Infect Dis 137:574, 1978.
15. Wilber RB, Doyle CA, Durham SJ, et al: Safety profile of cefprozil. Clin Infect Dis 14(Suppl):264S, 1992.
16. Steigbigel NH: Erythromycin, lincomycin, and clindamycin. *In* Mandell GL, Douglas RG Jr, Bennett JE (eds): Principles and Practice of Infectious Diseases, ed 3. New York, Churchill Livingstone, 1990, pp 308–317.
17. Bartlett JG: Antibiotic-associated diarrhea. J Infect Dis 15:573, 1992.
18. Hooton TM: A comparison of azithromycin and penicillin V for the treatment of streptococcal pharyngitis. Am J Med 91 (Suppl):23S, 1991.
19. Hardy DJ, Guay DRP, Jones RN: Clarithromycin, a unique macrolide. Diagn Microbiol Infect Dis 15:39, 1992.
20. Halkin H. Adverse effects of the fluoroquinolones. Rev Infect Dis 10(Suppl):5258S, 1988.
21. Murray DL, Singer DA, Singer AB: Cefaclor: A cluster of adverse reactions. N Engl J Med 303:1003, 1980.
22. Heckert SR, Stryker WS, Collin KL, Manson JE, Platt R: Serum sickness in children after antibiotic exposure: Estimates of occurrence and morbidity in a health maintenance organization population. Am J Epidemiol 132:336, 1990.
23. Hooton TM, Johnson C, Winter C, et al: Single-dose and three-day regimens of ofloxacin versus trimethoprim-sulfamethoxazole for acute cystitis in women. Antimicrob Agents Chemother 35:1479, 1991.
24. Boyko EJ, Iravani A, Silverman MH, et al: Randomized, controlled trial of a ten-day course of amifloxacin versus trimethoprim-sulfamethoxazole in the treatment of acute, uncomplicated urinary tract infection. Antimicrob Agents Chemother 34:665, 1990.
25. Iravani A: Comparative, double-blind, prospective, multicenter trial of temofloxacin versus trimethoprim-sulfamethoxazole in uncomplicated urinary tract infections in women. Antimicrob Agents Chemother 35:1777, 1991.
26. Sabbaj J, Hoagland VL, Shih WJ: Multiclinic comparative study of norfloxacin and trimethoprim-sulfamethoxazole for treatment of urinary tract infections. Antimicrob Agents Chemother 27:297, 1985.
27. Fihn SD, Johnson C, Roberts PL, et al: Trimethoprim-sulfamethoxazole for acute dysuria in women: A single-dose or 10-day course. Ann Intern Med 108:350, 1988.
28. Urinary Tract Infection Study Group: Coordinated multicenter study of norfloxacin versus trimethoprim sulfamethoxazole treatment of symptomatic urinary tract infections. J Infect Dis 155:170, 1987.
29. Wolfson JS, Hooper DC: Overview of fluoroquinolone safety. Am J Med 91(Suppl):153S, 1991.
30. Beam TR Jr, Gilbert DN, Kunin CM: General guidelines for the evaluation of anti-infective drug products. Clin Infect Dis 15(Suppl):5S, 1992.
31. Gilbert DN: Aspects of the safety profile of oral antibacterial agents. Infect Dis Clin Pract 4(Suppl 2):S103, 1995.
32. Saxon A: Immediate hypersensitivity reactions to β-lactam antibiotics. Rev Infect Dis 5(Suppl):368, 1983.
33. Sher TH: Penicillin hypersensitivity. A review. Pediatr Clin North Am 30:161, 1983.
34. Parry MF: Toxic and adverse reactions encountered with new β-lactam antibiotics. Bull N Y Acad Med 60:358, 1984.
35. Lin RY: A perspective on penicillin allergy. Arch Intern Med 152:930, 1992.
36. Levine BB, Redmond AP, Feller MF, et al: Penicillin allergy and the heterogeneous immune response of man to benzylpenicillin. J Clin Invest 45:1895, 1966.
37. Idosoe O, Gothe T, Wilcox RR, et al: Nature and extent of penicillin side reactions with particular reference to fatalities from anaphylactic shock. Bull WHO 38:159, 1968.
38. Sogn DD, Evans R 3rd, Shepherd GM, et al: Results of the National Institute of Allergy and Infectious Diseases Collaborative Clinical Trial to test the predictive value of skin testing with major and minor penicillin derivatives in hospitalized adults. Arch Intern Med 152:1025, 1992.
39. Shapiro S, Slone D, Siskind V, et al: Drug rash with ampicillin and other penicillins. Lancet 2:969, 1969.
40. Christ W, Esch B: Adverse reactions to fluoroquinolones in adults and children. Infect Dis Clin Pract 3(Suppl 3):S168, 1994.
41. Adam D, VonRosenstiel N: Adverse reactions to quinolones, potential toxicities, drug interactions, and metabolic effects. Infect Dis Clin Pract 3(Suppl 3):S177, 1994.
42. Murray DL, Singer DA, Singer AB: Cefaclor—A cluster of adverse reactions. N Engl J Med 303:1003, 1980.
43. Heckert SR, Stryker WS, Collin KL, et al: Serum sickness in children after antibiotic exposure: Estimates of occurrence and morbidity in a health maintenance organization population. Am J Epidemiol 132:336, 1990.
44. Saxon A, Gilden BN, Rohr AS, et al: Immediate hypersensitivity reactions to β-lactam antibiotics. Ann Intern Med 127:204, 1987.
45. Kishiyama JL, Adelman DC: The cross-reactivity and immunology of beta-lactam antibiotics. Drug Saf 10:318, 1994.
46. Sim E, Gill EW, Sim RR: Drugs that induce systemic lupus erythematosus inhibit complement component C4. Lancet 2:422, 1984.
47. Carroll OM, Bryan PA, Robinson RJ: Stevens-Johnson syndrome associated with long-acting sulfonamides. JAMA 195:691, 1966.
48. Selby CD, Ladusans EJ, Smith PG: Fatal multisystemic toxicity associated with prophylaxis with pyridomethamine and sulfadoxine (Fansidar). Br Med J 290:113, 1985.
49. Gibson JR: Recurrent trimethoprim-associated fixed skin eruption. Br Med J 284:1529, 1982.
50. Bartlett J: Medical Management of HIV Infection. Glenview, IL, Physicians & Scientists Publishing, 1994.
51. Ackerman BH, Bradsher RW: Vancomycin and red necks. Ann Intern Med 102:724, 1985.
52. Garrelts JC, Peterie JD: Vancomycin and the "red man" syndrome. N Engl J Med 312:245, 1985.
53. Bethell HJN: Photo-onycholysis caused by demethylchlortetracycline. Br Med J 2:96, 1977.
54. Mandell WF, Neu HC: Parasitic infections: Therapeutic considerations. Med Clin North Am 72:669, 1988.
55. Hooper DC, Wolfson JS: Adverse effects of quinolone antimicrobials. *In* Wolfson JS, Hooper DC (eds): Quinolone Antimicrobial Agents. Washington, DC, American Society for Microbiology, 1989.
56. Wallerstein RO, Condit PK, Kasper CK, et al: Statewide study of chloramphenicol therapy and fatal asplastic anemia. JAMA 208:2045, 1969.
57. Wilkinson JD, Pollack MM, Costello J: Chloramphenicol toxicity. Hemodynamic and oxygen utilization effects. Pediatr Infect Dis 4:69, 1985.

58. Stevens DC, Kleinman MB, Lietman PS, et al: Exchange transfusion in acute chloramphenicol toxicity. J Pediatr 99:651, 1981.
59. Freundlich M, Cynamon H, Tainer A, et al: Management of chloramphenicol intoxication in infancy by charcoal hemoperfusion. J Pediatr 103:485, 1983.
60. Brook I: Leukopenia and granulocytopenia after oxacillin therapy. South Med J 70:565, 1977.
61. Coucchonnal GJ, Hinthorn DR, Hodges GR, et al: Nafcillin-associated granulocytopenia. South Med J 71:1355, 1978.
62. Homayouni H, Gross PA, Setia U, et al: Leukopenia due to penicillin and cephalosporin homologues. Arch Intern Med 139:827, 1979.
63. Calandra GR, Brown KB, Grad CL, et al: Review of adverse experiences and tolerability in the first 2516 patients treated with imipenem-cilastatin. Am J Med 78:65, 1985.
64. Henry SA, Bendush CB: Aztreonam. Worldwide overview of the treatment of patients with gram-negative infections. Am J Med 78(Suppl 2A):57, 1985.
65. Lawson DH: Adverse effects of co-trimoxazole. *In* Hitchings GH (ed): Inhibition of Folate Metabolism in Chemotherapy. Berlin, Springer-Verlag, 1983.
66. Richman DD, Fischl MA, Grieco MH, et al: The toxicity of azidothymidine (AZT) in the treatment of patients with AIDS and AIDS-related complex. N Engl J Med 317:192, 1987.
67. Harris BE, Manning BW, Federle TW, et al: Conversion of 5-fluorocytosine to 5-fluorouracil by human intestinal microflora. Antimicrob Agents Chemother 29:44, 1986.
68. Beutler E: Glucose-6-phosphate dehydrogenase deficiency. *In* Stanbury JB, et al (eds): The Metabolic Basis of Inherited Disease, ed 5. New York, McGraw-Hill, 1983.
69. MacGregor RR, Bennett JE, Erslev AJ: Erythropoietin concentration in amphotericin B–induced anemia. Antimicrob Agents Chemother 14:270, 1978.
70. Rubin RN, Burka ER: Anticephalothin antibody and Coombs-positive hemolytic anemia. Ann Intern Med 86:64, 1977.
71. Meyers BR: Comparative toxicities of third-generation cephalosporins. Am J Med 79(Suppl 2A):96, 1985.
72. Miescher PA: Drug-induced thrombocytopenia. Semin Hematol 10:311, 1973.
73. Gentry LO, Jamsek JG, Natelson EA: Effect of sodium piperacillin on platelet function in normal volunteers. Antimicrob Agents Chemother 19:532, 1981.
74. Copeland EA, Kusumi RK, Miller L, et al: A comparison of the effects of mezlocillin and carbenicillin on hemostasis in volunteers. J Antimicrob Chemother 11(Suppl C):43, 1983.
75. Brown CH III, Natelson EA, Bradshaw MW, et al: Study of the effect of ticarcillin on blood coagulation and platelet function. Antimicrob Agents Chemother 7:652, 1975.
76. Bang NU, Kammer RB: Hematologic complications associated with β-lactam antibiotics. Rev Infect Dis 5(Suppl 2):380, 1983.
77. Andrassy K, Weischedel E, Ritz E, et al: Bleeding in uremic patients after carbenicillin. Thromb Haemost 36:115, 1976.
78. Andrassy K, Bechtold H, Ritz E: Hypoprothrombinemia caused by cephalosporins. J Antimicrob Chemother 15:133, 1985.
79. Lipsky JJ: *N*-Methyl-thio-tetrazole inhibition of gamma carboxylation of glutamic acid: Possible mechanism for antibiotic-associated hypoprothrombinaemia. Lancet 1:192, 1983.
80. Washington JA II, Wilson WR: Erythromycin: A microbial and clinical perspective after 30 years of clinical use. Mayo Clin Proc 60:271, 1985.
81. Fekety FR Jr: Gastrointestinal complications of antibiotic therapy. JAMA 203:210, 1968.
82. Tally FP, Desjardins RE, McCarthy EF, et al: Safety profile of cefixime. Pediatr Infect Dis J 6:976, 1987.
83. Lipman B, Neu HC: Imipenem. Med Clin North Am 72:567, 1988.
84. Silva J, Fekety R: Clostridial and antimicrobial colitis. Am Rev Med 32:327, 1981.
85. Bartlett JG: Antibiotic-associated colitis. Dis Mon 30:6, 1984.
86. Aronsson B, Mollby R, Nord C-E: Antimicrobial agents and *Clostridium difficile* enterocolitis in Sweden. J Antimicrob Chemother 14(Suppl D):85S, 1984.
87. Connor C: β-Lactamase inhibitors. Drug Intell Clin Pharm 19:475, 1985.
88. Campoli-Richards DM, Brodgen RN: Sulbactam-ampicillin: A review of its antibacterial activity, pharmacokinetic properties, and therapeutic use. Drugs 33:577, 1987.
89. Gordon AJ, Phyfferoen M: Cefoperazone sodium in the treatment of serious infections in 2100 adults and children: Multicentered trials in Europe, Latin America and Australia. Rev Infect Dis 5(Suppl 1):188, 1983.
90. Moskovitz BL: Clinical adverse effects during ceftriaxone therapy. Am J Med 77(Suppl 4C):84, 1984.
91. Jacobson ED, Faloon WN: Malabsorptive effects of neomycin in commonly used doses. JAMA 175:187, 1961.
92. Lindenbaum J, Maulitz RM, Butler VP Jr: Inhibition of digoxin absorption by neomycin. Gastroenterology 71:399, 1976.
93. Neu HC: Carbenicillin and ticarcillin. Med Clin North Am 66:61, 1982.
94. Neu HC: Antistaphylococcal penicillins. Med Clin North Am 66:51, 1982.
95. Shlock S: Drugs and the liver. Br Med J 1:227, 1986.
96. Tolman KG, Sannella JJ, Freston JW: Chemical structure of erythromycin and hepatotoxicity. Ann Intern Med 81:58, 1984.
97. Lepper MH, Wolfe CK, Zimmerman HJ, et al: Effect of large doses of aureomycin on human liver. Arch Intern Med 88:271, 1951.
98. Dujovne CA, Chan CH, Zimmerman HJ: Sulfonamide hepatic injury: Review of the literature and report of a case due to sulfamethoxazole. N Engl J Med 277:785, 1967.
99. Garibaldi RA, Drusin RE, et al: Isoniazid-associated hepatitis. Report of an outbreak. Am Rev Respir Dis 106:357, 1982.
100. Maddrey WC, Britnott JK: Isoniazid hepatitis. Ann Intern Med 79:1, 1973.
101. Bernstein RE: Isoniazid hepatotoxicity and acetylation during tuberculosis chemotherapy. Am Rev Respir Dis 121:429, 1980.
102. Horsburgh CR Jr, Kirkpatrick CH, Teutsch CB: Ketoconazole and the liver. Lancet 1:860, 1980.
103. Jannsen PAJ, Symoens JE: Hepatic reactions during ketoconazole treatment. Am J Med 74:80, 1983.
104. Sharp JR, Ishak KG, Zimmerman HJ: Chronic active hepatitis and severe hepatic necrosis associated with nitrofurantoin. Ann Intern Med 92:14, 1980.
105. Penn RG, Griffen JP: Adverse reactions to nitrofurantoin in the United Kingdom, Sweden, and Holland. Br Med J 284:1440, 1982.
106. Dawson RB: Pulmonary reactions to nitrofurantoin. N Engl J Med 274:522, 1966.
107. Robinson BWS: Nitrofurantoin-induced interstitial pulmonary fibrosis. Presentation and outcome. Med J Aust 1:72, 1983.
108. Wright DG, Robichaud KJ, Pizzo PA, et al: Lethal pulmonary reactions associated with the combined use of amphotericin B and leukocyte transfusions. N Engl J Med 304:1185, 1981.
109. Craven PC, Gremillion DH: Risk factors associated with ventricular fibrillation during rapid amphotericin B infusion. Antimicrob Agents Chemother 27:868, 1985.
110. Sands S, Kron MA, Brown RB: Pentamidine. A review. Rev Infect Dis 7:625, 1985.
111. Appel GB, Neu HC: The nephrotoxicity of antimicrobial agents. N Engl J Med 296:722, 1977.
112. Appel GB, Neu HC: Acute interstitial nephritis induced by β-lactam antibiotics. *In* Fillastre JP (ed): Nephrotoxicity-Ototoxicity of Drugs. Rouen, Inserm, 1981.
113. Stone WJ, Waldron JA, Dixon JH Jr, et al: Acute diffuse interstitial nephritis related to chemotherapy of tuberculosis. Antimicrob Agents Chemother 10:164, 1976.
114. Silverblatt F: Pathogenesis of nephrotoxicity of cephalosporins and aminoglycosides: A review of current concepts. Rev Infect Dis 49(Suppl):360, 1982.
115. McNeil JS, Jackson B, Nelson L, et al: The role of prostaglandins in gentamicin-induced nephrotoxicity in the dog. Nephron 33:202, 1983.
116. Leitman PS, Smith CR: Aminoglycoside nephrotoxicity in humans. J Infect Dis 5(Suppl 2):284, 1983.
117. Butler WT, Bennett JE, Alling DW, et al: Nephrotoxicity of amphotericin B. Early and late effects in 81 patients. Ann Intern Med 61:175, 1964.
118. Heidemann HT, Gerkins JF, Spickard WA, et al: Amphotericin B nephrotoxicity in humans decreased by salt repletion. Am J Med 75:475, 1983.
119. Trollfurs B, Wahl J, Alestig K: Cotrimoxazole, creatinine and renal function. J Infect 2:221, 1980.
120. Stahlmann R, Lode H: Safety overview: Toxicity, adverse effects

and drug interactions. *In* Andriole VT (ed): The Quinolones. London, Academic Press, 1988.
121. Kenney RE, Kirk LE, Bridgen D: Acyclovir tolerance in humans. Am J Med 73(Suppl):176, 1982.
122. Finegold SM: Metronidazole. Ann Intern Med 91:535, 1980.
123. Wolinsky E, Hines JD: Neurotoxic and nephrotoxic effects of colistin in patients with renal disease. N Engl J Med 266:759, 1962.
124. McQuillen MP, Cantor HE, O'Rourke JR: Myasthenic syndrome associated with antibiotics. Arch Neurol 18:402, 1968.
125. Caputy AJ, Kin YI, Sanders DB: The neuromuscular blocking effects of therapeutic concentration of various antibiotics on normal rat skeletal muscle. A quantitative comparison. J Pharmacol Exp Ther 217:369, 1981.
126. Snider DE Jr: Pyridoxine supplementation during isoniazid therapy. Tubercle 61:191, 1980.
127. Norrby R: Penetration of antimicrobial agents into cerebrospinal fluid. Pharmacokinetic and clinical aspects. *In* Wood JH (ed): Neurobiology of Cerebrospinal Fluid, Vol 1. New York, Plenum Publishing, 1988.
128. Schliamser SE, Broholm KA, Liljedahl AL, et al: Comparative neurotoxicity of benzylpenicillin, imipenem-cilastin and FCE 22101, a new injectable penem. J Antimicrob Chemother 22: 687, 1988.
129. Calandra GB, Wang C, Aziz M, Brown KR: The safety profile of imipenem/cilastatin: Worldwide clinical experience based on 3470 patients. J Antimicrob Chemother 18(Suppl E):193S, 1986.
130. Calandra GB, Lydick E, Carrigan J, et al: Factors predisposing to seizures in seriously ill infected patients receiving antibiotics: Experience with imipenem/cilastatin. Am J Med 84:911, 1988.
131. Norrby SR, Newell PA, Faulkner KL, Lesky W: Safety profile of meropenem: International clinical experience based on the first 3125 patients treated with meropenem. J Antimicrob Chemother 36(Suppl A):207, 1995.
132. Pearlman JT, Kadish AH, Ramseyer JC: Vision loss associated with amantadine hydrochloride use. JAMA 237:1200, 1977.
133. Lees AW, Allan GW, Smith J, et al: Toxicity from rifampin plus isoniazid and rifampicin plus ethambutol therapy. Tubercle 52:182, 1971.
134. Lerner SA, Matz GJ, Hawkins JE (eds): Aminoglycoside Ototoxicity. Boston, Little, Brown, 1981.
135. Bendush CL: Ototoxicity. Clinical considerations and comparative information. *In* Whelton A, Neu HC (eds): The Aminoglycosides. New York, Marcel Dekker, 1982.
136. Sorrell TC, Collignon PJ: A prospective study of adverse reactions associated with vancomycin therapy. J Antimicrob Chemother 16:235, 1985.
137. Igarashi M: Vestibular ototoxicity in primates. Audiology 12:337, 1973.
138. Fanning WL, Gump DW, Sofferman RA: Side-effects of minocycline. A double-blind study. Antimicrob Agents Chemother 11:712, 1977.

38

Strategies for the Cost-Effective Use of Antibiotics

Richard Quintiliani

Because of the proliferation of antibiotics and the attitude of many physicians that they should be able to use any antibiotic whenever they wish, control of antibiotic use and correction of misuse have been difficult to achieve. Inadequate control has led to excessive expenditure for antibiotics and improper prescription for many patients, and it may also result in the emergence of multidrug-resistant bacteria that threaten both the patient receiving the antibiotic and other patients in the hospital. Despite major constraints on health care costs, proper care of patients must always come first, and there are many ways to reduce costs and still provide proper care for the patient.

Devising a Strategy for Hospital Management of Antibiotics

To control antibiotic use and to carry out any policy effectively and efficiently, the skill and cooperation are required of persons trained in one or more of the various disciplines that affect antibiotic selection and use—pharmacists, microbiologists, hospital epidemiologists, and clinical infectious disease physicians. Moreover, to develop restrictions and limitations on the availability of a number of antibiotics and to obtain compliance with these control measures, the cooperation of the entire staff is required. It can be predicted that a sizable number of physicians will mistrust any type of control and oppose any recommendations regardless of how thoroughly they are explained. Some physicians insist on giving whatever antibiotic they choose whenever and however they want. Even if physicians with this prescribing style are few, they can disrupt any control program for appropriate antibiotic use. Once guidelines have been established by the therapeutics committee and approved by the executive committee of the medical staff, it is crucial that all physicians practicing in the hospital, including infectious disease physicians, follow the recommendations of the therapeutics committee without exception.

The Strategy in Operation

Integration of Pharmacokinetic Properties and Antimicrobial Activity of Antibiotics in the Determination of Appropriate Dose and Dosing Interval

In the early 1940s, when penicillin was scarce, it was administered in the smallest dose and as infrequently as possible. For instance, the standard dose to treat pneumococcal pneumonia in that decade was 300,000 units of aqueous procaine penicillin administered intramuscularly every 12 hours. By integrating the microbiologic and pharmacokinetic properties of penicillin, it could be predicted that this dose should be effective against infections by this type of organism, because the serum levels of penicillin remained above the usual minimal inhibitory concentration (MIC) or minimal bactericidal concentration for penicillin-sensitive *Streptococcus pneumoniae* (0.01 μg/mL) for more than 12 hours. In fact, there is no evidence that the massive doses of penicillin that are now often employed for this same infection achieve a better clinical outcome than the traditional dosage method. Unfortunately, dosing methods changed drastically with time, especially before the current era of cost containment, when there appeared to be unlimited hospital and financial resources.

Ever since antibiotics became available, there has been considerable controversy regarding the most appropriate way to administer them to maximize bacterial killing, minimize toxicity, and reduce costs. In only the past several years has adequate scientific information emerged from animal models of infection, in vitro pharmacodynamic studies, and clinical trials that has enabled establishment of the best mode of drug administration to achieve these goals.

Aminoglycosides (e.g., gentamicin, tobramycin, netilmicin, and amikacin) and fluoroquinolones (e.g., ofloxacin, ciprofloxacin) eliminate bacteria most rapidly when their concentrations are appreciably above their MICs for organisms; hence, their type of killing is referred to as concentration-dependent or dose-dependent killing.[1] For these drugs, the rate of bacterial killing increases with increasing concentration up to about 10 times above their MIC for an organism (i.e., a peak serum concentration/MIC ratio ≥ 10). In neutropenic animal models of infection, many more animals survive a potentially lethal challenge of bacteria if the aminoglycosides are given as a single large daily dose compared with the same amount of drug divided and given on a schedule of every 8 hours. Moreover, pathologic examination of tissue, such as the organ of Corti or renal tubular cells, has shown less rather than more damage. Ototoxicity and nephrotoxicity of aminoglycosides correlate with tissue accumulation and not with peak serum concentrations. With the once-daily dosing method of aminoglycosides, there is a much longer period of time during the 24 hours (approximately 12 hours in patients with normal renal function) that serum levels are low or undetectable, which allows more drug to egress from ears and kidneys, compared with the intermittent dosing technique. Because of these observations, there is a growing interest in once-daily aminoglycoside dosing with gentamicin and tobramycin so that one can obtain the preferable peak serum concentration/MIC ratios and reduce toxicity. Nicolau and coworkers[2] reported experience with 2184 adult patients treated with once-daily aminoglycoside dosing and, as predicted, observed excellent clinical outcomes with the lowest incidence (1.2%) of nephrotoxicity reported in the hospital compared with historical data, for which the incidence was 3% to 5%. Moreover, this approach was cost-effective owing to reduction in ancillary service time, the number of serum aminoglycoside determinations needed, and the costs associated with toxicity. Administration of aminoglycosides once a day permits many more patients to be treated on a home care basis.

Although fluoroquinolones such as ciprofloxacin and ofloxacin demonstrate concentration-dependent killing, excessively high serum concentrations can produce seizures. To obtain a serum concentration 10 times above the usual MIC of 2 μg/mL for *S. pneumoniae* or *Streptococcus pyogenes* would require a serum concentration of 20 μg/mL, which would be associated with excessive neurotoxicity. The only way to obtain peak serum concentration/MIC ratios of 10 or higher is to target these agents against sensitive organisms such as Enterobacteriaceae with typical MICs below 0.1 μg/mL. New fluoroquinolones (e.g., levo-ofloxacin, trovafloxacin, sparfloxacin) are under investigation that have appreciably lower MICs for streptococci, so in time it may be possible to achieve favorable ratios against these organisms.

One of the most important pharmacodynamic observations is that β-lactam antibiotics, such as cephalosporins and penicillins, kill bacteria in a manner essentially the opposite of that of the quinolones and aminoglycosides. In fact, β-lactams are said to exhibit concentration-independent or time-dependent killing, indicating that they inhibit the growth of bacteria equally well at high or low concentrations in serum and interstitial fluid as long as these levels are above the MIC for the target organism.[3] In brief, for β-lactam antibiotics, the treatment goal is to keep the drug level above the MIC for as long as possible in any one dosing interval. The length of time above the MIC is the pharmacodynamic parameter that correlates with clinical response, and not the magnitude of the concentration above the MIC.[4] For instance, β-lactams maintaining the drug level above the MIC for more than 50% of the dosing interval has been associated with the highest frequency of clinical cure.

For antibiotics with concentration-dependent killing, the often-mentioned advice in package inserts that antibiotics should be given in larger and more frequent doses for infections considered to be severe compared with those that are deemed mild makes little, if any, pharmacodynamic or pharmacoeconomic sense. It should be remembered that the high serum levels of β-lactam antibiotics do not result in higher intracellular or tissue concentrations because these agents have insignificant intracellular penetration. The higher serum levels merely result in similar levels in the interstitial fluid that surrounds the cells, and the same pharmacodynamic concepts that apply to serum levels also apply to interstitial concentrations. Although there typically exists a brief lag period before interstitial and serum levels attain equilibrium, for β-lactams there is a close parallel between their concentrations in serum and those in interstitial compartments.[5] High serum levels may improve a clinical response only for infection in compartments, such as cerebrospinal fluid or eye, because these high concentrations may provide a greater penetration of such sites.

Transitional Antibiotic Therapy

Conversion from intravenous to oral antibiotics results in important clinical and economic gains. Significant cost reductions occur because of lower drug acquisition costs, a reduction in pharmacy time for the preparation and mixing of drugs, the ability to deliver a drug without the intervention of intravenous technicians, and a reduction in the length of hospital stay. Perhaps the most important benefit derived from oral therapy is the elimination of the use of intravenous catheters, which are the major source of nosocomial bacteremias, especially those caused by staphylococci.[6] It has been estimated that there are more than 20 million vascular catheters inserted annually in patients admitted to hospitals in the United States, resulting in more than 50,000 episodes of bacteremia or line sepsis.[7] The frequency of these infections is directly correlated with the duration of their use.[8] In a cost analysis of 104 patients with line sepsis, it was noted that the average additional cost from each episode of line sepsis was $3,707 and even higher ($6,064) if it was caused by *Staphylococcus aureus*.[9]

Because of the absence of cumbersome intravenous delivery systems, patients are more easily mobilized with oral therapy, again reducing the possibility of other hospital-related problems such as deep venous thrombophlebitis, pulmonary emboli, depression, and adverse drug reactions. If there is no malabsorption problem, an attempt is made to replace intravenous drugs with oral agents after 2 to 3 days as long as the patient is clinically stable and shows a decreasing temperature and white cell count.[10] If one waits for the white cell count and temperature to become normal, the patient is usually cured and hence no longer requires antibiotic.

In an approach similar to our streamlining program, Kunin[11] has recommended that infectious disease consultation be obtained automatically when the first three doses of an expensive, potentially toxic antibiotic are ordered, and he has shown that this approach improves prescribing practices and reduces costs. His approach also recognizes that no restrictive policy should delay prompt initiation of antibiotic therapy, for that in itself would be inappropriate for patients with bacteremia, a disease in which it has been shown repeatedly that rapid introduction of an antibiotic decreases the chances of shock and death.

Reviewing the charts of patients taking antibiotics during their illness allows one to assess the appropriateness of antibiotic selection and dosage and whether appropriate tests are being done to avoid toxic effects. The antibiotic team provides another important quality assurance service down to the level of the individual physician. This has now become a requirement of the Joint Commission on Accreditation of Hospitals.

Role of the Pharmacist in Antibiotic Control

It is important to revise our ideas about the place of the pharmacist in management of the patient. What must now be recognized is that the proper dose of antibiotic—or any drug—is not easy to determine or remember, particularly for elderly or young patients and those with organ dysfunction. Here pharmacists can be instrumental in correcting overdosing or underdosing, one of their long-recognized responsibilities.

Once the therapeutics committee has developed specific guidelines for the use of antibiotics, including proper dose levels and intervals, many of these recommendations can be implemented by the pharmacy through automatic conversions. The conversion of prescriptions for cefoxitin to cefotetan, cephalothin to cefazolin, and cefamandole to cefuroxime represents the selection of a drug with preferable pharmacokinetics that allows less frequent dosing, which in turn reduces the burden on ancillary services. Conversion to drugs that are no different clinically in antimicrobial activity or toxicity but only in rate of elimination from the body is a safe practice and usually cost-effective, as long as (1) physicians are willing to comply with the recommended dose and dosing intervals and (2) the acquisition cost of the drug with the preferable pharmacokinetics is not excessive. For instance, for ceftriaxone (half-life of about 8 hours) to be a cost-effective alternative to cefotaxime or ceftizoxime (half-lives of about 1 hour and 1.6 hours, respectively), a 1- to 2-g once-daily dose of ceftriaxone must replace 1- to 2-g doses of cefotaxime every 8 hours because the pharmacy acquisition cost of ceftriaxone ($25 per gram) is about three times that of ceftizoxime or cefotaxime ($7 per gram). This kind of pharmacokinetic conversion makes good economic and clinical sense for the treatment of organisms that are equally susceptible to both drugs, such as Enterobacteriaceae, *Neisseria* species, and streptococci. Their MIC values for methicillin-susceptible staphylococci are significantly different, however (cefotaxime, 2 to 4 μg/mL; ceftriaxone, 16 to 32 μg/mL).[12] Thus, ceftriaxone's pharmacokinetic edge over cefotaxime is negated by its reduced antimicrobial activity against staphylococci, in consequence of which both drugs must be dosed in a similar fashion to treat infections from these bacteria. In such cases, the cost of ceftriaxone is appreciably greater. Complicating any once-daily dosing regimen is the tendency of physicians to give large, frequent doses of an antibiotic to any clinically unstable patient with a life-threatening illness out of fear that the single dose may inadvertently be omitted. In our hospital, we solved this problem by using cefotaxime for clinically unstable patients and shifting to ceftriaxone once a patient's condition has stabilized and the responsible pathogen has been identified as an organism that is equally susceptible to both drugs. In many cases, ceftriaxone can be replaced with oral doses of either ciprofloxacin or trimethoprim-sulfamethoxazole (TMP-SMX).

When a number of old antibiotics were introduced, the recommended doses and dosing intervals were excessive in view of the susceptibility of the bacteria they usually target. Clindamycin, 600 mg every 8 hours, and vancomycin, 1 g every 12 hours, provide serum levels in excess of their MICs for *Bacteroides fragilis* and *S. aureus*, respectively, for the entire dosing interval. No difference in clinical outcome has been noted in patients who have received clindamycin on dosing schedules of 600 mg every 6 hours to 600 mg intravenously every 8 hours.[13] Similarly, metronidazole at a dose of 500 mg intravenously every 12 hours achieves peak serum levels of about 23 μg/mL and trough levels of about 7 μg/mL, appreciably above the usual MIC for *B. fragilis* (no more than 1 μg/mL).[14] Even a single 400-mg oral dose of metronidazole achieves peak (about 17 μg/mL) and trough (about 6 μg/mL) levels, 12 hours after administration, that are close to those achieved with the intravenous formulation, so conversion from parenteral to oral therapy should be possible with little sacrifice of therapeutic action.

In a multidisciplinary approach involving the pharmacy and infectious disease services, we initiated a program to promote oral metronidazole for antibiotic-associated colitis that was implemented in three phases.[15] In the first phase, a detailed review of the literature comparing the therapeutic efficacy of metronidazole and oral vancomycin in the treatment of antibiotic-associated colitis determined that metronidazole was equally efficacious yet considerably less expensive.[16] Once therapeutic equivalence was established, the pharmacy department conducted a 1-year retrospective drug use review of patients with antibiotic-associated colitis treated with oral vancomycin to determine the average cost of therapy. In the third phase, the use of oral metronidazole for initial treatment of antibiotic-associated colitis was promoted by using in-service education programs and by restricting the use of oral vancomycin to patients whom oral metronidazole had failed to cure. Six months after implementation of the program, the average cost of drug therapy for antibiotic-associated colitis had dropped 89% from $343.24 per patient to $37.50 per patient. Projected annual savings are $38,829.

Allowing the pharmacy to request competitive bids from different pharmaceutical companies for similar antibiotics is another effective cost-containment strategy. A number of companies now market cefazolin, cephalexin, clindamycin, doxycycline, vancomycin, cefuroxime, ceftazidime, TMP-SMX, gentamicin, erythromycin, cephradine, tetracycline, and semisynthetic penicillins. These drugs should be selected solely in response to competitive bidding, regardless of confounding issues such as "free" goods, educational grants, and other enticements.

Certain antibiotics that are not identical are so similar in antimicrobial activity, pharmacokinetics, and toxicity that it is reasonable to consider them equivalent and subject them to competitive bidding. Two examples are oral cephradine and oral cephalexin, and cefotaxime and ceftizoxime. For susceptible pathogens, gentamicin represents an inexpensive alternative to tobramycin, for it has similar pharmacokinetics and no great difference in toxicity.

Restriction of Antibiotics to Approval by Infectious Disease Physicians

Antibiotics on the restricted list should be those reserved for patients with complicated problems of infectious disease and those that can produce serious toxic reactions if given improperly. It therefore seems unreasonable that approval for these types of agents can be obtained merely by a telephone consultation with an infectious disease physician. Telephone approval takes up too much time for the infectious disease consultants and the private practitioner and sullies the pedagogic goals they are ostensibly employed to serve: quality assurance, proper cost-effective use of antibiotics, and education of the physician. It makes little scientific sense that infectious disease physicians seldom disapprove an antibiotic from information obtained in a telephone conversation, knowing that they lack substantial clinical information to make this type of restrictive decision, yet they often think that the information is adequate to allow them to approve it. An infectious disease physician should examine the patient and provide a formal consultation before an antibiotic in this category is prescribed.

Antibiotic Order Form

There is considerable controversy over the value of the antibiotic order form as a method of cost containment and quality assurance. A form that is easy and quick to complete usually fails to provide sufficient clinical information for accurate analysis of its appropriateness for the intended use. For an antibiotic order form to supply all necessary information, it would have to be so elaborate that few prescribing physicians would take the time to fill it out. The retrospective nature of the analysis further reduces the usefulness of an order form. Like the telephone procedure, it may merely serve as a smoke screen to any meaningful antibiotic control policy. Yet some hospitals claim success in controlling antibiotic use by this means.[16]

Role of the Therapeutics Committee

Certainly one of the most important ways to establish the appropriate and cost-effective use of antibiotics is to have a therapeutics committee that makes decisions based only on scientific information obtained from peer-reviewed journals and not from personal testimonials, marketing brochures, and other unreliable sources. To make the best formulary decisions, hospitals should have an antibiotic subcommittee of the therapeutics committee with representatives from infectious diseases, microbiology, and pharmacy that advises the therapeutics committee about which antibiotics should be on or off the formulary and which should be restricted in some fashion, including dosing restrictions. Formulary decisions made in this fashion and approved by the executive committee of the medical staff should be followed by all staff members. At our hospital, a physician must obtain permission of both the department chair and the chair of the therapeutics committee to make an exception to the recommendations of the formulary committee. Hospitals cannot maintain the illusion of having a formulary if they allow physicians to bypass it easily.

Developing Guidelines for Antibiotic Prophylaxis

The decision to intervene with an antibiotic to prevent an infection must be based on several considerations. First, if natural defense mechanisms are normal, prophylactic antibiotics are seldom needed unless the extent of contamination is excessive. Second, in most of the well-established and successful applications of antibiotic prophylaxis, the drug is aimed with precision at specific organisms when the time of the contamination of tissue or invasion of blood can be predicted with reasonable accuracy. Third, protection is most evident when the prophylactic antibiotic is introduced shortly before or after the time of maximal tissue contamination. There is no evidence that continuing to give the antibiotic beyond the completion of the operation achieves any better protection against infection than one dose given at the proper time before the operation, so long as it maintains adequate tissue and serum levels during the perioperative period. In fact, in addition to adding unnecessarily to costs, continuing prophylactic antibiotics beyond 2 days may select resistant organisms or increase the chances for an adverse drug reaction. Considerable cost savings for hospitals can be realized by restricting dosing of prophylactic antibiotics to 2 days after an operation. In a random sample of hospitals in Pennsylvania, Shapiro and coworkers[17] noted that about 80% of patients received prophylactic antibiotics for too long.

Modes of Administration that Reduce the Burden on Ancillary Services

Clinical experience with the use of oral antibiotics to treat serious infections remains limited. Nevertheless, examination of the pharmacokinetics and antimicrobial activity of a number of oral antibiotics suggests that some should be able to duplicate the clinical activity of parenteral agents. The excellent serum levels achieved after oral administration of cephalexin, cephradine, and cefadroxil may make these drugs useful substitutes for some cephalosporins in the treatment of deep-seated infection such as staphylococcal osteomyelitis. After the administration of a 1-g oral dose of cephradine, cephalexin, or cefadroxil, for instance, peak levels are higher (approximately 30 μg/mL) than those achieved with an equal dose of intramuscular cephalothin (6 to 33 μg/mL) or cephapirin (15 to 24 μg/mL).[18] Clinical success has also been observed in treatment of staphylococcal bone and joint infections with oral semisynthetic penicillins, such as dicloxacillin and oral clindamycin.[19]

Another potential oral antibiotic for deep-seated infection that can replace parenteral agents, at least in clinically stable patients, is TMP-SMX. After a single dose of 160 mg of TMP and 800 mg of SMX, mean serum levels are about 75% and 60%, respectively, of concentrations that would be achieved by the same amount of drug given by the intravenous route. Six hours after a single oral dose of 160 mg of TMP and 800 mg of SMX, respective peak serum levels of are 1.1 μg/mL and 20.3 μg/mL.[20] Beyond the broad-spectrum effect of TMP-SMX used alone, giving it with metronidazole creates an antibiotic combination that is active against many microorganisms, surpassing the activity of a third-generation cephalosporin. Like TMP-SMX, metronidazole has excellent bioavailability when it is administered by the oral route (absorption 90% to 95%). Supporting the potential usefulness of TMP-SMX and metronidazole by the oral route in deep-seated infection has been the cure of some cases of meningitis with oral TMP-SMX and of anaerobic brain abscesses with metronidazole.[21]

Ciprofloxacin and ofloxacin have attracted considerable attention because of their potential for treating serious infections by the oral route, both in and outside the hospital. They are absorbed well, penetrate readily into tissues, exhibit a high degree of antimicrobial activity against many unusual and common pathogens, have long half-lives (3 to 4 hours), and have been therapeutically successful for a number of refractory infections including those traditionally treated with parenteral antibiotics for prolonged periods.

The spectrum of antimicrobial activity of ciprofloxacin and ofloxacin is even greater than that of aminoglycosides, so there is the potential for using them to replace combination therapy once a patient's clinical condition stabilizes, which may often be as early as several days into hospitalization. Like TMP-SMX, oral metronidazole could be given along with oral ciprofloxacin to create an antibiotic regimen that may be useful in polymicrobial infections with coverage for most Enterobacteriaceae, *P. aeruginosa*, staphylococci, and anaerobes. An even more potent oral combination may be obtained by combining ciprofloxacin or ofloxacin with oral clindamycin, because clindamycin is also well absorbed by the oral route and is active against anaerobes and streptococci. However, a number of agents can interfere with the absorption of ciprofloxacin and ofloxacin, including compounds that contain divalent or trivalent cations such as calcium, magnesium, aluminum, iron, and even multivitamins with zinc. As a result, patients taking antacids, sucralfate, iron, and even multivitamins may show unexpectedly low levels after oral administration of this drug. A number of new fluoroquinolones that may not have interaction problems of this type are under active study.

Most physicians tend to think of oral antibiotics as a way of keeping patients out of the hospital, but it is now possible to think of them also as a way to get patients out of the hospital. Although more studies comparing the outcome of therapy with parenteral and oral antibiotics are needed, early results with oral therapy look promising for hospital cost containment.

Too little attention has been given to other modes of drug administration that avoid the parenteral route, such as nasogastric, nasoduodenal, and rectal. The absorption of crushed tablets of ciprofloxacins administered by nasogastric and nasoduodenal instillation, even in the presence of enteric feeding, has been shown to be the same as from the drugs given by mouth. Identical levels of metronidazole are achieved whether the drug is given intravenously or by rectal suppository.

Dose-Dependent Pharmacokinetics

Although most antibiotics display linear pharmacokinetics (serum half-life does not change with dose size), the pharmacokinetics of the ureidopenicillins (azlocillin, mezlocillin, piperacillin) exhibits, dose dependency (half-life increases with dose) because the rate of renal elimination is reduced at the higher dosages. Because the half-life of mezlocillin changes from about 0.7 hour after a 3-g intravenous dose to about 1.2 hours after a 5-g intravenous dose, the areas under the concentration curve for a 24-hour period are similar for 3 g every 4 hours and 5 g every 8 hours.[22] Because of this observation, the therapeutics committee recommended that for any patient receiving a 3-g dose every 4 hours, therapy could automatically be changed to 5 g every 8 hours, which has resulted in an average cost saving of $50.98 per patient. It is possible that a similar approach could be taken with other ureidopenicillins. The pharmacokinetics of carboxypenicillins (ticarcillin or carbenicillin) is not dose dependent.[23]

Role of the Clinical Microbiology Laboratory in Antibiotic Selection

Control of inappropriate and excessive use of antibiotics is often most difficult in small hospitals owing to the absence of infectious disease clinicians, the lack of reliable and accurate microbiology services, and the uncontrolled pressure from pharmaceutical representatives. Paradoxically, even though these small hospitals have fewer and less complicated infections, often the expensive, new expanded-spectrum antibiotics become the popular choices to compensate indirectly for these problems. In small hospitals, most pathogens are common ones that have remained highly susceptible to inexpensive antibiotics such as first-generation cephalosporins (e.g., cefazolin), and most patients have adequate natural host defenses against infection. The clinical microbiology laboratory must familiarize physicians with the number and types of nosocomial infections and the usual antibiotic susceptibility patterns of responsible pathogens in their hospitals.

Many established microbiology laboratory practices produce substantial delay in reporting information and unnecessary expenditure of laboratory labor and materials. In most clinical situations, the antimicrobial susceptibility of anaerobic bacteria can be tested on a batch basis, and this information can be reported along with the susceptibility of aerobic bacteria in a table to be issued to all staff as a guide to choosing therapy.

The clinical microbiology laboratory can also assist considerably in cost containment and appropriate use of antibiotics by using algorithms and antibiotic susceptibility reporting that encourages single-drug therapy with the least expensive, least toxic agent. In a multidisciplinary project with pharmacy, infectious diseases, and microbiology specialists, we have developed an algorithmic approach to pneumonia based on the findings of the initial Gram stain examination of a good-quality sputum specimen and subsequent cultures. As more specific culture information appears, the recommendation changes accordingly. In all instances, the results of the Gram stain, culture, and recommended antibiotics are provided on video screens on the wards. To assist the physician further, the dose and dosing interval of the recommended drug are provided along with an oral agent that can replace it. This approach is only one of several that can be used in this clinical situation. For instance, on the basis of microbiologic activity, ticarcillin-clavulanate could be used in place of a third-generation cephalosporin, ampicillin-sulbactam in place of cefuroxime, and ticarcillin-clavulanate plus an aminoglycoside or a ureidopenicillin plus an aminoglycoside in place of ceftazidime with an aminoglycoside.

Unfortunately, culture reports of most seriously ill hospitalized patients are polymicrobial, so the microbiology reporting system must respond to this observation. Reporting susceptibility data or only a limited number of antibiotics for each isolate may actually add to costs if it encourages physicians to choose combination rather than single-drug therapy. Selected reporting makes sense when only one organism is isolated. It has also become important to report susceptibility data for oral drugs as well as for parenteral ones so that therapy can be streamlined as soon as possible to the most cost-effective mode of administration.

Use of Educational Programs and Pharmaceutical Representation in Antibiotic Selection

Hospitals have traditionally used a number of educational devices such as newsletters and lectures to encourage proper antibiotic use. Although these approaches have been helpful in reinforcing decisions made by the therapeutics committee, by themselves they have been, at best, only temporarily effective. Lectures and symposiums sponsored by pharmaceutical companies can be beneficial as long as the presentations are given by recognized authorities in the field who have published extensively in the area of their presentations. Lectures by biased or poorly informed speakers, on the other hand, may be detrimental to any antibiotic program.

If a recommendation of the therapeutics committee interferes with the sales of an antibiotic, that company's representative often resorts to the tactics that should never affect decision-making: testimonials from physicians or patients, anecdotal observations, information from material (abstracts, promotional literature, data on file) that cannot be scientifically evaluated. To avoid this problem, we have tried to persuade the pharmaceutical sales people to promote their drugs only according to the recommendations of the therapeutics committee, even if their views conflict with those of the companies.

Use of Home Intravenous Therapy Services

Because about half of hospital costs are attributable to board and care, measures that can shorten a hospital stay without interfering with the therapeutic outcome will have a major impact on reducing hospital costs. Early discharge not only eliminates expensive charges for room and board and for diagnostic and laboratory tests but also avoids the risk of a serious hospital-acquired infection. More important, the bed is available to treat another patient, who may have a more pressing need for hospital services.

Although home intravenous therapy remains an obviously cost-effective way to treat patients with infections that require prolonged therapy (e.g., osteomyelitis, bacterial endocarditis, Lyme disease) with parenteral antibiotics, its popularity has paradoxically been dampened by the lack of adequate reimbursement to patients, home intravenous therapy services, and physicians by many insurance carriers, including Medicare. For home intravenous therapy to be as successful as traditional parenteral therapy in a hospital, both the patient and the home therapy service must be carefully screened to be certain that they meet important criteria. For instance, patients should be clinically stable, be able to understand and cope with the intravenous program, be accessible by telephone, have no history of substance abuse, and have financial coverage for the expenses. The home care intravenous therapy service should have daily 24-hour coverage and well-trained intravenous technicians who consult frequently with the patient's physician about the patient's progress. It is also sensible for the physician to see the patient at least once a week.

Summary

Hemmed in between the fiscal constraints of the hospital and the obligation to deliver the best possible care, physicians should accept the assistance of specialists well trained in the best possible use of antiinfective drugs: pharmacists, microbiologists, and infectious disease physicians. Full staff compliance with the recommendations of the therapeutics committee is crucial to any antibiotic management program. There are a number of strategic ways to control antibiotic use and still obtain the best possible clinical outcome. In our hospital, the most effective approaches have been those that reduce the chances for the physician's error through the automatic correction of dose and dosing interval of antibiotics and their conversion to cost-effective alternative agents by pharmacy, daily review of the charts of patients receiving antibiotics by an antibiotic team, and an antibiotic reporting system that encourages single-drug and oral therapy.

References

1. Gilbert DN: Once-daily aminoglycoside therapy. Antimicrob Agents Chemother 35:399, 1991.
2. Nicolau DP, Freeman CD, Belliveau PP, et al: Experience with a once-daily aminoglycoside program administered to 2,184 adult patients. Antimicrob Agents Chemother 39:650, 1995.
3. Nishida M, Murakawa T, Kaminura T, et al: Bactericidal activity of cephalosporins in an in-vitro model simulating serum levels. Antimicrob Agents Chemother 14:6, 1978.
4. Craig WA: Interrelationship between pharmacokinetics and pharmacodynamics in determining dosing regimens for broad-spectrum cephalosporins. Diagn Microbiol Infect Dis 22:89, 1995.
5. Nicolau PD, Quintiliani R, Nightingale CH: Antibiotic kinetics and dynamics for the clinician. Med Clin North Am 79:477, 1995.
6. Quintiliani R, Cooper BW, Briceland LL, Nightingale CH: Economic impact of streamlining antibiotic àdministration. Am J Med 82(Suppl 4A):391, 1987.
7. Maki DG: Infection due to infusion therapy. *In* Bennett JV, Brachman PA (eds): Hospital Infection. Boston, Little, Brown, 1986, pp 561–580.
8. Read I, Body GP: Infectious complications of indwelling vascular catheters. Clin Infect Dis 15:197, 1992.
9. Arnow PM, Quimosing EM, Beach M: Consequences of intravascular catheter sepsis. Clin Infect Dis 16:778, 1993.
10. Quintiliani R: Transitional antibiotic therapy. Can J Infect Dis 6(Suppl A):6, 1995.
11. Kunin CM: Problems in antibiotic usage. *In* Mandell GL, Douglas RG, Barnett JE (eds): Principles and Practice of Infectious Diseases. New York, John Wiley & Sons, 1989.
12. Jones RN, Barry AL: Antimicrobial activity of ceftriaxone, cefotaxime, desacetylcefotaxime, and cefotaxime-desacetylcefotaxime in the presence of human serum. Antimicrob Agents Chemother 31:818, 1987.
13. Buchwald D, Sounerai SB, Vandevanter N, et al: Effects of hospital-wide change in clindamycin dosing schedule on clinical outcome. Rev Infect Dis 2:619, 1989.
14. Earl P, Sisson PR, Ingham HR: Twelve-hourly dosage schedule for oral and intravenous metronidazole. J Antimicrob Chemother 24:619, 1989.
15. Briceland LL, Quintiliani R, Nightingale CH: Multidisciplinary cost-containment program promoting oral metronidazole for treatment of antibiotic-associated colitis. Am J Hosp Pharm 45:122, 1988.
16. Teasley DG, Olson MM, Gebhard RL, et al: Prospective randomized trial of metronidazole versus vancomycin for *Clostridium difficile*–associated colitis. Lancet 2:1043, 1978.
17. Shapiro M, Townsend TR, Rosener B, et al: Use of antimicrobial drugs in general hospitals. N Engl J Med 301:351, 1979.
18. Chow M, Quintiliani R, Cunha BA, et al: Pharmacokinetics of high-dose oral cephalosporins. J Clin Pharmacol 19:185, 1979.
19. Nelson JD: A critical review of the role of oral antibiotics in the management of hematogenous osteomyelitis. *In* Remington JS, Swartz MN (eds): Current Clinical Topics in Infection. New York, McGraw-Hill, 1983.
20. Kremers P, Duvivier J, Heusghem C: Pharmacokinetic studies of cotrimoxazole in man after single and repeat doses. J Clin Pharmacol 14:112, 1974.
21. Wainer JF, Perkins RL, Cordero L: Metronidazole therapy of anaerobic bacteremia, meningitis, and brain abscess. Arch Intern Med 139:167, 1979.
22. Gundert-Remy U, Hildebrandt R, Stiehl A, Weber E: Nonlinear mezlocillin kinetics due to dose-dependent metabolism. Clin Pharmacol Ther 33:656, 1983.
23. Guglilmo BJ, Flaherty JF, Batman R, et al: Comparative pharmacokinetics of low- and high-dose ticarcillin. Antimicrob Agents Chemother 30:359, 1986.

39

Outpatient Parenteral Therapy

Donald M. Poretz

Traditionally, the treatment of certain infections such as osteomyelitis, infective endocarditis, and severe wound infections has required hospitalization for up to several weeks to administer parenteral antibiotics. Extensive experience in the past several years has shown that the intravenous administration of antibiotics and other medications in the home or outpatient setting is both safe and cost-effective when compared with similar therapy in the hospital. For many diseases, the parenteral administration of antibiotics on an outpatient basis has become the standard of care.

History of Intravenous Infusions

The first intravenous injection of medication was made in approximately 1660, when Sir Christopher Wren and Robert

Boyle, a chemist, used a hypodermic needle to inject medication into a dog. In the many years following, several attempts were made to inject material into human beings without significant success. In 1911, the first intravenous glucose solution was administered for nutritional support during surgery. Until 1925, normal saline was the major parenteral fluid used for infusion, but as late as the 1930s, intravenous fluid replacement was still considered a major procedure. In 1931, Thomas Latta administered saline solutions to treat the diarrhea associated with cholera. During subsequent years, many types of fluids, nutrients, antibiotics, and other medications were adapted for intravenous use. The development of various types of infusion devices, some of which could be left in place for a considerable time, allowed for ease of administration of many types of fluids and medications. In the late 1970s and 1980s, methods were adapted for use in the outpatient setting. Various types of delivery systems and miniaturization of pumps and other devices that had previously been used only in hospitals were adapted to the outpatient arena.

The first experience with intravenous antibiotics in the outpatient setting was published by Antoniskis and coworkers in 1978,[1] when they reported the results of 13 patients who administered parenteral antibiotics to themselves primarily for osteomyelitis. Subsequently, several other articles appeared in the literature that demonstrated the efficacy, safety, and cost savings of outpatient intravenous antibiotic therapy throughout different centers in the United States.[2–18] Most of these studies focused on bone and joint infections,[19–23] but as experience grew, a wide variety of other infectious processes were shown to be amenable to outpatient intravenous antibiotic therapy. In addition to the usage of intravenous antibiotics, it is now commonplace to administer total parenteral nutrition, intravenous fluid replacement, continuous narcotic infusions for pain, blood product and coagulation factor replacement, corticotropin, immune serum globulin, and other medications on an outpatient basis. Programs have been developed that teach family members to administer medications intramuscularly,[24] and pharmaceutical manufacturers have developed newer drugs with longer half-lives that will allow for once- or twice-daily administration. Under appropriate circumstances, chemotherapy patients with fever and neutropenia have been treated with parenteral antibiotic therapy on an outpatient basis.[25] In addition, elderly individuals who are medically stable and require prolonged parenteral antibiotic therapy have been shown to be safely treated outside of the hospital.[26, 27] Patients with acquired immunodeficiency syndrome, who often need infusions of multiple medications, are commonly treated outside of the hospital. Several reviews have been published concerning various aspects of outpatient intravenous antibiotic therapy.[28–30]

Development of a Home Intravenous Program

Regardless of where patients are treated—be it in the home, clinic, physician's office, specialized infusion center, or outpatient facility associated with a hospital—all studies have shown the need for a team approach.[5, 6, 9, 30] Physicians, nurses, pharmacists, other ancillary personnel, and administrators are necessary for a successful program. Wherever the patient is treated, a physician with training in outpatient intravenous infusion therapy is usually responsible for the care of the patient. Physicians need to be familiar with the particular infectious process being treated in addition to the relationship between the infection and other possible illnesses that the patient may have. Often, patients are receiving multiple medications, and the interaction between antimicrobial agents and these other medicines needs careful monitoring. The importance of communication with other physicians attending the patient cannot be overemphasized.

A registered nurse with expertise in the use of intravenous devices and vascular access is vital to the success of an outpatient program. It is common for nurses who had previously been on a hospital's intravenous team and are familiar with various types of vascular devices to become involved with outpatient programs. Guidelines for nurses involved with intravenous devices have been set up by the National Intravenous Therapy Association.[31] The nurse is responsible for training the patient, family member, or significant other in the management of the vascular access and medication delivery. Potential complications concerning a particular therapy need to be discussed by the nurse and explained to the patient and, if necessary, to a family member. The nurse is responsible for demonstrating to the patient the daily care of the intravenous device and ensuring that the patient is competent and proficient in intravenous procedures as well as good aseptic practices. The initial dose of any medication should be witnessed by the nurse to make sure that no untoward side effects occur.

A pharmacist is an additional integral part of an outpatient intravenous program and serves several functions.[32, 33] Because of the pharmacist's expertise in parenteral compounding and intravenous admixture services, familiarity with vendors of intravenous solutions, and multidisciplinary contacts within a hospital institution, the pharmacist's experience lends itself quite nicely for participation in an outpatient intravenous program. The pharmacist often assists the nurse in the training of patients, particularly noting any potential adverse drug reactions. The pharmacist's function may also include supervising the day-to-day operation of the outpatient program as well as preparing medications. The pharmacist may be responsible for preparation of materials used for training of patients, monitoring clinical results, and consulting with members of the health care team with regard to medications and supplies to be utilized. The pharmacist can act as a liaison between insurance companies and other providers, often explaining the details of an outpatient program, including its relative cost savings. Equipment should be regularly inspected and approved by the pharmacist. In addition, the traditional role of dispensor is obviously required of the pharmacist in a home intravenous antibiotic program. This includes overseeing the ordering of supplies, preparing prescriptions, evaluating new products and procedures, and supplying information on new drugs and products to other members of the health care team.

Pharmacists and nurses need to work closely together while carefully monitoring the patient's progress. They can significantly reduce the time demands on the physician who is overseeing the patient's care. All individuals involved need to be aware of adverse drug reactions and other potential side effects of medications. Infiltration of intravenous lines, phlebitis, gastrointestinal symptoms, and inflammation around venous access sites are other possible problems that need to be monitored closely. It is common for physician, nurse, and pharmacist to make rounds together when patients are examined so that all aspects of the patient's care can be discussed, wounds examined, vascular access sites inspected and changed, and any adverse drug reactions noted.

Criteria for Selection of Patients

Experience has shown that certain selection criteria are necessary to evaluate a candidate for an outpatient intravenous program. First, the patient's medical condition must be stable; the patient should be afebrile and, if a wound is present, the drainage contained in a bandage that is easily manipulated by the patient, the patient's family member, or a health care provider. If a patient has infective endocarditis, there

TABLE 39–1 ■ Selection Criteria for Outpatient Intravenous Antibiotics

A condition amenable to outpatient treatment
Reliable and compliant patient
Educable patient
Psychosocial conditions
Adequate venous access
Financial considerations
Medicolegal aspects

should be no recent evidence of embolic phenomena and the patient should not have congestive heart failure. Patients should be ambulatory and have a reasonable nutritional status. Patients must be compliant with all aspects of intravenous administration of outpatient drugs. Consideration should be given to family responsibilities such as small children or elderly parents who could hinder compliance. In addition, the patient or family member should be educable and have the ability to comprehend aseptic technique and the maintenance of intravascular access as well as specific instructions regarding medication. An adequate venous access must be available. Economic considerations in the form of third-party reimbursement must be acknowledged before the initiation of outpatient treatment (Table 39–1).

Factors that usually exclude a patient from participating in an outpatient intravenous program include current substance abuse, impaired vision with no one available to be trained in intravenous techniques, and a home environment that would prohibit proper treatment because of lack of electricity, running water, refrigeration, or adequate cleanliness.

Equipment Required

Several intravenous access devices are available to treat individuals on an outpatient basis.

A butterfly needle, also called a winged infusion needle, is short, inserts easily, and is good for short-term therapy such as a 30- to 60-minute infusion. In patients with poor venous access, it can be utilized in a hand vein. It infiltrates easily and is difficult to stabilize. It is infrequently used in individuals who require prolonged courses of therapy.

A heparin lock, also called an over-the-needle catheter or angiocatheter, is good for short-term therapy lasting from a few days to a couple of weeks. It can be difficult to insert in patients with poor venous access who require long-term therapy. The heparin lock site needs to be changed every 48 to 72 hours, which may be a problem in individuals needing long courses of therapy.

Midline catheters made of elastomeric hydrogel (Aquavene) soften and expand when in contact with the venous system. The catheter expands approximately two gauge sizes 90 minutes after placement. It must be maintained with heparin, and sterile dressing changes are recommended. It is good for long-term therapy.[34] There have been reports of anaphylactic-type reactions associated with these catheters.

Peripherally inserted central venous catheters, also known as PICC lines, are used for long-term therapy in individuals with poor venous access. These lines are particularly valuable when irritating solutions are used. Sterile dressing changes are required and maintenance with heparin is necessary. A chest x-ray film is required after placement. The PICC lines are easier to insert and have fewer complications than a central line; also, they do not involve the extra cost of a surgeon's fee, as they are usually placed by an intravenous nurse at the bedside.[35]

Indwelling catheters such as Groshong, Hickman,[36] and Broviac[37] are good for long-term therapy (up to years) and irritating fluids. They have Dacron cuffs and are surgically inserted. Hickman catheters usually require daily maintenance with heparin; Groshong catheters require weekly maintenance with saline. They both require frequent dressing changes. Potential complications on insertion of these devices include pneumothorax, hemohydrothorax, brachial plexus injury, hemorrhage, air embolism, venous thrombosis, catheter thrombosis, catheter tip migration, and catheter sepsis.

Implanted ports (commercially known as Port-a-Cath, P.A.S. Port, and Mediport) are devices whereby the entire access system is placed under the skin. There is a self-sealing injection port in a silicone catheter. These devices are good for long-term therapy and irritating solutions. Less maintenance is required—only monthly flushes with heparin when they are not in use. The devices are surgically placed and are accessed for intravenous therapy with a Huber needle. Some patients prefer these devices because they are cosmetically more acceptable[38] (Table 39–2).

Antibiotics are usually reconstituted and mixed by the pharmacist under a laminar flow hood. Most antibiotics are stable in solution for at least 48 hours and many are stable for several days. Various infusion devices are available for outpatient use. The simplest, least expensive method is a gravity drip bag. This is often used in conjunction with a lyophilized antibiotic that is mixed with sterile precautions, into the bag before infusion. There are also fixed-rate infusion pumps that include an elastomeric reservoir whereby a distended balloon forces the medication through a capillary tube with a fixed resistance, allowing for a fixed rate of drug infusion no matter where the device is placed in relation to the body. Bioelectric membrane pumps and electrovoltaic pumps are occasionally used. In addition, programmable pumps allow drugs to be administered from a cassette or external reservoir at a fixed rate and time interval. These devices, while offering accuracy and convenience to ambulatory patients, add to the cost of infusions.[39, 40]

Types of Treatable Infections

Experience from many centers has shown that a wide variety of infections requiring parenteral antibiotics can be treated on an outpatient basis. Osteomyelitis and skin and soft tissue infections are the most common entities treated, with diabetes mellitus often an associated condition seen in up to one third of patients with chronic osteomyelitis of the lower extremities. Many of these patients require up to 6 weeks of intravenous antibiotic therapy. Patients may require rehospitalization for débridement of wounds and removal of sequestra, but outpatient therapy can be resumed a few days after such procedures are performed. Although children with osteomyelitis are often treated with oral antibiotics, they can, when necessary, be treated safely with outpatient intravenous therapy.[10] The newer fluoroquinolone antimicrobials have allowed for some individuals with gram-negative osteomyelitis to be treated orally rather than receiving a protracted course of intravenous medications.[41]

Genitourinary infections are also commonly treated on an

TABLE 39–2 ■ Intravenous Access Devices

Butterfly needles
Heparin lock
Midline catheter
Peripherally inserted central venous catheter
Indwelling catheters
Implanted ports

outpatient basis. Acute uncomplicated urinary tract infection can most often be handled with an oral antimicrobial but patients with chronic urinary tract problems—including those with neurogenic bladders, recurrent prostatic disease, congenital abnormalities of the urinary tract, and other chronic conditions—often have infections caused by microorganisms that are susceptible only to drugs that must be given parenterally. It is not uncommon for many patients to be retreated on several occasions because of acute exacerbations of chronic urinary tract infections. These patients may not need to be admitted to the hospital but can be started with either an aminoglycoside or a third-generation cephalosporin pending the results of cultures.

Pelvic inflammatory disease is also well suited to outpatient intravenous antibiotic therapy, because the majority of these patients are young, otherwise healthy women without additional medical problems. Previously, many of these patients with relapsing infections were often admitted to the hospital to undergo significant pelvic surgery. A prolonged course of intravenous antibiotic therapy is often associated with less chance of recurrence; if there is a recurrence, the surgery performed is usually less radical.

Various pulmonary infections are quite amenable to outpatient intravenous antibiotic therapy. It is not uncommon for a patient with an acute exacerbation of chronic pulmonary disease to require a course of an aminoglycoside or third-generation cephalosporin; many patients can begin therapy when acute symptoms occur rather than waiting until the infection has advanced. In children and young adults with cystic fibrosis, acute exacerbations of infection can be treated on an outpatient basis rather than hospitalizing the patient.[42–44] Therapy in these individuals often depends on the patient's symptoms rather than new pulmonary infiltrates or other signs of infection. Patients with *Pneumocystis carinii* pneumonia—as well as those with other pulmonary infections commonly seen in association with immunodeficiency states—can also be treated as outpatients using trimethoprim-sulfamethoxazole or pentamidine[45] or other appropriate antimicrobials.

Ear, nose, and throat infections such as acute and chronic sinusitis that does not respond to oral antibiotic therapy and often needs several weeks of intravenous antibiotics are conditions that can easily be treated on an outpatient basis. Children with severe bouts of otitis media requiring a prolonged course of antibiotic therapy can have most of their therapy given on an outpatient basis. Infections caused by *Pseudomonas*—including otitis media, malignant external otitis, and mastoiditis—have been treated effectively outside of the hospital.

Endothelial surface infections such as infective endocarditis and infected vascular grafts often require up to 6 weeks of intravenous antibiotic therapy. Most experience has been with streptococcal endocarditis, but infection with other organisms has also been treated on an outpatient basis.[46] Assuming that the patient does not have significant congestive heart failure and is free of embolic events, the administration of outpatient intravenous antibiotics has reduced hospital costs considerably and enabled such patients to be at home.

Infected prosthetic devices that require prolonged courses of intravenous antibiotic therapy are often treated on an outpatient basis. In the past, it was common to remove all infected prosthetic devices, but it is now possible to treat many patients with long courses of intravenous antibiotics without removing the device.

A variety of miscellaneous infections can be treated outside of the hospital. Of particular note are the infections associated with acquired immunodeficiency syndrome, for which antiviral drugs such as acyclovir, ganciclovir, cidofovir, and foscarnet can be given effectively on an outpatient basis if careful monitoring is ensured. Amphotericin B, which often requires a prolonged infusion, can be safely infused on an outpatient basis. Infections in individuals who have received organ transplants can similarly be treated on an outpatient basis (Table 39–3).

Antibiotics Used in the Outpatient Setting

A variety of parenteral antimicrobials have been used to treat patients in the outpatient setting. The advent of newer cephalosporins with extended half-lives and the ability to treat a patient once or twice daily have made the delivery of these antibiotics much easier and convenient for patients and their families.

The antimicrobials used must obviously be active against the offending organism and have the fewest potential side effects, with minimal venous irritation. Because semisynthetic penicillin antibiotics can be quite irritative to the veins, cephalosporins have become popular in outpatient programs. Considerable experience has been gathered with newer cephalosporins such as ceftriaxone[9, 19–21, 24] and cefonicid,[23] which can be administered once daily, whereas other cephalosporins—such as cefoperazone, ceftizoxime, and cefotetan—can be given twice daily. Cefotaxime has been given via a portable infusion pump for a wide variety of infections.[28]

Aminoglycosides are easily administered on an outpatient basis both intravenously and intramuscularly. With the trend toward once-daily high-dose aminoglycoside therapy, there is less toxicity and more convenience for the patient. Monitoring renal function and serum levels is necessary, especially in patients with poor renal function. In general, if the medical condition warrants, almost any antimicrobial can be used on an outpatient basis.

The most common side effects seen with parenteral antibiotics include mild gastrointestinal complaints such as loose stools, nausea, and vague abdominal discomfort. Occasionally, significant diarrhea occurs, which may be related to *Clostridium difficile* toxin positivity. Changing to a different antibiotic and adding oral metronidazole or vancomycin can easily be done and do not usually indicate a need for rehospitalization. Because of the extreme expense of oral vancomycin, many physicians tend to favor oral metronidazole for antibiotic-related colitis. Other common reactions to antimicrobials include a variety of rashes, which may necessitate discontinuing the drug and using one of a different class. The first dose of a new antibiotic should always be given in the presence of either medical or nursing personnel to make sure that an acute accelerated allergic reaction does not occur. A peculiar disulfiram-like reaction to cephalosporins with a methylthiotetrazole side chain (cefamandole, cefoperazone, moxalactam) occurs when alcohol is taken concurrently with one of these drugs; therefore all patients should be told that they cannot consume alcohol while they are taking these medications.

TABLE 39–3 ■ Infections Treatable with Outpatient Intravenous Antibiotics

Antibiotics
Bone, joint, and soft tissue infections
Genitourinary infections
Ear, nose, and throat infections
Pulmonary infections
Intraabdominal infections
Endovascular infections
Prosthetic device infections
Infections associated with immunodeficiency states and organ transplantation

It has been uncommon to see infections at the intravenous catheter site when the heparin locks are used and changed twice weekly. Midline catheters and central venous catheters can cause localized inflammation at the insertion site and occasionally bacteremias.[47] Paying particular attention to renal function is necessary when patients are receiving vancomycin or aminoglycosides. The possibility of drug interactions is important, and one needs to be aware of all medications that the patient is taking. Occasionally, vitamin K supplementation may be necessary. The most common laboratory abnormality noted during infusions of β-lactam antibiotics, but also seen in patients who are receiving clindamycin and vancomycin, is leukopenia, which is dose related and usually reverses within a few days after the drug is discontinued. Elevation of liver enzyme values may be nonspecific or related to the antibiotic (Table 39–4).

Many of the newer expanded half-life cephalosporins are expensive per unit dose; however, when the cost of extra tubing, pharmacy preparation, time, minibags, infusion devices, and other supplies is added—plus the fact that patients can often go to work or school without having to administer extra infusions—there is often a total cost savings. Physicians need to be aware of the expense of the antimicrobials being used (Table 39–5).

Monitoring of Patients

Patients receiving outpatient intravenous antibiotic therapy can be treated in a variety of locations. No matter where they are treated, however, careful monitoring is mandatory. Protocols and teaching guides that include explanations of parenteral antibiotic therapy, aseptic technique, equipment and supplies, follow-up processes, and emergency procedures should be written and followed carefully by nurses, pharmacists, and physicians administering the program. Whenever patients are seen by either the nurse or physician, a notation should be made in the patient's chart. These notes should include pertinent physical findings and information about the venous access site. All laboratory studies should be maintained on a flow sheet for rapid review. Any manipulations performed and all equipment and drugs dispensed need to be documented. If a patient is referred by another physician, periodic updates regarding the patient's progress should be sent to the referring physician. Ongoing quality improvement should be routine.

Financial and Legal Considerations

There has been a dramatic growth in the home health care industry, including outpatient intravenous antibiotic therapy. In 1994 the total amount spent for home care was $15 billion, of which $4.3 billion was for intravenous infusions; of this amount, $1.6 billion was for antibiotics. Several studies have documented cost savings for home intravenous antibiotic therapy.[48, 49] Most studies have demonstrated between a 50% and 75% reduction when compared with in-hospital care. Many third-party payers have recognized these dramatic financial savings and have routinely included this type of care in their policies. Managed care programs have particularly embraced these types of programs. Although cost savings have been demonstrated in the Medicare population,[50] reimbursement is not generally the rule.

As the number of hospitals, physicians, nurses, and pharmacists involved in home health care continues to increase, medicolegal liability will also become an important issue. It is not uncommon for home health care agencies and physicians to have patients sign waivers when they are being treated at home with intravenous medications. The actual legal status of these waivers is not known. There have been a few instances of litigation by patients who have experienced adverse events while being treated as outpatients, the most common being ototoxicity from gentamicin. It is imperative

TABLE 39–4 ■ Adverse Effects of Outpatient Intravenous Antibiotics

Phlebitis
Infections at the intravenous access site
Drug interactions
Gastrointestinal symptoms
Disulfiram-like reactions
Vasovagal reactions
Leukopenia
Elevation of liver enzyme values
Renal toxicity
Clotting abnormalities
Interactions with other medications

TABLE 39–5 ■ Commonly Used Parenteral Antibiotics and Their Average Wholesale Prices

ANTIMICROBIAL AGENT	DOSE	AWP*/PER DOSE
Penicillin G, potassium	1 × 10⁶ units	$ 1.45
Ampicillin	1 g	1.54
Ampicillin-sulbactam	3 g	12.90
Nafcillin	2 g	4.40
Ticarcillin	3 g	9.76
Ticarcillin-clavulanate	3.1 g	13.88
Piperacillin	3 g	15.35
Piperacillin-tazobactam	4.5 g	20.41
Cefazolin	1 g	3.78
Cefamandole	1 g	9.06
Cefoxitin	1 g	9.90
Cefonicid	1 g	26.10
Cefotetan	1 g	11.16
Cefoperazone	2g	32.84
Cefotaxime	1 g	11.48
Cefuroxime	1.5 g	13.46
Ceftazidime	1 g	14.23
Ceftriaxone	1 g	34.92
Ceftizoxime	1 g	13.00
Cefepime	1 g	15.30
Imipenem	500 mg	27.32
Meropenem	1 g	51.84
Aztreonam	1 g	14.90
Gentamicin	80 mg	1.65
Tobramycin	80 mg	7.28
Amikacin	500 mg	32.89
Clindamycin	600 mg	13.84
Chloramphenicol	1 g	4.32
Doxycycline	100 mg	16.80
Erythromycin	500 mg	11.59
Metronidazole	500 mg	7.81
Trimethoprim-sulfamethoxazole	160 mg/800 mg	12.69
Vancomycin	1 g	15.60
Amphotericin B	50 mg	17.29
Fluconazole	200 mg	81.25
Pentamidine	300 mg	94.50
Acyclovir	500 mg	56.60
Ganciclovir	500 mg	34.80
Cidofovir	375 mg	117.80
Foscarnet	6 g	73.28
Ofloxacin	400 mg	27.60
Ciprofloxacin	400 mg	30.01

*AWP, Average wholesale price (in 1996, as quoted by individual manufacturers).

that physicians continue to take a leadership position in the outpatient treatment of their patients. The Joint Commission on Accreditation of Hospitals and Outpatient Facilities, in addition to federal and state authorities, will be carefully evaluating these programs for appropriateness, quality control, and cost containment.

References

1. Antoniskis A, Anderson BC, Van Volkinburg EJ, et al: Feasibility of outpatient self-administration of parenteral antibiotics. West J Med 128:203–206, 1978.
2. Stiver HG, Telford GO, Mossey JM, et al: Intravenous antibiotic therapy at home. Ann Intern Med 89:690–693, 1978.
3. Stiver HG, Trosky SK, Cote DD, et al: Self-administration of intravenous antibiotics: An efficient, cost-effective home care program. Can Med Assoc J 127:207–211, 1982.
4. Kind AC, Williams DN, Persons G, Gibson JA: Intravenous antibiotic therapy at home. Arch Intern Med 139:413–415, 1979.
5. Rehm SJ, Weinstein AJ: Home intravenous antibiotic therapy: A team approach. Ann Intern Med 99:388–392, 1983.
6. Poretz DM, Eron LJ, Goldenberg RI, et al: Intravenous antibiotic therapy in an outpatient setting. JAMA 248:336–339, 1982.
7. Eisenberg JM, Kitz DS: Savings from outpatient antibiotic therapy for osteomyelitis. Economic analysis of a therapeutic strategy. JAMA 255:1584–1588, 1986.
8. McCue JD: Outpatient IV antibiotic therapy: Practical and ethical considerations. Hosp Pract 23:208–211, 1988.
9. Poretz DM: Home management of intravenous antibiotic therapy. Bull N Y Acad Med 64:570–576, 1988.
10. Goldenberg RI, Poretz DM, Eron LJ, et al: Intravenous antibiotic therapy in ambulatory pediatric patients. Pediatr Infect Dis 3:514–517, 1984.
11. Smego RA Jr: Home intravenous antibiotic therapy. Arch Intern Med 145:1001–1002, 1985.
12. Sutker WL: Home intravenous antibiotic therapy. Infect Med 5:350–358, 1988.
13. Kind AC, Williams DN, Gibson J: Outpatient intravenous antibiotic therapy. Ten years' experience. Postgrad Med 77(2):105–111, 1985.
14. Williams DN, Kind AC, Gibson JA, et al: Outpatient intravenous antibiotics experience with 65 patients. Am J IV Ther Clin Nutr 9:33–40, 1982.
15. Frame PT: Outpatient intravenous antibiotic therapy (Editorial). JAMA 248:356, 1982.
16. Williams DN, Gibson JA, Kind AC: Outpatient intravenous antibiotic therapy. J Antimicrob Chemother 14:102–104, 1984.
17. Poretz DM: Outpatient intravenous antibiotic therapy. Outpatient Ther Med 2(4):1, 12–14, 1987.
18. Powell KR, Mawhorter SD: Outpatient treatment of serious infections in infants and children with ceftriaxone. J Pediatr 110:898–901, 1987.
19. Denny L, Eron LJ, Toy C, et al: Ceftriaxone therapy of osteomyelitis. Presented at the 13th International Congress of Chemotherapy; 1983; Vienna, Austria.
20. Eron LJ, Goldenberg RI, Poretz DM: Combined ceftriaxone and surgical therapy for osteomyelitis in hospital and outpatient settings. Am J Surg 148(4A):1–4, 1984.
21. Eron LJ, Park CH, Hixon DL, et al: Ceftriaxone therapy of bone and soft tissue infections in hospital and outpatient settings. Antimicrob Agents Chemother 23:731–737, 1983.
22. Ingram C, Eron LJ, Goldenberg RI, et al: Antibiotic therapy of osteomyelitis in outpatients. Med Clin North Am 72:723–738, 1988.
23. Kunkel MJ, Iannini PB: Cefonicid in a once-daily regimen for treatment of osteomyelitis in an ambulatory setting. Rev Infect Dis 4:S865–S869, 1984.
24. Russo TA, Cook S, Gorbach SL: Intramuscular ceftriaxone in home parenteral therapy. Antimicrob Agents Chemother 32:1439–1440, 1988.
25. Talcott JA, Whalen A, Clark J, et al: Home antibiotic therapy for low risk cancer patients with fever and neutropenia: A pilot study of 30 patients based on a validated prediction rule. J Clin Oncol 12:107–114, 1994.
26. Poretz DM: Home intravenous antibiotic therapy. Clin Geriatr Med 7:749–763, 1991.
27. Bernstein LH: An update on home intravenous antibiotic therapy. Geriatrics 46(6):47–54, 1991.
28. Poretz DM (ed): Outpatient use of intravenous antibiotics. Am J Med 97(Suppl 2A):34–42, 1994.
29. Tice AD: Outpatient parenteral antibiotic therapy. Management of serious infections. Hosp Pract 28(Suppl 1 and 2):6–10, 36–39, 1993.
30. McCloskey R (ed): The Home Care Symposium. Snowbird, Utah, 10–11 January 1989. Rev Infect Dis 13(Suppl 2):S141–S195, 1991.
31. Home I.V. therapy. NITA 8(2):93, 1984.
32. Swensen JP: Training patients to administer intravenous antibiotics at home. Am J Hosp Pharm 38:1480–1483, 1981.
33. Schneider PJ, Simon GI, Rising J: Home intravenous antibiotic therapy. *In* Wyant S (ed): The Home Advantage: Opportunities in Hospital Pharmacy, Vol 1, No 2. Fairfax, VA, Christopher Parios, 1986.
34. Fontaine PJ: Performance of a new softening expanding midline catheter in home intravenous therapy patients. J Intravenous Nurs 14:91–99, 1991.
35. Brown JM: Peripherally inserted central catheters—Use in the home. J Intravenous Nurs 12:144–147, 1989.
36. Hickman RO, Buckner CD, Clift RA, et al: A modified right atrial catheter for access to the venous system in marrow transplant recipients. Surg Gynecol Obstet 148:871–875, 1979.
37. Broviac JW, Cole BS, Scribner BH: A silicone rubber atrial catheter for prolonged parenteral alimentation. Surg Gynecol Obstet 136:602–606, 1973.
38. Bonstell R: What's new in implanted ports. Outpatient Intravenous Infusion Ther Assoc Newsl 3:6, 1992.
39. Kwan V: High-technology IV infusion devices. Am J Hosp Pharm 46:320–335, 1989.
40. Neu PB, Swanson CF, Bulich RG, et al: Ambulatory antibiotic infusion devices: Extending the spectrum of outpatient therapies. Am J Med 91:455–461, 1991.
41. Neu H: Quinolones. Med Clin North Am 72:623–636, 1992.
42. Winter RJD, George RJD, Deacock SJ, et al: Self-administered home intravenous antibiotic therapy in bronchiectasis and adult cystic fibrosis. Lancet 1:1338–1339, 1984.
43. Gilbert J, Robinson T, Littlewood JM: Home intravenous antibiotic treatment in cystic fibrosis. Arch Dis Child 63:512–517, 1988.
44. Strandvik B, Hjelte L, Malmborg AS, et al: Home intravenous antibiotic treatment of patients with cystic fibrosis. Acta Paediatr 81:340–344, 1992.
45. Morrison A, Eron L, Poretz D, et al: Outpatient intravenous therapy of nonbacterial infections in immunocompromised patients: New directions for cost containment (Abstr). Presented at the 27th International Conference on Antimicrobial Agents and Chemotherapy; 1987; New York.
46. Francioli P, Etienne J, Hoigne R, et al: Treatment of streptococcal endocarditis with a single daily dose of ceftriaxone sodium for four weeks. JAMA 26:264–267, 1992.
47. White MC, Ragland KE: Surveillance of intravenous catheter-related infections among home care clients. Am J Infect Control 22:231–235, 1994.
48. Bolinsky U, Nesbitt S: Cost effectiveness of outpatient parenteral antibiotics: A review of the literature. Am J Med 87:301–309, 1989.
49. Williams DN, Bosch D, Boots J, et al: Safety, efficacy, and cost-savings in an outpatient intravenous antibiotic program. Clin Ther 15:169–179, 1993.
50. Hindes R, Winkler C, Kane P, et al: Outpatient intravenous antibiotic therapy in Medicare patients: Cost-savings analysis. Infect Dis Clin Pract 4:211–217, 1995.

40

Tables of Antimicrobial Agents

John G. Bartlett

TABLE 40–1 ■ Preparations and Recommended Adult Dosing Regimens for Antimicrobial Agents*

AGENT	TRADE NAME	DOSE FORM	DAILY DOSE, ROUTE, DOSE INTERVAL
Acyclovir	Zovirax	5% ointment; 3-, 15-g tubes	Topical q 3 h
		200-mg caps; 800-mg tabs; 200 mg/5 mL susp	200–800 mg PO × 2–5/d
			15–36 mg/kg/d
		500-mg vials (IV)	IV in 1–3 h q 8 h
Albendazole	Zentel	400-mg tabs	400–800 mg PO × qd or bid
Amantadine	Symmetrel	100-mg caps, tabs; 50 mg/5 mL syrup	100–200 mg/d PO q 12–24 h
Amdinocillin	Coactin	0.5-, 1-g vials	40–60 mg/kg/d IM or IV q 4–6 h
Amikacin	Amikin	0.1-, 0.5-, 1-g vials	15 mg/kg/d IV × 1 or q 8–12 h
Aminosalicylic acid	PAS	0.5-g tabs	150 mg/kg/d PO q 6–12 h
Amoxicillin	Amoxil, Trimox, Wymox	250-, 500-mg caps; 125, 250 mg/5 mL syrup	0.75–2 g/d PO q 6–8 h
Amoxicillin-clavulanate	Augmentin	125/31 mg and 250/62 mg/5 mL; 125/31-, 250/125-, and 500/125-mg tabs	0.75–1.5 g/d PO q 8 h (amoxicillin)
Amphotericin B	Fungizone	50-mg vials	0.3–1 mg/kg/d IV in 4–8 h q 1–2 d
Amphotericin B lipid complex	Abelcet	100-mg vials	5 mg/kg/d IV
Ampicillin	Omnipen, Principen, Totacillin	250-, 500-mg caps; 125, 250, 500 mg/5 mL susp	1–2 g/d PO q 6 h
Ampicillin	Omnipen-N, Polycillin-N, Totacillin-N	0.125-, 0.25-, 0.5-, 1-, 2-, 10-g vials	2–8 g/d IV q 4–6 h
Ampicillin-sulbactam	Unasyn	1/0.5-, 2/1.0-g vials	4–8 g/d ampicillin IV or IM q 6 h
Atovaquone	Mepron	750 mg/5 mL susp	750 mg PO bid with food
Azlocillin	Azlin	2-, 3-, 4-g vials	8–24 g/d IV q 6–8 h
Aztreonam	Azactam	0.5-, 1-, 2-g vials	1.5–6 g/day IV or IM q 6–8 h
Bacampicillin	Spectrobid	400-mg tabs (equiv to 280 mg ampicillin); 125 mg/5 mL syrup (equiv to 87 mg ampicillin)	0.8–1.6 g/d PO q 12 h
Bacitracin	Baci-IM, Baciguent	50,000-unit vials	10,000–25,000 units IM q 6 h;
		500 units/g ointment	25,000 units PO q 6 h
Capreomycin	Capastat	1-g vials	1 g/d IM
Carbenicillin disodium	Geopen, Pyopen	1-, 2-, 5-, 10-, 30-g vials	8–40 g/d IV q 4–6 h
Carbenicillin indanyl sodium	Geocillin	382-mg tabs	382–764 mg PO q 6 h
Cefaclor	Ceclor	250-, 500-mg caps; 125, 187, 250, 375 mg/5 mL susp	1–2 g/d PO q 8 h
Cefadroxil	Duricef, Ultracef	500-mg caps; 1-g tabs; 125, 250, 500 mg/5 mL susp	1–2 g/d PO, single dose or bid
Cefamandole	Mandol	0.5-, 1-, 2-, 10-g vials	2–18 g/d IM or IV q 4–6 h
Cefazolin	Ancef, Kefzol, Zolicef	0.25-, 0.5-, 1-, 5-, 10-, 20-g vials	2–6 g/d IV or IM q 8 h
Cefepine	Maxipime	0.5-, 1-, 2-g vials	0.5–2 g IV q 12 h
Cefixime	Suprax	200-, 400-mg tabs, 100 mg/5 mL susp	400 mg/d PO, single dose or bid
Cefmetazole	Zefazone	1-, 2-g vials	4–8 g/d IV q 6–12 h
Cefonicid	Monocid	0.5-, 1-, 10-g vials	1–2 g/d IV or IM in 1 dose
Cefoperazone	Cefobid	0.5-, 1-, 2-g vials	2–8 g/d IM or IV q 12 h
Ceforanide	Precef	0.5-, 1-, 10-g vials	1–3 g/d IV or IM q 12 h
Cefotaxime	Claforan	0.5-, 1-, 2-, 10-g vials	2–12 g/d IV or IM q 6 h
Cefotetan	Cefotan	1-, 2-, 10-g vials	2–4 g/d IV or IM q 12 h
Cefoxitin	Mefoxin	1-, 2-, 10-g vials	2–18 g/d IV or IM q 4–6 h
Cefpodoxime proxetil	Vantin	100-, 200-mg tabs; 50, 100 mg/5 mL susp	200–800 mg/d PO q 12 h
Cefprozil	Cefzil	250-, 500-mg tabs; 125, 250 mg/5 mL susp	0.5–2 g/d PO q 12–24 h, usually 500 mg qd or bid

TABLE 40–1 ■ Preparations and Recommended Adult Dosing Regimens for Antimicrobial Agents* *Continued*

AGENT	TRADE NAME	DOSE FORM	DAILY DOSE, ROUTE, DOSE INTERVAL
Ceftazidime	Fortaz, Tazidime, Tazicef	0.5-, 1-, 2-, 6-g vials	3–6 g/d IV or IM q 8–12 h
Ceftibuten	Cedax	400-mg tabs	400 mg/d PO
Ceftizoxime	Cefizox	1-, 2-, 10-g vials	2–12 g/d IV or IM q 6–8 h
Ceftriaxone	Rocephin	0.25-, 0.5-, 1-, 2-, 10-g vials	1–4 g IV or IM q 24 h
Cefuroxime	Zinacef, Kefurox	0.75-,1.5-g vials	2.25–4.5 g/d IV or IM q 6–8 h
Cefuroxime axetil	Ceftin	0.125-, 0.25-, 0.5-g tabs	0.5–1.0 g/d PO q 12 h
Cephalexin	Keflex, Keftab, Cefanex, Zartan	0.25-, 0.5-g caps; 0.25-, 0.5-g tabs; 125, 250 mg/5 mL susp	1–2 g/d PO q 6 h
Cephalothin	Keflin	1-, 2-, 4-, 20-g vials	2–12 g/d IV q 4–6 h
Cephapirin	Cefadyl	0.5-, 1-, 2-, 4-g vials	2–4 g/d IV q 6 h
Cephradine	Anspor	250-, 500-mg caps; 125, 250 mg/5 mL susp	1–2 g/d PO q 6 h
	Velosef	0.25-, 0.5-, 1-g vials	2–8 g/d IV or IM q 6 h
Chloramphenicol	Chloromycetin	250-mg caps	1–2 g/d PO q 6 h
Chloramphenicol palmitate	Chloromycetin	150 mg/5 mL syrup	1–2 g/d PO q 6 h
Chloramphenicol sodium succinate	Chloromycetin sodium succinate	1-g vial	2–4 g/d IV q 6 h
Chloroquine HCl	Aralen HCl	250-mg ampules (200 mg base)	160–200 mg base IM q 6 h
Chloroquine PO_4	Aralen PO_4	500-mg tabs (300 mg base); 250-mg tabs (150 mg base)	300–600 mg (base) PO qd or once/wk
Chloroquine	Plaquenil	200-mg tabs (155 mg base)	10 mg/kg/d PO q 24 h
Cidofovir	Vistide	375-mg vials	5 mg/kg IV q 1–2 wk
Cinoxacin	Cinobac	250-, 500-mg caps	1 g/d PO q 6–12 h
Ciprofloxacin	Cipro	250-, 500-, 750-mg tabs	0.5–1.5 g/d PO q 12 h
	Cipro IV	200-, 400-mg vials	400–800 mg/d IV q 12 h
Clarithromycin	Biaxin	250-, 500-mg tabs	0.5–1 g/d PO q 12 h
Clindamycin HCl	Cleocin HCl	75-, 150-, 300-mg caps	0.6–1.8 g/d PO q 6–8 h
Clindamycin PO_4	Cleocin PO_4	150 mg/mL in 2-, 4-, 6-mL vials	1.8–2.7 g/d IV q 6–8 h
Clindamycin palmitate HCl	Cleocin Pediatric	75 mg/5 mL solution	0.6–1.8 g/d PO q 6–8 h
Clindamycin topical gel, solution	Cleocin T	1% gel, 0.30 g; 1% solution, 30, 60 mL	Topical 1 × /d
Clindamycin vaginal cream	Cleocin VC	2% 40-g tube	Topical 1 × /d × 7 d
Clofazimine	Lamprene	50-, 100-mg caps	50–100 mg/d PO q 8–24 h
Clotrimazole	Mycelex, Lotrimin	1% cream; 1% lotion; 10-mg troches; 500-mg vaginal tabs	Topical 1–5 × /d
Cloxacillin	Tegopen, Cloxapen	250-, 500-mg caps; 125 mg/5 mL solution	1–2 g/d PO q 6 h
Colistimethate	Coly-Mycin	150-mg (IM or IV) vials	2.5–5.0 mg/kg IV or IM q 6–12 h
Colistimethate	Coly-Mycin S	25 mg/5 mL susp; 150-mg vials (IV)	2.5–5.0 mg/kg/d IV or IM q 6–12 h
Cyclacillin	Cyclapen-W	250-, 500-mg caps; 125, 250 mg/5 mL susp	1–2 g/d PO q 6 h
Cycloserine	Seromycin	250-mg caps	0.5–1 g/d PO in 2 doses
Dapsone		25-, 100-mg tabs	100 mg PO q 24 h
Demeclocycline	Declomycin	150-, 300-mg caps	600 mg/d PO q 6–12 h
Dicloxacillin	Dycill, Dynapen, Pathocil	125-, 250-, 500-mg caps; 62.5 mg/5 mL susp	1–2 g/d PO q 6 h
Didanosine (ddI)	Videx	25-, 50-, 100-, 150-mg tabs; 167-, 250-, 375-mg powder packets	>60 kg: 200 mg tab PO or 250 mg powder PO bid <60 kg: 125 mg tab PO or 167 mg powder PO bid
Dideoxycytidine (ddC)	HIVID	0.375-, 0.75-mg tabs	0.75 mg PO q 8 h
Diethylcarbamazine	Hetrazan	50-mg tabs	6–13 mg/kg/d PO in 1–3 doses
Dirithromycin	Dynabac	500-mg tabs	500 mg/d PO qd
Doxycycline	Vibramycin, Doxy caps, Doxychel	50 mg/5 mL susp; 100-mg tabs; 50-, 100-mg caps	200 mg/d PO q 12 h
		100-, 200-mg vials	200 mg/d IV q 12 h
Emetine HCl	(Available from CDC)	65 mg/mL, 1-mL vial	1–1.5 mg/kg/d up to 90 mg/d, IM or deep SC injection
Enoxacin	Penetrex	200-, 400-mg tabs	400–800 mg/d PO bid
Erythromycin	E-Mycin, ERYC, Ery-Tab, Erythromycin Base, Ilotycin, RP-Mycin, Robimycin	125-, 250-mg caps; 250-, 333-, 500-mg tabs; 2% topical	1–2 g/d PO q 6 h (topical for acne)
Erythromycin estolate	Ilosone	250-mg caps; 125-, 250-, 500-mg tabs; 125, 250, 500 mg/5 mL susp	1–2 g/d PO q 6 h
Erythromycin ethylsuccinate	E.E.S., E-Mycin, EryPed, Pediamycin, Wyamycin	200-, 400-mg tabs; 100, 200, 400 mg/5 mL susp	1.6–3.2 g/d PO q 6 h
Erythromycin gluceptate	Ilotycin Gluceptate	0.25-, 0.5-, 1-g vials	2–4 g/d IV q 6 h

Table continued on following page

TABLE 40–1 ■ Preparations and Recommended Adult Dosing Regimens for Antimicrobial Agents* *Continued*

AGENT	TRADE NAME	DOSE FORM	DAILY DOSE, ROUTE, DOSE INTERVAL
Erythromycin lactobionate	Erythrocin lactobionate	0.5-, 1-g vials	1–4 g/d IV q 6 h
Erythromycin stearate	Eramycin, Erypar, Erythrocin Stearate, Ethril, SK-Erythromycin	250-, 500-mg tabs	1–2 g/d PO q 6 h
Ethambutol hydrochloride	Myambutol	100-, 400-mg tabs	15–25 mg/kg/d PO q 24 h
Ethionamide	Trecator-SC	250-mg tabs	0.5–1 g/d PO in 1–3 doses
Famciclovir	Famvir	500-mg tabs	500 mg PO q 8 h
Fluconazole	Diflucan	50-, 100-, 200-mg tabs; 100-, 200-mg vials	100–200 mg/d PO or IV in 1 dose
Flucytosine	Ancobon	250-, 500-mg caps	50–150 mg/kg/d PO q 6 h
Foscarnet	Foscavir	24 mg/mL, 500 mL	40–120 mg/kg/d IV qd or tid
Furazolidone	Furoxone	100-mg tabs; 50 mg/15 ml susp	100 mg PO q 6 h
Ganciclovir sodium	Cytovene	0.5-g vials	5 mg/kg IV in 2 doses (induction) or 1 dose (maintenance)
Gentamicin SO_4	Garamycin Gentamicin SO_4 Injection Isotonic (NaCl), Gentamicin SO_4, ADD-Vantage Gentamicin SO_4 in 5% dextrose piggyback	0.4–2.4 mg/mL in 40-, to 120-mg vials; 10, 40 mg/mL in 60-, 80-, 100-mg vials; 2 mg/mL for intrathecal use	3–5 mg/kg/d IV or IM q 8 h or qd
Griseofulvin	Grisactin, Fulvicin U/F, Grifulvin V, Gris-PEG, Grisactin Ultra, Fulvicin P/G	Microsize: 125-, 250-mg caps; 250-, 500-mg tabs; 125 mg/5 mL susp	500 mg–1 g/d PO
		Ultramicrosize: 125-, 165-, 250-, 330-mg tabs	330–750 mg/d PO
Imipenem-cilastatin	Primaxin	0.25-, 0.5-g vials	1–4 g/d IV q 6 h
Indinavir	Crixivan	200-, 400-mg caps	800 mg PO tid
Iodoquinol	Yodoxin	210-, 650-mg tabs	650 mg/d PO q 8 h
Isoniazid	Laniazid	50-, 100-, 300-mg tabs; 50 mg/5 mL (oral solution)	300 mg/d IM q 24 h
	Nydrazid	1-g vials (IM)	300 mg/d IM q 12–24 h
Kanamycin	Kantrex, Klebcil	0.075-, 0.5-, 1-g vials 500-mg caps	15 mg/kg/d IV q 8 h
Ketoconazole	Nizoral	200-mg tabs	200–400 mg/d PO q 12–24 h up to 1.6 g/d
Lamivudine (3TC)	Epivir	150-mg tab; 10 mg/mL susp	300 mg/d PO q 12 h
Lomefloxacin	Maxaquin	400-mg tabs	400 mg/d PO q 12 h
Loracarbef	Lorabid	200-, 400-mg parvules 100-, 200-mg/5-mL susp	400–800 mg/d PO q 12 h
Mafenide	Sulfamylon	2-, 4-oz tubes	Topical qd or bid
Mebendazole	Vermox	100-mg tabs	100 mg PO × 1–2 up to 2 g/d
Mefloquine	Lariam	250-mg tabs	1250 mg PO once (treatment); 250 mg PO q wk (prophylaxis)
Meropenem	Merrem	0.5-, 1-g vials	1 g IV q 8 h
Methenamine hippurate	Hiprex	1-g tabs	1–2 g/d PO q 12 h
Methenamine mandelate	Mandelamine	0.35-, 0.5-, 1-g tabs; 250, 500 mg/5 mL syrup; 0.5-, 1-g granules	1–4 g/d PO q 6 h
Methicillin	Celbenin, Staphcillin	1-, 4-, 6-, 10-g vials	4–12 g/d IV or IM q 6 h
Metronidazole	Flagly, Metryl, Metizol, Protostat, Metric 21, Satric	250-, 500-mg tabs 500-mg vials	0.75–2 g/d PO q 12 h 0.75–2 g/d IV q 6–12 h
Mezlocillin Na	Mezlin	1-, 2-, 3-, 4-g vials	6–24 g/d IV q 4–6 h
Miconazole	Monistat	200-mg ampule	0.6–3.6 g/d IVq 8 h
Minocycline HCl	Minocin	50-, 100-mg caps; 50 mg/5 mL syrup	200 mg/d PO q 12 h
		100-mg vials	200 mg/d IV q 6–8 h
Moxalactam	Moxam	1-, 2-, 10-g vials	2–8 g/d IV q 6–8 hr
Nafcillin Na	Unipen	250-mg caps; 500-mg tabs; 250 mg/5 mL solution	1–2 g/d PO q 6 h
	Nafcil, Nallpen, Unipen	0.5-, 1-, 2-g vials	2–12 g/d IV or IM q 4–6 h
Nalidixic acid	NegGram	0.25-, 0.5-, 1-g tabs; 250 mg/5 mL susp	1 g PO q 6 h
Neomycin SO_4	Mycifradin	500-mg tabs; 125 mg/5 mL solution 500-mg vial for IM	3–12 g/d PO
Netilmicin	Netromycin	50-, 150-mg vials	4–6.5 mg/kg/d IV or IM q 8 h
Niclosamide	Niclocide	500-mg tabs	2 g (single dose)
Nitrofurantoin	Macrodantin, Furantoin, Furaton, Furalan, Faran	Macrocrystals: 25-, 50-, 100-mg caps Microcrystals: 50-, 100-mg caps/tabs; 25 mg/5 mL susp	50–100 mg PO q 6 h
Norfloxacin	Noroxin	400-mg tabs	400 mg PO bid
Novobiocin	Albamycin	250-mg caps	1–2 g/d PO q 6–12 h
Nystatin	Mycostatin, Nystex, Nilstat	100,000-units, 500,000-unit tabs	0.5–1 million units PO 3–5 ×/d

TABLE 40–1 ■ Preparations and Recommended Adult Dosing Regimens for Antimicrobial Agents* *Continued*

AGENT	TRADE NAME	DOSE FORM	DAILY DOSE, ROUTE, DOSE INTERVAL
Ofloxacin	Floxin	200-, 300-, 400-mg tabs	200–400 mg PO q 12 h
	Floxin IV	400-mg vials	200–400 mg IV q 12 h
Oxacillin	Bactocill, Prostaphlin	250–500-mg caps; 250 mg/5 mL solution	2–4 g/d PO q 6 h
		0.25-, 0.5-, 1-, 2-, 4-, 10-g vials	2–12 g/d IV or IM q 4–6 h
Paromomycin	Humatin	250-mg caps	3-4 PO in 2–4 doses
Penicillin			
Crystalline G potassium		0.2-, 0.25-, 0.4-, 0.5-, 0.8–million unit tabs; 0.2, 0.25, 0.4 million units/5 mL	1–2 g/d PO q 6 h
	Penicillin G for injection	0.2-, 0.5-, 1-, 5-, 10-, 20–million unit vials	2–20 million units IV q 4–6 h
Crystalline G sodium	Penicillin G sodium for injection	5–million unit vials	2–20 million units IV q 4–6 h
Benzathine	Bicillin, Bicillin L-A, Permapen	200,000-unit tabs; 300,000, 600,000 units/mL vials	Not recommended PO; 1.2–2.4 million units IM
Benzathine + procaine	Bicillin C-R	Benzathine: procaine/mL 150,000:150,000 units (10 mL) 300,000:150,000 (1, 2, 4 mL) 450,000:150,000 units (2 mL)	1.2–2.4 million units IM
Phenoxymethylpenicillin (V)	Beepen, Betapen, Pen-Vee K, V-Cillin K, Veetids, Ledercillin	125-, 250-, 500-mg tabs; 125, 250 mL/5 mL susp	1–2 g/d PO q 6 h
Procaine	Crysticillin, Duracillin, Wycillin	3 million units (10 mL); 500,000 units (12 mL); 600,000 units (1-, 2-, 4-mL syringe)	0.6–4.8 million units/d IM q 6–12 h
Pentamidine	Pentam 300, NebuPent	300-mg vials	4 mg/kg/d IV
	NebuPent	300 mg aerosol	300 mg/mo (prophylaxis)
Piperacillin	Pipracil	2-, 3-, 4-, 40-g vials	6–24 g/d IV q 4–6 h
Piperacillin-tazobactam	Zosyn	2-, 3-, 4-g vials	12 g/d IV q 6 h
Piperazine	Antepar	250-mg tabs; 500 mg/5 mL	3.5–5 g/d PO
Polymyxin B	Aerosporin	500,000-unit vials (1 mg = 1000 units)	1.5–2.5 mg/kg/d IM or IV q 4–6 h
Praziquantel	Biltricide	600-mg tabs	20–75 mg/kg/d PO in 3 doses
Primaquine		15-mg (base) tabs	15 mg/d PO
Primaquine-chloroquine		45 mg primaquine + 300 mg chloroquine tabs	45/300-mg tab weekly
Pyrantel	Antiminth	50 mg/mL susp	11 mg/kg PO in 1 dose
Pyrazinamide		500-mg tabs	15–30 mg/kg/d PO in 6–8 doses
Pyrimethamine	Daraprim	25-mg tabs	25 mg PO q wk or d up to 200 mg/d
Pyrimethamine-sulfadoxine	Fansidar	25 mg pyrimethamine + 500 mg sulfadoxine	1 tab/wk; 3 tabs PO (1 dose)
Quinacrine	Atabrine	100 mg	300–800 mg/d PO
Quinine	Legatrin, Quine 200, Quine 300, Quin-260	130-, 200-, 300-, 325-mg caps; 162-, 260-, 325-mg tabs	325 mg bid (650 mg q 8 h PO)
Quinine dihydrochloride		IV (available from CDC)	600 mg IV q 8 h
Ribavirin	Virazole	6 g	Mist with 190 μg/L by SPAG-2 at 12.5 L/min
Rifabutin	Mycobutin	150-mg caps	300 mg/d PO
Rifampin	Rifadin	150-, 300-mg caps	600 mg/d PO (tuberculosis); 600–1200 mg/d PO (other indications)
		600-mg vials	600 mg/d IV qd
Ritonavir	Norvir	100-mg caps; 80 mg/mL, 240 mL	600 mg PO bid
Saquinavir	Invirase	200-mg caps	600 mg PO tid
		600-mg vials	600 mg/d IV
Spectinomycin	Trobicin	2-, 4-g vials	2 g IM once
Stavudine (d4T)	Zerit	15-, 20-, 30-, 40-mg tabs	80 mg/d PO bid
Streptomycin		1-, 5-g vials	1–2 g/d IM
Sulfonamides			
Trisulfapyrimidines	Triple Sulfa, Neotrizine (sulfadiazine, sulfamerazine, sulfamethazine)	167-mg tabs; 167 mg/5 mL susp	2–4 g/d PO q 4–8 h
Sulfadiazine	Microsulfon	0.5-g tabs	2–4 g/d PO q 4–8 h
Sulfamethoxazole	Gantanol	0.5-, 1-g tabs	1 g PO q 8–12 h
Sulfapyridine		0.5-g tabs	1–4 g/d PO q 6 h
Sulfasalazine	Azulfidine	0.5-g tabs; 0.25 mg/5 mL susp	3–4 g/d PO q 6 h
Sulfisoxazole	Gantrisin	0.5-g tabs	4–8 g/d PO q 4–6 h

Table continued on following page

TABLE 40–1 ■ Preparations and Recommended Adult Dosing Regimens for Antimicrobial Agents* *Continued*

AGENT	TRADE NAME	DOSE FORM	DAILY DOSE, ROUTE, DOSE INTERVAL
Tetracyclines			
Demeclocycline	Declomycin	150-mg caps; 150-, 300-mg tabs	600 mg/d PO q 6–12 h
Doxycycline	Vibramycin	50-, 100-mg tabs; 50-, 100-mg caps; 50 mg/5 mL susp	100–200 mg/d PO q 12–24 h
		100-mg vials	200 mg/d IV q 12–24 h
Minocycline	Minocin	50-, 100-mg caps; 50-, 100-mg tabs; 100-mg vials	100 mg/d PO or IV q 6–12 h
Oxytetracycline	Terramycin	250-mg caps	1–2 g/d PO q 12 h
		500-mg vial (IV)	0.5–1 g/d PO q 6 h
		50, 125 mg/mL with lidocaine (IM)	0.5–1 g/d IM q 12 h
Tetracycline	Achromycin, Brodspec, Cyclopar	100-, 250-, 500-mg caps; 250-, 500-mg tabs; 125 mg/5 mL susp	1–2 g/d PO q 6 h
	Sumycin	250-, 500-mg vials (IV)	0.5–1 g/d IV q 12 h (up to 4 g/d)
Thiabendazole	Mintezol	500-mg tabs, 500 mg/5 mL susp	1–3 g/d PO
Ticarcillin	Ticar	1-, 3-, 6-, 20-, 30-g vials	4–24 g/d IV q 4–6 h
Ticarcillin-clavulanate	Timentin	3 g ticarcillin + 100 mg clavulanate vials	3 g (ticarcillin) IV q 4–6 h
Tobramycin	Nebcin	20-, 60-, 80-, 1200-mg vials	3–5 mg/kg/d IV or IM q 8 h or qd
Tolnaftate	Aftate, Tinactin	1% gel, 15 g; 1% cream, 15 g; 1% powder, 45, 150 g; 1% liquid, 10, 45, 120 mL	Topical bid
Trifluridine	Viroptic	1% ophthalmic solution, 7.5 mL	Topical
Trimethoprim	Proloprim, Trimpex	100-, 200-mg tabs	200 mg/d PO q 12–24 h
Trimethoprim-sulfamethoxazole (TMP–SMX)	Bactrim, Septra, Cotrim, Sulfatrim, Triazole, Uroplus	TMP:SMX 40:200 mg/5 mL susp; 80:400 mg, 160:800 mg tabs; 16:80 mg/mL (IV)	2–20 mg/kg/d TMP PO or IV q 6–8 h
Trimetrexate	Neutrexin	25-mg vial	45 mg/m² q 24 h
Valacyclovir	Valtrex	500-mg caps	1000 mg PO tid
Vancomycin	Vancocin pulvules	125-, 250-mg caps	0.5–2 g/d PO q 6 h
	Vancocin HCl (oral solution)	1-, 10-g vials	
	Vancocin HCl IV, Lyphocin	0.5-, 1-g vials (IV)	1–2 g/d IV q 6–12 h
Vidarabine	Vira-A, Ara-A	200 mg/mL	15 mg/kg/d IV
Zidovudine	Retrovir, AZT	100-mg caps; 50 mg/5 mL syrup, 240 mL	100 mg PO q 4 h
		Infusion, 10 mg/mL (20 mL)	1–2 mg/kg IV q 4 h

*CDC, Centers for Disease Control and Prevention; IM, intramuscular; IV, intravenous; PO, oral; SC, subcutaneous; bid, twice daily; qd, every day; tid, three times a day; caps, capsules; tabs, tablets; susp, suspension.

Adapted from Bartlett JG: 1996 Pocketbook of Infectious Disease Therapy. Baltimore, Williams & Wilkins, 1996, pp 1–15.

TABLE 40–2 ■ Preferred Antimicrobial Agents for Specific Pathogens

ORGANISM	USUAL DISEASE	PREFERRED AGENT*	ALTERNATIVES
Achromobacter xylosoxidans	Meningitis, septicemia	Imipenem	Ceftazidime, trimethoprim-sulfamethoxazole (TMP-SMX), antipseudomonad penicillin, ticarcillin-clavulanate, doxycycline
Acinetobacter calcoaceticus var *antitratus (Herellea vaginicola)*; var *lwoffi (Mima polymorpha)*	Sepsis (especially line sepsis), pneumonia	Imipenem, fluoroquinolone + ceftazidime or amikacin	Fluoroquinolone, tetracycline, TMP-SMX
Actinobacillus actinomycetemcomitans	Actinomycosis	Pencillin	Clindamycin, tetracyclines, erythromycin, cephalosporins
	Endocarditis	Penicillin + aminoglycoside	Cephalosporin + aminoglycoside
Actinomyces israelii (also *Actinomyces naeslundii, Actinomyces viscosus, Actinomyces odontolyticus,* and *Arachnia propionica*)	Actinomycosis	Penicillin G	Clindamycin, tetracylines, erythromycin
Aeromonas hydrophila	Diarrhea	Fluoroquinolone, TMP-SMX	Tetracyclines
	Bacteremia		TMP-SMX
	Cellulitis, myositis, osteomyelitis	Ciprofloxacin	Aminoglycosides, tetracyclines, imipenem, aztreonam, amoxicillin-clavulanate, ticarcillin-clavulanate
Bacillus anthracis	Anthrax	Penicillin G	Erythromycin, tetracyclines, chloramphenicol, fluoroquinolone
Bacillus cereus	Food poisoning	Not treated	
Bacillus species	Septicemia (compromised host)	Vancomycin	Imipenem, aminoglycosides

TABLE 40–2 ■ Preferred Antimicrobial Agents for Specific Pathogens *Continued*

ORGANISM	USUAL DISEASE	PREFERRED AGENT*	ALTERNATIVES
Bacteroides bivius	Female genital tract infections	Metronidazole, clindamycin, cefoxitin, cefotetan	Chloramphenicol, antipseudomonad penicillin, imipenem, ticarcillin-clavulanate, ampicillin-sulbactam, cefmetazole
Bacteroides fragilis group	Abscesses, bacteremia, intraabdominal sepsis	Metronidazole, clindamycin, cefoxitin	Cefotetan, chloramphenicol, antipseudomonad penicillin, imipenem, ampicillin-sulbactam, ticarcillin-clavulanate, cefmetazole
Bartonella bacilliformis	Bartonellosis	Chloramphenicol, penicillin	Tetracycline + streptomycin
Bartonella henselae	Cat-scratch disease	Ciprofloxacin	TMP-SMX, gentamicin
	Trench fever	Tetracycline, chloramphenicol	
	Bacillary angiomatosis	Erythromycin	Doxycycline, chloramphenicol, TMP-SMX, azithromycin ciprofloxacin
Bordetella pertussis	Pertussis	Erythromycin	TMP-SMX, tetracyclines
Borrelia burgdorferi	Lyme disease	Tetracycline (early disease), ceftriaxone (late complications)	Penicillin G oral or intravenous, amoxicillin, erythromycin
Borrelia recurrentis	Relapsing fever	Tetracycline	Penicillin G, erythromycin, chloramphenicol
Branhamella (Moraxella) catarrhalis	Otitis, sinusitis, pneumonitis	TMP-SMX	Amoxicillin-clavulanate, erythromycin, tetracyclines, cefaclor, cephalosporins (3rd generation), cefuroxime, fluoroquinolone, cefixime
Brucella species	Brucellosis	Doxycycline + rifampin Doxycycline + gentamicin	Doxycycline + streptomycin, TMP-SMX; rifampin + doxycycline or cephalosporin (3rd generation) (central nervous system involvement)
Burkholderia (formerly *Pseudomonas*) *cepacia*	Septicemia, pneumonia	TMP-SMX	Chloramphenicol, ceftazidime
Calymmatobacterium granulomatis	Granuloma inguinale	Tetracycline	TMP-SMX, erythromycin (pregnancy), gentamicin, chloramphenicol
Campylobacter fetus	Septicemia, vascular infections, meningitis	Imipenem	Chloramphenicol, erythromycin, clindamycin, tetracyclines
Campylobacter jejuni	Diarrhea	Erythromycin, fluoroquinolone	Tetracylines, furazolidone
Capnocytophaga ochraceus	Periodontal disease, bacteremia in neutropenic host, tonsillitis (?)	Clindamycin, erythromycin	Amoxicillin-clavulanate, imipenem, cefoxitin, cephalosporins (3rd generation) ciprofloxacin, tetracyclines
Cardiobacterium species	Bacteremia, endocarditis	Penicillin + aminoglycoside	Cephalosporin ± aminoglycoside
Chlamydia pneumoniae (TWAR agent)	Pneumonia	Tetracycline, erythromycin	
Chlamydia psittaci	Psittacosis	Tetracycline	Chloramphenicol
Chlamydia trachomatis	Urethritis, endocervicitis, pelvic inflammatory disease, epididymitis, urethral syndrome	Tetracycline, azithromycin	Erythromycin, ofloxacin, sulfisoxazole
	Trachoma	Tetracycline (topical + oral)	Sulfonamide (topical + oral)
	Lymphogranuloma venereum	Tetracycline	Erythromycin
	Inclusion conjunctivitis	Erythromycin (topical or oral)	Sulfonamide
Citrobacter diversus	Urinary tract infections, pneumonia	Aminoglycoside, cephalosporin (2nd and 3rd generation), TMP-SMX	Tetracyclines, fluoroquinolone, imipenem, piperacillin
Citrobacter freundii	Urinary tract infection, wound infection, septicemia, pneumonia	Imipenem, TMP-SMX, aminoglycoside	Tetracyclines, cephalosporins (3rd generation), antipseudomonad penicillin
Clostridium difficile	Antibiotic-associated colitis	Vancomycin (oral), metronidazole (oral)	Bacitracin (oral), cholestyramine, lactobacilli, vancomycin + rifampin
Clostridium species	Gas gangrene, sepsis, tetanus, botulism, crepitant cellulitis	Penicillin G	Chloramphenicol, metronidazole, erythromycin, antipseudomonad penicillin, clindamycin
Corynebacterium diphtheriae	Diphtheria	Penicillin *or* erythromycin + antitoxin	
Corynebacterium JK strain	Septicemia	Vancomycin	Fluoroquinolone
Corynebacterium ulcerans	Pharyngitis	Erythromycin	
Coxiella burnetii	Q fever	Tetracycline	Chloramphenicol, ciprofloxacin, rifampin, erythromycin
Dysgonic fermenter type 2 (DF-2)	Septicemia (dog bite), wound infection	Penicillins	Cephalosporins, imipenem, vancomycin, fluoroquinolone, erythromycin

Table continued on following page

TABLE 40–2 ■ Preferred Antimicrobial Agents for Specific Pathogens *Continued*

ORGANISM	USUAL DISEASE	PREFERRED AGENT*	ALTERNATIVES
Edwardsiella tarda	Gastroenteritis (usually not treated), wound infection, bacteremia, liver abscess	Ampicillin	Tetracyclines, cephalosporins, aminoglycosides, chloramphenicol
Ehrlichia species	Ehrlichiosis	Tetracycline	Chloramphenicol
Eikenella corrodens	Oral infections, bite wounds	Ampicillin-amoxicillin, penicillin G	Tetracyclines, erythromycin, amoxicillin-clavulanate, cephalosporins, imipenem
Enterobacter aerogenes and *E. cloacae*	Sepsis, pneumonia, wound infections	Aminoglycoside, TMP-SMX, ciprofloxacin, imipenem	Aztreonam, antipseudomonad penicillin, cephalosporins (3rd generation)
	Urinary tract infection	TMP-SMX, cephalosporin (3rd generation)	Antipseudomonad penicillin, aminoglycoside, ciprofloxacin-norfloxacin, imipenem
Enterococcus faecalis	Urinary tract infection	Ampicillin-amoxicillin	Penicillin + aminoglycoside, nitrofurantoin, fluoroquinolone
	Wound infections, intraabdominal sepsis	Ampicillin	Penicillin + aminoglycoside, imipenem (*E. faecalis*), vancomycin
	Endocarditis	Penicillin G–ampicillin + gentamicin or streptomycin	Vancomycin + gentamicin or streptomycin
Enterococcus faecium, vancomycin resistant		Streptogramin	Chloramphenicol, tetracyclines, fluoroquinolone
Erwinia herbicola	Urinary tract infections, bacteremia, pneumonia	Aminoglycosides	Fluoroquinolone, chloramphenicol, cephalosporins
Erysipelothrix rhusiopathiae	Localized cutaneous erysipelas	Penicillin	Erythromycin
	Disseminated endocarditis	Penicillin	Cephalosporins
Escherichia coli	Septicemia, intraabdominal sepsis, wound infection	Aminoglycoside, cephalosporin, ampicillin (if sensitive)	TMP-SMX, imipenem, aztreonam, fluoroquinolone
	Urinary tract infection	Ampicillin (if sensitive), tetracycline, TMP-SMX, aminoglycoside, cephalosporin, antipseudomonad penicillin	Imipenem, aztreonam, sulfonamide, fluoroquinolone
Flavobacterium meningosepticum	Sepsis	Vancomycin	TMP-SMX, clindamycin, imipenem, fluoroquinolone
Francisella tularensis	Tularemia	Streptomycin, gentamicin	Tetracycline (?), chloramphenicol (?)
Fusobacterium species	Oral, dental, pulmonary infections, liver abscess	Penicillin G, metronidazole, clindamycin	Cefoxitin-cefotetan, chloramphenicol, imipenem
Gardnerella vaginalis	Vaginitis	Metronidazole	Clindamycin
Haemophilus aphrophilus	Sepsis, endocarditis	Penicillin G + aminoglycoside	Cephalosporin (3rd generation) + aminoglycoside
Haemophilus ducreyi	Chancroid	Ceftriaxone, erythromycin, azithromycin	Amoxicillin-clavulanate, ciprofloxacin
Haemophilus influenzae	Meningitis	Cephalosporin—cefotaxime, ceftriaxone	Chloramphenicol
	Epiglottitis, pneumonia, arthritis, cellulitis, otitis, sinusitis, bronchitis	Cephalosporin (3rd generation), TMP-SMX, cefamandole-cefuroxime, ampicillin (if sensitive), ampicillin-amoxicillin (if sensitive), amoxicillin-clavulanate	Chloramphenicol ± ampicillin, ampicillin-clavulanate, fluoroquinolone, erythromycin-sulfonamide, oral cephalosporin, tetracyclines
Hafnia alvei	Pneumonia, wound infection, urinary tract infection	Aminoglycosides	Fluoroquinolone, chloramphenicol, antipseudomonad, penicillin
Helicobacter pylori (*Campylobacter pylori*)	Gastritis, recurrent duodenal ulcer disease	Bismuth subcitrate + metronidazole + tetracycline (or amoxicillin)	Clarithromycin + omeprazole
Kingella species	Endocarditis, septic arthritis	Penicillin + aminoglycoside	Cephalosporin + aminoglycoside
Klebsiella pneumoniae and *K. oxytoca*	Septicemia, pneumonia, intraabdominal sepsis	Cephalosporin ± aminoglycoside, imipenem	Aminoglycoside, TMP-SMX, piperacillin-mezlocillin, imipenem, ticarcillin-clavulanate, aztreonam, ampicillin-sulbactam, fluoroquinolone
	Urinary tract infection	TMP-SMX, cephalosporin, tetracycline	Aminoglycoside, amoxicillin-clavulanate, ticarcillin-clavulanate, piperacillin-tazobactam, piperacillin, fluoroquinolone, piperacillin-mezlocillin, imipenem
Legionella species	Legionnaires' disease	Erythromycin ± rifampin, ciprofloxacin ± rifampin	TMP-SMX + rifampin
Leptospira species	Leptospirosis	Penicillin G or ampicillin	Tetracyclines
Leptotrichia buccalis	Orodental infections	Penicillin G	Tetracyclines, clindamycin
Listeria monocytogenes	Meningitis, septicemia	Ampicillin or penicillin ± gentamicin (systemic and intrathecal)	TMP-SMX, erythromycin, vancomycin (?)

TABLE 40–2 ■ Preferred Antimicrobial Agents for Specific Pathogens *Continued*

ORGANISM	USUAL DISEASE	PREFERRED AGENT*	ALTERNATIVES
Moraxella species	Ocular infections, bacteremia	Aminoglycoside, penicillins, TMP-SMX, cephalosporins (2nd and 3rd generation)	Cephalosporin (3rd generation), imipenem, ciprofloxacin, antipseudomonad penicillin, erythromycin, clarithromycin
Moraxella catarrhalis (see *Branhamella catarrhalis*)			
Morganella morganii	Bacteremia, urinary tract infection, pneumonia, wound infection	Aminoglycoside, fluoroquinolone	Imipenem, cephalosporin (3rd generation), TMP-SMX, aztreonam, antipseudomonad penicillin, ticarcillin-clavulanate, amoxicillin-clavulanate, tetracyclines
Mycobacterium avium-intracellulare	Pulmonary infection Disseminated infection	Clarithromycin + ethambutol ± rifampin	Capreomycin, ethionamide, amikacin, imipenem, cycloserine, ofloxacin, ciprofloxacin, azithromycin
Mycobacterium chelonae	Pulmonary, cutaneous	Clarithromycin	Amikacin ± cefoxitin, clofazimine, or clarithromycin
Mycobacterium fortuitum	Soft tissue and wound infections	Amikacin + cefoxitin	Rifampin, erythromycin, sulfonamide, cefoxitin, doxycycline, ciprofloxacin
Mycobacterium kansasii	Pulmonary infection	Isoniazid + rifampin + ethambutol or streptomycin	Ethionamide, cycloserine, streptomycin, amikacin, TMP-SMX
Mycobacterium leprae	Leprosy, paucibacillary	Dapsone + rifampin	Minocycline or ofloxacin
	Multibacillary	Clofazimine + rifampin + dapsone	Clarithromycin, protionamide
Mycobacterium marinum	Soft tissue infections	Rifampin + ethambutol, TMP-SMX, tetracycline	Erythromycin, ciprofloxacin
Mycobacterium tuberculosis	Tuberculosis	Isoniazid + rifampin + pyrazinamide	Cycloserine, ciprofloxacin, ofloxacin, ethambutol, ethionamide, kanamycin, capreomycin, aminosalicylic acid
Mycoplasma pneumoniae	Pneumonia	Erythromycin, tetracycline	Clarithromycin, azithromycin, fluoroquinolones
Neisseria gonorrhoeae	Urethritis, salpingitis, cervicitis, arthritis-dermatitis	Ceftriaxone, cefixine, fluoroquinolone	Spectinomycin, cefuroxime axetil, cefotaxime, ceftizoxime, cefpodoxime, TMP-SMX
Neisseria meningitidis	Meningitis, bacteremia, pericarditis, pneumonia	Penicillin G	Ampicillin, chloramphenicol, TMP-SMX, cephalosporin-cefotaxime, ceftizoxime, ceftriaxone, cefuroxime
Nocardia asteroides	Nocardiosis: pulmonary infection; abscesses of skin, lung, brain	Sulfonamide (usually sulfadiazine) or TMP-SMX	Minocycline ± sulfonamide, amikacin ± imipenem, ceftriaxone, cefuroxime, imipenem + cefotaxime or TMP-SMX
Pasteurella multocida	Animal bite wound	Penicillin G	Tetracyclines, cephalosporins, amoxicillin-clavulanate
	Septicemia, septic arthritis, osteomyelitis	Penicillin	Cephalosporins, ampicillin-sulbactam, chloramphenicol
Peptostreptococcus	Oral, dental, or pulmonary infection; intraabdominal sepsis; gynecologic infection	Penicillin G, ampicillin-amoxicillin	Clindamycin, metronidazole, cephalosporin, chloramphenicol, erythromycin, vancomycin, imipenem
Plesiomonas shigelloides	Diarrhea (usually not treated)	Fluoroquinolone, TMP-SMX	Tetracycline
	Extraintestinal infection	Cephalosporin (3rd generation), aminoglycoside	TMP-SMX, imipenem, fluoroquinolone
Prevotella melaninogenica (*Bacteroides melaninogenicus*) group	Oral-dental, pulmonary, female genital tract infections	Metronidazole, clindamycin, cefoxitin	Chloramphenicol, ampicillin-sulbactam, amoxicillin-clavulanate, ticarcillin-clavulanate, imipenem, cefotetan, cefmetazole
Propionibacterium acnes	Acne	Tetracycline	Clindamycin (topical)
Proteus mirabilis	Septicemia, urinary tract infection, intraabdominal sepsis, wound infection	Ampicillin, cephalosporins (1st, 2nd, 3rd generation)	Aminoglycosides, cephalosporins, TMP-SMX, antipseudomonad penicillin, aztreonam, imipenem, fluoroquinolone
Proteus vulgaris	Septicemia, urinary tract infection	Cephalosporin (3rd generation), aminoglycoside, imipenem	TMP-SMX, antipseudomonad penicillin, aztreonam, amoxicillin-clavulanate, ticarcillin-clavulanate, fluoroquinolone
Providencia rettgeri	Septicemia, urinary tract infection	Cephalosporin (3rd generation), imipenem	Antipseudomonad penicillin, aztreonam, TMP-SMX, aminoglycoside
Providencia stuartii	Septicemia, urinary tract infection	Aminoglycoside, cephalosporin (3rd generation)	Antipseudomonad penicillin, TMP-SMX, imipenem, aztreonam, fluoroquinolone
Pseudomonas aeruginosa	Septicemia, pneumonia, intraabdominal sepsis	Aminoglycoside (tobramycin) ± antipseudomonad penicillin	Aminoglycoside ± cefoperazone, imipenem, ceftazidime or aztreonam, ciprofloxacin
	Urinary tract infection	Aminoglycoside, antipseudomonad penicillin, ciprofloxacin	Imipenem, ceftazidime, cefoperazone, aztreonam
Pseudomonas mallei	Glanders	Streptomycin + tetracycline	Chloramphenicol ± streptomycin

Table continued on following page

TABLE 40–2 ■ Preferred Antimicrobial Agents for Specific Pathogens *Continued*

ORGANISM	USUAL DISEASE	PREFERRED AGENT*	ALTERNATIVES
Pseudomonas pseudomallei	Melioidosis	Ceftazidime	Tetracycline ± chloramphenicol; imipenem, TMP-SMX, amoxicillin-clavulanate
Pseudomonas putida	Septicemia, pneumonia, urinary tract infection	Aminoglycosides, fluoroquinolone	
Rickettsia species	Rocky Mountain spotted fever, Q fever, tick fever, murine typhus, scrub typhus, typhus, trench fever	Tetracycline (>8 y)	Chloramphenicol, fluoroquinolone
Salmonella typhi	Typhoid fever	Ceftriaxone, fluoroquinolone	Chloramphenicol, TMP-SMX, ampicillin-amoxicillin, cefotaxime, cefoperazone
Salmonella species (nontyphoid)	Enteric fever, mycotic aneurysm	Fluoroquinolone, cefotaxime, cefoperazone, ceftriaxone	Chloramphenicol, ampicillin, TMP-SMX
Serratia marcescens	Septicemia, urinary tract infection, pneumonia	Cephalosporin (3rd generation) ± gentamicin or amikacin ± fluoroquinolone, imipenem	Antipseudomonad penicillin ± gentamicin or amikacin, aztreonam
Shigella flexneri	Colitis	TMP-SMX, fluoroquinolone	Ampicillin, tetracyclines, ceftriaxone, cefixime
Spirillum minus	Rat-bite fever	Penicillin G	Tetracyclines, streptomycin
Staphylococcus aureus, methicillin resistant	Septicemia, pneumonia, wound infection	Vancomycin ± rifampin or gentamicin	TMP-SMX, fluoroquinolone (if sensitive), minocycline
Staphylococcus aureus, methicillin sensitive	Septicemia, pneumonia, wound infection	Penicillinase-resistant penicillin ± rifampin or gentamicin, cephalosporins (1st generation), cefuroxime-cefamandole, vancomycin ± rifampin or gentamicin	Erythromycin, clindamycin, vancomycin, amoxicillin-clavulanate, ticarcillin-clavulanate, imipenem, ciprofloxacin, ampicillin-sulbactam, TMP-SMX, ciprofloxacin
Staphylococcus epidermidis	Septicemia, infected prosthetic devices	Vancomycin	TMP-SMX, penicillinase-resistant penicillin, cephalosporin, fluoroquinolone
Staphylococcus saprophyticus	Urinary tract infection	TMP-SMX, ampicillin-amoxicillin, fluoroquinolone	Cephalosporins, tetracyclines
Stenotrophomonas (formerly *Xanthomonas*) *maltophilia*	Septicemia	TMP-SMX	Ticarcillin-clavulanate
Streptobacillus moniliformis	Rat-bite fever, Haverhill fever	Penicillin G	Tetracyclines, streptomycin
Streptococcus groups A, B, C, G; *S. bovis*, *S. milleri*, viridans, anaerobic, penicillin-sensitive *S. pneumoniae*	Pharyngitis, soft tissue infection, pneumonia, abscesses	Penicillin G	Cephalosporin, (1st generation), cefuroxime, cefotaxime, ceftriaxone, clindamycin, vancomycin, erythromycin, clarithromycin, azithromycin
	Endocarditis	Penicillin G ± streptomycin or gentamicin	Cephalosporin, vancomycin
	Meningitis	Penicillin G, cefotaxime, ceftriaxone	Chloramphenicol, vancomycin + rifampin
Streptococcus group D, *Enterococcus faecalis* and *E. faecium*	Urinary tract infection	Ampicillin-amoxicillin	Penicillin + aminoglycoside, vancomycin, nitrofurantoin, ciprofloxacin-norfloxacin
	Wound infection, intraabdominal sepsis	Ampicillin-amoxicillin	Vancomycin, penicillin + aminoglycoside, imipenem (not for *E. faecium*)
	Endocarditis	Penicillin G–ampicillin + gentamicin or streptomycin	Vancomycin + gentamicin or streptomycin
Streptococcus pneumoniae, penicillin resistant	Pneumonia, septicemia, septic arthritis	Vancomycin	Fluoroquinolones, cefotaxime, ceftriaxone, cefpodoxime, clindamycin, macrolide
	Meningitis	Vancomycin + cefotaxime or ceftriaxone ± rifampin	
Treponema carateum	Pinta	Penicillin G	Tetracyclines
Treponema pallidum	Syphilis	Penicillin G	Tetracyclines, ceftriaxone
Treponema pallidum subsp *endemicum*	Bejel	Penicillin	
Treponema pallidum subsp *pertenue*	Yaws	Penicillin G	Tetracyclines
Tropheryma whippelii	Whipple's disease	TMP-SMX (2 double-strength/d × 1 y)	Tetracycline, penicillin V
Ureaplasma urealyticum	Urethritis, endocervicitis, pelvic inflammatory disease (?)	Erythromycin	Tetracyclines, clarithromycin
Vibrio cholerae	Cholera	Tetracycline	Ampicillin, TMP-SMX, furazolidone, fluoroquinolone, erythromycin
Vibrio vulnificus	Septicemia, wound infection	Tetracycline	Chloramphenicol, penicillin G
Yersinia enterocolitica	Enterocolitis (usually not treated), mesenteric adenitis (usually not treated)	TMP-SMX	Cephalosporin (3rd generation), fluoroquinolone

TABLE 40–2 ■ Preferred Antimicrobial Agents for Specific Pathogens *Continued*

ORGANISM	USUAL DISEASE	PREFERRED AGENT*	ALTERNATIVES
	Septicemia	Aminoglycoside (gentamicin)	Chloramphenicol, cephalosporins (3rd generation), TMP-SMX
Yersinia pestis	Plague	Streptomycin	Chloramphenicol, tetracyclines, gentamicin
Yersinia pseudotuberculosis	Mesenteric adenitis (usually not treated), septicemia	Aminoglycoside, ampicillin	TMP-SMX, tetracyclines

**Aminoglycosides* are gentamicin, tobramycin, amikacin, and netilmicin. *Antipseudomonad penicillins* are carbenicillin, ticarcillin, piperacillin, mezlocillin, and azlocillin. *Penicillinase-resistant penicillins* are nafcillin, oxacillin, methicillin, cloxacillin, and dicloxacillin. *Tetracyclines* are tetracycline, doxycycline, and minocycline. *Cephalosporins:* first generation are cefadroxil, cefazolin, cephalexin, cephalothin, cephapirin, and cephradine; second generation are cefaclor, cefamandole, cefonicid, ceforanide, cefotetan, cefoxitin, cefuroxime, and cefmetazole; third generation are cefotaxime, ceftizoxime, ceftazidime, cefoperazone, ceftriaxone, moxalactam, and cefixime. *Fluoroquinolones* are norfloxacin (primarily urinary tract infections and enteric infections), ciprofloxacin, enoxacin, ofloxacin, and lomefloxacin (spectrum: *P. aeruginosa*—ciprofloxacin; mycobacteria—ciprofloxacin, lomefloxacin, ofloxacin; *C. trachomatis*—ofloxacin; penicillin-resistant *S. pneumoniae*—ofloxacin; staphylococcus—class resistance).

Adapted from Bartlett JG: 1996 Pocketbook of Infectious Disease Therapy. Baltimore, Williams & Wilkins, 1996, pp 20–40.

TABLE 40–3 ■ Drug Dosage Guidelines*

DRUG	PRINCIPAL EXCRETION ROUTE	HALF-LIFE (h)		USUAL REGIMEN		MAINTENANCE REGIMEN FOR RENAL FAILURE†		
		Normal	Anuria	Oral	Parenteral	GFR of 50–80 mL/min	GFR of 10–50 mL/min	GFR of <10 mL/min
Acyclovir	Renal	2–2.5	20	200 mg 2–5 × d	—	Usual	Usual	200 mg q 12 h
				800 mg 5 ×/d	—	Usual	800 mg tid	800 mg bid
				—	5–12 mg/kg q 8 h	Usual	5–12 mg/kg q 12–24 h	2.5–6 mg/kg 24 h
Albendazole	Hepatic	8	8	400–800 mg bid	—	Usual	Usual	Usual
Amantadine	Renal	15–20	170	100 mg bid	—	100–150 mg/d	100–200 mg 2–3 ×/wk	100–200 mg/wk
Amdinocillin	Renal	1.0	3.3	—	10 mg/kg q 4–6 h	Usual	10 mg/kg q 6 h	10 mg/kg q 8 h
Amikacin	Renal	2	30	—	7.5 mg/kg q 8 h	Loading dose, then 0.12 × C_{cr} = mg/kg/8 h†		
Amoxicillin	Renal	1	15–20	250–500 mg q 8 h	—	0.25–0.5 g q 12 h	0.25–0.5 g q 12–24 h	0.25–0.5 g q 12–24 h
Amoxicillin-clavulanate	Renal	1	8–16	250–500 mg q 8 h	—	Usual	0.25–0.5 g q 12 h	0.25–0.5 g q 20–36 h
Amphotericin B	Nonrenal	24	24	—	0.3–1.0 mg/kg/d	Usual	Usual	Usual
Amphotericin B lipid complex	Nonrenal	8 d	8 d	—	5 mg/kg	Usual	No guidelines	
Ampicillin	Renal	1.0	8–12	0.25–0.5 g q 6 h	—	Usual	Usual	Usual
					1–3 g q 4–6 h	Usual	1–2 g IV q 8 h	1–2 g IV q 12 h
Ampicillin-sulbactam	Renal	1.0	8–12	—	1–2 g q 6 h	1–2 g IV q 8 h	1–2 g IV q 8 h	1–2 g IV q 12 h
Atovaquone	Gut	70	70	750 mg bid	—	Usual	Usual	No data
Azithromycin	Hepatic	68	68	250 mg/d	—	Usual	No data	No data
Azlocillin	Renal	1	5	—	2–4 g q 4–6 h	Usual	1.5–2 g q 8 h	1.5–3 g q 12 h
Aztreonam	Renal	1.7–2	6–9	—	1–2 g q 6 h	1–2 g q 8–12 h	1–2 g q 12–18 h	1–2 g q 24 h
Bacampicillin	Renal	—	—	0.4–0.8 g q 12 h	—	Usual	Usual	—
Capreomycin	Renal	4–6	50–100	1 g/d 2 ×/wk	—	Usual	7.5 mg/kg q 1–2 d	7.5 mg/kg 2 ×/wk
Carbenicillin	Renal	1.0	13–16	0.5–1 g q 6 h	—	Usual	Usual	Avoid
				—	5–6 g IV q 4 h	Usual	2–3 g q 6 h	2 g q 12 h
Cefaclor	Renal	0.75	2.8	0.25–0.5 g q 8 h	—	Usual	Usual	Usual
Cefadroxil	Renal	1.4	20–25	0.5–1 g q 12–24 h	—	Usual	0.5 q 12–24 h	0.5 g q 36 h
Cefamandole	Renal	0.5–1.0	10	—	0.5–2 g q 4–8 h	0.5–2 g q 6 h	1–2 g q 8 h	0.5–1 g q 12 h
Cefazolin	Renal	1.8	18–36	—	0.5–2 g q 8 h	0.5–1.5 g q 8 h	0.5–1 g q 8–12 h	0.25–0.75 g q18–24h
Cefixime	Renal	3–4	12	400 mg/d	—	Usual	300 mg/d	200 mg/d
Cefmetazole	Renal	1.2	—	—	2 g q 6–12 h	1–2 g q 12 h	1–2 g q 16–24 h	1–2 g q 48 h
Cefonicid	Renal	4–5	50–60	—	0.5–2 g q 24 h	8–25 mg/kg q 24 h	4–15 mg/kg q 24–48 h	3–15 mg/kg q 3–5 d
Cefoperazone	Gut	1.9–2.5	2–2.5	—	1–2 g q 6–12 h	Usual	Usual	Usual
Ceforanide	Renal	3	20–40	—	0.5–1 g q 12 h	Usual	0.5–1 g q 24 h	0.5–1 g q 48–72 h
Cefotaxime	Renal	1.1	3	—	1–2 g q 8–12 h	Usual	1–2 g q 12–24 h	1–2 g q 24 h
Cefotetan	Renal	3–4	12–30	—	1–2 g q 12 h	Usual	1–2 g q 24 h	1–2 g q 48 h
Cefoxitin	Renal	0.7	13–22	—	1–2 g q 6–8 h	1–2 g q 8–12 h	1–2 g q 12–24 h	0.5–1 g q 12–48 h
Cefpodoxime	Renal	2.4	—	200–400 mg bid	—	Usual	200–400 mg 3 ×/wk	200–400 mg/wk

Table continued on following page

TABLE 40–3 ■ Drug Dosage Guidelines* *Continued*

DRUG	PRINCIPAL EXCRETION ROUTE	HALF-LIFE (h)		USUAL REGIMEN		MAINTENANCE REGIMEN FOR RENAL FAILURE†		
		Normal	Anuria	Oral	Parenteral	GFR of 50–80 mL/min	GFR of 10–50 mL/min	GFR of <10 mL/min
Cefprozil	Renal	1.3	5–6	0.25–0.5 g q 12 h	—	Usual	0.25–0.5 g q 24 h	0.25 g q 12–24 h
Ceftazidime	Renal	1.5–2	15–25	—	1–2 g q 8–12 h	Usual	1 g q 12–24 h	0.5 g q 24–48 h
Ceftibuten	Renal	2.4	—	400 mg/d	—	Usual	200 mg/d	100 mg/d
Ceftizoxime	Renal	1.4–1.8	25–35	—	1–3 g q 6–8 h	0.5–1.5 g q 8 h	0.25–1 g q 12 h	0.25 g q 24 h
Ceftriaxone	Renal, enteric	6–9	12–15	—	0.5–1 g q 12–24 h	Usual	Usual	Usual
Cefuroxime	Renal	1.3–1.7	20	—	0.75–1.5 g q 8 h	Usual	0.75–1.5 g q 8–12 h	0.75 g q 24 h
Cefuroxime axetil	Renal	1.2	20	250 mg q 12 h	—	Usual	Usual	250 mg q 24 h
Cephalexin	Renal	0.9	5–30	0.25–1.0 g q 6 h	—	Usual	0.25–1.0 g q 8–12 h	0.25–1 g q 24–48 h
Cephalothin	Renal	0.5–0.9	3–8	—	0.5–2 g q 4–6 h	Usual	1.0–1.5 g q 6 h	0.5 g q 8 h
Cephapirin	Renal	0.6–0.9	2.4	—	0.5–2 g q 4–6 h	0.5–2 g q 6 h	0.5–2 g q 8 h	0.5–2 g q 12 h
Cephradine	Renal	0.7–1	8–15	0.25–1.0 g q 6 h	—	Usual	0.5 g q 6 h	0.25 g q 12 h
				—	0.5–2 g q 4–6 h	0.5–1 g q 6 h	0.5–1 g q 6–24 h	0.5–1 g q 24–72 h
Chloramphenicol	Hepatic	2.5	3–7	0.25–0.75 g q 6 h	0.25–1 g q 6 h	Usual	Usual	Usual
Chloroquine	Renal metabolism	48–120	?	300–600 mg/d PO	—	Usual	Usual	150–300 mg/d PO
Cinoxacin	Renal	1.5	8.5	0.25–0.5 g q 12 h	—	0.25 g q 8 h	0.25 g q 12 h	0.25 g q 24 h
Ciprofloxacin	Renal, hepatic	4	5–10	0.25–0.75 g q 12 h	—	Usual	0.25–0.5 g q 12 h	0.25–0.5 g q 18 h
Clarithromycin	Hepatic, renal	4	Slight	250–500 q 12 h	—	Usual	Usual	250–500 q 24 h
Clindamycin	Hepatic	2–2.5	2–3.5	150–300 mg q 6 h	300–900 mg q 6–8 h	Usual	Usual	Usual
Clofazimine	Hepatic	8 d	8 d	50 mg/d–100 mg tid	—	Usual	Usual	Usual
Cloxacillin	Renal	0.5	0.8	0.5–1.0 g q 6 h	—	Usual	Usual	Usual
Colistin	Renal	3–8	10–20	—	1.5 mg/kg q 6–12 h	2.5–3.8 mg/kg/d	1.5–2.5 mg/kg q 24–36 h	0.6 mg/kg/d
Cycloserine	Renal	8–12	?	250–500 mg bid	—	Usual	250–500 mg/d	250 mg/d
Dapsone	Hepatic metabolism	30	Slight	50 mg/d–100 mg tid	—	Usual	Usual	No data
Dicloxacillin	Renal	0.5–0.9	1–1.6	0.25–0.5 g q 6 h	—	Usual	Usual	Usual
Dideoxycytidine (ddC)	Renal	2	8	0.75 mg tid	—	Usual	0.75 mg bid	0.75 mg qd
Dideoxyinosine (ddI)	Renal, nonrenal	1.3–1.6	?	200 mg bid	—	Usual	Consider dose reduction; note Na and Mg load	
Doxycycline	Renal, enteric	14–25	15–36	100 mg bid	100 mg bid	Usual	Usual	Usual
Enoxacin	Renal, hepatic	2–6	—	200–400 mg bid	—	Usual	½ usual dose	½ usual dose
Erythromycin	Hepatic	1.2–2.6	4–6	0.25–0.5 g q 6 h	1 g q 6 h	Usual	Usual	Usual
Ethambutol	Renal	3–4	8	15–25 mg/kg q 24 h	—	15 mg/kg/d	15 mg/kg q 24–36 h	15 mg/kg q 48 h
Ethionamide	Metabolic	4	9	0.5–1 g/d 1–3 doses	—	Usual	Usual	5 mg/kg q 24 h
Famciclovir	Renal	2.3	13	0.5 g q 8 h	—	Usual	0.5 g qd	No data
Fluconazole	Renal	20–50	—	100–200 mg/d	100–200 mg/d	Usual	50–100 mg/d	25–50 mg/d
Flucytosine	Renal	3–6	70	37 mg/kg q 6 h	—	Usual	37 mg/kg q 12–24 h	Adjust to keep 2-h level at 50–100 µg/mL
Foscarnet	Renal	3	8	—	60 mg/kg q 8 h	40–50 mg/kg q 8 h	20–30 mg/kg q 8 h	Contraindicated
				—	90 mg/kg qd	60–70 mg/kg qd	50–70 mg/kg qd	Contraindicated
Ganciclovir, oral	Gastro-intestinal	3–7	10	1 g tid	—	500 mg tid	500 mg/d	500 mg 3 ×/wk
Ganciclovir, parenteral	Renal	2.5–3.6	10	—	5.0 mg/kg IV bid	2.5 mg/kg/d	2.5 mg/kg/d	1.25 mg/kg/d
					Maintenance: 5.0 mg/kg IV qd	2.5 mg/kg/d	1.2 mg/kg/d	0.6 mg/kg/d
Gentamicin	Renal	2	48	—	1.7 mg/kg q 8 h	Loading dose, then 0.03 × C_{cr} = mg/kg/8 h†		
Griseofulvin								
Microsize	Hepatic metabolism	24	24	0.5–1 g/d	—	Usual	Usual	Usual
Ultramicrosize	Hepatic metabolism	24	24	0.33–0.66 g/d	—	Usual	Usual	Usual
Imipenem	Renal	0.8–1	3.5	—	0.5–1 g q 6 h	0.5 g q 6–8 h	0.5 g q 8–12 h	0.25–0.5 mg q 12 h
Indinavir	Hepatic	1.5–2	—	800 mg tid	—	Usual	Usual	Usual
Isoniazid	Hepatic	0.5–4	2–10	300 mg q 24 h	300 mg q 24 h	Usual	Usual	For slow acetylators, ½ dose
Kanamycin	Renal	2–3	27–30	—	7.5 mg/kg	Loading dose, then 0.12 × C_{cr} = mg/kg/8 h†		

TABLE 40–3 ■ Drug Dosage Guidelines* *Continued*

DRUG	PRINCIPAL EXCRETION ROUTE	HALF-LIFE (h)		USUAL REGIMEN		MAINTENANCE REGIMEN FOR RENAL FAILURE†		
		Normal	Anuria	Oral	Parenteral	GFR of 50–80 mL/min	GFR of 10–50 mL/min	GFR of <10 mL/min
Ketoconazole	Hepatic metabolism	1–4	1–4	200–400 mg q 12–24 h	—	Usual	Usual	Usual
Lamivudine (3TC)	Renal	3–6	—	150 mg bid	—	Usual	100–150 mg/d	25–50 mg/d
Lomefloxacin	Renal	8	45	400 mg qd	—	Usual	400 mg, then 200 mg/d	No data
Loracarbef	Renal	1	32	200–400 mg q 12 h	—	Usual	200–400 mg q 24 h	200–500 mg q 3–5 d
Mefloquine	Hepatic	2–4 wk	2–4 wk	1250 mg once, 250 mg/wk	—	Usual	Usual	Usual
Methenamine hippurate	Renal	3–6	?	1 g q 12 h	—	Usual	Avoid	Avoid
Methenamine mandelate	Renal	3–6	?	1 g q 12 h	—	Usual	Avoid	Avoid
Methicillin	Renal (hepatic)	0.5	4	—	1–2 g q 4–6 h	1–2 g q 6 h	1–2 g q 8 h	1–2 g q 12 h
Metronidazole	Hepatic	6–14	8–15	0.25–7.5 g tid	0.5 g q 6 h	Usual	Usual	Usual
Mezlocillin	Renal	1	1.5	—	3–4 g q 4–6 h	Usual	3 g q 8 h	2 g q 8 h
Miconazole	Hepatic	0.5–1	0.5–1	—	0.4–1.2 g q 8 h	Usual	Usual	Usual
Minocycline	Hepatic metabolism	11–26	17–30	100 mg q 12 h	100 mg q 12 h	Usual	Usual	Usual or slightly less
Moxalactam	Renal	2	20	—	1–4 g q 8–12 h	3 g q 8 h	2–3 g q 12 h	1 g q 12–24 h
Nafcillin	Hepatic metabolism	0.5	1.2	0.5–1 g q 6 h	0.5–2 g q 4–6 h	Usual	Usual	Usual
Nalidixic acid	Renal metabolism	1.5	21	1 g q 6 h	—	Usual	Usual	Avoid
Netilmicin	Renal	2.5	35	—	2.0 mg/kg q 8 h	Loading dose, then 0.03 × C_{cr} = mg/kg/8 h†		
Nitrofurantoin	Renal	0.3	1	50–100 mg q 6–8 h	—	Usual	Avoid	Avoid
Norfloxacin	Renal metabolism	3.5	8	400 mg bid	—	Usual	400 mg/d	400 mg/d
Nystatin	Not absorbed	—	—	0.4–1 million units 3–5 × /d	—	Usual	Usual	Usual
Ofloxacin	Renal	6	40	200–400 mg bid	—	Usual	200/400 mg qd	100–200 mg qd
				—	200–400 mg q 12 h	Usual	200–400 mg qd	100–200 mg qd
Oxacillin	Renal	0.5	1	0.5–1 g q 6 h	0.5–2 g q 4–6 h	Usual	Usual	Usual
Penicillin G								
Crystalline	Renal	0.5	7–10	0.4–0.8 million units q 6 h	1–4 million units q 4–6 h	Usual	Usual	½ usual dose
Procaine	Renal	24	—	—	0.6–1.2 million units IM q 12 h	Usual	Usual	Usual
Benzathine	Renal	Days	—	—	0.6–1.2 million units IM	Usual	Usual	Usual
V	Renal	0.5	7–10	0.4–0.8 million units q 6 h	—	Usual	Usual	Usual
Pentamidine	Nonrenal	6	6–8	—	4 mg/kg/d	Usual	4 mg/kg q 24–36 h	4 mg/kg q 48 h
Piperacillin	Renal	1.0	3.0	—	3–4 g q 4–6 h	Usual	3 g q 8 h	3 g q 12 h
Piperacillin-tazobactam	Renal	1	3	—	3 g q 6 h	Usual	2 g q 6 h	2 g q 8 h
Polymyxin B	Renal	6	48	—	0.8–1.2 g IV q 12 h	1–1.5 mg/kg/d	1–1.5 mg/kg q 2–3 d	1 mg/kg q 5–7 d
Praziquantel	Hepatic metabolism	0.8–1.5	?	10–25 mg/kg tid	—	Usual	Usual	Usual
Pyrazinamide	Metabolic	10–16	?	15–35 mg/kg/d	—	Usual	Usual	12–20 mg/kg/d
Pyrimethamine	Nonrenal	1.5–5 d	?	25–75 mg/d	—	Usual	Usual	Usual
Quinine	Hepatic metabolism	4–5	4–5	650 mg tid	7.5–10 mg/kg q 8 h	Usual	Usual	Usual
Quinacrine	Renal	5 d	—	100–200 mg q 6–8 h	—	Usual	?	?
Rifabutin	Hepatic	2–5	2–5	300 mg/d	—	Usual	Usual	Usual
Rifampin	Hepatic	2–5	2–5	600 mg/kg/d	600 mg/d	Usual	Usual	Usual
Ritonavir	Hepatic	3–4	—	600 mg bid	—	Usual	Usual	Usual
Saquinavir	Hepatic	1–2	1–2	600 mg tid	—	Usual	Usual	Usual
Spectinomycin	Renal	1–3	?	—	2 g/day IM	Usual	Usual	Usual
Stavudine	Renal, hepatic	1	—	40 mg bid	—	Usual	20 mg bid	No data
Streptogramin	Hepatic	1.5	—	—	7.5 mg/kg q 8 h	Usual	Usual	Usual (no data)
Streptomycin	Renal	2.5	100–110	—	500 mg q 12 h	7.5 mg/kg q 24 h	7.5 mg/kg q 24–72 h	7.5 mg/kg q 72–96 h

Table continued on following page

TABLE 40–3 ■ Drug Dosage Guidelines* *Continued*

DRUG	PRINCIPAL EXCRETION ROUTE	HALF-LIFE (h)		USUAL REGIMEN		MAINTENANCE REGIMEN FOR RENAL FAILURE†		
		Normal	Anuria	Oral	Parenteral	GFR of 50–80 mL/min	GFR of 10–50 mL/min	GFR of <10 mL/min
Sulfadiazine	Renal	17	?	0.5–1.5 g q 4–6 h	—	Usual	0.5–1.5 g q 8–12 h	0.5–1.5 g q 12–24 h
					30–50 mg/kg q 6–8 h	Usual	30–50 mg/kg q 12–18 h	30–50 mg/kg q 18–24 h
Sulfisoxazole	Renal	3–7	6–12	1–2 g q 6 h	—	Usual	1 g q 8–12 h	1 g q 12–24 h
Teicoplanin	Renal	6	41	—	6–12 mg/kg/d	Usual	½ dose	⅓ dose
Tetracycline	Renal	8	50–100	0.25–0.5 g q 6 h	0.5–1 g q 12 h	Usual	Use doxycycline	
Ticarcillin	Renal	1–1.5	16	—	3 g q 4 h	Usual	2–3 g q 6–8 h	2 g q 12 h
Ticarcillin-clavulanate	Renal	1–1.5	16	—	3 g q 4 h	Usual	2–3 g q 6–8 h	2 g q 12 h
Tobramycin	Renal	2.5	56	—	1.7 mg/kg q 8 h	Loading dose, then 0.03 × C_{cr} = mg/kg/8 h†		
Trimethoprim	Renal	8–15	24	100 mg q 12 h	—	Usual	100 mg q 18–24 h	Avoid
Trimethoprim-sulfamethoxazole (TMP-SMX)	Renal	TMP: 8–15 SMX: 7–12	TMP: 24 SMX: 22–50	2–4 tablets (1–2 if double-strength)	—	Usual	Half-dose	1 tablet bid
					3–5 mg/kg q 6–12 h	3–5 mg/kg q 18 h	3–5 mg/kg/d	Avoid
Trimetrexate	Metabolized	11	—	—	45 mg/m²/d	Usual	No data	No data
Valacyclovir	Renal	1	3	1000 mg tid	—	Usual	1 g q 12–24 h	500 mg q 24 h
				500 mg bid	—	Usual	500 mg q 12–24 h	500 mg q 24 h
Vancomycin	Renal	6–8	200–250	0.125–0.5 g q 6 h	—	Usual dose	Usual dose	0.125 mg PO
				—	15 mg/kg q 12 h	1 g q 24 h	1 g q 3–10 d	1 g q 5–d
Vidarabine	Renal	3.5	—	—	15 mg/kg/d	Usual	Usual	10 mg/kg/d
Zidovudine (AZT)	Hepatic	1	1.4	100 mg q 4 h	—	Usual	Usual	100 mg q 6 h

*GFR, glomerular filtration rate; IM, intramuscular; IV, intravenous; PO, oral; bid, twice daily; qd, every day; tid, three times a day; C_{cr}, creatinine clearance.

†Dose for once-daily dosing (creatinine clearance > 80 mL/min: amikacin: 15 mg/kg/d; tobramycin, gentamicin, and netilmicin: 5–6 mg/kg/d. In renal failure, the dose adjustments are for amikacin and kanamycin: 8 mg/kg loading dose, then 0.12 × creatinine clearance = mg/kg q 8 h; for gentamicin, tobramicin, and netilmicin: 1.7–2 mg/kg loading dose, then 0.03 × creatinine clearance = mg/kg q 8 h.

Data from Bennett WM, Muther RS, Parker RA, et al: Drug therapy in renal failure: Dosing guidelines for adults. Part I: Antimicrobial agents, analgesics. Ann Intern Med 93:62, 1980; Drug Evaluations, ed 6. Chicago, American Medical Association, 1986; and McEvoy GK, Litvak K, Welsh OH Jr, et al (eds): AHFS 96 Drug Information. American Hospital Formulary Service. Bethesda, MD, American Society of Health-System Pharmacists, 1996, pp 39–611.

TABLE 40–4 ■ Antimicrobial Dosage Regimens During Dialysis

DRUG	HEMODIALYSIS	PERITONEAL DIALYSIS
Acyclovir	2.5–5.0 mg/kg/d + extra dose after dialysis	2.5 mg/kg/d
Amdinocillin	No extra dose	—
Amikacin	2.5–3.75 mg/kg after dialysis	Loading dose before dialysis, 9–20 mg/L dialysate
Amoxicillin	0.25 g after dialysis	Usual regimen
Amoxicillin-clavulanate	0.50 g (amoxicillin) + 0.125 g (clavulanate) halfway through dialysis and another dose at end	Usual regimen
Amphotericin B	Usual regimen	Usual regimen
Ampicillin	Usual dose after dialysis	Usual regimen
Ampicillin-sulbactam	2 g ampicillin after dialysis	Usual regimen
Azithromycin	Usual regimen	Usual regimen
Azlocillin	3 g after dialysis, then 3 g q 12 h	3 g q 12 h
Aztreonam	⅛ initial dose (60–250 mg) after dialysis	Usual loading dose, then ¼ usual dose at usual intervals
Carbenicillin	0.75–2.0 after dialysis	2 g 6–12 h
Cefaclor	Repeat dose after dialysis	Usual regimen
Cefadroxil	0.5–1 g after dialysis	0.5 g/d
Cefamandole	Repeat dose after dialysis	0.5–1 g q 12 h
Cefazolin	0.25–0.5 g after dialysis	0.5 g q 12 h
Cefixime	300 mg/d	200 mg/d
Cefonicid	No extra dose	Usual regimen
Cefoperazone	Schedule dose after dialysis	Usual regimen
Cefotaxime	0.5–2 g daily plus supplemental dose after dialysis	1–2 g/d
Cefotetan	¼ usual dose q 24 h on nondialysis days and ½ dose on dialysis days	1 g/d
Cefoxitin	1–2 g after dialysis	1 g/d
Cefpodoxime	200–400 mg 3 ×/wk	—
Cefprozil	250–500 mg after dialysis	0.25 g q 12–24 h

TABLE 40–4 ■ Antimicrobial Dosage Regimens During Dialysis *Continued*

DRUG	HEMODIALYSIS	PERITONEAL DIALYSIS
Ceftazidime	1 g loading dose, 1 g after dialysis	0.5–1 g loading dose, then 0.5 g q 24 h or 250 mg in each 2 L dialysate
Ceftibuten	400 mg after dialysis	—
Ceftizoxime	Schedule dose after dialysis	1 g/d
Ceftriaxone	No extra dose	Usual regimen
Cefuroxime	Repeat dose after dialysis	15 mg/kg after dialysis or 750 mg/d
Cephalexin	0.25–1 g after dialysis	250 mg 3 ×/d
Cephalothin	Supplemental dose after dialysis	Option to add ≤6 mg/dL to dialysate
Cephapirin	7.5–15 mg/kg before dialysis and q 12 h afterward	—
Cephradine	250 mg before dialysis, then at 12 and 36–48 h later	0.5 g q 6 h
Chloramphenicol	Schedule dose after dialysis	Usual regimen
Ciprofloxacin	250–500 mg q 24 h after dialysis	250–500 mg q 24 h
Clindamycin	Usual regimen	Usual regimen
Cloxacillin	Usual regimen	Usual regimen
Dicloxacillin	Usual regimen	Usual regimen
Doxycycline	Usual regimen	Usual regimen
Erythromycin	Usual regimen	Usual regimen
Ethambutol	15 mg/kg/d after dialysis	15 mg/kg/d
Flucytosine	20–37.5 mg/kg after dialysis	½ usual dose
Ganciclovir, oral	500 mg after dialysis 3 ×/wk	—
Ganciclovir, parenteral	1.25 mg/kg q 24 h after dialysis on dialysis days	—
Gentamicin	1.0–1.7 mg/kg after dialysis	Loading dose before dialysis, 2–4 mg/L dialysate
Isoniazid	5 mg/kg after dialysis	Daily dose after dialysis
Imipenem	Supplemental dose after dialysis and q 12 h thereafter	500 mg/d
Kanamycin	4–5 mg/kg after dialysis	3.75 mg/kg/d
Ketoconazole	Usual regimen	Usual regimen
Metronidazole	Usual regimen	Usual regimen
Mezlocillin	2–3 g after dialysis, then 3–4 g q 12 h	3 g q 12 h
Minocycline	Usual dose (100 mg bid)	Usual regimen
Moxalactam	1–2 g after dialysis	Usual regimen
Nafcillin	Usual regimen	Usual regimen
Netilmicin	2 mg/kg after dialysis	Loading dose before dialysis, 3–5 mg/L dialysate
Oxacillin	200 mg then 100 mg/d	Usual regimen
Penicillin G	500,000 units after dialysis	—
Penicillin V	0.25 g after dialysis	—
Pentamidine	Usual regimen	Usual regimen
Piperacillin	1 g after dialysis then 2 g q 8 h	3–6 g/d
Streptomycin	0.5 g after dialysis	—
Tetracycline	500 mg after dialysis	Use doxycycline
Ticarcillin	3 g after dialysis, then 2 g q 12 h	3 g q 12 h
Ticarcillin-clavulanate	3 g (ticarcillin) after dialysis, then 2 g q 12 h	3 g (ticarcillin) q 12 h
Tobramycin	1 mg/kg after dialysis	Loading dose before dialysis, 2–4 mg/L dialysate
Trimethoprim-sulfamethoxazole	4–5 mg/kg (as TMP) after dialysis	0.16/0.8 q 48 h
Valacyclovir	1 g after dialysis	Usual regimen
Vancomycin	1 g/wk	0.5–1 g/wk
Vidarabine	Scheduled dose after dialysis	—
Zidovudine (AZT)	300 mg/d	300 mg/d

Adapted from Norris S, Nightengale CH, Mandell GL: Tables of antimicrobial agent pharmacology. *In* Mandell GL, Bennett J, Dolin R (eds): Principles and Practice of Infectious Diseases, ed 4. Churchill Livingstone, New York, 1995, pp 492–528; and McEvoy GK, Litvak K, Welsh OH Jr, et al (eds): AHFS Drug Information 96. American Hospital Formulary Service. Bethesda, MD, American Society of Health-System Pharmacists, 1996, pp 39–611.

41

Immunization of Children and Adults

Jerome O. Klein

Immunization may be achieved by active or passive means. Active immunity is achieved when an appropriate antigen stimulates immune cells to produce protective antibodies. Passive immunity is achieved by introduction of preformed protective antibodies.

The vaccine products available in the United States (as of March 1997) are listed in Table 41–1. Ten products are considered for universal immunization of children, including diphtheria and tetanus toxoids and pertussis whole-cell vaccine (DTP) or accellular vaccine (DTaP); measles, mumps, and rubella live virus vaccines (MMR); oral live poliovirus vaccine (OPV) or inactivated poliovirus vaccine (IPV); hepatitis B virus (HBV) vaccine; varicella virus vaccine; and conjugate *Haemophilus influenzae* type b (Hib) vaccine. Twelve vaccines are available for special circumstances: five virus vaccines—Japanese B encephalitis, hepatitis A, influenza, rabies, and yellow fever vaccines; and seven bacterial vaccines—anthrax, bacille Calmette-Guérin (BCG), cholera, meningococcal, pneumococcal, and typhoid vaccines. Combined products include DTP, DTaP, MMR, and conjugate *H. influenzae* vaccine plus DTP or DTaP and HBV plus conjugate *H. influenzae* vaccine.

Products available in 1997 for protection by passive immunization include immune globulin (IG) prepared from pooled plasma of adults and used for replacement therapy in antibody deficiency disorders, hepatitis A prophylaxis, and measles prophylaxis. Specific IGs are prepared from blood of donors with high titers of the desired antibodies. Current specific IGs include hepatitis B IG (HBIG), rabies IG (RIG), tetanus IG (TIG), varicella-zoster IG (VZIG), and respiratory syncytial virus IG (RSVIG).

Recommendations for use of new vaccines and modifications of use of old ones are frequent, so health care personnel must be alert for changes. Important sources of vaccine information include *Morbidity and Mortality Weekly Reports (MMWR)* published weekly by the Centers for Disease Control and Prevention (CDC), which also publishes regular and special recommendations of the Advisory Committee on Immunization Practices (ACIP) of the U. S. Public Health Service. Guidelines for use of vaccines in children and adults are published at regular intervals by the American Academy of Pediatrics (AAP) *(Report of the Committee on Infectious Diseases)*, the American College of Physicians *(Guide for Adult Immunization)*, the American College of Obstetricians and Gynecologists (technical bulletins), state and local health departments, and the Division of Immunization of the CDC. Addresses and telephone numbers for these sources are provided in the *MMWR* (38:205, 1989). A textbook by Plotkin and Mortimer provides extensive discussions of available vaccines.[1]

General Issues of Administration of Vaccines

Constituents of Vaccines

Vaccines consist of an antigen that elicits production of protective antibody; a suspending fluid, which may include materials derived from the system used to produce the vaccine; preservatives to prevent bacterial contamination or stabilize the antigen; and sometimes adjuvants that amplify the immunogenic effect. Patients may have allergic reactions to a constituent of the vaccine: egg proteins are present in measles, mumps, influenza, and yellow fever vaccines, and patients who have demonstrated severe allergy to eggs should not receive these products; trace amounts of antibiotics present in OPV (streptomycin and neomycin) and MMR (neomycin) vaccines may provoke reactions in persons allergic to the drugs.

Route and Schedule of Immunization

The package insert should be consulted to determine the optimal site for administration of the vaccine (see Table 41–1). Vaccine schedules (Table 41–2) are constructed to take into account the earliest time a person can respond to the antigen and the time of life when protection is needed (i.e., age of highest incidence and morbidity of the disease). For some vaccines, a compromise is necessary to provide maximal protection for most persons; pertussis vaccine is less immunogenic in early infancy, but young infants are the group at greatest risk from natural infection. Other schedules need to be considered for children not immunized in the first year of life or for children living in developing countries with limited medical facilities.

Vaccine schedules are changed at periodic intervals; the interested reader should consult current reports from the ACIP published in the *MMWR* and the reports of the Committee on Infectious Diseases of the AAP. The two advisory groups work together to develop uniform recommendations. The current recommended childhood immunization schedules were published in January 1997.[2]

Adverse Reactions

No vaccine is completely safe. Adverse reactions of varying severity, both local and systemic, are relatively frequent with some vaccines (pertussis, parenteral typhoid) and infrequent with others (polysaccharide vaccines). Contraindications to the first or repeated immunization are identified in the reports of the Committee on Infectious Diseases of the AAP and in statements of the ACIP in *MMWR* and are outlined later in the sections on special populations and in discussions of the vaccines. Because of misconceptions about reasons to withhold vaccines, the ACIP included a review[3] of conditions that were not contraindications to immunization, including mild acute illness, current antimicrobial therapy, prematurity, exposure to an infectious disease, breast-feeding, history of non–vaccine-associated allergies, and family history of convulsions or sudden infant death. Reporting of specific adverse events (Table 41–3) is mandated by the National Childhood Vaccine Injury Act, which became effective in March 1988.

Allergy to egg or egg products should be considered when administering measles, mumps, influenza, or yellow fever vaccines. Severe reactions due to egg antigens are rare after administration of these vaccines, but the products should be

TABLE 41–1 ■ Vaccine Products Available in the United States, by Type and Recommended Routes of Administration

VACCINE	TYPE	ROUTE
Anthrax	Inactivated bacteria	Subcutaneous
BCG (bacille Calmette-Guérin)	Live bacteria	Intradermal or subcutaneous
Cholera	Inactivated bacteria	Subcutaneous or intradermal*
DTaP (diphtheria, tetanus, and acellular pertussis)	Toxoids and bacterial products	Intramuscular
DTP (diphtheria, tetanus, pertussis)	Toxoids and inactivated bacteria	Intramuscular
HB (hepatitis B)	Inactive viral antigen	Intramuscular
Haemophilus influenzae b		
Polysaccharide (HbPV)	Bacterial polysaccharide or	Subcutaneous or intramuscular†
or conjugate (HbCV) (Hib)	polysaccharide conjugated to protein	Intramuscular
HbCV + DTP	Combined product	Intramuscular
HbCV + DTaP‡	Combined product	Intramuscular
HB + HbCV	Combined product	Intramuscular
Hepatitis A	Inactivated virus	Intramuscular
Influenza	Inactivated virus or viral components	Intramuscular
IPV (inactivated poliovirus vaccine)	Inactivated viruses of all three serotypes	Subcutaneous
Japanese encephalitis	Inactivated virus	Subcutaneous
Measles	Live virus	Subcutaneous
Meningococcal	Bacterial polysaccharides of serotypes A/C/Y/W-135	Subcutaneous
MMR (measles, mumps, rubella)	Live viruses	Subcutaneous
Mumps	Live virus	Subcutaneous
OPV (oral poliovirus vaccine)	Live viruses of all three serotypes	Oral
Pertussis, acellular	Bacterial products	Intramuscular
Plague	Inactivated bacteria	Intramuscular
Pneumococcal	Bacterial polysaccharides of 23 pneumococcal types	Intramuscular or subcutaneous
Rabies	Inactivated virus	Subcutaneous or intradermal§
Rubella	Live virus	Subcutaneous
Tetanus	Inactivated toxin (toxoid)	Intramuscular‖
Td or DT¶ (tetanus, diphtheria)	Inactivated toxins (toxoids)	Intramuscular‖
Typhoid, oral	Live bacteria	Oral
Typhoid, parenteral	Inactivated bacteria	Subcutaneous**
Typhoid polysaccharide	Capsular polysaccharide	Intramuscular
Varicella	Live virus	Subcutaneous
Yellow fever	Live virus	Subcutaneous

*The intradermal dose is lower.
†Route depends on the manufacturer; consult package insert for recommendation for specific product used.
‡Available only for administration as the fourth dose in the DTaP series for children ≥15 mo.
§Intradermal dose is lower and used only for preexposure vaccination.
‖Preparations with adjuvants should be given intramuscularly.
¶DT, Tetanus and diphtheria toxoids for use in children aged <7 y; Td, tetanus and diphtheria toxoids for use in persons aged ≥7 y. Td contains the same amount of tetanus toxoids as DTP or DT but a reduced dose of diphtheria toxoid.
**Boosters may be given intradermally unless acetone-killed and dried vaccine is used.

avoided in patients with histories of anaphylactic reactions to egg or egg products.

Simultaneous Administration of Vaccines

Use of multiple products in a single-dose form and simultaneous administration of vaccines is the rule (see Table 41–2). For infants who may not return for well-child care and for those who have not received vaccines or are behind schedule, administration of all vaccines appropriate for age is warranted and appears to be satisfactory in terms of immune response. As an example, DTP, MMR, Hib vaccine, HBV, and OPV or IPV may be administered at the same visit.

Immunization After Exposure to Disease

Because of the prolonged incubation period, immunization may be valuable for unimmunized patients after exposure to rabies, measles (within 3 days of exposure), hepatitis B, and tetanus (if the primary series was incomplete). Administration of rabies and hepatitis vaccines and tetanus toxoids should be accompanied by the specific IG. Rubella and mumps vaccines are ineffective when given after the exposure.

Special Patients

PREGNANT WOMEN

Because of the paucity of data about effects of vaccines on the fetus, pregnant women should receive immunizing products only for approved indications. Live virus vaccines are contraindicated except for yellow fever vaccine, which may be administered to susceptible women who must travel to endemic areas. If exposure to poliovirus is anticipated, IPV should be used. In the United States, tetanus and diphtheria-tetanus vaccines are recommended for nonimmunized pregnant women. Influenza vaccine should be considered for women who have a cardiorespiratory disorder that would place them at risk if infected.

IMMUNODEFICIENT PATIENTS

Live virus and live bacterial vaccines are contraindicated for patients who are immunodeficient. Household contacts of

TABLE 41–2 ■ Recommended Schedule for Active Immunization of Normal Infants and Children—1995*†

RECOMMENDED AGE	IMMUNIZATIONS‡	COMMENTS
Birth	HBV	Acceptable for immunization infants of hepatitis B virus antigen–negative mothers at 0–2 mo, dose 2 at 4 mo, and dose 3 at 6–18 mo.
1–2 mo	HBV	
2 mo	DTP or DTaP, Hib, OPV or IPV	2-mo interval (minimum, 6 wk) recommended for OPV.
4 mo	DTP or DTaP, Hib, OPV or IPV	
6 mo	DTP or DTaP, Hib, HBV, HBV	HBV may be given as third dose at 6–18 mo of age.
12–15 mo	Hib	
12–18 mo	Varicella	
15–18 mo	DTP or DTaP	
6–18 mo	OPV	IPV may be substituted for third dose at 12–18 mo.
12–15 mo	MMR	
4–6 y	DTP or DTaP, OPV	IPV may be substituted for fourth dose at 4–6 y.
11–12 y	MMR Td	MMR alternatively may be administered at 4–6 y.

*Approved by the Advisory Committee on Immunization Practices, American Academy of Pediatrics and the American Academy of Family Physicians.

†For all products used, consult manufacturer's package insert for instructions for storage, handling, dosage, and administration. Biologics prepared by different manufacturers may vary, and package inserts of the same manufacturer may change from time to time. Therefore, the physician should be aware of the contents of the current package insert.

‡DTP, diphtheria and tetanus toxoids with pertussis vaccine; DTaP, diphtheria and tetanus toxoids and acellular pertussis vaccine; HBV, hepatitis B virus vaccine; OPV, oral poliovirus vaccine containing attenuated poliovirus types 1, 2, and 3; IPV, inactivated poliovirus vaccine containing poliovirus types 1, 2, and 3; MMR, live measles, mumps, and rubella viruses in a combined vaccine (see text for discussion of single vaccines versus combination); Hib, *Haemophilus influenzae* type b conjugate vaccine; Td, adult tetanus toxoid (full dose) and diphtheria toxoid (reduced dose) for adult use.

immunodeficient patients should not receive OPV because of the possibility of transmission of vaccine virus to the patient. Inactivated vaccines may be used for immunodeficient patients, although their efficacy varies with the stage of the disease.

Patients with asymptomatic or symptomatic human immunodeficiency virus (HIV) infection should receive inactivated vaccines on schedule.[4] Children aged 2 years and older with HIV infection should receive, in addition, pneumococcal, meningococcal, and Hib vaccines. Live vaccines with the exception of MMR are contraindicated for children with symptomatic HIV infection. Because measles in children with acquired

TABLE 41–3 ■ Reportable Events After Vaccination

VACCINE/TOXOID	EVENT	INTERVAL FROM VACCINATION
DTP, P, DTP/polio combined	A. Anaphylaxis or anaphylactic shock	24 h
	B. Encephalopathy (or encephalitis)	7 d
	C. Shock-collapse or hypotonic-hyporesponsive collapse	7 d
	D. Residual seizure disorder	
	E. Any acute complication or sequela (including death) of above events	No limit
	F. Events in vaccinees described in manufacturer's package insert as contraindication to additional doses of vaccine (such as convulsions)	See package insert
MMR, DT, Td, tetanus toxoid	A. Anaphylaxis or anaphylactic shock	24 h
	B. Encephalopathy (or encephalitis)	15 d for measles, mumps, and rubella vaccines; 7 d for DT, Td, and T toxoids
	C. Residual seizure disorder	
	D. Any acute complication or sequela (including death) of above events	No limit
	E. Events in vaccinees described in manufacturer's package insert as contraindications to additional doses of vaccine	See package insert
OPV	A. Paralytic poliomyelitis	
	In a nonimmunodeficient recipient	30 d
	In an immunodeficient recipient	6 mo
	In a vaccine-associated community case	No limit
	B. Any acute complication or sequela (including death) of above events	No limit
	C. Events in vaccinees described in manufacturer's package insert as contraindications to additional doses of vaccine	See package insert
IPV	A. Anaphylaxis or anaphylactic shock	24 h
	B. Any acute complication or sequela (including death) of above event	No limit
	C. Events in vaccinees described in manufacturer's package insert as contraindications to additional doses of vaccine	See package insert

From Centers for Disease Control: Update on adult immunization: Recommendations of the Immunization Practices Advisory Comittee (ACIP). MMWR Morbid Mortal Wkly Rep 40(RR-12):53–54, 1991.

immunodeficiency syndrome tends to be severe, the ACIP suggests that both symptomatic and asymptomatic children with HIV infection be given MMR.

ADOLESCENTS AND COLLEGE STUDENTS

Adolescents and young adults may be incompletely protected from diseases for which vaccines are available because vaccines were never provided, were ineffective, or were administered at inappropriate ages or by inappropriate routes, or because protection has waned over time. Outbreaks of measles, mumps, rubella, and pertussis in high schools and colleges have underlined the need for systems to identify appropriate vaccine histories and to initiate primary or repeated immunization. Adolescent immunization is part of a program of comprehensive health services for adolescents. The vaccine initiative is directed to those who are 11 to 12 years of age and includes booster doses of MMR, tetanus and diphtheria toxoids, and HBV immunization for those who have not completed the series previously, and varicella vaccine for those who do not have protective antibody from immunization or prior infection.

HEALTH CARE PROFESSIONALS

For adults whose occupations place them in contact with patients with contagious diseases, protection by immunization is important to them and to their patients. Hospitals, clinics, and private offices should have policies for immunizing health care workers against measles, rubella, influenza, hepatitis B, and varicella.

REFUGEES

Refugees' vaccine histories usually are unavailable. In addition, vaccines used in the home country may not have been adequate for durable protection. Vaccines may be administered in camps or at the sites of embarkation before arrival in the United States. In the absence of documentation, the physician must assume that the patient received no prior immunization. Patients may be given multiple vaccines simultaneously to bring them up to standard schedules for age.

FOREIGN TRAVELERS

Because endemic and epidemic disease may vary in time and place, travelers must be provided with information and appropriate vaccines by the responsible physician. Current information available from the CDC is published in the annual booklet *Health Information for International Travel* (available from the Superintendent of Documents, U.S. Government Printing Office, Washington, DC 20402).

Diphtheria and Tetanus Toxoids and Pertussis Vaccine

DTP vaccine has been used widely for routine immunization of children in the United States since about 1945. The primary series of DTP is administered at 2, 4, and 6 months, with a booster dose administered at 18 months and between 4 and 6 years. If pertussis immunization is contraindicated, the child should be immunized with DT vaccine instead of DTP (the introduction of acellular pertussis vaccine may resolve this issue in most children). Outbreaks of pertussis and diphtheria and decreased protective levels of antibody to DTP in adolescents and adults indicate the need for repeated immunization. After the seventh birthday, primary immunization should consist of adult-type tetanus toxoid and a reduced dose of diphtheria toxoid (Td); boosters should be administered every 10 years throughout life at middecade ages (15 years, 25 years, and so on).

Diphtheria Toxoid

Diphtheria toxoid is prepared from a strain of *Corynebacterium diphtheriae* that is known to produce large amounts of toxin and grown in a liquid medium to enhance toxin production. The toxin is incubated with formalin to prepare the toxoid and is subsequently adsorbed onto an aluminum salt with thimerosal as a preservative.

Although no controlled trials have been performed to evaluate the efficacy of diphtheria toxoid in preventing disease, efficacy is believed to be in excess of 80% and disease is milder in immunized patients. Universal immunization likely contributes to the low incidence of disease now in the United States; fewer than five cases of diphtheria per year have been reported since 1980.[5] However, many adults lack protective antibody. A serologic survey in north London showed that 25% of those aged 20 to 29 years were susceptible and 52.8% of those aged 50 to 59 years.[6]

Epidemic diphtheria began in 1990 in the New Independent States of the former Soviet Union; cases of diphtheria in this area increased from 839 in 1989 to 39,703 in 1994. An important factor in the outbreak was the presence of a large number of susceptible children and adults, which enabled the spread of toxigenic strains of *C. diphtheriae.*[7] Since the epidemic began, cases of diphtheria associated with the outbreak have been reported in patients in eastern and western Europe and in U.S. citizens working in or visiting the former Soviet Union. The epidemic underlines the need for renewed efforts to maintain diphtheria immunization schedules throughout life.

Tetanus Toxoid

Like diphtheria toxoid, tetanus toxoid is prepared by formalin inactivation of the toxin. Although tetanus is a completely preventable disease, 70 to 100 cases occur in the United States each year,[8] principally in older adults. A population-based serologic survey of immunity to tetanus in the United States identified decreased protective levels of tetanus antibodies in adolescents and adults; the rate decreased from 87.7% among those 6 to 11 years of age to 27.8% among those 70 years of age or older.[9] After the primary series, protection against tetanus (and diphtheria) is sustained by scheduling booster doses routinely every 10 years.

Postexposure wound management includes consideration of both tetanus toxoid (administered as DTP or DTaP for children younger than 7 years of age and tetanus and diphtheria toxoid Td to older persons) and TIG. If the wound occurs within 10 years of the third of a series of doses of tetanus toxoid, neither toxoid nor TIG is necessary. If more than 10 years has elapsed since the last dose or if the immunization history is unknown or consisted of fewer than three doses, tetanus toxoid is administered for both clean, minor wounds and contaminated, severe wounds. In patients with unknown or incomplete history of tetanus toxoid immunization, TIG is added for contaminated wounds.

Pertussis Vaccine

A whole-cell pertussis vaccine has been documented to be 80% to 90% effective in preventing disease and to reduce the morbidity of disease in vaccinees who develop whooping cough. The major concern has been local and systemic reactions. Neurologic reactions include brief seizures that occur in association with approximately 1 per 1750 doses administered, usually within 12 to 24 hours of immunization and frequently associated with fever[10]; it is estimated that the association of acute encephalopathy with permanent neurologic sequelae is 1 in 310,000 doses.[11]

To maintain the immunogenicity of the whole-cell vaccine but limit reactivity, investigators have sought a safe and effective acellular, or subunit, vaccine. Four pertussis antigens have been identified that are believed to contribute to the development of antibodies for pertussis protection: lymphocytosis-promoting factor, or pertussis toxin, plays a role in attachment of the organism to ciliated respiratory cells and in propagation of the infection; filamentous hemagglutinin is associated with attachment of organisms to the host cell; agglutinogens induce agglutinating antibodies, which correlate with clinical protection; and pertactin, a 69-kD outer membrane protein, is immunogenic in humans. In 1991 and 1992, the U.S. Food and Drug Administration (FDA) approved two acellular pertussis vaccines (two-antigen and four-antigen formulations) for the fourth and fifth doses. In 1996 and 1997, these two products and a third acellular vaccine composed of three antigens were approved for the infant immunization series. Additional acelluar pertussis vaccines are likely to be licensed for use in infants in the future. In clinical trials, the acellular pertussis vaccines were equivalent to or more effective than the whole-cell vaccines. Significantly fewer local and systemic reactions occurred after the acellular pertussis vaccines compared with the whole-cell vaccines. Because of the lesser reactivity and comparable efficacy, it is likely that acellular pertussis vaccines will replace whole-cell vaccines for primary series and boosters.[12]

Outbreaks of pertussis in junior and senior high schools and colleges suggest waning immunity to pertussis in adolescents and young adults and the need to reconsider booster doses with the acellular pertussis vaccines in this population. Although the disease is relatively mild in adults, with the major sign being persistent cough,[13] adults serve as a reservoir for spread of infection to infants and young children.

Studies of the safety of acellular vaccines in adolescents and young adults are in progress. Booster doses in adolescent and adult groups may prevent or diminish morbidity of the disease and reduce transmission of infection to infants and young children.[14]

Measles, Mumps, and Rubella

The MMR live virus vaccines are administered in one preparation at 15 months of age. A second dose of vaccine is now recommended for measles only but is for practical purposes administered as MMR. Contraindications to MMR include known pregnancy, anaphylaxis to egg ingestion, anaphylactic allergy to neomycin, compromised immunity (except for HIV infection) and recent administration of IG. Suggested intervals between IG and administration of MMR depend on the indication for IG, varying between 3 months after intramuscular IG for hepatitis A prophylaxis to 11 months for intravenous IG administered for idiopathic thrombocytopenia or Kawasaki disease.

Measles

Live attenuated measles vaccine is prepared by multiple passage in chick embryos. The vaccine was introduced in the United States in 1966 and has been responsible for a decline in cases of more than 98%. An increase in incidence of measles was apparent beginning in 1986, when measles cases were reported from 46 states. Although a majority of cases occurred in preschool-aged children who had not been immunized, many of those affected were immunized teenagers and young adults who contracted the disease in outbreaks in high schools and colleges. The increased incidence of measles in persons who had been properly immunized prompted the AAP and ACIP to recommend a second dose of vaccine.[15] Their recommendations include the following measures:

1. Two doses of measles vaccine for all children after the first birthday, the first dose to be administered as MMR at 12 to 15 months of age and the second on entrance to grade or junior high school. Age for initial vaccination should be lowered to 6 months in outbreak areas if cases are occurring in children younger than 1 year of age.
2. Colleges and other institutions beyond high school should require documentation of two doses of measles-containing vaccines before entry of students.
3. Health care workers born after January 1, 1957, should receive two doses of MMR or measles vaccine (if there is no history of measles or laboratory evidence of measles immunity). The 1957 date was chosen because of the assumption that virtually all children born before that date had had natural measles.

In contrast to those with other disorders that are accompanied by immunologic defects, children with HIV infection should receive live measles vaccine (given as MMR). The live vaccine is suggested for these patients because of reports of severe and often fatal natural measles in children with HIV infection and disease and the lack of complications from the live virus vaccine in these patients.

Mumps

Live mumps virus vaccine is prepared in chick embryo cell cultures. The vaccine was licensed in 1967 and is believed to be more than 98% effective in providing durable protection. An increase in the number of mumps cases has been noted since 1986 by the CDC.[16] The relative increase in mumps cases is believed to be due to failure to vaccinate susceptible persons, particularly teenagers.

Rubella

Live rubella virus vaccine was licensed in 1969. The current product in the United States is produced in human diploid cell culture. Serum antibody is produced in almost all recipients and provides durable, perhaps lifelong, immunity. Viremia occurs after immunization, and virus has been recovered from placental and fetal tissues. To investigate potential teratogenicity, the CDC in 1971 established a registry of women who had received a rubella vaccine within 3 months before or after conception. None of 212 live-born infants of susceptible women who received the currently used (human diploid) rubella vaccine had signs of congenital rubella syndrome.[17] Because of the theoretical risk of teratogenicity, the CDC continues to recommend that rubella vaccine not be given to pregnant women, but it is not necessary to screen for pregnancy before administering the vaccine.

Susceptible postpubertal girls and women in the childbearing years should be encouraged to receive rubella vaccine (when not pregnant). Both male and female college students, daycare personnel, health care workers, and military recruits should be immunized for their protection and to limit spread of infection to contacts.

Arthritis (usually of small, peripheral joints) has been reported in up to 15% of susceptible postpubertal females who were immunized with the human diploid vaccine. Chronic arthritis and neuropathies have been reported after vaccination of adult women. Other side effects include a mild rubella-like illness with rash, fever, and lymphadenopathy.

Live Oral and Killed Parenteral Polio Vaccines

IPV was introduced in the United States in 1955 and was used extensively until OPV was licensed in 1961; OPV became the standard material for primary immunization of all but immunocompromised patients, and IPV use rapidly declined to a level of less than 1% of polio vaccines used in the United States. Extensive use of OPV has been extraordinarily successful. The Western Hemisphere is now free of paralytic polio caused by wild poliovirus; the last case of paralytic disease occurred in 1991 in Peru. Poliovirus infection remains endemic in most countries of West and Central Africa and in Southeast Asia. The World Health Organization has set a goal of worldwide eradication of wild poliovirus disease by the year 2000. Because of the continued incidence of OPV-associated paralytic disease, the American Academy of Pediatrics and the Advisory Committee on Immunization Practices in January 1997 suggested a new schedule of combined IPV/OPV: IPV to be administered as the first two doses at 2 and 4 months of age followed by booster doses of OPV at 12 to 18 months and 4 to 6 years. Four doses of IPV or four doses of OPV are acceptable alternatives.[18]

OPV provides lifelong protection against paralytic disease. The vaccine induces intestinal immunity against poliovirus reinfection, which is effective in controlling wild virus circulation. OPV is prepared in monkey kidney tissue culture. Although the immunization policy in the United States has resulted in elimination of endemic poliomyelitis, cases of paralytic poliomyelitis occur associated with OPV. The approximate risk of vaccine-associated paralytic disease in the United States is 1 case among 6.2 million immunologically normal recipients of OPV vaccine and 1 case of paralytic disease among household and community contacts per 7.6 million vaccinees.[18] The greatest risk of paralysis in recipients occurs after the first dose: the risk was 1 case in 1.4 million first doses and 1 case per 27.2 million subsequent doses. Patients with an immunodeficiency are at risk for acquiring paralytic disease if exposed to the vaccine virus as recipients or contacts and should receive only IPV.

A more potent IPV was licensed by the the FDA in April 1988. The new IPV is produced in a human diploid cell line grown on microcarriers in suspension culture and has been termed enhanced-potency IPV. No serious adverse events, including vaccine-associated paralytic disease, have been associated with IPV. IPV is the only poliovirus vaccine recommended for immunocompromised persons and their household contacts.

The new combined schedule of two doses of IPV followed by two booster doses of OPV is based on the following considerations: vaccine-associated paralytic disease is diminished by the first dose administered as the inactivated vaccine (IPV); intestinal immunity is provided by the third and fourth doses administered as OPV. Because the new schedule necessitates two additional parenteral doses in a crowded schedule and because of increased cost, some parents may choose to continue a schedule of OPV only. Other parents may be concerned about any possibility of vaccine-associated paralytic disease and choose a schedule of IPV only. Each of the three schedules, IPV/OPV, IPV only, and OPV only, is approved by the expert groups.[18]

Varicella Vaccine

In March 1995, the FDA approved a live attenuated varicella virus vaccine for individuals 12 months of age and older who have not had varicella. The OKA strain of virus used in the vaccine is attenuated by passage in human and embryonic guinea pig cell cultures. More than 2 million doses had been given in Japan and Korea before approval by the FDA in the United States. The development of the live attenuated varicella vaccine and current recommendations for vaccine use were reviewed by the Committee on Infectious Diseases of the AAP.[19]

A single dose of the vaccine resulted in seroconversion in more than 95% of children 1 to 12 years of age. Seroconversion in 13- to 17-years-olds was 79% and in adults was 82% after one dose and 94% after two doses. In children, the vaccine was approximately 70% effective in prevention of disease but more than 95% effective against more severe disease. Approximately 70% of adults who converted after immunization are protected against varicella; the remaining 30% of these adults usually developed attenuated disease after close exposure.

Adverse events are minimal. Maculopapular rash or vesicular lesions may occur in 7% of susceptible children and 8% of susceptible adolescents and adults. The frequency of zoster is less in vaccinated individuals than after natural infection. Transmission of the vaccine virus from healthy vaccinees to susceptible contacts is possible, because virus has been recovered from skin lesions of vaccinees, but no clinical cases of varicella from contact with healthy vaccinees have been reported.

A single subcutaneous dose is recommended for healthy children between 1 and 12 years of age. Two doses of varicella vaccine 4 to 8 weeks apart are recommended for healthy adolescents and adults with no history of varicella. The vaccine should not be given routinely to patients who are immunocompromised or patients in households with potentially immunocompromised contacts. Pregnant women should not receive this live virus vaccine because the effects on fetal development are unknown.

Polysaccharide Vaccines: *Haemophilus influenzae* Type b, *Streptococcus pneumoniae*, and *Neisseria meningitidis*

The capsular polysaccharides of Hib, *S. pneumoniae,* and *N. meningitidis* produce protective antibodies in patients older than 2 years of age. Because the highest age-specific attack rates for invasive disease due to these three encapsulated species occur in infants younger than 2 years of age, a more effective immunogen is needed to provide consistent concentrations of protective antibody. Conjugated polysaccharide vaccines using proteins to amplify the immune response stimulated protective levels of antibody in infants as young as 2 months. Conjugate Hib vaccine was introduced in October 1990 and has virtually eliminated invasive disease in areas where the vaccine has been extensively used. Conjugate pneumococcal and meningococcal vaccines are now in clinical trials. Worldwide concern about the decreased susceptibility of pneumococci to antimicrobial agents increases the importance of a pneumococcal vaccine that will protect infants as well as older children and adults.

Pneumococcal Vaccines

A 23-type vaccine composed of capsular polysaccharide antigens was licensed in the United States in 1983, replacing a 14-type vaccine licensed in 1977. Each polysaccharide antigen is prepared separately and stimulates a type-specific immune response. The current vaccine includes capsular antigens for approximately 90% of the types responsible for bacteremic pneumococcal disease in the United States. Protective levels of antibody are available for 5 to 10 years in adults. In children who have sickle cell disease, have had the spleen removed, or have nephrosis, antibody titers for some types will fall to unprotective levels in 3 to 5 years. Based on these serologic data, the AAP recommends reimmunization after 3 to 5 years for children older than 10 years of age and adults who remain at high risk for invasive pneumococcal disease.

Currently available polysaccharide pneumococcal vaccine is recommended for use in the following situations:

1. Children 2 years of age and older who are at increased risk for serious disease if they become infected. High-risk categories include patients with sickle cell disease, functional or anatomic asplenia, HIV infection, or nephrotic syndrome; those about to have cytoreduction therapy for Hodgkin's disease; and those who have cerebrospinal fluid leaks
2. Immunocompetent adults who are at increased risk for pneumococcal disease because of chronic illnesses (cardiovascular disease, pulmonary disease, diabetes mellitus, alcoholism, cirrhosis) or who are 65 years of age or older
3. Immunoincompetent adults with splenic dysfunction or anatomic asplenia, Hodgkin's disease, lymphoma, multiple myeloma, chronic renal failure, nephrotic syndrome, organ transplantation associated with immunosuppression, or symptomatic or asymptomatic HIV infection

Meningococcal Vaccine

With the success of the *H. influenzae* type of vaccine, *N. meninigitidis* and *S. pneumoniae* are the leading causes of bacterial meningitis in all age groups. A quadrivalent vaccine against groups A, C, Y, and W-135 is available in the United States. No vaccine is available for group B. Development of an immunogenic group B vaccine is of particular importance because this group remains the major cause of meningococcal disease in the United States. Group A vaccine is immunogenic in children as young as 5 months, but the other meningococcal group vaccines are poor immunogens in children younger than 2 years of age. The vaccine is given to all U.S. military personnel and has significantly reduced the incidence of endemic and epidemic disease at military bases.

Current applications of meningococcal vaccine include the following:

1. Immunoincompetent children and adults, including those with functional or anatomic asplenia and those with terminal complement deficiencies
2. Contacts of a patient with invasive meningococcal disease (secondary cases may occur several weeks after the index case)
3. Travelers to countries with epidemic disease

Haemophilus influenzae *Type b Vaccines*

In April 1985, the FDA licensed a polysaccharide vaccine for Hib infections. Because it was a poor immunogen in children 2 years of age and younger, the vaccine could be recommended only for children at least 2 years old. The vaccine's efficacy was less in the United States than the 90% protection that had been anticipated from results of Finnish trials. In retrospective studies, the efficacy of Hib vaccine in the United States varied between 45% and 88%,[20] but a study of Hib vaccine use in Minnesota indicated absence of *any* protective effect.[21]

On October 4, 1990, the FDA approved use of the oligosaccharide nontoxic mutant diphtheria toxin protein vaccine for infants at 2, 4, and 6 months of age, with a booster at 12 to 15 months. The approval was based on the results of a single study in northern California that enrolled more than 30,000 children and identified a decrease in invasive disease of more than 90% in those who received two or more doses.[22] Subsequent approval was given for a conjugate vaccine incorporating an outer membrane protein of group B meningococcus to be administered on a schedule of 2, 4, and 12 months of age. The conjugate vaccines have been extraordinarily successful: in areas with high rates of immunization, invasive disease caused by Hib is now a rare occurrence. The success of the vaccine in populations with partial immunization was believed to be due to reduction in nasopharyngeal carriage of Hib, thereby interrupting transmission of infection.[23]

Virus Vaccines for Specific Populations or Special Indications

Influenza Virus Vaccines

Influenza virus vaccines are prepared in embryonated eggs and are subsequently inactivated. The vaccines contain different viral subtypes; the types are chosen each spring in anticipation of the expected strains the following winter. The optimal time for immunization is the fall of the year, but immunization is effective to the end of the influenza season.

Three preparations are used in the United States: a whole-virus vaccine prepared from intact, purified virus particles; a "split" virus vaccine prepared by an additional step of disrupting the lipid-containing membrane of the virus; and a purified surface antigen vaccine. Only the split virus and purified surface antigen formulations are to be used in children to age 13 years. After vaccination, most young adults develop hemagglutination inhibition titers that are likely to protect them against infection. Children who have not had experience with influenza virus infection or vaccine require two doses of vaccine administered 1 month apart. Annual vaccination is recommended because immunity is limited in duration and infectious strains vary from year to year. Because influenza vaccine is prepared in eggs, it should not be administered to patients with a history of significant allergy to eggs. A review of prevention and control of influenza was prepared by the CDC in 1995.[24]

Vaccination is directed toward persons who are likely to suffer severe morbidity if infected with influenza virus or who are at high or moderate risk for infection.

PATIENTS AT HIGH RISK IF THEY CONTRACT INFLUENZA

This group includes children (6 months of age or older) and adults with chronic respiratory or cardiovascular disease (defined as requiring regular medical follow-up or hospitalization during the previous year) and residents (of any age) of nursing homes and other chronic care facilities who have chronic medical conditions.

PATIENTS AT MODERATE RISK IF THEY CONTRACT INFLUENZA

Those at moderate risk include healthy persons older than 65 years, adults and children who have had regular medical follow-up or hospitalization during the previous year because of chronic metabolic diseases (including diabetes mellitus), renal disease, hemoglobinopathies, or immunosuppression; also children and teenagers who are receiving long-term aspirin therapy and therefore may be at risk for contracting Reye's syndrome after influenza. Health care workers and personnel in nursing homes and chronic care facilities should also be immunized against influenza to prevent nosocomial transmission to patients at risk.

Hepatitis B Vaccine

In 1982, a safe and effective HBV vaccine derived from plasma of infected patients and subsequently inactivated was licensed in the United States; this vaccine is no longer available in the United States but is available in other countries. In 1986, the first of two currently available genetically engineered HBV vaccines was licensed in the United States; its immunogenicity was comparable to that of the plasma-derived vaccine. The recombinant vaccine is produced in *Saccharomyces cerevisiae* (bakers' yeast) into which a plasmid containing the gene for the HBV surface antigen has been inserted. When it is administered in a three-dose series, protective antibodies develop in more than 95% of healthy young adults. The schedule of administration includes an interval of 1 month between the first two doses and 5 months after the second.

Candidates to receive HBV vaccine include health care workers who were exposed through blood or needlesticks, patients and staff in institutions for developmentally disabled persons, hemodialysis patients, homosexually active men, users of illicit injectable drugs, recipients of certain blood products, and household members and sexual contacts of HBV carriers. Vaccine should be considered for prisoners, heterosexually active persons, and international travelers to HBV endemic areas.

In November 1991, the ACIP determined that routine infant HBV vaccination would be the most effective means to prevent HBV spread in the United States.[25] The committee recommended that HBV vaccine be universally administered to infants born to HBV surface antigen–negative mothers. Three doses of vaccine before 18 months of age are recommended: the first dose is given between birth and 2 months of age; the second, 1 to 2 months later; and the third, at 6 to 18 months of age. Vaccination is recommended for all 11- to 12-year-old children who have not previously received HBV vaccine.

A combination of HBIG and HBV vaccine provides immediate and durable protection for exposed persons. Transmission of perinatal HBV infection can be prevented in infants born to HBV surface antigen–positive mothers if HBIG is given within 12 hours after birth followed by HBV vaccine shortly after birth. A combination of HBIG and HBV vaccine should be administered to previously unvaccinated persons who have percutaneous exposure to blood that contains or might contain this antigen.

Hepatitis A Vaccine

Hepatitis A vaccine was approved by the FDA in February 1995. The vaccine is prepared in human cell culture, purified, and inactivated with formalin. The adult schedule is an initial intramuscular injection followed by a booster 6 to 12 months later. The pediatric formulation recommended for children 2 to 18 years of age is two intramuscular doses 1 month apart followed by a booster dose 6 to 12 months after the first dose. In clinical trials in Thailand and the United States, the vaccine was 90% and 100% effective.[26] Local reactions may occur but systemic reactions are rare. The vaccine should prove of value for military personnel, travelers to endemic areas, and groups in endemic areas such as Alaskan Natives, Native Americans, intravenous drug users, daycare center employees, health care personnel, workers at institutions for people with mental retardation, and possibly other workers in high-risk areas such as prisons, sewerage, and dietary professions. If immediate protection is needed against hepatitis A, intramuscular IG, 0.02 mL/kg, should be administered. The vaccine should displace the periodic use of IG for travelers and military personnel who spend variable periods in endemic areas.

Rabies Vaccine

Although the number of human rabies cases in the United States has ranged from zero to five per year, approximately 25,000 persons receive rabies prophylaxis. The rabies vaccine currently available in the United States is prepared by growing fixed rabies virus in human diploid cell cultures and subsequently inactivating it. Vaccine induces an active immune response that requires about 7 to 10 days to develop and persists for a year or more. Postexposure prophylaxis consists of local treatment of wounds, vaccination, and use of rabies-specific IG.

Physicians should consult local or state public health officials for current information about endemic rabies in the area. Use of rabies vaccine depends on the species of biting animal, the circumstances of the bite (penetration of the skin), and the type of exposure (provoked or not). In the United States, carnivorous wild animals (skunks, raccoons, foxes, and coyotes) are the animals most often infected. The chance of a domestic dog or cat being infected varies by region. Rodents (squirrels, hamsters, guinea pigs, gerbils, rats, and mice) are rarely infected and have not been known to cause human rabies in the United States. Rabies vaccine is used prophylactically by members of high-risk populations such as veterinarians. Because of the long incubation period, vaccine is also effective when given after exposure.

Yellow Fever Vaccine

Yellow fever is enzootic in some sylvatic areas in South America, and virus has been isolated from mosquitoes on Trinidad. Yellow fever vaccine is recommended for travelers 9 months of age or older who are likely to visit endemic areas. The vaccine is prepared in eggs; precautions noted before for measles, mumps, and influenza virus vaccines should be considered for patients with egg allergy.

Bacterial Vaccines for Special Populations and Special Indications

Anthrax Vaccine

A cell-free vaccine is available for persons at risk of acquiring anthrax. The vaccine is prepared from sterile filtrates of cultures of an attenuated unencapsulated strain of *Bacillus anthracis*. The current product induces an immune response in more than 90% of those who receive two doses, but the duration of immunity is relatively brief; three boosters at 6-month intervals followed by annual boosters is recommended. Routine immunization is recommended for workers who handle potentially contaminated animal products, including wool, goat hair, hides, and bones from countries in which animal anthrax is present. Laboratory workers who come in contact with *B. anthracis* should be immunized. The vaccine is available from the Division of Biologic Products of the Michigan Department of Public Health in Lansing.

Bacille Calmette-Guérin

BCG prepared from a strain of *Mycobacterium bovis* attenuated through serial passage in culture was first administered to humans in 1921. Current vaccines vary because of changes in the bacterial strains and different methods of production. Vaccines available in the United States have been evaluated only for their ability to produce delayed hypersensitivity. Vaccine efficacy remains a subject of controversy. A large controlled trial in Madras, India, with a 15-year follow-up failed to identify any difference in the rate of pulmonary tuberculosis among persons who were immunized with BCG and those who received placebo.[27]

In the United States, the ACIP recommends that tuberculosis is best controlled by effective case detection, chemotherapy, and preventive therapy. Although in prior years BCG had been recommended for health care workers in endemic areas, current policy is to provide protection by periodic skin testing rather than BCG. BCG should be considered for certain infants and children whose skin test results are negative and who are likely to be exposed to infectious contacts who may not have received adequate therapy. In addition, BCG should be considered for infants and children of groups in which the rate of new infection exceeds 1% per year and for whom usual surveillance and treatment programs have limited efficacy. Because rare complications of osteomyelitis and disseminated BCG infection have been reported in patients with HIV and other forms of immunodeficiency, BCG should be administered to these patients.

Cholera Vaccine

Cholera vaccines prepared from classic or *eltor* strains provide limited protection. Current vaccines provide only about 50% efficacy in reducing the incidence of clinical illness, and protection is limited to 3 to 6 months after immunization. Immunization does not prevent transmission of infection.

Because of its minimal efficacy, the World Health Organization no longer recommends cholera vaccination for travelers to or from cholera-affected areas. Some countries still require cholera vaccination for entry.

Plague Vaccine

A plague vaccine was prepared before 1900. Today, an inactivated whole-cell bacterial vaccine is used in persons whose vocations (geologist, laboratory worker) are likely to bring them into contact with infected rodents or their fleas, and it is recommended for travelers to areas where plague is occurring and domestic rats are known to be infected.

Salmonella typhi *Vaccine*

Three typhoid vaccines are available for use in the United States. A parenteral vaccine that is a heat- and phenol-inactivated whole-cell *S. typhi* vaccine (initially developed in the 1890s) produces protective serum antibodies. An orally administered live attenuated vaccine is available for children 6 years of age and older (data about efficacy in children younger than age 6 years are unavailable) and adults. The oral vaccine is derived from a stable mutant of the Ty21a strain of *S. typhi* and induces both intestinal and serum antibodies to *S. typhi* lipopolysaccharide. The third vaccine is a newly licensed capsular polysaccharide vaccine for parenteral administration. An acetone-inactivated parenteral vaccine is available but is used only in the armed forces.

The vaccines produce a comparable but limited degree of protection, which can be overcome by the ingestion of a large inoculum of *S. typhi.* For example, two trials of the oral vaccine in Chilean schoolchildren resulted in reduction of infection by 66% during 5 years in one trial but only 33% during 3 years in a second trial.[28]

Side effects of the heat-inactivated parenteral vaccine, including fever and local pain and swelling, are frequent, and the efficacy is not greater than that of the oral vaccine or the vaccine prepared from capsular polysaccharide. Thus, the latter two products with fewer reported side effects are the more acceptable ones. Indications for vaccination include travel to areas where typhoid fever is endemic and a recognized risk of exposure will occur, intimate exposure to a documented typhoid fever carrier, and frequent contact with the organism in laboratory work.

The schedule for the oral vaccine is one capsule taken four times on alternate days. The primary vaccination with the polysaccharide vaccine is one dose intramuscularly. The vaccine is not recommended for children younger than 2 years of age. The schedule for the parenteral inactivated vaccine consists of two subcutaneous injections separated by 4 weeks. Thus, for travelers who are leaving for endemic areas in the near future, the schedule for the oral vaccine and the parenteral polysaccharide vaccine is more useful. Because the oral vaccine is prepared with live bacteria, it is not recommended for persons who are immune deficient.

Immune Globulins

Intramuscular Immune Globulin

IG is derived from the pooled plasma of adults and consists principally of immunoglobulin G with trace amounts of immunoglobulins A and M. At least 1000 donors contribute to the final product, and the specific antibodies of each lot reflect the infectious and immunization experience of the donors. IG is administered by the intramuscular route and achieves peak serum levels within 72 hours after inoculation. The half-life of IG is about 23 days. It has demonstrated efficacy when used early enough to prevent infection or ameliorate disease due to measles and hepatitis A and for replacement therapy in patients with antibody-deficiency disorders.

Intravenous Immune Globulin

Intravenous IG is prepared from pooled adult plasma and is modified to make it suitable for intravenous use. Current indications include replacement therapy in antibody deficiency disorders, idiopathic thrombocytopenic purpura, and Kawasaki disease as well as for prophylaxis in patients with chronic lymphocytic leukemia and bone marrow transplantation. Conflicting or incomplete data for prophylactic use of intravenous IG are available for neonates, pediatric patients with acquired immunodeficiency syndrome, and critical care and surgery patients.[29] Although this product is considered safe, cases of hepatitis C associated with the administration of commercially available intravenous IG indicate that use of all human-derived products entails some risk.[30]

Specific Immune Globulins

Specific IGs are prepared from donors known to have high titers of the desired antibody. Available specific IGs are HBIG, rabies IG, TIG, varicella-zoster IG, and respiratory syncytial virus IG.

HBIG is administered as soon as possible after birth to infants of mothers who are "HB antigen–positive." Simultaneous administration of HBIG and hepatitis vaccine does not diminish the infant's response to the vaccine. Other uses of HBIG include percutaneous (needlestick) inoculation of a susceptible individual from a known carrier.

Rabies IG is administered with rabies vaccine as soon as possible after exposure (regardless of the interval between exposure and treatment). One dose is administered to provide immediate antibodies until the patient responds to the vaccine.

TIG is used to manage severe and contaminated wounds of patients whose primary immunization series with tetanus toxoid is either unknown or incomplete.

Administration of varicella-zoster IG is recommended after a significant exposure: household contact, playmate contact of more than 1 hour indoors, hospital exposure of prolonged face-to-face contact, or newborn infant of mother with onset of varicella 5 days or less before delivery or within 48 hours after delivery. Its use should be considered after such exposures for the following groups: immunodeficient children, normal susceptible adolescents and adults, newborn infants of mothers who had onset of varicella within 5 days of delivery or within 4 hours after delivery, premature infants of more than 28 weeks' gestational age whose mothers lack a history of varicella, and premature infants of less than 28 weeks' gestational age regardless of maternal history.

Respiratory syncytial virus IG has been demonstrated to be valuable for prophylaxis of but not therapy for respiratory syncytial virus disease. Children who received respiratory syncytial virus IG monthly during the respiratory syncytial virus season had fewer infections, hospitalizations, and hospital days.[31, 32] Respiratory syncytial virus IG was not effective for therapy of children who were hospitalized with respiratory syncytial virus lower respiratory tract infection.[33]

References

1. Plotkin SA, Mortimer EA Jr (eds): Vaccines, ed 2. Philadelphia, WB Saunders, 1994.
2. Immunization Practices Advisory Committee: Recommended childhood immunization schedule—United States, 1997. MMWR Morbid Mortal Wkly Rep 46:35–40, 1997.
3. Immunization Practices Advisory Committee: General recommendations on immunization. MMWR Morbid Mortal Wkly Rep 38:223, 1989.
4. Immunization Practices Advisory Committee: Immunization of children infected with human immunodeficiency virus—Supplementary ACIP statement. MMWR Morbid Mortal Wkly Rep 37:181–183, 1988.
5. Centers for Disease Control and Prevention: Summary of notifiable diseases, United States, 1987. MMWR Morbid Mortal Wkly Rep 36:5–59, 1989.
6. Maple PA, Efstratiou A, George RC, et al: Diphtheria immunity in UK blood donors. Lancet 345:936–965, 1995.
7. Centers for Disease Control and Prevention: Diphtheria epidemic—New independent states of the former Soviet Union, 1990–1994. MMWR Morbid Mortal Wkly Rep 44(10):177–181, 1995.
8. Centers for Disease Control and Prevention: Tetanus—United States, 1985–1986. MMWR Morbid Mortal Wkly Rep 36:477–481, 1987.
9. Gergen PJ, McQuillan GM, Kiely M, et al: A population-based serologic survey of immunity to tetanus in the United States. N Engl J Med 332:761–766, 1995.
10. Cody CL, Baraff LJ, Cherry JD, et al: Nature and rates of adverse reactions associated with DTP and DT immunizations in infants and children. Pediatrics 68:650–660, 1981.
11. Mortimer EA Jr: Pertussis vaccine. *In* Plotkin SA, Mortimer EA Jr (eds): Vaccine. Philadelphia, WB Saunders, 1988.
12. Committee on Infectious Diseases: Acellular pertussis vaccine: Recommendations for use as the initial series in infants and children. Pediatrics 99:282–288, 1997.
13. Wright SW, Edwards KM, Decker MD, Zeldin MH: Pertussis infection in adults with persistent cough. JAMA 273:1044–1046, 1995.
14. Edwards KM, Decker MD, Graham BS, et al: Adult immunization with acellular pertussis vaccine. JAMA 269:53–56, 1993.
15. Immunization Practices Advisory Committee: Measles prevention: Recommendations of the Immunization Practices Advisory Committee (ACIP). MMWR Morbid Mortal Wkly Rep 38(Suppl 9):1–18, 1989.
16. Cochi SL, Preblud SR, Orenstein WA: Perspectives on the relative resurgence of mumps in the United States. Am J Dis Child 142:499–507, 1988.
17. Centers for Disease Control and Prevention: Rubella vaccination during pregnancy—United States, 1971–1988. MMWR Morbid Mortal Wkly Rep 38:289–293, 1989.
18. Committee on Infectious Diseases, American Academy of Pediatrics: Poliomyelitis prevention: Recommendations for the use of inactivated poliovirus vaccine and live oral poliovirus vaccine. Pediatrics 99:300–305, 1997.
19. Committee on Infectious Disease: Recommendations for the use of live attenuated varicella vaccine. Pediatrics 95:791–796, 1995.
20. Mortimer EA: Efficacy of *Haemophilus* b polysaccharide vaccine: An enigma. JAMA 260:1454–1455, 1988.
21. Osterholm MT, Rambeck JH, White KE, et al: Lack of efficacy of *Haemophilus* b polysaccharide vaccine in Minnesota. JAMA 260:1423–1428, 1988.
22. Murphy TV, Granoff DM, Chrane RN, et al: Pharyngeal colonization with *Haemophilus influenzae* type b in children in a day care center without invasive disease. J Pediatr 106:712–716, 1985.
23. Mohle-Boetani JC, Ajello G, Breneman E, et al: Carriage of *Haemophilus influenzae* type b in children after widespread vaccination with conjugate *Haemophilus influenzae* type b vaccines. Pediatr Infect Dis J 12:589–593, 1993.
24. Centers for Disease Control and Prevention: Prevention and control of influenza: Recommendations of the Advisory Committee on Immunization Practices (ACIP). MMWR Morbid Mortal Wkly Rep 44(RR-3):1–22, 1995.
25. ACIP: Hepatitis B virus: A comprehensive strategy for eliminating transmission in the United States through universal childhood vaccination. MMWR Morbid Mortal Wkly Rep 40(RR-13):1–19, 1991.
26. Innis BL, Snitbhan R, Kunasol P, et al: Protection against hepatitis A by an inactivated vaccine. JAMA 271:1328–1334, 1994.
27. Tripathy SP: Fifteen-year follow-up of the Indian BCG prevention trial. Proceedings of the XXVIth IUAT World Conference on Tuberculosis and Respiratory Diseases. Singapore, Professional Postgraduate Services, International, 1987. (Cited in MMWR Morbid Mortal Wkly Rep 37:674, 1988.)
28. Levine MM, Ferreccio C, Black RE, et al: Large-scale field trial of Ty21a live oral typhoid vaccine in enteric-coated capsule formulation. Lancet 329:1049–1052, 1987.
29. Pennington JE: Newer uses of intravenous immunoglobulins as anti-infective agents. Antimicrob Agents Chemother 34:1463–1466, 1990.
30. Bjoro K, Frøland SS, Yun Z, et al: Hepatitis C infection in patients with primary hypogammaglobulinemia after treatment with contaminated immune globulin. N Engl J Med 331:1607–1611, 1994.
31. Groothuis JR, Simoes EAF, Levin MJ, et al: Prophylactic administration of respiratory syncytial virus immune globulin to high-risk infants and young children. N Engl J Med 329:1524–1530, 1993.
32. PREVENT Study Group: Reduction of respiratory syncytial virus hospitalization among premature infants and infants with bronchopulmonary dysplasia using respiratory syncytial virus immune globulin prophylaxis. Pediatrics 99:93–99, 1997.
33. Rodriguez WJ, Gruber WC, Welliver RC, et al: Respiratory syncytial virus (RSV) immune globulin intravenous therapy for RSV lower respiratory tract infection in infants and young children at high risk for severe RSV infection. Pediatrics 99:454–461, 1997.

42

Control of Nosocomial Infections

Donald A. Goldmann
Richard Platt
Cyrus C. Hopkins

Organization and Responsibilities of the Infection Control Program

Controlling nosocomial infection is not easy, as any hospital epidemiologist or infection control practitioner would attest.

Anyone can write policies. Implementation is another matter altogether, requiring at least as much art and cunning as science and epidemiology. Practitioners of this art must be confident yet humble, watchful yet unobtrusive, ready to act but patient, strong yet flexible. They must be eager to teach but willing to listen, bold enough to be critical yet willing to accept criticism. Seldom are they thanked; frequently they are blamed. Their beeper batteries wear out fastest, and so do the soles of their shoes.

To be effective, the infection control team must weave itself into the fabric of the hospital. Perhaps more than any other hospital department, infection control involves everyone, from the president to the housekeeper, from the chief of surgery to the central supply worker who washes surgical instruments, from the head of fiscal affairs to the discharge diagnosis coder. A successful infection control program usually reflects a well-governed hospital; a poorly governed hospital makes infection control difficult and prone to failure. Increasingly, infection control is being viewed as part of the hospital's overall quality improvement program. Infection control's emphasis on multidisciplinary, interdepartmental teamwork and data-driven improvement provides a useful model for hospital quality improvement programs, and many infection control professionals have expanded their responsibilities to include outcomes of care other than nosocomial infections.

These days, the task of infection control professionals is even more difficult because, like almost everyone else in the modern hospital, they are likely to be judged by their impact on the financial bottom line. Hospital administrators are increasingly requiring fiscal accountability and objective measures of success. The infection control profession itself has increasingly emphasized the need to set goals and measure outcomes, but it may be extremely difficult to document the benefits and savings conferred by an effective infection control program in an individual hospital. For example, it is impossible to quantitate accurately savings from problems that do not occur, such as lawsuits, epidemics, and days lost by personnel because of exposure to contagious diseases. Moreover, apparent reductions in infection rates may be difficult to attribute to specific infection control interventions without performing time-consuming, complex clinical studies, which themselves would be costly. Even if adequate resources and expertise are available for such investigations, many studies require sample sizes that are unrealistic for most institutions. Fortunately, compelling evidence for the overall cost-effectiveness of infection control programs is available in the literature.[1] Nevertheless, as the pressure to produce tangible evidence of success intensifies, one fears that precious resources will be diverted from protecting patients from infection to nonproductive activities, such as defending turf from administrators and justifying the value of the program. At its worst, overly aggressive fiscal scrutiny encourages defensive practices and selective reporting of data rather than innovative, cost-conscious initiatives and solutions.

Structure

The structure and responsibilities of the infection control program have been described in detail in standard references,[2–6] so only the most important features are summarized here. The program must first be empowered by the hospital administration and medical staff executive committee. The Joint Commission on Accreditation of Health Care Organizations (JCAHO) recommends that the authority of the infection control program be delineated clearly in the hospital bylaws. Specifically, the infection control team should be able to initiate whatever actions are necessary to reduce the risk of nosocomial infection. These include measures as simple as obtaining cultures from patients or removing employees with contagious diseases from the workplace to those as dramatic as closing a ward to stem an epidemic.

In general, the infection control program should be headed by a physician with specific training in infection control and hospital epidemiology. Physician leadership is critical for implementation of control measures that involve the medical staff, as nonphysician infection control personnel who have locked horns with a stubborn department chairperson know well. Training in epidemiology is becoming increasingly important, not only to design studies and to interpret data but also to supervise today's sophisticated infection control practitioners. Regrettably, only a small minority of programs are headed by a physician with any formal training whatsoever in hospital epidemiology, and there is little evidence that medical training programs are taking the steps required to rectify this situation.

Contemporary infection control programs have a wide range of responsibilities that may be supported most efficiently by a committee representing a broad spectrum of hospital departments. Two formats of committee structure are commonly encountered. In one, a large, multidisciplinary committee assembles for every meeting. This arrangement promotes dialogue and educates members about issues outside their area of expertise, but meetings can be inefficient and difficult to manage unless carefully planned by a smaller "executive" group, usually including the infection control personnel. Alternatively, this smaller executive group is itself defined as the committee and meets regularly to review general epidemiologic data and routine activities but supplements its membership ad hoc with personnel as required by specific topics on the agenda. Such committees tend to be focused and efficient but may lack the democratic atmosphere and unexpected insights that come with broad representation. Whichever format is chosen, permanent or ad hoc committee members should include representatives from the major clinical services, the nursing department, central supply, hospital engineering, environmental services, the dietary department, diagnostic microbiology, quality improvement and risk management, administration, pharmacy, employee health service, and others as dictated by local circumstances. Because active dialogue with individuals representing all facets of the hospital is essential, members of the infection control team should also serve on a variety of other key committees, such as nursing policy and practice, quality improvement, pharmacy and therapeutics, and product evaluation and procurement. Infection control personnel should also provide consultation and direction for relevant activities of the employee health service, as outlined later in this chapter. The infection control committee should participate in the drafting of general visitation policy and may have to impose additional restrictions on visitors in the event of an outbreak of measles, rubella, or other highly contagious disease in the community or hospital. No renovation or construction activity should commence in the hospital and its immediate environs without prior review by infection control to evaluate the potential risk of airborne fungal disease to the population of immunosuppressed patients. Participation in planning and implementation of hospital information systems is critical, particularly as infection control needs tend to be, at best, an afterthought. A strong liaison with public relations is important in the event that news of a hospital infection control problem reaches the ear of the press.

A formal, ongoing relationship with the microbiology laboratory is essential, as microbiology is the backbone of many surveillance and control activities.[7–9] Laboratory policies and procedures should be developed with the specific needs of infection control in mind, and reports must be both timely and relevant. Criteria should be developed for immediate ("stat") reporting of specific isolates to infection control. The laboratory director should be consulted about the selection of customized screening tests or special typing systems to assist in case finding during epidemic investigations. It is prudent to establish policies for saving specific strains of epidemiologic interest (for example, *Staphylococcus aureus* isolates from surgical wound infections or bacteria resistant to multiple antibiotics) in case more sophisticated microbiologic characterization is necessary at a later date. The laboratory director should ensure that sufficient fiscal and technical resources are available in the event that unexpected infection control problems place additional burdens on the laboratory.

Surveillance

(Table 42–1)

Traditionally, infection control programs have been obsessed with surveillance. This preoccupation can be explained in large measure by the powerful influence of the Centers for Disease Control and Prevention (CDC), which imposed a public health model of surveillance onto a hospital base. Further support for surveillance, which hospital administrators could hardly resist, came from the JCAHO. It was JCAHO standards that forced many hospitals to create an infection control program in the first place, and in the formative years of the profession, JCAHO inspectors placed much emphasis on comprehensive surveillance. According to guidelines disseminated by the CDC and adopted by the JCAHO, infection control practitioners were exhorted to go to the bedside to be certain that only clinically verifiable infections, as opposed to colonizing organisms, were counted. Postdischarge surveillance has been added to the practitioner's plate as lengths of stay have shortened and ambulatory surgery has increased.

The assumption underlying this inordinately labor-intensive surveillance was that knowledge of the specific nosocomial infection patterns in an institution would suggest avenues for intervention and control. Although this may have been true in part, surveillance tended to become an end in itself, and the resulting unmanageable volume of data often proved no more valuable than the culturing of countertops, carpets, and noses that it replaced. In retrospect, those who gathered and regurgitated this information at monthly infection control meetings have been criticized as being incredibly naive, particularly if they did not develop a strategic plan for translating their notebooks full of data into effective control activities.

The perceived role of surveillance as a guide to infection control has undergone considerable evolution. It is now recognized that one of the major benefits of surveillance has little to do with the detection of infections. Rather, surveillance provides an excuse for infection control practitioners to visit the wards on a regular basis. This greatly facilitates informal continuing education of clinical personnel, permits unobtrusive monitoring of compliance with infection control policies and procedures, and provides staff with an opportunity to ask questions.

Although surveillance of all areas of the hospital does bring practitioners onto the wards, few programs have the resources to perform such comprehensive total surveillance, particularly in an era of shrinking health care resources. The trick is to target specific groups of patients for intensive surveillance. Sophisticated computerized systems have been described that can accomplish this task,[10] but these systems are not available in the vast majority of hospitals. As described in Chapter 11, surveillance ofnosocomial pneumonia is important because this infection occurs frequently, increases length of stay and hospital costs, and is associated with high morbidity and mortality rates. Moreover, it is clear that the patients at highest risk for nosocomial pneumonia are those who require mechanical ventilation in an intensive care unit (ICU). Further exploration of risk factors for pneumonia might suggest additional criteria for focused surveillance, such as thoracoabdominal surgery or immunosuppressive therapy. The development of scoring systems for assessing severity of illness may provide future information about potential risk, although most of these systems have

TABLE 42–1 ■ Surveillance Strategies

STRATEGY	DATA SOURCES	ADVANTAGES	DISADVANTAGES
Comprehensive, total hospital-wide surveillance	Medical records, nursing notes or Kardex, staff interviews, bedside examination, laboratory results	Gives view of whole hospital, revealing areas of greatest concern Provides baseline data for all areas Brings infection control team to all wards, increasing visibility and facilitating education	Extremely labor-intensive Detracts from ability to perform intensive surveillance, intervention, and control efforts in specific problem areas
Targeted surveillance	Same as for comprehensive surveillance	Concentrates resources on highest risk patients, most costly or serious infections, and alterable problems Facilitates careful, thorough data collection on selected problems, permitting evaluation of impact of interventions	New problems in previously quiescent areas may be missed Visibility of infection control in nontargeted areas is decreased Overall performance of the hospital's infection control effort may be difficult to document
Laboratory-based surveillance	Microbiology records, other diagnostic tests (e.g., results of urinalyses, chest films)	Permits detection of the emergence of new pathogens or antibiotic resistance before clinical infection is widespread Facilitates selective surveillance	Relies on adequate culturing of patients Requires computerization for maximal efficiency If overemphasized, places personnel behind a desk instead of on the wards

not been validated extensively as predictors for nosocomial infections per se.[11] Thus, it should be possible to narrow the focus of surveillance considerably. However, even with focused surveillance, the goal must remain prevention of disease, not just counting infections.

Progressive reductions in the length of hospital stay have complicated nosocomial infection surveillance, particularly for surgical wound infections.[12] More than 50% of infections complicating clean surgery occur after discharge. Such infections can be difficult and labor-intensive to track. Similarly, the incubation period for neonatal nosocomial staphylococcal infection is considerably longer than a 1- to 2-day hospital stay for well infants.

Objective, consistent, workable definitions of infection are fundamental to good surveillance. If the case definition is chosen casually or applied haphazardly, the most compulsive data collection and the most sophisticated data analysis are incapable of rescuing the surveillance project. Generally accepted definitions, along with comments regarding their reliability and limitations, are discussed in Chapter 11.

Impact of Surveillance on Control of Infections

Even if the infection control team arrives at a sound definition and conducts surveillance according to the strictest standards, it may not be possible to translate the results of this surveillance into effective infection control activities. For example, results of the Study on the Efficacy of Nosocomial Infection Control (SENIC) suggest that although nosocomial pneumonia may have the most serious consequences for hospitalized patients, it is the least amenable to intensive surveillance and control efforts.[13] In addition, patients in the highest risk groups often have serious underlying diseases, the longest lengths of stay, and the greatest dependence on the devices and procedures that increase their risk. Such patients are not likely to be responsive even to the most aggressive control measures.

Despite these caveats concerning the global impact of surveillance programs on some types of nosocomial infection, it is still possible for careful analysis of surveillance data to suggest targets for specific infection control action. This process of setting new goals based on analysis of surveillance data has been called "surveillance by objectives."[14] The parallel assumption that rational, focused surveillance will lead to effective intervention and control is at the heart of contemporary quality improvement philosophy as expounded by the JCAHO in its agenda for change, which advocates universal monitoring of key outcome indicators, such as ICU pneumonia, wound infections after clean surgery, and nosocomial bacteremia.[15] Theoretically, the resulting rates can be compared with some standard or threshold rate, although in practice it may be difficult to define an acceptable or ideal goal for an individual hospital based only on results from other institutions, and this should be considered only if careful consideration of adjustment for severity of illness or other risk factors is included.[6, 11, 16]

Surely, however, if focused surveillance demonstrates a dramatic increase in the incidence of *Pseudomonas* pneumonia among patients in a respiratory ICU, further investigation might uncover contamination of nebulized medications. This common-source outbreak could then be terminated by simple, well-documented control measures, such as using unit-dose medication vials. Unfortunately, this kind of "soap-opera" epidemiology probably occurs rarely. Many outbreaks are immediately recognized by the nurses and physicians who care for the affected patients and who have an informal but highly sensitive system for comparing their current experience with their own expectations. Moreover, most nosocomial infection problems are endemic. Cases tend to occur sporadically and in relatively low numbers. Except in the largest institutions, such problems may be difficult to recognize, even assuming that the appropriate epidemiologic and biostatistical tools are available. Small deviations from the baseline infection rate may not be recognized as significant unless the baseline period of observation is quite long and the number of events is relatively large. Recognition of this critical limitation of surveillance cuts to the quick of the current quality improvement strategy, which assumes that continuous monitoring of key indicators detects events that are occurring at a rate greater than the expected variance in the baseline rate. In addition, important trends can be overlooked unless the data being captured are sufficiently specific. For example, detection of a nationwide epidemic of *Enterobacter agglomerans* bacteremia caused by contaminated intravenous fluid was delayed substantially both by failure of laboratories to identify this unusual pathogen correctly and by failure of infection control teams to look beyond the overall incidence of bacteremia to pathogen-specific bacteremia rates.[17] In our own neonatal ICUs, the role of lipids in the pathogenesis of coagulase-negative staphylococcal bacteremia would not have been appreciated had infection control personnel concentrated on collecting data about the most widely publicized risk factor for such infections, central venous catheterization.[18] Even if data on hyperalimentation had been recorded, the critical association would have been missed unless intravenous nutritional supplementation was subdivided into protein or lipid infusions for analysis. Regardless of the nature of the specific problem under investigation, exquisite analysis of raw data is often required, along with adjustment for severity of illness and consideration of potential confounding variables[11] (see Chapter 11).

Effect of Feedback of Surveillance Data to Caregivers

The SENIC study suggested that publicizing surveillance data can have a salutary effect on infection rates and that it is the process itself of feeding back the data that leads to the benefit, not a specific outcome-based control strategy.[13] Even if this is true, there may be many alternative reasons why infection control problems seem to wane with time, and the SENIC thesis is not universally accepted. In any case, it seems clear that the impact of surveillance data on clinical practice can be maximized by discussing the methodology and goals of the surveillance program with the relevant clinical services in advance and organizing the data in a clear and palatable format. Conversely, the infection control program that fails to respond to the requests and preferences of the clinical staff or to work with them collaboratively is inviting disaster. The Surgical Infection Society, for example, has suggested that surgeon-specific infection rates would be generated in a more timely fashion if the surgeons themselves controlled the surveillance process.[19, 20] This might improve ascertainment of infections that occur after discharge and promote involvement of surgeons in the infection control process, but it clearly does not provide an unbiased source of data.

All agree, however, that dialogue is paramount. Without it, surveillance by objectives and outcome measurement may be seen as nothing more than the tools for administrative policing. With it, there is hope for consensus, cooperation, and improvement in quality of care. Indeed, the so-called total quality management model is oriented toward a continuous systematic, multidisciplinary, interactive search for solutions to shared problems.[21] It recognizes that institutional problems, including nosocomial infections, are likely to be complex and multifactorial and be solved best by a collaborative effort that crosses the usual institutional hierarchical reporting lines. In industrial terms, the goal is not to keep trying to extirpate defects after they occur but to engage the energies and intellects of the entire work force in trying to prevent defects from occurring in the first place.

Role of Microbiology in Surveillance and Control

Laboratory-Based Surveillance

If the object of surveillance is to permit control of the spread of nosocomial organisms at the earliest possible moment, microbiology laboratory–based surveillance may be an important supplement to patient-oriented surveillance of clinically verifiable infections.[22] A decade ago, when there was evidence that many infectious agents remained uncultured, this strategy would have been heresy. Today, the problem is not too few cultures but rather too many, particularly from sites such as wounds and the respiratory tract. Of course, many of the organisms isolated from these cultures do not reflect infections but represent only contaminants, saprophytes, or components of the normal microbial flora; however, intelligent review of these data may permit the alert epidemiologist to spot the emergence and spread of bacteria that may later turn out to be significant problems for the infection control team. Timely detection of bacteria that have acquired resistance to antibiotics that are generally used empirically at a given institution is particularly important. For example, it is considerably easier to contain a strain of ceftazidime-resistant *Klebsiella*, methicillin-resistant *S. aureus*, or vancomycin-resistant enterococcus if it has colonized only a few patients. Were the epidemiologist to wait for an outbreak of clinical infections to occur, the antimicrobial-resistant pathogen may well have spread throughout the ward and perhaps to other areas of the hospital, making control an expensive, disruptive, and possibly fruitless pursuit.

If a specific problem of antibiotic resistance is under investigation, an efficient way to facilitate detection of resistant bacteria is to use selective, antibiotic-containing media. In some cases, routine surveillance for the emergence of strains resistant to critical antibiotics that are components of empirical regimens may be considered, especially in intensive care and other high-risk areas of the hospital. For example, methicillin-resistant staphylococci can usually be detected by using mannitol salt agar containing oxacillin at 6 μg/mL. Alternatively, cultures can be enriched by inoculating a nutrient broth before plating on the selective agar. Either method is considerably less expensive than conventional cultures, in terms of both media and labor. In the event of an outbreak, the hospital microbiologist may be able to suggest selective screening media that take advantage of the antibiotic resistance or metabolic requirements of a specific strain.

Advances in Epidemiologically Useful Microbiology Techniques

Advances in microbiology have had a large impact on the nature of surveillance. This has been particularly striking in virology. A decade ago, surveillance for viral disease was based almost entirely on clinical criteria. Few hospitals had clinical virology laboratories, and the available virologic techniques were labor-intensive, slow, and relatively insensitive in most cases. If the best an infection control practitioner had to offer was "Looks like a respiratory viral infection," it is no wonder that documentation of viral nosocomial infection was eschewed. However, exquisitely sensitive, technically straightforward, rapid viral diagnostic tests have become commercially available for many of the agents that commonly cause nosocomial infection. This technologic revolution makes surveillance for nosocomial viral infections practical for the first time. Such viral surveillance is more than just a novel luxury for some areas of the hospital, such as infant wards of pediatric services where respiratory syncytial virus (RSV) and rotavirus may account for the large majority of infections and considerable infection-related morbidity.

New molecular microbiology techniques, although generally available only in reference centers, have also facilitated the control of nosocomial infection.[9, 22] Previously, the armamentarium of microbiologic tools available to the hospital epidemiologist to define the spread of pathogens in the hospital was somewhat limited. Conventional phenotyping techniques, such as speciation, antibiograms, biotyping, serotyping, phage typing, and bacteriocin typing, were useful in some situations but certainly not all. For example, antibiograms and biotyping were not useful in characterizing strains of *Staphylococcus epidermidis* in an outbreak of nosocomial prosthetic valve endocarditis at the Seattle Veterans Administration Hospital[23]; however, plasmid typing, coupled with a newly described system for phage typing of *S. epidermidis*, indicated that four patients had been infected by the same strain. Genotyping techniques may be even more helpful in answering complex epidemiologic questions. Plasmid typing by agarose gel electrophoresis and restriction endonuclease analysis demonstrated that a plasmid mediating aminoglycoside resistance in gram-negative bacilli not only had spread in the Veterans Administration Hospital but also could be detected in a number of hospitals in the United States and abroad.[24, 25] The genes mediating production of the aminoglycoside-inactivating enzyme had been picked up by a transposon that had transferred them to a variety of plasmids carried by a broad range of gram-negative bacteria. The genes were cryptic in some strains, so that aminoglycoside-inactivating enzyme was not produced and antibiotic susceptibility testing could not betray the presence of the promiscuous transposon. Without probe technology, the extent of this "transposon epidemic" would not have been recognized. Pulsed-field gel electrophoresis of chromosomal DNA, random primer polymerase chain reaction, and ribotyping have emerged as powerful techniques for discriminating among nosocomial strains. Outbreaks of many viral illnesses can be similarly evaluated,[26] although such detailed analyses are infrequently necessary.

Fundamentals of Infection Control

Hand Washing

Efforts to control the transmission of infections in the hospital require a keen appreciation of how the infecting agents are spread. The principal mechanisms of transmission for key nosocomial pathogens are reviewed in Chapter 11. The most important factor in the spread of many nosocomial pathogens is contamination of the hands of hospital personnel. It follows that hand washing is at the heart of efforts to prevent cross-infection in the hospital. Most of the microorganisms that contaminate the hands of personnel are transient inhabitants of the skin and are removed by a brief hand wash. Occasionally, however, nosocomial bacteria, including gram-negative rods as well as gram-positive organisms, take up more long-lasting residence on the skin of the hands and become part of the resident cutaneous flora.[27] Hand washing may cleanse the surface of the skin in such cases, but it is not likely to terminate the carrier state.

Because hand washing plays a pivotal role in infection control, the choice of hand-washing agents and procedures is hotly debated, and detailed recommendations have been issued by the CDC[28] and by the Association for Professionals in Infection Control.[29] Hand washing after every contact with every patient is so time-consuming as to be impractical, and even the mildest hand-washing agent irritates the skin if used excessively. This is a substantial problem, not only because skin irritation reduces compliance but also because dermatitis probably encourages colonization of the skin of the hands with nosocomial pathogens. Caregivers must, therefore, exercise some degree of clinical judgment. For example, brief contact (such as taking a blood pressure reading) with a patient who has been admitted for elective surgery does not routinely require hand washing. On the other hand, even casual contact with a patient with dermatitis who is colonized with methicillin-resistant staphylococci clearly mandates hand washing. A trip to the sink is probably in order even if the caregiver touches only objects in the colonized patient's environment, because they are likely to be contaminated with methicillin-resistant staphylococci shed by the patient. Other pathogens likely to contaminate the environment of colonized or infected patients include vancomycin-resistant enterococci, *Clostridium difficile*, and RSV. Even when gloves are worn by the provider, the hands should be washed after removing the gloves, because pathogens can be found on the hands after removal of the gloves, even without a detectable leak.[30]

As for the hand-washing agent, plain soap and water are sufficient for general use because they remove most of the transient microbial flora. In critical care units, where the stakes are high and antibiotic-resistant bacteria may be prevalent, most authorities recommend using an antiseptic preparation, because bland soap is much less effective than antiseptic soap in killing antibiotic-resistant bacteria contaminating the hands.[31] The general recommendation that antiseptics should be used before performing invasive procedures or surgery has a strong rationale, if not convincing proof. Hexachlorophene should no longer be used, except perhaps for the specific control of a staphylococcal outbreak, because it is not effective against nosocomial gram-negative rods. Iodophors have excellent, prolonged antimicrobial activity against a broad spectrum of nosocomial pathogens but may product unacceptable skin irritation with frequent use. Contamination of iodophors with pseudomonads has been reported, but this problem does not occur frequently enough to discourage their use. Chlorhexidine gluconate in alcohol has excellent bactericidal activity as well as considerable residual activity on the skin. It appears to be much better tolerated than iodophors.[32] Triclosan also has a broad spectrum of bactericidal activity and a residual antibacterial effect.[33] The same properties that make iodophors and chlorhexidine gluconate in alcohol effective hand-washing agents have made them the favorites of surgeons for preoperative preparation of patients' skin.

Of course, a major impediment to hand washing is the lack of conveniently located sinks. Despite the obvious importance of hand washing to good care of patients, this remains a substantial problem on many wards. In such circumstances, "sinkless" hand-washing agents, such as alcohol or chlorhexidine gluconate with emollients, provide a satisfactory alternative to traditional hand-washing procedures. However, sinks should be a principal focus of any renovation project or new construction.

Isolation Systems

PREVIOUS CDC GUIDELINES

Formerly, most hospitals used an isolation system recommended by the CDC.[34] The original CDC guidelines recommended that hospitals adopt one of two general strategies for containing contagious diseases. In the category-specific system, diseases were grouped into categories of isolation based on their usual mode of transmission: strict isolation for diseases spread by both contact and the air (droplet nuclei); contact isolation for diseases spread by contact with the patient or the patient's contaminated environment; respiratory isolation for disease spread by close contact with large contaminated respiratory droplets; tuberculosis isolation for infections, such as tuberculosis, that are transmitted by airborne droplet nuclei; enteric precautions for diseases spread by the fecal-oral route; drainage-secretion precautions for infections spread by contact with purulent infective material; and blood and body fluid precautions for blood-borne diseases. Protective isolation was eventually deleted because a clinical trial showed no benefit for immunosuppressed patients.[35] In the disease-specific system, precautions were based on the known or suspected mode of transmission of individual infectious diseases, providing a more customized approach to isolation once the clinical picture and/or cultures suggested a specific diagnosis.

BODY SUBSTANCE ISOLATION

Some infection control specialists believed that the traditional CDC systems did not provide a mechanism for interrupting spread of pathogens from patients who did not have recognized infections or culture-demonstrated colonization. They noted that infection control practitioners spend an inordinate proportion of their professional lives trying to persuade their colleagues to wash their hands, often without success, even in high-risk areas of the hospital.[36] An alternative system of isolation, body substance isolation (BSI), represented a novel effort to cope with some of the difficulties presented by the traditional CDC systems.[37] In the BSI system, personnel are required to wear gloves when having contact with any potentially contaminated substance (e.g., excreta, secretions, fluids), as well as mucous membranes and nonintact skin of all hospitalized patients. Hand washing is still recommended after removal of the gloves but not after routine contacts with patients that do not require the use of gloves. If soiling of the clothes is likely, a gown is also donned, and suitable barriers are used if a splash in the face seems possible.

Theoretically, BSI has several advantages. First, gloves provide a barrier between the hands and nosocomial contaminants, so even if hand washing is neglected, there is a margin of safety. Second, BSI supplants most traditional isolation procedures, such as contact and enteric precautions, which basically rely on barrier techniques. Only airborne pathogens, such as *Mycobacterium tuberculosis*, and pathogens spread by large respiratory droplets, such as *Bordetella pertussis* and *Neisseria meningitidis*, require special precautions if BSI is employed. Third, compliance with gloving while personnel are in contact with patients should be much easier to monitor than compliance with hand washing, which is customarily performed after the fact and at a distance from the patient. Finally, if properly taught and implemented, BSI incorporates most of the standards mandated under universal precautions, as described in the following.

The efficacy of BSI remains to be demonstrated by appropriate investigations in a broad range of clinical settings. So far, evidence in support of this general concept is confined to a study in a pediatric ICU in which procedures similar to BSI—routine use of gloves and gowns for contact with patients—significantly reduced nosocomial bacterial colonization and infection.[38] However, gloves may provide a false sense of security and result in even less hand washing. Worse, caregivers might neglect to change gloves between patients. Because some pathogens, such as RSV, probably survive better on gloves than on skin[39] and bacteria may be difficult to remove from gloves even if the caregiver tries to wash the gloved hands,[40] nosocomial transmission of organisms could be facilitated.

UNIVERSAL PRECAUTIONS

Universal precautions are now mandated by the Occupational Safety and Health Administration (OSHA), largely to protect health care workers from blood-borne agents, especially the human immunodeficiency virus and hepatitis B and C viruses. Universal precautions were originally designed to apply CDC's previous blood and body fluid precautions universally to all patients, but CDC recommendations[41] broadened the scope of these guidelines to apply to nonintact skin and mucosal surfaces and to many other body fluids, such as pleural, pericardial, and cerebrospinal fluids and any fluid that contains visible blood. Like BSI, universal precautions rely on the use of barrier techniques. They have specifically been shown to decrease the risk of exposure to blood and body fluids.[42]

It is important to note that universal precautions were implemented to protect personnel, not to prevent the transmission of nosocomial pathogens from patient to patient. If this is the message and caregivers think of gloves only in terms of self-protection, they may be less inclined to worry about cross-infection and the importance of changing gloves between contacts with patients. Rigorous adherence to BSI might bring the focus back to the patient while still protecting personnel and satisfying regulators. Moreover, BSI would protect workers concerned about exposure to microscopic amounts of blood in urine or feces or leukocytes present in a draining wound, although there has been no evidence to date that such exposures are hazardous.

CURRENT CDC RECOMMENDATIONS

A new set of recommendations from the CDC may lead to greater consensus.[43] In the new guidelines for isolation precautions, which are likely to become widely accepted, a category of "standard precautions" is described, which is applied to all patients and is the "primary strategy for successful nosocomial infection control." This category synthesizes the major features of the previously defined universal precautions (for blood and body fluids) and BSI. These precautions apply to blood, all body fluids, secretions and excretions, nonintact skin, and mucous membranes and are applied equally regardless of test results, thus potentially reducing the risk of transmission from both recognized and unrecognized sources.

In addition, three categories of specific "transmission precautions" are applied to patients shown to be or suspected of being either infected or colonized with certain epidemiologically important pathogens. These are airborne precautions, used for agents widely dispersible and transmissible by airborne droplet nuclei (5 μm or less in diameter), such as the agents of tuberculosis, varicella, and measles; droplet precautions, used for pathogens transmitted via large-particle droplets, conveyed generally over short distances (approximately 3 feet), such as *Haemophilus influenzae* type b, meningococci, and certain other serious bacterial and viral agents; and contact precautions, to reduce the risk of direct physical contact with the organism, either directly between persons or via an intermediate object, usually inanimate (fomite) (Table 42–2). Depending on the specific situation, these specific types of precautions can be added either individually or in combinations to standard precautions. Transmission precautions may be triggered when patients present with distinctive clinical syndromes even before the putative etiologic agent can be demonstrated by microbiological testing (Table 42–3).

TABLE 42–2 ■ Synopsis of Indications of Transmission Precautions

TRANSMISSION PRECAUTION CATEGORY	MODE OF TRANSMISSION	MAJOR EXAMPLES
Airborne	Droplet nuclei—long distances	Measles paramyxovirus Varicella-zoster virus (varicella) Tuberculosis mycobacteria
Droplet	Large-particle droplets—short distances	*Haemophilus influenzae* type b *Neisseria meningitidis* Other important pathogens
Contact	Direct contact with patient or fomites	Multidrug-resistant bacteria Selected enteric pathogens Selected viral pathogens in children‡ Others§

*Including *Corynebacterium diphtheriae, Mycoplasma pneumoniae*, pertussis (*Bordetella* spp.), *Yersinia pestis* (pneumonic plague), group A streptococcus, adenovirus, influenza virus, mumps virus, parvovirus B19, and rubella virus.

†Including *Clostridium difficile*, enterohemorrhagic *Escherichia coli* O157:H7, *Shigella*, rotarivus, and hepatitis A virus.

‡RSV, parainfluenza virus, enterovirus.

§Including highly contagious skin pathogens, viral conjunctivitis agents, hemorrhagic fever viruses.

Education and Compliance

Whichever system of precautions is used, teaching and implementation are critical. It is a relatively easy task to prepare a handsome precautions manual and to place it in a prominent position on the ward of the hospital, ready for the JCAHO inspector. Enlisting compliance with the precautions policies is another matter altogether. In one author's (DAG's) hospital, surreptitious monitoring of compliance with gown and glove precautions for RSV infection on the infant and toddler ward revealed a compliance rate of only 39%, despite

TABLE 42–3 ■ Selected Clinical Syndromes Warranting Empirical Addition of Transmission Precautions

CLINICAL SYNDROME	POTENTIAL OR SUSPECTED PATHOGENS	EMPIRICAL PRECAUTIONS
Diarrhea	Enteric pathogens	Contact
	Clostridium difficile	
Meningitis	*Neisseria meningitidis*	Droplet
Rash, generalized	*N. meningitidis*	Droplet
	Varicella-zoster virus	Airborne and contact
	Measles virus	Airborne
Respiratory infections	*Mycobacterium tuberculosis*	Airborne
	Bordetella pertussis	Droplet
	RSV or parainfluenza virus	Contact
Abscess, draining wound	*Staphylococcus aureus*	Contact
	Group A streptococcus	

the staff's realization that RSV was the major cause of nosocomial infection on their ward each winter.[44] Open monitoring of compliance with surveillance procedures coupled with an intensive educational campaign increased compliance to greater than 90% and had a profound impact on the incidence of nosocomial RSV infection, even at a time when the ward was jammed with infants admitted for community-acquired RSV infection. Interestingly, compliance remained at a high level for more than a year after the period of open monitoring, suggesting that continuing education is likely to be more effective when personnel have been galvanized by the obvious impact of a successful intervention on an important nosocomial infection program.

Limitation of Barrier Techniques

Reviews on the transmission of nosocomial pathogens invariably cite the importance of "endogenous infection" or "autoinfection," in other words, nosocomial infection caused by organisms from the patient's own microbial flora. It must be emphasized, however, that many endogenous infections are caused not by the bacteria that the patient brings into the hospital but rather by nosocomial strains that are acquired from other patients after admission and become part of a new endogenous nosocomial flora. Such colonization can occur remarkably quickly. For example, 22% of patients admitted for medical intensive care in one study developed pharyngeal colonization with gram-negative bacilli after just 24 hours' hospitalization, and 45% were colonized by 10 days.[45] The stool may also serve as an important reservoir of gram-negative nosocomial pathogens,[46, 47] and the skin may be colonized by gram-positive organisms such as methicillin-resistant staphylococci.

Theoretically, barrier precautions should control the transmission of these pathogens and prevent subsequent colonization and infection of newly admitted patients. Surprisingly, however, traditional infection control barrier techniques have had little impact on colonization and infection with some organisms, such as *Pseudomonas*.[48] Faced with this puzzling observation, Weinstein's group[49, 50] performed a series of detailed investigations of their ICU population and showed that the majority of patients who were colonized with *Pseudomonas* actually brought their strains with them, although their bacteria may have become more resistant to antibiotics under the selective pressure of broad-spectrum therapy. Patients were particularly likely to have preexisting colonization with *Pseudomonas* if they had spent time elsewhere in the hospital or in a chronic care facility, but some apparently had acquired this organism in the community. Similarly, colonization and infection with *Enterobacter* in patients undergoing coronary artery surgery could be attributed to outgrowth of *Enterobacter* that had been present in small concentrations before surgery and emerged under the selective pressure of cephalosporin prophylaxis.[51] Thus, intensive efforts to prevent cross-infection by using barrier techniques must be implemented with realistic expectations and can never be expected to eliminate all infections.

Control of Epidemic Infections

Prevention of disease by implementation of appropriate policies and control of sporadic, endemic nosocomial infection problems occupy a major portion of an infection control program's day-to-day activities. Handling chickenpox exposures, containing antibiotic-resistant bacteria, reinforcing good technique in the insertion and maintenance of urinary and intravenous catheters—such are the routine, often humdrum mainstays of an infection control practitioner's career. Outbreaks of nosocomial infection, on the other hand, spawn apprehension and challenge the intellect, organization, and interpersonal skills of the infection control team[52] (Table 42–4).

In essence, there are several phases to outbreak control. First, the infection control team must confirm that an outbreak exists, because many false alarms are raised by concerned nurses and physicians. The next phase merely represents an intensification of routine procedures, including a review of current practices, clarification of existing recommendations, assessment of barriers to compliance, and correction of any immediately apparent problems. Concurrently, a case definition must be drafted and tested, then the extent of the outbreak gauged. Every effort should be made to identify as many cases as possible, as this facilitates both epidemiologic investigation and outbreak control. For many pathogens, comprehensive case finding requires detection of carriers as well as infected individuals, and the hospital microbiologist should be consulted about the most efficient screening procedures. Published information concerning the usual mode of spread of the epidemic pathogen (see Chapter 11) should help narrow the focus of the investigation. In practice this is critical, because the pressure to institute control measures is usually so intense that there is insufficient time to explore every conceivable epidemiologic scenario, and simple interventions can often be applied before all of the facts are available; however, the investigators must exercise judgment and restraint before implementing any control measure. In particular, the infection control team should avoid premature attempts to blame a single employee. Rarely is one individual responsible for dissemination of an epidemic pathogen, and finger pointing is almost always counterproductive—and devastating to morale. It is much more desirable to develop data in a systematic fashion while having an open dialogue with staff concerning alternative explanations for a problem. In the event that an individual is implicated by a thorough epidemiologic investigation, all of the political and interpersonal skills of the infection control team should be marshaled in an effort to prevent permanent scars.

Some outbreaks can be traced to a common source, such as a faulty air-handling system, an environmental reservoir, a carrier on the hospital staff, or a contaminated device or solution. Accordingly, review of new policies or procedures for new devices is important and may be particularly relevant for equipment.[53] However, most outbreaks are attributable to a breakdown in routine aseptic procedures and person-to-person spread. When person-to-person transmission is thought to be the principal source of the problem, appropriate precautions should be instituted and barrier techniques intensified. The single most important intervention in such cases is likely to be cohorting of all patients who are either infected or colonized with the outbreak strain. Physical

TABLE 42–4 ■ Steps in Outbreak Control

Confirm that an outbreak exists.
Review current practices, clarify recommendations, assess barriers to compliance, and correct apparent problems.
Draft and test a case definition.
Perform intensive case finding.
Review mode of spread of epidemic pathogen and narrow focus of investigation accordingly.
Avoid premature conclusions and assigning blame.
Collect, review, and analyze data and develop a hypothesis.
Design a control strategy.
Implement control measures.
Monitor impact of control measures.

cohorting of patients in the same location should be complemented by cohorting of caregivers if staffing permits. Architectural limitations of many hospital facilities and staffing shortages may make effective cohorting difficult, but no effort should be spared to attain this ideal.

Control Measures for Specific Device- and Procedure-Related Infections

As outlined in Chapter 11, the four major types of nosocomial infection are bacteremia, pneumonia, urinary tract infection, and postoperative infection, and it is not surprising that intensive efforts have been directed toward preventing these device- and procedure-related problems. Great caution is needed in evaluating the enormous number of published recommendations that have appeared over the years. Many may appear to be logical and rational, but experience has shown that uncritical acceptance of published standards can lead to ineffective, extremely costly interventions. The following recommendations, now discredited, all were once received enthusiastically:

- Experience with contaminated intravenous fluids in the early 1970s suggested that frequent changes of intravenous tubing could reduce the concentration of organisms inoculated into patients when intrinsically contaminated bottles of fluid were used.[17] Institution of this control measure at the height of the outbreak of *Enterobacter* bacteremias associated with infusion of dextrose solutions produced by one manufacturer dramatically reduced clinical sequelae, even though the full nature of the contamination problem had not been elucidated at the time. This experience led to a CDC recommendation to change intravenous tubing every 24 hours for all patients receiving infusions.[54, 55] Subsequent studies revealed that contamination of intravenous fluid is quite unusual and that the organisms that tend to be recovered are notable for not proliferating rapidly in these fluids.[56] Comparisons of 24-hour and 48- or 72-hour changes of tubing demonstrated no increased risk of infection and resulted in savings of more than $100,000 for many hospitals.[57–60] What may have been reasonable temporary recommendations in response to an epidemic were clearly inappropriate in the endemic situation.
- Similarly, comparative trials have demonstrated that CDC recommendations that respirator breathing circuits be changed every 24 hours[61] are too stringent and that tubing can be changed at intervals as long as 1 week or more.[62] Again, considerable savings were achieved without harm to patients.
- Migration of periurethral bacteria along the outside of drainage catheters into the bladder is thought to be important in the pathogenesis of nosocomial urinary tract infection.[63, 64] Although cleansing the urethral meatus with an antiseptic seemed to be an appropriate intervention, twice-daily cleaning with povidone-iodine, polyantibiotic ointment, or soap and water did not reduce the infection rate.[65, 66] Similarly, retrograde flow of contaminated urine from the drainage bag to the bladder may be responsible for some infections, but initial reports of decreased infection rates associated with instillation of antiseptics into the bag[67] could not be confirmed in prospective clinical trials.[68–70]

Skepticism is particularly important when evaluating expensive new medical devices that are promoted aggressively for their infection control features. Historically, most of these products have increased the hospital's supply expenditures without yielding the advertised reduction in infection rate. Antireflux valves for urinary drainage tubing, air filters for ventilators, and microbial filters for intravenous tubing are but a few of the products that fall into this category.

Studies of new devices and technologies have begun to focus on cost-benefit aspects. For example, evaluation of silver-impregnated collagen cuffs for central venous catheters demonstrated overall cost savings when cuffed catheters were used in populations with relative high catheter-associated bacteremia rates.[71] However, new devices are being introduced at such a fast pace that it is exceedingly difficult to design, perform, and report rigorous epidemiologic evaluations in a timely fashion.

The CDC has reinstituted its practice of developing and disseminating guidelines for the prevention and control of nosocomial infections though its Hospital Infection Control Practices Advisory Committee (HICPAC).[72] HICPAC members include CDC representatives and national infection control experts. The process for developing guidelines represents a major improvement over the CDC's previous guideline process and in general follows recommendations promulgated by the Institute of Medicine.[73] Guidelines are based on a thorough and rigorous evaluation of evidence, and there is extensive opportunity for commentary by professional societies, outside experts, industry, and the public. As before, an attempt has been made to grade each recommendation for validity on the basis of published data and applicability to some or all hospital settings. A "no recommendation" rating is given for guidelines for which data are conflicting or inadequate—a category that, unfortunately, includes many of the most controversial and novel aspects of infection control. Guidelines have been published for isolation precautions,[43] nosocomial pneumonia,[62] vancomycin resistance,[74] and intravascular device–related infections.[75]

The advantage of these reviews is that they can both encourage the practitioner to eliminate the least well accepted practices and allow the reader to see which measures have general acceptance, even if not yet definitively demonstrated. Some selected, generally advocated control measures are described in the following, along with a few promising developments that require further research.

Intravenous Catheters

The management of intravascular catheters and fluid has been reviewed by HICPAC.[75] Improvements in intravenous catheter design appear to have had a substantial impact on the risk of infection and bacteremia associated with intravenous devices. Replacing rigid plastic peripheral intravenous cannulas with catheters made of Teflon or polyurethane has reduced the risk of phlebitis and minimized the incidence of infection, especially when catheters are changed every 2 to 3 days.[76, 77] Tunneled central lines, such as Broviac and Hickman catheters, have a remarkably low per-day risk of infection if inserted and maintained with scrupulous technique, and the newer implantable catheters with subcutaneous injection ports appear to have even lower infection ratios.[78] Silver-impregnated cuffs may reduce the risk of contamination of central lines by skin flora in high-risk patients.[71, 79] Catheters impregnated with antimicrobials[80] or made of materials that impede bacterial attachment can be expected in the future but must be tested rigorously and established to be effective before they are accepted. Peripherally inserted catheters made of pliable plastics are being used with increasing frequency for both in-hospital and home care. Although these devices by and large appear to be associated with low infection rates even when left in place for a week or more, further study is needed.[81]

Preparation of the skin with chlorhexidine-containing antiseptics had a beneficial effect on central venous catheter infection in one study,[82] although the specific preparation used by the investigators is not available in the United States. Chlorhexidine skin preparation in newborns reduced the risk of intravenous catheter colonization.[83] A chlorhexidine-containing skin-catheter junction patch requires further evaluation. Semipermeable transparent dressings remain controversial. Although a metaanalysis suggested an increase in microbial proliferation under such dressings, as well as an increased infection risk,[84] conflicting results have been reported in individual studies, new dressing materials have not been well studied, and many caregivers use a gauze plus transparent dressing technique that has not been scrutinized. Insertion of central catheters using maximal barrier technique appears to be extremely important, regardless of whether catheters are inserted in the operating room or on the ward.[85]

Ventilatory Support Systems

Sound epidemiologic analyses of risk factors, coupled with improved understanding of the pathogenesis of these infections, have resulted in some important advances in this area.[86] Shortly after mechanical ventilation revolutionized intensive care, it was recognized that gram-negative bacillary pneumonia was a frequent, often fatal, complication of this new technology.[87–89] Pioneering work by Reinarz and colleagues[90] demonstrated that large-volume, in-line nebulizers generated aerosols that were frequently contaminated with gram-negative rods. Substitution of cascade humidifiers for these nebulizers, coupled with universal institution of effective disinfection procedures for respiratory therapy equipment, had a major impact on ventilator-associated pneumonia. Attention to proper use and disinfection of medication nebulizers, proper dispensing and storage of nebulized solutions, and appropriate handling of condensation in the respiratory tubing can reduce to practically zero the risk of infection directly attributable to the respirator itself.[91] Nosocomial pneumonia has continued to be a major cause of morbidity and mortality, particularly in ventilated postoperative patients whose stay in the ICU is protracted. Because these infections are among the most important in terms of impact on the patient and cost to the hospital, a vigorous search for novel control measures is mandatory.

A number of investigators have noted that gastric colonization with nosocomial pathogens occurs commonly in ICU patients and that concentrations of bacteria often exceed 10^5 per mL.[92–94] Normally, gastric acidity ensures near-sterility of the stomach, but loss of this protective barrier, whether related to achlorhydria or, more commonly, to prophylaxis against stress bleeding with histamine H_2 blockers or antacids, permits exuberant bacterial growth. Reflux into the nasopharynx, aided and abetted by the gastric tubes that are almost always placed in intubated patients, leads to colonization of the oropharynx. Alternatively, organisms can reach the nasopharynx by direct inoculation via the hands of caregivers. Aspiration of nasopharyngeal secretions occurs in the majority of patients, even if an attempt is made to keep the cuff of the endotracheal tube inflated, ultimately leading to pneumonia with the same pathogens that previously colonized the stomach and oropharynx.[95–96] Pooling of fluid just above the cuff of the endotracheal tube is nearly unavoidable, although some methods for decreasing this deserve further study.[96] Faced with these observations, some investigators have tried to prevent colonization of the stomach and oropharynx by instilling antibiotics, in much the same way that oncologists attempt to prevent colonization of neutropenic patients with antimicrobial mouth care and bowel preparations. In the earliest trials, aerosolized antibiotic (polymyxin) was introduced into the tracheobronchial tree via the endotracheal tube during an outbreak of *Pseudomonas aeruginosa* pneumonia.[97, 98] Constant use reduced the threat of *Pseudomonas* infection but led to pneumonia caused by polymyxin-resistant organisms. Intermittent use also reduced the incidence of *Pseudomonas* pneumonia but did not lead to a substantial increase in resistance. Subsequently, more aggressive regimens of oral, endotracheal, and gastric antibiotic prophylaxis have been studied, often (but not always) with surprisingly large reductions in the risk of pneumonia.[99–102] However, the impact of such regimens on ICU mortality has not been demonstrated, the long-term effect on antibiotic resistance remains a concern, and cost-effectiveness requires further study.

On another tack, some investigators have tried to maintain gastric acidity as a deterrent to proliferation of organisms in the stomach by using sucralfate instead of acid neutralization to prevent gastric bleeding. Some studies have demonstrated a reduction in the incidence of pneumonia,[103–105] but it does not appear that this strategy would benefit elderly, debilitated patients, who are at particularly high risk for pneumonia and already have a high gastric pH owing to poor acid production.

Recommended procedures for control of two other major categories of nosocomial infection, catheter-associated urinary tract infections and surgical site infections, were first summarized by the CDC some years ago[106, 107] but have not yet been updated by a formal HICPAC review.

Urinary Drainage Systems

Maintenance of a sterile closed urinary drainage system is the single most important measure in controlling catheter-associated urinary tract infections.[108] Breaking the system to obtain urine samples or to irrigate the bladder clearly increases infection risk, whereas design features such as "tamper-evident" drainage systems and urine sampling ports decrease the risk.[109, 110] Systemic antimicrobial drugs may reduce the risk of catheter-associated infection in the short term, but ultimately they lead to breakthrough infection with resistant organisms. It is unclear whether short-term prophylaxis (for 2 or 3 days) would have a net benefit.

Surgery

Surgical practice is particularly bound by tradition, and few of its rituals are supported by well-designed clinical trails. Nonetheless, a consensus has emerged regarding a number of control measures, including short preoperative hospital stays, preoperative treatment of active infections, avoidance of shaving the wound site (especially the night before surgery), preparation of the operative site and surgical hand scrub with a broad-spectrum antiseptic (preferably one with residual antimicrobial activity), limitation of operating room traffic, high-efficiency air filtration with frequent (20 or more) air exchanges per hour (but not laminar airflow or ultraviolet light, which remain controversial), and proper barrier and dress procedures.[107, 111–113] Assuming that these basic recommendations are followed, the most important determinant of infection risk by far is the technique of the surgeon. Unnecessarily lengthy surgery, excessive trauma to tissues and use of cautery, failure to eradicate dead space and establish drainage, unnecessary or excessive use of foreign materials, and accidental contamination of the wound all predispose the patient to infection. Fortunately, prophylactic antibiotics can compensate for many surgical problems. The most clear-cut and dramatic effect of prophylaxis is seen in clean-contaminated and contaminated procedures, in which the risk of infection is highest. Prophylactic antibiotics have been shown to be effective for a number of clean procedures and are almost always used when prosthetic materials and devices are implanted, cases in which wound infection would have catastrophic consequences (see Chapter 44). It is clear that the timing of the administration of prophylactic antibiotics is critical. Data on both animals and patients support the need to deliver antibiotics just before surgery.[114] If antibiotics are delivered more than 2 hours before surgery or after the operation has commenced, the risk of infection is increased. Unfortunately, when carefully examined, many routine hospital systems do not ensure timely antibiotic administration; quality improvement efforts may be necessary to do so.

Employee Health

Efforts to control the transmission of infections in the hospital must include the employee. The infection control aspects of employee health involve both protecting personnel from contagious disease encountered in the workplace and protecting patients from infected employees. Employee health programs have progressed a long way since the days when screening of food handlers for *Salmonella* (a ritual of little, if any, value) was the principal activity. Comprehensive reviews may be found in the general infection control textbooks and in guidelines issued by the CDC.[115–119] Specific elements for the protection of employees are now often mandated by OSHA, particularly for blood-borne pathogens. OSHA will also be enforcing compliance with CDC recommendations for control of tuberculosis,[120] whether or not OSHA ultimately issues its own standard. The major elements of contemporary programs include the following.

Identification of Susceptible Employees

Prospective employees should undergo an initial screening history and physical examination. From an infection control point of view, this process can be focused, placing emphasis on detecting immunosuppressed persons who might have increased susceptibility to infection and personnel with dermatitis or chronic infections who might be more likely to transmit bacteria to patients. Evidence of immunity to childhood viral diseases, particularly chickenpox, rubella, and measles, should be elicited.[121]

If there is no history of chickenpox, serologic testing may be indicated, especially if clinical responsibilities would involve contact with pediatric or immunosuppressed patients, to avoid the chaos that usually accompanies unanticipated exposures to chickenpox on the wards. Because reliable varicella serology is relatively expensive, the costs and potential benefits of screening should be weighed carefully. Some programs may choose to wait for exposures to occur and test only personnel who have been exposed and do not have a history of chickenpox. This strategy is possible because several days usually elapse between an exposure and the period of communicability when the individual would have to be removed from the workplace. Now that varicella vaccine is available, many institutions are immunizing susceptible employees, although there remains some controversy about the specific merits of various strategies. Guidelines have been published by the Advisory Committee on Immunization Practices (ACIP).[121a]

Immunity to rubella should not be assumed unless vaccine has been administered following the recommendations of the ACIP or results of rubella serology are available. If the prospective employee cannot produce evidence of immunity, some hospital epidemiologists recommend serologic testing and immunization of seronegative individuals, whereas others administer the vaccine and forgo the expense of testing.

Persons born before 1957 are almost always immune to measles, but younger employees should be vaccinated routinely unless they have already been immunized at the appropriate age or serologically tested. A history of clinical measles is not completely reliable, although most authorities would accept a written, physician-documented history. Because some persons who were appropriately immunized in infancy nonetheless developed measles in the setting of an outbreak, the American Academy of Pediatrics and the ACIP have advocated reimmunization on entering school or later in an effort to reduce the risk of infection.[122] If either measles or rubella vaccination is required, the use of measles, mumps, rubella vaccine should be considered because it ensures immunity against all three diseases, albeit at a considerably greater cost.

The recommended program for protecting employees for tuberculosis includes several different components: risk stratification of different groups based on skin test conversion rates or exposure rates, the provision of negatively pressurized isolation rooms for patients with known or suspected tuberculosis, the provision of carefully fitted approved personal protective respirators (masks), and early therapeutic and prophylactic intervention.[120]

Tuberculin status of all employees should be first determined during preemployment screening. A skin test (preferably using purified protein derivative) should be done unless there is documentation of a previous reaction of 10 mm or more. A history of bacille Calmette-Guérin vaccination does not obviate skin testing, although a 1:5 dilution of purified protein derivative can be used initially in individuals vaccinated after infancy to avoid severe skin reactions. In some regions of the country, a two-step skin testing procedure has been advocated to boost immune system "memory" and eliminate false-negative results on baseline tests.[120] If the skin test is positive for the first time, chest radiography should generally be performed and counseling about prophylaxis provided on an individual basis. If results of the skin test are negative, the frequency of routine follow-up testing depends on the likelihood of exposure to infected patients. After known unprotected exposure, the skin test status of those exposed should be reassessed. Skin test conversion after exposure to multidrug-resistant tuberculosis may require specially designed prophylaxis programs.

Personnel should be questioned about a history of hepatitis. Active immunization for hepatitis B is mandated for employees who are at risk for exposure to the virus because of the nature of their clinical or laboratory responsibilities. Many institutions offer serologic testing before considering immunizations, although this may not be cost-effective in some settings. A program for evaluation, support, and intervention for employees who have had exposure to blood or body fluids must be defined, in conjunction with employee health services. Such a program must include provision for identifying, and evaluating or treating, exposures to hepatitis B virus, hepatitis C virus, and human immunodeficiency virus. Guidelines for postexposure prophylaxis for human immunodeficiency virus have been published by the CDC.[122a]

Institutions may choose to offer other serologic tests or vaccines as employee benefits, but these cannot be justified on an infection control basis. For example, cytomegalovirus serologic testing is often requested by women of childbearing age, but because the risk of acquiring cytomegalovirus in the workplace is negligible[123, 124] testing is more appropriately performed at the discretion of the employee's obstetrician.

Protection of Employees from Hazardous Exposures on the Job

The importance of prompt reporting of exposure to potentially communicable agents or hazardous materials should be stressed so that if therapy is available or diagnostic tests are required, they can be administered in a timely fashion. For example, prompt administration of hepatitis B immune globulin can prevent clinical disease, whereas later administration cannot. In addition, workers' compensation claims may be compromised if the exposure that allegedly resulted in an infection is not reported to the employee health service. Under no circumstances should personnel seek treatment informally from colleagues on the medical staff, as this can lead to irrational treatment based on fear rather than fact. For example, scores of personnel in the authors' institutions received rifampin prophylaxis for trivial meningococcal exposures before a policy was implemented that required approval by a member of the infection control or infectious disease staff before prescriptions for employees would be filled by the hospital pharmacy.

Prevention of Secondary Spread of Contagious Diseases

Personnel should also be told when to report their own illnesses to employee health. It is critically important to reassure employees that they will not suffer in terms of pay or vacation time if they are forced to stay out of work because they have reported their contagious disease. Detailed guidelines for personnel with specific diseases have been published. Some of these guidelines are arbitrary, and a flexible policy is required in many cases, particularly when patients' care might be compromised by keeping a caregiver at home.

Education

Employment provides an unparalleled opportunity to teach personnel basic infection control principles. The educational program should include information about potential infectious hazards in the workplace, particularly in the environment to which the employee will be assigned, as well as a general discussion of barrier and isolation techniques. Education should be made available not only at hiring but also periodically thereafter. Generally, if it is appropriately performed and documented, education can also fulfill recommendations and mandates proposed by the CDC, OSHA, and JCAHO. Women of childbearing age tend to be especially concerned about possible encounters with infectious agents. Even though good hand-washing practices and standard isolation procedures provide sufficient protection against the few infections that might harm the fetus, needless anxiety can be avoided by providing timely, accurate information concerning pathogens such as cytomegalovirus, herpes zoster virus, parvovirus, enterovirus, hepatitis virus, and human immunodeficiency virus.

Conclusion

Specialists in hospital epidemiology and infection control ultimately must face the inherent limitations of their science. As patients in hospitals become increasingly fragile and are subjected to increasingly aggressive and invasive therapies and procedures, nosocomial infection remains inevitable for many patients. Improved understanding of risk factors may permit specific new control measures, but major breakthroughs require innovative basic and applied research.

References

1. Haley RW: Cost benefit analysis of infection control programs. *In* Bennett JV, Brachman PS (eds): Hospital Infections, ed 3. Boston, Little, Brown, 1992, pp 507–532.
2. Haley RW, Gaynes RP, Aber RC, Bennett JV: Surveillance of nosocomial infections. *In* Bennett JV, Brachman PS (eds): Hospital Infections, ed 3. Boston, Little, Brown, 1992, pp 79–108.
3. Centers for Disease Control: Outline for Surveillance and Control of Nosocomial Infections. Washington, DC, US Department of Health and Human Services, 1972.
4. Perl TM: Surveillance, reporting and use of computers. *In* Wenzel RP (ed): Prevention and Control of Nosocomial Infections, ed 2. Baltimore, Williams & Wilkins, 1993, pp 139–176.
5. Yamauchi T: Roles of the infection control professional. *In* Donowitz LG (ed): Hospital-Acquired Infection in the Pediatric Patient. Baltimore, Williams & Wilkins, 1988, pp 351–368.
6. Gaynes RP, Culver DH, Emori TG, et al: The national nosocomial infections surveillance system: Plans for the 1990s and beyond. Am J Med 91(Suppl 3B):116S, 1991.
7. Goldmann DA: Microbiological aspects of infection control. *In* Donowitz LG (ed): Hospital-Acquired Infection in the Pediatric Patient. Baltimore, Williams & Wilkins, 1988, pp 369–385.
8. McGowan JE Jr, Metchock B: Infection control epidemiology and clinical microbiology. *In* Murray PR (ed): Manual of Clinical Microbiology, ed 6. Washington, DC, ASM Press, 1995, pp 182–189.
9. Arbeit RD: Laboratory procedures for the epidemiologic analysis of microorganisms. *In* Murray PR (ed): Manual of Clinical Microbiology, ed 6. Washington, DC, ASM Press, 1995, pp 190–208.
10. Evans RS, Burke JP, Classen DC, et al: Computerized identification of patients as high risk for hospital-acquired infection. Am J Infect Control 20:4, 1992.
11. Gross PA: Striving for benchmark infection rates: Progress in control for patient mix. Am J Med 91(Suppl 3B):16S, 1991.
12. Sands K, Vineyard G, Platt R: Surgical site infections occurring after hospital discharge. J Infect Dis 173:963, 1996.
13. Haley RW, Culver DH, White JR, et al: The efficacy of infection surveillance and control programs in preventing nosocomial infections in US hospitals. Am J Epidemiol 121:182, 1985.
14. Haley RW: Managing Hospital Infection Control for Cost Effectiveness. Chicago, American Hospital Association, 1986.
15. Technical Briefing: The Joint Commission Quality Assurance Model. Chicago, American Hospital Association, 1989.
16. Gaynes RP, Martone WJ, Culver DH, et al: Comparison of rates of nosocomial infections in neonatal intensive care units in the United States. Am J Med 91(Suppl 3B):192S, 1991.
17. Maki DG, Rhame FS, Mackel DC, et al: Nationwide epidemic of septicemia caused by contaminated intravenous products. I. Epidemiologic and clinical features. Am J Med 60:471, 1976.
18. Freeman J, Goldmann D, Smith N, et al: Association of intravenous lipid emulsion and bacteremia in neonatal intensive care units. N Engl J Med 323:301, 1990.
19. Bryan CS: Surgeon-specific wound surveillance: The family or the bean counters? Infect Control Hosp Epidemiol 10:376, 1989.
20. The Society for Hospital Epidemiology of America, the Association for Practitioners in Infection Control, the Centers for Disease Control, the Surgical Infection Society: Consensus paper on the surveillance of surgical wound infections. Infect Control Hosp Epidemiol 13:599, 1992.
21. Berwick DM: Continuous improvement as an ideal in health care. N Engl J Med 320:53, 1989.
22. Goldmann DA: New microbiological techniques for hospital epidemiology. Eur J Clin Microbiol 6:344, 1987.
23. Mickelsen PA, Plorde JJ, Gordon KP, et al: Instability of antibiotic resistance in a strain of *Staphylococcus epidermidis* isolated from an outbreak of prosthetic valve endocarditis. J Infect Dis 152:50, 1985.
24. O'Brien TF, Mayer KH, Kishi H, et al: Intercontinental spread of a new antibiotic resistance gene on an epidemic plasmid. Lancet 2:87, 1985.
25. Tenover FC, Gootz TB, Gordon KP, et al: Development of a DNA probe for the structural gene of the 2'-*O*-adenyltransferase aminoglycoside-modifying enzyme. J Infect Dis 50:678, 1984.
26. Zuckerman MA, Hawkins AE, Briggs M, et al: Investigation of hepatitis B virus transmission in a health care setting: Application of direct sequence analysis. J Infect Dis 172:1080, 1995.
27. Knittle MA, Eitzman DV, Baer H: Role of hand contamination of personnel in the epidemiology of gram-negative nosocomial infection. J Pediatr 86:433, 1975.

28. Garner JS, Favero MS: Guideline for Handwashing in Hospital Environmental Control. Atlanta, Centers for Disease Control, 1985.
29. Larson EL: APIC guideline for handwashing and hand antisepsis in health care settings. Am J Infect Control 23:251, 1995.
30. Olsen RJ, Lynch P, Coyle MB, et al: Examination gloves as barriers to hand contamination in clinical practice. JAMA 270:350, 1993.
31. Ehrenkranz J: Bland soap handwash or hand antisepsis? The pressing need for clarity. Infect Control Hosp Epidemiol 13:299, 1992.
32. Newman JL, Seitz JC: Intermittent use of an antimicrobial hand gel for reducing soap-induced irritation of health care personnel. Am J Infect Control 18:194, 1990.
33. Bartzokas CA, Corkill JE, Makin T, et al: Assessment of the remanent antibacterial effect of a 2% triclosan-detergent preparation on skin. J Hyg 91:521, 1983.
34. Garner JS, Simmons BP: CDC Guideline for Isolation Precautions in Hospitals. Atlanta, Centers for Disease Control, 1983.
35. Nauseef WM, Maki DG: A study of the value of simple protective isolation in patients with granulocytopenia. N Engl J Med 304:448, 1981.
36. Albert RK, Condie F: Hand-washing patterns in medical intensive care units. N Engl J Med 304:1465, 1981.
37. Lynch P, Jackson MM, Cummings MJ, et al: Rethinking the role of isolation practices in the prevention of nosocomial infections. Ann Intern Med 107:243, 1987.
38. Klein BS, Perloff WH, Maki DG: Reduction of nosocomial infection during pediatric intensive care by protective isolation. N Engl J Med 320:1714, 1989.
39. Hall CB, Douglas KG Jr, Geiman JM: Possible transmission by fomites of respiratory syncytial virus. J Infect Dis 141:98, 1980.
40. Doebbeling BN, Pfaller MA, Houston AK, et al: Removal of nosocomial pathogens from the contaminated glove: Implications for glove reuse and handwashing. Ann Intern Med 109:394, 1988.
41. Update: Universal precautions for prevention of transmission of human immunodeficiency virus, hepatitis B virus, and other bloodborne pathogens in health-care settings. MMWR Morbid Mortal Wkly Rep 37:377, 1988.
42. Kristensen MS, Wernberg NM, Anker-Moller E: Healthcare workers' risk of contact with body fluids in a hospital: The effect of complying with the universal precautions policy. Infect Control Hosp Epidemiol 13:719, 1992.
43. Garner JS: The Hospital Infection Control Practices Advisory Committee guidelines for isolation precautions in hospitals. Infect Control Hosp Epidemiol 17:53, 1996.
44. Leclair JM, Freeman J, Sullivan LBF, et al: Prevention of nosocomial respiratory syncytial virus infections through compliance with glove and gown isolation precautions. N Engl J Med 317:329, 1987.
45. Johanson WG Jr, Pierce AK, Sanford JP, et al: Nosocomial respiratory infections with gram-negative bacilli. The significance of colonization of the respiratory tract. Ann Intern Med 77:701, 1972.
46. Selden R, Lee S, Wang WLL, et al: Nosocomial klebsiella infections: Intestinal colonization as a reservoir. Ann Intern Med 74:657, 1971.
47. Goldmann DA, Leclair J, Macone A: Bacterial colonization of neonates admitted to an intensive care environment. J Pediatr 93:288, 1978.
48. Weinstein RA, Kabins SA: Strategies for prevention and control of multiple drug–resistant nosocomial infection. Am J Med 70:449, 1981.
49. Olson B, Weinstein RA, Nathan C, et al: Epidemiology of endemic *Pseudomonas aeruginosa:* Why infection control efforts have failed. J Infect Dis 150:808, 1984.
50. Olson B, Weinstein RA, Nathan C, et al: Occult aminoglycoside resistance in *Pseudomonas aeruginosa:* Epidemiology and implications for therapy and control. J Infect Dis 152:679, 1985.
51. Flynn DM, Weinstein RA, Nathan C, et al: Patients' endogenous flora as the source of "nosocomial" *Enterobacter* in cardiac surgery. J Infect Dis 156:363, 1987.
52. Doebbeling BN: Epidemics: Identification and management. *In* Wenzel RP (ed): Prevention and Control of Nosocomial Infections, ed 2. Baltimore, Williams & Wilkins, 1993, pp 177–206.
53. Flaherty JP, Garcia-Houchins S, Chudy R, et al: An outbreak of gram-negative bacteremia traced to contaminated O-rings in reprocessed dialyzers. Ann Intern Med 119:1072, 1993.
54. Simmons BP, Hooten TM, Wong ES, Allen JR: Guidelines for Prevention of Intravascular Infections. Atlanta, Centers for Disease Control, 1981.
55. Maki DG: Pathogenesis, prevention, and management of infections due to intravascular devices used for infusion therapy. *In* Bisno AL, Waldvogel FA (eds): Infections Associated with Indwelling Medical Devices. Washington, DC, American Society for Microbiology, 1989, pp 161–177.
56. Maki DG: Sepsis arising from intrinsic contamination of the infusion and measures for control. *In* Phillips I (ed): Microbiological Hazards of Infusion Therapy. Lancaster, England, MTP Press, 1977, pp 99–141.
57. Band JD, Maki DG: Safety and efficacy of changing intravenous delivery systems at longer than 24 hour intervals. Ann Intern Med 91:173, 1979.
58. Buxton AE, Highsmith AK, Garner JS, et al: Contamination of intravenous fluid: Effects of changing administration sets. Ann Intern Med 90:764, 1979.
59. Gorbea HF, Snydman DR, Delaney A, et al: Intravenous tubing with burettes can be safely changed at 48-hour intervals. JAMA 251:2112, 1984.
60. Maki DG, Botticelli JT, LeRoy ML, Thielke TS: Prospective study of replacing administration sets for intravenous therapy at 48- vs 72-hours intervals. 72 hours is safe and cost-effective. JAMA 258:1777, 1987.
61. Simmons BP, Wong ES: CDC guidelines for the prevention and control of nosocomial pneumonia. Am J Infect Control 11:230, 1983.
62. Tablan OC, Anderson LJ, Arden NH: Guideline for prevention of nosocomial pneumonia. Part I. Issues on prevention of nosocomial pneumonia, 1994. Infect Control Hosp Epidemiol 15:588, 1994.
63. Kass EH, Schneiderman LJ: Entry of bacteria into the urinary tract of patients with inlying catheters. N Engl J Med 256:556, 1957.
64. Garibaldi RA, Burke JP, Britt MR, et al: Meatal colonization and catheter-associated bacteriuria. N Engl J Med 303:316, 1980.
65. Burke JP, Garibaldi RA, Britt MR, et al: Prevention of catheter-associated urinary tract infections. Efficacy of daily meatal care regimens. Am J Med 70:655, 1981.
66. Burke JP, Jacobson JA, Garibaldi KA, et al: Evaluation of daily meatal care with poly-antibiotic ointment in prevention of urinary catheter–associated bacteriuria. J Urol 129:331, 1983.
67. Maizels M, Schaeffer AJ: Decreased incidence of bacteriuria associated with periodic instillation of hydrogen peroxide into the urethral catheter drainage bag. J Urol 123:841, 1980.
68. Southampton Infection Control Team: Evaluation of aseptic techniques and chlorhexidine on the rate of catheter-associated urinary tract infection. Lancet 1:89, 1982.
69. Gillespie WA, Simpson RA, Jones JE, et al: Does the addition of disinfectant to urine drainage bags prevent infection in catheterised patients? Lancet 1:1037, 1983.
70. Thompson RL, Haley CE, Searcy MA, et al: Catheter-associated bacteriuria. Failure to reduce attack rates using periodic instillation of a disinfectant into urinary drainage systems. JAMA 251:747, 1984.
71. Maki DG, Cobb L, Garman JK, et al: An attachable silver-impregnated cuff for prevention of infection with central venous catheters: A prospective randomized trial. Am J Med 85:307, 1988.
72. Garner JS: The CDC Hospital Infection Control Practices Advisory Committee. Am J Infect Control 21:160, 1993.
73. Field MJ, Lohr KN (eds): Guidelines for Clinical Practice: From Development to Use. Washington, DC, Institute of Medicine, National Academy of Sciences, 1992.
74. Centers for Disease Control and Prevention: Recommendations for preventing the spread of vancomycin resistance: Recommendations of the Hospital Infection Control Practices Advisory Committee (HICPAC). MMWR Morbid Mortal Wkly Rep 44(RR-12):1, 1995.
75. Pearson ME, Hospital Infection Control Advisory Committee: HICPAC guidelines for prevention of intravascular device-related infections. Am J Infect Control 24:262, 1996.

76. Tully JL, Friedland GH, Baldini IM, et al: Complications of intravenous therapy with steel needles and Teflon catheters: A comparative study. Ann J Med 70:702, 1981.
77. Toltzis P, Goldmann D: Current issues in central venous catheter infection. *In* Creger WP, Coggins CH, Hancock EW (eds): Annual Review of Medicine. Palo Alto, CA, Annual Reviews, 1990, pp 169–176.
78. Ross MN, Haase GM, Poole MA, et al: Comparison of totally implanted reservoirs with external catheters as venous access devices in pediatric oncologic patients. Surg Gynecol Obstet 167:141, 1988.
79. Flowers RH III, Schwenzer KJ, Kopel RF, et al: Efficacy of an attachable subcutaneous cuff for the prevention of intravascular catheter–related infection. JAMA 261:876, 1989.
80. Trooskin SZ, Donetz AP, Harvey RA, et al: Prevention of catheter sepsis by antibiotic bonding. Surgery 97:548, 1985.
81. Raad I, Davis S. Becker M, et al: Low infection rate and long durability of nontunneled Silastic catheters. A safe cost-effective alternative for long-term venous access. Arch Intern Med 153:1791, 1993.
82. Maki DG, Ringer M, Alvarado CJ: Prospective randomised trial of povidone-iodine, alcohol, and chlorhexidine for prevention of infection associated with central venous and arterial catheters. Lancet 338:339, 1991.
83. Garland JS, Dunne WM, Havens P, et al: Peripheral intravenous catheter complications in critically ill children: A prospective study. Pediatrics 89:1145, 1992.
84. Conty JM, Grieve K, Peters B: A prospective randomized study comparing transparent and dry gauze dressings for central venous catheters. J Infect Dis 159:310, 1989.
85. Raad II, Hohn DC, Gilbreath BJ, et al: Prevention of central venous catheter–related infections by using maximal sterile barrier precautions during insertion. Infect Control Hosp Epidemiol 15:231, 1994.
86. Zucker JR, Goldmann DA: Nosocomial pneumonia in the immunocompromised host. *In* Shelhamer J, Pizzo PA, Parillo JE, Masur H (eds): Respiratory Disease in the Immunosuppressed Host. Philadelphia, JB Lippincott, 1989, pp 255–276.
87. Phillips L: *Pseudomonas aeruginosa* respiratory tract infections in patients receiving mechanical ventilation. J Hyg 65:229, 1967.
88. Ringrose RE, McKown B, Felton FG, et al: A hospital outbreak of *Serratia marcescens* associated with ultrasonic nebulizers. Ann Intern Med 69:719, 1968.
89. Mertz JJ, Scharer L, McClement JH: A hospital outbreak of *Klebsiella pneumoniae* from inhalation therapy with contaminated aerosol solution. Am Rev Respir Dis 95:454, 1967.
90. Reinarz JA, Pierce AK, Mays BB, et al: The potential role of inhalation equipment in nosocomial pulmonary infection. J Clin Invest 44:831, 1965.
91. Craven DE, Steger KA: Nosocomial pneumonia in the intubated patient. New concepts on pathogenesis and prevention. Infect Dis Clin North Am 3:843, 1989.
92. du Moulin GC, Paterson DG, Hedley-Whyte J, et al: Aspiration of gastric bacteria in antacid-treated patients: A frequent cause of postoperative colonisation of the airway. Lancet 1:242, 1982.
93. Atherton ST, White DJ: Stomach as source of bacteria colonising respiratory tract during artificial ventilation. Lancet 2:968, 1978.
94. Craven DE, Daschner FD: Nosocomial pneumonia in the intubated patient: Role of gastric colonization. Eur J Clin Microbiol Infect Dis 8:40, 1989.
95. Wenzel RP: Hospital-acquired pneumonia: An overview of the current state of the art for prevention and control. Eur J Clin Microbiol Infect Dis 8:56, 1989.
96. Valles J, Artigas A, Rello J, et al: Continuous aspiration of subglottic secretions in preventing ventilator-associated pneumonia. Ann Intern Med 122:179, 1995.
97. Klick JM, du Moulin GC, Hedley-Whyte J, et al: Prevention of gram-negative bacillary pneumonia using polymyxin aerosol as prophylaxis. II. Effect on the incidence of pneumonia in seriously ill patients. J Clin Invest 55:514, 1975.
98. Feeley TW, du Moulin GC, Hedley-Whyte J, et al: Aerosol polymyxin and pneumonia in seriously ill patients. N Engl J Med 293:471, 1975.
99. Johanson WG Jr, Seidenfeld JJ, De Los Santos R, et al: Prevention of nosocomial pneumonia using topical and parenteral antimicrobial agents. Am Rev Respir Dis 137:265, 1988.
100. Stoutenbeek CP, van Saene HKF, Miranda DR, et al: The effect of oropharyngeal decontamination using topical nonabsorbable antibiotics on the incidence of nosocomial respiratory tract infections in multiple trauma patients. J Trauma 27:357, 1987.
101. Ledingham IM, Alcock SR, Eastaway AT, et al: Triple regimen of selective decontamination of the digestive tract, systemic cefotaxime, and microbiological surveillance for prevention of acquired infection in intensive care. Lancet 1:785, 1988.
102. Unertl K, Ruckdeschel G, Selbmann HK, et al: Prevention of colonization and respiratory infections in long-term ventilated patients by local antimicrobial prophylaxis. Intensive Care Med 13:106, 1987.
103. Driks MR, Craven DE, Celli BR, et al: Nosocomial pneumonia in intubated patients given sucralfate as compared with antacids or histamine type 2 blockers. N Engl J Med 317:1376, 1987.
104. Daschner F, Kappstein I, Engels I, et al: Stress ulcer prophylaxis and ventilation pneumonia: Prevention of antibacterial cytoprotective agents? Infect Control Hosp Epidemiol 9:59, 1988.
105. Trybe M: Risk of acute stress bleeding and nosocomial pneumonia in ventilated intensive care unit patients: Sucralfate versus antacids. Am J Med 83(Suppl 3B):117, 1987.
106. Wong ES, Hooten TM: Guidelines for Prevention and Control of Nosocomial Infections: Guidelines for Prevention of Catheter-Associated Urinary Tract Infection. Atlanta, Centers for Disease Control, 1981.
107. Garner JS: Guideline for Prevention of Surgical Wound Infections. Atlanta, Centers for Disease Control, 1985.
108. Garibaldi RA: Hospital-acquired urinary tract infections: Epidemiology and prevention. *In* Wenzel RP (ed): Prevention and Control of Nosocomial Infections, ed 2. Baltimore, Williams & Wilkins, 1993, pp 600–613.
109. Platt R, Polk BF, Murdock B, et al: Prevention of catheter-associated urinary tract infection: A cost-benefit analysis. Infect Control Hosp Epidemiol 10:60, 1989.
110. Platt R, Polk BF, Murdock B, et al: Reduction of mortality associated with nosocomial urinary tract infection. Lancet 1:893, 1983.
111. Mayhall CG: Surgical infections including burns. *In* Wenzel RP: Prevention and Control of Nosocomial Infections, ed 2. Baltimore, Williams & Wikins, 1993, pp 614–664.
112. Ehrenkranz NJ, Meakins JL: Surgical infections. *In* Bennett JV, Brachman PS (eds): Hospital Infections, ed 3. Boston, Little, Brown, 1992, pp 685–710.
113. American College of Surgeons Committee on Control of Surgical Infections: Manual on Control of Infection in Surgical Patients, ed 2. Philadelphia, JB Lippincott, 1984.
114. Classen DC, Evans RS, Pestotnik SL, et al: The timing of prophylactic administration of antibiotics and the risk of surgical-wound infection. N Engl J Med 326:281, 1992.
115. Williams WW: Guideline for infection control in hospital personnel. Infect Control 4(Suppl):326, 1983.
116. Fedson D: Immunizations for health care workers and patients in hospitals. *In* Wenzel RP (ed): Prevention and Control of Nosocomial Infections, ed 2. Baltimore, Williams & Wilkins, 1993, pp 214–294.
117. Sheretz RJ, Marosok RD, Streed SA: Infection control aspects of hospital employee health. *In* Wenzel RP (ed): Prevention and Control of Nosocomial Infections, ed 2. Baltimore, Williams & Wilkins, 1993, pp 295–332.
118. Yamauchi T: Roles of the infection control professional. *In* Donowitz LG (ed): Hospital-Acquired Infection in the Pediatric Patient. Baltimore, Williams & Wilkins, 1988, pp 351–368.
119. Polder JA, Tablan OC, Williams WW, et al: Personnel health services. *In* Bennett JV, Brachman PS (eds): Hospital Infections, ed 3. Boston, Little, Brown, 1992, pp 31–61.
120. Centers for Disease Control and Prevention: Guidelines for preventing the transmission of *Mycobacterium tuberculosis* in health-care facilities, 1994. MMWR Morbid Mortal Wkly Rep 43(RR-13):1, 1994.
121. Centers for Disease Control: General recommendations on immunization. MMWR Morb Mortal Wkly Rep 38:205, 1989.
121a. Centers for Disease Control and Prevention: Prevention of varicella: Recommendations of the Advisory Committee on Immunization Practices (ACIP). MMWR Morbid Mortal Wkly Rep 45(RR-11):1, 1996.
122. Measles prevention: Recommendations of the Immunization

Practices Advisory Committee (ACIP). MMWR Morbid Mortal Wkly Rep 38(Suppl 9):1, 1989.
122a. Centers for Disease Control and Prevention: Update: Provisional Public Health Service recommendations for chemoprophylaxis after occupational exposure to HIV. MMWR Morbid Mortal Wkly Rep 45:468, 1996.
123. Goldmann DA: Prevention and management of neonatal infections. Infect Dis Clin North Am 3:779, 1989.
124. Adler SP: Nosocomial transmission of cytomegalovirus. Pediatr Infect Dis J 5:239, 1986.

43

Management of Urinary Catheters

Calvin M. Kunin

Urinary catheters are an essential part of medical care. They are widely used to provide temporary relief of anatomic or physiologic obstruction, to facilitate surgical repair of the urethra and surrounding structures, to provide a dry environment for a comatose or incontinent patient, and to permit accurate measurement of urine output in severely ill patients. Unfortunately, when used inappropriately or left in place too long, they can present a hazard to the very patients they are designed to protect. They are the leading cause of nosocomial urinary tract infections and the most common predisposing factor for preventable gram-negative sepsis in hospitals.[1]

Risks of Catheterization

The risk of acquisition of urinary tract infection from catheterization depends on host factors, how long the catheter is left in place, and how well it is managed once in place.

Single Catheterization

Indications

1. To relieve temporary obstruction or inability to void
2. To obtain urine from patients who cannot give a clean-voided specimen because of weakness, obesity, or major medical problems
3. To determine the volume of residual urine (other methods include postvoiding films after intravenous urograms, bladder ultrasonography, and dye studies)
4. To permit examination of the anatomy of the urethra
5. For intermittent catheterization

The rate of acquisition of urinary tract infections in healthy persons after a single catheterization is relatively low, on the order of 1% to 2%.[2] There may be several reasons: (1) the enteric gram-negative bacteria that commonly adhere to the vesical mucosa and produce urinary tract infections are not ordinarily present in the periurethral area[3]; (2) the few organisms that are introduced at the time of catheterization are washed out by the flow of urine; and (3) a foreign body is not left in place. Certain groups seem to be more susceptible to infection—mothers who are catheterized shortly before delivery or immediately post partum. The rate of infection may exceed 20% in women post partum.[4, 5] This may be due to incomplete emptying of the bladder after prolonged labor. Other groups at risk include males with prostatic obstruction, diabetic patients, elderly and debilitated persons, and those who retain significant residual urine in the bladder.[2]

Antimicrobial Prophylaxis

Prophylactic antimicrobial therapy to prevent acquisition of infection after single catheterizations in patients at high risk appears to be reasonable, although proof of efficacy is difficult to find in the literature. A single dose of an effective agent such as trimethoprim, trimethoprim-sulfamethoxazole, nitrofurantoin, or a quinolone may be useful in high-risk patients. Another approach is to irrigate the bladder with an antimicrobial solution such as neomycin-polymyxin or chlorhexidine. Gillespie and colleagues[5] reported that a chlorhexidine flush markedly reduced the frequency of bacteriuria in women who were catheterized post partum.

Antimicrobial prophylaxis may temporarily delay the onset of bacteriuria in patients with indwelling catheters, but it predisposes to superinfection with resistant microorganisms. For example, prophylactic use of a fluoroquinolone has been shown to reduce the rate of gram-negative but not gram-positive bacteriuria in patients catheterized for several weeks.[6, 7] However, excessive use of fluoroquinolones in catheterized patients is associated with the emergence of ciprofloxacin-resistant *Escherichia coli*.[8] The rate of nosocomial urinary tract infection at a university medical center doubled between 1982 and 1991.[9] This was associated with an increase in infections caused by yeasts, *Klebsiella pneumoniae,* and group B streptococci because of the selective pressure of antibiotic use. Harding and colleagues[10] found that bacteriuria resolved spontaneously in about a third of women after an indwelling catheter had been removed. Those who remained bacteriuric often developed symptomatic infection. A single dose of trimethoprim-sulfamethoxazole, given to those who were still bacteriuric at 48 hours after removal of the catheter, was as effective as a 10-day course. *It is recommended that prophylactic antibiotics not be used in catheterized patients. Treatment should be reserved for documented infection after the catheter is removed.*

The most important message, however, is to avoid unnecessary instrumentation.

Intermittent Catheterization

About 40 years ago, Sir Ludwig Guttmann introduced the concept of intermittent catheterization for the early treatment of patients with traumatic paraplegia.[11] Tribe and Silver,[12] working at the same institution in Stoke Mandeville, England, had found that urinary sepsis and pyelonephritis, complicated by hypertension and renal failure, were the chief causes of febrile illness and death among their patients. Guttmann reasoned that aseptic, intermittent catheterization would eliminate the foreign body and mimic the normal cycle of bladder emptying. This technique was a major advance in long-term care, reducing markedly the incidence of urinary tract infections and morbidity among paraplegic patients. These observations led Lapides and colleagues[13] to introduce clean, but not necessarily aseptic, "self-catheterization" as an effective measure for children with neurogenic disorders of bladder function. Urinary diversion procedures are needed much less often now than in the past. Advantages and disadvantages of intermittent catheterization are described in Table 43–1.

TABLE 43–1 ■ Advantages and Disadvantages of Intermittent Catheterization

ADVANTAGES
Mimics normal emptying of the bladder
Eliminates a persistent foreign body
Prevents overflow incontinence
Improves patients' self-esteem
Allows antimicrobial therapy to be more effective
Decreases complications of catheter care (fewer episodes of sepsis, less stone formation), protects the upper tract, and decreases the need for urinary diversion procedures
DISADVANTAGES
Requires more nursing time in hospitals
Requires cooperation of patients or assistance at home
May produce strictures and false passages
May ultimately require bladder neck surgery for males
UNRESOLVED ISSUES
Do antimicrobial irrigation solutions decrease infections?
Should asymptomatic bacteriuria be treated?

From Kunin CM: Urinary Tract Infections: Detection, Prevention, and Management, ed 5. Baltimore, Williams & Wilkins, 1997.

The frequency of urinary tract infections is decreased but not eliminated by intermittent catheterization. Nevertheless, infection is much more readily treated in the absence of a persistent foreign body. The major points of controversy relate to the optimal method for preventing bacteriuria in patients who undergo prolonged intermittent catheterization. This should be individualized because patients are highly variable. Some may develop infection rarely, and each infection may be treated with a brief course of antimicrobial therapy. Others may develop persistent, symptomatic infection and may require long-term prophylaxis with an effective agent. Various methods have been claimed to be effective for paraplegic patients—instillation of a solution of neomycin-polymyxin into the bladder at the termination of each catheterization,[14] oral prophylaxis with nitrofurantoin,[15] and methenamine mandelate combined with ammonium chloride to acidify the urine.[16] Bladder irrigations with polymyxin-neomycin may be complicated by superinfection with yeasts and enterococci. In one controlled trial, neomycin irrigation was found to be ineffective.[17] Intermittent catheterization in males may be complicated by bleeding and development of urethral strictures, false urethral passages, and epididymitis. These problems may be overcome in patients with detrusor-external sphincter dyssynergia by performing a sphincterotomy[18] or inserting an endoluminal urethral stent.[19] The patient then has external condom drainage. An alternative approach is to insert a suprapubic catheter. Urethral stents and suprapubic catheters may also be useful for avoiding urethral complications in males with prostatic obstruction.

Postoperative Urinary Catheterization

Catheterization need not be used routinely in postoperative patients who have difficulty voiding. It is not uncommon for a male patient to trace the onset of recurrent prostatitis or a female patient to relate recurrent urinary infections to postoperative or postpartum catheterization. The patient should be given adequate time, placed in a comfortable position to void, and, most important, have the privacy to relieve inhibitions. A single or several intermittent catheterizations may suffice for the patient who cannot void after several hours. The surgeon may elect to use an indwelling catheter for 1 or 2 days instead of intermittent catheterization. In one study,[20] short-term use of the indwelling catheter reduced the occurrence of urine retention and bladder distention without increasing the rate of urinary tract infection.

Regardless of the method used to relieve postoperative urinary retention, it is recommended that microscopic examination of the urine or culture be done after the catheter is removed and that infection be eradicated by a short course of antimicrobial therapy.

The Indwelling Urinary Catheter

The urethral indwelling catheter is one of the most commonly used instruments in hospitals. It is inserted in about 10% of all patients admitted to general hospitals and is used commonly in the care of elderly, incontinent women in nursing homes. According to the National Nosocomial Infections Study, 40% of the 2,000,000 hospital-acquired infections arise from the urinary tract each year in the United States. About 800,000 of these patients per year develop nosocomial urinary infections, mainly from indwelling catheters. It is estimated that at least 50,000 cases of nosocomial urinary infections per year are associated with bacteremia and potentially life-threatening illness.[1, 21] Givens and Wenzel[22] estimated that Foley catheter–associated urinary tract infections after five common surgical procedures extended hospital stays an average of 2.4 days. Rubinstein and colleagues[23] calculated that urinary tract infections from catheters used in general and orthopedic surgery prolonged the average length of stay to 5.1 days. Platt and associates,[24] working in an acute care general hospital, reported a threefold increase in mortality among catheterized patients who became infected. It is not uncommon to encounter patients with severe sepsis and gram-negative bacteremia who are admitted with an indwelling urinary catheter from long-term care facilities. These are usually elderly female patients transferred from nursing homes or paraplegic patients who are not managed by intermittent catheterization. We noted in a study of elderly patients in nursing homes that there was a stepwise increase in mortality with duration of catheterization.[25] This was independent of other risk factors for death. Patients who were catheterized for 76% or more of their days in the nursing homes were three times more likely to die within a year. The number of hospitalizations, duration of hospitalization, and use of antimicrobial drugs were three times greater among catheterized patients. In a randomized, prospective clinical trial comparing catheterization with incontinence pads among elderly female patients, McMurdo and colleagues[26] found that asymptomatic bacteriuria was common among both groups, but 73% of catheterized patients received treatment for clinical signs of infection, compared with 40% of patients managed with pads. Catheterized patients required less nursing time, but costs for catheter care were greater. Nordqvist and coworkers[27] compared catheter and noncatheter care in two different wards and found no differences in mortality at 4 years. Nevertheless, they were favorably impressed by the advantages of noncatheter care—the relative ease of removing catheters from most patients, the spontaneous disappearance of bacteriuria and ease of eradicating infection with oral antimicrobial agents, improved contact with the staff, decrease in odors, absence of pressure sores, reduction in the number of gram-negative nosocomial strains of bacteria, marked reduction in the use of antibiotics, and, paradoxically, lower laundry costs. The last observation is difficult to understand based on experiences in this country of other groups.[28]

The risk of infection and its sequelae depend on the duration of catheterization, age, sex, type of service, and the presence of associated diseases. For example, females tend to acquire induced infections more readily than do males.[29, 30] Males more frequently suffer from local suppurative complications. *Long-term placement of a suprapubic catheter in males is useful for preventing urethral strictures, epididymitis, and orchitis, but it does not prevent acquisition of urinary tract infections.*

Effect of Catheters on the Voiding Mechanism

Progress in this field has been remarkably slow. It took more than 30 years before the work of Dukes[31] on closed drainage was reintroduced by Miller and colleagues.[32] The use of closed drainage bags was not adopted widely in the United States until almost 10 years later.[29, 33] The technical issues can be summarized briefly.[34] The bladder is a smooth-walled, distensible structure that contracts once the internal pressure exerted by the expanding volume of urine reaches a critical point. This detrusor activity is synchronized with a combination of voluntary and involuntary relaxation of the external sphincter. The flow of urine then distends the normally collapsed urethral passage, allowing virtually complete emptying of the bladder. This cyclic process is the bladder's chief mechanical defense against infection.[35]

The indwelling catheter violates this defense altogether. With the catheter, the cycle of filling, expansion, and emptying of the bladder is altered to produce continuous flow. The bladder cannot empty completely because of the presence of the retention balloon, pressure from which erodes the smooth mucosal surface. The urethra is distended, its blood supply is attenuated by lateral pressure, and the lubricating periurethral glands are blocked. There is a continuous open channel that permits microorganisms to flow upstream into the bladder and a stressed periurethral surface that offers a second channel for bacterial colonization around the urethra. In essence, a foreign body converts a dynamic system to a static state. *Antimicrobial therapy may delay infection, but it is ultimately ineffectual. The use of antibiotics alters the bacterial flora and favors colonization with resistant microbes, including urease-producing* Proteus *and* Providencia *species.*[36] Alkaline urine produced by the breakdown of urea to ammonia causes precipitation of struvite crystals. The crystals aggregate by mechanisms not yet fully understood to form encrustations that block the channel and lead to obstruction and septic episodes.

Management of Sepsis in Patients with an Indwelling Catheter

Patients with indwelling catheters may suffer acute episodes of fever and chills, sometimes accompanied by septic shock. Detecting sepsis may be difficult in elderly patients, who may have only low-grade fever, appear to be dehydrated, and develop mental confusion. The first step should be to remove the catheter, which may be kinked or blocked. The urine should be examined by Gram stain to obtain a preliminary assessment of the possible causative organisms. Ordinarily one suspects gram-negative bacteria, but gram-positive bacteria (staphylococci and enterococci) or yeasts may be seen. Blood cultures and standard laboratory tests should be conducted and attention directed at managing hypotension and repletion of fluids and electrolytes. Although antibiotics directed at resistant gram-negative bacteria customarily are administered, how long they should be given is not well understood. Bacteremia is often transient and rarely metastatic.

Advances in Management of Indwelling Urinary Catheters

Closed Drainage. Attempts to improve indwelling catheter care are summarized in Table 43–2. All indwelling catheters should be attached to closed drainage. This delays colonization of the bladder in most patients by about 1 to 2 weeks. Thereafter, microbes ascend around the catheter in the periurethral space.[29] This does not appear to be preventable by using antimicrobial lubricants or povidone-iodine ointment at the time of insertion[37] or by applying silver sulfadiazine cream twice daily to the urethral meatus.[38] Even washing the periurethral area has not been shown to be beneficial. Continuous irrigation of the bladder with neomycin-polymyxin solutions does not appear to be any more effective than closed drainage and probably is not additive. Care needs to be taken to avoid breaking the junction between the catheter and drainage tube. Sealed joints are preferred by some workers,[39] but use of a tape seal applied to the catheter–drainage tubing junction within 24 hours of catheter insertion was not associated with significantly lower rates of bacteriuria or mortality in patients undergoing short-term catheterization.[40]

Wille and colleagues[41] found no difference in the time of onset and incidence of nosocomial urinary infection in patients managed with a simple closed drainage bag with an antireflux valve compared with a more complex system that included a preconnected, coated catheter, a tamper seal at the catheter-drainage junction, a drip chamber, an antireflux valve, a hydrophobic drainage vent, and a povidone-iodine–releasing cartridge in line with the outlet tube of the urine collection bag. Adding an antimicrobial agent such as hydrogen peroxide or chlorhexidine to the drainage bag is not beneficial.[42, 43]

Catheter Materials. Latex catheters are least expensive and usually suffice. They need not be changed routinely unless

TABLE 43–2 ■ Attempts to Improve Indwelling Catheter Care

SITE	METHOD*
Urethra	Aseptic method of insertion[c]
	Antimicrobial lubricants[d]
	Washing the perineum[d]
	Applications of antimicrobial ointments[d]
	Chlorhexidine-soaked sponges[b]
Bladder	Irrigation with antimicrobial solutions[a*]
Catheter	New materials (silicone versus latex)[a**]
	Hydrophilic catheters[d]
	Conformable catheters[a***]
	Impregnation with antimicrobial agents[d]
	The "silver" catheter[c]
	Vented catheters[d]
Drainage tube junction	Preattached collecting systems[c]
	Construction (hanging characteristics,[b] leg bands,[b] vents,[a] drip chambers, valves, spigots[d])
Drainage bag	Antimicrobial additives[d] (povidone-iodine, hydrogen peroxide, chlorhexidine)
Systemic	Antimicrobial prophylaxis or therapy[d]
Epidemiologic	Geographic separation, sterilization of urine outflow from bags[a]
	Washing hands between patients[b]
	Sterilization of urine drained from bags[c]
	Measures that restrict use of common devices and irrigation syringes[a]
General	Proper positioning of the drainage system[a]
	Avoidance of breaking the closed system[a]

*Key: a, effective (*no more effective than closed drainage; **silicone catheters tend to become less encrusted during chronic use; ***appear to be more comfortable, but there is no evidence that the rate of infection is altered); b, probably effective; c, possibly effective; d, not effective.

From Kunin CM: Urinary Tract Infections: Detection, Prevention, and Management, ed 5. Baltimore, Williams & Wilkins, 1997.

they become blocked by encrustations. In general, patients who form encrustations ("blockers")[44] may be managed effectively by changing the catheter at 1- to 2-week intervals. Silicone catheters tend to become encrusted less frequently, but because of their greater cost should be reserved for special situations, such as for blockers.[45] There is insufficient evidence that "hydrophilic" coated catheters prevent infection. Indeed, one report[46] suggests that they may be associated with an increased incidence of infection.

New Catheter Designs. Two new advances deserve special mention: catheters coated with silver oxide[47–49] and a conformable catheter constructed with a flexible, thin rubber urethral portion.[50] Short-term use of the silver catheter was found to reduce the frequency of urinary infections in a subgroup of women not receiving antibiotics,[49] but it is doubtful that it will prove cost-effective for long-term care. The conformable catheter is reported to be more comfortable, to stay in place several days longer, and to be less often obstructed by struvite. There is no evidence, however, that it prevents acquisition of infection.

Other approaches to prevent infection and delay formation of biofilms and encrustations on the catheter surface include impregnating catheters with antimicrobial drugs,[51] salicylic acid,[52] or heparin[53]; irrigating with acidic solutions[54]; or applying electric currents to kill microbes within the catheter urine.[55] Although some of these measures may eventually be shown to be effective, it is easier and more cost-effective to simply change to a fresh catheter or remove it as soon as possible. *It must be emphasized that sterilizing urine within the catheter or the periurethral space might delay acquisition of infection in the short term but would not be expected to eradicate infection within the bladder.*

The challenge for the future is to produce an instrument that matches as closely as possible the normal physiologic and mechanical characteristics of the voiding system. It seems to me that this will require the construction of a thin-walled, continuously lubricated, collapsible catheter to restore the integrity of the urethra; a system to hold the catheter in place without a balloon; and measures to imitate the intermittent washing of the bladder urine. The efficacy of each component of the system will need to be evaluated in carefully conducted, controlled clinical trials. Catheters of the future may be more expensive but should be well worth the investment.

References

1. Kunin CM: Urinary Tract Infections: Detection, Prevention, and Management, ed 5. Baltimore, Williams & Wilkins, 1997.
2. Turck M, Goffe B, Pertersdorf RG: The urethral catheter and urinary tract infection. J Urol 88:834, 1962.
3. Daifuku R, Stamm WE: Bacterial adherence to bladder uroepithelial cells in catheter-associated urinary tract infection. N Engl J Med 314:1208, 1986.
4. Brumfitt W, Davies BI, Rosser E: Urethral catheter as a cause of urinary tract infection in pregnancy and puerperium. Lancet 2:1059, 1961.
5. Gillespie WA, Lennon GG, Linton KB, Slade N: Prevention of urinary infection in gynaecology. Br Med J 2:423, 1964.
6. Vollaard EJ, Clasener AL, Zambon JV et al: Prevention of catheter-associated gram-negative bacilluria with norfloxacin by selective decontamination of the bowel and high urinary concentration. J Antimicrob Chemother 23:915, 1989.
7. Van der Wall E, Verkooyen RP, Mintjes-De Groot J, et al: Prophylactic ciprofloxacin for catheter-associated urinary-tract infection. Lancet 339:946, 1992.
8. Ena J, Amador C, Martinez C, et al: Risk factors for acquisition of urinary tract infections caused by ciprofloxacin resistant *Escherichia coli.* J Urol 153:117, 1995.
9. Bronsema DA, Adams JR, Pallares R, et al: Secular trends in rates and etiology of nosocomial urinary tract infections at a university hospital. J Urol 150:414, 1993.
10. Harding GKM, Nicolle LE, Ronald AR, et al: How long should catheter-acquired urinary tract infection in women be treated? Ann Intern Med 114:713, 1991.
11. Guttmann L, Frankel H: The value of intermittent catheterisation in the early management of traumatic paraplegia and tetraplegia. Paraplegia 4:63, 1966.
12. Tribe CR, Silver JR: Renal Failure in Paraplegia. London, Pitman, 1969.
13. Lapides J, Diokno AC, Silber SJ, Lowe BS: Clean, intermittent self-catheterization in the treatment of urinary tract disease. J Urol 107:458, 1972.
14. Rhame FS, Perkash I: Urinary tract infections occurring in recent spinal cord injury patients on intermittent catheterization. J Urol 122:669, 1979.
15. Anderson R: Prophylaxis of bacteriuria during intermittent catheterization of the acute neurogenic bladder. J Urol 123:364, 1980.
16. Kevorkian CG, Merritt JL, Ilstrup DM: Methenamine mandelate with acidification: An effective urinary antiseptic in patients with neurogenic bladder. Mayo Clin Proc 59:523, 1984.
17. Haldorson AM, Keys TF, Maker MD, Opitz JL: Nonvalue of neomycin instillation after intermittent urinary catheterization. Antimicrob Agents Chemother 14:368, 1978.
18. Vapnek JM, Couillard DR, Stone AR: Is sphincterotomy the best management of the spinal cord injured bladder? J Urol 151:961, 1994.
19. Chancellor MB, Rivas DA, Linsenmeyer T, et al: Multicenter trial in North America of UroLume urinary sphincter device. J Urol 152:924, 1994.
20. Michelson JD, Lotke PA, Steinberg ME: Urinary bladder management after total joint surgery. N Engl J Med 319:321, 1988.
21. Pittet D, Wenzel RP: Nosocomial blood stream infections. Secular trends in rates, mortality, and contributions to hospital deaths. Arch Intern Med 155:1177, 1995.
22. Givens CD, Wenzel RP: Catheter-associated urinary tract infections in surgical patients: A controlled study on the excess morbidity and costs. J Urol 124:646, 1980.
23. Rubinstein E, Green M, Modan M, et al: The effects of nosocomial infection on the length of stay and hospital costs. J Antimicrob Chemother 9(Suppl A):93, 1982.
24. Platt R, Polk F, Murdock B, et al: Mortality associated with nosocomial urinary tract infection. N Engl J Med 307:637, 1982.
25. Kunin CM, Douthitt S, Dancing J, et al: The association between the use of urinary catheters and morbidity and mortality among elderly patients in nursing homes. Am J Epidemiol 135:291, 1992.
26. McMurdo ME, Davey PG, Elder MA, et al: The cost-effectiveness of the management of intractable urinary incontinence by urinary catheterization or incontinence pads. J Epidemiol Community Health 46:222, 1992.
27. Nordqvist P, Ekelund P, Edouard L, et al: Catheter-free geriatric care. Routines and consequences for clinical infection, care and economy. J Hosp Infect 5:298, 1984.
28. Ouslander JG, Kane RL: The costs of urinary incontinence in nursing homes. Med Care 22:69, 1984.
29. Kunin CM, McCormack RC: Prevention of catheter-induced urinary tract infections by sterile closed drainage. N Engl J Med 274:1155, 1966.
30. Garibaldi RA, Burke JP, Britt MR, et al: Meatal colonization and catheter-associated bacteriuria. N Engl J Med 303:216, 1980.
31. Dukes C: Urinary tract infections after excision of the rectum: Their causes and prevention. Proc R Soc Med 22:1, 1928.
32. Miller A, Gillespie WA, Linton KB, et al: Prevention of urinary infection after prostatectomy. Lancet 2:886, 1960.
33. Desautels RE, Walter CW, Graves RC, et al: Technical advances in the prevention of urinary tract infection. J Urol 87:487, 1962.
34. Kunin CM: Can we build a better urinary catheter? N Engl J Med 319:365, 1988.
35. O'Grady F, Cattell WR: Kinetics of urinary infection. II. The bladder. Br J Urol 38:156, 1966.
36. Warren JW: *Providencia stuartii:* A common cause of antibiotic-resistant bacteriuria in patients with long-term indwelling catheters. Rev Infect Dis 8:61, 1986.
37. Burke JP, Jacobson JA, Garibaldi RA, et al: Evaluation of daily meatal care with poly-antibiotic ointment in prevention of urinary catheter-associated bacteriuria. J Urol 129:331, 1983.

38. Huth, TS, Burke JP, Larsen RA, et al: Randomized trial of meatal care with silver sulfadiazine cream for the prevention of catheter-associated bacteriuria. J Infect Dis 165:14, 1992.
39. Platt R, Murdock B, Polk BF, et al: Reduction of mortality associated with nosocomial urinary tract infection. Lancet 1:893, 1983.
40. Huth TS, Burke JP, Larsen RA, et al: Clinical trial of junction seals for the prevention of urinary catheter–associated bacteriuria. Arch Intern Med 152:807, 1992.
41. Wille JC, Blusse van Oud Alblas A, Thewessen EA: Nosocomial catheter-associated bacteriuria: A clinical trial comparing two closed urinary drainage systems. J Hosp Infect 25:191, 1993.
42. Thompson RL, Haley CE, Searcy MA, et al: Catheter-associated bacteriuria. Failure to reduce attack rates using periodic instillations of a disinfectant into urinary drainage systems. JAMA 151:747, 1984.
43. Gillespie WA, Simpson RA, Jones JE, et al: Does the addition of disinfectant to urine drainage bags prevent infection in catheterised patients? Lancet 1:1037, 1983.
44. Kunin CM, Chin QF, Chambers ST: Indwelling urinary catheters in the elderly. Relation of "catheter life" to formation of encrustations in patients with and without blocked catheters. Am J Med 82:405, 1987.
45. Kunin CM, Chin QF, Chambers ST: Formation of encrustations on indwelling catheters in the elderly: A comparison of different types of catheter materials in "blockers" and "nonblockers." J Urol 138:899, 1987.
46. Dailey MP, Axtell J: Increased incidence of urinary tract infections related to the hydrophilic coated catheter (Abstr 1145). *In* Program and Abstracts of the 28th Interscience Conference on Antimicrobial Agents and Chemotherapy. Washington, DC, American Society for Microbiology, 1988.
47. Schaeffer AJ, Story KO, Johnson SM: Effect of silver oxide trichloroisocyanuric acid antimicrobial urinary drainage system on catheter-associated bacteriuria. J Urol 139:69, 1988.
48. Lundeberg T: Prevention of catheter-associated urinary tract infections by use of silver-impregnated catheters. Lancet 1:1031, 1986.
49. Johnson JR, Roberts PL, Olsen RJ, et al: Prevention of catheter-associated urinary tract infection with a silver oxide–coated urinary catheter: Clinical and microbiologic correlates. J Infect Dis 162:1145, 1990.
50. Brocklehurst C, Hickey DS, Davies I, et al: A new urethral catheter. Br Med J 296:1691, 1988.
51. Reid G, Sharma S, Advikolanu K, et al: Effects of ciprofloxacin, norfloxacin, and ofloxacin on in vitro adhesion and survival of *Pseudomonas aeruginosa* AK1 on urinary catheters. Antimicrob Agents Chemother 38:1490, 1994.
52. Farber BF, Wolff AG: Salicylic acid prevents the adherence of bacteria and yeast to Silastic catheters. J Biomed Mater Res 27:599, 1993.
53. Fuse H, Ohkawa M, Nakashima T, et al: Crystal adherence to urinary catheter materials in rats. J Urol 151:1703, 1994.
54. Getliffe KA: The use of wash-outs to reduce urinary catheter encrustation. Br J Urol 73:696, 1994.
55. Davis CP, Wagle N, Anderson MD, et al: Iontophoresis generates an antimicrobial effect that remains after iontophoresis ceases. Antimicrob Agents Chemother 36:2552, 1992.

44

Prophylaxis for Surgical Infections

Ronald Lee Nichols

Postoperative wound infection remains the major source of infectious morbidity in the surgical patient.[1] In a nationwide study conducted during a 12-month period, reported in 1985, it was estimated that wound infections accounted for about one fourth of all nosocomial infections.[2] This number represented more than 500,000 wound infections, or about 2.8 per 100 operations performed. Many perioperative techniques have been shown to influence the development of surgical wound infection, including the use of antibiotic prophylaxis.[3]

Classification of Surgical Wounds

The best predictor of wound infection was previously thought to be the type of operative procedure. A description of the widely accepted classification of operative procedures follows.

Clean Wounds. Clean wounds are uninfected operative wounds in which no inflammation is encountered and the respiratory, alimentary, genital, and uninfected urinary tracts have not been entered.

Clean-Contaminated Wounds. Clean-contaminated wounds are those from operations in which the respiratory, alimentary, genital, or urinary tract is entered under controlled conditions and without unusual contamination.

Contaminated Wounds. Contaminated wounds include open, fresh, accidental wounds; those produced during operations in which there is a major break in sterile technique or gross spillage from the gastrointestinal tract; and incisions marked by acute, acute nonpurulent inflammation.

Dirty or Infected Wounds. Dirty wounds include old trauma wounds in which devitalized tissue is retained and those that involve existing clinical infection or perforated viscera.

The wound infection in clean operations by definition is due to airborne exogenous or skin microorganisms such as *Staphylococcus aureus*, whereas in the other categories of surgery the agent or agents usually originate from the endogenous polymicrobial aerobic and facultative anaerobic flora. The often-quoted infection rates for the different types of operative procedures are as follows: clean, 1% to 5%; clean-contaminated, 3% to 11%; contaminated, 10% to 17%; and dirty, more than 27%.[4]

The Patient as a Risk for Infection

Although this observation is unproved, the greatest risk factor for postoperative infection appears to be the patient's physical status. Weight loss of more than 10% with clear evidence of physiologic dysfunction of two or more organ systems at the time of operation has been associated with significantly more postoperative complications, including septic ones, than when patients have not lost weight or have done so but have suffered no obvious physiologic impairment.[5] This suggests that adequate body protein stores are necessary to normal body function and to minimize the risks of surgery. A similar observation by the same investigators has shown that the incidence of major complications and pneumonia after major surgery was significantly higher for protein-depleted patients (39% mean protein loss) and their duration of hospital stay longer than those for protein-replete patients (4% mean protein loss).[6]

Immunocompetence, as measured by the degree of hypersensitivity response (cell-mediated immunity) evoked by the injection of seven antigens, was compared in patients who had gastric cancer during the preoperative period.[7] The sum of the mean responses to the antigens constituted each patient's score; anergy was defined as induration of less than 2 mm. The postoperative course of the anergic patients was marked by significantly more septic complications than a comparable group of immunocompetent patients experienced.

Other evidence of the importance of individual patient-related risks include an overall lower infection rate for operative procedures of all categories in the pediatric age group than in adults.[8] Presumably, these young patients as a group have a better overall health status than older adults. Different rates of surgical wound infection in public hospitals (5.4%) and private hospitals (2.8%) were reported in a national study of the predictors of surgical wound infection in Australia.[9] The authors of that report believed that these differences may be explained by the fact that patients who are more ill and who require more complex surgery are more likely to be sent to public rather than private hospitals. Higher wound infection rates were also observed in patients older than 55 years of age.

Haley and colleagues[10] were the first to publish on the importance of identifying individual patients who are at high risk of surgical wound infection for each category of operative procedure. To predict the likelihood of surgical wound infection from several risk factors, the authors used information collected from 58,498 patients undergoing operations in 1970 to develop a simple multivariate risk index. Analyzing 10 possible risk factors by stepwise multiple logistic regression techniques, they developed a model containing four risk factors: (1) abdominal operation, (2) operation lasting longer than 2 hours, (3) contaminated or dirty infected operation by traditional wound classification system, and (4) patient having three or more different diagnoses. They utilized the resulting formula to predict an individual patient's probability of developing a postoperative wound infection. When this approach was tested on another group of 59,352 surgical patients admitted in 1975 and 1976, it was found to be a valid predictor of surgical wound infection. The authors concluded that their simplified index predicts surgical wound infection risk about twice as well as the traditional classification of wound contamination. Utilizing this model, low-, medium-, and high-risk factors for developing wound infection were identified in the different categories of the traditional wound classification. In this study, the overall wound infection rate progressively increased from clean (2.9%), to clean-contaminated (3.9%), to contaminated (8.5%), to dirty or infected (12.6%). The range of infection risk in patients in each category was wide: in clean operations, 1.1% in persons at low risk to 15.8% in those at high risk; in clean-contaminated operations, 0.6% to 17.7%; in contaminated operations, 4.5% (medium risk) to 23.9%; and in dirty or infected operations, 6.7% (medium risk) to 27.4%. For contaminated and dirty or infected operations, no patients at low risk were identified.

Centers for Disease Control and Prevention investigators have reported on a composite risk index used in the National Nosocomial Infections Surveillance System.[11] This index uses a dichotomization of the American Society of Anesthesiology score to identify host factors as a risk for infection instead of three or more discharge diagnoses.[12] This change facilitates data collection and apparently increases objectivity. Second, in the new risk index "prolonged surgery" is defined individually for each procedure, rather than being 2 hours for all operations. For some procedures, such as cesarean section, the cutoff point is 1 hour; for others, such as coronary artery bypass graft operation, it is 5 hours. This adjustment makes the index more discriminating. This study is detailed in Chapter 101.

Factors Other Than Antibiotics That Help Control the Incidence of Surgical Wound Infection

Many perioperative factors have been proved to have a significant influence on the development of postoperative wound infection, especially in clean surgical procedures, in which the infection rate is generally expected to be lower than 3%, owing to the fact that only airborne exogenous microorganisms are involved.[3, 4, 13] These perioperative measures are aimed at preventing microbial contamination of the wound at the onset of operation as well as during the period of operative manipulation.

Preoperative Stay in Hospital

A direct correlation is seen in the relationship between the duration of preoperative hospitalization and the development of postoperative wound infections. Cruse and Foord[13] reported that the overall infection rate was 1.1% for patients whose preoperative stay was 1 day; this rate doubled with each week that the patient remained in the hospital before surgery. Most patients who undergo elective operation today are admitted to the hospital on the morning of surgery or on the day before the operation. This greatly decreases the chance for colonization with hospital bacteria and the chance of subsequent infection. Patients admitted for other medical problems should not undergo elective operations later in the same hospital stay as they are at significant risk of infection due to hospital-acquired bacteria.

Preoperative Shave

Preoperative razor shaving 1 day before surgery is associated with significantly higher wound infection rates.[13] Seropian and Reynolds[14] documented an infection rate of 0.6% when a depilatory agent was used for hair removal and a rate of 5.6% for razor shaving done the day before surgery. It was postulated that even skillful razor preparation causes microscopic injury, which provides portals of exit from and entry to injured tissue, which in turn serves as a substrate for bacterial growth. Although the lowest infection rate found by Cruse and Foord[13] was in patients who had not been shaved, all surgeons prefer to operate in a "deforested" field. The investigators proposed the alternative of hair clipping, which has an acceptably low infection rate of 1.7%. Subsequently, this approach was found to be a viable alternative to shaving.[15]

Preoperative Cleansing

Preoperative showering or bathing with a hexachlorophene antiseptic on the evening before surgery is associated with a lower rate of postoperative wound infection than bathing with regular soap.[13] Today, many other antiseptic soaps are available that appear to offer similar protection. One large multihospital study of clean operative procedures showed no fewer wound infections when patients bathed twice preoperatively with chlorhexidine-detergent than when they used detergent alone.[16]

Presence of Remote Infections

The presence of an active remote infection at the time of elective operation has been shown to greatly influence the development of subsequent postoperative wound infections.[17, 18] In order of frequency, these infections occur in the urinary tract, skin, and respiratory tract. Antibiotic prophylaxis or surgical incision of a skin abscess on the night prior to surgery does not reduce the incidence of subsequent wound infections, but preoperative treatment (more than 24 hours before surgery) has been shown to reduce it significantly to a level similar to that for patients who have no remote infection.[18]

Length of Operation

With each hour of operation, the infection rate almost doubles. Shapiro and coworkers[19] reported that an increasing duration of hysterectomy was associated with a decreasing effect of antibiotic prophylaxis in preventing infection at the operative site. This finding undoubtedly relates to the pharmacokinetics of the antibiotic prophylaxis as well as to the greater bacterial wound contamination that occurs in lengthy, complicated operative procedures.

In another study of postoperative wound infection in 676 pediatric patients, an increased rate of wound infection was associated with operative procedures of longer than 1 hour.[8] These studies have undoubtedly influenced the current practice of repeating the dose of prophylactic antibiotics when adults' operations exceed 2 to 3 hours, although the exact risk associated with the duration of operation differs from procedure to procedure.[11, 20]

Use of Prophylactic Abdominal Drainage

Nora and coworkers[21] reported both clinical and experimental studies of the dangers of using prophylactic drains in abdominal surgery. On the basis of their frequent findings of skin bacteria in the interior of the abdominal drains, these investigators stressed the "two-way street" concept. Cerise and associates[22] reported increased infection rates after splenectomy when drains were employed. Magee[23] demonstrated that the presence of either Silastic or latex Penrose drains in experimental wounds dramatically enhanced the wound infection rate, even in the presence of subinfective doses of bacteria. On the basis of these experimental and clinical studies, it appears safe to conclude that the prophylactic use of abdominal drains is unwarranted and, indeed, may be a dangerous practice. When drains are required to empty localized collections, they should be placed through sites other than the primary surgical incision, to decrease the incidence of subsequent wound infection. Closed suction drainage, as suggested by Alexander and coworkers,[24] is the method of choice when abdominal drainage is indicated.

Operating Suite Design and Ventilation Systems

It appears that in most operative procedures the patient and personnel are the chief factors in the control of wound infections, but architectural design concepts have evolved that also play a role in modern operating suites. Laufman[25] has reviewed the key features of design. These include the isolation of the surgical suite from the mainstream of common corridor traffic and the development of the "clean central core," which serves as the supply center and supposedly offers the cleanest environment. The inner corridors that surround the clean core are designed for use by clean traffic, which includes the preoperative patient, nurses, and surgeons. The peripheral corridors are designated for traffic that includes the postoperative patient as well as surgeons and nurses after the operation or between cases. Infected patients should be transferred through the peripheral corridors before and after operation. Floors in the operating room should be nonporous, and other surfaces as dirt resistant as possible. The use of tacky or antiseptic mats at the entrance of the operating room is contraindicated.[4]

The optimal size for most routine operating rooms is 20 by 20 feet with 10-foot ceilings, which allows for easy gowning, draping, circulation of personnel, and the use of equipment without the risk of contact contamination. The door of each operating room should be kept closed except to allow passage of equipment, personnel, and the patient. The number of personnel allowed to enter each operating room should be kept to an absolute minimum, because the origin of infecting bacteria can sometimes be traced to shedding that occurs during their movement in the operating room. Limiting the number of people in attendance, excessive conversation, and the number of times the doors are opened and monitoring the pattern of antibiotic prophylaxis have reduced the infection rate after implant surgery.[26]

Today, most conventional operating rooms in the United States are ventilated with 20 to 25 changes per hour of high-efficiency filtered air delivered in unidirectional vertical flow.[27] The most common system is high-efficiency particulate air filtration, which removes most bacteria that measure 0.5 to 5.0 μm. Therefore, the first air downstream from the high-efficiency particulate air filter is virtually bacteria free. Bacteria released in the operating room environment remain unaffected by the filter system. At least 20% of the air changes each hour should be fresh air. The air delivered should be at temperatures between 18°C and 24°C (65°F and 75°F) and at 50% to 55% humidity. Inlets should be located as high above the floor as possible and remote from the active exhaust outlets, which are located low on the walls. This arrangement allows for the unidirectional airflow. The operating room also should be under higher pressure than the surrounding corridors, to minimize the flow into the operating room when the doors are opened. Careful maintenance of such a ventilation system offers an environment that is virtually as clean as more costly special chambers unless abuses by personnel occur.[25] The use of this type of air-handling system is clearly indicated for most clean surgical procedures and for all procedures where the patient's endogenous microflora are released during the surgical procedure. The debate continues as to whether additional highly specialized laminar flow ventilation systems are advantageous when major implant surgery is to be undertaken.[28]

Other Factors

Many other factors have been thought to influence postoperative wound infection—preoperative scrub technique, surgical glove damage, barrier materials—but there is no convincing evidence. Anecdotal experience and commercial interests, rather than scientific studies, usually account for these associations. A thoughtful review by Sebben[29] offered recommendations that I believe to be essential elements of infection control for office-based surgical practice: modern concepts of instrument sterilization, skin cleansing, and insights into the use of prophylactic antibiotics.

Antibiotic Prophylaxis

Great strides have been accomplished in the last decade in the rational use of antibiotic prophylaxis.[30–32] To better understand the current state of this art, it appears necessary to review a few of the historical milestones of the last three decades.

Historical Considerations

Confusing and heated debate concerning the efficacy of prophylactic antibiotics in surgery followed the publication of clinical trial results during the 1950s. Errors in study design of these early efforts included nonrandomization, lack of "blinding," faulty timing of initial antibiotic administration, prolonged antibiotic use, and incorrect choices of antimicrobial agents.

Experimental studies published during the early 1960s helped to clarify many of these problems and resulted in a more scientifically accurate approach to antimicrobial prophylaxis. Most significant was the report by Burke[33] that demonstrated the crucial relationship between timing of antibiotic administration and its prophylactic efficacy. His experimental studies showed that to greatly reduce experimental skin infection produced by penicillin-sensitive *S. aureus,* the penicillin must be in the skin shortly before or at the time of bacterial inoculation. Critical delays in antibiotic administration after bacterial inoculation of just 3 to 4 hours resulted in infected lesions that were indistinguishable in size and histologic appearance from those of animals that had received no prophylaxis. This study and others that followed helped to develop the attitude that to prevent subsequent infection the antibiotic must be in the tissues before or at the time of bacterial contamination. This important change in strategy avoided the common error of administering the first prophylactic antibiotic in the recovery room after the operation was completed.

As early as 1964, Bernard and Cole[34] were the first to report on the successful use of prophylactic antibiotics in a randomized, prospective placebo-controlled clinical study of gastrointestinal tract operations. Their study design utilized a total of three intramuscular doses of antibiotics of appropriate size given shortly before, during, and shortly after operation. Sixty-six patients who received the antibiotics had a significantly reduced postoperative infection rate of 8%, compared with the 27% infection rate observed in 79 placebo-treated patients. The success of antibiotic prophylaxis noted in this early study was clearly due to the investigators' appropriate selection of patients and wise choice of available agents as well as to appropriate timing of their administration.

Further advances in our understanding of antibiotic prophylaxis in abdominal surgery occurred in the 1970s, when the qualitative and quantitative nature of the endogenous gastrointestinal flora in health and in disease was accurately defined.[35] Despite these early advances, skepticism about the efficacy of antibiotic prophylaxis continued into the 1980s.[36]

Principles of Antibiotic Prophylaxis

Many authoritative reviews of countless clinical studies of surgical prophylaxis have identified which patients may be expected to benefit from perioperative antibiotics.[37, 38] Heretofore, prophylactic antibiotics were clearly indicated for *clean* operations that involved a foreign body implant and for all *clean-contaminated* procedures, but certain data suggest that prophylactic antibiotics are of value for some patients undergoing clean procedures *without* foreign implants, such as inguinal hernia repair or breast surgery.[39] For patients with established infection (*dirty* cases), the use of antibiotics is considered to be therapeutic and is not discussed in this chapter.

CHOICE OF AGENTS

No single antibiotic agent or combination should be relied on for effective prophylaxis in all operations. The agent or agents should be chosen principally on the basis of their efficacy against the usual exogenous and endogenous microorganisms known to cause infectious complications in each clinical setting, as well as on their safety profile and cost. When several drugs or regimens are equally efficacious and safe, local hospital cost analyses and utilization studies may result in use of the agent that is least expensive overall.[40] Usual infecting microorganisms and antibiotic recommendations for each surgical procedure are listed in Table 44–1. Worldwide, the cephalosporins are the most widely used antibiotics for surgical prophylaxis.[32] It has been stressed that antibiotic coverage for all the potential pathogens is not a desired feature of a prophylactic regimen. Nevertheless, it is important to maintain an up-to-date local hospital analysis of the antimicrobial susceptibilities of wound isolates to detect important shifts in patterns of resistance.[41] Routine use of second- or third-generation cephalosporins has not improved the clinical results over those achieved with first-generation cephalosporins.[42] Until there is evidence of their superiority, these agents should be reserved for procedures that require special coverage, such as the anaerobic coverage required in appendectomy and in other colon procedures.[31]

TIMING OF PROPHYLAXIS

The effective use of prophylactic antibiotics depends to a great extent on the appropriate timing of their administration. Historically, the most common errors in prophylaxis, which undoubtedly dulled the luster of this technique, were the faulty timing of the initial administration and the common practice of continuing to administer the antibiotic beyond 72 hours.[43]

Current recommendations call for the parenteral antibiotic used in prophylaxis to be given in a sufficient dose within 30 minutes of incision.[30, 31, 37, 38] This can be facilitated by having the anesthesiologist administer the drug in the operating room shortly before operative incision when the intravenous lines are started. The former practice of giving the antibiotic "on-call" to the operating room frequently meant that it was given 3 to 4 hours before the incision was made, with the result that levels of antibiotic in tissue and serum at the time of operation were low or undetectable. Starting the antibiotic agent within 30 minutes of incision results in therapeutic drug levels in the wound and surrounding tissues during the operation. Evidence from clinical trials is mounting that supports the assertion that this single preoperative dose of antibiotic is as efficacious as multiple doses of prophylactic antibiotics given during the perioperative course.[44] Advocates of single-dose prophylaxis generally recommend that another dose be given when the operation lasts longer than 2 or 3 hours. It also appears that no additional benefit can be derived from longer courses of antibiotic prophylaxis (more than 24 hours), even for immunosuppressed patients.[45]

For oral preoperative antibiotic preparations commonly utilized before elective colon resection, the chosen agents should be given during the 24 hours before operation to attain significant intraluminal (local) and serum (systemic) levels.[46] With oral neomycin and erythromycin base, it is necessary to give only three doses of each agent during the 19 hours before operative incision to accomplish these ends.[47]

TABLE 44–1 ■ Infecting Microorganisms Usually Associated with Certain Operative Procedures and Prophylactic Antibiotic Recommendations

	INFECTING MICROORGANISMS					
SURGICAL PROCEDURE	Facultative	Anaerobic	RECOMMENDED AGENTS	ROUTE[a]	DOSE (g)[b]	ALTERNATIVE
Clean[c]	*Staphylococcus* *Staphylococcus epidermidis*	—	1st-generation[d] cephalosporin (cefazolin)	IV	1–2	2nd- or 3rd-generation cephalosporin (IV)[e] or vancomycin (IV)[f]
Gastroduodenal	Streptococci Coliforms	*Bacteroides* (other than *B. fragilis*) Peptostreptococci	Cefazolin	IV	1–2	2nd- or 3rd-generation cephalosporin (IV)
Cholecystectomy	Coliforms Enterococci	Clostridia	Cefazolin	IV	1–2	2nd- or 3rd-generation cephalosporin (IV)
Elective colon resection	Coliforms	*B. fragilis* Peptostreptococci Clostridia	Neomycin–erythromycin base[g]	PO	1 each × 3[h]	Aminoglycoside (PO) + metronidazole (PO) or tetracycline (PO)
Small intestine resection	Coliforms	*B. fragilis* Peptostreptococci	Neomycin–erythromycin base[g]	PO	1 each × 3	IV antibiotic with aerobic and anaerobic coverage (see Table 44–3)[i]
Appendectomy	Coliforms	*B. fragilis* Peptostreptococci	Cefoxitin or ceftizoxime	IV	1–2	Other IV agents (see Table 44–3)
Penetrating abdominal trauma	Coliforms[j]	*B. fragilis*[j] Clostridia Peptostreptococci	Cefoxitin	IV	2[k]	Other IV agents (see Table 44–3)
Vaginal or abdominal hysterectomy	Coliforms Enterococci Group B streptococci	*B. fragilis* Clostridia	Cefazolin	IV	1	Other IV agents (see Table 44–3)
Cesarean section	Same as hysterectomy		Cefazolin	IV	1[l]	Other IV agents (see Table 44–3)
Abortion	Same as hysterectomy		Cefazolin[m]	IV	1	Other IV agents (see Table 44–3)
Prostatectomy[n]	Coliforms	—	Cefazolin[o]	IV	1	Based on sensitivity of infecting microorganisms
Traumatic hemopneumothorax[p]	*S. aureus* Streptococci	— —	Cefazolin or cefonicid	IV	0.5–1.0[q]	—

[a]IV, Intravenous; PO, oral.
[b]Single-dose prophylaxis is preferred unless operative time is longer than 2 h, in which case an additional intraoperative dose is indicated.
[c]Includes cardiac, vascular, and orthopedic procedures that utilize a prosthetic implant or device. Some recommend same approach in clean procedures such as hernia repair or breast surgery.[39]
[d]Cephalothin and cephapirin are alternatives to cefazolin, but cefazolin is preferred because of its longer half-life and higher tissue levels.
[e]Some prefer agents such as cefuroxime, cefamandole, or ceftriaxone.
[f]Vancomycin is utilized in patients allergic to penicillins or cephalosporins or in hospitals where methicillin-resistant *S. aureus* and *S. epidermidis* frequently cause wound infection.
[g]Most also utilize an additional IV dose of antibiotic at time of operation with efficacy against facultative coliforms and anaerobic *Bacteroides* (see Table 44–3).
[h]Mechanical cleansing (see Table 44–2) precedes oral antibiotic intake. Timing of oral antibiotics also noted in Table 44–2.
[i]In nonelective small intestine surgery (bleeding or obstruction), systemic antibiotics alone are utilized.
[j]Intestinal flora expected in cases with observed leakage. If no perforation is noted, infecting flora is usually facultative gram-positive cocci (staphylococci).
[k]Single preoperative dose suffices when no intestinal leakage is observed at operation. When intestinal leakage is present, dosing continues 2–5 d.
[l]In high-risk sections only; to be given after cord is clamped.
[m]IV cefazolin is utilized in second-trimester abortions. In first-trimester abortions in patients with previous pelvic inflammatory disease, aqueous penicillin, 1 million units IV, or doxycycline, 300 mg PO, is recommended.
[n]In the presence of infected urine in the patient undergoing transurethral prostatic resection.
[o]If preoperative urine culture shows sensitive microorganism.
[p]Requiring placement of closed tube thoracostomy.
[q]Regimens vary from dosing every 8 h for 24 h to 1g daily until chest tube removal.

Longer periods of preoperative preparation are unnecessary and have been associated with the isolation of resistant organisms within the colon lumen at the time of resection.[37]

ROUTE OF ADMINISTRATION

Intravenous administration of the prophylactic antibiotic is preferred for most operative procedures. When this is accomplished in a relatively small volume over a short period (20 to 30 minutes), high serum and tissue levels are the rule. The pharmacokinetics of each individual antibiotic largely determine how long efficacious serum levels will be sustained. Doses of short–half-life agents (less than 1 hour) should be repeated every 2 to 3 hours during the operation. The study of different half-life agents in surgical antibiotic prophylaxis in long-duration procedures has not been done. At this time orally administered antibiotics have a major role only in the preparation of patients for elective colon operations.[46]

Antibiotic Prophylaxis in Specific Surgical Procedures

There appears to be a clear consensus that antibiotic prophylaxis is necessary and helpful in clean-contaminated procedures that involve mucous membranes harboring an endogenous microflora and in clean procedures that involve the implantation of grafts or prosthetic devices. When infection is presumed to be present at the time of surgery, as in contaminated or dirty procedures, antibiotics are given with therapeutic intent. Perforation of the gastrointestinal tract, whether by penetrating trauma or a disease process (e.g., ruptured appendix, perforated colonic diverticulum), permits the escape of endogenous microflora resulting in direct contamination of the peritoneal cavity and of the operative incision at the time of operation. These clinical settings constitute high-risk situations for the development of postoperative infection; however, the use of perioperative antibiotic prophylaxis within a few hours of perforation appears to be efficacious. Longer delays, which are associated with the development of systemic sepsis or severe intraabdominal infections including abscess formation or diffuse peritonitis, require therapeutic antibiotic and surgical approaches. Operative procedures not specified in this chapter include ocular, neurosurgical, and head and neck operations and pulmonary resection. Few data are available on the efficacy of antibiotic prophylaxis in these clinical settings, and some recommendations have been made.[38]

Clean Surgical Procedures

Currently, antibiotic prophylaxis is indicated in clean surgical procedures that utilize a foreign material, grafts, or prosthetic devices—many vascular, cardiac, and orthopedic operations, among others.[30, 37, 38] In these settings the prophylactic drug regimen is often continued as long as 24 to 48 hours postoperatively despite lack of clear evidence that this practice is effective.[32] Continuing the prophylactic antibiotic regimen beyond the immediate perioperative period dramatically increases the cost[48] and has been associated with the development of *Clostridium difficile* colitis[49] and also with a high level of colonization with methicillin-resistant *Staphylococcus epidermidis.*[50] Although the experience with single-dose prophylaxis in cardiovascular surgery is somewhat limited, it appears this approach is effective when a long-acting drug such as ceftriaxone is utilized.[32, 51]

When infection does occur postoperatively in these procedures the pathogen is usually *S. aureus* (antibiotic recommendations are offered in Table 44–1). Several cephalosporin agents of different generations have been utilized; none shows clear evidence of superiority.[32] Vancomycin may be employed instead of the cephalosporin agents if a high degree of methicillin resistance has been noted in the individual hospital centers or in postoperative infections. The routine use of vancomycin prophylaxis in these cases is clearly not necessary and if done will lead to increasing bacterial resistance.

The use of antibiotic prophylaxis for clean surgical procedures that do not involve prostheses or other foreign materials is presently under debate. Platt and coauthors[39] have shown the apparent benefit of the use of one dose of cephalosporin over placebo in reducing wound infections after breast or hernia surgery. Future studies will undoubtedly indicate which groups of patients are at high risk for infection in other clean procedures in which a synthetic material is not implanted. These studies will also reveal whether antibiotic prophylaxis proves to be efficacious for patients at such high risk.

Gastroduodenal Procedures

The most common indication for gastroduodenal operation before 1975 was for the treatment of chronic nonobstructing duodenal ulcer.[52] The rarity of associated postoperative infectious complications fostered the belief that the stomach contents were often sterile and that antibiotic prophylaxis was not indicated. With the advent of modern medical treatment for chronic duodenal ulcer, surgeons are called on less frequently to operate for this indication. Gastroduodenal operations are now frequently performed for the complications of duodenal ulcer, gastric ulcer, and malignancy. The frequency of postoperative infection in such cases prompted a reappraisal of the role of antibiotic prophylaxis for gastroduodenal surgery.

RISK OF INFECTION

Published studies have defined two risk groups for infections after gastric surgery.[52] Patients at low risk (less than 5%) are those who undergo operation for chronic nonobstructing duodenal ulcer and have high or normal levels of gastric acid and normal motility. These patients have few microorganisms, if any, in the gastric lumen at the time of resection. Another low-risk category includes patients operated on for perforating duodenal ulcer disease.[53] The peritonitis encountered at operation in these cases is largely chemical, and a bacterial pathogen is found only if surgical intervention is long delayed.

Patients at high risk (more than 10%) of postoperative infection are those who undergo operation for bleeding or obstructing duodenal ulcer, gastric ulcer, or malignancy. Gastric colonization with organisms entering the stomach from saliva or refluxing through the pylorus is routinely observed in these cases.

PROPHYLACTIC ANTIBIOTIC RECOMMENDATIONS

Antibiotic prophylaxis is indicated for every patient at high risk (see Table 44–1). Prospective randomized clinical trials have shown the benefit to these patients of prophylaxis with a parenteral first- or second-generation cephalosporin.[54] The optimal regimen would utilize a 1- to 2-g dose of the cephalosporin given intravenously within 30 minutes of incision. The administration of additional doses during the 24 hours after the start of operation appears to be unnecessary unless the operative procedure is quite complex and protracted. Intermittent intraoperative local wound irrigation with antibiotic solution instead of parenteral antibiotic prophylaxis has been recommended by one author.[55]

Elective Cholecystectomy

Cholecystectomy for chronic calculous cholecystitis is the only biliary tract operation for which antibiotic prophylaxis is employed. Operations for acute cholecystitis, empyema of the gallbladder, ascending cholangitis, or liver abscess require antibiotic treatment rather than prophylaxis.

The healthy human biliary tract rarely harbors significant concentrations of bacteria. In the presence of chronic calculous cholecystitis, bacteria have been isolated from bile in 15% to 30% of cases. The bacteria isolated are predominantly gram-negative bacilli. *Escherichia coli,* alone or mixed with another organism, is present in 50% of cultures that propagate an organism. Other coliforms—*Klebsiella, Enterobacter, Proteus*—are isolated less often. Anaerobic microorganisms are isolated in less than 20% of the cases, *Clostridium perfringens* and *Bacteroides fragilis* being the most common. A polymicrobial infection by both facultative aerobes and anaerobes may be associated with liver abscess or long-standing common duct obstruction due to choledocholithiasis.

RISK OF INFECTION

Propagation in cultures of organisms collected at the time of cholecystectomy are associated with a high risk of postoperative infection. Several studies have defined the clinical factors that favor bacterbilia and, therefore, a correspondingly greater risk of postoperative infection: age more than 70 years; history or presence of jaundice; previous biliary tract surgery; chills or fever within 1 week of operation; common duct disease; operations done within 1 month of an acute attack of cholecystitis; and diabetes mellitus.[56]

PROPHYLACTIC ANTIBIOTIC RECOMMENDATIONS

Placebo-controlled studies have shown decreased rates of postoperative infection when antibiotic prophylaxis is used for cholecystectomy in high-risk patients (those who have one or more clinical risk factors).[31] Most studies have employed a first- or second-generation cephalosporin. No comparative studies of these different regimens are available, but in a large multicenter study of elective cholecystectomy single-dose prophylaxis with cefazolin, cefamandole, or cefuroxime provided similar satisfactory results.[57]

The principal controversy is whether only patients who have a clinical risk factor or positive intraoperative Gram stain examination should receive antibiotic prophylaxis before elective cholecystectomy. One clinical study recommended a single dose of cephalosporin for all patients undergoing cholecystectomy, regardless of clinical risk factors or Gram stain results.[58] This study revealed a high wound infection rate (18%) after intraoperative administration of antibiotics when organisms were seen in gram-stained preparations of bile from patients who had no clinical risk factors.

Elective Colon Resection

The human colon and distal small intestine contain an enormous reservoir of facultative aerobic and anaerobic bacteria that are sequestered from the rest of the body by the mucous membrane. Experimental studies from our laboratory have defined both a luminal microflora and a mucosal related microflora in animals and humans that are qualitatively and quantitatively similar.[59, 60] When the mucous membrane barrier is disturbed by disease or trauma or if the colon is opened to the peritoneal cavity during surgery, escape of bacteria into adjacent tissues may result in a serious infection. For this reason, finding a reliable method of sterilizing the colonic contents has been a goal of surgeons throughout this century. In the past 20 years, results of clinical trials have clearly shown that to significantly reduce septic complications after elective colon surgery it is necessary to employ antibiotics that are active against both colonic facultative aerobes (e.g., *E. coli*) and anaerobes (e.g., *B. fragilis*). Controversy exists, however, over the optimal antibiotic regimen and route of administration.

Before the 1970s the majority of surgeons utilized mechanical cleansing alone before elective colon surgery.[61] The oral antibiotics that had been utilized up to that time (neomycin, kanamycin, streptomycin, sulfonamides) most often only suppressed the facultative aerobic colon flora and were associated with high rates of clinical failure. In addition, use of these oral antibiotics for 3 to 5 days before elective colon resection was frequently associated with overgrowth of staphylococci and yeast in the patient's gastrointestinal tract, a development that rarely follows a 1-day course of oral antibiotic operative preparation.

RISK OF INFECTION

All patients undergoing elective colon resection are at significant risk of developing postoperative infection because of the great number of bacteria in the colon microflora, which increases in protracted operations and in those done on the extraperitoneal rectum.[46]

Kaiser and colleagues[62] studied different approaches to preoperative antibiotic prophylaxis for elective colon resection and showed a direct correlation between the duration of operation and the postoperative infection rate. In operations of less than 3 hours, no infections were identified when antibiotic prophylaxis was accomplished with a parenteral agent alone or a combination of oral and parenteral agents; however, in operations that lasted more than 4 hours significantly fewer infections were observed in patients who received the combination prophylactic regimen. In a similar study of elective colon resection, Coppa and Eng[63] stressed that postoperative wound infections are associated with the duration of operation and the location of the colon resection (intraperitoneal versus rectal). These authors showed that the wound infection rate for high-risk patients who have operations longer than 215 minutes that involve rectal resection could benefit significantly from the use of a combination of oral and parenteral prophylactic antibiotics.

MECHANICAL PREPARATION

Mechanical cleansing of the colon lumen before elective colon resection is a time-tested procedure that, when done properly, reduces the total fecal luminal mass, allowing easier operative manipulation of the colon. The cleansing also facilitates the action of oral antibiotics. Vigorous mechanical cleaning alone, utilizing either lavage techniques or the classic approach of dietary restriction, enemas, and cathartics, has not significantly reduced the number of microorganisms in the residual colonic material. This microbiologic failure of mechanical cleansing alone also equates with clinical failure. In two large prospective, randomized, double-blind clinical trials investigating the efficacy of oral antibiotic prophylaxis, more than 40% of patients undergoing elective colon resection who were given mechanical cleansing alone developed septic complications.[64, 65]

Today, approaches to mechanical cleansing vary considerably.[46, 66] The time-honored 5-day preoperative preparation utilizing dietary restriction, enemas, and cathartics was long ago abandoned, for many good reasons. At the top of this list were the severe iatrogenically induced metabolic abnormalities that were reported more than 20 years ago. Modern approaches include standard mechanical cleansing utilizing dietary restriction, cathartics, and enemas for 2 days, or, on the day preceding operation, whole-gut lavage with an electrolyte solution, 10% mannitol, sodium phosphate solution, or polyethylene glycol. A suggested schema for mechanical preparation is offered in Table 44–2 and Figure 44–1.

ANTIBIOTIC PREPARATION

Today the vast majority of surgeons employ antibiotics as well as mechanical cleansing as preparation for elective colon resection.[46, 66] The chosen antibiotics should be effective in suppressing both colonic facultative aerobes and anaerobes.[67, 68] Debate continues as to which agents are ideal and which route of administration is preferred. Investigators who advocate oral antibiotics generally stress the importance of

TABLE 44–2 ■ Recommended Approach to Preoperative Colon Preparation

Two days before surgery (at home):
Dietary restriction: low-residue or liquid diet
Magnesium citrate, 30 mL of a 50% solution (15 g) PO at 10:00 AM, 2:00 PM, and 6:00 PM
Fleet enemas until clear in the evening
Day of hospitalization (preoperative day) (admit in the morning):
Clear liquid diet, IV fluids as needed
Magnesium citrate, dose as above, at 10:00 AM and 2:00 PM OR
Whole-gut lavage with polyethylene glycol electrolyte solution (GoLYTELY or Colyte), 1 L/h for 2–4 h until effluent is clear, before administration of oral antibiotic at 1:00 PM (usually commencing at 7:00 or 8:00 AM)
No enemas
Neomycin–erythromycin base, 1 g each PO at 1:00 PM, 2:00 PM, and 11:00 PM
Day of surgery:
Operation at 8:00 AM
One dose of antibiotic with facultative aerobic-anaerobic activity given IV by anesthesiologist in the operating room just before incision (see Table 44–3)

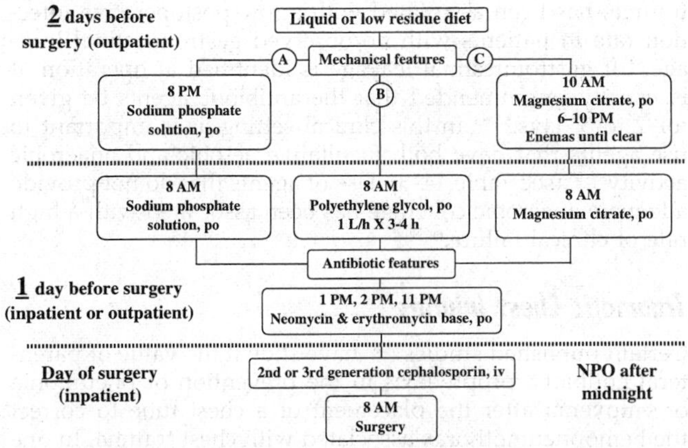

FIGURE 44–1 ▫ Preoperative bowel preparation.

reducing the number of microorganisms in the colon lumen before opening the colon; those who rely on parenteral agents stress the importance of adequate tissue levels of antibiotics.

Oral Antibiotic Agents. At the present time, three regimens of oral agents are utilized, which combine neomycin with either erythromycin base, metronidazole, or tetracycline.[46] The greatest experience in the United States has been with the neomycin–erythromycin base preparation, which was introduced in 1972,[67] whereas metronidazole plus either kanamycin or neomycin is popular in Great Britain.[46] Authoritative reviews of antibiotic prophylaxis for colon surgery continue to support the value of oral neomycin–erythromycin base in preventing infections after elective colon resection.[31, 37, 38, 46, 66] No convincing data are available to recommend the use of metronidazole over erythromycin base in this clinical setting. The pharmacokinetics of the oral neomycin–erythromycin base bowel preparation has been studied in healthy volunteers and in patients undergoing elective colon resection.[47, 69] The studies suggest that when adequate mechanical preparation is used, intraluminal (local) levels of both antibiotics and the serum (systemic) level of erythromycin are significant and that both mechanisms may play a role in preventing infection after colon surgery. The timing of administration of these oral agents appears to be critical. It is recommended that only 1 g of each agent, neomycin and erythromycin base, be given at 1:00 PM, 2:00 PM, and 11:00 PM on the day before surgery (6 g total; see Table 44–2). Surgery should be planned for about 8:00 AM when this schedule is followed. If the operation is scheduled for later in the day, the timing of the doses should be adjusted to preserve the 19 hours' preparation.

Parenteral Antibiotic Agents. The first prospective, randomized, double-blind study on parenteral antibiotic prophylaxis in elective colon resection (published in 1969) utilized perioperative intramuscular cephaloridine.[70] This study revealed a significant reduction in postoperative infections (7% versus 30%) in the group of patients who received antibiotics in addition to mechanical preparation as compared with those who had mechanical preparation alone, but other clinical studies utilizing the same or similar first-generation cephalosporins for prophylaxis failed to show the superiority of this approach over placebo (mechanical preparation alone) or oral neomycin–erythromycin base.[71, 72] Clinical studies comparing parenteral cephalosporin alone in this setting showed a lack of efficacy unless the antibiotic was active against facultative aerobic and anaerobic organisms.[73] Parenteral agents that have shown efficacy alone or in combination with an aminoglycoside include cefoxitin, cefotetan, metronidazole, and doxycycline.[46] Most investigators recommend perioperative administration of one to five doses of parenteral agent during a 24-hour period starting shortly before operation; however, one multicenter study showed that a single intravenous dose of cefotetan resulted in a 14% infection rate, which was thought to be comparable to an 11% rate among patients who received multiple doses of intravenous cefoxitin.[74] It should be noted, however, that the total infection rates in this study were higher than those reported in the Veterans Administration study using oral neomycin and erythromycin alone (6% to 9%).[64, 75] In my opinion, potent therapeutic antibiotic agents such as imipenem, which was more recently advocated, have no place in prophylactic antibiotic regimens used before elective colon resection.[76]

Combination of Parenteral and Oral Antibiotic Agents. Most surgeons presently utilize both oral and parenteral antibiotic agents and mechanical cleansing as preoperative preparation before elective colon resection in the hope of reducing the postoperative infection rate.[66] In a survey of more than 500 surgeons reported in 1979, only 8% used systemic antibiotics alone before colon surgery, 37% oral antibiotics alone, and 49% oral plus systemic antibiotics.[77] In one survey of more than 350 board-certified colon and rectal surgeons, all used antibiotics in addition to mechanical cleansing.[66] Three percent used oral agents alone, 8% systemic agents alone, and the remaining 89% a combination of both oral and parenteral agents. Parenteral antibiotics that are active against both facultative aerobic and anaerobic organisms (e.g., cefotetan, cefoxitin, ceftizoxime) given in addition to oral neomycin–erythromycin base have been shown to be associated with a low incidence of infection.[46] It appears at this time that the addition of one dose of parenteral antibiotic such as that already mentioned, given within 30 minutes of incision to the oral and mechanical bowel preparation, may be beneficial (see Table 44–2). A complete review of all agents utilized and recommended for preoperative antibiotic preparation throughout the world was updated.[46]

Small Intestinal Operations

Because the contents of the small intestine are liquid and transit time is rapid, extensive preoperative mechanical preparation for elective surgery is unnecessary. There are no antibiotic prophylaxis studies on surgery of the ileum, the site of most apparent risk for infection, because of the complex intestinal flora present at this level.[78] It seems prudent, however, to use the neomycin–erythromycin base oral bowel preparation for such elective procedures. Parenteral agents effective against fecal facultative aerobes and anaerobes are recommended for emergency procedures such as small bowel obstruction (Table 44–3).

Appendectomy

The bacteriology of perforated and gangrenous appendicitis is extremely complex. Bennion and colleagues[79] have isolated in these cases an average of 11 different bacteria from each specimen, including three facultative aerobes and eight anaerobes. As in the other postcolonic resection infections, *B. fragilis* was the most commonly isolated anaerobe and *E. coli* the most common facultative aerobe.

RISK OF INFECTION

The pathologic state of the appendix is the most important determinant of postoperative infection.[80–82] The wound infection rate after appendectomy for perforated or gangrenous appendicitis is four to five times higher than for early disease. A prospective study of nonperforated appendicitis that utilized a logistic regression analysis of risk factors has

TABLE 44–3 ■ Selected Single and Combination Antibiotic Agents That Cover Facultative and Anaerobic Colonic Microflora for Surgical Prophylaxis

Facultative coverage (to be combined with a drug having anaerobic activity)
Amikacin
Aztreonam
Ceftriaxone
Ciprofloxacin
Gentamicin
Tobramycin
Anaerobic coverage (to be combined with a drug having facultative activity)
Chloramphenicol
Clindamycin
Metronidazole
Single agents that provide facultative and anaerobic coverage
Ampicillin-sulbactam
Cefotetan
Cefoxitin
Ceftizoxime
Piperacillin-tazobactam
Ticarcillin-clavulanate

shown that the risk of postoperative wound infection is related only to failure to use perioperative antibiotics and the surgeon's determination of the appendix as being gangrenous.[81] The highest rate of infection (77%) was predicted for patients who received placebo and had a gangrenous appendix, and the lowest rate (2%) for those who received an antibiotic perioperatively and did not have a gangrenous appendix at surgery. Perioperative antibiotic prophylaxis had a beneficial effect in decreasing hospital stay.

ANTIBIOTIC RECOMMENDATIONS

Because it is often impossible to determine the pathologic state of the appendix before, or even during, operation,[81] it is recommended that a parenteral antibiotic agent be given prophylactically in all cases. Agents that are active against both aerobic gram-negative bacilli and anaerobes are more effective than those that are active only against the anaerobes[80] (see Table 44–3). It appears that the prophylactic regimen can be a single dose[82] or three doses.[81] For perforated appendicitis with evidence of local or general peritonitis or intraabdominal abscess, the use of antimicrobials should be considered therapeutic, not prophylactic.

Penetrating Abdominal Trauma

RISK OF INFECTION

Hollow viscus damage with the associated escape of endogenous microorganisms is the principal risk factor for the development of postoperative infectious complications after exploratory laporatomy for penetrating abdominal trauma.[83–85] Utilizing a logistic regression analysis of such patients, we showed that a statistically higher risk of infection was also associated with increasing age of the patient, associated injury to the left colon necessitating colostomy, many units of blood or blood products administered at surgery, and a large number of injured organs identified at operation.[83] Leaving the operative wound packed open with saline-soaked gauze decreases the frequency of postoperative wound infection in high-risk patients.[86]

ANTIBIOTIC RECOMMENDATIONS

The use of one parenteral dose of antibiotic alone, given just before abdominal exploration for penetrating abdominal trauma, has been associated with a low postoperative infection rate in patients with no observed gastrointestinal leakage.[83] If gastrointestinal leakage is identified at operation, it is usually recommended that the antibiotic agents be given for 2 to 5 days.[83–85] In this clinical setting, it is important to use agents that have both facultative aerobic and anaerobic activity[83–85] (see Table 44–3). Use of agents that do not provide adequate anaerobic coverage has been associated with a high rate of clinical failure.[84, 85]

Traumatic Chest Injuries

Certain published studies[87, 88] have shown the value of parenteral antibiotic prophylaxis in the prevention of pneumonia or empyema after the placement of a chest tube to correct the hemopneumothorax associated with chest trauma. In one study,[87] 500 mg of cefazolin was given intravenously every 8 hours for 24 hours. In the other study,[88] 1 g of cefonicid was administered every 24 hours until the time of chest tube removal. Significantly reduced infection rates were observed in both studies in the patients receiving antibiotics compared with the patients receiving placebo.

Gynecologic and Obstetric Infections

Parenteral antibiotic prophylaxis has been shown to decrease significantly the incidence of postoperative infections after vaginal hysterectomy and after emergency cesarean section[32, 38] and may be of benefit in abdominal hysterectomy.[38]

RISK OF INFECTION

In 1982, Shapiro and coinvestigators[19] were the first to utilize logistic regression analysis to identify the risk factors for operative site infections after abdominal or vaginal hysterectomy. They observed that increasing duration of operative time was associated with decreasing effect of antibiotic prophylaxis for operative site infection. The statistically significant benefit of antibiotic prophylaxis in procedures that lasted 1 hour or less was lost in operations that lasted more than 3.3 hours.

In one large single hospital study of post–cesarean section wound infections, significantly higher rates of infections were observed among clinic patients (15.8%) than among private patients (6.0%).[89] All the significant individual risk factors for infection—including emergency versus elective operation, number of vaginal examinations before operation, duration of operation, vertical skin incision, and category of surgeon—were overrepresented in the clinic group.

ANTIBIOTIC RECOMMENDATIONS

A single intravenous dose of parenteral cefazolin given shortly before incision for abdominal or vaginal hysterectomy or after cord clamping in high-risk cesarean section is currently recommended.[32, 38] Many other second- or third-generation cephalosporin agents have also proved efficacious in a single-dose regimen; however, evidence of their clinical superiority is lacking.[32, 38] Oral doxycycline or intravenous penicillin G is utilized for first-trimester abortion for patients with a history of pelvic inflammatory disease; intravenous cefazolin is given to patients undergoing second-trimester abortion.[38, 90]

Urologic Procedures

Antimicrobial prophylaxis is not recommended before urologic operations if the patient has sterile urine.[38] If culture of urine propagates organisms, the patient should be treated with appropriate antimicrobial agents before operation to sterilize the urine. Before prostatectomy, a single dose of intravenous prophylactic antibiotic is utilized immediately before operation if the urine is not sterile.[38]

Overview of Antibiotic Prophylaxis in Surgery

Improvements in antibiotic prophylaxis, including the timing of initial administration, appropriate choice of antibiotic agents in each clinical setting, and short duration of administration, have proved the value of the use of prophylactic antibiotics and are currently recommended by authoritative groups. A computer-generated reminder of appropriate perioperative antibiotic treatment, placed in the patient's chart before operation, has been shown to improve prescribing habits and to produce a concurrent decline in the number of postoperative wound infections.[91] Future studies of antibiotic prophylaxis should strongly consider risk factors of the individual patient in addition to testing new antibiotic agents and administration approaches.

References

1. Nichols RL: Postoperative wound infection. N Engl J Med 307:1701, 1982.
2. Haley RW, Culver DH, White JW, et al: The nationwide nosocomial infection rate: A new need for vital statistics. Am J Epidemiol 121:159, 1985.
3. Nichols RL: Techniques known to prevent postoperative wound infection. Infect Control 3:34, 1982.
4. Garner JS: CDC guidelines for the prevention and control of nosocomial infections: Guideline for prevention of surgical wound infections, 1985. Am J Infect Control 14:71, 1986.
5. Windsor JA, Hill GL: Weight loss with physiologic impairment: A basic indicator of surgical risk. Ann Surg 207:290, 1988.
6. Windsor JA, Hill GL: Protein depletion and surgical risk. Aust N Z J Surg 58:711, 1988.
7. Cainzos M, Alcalde JA, Potel J, et al: Anergy in patients with gastric cancer. Hepatogastroenterology 36:36, 1989.
8. Bhattacharyya N, Kosloske AM: Preoperative wound infection in pediatric surgical patients: A study of 676 infants and children. J Pediatr Surg 25:125, 1990.
9. McLaws ML, Irwig LM, Mock P, et al: Predictors of surgical wound infection in Australia: A national study. Med J Aust 149:591, 1988.
10. Haley RW, Culver DH, Morgan WM, et al: Identifying patients at high risk of surgical wound infection. Am J Epidemiol 121:206, 1985.
11. Culver DH, Horan TC, Gaynes RP and the National Nosocomial Infections Surveillance Systems (NNIS): Surgical wound infection rates by wound class, operation, and risk index in U.S. hospitals. Am J Med 91(Suppl 3B):152S, 1991.
12. Keats AS: The ASA classifications of physical status—A recapitulation. Anesthesiology 49:233, 1978.
13. Cruse PJE, Foord R: A five-year prospective study of 23,649 surgical wounds. Arch Surg 107:206, 1973.
14. Seropian R, Reynolds BM: Wound infections after preoperative depilatory versus razor preparation. Am J Surg 121:251, 1971.
15. Balthazar ER, Colt J, Nichols RL: Preoperative hair removal: A random, prospective study. South Med J 75:799, 1982.
16. Rotter ML, Larsen SO, Cooke EM, et al: A comparison of the effects of preoperative whole-body bathing with detergent alone and with detergent containing chlorhexidine gluconate on the frequency of wound infections after clean surgery. J Hosp Infect 11:310, 1988.
17. Edwards LD: The epidemiology of 2056 remote site infections and 1966 surgical wound infections occurring in 1865 patients: A four-year study of 40,923 operations at Rush-Presbyterian-St. Luke's Hospital, Chicago. Ann Surg 184:758, 1976.
18. Valentine RJ, Weigelt JA, Dryer D, et al: Effect of remote infections on clean wound infection rates. Am J Infect Control 14:64, 1986.
19. Shapiro M, Munoz A, Tager IB, et al: Risk factors for infection at the operative site after abdominal or vaginal hysterectomy. N Engl J Med 307:1661, 1982.
20. Gorbach SL, Condon RE, Conte JE Jr, et al: Evaluation of new anti-infective drugs for surgical prophylaxis. Clin Infect Dis 15(Suppl 1):S313, 1992.
21. Nora PF, Vanecko RM, Bransfield JJ: Prophylactic abdominal drains. Arch Surg 106:173, 1972.
22. Cerise EJ, Pierce WA, Diamond DL: Abdominal drains: Their role as a source of infection following splenectomy. Ann Surg 171:764, 1970.
23. Magee C: Potentiation of wound infection by surgical drains. Am J Surg 131:547, 1976.
24. Alexander JW, Koorelitz J, Alexander NS: Prevention of wound infections: A case for closed suction drainage to remove wound fluids deficient in opsonic proteins. Am J Surg 132:59, 1976.
25. Laufman H: The operating room. *In* Bennett JV, Brachman PS (eds): Hospital Infections, ed 2. Boston, Little, Brown, 1986, pp 315–324.
26. Borst M, Collier C, Miller D: Operating room surveillance: A new approach in reducing hip and knee prosthetic wound infections. Am J Infect Control 14:161, 1986.
27. LoCicero III J, Quebbeman EJ, Nichols RL: Health hazards in the operating room: An update. Bull Am Coll Surg 72:4, 1987.
28. Lidwell OM, Lowbury EJL, Whyte W, et al: Effect of ultraclean air in operating rooms on deep sepsis in the joint after total hip or knee replacement: A randomised study. Br Med J 285:10, 1982.
29. Sebben JE: Sterile technique and the prevention of wound infection in office surgery—Part II. J Dermatol Surg Oncol 15:38, 1989.
30. Nichols RL: Current approaches to antibiotic prophylaxis in surgery. Infect Dis Clin Pract 2:149, 1993.
31. Nichols RL: Antibiotic prophylaxis in surgery. Curr Opin Infect Dis 7:647, 1994.
32. Gorbach SL: The role of cephalosporins in surgical prophylaxis. J Antimicrob Chemother 23(Suppl D):61, 1989.
33. Burke JF: The effective period of preventive antibiotic action in experimental incision and dermal lesions. Surgery 50:161, 1961.
34. Bernard HR, Cole WR: The prophylaxis of surgical infection: The effect of prophylactic antimicrobial drugs on the incidence of infection following potentially contaminated operations. Surgery 56:151, 1964.
35. Nichols RL: Surgical bacteriology: An overview. *In* Nyhus LM (ed): Surgery Annual, Vol 13. New York, Appleton-Century-Crofts, 1981, pp 205–238.
36. Finland M, McGowan JE Jr: Nosocomial infections in surgical patients. Arch Surg 111:143, 1976.
37. American Medical Association: Antimicrobial chemoprophylaxis for surgical patients. *In* Drug Evaluations Annual 1995, Vol 62. Chicago, American Medical Association, 1995, p 1369.
38. Antimicrobial prophylaxis in surgery. Med Lett 35:91, 1993.
39. Platt R, Zaleznik DF, Hopkins CC, et al: Perioperative antibiotic prophylaxis for herniorrhaphy and breast surgery. N Engl J Med 322:153, 1990.
40. Westererman EL: Antibiotic prophylaxis in surgery. Historical background, rationale, and relationship to prospective payment. Am J Infect Control 12:339, 1984.
41. Kernodle DS, Classen DC, Burke JP, et al: Failure of cephalosporins to prevent *Staphylococcus aureus* surgical wound infections. JAMA 263:961, 1990.
42. DiPiro JT, Bowden TA Jr, Hooks VH III: Prophylactic parenteral cephalosporins in surgery: Are the newer agents better? JAMA 252:3277, 1984.
43. Shapiro M, Townsend TR, Rosner B, et al: Use of antimicrobial drugs in general hospitals: Patterns of prophylaxis. N Engl J Med 301:351, 1979.
44. DiPiro JT, Cheung RPF, Bowden TA Jr, et al: Single dose systemic antibiotic prophylaxis of surgical wound infections. Am J Surg 152:552, 1986.
45. Moesgaard F, Lykkegaard-Nielsen L: Preoperative cell-mediated immunity and duration of antibiotic prophylaxis in relation to postoperative infectious complications. Acta Chir Scand 155:281, 1989.
46. Nichols RL: Bowel preparations. *In* Meakins J (ed): Care of the Surgical Patient, ed 2. New York, Scientific American, 1990, pp 1–10.
47. Nichols RL, Condon RE, DiSanto AR: Preoperative bowel preparation. Arch Surg 112:1493, 1977.

48. Moleski RJ, Andriole VT: Role of the infectious disease specialist in containing costs of antibiotics in the hospital. Rev Infect Dis 8:488, 1986.
49. Cannon SR, Dyson PH, Sanderson PJ: Pseudomembranous colitis associated with antibiotic prophylaxis in orthopedic surgery. J Bone Joint Surg Br 70:600, 1988.
50. Kernodle DS, Barg NL, Kaiser AB: Low-level colonization of hospitalized patients with methicillin-resistant coagulase-negative staphylococci and emergence of the organisms during surgical antimicrobial prophylaxis. Antimicrob Agents Chemother 32:202, 1988.
51. Hall JC, Christiansen K, Carter MJ, et al: Antibiotic prophylaxis in cardiac operations. Ann Thorac Surg 56:916, 1993.
52. Nichols RL, Smith JW: Intragastric microbial colonization in common disease states of the stomach and duodenum. Ann Surg 182:557, 1975.
53. LoCicero J, Nichols RL: Sepsis after gastroduodenal operations: Relationship to gastric acid, motility, and endogenous microflora. South Med J 73:878, 1980.
54. Nichols RL, Webb WR, Jones JW, et al: Efficacy of antibiotic prophylaxis in high risk gastroduodenal operations. Am J Surg 143:94, 1982.
55. Lord JW Jr, LaRaja RD, Daliana M, et al: Prophylactic antibiotic wound irrigation in gastric, biliary, and colonic surgery. Am J Surg 145:209, 1983.
56. Keighley MRB, Flinn R, Alexander-Williams J: Multivariate analysis of clinical and operative findings associated with biliary sepsis. Br J Surg 63:528, 1976.
57. Hurlow RA, Strachan CJL, Wise R: Comparative study of the efficacy of cefuroxime for preventing wound sepsis after cholecystectomy. *In* Wood C, Rue Y (eds): Cefuroxime Update, Royal Society of Medicine International Congress Symposium Series No. 38, 1980, pp 1–7.
58. Murray WR, Bradley JA: Antibiotic prophylaxis in elective biliary surgery. Res Clin Forums 5:97, 1983.
59. Lindsey JT, Smith JW, McClugage SG Jr, et al: Effects of commonly used bowel preparations on the large bowel mucosal-associated and luminal microflora in the rat model. Dis Colon Rectum 33:554, 1990.
60. Smith MB, Goradia VK, Holmes JW, et al: Suppression of the human mucosal-related microflora with prophylactic parenteral and/or oral antibiotics. World J Surg 14:636, 1990.
61. Nichols RL, Condon RE: Preoperative preparations of the colon. Surg Gynecol Obstet 132:323, 1971.
62. Kaiser AB, Herrington JL Jr, Jacobs JK, et al: Cefoxitin versus erythromycin, neomycin, and cefazolin in colorectal operations. Ann Surg 198:525, 1983.
63. Coppa GF, Eng K: Factors involved in antibiotic selection in elective colon and rectal surgery. Surgery 104:853, 1988.
64. Clarke JS, Condon RE, Bartlett JG, et al: Preoperative oral antibiotics reduce septic complications of colon operations: Results of prospective, randomized, double-blind clinical study. Ann Surg 186:251, 1977.
65. Washington JA II, Dearing WH, Judd ES, et al: Effect of preoperative antibiotic regimen on development of infection after intestinal surgery: Prospective, randomized, double-blind study. Ann Surg 180:567, 1974.
66. Solla JA, Rothenberger DA: Preoperative bowel preparation—A survey of colon and rectal surgeons. Dis Colon Rectum 33:154, 1990.
67. Nichols RL, Condon RE, Gorbach SL, et al: Efficacy of preoperative antimicrobial preparation of the bowel. Ann Surg 176:227, 1972.
68. Nichols RL, Broido P, Condon RE, et al: The effect of preoperative neomycin-erythromycin intestinal preparation on the incidence of infectious complications following colon surgery. Ann Surg 178:453, 1973.
69. DiPiro JT, Patrias JM, Townsend RJ, et al: Oral neomycin sulfate and erythromycin base before colon surgery: A comparison of serum and tissue concentrations. Pharmacotherapy 5:91, 1985.
70. Polk HC Jr, Lopez-Mayor JF: Postoperative wound infections. A prospective study of determinant factors and prevention. Surgery 66:97, 1969.
71. Edmondson HT, Rissing JP: Prophylactic antibiotics in colon surgery. Arch Surg 118:227, 1983.
72. Panichi G, Pantosti A, Giunchi G, et al: Cephalothin, cefoxitin, or metronidazole in elective colonic surgery? A single-blind randomized trial. Dis Colon Rectum 25:783, 1982.
73. Slama TG, Carey LC, Fass RJ: Comparative efficacy of prophylactic cephalothin and cefamandole for elective colon surgery. Am J Surg 137:593, 1979.
74. Jagelman PG, Fabian TC, Nichols RL, et al: Single-dose cefoxitin versus multiple-dose cefoxitin as prophylaxis in colorectal surgery. Am J Surg 155(5A):71, 1988.
75. Condon RE, Bartlett JG, Greenlee H, et al: Efficacy of oral and systemic antibiotic prophylaxis in colorectal operations. Arch Surg 118:496, 1983.
76. Karran SJ, Sutton G, Gartell P, et al: Imipenem prophylaxis in elective colorectal surgery. Br J Surg 80:1196, 1993.
77. Condon RE, Bartlett JG, Nichols RL, et al: Preoperative prophylactic cephalothin fails to control septic complications of colorectal operations: Results of controlled clinical trial—A Veterans Administration Cooperative Study. Am J Surg 137:68, 1979.
78. Nichols RL, Condon RE, Bentley DW, et al: Ileal microflora in surgical patients. J Urol 105:351, 1971.
79. Bennion RS, Thompson JE, Baron EJ, et al: Gangrenous and perforated appendicitis with peritonitis: Treatment and bacteriology. Clin Ther 12:1, 1990.
80. Krukowski ZH: Preventing wound infection after appendectomy: A review. Br J Surg 75:1023, 1988.
81. Browder W, Smith JW, Vivoda L, et al: Nonperforative appendicitis: A continuing surgical dilemma. J Infect Dis 159:1088, 1989.
82. Bauer T, Vennits BO, Holm B, et al: Antibiotic prophylaxis in acute non-perforated appendicitis. Ann Surg 209:307, 1989.
83. Nichols RL, Smith JW, Klein DB, et al: Risk of infection after penetrating abdominal trauma. N Engl J Med 311:1065, 1984.
84. Gentry LO, Feliciano DV, Lea AS, et al: Perioperative antibiotic therapy for penetrating injuries of the abdomen. Ann Surg 200:562, 1984.
85. Jones RD, Thal ER, Johnson NA, et al: Evaluation of antibiotic therapy following penetrating abdominal trauma. Ann Surg 201:576, 1985.
86. Nichols RL, Smith JW, Robertson GD, et al: Prospective alterations in therapy in penetrating abdominal trauma. Arch Surg 128:55, 1993.
87. Cant PJ, Smyth S, Smart DO: Antibiotic prophylaxis is indicated for chest stab wounds requiring closed tube thoracostomy. Br J Surg 80:464, 1993.
88. Nichols, RL, Smith JW, Muzik AC, et al: Preventive antibiotic usage in traumatic thoracic injuries requiring closed tube thoracostomy. Chest 106:1493, 1994.
89. Webster J: Post-caesarean wound infection: A review of the risk factors. Aust N Z J Obstet Gynaecol 28:201, 1988.
90. Darj E, Stralin EB, Nilsson S: The prophylactic effect of doxycycline on postoperative infection rate after first trimester abortion. Obstet Gynecol 70:755, 1987.
91. Larsen RA, Evans RS, Burke JP, et al: Improved perioperative antibiotic use and reduced surgical wound infection through use of computer decision analysis. Infect Control Hosp Epidemiol 10:316, 1989.

45

Antimicrobial Prophylaxis for Nonsurgical Infections

Jan V. Hirschmann

Physicians have applied the term antimicrobial prophylaxis to four different situations:

1. *Preventing infection by exogenous pathogens.* The target organisms are not members of the host's normal flora, and the antimicrobial agent, given before exposure, promptly eradicates the pathogens when they enter the blood stream or tissues. An example of this type of prophylaxis is the continuous administration of penicillin to prevent streptococcal pharyngeal infections in patients with rheumatic heart disease.
2. *Preventing the host's resident flora from infecting a normally sterile site.* The antimicrobial agent, present in the tissues or body fluids, prevents infection in these sites caused by the host's own organisms, usually colonizing a contiguous cutaneous or mucosal surface. An example is the use of antimicrobials in predisposed females to prevent recurrent urinary tract infections by bacteria that originate from adjacent vaginal or fecal flora.
3. *Preventing disease by a dormant pathogen that is already infecting the host.* The infection occurred long ago, and the organism remains alive but dormant in the asymptomatic host. An example is the use of isoniazid to prevent reactivation of tuberculosis in a previously infected but untreated patient. Because infection has already occurred, the term treatment of asymptomatic infection may be more accurate than prophylaxis in this setting.
4. *Preventing disease by pathogens that recently infected the host who does not yet exhibit clinical manifestations.* An example is the use of antimicrobial agents shortly after an animal bite is sustained but before clinical signs of infection have emerged. Because the organisms have already entered normally sterile tissues before the administration of the antimicrobials, early therapy is probably a more accurate term than prophylaxis.

In this chapter I discuss oral or parenteral antimicrobial prophylaxis used in the first two senses just mentioned in nonsurgical settings; I have organized the discussion by the anatomic sites at which the prophylaxis is directed. It will be confined to prophylaxis against bacterial and fungal infections and will summarize the most important uses; other chapters provide more detailed information about some of these.

In general, antimicrobial prophylaxis is most likely to be successful if the target organisms have a stable pattern of susceptibility and the duration of use is short. Otherwise, resistance to the administered agent may develop. Demonstrating the efficacy of prophylaxis requires carefully controlled trials with clearly defined outcomes. Even when these studies show that prophylaxis is effective, however, the benefits should clearly exceed the liabilities, which include costs, adverse effects, and the potential for the emergence of antimicrobial-resistant organisms, both in the individual recipients and in the environment at large. Widespread use of antibiotics to prevent otitis media in children has probably contributed significantly to the increasing antimicrobial resistance of *Streptococcus pneumoniae* and *Haemophilus influenzae*, for example, and substantial use of prophylactic antibiotics in intensive care unit settings may eventuate in the emergence of infections due to multidrug-resistant bacteria. Clinicians, therefore, have to be cautious in using antimicrobials to prevent infections.

Respiratory Tract

Group A Streptococcal Pharyngitis in Patients with Previous Rheumatic Fever

Because protracted antimicrobial administration may encourage drug-resistant organisms to flourish in the host, prophylactic agents are most likely to be effective if their use is brief or the target organisms have a stable susceptibility. The latter is true for group A streptococci, which have consistently remained sensitive to penicillin, an antibiotic that continues to be effective in preventing streptococcal pharyngeal infections in patients with previous rheumatic fever. These infections, often asymptomatic, may provoke recurrences of rheumatic fever, the consequences of which are particularly serious for those who have had carditis, because each episode can cause further heart damage. A carefully controlled trial in patients with previous rheumatic fever has convincingly demonstrated that a monthly intramuscular dose of benzathine penicillin is superior to daily oral doses of penicillin or sulfadiazine in reducing the frequency of recurrent streptococcal infections and subsequent attacks of rheumatic fever in patients with previous rheumatic fever.[1] Benzathine penicillin is more effective, partly because compliance is better with a single monthly injection than with daily oral doses.

Streptococcal Pharyngitis in Military Recruits

In the mid-1940s a controlled trial demonstrated that oral sulfadiazine substantially reduced the incidence of streptococcal infections in military recruits in whom large outbreaks of pharyngitis occurred. The emergence of sulfadiazine-resistant strains, however, rendered prophylaxis ineffective. Later programs administering benzathine penicillin to all recruits at centers with previous high rates of streptococcal infections markedly diminished their frequency. When routine prophylaxis ended, outbreaks of streptococcal disease recurred.[2] In this setting, the long-acting penicillin presumably eradicated pharyngeal infection in those already infected (treatment of asymptomatic carriers) and prevented acquisition of the organism by those who were not (prophylaxis).

All members of the group require prophylaxis, however, because those who do not receive it may serve as a reservoir for transmitting the organism to the penicillin recipients as their drug levels fall and protection wanes.[3] For penicillin-allergic recruits, oral erythromycin, which appears to be as effective as benzathine penicillin, should be used to ensure prophylaxis throughout the population.[4]

Meningococcal Infection and Haemophilus influenzae Infection

Epidemics of meningococcal disease in military installations in World War II also led to trials of sulfadiazine prophylaxis, which was quite effective.[5] The subsequent development of sulfadiazine resistance has made this agent useful only when the epidemic strain is known to be susceptible. Antimicrobial prophylaxis is now directed mainly at household contacts of patients with meningococcal disease, in whom the medication used (usually oral rifampin) functions principally to eradicate asymptomatic colonization already present rather than to prevent acquisition of the organism. Administering antibiotics to contacts in households or daycare centers of children with invasive *H. influenzae* type b infections serves the same purpose of eradicating the organism from asymptomatic carriers who are at increased risk of developing serious disease.[6]

Otitis Media

Controlled trials have shown that sulfisoxazole,[7, 8] ampicillin,[9] or amoxicillin[10] reduces the incidence of recurrent episodes of acute otitis media in children. Although the criteria for the studies differed, prophylaxis may be most reasonable for those who have had at least three episodes in 6 months or four in 1 year.[11]

Bacterial Superinfections of Viral Respiratory Diseases

Several studies have shown no benefit for antimicrobials in preventing bacterial superinfections of viral upper respiratory diseases. These include colds, influenza, and measles.[12]

Bacterial Pneumonia

Administration of antibiotics to unconscious patients[13] or those with acute heart failure[14] does not reduce the incidence of bacterial pneumonia. Similarly, prophylactic tetracycline or minocycline given to Air Force trainees with nonbacterial pneumonia did not reduce the incidence of bacterial pneumonias (superinfections).[15]

To reduce the frequency of bacterial pneumonia and possibly other infections in critically ill patients, several studies have evaluated "selective decontamination" of the digestive tract. The goal is to prevent potential pathogens, primarily facultative gram-negative bacilli and yeasts, from colonizing the oropharynx and gastrointestinal tract, the presumed sites of origin from which these organisms migrate to cause pneumonias and other infections. Most trials have included patients in intensive care units receiving mechanical ventilation and have employed three types of antibiotics applied as a topical oropharyngeal paste and administered orally: polymyxin E or colistin, tobramycin or gentamicin, and amphotericin B. Most have also given a parenteral cephalosporin, usually cefotaxime, for the first 3 to 5 days, based on the assumption that achieving decontamination takes several days and the systemic agents should prevent infection during that period of inadequate protection. The quality of the studies has varied; most but not all of the rigorously performed trials show a dramatic reduction in the occurrence of pneumonia, especially from gram-negative bacilli.[16] The diagnosis of pneumonia in ventilated patients is difficult, however, and definitions have varied. Those with the most stringent criteria have shown significant but less impressive effects.[17] Overall, the studies have demonstrated no decreased mortality, length of hospital stay, or costs. Because of the expense and adverse effects, particularly the emergence of antibiotic-resistant organisms, selective decontamination does not seem prudent unless more convincing evidence demonstrates that its benefits clearly outweigh its liabilities, even when used on a long-term basis.[17]

Pneumocystis carinii *Pneumonia*

Children with acute lymphoblastic leukemia or rhabdomyosarcoma receiving certain forms of cancer chemotherapy are at high risk of developing *P. carinii* pneumonia. Daily or thrice-weekly oral trimethoprim-sulfamethoxazole (TMP-SMX) markedly reduces this infectious complication.[18, 19] Similarly, daily TMP-SMX diminishes the frequency of *P. carinii* pneumonia in patients with the acquired immunodeficiency syndrome.[20]

Some prophylactic regimen against *P. carinii* pneumonia is recommended in patients with human immunodeficiency virus infection who have had a previous episode or whose $CD4^+$ T-lymphocyte count is less than 200/mm^3. Alternatives to daily TMP-SMX include three-times-weekly TMP-SMX doses, daily dapsone, or monthly aerosolized pentamidine.[21]

Urinary Tract

Daily doses of nitrofurantoin,[22, 23] methenamine mandelate with asorbic acid,[24] TMP-SMX,[23, 24] or TMP alone[23, 25] reduce the frequency of urinary tract infections in women with recurrent episodes. Mandelamine, however, seems less effective than the other agents.[24] TMP-SMX used thrice weekly works as well as daily doses[26] and continues to be effective for at least as long as 5 years of uninterrupted administration.[27] An analysis of costs suggests that antimicrobial prophylaxis is worthwhile for women who have three or more urinary tract infections per year.[28]

For those with infections temporally related to intercourse, or in whom sexual activity is infrequent or sporadic, postcoital administration of TMP-SMX is an alternative to three-times-weekly doses.[29]

Patients with neurogenic bladder dysfunction pursuing a bladder retraining program with intermittent urethral catheterization had significantly fewer episodes of bacteriuria when given methenamine mandelate and ammonium chloride for 21 days than did a group who received placebo.[30] Another study demonstrated that TMP-SMX delayed the onset of bacteriuria, decreased its frequency, and reduced symptomatic episodes. Subsequent bacteriuria with resistant organisms was common, however, seriously limiting the usefulness of this approach.[31]

Gastrointestinal Tract

Traveler's Diarrhea

Controlled trials have demonstrated the efficacy of doxycycline,[32, 33] TMP-SMX,[34, 35] TMP alone,[35] norfloxacin,[35] ciprofloxacin,[36] and bicozamycin[37] in reducing the frequency of traveler's diarrhea by 50% to 85% in persons visiting high-risk areas. The common pathogen is apparently enterotoxigenic *Escherichia coli*, but many cases are due to viruses, parasites, or other bacteria. Some have argued that antimicrobial prophylaxis is more cost-effective than treating the diarrhea when it occurs[38]; others have asserted that antimicrobial prophylaxis is not warranted for any group because of the possible (although rare) adverse effects, the infrequency of moderate to severe disease (less than 30%), and the prompt response to antimicrobial treatment.[39] Prophylaxis is probably most appropriate for patients in whom diarrhea exacts a heavy toll: those with significant underlying disorders, such as inflammatory bowel disease, insulin-dependent diabetes mellitus, acquired immunodeficiency syndrome, and serious cardiac disorders.[40]

Acute Pancreatitis

Two studies, one of 58 patients[41] and the other of 86 patients,[42] failed to show that prophylactic ampicillin reduced infectious complications of acute pancreatitis. The duration of fever or hospitalization was not diminished, and the frequency of pancreatic abscess in both treated and control groups was quite low, but most of the patients had mild to moderately severe pancreatitis.

In a study including only patients with necrotizing pancreatitis, defined by computed tomographic criteria, a 14-day course of imipenem significantly reduced the incidence of pancreatic sepsis.[43] The frequency of surgical intervention and the mortality rates, however, did not differ between the antibiotic recipients and the control group. One reasonable inference from these studies is that patients with nonnecrotic (edematous) pancreatitis do not benefit from prophylaxis. Further studies are necessary, however, to support the routine use of antibiotics in necrotizing pancreatitis.

Infections with Granulocytopenia

Attempts to prevent infections in patients with neutropenia from an underlying disease or from cancer chemotherapy have included antimicrobial agents aimed at "total decontamination" of the alimentary tract and a more selective regimen directed primarily at the enteric gram-negative bacilli. The underlying assumption is that organisms that cause infection in granulocytopenic patients usually originate from their gastrointestinal tract. The total decontamination program uses broad-spectrum oral nonabsorbable agents like vancomycin, nystatin, polymyxin B, and gentamicin, often in conjunction with protective isolation in units that employ laminar flow ventilation. Results of the studies are conflicting but in general suggest that the combination of prophylactic antimicrobials and strict isolation reduces the frequency of infections compared with antimicrobials alone, isolation alone, or neither.[44] Overall, the survival rates and the incidence of complete remission in those with acute leukemia have not increased, despite the reduction in frequency of infections.

Because of the great expense of protective isolation, the high cost of the antimicrobial agents, and their frequent gastrointestinal side effects, selective decontamination, which is directed predominantly at enteric gram-negative bacilli, has replaced the total decontamination program. This approach, which employs no protective isolation, assumes that anaerobic bowel flora help prevent colonization by potential pathogens and should not be eradicated. The agents most frequently used have been TMP-SMX and the quinolones.

When compared with placebo recipients or untreated control subjects, patients receiving TMP-SMX have consistently had a marked reduction in the number of enteric gram-negative bacilli in stool cultures,[45–50] but sometimes colonization with resistant gram-positive[48] or gram-negative[47–51] organisms has occurred. In general, fungi have not increased. The clinical outcome of prophylaxis, however, has varied strikingly in these studies: some have shown a significant reduction in the incidence of fever,[45, 46, 52, 53] whereas others have not[47, 48, 51, 54]; in most[46, 48, 50, 51, 54, 55] but not all,[45, 47] TMP-SMX has reduced the frequency of documented infections. It usually has not diminished the number of deaths due to infection,[46, 47, 49, 53, 54] and an equal number of studies have reported a decrease[46, 48, 49] or no difference[47, 51, 54] in intravenous antibiotic use in those receiving TMP-SMX. In some trials the infections in those receiving TMP-SMX have often been from resistant organisms,[46, 50] and this agent has sometimes significantly prolonged the duration of granulocytopenia.[46, 53] Antimicrobial prophylaxis does not seem to be effective when the neutropenia is short-lived[47]; in nearly all studies that show any benefit the average duration of granulocytopenia has been at least 3 weeks.

The remarkable diversity in the reported efficacy of TMP-SMX probably relates to several factors—differences in doses, bacterial susceptibility at the sites of the trials, definitions of criteria for outcomes, number of patients studied, and populations of patients studied. Many studies are small, some include patients with granulocytopenia associated with both malignant and benign conditions, some involve only one type of cancer (e.g., leukemia, small cell carcinoma), and many fail to report certain important details (e.g., intravenous antibiotic use, antimicrobial susceptibility of the infecting organisms). One consistent finding, however, is that antimicrobial prophylaxis does not decrease the *overall fatality* rate even in those studies in which it reduces *infectious* mortality. Furthermore, although many trials show a diminution in infections among those who receive cancer chemotherapy, this benefit does not translate into an increased remission rate for the underlying malignancy.

Compared with oral nonabsorbable antimicrobials, TMP-SMX was better than neomycin and colistin in reducing fever and the use of other antibiotics[56]; it was equivalent to oral gentamicin in reducing infection rates but was tolerated better.[57] The addition of oral nonabsorbable antibiotics (framycetin and colistin) to TMP-SMX had no advantage over TMP-SMX alone.[58] Compared with oral nalidixic acid, TMP-SMX caused more protracted neutropenia but also significantly delayed the appearance of infection.[59] Granulocytopenia was also more prolonged with TMP-SMX than with TMP alone, although the infection rates were similar and colonization with resistant gram-negative bacilli was greater with TMP.[60]

One study has compared the quinolone norfloxacin with placebo in patients with acute leukemia and granulocytopenia.[61] Norfloxacin significantly delayed the onset and decreased the duration of fever, diminished the frequency of gram-negative bacillary infections, and reduced the colonization of the stool with aerobic organisms. Mortality due to infections was not affected. Other trials have compared the quinolones with other forms of prophylaxis. Norfloxacin was tolerated better than oral vancomycin and polymyxin; it was also effective in reducing documented infections, including gram-negative bacteremia, and in decreasing the acquisition of resistant gram-negative organisms in the stool.[62] When compared with TMP-SMX, norfloxacin was better in preventing acquisition of resistant gram-negative bacilli in stool cultures; there was no difference in infection rates, but gram-positive bacteremias were significantly more frequent with norfloxacin.[63] Another quinolone, ciprofloxacin, was superior to TMP-SMX plus colistin in reducing bacteriologically documented infections, including those due to gram-negative bacilli, and in preventing colonization by resistant gram-negative bacilli.[64] A study comparing norfloxacin with ciprofloxacin showed that the latter was more effective.[65] Experience with these agents is limited, however, and the emergence of resistant organisms because of overuse could easily destroy their potential as both therapeutic and prophylactic agents.[66]

In summary, the efficacy of antimicrobial prophylaxis for patients with granulocytopenia remains unclear. Certainly, it does not seem worthwhile unless the neutropenia is prolonged (at least 3 weeks). Its utility probably is also related in part to the nature of the nosocomial flora of the medical center where the patients receive treatment. Because antibiotic prophylaxis does not decrease mortality or improve response to cancer chemotherapy and because resistant organisms may develop, the risks of giving these agents probably exceed their benefits in most circumstances.

Skin

Recurrent Cellulitis and Staphylococcal Abscesses

In patients with lymphedema and recurrent episodes of cellulitis, monthly intramuscular doses of benzathine penicillin or daily oral doses of either penicillin or erythromycin for 1 week each month reduce the frequency of subsequent attacks.[67] A study of patients with two or more episodes of erysipelas or cellulitis in the previous year demonstrated that daily erythromycin or penicillin prevented any recurrences, compared with a frequency of 50% in the control group.[68] In a trial involving 22 patients with a history of recurrent staphylococcal skin abscesses, oral daily clindamycin for 3 months significantly reduced the frequency of this infection when compared with placebo.[69]

Miscellaneous Infections

Group B Streptococcal Infection in Neonates

Colonization of neonates with group B streptococci acquired from the mother during birth can cause sepsis and meningitis. Antibiotic therapy of colonized women in the third trimester of pregnancy before delivery—even when their male partners are treated concurrently—is not always effective in eradicating the organism, which usually returns shortly after the antimicrobial drug is discontinued.[70, 71] When benzathine penicillin is used, however, colonization at delivery is diminished.[72] Two alternative approaches are to treat the mother at delivery or to give antibiotics to the infant afterward. The effect of intrapartum antibiotics may be to reduce the number of organisms in the mother's genital tract at birth and, by crossing the placenta, to protect the child against invasive disease in utero and during the first hours of life. When given at delivery, intravenous ampicillin[73, 74] and penicillin or erythromycin, either intramuscular[75] or oral,[76] markedly reduce the frequency of colonization of the infant at birth. The effect is sustained throughout hospitalization, but colonization of the infants at 6 weeks is common.[75]

In one trial in which all neonates received penicillin shortly after birth, the frequency of early-onset group B streptococcal infection decreased but disease from penicillin-resistant organisms increased, and the overall mortality rate from infection did not differ in penicillin recipients and untreated control subjects.[77] In another study, infants weighing 2000 g or less given penicillin did not have fewer early-onset group B streptococcal infections.[78] In most cases the infants were symptomatic at birth or within 4 hours afterward, and results of their initial blood cultures were positive, suggesting that infection had occurred in utero or during birth, before penicillin administration. These studies indicate that intrapartum antibiotics are the most effective regimen for decreasing group B streptococcal colonization in the neonate.

One recommended approach to decreasing the frequency of group B streptococcal perinatal infections is to screen all pregnant women at 26 to 28 weeks' gestation for anogenital colonization and to give intrapartum antibiotics to all those with positive cultures and one or more of the following: (1) intrapartum temperature of 37.5°C or higher that is not attributable to an extrauterine source; (2) membrane rupture or onset of labor before 37 weeks' gestation; and (3) membrane rupture for more than 24 hours. Prophylactic antibiotics would also be given to women with any of the previous characteristics who did not have prenatal cultures and to all with a history of giving birth to an infant with early-onset group B streptococcal disease.[79]

Staphylococcus aureus Infections with Hemodialysis

Patients undergoing hemodialysis who were nasal carriers of *S. aureus* were randomly assigned to receive no treatment or topical bacitracin four times a day for 7 days and oral rifampin for 5 days every 3 months if results of the nasal culture were positive.[80] The frequency of *S. aureus* infections, including bacteremia, access site infections, and cutaneous abscesses, during the 3.5 years of study was significantly lower in those receiving prophylaxis. Rifampin-resistant *S. aureus*, however, did emerge, although these organisms neither persisted in the nares nor caused infection.

Skull Fractures with Cerebrospinal Fluid Leak

A trial of penicillin in patients with skull fractures and cerebrospinal fluid rhinorrhea or otorrhea failed to demonstrate that the antibiotic prevented meningitis, although the incidence of this infection was quite low in both treated and untreated patients.[81] A study including both open and basilar skull fractures also failed to demonstrate a reduction in meningitis when patients received 3 days of ceftriaxone or combined ampicillin-sulfadiazine.[82]

Pneumococcal Infections in Sickle Cell Anemia

A trial of daily oral penicillin in children younger than 3 years of age with sickle cell anemia demonstrated a significant reduction in the frequency of pneumococcal septicemia compared with a placebo group.[83] In another trial, monthly benzathine penicillin was markedly superior to the pneumococcal vaccine in preventing bacteremia and meningitis.[84]

Systemic Infections in Acquired Immunodeficiency Syndrome

Daily fluconazole decreases the frequency of superficial fungal infections and invasive disease caused by *Cryptococcus neoformans* and *Candida* species in patients with $CD4^+$ T-lymphocyte counts of less than 200/mm³.[85] The most benefit occurs in those with counts lower than 50/mm³, but the potential for emergence of resistant organisms is worrisome.

Daily rifabutin decreases the frequency of bacteremia with *Mycobacterium avium* complex in patients with acquired immunodeficiency syndrome and $CD4^+$ T-lymphocyte counts lower than 200/mm³.[86] The mortality rate is not reduced, and the long-term effect on the organism's antimicrobial susceptibility is unknown.

Spontaneous Bacterial Peritonitis in Cirrhosis

In patients with cirrhosis and gastrointestinal hemorrhage, oral nonabsorbable antibiotics, consisting of gentamicin-nystatin or neomycin-colistin-nystatin, decreased the frequency of spontaneous bacteremia or peritonitis from about 21% to about 9% when given until 48 hours after the hemorrhage ceased.[87] Although infectious mortality was significantly diminished, the mortality rate for the whole hospitalization was unaffected. In another study, patients with cirrhosis and a total protein concentration of less than 1.5 g/dL in the ascitic fluid received norfloxacin throughout their hospitalization, which averaged nearly a month in duration. Spontaneous bacterial peritonitis was reduced from about 40% to about 3%, but no difference in mortality occurred in this study of 63 patients.[88] Routine use of intravenous cefotaxime before emergency endoscopic variceal sclerotherapy for variceal bleeding did not reduce the frequency of peritonitis.[89] Unless more convincing evidence of substantial benefit accrues, the use of prophylactic antibiotics to prevent peritonitis does not seem warranted.

Summary

Table 45–1 summarizes the situations in which studies have demonstrated the efficacy of antibacterial prophylaxis with

TABLE 45–1 ■ Regimens for Recommended Medical Antimicrobial Prophylaxis

CONDITION	INDICATION	REGIMEN*
Streptococcal pharyngitis (and rheumatic fever)	Military recruits	Benzathine penicillin G IM 1.2 million units about day 14 of training, repeat in 30 d *or* Erythromycin PO 250 mg bid for 60 d
Streptococcal pharyngitis (and rheumatic fever) recurrence	Recent rheumatic fever or rheumatic heart disease	Benzathine penicillin G IM 1.2 million units every 4 wk *or* Penicillin V PO 250 mg bid *or* Erythromycin PO 250 mg bid
Meningococcal disease	Household contact with meningococcal disease	Rifampin PO: adults 600 mg bid for 2 d; children younger than 1 y, 9 mg/kg bid for 2 d; for those 1–12 y old, 10 mg/kg bid for 2 d
Haemophilus influenzae disease	Household or daycare center contact with patient younger than 2 y with *H. influenzae* type b disease	Rifampin PO 20 mg/kg qd for 4 d (maximal daily dose 600 mg)
Recurrent otitis media	At least three episodes in 6 mo or four in 1 y	Sulfisoxazole PO 50 mg/kg qd *or* Ampicillin PO 125 mg qd for those younger than 2.5 y, 250 mg qd for those older than 2.5 y *or* Amoxicillin 20 mg/kg qd
Pneumocystis carinii pneumonia	Cancer chemotherapy in certain high-risk patients	TMP-SMX PO (150 mg/m² of TMP, 750 mg/m² of SMX) in two doses per day for 3 consecutive days per week (maximal daily dose: SMX, 1600 mg; TMP, 320 mg)
	Acquired immunodeficiency syndrome	TMP-SMX PO (160 mg of TMP, 800 mg of SMX) qd or three times a week *or* Dapsone 50 mg bid *or* Inhaled pentamidine 300 mg q 4 wk
Recurrent urinary tract infections in women	At least three infections per year	TMP-SMX 200 mg; 40 mg three times a week or nitrofurantoin PO 100 mg qhs
	Related to coitus	TMP-SMX PO 200 mg/40 mg after coitus
Neurogenic bladder	Intermittent catheterization; bladder retraining	Methenamine mandelate PO 1 g q 6 h
Traveler's diarrhea	Serious underlying diseases	Doxycycline PO, 100 mg qd *or* TMP-SMX PO (800 mg; 160 mg) qd *or* Norfloxacin PO 400 mg qd *or* Ciprofloxacin 500 mg qd
Recurrent cellulitis	Multiple episodes	Benzathine penicillin IM 1.2 million units/mo *or* Erythromycin or penicillin V 250 mg bid
Recurrent staphylococcal skin infections	Multiple episodes	Clindamycin PO 150 mg qd for 3 mo
Group B streptococcal disease in neonates	See text	Aqueous penicillin G IV 5 million units q 6 h or ampicillin IV 2 g initially, then q 6 h until delivery *or* Clindamycin IV 600 mg q 8 h until delivery if penicillin allergic
Staphylococcus aureus infection in patients undergoing long-term hemodialysis	Recurrent infection and nasal colonization	Rifampin PO 600 mg bid for 5 d plus topical bacitracin to nares qd for 7 d every 3 mo if positive nasal cultures for *S. aureus*
Streptococcus pneumoniae infections	Children with sickle-cell anemia	Penicillin V PO 250 mg bid

*IM, Intramuscularly; PO, orally; IV, intravenously; bid, twice daily; qd, daily; qhs, every day at bedtime.

systemic antimicrobial agents and delineates the doses employed. Some of the indications, particularly for traveler's diarrhea and granulocytopenia, are controversial. Physicians considering the use of prophylaxis in these circumstances should carefully evaluate the original articles and thoughtfully weigh both the potential benefits and the liabilities involved.

References

1. Wood HF, Feinstein AR, Taranta A, et al: Rheumatic fever in children and adolescents. III. Comparative effectiveness of three prophylaxis regimens in preventing streptococcal infections and rheumatic recurrences. Ann Intern Med 60(Suppl 5):31, 1964.
2. Thomas RJ, Conwill DE, Morton DE, et al: Penicillin prophylaxis for streptococcal infections in United States Navy and Marine Corps Recruit Camps, 1951–1985. Rev Infect Dis 10:125, 1988.
3. Gray GC, Escamilla J, Hyams KC, et al: Hyperendemic *Streptococcus pyogenes* infection despite prophylaxis with penicillin G benzathine. N Engl J Med 325:92, 1991.
4. Fujikawa J, Struewing JP, Hyams KC, et al: Oral erythromycin prophylaxis against *Streptococcus pyogenes* infection in penicillin-allergic military recruits: A randomized clinical trial. J Infect Dis 166:162, 1992.
5. Kuhns DM, Nelson CT, Feldman HA, Kuhn LR: Prophylactic

value of sulfadiazine in control of meningococci meningitis. JAMA 123:335, 1943.
6. Broome CV, Mortimer EA, Katz SL, et al: Use of chemoprophylaxis to prevent the spread of *Haemophilus influenzae* b in day care facilities. N Engl J Med 316:1226, 1987.
7. Perrin JM, Charney E, MacWhinney TK, et al: Sulfisoxazole as chemoprophylaxis for recurrent otitis media. A double-blind crossover study in pediatric practice. N Engl J Med 291:644, 1974.
8. Liston TE, Foshee WS, Pierson WD: Sulfisoxazole chemoprophylaxis for frequent otitis media. Pediatrics 71:524, 1983.
9. Maynard JE, Fleshman JK, Tschopp CF: Otitis media in Alaskan Eskimo children: Prospective evaluation of chemoprophylaxis. JAMA 219:597, 1972.
10. Casselbrant ML, Kaleida PH, Rockette HE, et al: Efficacy of antimicrobial prophylaxis and of tympanostomy tube insertion for prevention of recurrent otitis media: Results of a randomized clinical trial. Pediatr Infect Dis 11:278, 1992.
11. Klein JO: Otitis media. Clin Infect Dis 19:823, 1994.
12. Davis SD, Wedgwood RJ: Antibiotic prophylaxis in acute viral respiratory diseases. Am J Dis Child 109:544, 1965.
13. Petersdorf RG, Curtin JA, Hoeprich PD, et al: A study of antibiotic prophylaxis in unconscious patients. N Engl J Med 257:1001, 1957.
14. Petersdorf RG, Merchant RK: Study of antibiotic prophylaxis in patients with acute heart failure. N Engl J Med 260:565, 1959.
15. Ellenbogen C, Graybill JR, Silva J, Homme PJ: Bacterial pneumonia complicating adenoviral pneumonia. A comparison of respiratory bacterial culture sources and effectiveness of chemoprophylaxis against bacterial pneumonia. Am J Med 56:169, 1974.
16. Heyland DC, Cook DJ, Jaeschke R, et al: Selective decontamination of the digestive tract. An overview. Chest 105:1221, 1994.
17. Brun-Buisson C: Selective decontamination in critical care. Interpreting the synthesized evidence. Chest 105:978, 1994.
18. Hughes WT, Kuhn S, Chaudhany S, et al: Successful chemoprophylaxis for *Pneumocystis carinii* pneumonitis. N Engl J Med 297:1419, 1977.
19. Hughes WT, Rivera GK, Schell MJ, et al: Successful intermittent chemoprophylaxis for *Pneumocystis carinii* pneumonia. N Engl J Med 316:1627, 1987.
20. Fischl MA, Dickinson GM, LaVoie L: Safety and efficacy of sulfamethoxazole and trimethoprim chemoprophylaxis for *Pneumocystis carinii* pneumonia in AIDS. JAMA 259:1185, 1988.
21. Bozzette SA, Finkelstein DM, Spector SA, et al: A randomized trial of three antipneumocystis agents in patients with advanced human immunodeficiency virus infection. N Engl J Med 332:693, 1995.
22. Bailey RR, Roberts AP, Gower PE, DeWardener HE: Prevention of urinary tract infection with low-dose nitrofurantoin. Lancet 2:1112, 1971.
23. Stamm WE, Counts GW, Wagner KF, et al: Antimicrobial prophylaxis of recurrent urinary tract infections. A double-blind, placebo-controlled trial. Ann Intern Med 92:770, 1980.
24. Harding GKM, Ronald AR: A controlled study of antimicrobial prophylaxis of recurrent urinary infection in women. N Engl J Med 291:597, 1974.
25. Light RB, Ronald AR, Harding GKM, et al: Trimethoprim alone in the treatment and prophylaxis of urinary tract infection. Arch Intern Med 141:1807, 1981.
26. Harding GKM, Buckwold FJ, Marrie TJ, et al: Prophylaxis of recurrent urinary tract infection in female patients. Efficacy of low-dose, thrice-weekly therapy with trimethoprim-sulfamethoxazole. JAMA 242:1975, 1979.
27. Nicolle LE, Harding GKM, Thomson M, et al: Efficacy of five years of continuous low-dose trimethoprim-sulfamethoxazole prophylaxis for urinary tract infection. J Infect Dis 157:1239, 1988.
28. Stamm WE, McKevitt M, Counts GW, et al: Is antimicrobial prophylaxis of urinary tract infections cost effective? Ann Intern Med 94:251, 1981.
29. Stapleton A, Latham RH, Johnson C, et al: Postcoital antimicrobial prophylaxis for recurrent urinary tract infection. A randomized, double-blind, placebo-controlled trial. JAMA 264:703, 1990.
30. Kevorkian CG, Merritt JL, Ilstrup DM: Methenamine mandelate with acidification: An effective urinary antiseptic in patients with neurogenic bladder. Mayo Clin Proc 59:523, 1984.
31. Gribble MJ, Puterman ML: Prophylaxis of urinary tract infection in persons with recent spinal cord injury: A prospective, randomized, double-blind, placebo-controlled study of trimethoprim-sulfamethoxazole. Am J Med 95:141, 1993.
32. Sack DA, Kaminsky DC, Sack RB, et al: Prophylactic doxycycline for travelers' diarrhea. Results of a prospective double-blind study of Peace Corps volunteers in Kenya. N Engl J Med 298:758, 1978.
33. Sack RB, Froehich JL, Zulich AW, et al: Prophylactic doxycycline for travelers' diarrhea. Results of a prospective double-blind study of Peace Corps volunteers in Morocco. Gastroenterology 76:1368, 1979.
34. DuPont HL, Evans DG, Rios N, et al: Prevention of travelers' diarrhea with trimethoprim-sulfamethoxazole. Rev Infect Dis 4:533, 1982.
35. DuPont HL, Galindo E, Evans DG, et al: Prevention of travelers' diarrhea with trimethoprim-sulfamethoxazole and trimethoprim alone. Gastroenterology 84:75, 1983.
36. Rademaker CM, Hoepelman IM, Wolfhagen MJ, et al: Results of a double-blind placebo-controlled study using ciprofloxacin for prevention of traveler's diarrhea. Eur J Clin Microbiol Infect Dis 8:690, 1989.
37. Ericsson CD, DuPont HL, Galindo E, et al: Efficacy of bicozamycin in preventing travelers' diarrhea. Gastroenterology 88:473, 1985.
38. Reves RR, Johnson PC, Ericsson CD, DuPont HL: A cost-effectiveness comparison of the use of antimicrobial agents for treatment or prophylaxis of travelers' diarrhea. Arch Intern Med 148:2421, 1988.
39. Gorbach SL, Carpenter CCJ, Grayson R, et al: Consensus development conference statement. Rev Infect Dis 2(Suppl):S227, 1986.
40. DuPont HL, Ericsson CD: Prevention and treatment of traveler's diarrhea. N Engl J Med 328:1821, 1993.
41. Finch WT, Sawyers JL, Schencker S: A prospective study to determine the efficacy of antibiotics in acute pancreatitis. Ann Surg 183:667, 1976.
42. Howes R, Zuidema GD, Cameron JL: Evaluation of prophylactic antibiotics in acute pancreatitis. J Surg Res 18:197, 1975.
43. Pederzoli P, Bassi C, Vesentini S, et al: A randomized multicenter clinical trial of antibiotic prophylaxis of septic complications in acute necrotizing pancreatitis with imipenem. Surg Gynecol Obstet 176:480, 1993.
44. Henry SA: Chemoprophylaxis of bacterial infections in granulocytopenic patients. Am J Med 76:645, 1984.
45. Gurwith MJ, Brunton JL, Lank BA, et al: A prospective controlled investigation of prophylactic trimethoprim-sulfamethoxazole in hospitalized granulocytopenic patients. Am J Med 66:248, 1979.
46. Dekker AW, Rozenberg-Arska M, Sixma JJ, Verhoef J: Prevention of infection by trimethoprim-sulfamethoxazole plus amphotericin B in patients with acute nonlymphocytic leukaemia. Ann Intern Med 95:555, 1981.
47. Weiser B, Lange M, Fialk MA, et al: Prophylactic trimethoprim-sulfamethoxazole during consolidation chemotherapy for acute leukemia: A controlled trial. Ann Intern Med 95:436, 1981.
48. Kauffman CA, Liepman MK, Bergman AG, Mioduszewski J: Trimethoprim-sulfamethoxazole prophylaxis in neutropenic patients. Am J Med 74:599, 1983.
49. DeJongh CA, Wade JC, Finley RS, et al: Trimethoprim-sulfamethoxazole versus placebo: A double-blind comparison of infection prophylaxis in patients with small cell carcinoma of the lung. J Clin Oncol 1:302, 1983.
50. EORTC International Antimicrobial Therapy Project Group: Trimethoprim-sulfamethoxazole in the prevention of infection in neutropenic patients. J Infect Dis 150:372, 1984.
51. Gualtieri RJ, Donowitz GR, Kaiser DL, et al: Double-blind randomized study of prophylactic trimethoprim-sulfamethoxazole in granulocytopenic patients with hematologic malignancies. Am J Med 74:934, 1983.
52. Martino P, Venditti M, Petti MC, et al: Cotrimoxazole prophylaxis in patients with leukemia and prolonged granulocytopenia. Am J Med Sci 287:7, 1984.
53. Kovatch AL, Wald ER, Albo VC, et al: Oral trimethoprim-sulfamethoxazole for protection of bacterial infection during the induction phase of cancer chemotherapy in children. Pediatrics 76:754, 1985.
54. Henry SA, Armstrong D, Kempin S, et al: Oral trimethoprim-sulfamethoxazole in attempt to prevent infection after induction chemotherapy for acute leukemia. Am J Med 77:663, 1984.

55. Estey E, Maksymiuk A, Smith T, et al: Infection prophylaxis in acute leukemia—comparative effectiveness of sulfamethoxazole and trimethoprim, ketoconazole, and a combination of the two. Arch Intern Med 144:1562, 1984.
56. Watson JG, Powles RL, Lason DN, et al: Co-trimoxazole versus nonabsorbable antibiotics in acute leukaemia. Lancet 1:6, 1982.
57. Wade JC, Schimpff SC, Hargadon MT, et al: A comparison of trimethoprim-sulfamethoxazole plus nystatin with gentamicin plus nystatin in the prevention of infections in acute leukemia. N Engl J Med 304:1057, 1981.
58. Starke ID, Catovsky D, Johnson SA, et al: Co-trimoxazole alone for prevention of bacterial infection in patients with acute leukaemia. Lancet 1:5, 1982.
59. Wade JC, deJongh CA, Newman KA, et al: Selective antimicrobial modulation as prophylaxis against infection during granulocytopenia: Trimethoprim-sulfamethoxazole vs nalidixic acid. J Infect Dis 147:624, 1983.
60. Bow EJ, Louie TJ, Riben PD, et al: Randomized controlled trial comparing trimethoprim-sulfamethoxazole and trimethoprim for infection prophylaxis in hospitalized granulocytopenic patients. Am J Med 76:223, 1984.
61. Karp JE, Merz WG, Hendricksen C, et al: Oral norfloxacin for prevention of gram-negative bacterial infections in patients with acute leukemia and granulocytopenia. A randomized, double-blind, placebo-controlled trial. Ann Intern Med 106:1, 1987.
62. Winston DJ, Ho WG, Nakao SL, et al: Norfloxacin versus vancomycin/polymyxin for prevention of infections in granulocytopenic patients. Am J Med 80:884, 1986.
63. Bow EJ, Raynor E, Louie TJ: Comparison of norfloxacin with cotrimoxazole for infection prophylaxis in acute leukemia. The trade-off for reduced gram-negative sepsis. Am J Med 84:847, 1988.
64. Dekker AW, Rozenberg-Arska M, Verhoef J: Infection prophylaxis in acute leukemia: A comparison of ciprofloxacin with trimethoprim-sulfamethoxazole and colistin. Ann Intern Med 106:7, 1987.
65. GIMEMA Infection Program: Prevention of bacterial infections in neutropenic patients with hematologic malignancies. A randomized, multicenter trial comparing norfloxacin with ciprofloxacin. Ann Intern Med 115:7, 1991.
66. Young LS: The new fluorinated quinolones for infection prevention in acute leukemia. Ann Intern Med 106:144, 1987.
67. Babb RR, Spittell JA, Martin WJ, Schirger A: Prophylaxis of recurrent lymphangitis complicating lymphedema. JAMA 195:871, 1966.
68. Kremer M, Zuckerman R, Avraham Z, et al: Long-term antimicrobial therapy in the prevention of recurrent soft-tissue infections. J Infect 22:37, 1991.
69. Klempner MS, Styrt B: Prevention of recurrent staphylococcal skin infections with low-dose oral clindamycin therapy. JAMA 260:2682, 1988.
70. Gardner SE, Yow MD, Leeds LJ, et al: Failure of penicillin to eradicate group B streptococcal colonization in the pregnant woman: A couple study. Am J Obstet Gynecol 135:1062, 1979.
71. Hall RT, Barnes W, Krishnan L, et al: Antibiotic treatment of parturient women colonized with Group B streptococci. Am J Obstet Gynecol 124:630, 1976.
72. Lewin EB, Amstey MS: Natural history of group B streptococcus colonization and its therapy during pregnancy. Am J Obstet Gynecol 139:512, 1981.
73. Yow MD, Mason EO, Leeds LJ, et al: Ampicillin prevents intrapartum transmission of group B streptococci. JAMA 241:1245, 1979.
74. Boyer KM, Gadzala CA, Kelly PD, Gotoff SP: Selective intrapartum chemoprophylaxis of neonatal Group B streptococcal early onset disease. III. Interruption of mother-to-infant transmission. J Infect Dis 148:810, 1983.
75. Easmon CSF, Hastings MJG, Deeley J, et al: The effect of intrapartum chemoprophylaxis on the vertical transmission of group B streptococci. Br J Obstet Gynecol 90:633, 1983.
76. Merenstein GB, Todd WA, Brown G, et al: Group B β-hemolytic streptococcus: Randomized controlled treatment study at birth. Obstet Gynecol 55:315, 1980.
77. Siegel JD, McCracken GH, Threlkeld N, et al: Single-dose penicillin prophylaxis of neonatal group B streptococcal disease. Conclusion of a 41-month controlled trial. Lancet 1:1426, 1982.
78. Pyati SP, Pildes RS, Jacobs NM, et al: Penicillin in infants weighing 2 kilograms or less with early-onset group B streptococcal disease. N Engl J Med 308:1383, 1983.
79. Centers for Disease Control: Prevention of group B streptococcal diseases: A public health perspective. Fed Reg 59:64764, 1994.
80. Yu VL, Goetz A, Wagener M, et al: *Staphylococcus aureus* nasal carriage and infection in patients on hemodialysis. Efficacy of antibiotic prophylaxis. N Engl J Med 315:91, 1986.
81. Klastersky J, Sadeghi M, Brihaye J: Antimicrobial prophylaxis in patients with rhinorrhea or otorrhea. A double-blind study. Surg Neurol 6:111, 1976.
82. Demetriades D, Charalambides D, Lakhoo M, et al: Role of prophylactic antibiotics in open and basilar fractures of the skull: A randomized study. Injury 23:377, 1992.
83. Gaston MH, Verter JI, Woods G, et al: Prophylaxis with oral penicillin in children with sickle cell anemia. A randomized trial. N Engl J Med 314:1593, 1986.
84. John AB, Ramlal A, Jackson H, et al: Prevention of pneumococcal infection in children with homozygous sickle cell disease. Br Med J 288:1567, 1984.
85. Powderly WG, Finkelstein DM, Feinberg J, et al: A randomized trial comparing fluconazole with cotrimoxazole troches for the prevention of fungal infections in patients with advanced human immunodeficiency virus. N Engl J Med 332:700, 1995.
86. Nightengale SD, Cameron DW, Gordin FM, et al: Two controlled trials of rifabutin prophylaxis against *Mycobacterium avium* complex infection in AIDS. N Engl J Med 329:828, 1993.
87. Romola A, Bory F, Teres J, et al: Oral, nonabsorbable antibiotics prevent infection in cirrhotics with gastrointestinal hemorrhage. Hepatology 5:463, 1985.
88. Soriano G, Guarner C, Teixido M, et al: Selective intestinal decontamination prevents spontaneous bacterial peritonitis. Gastroenterology 100:477, 1991.
89. Selby WS, Norton ID, Pokorny CS, Benn RA: Bacteremia and bacterascites after endoscopic sclerotherapy for bleeding esophageal varices and prevention by intravenous cefotaxime: A randomized trial. Gastrointest Endosc 40:680, 1994.

46

Advice to Travelers

Mary E. Wilson

Epidemiology of Travel-Associated Infections

Travel has become fast and frequent and shows no signs of waning. In the early 1990s, more than 500 million persons annually crossed international borders on commercial airplane flights (World Tourism Organization, Madrid, unpublished data). In 1994, air passenger traffic worldwide exceeded two billion passengers (Survey from Airports Council International, unpublished data). Persons entering a new environment often encounter threats to health that differ from those at home.[1] The risk profile of an area has many dimensions; some risks are typically greater whereas others are less than at home. The act of travel itself poses other risks. This chapter reviews the epidemiology of illnesses in travelers, describes various strategies to reduce risk, discusses briefly the evaluation of the symptomatic returned traveler, and identifies key sources for information and assistance. Although many psychologic and medical problems beset travelers, the main focus of this section is on infectious diseases related to travel.

Overview

The thought of travel to remote areas conjures up images of exotic, sometimes lethal infections such as African sleeping sickness, Lassa fever, and tsutsugamushi fever. It may come as a surprise to learn that infections are a rare cause of travel-related death and that most infections acquired during travel are caused by pathogens that are widely distributed but are more commonly encountered in tropical and developing areas of the world. Numerous studies have assessed the epidemiology of illness in travelers.[2–4] Results vary by destination and other circumstances, although common findings emerge. Among the largest and most informative studies of travel-related illness were those done in Swiss travelers.[2] Figure 46–1 depicts quantitative estimates of many problems encountered by travelers.[3] The incidence rate is calculated per month of stay in developing countries. As has been confirmed by multiple studies to many areas of the world, diarrhea is the most common illness leading to disruption during travel. A study of 3049 travelers from the United Kingdom who became ill during travel found that 1% required hospitalization on return home and 14% consulted a physician.[5] A surveillance system that collected information about health problems in Peace Corps workers in Africa in 1990 found that the most commonly reported health problems were diarrhea, skin problems, amebiasis, injuries, dental problems, emotional problems, fevers, malaria, and giardiasis.[6] This is a population that presumably was well protected by malaria chemoprophylaxis and immunizations.

Other Risks During Travel

Preparation for travel frequently focuses on preventing infectious diseases. As a consequence, travelers often seek assistance from infectious disease physicians. Physicians and travelers should recognize the wide range of risks incurred by travelers, including many noninfectious diseases. Physicians should inquire about anticipated activities, such as hiking at high altitudes[7] and spending time in extreme environments (e.g., heat, cold, deep-sea diving) that may require special attention or preparation.[8] Sunburns and phototoxic skin reactions are especially common among travelers from northern latitudes who visit tropical areas during winter months.

Although infection is a common cause of disruption during travel, it rarely kills. In young adults, injury is by far the most common cause of death during travel.[9] Rates of death from injury are higher in developing countries than in the United States.[10] The majority of deaths in young travelers are a result of motor vehicle crashes, drownings, aircraft crashes, homicides, and burns. For most destinations, injuries are the most common cause of travel-related death and the most common reason for air medical evacuation.[11]

Diarrhea

Diarrhea occurs in 20% to 40% or more of short-term travelers from industrialized countries who visit developing countries.[2, 12, 13] Studies that have analyzed data by age have found that younger persons experience higher rates of gastrointestinal illness. The term traveler's diarrhea describes the circumstances of acquisition rather than the etiology. Although most often caused by toxigenic *Escherichia coli*,[14] traveler's diarrhea has been associated with a wide range of organisms, including bacteria, viruses, and protozoa.[12] Bacterial enteropathogens cause about 80% of traveler's diarrhea. The incidence of disease and relative proportion of disease caused by each pathogen vary by geographic region, by season, and over time and to some extent is influenced by host factors.[15] The principal agents in most areas are enterotoxigenic *E. coli*, *Shigella* species, *Campylobacter jejuni*, *Aeromonas* species, *Plesiomonas shigelloides*, *Salmonella* species, and noncholera vibrios.[12] Norwalk virus and rotavirus may cause up to 10% of diarrhea in some areas. *Giardia* and *Cryptosporidium* are the most commonly diagnosed protozoa causing diarrhea in travelers, although *Cyclospora* has been an important cause of diarrhea in Nepal.[16] The epidemiology of *Cyclospora* infections is not yet fully defined, although infections appear to be widely distributed.[17] Diarrhea caused by *Entamoeba histolytica* (amebic colitis or dysentery) is rare among short-term travelers.

Factors that have been associated with increased risk for diarrhea among persons traveling from an industrialized country include living close to local residents during the travel, failure to adhere to strict principles in choosing food and drink, young age, reduced gastric acidity, underlying

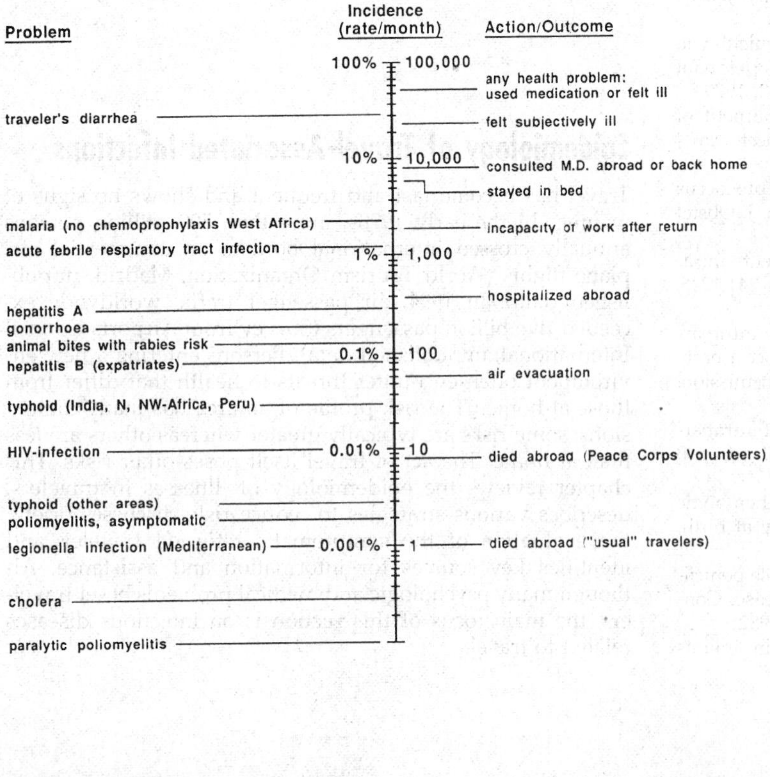

FIGURE 46–1 □ Epidemiology of travel-related infections. Incidence rate per month of health problems during a stay in developing countries. (From Steffen R, DuPont HL: Travel medicine: What's that? J Travel Med 1:1–3, 1994.)

gastrointestinal disease, and immunodeficiency disorders.[12] For a more complete discussion of traveler's diarrhea, see Chapter 81.

Malaria

Malaria remains a threat to travelers in tropical regions.[18] It is estimated that 25 to 30 million persons from nonendemic areas visit malarious countries each year. Risk of infection varies widely by geographic region, season of year, activities, and duration of stay. The malaria attack rate exceeded 1% in travelers to West Africa in the early 1990s.[19] The relative risk for infection increases with longer stays. For example, for British travelers returning from West Africa, the attack rates per 100,000 travelers for malaria were 61 after a 1-week stay but reached almost 4899 after visits of 6 months to 1 year (an 80-fold increase in the relative risk).[19] Malaria is discussed in detail in Chapter 287.

Hepatitis

Viral hepatitis has been an important cause of morbidity and mortality in travelers. Among Swiss travelers, hepatitis accounted for more days of inability to work (mean of 33 days) than any other travel-related infection.[2] Well-documented agents include hepatitis viruses A, B, C, D, and E. Swiss travelers returning from Africa, Latin America, and Asia with acute hepatitis, studied at a time when only tests for hepatitis A and B were available, were found to have predominantly hepatitis A (60%).[20] Only 15% were found to have hepatitis B, and the remaining 25% were categorized as non-A, non-B hepatitis or unclassified. Hepatitis E has been documented in travelers now that diagnostic tests to detect hepatitis E virus are available.[21] The estimated risk of symptomatic hepatitis A for a nonimmune person per month of travel in a developing country is 3 per 1000, although it may be as high as 20 per 1000 per month for backpackers and persons who eat and drink under poor hygienic conditions.[20] Many other infections that can cause prominent hepatic dysfunction (e.g., leptospirosis, yellow fever, typhoid fever, *Hantavirus* infections, dengue, rickettsial infections, and Q fever, among others)[1] are also seen in travelers but typically after a shorter incubation period than for most of the hepatitis viruses.

Sexually Transmitted Diseases

Sexual activity is common during travel, and sexually transmitted infections have been prominent among travel-related infections.[22, 23] Tours arranged specifically to facilitate sexual contacts (sexual tourism) are popular in some areas. Among short-term Swiss tourists traveling to tropical Africa, Asia, and Latin America, almost 60% of those identified in a high-risk group reported casual sexual contacts during their trip.[24] Among Danish Volunteer Service personnel who worked in Kenya, Tanzania, and Zambia for 11 to 41 months, 48% (53 of 110) of the men and 29% (32 of 112) of the women reported heterosexual contact with local residents.[25] In the mid-1980s, of American college students who traveled in the tropics (mean duration 74 days), 29% reported contact with a new partner, 44% without the use of condoms.[26]

Systemic infections, such as hepatitis B, human immunodeficiency virus (HIV) infection, and cytomegalovirus infection, as well as infections causing only or primarily genital lesions, follow sexual contact. Although sexually transmitted diseases have a worldwide distribution, the incidence, locally prevalent infections, and antimicrobial resistance patterns of bacterial pathogens vary by geographic regions. For example, chancroid, an uncommon or rare sexually transmitted disease in the United States, is the cause of more than half of genital ulcers in parts of Southeast Asia and Africa.[27] Serologic studies found that 6% of American troops stationed in Korea for 4 to 12 months became infected with hepatitis B. Although unrecognized intravenous drug use may have accounted for some of the transmission, 83% of those with acute hepatitis B infection gave a history of Korean sexual partners, each reporting a mean number of 6.32 partners.[28]

Host Factors and Risk of Infection

Short-term travelers infrequently acquire helminthic infections, such as cysticercosis, strongyloidiasis, hookworm disease, and filarial infections (such as onchocerciasis, loiasis, bancroftian filariasis). Although schistosomiasis is much more common in persons with prolonged exposures, many cases and clusters have occurred in short-term travelers who have had the misfortune of swimming in cercariae infested waters. Among 30 Dutch travelers returning from Mali, West Africa, 28 of 29 who swam in freshwater pools became ill with schistosomiasis.[29] The duration of exposure to the fresh water ranged from a few minutes to several hours. African trypanosomiasis, which can result from a single bite of an infective tsetse fly, is occasionally seen in persons who have been on safaris in Africa. In the United States between 1968 and 1985, only 13 cases of African trypanosomiasis were reported to the Centers for Disease Control and Prevention.[30]

Characteristics of the human host affect the risk of exposure to pathogens and expression of infection. Most of the relevant host factors can be broadly categorized as behavioral, immunologic, and genetic. Factors that are associated with increased risk for exposure to many infections during travel include prolonged duration of stay; travel to remote and rural areas; living under poor hygienic conditions; close contact with animals, water, and soil as might occur during field work; sexual contacts with local residents; and consumption of food prepared by street vendors. At the same time, it is important to recognize that persons who stay entirely in first-class or deluxe hotels and sleep in screened or air-conditioned rooms can acquire infections. Food- and water-borne infections still spread in sumptuous surroundings.

Immunologic and genetic factors may determine susceptibility to infection and expression of disease. Immunity to infection may come from past infection or from active or passive immunization. Persons who have always lived under good hygienic conditions lack immunity to many pathogens that commonly contaminate food and water in developing countries (e.g., hepatitis A virus, many other enteric pathogens). Several key concepts about travel-related illness are summarized in Table 46–1.

Sources and Acquisition of Infection During Travel

To prevent infection during travel, it is essential to have a basic understanding of the sources of pathogens. The major sources are food and drink, soil and water, animals and arthropods, and other humans. A few comments about each will help inform thinking about risks during travel.

Food and Drink

Fecally contaminated food and drink are the sources of traveler's diarrhea, hepatitis A, typhoid fever, poliomyelitis, cholera, and many other infections. Foods can also harbor parasites (e.g., eggs, larvae, or other forms) and pathogens

TABLE 46–1 ■ Key Concepts: Travel-Related Illness and Death

Injuries are an important cause of travel-related deaths.
Most infections acquired during travel to tropical and developing countries are caused by pathogens that are widely distributed.
Risk for infection from exposure to many widely distributed pathogens (e.g., hepatitis A, typhoid fever, salmonellosis, amebiasis) is substantially higher during travel to developing countries than during life at home.
Unusual infections can be found in temperate and industrialized countries, including the United States.
Vacation activities (e.g., swimming, hiking) facilitate exposure to many pathogens.
Activities that pose no risk at home may be hazardous in another environment (e.g., eating raw foods, swimming in fresh water, going barefooted, sustaining mosquito bites, petting stray animals).
Expensive hotels and posh restaurants are no guarantee of safe food and beverages.
Disease during and immediately after travel may be unrelated to exposures during travel (e.g., acute appendicitis, pyelonephritis).
Infections can be acquired en route and on brief layovers.
Travel-associated diseases include noninfectious diseases (e.g., pulmonary emboli related to prolonged sitting, drug reactions).

from animals (e.g., *Brucella, Salmonella*). Contaminated water can be hidden in many forms, such as in ice cubes,[31] reconstituted orange juice and other beverages, iced tea, shower water (that some persons drink while showering), and water sprayed on fresh fruits and vegetables. Produce may be contaminated in the fields when night soil or fecally contaminated water is used on crops, or it may become contaminated during shipping and processing. In many developing countries where energy supplies are limited, refrigeration is unavailable or erratic. Energy is also required to cook foods and to keep them hot. The warm, humid environment provides a milieu conducive to the rapid proliferation of bacteria that contaminate foods. In some places, bottled water consists of bottles refilled with water from a source of questionable purity.

Soil and Water

Sandy beaches may be contaminated with parasites from feces of humans and animals. Going barefooted or having direct contact between skin and sand or soil places persons at risk for cutaneous larva migrans,[32] hookworm, and other parasites that can penetrate the skin. Recreational water can be a source of enteric pathogens as outbreaks of shigellosis, hemorrhagic colitis, and cryptosporidiosis in the United States have demonstrated.[33, 34] Polluted marine bathing water can be a source of pathogens that cause acute gastroenteritis as well as conjunctivitis.[35] Cercarial dermatitis (caused by animal schistosomes unable to complete their life cycle in humans) can result from exposures to fresh and salt water in many areas of the world. Although unpleasant, the disease does not cause late sequelae. Of greater importance is schistosomiasis, transmitted by contact with fresh water infested with cercariae that can penetrate intact human skin in a period of 30 seconds to 10 minutes and mature in the human host. Water exposures during bathing and wading and getting splashed during boating and rafting have been associated with transmission of schistosomiasis. Leptospirosis is another infection that is more common in tropical areas and can be acquired by contact with water.[36] Larvae of coelenterates, such as jellyfish and sea anemones, can penetrate intact skin during swimming and cause an annoying pruritic skin eruption known as seabather's eruption.[37, 38]

Animals and Arthropods

Animals can transmit infection by biting the human host. An underappreciated threat during travel is rabies, which is common in animals (especially dogs) in many parts of Asia, Africa, and Central and South America. For example, studies in Thailand have found rabies virus in 3% to 6% of stray dogs. In India, an estimated 40,000 to 50,000 persons die annually of rabies.[39, 40] More often animals play a role in human disease through indirect means. Humans eat animal flesh or animal products that are infected or contaminated with pathogens, including parasites. Animal excreta and tissues contain pathogens (e.g., *Hantavirus*, Lassa virus) that can reach humans by a variety of routes. Animals may be the site of an essential developmental step in the life cycle of the pathogen or serve as the reservoir host from which an arthropod vector carries the pathogen to humans. Many arthropods important for human disease are closely associated with animals. Among the most important infections in travelers, many are arthropod borne (e.g., malaria, dengue, rickettsial infections, leishmaniasis, Japanese encephalitis, yellow fever, and many others).

Other Humans

Humans are a source of infections that are transmitted by aerosols and droplets, sexual and other close contact, and fecal-oral spread. In many parts of the world, sterile needles and syringes are not consistently available, and blood and blood products used for transfusion may not be screened. Contact with needles (including tattooing, acupuncture), medical and dental care, and transfusions can be a source of infection. Blood transfusion can be a source of malaria, *Trypanosoma cruzi* infection, and other parasitic infections in some regions of the world in addition to the more familiar risks, such as HIV infection, hepatitis B, hepatitis C, human T-cell lymphotropic virus infection, and syphilis.[1]

Air Travel

The immobility associated with prolonged travel can predispose to venous thrombosis and pulmonary emboli.[41] Several features of air travel predispose to respiratory illness: low humidity of air in aircraft, crowding of persons in a closed space with limited infusions of fresh air, and changes in air pressure with ascent and descent. Moreover, aircraft cabins are pressurized to the equivalent of 6000 to 8000 feet above sea level.[42] Persons with underlying chronic lung disease who are marginally compensated at sea level may suffer from reduced partial pressure of oxygen while flying. Changes in air pressure associated with flying may exacerbate chronic ear and sinus problems or precipitate acute problems, especially in persons with upper respiratory infections.

Although most of the reports of respiratory infections after air travel are anecdotal, transmission of infections, such as influenza, aboard aircraft has been well documented.[43] Epidemiologic studies suggest that tuberculosis may occasionally be transmitted on aircraft.[44]

Infections Acquired En Route

Although preparation for travel tends to focus on the destination, the vehicle of transportation can be the site for transmission of infection. Examples include legionellosis transmitted on cruise ships,[45] cholera on aircraft, shigellosis from food served on multiple flights,[46] malaria thought to have been transmitted by a "commuter mosquito," and many other infections transmitted primarily by food or drink. Food and ice served on aircraft and ships generally come from the port of departure and may reflect conditions in that country.

Infections Acquired in Temperate and Industrialized Areas

Whereas tropical and developing countries may have a greater array and abundance of exotic pathogens, temperate and industrialized countries, including the United States, can also be the site for transmission of unfamiliar infections with geographically focal distributions. Some examples are listed in Table 46–2. The intent is not to provide an exhaustive list of such infections but to remind physicians that travel to a seemingly familiar place can result in unusual infections. These include bacterial, fungal, protozoan, helminthic, and viral infections.

Preventive Strategies

Preparation for travel should include a review of the entire itinerary, including intermediate stops and layovers. Persons planning prolonged stays in developing countries should undergo a complete medical evaluation. The pretravel evaluation is the time to identify specific geographic regions, planned activities, and host factors that require special attention or interventions.

Overview

Several approaches can be used to reduce the risk of disruption and death related to travel. These generally fall into three broad categories: education that leads to a change in behavior, chemoprophylaxis, and immunization. Although immunizations have an important role in the prevention of travel-related infections, most infections acquired during travel are not vaccine preventable (with currently available vaccines), and vaccines are not the only means available to prevent vaccine-preventable infections.[46a] Several interventions are disease specific (e.g., yellow fever vaccine); many others are more broadly applicable (e.g., use of repellent to prevent insect bites).

The burden of disease can be reduced by interventions at three points: preventing exposure to the pathogen, preventing infection after exposure has occurred (e.g., through protective immunity of host; preventive chemotherapy or immunoprophylaxis), and limiting the impact or severity of infection (e.g., by partial immunity to infection; early diagnosis and treatment; prevention of spread to others). Prevention of exposure is typically accomplished by specific behavior (e.g., avoiding person, place, or activity) or by use of physical (barrier) or chemical protection. Table 46–3 lists general recommendations that can protect against multiple diseases.

TABLE 46–2 ■ Geographically Focal Infections in Temperate and Industrialized Areas (Examples)

UNITED STATES
Colorado tick fever
Relapsing fever
Plague
Babesiosis
Eastern equine encephalitis
Coccidioidomycosis
WESTERN AND SOUTHERN EUROPE
Lyme disease
Hemorrhagic fever with renal syndrome
Nephropathica hemorrhagica
Visceral leishmaniasis
Spotted fever due to *Rickettsia conorii* (boutonneuse fever)
AUSTRALIA
Angiostrongyliasis due to *Angiostrongylus cantonensis*
Dengue fever
Murray Valley encephalitis (Australian encephalitis)
Ross River fever
Spotted fever due to *Rickettsia australis* (north Queensland tick typhus)

Medical Kit

Travelers should carry basic medical supplies with them. The composition of their personal medical kit will vary depending on duration of travel, destination, and planned activities. Prescription drugs should be packed in their original containers. Sunscreens and insect repellents are essential for many destinations. Many other items may be included: acetaminophen, ibuprofen, or aspirin; diphenhydramine or other antihistamine; extra pair of prescription glasses and sunglasses; thermometer, tweezers, small scissors, and safety pins; small flashlight; adhesive bandages and Steri-Strips; antimicrobial and antimotility agent; antimalarial drugs, if needed; alcohol wipes; condoms; and personal supplies, such as tampons or sanitary napkins for menstruating women. Depending on destination and circumstances, the traveler may need to take materials for water purification, bed nets, sterile needles and syringes, and permethrin-impregnated clothing. Other references provide practical advice about how to put together a personal medical kit.[47]

Insurance

Before departure, travelers should determine whether their medical insurance will cover them if they become ill abroad. If it does not, they should obtain special trip insurance. Persons planning extended stays in remote areas and those with underlying diseases should seriously consider getting insurance that will cover medical evacuation, should that be necessary. A number of companies now offer these services.

Injury

There is a tendency to think of injury as unpredictable and thus not preventable. Although it is impossible to avoid all injuries, it is possible to anticipate many risks and to find ways to reduce them. This involves actions taken before and during the travel. Strategies include selecting cars that are in good repair and are equipped with seat belts, driving during daylight hours, avoiding driving and swimming when fatigued or after drinking, avoiding use of mopeds (use helmets to ride mopeds, bicycles, and motorcycles—a helmet may need to be taken along), arranging for a driver familiar with the roads in some instances, and obtaining good road maps of areas to be visited. Injury is the leading reason for blood transfusion in travelers visiting developing countries.

Prevention of Traveler's Diarrhea

Paying strict attention to choice of food and drink during travel can reduce but does not eliminate the risk of traveler's diarrhea.[48] Thus, it is recommended that travelers to developing countries be prepared to deal with diarrhea by taking medications with them to use for early therapy should diarrhea develop. Prophylactic antimicrobials against traveler's diarrhea are not routinely advised. Circumstances that might lead to the consideration of prophylactic antimicrobials include underlying diseases (such as insulin-dependent diabetes mellitus, active inflammatory bowel disease, acquired immunodeficiency syndrome, others) or extreme inconvenience if the trip were interrupted by traveler's diarrhea.[12]

TABLE 46–3 ■ General Recommendations for Travelers*

MODE OF TRANSMISSION	PREVENTIVE STRATEGY	SUPPLEMENTAL PROTECTION
Sexually transmitted	Avoid sexual contact	Use condoms; see also vaccines for specific diseases
Vector-borne	Varies with vector; multiple possible interventions include Stay in screened or air-conditioned rooms Use bed nets (preferably impregnated with repellents) in malarious areas Avoid outdoor exposure at biting time for vectors Use insect repellents Use protective clothing (some insects can bite through clothing) Inspect skin for ticks in areas with tick-borne infections Avoid scented soaps, perfumes	See also vaccines (yellow fever and Japanese encephalitis) and Chemoprophylaxis Against Malaria
Food- and beverage-borne	Choose foods and fluids that are generally safe, e.g., steaming hot food, coffee and tea, wine and beer, bottled carbonated water or beverages, fruits that can be peeled by the consumer, bread (without fillings) Avoid raw and undercooked seafood and animal flesh Avoid raw fruits and vegetables (unless peeled by consumer) Avoid ice, tap water and beverages made with it Avoid buffets and foods held in open areas especially if abundant flies Avoid foods, ices, and beverages sold by street vendors Avoid unpasteurized milk and milk products	See also vaccines See also Prevention of Traveler's Diarrhea
Water and soil associated	Avoid skin contact with fresh water in endemic schistosomiasis areas Avoid direct skin contact with soil and sand contaminated with feces Avoid going barefooted Avoid swimming in beaches near sewage outflow tracts Avoid swimming in ponds near where animals graze and wade Avoid ingesting water while swimming	

*These recommendations protect against multiple diseases, although the specific diseases may vary from one geographic area to another. How carefully the recommendations need to be followed will vary with the geographic region and the host.

Prophylactic agents that have been shown effective in clinical studies include bismuth subsalicylate, the fluoroquinolones, trimethoprim-sulfamethoxazole (160 mg of trimethoprim and 800 mg of sulfamethoxazole once daily), and doxycycline 100 mg daily.[49, 50] Enteric pathogens in many parts of the world are now resistant to doxycycline and increasingly to trimethoprim-sulfamethoxasole.[51]

The approach preferred by most travelers to developing countries is to carry an antimotility agent and antimicrobials to take for self-therapy for specified symptoms. Travelers who develop watery diarrhea without blood in stools have shown good response to an antibacterial agent (quinolone or trimethoprim-sulfamethoxasole) plus loperamide.[52, 53] Travelers with fever or bloody stools should take an antimicrobial alone (without an antimotility agent). Given the increasing rates of resistance to many antimicrobials, the most reliable agents currently are the quinolones (norfloxacin, 400 mg twice daily; ciprofloxacin, 500 mg twice daily; or ofloxacin 300 mg twice daily, each for 3 days). A single dose may be effective for mild disease. Bismuth subsalicylate is a reasonable choice for mild disease (e.g., mild diarrhea with no fever or bloody stools).[54] Travelers should be reminded of the need to maintain adequate hydration as an essential part of the therapy for any diarrheal illness and be cautioned to seek medical attention if diarrhea persists despite treatment or is associated with high fevers. This is especially important advice to persons traveling to endemic malaria regions, because malaria can cause gastrointestinal symptoms that can be misinterpreted as an enteric infection.

Chemoprophylaxis Against Malaria

Chemoprophylaxis should be provided for persons traveling to endemic malaria regions along with instructions for personal protective measures to reduce the risk of bites from infective mosquitoes.[55–57] Malaria persists in many tropical regions of the world. Occurrence has risen in some areas owing to increasing drug resistance, reduction in vector control programs, changes in land use, and migration of human populations. Malaria remains an important cause of potentially lethal infection in travelers.[18] Its protean clinical manifestations can delay recognition and appropriate treatment. Malaria is discussed in Chapter 287.

Immunoprophylaxis

Preparation for travel provides an opportunity to review and update routine vaccines along with assessing the need for special vaccines.[58] Simply looking at what vaccines are required for entry into a country is insufficient. It is useful to think about the vaccines in three general groups: those that are required by the country; those that are prudent, given the risks the person will undergo; and routine vaccines that should be updated. Vaccines commonly used for adult travelers are listed in Table 46–4.

Vaccines used to prevent many of the common childhood infections save more money than they cost (e.g., measles, mumps, rubella, pertussis, *Haemophilus influenzae* infection).[59–62] In contrast, many of the vaccines used to prevent infections in travelers are extremely expensive per death averted or case prevented.[63–65] This does not mean that these vaccines should not be used. Travelers have special characteristics that are pertinent in making decisions about vaccines.[46a] The cost of travel is high and the value placed on a day during a trip may greatly exceed the value of a day at home. Disruption during travel can be expensive as well as inconvenient, especially if it involves a change in itinerary or hospitalization. The availability and quality of medical treatment in many parts of the world are uncertain. Some of the vaccines given before travel also have benefit that extends beyond the individual trip. Preventing infection in the traveler may also eliminate a potential source of spread of infec-

TABLE 46–4 ■ Vaccines for Adult Travelers

ROUTINE	
Updated as needed	
Diphtheria-tetanus	
Measles-mumps-rubella	
Routine for Defined Groups	
Influenza virus	
Pneumococcal	
REQUIRED BY SOME COUNTRIES (CHECK CURRENT REQUIREMENTS)	
Yellow fever	
Meningococcal	
RECOMMENDED FOR TRAVELERS TO DEVELOPING COUNTRIES	
Standard for Travelers to Developing Countries	
Hepatitis A vaccine or immune globulin	
Typhoid	
Poliovirus	
Special for Travelers to Developing Countries	
Cholera	
Hepatitis B	
Meningococcal	
Japanese encephalitis	
Plague	
Rabies	

tion to family and friends on return (e.g., hepatitis A, typhoid fever).

ROUTINE VACCINES

Travelers to developing countries are at risk for exposure to many infections that have been largely controlled with improved living conditions and vaccines in the United States. These include poliomyelitis, pertussis, diphtheria, tetanus, measles, rubella, and mumps. Persons who are not up to date on any of these should receive the appropriate boosters (note that pertussis vaccine is not currently recommended in adults).[66] Tetanus boosters should be updated so that travelers will not run the risk of needing a tetanus booster during travel in a setting where injections may be unsafe. Many persons, particularly older adults, lack immunity to vaccine-preventable infections. A study of serum levels of antibody against tetanus in a representative noninstitutionalized population in the United States found that only 69.7% had protective levels of antibodies. Among persons 70 years of age and older, only 27.8% had protective levels of antibodies.[67] A study of London blood donors done in 1993 found that 37.6% were susceptible to diphtheria according to internationally accepted definitions of immunity. More than half of those in the age group 50 to 59 years were susceptible to diphtheria.[68] The risk from waning levels of immunity to diphtheria is reinforced by events since the early 1990s in the New Independent States of the former Soviet Union where outbreaks of diphtheria have occurred, reaching almost 50,000 reported cases in 1994.[69] Throughout the epidemic, about 70% of the cases have been in persons 15 years of age and older.

The elderly population constitutes a growing percentage of the traveling public. Persons in risk groups for whom pneumococcal and influenza vaccines are advised should receive these vaccines. Risk of these infections may not be increased during travel, but illness during travel is especially unpleasant and inconvenient. Influenza occurs in all months of the year in tropical areas and appears mainly in our summer months in the Southern Hemisphere.

YELLOW FEVER VACCINE

Yellow fever vaccine is required for entry into many countries.[70, 71] The certificate of vaccination becomes valid 10 days after receipt of the vaccine. Decisions about the yellow fever vaccine must take into account the risk of infection, immunogenicity and potential side effects from this live virus vaccine, and requirements of the countries to be visited. To be valid, the vaccine must be given at an official Yellow Fever Vaccination Center and recorded on the International Certificate of Vaccination, signed by a licensed physician or by a person designated by the physician. Persons without a valid certificate who try to enter a country requiring yellow fever vaccination may be denied entry into a country, quarantined, or revaccinated at that site.

Information about individual country requirements is updated each year in the yellow booklets published by the World Health Organization and the Centers for Disease Control and Prevention. The country codes should be reviewed with care; some countries outside of the yellow fever endemic zones require the yellow fever vaccine (because they may have mosquitoes that could allow introduction of the virus), and some countries within the endemic zone do not require travelers to be immunized. The regulations are designed to prevent introductions and epidemics of yellow fever, not necessarily for the protection of the individual traveler. A number of countries, for example, Australia and Bangladesh, require a valid yellow fever certificate from travelers arriving from countries with yellow fever (even if they only passed briefly through that country) even though there is no yellow fever in Australia or Bangladesh. Many countries where yellow fever is endemic or epidemic do not require persons arriving from the United States to have the vaccine, even though the Centers for Disease Control and Prevention and other groups recommend that travelers receive the vaccine.

Because it is a live vaccine, there are concerns about use of yellow fever vaccine in young infants, pregnant women, and persons who are immunocompromised. Pregnant women and infants younger than 9 months should not be given the vaccine unless risk of infection is high. Yellow fever vaccine virus can infect the developing fetus, although the magnitude of risk for congenital defects from vaccine-associated infection is unknown.[72] HIV-infected persons may be at increased risk for complications from the vaccine (although a few data suggest it has been well tolerated) and may not develop protective immunity to infection after receiving vaccine. Vaccine-induced immunity may wane faster than in persons with normal immunity. If risk of infection is high, it may be wise to assess adequacy of immune response by checking serum antibody titers.

MENINGOCOCCAL VACCINE

Meningococcal vaccine has been required during more recent years by Saudi Arabia for pilgrims to Mecca for the annual hajj. The polysaccharide vaccine, available as a quadrivalent vaccine against A, C, Y, and W-135, is sometimes recommended for other selected persons, such as travelers to parts of Africa, trekkers to Nepal, and persons traveling to areas experiencing meningitis outbreaks.

CHOLERA VACCINE

Although no country has a formal requirement for cholera vaccine, travelers report occasional demands for vaccine documentation when international borders are crossed. The currently available vaccine has limited efficacy (50% to 60%) of brief duration. Risk of cholera to travelers on usual itineraries is extremely low. The current vaccine has a limited role in travelers, although it might be considered for persons who will be living or working in an area experiencing cholera epidemics, especially if they are living under conditions of crowding and poor sanitation.

HEPATITIS A PREVENTION

Two options are now available for the prevention of hepatitis A, immune globulin and the inactivated hepatitis A vaccine.[20] Both are highly effective in preventing hepatitis A. Advantages of immune globulin are that it provides immediate protection and is relatively inexpensive. Advantages of the hepatitis A vaccine are that it has been highly efficacious in clinical trials, and a vaccine series (two or three doses, depending on vaccine formulation) will probably provide protection for 10 years or longer. It is well tolerated and has been given simultaneously with other vaccines without apparent adverse effect on immunogenicity. Because it is an inactivated vaccine, it can be used safely in persons who are immunocompromised. A number of papers have analyzed use of the vaccine versus immune globulin.[65, 73] Persons who have antibodies to hepatitis A because of prior natural infection will derive no benefit from the vaccine (but also experience no apparent harm from the vaccine). Travelers for whom the vaccine is most cost effective are persons who travel frequently to developing countries or who expect to spend prolonged periods living in developing countries. There is no evidence that the immune globulin available in the United States protects against hepatitis E.

TYPHOID FEVER VACCINES

Three different typhoid vaccines are now available in the United States: a parenteral, heat-phenol–inactivated vaccine, used for many years; an oral live-attenuated vaccine made from the Ty21a strain of *Salmonella typhi;* and capsular polysaccharide vaccine for parenteral use (Typhim Vi).[74] No direct comparative studies have assessed relative efficacy of the three. All have shown efficacy in field trials, typically in the range of 50% to 75%. The parenteral, inactivated vaccine causes frequent side effects, and for that reason the newer preparations are preferred by most persons who are given a choice of vaccines. The oral vaccine is attractive to persons who dislike injections. Because it is a live vaccine, it requires careful attention to handling and administration (e.g., it requires refrigeration and cannot be given with antibiotics). Four doses are taken in a period of 6 days. The polysaccharide vaccine has the advantage of requiring a single injected dose with recommendation for a booster every 2 years. Geographic areas reporting the highest frequency of typhoid fever in travelers are the Indian subcontinent including Nepal, parts of South America, Asia, and Africa. Persons who plan extended low-budget trips in remote and rural areas are at greatest risk.

JAPANESE ENCEPHALITIS VACCINE

The Japanese encephalitis vaccine available in the United States is an inactivated vaccine (virus grown in mouse brain) manufactured by Biken, Japan, and distributed by Connaught. Because symptomatic infections have been rare in travelers and adverse reactions to the vaccine, sometimes severe, occur in 1 to 104 per 10,000 vaccinees, use of the vaccine is recommended only for persons planning prolonged stays in rural areas during the transmission season. The vaccine is not recommended for short-term travelers (less than 30 days) unless their itineraries place them at especially high risk.[75] The vaccine series is given in three doses in a period of 30 days. The last dose should be given at least 10 days before departure so that adverse reactions can be handled before travel. Efficacy of the vaccine in children in endemic areas has been 80% to 90%.

RABIES VACCINE

Decisions about use of rabies vaccine can be difficult for several reasons: vaccine is extremely expensive; rabies in travelers is rare; infection is lethal; and postexposure treatment in developing countries varies greatly in accessibility, efficacy, and safety. Risk for exposure in many areas is much higher than in the United States but is still low relative to the risk for other infections, such as malaria and typhoid fever. Whether or not the rabies vaccine is given, the prospective traveler needs to be educated about the risk for animal bites and licks. Dogs are the most important reservoir of rabies in most countries and are the source of about 90% of the human cases. Monkeys and other animals can also carry rabies, and travelers may be unaware of this risk. Travelers must be informed about the need to seek care if a bite occurs. Persons for whom preexposure prophylaxis should be considered are those spending prolonged periods in developing countries where animal rabies is common (especially if safe, effective vaccines and rabies immune globulin will be unavailable locally), particularly if the person will be biking, working with animals, or traveling to remote areas where access to medical care will be difficult.[76]

HEPATITIS B VACCINE

A growing segment of the population has received the hepatitis B vaccine. The primary modes of transmission of hepatitis B are through sex and percutaneous injuries (e.g., needlesticks, medical care). Rates of chronic hepatitis B infection reach 8% to 15% or higher in parts of China, Southeast Asia, Africa, the Pacific Islands, and the Amazon Basin in South America. Persons planning prolonged stays in areas where infection is highly endemic should receive the vaccine. It is especially important for persons who plan to work in a health care setting or plan to have sexual contact with local residents.

Integrating Multiple Vaccines

Integration of multiple vaccines requires careful planning. Administration of antimicrobials and antimalarials influences the timing or route of administration of some vaccines. For example, persons taking chloroquine who are given the rabies vaccine have a lower antibody response than those who are not receiving the drug. Most inactivated vaccines do not interfere with the immune response to other vaccines (inactivated or live), so these vaccines can be given simultaneously or before or after other vaccines. A few data suggest that the immune response to yellow fever and cholera vaccines is reduced if the vaccines are given simultaneously or separated by 1 to 3 weeks. If possible, the vaccines should be given at least 3 weeks apart. This rarely creates a problem because the current cholera vaccine is rarely indicated. Immune globulin can impair antibody response to some live vaccines (e.g., measles-mumps-rubella) but does not affect response to either oral live polio or yellow fever vaccines. Measles-mumps-rubella vaccination should be delayed at least 3 months after administration of immune globulin. Immune globulin should be deferred until at least 14 days after the measles-mumps-rubella vaccine is given. Physicians should also review the history for any other sources of antibodies (e.g., in blood or blood products, hepatitis B immune globulin, rabies immune globulin) because these will also interfere with immune response.

Special Groups

HIV-INFECTED TRAVELERS

Pretravel preparation for HIV-infected travelers requires special attention for several reasons: travel-related infections may be more common and more severe; manifestations of infection may be atypical; usual forms of therapy may fail to cure infections; reactions to drugs are common and may mimic infectious diseases; immune response to vaccines may be diminished; informed treatment and special drugs may be difficult to obtain should illness develop during travel; and legal and social issues may inhibit free movement of HIV-infected persons across international borders.[77] In addition, HIV-infected persons may be taking multiple medications that must be considered when immunization and chemoprophylactic regimens are planned.[78] A study in California found that travel was common in HIV-infected persons, despite advanced disease. Destinations included tropical and developing countries.[79] Physicians must be able to identify risks, assess their magnitude, and review options to reduce risk with HIV-infected persons who wish to travel.

PREGNANT WOMEN

Pregnant women also require special attention. Some vaccines and chemoprophylactic agents are contraindicated during pregnancy. Reviews have outlined approaches to management.[80, 81]

CHRONIC MEDICAL PROBLEMS

The expanding population traveling includes many persons with chronic medical conditions, such as diabetes mellitus and cardiac disease; those who are confined to wheelchairs; and persons on chronic renal dialysis. A variety of organizations, newsletters, books, and other resources are now available to help such persons arrange their travel.[82]

TABLE 46–5 ■ Sources of Information

Centers for Disease Control and Prevention: Health Information for International Travel.
U.S. Department of Health and Human Services. Revised annually. For sale by the Superintendent of Documents, U.S. Government Printing Office, Washington, DC 20402, 202-783-3238. HHS publication (CDC) 95-8280.
CDC International Travelers Hotline: 404-332-4559
CDC fax information: 404-332-4565
CDC Parasitic Diseases Drug Service: 404-639-3670
CDC main switchboard: 404-639-3311
CDC WebServer http://www.cdc.gov

International Association for Medical Assistance to Travellers (IAMAT), 40 Regal Road, Guelph, Ontario N1K 1B5F. Publishes regularly updated summaries on immunizations, malaria prophylaxis, schistosomiasis, and American trypanosomiasis. World climate charts are also available.

Travel Medicine Advisor, published by American Health Consultants Inc. Uses loose-leaf format to allow regular updating of sections. Provides newsletter every 2 months. Telephone 1-800-688-2421.

World Health Organization: International Travel and Health. Vaccination Requirements and Health Advice. World Health Organization, 1211 Geneva, Switzerland. Revised annually.

In addition to the Infectious Diseases Society of America and the American Society for Microbiology, the following organizations have regular scientific meetings that focus at least in part on infections in travelers:
International Society of Travel Medicine (publishes *Journal of Travel Medicine*)
Wilderness Medical Society (publishes a journal, *Wilderness and Environmental Medicine*)
American Committee on Clinical Tropical Medicine and Traveler's Health, within the American Society of Tropical Medicine and Hygiene (*American Journal of Tropical Medicine and Hygiene*)

Current information can also be accessed through the Internet.

Evaluation of the Returned Traveler

Evaluation of the patient after travel should begin with a consideration of what is possible had the person not traveled. The differential diagnosis should then be expanded to include diseases that may have been acquired during travel. Patients with fever need immediate attention. Initial focus should be on infections that are treatable, transmissible, or both. The geographic areas of travel, the types of exposures, and the time elapsed since the exposures along with the clinical findings are all key bits of data that allow construction of an informed differential diagnosis. It is essential to evaluate for malaria in persons who have spent time in endemic malaria regions. Malaria can occur even if persons took malaria prophylaxis as prescribed. Dengue fever is spreading in tropical areas and occurs in urban areas frequently visited by tourists.[83] Dengue, typhoid fever, malaria, and rickettsial infections share some clinical and laboratory features. Specific laboratory studies must be carried out to make a specific diagnosis so that appropriate therapy can be given.

Skin lesions are common in returned travelers. Although skin diseases rarely lead to hospitalization, they are a common reason for medical attention after travel.[84] Many reflect superficial infections, reactions to insect bites, or other easily managed problems. Skin findings can also provide important clues to systemic infections or processes that may cause late complications (e.g., leishmaniasis).

The distribution of diseases changes over time, making it important to obtain current information about what diseases occur in which geographic areas. Resistance patterns to antimicrobials and serotypes of pathogens may vary from one region to another. Table 46–5 lists several sources of information that are regularly updated. Although this chapter focuses on helping the traveler avoid disease and disruption, we should also recognize that the massive movement of humans today affects the distribution of infectious diseases and their impact on populations.[85]

References

1. Wilson ME: A World Guide to Infections: Diseases, Distribution, Diagnosis. New York, Oxford University Press, 1991.
2. Steffen R, Rickenbach M, Wilhelm U, et al: Health problems after travel to developing countries. J Infect Dis 156:84–91, 1987.
3. Steffen R, DuPont HL: Travel medicine: What's that? J Travel Med 1:1–3, 1994.
4. Steffen R: Travel medicine—Prevention based on epidemiologic data. Trans R Soc Trop Med Hyg 85:156–162, 1991.
5. Reid D, Cossar JH: Epidemiology of travel. Br Med Bull 49:257–268, 1993.
6. Eng TR, Bernard KW, Banks D, et al: Epidemiologic surveillance of health conditions among temporary residents of developing countries: The Peace Corps experience. *In* Lobel HO, Steffen R, Kozarsky PE (eds): Travel Medicine 2. Atlanta, International Society of Travel Medicine, pp 16–19, 1991.
7. Honigman B, Theis MK, Koziol-McLain J, et al: Acute mountain

sickness in a general tourist population at moderate altitude. Ann Intern Med 118:587–592, 1993.
8. Auerbach PS: Marine envenomations. N Engl J Med 325:486–493, 1991.
9. Guptill KS, Hargarten SW, Baker TD: American travel deaths in Mexico. Causes and prevention strategies. West Med J 154:169–171, 1991.
10. Baker TD, Hargarten SW, Guptill KS: The uncounted dead—American civilians dying overseas. Public Health Rep 107:155–160, 1992.
11. Hargarten SW: Injury prevention: A crucial aspect of travel medicine. J Travel Med 1:48–50, 1994.
12. DuPont HL, Ericsson CD: Prevention and treatment of traveler's diarrhea. N Engl J Med 328:1821–1827, 1993.
13. Ericsson CD, DuPont HL: Travelers' diarrhea: Approaches to prevention and treatment. Clin Infect Dis 16:616–626, 1993.
14. Gorbach SL, Kean BH, Evans DG, et al: Travelers' diarrhea and toxigenic *Escherichia coli.* N Engl J Med 292:933–937, 1975.
15. Mattila L, Siitonen A, Kyronseppa H, et al: Seasonal variation in etiology of travelers' diarrhea. J Infect Dis 165:383–388, 1992.
16. Hoge CW, Shlim DR, Rajah R, et al: Epidemiology of diarrhoeal illness associated with coccidian-like organism among travellers and foreign residents in Nepal. Lancet 341:1175–1179, 1993.
17. Ortega YR, Sterling CR, Gilman RH, et al: *Cyclospora* species—a new protozoan pathogen of humans. N Engl J Med 328:1308–1312, 1993.
18. Lackritz EM, Lobel HO, Howell JB, et al: Imported *Plasmodium falciparum* malaria in American travelers to Africa—Implications for prevention strategies. JAMA 265:383–385, 1991.
19. Phillips-Howard PA, Radalowicz J, Mitchell J, Bradley DJ: Risk of malaria in British residents returning from malarious areas. BMJ 300:499–503, 1990.
20. Steffen R, Kane MA, Shapiro CN, et al: Epidemiology and prevention of hepatitis A in travelers. JAMA 272:885–889, 1994.
21. Centers for Disease Control and Prevention: Hepatitis E among U.S. travelers, 1989–1992. MMWR Morbid Mortal Wkly Rep 42:1–4, 1993.
22. De Schryver A, Meheus A: International travel and sexually transmitted diseases. World Health Stat Q 42:90–99, 1989.
23. Mulhall BP: Sexually transmissible diseases and travel. Br Med Bull 49:394–411, 1993.
24. Stricker M, Steffen R, Gutzwiller F, Eichmann A: Casual sexual contacts of Swiss tourist in tropical Africa, the Far East and Latin America. *In* Lobel HO, Steffen R, Kozarsky PE (eds): Travel Medicine 2. Atlanta, International Society of Travel Medicine, pp 220–221, 1991.
25. Nielsen NJ, Lindhardt BO, Ulrich K: HIV antibodies in Danish Volunteer Service personnel in Kenya, Tanzania and Zambia. Trans R Soc Trop Med Hyg 81:680, 1987.
26. Smith RP, Smith D, Bern K, et al: Health risks of international travel among United States college students. *In* Steffen R, Lobel HO, Bradley DJ (eds): Travel Medicine. Berlin, Springer-Verlag, 1989, pp 67–80.
27. Taylor DN, Duangmani C, Suvongse C, et al: The role of *Haemophilus ducreyi* in penile ulcers in Bangkok, Thailand. Sex Transm Dis 11:148–151, 1984.
28. Aronson NE, Palmer BF: Acute viral hepatitis in American soldiers in Korea. South Med J 81:949–951, 1988.
29. Visser LG, Polderman AM, Stuiver PC: Outbreak of schistosomiasis among travelers returning from Mali, West Africa. Clin Infect Dis 20:280–285, 1995.
30. Panosian CB, Cohen L, Bruckner D, et al: Fever, leukopenia, and a cutaneous lesion in a man who had recently traveled to Africa. Rev Infect Dis 13:1130–1138, 1991.
31. Dickens DL, DuPont HL, Johnson PC: Survival of bacterial enteropathogens in the ice of popular drinks. JAMA 253:3141–3143, 1985.
32. Davies HD, Sakuls P, Keystone JS: Creeping eruption. A review of clinical presentation and management of 60 cases presenting to a tropical disease unit. Arch Dermatol 129:588–591, 1993.
33. Keene WE, McAnulty JM, Hoesly RC, et al: A swimming-associated outbreak of hemorrhagic colitis caused by *Escherichia coli* O157:H7 and *Shigella sonnei.* N Engl J Med 331:579–584, 1994.
34. McAnulty JM, Fleming DW, Gonzalez AH: A community-wide outbreak of cryptosporidiosis associated with swimming at a wave pool. JAMA 272:1597–1600, 1994.
35. Cabelli VJ, Dufour AP, McCabe LJ, Levin MA: Swimming-associated gastroenteritis and water quality. Am J Epidemiol 115:606–616, 1982.
36. Van Crevel R, Speelman P, Gravekamp C, et al: Leptospirosis in travelers. Clin Infect Dis 19:132–134, 1994.
37. Tomchik RS, Russell MT, Szmant AM, Black NA: Clinical perspectives on seabather's eruption, also known as 'sea lice.' JAMA 269:1669–1672, 1993.
38. Freudenthal AR, Joseph PR: Seabather's eruption. N Engl J Med 329:542–544, 1993.
39. World Health Organization, Veterinary Public Health Unit: World Survey of Rabies 25 (for year 1989). Geneva, World Health Organization, 1992. Rabies/92.203.
40. Wilkerson JA. Rabies: Epidemiology, diagnosis, prevention, and prospects for worldwide control. Wilderness Environ Med 6:48–96, 1995.
41. AMA Commission on Emergency Medical Services: Medical aspects of transportation aboard commercial aircraft. JAMA 247:1007–1011, 1982.
42. Dillard TA, Berg BW, Rajagopal KR, et al: Hypoxemia during air travel in patients with chronic obstructive pulmonary disease. Ann Intern Med 111:362–367, 1989.
43. Moser MR, Bender TR, Margolis HS, et al: An outbreak of influenza aboard a commercial airliner. Am J Epidemiol 110:1101–1106, 1979.
44. Driver CR, Valway SE, Margan WM, et al: Transmission of *Mycobacterium tuberculosis* associated with air travel. JAMA 272:1031–1035, 1994.
45. Centers for Disease Control and Prevention: Update: Outbreak of Legionnaires' disease associated with a cruise ship. MMWR Morbid Mortal Wkly Rep 43:574–575, 1994.
46. Hedberg CW, Levine WC, White KE, et al: An international foodborne outbreak of shigellosis associated with a commercial airline. JAMA 268:3208–3212, 1992.
46a. Wilson ME: Critical evaluation of vaccines for travelers. J Travel Med 2:239–243, 1996.
47. Jong EC: The travel medical kit and emergency medical care abroad. *In* Jong EC, McMullen R: The Travel and Tropical Medicine Manual, ed 2. Philadelphia, WB Saunders, 1995, pp 17–27.
48. Blaser MJ: Environmental interventions for the prevention of travelers' diarrhea. Rev Infect Dis 8:S142–S150, 1986.
49. Sack DA, Kaminsky DC, Sack RB, et al: Prophylactic doxycycline for travelers' diarrhea: Results of a prospective double-blind study of Peace Corps volunteers in Kenya. N Engl J Med 298:758–763, 1978.
50. DuPont HL, Ericsson CD, Johnson PC, et al: Prevention of travelers' diarrhea by the tablet formulation of bismuth subsalicylate. JAMA 257:1347–1350, 1987.
51. Tauxe RV, Tuhr ND, Wells JG, et al: Antimicrobial resistance of *Shigella* isolates in the USA: The importance of international travelers. J Infect Dis 162:1107–1111, 1990.
52. Murphy GS, Bodhidatta L, Echeverria P, et al: Ciprofloxacin and loperamide in the treatment of bacillary dysentery. Ann Intern Med 118:582–586, 1993.
53. Taylor DN, Sanchez JL, Candler W, et al: Treatment of travelers' diarrhea: Ciprofloxacin plus loperamide versus ciprofloxacin alone. A placebo-controlled, randomized trial. Ann Intern Med 114:731–734, 1991.
54. Johnson PC, Ericsson CD, DuPont HL, et al: Comparison of loperamide with bismuth subsalicylate for the treatment of acute travelers' diarrhea. JAMA 255:757–760, 1986.
55. Wyler DJ: Malaria chemoprophylaxis for the traveler. N Engl J Med 328:31–37, 1993.
56. Steffen R, Heusser R, Machler R, et al: Malaria chemoprophylaxis among European tourists in tropical Africa: Use, adverse reactions, and efficacy. Bull World Health Organ 68:313–322, 1990.
57. Lobel H, Miani M, Eng T, et al: Long-term malaria prophylaxis with weekly mefloquine. Lancet 341:848–851, 1993.
58. Hilton E, Singer C, Kozarsky P, et al: Status of immunity to tetanus, measles, mumps, rubella, and polio among U.S. travelers. Ann Intern Med 115:32–33, 1991.
59. White CC, Koplan JP, Orenstein WA: Benefits, risks and costs of immunization for measles, mumps and rubella. Am J Public Health 75:739–744, 1985.
60. Koplan JP, Schoenbaum SC, Weinstein MC, Fraser DW: Pertussis vaccine—Analysis of benefits, risks and costs. N Engl J Med 301:906–911, 1979.

61. Hinman AR, Koplan JP: Pertussis and pertussis vaccine—Reanalysis of benefits, risks and costs. JAMA 251:3109–3113, 1984.
62. Hay JW, Daum RS: Economic analysis of *Haemophilus influenzae* type b vaccination. Pediatr Infect Dis J 9:246–252, 1990.
63. MacPherson DW, Tonkin M: Cholera vaccination: A decision analysis. Can Med Assoc J 146:1947–1952, 1992.
64. Wilson ME, Fineberg HV: Rabies vaccine in travelers: A decision analysis (Abstr 4). Am J Trop Med Hyg 45(Suppl):95, 1991.
65. Behrens RH, Roberts JA: Is travel prophylaxis worthwhile: Economic appraisal of prophylactic measures against malaria, hepatitis A, and typhoid in travellers. BMJ 309:918–922, 1994.
66. Herwaldt LA: Pertussis and pertussis vaccines in adults. JAMA 269:93–94, 1993.
67. Gergen PJ, McQuillan GM, Kiely M, et al: A population-based serologic survey of immunity to tetanus in the United States. N Engl J Med 332:761–766, 1995.
68. Maple PA, Efstratiou A, George RC, et al: Diphtheria immunity in UK blood donors. Lancet 345:963–965, 1995.
69. Centers for Disease Control and Prevention: Diphtheria epidemic—New Independent States of the former Soviet Union, 1990–1994. MMWR Morbid Mortal Wkly Rep 44:177–181, 1995.
70. Centers for Disease Control and Prevention: Health Information for International Travel. Washington, DC, US Department of Health and Human Services, 1997.
71. World Health Organization: International Travel and Health. Vaccination Requirements and Health Advice. Geneva, World Health Organization, 1996.
72. Tsai T, Paul R, Lynberg MC, Letson GW: Congenital yellow fever virus infection after immunization in pregnancy. J Infect Dis 168:1520–1523, 1993.
73. Tormans G, Van Damme P, Van Doorslaer E: Recommendations for prevention of hepatitis A based on a cost-effectiveness analysis. J Travel Med 1:127–135, 1994.
74. Centers for Disease Control and Prevention: Typhoid immunization—Recommendations of the Advisory Committee on Immunization Practices (ACIP). MMWR Morbid Mortal Wkly Rep 43(RR-14):1–7, 1994.
75. Centers for Disease Control and Prevention: Inactivated Japanese encephalitis virus vaccine. Recommendations of the Advisory Committee on Immunization Practices (ACIP). MMWR Morbid Mortal Wkly Rep 42(RR-1):1–15, 1993.
76. Centers for Disease Control: Rabies prevention—United States. Recommendations of the Immunization Practices Advisory Committee (ACIP). MMWR Morbid Mortal Wkly Rep 40(RR-3):1–19, 1991.
77. Wilson ME: Travel and HIV infection. *In* Jong EC, McMullen R: The Travel and Tropical Medicine Manual, ed 2. Philadelphia, WB Saunders, pp 166–176, 1995.
78. Wilson ME, von Reyn CF, Fineberg HV: Infections in HIV-infected travelers: Risks and prevention. Ann Intern Med 114:582–592, 1991.
79. Klemper CA, Linett A, Kane C, Deresinski SC: Frequency of travel of adults infected with HIV. J Travel Med 2:85–88, 1995.
80. Bia FJ: Medical considerations for the pregnant traveler. Infect Dis Clin North Am 6:371–388, 1992.
81. Barry M, Bia F: Pregnancy and travel. JAMA 261:728–731, 1989.
82. Jong EC, Benson EA: Travel with chronic medical conditions. *In* Jong EC, McMullen R: The Travel and Tropical Medicine Manual, ed 2. Philadelphia, WB Saunders, 1995, pp 142–150.
83. Centers for Disease Control and Prevention: Imported dengue—United States, 1993–1994. MMWR Morbid Mortal Wkly Rep 44:353–356, 1995.
84. Caumes E, Carriere J, Guermonprez G, et al: Dermatoses associated with travel to tropical countries: A prospective study of the diagnosis and management of 269 patients presenting to a tropical disease unit. Clin Infect Dis 20:542–548, 1995.
85. Wilson ME: Travel and the emergence of infectious diseases. Emerging Infect Dis 1:39–46, 1995.

HEAD AND NECK

47

Dental Infections

Walter J. Loesche

Dental infections such as dental caries and periodontal disease occur in and around the teeth. Dental caries or dental decay is unique among human infections, as it involves the destruction of hard acellular tissue, the enamel and dentine of the tooth, and does not provoke an inflammatory response until the decay impinges on the pulp. Among the estimated 200 to 300 bacterial species that colonize the tooth surface in bacterial communities known as dental plaque, only the mutans streptococci, lactobacilli, and possibly yeast have been etiologically associated with dental decay. A different group of bacteria comprising mainly gram-negative anaerobes are associated with periodontal disease. These anaerobes accumulate in the plaque that forms at the gingival margin (Fig. 47–1) and produce an array of biologically active products that diffuse into and provoke an inflammatory response in the adjacent host tissue. These responses result in a loss of periodontal fibers that attach the tooth to the bone; a defect, known as a periodontal pocket, forms between the root surface of the tooth and the surrounding host tissue.

Possible Association of Dental Infections with Cardiovascular Disease

Dental caries and periodontal disease have been the domain of the dentist and have been mostly ignored by the medical community. This may need to change if observations showing a statistically significant positive association between dental infections and cardiovascular disease can be confirmed.

In 1989 Finnish investigators reported that poor dental health could be associated with both an acute myocardial infarction[1] and a cerebrovascular accident.[2] These investigators developed two measurements of dental disease, one based on radiographs of the teeth and jaws and the second based on a clinical examination that gave a cumulative score called the total dental index for the amount of missing, decayed, and/or periodontally involved teeth. Subsequently, in a 7-year prospective study, the total dental index (P = .007) and the number of previous myocardial infarctions (P = .003) were associated with a risk of developing a new and often fatal myocardial infarction.[3] Traditional risk factors such as diabetes, hypertension, smoking, total cholesterol levels, high-density lipoprotein cholesterol levels, triglyceride levels, socioeconomic status, gender, and age were not significant predictors of a coronary event.

Other studies have generally confirmed this link between dental disease and coronary heart disease. A prospective cohort design study involving data for 9760 U.S. men examined three times between 1971 and 1987 found a slight but significant relationship between either periodontitis or edentulism (missing all teeth) and coronary heart disease, after adjusting for 13 known risk factors.[4] A representative sample of 1384 Finnish men, 45 to 64 years old, showed that the number of missing teeth, along with hypertension, geographic area, and educational level, were independent explanatory factors for the presence of ischemic heart disease.[5] Among U.S. veterans, a significant association between periodontal disease and coronary heart disease and stroke could be demonstrated after adjusting for various cardiovascular risk factors.[6]

Collectively, these studies imply that dental infections may be important contributors to cardiovascular pathology. Although no causal link between dental disease and cardiovascular pathology has been demonstrated, several hypotheses have been proposed.[6–8] The ones most relevant in the present context are those related to dental infections causing asymptomatic bacteremias, a generalized increase in white cell counts in the normal range, a generalized increase in inflammatory mediators, and possibly specific effects on coagulation. These hypotheses are not discussed further in this chapter, but they form the basis for a better understanding

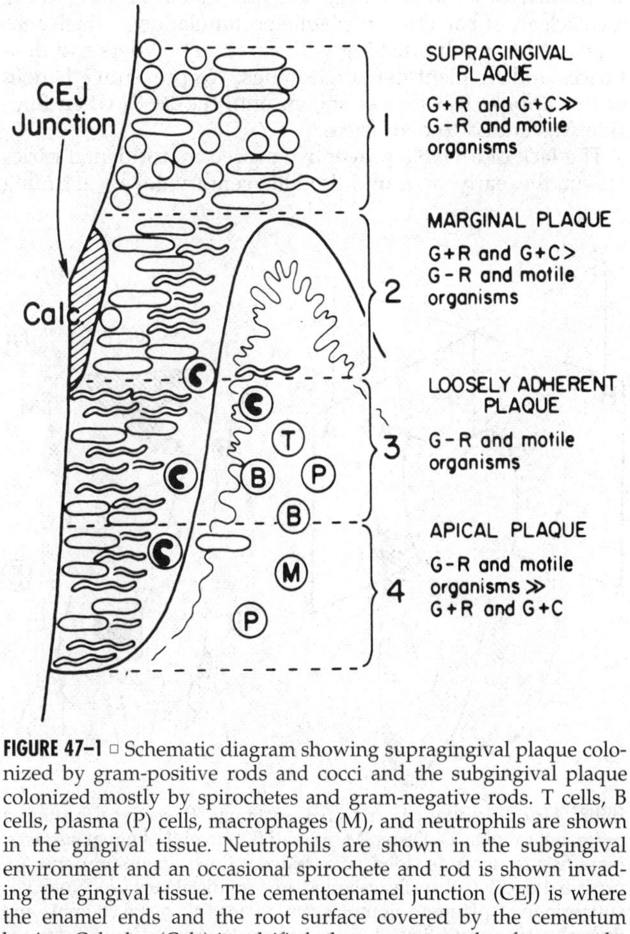

FIGURE 47–1 □ Schematic diagram showing supragingival plaque colonized by gram-positive rods and cocci and the subgingival plaque colonized mostly by spirochetes and gram-negative rods. T cells, B cells, plasma (P) cells, macrophages (M), and neutrophils are shown in the gingival tissue. Neutrophils are shown in the subgingival environment and an occasional spirochete and rod is shown invading the gingival tissue. The cementoenamel junction (CEJ) is where the enamel ends and the root surface covered by the cementum begins. Calculus (Calc) is calcified plaque or tartar that forms on the teeth where stagnant conditions exist.

of the pathophysiology of dental caries and periodontal disease by all health professionals.

Dental Caries

History

Dental caries is both an ancient and a modern infection. Fossil records of teeth from ancient humans have been used to describe the lineage of dental decay in the English from the Iron Age to modern times.[9] The modern era of dental caries can be traced to the repeal by Parliament of the Corn Laws in 1850, which allowed the duty-free entry of cane sugar into the United Kingdom. Within 15 years there was a sudden increase in dental caries, a phenomenon that has been observed in many cultures, including the African Bushmen, the Eskimos, the Tahitians, and currently the Nigerians, soon after the introduction of sugar.[10]

The connection between dietary carbohydrates and bacteria was the basis of a 19th century theory, known as the chemoparasitic theory on the causation of caries.[11] Miller's[11] concepts have dominated the treatment of dental decay until the present time. He sought assiduously to find the etiologic agent of dental decay but, lacking the technical procedures that in the 1960s led to the successful cultivation of the dominant microflora found on the teeth,[10, 12] was unable to find any consistent microbial association and concluded that decay was bacteriologically nonspecific. Miller noted that decay occurred almost uniformly in the retentive areas of the tooth, such as the occlusal fissures on the tops of the teeth and in the approximal surfaces where the teeth made contact with each other (Fig. 47–2). He advocated keeping these areas clean of bacterial or plaque accumulations, which was translated to tooth brushing with abrasive powders and dentifrices and frequent dental cleanings. No preventive benefit of this approach was ever shown until the 1960s when fluoride was added to dentifrices.[10]

The lack of a viable preventive procedure for dental caries led in the early and middle 20th century to an alarming dental morbidity among U.S. citizens. Dental caries and tooth loss were the most common cause of rejection for military service in World War I, World War II, the Korean War, and the early days of the Vietnam War. (Apparently a certain number of teeth are required to remove a pin from a grenade.) In 1960, approximately 60% of adults older than 65 years of age were without teeth. The cost of dental treatment, which was given mostly in response to symptoms, was enormous. In 1994, the cost of treatment in the United States was estimated to be about $34 billion to $36 billion; as about 85% of this cost is caries related, this would make dental caries the most expensive infection described in this textbook.

Despite these staggering costs, this dental morbidity has been contained by the use of fluoride in drinking water, salt, and dentifrices. In the future, further cost containment should follow from the elucidation of the specific role of the mutans streptococci in dental caries that was first shown in animal models.[13, 14] Keyes[12] showed that penicillin could convert an animal from being caries susceptible to caries resistant and that the infection could be transmitted by inoculation of an uninfected animal with infected feces, by caging infected animals with noninfected animals, and by direct inoculation of the mutans streptococci into the noninfected animal. These experiments ushered in the age of the specific plaque hypothesis[10, 15] and provided the dental profession, for the first time, with the knowledge to control the level of dental caries in a population and in the individual.

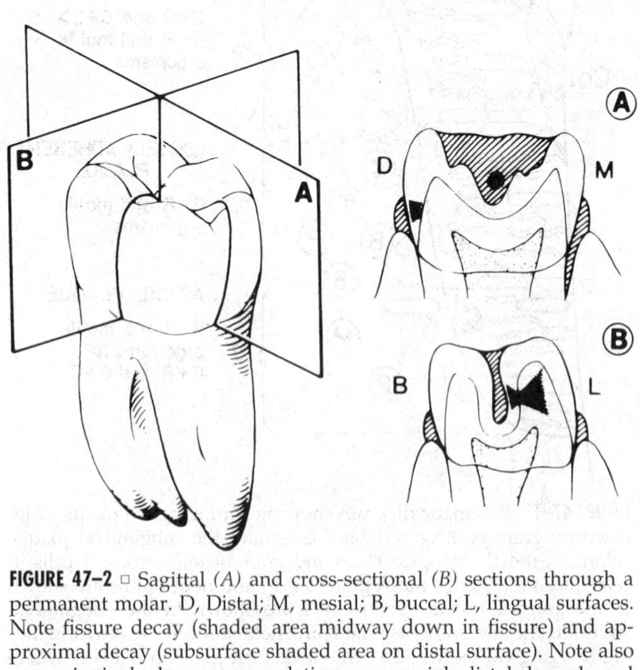

FIGURE 47–2 □ Sagittal *(A)* and cross-sectional *(B)* sections through a permanent molar. D, Distal; M, mesial; B, buccal; L, lingual surfaces. Note fissure decay (shaded area midway down in fissure) and approximal decay (subsurface shaded area on distal surface). Note also supragingival plaque accumulations on mesial, distal, buccal, and lingual surfaces and the extension of the plaque subgingivally in the mesial surface.

Characteristics of Odontopathogens: Mutans Streptococci

CLASSIFICATION

The mutans streptococci are the streptococci that ferment mannitol and sorbitol, produce extracellular glucans (glucose polymers) from sucrose, and are cariogenic in animal models. In 1924, Clarke[16] isolated such organisms from human carious lesions and called them *Streptococcus mutans* because their pleomorphic coccal shape suggested a mutant form of a streptococcus. When *S. mutans* strains were collected from different sources, it became apparent that considerable serologic and genetic heterogenicity existed. Eight serotypes could be recognized on the basis of carbohydrate antigens,[17] and DNA hybridization studies revealed four genetic groups. These genetic groups were given species names that reflected their original mammalian source of isolation.[18] *S. mutans* was assigned to the predominant human isolates, whereas other human isolates were called *Streptococcus sobrinus*. *Streptococcus rattus* and *Streptococcus cricetus* were assigned to the mutans streptococci isolated from laboratory-bred rats and hamsters, respectively. Subsequently, new species of mutans streptococci were isolated from wild rats *(Streptococcus ferus)* and the macaque monkey *(Streptococcus macacae)*. Thus, six distinct species have been identified as mutans streptococci, but only two species, *S. mutans* and *S. sobrinus*, have been studied for their virulence mechanisms.

BIOLOGIC AND BIOCHEMICAL PROPERTIES

For *S. mutans* and *S. sobrinus* to be uniquely associated with dental caries there would need to be a special relationship between these species and sucrose. This would have to be something other than the ability to ferment sucrose, as many of the other 200 species that can be isolated from plaque can also ferment sucrose. In fact, when germ-free rats were monoassociated with various acidogenic species and fed high-sucrose diets, there was usually no decay.[19] This means that something besides acid production per se was needed for decay to occur.

A clue to what one of these factors was came from hamster studies in which these animals were fed, at weaning, a diet containing either 56% sucrose or 56% glucose and then were inoculated with an Str^R strain of *S. mutans*.[20] In the sucrose-fed animals, *S. mutans* became established on the teeth in high numbers, and the animals developed extensive decay. In the glucose-fed animals, *S. mutans* was recovered in low numbers, and the level of decay was similar to that found in the uninoculated control animals.

Studies soon showed that in the presence of sucrose, *S. mutans* and *S. sobrinus* formed adhesive colonies that stuck to the surfaces of culture vessels.[21] Chemical analysis indicated that the adhesive material was a glucose homopolymer or glucan composed of two classes of compounds, an α-1,6 core–linked polymer classified as a dextran and a unique α-1,3–rich polymer classified as a mutan. The α-1,3–rich polymer was water insoluble and cell associated and was involved in smooth-surface decay, whereas the α-1,6–rich polymer was water soluble and was not associated with smooth-surface decay.[10] These glucans apparently provided a mechanism by which the mutans streptococci extended their niche from the retentive fissure site to the nonretentive smooth tooth surface. However, these studies did not explain why *S. mutans* was the more cariogenic of the two species in humans.

Insight into this mechanism was provided by a mutant of *S. mutans* that exhibited less decay than the wild type on both smooth and occlusal fissures and that possessed reduced aciduricity or the ability to grow in a low-pH environment.[22] The pH in plaque can drop below 5.0 for 30 to 120 minutes after exposure to a fermentable dietary carbohydrate.[23] *S. mutans* and, to a lesser extent, *S. sobrinus* have a pH optimum at about 5.0 to 5.5[24] and can survive and actually grow at these low pH values found in plaque during and after eating. Because of their aciduricity, these mutans streptococci become dominant in the plaques, and because of their acid production, they lead to the demineralization of the tooth that, if unchecked, results in dental decay.

Pathogenesis of Decay

The saliva is a remarkably protective fluid for the tooth surface, as it contains buffers and is supersaturated with calcium and phosphate ions, which favor remineralization of the tooth surface.[25] When the plaque is exposed to fermentable dietary carbohydrates, there is an immediate and persistent drop in the pH. At a pH of about 5.0 to 5.5, known as the critical pH, the salivary buffers are overwhelmed; a second buffer system, the hydroxyapatite of the tooth, acts as a buffer so that further pH drops are not encountered. But why would the tooth act as a buffer to maintain the pH in the vicinity of 5.0? If the pH dropped to 3 or 4, the enamel surface layer would be irreversibly lost, as occurs when a tooth is exposed to acid in vitro. However, at pH 5.0 the mineral is lost from the subsurface layers in such a way that repair, in the form of remineralization, can proceed once the pH returns to values above the critical pH. It is in this situation that the supersaturated levels of calcium and phosphate diffuse into the teeth and promote remineralization.

This remarkable dissolution pattern has great significance with regard to the development of dental decay. Whenever a fermentable dietary substrate diffuses into the plaque and is converted to acid end products, some degree of subsurface demineralization occurs. Then between meals or snacks, the pH in the plaque returns to neutrality and the supersaturated levels of calcium and phosphate ions promote remineralization. Demineralization that progresses to cavitation occurs if the frequency and magnitude of acid production overwhelm the repair process. This occurs with frequent eating[26] or if the repair process is compromised by xerostomia.[27] In both situations, there would be a selection for aciduric organisms such as *S. mutans* and lactobacilli. This sequence of events can be illustrated by a situation in which sucrose availability is frequent and by one in which salivary flow is reduced.

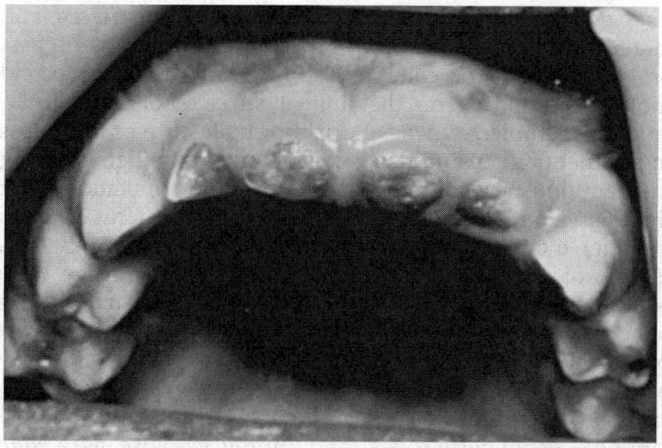

FIGURE 47–3 □ Nursing bottle caries. Note that the crowns of the four maxillary anterior teeth are completely decayed, whereas the adjacent teeth are intact.

Nursing bottle caries is extensive decay of the maxillary anterior teeth (Fig. 47–3) that is associated with prolonged and frequent bottle feeding or breast-feeding.[28] Liquid from the mother's breast or nursing bottle may bathe all of the teeth except the lower incisors. The bacteria on these teeth have prolonged access to any fermentable substrates such as lactose or sucrose in the liquid. In one study, *S. mutans* accounted for more than 50% and lactobacilli for 5% of the flora on the teeth.[29] These are the highest values for *S. mutans* and lactobacilli that have been reported for human teeth.

Rampant caries is also found where salivation is reduced for various reasons. Rampant decay in patients receiving radiation treatment for head and neck cancer is so predictable that these individuals have been studied in a prospective fashion. In one such study, during the development of decay a pronounced shift to *S. mutans* and lactobacilli occurred at the expense of noncariogenic organisms such as *Streptococcus sanguis*, *Bacteroides*, *Fusobacterium*, and *Neisseria* species. Three to four months after radiation therapy, the proportions of *S. mutans* peaked at 18% of the plaque flora and five new carious lesions were present. Thereafter, the lactobacilli became the dominant aciduric species coincident with the lesions' becoming larger and more numerous.[30]

This sequence of events indicated that *S. mutans* was involved with the initiation of decay, whereas the lactobacilli were associated with progression of the lesion. This was also suggested by a study in which the incipient lesion was monitored to determine whether it would progress to the stage of cavitation.[31] *S. mutans* was the numerically dominant organism in the plaques but was isolated with equal frequency from progressive and nonprogressive lesions. *Lactobacillus casei* was present in 85% of the progressive lesions before the clinical diagnosis of progression was made and was never isolated from nonprogressive lesions. These findings indicate that dental decay is a two-stage process in which *S. mutans* is associated with the initial lesion and lactobacilli, especially *L. casei*, are associated with its progression.

Epidemiology

Epidemiologic surveys indicate that dental decay is mainly a disease of youth, occurs in teeth shortly after their eruption, does not occur uniformly on all teeth or tooth surfaces, and tends to be symmetric.[10] The prevalence of decay is highest on the occlusal (or chewing) surfaces of first and second molars and lowest on the lingual surfaces of mandibular anterior teeth. Decay was and is the chief cause of tooth loss in populations consuming a sucrose-containing diet, resulting in edentulousness for more than 50% of the population older than 65 years. This pattern is changing: now many children younger than 10 years of age are caries free, and only 12% to 14% of Americans between 55 and 64 years of age were edentulous in 1985.[32] This means that more older individuals have more teeth and require more dental health care than previously. These teeth may be at increased risk of decay because so many medications that are prescribed by physicians on a continuing basis, such as antidepressants, antihistamines, antihypertensives, and diuretics, cause as a side effect a reduction in salivary flow.[33] When this reduction is combined with a tendency to snack and a reduced ability to perform oral hygiene, dental caries manifests itself as a disease of the elderly.

Clinical Manifestations

Dental caries begins as a subsurface demineralization of the enamel that may be detected on visual examination; most clinicians, however, wait until there is radiographic evidence of decay or obvious cavitation of the tooth that extends into the dentine before placing a dental restoration. If these lesions are not detected and treated, the decay extends deeper into the dentine and encroaches on the pulp. This stage is often painful and causes the patient to seek treatment. If the pulp is involved, extirpation of the pulp and filling of the pulp canal are recommended. However, because of cost, most individuals choose extraction, starting down the road toward complete edentulousness.

Diagnosis

Diagnosis of dental decay is usually a post facto event and devoid of any bacteriologic testing. Any procedure that is intended to show an *S. mutans* infection is complicated by the fact that most individuals harbor *S. mutans* on their teeth. However, the level and persistence of the *S. mutans* colonization seem to determine the risk of decay.[34, 35] This level has been empirically determined for the saliva, as individuals with salivary *S. mutans* levels above 10^6 colony-forming units per milliliter of saliva are at a high caries risk.[36] The ability to detect *S. mutans* in saliva is dependent on the use of a selective medium that employs bacitracin and 20% sucrose.[37] Several variants of this medium have been described, and individuals have developed various kits for office use.[38] Similar kits exist for the detection of lactobacilli in saliva.[39]

Treatment

The treatment of dental caries has been mechanical and symptomatic. The decayed tooth substance is completely removed and replaced with a metal or plastic material that is strong, has thermal characteristics similar to those of the tooth itself, and is aesthetically acceptable to the patient. The most common filling material is amalgam, so called because it is an amalgamation of silver, tin, and mercury, although lesser amounts of zinc and copper may be present. The amalgam is not an ideal restoration and has a half-life of about 4 to 7 years in a caries-active mouth.[40] The main reason for failure is the appearance of decay about the margin of the filling. Whether this is a new episode of an *S. mutans* infection or a residual infection resulting from failure of the clinician to treat the *S. mutans* infection that was present at the time of the replacement of the restoration is not known.

Prevention

The prevention of an *S. mutans* infection is now a practical procedure. The tooth surface is the natural habitat of *S. mutans*. This has important implications for antimicrobial therapy, as the agent need only be applied to the teeth; if it eliminates *S. mutans* from the tooth, there may be a prolonged period before a reinfection with *S. mutans* can occur. Also, the occlusal fissure that appears to be the preferential niche for *S. mutans* on the tooth (see Fig. 47–2) is available for colonization in its depth only during a finite time period after the tooth erupts. These considerations have led to the development of two strategies to prevent an *S. mutans* infection from occurring or recurring: namely, to interrupt or delay the acquisition of *S. mutans* by infants and to suppress an existing *S. mutans* infection once it has been diagnosed.

INTERFERENCE WITH TRANSMISSION

Colonization by *S. mutans* occurs at about the time that teeth erupt in infants.[41] Early colonization may be a reliable predictor of subsequent caries activity. In one study, children who harbored *S. mutans* by age 2 years developed 10.6 decayed surfaces by age 4 years. In contrast, children in whom *S. mutans* was detected between 2 and 4 years developed 3.4 decayed surfaces; children in whom *S. mutans* could not be detected were essentially caries free by age 4, that is, had 0.3 decayed surfaces.[42] Several investigators have demonstrated a significant relationship between maternal salivary levels of *S. mutans* and the salivary levels of *S. mutans* in their children.[43] This suggested that treatment of the mothers could interfere with or delay the bacterial colonization of the children.

Kohler and associates[44, 45] have interrupted this passage of *S. mutans* from mother to child by aggressively treating only mothers who had salivary *S. mutans* levels above 10^6 colony-forming units per milliliter of saliva and whose infants had no erupted teeth. An intensive preventive program involving dietary counseling, professional tooth cleaning with a fluoride paste, topical fluoride treatments, and excavation of carious lesions was employed to get the mother's salivary levels of *S. mutans* below 2.5×10^5 colony-forming units per milliliter of saliva. In 60% of the mothers this goal was achieved. In the remaining mothers, a topical gel containing 1% chlorhexidine (Hibitane) used once a day for 2 weeks was able to reduce the *S. mutans* organisms to this level. At 3 years of age, only 16% of the children of the treated mothers had decay, compared with 43% of the children of the untreated mothers. There was also a comparable decrease in the prevalence of *S. mutans* among the children of the treated mothers. These findings show that intensive measures directed toward the mother can delay or prevent the acquisition of *S. mutans* in the child and that this can be associated with a reduced incidence of decay.

SUPPRESSION OF AN EXISTING INFECTION

Many agents, such as iodine, fluoride, chlorhexidine, vancomycin, and kanamycin, have reduced for a finite period the plaque and saliva proportions and/or levels of *S. mutans*. The universality of the response pattern, that is, decline in *S. mutans* followed by its eventual return, suggested that the antimicrobial agents used were unable to penetrate all the niches in which *S. mutans* exists on the tooth. Paramount among these would be the depths of the fissure and the incipient carious lesions. Stannous fluoride and chlorhexidine seem to penetrate the fissure, and fluoride penetrates the incipient lesion.[10] Both fluoride and chlorhexidine exhibit substantivity on the tooth surfaces, as there is a persistent antimicrobial activity. The fluoride effect can come about as the plaque pH drop after ingestion of the food can release bound fluoride from the enamel. The chlorhexidine effect comes from the calcium ions in the saliva eluting any bound chlorhexidine from the tooth surface. The effectiveness of both antimicrobials can be enhanced by the use of slow-release delivery systems, in which the agents are painted onto the tooth surface as a varnish.[46, 47]

Periodontal Disease

History

The treatment of periodontal disease has generally been neglected by the dental profession. As recently as 1977, dentists in general practice reported that less than 1% of their income was derived from the treatment of periodontal disease.[48] This situation has changed owing to the decline of dental caries, and dentists are now free to address this other major dental infection.

Microbial specificity in periodontal disease has taken longer to demonstrate because before 1968 most investigators focused their attention on supragingival plaque, which is the plaque above the gingival margin, and did not examine the subgingival plaque, which is below the gingival margin (see Fig. 47–1). Also, the subgingival flora is composed mainly of anaerobic species, most of which could not be cultured and, when they could be cultured, could not be assigned to known species. The use of quantitative anaerobic culturing procedures has led to the isolation of many new species and, at times, what seems to be a bewildering array of putative periodontal pathogens. Clinical criteria have improved to the point at which several distinct clinical entities are recognized, whereas formerly the condition was considered to be either gingivitis or periodontitis. Thus, the relationship between periodontal disease and specific microbes is more complicated than that observed between *S. mutans* or *Lactobacillus* and dental caries (Table 47–1).

TABLE 47–1 ■ Relationship Between Clinical Forms of Periodontal Disease and Various Bacterial Species

CLINICAL ENTITY	BACTERIAL FACTOR
Gingivitis	
Experimental	Plaque accumulation, streptococci, actinomycetes
Pregnancy	*Prevotella intermedia*
Puberty	*P. intermedia ?*
Stress (acute necrotizing ulcerative gingivitis)	*P. intermedia*, spirochetes
Simple	Plaque accumulation, spirochetes
Generalized severe	Spirochetes
Periodontitis	
Prepuberty	Spirochetes, black-pigmented species
Localized juvenile	*Actinobacillus actinomycetemcomitans*
Early onset	Spirochetes, *Porphyromonas gingivalis*, *A. actinomycetemcomitans*
Adult	Spirochetes, black-pigmented species, *A. actinomycetemcomitans*
Progressive	*Bacteroides forsythus*, *Campylobacter rectus* (formerly *Wolinella recta*)

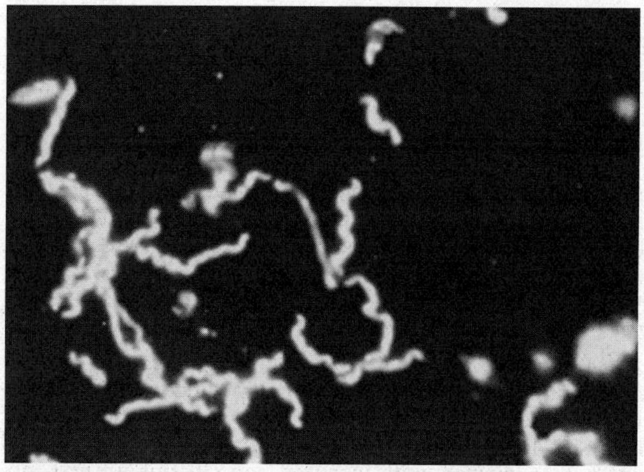

FIGURE 47–4 □ Darkfield microscopic examination of plaque showing small spirochetes.

Characteristics of Putative Periodontal Pathogens

SPIROCHETES

Many spirochetes are evident in subgingival plaque samples taken from periodontal pockets. They are classified as *Treponema* species, but owing to difficulties in their isolation and cultivation, little taxonomic information is available. They are easily recognizable because of their helical shape (Fig. 47–4) and vigorous motility when observed by either darkfield or phase-contrast microscopy. The spirochetes have the highest surface/volume ratio of any plaque species, leading to speculation that this morphology facilitates the uptake of nutrients from their environment. Many spirochetes are less than 0.2 μm in diameter and have been shown to invade the soft tissue adjacent to the plaque.[49] *Treponema denticola* possesses a wide array of proteolytic enzymes, which makes it a prime suspect in periodontal pathogenesis.[50] Spirochetes are usually not detected or are present in low number in plaques removed from healthy periodontal sites in children. They increase in numbers and proportions in plaque associated with gingivitis and reach their highest absolute and relative values in plaques removed from sites with periodontitis, where they can constitute almost half the total flora.

BLACK-PIGMENTED SPECIES

Black-pigmented colonies isolated from dental plaque were initially called *Bacteroides melaninogenicus* (now *Prevotella melaninogenica*). Taxonomic studies, including DNA analysis, have shown that these black-pigmented species are composed of at least nine types of bacteria and are distinctly different from intestinal gram-negative rods classified as *Bacteroides*. Two new genera were proposed in which the non–carbohydrate-fermenting or asaccharolytic organisms were assigned to the new genus *Porphyromonas*, whereas the species capable of fermenting both carbohydrates and peptides were assigned to the genus *Prevotella*.[51]

Only three black-pigmented species have been associated with dental infections. *Porphyromonas gingivalis* is frequently isolated in high proportions from the more aggressive forms of periodontitis such as early-onset forms[52] and those refractory to treatment.[52] *Porphyromonas endodontalis* is frequently isolated from infections of the dental pulp. *Prevotella intermedia* is uniquely associated with acute necrotizing ulcerative gingivitis and with pregnancy gingivitis[53] (see Table 47–1). The black-pigmented species could contribute to periodontal disease by releasing endotoxin, various organic acids such as butyric acid, and low-molecular-weight compounds such as hydrogen sulfide and ammonia into the pocket microenvironment.

BACTEROIDES FORSYTHUS

B. forsythus is an anaerobic, gram-negative, pleomorphic, nonmotile, long thin rod[54] that has been isolated from some but not all lesions that are actually breaking down.[55]

ACTINOBACILLUS ACTINOMYCETEMCOMITANS

A. actinomycetemcomitans is a small, gram-negative, microaerophilic coccobacillus. There is compelling but circumstantial evidence that *A. actinomycetemcomitans* is the etiologic agent of localized juvenile periodontitis, a unique clinical entity that presents with localized bone loss about first molars and incisor teeth of teenagers.[56] This organism is rarely found in plaques taken from healthy sites in these patients, but it can usually be found in other members of the family who also have or have had localized juvenile periodontitis or periodontal disease. What is particularly supportive of the etiologic role of *A. actinomycetemcomitans* is the production of a leukotoxin that inhibits neutrophils in vitro.[57] If the leukotoxin is produced in vivo, as is likely given the presence of antibodies to this toxin in the patient's serum,[56, 58] it could locally disarm the neutrophils in the pocket. The host's main protective barrier would thereby be removed,[59] allowing *A. actinomycetemcomitans* to penetrate into the connective tissue,[60] causing destruction of the periodontal attachment.

Epidemiology

The precise epidemiology of periodontal disease is not known, primarily because the disease is so chronic and insidious that long-term studies are not practical. In its earliest forms, the disease is a simple inflammatory response to the accumulation of plaque at the dental gingival margin. The events surrounding this inflammation have been widely investigated using the experimental gingivitis model.[61] The accumulation of plaque containing mainly streptococci and actinomyces elicits a T-cell response in the gingival tissue[62] that can also be detected in the peripheral blood.[63] It is not known whether this gingivitis, if left alone, would progress to the type of gingivitis seen clinically, in which spirochetes account for about 10% of the flora. Likewise, it is not known whether any of the types of gingivitis progress to periodontitis, or whether periodontitis develops directly after infection with organisms such as *A. actinomycetemcomitans,* a sequence that is suspected to occur in localized juvenile periodontitis (Fig. 47–5).

The traditional view, based on cross-sectional epidemiologic surveys, has been that gingivitis and periodontitis are a continuum with periodontal attachment and bone loss occurring slowly with age. Longitudinal studies in Sri Lanka suggested that, at least in some individuals, attachment loss began in adolescence and proceeded at a rapid rate, whereas in the majority of the subjects the loss of attachment occurred slowly.[64] In other studies, patients with advanced periodontal disease were examined at 2-month intervals but were otherwise left untreated.[65] During the monitoring period, about 5% of the sites showed attachment loss of 2 mm or more that occurred within 2 months, whereas the majority of sites exhibited no change. This suggested that in a few sites, periodontal destruction could be acute and episodic.

Pathogenesis

The pathogenesis of periodontal disease is not known, except in general terms. The bacterial species associated with the disease (see Table 47–1), with the possible exception of *A. actinomycetemcomitans,* are members of the normal plaque flora, so the mere presence of these organisms has no diagnostic implications. Each of these putative periodontal pathogens produces such a large array of biologically active molecules that it is surprising that so many teeth are retained by the host. This implies that under normal circumstances the

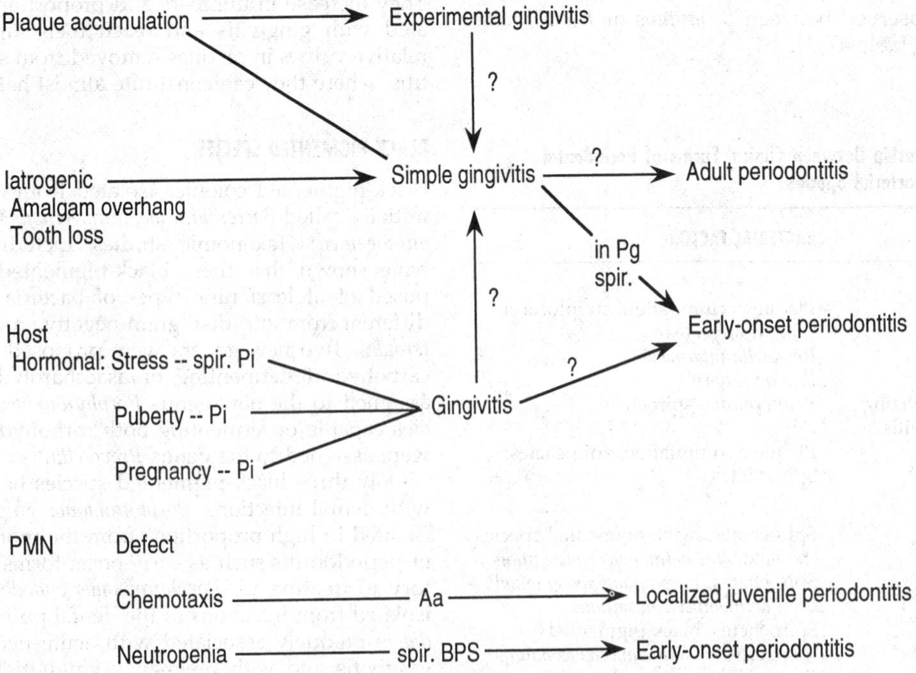

FIGURE 47–5 □ Possible sequence of events in periodontal disease. ?, Pathway not known; Bf, *Bacteroides forsythus*; spir., spirochetes; Pg, *Porphyromonas gingivalis*; Pi, *Prevotella intermedia*; Aa, *Actinobacillus actinomycetemcomitans.*

host's defensive barriers to bacterial invasion and inflammatory response to biologically active molecules are more than adequate to retain the teeth in the mouth. When these defenses are compromised, and especially when there are neutrophil defects, periodontal disease is severe and generalized.[66] In fact, symptoms related to periodontal problems can be one of the chief complaints given by patients with cyclic neutropenia and chronic granulomatous disease. Not surprisingly, individuals with human immunodeficiency virus infection often present with aggressive forms of periodontal disease.[67] However, nowhere is the relationship between neutrophils and plaque microbes better understood than in localized juvenile periodontitis.

Localized juvenile periodontitis occurs with a prevalence of about 0.1%[68] in young subjects. Because the degree of bone loss about the molars and incisors was incompatible with local plaque factors, such as gingivitis or calculus (tartar or mineralized plaque), this entity was called periodontosis, and an unidentified host factor was believed to be involved. Thus, it came as no surprise when a neutrophil defect in chemotaxis was found[69] that appeared to be due to a reduced number of available binding sites for chemotactic peptides.[70] This would lead in vivo to fewer neutrophils being recruited to the gingival and periodontal tissue in response to the chemotactic molecules produced by the plaque flora. However, this phenomenon should affect all teeth and not just the molars and incisors. Clearly, something else was needed to explain the localization to these teeth.

The missing element appears to be the involvement of *A. actinomycetemcomitans* and especially its leukotoxin. If *A. actinomycetemcomitans* overgrows in the pockets of molars and incisors, the resulting production of leukotoxin negates the protective effects of the neutrophils that eventually migrate to these sites. With time, *A. actinomycetemcomitans* invades the tissue, releasing its complement of cytotoxic factors, including the leukotoxin. The host mounts a containing response, including the production of antibodies to the *A. actinomycetemcomitans* antigens, including the leukotoxin. The amount of antibody formed to the leukotoxin is so great that it can easily be detected in the peripheral circulation[58] and most likely would be present in the gingival crevicular fluid about the teeth. If *A. actinomycetemcomitans* had not yet colonized a sulcus or overgrown in a site, this antibody could protect that site from subsequent colonization or infection. Hence, the *A. actinomycetemcomitans* infection is confined to the original sites of colonization or infection, which in most instances are the molars and incisors. Although the pathogenesis of the more typical forms of periodontal disease is not this apparent, most investigators suspect that this type of neutrophil-antibody-microbe interaction is responsible for tissue loss.

Clinical Manifestations

Periodontal disease is usually asymptomatic until the late stages, when frank periodontal abscesses cause pain and discomfort. Bleeding while brushing the teeth is the most common indicator of an underlying problem and one that usually brings an individual to the dentist. Halitosis is a less common reason for the patient's seeking treatment. Most dentists examine for the degree of periodontal pocketing about the teeth and, when depths are consistently greater than 4 mm, recommend some form of mechanical débridement. Radiographs taken over time can document the amount and rate of bone loss. On some occasions the patient seeks treatment because the teeth have shifted, with spacing being apparent between the anterior teeth (Fig. 47–6).

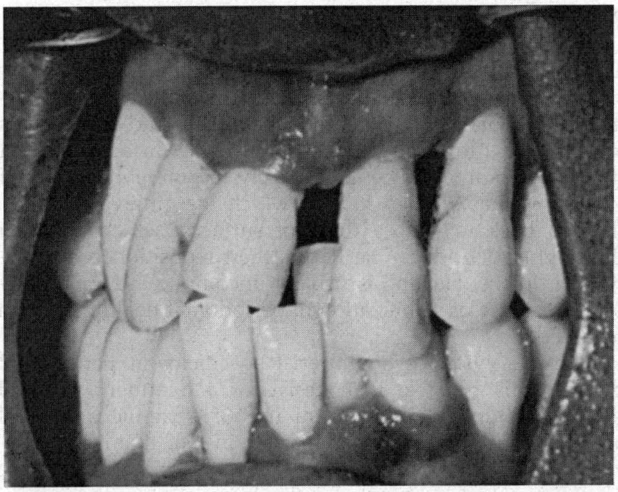

FIGURE 47–6 □ Early-onset periodontitis in a young adult. Note that teeth are separated because of bone loss.

Diagnosis

Diagnosis is usually made by documenting the probing depths about the teeth and by the amount of bone support that has been lost. Probing depths greater than 6 mm are always indicative of disease, but whether it is an active process of attachment loss or loss that occurred years ago cannot be ascertained without some sort of longitudinal measurements or radiographs. It is in this situation that microbiologic monitors can be helpful.

The simplest procedure would be to remove the subgingival plaque and examine it under the phase-contrast or darkfield microscope for the presence of motile organisms including spirochetes.[71] In healthy sites the plaques are usually devoid of spirochetes, whereas in diseased sites these organisms are abundant (see Fig. 47–4). It is also possible to examine these plaque smears with polyclonal or monoclonal antibodies that are directed toward one or more of the putative periodontal pathogens. These immunologic reagents are usually tagged with either a fluorescein dye or an enzyme such as alkaline phosphatase.[72] DNA probes have been made to *P. gingivalis, P. intermedia,* and *A. actinomycetemcomitans* and have been successfully evaluated for the detection of these species in plaque samples.[73]

Another approach is the detection of either bacterial or host enzymes that are present or are increased in sites of periodontal inflammation. One such bacterial enzyme that hydrolyzes the synthetic trypsin substrate benzoylarginine-2-naphthylamide (BANA) is possessed by *T. denticola, P. gingivalis,* and *B. forsythus.*[74] As all three species have been associated with periodontal disease[75–77] and all are anaerobes, the presence of this enzyme could be used as a marker for diagnosis of an anaerobic infection. Several studies have shown that BANA hydrolysis reflects primarily the spirochete levels in plaque and corresponds to increasing probing depth of the pockets.[76] The BANA test has a diagnostic accuracy comparable to that obtained with either DNA probes or immunologic reagents to *P. gingivalis, T. denticola,* or *B. forsythus.*[77] However, because these species are members of the normal flora, the BANA test has low specificity. It should not be used as a screening instrument, as it often gives a positive reaction in plaque samples removed from healthy tooth sites.[78] The ability to objectively diagnose periodontal infections with these species has clearly moved beyond the theory stage.

Treatment

Treatment of periodontal disease has relied almost exclusively on mechanical débridement of the tooth surfaces. This involves labor-intensive débridement with hand instruments and, if access to these surfaces is difficult, various forms of periodontal surgery. The most widely recommended form of surgery is the Widman flap, in which the gingival tissue is flapped back to expose the root surfaces, which are then thoroughly débrided. The flap is then repositioned and sutured in place. Healing is usually uncomplicated, and long-term evidence of stabilization of periodontal health has been obtained.[79]

With the evidence of bacterial specificity in periodontal disease it is possible to conceive of a treatment protocol that would include short-term use of systemic and local antimicrobial agents. Shinn[80] reported in 1962 that metronidazole quickly improves cases of acute necrotizing ulcerative gingivitis, which eventuated in the demonstration that metronidazole is a specific inhibitor of anaerobic bacteria.[81] Subsequently, metronidazole was shown to reduce the plaque levels of spirochetes and *P. intermedia* in cases of acute necrotizing ulcerative gingivitis.[53] The similarity of the anaerobic flora in acute necrotizing ulcerative gingivitis to the anaerobic flora found in adult periodontitis suggested that metronidazole could be effective in the treatment of adult periodontitis. Two double-blind studies have shown that metronidazole was effective in reducing probing depths and in increasing attachment levels about the most severely involved teeth.[82, 83]

In additional double-blind studies, a 1-week treatment with metronidazole in combination with débridement of the tooth surfaces was able to significantly reduce the need for periodontal surgery compared with placebo plus débridement.[84, 85] In a double-blind study, if patients were retreated with either systemic or locally delivered antimicrobials, about 88% of the initially recommended surgical needs, in some cases tooth extractions, could be avoided.[86] This indicated that most forms of periodontal disease that are diagnosed as anaerobic infections (about 90% in our experience) could be treated with short-term use of antimicrobial agents.

Treatment with metronidazole is compromised by noncompliance of patients, especially with a label attached to the bottle warning not to drink alcoholic beverages. When noncompliance is suspected, comparable results may be achieved with doxycycline, which needs to be taken only once per day.[86] An alternative approach is to use devices that deliver the antimicrobial agent directly to the periodontal pocket. A variety of devices, including a cord that can be wrapped around the tooth,[87] gels that can be placed into the pocket,[88] or films that can be attached to the tooth,[86] have been developed. One involving a tetracycline-impregnated cord has been approved by the U.S. Food and Drug Administration.[87]

These studies with metronidazole, doxycycline, and slow-release delivery devices suggest that in the future, periodontal disease can be controlled by the judicious usage of short-term antimicrobial therapy combined with the traditional débriding procedures. The use of the systemic antimicrobials should be based on the microbiologic diagnosis of either an anaerobic or a microaerophilic infection.

Prevention

The prevention of periodontal disease would be based on the control of gingivitis, on the assumption that most gingivitis leads to periodontitis. This is done by practicing good home oral hygiene and by the judicious use of antigingivitis agents such as chlorhexidine.

Summary

Dental caries and periodontal disease are the two most common infections in humans. Although they represent a collection of infections, it is apparent that most can be treated as if they are specific *S. mutans* infections in the case of dental caries and as anaerobic infections in the case of adult periodontitis. This recognition provides the clinician, for the first time, with the ability to control the severity of the morbidity in patients; if patients present before morbidity occurs, the clinician may be able to keep them caries free and periodontally healthy for a lifetime. This in turn may have profound implications for the medical health of the individual, especially cardiovascular health.

References

1. Mattila KJ, Nieminen MS, Valtonen VV, et al: Association between dental health and acute myocardial infarction. BMJ 298:779–781, 1989.
2. Syrjänen J, Peltola J, Valtonen V, et al: Dental infections in association with cerebral infarction in young and middle-aged men. J Intern Med 225:179–184, 1989.
3. Mattila KJ, Valtonen VV, Nieminen M, et al: Dental infection and the risk of new coronary events: Prospective study of patients with documented coronary artery disease. Clin Infect Dis 20:588–592, 1995.
4. DeStefano F, Anda RF, Kahn HS, et al: Dental disease and risk of coronary heart disease and mortality. BMJ 306:688–691, 1993.
5. Paunio K, Impivaara O, Tiekso J, et al: Missing teeth and ischaemic heart disease in men aged 45–64 years. Eur Heart J 14(Suppl K):54–56, 1993.
6. Beck JD, Garcia RI, Heiss G, et al: Periodontal disease and cardiovascular disease. J Periodontol 67(Suppl) (in press).
7. Loesche WJ: Periodontal disease as a risk factor for heart disease. Compend Contin Educ Dent 15:976–991, 1995.
8. Loesche WJ: Association of the oral flora with important medical diseases. Curr Opin Periodontol (in press).
9. Corbett ME, Moore WJ: Distribution of dental caries in ancient British populations. IV. 19th century. Caries Res 10:401–414, 1976.
10. Loesche WJ: Dental Caries: A Treatable Infection. Grand Haven, MI, ADQ Publications, 1993.
11. Miller WD: The Micro-organisms of the Human Mouth. Philadelphia, SS White Manufacturing, 1890.
12. Gibbons RJ, van Houte J: On the formation of dental plaque. J Periodontol 44:347–360, 1973.
13. Keyes PH: The infectious and transmissible nature of experimental dental caries. Findings and implications. Arch Oral Biol 1:304–320, 1960.
14. Fitzgerald RJ, Keyes PH: Demonstration of the etiologic role of streptococci in experimental caries in the hamster. J Am Dent Assoc 61:9–19, 1960.
15. Loesche WJ: Chemotherapy of dental plaque infections. Oral Sci Rev 9:65–107, 1976.
16. Clarke JK: On the bacterial factor in the aetiology of dental caries. Br J Exp Pathol 5:141–146, 1924.
17. Perch B, Kjems E, Ravn T: Biochemical and serological properties of *Streptococcus mutans* from various human and animal sources. Acta Pathol Microbiol Scand [B] Microbiol Immunol 82:357–370, 1974.
18. Coykendall AL: Proposal to elevate the subspecies of *Streptococcus mutans* to species status, based on their molecular composition. Int J Syst Bacteriol 27:26–30, 1977.
19. Fitzgerald RJ: Dental caries research in gnotobiotic animals. Caries Res 2:139–146, 1968.
20. Krasse B: Human streptococci and experimental caries in hamsters. Arch Oral Biol 11:429–436, 1966.
21. Gibbons RJ, Berman KS, Knoettner P, et al: Dental caries and alveolar bone loss in gnotobiotic rats infected with capsule-forming streptococci of human origin. Arch Oral Biol 11:549–560, 1966.
22. Donoghue HD, Newman NH: Effect of glucose and sucrose on survival in batch culture of *Streptococcus mutans* C67–25. Infect Immun 13:16–21, 1976.

23. Stephan RM: Intra-oral hydrogen-ion concentrations associated with dental caries activity. J Dent Res 23:257–266, 1944.
24. Harper DS, Loesche WJ: Growth and acid tolerance of human dental plaque bacteria. Arch Oral Biol 29:843–848, 1984.
25. Hay DI, Moreno EC: Macromolecular inhibitors of calcium phosphate precipitation in human saliva. Their roles in providing a protective environment for the teeth. *In* Kleinberg I, Ellison SA, Mandel ID (eds): Saliva and Dental Caries. Washington, DC, Information Retrieval, 1979, pp 45–58. Special Supplement Microbiology Abstracts.
26. Gustafsson BE, Quensel CE, Lanke LS, et al: The Vipeholm dental caries study. The effect of different levels of carbohydrate intake on caries activity in 436 individuals observed for five years. Acta Odontol Scand 11:232–364, 1954.
27. Mandel ID, Ellison SA: Naturally occurring defense mechanisms in saliva. *In* Tanzer JM (ed): Animal Models in Cariology. Washington, DC, Information Retrieval, 1981, pp 367–379. Special Supplement Microbiology Abstracts.
28. Ripa LW: Nursing habits and dental decay in infants: "Nursing bottle caries." J Dent Child 45:274–275, 1978.
29. Berkowitz RJ, Turner J, Hughes C: Microbial characteristics of the human dental caries associated with prolonged bottle feeding. Arch Oral Biol 29:949–951, 1984.
30. Brown LR, Dreizen S, Handler S: Effects of selected caries preventive regimens on microbial changes following irradiation-induced xerostomia in cancer patients. *In* Stiles M, Loesche WJ, O'Brien T (eds): Proceedings of the Microbial Aspects of Dental Caries, Vol 1. Washington, DC, Information Retrieval, 1976, pp 275–290. Special Supplement Microbiology Abstracts.
31. Boyar RM, Bowden GH: The microflora associated with the progression of incipient carious lesions in teeth of children living in a water-fluoridated area. Caries Res 19:298–306, 1985.
32. Miller AJ, Brunelle JA, Carlos JP: Oral Health of United States Adults. Bethesda, MD, National Institutes of Health, 1987. DHHS publication 87-2868.
33. Fox PC, van der Ven PF, Sonies BC, et al: Xerostomia: Evaluation of a symptom with increasing significance. J Am Dent Assoc 110:519–525, 1985.
34. Zickert I, Emilson CG, Krasse B: Correlation of level and duration of *Streptococcus mutans* infection with incidence of dental caries. Infect Immun 39:982–985, 1983.
35. Loesche WJ: Role of *Streptococcus mutans* in human dental decay. Microbiol Rev 50:353–380, 1986.
36. Krasse B: Caries Risk. A Practical Guide for Assessment and Control. Chicago, Quintessence Publishing, 1985.
37. Gold OC, Jordan HV, van Houte J: A selective medium for *Streptococcus mutans*. Arch Oral Biol 18:1356–1364, 1973.
38. Jensen B, Bratthall D: A new method for the estimation of mutans streptococci in human saliva. J Dent Res 68:468–471, 1989.
39. Larmas M: A new dip-slide method for the counting of salivary lactobacilli. Proc Finn Dent Soc 71:31–35, 1975.
40. Thylstrup A, Qvist V: Is health promotion the main issue of preventive dentistry? *In* Guggenheim B (ed): Cariology Today. Basel, S Karger, 1984, p 321.
41. Berkowitz R, Jordan H, White G: The early establishment of *Streptococcus mutans* in the mouths of infants. Arch Oral Biol 20:171–174, 1975.
42. Alaluusua S: *Streptococcus mutans* establishment and changes in salivary IgA in young children with reference to dental caries. Longitudinal studies and studies on associated methods. Proc Finn Dent Soc 79(Suppl 3):1–55, 1983.
43. Kohler B, Bratthall D: Intrafamilial levels of *Streptococcus mutans* and some aspects of the bacterial transmission. Scand J Dent Res 86:35–42, 1978.
44. Kohler B, Bratthall D, Krasse B: Preventive measures in mothers influences the establishment of the bacterium *Streptococcus mutans* in their infants. Arch Oral Biol 28:225–231, 1983.
45. Kohler B, Andreen I, Jonsson B: The effect of caries-preventive measures in mothers on dental caries and the oral presence of the bacteria *Streptococcus mutans* and lactobacilli in their children. Arch Oral Biol 29:879–883, 1984.
46. Sandham HJ, Brown J, Phillips HI, et al: A preliminary report of long-term elimination of detectable mutans streptococci in man. J Dent Res 67:9–14, 1988.
47. Friedman M, Golomb G: New sustained release dosage form of chlorhexidine for dental use. I. Development and kinetics of release. J Periodontal Res 17:323–328, 1982.
48. Douglas CW, Day JM: Cost and payment of dental services in the United States. J Dent Educ 43:330–348, 1979.
49. Saglie R, Newman MG, Carranza FA Jr, et al: Bacterial invasion of gingiva in advanced periodontitis in humans. J Periodontol 53:217–222, 1982.
50. Loesche WJ: The role of spirochetes in periodontal disease. Adv Dent Res 2:275–283, 1988.
51. Shah HN, Collins DM: *Prevotella*, a new genus to include *Bacteroides melaninogenicus* and related species formerly classified in the genus *Bacteroides*. Int J Syst Bacteriol 40:205–208, 1990.
52. Loesche WJ, Syed SA, Schmidt E, et al: Bacterial profiles of subgingival plaques in periodontitis. J Periodontol 56:447–456, 1985.
53. Loesche WJ, Syed SA, Laughon B, et al: The bacteriology of acute necrotizing ulcerative gingivitis. J Periodontol 53:223–230, 1982.
54. Tanner ACR, Listgarten MA, Ebersole JL, et al: *Bacteroides forsythus* sp. nov., a slow-growing, fusiform *Bacteroides* sp. from the human oral cavity. J Syst Bacteriol 36:213–221, 1986.
55. Dzink JL, Socransky SS, Haffajee AD: The predominant cultivable microbiota of active and inactive lesions of destructive periodontal diseases. J Clin Periodontol 15:316–323, 1988.
56. Zambon JJ: *Actinobacillus actinomycetemcomitans* in human periodontal disease. J Clin Periodontol 12:1–20, 1985.
57. Baehni P, Tsai CC, McArthur W, et al: Interaction of inflammatory cells and oral microorganisms. VIII. Detection of leukotoxic activity of a plaque-derived gram negative microorganism. Infect Immun 24:233–243, 1979.
58. Tsai CC, McArthur WP, Baehni PC, et al: Serum neutralizing activity against *Actinobacillus actinomycetemcomitans* leukotoxin in juvenile periodontitis. J Clin Periodontol 8:338–348, 1981.
59. Page RC, Schroeder HE: Periodontitis in Man and Other Animals. A Comparative Review. Basel, S Karger, 1982.
60. Christersson LA, Albini B, Zambon J, et al: Demonstration of *Actinobacillus actinomycetemcomitans* in gingiva of localized periodontitis lesions. J Dent Res 62:198–204, 1983.
61. Löe H, Theilade E, Jensen SB: Experimental gingivitis in man. J Periodontol 36:177–185, 1965.
62. Seymour GJ: Possible mechanisms involved in the immunoregulation of chronic inflammatory periodontal disease. J Dent Res 66:2–9, 1987.
63. Lang NP, Smith FN: Lymphocyte blastogenesis to plaque antigens in human periodontal disease. I. Populations of varying severity of disease. J Periodontal Res 12:298–309, 1977.
64. Löe H, Anerud A, Boysen H, et al: Natural history of periodontal disease in man. Rapid, moderate and no loss of attachment in Sri Lankan laborers 14 to 46 years of age. J Clin Periodontol 13:431–440, 1986.
65. Goodson JM, Tanner ACR, Haffajee AD, et al: Patterns of progression and regression of advanced destructive periodontal disease. J Clin Periodontol 9:472–481, 1982.
66. Genco RJ, Van Dyke TE, Levine MJ, et al: 1985 Kreshover Lecture: Molecular factors influencing neutrophil defects in periodontal disease. J Dent Res 65:1379–1391, 1986.
67. Masouredis CM, Katz MH, Greenspan D, et al: Prevalence of HIV-associated periodontitis and gingivitis in HIV-infected patients attending an AIDS clinic. J Acquir Immune Defic Syndr 5:479–483, 1992.
68. Saxen L, Murtomas H: Age-related expression of juvenile periodontitis. J Clin Periodontol 12:21–26, 1985.
69. Van Dyke TE, Horoszewicz HU, Genco RJ: The polymorphonuclear leukocyte (PMNL) locomotor defect in juvenile periodontitis. Study of random migration, chemokinesis and chemotaxis. J Periodontol 53:682–687, 1982.
70. Van Dyke TE, Levine MJ, Tabak LA, et al: Reduced chemotaxic peptide binding in juvenile periodontitis: A method for neutrophil function. Biochem Biophys Res Commun 100:1278–1284, 1981.
71. Keyes PH, Rams TE: A rationale for the management of periodontal diseases: Rapid identification of microbial "therapeutic targets" with phase-contrast microscopy. J Am Dent Assoc 106:803–812, 1983.
72. Zambon JJ, Reynolds HS, Chen P, et al: Rapid identification of periodontal pathogens in subgingival dental plaque. Comparison of indirect immunofluorescence microscopy with bacterial culture for detection of *Bacteriodes gingivalis*. J Periodontol 56(11 Suppl):32–40, 1985.

73. Savitt ED, Strzempko MN, Vaccaro KK, et al: Comparison of cultural methods and DNA probe analyses for the detection of *Actinobacillus actinomycetemcomitans, Bacteroides gingivalis,* and *Bacteroides intermedius* in subgingival plaque samples. J Periodontol 59:431–438, 1988.
74. Loesche WJ: The identification of bacteria associated with periodontal disease and dental caries by enzymatic methods. Oral Microbiol Immunol 1:65–70, 1986.
75. Grossi SG, Genco RJ, Marthei EE, et al: Assessment of risk for periodontal disease. II. Risk indicators for alveolar bone loss. J Periodontol 66:23–29, 1995.
76. Loesche WJ, Syed SA, Stoll J: Trypsin-like activity in subgingival plaque: A diagnostic marker for spirochetes and periodontal disease? J Periodontol 58:266–273, 1987.
77. Loesche WJ, Lopatin DE, Giordano J, et al: Comparison of the BANA test, DNA probes and immunological reagents for their ability to detect anaerobic periodontal infections due to *Porphyromonas gingivalis, Treponema denticola* and *Bacteroides forsythus.* J Clin Microbiol 30:427–433, 1992.
78. Amalfitano J, de Fillippo AB, Bretz WA, et al: The effects of incubation length and temperature on the specificity and sensitivity of the BANA (*N*-benzoyl-DL-arginine-naphthylamide) test. J Periodontol 64:848–852, 1993.
79. Knowles JW, Burgett FG, Nissle RR, et al: Results of periodontal treatment related to pocket depth and attachment level. J Periodontol 50:225–233, 1979.
80. Shinn DLS: Metronidazole in acute ulcerative gingivitis. Lancet 1:1191–1193, 1962.
81. Tally FP, Sutter VL, Finegold SM: Metronidazole versus anaerobes. In vitro data and initial clinical observations. Calif Med 117:22–26, 1972.
82. Loesche WJ, Syed SA, Morrison EC, et al: Metronidazole in periodontitis. I. Clinical and bacteriological results after 15 to 30 weeks. J Periodontol 55:325–335, 1984.
83. Joyston-Bechal S, Smales FC, Duckworth R: Effect of metronidazole on chronic periodontal disease in subjects using a topically applied chlorhexidine gel. J Clin Periodontol 11:53–62, 1984.
84. Loesche WJ, Schmidt E, Smith BA, et al: Effect of metronidazole on periodontal treatment needs. J Periodontol 62:247–257, 1991.
85. Loesche WJ, Giordano JR, Hujoel, P, et al: Metronidazole in periodontitis. III. Reduced need for surgery. J Clin Periodontol 19:103–112, 1992.
86. Loesche WJ, Giordano J, Soehren S, et al: The non-surgical treatment of periodontal patients. Oral Surg Oral Med Oral Pathol 81:533–543, 1996
87. Goodson JM, Tanner A, McArdle S, et al: Multicenter evaluation of tetracycline fiber therapy. III. Microbiological response. J Periodontol 62:440–451, 1991.
88. Ainamo J, Lie T, Ellingsen BH, et al: Clinical response to subgingival application of a metronidazole 25% gel compared to the effect of subgingival scaling in adult periodontitis. J Clin Periodontol 19:723–729, 1992.

48

Infections of Head and Neck Spaces and Salivary Glands

*Ann Sullivan Baker**
Gerard J. Nau

Deep neck infections are most often secondary to contiguous spread of local pharyngeal or dental foci. If not recognized and drained, they have the potential for life-threatening complications.[1]

Anatomy

Knowledge of the cervical compartments and interfascial spaces is essential to an understanding of the pathogenesis of infections in these spaces (Fig. 48–1).

Cervical Fascia

The muscles, vessels, and visceral structures of the neck are enveloped in fascia; interfascial spaces are potential areas between fascial compartments. Two layers, superficial and deep, constitute the cervical fascia. The superficial fascia consists of the subcutaneous tissues of the neck, which completely enclose it and are continuous with the platysma anteriorly. The deep cervical fascia can be thought of as defining a series of cylindrical compartments that extend longitudinally from the base of the skull to the mediastinum. The superficial or investing layer of the deep cervical fascia encloses all the deeper parts of the neck. It begins at the nuchal line and extends anteriorly, dividing to enclose the trapezius, sternocleidomastoid, and strap muscles as well as the submaxillary and parotid glands. The middle or pretracheal fascia encloses the cervical viscera, including the pharynx, esophagus, larynx, trachea, and thyroid and parathyroid glands. The deep or prevertebral fascia arises from the nuchal ligament and encloses the vertebral column and muscles of the spine. It is continuous inferiorly with the posterior mediastinum. All three layers of the deep cervical fascia contribute to the carotid sheath, which forms a neurovascular compartment that encloses the carotid artery, the internal jugular vein, and the vagus nerve (see Fig. 48–1*B*).

Fascial Spaces

Three major spaces of clinical importance lie between the planes of deep cervical fascia.[2] The parapharyngeal (or lateral pharyngeal) or pharyngomaxillary space is located in the upper portion of the neck above the hyoid bone between the pretracheal fascia of the visceral compartment medially and the superficial fascia, which invests the parotid gland, internal pterygoid muscle, and mandible laterally (see Fig. 48–1*A*). Its shape is an inverted cone, the base bounded superiorly by the skull and the apex directed inferiorly toward the hyoid bone. The carotid sheath, which runs in the posterior

*Deceased.

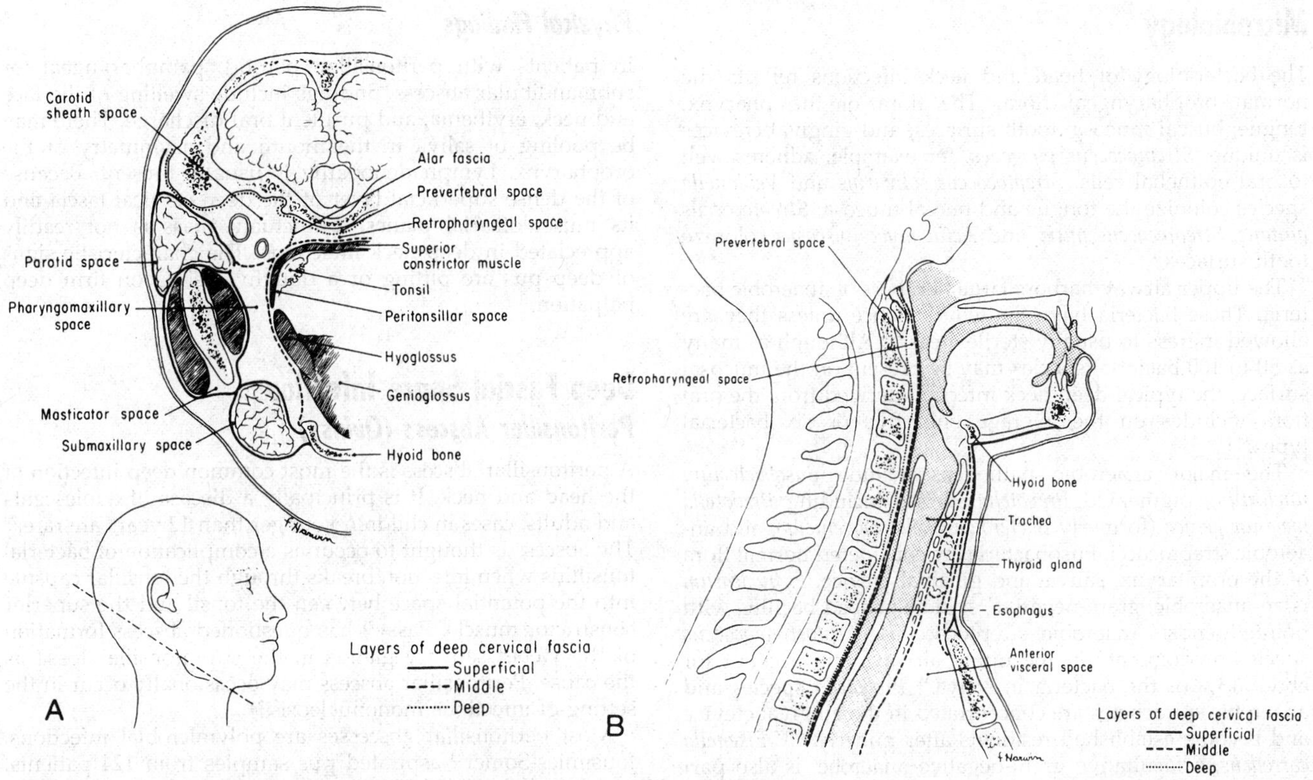

FIGURE 48–1 □ *A*, Midsagittal section of the neck illustrating the anterior visceral space, retropharyngeal space, and prevertebral space. (From Levitt GW: Cervical fascia and deep neck infections. Laryngoscope 80:409–435, 1970.) *B*, Oblique section through the head. (From Langenbrunner DJ, Dajani S: Pharyngomaxillary space abscess with carotid artery erosion. Arch Otolaryngol 94:447–457, 1971. Copyright 1971, American Medical Association.)

aspect of the parapharyngeal space, pierces the cone at its apex to enter the mediastinum.

The second space lies within the submental and submandibular triangles between the mucosa of the floor of the mouth and the superficial layer of deep fascia of these regions. This space is subdivided by the mylohyoid muscle into the submandibular space (which contains the submandibular salivary gland and lymph nodes) and the sublingual space (which contains sublingual gland, hypoglossal nerve, part of the submandibular gland, and loose connective tissue). The two divisions communicate around the mylohyoid muscle.

The third clinically important space is the retropharyngeal space, which runs longitudinally from the base of the skull to the posterior mediastinum between the prevertebral fascia posteriorly and the posterior aspect of the pretracheal fascia anteriorly (see Fig. 48–1*A* and *B*). It communicates with the parapharyngeal space laterally, where it is bounded by the carotid sheaths. The retropharyngeal space is the most important communication between the neck and the chest.

Potential spaces such as the masticator, pterygopalatine, temporal, and prevertebral spaces are discussed in relation to clinical infections in those areas.

Lymph Nodes

The lymph nodes of the head and neck may be divided into 10 principal groups. Six groups (occipital, mastoid, parotid, facial, submandibular, and submental nodes) form a collar at the junction of the head and neck. Within this collar near the base of the tongue lie the sublingual and retropharyngeal nodes. The anterior and lateral cervical nodes form a chain along the front and side of the neck, respectively. The lateral cervical chain serves as a common root for drainage. The final conduit from all lymphatics in the head and neck is the large deep chain situated along the carotid sheath. When inflamed, these nodes become adherent to the fascial sheath of the vessels, and it is understandable that the blood stream is frequently infected by contiguous spread.

Radiologic Investigation of the Head and Neck

The most valuable plain radiograph for detecting soft tissue swelling in the neck is the lateral cervical view exposed for soft tissue detail. The soft tissues of the posterior wall of the hypopharynx are approximately 5 mm deep, less than one third the diameter of the fourth cervical vertebra (C-4). The retrolaryngeal soft tissues should be approximately two thirds the width of C-4, and the retrotracheal space slightly less. Dental films are indicated when a periapical abscess is suspected.

The axial imaging format of computed tomography (CT) is particularly well suited to the head and neck. CT allows the critical evaluation of soft tissues and especially bone from a single exposure. Because CT can localize a process and define its extent, particularly extension into the mediastinum or into the cranial vault, it is an invaluable tool for planning and guiding aspiration for culture or open drainage.

Magnetic resonance imaging (MRI) has assumed the premier role in the radiologic evaluation of head and neck infection. MRI is more sensitive than CT and probably the bone scan in detecting bone involvement. T2-weighted images may identify and localize areas of pus for drainage or aspiration. Gadolinium enhancement is important to accurately define the soft tissue component. Finally, MRI is useful for imaging vascular lesions, such as jugular thrombophlebitis.[3]

Microbiology

The bacteriology of head and neck infections reflects the normal oropharyngeal flora. The flora of the pharynx, tongue, buccal mucosa, tooth surfaces, and gingival crevices is unique. *Streptococcus pyogenes*, for example, adheres well to oral epithelial cells. *Streptococcus salivarius* and *Veillonella* species colonize the tongue and buccal mucosa; *Streptococcus mutans*, *Streptococcus mitis*, and *Actinomyces viscosus* colonize tooth surfaces.[4, 5]

The upper airway harbors large numbers of anaerobic bacteria. These bacteria have limited virulence unless they are allowed ingress to usually sterile areas.[6–8] Although as many as 50 to 100 bacterial species may be present on the mucosal surface, the typical deep neck infection derived from the oral flora includes on the average only five or six bacterial types.[9, 10]

The major anaerobic pathogens include *Fusobacterium nucleatum*, pigmented *Prevotella* species including *Prevotella melaninogenica* (formerly *Bacteroides melaninogenicus*), and anaerobic streptococci. Fusobacteria are considered normal flora of the oropharynx, saliva, and gingival crevice. *F. nucleatum* is an anaerobic, gram-negative, spindle-shaped bacillus with pointed ends. Anaerobic streptococci or *Peptostreptococcus* species predominate in the upper airways and account for about 13% of the bacteria in saliva.[11] *Prevotella* species and anaerobic spirochetes are concentrated in the gingival crevice and become established residents after puberty.[12, 13] *Eikenella corrodens*, a facultative gram-negative anaerobe, is also part of the usual oral flora.[14, 15] A combination of aerobic streptococci and gram-negative organisms such as *Proteus* species may produce synergistic necrotizing cellulitis.[16]

Actinomyces species are filamentous, branching gram-positive coccobacilli that live on dental plaque. *Actinomyces israelii* is the most common pathogen; less common are *Arachnia propionica* and *Actinomyces naeslundii*, *Actinomyces viscosus*, and *Actinomyces odontolyticus*.[17, 18] All of these organisms are part of the oral flora and produce similar infections. *Actinobacillus actinomycetemcomitans*, a fastidious capnophilic gram-negative coccobacillus, is commonly associated with the actinomyces. Other commonly associated bacteria include streptococci and many gram-negative bacilli such as *Bacteroides ureolyticus*.[19]

The bacteriologic diagnosis of particular space infections may be anticipated from the microbial flora of the originating focus. Thus, most abscesses originating about the teeth harbor four or five organisms, mainly oral anaerobes, whereas infections arising from the pharynx contain oral anaerobes and *S. pyogenes*.

Clinical Manifestations

Symptoms

In general, patients with peritonsillar, parotid, parapharyngeal, and submandibular abscesses complain of sore throat or pain and trismus. Trismus, the inability to open the jaw, indicates pressure or infection of the muscles of mastication (the masseter and the pterygoids) or involvement of the motor branch of the trigeminal nerve.

Dysphagia and odynophagia are secondary to inflammation about the cricoarytenoid joints. Dysphonia and hoarseness are late findings in neck infections and may indicate involvement of the 10th cranial nerve; unilateral tongue paresis indicates involvement of the 12th cranial nerve. Stridor and dyspnea may be manifestations of local pressure or spread of infection to the mediastinum.

Physical Findings

In patients with peritonsillar, parotid, parapharyngeal, or submandibular abscess, findings include swelling of the face and neck, erythema, and purulent oral discharge. There may be pooling of saliva in the mouth and asymmetry of the oropharynx. Lymphadenopathy is usually present. Because of the dense superficial layer of the deep cervical fascia and its musculofascial planes, a fluctuant mass is not readily appreciated in deep neck infections. The characteristic signs of deep pus are pitting or a doughy feeling on firm deep palpation.

Deep Fascial Space Infections

Peritonsillar Abscess (Quinsy)

A peritonsillar abscess is the most common deep infection of the head and neck. It is principally a disease of adolescents and adults; cases in children younger than 12 years are rare.[20] The abscess is thought to occur as a complication of bacterial tonsillitis when infection breaks through the tonsillar capsule into the potential space between the tonsil and the superior constrictor muscle. Passy[21] has questioned abscess formation of the Weber salivary glands in the supratonsillar fossa as the cause. Peritonsillar abscess may occasionally occur in the setting of infectious mononucleosis.[22]

Most peritonsillar abscesses are polymicrobial infections. Jousimies-Somer[23] aspirated pus samples from 124 patients, which included 143 aerobes and 407 anaerobes. Aerobes were isolated from 86% of patients—alone in 20 cases and together with anaerobes in 87 cases. *S. pyogenes* was most prominent (45%), followed by *Streptococcus milleri* (27%), *Haemophilus influenzae* (11%), and viridans streptococci (11%). Anaerobes were isolated from 82% of the samples and were the sole finding in 15 abscesses. *Fusobacterium necrophorum* and *P. melaninogenica* were both isolated from 38% of patients, *Prevotella intermedia* from 32%, *Peptostreptococcus micros* from 27%, *F. nucleatum* from 26%, and *A. odontolyticus* from 23%. Recurrences were more common with *F. necrophorum*.

The classic clinical presentation of peritonsillar abscess is gradually increasing pharyngeal discomfort and ipsilateral otalgia followed by trismus and dysarthria. Dysphagia is less common but is often accompanied by drooling.[24] Edema and pain produce characteristic muffled or "hot potato in the mouth" speech. The patient is usually in a mildly toxic condition; a temperature above 39°C suggests bacteremia or extension of the abscess into the parapharyngeal space.

Physical examination reveals a tender, exudative peritonsillar mass with edema of the soft palate and uvula. Displacement of the soft palate medially and of the uvula to the opposite side differentiates peritonsillar abscess from other pharyngeal abscesses. Sloughing in the crypts of the tonsil or large necrotic ulcers of the tonsil may occasionally occur. Ipsilateral tender anterior cervical adenopathy is usually present.

Treatment with needle aspiration combined with administration of parenteral antibiotics is the simplest, most cost-effective therapy for peritonsillar abscess.[25–28] Intravenous antibiotic therapy (penicillin at 1 to 2 million units every 4 hours plus metronidazole at 500 mg every 6 hours; or clindamycin at 600 mg every 8 hours) should be followed by a total of 10 to 14 days' oral therapy (penicillin plus metronidazole; or clindamycin).[29, 30] Interval tonsillectomy is indicated only when there is a history of recurrent tonsillitis or of peritonsillar abscess.[31, 32]

Complications result from extension beyond the peritonsillar space. As soon as the infection penetrates the muscle bed of the tonsillar fossa, it becomes a parapharyngeal space infection (see later). A peritonsillar abscess frequently spreads by this route. Necrotizing fasciitis has been described as a rare but lethal complication of peritonsillar abscess.[33]

Submandibular Space Infections

Ludwig Angina. The process first described in 1836 by Frederick Wilhelm von Ludwig[34] is a rapidly spreading phlegmon or cellulitis—not an abscess—involving the floor of the mouth and the loose areolar tissue above the mylohyoid diaphragm. The disease usually occurs in patients between the ages of 20 and 50 years who have abscessed teeth or pyorrhea.[35] Apical infection from incisors, canines, and third molars perforates this sublingual space above the mylohyoid muscle. Inflammation from the tongue and the floor of the mouth, lingual tonsillitis, and local tonsillectomy are other less likely causes.

Ludwig angina begins as a localized cellulitis of the loose areolar tissue of the floor of the mouth. A fulminating swelling develops, with pouting of the tissue over the edges of the lower teeth. Later, necrosis and pus formation accompany local lymphadenitis. At this time, manifestations of sepsis are evident. The infection may break through the deep cervical fascia to produce a cellulitis that extends from the clavicle up over the face.

Oral bacteria, in particular streptococci and anaerobic organisms, are the predominant bacterial pathogens in Ludwig angina. In a study of 21 perimandibular closed space infections, Bartlett[36] found an average of six microbial species per specimen. The predominant aerobes were α-hemolytic and nonhemolytic streptococci; the predominant anaerobes were peptostreptococci, *Prevotella* species, and *F. nucleatum*. By contrast, organisms such as *Staphylococcus aureus* are not of primary importance in Ludwig angina.

The patient may complain of a foul taste in the mouth, crepitus in the temporomandibular joint, or unilateral pharyngitis. A history of recent tooth extraction should be sought.[37] With the full-blown syndrome, the patient is in acute distress. Edema and induration elevate the floor of the mouth, thrusting the tongue upward and backward toward the palate (Fig. 48–2*A*). There is trismus as well as brawny induration of the submandibular area. Pain, redness, heat, and swelling—the classic picture of a phlegmon—are followed by dysphagia, dyspnea, and spiking fevers.

The peripheral white cell count is usually elevated, with a predominance of polymorphonuclear leukocytes. CT often illustrates increased soft tissue swelling or, rarely, an accumulation of pus in the sublingual-submandibular area (Fig. 48–2*B*). Panradiographic views of the teeth and jaws should be obtained to look for an apical abscess.

Treatment is aimed first at securing the airway and then at controlling the infection.[38] Equipment for emergency endotracheal intubation or tracheostomy should be available at the bedside. Penicillin G and metronidazole, clindamycin, or ampicillin-sulbactam should be administered intravenously. If sepsis and respiratory compromise are both present, endotracheal intubation or tracheostomy should be performed, followed by surgical decompression. If sepsis is not present, a more conservative approach may be used.[39, 40]

Complications of Ludwig angina include spread of infection into the parapharyngeal and retropharyngeal spaces and on into the superior mediastinum. In addition, submucosal swelling in the floor of the mouth has the added danger of producing asphyxiation.

Submandibular and Submental Abscesses. A submandibular abscess can develop after suppuration of the submandibular lymph nodes, an infection of the submandibular salivary gland, or apical infections of second and third molar teeth below the mylohyoid muscle. The fluctuant quality is

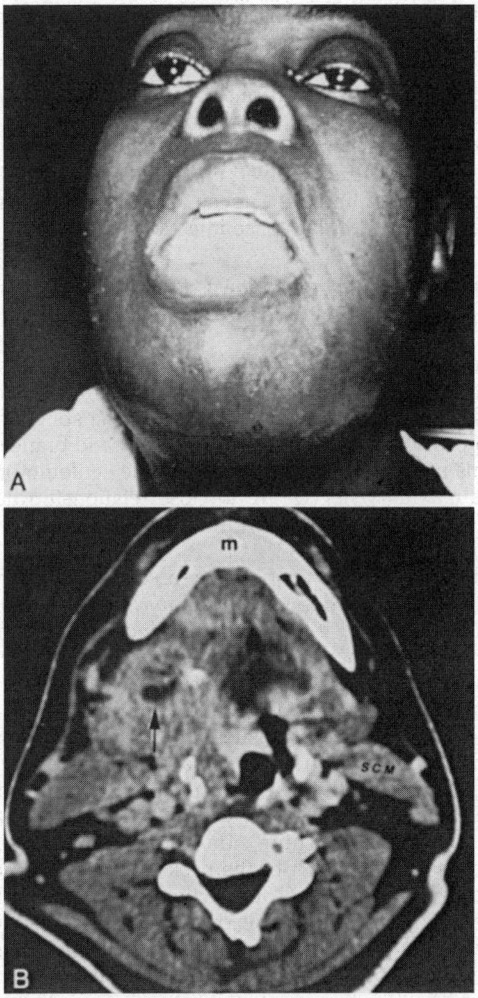

FIGURE 48–2 □ *A,* Patient with Ludwig angina revealing massive sublingual swelling with upward protrusion of the tongue and bilateral neck swelling. *B,* Axial CT view of patient with Ludwig angina revealing lucent zone *(arrow)* in submandibular space posterior to mylohyoid muscle. m, Mandible; SCM, sternocleidomastoid muscle. (*A* and *B* courtesy of Dr. A. Weber, Massachusetts Eye and Ear Infirmary, Boston, MA.)

more apt to be appreciated here than in other deep neck infections because there is no overlying musculature and the fascia is not so dense. Submental abscesses usually result from spread of an apical abscess of the lower incisors through the thin buccolabial areolar plate and below the mylohyoid muscle. Suppuration of a submental lymph node may be another source of infection. There may be moderate elevation of the floor of the mouth, but the exuberant swelling of the soft tissues of the mouth, as seen in Ludwig angina, is lacking. Abscesses in submandibular or submental spaces are treated by incision and drainage.

Masticator Space Infections

The masticator space lies between the subperiosteal region of the mandible and the fascial sling containing the masseter and pterygoid muscles. Infection of this space usually follows extraction of a lower second or an impacted third molar tooth or curettage of an infected dental socket. Patients present with pain and fever of acute onset. There is broad induration over the angle and ramus of the mandible. The swelling often extends down the neck and occasionally across the midline. Marked trismus develops because of the muscles involved. There is pharyngeal swelling over the medial aspect of the involved mandible. The tonsils are pushed toward the midline, but the lateral pharyngeal wall posterior to the tonsil is not swollen (in contrast to parapharyngeal space infections).

Radiography of the involved mandible and teeth is helpful to reveal a hidden initiating focus. Treatment is the same as for other submandibular space infections.

Pterygopalatine, Infratemporal, and Temporal Fossa Infections

The pterygopalatine fossa is behind the maxillary antrum and below the orbital apex. It contains three important structures: the maxillary nerve and branches, the sphenopalatine ganglion, and the internal maxillary artery and branches. The abducens nerve, the inferior branch of the oculomotor nerve, and the maxillary nerves are in close relationship here and are often involved together in infection of the maxillary and sphenoid sinuses.

Infections of the pterygopalatine fossa and adjacent spaces usually follow extraction of a maxillary molar tooth or result from introduction of infection during local anesthesia of the superior alveolar nerve. A fulminating cellulitis develops, progressively involving the upper molar gingiva and the pterygopalatine, infratemporal, and temporal fossae; abscess formation in these spaces ensues.

On clinical presentation, there is painful swelling of the maxillary gingival tissues that spreads in a few days to involve the cheek (Fig. 48–3). Unchecked, the cellulitis progresses to involve the entire side of the head, including the nose, ear, and upper part of the neck. Proptosis of the globe may result from extension of infection into the orbit through the inferior orbital fissure. Vision may be threatened by the development of optic neuritis. If osteomyelitis of the maxilla is present, the maxillary sinus may become secondarily infected.

CT or MRI of the pterygopalatine fossa and the orbit is crucial in the evaluation and localization of the cellulitis or abscess.

If diagnostic evaluation reveals a mass, surgical drainage of both the pterygopalatine abscess and any orbital abscess should be initiated immediately. Intravenous penicillin remains the antibiotic of choice for treating deep oropharyngeal infections of odontogenic origin. Metronidazole (500 mg every 6 hours) is added or intravenous clindamycin (600 mg every 8 hours) or ampicillin-sulbactam is substituted in place of penicillin to cover mixed anaerobic infections, resistant anaerobes such as *Prevotella* species, gram-negative organisms, and *H. influenzae*.

Parapharyngeal Abscess

Parapharyngeal abscess most often arises as a complication of a peritonsillar abscess, but infections of the parotid gland, dental roots, and petrous pyramid or infections secondary to dental or pharyngeal surgery may extend into the parapharyngeal space. A cause is not always apparent, however, in spite of a detailed evaluation.[41] Before the advent of antimicrobial chemotherapy, 50% of neck infections occurred in the parapharyngeal space; the most frequent cause was infection from the tonsils and pharynx (adenoids).[42] Antibiotic therapy has reduced the frequency to less than 30%.[43] More recently, Ungkanont and coworkers[44] found parapharyngeal abscesses to be one of the least frequent (2%) of the deep neck infections in children.

The triad of (1) tonsillar prolapse with swelling of the lateral pharyngeal wall, (2) trismus, and (3) parotid swelling

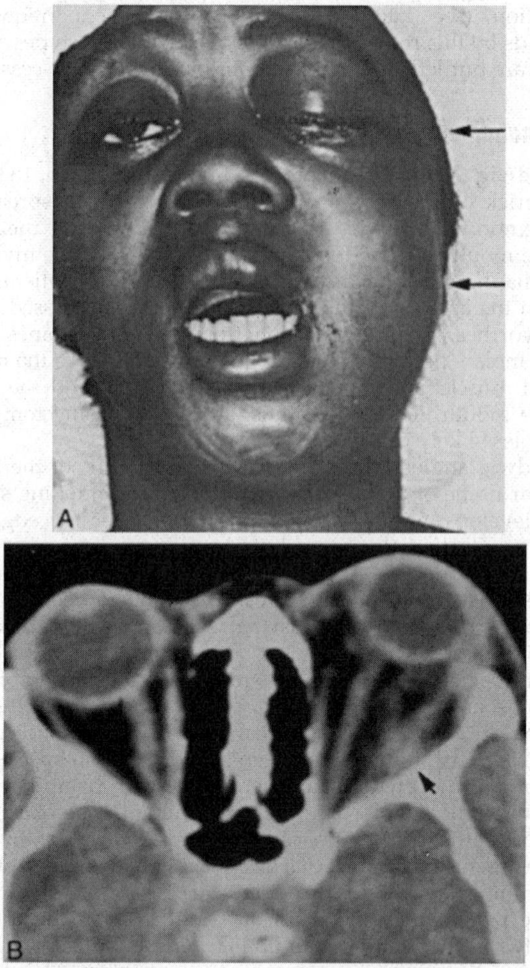

FIGURE 48–3 □ *A*, Pterygopalatine space and temporal space infection with an orbital abscess in a patient with an upper molar tooth abscess. *B*, Extension of pterygopalatine space infection into the left orbit; soft tissue mass is evident *(arrow)*. (*A* and *B* courtesy of Dr. A. Weber, Massachusetts Eye and Ear Infirmary, Boston, MA.)

indicates an abscess in the parapharyngeal space (Fig. 48–4). The first clinical symptoms and signs are fever and painful swallowing. If the abscess is located in the anterior muscle compartment of the parapharyngeal space, inflammation of the internal pterygoid muscles results in trismus. Dyspnea is a consequence of invasion of the pretracheal fascia; otalgia and odynophagia may also be present. Inflammation of the lymph nodes under the sternocleidomastoid muscle produces torticollis toward the side opposite the abscess. Continued signs of sepsis after drainage of the peritonsillar space usually indicate concomitant undrained parapharyngeal space infection.

An abscess localized to the posterior neurovascular compartment of the parapharyngeal space is manifested by sepsis and cranial nerve involvement (e.g., Horner syndrome, hoarseness, unilateral tongue paresis) but with minimal trismus. The posterior tonsillar pillar is displaced. Swelling and displacement of the parotid gland usually occur with infection in either the anterior or posterior parapharyngeal space. Upper airway bleeding, secondary to erosion of the great vessels, is a late finding in untreated cases.

The site and extent of infection are best evaluated by CT or MRI; external drainage is mandatory for frank abscess. Internal drainage is contraindicated owing to the proximity of the great vessels.

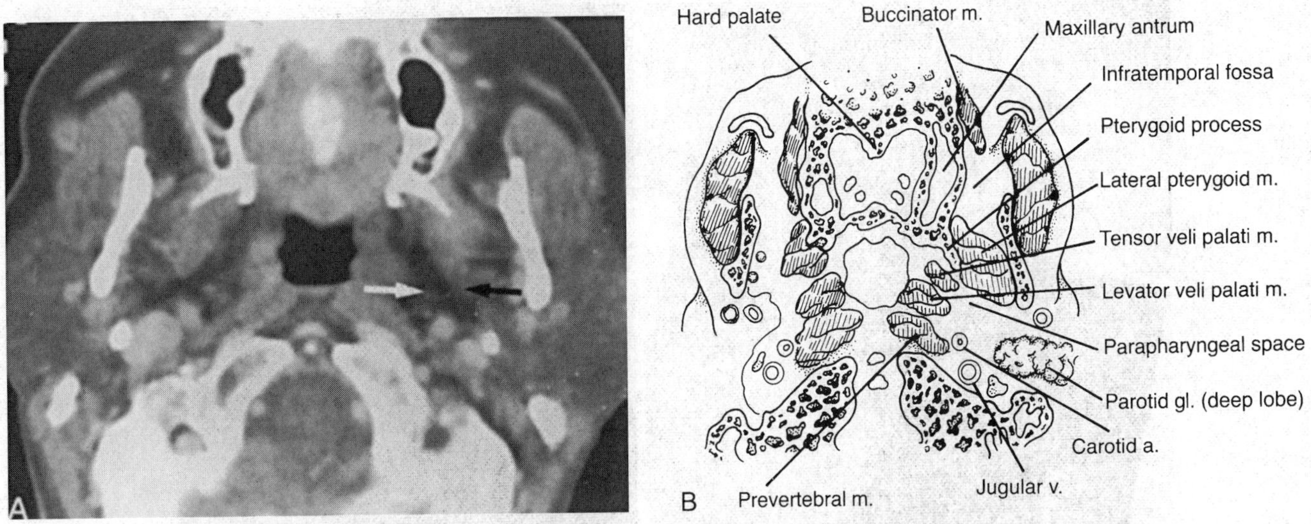

FIGURE 48–4 ▫ Parapharyngeal space. *A*, CT view *(arrows)*. *B*, Anatomy.

Infection of the carotid sheath is a frequent complication of parapharyngeal abscess. Erosion of the internal carotid artery can cause fatal hemorrhage and was the major cause of death from infection of this space in the preantibiotic era. Thrombophlebitis of the internal jugular vein with intracranial extension is another vascular complication. Intracranial involvement may also occur by superior extension of the abscess to the base of the skull. Inferior extension to the piriform sinus may result in upper airway obstruction. Mediastinitis may occur by extension from the retropharyngeal space or carotid sheath.

Retropharyngeal Abscess

An acute retropharyngeal abscess may involve the space between the pharyngeal wall and the visceral fascia, the space between the visceral and alar fasciae, or the space between the alar and prevertebral fasciae (the danger space) (see Fig. 48–1*A* and *B*). A retropharyngeal space infection often results from lymphatic spread of infection in the pharynx or sinuses to the retropharyngeal lymph nodes. The lymph nodes usually suppurate, which leads to abscess development. Retropharyngeal infections are most common in children, because the lymph nodes atrophy by age 3 or 4 years.[45, 46] In children or adults, infections in this space may be secondary to accidental perforation of the pharynx or esophagus, for example, by a lollipop stick or other foreign body, by endoscopic trauma, or by surgery.[41, 47–50] Alternatively, a retropharyngeal abscess may extend from cervical vertebral osteomyelitis.[51] Infections of the retropharyngeal space are usually polymicrobial, with anaerobes, streptococci, and staphylococci predominating.[52–54]

The classic presentation of retropharyngeal abscess is chills and fever after pharyngitis, but no antecedent illness is identified in many patients.[55] Adults may complain of dysphagia, neck pain, dyspnea, and regurgitation. In the child, the onset may be insidious, manifested primarily by irritability and refusal to eat.[56] On physical examination, the neck may be rigidly hyperextended with local tenderness. As swelling increases, a muffled voice (dysphonia) and drooling are followed by tachypnea and stridor. The oropharynx should be examined carefully by indirect (mirror) hypopharyngeal inspection and gentle digital palpation. Bulging of the posterior pharyngeal wall may be noted, usually to one side of the midline. Cervical lymphadenopathy is usually present.

Differential diagnosis of retropharyngeal abscess includes cervical osteomyelitis, Pott disease, meningitis, and calcific tendinitis of the long muscle of the neck.[57, 58] A lateral radiograph is the most important diagnostic procedure in the initial evaluation of a patient with suspected retropharyngeal abscess (Fig. 48–5). The neck should be fully extended during deep inspiration while the film is taken. The radiograph should be evaluated for increased thickness of the prevertebral soft tissues, air or air-fluid levels in the soft tissues, and the presence of foreign bodies. A chest radiograph should be obtained to identify mediastinal extension.

Treatment consists of expeditious drainage of the abscess and intravenous high-dose penicillin (2 to 4 million units every 4 hours) and metronidazole (500 mg every 6 hours) or ampicillin-sulbactam (3 g intravenously every 6 hours) for a minimum of 5 days. Antibiotics should be adjusted as culture data become available, and oral therapy is continued to complete at least a 14-day course.

Untreated retropharyngeal abscess may rupture spontaneously into the pharynx. Aspiration of the purulent drainage can lead to pneumonia and empyema. An abscess in the danger space between the alar and prevertebral fasciae may drain by gravity into the posterior mediastinum, resulting in mediastinitis that may include empyema.[59–62] In the past, 70% of cases of mediastinitis were the result of infection spread in this manner.[63] With the introduction of antibiotics, mediastinal extension has become uncommon,[52, 55] and most cases of mediastinitis result from esophageal perforation.[64] Extension of infection into the mediastinum is characterized by chest pain, dyspnea, persistent fever, and radiographic evidence of a widened mediastinum. In children, stridor is suggestive of airway compromise from physical obstruction and is evidence of later stage disease.[65]

Hemorrhage in the setting of retropharyngeal infection suggests involvement of the major vessels in the neck.[66] Another important vascular complication is phlebitis or thrombosis of the internal jugular vein, which should be suspected when retropharyngeal abscess is associated with a septic clinical course[67] (see the next section).

Vascular Complications of Deep Neck Infections

Carotid Sheath Infections

The carotid sheath abuts all three layers of deep cervical fascia. Infection may therefore arise by spread from the parapharyngeal space, Ludwig angina, or suppuration of deep

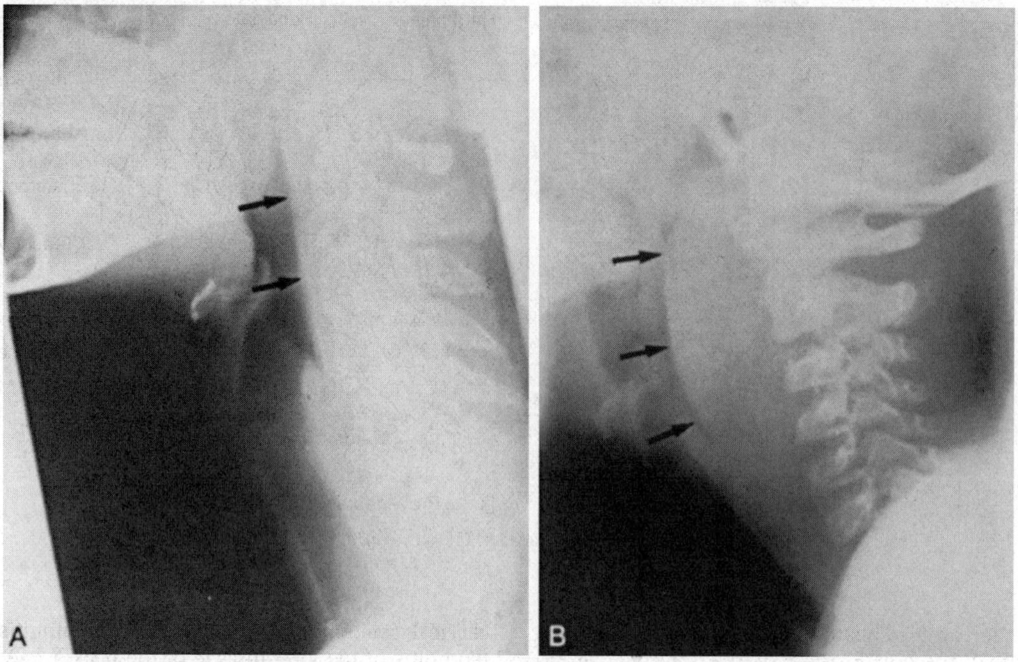

FIGURE 48–5 ▫ Retropharyngeal space. *A*, Normal lateral cervical view. *B*, Expansion of prevertebral soft tissues by retropharyngeal abscess. (*A* and *B* courtesy of Dr. A. Weber, Massachusetts Eye and Ear Infirmary, Boston, MA.)

cervical nodes.[68] There are no characteristic symptoms or signs of carotid sheath infections. In some patients, there is diffuse swelling along the sternocleidomastoid muscle with marked tenderness and torticollis to the opposite side. Erosion of the carotid artery may be heralded by minor episodes of oral bleeding. Ligation of the carotid artery may be necessary in cases of major hemorrhage, but the mortality rate remains high and the risk of stroke is significant.[69]

Septic Jugular Thrombophlebitis (Postanginal Sepsis)

Postanginal sepsis was first described by Long[70] in 1912 and Mosher[71] in 1920. The term, also known as Lemierre syndrome, refers to septic thrombophlebitis of the internal jugular vein after oropharyngeal infection complicated by spread to the parapharyngeal space.[70–74]

There is . . . a more lingering type of infection in the neck. . . . There may have been frank pus, . . . about the tonsil. This is soon evacuated by surgery or nature, but the patient sinks into a long drawn-out septicemia and dies.[67]

Symptoms of jugular vein thrombosis include pain in the neck made worse by turning the head away from the involved side. This motion causes the sternocleidomastoid muscle to compress the inflamed mass. Dysphagia and dysphonia may also occur.

On examination, the tonsil is displaced medially. Vocal cord paralysis on the same side occurs together with edema of the lateral pharyngeal wall. Chills and sweats may indicate blood stream infection. Septic emboli from the jugular venous system travel to the lung, followed by blood-borne dissemination of infection to other organs.[37, 74] Diagnosis and treatment of postanginal sepsis may be delayed because of the lack of an obvious source for the infection. In the absence of a demonstrable cause for sepsis, careful efforts should be made to elicit a history of pharyngitis. Contrast-enhanced CT may show the normal carotid artery and an enlarged jugular venous wall surrounding a more lucent intraluminal clot (Fig. 48–6). Thrombosis of the jugular vein can also be demonstrated by magnetic resonance angiography.

The organisms most frequently involved in postanginal sepsis are anaerobic streptococci and *Bacteroides* (now including *Prevotella*) species and *Fusobacterium* species.[75, 76] Less common are α-hemolytic and group A β-hemolytic strepto-

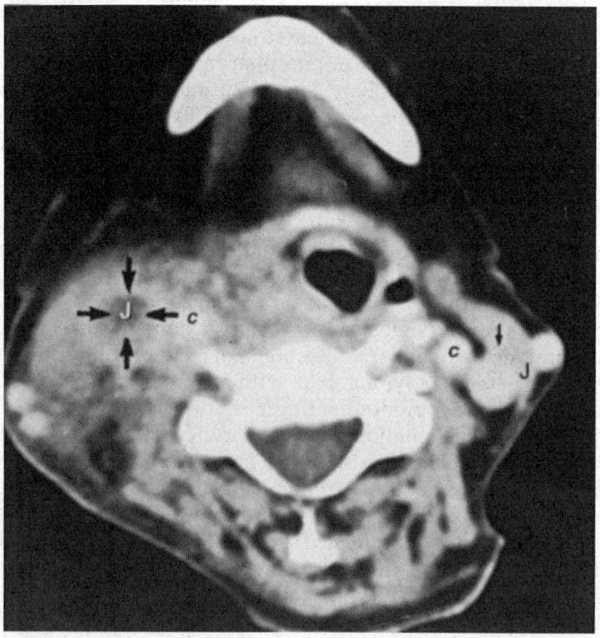

FIGURE 48–6 ▫ Jugular venous thrombosis. *A*, Contrast-enhanced axial CT scan at C-3 shows the normal left carotid (c) and jugular (J) vessels *(arrow)*. The right common carotid is normal, but the jugular vein is enlarged with a dense or enhancing wall *(arrows)* that surrounds the more lucent intraluminal clot. (Courtesy of Dr. A. Weber, Massachusetts Eye and Ear Infirmary, Boston, MA.)

cocci, the pneumococcus, *S. aureus*, and *E. corrodens*.[77] Treatment usually consists of external drainage of the lateral pharyngeal space.

Infections of the Salivary Glands

Suppurative Parotitis

Acute bacterial parotitis typically occurs in an elderly, dehydrated, intubated, or postoperative inpatient, although this condition is also commonly seen in outpatients.[78, 79] Other predisposing factors include recent intensive teeth cleaning, use of anticholinergic drugs, and salivary calculi with obstruction. Salivary stasis permits retrograde seeding of the duct of Stensen with virulent oral flora.[80, 81] Raad and colleagues[78] found *S. aureus* to be the most common pathogen, followed by viridans streptococci and with only one gram-negative isolate in their study. However, acute parotitis resulting from anaerobes, enteric gram-negative bacilli, *Pseudomonas aeruginosa*, and *E. corrodens* has been documented.[82–85]

Patients present with complaints of pain, swelling, and dysphagia. On examination, tense swelling over the parotid area, tenderness, and pain on opening the mouth are seen. A fluctuant quality is generally not appreciated because of the dense parotid fascia that overlies the gland. Purulent material may be expressed from the orifice of the Stensen duct and should be examined by Gram stain and culture. Treatment includes hydration and intravenous antibiotics directed against staphylococci and mouth flora, with coverage adjusted in response to culture results.

Viral Parotitis

In the prevaccine era, mumps virus was the most common cause of viral parotitis. Other viruses that are associated with parotitis include coxsackievirus,[86] influenza virus,[87] parainfluenza virus types 1[88] and 3,[89] lymphocytic choriomeningitis virus,[90] and cytomegalovirus.[91] Parotitis is associated with human immunodeficiency virus infection, both in children[92, 93] and in seropositive, asymptomatic adults,[94] but it is also due to opportunistic infection.[95] Patients with viral parotitis present with tender swelling of the parotid glands bilaterally along with fever, headache, and myalgias. Swelling is occasionally unilateral. The extreme parotid tenderness and systemic toxic effects of suppurative infection are absent in viral parotitis. For infections not related to human immunodeficiency virus, symptoms usually resolve within 5 to 10 days, and treatment—hydration and relief of pain and fever—is directed at the symptoms. Specific therapy for human immunodeficiency virus–related infections is dictated by the diagnosis.

Chronic Parotitis

Recurrent or persistent swellings of the parotid gland, which may or may not be painful, are loosely grouped as chronic parotitis. Whereas noninfectious entities such as Sjögren syndrome, sarcoidosis, and even hyperuricemia[96] should be considered, obstruction and abnormal duct architecture can lead to recurrent infections. Chronic pyogenic infections have bacteriologic diagnoses similar to those of acute infections; Iko[97] found *S. aureus*, viridans streptococci, *Streptococcus pneumoniae*, and *Klebsiella* to be the most common etiologic agents in a group of patients with chronic pyogenic parotitis. *Mycobacterium tuberculosis*,[98] *A. actinomycetemcomitans*,[99] and actinomycosis[79] can also cause chronic parotid swelling that can be confused with a parotid tumor.[98, 99] Human immunodeficiency virus infection has been associated with parotid swelling of years in duration.[100] The evaluation of chronic parotitis should include a search for parotid stones, ductal strictures, or other predisposing factors. Antimicrobials should be directed at the causative organism. Subtotal or total parotidectomy has been advocated for intractable recurrent infections.[101, 102]

References

1. Baker AS, Montgomery WW: Oropharyngeal space infections. Curr Clin Top Infect 8:227, 1987.
2. Grodinsky M: Ludwig's angina, retropharyngeal abscess, and other deep abscesses of the head and neck. JAMA 114:18, 1940.
3. Council on Scientific Affairs of the AMA: Magnetic resonance imaging of the head and neck region. Present status and future potential. JAMA 260:3313, 1988.
4. Ellen RP, Gibbons RJ: Parameters affecting the adherence and tissue tropisms of *Streptococcus pyogenes*. Infect Immun 9:85, 1974.
5. Gibbons RJ, VanHoute J: Bacterial adherence in oral microbiological ecology. Annu Rev Med 29:19, 1975.
6. Bartlett JG, Gorbach SJ: Anaerobic infections of the head and neck. Otolaryngol Clin North Am 9:655, 1976.
7. Newman MG, Goodman AD: Oral and dental infections. *In* Finegold SM, George WL (eds): Anaerobic Bacteria in Human Disease. New York, Academic Press, 1989, p 234.
8. Busch DF: Anaerobes in infections of the head, neck, ear, nose, and throat. Rev Infect Dis 6(Suppl):S115, 1984.
9. Bartlett JG, O'Keefe P: The bacteriology of perimandibular space infections. J Oral Surg 37:407, 1979.
10. Tanner A, Stillman N: Oral and dental infections with anaerobic bacteria: Clinical features, predominant pathogens, and treatment. Clin Infect 16(Suppl 4):S304, 1993.
11. Gordon DF, Jong BB: Indigenous flora from human saliva. Appl Microbiol 61:428, 1968.
12. Hampp EG, Mergenhagen SEL: Experimental infections with oral spirochetes. J Infect Dis 109:43, 1961.
13. Newman MG: The role of *Bacteroides melaninogenicus* and other anaerobes in periodontal infections. Rev Infect Dis 1:313, 1979.
14. Jones JL, Romig DA: *Eikenella corrodens*: A pathogen in head and neck infections. Oral Surg Oral Med Oral Pathol 48:501, 1979.
15. Tami TA, Parker GS: *Eikenella corrodens*: An emerging pathogen in head and neck infections. Arch Otolaryngol 110:752, 1984.
16. Pizzo LJ: Synergistic necrotizing cellulitis of the head and neck. Am J Otolaryngol 3:452, 1982.
17. Newman MG: Anaerobic oral and dental infections. Rev Infect Dis 1(Suppl):S107, 1984.
18. George LK: The agents of actinomycosis. *In* Balows A, DeHaan RM, Dowell VR Jr (eds): Anaerobic Bacteria: Role in Disease. Springfield, IL, Charles C Thomas, 1974, pp 237–256.
19. Holm P: Studies on the aetiology of human actinomycosis. I. The "other microbes" of actinomycosis and their importance. Acta Pathol Microbiol Scand 27:736, 1950.
20. Holt GR, Tinsley PP Jr: Peritonsillar abscesses in children. Laryngoscope 91:1226, 1981.
21. Passy V: Pathogenesis of peritonsillar abscess. Laryngoscope 104:185, 1994.
22. Portman M, Ingall D, Westenfelder G, et al: Peritonsillar abscess complicating infectious mononucleosis. J Pediatr 104:742, 1984.
23. Jousimies-Somer H, Savolainen S, Ylikoski J: Bacteriologic findings in peritonsillar abscess. Clin Infect Dis 16(Suppl 4):S292, 1993.
24. Brodsky L, Sobie SR, Korwin D, et al: A clinical prospective study of peritonsillar abscess in children. Laryngoscope 98:780, 1988.
25. Savolainen S, Jousimies-Somer HR, Makitie AA, Ylikoski JS: Peritonsillar abscess. Clinical and microbiologic aspects and treatment regimens. Arch Otolaryngol Head Neck Surg 119:521, 1993.
26. Herzon FS, Aldrige JM: Peritonsillar abscess: Needle aspiration. Otolaryngol Head Neck Surg 89:910, 1981.
27. Schechter GL, Sly DE, Roper AL, et al: Changing face of treatment of peritonsillar abscess. Laryngoscope 92:657, 1982.
28. Spires JR, Owens JJ, Woodson GE, et al: Treatment of peritonsil-

lar abscess. A prospective study of aspiration vs. incision and drainage. Arch Otolaryngol Head Neck Surg 113:984, 1987.
29. Stringer SP, Schaefer SD, Close LG: A randomized trial for outpatient management of peritonsillar abscess. Arch Otolaryngol Head Neck Surg 114:298, 1988.
30. Maisel RH: Peritonsillar abscess: Tonsil antibiotic levels in patients treated by acute abscess surgery. Laryngoscope 92:80, 1982.
31. Wolf M, Even-Chen I, Kronenberg J: Peritonsillar abscess: Repeated needle aspiration versus incision and drainage. Ann Otol Rhinol Laryngol 103:554, 1994.
32. Herbild O, Barding P: Peritonsilar abscess: Recurrence rate and treatment. Arch Otolaryngol 107:540, 1981.
33. Wenig BL, Shikowitz MJ, Abramson AL: Necrotizing fasciitis as a lethal complication of peritonsillar abscess. Laryngoscope 94:1576, 1984.
34. von Ludwig FW: Eine neue Art von Halsentzuendung. Med Correspond Blatt Wurtemberg Arztl Ver 6:21, 1836.
35. Moreland LW, Corey J, McKenzie R: Ludwig's angina. Report of a case and review of the literature. Arch Intern Med 148:461, 1988.
36. Bartlett JG: Bacteriologic patterns in infections of the head and neck. *In* Finegold SM (ed): First United States Metronidazole Conference—Proceedings from a Symposium. Tarpon Springs, FL, Biochemical Information Corporation, 1982.
37. Horn J, Bender BS, Bartlett JG: Role of anaerobic bacteria in perimandibular space infections. Ann Otol Rhinol Laryngol Suppl 154:34, 1991.
38. Williams AC, Guralnick WC: The diagnosis and treatment of Ludwig's angina. A report of twenty cases. N Engl J Med 228:443, 1943.
39. Juang YC, Cheng DL, Wang LS, et al: Ludwig's angina: An analysis of 14 cases. Scand J Infect Dis 21:121, 1989.
40. Allen D, Loughnan TE, Ord RA: A re-evaluation of the role of tracheostomy in Ludwig's angina. J Oral Maxillofac Surg 43:436, 1985.
41. Sethi OS, Stanley RE: Deep neck abscesses—Changing trends. J Laryngol Otol 108:138, 1994.
42. Beck AL: Deep neck infections. Ann Otol Rhinol Laryngol 56:439, 722, 1947.
43. Beck AL: Influence of chemotherapeutic and antibiotic drugs on incidence and course of deep neck infections. Ann Otol Rhinol Laryngol 61:515, 1952.
44. Ungkanont K, Yellon RF, Weissman JL, et al: Head and neck space infections in infants and children. Otolaryngol Head Neck Surg 112:375, 1995.
45. Brown JM: Acute retropharyngeal abscess in children. Laryngoscope 29:9, 1919.
46. Smith JE: Retropharyngeal abscess with reference to abnormally large percentage of adult cases. Ann Otol Rhinol Laryngol 47:490, 1940.
47. Bryan CS, King BG Jr, Bryant RE: Retropharyngeal infection in adults. Arch Intern Med 134:126, 1974.
48. Davidson M: Abscesses of the retropharyngeal spaces in adults. Laryngoscope 59:1146, 1949.
49. Heath LK, Peirce TH: Retropharyngeal abscess following endotracheal intubation. Chest 72:776, 1977.
50. Prado VM, Garcia M, De Sousa RM, Formigoni GG: Retropharyngeal abscess after adenoidectomy. Ear Nose Throat J 74:54, 1995.
51. Faidas A, Ferguson JV, Nelson JE, et al: Cervical vertebral osteomyelitis presenting as retropharyngeal abscess. Clin Infect Dis 18:992, 1994.
52. Barrat GE, Koopman CF Jr, Coulthard SW: Retropharyngeal abscess—A ten-year experience. Laryngoscope 94:455, 1984.
53. Brook I: Microbiology of retropharyngeal abscess in children. Am J Dis Child 141:202, 1987.
54. Har-El G, Aroesty JH, Shaha A, Lucente FE: Changing trends in deep neck abscess: A retrospective study of 110 patients. Oral Surg Oral Med Oral Pathol 77:446, 1994.
55. Thompson JW, Cohen SR, Reddix P: Retropharyngeal abscess in children: A retrospective and historical analysis. Laryngoscope 98:589, 1988.
56. Gaglani MJ, Edwards MS: Clinical indicators of retropharyngeal abscess. Am J Emerg Med 13:333, 1995.
57. Kaplan MJ, Eavey RD: Calcific tendinitis of the longus colli muscle. Ann Otol Rhinol Laryngol 93:215, 1984.
58. Ring D, Vaccaro AR, Scuderi G, et al: Acute calcific retropharyngeal tendinitis. Clinical presentation and pathological characterization. J Bone Joint Surg Am 76:1636, 1994.
59. Takao M, Ido M, Hamaguchi K, et al: Descending necrotizing mediastinitis secondary to retropharyngeal abscess. Eur Respir J 7:1716, 1994.
60. al-Ebrahim KE: Descending necrotizing mediastinitis: A case report and review of the literature. Eur J Cardiothorac Surg 9:161, 1995.
61. Civen R, Vaisman ML, Finegold SM: Peritonsillar abscess, mediastinitis, and non-clostridial anaerobic myonecrosis: A case report. Clin Infect Dis 16(Suppl 4):S299, 1993.
62. Watanabe M, Ohshika U, Aoki T, et al: Empyema and mediastinitis complicating retropharyngeal abscess. Thorax 49:1179, 1994.
63. Pearse HE: Mediastinitis following cervical suppuration. Ann Surg 108:588, 1938.
64. Howell HS, Prinz RA, Pickelman JR: Anaerobic mediastinitis. Surg Gynecol Obstet 143:353, 1976.
65. Thompson JW, Cohen SR, Reddix P: Retropharyngeal abscess in children: A retrospective and historical analysis. Laryngoscope 98:589, 1988.
66. Salinger S, Pearlman SJ: Hemorrhage from pharyngeal and peritonsillar abscesses. Arch Otolaryngol 18:464, 1933.
67. Mosher HP: The submaxillary fossa approach to deep pus in the neck. Trans Am Acad Ophthalmol Otolaryngol 34:19, 1929.
68. Alexander DW, Leonard JR, Trail ML: Vascular complications of deep neck abscesses. Laryngoscope 78:361, 1968.
69. McCurdy JA, MacInnis EL, Hays LL: Fatal mediastinitis after a dental infection. J Oral Surg 35:726, 1977.
70. Long JW: Excision of internal jugular vein for streptococci: Thrombosis of vein and cavernous sinus causing paralysis of orbital muscles. Surg Gynecol Obstet 14:86, 1912.
71. Mosher HP: Deep cervical abscess and thrombosis of the internal jugular vein. Laryngoscope 30:365, 1920.
72. Boharas S: Postanginal sepsis. Arch Intern Med 71:844, 1943.
73. Lustig LR, Cusick BC, Cheung SW, Lee KC: Lemierre's syndrome: Two cases of postanginal sepsis. Otolaryngol Head Neck Surg 112:767, 1995.
74. Hughes CE, Spear RK, Shinabarger CE, Tuna IC: Septic pulmonary emboli complicating mastoiditis: Lemierre's syndrome revisited. Clin Infect Dis 18:633, 1994.
75. Seidenfeld SM, Sutker WL, Luby JP: *Fusobacterium necrophorum* septicemia following oropharyngeal infection. JAMA 248:1348, 1982.
76. Goldhagen J, Alford BA, Prewitt LH, et al: Suppurative thrombophlebitis of the internal jugular vein: Report of three cases and review of the pediatric literature. Pediatr Infect Dis J 7:410, 1988.
77. Celikel TH, Mhuthuswamy PP: Septic pulmonary emboli secondary to internal jugular vein phlebitis (postanginal sepsis) caused by *Eikenella corrodens*. Am Rev Respir Dis 130:510, 1984.
78. Raad II, Sabbagh MF, Caranasos GJ: Acute bacterial sialadenitis: A study of 29 cases and review. Rev Infect Dis 12:591, 1990.
79. Lamey PJ, Boyle MA, MacFarlane TW, et al: Acute suppurative parotitis in outpatients: Microbiologic and posttreatment sialographic findings. Oral Surg Oral Med Oral Pathol 63:37, 1987.
80. Krippaehne WW, Hunt TK, Dunphy JE: Acute suppurative parotitis: A study of 161 cases. Ann Surg 156:251, 1962.
81. Carlson RG, Glas WW: Acute suppurative parotitis. Twenty-eight cases at a county hospital. Arch Surg 86:659, 1963.
82. Brook I, Finegold SM: Acute suppurative parotitis caused by anaerobic bacteria: Report of two cases. Pediatrics 62:1019, 1978.
83. Anthes WH, Blaser MJ, Reller LB: Acute suppurative parotitis associated with anaerobic bacteremia. Am J Clin Pathol 75:260, 1981.
84. Pruett TL, Simmons RL: Nosocomial gram-negative bacillary parotitis. JAMA 251:252, 1984.
85. Bissell P, Glew RH, Liland JB: Parotitis associated with *Eikenella corrodens* in a healthy adult. Arch Otolaryngol 109:772, 1983.
86. Howlett JG, Somlo F, Kalz F: A new syndrome of parotitis with herpangina caused by coxsackie virus. Can Med Assoc J 77:5, 1957.
87. Krilov LR, Swenson P: Acute parotitis associated with influenza A infection. J Infect Dis 152:853, 1985.
88. Bloom HH, Johnson KM, Jacobsen R, Chanock RM: Recovery

of parainfluenza viruses from adults with upper respiratory illness. Am J Hyg (Epidemiol) 74:50, 1961.
89. Zollar LM, Mufson MA: Acute parotitis associated with parainfluenza 3 virus infection. Am J Dis Child 119:147, 1970.
90. Lewis JM, Utz JP: Orchitis, parotitis and meningoencephalitis due to lymphocytic choriomeningitis virus. N Engl J Med 265:776, 1961.
91. Henson D, Siegel SE, Fucillo DA, et al: Cytomegalovirus infections during acute childhood leukemia. J Infect Dis 126:469, 1972.
92. Rubinstein A, Sicklick M, Gupta A, et al: Acquired immunodeficiency with reversed T4/T8 ratios in infants born to promiscuous and drug-addicted mothers. JAMA 249:2350, 1983.
93. Lepage P, Van de Perre P, Van Vliet G, et al: Clinical and endocrinologic manifestations in perinatally human immunodeficiency virus type 1–infected children aged 5 years or older. Am J Dis Child 145:1248, 1991.
94. Colebunders R, Francis H, Mann JM, et al: Parotid swelling during human immunodeficiency virus infection. Arch Otolaryngol Head Neck Surg 114:330, 1988.
95. Redleaf MI, Bauer CA, Robinson RA: Fine-needle detection of cytomegalovirus parotitis in a patient with acquired immunodeficiency syndrome. Arch Otolaryngol Head Neck Surg 120:414, 1994.
96. Eilon A, Deutsch E, Zelig S: Hyperuricemia: A possible etiologic factor in chronic recurrent parotitis. Laryngoscope 92:1181, 1982.
97. Iko BO: Computed tomography and sialography of chronic pyogenic parotitis. Br J Radiol 57:1083, 1984.
98. O'Connell JE, George MK, Speculand B, Pahor AL: Mycobacterial infection of the parotid gland: An unusual cause of parotid swelling. J Laryngol Otol 107:561, 1993.
99. Patel PK, Seitchik MW: *Actinobacillus actinomycetemcomitans*: A new cause for granuloma of the parotid gland and buccal space. Plast Reconstr Surg 77:476, 1986.
100. Jonckheer T, Dab I, Van de Perre P, et al: Cluster of HTLV-III/LAV infection in an African family (Letter). Lancet 1:400, 1985.
101. Arriaga MA, Myers EN: The surgical management of chronic parotitis. Laryngoscope 100:1270, 1990.
102. Schultz PW, Woods JE: Subtotal parotidectomy in the treatment of chronic sialadenitis. Ann Plast Surg 11:459, 1983.

49

Infections of the Sinuses and Parameningeal Structures

Anthony W. Chow

SINUS INFECTIONS

Sinusitis, an inflammation of the mucosal lining of the paranasal sinuses, is a common disorder in both children and adults. Approximately 0.5% of upper respiratory tract infections of children are complicated by acute sinusitis,[1] and 0.02% of the adult population have chronic sinusitis.[2] A clear understanding of the anatomy, pathophysiology, manifestations, and etiology is essential for early diagnosis and effective treatment of sinusitis and for the prevention of life-threatening complications and chronic sequelae.

Anatomic Considerations and Pathophysiology

The paranasal sinuses are air-filled cavities lined by ciliated pseudocolumnar epithelium. They are connected one to another through small tubular openings, the sinus ostia, which drain into various regions of the nasal cavity (Fig. 49–1). The frontal, anterior ethmoidal, and maxillary sinuses open into the middle meatus; the posterior ethmoidal and sphenoidal sinuses open into the superior meatus.

The ostium of the maxillary sinus is at an obtuse angle toward the roof (see Fig. 49–1), so this sinus does not empty well in the erect posture but drains best when the patient is lying on the side opposite the affected sinus. The floor of the maxillary sinus directly adjoins the maxillary bone in which reside the apices of the first, second, and third molar teeth; hence, extraction or root infection of these teeth is a frequent cause of maxillary sinusitis. Furthermore, because the superior alveolar nerves (branches of the maxillary nerve) supply both the molar teeth and the mucous membranes of the sinus, maxillary sinusitis may frequently present as a toothache. Extension of infection from the maxillary sinus into the adjacent structures may result in osteomyelitis of the facial bones, including prolapse of the orbital antral wall with retroorbital cellulitis, proptosis, and ophthalmoplegia. Direct intracranial extension from the maxillary sinus is rare, except in rhinocerebral mucormycosis and other invasive fungal sinusitides.

The frontal sinus is supplied by the supraorbital branch of the ophthalmic division of the trigeminal nerve. Thus, headache is a prominent symptom of frontal sinusitis. Owing to the rich vascular supply in this area, infection may readily extend intracranially by the diploic veins to result in epidural abscess, subdural empyema, brain abscess, meningitis, or cavernous sinus thrombosis (Fig. 49–2). Frontal sinusitis may also result in thrombosis of the superior sagittal sinus, which arises in the roof of the frontal air sinuses. Extension of infection into bone can lead to Pott puffy tumor, whereas orbital extension may lead to periorbital cellulitis.

The ethmoidal sinuses are separated from the orbital cavity

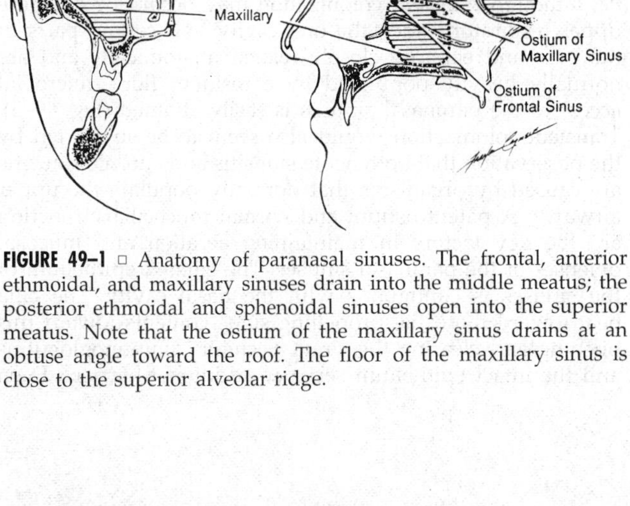

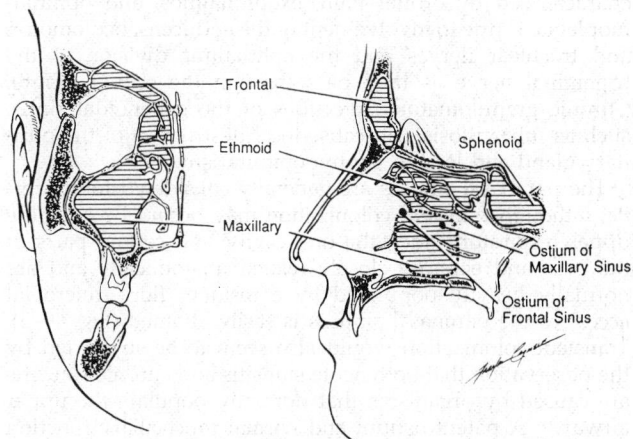

FIGURE 49–1 □ Anatomy of paranasal sinuses. The frontal, anterior ethmoidal, and maxillary sinuses drain into the middle meatus; the posterior ethmoidal and sphenoidal sinuses open into the superior meatus. Note that the ostium of the maxillary sinus drains at an obtuse angle toward the roof. The floor of the maxillary sinus is close to the superior alveolar ridge.

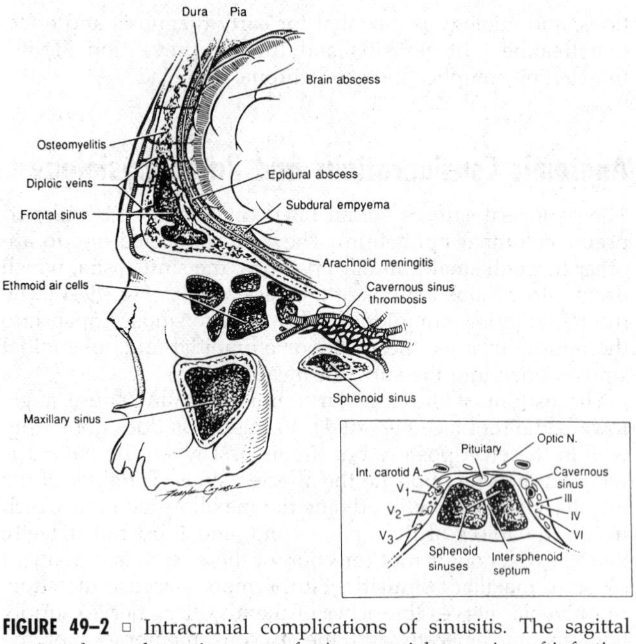

FIGURE 49–2 ▫ Intracranial complications of sinusitis. The sagittal section shows the major routes for intracranial extension of infection either directly or by the vascular supply. Note the proximity of the diploic veins to the frontal sinus and of the cavernous sinuses to the sphenoidal sinus. The coronal section demonstrates the structures adjoining the sphenoidal sinus.

by a paper-thin orbital plate. Perforation of the plate allows direct spread of infection into the retroorbital space. Ethmoidal sinusitis can also spread to the superior sagittal vein or the cavernous venous sinus (see Fig. 49–2).

The sphenoidal sinus also drains through an opening at an obtuse angle anteriorly (see Fig. 49–2). Thus, this sinus empties only when the head is bent forward and does not drain well in the erect posture. The sphenoidal sinus occupies the body of the sphenoid bone in proximity to the pituitary gland above; the optic nerve and optic chiasma in front; and the internal carotids, the cavernous sinuses, and the temporal lobes of the brain on each side (see Fig. 49–2). Thus, sphenoidal sinusitis can spread locally to cause cavernous sinus thrombosis, meningitis, temporal lobe abscess, and orbital fissure syndromes. The superior orbital fissure syndrome, characterized by orbital pain, exophthalmos, and ophthalmoplegia, is due to involvement of the abducens, oculomotor, and trochlear nerves and the ophthalmic division of the trigeminal nerve as they pass through the orbital fissure. Chronic granulomatous infections of the sphenoidal sinus, such as tuberculosis, can cause local destruction of the pituitary gland and lead to panhypopituitarism.

The paranasal sinuses are generally considered to be sterile, although transient colonization may occur.[3] Because the upper respiratory tract, the oral cavity, and certain parts of the eyes and ears are closely related anatomically and are normally heavily populated by a resident flora, microbial access to the paranasal sinuses is easily attained (Fig. 49–3). Transient colonization would also seem to be supported by the observation that both acute sinusitis and chronic sinusitis are caused by organisms that normally populate the upper airway.[4–6] A patent ostium and normal mucociliary function are the key factors in maintaining aeration and mucosal defenses of the paranasal sinuses. The ciliated epithelium of the sinuses is contiguous with the nasal cavity. The cilia beat toward the ostia, propelling sinus contents toward this opening and clearing the sinus. Secretory immunoglobulins and the intact epithelium serve as additional barriers. Even

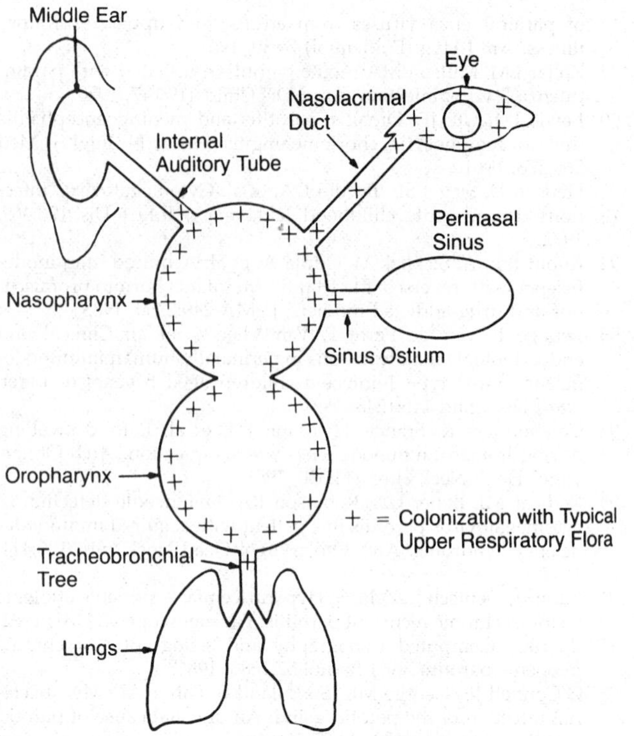

FIGURE 49–3 ▫ Diagrammatic illustration of the anatomic relationship of head and neck structures and distribution of the indigenous flora. (From Todd JK: Bacteriology and clinical relevance of nasopharyngeal and oropharyngeal cultures. Pediatr Infect Dis 3:159–163, 1984.)

if microorganisms have adhered to and penetrated the epithelium, continuous shedding of the epithelial cells serves to further deter microbial invasion and contributes to mucosal self-cleaning. Conditions that affect the patency of the sinus ostia, the normal mucociliary function of the sinus epithelium, or immune defenses of the upper airways or events that facilitate direct introduction of microorganisms into the paranasal sinuses are the key predisposing factors to sinus infection (Table 49–1). Such factors include viral upper respi-

TABLE 49–1 ■ Factors That Predispose to Sinusitis

Impaired mucociliary function
Viral upper respiratory tract infection
Cold or dry air
Chemicals, drugs
Cystic fibrosis
Ciliary dysmotility syndrome
Obstruction of sinus ostia
Viral upper respiratory tract infection
Allergic rhinitis
Rhinitis medicamentosa
Anatomic abnormalities (e.g., nasal polyps, deviated nasal septum, foreign body, tumors)
Immune defects
Immunoglobulin A deficiency
Immunoglobulin G2 or G4 subclass deficiency
Acquired immunodeficiency syndrome
Wegener granulomatosis
Diabetes mellitus
Increased risk of microbial invasion of the sinuses
Odontogenic infections
Nasotracheal intubation
Head trauma
Swimming or diving
Cocaine sniffing

ratory tract infections,[7] allergies,[8] the immotile cilia syndrome, alterations in mucus (as in cystic fibrosis), selective immunoglobulin deficiencies (IgG2, IgG4 subclass, or IgA), and acquired immunodeficiency syndrome.[9, 10]

Obstruction or reduction in the patency of the ostia appears to be the most important predisposing factor. The size of the ostia decreases in recumbency.[11] In addition, mucosal inflammation and anatomic abnormalities (e.g., polyps and deviated septum) can influence ostia size. Gas exchange and oxygen content of the sinus cavity are dependent on the patency and size of the ostium.[12] With obstruction and reduced ventilation, the oxygen tension falls and there is a concomitant rise in carbon dioxide tension. Growth of anaerobic and facultative bacteria is favored under these conditions, and polymorphonuclear and phagocytic cell function is impaired. When the ostia are obstructed, as during upper respiratory tract infections, ventilation and drainage are impaired. The retained secretions provide an ideal environment for microbial replication. Further, proteolytic products released by granulocytes and other inflammatory exudates lead to mucosal destruction and disrupt the normal epithelial barrier. After repeated infections, the ciliated epithelium of the sinuses becomes irreversibly replaced by stratified squamous epithelium. Thus, an effective clearance mechanism by mucociliary activity is lost, and chronic or recurrent infection may ensue.

Certain activities or events may repeatedly traumatize the nasal mucosa and facilitate microbial invasion of the paranasal sinuses. These include head trauma, swimming and diving, cocaine sniffing, and nasotracheal or nasopharyngeal intubation. Transnasal intubation is an important cause of nosocomial sinusitis.[13–15] Dental extraction and periapical infections of the maxillary molar teeth are particularly important causes of maxillary sinusitis. Odontogenic sources may account for 5% to 10% of acute maxillary sinusitis[16] and more than 40% of chronic maxillary sinusitis.[2]

Clinical Manifestations and Diagnosis

The clinical manifestations of sinusitis vary greatly, depending on duration of infection (i.e., acute or chronic) and age of the patient (i.e., child or adult).

Acute Sinusitis

Acute sinusitis is defined as inflammation of the sinuses associated with symptoms lasting 4 weeks or less.[17] Symptoms of acute sinusitis are often difficult to distinguish from those of the common cold or allergic (vasomotor) rhinitis. This is further complicated in that there appears to be an association between allergic rhinitis and sinusitis,[18, 19] raising the possibility that chronic allergic rhinitis may predispose to sinus disease and that some patients with symptoms of sinusitis may have been misdiagnosed as having allergic rhinitis. The clinical manifestations of acute sinusitis in children may be distinct from those of adults. Wald and coworkers[20] prospectively evaluated 30 children with radiographic evidence of acute maxillary sinusitis. The most common symptoms were cough (80%) and nasal discharge (76%). These symptoms were the chief complaint in approximately 30% of cases. Fever was present in 63%. Headache, pain, and swelling, common presentations in adults, were present in only 30% to 33% of these children. Sore throat was a major complaint in 23%. Parents often noticed malodorous breath in preschoolers (50% of cases) who had neither signs of pharyngitis nor poor dental hygiene. In adults, purulent postnasal discharge and facial pain over the affected sinus that worsens with movement or percussion are the cardinal symptoms.[11, 16] Fever occurs in less than 50% of cases.

The combination of certain clinical findings, particularly history of maxillary toothache, colored nasal discharge and poor response to decongestants, and physical signs of purulent nasal secretions and abnormal transillumination findings, greatly enhances the diagnostic probability of acute sinusitis.[21] Hyposmia, jaw pain with mastication, nasal congestion, and a history of recent upper respiratory tract infection are other manifestations. Pain on percussion of all the molar teeth of the upper jaw is characteristic of maxillary sinusitis; more localized tooth tenderness points to an odontogenic source of infection. In ethmoidal sinusitis, edema of the eyelids and excessive tearing may be a prominent feature. Retroorbital pain and proptosis indicate extension of infection into the orbit. Anterior rhinoscopy may reveal hyperemic and edematous nasal turbinates, often with purulent discharge from the middle meatus where the orifices of the maxillary, frontal, and anterior ethmoidal sinuses enter the intranasal cavity. Severe intractable headache is dominant in sphenoidal sinusitis and can mimic ophthalmic migraine or trigeminal neuralgia. Neurologic deficit with hypoesthesia or hyperesthesia of the ophthalmic or maxillary dermatomes of the trigeminal nerve may be detected in one third of the patients.[22] A depression of the mental status accompanied by clinical signs of meningeal irritation, ptosis, chemosis, proptosis, and paralysis of the third, fourth, and sixth cranial nerves suggests that the infection has extended to the cavernous sinus.

In patients with nosocomial sinusitis secondary to prolonged nasotracheal intubation, the clinical features, apart from unexplained fever, may be relatively silent. The presence of purulent rhinorrhea or a middle-ear effusion, as determined by pneumatic otoscopy, may be the only physical finding. A high index of suspicion and appropriate diagnostic procedures are required for early recognition of this entity.[13, 15] Sinusitis in patients infected with human immunodeficiency virus is relatively common. Patients with $CD4^+$ cell counts less than 200/mm^3 are susceptible to infection involving multiple sinuses that responds incompletely to antibiotic therapy, often resulting in chronic sinusitis.[9]

Subacute and Chronic Sinusitis

Subacute sinusitis is defined as inflammation of the sinuses associated with symptoms lasting between 1 and 3 months; chronic sinusitis is associated with symptoms of more than 3 months' duration.[17] Symptoms associated with subacute or chronic sinusitis are usually less intense but more protracted than are those of acute sinusitis. Fever is uncommon. Fatigue, general malaise, and an ill-defined feeling of unwellness and irritability can be more prominent than local symptoms of nasal congestion, facial pain, or postnasal drip. Chronic sinusitis may mimic asthma, allergic rhinitis, or chronic bronchitis. Physical findings may be subtle. Results of anterior rhinoscopy and mirror examination may be normal, although often there is evidence of posterior nasal discharge. Melen and colleagues[2] observed that 40% of 198 patients with chronic maxillary sinusitis had a dental cause. Marginal periodontitis and periapical granuloma together accounted for 83% of their cases of chronic odontogenic sinusitis. Nasal polyps were found in 16% of all patients with chronic maxillary sinusitis.

Diagnostic Procedures

Because the symptoms and signs of sinusitis are often nonspecific, additional diagnostic procedures may be helpful.

Transillumination

Transillumination should be performed in a completely darkened room. The frontal sinus is examined by placing a high-intensity light source inferior to the medial border of the supraorbital ridge to evaluate the symmetry of the blush bilaterally. Examination of the maxillary sinus is accomplished by placing the light source over the midpoint of the inferior orbital rim and examining for transmission of light through the hard palate with the patient's mouth open. The finding of complete opacity is highly indicative of infection. Conversely, normal light transmission indicates that no infection is present. The finding of reduced or "dull" transmission is less helpful, because only a quarter of such patients are found to have active infection as determined by sinus puncture.[23] Transillumination is less useful for chronic sinusitis because of persistent mucosal abnormalities. Transillumination is also less informative in children younger than 6 years. Wald and colleagues[24] found that the procedure could not be performed in 24% of cases, and the results were equivocal in another 15%. Overall, there was concordance with radiographic findings in 41% of cases and discordance in 20%.

Radiography

Radiographic examination is a sensitive method for diagnosing acute sinusitis in adults and in children older than 1 year (Fig. 49–4). Abnormal radiographic findings (e.g., complete opacification, air-fluid level, or mucosal thickening of 4 mm or more in children and 5 mm or more in adults) are predictive of infection as determined by sinus puncture in 75% of cases, whereas a normal radiograph correlates with a normal aspirate in 80% of cases.[23] Four standard radiographic views are used: occipitomental (Waters) projection for the maxillary sinus, posteroanterior (Caldwell) projection for the ethmoidal and frontal sinuses, and lateral and submentovertex projections for the sphenoidal sinus. Radiographic examination is less useful in chronic sinusitis because of persistent abnormalities,[2] and in infants before age 1 year because of redundant sinus mucosa and asymmetry of facial bone or sinus development.[1] An orthopantograph is indicated if odontogenic infection is suspected.

Ultrasonography

The alleged advantages of ultrasonography over radiography are its nonionizing radiation and ability to better discriminate between mucosal thickening and retained secretions.[25] Ultrasonography may be particularly useful in predicting the presence of fluid in patients whose radiographs show partial or complete opacification. In general, however, ultrasonography is no better than radiography. Furthermore, young children present technical and diagnostic difficulties.[20] More experience is required to assess the diagnostic value of ultrasonography in children younger than 3 years.

Computed Tomography and Magnetic Resonance Imaging

Both computed tomography (CT) (see Fig. 49–4) and magnetic resonance imaging (MRI) are extremely sensitive radiographic techniques for diagnosing sinus disease.[26, 27] MRI has been shown to give better paranasal sinus detail than CT, but both are excellent for delineating masses in the sinuses and adjoining structures. These procedures are best reserved for the investigation of intracranial suppurative complications of both acute and chronic sinusitis.

Sinus Aspiration

A sinus puncture with aspiration is the only means to obtain reliable material for microbiologic evaluation. It should be performed in ill or immunocompromised patients and in those who have complicated sinusitis when precise identification of the microorganism is necessary (Table 49–2). Through a puncture, the maxillary sinus can be accessed intranasally below the inferior turbinate and the frontal sinus below the infraorbital rim of the eye. Thorough cleansing of the puncture site with an antiseptic such as povidone-iodine is important to avoid contaminating the specimen with surface bacteria. If no fluid is obtained, 1 mL of sterile normal saline solution without bactericidal preservative is instilled, and the washings are reaspirated. Specimens should be sent for leukocyte count, Gram stain, and cultures of aerobes, anaerobes, fungi, and mycobacteria. Viral cultures should be

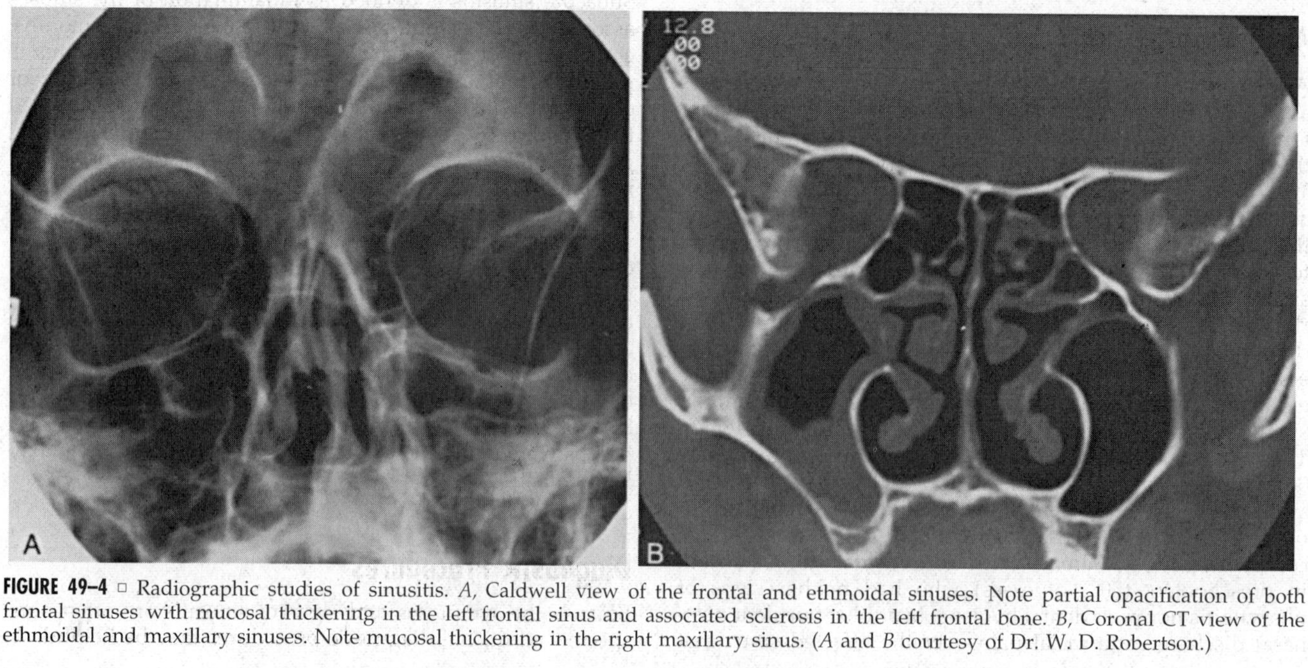

FIGURE 49–4 □ Radiographic studies of sinusitis. *A,* Caldwell view of the frontal and ethmoidal sinuses. Note partial opacification of both frontal sinuses with mucosal thickening in the left frontal sinus and associated sclerosis in the left frontal bone. *B,* Coronal CT view of the ethmoidal and maxillary sinuses. Note mucosal thickening in the right maxillary sinus. (*A* and *B* courtesy of Dr. W. D. Robertson.)

TABLE 49–2 ■ Indications for Sinus Aspiration

Severe symptoms or toxic condition
Failure of adequate or appropriate antimicrobial therapy to improve patient's condition
Suppurative complications
Immunocompromised host
Nosocomial sinusitis
Diagnostic uncertainty (e.g., opacification of sinus in a patient with fever of undetermined origin and no other findings)

obtained when they are available and indicated. With the appropriate technique, more than 76% of such specimens yield positive cultures in acute maxillary sinusitis.[6] Quantitative cultures are useful in distinguishing between colonization and contamination from true infection. Bacterial counts of 10^3 colony-forming units per milliliter correlate strongly with antral leukocyte counts of $5000/mm^3$ or more than 20 cells per oil-immersion field.[6, 28] If organisms are seen with a Gram stain of antral secretions, the bacterial morphotype can give a presumptive diagnosis in up to 90% of cases.[6] A diluted injection aspirate has a higher probability of nasal contamination.

Endoscopic Sinoscopy

Sinoscopy allows direct visualization of the sinonasal tract as well as of the sinus mucosa.[29] A flexible endoscope provides a detailed examination of the upper nasal cavities and the posterior nasopharynx. The application of local anesthetic and decongestants to the natural ostium of the maxillary sinus and anterior ethmoids can also reduce edema and further encourage drainage. The maxillary ostium is rarely visualized during endoscopy, however, because it is hidden in the ethmoid infundibulum located posterolateral to the uncinate process. Accessory sinus ostia, which are located in the anterior portion of the middle meatus, are readily seen, as are the eustachian tube orifices.[30] A rigid endoscope is more suited for endoscopic sinus surgery. Thus, sinoscopy offers the added advantage of accessibility to mucosal biopsy for histopathologic confirmation of diagnosis and removal of localized ostial obstructions.[31] It is an invaluable tool in the management of chronic sinusitis.

Causal Agents

The precise microbial agent of sinusitis can be determined only by direct aspiration or injection wash of the sinus cavity. Surface cultures of the nasal vestibule or the nasopharynx are unreliable owing to regular contamination by the resident microflora.[1, 18, 32] Cultures obtained directly from the middle meatus during sinus endoscopy have a low positive predictive value (38%) and overall accuracy (49%) compared with sinus aspiration[33] and are inadequate to guide antimicrobial therapy.

The agents of sinusitis vary according to the chronicity of infection and the patient's age and underlying conditions.[5, 16] *Streptococcus pneumoniae* and nonencapsulated *Haemophilus influenzae* are responsible for approximately 70% of cases of acute sinusitis in adults; *Branhamella (Moraxella) catarrhalis* in addition to *S. pneumoniae* and *H. influenzae* accounts for two thirds of cases in children (Table 49–3). Anaerobes are uncommonly isolated in acute sinusitis[6] but are the predominant flora in chronic sinusitis.[34, 35] Anaerobes recovered during acute sinusitis suggest an odontogenic source. *Staphylococcus aureus* is a common nasal contaminant and an infrequent cause of acute maxillary sinusitis. In contrast, *S. aureus* together with viridans streptococci and *S. pneumoniae* are the predominant isolates in acute sphenoidal sinusitis.[22] The role of *Chlamydia pneumoniae* (TWAR agent) in acute sinusitis is unclear, but it appears to account for only a small proportion of purulent maxillary sinusitis cases.[36, 37] *Mycoplasma pneumoniae* is an uncommon pathogen in acute sinusitis. Rarely, paranasal sinuses can serve as a cryptic focus of *S. aureus* infection causing toxic shock syndrome.[38] Although antecedent viral upper respiratory tract infection is an important cause of acute sinusitis, viruses (e.g., rhinovirus, influenza virus, parainfluenza virus, adenovirus) are isolated from only 15% of antral aspirates.[5, 39]

Nosocomial sinusitis secondary to head trauma or prolonged nasotracheal intubation is commonly caused by polymicrobial gram-negative bacteria, *S. aureus,* and anaerobes.[13, 40] In patients with cystic fibrosis, *Pseudomonas aeruginosa* and nontypable *H. influenzae* are the most frequent pathogens.[41] Sinusitis in patients infected with human immunodeficiency virus is often due to unusual pathogens, such as *Legionella pneumoniae* and *P. aeruginosa,* and may be more difficult to eradicate.[9, 10]

The bacteriology of chronic sinusitis in both adults and children is characterized by a predominance of respiratory tract anaerobes, including *Bacteroides, Peptostreptococcus, Fusobacterium,* and *Veillonella.*[35] The infection is usually polymicrobial, viridans streptococci and nonencapsulated *H. influenzae* being the major aerobic isolates. Fungal sinusitis is rare, but *Aspergillus, Mucor, Candida* species, *Pseudoallescheria boydii,* and other saprophytic fungi can cause invasive disease in the debilitated host.[11, 42, 43]

Treatment

The goals of therapy for sinusitis are to eradicate the causative pathogens, restore and improve sinus function, provide symptomatic relief, and prevent intracranial complications and chronic sequelae. Although many management options are available (Table 49–4), antibiotics are the mainstay of treatment.

TABLE 49–3 ■ Microbial Causes of Acute Maxillary Sinusitis

MICROBIAL AGENT	PREVALENCE MEAN (RANGE) Adults (%)	Children (%)
Bacteria		
Streptococcus pneumoniae	31 (20–35)	36
Haemophilus influenzae (nonencapsulated)	21 (6–26)	23
S. pneumoniae and *H. influenzae*	5 (1–9)	—
Anaerobes *(Bacteroides, Fusobacterium, Peptostreptococcus, Veillonella)*	6 (0–10)	—
Staphylococcus aureus	4 (0–8)	—
Streptococcus pyogenes	2 (1–3)	2
Branhamella (Moraxella) catarrhalis	2	19
Gram-negative bacteria	9 (0–24)	2
Viruses		
Rhinovirus	15	—
Influenza virus	5	—
Parainfluenza virus	3	2
Adenovirus	—	2

Adapted from Gwaltney JM Jr: Sinusitis. *In* Mandell GL, Douglas RG Jr, Bennett JE (eds): Principles and Practice of Infectious Diseases, ed 3. Churchill Livingstone, New York, 1990.

TABLE 49–4 ■ Management Options for the Treatment of Sinusitis

MEDICAL
- Antimicrobials (oral and parenteral)
- Decongestants (topical and systemic)
- Analgesics
- Antihistamines
- Cromolyn sodium
- Corticosteroids
- Humidification and hydration
- Sinus irrigation (Poretz procedure)

SURGICAL
- Promote drainage
  - Intranasal endoscopic sinoscopy
  - Intranasal antrostomy
  - Ethmoidotomy
  - Frontal sinus trephination
- Remove diseased tissue
  - Caldwell-Luc operation
  - Ethmoidectomy
  - Frontal sinus obliteration
  - Sphenoidectomy
- Correct intranasal, ostial, or other abnormalities
  - Turbinectomy
  - Septal surgery
  - Polypectomy
  - Adenoidectomy
  - Tonsillectomy

Antimicrobial Therapy

The efficacy of antimicrobials for the treatment of acute sinusitis has been established by placebo-controlled clinical trials[24] and by studies that employed pretreatment and posttreatment sinus aspiration.[4] Pretreatment sinus aspirations may not yield a bacterial pathogen in approximately 30% to 40% of patients with acute sinusitis.[4] It is also known that children with acute sinusitis may have a spontaneous clinical cure rate of 40% to 45%.[1] These factors make it difficult to accurately assess the efficacy of any antimicrobial regimen for the treatment of acute sinusitis. The initial choice of antibiotic treatment for acute sinusitis should be selected on an empirical basis, because routine sinus aspiration for specific microbiologic diagnosis is not indicated.[44] In adults, antibiotic therapy is primarily directed against *H. influenzae* and *S. pneumoniae*; in children, therapy should be directed against *B. catarrhalis* in addition. A 10- to 14-day course of ampicillin or amoxicillin may be used initially (Table 49–5). Trimethoprim-sulfamethoxazole and erythromycin-sulfisoxazole are suitable alternatives for penicillin-allergic patients. Tetracycline or erythromycin alone is inadequate for initial treatment of acute sinusitis. Because β-lactamase–producing bacteria among respiratory pathogens have become increasingly common in the United States and Canada (up to 40% among *H. influenzae*, 80% among *B. catarrhalis*, and 30% among respiratory tract anaerobes[5, 45–47]), a case may be made for the selection of a β-lactamase–resistant antibiotic for the initial empirical therapy of acute sinusitis. β-Lactamase–resistant antibiotics, such as amoxicillin-clavulanate, cefaclor, cefuroxime axetil, cefdinir, cefixime, loracarbef, and newer macrolides and quinolones, are also being used with increasing frequency because of the emerging problem of penicillin-resistant pneumococci in different cities within the United States and Canada.[48–52] Nevertheless, several randomized double-blind trials in the recent past have shown similar therapeutic response rates (greater than 80%) comparing ampicillin or amoxicillin with a β-lactamase–resistant antibiotic.[4, 24, 53] Therefore, until the need is clearly demonstrated by further controlled clinical trials, ampicillin or amoxicillin has remained the most commonly prescribed antimicrobial agent during initial therapy of presumed acute bacterial sinusitis in North America. β-Lactamase–resistant antibiotics should be reserved for patients with severe symptoms, patients who are immunocompromised, or those who have failed to respond to other agents despite 48 to 72 hours of antimicrobial therapy. Cefaclor has been associated with inadequate response rates for acute sinusitis in several controlled clinical trials[4] and cannot be recommended as initial empirical therapy. In patients with acute maxillary sinusitis of dental origin, treatment should be directed at mixed anaerobes and streptococci, the common causative organisms,[54] and penicillin and clindamycin are suitable agents.

TABLE 49–5 ■ Antimicrobial Regimens for Acute Sinusitis*

AGENT	ADULTS (ORAL DOSE)	CHILDREN (mg/kg/d)
Ampicillin	500 mg qid	50–100
Amoxicillin	500 mg tid	40
Trimethoprim (80 mg)–sulfamethoxazole (40 mg)	160–800 mg bid	8–40
Erythromycin plus sulfisoxazole	500 mg qid	50
	500 mg qid	150
Amoxicillin clavulanate	500 mg tid	40
Cefuroxime axetil	250 mg bid	45–60
Cefixime	200 mg bid	8
Cefpodoxime proxetil	400 mg bid	10
Loracarbef	400 mg bid	15

*Cefaclor is associated with suboptimal response rates and is not recommended for the empirical treatment of acute bacterial sinusitis; bid, twice daily; qid, four times a day; tid, three times a day.

Patients in whom symptoms persist despite a 10- to 14-day course of first-line antibiotic therapy should receive an additional course of treatment with a β-lactamase–resistant agent. If this regimen fails, a sinus aspirate should be obtained, and further antimicrobial therapy should be guided by culture and sensitivity data. Patients with subacute or recurrent symptoms that fail to respond to this approach should be examined for an underlying disorder (e.g., by endoscopic sinoscopy) and treated with repeated antral lavage in addition to antibiotics before consideration of a surgical approach.

Nosocomial sinusitis should be strongly suspected in patients with prolonged transnasal intubation and presumed to be present if there is also concurrent purulent rhinorrhea or otitis media.[55] In such patients, the nasal tube should be removed and nasal decongestants as well as broad-spectrum antibiotics initiated to cover aerobic gram-negative rods, *S. aureus*, and anaerobes (e.g., cefotaxime, ceftizoxime, imipenem, or piperacillin-tazobactam) while the search is continued for other causes of fever. If fever persists and no other cause is found, CT of the paranasal sinuses should be performed. If CT reveals evidence of sinusitis, maxillary sinus aspiration should be performed and additional antibiotic therapy tailored according to culture results (Fig. 49–5).

Treatment of chronic sinusitis requires surgery to facilitate sinus drainage by creation of an artificial ostium and submucosal resection of diseased tissue.[56] Conservative management with antibiotics alone together with sinus irrigations has yielded satisfactory results in only 34% of cases.[57] Acute exacerbations of infection should be treated in the same way as described before for acute sinusitis.

Specific antimicrobial therapy for fungal sinusitis is required only if the disease is invasive or the patient is severely immunocompromised and the risk for progressive disease is high. Noninvasive disease usually responds to surgical débridement alone. Most patients with invasive disease

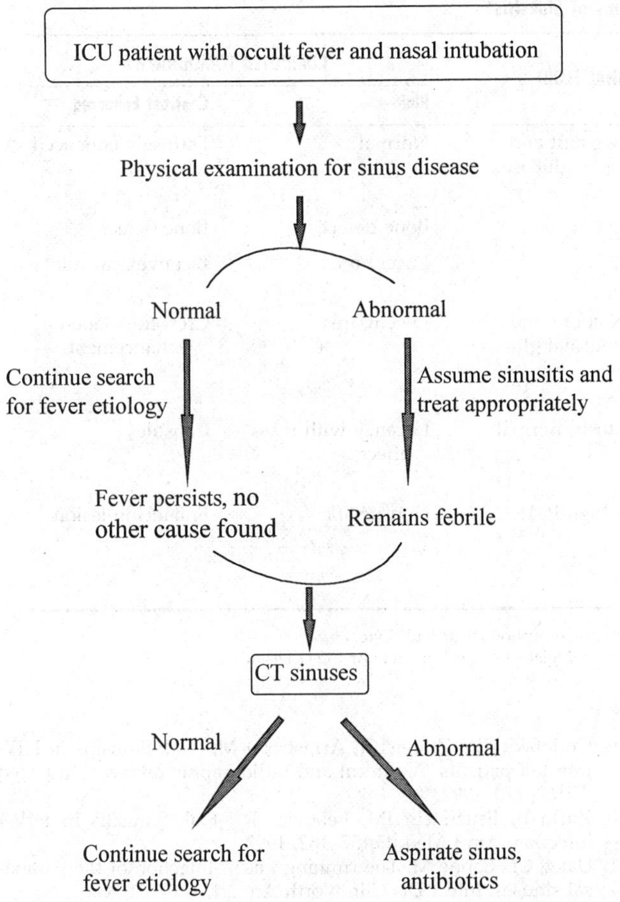

FIGURE 49–5 □ Algorithm for the management of intensive care unit (ICU) patients with occult fever and nasal intubation. (From Deresinski S: Sinusitis in surgical ICU patients. Infect Dis Alert 12:66, 1993.)

should be treated with amphotericin B in cumulative doses exceeding 2 g. The role of azole antifungal agents, such as fluconazole or itraconazole, for invasive fungal sinusitis remains unclear at present.

Supportive Therapy

The role of oral or topical decongestants and antihistamines in the treatment of acute and chronic sinusitis has not been adequately evaluated.[58] Systemic decongestants (e.g., phenylpropanolamine) have been found to increase ostial diameter and reduce symptoms of nasal congestion.[59] Topical decongestants (e.g., phenylephrine or oxymetazoline nose drops) shrink the nasal mucous membrane and provide symptomatic improvement, but use beyond 5 to 7 days may lead to rebound vasodilation and nasal obstruction (rhinitis medicamentosa) and should be avoided.[60] Intranasal steroids, such as beclomethasone or flunisolide, one or two sprays to each nostril three times daily, appear to be useful for chronic or recurrent sinusitis. Use of antihistamines may lead to inspissation of secretions and impair drainage. They should be prescribed only if an allergic component is present. Of interest, studies have suggested that patients with a history of allergic rhinitis or bronchial asthma tend to have more severe sinus disease and that aggressive treatment of sinusitis in such patients may enhance the symptomatic control of asthma.[18, 19, 61] Intranasal spray with cromolyn sodium prevents allergic mediator release and may be associated with fewer side effects than are antihistamines. Repeated sinus irrigation by the Poretz procedure is useful for subacute or chronic sinusitis. The patient is placed in the Trendelenburg position. The nose is first partially filled with normal saline solution, which is then removed by suction through one nostril while the other nostril is occluded. The intent is to irrigate sinuses with partially patent ostia. It is not recommended for untreated acute disease, because there is a potential risk for hematogenous spread of infection.

Surgical Therapy

The surgical treatment of sinusitis is directed toward restoring sinus drainage and removing diseased tissue. It should be reserved for patients who have failed to respond to medical therapy, patients with chronic sinusitis, and patients with life-threatening or established complications. The wide spectrum of surgical procedures available includes intranasal antrostomy, Caldwell-Luc operation, intranasal sphenoethmoidectomy, transantral ethmoidectomy, frontal sinus trephination and obliteration, and endoscopic sinus surgery.[31, 56] In addition, indirect surgical measures to correct intranasal disease and improve sinus drainage include septal and turbinate surgery, polypectomy, adenoidectomy, and tonsillectomy.

Intranasal antrostomy creates a permanent opening through the inferior meatus and provides gravitational drainage of the maxillary sinus. This procedure can be performed with local anesthesia; however, visualization of the antrum is limited, and ability to remove diseased tissue is incomplete. The Caldwell-Luc procedure provides a more direct approach to the antrum as well as to the ethmoidal sinuses and is recommended for more severe disease. An anterior maxillary antrostomy is performed through a sublabial incision. When the interior of the maxillary sinus is visualized and most of the anterior wall resected, the upper medial wall of the maxillary sinus is then approached at a point halfway along the border between the medial and superior walls. A transantral ethmoidectomy can be accomplished at the same time. Bilateral intranasal sphenoethmoidectomy is particularly beneficial in patients with pansinusitis. External approaches to the sinuses allow a more comprehensive procedure, but they require general anesthesia and not uncommonly (3%) are complicated by postoperative facial paresthesias. External sphenoethmoidectomy is an effective operation for the posterior ethmoidal and sphenoidal sinuses. Trephination or obliteration of the frontal sinuses is useful for patients with chronic frontal sinusitis and for those with suppurative complications and intracranial extension of infection.

Intranasal endoscopic sinus surgery has become a treatment of choice for chronic and recurrent sinusitis.[62] It allows improved visualization of the sinuses and removal of localized diseased tissue without unnecessary curettage of normal mucosa. It can be performed with local anesthesia, and relatively inaccessible areas such as the infundibulum of the anterior ethmoidal sinus can be easily visualized. The introduction of endoscopic sinoscopy has precipitated a drastically different approach to the surgical management of recurrent and chronic sinusitis. The contemporary emphasis is clearly on preservation of sinus function by retaining sinus mucosa rather than the conventional practice of radical mucosal resections. It remains to be seen whether the long-term outlook for these infections can be further improved by this approach.

With a combination of medical and surgical treatment, the success rate for chronic maxillary sinusitis is more than 60% of cases after 3.5 years' follow-up.[57]

Complications and Prevention

Fortunately, the suppurative and life-threatening complications of acute and chronic sinusitis have become relatively

TABLE 49–6 ■ The Clinical Spectrum and Investigation of Intracranial Complications of Sinusitis*

COMPLICATION	CLINICAL SIGNS	CEREBROSPINAL FLUID FINDINGS	COMPUTED TOMOGRAPHY	
			Plain	Contrast Enhanced
Meningitis	Headache, fever + + Stiff neck, lethargy + + Rapid death + +	High PMN count and protein; low glucose	Normal	Diffusely enhanced
Osteomyelitis	Pott puffy tumor ±	Normal	Bone defect	Bone defect
Epidural abscess or mucocele	Headache ± Fever ±	Normal	Lucent area	Biconvex capsule
Subdural empyema	Headache + + Convulsions + + Hemiplegia + + Rapid death + +	High PMN count and protein; normal glucose	Lucent area	Crescent-shaped enhancement
Cerebral abscess	Convulsions + Headache + Personality change +	Lymphocytosis; normal glucose	Lucency with mass effect	Capsule
Venous sinus thrombosis (cavernous)	"Picket-fence" fever + + Rapid death + + (orbital edema + +, ocular palsies + +)	Normal or high PMN count	Nonspecific	Enhancing lesion

*±, May or may not be seen; +, seen frequently; + + seen characteristically; PMN, polymorphonuclear leukocyte.
Modified from Fairbanks DNF, Milmoe GJ: Complications and sequelae—An otolaryngologist's perspective. Pediatr Infect Dis 4(Suppl 6):S75, 1985.

infrequent in the postantibiotic era.[63] Owing to the anatomic locations (see Fig. 49–2), the clinical spectrum of such complications is varied (Table 49–6). Management of these suppurative complications requires an aggressive approach, including CT and examination of the cerebrospinal fluid. Antimicrobial therapy should be guided by examination of sinus aspirates and administered parenterally and in high doses to optimize penetration of bone and the blood-brain barrier. A multidisciplinary approach, including specialists in radiology, otolaryngology, neurology, and neurosurgery, is generally required.

Apart from pneumococcal and *H. influenzae* vaccines, there are currently no effective preventive measures for acute or chronic sinusitis. Efforts should be directed to early and aggressive treatment of acute sinusitis, surgical correction of anatomic deformities of the sinus ostia and intranasal structures, promotion of good dental hygiene, and effective control of underlying allergic manifestations.

References

1. Wald ER: Sinusitis in children. N Engl J Med 326:319–323, 1992.
2. Melen I, Lindahl L, Andreasson L, Rundcrantz H: Chronic maxillary sinusitis. Definition, diagnosis and relation to dental infections and nasal polyposis. Acta Otolaryngol 101:320–327, 1986.
3. Sobin J, Engquist S, Nord CE: Bacteriology of the maxillary sinus in healthy volunteers. Scand J Infect Dis 24:633–635, 1992.
4. Gwaltney JM Jr, Scheld WM, Sande MA, Sydnor A: The microbial etiology and antimicrobial therapy of adults with acute community-acquired sinusitis: A fifteen-year experience at the University of Virginia and review of other selected studies. J Allergy Clin Immunol 90:457–462, 1992.
5. Wald ER: Microbiology of acute and chronic sinusitis in children. J Allergy Clin Immunol 90:452–460, 1992.
6. Jousimies-Somer HR, Savolainen S, Ylikoski JS: Bacteriological findings of acute maxillary sinusitis in young adults. J Clin Microbiol 26:1919–1925, 1988.
7. Turner BW, Cail WS, Hendley JO, et al: Physiologic abnormalities in the paranasal sinuses during experimental rhinovirus colds. J Allergy Clin Immunol 90:474–478, 1992.
8. Rossi OV, Pirila T, Laitinen J, Huhti E: Sinus aspirates and radiographic abnormalities in severe attacks of asthma. Intern Arch Allergy Immunol 103:209–213, 1994.
9. Godofsky EW, Zinreich J, Armstrong M, et al: Sinusitis in HIV-infected patients. A clinical and radiographic review. Am J Med 93:163–170, 1992.
10. Zurlo JJ, Feuerstein IM, Lebovics R, et al: Sinusitis in HIV-1 infection. Am J Med 93:157–162, 1992.
11. Daley CL, Sande M: The running nose—Infection of the paranasal sinuses. Infect Dis Clin North Am 2:131–147, 1988.
12. Wagenmann M, Naclerio RM: Anatomic and physiologic considerations in sinusitis. J Allergy Clin Immunol 90:419–423, 1992.
13. Humphrey MA, Simpson GT, Grindlinger GA: Clinical characteristics of nosocomial sinusitis. Ann Otol Rhinol Laryngol 96:687–690, 1987.
14. Holzapfel L, Chevret S, Madinier G, et al: Influence of long-term oro- or nasotracheal intubation on nosocomial maxillary sinusitis and pneumonia: Results of a prospective, randomized, clinical trial. Crit Care Med 21:1132–1138, 1993.
15. Rouby JJ, Laurent P, Gosnach M, et al: Risk factors and clinical relevance of nosocomial maxillary sinusitis in the critically ill. Am J Respir Crit Care Med 150:776–783, 1994.
16. Gwaltney JM Jr: Sinusitis. *In* Mandell GL, Bennett JE, Dolin R (eds): Principles and Practice of Infectious Diseases, ed 4. New York, Churchill Livingstone, 1995, pp 585–590.
17. Bluestone CD: The diagnosis and management of sinusitis in children—Proceedings of a closed conference. Pediatr Infect Dis 4(Suppl 6):S49–S51, 1985.
18. Shapiro GG: Role of allergy in sinusitis. Pediatr Infect Dis 4(Suppl 6):S55–S60, 1985.
19. Spector SL: The role of allergy in sinusitis in adults. J Allergy Clin Immunol 90:518–520, 1992.
20. Wald ER, Milmoe GJ, Bowen AD, et al: Acute maxillary sinusitis in children. N Engl J Med 304:749–754, 1981.
21. Williams JW Jr, Simel DL, Roberts L, Samsa GP: Clinical evaluation for sinusitis: Making the diagnosis by history and physical examination. Ann Intern Med 117:705–710, 1992.
22. Lew D, Southwick FS, Montgomery WW, et al: Sphenoid sinusitis. A review of 30 cases. N Engl J Med 309:1149–1154, 1983.
23. Gwaltney JM Jr, Sydnor A Jr, Sande MA: Etiology and antimicrobial treatment of acute sinusitis. Ann Otol Rhinol Laryngol 90(Suppl 84):68–71, 1981.
24. Wald ER, Chipnonis D, Ledesma-Medina J: Comparative effectiveness of amoxicillin and amoxicillin-clavulanate potassium in acute paranasal sinus infections in children. A double-blind, placebo-controlled trial. Pediatrics 77:795–800, 1986.
25. Bruce HM: Diagnosis of sinusitis in adults: History, physical examination, nasal cytology, echo, and rhinoscope. J Allergy Clin Immunol 90:436–441, 1992.

26. Diament MJ: The diagnosis of sinusitis in infants and children: X-ray, computed tomography, and magnetic resonance imaging. J Allergy Clin Immunol 90:442–444, 1992.
27. Zinreich SJ: Imaging of chronic sinusitis in adults: X-ray, computed tomography, and magnetic resonance imaging. J Allergy Clin Immunol 90:445–451, 1992.
28. Evans FO Jr, Sydnor JB, Moore WEC, et al: Sinusitis of the maxillary antrum. N Engl J Med 293:735–739, 1975.
29. Woodham JD, Doyle PW: Endoscopic diagnosis, medical treatment and a working classification for chronic sinusitis. J Otolaryngol 20:438–441, 1991.
30. Yanagisawa E, Yanagisawa K: Endoscopic view of maxillary sinus ostia. Ear Nose Throat J 72:518–519, 1993.
31. Schaefer SD, Manning S, Close LG: Endoscopic paranasal sinus surgery. Laryngoscope 99:1–5, 1989.
32. Axelsson A, Brorson JE: The correlation between bacteriological findings in the nose and maxillary sinus in acute maxillary sinusitis. Laryngoscope 83:2003–2011, 1973.
33. Talbot G, Kennedy D, Scheld WM, et al: Correlation of sinus endoscopy vs. sinus aspiration for microbiologic documentation of acute maxillary sinusitis (Abstr). Presented at the 35th International Conference on Antimicrobial Agents and Chemotherapy; September 17–20, 1995; San Francisco.
34. Su WY, Liu C, Hung SY, Tsai WF: Bacteriological study in chronic maxillary sinusitis. Laryngoscope 93:931–934, 1983.
35. Brook I: Bacteriology of chronic maxillary sinusitis in adults. Ann Otol Rhinol Laryngol 98:426–428, 1989.
36. Hammerschlag MR, Chirgwin K, Roblin PM, et al: Persistent infection with *Chlamydia pneumoniae* following acute respiratory illness. Clin Infect Dis 14:178–182, 1992.
37. Grayston JT: Infections caused by *Chlamydia pneumoniae* strain TWAR. Clin Infect Dis 15:757–763, 1992.
38. Ferguson MA, Todd JK: Toxic shock syndrome associated with *Staphylococcus aureus* sinusitis in children. J Infect Dis 161:953–955, 1990.
39. Hamory BH, Sande MA, Sydnor A Jr, et al: Etiology and antimicrobial therapy of acute maxillary sinusitis. J Infect Dis 139:197–202, 1979.
40. Linden BE, Aguilar EA, Allen SJ: Sinusitis in the nasotracheally intubated patient. Arch Otolaryngol Head Neck Surg 114:860–861, 1988.
41. Shapiro ED, Milmoe GJ, Wald ER, et al: Bacteriology of the maxillary sinuses in patients with cystic fibrosis. J Infect Dis 146:589–593, 1982.
42. Zieske LA, Kopke RD, Hamill R: Dermatiaceous fungal sinusitis. Otolaryngol Head Neck Surg 105:567–577, 1991.
43. Corey JP: Allergic fungal sinusitis. Ann Otol Rhinol Laryngol 25:225–230, 1992.
44. Chow AW, Hall CB, Klein JO, et al: Evaluation of new anti-infective drugs for the treatment of respiratory tract infections. Clin Infect Dis 15(Suppl 1):S62–S88, 1992.
45. Camacho AE, Cobo R, Otte J, et al: Clinical comparison of cefuroxime axetil and amoxicillin/clavulanate in the treatment of patients with acute bacterial maxillary sinusitis. Am J Med 93:271–276, 1992.
46. Brook I: Beta-lactamase producing bacteria in head and neck infection. Laryngoscope 98:428–431, 1988.
47. Brook I: Infections caused by β-lactamase–producing *Fusobacterium* spp. in children. Pediatr Infect Dis 12:532–533, 1993.
48. Giebink GS: Childhood sinusitis: Pathophysiology, diagnosis and treatment. Pediatr Infect Dis 13:S55–S58, 1994.
49. Scandinavian Study Group: Loracarbef versus doxycycline in the treatment of acute maxillary sinusitis. J Antimicrob Chemother 31:949–961, 1993.
50. Bamberger DM: Antimicrobial treatment of sinusitis. Semin Respir Infect 6:77–84, 1991.
51. Fiscella RG, Chow JM: Cefixime for treatment of maxillary sinusitis. Am J Rhinol 5:193–197, 1991.
52. Karma P, Pukander J, Penttila M, et al: The comparative efficacy and safety of clarithromycin and amoxycillin in the treatment of outpatients with acute maxillary sinusitis. J Antimicrob Chemother 27(Suppl A):83–90, 1991.
53. Wald ER, Reilly JS, Casselbrant M, et al: Treatment of acute maxillary sinusitis in childhood—A comparative study of amoxicillin and cefaclor. J Pediatr 104:297–302, 1984.
54. Chow AW: Infections of the oral cavity, neck and head. *In* Mandell GL, Bennett JE, Dolin R (eds): Principles and Practice of Infectious Diseases, ed 4. New York, Churchill Livingstone, 1995, pp 593–606.
55. Borman KR, Brown PM, Mezera KK, Phaveri H: Occult fever in surgical intensive care unit patients is seldom caused by sinusitis. Am J Surg 164:412–416, 1992.
56. Lanza DC, Kennedy DW: Current concepts in the surgical management of chronic and recurrent acute sinusitis. J Allergy Clin Immunol 90:505–511, 1992.
57. Melen I, Lindahl L, Andreasson L: Short and long-term treatment results in chronic maxillary sinusitis. Acta Otolaryngol 102:282–290, 1986.
58. Anggard A, Malm L: Orally administered decongestant drugs in disorders of the upper respiratory passages. A survey of clinical results. Clin Otolaryngol 9:43–49, 1984.
59. Axelsson A, Jensen C, Melin O, et al: Treatment of acute maxillary sinusitis. V. Amoxicillin, azidocillin, phenylpropanolamine and pivampicillin. Acta Otolaryngol 91:313–318, 1981.
60. Toohill RJ, Lehman RH, Grossman TW, Belson TP: Rhinitis medicamentosa. Laryngoscope 91:1614–1621, 1981.
61. Cummings NP, Lere JL, Wood R, et al: Effect of treatment of sinusitis on asthma and bronchial reactivity. Results of a double-blind study (Abstr). J Allergy Clin Immunol 73(Suppl):143, 1984.
62. Woodham J, Strecker H, Parikh S: Conservative endoscopic sinus surgery for chronic sinusitis. B C Med J 35:246–249, 1993.
63. Chow AW: Life-threatening infections of the head and neck. Clin Infect Dis 14:991–1004, 1992.

INFECTIONS OF THE PARAMENINGEAL STRUCTURES

Infections of the parameningeal structures include subdural empyema, cranial and spinal epidural abscess, and cranial septic venous thrombosis. These infections most frequently arise by direct extension from a pericranial focus, such as chronic sinusitis, otitis media, mastoiditis, or petrous osteomyelitis.[1, 2] Hematogenous infection is more common with spinal epidural abscess, although contiguous spread from vertebral osteomyelitis, infection after epidural anesthesia or laminectomy, and extension of pressure sores are not uncommon.[3, 4] These suppurative infections carry a high rate of mortality and morbidity and should be considered both medical and surgical emergencies. Early diagnosis and effective therapy are the only means of preventing death and long-term neurologic sequelae, yet the necessary diagnostic measures and therapeutic interventions are often delayed. This may be related in part to the complexity of the clinical problem: key and important medical history may be unobtainable in a comatose patient, and the differential diagnoses may be uncertain if the primary source of infection is unrecognized. A systematic approach with rapid mobilization and assistance from various specialists (such as neurologist, neurosurgeon, neuroradiologist, infectious disease specialist, and microbiologist) is essential for optimal management.

Anatomic Considerations

Dura Mater

The cranial dura mater adheres tightly to the periosteum of the skull except where it invaginates into the cranial cavity to form the falx cerebri, falx cerebelli, tentorium cerebelli, and diaphragma sellae (Fig. 49–6). Infection in the extradural space, therefore, tends to be localized. Cranial extradural abscess is rare but may occur after spread of infection from an adjacent purulent frontal or ethmoidal sinusitis or chronic suppurative otitis media. More commonly, loculation of in-

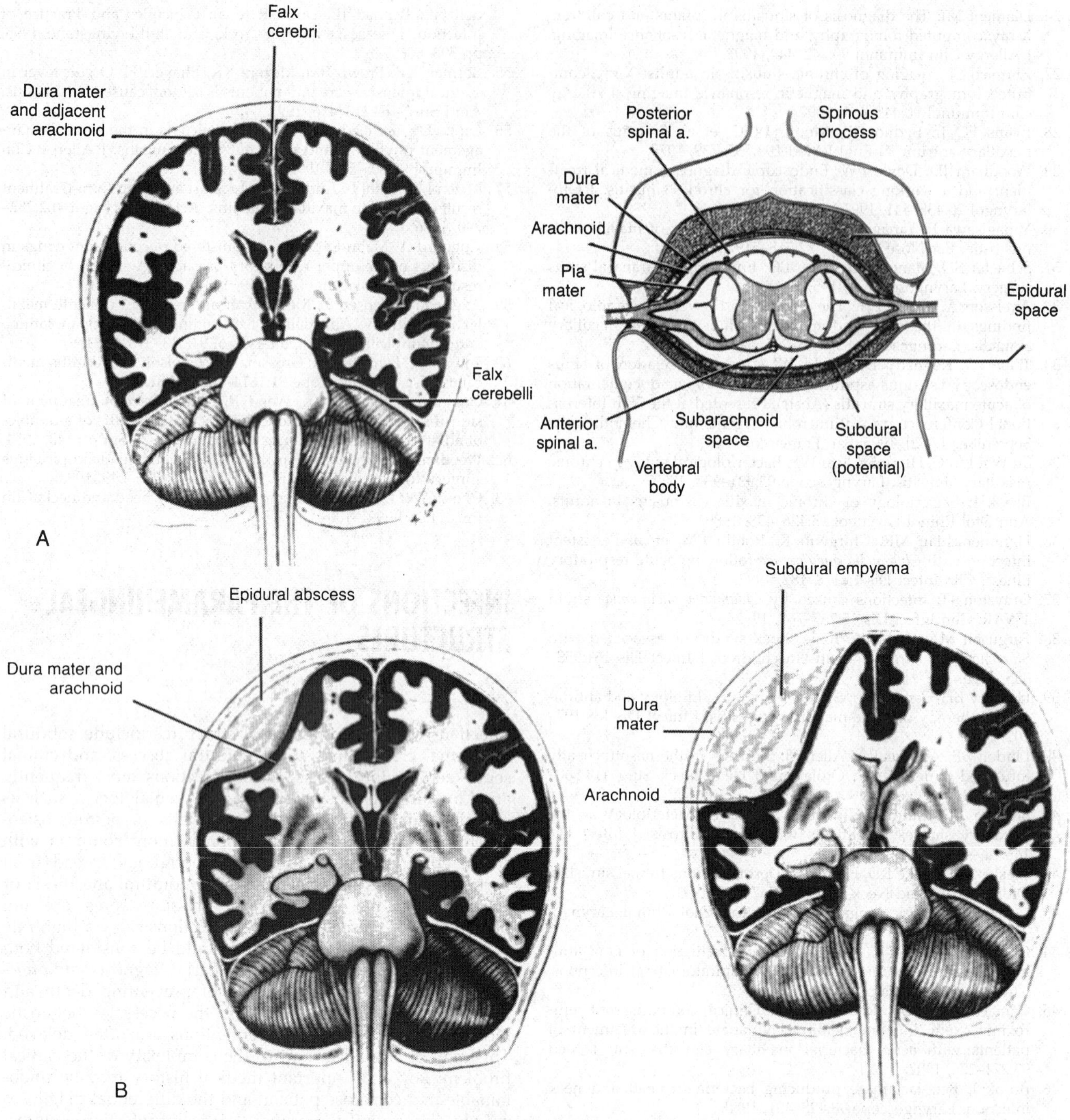

FIGURE 49–6 □ Anatomic relationships of normal cranial and spinal meninges *(A)* and cranial epidural abscess and subdural empyema *(B)*. (Adapted from Greenlee JE: Anatomic considerations in central nervous system infections. *In* Mandell GL, Douglas RG Jr, Bennett JE [eds]: Principles and Practice of Infectious Diseases, ed 4. Churchill Livingstone, New York, 1994, pp 821–831. Drawing in *A* modified from Baker AS, Ojeman RG, Swartz MN, Richardson EP Jr: Spinal epidural abscess. N Engl J Med 293:463–468, 1975. Copyright © 1975 Massachusetts Medical Society. All rights reserved.)

fection occurs between the arachnoid and dura mater, resulting in a subdural empyema. Because the arachnoid and dura are only loosely attached, subdural infection tends to spread rapidly over the surface of the cerebral hemisphere. This infection is usually unilateral; further spread is restricted medially by the falx cerebri and inferiorly by the tentorium cerebelli.

In contrast to the cranial dura, the spinal dura mater and periosteum are separated by a fat-filled epidural space from the foramen magnum to the level of the seventh cervical vertebra. Thus, both spinal subdural empyema and spinal epidural abscess may extend over many vertebral segments and are usually posterior to the cord.

Cranial Venous Sinuses

The cranium is drained by a network of superficial veins (external portions of the cerebrum and brain stem), deep veins (central white matter, basal ganglia, and thalamus), and venous sinuses within the dura mater.[5] The superficial veins and venous sinuses also communicate extensively with the extracranial venous system through numerous emissary veins that cross the skull and meninges. The cortical venous sinuses also resorb cerebrospinal fluid through the arachnoid villi, most of which are located along the anterior third of the superior sagittal sinus. Thus, obstruction of venous outflow caused either by thrombosis of the superior sagittal sinus or by occlusion of both lateral sinuses may result in communicating hydrocephalus. The intracranial venous system and sinuses lack valves and allow bidirectional blood flow. Because of extensive anastomosis, cortical venous thrombosis or occlusion of venous sinuses often produces only transient neurologic manifestations and at times may be silent.

Cranium and Contiguous Structures

Knowledge of the anatomic relationship of the cranium and adjacent structures is essential for early recognition and management of parameningeal infections caused by contiguous spread (see Fig. 49–2). The understructures of the brain rest within the anterior, middle, and posterior cranial fossae. The anterior fossa forms the roof of the frontal and ethmoidal sinuses; infection within either sinus may produce a frontal epidural abscess, a subdural empyema, or a frontal lobe brain abscess. The sphenoidal sinus occupies the body of the sphenoid bone close to the pituitary gland above; the optic nerve and optic chiasma in front; and the internal carotids, the cavernous sinuses, and the temporal lobes of the brain on each side (see Fig. 49–2). Thus, infection originating from the sphenoidal sinus may extend locally to cause cavernous sinus thrombosis, anteriorly to involve the frontal lobe, and posteriorly to involve the temporal lobe.[6] Infections of the middle ear or mastoid within the petrous bone may extend into the middle fossa to involve the temporal lobe or into the posterior fossa to involve the cerebellum or brain stem. The skull overlying the dura of the cerebrum is covered extracranially by the galea aponeurotica. Pericranial infections, secondary to head trauma or a craniotomy, may result in subgaleal abscess and cranial osteomyelitis, with possible retrograde spread through the emissary veins to the epidural, subdural, and subarachnoid spaces.

Both cranial and spinal nerve roots may be involved either directly, owing to contiguous infection, or indirectly, owing to increased intracranial pressure. Of particular importance is the close relationship of the third cranial nerve to the tentorium (uncal herniation of the temporal lobe); the third, fourth, fifth, and sixth cranial nerves to the cavernous sinus (septic cavernous sinus thrombosis); the fifth and sixth cranial nerves to the petrous portion of the temporal bone (chronic otitis media and petrous osteomyelitis); and the ninth and eleventh cranial nerves to the jugular foramen (septic jugular thrombophlebitis).

Clinical Syndromes and Diagnosis

Subdural Empyema

Intracranial subdural empyema in the adult usually results from a suppurative infection of the paranasal sinuses, mastoid, or middle ear.[7–9] Local pain, increase in purulent nasal or aural discharge, generalized headache, and high fever are the first indications of intracranial spread. This acute flare-up is followed within days by focal neurologic findings such as unilateral motor seizures, hemiplegia, hemianesthesia or aphasia, and signs of increased intracranial pressure with progressive lethargy and coma.[10, 11] The neck is stiff, but cerebrospinal fluid examination is more consistent with an aseptic meningitis syndrome. In infants and young children, however, an intracranial subdural empyema is almost invariably a complication of bacterial meningitis. Early signs such as irritability, poor feeding, and increased head size are nonspecific, but hemiparesis, convulsions, stupor, and coma may ensue rapidly.[12]

Plain radiographs and tomograms of the paranasal sinuses, mastoids, and petrous portion of the temporal bone may provide invaluable clues to contiguous foci of suppurative infection. However, CT is the procedure of choice for the diagnosis of subdural empyema.[13] CT can also detect cerebral edema, hydrocephalus, an associated mass effect, and the presence of extracranial infection. In subdural empyema, CT reveals inward displacement of cerebral substance due to an extracerebral mass and a crescent-shaped area of low density directly between the inner table of the skull and cerebral cortex or adjacent to the falx cerebri. With use of a contrast agent, there is fine, irregular enhancement of the peripheral margins of the subdural empyema. Occasionally, CT may be inconclusive because density of the lesion may be similar to that of cerebral tissue, and the decreased attenuation may not be evident. MRI may offer an advantage over CT in such cases.[14] Angiography is recommended on an emergency basis if CT results are normal and facilities for MRI are not available. As with brain abscess, lumbar puncture should be avoided in patients suspected of having a subdural empyema.

Cranial Epidural Abscess

Intracranial epidural abscess is usually associated with a postcraniotomy infection or a cranial osteomyelitis secondary to chronic sinusitis or middle-ear infection.[7, 15] The onset of symptoms may be insidious and overshadowed by the localized inflammatory process. Focal neurologic findings are less common than in subdural empyema. Rarely, a fifth and sixth cranial nerve palsy may develop in association with infections of the petrous portion of the temporal bone (Gradenigo syndrome).

CT demonstrates a thick and circumscribed area of diminished density associated with extracerebral displacement and contiguous cranial osteomyelitis.[13, 16, 17] As with subdural empyema, angiography may occasionally be required in highly suggestive cases when CT results are normal. The possibility of a coexistent intracranial suppurative process must be evaluated carefully.

Septic Intracranial Thrombophlebitis

Intracranial thrombophlebitis most frequently follows infection of paranasal sinuses, middle ear, mastoid, or oropharynx.[18, 19] If collateral venous drainage is adequate, septic venous thrombosis may produce only transient neurologic findings or may be silent. If the thrombus outstrips collateral flow, however, progressive neurologic deficits will lead to impairment of consciousness, focal or generalized seizures, and increased intracranial pressure. The clinical findings vary with the location of cortical veins or dural sinuses involved. Cavernous sinus thrombosis is characterized by abrupt onset with diplopia, photophobia, orbital edema, and progressive exophthalmos.[20, 21] Involvement of the third, fourth, fifth, and sixth cranial nerves produces ophthalmoplegia, a midposition fixed pupil, loss of corneal reflex, and diminished sensation over the upper face. Obstruction of venous return from the retina results in papilledema, retinal hemorrhage, and visual loss. Thrombosis of the superior sagittal sinus produces bilateral leg weakness and may cause communicating hydrocephalus.[18] Occlusion of the lateral sinus produces pain over the ear and mastoid and may cause edema over the mastoid (Griesinger sign).

Involvement of the fifth and sixth cranial nerves produces ipsilateral facial pain and lateral rectus weakness (Gradenigo syndrome). The danger of septic pulmonary embolization is always present.

Septic intracranial thrombophlebitis is fortunately rare in the postantibiotic era. Skull radiographs may show pineal shift and evidence of sinusitis or mastoiditis. Lumbar puncture reveals increased intracranial pressure, a slight lymphocytic pleocytosis, and slightly elevated protein level. MRI is the preferred diagnostic procedure because of its ability to differentiate between flowing blood and thrombus.[22] Its sensitivity can be further increased by magnetic resonance angiography. CT is useful and should be employed when MRI is not available.[16, 23] Angiography with close attention to the venous phase or retrograde jugular venography may prove useful in cases suggestive of lateral sinus thrombosis if CT or MRI findings are normal.[19]

Spinal Epidural Abscess

Spinal epidural abscess usually arises hematogenously or by contiguous spread from vertebral osteomyelitis, extension of pressure sores, or infection after epidural anesthesia or penetrating injury.[3, 4] Distant sources of infection include infective endocarditis, pneumonia, intraabdominal or pelvic sepsis, and urinary tract infection with entry of organisms through the paravertebral venous plexus. Spinal epidural abscess may span several vertebrae and may be inadvertently entered during a lumbar puncture. The abscess may develop acutely or follow a more chronic course. Four stages in the clinical presentation can be recognized. The first phase is usually accompanied by fever and back pain, and the second phase involves progression to root pain. Symptoms developing in the cervical or lumbar area suggest nerve root compression due to a ruptured disk. In the third phase, there is progression to motor weakness, sensory changes, and bowel or bladder dysfunction, signaling spinal cord compression. The fourth phase involves total paralysis, which may occur within hours after the onset of motor weakness. If the cervical cord is involved, respiratory function may be impaired.

MRI is the diagnostic method of choice because it can visualize the cord and epidural space in both sagittal and transverse sections and can also identify an associated vertebral osteomyelitis or joint space infection.[24, 25] Myelography should be employed if MRI is not available or cannot be performed. CT with contrast enhancement may be helpful in differentiating subdural from epidural infection or in identifying osteomyelitis. Analysis of cerebrospinal fluid is usually nondiagnostic unless the abscess has ruptured into the subarachnoid space or the spinal needle has inadvertently entered the epidural abscess during the lumbar puncture.

Antimicrobial and Adjunctive Therapy

Subdural Empyema and Cranial Epidural Abscess

Early surgical evacuation is the cornerstone of therapy for both subdural and cranial epidural empyemas. The frequency of mortality and neurologic sequelae varies directly with elapsed time to surgical drainage.[26] In addition, the primary focus of infection, such as chronic sinusitis, mastoiditis, or petrous osteomyelitis, should be explored and debrided. The choice of initial empirical antimicrobial therapy is based on the suspected source of infection, the immunologic status of the patient, and the most likely causative organisms (Table 49–7). In rhinogenic causes associated with chronic sinusitis, anaerobic or microaerophilic streptococci (*Peptostreptococcus* sp., viridans streptococci, *Streptococcus anginosus*) and *Bacteroides* and *Prevotella* species predominate, often as mixed infections.[27–29] In otogenic infection associated with chronic otitis media or mastoiditis, enteric gram-negative bacilli, such as *Pseudomonas aeruginosa* and *Proteus mirabilis*, as well as anaerobic organisms are most common.[2, 7] Epidural abscesses secondary to penetrating cranial trauma or postoperative infection are most commonly caused by *S. aureus* and enteric gram-negative bacilli.[3, 4, 27]

When anaerobes and microaerophilic streptococci are implicated, penicillin G remains the antibiotic of first choice even though β-lactamase–producing organisms are increasingly isolated in such infections.[30, 31] Chloramphenicol and metronidazole are useful alternatives in the penicillin-allergic

TABLE 49–7 ■ Empirical Antimicrobial Regimens for Suppurative Parameningeal Infections

SOURCE OR ASSOCIATED INFECTION	ANTIMICROBIAL REGIMENS: Normal Host	ANTIMICROBIAL REGIMENS: Compromised Host
Cranial Parameningeal Infections*		
Otogenic	Penicillin G 2–4 million units intravenously (IV) q 4–6 h *or* Ciprofloxacin 0.2 g q 12 h *plus* Metronidazole 0.5 g IV q 6 h *or* Chloramphenicol 0.5 g IV q 6 h	Cefotaxime 2 g IV q 6 h *or* Ceftizoxime 4 g IV q 8 h *or* Imipenem 500 mg IV q 6 h
Rhinogenic	Penicillin G 2–4 million units IV q 4–6 h *plus* Metronidazole 0.5 g IV q 6 h *or* Chloramphenicol 0.5 g IV q 6 h	Same as for otogenic
Odontogenic	Same as for rhinogenic	Same as for otogenic
After cranial surgery	Nafcillin 1.5 g IV q 4–6 h *plus* Tobramycin 2 mg/kg IV q 8 h *or* Ciprofloxacin 0.2 g q 12 h	Vancomycin 0.5 g IV q 6 h *plus* Cefotaxime, ceftizoxime, *or* imipenem
Hematogenous from distant site	Choice based on suspected organism from primary site	
Spinal Epidural Abscess		
Extension of osteomyelitis or paravertebral infection	Nafcillin 1.5 g IV q 4–6 h *plus* Tobramycin 2 mg/kg IV q 8 h *or* Ciprofloxacin 0.2 g q 12 h	Vancomycin 0.5 g IV q 6 h *plus* Cefotaxime, ceftizoxime, *or* imipenem

*Includes subdural empyema, cranial epidural abscess, and septic venous thrombosis.

patient. Metronidazole is particularly active against *Bacteroides.* Lack of activity against gram-positive anaerobic cocci, such as *Peptostreptococcus,* and facultative organisms, such as streptococci, precludes the use of metronidazole as monotherapy for otogenic or odontogenic intracranial suppuration.[32] Combination of penicillin with metronidazole or chloramphenicol is recommended. Clindamycin penetrates the blood-brain barrier poorly and is generally not recommended in central nervous system infections. For immunocompromised and critically ill patients, broad coverage of aerobic gram-negative bacilli, *S. aureus,* and anaerobes with extended-spectrum β-lactams (e.g., cefotaxime, ceftizoxime, imipenem) is indicated (see Table 49–7). The final antibiotic selection should be guided by culture results and susceptibility data.

Maximal doses of systemic antimicrobials are required for the treatment of subdural empyema and epidural abscess. Therapy should generally be continued for at least 4 to 6 weeks. Patients should be carefully monitored both clinically and by repeated CT. Follow-up for up to 1 year is required to ensure against recurrence. In addition to antibiotic therapy, corticosteroids or osmotic diuretics are used frequently to decrease intracranial edema and pressure. External or ventriculoperitoneal shunting may be required if hydrocephalus is present.

Septic Cranial Venous Sinus Thrombosis

Antimicrobial therapy for cranial septic venous thrombosis is similar to that for subdural empyema (see Table 49–7). High-dose intravenous antibiotics and surgical decompression of the underlying predisposing infection are essential. Before the antibiotic era, septic cavernous sinus thrombosis was virtually always fatal. Mortality since 1970 has been markedly reduced to between 15% and 30%.[20] Intracranial hypertension may require corticosteroids or osmotic diuresis. The use of anticoagulants or thrombolytic therapy is controversial.[33, 34] Internal jugular vein ligation has been used in lateral sinus thrombosis, and in a few instances thrombectomy has been successful.[19, 29, 35]

Spinal Epidural Abscess

Discovery of a spinal epidural abscess is an indication for immediate intravenous antibiotic therapy and surgical evacuation unless the abscess is located below the spinal cord. In selected cases, CT-guided needle aspiration may be used in place of laminectomy; if localized pain or radicular symptoms are present without neurologic deficit, antibiotic therapy alone, with meticulous serial neurologic examinations and repeated MRI or CT studies, may be considered.[36] The appearance of neurologic deficit, worsening pain, and increasing temperature and leukocytosis while the patient is receiving antibiotic therapy are indications for surgery.[37] The initial empirical antimicrobial therapy should be directed at both *S. aureus* (found in approximately 50% of cases) and enteric gram-negative bacilli (see Table 49–7). Thus, oxacillin or nafcillin plus an aminoglycoside, a third-generation cephalosporin (e.g., cefotaxime, ceftizoxime, ceftriaxone, or ceftazidime), or a systemic quinolone may be suitable. If infection with *S. aureus* is suspected, nafcillin, 2 g every 4 hours, may be added. If the *S. aureus* strain is methicillin resistant, nafcillin should be replaced by vancomycin. An extended-spectrum penicillin (e.g., piperacillin, ticarcillin-clavulanate, imipenem, mezlocillin, or azlocillin) plus an aminoglycoside is appropriate if *P. aeruginosa* is suspected. Intravenous quinolone (e.g., ciprofloxacin) or trimethoprim-sulfamethoxazole (5 to 10 mg/kg per day and 25 to 50 mg/kg per day, respectively, every 6 hours intravenously) may also be considered in the penicillin-allergic patient. Intravenous therapy should be continued for 4 to 6 weeks after surgical drainage.

Prevention

Parameningeal infections can be prevented only by early, appropriate treatment of the underlying conditions, such as sinusitis, otitis media, mastoiditis, and vertebral osteomyelitis.

References

1. Yoshikawa TT, Quinn W: The aching head—Intracranial suppuration due to head and neck infections. Infect Dis Clin North Am 2:265–277, 1988.
2. Altman NR: Intracranial infection in children. Top Magn Reson Imaging 5:143–160, 1993.
3. Nussbaum ES, Rigamonti D, Standiford H, et al: Spinal epidural abscess: A report of 40 cases and review. Surg Neurol 38:225–231, 1992.
4. Darouiche RO, Hamill RJ, Greenberg SB, et al: Bacterial spinal epidural abscess. Review of 43 cases and literature survey. Medicine (Baltimore) 71:369–385, 1992.
5. Greenlee JE: Anatomic considerations in central nervous system infections. *In* Mandell GL, Bennett JE, Dolin R (eds): Principles and Practice of Infectious Diseases, ed 4. New York, Churchill Livingstone, 1995, pp 821–831.
6. Lew D, Southwick FS, Montgomery WW, et al: Sphenoid sinusitis. A review of 30 cases. N Engl J Med 309:1149–1154, 1983.
7. Chow AW: Life-threatening infections of the head and neck. Clin Infect Dis 14:991–1004, 1992.
8. Munz M, Farmer JP, Auger L, et al: Otitis media and CNS complications. J Otolaryngol 21:224–226, 1992.
9. Goldstein EJC, Citron DM, Wield B, et al: Bacteriology of human and animal bite wounds. J Clin Microbiol 8:667–672, 1978.
10. Wackym PA, Canalis RF, Feuerman T: Subdural empyema of otorhinological origin. J Laryngol Otolaryngol 104:118–122, 1990.
11. Skelton R, Maixner W, Isaacs D: Sinusitis-induced subdural empyema. Arch Dis Child 67:1478–1480, 1992.
12. Fairbanks DNF, Milmoe GJ: Complications and sequelae—An otolaryngologist's perspective. Pediatr Infect Dis 4(Suppl 6):S75–S78, 1985.
13. Kaufman DM, Leeds NE: Computed tomography (CT) in the diagnosis of intracranial abscesses. Brain abscess, subdural empyema, and epidural empyema. Neurology 27:1069–1073, 1977.
14. Komori H, Takagishi T, Otaki E, et al: The efficacy of MR imaging in subdural empyema. Brain Dev 14:123–125, 1992.
15. Maniglia AJ, Goodwin WJ, Arnold JE, et al: Intracranial abscesses secondary to nasal, sinus, and orbital infections in adults and children. Arch Otolaryngol Head Neck Surg 115:1424–1429, 1989.
16. Latchaw RE, Hirsch WL Jr, Yock DH Jr: Imaging of intracranial infection. Neurosurg Clin North Am 3:303–322, 1992.
17. Smith RR: Neuroradiology of intracranial infection. Pediatr Neurosurg 18:92–104, 1992.
18. Southwick FS, Richardson EP, Swartz MN: Septic thrombosis of the dural venous sinuses. Medicine (Baltimore) 65:82–106, 1986.
19. Teichgraeber JF, Per-Lee JH, Turner JS: Lateral sinus thrombosis—A modern perspective. Laryngoscope 92:744–751, 1982.
20. Harbour RC, Trobe JD, Ballinger WE: Septic cavernous sinus thrombosis associated with gingivitis and parapharyngeal abscess. Arch Ophthalmol 102:94–97, 1984.
21. Yarington CT Jr: Cavernous sinus thrombosis revisited. Proc R Soc Med 70:456–459, 1977.
22. Medlock MD, Olivero WC, Hanigan WC, et al: Children with cerebral venous thrombosis diagnosed with magnetic resonance imaging and magnetic resonance angiography. Neurosurgery 31:870–876, 1992.
23. Virapongse C, Cazenave C, Quisling R, et al: The empty delta sign: Frequency and significance in 76 cases of dural sinus thrombosis. Radiology 162:779–785, 1987.
24. Teman AJ: Spinal epidural abscess. Early detection with gadolinium magnetic resonance imaging. Arch Neurol 49:743–746, 1992.

25. Post MJ, Bowen BC, Sze G: Magnetic resonance imaging of spinal infection. Rheum Dis Clin North Am 17:773–794, 1991.
26. Mauser HW, Van Houwelingen HC, Tulleken CAF: Factors affecting the outcome in subdural empyema. J Neurol Neurosurg Psychiatry 50:1136–1141, 1987.
27. Brook I: Aerobic and anaerobic bacteriology of intracranial abscesses. Pediatr Neurol 8:210–214, 1992.
28. Rosenfeld EA, Rowley AH: Infectious intracranial complications of sinusitis, other than meningitis, in children: 12 year review. Clin Infect Dis 18:750–754, 1994.
29. Pallares R, Santamaria J, Ariza X, et al: Polymicrobial anaerobic septicemia due to lateral sinus thrombophlebitis. J Laryngol Otolaryngol 98:895–899, 1984.
30. Brook I: Beta-lactamase producing bacteria in head and neck infection. Laryngoscope 98:428–431, 1988.
31. Akova M, Akalin HE, Korten V, et al: Treatment of intracranial abscesses: Experience with sulbactam/ampicillin. J Chemother 5:181–185, 1993.
32. Sjolin J, Lilja A, Eriksson N, et al: Treatment of brain abscess with cefotaxime and metronidazole: Prospective study in 15 consecutive patients. Clin Infect Dis 17:857–863, 1993.
33. Einhaupl KM, Villringer A, Meister W, et al: Heparin treatment in venous sinus thrombosis. Lancet 338:597–600, 1991.
34. Alexander LF, Yamamota Y, Ayoubi S, et al: Efficacy of tissue plasminogen activator in the lysis of thrombosis of the cerebral venous sinus. Neurosurgery 26:559–564, 1990.
35. Persson L, Anders L: Extensive dural sinus thrombosis treated by surgical removal and local streptokinase infusion. Neurosurgery 26:117–121, 1990.
36. Wheeler D, Keiser P, Rigamonti D, et al: Medical management of spinal epidural abscesses; case report and review. Clin Infect Dis 15:22–27, 1992.
37. Rea GL, McGregor JM, Miller CA, et al: Surgical treatment of the spontaneous spinal epidural abscess. Surg Neurol 37:274–279, 1992.

50

Ear and Mastoid Infections

Charles D. Bluestone

Currently, otitis media is the most common diagnosis for office visits to physicians in the United States. This finding was reported by the National Center for Health Statistics,[1] which also found that the diagnosis had increased from about 10 million visits in 1975 to 25 million in 1990; most likely, even more patients have the diagnosis today. Although common in adults, the disease affects primarily infants and children. As reported by the National Center for Health Statistics, the annual visit rate for children younger than 2 years statistically increased by 224% during the period of the study, and significant increases occurred in older children, but not as dramatically. In Boston, a survey of about 17,000 office visits during the first year of life revealed that otitis media was the diagnosis in approximately one third of visits for illness and one fifth of all office visits.[2] It is likely that the increase in daycare attendance, a known risk factor, during this same period has been related to this rise in the disease in infants and young children.

It is estimated that more than $5 billion is spent annually for the care of otitis media in the United States.[3] Of the estimated 120 million prescriptions written for oral antimicrobial agents each year in this country, more than one fourth are for the treatment of otitis media.[4] Myringotomy with insertion of tympanostomy tube is the most common surgical procedure performed in children for which a general anesthetic is required, and tonsillectomy and adenoidectomy are still the most common major surgical procedures performed in children, many of which are for the prevention of otitis media. Otitis media is, indeed, a major health problem.

Acute Otitis Media

Diagnosis

The rapid, brief onset of signs and symptoms of infection in the middle ear is termed acute otitis media. Synonyms such as acute suppurative or purulent otitis media are acceptable. One or more of the following are present: otalgia (or pulling of the ear in the young infant), fever, or irritability of recent onset. The tympanic membrane is full or bulging and opaque, and it has limited mobility or none to pneumatic otoscopy, all of which are indicative of a middle-ear effusion. The acute onset of ear pain, fever, and a purulent discharge (otorrhea) through a perforation of the tympanic membrane (or tympanostomy tube) would also be evidence of acute otitis media.

When the diagnosis of acute otitis media is in doubt or when determination of the etiologic agent is desirable, aspiration of the middle ear should be performed by the clinician; if he or she is not skilled in this procedure, the patient can be referred to an otolaryngologist.[5] Today, with the emergence of resistant bacterial organisms causing otitis media, such as β-lactamase–producing *Haemophilus influenzae* and *Branhamella* (formerly *Moraxella) catarrhalis,* and the more recent troublesome rise in penicillin- as well as multidrug-resistant pneumococcus,[6,7] tympanocentesis is an evermore important diagnostic procedure. Indications for tympanocentesis (or myringotomy) include the following ones:

1. Otitis media in patients who have severe otalgia, are seriously ill, or appear toxic
2. Unsatisfactory response to antimicrobial therapy
3. Onset of otitis media in a child who is receiving appropriate and adequate antimicrobial therapy
4. Otitis media associated with a confirmed or potential suppurative complication
5. Otitis media in a newborn infant, an ill neonate, or an immunologically deficient patient, any of whom might harbor an unusual organism[8]

Unfortunately, nasopharyngeal cultures do not accurately identify the causative organism in children with acute otitis media.

Characteristics of the Pathogen

Effective treatment of acute otitis media in infants, children, and adults should be based on a knowledge of the bacterial etiology. Figure 50–1 shows the distribution of bacteria from middle-ear aspirates isolated from 1980 to 1989 at our Otitis Media Research Center.[9] *Streptococcus pneumoniae* was the predominant pathogen cultured (35%) from aspirates of patients who had acute otitis media during this 10-year period; however, this rate significantly increased from 29% in 1980 to 44% in 1989 (Fig. 50–2). *H. influenzae* was the second most common pathogen isolated in acute ear infections (23%). Before 1980, the frequency of *M. catarrhalis* was less than 10%, but it is now present in 14% of acute effusions. Group A β-hemolytic streptococcus, *Staphylococcus aureus,* anaerobic bacteria, and viruses were infrequently cultured from middle-ear aspirates of these children.

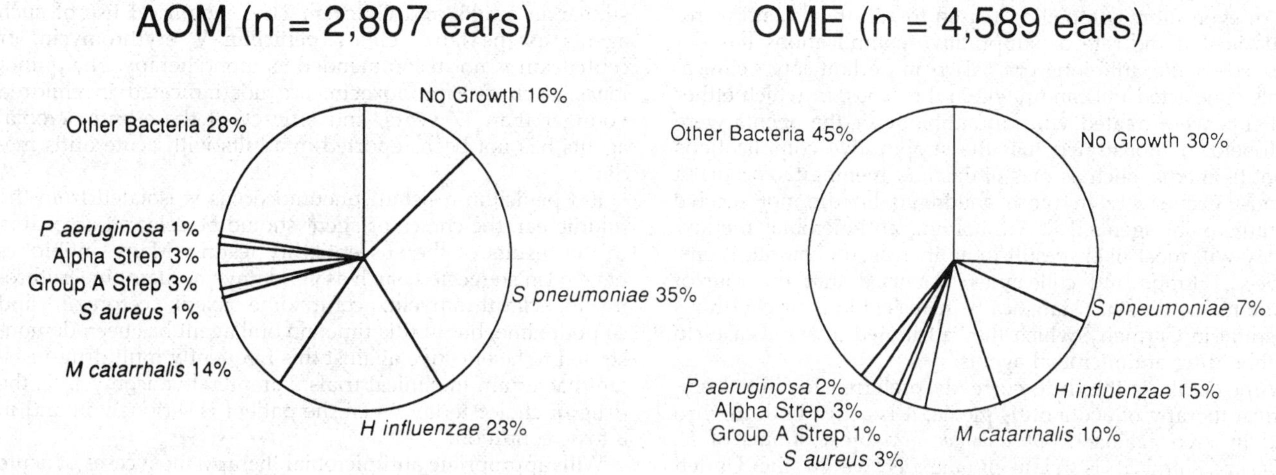

FIGURE 50–1 ▫ Comparison of bacteria from middle-ear aspirates obtained by tympanocentesis in infants and children with acute otitis media (AOM) or otitis media with effusion (OME), the latter immediately before insertion of tympanostomy tubes. Totals may add up to more than 100% because of the presence of multiple pathogens. (From Bluestone CD, Stephenson JS, Martin LM: Ten-year review of otitis media pathogens. Pediatr Infect Dis J 11:S7–S11, 1992.)

Figure 50–3 shows that the percentage of β-lactamase–producing *H. influenzae* (primarily nontypable in otitis media) is now more than 30% in the Pittsburgh area. This percentage has increased during the 1980s, as has that for *M. catarrhalis.* Currently, most if not all strains of *M. catarrhalis* produce β-lactamase. In 1993, we isolated *S. pneumoniae* from 120 middle-ear effusions; of these, 17% were relatively resistant, and 13% were resistant to penicillin (unpublished data). Mason and colleagues[10] reported that the middle ear was the most common site in which resistant pneumococcus was isolated at their children's hospital in Houston. Reichler and colleagues[11] reported a high rate of resistant pneumococcus in daycare centers. The change in the frequency of these pathogens and the increasing emergence of β-lactamase–producing organisms has an important impact on management today.

Many have thought that *H. influenzae* is an uncommon etiologic agent in acute otitis media in adults. However, in a study conducted at our center that involved 34 adults who had an episode of acute otitis media, we found that 26% of acute middle-ear effusions demonstrated isolates of this organism, and 22.5% of *H. influenzae* produced β-lactamase.[12] In only 21% of the aspirates was *S. pneumoniae* recovered; both *M. catarrhalis* (β-lactamase producing) and *Streptococcus pyogenes* were isolated in 3%. Overall, 9% of the subjects had β-lactamase–producing organisms.

Management

Most experts in the United States agree that patients who have the signs and symptoms of acute otitis media should receive antimicrobial therapy; however, several reports have questioned the need for antimicrobial agents in all cases.[13–15] Nevertheless, in a clinical trial by Howie and Ploussard,[16] antimicrobial agents were shown to be superior to placebo in "sterilizing" the middle-ear effusion. In addition, a large clinical trial by Kaleida and colleagues[17] found that subjects who had "severe" acute otitis media and who had been randomized to receive myringotomy without antibiotic had statistically more initial treatment failures than those children who received an antimicrobial agent with or without the adjunctive use of a myringotomy. As part of that trial, another group of children who had "nonsevere" acute otitis media were randomized to receive either antibiotic or placebo, and those in the placebo group also had more treatment failures as well as more time with middle-ear effusion than those in the antibiotic group.

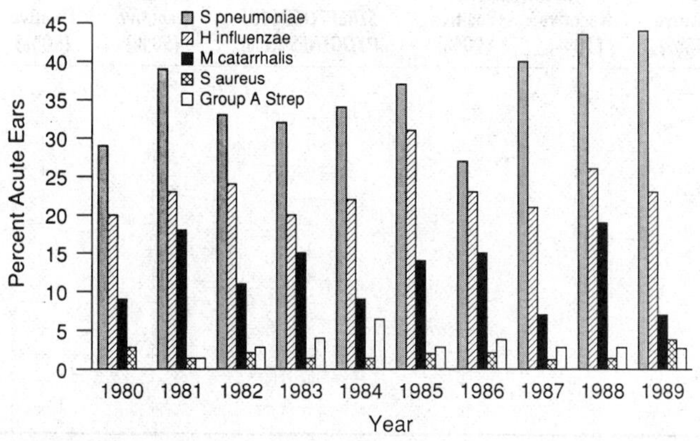

FIGURE 50–2 ▫ Frequency of the most common pathogens causing acute otitis media during the decade of the 1980s. (From Bluestone CD, Stephenson JS, Martin LM: Ten-year review of otitis media pathogens. Pediatr Infect Dis J 11:S7–S11, 1992.)

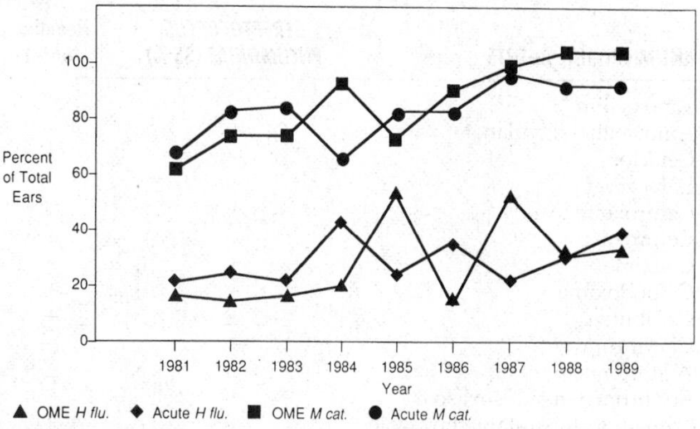

FIGURE 50–3 ▫ Percentage of β-lactamase–producing *H. influenzae* and *M. catarrhalis* in acute otitis media (AOM) and otitis media with effusion (OME), 1981 to 1989. (From Bluestone CD, Stephenson JS, Martin LM: Ten-year review of otitis media pathogens. Pediatr Infect Dis J 11:S7–S11, 1992.)

An even more compelling reason to administer antimicrobials is that the rate of suppurative complications has decreased in the antibiotic era.[18] Two important large clinical trials conducted in Scandinavia in the 1950s, in which either patients were treated with an antibiotic or the agents were withheld, demonstrated that the suppurative complications of otitis media, such as mastoiditis and meningitis, occurred almost exclusively in those children who did not receive antimicrobial agents.[19, 20] Withholding antimicrobial therapy today will most likely result in an increase in complications. Indeed, Hoppe and colleagues[21] reported that the rate of acute mastoiditis has statistically increased in their children's hospital in Germany, which they attributed in some cases to withholding antimicrobial agents.

Amoxicillin is the drug currently preferred for initial empirical therapy of acute otitis media; it is active both in vitro and in vivo against *S. pneumoniae* and most strains of *H. influenzae,* and it is relatively inexpensive in the United States.[22] Amoxicillin is recommended because it can be given in three divided doses and produces fewer adverse reactions than ampicillin; 10 days' treatment is recommended.[23] If the patient is allergic to the penicillins, a combination of erythromycin and sulfisoxazole, or one of the new macrolides, azithromycin or clarithromycin, is advocated; as an alternative, one of the newer cephalosporins could be used if the patient does not have hypersensitivity to these agents and does not have an immediate hypersensitivity reaction to the penicillins. If β-lactamase–producing *H. influenzae* or *M. catarrhalis* organisms are isolated by tympanocentesis or from otorrhea fluid—in which case amoxicillin would not be appropriate—then the choices would also be these antimicrobials or amoxicillin-clavulanate. Six cephalosporins are currently effective for treatment of acute otitis media: the second-generation agents cefaclor, loracarbef, cefuroxime axetil, and cefprozil, and the third-generation drugs cefpodoxime and cefixime. Trimethoprim-sulfamethoxazole would also be an appropriate alternative. The clinical efficacy of these antimicrobial agents is summarized in Table 50–1. Even though no data are available on the efficacy of these antimicrobial agents for treatment of adults with acute otitis media, the recommendations discussed before should be applied to adults as well, because the causative organisms are probably similar in adults and children. Thus, empirical use of such agents as the tetracyclines, penicillin V, erythromycin, or cephalexin is not recommended as monotherapy. The quinolones, such as ciprofloxacin, are not indicated in children younger than 17 years, and efficacy of these antimicrobial agents has not been reported in adults with acute otitis media.

If a penicillin-resistant pneumococcus is isolated from the middle ear, the choice of agent should be selected according to the results of the susceptibility testing. Many antibiotics have been suggested, such as clindamycin, rifampin, erythromycin, clarithromycin, cefuroxime axetil, cefprozil, and cefpodoxime, but at this time, no oral agent has been demonstrated to be effective against this frequently multidrug-resistant bacterium in clinical trials. Parenteral vancomycin is the drug of choice today when the patient is seriously ill and in a toxic condition.

With appropriate antimicrobial therapy, most cases of acute bacterial otitis media improve significantly within 48 to 72 hours; if signs and symptoms of infection progress despite antimicrobial therapy, the patient should be reevaluated within 24 hours; a suppurative complication may have developed, or there may be a concurrent serious infection (e.g., an infant may have meningitis). Persistent or recurrent pain or fever, or both, during treatment would signal the need for tympanocentesis and myringotomy (for Gram stain, culture, and susceptibility testing), selection of another antimicrobial agent, or both. As stated before, tympanocentesis should be more frequently employed when appropriate and adequate antimicrobial therapy fails, because resistant organisms may be the cause of the antibiotic treatment failure. If a middle-ear aspirate is not obtained for culture and susceptibility testing, the agent chosen should be effective against whatever resistant bacteria have been found to be in the community that have been associated with symptomatic treatment failures.

The new antimicrobial agent should be effective against β-lactamase–producing bacteria such as *H. influenzae* or *M. catarrhalis.* If ampicillin or amoxicillin was given initially, then the combination of erythromycin-sulfisoxazole or trimethoprim-sulfamethoxazole should be effective when these organisms are present; however, trimethoprim-sulfamethoxa-

TABLE 50–1 ■ Comparative Efficacy of Selected Oral Antimicrobial Agents for Common Pathogens in Acute Otitis Media*

ANTIMICROBIAL AGENTS	*STREPTOCOCCUS PNEUMONIAE* (35%)	*HAEMOPHILUS INFLUENZAE* (23%) β-Lactamase Negative (66%)	*HAEMOPHILUS INFLUENZAE* (23%) β-Lactamase Positive (34%)	*MORAXELLA CATARRHALIS* (14%) β-Lactamase Negative (10%)	*MORAXELLA CATARRHALIS* (14%) β-Lactamase Positive (90%)	*STREPTOCOCCUS PYOGENES* (3%)	*STAPHYLOCOCCUS AUREUS* (1%) β-Lactamase Negative (50%)	*STAPHYLOCOCCUS AUREUS* (1%) β-Lactamase Positive (50%)
Amoxicillin	+†	+	−	+	−	+	+	−
Amoxicillin-clavulanate	+	+	+	+	+	+	+	+
Cefaclor	+	+	+	+	±	+	+	+
Loracarbef	+	+	+	+	+	+	+	+
Cefuroxime axetil	+	+	+	+	+	+	+	+
Cefprozil	+	+	+	+	+	+	+	+
Cefixime	±	+	+	+	+	+	−	−
Cefpodoxime	+	+	+	+	+	+	+	+
Ceftibuten	±	+	+	+	+	+	−	−
Clarithromycin	+	+	+	+	+	+	+	+
Azithromycin	+	+	+	+	+	+	+	+
Erythromycin-sulfisoxazole	+	+	+	+	+	+	+	+
Trimethoprim-sulfamethoxazole	+	+	+	+	+	−	+	+

*Based on available data from clinical trials and laboratory studies. Percentages represent distribution of bacteria found in middle-ear aspirates of acute otitis media (Pittsburgh Otitis Media Research Center). +, Effective/susceptible; −, not effective/not susceptible; ± marginally effective/susceptible.

†In 1993, 17% of *S. pneumoniae* strains were relatively resistant and 13% were resistant to penicillin at the Pittsburgh Otitis Media Research Center (unpublished data).

zole is apparently not effective when *S. pyogenes* is the causative organism (this drug combination is not indicated if an associated streptococcal pharyngitis is present). In addition, both of these drug combinations contain a sulfonamide, which is associated with a high rate of adverse side effects and which on rare occasion can be serious, and even fatal, to children.[24] Cefaclor is probably effective against all the β-lactamase–producing organisms, except possibly some strains of *M. catarrhalis,* and it has been associated with serum sickness–like reactions in children.[25] Amoxicillin-clavulanate would be another choice at this stage; comparative trials in the United States have shown this combination to be an effective antimicrobial treatment for middle-ear infection caused by resistant bacteria.[26–28] Cefuroxime axetil would also be appropriate.[29–31] Cefixime is also effective for β-lactamase–producing *H. influenzae* and *M. catarrhalis* but is not effective if *S. aureus* is the causative organism.[32, 33] The new cephalosporins, loracarbef, cefprozil, and cefpodoxime, would also be appropriate at this stage, as would be one of the new macrolides, azithromycin and clarithromycin.

Patients should probably be reexamined at the end of the course of antibiotic therapy (i.e., after 10 to 14 days), at which time some patients (approximately 50%) will have a persistent middle-ear effusion. The presence of persistent effusion after a 10-day trial of an antimicrobial agent is common, and it is usually asymptomatic in infants and children; myringotomy can be helpful in older patients if symptoms are present, such as fullness in the ear, hearing loss, tinnitus, or vertigo. However, Mandel and colleagues[34] conducted a clinical trial in children in which 20-day therapy was compared with the traditional 10-day course. They recommended having children who are asymptomatic return for their first follow-up visit in 4 weeks, because further treatment with antimicrobial therapy immediately after 10-day treatment in the trial provided no long-term advantage. However, patients who still have any signs or symptoms of acute infection should be reevaluated during or at the end of the initial course of treatment.

Additional supportive therapy at the onset of the illness may be helpful, such as analgesics or antipyretics. An oral decongestant, such as pseudoephedrine hydrochloride, may relieve nasal congestion, and antihistamines may help patients with known or suspected nasal allergy; however, the use of antihistamines for treatment of upper respiratory tract infections is not recommended.[35] Administration of antihistamines and decongestants in the treatment of acute otitis media has not been shown to be effective in children. If complete resolution has occurred and the episode represents the only known attack, the patient may be discharged; however, periodic follow-up is indicated for infants and children who have had recurrent episodes.

Persistent Middle-Ear Effusion

If the middle-ear effusion persists after the initial 10 days' antimicrobial therapy, one or more of the following treatment options have been advocated to hasten the resolution of the effusion during the next *subacute* phase:

1. Another 10-day course of therapy with the same antimicrobial agent that was used initially, because the optimal duration of antibiotic treatment for acute otitis media has not been defined
2. If amoxicillin was given initially, a course of an antimicrobial agent that is effective against resistant organisms
3. A topical or systemic nasal decongestant or systemic antihistamine, or a combination of these drugs
4. Administration of systemic corticosteroids
5. Inflation of the eustachian tube–middle ear by using the method of Valsalva or Politzer

Unfortunately, none of these commonly employed methods has been shown to be effective in randomized, controlled trials of children with subacute middle-ear effusions. As described before, Mandel and coworkers[34] found no long-term advantage in re-treating asymptomatic children with an antimicrobial agent at this stage. Also, two Pittsburgh studies demonstrated inefficacy of a combination of an oral decongestant and antihistamine, with and without amoxicillin, in eliminating persistent middle-ear effusion that involved more than 1000 infants and children, although these studies did not test the efficacy of this combination in patients older than 12 years or in those children who had documented nasal allergy.[36, 37] With our current understanding of this stage of otitis media, clinicians do not have to treat patients who have asymptomatic (except for hearing loss) persistent middle-ear effusion still present after 2 weeks, because most patients will be effusion free at the end of 3 or 4 months without further treatment.[38] However, the patient should be reexamined during this period to determine whether the effusion has persisted for 3 months or longer, at which point the effusion is chronic and should be treated as described later for otitis media with effusion. Also, some patients may benefit from further treatment at an earlier time, which is also described later.

Recurrent Acute Otitis Media

Recurrent acute otitis media is a common problem of infants and young children. The child with recurrent acute otitis media whose infection clears completely between episodes may be treated as outlined previously. The bacteriology of middle-ear infection in children who have recurrent episodes of acute otitis media separated by a month or more is similar to that found in first episodes: the predominant pathogens are *S. pneumoniae* and nontypable strains of *H. influenzae.* When patients initially receive amoxicillin and then develop a recurrence soon after the course of amoxicillin is completed, resistant organisms are more frequently present; such patients might benefit from a broader spectrum antimicrobial agent.[39]

If the episodes of acute otitis media are frequent and close together, which is common in infants, prevention of further attacks is desirable. When this occurs, the child requires further evaluation. Several avenues of investigation are open: a search for respiratory allergy may prove fruitful; roentgenograms of the paranasal sinuses may reveal sinusitis; immunologic studies may be of value in the infant and young child if other organs are involved (i.e., the lung), but if the child is 5 or 6 years of age or older, an evaluation of immune function might be helpful even if recurrent or chronic ear disease is the only apparent problem. If none of these conditions is present, one or more of the popular methods of prevention may be attempted. For infants and children who have frequent episodes of acute otitis media, without middle-ear effusion between the bouts, the most common nonsurgical and surgical methods currently employed for prevention are (1) chemoprophylaxis with an antimicrobial agent, (2) myringotomy with insertion of a tympanostomy tube, (3) adenoidectomy with or without tonsillectomy, and (4) pneumococcal vaccine in children who are 18 to 24 months of age or older.

Prophylaxis

Several clinical trials conducted in the past have shown antimicrobial prophylaxis to be effective.[40–42] A metaanalysis con-

TABLE 50–2 ■ Outcome of Randomized 2-Year Clinical Trial of Amoxicillin Prophylaxis and of Tympanostomy Tube Insertion Versus Placebo for Prevention of Recurrent Acute Otitis Media in 264 Pittsburgh Children, 7 to 35 Months of Age*

OUTCOME MEASURE	TREATMENT GROUPS 1 Amoxicillin	2 Placebo	3 Tympanostomy Tube	P VALUE GROUPS 1 vs. 2	3 vs. 2	1 vs. 3
Rates of AOM or AOM-otorrhea (child-years)	0.60	1.08	1.02	<.001	NS	.001
Mean percent time with OM	10.0	15.0	6.6	.03	<.001	NS
Median time to first episode of AOM-otorrhea (mo)	22.1	8.2	11.2	.002	NS	—

*AOM, Acute otitis media; OM, otitis media; NS, not significant.
Adapted from Casselbrant ML, Kaleida PH, Rockette HE, et al: Efficacy of antimicrobial prophylaxis and of tympanostomy tube insertion for prevention of recurrent acute otitis media: Results of a randomized clinical trial. Pediatr Infect Dis J 11:278–286, 1992.

firmed the beneficial effect of antibiotic prophylaxis.[43] For the child who has repeated episodes of otitis media (e.g., three episodes in 6 months or four or five episodes in 12 months, with at least one episode being present during the preceding 6 months), it seems reasonable to recommend amoxicillin at 20 mg/kg in one dose (given at bedtime).[44] If the child is allergic to the penicillins, a daily dose of sulfisoxazole at 50 mg/kg may be substituted. This prophylactic regimen should be continued during the respiratory season. As a note of caution, trimethoprim-sulfamethoxazole is not recommended for prophylaxis of otitis media for any age group.[45]

Children receiving prophylaxis should be examined at frequent and regular intervals (every 6 to 8 weeks) to be certain that inapparent middle-ear effusion, which might become chronic, does not occur. Prolonged antimicrobial prophylaxis is inappropriate if long-standing persistent middle-ear effusion is present. In this case, surgical intervention should be considered, such as myringotomy and tympanostomy tube insertion, with or without adenoidectomy. Today, with the emergence of resistant bacteria, myringotomy and tube insertion may be a reasonable alternative to antimicrobial prophylaxis.

At present, there is no evidence that a topical or systemic nasal decongestant or antihistamine, either alone or in combination, administered daily or at the onset of an upper respiratory tract infection, prevents recurrent acute otitis media. Therefore, the use of such medications for prophylaxis is not recommended until their efficacy is proved.

Surgical Treatment

Because studies reported in the past have shown that some children still have recurrent episodes of acute otitis media despite use of the preventive dose of an antibiotic, myringotomy and tympanostomy tube placement should be considered for patients whose prophylaxis fails. Myringotomy with tympanostomy tube insertion has been shown to be effective, compared with nonsurgical control groups, for prevention of recurrent acute otitis media in otitis-prone infants.[46, 47] A clinical trial reported by Casselbrant and coworkers[44] has shown that both amoxicillin prophylaxis and myringotomy with tympanostomy tube insertion were more effective than placebo in the prevention of recurrent acute otitis media; antimicrobial prophylaxis was recommended as the initial method, and for those children whose prophylaxis failed, tubes were then suggested as an alternative (Table 50–2). Adenoidectomy, with or without tonsillectomy, is frequently advocated for the prevention of recurrent acute otitis media, but only one randomized, controlled study has been reported that has shown the efficacy of adenoidectomy, albeit limited, for this condition. Paradise and coworkers[48] did demonstrate a significant difference in the attack rate of acute otitis media in children who had been randomized to receive adenoidectomy compared with those who did not receive this operation; all subjects in this clinical trial had at least one myringotomy and tympanostomy tube insertion before random assignment (Table 50–3). However, as a note of caution, adenoidectomy in infants should be recommended only selectively (such as in those who also have severe nasal obstruction due to obstructive adenoids), because the operation carries some degree of increased risk in this age group.

In cases of recurrent otitis media, the decision should be between administering an antibiotic in a prophylactic dose and a myringotomy with insertion of a tympanostomy tube, and adenoidectomy in selected patients.

In some patients, insertion of tympanostomy tubes prevents the severe symptoms of acute otitis media, but recurrent episodes of otorrhea still occur. A systemic antimicrobial agent or ototopical antibiotic-cortisone medication or both are usually effective in resolving the otitis media. Caution is

TABLE 50–3 ■ Efficacy of Adenoidectomy for Recurrent Otitis Media in Children Previously Treated with Tympanostomy Tube Placement

	TREATMENT GROUP	NUMBER OF SUBJECTS	MEAN NUMBER EPISODES OF OTITIS MEDIA	P VALUE*	PROPORTION OF DAYS OTITIS MEDIA PRESENT	P VALUE*
First year	Adenoidectomy	48	1.06	.51	15.0	.04
	Control	38	1.45		28.5	
Second year	Adenoidectomy	45	1.09	.01	17.8	.005
	Control	27	1.67		28.4	

*P values by χ^2 test.
Adapted from Paradise JL, Bluestone CD, Rogers KD, et al: Efficacy of adenoidectomy for recurrent otitis media in children previously treated with tympanostomy-tube placement. Results of parallel randomized and nonrandomized trials. JAMA 263:2066–2073, 1990. Copyright 1990, American Medical Association.

advised in prescribing ototopical agents owing to their potential ototoxicity.

For the rare child whose tympanostomy tubes fail to prevent frequently recurrent acute otitis media (who have otorrhea through the tube), the combination of antimicrobial prophylaxis and tympanostomy tube insertion is usually effective in preventing the recurrent episodes.

These management options should be offered only to children who do not have chronic middle-ear effusion. If recurrent bouts of acute otitis media are superimposed on the chronic condition, the child should be treated as described in the following section for management of chronic otitis media with effusion.

Otitis Media with Effusion

Diagnosis

The presence of a relatively asymptomatic middle-ear effusion has many synonyms, such as secretory, nonsuppurative, or serous otitis media, but the most acceptable term is otitis media with effusion. Pneumatic otoscopy frequently reveals either a retracted or concave tympanic membrane, the mobility of which is limited or absent. However, fullness or even bulging may be visualized. In addition, an air-fluid level or bubbles or both may be observed through a translucent tympanic membrane. The duration (not the severity) of the effusion can be classified as acute (less than 3 weeks), subacute (3 weeks to 3 months), or chronic (longer than 3 months). The most important distinction between this type of disease and acute otitis media is that the signs and symptoms of acute infection are lacking in otitis media with effusion (e.g., otalgia, fever), but hearing loss is usually present in both conditions.

Microbiology

For decades, otitis media with effusion was assumed to be sterile, because several reports described unsuccessful attempts to culture bacteria[49, 50]; however, studies reported during the past 15 years identified bacteria by means of smears and cultures.[51–54] A study was conducted in Pittsburgh by Riding and coworkers[54] of 179 children aged 1 to 16 years who had chronic middle-ear effusions. Of 179 ears, bacteria were cultured from 86 (48%) chronic middle-ear effusions. Bacteria were present in serous and mucoid effusions as well as in the purulent type.

More recent findings from our center (see Fig. 50–1) show that of middle-ear aspirates from ears with chronic otitis media with effusion, about two thirds had bacteria isolated; of the one third that were considered to be pathogens, the most common bacteria were *H. influenzae, M. catarrhalis,* and *S. pneumoniae,* which are the common pathogens found in middle-ear aspirates from children with acute otitis media. In addition, *Staphylococcus epidermidis* was cultured from many middle ears when it was not cultured from the external canal of the same ear. (A culture preceded sterilization and tympanocentesis.) β-Lactamase activity was similar to that reported for isolates from ears with acute otitis media; anaerobic bacteria were also isolated in about 10%.

Post and colleagues[55] found that 78% of middle-ear effusions had evidence of the three major organisms (i.e., *H. influenzae, M. catarrhalis,* and *S. pneumoniae*) by polymerase chain reaction, whereas only 28% of the aspirates were culture-positive. The investigators postulated that bacteria may have a larger role in the inflammatory process than previously believed.

Unfortunately, information concerning the microbiology of otitis media with effusion that occurs in adults is not available.

Infants and children who have otitis media with effusion most likely have a condition that is an extension of an upper respiratory tract infection, which should resolve spontaneously without active treatment.[56] Casselbrant and coworkers[57] reported that approximately 80% of preschool children who developed otitis media with effusion while attending a day-care center in a Pittsburgh suburb had their effusions clear without treatment within 2 months. Treatment may be indicated in some children, however, because there are possible complications and sequelae associated with this condition. Because little information is presently available regarding the frequency of these complications and sequelae, some clinicians advocate taking a watch-and-wait position and not actively treating such a child.[58] However, hearing loss of some degree usually accompanies a middle-ear effusion.[59] Although the significance of this hearing loss is still uncertain, such a loss may impair cognitive and language function and result in disturbances in psychosocial adjustment.[60] With these uncertainties in mind, the clinician should decide whether to treat or to watch and, if treatment is decided on, which treatment options appear to be most appropriate in eliminating the middle-ear effusion in the individual child.

Important factors other than hearing loss that should be considered in deciding whether to treat (and which treatment) include (1) occurrence in infants, because they are unable to communicate about their symptoms and may have suppurative disease; (2) an associated acute purulent upper respiratory tract infection; (3) concurrent permanent conductive or sensorineural hearing loss, or both; (4) vertigo or tinnitus; (5) alterations of the tympanic membrane, such as severe atelectasis, especially a deep retraction pocket in the posterosuperior quadrant or the pars flaccida, or both; (6) middle-ear changes, such as adhesive otitis or ossicular involvement; (7) effusion that persists for 3 months or longer (i.e., chronic otitis media with effusion); or (8) when the episodes recur frequently, such as in 6 of the preceding 12 months.

Management

Before the clinician embarks on a nonsurgical or surgical method of management of children with frequently recurrent or chronic effusions, a thorough search for an underlying cause should be attempted. Probably the most popular method of management—a trial with an orally administered combination of a decongestant and antihistamine—was shown to be ineffective in the Pittsburgh study of infants and children with acute, subacute, and chronic otitis media with effusion.[36] In contrast, the efficacy of systemic corticosteroid therapy for treatment of otitis media with effusion has been tested in clinical trials, most of which showed some benefit.[61] However, some clinicians consider the risks of corticosteroid therapy for otitis media with effusion in children to outweigh its possible benefits.[56] As of yet, clinical trials have not been reported that have tested the efficacy of topical nasal treatment, immunotherapy, and control of allergy in children who have nasal allergy and middle-ear disease. However, this method of management seems reasonable in children who have frequently recurrent or chronic otitis media with effusion and evidence of upper respiratory tract allergy. Inflation of the eustachian tube–middle ear by use of the Politzer method or Valsalva maneuver has been advocated for more than a century for this condition. However, a randomized controlled trial by Chan and Bluestone[62] found a lack of efficacy of middle-ear inflation for chronic otitis media with effusion, and therefore it is not recommended in children. However, inflation may be effective for adults and

TABLE 50–4 ■ Morbidity for First Year of Randomized Trial of Myringotomy, Myringotomy and Tympanostomy Tube, and No Surgery (Control) in 111 Pittsburgh Infants and Children with Chronic Otitis Media with Effusion

	TREATMENT GROUPS			
OUTCOME MEASURE	1 No Surgery (N = 35)	2 Myringotomy (N = 38)	3 Myringotomy and Tympanostomy Tube (N = 36)	STATISTICALLY SIGNIFICANT DIFFERENCE
Treatment failure (proportion of subjects)	0.56	0.70	0.06	Yes*
Acute otitis media (episodes/person-year)	0.95	0.81	0.23	$P < .001$†
Middle-ear effusion (proportion of time)	0.64	0.61	0.17	$P < .001$†

*Actuarial rate; 90% confidence intervals for group 1–group 2 (−0.33,0.05); group 1–group 3 (0.35,0.66); group 2–group 3 (0.50,0.78).
†For groups 1 versus 2 versus 3.
Adapted from Mandel EM, Rockette HE, Bluestone CD, et al: Efficacy of myringotomy with and without tympanostomy tubes for chronic otitis media with effusion. Pediatr Infect Dis J 11:270–277, 1992.

all age groups for the management of middle-ear effusion that follows barotrauma (e.g., by air travel or scuba diving).

Antimicrobial Treatment

Of all the medical treatments that have been advocated, a trial of an antimicrobial agent would appear to be most appropriate in those children who have not received an antibiotic recently. Because bacteria similar to those found in acute otitis media have been isolated from a significant proportion of middle-ear aspirates in children with chronic otitis media with effusion, the antibiotic chosen for treatment should be the same as that recommended for children who have acute otitis media. As in acute otitis media, amoxicillin is a reasonable choice for treating otitis media with effusion, because a study reported by Mandel and associates[37] demonstrated its efficacy for some, although not all, of the 518 infants and children with otitis media with effusion who participated in the study. If the effusion is chronic and unresponsive to amoxicillin therapy, a trial with an antimicrobial agent effective against ampicillin-resistant bacteria may be helpful before surgery is considered.

Of the other possible antimicrobial agents currently available, such as erythromycin and sulfisoxazole, trimethoprim-sulfamethoxazole, cefaclor, cefuroxime axetil, cefixime, or amoxicillin-clavulanate, only amoxicillin-clavulanate, given for 10 days, has been shown to be marginally more effective than a 10-day course of amoxicillin for otitis media with effusion.[63] Thomsen and colleagues[64] also demonstrated the efficacy of amoxicillin-clavulanate in a placebo-controlled study of children who had chronic otitis media with effusion, but both the drug and its placebo were given for 30 days in this trial. Mandel and colleagues[65] compared a 2-week course of cefaclor and erythromycin-sulfisoxazole with amoxicillin and failed to demonstrate an increased effect of these other agents over amoxicillin. Although no trial has been reported in which the efficacy of a course of amoxicillin longer than 10 days has been tested for chronic otitis media with effusion, it is possible that longer therapy is more effective than shorter therapy. A metaanalysis of the effect of antimicrobial agents in the treatment of otitis media with effusion was reported by Rosenfeld and Post,[66] which confirmed the efficacy of this treatment. Another metaanalysis also confirmed the short-term effect in otitis media and tubes[43] but, as expected, not a long-term effect. Other strategies, such as antimicrobial prophylaxis or surgery, are required for long-term control of this disease, because the disease frequently recurs owing to repeated exposure to upper respiratory tract infections.

Surgical Treatment

If nonsurgical methods of management fail and the effusion is chronic, surgical intervention should be considered, and referral of the patient to an otolaryngologist is appropriate. In 109 Pittsburgh children with chronic otitis media with effusion that was unresponsive to amoxicillin, myringotomy with tympanostomy tube insertion was shown to be more effective than myringotomy without tube insertion or no surgery.[67] After spontaneous extubation of the tympanostomy tube, reinsertion for recurrent effusion is indicated only after antimicrobial therapy has failed and the effusion has persisted for 3 months or longer. The outcome of this study was confirmed in a clinical trial conducted by the same group, which was similar in design to the first one and involved 111 subjects who were also observed monthly for 3 years[68] (Table 50–4). In some children, the procedure must be repeated for several years until the child grows older; the occurrence of otitis media with effusion is less frequent after 5 years of age.[69]

Table 50–5 shows the current indications for insertion of tympanostomy tubes in children.[70] These indications are derived from clinical trials as well as from long experience with otitis media in children, in whom the occurrence is vastly more common than in adults. Unfortunately, there are no

TABLE 50–5 ■ Indications for Tympanostomy Tube Insertion in Children

Chronic otitis media with effusion unresponsive to medical management, 3 mo or more bilateral, or 6 mo or more unilateral; earlier when significant hearing loss (e.g., >25 dB), speech-language delay, severe retraction pocket, disequilibrium-vertigo, or tinnitus is present
Recurrent episodes of middle-ear effusion not meeting criteria for chronic disease, but cumulative duration excessive, e.g., 6 of 12 mo
Recurrent acute otitis media, especially when antimicrobial prophylaxis fails to reduce frequency, severity, and duration of attacks; minimal frequency: 3 or more episodes in 6 mo, or 4 or more in 12 mo, with 1 recent
Eustachian tube dysfunction (with or without effusion), when persistent or recurrent signs and symptoms—e.g., hearing loss (usually fluctuating), disequilibrium-vertigo, tinnitus, or a severe retraction pocket—are not relieved by medical treatment
Tympanoplasty when eustachian tube function is poor, e.g., surgery for cholesteatoma
Suppurative complication present or suspected

Adapted from Bluestone CD, Klein JO, Gates GA: "Appropriateness" of tympanostomy tubes. Setting the record straight. Arch Otolaryngol Head Neck Surg 120:1051–1053, 1994. Copyright 1994, American Medical Association.

TABLE 50–6 ■ Effectiveness of Various Treatments in 578 Children with Chronic Otitis Media with Effusion

OUTCOME*	MYRINGOTOMY	MYRINGOTOMY AND TUBE INSERTION	ADENOIDECTOMY AND MYRINGOTOMY	ADENOIDECTOMY, MYRINGOTOMY, AND TUBE INSERTION
Percentage of time with effusion	49.1	34.9	30.2	25.8
Percentage of time with hearing loss†	37.5	30.4	22.0	22.4
Median time to first recurrence (d)	54	222	92	240
Number of surgical retreatments	66	36	17	17

*During 2-y follow-up.
†Hearing loss equal to or greater than 20 dB.
Adapted with permission from Gates GA, Avery CA, Prihoda TJ, Cooper JC Jr: Effectiveness of adenoidectomy and tympanostomy tubes in the treatment of chronic otitis media with effusion. N Engl J Med 317:1444–1451, 1987.

similar published clinical trials that have been conducted in adults, but the clinician can use the outcomes of the studies in children as a guide to treating adults. However, there are some important differences, such as the usual intolerance of adults when even relatively asymptomatic middle-ear effusion of short duration is present and the feasibility of performing myringotomy, with or without tympanostomy tube insertion, by use of local anesthesia in teenagers and adults. Thus, surgical intervention should be considered at a much earlier stage in the natural history of acute otitis media, persistent middle-ear effusion, recurrent acute otitis media, and otitis media with effusion in older patients.

Adenoidectomy, in conjunction with myringotomy and tympanostomy tube insertion or myringotomy alone, can benefit some children. However, others improve without removal of the adenoids, and still others will have persistent disease despite adenoidectomy[48, 71, 72] (see Table 50–3). Table 50–6 shows the outcomes of the clinical trial conducted by Gates and colleagues.[72] Because the effectiveness of adenoidectomy for chronic otitis media with effusion is apparently unrelated to adenoid size,[48, 73, 74] the selection of children who might benefit from adenoidectomy at present must be based on the potential benefits weighed against the costs and potential risks. For children who have recurrent or chronic otitis media with effusion and who have had one or more myringotomy and tympanostomy tube operations in the past, adenoidectomy is a reasonable option. The presence of upper airway obstruction (due to obstructive adenoids), recurrent acute or chronic adenoiditis, or both conditions would also be more compelling indications to consider adenoidectomy.

Chronic Suppurative Otitis Media with and Without Cholesteatoma

Chronic suppurative otitis media is a stage of ear disease in which there is chronic infection of the middle ear and mastoid and in which a "central" perforation of the tympanic membrane (or a patent tympanostomy tube) and discharge (otorrhea) are present. Mastoiditis is invariably a part of the pathologic process. The condition has been called chronic otitis media, but this term can be confused with chronic otitis media with effusion, which is not characterized by perforation. It is also called chronic suppurative otitis media and mastoiditis, chronic purulent otitis media, and chronic otomastoiditis. The most descriptive term is chronic otitis media with perforation, discharge, and mastoiditis, but this is not common usage. When a cholesteatoma is also present, the term chronic suppurative otitis media with cholesteatoma is used; however, an acquired aural cholesteatoma does not have to be associated with chronic suppurative otitis media.

Microbiology

Chronic suppurative otitis media develops from a chronic bacterial infection; however, the bacteria that caused the initial episode of acute otitis media with perforation and otorrhea may not be those that are isolated from the discharge when there is chronic infection in the middle ear and mastoid. In fact, Mandel and associates[75] reported that infants and young children who had the acute onset of otorrhea through a tympanostomy tube usually had the common organisms that cause acute otitis media when the tympanic membrane is intact, whereas in older children, especially in the summer, the predominant organism was frequently *Pseudomonas*, presumably as a result of contamination of the middle ear during swimming. Thus, the antimicrobial therapy recommended for acute otitis media may not be effective for most cases of chronic suppurative otitis media. The microbiology of chronic suppurative otitis media without cholesteatoma in children has been reported by Kenna and coworkers.[76] From the 51 ear cultures obtained from the 36 children, 23 microbiologic species were isolated. One organism was isolated from 18 ears, two from 20 ears, three from 3 ears, four from 4 ears, and five from 2 ears. The most common bacterial species isolated was *Pseudomonas aeruginosa,* which was present in 34 ears (67%) and was the only isolate in 16 ears (31%). Of the 15 children who had bilateral otorrhea, 11 (73%) had the same organism identified in both middle ears: 7 children had *P. aeruginosa* isolated; 4 had *S. aureus*; and 1 each had *S. epidermidis, Candida albicans,* and diphtheroids.

The bacteriology of chronic suppurative otitis media with cholesteatoma in children and adults has been reported. The most common aerobic microbiologic organisms isolated were *P. aeruginosa* and *S. aureus*; the most frequent anaerobic organisms were *Bacteroides, Peptostreptococcus,* and *Peptococcus* species. It is important to make the distinction between chronic suppurative otitis media with and without cholesteatoma; tympanomastoid surgery is indicated when cholesteatoma is present, whereas medical management may be effective when it is not.

Management

Medical management of chronic suppurative otitis media without cholesteatoma is directed toward eliminating the infection from the middle ear and mastoid. Because the bacteria most frequently cultured are gram-negative, antimicrobial agents should be selected to be effective against these organisms. A suspension that contains polymyxin B, neomycin, and hydrocortisone (Cortisporin), or one that has neomycin, polymyxin E, and hydrocortisone (Coly-Mycin), has been advocated, but owing to concern about the potential ototoxicity of these agents, caution is advised. In children, orally administered antibiotics are usually not effective unless an organism is seen by Gram stain or is cultured from the discharge that will be susceptible, such as *S. aureus.* Oral antibiotics are also effective against the organisms that commonly cause acute otitis media, such as pneumococcus and *H. influenzae*; ciprofloxacin, an oral antimicrobial agent with activity against most of the organisms that cause chronic suppurative disease, may be effective, although randomized clinical trials demonstrating efficacy for this infection have not been reported. However, treatment of adults who have chronic suppurative otitis media with the quinolones when the causative organism is *Pseudomonas* seems reasonable; these drugs are *not* indicated for patients younger than 17 years.

If topical antibiotic medication is elected, the patient should return to the outpatient facility daily so that the discharge can be aspirated thoroughly. Frequently, the discharge resolves rapidly with this type of treatment, within a week or two.

If ototopical agents are used, patients (and parents) should be informed of the potential for toxic effects. As an alternative, we hospitalize our children and administer a parenteral β-lactam antipseudomonal drug, such as ticarcillin. The middle ear is aspirated daily. In most children, the middle ear will be free of discharge within 7 to 10 days, and the signs of otitis media will be greatly improved or absent.

When the discharge fails to respond to intensive medical therapy, surgery on the middle ear and mastoid is indicated. In the Kenna group's study[76] of 36 pediatric patients with chronic suppurative otitis media, all of whom received parenteral antimicrobial therapy and daily otic toilet, 32 children (89%) experienced resolution of their initial infection with medical therapy alone; 4 children required tympanomastoidectomy.

In a follow-up of that study, 51 of the original 66 were evaluated for their long-term outcomes.[77] Of these 51 children, 40 (78%) had resolution of their initial or recurrent infection after medical treatment; 11 (22%) had to have mastoid surgery eventually. Failure was associated with older children and an early recurrence. Even though similar large-scale clinical trials of parenteral antimicrobial therapy have not been reported for adults, this management option also seems reasonable before mastoid surgery is performed in this age group.

If the infection can be eliminated by the methods described, recurrence can usually be prevented by one of the following measures: prophylactic antimicrobial therapy; removal of the tympanostomy tube; or surgical repair of the tympanic membrane defect. The choice depends on the age of the patient and the function of the eustachian tube.[78]

When chronic suppurative otitis media is present with cholesteatoma, tympanomastoid surgery is indicated. Preoperative antimicrobial therapy, and possibly perioperative prophylaxis, may be helpful in reducing postoperative infection and should promote better healing.

Acknowledgment

Ms. Deborah A. Hepple helped with the preparation of this manuscript.

References

1. Shappert SM: Office visits for otitis media: United States, 1975–90. Vital Health Stat 214:1, 1992.
2. Teele DW, Klein JO, Rosner B, et al: Middle ear disease and the practice of pediatrics: Burden during the first 5 years of life. JAMA 249:1026, 1983.
3. Gates GA: Cost benefit analysis for otitis media (Abstr). *In* Lim DJ, et al (eds): Sixth International Symposium in Recent Advances in Otitis Media. Fort Lauderdale, FL, 1995, p 2.
4. Nelson WL, Kuritsky JN, Kennedy DL, et al: Outpatient pediatric antibiotic use in the U.S.: Trends and therapy for otitis media, 1977–1986. *In* Program and Abstracts of the 27th Interscience Conference on Antimicrobial Agents and Chemotherapy. Washington, DC, American Society for Microbiology, 1987.
5. Bluestone CD, Klein JO: Otitis Media in Infants and Children, ed 2. Philadelphia, WB Saunders, 1995, p 103.
6. Spika JS, Facklam RR, Plikaytis BD, et al: Antimicrobial resistance of *Streptococcus pneumoniae* in the United States, 1979–1987. J Infect Dis 163:1273, 1991.
7. Welby PL, Keller DS, Cromien JL, et al: Resistance to penicillin and non–beta-lactam antibiotics of *Streptococcus pneumoniae* at a children's hospital. Pediatr Infect Dis J 13:281, 1994.
8. Bluestone CD, Klein JO: Otitis media, atelectasis, and eustachian tube dysfunction. *In* Bluestone CD, Stool SE, Kenna MA (eds): Pediatric Otolaryngology, ed 3. Philadelphia, WB Saunders, 1995, p 470.
9. Bluestone CD, Stephenson JS, Martin LM: Ten-year review of otitis media pathogens. Pediatr Infect Dis J 11:S7, 1992.
10. Mason EO, Kaplan SL, Lamberth LB, et al: Increased rate of isolation of penicillin-resistant *Streptococcus pneumoniae* in a children's hospital and in vitro susceptibilities to antibiotics of potential use. Antimicrob Agents Chemother 36:1703, 1992.
11. Reichler MR, Allphin AA, Breiman RF, et al: The spread of multiply resistant *Streptococcus pneumoniae* at a day care center in Ohio. J Infect Dis 166:1346, 1992.
12. Celin SE, Bluestone CD, Stephenson J, et al: Bacteriology of acute otitis media in adults. JAMA 266:2249, 1991.
13. Diamant M, Diamant B: Abuse and timing of use of antibiotics in acute otitis media. Arch Otolaryngol 100:226, 1974.
14. van Buchem FL, Dunk JHM, van't Hof MA: Therapy of acute otitis media: Myringotomy, antibiotics, or neither? A double-blind study in children. Lancet 2:883, 1981.
15. van Buchem FL, Peeters MF, van't Hof MA: Acute otitis media: A new treatment strategy. Br Med J 290:1033, 1985.
16. Howie VM, Ploussard JH: Efficacy of fixed combination antibiotics versus separate components in otitis media. Clin Pediatr 11:205, 1972.
17. Kaleida PH, Casselbrant ML, Rockette HE, et al: Amoxicillin or myringotomy or both for acute otitis media: Results of a randomized clinical trial. Pediatrics 87:466, 1991.
18. Sorenson H: Antibiotics in suppurative otitis media. Otolaryngol Clin North Am 10:45, 1977.
19. Rudberg RD: Acute otitis media: Comparative therapeutic results of sulfonamide and penicillin administered in various forms. Acta Otolaryngol (Stockh) 113:1, 1954.
20. Lahikainen EA: Clinico-bacteriologic studies on acute media: Aspiration of tympanum as diagnostic and therapeutic method. Acta Otolaryngol (Stockh) 107(Suppl):1, 1953.
21. Hoppe JE, Koster S, Bootz F, Niethammer D: Acute mastoiditis—Relevant once again. Infection 22:180, 1994.
22. Drugs for treatment of acute otitis media in children. Med Lett 36:19, 1994.
23. Bluestone CD: The ear. *In* Behrman RE, Vaughan VC III (eds): Nelson Textbook of Pediatrics, ed 14. Philadelphia, WB Saunders, 1990, p 1610.
24. Serious adverse reactions with sulfonamides. FDA Drug Bull 14:5, 1984.
25. Levine LR: Quantitative comparison of adverse reactions to cefaclor vs. amoxicillin in a surveillance study. Pediatr Infect Dis J 4:358, 1985.
26. Odio CM, Kusmiesz H, Shelton S, et al: Comparative treatment trial of Augmentin versus cefaclor for acute otitis media with effusion. Pediatrics 75:819, 1985.
27. Kaleida PH, Bluestone CD, Rockette HE, et al: Amoxicillin–clavulanate potassium comparison with cefaclor for acute otitis media in infants and children. Pediatr Infect Dis J 6:265, 1987.
28. Marchant CD, Shurin PA, Johnson CE, et al: A randomized controlled trial of amoxicillin plus clavulanate compared with cefaclor for treatment of acute otitis media. J Pediatr 109:891, 1986.
29. Aronovitz GH: Treatment of otitis media with cefuroxime axetil. South Med J 81:978, 1988.
30. Kenna MA, Bluestone CD, Fall P, et al: Cefuroxime axetil versus

cefaclor in the treatment of acute otitis media. *In* Lim DJ, Bluestone CD, Klein JO, Nelson JD (eds): Proceedings of the Fourth International Symposium. Recent Advances in Otitis Media. Philadelphia, BC Decker, 1988, p 214.
31. McLinn SE, Werner K, Cocchetto DM: Clinical trial of cefuroxime axetil versus cefaclor for acute otitis media with effusion. Curr Ther Res 43:1, 1988.
32. Hotaling AJ, Doyle WJ, Cantekin EI: Efficacy of a new cephalosporin for acute otitis media. Arch Otolaryngol 113:370, 1987.
33. Kenna MA, Bluestone CD, Fall P, et al: Cefixime vs. cefaclor in the treatment of acute otitis media in infants and children. Pediatr Infect Dis J 6:992, 1987.
34. Mandel EM, Casselbrant ML, Rockette HE, et al: Efficacy of 20- vs. 10-day antimicrobial treatment for acute otitis media. Pediatrics 96:5, 1995.
35. Bluestone CD, Connell JT, Doyle WJ, et al: Symposium: Questioning the efficacy and safety of antihistamines in the treatment of upper respiratory infection. Pediatr Infect Dis J 7:239, 1988.
36. Cantekin EI, Mandel EM, Bluestone CD, et al: Lack of efficacy of a decongestant-antihistamine combination for otitis media with effusion ("secretory" otitis media) in children. N Engl J Med 308:297, 1983.
37. Mandel EM, Rockette HE, Bluestone CD, et al: Efficacy of amoxicillin with and without decongestant-antihistamine for otitis media with effusion in children. N Engl J Med 316:432, 1987.
38. Kaleida PH, Bluestone CD, Rockette HE, et al: Amoxicillin–clavulanate potassium compared with cefaclor for acute otitis media in infants and children. Pediatr Infect Dis J 6:265, 1987.
39. Harrison CJ, Marks MI, Welch PF: Microbiology of recently treated acute otitis media compared with previously untreated acute otitis media. Pediatr Infect Dis J 4:641, 1985.
40. Liston TE, Foshee WS, Pierson WD: Sulfisoxazole chemoprophylaxis for frequent otitis media. Pediatrics 71:524, 1983.
41. Maynard JE, Fleshman JK, Tschopp CF: Otitis media in Alaskan Eskimo children: Prospective evaluation of chemoprophylaxis. JAMA 219:597, 1972.
42. Perrin JM, Charney E, MacWhinney JB Jr, et al: Sulfisoxazole as chemoprophylaxis for recurrent otitis media: A double-blind crossover study in pediatric practice. N Engl J Med 291:664, 1974.
43. Williams RL, Chalmers TC, Stange KC, et al: Use of antibiotics in preventing recurrent acute otitis media and in treating otitis media with effusion. JAMA 270:1344, 1993.
44. Casselbrant ML, Kaleida PH, Rockette HE, et al: Efficacy of antimicrobial prophylaxis and of tympanostomy tube insertion for prevention of recurrent acute otitis media: Results of a randomized clinical trial. Pediatr Infect Dis J 11:278, 1992.
45. Physicians' Desk Reference, ed 49. Montvale, NJ, Medical Economics Data Production, 1995, pp 816, 2028.
46. Gebhart DE: Tympanostomy tubes in the otitis media prone child. Laryngoscope 91:849, 1981.
47. Gonzalez C, Arnold JE, Woody EA, et al: Prevention of recurrent acute otitis media: Chemoprophylaxis versus tympanostomy tubes. Laryngoscope 96:1330, 1986.
48. Paradise JL, Bluestone CD, Rogers KD, et al: Efficacy of adenoidectomy for recurrent otitis media in children previously treated with tympanostomy-tube placement. Results of parallel randomized and nonrandomized trials. JAMA 263:2066, 1990.
49. Harcourt FL, Brown AK: Hydrotympanum (secretory otitis media). Arch Otolaryngol 57:12, 1953.
50. Robinson JM, Nicholas HO: Catarrhal otitis media with effusion—A disease of a retropharyngeal and lymphatic system. South Med J 44:777, 1951.
51. Healy GB, Teele DW: The microbiology of chronic middle ear effusions in young children. Laryngoscope 87:1472, 1977.
52. Liu YS, Lim DJ, Lang R, et al: Microorganisms in chronic otitis media with effusion. Ann Otol Rhinol Laryngol 85:245, 1976.
53. Senturia BH, Gessert CF, Carr CD, et al: Studies concerned with tubotympanitis. Ann Otol Rhinol Laryngol 67:440, 1958.
54. Riding KH, Bluestone CD, Michaels RH, et al: Microbiology of recurrent and chronic otitis media with effusion. J Pediatr 93:739, 1978.
55. Post JC, Preston RA, Aul JJ, et al: Molecular analysis of bacterial pathogens in otitis media with effusion. JAMA 273:1598, 1995.
56. Stool SE, Berg AO, Carney CJ, et al: Otitis Media with Effusion in Young Children. Clinical Practice Guideline 12. Rockville, MD, Agency for Health Care Policy and Research, Public Health Service, U.S. Department of Health and Human Services, July 1994. AHCPR publication 94-0622.
57. Casselbrant ML, Brostoff LM, Cantekin EI, et al: Otitis media with effusion in preschool children. Laryngoscope 95:428, 1985.
58. Bluestone CD: Otitis media in children: To treat or not to treat? N Engl J Med 306:1399, 1982.
59. Fria TH, Cantekin EI, Eichler JA: Hearing acuity of children with otitis media with effusion. Arch Otolaryngol 111:10, 1985.
60. Teele DW, Klein JO, Rosner BA, et al: Otitis media with effusion during the first three years of life and development of speech and language. Pediatrics 74:282, 1984.
61. Rosenfeld RM, Mandel EM, Bluestone CD: Systemic steroids for otitis media with effusion in children. Arch Otolaryngol Head Neck Surg 117:984, 1991.
62. Chan KH, Bluestone CD: Lack of efficacy of middle-ear inflation: Treatment of otitis media with effusion in children. Otolaryngol Head Neck Surg 100:317, 1989.
63. Chan KH, Mandel EM, Rockette HE, et al: A comparative study of amoxicillin-clavulanate and amoxicillin. Arch Otolaryngol 114:142, 1988.
64. Thomsen J, Sederberg-Olsen J, Balle V, et al: Antibiotic treatment of children with secretory otitis media. Arch Otolaryngol Head Neck Surg 115:447, 1989.
65. Mandel EM, Rockette HE, Paradise JL, et al: Comparative efficacy of erythromycin-sulfisoxazole, cefaclor, amoxicillin or placebo for otitis media with effusion in children. Pediatr Infect Dis J 10:899, 1991.
66. Rosenfeld RM, Post JC: Meta-analysis of antibiotics for the treatment of otitis media with effusion. Otolaryngol Head Neck Surg 106:378, 1992.
67. Mandel EM, Rockette HE, Bluestone CD, et al: Myringotomy with and without tympanostomy tubes for chronic otitis media with effusion. Arch Otolaryngol Head Neck Surg 115:1217, 1989.
68. Mandel EM, Rockette HE, Bluestone CD, et al: Efficacy of myringotomy with and without tympanostomy tubes for chronic otitis media with effusion. Pediatr Infect Dis J 11:270, 1992.
69. Casselbrant ML, Brostoff LM, Cantekin EI, et al: Otitis media in children in the United States. *In* Sade J (ed): Proceedings of the International Conference on Acute and Secretory Otitis Media. Amsterdam, Kugler Publications, 1986, p 161.
70. Bluestone CD, Klein JO, Gates GA: "Appropriateness" of tympanostomy tubes. Setting the record straight. Arch Otolaryngol Head Neck Surg 120:1051, 1994.
71. Maw AR: Chronic otitis media with effusion (glue ear) and adenotonsillectomy: Prospective randomised controlled study. Br Med J 287:1586, 1983.
72. Gates FA, Avery CA, Prihoda TJ, Cooper JC Jr: Effectiveness of adenoidectomy and tympanostomy tubes in the treatment of chronic otitis media with effusion. N Engl J Med 317:1444, 1987.
73. Maw AR: Age and adenoid size in relation to adenoidectomy in otitis media with effusion. Am J Otolaryngol 6:245, 1985.
74. Gates GA, Avery CA, Prihoda TJ: Effect of adenoidectomy upon children with chronic otitis media with effusion. Laryngoscope 98:58, 1988.
75. Mandel EM, Casselbrant ML, Kurs-Lasky M: Acute otorrhea: Bacteriology of a common complication of tympanostomy tubes. Ann Otol Rhinol Laryngol 103:713, 1994.
76. Kenna MA, Bluestone CD, Reilly JS, et al: Medical management of chronic suppurative otitis media without cholesteatoma in children. Laryngoscope 96:146, 1986.
77. Kenna MA, Rosane BA, Bluestone CD: Medical management of chronic suppurative otitis media without cholesteatoma in children—Update 1992. Am J Otol 14:469, 1993.
78. Bluestone CD: Otologic surgical procedures. *In* Bluestone CD, Stool SE (eds): Atlas of Pediatric Otolaryngology. Philadelphia, WB Saunders, 1995, pp 27–128.

51

Infections of the Pharynx, Larynx, Epiglottis, Trachea, and Thyroid

*Ann Sullivan Baker**
Irmgard Behlau
Maureen R. Tierney

Pharyngitis

Pharyngitis or pharyngotonsillitis is defined as an inflammation in the area of the posterior oral cavity involving lymphoid tissues of the posterior pharynx and lateral pharyngeal bands. Scarlatina anginosa, or sore throat, was described by James Sims[1] in 1803 in Boston and London.

Anatomy

The lymphoid tissues of the nasopharynx and pharynx, known as the Waldeyer ring, include the adenoid, palatine, and lingual tonsils.[2] The lymphoid tissues are present at birth, enlarge in infancy and childhood, and undergo atrophy shortly after puberty. The adenoid, known as the pharyngeal tonsil or Luschka tonsil, is lymphoid tissue of the nasopharynx. It drains into the lymphatics of the retropharyngeal and pharyngomaxillary spaces and from there into the neck. The faucial or palatine tonsil is a cryptic, subepithelial encapsulated lymph node that lies in the tonsillar fossa. The fossa is formed by three muscles: the palatoglossus forms the anterior pillar, the palatopharyngeal forms the posterior pillar, and the superior pharyngeal constrictor forms the bed. The lingual tonsil covers the base of the tongue; it is located behind the circumvallate papillae and may extend to the base of the epiglottis. The lingual tonsil's lymphatics drain into the suprahyoid, submaxillary, and deep cervical lymphatic chains. Whereas the other lymphoid tissue becomes atrophic after puberty, the lingual tonsil often becomes hypertrophic. The cervical lymph nodes effectively drain and filter microorganisms from the structures of Waldeyer ring. The two potential spaces important in the spread of infection from the lymphatic structures of Waldeyer ring are the pharyngomaxillary fossa and the retropharyngeal space (see Chapter 48).

Microbiology

Organisms responsible for acute pharyngitis and tonsillitis include viruses, bacteria, and less often mycoplasmas, spirochetes, and chlamydiae.

The most common viral agents of sore throat are rhinovirus, coronavirus, adenovirus, influenza A and B viruses, and parainfluenza viruses.[3–7] Other viruses associated with pharyngitis include herpes simplex virus (types 1 and 2), coxsackievirus A (types 2, 4, 5, 6, 8, 10), Epstein-Barr virus (EBV), cytomegalovirus, and human immunodeficiency virus.[8, 9]

Of the bacterial organisms, group A β-hemolytic streptococci are estimated to cause approximately 15% of all cases of pharyngitis or pharyngotonsillitis. *Streptococcus pyogenes* is important to diagnose as an agent of pharyngitis because of the possibility of serious suppurative and nonsuppurative sequelae. Less often, groups B, C, and G β-hemolytic streptococci are responsible for sore throat.[7, 10–17] Group C streptococci have been associated with endemic pharyngitis among adults.[12] Corynebacteria including *Corynebacterium diphtheriae* and *Corynebacterium ulcerans, Arcanobacterium haemolyticum* (formerly *Corynebacterium haemolyticum*), *Yersinia enterocolitica, Neisseria gonorrhoeae,* mixed anaerobic infection (Vincent angina), and *Treponema pallidum* are less common causes of pharyngitis.[18–31] In patients with recurrent pharyngotonsillitis, the possibility of β-lactamase–producing bacteria (*Staphylococcus aureus, Haemophilus influenzae, Branhamella (Moraxella) catarrhalis, Bacteroides* species, *Prevotella, Porphyromonas,* and *Fusobacterium*) should be considered. Anaerobes are a major component of tonsil surface and core bacterial flora in patients with recurrent tonsillitis.[32]

Mycoplasma pneumoniae may cause up to 10% of pharyngitis in adults.[7, 33] A less common cause of pharyngitis is *Mycoplasma hominis.* Mufson and colleagues[34, 35] introduced this organism into the nasopharynx of healthy volunteers and induced pharyngitis in 50%, but they were unable to isolate the organism from the pharynx of adults with "natural" pharyngitis. *M. hominis* has also been reported to be the cause of submandibular adenitis in an infant.[36] The role of *Chlamydia trachomatis* is even less firmly established.[37–40] It may be a cause of pharyngitis in the sexually active population seen in sexually transmitted disease clinics, although data are conflicting.[41] *Chlamydia pneumoniae,* previously a TWAR strain of *Chlamydia psittaci,* is associated with cases of pharyngitis, bronchitis, and pneumonia.[42–45]

Epidemiology

In temperate climates, pharyngitis occurs during the respiratory season or during colder months of the year. The peak prevalence of rhinoviruses is during spring and fall, of coronaviruses and adenoviruses (acute respiratory disease) mainly during the colder months, and of other adenoviruses (pharyngoconjunctival fever) in the early summer. Streptococcal pharyngitis occurs during the colder months of the year in temperate climates, and infection rates are higher in late winter and early spring. Fifteen percent to 20% of schoolchildren carry group A streptococci in their throat, but less than 10% have a sore throat. The disease is ordinarily spread by direct person-to-person contact, most likely by droplets of saliva or nasal secretions. Patients who do not receive antibiotic therapy develop type-specific antibodies that are detectable in serum between 4 and 8 weeks after infection; these opsonic antibodies protect against later infection.

Pathogenesis and Pathology

Coronavirus and adenovirus may invade the pharyngeal mucosa directly. Physical findings in viral pharyngitis include hyperemia and edema of the tonsils and pharyngeal mucosa; adenovirus and EBV may produce an inflammatory exudate. Streptococcal invasion may involve natural and acquired host immunity. *S. pyogenes* elaborates several factors—streptokinase, hemolysins, erythrogenic toxin, deoxyribonuclease, proteinase, hyaluronidase—that may play a role in invasion. *S. pyogenes* infection causes edema, hyperemia with exudate, and hemorrhage of pharyngeal walls and tonsils. *C. diphtheriae* may in addition cause a fibrinous membrane of leukocytes, necrotic cells, and bacteria. Increased adherence of *S. aureus, Streptococcus pneumoniae* type I, and *H. influenzae* to pharyngeal cells early during experimental infection with influenza virus suggests that mucosal cell changes leading to

*Deceased.

increased adherence of selected bacteria may also contribute to the pathogenesis of these secondary infections.[46]

Clinical Manifestations

Adenoviral pharyngitis is marked by severe sore throat, malaise, headache, chills, myalgia, and fever. On examination, pharyngeal erythema and exudate are present; conjunctivitis (follicular) may also be present in 25% to 50% of cases. With influenzal pharyngitis, severe sore throat is present with myalgia, headache, cough, coryza, and temperature elevation, but erythema of the pharynx is mild. Only mild pharyngeal irritation is found with rhinovirus infection (common cold); on examination, the pharynx is only slightly inflamed. Primary infection with herpes simplex virus may present as acute painful pharyngitis with erythema and exudate; vesicles and shallow ulcers of both posterior (buccal) and anterior (labial) mucosa are helpful in the diagnosis if associated with gingival stomatitis. Chronic herpes simplex infection in immunocompromised hosts is characterized by progressive large, shallow, painful ulcers. Herpangina (coxsackievirus A) is more common in children and may present as severe sore throat; small vesicles (1 to 2 mm) are typically seen in the posterior pharynx only (soft palate, uvula, and anterior tonsillar pillars). Pharyngitis or exudative tonsillitis occurs in half of patients with infectious mononucleosis (EBV); usually fatigue, malaise, headache, adenopathy, and fever are all present. Pharyngitis with fever, myalgia, lethargy, and truncal maculopapular rash is characteristic of primary infection with human immunodeficiency virus.[9, 47]

The clinical pattern of pharyngitis with *S. pyogenes* ranges from abrupt onset of marked pain, headache, malaise, dysphagia, and fever (temperature higher than 39.4°C) with pharyngeal inflammation, edema, and gray-white tonsillar exudate and tender submandibular lymph nodes to only mild sore throat; pharyngitis due to strains of groups C and G streptococci may present in similar fashion. The disease is self-limited; all acute signs subside within a week. Rare cases of toxic shock syndrome have been described with noninvasive streptococcal pharyngitis.[48] Sore throat, diffuse maculopapular rash, and pharyngeal exudate and erythema may be seen in children and young adults with *A. haemolyticum* infection.[24, 25] *M. pneumoniae* usually produces mild pharyngitis, which may be associated with bronchitis or pneumonia.[49] *C. pneumoniae* may be associated with chronic pharyngitis.[44, 45]

Diagnosis

A definitive diagnosis of pharyngitis may be difficult to make on clinical grounds alone, although the presence of pharyngeal or tonsillar exudate, tender lymph nodes at the angle of the mandible, rash, or conjunctivitis is helpful. Pharyngeal exudate is usually present with group A, C, or G streptococci, *C. diphtheriae, A. haemolyticum, Y. enterocolitica,* anaerobic bacteria, adenovirus, herpes simplex virus, and EBV. Pharyngeal exudate is not usually present with influenza or rhinovirus. Rash may suggest infection with *S. pyogenes, A. haemolyticum,* human immunodeficiency virus, or EBV. The presence of conjunctivitis suggests adenovirus infection or less commonly diphtheria or chlamydia infections. Diagnosis of group A streptococcal infections depends on recognizing the clinical syndrome and culturing the bacterium from a deep throat culture onto a blood agar plate. Tests are available that allow rapid diagnosis of streptococcal pharyngitis by detecting group A streptococcal antigen on throat swab specimens. Latex agglutination and other rapid systems are highly specific (95% to 99%) and moderately sensitive (70% to 90%) compared with throat cultures. Throat cultures should be obtained in clinically suspected cases with negative antigen test results.[50, 51] Most strains of group C and G are β-hemolytic and some are bacitracin sensitive; bacteria in both groups can produce many of the same enzymes and toxins produced by group A streptococci. Serologic tests are also useful in documenting recent streptococcal infection. Many of the enzymes and toxins produced by group A streptococci are antigenic; a variety of antibody tests are available. The most widely used is the antistreptolysin O titer, which is elevated after most respiratory tract infections. Anti-DNase titers are also elevated after streptococcal pharyngitis.

A throat culture plated on Loeffler medium is necessary for any suspected case of diphtheria. The hemolysis associated with *A. haemolyticum* is maximal at 48 to 72 hours and is more prominent on rabbit and human blood agar.[24] Diagnosis of *Mycoplasma* infection depends either on isolation of the organism in culture or on demonstration of a rise in antibody titer. Throat or sputum cultures are placed on SP-4 medium. A report has evaluated a commercially available nucleic acid probe test for *M. pneumoniae* detection in sputum.[52] The diagnosis of *Chlamydia* infections in the acute phase, especially by culture, is often difficult, and the technology is expensive and not widely available. Serologic methods, particularly for *C. pneumoniae,* are helpful in retrospect.[38–42]

Therapy

Group A streptococci continue to be uniformly sensitive to penicillin V potassium, which remains the drug of choice. The dose, schedule, and duration vary; adults usually receive 10 days of oral therapy (500 mg every 6 to 8 hours), and children receive 25 to 50 mg/kg per day in three or four equal doses.[53, 54] A single intramuscular dose of 1.2 million units of benzathine penicillin is an excellent form of therapy because it does not require the patient's compliance. For penicillin-allergic patients, erythromycin, 500 mg four times daily for 10 days, is a good alternative. Instituting treatment within 1 week of the onset of streptococcal pharyngitis prevents subsequent acute rheumatic fever[55]; either approach—waiting for the results of throat culture before starting treatment or beginning therapy and discontinuing it if the culture is negative—is reasonable. In addition to the benefit in rheumatic fever prevention and reduction of acute morbidity, treatment of streptococcal pharyngitis is also important to prevent suppurative complications such as peritonsillar abscess, bacteremia, and rarely postangina sepsis.[56, 57] Multiple M types, most belonging to Fischetti "class I" proteins, have been implicated in acute rheumatic fever. Whether mucoid strains, and especially M type 18, are responsible for the resurgence of acute rheumatic fever remains to be evaluated.[58, 59] Studies have documented failure rates of 25% or more in patients treated with penicillin for acute tonsillitis and even higher for chronic tonsillitis.[60] Factors include reinfection, carrier state, noncompliance, and possible selection of β-lactamase–producing strains of *Haemophilus, Bacteroides, Fusobacterium,* pigmented *Prevotella* and *Porphyromonas* species, and *B. catarrhalis.* In the case of recurrent streptococcal tonsillitis, clindamycin, amoxicillin-clavulanate, or penicillin and metronidazole or a macrolide and metronidazole are reasonable. *Mycoplasma* and chlamydial upper respiratory tract infections respond to erythromycin, 500 mg orally four times daily, or tetracycline, 500 mg orally qid, for 14 days. Viral pharyngitis or chronic oral pharyngeal herpetic infection in an immunosuppressed patient should be treated with acyclovir; therapy is not necessary for acute herpetic pharyngitis in normal hosts. Symptomatic therapy is directed at relieving pharyngeal discomfort. Warm saline gargles, rest, acetaminophen, aspirin, and liquids are sufficient in most cases of viral pharyngitis.

Vincent Angina

Vincent angina is an acute pseudomembranous involvement of the pharynx or tonsils. Acute necrotizing ulcerative gingivitis, or trench mouth, is an ulcerative necrosis of the interdental papillae in the marginal gingivae. If the disease spreads to other oral structures, the term acute necrotizing ulcerative mucositis, or Vincent stomatitis, is used. Acute necrotizing ulcerative gingivitis, acute necrotizing ulcerative mucositis, and Vincent angina are all classified as Vincent disease or Vincent infection.

Etiology

Poor oral hygiene, local irritation from food impaction, and smoking are important local factors; malnutrition, fatigue, stress, trauma, and endocrine or metabolic disturbances are other predisposing factors.[61, 62] The disease is most likely secondary to a combination of fusospirochetal organisms and gram-negative anaerobic organisms (*Bacteroides* species); the fusiform organism most often identified is *Fusobacterium nucleatum*.[63, 64]

Pathogenesis and Pathology

Loesche and coworkers[65] cultured *Prevotella (Bacteroides) intermedius* and *Fusobacterium* species from most patients. Cardocci and Clarke[66] in 1974 postulated that the disease may start as aseptic necrosis secondary to capillary stasis due to poor oral hygiene, smoking, trauma, or stress. Poor oral hygiene may also contribute to stasis by releasing bacterial products from the accumulating dental plaque.

Clinical Manifestations

The disease begins abruptly with pain, fetid odor of the breath, and gingival or tonsillar bleeding. There is necrosis, pseudomembrane, lymphadenopathy, and excessive salivation; fever and anorexia may also occur. The disease may spread to other mucosa and may lead to noma, a gangrenous stomatitis, beginning in the corner of the mouth or cheek and rapidly involving the entire thickness of the lips and cheeks with necrosis and tissue sloughing.[67] Transient bacteremia or septicemia may develop from the massive bacterial flora at bleeding sites.

Diagnosis

Gram-stained specimens of the affected mucosa should be examined for gram-positive cocci, gram-negative bacilli, and fusospirochetal gram-negative organisms. Débrided material is optimal for anaerobic culture.

Therapy

Penicillin at 500 mg four times daily, metronidazole at 500 mg three times daily, and clindamycin at 600 mg three times daily are reasonable therapeutic options.

Laryngitis

The larynx rests in the hypopharynx anterior to the fourth, fifth, and sixth cervical vertebrae. The supraglottic larynx includes the laryngeal inlet formed by the epiglottis anteriorly and the arytenoepiglottic folds bilaterally, all merging inferiorly into false cords. The glottic larynx consists of the true vocal folds; the space between the folds is termed the glottis. Respiratory viruses such as influenza virus, parainfluenza virus, rhinovirus, and adenovirus are most often isolated in cases of laryngitis.[68, 69] *B. catarrhalis* has been recovered from the nasopharynx of 50% to 55% and *H. influenzae* from 14% of adults with acute laryngitis; whether these represent secondary bacterial invasion is not clear.[70] *M. hominis* is an uncommon but important pathogen as a cause of granulomatous laryngitis. The spread may occur contiguously from the pulmonary infection or hematogenously.[71, 72] Hoarseness in the patient with pulmonary lesions and productive cough should prompt biopsy of the larynx. Other causes of granulomatous laryngitis include fungal infections such as histoplasmosis, coccidioidomycosis, blastomycosis, and candidiasis. *Candida* infection commonly accompanies esophageal infection in compromised hosts.[73–77] *T. pallidum*, herpes simplex virus, and herpes zoster virus may be isolated from the larynx[78]; finally, Wegener granulomatosis, sarcoid, and rhinoscleroma should be considered.[71]

Symptoms of acute laryngitis include hoarseness, odynophagia, and pain, which may be referred to other branches of the vagus and manifested by otalgia. Examination of the larynx reveals inflammation, edema, and secretions; there may be superficial mucosal ulcerations. The presence of an exudate or membrane on the pharyngeal or laryngeal mucosa should raise the suspicion of streptococcal infection, mononucleosis, or diphtheria; granulomatous infiltration is compatible with tuberculosis, fungal infection, syphilis, or sarcoid. Treatment consists of resting the voice, inhaling moistened air, and appropriate antibiotic therapy.

Acute Supraglottitis (Epiglottitis)

Supraglottitis (epiglottitis), first described in 1900 by Theisen,[79] is characterized by a severe upper respiratory tract infection with fever, sore throat, hoarseness, dysphagia, and drooling that may rapidly progress to fatal airway obstruction. Despite that LeMierre and coworkers[80] in 1936 were among the first clinicians to describe adult epiglottitis and the association with *H. influenzae* infection, it was not until the late 1960s and reports by Johnstone and Lawy[81] and Gorfinkel and colleagues[82] that supraglottitis was increasingly recognized in adults.

Epiglottitis, which most commonly affects children 2 to 7 years of age, is undergoing a dramatic and changing epidemiologic pattern since the introduction of the *H. influenzae* type b (Hib) vaccines in the middle to late 1980s. With continued widespread vaccination of younger children with the conjugate Hib vaccines, *H. influenzae* type b epiglottitis in young children should soon become a rarity. Epiglottitis will become a disease of older children and adults, and it will be due predominantly to microbial pathogens other than *H. influenzae* type b.

Microbiology

The bacterium in most cases of acute supraglottitis in children is *H. influenzae* type b, but other pathogens have included *S. pneumoniae*, *S. aureus*, other streptococci, *H. influenzae* type non-b, and *Haemophilus parainfluenzae*.[83] The isolation rate for *H. influenzae* from blood cultures is between 80% and 100%.[83, 84] The bacteriology of adult epiglottitis is less well defined, but *H. influenzae* type b is a principal agent, in some reports accounting for 26%.[85] The presence of *H. influenzae* bacteremia is associated with a more fulminant course, with the development of respiratory obstruction.[85, 86] In adults, infection may also occur with organisms other than *H. influenzae* type b, including *S. pneumoniae*, β-hemolytic streptococci, *H. influenzae* of unspecified type, *H. parainfluenzae*, and *Pasteurella multocida*.[87, 88] The role of respiratory tract viruses as pathogens in adults and children remains unclear. In many adult cases, an agent is not found.[88]

Epidemiology

Supraglottitis is responsible for 1 of every 1000 to 2000 admissions to a pediatric hospital[89]; for adults, the frequency is much lower, approximately 10 cases per million.[86]

Pathophysiology

Supraglottitis is characterized by inflammation and edema of the supraglottic structures, including the epiglottis, arytenoepiglottic folds, arytenoids, and false vocal cords; paradoxically, the epiglottis may be spared. The mechanism of supraglottic infection is unknown. Supraglottitis may arise from direct invasion by *H. influenzae* or other pathogens. It is possible that mucosal surface trauma secondary to eating or antecedent viral infection may lead to a secondary bacterial infection, but the role of virus as a primary pathogen has not been demonstrated. It is also not clear whether bacteremia, which is seen frequently in children, may be a primary event, with seeding of the supraglottis, or a secondary event.

Clinical Manifestations

In children, acute supraglottitis is typically characterized as a fulminating course of severe sore throat, high fever, dysphagia, drooling, and airway obstruction, which, left untreated, leads to death. Low-pitched inspiratory stridor is due to the approximation of the swollen supraglottic structures. On physical examination, the child looks toxic and apprehensive and frequently assumes an airway-preserving posture—sitting upright, with the jaw protruding forward, while drooling. Respirations are deliberate without marked tachypnea. Tachycardia out of proportion to the amount of pyrexia is a reflection of the hypoxia. Should stridor be absent, an unwary physician might underestimate the severity and rapidity of progression of the patient's worsening air exchange, which may result in cardiopulmonary arrest if it is left untreated.

The presentation of acute supraglottitis in adults is more variable; most adults have mild illness with a prolonged prodrome.[88] Some may not seek medical attention or may be treated for presumed pharyngitis. This does not mean that the disease is any less serious; in some studies, it carries a mortality risk of 7.1%.[88] In immunocompromised hosts, the clinical presentation may be less typical. In a report of five patients with the acquired immunodeficiency syndrome,[90] the clinical presentation was notable for a paucity of physical findings. Laryngoscopy revealed a large, pale, boggy epiglottis with an edematous supraglottis and cervical adenopathy coupled with rapidly progressing airway obstruction. Local complications of supraglottitis include spread into the retropharyngeal area and epiglottic abscess formation; systemic complications include bacteremia, pneumonia (in up to 25% of cases),[91] meningitis, arthritis, and cellulitis.

Diagnosis

Definitive diagnosis is made by examination of the epiglottis and supraglottic structures. No attempt should be made to visualize the epiglottis in an awake young child, so a severely ill child must often be examined in the operating room at the time of control of the airway. In adults, awake indirect laryngoscopy is usually sufficient to make the diagnosis. This examination should be performed only when it is possible to establish an artificial airway if necessary. In children, the epiglottis is typically fiery red and extremely swollen, but occasionally the major inflammation involves the ventricular bands and arytenoepiglottic folds, and the epiglottis appears relatively normal. In adults, the supraglottic structures may appear pale with watery edema.

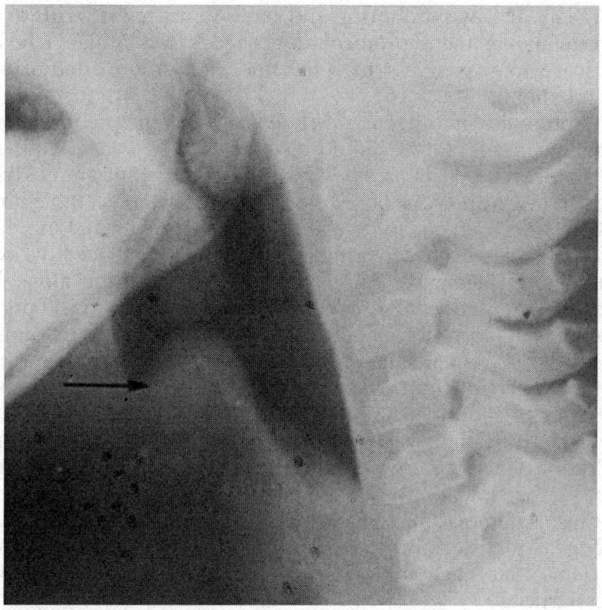

FIGURE 51–1 □ Thickened epiglottis *(arrow)* in patient with epiglottitis. (Courtesy of Dr. A. Weber, Massachusetts Eye and Ear Infirmary, Boston, MA.)

Laboratory findings include leukocytosis. Blood and supraglottic specimens should be obtained for culture; serum and urine samples for *H. influenzae* type b antigen may be useful. Lateral soft tissue radiographs may reveal the classic thumb sign (Fig. 51–1) and, in some, swelling of the arytenoepiglottic folds and arytenoids, with a sensitivity of approximately 79%.[83, 86]

Major causes of upper airway obstruction can be classified by the anatomic level of involvement, using the glottis as the dividing line. Other supraglottic conditions are peritonsillar and retropharyngeal abscesses, severe tonsillitis, and adenotonsillar hypertrophy associated with infectious mononucleosis. Subglottic obstruction may be from croup (laryngotracheitis), laryngotracheobronchitis, diphtheria, angioedema (allergic laryngeal edema), foreign body aspiration, or neoplasm.

Treatment

Treatment of acute supraglottitis is directed at establishment of an airway and administration of appropriate antibiotics. The mortality rates of supraglottitis vary greatly; most deaths occur within the first few hours after arrival at a hospital. Children with epiglottitis should routinely have an artificial airway established; observation cannot be recommended, because the associated mortality rate is 6% to 25%, and it increases to 33% to 80% for those who develop obstruction.[92, 93] The use of a "prophylactic airway" has reduced mortality in children from 6% to less than 1%.[94] An endotracheal tube is preferred by most authors over a tracheotomy for provision of the artificial airway.[94–96] Advantages of nasotracheal intubation are (1) the ease of removal of the tube 2 or 3 days after edema has subsided, thereby shortening hospitalization[95, 96]; (2) no surgery; and (3) mortality and complication rates equal to or lower than those for tracheotomy. If accidental extubation should occur, there is a grace period of 30 to 60 minutes caused by the ballooning effect of the endotracheal tube,[95, 97] which is not afforded by tracheotomy. Once the tube is in place, accidental extubation is uncommon (9%).[95] The management of airway in adult epiglottitis reflects the greater variability of clinical presentation and course; the range of mortality rates is 10% to 32%.[84, 86, 98–101]

Vigilant airway monitoring and continuous staging with uniform management protocols are needed for adults, whose disease may progress to respiratory compromise requiring intubation.[102–104]

Antibiotics are directed at *H. influenzae* as the predominant organism; antibiotics should also cover *S. pneumoniae*, other streptococci, and *H. parainfluenzae*. With a risk of ampicillin-resistant *H. influenzae* of 15% to 25%,[83] intravenous ampicillin, 200 mg/kg per day, plus chloramphenicol, 75 to 100 mg/kg per day, has been conventional therapy. When negative results of β-lactamase tests are available, ampicillin alone is given. Alternatively, intravenous cefuroxime, 100 to 200 mg/kg per day, or a third-generation cephalosporin active against *H. influenzae* is also effective as initial therapy. The condition of most patients improves by 48 hours, but antibiotic therapy should be continued for 10 to 14 days.

The artificial airway can usually be removed by 48 hours. Criteria for safe removal of the airway are clinical response and either a leak around the endotracheal tube or evidence of resolution on direct visualization with a fiberoptic laryngoscope. An air leak has proved to be a reliable indicator of the extent of laryngeal inflammation, making direct visualization less crucial.[97]

Prevention

Rifampin prophylaxis,[105] a single daily dose for 4 days (20 mg/kg, not to exceed 600 mg/d)[105] is recommended for (1) all household contacts when there are susceptible members younger than 4 years, (2) daycare and nursery school classroom contacts (including adults), and (3) the patient, who should receive rifampin in the same dosage before discharge to prevent reintroduction of the organism into the household.

Promise for the prevention of invasive disease due to *H. influenzae* was heralded by the development of a polysaccharide Hib vaccine first marketed in the United States in 1985[106, 107] and newer, more effective conjugated vaccines licensed in 1987.[108] Since 1990, two Hib conjugate vaccines have been available in the United States for infants beginning at 2 months of age, and Hib vaccination has become more widespread. Completed vaccination levels in children aged 19 to 35 months were 28.2% in 1992 and 55.0% in 1993.[109] With this limited vaccination, we are already witnessing a marked decline in the incidence of all invasive diseases caused by *H. influenzae* type b in the United States from 41 per 100,000 population in 1987 to 2 per 100,000 in 1993, a 95% decrease.[110]

As of yet, there have not been any large-scale studies published that analyze effects of a vigorous immunization program on the incidence of epiglottitis representative of the U.S. population at large. In Finland, large-scale vaccination of 94% to 98% of infants with the Hib conjugate vaccine was begun in 1986.[111] In the next 5 years, the incidence of *H. influenzae* type b epiglottitis decreased by 50 to 60 cases annually in 1985 and 1986 to 2 cases in 1992. There was no increase in the occurrence of epiglottitis caused by other pathogens. In limited U.S. population studies, the incidence of epiglottitis appears to have also declined dramatically. In one larger study, Gorelick and Baker[112] reported an 84% decline in the incidence of epiglottitis from 10.9 per 10,000 admissions to the Children's Hospital of Philadelphia from 1979 to 1989 to an average annual incidence of 1.8 per 10,000 during 1990 to 1992. With continued widespread immunization with the Hib conjugate vaccine, we can hope for near-eradication of *H. influenzae* type b epiglottitis in children.

Tracheitis

Whether George Washington died of bacterial laryngotracheitis, supraglottitis, or peritonsillar abscess is unclear; his physician's description was that of "cynanche trachealis."[113] The classic description of "angina suffocativa" fits well with the entity described as bacterial tracheitis.[114] Cases of probable bacterial tracheitis (laryngotracheobronchitis) with marked exudate were described in the 1940s by Orton and coworkers[115] and Neffson.[116] This entity affects both children and adults. The syndrome develops as a sequela of injury to the trachea, as from a viral infection (most commonly parainfluenza) or intubation.[117–120] The acute onset is marked by high fever, stridor, and dyspnea, with copious amounts of purulent sputum. The clinical picture may resemble that of epiglottitis and may progress rapidly, requiring endotracheal intubation.

The organisms most commonly recovered from the tracheal exudate are *S. aureus*, group A β-hemolytic streptococci, and *H. influenzae* type b.[121]

The rapidly progressive course demands prompt diagnosis and differentiation from epiglottitis and croup. Relapsing polychondritis develops more slowly. Endoscopic examination demonstrates a normal glottic larynx with purulent debris, ulceration, and edema of the subglottis and trachea. The lateral soft tissue radiograph of the neck characteristically reveals a normal epiglottis with subglottic narrowing (pencil sign). Gram stain examination and culture of the tracheal secretions are necessary to identify the pathogen. Initial antibiotic therapy should cover streptococci, *S. aureus*, and *H. influenzae*; ampicillin-sulbactam or nafcillin and cefuroxime are reasonable antibiotics.

Thyroiditis

Infections of the thyroid gland range from acute suppurative thyroiditis due to bacterial or fungal disease[122, 123] to the more subtle forms of subacute thyroiditis that may be related in some cases to recent viral infections. Other indolent forms of thyroiditis that are believed to be autoimmune in etiology may also be triggered by previous bacterial or viral infections.

Etiology and Pathogenesis

Acute suppurative thyroiditis is a rare occurrence and was so even in the preantibiotic era. The thyroid is fairly resistant to infection, owing to its capsule, its high iodine content, and the lack of direct communication with neighboring structures.[124, 125] In children, thyroiditis often develops in a persistent thyroglossal duct or in a third or fourth branchial arch anomaly arising from the left piriform sinus; a congenital fistula from the piriform sinus apex to the thyroid gland has been identified in approximately 23 cases of suppurative thyroiditis. Less common causes in children, but more common in adults, are blood-borne infections, direct or blunt trauma, and contiguous spread from infected adjacent structures.[122–128]

Because suppurative infections of the thyroid gland usually accompany infections of the upper respiratory tract or nearby head and neck structures, the usual organisms involved include oral flora, *S. aureus*, *S. pyogenes*, and *S. pneumoniae*. On needle aspiration, anaerobes are obtained approximately half the time, either alone or as part of a mixed infection.[124, 125] A few cases of emphysematous or gangrenous thyroiditis secondary to *Clostridium* species have been reported.[129] Unusual agents of thyroiditis—*Pseudallescheria (Petriellidium) boydii, Candida, Aspergillus, Coccidioides immitis, Pneumocystis carinii,* and *Actinomyces* organisms—have been reported occasionally.[130–136] These atypical cases are usually opportunistic infections in immunocompromised patients; they may follow either a subacute or a fulminant course.

Rarely, mycobacterial infections have been reported to cause suppurative thyroiditis.[137]

Subacute thyroiditis is either of two entities: subacute granulomatous thyroiditis or subacute lymphocytic thyroiditis.[138] Subacute granulomatous thyroiditis is about one fortieth as common as Hashimoto thyroiditis and was originally described by de Quervain in 1904. It has been associated with recent infection by mumps, measles, influenza, adenovirus, EBV, or coxsackievirus.[139, 140] Cytomegalovirus involvement of the thyroid has also occurred with disseminated cytomegalovirus infection in immunocompromised hosts.[141] Studies have also suggested a serologic association between *Yersinia* infections and subacute thyroiditis as well as other forms of thyroid disease.[142, 143] Subacute lymphocytic thyroiditis was previously thought to be a variant of Hashimoto thyroiditis or subacute granulomatous thyroiditis. Although rare, it usually affects women post partum and is probably an autoimmune disease.[144]

Clinical Manifestations

Acute suppurative thyroiditis presents with the sudden onset of painful, tender swelling in the area of the thyroid and is accompanied by fever, sore throat, and occasionally hoarseness and dysphagia. Many patients, especially children, have a recent history of upper respiratory tract infection or otitis media. Examination reveals a tender neck mass, erythema, and a fluctuant mass in the case of abscess formation.[124, 125] Actinomycosis and other fungal infections of the thyroid progress slowly and may mimic subacute thyroiditis.[130–136] Crepitus is suggestive of emphysematous thyroid infections and demands a more urgent course of action. Only in rare cases does thyroid storm occur as a result of acute suppuration of the thyroid.

Pain, enlargement, and tenderness of the thyroid, often in the absence of fever, are typical of subacute granulomatous thyroiditis. Other constitutional symptoms may accompany the local manifestations.[138, 139, 144] Subacute lymphocytic thyroiditis, however, is manifested by painless enlargement of the thyroid with minimal tenderness.[138] Both forms of subacute inflammation are accompanied by an early period of transient hyperthyroidism, usually followed by a temporary hypothyroid phase. Subacute thyroiditis may relapse one or more times before recovery is complete.[144] Any form of thyroiditis may rarely present as a fever of unknown origin; this is less common with the acute suppurative thyroiditis, which is usually accompanied by other symptoms.

Diagnosis

The diagnosis of acute suppurative thyroiditis may be evident on clinical grounds alone; however, similar signs may herald cervical adenitis, Ludwig angina, perichondritis of the laryngeal cartilage, and cellulitis of the anterior neck.[124, 125] Findings of thyroid function tests are rarely abnormal, and they may be either elevated or depressed. Thyroid nuclear imaging usually demonstrates diminished uptake, or none, in the involved lobe or pole. Soft tissue films can determine roughly the extent of the mass and whether tracheal compression or any air is present. Computed tomography may help if the presence of an abscess is suggested by physical examination. Needle aspiration or biopsy should be done to identify the pathogen.[122–125]

All children and most adults with acute suppurative thyroiditis should have a barium swallow examination to evaluate for persistent thyroglossal duct or piriform sinus anomaly. Endoscopic examination of the hypopharynx is useful to confirm the diagnosis.[126]

Subacute granulomatous thyroiditis is also suggested by the presence of a painful, tender neck mass. It should be considered in certain patients with nonpainful neck mass and low-grade fever or accelerated erythrocyte sedimentation rate. Evaluation includes thyroid function tests, antimicrosomal antibodies, and a radionuclide-enhanced thyroid scan, which will reveal diffuse low uptake. Needle biopsy is performed to differentiate subacute thyroiditis from lymphoma, thyroid carcinoma, indolent fungal infection, and the occasional case of Hashimoto thyroiditis that presents with either fever or a tender goiter.[138]

Therapy and Prognosis

Therapy for suppurative thyroiditis depends on the organism isolated. Initial empirical antibiotic therapy includes coverage for *S. aureus*, *S. pneumoniae*, and oral flora. *H. influenzae* should also be considered when thyroiditis accompanies otitis or supraglottitis. If air or abscess formation is present, then a more extensive surgical approach and antibiotic coverage for clostridia are necessary.[124, 125]

Patients with subacute thyroiditis often need no therapy. If fever or pain persists, antiinflammatory agents may be useful. In extreme cases, steroid therapy may be necessary. The patient should be informed that recurrences are possible but do not indicate a poorer prognosis. Thyroid function is monitored to detect the 10% of patients who develop hypothyroidism.[138]

References

1. Sims J: Scarlatina anginosa, commonly called sore throat. *In* Observations, ed 3. London, Hall and Hiller, 1803.
2. Pratt LW: Infections of the lymphoid tissue. Otolaryngology 3:27, 1990.
3. MacMillan JA, Sandstrom C, Weiner LB, et al: Viral and bacterial organisms associated with acute pharyngitis in a school-aged population. J Pediatr 109:747, 1986.
4. Hendley JO, Fishburne HB, Gwaltney JM Jr: Coronavirus infections in working adults. Am Rev Respir Dis 105:805, 1972.
5. Wenzel RP, Hendley JO, Davies JA, et al: Coronavirus infections in military recruits. Three-year study with coronavirus strains OC43 and 229E. Am Rev Respir Dis 109:621, 1974.
6. Evans AS, Dick EC: Acute pharyngitis and tonsillitis in University of Wisconsin students. JAMA 190:699, 1964.
7. Glezen WP, Clyde WA Jr, Senior RJ, et al: Group A streptococci, mycoplasmas, and viruses associated with acute pharyngitis. JAMA 202:455, 1967.
8. Glezen WP, Fernald GW, Lohr JA: Acute respiratory disease of university students with special reference to the etiologic role of *Herpesvirus hominis*. Am J Epidemiol 101:111, 1975.
9. Valle SOL: Febrile pharyngitis as the primary sign of HIV infection in a cluster of cases linked by sexual contact. Scand J Infect Dis 19:13, 1987.
10. Paradise JL: Etiology, diagnosis and antimicrobial treatment of pharyngitis and pharyngotonsillitis. Ann Otol Rhinol Laryngol 90(Suppl):75, 1981.
11. Chretien JH, McGinniss CG, Thompson J, et al: Group B β-hemolytic streptococci causing pharyngitis. J Clin Microbiol 10:263, 1979.
12. Meier FA, Centor RM, Graham L Jr, Dalton HP: Clinical and microbiological evidence for endemic pharyngitis among adults due to group C streptococci. Arch Intern Med 150:825, 1990.
13. Turner JC, Hayden GF, Kiselica D, et al: Association of group C β-hemolytic streptococci with endemic pharyngitis among college students. JAMA 264:2644, 1990.
14. Turner JC, Fox A, Fox K, et al: Role of group C beta-hemolytic streptococci in pharyngitis: Epidemiologic study of clinical features associated with isolation of group C streptococci. J Clin Microbiol 31:808, 1993.
15. Stryker WS, Fraser DW, Facklam RR: Food-borne outbreak of group G streptococcal pharyngitis. Am J Epidemiol 116:533, 1982.

16. Cohen D, Ferne M, Rouach T, et al: Food-borne outbreak of group G streptococcal sore throat in an Israeli military base. Epidemiol Infect 99:249, 1987.
17. Gerber MA, Randolph MF, Martin NJ, et al: Community-wide outbreak of group G streptococcal pharyngitis. Pediatrics 87:598, 1991.
18. Tacket CO, Davis BR, Carter GP, et al: *Yersinia enterocolitica* pharyngitis. Ann Intern Med 99:40, 1983.
19. Harnisch JP, Tronca E, Nolan CM, et al: Diphtheria among alcoholic urban adults. Ann Intern Med 111:71, 1989.
20. Seidenfeld SM, Sutker WL, Luby JP: *Fusobacterium necrophorum* septicemia following oropharyngeal infection. JAMA 248:1348, 1982.
21. Hutt DM, Judson FN: Epidemiology and treatment of oropharyngeal gonorrhea. Ann Intern Med 105:655, 1986.
22. Green SL, LaPeter KS: Pseudodiphtheritic membranous pharyngitis caused by *Corynebacterium hemolyticum.* JAMA 245:2330, 1981.
23. Kovatch AL, Schuit KE, Michaels RH: *Corynebacterium hemolyticum* peritonsillar abscess mimicking diphtheria. JAMA 249:1757, 1983.
24. Miller RA, Brancato F, Holmes KK: *Corynebacterium hemolyticum* as a cause of pharyngitis and scarlatiniform rash in young adults. Ann Intern Med 105:867, 1986.
25. Karpathios T, Drakonaki S, Zervoudaki A, et al: *Arcanobacterium haemolyticum* in children with presumed streptococcal pharyngotonsillitis or scarlet fever. J Pediatr 12:735, 1992.
26. Greenman JL: *Corynebacterium hemolyticum* and pharyngitis. Ann Intern Med 106:633, 1987.
27. Hart RJC: *Corynebacterium ulcerans* in humans and cattle in North Devon. J Hyg 92:161, 1984.
28. Banck G, Nyman M: Tonsillitis and rash associated with *Corynebacterium haemolyticum.* J Infect Dis 154:1037, 1986.
29. Carlson P, Renkonen OV, Kontiainen S: *Arcanobacterium haemolyticum* and streptococcal pharyngitis. Scand J Infect Dis 26:283, 1994.
30. Rose FB, Camp CJ, Antes EJ: Family outbreak of fatal *Yersinia enterocolitica* pharyngitis. Am J Med 82:636, 1987.
31. Shimizu T, Shinogi J, Majima Y, Sakakura Y: Secondary syphilis of the tonsil. Arch Otorhinolaryngol 246:117, 1989.
32. Mitchelmore IJ, Reilly PG, Hay AJ, Tabaqchali S: Tonsil surface and core cultures in recurrent tonsillitis: Prevalence of anaerobes and beta-lactamase producing organisms. Eur J Clin Microbiol Infect Dis 13:542, 1994.
33. Foy HM, Grayston JR, Kenny GE, et al: Epidemiology of *Mycoplasma pneumoniae* infections in families. JAMA 197:859, 1966.
34. Mufson MA, Ludwig WM, Purcell RH, et al: Exudative pharyngitis following experimental *Mycoplasma hominis* type I infection. JAMA 192:1146, 1965.
35. Mufson MA: *Mycoplasma hominis*: A review of its role as a respiratory tract pathogen of humans. Sex Transm Dis 10:335, 1983.
36. Powell DA, Miller K, Clyde WA Jr: Submandibular adenitis in a newborn caused by *Mycoplasma hominis.* Pediatrics 63:798, 1979.
37. Reed BD, Huck W, Lutz LJ, et al: Prevalence of *Chlamydia trachomatis* and *Mycoplasma pneumoniae* in children with and without pharyngitis. J Fam Pract 26:387, 1988.
38. Komaroff AL, Aronson MD, Pass TM, et al: Serologic evidence of chlamydial and mycoplasmal pharyngitis in adults. Science 222:927, 1983.
39. Gerber MA, Ryan RW, Tilton RC, et al: Role of *Chlamydia trachomatis* in acute pharyngitis in adults. J Clin Microbiol 20:993, 1984.
40. Huss H, Jungkind D, Amadio P, et al: Frequency of *Chlamydia trachomatis* as the cause of pharyngitis. J Clin Microbiol 22:858, 1985.
41. Jones RB, Rabinovitch RA, Katz BP, et al: *Chlamydia trachomatis* in the pharynx and rectum of heterosexual patients at risk of genital infection. Ann Intern Med 102:757, 1985.
42. Grayston JT, Juo C-C, Wan S-P, et al: A new *Chlamydia psittaci* strain, TWAR, isolated in acute respiratory tract infections. N Engl J Med 315:161, 1986.
43. Grayston JT: Infections caused by *Chlamydia pneumoniae* strain TWAR. Clin Infect Dis 15:757, 1992.
44. Hammerschlag WR, Chirgwin K, Roblin PW, et al: Persistent infection with *Chlamydia pneumoniae* following acute respiratory illness. Clin Infect Dis 14:178, 1992.
45. Falck G, Heyman L, Gnarpe J, Gnarpe H: *Chlamydia pneumoniae* and chronic pharyngitis. Scand J Infect Dis 27:179, 1995.
46. Fainstein V, Musher DM, Cate TR: Bacterial adherence to pharyngeal cells during viral infection. J Infect Dis 141:2, 1980.
47. Kessler HA, Blaauw B, Spear J, et al: Diagnosis of human immunodeficiency virus infection in seronegative homosexuals presenting with an acute viral syndrome. JAMA 258:1196, 1987.
48. Chapnick EK, Gradon JO, Lutwick LI, et al: Streptococcal toxic shock syndrome due to noninvasive pharyngitis. Clin Infect Dis 14:1074, 1992.
49. Murray HW, Masur H, Senterfit L, Roberts R: The protean manifestations of *Mycoplasma pneumoniae* in adults. Am J Med 58:229, 1975.
50. Bisno AL, Ofek I: Serologic diagnosis of streptococcal infection: Comparison of a rapid hemagglutination technique with conventional antibody tests. Am J Dis Child 127:676, 1974.
51. Centor RM, Meier FA, Dalton HP: Throat cultures and rapid tests for diagnosis of group A streptococcal pharyngitis. Ann Intern Med 105:892, 1986.
52. Kleemola SRM, Karjalainen JE, Raty RKH: Rapid diagnosis of *Mycoplasma pneumoniae* infection: Clinical evaluation of a commercial Probe Test. J Infect Dis 162:70, 1990.
53. Denny FW: Current management of streptococcal pharyngitis. J Fam Pract 35:619, 1992.
54. Peter G: Streptococcal pharyngitis: Current therapy and criteria for evaluation of new agents. Clin Infect Dis 14(Suppl):S218, S231, 1992.
55. Massell BF: Prophylaxis of streptococcal infections and rheumatic fever. JAMA 241:1589, 1979.
56. Shapiro J, Strome M, Fried MP: Postanginal sepsis. Head Neck Surg 11:164, 1989.
57. Alvarez A, Schreiber JR: Lemierre's syndrome in adolescent children—Anaerobic sepsis with internal jugular vein thrombophlebitis following pharyngitis. Pediatrics 96(pt 1):354, 1995.
58. Veasy LG, Wiedmeier SE, Orsmond GS, et al: Resurgence of acute rheumatic fever in the intermountain area of the United States. N Engl J Med 316:421, 1987.
59. Stollerman GH: Rheumatogenic group A streptococci and the return of rheumatic fever. Adv Intern Med 35:1, 1990.
60. Orrling A, Stjernquist-Desatnik A, Schalen C, Kamme C: Clindamycin in persisting streptococcal pharyngotonsillitis after penicillin treatment. Scand J Infect Dis 26:535, 1994.
61. Barnes PB, Bowles WF III, Carter HG: Acute necrotizing ulcerative gingivitis: A survey of 218 cases. J Periodontol 44:35, 1973.
62. Russell AL: Epidemiology of periodontal disease. Int Dent J 17:282, 1967.
63. Uohara GI, Knapp MJ: Oral fusospirochetosis and associated lesions. Oral Surg Oral Med Oral Pathol 24:113, 1967.
64. Listgarten MA, Lewis DW: The distribution of spirochetes in the lesion of acute necrotizing ulcerative gingivitis. An electron microscopic and statistical survey. J Periodontol 38:379, 1967.
65. Loesche WJ, Syed SA, Laughon BE, Stoll J: The bacteriology of acute necrotizing ulcerative gingivitis. J Periodontol 53:223, 1982.
66. Cardocci BJ, Clarke NG: Aetiology of acute necrotizing ulcerative gingivitis: A hypothetical explanation. J Periodontol 45:830, 1974.
67. Ryan ME, Hopkins K, Wilbur RB: Acute necrotizing ulcerative gingivitis in children with cancer. Am J Dis Child 137:592, 1983.
68. Dingle JH, Badger GF, Jordan WS Jr: Illness in the Home. A Study of 25,000 Illnesses in a Group of Cleveland Families. Cleveland, The Press of Western Reserve University, 1964, p 66.
69. McNamara MJ, Pierce WE, Crawford YE, et al: Patterns of adenovirus infection in the respiratory diseases of naval recruits, a longitudinal study of two companies of naval recruits. Am Rev Respir Dis 86:485, 1962.
70. Schalen L, Christensen P, Kamme C, et al: High isolation rate of *Branhamella catarrhalis* from the nasopharynx in adults with acute laryngitis. Scand J Infect Dis 12:277, 1980.
71. Case records of the Massachusetts General Hospital. N Engl J Med 309:1569, 1983.
72. Thaller SR, Gross JR, Pilch BZ, et al: Laryngeal tuberculosis as manifested in the decades 1963–1983. Laryngoscope 97:848, 1987.
73. Dudley JP, Byrne WJ, Kobayashi R, et al: *Candida* laryngitis in chronic mucocutaneous candidiasis. Its association with *Candida* esophagitis. Ann Otol Rhinol Laryngol 89:574, 1980.

74. Lawson R, Bodey G, Luna M: *Candida* infection presenting as laryngitis. Am J Med Sci 280:173, 1980.
75. Donegan JO, Wood MD: Histoplasmosis of the larynx. Laryngoscope 94:206, 1984.
76. Platt M: Laryngeal coccidioidomycosis. JAMA 237:1234, 1977.
77. Suen JY, Wetmore SJ, Wetzel WJ, Craig RD: Blastomycosis of the larynx. Ann Otol Rhinol Laryngol 89:563, 1980.
78. Karnauchow PN, Kaul WH: Chronic herpetic laryngitis with oropharyngitis. Ann Otol Rhinol Laryngol 97:286, 1988.
79. Theisen CF: Angina epiglottidea anterior: Report of 3 cases. Albany Med Ann 21:395, 1900.
80. LeMierre A, Meyer A, Laplone R: Les septicimies à bacille de Pfeiffer. Ann Med 39:97, 1936.
81. Johnstone JM, Lawy HS: Acute epiglottitis in adults due to infection with *Haemophilus influenzae* type b. Lancet 2:134, 1967.
82. Gorfinkel HJ, Brown R, Kabin SA: Acute infectious epiglottitis in adults. Ann Intern Med 70:289, 1969.
83. Crysdale WS, Sendi K: Evolution in the management of acute epiglottitis: A 10-year experience with 242 children. Int Anesthesiol Clin 26:32, 1988.
84. Butt W, Shann F, Walker C, et al: Acute epiglottitis: A different approach to management. Crit Care Med 16:43, 1988.
85. Mustoe T, Strome M: Adult epiglottitis. Am J Otolaryngol 4:393, 1983.
86. Mayosmith MF, Hirsch PJ, Wodzinski SF, et al: Acute epiglottitis in adults: An eight-year experience in the state of Rhode Island. N Engl J Med 314:1133, 1986.
87. Carenfelt C: Etiology of acute infectious epiglottitis in adults: Septic vs. local infection. Scand J Infect Dis 21:53, 1989.
88. Shapiro J, Eavey RD, Baker AS: Adult supraglottitis: A prospective analysis. JAMA 259:563, 1988.
89. Takala AK, Eskola J, Peltola H, Makela PH: Epidemiology of invasive *Haemophilus influenzae* type b disease among children in Finland before vaccination with *Haemophilus influenzae* type b conjugate vaccine. Pediatr Infect Dis J 8:297, 1989.
90. Rothstein SG, Persky MS, Edelman BA, et al: Epiglottitis in AIDS patients. Laryngoscope 99:389, 1989.
91. Molteni RA: Epiglottitis: Incidence of extraepiglottic infection: Report of 72 cases and review of the literature. Pediatrics 58:526, 1976.
92. Bass JW, Steele RW, Weibe RA: Acute epiglottitis: A surgical emergency. JAMA 229:671, 1974.
93. Baines DB, Wark H, Overton JH: Acute epiglottitis in children. Anaesth Intensive Care 13:25, 1984.
94. Cantrell RW, Bell RA, Morioka WT: Acute epiglottitis: Intubation versus tracheotomy. Laryngoscope 88:994, 1978.
95. Crockett DM, Healy GB, McGill TJ, Friedman EM: Airway management of acute supraglottitis at the Children's Hospital, Boston: 1980–1985. Ann Otol Rhinol Laryngol 97:114, 1988.
96. Oh TH, Motoyama ED: Comparisons of nasotracheal intubation and tracheotomy in management of acute epiglottitis. Anesthesiology 46:214, 1983.
97. Arndal H, Andreassen UK: Acute epiglottitis in children and adults. Nasotracheal intubation, tracheostomy or careful observation? Current status in Scandinavia. J Laryngol Otol 102:1012, 1988.
98. Robbins JP, Fitz-Hugh GS: Epiglottitis in the adult. Laryngoscope 81:700, 1971.
99. Hawkins DB, Miller AH, Sachs GB, et al: Acute epiglottitis in adults. Laryngoscope 83:1211, 1973.
100. Khilanani U, Khatib R: Acute epiglottitis in adults. Am J Med Sci 287:65, 1984.
101. Baker AS, Eavey R: Adult supraglottitis (epiglottitis). N Engl J Med 314:1185, 1986.
102. Stanley RE, Liang TS: Acute epiglottitis in adults (the Singapore experience). J Laryngol Otol 102:1017, 1988.
103. Shih L, Hawkins DB, Stanley RB: Acute epiglottitis in adults. A review of 48 cases. Ann Otol Rhinol Laryngol 97:527, 1988.
104. Friedman M, Toriumi DM, Grybauskas V, Applebaum EI: A plea for uniformity in the staging and management of adult epiglottitis. Ear Nose Throat J 67:873, 1988.
105. Committee on Infectious Disease, American Academy of Pediatrics: Redbook Report. Evanston, IL, American Academy of Pediatrics, 1988, p 11.
106. Granoff DM, Sheetz K, Pandey JP, et al: Host and bacterial factors associated with *Haemophilus influenzae* type b disease in Minnesota children vaccinated with type b polysaccharide vaccine. J Infect Dis 159:908, 1989.
107. ACIP: Update: Prevention of *Haemophilus influenzae* type b disease. MMWR Morbid Mortal Wkly Rep 35:170, 1986.
108. Committee on Infectious Diseases: *Haemophilus influenzae* type B conjugate vaccine. Pediatrics 81:908, 1988.
109. Centers for Disease Control and Prevention: Vaccination coverage of 2-year-old children—United States, 1993. MMWR Morbid Mortal Wkly Rep 43:705, 1994.
110. Centers for Disease Control and Prevention: Progress toward elimination of *Haemophilus influenzae* type b disease among infants and children—United States, 1987–1993. MMWR Morbid Mortal Wkly Rep 43:144, 1994.
111. Takala AK, Peltola H, Eskola J: Disappearance of epiglottitis during large-scale vaccination with *Haemophilus influenzae* type b conjugate vaccine among children in Finland. Laryngoscope 104:73, 1994.
112. Gorelick MH, Baker D: Epiglottitis in children, 1979 through 1992: Effects of *Haemophilus influenzae* type b immunization. Arch Pediatr Adolesc Med 148:47, 1994.
113. Reece R: George Washington: His death and his doctors. Minn Med 49:1185, 1966.
114. Bard S: An enquiry into the nature, cause and cure of the angina suffocativa, or, sore throat distemper. New York, S. Inslee and A. Car, 1771.
115. Orton HB, Smith EL, Bell HO, et al: Acute laryngotracheobronchitis: Analysis of sixty-two cases with report of autopsies in eight cases. Arch Otolaryngol 33:926, 1941.
116. Neffson AL: Acute laryngotracheobronchitis: A 25 year review. Am J Med Sci 208:524, 1944.
117. Nelson WE: Bacterial croup: A historical perspective. J Pediatr 105:52, 1984.
118. Liston SL, Gehrz RC, Jarvis CW: Bacterial tracheitis. Arch Otolaryngol 107:561, 1981.
119. Johnson JT, Liston SL: Bacterial tracheitis in adults. Arch Otolaryngol Head Neck Surg 113:204, 1987.
120. Miller BP, Arthur JD, Parry WH, et al: Atypical croup and *Chlamydia trachomatis* (Letter). Lancet 1:1022, 1982.
121. Donnelly BW, McMillan JA, Weiner LB: Bacterial tracheitis: Report of eight new cases and review. Rev Infect Dis 12:729, 1990.
122. Hazard JB: Thyroiditis: A review. Am J Clin Pathol 25:289, 1955.
123. Singer PA: Thyroiditis: Acute, subacute and chronic. Med Clin North Am 75:61, 1991.
124. Abe K, Taguchi T, Okano A, et al: Acute suppurative thyroiditis in children. J Pediatr 94:912, 1979.
125. Tayler WE, Myer CM, Hays LL, Cotton RT: Acute suppurative thyroiditis in children. Laryngoscope 92:1269, 1982.
126. Ueda J, Kobayashi Y, Harra K, et al: Routes of infection of acute suppurative thyroiditis diagnosed by barium examination. Acta Radiol Diagn 27:209, 1986.
127. DeLozier H: Pyriform sinus fistula: An unusual cause of recurrent retropharyngeal abscess and cellulitis. Ann Otol Rhinol Laryngol 95:377, 1986.
128. Har-el G, Sasaki CT, Prager D, Krespi YP: Acute suppurative thyroiditis and the branchial apparatus. Am J Otolaryngol 12:6, 1991.
129. Gigot JF, Mannell A: Acute emphysematous thyroiditis. Br J Surg 70:256, 1983.
130. Walker DH, Adamec T, Krigman M: Disseminated petriellidosis (allescheriosis). Arch Pathol Lab Med 102:158, 1978.
131. Robinson MF, Forgan-Smith WR, Craswell DW: *Candida* thyroiditis treated with 5 fluorocytosine. Aust N Z J Med 5:472, 1974.
132. Fernandez JF, Anaissie EJ, Vassilopoulou-Sellin R, Samaan HA: Acute fungal thyroiditis in a patient with acute myelogenous leukaemia. J Int Med 230:539, 1991.
133. Halazun JF, Anast CS, Lukens JM: Thyrotoxins associated with *Aspergillus* in chronic granulomatous disease. J Pediatr 80:106, 1972.
134. Loeb JM, Livermore BM, Wofsy D: Coccidioidomycosis of the thyroid. Ann Intern Med 91:409, 1979.
135. Guttler R, Singer PA, Axline SG, et al: *Pneumocystis carinii* thyroiditis. Report of three cases and review of the literature. Arch Intern Med 153:1002, 1993.
136. Leers WD, Dussault J, Mullens JE, Volpe R: Suppurative thyroiditis: An unusual case caused by *Actinomyces naeslundi*. Can Med Assoc J 101:56, 1969.

137. Das DK, Pant CS, Chachra KL, Gupta AK: Five needle aspiration cytology diagnosis of tuberculous thyroiditis: A report of eight cases. Acta Cytol 36:517, 1992.
138. Hamburger JI: The various presentations of thyroiditis. Ann Intern Med 104:219, 1986.
139. Volpe R: Thyroiditis: Current views of pathogenesis. Med Clin North Am 59:1163, 1975.
140. Srinivasappa J, Garrelli C, Orodera T, et al: Virus-induced thyroiditis. Endocrinology 122:563, 1988.
141. Frank TS, LiVolsi VA, Conner AM: Cytomegalovirus infection of the thyroid gland in immunocompromised adults. Yale J Biol Med 60:1, 1987.
142. Shenkman L, Bottone EJ: Antibodies to *Yersinia enterocolitica* in thyroid disease. Ann Intern Med 85:735, 1976.
143. Valtinen V, Ruutu P, Varis K, et al: Serological evidence for the role of bacterial infections in the pathogenesis of thyroid diseases. Acta Med Scand 219:105, 1986.
144. Greene J: Subacute thyroiditis. Am J Med 51:97, 1971.

52

The Common Cold

W. Paul Glezen

The common cold is aptly named because it is one of the most common human maladies, and it is the common clinical manifestation of infection of the upper respiratory tract with many different viruses. Contributing to its commonness is the fact that there is no specific therapy for most of its causes, and there are no specific preventive measures.

History

The common cold has received notice since earliest recorded history.[1] Hippocrates rejected therapeutic bleeding as a treatment for colds. In the first century AD, Pliny the Younger recommended kissing the hairy muzzle of a mouse as therapy. Benjamin Franklin was a strong believer in fresh air for prevention of colds, for he observed that colds were contracted by close contact with other cold sufferers. He therefore was against the idea that exposure to cold and dampness was responsible for susceptibility to colds.

Early in this century, volunteers in a study who were inoculated with filtered nasal secretions from patients with colds developed colds themselves. The nasal secretions had been passed through filters that excluded bacteria, leading to the theory that an organism other than a bacterium, one small enough to pass through a bacterial filter, was the etiologic agent of the common cold.[2] Systematic studies of experimental colds in human volunteers were carried out by Andrewes[3] at the Common Cold Research Unit at Harvard Hospital in Salisbury, England, beginning in 1946. In the United States, Jackson and coworkers[4] used student volunteers to attack the problem during the next decade. These studies were all performed without knowledge of the specific agents; although several respiratory viruses including influenza viruses and adenoviruses were known at the time, the requirements for cultivating rhinoviruses and other agents of the common cold had not yet been described. It was subsequently learned that many of the filtered nasal secretions used to inoculate volunteers contained rhinoviruses.

These studies were also important for describing some of the conditions that favored the transmission of cold viruses and for determining some host factors related to susceptibility and resistance. Specifically, they showed that immunity to reinfection with the same secretion pool was acquired by primary infection,[5] that moderate exposure to cold and dampness did not increase the risk of infection,[6] and that women in the middle third of the menstrual cycle were more susceptible to infection.[7]

Virology

More than 200 viruses have been associated with the common cold syndrome. These include specific serotypes of all of the respiratory virus groups listed in Table 52–1. Without question, the rhinoviruses of the Picornaviridae family are the most important etiologic agents of the common cold, but even these are not associated with the majority of colds in most studies. To date, 100 distinct serotypes have been accepted, but more than 100 have been described and others await discovery. The evidence suggests that antigenic variation is driven by immunity, which leads to the emergence of new strains.[8] The important biologic characteristic that separates rhinoviruses from enteroviruses is acid lability; rhinoviruses are inactivated rapidly at pH 3.0, whereas enteroviruses are not. Rhinoviruses are relatively stable in the environment and will survive for long periods on surfaces and fomites. This stability is important for the dissemination of these viruses in human populations, as seen in the next section.

Human coronaviruses are also important causes of the common cold, but much less is known about their role because of the difficulty of isolating these viruses from clinical specimens and preparing reagents for diagnostic tests.[9] Some new technologies have been brought to bear on the problem, and these will provide new information. At least two distinct serotypes cause upper respiratory illnesses (URIs) in humans, and reinfections—some of which are symptomatic—are common. These viruses have lipid envelopes and are less stable in the environment than are rhinoviruses.

Adenoviruses, parainfluenza viruses, respiratory syncytial (RS) viruses, and influenza viruses also contribute to the burden of URI. Adenoviruses are DNA-containing viruses with a protein coat that provides relative environmental stability. Adenovirus types 1, 2, 5, and 6 are common causes of febrile, undifferentiated URI in children. The other adenovirus types are more specialized in their manifestations and settings. Types 3 and 7 cause pharyngoconjunctival fever in

TABLE 52–1 ■ Viruses Associated with the Common Cold

VIRUS TYPE	NUMBER OF SEROTYPES
Adenoviridae	
Adenoviruses	41
Coronaviridae	
Coronaviruses	2
Orthomyxoviridae	
Influenza viruses	3
Paramyxoviridae	
Parainfluenza viruses	4
Respiratory syncytial virus	1
Picornaviridae	
Rhinoviruses	100+
Enteroviruses	60+

civilian populations; types 4, 7, and 21 cause particular problems for military recruits. Type 8 has been associated with epidemic keratoconjunctivitis. All of these and type 11 have been associated with viral pneumonia.

Parainfluenza and RS viruses belong to the Paramyxoviridae family. They are noted more for their propensity to cause lower respiratory tract illness in infants and young children but are also important etiologic agents of URI. For instance, virtually all children have been infected with parainfluenza virus type 3 and RS virus by 3 years of age, and at least half of these infections involve only the upper tract. Infections with parainfluenza virus types 1 and 2 occur at a slightly later age when an even higher proportion of infections may involve the upper tract. Less is known about type 4, but most documented infections have involved the upper tract. Reinfections with all of these paramyxoviruses continue to occur throughout life, producing the common cold syndrome.

Influenza viruses must also be considered important causes of the common cold. Influenza C virus, the orthomyxovirus about which we know the least, infects most persons by adulthood and has usually been associated with URI. This virus grows in embryonated eggs, but it has different growth requirements than A and B viruses, and it is not as mutable as influenza viruses A and B. Our understanding of influenza C virus is incomplete, but it probably is an important cause of colds.

Primary infection with any of the three influenza virus A subtypes or with influenza B virus usually produces an influenza-like illness with appreciable systemic symptoms as well as upper or even lower tract findings. However, after the first infection, subsequent reinfections with the same virus or related variants may result in an afebrile URI. Longitudinal observations of the Houston Family Study revealed that about 30% of influenza virus infections were manifested by afebrile URI.[10, 11] Afebrile URI may be an important mechanism for spread of influenza, because persons so affected usually do not limit their activity and therefore may have many contacts. Afebrile URI may not only be the result of infection confronting partial immunity, it may also have to do with the site of inoculation. An appreciable proportion of volunteers with low or undetectable specific antibodies developed colds after being inoculated with influenza virus by nose drops.[12] The dose of virus required to infect volunteers by this route is relatively large, usually at least 300 $TCID_{50}$ (median tissue culture infective dose units). In contrast, less than 10 $TCID_{50}$ administered by small-particle aerosol and deposited in the lower respiratory tract may produce an influenza-like illness with tracheitis.[13] Therefore, URI caused by influenza-like viruses may result from direct contact inoculation, whereas influenza-like illness may occur more frequently after exposure to natural aerosol.

By the sheer weight of their numbers, the picornaviruses are the most important causes of colds; however, adenoviruses, coronaviruses, and especially reinfections with myxoviruses and paramyxoviruses contribute out of proportion to their small numbers. Table 52–2 shows the proportions by which each of the virus groups contributed to the cause of acute respiratory illnesses of persons in three different studies carried out during several years in different geographic areas. The Tecumseh study provided data that are most representative of the general population.[14] The Chapel Hill data are derived from intensive surveillance of children in daycare,[15] and the Cirencester study was carried out in the setting of a general practice in the United Kingdom.[16] The proportions reflect the structure of the study and the populations involved; the contribution of coronaviruses is underestimated because of the difficulty in diagnosing infection with these viruses. The plethora of agents involved makes any proposals for immunoprophylaxis assume awesome proportions.

TABLE 52–2 ■ Frequency of Association of Respiratory Agents with Acute Respiratory Illnesses in Ambulatory Settings

AGENTS	PERCENTAGE OF TOTAL AGENTS: Tecumseh[14]	Chapel Hill Daycare[15]	Cirencester[16]
Rhinovirus	38.5	9.5	26.2
Parainfluenza virus	16.9	24.1	7.8
Influenza virus	11.9	4.7	24.4
Respiratory syncytial virus	5.9	9.5	2.6
Adenovirus	4.5	22.0	6.3
Enterovirus	4.3	13.6	7.3
Coronavirus	c. 4.0*	NT†	0.4‡
Other viruses	4.7	6.1	9.6
Streptococci	13.3	8.8	15.4§

*Serologic test only.
†NT, Not tested.
‡Virus isolation only.
§Includes groups C and G in addition to group A.

Epidemiology

Incidence

Respiratory infections are the most common acute conditions experienced by persons in the United States. Monto and Ullman[14] found that a representative population living in a small town reported an average of three acute respiratory illnesses a year, with a range of six per year for infants and about one per year for persons older than 60 years. Illnesses were more common among boys younger than 3 years, but for older persons, females had higher rates. Only a portion of these illnesses would be classified as colds.

In the National Health Survey, about one third of acute respiratory conditions reported by a representative sample of respondents are classified as common cold.[17] In 1992, about one fourth of the population reported a common cold that altered their usual activities or caused them to seek medical care (Table 52–3). It was estimated that almost 65 million colds met that definition. Less than half of these colds were reported for children, and more than 10 million were reported by older adults (45 years and older). The 65 million colds resulted in more than 150 million days of restricted activity, and more than 24 million episodes were medically

TABLE 52–3 ■ Frequency of Acute Respiratory Conditions That Alter Usual Activities, United States, 1992

TYPE OF CONDITION	NUMBER	RATE PER 100 PERSONS
Common cold	64,604,000	25.7
Other upper respiratory illness	24,812,000	9.9
Influenza	107,309,000	42.7
Bronchitis	10,257,000	4.1
Pneumonia	3,910,000	1.6
Ear infections	26,036,000	10.4
Other	4,465,000	1.8
Total	241,393,000	96.2

Data from the National Center for Health Statistics: Current Estimates from the National Health Interview Survey, United States, 1992. No. 189. Washington, DC, U.S. Department of Health and Human Services, 1994. DHHS publication (PHS) 94-1517.

attended. As a result, about 18 million days were lost from work and 22 million school days were missed by students 5 to 17 years of age. From these statistics, it can be seen that the economic burden imposed by colds is more than $1 billion each year.

The contribution of rhinoviruses to total acute respiratory illness is considerable. For children younger than 10 years, about one illness per year can be attributed to rhinovirus infection; however, because young children have high total illness rates, the rhinovirus infections account for only about one fourth or one fifth of their URIs. For employed young adults and mothers of young children who experience about one illness per year, rhinoviruses may be responsible for about half of their URIs.

Transmission

Most respiratory infections are spread by direct contact with the respiratory secretions of infected persons.[18] This usually results from hand-to-hand transmission or transmission from hand to environmental surface to hand, with inoculation of the recipient's eye or nose. Inoculation by mouth is usually a less effective route. Direct contact spread explains the high secondary infection rates within households. Spread by aerosol has been documented for influenza viruses,[19] and some experimental evidence for this has been reported for enteroviruses[20] and rhinoviruses[21]; however, most studies favor spread by direct contact. The stability of rhinoviruses facilitates contact spread, because the virus may remain infectious on environmental surfaces for hours or even days.

In temperate climates, the spread of respiratory viruses increases during the cooler months of the year. However, the midwinter peak of respiratory illness does not result from the overlayering of an increasing number of agents. In fact, each of the major groups of viruses has a relatively distinct seasonal niche to fill. As enterovirus activity is declining in the autumn, rhinovirus activity increases. Parainfluenza virus types 1 and 2 produce outbreaks in the autumn but only every other year. RS viruses and influenza viruses usually constitute the midwinter peak. Coronaviruses are active in late winter and spring. Rhinoviruses and parainfluenza virus type 3 also have increased activity in the spring. The pattern of seasonal occurrence, illustrated in Figure 52–1, suggests an interference phenomenon, but there is no complete explanation for the seasonality of the various respiratory viruses.[22]

Increasing virus activity always accompanies the return of children to school. Many studies have demonstrated the importance of schoolchildren in the spread of respiratory

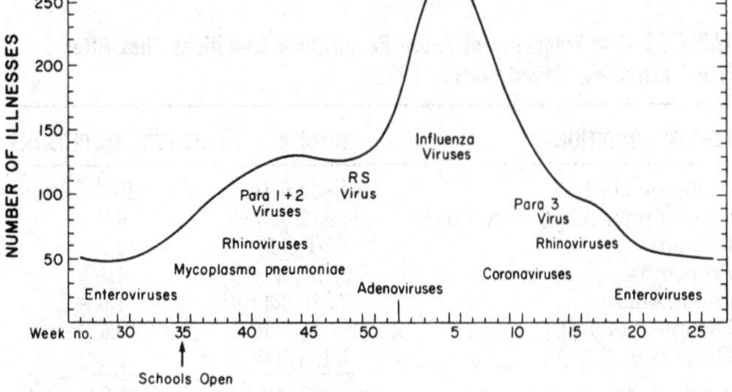

FIGURE 52–1 □ The 5-week running average of visits for acute respiratory illnesses to sentinel primary care facilities in Houston, 1975 to 1981. Superimposed are the respiratory agents contributing to illness during different seasons. Para, Parainfluenza; RS, respiratory syncytial.

viruses in the community and in the introduction of these viruses into the home.[23] The increasing proportion of preschool children in group daycare also increases the opportunity for spread of respiratory viruses and increases the number of agents to which young children are exposed.

The role of climate and temperature change is not understood; lower temperature may increase congregation of persons indoors, resulting in more effective contact. Changes in the relative humidity may also be important. Viability of rhinoviruses may be favored by relative humidities in the range of 40% to 50%, which are common in the autumn and spring.[18] Influenza and parainfluenza viruses remain viable in aerosol for longer periods in low relative humidity such as occurs in midwinter.[24]

Pathogenesis

The incubation period for most respiratory viruses ranges from 1 to 4 days. The site of virus replication is the ciliated epithelium of the nasal turbinates and the nasopharynx. Viremia is not a regular feature of respiratory virus infection other than for enteroviruses; if it occurs with other viruses, it is transient and is not an important pathogenic feature. Systemic symptoms that accompany colds result from the inflammatory response to the surface infection, which produces variable destruction of the cells of the epithelium. Infection usually commences in the posterior pharynx and progresses toward the nose and glottis. Virus shedding usually peaks on the third or fourth day and may be undetectable by the fifth to the seventh day; virus excretion tends to be longer in children than in adults. Infection is limited by endogenous production of interferon and by mobilization of cytotoxic cells—both nonspecific natural killer cells and specific T lymphocytes.

Although there is some destruction of epithelial cells, the more impressive histopathologic picture consists of edema of the submucosa accompanied by hyperemia with some subepithelial infiltration of inflammatory cells. The airways are narrowed by the swelling of the mucosa and filled by exudation of seromucinous fluid. Chemical mediators of inflammation can be detected in the nasal secretions, including interleukin-1,[25] kinins,[26] the vasoactive peptides, and—especially in atopic individuals—histamine[27] and leukotrienes.[28] Symptoms usually peak within 5 days, and recovery usually requires another 5 days.

Clinical Manifestations

Some colds are preceded by a prodrome consisting of chilly sensations and some vague symptoms of non–well-being. (This prodrome is probably the source of the strong belief that chilling causes a cold.) The first symptom is usually a dry, scratchy sore throat, and this is soon followed by sneezing, nasal stuffiness, and rhinorrhea. Some systemic symptoms may occur, such as feverishness, malaise, myalgias, and headache, but temperature elevation is not common, and if it occurs, it is low grade. Hoarseness and cough may also occur; the cough, which is dry and annoying, results from irritation in the glottic region.

Complications

From the previous description of the pathologic factors, it is logical to propose that the inflammation produced by common cold viruses will occlude the ostia of the paranasal sinuses and cause dysfunction of the eustachian tubes, leading to acute sinusitis and otitis media.[29] This obstruction may trap bacteria in the closed space, resulting in suppuration. Sinusitis and otitis media are the most common complications of URIs. Children average about one episode of otitis media per year during the early years of life. These complications should be suspected if the patient develops fever 3 to 5 days after onset of a cold. Children with otitis media may complain of ear pain, and patients with sinusitis will have facial pain over the involved sinus. *Streptococcus pneumoniae* is the most common secondary invader. *Haemophilus influenzae,* usually nontypable, is the next most frequent cause, followed by *Branhamella (Moraxella) catarrhalis.*

Less common complications include bacteremias, bacterial meningitis, pneumonia, and other systemic bacterial infections.[30] It is assumed that the inflammation in the upper respiratory tract allows the bacterial pathogens in the nasopharynx to invade the blood stream, resulting in systemic infections at distant sites. URIs also appear to be a common triggering event for Guillain-Barré syndrome.[31]

For children with reactive airway disease, respiratory virus infections are common initiators of asthma attacks.[32] Welliver and colleagues[33] have found that young children with wheezing may have immunoglobulin E antibodies specific for RS or parainfluenza viruses in their nasal secretions. Rhinovirus and influenza virus infections commonly precede asthma attacks in older children. Many studies have found evidence that these virus infections may stimulate the production of chemical mediators of bronchospasm in atopic children. Because the frequency of severe asthma resulting in hospitalization and death of children is increasing, this may be one of the most urgent reasons for searching for methods to prevent colds.

Diagnosis

The diagnosis is presumed from the clinical presentation. Specific etiologic diagnosis is usually not warranted. For patients with sore throat, it is important to rule out the presence of group A streptococcus by culture or a rapid antigen detection test. This is the only uncomplicated upper respiratory infection that requires specific therapy.

Knowledge of the seasonal occurrence of the major virus groups provides a basis for assigning the presumptive etiologic diagnosis. Rhinoviruses usually predominate in the autumn and early spring. Parainfluenza virus types 1 and 2 have been epidemic in the autumn of odd-numbered years since 1973.[22] Reinfection colds caused by parainfluenza viruses may include hoarseness; the signal illness for the presence of these viruses is croup, or laryngotracheobronchitis, which occurs with primary infection of young children. RS virus and influenza viruses are epidemic in midwinter. RS virus produces annual epidemics, which are clinically evident by the occurrence of bronchiolitis and pneumonia in infants. During this time, many of the URIs of older children and adults may be caused by RS virus. The arrival of influenza in the community is heralded by the sudden appearance at primary care facilities of school-age children with febrile respiratory illnesses. During influenza epidemics, many afebrile URIs will occur in partially immune schoolchildren and adults.

Rapid diagnosis of the causes of URIs during midwinter epidemics may be indicated under certain circumstances for epidemiologic reasons. Influenza A infections can be aborted by early treatment with amantadine, which has been shown to reduce virus shedding and therefore the risk of spreading the infection to vulnerable contacts. RS virus, as well as influenza virus, may produce life-threatening infections in chronically ill or immunocompromised patients. Therefore, timely information about their occurrence may be important.

Differential Diagnosis

Allergic rhinitis, or hay fever, may be confused with the common cold. A nasal smear may aid in differentiating allergic rhinitis from URIs. Eosinophils may be present in the nasal secretions of patients with allergic rhinitis. As mentioned before, group A streptococcal infection must be ruled out by throat culture or an antigen detection test for patients with sore throat. The clinical finding of hoarseness is negatively correlated with group A streptococcal infection. A reminder that continuous rhinorrhea (which may soak the pillow at night) may be the result of a spontaneous leak of cerebrospinal fluid is in order. In this situation, the nasal secretions should be tested for glucose, which is present in cerebrospinal fluid.

Treatment

There is no specific treatment for the common cold. Treatment of colds with amantadine should be considered for certain persons during influenza A epidemics. Persons recommended for treatment are members of the health care team and those who are household contacts of high-risk patients. The purpose is to abort influenza A infections and reduce the risk that vulnerable patients will be exposed to infection.

Many drugs have been tested for effect against rhinoviruses. One drug, enviroxime, has been shown to have antiviral effect in vitro; however, the drug is insoluble in water, and clinical use has not been possible. Enviroxime has been incorporated into liposomes and administered by aerosol. In vitro tests and limited clinical testing suggest that this method of delivery could be promising.[34, 35]

The structure of rhinoviruses has been completely described, including the cell attachment site.[36] In addition, the specific receptor for rhinoviruses on human cells has been defined.[37] Furthermore, antiviral drugs have been designed that block the attachment site of rhinoviruses in vitro, but clinical studies have been disappointing.[38]

The use of antibiotics is not warranted for viral URIs. Double-blind studies have shown no benefit for treated subjects.[39] Antibiotics do not reduce the frequency of bacterial complications but may alter the bacterial flora of the nasopharynx, allowing the emergence of resistant organisms.

Nonspecific Therapy

Relief of some symptoms of a cold can be achieved by administration of over-the-counter remedies. Aspirin may relieve some of the systemic symptoms, but its use should be limited; one study demonstrated prolonged excretion of rhinoviruses from persons who were given aspirin.[40] Experimental studies of influenza virus infection have shown similar results.[41] Aspirin is contraindicated for influenza infections in children because its use has been associated with increased risk of Reye's syndrome.[42] Acetaminophen is probably a better choice for this purpose but should be used judiciously and only as necessary, because the antipyretic effect probably does not favor recovery from infection.

Oral decongestants may relieve nasal stuffiness; pseudoephedrine is effective. Use of topical decongestants may be helpful also, but frequent use can lead to a distressing rebound phenomenon. Antihistamines have a drying effect on secretions and may be helpful if used in combination with decongestants. Newer antihistamines are available that do not produce the drowsiness that accompanied many of the earlier products.

A persistent dry cough may be troublesome and can be

relieved by administration of a cough suppressant such as dextromethorphan. Caution should be used in administering such preparations to young children, for whom cough may be important for keeping the airways clear of upper tract secretions.

Prevention

The only vaccines available for respiratory viruses are inactivated influenza vaccines and a live virus vaccine for adenovirus types 4 and 7, which is administered in an enteric-coated capsule to military recruits. These vaccines would prevent only a small proportion of colds in civilian populations and are not recommended generally for this indication. In addition to the recommendation for patients with chronic underlying conditions, influenza vaccine is recommended for all members of the health care team and for household contacts of high-risk patients to reduce the risk of exposing vulnerable patients to influenza virus infection.

The large number of rhinovirus serotypes and the fact that no effective cross-protection is evident after infection with a given serotype make it unlikely that immunoprophylaxis will work. Furthermore, it appears that antigenic variation and the emergence of new types are driven by immunity. This makes it even less likely that vaccine development would be practical.

Endogenous interferon production appears to be the important limiting factor for rhinovirus infection. Experimental studies with human volunteers have demonstrated that nasal instillation of interferon will prevent rhinovirus colds.[43, 44] Studies have also shown that secondary rhinovirus infections can be prevented in household contacts of persons with natural rhinovirus colds by intranasal administration of recombinant interferon.[45, 46] The problem is that regular use of the interferon spray excites an inflammatory response in the nose, which results in a nasal obstruction and bloody nasal discharge. Therefore, the treatment is almost as annoying as the disease. Furthermore, interferon does not prevent infections with the other viruses associated with the common cold. At this juncture, the most promising prospect for cure (or prevention) of the common cold lies with development of more effective antiviral therapy. An antiviral preparation combined with products that block the mediators of inflammation may be the treatment of the future.[47]

References

1. Gwaltney JM Jr: Rhinoviruses. *In* Evans AS (ed): Viral Infections of Humans, ed 2. New York, Plenum Publishing, 1982, pp 491–517.
2. Kruse W: Die Erregen von Husten und Schupfen [the etiology of cough and nasal catarrh]. Munch Med Wochenschr 61:1574, 1914.
3. Andrewes C: In Pursuit of the Common Cold. London, William Heinemann Medical Books, 1973.
4. Jackson GG, Dowling HF, Spiesman EG, Boand AV: Transmission of the common cold to volunteers under controlled conditions. I. The common cold as a clinical entity. Arch Intern Med 101:267, 1958.
5. Jackson GG, Dowling HF: Transmission of the common cold to volunteers under controlled conditions. IV. Specific immunity to the common cold. J Clin Invest 38:762, 1959.
6. Dowling HF, Jackson GG, Spiesman IG, Inouye T: Transmission of the common cold to volunteers under controlled conditions. III. The effect of chilling of the subjects upon susceptibility. Am J Hyg 68:59, 1958.
7. Dowling HF, Jackson GG, Inouye T: Transmission of the experimental common cold in volunteers. II. The effect of certain host factors upon susceptibility. J Lab Clin Med 50:516, 1957.
8. Couch RB: Rhinoviruses. *In* Fields BN, Knipe DM (eds): Fields Virology, ed 2. New York, Raven Press, 1990, pp 607–629.
9. Monto AS: Coronaviruses. *In* Evans AS (ed): Viral Infections of Humans, ed 2. New York, Plenum Publishing, 1982, pp 151–165.
10. Frank AL, Taber LH, Glezen WP, et al: Influenza B virus infections in the community and the family. Am J Epidemiol 118:313, 1983.
11. Frank AL, Taber LH, Wells JM: Comparison of infection rates and severity of illness for influenza A subtypes H1N1 and H3N2. J Infect Dis 151:73, 1985.
12. Douglas RG Jr: Influenza in man. *In* Kilbourne ED (ed): The Influenza Viruses and Influenza. New York, Academic Press, 1975, pp 395–447.
13. Alford RH, Kasel JA, Geron PJ, Knight V: Human influenza resulting from aerosol inhalation. Proc Soc Exp Biol Med 122:800, 1966.
14. Monto AS, Ullman BM: Acute respiratory illness in an American community. JAMA 227:264, 1974.
15. Denny FW: Acute respiratory infections in children: Etiology and epidemiology. Pediatr Rev 9:135, 1987.
16. Higgins PG: Viruses associated with acute respiratory infections 1961–71. J Hyg (Camb) 72:425, 1974.
17. National Center for Health Statistics: Current Estimates from the National Health Interview Survey, United States, 1992. No. 189. Washington, DC, U.S. Department of Health and Human Services, 1994. DHHS publication (PHS) 94-1517.
18. Hendley JO, Gwaltney JM Jr: Mechanisms of transmission of rhinovirus infections. Epidemiol Rev 10:242, 1988.
19. Glezen WP, Couch RB: Influenza viruses. *In* Evans AS (ed): Viral Infections of Humans, ed 3. New York, Plenum Publishing, 1989.
20. Couch RB, Douglas RG Jr, Lindgren KM, et al: Airborne transmission of respiratory infection with coxsackie virus A type 21. Am J Epidemiol 91:78, 1970.
21. Dick EC, Jennings LC, Mink KA, et al: Aerosol transmission of rhinovirus colds. J Infect Dis 156:442, 1987.
22. Glezen WP, Frank AL, Taber LH, Kasel JA: Parainfluenza virus type 3: Seasonality and risk of infection and reinfection in young children. J Infect Dis 150:851, 1984.
23. Glezen WP: Consideration of the risk of influenza in children and indications for prophylaxis. Rev Infect Dis 2:408, 1980.
24. Glezen WP, Loda FA, Denny FW: Parainfluenza viruses. *In* Evans AS (ed): Viral Infections of Humans, ed 3. New York, Plenum Publishing, 1989.
25. Proud D, Gwaltney JM Jr, Hendley JO, et al: Increased levels of interleukin-1 are detected in nasal secretions of volunteers during experimental rhinovirus colds. J Infect Dis 169:1007, 1994.
26. Naclerio RM, Proud D, Lichtenstein LM, et al: Kinins are generated during experimental rhinovirus cold. J Infect Dis 157:133, 1988.
27. Smith TF, Remigio LK: Histamine in nasal secretions and serum may be elevated during viral respiratory tract infections. Int Arch Allergy Appl Immunol 67:380, 1982.
28. Volovitz B, Faden H, Ogra PL: Release of leukotriene C4 in respiratory tract during acute viral infection. J Pediatr 112:218, 1988.
29. Buchman CA, Doyle WJ, Skoner D, et al: Otologic manifestations of experimental rhinovirus infection. Laryngoscope 104:1295, 1994.
30. Kaplan SL, Taber LH, Frank AL, Feigin RD: Nasopharyngeal viral isolates in children with *Haemophilus influenzae* type b meningitis. J Pediatr 99:591, 1981.
31. Leneman F: The Guillain-Barré syndrome. Arch Intern Med 118:139, 1966.
32. Glezen WP: Reactive airway disorders in children: Role of respiratory virus infections. Clin Chest Med 5:635, 1984.
33. Welliver RC, Wong DT, Middleton E Jr, et al: Role of parainfluenza virus–specific IgE in pathogenesis of croup and wheezing subsequent to infection. J Pediatr 101:889, 1982.
34. Wyde PR, Six HR, Wilson SZ, et al: Activity against rhinoviruses, toxicity, and delivery in aerosol of enviroxime in liposomes. Antimicrob Agents Chemother 32:890, 1988.
35. Gilbert BE, Six HR, Wilson SZ, et al: Small particle aerosols of enviroxime-containing liposomes. Antiviral Res 9:355, 1988.
36. Rossman MG, Arnold E, Erickson JW, et al: Structure of a human common cold virus and functional relationship to other picornaviruses. Nature 317:145, 1985.

37. Colonno RJ, Condra JH, Muzutani S: Interaction of cellular receptors with the canyon structure of human rhinoviruses. *In* Compans RW, Helenius A, Oldstone MBS (eds): Cell Biology of Virus Entry, Replication, and Pathogenesis. New York, Alan R Liss, 1989, pp 75–83.
38. McKinlay MA, Pevear DC, Rossman MG: Treatment of the picornavirus common cold by inhibitors of viral uncoating and attachment. Annu Rev Microbiol 46:635, 1992.
39. Soyka LF, Robinson DS, Lachant N, Monaco J: The misuse of antibiotics for treatment of upper respiratory tract infections in children. Pediatrics 55:552, 1975.
40. Stanley ED, Jackson GG, Panusarn C, et al: Increased virus shedding with aspirin treatment of rhinovirus infection. JAMA 231:1247, 1975.
41. Husseini RH, Sweet C, Collie MH, Smith H: Elevation of nasal viral levels in suppression of fever in ferrets infected with influenza viruses of different virulence. J Infect Dis 145:520, 1982.
42. Hurwitz ES, Barrett MJ, Bregman D, et al: Public Health Service Study on Reye's syndrome and medications. N Engl J Med 313:849, 1985.
43. Samo TC, Greenberg SB, Couch RB, et al: Efficacy and tolerance of intranasally applied recombinant leukocyte A interferon in normal volunteers. J Infect Dis 148:535, 1983.
44. Samo TC, Greenberg SB, Palmer JM, et al: Intranasally applied recombinant leukocyte A interferon in normal volunteers. II. Determination of minimal effective dose and tolerable dose. J Infect Dis 150:181, 1984.
45. Douglas RM, Moore BW, Miles HB, et al: Prophylactic efficacy of intranasal alpha$_2$-interferon against rhinovirus infections in the family setting. N Engl J Med 314:65, 1986.
46. Hayden FG, Albrecht JK, Kaiser DL, Gwaltney JM Jr: Prevention of natural colds by contact prophylaxis with intranasal alpha$_2$-interferon. N Engl J Med 314:71, 1986.
47. Gwaltney JM Jr: Combined antiviral and antimediator treatment of rhinovirus colds. J Infect Dis 166:776, 1992.

PLEUROPULMONARY

53

Approach to the Patient with Pneumonia

John G. Bartlett

Pneumonia occurs in an estimated 3 to 4 million patients in the United States each year, of whom approximately 1 million require hospitalization. Pneumonia also accounts for about 15% of all nosocomial infections. The total cost of these infections is estimated at about $4 billion per year.[1,2] Pneumonia is the sixth most common cause of death in the United States, accounting for approximately 30 deaths per 100,000 populations or 75,000 deaths per year.[3] This represents 3.5% of all deaths in the United States and 46% of those directly due to infectious disease.[3] Comparative data for the prepenicillin era are summarized in Table 53–1.[3–5] One of the most striking changes noted is the frequency with which the pneumococcus is implicated. There have been substantial additional changes relating to the other implicated pathogens, the host, and the treatment options. The purpose of this chapter is to provide a guideline for the approach to the patient with suspected pneumonia.

Definitions and Terms

Pneumonia indicates inflammation of the lung parenchyma that is usually caused by a microbial agent. In many cases, the term is modified to indicate a specific clinical setting, such as community-acquired pneumonia, nursing home pneumonia, nosocomial pneumonia, pneumonia in the immunocompromised host, and aspiration pneumonia, among others. These terms are important because of differences in likely microbial agents, prognosis, and diagnostic evaluation. Other classifications are based on the tempo of the disease, such as acute, subacute, or chronic pneumonia. Classification may also be based on observations with radiographs or scans to characterize the changes as lobar pneumonia, bronchopneumonia, interstitial pneumonia, or lung abscess and accompanying findings, such as hilar adenopathy, pleural fluid, or atelectasis.

Diagnosis

Clinical Features

Symptoms suggesting pneumonia include fever combined with respiratory complaints including cough, dyspnea, sputum production, and pleurisy. Patients with chronic pneumonia often complain of unintentional weight loss, chronic fa-

TABLE 53–1 ■ Pneumonia: Comparison of Data for the Prepenicillin Era and the Modern Era

PARAMETER	PREPENICILLIN ERA (ANNUAL, U.S.)*	CURRENT ERA (ANNUAL, U.S.)†
Incidence (hospitalized patients/1000 population)	3/1000	2.5/1000
Mortality rate (hospitalized patients)	33%	13.7%
Mortality (incidence/100,000 population)	90–110/100,000	25–30/100,000
Mortality as percentage of all deaths	8.5%	3.5%
Cases due to *Streptococcus pneumoniae*	81%	25%

*Data for prepenicillin era from Heffron R: Pneumonia. Cambridge, MA, Harvard University Press, 1939. Mortality data are based on metaanalysis of 18,540 cases reported from 1905 to 1937 (pp 656–663); recovery rate of *S. pneumoniae* is based on experience of Bullowa with 4416 cases from 1928 to 1936 (p 2); rates are for major metropolitan areas from 1931 to 1933 (p 276).

†Data for mortality from Pinner RW, Teutsch SM, Simonsen L, et al: Trends in infectious diseases mortality in the United States. JAMA 275:189–193, 1996; based on analysis of tapes from National Center for Health Statistics for 1980 to 1992. Data for mortality rate and bacteriology are from Fine MJ, Smith MA, Carson CA, et al: Prognosis and outcomes of patients with community-acquired pneumonia. JAMA 274:134–141, 1995; based on metaanalysis of 33,148 patients reported in 122 English language reports published from 1966 to 1995.

TABLE 53–2 ■ Chest Radiography: Differential Diagnosis

IMMUNOCOMPETENT	IMMUNOSUPPRESSED (ACQUIRED IMMUNODEFICIENCY SYNDROME)
Focal Opacity	**Focal Opacity**
Streptococcus pneumoniae	Pyogenic bacteria (as with immunocompetent)
Haemophilus influenzae	*Cryptococcus neoformans*
Mycoplasma pneumoniae	*Nocardia*
Legionella	*Mycobacterium tuberculosis*
Chlamydia pneumoniae	Kaposi's sarcoma
Staphylococcus aureus	
Mycobacterium tuberculosis	
Gram-negative bacteria	
Anaerobes	
Interstitial-Miliary	**Interstitial-Miliary**
Viruses	*Pneumocystis carinii*
Mycoplasma pneumoniae	*Mycobacterium tuberculosis*
Mycobacterium tuberculosis	Pathogenic fungi*
Pathogenic fungi*	*Leishmania donovani*
	Cytomegalovirus
Hilar Adenopathy ± Infiltrate	**Hilar Adenopathy**
Epstein-Barr virus	*Mycobacterium tuberculosis*
Francisella tularensis	*Cryptococcus neoformans*
Chlamydia psittaci	Pathogenic fungi*
Mycoplasma pneumoniae	Lymphoma
Mycobacterium tuberculosis	Kaposi's sarcoma
Pathogenic fungi*	
Atypical rubella	
Cavitation	**Cavitation**
Anaerobes	Gram-negative bacilli
Mycobacterium tuberculosis	*Mycobacterium tuberculosis*
Pathogenic fungi*	*Mycobacterium kansasii*
Gram-negative bacilli	*Cryptococcus neoformans*
Staphylococcus aureus	Pathogenic fungi*
	Rhodococcus equi
	Staphylococcus aureus (injection drug use)

*Pathogenic fungi: *Histoplasma capsulatum, Coccidioides immitis,* and *Blastomyces dermatitidis.*

tigue, and night sweats. Physical examinations in patients with pneumonia show fever in the great majority; crackles are heard by auscultation in 80%, and 15% to 30% of patients have findings of lobar consolidation by radiography and physical examination.[2]

Chest Radiography

An important diagnostic test is the chest radiograph, because this is usually necessary for a confirmed diagnosis. The distinction between bronchitis and pneumonia may be difficult on the basis of clinical observations. The issue is not trivial because most patients with pneumonias are treated with antimicrobial agents, whereas those with bronchitis generally derive no benefit from antimicrobial agents. This point notwithstanding, some have argued in the era of managed care that routine administration of oral antibiotics to all patients with cough and fever is less expensive than a chest radiograph to identify the subset expected to benefit from antibiotics.

False-positive results on x-ray examination may be noted with a multitude of clinical conditions, including pulmonary infarct; congestive heart failure; carcinoma; and primary lung conditions such as sarcoidosis, interstitial lung disease, atelectasis, vasculitis, Wegener granulomatosis, and others. False-negative x-ray results are rare and include dehydration, neutropenia, early disease, and pneumonia caused by *Pneumocystis carinii.* Dehydration is an especially rare cause of false-negative results and may actually represent an erroneous concept, because animal studies show only modest reductions in infiltrates based on hydration status. Neutropenia is also a relatively rare cause of false-negative results. Studies in the preantibiotic era showed that up to 24 hours may be required for a demonstrable infiltrate on the chest film after the inception of symptoms; again, this is rare. One of the most common causes of a false-negative x-ray result is *Pneumocystis* pneumonia, which may occur in up to 40% of patients in some series.[6] It is generally thought that radiographs do not distinguish bacterial from nonbacterial infection. Nevertheless, some findings on chest radiography strongly support selected diagnoses (Table 53–2). Changes on the chest film may also indicate the severity of the illness and guide management decisions.

TABLE 53–3 ■ Routine Tests in Hospitalized Patients with Community-Acquired Pneumonia

Chest radiograph
Arterial blood gas analysis
Complete blood count
Chemistry profile including kidney and liver function tests and electrolyte determinations
Human immunodeficiency virus serology (age 15–54 y)
Blood culture
Sputum Gram stain and culture ± acid-fast stain and culture, *Legionella* test (culture, direct fluorescent antibody stain, or urinary antigen assay), *Mycoplasma* immunoglobulin M
Pleural fluid analysis (if present): white cell count and differential, lactate dehydrogenase, pH, protein, glucose; Gram stain, acid-fast stain; and culture for bacteria (aerobes and anaerobes), fungi, and mycobacteria

Laboratory Tests

Laboratory tests that are commonly advocated in patients who are candidates for hospitalization are summarized in Table 53–3. The goal is to determine the severity of illness, possible complications, and the status of underlying or associated conditions. Results, coupled with clinical observations, often dictate the need for hospitalization in community-acquired cases or may indicate the need for care in the intensive care unit.[7] Table 53–4 enumerates the indications for hospitalization and their frequency of application for patients hospi-

TABLE 53–4 ■ Indications for Hospitalization

Severe vital sign abnormality
Pulse >140/min, systolic blood pressure <90 mm Hg, respiratory rate >30/min (46%)*
Altered mental status (newly diagnosed)
Disorientation to person, place, or time; stupor or coma (20%)
Arterial hypoxemia
Partial pressure of oxygen <60 mm Hg on room air (51%)
Suppurative pneumonia-related infection
Empyema, septic arthritis, meningitis, endocarditis (1%)
Severe electrolyte, hematologic, or metabolic laboratory value not known to be chronic
Serum Na^+ <130 mEq/L, hematocrit <30%, absolute neutrophil count <1000/mm³, blood urea nitrogen >50 mg/dL, or creatinine >2.5 mg/dL (13%)
Acute coexistent medical condition requiring admission (23%)

*Indicates the percentage of patients hospitalized for community-acquired pneumonia with this observation.

Adapted and reprinted by permission of the publisher from Fine MJ, Smith DN, Singer DE: Hospitalization decision in patients with community-acquired pneumonia: A prospective cohort study. Am J Med 89:713–721, 1990. Copyright 1990 by Excerpta Medica Inc.

talized in a representative series from Massachusetts General Hospital.

Anemia often indicates chronic disease, complicated pneumonia, or mycoplasma infection. The peripheral white cell count is generally not useful for distinguishing etiologic agents, although a count higher than 15,000/mm^3 suggests bacterial infection, and counts lower than 3000 or higher than 25,000/mm^3 appear to be prognostic indicators. Blood gas determination is a particularly important prognostic indicator. Hypoxemia with a partial pressure of oxygen of less than 60 mm Hg on room air represents a standard criterion for hospitalization and consideration for an intensive care unit.[7] Serologic testing for human immunodeficiency virus is often suggested with community-acquired pneumonia in patients aged 15 to 54 years who require hospitalization.[8] In the absence of the availability of serologic testing or when there is a delay in reporting, there may be a clue to the diagnosis if the absolute lymphocyte count is less than 1000/mm^3. A preferred test is the CD4$^+$ cell count, which is usually lower than 200/mm^3 in most patients with human immunodeficiency virus–associated complications including pneumonia, and this level of CD4$^+$ cell depletion is rarely due to other causes.

Pleural effusions are found in up to 30% of patients with pneumonia. Indications for a thoracocentesis are arbitrary, but it should be done if there is a delay in resolution, a large collection, or no diagnosis. The definition of large collection is also arbitrary, but one recommendation is to perform thoracocentesis on effusions that exceed 10 mm on a lateral decubitus film, which will be the great majority.[9] Pleural fluid that is grossly purulent is diagnostic of empyema and requires drainage. When the fluid is thin and free flowing, it should be analyzed for pH, glucose, protein, and lactate dehydrogenase; white cell count and differential; Gram stain and acid-fast stain; and cultures for aerobic and anaerobic bacteria, fungi, and mycobacteria. A pH greater than 7.3 predicts response to antibiotic treatment; a pH below 7.1 predicts the necessity for drainage. A metaanalysis suggested that pleural fluid pH is the most useful test to determine effusions that require drainage.[10]

Etiologic Diagnosis

The management of pneumonia is notably simplified if the etiologic agent is accurately identified. A probable pathogen is detected in 40% to 50% of cases in published reports, although even this relatively poor yield may exaggerate the yield because of false-positive cultures of expectorated sputum. Relatively few patients have a clearly documented pathogen as defined by the following:

1. A likely pulmonary pathogen is recovered from uncontaminated sources such as blood, pleural fluid, metastatic sites, or transtracheal aspirates.
2. The organism is considered pathogenic regardless of the specimen source because it does not colonize the respiratory tract in the absence of disease. Microbes in this category are summarized in Table 53–5.[11]
3. There is positive serology by standard criteria for selected pathogens.

In practice, the physician is usually required to interpret the results of less definitive studies, most commonly the results of Gram stain and culture of expectorated sputum. Alternative specimen sources, such as transtracheal aspiration, transthoracic needle aspiration, or bronchoscopy, are usually reserved for patients who have atypical presentation, severe disease, or disease in a specific host setting and for patients who fail to respond to treatment. Diagnostic tests of choice by microbial pathogen are summarized in Table 53–6. The diagnostic yield from any specimen source is notably reduced by antecedent antibiotic use; fragile organisms such as *Streptococcus pneumoniae, Haemophilus influenzae,* and anaerobes are especially a problem.

TABLE 53–5 ■ Microbial Pathogens Recovered from Respiratory Secretions

DIAGNOSTIC OF PATHOGENIC ROLE REGARDLESS OF SPECIMEN SOURCE	NONDIAGNOSTIC IF RECOVERED FROM USUAL RESPIRATORY SPECIMENS*
Bacteria	
Legionella	Virtually all other bacteria
Mycobacteria	
Mycobacterium tuberculosis	Mycobacteria other than tuberculosis
Viruses	
Influenza virus	Cytomegalovirus
Respiratory syncytial virus	Herpes simplex virus
Parainfluenza virus	
Adenovirus	
Coxsackievirus	
Parasites	
Strongyloides	—
Toxoplasma gondii	
Fungi	
Pneumocystis carinii	*Candida* sp.
Histoplasma capsulatum	*Cryptococcus neoformans*
Coccidioides immitis	*Aspergillus* sp.
Blastomyces dermatitidis	

*Sputum, bronchoscopy, nasotracheal suction, and others.

Expectorated Sputum

The diagnostic utility of expectorated sputum and culture has been debated for decades. In the late 1960s and early 1970s, multiple studies showed that the yield of *S. pneumoniae* in expectorated sputum from patients with bacteremic pneumonia was only about 50%.[12, 13] The conclusion was that the usual specimen source for detecting *S. pneumoniae*, the most common identifiable agent of lower respiratory tract infections, was complicated by a high frequency of false-negative results, and the outcome was an intensive effort in the 1970s to deal more effectively with pathogen detection by using two approaches. The first was an attempt to obtain specimens that were not contaminated by the upper airway flora with use of transtracheal aspiration, transthoracic needle aspiration, or bronchoscopy. The second tactic was fostered by the impression that the only practical specimen was the expectorated sputum, and the need was to deal with the problem of contamination during passage through the upper airways by use of alternative methods to process sputum: wash procedures, quantitation of bacteria, and cytologic screening. From these studies, the only technique that has withstood the test of time and has subsequently been incorporated into standard laboratory practice is cytologic screening of expectorated sputum.[14, 15]

Many authorities[16] now believe that Gram stain and culture of expectorated sputum are important diagnostic tests that account for less than 1% of hospital charges, but with the following caveats: (1) the specimen must be obtained before antibiotic treatment; (2) there need to be good efforts in quality control for specimen procurement, expeditious transport to the laboratory, and proper processing; and (3) there needs to be cytologic screening to demonstrate the presence of secretions from the lower airway with limited upper air-

TABLE 53–6 ■ Pulmonary Infections: Specimens and Tests for Detection of Lower Respiratory Tract Pathogens

ORGANISM	PULMONARY SPECIMEN*	MICROSCOPY†	CULTURE	SEROLOGY†	OTHER†
Bacteria					
Aerobic and facultatively anaerobic	Expectorated sputum, quant bronch, blood, TTA, empyema fluid	Gram stain	X	—	
Anaerobic	TTA, empyema fluid, quant bronch	Gram stain	X	—	
Legionella sp.	Sputum, lung biopsy, pleural fluid, TTA, bronch, blood	FA (*L. pneumophila*)	X	IFA, EIA	Urinary antigen (*L. pneumophila* serogroup 1)‡
Nocardia sp.	Expectorated sputum, TTA, lung biopsy, BAL	Gram stain and modified carbolfuchsin stain	X	—	
Chlamydia sp.	Nasopharyngeal swab, expectorated sputum, bronch	Negative	X‡	CF for *C. psittaci* MIF for *C. pneumoniae*‡	PCR for *C. pneumoniae*‡ (experimental)
Mycoplasma sp.	Expectorated sputum, nasopharyngeal swab	Negative	X‡	CF, EIA	PCR‡ (experimental) Cold agglutinins (titer ≥1:32)
Mycobacteria	Expectorated or induced sputum, TTA, bronch	Fluorochrome stain or carbolfuchsin stain	X	—	PPD skin test PCR‡ (experimental)
Fungi					
Deep-seated *Blastomyces* sp., *Coccidioides* sp.	Expectorated or induced sputum, bronch, biopsy	Potassium hydroxide with phase contrast	X X	CF, ID CF, ID, LA	
Histoplasma sp.		GMS stain	X	CF, ID	Antigen assay: BAL, blood, urine‡
Opportunistic *Pneumocystis carinii*	Induced sputum or bronch	Toluidine blue, Giemsa, FA, or GMS stain	—	—	Lactate dehydrogenase elevated in >90%
Aspergillus sp.	Lung biopsy	H&E, GMS stain	X	ID‡	Computed tomography
Candida sp.	Lung biopsy	H&E, GMS stain	X	—	
Cryptococcus sp.	Expectorated sputum, serum, transbronchial biopsy, or BAL	H&E, GMS stain, calcofluor white	X	—	Serum or BAL antigen assay
Zygomycetes	Expectorated sputum, tissue	H&E, GMS stain	X	—	
Viruses					
Influenza virus, parainfluenza virus, respiratory syncytial virus, cytomegalovirus	Nasal washings, nasopharyngeal aspirate or swab, bronch	FA: influenza and respiratory syncytial viruses	X‡	CF, EIA, LA, FA	Cytomegalovirus: shell viral culture, FA stain of BAL or biopsy specimen
Hantavirus		Negative	—	EIA for immunoglobulins G and M‡	PCR‡ (experimental) complete blood count: thrombocytopenia, leukocytosis, left shift, and >10% immunoblasts

*Specimens: BAL, bronchoalveolar lavage; bronch, bronchoscopy specimen including aspirate, brushing, BAL, or biopsy; quant bronch, quantitative bronchoscopy culture including quantitative brush catheter or BAL; TTA, transtracheal aspirate or transthoracic aspirate; biopsy, transbronchial, transthoracic, or open lung biopsy.

†CF, Complement fixation; CIE, counterimmunoelectrophoresis; EIA, enzyme immunoassay; FA, fluorescent antibody stain; GMS, Gomori methenamine–silver nitrate; H&E, hematoxylin and eosin; ID, immunodiffusion; IFA, indirect fluorescent antibody; LA, latex agglutination; MIF, microimmunofluorescence test; PCR, polymerase chain reaction; PPD, purified protein derivative.

‡Few clinical microbiology laboratories offer these tests.

way contamination. The "classic" criterion for the last is a low-power examination (×100) showing more than 25 polymorphonuclear leukocytes per field or less than 10 epithelial cells per field,[14] but most laboratories require simply a predominance of polymorphonuclear leukocytes or sparse epithelial cells.[15, 16] Cytologic screening is not necessary for detection of *Mycobacterium tuberculosis* and *Legionella*. Interpretation of Gram stain and culture must be based on clinical correlations. Specialized tests are required for detection of mycobacteria, chlamydiae, mycoplasmas, fungi, and viruses, and some laboratories offer specialized tests for detection of pneumococci (Quellung stain or tests for pneumococcal capsular polysaccharide).[17]

Transtracheal Aspiration

This technique was originally reported in 1963[18] and subsequently became popular during the period 1968 to about 1980.[19] During this time, there were many large series using transtracheal aspiration in diverse settings, but there were also several reports of complications.[20] The technique consists of the insertion of a catheter through the cricoid membrane to the carina with suction aspiration to obtain specimens from the level of the carina. Our experience with 488 patients included 383 who satisfied clinical criteria for probable bacterial pneumonia; a likely pathogen was recovered in 235, and 44 of 48 false-negative cultures were from patients who had previously received antibiotics.[21] With restriction of analysis to untreated patients, the true frequency of false-negative cultures was only about 1%. There were 23 patients with bacteremic pneumococcal pneumonia, and all 23 had positive transtracheal aspiration cultures for this organism. False-positive cultures are occasionally encountered, primarily from patients with chronic bronchitis or bronchiectasis who represent a subset of patients with airway colonization by bacteria below the level of the larynx.[22] This procedure is almost never done at the present time owing to the lack of physicians trained in the technique, concern for side effects, and decreased emphasis on microbial diagnoses.

Transthoracic Needle Aspiration

The most extensive experience with this technique was in the prepenicillin era when the major indication was to recover *S. pneumoniae* to provide the necessary information for administration of type-specific antisera, which was the only therapy available at the time.[23] More recently, this has been done primarily for cytologic evaluation in suspected malignant disease and in occasional patients for a microbial diagnosis. In brief, the area of involvement is determined radiographically, and this site is sampled by percutaneous insertion of an 18- to 22-gauge thin-walled spinal needle or the "skinny" 25-gauge needle.[19, 24] A review of 19 reported series showed that the diagnostic yield with suspected bacterial pneumonia is 35% to 50%.[19] Possibly the most accurate definition of the frequency of false-negative cultures is the experience with 211 patients with bacteremic pneumococcal pneumonia by Bullowa[23] in the prepenicillin era, which showed positive results for this organism in 165 (78%). The presumed explanation is improper placement of the needle or nonviable organisms. The most common complication is pneumothorax in 20% to 30%, but a chest tube is required in only 1% to 10%.[19] A review of 105 institutions with transthoracic needle aspiration in 1562 patients showed a mortality rate of 0.1%, major hemorrhage in 0.2%, and pneumothorax requiring a chest tube in 7%.[25] At present, transthoracic needle aspiration is generally restricted to tertiary medical centers with appropriate expertise for use in selected clinical settings, primarily immunocompromised patients or patients with atypical presentation in which the usual diagnostic specimen sources are either contraindicated or negative.

Bronchoscopy Specimens

Bronchoscopy with the rigid bronchoscope was developed in the late 1930s, and fiberoptic techniques were introduced in the late 1960s. Cultures obtained by suction aspiration through the inner channel for the usual bacteria are generally no better than the results with expectorated sputum.[26] The reason is that the inner channel becomes filled with saliva during instrument passage through the upper airways. The result is that bronchoscopy is now generally reserved either for the recovery of specific microbes or for the detection of common bacterial pathogens by use of quantitative techniques to distinguish colonization and infection. With regard to specific microbes, the best data are for *M. tuberculosis* and *P. carinii*. The types of specimens available are fixed tissue specimens, touch imprints of tissue from transbronchial biopsy, bronchoalveolar specimens, and brush biopsy specimens. For tuberculosis, bronchoscopy is an appropriate specimen source for patients who cannot provide expectorated specimens; contrary to popular opinion, the yield with both acid-fast stain and culture is superior with expectorated sputum.[27]

The utility of bronchoscopy for detecting the usual bacterial pathogens in the lower airways has been pursued by adding quantitation to the analysis. Theoretical support for quantitative cultures is based on the assumption that bacterial pathogens are invariably present in concentrations exceeding 10^5 per dL at the infected site; contaminants or colonizing bacteria are generally present in lower concentrations. This principle applies to specimens obtained at virtually any anatomic site (e.g., bile cultures, burn wounds, urine) and may be applied to expectorated sputum after liquefaction as well.[28] The usual techniques for obtaining bronchoscopic specimens for quantitative culture are with bronchoalveolar lavage or a double-lumen catheter with a distal occluding plug.[19, 29–32] Brush specimens must be placed in a diluent, and serial dilutions are done for quantitative culture. Specific techniques are described elsewhere, but they are critically important for accurate results. This requires a commitment to follow precise methodology by the bronchoscopist for specimen procurement and by the microbiologist for performing cultures. Major uses of this technique are for nosocomial pneumonia, particularly pneumonia in the intensive care unit and in intubated patients.[19, 31, 32]

Alternative Specimens

The use of specimen sources is commonly based on the likely pathogen as summarized in Table 53–6.

Community-Acquired Pneumonia

Microbiology

Major pathogens encountered in community-acquired pneumonia are summarized in Table 53–7. These results are based on three analyses: the author's review of 15 publications dealing with community-acquired pneumonia,[13, 33–48] primarily from the United States; a metaanalysis[4] of 122 reports of community-acquired pneumonia in the English language literature for 1966 to 1996; and estimates by The British Thoracic Society[49] based on their study involving 25 hospitals in England in the early 1980s. There is a notable bias in all three analyses because most of the patients are from hospital-based experiences in academic centers. In addition, there is a substantial variation in attempts to recover some microbes, especially those requiring nonroutine microbiologic techniques, such as *Legionella, Chlamydia pneumoniae, Mycoplasma pneumoniae*, and viruses. Of particular interest is the observation that even with extensive diagnostic studies, nearly all reports show no likely etiologic diagnosis in 30% to 50% of cases. This relatively sparse yield is ascribed to four problems: first, 20% to 30% of patients do not provide sputum samples; second, 20% to 30% have received antibiotics before evaluation; third, some pathogens require specialized techniques for detection that are not routinely done; and fourth, microbiologic methods are often substandard. The relatively low yield in many studies and skepticism about results have prompted vigorous debate about the value of expectorated sputum for stain and culture. The American Thoracic Society position paper opposes any diagnostic studies unless there is failure to respond to empirical treatment[50]; others are much more proactive for pretreatment diagnostic studies to simplify antibiotic decisions and help track the epidemiology of selected agents, such as penicillin-resistant *S. pneumoniae* and *Legionella*.[16, 48]

A historical perspective on studies of community-acquired

TABLE 53–7 ■ Microbiology of Community-Acquired Pneumonia

MICROBIAL AGENTS	LITERATURE REVIEW* (%)	THE BRITISH THORACIC SOCIETY† (%)	METAANALYSIS‡ Cases (%)	METAANALYSIS‡ Deaths (%)
Bacteria				
Streptococcus pneumoniae	20–60	60–75	65	66
Haemophilus influenzae	3–10	4–5	12	7
Staphylococcus aureus	3–5	1–5	2	6
Gram-negative bacilli	3–10	Rare	1	3
Miscellaneous agents§	3–5	(Not included)	4	9
Atypical agents	10–20	—	12	6
Legionella sp.	2–8	2–5	4	5
Mycoplasma pneumoniae	1–6	5–18	7	1
Chlamydia pneumoniae	4–6	(Not included)	1	<1
Viral	2–15	8–16	3	<1
Aspiration pneumonia	6–10	(Not included)	—	—
No diagnosis	30–60	—	—	—

*Based on 15 published reports from North America. Low and high values are deleted.[33–48]
†Estimates are based on analysis of 453 adults in prospective study of community-acquired pneumonia in 25 British hospitals.[46]
‡Metaanalysis of 122 published studies of community-acquired pneumonia in the English language literature 1966 to 1995; data are limited to 7057 patients who had an etiologic diagnosis.[4] Percentage in death column refers to percentage of all deaths attributed to the designated pathogen.
§Includes *Branhamella* (formerly *Moraxella*) *catarrhalis*, group A streptococcus, and *Neisseria meningitidis* (each 1%–2%).

pneumonia is of particular interest with regard to *S. pneumoniae*. In the prepenicillin era, *S. pneumoniae* accounted for more than 80% of pneumonias and 96% of lobar pneumonias.[5, 23] There has subsequently been a gradual reduction of the yield in various series so that nearly all studies reported during the past decade indicate a yield of only 10% to 22%. The implication is that this organism is disappearing, other agents are becoming more prevalent, or laboratory techniques for its recovery are now relatively poor. The truth is probably some combination of these observations. Many think that *S. pneumoniae* may account for a substantial portion of these enigmatic cases on the basis of the following: (1) studies using more aggressive methods to obtain uncontaminated specimens, such as transtracheal aspiration, show much higher yields[19–21, 51, 52]; (2) multiple studies show that the frequency of *S. pneumoniae* from sputum culture in patients with bacteremic pneumococcal pneumonia is only 40% to 50%,[12, 13] suggesting that the yield in most studies should be at least doubled; and (3) an analysis by The British Thoracic Society Pneumonia Research Committee based on a review of 148 patients with no identifiable pathogens concluded that most of these cases were probably due to *S. pneumoniae*.[53] Anaerobic bacteria are an additional category of organisms that have been conspicuously absent in virtually all studies since 1980. This reflects the fact that transtracheal aspirations are no longer done. Our prior studies using transtracheal aspiration indicated that anaerobic bacterial pneumonitis could not be easily distinguished from other common forms of bacterial pneumonia on the basis of clinical observations.[54] In addition, studies by Ries and colleagues[55] using transtracheal aspiration in unselected patients with community-acquired pneumonia showed anaerobic bacteria in 29 of 89 patients (33%). A similar yield was found by Pollock and colleagues[56] using quantitative cultures of fiberoptic bronchoscopy aspirates; here the yield was 38 of 172 patients (22%). These observations suggest that anaerobic bacteria probably account for a significant number of enigmatic pneumonias.

The term atypical agents was initially used to indicate *M. pneumoniae*,[57, 58] but it subsequently came to include *Legionella* and *C. pneumoniae* as well. These three organisms collectively account for 10% to 20% of all cases according to most studies that use aggressive techniques for their detection. Methods used to detect *Legionella* include culture, direct fluorescent antibody stain, urinary antigen assay, and serology.[17] All of these tests are reasonably specific but lack sensitivity. Culture and direct fluorescent antibody stain are technically demanding, so that the yield by different laboratories is highly variable. By contrast, urinary antigen assays are technically easy but are limited to the detection of *Legionella pneumophila* serogroup 1, which accounts for about 70% of cases.[59] *M. pneumoniae* has been found in 1% to 8% of patients with community-acquired pneumonia who require hospitalization; the rates are much higher for young adults with "walking pneumonia," and some report *Mycoplasma* species in up to 10% of elderly patients who require hospitalization.[45] The problem with *Mycoplasma* diagnostic studies is that most laboratories do not offer tests that provide useful information at the time that therapeutic decisions are made. Cultures are difficult to perform and are not offered by most laboratories. Measurement of cold agglutinins is somewhat nonspecific but may support this diagnosis in patients with a compatible clinical illness and a titer of 1:64 or higher. The same problem with diagnostic testing applies to *C. pneumoniae*, which allegedly accounts for 5% to 10% of cases of community-acquired pneumonia,[2, 39, 60] but diagnostic tests are not generally offered. The standard test for most prior studies has been serology, which is viewed by many authorities as nonspecific.[61] It is likely that improved diagnostic methods will be available for detection of these three atypical agents in the future, presumably using polymerase chain reaction technology.

Viral agents are detected in 2% to 15% of cases, most frequently influenza virus and less commonly parainfluenza virus and adenovirus. Viruses probably account for a substantial number of pneumonia cases in young, otherwise healthy adults and most children. The problem is the paucity of studies using appropriate diagnostic techniques in diverse populations of patients, and there are doubts regarding the sensitivity of current techniques for detecting viral agents that may be fastidious or unknown. Influenza virus is an important exception because this is a major cause of epidemics, and these viruses are associated with an increase of at least 20,000 pneumonia deaths per year for most years.[3, 62] The great majority of these are in elderly patients.[63]

Diagnostic Evaluation

There is no consensus about the use of laboratory resources to make a microbiologic diagnosis in outpatients with community-acquired pneumonia. Young and previously healthy adults who do not require hospitalization can usually be treated empirically with antibiotics. Patients who require hospitalization should probably have Gram stain and culture of expectorated sputum samples and should also have blood cultures if the course is acute. Most studies report the blood culture yield to be 5% to 20%; the mean for all reported cases is 12%, and *S. pneumoniae* accounts for two thirds of these.[4] Although it is admittedly arbitrary, we recommend Gram stain and culture of expectorated secretions using the guidelines noted before for obtaining purulent secretions before antibiotic treatment. In our experience, a likely microbial pathogen can be detected with Gram stain of expectorated sputum in about 50% of cases, the organism identified by Gram stain can be cultured in approximately 90% of cases, and the yield with culture is doubled by obtaining the specimen before antibiotic administration (64% versus 32%).[43, 44, 48] As noted earlier, diagnostic resources for atypical agents are controversial and limited. Edelstein[17] recommended diagnostic studies for *Legionella* as routine in epidemics caused by this organism, with pneumonia in the compromised host and for patients who fail to respond to antibiotics.

Therapy

Decisions regarding the selection of antibiotics are obviously simplified if a microbial diagnosis is strongly suspected or established by stains and culture. Guidelines for the empirical treatment of pneumonia have been provided by the American Thoracic Society[50] and The British Thoracic Society[49] (Table 53–8). These guidelines from authoritative sources are based on analysis of similar published data. They were both published in 1993, and each reflects a consensus opinion of authorities in the field; nevertheless, they are quite different. The British Thoracic Society emphasizes the paramount position of *S. pneumoniae* as the most common agent of pneumonia and the most common cause of life-threatening pneumonia, making penicillin and amoxicillin the preferred agents at that time. The more recent experience with penicillin-resistant *S. pneumoniae* may require an appropriate modification in geographic areas with high rates of resistant pneumococci.[64–67]

The recommendations of the American Thoracic Society are in four categories based on the severity of illness, age, and associated diseases. The preferred drug for outpatients younger than 60 years with no comorbidity is erythromycin because of its activity against *Mycoplasma, C. pneumoniae,* and *S. pneumoniae.* Alternatives include other macrolides (clarithromycin and azithromycin) because of better gastrointestinal tolerance and superior activity against *H. influenzae.* Outpatients older than 60 years or those with comorbid conditions should receive a second-generation cephalosporin, trimethoprim-sulfamethoxazole, or amoxicillin-clavulanate. There is the option to add erythromycin if *Legionella* is suspected. For patients who require hospitalization, the recommendation is based on the severity of illness. For those who are not critically ill, the recommendation is a second- or third-generation cephalosporin or a β-lactam–β-lactamase inhibitor with the option of adding erythromycin if *Legionella* is suspected. For patients who are critically ill, the recommendation is for a macrolide plus therapy for *Pseudomonas aeruginosa* infection. A concern for this last recommendation is the infrequency of *Pseudomonas* as an important cause of community-acquired pneumonia in patients other than those in settings where this risk is evident (i.e., patients with cystic fibrosis, bronchiectasis, advanced acquired immunodeficiency syndrome, or neutropenia). A metaanalysis of 19,095 reported cases of community-acquired pneumonia showed that *P. aeruginosa* was detected in only 18 (0.1%).[4] On the basis of problems associated with penicillin-resistant *S. pneumoniae* and the observation that *S. pneumoniae* and *Legionella* are responsible for most lethal pneumonias, many authorities prefer a macrolide plus either cefotaxime or ceftriaxone for empirical use in seriously ill patients with community-acquired pneumonia.

TABLE 53–8 ■ Recommendations for Empirical Treatment of Community-Acquired Pneumonia

THE BRITISH THORACIC SOCIETY[49]

1. Uncomplicated pneumonia of unknown etiology without features indicating severe or nonpneumococcal disease
   Preferred: An aminopenicillin: amoxicillin, 500 mg orally (PO) three times daily (tid), or ampicillin, 500 mg intravenously (IV) four times daily (qid), or benzylpenicillin, 1.2 g IV qid
   Alternatives: Erythromycin, 500 mg PO or IV qid, or second- or third-generation cephalosporin (cefuroxime or cefotaxime)
2. Severe pneumonia of unknown etiology
   Preferred: Erythromycin, 1 g IV qid, plus second- or third-generation cephalosporin (cefuroxime, 1.5 g, or cefotaxime, 2 g IV tid)
   Alternative: Ampicillin, 1 g, flucloxacillin, 2 g, and erythromycin, 1 g, all IV qid

AMERICAN THORACIC SOCIETY[50]

1. Outpatient pneumonia without comorbidity* and age ≤60 y
   Preferred: Macrolide—erythromycin; alternative (clarithromycin or azithromycin) with erythromycin intolerance and smokers (to treat *Haemophilus influenzae*)
   Alternative: Tetracycline
2. Outpatient pneumonia with comorbidity* and age ≥60 y
   Second-generation cephalosporin, trimethoprim-sulfamethoxazole, or β-lactam–β-lactamase inhibitor ± erythromycin or other macrolide if *Legionella* is suspected
3. Hospitalized patients
   Second- or third-generation cephalosporin or β-lactam–β-lactamase inhibitor ± erythromycin if legionellosis is a concern; rifampin may be added if *Legionella* is documented
4. Severe community-acquired pneumonia
   Macrolide (with rifampin for legionellosis) + third-generation antipseudomonal cephalosporin or other antipseudomonal therapy including imipenem or ciprofloxacin + aminoglycoside × ≥3 d

*Chronic lung disease, diabetes mellitus, renal failure, congestive heart failure, chronic alcohol abuse, malnutrition.

Nosocomial Pneumonia

Risk Factors and Rates

Risks for nosocomial pneumonia may be considered patient related, infection control related, or intervention related. Patient-related risks are associated with underlying disease that predisposes to upper airway colonization by gram-negative bacilli (discussed later), predisposition to aspiration, and predisposition to opportunistic infection (immunocompromised). Infection control–related risks relate to transmissible airborne pathogens (such as in tuberculosis, legionellosis, aspergillosis, and influenza) and contact transmission (as with *Staphylococcus aureus*, Enterobacteriaceae, *P. aeruginosa*, and *Acinetobacter*). The third risk is intervention related, such as surgery (especially thoracoabdominal surgery), medications (antibiotics, gastric pH neutralization, immunosuppressive agents, sedatives), and tubes (nasogastric intubation, tracheostomy, endotracheal intubation).

The rate of nosocomial pneumonia is 0.5% to 1.0% of all hospitalized persons. For intensive care units, the rate is reported at 15% to 20%; for mechanically ventilated patients, it is 18% to 60%. Fagon and colleagues[68] have challenged some of these incidence data by showing that many hospitalized patients who satisfy standard criteria (x-ray evidence of infiltrate combined with cough and fever) do not appear to have bacterial pneumonia on the basis of quantitative cultures of bronchoscopic aspirates.

Pathophysiology

The dominant organisms in nosocomial pneumonia are gram-negative bacteria, which presumably reach the lower airways by aspiration of gastric contents or by "microaspiration" of upper airway secretions.[69–74] This microbiologic pattern is distinctly different from that of community-acquired pneumonia, in which gram-negative bacteria play essentially no role except for precisely defined and unusual settings. The presumed explanation for the distinction is the high rates of colonization of the upper airways by gram-negative bacteria as a reflection of serious illness. The classic study to examine this association used throat cultures to determine the rate of asymptomatic carriage of gram-negative bacilli in various populations.[75] Healthy persons, physicians, medical students, and psychiatric patients, all exposed to a common hospital environment, had colonization rates of 2% to 3%. The rate in patients who were moderately ill was 30% to 40%; in the intensive care unit, it was 60% to 70%. These studies were done in patients who were not receiving antibiotics, but this type of treatment would also favor colonization by gram-negative bacilli. The presumed source of bacteria is the patient's own colonic flora. Thus, the postulated mechanism is colonization of the upper airways in a patient rendered vulnerable by severe disease with microaspiration as the mechanism for seeding of the lower airways. Aspiration and airway entry are promoted by violations of airway integrity, such as tracheostomy or intubation. Other pathophysiologic mechanisms for nosocomial pneumonia involve inhalation of selected pathogens responsible for epidemic or sporadic cases, including tuberculosis, legionellosis, and aspergillosis.

Bacteriology

Studies of nosocomial pneumonia indicate that gram-negative bacteria account for 50% to 70% of cases[69–74] (Table 53–9). The most common is *P. aeruginosa*, followed by a diverse array of Enterobacteriaceae. *S. aureus* is second to gram-negative bacteria in most studies and accounts for 15% to 30%.[68–74] Anaerobic bacteria may be found in up to 10% to 30% of cases but are not generally sought with use of appropriate diagnostic specimen sources.[69, 70] When they are found, there is usually the concurrent presence of aerobic gram-negative bacilli or *S. aureus*, and the role of anaerobes is somewhat unclear. Other organisms found in 5% to 20% of cases include *S. pneumoniae, H. influenzae*, and possibly *C. pneumoniae*. *Legionella* has been responsible for about 4% of all lethal nosocomial infections, but there have been multiple large outbreaks of Legionnaires' disease in hospitals that are usually traced to water supplies with distribution through cooling systems of air conditioners or showerheads.[17, 76] Tuberculosis accounts for a relatively small number of nosocomial infections but obviously represents an important public health problem.[77] Aspergillosis may occur in epidemics among patients who are vulnerable, usually those who have suppressed cell-mediated immunity or neutropenia. This infection should be suspected when a patient at risk develops a pleura-based lesion that shows characteristic features at computed tomography.

TABLE 53–9 ■ Nosocomial Pneumonia: Microbiology

MICROBIAL AGENT	%
Bacterial	
Gram-negative bacilli	50–70
*Pseudomonas aeruginosa**	
Enterobacteriaceae*	
*Staphylococcus aureus**	15–30
Anaerobic bacteria	10–30
Haemophilus influenzae	10–20
Streptococcus pneumoniae	10–20
*Legionella**	4
Viral	10–20
Cytomegalovirus	
Influenza virus*	
Respiratory syncytial virus*	
Fungal	<1
*Aspergillus**	

*May cause nosocomial epidemics.

Diagnosis

Pulmonary infection is usually suspected in hospitalized patients with fever, respiratory symptoms, and a new infiltrate on chest x-ray examination. However, studies by Fagon and coworkers[68] suggested that most of these patients have alternative diagnoses. These investigators used quantitative culture of fiberoptic bronchoscopy aspirates in patients with the characteristic clinical features and found positive results with quantitative cultures in only about 40%; the majority of patients with negative results were not treated with antibiotics and subsequently recovered.

The usual specimen for a microbiologic diagnosis is expectorated sputum for Gram stain and culture. This usually yields gram-negative bacilli and *S. aureus* in large concentrations if they are involved in the pulmonary infection. The most frequent problem here is false-positive cultures for these microbes. Patients with pneumonia in the intensive care unit, and especially those who are intubated, often undergo fiberoptic bronchoscopy with quantitative culture.[29–32, 78] This is regarded as a controversial issue among pulmonary physicians who appear divided over the role of bronchoscopy to evaluate pneumonia in the intensive care unit.[74]

Therapy

The predominant organisms are gram-negative bacteria and *S. aureus*. These organisms require in vitro sensitivity tests to define optimal therapy and are readily recovered from most patients with expectorated sputum, nasotracheal suction, or endotracheal tube aspiration. Empirical treatment decisions should be based on Gram stains of these specimens pending culture and in vitro sensitivity test results. Guidelines for empirical antibiotic selection from the American Thoracic Society[74] are provided in Table 53–10.

Prevention

The high risk for pneumonia in intensive care units has prompted aggressive methods to prevent this complication (Table 53–11). The most important recommendations are the use of the semiupright position to reduce the risk of aspiration[79] and the use of appropriate precautions to prevent secondary cases by airborne spread or contact. It is common practice in intensive care units to give prophylaxis to prevent peptic ulceration, but neutralization of gastric acid eliminates the gastric barrier, the acid defense mechanism that prevents

TABLE 53–10 ■ Treatment of Nosocomial Pneumonia

MILD TO MODERATELY SEVERE EARLY ONSET NO RISK FACTORS	SEVERE LATE ONSET RISK
Cephalosporin: second or third generation (nonpseudomonal)	Aminoglycoside or ciprofloxacin *plus*
β-Lactam–β-lactamase inhibitor	Antipseudomonal penicillin β-Lactam–β-lactamase inhibitor
Penicillin: fluoroquinolone or clindamycin + aztreonam	Antipseudomonal cephalosporin Imipenem or Aztreonam *with or without* Vancomycin

Data from American Thoracic Society: Hospital-acquired pneumonia in adults: Diagnosis, assessment of severity, initial antimicrobial therapy and preventative strategies. A consensus statement. Am Rev Respir Crit Care Med 153:1711–1725, 1996.

colonization of the stomach by various bacteria including gram-negative bacilli. Sucralfate is advocated as a substitute for histamine H_2 blockers or antacids, and preliminary evidence suggests efficacy.[80, 81] A relatively recent procedure advocated to prevent pneumonia in ventilated patients is continuous aspiration of subglottic secretions.[82] Selective decontamination has been a popular method to interrupt the cycle of colonization of the colon by gram-negative bacilli followed by colonization of the pharynx with subsequent aspiration from either an upper airway source or gastric contents. The goal of selective decontamination is to eliminate or reduce gram-negative bacilli (and sometimes *S. aureus* and *Candida*) in the gastrointestinal tract with antibiotics that select for these organisms but preserve the anaerobic bacteria that appear critical for population control of flora in the colon. An extensive experience with this technique including 12 controlled trials with more than 4000 participants showed that this tactic effectively reduces the frequency of pneumonia in intensive care units, but there is no substantial impact on mortality rates.[83, 84] Major concerns are the failure to reduce mortality, excessive costs of the regimens, and the concern of antibiotic abuse with its impact on bacterial resistance. Most authorities consequently no longer recommend selective decontamination in this setting.

TABLE 53–11 ■ Prevention of Nosocomial Pneumonia

STRONGLY RECOMMENDED

Semiupright position to reduce risk of aspiration

Contact precautions with mask for the following respiratory tract pathogens

- Bacteria: *Staphylococcus aureus*, group A streptococci, *Neisseria meningitidis, Bordetella pertussis, Yersinia pestis* (plague), penicillin-resistant *Streptococcus pneumoniae*, multidrug-resistant gram-negative bacilli
- Bacteria-like: *Mycoplasma pneumoniae*
- Mycobacteria: *Mycobacterium tuberculosis*
- Viruses: Viral exanthems (measles, rubella, chickenpox, mumps), influenza virus, enterovirus
- Fungi: None

ENCOURAGED

Use of sucralfate in place of histamine H_2 agonists or antacids to preserve the gastric barrier

EXPERIMENTAL

Continuous aspiration of subglottic secretions in ventilated patients

NOT RECOMMENDED

Selective decontamination of gastrointestinal tract

Topical administration (intratracheal instillations or aerosolized administration) of antimicrobial agents

Topical antibiotics have also been tested by instillation of drugs through tracheostomies or endotracheal tubes or by aerosolization. Drugs that are usually given by these routes are polymyxin or aminoglycosides, although multiple different agents have been used. The most extensive experience is by Feeley and colleagues[85] using polymyxin in an attempt to prevent nosocomial infections with *P. aeruginosa*. They were able to reduce the frequency of *P. aeruginosa*, but there was no impact on mortality rates, and there was an associated risk of infection involving resistant strains, primarily *Proteus* infections. Most authorities discourage the use of topical agents except for the single clinical setting in which efficacy seems established: cystic fibrosis.

Pneumonia in the Immunocompromised Host

The immunocompromised host now represents an enlarging component of the population of hospitalized patients and outpatients. A review of 385 consecutive patients hospitalized at Johns Hopkins Hospital with community-acquired pneumonia in 1991 showed that 56% were considered immunocompromised.[43] The majority of these were patients with human immunodeficiency virus infection, but there were also a large number who were receiving immunosuppressive therapy for organ transplantation or cancer chemotherapy. Etiologic agents are highly variable and largely dependent on the nature of the host defect. The reader is referred to Chapter 54 for the approach to the immunocompromised host with suspected pneumonia; pneumonia in patients with human immunodeficiency virus infection is discussed in Chapter 122.

Response to Therapy

The response and outcome of patients with community-acquired pneumonia depend to a large extent on the microbial agent involved and the host status. Factors suggesting poor prognosis based on host status, clinical features, laboratory findings, and microbial pathogens for community-acquired pneumonia are summarized in Table 53–12.[4, 7, 40, 50] The overall mortality of patients hospitalized with community-acquired pneumonia according to a metaanalysis of 25,629 patients from 80 cohort studies reported from 1966 to 1995 was 13.6%; it was 17.6% for elderly patients, 19.6% for bacteremic patients, and 36.5% for patients hospitalized in the intensive care unit.[4] Factors related to poor prognosis were hypothermia (odds ratio [OR] = 5.0), hypotension (OR = 4.8), tachypnea (OR = 2.9), neoplastic disease (OR = 2.8), neurologic disease (OR = 4.6), bacteremia (OR = 2.8), leukopenia (OR = 2.5), and multiple lobe infiltrates (OR = 3.1).[4]

With regard to response by microbial pathogens, the greatest experience is with pneumococcal pneumonia. After initiation of penicillin treatment with penicillin-sensitive *S. pneumoniae*, most patients show clinical improvement within 24 to 48 hours with a decrease in temperature and reduction in systemic toxic effects.[86] The mean duration of fever in bacteremic pneumococcal pneumonia is approximately 6 days.[4] The time to resolution of changes on the chest film depends largely on the host.[87] Young and previously healthy adults show a mean time to radiographic clearing of 3 weeks; older patients and those with complicated infections show an average of 12 weeks to radiographic clearing. A subset of pneumococcal pneumonia patients does poorly. Features of poor prognosis include multiple lobe involvement, bacteremia, age older than 60 years, concomitant disease, and neutropenia.

TABLE 53–12 ■ Factors Related to Poor Prognosis for Patients with Pneumonia

Age >65 y
Coexisting disease
Diabetes, renal failure, heart failure, chronic lung disease, chronic alcoholism
Hospitalization within 1 y previously
Immunosuppression
Neoplastic disease
Clinical findings
Respiratory rate >30/min
Systolic pressure <90 mm Hg or diastolic pressure <60 mm Hg
Temperature >38.3°C or hypothermia
Altered mental status (lethargy, stupor, disorientation, coma)
Extrapulmonary site of infection: e.g., meningitis, septic arthritis
Laboratory tests
White cell count <4000/mm³ or >30,000/mm³
Partial pressure of oxygen, arterial, <60 mm Hg on room air
Renal failure
Chest radiograph showing multiple lobe involvement, rapid spread, or pleural effusion
Hematocrit <30%
Bacteremia
Microbial pathogens
Streptococcus pneumoniae
Legionella

Data from American Thoracic Society: Guidelines for initial management of adults with community-acquired pneumonia. Am Rev Respir Dis 148:1418–1426, 1993; Fine MJ, Smith DN, Singer DE: Hospitalization decision in patients with community-acquired pneumonia. Am J Med 89:713–721, 1990; Farr BM, Sloman AJ, Fisch MJ: Predicting death in patients hospitalized for community-acquired pneumonia. Ann Intern Med 115:428–436, 1991; Fine MJ, Smith MA, Carson CA, et al: Prognosis and outcomes of patients with community-acquired pneumonia. JAMA 274:134–141, 1995.

Studies since the introduction of penicillin have shown that this drug has obviously had a notable impact on outcome; nevertheless, there is also good evidence that penicillin and other antibiotics have had little impact on the mortality rate during the first 5 days of treatment in patients with bacteremic pneumococcal pneumonia. The overall mortality rate of pneumococcal pneumonia among 4432 patients hospitalized with this diagnosis was 12.3%; for 1145 patients with bacteremic pneumococcal pneumonia, it was 19%.[4]

Patients with *Mycoplasma* pneumonia usually become afebrile within 1 to 2 days after treatment with tetracycline or a macrolide. Extrapulmonary signs and symptoms usually respond more slowly, and the role of antibiotics for these complications is unclear. The mortality rate is virtually nil,

TABLE 53–13 ■ Causes of Failure to Respond to Treatment

Disease is too far advanced at time of treatment or treatment is delayed too long: most common with pneumonia due to *Streptococcus pneumoniae*, *Legionella*, or gram-negative bacilli
Wrong antibiotic selection: uncommon
Inadequate dose of antibiotic: most common with aminoglycosides owing to failure to use adequate dose or to monitor serum levels
Wrong diagnosis: noninfectious disease such as pulmonary embolism with infarction, congestive failure, Wegener granulomatosis, sarcoidosis, atelectasis, chemical pneumonitis
Wrong microbial diagnosis
Inadequate host: debilitated, severe associated disease, immunosuppressed
Complicated pneumonia with undrained empyema, metastatic site of infection (meningitis), or bronchial obstruction (foreign body, carcinoma)
Pulmonary superinfection: most patients respond and then deteriorate with new fever

TABLE 53–14 ■ Definition of Severe Hospital-Acquired Pneumonia

Admission to the intensive care unit
Respiratory failure, defined as the need for mechanical ventilation or the need for >35% oxygen to maintain an arterial oxygen saturation at >90%
Rapid radiographic progression, multilobar pneumonia, or cavitation of a lung infiltrate
Evidence of severe sepsis with hypotension or end organ dysfunction
Shock (systolic blood pressure <90 mm Hg, or diastolic blood pressure <60 mm Hg)
Requirement for vasopressors for more than 4 h
Urine output <20 mL/h or total urine output <80 mL in 4 h (unless another explanation is available)
Acute renal failure requiring dialysis

although some patients with sickle cell disease and some elderly patients may have relatively severe disease.[4, 58]

Legionella pneumonia is like serious pneumococcal pneumonia in the sense that many patients have progressive disease despite appropriate antibiotic therapy. The reported mortality is 15% to 25% even with erythromycin treatment.[4, 17]

Patients with persistent fever and progressive symptoms after 3 to 5 days of treatment must be considered possible therapeutic failures if no etiologic diagnosis was established. Diagnostic considerations in this clinical setting are summarized in Table 53–13. In many instances, the infection has progressed too far by the time treatment is initiated, or else the patient is an inadequate host because of debility, immunosuppression, or associated diseases that preclude clinical response. Nevertheless, a diagnostic evaluation is necessary to exclude alternative treatable conditions. This evaluation often consists of sequential cultures of expectorated sputum or some other specimen from the respiratory tract, but these cultures are likely to be misleading because of the inherent problem of the antibiotic effect on fragile, susceptible microbes and the probability of "sputum superinfection" reflecting colonization of the airways. Most studies show that the yield of gram-negative bacilli of *S. aureus* is 25% to 50% when specimens are collected after common forms of antibiotic treatment. Unfortunately, it is often difficult for physicians to resist the temptation to add new antibiotics with each new organism that represents a potential pathogen in the lower airways.

A diagnostic study that may be useful is fiberoptic bronchoscopy, which may detect conditions other than infections by conventional pathogens (such as *M. tuberculosis*, pathogenic fungal, and *P. carinii* infections) and noninfectious conditions (such as bronchogenic neoplasms, atelectasis, chemical pneumonitis, interstitial lung disease, and sarcoidosis). An additional diagnostic test to consider is computed tomography to detect pleural effusions, cavitary lung disease, adenopathy, and other anatomic changes that may alter the differential diagnosis. If pulmonary embolism is a diagnostic consideration, a reasonable next step is a lung scan or pulmonary angiography.

For nosocomial pneumonia, especially for cases in the intensive care unit, the mortality rate is often reported at 20% to 30%.[74] In many cases, there are multiple contributing factors in addition to the pulmonary infection. Nevertheless, nosocomial pneumonia is regarded as a devastating disease associated with an extraordinarily high mortality rate, primarily in the intensive care unit and in intubated patients. The definition of severe nosocomial pneumonia is summarized in Table 53–14.[74]

References

1. Dixon RE: Economic costs of respiratory tract infections in the United States. Am J Med 78(Suppl 6B):45–51, 1985.

2. Marrie TJ: Community-acquired pneumonia. Clin Infect Dis 18:501–515, 1994.
3. Pinner RW, Teutsch SM, Simonsen L, et al: Trends in infectious diseases mortality in the United States. JAMA 275:189–193, 1996.
4. Fine MJ, Smith MA, Carson CA, et al: Prognosis and outcomes of patients with community-acquired pneumonia. JAMA 274:134–141, 1995.
5. Heffron R: Pneumonia. Cambridge, MA, Harvard University Press, 1939, pp 302–308.
6. Opravil M, Marincek B, Fuchs WA, et al: Shortcomings of chest radiography in detecting *Pneumocystis carinii* pneumonia. J Acquired Immune Defic Syndr 7:39–45, 1994.
7. Fine MJ, Smith DN, Singer DE: Hospitalization decision in patients with community-acquired pneumonia: A prospective cohort study. Am J Med 89:713–721, 1990.
8. Janssen RS, St. Louis ME, Statten GA, et al: HIV infection among patients in U.S. acute care hospitals: Strategies for the counseling and testing of hospital patients. N Engl J Med 327:445–452, 1992.
9. Light RW: A new classification of parapneumonic effusions and empyema. Chest 108:299–306, 1995.
10. Heffner JE, Brown LK, Barbieri C, et al: Pleural fluid chemical analysis in parapneumonic effusions. Am J Respir Crit Care Med 151:1700–1708, 1995.
11. American Thoracic Society: Clinical role of bronchoalveolar lavage in adults with pulmonary disease. Am Rev Respir Dis 142:481–486, 1990.
12. Barrett-Conner E: The nonvalue of sputum culture in the diagnosis of pneumococcal pneumonia. Am Rev Respir Dis 103:845–848, 1971.
13. Mufson MA, Chang V, Gill V, et al: The role of viruses, mycoplasmas and bacteria in acute pneumonia in civilian adults. Am J Epidemiol 86:526–544, 1967.
14. Murray PR, Washington JA II: Microscopic and bacteriologic analysis of expectorated sputum. Mayo Clin Proc 50:339–344, 1975.
15. Van Scoy RE: Bacterial sputum cultures: A clinician's viewpoint. Mayo Clin Proc 52:39–41, 1977.
16. Rein MF, Gwaltney JM Jr, O'Brien WM, et al: Accuracy of Gram's stain in identifying pneumococci in sputum. JAMA 239:2671–2673, 1978.
17. Edelstein PH: Legionnaires' disease. Clin Infect Dis 16:741–749, 1993.
18. Pecora DV: A comparison of transtracheal aspiration with other methods of determining the bacterial flora of the lower respiratory tract. N Engl J Med 296:664–666, 1963.
19. Bartlett JG: Invasive diagnostic techniques in pulmonary infections. *In* Pennington JE (ed): Respiratory Infections: Diagnosis and Management, ed 3. New York, Raven Press, 1994, pp 73–99.
20. Bartlett JG: The technique of transtracheal aspiration. J Crit Ill 1:43–49, 1986.
21. Bartlett JG: Diagnostic accuracy of transtracheal aspiration bacteriology. Am Rev Respir Dis 115:777–782, 1977.
22. Bjerkestrand G, Digranes A, Schreiner A: Bacteriological findings in transtracheal aspirates from patients with chronic bronchitis and bronchiectasis. Scand J Respir Dis 56:201–207, 1975.
23. Bullowa JGM: The reliability of sputum typing and its relation to serum therapy. JAMA 105:1512–1523, 1935.
24. American Thoracic Society: Guidelines for percutaneous transthoracic needle aspiration. Am Rev Respir Dis 140:255–256, 1989.
25. Herman PG, Hessel SJ: The diagnostic accuracy and complications of closed lung biopsies. Radiology 125:11–14, 1977.
26. Bartlett JG, Alexander J, Mayhew J, et al: Should fiberoptic bronchoscopy aspirates be cultured? Am Rev Respir Dis 114:73–78, 1976.
27. Jett JR, Cortese DA, Dines DE: The value of bronchoscopy in the diagnosis of mycobacterial disease. Chest 80:575–578, 1981.
28. Bartlett JG, Finegold SM: Bacteriology of expectorated sputum with quantitative culture and wash technique compared to transtracheal aspirates. Am Rev Respir Dis 117:1010–1027, 1978.
29. Wimberly N, Faling J, Bartlett JG: A fiberoptic bronchoscopy technique to obtain uncontaminated lower airway secretions for bacterial culture. Am Rev Respir Dis 119:337–343, 1979.
30. Wimberly NW, Bass JB, Boyd BS, et al: Use of a bronchoscopic protected catheter brush for the diagnosis of pulmonary infections. Chest 81:556–562, 1982.
31. Papazian L, Thomas P, Garbe L, et al: Bronchoscopic or blind sampling techniques for the diagnosis of ventilator-associated pneumonia. Am J Respir Crit Care Med 152:1982–1991, 1995.
32. Chastre J, Fagon JY, Lamer CH: Procedures for the diagnosis of pneumonia in ICU patients. Intensive Care Med 18:S10–S17, 1992.
33. Fekety FR Jr, Caldwell J, Gump D, et al: Bacteria, viruses and mycoplasmas in acute pneumonia in adults. Am Rev Respir Dis 104:499–507, 1971.
34. Sullivan RJ Jr, Dowdle WR, Marine WM, et al: Adult pneumonia in a general hospital: Etiology and host risk factors. Arch Intern Med 129:935–942, 1972.
35. Bisno AL, Griffin JR, Van Epps KA, et al: Pneumonia and Hong Kong influenza: A prospective study of the 1968–1969 epidemic. Am J Med Sci 261:251–263, 1971.
36. Dorff GJ, Rytel MW, Farmer SG, et al: Etiologies and characteristic features of pneumonias in a municipal hospital. Am J Med Sci 266:349–358, 1973.
37. Fick RB Jr, Reynolds HY: Changing spectrum of pneumonia—News media creation or clinical reality? Am J Med 74:1–8, 1983.
38. Larsen RA, Jacobson JA: Diagnosis of community-acquired pneumonia: Experience at a community hospital. Compr Ther 10:20–25, 1984.
39. Marrie TJ, Durant H, Yates L: Community-acquired pneumonia requiring hospitalization: 15 year prospective study. Rev Infect Dis 11:586–599, 1989.
40. Farr BM, Sloman AJ, Fisch MJ: Predicting death in patients hospitalized for community-acquired pneumonia. Ann Intern Med 115:428–436, 1991.
41. Bates JH, Campbell GD, Barron AL, et al: Microbial etiology of acute pneumonia in hospitalized patients. Chest 101:1005–1012, 1992.
42. Fang GD, Fine M, Orloff J, et al: New and emerging etiologies for community-acquired pneumonia with implication for therapy. A prospective multicenter study of 359 cases. Medicine (Baltimore) 69:307–316, 1990.
43. Mundy LM, Auwaerter PG, Oldach D, et al: Community-acquired pneumonia: Impact of immune status. Am J Respir Crit Care Med 152:1309–1315, 1995.
44. Dans P, Charache PC, Fahey M, et al: Management of pneumonia in the prospective payment era. Arch Intern Med 144:1392–1397, 1984.
45. Marston BJ, Plouffe JF, Breiman RF, et al: Preliminary findings in a community-based pneumonia incidence study. *In* Barbaree JM, Breiman RF, Dufour AP (eds): Legionella. Washington, DC, American Society for Microbiology, 1993, pp 36–37.
46. Research Committee of the British Thoracic Society and the Public Health Laboratory Service: Community-acquired pneumonia in adults in British hospitals in 1982–1983: A survey of aetiology, mortality, prognostic factors and outcome. Q J Med 239:195–220, 1987.
47. Lim I, Shaw DR, Stanley DP, et al: A prospective hospital study of the aetiology of community-acquired pneumonia. Med J Aust 151:87–91, 1989.
48. Bartlett JG, Mundy LM: Community-acquired pneumonia. N Engl J Med 333:1618–1624, 1995.
49. The British Thoracic Society: Guidelines for the management of community-acquired pneumonia in adults admitted to hospital. Br J Hosp Med 49:346–350, 1993.
50. American Thoracic Society: Guidelines for the initial management of adults with community-acquired pneumonia: Diagnosis, assessment of severity, and initial antimicrobial therapy. Am Rev Respir Dis 148:1418–1426, 1993.
51. Kalinske RW, Parker RH, Brandt E: Diagnostic usefulness and safety of transtracheal aspiration. N Engl J Med 276:604–608, 1970.
52. Hoeprich PD: Etiologic diagnosis of lower respiratory tract infections. Calif Med 112:1–8, 1970.
53. Farr BM, Kaiser DL, Harrison BDW, Connolly CK: Prediction of microbial aetiology at admission to hospital for pneumonia from the presenting clinical features. Thorax 44:1031–1035, 1989.
54. Bartlett JG: Anaerobic bacterial pneumonitis. Am Rev Respir Dis 119:19–23, 1979.
55. Ries K, Levison ME, Kaye D: Transtracheal aspiration in pulmonary infection. Arch Intern Med 133:453–458, 1974.
56. Pollock HM, Hawkins EL, Bonner JR, et al: Diagnosis of bacterial pulmonary infections during quantitative protected catheter cultures obtained during bronchoscopy. J Clin Microbiol 17:255–259, 1983.

57. Chanock RM, Mufson MA, Bloom HH, et al: Eaton agent pneumonia. JAMA 175:213–220, 1961.
58. Foy HM: Infections caused by *Mycoplasma pneumoniae* and possible carrier state in a different population of patients. Clin Infect Dis 17(Suppl):S37–S46, 1993.
59. Marston BJ, Lipman HB, Breiman RF: Surveillance for Legionnaires' disease. Risk factors for morbidity and mortality. Arch Intern Med 154:2417–2422, 1994.
60. Grayston JT, Campbell LA, Kuo CC, et al: A new respiratory tract pathogen: *Chlamydia pneumoniae*, strain TWAR. J Infect Dis 161:618–625, 1990.
61. Hyman CL, Roblin PM, Gaydos CA, et al: Prevalence of asymptomatic nasopharyngeal carriage of *Chlamydia pneumoniae* in subjectively healthy adults: Assessment by polymerase chain reaction–enzyme immunoassay and culture. Clin Infect Dis 20:1174–1178, 1995.
62. Sullivan KM, Monto AS, Longini IM Jr: Estimates of the U.S. health impact of influenza. Am J Public Health 83:1712–1716, 1993.
63. Mullooly JP, Bennett MD, Hornbrook MC, et al: Influenza vaccination programs for elderly persons: Cost-effectiveness in a health maintenance organization. Ann Intern Med 121:947–952, 1994.
64. Austrian R: Confronting drug-resistant pneumococci. Ann Intern Med 121:807–809, 1994.
65. Breiman RF, Butler JC, Tenover FC, et al: Emergence of drug-resistant pneumococcal infections in the United States. JAMA 271:1831–1835, 1994.
66. Doern GV, Brueggemann A, Holley HP Jr, Rauch AM: Antimicrobial resistance of *Streptococcus pneumoniae* recovered from outpatients in the United States during the winter months of 1994 to 1995: Results of a 30-center national surveillance study. Antimicrob Agents Chemother 40:1209–1213, 1996.
67. Hofmann J, Cetron MS, Farley MM, et al: The prevalence of drug-resistant *Streptococcus pneumoniae* in Atlanta. N Engl J Med 333:481–486, 1995.
68. Fagon JY, Chastre J, Hance AJ, et al: Detection of nosocomial lung infection in ventilated patients: Use of a protected specimen brush and quantitative culture techniques in 147 patients. Am Rev Respir Dis 138:110–116, 1988.
69. Bartlett JG, O'Keefe P, Tally FP, et al: Bacteriology of hospital-acquired pneumonia. Arch Intern Med 146:868–871, 1986.
70. Dore P, Robert R, Grollier G, et al: Incidence of anaerobes in ventilator-associated pneumonia with use of a protected specimen brush. Am J Respir Crit Care Med 153:1292–1298, 1996.
71. Rouby JJ, Martin De Lassale E, Poete P, et al: Nosocomial bronchopneumonia in the critically ill. Histologic and bacteriologic aspects. Am Rev Respir Dis 146:1059–1066, 1992.
72. Horan TC, White JW, Jarvis WR, et al: Nosocomial infection surveillance, 1984. MMWR CDC Surveill Summ 35:17SS–29SS, 1986.
73. Schleupner CJ, Cobb DK: A study of the etiologies and treatment of nosocomial pneumonia in a community-based teaching hospital. Infect Control Hosp Epidemiol 13:515–525, 1992.
74. American Thoracic Society: Hospital-acquired pneumonia in adults: Diagnosis, assessment of severity, initial antimicrobial therapy and preventative strategies. A consensus statement. Am Rev Respir Crit Care Med 153:1711–1725, 1996.
75. Johanson WG, Pierce AK, Sanford JP: Changing pharyngeal bacterial flora of hospitalized patients: Emergence of gram-negative bacilli. N Engl J Med 281:1137–1140, 1969.
76. Carratala J, Gudiol F, Pallares R, et al: Risk factors for nosocomial *Legionella pneumophila* pneumonia. Am J Respir Crit Care Med 149:625–629, 1994.
77. McGowan JE Jr: Nosocomial tuberculosis: New progress in control and prevention. Clin Infect Dis 21:489–505, 1995.
78. Torres A, Puig de la Bellacasa JP, Xaubet A, et al: Diagnostic value of quantitative cultures of bronchoalveolar lavage and telescoping plugged catheters in mechanically ventilated patients with bacterial pneumonia. Am Rev Respir Dis 140:306–310, 1989.
79. Torres A, Serra-Batlles J, Ros E, et al: Pulmonary aspiration of gastric contents in patients receiving mechanical ventilation: The effect of body position. Ann Intern Med 116:540–543, 1992.
80. Driks MR, Craven DE, Celli BR, et al: Nosocomial pneumonia in intubated patients given sucralfate as compared with antacids or histamine type 2 blockers: The role of gastric colonization. N Engl J Med 317:1376–1382, 1987.
81. Prod'hom G, Leuenberger P, Koerfer J, et al: Nosocomial pneumonia in mechanically ventilated patients receiving antacid, ranitidine, or sucralfate as prophylaxis for stress ulcer. A randomized controlled trial. Ann Intern Med 120:653–662, 1994.
82. Valles J, Artigas A, Rello J, et al: Continuous aspiration of subglottic secretions in preventing ventilator-associated pneumonia. Ann Intern Med 122:179–186, 1995.
83. Gastinne H, Wolff M, Delatour F, et al: A controlled trial in intensive care units of selective decontamination of the digestive tract with nonabsorbable antibiotics. N Engl J Med 326:594–599, 1992.
84. Selective Decontamination of the Digestive Tract Trialists' Collaborative Group: Meta-analysis of randomised controlled trials of selective decontamination of the digestive tract. Br Med J 307:525–532, 1993.
85. Feeley TW, Du Moulin GC, Hedley-Whyte J, et al: Aerosol polymyxin and pneumonia in seriously ill patients. N Engl J Med 293:471–475, 1975.
86. Austrian R, Winston AL: The efficacy of penicillin V in the treatment of mild or moderately severe pneumococcal pneumonia. Am J Med Sci 232:624–628, 1956.
87. Jay SJ, Johanson WG, Pierce AK: The radiographic resolution of *Streptococcus pneumoniae* pneumonia. N Engl J Med 293:798–801, 1975.

54

Pneumonias in Immunocompromised Hosts

James E. Pennington
Christopher H. Fanta

The Dilemma

Fever and the appearance of new infiltrates on chest radiographs are dreaded complications in immunocompromised patients. In fact, the lung is the most common target organ for infectious complications in such patients, with associated mortalities often exceeding 50%. Furthermore, a presentation with fever and new lung infiltrates may mimic infectious pneumonia but actually result from noninfectious causes. To the constant frustration of the clinician, the diagnostic methods employed in the traditional work-up of pneumonia, such as sputum examination and culture, serologic studies, and radiographic clues, are often of little or no use in immunocompromised patients.

Thus, the clinician confronted with an immunocompromised host who has new fever and lung infiltrate faces a dilemma. The situation is urgent, calling for rapid institution of correct therapy, yet noninvasive diagnostic tools are often unhelpful. Furthermore, the list of etiologic possibilities is immense, with many requiring considerably different therapies. This dilemma usually leads to a choice of either empirical treatment, based on clinical assessment of the most likely etiologic possibilities, or aggressive deployment of invasive diagnostic procedures, such as bronchoscopic lavage and biopsy or open lung biopsy. Both approaches are hazardous, and the proper management decision is generally based on the clinician's own experience as well as the local expertise in biopsy techniques. This chapter reviews the clinical considerations leading up to this critical decision point so that a logical rather than a "shotgun" approach may be taken.

The Problem

The attack rate of pneumonia among various types of immunocompromised patients depends on the underlying condition. The frequency of pneumonia is highest among patients with hematologic malignant neoplasms, bone marrow transplant recipients, and patients with acquired immunodeficiency syndrome. For example, in patients with lymphoma who are receiving intensive chemotherapy, the lung is the most common site of serious infections, and deaths from infection are most often associated with pneumonia.[1] Patients with acute leukemia in relapse suffer an episode of pneumonia once every 60 days of risk.[2] Interstitial pneumonias occur in as many as 55% of bone marrow transplant recipients who survive 30 days after transplantation, with an associated mortality of approximately 60%.[3, 4] Finally, among patients with acquired immunodeficiency syndrome, the most frequent cause of death is opportunistic infection of the lungs (usually with *Pneumocystis carinii*).[5]

There is some evidence that pneumonia-related mortality among certain groups of patients may be falling. For example, one renal transplant center reported a 24% incidence of pneumonia among renal graft recipients between 1966 and 1978. A mortality of 50%, often due to pulmonary superinfections, was noted.[6] In a later series (1977 to 1979), however, the incidence of pneumonia among renal transplant recipients was 12%, and all survived their infection.[7]

In another report dealing with a mixed population of immunosuppressed patients, mortality associated with diffuse interstitial infiltrates was 38%; mortality for focal pneumonias was 21%.[8] There is also evidence that mortalities associated with cytomegalovirus (CMV) in bone marrow transplantation patients may be reduced from the usual 80% to 90% to 50% if combinations of chemotherapy and immunotherapy are employed.[9, 10] Despite some encouraging trends, however, pneumonia remains a potentially fatal complication among all types of immunosuppressed patients. Any hope for improved clinical management must be associated with aggressive and rational employment of diagnostic and therapeutic tools.

Etiologic Mechanisms

The causes for new fever and lung infiltrate in immunocompromised hosts can generally be divided into infectious (Table 54–1), noninfectious (Table 54–2), and idiopathic categories. Identification of the precise cause is an obvious goal of clinical management, and appropriate therapies are well defined (see Table 54–1). However, information to guide therapy is often lacking. A particularly frustrating diagnostic category is nonspecific interstitial pneumonitis. This "diagnosis" may account for 20% to 25% of all lung biopsy results.[11] Needless to say, management of nonspecific interstitial pneumonitis is controversial. In view of the long list of treatments for different infectious causes, as well as the possible use of corticosteroids for toxic drug effects or even antineoplastic agents if progressive lymphoma is suspected, it is not unusual for the empirically treated patient to receive four to six different drugs.

Clinical Approach

Two Important Clues

How, then, should the clinician approach this situation? By far the two most useful clues to management of pneumonia in the immunocompromised host are the underlying host defect (Table 54–3) and the radiographic pattern of the lung infiltrate (Table 54–4). The most common causes in granulocytopenic patients result in focal infiltrates. Not unexpectedly, among the common etiologic categories for focal infiltrates (see Table 54–4) are the causes that are most often seen in granulocytopenic patients. *Nocardia* and *Cryptococcus* spp. are the only exceptions, in that these pathogens usually cause focal infiltration but are much more common in cell-mediated immunodeficiency states. In patients with cell-mediated immunodeficiency, diffuse infiltrates are most common. The common category for diffuse infiltrates (see Table 54–4) includes two etiologic agents (*Pneumocystis* spp. and CMV) commonly encountered in such patients (see Table 54–3).

However, care must be used in coordinating these two clues. For example, a focal infiltrate in a patient with cell-mediated immunodeficiency is more likely to be caused by *Nocardia* or *Cryptococcus* spp. than by the usual bacteria, whereas a diffuse infiltrate in a granulocytopenic patient is more likely to be caused by *Aspergillus* spp. rather than by *Pneumocystis* spp. or CMV. It thus appears that the underlying host defect is the single most important etiologic clue.

Traditional Evaluation

Although symptomatologic history, physical examination, and laboratory evaluation are obviously recommended in a case of pneumonia in the immunocompromised host, these procedures usually yield nonspecific information. Dyspnea and cough are the most common complaints in patients with symptoms caused by pulmonary infiltrates. Most patients with pulmonary infections, even in the presence of neutropenia, manifest a fever; however, fever is by no means a reliable sign of infection. Many noninfectious processes elicit fever as part of the inflammatory response, including radiation pneumonitis, cytotoxic drug–induced lung disease, and nonspecific interstitial pneumonitis. Furthermore, fever may be caused by the underlying neoplasm (particularly Hodgkin's disease and some non-Hodgkin's lymphomas) or by occult infection unrelated to the pulmonary process. The absence of fever, however, lessens the chance of an infectious pneumonia.

The time of onset as well as the tempo of illness may also focus the differential diagnosis. CMV pneumonia occurs 1 to 6 months after renal transplantation but is uncommon before or after this period.[12, 13] Among the noninfectious pulmonary diseases, certain entities also have a predictable time for their radiographic appearance. Radiation pneumonitis typically develops approximately 8 weeks after completion of a course of radiation therapy and roughly 1 week earlier for every 1000 rad above a total dose of 4000 rad.[14] Radiation pneumonitis is generally not seen within the first month after irradiation, except in reirradiated lung.[14] Certain cytotoxic and other chemotherapeutic drugs are clearly associated with febrile lung reactions,[15, 16] and a careful history of drug exposure may offer important etiologic clues. Bleomycin is particularly a problem. Bleomycin-induced interstitial pneumonitis is in large part dose related. Life-threatening lung damage appears only after cumulative doses greater than 150 mg[17]; however, toxic reactions to the drug have been observed at lower doses, especially when it is used as part of combination chemotherapy programs.[18] Thus, no minimal dose completely excludes the diagnosis of bleomycin lung injury.[19] Leukoagglutinin reaction is a sudden diffuse vascular endothelial injury that appears to result from the interaction of antibodies in transfused blood products with the recipient's white blood cells. A pattern of pulmonary edema develops within minutes to hours of transfusion.[20]

Another important historical observation is the tempo of

TABLE 54–1 ■ Infectious Causes of Pneumonia in Immunocompromised Patients

ETIOLOGY	USUAL UNDERLYING CONDITIONS	USUAL DIAGNOSTIC METHODS	TREATMENT
Bacteria			
Gram-negative bacilli (e.g., *Klebsiella, Escherichia coli, Pseudomonas*)	Hematologic neoplasia with neutropenia	Blood culture, sputum culture, empirical ("response" to antibiotics)	Cephalosporins or ticarcillin, plus an aminoglycoside
Staphylococcus	Hematologic neoplasia	Same	Semisynthetic penicillin or cephalosporins
Pneumococcus	Transplants (especially bone marrow) and splenectomy	Sputum or blood culture	Penicillin
Nocardia	Transplants, lymphoma, AIDS*	Invasive procedures (rarely, sputum examination)	Sulfonamides or co-trimoxazole
Legionella	Transplants, corticosteroid therapy, lymphoma, AIDS	Indirect fluorescent antibody titer, direct fluorescent antibody preparation, charcoal–yeast extract media culture	Erythromycin alone or with rifampin
Mycobacterium tuberculosis	Transplants, AIDS	Sputum culture, lung biopsy	Isoniazid, rifampin, ethambutol
Mycobacterium avium-intracellulare complex	AIDS	Sputum or blood culture, lung biopsy	Rifabutin, clofazimine, clarithromycin; ± amikacin
Fungi			
Aspergillus, Phycomycetes	Neutropenia, transplants	Lung aspirate or biopsy	Amphotericin B; ± itraconazole
Cryptococcus	Transplants, lymphoma, AIDS	Lung aspirate or biopsy, cerebrospinal fluid examination, serum latex agglutination test	Amphotericin B plus flucytosine; or fluconazole
Parasites			
Pneumocystis carinii	Transplants, corticosteroid therapy, AIDS	Lung biopsy or aspirate	Co-trimoxazole or pentamidine
Toxoplasma gondii	Transplants	Lung biopsy, serology	Pyrimethamine plus sulfadiazine
Strongyloides	High-dose corticosteroids	Sputum and stool examination or duodenal aspirates	Thiabendazole
Viruses			
Cytomegalovirus	Transplants, lymphoma, AIDS	Lung biopsy, serology, and culture	Ganciclovir plus intravenous immunoglobulin (investigational)
Varicella-zoster virus	Hodgkin's disease, renal and bone marrow transplant	Clinical appearance, lesion cultures	Acyclovir
Herpes simplex	Bone marrow transplant	Lung biopsy and culture	Acyclovir
Human herpesvirus 6	Bone marrow transplant	Lung biopsy, polymerase chain reaction	Uncertain
Parainfluenza virus	Bone marrow transplant	Lung aspirates, cultures	Uncertain

*AIDS, Acquired immunodeficiency syndrome.
Modified from Fanta CH, Pennington JE: Oxford Textbook of Medicine, ed 2. Oxford, UK, Oxford Medical Publications, 1987.

disease (Table 54–5). Pulmonary infections in immunocompromised patients can be differentiated according to their rate of progression.[13] The acute, often fulminant, onset of *Pneumocystis* pneumonia is notorious; the disease may progress from mild breathlessness and a minimally abnormal

TABLE 54–2 ■ Noninfectious Causes of Fever and Pulmonary Infiltrates in Immunocompromised Patients

Tumor	Drug reactions
Radiation pneumonitis	Bleomycin
Pulmonary hemorrhage	Cyclophosphamide
Pulmonary infarction	Busulfan (after long periods of treatment)
Leukoagglutinin reaction	
Nonspecific interstitial pneumonitis	Methotrexate
Leukemic cell lysis	Carmustine
Pulmonary edema	Lomustine
Leukostasis	Mitomycin
	Chlorambucil
	Melphalan
	Procarbazine

Modified from Fanta CH, Pennington JE: Oxford Textbook of Medicine, ed 2. Oxford, UK, Oxford Medical Publications, 1987.

TABLE 54–3 ■ Association Between Immune Defect and Causes of Pneumonia

IMMUNE DEFECT	USUAL CAUSES
Granulocytopenia	Gram-negative rods (e.g., *Escherichia coli, Klebsiella, Pseudomonas*) *Staphylococcus aureus* *Aspergillus* spp. *Mucor* spp.
Cell-mediated immune deficiency	Herpes group viral agent (e.g., CMV) *Pneumocystis carinii* *Nocardia* spp. *Cryptococcus* spp. *Legionella* spp. *Mycobacterium* spp. *Aspergillus* spp.
Hypogammaglobulinemia or splenectomy	*Pneumococcus* spp. *Haemophilus influenzae*

Modified from Fanta CH, Pennington JE: Oxford Textbook of Medicine, ed 2. Oxford, UK, Oxford Medical Publications, 1987.

TABLE 54–4 ■ Radiographic Patterns of Pulmonary Infiltrates in Immunocompromised Patients

DIFFUSE	NODULAR OR CAVITARY	FOCAL
	Common	
Pneumocystis spp. CMV Pulmonary edema Nonspecific interstitial pneumonitis Drug induced Lymphangitic carcinomatosis	*Cryptococcus* spp. *Nocardia* spp. Bacterial lung abscess Neoplastic *Aspergillus* spp.	Bacteria, including *Nocardia* spp. *Cryptococcus* spp. *Aspergillus* spp. *Mucor* spp. Nonspecific interstitial pneumonitis
	Uncommon	
Cryptococcus spp. *Aspergillus* spp. *Candida* spp. Hemorrhage Leukemic involvement	*Legionella* spp. Septic emboli	Tuberculosis Viral *Legionella* spp.

Modified from Fanta CH, Pennington JE: Respiratory Infections: Diagnosis and Management, ed 2. New York, Raven Press, 1989.

chest radiograph to overwhelming dyspnea, hypoxemia, and diffuse pulmonary infiltrates within a few days. An indolent form of *Pneumocystis* pneumonia, with symptoms extending for many days to weeks, appears to be unique to patients with acquired immunodeficiency syndrome.[21] Bacterial infections (including Legionnaires' disease), particularly in the neutropenic host, can also spread to multilobe involvement within days. Although CMV pneumonia may have an explosive onset as well, it more often evolves in 1 to 2 weeks, a tempo similar to that for *Aspergillus* or *Mucor* pneumonia. Nocardiosis, tuberculosis, and the more slowly growing fungal infections (e.g., cryptococcosis) usually follow a more insidious course. Their development during several weeks or more may mimic noninfectious pulmonary processes, such as growth of metastatic malignant neoplasms, drug-induced lung injury, or the appearance of radiation fibrosis.

Finally, a careful review of fluid balance is important in the immunocompromised patient with diffuse pulmonary infiltrates. Large-volume loads are often given in conjunction with certain chemotherapeutic agents or for resuscitation of the hypotensive, septic patient. Impaired renal function, atherosclerotic heart disease, cardiotoxic effects of doxorubicin, or other poorly defined factors may impair the ability to compensate for large infusions of fluids, with the resultant development of pulmonary edema. Early interstitial-phase pulmonary edema may resemble interstitial inflammatory processes such as mycoplasmal or viral pneumonia, cytotoxic drug–induced lung disease, or nonspecific idiopathic interstitial pneumonitis. The late alveolar filling phase of pulmonary edema may be difficult to differentiate radiographically from *Pneumocystis* or CMV pneumonia.

Physical examination of the immunocompromised patient with pneumonia may be frustratingly unrevealing. Even in the face of life-threatening dyspnea and hypoxemia, with widespread infiltrates on the chest radiograph, auscultation of the lungs may be normal or reveal only minimal end-inspiratory rales.[22] Particularly in neutropenic patients, with their impaired inflammatory response to infection, the usual physical findings in chest infection may be lacking. Chest examination may offer some useful information, however. For example, rales may become audible even before infiltrates appear radiographically and may be the first clue to an infiltrative lung process. Also, when the chest radiograph shows an early unilateral infiltrate, examination may reveal the presence of bilateral disease, altering diagnostic considerations. A pleural friction rub may be the only sign of active pleural inflammation. Its presence along with a rapidly progressing pulmonary infiltrate suggests a virulent bacterial or fungal (usually *Aspergillus*) infection, whereas a pleural friction rub is strong evidence against a *Pneumocystis* organism as the sole etiologic agent. Finally, and perhaps most important, physical examination is often superior to chest radiography in suggesting the overall severity of the illness. Respiratory rate alone may provide critical information about the extent of physiologic derangement, thereby directing the rapidity and course of the diagnostic evaluation. In the patient with diffuse, bilateral pulmonary infiltrates, physical examination may be the best test for the presence of congestive heart failure. Detection of a laterally displaced cardiac impulse, jugular venous distention, and early diastolic gallop has spared more than one patient an unnecessary lung biopsy for pulmonary edema.

Traditional diagnostic laboratory procedures for pneumonia in the immunocompromised host are frequently unhelpful. In one prospectively studied group of 80 immunocompromised patients with diffuse pulmonary infiltrates, a specific etiologic diagnosis was made by blood and sputum cultures in only 4 patients and by serologic methods in another 4 (total of 10%).[23] In fact, sputum is often not available for examination, especially in neutropenic patients. Skin testing is of little or no value in the diagnosis of acute infections in the immunocompromised host. This includes skin tests

TABLE 54–5 ■ Tempo of Pulmonary Infections in Immunocompromised Patients

RAPID	SUBACUTE	INSIDIOUS
Pneumocystis carinii Bacterial (especially gram-negative, *Staphylococcus aureus, Legionella* spp.) CMV	CMV *Aspergillus/Mucor* spp. *Cryptococcus* spp.	*Nocardia* spp. *Cryptococcus* spp. *Mycobacterium tuberculosis* *Pneumocystis carinii**

*In patients with acquired immunodeficiency syndrome.
Modified from Fanta CH, Pennington JE: Respiratory Infections: Diagnosis and Management, ed 2. New York, Raven Press, 1989.

that under other circumstances may provide valuable information about the presence of disease, such as the *Aspergillus* skin test in allergic bronchopulmonary aspergillosis. Even patients with active tuberculosis are generally nonreactive to standardized purified protein derivative antigen when they are undergoing immunosuppressive chemotherapy.

Serologic tests may prove of value in certain limited clinical situations. In renal, bone marrow, or cardiac transplant recipients in whom diffuse interstitial pulmonary infiltrates develop, fourfold elevation in enzyme-linked immunosorbent assay or complement fixation titer against CMV above pretransplant levels would suggest a diagnosis of CMV pneumonia.[24] CMV pneumonia may occur, however, in the absence of seroconversion, a situation with a particularly poor prognosis.[24] Circulating cryptococcal antigen, detectable in serum by a latex agglutination test, has been reported in some cases of diffuse cryptococcal pneumonia.[25] Although highly specific (in the absence of latex fixation–positive rheumatoid arthritis), its sensitivity is low. Indirect fluorescent antibody tests are available for diagnosis of Legionnaires' disease, but they require acute and convalescent blood samples and testing for antibodies against multiple serotypes. Research continues on serologic tests to distinguish invasive from noninvasive fungal infections. Immunodiffusion and counterimmunoelectrophoresis techniques have been applied in *Aspergillus* infection.[26] Gas-liquid chromatography and other techniques have been used to detect invasive candidiasis.[27] As yet, none of these serologic tests appears entirely reliable, nor are the tests widely available. Finally, the role of polymerase chain reaction methodology in diagnosis of lung infection remains speculative. One report, however, suggested that occult viral infections might be diagnosed with use of this method.[28]

Special staining and culture procedures should be employed if a high-quality sputum specimen is obtained. For example, methenamine–silver nitrate or toluidine blue O stains of air-dried sputum smears may reveal the cyst walls of *Pneumocystis* organisms, especially when specimens of sputum have been induced with the inhalation of hypertonic saline by ultrasonic nebulization. Table 54–6 reviews the recommended staining and culture methods for evaluation of high-quality sputum specimens as well as for work-up of materials obtained by invasive diagnostic methods.

Invasive Diagnostic Methods

There is no question that diagnostic accuracy in the immunocompromised host with pneumonia is improved when invasive diagnostic methods are used.[8, 11, 29, 30] The major question is whether the usefulness of the information obtained warrants the risk and expense of thoracotomy or bronchoscopy.[31] It is clear that management is improved by invasive procedures in certain instances,[29] whereas benefit is not clear in other instances.[32, 33] A number of retrospective studies have analyzed the effect of lung biopsy by comparing the outcome of patients who had a specific diagnosis established by lung biopsy with the outcome of patients who had a nonspecific result.[34–36] In general, patients who had a specific diagnosis after lung biopsy had no better chance of survival than did patients with nonspecific findings. This is not the same as saying that survival is not improved by making a specific diagnosis, however. Until clear-cut prospective studies indicate that the risk/benefit ratio of invasive diagnostic procedures cannot be shown, we believe that lung sampling procedures are indicated whenever there is a reasonable possibility of establishing a treatable diagnosis for which empirical therapy cannot safely be given. The risks of multidrug empirical (and potentially inappropriate) therapy must be weighed against the morbidity and mortality of the lung sampling procedure. Fortunately, for bronchoalveolar lavage with or without transbronchial lung biopsy,[13, 37] as well as for open lung biopsy,[8] the morbidity and mortality are low.

A variety of invasive methods have been employed in immunocompromised hosts to obtain lung tissue or lung washings for diagnostic purposes. Table 54–7 lists those procedures offering the highest yield. The choice of initial procedure for a given patient will be dictated by the type of infiltrate, the tempo of disease, and the local expertise. In more slowly moving illness, less invasive procedures (e.g., bronchoalveolar lavage) may be attempted before the greater yielding but more invasive procedure of open lung biopsy. In a critically ill patient, however, open lung biopsy may be

TABLE 54–6 ■ Staining and Cultivation Techniques Recommended for Sputum Specimens and Specimens Obtained by Invasive Techniques

	STAINING TECHNIQUES*		CULTURE TECHNIQUES	
POTENTIAL ETIOLOGIC AGENT	**Fresh Material**	**Fixed Tissue**	**Medium**	**Period of Incubation (Time to Preliminary Identification)**
Legionella spp.	Direct immunofluorescent antibody	Dieterle, acid-fast (*L. micdadei*)	Charcoal–yeast extract	3–5 d, sometimes up to 10 d
Nocardia spp.	Modified acid-fast, Gram	Modified acid-fast, Gram	Sabouraud	Minimum of 5 d, up to 4 wk
Cryptococcus spp.	India ink	H&E, PAS, MSS, mucicarmine	Sabouraud	4–7 d, occasionally up to 4–6 wk
Aspergillus spp.	Potassium hydroxide	H&E, PAS, MSS	Blood agar, Sabouraud	1–2 wk
Mucor spp. (Phycomycetes)	Potassium hydroxide	H&E, MSS	Sabouraud	1–2 wk
Mycobacterium spp.	Acid-fast (Ziehl-Neelson, Kinyoun)	Acid-fast stains	Löwenstein-Jensen	Up to 4–6 wk
Pneumocystis	MSS, toluidine blue	MSS	—	—
CMV	Tzanck preparation, in situ DNA hybridization, immunofluorescence (monoclonal antibodies)	H&E, in situ DNA hybridization	Cell culture (fibroblasts)	2–10 d when inoculum high, up to 6 wk Shell vial method, 1–3 d

*H&E, Hematoxylin and eosin; MSS, methenamine silver stain; PAS, periodic acid–Schiff.
Modified from Fanta CH, Pennington JE: Oxford Textbook of Medicine, ed 2. Oxford, UK, Oxford Medical Publications, 1987.

TABLE 54–7 ■ Invasive Diagnostic Techniques for Immunocompromised Patients with Pneumonia

PROCEDURE	SPECIMENS PROVIDED	YIELD	COMPLICATIONS	COMMENTS
Percutaneous needle aspiration	Fluid aspirate Sometimes a small core of tissue	For localized pulmonary infections = 70%–80%	Pneumothorax requiring evacuation (10%) Hemoptysis (2%–5%) Empyema (rare)	Particularly useful for peripheral nodules or cavitary infiltrates
Fiberoptic bronchoscopy	Bronchial washings, bronchial brushings, transbronchial lung biopsy (approximately 1.0–1.5 mm in diameter) Bronchoalveolar lavage	Overall yield = 40%–50% In certain infections (e.g., *Pneumocystis*), yield exceeds 90%	Hemoptysis (5%) Pneumothorax requiring evacuation (5%)	Particularly useful for focal or diffuse infiltrates suspected of being infectious in etiology
Open lung biopsy	Lung tissue (approximately 2–4 cm in size)	Approximately 90%	Delayed pneumothorax Wound complication Prolonged ventilator dependence	Necessary to establish diagnosis based on histopathology, such as radiation pneumonitis, drug-induced lung disease, or nonspecific interstitial pneumonitis

Modified from Fanta CH, Pennington JE: Oxford Textbook of Medicine, ed 2. Oxford, UK, Oxford Medical Publications, 1987.

selected immediately because the chance of a false-negative result with open lung biopsy is the lowest among all invasive procedures (i.e., 5% to 10%).[30] The major drawbacks of the open biopsy procedure are the requirement for general anesthesia, the pain of the operative incision, and occasional surgical complications, particularly delayed pneumothorax and prolonged need for assisted ventilation. Despite the grave medical condition of many of the patients who undergo surgery, however, overall surgical mortality from open lung biopsy is less than 5%.[8, 38, 39] At least in one series, the results of open biopsy led to a change in therapy in as many as one half of the patients.[38] Nevertheless, these considerations have led to a search for simpler, less invasive means of sampling lung tissue. A number of techniques have evolved, including percutaneous needle aspiration and biopsy,[40] fluoroscopically guided bronchial brushing,[41] thorascopic lung biopsy,[42] and transbronchial lung biopsy and bronchoalveolar lavage through the fiberoptic bronchoscope.[13, 37, 43–45]

The introduction of a relatively simple diagnostic technique, bronchoalveolar lavage performed through the fiberoptic bronchoscope, has had a major impact on the evaluation of infiltrates in immunocompromised hosts. The procedure involves wedging the tip of the bronchoscope into a subsegmental bronchial lumen and then instilling approximately 100 to 150 mL of normal saline into the lung in 20- to 50-mL aliquots and aspirating the lavage fluid after each aliquot. Usually, approximately half of the instilled volume is retrieved. The procedure can be completed easily within 10 to 15 minutes. It can be safely performed in patients who are intubated and receiving positive-pressure ventilation without risk of pneumothorax and bronchopleural fistula. Likewise, the risk of hemorrhage is far less than with biopsy techniques.

Extensive experience with bronchoalveolar lavage has been obtained in patients with acquired immunodeficiency syndrome, in whom the sensitivity of the technique for diagnosing *Pneumocystis* pneumonia exceeds 90%. Fewer reports have described the results of bronchoalveolar lavage in the diagnosis of pulmonary infiltrates in patients with other immunocompromising illnesses. Stover and colleagues[45] reported making a specific diagnosis by analysis of bronchoalveolar lavage fluid alone in 66% of 97 patients with diffuse pulmonary infiltrates and a variety of causes for immunosuppression. Thirty-eight of 46 opportunistic infections (83%) were correctly diagnosed by examination and culture of the lavage fluid. Other studies have documented the utility of bronchoalveolar lavage among recipients of bone marrow[44] and renal[46] transplants. In one report, 100 immunosuppressed patients with various underlying diseases and with suspected lung infection were evaluated by bronchoalveolar lavage.[37] Infectious etiologic agents were found in 30 patients. Follow-up open lung biopsy was carried out in 23 patients with negative lavage result, and a specific etiologic agent was found in 11. In another report, a review of bronchoalveolar lavage in 327 immunosuppressed patients yielded specific diagnoses in 55% and false-negative results in 22% of procedures.[30] Thus, the false-negative rate for bronchoalveolar lavage in certain categories of immunocompromised patients may be high.

New methods for rapid identification of pathogens in the lavage fluid are being explored to improve sensitivity. These include nucleic acid probes for in situ hybridization, used to detect CMV, *Legionella* spp.,[47, 48] and monoclonal antibodies to early antigens expressed by CMV in cell culture.[49] Also, shell vial cultures for CMV offer more rapid cultural identification.[50] In one report, specific cultures for parainfluenza virus revealed a surprising diagnostic yield among bone marrow transplant patients.[51] Complications of bronchoalveolar lavage are few; the most common complication is arterial oxygen desaturation, which can be effectively monitored by means of oximetry. Because of the sensitivity and safety of the procedure, fiberoptic bronchoscopy with bronchoalveolar lavage is probably the initial procedure of choice for patients with diffuse infiltrates in whom infection is likely.

Management Scheme

Figure 54–1 provides an overview for management of the immunocompromised patient with new fever and lung infiltrate. Not illustrated on this scheme, however, is the critical issue of the underlying host defect. For example, if the patient has a focal infiltrate and cell-mediated immunodeficiency, earlier use of erythromycin (i.e., for *Legionella* spp. coverage) may be considered. The cardinal rule of management, however, must be that virtually any etiologic agent can occasionally cause any radiographic pattern. Thus, an empirical approach is always based on "clinical odds" rather than certainty of judgment.

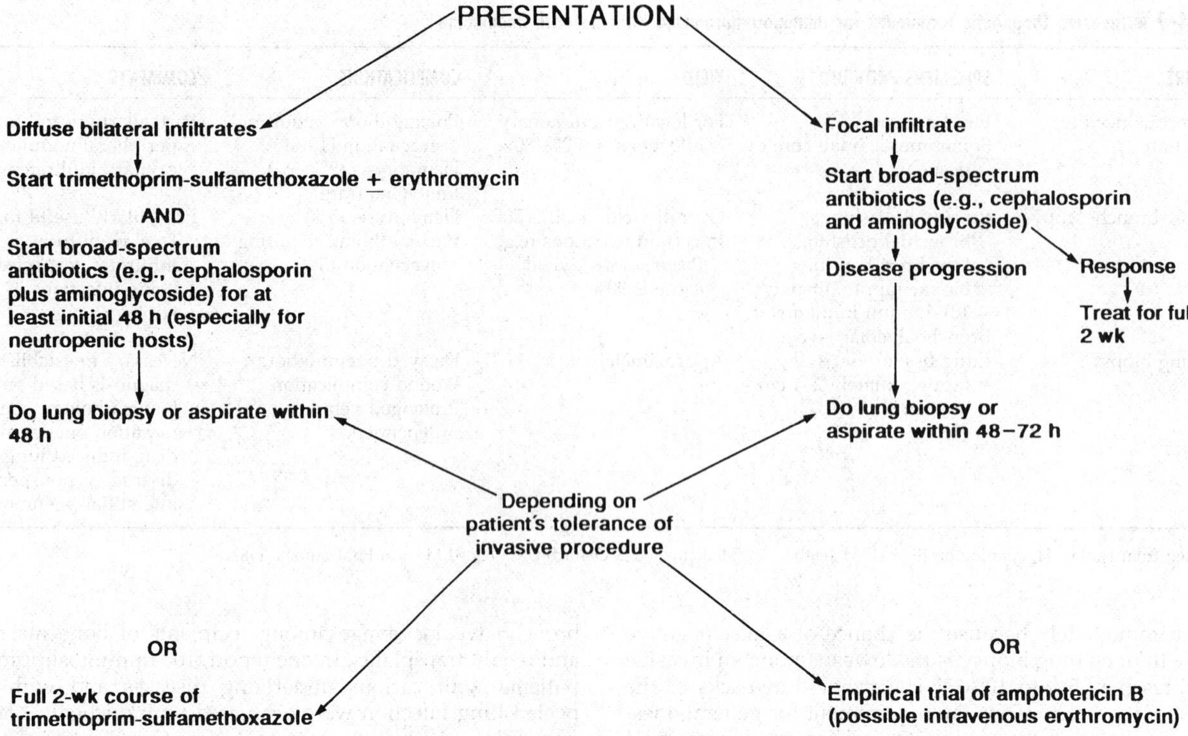
PRESENTATION
Diffuse bilateral infiltrates
Start trimethoprim-sulfamethoxazole ± erythromycin
AND
Start broad-spectrum antibiotics (e.g., cephalosporin plus aminoglycoside) for at least initial 48 h (especially for neutropenic hosts)
Do lung biopsy or aspirate within 48 h
Focal infiltrate
Start broad-spectrum antibiotics (e.g., cephalosporin and aminoglycoside)
Disease progression
Response
Treat for full 2 wk
Do lung biopsy or aspirate within 48–72 h
Depending on patient's tolerance of invasive procedure
OR
Full 2-wk course of trimethoprim-sulfamethoxazole
OR
Empirical trial of amphotericin B (possible intravenous erythromycin)

FIGURE 54–1 □ Management schema for fever and pulmonary infiltrates in the immunocompromised host. (Modified from Fanta CH, Pennington JE: Respiratory Infections: Diagnosis and Management, ed 2. New York, Raven Press, 1989.)

References

1. Bishop JF, Schimpff SC, Diggs CH, Wiernik PH: Infections during intensive chemotherapy for non-Hodgkin's lymphoma. Ann Intern Med 95:549, 1981.
2. Sickles EA, Young VM, Greene WH, Wiernik PH: Pneumonia in acute leukemia. Ann Intern Med 79:528, 1973.
3. Winston DJ, Gale RP, Meyer DV, Young LS: UCLA bone marrow transplantation group: Infectious complications of human bone marrow transplantation. Medicine (Baltimore) 58:1, 1979.
4. Crawford SW, Hackman RC: Clinical course of idiopathic pneumonia after bone marrow transplantation. Am Rev Respir Dis 147:1393, 1993.
5. Murray JF, Felton CP, Garay SM, et al: Pulmonary complications of the acquired immunodeficiency syndrome. N Engl J Med 310:1682, 1984.
6. Ramsey PG, Rubin RH, Tolkoff-Rubin NE, et al: The renal transplant patient with fever and pulmonary infiltrates: Etiology, clinical manifestations, and management. Medicine (Baltimore) 59:206, 1980.
7. Masur H, Cheigh JS, Stubenbord WT: Infection following renal transplantation: A changing pattern. Rev Infect Dis 4:1208, 1982.
8. Cockerill FR III, Wilson WR, Carpenter HA, et al: Open lung biopsy in immunocompromised patients. Arch Intern Med 145:1398, 1985.
9. Emanuel D, Cunningham I, Jules-Elysee K, et al: Cytomegalovirus pneumonia after bone marrow transplantation successfully treated with the combination of ganciclovir and high-dose intravenous immune globulin. Ann Intern Med 109:777, 1988.
10. Reed EC, Bowden RA, Dandliker PS, et al: Treatment of cytomegalovirus pneumonia with ganciclovir and intravenous cytomegalovirus immunoglobulin in patients with bone marrow transplants. Ann Intern Med 109:783, 1988.
11. Pennington JE, Feldman NT: Pulmonary infiltrates and fever in patients with hematologic malignancy: Assessment of transbronchial biopsy. Am J Med 62:581, 1977.
12. Fanta CH, Pennington JE: Pulmonary infections in the transplant patient. *In* Morris PJ, Tilney NL (eds): Progress in Transplantation, Vol 2. New York, Churchill Livingstone, 1985, pp 207–230.
13. Rubin RJ, Wolfson JS, Cosimi AB, Tolkoff-Rubin NE: Infection in the renal transplant recipient. Am J Med 70:405, 1981.
14. Gross NJ: Pulmonary effects of radiation therapy. Ann Intern Med 86:81, 1977.
15. Cooper JAD Jr, White DA, Matthay RA: Drug-induced pulmonary disease. Am Rev Respir Dis 133:321, 1986.
16. Rosenow EC: The spectrum of drug-induced pulmonary disease. Ann Intern Med 77:977, 1972.
17. Sostman HD, Matthay RA, Putman CE: Cytotoxic drug–induced lung disease. Am J Med 62:608, 1977.
18. Bauer KA, Skarin AT, Balikian JP, et al: Pulmonary complications associated with combination chemotherapy programs containing bleomycin. Am J Med 74:557, 1983.
19. Richman SD, Levensohn SM, Bunn PA, et al: Ga^{67} accumulation in pulmonary lesions associated with bleomycin toxicity. Cancer 36:1966, 1975.
20. Ward HN: Pulmonary infiltrates associated with leukoagglutinin transfusion reaction. Ann Intern Med 73:689, 1970.
21. Kovacs JA, Hiemenz JW, Macher AM, et al: *Pneumocystis carinii* pneumonia: A comparison between patients with the acquired immunodeficiency syndrome and patients with other immunodeficiencies. Ann Intern Med 100:663, 1984.
22. Hughes WT, Sanyal SK, Price RA: Signs, symptoms, and pathophysiology of *Pneumocystis carinii* pneumonitis. Natl Cancer Inst Monogr 43:77, 1976.
23. Singer C, Armstrong D, Rosen PP, et al: Diffuse pulmonary infiltrates in immunosuppressed patients: Prospective study of 80 cases. Am J Med 66:110, 1979.
24. Neiman PE, Reeves W, Ray G, et al: A prospective analysis of interstitial pneumonia and opportunistic viral infection among recipients of allogeneic bone marrow grafts. J Infect Dis 136:754, 1977.
25. Fisher BD, Armstrong D: Cryptococcal interstitial pneumonia: Value of antigen determination. N Engl J Med 297:1440, 1977.
26. Ma P: The microbiology laboratory in diagnosis and therapy. *In* Grieco MH (ed): Infections in the Abnormal Host. New York, Yorke Medical Books, 1980, pp 797–847.
27. Kiehn TE, Bernard EM, Gold JWM, Armstrong D: Candidiasis: Detection by gas-liquid chromatography of *d*-arabinitol, a fungal metabolite, in human serum. Science 206:577, 1979.
28. Cone RW, Hackman RC, Huang M-LW, et al: Human herpesvirus 6 in lung tissue from patients with pneumonitis after bone marrow transplantation. N Engl J Med 329:156, 1993.

29. Catterall JR, McCabe RE, Brooks RG, Remington JS: Open lung biopsy in patients with Hodgkin's disease and pulmonary infiltrates. Am Rev Respir Dis 139:1274, 1989.
30. Shelhamer JH, Toews GB, Masur H, et al: Respiratory disease in the immunosuppressed patient. Ann Intern Med 117:415, 1992.
31. Robin ED, Burke CM: Lung biopsy in immunosuppressed patients. Chest 89:276, 1986.
32. McCabe RE, Brooks RG, Mark JBD, Remington JS: Open lung biopsy in patients with acute leukemia. Am J Med 78:609, 1985.
33. Potter D, Pass HI, Brower S, et al: Prospective randomized study of open lung biopsy versus empirical antibiotic therapy for acute pneumonitis in nonneutropenic cancer patients. Ann Thorac Surg 40:422, 1985.
34. Haverkos HW, Dowling JN, Pasculle AW, et al: Diagnosis of pneumonitis in immunocompromised patients by open lung biopsy. Cancer 52:1093, 1983.
35. Puksa S, Hutcheon MA, Hyland RH: Usefulness of transbronchial biopsy in immunosuppressed patients with pulmonary infiltrates. Thorax 38:146, 1983.
36. Williams D, Yungbluth M, Adams G, Glassroth J: The role of fiberoptic bronchoscopy in the evaluation of immunocompromised hosts with diffuse pulmonary infiltrates. Am Rev Respir Dis 131:880, 1985.
37. Martin WJ II, Smith TF, Brutinel WM, et al: Role of bronchoalveolar lavage in the assessment of opportunistic pulmonary infections: Utility and complications. Mayo Clin Proc 62:549, 1987.
38. Rossiter SJ, Miller DC, Churg AM, et al: Open lung biopsy in the immunosuppressed patient: Is it really beneficial? J Thorac Cardiovasc Surg 77:338, 1979.
39. Toledo-Pereyna LH, DeMeester TR, Kinealey A, et al: The benefits of open lung biopsy in patients with previous non-diagnostic transbronchial lung biopsy: Guide to appropriate therapy. Chest 77:647, 1980.
40. Bandt PD, Blank N, Castellino RA: Needle diagnosis of pneumonitis: Value in high-risk patients. JAMA 220:1578, 1972.
41. Finley R, Kieff E, Thomsen S, et al: Bronchial brushing in the diagnosis of pulmonary disease in patients at risk for opportunistic infection. Am Rev Respir Dis 109:379, 1974.
42. Dijkman JH, van der Meer JWM, Bakker W, et al: Transpleural lung biopsy by the thorascopic route in patients with diffuse interstitial pulmonary disease. Chest 82:76, 1982.
43. Feldman NT, Pennington JE, Ehrie MG: Transbronchial lung biopsy in the compromised host. JAMA 238:1377, 1977.
44. Springmeyer SC, Hackman RC, Holle R, et al: Use of bronchoalveolar lavage to diagnose acute diffuse pneumonia in the immunocompromised host. J Infect Dis 154:604, 1986.
45. Stover DE, Zaman MB, Hajdu SI, et al: Bronchoalveolar lavage in the diagnosis of diffuse pulmonary infiltrates in the immunosuppressed host. Ann Intern Med 101:1, 1984.
46. Hopkin JM, Turney JH, Young JA, et al: Rapid diagnosis of obscure pneumonia in immunosuppressed renal patients by cytology of alveolar lavage fluid. Lancet 2:299, 1983.
47. Edelstein PH, Bryan RN, Enns RK, et al: Retrospective study of Gen-Probe rapid diagnostic system for detection of legionellae in frozen clinical respiratory tract samples. J Clin Microbiol 25:1022, 1987.
48. Myerson D, Hackman RC, Meyers JD: Diagnosis of cytomegaloviral pneumonia by in situ hybridization. J Infect Dis 150:272, 1984.
49. Crawford SW, Bowden RA, Hackman RC, et al: Rapid detection of cytomegalovirus pulmonary infection by bronchoalveolar lavage and centrifugation culture. Ann Intern Med 108:180, 1988.
50. Martin WJ II, Smith TF: Rapid detection of cytomegalovirus in bronchoalveolar lavage specimens by a monoclonal antibody method. J Clin Microbiol 23:1006, 1986.
51. Wendt CH, Weisdorf DJ, Jordan MC, et al: Parainfluenza virus respiratory infection after bone marrow transplantation. N Engl J Med 326:921, 1992.

55

Bacterial Pneumonia

John G. Bartlett

Lower respiratory tract infections are the major cause of death due to infectious diseases in the world. Current estimates are 395,000,000 infections annually with 4,400,000 deaths accounting for approximately 8% of all deaths. In the United States, the death rate per 100,000 population was 30 in 1992, and this represented a 20% increase from 1980.[1] The most common identifiable cause of pneumonia is bacterial infection. This chapter reviews bacterial pneumonia by microbe for the most frequently implicated bacterial agents. Other related topics discussed elsewhere include the approach to the patient with pneumonia (Chapter 53), pneumonia in immunocompromised hosts (Chapter 54), viral pneumonia (Chapter 57), *Mycoplasma* pneumonia (Chapter 58), aspiration pneumonia (Chapter 63), Legionnaires' disease (Chapter 61), *Chlamydia* pneumonia (Chapter 62), *Streptococcus pneumoniae* (Chapter 193), *Haemophilus influenzae* (Chapter 212), *Branhamella* (Chapter 203), and pulmonary infections in patients with human immunodeficiency virus (HIV) infection (Chapter 122).

History

S. pneumoniae plays a prominent role in the history of microbiology and pneumonia. It was originally described in 1881 by Pasteur in France and Sternberg in the United States, and both showed its pathogenic potential by injection of saliva into rabbits.[2] The organism was subsequently referred to as pneumococcus in 1886, reflecting its role in pulmonary infections,[3] and was named *Diplococcus pneumoniae* in 1920 in reference to the Gram stain appearance[4]; it was renamed as a *Streptococcus* in 1974.[5] The organism was one of the first to be described in the development of the Gram stain in 1884.[6] Capsular serotypes and the role of type-specific antibody in opsonization were reported at the turn of the century by Neufeld and Haendel.[7] The prominent role of *S. pneumoniae* in pulmonary infection was recognized by Frankel in 1884.[8] A classic description of pneumococcal pneumonia in these early reviews was provided by Lord[9]:

> *Pneumonia due to the pneumococcus differs from pulmonary infection with other organisms in that it has an explosive onset, usual massive lung involvement, short course, abrupt termination and relatively rapid restoration of the involved area to normal.*

Serotherapy with type-specific antisera from sensitized horses became a popular method of treatment in the 1930s[10]; this prompted a period in history when microbiology studies were at their finest, reflecting that treatment required retrieval of the pathogen to permit serotyping. The role of penicillin therapy was reported in 1941,[11] and dramatic results in 500 cases were reported by Keefer and coworkers[12] in 1943.

Pneumococcal Pneumonia

Frequency

S. pneumoniae is the major identifiable cause of pneumonia in virtually all studies of community-acquired pneumonia in patients who require hospitalization. In the prepenicillin era, this organism accounted for approximately 80% of all pneumonias and 96% of lobar pneumonias.[13] During the ensuing decades, there has been a gradual decline in the frequency of recovery of *S. pneumoniae* so that most studies in the 1990s show a yield of only 10% to 20%.[14, 15] This decline is ascribed to multiple factors including the impact of antecedent antibiotic treatment on recovery in respiratory secretions, failure to produce sputum, recognition of alternative agents of pneumonia, and sloppy microbiology. A metaanalysis of 122 reports in the English literature of community-acquired pneumonia from 1966 through 1995 showed that approximately 6000 had a bacterial pathogen defined; *S. pneumoniae* accounted for 73% of all cases in this category and also accounted for 66% of those with a lethal outcome[14] (Table 55–1). The estimated annual rate of pneumococcal pneumonia is 1 to 10 per 1000 in the United States, with an annual total of about 500,000.[16–18]

Microbiology

S. pneumoniae is a gram-positive coccus that usually appears in pairs with tapered ends referred to as lancet shaped. It is relatively fastidious and easily overgrown by other bacteria or overlooked because of confusion with other α-hemolytic streptococci. Identification is by susceptibility to ethylhydrocupreine hydrochloride (Optochin). Pathogenicity is related to the polysaccharide capsule with at least 84 identified serotypes. The capsular polysaccharide may be used for detection in the Quellung reaction or by antigen detection with use of blood, urine, or respiratory secretions. Most laboratories rely on conventional Gram stain and culture. The individual serotypes show differences in frequency, pathogenicity, and susceptibility to penicillin.[19] The major use of serotyping is for epidemiologic investigation and for implementing strategies for disease control with pneumococcal vaccine, which contains polysaccharides of the 23 serotypes that account for 89% of invasive infections caused by *S. pneumoniae.*

Pathogenesis

The usual mechanism of pneumonia is by aspiration of *S. pneumoniae* that is harbored in the nasopharynx. Colonization rates are highly variable but usually reported at 5% to 30% among healthy adults.[20] Antibody is type specific and appears to play an important role in susceptibility to infection but does not prevent colonization. Virtually all patients are susceptible, and *S. pneumoniae* is clearly the most common pathogen in previously healthy adults requiring hospitalization for community-acquired pneumonia.[14] Nevertheless, a variety of risk factors have been identified for both frequency and severity of pneumococcal pneumonia. One of the most common risk factors is age. Studies in the prepenicillin era showed a linear correlation between the frequency of pneumococcal pneumonia and age 20 through 80 years.[21(pp656–726)] Other common associated risk factors include chronic lung disease, cigarette use, congestive heart failure, neurologic conditions that predispose to aspiration, and alcoholism.[21–23] Patients with compromised B-cell function have high rates of pneumococcal pneumonia, including conditions such as common variable immunodeficiency, X-linked agammaglobulinemia, multiple myeloma, and chronic lymphocytic leukemia. The rate of pneumococcal pneumonia is at least 100-fold greater among patients with HIV infection.[24] Clustering may also be a factor, with high rates of pneumococcal pneumonia, sometimes in epidemic form, in South African miners; in military personnel in closed quarters; or in association with daycare centers, jails, and homeless shelters. Miscellaneous risks are found in patients who have undergone splenectomy; in Native Americans living on reservations; and with selected occupations, such as painters and welders.

TABLE 55–1 ■ Bacteriology of Community-Acquired Pneumonia: Metaanalysis of 59 Reports, 1966 to 1995*

Total number of cases with bacterial pathogen	6104
Streptococcus pneumoniae	4432 (73%)
Haemophilus influenzae	833 (14%)
Legionella	272 (4%)
Staphylococcus aureus	157 (3%)
Gram-negative bacilli	103 (2%)
Klebsiella	56
Pseudomonas aeruginosa	18

*Analysis is restricted to cases with a bacterial pathogen. No likely etiologic agent was detected in 11,229 cases.

Data from Fine MJ, Smith MA, Carson CA, et al: Prognosis and outcomes of patients with community-acquired pneumonia: A meta-analysis. JAMA 275:134–141, 1996.

Clinical Features

The classic presentation of pneumococcal pneumonia is a dramatic illness characterized by abrupt onset with a rigor followed by high fever, cough productive of sputum that is purulent and often rust colored, dyspnea, and in most cases pleuritic pain. In the absence of treatment, the classic description includes high fever, tachypnea, and severe toxic effects for 7 to 10 days.[9, 12, 13, 21(pp656–726)] The development of antibody is accompanied by abrupt lysis of fever with dramatic clinical recovery despite the persistence of consolidation on chest radiographs. Many patients with pneumococcal pneumonia as seen in current practice have a less dramatic evolution of disease, and most have intervening antibiotic treatment that alters the natural course. Laboratory studies usually show leukocytosis with a leftward shift, mild to moderate hypoxemia, and characteristic changes on chest radiographs. There is a direct correlation between the extent of leukocytosis and mortality, although leukopenia is also viewed as a finding related to poor prognosis.[21(pp656–726)] The classic chest film finding is lobar consolidation, and the majority of patients with lobar consolidation have *S. pneumoniae* as the putative agent.[13, 21(pp656–726)] Nevertheless, many or most patients show changes described as bronchopneumonic or even interstitial.[25]

Diagnosis

An established diagnosis requires recovery of *S. pneumoniae* from an uncontaminated specimen source including blood, pleural fluid, transtracheal aspirate, or transthoracic needle aspirate. *S. pneumoniae* accounts for 65% of bacteremic pneumonias, and about 5% to 12% of hospitalized patients with community-acquired pneumonia have *S. pneumoniae* bacteremia.[14] For the majority of patients, the diagnosis is established with Gram stain and culture of expectorated sputum. Culture of sputum is fraught with problems for both false-positive and false-negative results. False-positive results reflect contamination of the specimen in the 5% to 30% of patients who are colonized with *S. pneumoniae* in the nasopharynx. The rate of false-negative cultures based on studies of bacteremic pneumonia is estimated at approximately 50%.[26, 27] That is, *S. pneumoniae* is recovered in expectorated sputum cultures from about 50% of patients who have positive blood cultures accompanied by a pulmonary infiltrate on chest radiographs. The low yield of only 10% to 20% for *S. pneumoniae* in expectorated sputum cultures among all hospitalized patients with community-acquired pneumonia is ascribed to (1) absence of productive cough in 20% to 30% of patients; (2) antecedent antibiotic exposure, which usually precludes recovery of this fastidious pathogen in 20% to 30%; (3) delays in transport of specimens to the laboratory for prompt microbiologic processing; and (4) reduced competence or commitment of laboratory personnel for detection with routine methods of processing specimens. An analysis of cases of enigmatic pneumonia by the British Thoracic Society suggested that the majority were due to this pathogen.[28] Alternative methods that have been used to increase the yield include the Quellung reaction with expectorated sputum and detection of pneumococcal polysaccharide by latex agglutination or counterimmunoelectrophoresis.[29–32] Antigen detection is routinely employed in many laboratories in Europe and Scandinavia, which presumably accounts for higher yields of the pneumococcus in studies of community-acquired pneumonia in those areas; many authorities think that these antigen detection techniques lack sufficient specificity for routine laboratory use.

Treatment

Penicillin has generally been regarded as the drug of choice for pneumococcal infections, and the standard dose for uncomplicated cases was 600,000 units of aqueous procaine penicillin given intramuscularly every 12 hours or oral penicillin V in a dose of 1 to 2 g/d.[33] In the 1960s, this therapy was successful in the majority of uncomplicated cases of pneumococcal pneumonia. Patients with bacteremia or more complicated cases were generally treated with intravenous aqueous penicillin G in a daily dose of 2 million units, and higher doses were of no therapeutic benefit.[34] These recommendations are now antiquated because of the evolution of penicillin resistance.[35–37] Studies of *S. pneumoniae* in 1994 from multiple centers in the United States showed that approximately 25% of strains had reduced sensitivity to penicillin (minimal inhibitory concentration exceeding 0.1 μg/mL), and 10% to 15% showed relatively high resistance (minimal inhibitory concentration exceeding 2 μg/mL)[35] (Table 55–2). Furthermore, strains of *S. pneumoniae* resistant to penicillin were often resistant to multiple other antimicrobial agents as well (see Table 55–1). The evolution of resistance has confounded treatment options for empirical decisions for suspected or established infection involving this microbe. The result is increased emphasis on recovery of the pathogen, routine susceptibility testing of all clinically significant isolates of *S. pneumoniae*, knowledge of sensitivity profiles within the community, restraint in antibiotic abuse to reduce the problem, and use of pneumococcal vaccine.[36] The probability of penicillin resistance is increased in children and in patients who have had recent hospitalization, exposure to daycare centers, extensive exposure to antibiotics, and residency or recent travel in areas that have high rates of resistance. Penicillin is regarded as the preferred agent for penicillin-sensitive strains, and this drug may be used in higher concentrations (10 to 12 million units/d intravenously) for strains showing intermediate susceptibility. Alternative drugs that are often active include cefotaxime, ceftriaxone, macrolides, doxycycline, carbapenems, and fluoroquinolones.[35–37] The only drug that is uniformly active is vancomycin, although there is concern for abuse of this drug because of the evolving resistance of *Enterococcus*. Erythromycin has usually been considered the standard alternative agent for patients with contraindications to β-lactams. This option is confounded by high rates of intolerance to erythromycin and by reduced susceptibility primarily in penicillin-resistant strains. Alternative macrolides including clarithromycin, dirithromycin, and azithromycin are better tolerated, but strains of *S. pneumoniae* resistant to erythromycin generally show class resistance. Among the oral cephalosporins, the most active in vitro are cefpodoxime, cefprozil, and cefuroxime.[37] Particularly promising for penicillin-resistant strains are fluoroquinolones including new agents in this class such as levofloxacin, trovafloxacin, and sparfloxacin.[35, 38]

TABLE 55–2 ■ Antimicrobial Susceptibility of *Streptococcus pneumoniae*: Analysis of 1527 Strains from 30 Medical Centers, United States, 1994 to 1995

AGENT	% RESISTANT
Penicillin G	24
Intermediate	14
High level	10
Cephalosporins*	
Cefuroxime	12
Ceftriaxone	5
Cefotaxime	3
Erythromycin	10
Tetracycline	8
Chloramphenicol	4
Vancomycin	0

*Rank order of cephalosporins was cefotaxime = ceftriaxone ≥ cefpodoxime ≥ cefuroxime > cefprozil ≥ cefixime > cefaclor = loracarbef > cefadroxil = cephalexin.

Adapted from Doern GV, Brueggemann A, Holley HP Jr, Rauch AM: Antimicrobial resistance of *Streptococcus pneumoniae* recovered from outpatients in the United States during the winter months of 1994 to 1995: Results of a 30-center national surveillance study. Antimicrob Agents Chemother 40:1209–1213, 1996.

Complications and Response to Therapy

The major complications of patients hospitalized with pneumococcal pneumonia are bacteremia in 12% of cases, empyema in 0.5% to 1%, and meningitis in 0.3% to 0.5%.[14, 21(pp656–726)] Other infrequent complications include purulent pericarditis and septic arthritis. The overall mortality rate in hospitalized patients is 12%.[14] Factors associated with a poor prognosis include age extremes, multilobar involvement, bacteremia, neutropenia, selected serotypes, alcoholism, and asplenia. The impact of age was well studied in the prepenicillin era when it was noted that pneumococcal pneumonia was lethal in 24% of patients 20 to 39 years of age, in 36% of those 40 to 49 years of age, in 50% of persons 50 to 59 years of age, and in 72% of those who were older than 60 years.[21(pp656–726)] It was also observed that the mortality rate was 13% without bacteremia and increased to 62% in those with bacteremia. Later studies have shown that the mortality rate of pneumococcal pneumonia has been substantially reduced by the impact of antibiotics. Nevertheless, there has been no significant decrease in mortality rates during the first 5 days of treatment, and the mortality rate for bacteremic pneumococcal pneumonia continues at the high rate of 25% to 30%.[39] Studies of patients with pneumonia involving penicillin-resistant strains often fail to show increased mortality even when these patients are treated with β-lactam antibiotics.[40] The mean time to resolution of fever is 3 to 5 days among patients who respond to antibiotics and 6 to 7 days in those with bacteremic pneumonia. Chest radiographs may normalize within 3 to 4 weeks in young, previously healthy adults, but this clearing is delayed to a mean of 13 weeks in older patients and in patients who have pneumococcal bacteremia, structural abnormalities of the lung, or coexisting medical conditions.[41–44]

Prevention

The major preventive measure is the polyvalent pneumococcal vaccine that includes 23 serotypes of *S. pneumoniae* that account for about 89% of cases of pneumococcal disease. This vaccine is recommended for persons older than 65 years or in the presence of HIV infection, a cerebrospinal fluid leak, chronic renal failure, alcoholism, asplenia, diabetes, malignant neoplasia, chronic obstructive lung disease, and chronic cardiovascular disease. Revaccination is recommended at 5 years in those at high risk. Many recommend routine pneumococcal vaccine at the time of hospitalization for vaccine candidates because most with serious pneumococcal infections have been hospitalized within the prior 5 years.[45]

Haemophilus influenzae Pneumonia

History

H. influenzae was initially described in 1892 by Pfeiffer,[46] who erroneously thought this to be the agent responsible for influenza. Support for this notion was based on high recovery rates in expectorated sputum as well as on experimental animal studies showing that intratracheal challenge to monkeys produced tracheobronchitis, bronchiolitis, or bronchopneumonia.[47, 48] The etiology of influenza became clarified with the description of a filterable virus in 1933[49]; the role of "the influenza bacillus" as a pulmonary pathogen was then disputed because most patients with lobar pneumonia or bronchopneumonia had other bacterial pathogens recovered concurrently in expectorated sputum.[21(pp8–9)] In 1931, Pittman[50] described encapsulated and unencapsulated forms and identified the six encapsulated types of *H. influenzae* on the basis of antigenically distinct capsular polysaccharides. It was noted that type b was the most virulent pathogen and the organism responsible for serious infections, including pneumonia, in young children. The role of *H. influenzae* as a cause of pneumonia in adults was clearly established in 1942 by Keefer and Rammelkamp,[51] who described the recovery of *H. influenzae* from both blood and sputum cultures of a 30-year-old patient with lobar pneumonia. Since that time, *H. influenzae* has been implicated in 10% to 20% of bacterial pneumonias.[14, 15, 27] The best established cases have been type b infections in children,[52, 53] but this form of *H. influenzae* disease has nearly disappeared since the implementation of the protective vaccine. *H. influenzae* disease with nontypeable and type b strains has been much more difficult to define in adults. This organism is second only to the pneumococcus as a pathogen recovered in expectorated sputum samples in adults with pneumonia, and it is a particularly prevalent isolate in patients with chronic bronchitis. Nevertheless, the number of well-confirmed cases of *H. influenzae* pneumonia in adults based on recovery from uncontaminated specimen sources is relatively sparse.

Frequency

H. influenzae is implicated in approximately 10% of all patients with a likely etiologic agent of community-acquired pneumonia sufficiently severe to require hospitalization, according to a review of 122 reports published from 1966 to 1995.[14] Because the yield of any pathogen is only 30% to 50% in most series, the overall recovery rate is 3% to 5% among all patients, and it is 10% to 15% in those with an identified bacterial pathogen (see Table 55–1). This figure is confounded by the lack of diagnostic precision because of frequent false-positive and false-negative results. Bacteremia and recovery from extrapulmonary sites reflecting disseminated disease are unusual.

Microbiology

The organism is a small, somewhat pleomorphic gram-negative bacillus with fastidious growth requirements. There is an outer membrane polysaccharide that provides the basis for grouping into serotypes designated A to F.[50] Most cases complicated by bacteremia or empyema in the past were due to serotype b, but this is now virtually eliminated owing to widespread use of the vaccine.[54] Most uncomplicated infections involving the respiratory tract are due to "rough" strains that are unencapsulated or nontypeable. The organism is difficult to recover, and only 30% to 50% of patients with bacteremic pneumonia have positive sputum cultures.[55–60] Growth is optimal on enriched media such as chocolate agar. Colonization rates are variable but are higher in young persons and may reach rates of 25% to 85% in healthy adults.[61, 62] Only 4% to 10% of these are typeable strains. This organism must be distinguished from *Haemophilus parainfluenzae*, which is regarded as a nonpathogen when it is recovered in respiratory secretions.

Clinical Features

Analysis of *H. influenzae* pneumonia in reported cases in adults is confusing because of concerns about improper diagnosis based on reliance on expectorated sputum cultures. Clinical features of 151 cases reported in four series[55, 56, 59, 62] are summarized in Table 55–3. The role of *H. influenzae* in most of these cases was verified by recovery in uncontaminated specimen sources; this will bias the findings but also limits analysis to patients with well-confirmed bacteriologic findings. The results showed that pneumonia ascribed to *H. influenzae* is not unique but resembles pneumonia due to multiple other bacterial pathogens. Some patients have a preceding upper respiratory tract infection, but this is unusual. Pneumonia due to *H. influenzae* appears to be more frequent in patients with chronic obstructive lung disease or chronic bronchitis. Patients with HIV infection are predisposed to *H. influenzae* pulmonary infections,[63] predominantly with nontypeable strains. Patients with humoral immune defects are predisposed to *H. influenzae* infections with type b

TABLE 55–3 ■ Clinical Features of Pneumonia Caused by *Haemophilus influenzae* in Adults

CLINICAL FEATURE	FOUR REPORTS*	RANGE*
Age (mean)	53 y	50–55 y
Associated conditions		
Alcoholism	42/133 (32%)	27%–37%
Chronic lung disease	91/151 (60%)	44%–80%
Temperature >37.5°C	81/92 (88%)	87%–90%
Peripheral leukocyte count >10,000/mm^3	63/110 (57%)	30%–69%
Radiographic changes		
Consolidated	30/92 (33%)	23%–37%
More than one lobe involved	85/121 (70%)	39%–74%
Abscess formation	1/121 (1%)	0%–2%
Pleural effusion	32/121 (26%)	10%–49%
Mortality rate	31/151 (20%)	0%–37%

*Analysis of 151 cases in four reports[55, 56, 59, 62] with 18–62 cases each. The majority were established with bacteriologic confirmation based on positive cultures of blood, pleural fluid, or transtracheal aspirate. The denominator varies because of variation in the data reported.

strains. The usual findings with either type b or nontypeable strains are fever, cough, sputum production, and dyspnea. The chest radiograph usually shows bronchopneumonia, but lobar consolidation is reported in 23% to 37% of cases. As noted, *H. influenzae* pneumonia complicated by bacteremia, abscess formation, or empyema has historically been most common in children younger than 5 years and usually due to type b strains. These complications are unusual in adults.

Diagnosis

The usual diagnosis is based on Gram stain and culture of expectorated sputum. The difficulties encountered are the high rates of false-positive cultures reflecting the high rates of colonization of *H. influenzae* in the upper airways[61, 62, 64] and high rates of false-negative cultures due to the fastidious growth requirements. There is also difficulty in recognition on Gram stain even with transtracheal aspirates.[56] Complicated disease with bacteremia, meningitis, empyema, or lung abscess previously associated with type b strains has now become infrequent in clinical practice. The majority of reported cases are based on presumptive diagnoses with expectorated sputum, a tenuous conclusion. As noted, colonization by nontypeable strains in the upper airways is common in healthy adults; *H. influenzae* is also commonly found in large concentrations in the expectorated sputum of patients with chronic bronchitis (10^5 organisms per mL or higher) during periods of stability and during exacerbations.[65] Again, the majority are nontypeable. In my experience with 488 transtracheal aspirates in patients with acute community-acquired pneumonia, *H. influenzae* was recovered in 28 (5.5%).[66] Even this figure is possibly deceptive because patients with chronic lung disease often have *H. influenzae* colonization of the lower airways.[67]

Treatment

Ampicillin was generally considered the preferred drug for infections involving *H. influenzae* until the early 1970s, when β-lactamase production complicated this treatment. At present, approximately 25% to 35% of strains of both typeable and nontypeable *H. influenzae* strains are resistant to ampicillin. Alternative drugs that are active in vitro against most strains include second- and third-generation cephalosporins, trimethoprim-sulfamethoxazole, doxycycline, carbapenems, fluoroquinolones, any combination of a β-lactam and a β-lactamase inhibitor, and azithromycin; drugs that are usually inactive include erythromycin, clindamycin, and vancomycin.

Staphylococcus aureus Pneumonia

History

S. aureus has been a recognized pulmonary pathogen since the turn of the century, when it was responsible for a fulminant pneumonia that occurred in influenza epidemics.[68, 69] The classic description is ascribed to Chickering and Park,[70] who reported 153 cases during the influenza pandemic of 1918 at Camp Jackson. During this outbreak, there were 151 cases with only two survivors. Autopsy examinations showed circumscribed abscesses of 1 to 10 mm scattered throughout congested lung tissue. Subsequent reports also emphasized the association between influenza A and staphylococcal pneumonia during the Asian influenza epidemic in 1957 to 1958[71] and the Hong Kong influenza epidemic in 1968 to 1969.[72] In 1933, Relman[73] implicated *S. aureus* in approximately 9% of atypical pneumonias that occurred sporadically in the absence of influenza. The initial and classic studies of staphylococcal pneumonia fostered a prevalent opinion that this usually occurs in association with influenza epidemics, follows a fulminant course, is usually complicated by tissue necrosis with abscess formation, and carries an extraordinary mortality rate even with appropriate antibiotic treatment. Subsequent reports have shown considerable variations from this pattern. In some of the settings in which staphylococcal pneumonia is likely to occur, the course shows substantial variation and the mortality rate ranges from 0% to 65% depending, to a large extent, on the host's status.

Frequency

S. aureus is recovered from respiratory secretions of about 1% of all patients with community-acquired pneumonia, 3% of patients with a bacteriologic diagnosis[14] (see Table 55–1), and 10% to 30% of patients with nosocomial pneumonia. Staphylococcal pneumonia is rare in adults without specifically defined defects, as follows:

1. Nosocomial pneumonia, in which this organism is second only to gram-negative bacilli in frequency[74–76]; *S. aureus* is especially common in ventilator-associated pneumonia and in some series is the most common pathogen in this setting[76]
2. Postinfluenza pneumonia, in which this organism is second only to *S. pneumoniae* in frequency[70–72]
3. Septic pulmonary emboli, especially with tricuspid valve endocarditis associated with parenteral drug abuse[77]
4. Structural disease of the lung, including cystic fibrosis and bronchiectasis[78]
5. Specific defects in host defenses such as chronic granulomatous disease or structural disease such as cystic fibrosis
6. Other associations that are less clearly established, including corticosteroid administration, HIV infection, laryngeal or bronchogenic carcinoma, trauma, chronic bronchitis, central nervous system disease, and age older than 50 years[79]

Staphylococcal pneumonia can be seen in neonates, especially when it is complicated by pneumatoceles.[80–82]

Microbiology

This organism grows readily on standard laboratory media such as blood agar and on selective agar such as mannitol salt agar. It is easily recovered and identified in common clinical specimens including sputum, bronchoscopy specimens, and blood. It must be distinguished from coagulase-negative staphylococci and *Staphylococcus epidermidis*, which have not been clearly implicated as etiologic agents of pneumonia.

Pathogenesis

Nasal cultures show colonization by *S. aureus* in 25% to 40% of healthy adults, but pharyngeal cultures show this organism in only 5% to 10%.[83, 84] The colonization rate is increased in injection drug users, insulin-dependent diabetic individuals, and hemodialysis patients. Colonization of the pharynx is promoted by viral pharyngitis, which may be a contributing factor in the association with influenza.[85] The usual route of transmission is by aspiration of the organism in the upper airways. A less common mechanism is by the hematogenous route, as with staphylococcal pneumonia occurring in association with tricuspid valve endocarditis, pelvic vein septic thrombophlebitis, hemodialysis access site infection, and rare cases of intravenous catheter–associated septicemia.[86–88] According to the mouse model, the likelihood of pneumonia is directly related to the inoculum size of the organism; on experimental challenge, 10^5 organisms are easily cleared, 10^6

are cleared slowly, and 10^7 or higher generally result in pneumonia.[89]

Clinical Features

The classic studies of staphylococcal pneumonia[70–72] suggested a distinctive clinical syndrome characterized by fulminant onset, high rates of tissue necrosis, and high fatality rates. Later studies suggested great variation in both the initial presentation and the subsequent course.[79, 90–93] Pneumonia due to *S. aureus* may be acute or chronic.[94] The usual features are cough and fever that may be abrupt in onset or more subtle with a slowly evolving clinical presentation (Table 55–4). Most patients produce purulent sputum. The frequency of this infection among all patients with postinfluenza bacterial pneumonia is 6% to 20%.[72] The illness classically occurs in two phases: there is the initial influenza syndrome with respiratory symptoms and constitutional complaints followed by improvement and then deterioration with the features of staphylococcal pneumonia after 1 to 2 weeks. Patients with tricuspid valve endocarditis present with the usual features of injection drug use combined with a febrile illness and *S. aureus* bacteremia.[77] The most characteristic feature of this and other embolic forms of staphylococcal pneumonia is multiple round densities with or without cavitation involving multiple pulmonary segments on chest radiographs.[77] The lung is also a common site of secondary infection in patients with *S. aureus* bacteremia, but this may present with diverse changes on chest radiographs.[86–88] In these cases, it is often difficult to determine whether the pneumonia is the primary event or a secondary feature of bacteremia. Reviews of *S. aureus* bacteremia showed that the lung is considered the primary portal of entry for 5% to 10%.[88] The most common setting for staphylococcal pneumonia in more recent years has been with nosocomial acquisition, for which risk factors include antimicrobial exposure, advanced age, chronic lung disease, mechanical ventilation, and recent surgical procedures.[74–76] Many of these same risk factors apply to the nursing home setting, where *S. aureus* is also relatively common as a cause of pneumonia.[95] The clinical features of nosocomial *S. aureus* pneumonia are similar to those of nosocomial pneumonia in general, with cough, fever, and purulent sputum. Chest radiographs in nonembolic staphylococcal pneumonia in both the nosocomial and the postinfluenza settings show a bronchopneumonic pattern. Lobar consolidation is relatively rare, and cavitation, contrary to popular opinion, is also a relatively unusual complication.[93] Empyema was once reported as a complication in 8% to 30% of cases,[90, 91, 96, 97] but this is now less frequent, presumably reflecting the impact of effective antimicrobial treatment.[93] *S. aureus* now accounts for 10% to 40% of all empyemas; it is most common in the settings described, and this is the most common pathogen encountered in empyema as a complication of thoracic surgery[98] (see Table 67–1). Pneumatocele is a characteristic feature of staphylococcal pneumonia in children but is an unusual feature in adults.

TABLE 55–4 ■ Clinical Features of Staphylococcal Pneumonia in Adults (29 Cases)*

Age	
Mean	61.3 y
Range	28–83 y
Associated major underlying conditions	29 (100%)
Hospital acquired	20 (69%)
Peak temperature	
Mean	102.9°F
Range	100°F–105.6°F
Peripheral leukocyte count (mean)	18,900/mm³
Radiographic changes	
Abscess	3 (10%)
Effusion	14 (48%)
Multiple lobe involvement	14 (48%)
Bilateral	11 (38%)
Mortality rate	10 (34%)

*Etiologic diagnosis is based on recovery of *S. aureus* in pure culture from transtracheal aspirate (13 cases), pleural fluid (7), lung aspirate (2), and blood culture (9).

Diagnosis

The diagnosis is best established by the usual clinical features of pneumonia accompanied by recovery of *S. aureus* in an uncontaminated specimen source such as blood or pleural fluid. With expectorated sputum or bronchoscopic aspirates, there should be a compatible Gram stain showing typical gram-positive cocci in "bowling pin" arrangements combined with recovery of *S. aureus* in moderate to heavy growth or, with quantitative bronchoscopic cultures, concentrations exceeding 10^3 to 10^4 organisms per mL, depending on laboratory standards. False-positive cultures are common owing to the frequency of colonization of *S. aureus* in the upper airways, especially in hospitalized patients and those who have received prior antibiotic treatment. False-negative cultures of respiratory secretions are unusual so that the failure to recover *S. aureus* with standard microbiology techniques is strong evidence against the role of these organisms in the pulmonary infection.

Complications and Course

Staphylococcal pneumonia is regarded as a serious infection; mortality rates as high as 67% are reported even in the antibiotic era.[90] This is highly variable and depends to a large extent on the setting and the host's health status.[91, 93] The prognosis for injection drug users with tricuspid valve endocarditis is usually good, with mortality rates of less than 5% to 10% in most series.[77] Postinfluenza staphylococcal pneumonia shows a relatively high mortality rate in young, previously healthy adults when this complication is accompanied by the clinical features of toxic shock syndrome.[99] With nosocomial pneumonia, the mortality rate is high; when it is accompanied by bacteremia, the mortality rate is often reported at 30% to 50%.[74–76] Complications include toxic shock syndrome, extension to contiguous sites with purulent pericarditis, and, more commonly, pulmonary necrosis with abscess formation or a bronchopleural fistula leading to empyema. Chronic pneumonitis with a slowly evolving course is a feature in occasional cases.[94]

Treatment

The standard treatment is oxacillin or nafcillin in doses up to 12 g/d intravenously. Alternative drugs include selected cephalosporins (such as cefazolin or cefuroxime), vancomycin, clindamycin, trimethoprim-sulfamethoxazole, and fluoroquinolones. The specific agent used should be selected by in vitro sensitivity test results. With nosocomial infections, vancomycin is often required because 20% to 35% of nosocomial isolates of *S. aureus* are methicillin resistant. Methicillin resistance is unusual in community-acquired strains of *S. aureus*, but some studies are reporting increasing rates of 5% to 10%. Rifampin may be used to reduce nasopharyngeal carriage and is sometimes used to enhance antimicrobial activity of other agents such as oxacillin or a fluoroquinolone. The combination of ciprofloxacin plus rifampin has established merit in staphylococcal tricuspid valve endocarditis with septic pulmonary emboli, but use of this regimen requires documentation of in vitro activity of ciprofloxacin because of escalating resistance of *S. aureus* to the fluoroquinolone class. The duration of treatment is arbitrary and depends to a large extent on complications and course. Most authorities recommend 2 to 4 weeks of treatment, some of which can be accomplished with oral agents on an outpatient basis.

Neisseria meningitidis Pneumonia

History

N. meningitidis became well established as a pulmonary pathogen when these organisms were recovered from lung tissue at autopsy during the 1918 to 1919 influenza pandemic.[100–102] The majority of cases involved military personnel. Since World War II, there have been fewer than 50 cases of meningococcal pneumonia reported and only about 11 involving civilians.[14, 103–112] The earlier studies emphasized the role of the meningococcus as a superinfecting organism in patients with viral respiratory tract infections, especially influenza[100–102]; the more recent work has also emphasized the role of this organism as a transmissible agent in the hospital setting.[109–112] Although the number of reported cases is relatively sparse, the true frequency of the disease is unknown.

Microbiology

N. meningitidis is subdivided into polysaccharide-specific serogroups designated A, B, C, D, X, Y, Z, 29E, and W135. Meningococcal disease, including pneumonia, often occurs in epidemics in military populations, and occurrence of the pathogen is more likely to be sporadic in civilians. Organisms belonging to group Y have become the major cause of meningococcal disease, including pneumonia among military personnel.[107, 108] These organisms replaced group C as the major cause of meningococcal disease in military recruits in the early 1970s, a shift ascribed to routine vaccination of basic trainees against *N. meningitidis* groups A and C.[113] In civilians, group Y strains are the ususal cause of pulmonary infections.

Clinical Features

Most reports, especially those from military populations, emphasize the predisposing role of respiratory tract infections, the most common being influenza,[100, 102, 113] measles,[101] and adenovirus infection.[114] Experimental support for this association is available from a mouse model in which the rodent was rendered susceptible to an aerosol containing *N. meningitidis* after exposure to an avirulent encephalomyocarditis virus.[115] Occasional cases occur in the context of an outbreak of meningococcal disease without a preceding viral infection. Nosocomial acquisition is occasionally suggested.[109, 111, 112] There is nothing particularly distinctive about meningococcal pneumonia. Most patients do not have evidence of extrapulmonary involvement, such as meningitis or clinical signs of meningococcemia. Usual findings are cough, sputum production, fever, and leukocytosis. Chest radiographs typically show bronchial pneumonia or lobar consolidation; empyema is unusual, and lung abscess has not been reported. The prognosis is excellent. Although meningococcal pneumonia superimposed on influenza was often lethal in the early reports from military hospitals, nearly all patients described during the antibiotic era have survived.

Diagnosis

Expectorated sputum, the usual specimen source in patients with bacterial pneumonia, has proved to be particularly unrewarding in the detection of meningococcal pneumonia. This point is emphasized by a review of the specimen sources used to establish this diagnosis: only 5 of 39 cases reported since 1970 used expectorated sputum cultures.[106–114, 116–118] One problem is that *N. meningitidis* may be easily overgrown by the normal respiratory tract flora so that false-negative cultures are common. Some have suggested that selective media, such as Thayer-Martin media, be used to facilitate recovery and identification.[117] The problem is the potential for false-positive cultures as a result of asymptomatic carriage of *N. meningitidis,* which has been found in throat cultures from 5% to 15% of healthy persons.[119, 120] Using selective media for sputum cultures, Putsch and colleagues[119] recovered this organism from 30% of patients with acute pneumonia, but the recovery rate was approximately the same using sputum from patients without pneumonia. Lewis and coworkers[118] cultivated 2604 sputum samples on Thayer-Martin media, recovered meningococci in 48, and concluded that 6 of these were consistent with meningococcal pneumonia. Laboratory detection is further complicated because most authorities do not recommend speciation of *Neisseria* isolates that are recovered in expectorated sputum samples and do not endorse the routine use of Thayer-Martin or other selected media. Thus, the usual method to establish diagnosis is by recovering the organism from uncontaminated specimens such as transtracheal aspirate, transthoracic aspirate, blood, pleural fluid, or extrapulmonary sources such as cerebrospinal fluid. Gram stain of expectorated sputum shows typical large gram-negative cocci that are often within leukocytes, providing an important clue. Other *Neisseria* species and *Branhamella (Moraxella) catarrhalis* have nearly identical morphologic characteristics and are far more common pulmonary pathogens. The distinction is important because *B. catarrhalis* is usually resistant to penicillin.

Treatment

N. meningitidis is susceptible to a variety of antibiotics including penicillin, cephalosporins, tetracycline, erythromycin, and chloramphenicol. Penicillin G is generally regarded as the preferred drug. Respiratory precautions should be prescribed for patients with meningococcal pneumonia when the diagnosis is either established or strongly suspected. This should be continued until the organism has been eradicated from the respiratory tract or after treatment for 24 hours. Prophylaxis is recommended for close contacts, primarily those with exposure to respiratory secretions, using a fluoroquinolone or rifampin. This includes hospital personnel with the usual types of airborne exposure.

Pulmonary Infections Involving Other Species of *Neisseria*

Neisseria gonorrhoeae is not generally regarded as a pulmonary pathogen, although a case of lobar pneumonia with empyema involving this organism has been reported.[121] Other species of *Neisseria* are generally regarded as components of the normal flora of the upper airways. Occasional cases of pulmonary infection involve *Neisseria sicca*. *B. catarrhalis* (formerly *Neisseria catarrhalis*) has been reported in up to 2% to 3% of community-acquired pneumonias.[122, 123]

Gram-Negative Bacillary Pneumonia

History

The history of gram-negative bacillary pneumonia in the prepenicillin era is largely restricted to the studies of *Klebsiella pneumoniae*. This organism was initially described in 1882 by Friedländer, who believed it to be the exclusive cause of pneumonia.[124] The proposal was subsequently rejected with the discovery of the pneumococcus, although *Klebsiella* remained a well-established if infrequent cause of pneumonia in the preantibiotic era. Two forms of the disease were recognized. An acute form known as Friedländer pneumonia resembled pneumococcal lobar pneumonia except for its occurrence almost exclusively in debilitated subjects and a possibly more fulminant course.[125–127] The second form of the disease was a chronic infection that persisted for weeks or months and was, at times, confused with pulmonary tuberculosis.[128] Both the acute and the chronic forms of the disease showed a distinct propensity for tissue necrosis with abscess formation.[129] *Klebsiella* was never a common cause of pneumonia in the preantibiotic era, accounting for about 0.6% to 1.1% of cases reported at that time.[21(p2), 127, 130, 131] This organism continues to be a rare cause of community-acquired pneumonia, still accounting for about 1% of cases (see Table 55–1); cases conforming to the classic clinical descriptions are especially rare. Gram-negative bacillary pneumonia involving organisms other than *K. pneumoniae* is largely a product of the antibiotic era. These organisms were occasionally encountered in community-acquired pneumonia, but rates of recovery were always low; even when they were found, the source was usually respiratory secretions, raising questions about the validity of the results. In the 1960s, Tillotson and Lerner[132] published a series of reports on pneumonia caused by various gram-negative bacilli. The scientific community was divided on the validity of these studies, and many remained skeptical despite the authors' claim of stringent diagnostic criteria requiring the same gram-negative bacillus as the dominant potential pathogen in at least two expectorated sputum samples. Problems included the lack of confirmation with uncontaminated specimen sources such as blood or pleural fluid. Also, transtracheal aspiration that was commonly done at that time almost never yielded gram-negative bacilli to the exclusion of other well-recognized pulmonary pathogens.[66] The notable exception was the evolution of gram-negative bacteria as the major cause of hospital-acquired pneumonia, especially when it was acquired in intensive care units and in patients receiving mechanical ventilation. Another new setting in which these organisms play a prominent role is the compromised host, including transplant recipients, patients receiving chemotherapy, and patients with advanced acquired immunodeficiency syndrome.

Frequency

Gram-negative bacteria (Enterobacteriaceae and *Pseudomonas* species) are rare causes of community-acquired pneumonia. A metaanalysis of 122 reports of community-acquired pneumonia in the English medical literature from 1966 through 1995 showed that this category of bacteria accounted for only about 103 of the approximately 6100 cases (2%) in which a microbial etiology was defined[14] (see Table 55–1). By contrast, these organisms are the major causes of nosocomial pneumonia, accounting for 30% to 60% of cases in most series.[133–138] Confirmation of their etiologic role based on specimen source is the high yield of these organisms in bacteremic patients,[137] in transtracheal aspirates,[135] and by quantitative cultures of bronchoscopic aspirates.[136, 138] In addition to nosocomial acquisition, other predisposing factors for infection involving gram-negative bacilli include neutropenia, structural disease of the lung such as bronchiectasis and cystic fibrosis, prior antibiotic treatment with pulmonary superinfection, and advanced acquired immunodeficiency syndrome. Gram-negative bacilli are also frequently encountered in "nursing home pneumonia."

Pathogenesis

Gram-negative bacillary pneumonia usually follows aspiration of these organisms when they reside in the upper airways or stomach.[139–141] Previous studies indicated that colonization rates are highly variable, depending on the host's status. Pharyngeal cultures infrequently yield gram-negative bacilli in healthy adults, even when they are exposed to the hospital environment through employment or with hospitalization for relatively minor medical diseases or for psychiatric conditions.[139] The frequency of colonization increases substantially in direct relationship to severity of associated conditions. Thus, patients classified as moderately ill show colonization rates of 30% to 40%, and those who are categorized as severely ill requiring placement in intensive care units have colonization rates that often exceed 60%.[139, 141] These associations are independent of antibiotic exposure, although antibiotic exposure favors this type of colonization as well.[141] The conditions that are associated with increased colonization include advanced age, neutropenia, coma, renal failure, hypotension, ketoacidosis, physical impairment for daily living activities, alcoholism, diabetes mellitus, and viral respiratory tract infections. The usual source of gram-negative bacilli in the pharynx is the patient's colon, although these organisms are occasionally transmitted from patient to patient or through hospital personnel.

Microbiology

Enterobacteriaceae species that are frequently implicated in pneumonia, primarily nosocomial pneumonia, are *Klebsiella* species (primarily *K. pneumoniae* and, less frequently, *Klebsiella oxytoca*), *Enterobacter* species (*Enterobacter aerogenes*, *Enterobacter cloacae*, and *Enterobacter agglomerans*), *Escherichia coli*, *Serratia marcescens*, and *Proteus mirabilis*. The Enterobacteriaceae species contain a common antigen in the outer membrane (enterobacterial common antigen) composed of endotoxin and phospholipid.[142] A capsule attached to the outer membrane is composed of dense polysaccharide bundles of varying thickness that are attached to the outer membrane. The capsule thickness varies from 10 nm in *E. coli* to 160 nm in *K. pneumoniae*. *K. pneumoniae* has been the most frequent pathogen in this category isolated in both community-acquired pneumonia[14] and nosocomial pulmonary infection.[135] These organisms may be serotyped on the basis of composition of the capsular or K antigen.[143, 144] At least 77 different K serotypes have been identified. Virulence ascribed to endotoxin is characterized by endotoxic shock and is not different for the various members of Enterobacteriaceae. The polysaccharide capsule of *Klebsiella* in animal studies and in vitro assays appears to inhibit migration of phagocytic cells, inhibit phagocytosis, and retard killing by serum.[144–146] The classic studies of *K. pneumoniae* in the prepenicillin era showed that capsular serotypes K1 through K6 were most frequent, especially K2.[129–131, 147, 148] An attractive thesis is that this organism demonstrated unique pathogenic potential for the lung by virtue of the capsule of these specific serotypes. The gene encoding the K2 serotype polysaccharide has been cloned and transformed to unencapsulated strains, but this did not confer unique virulence properties, casting doubt on the thesis.[149] *Klebsiella* also produced fimbriae that may account for unique pathogenic potential including adherence to respiratory epithelium,[150] but this has not been clearly demonstrated. Although older studies showed that serotypes K1 to K6 predominated, these serotypes have become far less frequent, and the classic features of *Klebsiella* pulmonary infections also appear to be much less frequent. In fact, it has become difficult to define clinical features that distinguish pneumonia due to different members of Enterobacteriaceae and also difficult to implicate organism-specific differences in virulence factors. Of particular importance is the resistance profile of these microbes, which will obviously influence recovery rates among patients who develop pneumonia in the presence of antibiotic exposure.

Pseudomonads resemble Enterobacteriaceae species morphologically but are found most frequently in extraintestinal sources, including water habitats. They are strict aerobes that will not grow anaerobically; they have only polar flagella; and, with few exceptions, they are oxidase-positive. These organisms cannot be distinguished from Enterobacteriaceae species by Gram stain, and they also contain endotoxin as a major identifiable virulence factor. Other virulence factors include a polysaccharide capsule, fimbriae, exotoxin A, and leukocidin[151] (see Chapter 210). The mucoexopolysaccharide capsule may serve as an important virulence factor predisposing to colonization and infection because of binding to surface epithelial cells.[152, 153] *Pseudomonas aeruginosa* is uniquely associated with pulmonary infections in patients with cystic fibrosis (mucoid strains), bronchiectasis, advanced acquired immunodeficiency syndrome, and neutropenia. Other species of the Pseudomonadaceae family include *Burkholderia* (formerly *Pseudomonas*) *cepacia* (an important pathogen in cystic fibrosis), *Pseudomonas mallei* (nodular necrotizing lung infections in developing countries), and *Pseudomonas pseudomallei* (pulmonary disease often with cavity formation in residents from or travelers to Southeast Asia).

Clinical Features

Gram-negative bacillary pneumonia was classically described by Friedländer in 1882 and subsequent authors in the prepenicillin era as summarized earlier.[124] Classic features included an abrupt onset with high fever and cough productive of copious amounts of bloody sputum that had the appearance of currant jelly. Chest radiography typically showed lobar consolidation, often with a bulging interlobar fissure (bulging fissure sign), indicating an expanding necrotic lesion with abscess formation. There was a propensity for involvement of an upper lobe.[124–131] This classic presentation is infrequently encountered in the current era, possibly reflecting involvement of different serotypes of *K. pneumoniae* as summarized before. Instead, gram-negative bacillary pneumonia usually presents with no unique clinical features that would easily distinguish this infection from pneumonia caused by other microbial pathogens, and no clinical features distinguish gram-negative bacillary pneumonia due to different species of Enterobacteriaceae or pseudomonads. The most common form is nosocomial pneumonia, most of the patients are severely compromised by associated medical conditions, most have antecedent colonization of the respiratory tract by the same species of gram-negative bacilli, the prognosis is often poor owing to both the pneumonia and the associated condition, and the mortality rates are high.

Diagnosis

The etiologic diagnosis is established by recovery of gram-negative bacilli from an uncontaminated specimen source (blood, pleural fluid, transtracheal aspirate) in association with a compatible clinical illness. This diagnosis is supported by the demonstration of gram-negative bacilli with the characteristic morphologic features on Gram stain combined with recovery of these organisms in moderate or heavy growth in culture from respiratory secretions. Gram-negative bacilli are easily detected in respiratory secretions because they grow readily on selective and nonselective media that are routinely used in microbiology laboratories. Thus, false-negative cultures with adequate specimens are rare. The main problem is false-positive cultures, especially in patients with prior antibiotic exposure. It is important in such cases to distinguish "sputum superinfection" from superinfection of the patient.

Treatment

Treatment of gram-negative bacillary pneumonia consists of supportive measures and antibiotic directed against the implicated pathogens. The selection of agents is optimally based on in vitro sensitivity testing, which is usually easily accomplished with culture of blood or pulmonary secretions. Recommendations for empirical use[134] in patients who are seriously ill are directed toward relatively resistant agents commonly encountered in the hospital environment and include a carbapenem (imipenem or meropenem), any combination of a β-lactam and a β-lactamase inhibitor (primarily piperacillin-tazobactam or ticarcillin-clavulanate), ciprofloxacin (the preferred fluoroquinolone based on activity against *P. aeruginosa*), or an antipseudomonad β-lactam (ceftazidime, cefoperazone, ticarcillin, piperacillin, or mezlocillin). Any of these may be given in combination with an aminoglycoside, usually gentamicin or tobramycin.

References

1. Pinner RW, Teutsch SM, Simonsen L, et al: Trends in infectious diseases mortality in the United States. JAMA 275:189–193, 1996.
2. Watson DA, Musher DM, Jacobson JW, Verhoff J: A brief history of the pneumococcus in biomedical research: A panoply of scientific discovery. Clin Infect Dis 17:913–924, 1993.
3. Fraenkel A: Weitere Beitrage zur Lehre von den Mikrococcen der genuinen fibrinosen Pneumonie. Z Klin Med 11:437–458, 1886.
4. Winslow CEA, Broadhurst J, Buchanan RE, et al: The families and genera of the bacteria: Final report of the committee of the Society of American Bacteriologists on characterization and classification of bacterial types. J Bacteriol 5:191–229, 1920.
5. Deibel RH, Seeley HW Jr: Family II. Streptococcaceae fam. nov. *In* Buchanan RE, Gibbons NE (eds): Bergey's Manual of Determinative Bacteriology, ed 8. Baltimore, Williams & Wilkins, 1974, pp 490–517.
6. Gram C: Über die isolierte Farbung der Schizomyceten in Schnittund Trockenpraparaten. Fortschr Med 2:185–189, 1884.
7. Neufeld F, Haendel L: Weitere Untersuchungen über Pneumokokken-Heilsera. III. Mitteilung. Arb Kaiserlich Gesundh 34:293–304, 1910.
8. White B, with the collaboration of Robinson ES, Barnes LA: The Biology of Pneumococcus. The Bacteriological, Biochemical, and Immunological Characters and Activities of *Diplococcus pneumoniae*. New York, The Commonwealth Fund, 1937.
9. Lord FT: Immunity factors in recovery from lobar pneumonia and results of specific treatment in type I pneumococcus pneumonia. N Engl J Med 205:854, 1931.
10. Finland M, Sutliff WD: Specific cutaneous reactions and circulating antibodies in the course of lobar pneumonia: II. Cases treated with antipneumococcic sera. J Exp Med 54:653–667, 1931.
11. Abraham EP, Gardner AD, Chain E, et al: Further observations on penicillin. Lancet 2:177–189, 1941.
12. Keefer CS, Blake FG, Marshall EK Jr, et al: Penicillin in the treatment of infections: A report of 500 cases. JAMA 122:1217–1224, 1943.
13. Bullowa JGM: The reliability of sputum typing and its relation to serum therapy. JAMA 105:1512–1523, 1935.

14. Fine MJ, Smith MA, Carson CA, et al: Prognosis and outcomes of patients with community-acquired pneumonia: A meta-analysis. JAMA 275:134–141, 1996.
15. Mundy LM, Auwaerter PG, Oldach D, et al: Community-acquired pneumonia: Impact of immune status. Am J Respir Crit Care Med 152:1309–1315, 1995.
16. Centers for Disease Control and Prevention: Nosocomial infections surveillance, 1984. MMWR CDC Surveill Summ 35:17–29, 1986.
17. Mufson MA, Oley G, Hughey D: Pneumococcal disease in a medium-sized community in the United States. JAMA 248:1486–1489, 1982.
18. Austrian R: Some observations on the pneumococcus and on the current status of pneumococcal disease and its prevention. Rev Infect Dis 3(Suppl):1–17, 1981.
19. Scott JAG, Hall AJ, Dagan R, et al: Serogroup-specific epidemiology of *Streptococcus pneumoniae*: Associations with age, sex, and geography in 7,000 epidosdes of invasive disease. Clin Infect Dis 22:973–981, 1996.
20. Hendley JO, Sande MA, Steward PM, et al: Spread of *Streptococcus pneumoniae* in families. I. Carriage rates and distribution of types. J Infect Dis 132:55–61, 1975.
21. Heffron R: Pneumonia with Special Reference to Pneumococcus Lobar Pneumonia. New York, The Commonwealth Fund, 1939.
22. Lipsky BA, Boyko EJ, Inui TS, et al: Risk factors for acquiring pneumococcal infections. Arch Intern Med 146:2179–2185, 1986.
23. Grandsden WR, Eykyn SJ, Phillips I: Pneumococcal bacteremia: 325 episodes diagnosed at St. Thomas' Hospital. Br Med J 290:505–508, 1985.
24. Janoff EN, Breiman RF, Daley CL, Hopewell PC: Pneumococcal disease during HIV infection: Epidemiologic, clinical, and immunologic perspectives. Ann Intern Med 117:314–324, 1992.
25. Kantor HG: The many radiologic faces of pneumococcal pneumonia. Am J Radiol 13:1213–1220, 1981.
26. Barrett-Connor E: The nonvalue of sputum culture in the diagnosis of pneumococcal pneumonia. Am Rev Respir Dis 103:845–848, 1971.
27. Bartlett JG, Mundy LM: Community-acquired pneumonia. N Engl J Med 333:1618–1624, 1995.
28. Farr BM, Kaiser DL, Harrison BDW, Connolly CK: Prediction of microbial aetiology at admission to hospital for pneumonia from the presenting clinical features. Thorax 44:1031–1035, 1989.
29. Levy M, Dromer F, Brion W, et al: Community-acquired pneumonia. Importance of initial noninvasive bacteriologic and radiographic investigations. Chest 92:43–48, 1988.
30. Merrill CW, Gwaltney JM, Hendley JO, et al: Rapid identification of pneumococci. N Engl J Med 288:510–512, 1973.
31. Perlino CA: Laboratory diagnosis of pneumonia due to *Streptococcus pneumoniae*. J Infect Dis 150:139–144, 1984.
32. Dans P, Charache PC, Fahey M, et al: Management of pneumonia in the prospective payment era. Arch Intern Med 144:1392–1397, 1984.
33. Austrian R, Winston AL: The efficacy of penicillin V (phenoxymethyl penicillin) in the treatment of mild and moderately severe pneumococcal pneumonia. Am J Med Sci 232:624–628, 1958.
34. Brewin A, Arango L, Hadley WK, Murray JF: High-dose penicillin therapy and pneumococcal pneumonia. JAMA 230:409–413, 1974.
35. Hofmann J, Cetron MS, Farley MM, et al: The prevalence of drug-resistant *Streptococcus pneumoniae* in Atlanta. N Engl J Med 333:481–486, 1995.
36. Gold HS, Moellering RC Jr: Antimicrobial drug resistance. N Engl J Med 335:1445–1453, 1996.
37. Doern GV, Brueggemann A, Holley HP Jr, Rauch AM: Antimicrobial resistance of *Streptococcus pneumoniae* recovered from outpatients in the United States during the winter months of 1994 to 1995: Results of a 30-center national surveillance study. Antimicrob Agents Chemother 40:1209–1213, 1996.
38. Spangler SK, Jacobs MR, Appelbaum PC: Susceptibilities of penicillin-susceptible and -resistant strains of *Streptococcus pneumoniae* to RP 59500, vancomycin, erythromycin, PD 131628, sparfloxacin, temafloxacin, Wm 57273, ofloxacin and ciprofloxacin. Antimicrob Agents Chemother 36:856–859, 1992.
39. Austrian R, Gold J: Pneumococcal bacteremia with especial reference to bacteremic pneumococcal pneumonia. Ann Intern Med 60:759–776, 1964.
40. Pallares R, Linares J, Vadillo M, et al: Resistance to penicillin and cephalosporin and mortality from severe pneumococcal pneumonia in Barcelona, Spain. N Engl J Med 333:474–480, 1995.
41. Marrie TJ: Normal resolution of community-acquired pneumonia. Semin Respir Infect 7:256–270, 1992.
42. Meeker DP, Longworth DL: Community-acquired pneumonia: An update. Cleve Clin J Med 63:16–30, 1996.
43. Rello J, Quintana E, Ausina V, et al: A three-year study of severe community-acquired pneumonia with emphasis on outcome. Chest 103:232–235, 1993.
44. Mittl RL Jr, Schwab RJ, Duchin JS, et al: Radiographic resolution of community-acquired pneumonia. Am J Respir Crit Care Med 149:630–635, 1994.
45. Fedson DS: Improving the use of pneumococcal vaccine through a strategy of hospital based immunization. J Am Geriatr Soc 33:142–150, 1985.
46. Pfeiffer R: Vorlaufige Mitteilungen über die Effeger der Influenza. Dtsch Med Wochenschr 18:28, 1892.
47. Blake FG, Cecil RL: Studies on experimental pneumonia. J Exp Med 32:691, 1920.
48. Cecil RL, Blake FG: Studies on experimental pneumonia. Pathology of experimental influenza and of *Bacillus influenzae* pneumonia in monkeys. J Exp Med 32:719, 1920.
49. Smith W, Andrews CH, Laidlaw PP: A virus obtained from influenza patients. Lancet 2:66, 1933.
50. Pittman M: Variation and type specificity in the bacterial species *Hemophilus influenzae*. J Exp Med 53:471, 1931.
51. Keefer CS, Rammelkamp CH: *Hemophilus influenzae* bacteremia. Ann Intern Med 16:1221, 1942.
52. Ginsberg CM, Howard JB, Nelson JD: Report of 65 cases of *Haemophilus influenzae* b pneumonia. Pediatrics 64:283–286, 1979.
53. Jacobs NM, Harris VJ: Acute *Haemophilus* pneumonia in childhood. Am J Dis Child 133:603–605, 1979.
54. Centers for Disease Control and Prevention: Progress toward elimination of *Haemophilus influenzae* type b disease among infants and children—United States, 1987–1995. MMWR Morbid Mortal Wkly Rep 45:901–905, 1996.
55. Wallace RJ Jr, Musher DM, Martin RR: *Hemophilus influenzae* pneumonia in adults. Am J Med 64:87–93, 1978.
56. Everett ED, Rahm AE, Aaniya MR, et al: *Haemophilus influenzae* pneumonia in adults. JAMA 238:319–321, 1977.
57. Goldstein E, Daly AK, Seamans C: *Haemophilus influenzae* as a cause of adult pneumonia. Ann Intern Med 66:35–40, 1967.
58. Johnson WD, Kaye D, Hook EW: *Hemophilus influenzae* pneumonia in adults. Report of five cases and review of the literature. Am Rev Respir Dis 97:1112–1117, 1968.
59. Levin DC, Schwarz MI, Matthay RA, LaForce FM: Bacteremic *Hemophilus influenzae* pneumonia in adults. A report of 24 cases and a review of the literature. Am J Med 62:219–224, 1977.
60. Weinstein L: Type b *Haemophilus influenzae* infections in adults. N Engl J Med 282:221–222, 1970.
61. Austrian R: The bacterial flora of the respiratory tract: Some knowns and unknowns. Yale J Biol Med 40:400–413, 1968.
62. Holdaway MD, Turk DC: Capsulated *Haemophilus influenzae* and respiratory tract disease. Lancet 1:358–360, 1967.
63. Steinhart R, Reingold AL, Taylor F, et al: Invasive *Haemophilus influenzae* infections in men with HIV infection. JAMA 268:3350–3352, 1992.
64. Mulder J, Goslings WRO, Van der Plas MC, Cardozo PL: Studies on the treatment with antibacterial drugs of acute and chronic mucopurulent bronchitis caused by *Haemophilus influenzae*. Acta Med Scand 143:32–48, 1952.
65. Gump DW, Phillips CA, McIntosh K, et al: Role of infection in chronic bronchitis. Am Rev Respir Dis 113:465–474, 1976.
66. Bartlett J: Diagnostic accuracy of transtracheal aspiration bacteriologic studies. Am Rev Respir Dis 115:777–782, 1977.
67. Bjerkestrand G, Digranes A, Schreiner A: Bacteriological findings in transtracheal aspirates from patients with chronic bronchitis and bronchiectasis. Scand J Respir Dis 56:201–207, 1975.
68. Fraenkel A: Spezielle Pathologie und Therapie der Lungenkrankheiten. Berlin, Urban and Schwarzenberg, 1904.
69. Netter R: Étude bacteriologique de la bronchopneumonie chez l'adulte et chez l'enfant. Arch Med Exp 4:28–65, 1882.
70. Chickering HT, Park JH Jr: *Staphylococcus aureus* pneumonia. JAMA 72:617–626, 1919.
71. Martin CM, Kunin CM, Gottleib LS, et al: Asian influenza A in Boston, 1957–1958. Arch Intern Med 103:532, 1959.

72. Schwarzmann SW, Adler JL, Sullivan RJ, et al: Bacterial pneumonia during the Hong Kong influenza epidemic of 1968–1969. Arch Intern Med 127:1037–1041, 1971.
73. Relman HA: Primary staphylococcus pneumonia. JAMA 101:514–520, 1933.
74. Niederman MS: Gram-negative colonization of the respiratory tract: Pathogenesis and clinical consequences. Semin Respir Infect 5:173–181, 1990.
75. Fagon JY, Chastre J, Hance AJ, et al: Detection of nosocomial lung infection in ventilated patients: Use of a protected specimen brush and quantitative culture techniques in 147 patients. Am Rev Respir Dis 138:110–116, 1988.
76. Espersen F, Gabrielsen J: Pneumonia due to *Staphylococcus aureus* during mechanical ventilation. J Infect Dis 144:19–23, 1981.
77. Heldman AW, Hartert TV, Ray SC, et al: Oral antibiotic treatment of right-sided staphylococcal endocarditis in injection drug users: Prospective randomized comparison with parenteral therapy. Am J Med 101:68–76, 1996.
78. Fick RB Jr, Sonoda F, Hornick DB: Emergence and persistence of *Pseudomonas aeruginosa* in the cystic fibrosis airway. Semin Respir Infect 7:168–178, 1992.
79. Hirschtick RE, Glassroth J: *Staphylococcus aureus* pneumonia: When to suspect—How to treat. J Crit Illness 7:1576–1586, 1992.
80. Victoria MS, Steiner P, Rao M: Persistent post pneumonic pneumatoceles in children. Chest 79:359–361, 1981.
81. Warner JO, Gordon I: Pneumatoceles following *Haemophilus influenzae* pneumonia. Clin Radiol 32:99–105, 1981.
82. Kanof A, Kramer B, Carnes M: *Staphylococcus* pneumonia. J Pediatr 14:712, 1939.
83. Kirmani N, Tuazon CU, Murray HW, et al: *Staphylococcus aureus* carriage rate of patients receiving long-term hemodialysis. Arch Intern Med 138:1657, 1978.
84. Tuazon CU, Sheagren JN: Increased rate of carriage of *Staphylococcus aureus* among narcotic addicts. J Infect Dis 129:725–727, 1974.
85. Fainstein V, Musher DM, Cate TR: Bacterial adherence to pharyngeal cells during viral infection. J Infect Dis 141:172–176, 1980.
86. Narqi S, McDonnell G: Hematogenous staphylococcal pneumonia secondary to soft tissue infection. Chest 79:173–175, 1981.
87. Tsao TCY, Tsai YH, Lan RS, et al: Pulmonary manifestations of *Staphylococcus aureus* septicemia. Chest 101:574–576, 1992.
88. Mylotte JM, McDermott C, Spooner JA: Prospective study of 114 consecutive episodes of *Staphylococcus aureus* bacteremia. Rev Infect Dis 9:891–907, 1987.
89. Onofrio JM, Toews GB, Lipscomb MF, et al: Granulocyte-alveolar-macrophage interaction in the pulmonary clearance of *Staphylococcus aureus*. Am Rev Respir Dis 127:335–341, 1983.
90. Fisher AM, Trever RT, Curtin JA, et al: Staphylococcal pneumonia. A review of 21 cases in adults. N Engl J Med 258:919, 1958.
91. Rebhan AW, Edwards HE: Staphylococcal pneumonia: A review of 329 cases. Can Med Assoc J 82:513–517, 1960.
92. Watanakunakorn C: Bacteremic *Staphylococcus aureus* pneumonia. Scand J Infect Dis 19:623–627, 1987.
93. Kaye MG, Fox MJ, Bartlett JG, et al: The clinical spectrum of *Staphylococcus aureus* pulmonary infection. Chest 97:788–792, 1990.
94. Kuberman AS, Fernandez RB: Subacute staphylococcal pneumonia. Am Rev Respir Dis 101:95–99, 1970.
95. Garb JL, Brown RB, Garb JR, Tuthill RW: Differences in the etiology of pneumonias in nursing home and community patients. JAMA 240:2169–2172, 1978.
96. Weese WC, Shindler ER, Smith IM, et al: Empyema of the thorax then and now. Arch Intern Med 131:516–520, 1973.
97. Ede S, Davis GM, Holmes FH: Staphylococcic pneumonia. JAMA 170:638–643, 1959.
98. Bartlett JG: Bacterial infections of the pleural space. Semin Respir Infect 3:308–321, 1988.
99. Kain KC, Schulzer M, Chow AW: Clinical spectrum of nonmenstrual toxic shock syndrome (TSS): Comparison with menstrual TSS by multivariate discriminant analysis. Clin Infect Dis 16:100–106, 1993.
100. Fletcher W: Meningococcus broncho-pneumonia in influenza. Lancet 1:104–105, 1919.
101. Herrick WW: Extra-meningeal meningococcus infections. Arch Intern Med 23:409–419, 1919.
102. Holm ML, Davidson WC: Meningococcus pneumonia. Bull Hopkins Hosp 30:324–329, 1919.
103. Brick IB: Meningococcal pneumonia. Report of two cases with meningococcal effusion in one. N Engl J Med 238:289–291, 1948.
104. Meltzer JI, Kneeland Y Jr: Primary meningococcal lobar pneumonia without meningitis. Ann Intern Med 46:183–186, 1959.
105. Paine TF Jr, Garrard CL, Walker PJ: Meningococcal pneumonia. Arch Intern Med 119:111–112, 1967.
106. Ball JH, Young DA: Primary meningococcal pneumonia. Am Rev Respir Dis 109:480–483, 1974.
107. Irwin RS, Woelk WK, Coudon WL III: Primary meningococcal pneumonia. Ann Intern Med 82:493–498, 1975.
108. Reinecke ME: Group-Y meningococcal disease. Ann Intern Med 82:719–720, 1975.
109. Barnes RV, Dopp AC, Gelberg HJ, Silva J Jr: *Neisseria meningitidis*: A cause of nosocomial pneumonia. Am Rev Respir Dis 111:229–231, 1975.
110. Galpin JE, Chow AW, Yoshikawa TT: Meningococcal pneumonia. Am J Med Sci 269:247–250, 1975.
111. Cohen MS, Steere AC, Baltimore R, et al: Possible nosocomial transmission of group Y *Neisseria meningitidis* among oncology patients. Ann Intern Med 91:7–12, 1979.
112. Rose HD, Lenz IE, Sheth NK: Meningococcal pneumonia: A source of nosocomial infection. Arch Intern Med 141:575–577, 1981.
113. Young LS: A simultaneous outbreak of meningococcal and influenza infections. N Engl J Med 287:5–8, 1972.
114. Reinarz TA, Sande MA, Silva J Jr: Bacterial pneumonia complicating adenoviral pneumonia. Am J Med 56:169–178, 1974.
115. Goldstein E: Murine resistance to inhaled *Neisseria meningitidis* after infection with an encephalomyocarditis virus. Infect Immun 6:398–402, 1972.
116. Nikoskelainen J, Leino A, Lahtonen E, et al: Is group specific meningococcal vaccination resulting in epidemics caused by groups of virulent meningococci? Lancet 2:403–405, 1978.
117. Jacobs SA, Norden CW: Pneumonia caused by *Neisseria meningitidis*. JAMA 227:67–68, 1974.
118. Lewis JF, Arnold C, Alexander J: Meningococcal pneumonia. Am J Clin Pathol 59:388–390, 1973.
119. Putsch RW, Hamilton JD, Wolinsky E: *Neisseria meningitidis*, a respiratory pathogen? J Infect Dis 121:48–54, 1970.
120. Farrell DG, Dahl EV: Nasopharyngeal carriers of *Neisseria meningitidis*: Studies among Air Force recruits. JAMA 198:1189–1192, 1966.
121. Enos WF, Beyer JC, Zimmet SM, Kiesel JA: Unilateral lobar pneumonia with empyema caused by *Neisseria gonorrhoeae*. S Med J 73:266–267, 1980.
122. Johnson MA, Drew WL, Roberts M: *Branhamella (Neisseria) catarrhalis*—A lower respiratory tract pathogen? J Clin Microbiol 13:1066–1069, 1981.
123. Srinivasan G, Raff MJ, Templeton WC, et al: *Branhamella catarrhalis* pneumonia: Report of two cases and review of the literature. Am Rev Respir Dis 123:553–555, 1981.
124. Friedländer C: Über die Schizomyceter bei der acuten fibrosen Pneumonie. Virchows Arch Pathol Anat 87:319, 1882.
125. Belk WP: Pulmonary infections by Friedländer's bacillus. J Infect Dis 38:115, 1926.
126. Fremmel F, Henrichsen KJ, Sweany HC: Pulmonary infections by Friedländer's bacillus. Ann Intern Med 5:886, 1932.
127. Bullowa JGM, Chess J, Friedman NB: Pneumonia due to *Bacillus friedländeri*. Arch Intern Med 9:735–752, 1937.
128. Collins LH Jr: Chronic pulmonary infection due to the Friedländer bacillus. Arch Intern Med 58:235, 1936.
129. Olcott CT: Pneumonia due to Friedländer's bacillus. Arch Pathol 16:471, 1933.
130. Solomon S: Primary Friedländer pneumonia. JAMA 108:937, 1937.
131. Bullowa JGM: Management of the Pneumonias. New York, Oxford University Press, 1937, p 508.
132. Tillotson JR, Lerner AM: Pneumonias: Caused by gram negative bacilli. Medicine (Baltimore) 45:65–76, 1966.
133. Celis R, Torres A, Gatell JM, et al: Nosocomial pneumonia. A multivariate analysis of risk and prognosis. Chest 93:318–324, 1988.
134. American Thoracic Society: Hospital-acquired pneumonia in adults: Diagnosis, assessment of severity, initial antimicrobial

therapy and preventative strategies. Am J Respir Crit Care Med 153:1711–1725, 1995.
135. Bartlett JG, O'Keefe P, Tally FP, et al: Bacteriology of hospital-acquired pneumonia. Arch Intern Med 146:868–871, 1986.
136. Fagon JY, Chastre J, Hance A, et al: Nosocomial pneumonia in ventilated patients: A cohort study evaluating attributable mortality and hospital stay. Am J Med 94:281–288, 1993.
137. Bryan CS, Reynolds KL: Bacteremic nosocomial pneumonia. Am Rev Respir Dis 129:668–671, 1984.
138. Torres A, Puig de la Bellacasa JP, Xaubet A, et al: Diagnostic value of quantitative cultures of bronchoalveolar lavage and telescoping plugged catheters in mechanically ventilated patients with bacterial pneumonia. Am Rev Respir Dis 140:306–310, 1989.
139. Johanson WG, Pierce AK, Sanford JP: Changing pharyngeal bacterial flora of hospitalized patients: Emergence of gram-negative bacilli. N Engl J Med 281:1137–1140, 1969.
140. Montgomerie JZ: Epidemiology of *Klebsiella* and hospital-associated infections. Rev Infect Dis 1:736–752, 1979.
141. Tillotson JR, Finland M: Bacterial colonization and clinical superinfection of the respiratory tract complicating antibiotic treatment of pneumonia. J Infect Dis 119:597–624, 1969.
142. Kuhn HM, Meier-Dieter U, Mayer H: ECA, the enterobacterial common antigen. FEMS Microbiol Rev 4:195–222, 1988.
143. Edwards PP, Fife MA: Capsule types of *Klebsiella*. J Infect Dis 91:92–104, 1952.
144. Benge GR: Bactericidal activity of human serum against strains of *Klebsiella* from different sources. J Med Microbiol 27:11–15, 1988.
145. Coonrod JD: Pulmonary opsonins in *Klebsiella pneumoniae* pneumonia in rats. Infect Immun 33:533–539, 1981.
146. Domenico P, Johanson WG, Straus DC: Lobar pneumonia in rats produced by clinical isolates of *Klebsiella pneumoniae*. Infect Immun 37:327–335, 1982.
147. Julianelle LA: Biological classification of *Encapsulatus pneumoniae* (Friedländer's bacillus). J Exp Med 44:113, 1926.
148. Nowotny A: Review of the molecular requirements of endotoxic actions. Rev Infect Dis 9(Suppl 5):S503–S511, 1987.
149. Arakawa Y, Ohta M, Wacharotayankun R, et al: Biosynthesis of *Klebsiella* K2 capsular polysaccharide in *Escherichia coli* HB101 requires the functions of rmpA and the chromosomal cps gene cluster of the virulent strain *Klebsiella pneumoniae* Chedid (O1:K2). Infect Immun 59:2043–2050, 1991.
150. Fader RC, Gondesen K, Tolley B, et al: Evidence that in vitro adherence of *Klebsiella pneumoniae* to ciliated hamster tracheal cells is mediated by type 1 fimbriae. J Bacteriol 56:3011–3013, 1988.
151. Hata JS, Fick RB: Airway adherence of *Pseudomonas aeruginosa*: Mucoexopolysaccharide binding to human and bovine airway proteins. J Lab Clin Med 117:410–422, 1991.
152. Ramphal R, Pier GB: Role of *Pseudomonas aeruginosa* mucoid exopolysaccharide in adherence to tracheal cells. Infect Immun 47:1–7, 1985.
153. Woods DE, Straus DC, Johanson WG Jr, Bass JA: Role of salivary protease activity in adherence of gram-negative bacilli to mammalian buccal epithelial cells in vivo. J Clin Invest 68:1435–1440, 1981.

56

Bronchitis

John G. Bartlett

Bronchitis is one of the most common conditions encountered in clinical practice. In general, there are two main categories: acute bronchitis and exacerbations of chronic bronchitis. Related syndromes based on the common clinical feature of cough include "postnasal drip syndrome," asthma, gastroesophageal reflux, chronic bronchitis, bronchiectasis, and selected miscellaneous conditions (sarcoidosis, lung cancer, heart failure, and Zenker diverticulum).[1] There are multiple causes of bronchitis, and infection is only one of many. This review deals with the clinical features of acute bronchitis and exacerbations of chronic bronchitis with guidelines for medical management.

Acute Bronchitis

Incidence

Bronchitis has been known throughout the history of medicine but is clearly more common since the industrial revolution and widespread use of cigarettes. It is most common during acute respiratory tract infections, especially during winter months. Annual attack rates of bronchitis in surveys of general practice in Great Britain are 40% to 50% and are four to five times higher in the winter than in the summer.[2] Approximately 30% to 50% of all cases of common upper respiratory tract infections are accompanied by cough.[3–6]

Definition

Acute bronchitis is an isolated event characterized by inflammation of the tracheobronchial tree. Anatomic studies of the tracheobronchial tree show hyperemia and edema with increased bronchial secretions. There may be destruction of the respiratory epithelium, which is most extensive with influenza[7] but minimal with other viral infections, such as those caused by rhinovirus.[8] Mucociliary function may be diminished even when mucosal damage is minimal.[9] The usual clinical expression is cough that is commonly accompanied by sputum production, and there may be associated fever and constitutional complaints. The severity of symptoms may be increased with exposure to cigarette smoke and air pollution. Studies of pulmonary function show an increase in airway resistance and reactivity.[10, 11] A major sequela is asthma, including previously undiagnosed asthma.[12, 13] It is possible that acute bronchitis may be a contributing factor to chronic obstructive lung disease.[14, 15] The major considerations in the differential diagnosis are pneumonia and upper respiratory tract conditions such as sinusitis or allergic rhinitis with bronchial drainage. Pneumonia can be distinguished with a chest radiograph showing the absence of a pulmonary infiltrate. Upper respiratory tract conditions can often be distinguished by the symptom complex, including the patient's perception of postnasal drainage.

Etiology

Infectious causes of acute bronchitis are primarily viral and include influenza A and B viruses, parainfluenza virus, rhinovirus, coronavirus, adenovirus, and respiratory syncytial virus (Table 56–1). Potentially treatable causes of acute bronchitis are *Mycoplasma pneumoniae, Chlamydia pneumoniae*, influenza A virus, and *Bordetella pertussis*.[16–19]

M. pneumoniae infection is a common one in young adults with clinical features that include pharyngitis, fever, constitutional symptoms, and relatively high rates of extrapulmonary complications.[16] The course is self-limited, usually with recovery in 1 to 2 weeks, but occasional cases are relatively chronic with persistent symptoms for up to 4 to 6 weeks. The cough is usually accompanied by production of mucoid sputum. The diagnosis may be established by recovery of *M. pneumoniae*, serial serologic studies showing a fourfold rise in titer, an elevated serum immunoglobulin M titer, or gene amplification with polymerase chain reaction.[20, 21]

C. pneumoniae is a relatively newly recognized agent of respiratory tract infections that is most common in young adults.[17] Common clinical features include pharyngitis, laryngitis, and bronchitis expressed with hoarseness, low-grade fever, and a cough that may persist for several weeks. This agent has been implicated in new-onset asthma and asthmatic bronchitis.[18] Diagnostic studies include serology, tissue culture, and polymerase chain reaction.[22, 23] These laboratory studies are controversial, and for practical purposes, most physicians do not have access to laboratories with appropriate diagnostic resources to detect *C. pneumoniae*.

Pertussis is a disease with substantial potential morbidity and mortality that has been notably reduced since the vaccine was introduced in the 1940s. The epidemiology of this disease since the early 1980s shows periodic increases in reported cases. Current rates in the United States are 1.5 to 3.0 cases per 100,000 population.[24] This is primarily a disease of children, but about 30% of pertussis cases are reported in persons older than 10 years. The experience with the current vaccine shows 64% protection against mild disease and 95% protection against serious disease.[25] Patients at greatest risk are those who have not received the vaccine, primarily infants but also some adults. Exposure is obviously necessary so that an infected infant may become the source of infection for close contacts including family members, schoolmates, other persons in daycare centers, and the like. The major clinical feature in adults is a barking cough that is often so prominent and severe that the patient has difficulty completing a sentence. Another common feature is the persistence of this cough for more than 3 weeks, which applies to 80% of adults with pertussis.[26] Diagnosis is established with the traditional cough plate, in which the agar plate appropriate for culture of *B. pertussis* is held before the patient's mouth for aerosolized inoculation during a typical coughing bout.

TABLE 56–1 ■ Acute Bronchitis: Infectious Agents and Treatment

AGENT	TREATMENT
Viral	
Influenza A virus	Amantadine or rimantadine
Influenza B virus	—
Parainfluenza virus	—
Coronavirus	—
Respiratory syncytial virus	—
Rhinovirus	—
Adenovirus	—
Bacterial and Bacteria-Like	
Mycoplasma pneumoniae	Doxycycline or macrolide*
Chlamydia pneumoniae	Doxycycline or macrolide*
Bordetella pertussis	Erythromycin

*Macrolides are erythromycin, azithromycin, and clarithromycin.

An alternative is nasopharyngeal aspirate or, possibly in the near future, polymerase chain reaction.[27, 28]

Influenza is another potentially treatable cause of bronchitis. The usual clinical features are respiratory tract complaints accompanied by bronchitis; the production of mucoid or purulent sputum; and constitutional symptoms that may be profound and include fever, fatigue, and malaise. Many patients have prolonged periods in which there is reduced pulmonary function after apparent clinical recovery.[29, 30] The diagnosis is established by viral culture, fluorescent stain of respiratory secretion, or demonstration of seroconversion. For practical purposes, the diagnosis is generally based on the observation of typical symptoms with an exposure history in a location associated with an influenza epidemic.

There is often suspicion that acute bronchitis may be caused by common bacterial pathogens of the upper airways, including *Streptococcus pneumoniae, Haemophilus influenzae*, or *Staphylococcus aureus*. Nevertheless, there is sparse support of this assumption with the possible exception of neonates, patients with airway violations such as tracheostomy or endotracheal intubation, or immunosuppressed hosts. These bacteria may be responsible for pulmonary superinfections in patients with influenza, and possibly other viral respiratory tract infections, but these appear to be inevitably associated with a pulmonary infiltrate indicating pneumonia rather than bronchitis.[31]

Clinical Presentation

Cough is the prominent feature in patients with acute bronchitis. This is noted in 70% to 90% of patients with influenza and 30% to 50% of patients with other common viral infections of the upper airways.[3–6] The cough is usually nonproductive initially and then becomes productive of mucoid or purulent sputum. The cough resolves spontaneously within 2 weeks in approximately half of patients. Prolonged cough often suggests *C. pneumoniae* infection or pertussis, but cough may last 3 weeks or longer in patients with common viral infections of the upper airways including rhinovirus infection.[32] A review by Kaiser Permanente in San Francisco from 1994 to 1995 showed that 12% of 154 adult patients complaining of cough persisting longer than 2 weeks had serologic evidence of pertussis.[33] The diagnosis of pertussis was not suspected by the clinician in any of these cases. Dyspnea is unusual with acute bronchitis except for patients with chronic obstructive lung disease. Fever is common in patients with influenza virus, adenovirus, *M. pneumoniae*, and *C. pneumoniae* infections; fever is unusual with common viral infections of the upper airways. Physical examination often reveals rhonchi but no rales or signs of consolidation. Wheezing is relatively common in patients with asthma.

Most patients with bronchitis do not undergo diagnostic studies except for a possible chest radiograph to exclude pneumonia, which is best justified in patients with rales, severe symptoms, and fever. Diagnostic studies may be done for detection of influenza virus, *M. pneumoniae, B. pertussis*, or *C. pneumoniae*. Guidelines for these tests are noted earlier, but the availability of appropriate diagnostic technology is often limited, and this would not be considered cost-effective in the majority of cases.

Cough is defined as chronic when it persists for 3 weeks. For nonsmoking patients with normal findings on a chest radiograph, the most common cause is the postnasal drip syndrome followed by asthma and gastroesophageal reflux (Table 56–2). Chronic bronchitis ascribed to smoking or to environmental pollutants ("industrial asthma") is the most common cause of chronic cough. Other causes are tuberculosis, bronchiectasis, angiotensin-converting enzyme inhibitors, congestive heart failure, sarcoidosis, Zenker diverticulum,

TABLE 56–2 ■ Major Causes of Chronic Cough in Nonsmoking Patients with Normal Findings on Chest Radiography

CONDITION	FREQUENCY (%)	PRESUMPTIVE DIAGNOSIS
Postnasal drip syndrome	41	Sensation of posterior drainage Frequent clearing of throat Examination of nasopharynx shows mucoid or mucopurulent secretions Radiography shows sinusitis
Asthma	24	Episodic wheezing, dyspnea with cough Physical examination shows wheezing Pulmonary function tests show reversible airway obstruction
Gastroesophageal reflux	21	Heartburn or sour taste in mouth Demonstration of reflux with radiography, endoscopy, or esophageal monitoring
Chronic bronchitis	5	Satisfy definition Pulmonary function tests show irreversible airway obstruction
Bronchiectasis	4	Cough with >30 mL discolored sputum per day Radiography or high-resolution computed tomography shows typical changes

Adapted from Irwin RS, Curley FJ, French CL: Chronic cough. The spectrum and frequency of causes, key components of the diagnostic evaluation, and outcome of specific therapy. Am Rev Respir Dis 141:640–647, 1990.

and carcinoma. The postnasal drip syndrome is an unscientific term referring to a number of clinical conditions of the upper respiratory tract characterized by postnasal drainage. Most of these patients describe the sensation of postnasal drainage with chronic cough or a perceived need to clear the throat. The usual causes include the common cold, allergic rhinitis, vasomotor rhinitis, postinfectious rhinitis, sinusitis, drug-induced conditions (primarily angiotensin-converting enzyme inhibitors), and environmental irritants. The relative frequency of these conditions among patients with chronic cough (defined as cough lasting longer than 3 weeks) who do not smoke and who have normal findings at chest radiography is summarized in Table 56–2. A diagnosis may be established in more than 90% of these patients.[1] The usual diagnostic evaluation includes a history, physical examination, and chest radiography; this evaluation is followed by appropriate tests based on initial observations in terms of probabilities. With identification of the cause, therapy successfully eliminates the cough in more than 90% of patients.

Treatment

The major treatment for constitutional symptoms including fever is aspirin or acetaminophen and restricted activity with appropriate precautions for preventing transmission. Cough suppressants (dextromethorphan, 15 mg orally every 6 hours) or, for more severe cough, cough suppressants containing codeine have established efficacy.[34] Expectorants are not advocated; virtually all contain guaifenesin and have failed to provide benefit in controlled trials.[35] In patients with wheezing, the treatment should include bronchodilators.[36] Patients with serious associated chronic lung disease may require ventilatory support and oxygen therapy. Antibiotics play a limited role in acute bronchitis because most cases are due to viral infections. Occasional exceptions are *M. pneumoniae* or *C. pneumoniae* infections that may be responsive to doxycycline or a macrolide, pertussis treated with erythromycin, or influenza treated with rimantadine or amantadine. Several trials have demonstrated that oral β-lactam drugs with activity against *S. pneumoniae, H. influenzae,* and *Branhamella (Moraxella) catarrhalis* will effectively eliminate these suspected pathogens in patients with acute bronchitis, but these are not placebo-controlled trials that would be necessary to document clinical benefit.[37–40] The assumption is that these organisms, when found in expectorated secretions in patients with acute bronchitis, merely reflect colonization of the upper airways. Properly controlled trials have demonstrated that doxycycline, tetracycline, and erythromycin confer no benefit in terms of the duration of cough, duration of sputum production, and loss of work.[41–44] Another trial suggested that doxycycline was associated with a modest benefit in patients older than 55 years with frequent cough and systemic complaints,[45] but this report has been criticized because of methodologic problems.[31] Despite these findings, surveys of physicians indicate that 50% to 70% of patients with acute bronchitis are treated with antibiotics,[46, 47] leading to the conclusion that this is a syndrome associated with substantial antibiotic abuse.[31]

Exacerbations of Chronic Bronchitis

Definition

Chronic bronchitis is characterized by cough and sputum production for an extended time. The standard definition is arbitrarily a productive cough and sputum production for at least 3 months per year for at least 2 years that is not caused by other conditions such as tuberculosis or bronchiectasis.[48] Many patients have emphysema, and the two conditions are commonly combined with the appellation "chronic obstructive lung disease with bronchitis and emphysema." Chronic bronchitis associated with wheezing is often referred to as chronic or recurrent asthmatic bronchitis.

Incidence

Chronic bronchitis is noted in 10% to 25% of the adult population, is more common in men than in women, and is most common in persons older than 40 years. Chronic obstructive lung disease represents the fifth leading cause of death in the United States.

Etiology

The major contributing factors in chronic bronchitis are cigarette smoking, infection, and environmental pollution. Industrial bronchitis is the term commonly used for bronchitis resulting from occupational exposure to dust, gas, or fumes.[49, 50] A small subset of these patients have congenital defects or immunodeficiency syndromes, such as cystic fibrosis, immunoglobulin A or selective immunoglobulin G subclass deficiency, abnormal polymorphonuclear function, primary ciliary dyskinesia, or α_1-globulin deficiency. The major culprit is cigarette smoking, and the frequency depends on the extent of smoking exposure. For patients with a history of 40 to 60 packs per year, the frequency of chronic bronchitis approaches 50%.[51] The usual pathologic change noted in the lungs of patients with chronic bronchitis is an increase in the number of goblet cells on the surface epithelium of the bronchi with an increase in mucous glands.[52, 53]

Clinical Presentation

The hallmark of chronic bronchitis is the chronic cough, which is often accompanied by tenacious, mucoid sputum. Exacerbation may be ascribed to any of the following: smoking, air pollution, allergens, occupational exposure, and preclinical or subclinical asthma. Infection is thought to be an important cause, but this has been difficult to prove on the basis of microbiologic studies or with clinical trials. The organisms most commonly implicated are viral agents that cause upper respiratory tract infections and two commonly found bacterial species: *S. pneumoniae* and *H. influenzae*. Exacerbation of chronic bronchitis is one of the conditions in medicine that has been most extensively studied, but the role of infection as a major cause or as a factor in promoting progression of the underlying condition remains inconclusive. The following conclusions can be made on the basis of multiple studies:

1. Viral infections are found in association with exacerbations in 7% to 64% of cases.[54–58] Perhaps the best studies have been done by Gump and colleagues,[55] who found viral infections in 32% of patients during exacerbations compared with 1% during remissions. Most commonly implicated are influenza A or B virus, parainfluenza virus, coronavirus, and rhinovirus.[54–60]

2. The role of bacterial infection in exacerbations and in progression of chronic obstructive lung disease has been examined with sequential cultures, response rates to antibiotics in controlled trials, and sputum cytology. Sputum cytology is based on quantitative assessment of expectorated secretions obtained sequentially for a period of years during exacerbations and during periods of relative quiescence.[61, 62] Results indicate high concentrations of polymorphonuclear cells throughout the course of chronic bronchitis without notable changes during exacerbations. Thus, the perception of increased purulence cannot be confirmed by the concentration of leukocytes. Biopsies of bronchi show increased mucosal and mural inflammation with increased numbers of macrophages, CD4$^+$ lymphocytes, and CD8$^+$ lymphocytes.[63, 64]

3. Bacterial cultures of expectorated sputum in patients with chronic bronchitis show a high yield of potential respiratory tract pathogens during both exacerbations and remissions. One of the most comprehensive studies was by Gump and coworkers,[55] who periodically obtained sputum from patients with chronic bronchitis for a period of years and performed quantitative cultures using serial dilutions. This work showed high counts of potential pathogens, primarily *S. pneumoniae* and *H. influenzae*, during both exacerbations and remissions; the mean count was about 10^7 per mL. The yield of *S. pneumoniae* in culture is 15% to 50%, but it is no higher during exacerbations than in remissions.[55, 65, 66] Similar data apply to *H. influenzae*.[55, 65–67] Nearly all strains of *H. influenzae* are nontypable.[67] Transtracheal aspirates from many patients with chronic obstructive lung disease and chronic bronchitis show high rates of lower airway colonization by bacteria that are not seen in healthy control subjects; the dominant organisms are *S. pneumoniae*, *H. influenzae*, and nonpathogens such as α-hemolytic streptococci and *Haemophilus parainfluenzae*.[65, 68, 69] These studies show that patients with chronic bronchitis have high rates of colonization by multiple bacteria that extends to the tracheobronchial tract below the level of the larynx. Further, this work suggests that exacerbations cannot be distinguished from relatively quiescent periods in patients with chronic bronchitis by bacteriology studies using transtracheal aspirates or quantitative cultures of expectorated sputum.

4. There are multiple studies of antibiotics given for the treatment of exacerbations of chronic bronchitis, but relatively few have an appropriate study format with a placebo control.[70–80] Antibiotics used in the studies that are considered optimal in terms of trial design include amoxicillin, tetracyclines, trimethoprim-sulfamethoxazole, and chloramphenicol. One of the largest studies was a double-blind, placebo-controlled trial of 173 patients with 362 exacerbations.[73] This showed an accelerated clinical recovery in 68% of antibiotic recipients compared with 55% in the placebo group, a difference that was statistically significant. Saint and colleagues[72] have provided a metaanalysis of published trials to address this issue. A review of published reports from 1955 to 1994 showed that only 9 of 214 reports satisfied the selection criteria for a randomized trial with antibiotic treatment versus placebo (Table 56–3). The outcome parameters were diverse and included days of illness, symptom score, physician's evaluation, and peak expiratory flow rates. Results were variable, but seven of the nine studies showed a benefit of treatment, and the overall results demonstrated a small but statistically significant improvement. Analysis of six studies that measured peak expiratory flow rates showed

TABLE 56–3 ■ Antibiotics for Exacerbations of Chronic Obstructive Lung Disease: Metaanalysis

STUDY	NUMBER	SETTING	ANTIBIOTIC	OUTCOME	RESULT*
Elmes et al,[74] 1957	113	Outpatients	Tetracycline	Days of illness	Benefit; NS
Berry et al,[78] 1960	33	Outpatients	Tetracycline	Symptom score	Benefit; Sig
Fear and Edwards,[79] 1962	119	Outpatients	Tetracycline	Symptom score	Benefit; NS
Elmes et al,[75] 1965	56	Hospitalized patients	Ampicillin	PEFR†	Benefit; NS
Peterson et al,[80] 1967	19	Hospitalized patients	Chloramphenicol	PEFR	No benefit; NS
Saint et al,[72] 1995	149	Hospitalized patients	Tetracycline	Symptom score, PEFR	Benefit; Sig
Nicotra et al,[76] 1982	40	Hospitalized patients	Tetracycline	Days of illness, PEFR	Benefit; NS
Anthonisen et al,[73] 1987	310	Outpatients	TMP-SMX,† amoxicillin, or doxycycline	Days of illness, PEFR	Benefit; Sig
Jorgensen et al,[81] 1992	262	Outpatients	Amoxicillin	Symptom score, PEFR	No benefit; NS

* Results show benefit favoring antibiotic treatment. Individual studies evaluated for significance of difference for outcome measured. NS, Not statistically significant; Sig, statistically significant. The overall results showed a small but statistically significant benefit with antibiotic treatment.
† PEFR, Peak expiratory flow rates; TMP-SMX, trimethoprim-sulfamethoxazole.

an improvement of 10.75 L/min favoring antibiotic treatment.

Diagnosis

Patients with exacerbations of bronchitis need to be evaluated for the severity of symptoms to determine the need for hospitalization, supportive care, and possible antibiotic treatment. A chest radiograph is often required to evaluate for pneumonitis. The role of Gram stains and culture of expectorated sputum is debated.[81] A potential advantage is the detection of eosinophils on direct stain (or peripheral blood eosinophilia) suggestive of an allergic component.[82] Pulmonary function tests and blood gas analysis may indicate the severity of illness.

Treatment

The major treatment modality in patients who are seriously ill is respiratory support. Many patients have copious secretions and benefit from postural drainage. Treatment with a bronchodilator may be important in any patient with bronchospasm. In general, mucolytic agents and intermittent positive-pressure breathing are generally not indicated. Occasional patients with refractory symptoms benefit from systemic corticosteroid treatment.[83]

The utility of short-term antibiotic treatment is controversial, although most clinicians use these agents. The usual treatment is a 7- to 10-day course of trimethoprim-sulfamethoxazole, amoxicillin, or doxycycline based on the studies summarized before. Owing to the evolution of resistance, some now prefer oral cephalosporins, fluoroquinolone, or a macrolide directed at *S. pneumoniae* and *H. influenzae*. Potential disadvantages of these newer agents are cost and the lack of adequately controlled studies to demonstrate superiority over the alternatives suggested.

References

1. Irwin RS, Curley FJ, French CL: Chronic cough: The spectrum and frequency of causes, key components of the diagnostic evaluation, and outcome of specific therapy. Am Rev Respir Dis 141:640, 1990.
2. Ayres JG: Seasonal pattern of acute bronchitis in general practice in the United Kingdom. Thorax 41:107, 1986.
3. Dingle JH, Badger GF, Jordon WS Jr: Illness in the home: A study of 25,000 illnesses in a group of Cleveland families. Cleveland, OH, The Press of Western Reserve University, 1964, p 68.
4. Gwaltney JM Jr: Rhinoviruses. *In* Evans AS (ed): Viral Infections of Humans: Epidemiology and Control, ed 3. New York, Plenum Publishing, 1989, p 593.
5. Hendley JO, Fishburne HB, Gwaltney JM Jr: Coronavirus infections in working adults. Eight-year study with 229E and OC43. Am Rev Respir Dis 105:805, 1972.
6. Knight V, Kapikian AZ, Kravetz MH, et al: Ecology of a newly recognized common respiratory agent RS-virus. Ann Intern Med 55:507, 1961.
7. Douglas RG Jr, Alford BR, Cough RB: Atraumatic nasal biopsy for studies of respiratory virus infection in volunteers. Antimicrob Agents Chemother 8:340, 1968.
8. Winther B, Farr B, Turner RB, et al: Histopathologic examination and enumeration of polymorphonuclear leukocytes in the nasal mucosa during experimental rhinovirus colds. Acta Otolaryngol Suppl (Stockh) 413:19, 1984.
9. Sasaki Y, Togo Y, Wagner NJ Jr, et al: Mucociliary function during experimentally induced rhinovirus infection in man. Ann Otol 82:203, 1973.
10. Hall WJ, Hall CB, Speers DM: Respiratory syncytial virus infection in adults. Clinical, virologic, and serial pulmonary function studies. Ann Intern Med 88:203, 1978.
11. Boldy DAR, Skidmore SJ, Ayres JG: Acute bronchitis in the community: Clinical features, infective factors, changes in pulmonary function and bronchial reactivity to histamine. Respir Med 84:377, 1990.
12. Hallett JS, Jacobs RL: Recurrent acute bronchitis: The association with undiagnosed bronchial asthma. Ann Allergy 55:568, 1985.
13. Williamson HA Jr, Schultz P: An association between acute bronchitis and asthma. J Fam Pract 24:35, 1987.
14. Lebowitz MD, Burrows B: The relationship of acute respiratory illness history to the prevalence and incidence of obstructive lung disorders. Am J Epidemiol 105:544, 1977.
15. Monto AS, Ross HW: The Tecumseh study of respiratory illness. X. Relation of acute infections to smoking, lung function and chronic symptoms. Am J Epidemiol 107:57, 1978.
16. Denny FW, Clyde WA, Glenzen WP: *Mycoplasma pneumoniae* disease. Clinical spectrum, pathophysiology, epidemiology and control. J Infect Dis 123:74, 1971.
17. Grayston JT, Kuo C-C, Wang S-P, et al: A new *Chlamydia psittaci* strain, TWAR, isolated in acute respiratory tract infections. N Engl J Med 315:161, 1986.
18. Hahn DL, Dodge RW, Golubjatnikov R: Association of *Chlamydia pneumoniae* (strain TWAR) infection with wheezing, asthmatic bronchitis, and acute onset asthma. JAMA 266:225, 1991.
19. Herwaldt LA: Pertussis in adults. What physicians need to know. Arch Intern Med 151:1510, 1991.
20. Uldum SA, Jensen JS, Sondergard-Anderson J, et al: Enzyme immunoassay for detection of immunoglobulin M (IgM) and IgG antibodies to *Mycoplasma pneumoniae*. J Clin Microbiol 30:1198, 1992.
21. Dular R, Kajioka R, Kasatiya S: Comparison of Gen-Probe commercial kit and culture technique for the diagnosis of *Mycoplasma pneumoniae* infection. J Clin Microbiol 26:1068, 1988.
22. Campbell LA, Perez-Melgosa M, Hamilton DJ, et al: Detection of *Chlamydia pneumoniae* by polymerase chain reaction. J Clin Microbiol 30:434, 1992.
23. Gaydos CA, Quinn TC, Eiden JJ: Identification of *Chlamydia pneumoniae* by DNA amplification of the 16S rRNA gene. J Clin Microbiol 30:796, 1992.
24. Christie CDC, Marx ML, Marchant CD, Reising SF: The 1993 epidemic of pertussis in Cincinnati. N Engl J Med 331:16, 1994.
25. Jenkinson D: Duration of effectiveness of pertussis vaccine: Evidence from a 10 year community study. Br Med J 296:612, 1988.
26. Postels-Multani S, Schmitt HJ, Wirsing von Konig CH, et al: Symptoms and complications of pertussis in adults. Infection 23:139, 1995.
27. Hoppe JE: Methods for isolation of *Bordetella pertussis* from patients with whooping cough. Eur J Clin Microbiol Infect Dis 7:616, 1988.
28. Meade BD, Bollen A: Recommendations for use of the polymerase chain reaction in the diagnosis of *Bordetella pertussis* infections. J Med Microbiol 41:51, 1994.
29. Little JW, Hall WJ, Douglas RG Jr, et al: Airway hyperactivity and peripheral airway dysfunction in influenza A infection. Am Rev Respir Dis 118:295, 1978.
30. Horner GJ, Gray FD Jr: Effect of uncomplicated presumptive influenza on the diffusing capacity of the lung. Am Rev Respir Dis 108:866, 1973.
31. Gonzales R, Sande M: What will it take to stop physicians from prescribing antibiotics in acute bronchitis? Lancet 345:665, 1995.
32. Gwaltney JM Jr, Hendley JO, Simon G, et al: Rhinovirus infections in an industrial population. II. Characteristics of illness and antibody response. JAMA 202:494, 1967.
33. Nennig ME, Shinefield HR, Edwards KM, et al: Prevalence and incidence of adult pertussis in an urban population. JAMA 275:1672, 1996.
34. Eddy NB: Codeine and its alternates for pain and cough relief. Ann Intern Med 71:1209, 1969.
35. Kuhn JJ, Hendley JO, Adams KF: Antitussive effect of guaifenesin in young adults with natural colds. Objective and subjective assessment. Chest 82:713, 1982.
36. Hueston WJ: A comparison of albuterol and erythromycin for the treatment of acute bronchitis. J Fam Pract 33:476, 1991.
37. Henry D, Ruoff GE, Rhudy J: Effectiveness of short-course therapy with cefuroxime axetil in treatment of secondary bacterial infections of acute bronchitis. Antimicrob Agents Chemother 39:2528, 1995.
38. Hebblethwaite EM, Brown GW, Cox DM: A comparison of the

efficacy and safety of cefuroxime axetil and Augmentin in the treatment of upper respiratory tract infections. Drugs Exp Clin Res 2:91, 1987.
39. Nolen TM, Phillips HL, Hutchison J, Cocchetto DM: Comparison of cefuroxime axetil and cefaclor for patients with lower respiratory tract infections presenting to a rural family practice clinic. Curr Ther Res Clin Exp 44:821, 1988.
40. Schleupner CJ, Anthony WC, Tan J, et al: Blinded comparison of cefuroxime to cefaclor for lower respiratory tract infections. Arch Intern Med 148:343, 1988.
41. Howie JGR, Clark GA: Double-blind trial of early dimethylchlortetracycline in minor respiratory illness in general practice. Lancet 2:1099, 1970.
42. Stott NCH, West RR: Randomised controlled trial of antibiotics in patients with cough and purulent sputum. Br Med J 2:556, 1976.
43. Williamson HA: A randomized, controlled trial of doxycycline in the treatment of acute bronchitis. J Fam Pract 19:185, 1984.
44. Brickfield FX, Carter WH, Johnson RE: Erythromycin in the treatment of acute bronchitis in a community practice. J Fam Pract 23:119, 1986.
45. Verheij TJM, Hermans J, Mulder JD: Effects of doxycycline in patients with acute cough and purulent sputum: A double blind placebo controlled trial. Br J Gen Pract 44:400, 1994.
46. Franks P, Gleiner JA: The treatment of acute bronchitis with trimethoprim and sulfamethoxazole. J Fam Pract 19:185, 1984.
47. Verheij TJM, Hermans J, Kaptein AA, Mulder JD: Acute bronchitis: General practitioners' views regarding diagnosis and treatment. Fam Pract 7:175, 1990.
48. Dantzker DR, Pingleton SK, Pierce JA, and other Task Force Members: Standards for the diagnosis and care of patients with chronic obstructive pulmonary disease and asthma—American Thoracic Society. Am Rev Respir Dis 136:225, 1987.
49. Minette A: Is chronic bronchitis also an industrial disease? Eur J Respir Dis 69(Suppl 146):87, 1986.
50. Speizer FE, Tager B: Epidemiology of chronic mucus hypersecretion and obstructive airways disease. Epidemiol Rev 1:124, 1979.
51. Linden M, Rasmussen JB, Piitulainen E, et al: Airway inflammation in smokers with nonobstructive and obstructive chronic bronchitis. Am Rev Respir Dis 148:1226, 1993.
52. Gail DB, Lenfant CJM: Cells of the lung: Biology and clinical implications. Am Rev Respir Dis 127:366, 1983.
53. Reid L: Measurement of the bronchial mucous gland layer: A diagnostic yardstick in chronic bronchitis. Thorax 15:132, 1960.
54. Eadie MB, Stott EJ, Grist NR: Virological studies in chronic bronchitis. Br Med J 2:671, 1966.
55. Gump DW, Phillips CA, Forsyth BR, et al: Role of infection in chronic bronchitis. Am Rev Respir Dis 113:465, 1976.
56. Lamy ME, Pouthier-Simon F, Debacker-Willame E: Respiratory viral infections in hospital patients with chronic bronchitis. Chest 63:336, 1973.
57. McNamara MJ, Phillips IA, Williams OB: Viral and *Mycoplasma pneumoniae* infections in exacerbations of chronic lung disease. Am Rev Respir Dis 100:19, 1969.
58. Stark JE, Heath RB, Curwen MP: Infection with parainfluenza viruses in chronic bronchitis. Thorax 20:124,1965.
59. Buscho RO, Saxtan D, Shultz PS, et al: Infections with viruses and *Mycoplasma pneumoniae* during exacerbations of chronic bronchitis. J Infect Dis 137:377, 1978.
60. Carilli AD, Gohd RS, Gordon W: A virologic study of chronic bronchitis. N Engl J Med 270:123, 1964.
61. Chodosh S: Treatment of acute exacerbations of chronic bronchitis: State of the art. Am J Med 91(Suppl 6A):87S, 1991.
62. Chodosh S: Examination of sputum cells. N Engl J Med 282:854, 1970.
63. Fournier M, Lebargy F, Leroy Ladurie F, et al: Intraepithelial T-lymphocyte subsets in the airways of normal subjects and/or patients with chronic bronchitis. Am Rev Respir Dis 140:737, 1989.
64. Saetta M, DiStefano A, Maestrelli P, et al: Activated T-lymphocytes and macrophages in bronchia mucosa of subjects with chronic bronchitis. Am Rev Respir Dis 147:301, 1993.
65. Lees AW, McNaught W: Bacteriology of lower respiratory tract secretions, sputum, and upper respiratory tract secretions in "normals" and chronic bronchitis. Lancet 2:1112, 1959.
66. Miller DL, Jones R: The bacterial flora of the upper respiratory tract and sputum of working men. J Pathol Bacteriol 87:182, 1964.
67. Murphy TF, Apicella MA: Nontypable *Hemophilus influenzae:* A review of clinical aspects, surface antigens, and the human immune response to infection. Rev Infect Dis 9:1, 1987.
68. Bjerkestrand G, Digranes A, Schreiner A: Bacteriological findings in transtracheal aspirates from patients with chronic bronchitis and bronchiectasis. Scand J Respir Dis 56:201, 1975.
69. Bartlett J: Diagnostic accuracy of transtracheal aspiration bacteriologic studies. Am Rev Respir Dis 115:777, 1977.
70. Rodnick JE, Gude JK: The use of antibiotics in acute bronchitis and acute exacerbations of chronic bronchitis. West J Med 149:347, 1988.
71. Murphy TF, Sethi S: Bacterial infection in chronic obstructive pulmonary disease. Am Rev Respir Dis 146:1067, 1992.
72. Saint S, Bent S, Vittinghoff E, Grady D: Antibiotics in chronic obstructive pulmonary disease exacerbations: A meta-analysis. JAMA 273:957, 1995.
73. Anthonisen NR, Manfreda J, Warren CPW, et al: Antibiotic therapy in exacerbations of chronic obstructive pulmonary disease. Ann Intern Med 106:196, 1987.
74. Elmes PC, Fletcher CM, Dutton AAC: Prophylactic use of oxytetracycline for exacerbations of chronic bronchitis. Br Med J 2:1272, 1957.
75. Elmes PC, King TKC, Langlands JHM, et al: Value of ampicillin in the hospital treatment of exacerbations of chronic bronchitis. Br Med J 2:904, 1965.
76. Nicotra MB, Rivera M, Awe RJ: Antibiotic therapy of acute exacerbations of chronic bronchitis. Ann Intern Med 97:18, 1982.
77. Pines A, Raafat H, Plucinski K, et al: Antibiotic regimens in severe and acute patient exacerbations of chronic bronchitis. Br Med J 2:735, 1968.
78. Berry DG, Fry J, Hindley CP, et al: Exacerbations of chronic bronchitis treatment with oxytetracycline. Lancet 1:137, 1960.
79. Fear EC, Edwards G: Antibiotic regimes in chronic bronchitis. Br J Dis Chest 56:153, 1962.
80. Petersen ES, Esmann V, Honcke P, Munkner C: A controlled study of the effect of treatment on chronic bronchitis: An evaluation using pulmonary function tests. Acta Med Scand 182:293, 1967.
81. Jorgensen AF, Coolidge J, Pedersen PA, et al: Amoxicillin in treatment of acute uncomplicated exacerbations of chronic bronchitis. A double-blind, placebo-controlled multicentre study in general practice. Scand J Prim Health Care 10:7, 1992.
82. Corrao WM, Bramen SS, Irwin RS: Chronic cough as the sole presenting manifestation of bronchial asthma. N Engl J Med 300:633, 1979.
83. Mendella LA, Manfreda J, Warren CPW, et al: Steroid response in stable chronic obstructive lung disease. Ann Intern Med 96:17, 1982.

57

Viral Pneumonia

Stephen G. Baum
David C. Perlman

Viral pneumonia is a subset of those pneumonitides that were previously referred to as atypical pneumonia. This term arose at the beginning of the antibiotic era to describe a group of lower respiratory tract infections in which no bacterial pathogen could be identified by Gram stain or culture and that did not respond to the antibiotics then available. With the advent of cell culture techniques, it became possible to isolate viruses and thereby establish the viral etiology of many of these infections.

Numerous viruses are capable of causing pneumonia. Some, such as influenza virus, respiratory syncytial virus (RSV), and adenovirus, do so as their primary disease manifestation; some, such as paramyxovirus (measles) and varicella-zoster virus, do so as only one aspect of a multisystem disease syndrome. Although viral respiratory syndromes are generally thought to be mild and self-limited, some (such as influenza) are responsible for thousands of deaths annually and can, under epidemic conditions, kill millions of people throughout the world in a matter of a few years. An increase in the number of people who are immunocompromised by virtue of age, cancer chemotherapy, organ transplantation, and acquired immunodeficiency syndrome (AIDS) has resulted in a corresponding increase in the incidence and severity of viral pneumonias. On the other hand, effective vaccines are available to protect against several pneumotropic viruses, and only the incomplete implementation of vaccine programs prevents widespread use and the resultant reduction of morbidity, mortality, and financial cost.

Pathogens

The viruses to be discussed that are primary causes of the atypical pneumonia syndrome are influenza virus, adenovirus, RSV, parainfluenza viruses (PIVs), hantaviruses, and cytomegalovirus (CMV). Influenza virus, RSV, PIVs, and hantaviruses are single-stranded RNA viruses; adenovirus and CMV are double-stranded DNA viruses. Both adenovirus and CMV are capable of establishing latent infections that can undergo reactivation to a cellulytic cycle. Chapters on the individual viruses should be consulted for more detailed information.

Epidemiology

The epidemiology of the various pneumotropic viruses is varied, and knowledge of the epidemiology can provide the best clue as to the specific cause of the atypical pneumonia syndrome in a given patient.

Influenza is an age-old disease of worldwide distribution that received its name because the renaissance Italians thought the malady, which has a great seasonal variation in occurrence, was under the *influence* of the planets. Many if not all of the viruses discussed in this chapter can cause an influenza-like syndrome consisting of fever, malaise, cough, and myalgia. In fact, it is often difficult to differentiate disease caused by one virus from another on clinical grounds alone. Of all the agents, however, only influenza virus appears capable of the widespread epidemics and pandemics, which in turn can produce excess mortality of tens of thousands.[1]

There are three serologic types of influenza virus (A, B, and C), and these serotypes have different propensities for causing major epidemics. Type A is the cause of most epidemic disease; type B causes clusters of infection in relatively closed populations, such as boarding schools; and type C is far less common and seems to cause primarily isolated cases. Type A epidemics have historically occurred in triennial cycles, with major pandemics occurring about once every decade or two.[2] Between epidemics, this agent is also the cause of most sporadic cases of influenza throughout the world. The ability of type A virus to alter its surface antigens (hemagglutinin and neuraminidase) and its ability to infect agricultural animals, providing a reservoir of infection,[3] appears to be responsible for the periodicity of epidemics. The alteration of surface antigens is known as antigenic drift when minor changes occur and antigenic shift when these changes are more pronounced. These phenomena and the molecular biologic basis for them are described more fully in Chapter 250.

The PIVs are second only to rhinoviruses as causes of respiratory tract illnesses in humans. After RSV, PIVs are the most common cause of lower respiratory tract disease in infants throughout the world.[4] Outbreaks due to PIVs are associated with increased emergency department visits, hospitalizations, and substantial cost.[5, 6]

There are four major PIV serotypes, designated types 1 to 4, that are delineated by neutralization assays. Shared antigens, however, result in heterotypic in vivo antibody responses. PIV-4 has two major antigenic subtypes (A and B), but antigenic and genetic heterogeneity has been increasingly recognized among all four PIVs.[7–10] Antigenic drift, such as is seen with influenza A virus, has not been observed with the PIVs.[7, 8]

The PIVs have a worldwide distribution.[4] Whereas they are related to several animal paramyxoviruses, there are no known animal reservoirs for the human PIVs. PIV-1 and PIV-2 cause epidemics that occur in alternate years in the fall.[5, 6, 11] Activity of PIV-1 and PIV-2 often declines as activity of RSV rises in the late fall.[5] PIV-3 occurs throughout the year, but epidemics occurring in the spring have been observed in the United States.[5, 11, 12] The epidemiology of PIV-4 is less well characterized, in part because of technical difficulties with viral isolation, weak hemadsorption, and the lack, until recently, of a rapid immunofluorescence method.[13] Passively acquired antibody probably provides some protection to PIV-1 and PIV-2, because most severe disease is seen in children after 6 months of age.[6, 7, 9] PIV-3 resembles RSV in its capacity to cause severe disease at a time when maternally acquired antibody is present.[7, 11, 12] Seroprevalence data suggest that PIV-4 infection is common but disease is usually mild.[13] By age 8 years, the majority of children have serologic evidence of prior infection with PIV types 1, 2, 3, and 4.[4, 9]

The mode of transmission appears to be primarily by person-to-person aerosol droplet spread. PIV-3 has been shown to survive only briefly on human fingers, and transfer from finger to finger or environmental surface is inefficient. On the other hand, transfer from environmental surface to fingers is more readily accomplished, supporting a role for fomites in transmission.[14] Nosocomial transmission has been reported, most commonly with PIV-3, but outbreaks due to PIV-1 and PIV-2 have also been reported.[11, 15]

RSV is the most common cause of pneumonia in infants and children both in the United States and throughout the world.[4, 16] In this population, it causes approximately 90,000 hospitalizations and 4500 deaths annually from lower respiratory tract disease in the United States.[17] RSV outbreaks occur annually with seasonal periodicity. In the United States, RSV activity rises in the late fall, peaks in the winter, and returns to baseline levels in the spring.[16, 17] RSV outbreaks are associated with excess deaths related to lower respiratory tract disease in infants.[18] Both strains A and B usually cocirculate in an outbreak, although their relative proportions may vary.[19] There is often a decline in PIV-1 and PIV-2 activity as RSV activity increases.[5] Influenza virus activity may rise during or subsequent to peak RSV activity.

Infection with RSV is nearly universal. Peak attack rates occur in children younger than 6 months, at a time when they still have specific maternally derived antibody. Immunity from natural infection is incomplete, and reinfections with both heterologous and homologous strains occur.[20, 21] Both attack rates and the severity of disease decrease with subsequent infections; however, in a longitudinal study, attack rates among normal children for second and third infections were still 75% and 65%, respectively.[20] Comparable attack rates have been seen among the institutionalized elderly[22]; rates among older children and adults have been between 38% and 47%.[23] Transmission of RSV is by inoculation of virus, from secretions or fomites, through nasal or ocular mucosa. Virus may survive on hands for up to a half-hour, on gloves for up to 2 hours, and on environmental surfaces for up to 7 hours.[24]

Primary infection with adenoviruses most often occurs in childhood.[25] Although there are about 50 adenovirus serotypes, types 1 to 7 cause the majority of respiratory infection, and three types (3, 4, and 7) cause most cases of adenoviral pneumonia. These three serotypes affect young adults, and there have been numerous outbreaks among military recruits.[26] Spread is from person to person by aerosols. In immunocompromised patients, especially renal or bone marrow transplant recipients, types 31, 34, and 35 have caused overwhelming pneumonia.[27, 28]

CMV is transmitted transplacentally, during delivery in vaginal and cervical secretions, and postnatally in breast milk. It is transmitted among young children in daycare, where CMV has been shown to persist on toys and environmental surfaces for up to 30 minutes.[29] CMV is found in high concentrations in semen and vaginal secretions, and sexual transmission is an important mode of spread. CMV may be transmitted by blood products and organ transplants. The prevalence of CMV infection continues to rise throughout life, and by age 60 years, 80% to 100% of the U.S. population is infected.[29, 30]

The hantavirus pulmonary syndrome (HPS) is a recently recognized entity caused by one or more newly identified viruses of the *Hantavirus* genus.[31] Illness associated with previously isolated hantaviruses (Hantaan, Seoul, Puumula) has consisted of various degrees of fever, renal disease, and hemorrhage without prominent pulmonary involvement. HPS differs from other *Hantavirus* illness in causing disease with primarily respiratory manifestations and with a higher mortality rate.

Sin Nombre virus appears to be the primary agent of HPS.[32] The agent was initially implicated by finding immunoglobulin M or G antibodies in patients with HPS that cross-reacted with previously recognized hantaviruses. Later, the agent was detected in tissue by immunohistochemical testing and by reverse transcriptase polymerase chain reaction amplification of the viral genome. The virus has subsequently been isolated in cell culture.[33] The natural reservoir for Sin Nombre virus is the deer mouse, *Peromyscus maniculatus*, an indigenous North American species.[34] This rodent has a broad geographic range throughout North America and occurs in most habitats. In Arizona, New Mexico, and Colorado, between 29% and 33% of *P. maniculatus* have serologic evidence of Sin Nombre virus infection.[34] Whereas the majority of cases of HPS have occurred in the southwestern states of Arizona, Colorado, New Mexico, and Utah, cases have been identified in Texas, Nevada, Louisiana, Indiana, and Rhode Island. Viral genomic sequences can be amplified from seropositive rodents by reverse transcriptase polymerase chain reaction analyses, suggesting a persistent viral infection despite a significant antibody response. This has been seen with other hantaviruses with which the primary reservoir rodents remain asymptomatically infected for life, shedding virus in urine, feces, and saliva.

Increased domestic rodent infestation and activities such as cleaning of barns and other outdoor structures, cleaning food storage areas, and plowing with hand tools, which increase the likelihood of exposure to infected rodents and their secretions or excreta, may be associated with acquisition of disease.[35] Transmission is thought to occur primarily through the inhalation of infected excreta, although the presence of virus in saliva allows transmission by rodent bites. Neither arthropod vectors nor person-to-person transmission has been implicated in HPS or in illnesses caused by related hantaviruses. Serologic data suggest that clinically mild or asymptomatic disease is uncommon. Although newly recognized, the syndrome is probably not new. The significant sequence diversity found among rodent Sin Nombre virus isolates suggests that this diversity accumulated over time,[34] and retrospective cases have been identified from stored sera.[36, 37]

When pneumonia occurs as a complication of other systemic virus infections, such as varicella or rubeola, the epidemiology is that of the underlying infection.

Pathophysiology

The viruses described in this chapter gain access to the body through the respiratory route. In addition, they have evolved receptors that have primary affinity for respiratory epithelial cells. In the case of influenza, the virus adsorbs to ciliated epithelial cells using the hemagglutinin glycoprotein on the virus surface.[38] This results first in cessation of ciliary motility and later in desquamation of cells, thereby triggering cough. If the lower respiratory tract is involved, hyperemia and invasion by both polymorphonuclear and mononuclear cells occur. The alveoli may become involved, and formation of a hyaline membrane lining alveoli has been noted. This may be responsible for the profound hypoxemia that can result and this, in turn, for the relatively high morbidity and mortality in otherwise healthy adults.

PIVs enter through the mucosa of the nose and mouth. The incubation period is 2 to 6 days.[7] PIVs may have a tropism for the epithelial cells of the subglottic region.[4, 12] Cell damage results from both direct viral effects and effects of the host immune response.[7, 9] Humoral immunity appears to play some role in host defense as evidenced by the general protection against PIV-1 and PIV-2 afforded by maternal antibody and by the fact that infants with high titers of passively acquired antibody to PIV-3 also have relative protection.[7] However, the immunity conferred by homologous virus is incomplete, and as with RSV, reinfection with PIVs can occur, albeit with decreased frequency and severity.[12]

After initial RSV infection in the respiratory epithelium, there is an average incubation of 5 days. Spread of the virus to the lower respiratory tract results in a lymphocytic peribronchiolar infiltration and edema, which may be followed by bronchiolar epithelial proliferation and necrosis. The resultant impedance of airflow, especially on expiration, results in the air trapping and hyperinflation seen in bronchiolitis. Pneumonia, with a mononuclear cell interstitial infiltration, edema, and necrosis with alveolar space filling, frequently coexists with pathologic findings of bronchiolitis.

The occurrence of lower respiratory tract RSV disease at a time when maternal antibody is still present and the exaggerated disease that was seen in recipients of a candidate inactivated RSV vaccine have led to the hypothesis that the host immunologic response may contribute to disease pathogenesis.[39] Local production of immunoglobulin E, leukotriene C_4, and eosinophilic cationic protein may play an important role in virus-induced airway obstruction.[39, 40] The occurrence of severe RSV disease in patients with defects in host defenses due to either respiratory tract anatomic abnormalities or defects in cellular immunity suggests that these factors are important in the host's ability to resolve RSV infection.[41]

Adenoviruses are spread by the respiratory route as well but can establish latency in oropharyngeal lymphoid tissue.[42] The adenovirus pneumonia that typically occurs in young healthy adults is probably the result of primary infection, but adenovirus pneumonia in the immunocompromised patient is almost certainly the result of activation of latent infection.[27, 28] Adenoviruses adsorb to cells using the fiber protein that extends from the 12 corners of the capsid coat.[25] (see Chapter 239).

The pathogenic potential and specific pathogenic mechanisms of CMV disease differ in different hosts and settings. Further, given the ubiquitous nature of CMV infection, the distinction between disease and infection without pathogenicity is sometimes difficult.[43, 44] Higher rates of CMV infection among CMV seropositive organ recipients than among seronegative organ recipients suggest that the reactivation of latent infection is an important process.[30, 44, 45] However, substantial rates of infection also occur among seronegative recipients of seropositive organs, and reinfections of seropositive recipients of seropositive organs has been documented. Each of these pathways to active CMV infection has been documented by restriction endonuclease analysis of viral DNA.[46]

The response of CMV pneumonia in renal transplant recipients and in infants with congenital CMV disease to antiviral therapy has been taken to suggest a prime role for direct viral replication in pathogenesis.[44] Among recipients of allogeneic bone marrow transplants, the clinical response of CMV pneumonia to antiviral therapy has been limited, despite a clear impact on viral titers, implicating an immunopathogenic mechanism. The higher rate of CMV pneumonitis among allogeneic bone marrow recipients than among autologous recipients, despite comparable CMV infection rates and comparable immunosuppression,[47] and the identification of graft-versus-host disease as a significant risk factor for CMV pneumonia suggest a role for transplanted allogeneic cells in disease pathogenesis.[44, 45] A T-cell–mediated response to a virally induced antigen in the lung has been implicated.[4, 30] The primary sites of CMV latency are not completely known. Peripheral blood mononuclear cells have been shown to harbor latent virus; bone marrow, spleen, and lung are potential organ reservoirs of latent virus.[30, 43]

In HPS, there appears to be a tropism of Sin Nombre virus for capillary endothelial cells in general, and for the pulmonary capillary endothelium in particular, as detected by immunohistochemical staining for viral antigens. In fatal cases, most of the cells of the pulmonary microcirculation may contain Sin Nombre virus antigen.[33] Lung specimens reveal variable degrees of edema, congestion, focal hyaline membranes, and a mononuclear cell infiltrate consisting of small and enlarged mononuclear cells and immunoblasts. Hantaviral inclusions have been demonstrated in pulmonary endothelial cells by electron microscopy. However, despite the high viral load in the pulmonary microvasculature, there is a paucity of necrosis, and pneumocytes and endothelial cells usually appear morphologically intact. These findings have led to the hypothesis that local immune responses to viral antigen may induce a functional derangement of the vascular endothelium that contributes to the severe pulmonary edema observed clinically.[33]

Each of the respiratory viruses has also evolved a special mechanism to permit infection of neighboring cells. Influenza virus employs its other main surface glycoprotein, neuraminidase, to cleave the budding virus from the cell surface, allowing the daughter virions to infect other cells.[48] RSV and PIVs form syncytia, which facilitate cell-to-cell spread. Adenovirus replicates by a lytic cycle in which the infected cell bursts at the end of replication with the production of free daughter virions.[25]

Clinical Manifestations

Influenza Virus

Clearly, disease caused by influenza virus is the paradigm for so-called influenza-like illness. After an incubation period of 1 to 3 days, there is the rapid onset of chills, fever, cough, and prominent malaise and myalgia. These last two symptoms have given rise to the concept that the patient is experiencing viremia, but with rare exception,[49, 50] attempts to isolate influenza virus from the blood stream at any stage of the disease have been unsuccessful. Experience using the interferons as therapeutic agents has shown that they produce similar symptoms, and it may be the induction of endogenous interferon in the course of influenza and other viral infections that is the cause of these symptoms.

Influenza upper respiratory infection, which takes the form of tracheobronchitis, is far more common than is pneumonia. This is a self-limited disease with a 5- to 7-day duration. During the severe epidemic of Asian (A2) influenza in 1957 to 1958, Louria and colleagues[51] described several distinct clinical patterns of disease. The first and most common was influenza upper respiratory infection. The virus was culturable from the sputum during the week-long illness. Most of these patients were adults with no underlying illness, and most recovered with no sequelae. In a second group of patients, pneumonia supervened, the patients' conditions worsened about the third day, and severe hypoxia and obtundation occurred. This group had influenza viral pneumonia, and virus could also be cultured from their sputum. This pattern of the disease was more common among patients with underlying cardiopulmonary disease, including those with rheumatic disease and mitral stenosis, especially in late pregnancy. A third group, while in the throws of influenza, developed a superinfecting bacterial pneumonia. This syndrome again was seen predominantly in patients with underlying disease and carried with it a high mortality. The fourth group of patients identified had influenza and, after a period of 1 to 2 weeks when they appeared to be recovering, developed bacterial pneumonia. This occurred primarily in the oldest of the patients. In the last two groups, influenza virus could not be isolated at the time that bacterial superinfection was occurring. The total number of patients in this study was small, but evidence from subsequent epidemics substantiates these patterns.[52] Numerous studies have elucidated the mechanisms whereby influenza virus infection predisposes to bacterial superinfection of the lung. These include interruption of ciliary motility, denudation of mucosa, decrease in polymorphonuclear leukocyte and macrophage chemotaxis, and impaired humoral and cellular immunity.

These studies have further emphasized the need to be aware that *Staphylococcus aureus* can cause postinfluenzal bacterial pneumonia. Staphylococcal pneumonia is far more common after outbreaks of influenza[50, 51] than it is in years of low influenza prevalence. However, the most common cause of postinfluenzal pneumonia is *Streptococcus pneumoniae*, followed in frequency by *Haemophilus influenzae*, as is the case in patients who have not had recent influenza. In fact, *H. influenzae* was so named because it was thought to be the cause of the 1918 influenza pandemic.

The primary life-threatening aspect of influenza pneumonia is the development of diffuse alveolar involvement leading to the adult respiratory distress syndrome (ARDS). Other organ systems can be affected during influenza pneumonia, including the heart and pericardium,[53] brain,[54] and spinal cord (Guillain-Barré syndrome).[55] The pathophysiologic mechanisms of these complications are unclear. If the attendant bacterial pneumonia is due to toxigenic *S. aureus*, the toxic shock syndrome may supervene.[56]

One fascinating complication of influenza as well as of varicella-zoster virus infection is Reye's syndrome. After recovery from influenza or chickenpox, some children develop encephalopathy and coma complicated by hepatic failure. The syndrome was first described at autopsy and was thought to be invariably fatal. Although mortality is high, some children spontaneously recover. Hepatic enzyme levels are elevated, as are the serum ammonia and creatine kinase levels; jaundice is unusual. Examination of the cerebrospinal fluid shows few mononuclear cells and a striking hypoglycorrhachia, sometimes as low as 0 mg/dL. Influenza type B has most often been reported as the preceding event, and the chances of developing Reye's syndrome seem to be enhanced by treatment of the antecedent viral infection with salicylates.[57, 58] See Chapters 165 and 250 for further description.

Parainfluenza Viruses

All the PIVs cause upper respiratory tract illnesses, including rhinitis, pharyngitis, and bronchitis. PIV-1, PIV-2, and PIV-3 are important causes of croup.[6, 9, 12] PIV-3 is the second leading cause of hospitalization for acute respiratory infection and pneumonia in infants.[4, 9, 12] PIV-4A and PIV-4B can cause severe lower respiratory tract disease but appear to do so infrequently.[13] Syndromes caused by PIVs and RSV can be difficult to distinguish clinically. No characteristic radiographic pattern has been noted in PIV pneumonia. In the normal host, secondary bacterial infection after PIV infection is unusual.[4] PIVs are rare causes of pneumonia in immunocompetent adults.[59] Severe PIV disease manifestations, including giant cell pneumonia, respiratory failure, and death, have been reported in immunocompromised children and adults, including patients with severe combined immunodeficiency, solid organ transplants, and leukemia.[60–62] Prolonged virus shedding has also been reported in immunocompromised hosts including children with human immunodeficiency virus (HIV) infection.[62, 63] PIV-3 is the type most frequently isolated from immunocompromised hosts with lower respiratory tract disease.

Lower respiratory tract PIV disease is usually preceded by upper respiratory tract signs and symptoms, such as nasal congestion and pharyngitis. Fever and cough are usually present. Rales, rhonchi, wheezing, and intercostal muscle retractions may be present on physical examination. Chest radiographs may reveal interstitial infiltrates and hyperinflation, with consolidation present in up to 25% of cases, usually in the right upper or middle lobe. Severe hypoxemia may be present, often without cyanosis.

Respiratory Syncytial Virus

Whereas the most common manifestations of RSV infection occur in the upper respiratory tract, the most serious are those of the lower respiratory tract. Lower respiratory tract involvement may occur in 30% to 70% of first infections. Bronchiolitis accounts for a greater proportion of lower respiratory tract RSV involvement in children than does pneumonia. However, pneumonia may occur in 5% to 40% and the two may be difficult to differentiate and may coexist.[41]

Children with bronchopulmonary dysplasia, cystic fibrosis, prematurity, cyanotic or complicated congenital heart disease, congenital combined immunodeficiencies, and malignant neoplasms are at increased risk for severe RSV lower respiratory tract disease.[64] Children receiving steroid therapy for other chronic conditions may not have more severe disease, but they have more prolonged virus shedding than do normal children. Children with HIV-1 infection may have prolonged virus shedding and may be at increased risk for lower respiratory tract disease, particularly pneumonia.[65, 66] In the normal child with RSV pneumonia, early bacterial superinfection may occur, but late bacterial secondary infections are unusual.[4]

RSV infections in adults, by virtue of the near universality of childhood infection, are essentially all reinfections. These reinfections are more often limited to the upper respiratory tract. However, lower respiratory tract involvement, usually tracheobronchitis or pneumonia rather than bronchiolitis, may occur in both healthy and immunocompromised adolescents and adults.[22, 23, 67] Outbreaks in the elderly have been associated with particularly high rates of bronchopneumonia with substantial morbidity and mortality.[22] Bone marrow transplant recipients are at high risk for severe disease, with mortality rates up to 78% reported.[68, 69] RSV upper respiratory tract disease may be underrecognized in immunocompromised patients. Therefore, it may be important to consider RSV early in susceptible hosts, such as bone marrow transplant recipients, who present with upper respiratory tract symptoms.[41, 68, 69]

Adenovirus

Adult pneumonia caused by adenovirus has no particular distinguishing features. The clinical picture is much like that of influenza, and diagnosis would rest on the epidemiologic setting of a young adult entering a new closed population group. In children, in whom the adenoviruses are the single most common cause of upper respiratory infection, adenoviruses should always be suspected. One of the more common syndromes in this age group is pharyngoconjunctival fever due to infection with type 3 adenovirus. This often occurs in small epidemics in summer camps, where swimming pool water is the probable reservoir. Keratoconjunctivitis is another common adenovirus syndrome but is not associated with adenovirus pneumonia.

Cytomegalovirus

CMV pneumonia is rare in immunocompetent adults[70] but may occur in up to 6% of cases of CMV-induced mononucleosis.[71] Patients may be asymptomatic or symptomatic. Radiographic findings and symptoms, when present, usually resolve spontaneously. CMV pneumonia develops in 50% of infants with CMV inclusion disease. Up to 20% of episodes of hospitalized pneumonia in infants between 1 and 3 months old may be due to CMV.[72]

Interstitial pneumonia is a common and important complication of organ transplantation, particularly bone marrow transplantation. It presents with tachypnea, hypoxemia, fever, and interstitial infiltrates on chest radiograph. Specific microbiologic diagnosis usually requires bronchoscopy or surgical lung biopsy. Fifteen percent to 40% of allogeneic marrow transplant recipients develop interstitial pneumonitis.[30, 45, 73] CMV accounts for approximately one half of transplant interstitial pneumonitis cases, with the other half being due to *Pneumocystis carinii*, adenovirus, other viruses, or toxicity effects of radiation or chemotherapeutic agents. The mortality from CMV pneumonia in this setting has been as high as 80% to 90%.

Heart-lung transplant recipients, in particular seronegative recipients of donor-positive organs, are at greater risk for CMV pneumonia than are other solid organ recipients.[30, 74] However, as previously mentioned, disease may occur in seropositive recipients through either reactivation of latent CMV strains or reinfection with a new strain.

Patients with AIDS are at substantial risk for the development of CMV disease, especially as $CD4^+$ lymphocyte counts fall below $100/mm^3$. Patients with AIDS and advanced immunosuppression frequently shed CMV in urine and semen and frequently have viremia without clinically apparent end organ disease. The most common sites of CMV disease in persons with AIDS are the retina and the gastrointestinal tract. Disease may be due to both viral reactivation and reinfection, and coinfections with multiple strains have been reported. The response of CMV retinitis in AIDS to antiviral therapy is consistent with viral replication as the pathogenetic mechanism in these hosts.[44] Despite the clear significance of CMV retinitis and gastrointestinal disease among HIV-infected persons, the significance of CMV pulmonary disease has been less clear.[75, 76] Among AIDS patients with symptomatic pneumonitis, in most instances in which CMV is identified ante mortem by culture or by characteristic cytopathic effects in bronchoscopic washings, coexistent pathogens such as *P. carinii* are also found.[75] The presence of culturable CMV from bronchoscopy specimens has been shown not to affect the short-term morbidity or mortality of patients with first-episode *P. carinii* pneumonia.[76] However, evidence of CMV pneumonia with viral inclusions present is frequently seen at autopsy,[77] and there are reports of CMV pneumonia with CMV identified as a sole pathogen by the presence of numerous viral inclusions in alveolar cells in transbronchial biopsy specimens.[78, 79]

Hantavirus Pulmonary Syndrome

HPS begins with a prodromal illness (median, 3 to 4 days) consisting primarily of fever (in 98% to 100%) and myalgias (in 57% to 100%).[33, 35, 80] Cough, nausea, vomiting, headache, and other symptoms are variably present initially. The presentation may be difficult to distinguish from influenza, aseptic meningitis, or other viral illnesses; however, coryza, conjunctivitis, meningismus, and sore throat are usually not present in HPS.

As the illness proceeds, patients develop progressive cough, dyspnea, tachypnea, tachycardia, and hypotension. Laboratory findings include hemoconcentration, thrombocytopenia, a prolonged partial thromboplastin time, and elevated serum lactate dehydrogenase levels. A marked leukocytosis is common, frequently with an increased proportion of immature forms and a mild atypical lymphocytosis.[80]

Chest radiograph findings may differ from those of either cardiogenic or noncardiogenic pulmonary edema. Initial chest radiographs frequently reveal interstitial edema with Kerly B lines and peribronchial cuffing (such as seen in cardiogenic pulmonary edema and not ARDS) but with a normal heart size (such as seen in ARDS and not cardiogenic pulmonary edema).[80, 81] Pleural effusions and airspace disease may develop rapidly, and the airspace disease may lack the peripheral distribution typical of ARDS.[80, 81] Many patients require mechanical ventilation. The systemic vascular resistance may be normal or elevated, the pulmonary capillary wedge pressure normal or low, and the cardiac index depressed.[35, 80]

Resolution of the respiratory and hemodynamic manifestations may occur spontaneously and rapidly. However, the mortality rate may be as high as 52%.[37] Increases in the hematocrit, lactate dehydrogenase level, partial thromboplastin time, and white cell count are poor prognostic indicators.[80]

Diagnosis

The etiologic diagnosis of viral pneumonia on clinical grounds alone is inaccurate. During an epidemic, influenza etiology is probably overdiagnosed; at other times, sporadic cases of true influenza are often unrecognized. Much of the influenza-like illness that is seen in nonepidemic periods may be caused by some of the other viruses discussed in this chapter as well as by *Mycoplasma pneumoniae, Chlamydia psittaci, Chlamydia pneumoniae, Legionella pneumophila*, and *P. carinii*. Although adenovirus pneumonia can evolve into ARDS,[26] this is relatively uncommon in immunocompetent patients. If ARDS occurs in the course of an influenza-like illness in an adult, the likely viral causes are influenza virus or hantavirus. The differentiation would be made acutely by lack of a history of rodent exposure in influenza. Clinical factors that may aid in establishing the etiology in a case of atypical pneumonia syndrome are shown in Table 57–1.

Diagnosis can be confirmed in a reference laboratory by viral culture enhanced by immunofluorescence assays of the infected cell culture and by demonstrating a rise in titer of complement-fixing or other antibodies. None of these tests is performed routinely. For adenovirus and PIV, the importance of a specific diagnosis is primarily in documenting the start of an outbreak. For influenza virus, RSV, CMV, and hantavirus, arriving at a specific etiologic diagnosis is important both because of the severity of disease that may prevail in these infections and because therapeutic modalities (with variable efficacy) may be required.

A presumptive diagnosis of lower respiratory tract RSV disease can often be made clinically in children in the RSV season, with or without subsequent laboratory confirmation. The diagnosis in adolescents and adults, in whom the role of RSV as a pathogen is not as well recognized, usually requires specific laboratory methods. Nasal washes are superior to swabs of the throat and nasopharynx for viral isolation in cell culture.[39, 41] The two most widely used methods for rapid diagnosis with nasal washings are immunofluorescence staining for RSV antigen and enzyme-linked immunosorbent assays.[39] Immunofluorescence assays of washings are sensitive, are rapid, and may allow simultaneous screening for other respiratory pathogens but require a trained technician, labile reagents, and a fluorescence microscope. Enzyme-linked immunosorbent assays may be slightly less sensitive than immunofluorescence techniques but are considered sensitive enough to be used in the clinical laboratory, are less operator dependent, and require no special equipment.[39, 81]

Given the high prevalence of CMV infection in the population, serologic testing is of limited value in the diagnosis of CMV disease in adults. CMV can be identified in culture, but this finding correlates poorly with the presence of CMV disease.[30, 44, 75, 76, 82] The diagnosis of CMV end organ disease usually requires the presence of the characteristic intranuclear ("owl's eye") and intracytoplasmic viral inclusion bodies on tissue specimens.

Among HIV-infected persons, the presence of CMV viruria or CMV viremia suggests an increased likelihood of developing CMV end organ disease. However, the positive predictive values for CMV viremia (35%) and CMV viruria (28%) in predicting CMV end organ disease within 6 months are low, the costs associated with surveillance viral cultures are not insignificant, and $CD4^+$ lymphocyte counts ($\leq$100 cells per mm^3) are more potent predictors of CMV disease risk.[82]

The distinction between situations in which evidence of active CMV infection reflects nonpathogenic virus shedding and those in which it reflects a pathogenic process can be difficult and has obvious therapeutic implications. The presence and abundance of CMV viral inclusions on lung biopsy specimens and the finding of CMV as a sole pathogen may suggest a role for antiviral therapy; the decision can occasionally be simplified by the identification of other concomitant CMV end organ diseases (e.g., retinitis) that clearly require therapy.

The diagnosis of HPS may be difficult because of the lack of specificity of the initial symptoms.[35] The diagnosis should be considered when severe respiratory symptoms follow a nonspecific febrile prodrome, especially if there is reason to suspect rodent exposure. Subsequently, the radiographic and laboratory findings may suggest the diagnosis.

Confirmatory enzyme-linked immunosorbent assays and Western blot assays have been developed.[35, 83] Diagnosis may be made by detecting immunoglobulin M antibody to Sin Nombre virus or a fourfold or greater rise in immunoglobu-

TABLE 57–1 ■ Clinical Aids to the Etiologic Diagnosis of the Atypical Pneumonia Syndrome*

PATHOGEN	SYMPTOMS	SIGNS	HISTORY	LABORATORY
Influenza virus	Myalgia, severe respiratory distress	ARDS	Epidemic	↓ Po_2
Respiratory syncytial virus	Wheezing, persistent cough	Bronchospasm	—	—
Hantavirus	Severe respiratory distress	ARDS	Exposure to rodents or their excreta	Hemoconcentration, ↑ LDH, ↓ platelets
Adenovirus	—	—	Military, school, AIDS, transplant	—
Cytomegalovirus	—	Retinitis, colitis	AIDS, transplant	—
Chlamydia psittaci	—		Bird exposure	—
Mycoplasma pneumoniae	Insidious onset, cough	Negative chest examination findings	School, military	Cold agglutinins
Pneumocystis carinii	—	—	AIDS risk activity	↓ Po_2, ↑ LDH

*ARDS, Adult respiratory distress syndrome; AIDS, acquired immunodeficiency syndrome; LDH, lactate dehydrogenase; Po_2, oxygen tension.

lin G antibody in serum. Immunohistochemical staining has been used to identify Sin Nombre virus antigens in tissue, and reverse transcriptase polymerase chain reaction amplification has been used to identify the viral genome in tissue.[33, 35]

Treatment

Faced with a patient with apparent viral pneumonia, the physician's first task would be to attempt to identify and exclude some of the more readily treatable etiologic agents that can cause a similar syndrome. These again include *M. pneumoniae* and *L. pneumophila,* which respond to treatment with a macrolide antibiotic such as erythromycin; *C. psittaci,* which can be treated with a tetracycline; and *P. carinii,* which should be treated with trimethoprim-sulfamethoxazole or pentamidine.

The therapy for most cases of influenza is supportive. Milder cases are treated with bed rest, high intake of oral fluids, and antipyretic analgesic medications such as acetaminophen. Aspirin should be avoided.

Amantadine has been licensed for use as a prophylactic agent to prevent infection with influenza type A virus. It appears to act at an early step in viral replication, probably uncoating of the RNA genome.[84] Rimantadine, more recently licensed in the United States, has the same therapeutic effect as amantadine with a lower rate of side effects such as drowsiness and confusion.[85, 86] Amantadine has been used to treat influenza A with resultant shortening and decreased severity of symptoms.[87] Because viral syndromes probably result from multiple rounds of virus replication, it would be reasonable to expect that a drug that interferes with an early replication step would curtail the syndrome. Therefore, in patients at high risk for serious complications of influenza who have not been immunized, not only prophylaxis but also therapy with amantadine or rimantadine should be contemplated.[87]

Treatment of PIV infection is generally supportive, particularly in healthy hosts. There are currently no antiviral agents with documented clinical efficacy in the treatment of PIV infection. Ribavirin, a synthetic nucleoside analog that appears to inhibit viral messenger RNA formation and to alter cellular nucleotide pools, has in vitro activity against PIVs. There are anecdotal reports of clinical benefit of aerosolized ribavirin for PIV infection in infants with severe combined immunodeficiency.[60, 61] In an uncontrolled series, use of aerosolized ribavirin did not alter mortality among bone marrow transplant recipients with PIV infection, although delayed diagnoses and treatment may have contributed to this outcome.[62]

Ribavirin also has in vitro activity against RSV.[88] Ribavirin is administered by an oxygen mask or in a hood or tent. A small-particle generator is employed to create aerosols with a median diameter of 1 to 2 μm to allow distribution to the lower respiratory tract. Controlled studies have documented some beneficial effects on clinical signs, such as retractions and rales, and some significant improvements in arterial oxygen saturation. Treatment is indicated both for infants with severe lower respiratory tract RSV disease and for those with milder disease and coexisting medical conditions that increase the risk of severe disease.

Ribavirin may infrequently cause reversible irritation of mucous membranes of staff exposed during its aerosol administration. Reproductive and teratogenic toxic reactions have been observed in rodents but not in baboons and have not been reported in humans. Ribavirin has rarely been detected in the urine of exposed staff.[88] Despite the lack of any clear suggestion of toxicity in humans, because of the embryopathy observed in nonprimate animals, it has been recommended that pregnant women not care directly for patients receiving aerosolized ribavirin, that it be administered in a well-ventilated room, and that its administration be interrupted when the hood or tent is opened.

Acyclovir and famciclovir have limited activity against CMV. Ganciclovir and foscarnet have in vitro activity, and ganciclovir-resistant isolates retain susceptibility to foscarnet. Both ganciclovir and foscarnet have been demonstrated to be effective in the treatment of CMV retinitis in persons with AIDS.[89] Anecdotal reports suggest a potential role for antiviral therapy in the management of congenital and neonatal CMV disease.[90] Significant cumulative, uncontrolled experience with ganciclovir speaks for efficacy in renal transplant recipients with CMV pneumonia. However, the response of CMV pneumonia among bone marrow transplant recipients to ganciclovir has been more limited and appears to be enhanced by the addition of high-dose intravenous immunoglobulin.[91]

The duration of therapy required for CMV pneumonia in patients with AIDS and in transplant recipients is not well delineated. To prevent relapse, AIDS patients with CMV retinitis require ongoing antiviral therapy with parenteral ganciclovir or foscarnet or, particularly in situations in which long-term intravenous access is a problem, with oral ganciclovir.

The treatment of HPS has primarily been supportive, with measures appropriate for noncardiogenic pulmonary edema.[35, 80] Both Sin Nombre virus and Hantaan virus, the cause of hemorrhagic fever with renal syndrome, are sensitive in cell culture to ribavirin. Intravenous ribavirin has been shown, in a placebo-controlled trial, to have a beneficial effect on the renal and hemorrhagic manifestations of hemorrhagic fever with renal syndrome and to reduce mortality.[92] There are also data from a controlled trial suggesting that corticosteroids may diminish some of the morbidity of hemorrhagic fever with renal syndrome.[93] Intravenous ribavirin has been employed in the United States for patients with suspected HPS through an open-label trial. However, there were no clearly beneficial effects on outcomes.[94] No data regarding the effect of corticosteroids on outcomes of HPS exist.

There is no specific antiviral therapy for adenovirus infection.

Prevention

One of the greatest advances in public health is the development of influenza vaccination. One of the greatest failures in public health is that only about one fifth of the people who should receive influenza vaccine get it.[95] The U.S. Public Health Service has stated that all people older than 65 years should be vaccinated. In addition, patients with cardiopulmonary disease, diabetes, chronic renal disease, or requirements for ongoing salicylate therapy and residents of nursing homes and chronic care facilities as well as all health care workers should be vaccinated.

Influenza virus was isolated in 1933, and by the 1950s, vaccine virus had been produced by inoculation of embryonated hen eggs. This remains the most productive method of growing the virus, but fragmentation and purification procedures have been introduced to decrease the amount of egg protein in the vaccine. The most commonly used vaccine is a subvirion or split-virus product that has been enriched for the hemagglutinin and neuraminidase antigens. The vaccine is trivalent, containing two strains of type A and one strain of type B influenza virus chosen each year on the basis of those strains that emerge as the most prevalent at the end of the previous year. The vaccine must be given annually because of the phenomena of antigenic shift and drift and because immunity conferred by this killed subunit vaccine is short-lived. The optimal time for vaccination is in the late fall, and protection is in the range of 70%. The vaccine is safe for pregnant and immunocompromised patients, but the immunocompromised patient may not mount a protective antibody response. The only specific contraindication is allergy to egg protein.[96]

Amantadine and rimantadine are about 70% effective in preventing influenza type A infections. In the face of an impending influenza A outbreak, one of these drugs should be given to any member of the high-risk populations named before who were not vaccinated in that year. Prophylaxis should be continued for the duration of the outbreak. If it is early in the influenza season, vaccination can be carried out at the same time, because these drugs do not interfere with the normal antibody response.[96]

There are currently no effective vaccines for the PIVs. Inactivated vaccines were poorly immunogenic, and no protection was afforded. Live attenuated and subunit vaccines are being evaluated.[7, 9]

Prevention of RSV infection in nosocomial settings requires adherence to infection control measures intended to reduce contact with infectious secretions and contaminated fomites. There is currently no vaccine available to prevent RSV. Trials of an inactivated RSV vaccine were conducted in the 1960s. Despite high antigenicity and the production of complement-fixing and neutralizing antibodies, many vaccinated children exposed to natural RSV infection developed enhanced disease, presumably owing to formation of antigen-antibody complexes on alveolar membranes.[97] Alternative vaccine strategies including the use of specific viral proteins and adjuvant systems are being evaluated.

Breast-feeding may provide infants some protection against severe RSV disease.[98] Epidemiologic data suggest that breast-fed infants may have a lower risk of hospitalization for lower respiratory tract RSV infection. However, the risk reduction is by no means complete, and the specific mechanism through which protection may be conferred is uncertain.

The prophylactic monthly administration of intravenous immune globulin with high titers of RSV-neutralizing antibody has been shown to reduce the frequency and severity of lower respiratory tract RSV disease among premature infants and young children with congenital heart disease or bronchopulmonary dysplasia.[99]

Transmission of RSV in the nosocomial setting may be diminished through implementation of and compliance with infection control measures designed to deter spread of virus from patient to patient, visitor to patient, and staff to patient. Such measures may include glove and gown precautions, the use of eye-nose goggles, the isolation or grouping of infected patients, and the use of cohort nursing.[100–102] The potential for spread by gloves or hands contaminated by touching infectious secretions or environmental surfaces makes changing gloves and hand washing key means of interrupting nosocomial transmission.

Effective vaccines to prevent adenovirus infection with types 3, 4, and 7 were developed 30 years ago for use in the military population, where they are still used.[26] They have not been licensed for use in the general population.

The prevention of CMV pneumonia in transplant recipients has been the focus of substantial investigation. Acyclovir, despite its limited therapeutic activity against CMV, when given intravenously or at high oral doses, has been shown to reduce the frequency of CMV disease among bone marrow and renal transplant recipients but not among liver or lung transplant patients.[103, 104] CMV immune globulin can reduce the rate of severe CMV disease among recipients of renal, bone marrow, and liver transplants but not among seronegative recipients of seropositive liver transplants.[30, 44, 105] Prophylactic intravenous ganciclovir has been shown to significantly reduce the occurrence of CMV disease among allogeneic bone marrow transplant recipients, but neutropenia is a frequent complication.[106] The strategy of obtaining surveillance cultures of buffy coat and urine for CMV and instituting "preemptive" intravenous ganciclovir if cultures are positive appears to be effective and well tolerated.[104] The efficacy of oral ganciclovir for prophylaxis against CMV infection and disease in transplant recipients is under evaluation. Among HIV-infected persons with $CD4^+$ lymphocyte counts less than $100/mm^3$, oral ganciclovir has been shown to reduce the frequency of CMV disease.[107] The frequency with which prophylactic antiviral therapy may select for resistant CMV isolates is not fully known, and the potential for its doing so remains a significant concern. Whether surveillance cultures play a role in the decision to institute prophylactic (or preemptive) ganciclovir is not yet known.

Measures to prevent HPS consist of rodent control and of attempts to reduce the likelihood of exposure to infected rodents and their secretions.[35, 108] Rodent infestation may be prevented or eliminated through the use of traps and rodenticides and by altering potential rodent habitats to make them less accessible. The risk to those potentially exposed during occupational and leisure activities may be diminished through avoiding rodent burrows, infested shelters, or potentially contaminated water; by using masks with high-efficiency particulate air filters when cleaning out potentially rodent-infested areas; and by burying, burning, or disposing of all trash in sealed containers to limit rodent food sources.

There is no hantavirus vaccine, and there is no information on postexposure prophylaxis. Universal precautions are appropriate in handling specimens from potentially infected patients. Biosafety level 3 containment facilities should be employed for cell cultures, and biosafety level 4 facilities should be used for viral concentrates and work with infected host species.[109]

References

1. Choi K, Thacker SB: Mortality influenza epidemics in the United States, 1967–1978. Am J Public Health 72:1280–1283, 1982.
2. Kilbourne ED: Epidemiology of influenza. *In* Kilbourne ED (ed): Influenza Viruses and Influenza. New York, Academic Press, 1975, p 483.
3. Wells DL, Hopfensperger DJ, Arden NH, et al: Swine influenza virus infections. Transmission from ill pigs to humans at a Wisconsin agricultural fair and subsequent probable person-to-person transmission. JAMA 265:478–481, 1991.
4. McIntosh K: Pathogenesis of severe acute respiratory infections in the developing world: Respiratory syncytial virus and parainfluenza viruses. Rev Infect Dis 131(Suppl 6):S492–S500, 1991.
5. Centers for Disease Control: Respiratory syncytial virus and parainfluenza virus surveillance—United States, 1989–90. MMWR Morbid Mortal Wkly Rep 39:832–833, 839, 1990.
6. Henrickson KJ, Kuhn SM, Savatski LM: Epidemiology and cost of infection with human parainfluenza virus types 1 and 2 in young children. Clin Infect Dis 18:770–779, 1994.
7. Vainionpaa R, Hyypia T: Biology of parainfluenza viruses. Clin Microbiol Rev 7:265–275, 1994.
8. Warner JL: Parainfluenza viruses. *In* Balows A, Hausler WJ, Herrmann KL, et al (eds): Manual of Clinical Microbiology, ed 5. Washington, DC, American Society for Microbiology, 1991, pp 878–882.
9. Henrickson K, Ray R, Belshe R: Parainfluenza viruses. *In* Mandell GL, Bennett JE, Dolin R (eds): Mandell, Douglas and Bennett's Principles and Practice of Infectious Diseases, ed 4. New York, Churchill Livingstone, 1995, pp 1489–1496.
10. Henrickson KJ, Savtski LL. Genetic variation and evolution of human parainfluenza virus type 1 hemagglutinin neuraminidase: Analysis of 12 clinical isolates. J Infect Dis 166:995–1005, 1992.
11. Knott AM, Long CE, Hall CB: Parainfluenza viral infections in pediatric outpatients: Seasonal patterns and clinical characteristics. Pediatr Infect Dis J 13:269–273, 1994.
12. Glezen WP, Frank AL, Taber LH, Kasel JA: Parainfluenza virus type 3: Seasonality and risk of infection and reinfection in young children. J Infect Dis 150:851–857, 1984.
13. Rubin EE, Quennec P, McDonald JC: Infections due to parainfluenza virus type 4 in children. Clin Infect Dis 17:998–1002, 1993.
14. Ansari SA, Springthorpe VS, Sattar SA, et al: Potential role of hands in the spread of respiratory viral infections: Studies with human parainfluenza virus 3 and rhinovirus 14. J Clin Microbiol 29:2115–2119, 1991.
15. Karron RA, O'Brien KL, Froehlich JL, Brown VA: Molecular epidemiology of a parainfluenza type 3 virus outbreak on a pediatric ward. J Infect Dis 167:1441–1445, 1993.
16. Gilchrist S, Torok TJ, Gary HE, et al: National surveillance for respiratory syncytial virus, United States, 1985–1990. J Infect Dis 170:986–990, 1994.
17. Centers for Disease Control and Prevention: Update: Respiratory syncytial virus activity—United States, 1994–1995 season. MMWR Morbid Mortal Wkly Rep 43:920–922, 1994.
18. Anderson LJ, Parker RA, Strikas RL: Association between respiratory syncytial virus outbreaks and lower respiratory tract deaths of infants and young children. J Infect Dis 161:640–646, 1990.
19. Anderson LJ, Hendry RM, Pierik LT, et al: Multicenter study of strains of respiratory syncytial virus. J Infect Dis 163:687–692, 1991.
20. Henderson FW, Collier AM, Clyde WA, Denny FW: Respiratory-syncytial-virus infections, reinfections and immunity: A prospective, longitudinal study in young children. N Engl J Med 300:530–534, 1979.
21. Glezen WP, Taber LH, Frank AL, Kassel JA: Risk of primary infection and reinfection with respiratory syncytial virus. Am J Dis Child 140:543–546, 1986.
22. Agius G, Dindinaud G, Biggar RJ, et al: An epidemic of respiratory syncytial virus (RSV) in elderly people: Clinical and serologic findings. J Med Virol 30:117–127, 1990.
23. Hall CB, Geiman JM, Biggar R, et al: Respiratory syncytial virus infections within families. N Engl J Med 294:414–419, 1976.
24. Hall CB, Douglas RG Jr, Geiman JM: Possible transmission by fomites of respiratory syncytial virus. J Infect Dis 141:98–102, 1980.
25. Baum SG: Adenovirus. *In* Mandell GL, Bennett JE, Dolin R (eds): Mandell, Douglas and Bennett's Principles and Practice of Infectious Diseases, ed 4. New York, Churchill Livingstone, 1995, pp 1382–1387.
26. Dudding BA, Top FH Jr, Winter PE, et al: Acute respiratory disease in military trainees: The adenovirus surveillance program 1966–1971. Am J Epidemiol 97:187–198, 1973.
27. Stalder H, Hierholzer JC, Oxman MN: New human adenovirus (candidate adenovirus type 35) causing fatal disseminated infection in a renal transplant recipient. J Clin Microbiol 6:257–265, 1977.
28. Hierholzer JC, Wigand R, Anderson LJ: Adenoviruses from patients with AIDS: A plethora of serotypes and a description of five new serotypes of subgenus D (types 43–47). J Infect Dis 158:804–813, 1988.
29. Forbes BA: Acquisition of cytomegalovirus infection: An update. Clin Microbiol Rev 2:204–216, 1989.
30. Ho M: Cytomegalovirus. *In* Mandell GL, Bennett JE, Dolin R (eds): Mandell, Douglas and Bennett's Principles and Practice of Infectious Diseases, ed 4. New York, Churchill Livingstone, 1995, pp 1351–1364.
31. Centers for Disease Control and Prevention: Outbreak of acute illness—Southwestern United States, 1993. MMWR Morbid Mortal Wkly Rep 42:421–424, 1993.
32. Nichol ST, Spiropoulou CF, Morzunov S, et al: Genetic identification of a hantavirus associated with an outbreak of acute respiratory illness. Science 262:914–917, 1993.
33. Zaki SR, Greer PW, Coffield LM, et al: Hantavirus pulmonary syndrome: Pathogenesis of an emerging infectious disease. Am J Pathol 146:552–579, 1995.
34. Childs JE, Ksiazek TG, Spiropoulou CF, et al: Serologic and genetic identification of *Peromyscus maniculatus* as the primary rodent reservoir for a new hantavirus in the Southwestern United States. J Infect Dis 169:1271–1280, 1994.
35. Butler JC, Peters CJ: Hantaviruses and hantavirus pulmonary syndrome. Clin Infect Dis 19:387–395, 1994.
36. Zaki SR, Albers RC, Greer PW, et al: Retrospective diagnosis of a 1983 case of fatal hantavirus pulmonary syndrome. Lancet 343:1037–1038, 1994.
37. Centers for Disease Control and Prevention: Hantavirus pulmonary syndrome—Virginia, 1993. MMWR Morbid Mortal Wkly Rep 43:876–877, 1994.
38. Schulze IT: The biologically active proteins of influenza virus: The hemagglutinin. *In* Kilbourne ED (ed): The Influenza Viruses and Influenza. New York, Academic Press, 1975, p 53.
39. Welliver RC: Detection, pathogenesis, and therapy of respiratory syncytial virus infections. Clin Microbiol Rev 1:27–39, 1988.
40. Garofalo R, Kimpen JLL, Welliver RC, Ogra PL: Eosinophil degranulation in the respiratory tract during naturally acquired respiratory syncytial virus infection. J Pediatr 120:28–32, 1992.
41. Hall CB, McCarthy CA: Respiratory syncytial virus. *In* Mandell GL, Bennett JE, Dolin R (eds): Mandell, Douglas and Bennett's Principles and Practice of Infectious Diseases, ed 4. New York, Churchill Livingstone, 1995, pp 1501–1519.
42. Rowe WP, Huebner RJ, Gillmore LK, et al: Isolation of a cytopathogenic human adenoids undergoing spontaneous degeneration in tissue culture. Proc Soc Exp Biol Med 84:570–573, 1953.
43. Balthesen M, Messerle M, Reddehase MJ: Lungs are a major organ site of cytomegalovirus latency. J Virol 67:5360–5366, 1993.
44. Grundy JE: Virologic and pathogenic aspects of cytomegalovirus infection. Rev Infect Dis 12(Suppl 7):S711–S719, 1990.

45. Meyers JD, Flournoy N, Thomas ED: Risk factors for cytomegalovirus infection after human marrow transplantation. J Infect Dis 153:478–488, 1986.
46. Chou S: Acquisition of donor strains of cytomegalovirus by renal-transplant recipients. N Engl J Med 314:1418–1423, 1986.
47. Wingard JR, Mellitis ED, Sostrin MB, et al: Interstitial pneumonitis after allogeneic bone marrow transplantation. Nine year experience at a single institution. Medicine (Baltimore) 67:175–186, 1988.
48. Palese P, Tobita K, Ueda M, et al: Characterization of temperature sensitive influenza virus mutants defective in neuraminidase. Virology 61:397–410, 1974.
49. Naficy K: Human influenza with proved viremia. N Engl J Med 269:964–966, 1963.
50. Stanley ED, Jackson GG: Viremia in Asian influenza. Trans Assoc Am Physicians 79:376–387, 1966.
51. Louria DB, Blumenfield HL, Ellis JT, et al: Studies on influenza in the pandemic of 1957–1958. II. Pulmonary complications of influenza. J Clin Invest 38:213–265, 1959.
52. Schwarzmann SW, Adler JL, Sullivan RF Jr, et al: Bacterial pneumonia during the Hong Kong influenza epidemic of 1968–1969. Arch Intern Med 127:1037–1041, 1971.
53. Proby CM, Hackett D, Gupta S, et al: Acute myopericarditis in influenza A infection. Q J Med 60:887–892, 1986.
54. Flewett TH, Hoult JG: Influenzal encephalopathy and postinfluenzal encephalitis. Lancet 2:11–15, 1958.
55. Wells CEC, James WRL, Evans AD: Guillain-Barré syndrome and virus of influenza A (Asian strain). Arch Neurol Psychiatry 81:699–705, 1959.
56. Sperber SJ, Francis JB: Toxic shock syndrome during an influenza outbreak. JAMA 257:1086–1087, 1987.
57. Forsyth BW, Horwitz RI, Acampora D, et al: New epidemiologic evidence confirming that bias does not explain the aspirin–Reye's syndrome association. JAMA 261:2517–2524, 1989.
58. Hurwitz ES, Nelson DB, Davis C, et al: National surveillance for Reye syndrome: A five-year review. Pediatrics 6:895–900, 1982.
59. Wenzel RP, McCormick DP, Beam WE: Parainfluenza pneumonia in adults. JAMA 221:294–295, 1971.
60. Gelfand EW, McCurdy D, Rao CP, Middleton PJ: Ribavirin treatment of viral pneumonitis in severe combined immunodeficiency syndrome. Lancet 2:732–733, 1983.
61. McIntosh K, Kurachek SC, Cairns LM, et al: Treatment of respiratory viral infection in an immunodeficient infant with ribavirin aerosol. Am J Dis Child 138:305–308, 1984.
62. Wendt CH, Weisdorf DJ, Jordan C, et al: Parainfluenza virus respiratory infection after bone marrow transplantation. N Engl J Med 326:921–926, 1992.
63. Josephs S, Kim HW, Prandt CD, Parrott RH: Parainfluenza 3 virus and other common respiratory pathogens in children with human immunodeficiency virus infection. Pediatr Infect Dis J 7:207–209, 1988.
64. Groothuis JR, Gutierrez KM, Lauer BA: Respiratory syncytial virus infection in children with bronchopulmonary dysplasia. Pediatrics 82:199–203, 1988.
65. Chandwani S, Borkowsky W, Krasinski K, et al: Respiratory syncytial virus infection in human immunodeficiency virus–infected children. J Pediatr 117:251–254, 1990.
66. King JC Jr, Burke AR, Clemens JD, et al: Respiratory syncytial virus illnesses in human immunodeficiency virus- and noninfected children. Pediatr Infect Dis J 12:733–739, 1993.
67. Englund JA, Sullivan CJ, Jordan C, et al: Respiratory syncytial virus infection in immunocompromised adults. Ann Intern Med 109:203–208, 1988.
68. Hertz MI, Englund JA, Snover D, et al: Respiratory syncytial virus–induced acute lung injury in adult patients with bone marrow transplants: A clinical approach and review of the literature. Medicine (Baltimore) 68:269–281, 1989.
69. Harrington RD, Hooton TM, Hackman RC, et al: An outbreak of respiratory syncytial virus in a bone marrow transplant center. J Infect Dis 165:987–993, 1992.
70. Klemola E, Stenstrom R, von Essen R: Pneumonia as a clinical manifestation of cytomegalovirus infection in previously healthy adults. Scand J Infect Dis 4:7–10, 1972.
71. Cohen JI, Corey GR: Cytomegalovirus infection in the normal host. Medicine (Baltimore) 64:100–114, 1985.
72. Stagno S, Brasfield DM, Brown MB, et al: Infant pneumonitis associated with cytomegalovirus, *Chlamydia, Pneumocystis*, and *Ureaplasma*: A prospective study. Pediatrics 68:322–329, 1981.
73. Smith CB: Cytomegalovirus pneumonia: State of the art. Chest 95:182S–187S, 1989.
74. Smyth RL, Scott JP, Borysiewicz LK, et al: Cytomegalovirus infection in heart-lung transplant recipients: Risk factors, clinical associations, and response to treatment. J Infect Dis 164:1045–1050, 1991.
75. Millar AB, Patou G, Miller RF, et al: Cytomegalovirus in the lungs of patients with AIDS: Respiratory pathogen or passenger? Am Rev Respir Dis 141:1474–1477, 1990.
76. Jacobson MA, Mills J, Rush J, et al: Morbidity and mortality of patients with AIDS and first-episode *Pneumocystis carinii* pneumonia unaffected by concomitant pulmonary cytomegalovirus infection. Am Rev Respir Dis 144:6–9, 1991.
77. Wallace JM, Hannah J: Cytomegalovirus pneumonitis in patients with AIDS: Findings in an autopsy series. Chest 92:198–203, 1987.
78. Squire SB, Lipman MCI, Bagdades EK, et al: Severe cytomegalovirus pneumonitis in HIV infected patients with higher than average CD4 counts. Thorax 47:301–304, 1992.
79. Lundgren JD, Vestbo J, Junge J, Mathiesen LR: CMV pneumonia and response to ganciclovir treatment in an AIDS patient. Respir Med 85:437–439, 1991.
80. Duchin JS, Koster FT, Peters CJ, et al: Hantavirus pulmonary syndrome: A clinical description of 17 patients with a newly recognized syndrome. N Engl J Med 330:949–955, 1994.
81. Ketai LH, Williamson MR, Telepak RJ, et al: Hantavirus pulmonary syndrome: Radiographic finding in 16 patients. Radiology 191:665–668, 1994.
82. Zurlo JJ, O'Neill D, Polis MA, et al: Lack of utility of cytomegalovirus blood and urine cultures in patients with HIV infection. Ann Intern Med 118:12–17, 1993.
83. Centers for Disease Control and Prevention: Progress in the development of *Hantavirus* diagnostic assays—United States. MMWR Morbid Mortal Wkly Rep 42:770–771, 1993.
84. Skehel JJ, Hay AJ, Armstrong JA: On the mechanism of inhibition of influenza virus replication by amantadine hydrochloride. J Gen Virol 38:97–110, 1977.
85. Dolin R, Reichman RC, Madore HP, et al: A controlled trial of amantadine and rimantadine in the prophylaxis of influenza A infection. N Engl J Med 307:580–584, 1982.
86. Hayden FG, Gwaltney JM Jr, Van de Castle RL: Comparative toxicity of amantadine hydrochloride and rimantadine hydrochloride in healthy adults. Antimicrob Agents Chemother 19:226–233, 1981.
87. Younkin SW, Betts RF, Roth FK, Douglas RG Jr: Reduction in fever and symptoms in young adults with influenza A/Brazil/78 H1N1 infection after treatment with aspirin or amantadine. Antimicrob Agents Chemother 23:577–582, 1983.
88. Committee on Infectious Diseases: Use of ribavirin in the treatment of respiratory syncytial virus infection. Pediatrics 92:501–504, 1993.
89. AIDS Clinical Trials Group: Mortality in patients with the acquired immunodeficiency syndrome treated with either ganciclovir or foscarnet for cytomegalovirus retinitis. N Engl J Med 326:213–220, 1992.
90. Hocker JR, Cook LN, Adams G, Rabalais GP: Ganciclovir therapy of congenital cytomegalovirus pneumonia. Pediatr Infect Dis J 9:743–745, 1990.
91. Emanuel D, Cunningham I, Jules-Elysee K, et al: Cytomegalovirus pneumonia after bone marrow transplantation successfully treated with the combination of ganciclovir and high-dose intravenous immune globulin. Ann Intern Med 109:777–782, 1988.
92. Huggins JW, Hsiang CM, Cosgriff TM, et al: Prospective, double-blinded, concurrent, placebo-controlled clinical trial of intravenous ribavirin therapy of hemorrhagic fever with renal syndrome. J Infect Dis 164:1119–1127, 1991.
93. Sayer WJ, Entwhisleg, Uyeno B, et al: Cortisone therapy of early epidemic hemorrhagic fever: A preliminary report. Ann Intern Med 42:839–851, 1955.
94. Centers for Disease Control and Prevention: Hantavirus pulmonary syndrome—Northeastern United States, 1994 [published erratum in MMWR Morbid Mortal Wkly Rep 43:638, 1994]. MMWR Morbid Mortal Wkly Rep 43:548–549, 555–556, 1994.
95. Nichol KL, Margolis KL, Wourenma J, Von Sternberg J: The

efficacy and cost effectiveness of vaccination against influenza among elderly persons living in the community. N Engl J Med 331:778–784, 1994.
96. Centers for Disease Control and Prevention: Prevention and control of influenza recommendations of the Advisory Committee on Immunization Practices (ACIP). MMWR Morbid Mortal Wkly Rep 44(RR-3):1–22, 1995.
97. Kapikian AZ, Mitchell RH, Chanock RM, et al: An epidemiologic study of altered clinical reactivity to respiratory syncytial (RS) virus infection in children previously vaccinated with an inactivated RS vaccine. Am J Epidemiol 89:405–421, 1969.
98. Pullan CR, Toms GL, Martin AJ, et al: Breast feeding and respiratory syncytial virus infection. Br Med J 281:1034–1036, 1980.
99. Groothius JR, Simoes EAF, Levin MJ, et al: Prophylactic administration of respiratory syncytial virus immune globulin to high risk infants and young children. N Engl J Med 329:1524–1530, 1993.
100. Leclair JM, Freeman J, Sullivan BF, et al: Prevention of nosocomial respiratory syncytial virus infections through compliance with glove and gown isolation precautions. N Engl J Med 317:329–334, 1987.
101. Madge P, Paton JY, McColl JH, Mackie PLK: Prospective controlled study of four infection-control procedures to prevent nosocomial infection with respiratory syncytial virus. Lancet 340:1079–1083, 1992.
102. Gala CL, Hall CB, Schnabel KC, et al: The use of eye-nose goggles to control nosocomial respiratory syncytial virus infection. JAMA 256:2706–2708, 1986.
103. Meyers JD, Reed EC, Shepp DH, et al: Acyclovir for prevention of cytomegalovirus infection and disease after allogeneic marrow transplantation. N Engl J Med 318:70–71, 1988.
104. Singh N, Yu VL, Mieles L, et al: High-dose acyclovir compared with short-course preemptive ganciclovir therapy to prevent cytomegalovirus disease in liver transplant recipients: A randomized trial. Ann Intern Med 120:375–381, 1994.
105. Winston DJ, Ho WG, Cheng-Hsien L, et al: Intravenous immune globulin for prevention of cytomegalovirus infection and interstitial pneumonia after bone marrow transplantation. Ann Intern Med 106:12–18, 1987.
106. Goodrich JM, Bowden RA, Fisher L, et al: Ganciclovir prophylaxis to prevent cytomegalovirus disease after allogeneic marrow transplant. Ann Intern Med 118:173–178, 1993.
107. Spector SA, McKinley GF, Lalezari JP, et al: Oral ganciclovir for the prevention of cytomegalovirus disease in persons with AIDS. N Engl J Med 334:1491–1497, 1996.
108. Centers for Disease Control and Prevention: Hantavirus infection—Southwestern United States. Interim recommendations for risk reduction. MMWR Morbid Mortal Wkly Rep 42(RR-11):1–13, 1993.
109. Centers for Disease Control and Prevention: Laboratory management of agents associated with hantavirus pulmonary syndrome: Interim biosafety guidelines. MMWR Morbid Mortal Wkly Rep 43(RR-7):1–7, 1994.

58

Mycoplasma Pneumonia

Maurice A. Mufson

History

In the 1960s, 20 years after Eaton first attempted to isolate a causative organism from persons with "primary atypical pneumonia," *Mycoplasma pneumoniae* was recognized as the etiologic agent of mycoplasmal pneumonia. Primary atypical pneumonia encompassed the nonbacterial pneumonias of undefined cause that failed to respond to the antimicrobial drugs available in the 1940s. Eaton succeeded in producing pneumonia in cotton rats by intranasal administration of infectious sputum specimens from persons with "primary atypical pneumonia," but he was unable to isolate an etiologic organism.[1, 2] Ten years later, Eaton and Liu demonstrated the organism (the Eaton agent) in experimentally infected embryonated eggs using an indirect immunofluorescence procedure.[3, 4] In the following years, Chanock and coworkers[5–7] isolated *M. pneumoniae* from the sputum of persons with mycoplasmal pneumonia and established that it was the first *Mycoplasma* species that was pathogenic for humans.

Microbiology

M. pneumoniae belongs to the class Mollicutes, order Mycoplasmatales, family Mycoplasmataceae, and genus *Mycoplasma*.[8] The smallest organisms capable of replicating on complex cell-free medium, mycoplasmas lack a cell wall and require cholesterol for growth. *M. pneumoniae* also metabolizes glucose, exhibits hemadsorption, and produces hydrogen peroxide and superoxide anion.[9] The GC content of *M. pneumoniae* is about 40%, higher than for any other *Mycoplasma* species. All isolates tested of *M. pneumoniae* appear identical.[10]

The genome of *M. pneumoniae* comprises about 800 to 850 kilobase pairs.[11] It contains one ribosomal RNA operon, and its RNA gene order is 5′-16S-23S-5S-3′.[12] *M. pneumoniae* contains several specific proteins of molecular masses 168/170, 130, 110, 92, 90, 45, and 35 kDa, of which two are adhesins.[10] The P1 adhesin protein (168/170 kDa) and a second adhesin mediate attachment to cells by recognition of either sulfated glycolipids or α_{2-3}-linked sialyloligosaccharides on glycoproteins.[13–15] Erythrocyte binding requires only the α_{2-3}-linked sialyloligosaccharide receptor; sialoglycolipids inhibit adhesion of *M. pneumoniae* to erythrocytes.[15, 16] Two distinct groups of *M. pneumoniae* have been reported on the basis of variation of the gene encoding P1 adhesin protein.[17] The two groups differ by a single 12-kb fragment that was detected in group 1 (few isolates) and absent in group 2 (most, including prototype, isolates). The P1 adhesin resides on the tiplike configuration of *M. pneumoniae*. The gene for the P1 protein has been cloned, the amino acid sequence deduced, and a single 13–amino acid site-specific epitope synthesized that reacts with a cytadherence-blocking monoclonal antibody.[18, 19] In *M. pneumoniae*, cytadherence undergoes spontaneous reversible switching involving five high-molecular-weight proteins.[12]

Epidemiology

M. pneumoniae occurs endemically, occasionally epidemically, and among all age groups. Epidemics occur at 4- to 7-year intervals.[20] Pneumonia develops in 3% to 10% of persons infected with *M. pneumoniae*. It accounts for about 5% to 15% of all pneumonia illnesses, although the rate may be two to three times higher in high-risk groups. Less than 5% of patients with mycoplasmal pneumonia require in-hospital care. Mycoplasmal pneumonia occurs commonly in children and young adults, causing about one third to two thirds of pneumonias in these groups. Peak incidence of *M. pneumoniae* pneumonia occurs among teenagers; the annual rate is 2 to 5 per 1000.[20]

M. pneumoniae spreads slowly in families and in semiclosed populations during several months. The organism enters a household by school-age children and eventually spreads to all susceptible family members. As many as one half of family members may develop pneumonia. The incubation period is 3 weeks. *M. pneumoniae* spreads by infectious droplets; the larger droplets deposit on the nasal and upper respiratory tract passages; the particles less than 5 nm in diameter reach the lungs.

Pathogenesis

The pathogenic mechanisms of *M. pneumoniae* involve several components, including the attachment of cytadhesins, the secretion of hydrogen peroxide and superoxide anion, and the formation of autoantibodies.[14, 15, 21–25] *M. pneumoniae* attaches to the ciliated epithelium of the respiratory tract by two adhesins, one of which is the P1 protein, that bind to α_{2-3}-linked sialyloligosaccharides of glycoproteins and to Gal($3SO_4$)β1 residues of sulfated glycolipids. These sites are abundant in the bronchial epithelium.[14, 15, 21] The close attachment of the organism through these cytadherence receptors probably promotes its destructive effects on ciliated cells. The P1 protein evokes a homologous antibody response.[26] The formation of complexes between the receptors of host cells and the organism may be the stimulus for the formation of a number of autoantibodies in *M. pneumoniae* infection.[14, 15, 21, 25] *M. pneumoniae* attaches to erythrocytes also by means of the α_{2-3}-linked sialyloligosaccharides of Ii antigen, and these complexes may induce the formation of cold hemagglutinins.[16, 25] Circulating autoantibodies may be involved in the pulmonary and extrapulmonary manifestations of *M. pneumoniae* infection.[27]

Hydrogen peroxide and superoxide anion produced by *M. pneumoniae* damage respiratory tract cells and erythrocytes.[22–24] Viable organisms inhibit catalase activity of host cells, thus averting inactivation of the peroxide and superoxide anion.[23] Circulating and cell surface antibodies may also influence recovery from *M. pneumoniae* infection.[6] Cellular immunity may be implicated in recovery from infection, because *M. pneumoniae* induces release of interferon from human lymphocytes.[22, 28]

Clinical Manifestations

Mycoplasmal pneumonia begins insidiously, with fever, nonproductive cough, chills, headache, and malaise. Several days elapse before the patient seeks medical care (Table 58–1). More than half of patients suffer all of these symptoms.[29–33] Nearly all patients experience fever, usually a temperature between 100°F and 103°F, accompanied by a chilly sensation; frank shaking chills do not occur.[30] After a few days, the cough produces small amounts of white mucoid or watery sputum. Hemoptysis rarely occurs. The paucity of physical findings at the beginning of the pneumonia contrasts with its apparent severity. Rales and rhonchi develop in more than three fourths of patients, often appearing several days after the onset. Rhinorrhea, myalgias, chest pain, sore throat, and hoarseness occur in one fourth to one half of patients. Few patients develop tympanitis or bullous myringitis.[6, 32]

Untreated mycoplasmal pneumonia usually abates in 10 to 14 days; in a minority of patients, the course of illness may be protracted, lasting as long as 6 weeks.[7, 31, 33] Some patients experience persistent cough, and about one fifth of patients manifest radiographic abnormalities for up to 4 months.[7, 31] In nearly all instances, mycoplasmal pneumonia heals without pulmonary sequelae.[7, 31] Rare complications include residual pleural abnormalities, lung abscesses, lobar consolidation, severe respiratory failure, and adult respiratory distress syndrome.[34]

TABLE 58–1 ■ Salient Clinical Features of Mycoplasmal Pneumonia

Onset is insidious with cough, fever, headache, chills, and malaise.
Mucoid sputum develops several days later.
Sputum is rarely blood tinged.
Rhonchi and rales appear, usually several days after first physical examination.
On radiographic examination, pneumonic infiltrates appear diffusely reticulonodular or interstitial, often leading from the hilum to the lung base.
The pneumonia is unilateral in most cases; in about one fourth of cases, it is bilateral.
Pleural effusion may be present in about one fifth of cases.
Leukocytosis occurs in about one fourth of cases.
Cold hemagglutinins develop in about one half of cases, usually in the more serious illnesses.
Other organ systems are infrequently involved.
Treatment with tetracycline or erythromycin effectively reduces the duration of symptoms and signs and shortens the duration of illness; however, shedding of *M. pneumoniae* continues for 1 or 2 wk after antibiotic treatment is begun.
Fatalities rarely occur.

Mycoplasmal pneumonia tends to occur in one lung, more often the right lung, and in the lower lobes. The infiltrates appear diffusely reticulonodular or interstitial, often appearing as streaks from the hilum to the base.[30, 31] One fourth of patients develop bilateral pneumonias, sometimes involving both hilar regions and producing a "butterfly-like" infiltrate. Small pleural effusions are found at radiography in about one fourth of cases, but an associated pleuritis occurs uncommonly.

The results of routine laboratory tests are normal in the majority of cases of mycoplasmal pneumonia. Leukocytosis develops in about one fourth of patients, and an elevated erythrocyte sedimentation rate develops in about one third.[30]

Serious extrapulmonary complications of *M. pneumoniae* infection occur at exceedingly low rates. About 1 per 1000 *M. pneumoniae* infections becomes complicated by central nervous system disease.[35] The leading complications involve diverse central nervous system diseases, mainly meningoencephalitis, meningitis, and encephalitis and rarely acute cerebellar ataxia, cranial nerve neuritis, Guillain-Barré syndrome, and mononeuritis multiplex with brachial plexus neuropathy.[36–42] Uncommon complications include pericarditis, Stevens-Johnson syndrome, erythema nodosum, and cold hemagglutinin–mediated hemolytic anemia.[34] The altered immune reactivity in *M. pneumoniae* infection may contribute to the pathogenesis of extrapulmonary involvement.[43] Fatal infection rarely occurs.

Diagnosis

A specific laboratory diagnosis of *M. pneumoniae* infection can be made by isolation on agar of the organism from sputum, throat swab, pleural fluid, or tissue; demonstration of a diagnostic rise in antibody to *M. pneumoniae* during convalescence by complement fixation or enzyme-linked immunosorbent assay; detection of a high-titer immunoglobulin M– or immunoglobulin A–specific antibody to *M. pneumoniae* in an acute-phase serum specimen; or amplification of genomic sequences in sputum specimens by polymerase chain reaction using primer sets from variable regions of 16S ribosomal RNA specific for *M. pneumoniae.* Detection of high levels (above 1:40) of cold hemagglutinin antibody in a single serum specimen provides presumptive evidence of *M. pneumoniae* infection, although this antibody can clearly be present in other clinical conditions. Without the ready availability of specific antibody tests, a positive test result for cold hemagglutinins provides a rational basis for initiating antibiotic treatment.

The isolation of *M. pneumoniae* from clinical specimens usually requires about 10 to 14 days. On mycoplasma agar plates, the organism grows as small colonies that can be seen adequately only by low-power microscopy. Colonial morphology does not differentiate *M. pneumoniae* from other nonpathogenic mycoplasmas that inhabit the oropharynx. The colonies can be identified by metabolic characteristics or growth (disk) neutralization employing antibody-impregnated disks. In SP-4 diphasic medium, growth of the organism produces acid metabolites that change the indicator from blue to yellow or cause turbidity in the liquid. Isolates in SP-4 diphasic medium must be subcultured onto agar and identified either by a rapid direct plate immunofluorescence antibody test or by disk neutralization procedures.[44]

Although culture of *M. pneumoniae* from clinical specimens represents the "gold standard" for diagnosis of infection, it is much less rapid than serologic methods or polymerase chain reaction for *M. pneumoniae*. Rapid identification of *M. pneumoniae* infection facilitates early appropriate antibiotic treatment. Polymerase chain reaction applied to sputum specimens holds promise as a rapid albeit complex procedure of high sensitivity and specificity.[45–49] Different primer sets of the variable region of 16S ribosomal RNA successfully amplify genomic sequences specific to *M. pneumoniae* (and not to *Mycoplasma genitalium*, another human pathogen).[50] These procedures can detect 5 to 50 fg of *M. pneumoniae* DNA or about 100 colony-forming units/mL.[51] Polymerase chain reaction can rapidly identify *M. pneumoniae* DNA in cerebrospinal fluid of persons with central nervous system infections.[52] The determination of immunoglobulin A– and immunoglobulin M–specific antibody also has the advantage of quickly identifying *M. pneumoniae* as the infecting organism. The detection of immunoglobulin A– and immunoglobulin M–specific antibody in high titers measured by enzyme-linked immunosorbent assay in single serum specimens collected 8 to 14 days after the onset of illness provides a sensitive and specific means of serologic diagnosis.[53] Immunoglobulin A–specific antibody to *M. pneumoniae* occurs in reinfection. Peak titers of these antibodies develop about 1 week later. Immunoglobulin M anti-P1 antibody detected by immunoblotting can also be used as a rapid test for the diagnosis of *M. pneumoniae* infection.[54]

Routine antibody tests for detection of *M. pneumoniae* infection include complement fixation, enzyme-linked immunosorbent assay, and growth inhibition. These procedures are sensitive and specific and command wide use in clinical laboratories and in epidemiologic studies. However, serologic diagnosis of infection requires the demonstration of a rise in antibody level by testing paired serum specimens obtained during the acute and convalescent phases of illness. In these cases, the convalescent-phase serum specimen should be obtained 18 to 21 days after the acute-phase serum specimen. Other antibody assays, such as immunofluorescence and indirect hemagglutination, are less often employed routinely for the diagnosis of infection (Table 58–2).

The differential diagnosis of mycoplasmal pneumonia includes psittacosis; Q fever; common viral pneumonias, especially influenza virus pneumonia; and *Legionella* pneumonia. These pneumonias can cause similar clinical features and radiographic findings. Bacterial pneumonia should be considered in the differential diagnosis, because mycoplasmal pneumonia uncommonly shows a lobar pattern at radiography. Mycoplasmal pneumonia may present as an apical pneumonia mimicking pulmonary tuberculosis.

Treatment

The treatment of mycoplasmal pneumonia consists of the administration of appropriate antibiotics and supportive therapy to lessen the discomfort of the illness. Among adults, the recommended antibiotics are tetracycline, 2 g daily in four divided doses, or erythromycin, 2 g daily in divided doses for at least 10 to 14 days.[7, 55] Both antibiotics are effective; the choice may depend on secondary circumstances. Tetracycline must not be given to children or to pregnant women, because it mottles the teeth of infants and children. Administer erythromycin in a dose of 30 to 50 mg/kg per day to infants and children weighing less than 25 kg and 1 g daily in divided doses to children weighing more than 25 kg. Alternatively, one of the newer macrolides, clarithromycin and azithromycin, can be used; however, no controlled trial of the treatment of *M. pneumoniae* infection with these antibiotics has been conducted.[56] In vitro tests show that *M. pneumoniae* is sensitive to both antibiotics. The dose is 500 mg of clarithromycin twice a day and 500 mg of azithromycin on the first day and 250 mg daily thereafter in adults only.

TABLE 58–2 ▪ Laboratory Diagnosis of *Mycoplasma pneumoniae* Infection

TARGET	PROCEDURE	REAGENT	USE AS ROUTINE TEST	SIGNIFICANCE
Isolation	Culture on agar	—	Yes	Gold standard for diagnosis
Direct	Polymerase chain reaction	Primer sets	No	Rapid detection of amplification is diagnostic
Specific antibody	Complement fixation	Glycolipid	Yes	Rise is diagnostic
	Metabolic inhibition	Whole organism	Yes	Rise is diagnostic
	Enzyme immunoassay	Protein; purified P1 protein	Yes	Rise is diagnostic
	Mycoplasmacidal assay	Whole organism	No	Rise is diagnostic
	Immunofluorescence	Membrane	No	Rise is diagnostic
	Indirect hemagglutination	Whole organism	No	Rise is diagnostic
	Immunoblotting	Sonicated, solubilized organism	No	Specific peptide lines diagnostic
Nonspecific antibody	Cold hemagglutination	Anti-I agglutinins	Yes	Rise is presumptive
	Venereal Disease Research Laboratory test	False-positive serologic test for syphilis	No	None
	Streptococcus agglutination	Streptococcus MG	No	None
	Complement fixation	Autoantibodies	No	None
		Rheumatoid factor	No	False-positive

Use erythromycin when the clinical features suggest mycoplasmal or *Legionella* pneumonia; use tetracycline (unless contraindicated) when psittacosis or Q fever cannot be ruled out. Bed rest, ample fluids, bronchodilators, antipyretic medications (avoid aspirin in infants and children), and antitussive syrups also make the patient more comfortable.

Prevention

Recommended general preventive measures are hand washing and use of disposable paper tissues, rather than handkerchiefs, to wipe the nose and hands.

There is no commercially available vaccine for *M. pneumoniae*. During the past two decades, experimental inactivated whole-organism vaccines and live attenuated vaccines were tested in volunteers for antigenicity and efficacy.[57, 58] However, they failed to produce the levels of protection necessary for use in high-risk groups or the general population. Studies of vaccines center on the use of purified components of the organism as vaccines, principally the P1 adhesin.[18, 19, 58] An acellular extract vaccine composed of several *M. pneumoniae* proteins including the P1 adhesin protein administered to chimpanzees protected them from serious illness during subsequent challenge.[59]

References

1. Eaton MD, Meiklejohn G, Van Herick W: Studies on the etiology of primary atypical pneumonia: A filterable agent transmissible to cotton rats, hamsters, and chick embryos. J Exp Med 79:649, 1944.
2. Eaton MD, Meiklejohn G, Van Herick W, et al: Studies on the etiology of primary atypical pneumonia. II. Properties of the virus isolated and propagated in chick embryos. J Exp Med 82:317, 1945.
3. Liu C: Studies on primary atypical pneumonia. I. Localization, isolation, and cultivation of a virus in chick embryos. J Exp Med 106:455, 1957.
4. Liu C, Eaton MD, Heyl JT: Studies on primary atypical pneumonia. II. Observations concerning development and immunological characteristics of antibody in patients. J Exp Med 109:545, 1959.
5. Chanock RM, Hayflick L, Barile MF: Growth on artificial medium of an agent associated with atypical pneumonia and its identification as a PPLO. Proc Natl Acad Sci USA 48:41, 1962.
6. Rifkind D, Chanock R, Kravetz H, et al: Ear involvement (myringitis) and primary atypical pneumonia following inoculation of volunteers with Eaton agent. Am Rev Respir Dis 85:479, 1962.
7. Kingston JR, Chanock RM, Mufson MA, et al: Eaton agent pneumonia. JAMA 176:118, 1961.
8. Freundt EA, Edward DG: Classification and taxonomy. *In* Barile MF, Razin S (eds): The Mycoplasmas, Vol 1. New York, Academic Press, 1979, pp 1–41.
9. Gardella RS, DelGiudice RA: Hemagglutination, hemadsorption, and hemolysis. *In* Razin S, Tully JG (eds): Methods in Mycoplasmology, Vol I: Mycoplasma Characterization. New York, Academic Press, 1983, pp 379–384.
10. Cong Vu A, Foy HM, Cartwright FD, et al: The principal protein antigens of isolates of *Mycoplasma pneumoniae* as measured by levels of immunoglobulin G in human serum are stable in strains collected over a 10-year period. Infect Immun 55:1830, 1987.
11. Wenzel R, Herrmann R: Cloning of the complete *Mycoplasma pneumoniae* genome. Nucleic Acids Res 17:7029, 1989.
12. Bove JM: Molecular features of Mollicutes. Clin Infect Dis 17:S10, 1993.
13. Collier AM, Hu PC, Clyde WA: Localization of attachment moiety on *Mycoplasma pneumoniae*. Yale J Biol Med 56:671, 1983.
14. Krivan HC, Olson LD, Barile MF, et al: Adhesion of *Mycoplasma pneumoniae* to sulfated glycolipids and inhibition by dextran sulfate. J Biol Chem 264:9283, 1989.
15. Roberts DD, Olson LD, Barile MF, et al: Sialic acid–dependent adhesion of *Mycoplasma pneumoniae* to purified glycoproteins. J Biol Chem 264:9289, 1989.
16. Loomes LM, Uemura KI, Feizi T: Interaction of *Mycoplasma pneumoniae* with erythrocyte glycolipids of I and i antigen types. Infect Immun 47:15, 1985.
17. Su CJ, Dallo SF, Baseman JB: Molecular distinctions among clinical isolates of *Mycoplasma pneumoniae*. J Clin Microbiol 28:1538, 1990.
18. Su CJ, Tryon VV, Baseman JB: Cloning and sequence analysis of cytadhesin P1 gene from *Mycoplasma pneumoniae*. Infect Immun 55:3203, 1987.
19. Dallo SF, Su CJ, Horton JR, et al: Identification of P1 gene domain containing epitope(s) mediating *Mycoplasma pneumoniae* cytadherence. J Exp Med 167:718, 1988.
20. Foy HM: Infections caused by *Mycoplasma pneumoniae* and possible carrier state in different populations of patients. Clin Infect Dis 17(Suppl 1):S37, 1993.
21. Loveless RW, Feizi T: Sialo-oligosaccharide receptors for *Mycoplasma pneumoniae* and related oligosaccharides of poly-*N*-acetyllactosamine series are polarized at the cilia and apical-microvillar domains of the ciliated cells in human bronchial epithelium. Infect Immun 57:1285, 1989.
22. Arai S, Munakata T, Kuwano K: Mycoplasma interaction with lymphocytes and phagocytes: Role of hydrogen peroxide released from *M. pneumoniae*. Yale J Biol Med 56:631, 1983.
23. Almagor M, Yatziv S, Kahane I: Inhibition of host cell catalase by *Mycoplasma pneumoniae*: A possible mechanism for cell injury. Infect Immun 41:251, 1983.
24. Almagor M, Kahane I, Yatziv S: Role of superoxide anion in host cell injury induced by *Mycoplasma pneumoniae* infection: A study in normal and trisomy 21 cells. J Clin Invest 73:842, 1984.
25. Konig AL, Kreft H, Hengg U: Coexisting anti-I and anti-Fl/Gd cold agglutinins in infections by *Mycoplasma pneumoniae*. Vox Sang 55:176, 1988.
26. Leith DK, Trevino LB, Tully JG, et al: Host discrimination of *Mycoplasma pneumoniae* proteinaceous immunogens. J Exp Med 157:502, 1983.
27. Hodson ME, Taylor P: Autoantibodies in infections of the respiratory tract with *Mycoplasma pneumoniae* or influenza virus A. Eur J Respir Dis 71:86, 1987.
28. Whittlestone P: Immunity to mycoplasma causing respiratory diseases in man and animals. Adv Vet Sci Comp Med 20:277, 1976.
29. Ponka A: The occurrence and clinical picture of serologically verified *Mycoplasma pneumoniae* infections with emphasis on central nervous, cardiac and joint manifestations. Ann Clin Res 11(Suppl 24):1, 1979.
30. Mansel JK, Rosenow EC III, Smith TF, et al: *Mycoplasma pneumoniae* pneumonia. Chest 95:639, 1989.
31. Mufson MA, Manko MA, Kingston JR, et al: Eaton agent pneumonia: Clinical features. JAMA 178:369, 1961.
32. Foy HM, Grayston JT, Kenny GE, et al: Epidemiology of *Mycoplasma pneumoniae* infection in families. JAMA 197:859, 1966.
33. Izumikawa K, Hara K: Clinical features of mycoplasmal pneumonia in adults. Yale J Biol Med 56:505, 1983.
34. Cassell GH, Cole BC: Mycoplasmas as agents of human disease. N Engl J Med 304:80, 1981.
35. Koskiniemi M: CNS manifestations associated with *Mycoplasma pneumoniae* infections: Summary of cases at the University of Helsinki and review. Clin Infect Dis 17(Suppl 1):S52, 1993.
36. Sterner G, Biberfeld G: Central nervous system complications of *Mycoplasma pneumoniae* infections. Scand J Infect Dis 1:203, 1969.
37. Lind K: Manifestations and complications of *Mycoplasma pneumoniae* disease: A review. Yale J Biol Med 56:461, 1983.
38. Mardh P-A, Ursing BO, Lind K: Persistent cerebellar syndrome after infection with *Mycoplasma pneumoniae*. Scand J Infect Dis 7:157, 1975.
39. Rothstein R, Kenny GE: Cranial neuropathy, myeloradiculopathy and myositis: Complications of *Mycoplasma pneumoniae* infection. Arch Neurol 36:476, 1979.
40. Laarman GJ, Hoekstra JBL, Donker DNJ, et al: Meningoencephalitis and Guillain-Barré type ascending sensorimotor paralysis associated with *Mycoplasma pneumoniae* infection. Neth J Med 31:66, 1987.
41. Abramovitz P, Schvartzman P, Harel D, et al: Direct invasion of the central nervous system by *Mycoplasma pneumoniae*: A report of two cases. J Infect Dis 155:482, 1987.

42. Kidron D, Barron SA, Mazliah J: Mononeuritis multiplex with brachial plexus neuropathy coincident with *Mycoplasma pneumoniae* infection. Eur Neurol 29:90, 1989.
43. Fernald GW: Immunologic mechanisms suggested in the association of *M. pneumoniae* infection and extrapulmonary disease: A review. Yale J Biol Med 56:475, 1983.
44. Tully JG: New laboratory techniques for isolation of *Mycoplasma pneumoniae*. Yale J Biol Med 56:511, 1983.
45. Bernet C, Garret M, Barbeyrac B, et al: Detection of *Mycoplasma pneumoniae* by using the polymerase chain reaction. J Clin Microbiol 27:2492, 1989.
46. van Kuppeveld FJ, Johansson KE, Galama JM, et al: 16S rRNA based polymerase chain reaction compared with culture and serological methods for diagnosis of *Mycoplasma pneumoniae* infection. Eur J Clin Microbiol Infect Dis 13:401, 1994.
47. Lüneberg E, Jensen JS, Frosch M: Detection of *Mycoplasma pneumoniae* by polymerase chain reaction and nonradioactive hybridization in microtiter plates. J Clin Microbiol 31:1088, 1993.
48. Leng Z, Kenny GE, Roberts MC: Evaluation of the detection limits of PCR for identification of *Mycoplasma pneumoniae* in clinical samples. Mol Cell Probes 8:125, 1994.
49. Tjhie JH, van Kuppeveld FJ, Roosendaal R, et al: Direct PCR enables detection of *Mycoplasma pneumoniae* in patients with respiratory tract infections. J Clin Microbiol 32:11, 1994.
50. Sasaki Y, Shintani M, Shimada T, et al: Detection and discrimination of *Mycoplasma pneumoniae* and *Mycoplasma genitalium* by the in vitro DNA amplification. Microbiol Immunol 36:21, 1992.
51. Kai M, Kamiya S, Yabe H, et al: Rapid detection of *Mycoplasma pneumoniae* in clinical samples by the polymerase chain reaction. J Med Microbiol 38:166, 1993.
52. Narita M, Matsuzono Y, Togashi T, et al: DNA diagnosis of central nervous system infection by *Mycoplasma pneumoniae*. Pediatrics 90:250, 1992.
53. Granstrom M, Holme T, Sjogren AM, et al: The role of IgA determination by ELISA in the early serodiagnosis of *Mycoplasma pneumoniae* infection, in relation to IgG and mu-capture IgM methods. J Med Microbiol 40:288, 1994.
54. Cimolai N, Cheong AC: IgM anti-P1 immunoblotting. A standard for the rapid serologic diagnosis of *Mycoplasma pneumoniae* infection in pediatric care. Chest 102:477, 1994.
55. Shames JM, George RB, Holliday WB, et al: Comparison of antibiotics in the treatment of mycoplasmal pneumonia. Arch Intern Med 125:680, 1970.
56. BéBéar C, Dupon M, Renaudin H, et al: Potential improvements in therapeutic options for mycoplasmal respiratory infections. Clin Infect Dis 17:S202, 1993.
57. Wenzel RP, Craven RB, Davies JA, et al: Field trial of an inactivated *Mycoplasma pneumoniae* vaccine. I. Vaccine efficacy. J Infect Dis 134:571, 1976.
58. Barile MF: Immunization against *Mycoplasma pneumoniae* disease: A review. Isr J Med Sci 20:912, 1984.
59. Barile MF, Grabowski MW, Kapatais-Zoumbois K, et al: Protection of immunized and previously infected chimpanzees challenged with *Mycoplasma pneumoniae*. Vaccine 12:707, 1994.

59

Pneumocystis carinii Pneumonia

Walter T. Hughes

Unlike the usual pneumonia caused by bacteria and viruses, that due to *Pneumocystis carinii* is unique in several ways. It occurs almost exclusively in patients whose immune systems are compromised. Even so, the organism and the disease remain localized to the lung parenchyma, whereas other infections in the immunocompromised host undergo systemic spread. This localized but complex infection requires a multidisciplinary approach by physician specialists. Because the patient almost assuredly has some underlying disease, an oncologist, organ transplanter, or clinical immunologist may be the primary physician who elicits the help of an infectious disease specialist. The diagnosis requires an invasive procedure, such as endoscopy and bronchoalveolar lavage done by the pulmonologist or thoracic surgeon, or an open lung biopsy under general anesthesia in some cases. Specimens are processed and interpreted by the pathologist. Patients with *P. carinii* pneumonitis often require assisted ventilation and the services of an intensive care unit team. It is wise to alert those personnel who are likely to be involved in the management as soon as the diagnosis is suspected.

History

P. carinii was first shown to be a cause of infection in humans in the early 1940s, when it was associated with epidemics of infantile interstitial plasma-cell pneumonitis in Europe. By the mid-1950s, it was recognized as a cause of diffuse alveolar disease in children and adults who had an underlying immunodeficiency disorder. As immunosuppressive therapy came to be used more extensively in cancer patients and organ transplant recipients, the prevalence of *P. carinii* pneumonitis increased. However, by far the greatest impact has been the epidemic of human immunodeficiency virus (HIV) infection (see also Chapter 122). In fact, the acquired immunodeficiency syndrome (AIDS) was first discovered because of the occurrence of *P. carinii* pneumonitis in young men with no obvious underlying disease.[1,2] Today, *P. carinii* pneumonitis causes more deaths in the United States than any other infectious disease.

Characteristics of the Pathogen

See Part VII, Microbial Agents.

Epidemiology

P. carinii has been found only in the lungs of humans and lower mammals. No natural habitat outside the lung has been identified. Studies in the United States and Europe show that more than 75% of normal healthy individuals have acquired antibody to *P. carinii* by 4 years of age.[3, 4] Furthermore, rats, mice, ferrets, and rabbits are latently infected to the extent that when they are immunosuppressed, overt *P. carinii* pneumonia ensues. In most parts of the world, both humans and lower animals are infected, with no areas of predominance or clustering.

The mode of transmission of *P. carinii* to humans is not known, but experimental studies in rats have shown that the organism can be airborne from animal to animal.[5] It is believed that *P. carinii* is acquired early in life and unassociated with discernible illness and that the organism persists in a latent subclinical state in the immunocompromised host. However, if the immune system becomes profoundly impaired, the organisms replicate and pneumonitis becomes evident. *P. carinii* pneumonitis occurs in about 75% of patients with AIDS and 43% of patients with severe combined immunodeficiency syndrome.

Pathogenesis

It is most likely that the trophozoite, the cyst, or both forms of *P. carinii* are inhaled and reach the alveolar lumen. From this point, the type and extent of the disease process, if any, depend on the immune response of the host and the replication of the organism. Because evidence of disease is rarely found in normal immunocompetent individuals, it is believed that the quantity of organisms is maintained at a low number. This could be explained by continuous surveillance and phagocytosis of replicating organisms at a rate sufficient to maintain a disease-free state. An alternative hypothesis is that one is exposed frequently to the organism, that immunity does not develop from asymptomatic infection, and that reinfection occurs in the absence of adequate host defense when the host becomes immunocompromised. In fact, data support the latter hypothesis. Animal studies show that *P. carinii* is spontaneously cleared from the lungs after the pneumonitis during a period of several months when the animals are maintained in *P. carinii*–free isolators[6] and that immune reconstitution of immunodeficient mice is associated with clearing of naturally acquired *P. carinii* infection.[7] With use of molecular methods to identify specific strains of *P. carinii*, laboratory animals were found to have more than one strain in the same lung, suggesting replenishment of the organism from the environment.[8] *P. carinii* DNA sequences can readily be found in air samples.[9]

The most effective component of the immune system in defense against *P. carinii* is the cell-mediated response. This has been most vividly exemplified by the results of retroviral infection and destruction of the important $CD4^+$ lymphocyte (helper T cell) by HIV. Under these circumstances, *P. carinii* pneumonia is highly prevalent, affecting more than 75% of such patients. The attack rate of *P. carinii* pneumonitis can be related directly to the quantity of $CD4^+$ cells.[11] Once the $CD4^+$ cell count reaches $200/mm^3$ or less, the risk for developing the pneumonitis is greatly enhanced, as has been demonstrated in HIV-infected patients. However, episodes may occur infrequently with $CD4^+$ lymphocyte counts of 200 to $500/mm^3$.[11]

The immune defect permissive to *P. carinii* pneumonitis is not limited to impaired cell-mediated response. Cases have been associated with classic X-linked agammaglobulinemia. Broad-spectrum immunodeficiency induced by corticosteroids and other immunosuppressive drugs effectively provokes the pneumonitis. Factors that enhance replication of *P. carinii* in vivo or in vitro are unknown.

Once in the alveolus, *P. carinii* attaches to the alveolar wall. As the disease evolves, an increase in trophozoites and cysts is seen, reactive alveolar macrophages appear, and organisms may be found in the cytoplasm of the phagocytes in varying stages of digestion. No intracellular phase of the life cycle has been demonstrated. Eventually, the alveolar lumen becomes filled with a proteinaceous exudate. The extensive diffuse desquamative alveolopathy is usually found throughout all lobes of the lungs. Rarely, atypical localized lesions occur. The interstitial tissue may show mononuclear cell infiltrates. In the infantile form, an interstitial plasma cell pneumonitis predominates, but this is rarely found in the immunocompromised child and adult. Although the organism and the disease remain localized to the pulmonary parenchyma in more than 99% of cases, extrapulmonary lesions may rarely be encountered. Lesions with *P. carinii* have been described in the bone marrow, skin, liver, heart, spleen, lymph nodes, eye, ear, thyroid, and mastoid.

Clinical Manifestations

Although the symptoms and signs of *P. carinii* pneumonitis are limited to cough, shortness of breath, fever, tachypnea, dyspnea, flaring of the nasal alae, cyanosis, and occasionally chest pain, the number and extent of these manifestations vary from patient to patient. The underlying condition of the host may indicate the clinical pattern to be expected. For example, in the infantile type, seen in patients younger than 6 months, fever is usually absent and the onset is subtle; rales are usually abundant. In the immunosuppressed child or adult with cancer, the onset is usually abrupt with fever and tachypnea in the absence of rales. In patients with AIDS, the onset is more subtle than with the cancer patient, although fever, cough, tachypnea, and dyspnea are prominent manifestations.

The chest radiograph reveals a bilateral diffuse alveolar disease in 90% or more of cases. The infiltrates become apparent first in the perihilar area, spreading peripherally but sparing the apical areas until the disease is far advanced. The hilar nodes are not enlarged. Spontaneous pneumothorax is occasionally seen even without an invasive diagnostic procedure. Atypical forms of *P. carinii* pneumonitis, seen uncommonly, include lobar pneumonia, single-coin lesions, unilateral infiltrates, and hyperexpanded lung.

A gallium scan of the lung may reveal diffuse uptake even before the abnormalities are discernible by radiography. However, this technique does not provide more specific etiologic information than does the chest radiograph.

Studies of arterial blood gases are especially helpful in identifying the presence of pulmonary disease before radiographic tests can detect infiltrates and also for assessing the extent of established pneumonitis. Although not specific for *P. carinii* pneumonitis, the presence of reduced arterial oxygen tension (PaO_2) and increased alveolar-arterial oxygen gradient is characteristic. These changes may be evident before abnormalities are seen radiographically but rarely before tachypnea occurs.

Serum lactate dehydrogenase activity may be increased and *P. carinii* antibody detectable, but these are not of diagnostic help.

The course of the pneumonitis is progressive, worsening with increasing hypoxia if no specific therapy is given. Once the pneumonitis has become evident radiographically, few patients if any will survive without treatment.

Diagnosis

A definitive diagnosis requires the demonstration of *P. carinii* in lung tissue or fluids aspirated from the lung or lower airways. Specimens may be obtained by one or more of the following procedures.

Open Lung Biopsy. This procedure provides the greatest amount of dependable information about the pulmonary disease. Adequate samples are available for cultures and histologic stains. If no *P. carinii* organisms are seen in an adequate biopsy specimen, one can reliably conclude that the pneumonitis is not due to this organism. Also, concomitant infections may be detected by this method. Although this may be the most sensitive method and the "gold standard," it may not necessarily be the most appropriate for a given patient, because a general anesthetic is required and the operative procedure may jeopardize pulmonary function at a critical time in the course of the disease.

Bronchoscopy and Bronchoalveolar Lavage. This procedure is especially useful for the diagnosis of *P. carinii* pneumonitis in AIDS patients, because organisms seem generally to be more abundant than in non-AIDS patients. Organisms may be missed in about 10% of cases, and complications of pneumothorax, bleeding, and transient impairment of pulmonary functions are undesirable features.

Transbronchial Biopsy. Transbronchial biopsy may be done with bronchoscopy and bronchoalveolar lavage, adding information to that from the lavage specimen. This should be done when the patient's condition will permit it without undue risk. The complications of bleeding and pneumothorax are more likely than with bronchoalveolar lavage alone.

Induced Sputum. This has been of diagnostic help when organisms are found, but the failure to find *P. carinii* in sputum samples does not exclude the diagnosis. The success of this procedure varies from institution to institution and probably depends on the development of skills in inducing the production of adequate sputum samples.

One study showed that *P. carinii* could be obtained from gastric aspirate and that its presence was associated with *P. carinii* pneumonitis.[12] However, this approach has not been pursued by others.

Specimens should be stained by methods that will identify the cyst and the trophozoite forms. The Gomori-Grocott methenamine–silver nitrate stain or toluidine blue O identifies the cyst form. Giemsa and Wright-Giemsa stains are preferred for the trophozoite forms (see Part VII, Microbial Agents). An immunofluorescence stain using a monoclonal antibody to *P. carinii* has been used successfully.

Differential Diagnosis

The differential diagnosis includes infections due to *Mycobacterium avium-intracellulare*, cytomegalovirus, Epstein-Barr virus, *Toxoplasma gondii*, and *Chlamydia trachomatis*; acute bacterial pneumonia (pneumococcal, streptococcal, and so forth); pulmonary mycosis *(Cryptococcus, Histoplasma, Coccidioides)*; and acute viral pneumonia (parainfluenza virus respiratory syncytial virus).

In infants and children with AIDS, lymphoid interstitial pneumonitis resembles *P. carinii* pneumonitis.

Treatment

Four drugs are approved by the U.S. Food and Drug Administration for the treatment of *P. carinii* pneumonitis. These are trimethoprim-sulfamethoxazole, pentamidine isethionate, atovaquone, and trimetrexate with leucovorin. Two other drugs in general use are dapsone plus trimethoprim and clindamycin plus primaquine. Trimethoprim-sulfamethoxazole is the drug of first choice.

Trimethoprim-Sulfamethoxazole

Trimethoprim alone has no effect on *P. carinii*, and sulfamethoxazole alone is effective; however, the combination is presumed to be synergistic, and approximately 75% of patients will recover with treatment.[13, 14] The dosage for intravenous administration is trimethoprim at 15 mg/kg and sulfamethoxazole at 75 mg/kg per day in three or four equally divided doses. Orally, the dosage is based on trimethoprim at 20 mg/kg and sulfamethoxazole at 100 mg/kg per day in three or four divided doses. If treatment is initiated with the oral preparation, it is often advisable to give the first dose as half the total daily quantity as a loading dose. The subsequent total daily doses, oral or intravenous, should not exceed 640 mg of trimethoprim and 3200 mg of sulfamethoxazole. In general, doses may be modified as needed to maintain peak serum levels of trimethoprim of about 5 to 8 μg/mL and sulfamethoxazole of 100 to 150 μg/mL. A course of 10 days is usually adequate in non-AIDS patients. Those with AIDS generally require 2 to 3 weeks of treatment.

Adverse reactions to trimethoprim-sulfamethoxazole include rashes, fever, leukopenia, elevated transaminase values, and gastrointestinal symptoms. AIDS patients have a unique susceptibility to react adversely to this drug. More than half of AIDS patients may have such reactions; a maculopapular erythematous rash is the most frequent effect.[15, 16] Less than 5% of non-AIDS patients have adverse reactions.

For patients who have no history of sulfonamide allergy, trimethoprim-sulfamethoxazole is the drug of choice for initial therapy.

Pentamidine Isethionate

Pentamidine is available only for intravenous or intramuscular administration. Aerosolized pentamidine is undergoing evaluation for therapy, but this is not the route of preference. A dose of 4.0 mg/kg per day administered intravenously in a period of 1 hour is preferred. The same dose can be used as a single daily intramuscular injection, but local injection site reactions are frequent and severe.

Adverse reactions to pentamidine occur in more than 50% of both AIDS and non-AIDS patients.[14, 17] These include renal dysfunction, hypoglycemia, hypertension, neutropenia, and thrombocytopenia. The duration of treatment is the same as for trimethoprim-sulfamethoxazole. Recovery can be expected in about 75% of cases.

Atovaquone

In mild and moderately severe cases of *P. carinii* pneumonitis (alveolar-arterial oxygen gradient less than 45 mm Hg), the overall therapeutic success with atovaquone was found to be equal to that of trimethoprim-sulfamethoxazole. This was due to a significantly lower rate of treatment-limiting adverse effects balanced by a lower rate of antimicrobial efficacy from atovaquone.[18] Similar results were obtained when atovaquone was compared with intravenous pentamidine.[19] Atovaquone is available only for oral administration. The original formulation was tablets, but a suspension has become available. Greater absorption occurs with the suspension. The dosage of atovaquone is 750 mg three times daily with meals. No significant adverse effects have been associated with atovaquone therapy.

Trimetrexate and Leucovorin

Trimetrexate inhibits the dihydrofolate reductase of *P. carinii*. Leucovorin must be administered concomitantly to prevent antifolate toxicity in the host. In moderate to severe cases of

P. carinii pneumonitis, this drug regimen was found effective, but it was less effective than trimethoprim-sulfamethoxazole.[20] The dose is 45 mg (base)/m^2 once daily for 21 days. The drug is administered intravenously in 30 to 60 minutes. Leucovorin may be given orally or intravenously at a dose of 20 mg/m^2 every 6 hours. Treatment-limiting adverse reactions are less frequent with trimetrexate than with trimethoprim-sulfamethoxazole.

Dapsone and Trimethoprim

Although dapsone alone is effective therapy for *P. carinii* pneumonitis, the addition of trimethoprim provides a synergistic effect. The drug combination has efficacy similar to that of trimethoprim-sulfamethoxazole or pentamidine.[21] The usual dose is dapsone at 100 mg/d and trimethoprim at 20 mg/kg per day. The adverse effects are similar to those of trimethoprim-sulfamethoxazole; however, about two thirds of patients who have adverse reactions to trimethoprim-sulfamethoxazole are able to tolerate dapsone.

Clindamycin Plus Primaquine

The combination of 600 mg of clindamycin every 8 hours and 30 mg of primaquine once daily orally is effective therapy.[22] The adverse effects include rash, diarrhea, and vomiting. Clinical studies have been limited at this time.

Other Therapeutic Modalities

Corticosteroid treatment is recommended for AIDS patients with moderately severe or severe *Pneumocystis* pneumonia, as indicated by a Po_2 less than 70 mm Hg.[23] A study suggested that oral corticosteroids prevent early deterioration in AIDS patients with mild *P. carinii* pneumonitis.[24]

Prevention

P. carinii pneumonitis can be prevented by chemoprophylaxis. Several drugs are available for this purpose. Trimethoprim-sulfamethoxazole is the drug of first choice. The dose of 160 mg of trimethoprim and 800 mg of sulfamethoxazole may be given orally in single or divided doses daily or only 3 days a week.[25–28] For patients who have mild to moderate adverse reactions to trimethoprim-sulfamethoxazole, it is often possible to rechallenge or attempt desensitization to the drug,[29] or an alternative drug may be selected. Dapsone alone in the dose of 100 mg/d is effective. Studies have shown that 50 mg of dapsone daily plus 50 mg of pyrimethamine per week plus 25 mg of leucovorin per week, or 200 mg of dapsone plus 75 mg of pyrimethamine plus 25 mg of leucovorin once a week, provides effective prophylaxis against toxoplasmosis as well as *P. carinii* pneumonitis.[30–32]

Aerosolized pentamidine is also effective in the prevention of the pneumonitis and is safe.[33, 34] The dosage of 300 mg of pentamidine delivered in a Respirgard II–like nebulizer given in a period of 30 to 40 minutes once monthly will prevent *P. carinii* pneumonitis in about 90% of AIDS patients. Adverse effects are predominantly cough, wheezing, and bronchospasm. Other dosage schemes and nebulizers are currently under study.

Recommendations for prophylaxis of *P. carinii* in AIDS patients have been proposed by a panel of experts.[10] They include the following:

1. Give prophylaxis to patients who have had one or more episodes of *P. carinii* pneumonia and others who have a CD4+ lymphocyte count less than 200/mm^3.

2. HIV-positive patients who do not qualify for prophylaxis should have CD4+ lymphocyte counts done every 6 months; when the count is confirmed to be less than 200/mm^3, a program for prophylaxis should be started.

References

1. Masur H, Michelis MA, Greene JB, et al: An outbreak of community-acquired *Pneumocystis carinii* pneumonia: Initial manifestation of cellular immune dysfunction. N Engl J Med 305:1431, 1981.
2. Gottlieb MS, Schroff R, Schanker HM, et al: *Pneumocystis carinii* pneumonia and mucosal candidiasis in previously healthy homosexual men: Evidence of a new acquired cellular immunodeficiency. N Engl J Med 305:1425, 1985.
3. Pifer LL, Hughes WT, Stagno S, et al: *Pneumocystis carinii* infection: Evidence for high prevalence in normal and immunosuppressed children. Pediatrics 61:35, 1978.
4. Meuwissen JH, Tauber I, Leeuwenberg AD, et al: Parasitologic and serologic observations of infection with *Pneumocystis* in humans. J Infect Dis 136:43, 1977.
5. Hughes WT: Natural mode of acquisition for de novo infection with *Pneumocystis carinii*. J Infect Dis 145:843, 1982.
6. Vargas SL, Hughes WT, Wakefield AE, Oz H: Limited persistence in and subsequent elimination of *Pneumocystis carinii* from the lungs after *P. carinii* pneumonia. J Infect Dis 172:506, 1995.
7. Cheu W, Gigliotti F, Harmsen AG: Latency is not an inevitable outcome of infection with *Pneumocystis carinii*. Infect Immun 61:5405, 1993.
8. Armstrong MYH, Cushion MT: Animal models. *In* Walzer PD (ed): *Pneumocystis carinii* Pneumonia; ed 2. New York, Marcel Dekker, 1993, pp 181–222.
9. Wakefield A: Detection of DNA sequences identical to *Pneumocystis carinii* in samples of ambient air. J Eukaryot Microbiol 41:116S, 1994.
10. Centers for Disease Control: Guidelines for the prevention of opportunistic infections in persons with human immunodeficiency virus: A summary. MMWR Morbid Mortal Wkly Rep 44(RR-8):1, 1995.
11. Phair J, Muñoz A, Retels R, et al: The risk of *Pneumocystis carinii* pneumonia among men infected with human immunodeficiency virus type 1. N Engl J Med 322:161, 1990.
12. Chan H, Pifer L, Hughes WT, et al: Comparison of gastric contents to pulmonary aspirates for the cytological diagnosis of *Pneumocystis carinii* pneumonia. J Pediatr 90:243, 1977.
13. Hughes WT, Feldman S, Chaudhary SC, et al: Comparison of pentamidine isethionate and trimethoprim-sulfamethoxazole in the treatment of *Pneumocystis carinii* pneumonia. J Pediatr 92:285, 1978.
14. Sattler FR, Cowan R, Nielsen DM, et al: Trimethoprim-sulfamethoxazole compared with pentamidine for treatment of *Pneumocystis carinii* pneumonia in the acquired immunodeficiency syndrome: A prospective, noncrossover study. Ann Intern Med 109:280, 1988.
15. Jaffe HS, Abrams DI, Ammann AJ, et al: Complications of cotrimoxazole in treatment of AIDS-associated *Pneumocystis carinii* pneumonia in homosexual men. Lancet 2:1109, 1983.
16. Gordin FM, Simon GL, Mills J, et al: Adverse reactions to trimethoprim-sulfamethoxazole in patients with acquired immune deficiency syndrome. Ann Intern Med 100:495, 1984.
17. Young RD, DeVita VT Jr: Treatment of *Pneumocystis carinii* pneumonia: Current status of the regimens of pentamidine isethionate and pyrimethamine-sulfadiazine. Natl Cancer Inst Monogr 43:193, 1976.
18. Hughes WT, Leoung G, Kramer F, et al: Comparison of atovaquone (566C80) with trimethoprim-sulfamethoxazole to treat *Pneumocystis carinii* pneumonia in patients with AIDS. N Engl J Med 328:1521, 1993.
19. Dohn MN, Weinberg WG, Torres RA, et al: Oral atovaquone compared with intravenous pentamidine for *Pneumocystis carinii* pneumonia in patients with AIDS. Ann Intern Med 121:174, 1994.
20. Sattler FR, Frame P, Davis R, et al: Trimetrexate with leucovorin versus trimethoprim-sulfamethoxazole for moderate to severe episodes of *Pneumocystis carinii* pneumonia in patients with AIDS: A prospective, controlled multicenter investigation of the

AIDS Clinical Trials Group Protocol 029/031. J Infect Dis 170:165, 1994.
21. Leoung GS, Mills J, Hopewell PC, et al: Dapsone-trimethoprim for *Pneumocystis carinii* pneumonia in the acquired immunodeficiency syndrome. Ann Intern Med 105:45, 1986.
22. Black JR, Heinberg J, Murphy RL: Clindamycin and primaquine therapy for mild-to-moderate episodes of *Pneumocystis carinii* pneumonia in patients with AIDS: AIDS Clinical Trials Group 044. Clin Infect Dis 18:905, 1994.
23. Kovacs JA, Masur H: Are corticosteroids beneficial as adjunctive therapy for *Pneumocystis carinii* pneumonia in AIDS? Ann Intern Med 113:1, 1990.
24. Montaner JSG, Guillerni S, Quieffin J, et al: Oral corticosteroids in patients with mild *Pneumocystis carinii* pneumonia and the acquired immune deficiency syndrome. Tuber Lung Dis 74:173, 1993.
25. Simonds RJ, Hughes WT, Feinberg J, Navin TR: Preventing *Pneumocystis carinii* pneumonia in persons with HIV infection. Clin Infect Dis 21(Suppl 1):S44, 1995.
26. Schneider MME, Hoepelman AIM, Schattenkerk JKME, et al: A controlled trial of aerosolized pentamidine or trimethoprim-sulfamethoxazole as primary prophylaxis against *Pneumocystis carinii* pneumonia in patients with human immunodeficiency virus infection. N Engl J Med 327:1836, 1992.
27. Hardy WD, Feinberg J, Finkelstein DM, et al: A controlled trial of trimethoprim-sulfamethoxazole or aerosolized pentamidine for secondary prophylaxis of *Pneumocystis carinii* pneumonia in patients with acquired immunodeficiency syndrome. N Engl J Med 327:1842, 1992.
28. Hughes WT, Rivera GK, Schell MJ, et al: Successful intermittent chemoprophylaxis for *Pneumocystis carinii* pneumonitis. N Engl J Med 316:1627, 1987.
29. Gluckstein D, Ruskin J: Rapid oral desensitization to trimethoprim-sulfamethoxazole (TMP-SMZ) use in prophylaxis for *Pneumocystis carinii* pneumonia in patients with AIDS who were previously intolerant to TMP-SMZ. Clin Infect Dis 20:849, 1995.
30. Girard PM, Landman R, Gandebout C, et al: Dapsone-pyrimethamine compared with aerosolized pentamidine as primary prophylaxis against *Pneumocystis carinii* pneumonia and toxoplasmosis in HIV infection. N Engl J Med 328:1514, 1993.
31. Mallolas J, Zamora L, Gatell JM, et al: Primary prophylaxis for *Pneumocystis carinii* pneumonia: A randomized trial comparing cotrimoxazole, aerosolized pentamidine and dapsone plus pyrimethamine. AIDS 7:59, 1993.
32. Opravil M, Heald A, Lazzarin A, et al: Once-weekly administration of dapsone-pyrimethamine vs. aerosolized pentamidine for *Pneumocystis carinii* pneumonia and toxoplasmic encephalitis in human immunodeficiency virus–infected patients. Clin Infect Dis 20:531, 1995.
33. Bernard EM, Schmit HJ, Litton A, et al: Prevention of *Pneumocystis carinii* pneumonia with aerosol pentamidine (Abstr). Presented at the IV International Conference on AIDS; June 13–14, 1988; Stockholm; p 420.
34. Leoung GS, Feigal DW Jr, Montgomery AB, et al: Aerosolized pentamidine for prophylaxis against *Pneumocystis carinii* pneumonia. N Engl J Med 323:769, 1990.

60

Fungal Pneumonias

Donald B. Louria

I divide fungal, yeast, and higher bacterial infections of the lung arbitrarily into three categories: those arising for the most part in normal hosts; those in which there is an approximately even distribution between apparently normal and immunocompromised hosts; and those confined for the most part to those whose susceptibility is increased by specific underlying diseases or host defense abnormalities (Table 60–1).

Infections Arising Primarily in Normal Hosts

Histoplasmosis

Histoplasma capsulatum was originally described in Panama by Darling and was long thought to be confined to the midwestern and central-eastern parts of the United States. Now it is known that this soil-residing dimorphic fungus has a worldwide distribution. It is puzzling that despite the wide geographic soil habitat for *H. capsulatum*, the preponderance of clinical cases occur in a limited area of the continental United States, Mexico, and Puerto Rico. In part, this may represent underdiagnosis in many areas of the world. Although histoplasmosis remains a predominantly rural disease, numerous outbreaks have occurred in urban environments, most of them associated with exposure to droppings of urban-living birds, particularly starlings. Histoplasmosis is also a hazard to spelunkers who explore caves laden with bat and bird guano. There have been more than 40 cave-associated outbreaks; the majority of spelunkers in many areas should expect to have a positive histoplasmin skin test result.[1] Because delayed-type immunity is the major defense against *H. capsulatum*, those with underlying diseases characterized by defects in delayed-type immunity, such as Hodgkin's disease or acquired immunodeficiency syndrome (AIDS), are inordinately susceptible to *Histoplasma* infection. Indeed, in some geographic areas, histoplasmosis is a major cause of morbidity and death in AIDS patients.[2]

In soil, *H. capsulatum* is mycelial in form, possessing characteristic tuberculate chlamydospores. After the spores are inhaled, there is prompt phagocytosis by in situ lung mononuclear phagocytes and thereafter a rapid morphologic metamorphosis to the tissue yeast form. Mycelia are found only within chronic lung cavities and rarely on the surface of cardiac vegetations. Medoff and colleagues[3] demonstrated that the temperature shift after inhalation of spores triggers transformation from the mycelial to the yeast phase, presumably by gene stimulation, and that this transformation is sulfhydryl enzyme dependent.

Once within mononuclear phagocytes, *H. capsulatum*, now in the yeast phase, survives. The balance between intracellular germination and intracellular control is determined by the efficacy of delayed immune mechanisms.[4] T-cell activation of macrophages is essential for such control.[5] Experimentally, protective immunity can be transferred with a $CD4^+$ clone.[6]

Multiple clinical patterns appear after the inhalation of *H. capsulatum.*

Mild Pneumonitis with Minimal Parenchymal Infiltrates Followed by Either Complete Healing or Residual Calcification. This is the most prevalent clinical form of the disease. In the majority of cases, the infection is so mild that it comes to the attention of physicians relatively infrequently. Chest radiographs during healing may show one or more round, oval, or irregular lesions with varying degrees of calcification that typically have a laminated or stippled appearance. No antihistoplasma treatment is required.

Progressive Primary Infection. This is characterized by the presence of one or more nodules accompanied by fever, sweats, cough, weakness, fatigue, and, in some cases, sputum production or dyspnea. There may be a large number of nodules. In most cases, the nodules heal with residual fibrosis or calcification, but in some cases the nodules persist, accompanied by evidence of extrapulmonary dissemination. In still

TABLE 60–1 ■ Fungi, Yeasts, and Higher Bacteria That Cause Pneumonia

MOSTLY IN NORMAL HOSTS	ABOUT EQUALLY IN NORMAL AND COMPROMISED PERSONS	MOSTLY IN COMPROMISED HOSTS
Histoplasma capsulatum	*Cryptococcus neoformans*	*Aspergillus* sp.
Blastomyces dermatitidis	*Nocardia asteroides*	Zygomycetes
Coccidioides immitis	*Sporothrix schenckii*	*Pseudallescheria boydii*
Actinomyces sp.	*Penicillium marneffei*	*Curvularia lunata*
	Geotrichum sp.	*Scopulariopsis* sp.
		Fusarium sp.
		Paecilomyces varioti
		Candida sp.
		Trichosporon sp.
		Candida (Torulopsis) glabrata

other cases, the nodules persist for prolonged periods, increasing and decreasing in size; the radiographic worsening is usually accompanied by an increase in fever, cough, and dyspnea. Although most of the lesions heal after months or even years, treatment with amphotericin B or oral imidazoles is usually indicated.

Pneumonic Histoplasmosis. Infiltrates range from limited segmental to diffuse multilobar involvement and may be primarily interstitial, nodular, fluffy, or dense. The infiltrate is occasionally lobar, mimicking lobar bacterial pneumonia. Symptoms include fever, chills, sweats, anorexia, and weakness. The cough is often productive of mucopurulent sputum; with both pneumonic histoplasmosis and progressive primary histoplasmomas, there may be substantial amounts of hemoptysis.[7] Chest pain is not infrequent and may be pleuritic. Physical findings are variable. There may be no abnormalities or only sticky inspiratory rales or areas with dullness to percussion and altered breath sounds; occasionally, there may be evidence of frank consolidation. Pleural rubs are observed infrequently. In a small number of cases, there may be a pleural effusion; in such cases, the fluid can be serous, serosanguineous, or even frankly bloody. The predominant cell type in the effusion is usually the lymphocyte, but there can be a striking number of eosinophils.[8] Chest radiographs show one or more areas of soft infiltrates, patchy or coalescent densities, or consolidation. Hilar adenopathy is frequently present, and the pneumonia may be accompanied by evidence of pericarditis.

Other Forms of Acute Pulmonary Involvement. Occasionally there are infiltrates in one part of the lung that improve markedly or even resolve, only to be followed by new infiltrates in a different lung segment. This pattern may be repeated for a period of months or even years, resolving either spontaneously or after treatment. Rarely, pulmonary histoplasmosis is manifested as a pneumonic infiltrate accompanied by striking peripheral eosinophilia, a pattern consistent with Löffler syndrome. The disease may also be manifested radiographically as hilar adenopathy in the absence of parenchymal infiltrates. Particularly in the compromised host, miliary infiltrates can be seen.

Chronic Disease. The majority of patients suffering from chronic (or reinfection) histoplasmosis have radiographic evidence of one or more cavities, usually in the upper lobes. These may rupture into the pleural space with resultant empyema or bronchopleural fistula. Symptoms include cough, dyspnea, fever, and hemoptysis. Physical examination shows rales and diminished breath sounds, sometimes accompanied by percussion dullness.

Calcified nodes can erode into the bronchus; these broncholiths can cause either hemoptysis or recurrent pneumonia and may require surgical intervention. They can also obstruct major bronchi, with resultant localized wheeze. There has been increased interest in *Histoplasma*-induced mediastinal fibrosis.[9, 10] Manifestations include dyspnea, hemoptysis, and postobstructive pneumonia resulting from tracheal or bronchial stenosis. Superior vena caval or pulmonary artery occlusion may occur. Fibrosing mediastinitis may also affect the esophagus, with the potential for traction diverticula or fistulae; symptoms include dysphagia, chest pain, and odynophagia.[11] Dysphagia can also result from extrinsic lymph node pressure. The nodes on the right side of the mediastinum are involved more frequently than those on the left side.

Diagnosis of pulmonary histoplasmosis is best made by culture of expectorated sputum or, if required, by culture of bronchoalveolar lavage fluid.[12] During acute pneumonic episodes, fungemia may be detected by using lysis-centrifugation techniques.[13] In most cases, however, diagnosis is made serologically using precipitation, immunodiffusion, complement fixation, and latex agglutination tests. Unfortunately, the precipitation test suffers from inadequate sensitivity. *Histoplasma* antigens can also be detected in serum and urine.[14]

No treatment is required for most cases of acute pulmonary histoplasmosis. Treatment is advisable for those with severe, persistent, or progressive disease and for those who are immunocompromised and do not improve rapidly without treatment. Amphotericin B is fungicidal for *H. capsulatum* and remains the most predictable agent in severe or life-threatening disease, especially in immunocompromised hosts. Itraconazole is the alternative agent; a dosage of 200 to 400 mg/d given for 1 to 12 months depending on the clinical circumstances is usually effective in pulmonary and disseminated histoplasmosis, particularly in nonimmunocompromised hosts. Those with chronic cavitary disease should almost always be treated with either amphotericin B or itraconazole; treatment must often be prolonged (6 to 12 months). Fluconazole by mouth is used primarily for follow-up after amphotericin B or for long-term prophylaxis in AIDS patients who have recovered from acute histoplasmosis. The efficacy of treatment can be evaluated in many cases by monitoring blood and urine *Histoplasma* antigen levels.[15] Patients with mediastinal fibrosis, obstructing nodes, obstructing histoplasmomas, broncholith-induced bleeding, or esophageal diverticula or fistulae frequently require surgical intervention.[9]

Blastomycosis

Described by Gilchrist in 1896, blastomycosis is an acute or chronic disease caused by the dimorphic fungus *Blastomyces dermatitidis*. Although soil is clearly the reservoir during the infectious mycelial phase, it has been remarkably difficult to recover *B. dermatitidis* from soil samples. However, in an outbreak in Wisconsin, the fungus was isolated repeatedly from environmental samples, and the attack rate of exposed persons was a surprisingly high 51%; about half were symptomatic after an incubation period ranging from 21 to 106 days.[16, 17] For 70 years, blastomycosis was thought to be confined geographically to the central and southeastern United States. Now the disease appears to have a more global distribution; cases have been reported from Canada, Mexico, the Middle East, Africa, and India.[18] The disease pattern appears to vary according to geographic region. Studies of African isolates suggest that differences in clinical patterns may be related to differences in the serotypes responsible for disease.[19] Although most of those acquiring *B. dermatitidis* infection are immunocompetent, those suffering from human immunodeficiency virus (HIV) infection are inordinately susceptible.

In the United States, the lung is the major target organ. Experimental data indicate that lung macrophages have some ability to ingest and kill *B. dermatitidis*, as do polymorphonuclear cells.[20] Transformation from the mycelial to the yeast phase appears to result from temperature-dependent changes in oxidative phosphorylation and respiratory rates.[21] The critical shunt pathways are sulfhydryl dependent. The tissue response to the yeast forms consists of both polymorphonuclear cells (abscesses) and macrophages (granulomata).

The Wisconsin epidemic involved enough persons to permit a better understanding of symptom and sign frequency.[16] In decreasing frequency, the following occurred in the 26 symptomatic persons: cough, headache, chest pain, weight loss, fever, abdominal pain, night sweats, chills, and anorexia. The onset of illness is usually abrupt (but may be insidious), and the cough is frequently productive of mucopurulent sputum. Myalgias and arthralgias may accompany the pulmonary manifestations, producing an influenza-like clinical picture. On occasion, the pulmonary infection may be overwhelming, mimicking severe acute bacterial pneumonia; the adult respiratory distress syndrome has also been noted.[22]

Physical findings on lung examination range from none to inspiratory rales to evidence of frank consolidation. Radiographic findings are likewise variable, including consolidation of part or all of a lobe, multilobar infiltrates, perihilar infiltrates, multiple nodules, and mediastinal node involvement. Miliary infiltrates are occasionally noted. Pleural effusion occurs infrequently. In HIV-positive individuals, the characteristic findings are diffuse or miliary infiltrates.

Acute involvement may resolve spontaneously, persist, or progress. Chronic lesions are characterized by fibrosis and cavitation.

The fungus may be seen in sputum or bronchoalveolar lavage specimens as spherical 5- to 20-μm cells with a thick double-contoured refractile wall. The fungus grows slowly; colonies appear 3 to 35 days after incubation. Serologic tests are not entirely satisfactory. Enzyme immunoassay appears to have greater sensitivity than either immunodiffusion or complement fixation, but test results of a significant percentage of those who are infected remain negative.[23] The immunodiffusion and complement fixation tests have greater specificity.

Amphotericin B is clearly an effective agent in both acute and chronic pulmonary blastomycosis and should be used in overwhelming or life-threatening infection. In disease of mild to moderate severity, itraconazole appears equally effective.[24] Fluconazole may also be useful.[25]

Coccidioidomycosis

Originally described in 1892, the disease has a variety of sobriquets—valley fever, desert rheumatism, San Joaquin fever. The major endemic area is confined to the lower Sonoran life zone in the United States, where the soil is arid and alkaline and the ambient temperature is usually in the 80°F to 100°F range. Parts or all of California, Nevada, Arizona, Texas, Utah, and New Mexico lie in this zone, but coccidioidal infections are not limited to this area. Some desert regions of Mexico are also endemic areas, and small numbers of cases have been reported from Central America, South America, Italy, Australia, and Japan.

In endemic areas, the attack rate is high. At least 15% of persons entering such an area can expect to have a positive skin test result within a year, and 30% to more than 50% will have a positive skin test result after 2 to 4 years of residence.[26–28] Those suffering from AIDS or lymphomas, those receiving adrenal steroids or immunosuppressive treatments, and persons undergoing organ transplantation show increased susceptibility to coccidioidal infection.[26–29] Host control after *Coccidioides immitis* invasion appears to be dependent on activated T lymphocytes.[30] Diabetic patients and women in the third trimester of pregnancy suffer more severe infection.[26–28]

In at least 95% and probably more than 99% of cases of acute pneumonia, coccidioidomycosis is a self-limited disease, requiring no treatment and having no sequelae. Symptoms include, in descending order of frequency, cough, fever, chest pain, headache, chills, shortness of breath, malaise, myalgias, and rash (erythema nodosum or erythema multiforme). The chest pain may be pleuritic, may be centrally located and severe on occasion, and may mimic acute costochondritis. The pulmonary infection can occasionally be overwhelming, can mimic bacterial septic shock, and can be accompanied by adult respiratory distress syndrome.[31]

Physical examination is often unrewarding. In some cases, rales, rhonchi, or wheezes are heard; in others, there is evidence of frank consolidation. Evidence of pleural effusion may also be detected.

Radiographs may show only hilar adenopathy (on occasion massive), or there may be a variety of soft or nodular infiltrates, most frequently found in the upper lobes.

In those with persistent or progressive disease, infiltrates are most often bilateral in the upper lobes (often apical), are fibronodular and contain multiple cavities that are characteristically thin walled, and may have air-fluid levels. These cavities may close spontaneously. Chronic cavitary diseases may be complicated by bacterial or fungal superinfection, significant hemoptysis, pyopneumothorax, or bronchopleural fistulae. Those suffering from HIV infection usually develop *C. immitis* infection after $CD4^+$ lymphocyte counts are less than 200/mm^3; their pulmonary disease may manifest as focal pneumonic infiltrates but is usually characterized by diffuse reticulonodular or nodular patterns.

In some cases, solitary nodules—coccidioidomas—may be the only manifestation of lung involvement; some of these may calcify. Miliary disease is seen in a small percentage of those with primary lung involvement, usually in patients suffering from severe underlying diseases, such as diabetes or AIDS, or in those being treated with immunosuppressive agents or corticosteroids. On rare occasions, lung lesions may be accompanied by striking tissue eosinophilia and some peripheral eosinophilia.[32]

Dissemination from the lungs ordinarily occurs early during the course of the acute infection; only rarely does dissemination occur after several months of infection in those with chronic pulmonary coccidioidomycosis. The lung lesion can be complicated by fistula formation that is not necessarily restricted to the thorax; extraordinary examples have been reported of pulmonary-gluteal or pulmonary-thigh fistulae.

The diagnosis can be established by isolation of the fungus and by serologic tests. In some cases, examination of sputum treated with sodium hydroxide will demonstrate the yeast phase, the spherule, which ranges from 20 to 80 μm in diameter and may contain small (2- to 4-μm) endospores. *C. immitis* grows readily in culture, producing white cottony mycelia in 2 to 8 days; the hyphae contain characteristic rectangular arthrospores. Serologic studies include precipitation, latex agglutination, complement fixation, immunodiffusion, counterimmunodiffusion, and enzyme immunoassay. The precipitation test, reflecting immunoglobulin M early in the course of the infection, and the complement fixation test, reflecting immunoglobulin G somewhat later, are still the two most useful studies. In coccidioidomycosis limited to the lungs, the complement fixation titers usually do not exceed 1:16. Complement fixation titers are often deceptively low in patients with chronic cavitary disease and in those with coccidioidomas.

Most patients with acute pulmonary coccidioidomycosis do not require therapy. In persistent or progressive disease or in chronic cavitary disease, amphotericin B remains the agent of choice. The imidazoles fluconazole and itraconazole given in a dosage of at least 400 mg/d appear to be reasonable alternatives for non–life-threatening disease.[28] Surgery may be required for severe hemoptysis, cavities that rupture or enlarge despite treatment, empyema, or fistulae.

Actinomycosis

Pulmonary actinomycosis usually affects otherwise normal hosts; there is no underlying disease particularly associated with it. The manifestations include pneumonic infiltrates, one or more lung abscesses, and empyema. On occasion, cough and sputum production are accompanied by hemoptysis. The pneumonia or lung abscess is usually subacute or chronic, with no evidence of spread to adjacent tissues. However, invasion of contiguous structures is not uncommon. Osteomyelitis and skin fistulae occur relatively frequently, but invasion of the pericardium or through the diaphragm into the liver is seen only rarely. Empyema fluid is often thick, almost invariably shows a polymorphonuclear leukocyte predominance, and sometimes has a putrid odor.

Pulmonary actinomycosis usually arises from aspiration; teeth are often in poor repair or there is clinically apparent periodontal disease, but this is not always so. Infection is usually caused by *Actinomyces israelii*, but other species may be involved, including *Actinomyces naeslundii*, *Actinomyces odontolyticus*, and *Actinomyces viscosus*. The treatment of choice continues to be penicillin G, given in large dosage for periods ranging from 4 to 12 weeks. Tetracyclines, erythromycin, clindamycin, and imipenem are alternative agents.

Infections Arising in Both Normal and Abnormal Hosts

Cryptococcosis

Cryptococci reside in soil and ordinarily infect through the respiratory route. Cryptococcal pneumonia not infrequently arises in ostensibly healthy persons; more often, however, the yeast attacks those with defects in delayed immune mechanisms, those receiving adrenal steroids, and those being treated simultaneously with immunosuppressive drugs and adrenal glucocorticoids as therapy for malignant neoplasms or after organ or tissue transplantation. Those suffering from lymphomas or chronic lymphatic leukemia are susceptible in the absence of therapy, but that susceptibility is markedly increased during treatment. Other less well established risk factors include the presence of sarcoidosis, diabetes, and hepatic cirrhosis. Of course, AIDS is now a major risk factor; as many as 10% of AIDS patients develop *Cryptococcus neoformans* infection.[33, 34]

The symptoms and signs of pulmonary cryptococcal infection are variable and lack specificity. Indeed, there may be no symptoms referable to the chest. Mild temperature elevation and nonproductive or slightly productive cough are found frequently, but there may also be chest pain, and substantial hemoptysis has been reported rarely. The sputum may rarely appear purulent. Although the clinical pattern is usually characterized by insidious onset and slow progression, the disease can be fulminating[35]; this pattern is found with considerable frequency in those with AIDS. Cryptococcosis can also be a nosocomial infection,[36] but it is unclear in such cases whether the infection arises from the hospital environment or the patient's own respiratory tract. Rarely, endobronchial lesions have caused obstructive phenomena.

Chest radiographs are variable. Patterns include one or more nodular lesions that are often round and devoid of surrounding inflammation, patchy infiltrates, lobar or lobular consolidation, pneumonia with cavitation, diffuse reticulonodular or interstitial infiltrates, and miliary disease (Fig. 60–1). Pleural effusions occur infrequently. Focal lesions can mimic lung carcinoma.

The diagnosis is best made by isolating the organism from cultures of sputum, bronchoscopy washings, bronchoalveolar lavage fluid, or blood. In some cases, lung biopsy is necessary. Serologic studies may be helpful if antigen titers exceed 1:8, but titers of less than 1:8 may represent false-positive findings. Serum antibody determinations are not useful. Dual pulmonary infection is not infrequent; pneumonias due concomitantly to *C. neoformans* and *Mycobacterium tuberculosis*, *H. capsulatum*, *Nocardia asteroides*, or *Legionella pneumophila*[37] are well described.

Some advocate no treatment for isolated pulmonary cryptococcosis in an apparently healthy host.[38] Others, concerned by reports of persistence of the infection or spread to the central nervous system, recommend treatment for all those suffering from pulmonary cryptococcal infection.[39] There is no debate about immunocompromised patients—all should be treated. Amphotericin B is the most effective agent; there are no data documenting the need to add a second agent in isolated pulmonary disease. Some would treat with two agents, particularly lower doses of amphotericin B plus 5-fluorocytosine. Fluconazole is an alternative agent but the optimal dose and route of administration have not been fully established. Itraconazole has been effective in some cases, but data at present are meager.

Nocardiosis

The histologic reaction to *N. asteroides* appears to be both polymorphonuclear and mononuclear. Limited clinical and experimental evidence points to the primacy of delayed immune mechanisms.[40] Studies by Felice and Niewoehner[41] in mice showed impressively that the initial response was polymorphonuclear, followed in 4 to 7 days by predominance of a mononuclear reaction; ablation of either the polymorph or the cell-mediated (monocyte) component of the response resulted in augmented tissue invasion, as did the administration of adrenal glucocorticoids.

Nocardial infection arises in those with hematologic malignant neoplasms that sunder delayed-type immunity (especially during therapy)[42]; during immunosuppression after organ or tissue transplantation (especially after periods of threatened rejection); during steroid treatment for a variety of diseases[42] (Fig. 60–2); and in those with HIV infection.[43] In addition, persons with alveolar proteinosis, sarcoidosis, and chronic granulomatous disease may suffer from nocardial

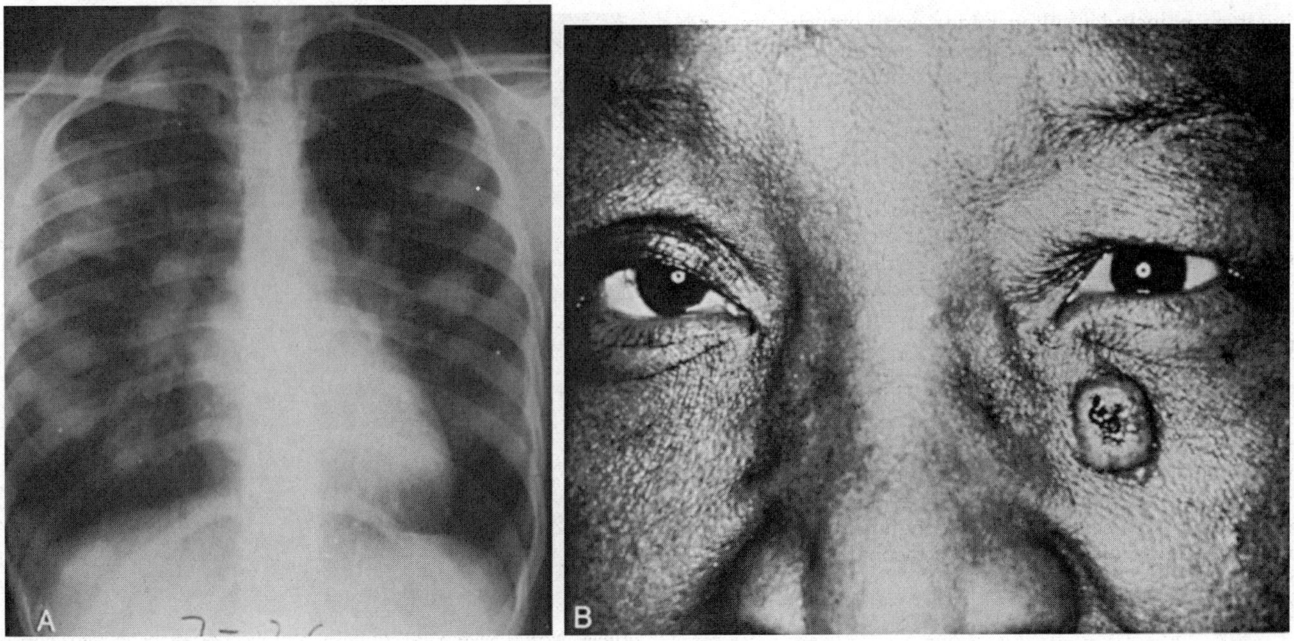

FIGURE 60–1 ▫ Cryptococcal nodular lung lesions *(A)* and ulcerating skin nodules *(B)* in a 72-year-old woman during steroid treatment for chronic lymphatic leukemia.

superinfection. A significant percentage of patients have no demonstrable underlying disease.

Pulmonary manifestations are variable and include cough, purulent or bloody sputum, pleuritic pain, and dyspnea. Fever and occasionally chills characterize the infection. Although the onset is usually insidious, it may be fulminating and can result in adult respiratory distress syndrome.[44] Occasionally, obstructing endobronchial masses have been observed.[45]

Chest radiographic findings are also variable and include single or multiple nodules; patchy infiltrates; lobar or lobular infiltrates, particularly in the upper lobes; reticulonodular or alveolar infiltrates; one or more abscesses or cavities; and pleural effusions (at thoracocentesis, the fluid may be thin, thick, or sanguineous, and there is ordinarily a predominance of polymorphonuclear leukocytes).

There are no reliable serologic tests. The diagnosis is usually made by visualizing the organism or culturing it from sputum, bronchoscopy specimens, or bronchoalveolar lavage fluid. *N. asteroides* is often seen in Gram-stained specimens (Fig. 60–3), but some strains require a modified acid-fast stain. Pneumonia indistinguishable from that due to *N. asteroides* can be caused by other nocardial species, including *Nocardia brasiliensis, Nocardia caviae,* and *Nocardia nova.*

Although nocardial infection can resolve spontaneously, treatment is recommended, particularly because of the organism's proclivity to invade the brain. Trimethoprim-sulfamethoxazole is now considered the agent of choice, but about 20% of strains resist the combination in vitro. Alterna-

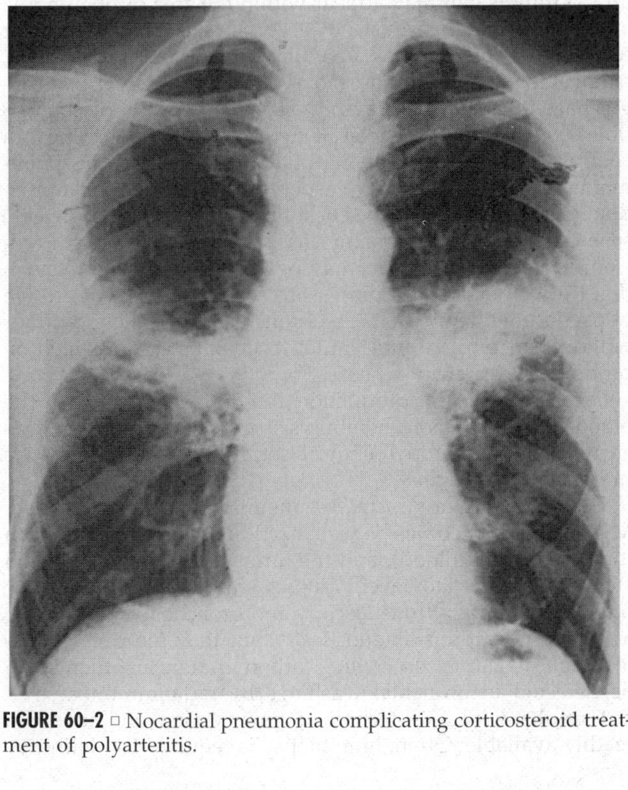

FIGURE 60–2 ▫ Nocardial pneumonia complicating corticosteroid treatment of polyarteritis.

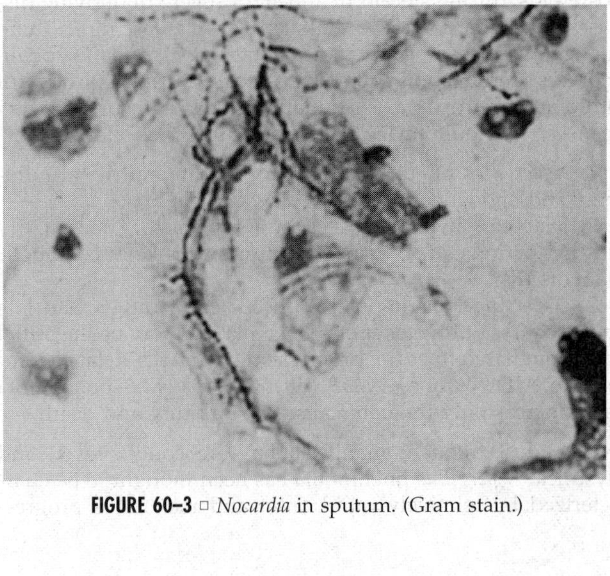

FIGURE 60–3 ▫ *Nocardia* in sputum. (Gram stain.)

tive therapy includes sulfonamides, erythromycin, amikacin, minocycline, and imipenem. In an experimental model of central nervous system disease, a combination of amikacin and imipenem appeared to be most efficacious.[46]

There is an increasing number of reports of dual infection, often with *N. asteroides* and *M. tuberculosis*. Failure of therapy or recurrent infection in patients with isolated pulmonary infection should suggest a serious underlying disease, including lymphoma, HIV infection, alveolar proteinosis, or chronic granulomatous disease. However, multiple relapses have been reported in apparently healthy individuals.[47]

Sporotrichosis

Pulmonary sporotrichosis may be primary in the lung in normal or compromised hosts or may arise from hematogenous dissemination. In primary disease, the upper lobes are most frequently involved, and cavitation often occurs in the pneumonic area. In cases of hematogenous spread, any area of the lung may be involved. Amphotericin B is the agent of choice; imidazoles, particularly itraconazole, may also be effective.[48, 49]

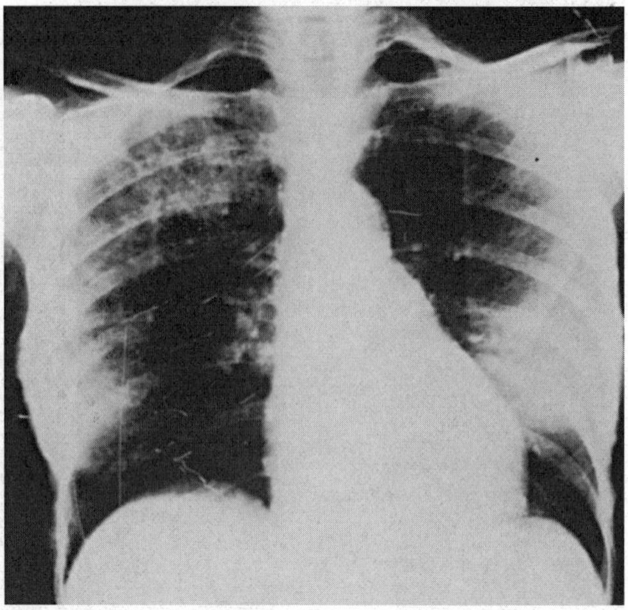

FIGURE 60–4 □ Severe aspergillosis complicating diabetic ketoacidosis in a 54-year-old woman, presenting as progressive hemoptysis.

Infections Ordinarily Arising in Immunocompromised Hosts

Aspergillosis

The face of *Aspergillus* pneumonia has changed dramatically in the last decade. *Aspergillus* pneumonia can occur in ostensibly healthy persons,[50] but this is rare. The evidence now indicates that pulmonary pneumocytes can ingest and kill spores of *Aspergillus*; for the most part, killing occurs after spore germination.[51, 52] Steroids inhibit this killing. Polymorphonuclear leukocytes also ingest and kill both spores and mycelia of *Aspergillus*; the killing is probably due both to the actions of cationic proteins and to the actions of the myeloperoxidase-halide system.[51, 53] It appears that both defense mechanisms (pulmonary phagocytes and polymorphonuclear leukocytes) are effective and that both cellular defenses are usually breached before clinical *Aspergillus* pneumonia supervenes.[54] The causative organism is usually *Aspergillus fumigatus*, but other species, particularly *Aspergillus flavus*, may be the etiologic agent.

In the past, aside from the few surprising cases in healthy hosts, most cases of *Aspergillus* pneumonia occurred as late events in patients with malignant neoplasms (especially hematologic) during treatment with antitumor agents and corticosteroids, during steroid treatment of severe underlying diseases, or after organ or tissue transplantation. In both malignant disease and transplantation, *Aspergillus* pneumonic superinfection occurs most often during episodes of profound neutropenia. The reported changes in susceptibility to *Aspergillus* pulmonary infection include the following:

1. *Aspergillus* pneumonia may complicate both viral influenza and endogenous Cushing's syndrome.[55,56]
2. Diabetes mellitus is clearly a risk factor, particularly during periods of ketosis but also in nonketotic diabetic patients (Fig. 60–4).
3. *Aspergillus* pneumonia can occur early rather than late in the course of myelogenous leukemia and may be the initial infection that defines the progression from AIDS-related complex to AIDS. Among AIDS patients, *Aspergillus* pneumonia is an increasingly frequent cause of morbidity and death.[57]

The most frequent manifestations are cough, fever, and dyspnea. *Aspergillus* pneumonia has been thought to be characterized by relatively rapid onset and inexorable progression. That is not always so, however. Onset may be surprisingly indolent; in some cases, the pneumonia may progress slowly or may appear to improve temporarily without treatment. Radiographic findings are variable, usually showing unilateral or bilateral dense or fluffy infiltrates that are segmental or lobar in distribution, with or without cavitation. In some cases, there may be single or multiple nodular lesions, sometimes with cavitation. Occasionally, there may be so many nodules that there is a miliary-nodular radiographic pattern. The fungus has a propensity to grow into blood vessels, resulting in infarct-like lesions that are often wedge shaped on radiographs (Fig. 60–5). These pneumonic areas may then undergo necrosis, producing cavitation, and thereafter a fungus ball may appear within the area of pneumonia and cavitation. This must not be construed as being similar to benign aspergillomas invading established tuberculous, neoplastic, or cystic lung lesions (Fig. 60–6). *Aspergillus* fungus balls in established cavities or cysts are ordinarily benign unless hemoptysis or bacterial superinfection supervenes. In contrast, a fungus ball arising in an area of *Aspergillus* pneumonia is part of progressive aspergillosis and requires immediate treatment. Rarely, the chest film appears normal despite severe dyspnea and, in some cases, low arterial oxygen tension; in such cases, there may be diffuse vascular invasion that can be detected by lung scans. In some cases, ulcerative or pseudomembranous tracheobronchial aspergillosis with or without concomitant lung infiltrates may be accompanied by prominent expiratory wheezes.[58]

Fever and sputum production are variable. Because of the blood vessel invasion, hemoptysis occurs frequently; its occurrence in the proper clinical setting should suggest the presence of *Aspergillus*.

The diagnosis of *Aspergillus* pneumonia is often difficult. Mycelia can sometimes be visualized in expectorated sputum (or expectorated blood), and the fungus can be cultivated on standard media. However, sputum smears and cultures are often unrevealing. Bronchoscopy and bronchoalveolar lavage are more rewarding diagnostically, but they too can be misleadingly negative. *Aspergillus* carbohydrate constituents can be detected in bronchial washings by radioimmunoassay,[59] but results with this technique have varied and it is not readily available. Often, lung biopsy is required for definitive diagnosis. Serum antibody can be determined by a variety of techniques including immunodiffusion and counterimmunoelectrophoresis. However, the available tests are not adequately sensitive or specific, and they are not reliable in early invasive aspergillosis.[60, 61] *Aspergillus* antigens in body fluids can also be detected by a variety of techniques; the usefulness of their detection in early diagnosis is currently being examined.[62]

It is important to establish the diagnosis because vigorous therapy may be effective. Amphotericin B is clearly the mainstay of treatment; itraconazole is alternative therapy.[63] Other agents may also be beneficial; these include flucytosine and rifampin. There are a few extraordinary anecdotes concerning response of fulminating disease on addition of flucytosine and rifampin or rifampin alone to amphotericin B.[64, 65] In severely neutropenic patients, improvement during antiaspergillus treatment appears to occur mostly in those who simultaneously show a significant increase in the number of circulating neutrophils.

No treatment is required for mycetoma arising in an established neoplastic or tuberculous cavity; if severe hemoptysis or bacterial superinfection occurs, surgical excision is the treatment of choice. There is also a form of allergic bronchopulmonary aspergillosis characterized by strikingly elevated serum immunoglobulin E levels; this usually responds well to corticosteroid treatment.

Zygomycosis (Mucormycosis)

Both pulmonary macrophages and polymorphonuclear leukocytes appear to be important in host defenses against spores and hyphae of Zygomycetes.[51, 53, 66] Spores are ingested by host defense cells and are killed or controlled by inhibition of germination. Hyphal elements either are ingested by host defense cells or are damaged extracellularly after attachment by macrophages or polymorphs. The major risk factors for pneumonic zygomycosis are diabetes, hematologic malignant neoplasms, and burns. Those suffering from hematologic malignant neoplasms ordinarily develop zygomycetic pneumonia during treatment, particularly during periods of profound neutropenia. In experimental models, diabetic mice show multiple defects in pulmonary macrophage function, including diminished capacity to attach to hyphal elements and reduced ability to prevent spore germination.[66] Although ketoacidosis increases susceptibility to zygomycetic superinfection, nonketotic diabetic patients are also susceptible; indeed, zygomycosis can occur before clinical manifestations of diabetes.[67] Profound and prolonged neutropenia from any cause (e.g., aplastic anemia, after treatment of solid tumors) can be followed by zygomycetic superinfection. Administration of deferoxamine for iron overload is also associated with zygomycetic superinfection.[68] Rarely, zygomycetic pneumonia occurs in those without any demonstrable underlying defect.[69, 70]

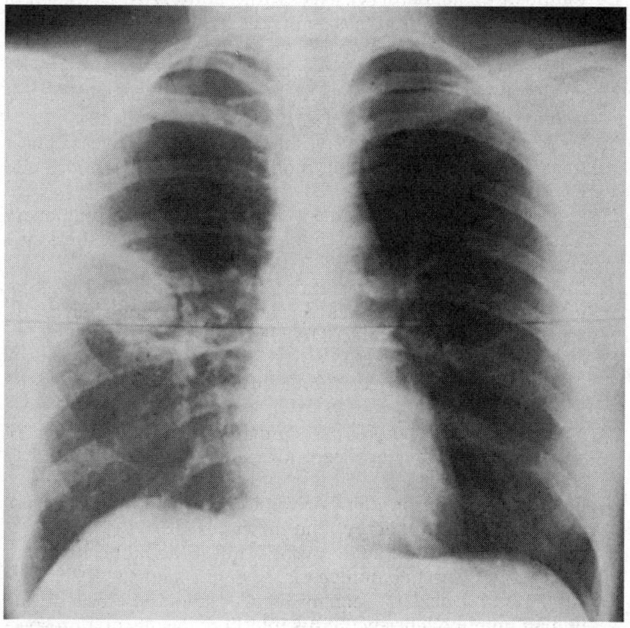

FIGURE 60–5 □ *Aspergillus* pneumonia presenting as an infarct-like lesion in a patient with subacute myelogenous leukemia after antileukemia therapy and multiple antibiotics for bacterial sepsis. (Courtesy of Dr. Donald Armstrong, Memorial Sloan-Kettering Cancer Center, New York.)

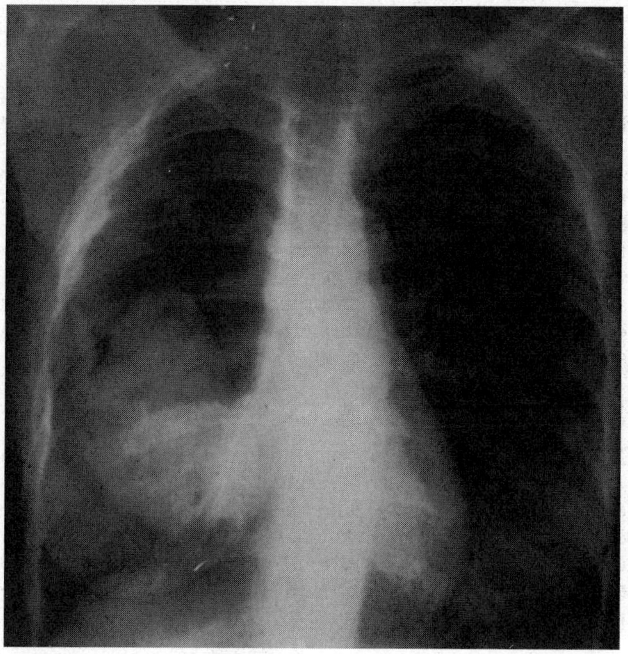

FIGURE 60–6 □ Huge aspergilloma within a lung cyst. (Courtesy of Dr. Baynard Tynes, University of Alabama School of Medicine, Birmingham, AL.)

Most cases are caused by species of *Rhizopus, Absidia,* or *Mucor,* but a small number have been caused by other Zygomycetes, including *Cunninghamella elegans, Cunninghamella bertholletiae, Conidiobolus incongruus,* and *Saksenaea vasiformis.*[69–73] There is no characteristic clinical pattern; cough, fever, dyspnea, and pleural pain are all noted frequently. Zygomycetes tend to grow into blood vessels; consequently, hemoptysis (sometimes massive) as well as infarct-like lesions may be observed on radiographic examination. In other cases, patchy lobular or lobar infiltrates are found.[74] Occasionally, despite extensive disease, standard chest films are normal but lung scans show diffuse involvement.[75] Bronchopleural fistula followed by fatal hemoptysis has also been described.[76]

There are no useful serologic tests. Diagnosis can sometimes be made at bronchoscopy, but lung biopsy is often required.

Treatment is often unsuccessful. Amphotericin B is the only potentially effective agent; unfortunately, Zygomycetes are not particularly sensitive to it in vitro. In addition to administration of amphotericin B, successful treatment often requires control of underlying diseases such as diabetes or return of the neutrophil count in peripheral blood to relatively normal levels.

Pseudallescheriasis

Although *Pseudallescheria boydii (Allescheria boydii, Petriellidium boydii)* has been described as the cause of necrotizing pneumonia in a normal host,[77] *Pseudallescheria* pneumonia almost always complicates severe underlying diseases, including sarcoidosis and malignant neoplasms during treatment with steroids or antitumor agents.[78, 79] The fungus has a proclivity to grow into blood vessels; consequently, in addition to lung infiltrates or abscesses, radiographs may show wedge-shaped, infarct-like lesions. The pneumonia can be acute, subacute, or chronic. At present, there is no predictably effective therapy, although imidazoles may be helpful in some cases.

Miscellaneous Fungi and Yeasts

Many other fungi and yeasts can cause pneumonia. South American blastomycosis may involve the lungs in the visceral form of the disease, but almost always there is evidence of extrapulmonary involvement. Chest films usually show diffuse nodular lesions, but focal pneumonic infiltrates may also be seen. The imidazoles are remarkably effective; amphotericin B is an alternative agent.

It is inevitable that as the pool of patients with severe underlying diseases—especially hematologic malignant neoplasms (during treatment) and AIDS—increases, there will be a small number of unusual pulmonary fungal and yeast infections.[80, 81] Such infections have been reported with strains of *Curvularia lunata*,[82, 83] *Scopulariopsis* species,[84] *Paecilomyces* sp.,[85] *Fusarium* sp.,[86] *Drechslera* sp.,[80, 87] *Scedosporium* sp.,[88] *Exophiala jeanselmei*,[89] and *Schizophyllum commune*.[90] *Penicillium marneffei* has caused pneumonia or pleural effusion in both normal and severely immunocompromised hosts.[91, 92] Pulmonary geotrichosis, either primary in the lung or hematogenous in origin, has also been described in both normal and immunocompromised hosts.[79]

A case of *Alternaria* granuloma of the lung in an apparently healthy man has been reported.[93]

Three yeasts or yeastlike fungi can also cause pneumonia. The most common of the three is *Candida*. This can be upper respiratory tract acquired in severely immunocompromised hosts during antibiotic, steroid, or antitumor therapy and appears radiographically as unilateral or bilateral lobar or segmental infiltrates. Alternatively, diffuse lesions can arise by hematogenous spread.[94, 95] *Candida* pneumonia occasionally supervenes in reasonably normal hosts after aspiration.[96, 97] *Trichosporon beigelii* and *T. capitatum (Blastoschizomyces pseudotrichosporon)* can produce bilateral infiltrates as part of systemic infection, particularly during treatment for underlying malignant disease.[98–101] *Candida (Torulopsis) glabrata* occasionally produces pneumonia or empyema in diabetic patients and in those suffering from immunosuppression or severe malnutrition.[102, 103] For each of these yeast infections, amphotericin B is the drug of choice.

References

1. Sacks JJ, Ajello L, Crockett LK: An outbreak and review of cave-associated histoplasmosis capsulati. J Med Vet Mycol 24:313, 1986.
2. Sarosi GA, Johnson PC: Disseminated histoplasmosis in patients infected with human immunodeficiency virus. Clin Infect Dis 14(Suppl 1):S60, 1992.
3. Medoff C, Kobayashi GS, Painter A, Travis S: Morphogenesis and pathogenicity of *Histoplasma capsulatum*. Infect Immun 55:1355, 1987.
4. Howard DH: Further studies on the inhibition of *Histoplasma capsulatum* within macrophages from immunized animals. Infect Immun 8:577, 1973.
5. Wu-Hsieh B, Zlotnik A, Howard DH: T cell hybridoma–produced lymphokine that activates macrophages to suppress intracellular growth of *Histoplasma capsulatum*. Infect Immun 43:380, 1984.
6. Gomez AM, Bullock WE, Taylor CL, Deepe GS Jr: Role of L3T4+ T cells in host defense against *Histoplasma capsulatum*. Infect Immun 56:1685, 1988.
7. Zeiss J, Woldenberg LS, Morgan R, Davis JT: Pulmonary histoplasmoma presenting as massive hemoptysis. Pediatr Infect Dis J 6:689, 1987.
8. Swinburne AJ, Fedullo AJ, Wahl GW, Farnand B: Histoplasmoma, pleural fibrosis and slowly enlarging pleural effusion in an asymptomatic patient. Am Rev Respir Dis 135:502, 1987.
9. Garrett EH Jr, Roper CL: Surgical intervention in histoplasmosis. Ann Thorac Surg 42:711, 1986.
10. Mathisen DJ, Grillo C: Clinical manifestation of mediastinal fibrosis and histoplasmosis. Ann Thorac Surg 54:1053, 1992.
11. Coss KC, Wheat LJ, Conses DJ Jr, et al: Esophageal fistula complicating mediastinal histoplasmosis. Am J Med 83:343, 1987.
12. Baughman RP, Kim CK, Bullock WE: Comparative diagnostic efficacy of bronchoalveolar lavage, transbronchial biopsy and open lung biopsy in experimental pulmonary histoplasmosis. J Infect Dis 153:376, 1986.
13. Paya CV, Roberts GD, Cockerill FR III: Transient fungemia in acute pulmonary histoplasmosis: Detection by new blood-culturing techniques. J Infect Dis 156:313, 1987.
14. Wheat LJ, Connolly-Stringfield P, Kohler RB, et al: *Histoplasma capsulatum* polysaccharide antigen detection in diagnosis and management of disseminated histoplasmosis in patients with acquired immune deficiency syndrome. Am J Med 87:396, 1989.
15. Wheat LJ, Connolly-Stringfield P, Blair R, et al: Effect of successful treatment with amphotericin B on *Histoplasma capsulatum* variety *capsulatum* polysaccharide antigen levels in patient with AIDS and histoplasmosis. Am J Med 92:153, 1992.
16. Klein B, Vergeront JM, Weeks RJ, et al: Isolation of *Blastomyces dermatitidis* in soil associated with a large outbreak of blastomycosis in Wisconsin. N Engl J Med 314:529, 1986.
17. Klein BS, Bradsher RW, Vergeront JM, Davis JP: Development of long-term specific cellular immunity after acute *Blastomyces dermatitidis* infection: Assessments following a large point-source outbreak in Wisconsin. J Infect Dis 161:97, 1990.
18. Berkowitz I, Diamond TH: Disseminated *Blastomyces dermatitidis* infection in a non-endemic area. S Afr Med J 71:717, 1987.
19. Kaufman L, Standard PG, Weeks RJ, Padhye AA: Detection of two *Blastomyces dermatitidis* serotypes by exoantigen analysis. J Clin Microbiol 18:110, 1983.
20. Sugar AM, Brummer E, Stevens DA: Fungicidal activity of murine bronchoalveolar macrophages against *Blastomyces dermatitidis*. J Med Microbiol 21:7, 1986.
21. Medoff G, Painter A, Kobayashi GS: Mycelial to yeast phase transitions of the dimorphic fungi *Blastomyces dermatitidis* and *Paracoccidioides brasiliensis*. J Bacteriol 169:4055, 1987.
22. Meyer KC, McManus EJ, Maki DG: Overwhelming pulmonary blastomycosis associated with the adult respiratory distress syndrome. N Engl J Med 329:1231, 1993.
23. Klein BS, Vergeront JM, Kaufman L, et al: Serological tests for blastomycosis: Assessments during a large point-source outbreak in Wisconsin. J Infect Dis 155:262, 1987.
24. Dismukes WE, Bradsher RW Jr, Cloud GC, et al: Itraconazole therapy for blastomycosis and histoplasmosis. Am J Med 93:489, 1992.
25. Pappas PG, Bradsher RW, Chapman SW, et al: Treatment of blastomycosis with fluconazole: A pilot study. Clin Infect Dis 20:267, 1995.
26. Einstein HE, Johnson RH: Coccidioidomycosis: New aspects of epidemiology and therapy. Clin Infect Dis 16:349, 1993.
27. Pappagianis D: Coccidioidomycosis. Infect Med 8:19, 1991.
28. Stevens DA: Coccidioidomycosis. N Engl J Med 332:1077, 1995.
29. Ampel NM, Dols CL, Galgiani JN: Coccidioidomycosis during human immunodeficiency virus infection: Results of a prospective study in a coccidioidal endemic area. Am J Med 94:235, 1993.
30. Beaman L, Pappagianis D, Benjamini E: Mechanisms of resistance to infection with *Coccidioides immitis* in mice. Infect Immun 23:681, 1979.

31. Larsen RA, Jacobson JA, Morris AH, Benowitz BA: Acute respiratory failure caused by primary pulmonary coccidioidomycosis. Am Rev Respir Dis 131:797, 1985.
32. Lombard CM, Tazelaar HD, Krasne DL: Pulmonary eosinophilia in coccidioidal infections. Chest 91:734, 1987.
33. Clark RA, Greer D, Atkinson W: Spectrum of *Cryptococcus neoformans* infection in 68 patients infected with human immunodeficiency virus. Rev Infect Dis 12:768, 1990.
34. Rozenbaum R, Goncalves AJR: Clinical epidemiological study of 171 cases of cryptococcosis. Clin Infect Dis 18:369, 1994.
35. Henson DJ, Hill AR: Cryptococcal pneumonia: A fulminant presentation. Am J Med Sci 288:221, 1984.
36. Kauffman CA, Severance PJ: Nosocomial cryptococcal infection. South Med J 73:267, 1980.
37. Korvick J, Yu VL: Simultaneous infection with *Cryptococcus neoformans* and *Legionella pneumophila*. Respiration 53:132, 1988.
38. Kerkering TM, Duma RJ, Shadomy S: The evolution of pulmonary cryptococcosis. Ann Intern Med 94:611, 1981.
39. Louria DB: Controversies in the treatment of cryptococcal infections. Infect Med 2:187, 1985.
40. Simpson GL, Stinson EB, Egger MJ, Remington JS: Nocardial infections in the immunocompromised host. Rev Infect Dis 3:492, 1981.
41. Felice GA, Niewoehner DE: Contribution of neutrophils and cell mediated immunity to control of *Nocardia asteroides* in murine lungs. J Infect Dis 156:113, 1987.
42. Berkey P, Bodey GP: Nocardial infection in patients with neoplastic disease. Rev Infect Dis 11:407, 1989.
43. Uttamchandani RB, Daikos GL, Reyes RR, et al: Nocardiosis in 30 patients with advanced human immunodeficiency virus infection: Clinical features and outcome. Clin Infect Dis 18:348, 1994.
44. Schulman LL, Enson Y: Nocardia pneumonitis and the adult respiratory distress syndrome. Am J Med Sci 293:315, 1987.
45. Henkle JQ, Nair SV: Endobronchial pulmonary nocardiosis. JAMA 256:1331, 1986.
46. Gombert ME, Aulicino TM, duBouchet L, et al: Therapy of experimental cerebral nocardiosis with imipenem, amikacin, trimethoprim-sulfamethoxazole and minocycline. Antimicrob Agents Chemother 30:270, 1986.
47. Stropes L, Bartlett M, White A: Multiple recurrences of nocardial pneumonia. Am J Med Sci 280:119, 1980.
48. Dall L, Salzman G: Treatment of pulmonary sporotrichosis with ketoconazole. Rev Infect Dis 9:795, 1987.
49. Sharkey-Mathis PK, Kauffman CA, Graybill JR, et al: Treatment of sporotrichosis with itraconazole. Am J Med 95:279, 1993.
50. Cook DJ, Achong MR, King DEL: Disseminated aspergillosis in an apparently healthy patient. Am J Med 88:74, 1990.
51. Levitz SM, Selsted ME, Ganz T, et al: In vitro killing of spores and hyphae of *Aspergillus fumigatus* and *Rhizopus oryzae* by rabbit neutrophil cationic peptides and bronchoalveolar macrophages. J Infect Dis 154:483, 1986.
52. Schaffner A, Douglas H, Braude A: Selective protection against conidia by mononuclear and against mycelia by polymorphonuclear phagocytes in resistance to *Aspergillus*. J Clin Invest 69:617, 1982.
53. Diamond RD, Clark RA: Damage to *Aspergillus fumigatus* and *Rhizopus oryzae* hyphae by oxidative and non-oxidative microbicidal products of human neutrophils in vitro. Infect Immun 38:487, 1982.
54. Schaffner A, Davis CE, Schaffner T, et al: In vitro susceptibility of fungi to killing by neutrophil granulocytes discriminates between primary pathogenicity and opportunism. J Clin Invest 78:511, 1986.
55. Lewis M, Kallenbach J, Zaltzman M, Zwi S: Invasive pulmonary aspergillosis complicating influenza A pneumonia in a previously healthy patient. Chest 87:691, 1985.
56. Graham BS, Tucker WS Jr: Opportunistic infections in endogenous Cushing's syndrome. Ann Intern Med 101:334, 1984.
57. Lortholary O, Meyohas M, Dupont B, et al: Invasive aspergillosis in patients with acquired immunodeficiency syndrome. Report of 33 cases. Am J Med 95:177, 1993.
58. Kemper CA, Hostetler JS, Follansbee SE, et al: Ulcerative and plaque-like tracheobronchitis due to infection with *Aspergillus* in patients with AIDS. Clin Infect Dis 17:344, 1993.
59. Andrews CP, Weiner MH: *Aspergillus* antigen detection in bronchoalveolar lavage fluid from patients with invasive aspergillosis and aspergillomas. Am J Med 73:372, 1982.
60. Holmberg K, Berdischewsky M, Young LS: Serologic immunodiagnosis of invasive aspergillosis. J Infect Dis 141:656, 1980.
61. Sabetta JR, Miniter P, Andriole VT: The diagnosis of invasive aspergillosis by an enzyme-linked immunosorbent assay for circulating antigen. J Infect Dis 152:946, 1985.
62. Andriole VT: Infections with *Aspergillus* species. Clin Infect Dis 17(Suppl 2):S481, 1993.
63. Denning DW, Lee JY, Hostetler JS, et al: NIAID mycoses study group multicenter trial of oral itraconazole therapy for invasive aspergillosis. Am J Med 97:135, 1994.
64. Yu VL, Wagner GE, Shadomy S: Sino-orbital aspergillosis treated with combination antifungal therapy. JAMA 244:814, 1980.
65. Ribner B, Keusch GT, Hanna BA, Perloff M: Combination amphotericin B–rifampin therapy for pulmonary aspergillosis in a leukemic patient. Chest 70:681, 1976.
66. Waldorf AR, Ruderman N, Diamond RD: Specific susceptibility to mucormycosis in murine diabetes and bronchoalveolar macrophage defense against *Rhizopus*. J Clin Invest 74:150, 1984.
67. Blankenberg HW, Verhoeff D: Mucormycosis of the lung: A case without significant predisposing factor. Am Rev Tuberc 79:357, 1959.
68. Rex JH, Ginsberg AM, Fries LF, et al: *Cunninghamella bertholletiae* infection associated with deferoxamine therapy. Rev Infect Dis 10:1187, 1988.
69. Hay RJ, Campbell CK, Marshall WM, et al: Disseminated zygomycosis (mucormycosis) caused by *Saksenaea vasiformis*. J Infect 7:162, 1983.
70. Ingram CW, Sennesh J, Cooper JN, Perfect JR: Disseminated zygomycosis: Report of four cases and review. Rev Infect Dis 11:741, 1989.
71. Ventura GJ, Kantarjian HM, Anaissie E, et al: Pneumonia with *Cunninghamella* species in patients with hematologic malignancies. Cancer 58:1534, 1986.
72. Walsh TJ, Renshaw G, Andrews J, et al: Invasive zygomycosis due to *Conidiobolus incongruus*. Clin Infect Dis 19:423, 1994.
73. Kontoyianis DP, Vartivarian S, Anaissie EJ, et al: Infections due to *Cunninghamella bertholletiae* in patients with cancer: Report of three cases and review. Clin Infect Dis 18:925, 1994.
74. Libshitz HI, Pagani JJ: Aspergillosis and mucormycosis: Two types of opportunistic fungal pneumonia. Radiology 140:301, 1981.
75. Aderka A, Sidi Y, Garfinkel A, et al: Roentgenologically invisible mucormycosis pneumonia. Respiration 44:158, 1983.
76. Watts WJ: Bronchopleural fistula followed by massive fatal hemoptysis in a patient with pulmonary mucormycosis. Arch Intern Med 143:1029, 1983.
77. Saadah HA, Dixon T: *Petriellidium boydii (Allescheria boydii)* necrotizing pneumonia in a normal host. JAMA 245:605, 1981.
78. Walker DH, Adamec T, Krigman M: Disseminated petriellidiosis (allescheriosis). Arch Pathol Lab Med 102:158, 1978.
79. Louria DB, Tynes B, Nuccio PA, et al: Fungi and yeasts isolated infrequently from the lower respiratory tract. *In* Von Graevenitz A, Sall T (eds): Pathogenic Microorganisms from Atypical Clinical Sources. New York, Marcel Dekker, 1975, p 65.
80. Anaissie E, Bodey GP, Kantarjian H, et al: New spectrum of fungal infections in patients with cancer. Rev Infect Dis 11:369, 1989.
81. Anaissie E: Opportunistic mycosis in the immunocompromised host—Experience at a cancer center and review. Clin Infect Dis 14(Suppl 1):S43, 1992.
82. De la Monte SM, Hutchins GM: Disseminated *Curvularia* infection. Arch Pathol Lab Med 109:872, 1985.
83. Brubaker LH, Steele JC Jr, Rissing JP: Cure of *Curvularia* pneumonia by amphotericin B in a patient with megakaryocytic leukemia. Arch Pathol Lab Med 112:1178, 1988.
84. Wheat LJ, Bartlett M, Ciccarelli M, Smith JW: Opportunistic *Scopulariopsis* pneumonia in an immunocompromised host. South Med J 77:1608, 1984.
85. Dharmasena FM, Davies GS, Catovsky D: *Paecilomyces varioti* pneumonia complicating hairy cell leukaemia. Br Med J 290:967, 1985.
86. Zach TL, Penn RG, Gnarra DJ, Bever JL: *Fusarium moniliforme* pneumonia. Nebr M J 72:6, 1987.

87. Dolon CT, Weed LA, Dines DE: Bronchopulmonary helminthosporiosis. Am J Clin Pathol 53:235, 1970.
88. Rabodonirina M, Paulus S, Thevenet F, et al: Disseminated *Scedosporium prolificans (S. inflatum)* infection after single lung transplantation. Clin Infect Dis 19:138, 1994.
89. Manian FA, Brischetto MJ: Pulmonary infection due to *Exophiala jeanselmei*: Successful treatment with ketoconazole. Clin Infect Dis 16:445, 1993.
90. Kamei K, Unno H, Nagao K, et al: Allergic bronchopulmonary mycosis caused by the basidiomycetous fungus *Schizophyllum commune*. Clin Infect Dis 18:305, 1994.
91. Deng Z, Ribas JL, Gibson DW, Connor DH: Infections caused by *Penicillium marneffei*: In China and Southeast Asia. Review of eighteen published cases and report of four more Chinese cases. Rev Infect Dis 10:640, 1988.
92. Supparatpinyo K, Chiewchanvit S, Hirunsri P, et al: *Penicillium marneffei* infection in patients infected with human immunodeficiency virus. Clin Infect Dis 14:871, 1992.
93. Lobritz RW, Roberts TH, Marraro RV, et al: Granulomatous pulmonary disease secondary to *Alternaria*. JAMA 241:596, 1979.
94. Masur H, Rosen PR, Armstrong D: Pulmonary disease caused by *Candida* species. Am J Med 63:914, 1977.
95. Buff SJ, McLelland R, Gallis HA, et al: *Candida albicans* pneumonia: Radiographic appearance. Am J Roentgenol 138:645, 1982.
96. Worthington M: Fatal *Candida* pneumonia in a non-immunosuppressed host. J Infect 7:159, 1983.
97. Ramirez G, Shuster M, Kozub W, Pribor HC: Fatal acute *Candida albicans* bronchopneumonia. JAMA 199:340, 1967.
98. Hoy J, Hsu K, Rolston K, et al: *Trichosporon beigelii* infection. Rev Infect Dis 8:959, 1986.
99. Saul SH, Khachatoorian T, Poorsattar A, et al: Opportunistic *Trichosporon* pneumonia. Arch Pathol Lab Med 105:456, 1981.
100. Walling DM, McGraw DJ, Merz WG, et al: Disseminated infection with *Trichosporon beigelii*. Rev Infect Dis 9:1013, 1987.
101. Martino P, Venditti M, Micozzi A, et al: *Blastoschizomyces capitatus*. An emerging cause of invasive fungal disease in leukemia patients. Rev Infect Dis 12:570, 1990.
102. Greenfield RA, Jones JM: *Torulopsis glabrata* pneumonia: Value of serologic testing. South Med J 76:504, 1983.
103. Sander LA, Young EJ, Musher DM, Clarridge JE: *Torulopsis glabrata* pneumonia in a malnourished woman. South Med J 72:1477, 1979.

61

Legionnaires' Disease

Robert R. Muder

Legionnaires' disease is a bacterial pneumonia caused by organisms of the genus *Legionella,* members of which are fastidious gram-negative aerobic bacilli. The disease and the genus take their name from an outbreak occurring at the American Legion convention in Philadelphia in 1976,[1] during which more than 200 people became ill and 34 died. The causative organism, *Legionella pneumophila,* was isolated from lung tissue by workers at the Centers for Disease Control and Prevention.[2] Although previous workers had isolated *Legionella* species in animals or embryonated eggs as early as 1943, isolation onto artificial media and phenotypic characterization did not occur until the investigation of the 1976 epidemic. Since that time, 40 species of *Legionella* have been described; 17 have been isolated in cases of human infection (Table 61–1). *Legionella* species may also cause a nonpneumonic, self-limited febrile illness known as Pontiac fever.

TABLE 61–1 ■ *Legionella* Species Isolated from Cases of Pneumonia

L. pneumophila	*L. maceachernii*
L. micdadei	*L. wadsworthii*
L. bozemanii	*L. birminghamensis*
L. dumoffii	*L. cincinnatiensis*
L. longbeachae	*L. tucsonensis*
L. jordanis	*L. anisa*
L. gormanii	*L. sainthelensi*
L. feeleii	*L. lansingensis*
L. hackeliae	

Epidemiology

Legionella species have a widespread distribution in both natural and artificial aquatic habitats, including freshwater,[3] cooling towers[4] and evaporative condensers,[5] whirlpool spas,[6] and potable water systems.[7, 8] Members of the genus grow well at 40°C to 50°C and can often be found readily in warm, nutrient-rich water.[9, 10] Humans acquire infection from environmental sources; there is no evidence for direct person-to-person transmission. Ninety percent of human infections are caused by *L. pneumophila;* of these, more than 80% are due to a single serogroup, serogroup 1.[11]

Legionnaires' disease was initially recognized after a point-source epidemic of *L. pneumophila* infection linked to a hotel.[1] Similar occurrences linked to hotels, hospitals, and other structures have subsequently been reported, with several to hundreds of persons affected. Most cases of community-acquired disease are not associated with recognized outbreaks. More recent studies have demonstrated that *Legionella* species are relatively common causes of community-acquired pneumonias occurring in an endemic or sporadic fashion (Table 61–2). The considerable difference in the frequency of legionellosis as a cause of pneumonia from study to study is based at least in part on differences in location, population, time, and use of culture in diagnosis among the various studies. A large, community-based pneumonia study estimated the annual incidence of Legionnaires' disease to be 6.1 per 100,000 adults per year; this extrapolates to 11,000 cases annually in the United States.[12] Although nosocomial legionellosis has been discovered in apparent outbreaks,[4, 13] when it is specifically sought, endemic disease has been found in a number of hospitals.[14, 15] Colonization of a hospital's potable water supply by *Legionella* may predict the occurrence of nosocomial infection.[15] The precise mode of transmission from aquatic habitats is often uncertain. A number of community outbreaks of *L. pneumophila* infection have been linked to point sources; studies of several of these have implicated aerosol-generating devices, such as cooling towers and evaporative condensers, contaminated with *Legionella.*[16] Other community outbreaks have been traced to a grocery store mist machine[17] and a decorative fountain[18] contaminated with *L. pneumophila.* Several community outbreaks have occurred in which no potential source of *Legionella* could be identified despite extensive investigation.[19, 20] Potable water systems of large buildings such as hospitals and hotels are often extensively colonized by *Legionella;* these systems may be associated with human infection.[7, 8, 21–23] Residential water systems have been implicated in community-acquired cases.[24, 25]

Nosocomial infection is particularly associated with colonization of hospital hot-water systems by *Legionella.*[7, 23] In addition to *L. pneumophila, Legionella micdadei,*[8] *Legionella dumoffii,*[26] and *Legionella bozemanii*[27] may cause nosocomial disease in the presence of colonized water. There are a number of potential mechanisms of transmission of the organism. Contamination of aerosol-generating respiratory therapy equipment by

TABLE 61–2 ■ Proportion of Community-Acquired Pneumonias Caused by *Legionella*

YEAR	LOCATION	NO. OF PATIENTS	DIAGNOSTIC METHOD* Culture	DFA	Serology	Urine	INCIDENCE (%)	REFERENCE
1974–1980	Bristol, UK	210	No	No	Yes	No	2.9	125
1980–1981	Nottingham, UK	127	No	No	Yes	No	15.0	126
1981	Hartford, CT	204	No	No	Yes	No	14.0	127
1981	Pittsburgh, PA	70	Yes†	Yes	Yes	No	16.0	14
1981–1984	Nova Scotia, Canada	301	No	No	Yes	No	6.3	128
1982–1983	France	274	Yes‡	No	Yes	No	10.6	129
1982–1983	United Kingdom	453	No	No	Yes	No	3.0	130
1982–1983	Sweden	147	No	No	Yes	No	2.7	131
1982–1983	Denmark	92	Yes§	Yes§	Yes	No	23.9	132
1983–1984	Paris, France	116	Yes§	Yes§	Yes	No	6.7	133
1984–1985	Nottingham, UK	236	No	Yes‖	Yes	No	1.0	89
1985	Israel	133	Yes¶	Yes¶	Yes¶	No	9.0	134
1985–1986	Pittsburgh, PA	359	Yes†	Yes	Yes	Yes	6.7	74
1987–1988	Australia	106	Yes	Yes	Yes	No	3.0	135

*Culture, *Legionella* culture; DFA, direct fluorescent antibody stain; Serology, antibody titer serology; Urine, *Legionella* urinary antigen.
†Buffered charcoal–yeast extract agar plus *Legionella*-selective, dye-containing media.
‡Buffered charcoal–yeast extract agar only.
§DFA and culture applied to selected cases only.
‖DFA applied to autopsy cases only.
¶Serology applied to selected cases; DFA and culture applied to tissue culture only.
Modified from Muder RR, Yu VL, Fang GD: Community-acquired Legionnaires' disease. Semin Respir Infect 4:32–39, 1989.

tap water has been implicated as a source.[28, 29] Aerosolization from showers and taps is a possible mode of transmission.[30, 31] Aspiration of contaminated water as a mode of transmission is supported by several epidemiologic studies.[32–34] Major oncologic surgery of the head and neck, in which postoperative aspiration is nearly universal, predisposes to *Legionella* infection.[35] Introduction of contaminated water into nasogastric tubes is also associated with nosocomial pneumonia,[36, 37] presumably due to aspiration of gastric contents. An outbreak of postoperative wound infection was associated with washing of the wound area with *Legionella*-contaminated tap water.[38]

Factors associated with an increased risk for infection include male sex, advanced age, cigarette smoking, chronic obstructive pulmonary disease, organ transplantation, use of immunosuppressive medications, malignant disease, and chronic renal failure.[11, 39] Patients with acquired immunodeficiency syndrome also have a markedly elevated risk for *Legionella* infection compared with the general population.[11] In addition, risk for nosocomial infection is further increased by general anesthesia and by endotracheal intubation.[14, 40, 41] Infection in children is rare but has been reported in both immunocompromised and immunocompetent children.[42] There are reports of nosocomial *Legionella* infection in premature neonates requiring mechanical ventilation.[43, 44]

Pontiac fever occurs after exposure to aerosols contaminated by *Legionella*. Implicated sources include air-conditioning systems,[45] industrial equipment,[46] and whirlpool spas.[47] In addition to *L. pneumophila, Legionella feeleii,*[46] *L. micdadei,*[48] and *Legionella anisa*[49] may cause Pontiac fever.

Pathogenesis

Although capable of multiplying freely in the environment and on artificial media, *Legionella* species are considered intracellular parasites. *Legionella* can multiply within freshwater amoebae and protozoa.[50] Although these protozoa have been found in potable water distribution systems,[51] it is unclear whether this growth in protozoa is related to pathogenesis.

The organisms enter the respiratory tract by aerosolization or aspiration. Human neutrophils have little capacity to kill *L. pneumophila* even in the presence of specific antibody and complement.[52] *L. pneumophila* is phagocytosed by monocytes and alveolar macrophages; uptake is mediated by complement fixed to the bacterial surface through the alternative pathway[53] and enhanced in the presence of specific antibody.[54] A major virulence determinant of *L. pneumophila* is the Mip protein, a 24-kDa molecule that promotes infection of mononuclear phagocytes.[55] Inside the phagocyte, *L. pneumophila* multiples within a ribosome-lined vacuole and inhibits phagosome-lysosome fusion.[56] Multiplication occurs until the phagocytic cell ruptures.

Cell-mediated immunity is the primary host defense. Lymphocyte proliferation and cutaneous delayed hypersensitivity to *L. pneumophila* occur in the first 2 weeks of infection.[51, 57, 58] Lymphocytes from patients and experimental animals surviving *Legionella* infection demonstrate proliferation and lymphokine production in the presence of the organism.[59, 60] Murine alveolar macrophages activated by interferon-γ kill ingested *L. pneumophila* in a dose-dependent manner.[61] Activated human mononuclear cells inhibit but do not kill the organism.[52] Interferon-γ causes down-regulation of transferrin receptors in human monocytes, limiting the availability of iron, an essential growth factor for *L. pneumophila*.[62]

The central role of cell-mediated immunity in host defense against *Legionella* infection is substantiated by the epidemiologic association with specific host immune defects, including corticosteroid therapy, organ transplantation, and acquired immunodeficiency syndrome. Patients with hairy cell leukemia, a disorder characterized by defective monocyte number and function, may have an increased risk for *Legionella* infection.[63]

Humoral immunity appears to have a limited role in host defense. Type-specific antibody, initially immunoglobulin M followed by immunoglobulin G, appears in the first weeks of infection. Immunized animals also develop a specific antibody response that may be protective.[64, 65] On the other hand, specific antibody stimulates uptake of *Legionella* by macrophages without inhibiting intracellular replication.[52]

Cytotoxins produced by the organism cause defective triggering of neutrophil oxidative metabolism.[66, 67] Virulent strains of *L. pneumophila* are directly toxic to alveolar macrophages.[68] A number of extracellular enzymes including proteases may be responsible for tissue damage.[69]

Although a variety of potential virulence factors have been identified, none, with the exception of the Mip protein, has been definitely shown to be a virulence determinant.[70]

Pathology

The characteristic pathologic presentation is a fibrinopurulent pneumonia with inflammatory cellular exudate composed of neutrophils and macrophages in the terminal airspaces. A characteristic lysis of the exudate has been described.[71] Diffuse alveolar damage especially to the capillaries and hyaline membrane formation are seen. *Legionella* can be demonstrated in phagocytes and alveolar spaces by Dieterle silver staining or direct immunofluorescence. Invasion of blood vessels and lymphatics can be seen by immunofluorescent staining. *Legionella* organisms have been seen in extrapulmonic tissues including spleen, liver, kidney, myocardium, brain, prostate, thyroid, and muscle,[72, 73] consistent with hematogenous spread.

Clinical Manifestations

The overwhelming majority of *Legionella* infections are caused by *L. pneumophila.* Pneumonia (Legionnaires' disease) is the major clinical manifestation of *Legionella* infection, although extrapulmonary infection and nonpneumonic disease (Pontiac fever) occur.

On the basis of data from point-source outbreaks, the incubation period of *Legionella* pneumonia is estimated to be 2 to 10 days after exposure.[1] There may be a prodrome of several days with the insidious onset of fever, malaise, and nonproductive cough. Nearly all patients will be febrile at presentation, and half will have a temperature of 103°F or greater.[74] Cough is usually nonproductive at first, but 50% to 75% of patients will produce sputum within several days of presentation. Chest pain and dyspnea occur in about 50% of patients.[75] Respiratory failure necessitating ventilatory support occurs in 15% to 50% of community-acquired cases.[74–77] Gastrointestinal symptoms including diarrhea and abdominal pain are common. Myalgias may be a prominent presenting feature. Initial reports emphasized the multisystemic nature of *Legionella* pneumonia. Confusion, hematuria, renal failure, and hepatic dysfunction were symptoms reported to be typical of Legionnaires' disease. However, *Legionella* infection does not appear to be distinguishable from other pneumonias on clinical grounds alone.[75, 78] Early reports included many patients given inadequate therapy; the multiorgan dysfunction reported is probably nonspecific and can be seen in overwhelming bacterial pneumonia of any cause. In later reports, multiorgan system failure appears to be associated with the requirement for mechanical ventilation or pressors during treatment of pneumonia.[79, 80]

Syndromes such as acute tubular necrosis, pancreatitis, cerebellar ataxia, peripheral neuropathy, rhabdomyolysis, hemolytic anemia, thrombotic thrombocytopenic purpura, and various rashes have been reported with *Legionella* infection.[81–84] The mechanism by which *Legionella* could cause these manifestations is unclear. Each of these sequelae occurs after infections due to other agents as well.

Extrapulmonary *Legionella* infection occurs infrequently. In most but not all cases, such infections have occurred during the course of pneumonia, presumably through hematogenous spread. Renal abscess, soft tissue infection, endocarditis, myocarditis, pericarditis, peritonitis, and hemodialysis fistula infection have been reported.[85]

In highly immunocompromised hosts (e.g., transplant recipients), the presentation of *Legionella* infection may not suggest bacterial pneumonia initially. The onset may be abrupt, and typical pneumonic symptoms may be absent; fever may be the only symptom.[86] Localized pleuritic pain and dyspnea may suggest the diagnosis of pulmonary embolism.[87]

Laboratory data are likewise nonspecific. The majority of patients have a polymorphonuclear leukocytosis on presentation. Early reports of Legionnaires' disease suggested elevated creatinine concentration, abnormal hepatic function, hypophosphatemia, and hematuria as characteristic manifestations. Subsequent comparative studies have concluded that the laboratory manifestations of *Legionella* infection are not distinctive compared with those of other bacterial pneumonias.[78, 88, 89] Hyponatremia appears to occur more frequently in Legionnaires' disease than in pneumonia of other causes.[78]

Radiography

Most patients present with abnormal chest radiographs, and essentially all have radiographic evidence of pneumonia by the third day of illness.[90] There is a slight predominance of lower lobe involvement, but any area may be affected. The infiltrates are alveolar and may be segmental, lobar, or diffuse on presentation. Pleura-based, rounded opacities with poorly defined margins may resemble pulmonary infarction or neoplasm (Fig. 61–1). Although the majority of cases present with single-lobe involvement, there is a notable tendency for the radiographic extent of pneumonia to increase during the first several days after presentation and to involve additional lobes in 25% to 50% of patients[91] (Fig. 61–2). This progression may occur in the face of appropriate antibiotic

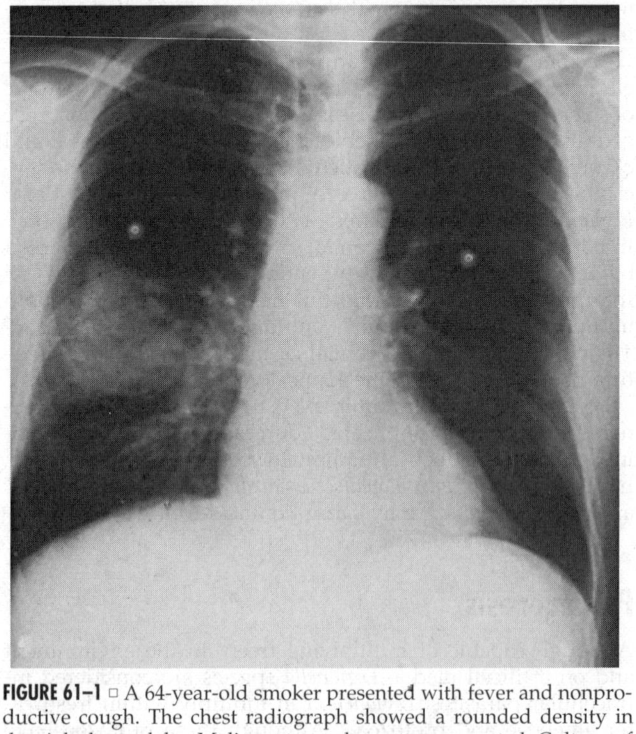

FIGURE 61–1 □ A 64-year-old smoker presented with fever and nonproductive cough. The chest radiograph showed a rounded density in the right lower lobe. Malignant neoplasm was suspected. Culture of respiratory secretions obtained at bronchoscopy yielded *L. pneumophila.* (From Muder RR, Yu VL, Fang GD: Community-acquired Legionnaires' disease. Semin Respir Infect 4:32–39, 1989.)

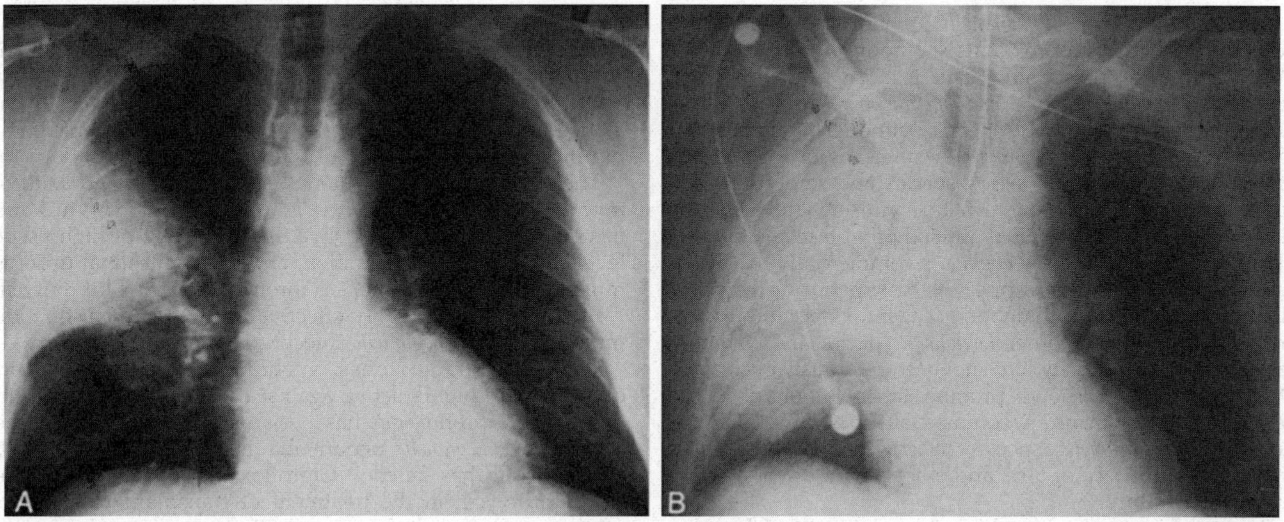

FIGURE 61–2 □ A 47-year-old man presented with chills and slightly productive cough. His history was remarkable only for cigarette smoking and essential hypertension. The chest radiograph showed a segmental infiltrate in the lower portion of the right upper lobe *(A)*. Cephalosporin therapy was begun. By the third hospital day, the infiltrate had progressed to the right upper lobe and the upper portion of the right lower lobe *(B)*. Sputum culture obtained on admission yielded heavy growth of *L. pneumophila*. Erythromycin and rifampin were begun, followed by clinical response and ultimate recovery. (From Muder RR, Yu VL, Parry M: Radiology of *Legionella* pneumonia. Semin Respir Infect 2:242–254, 1987.)

therapy and does not of itself predict clinical failure. The extent of radiologic involvement in *Legionella* infection bears little relationship to prognosis.[92] Small to moderate pleural effusions occur in at least one third of patients and can occasionally precede the appearance of the infiltrate; in a few patients, pleural effusion is the only radiographic abnormality.[90, 93] Loculated effusion and empyema occur occasionally and require drainage.

Cavitation is unusual in the immunologically intact patient but is frequent in the patient receiving corticosteroids or immunosuppressive medications.[90] In these patients, the initial infiltrate tends to appear as a rounded density that undergoes progressive central cavitation until a thin-walled cavity remains. The progression of cavitation may occur during the course of successful antibiotic therapy. The cavity usually closes spontaneously in time.

Radiographic clearing of infiltrates after *Legionella* infection tends to be slower than that seen in other bacterial pneumonias. Residual infiltrates are present in 30% to 40% at 3 months or beyond after illness.[90, 91]

Other *Legionella* Species

Sixteen *Legionella* species other than *L. pneumophila* have been isolated from cases of human infection.[93–96] Of the 10% of *Legionella* infections due to these other species, most are caused by four species: *L. micdadei*, *Legionella longbeachae*, *L. bozemanii*, and *L. dumoffii*. Patients with non-*pneumophila* infections appear more likely to be immunocompromised than patients infected with *L. pneumophila*.[94] Otherwise, the clinical and radiologic features are similar to those described for *L. pneumophila* infection. Cases of simultaneous infection by multiple *Legionella* species have been documented.[97, 98]

Pontiac Fever

Pontiac fever is an acute febrile illness occurring after exposure to aerosolized *L. pneumophila*,[45] *L. feeleii*,[46] *L. micdadei*,[48] or *L. anisa*.[49] The attack rate may exceed 90% in exposed individuals. The illness has a superficial resemblance to influenza, with associated chills, myalgia, headache, and malaise.[99] Although nonproductive cough and chest pain are present in about half of the patients, radiographic evidence of pneumonia does not develop. The symptoms occur 1 to 2 days after exposure and resolve spontaneously in 2 to 5 days. Isolation of *Legionella* in culture has never occurred, and diagnosis is established by seroconversion. It is not clear whether the symptoms are due to infection or to a hypersensitivity phenomenon. There is no specific therapy.

Diagnosis

Legionella species are fastidious and cannot be recovered on the usual bacteriologic media used in the diagnosis of pneumonia. Although gram-negative, they are generally not visible on Gram stain of respiratory specimens. *L. micdadei* is weakly acid fast and can be visualized in clinical specimens. Specialized microbiologic and immunologic techniques are needed for the diagnosis of *Legionella* infection.

Recovery from clinical specimens by culture is hampered by the tendency for overgrowth of commensal flora. The base medium is buffered charcoal–yeast extract agar. Antibacterial and antifungal agents are added to inhibit competing flora, and dyes are added to enhance visibility. *L. pneumophila* can be isolated from expectorated sputum in 70% of samples if multiple selective media are used.[100, 101] Specimens obtained by bronchoscopy probably do not give a significantly better yield than sputum. Transtracheal aspirate specimens that are free of contaminating oral flora give the highest yield (sensitivity of 90%). Acid washing of sputum samples reduces competing flora and improves sensitivity.[102] Characteristic ground-glass colonies can be identified in 48 to 72 hours with a dissecting microscope. Rapid speciation of the isolate is accomplished by direct fluorescent antibody staining or slide agglutination. Isolation of *Legionella* from the sputum of a patient with pneumonia is presumed to be diagnostic of infection because colonization of the oropharynx has not yet been demonstrated.

Legionella can be isolated from the blood of patients by specially supplemented media or by "blind" direct subculture of nonsupplemented aerobic blood culture media onto buffered charcoal–yeast extract agar.[103]

Direct visualization of *Legionella* in clinical specimens can be accomplished in approximately 2 hours by use of direct fluorescent antibody staining. This test has a sensitivity of 30% to 70% in detecting *L. pneumophila* in respiratory secretions.[100] The test is highly specific, although false-positive results due to cross-reactions with other species of bacteria have been reported. The test is species and serogroup specific; conjugates containing multiple antisera are commercially available. A monoclonal antibody that reacts with multiple serogroups of *L. pneumophila* is commercially available; sensitivity and specificity appear to be superior to the polyclonal direct fluorescent antibody reagent. Direct fluorescent antibody reagents for other *Legionella* species are available; sensitivity and specificity have not been rigorously evaluated. DNA amplification shows promise for detection of *Legionella* clinical specimens. A commercial kit designed for the detection of *Legionella* species in environmental samples showed a sensitivity of 90% and a specificity of 100% compared with culture.[104]

Rapid diagnosis can be achieved by detection of *L. pneumophila* antigens in the urine. Sensitivity is 80% by day 3 of illness, and specificity is 99%.[105, 106] The test is commercially available but limited to *L. pneumophila* serogroup 1. Antigenuria may persist for months after clinical illness.

Serologic diagnosis can be accomplished by a variety of methods, although the indirect fluorescent antibody assay and enzyme-linked immunosorbent assay are most widely used.[107, 100] Eighty percent of patients infected with *L. pneumophila* show a diagnostic rise in titer within 2 to 6 weeks. A fourfold rise to a titer of 1:128 by indirect fluorescent antibody assay is considered diagnostic; a single elevated titer of 1:256 accompanying a compatible clinical illness can be considered presumptive. The specificity of serology is estimated to be 95% in the diagnosis of *L. pneumophila.* Neither sensitivity nor specificity has been established for other species, and diagnosis of an infection with a *Legionella* species other than *L. pneumophila* based solely on serology should be made with caution.

Diagnostic of nonpneumonic legionellosis (Pontiac fever) is based on antibody seroconversion after a compatible clinical illness. *Legionella* organisms have not been demonstrated in clinical specimens by either culture or direct fluorescent antibody staining.

Therapy

In the 1976 Philadelphia outbreak, therapy with erythromycin or tetracycline was associated with markedly improved survival compared with treatment with β-lactam or aminoglycoside antibiotics.[1] Controlled trials of therapy for *Legionella* infection in humans have not been performed. Although *Legionella* organisms are sensitive in vitro to a variety of antibiotics, animal and egg model studies have demonstrated that agents that penetrate intracellularly have therapeutic efficacy. Erythromycin, rifampin, tetracycline, trimethoprim-sulfamethoxazole, and 5-fluoroquinolones have demonstrated in vitro and in vivo activity against *Legionella.*

The most extensive experience is with the use of erythromycin. In hospitalized patients, erythromycin, 1 g intravenously every 6 hours, is recommended. Once the patient has responded, the oral form may be given in a dose of 500 mg four times daily. The dosage of erythromycin should be reduced in hepatic or renal failure to prevent ototoxic effects.[108] Relapse has been reported in immunocompromised patients treated with shorter courses such that 3 weeks of therapy has been recommended. Fourteen days of therapy is adequate in nonimmunosuppressed patients who experience a prompt clinical response. Rifampin may be added to erythromycin in the treatment of patients who are immunocompromised, have multilobar involvement, or require mechanical ventilation. Although the combination of rifampin and erythromycin is more rapidly bactericidal than erythromycin alone, there is no clinical evidence that the addition of rifampin improves prognosis.

The newer macrolides such as clarithromycin and azithromycin have excellent activity against *Legionella* in vitro and in vivo.[109, 110] These agents have the advantage of high tissue levels after oral administration, and gastrointestinal upset is much less than with oral erythromycin. Oral azithromycin was reported to be highly effective in the treatment of community-acquired *Legionella* infection.[111]

The 5-fluoroquinolones, including ciprofloxacin and ofloxacin, are highly active against *Legionella* in vitro and in vivo.[112, 113] Ciprofloxacin has been used successfully in the treatment of *Legionella* pneumonia, including cases in which erythromycin has failed.[114] Ciprofloxacin may be preferable to erythromycin in the treatment of transplant patients receiving cyclosporine, because erythromycin interferes with cyclosporine metabolism.[115] Ciprofloxacin may also be preferable in patients with hepatic and renal failure, who are at risk for ototoxic effects of erythromycin.

Tetracycline,[116] trimethoprim-sulfamethoxazole,[117] and imipenem-cilastatin[118] have been used successfully in a limited number of patients.

Mortality of patients receiving erythromycin for treatment of community-acquired illness is about 10% and is dependent on the severity of underlying illness and the timing of initiation of specific antibiotic therapy. Risk for mortality is increased by advanced age and the presence of underlying conditions such as immunosuppression, malignant neoplasm, and end-stage renal disease. Mortality in nosocomially acquired disease approaches 40%,[11] reflecting the severity of the patients' underlying illnesses.

Prevention and Control

Colonization of a hospital water system with *L. pneumophila* predicts the occurrence of nosocomial legionellosis.[14, 15] Surveillance of hospital water systems for *Legionella* is a reasonable precaution. The isolation of *Legionella* from a hospital's water system mandates, at a minimum, surveillance for cases of nosocomial infection. One potential strategy is to apply diagnostic tests for *Legionella* infection to cases of nosocomial pneumonia among patients at highest risk, including patients receiving immunosuppressive therapy, undergoing general anesthesia, or suffering from chronic pulmonary disease.[119]

Various biocides have been used to decontaminate cooling towers, but microbiologic control has been inconsistent and clinical correlation has been lacking.[120] Several methods have been used successfully to decontaminate potable water systems linked to nosocomial infection; decrease in the frequency of *Legionella* isolation has been followed by decrease in the occurrence of disease. Periodic elevation of hot-water temperature to 70°C followed by flushing of distal sites (faucets, showerheads)[8, 120] is effective. Continuous hyperchlorination is likewise effective but may cause accelerated corrosion of pipes.[121] A system using electrodes that continuously generate copper and silver ions is highly effective in eliminating *Legionella*[122] from hospital water systems. Unlike chlorine, metal ions do not promote corrosion of pipes. Ultraviolet light treatment of water near the point of use[123] is a means of providing a locally disinfected water supply to a high-risk group of patients.

Both infection of guinea pigs by an avirulent strain of *L. pneumophila* and immunization with a major secretory protein of the organism afforded protection against aerosol infection by virulent *L. pneumophila.*[65] Immunization with the major cytoplasmic membrane protein of *L. pneumophila,* a genus common antigen, also provided protection against lethal aerosol challenge.[124] Thus, the development of a vaccine providing protection against infection with multiple *Legionella* species is possible.

References

1. Fraser DW, Tsai T, Ornstein W, et al: Legionnaires' disease: Description of an epidemic of pneumonia. N Engl J Med 297:1189–1197, 1977.
2. McDade J, Shepard C, Fraser D, et al: Legionnaires' disease: Isolation of a bacterium and demonstration of its role in other respiratory disease. N Engl J Med 297:1197–1203, 1977.
3. Fliermans CB, Cherry WB, Orrison LH, Thacker L: Ecological distribution of *Legionella pneumophila.* Appl Environ Microbiol 41:9–16, 1981.
4. Dondero TJ Jr, Rendtorff RC, Mallison GF, et al: An outbreak of Legionnaires' disease associated with a contaminated air-conditioning cooling tower. N Engl J Med 302:365–370, 1980.
5. Keys TF: Therapeutic considerations in the treatment of *Legionella* infection. Semin Respir Infect 2:270–273, 1987.
6. Groothius DG, Havelaar AH, Veenendaal HR: A note on legionellas in whirlpools. J Appl Bacteriol 58:479–482, 1985.
7. Stout JE, Yu VL, Vickers RM, et al: Ubiquitousness of *Legionella pneumophila* in the water supply of a hospital with endemic Legionnaires' disease. N Engl J Med 36:466–468, 1982.
8. Best M, Yu VL, Stout J, et al: Legionellaceae in the hospital water supply—Epidemiological link with disease and evaluation of a method of control of nosocomial Legionnaires' disease and Pittsburgh pneumonia. Lancet 2:307–310, 1983.
9. Wadowsky RM, Yee RB, Mezmar L, et al: Hot water systems as sources of *Legionella pneumophila* in hospital and nonhospital plumbing fixtures. Appl Environ Microbiol 43:1104–1110, 1982.
10. Tison DL, Baross JA, Seidler RJ: *Legionella* in aquatic habitats in the Mount Saint Helens blast zone. Curr Microbiol 9:345–348, 1983.
11. Marston BJ, Lipman HB, Breiman RF: Surveillance for Legionnaires' disease. Risk factors for morbidity and mortality. Arch Intern Med 154:2417–2422, 1994.
12. Marston BJ, Plouffe JF, Breiman RF, et al: Preliminary findings of a community-based pneumonia incidence study. *In* Barbaree J, Breiman RF, Dufour AP (eds.): *Legionella*—Current Status and Emerging Perspectives. Washington, DC, American Society for Microbiology 1993, pp 36–37.
13. Thacker SB, Bennet JV, Tsai T: An outbreak in 1975 of severe respiratory illness caused by Legionnaires' disease bacterium. J Infect Dis 238:512–519, 1978.
14. Muder RR, Yu VL, McClure J, Kominos S: Nosocomial Legionnaires' disease uncovered in a prospective pneumonia study: Implications for underdiagnosis. JAMA 249:3184–3188, 1983.
15. Yu VL, Beam TR Jr, Lumish RM, et al: Routine culturing for *Legionella* in the hospital environment may be a good idea: A three-hospital prospective study. Am J Med Sci 294:97–99, 1987.
16. Cordes L, Fraser D, Skaliy P, et al: Legionnaires' disease outbreak at Atlanta, Georgia, country club: Evidence for spread from an evaporative condenser. Am J Epidemiol 11:425–431, 1980.
17. Mahoney FJ, Hoge CW, Farley TA, et al: Community-wide outbreak of Legionnaires' disease associated with a grocery store mist machine. J Infect Dis 165:736–739, 1992.
18. Hlady WG, Mullen RC, Mintz CS, et al: Outbreak of Legionnaires' disease linked to a decorative fountain. Am J Epidemiol 138:555–562, 1993.
19. Mamolen M, Breiman RF, Barbaree JM: Use of multiple molecular subtyping techniques to investigate a Legionnaires' disease outbreak due to identical strains at two tourist lodges. J Clin Microbiol 31:2584–2588, 1993.
20. Redd SC, Yeng F, Lin C, et al: A rural outbreak of Legionnaires' disease linked to visiting a retail store. Am J Public Health 80:431–434, 1990.
21. Nolte FS, Conlin C, Roisin A: Plasmids as epidemiological markers in nosocomial Legionnaires' disease. J Infect Dis 149:251–256, 1984.
22. Schlech WF III, Gorman GW, Payne MD, Broome CV: Legionnaires' disease in the Caribbean: An outbreak associated with a resort hotel. Arch Internal Med 145:2076–2079, 1985.
23. Helms CM, Massanari R, Zeiter S, et al: Legionnaires' disease associated with a hospital water system. Ann Intern Med 99:172–178, 1983.
24. Stout JE, Yu VL, Muraca P, et al: Potable water as the cause of sporadic cases of community-acquired Legionnaires' disease. N Engl J Med 326:151–154, 1992.
25. Castellani Pastoris M, Vigano EF, Passi C: A family cluster of *Legionella pneumophila* infections. Scand J Infect Dis 20:489–493, 1988.
26. Joly JR, Diery P, Gauvrau L, et al: Legionnaires' disease caused by *Legionella dumoffi* in distilled water. Can Med Assoc J 135:1273–1277, 1986.
27. Parry MF, Stampleman L, Hutchinson J, et al: Waterborne *Legionella bozemanii* and nosocomial pneumonia in immunosuppressed patients. Ann Intern Med 103:205–210, 1985.
28. Arnow P, Chou T, Weil D, et al: Nosocomial Legionnaires' disease caused by aerosolized tap water from respiratory devices. J Infect Dis 146:460–467, 1982.
29. Mastro TD, Fields BS, Breiman RF, et al: Nosocomial Legionnaires' disease and use of medication nebulizers. J Infect Dis 163:667–671, 1991.
30. Bollin GE, Plouffe JF, Para MF, et al: *Legionella pneumophila* generated by shower heads and hot water faucets. Appl Environ Microbiol 50:1128–1131, 1986.
31. Woo AH, Goetz A, Yu VL: Transmission of *Legionella* by respiratory equipment aerosol generating devices. Chest 102:1586–1590, 1992.
32. Muder RR, Yu VL, Woo A: Mode of transmission of *L. pneumophila:* A critical review. Arch Intern Med 146:1607–1612, 1986.
33. Yu VL: Could aspiration be the major mode of transmission for *Legionella?* Am J Med 95:13–15, 1993.
34. Marrie TJ, Macdonald S, Clarke K, et al: Nasogastric tubes flushed with contaminated potable water are a risk factor for nosocomial Legionnaires' disease (Abstr 191). *In* Program and Abstracts of the 28th Interscience Conference on Antimicrobial Agents and Chemotherapy. Washington, DC, American Society for Microbiology, 1988.
35. Johnson JT, Yu VL, Best M, et al: Nosocomial legionellosis uncovered in surgical patients with head and neck cancer: Implications for epidemiologic reservoir and mode of transmission. Lancet 2:298–300, 1985.
36. Blatt SP, Parkinson M, Pace E, et al: Nosocomial Legionnaires' disease. Aspiration as a primary mode of transmission. Am J Med 95:16–22, 1993.
37. Venezia RA, Agresta MD, Hanley EM, et al: Nosocomial legionellosis associated with aspiration of nasogastric feedings diluted in tap water. Infect Control Hosp Epidemiol 15:529–533, 1994.
38. Lowry PW, Blankenship RJ, Gridley W, et al: A cluster of *Legionella* sternal wound infections due to postoperative topical exposure of contaminated tap water. N Engl J Med 324:109–112, 1991.
39. England AC, Fraser DW: Sporadic and epidemic nosocomial legionellosis in the United States. Am J Med 70:707–711, 1981.
40. Tompkins LS, Roessler BJ, Redd SC, et al: *Legionella* prosthetic-valve endocarditis. N Engl J Med 318:530–535, 1988.
41. Strebel P, Ramos J, Eidelman I, Tobiansky L: Legionnaires' disease in a Johannesburg teaching hospital. Investigation and control of an outbreak. S Afr Med J 19:329–333, 1988.
42. Brady M: Nosocomial Legionnaires' disease in a children's hospital. J Pediatr 15:46–50, 1989.
43. Womack S, Liang KC, Llagan N, et al: *Legionella pneumophila* in a preterm infant—A case report. J Perinatol 12:303–305, 1992.
44. Luck PC, Dinger D, Helbig JH, et al: Analysis of *Legionella pneumophila* strains associated with nosocomial pneumonia in a neonatal intensive care unit. Eur J Clin Microbiol Infect Dis 13:565–571, 1994.
45. Kaufman AF, McDade J, Patton C, et al: Pontiac fever: Isolation of the etiologic agent *(Legionella pneumophila)* and demonstration of its mode of transmission. Am J Epidemiol 114:337–347, 1981.
46. Herwaldt L, Gorman G, McGrath T, et al: A new *Legionella*

species, *Legionella feeleii* species nova, causes Pontiac fever in an automobile plant. Ann Intern Med 100:333–338, 1984.
47. Spitalny K, Voot R, Orciarl L, et al: Pontiac fever associated with a whirlpool spa. Am J Epidemiol 120:809–817, 1984.
48. Goldberg DJ, Wrench JG, Collier PW, et al: Lochgoilhead fever: Outbreak of non-pneumonic legionellosis due to *Legionella micdadei.* Lancet 1:316–318, 1989.
49. Fenstersheib M, Miller M, Diggins C, et al: Outbreak of Pontiac fever due to *Legionella anisa.* Lancet 336:35–37, 1990.
50. Fields BS: *Legionella* and protoza: Interaction of a pathogen and its natural host. *In* Barbaree JM, Breiman RF, Dufour AP (eds). *Legionella*—Current Status and Emerging Prospectives. Washington, DC, American Society for Microbiology, 1993, pp 129–136.
51. Breiman R, Fields B, Sanden G, et al: Association of shower use with Legionnaires' disease: Possible role of amoebae. JAMA 263:2924–2926, 1990.
52. Horwitz MA, Silverstein SC: Interaction of the Legionnaires' disease bacterium *(Legionella pneumophila)* with human phagocytes II. Antibody promotes binding of *L. pneumophila.* J Exp Med 153:398–406, 1981.
53. Payne NR, Horwitz MA: Phagocytosis of *Legionella pneumophila* is mediated by human monocyte complement receptors. J Exp Med 166:1377–1389, 1987.
54. Nash TW, Libby D, Horwitz MA: Interaction between the Legionnaires' disease bacterium *(L. pneumophila)* and human alveolar macrophages. Influence of antibody, lymphokine, and hydrocortisone. J Clin Invest 74:771–782, 1984.
55. Cianciotto NP, Eisenstein BI, Mody CH, et al: A *Legionella pneumophila* gene encoding a species-specific surface protein potentiates initiation of intracellular infection. Infect Immun 57:1255–1262, 1989.
56. Horwitz MA: The Legionnaires' disease bacterium *(Legionella pneumophila)* inhibits phagosome-lysosome fusion in human monocytes. J Exp Med 158:2108–2126, 1983.
57. Plouffe JF, Baird IM: Lymphocyte blastogenic responses to *Legionella pneumophila* in acute legionellosis. J Clin Lab Immunol 7:43–44, 1982.
58. Friedman H, Widen R, Lee I, Klein T: Cellular immunity to *Legionella pneumophila* in guinea pigs assessed by direct and indirect migration inhibition reactions in vitro. Infect Immun 41:1132–1137, 1983.
59. Horwitz MA, Silverstein SC: Intracellular multiplication of Legionnaires' disease bacteria *(Legionella pneumophila)* in human monocytes is reversibly inhibited by erythromycin and rifampin. J Clin Invest 1:15–26, 1983.
60. Skerrett SJ, Schmidt R, Martin TR: Impaired clearance of aerosolized *L. pneumophila* in corticosteroid treated rats: A model of Legionnaires' disease in the compromised host. J Infect Dis 160:261–268, 1989.
61. Skerrett SJ, Martin TR: Alveolar macrophage activation in experimental legionellosis. J Immunol 147:337–345, 1991.
62. Byrd TF, Horwitz MA: Interferon gamma–activated human monocytes downregulate transferrin receptors and inhibit the intracellular multiplication of *Legionella pneumophila* by limiting the availability of iron. J Clin Invest 83:1457–1465, 1989.
63. Cordonnier C, Farcet JP, Desforges L: Legionnaires' disease and hairy-cell leukemia. Arch Intern Med 144:2373–2375, 1984.
64. Rolstad B, Berdal B: Immune defenses against *Legionella pneumophila* in rats. Infect Immun 32:805–812, 1981.
65. Blander SJ, Breiman R, Horwitz MA: A live avirulent mutant *L. pneumophila* vaccine induces protective immunity against lethal aerosol challenge. J Clin Invest 83:810–815, 1989.
66. Summersgill JT, Raff MJ, Miller RD: Interactions of virulent and avirulent *Legionella pneumophila* with human polymorphonuclear leukocytes. Microb Pathog 4:41–47, 1988.
67. Lochner TC, Bigley R, Iglewski BH: Defective triggering of polymorphonuclear leukocyte oxidative metabolism by *L. pneumophila* toxin. J Infect Dis 151:42–46, 1985.
68. Caparon M, Johnson W: Macrophage toxicity and complement sensitivity of virulent and avirulent strains of *Legionella pneumophila.* Rev Infect Dis 10:S377–S384, 1988.
69. Conlan JW, Williams A, Ashworth L: In vivo production of a tissue-destructive protease by *Legionella pneumophila* in the lungs of experimentally infected guinea pigs. J Gen Microbiol 134:143–149, 1988.
70. Horwitz MA: Toward an understanding of host and bacterial molecules mediating *L. pneumophila* pathogenesis. *In* Barbaree JM, Breiman RF, Dufour AP (eds): *Legionella*—Current Status and Emerging Perspectives. Washington, DC, American Society for Microbiology, 1993, pp 55–62.
71. Winn WC, Myerowitz RL: The pathology of the *Legionella* pneumonias. Hum Pathol 12:401–422, 1981.
72. Monforte R, Maro F, Estruch R, Campo E: Multiple organ involvement by *L. pneumophila* in a fatal case of Legionnaires' disease (Letter). J Infect Dis 159:809, 1989.
73. White H, Felton W, Sun CN: Extrapulmonary histopathologic manifestations of Legionnaires' disease. Arch Pathol Lab Med 104:287–289, 1980.
74. Fang GD, Fine M, Orloff J, et al: New and emerging etiologies for community-acquired pneumonia with implications for therapy. A prospective multicenter study of 359 cases. Medicine (Baltimore) 69:307–316, 1990.
75. Woodhead MA, Macfarlane JT: Legionnaires' disease: A review of 79 community acquired cases in Nottingham. Thorax 41:635–640, 1986.
76. Falco V, Fernandez de Sevilla T, Alegre J, et al: *L. pneumophila*—A cause of several community acquired pneumonias. Chest 100:1007–1011, 1991.
77. Tsai TF, Finn DR, Plikaytis B, et al: Clinical features of the epidemic in Philadelphia. Ann Intern Med 90:509–517, 1979.
78. Yu VL, Kroboth FJ, Shonnard J, et al: Legionnaires' disease. New clinical perspective from a prospective pneumonia study. Am J Med 73:357–361, 1982.
79. Hubbard RB, Mathur RM, MacFarlan JT: Severe community-acquired legionella pneumonia: Treatment, complications and outcome. Q J Med 86:327–332, 1993.
80. Kociuba KR, Buist M, Munro R, et al: Legionnaires' disease outbreak in south western Sydney, 1992: Clinical aspects. Med J Aust 160:274–277, 1992.
81. Posner MR, Caudill A, Brass R, Ellis E: Legionnaires' disease associated with rhabdomyolysis and myoglobinuria. Arch Intern Med 140:848–850, 1980.
82. Fenves AZ: Legionnaires' disease associated with acute renal failure. A report of two cases and review of the literature. Clin Nephrol 23:96–100, 1985.
83. Johnson JD, Raff M, VanArsdall J: Neurologic manifestations of Legionnaires' disease. Medicine (Baltimore) 63:303–310, 1984.
84. Westblom T, Hamory BH: Acute pancreatitis caused by *Legionella pneumophila.* South Med J 81:1200–1201, 1988.
85. Lowry PW, Tompkins LS: Nosocomial legionellosis: A review of pulmonary and extrapulmonary syndromes. Am J Infect Control 21:21–27, 1993.
86. Fuller J, Levinson MD, Kline JR, Copeland J: Legionnaires' disease after heart transplantation. Ann Thorac Surg 39:308–311, 1985.
87. Moore EH, Webb WR, Gamsu G, Golden JA: Legionnaires' disease in the renal transplant patient: Clinical presentation and radiographic progression. Radiology 153:583–593, 1984.
88. Woodhead MA, Macfarlane JT: Comparative clinical and laboratory features of legionella with pneumococcal and mycoplasma pneumonias. Br J Dis Chest 81:133–139, 1987.
89. Woodhead MA, Macfarlane JT, McCracken JS, et al: Prospective study of the aetiology and outcome of pneumonia in the community. Lancet 1:671–674, 1987.
90. Muder RR, Yu VL, Parry M: Radiology of *Legionella* pneumonia. Semin Respir Infect 2:242–254, 1987.
91. Macfarlane JT, Miller AC, Roderick Smith WH: Comparative radiographic features of community acquired Legionnaires' disease, pneumococcal pneumonia, mycoplasma pneumonia, and psittacosis. Thorax 39:28–33, 1984.
92. Fairbank JT, Mamourian AC, Dietrich PA, Girod JC: The chest radiograph in Legionnaires' disease. Further observations. Radiology 147:33–34, 1983.
93. Bornstein N, Mercatello A, Marmet D, et al: Pleural infection caused by *Legionella anisa.* J Clin Microbiol 27:2100–2101, 1989.
94. Fang GD, Yu VL, Vickers RM: Disease due to Legionellaceae (other than *Legionella pneumophila*). Historical, microbiological, clinical and epidemiological review. Medicine (Baltimore) 68:116–139, 1989.
95. Benson RF, Thacker WL, Fang FC, et al: *Legionella sainthelensi* serogroup 2 isolated from patients with pneumonia. Res Microbiol 141:453–463, 1990.

96. Thacker WL, Dyke JW, Benson RF, et al: *Legionella lansingensis* sp. nov. isolated from a patient with pneumonia and underlying chronic lymphocytic leukemia. J Clin Microbiol 30:2398–2401, 1992.
97. Muder RR, Yu VL, Vickers R, et al: Simultaneous infection with *Legionella pneumophila* and Pittsburgh pneumonia agent—Clinical features and epidemiological implications. Am J Med 74:609–614, 1983.
98. Tompkins LS, Trout N, Wood ST, et al: Molecular epidemiology of *Legionella* species by restriction endonuclease and alloenzyme analysis. J Clin Microbiol 25:1875–1880, 1987.
99. Glick TH, Gregg MB, Berman B, et al: Pontiac fever. An epidemic of unknown etiology in a health department. I. Clinical and epidemiologic aspects. Am J Epidemiol 107:149–160, 1978.
100. Zuravleff JJ, Yu VL, Shonnard J, et al: Diagnosis of Legionnaires' disease: An update of laboratory methods with new emphasis on isolation by culture. JAMA 250:1981–1985, 1983.
101. Vickers RM, Stout JE, Yu VL, Rihs JD: Culture methodology for the isolation of *Legionella pneumophila* and other Legionellaceae from clinical and environmental specimens. Semin Respir Infect 2:274–279, 1987.
102. Bopp CA, Sumner JW, Morris GK, Wells JG: Isolation of *Legionella* spp from environmental water samples by low pH treatment and use of a selective medium. J Clin Microbiol 13:714–719, 1981.
103. Rihs JD, Yu VL, Zuravleff JJ, et al: Isolation of *Legionella pneumophila* from blood using the BACTEC: A prospective study yielding positive results. J Clin Microbiol 22:422–442, 1985.
104. Matsiota-Bernard P, Pitsouni E, Legakis N, Nauciel C: Evaluation of commercial amplification kit for detection of *Legionella pneumophila* in clinical samples. J Clin Microbiol 32:1503–1505, 1994.
105. Kohler RB, Winn WC Jr, Wheat LJ: Onset and duration of urinary antigen excretion in Legionnaires' disease. J Clin Microbiol 20:605–607, 1984.
106. Vickers RM, Yee YC, Rihs JD, et al: Prospective assessment of sensitivity, quantitation, and timing of urinary antigen, serology, and direct fluorescent antibody for diagnosis of Legionnaires' disease (Abstr C-17). *In* Program and Abstracts of the 94th Annual Meeting. Washington, DC, American Society for Microbiology, 1994.
107. Wilkinson H, Cruce D, Brome C: Validation of *Legionella pneumophila* indirect immunofluorescence assay with epidemic sera. J Clin Microbiol 13:139–146, 1981.
108. Swanson DJ, Sung RJ, Fine MJ, et al: Erythromycin ototoxicity. Prospective assessment with serum concentrations and audiograms in a study of patients with pneumonia. Am J Med 92:61–68, 1992.
109. Fitzgeorge RB, Featherstone ASR, Baskerville A: Efficacy of azithromycin in the treatment of guinea pigs infected with *Legionella pneumophila* by aerosol. J Antimicrob Chemother 25:101–108, 1990.
110. Edelstein PH, Edelstein MAC: In vitro activity of azithromycin against clinical isolates of *Legionella* species. Antimicrob Agents Chemother 35:180–181, 1991.
111. Kuzman I, Soldo I, Schonwald S, Culig J: Azithromycin and Legionnaires' disease. Scand J Infect Dis 27:503–505, 1995.
112. Sazito A, Koga H, Shigeno H, et al: The antimicrobial activity of ciprofloxacin against *Legionella* species and the treatment of experimental *Legionella* pneumonia in guinea pigs. J Antimicrob Chemother 18:251–260, 1986.
113. Saito A, Sawatari K, Fukuda Y, et al: Susceptibility of *Legionella pneumophila* to ofloxacillin in vitro and in experimental *Legionella* pneumonia in guinea pigs. Antimicrob Agents Chemother 28:15–20, 1985.
114. Unertl KE, Lenhart FL, Forst H, et al: Brief report. Ciprofloxacin in the treatment of legionellosis in critically ill patients including those cases unresponsive to erythromycin. Am J Med 87(Suppl 5A):128S–131S, 1989.
115. Hooper T, Gould F, Swinburn CR, et al: Ciprofloxacin. A preferred treatment for *Legionella* infection in patients receiving cyclosporin. J Antimicrob Chemother 6:952–953, 1988.
116. Miller AC: Erythromycin in Legionnaires' disease: A reappraisal. J Antimicrob Chemother 7:217–222, 1981.
117. Rudin JE, Evans TL, Wing EJ: Failure of erythromycin in treatment of *Legionella micdadei* pneumonia. Am J Med 76:318–320, 1984.
118. Farrell ID, Baher J, Chiodini PL, Hutchinson JGP: The activity of imipenem on *Legionella pneumophila,* with a note on the treatment of two cases. J Antimicrob Chemother 16:61–65, 1985.
119. Goetz A, Yu VL: Screening for nosocomial legionellosis by culture of the water supply and targeting of high-risk patients for specialized laboratory testing. Am J Infect Control 19:63–66, 1991.
120. Muraca P, Yu VL, Goetz A: Disinfection of water distribution systems for *Legionella:* A review of application procedures and methodologies. Infect Control Hosp Epidemiol 11:79–88, 1990.
121. Grosserode M, Helms C, Pfaller M, et al: Continuous hyperchlorination for control of nosocomial Legionnaires' disease: A ten year follow-up of efficacy, environmental effects, and cost. *In* Barbaree JM, Breiman RF, Dufour AP (eds): *Legionella*—Current Status and Emerging Perspectives. Washington, DC, American Society for Microbiology, 1993, pp 226–229.
122. Liu Z, Stout JE, Tedesco L, et al: Controlled evaluation of copper-silver ionization in eradicating *Legionella pneumophila* from a hospital water distribution system. J Infect Dis 169:919–922, 1994.
123. Farr BM, Bratz J, Tartaglino J, et al: Evaluation of ultraviolet light for disinfection of hospital works contaminated with *Legionella.* Lancet 2:669–672, 1988.
124. Blander SJ, Horwitz MA: Major cytoplasmic membrane protein of *L. pneumophila,* a genus common antigen and member of hsp 60 family of heat shock proteins, induces protective immunity in a guinea pig model of Legionnaires' disease. J Clin Invest 91:717–723, 1993.
125. White RJ, Blainey AD, Harrison KJ, Clarke SKR: Causes of pneumonia presenting to a district general hospital. Thorax 36:566–570, 1981.
126. Macfarlane JT, Finch RG, Ward MD, Macrae AD: Hospital study of adult community-acquired pneumonia. Lancet 2:255–258, 1982.
127. Klimek JJ, Ajemian E, Fonteccio S: Community-acquired bacterial pneumonia requiring admission to hospital. Am J Infect Control 11:79–82, 1983.
128. Marrie TJ, Grayston JT, Wang S, et al: Pneumonia associated with TWAR strain of chlamydia. Ann Intern Med 106:507–511, 1987.
129. Aubertin J, Dabis F, Fleurette J, et al: Prevalence of legionellosis among adults: A study of community-acquired pneumonia in France. Infection 15:328–331, 1987.
130. Research Committee of the British Thoracic Society and the Public Health Laboratory Service. Community-acquired pneumonia in adults in British hospitals in 1982–1983. Q J Med 62:195–220, 1987.
131. Holmberg H: Aetiology of community-acquired pneumonia in hospital patients. Scand J Infect Dis 19:491–501, 1987.
132. Fris-Moller A, Rechnitzer C, Blak F, et al: Prevalence of Legionnaires' disease in pneumonia patients admitted to a Danish department of infectious diseases. Scand J Infect Dis 18:321–328, 1986.
133. Levy M, Dromer F, Brion N, et al: Community-acquired pneumonia—Importance of initial noninvasive bacteriologic and radiographic investigation. Chest 92:43–48, 1988.
134. Maayan S, Morali G, Engelhard D, et al: Legionellosis at Hadassah University Hospital. A 1-year survey. Isr J Med Sci 27:145–149, 1991.
135. Lim R, Shaw DR, Stanley DP, et al: A prospective hospital study of the aetiology of community-acquired pneumonia. Med J Aust 151:87–91, 1989.

62

Chlamydia Pneumonia

Margaret R. Hammerschlag

The genus *Chlamydia* is a group of obligate intracellular parasites that have a unique developmental cycle with morphologically distinct infectious and reproductive forms. All members of the genus have a gram-negative envelope without peptidoglycan, share a genus-specific lipopolysaccharide (LPS) antigen, and use host adenosine triphosphate for the synthesis of chlamydial protein. The genus now contains four species, *Chlamydia trachomatis, Chlamydia pneumoniae* (TWAR strains), *Chlamydia psittaci*, and *Chlamydia pecorum*. The last was speciated from *C. psittaci* and infects cattle and sheep; human infection has not been reported so far.[1] The first three species are capable of causing pneumonia in humans; the routes of transmission, susceptible populations, and clinical presentations differ (Table 62–1). The microbiology of the genus is described in detail in Chapter 232.

Respiratory Infection Caused by *Chlamydia pneumoniae*

The first isolates of *C. pneumoniae* were serendipitously obtained during trachoma studies in the 1960s.[2] TW-183 was isolated from the eye of a child with suspected trachoma in Taiwan, and IOL-207 was isolated from the eye of another child with trachoma in Tehran. Subsequently, serologic studies of an outbreak of mild pneumonia among schoolchildren in rural Finland in the late 1970s suggested that an organism related to TW-183 was the cause.[3] After the recovery of a similar isolate from the respiratory tract of a college student with pneumonia in Seattle, Grayston and colleagues[4] applied the designation TWAR after their first two isolates, TW-183 and AR-39. On the basis of inclusion morphology and staining characteristics in cell culture, TWAR was initially considered a *C. psittaci* strain. Subsequent analyses, however, have demonstrated that this organism is distinct from both *C. psittaci* and *C. trachomatis*.[5] Only one serotype has been identified so far. Initial ultrastructural studies demonstrated that the elementary bodies of *C. pneumoniae* had a pear-shaped appearance caused by a loose periplasmic membrane, whereas the elementary bodies of *C. trachomatis* and *C. psittaci* are round.[6] However, ultrastructural studies of IOL-207 and other strains of *C. pneumoniae* isolated in Japan and Finland revealed round elementary bodies similar in appearance to those of the other two chlamydial species.[7, 8] Restriction endonuclease pattern analysis and nucleic acid hybridization studies suggest a high degree of genetic relatedness (greater than 95%) among the *C. pneumoniae* isolates examined so far.[8, 9]

Epidemiology

C. pneumoniae appears to be a primary human pathogen, and attempts to identify zoonotic reservoirs have been unsuccessful. The mode of transmission remains uncertain but probably occurs through infected respiratory secretions. Acquisition of infection by droplet aerosol was described during a laboratory accident.[10] *C. pneumoniae* can remain viable on Formica countertops for 30 hours and can survive small-particle aerosolization.[11, 12] Spread within families and enclosed populations such as military recruits has been described.[13, 14] Several serologic surveys have documented rising chlamydial antibody prevalence rates beginning in school-age children and reaching 30% to 45% by adolescence.[2] Seroprevalence of antibody, as determined by the microimmunofluorescence (MIF) method, can exceed 80% in some adult populations.[15, 16]

The proportion of community-acquired pneumonias associated with *C. pneumoniae* infection has ranged from 6% to 19%, varying with geographic location, the age group examined, and the methods used to determine infection (i.e., serologic or culture).[2, 17–21] Infection in children younger than 5 years has been rare in Seattle and Scandinavia,[2] whereas in a study of Filipino children younger than 5 years presenting with lower respiratory tract infection, nearly 10% had either acute or chronic antibody to *C. pneumoniae*.[18] In contrast, in a study from Brooklyn, the proportion of lower respiratory tract infections associated with *C. pneumoniae*, as determined by culture, increased from 9% in children younger than 5 years to 19% in the 5- to 16-year-old age category.[20]

In a multicenter antibiotic treatment study, cultures for *C. pneumoniae* were obtained from children 3 through 12 years of age with community-acquired pneumonia.[21] Forty-two (16%) of the 260 children enrolled were culture-positive. The prevalence of *C. pneumoniae* infection in children 3 through 6 years of age and those 6 through 12 years of age was similar. Seven children were coinfected with *C. pneumoniae* and *Mycoplasma pneumoniae*. The only child in the study who had a positive blood culture for *Streptococcus pneumoniae* was also culture-positive for *C. pneumoniae*. Chirgwin and coworkers[20] also reported several coinfections with *C. pneumoniae, S. pneumoniae*, and *Haemophilus influenzae* type b. In these cases, *C. pneumoniae* may not be the primary cause of the pneumonia but might disrupt the normal clearance mechanisms and enable other pathogens to invade. *C. pneumoniae* has been found to inhibit ciliary motion of bronchial epithelial cells.[22] Use of corticosteroids appears to cause protracted infection.[23, 24]

Approximately 50% of the children reported by Chirgwin

TABLE 62–1 ■ Epidemiologic and Clinical Characteristics of Respiratory Disease Caused by *Chlamydia*

FEATURE	*C. PNEUMONIAE*	*C. TRACHOMATIS*	*C. PSITTACI*
Natural host	Humans	Humans	Birds, mammals
Population	All ages	Infants, immunocompromised adults	Veterinarians, bird fanciers, poultry workers
Mode of transmission	Person to person: by aerosol droplets	Vertical: mother to infant	Bird to person: by aerosolized fecal material
Major respiratory diseases	Pneumonia, bronchitis, reactive airway disease	Pneumonia	Pneumonia

and colleagues and the pneumonia treatment study did not have or failed to develop any detectable antibody by MIF.[20, 21] This would suggest that serosurveys of pediatric populations may actually underestimate the prevalence of infection in young children.

In studies to date, acute infection with *C. pneumoniae* does not appear to vary by season. There are reports of cycles in Seattle and Scandinavia lasting several years during which the incidence of new infection with *C. pneumoniae* waxes and wanes. In contrast, the infection appears to be endemic in Brooklyn, which may be a function of the greater population density.

Prolonged culture positivity after acute infection, lasting several weeks to more than a year, has been described.[23] Asymptomatic respiratory infection may occur in 2% to 5% of adults and children.[15, 24] It is not known what role asymptomatic carriage plays in the epidemiology of *C. pneumoniae*.

Pathogenesis

The pathogenic mechanisms of *C. pneumoniae* infection in humans are largely unknown. Experimental infection has been produced in nonhuman primates and mice.[25–27] The infection in monkeys is largely asymptomatic, and the animals may shed the organism from the respiratory tract for 12 months or longer.[25] The infection in mice is also largely asymptomatic. The lung disorder is characterized by patchy interstitial pneumonitis with predominantly polymorphonuclear leukocyte infiltration in the early stage and mononuclear cell infiltration in the later stage of infection.[26, 27] *C. pneumoniae* can be isolated from the lungs for several weeks after inoculation as well as from other organs including the spleen. Administration of corticosteroids results in reactivation of lung infection in mice after apparent resolution.[28]

In vitro studies have demonstrated that elementary bodies of *C. pneumoniae* have a direct ciliastatic effect on human bronchial epithelium.[22]

Clinical Presentation

The spectrum of disease associated with *C. pneumoniae* is expanding. Most infections are probably mild or asymptomatic. Initial reports emphasized mild atypical pneumonia clinically resembling that associated with *M. pneumoniae*.[2] In several subsequent studies, however, pneumonia associated with *C. pneumoniae* has been clinically indistinguishable from other pneumonias.[17, 21] Coinfection with other pathogens, especially *M. pneumoniae*, can be frequent. Twenty percent of the children in the multicenter pediatric pneumonia study with positive *C. pneumoniae* cultures were coinfected with *M. pneumoniae*; they could not be distinguished from those who were infected with either organism alone.[21]

C. pneumoniae has been associated with severe illness and even death, although the role of preexisting chronic conditions as contributing factors in many of these patients is difficult to assess. In some cases, however, *C. pneumoniae* clearly appears to be implicated as a serious pathogen even in the absence of underlying disease. *C. pneumoniae* was isolated from the respiratory tract and the pleural fluid of a previously healthy adolescent boy with severe pneumonia complicated by respiratory failure and pleural effusions.[29]

The role of host factors remains to be determined. Although *C. pneumoniae* has been detected in bronchoalveolar lavage fluid from 10% of a group of patients with acquired immunodeficiency syndrome and pneumonia, its clinical role in these patients is uncertain because most were coinfected with other well-recognized pathogens such as *Pneumocystis carinii* and *Mycobacterium tuberculosis*.[30] Gaydos and colleagues[31] identified *C. pneumoniae* infection by polymerase chain reaction (PCR) in 11% of a group of immunocompromised adults with human immunodeficiency virus infection, malignant neoplasms, and other immune disorders including systemic lupus erythematosus, sarcoidosis, and common variable immunodeficiency. *C. pneumoniae* appeared to be responsible for 6 of 31 (19%) episodes of acute chest syndrome in children with sickle cell disease.[32] *C. pneumoniae* infection in these patients appeared to be associated with more severe hypoxia than was infection with *M. pneumoniae*.

C. pneumoniae may also act as an inflammatory trigger for asthma. There are several reports of patients with culture-documented *C. pneumoniae* infection who developed significant bronchospasm.[23] One patient was diagnosed as having asthmatic bronchitis and was receiving systemic and topical steroids. She did not improve until her chlamydial infection was treated. Hahn and colleagues[33] reported an association between serologic evidence of acute *C. pneumoniae* infection and wheezing in adults seen for lower respiratory tract illness. However, they were able to isolate the organism from only 1 of 365 patients. As part of a preliminary study in children, *C. pneumoniae* was isolated from 13 of 118 (11%) children 5 to 15 years of age who were initially evaluated for either new or acute exacerbations of asthma.[24] Treatment of the infection appeared to result in both clinical improvement and improvement in pulmonary function test scores. Only five of the children with confirmed infection had detectable immunoglobulin (Ig) G antibody to *C. pneumoniae*. One child who was noncompliant with his antibiotic therapy was culture-positive on five occasions in a 3-month period. In addition, no anti–*C. pneumoniae* antibody was ever able to be detected. However, specific anti–*C. pneumoniae* IgE was detected in 85.7% of the culture-positive asthmatic children compared with 9% of children with *C. pneumoniae* pneumonia who were not wheezing.[34] This suggests that bronchial reactivity seen with *C. pneumoniae* infection may be IgE mediated. The potential of *C. pneumoniae* to cause prolonged, persistent infection may produce chronic inflammation and trigger bronchospasm in susceptible individuals. Immune-mediated phenomena, including erythema nodosum and iritis, have also been described complicating *C. pneumoniae* infection.[35, 36]

Diagnosis

A specific laboratory diagnosis of *C. pneumoniae* infection can be made by isolation of the organism from nasopharyngeal swabs and pleural fluid. The nasopharynx appears to be the optimal site for isolation of the organism.[21] The organism can also be isolated from throat swabs and sputum, but the relative yield from these sites is not known. Most investigators to date have relied on serologic diagnosis using the MIF test and the complement fixation (CF) test. The CF test is genus specific and has mainly been used for the diagnosis of lymphogranuloma venereum and psittacosis.

The isolation of *C. pneumoniae* requires culture in tissue; the organism cannot be propagated in cell-free media. Initial studies suggested that *C. pneumoniae* was difficult to isolate in tissue culture compared with *C. trachomatis*. The same methods were originally used, HeLa or McCoy cells pretreated with diethylaminoethyl-dextran. Multiple passages were needed, the inclusions were small and difficult to see, and the yield in general was poor. *C. pneumoniae* grows more readily in other cell lines derived from respiratory tissue, specifically HEp-2 and HL cells.[37] Omission of pretreatment with diethylaminoethyl-dextran results in much larger inclusions, and specimens need be passed only once. Culture with an initial inoculation and one passage should take 4 to 7 days.

Nasopharyngeal cultures can be obtained with Dacron-tipped wire-shafted swabs. Specimens for culture should be placed in appropriate transport media, usually a sucrose-phosphate buffer with antibiotics and fetal calf serum, and stored immediately at 4°C for no longer than 24 hours. Viability decreases if specimens are held at room temperature. If the specimen cannot be processed within 24 hours, it should be frozen at −70°C until culture can be performed. After 72 hours of incubation, culture confirmation can be performed by staining with either a *C. pneumoniae* species-specific or a *Chlamydia* genus-specific (anti-LPS) fluorescein-conjugated monoclonal antibody.[38] Inclusions of *C. pneumoniae* do not contain glycogen; thus, they will not stain with iodine. Unfortunately, there is limited availability of commercially produced *C. pneumoniae*–specific reagents. If a genus-specific antibody is used, *C. pneumoniae* should be confirmed by differential staining with a specific *C. trachomatis* antibody; if this is negative, then the isolate is either *C. pneumoniae* or *C. psittaci*. If there was no avian exposure, psittacosis would be highly unlikely.

Because isolation of *C. pneumoniae* was difficult and initially limited, more emphasis was placed on serologic diagnosis. However, performance of the MIF test is also limited to a small number of research laboratories. The MIF was modified from the test for *C. trachomatis* by use of elementary bodies from TW-183 or other *C. pneumoniae* strains as the antigen. With the MIF test, one can detect IgG, IgM, and IgA antibodies. Grayston and colleagues[2] have proposed a set of criteria for serologic diagnosis of *C. pneumoniae* infection with the MIF test that is used by many laboratories and clinicians. For acute infection, the patient should have a fourfold rise in IgG titer, a single IgM titer of 1:16 or greater, or a single IgG titer of 1:512 or higher. Past or preexisting infection is defined as an IgG titer of 1:16 or higher but less than 1:512. It was further proposed that the pattern of antibody response in primary infection differed from that seen in reinfection. In initial infection, the IgM response appears about 3 weeks after the onset of illness, and the IgG response appears at 6 to 8 weeks. In reinfection, the IgM response may be absent and the IgG occurs earlier, within 1 to 2 weeks.[2] A fourfold titer rise or a titer of 1:64 or higher with the CF test is also thought to be diagnostic. Initially, Grayston and colleagues[4] found that less than one third of hospitalized patients with suspected *C. pneumoniae* infection had detectable CF antibody. However, in a report of a small outbreak of *C. pneumoniae* infections among University of Washington students, all seven patients with pneumonia had CF titers of 1:64 or greater.[39]

Because of the relatively long period until the development of a serologic response in primary infection, the antibody response may be missed if convalescent serum samples are obtained too soon, that is, earlier than 3 weeks after the onset of illness. Use of paired serum samples also affords only a retrospective diagnosis, which is of little help in terms of deciding how to treat the patient. The criteria for use of a single serum sample have not been correlated with the results of culture and are based mainly on data from adults. The antibody response in acute infection may take longer than 3 months to develop. Acute, culture-documented infection can also occur without seroconversion, especially in children.[19, 21, 24] Only 28% of the culture-positive children enrolled in the multicenter pneumonia treatment study had met the serologic criteria for acute infection; most had no detectable antibody by the MIF test even after 3 months of follow-up.[21] However, the results of immunoblotting revealed that these children do have antibody to a number of *C. pneumoniae* proteins but that less than 30% react with the major outer membrane protein, which is the antigen presented in the MIF test.[21] Although the major outer membrane protein has been demonstrated to be immunodominant in *C. trachomatis* infection, it does not appear to be so for *C. pneumoniae*.[40, 41]

Background rates of seropositivity can also be high in some populations. Hyman and coworkers,[15] as part of a study of asymptomatic *C. pneumoniae* infection among subjectively healthy adults in Brooklyn, New York, found 81% to have IgG or IgM titers of 1:16 or greater. Seventeen percent had evidence of "acute infection," IgG titer equal to or greater than 1:512, or IgM titer equal to or greater than 1:16. However, none of these individuals was culture- or PCR-positive. Similar results were reported by Kern and associates[16] among healthy firefighters and police officers in Rhode Island. The specificity of the MIF IgM assay can be affected by the presence of rheumatoid factor in the study. A study from the Netherlands found that an increased probability of false-positive results was due to rheumatoid factor with increasing age.[42] Sera should be routinely absorbed before MIF IgM testing. Hyman and colleagues absorbed all the IgM-positive sera; the titers did not change. Some IgG antibody may result from a heterotypic response to other chlamydial species because there are cross-reactions with the major outer membrane protein between the three species as well as cross-reactions due to the genus LPS antigen. Moss and colleagues[43] reported that antibodies to *C. pneumoniae* and *C. psittaci* accounted for up to half of all chlamydial IgG-positive persons attending a sexually transmitted disease clinic. This point is reinforced by the observation that studies from the early 1980s suggesting that *C. trachomatis* was a cause of community-acquired pneumonia and pharyngitis in adults were probably detecting antibody to *C. pneumoniae* rather than *C. trachomatis*.[44, 45]

Direct detection of *C. pneumoniae* elementary bodies in clinical specimens by fluorescent antibody stains is sometimes possible but is insensitive and frequently nonspecific.[2] There are also no commercially available reagents that have been evaluated or approved for this purpose. All the currently available chlamydial enzyme immunoassays (EIAs) will detect *C. pneumoniae* as well as *C. trachomatis* because they use polyclonal or genus-specific monoclonal antibodies. However, there are few data on the use of these assays in this setting, and data that are available also suggest that EIAs are insensitive for detection of *C. pneumoniae* in respiratory specimens. Chirgwin and coworkers[20] obtained nasopharyngeal specimens from 91 patients with pneumonia for testing with Chlamydiazyme (Abbott Diagnostics, North Chicago). Although there were no false-positive responses, the EIA detected only 2 of 15 (15%) patients who were culture-positive for *C. pneumoniae*.

It appears that the number of *C. pneumoniae* organisms present in the respiratory tract of individuals with pneumonia or other respiratory disease is less than the number found in genital *C. trachomatis* infection. DNA amplification methods (e.g., PCR) appear to be the most promising technology in the development of a rapid, nonculture means of detection of *C. pneumoniae*. Although there are no commercially available kits, several investigators have evaluated in-house PCRs. In general, PCR appears to be at least as sensitive as culture for detecting *C. pneumoniae* in throat and nasopharyngeal specimens.[46, 47]

Treatment

Chlamydia species are susceptible to tetracyclines, macrolides, and quinolones. *C. pneumoniae* and *C. psittaci* are resistant to sulfonamides.[48] To date, there have also been few published data describing the response of *C. pneumoniae* to antimicrobial therapy.[48] Most of the treatment studies of pneumonia caused by *C. pneumoniae* published so far have relied entirely on diagnosis by serology; thus, microbiologic efficacy could not be assessed. Anecdotal reports have suggested that prolonged courses (up to 3 weeks) of either tetracyclines or erythromycin may be needed to eradicate *C. pneumoniae* from the nasopharynx of adults with influenza-like illness and pharyngitis.[23] Results of a multicenter study comparing erythromycin suspension with clarithromycin suspension for 10 days in children 3 through 12 years of age with radiographically proven pneumonia found both drugs to be equally efficacious, eradicating the organism in 86% and 79% of the children, respectively.[21] Preliminary data examining azithromycin in adults with pneumonia and bronchitis found an eradication rate of 75%.[48]

On the basis of these few data, I can suggest the following regimens for respiratory infection due to *C. pneumoniae*: in adults, doxycycline at 100 mg twice daily for 14 to 21 days, tetracycline at 250 mg four times daily for 14 to 21 days, or azithromycin at 1.5 g in 5 days (some patients may need to be re-treated); for children, erythromycin suspension at 50 mg/kg per day for 10 to 14 days, or clarithromycin suspension at 15 mg/kg per day for 10 days.

Respiratory Infection Caused by *Chlamydia trachomatis*

Although *C. trachomatis* is primarily a sexually transmitted pathogen, it can cause respiratory tract infection, including pneumonia in specific circumstances. Pregnant women who have cervical infection with *C. trachomatis* can transmit the infection to their infants, who may subsequently develop neonatal conjunctivitis and pneumonia. Epidemiologic evidence strongly suggests that the infant acquires chlamydial infection from the mother during vaginal delivery.[49] Infection after caesarean section is rare and usually occurs after early rupture of the amniotic membrane. There is no evidence supporting postnatal acquisition from the mother or other family members. Approximately 50% to 75% of infants born to infected women become infected at one or more anatomic sites, including the conjunctiva, rectum, and vagina. The nasopharynx is by far the most frequent site of infection. Approximately 70% of infected infants have positive cultures from that site. Most of these nasopharyngeal infections are asymptomatic and may persist for 3 years or more.[50]

Pneumonia develops in only about 30% of infants with nasopharyngeal infection; the reasons are unknown. In those who develop pneumonia, the presentation and clinical findings are characteristic. The children are usually seen between 4 and 12 weeks of age; a few cases have been reported as early as 2 weeks of age, but no cases have been seen beyond 4 months. The infants frequently have a history of cough and congestion with an absence of fever. On physical examination, the infant is tachypneic, and rales are heard on auscultation of the chest; wheezing is distinctly uncommon. There are no specific radiographic findings except hyperinflation.[51, 52] Significant laboratory findings include peripheral eosinophilia (greater than 300 cells per mm^3) and elevated serum immunoglobulin levels.[51, 52]

Although asymptomatic perinatally acquired nasopharyngeal infection with *C. trachomatis* may persist for at least 2 years, respiratory tract infection in older children and adults appears to be distinctly uncommon. The reasons for this are not clear. Studies of the interaction of *C. trachomatis* and alveolar macrophages from normal healthy adults have demonstrated that these cells kill both biotypes of *C. trachomatis* efficiently.[53] *C. trachomatis* has been isolated from the pharynx of some adults, apparently related to certain sexual practices. These infections have been asymptomatic. Two earlier studies, based entirely on serology, suggested that *C. trachomatis* might be a cause of pharyngitis and community-acquired pneumonia in adults.[43, 44] Subsequent studies using cultural methods did not confirm this.[54, 55] It appears that the original studies may actually have detected cross-reacting antibody to *C. pneumoniae*.

There are two specific situations in which *C. trachomatis* can cause pneumonia in older children or adults. One is in immunosuppressed individuals. There have been several well-documented cases of pneumonia due to *C. trachomatis* in individuals with leukemia, bone marrow transplant recipients, and those with acquired immunodeficiency syndrome.[56–58] In all of these cases, *C. trachomatis* was isolated from biopsy specimens of lung tissue or bronchoalveolar lavage fluid. Several patients also had a serologic response that was diagnostic of acute *C. trachomatis* infection. Unfortunately, there was no characteristic clinical presentation. These adults had none of the findings that are characteristic of infantile chlamydial pneumonia.

There have also been several reports of pulmonary infection after exposure to *C. trachomatis* serotypes L_1 and L_2 in the laboratory.[59] The infections were probably acquired by inhalation of aerosolized organisms. These patients presented clinically with high fever, night sweats, and cough and were found to have mediastinal lymphadenopathy or pneumonitis and splenomegaly. In two cases, the diagnosis of lymphoma was considered seriously. These findings are not unexpected given the severity of lymphogranuloma venereum genital infection. Accidental exposure to aerosolized *C. trachomatis* trachoma biotype has not been associated with significant illness.

Diagnosis

The definitive diagnosis of *C. trachomatis* pneumonia in infants is made by isolation of the organism from nasopharyngeal wash or swab specimens. *C. trachomatis* culture is usually performed in cycloheximide-treated McCoy cells with culture confirmation by staining with a specific fluorescein-conjugated monoclonal antibody.[60] Some laboratories still use iodine staining, which is species specific but less sensitive than fluorescent antibody staining. *C. trachomatis* can also be identified in nasopharyngeal specimens by nonculture antigen detection methods. The two major types of test available are the direct fluorescent antibody and EIA. Both types of test appear to be good for the detection of *C. trachomatis* in nasopharyngeal specimens from infants with suspected *C. trachomatis* pneumonia, with sensitivities of 93% to 100% in comparison with culture.[61–63] Preliminary data with use of a commercially available PCR (Amplicor, Roche Molecular Diagnostics, New Jersey) suggest that this test may be more sensitive than culture in respiratory specimens from infants with *C. trachomatis* pneumonia and conjunctivitis.

Infants with pneumonia should have IgM titers of specific anti–*C. trachomatis* antibody equal to or greater than 1:32 as determined by the MIF method. The CF test is a genus-specific test and is not sensitive enough to detect antibody in infants with *C. trachomatis* pneumonia.

Treatment

The treatment of choice for *C. trachomatis* pneumonia in infants is oral erythromycin ethylsuccinate suspension, 50 mg/kg per day in three or four divided doses, for 10 to 14 days. There are no data on the treatment of *C. trachomatis* respiratory infections in adults, but one can extrapolate and assume that erythromycin, tetracycline, doxycycline, and ofloxacin in the dosage regimens recommended for genital infection may be effective. Azithromycin and clarithromycin may also be useful, but with use of dosage regimens suggested for *C. pneumoniae* infection.

Respiratory Infection Caused by *Chlamydia psittaci*

Human infection with *C. psittaci* was probably first described by Juergensen in 1874 or Ritter in 1876. Ritter described seven cases of an unusual pneumonia that appeared to be caused by parrots and finches that were caged in the study of his brother's home in Switzerland. After these reports, there were several outbreaks of a similar disease in Europe that established the association with an exposure to birds.[64] The term psittacosis was coined by Morange in 1892 from the Greek word for parrots, *psittakos*.[64]

Organism

C. psittaci is a diverse species that affects nonpsittacine birds and many mammalian species as well. The known host range includes 15 mammalian species and 130 avian species, representing 10 orders.[65] There is only 5% to 10% DNA homology between *C. psittaci* and *C. trachomatis* and *C. pneumoniae*. *C. psittaci*, like *C. pneumoniae*, lacks glycogen in its inclusions and is resistant to sulfonamides.

Strains of *C. psittaci* have been analyzed by pathogenicity patterns, growth characteristics, inclusion morphology in cell culture, DNA restriction endonuclease analysis, monoclonal antibodies, and numerous serologic tests, which indicate that there are nine mammalian serotypes, seven avian serotypes, and two koala biotypes.[65] The mammalian strains differ greatly from avian strains in their antigenic characteristics. Two of the avian serotypes, psittacine and turkey, are of major importance in the avian population of the United States. Each is associated with important host preferences and disease characteristics.[66] Strains of the turkey serotype have all been associated with a serious disease in either birds or human beings, with major epizootics in turkeys often resulting in disease in humans. The psittacine serotype has also been associated with serious disease in humans; however, human involvement is usually limited to sporadic cases after exposure to pet birds or pigeons. The pathogenicity of each *C. psittaci* strain to humans is unclear.

Epidemiology

According to a report from the Centers for Disease Control and Prevention (CDC), 1136 cases of psittacosis were reported in the United States from 1975 to 1984; 85% were associated with contact with birds.[67] Seventy percent of the cases were the result of exposure to caged pet birds. Those at highest risk for acquiring psittacosis included bird owners or fanciers, pet shop employees, and pigeon fanciers. Since 1984, there have been several major outbreaks of psittacosis in the United States in turkey-processing plants; approximately 300 individuals contracted the infection.[68, 69] Workers exposed to turkey viscera were at the highest risk for infection.[69] In Australia, outbreaks of psittacosis have been associated with duck farming.[70] An outbreak in Philadelphia was associated with an aviary.[71]

Inhalation of infectious aerosols derived from feces, fecal dust, or secretions of *C. psittaci*–infected animals is believed to be the primary route of infection. The source birds can be infected asymptomatically or can show signs of infection, such as anorexia, ruffled feathers, depression, and watery green droppings. Psittacosis is frequently a systemic infection in birds. The turkey strains can induce severe pericarditis. The gastrointestinal tract is also infected frequently. The psittacine serotype appears to be much less virulent in both turkeys and pigeons than in psittacine birds.[65, 66]

Clinical Manifestations

Infection with *C. psittaci* in humans may range from clinically inapparent to severe systemic infection involving multiple organs as well as pneumonia. Overall mortality now is low compared with that in the past: 0.7% in the CDC series[67] and none in a series of 135 patients reported by Yung and Grayston[72] from Australia. The mean incubation period is 15 days after exposure, and the range is 5 to 21 days. The onset is usually abrupt, with complaints of fever, cough, and headache. The fever is high and frequently associated with rigors and sweats. The headache can be so severe that meningitis can be considered a possibility; 33% of the patients in the Australian series had lumbar punctures.[72] The cough is usually nonproductive. Rales may be heard on auscultation. Chest radiographs are usually abnormal, with variable infiltrates. Pleural effusions may also be present.

The white cell count is usually not elevated, but there may be a mild leukocytosis. Almost 50% of the patients in the Australian series had abnormal liver function tests, including elevated levels of aspartate aminotransferase, alkaline phosphatase, and bilirubin.[72]

Psittacosis can be fulminant and has been associated with acute renal failure and acute thrombocytopenic purpura.[73, 74] *C. psittaci* has also been implicated as a cause of endocarditis.[75, 76] Patients may also present with fever of unknown origin.

Initial infection does not appear to be followed by long-term immunity. Reinfection and clinical disease can develop within 2 months of treatment; there are two well-documented cases of reinfection. A pet shop employee had two episodes of psittacosis 11 months apart.[77] The second episodes tend to be severe.

Diagnosis

Because of the varying clinical presentation, the diagnosis of psittacosis can be difficult. History of exposure to birds is important. However, as many as 20% of patients with psittacosis may not have a history of contact with birds.[67, 72] In the Australian series, 85% of the patients had a history of recent bird contact; 71% of these described a strong history of bird contact.[72] Exposure to poultry was found in only five patients. Eighty-five percent of the patients in the CDC series had a history of contact with birds, predominantly pet birds.[67] Pneumonia due to *C. pneumoniae* can also have a similar clinical presentation. Data from Sweden, Denmark, and England have suggested that many cases of "psittacosis" with no history of bird exposure are probably due to *C. pneumoniae*.[78–80] Infection with *C. pneumoniae* is more likely if there has been evidence of person-to-person spread, which is extremely unusual with human psittacosis. Other infections that can produce the syndrome of pneumonia with high fever, unusually severe headache, and myalgia include *M. pneumoniae* infection, tularemia, tuberculosis, fungal infections, Legionnaires' disease, and various bacterial infections.

Diagnosis of psittacosis in the human population is primarily based on clinical presentation, epidemiology, and serology. Although many laboratories are able to isolate *C. psittaci*, it is not a service provided by most clinical microbiology laboratories on a routine basis. The most frequently used and widely available serologic method is the CF test. The CDC has three classes of cases of psittacosis based on laboratory findings or exposures[67]:

1. Confirmed: a clinical specimen yielding *C. psittaci* or compatible clinical illness and a fourfold rise in CF antibody titer
2. Presumptive: compatible clinical illness and a single

serum sample titer of 1:32 or greater or a stable antibody titer of 1:32 or greater in two samples

3. Suspect: a case that does not meet the criteria in 1 or 2 but is associated with another case of avian chlamydiosis

The CF test is genus specific; thus, infection due to *C. pneumoniae* can give titers of 1:32 or greater. Early treatment with tetracycline may also suppress the antibody response. The CDC reported using a modification of the MIF test for serodiagnosis of human psittacosis.[81] Eight strains of *C. psittaci* were used to have a wide host range, including two psittacine and one each of pigeon, turkey, calf, sheep, cat, and guinea pig. The sera were also tested against *C. pneumoniae* and *C. trachomatis*. The 78 patients examined were diagnosed as having psittacosis on the basis of compatible clinical symptoms after exposure to sick birds. The conventional CF test result was positive in 36 (46%) of the patients. The MIF test detected diagnostic antibody responses in all the CF-positive patients and another 12 patients whose serum samples were negative or anticomplementary in the CF test. Seven other patients were thought to have *C. pneumoniae* infection on the basis of their MIF antibody responses.

Several reports have also examined the use of nonculture methods, including direct fluorescent antibody staining, EIA, and PCR, for the direct identification of *C. psittaci* in clinical specimens. Oldach and coworkers[82] described two patients in whom a rapid diagnosis of psittacosis was made by direct fluorescent antibody staining of sputum specimens with *Chlamydia* genus-specific monoclonal antibody. Chlamydial LPS antigen was also detected with a commercially available EIA kit. In one case, the diagnosis was confirmed by isolation of *C. psittaci* from sputum and a pharyngeal swab. Both patients had strong histories of exposure to sick birds. MIF serology was also performed for both patients, and serologic cross-reactivity was observed for *C. psittaci, C. pneumoniae,* and *C. trachomatis* in the sera. *C. psittaci* can also be detected by two-step PCR, using primers directed against a portion of the major outer membrane protein gene specific for *C. psittaci* and *C. pneumoniae* followed by amplification with primers targeted specifically at *C. pneumoniae*.[83] Tong and Sillis[83] used this method to detect *C. psittaci* in sputum samples from four of eight patients with suspected psittacosis. Six of the sputum samples were also positive by *Chlamydia* genus EIA, and all were positive by direct fluorescent antibody staining with an anti-LPS monoclonal antibody; two were culture-positive.

Treatment

The recommended treatment for psittacosis in humans is 500 mg of tetracycline every 6 hours, orally, for 7 to 10 days. Erythromycin, 2 g/d for 7 to 10 days, can also be used. The experience in the Australian series[72] and anecdotal reports suggest that tetracycline may be more effective than erythromycin. Both patients described by Oldach and colleagues[82] did not improve when they were initially prescribed erythromycin; after doxycycline or tetracycline was added, both defervesced within 48 hours.

References

1. Fukushi H, Hirai K: Proposal of *Chlamydia pecorum* sp. nov. for *Chlamydia* strains derived from ruminants. Int J Syst Bacteriol 42:306–308, 1994.
2. Grayston JT, Campbell LA, Kuo C-C, et al: A new respiratory tract pathogen: *Chlamydia pneumoniae* strain TWAR. J Infect Dis 161:618–625, 1990.
3. Saikku P, Wang S-P, Kleemola M, et al: An epidemic of mild pneumonia due to an unusual strain of *Chlamydia psittaci*. J Infect Dis 151:832–839, 1985.
4. Grayston JT, Kuo C-C, Wang S-P, et al: A new *Chlamydia psittaci* strain, TWAR, isolated in acute respiratory tract infections. N Engl J Med 315:161–168, 1986.
5. Grayston JT, Kuo C-C, Campbell LA, et al: *Chlamydia pneumoniae* sp. nov. for *Chlamydia* sp. strain TWAR. Int J Syst Bacteriol 39:88–90, 1989.
6. Chi EY, Kuo C-C, Grayston JT: Unique ultrastructure in the elementary body of *Chlamydia* sp. strain TWAR. J Bacteriol 169:3757–3763, 1987.
7. Carter MW, Al-Mahdawi SAH, Treharne JD, et al: Nucleotide sequence and taxonomic value of the major outer membrane protein gene of *Chlamydia pneumoniae* IOL-207. J Gen Microbiol 137:465–475, 1991.
8. Myashita A, Kanamoto Y, Matsumoto A: The morphology of *Chlamydia pneumoniae*. J Med Microbiol 38:418–425, 1993.
9. Campbell LA, Kuo C-C, Grayston JT: Characterization of the new *Chlamydia* agent, TWAR, as a unique organism by restriction endonuclease analysis and DNA-DNA hybridization. J Clin Microbiol 25:1911–1916, 1987.
10. Hyman CL, Augenbraun MH, Roblin PM, et al: Asymptomatic respiratory tract infection with *Chlamydia pneumoniae*. J Clin Microbiol 29:2082–2083, 1991.
11. Falsey AR, Walsh EE: Transmission of *Chlamydia pneumoniae*. J Infect Dis 168:493–496, 1993.
12. Theunissen HJH, Lemmens-den Toom NA, Burggraaf A, et al: Influence of temperature and relative humidity on the survival of *Chlamydia pneumoniae* in aerosols. Appl Environ Microbiol 59:2589–2593, 1993.
13. Yamazaki T, Nakada H, Sakurai N, et al: Transmission of *Chlamydia pneumoniae* in young children in a Japanese family. J Infect Dis 162:1390–1392, 1990.
14. Kleemola M, Saikku P, Visakorpi R, et al: Epidemics of pneumonia caused by TWAR, a new *Chlamydia* organism, in military trainees in Finland. J Infect Dis 157:230–236, 1988.
15. Hyman CL, Roblin PM, Gaydos CA, et al: Prevalence of asymptomatic nasopharyngeal carriage of *Chlamydia pneumoniae* in subjectively healthy adults: Assessment by polymerase chain reaction–enzyme immunoassay and culture. Clin Infect Dis 20:1174–1178, 1995.
16. Kern DG, Neill MA, Schachter J: A seroepidemiologic study of *Chlamydia pneumoniae* in Rhode Island. Chest 104:208–213, 1993.
17. Marrie TJ, Grayston JT, Wang SP, et al: Pneumonia associated with the TWAR strain of *Chlamydia*. Ann Intern Med 106:507–511, 1987.
18. Saikku P, Ruutu P, Leinonen M, et al: Acute lower-respiratory-tract infection associated with chlamydial TWAR antibody in Filipino children. J Infect Dis 158:1095–1097, 1988.
19. Grayston JT, Diwan VK, Cooney M, et al: Community and hospital acquired pneumonia associated with *Chlamydia* TWAR infection demonstrated serologically. Arch Intern Med 149:169–173, 1989.
20. Chirgwin K, Roblin PM, Gelling M, et al: Infection with *Chlamydia pneumoniae* in Brooklyn. J Infect Dis 163:757–761, 1991.
21. Block S, Hedrick J, Hammerschlag MR, et al: *Mycoplasma pneumoniae* and *Chlamydia pneumoniae* in pediatric community-acquired pneumonia: Comparative efficacy and safety of clarithromycin vs. erythromycin ethylsuccinate. Pediatr Infect Dis 14:471–477, 1995.
22. Shemer-Avni Y, Lieberman D: *Chlamydia pneumoniae*–induced ciliostasis in ciliated bronchial epithelial cells. J Infect Dis 171:1274–1278, 1995.
23. Hammerschlag MR, Chirgwin K, Roblin PM, et al: Persistent infection with *Chlamydia pneumoniae* following acute respiratory illness. Clin Infect Dis 14:178–182, 1992.
24. Emre U, Roblin PM, Gelling M, et al: The association of *Chlamydia pneumoniae* infection and reactive airway disease in children. Arch Pediatr Adolesc Med 148:727–732, 1994.
25. Holland SM, Taylor HR, Gaydos CA, et al: Experimental infection with *Chlamydia pneumoniae* in nonhuman primates. Infect Immun 58:593–597, 1990.
26. Yang ZP, Kuo CC, Grayston JT: A mouse model of *Chlamydia pneumoniae* strain TWAR pneumonitis. Infect Immun 61:2037–2040, 1993.
27. Kaukoranta-Tolvanen SS, Laurila AL, Saikku P, et al: Experimental infection of *Chlamydia pneumoniae* in mice. Microb Pathog 15:293–302, 1993.

28. Malinverni R, Kuo C-C, Campbell LA, et al: Reactivation of *Chlamydia pneumoniae* lung infection in mice by cortisone. J Infect Dis 172:593–594, 1995.
29. Augenbraun MH, Roblin PM, Mandel LJ, et al: *Chlamydia pneumoniae* pneumonia with pleural effusion: Diagnosis by culture. Am J Med 43:437–438, 1991.
30. Augenbraun MH, Roblin PM, Chirgwin K, et al: Isolation of *Chlamydia pneumoniae* from the lungs of patients infected with the human immunodeficiency virus. J Clin Microbiol 29:401–402, 1991.
31. Gaydos CA, Fowler CL, Gill VJ, et al: Detection of *Chlamydia pneumoniae* by polymerase chain reaction–enzyme immunoassay in an immunocompromised population. Clin Infect Dis 17:718–723, 1993.
32. Miller ST, Hammerschlag MR, Chirgwin K, et al: The role of *Chlamydia pneumoniae* in acute chest syndrome of sickle cell disease. J Pediatr 118:30–33, 1991.
33. Hahn DL, Dodge RW, Galubjatnikov R: Association of *Chlamydia pneumoniae* (strain TWAR) infection with wheezing, asthmatic bronchitis and adult-onset asthma. JAMA 266:225–230, 1991.
34. Emre U, Sokolovskaya N, Roblin PM, et al: Detection of anti-*Chlamydia pneumoniae* IgE in children with reactive airway disease. J Infect Dis 172:265–267, 1995.
35. Sundelof B, Gnarpe H, Gnarpe J: An unusual manifestation of *Chlamydia pneumoniae* infection: Meningitis, hepatitis, iritis and atypical erythema nodosum. Scand J Infect Dis 25:259–261, 1993.
36. Yamada S, Tsumura N, Nagai K, et al: A child with iritis due to *Chlamydia pneumoniae* infection. J Jpn Assoc Infect Dis 68:1543–1547, 1994.
37. Roblin PM, Dumornay W, Hammerschlag MR: Use of HEp-2 cells for improved isolation and passage of *Chlamydia pneumoniae*. J Clin Microbiol 30:1968–1971, 1992.
38. Montalban GS, Roblin PM, Hammerschlag MR: Performance of three commercially available monoclonal reagents for confirmation of *Chlamydia pneumoniae* in cell culture. J Clin Microbiol 32:1406–1407, 1994.
39. Grayston JT, Aldous MB, Easton A, et al: Evidence that *Chlamydia pneumoniae* causes pneumonia and bronchitis. J Infect Dis 168:1231–1235, 1993.
40. Black CM, Johnson JE, Farshy CE, et al: Antigenic variation among strains of *Chlamydia pneumoniae*. J Clin Microbiol 29:1312–1316, 1991.
41. Iljima Y, Miyashita N, Kishimoto T, et al: Characterization of *Chlamydia pneumoniae* species-specific proteins immunodominant in humans. J Clin Microbiol 32:583–588, 1994.
42. Verkooyen RP, Hazenberg MA, Van Haaren GH, et al: Age-related interference with *Chlamydia pneumoniae* microimmunofluorescence serology due to circulating rheumatoid factor. J Clin Microbiol 30:1287–1290, 1992.
43. Moss TR, Darougar S, Woodland RM, et al: Antibodies to *Chlamydia* species in patients attending a genitourinary clinic and the impact of antibodies to *C. pneumoniae* and *C. psittaci* on the sensitivity and the specificity of *C. trachomatis* serology tests. Sex Transm Dis 20:61–65, 1993.
44. Komaroff AL, Aronson MD, Schachter J: *Chlamydia trachomatis* infection in adults with community-acquired pneumonia. JAMA 245:1319–1322, 1981.
45. Komaroff AL, Aronson MD, Pass TM, et al: Serologic evidence of chlamydial and mycoplasmal pharyngitis in adults. Science 222:927–928, 1983.
46. Campbell LA, Melgosa MP, Hamilton DJ, et al: Detection of *Chlamydia pneumoniae* by polymerase chain reaction. J Clin Microbiol 30:434–439, 1992.
47. Gaydos CA, Roblin PM, Hammerschlag MR, et al: Diagnostic utility of PCR–enzyme immunoassay, culture, and serology for detection of *Chlamydia pneumoniae* in symptomatic and asymptomatic patients. J Clin Microbiol 32:903–905, 1994.
48. Hammerschlag MR: Antimicrobial susceptibility and therapy of infections caused by *Chlamydia pneumoniae*. Antimicrob Agents Chemother 38:1873–1878, 1994.
49. Hammerschlag MR: Chlamydial infections. J Pediatr 114:727–734, 1989.
50. Bell TA, Stamm WE, Wang SP, et al: Chronic *Chlamydia trachomatis* infections in infants. JAMA 267:400–402, 1992.
51. Beem MO, Saxon EM: Respiratory-tract colonization and a distinctive pneumonia syndrome in infants infected with *Chlamydia trachomatis*. N Engl J Med 296:306–310, 1977.
52. Harrison HR, English MG, Lee CK, et al: *Chlamydia trachomatis* infant pneumonitis: Comparison with matched controls and other infant pneumonitis. N Engl J Med 298:702–708, 1978.
53. Nakajo MN, Roblin PM, Hammerschlag MR, et al: Chlamydicidal activity of human alveolar macrophages. Infect Immun 58:3640–3644, 1990.
54. Gerber MA, Ryan RW, Tilton RC, et al: Role of *Chlamydia trachomatis* in acute pharyngitis in young adults. J Clin Microbiol 20:993–994, 1984.
55. Huss H, Jungkind D, Amodio P, et al: Frequency of *Chlamydia trachomatis* as the cause of pharyngitis. J Clin Microbiol 22:858–860, 1985.
56. Ito JI, Comess KA, Alexander ER, et al: Pneumonia due to *Chlamydia trachomatis* in an immunocompromised adult. N Engl J Med 307:95–98, 1982.
57. Meyers JD, Hackman RC, Stamm WE: *Chlamydia trachomatis* infection as a cause of pneumonia after human marrow transplantation. Transplantation 36:130–134, 1983.
58. Moncada JV, Schachter J, Wofsy C: Prevalence of *Chlamydia trachomatis* lung infection in patients with acquired immune deficiency syndrome. J Clin Microbiol 23:986, 1986.
59. Bernstein DI, Hubbard T, Wenman WM, et al: Mediastinal and supraclavicular lymphadenitis and pneumonitis due to *Chlamydia trachomatis* serovars L_1 and L_2. N Engl J Med 311:1543–1546, 1984.
60. Centers for Disease Control: Recommendations for the prevention and management of *Chlamydia trachomatis* infections, 1993. MMWR Morbid Mortal Wkly Rep 42(RR-12):1–39, 1993.
61. Paisley JW, Lauer BA, Melinkovich P, et al: Rapid diagnosis of *Chlamydia trachomatis* pneumonia in infants by direct immunofluorescence microscopy of nasopharyngeal secretions. J Pediatr 109:653–655, 1986.
62. Roblin PM, Hammerschlag MR, Cummings C, et al: Comparison of two rapid microscopic methods and culture for detection of *Chlamydia trachomatis* in ocular and nasopharyngeal specimens from infants. J Clin Microbiol 27:968–970, 1989.
63. Hammerschlag MR, Roblin PM, Gelling M, et al: Comparison of two enzyme immunoassays to culture for the diagnosis of chlamydial conjunctivitis and respiratory infection in infants. J Clin Microbiol 28:1725–1727, 1990.
64. MacFarlane JT, MacRae AD: Psittacosis. Br Med Bull 39:163–167, 1983.
65. van Buuren CE, Dorrestein GM, van Dijk JE: *Chlamydia psittaci* in birds: A review on the pathogenesis and histopathological features. Vet Q 16:38–41, 1994.
66. Andersen AA, Tappe JP: Genetic, immunologic and pathologic characterization of avian chlamydial strains. J Am Vet Med Assoc 195:1512–1516, 1989.
67. Centers for Disease Control: Psittacosis Surveillance 1975–1984. Atlanta, Centers for Disease Control, 1987, pp 1–60.
68. Centers for Disease Control: Psittacosis at a turkey processing plant—North Carolina, 1989. MMWR Morbid Mortal Wkly Rep 39:460–461, 467–469, 1990.
69. Hedberg K, White KE, Forfang JC, et al: An outbreak of psittacosis in Minnesota turkey industry workers: Implications for modes of transmission and control. Am J Epidemiol 130:569–577, 1989.
70. Hinton DG, Shipley A, Galvin JW, et al: Chlamydiosis in workers at a duck farm and processing plant. Aust Vet J 70:174–176, 1993.
71. Schlossberg D, Delgado J, Moore MM, et al: An epidemic of avian and human psittacosis. Arch Intern Med 153:2594–2596, 1993.
72. Yung AP, Grayson ML: Psittacosis—A review of 135 cases. Med J Aust 148:228–233, 1988.
73. Mason AB, Jenkins P: Acute renal failure in fulminant psittacosis. Respir Med 88:239–240, 1994.
74. Day CJ, Fawcett IW: Psittacosis and acute thrombocytopenia. J Rl Soc Med 85:360–361, 1992.
75. Shapiro DS, Kenney SC, Johnson M, et al: *Chlamydia psittaci* endocarditis diagnosed by blood culture. N Engl J Med 325:1192–1195, 1992.
76. Laumaury I, Sotto A, Le Quellec A, et al: *Chlamydia psittaci* as a cause of lethal bacterial endocarditis. Clin Infect Dis 17:821–822, 1993.
77. Cartwright KAV, Caul EO, Lamb RW: Symptomatic *Chlamydia psittaci* reinfection (Letter). Lancet 1:1004, 1988.
78. Fryden A, Kihlstrom E, Maller R, et al: A clinical and epidemiological study of "ornithosis" caused by *Chlamydia psittaci* and

Chlamydia pneumoniae (strain TWAR). Scand J Infect Dis 21:681–691, 1989.
79. Bruu AL, Haukenes G, Aasen S, et al: *Chlamydia pneumoniae* infections in Norway 1981–87 earlier diagnosed as ornithosis. Scand J Infect Dis 23:299–304, 1991.
80. Pether JVS, Wang SP, Grayston JT: *Chlamydia pneumoniae* strain TWAR, as the cause of an outbreak in a boys' school previously called psittacosis. Epidemiol Infect 103:395–400, 1989.
81. Wong KH, Skelton SK, Daugharty H: Utility of complement fixation and microimmunofluorescence assays for detecting serologic responses in patients with clinically diagnosed psittacosis. J Clin Microbiol 32:2417–2421, 1994.
82. Oldach DW, Gaydos CA, Mundy LM, et al: Rapid diagnosis of *Chlamydia psittaci* pneumonia. Clin Infect Dis 17:338–343, 1993.
83. Tong CYW, Sillis M: Detection of *Chlamydia pneumoniae* and *Chlamydia psittaci* in sputum samples by PCR. J Clin Pathol 46:313–317, 1993.

63

Aspiration Pneumonia

John G. Bartlett

Aspiration pneumonia refers to the pulmonary consequences that follow abnormal entry of fluid, particulate exogenous substances, or endogenous secretions into the lower airways. There are usually two requirements. First, there needs to be a compromise in the usual defenses that protect the tracheobronchial tree, such as glottic closure, cough reflex, or other clearing mechanisms of the lower airways. Second, the inoculum must be deleterious to the lower airways by a direct toxic effect, a bacterial inoculum sufficient to initiate an inflammatory process, or a sufficient volume to cause obstruction.

Predisposing Conditions

Numerous studies indicate that even healthy persons aspirate, but this is usually inconsequential. For example, Amberson[1] placed contrast material in the mouths of sleeping patients and showed by chest radiographs the following day that although the contrast material was regularly detected in the lower airways in the majority of patients, there was no apparent clinical disease. Similarly, dye markers placed in the stomachs of postoperative patients can be aspirated from the tracheobronchial tree at the time of surgery to demonstrate aspiration of gastric contents during general anesthesia in 7% to 16% of patients.[2, 3] Scintigraphic methods have been used to document frequent aspiration in patients with tracheostomies, endotracheal tubes, nasogastric tubes, gastrostomy tubes, and dysphagia.[4–10] In most studies, the frequency of aspiration of the marker placed in the stomach of patients with these conditions is 10% to 40%; elimination from the airways is complete or nearly complete by 3 hours. The frequency of aspiration during endoscopy of the upper gastrointestinal tract has been reported at 25%.[11–13] These observations show that aspiration is relatively common and usually resolves unrecognized without detectable sequelae. The decisive factor in the development of pulmonary complications appears to depend on the frequency, volume, and character of the material in the inoculum.

Conditions associated with an increased frequency of aspiration pneumonia include reduced levels of consciousness resulting in compromise of the cough reflex and glottic closure; dysphagia from neurologic deficits; disorders of the upper gastrointestinal tract including esophageal disease, surgery involving the upper airways or esophagus, and gastric reflux; mechanical disruption of the glottic closure or the cardiac sphincter due to tracheostomy, endotracheal tube, bronchoscopy, esophagogastroduodenoscopy, and nasogastric feeding; pharyngeal anesthesia; and miscellaneous conditions such as protracted vomiting, large-volume tube feedings, feeding gastrostomy, and the recumbent position (Table 63–1). The conditions cited predispose to more frequent aspiration or aspiration of large volumes, thus defining the population at greatest risk for pulmonary complications.

Prevention

Prevention of aspiration has been most extensively studied in patients hospitalized in intensive care units, patients with neurologic or esophageal conditions that predispose to aspiration, and patients who receive enteral feedings. The most convincing preventive measure in the intensive care unit is use of a semirecumbent or upright position.[14] Other methods to address this issue include tracheostomy, reduction of gastric volume by suction or metoclopramide, feedings by nasogastric tube or gastrostomy, and gastric acid neutralization by antacids or histamine H_2 blockers.[14–22] The effectiveness of these maneuvers is variable and often confounded by the fact that the remedy itself predisposes to aspiration. For example, inflation of the balloon on the tracheostomy tube may occlude the esophagus to promote aspiration. Neutralization of gastric acid effectively reduces the risk of chemical pneumonitis due to acid aspiration,[10, 16, 17, 21] but elimination of the gastric barrier promotes bacterial growth and bacterial pneumonia after gastric aspiration.[18, 22, 23] Percutaneous endoscopic gastroscopy has been extensively used and studied as a method to prevent aspiration pneumonia in patients rendered vulnerable by nasogastric feeding or oral feedings. Results are variable.[7, 15, 19, 24–26] An alternative is the feeding jejunostomy, which appears superior to percutaneous endoscopic gastroscopy.[15, 27, 28] Surgery is the major preventive method with some esophageal lesions, such as Zenker diverticula[29]; it is more controversial with gastroesophageal reflux.[30]

TABLE 63–1 ■ Conditions That Predispose to Aspiration

Altered consciousness
Alcoholism, seizures, cerebrovascular accident, head trauma, general anesthesia, drug overdose
Dysphagia
Esophageal disorder: stricture, neoplasm, diverticula, tracheoesophageal fistula, incompetent cardiac sphincter
Gastroesophageal reflux
Neurologic disorder
Multiple sclerosis, Parkinson disease, myasthenia gravis, pseudobulbar palsy
Mechanical disruption of the usual defense barriers
Nasogastric tube, endotracheal intubation, tracheostomy, upper gastrointestinal endoscopy, bronchoscopy
Protracted vomiting, gastric outlet obstruction, large-volume nasogastric tube feedings
Pharyngeal anesthesia
General debility
Recumbent position

Classification

Aspiration pneumonia refers to distinctive syndromes that may be distinguished on the basis of the character of the inoculum, pathogenesis of pulmonary complications, clinical presentation, and management guidelines[31] (Table 63–2). Although there may be overlap in individual cases and some patients are difficult to classify, this classification scheme provides a useful conceptual approach to a complex topic. The three syndromes include chemical pneumonitis, bacterial infection, and airway obstruction.

Incidence

Many population-based studies of pneumonia include a category of aspiration pneumonia that is variously defined, but common criteria are a predisposition to aspiration, an infiltrate involving a dependent pulmonary segment, and no competing diagnosis. These cases account for 5% to 10% of patients in most series; although the distribution of cases using the three categories of aspiration pneumonia is rarely attempted, most consider infections involving anaerobic bacteria to account for the majority.[32–34] In studies of selected populations of patients, the frequency of aspiration is probably much higher. These include the elderly, patients in nursing homes, victims of head trauma, multiple sclerosis patients, and patients with dysphagia.

Chemical Pneumonitis

Chemical pneumonitis refers to the aspiration of substances that are inherently toxic to the lower airways. These substances initiate an inflammatory reaction that is independent of bacterial infection and cannot be ascribed to bronchial obstruction. Examples include acid, animal fats such as milk and mineral oil, and volatile hydrocarbons such as gasoline or kerosene. The prototypic example and best studied of these is the chemical pneumonitis associated with aspiration of gastric acid, as classically described by Mendelson in 1946.[35]

Clinical Presentation

The classic study by Mendelson[35] concerned 61 obstetric patients who aspirated gastric contents during ether anesthesia. When the aspiratory event was witnessed, the onset of respiratory distress followed rapidly. Subsequent studies have shown that symptoms generally become apparent within 2 hours.[36] The major clinical features included the abrupt onset of cyanosis, dyspnea, tachypnea, and tachycardia. Nearly all patients had bronchospasm, leading Mendelson to compare this with an acute asthmatic attack. Chest radiographs showed infiltrates that were generally located in one or both lower lobes. Despite the severity of illness, including cyanosis in the majority of patients, all 61 recovered and most were clinically stable within 24 to 36 hours. Radiographs generally showed clearing of infiltrates within 4 to 7 days.

There have been extensive studies of acid pneumonitis since this original report. This later work has shown an increased frequency of fever, reduced frequency of observed bronchospasm, and a substantial mortality.[37–41] Acid aspiration is now recognized as one of the three most common causes of the adult respiratory distress syndrome.[41a] The most striking difference compared with Mendelson's experience concerns mortality, which later reports showed to be in the range of 30% to 60%. The best explanation is that the patients described by Mendelson were young, previously healthy obstetric patients, whereas those reviewed in the later reports were often debilitated and had multiple associated conditions. Analysis of blood gases, which was not available at the time of Mendelson's report, shows hypoxemia early in the course. Measurements of partial pressure of oxygen are often in the 35 to 50 mm Hg range, usually accompanied by a normal or low partial pressure of carbon dioxide and a respiratory alkalosis. If hypoxemia is severe, the partial pressure of carbon dioxide may be elevated with a metabolic acidosis. Factors contributing to the hypoxemia include pulmonary edema, reduced surfactant activity, reflex airway closure, alveolar hemorrhage, and hyaline membrane formation. Pulmonary function tests show decreased compliance, abnormalities of ventilation-perfusion, and reduced diffusing capacity. Many patients have hypotension owing to an immediate reflex reaction or fluid aggregation in the lung with intravascular volume depletion. Pulmonary artery pressure is usually low or normal because of reduced cardiac output with decreased intravascular volume. Patients with severe disease often progress to the adult respiratory distress syndrome. Another potential complication is superimposed infection because the acid-injured lung appears to be predisposed to bacterial infection.

TABLE 63–2 ■ Classification of Aspiration Pneumonia

INOCULUM	PULMONARY SEQUELAE	CLINICAL FEATURES	THERAPY
Acid	Chemical pneumonitis	Acute dyspnea, tachypnea, tachycardia; ± cyanosis, bronchospasm, fever Sputum: pink, frothy Radiograph: infiltrates in one or both lower lobes Hypoxemia	Positive-pressure breathing Intravenous fluids Tracheal suction
Oropharyngeal bacteria	Bacterial infection	Usually insidious onset Cough, fever, purulent sputum Radiograph: infiltrate involving dependent pulmonary segment or lobe ± cavitation	Antibiotics
Inert fluids	Mechanical obstruction Reflex airway closure	Acute dyspnea, cyanosis ± apnea Pulmonary edema	Tracheal suction Intermittent positive-pressure breathing with oxygen and isoproterenol
Particulate matter	Mechanical obstruction	Dependent on level of obstruction, ranging from acute apnea and rapid death to irritating chronic cough ± recurrent infections	Extraction of particulate matter Antibiotics for superimposed infection

Clinical features that specifically suggest chemical pneumonitis include the abrupt onset of symptoms, dyspnea, cyanosis, low-grade fever, diffuse rales, hypoxemia, and infiltrates in dependent pulmonary segments.[42] The course of the disease has been examined in a retrospective review of 50 cases by Bynum and Pierce.[36] These investigators divided patients into three categories. The first group accounted for 12% and was characterized by a fulminant course with death shortly after aspiration, presumably due to the adult respiratory distress syndrome. The second group accounted for 62% and had a rapid improvement of the chest radiograph in a fashion analogous to the course described by Mendelson[35]; in these patients, the radiographic changes cleared in a mean time of 4.5 days. The third group accounted for 26% and resembled the second group in terms of rapid improvement; however, these individuals subsequently had new or extending infiltrates on the chest radiograph associated with fever, which was ascribed to pulmonary superinfection.

Pathophysiology

Acid pneumonitis has been studied extensively in vivo or ex vivo using experimental animals with intratracheal instillations of acid.[43–50] There are two essential requirements in these experiments. First, challenge using graded acids indicates that the pH must be 2.5 or less to initiate an inflammatory reaction. Substances with a higher pH, including saline, saliva, buffered gastric acid, and so forth, demonstrate only a transient, self-limited period of respiratory distress, which is probably due to brief airway obstruction or reflex airway closure. The severity of the pneumonitis correlates with the pH of the inoculum at levels below 2.5. The second requirement is a relatively large inoculum, generally 1 to 4 mL/kg. Translation of these observations to the clinical setting indicates that aspiration of gastric contents in adult patients should involve at least 25 mL with a pH of 2.5 or lower. Smaller volumes may produce a more subtle process that either escapes clinical detection or causes a less fulminant form of pneumonitis. In support of this contention is the observation of frequent bouts of recurrent pneumonitis or otherwise unexplained pulmonary fibrosis in patients with esophageal disease or gastric reflux.[51–56]

The pathologic changes in acid pneumonitis occur with extraordinary rapidity.[47] Atelectasis is apparent within seconds and becomes extensive at 3 minutes. Additional early changes include peribronchial hemorrhage, pulmonary edema, and degeneration of bronchial epithelial cells. By 4 hours, the alveolar spaces are filled with polymorphonuclear leukocytes in fibrin. Hyaline membranes can be seen at 48 hours.[47] At this time, the lung is grossly edematous and hemorrhagic with alveolar consolidation. Resolution begins on the third day and may be complete or result in residual parenchymal scarring. Virtually all of these findings have been noted on autopsy studies of patients with fatal aspiration pneumonia. The pathophysiology of these events is now ascribed to the release of proinflammatory cytokines, especially tumor necrosis factor and interleukin-8, which are responsible for recruitment and activation of neutrophils.[56a] Long-term follow-up studies in patients who survive this condition show either complete recovery or radiographic evidence of pulmonary fibrosis with disturbances in gas exchange.[57, 58]

Diagnosis

Acid pneumonitis is usually a presumed diagnosis that is based on clinical observations and supported by radiographic findings. A highly characteristic feature of the disease is its precipitous onset and its rapid evolution to complete clearing within days, progression to the adult respiratory distress syndrome, or secondary bacterial infection. If the aspiratory event is observed, the chest radiograph will demonstrate pulmonary infiltrates within 1 to 2 hours.[36] The implication is that a normal chest radiograph 2 hours or longer after the aspiration event excludes chemical pneumonitis. It is not possible to confirm this diagnosis by measurement of the pH of tracheal secretions owing to the rapid neutralization of the inoculum by pulmonary edema fluid and bronchial secretions. On occasion, it may be useful to measure the pH of gastric contents or vomitus to establish the critical value noted previously. Bronchoscopy is sometimes advocated to remove particulate matter that may be aspirated concurrently. Bronchoscopy will demonstrate erythema of the bronchi, which suggests acid injury.

Treatment

Tracheal suction is often appropriate to clear fluids and particulate matter that may cause obstruction as a compounding feature. Intravenous fluid support is necessary to expand intravascular space. Tracheal inoculation of buffering solutions and pulmonary lavage in an attempt to neutralize the acid inoculum are generally futile because of the rapidity with which acid is neutralized by the normal defense mechanisms. This disease has been compared with a "flash burn" of the lung in which most of the damage has occurred by the time the patient is initially treated.

The major therapeutic modality is support of pulmonary function. Studies in dogs showed benefit with positive-pressure ventilation, high-molecular-weight colloids given intravenously, and sodium nitroprusside infused into the capillary artery.[49, 50, 59–64] The role of positive-pressure ventilation is to improve oxygenation and increase alveolar pressure to reduce the transduction of fluids. Colloids are given to restore circulating volume and osmotic pressure, although their benefit compared with intravenous saline or other nonosmotic fluid is not clear. The purpose of sodium nitroprusside is to decrease pulmonary arterial pressure. It is difficult to confirm the benefit of these therapeutic maneuvers in patients with appropriate controlled trials because of the infrequency of the syndrome. There is a consensus impression that ventilatory support is mandatory, but further recommendations using some of the techniques just described are controversial.

One of the previously controversial areas concerned the use of corticosteroids. In animals, these agents have given variable results,[39, 43, 45, 65–67] but their use in humans has been uniformly unsuccessful.[6, 36, 44] Similarly, these agents also appear to be contraindicated for the adult respiratory distress syndrome, which is a relatively frequent complication.[68] More recent studies in animals suggest a possible role for intratracheal instillation of antibodies to adhesion molecules including selectins and integrins.[56a] There is no good evidence that bacteria play any important role in the acute events in animal or clinical studies. Indeed, the pH of the inoculum necessary to initiate a chemical pneumonitis is inhospitable to bacterial survival. Antimicrobial agents are commonly given because it is difficult to eliminate bacterial infection as a contributing factor. Studies in experimental animals have shown that the acid-injured lung is highly susceptible to bacterial challenge.[69] Clinical studies indicated that 13% to 26% of patients acquire pulmonary superinfections during the course of recovery.[36, 37, 70] Nevertheless, available evidence does not support the use of prophylactic antibiotics in aspiration-prone patients.[36, 40]

Bacterial Infection

The most common form of aspiration pneumonia is bacterial infection due to aspiration of bacteria that normally reside in the upper airways or stomach. There is a potential problem here with semantics, because the majority of bacterial pneumonias probably occur as a result of aspiration, including cases caused by *Streptococcus pneumoniae, Haemophilus influenzae*, gram-negative bacilli, and *Staphylococcus aureus*. These are relatively virulent in the lower airways so that only a small inoculum is required. The process might be referred to as microaspiration, which is subtle and relatively common in the patient who is not aspiration prone. By contrast, aspiration pneumonia due to bacterial pathogens usually refers to pneumonia in a patient who is predisposed to aspiration of relatively large volumes, most commonly as a result of altered consciousness or dysphagia (see Table 64–1). This diagnosis is suspected when a susceptible host develops typical findings for a pulmonary infection, including fever, purulent sputum, and a pulmonary infiltrate in a dependent pulmonary segment.[31, 71, 72]

Clinical Features

The presenting findings are highly variable, depending to a large extent on the bacteria involved and the host's status. The predominant pathogens are anaerobic bacteria that normally reside in the gingival crevice. The tempo of the disease in this process tends to be relatively slow. The initial lesion is pneumonitis, which may be clinically similar to other forms of acute bacterial pneumonias. The patient has an acute episode of cough, fever, purulent sputum production, and dyspnea.[71–75] If the patient is less seriously ill and does not seek medical attention in this early stage, there is often progression to the late stages, which are characterized by suppuration including lung abscess, necrotizing pneumonia, or empyema associated with bronchopleural fistula.[31, 71–75]

Factors that specifically suggest that acute pneumonia is due to aspiration of anaerobic bacteria are the associated conditions predisposing to aspiration, lack of rigors, failure to recover likely pathogens with cultures of expectorated sputum, indolent course, sputum that is usually putrid, and a chest radiograph that shows evidence of tissue necrosis with abscess formation or empyema. Many of these patients show evidence of periodontal disease, because the organisms involved generally reside in the periodontal pockets. Radiographs show infiltrates with or without cavitation in the dependent pulmonary segments. The favored locations are the superior segment of the lower lobes or posterior segments of the upper lobes, which are dependent in the recumbent position. Basilar segments of the lower lobes are favored in patients who aspirate in the sitting or upright position.

Bacteriology

Aspiration of oropharyngeal or gastric contents usually results in an infection involving a polymicrobial flora. The major pathogens are anaerobic bacteria, which are found in 60% to 85% of cases according to studies using appropriate diagnostic methods.[31, 71–80] Expectorated sputum is unsuitable for anaerobic culture because of inevitable contamination by the normal flora of the upper airways. Preferred specimens to establish the microbiologic diagnosis are transtracheal aspirates, transthoracic needle aspirates, empyema fluid, and quantitative cultures of bronchoscopy specimens obtained with the protected brush or of bronchoalveolar lavage specimens.[36, 71, 72, 77, 78, 81–83] Most clinical studies that included uncontaminated specimens for bacteriologic analysis in aspiration pneumonia were done in the period 1970 to 1980, when transtracheal aspiration was common.[73–76, 79, 80] This procedure is now rarely performed; there is increasing interest in quantitative cultures of bronchoscopic specimens, although the experience with this technique in anaerobic bacterial infections of the lung is limited.[81, 82]

The major bacterial isolates in patients with aspiration pneumonitis or lung abscess include anaerobic streptococci (*Peptostreptococcus* spp.), *Fusobacterium nucleatum*, and *Prevotella melaninogenica* (formerly *Bacteroides melaninogenicus*).[36, 71–80] Most of these patients have multiple species of anaerobic bacteria in the lower airways, of which at least 15% to 25% are resistant to penicillin owing to penicillinase production.[71, 72, 84] Aerobic or microaerophilic bacteria are concurrently present in at least half of cases of pulmonary infections involving anaerobic bacteria. Gram-negative bacilli are especially common in patients with hospital-acquired aspiration pneumonia.[80, 85] These organisms are not considered to be components of the normal oral flora. However, studies indicate that the rate of colonization of the upper airways by gram-negative bacilli is directly correlated with the severity of associated conditions.[86] This observation presumably accounts for the marked difference in bacteriologic patterns between community-acquired and hospital-acquired aspiration pneumonia. It also appears that gastric contents may be the source of gram-negative bacteria in aspiration pneumonia, and this especially applies to patients who have lost the acid gastric barrier from medication (antacids or H_2-blocking agents) or aging.[22]

Treatment

The mainstay of treatment is antibiotics, and the selection of specific agents is obviously simplified if definitive bacteriologic studies have been done. As noted previously, the major pathogens are anaerobic bacteria, which require invasive diagnostic techniques that are generally not performed except for thoracocentesis in patients with empyema. As a consequence, antibiotics are usually selected empirically. Expectorated sputum cultures are often used to guide the selection of agents for aerobic bacteria that may be present concurrently.

The standard drug historically for aspiration pneumonia or lung abscess due to anaerobic bacteria has been penicillin given intravenously or high doses given orally.[87–91] Several trials performed from 1950 through 1975 showed that the great majority of patients responded. The occasional failures appeared to respond to substitution with tetracycline.[89–92] These recommendations have been confounded in more recent years by the observation that up to 40% of *Fusobacterium* spp. and 60% of non-*fragilis Bacteroides* sp. produce penicillinase.[36, 71, 72, 78, 84] In the only comparative therapeutic trials of lung abscess, clindamycin was significantly superior to intravenous penicillin in terms of response rates and time to defervescence.[92, 93] Alternative regimens in which the anecdotal experience is favorable include amoxicillin-clavulanate[94] and penicillin plus metronidazole.[95] Metronidazole should not be used as a single agent because extensive studies have shown that approximately 50% of patients do not respond, presumably owing to the contributing role of aerobic and microaerophilic streptococci.[96, 97] When penicillin is used, most advocate relatively large doses such as 10 to 12 million units daily, although oral penicillin V in doses of 3 g daily proved equally effective in older studies of lung abscess.[89] Patients with nosocomial aspiration pneumonia are likely to have a polymicrobial flora that includes aerobic gram-negative bacilli or *S. aureus* as well as anaerobic bacteria. The need to treat all components of a mixed flora in such cases is not well established. However, the high mortality for gram-negative bacillary pneumonia suggests that these organisms should clearly be treated in patients who are seriously ill and those who have hospital-acquired infection.

Mechanical Obstruction

Aspiration pneumonia may involve fluid or particulate matter that is not inherently toxic to the lung but may cause airway obstruction or reflux airway closure.

Fluids

Typical fluids that may be aspirated and are not inherently toxic to the lung include saline, barium, water, most ingested fluids, and gastric contents with a pH exceeding 2.5. When these fluids are instilled intratracheally into animals in limited quantities, the result is a transient, self-limited hypoxemia. This type of insult occasionally produces pulmonary edema with more severe hypoxemia and reduced compliance.[98] This reaction is reversible by vagotomy or administration of atropine or isoproterenol, suggesting intrinsic pulmonary reflex closure that is not related to the chemical composition of the inoculum.[48, 98, 99] A possible clinical counterpart of this observation in experimental animals is apparently seen in some drowning victims.[99, 100] Appropriate treatment consists of intermittent positive-pressure breathing with 100% oxygen combined with isoproterenol.

The major consequence of aspirating fluids is simple mechanical obstruction. Most patients tolerate aspiration of relatively large volumes well, as verified by tolerance of the large volumes used in pulmonary lavage with bronchoscopy. Patients at risk for mechanical obstruction are those who have profound neurologic deficit with no cough reflex, unconscious patients, or drowning victims. The obvious critical therapeutic intervention is tracheal suction. If a subsequent chest radiograph fails to show any pulmonary infiltrate, no additional therapy is required except that intended to prevent further episodes of aspiration.

Solid Particles

The severity of respiratory obstruction after aspiration of particulate matter depends on the relative size of the object aspirated and the caliber of the lower airways. Foreign body aspiration usually occurs in children during the oral stage of development, at approximately 1 to 3 years of age. The most common objects recovered from the lower airways are peanuts, other vegetable particles, inorganic materials, and teeth.[101–104] Vegetable materials including peanuts are especially a problem because they are not apparent on a radiograph, they tend to swell because of their hydroscopic properties, and the undigested cellulose acts as a local irritant to produce the inflammation.

The clinical consequences of aspiration depend to a large extent on the level of obstruction. Large objects that lodge in the larynx or trachea cause sudden respiratory distress, cyanosis, and aphonia and lead quickly to death if the obstruction is not immediately relieved. This has been referred to as the cafe coronary syndrome because the symptoms may simulate those of acute myocardial infarction and often involve a piece of meat that is aspirated during restaurant dining.[105] In these cases, there is little opportunity for diagnostic evaluation or even transfer to an acute care facility. The suggested maneuver is the Heimlich maneuver, consisting of firm, rapid pressure applied to the upper abdomen in an effort to force the diaphragm up and dislodge the particle.

Aspiration of smaller particles causes less severe obstruction or simply partial obstruction unless multiple small airways are involved. The usual initial symptom is an irritating cough. When major bronchi are involved, there may be cyanosis, dyspnea, wheezing, chest pain, and vomiting. Chest radiographs may show atelectasis or obstructive emphysema. When the obstruction is partial, there may be unilateral wheezing, and an expiration radiograph will often demonstrate a shift in the mediastinum. Bacterial infection is a frequent complication when obstruction or partial obstruction persists for more than 1 week.[103, 106] The usual pathogens are anaerobic bacteria from the upper airways, as described previously. This alleged bacteriologic pattern is supported only by anecdotal cases studied with appropriate diagnostic techniques and using uncontaminated specimens and by experimental animal studies. In the animal studies, cotton plugs were used to obstruct the lower airways in dogs; the subsequent pneumonia that occurred distal to the obstructing lesion involved anaerobic bacteria from the upper airways.[107] Patients with this complication may respond well to antibiotics, but infections are likely to recur. An important clue is that the infections tend to involve the same anatomic site as shown by chest radiography.

The primary therapeutic modality is removal of the foreign object from the lower airways. Fiberoptic bronchoscopy has been used successfully alone, but many authorities prefer the Jackson bronchoscope because of its superior visualization and larger channel, which facilitates mechanical removal.[108]

References

1. Amberson JB: Aspiration bronchopneumonia. Int Clin 3:126, 1937.
2. Berson W, Adiani J: "Silent" regurgitation and aspiration of gastric contents during anesthesia. Anesthesiology 15:644, 1954.
3. Gardner AMN: Aspiration of food and vomit. Q J Med 27:227, 1958.
4. Cameron JL, Reynolds J, Zuidema GD: Aspiration in patients with tracheostomies. Surg Gynecol Obstet 136:68, 1973.
5. Spray SB, Zuidema GD, Cameron JL: Aspiration pneumonia: Incidence of aspiration with endotracheal tubes. Am J Surg 121:701, 1976.
6. Stewardson RH, Nyhus LM: Pulmonary aspiration. Arch Surg 112:1192, 1977.
7. Cole MJ, Smith JT, Molnar C, Shaffer EA: Aspiration after percutaneous gastrostomy: Assessment by Tc-99m labeling of the enteral feed. J Clin Gastroenterol 9:90, 1987.
8. Coben RM, Weintraub A, DiMarino AJ Jr, et al: Gastroesophageal reflux during gastrostomy feeding. Gastroenterology 106:13, 1994.
9. Silver KH, Van Nostrand D: The use of scintigraphy in the management of patients with pulmonary aspiration. Dysphagia 9:107, 1994.
10. Martin BJ, Corlew MM, Wood H, et al: The association of swallowing dysfunction and aspiration pneumonia. Dysphagia 9:1, 1994.
11. Prout BJ, Metreweli C: Pulmonary aspiration after fibre-endoscopy of the upper gastrointestinal tract. Br Med J 4:269, 1972.
12. Vennes JA: Infectious complications of gastrointestinal endoscopy. Dig Dis Sci 26:60S, 1981.
13. Lipper B, Simon D, Cerrone F: Pulmonary aspiration during emergency endoscopy in patients with upper gastrointestinal hemorrhage. Crit Care Med 19:330, 1991.
14. Gipson SL, Stovall TG, Elkins TE, Crumrine RS: Pharmacologic reduction of the risk of aspiration. South Med J 79:1356, 1986.
15. Burtch GD, Shatney CH: Feeding gastrostomy: Assistant or assassin? Am Surg 51:204, 1985.
16. Kinni ME, Stout MM: Aspiration pneumonitis: Predisposing conditions and prevention. J Oral Maxillofac Surg 44:378, 1986.
17. Lam AM, Grace DM, Penny FJ, Vezina WC: Prophylactic intravenous cimetidine reduces the risk of acid aspiration in morbidly obese patients. Anesthesiology 65:684, 1986.
18. Mehta S, Archer JF, Mills J: pH-dependent bactericidal barrier to gram-negative aerobes: Its relevance to airway colonization and prophylaxis of acid aspiration and stress ulcer syndromes—Study in vitro. Intensive Care Med 12:134, 1986.
19. Ciocon JO, Silverstone FA, Graver LM, Foley CJ: Tube feedings in elderly patients: Indications, benefits, and complications. Arch Intern Med 148:429, 1988.
20. Chang JH, Coln CD, Stickland AD, Andersen JM: Surgical man-

agement of gastroesophageal reflux in severely mentally retarded children. J Ment Defic Res 31:1, 1987.
21. Kowalsky SF: Cimetidine in anesthesia: Does it minimize the complications of acid aspiration? Drug Intell Clin Pharmacol 18:382, 1984.
22. Driks MR, Craven DE, Celli BR, et al: Nosocomial pneumonia in intubated patients given sucralfate as compared with antacids or histamine type 2 blockers: The role of gastric colonization. N Engl J Med 317:1376, 1987.
23. Toung TJ, Rosenfeld BA, Yoshiki A, et al: Sucralfate does not reduce the risk of acid aspiration pneumonitis. Crit Care Med 21:1359, 1993.
24. Mathus-Vliegen LM, Louwerse LS, Merkus MP, et al: Percutaneous endoscopic gastrostomy in patients with amyotrophic lateral sclerosis and impaired pulmonary function. Gastrointest Endosc 40:463, 1994.
25. Park RH, Allison MC, Lang J, et al: Randomised comparison of percutaneous endoscopic gastrostomy and nasogastric tube feeding in patients with persisting neurological dysphagia. BMJ 304:1406, 1992.
26. Fay DE, Poplausky M, Gruber M, et al: Long-term enteral feeding: A retrospective comparison of delivery via percutaneous endoscopic gastrostomy and nasoenteric tubes. Am J Gastroenterol 86:1604, 1991.
27. Weltz CR, Morris JB, Mullen JL: Surgical jejunostomy in aspiration risk patients. Ann Surg 215:140, 1992.
28. MacFadyen BV Jr, Ghobrial R, Catalano M, et al: Concomitant placement of percutaneous endoscopic gastrostomy and jejunostomy. Surg Endosc 6:289, 1992.
29. Schmit PJ, Zuckerbraun L: Zenker's diverticula by cricopharyngeus myotomy under local anesthesia. Am Surg 58:710, 1992.
30. Kiviluoto T, Luukkonen P, Salo J: Laparoscopic gastro-oesophageal antireflux surgery. Ann Chir Gynaecol 83:101, 1994.
31. Bartlett JG, Gorbach SL: The triple threat of aspiration pneumonia. Chest 68:560, 1975.
32. Potgieter PD, Hammond JM: Etiology and diagnosis of pneumonia requiring ICU admission. Chest 101:199, 1992.
33. Fang G, Fine M, Orloff J, et al: New and emerging etiologies for community-acquired pneumonia with implications of therapy. Medicine (Baltimore) 69:307, 1990.
34. Mundy LM, Auwaerter PG, Oldach D, et al: Community-acquired pneumonia: Impact of immune status. Am J Respir Crit Care Med 152:1309, 1995.
35. Mendelson CL: The aspiration of stomach contents into the lungs during obstetric anesthesia. Am J Obstet Gynecol 52:191, 1946.
36. Bynum LJ, Pierce AK: Pulmonary aspiration of gastric contents. Am Rev Respir Dis 114:1129, 1976.
37. Cameron JL, Mitchell WH, Zuidema GD: Aspiration pneumonia. Arch Surg 106:49, 1973.
38. Awe WC, Fletcher WS, Jacob SW: The pathophysiology of aspiration pneumonitis. Surgery 50:232, 1966.
39. Broe PJ, Toung TJ, Cameron JL: Aspiration pneumonia. Surg Clin North Am 60:1551, 1980.
40. Hamelberg WV, Bosomworth PP: Aspiration Pneumonitis. Springfield, IL, Charles C Thomas, 1968.
41. Lewis RT, Burgess JH, Hampson LG: Cardiorespiratory studies in critical illness. Arch Surg 103:335, 1971.
41a. Doyle RL, Szarflarski N, Modin GW, et al: Identification of patients with acute lung injury. Am J Respir Crit Care Med 152:1818, 1995.
42. DePaso WJ: Aspiration pneumonia. Clin Chest Med 12:269, 1991.
43. Toung TJ, Bordos D, Benson DW, et al: Aspiration pneumonia: Experimental evaluation of albumin and steroid therapy. Ann Surg 183:179, 1976.
44. Wolfe JE, Bone RC, Ruth WE: Effects of corticosteroids in the treatment of patients with gastric aspiration. Am J Med 63:719, 1977.
45. Chapman RL Jr, Downs JB, Modell JH, Hood CI: The ineffectiveness of steroid therapy in treating aspiration of hydrochloric acid. Arch Surg 108:858, 1974.
46. Fisk RL, Symes JF, Aldridge LL, Couves CM: The pathophysiology and experimental therapy of acid pneumonitis in ex vivo lungs. Chest 57:364, 1970.
47. Greenfield LJ, Singleton RP, McCaffree DR, Coalson JJ: Pulmonary effects of experimental graded aspiration of hydrochloric acid. Ann Surg 170:74, 1969.
48. Halmagyi DJF: Lung changes and incidence of respiration arrest in rats after aspiration of sea and fresh water. J Appl Physiol 16:41, 1961.
49. Teabeaut J II: Aspiration of gastric contents: An experimental study. Am J Pathol 28:51, 1952.
50. Toung TJ, Cameron JL, Kimera T, Permutt S: Aspiration pneumonia: Treatment with osmotically active agents. Surgery 89:588, 1981.
51. Hiebert CA, Belsey R: Incompetency of the gastric cardia without radiologic evidence of hiatus hernia. J Thorac Cardiovasc Surg 42:352, 1961.
52. Mays EE, Dubois JJ, Hamilton GB: Pulmonary fibrosis with tracheobronchial aspiration. Chest 69:512, 1976.
53. Urschel HC Jr, Paulson DL: Gastroesophageal reflux and hiatal hernia. J Thorac Cardiovasc Surg 53:21, 1967.
54. Crausaz FM, Favez G: Aspiration of solid food particles into lungs of patients with gastroesophageal reflux and chronic bronchial disease. Chest 93:376, 1988.
55. Johnson LF, Rajagopal KR: Aspiration resulting from gastroesophageal reflux: A cause of chronic bronchopulmonary disease (Editorial). Chest 93:676, 1988.
56. Wynne JW, Modell JH: Respiratory aspiration of stomach contents. Ann Intern Med 87:466, 1977.
56a. Matthay MA, Rosen GD: Acid aspiration induced lung injury. Am J Respir Crit Care Med 154:277, 1996.
57. Sladen A, Zanca P, Hadnott WH: Aspiration pneumonitis: The sequelae. Chest 59:448, 1971.
58. Steiner J, Bachofen M, Bachofen H: Recovery from aspiration pneumonitis. Pneumologie 151:127, 1974.
59. Broe PJ, Toung TJ, Permutt S, Cameron JL: Aspiration pneumonia: Treatment with pulmonary vasodilators. Surgery 94:95, 1983.
60. Booth DJ, Zuidema GD, Cameron JL: Aspiration pneumonia: Pulmonary arteriography after experimental aspiration. J Surg Res 12:48, 1972.
61. Cameron JL, Mitchell WH, Zuidema GD: Aspiration pneumonia: Clinical outcome following documented aspiration. Arch Surg 106:49, 1973.
62. Cameron JL, Sebor J, Anderson PR, Zuidema GD: Aspiration pneumonia: Results of treatment by positive-pressure ventilation in dogs. J Surg Res 8:447, 1968.
63. Cameron JL, Caldini P, Toung JK, Zuidema GD: Aspiration pneumonia: Physiologic data following experimental aspiration. Surgery 72:238, 1973.
64. Peitzman AB, Shires GT III, Illner HK, Shires GT: Pulmonary acid injury: Effects of positive end-expiratory pressure and crystalloid vs. colloid fluid resuscitation. Arch Surg 117:662, 1982.
65. Lawson DW, Defalco AJ, Phelps JA, et al: Corticosteroids as treatment for aspiration of gastric contents: An experimental study. Surgery 59:845, 1966.
66. Lowrey LD, Anderson M, Calhoun J, et al: Failure of corticosteroid therapy for experimental acid aspiration. J Surg Res 32:168, 1982.
67. Peitzman AB, Shires GT III, Illner H, Shires GT: The effect of intravenous steroids on alveolar-capillary membrane permeability in pulmonary acid injury. J Trauma 22:347, 1982.
68. Bernard GR, Luce JM, Sprung CL, et al: High-dose corticosteroids in patients with the adult respiratory distress syndrome. N Engl J Med 317:1565, 1987.
69. Johanson WG Jr, Jay SJ, Pierce AK: Bacterial growth in vivo: An important determinant of the pulmonary clearance of *Diplococcus pneumoniae* in rats. J Clin Invest 53:1320, 1974.
70. Dines DE, Titus JL, Sessler AD: Aspiration pneumonitis. Mayo Clin Proc 45:347, 1970.
71. Bartlett JG: Anaerobic bacterial infections of the lung and pleural space. Clin Infect Dis 4:S248, 1993.
72. Finegold SM: Aspiration pneumonia. Rev Infect Dis 9:S737, 1991.
73. Bartlett JG, Finegold SM: Anaerobic infections of the lung and pleural space. Am Rev Respir Dis 110:56, 1974.
74. Bartlett JG: Anaerobic bacterial infections of the lung. Chest 6:901, 1987.
75. Bartlett JG: Anaerobic bacterial pneumonitis. Am Rev Respir Dis 119:19, 1979.

76. Yamashita Y, Kohno S, Tanaka K, et al: Anaerobic respiratory infection—Evaluation of methods of obtaining specimens. Kansenshogaku Zasshi 68:631, 1994.
77. Beerens H, Tahon-Castel M: Infection Humaines a Bacteries Anaerobies Non-toxigenes. Brussels, Presses Academiques Europeennes, 1965, p 91.
78. Finegold SM, George WL, Mulligan ME: Anaerobic infections. Dis Mon 31:8, 1985.
79. Brook I, Finegold SM: Bacteriology of aspiration pneumonia in children. Pediatrics 65:1115, 1980.
80. Lorber B, Swenson RM: Bacteriology of aspiration pneumonia. Ann Intern Med 81:329, 1974.
81. Wimberly NW, Bass JB, Boyd BW, et al: Use of a bronchoscopic protected catheter brush for the diagnosis of pulmonary infections. Chest 81:556, 1982.
82. Henriquez AH, Mendoza J, Gonzalez PC: Quantitative culture of bronchoalveolar lavage from patients with anaerobic lung abscesses. J Infect Dis 164:414, 1991.
83. Bartlett JG: Diagnostic accuracy of transtracheal aspiration bacteriologic studies. Am Rev Respir Dis 115:777, 1977.
84. Appelbaum PC, Spangler SK, Jacobs MR: Beta-lactamase production and susceptibilities to amoxicillin, amoxicillin-clavulanate, ticarcillin, ticarcillin-clavulanate, cefoxitin, imipenem and metronidazole of 320 non–*Bacteroides fragilis Bacteroides* isolates and 129 fusobacteria from 28 U.S. centers. Antimicrob Agents Chemother 34:1546, 1990.
85. Bartlett JG, O'Keefe P, Tally FP, et al: The bacteriology of hospital-acquired pneumonia. Arch Intern Med 146:868, 1986.
86. Johanson WG, Pierce AK, Sanford JP: Changing pharyngeal bacterial flora of hospitalized patients: Emergence of gram-negative bacilli. N Engl J Med 281:1137, 1969.
87. Bartlett JG: Treatment of anaerobic pleuropulmonary infections. Ann Intern Med 83:376, 1975.
88. Bartlett JG, Gorbach SL: A comparison of penicillin and clindamycin in the treatment of aspiration pneumonia and lung abscess. JAMA 234:935, 1975.
89. Weiss W: Oral antibiotic therapy of acute primary lung abscess: Comparison of penicillin and tetracycline. Curr Ther Res 12:154, 1970.
90. Weiss W: Delayed cavity closure in acute nonspecific primary lung abscess. Am J Med Sci 255:313, 1968.
91. Weiss W: Cavity behavior in acute, primary nonspecific lung abscess. Am Rev Respir Dis 108:1273, 1973.
92. Levison ME, Mangura CT, Lorber B, et al: Clindamycin compared with penicillin for the treatment of anaerobic lung abscess. Ann Intern Med 98:466, 1983.
93. Gudiol F, Manressa F, Pallares R, et al: Clindamycin vs. penicillin for anaerobic lung infections. Arch Intern Med 158:2525, 1990.
94. Germaud P, Poirier J, Jacqueme P, et al: Monotherapy using amoxicillin/clavulanic acid as treatment of first choice in community-acquired lung abscess. Apropos of 57 cases. Rev Pneumol Clin 49:137, 1993.
95. Eykyn SJ: Therapeutic use of metronidazole in anaerobic infection: Six years' experience in a London hospital. Surgery 93:209, 1983.
96. Perlino CA: Metronidazole vs clindamycin treatment of anaerobic pulmonary infection. Arch Intern Med 141:1424, 1981.
97. Sanders CV, Hanna BJ, Lewis AB: Metronidazole in the treatment of anaerobic infections. Am Rev Respir Dis 120:337, 1979.
98. Colebatch HJH, Halmagyi DFJ: Reflex airway reaction to fluid aspiration. J Appl Physiol 17:787, 1964.
99. Modell JH, Moya F, Newby EJ, et al: The effects of fluid volume in seawater drowning. Ann Intern Med 67:68, 1967.
100. Modell JH, Moya F, Williams HD, Welbley TC: Changes in blood gases and A-aDO_2 during near drowning. Anesthesiology 29:456, 1968.
101. Abdulmajid OA, Ebeid AM, Motaweh MM, Kleibo S: Aspirated foreign bodies in the tracheobronchial tree: Report of 250 cases. Thorax 31:635, 1976.
102. Brooks JW: Foreign bodies in the air and food passages. Ann Surg 175:720, 1972.
103. Clerf LH: Foreign bodies in the air and food passages. Surg Gynecol Obstet 70:328, 1940.
104. Kim IG, Brummitt WM, Humphry A, et al: Foreign body in the airway: A review of 202 cases. Laryngoscope 83:347, 1973.
105. Haugen RK: The cafe coronary: Sudden deaths in restaurants. JAMA 186:142, 1963.
106. Hedblom CA: Foreign bodies of dental origin in a bronchus pulmonary complication. Ann Surg 71:568, 1920.
107. Lansing AM, Jamieson WG: Mechanisms of fever in pulmonary atelectasis. Arch Surg 87:184, 1963.
108. Zavala DC, Rhodes ML: Foreign body removal: A new role for the fiberoptic bronchoscope. Ann Otol Rhinol Laryngol 84:650, 1975.

64

Lung Abscess and Necrotizing Pneumonia

John G. Bartlett

Lung abscess is described as necrosis of the pulmonary parenchyma caused by a microbial infection. Some authorities categorize necrotizing pneumonia and lung gangrene separately in reference to multiple small pulmonary abscesses in contiguous areas of the lung. Numerous microbiologic agents can be responsible for lung abscess, but the usual agents are bacteria other than mycobacteria. Before the era of penicillin, lung abscess was a relatively common infection with considerable morbidity and mortality. Since that time, the incidence of lung abscess has been decreased by about 10-fold, and the mortality has decreased from 30% to 40% to 5% to 10%. Despite the apparent progress, there continues to be considerable controversy regarding methods to determine microbial agents and select antimicrobial agents.

Classification

A number of criteria have been used to classify lung abscess. Many of these were developed decades ago, when the infection was far more common. Lung abscess may be classified as acute or chronic on the basis of the duration of symptoms before the patient seeks medical care. The usual dividing line is 4 to 6 weeks. Lung abscess may also be considered primary or secondary on the basis of associated conditions. Abscesses in patients prone to aspiration or in previously healthy individuals are considered primary; secondary lesions are a complication of a primary condition in the lungs, such as a bronchogenic neoplasm or systemic disease that compromises immune defenses. Nonspecific lung abscess refers to lung abscess with no likely pathogen recovered from expectorated sputum. The presumed pathogens in most of these cases are anaerobic bacteria. Putrid lung abscess indicates the offensive odor of sputum or breath that is considered diagnostic of anaerobic infection, although 30% to 40% of patients with lung abscess due to anaerobic bacteria do not have this characteristic feature. In extensive experience with more than 1000 reported cases of lung abscess during the antibiotic era, approximately 80% were considered primary, 60% putrid, 40% nonspecific, and 40% chronic.[1–20]

Clinical Features

The most frequent pathogens are anaerobic bacteria. Patients with this type of infection usually have indolent symptoms combined with associated conditions that predispose to aspiration (see Chapter 63). The most common associated conditions are those that compromise consciousness or cause dysphagia.[5, 21–23] A second characteristic associated condition is periodontal infection with pyorrhea or gingivitis. The dominant organisms are located in the gingival crevice or gingival pockets, which represent the space separating the gum and tooth. In my experience, approximately 10% to 15% of patients with lung abscesses due to anaerobic bacteria have no apparent predisposition to aspiration or periodontal disease.[5, 21–23]

Symptoms associated with lung abscesses due to anaerobic bacteria are usually chronic, with complaints dating for weeks or months. The usual symptoms are fever, fatigue, and cough with sputum production, often associated with pleuritic pain and sometimes hemoptysis. Weight loss and anemia are often present and provide testimony to the chronicity of these infections, even in patients who report an abbreviated illness. Studies using sequential radiographs in experimental animals or in patients who have a defined period of aspiration indicate that the initial lesion is pneumonitis followed by cavitation, which usually appears at least 7 to 14 days later. The sputum is usually purulent, and approximately 60% of those with lung abscesses due to anaerobic bacteria will have putrid sputum, empyema fluid, or breath. Most have leukocytosis with peripheral white cell counts of 15,000 to 20,000/mm^3. About one third of patients develop empyema.

Occasional patients have a more fulminant course characterized by high fever, high white cell count, rapid spread to involve contiguous lung segments, and early involvement of the pleural space. This process is usually caused by anaerobic bacteria and is sometimes referred to as pulmonary gangrene.

TABLE 64–1 ■ Differential Diagnosis of a Cavitary Lesion on Chest Radiograph

Necrotizing infections
Bacteria: anaerobes *Staphylococcus aureus*, enteric gram-negative bacteria, *Pseudomonas aeruginosa*, *Legionella* spp., *Haemophilus influenzae*, *Streptococcus pyogenes*, *Streptococcus pneumoniae (?)*, *Rhodococcus*, *Actinomyces*
Mycobacteria: *Mycobacterium tuberculosis*, *Mycobacterium kansasii*, *Myocbacterium avium-intracellulare*
Bacteria-like: *Nocardia* spp.
Fungi: *Coccidioides immitis*, *Histoplasma capsulatum*, *Blastomyces hominis*, *Aspergillus* spp., *Mucor* spp.
Parasitic: *Entamoeba histolytica*, *Paragonimus westermani*, *Echinococcus*
Cavitary infarction
Bland infarction (with or without superimposed infection)
Septic embolism
S. aureus, anaerobes, others
Vasculitis
Wegener granulomatosis, periarteritis
Neoplasms
Bronchogenic carcinoma, metastatic carcinoma, lymphoma
Miscellaneous lesions
Cysts, blebs, bullae, or pneumatocele with or without fluid collections
Sequestration
Empyema with air-fluid level
Bronchiectasis

Evaluation

The diagnosis of lung abscess is generally established with a chest radiograph showing an infiltrate in the pulmonary parenchyma with a cavity indicating necrosis of tissue, often in association with an air-fluid level. The differential diagnosis for radiographs with this finding is provided in Table 64–1. With the usual pyogenic bacteria, there is usually an irregular thick-walled mass containing gas with or without a fluid level. The infiltrate is usually confined to a pulmonary segment or lobe, and there is no associated lymphadenopathy. Associated pleural effusions are common and may represent empyema. Other diagnostic considerations with lucent areas on the chest radiograph are cysts, blebs, bullae, and pneumatoceles; all have walls with a thickness less than 1 mm, which distinguishes them from abscesses. Computed tomography is an especially sensitive method to detect lung abscesses. With computed tomography, compared with chest radiography, the abscess is apparent earlier and anatomic definition is better. Computed tomography is regarded as more sensitive, and it clearly distinguishes air-fluid levels in the pleural space from those due to lung abscess in the pulmonary parenchyma.[24–27] The usual anatomic locations of anaerobic lung abscesses are the segments that are dependent in the recumbent position, including the superior segments of the lower lobe and the posterior segments of the upper lobe.

Microbiologic studies in patients with cavitary lesions of the lung should include stains and culture of expectorated sputum for detecting fungi, mycobacteria, and aerobic bacteria. Thoracocentesis should be performed on patients with an associated pleural effusion; the fluid is used for aerobic and anaerobic culture. Other acceptable methods of obtaining specimens for anaerobic culture include transtracheal aspiration, transthoracic aspiration, and fiberoptic bronchoscopy using the protected brush or bronchoalveolar lavage and quantitative cultures.[28–32] Experience with quantitative cultures of bronchoscopy specimens for anaerobes is limited but promising.[31, 32] Blood cultures should be performed in patients with a "septic" clinical picture, but these are commonly positive only in infections due to pyogenic bacteria other than anaerobes. The typical presentation is a patient who is prone to aspiration with an abscess in a dependent pulmonary segment and putrid sputum. In such cases, a presumptive diagnosis of anaerobic infection can be made without the need for invasive diagnostic studies. When the etiologic agent is less apparent and other cultures (pleural fluid, blood, and expectorated sputum) are negative, invasive tests are better justified. The indications and the specific technique used are variable, depending to a large extent on the available resources and the likely pathogens according to the clinical setting. Any of these diagnostic tests for bacteria are considered relatively unreliable after antimicrobial agents are given; this especially applies to fragile organisms such as anaerobes.

A common recommendation in previous years was to perform bronchoscopy in virtually all patients with lung abscess to facilitate drainage and detect underlying pulmonary lesions. However, there has been no convincing evidence that this procedure is therapeutically beneficial, and the need to detect underlying pulmonary lesions in patients with typical presentations is not cost-effective. As a consequence, bronchoscopy is now generally reserved for patients who have an atypical presentation, who fail to respond to antibiotic treatment directed against likely pathogens, or in whom there is a specific reason to suspect a localized lesion, especially bronchogenic neoplasms.[33]

Bacteriology

The usual bacteria responsible for lung abscess are anaerobic bacteria that colonize the gingival crevice. The prominent role of these organisms in lung abscess was established by the pioneering work of David Smith[34–36] in the late 1920s.

My experience with bacteriologic studies of patients with lung abscess based on cultures of transtracheal aspirates, empyema fluid, thoracotomy aspirates, or positive blood cultures is summarized in Table 64–2. The results show that 89% of infections involved anaerobic bacteria. The major isolates were *Peptostreptococcus* spp., *Prevotella melaninogenica* (formerly *Bacteroides melaninogenicus*), and *Fusobacterium nucleatum*. Other investigators have found similar results regarding the frequency of recovery of anaerobic bacteria with uncontaminated specimens and the frequency of specific organisms.[37]

Other bacteria that occasionally cause lung abscess include *Staphylococcus aureus*,[38, 39] *Klebsiella pneumoniae*,[40] other gram-negative bacilli,[41] *Streptococcus pyogenes*,[42] *Pseudomonas pseudomallei*,[43] *Haemophilus influenzae* (primarily type b), *Legionella pneumophila*,[44] *Legionella micdadei*,[45] *Nocardia* spp., *Brucella*,[46] *Selenomonas*,[47] and *Actinomyces* spp. Parasites include *Paragonimus westermani* (lung fluke), *Entamoeba histolytica* (amebiasis), and *Echinococcus* (hydatid disease).[48, 49] There are occasional reports of *Streptococcus pneumoniae*, especially type 3, but some observers believe that this represents an anaerobic infection superimposed on pneumococcal pneumonia.[50] Multiple opportunistic pathogens have been reported in lung abscesses in patients with compromised cell-mediated immunity, including *Salmonella*,[51] *Rhodococcus*,[52–54] *Pseudomonas cepacia*,[55] and *Pneumocystis carinii*.[56] The most common bacterial causes of cavitation in patients with defective cell-mediated immunity are *Mycobacterium* and *Nocardia*. Fungi are also common causes of pulmonary cavitation in this population, including *Aspergillus*, *Cryptococcus*, and *Phycomycetes*, although these are not traditionally categorized as pyogenic lung abscesses. Cavitating septic emboli most often occur with tricuspid valve endocarditis in injection drug users, and *S. aureus* bacteremia is the usual cause. Occasional cases represent complications of septic thrombophlebitis due to jugular thrombophlebitis (Lemierre syndrome) or pelvic thrombophlebitis; the usual pathogens in these cases are anaerobes. Unique features of septic emboli are the associated conditions and the involvement of multiple noncontiguous areas of the lung.

Treatment

The natural history of pyogenic lung abscess was described by Allen and Blackman[57] in the prechemotherapeutic era.

TABLE 64–2 ■ Bacteriology of Lung Abscess

TOTAL CASES	93
Aerobic bacteria only	10 (11%)
Anaerobic bacteria only	43 (46%)
Mixed aerobes-anaerobes	40 (43%)
PREDOMINANT ISOLATES	
Aerobes	
Staphylococcus aureus	13 (4)*
Escherichia coli	9
Klebsiella pneumoniae	7 (3)
Pseudomonas aeruginosa	7 (1)
Streptococcus pneumoniae	6 (1)
Anaerobes	
Peptostreptococcus spp.	40 (12)
Fusobacterium nucleatum	34 (5)
Prevotella melaninogenica	32 (1)
Bacteroides fragilis group	14

*Frequency of isolation; number in parentheses is frequency of isolation in pure culture.

Adapted from Bartlett JG: Anaerobic bacterial infections of the lung. Chest 91:901, 1987.

These investigators reviewed 2114 cases reported before 1936, when there was nearly equal division between conservative management, bronchoscopic or postural drainage, and surgery. They noted a mortality of 32% to 34% with all three therapeutic approaches. Of the surviving patients, approximately half had persistent illness with recurrent abscesses, chronic empyema, debilitating bronchiectasis, and other sequelae. A subsequent review by Smith[36] of 1650 cases reported from 1935 to 1945, when sulfonamides were available, showed that these agents had no effect on outcome.

Resectional surgery was developed at the time that penicillin became available so that during the early 1950s, the relative merits of surgery and penicillin became the subject of great controversy. However, by the late 1950s, there was general agreement that most patients with primary lung abscess should be treated with a trial of antibiotics. The favored agent of the time was penicillin; tetracycline was used in patients who did not respond.[22, 23, 58–62] Important contributions were made by Weiss and Cherniack[62] at Philadelphia General Hospital, who showed that oral penicillin (750 mg of penicillin V four times daily) was as effective as high-dose intravenous penicillin G. Weiss showed that even patients with "delayed closure" (persistent cavity shown by chest radiograph after 4 to 6 weeks of treatment) would eventually respond to antibiotics,[58] that more than 90% of patients responded to penicillin,[58–62] and that the occasional penicillin failure generally responded to tetracycline.[59]

In more recent years, there has been concern about penicillin as the preferred agent. In vitro sensitivity data show that 15% to 25% of lung abscesses involve anaerobic bacteria that are resistant to this agent, primarily by the production of penicillinase. These include *P. melaninogenica, Bacteroides ruminicola, Campylobacter* (formerly *Bacteroides*) *gracilis, Bacteroides ureolyticus*, and others.[37, 63] More recent data suggest that up to 40% of fusobacteria and 60% of non-*fragilis Bacteroides* species may produce penicillinase.[64] Nevertheless, it is not clear that many or most patients with these strains will not respond to treatment with penicillins.

The only large-scale prospective studies in modern times that compared antibiotic regimens for anaerobic lung abscesses were reported by Levison and coworkers[65] in 1983 and Gudiol and colleagues[66] in 1990. Both groups compared clindamycin with high-dose intravenous penicillin and concluded that clindamycin was superior on the basis of rate of response, time to defervescence, time to resolution of putrid sputum, and rate of relapses. Another option is metronidazole combined with penicillin, which provides relatively low cost as well as excellent in vitro activity against anticipated pathogens. The published experience with metronidazole plus penicillin is favorable but limited[67]; however, the experience with metronidazole alone is poor despite excellent in vitro activity against virtually all anaerobes.[68, 69] The presumed explanation is that clinically important aerobic and microaerophilic streptococci are resistant to metronidazole, and this accounts for the recommendation for concurrent use of penicillin. Furthermore, care must be exercised in selecting this regimen for alcoholic patients because of the disulfiram reaction. A prospective but uncontrolled trial of ampicillin-clavulanate (4 g/d for 7 days or longer followed by 2 g/d for 14 days or longer) showed that 52 of 57 patients responded.[70]

Recommendations for the duration of therapy are variable and range from 3 weeks to several months. My practice is to continue these drugs according to serial chest radiographs.[22, 23] Drugs are discontinued when the radiograph is either clear or shows only a small stable residual lesion. The risk with premature discontinuation is relapse.

Many authorities emphasize the role of drainage, which is commonly viewed as the most important aspect in managing abscesses at virtually all anatomic sites. However, with lung

TABLE 64–3 ■ Mortality Rates for Lung Abscess

DATE OF REPORT	NUMBER OF PATIENTS	SURGICAL TREATMENT (%)	MORTALITY (%)
1889–1935	2114	49	34
1936–1945	1650	45	34
1946–1955	460	32	5
1956–1965	496	38	8
1966–1992	1709	14	10

Adapted from Bartlett JG: Anaerobic bacterial infections of the lung. Chest 91:901, 1987; and data from Bartlett JG: Anaerobic bacterial infections of the lung and pleural space. Clin Infect Dis 4:S248, 1993.

abscess, the air-fluid level that is characteristically found on the chest radiograph usually indicates communication with the bronchus, meaning that spontaneous drainage has already taken place. Improved drainage may be facilitated with physical therapy or bronchoscopy. However, as noted previously, initial studies with bronchoscopy in the prechemotherapeutic era showed no advantage. Aggressive attempts to drain substantial collections may result in spillage to other pulmonary segments with the immediate complication of airway obstruction.[71]

Surgery is reserved for a minority of patients, 10% to 12% in the cumulative literature experience for the past two decades (Table 64–3). The usual indications are failure to respond to medical management, suspected neoplasm, or hemorrhage. Failure to respond to antibiotics usually results from an obstructed bronchus, an extremely large abscess, an abscess that has been present long before treatment, and an abscess due to relatively resistant organisms such as *Pseudomonas aeruginosa*. The usual procedure in such cases is lobectomy or pneumonectomy. An alternative is percutaneous drainage, which is being used with increasing frequency, primarily in patients who fail to respond to medical therapy. This is often done under computed tomographic guidance, and the reported experience in about 30 patients showed nearly uniform response.[72–76] The aspirate should be submitted for microbiologic studies (bacteria, fungi, mycobacteria) and cytology.[77]

Response to Therapy

Patients with lung abscess usually show clinical improvement with decreased fever within 3 to 4 days of initiation of antibiotic treatment. Defervescence is expected within 7 to 10 days.[5, 58–62, 66, 67] Patients with fevers persisting for 7 to 14 days should undergo bronchoscopy or other diagnostic tests to better define anatomic changes and microbiologic findings. Cultures of expectorated sputum are not likely to be helpful at this juncture, except for detecting nonbacterial pathogens such as mycobacteria and fungi. The response to therapy by serial chest radiographs is delayed. In fact, infiltrates usually show progression during the first 3 days in approximately one half of patients, continuing for at least 1 week in about one third.[24] Pleural involvement is relatively common and may occur in an explosive fashion. The most frequent causes of failures with medical management include the failure to drain pleural collections; inappropriate choice of antimicrobial agents; an obstructed bronchus that prevents drainage; or refractory lesions due to an inadequate host, resistant organisms, or large cavity size.[78]

Mortality rates for primary lung abscess are generally reported at 5% to 15% (see Table 64–3). Clinical findings suggesting a poor prognosis include large cavity size, usually greater than 6 cm in diameter; symptoms that have persisted for 8 weeks or longer before presentation; necrotizing pneumonia or lung gangrene; elderly, debilitated, or immunologically compromised patients; abscesses that complicate bronchial obstruction; abscesses due to aerobic bacteria; and nosocomial acquisition. Perlman and colleagues[14] found only a single death among 57 patients with primary lung abscess, compared with a 75% mortality among patients who had abscesses associated with obstructing lesions or compromised host defense mechanisms. A review of lung abscess cases in Japan showed the mortality rate to be 2% in community-acquired cases and 67% for nosocomial cases.[79]

References

1. Abernathy RS: Antibiotic therapy of lung abscesses: Effectiveness of penicillin. Dis Chest 53:592, 1968.
2. Anderson MN, McDonald KE: Prognostic factors of results of treatment in pyogenic pulmonary abscess. J Thorac Surg 39:573, 1970.
3. Barnett TB, Herring CL: Lung abscess. Arch Intern Med 127:217, 1971.
4. Bartlett JG: Treatment of anaerobic pleuropulmonary infections. Ann Intern Med 83:376, 1975.
5. Bartlett JG, Gorbach SL, Tally FP, Finegold SM: Bacteriology and treatment of primary lung abscess. Am Rev Respir Dis 109:510, 1974.
6. Block JA, Wagley PF, Fisher MA: Delayed closure in lung abscess: A re-evaluation of the indications for surgery. Johns Hopkins Med J 126:19, 1969.
7. Collins HA, Guest JL, Daniel RA Jr: Primary lung abscess. J Thorac Cardiovasc Surg 47:383, 1964.
8. Drake EH, Stones FM Jr: The management of lung abscess with special reference to the place of antibiotics in therapy. Ann Intern Med 35:1218, 1951.
9. Fox JR, Hughes FA, Sutliff WD: Nonspecific lung abscess: Experience with fifty-five consecutive cases. J Thorac Surg 26:255, 1953.
10. Gopalakrishna KV, Lerner PI: Primary lung abscess. Cleve Clin Q 42:3, 1975.
11. Hagan JL, Hardy JD: Lung abscess revisited: A survey of 184 cases. Ann Surg 197:755, 1983.
12. Harber P, Terry PB: Fatal lung abscesses: Review of 11 years' experience. South Med J 74:281, 1981.
13. Jensen H, Amdrup E: Nonspecific abscesses of the lung 129 cases. Acta Chir Scand 127:487, 1964.
14. Perlman LV, Lerner E, D'Esopo N: Clinical classification and analysis of 97 cases of lung abscess. Am Rev Respir Dis 99:390, 1969.
15. Pohlson EC, McNamara J, Char C, Kurata B: Lung abscess: A changing pattern of the disease. Ann Surg 150:97, 1985.
16. Rambaugh IF, Prior JA: Lung abscess: A review of forty-one cases. Ann Intern Med 55:223, 1961.
17. Schweppe HI, Knowles JH, Kane L: Lung abscess: An analysis of the Massachusetts General Hospital cases from 1943 through 1956. N Engl J Med 265:1039, 1961.
18. Shafron RD, Tate CF Jr: Lung abscess: A five-year evaluation. Dis Chest 53:12, 1968.
19. Shoemaker EH, Yow EM, Byrd WC: Antibiotic therapy of primary pulmonary abscess. Arch Intern Med 96:683, 1955.
20. Wolcott MW, Coury OH, Baum GL: Changing concepts in the therapy of lung abscess: A twenty year survey. Dis Chest 40:1, 1961.
21. Bartlett JG, Finegold SM: Anaerobic infections of the lung and pleural space. Am Rev Respir Dis 110:56, 1974.
22. Bartlett JG: Lung abscess. Johns Hopkins Med J 150:141, 1982.
23. Bartlett JG: Anaerobic bacterial infections of the lung and pleural space. Clin Infect Dis 4:S248, 1993.
24. Landay MJ, Christensen EE, Bynum LJ, Goodman C: Anaerobic pleural and pulmonary infections. AJR 134:233, 1980.
25. Stark DD, Federle MP, Goodman PC, Webb WR: Differentiating lung abscess and empyema: Radiography and computed tomography. AJR 141:163, 1983.
26. Williford ME, Godwin JD: Computed tomography of lung abscess and empyema. Radiol Clin North Am 21:575, 1983.
27. Johnson JF, Shiels WE, White CB, Williams BD: Concealed pul-

monary abscess: Diagnosis by computed tomography. Pediatrics 78:283, 1986.
28. Bartlett JG: Diagnostic accuracy of transtracheal aspiration bacteriology. Am Rev Respir Dis 115:777, 1977.
29. Bartlett JG: The technique of transtracheal aspiration. J Crit Illness 1:43, 1986.
30. Bandt PD, Blank N, Casstellino RA: Needle diagnosis of pneumonitis: Value in high-risk patients. JAMA 220:1578, 1972.
31. Wimberley NW, Bass JB, Boyd BW, et al: Use of a bronchoscopic protected catheter brush for the diagnosis of pulmonary infections. Chest 81:556, 1982.
32. Henriquez AH, Mendoza J, Gonzalez PC: Quantitative culture of bronchoalveolar lavage from patients with anaerobic lung abscesses. J Infect Dis 164:414, 1991.
33. Sosenko A, Glassroth J: Fiberoptic bronchoscopy in the evaluation of lung abscesses. Chest 87:489, 1985.
34. Smith DT: Experimental aspiratory abscess. Arch Surg 14:231, 1927.
35. Smith DT: Fuso-spirochetal disease of the lungs. Tubercle 9:420, 1928.
36. Smith DT: Medical treatment of acute and chronic pulmonary abscesses. J Thorac Surg 17:72, 1948.
37. Finegold SM, George WL, Mulligan ME: Anaerobic infections. Dis Mon 31:8, 1985.
38. Wollenman OJ, Finland M: Pathology of staphylococcal pneumonia complicating clinical influenza. Am J Pathol 19:23, 1943.
39. Fisher AM, Trever RW, Curtin JA, et al: Staphylococcal pneumonia: A review of 21 cases in adults. N Engl J Med 258:919, 1958.
40. Bullowa JGM, Chess J, Friedman NJ: Pneumonia due to *Bacillus friedlanderi*. Arch Intern Med 60:735, 1937.
41. Williams DM, Krick JA, Remington JS: Pulmonary infections in the compromised host. Am Rev Respir Dis 114:359, 1976.
42. Frieden TR, Biebuyck J, Hierholzer WJ Jr: Lung abscess with group A beta-hemolytic streptococcus. Case report and review. Arch Intern Med 151:1655, 1991.
43. Howe C, Sampath A, Spotnitz M: The pseudomallei group: A review. J Infect Dis 124:596, 1971.
44. Senecal JL, St-Antoine P, Beliveau C: *Legionella pneumophila* lung abscess in a patient with systemic lupus erythematosus. Am J Med Sci 293:309, 1987.
45. Halberstam M, Isenberg HD, Hilton E: Abscess and empyema caused by *Legionella micdadei*. J Clin Microbiol 30:512, 1992.
46. Papiris SA, Maniati MA, Haritou A, Constantopoulou SH: *Brucella* haemorrhagic pleural effusion. Eur Respir J 7:1369, 1994.
47. Bisiaux-Salauze B, Perez C, Sebald M, Petit JC: Bacteremias caused by *Selenomonas artemidis* and *Selenomonas infelix*. J Clin Microbiol 28:140, 1990.
48. Woolf DC: Presentation of *Echinococcus* infection as lung abscess. Trop Geogr Med 43:297, 1991.
49. Lamy AL, Cameron BH, LeBlanc JG, et al: Giant hydatid lung cysts in the Canadian northwest: Outcome of conservative treatment in three children. J Pediatr Surg 28:1140, 1993.
50. Leatherman JW, Iber C, Davies SF: Cavitation in bacteremic pneumococcal pneumonia. Am Rev Respir Dis 129:317, 1984.
51. Ankobiah WA, Salehi F: *Salmonella* lung abscess in a patient with acquired immunodeficiency syndrome (Letter). Chest 100:591, 1991.
52. Harvey RL, Sunstrum JC: *Rhodococcus equi* infection in patients with and without human immunodeficiency virus infection. Rev Infect Dis 13:139, 1991.
53. Verville TD, Huycke MM, Greenfield RA, et al: *Rhodococcus equi* infections of humans. 12 cases and a review of the literature. Medicine (Baltimore) 73:119, 1994.
54. Shapiro JM, Romney BM, Weiden MD, et al: *Rhodococcus equi* endobronchial mass with lung abscess in a patient with AIDS. Thorax 47:62, 1992.
55. Snell GI, de Hoyos A, Krajden M, et al: *Pseudomonas cepacia* in lung transplant recipients. Chest 103:466, 1993.
56. Ungar JD, Rose HD, Unger GF: Gram-negative pneumonia. Radiology 107:283, 1973.
57. Allen CI, Blackman JF: Treatment of lung abscess with report of 100 consecutive cases. J Thorac Surg 6:156, 1936.
58. Weiss W: Delayed cavity closure in acute nonspecific primary lung abscess. Am J Med Sci 255:313, 1968.
59. Weiss W: Oral antibiotic therapy of acute primary lung abscess: Comparison of penicillin and tetracycline. Curr Ther Res 12:154, 1970.
60. Weiss W: Cavity behavior in acute, primary, nonspecific lung abscess. Am Rev Respir Dis 108:1273, 1973.
61. Weiss W: Letter to the editor. Chest 67:625, 1975.
62. Weiss W, Cherniack NS: Acute nonspecific lung abscess: A controlled study comparing orally and parenterally administered penicillin G. Chest 66:348, 1974.
63. Finegold SM, Rolfe RD: Susceptibility testing of anaerobic bacteria. Diagn Microbiol Infect Dis 1:33, 1983.
64. Appelbaum PC, Spangler SK, Jacobs MR: Beta-lactamase production and susceptibilities to amoxicillin, amoxicillin-clavulanate, ticarcillin, ticarcillin-clavulanate, cefoxitin, imipenem and metronidazole of 320 non–*Bacteroides fragilis Bacteroides* isolates and 129 fusobacteria from 28 U.S. centers. Antimicrob Agents Chemother 34:1546, 1990.
65. Levison ME, Mangura CT, Lorber B, et al: Clindamycin compared with penicillin for the treatment of anaerobic lung abscess. Ann Intern Med 98:466, 1983.
66. Gudiol F, Manressa F, Pallares R, et al: Clindamycin vs. penicillin for anaerobic lung infections. Arch Intern Med 158:2525, 1990.
67. Eykyn SJ: The therapeutic use of metronidazole in anaerobic infection: Six years' experience in a London hospital. Surgery 93:209, 1983.
68. Perlino CA: Metronidazole vs. clindamycin treatment of anaerobic pulmonary infection. Arch Intern Med 141:1424, 1981.
69. Sanders CV, Hanna BJ, Lewis AC: Metronidazole in the treatment of anaerobic infections. Am Rev Respir Dis 120:337, 1979.
70. Germaud P, Poirier J, Jacqueme P, et al: Monotherapy using amoxicillin/clavulanic acid as treatment of first choice in community-acquired lung abscess. Apropos of 57 cases. Rev Pneumol Clin 49:137, 1993.
71. Rasanen J, Bools JC, Downs JB: Endobronchial drainage of undiagnosed lung abscess during chest physical therapy: A case report. Phys Ther 68:371, 1988.
72. Vainrub B, Musher DM, Guinn GA, et al: Percutaneous drainage of lung abscess. Am Rev Respir Dis 117:153, 1978.
73. Weissberg D: Percutaneous drainage of lung abscess. J Thorac Cardiovasc Surg 87:308, 1984.
74. Ha HK, Kang MW, Park JM, et al: Lung abscess. Percutaneous catheter therapy. Acta Radiol 34:362, 1993.
75. VanSonnenberg E, D'Agostino HB, Casola G, et al: Lung abscess: CT-guided drainage. Radiology 178:347, 1991.
76. Shim C, Santos GH, Zelefsky M: Percutaneous drainage of lung abscess. Lung 168:201, 1990.
77. Aizumi K, Watanabe A, Saito A, et al: Yield of percutaneous needle lung aspiration in lung abscess. Chest 97:69, 1990.
78. Cordice JW Jr, Chitkara RK: The role of surgery in treating pleuropulmonary suppurative disease—Review of 77 cases managed at Queens Hospital Center between 1986 and 1989. J Natl Med Assoc 84:145, 1992.
79. Mori T, Ebe T, Takahashi M, et al: Lung abscess: Analysis of 66 cases from 1979 to 1991. Intern Med 32:278, 1993.

65

Empyema

John G. Bartlett

Empyema has been the subject of extensive study since the time of Hippocrates. Considerable differences have been noted in studies of empyema depending on the period of study and investigator bias regarding incidence, bacteriologic findings, and guidelines for management. Most empyemas represent complications of bacterial pneumonias; less common predisposing causes are prior thoracic surgery, chest trauma, esophageal rupture, subdiaphragmatic infection, and septicemia. About 40% of patients with bacterial pneumonias have pleural effusions, but less than 5% of these represent empyemas. The major challenge to clinicians is to determine which effusions require specific therapy, that is, which require drainage, which require chest tube drainage, and which require thoracic surgery.

Definition

Empyema means literally a purulent collection in a body cavity, but the term is often used synonymously with pleural empyema. The classic definition is pleural pus. Subsequent definitions used by various investigators include pleural fluid with a leukocyte count exceeding 25,000/mm^3 with a predominance of polymorphonuclear leukocytes, pleural fluid with microorganisms demonstrated by stain and/or culture, and physicochemical characteristics (low pH) of the pleural fluid. Particular attention has been paid to pleural fluid pH levels of 7.0 or lower, which strongly suggest empyema and the necessity for thoracostomy drainage.[1] Nevertheless, low pH levels may also be noted in pleural effusions associated with tuberculosis, malignancy, or rheumatoid arthritis.

Pathophysiology

The most common cause of empyema is extension of bacterial infection of the lung to the pleural space. This accounts for 40% to 60% of cases in most series.[2–20] Prior thoracic surgery accounts for 15% to 30% of cases, and extension from subdiaphragmatic infection accounts for 5% to 10%. Less frequent antecedent predisposing conditions are perforation of the esophagus, chest trauma (especially with hemothorax), embolic lesions (including tricuspid valve endocarditis), extension from perimandibular or neck space infection, inadvertent contamination of the pleura by drug users attempting injection into cervical veins, septicemia, and thoracentesis with inadequate sterile technique. These miscellaneous causes collectively account for 10% to 20%. Rare cases are idiopathic.[2–20]

Empyema after bacterial pneumonitis or lung abscess is the most common form. The usual mechanism is direct extension of the infection to an adjacent parapneumonic effusion. In the preantibiotic era, the dominant agent of pneumonia and empyema was clearly *Streptococcus pneumoniae.* Empyema was noted as a complication of pneumococcal pneumonia in 11% of 3131 cases reported by Finland[21] in 1939. A review of 3000 cases of empyema reported between 1934 and 1939 showed that 80% were associated with pneumonia; *S. pneumoniae* accounted for 64%.[22]

Another mechanism of postpneumonic empyema is by a bronchopleural fistula, which results when necrosis of tissue in the airways provides a direct conduit to the pleural cavity. Bronchopleural fistulae account for approximately 10% to 20% of all empyemas and are generally ascribed to the organisms most likely to cause pulmonary necrosis, most commonly anaerobic bacteria[1, 10, 17, 23]; less common causes of pulmonary necrosis are microaerophilic streptococci such as *Streptococcus milleri, Staphylococcus aureus,* Enterobacteriaceae, and pseudomonads.[24]

The host response to microorganisms in the pleural space is divided into three stages that merge indistinguishably. The time frame in this sequence largely accounts for the variations noted with analysis of pleural fluid and also dictates the appropriate methods of drainage.[2, 17] The initial stage is the exudated stage, in which there is a collection of thin, free-flowing fluid that shows a low number of leukocytes that are predominantly neutrophils, normal blood chemistries (pH higher than 7.2; lactate dehydrogenase values lower than 1000 IU/L), and negative microbial studies including Gram stain and culture. Adequate antibiotic treatment at this stage usually stops progression of the illness. The second stage is the fibropurulent stage in which a large number of polymorphonuclear leukocytes and fibrin accumulate. Pleural fluid analysis at this stage shows low pH, lactate dehydrogenase values higher than 1000 IU/L, and low glucose values; bacteria are seen on a Gram stain and cultures are positive. Fibrin is deposited in both the parietal and the visceral pleurae, at the site of involvement, causing loculation and fixation of the lung. These loculi make adequate drainage with chest tubes progressively difficult. The final stage is the organizing stage, in which fibroblasts produce a pleural peel of fibrous tissue. At this stage the empyema is regarded as chronic, the exudate is composed of thick pus, and the empyema may drain spontaneously through the chest wall (empyema necessitatis), or it may drain into the lung via a bronchopleural fistula. The lung at this stage is trapped and essentially nonfunctional.

Incidence

Empyema was once a relatively common complication of bacterial infections of the lung. In the prepenicillin era, it complicated 10% to 20% of cases of pneumococcal pneumonia.[21, 25, 26] Infection of the pleural space occurred relatively late in the disease course and was referred to as metapneumonic. This was in contrast to streptococcal empyema, which generally occurred early in the course of pneumonia and was referred to as synpneumonic.[27, 28] Since that time, there has been a notable decrease in the frequency of empyema and an even greater decrease in the frequency with which *S. pneumoniae* is recovered in pleural fluid. The implication is that previous antibiotic treatment successfully prevents this relatively late complication. Elfing[29] reviewed 21,000 cases of pulmonary infections between 1938 and 1952 and noted that the incidence of infections of the pulmonary parenchyma changed little during that period, whereas empyema nearly disappeared after antibiotics became available. Reports from thoracic surgery services also indicated a 5-fold to 10-fold decrease in rates of hospitalization for empyema.[30, 31] At present, the reported incidence of empyema is generally on the order of 0.5 to 0.8 per 1000 admissions.[4, 5, 7, 17] The frequency of empyema as a complication of lung resection is 1% to 5%[32, 33]; most of these empyemas are associated with a bronchopleural fistula.

Bacteriology

Microbiologic studies of empyema may be divided into three stages: the preantibiotic era, the early postantibiotic era, and the five decades of the antibiotic era (Table 65–1).

Preantibiotic Era

Multiple studies of empyema in the preantibiotic era showed that *S. pneumoniae* consistently accounted for 60% to 70% of all cases in adults; group A β-hemolytic streptococci accounted for 10% to 15%; and *S. aureus* accounted for 5% to 8%.[22, 25, 34–36] In a review of 5393 cases of pneumococcal pneumonia reported from 1926 to 1933, there were 286 with empyema, for a frequency of 5.3%.[26] Coliforms were so rare as to be the subject of anecdotal case reports. Anaerobic

TABLE 65–1 ■ Bacteriology of Empyema

LITERATURE SOURCE	YEARS REVIEWED	PATIENTS	NO. OF CASES	BACTERIOLOGIC FINDINGS* Sterile	SP	β-Streptococci	SA	GNB	Anaerobes	More Than One Species
Elher[22]	1934–1939	Literature review; all cases	3000	NS	1920 (64)	282 (9)	195 (7)	NS	5% putrid	NS
Novak[34]	1932–1939	All cases	500	NS	317 (63)	92 (16)	38 (5)	NS	7% putrid	NS
Hochberg and Kramer[35]	1929–1936	Children	267	NS	122 (46)	82 (31)	35 (13)	NS	NS	28 (10)
Yeh et al[3]	1956–1963	All cases	103	42 (4)	1 (2)	1 (2)	26 (43)	36 (59)	NS	16 (26)
Beerens and Tahon-Castel[37]	1948–1965	All cases	45	0	0	1 (2)	13 (29)	13 (29)	23 (51)	21 (47)
Stiles et al[38]	1955–1961	Children	152	84 (55)	6 (9)	NS	78 (51)	NS	NS	NS
Snider and Saleh[4]	1952–1967	Adults; VA hospital	79	15 (16)	7 (11)	6 (9)	42 (66)	36 (56)	6 (9)	25 (52)
Lutz et al[39]	1948–1962	All cases	638	NS	35 (5)	16 (3)	255 (40)	238 (37)	86 (13)	141 (22)
Simmons et al[6]	1957–1971	All cases	60	13 (22)	3 (6)	NS	11 (23)	23 (49)	0	29 (62)
Sullivan et al[40]	1950–1972	All cases	482	256 (53)	32 (13)	NS	31 (12)	16 (6)	42 (19)	58 (39)
Weese et al[5]	1967–1969	All cases	49	15 (31)	4 (12)	9 (26)	12 (35)	19 (56)	NS	6 (17)
Bartlett et al[10]	1971–1973	Adults	83	0	5 (6)	0	17 (20)	21 (25)	63 (76)	60 (72)
Varkey et al[7]	1969–1978	Adults	72	10 (14)	6 (10)	3 (5)	7 (11)	11 (18)	28 (39)	20 (32)
Benfield[11]	1968–1978	All cases	117	38 (32)	12 (15)	NS	20 (25)	23 (29)	9 (11)	NS
Mauroudis et al[8]	1970–1980	Adults	100	3 (3)	17 (17)	NS	33 (34)	35 (36)	25 (26)	42 (43)
Lemmer et al[12]	1978–1982	Adults	70	4 (6)	4 (6)	NS	27 (26)	13 (20)	20 (30)	41 (62)
Grant and Finley[9]	1970–1980	All cases	90	9 (10)	NS	NS	NS	NS	26 (32)	30 (37)
Mayo[13]	1955–1979	All cases	63	18 (29)	0	5 (11)	17 (38)	10 (22)	6 (13)	14 (31)
Caplan et al[41]	1982–1983	Trauma	31	0	0	3 (10)	14 (45)	11 (35)	3 (10)	14 (43)
Brook[42]	1974–1978	Children	72	0	13 (18)	3 (4)	10 (14)	8 (11)	24 (33)	14 (19)
Alfageme et al[18]	1984–1990	All cases	82	6 (7)	9 (11)	NS	11 (13)	21 (26)	32 (39)	30 (37)
Kelly and Morris[43]	1985–1993	Adults	60	13 (22)	5 (6)	NS	10 (17)	22 (27)	10 (17)	14 (17)
LeMense et al[20]	1989–1993	All cases	43	16 (37)	1 (2)	NS	11 (26)	1 (2)	5 (12)	7 (16)

*Numbers of cases, with percentage in parentheses, are given. SP, *Streptococcus pneumoniae;* SA, *Staphylococcus aureus;* GNB, gram-negative bacteria; NS, not specified.
Adapted from Bartlett JG: Bacterial infections of the pleural space. Semin Respir Infect 3:309, 1988.

cultures were infrequently done, but 5% to 7% of cases were noted to have putrid pleural fluid.

Early Antibiotic Era

Bacteriologic studies of empyema fluid after the introduction of penicillin in the mid-1940s through the late 1960s showed that 30% to 60% of cases were associated with sterile cultures of pleural fluid. Of those with positive cultures, *S. pneumoniae* accounted for only 5% to 10%, *S. aureus* accounted for 20% to 60%, and coliforms accounted for 30% to 60%.[3, 4, 37–39] Many of these infections were polymicrobial. Cultures for anaerobic bacteria were infrequently done, with the exception of the report by Beerens and Tahon-Castel[37] and periodic anecdotal case reports. Nevertheless, the frequency of negative cultures and polymicrobial infection suggested that these organisms were more prevalent than previously suspected.

More Recent Experience

During the past two decades increasing attention has been paid to the role of anaerobic bacteria, reflecting the heightened awareness of the role of anaerobic bacteria in diverse infections and the availability of GasPak jars, which permitted virtually all microbiology laboratories to cope with oxygen-sensitive bacteria. Nevertheless, the recovery rate of anaerobic bacteria in patients with empyema complicating community-acquired pneumonia or lung abscess is highly variable, ranging from 11% to 76%.[6–13, 20, 40, 42, 43] Important clues to these organisms are the presence of putrid pleural fluid, which is diagnostic of anaerobic infection, and a Gram stain showing a polymicrobial flora or a Gram stain showing bacteria with the morphologic characteristics of anaerobes. Important factors contributing to differences in bacteriology results are the host population, the associated conditions, the adequacy of anaerobic cultures, and the use of antibiotics before pleural fluid culture. Empyemas associated with thoracic surgery or chest trauma are usually caused by *S. aureus;* gram-negative bacteria are less frequent. Most infections involving anaerobes are polymicrobial; monomicrobial infections are most likely to involve *S. pneumoniae, S. aureus,* or gram-negative bacteria.

Clinical Features

The usual clinical presentation cannot be distinguished from that of pneumonitis or lung abscess. Common features include fever, cough, sputum production, and dyspnea. About 60% of patients complain of pleurisy. Physical examination usually shows evidence of pleural fluid with dullness and reduced breath sounds on the affected side. In general, it is not possible to distinguish patients with empyema from those with sterile parapneumonic effusions on the basis of history or physical examination. Chest radiographs show pleural effusions, which are most readily apparent at the costophrenic angles on the posteroanterior view and the posterior gutters on the lateral view. A lateral decubitus film will reveal smaller effusions. Some authorities consider the lateral decubitus film to be essential in the evaluation of small pleural effusions detected by blunting of a costophrenic angle.[2] If the distance from the inside chest wall to the bottom of the lung measures more than 10 mm, there should be a thoracentesis; smaller pleural effusions are considered insignificant. Computed tomography or ultrasonography is generally unnecessary but will distinguish pleural collections from parenchymal infiltrates.[44] The differential diagnosis of a pleural effusion includes pulmonary embolism, mycobacterial infection, viral infection, fungal infection, postcardiotomy syndrome, collagen-vascular disease (lupus or rheumatoid effusions), malignant effusion, drug-induced pulmonary disease, congestive heart failure, and sympathetic effusion reflecting subdiaphragmatic disease such as pancreatitis or subphrenic abscess. Patients with empyema usually show concurrent evidence of pneumonitis or lung abscess, but up to 25% show no evidence of infection of the pulmonary parenchyma.[45] Parapneumonic effusions are found in 30% to 40% of patients with bacterial pneumonias, but less than 5% satisfy the criteria for empyema.[2, 17, 46]

Diagnostic Studies

In suspected infection, analysis of pleural fluid is mandatory for diagnosis and treatment. Recommended routine tests include leukocyte count and differential, total protein, pH determination, levels of lactate dehydrogenase and glucose, Gram stain, and cultures for aerobic and anaerobic bacteria. Grossly purulent pleural fluid generally requires no diagnostic studies beyond culture. For patients without grossly purulent fluid, the findings on pleural fluid analysis often dictate management[2, 17] (Table 65–2). The utility of the diagnostic studies has been extensively reviewed but continues to be somewhat controversial.[45–48] A metaanalysis of seven studies reporting values for pH, lactate dehydrogenase, and glucose showed that pleural fluid pH had the highest diagnostic accuracy for identifying parapneumonic effusions that require drainage.[49] The decision threshold in this analysis varied between 7.21 and 7.29.

The Gram stain usually provides immediate information regarding the presence or absence of bacteria as well as morphologic features of the implicated organism to guide the initial selection of antimicrobial agents. Putrid odor to the fluid is considered diagnostic of anaerobic infection, although anaerobic organisms may be difficult to recover with culture due to faulty laboratory techniques or antecedent antibiotic treatment.

Therapy

The usual treatment for patients with empyema includes administration of antibiotics, supportive care, arbitrary use of thrombolytic agents, and drainage. The greatest controversy and most important decision concern the drainage procedure.

Antibiotic Selection

Antibiotic selection is obviously simplified if the bacteriologic diagnosis is established with a Gram stain and/or cultures of the empyema fluid. The majority of patients with empyema have positive cultures of pleural fluid if appropriate microbiologic processing is performed. The major exception concerns relatively fastidious organisms that may be difficult to recover after antibiotic treatment, such as *S. pneumoniae* and anaerobic bacteria. By contrast, *S. aureus* and aerobic gram-negative bacilli should be easily recovered. In vitro sensitivity tests are required as a guide to therapeutic agents. Antibiotics diffuse well into pleural fluid with or without infection so that local instillation is usually not advocated. Nevertheless, aminoglycosides and some β-lactam agents may be relatively inactive because of the presence of pus, low pH, and β-lactamase.[50]

Thrombolytic Agents

Streptokinase and urokinase are often advocated for patients with loculated effusions. The goal is to dissolve fibrin membranes to facilitate drainage. The usual regimen is 250,000 units of streptokinase or 100,000 units of urokinase in a volume of 100 mL delivered through the chest tube that is clamped for 1 to 2 hours. This may be given daily for up to 14 days. The reported experience is favorable but anecdotal.[51–53]

Drainage

The most controversial issue in the management of empyema concerns the timing and method of drainage. General guidelines are dictated largely by radiographic findings and analyses of pleural fluid that reflect the stage of the infection.[2, 9, 17, 54–63] Specific guidelines are summarized in Table 65–2. An alternative approach offered by LeMense and colleagues[20] is a decision tree based on chest computed tomography. If there are no multiple loculi the treatment is thoracentesis or thoracostomy drainage; if repeated computed tomography shows inadequate drainage at 24 hours, thrombolytics are added. If there are multiple loculi or an inadequate response to thrombolytics, the preferred treatment is thoracostomy drainage or decortication.

During the initial exudative phase, the fluid is thin and free flowing and the lung is easily reexpanded. This may resolve with antibiotic therapy for the associated pneumonia,

TABLE 65–2 ■ Classification and Therapy for Parapneumonic Effusions and Empyema

CLASS	DIAGNOSTIC CRITERIA	TREATMENT
Insignificant effusion	Small (<10 mm fluid on a lateral decubitus film; see text)	Antibiotics Thoracentesis usually unnecessary
Parapneumonic effusion	>10 mm thick on lateral decubitis film	Antibiotics Thoracentesis
Borderline complicated effusion	pH 7–7.2 and/or lactate dehydrogenase value >1000 IU/L; glucose level >40 mg/dL; negative Gram stain and culture	Antibiotics and serial thoracentesis Tube thoracostomy sometimes necessary
Simple complicated effusion	pH <7 and/or glucose value <40 mg/dL and/or positive Gram stain or culture	Antibiotics and tube thoracostomy
Complex complicated effusion	Above plus multiple loculi	Antibiotics Tube thoracostomy and thrombolytics
Simple empyema	Pus Single loculus or free-flowing fluid	Antibiotics Tube thoracostomy ± decortication
Complex empyema	Pus Multiple loculi	Antibiotics Tube thoracostomy and thrombolytics Thoracostomy or decortication

or repeated thoracentesis or tube thoracostomy drainage may be required. The necessity for thoracostomy drainage increases the lower the pH, the lower the glucose level, and the higher the lactate dehydrogenase level. Some authorities base the decision to perform thoracostomy in patients with nonpurulent effusions on the pleural fluid pH. Nearly all patients with a pH below 7.0 require tube drainage, and nearly all with a pH above 7.3 experience resolution without sequelae with appropriate antibiotics alone.[2, 17] Pleural fluid pH levels of 7.0 to 7.3 represent a gray zone; repeated pleural fluid analyses and careful clinical follow-up are required to evaluate the response to antibiotics.[2, 17, 20] Some authorities use repeated thoracentesis, resorting to thoracostomy only if there are persistent signs of sepsis after 3 or 4 days or rapid reaccumulation of fluid regardless of pleural fluid pH levels.

During the fibropurulent phase the fluid is too thick for adequate drainage by thoracentesis, so thoracostomy is required. Large-bore needles may be required to obtain diagnostic material. Drainage may be facilitated by fluoroscopic, computed tomographic, or ultrasonic guidance for catheter placement.[64–66] This type of closed drainage with suction is recommended as the initial procedure when the fluid is thick, there is evidence of a bronchopleural fistula, or the pleural fluid is putrid. The tubes are left in place until the cavity is obliterated by expansion of the lung, pleural drainage is small (less than 25 mL/d), infection is controlled with no fever (usually within 7 to 10 days), and any prior bronchopleural fistula is sealed airtight. Failure to respond with clinical improvement in 48 to 72 hours indicates inadequate drainage, occluded tube, improperly placed tube, debilitated host, inappropriate antibiotic selection, or severe pneumonia. The adequacy of tube placement may be evaluated with radiography or preferably computed tomography.

Open drainage with rib resection or decortication is required if the closed procedure fails. Indications are persistent signs of sepsis, failure to demonstrate reduction in cavity size, or inadequate removal of infected material despite reinsertion of tubes.[2, 17] Open drainage requires a pleural cavity with margins that are adherent to the chest wall. This usually occurs 1 to 2 weeks after thoracostomy drainage and can be demonstrated radiographically after the chest tube is opened. The procedure is performed in the operating room. Adhesions are lysed under direct vision and chest tubes are placed in appropriate sites, or a pleurocutaneous fistula is created (Eloesser procedure). Open drainage is seldom necessary when empyema is adequately treated early in its course.

During the late organizing phase, extensive fibrous material may compromise pulmonary function with a pleural peel and entrapment of the lung. This generally represents a complication of chronic empyema and is most common with anaerobic infections of the pleural space. Guidelines for management are controversial, as indicated by a survey at the 1991 American College of Chest Physicians Annual Scientific Assembly. The questions concerned management preference of an anaerobic multiloculated empyema. Of 339 respondents, 49% preferred decortication, 22% preferred open thoracotomy, 14% preferred a chest tube with streptokinase, 8% preferred a chest tube placed in the largest loculated area, and 7% preferred placement of multiple small-bore catheters with computed tomographic guidance.[63] Despite variations in opinion about the drainage procedure of choice, there is a consensus that delay in drainage contributes significantly to morbidity and mortality.[62]

Mortality

There is considerable variation in mortalities reported for empyema in different series. This variation is perhaps best ascribed to variations in the population studied the time of the report, studies from thoracic surgery versus medical services, the type of treatment used, and the distinction between mortality ascribed directly to empyema versus mortality with empyema as a contributing factor. However, even studies from the prepenicillin era, when 60% to 70% of cases were associated with pneumococcal pneumonia and involved patients with a relatively consistent demographic profile, mortalities ranged from 7% to 41%.[22, 34–37, 67] During the antibiotic era, most studies have indicated mortalities ranging from 8% to 20%[3–12, 68, 69]; these include series published in the 1990s.[18, 20, 43] Of particular note is the report by Finland and Barnes[70] of 452 patients seen at Boston City Hospital. Approximately half were seen in the prepenicillin era and half thereafter.[70] The overall mortality in this series was 49%. Empyema was generally considered directly responsible for the fatal outcome, and there was minimal change between the results before and after the availability of penicillin. Factors that bore an ominous prognosis included the presence of a bronchopleural fistula, chronic empyema, nosocomial acquisition, cases involving aerobic gram-negative bacilli, old age (or adults versus children), and association with malignant neoplasms. By excluding patients with serious or ultimately lethal associated conditions, some investigators have reported mortality rates of only 3% to 6%.[3, 4, 7, 16, 68]

References

1. Bartlett JG: Bacterial infections of the pleural space. Semin Respir Infect 3:309, 1988.
2. Light RW: A new classification of parapneumonic effusions and empyema. Chest 108:299, 1995.
3. Yeh T, Hall D, Ellison R: Empyema thoracis: A review of 110 cases. Am Rev Respir Dis 88:785, 1963.
4. Snider G, Saleh S: Empyema of the thorax in adults: Review of 105 cases. Dis Chest 54:12, 1968.
5. Weese W, Shindler E, Smith I, et al: Empyema of the thorax then and now. Arch Intern Med 131:516, 1973.
6. Simmons E, Sauer P, Elkadi A, et al: Review of nontuberculous empyema at the University of Missouri Medical Center from 1957 to 1971. J Thorac Cardiovasc Surg 64:578, 1972.
7. Varkey B, Rose H, Kutty K, et al: Empyema thoracis during a ten-year period. Arch Intern Med 141:1771, 1981.
8. Mauroudis C, Symmonds J, Minagi H, et al: Improved survival in management of empyema thoracis. J Thorac Cardiovasc Surg 82:49, 1981.
9. Grant D, Finley R: Empyema: Analysis of treatment techniques. Can J Surg 28:449, 1985.
10. Bartlett J, Thadepalli H, Gorbach S, et al: Bacteriology of empyema. Lancet 1:338, 1974.
11. Benfield G: Recent trends in empyema thoracis. Br J Dis Chest 75:358, 1981.
12. Lemmer J, Rotham M, Orringer M: Modern management of adult thoracic empyema. J Thorac Cardiovasc Surg 90:849, 1985.
13. Mayo P: Early thoracotomy and decortication for nontuberculous empyema in adults with and without underlying disease: A 25 year review. Am Surg 51:230, 1985.
14. LeBlanc K, Tucker W: Empyema of the thorax. Surg Gynecol Obstet 158:66, 1984.
15. Meyerovitch J, Shohet I, Rubinstein E: Analysis of 37 cases of pleural empyema. Eur J Clin Microbiol 4:337, 1985.
16. Geha A: Pleural empyema: Changing etiologic, bacteriologic, and therapeutic aspects. J Thorac Cardiovasc Surg 61:626, 1971.
17. Light RW: Pleural Diseases. Baltimore, Williams & Wilkins, 1995.
18. Alfageme I, Munoz F, Pena N, Umbria S: Empyema of the thorax in adults. Etiology, microbiologic findings, and management. Chest 103:839, 1993.
19. Wiedemann HP, Rice TW: Lung abscess and empyema. Semin Thorac Cardiovasc Surg 7:119, 1995.
20. LeMense GP, Strange C, Sahn SA: Empyema thoracis. Therapeutic management and outcome. Chest 107:1532, 1995.
21. Finland M: The significance of pneumococcal types in disease,

including types IV to XXXII (Cooper). Ann Intern Med 15:1531, 1939.

22. Ehler AA: Non-tuberculous thoracic empyema: Collective review of literature from 1934 to 1939. Int Abstr Surg 72:17, 1941.
23. Bartlett JG: Anaerobic bacterial infections of the lung and pleural space. Clin Infect Dis 16(Suppl 4):S248, 1993.
24. Molina JM, Leport C, Bure A, et al: Clinical and bacterial features of infections caused by *Streptococcus milleri*. Scand J Infect Dis 23:659, 1991.
25. Finland M, Brown J, Ruegegger J: Anatomic and bacteriologic findings in infections with specific types of pneumococci, including types I to XXXII. Arch Pathol 23:801, 1937.
26. Heffron R: Pneumonia. Cambridge, MA, Harvard University Press, 1939, pp 566–585.
27. Keefer C, Rantz L, Rammelkamp C: Hemolytic streptococcal pneumonia and empyema: A study of 55 cases with special reference to treatment. Ann Intern Med 14:1533, 1941.
28. Welch C, Tombridge T, Baker W, et al: Beta-hemolytic streptococcal pneumonia: Report of an outbreak in a military population. Am J Med Sci 242:157, 1961.
29. Elfing G: A comparison of the frequency of lung abscess, pneumonia, acute bronchitis and acute pleural empyema. Acta Clin Scand 107:454, 1954.
30. Lindskog GE: Present day management of pleural empyema in infants and adults. N Engl J Med 255:320, 1956.
31. Ravitch M, Fein R: The changing picture of pneumonia and empyema in infants and children. JAMA 175:1039, 1961.
32. Deschamps C, Allen MS, Trastek VA, Pairolero PC: Empyema following pulmonary resection. Chest Surg Clin North Am 4:583, 1994.
33. Bernard A, Pillet M, Goudet P, Viard H: Antibiotic prophylaxis in pulmonary surgery. A prospective randomized double-blind trial of flash cefuroxime versus forty-eight-hour cefuroxime. J Thorac Cardiovasc Surg 107:896, 1994.
34. Novak S: Empyema thoracis: An analytical study of 500 cases with general remarks. Med Clin North Am 23:1355, 1939.
35. Hochberg LA, Kramer B: Acute empyema of the chest in children: A review of 300 cases. Am J Dis Child 57:1310, 1939.
36. Shank P: Empyema of the lung: Review of literature and analysis. Am J Surg 66:224, 1944.
37. Beerens H, Tahon-Castel M: Infection Humaines à Bacteries Anaérobies Non-toxigènes. Brussels, Academiques Européennes, 1965, p 92.
38. Stiles QR, Lindesmith GG, Tucker BL, et al: Pleural empyema in children. Ann Thorac Surg 10:37, 1970.
39. Lutz A, Grooten O, Berger M: Considerations apropos of germs isolated in 638 cases of purulent pleurisy. Strasbourg Med 2:119, 1963.
40. Sullivan K, O'Toole R, Fisher R, et al: Anaerobic empyema thoracis. Arch Intern Med 131:521, 1973.
41. Caplan ES, Hoyt N, Rodrigues A, et al: Empyema occurring in the multiply traumatized patient. J Trauma 24:785, 1984.
42. Brook I: Microbiology of empyema in children and adolescents. Pediatrics 85:722, 1990.
43. Kelly JW, Morris MJ: Empyema thoracis: Medical aspects of evaluation and treatment. South Med J 87:1102, 1994.
44. Schabel SI: Imaging of pleural infections. Semin Respir Infect 3:298, 1988.
45. Sokolowski JW Jr, Burgher LW, Jones FL Jr, et al: Guidelines for thoracentesis and needle biopsy of the pleura. Am Rev Respir Dis 140:257, 1989.
46. Storey D, Dines D, Coles D: Pleural effusion: A diagnostic dilemma. JAMA 236:2183, 1976.
47. Sahn S, Targl DA, Good JT: Experimental empyema: Time course and pathogenesis of pleural fluid acidosis and low pleural fluid glucose. Am Rev Respir Dis 120:355, 1979.
48. Potts DE, Taryle DA, Sahn SA: The glucose-pH relationship in parapneumonic effusions. Arch Intern Med 138:1378, 1978.
49. Heffner JE, Brown LK, Barbieri C, DeLeo JM: Pleural fluid chemical analysis in parapneumonic effusions. A meta-analysis. Am J Respir Crit Care Med 151:1700, 1995.
50. Hughes CE, Van Scoy RE: Antibiotic therapy of pleural empyema. Semin Respir Infect 6:94, 1991.
51. Henke CA, Leatherman JW: Intrapleurally administered streptokinase in the treatment of acute loculated nonpurulent parapneumonic effusions. Am Rev Respir Dis 1-45:680, 1992.
52. Robinson LA, Moulton AL, Fleming WH, et al: Intrapleural fibrinolytic treatment of multiloculated thoracic empyemas. Ann Thorac Surg 57:803, 1994.
53. Pollak JS, Passik CS: Intrapleural urokinase in the treatment of loculated pleural effusions. Chest 105:868, 1994.
54. Frimodt-Moller P, Vejlsted H: Early surgical intervention in nonspecific pleural empyema. J Thorac Cardiovasc Surg 33:41, 1985.
55. Morgan JF: Surgical management of pleural space infections. Semin Respir Infect 3:383, 1988.
56. le Roux BT, Mohlala ML, Odell JA et al: Suppurative diseases of the lung and pleural space: Empyema thoracis and lung abscess. Curr Probl Surg 23:5, 1986.
57. Iioka S, Sawamura K, Mori T, et al: Surgical treatment of chronic empyema: A new one-stage operation. J Thorac Cardiovasc Surg 90:179, 1985.
58. Orringer MB: Thoracic empyema: Back to basics. Chest 93:901, 1988.
59. Kaplan DK: Treatment of empyema thoracis. Thorax 49:845, 1994.
60. Odell JA: Management of empyema thoracis. J R Soc Med 87:466, 1994.
61. Strange C, Sahn SA: The clinician's perspective on parapneumonic effusions and empyema. Chest 103:259, 1993.
62. Ashbaugh DG: Empyema thoracis. Factors influencing morbidity and mortality. Chest 99:1162, 1991.
63. Yim AP, HO JK, Lee TW, Chung SS: Thoracoscopic management of pleural effusions revisited. Aust N Z J Surg 65:308, 1995.
64. Hunnam GR, Flower CD: Radiologically-guided percutaneous catheter drainage of empyemas. Clin Radiol 39:121, 1988.
65. Stavas J, vanSonnenberg E, Casola G, Wittich GR: Percutaneous drainage of infected and noninfected thoracic fluid collections. J Thorac Imaging 2:80, 1987.
66. O'Moore PV, Mueller PR, Simeone JF, et al: Sonographic guidance in diagnostic and therapeutic interventions in the pleural space. AJR 149:1, 1987.
67. Maes U: Mortality of empyema analysis of 100 consecutive deaths from records of charity hospital in New Orleans. J Thorac Surg 4:615, 1935.
68. Jess P, Brynitz S, Friis Moller A: Mortality in thoracic empyema. Scand J Thorac Cardiovasc Surg 18:85, 1984.
69. Cohn L, Blaisdell E: Surgical treatment of nontuberculous empyema. Arch Surg 100:376, 1970.
70. Finland M, Barnes M: Changing ecology of acute bacterial empyema: Occurrence and mortality at Boston City Hospital during 12 selected years from 1935 to 1972. J Infect Dis 137:274, 1978.

CARDIOVASCULAR SYSTEM

66

Blood Stream Invasion

John E. McGowan, Jr.
Jonas A. Shulman

Blood stream invasion (which for the purposes of this chapter means the presence in the blood stream of bacteria, fungi, or mycobacteria) remains a major problem for patient and physician alike. Blood stream infections remain common, and new patterns of occurrence and cause have made it more difficult for the physician to provide appropriate treatment. Moreover, rates of bacteremia and fungemia are useful sentinel indicators for overall change in severe infections, as study of blood stream invasion avoids some of the difficulties involved in defining infection at other sites.[1]

This chapter reviews blood stream invasion by bacteria, fungi, and mycobacteria. Endocarditis is excluded from the discussion, as it is the subject of Chapter 68. Septic shock, which is often associated with blood stream invasion, is covered separately as well (Chapter 67).

Occurrence

Several investigators have defined a variety of sepsis syndromes, usually in association with trials of therapeutic agents given for a heterogeneous and broad range of severe illness. Systemic inflammatory response syndrome, sepsis, severe sepsis, and septic shock have all been defined and used in various studies.[2] This presentation focuses on the classic and more conservative entity of blood stream invasion as defined by demonstration of bacteremia, fungemia, or viremia. Such restriction may correlate with the definition of sepsis (a systemic inflammatory response syndrome caused by documented infection) in some studies and not in others, depending on whether documentation of the infection by culture from sources other than the blood stream is accepted by a given study's authors.

Approximately 300,000 to 500,000 cases of bacteremia occur annually in the United States, and between 20% and 30% of the affected patients die.[3] The rate of discharge diagnoses reporting blood stream invasion increased from 74 cases per 10,000 patients in 1979 to 176 per 10,000 in 1987.[4] Table 66–1 lists incidence rates of blood stream invasion for some hospitals reporting overall incidence rates for nosocomial or community-acquired infection or both since 1975. Incidence rates are expressed in terms of admissions or discharges from the hospital.[5–34] The hospitals represented reported markedly different characteristics and overall attack rates of nosocomial bacteremia and fungemia. The table shows that reported rates of nosocomial bacteremia have increased dramatically in the 1990s. An overall incidence of bacteremia for one major city was 80 cases per 100,000 population per year.[35]

Etiologic Factors

Major changes have occurred in the cause of septicemia in the past few decades.[34] The relative frequency of some organisms and organism groups in selected studies since 1991 is shown in Table 66–2.[13, 23, 36] Some of the changes are discussed in the following sections.

Polymicrobial Sepsis

In a longitudinal study of blood stream invasion at Boston City Hospital from 1935 to 1972,[37] single isolates from cases of nosocomial blood stream invasion were the rule in the early years. In succeeding years, the average number of isolates per case gradually increased. This trend has continued to the present.[4] Polymicrobial sepsis is as likely in community-acquired as in nosocomial blood stream invasion.[29] The likelihood of isolating multiple pathogens is particularly high for patients in intensive care, for children, for diabetic patients, for patients with burns, and for those with malignancies.[38] In a study from France, 43% of patients with sepsis acquired in the intensive care unit (ICU) had polymicrobial infection, compared with 31% of those outside the ICU.[2]

Sequential Episodes of Infection in the Same Patient and at Multiple Sites

Not only are more organisms being found in each episode, but many patients now have more than one episode of blood stream invasion.[39]

Gram-Positive Organisms

A dramatic increase has been noted in the cases of bacteremia caused by gram-positive cocci both in the United States and around the world.[4] Infections with gram-positive bacilli are now becoming more frequent as well. In large measure this is due to increasing occurrence of antimicrobial resistance. Among major organisms accounting for this change are

1. *Streptococcus pneumoniae*. The organism remains important in community-acquired infections, especially in association with pneumonia. Mortality has not changed significantly in the past few decades.[40] Bacteremic pneumococcal strains resistant to penicillin have been associated with occurrence and complicate treatment.[41, 42] These strains are often multidrug resistant.[43] This brings renewed interest in pneumococcal vaccine, which can reduce the risk of pneumococcal bacteremia in high-risk patients.[44]
2. Group A and group B streptococci. Endemic cases of sepsis caused by group A streptococci are seen in both adults and children.[45, 46] Toxic shock syndrome may be part of the presentation of adults with bacteremia caused by group A streptococci.[47] Group B streptococcal sepsis continues to occur with some frequency, especially in older persons and in those with serious underlying conditions.[48, 49]
3. *Enterococcus*. Enterococcal sepsis can have severe consequences; overall mortality is 30% or higher, with significantly higher mortality in burn patients and other immunocompromised patients.[50, 51] The appearance of resistance to vancomycin, added to resistance to aminoglycosides and β-lactam drugs, has made therapy for enterococcal bacteremia much more difficult.[52] For some of these strains no antimicrobial treatment is currently available. Prior use of broad-spectrum cephalosporins has been implicated as a risk factor for nosocomial bacteremia with *Enterococcus faecalis*.[53]
4. Nonenterococcal group D, group C, and group G streptococci. The ability of the hospital laboratory to perform routine serogrouping of streptococcal isolates has shed new

TABLE 66–1 ■ Occurrence of Bacteremia and Fungemia in Selected Incidence Studies Since 1975

		INCIDENCE (CASES PER 1000 ADMISSIONS OR DISCHARGES)			
YEAR	**LOCATION**	**Overall**	**Community Acquired**	**Nosocomial**	**REFERENCE**
1975	Copenhagen, Denmark	7.2	3.5	3.7	5
1976	London, UK	1.3–6.6*			6
1977	Hackensack, NJ	5.6	3.3	2.3	7
1977	Houston, TX	3.8			8
1977	Madison, WI	3.4	2.2	1.2	9
1977	Atlanta, GA	14.7	9.9	4.8	10
1977	New York City, NY			1.5	11
1977	Charlottesville, VA			4.0	12
1974–1979	Bergen, Norway	4.3	2.1	2.4	13
1979	London, UK	6.1–8.0†			14
1981	Columbia, SC	2.8–15.4‡	1.9–6.8	0.9–9.8	15
1981	Madison, WI			7.5	16
1981	Iowa City, IA			6.7	4
1982	Madison, WI	3.4			17
1983	Denver, CO	12.5	4.4	8.1	18
1984	Huddinge, Sweden	4.3	2.1	2.4	19
1985	Kuwait	10.9	6.8	4.1	20
1985	Newcastle, Australia	5.4	3.3	2.1	21
1985	Atlanta, GA			5.8	22
1970–1986	London, UK		4.3‖	2.9‖	23
1986	Columbia, SC	10.0§	4.9	5.1	24
1986	Virginia			2.6¶	25
1984–1987	Vancouver, Canada	14.6			26
1987	Madison, WI	10.3			17
1987	Nottingham, UK	7.1			27
1987	Gainesville, FL; Iowa City, IA	2.6			28
1988	Barcelona, Spain	19.1	11.5	7.6	29
1979–1989	Berlin, Germany	8.1	3.8	4.3	30
1988–1989	Bergen, Norway	8.7	4.2	4.5	13
1981–1990	Oviedo, Spain	15.7			31
1990–1991	Hadyai, Thailand			15.5	32
1991	Iowa City, IA			21.3	4
1989–1992	Newcastle, UK	11.7			33
1992	Iowa City, IA			18.4	4

*Range of annual figures for the 10-y period 1966–1975.
†Range of annual figures for the 5-y period 1972–1976.
‡Range of figures for four hospitals in one city during the 3-y period 1977–1979.
§Mean value for four hospitals in one city during the 5-y period 1977–1981.
‖Episodes of bacteremia from 1969 to 1989; rate was calculated by using discharges for 1988–1989.
¶Combined data for average of 44 hospitals reporting data for 6 mo or more during the period 1978–1984.
Adapted in part from McGowan JE Jr: Septicaemia: Changing patterns of causative organisms and underlying conditions. *In* Shanson DC (ed): Septicaemia and Endocarditis: Clinical and Microbiological Aspects. London, Oxford University Press, 1989, p 8, by permission of Oxford University Press.

light on these organisms as a source of sepsis. Group C streptococcal bacteremia affects primarily older patients with severe underlying diseases and has an underlying focus in skin or soft tissue.[54, 55] Group G streptococcal bacteremia is commonly a community-acquired infection, seen especially in parenteral drug abusers and older patients.[55, 56] Biotyping of *Streptococcus bovis* has distinguished strains closely associated with bacteremia and colonic neoplasm (biotype 1) from other bacteremic strains of the organism.[57]

5. *Streptococcus viridans*. Soft tissue, skin, and respiratory tract infections are the most prominent conditions associated with sepsis caused by this group of organisms.[58] Neutropenic patients, especially those undergoing bone marrow transplantation, are at higher risk.[59, 60] Treatment is complicated by the presence of high-level resistance to aminoglycosides and resistance to penicillins in some strains.[61]

6. *Staphylococcus aureus*. This organism has continued to be a frequent source of both community-acquired and nosocomial blood stream invasion in the United States and in other countries.[62] Mortality remains high in series of bacteremia, especially those associated with methicillin-resistant strains.[63] Methicillin-resistant strains are prominent in many hospitals in the United States and elsewhere.[62, 63] Intravenous narcotic addiction, presence of a foreign body (e.g., arterial sheath catheters), and occurrence of septic pulmonary embolism are highly associated with a staphylococcal cause.[64] The disease is especially likely in patients with acquired immunodeficiency syndrome (AIDS), who have a higher rate of metastatic complications than other patients.[65] When bacteremic episodes recur they are often associated with the presence of intravascular foreign bodies (e.g., catheters).[66]

7. Coagulase-negative staphylococci and other components of endogenous flora. Many isolates of coagulase-negative staphylococci from blood do not represent true pathogens.[67] Nevertheless, in the right host setting the organism must be considered virulent.[68] Occurrence is often related to the presence of indwelling vascular catheters.[69] Bacteremia related to this organism has been shown to increase mortality and duration of hospital stay.[70]

Other components of endogenous flora are now known to have a potential similar to that of coagulase-negative staphy-

TABLE 66–2 ■ Relative Frequency of Selected Organisms in Community-Acquired and Nosocomial Blood Stream Invasion from Two Studies Published Since 1991*

ORGANISM GROUP AND SELECTED ORGANISMS	RELATIVE FREQUENCY OF ORGANISM (RANGE) (%) Community-Acquired Cases†	Nosocomial Cases‡
Gram-positive cocci		
Staphylococcus aureus	7–9	18–19
Coagulase-negative staphylococci	<2–11	8–10
Enterococcal species	<2–2	5–7
Pneumococcus	7–13	0–2
Viridans streptococcus	2–10	0–4
β-Hemolytic streptococci	4–5	0–2
Gram-positive rods	0–3	0–3
Gram-negative aerobic bacilli and coccobacilli		
Escherichia coli	25–27	16–19
Klebsiella species	<2–4	9–12
Proteus species	3–4	5–6
Pseudomonas species	0–1	4–9
Haemophilus influenzae	4–6	<1
Neisseria meningitidis	3–6	<1
Anaerobes		
Bacteroides species	1–6	<1–5
Candida species	<2	1–4

*Does not include data from the National Nosocomial Infections Surveillance (NNIS) Study of the CDC[36] as the NNIS program uses a definition of "primary blood stream invasion" that differs from that in the included studies.

†Range of values for cases of community-acquired bacteremia in 1969–1989[23] and 1988–1989.[13]

‡Range of values for cases of nosocomial bacteremia in 1969–1989[23] and 1988–1989.[13]

lococci for infecting the patient whose host defenses are sufficiently impaired. For example, antibiotic-resistant corynebacteria cause bacteremia, especially in patients with compromised host defenses.[71, 72] Vancomycin-resistant gram-positive bacilli such as *Lactobacillus* spp. are usually community acquired.[73] In immunosuppressed patients, *Bacillus* spp. organisms can cause septicemia, especially in association with Hickman and other long-term indwelling catheters.[74]

Gram-Negative Bacilli

Bacteremia caused by these organisms remains common.[75] In large measure this is due to increasing occurrence of antimicrobial resistance. A French study found that 69% of ICU-associated bacteremias were due to gram-negative bacilli, compared with 56% outside the ICU.[2] Among major organisms causing bacteremia in this group are

1. Enterobacteriaceae. Organisms of this group (e.g., *Escherichia coli, Klebsiella* spp., *Enterobacter* spp., *Proteus mirabilis, Serratia marcescens*) continue to be a major cause of gram-negative aerobic bacillary bacteremia.[76] Blood stream invasion caused by gram-negative bacilli has increased, perhaps because the organisms translocate more efficiently from the gastrointestinal tract than do other bacteria.[77] Although antimicrobial resistance has been a problem in some areas, it has been less so in others.[78] *E. coli* is usually the most common blood culture isolate in community-acquired infections.[23] In some settings, antimicrobial resistance is as frequent in community-acquired bacteremic strains of *E. coli* as in those of nosocomial origin.[79] *Klebsiella pneumoniae* continues to be important in both nosocomial and community-acquired bacteremias.[80] *Enterobacter* spp. have accounted for a sizable proportion (between 3% and 10%) of nosocomial bacteremic infections since the 1970s in both the United States and Europe.[81, 82] The role of *Enterobacter* spp. has been enhanced by frequent resistance to multiple antimicrobial agents and by association with vascular catheters and prior antimicrobial therapy.[83, 84] *Salmonella* bacteremia remains prominent in developing nations, in children, and in patients with AIDS.[85, 86] *Shigella* bacteremia is rare in adults, but patients with human immunodeficiency virus (HIV) infection may be at increased risk.[65] The major contexts in which bacteremic Enterobacteriaceae have been noted are hospital outbreaks associated with intestinal colonization, urinary catheterization, and resistance to many different antimicrobials.

2. *Pseudomonas* spp. For decades, *Pseudomonas aeruginosa* has been an appreciable source of both community-acquired and nosocomial bacteremias. High case-fatality rates have characterized cases associated with this organism.[62] Factors especially important in fatal outcomes of *P. aeruginosa* infection are shock, granulocyte count less than 500/mm³, inappropriate antimicrobial therapy, development of secondary foci of infection, and presence of AIDS.[87, 88] Community-acquired cases of bacteremia caused by *Pseudomonas* species other than *P. aeruginosa* have been rare, but nosocomial infections with these organisms are seen with increased frequency.[89] Nosocomial infections with these organisms tend to appear in association with contamination of a commercial product such as respiratory therapy equipment, disinfectants, blood gas analyzers, or blood products.[90] *Burkholderia* (formerly *Pseudomonas*) *cepacia* is a multidrug-resistant organism; associated cases of bacteremia are usually seen in the hospital setting.[91] *Chryseomonas luteola* (formerly Centers for Disease Control and Prevention [CDC] group Ve-1) and *Flavimonas oryzihabitans* (formerly CDC group Ve-2) have caused sepsis in association with neurosurgery.[92]

3. Gram-negative bacilli other than *Pseudomonas*. So-called nonfermenters (gram-negative aerobic bacilli that do not ferment the sugars commonly tested in clinical laboratories) include *Pseudomonas* spp. as well as other organisms. Among the non-*Pseudomonas* isolates appearing in blood stream invasion cases, *Acinetobacter* spp. are probably the most prominent. Although the organism on occasion is found in community-onset disease, its major importance is as a nosocomial pathogen. The spectrum of illness caused by *Acinetobacter* spp. ranges from mild and possibly self-limiting to serious and life threatening. Life-threatening infection is especially likely in those with compromised host defenses, burns, and trauma, especially after antimicrobials have been given.[93] Nosocomial strains frequently demonstrate resistance to many antimicrobial agents. *Flavobacterium meningosepticum* has caused a variety of nosocomial infections, and bacteremia is one of the situations in which it has been found.[94] Most hospital outbreaks associated with *Flavobacterium* spp. have involved environmental contamination of fluids, notably solutions, medications for respiratory therapy, or antiseptics. *Aeromonas* spp. cause infection more frequently in patients with underlying hepatic cirrhosis.[95] Several pseudooutbreaks with *Stenotrophomonas* (formerly *Xanthomonas*) *maltophilia* frequently make it difficult to assess the clinical impact of blood isolates of this organism.[89]

Gram-Negative Coccobacilli

Occurrence of sepsis caused by *Haemophilus influenzae* in children has decreased in association with the introduction of an effective vaccine.[96, 97] *Haemophilus* bacteremia in adults occurs more frequently in the elderly and is usually due to nontypable strains of *H. influenzae*.[98]

Meningococcemia still occurs in epidemic as well as endemic fashion.[99] *Branhamella (Moraxella) catarrhalis* bacteremia is typically accompanied by pneumonia in adults but may present without an obvious focus in neutropenic patients.[100]

Anaerobes

Cases of bacteremia associated with anaerobes have declined in frequency in some centers.[101] This has been especially the case for anaerobic blood stream infections in children.[102] *Bacteroides fragilis* and *Clostridium* spp. remain the most frequently reported anaerobic organisms causing bacteremia. In part this may be due to a selection bias, as many laboratories identify only certain anaerobes and provide a morphologic description for the remainder. Cases are often associated with malignancy or localized intraabdominal abscess formation.[103] Mortality associated with organisms of the *B. fragilis* group is still appreciable.[104]

Fungi

Rates of fungemia have increased at many hospital centers.[4, 105] For blood stream invasion by *Candida* spp., attributable mortality is high and hospital stay is prolonged.[106] Prior antimicrobial therapy, indwelling intravascular catheters, parenteral alimentation, urinary catheterization, central intravascular lines, burns, and neutropenia are significant risk factors for candidal blood stream invasion.[107] Candidemia can follow candiduria in rapid and often severe fashion.[108] Catheter-associated sepsis has also increased the frequency with which formerly unusual fungi such as non-*albicans Candida* spp., *Hansenula anomala,* and *Malassezia furfur* are recovered from blood.[109]

Nontuberculous Mycobacteria

The recovery from blood of nontuberculous mycobacteria of the *Mycobacterium avium* complex has become common as the number of patients with AIDS has increased.[110] The likelihood of such bacteremia can be predicted fairly well by several features of clinical and laboratory evaluation.[111] The rapidly growing mycobacteria (*Mycobacterium chelonae* and *Mycobacterium fortuitum*) are occasionally found to produce blood stream invasion.[112]

Other Organisms

Improved methods for detection have increased documentation of viremia with organisms such as herpes simplex virus.[113] Spirochetal culture can identify blood stream invasion with *Borrelia burgdorferi*, the agent of Lyme disease, although use of polymerase chain reaction is more sensitive for this purpose.[114] However, much remains to be learned about these and other nonbacterial organisms.

Pathogenesis

Organisms frequently enter the blood stream. Usually, host defenses clear these invaders without adverse effects on the patient. When host defenses become compromised or the organism's virulence is enhanced, illness may result.[62, 115] Host defenses may be impaired by the patient's primary disease, but blood stream invasion today arises commonly in association with therapy (e.g., antimicrobial agents, immunosuppressives) or with instruments used for the patient's care.[23] Even when no underlying disorder is present, consequences of bacteremia may be severe.[115]

Infection may occur as a result of invasion by an exogenous source. Today, however, bacteremic infection is more frequently due to organisms that are usually among the endogenous flora of the patient or that have replaced or joined the usual microbial flora at one or more body sites. Changes in usual flora are especially frequent after hospitalization.

Bacteremia occurs more frequently in neonates and older persons than in persons in age groups in between.[116] Septicemia in children has different implications and a different pattern than that in adults.[116, 117] In the elderly, blood stream infection acquired in the community is often as severe as cases acquired in the hospital, in contrast to the greater hazard from nosocomial infection in most other age groups.[27]

The relationship between sepsis and hematologic malignancy is especially prominent,[13, 23] as is the link between sepsis and other neoplasms.[118] Intravenous drug abusers are at higher risk of septicemia than many other population groups.[56] Frequently associated infections include endocarditis, abscess, and cellulitis.

Although opportunistic infections are considered more characteristic of those infected with HIV, bacteremia and fungemia still occur with considerable frequency.[119] Moreover, the associated illness may be of relatively greater severity—for example, AIDS patients with *Salmonella* infection experience recurrent bacteremia despite therapy.[86] Infections associated with instrumentation, such as with Hickman catheters, have high rates of associated bacteremia in HIV-infected patients.[120] Bacteremia with *S. aureus* may have more severe complications in AIDS patients than in patients without HIV infection; these *S. aureus* bacteremias may be more common in HIV-positive patients, even in the absence of indwelling intravenous catheters.[121]

Other groups at high risk of blood stream invasion include patients with liver or splenic dysfunction,[122] patients with burns,[107, 123] patients in ICUs, patients in long-term care facilities,[124] patients with implanted foreign bodies, and patients with indwelling urinary catheters. In particular, the profusion of intravascular catheters used in providing modern medical care in both hospital and community settings has led to greater risks of sepsis than in the past.[125, 126] These features account in large part for the increased frequency of blood stream invasion in patients in ICUs.[2, 13]

Use of multilumen catheters, tunneled central intravenous lines, arterial sheath catheters, or pressure transducers entails increased infection risk, which requires special policies for prevention.[64, 125] Gram-positive cocci, especially the coagulase-negative staphylococci, are the most prominent isolates for all types of intravascular catheters.[126] Bacterial sepsis associated with transfusion has been noted more frequently than in the past.[120] An unknown source of bacteremia is independently associated with a greater likelihood of fatal outcome.[127]

Prior antimicrobial therapy is associated with the presence of antimicrobial resistance in blood stream isolates.[42, 53] However, the cause and effect relationship is by no means a general one and probably holds only for specific organism-drug combinations.[78, 128]

Clinical Manifestations

No specific clinical findings are diagnostic of bacteremia or fungemia.[129] Early signs of blood stream invasion are nonspecific: malaise, lethargy, confusion, nausea, vomiting, and/or hyperventilation. Progression to a more classic history of fever, sweating, and shivering (chills) may or may not be noted.[130] Hypothermia may occur and is a sign of a particularly bad prognosis. On occasion, the only subjective manifestation may be a general feeling of unease or apprehension.

Objective signs of blood stream invasion may be few. Fever may be absent, especially in the elderly, the newborn, and patients receiving immunosuppressive drugs. In the absence of septic shock (see Chapter 67), the patient may or may not have tachycardia or tachypnea. Various rashes, evidence of embolization, or bleeding and clotting abnormalities may be present, especially in association with certain invading organisms (meningococcus, *Salmonella typhi*, *P. aeruginosa*). Skin findings accompany some cases,[131] and gastrointestinal symptoms, mental confusion symptoms, and mental or other brain dysfunction may be noted in others. Acute respiratory distress syndrome (shock lung) may appear during the course. Renal manifestations become prominent as an acute or subacute process.[132]

More prominent may be the signs and symptoms related to an underlying site of infection from which the organisms reach the blood stream. Infections of the urinary tract, surgical wounds, and gastrointestinal tract (including the biliary tree) are especially likely sources for blood stream invasion; these often have associated local manifestations. Infants and children with fever of unclear etiology may have occult bacteremia, and their evaluation often includes blood culture.[96, 117]

Changes in the white cell differential count and sustained neutrophilia often accompany sepsis. However, neither vital signs nor white cell count may be abnormal in bacteremic patients with AIDS.[133] Leukopenia or neutropenia may be characteristic of some infections (e.g., typhoid fever); however, in cases related to other pathogens neutropenia sometimes occurs and often indicates a poor prognosis. Of course, many patients with nosocomial bacteremia have extremely low neutrophil counts because of cancer chemotherapy or immunosuppressive drugs. Isolated thrombocytopenia is more frequently observed than disseminated intravascular coagulation.[132] At times, however, clotting disturbances may produce serious sequelae.

Diagnosis

Early recognition of bacteremia and its complications is the most important part of care. The physician must maintain a healthy suspicion for blood stream invasion, by searching for the clinical clues that lead to culture of blood, ancillary diagnostic testing, and/or empirical therapy.[134] Blood culture results have had a measurable positive impact on antibiotic treatment.[135] However, the cost-effectiveness of blood culture in some settings remains unclear.[136] Studies have led to models that predict patients at high and low risk for bacteremia.[137, 138] These appear promising but have yet to be evaluated prospectively in clinical practice. This is true as well for algorithms developed to help determine whether or not a positive blood culture represents contamination.[139]

Microbiologic cultures must be done before antimicrobial agents are given. Blood cultures are the most important part of the process, but cultures of other potential sources of blood stream invasion are appropriate when present (concurrent urinary tract infection, surgical wound infection, pneumonia, skin sites of sepsis). Culture of other sites is also necessary when complications of sepsis (e.g., meningitis) are suspected. Gram staining of material from local sites of infection (e.g., sputum, wound exudate, abscess drainage) may be useful. Additional nonculture tests (e.g., buffy coat smears, polymerase chain reaction, or other amplification techniques) are sometimes helpful; however, their use has not been beneficial in most situations and is, in general, reserved for carefully selected cases.[114] False-positive blood cultures can lead to diagnostic confusion and incorrect treatment, with grave consequences for the patients.[140] Thus, care in use of any of these methods is important.[141]

The recovery of infecting organisms is crucially dependent on methods used for culture.[134] For example, recovery varies directly with the volume of blood cultured.[142] At least 20 and preferably 30 mL should be collected with each venipuncture.[143] Two separate venipunctures should be done as a routine practice. The blood for culture should be drawn separately from blood for other determinations, such as blood gas, blood chemistry, and hematologic studies; if this is not possible, the blood culture vials must be filled before the other containers. Failing to observe this order can lead to epidemics of pseudobacteremia.[141] Blood cultures should be obtained by separate venipunctures, but there is no evidence that any particular interval between the collections is more efficient in demonstrating bacteremia.[144] Likewise, drawing arterial rather than venous blood for cultures has little justification. The effectiveness of adding ion-exchange resins to blood culture media to remove antimicrobials in blood is still being evaluated. Likewise, the advantages of using iodine rather than iodophor antiseptics before the skin is punctured are still debated.[145]

A major change in the past decade has been marked and rapid improvements in laboratory techniques for isolating and identifying organisms from culture of blood.[146–148] These technologic advances alone may account for some of the absolute increase in frequency of septicemia seen in the past five decades. The classic way to detect organisms in blood cultures was to incubate a liquid medium; observe it for a number of days for hemolysis, gas bubbles, or other change in physical characteristics; and then subculture to solid media if evidence of the presence of microorganisms was found. Newer methods detect gas production or other metabolic activity by organisms. This can be signaled by a variety of methods (e.g., infrared spectroscopy, color change in an indicator, pressure measurement). Instrumented approaches for detecting these signals are now widely used.[146] Another approach to diagnosis is lysis-centrifugation, in which the initial blood culture is treated with chemical agents to lyse the blood cells, centrifuged to concentrate any organisms, and then plated on a variety of media specific for bacteria, fungi, mycobacteria, or other organisms. These different methods vary in their ability to detect different groups of organisms. Lysis-centrifugation is more sensitive for detection of noncandidal fungi and mycobacteria in blood and is regarded as the method of choice for recovering these organisms.[149] However, for bacterial infection this method is more labor-intensive than use of automated instruments.[150, 151] No single method is satisfactory in identifying the presence of all bacterial organisms in blood or in recovering detected organisms in culture. Thus, in most hospitals one system is designated as the standard set for routine use to detect most common blood pathogens; supplemental methods are made available for special circumstances.

Processing of cultures depends on the system used. Most systems provide for distribution of the blood from venipuncture among at least two vials, one for aerobic incubation and one vial for anaerobic incubation. The time for which vials must be incubated before the culture is called negative varies with the processing method; with most of the newer systems, a 72-hour period of incubation detects most of the common pathogens.[152] In view of the frequency with which polymicrobial cases now occur (discussed previously), the laboratory must continue to look for pathogens in a blood culture even after one organism is recovered. Further steps in the processing of the vials are crucial if the laboratory intends to obtain a good yield; these steps have been reviewed in detail.[148]

When a patient with blood stream invasion responds well clinically, follow-up blood cultures are rarely indicated. However, if the patient fails to improve despite what seems to be appropriate therapy, cultures must be repeated in an attempt to detect "breakthrough" bacteremia.[153] This condition may indicate inadequate antimicrobial therapy, an undrained focus of infection, or an infected prosthesis. Emergence of resistance to antimicrobials during therapy is perhaps more likely in patients with *Enterobacter* spp. bacteremia.[81] These patients must be monitored closely for this possibility.

Treatment

For most cases of blood stream invasion, prompt initiation of aggressive, appropriate therapy is vital.[129] Beginning correct therapy before complications develop can reduce the mortality in bacterial sepsis[154] and probably affects mortality in cases related to other organisms as well. Treatment includes several steps other than antimicrobial therapy.[155] Ancillary measures to manage complications such as hypovolemia, metabolic problems, and organ dysfunction (e.g., renal failure) must be started immediately. Intravenous fluids, oxygen, or β-adrenergic agents may be required.

Antimicrobials are important not only for clearing the blood stream but also for preventing secondary infection from developing as a result of blood stream invasion, especially in *S. aureus* bacteremia.[66] Dealing with blood stream invasion is easiest when information is available about the site of infection, the identity of the infecting agent, or results of susceptibility testing for the causative organism. The site of infection can often be determined and at times can help the physician plan initial antimicrobial therapy and adjunctive measures (e.g., drainage of pus, removal of a foreign body) when antibiotics are chosen. However, it is rare to have information about the exact infecting pathogen or its susceptibilities when initial therapy must be given. Thus, empirical therapy based on site of infection and results of immediate tests (e.g., Gram staining, discussed later) is the rule rather than the exception. Treatment regimens are empirically chosen to try to eradicate the most likely etiologic agents in the hope that the choice can be modified on the basis of culture results and other subsequent information. Appropriate smears and cultures must be obtained before antimicrobial therapy is begun.

No single antimicrobial regimen is adequate to deal with all episodes of blood stream invasion.[76] The choice depends on the range of organisms commonly encountered in a given institution and the susceptibility patterns prevalent in these organisms. These factors determine whether single or combination therapy is preferred.[156] Thus, empirical therapy for infection must be tailored for the individual patient, but a variety of suitable regimens should be available at most centers.

Therapy should cover the sites of infection that seem likely from initial examination of the patient. No symptom or sign can clearly differentiate infection caused by gram-negative bacilli from those caused by gram-positive cocci or other organism groups, although appropriate Gram stains from localized sites of infection may help make this distinction. Some laboratory data may assist the clinician at this point; for example, a suspected urinary tract infection may be treated more logically after a urine specimen is examined. This can help in determining whether organisms are present and (if they are) deciding whether the infecting organism is a gram-positive coccus (suggesting *Enterococcus* as the source of sepsis), a gram-negative rod (suggesting a different group of antibacterial drug choices to deal with gram-negative aerobic bacilli), or yeast (suggesting *Candida* spp. or other fungi). Therapy for several newer bacteremic pathogens (e.g., nontuberculous mycobacteria) is hindered by the lack of controlled clinical treatment trials.[110]

TABLE 66–3 ■ Case Fatality Rates Associated with Blood Stream Invasion in Selected Series Published Since 1975

YEAR PUBLISHED	LOCATION	CASE-FATALITY RATES (%) Overall	Community Acquired	Nosocomial	REFERENCE
1975	Copenhagen, Denmark	25	18	33	5
1977	Hackensack, NJ	35	37	32	7
1977	Madison, WI	20			9
1977	New York City, NY			17	11
1977	Charlottesville, VA			34	12
1979	London, UK	42*			14
1981	Columbia, SC		11–28†	23–58†	15
1981	Madison, WI			40	16
1981	Iowa City, IA			51	4
1982	Madison, WI	21			17
1983	Denver, CO	42	21	52	18
1984	Huddinge, Sweden	13			19
1985	Newcastle, Australia			29	21
1986	Columbia, SC	30‡	20‡	40‡	24
1986	Berlin, Germany	22			30
1987	Nottingham, UK	29	23	36	27
1987	Gainesville, FL; Iowa City, IA	20			28
1988	Barcelona, Spain			18	29
1989	Berlin, Germany	21			30
1989	Bergen, Norway	19			13
1990–1991	Hadyai, Thailand			37	32
1989–1992	Newcastle, UK	7	9	5	33
1992	Iowa City, IA			32	4
1995	Petah Tiqva, Israel		23	42	163

*Range of annual figures for the 5-y period 1972–1976.
†Range of figures for four hospitals in one city during the 3-y period 1977–1979.
‡Mean value for four hospitals in one city during the 5-y period 1977–1981.
Adapted in part from McGowan JE Jr: Septicaemia: Changing patterns of causative organisms and underlying conditions. *In* Shanson DC (ed): Septicaemia and Endocarditis: Clinical and Microbiological Aspects. London, Oxford University Press, 1989, p 9, by permission of Oxford University Press.

The status of the patient's host defenses is another major factor. A patient with defective defenses has less margin of error for tolerating an inappropriate drug regimen. The prescriber should err on the side of increasing the spectrum of coverage for a brief period in such patients. The possible emergence of antimicrobial resistance during the course of therapy must be considered when patients fail to respond.[157]

This point should also be considered when empirical therapy is selected for AIDS patients with apparent blood stream invasion.[129] In addition, the effect of other therapeutic agents on the etiologic agent must be considered; for example, treatment with interleukin-2 appears to have a major effect in increasing the likelihood of bacterial infections in the patient with AIDS.[158] Likewise, in children with cancer the local epidemiologic patterns should determine empirical treatment.[159]

Close cooperation among the pharmacy, the nursing department, and the attending physician is required to ensure that the patient receives appropriate therapy.[154]

Course

Blood stream infection increases mortality.[160] Nosocomial cases increase attributable mortality, lead to an alarming increase in length of acute hospital stay, and add extra costs for care of about $40,000 per patient.[161] The fearsome toll of septicemia is dramatically illustrated by Table 66–3, which portrays case-fatality rates from a variety of the studies reported in Table 66–1.

Patients in intensive care experience case-fatality rates in the neighborhood of 50%.[2] This holds true for both directly related mortality (24% case-fatality rate for nosocomial cases versus 13% in community-acquired sepsis) and unrelated deaths. Bacteremia associated with lower respiratory tract sites or abdominal wound infections is associated with the highest mortality rates and the highest costs.[162] Blood stream invasion arising from other sources can be dealt with more readily in today's medical practice. For example, mortality associated with burns has decreased in the past decade.[123] About half of the patients with gram-negative bacteremia died in a Turkish study between 1983 and 1989.[75]

Not only is bacteremia associated with high short-term mortality, it is also a sign of poor long-term prognosis, especially for patients with low serum albumin levels, high serum creatinine values, and malignancy.[163] In addition to risk of mortality, risk of physical dysfunction increases after an episode of blood stream invasion.[164]

Antibiotic resistance is thought to increase risk of death. However, neither vancomycin resistance nor gentamicin resistance has led to greater mortality in patients with bacteremic enterococcal infection in comparison with those bacteremic with susceptible strains, after adjustment for factors such as underlying illness.[51, 165]

Prevention

Rapid and effective attention to other sites of infection can prevent the infection from reaching a level of severity at which blood stream invasion can occur. The key to minimizing the occurrence of nosocomial blood stream invasion is effective control of initial infection, as many hospital-acquired infections may lead to sepsis. Proper use of instruments, especially intravascular catheters, is the key to preventing their infection and resultant blood stream invasion.[166] New vaccines against common agents of bacteremia are in clinical trial, but their effectiveness and cost-efficiency have not yet been established. Use of prophylactic antimicrobials to attempt to "decontaminate" the gut and other endogenous sites for nosocomial pathogens has been proposed, but carefully controlled studies have not documented a benefit for this.[167]

References

1. Freeman J, McGowan JE Jr: Methodologic issues in hospital epidemiology. I. Rates, case-finding, and interpretation. Rev Infect Dis 3:658, 1981.
2. Brun-Buisson C, Doyon F, Carlet J, et al: Incidence, risk factors, and outcome of severe sepsis and septic shock in adults. A multicenter prospective study in intensive care units. JAMA 274:968, 1995.
3. Wenzel RP: Anti-endotoxin monoclonal antibodies: A second look. N Engl J Med 326:1151, 1992.
4. Pittet D, Wenzel RP: Nosocomial bloodstream infections. Secular trends in rates, mortality, and contribution to total hospital deaths. Arch Intern Med 155:1177, 1995.
5. Jepsen OB, Korner B: Bacteremia in a general hospital: A prospective study of 102 consecutive cases. Scand J Infect Dis 7:179, 1975.
6. Williams GT, Houang ET, Shaw EJ, Tabaqchali S: Bacteraemia in a London teaching hospital 1966–75. Lancet 2:1291, 1976.
7. Setia U, Gross PA: Bacteremia in a community hospital. Arch Intern Med 137:1698, 1977.
8. Quadri SMH, Evans LJ, Wende RD, Williams RP: Bacteremia in a metropolitan teaching hospital. Tex Med 73:59, 1977.
9. Scheckler WE: Septicemia in a community hospital 1970 through 1973. JAMA 237:1938, 1977.
10. McGowan JE Jr, Parrott PL, Duty VP: Nosocomial bacteremia: Potential for prevention. JAMA 237:2727, 1977.
11. Holzman RS, Florman AL, Toharsky B: The clinical usefulness of an ongoing bacteremia surveillance program. Am J Med Sci 274:13, 1977.
12. Rose RC, Hunting KJ, Townsend TR, Wenzel RP: Morbidity/mortality and economics of hospital-acquired bloodstream infections: A controlled study. South Med J 70:1267, 1977.
13. Haug JB, Harthug S, Kalager T, et al: Bloodstream infections at a Norwegian university hospital, 1974–1979 and 1988–1989: Changing etiology, clinical features, and outcome. Clin Infect Dis 19:246, 1994.
14. Abeysundere RL, Bradley JM, Chipping P, et al: Bacteraemia in the Royal Free Hospital 1972–1976. J Infect 1:127, 1979.
15. Brenner ER, Bryan CS. Nosocomial bacteremia in perspective: A community-wide study. Infect Control 2:219, 1981.
16. Maki DG. Epidemic nosocomial bacteremias. *In* Wenzel RP (ed): CRC Handbook of Hospital-Acquired Infections. West Palm Beach, FL, CRC Press, 1981, p 371.
17. Scheckler WE, Scheibel W, Kresge D: Temporal trends in septicemia in a community hospital. Am J Med 91(Suppl 3B):90S, 1991.
18. Weinstein MP, Reller LB, Murphy JR, Lichtenstein KA: The clinical significance of positive blood cultures: A comprehensive analysis of 500 episodes of bacteremia and fungemia in adults. I. Laboratory and epidemiologic observations. Rev Infect Dis 5:35, 1983.
19. Ljungman P, Malmborg AS, Nystrom B, Tillegard A: Bacteremia in a Swedish university hospital: A one-year prospective study in 1981 and a comparison with 1975–76. Infection 12:243, 1984.
20. Elhag KM, Mustafa AK, Sethi SK: Septicaemia in a teaching hospital in Kuwait. I: Incidence and aetiology. J Infect 10:17, 1985.
21. Duggan JM, Oldfield GS, Ghosh HK: Septicaemia as a hospital hazard. J Infect 6:406, 1985.
22. McGowan JE Jr: Changing etiology of nosocomial bacteremia and fungemia and other hospital-acquired infections. Rev Infect Dis 7(Suppl):S357, 1985.
23. Gransden WR: Predictors for bacteraemia. J Hosp Infect 18(Suppl A):308, 1991.
24. Bryan CS, Reynolds KL, Brenner ER: Analysis of 1,186 episodes of gram-negative bacteremia in non-university hospitals: The effects of antimicrobial therapy. Rev Infect Dis 5:629, 1986.
25. Morrison AJ Jr, Freer CV, Searcy MA, et al: Nosocomial bloodstream infections: Secular trends in a statewide surveillance program in Virginia. Infect Control 7:550, 1986.

26. Roberts FJ, Geere IW, Coldman A: A three-year study of positive blood cultures, with emphasis on prognosis. Rev Infect Dis 13:34, 1991.
27. Ispahani P, Pearson NJ, Greenwood D: An analysis of community and hospital-acquired bacteraemia in a large teaching hospital in the United Kingdom. Q J Med 241:427, 1987.
28. Haddy RI, Klimberg S, Epting RJ: A two-center review of bacteremia in the community hospital. J Fam Pract 24:253, 1987.
29. Gatell JM, Trilla A, Latorre X, et al: Nosocomial bacteremia in a large Spanish teaching hospital: Analysis of factors influencing prognosis. Rev Infect Dis 10:203, 1988.
30. Geerdes HF, Ziegler D, Lode H, et al: Septicemia in 980 patients at a university hospital in Berlin: Prospective studies during 4 selected years between 1979 and 1989. Clin Infect Dis 15:991, 1992.
31. Vazquez F, Mendoza MC, Villar MH, et al: Survey of bacteraemia in a Spanish hospital over a decade (1981–1990). J Hosp Infect 26:111, 1994.
32. Jamulitrat S, Meknavin U, Thongpiyapoom S: Factors affecting mortality, outcome and risk of developing nosocomial bloodstream infection. Infect Control Hosp Epidemiol 15:163, 1994.
33. Gray J, Pedler SJ: The changing face of bacteraemia. J Hosp Infect 28:317, 1994.
34. McGowan JE Jr: Septicaemia: Changing patterns of causative organisms and underlying conditions. *In* Shanson DC (ed): Septicaemia and Endocarditis: Clinical and Microbiological Aspects. London, Oxford University Press, 1989, p 5.
35. Filice GA, Van Etta LL, Darby CP, Fraser DW: Bacteremia in Charleston County, South Carolina. Am J Epidemiol 123:128, 1986.
36. Horan TC, White JW, Jarvis WR, et al: Nosocomial infection surveillance, 1984. MMWR CDC Surveill Summ 35:17SS, 1986.
37. McGowan JE Jr, Barnes MW, Finland M: Bacteremia at Boston City Hospital: Occurrence and mortality during 12 selected years (1935–1972), with special reference to hospital-acquired cases. J Infect Dis 132:316, 1975.
38. Reuben AG, Musher DM, Hamill RJ, Broucke I: Polymicrobial bacteremia: Clinical and microbiologic patterns. Rev Infect Dis 11:161, 1989.
39. Capdevila JA, Almirante B, Pahissa A, et al: Incidence and risk factors of recurrent episodes of bacteremia in adults. Arch Intern Med 154:411, 1994.
40. Afessa B, Greaves WL, Frederick WR: Pneumococcal bacteremia in adults: A 14-year experience in an inner-city university hospital. Clin Infect Dis 21:345, 1995.
41. Moreno F, Crisp C, Jorgensen JH, Patterson JE: The clinical and molecular epidemiology of bacteremias at a university hospital caused by pneumococci not susceptible to penicillin. J Infect Dis 172:427, 1995.
42. Nava JM, Bella F, Garau J, et al: Predictive factors for invasive disease due to penicillin-resistant *Streptococcus pneumoniae*: A population-based study. Clin Infect Dis 19:884, 1994.
43. Verhaegen J, Glupczynski Y, Verbist L, et al: Capsular types and antibiotic susceptibility of pneumococci isolated from patients in Belgium with serious infections, 1980–1993. Clin Infect Dis 20:1339, 1995.
44. Farr BM, Johnston BL, Cobb DK, et al: Preventing pneumococcal bacteremia in patients at risk: Results of a matched case-control study. Arch Intern Med 155:2336, 1995.
45. Moses AE, Mevorach D, Rahav G, et al: Group A streptococcus bacteremia at the Hadassah Medical Center in Jerusalem. Clin Infect Dis 20:1393, 1995.
46. Demers B, Simor AE, Vellend H, et al: Severe invasive group A streptococcal infections in Ontario, Canada: 1987–1991. Clin Infect Dis 16:792, 1993.
47. Forni AL, Kaplan EL, Schlievert PM, Roberts RB: Clinical and microbiological characteristics of severe group A streptococcus infections and streptococcal toxic shock syndrome. Clin Infect Dis 21:333, 1995.
48. Jackson LA, Hilsdon R, Farley MM, et al: Risk factors for group B streptococcal disease in adults. Ann Intern Med 123:415, 1995.
49. Colford JM Jr, Mohle-Boetani J, Vosti KL: Group B streptococcal bacteremia in adults. Five years' experience and a review of the literature. Medicine (Baltimore) 74:176, 1995.
50. Noskin GA, Peterson LR, Warren JR: *Enterococcus faecium* and *Enterococcus faecalis* bacteremia: Acquisition and outcome. Clin Infect Dis 20:296, 1995.
51. Antalek MD, Mylotte JM, Lesse AJ, Sellick JA Jr: Clinical and molecular epidemiology of *Enterococcus faecalis* bacteremia, with special reference to strains with high-level resistance to gentamicin. Clin Infect Dis 20:103, 1995.
52. Edmond MB, Ober JF, Weinbaum DL, et al: Vancomycin-resistant *Enterococcus faecium* bacteremia: Risk factors for infection. Clin Infect Dis 20:1126, 1995.
53. Pallares R, Pujol M, Pena C, et al: Cephalosporins as risk factor for nosocomial *Enterococcus faecalis* bacteremia. A matched case-control study. Arch Intern Med 153:1581, 1993.
54. Carmeli Y, Schapiro JM, Neeman D, et al: Streptococcal group C bacteremia. Survey in Israel and analytic review. Arch Intern Med 155:1170, 1995.
55. Kristensen B, Schonheyder HC: A 13-year survey of bacteraemia due to β-haemolytic streptococci in a Danish county. J Med Microbiol 43:63, 1995.
56. O'Connor PG, Selwyn PA, Schottenfeld RS: Medical care for injection-drug users with human immunodeficiency virus infection. N Engl J Med 331:450, 1994.
57. Ruoff KL, Miller SI, Garner CV, et al: Bacteremia with *Streptococcus bovis* and *Streptococcus salivarius*: Clinical correlates of more accurate identification of isolates. J Clin Microbiol 27:305, 1989.
58. Jacobs JA, Pietersen HG, Stobberingh EE, Soeters PB: Bacteremia involving the "*Streptococcus milleri*" group: Analysis of 19 cases. Clin Infect Dis 19:704, 1994.
59. Carratala J, Alcaide F, Fernandez-Sevilla A, et al: Bacteremia due to viridans streptococci that are highly resistant to penicillin: Increase among neutropenic patients with cancer. Clin Infect Dis 20:1169, 1995.
60. Rolston KVI, Elting LS, Bodey GP: Bacteremia due to viridans streptococci in neutropenic patients. Am J Med 99:450, 1995.
61. Bochud P-Y, Calandra T, Francioli P: Bacteremia due to viridans streptococci in neutropenic patients: A review. Am J Med 97:256, 1994.
62. Mizushima Y, Kawasaki A, Hirata H, et al: An analysis of bacteraemia in a university hospital in Japan over a 10-year period. J Hosp Infect 28:285, 1994.
63. Romero-Vivas J, Rubio M, Fernandez C, Picazo JJ: Mortality associated with nosocomial bacteremia due to methicillin-resistant *Staphylococcus aureus*. Clin Infect Dis 21:1417, 1995.
64. Malanoski GJ, Samore MH, Pefanis A, Karchmer AW: *Staphylococcus aureus* catheter-associated bacteremia. Minimal effective therapy and unusual infectious complications associated with arterial sheath catheters. Arch Intern Med 155:1161, 1995.
65. Kaplan JE, Masur H, Holmes KK, et al: USPHS/IDSA guidelines for the prevention of opportunistic infections in persons infected with human immunodeficiency virus: Introduction. Clin Infect Dis 21(Suppl 1):S1, 1995.
66. Hartstein AI, Mulligan ME, Morthland VH, Kwok RYY: Recurrent *Staphylococcus aureus* bacteremia. J Clin Microbiol 30:670, 1992.
67. Viagappan M, Kelsey MC: The origin of coagulase-negative staphylococci isolated from blood cultures. J Hosp Infect 30:217, 1995.
68. Rupp ME, Archer GL: Coagulase-negative staphylococci: Pathogens associated with medical progress. Clin Infect Dis 19:231, 1994.
69. Dahmash NS, Chowdhury MN, Fayed DF: Coagulase-negative staphylococcal bacteraemia with special reference to septic shock: Experience in an intensive care unit. J Infect 29:295, 1994.
70. Martin MA, Pfaller MA, Wenzel RJ: Coagulase-negative staphylococcal bacteremia: Mortality and hospital stay. Ann Intern Med 110:9, 1989.
71. Tumbarello M, Tacconelli E, Del Forno A, et al: *Corynebacterium striatum* bacteremia in a patient with AIDS. Clin Infect Dis 18:1007, 1994.
72. Wood CA, Pepe R: Bacteremia in a patient with non–urinary-tract infection due to *Corynebacterium urealyticum*. Clin Infect Dis 19:367, 1994.
73. Woodford N, Johnson AP, Morrison D, Speller DCE: Current perspectives on glycopeptide resistance. Clin Microbiol Rev 8:585, 1995.
74. Blue SR, Singh VR, Saubolle MA: *Bacillus licheniformis* bacteremia: Five cases associated with indwelling central venous catheters. Clin Infect Dis 20:629, 1995.
75. Uzun O, Akalin HE, Hayran M, Unal S: Factors influencing

prognosis in bacteremia due to gram-negative organisms: Evaluation of 448 episodes in a Turkish university hospital. Clin Infect Dis 15:866, 1992.
76. Chamberland S, L'Ecuyer J, Lessard C, et al: Antibiotic susceptibility profiles of 941 gram-negative bacteria isolated from septicemic patients throughout Canada. Clin Infect Dis 15:615, 1992.
77. Steffen EK, Berg RD, Deitch EA: Comparison of translocation rates of various indigenous bacteria from the gastrointestinal tract to the mesenteric lymph node. J Infect Dis 157:1032, 1988.
78. McGowan JE Jr: Do intensive hospital antibiotic control programs prevent the spread of antibiotic resistance? Infect Control Hosp Epidemiol 17:478, 1994.
79. Gransden WR, Eykyn SJ, Phillips I, Rowe B: Bacteremia due to *Escherichia coli*: A study of 861 episodes. Rev Infect Dis 12:1008, 1990.
80. Lee KH, Hui KP, Tan WC, Lim TK: *Klebsiella* bacteraemia: A report of 101 cases from National University Hospital, Singapore. J Hosp Infect 27:299, 1994.
81. Chow JW, Fine MJ, Shlaes DM, et al: *Enterobacter* bacteremia: Clinical features and emergence of antibiotic resistance during therapy. Ann Intern Med 115:585, 1991.
82. Andresen J, Asmar BI, Dajani AS: Increasing *Enterobacter* bacteremia in pediatric patients. Pediatr Infect Dis J 13:787, 1994.
83. Al Ansari N, McNamara EB, Cunney RJ, et al: Experience with *Enterobacter* bacteraemia in a Dublin teaching hospital. J Hosp Infect 27:69, 1994.
84. Weischer M, Kolmos HJ: Retrospective 6-year study of *Enterobacter* bacteraemia in a Danish university hospital. J Hosp Infect 20:15, 1992.
85. Ramos JM, Garcia-Corbiera P, Aguado JM, et al: Clinical significance of primary vs. secondary bacteremia due to nontyphoid *Salmonella* in patients without AIDS. Clin Infect Dis 19:777, 1994.
86. Galofre J, Moreno A, Mensa J, et al: Analysis of factors influencing the outcome and development of septic metastasis or relapse in *Salmonella* bacteremia. Clin Infect Dis 18:873, 1994.
87. Fergie JE, Shema SJ, Lott L, et al: *Pseudomonas aeruginosa* bacteremia in immunocompromised children: Analysis of factors associated with a poor outcome. Clin Infect Dis 18:390, 1994.
88. Mendelson MH, Gurtman A, Szabo S, et al: *Pseudomonas aeruginosa* bacteremia in patients with AIDS. Clin Infect Dis 18:886, 1994.
89. Aoun M, Van der Auwera P, Devleeshouwer C, et al: Bacteraemia caused by non-*aeruginosa Pseudomonas* species in a cancer centre. J Hosp Infect 22:307, 1992.
90. Henderson DK, Baptiste R, Parrillo J, Gill VJ: Indolent epidemic of *Pseudomonas cepacia* bacteremia and pseudobacteremia in an intensive care unit traced to a contaminated blood gas analyzer. Am J Med 84:75, 1988.
91. Pegues DA, Carson LA, Anderson RL, et al: Outbreak of *Pseudomonas cepacia* bacteremia in oncology patients. Clin Infect Dis 16:407, 1993.
92. Kostman JR, Solomon F, Fekete T: Infections with *Chryseomonas luteola* (CDC group Ve-1) and *Flavimonas oryzihabitans* (CDC group Ve-2) in neurosurgical patients. Rev Infect Dis 13:233, 1991.
93. Tilley PAG, Roberts FJ: Bacteremia with *Acinetobacter* species: Risk factors and prognosis in different clinical settings. Clin Infect Dis 18:896, 1994.
94. Pokrywka M, Viazano K, Medvick J, et al: A *Flavobacterium meningosepticum* outbreak among intensive care patients. Am J Infect Control 21:139, 1993.
95. Ko W-C, Chuang Y-C: *Aeromonas* bacteremia: Review of 59 episodes. Clin Infect Dis 20:1298, 1995.
96. Saarinen M, Takala AK, Koskenniemi E, et al: Spectrum of 2,836 cases of invasive bacterial or fungal infections in children: Results of prospective nationwide five-year surveillance in Finland. Clin Infect Dis 21:1134, 1995.
97. Bothner J, Lelyveld S, Losek JD, Cunningham SJ: *Haemophilus influenzae* bacteremia: A vanishing entity. Pediatr Emerg Care 11:127, 1995.
98. Najm WI, Cesario TC, Spurgeon L: Bacteremia due to *Haemophilus* infections: A retrospective study with emphasis on the elderly. Clin Infect Dis 21:213, 1995.
99. Powars D, Larsen R, Johnson J, et al: Epidemic meningococcemia and purpura fulminans with induced protein C deficiency. Clin Infect Dis 17:254, 1993.
100. Ioannidis JPA, Worthington M, Griffiths JK, Snydman DR: Spectrum and significance of bacteremia due to *Moraxella catarrhalis*. Clin Infect Dis 21:390, 1995.
101. Dorsher CW, Rosenblatt JE, Wilson WR, Ilstrup DM: Anaerobic bacteremia: Decreasing rate over a 15-year period. Rev Infect Dis 13:633, 1991.
102. Zaidi AK, Knaut AL, Mirrett S, Reller LB: Value of routine anaerobic blood cultures for pediatric patients. J Pediatr 127:263, 1995.
103. Arzese A, Trevisan R, Menozzi MG: Anaerobe-induced bacteremia in Italy: A nationwide survey. Clin Infect Dis 20(Suppl 2):S230, 1995.
104. Redondo MC, Arbo MDJ, Grindlinger J, Snydman DR: Attributable mortality of bacteremia associated with the *Bacteroides fragilis* group. Clin Infect Dis 20:1492, 1995.
105. Beck-Sague CM, Jarvis WR, National Nosocomial Infections Surveillance System: Secular trends in the epidemiology of nosocomial fungal infection in the United States, 1980–1990. J Infect Dis 167:1247, 1993.
106. Guiot HFL, Fibbe WE, van't Wout JW: Risk factors for fungal infection in patients with malignant hematologic disorders: Implications for empirical therapy and prophylaxis. Clin Infect Dis 18:525, 1994.
107. Ekenna O, Sherertz RJ, Bingham H: Natural history of bloodstream infections in a burn patient population: The importance of candidemia. Am J Infect Control 21:189, 1993.
108. Orenstein R: Candidemia following candiduria: Not so benign and not so delayed. Clin Infect Dis 19:207, 1994.
109. Dube MP, Heseltine PNR, Rinaldi MG, et al: Fungemia and colonization with nystatin-resistant *Candida rugosa* in a burn unit. Clin Infect Dis 18:77, 1994.
110. Chin DP, Hopewell PC: How to treat bacteraemic *Mycobacterium avium* complex disease. Lancet 346:920, 1995.
111. Chin DP, Reingold AL, Horsburgh CR Jr, et al: Predicting *Mycobacterium avium* complex bacteremia in patients infected with human immunodeficiency virus: A prospectively validated model. Clin Infect Dis 19:668, 1994.
112. Ingram CW, Tanner DC, Durack DT, et al: Disseminated infection with rapidly growing mycobacteria. Clin Infect Dis 16:463, 1993.
113. Stanberry LR, Floyd-Reising SA, Connelly BL, et al: Herpes simplex viremia: Report of eight pediatric cases and review of the literature. Clin Infect Dis 18:401, 1994.
114. Goodman JL, Bradley JF, Ross AE, et al: Bloodstream invasion in early Lyme disease: Results from a prospective, controlled, blinded study using the polymerase chain reaction. Am J Med 99:6, 1995.
115. Amit M, Pitlik SD, Samra Z, et al: Bacteremia in patients without known underlying disorders. Scand J Infect Dis 26:605, 1994.
116. Gransden WR, Eykyn SJ, Phillips I: Septicaemia in the newborn and elderly. J Antimicrob Chemother 34(Suppl A):101, 1994.
117. Baker MD, Bell LM, Avner JR: Outpatient management without antibiotics of fever in selected infants. N Engl J Med 329:1437, 1993.
118. Beebe JL, Koneman EW: Recovery of uncommon bacteria from blood: Association with neoplastic disease. Clin Microbiol Rev 8:336, 1995.
119. Vugia DJ, Kiehlbauch JA, Yeboue K, et al: Pathogens and predictors of fatal septicemia associated with human immunodeficiency virus infection in Ivory Coast, West Africa. J Infect Dis 168:564, 1993.
120. Wagner SJ, Friedman LI, Dodd RY: Transfusion-associated bacterial sepsis. Clin Microbiol Rev 7:290, 1994.
121. Jacobson MA, Gellermann H, Chambers H: *Staphylococcus aureus* bacteremia and recurrent staphylococcal infection in patients with acquired immunodeficiency syndrome and AIDS-related complex. Am J Med 85:172, 1988.
122. Jong GM, Hsiue TR, Chen CR, et al: Rapidly fatal outcome of bacteremic *Klebsiella pneumoniae* pneumonia in alcoholics. Chest 107:214, 1995.
123. McManus AT, Mason AD Jr, McManus WF, Pruitt BA Jr: A decade of reduced gram-negative infections and mortality associated with improved isolation of burned patients. Arch Surg 129:1306, 1994.
124. Richardson JP: Bacteremia in the elderly. J Gen Intern Med 8:89, 1993.

125. Brown RB, Cipriani D, Schulte M, et al: Community-acquired bacteremias from tunneled central intravenous lines: Results of studies of a single vendor. Am J Infect Control 22:149, 1994.
126. Collignon PJ: Intravascular catheter associated sepsis: A common problem. The Australian Study on Intravascular Catheter Associated Sepsis. Med J Aust 161:374, 1994.
127. Leibovici L, Konisberger H, Pitlik SD, et al: Bacteremia and fungemia of unknown origin in adults. Clin Infect Dis 14:436, 1992.
128. Tenover FC, McGowan JE Jr: Reasons for the emergence of antibiotic resistance. Am J Med Sci 311:9, 1996.
129. Cunha BA: Antibiotic treatment of sepsis. Med Clin North Am 79:551, 1995.
130. Finch RG: Septicaemia: Clinical features. *In* Shanson DC (ed): Septicaemia and Endocarditis: Clinical and Microbiological Aspects. London, Oxford University Press, 1989, p 49.
131. Kingston ME, Mackey D: Skin clues in the diagnosis of life-threatening infections. Rev Infect Dis 8:1, 1986.
132. Harris RL, Musher DM, Bloom K, et al: Manifestations of sepsis. Arch Intern Med 147:1895, 1987.
133. Saviteer SM, Samsa GP, Rutala WA: Nosocomial infections in the elderly. Increased risk per hospital day. Am J Med 84:661, 1988.
134. Chandrasekar PH, Brown WJ: Clinical issues of blood cultures. Arch Intern Med 154:841, 1994.
135. Schonheyder HC, Hojbjerg T: The impact of the first notification of positive blood cultures on antibiotic therapy. A one-year survey. APMIS 103:37, 1995.
136. Chalasani NP, Valdecanas MA, Golpal AK, et al: Clinical utility of blood cultures in adult patients with community-acquired pneumonia without defined underlying focus. Chest 108:932, 1995.
137. Mylotte JM, Pisano MA, Ram S, et al: Validation of a bacteremia prediction model. Infect Control Hosp Epidemiol 16:203, 1995.
138. Pfitzenmeyer P, Decrey H, Auckenthaler R, Michel JP: Predicting bacteremia in older patients. J Am Geriatr Soc 43:230, 1995.
139. Bates DW, Lee TH: Rapid classification of positive blood cultures. Prospective validation of a multivariate algorithm. JAMA 267:1962, 1992.
140. Emmanuel FXS, Aucken H, Watt B, et al: False-positive blood-cultures from contaminated ESR tubes. Lancet 341:111, 1993.
141. Jumaa PA, Chattopadhyay B: Pseudobacteraemia. J Hosp Infect 27:167, 1994.
142. Mermel LA, Maki DG: Detection of bacteremia in adults: Consequences of culturing an inadequate volume of blood. Ann Intern Med 119:270, 1993.
143. Kellogg JA, Bankert DA, Manzella JP, et al: Occurrence and documentation of low-level bacteremia in a community hospital's patient population. Am J Clin Pathol 104:524, 1995.
144. Li J, Plorde JJ, Carlson LG: Effects of volume and periodicity on blood cultures. J Clin Microbiol 32:2829, 1994.
145. Strand CL, Wajsbort RR, Sturmann K: Effect of iodophor vs iodine tincture skin preparation on blood culture contamination rate. JAMA 269:1004, 1993.
146. Schwabe LD, Thomson RB Jr, Flint KK, Koontz FP: Evaluation of BACTEC 9240 blood culture system by using high-volume aerobic resin media. J Clin Microbiol 33:2451, 1995.
147. Wilson ML, Weinstein MP, Mirrett S, et al: Controlled evaluation of BacT/Alert standard anaerobic and FAN anaerobic blood culture bottles for the detection of bacteremia and fungemia. J Clin Microbiol 33:2265, 1995.
148. Strand CL, Shulman JA: Bloodstream Infections—Laboratory Detection and Clinical Considerations. Chicago, ASCP Press, 1988.
149. Lyon R, Woods G: Comparison of the BacT/Alert and Isolator blood culture systems for recovery of fungi. Am J Clin Pathol 103:660, 1995.
150. Cockerill FR, Torgerson CA, Reed GS, et al: Clinical comparison of Difco ESP, Wampole Isolator, and Becton Dickinson Septi-Chek aerobic blood culturing systems. J Clin Microbiol 34:20, 1996.
151. Pohlman JK, Kirkley BA, Easley KA, Washington JA: Controlled clinical comparison of Isolator and BACTEC 9240 Aerobic/F resin bottle for detection of bloodstream infections. J Clin Microbiol 33:2525, 1995.
152. Masterson KC, McGowan JE Jr: Detection of positive blood cultures by the Bactec NR660. The clinical importance of five versus seven days of testing. Am J Clin Pathol 90:91, 1988.
153. Weinstein MP, Reller LB: Clinical importance of "breakthrough" bacteremia. Am J Med 76:175, 1984.
154. Gross PA, Barrett TL, Dellinger EP, et al: Quality standard for the treatment of bacteremia. Clin Infect Dis 18:428, 1994.
155. Lynn WA, Cohen J: Adjunctive therapy for septic shock: A review of experimental approaches. Clin Infect Dis 20:143, 1995.
156. Korvick JA, Bryan CS, Farber B, et al: Prospective observational study of *Klebsiella* bacteremia in 230 patients: Outcome for antibiotic combinations versus monotherapy. Antimicrob Agents Chemother 36:2639, 1992.
157. Siebert JD, Thomson RB Jr, Tan JS, Gerson LW: Emergence of antimicrobial resistance in gram-negative bacilli causing bacteremia during therapy. Am J Clin Pathol 100:47, 1993.
158. Murphy PM, Lane HC, Gallin JI, Fauci AS: Marked disparity in incidence of bacterial infections in patients with the acquired immunodeficiency syndrome receiving interleukin-2 or interferon-gamma. Ann Intern Med 108:36, 1988.
159. Aquino VM, Pappo A, Buchanan GR, et al: The changing epidemiology of bacteremia in neutropenic children with cancer. Pediatr Infect Dis J 14:140, 1995.
160. Bates DW, Pruess KE, Lee TH: How bad are bacteremia and sepsis? Outcomes in a cohort with suspected bacteremia. Arch Intern Med 155:593, 1995.
161. Pittet D, Tarara D, Wenzel RP: Nosocomial bloodstream infection in critically ill patients. Excess length of stay, extra costs, and attributable mortality. JAMA 271:1598, 1994.
162. Pinner RW, Haley RW, Blumenstein BA, et al: High cost nosocomial infections. Infect Control 3:143, 1982.
163. Leibovici L, Samra Z, Konigsberger H, et al: Long-term survival following bacteremia or fungemia. JAMA 274:807, 1995.
164. Perl TM, Dvorak L, Hwang T, Wenzel RP: Long-term survival and function after suspected gram-negative sepsis. JAMA 274:338, 1995.
165. Shay DK, Maloney SA, Montecalvo M, et al: Epidemiology and mortality risk of vancomycin-resistant enterococcal bloodstream infection. J Infect Dis 172:993, 1995.
166. Maki DG: Yes, Virginia, aseptic technique is very important: Maximal barrier precautions during insertion reduce the risk of central venous catheter–related bacteremia. Infect Control Hosp Epidemiol 15:227, 1994.
167. Wiener J, Itokazu G, Nathan C, et al: A randomized, double-blind, placebo-controlled trial of selective digestive decontamination in a medical-surgical intensive care unit. Clin Infect Dis 20:861, 1995.

67

Sepsis

David W. Hines
Jeffrey M. Lisowski
Roger C. Bone

Sepsis, the inflammatory response to an infection, is a leading cause of death in intensive care units.[1] Mortality rates range from 20% to 90% despite both our growing understanding of the pathogenesis of sepsis and advances in its therapy.[1–6] Every year in the United States, there are an estimated 400,000 cases of sepsis; half of these are severe enough to result in shock, and they are responsible for more than 100,000 deaths.[6–9] Clearly, early recognition of sepsis and appropriate therapy before shock ensues are paramount in reducing the high mortality.[4, 10–12]

This chapter reviews some of the microbiologic and host factors related to sepsis, its pathogenesis, and its protean clinical manifestations. The chapter also provides practical recommendations on optimal therapy for this medical emergency as well as a brief review of potentially useful adjunctive therapies involving the various mediators of sepsis that are currently under investigation.

Definitions

As investigators delineate the pathogenesis of sepsis and the inflammatory response to it, new and confusing terms have arisen to describe disease states that defy pigeonholing into separate and discrete categories. Sepsis, septic shock, sepsis syndrome, systemic inflammatory response syndrome (SIRS), and other terms have been applied to various groups of patients whose responses to therapy may be divergent.

To better understand sepsis, and therefore better treat patients, it is imperative that consistent definitions be employed.[13] To this end, a consensus conference met in August 1991 to agree on a set of definitions that could be applied to patients with sepsis and its sequelae.[14] At that conference, the use of SIRS was agreed on, and its relation to sepsis is depicted in Figure 67–1.

SIRS may be associated with either infectious or noninfectious injuries (e.g., pancreatitis, trauma, burns) and can be identified by the presence of at least two of the following manifestations:

1. Body temperature greater than 38°C or less than 36°C
2. Heart rate greater than 90 beats per minute
3. Tachypnea greater than 20 breaths per minute, or arterial carbon dioxide tension (Pa_{CO_2}) less than 32 mm Hg
4. White cell counts greater than 12,000/mm^3, or less than 4000/mm^3, or greater than 10% immature forms (bands)

These criteria are by no means specific in identifying septic patients, but they are quite sensitive.[15]

The patient with sepsis meets all the criteria for SIRS, of which it is a subset; however, it is the result of an infection. Severe sepsis is defined as sepsis associated with organ dysfunction, perfusion abnormalities, or hypotension (Table 67–1). Septic shock is sepsis with hypotension despite adequate fluid resuscitation. Multiorgan dysfunction syndrome emphasizes the search for early signs of organ dysfunction rather than waiting for its failure.

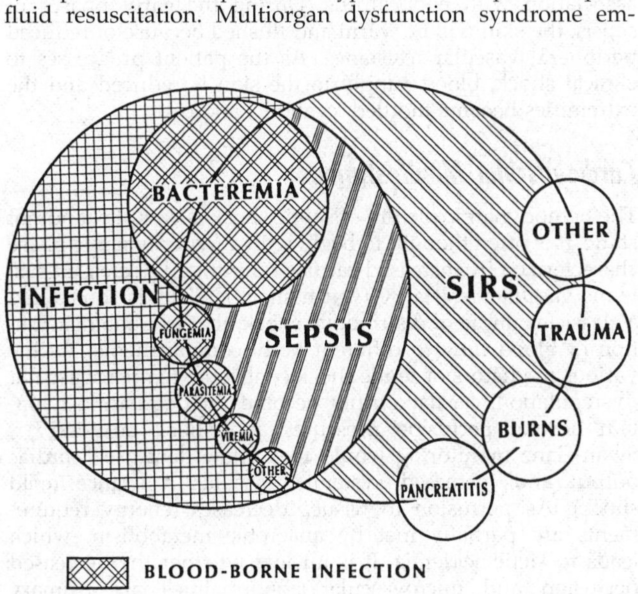

FIGURE 67–1 □ The interrelationship among systemic inflammatory response syndrome (SIRS), sepsis, and infection.

From one large prospective epidemiologic study, it was evident that there is a clinical progression from SIRS to sepsis to severe sepsis and septic shock.[15] There was also a progressive increase in mortality rates along this continuum, from 7% to 16% to 20% and 46%, respectively. In subgroups of patients meeting two, three, and all four criteria for SIRS, mortality rates increased directly with the number of criteria present.

Others have suggested using severity of illness scales to predict outcome more accurately.[16] Given the protean manifestations of sepsis and the unpredictable response in an individual patient, these scoring systems are perhaps more useful to compare groups of patients in clinical trials.

The rationale for making the new definitions broad based and standardized is twofold. Foremost is the rapid identification and treatment of potentially septic patients, and second is to improve research efforts in comparative trials of new therapies for septic patients.

Microbiology and Host Factors

Sepsis may complicate infections with bacteria, viruses, rickettsiae, mycobacteria, fungi, and parasites. Gram-positive organisms were responsible for most cases of bacteremias in the preantibiotic era.[9] Gram-negative infections emerged during the antibiotic era and eventually surpassed bacteremias with gram-positive organisms.[7–10, 12] The reasons for this may be related to (1) antibiotic pressures on normal flora; (2) use of invasive devices in a hostile nosocomial environment (urinary catheters, central lines); and (3) our ever-increasing ability to suppress the immune system with steroids, chemotherapy, radiation, and antirejection therapies in transplant recipients. Gram-negative sepsis and septic shock became synonymous, which has in part contributed to the confusion surrounding sepsis.

More recently, gram-positive organisms have reemerged as important pathogens in sepsis.[17–19] In a review of several studies of sepsis, gram-positive infections accounted for one third to one half of the cases.[20] Factors that predispose patients to infections with gram-positive organisms include (1) the aggressive use of catheters, (2) prosthetic devices, (3) history of intravenous drug use, and (4) immunosuppressed states and chemotherapy.[20]

Although it is impossible to clinically distinguish gram-negative or gram-positive bacterial sepsis from that caused by other pathogens, knowledge of predisposing host factors can give valuable clues to organisms of particular importance[21, 22] (Table 67–2).

The nature of the underlying illness markedly influences the likelihood of surviving an episode of gram-negative bacteremia.[2, 3, 5, 10, 11] In patients with rapidly fatal diseases, it is difficult even to show that antibiotics increase survival at all.[11] In patients with nonfatal or ultimately fatal conditions, however, appropriate antibiotic use seems to correlate with improved survival.[2, 4, 10–12] Infections with some organisms, for example, *Pseudomonas* spp., may have a higher mortality.[10, 11] Whether this is related to properties of the bacteria or is just an association with an underlying disease remains to be proved.

Other factors that seem to be associated with an increased mortality are listed in Table 67–3.

Clinical Manifestations

Classic Signs

Fever, chills, and hypotension are classic signs of septic shock and should prompt cultures of blood and other likely sources

TABLE 67–1 ■ New Definitions for Sepsis and Related Disorders*

Infection	A microbial phenomenon characterized by an inflammatory response to the presence of microorganisms or the invasion of normally sterile host tissue by those organisms.
Bacteremia	The presence of viable bacteria in the blood (the presence of other organisms in the blood should be described in a similar manner—viremia, fungemia, and so on).
Systemic inflammatory response syndrome (SIRS)	The systemic inflammatory response to a variety of severe clinical insults, including infection, pancreatitis, ischemia, multiple trauma and tissue injury, hemorrhagic shock, immune-mediated organ injury, and exogenous administration of inflammatory mediators such as tumor necrosis factor or other cytokines. SIRS is manifested by (but not limited to) two or more of the following conditions: • Temperature: >38°C or <36°C • Heart rate: >90 beats/min • Respiratory rate: >20 breaths/min or arterial carbon dioxide tension of <32 mm Hg • White cell count: >12,000 cells/mm³, <4000 cells/mm³, or >10% immature (band) forms These changes should represent an acute alteration from baseline in the absence of another known cause for the abnormalities.
Sepsis	The systemic response to infection. This response is identical to SIRS, except that it must result from infection.
Severe sepsis	Sepsis associated with organ dysfunction, perfusion abnormalities, or hypotension. Perfusion abnormalities may include (but are not limited to) lactic acidosis, oliguria, and an acute alteration in mental status. Hypotension is defined as a systolic blood pressure <90 mm Hg or a reduction of >40 mm Hg from baseline in the absence of another known cause for hypotension.
Septic shock	Sepsis with hypotension (as defined above) despite adequate fluid resuscitation, in conjunction with perfusion abnormalities (as defined above). Patients who are receiving inotropic or vasopressor agents may not be hypotensive at the time that perfusion abnormalities are measured, yet they may still be considered to have septic shock.
Multiorgan dysfunction syndrome (MODS)	Presence of altered organ function in an acutely ill patient, such that homeostasis cannot be maintained without intervention. Primary MODS is the direct result of a well-defined insult in which organ dysfunction occurs early and can be directly attributable to the insult itself. Seconary MODS develops as a consequence of a host response and is identified within the context of SIRS.

*These definitions were developed at a consensus conference jointly sponsored by the American College of Chest Physicians and the Society for Critical Care Medicine held in August 1991.

Reprinted by permission of the publisher from Why new definitions of sepsis and organ failure are needed, by Bone RC, American Journal of Medicine, Vol 95, Pages 348–350. Copyright 1993 by Excerpta Medica Inc.

of infection. Two and three sets of blood cultures from a bacteremic patient will yield the organism 89% and 99% of the time, respectively.[23] Many patients, especially the elderly and debilitated, may not manifest the classic symptoms. Hypothermia may be seen with gram-negative sepsis and usually indicates a poorer prognosis.[4, 11, 12] Hyperventilation may precede any other changes in vital signs and can lead to respiratory alkalosis. Diaphoresis, apprehension, and a change in mental status, none of which is specific for sepsis, may also occur early.

Skin Findings

Cutaneous manifestations of sepsis due to gram-negative bacilli are varied and include cellulitis, erythema multiforme, diffuse bullous lesions, symmetric peripheral gangrene with disseminated intravascular coagulation (DIC), and the classic lesions associated with endocarditis (Janeway lesions, Osler nodes).[24] A peculiar lesion most frequently seen in neutropenic patients with *Pseudomonas* sepsis is ecthyma gangrenosum.[25, 26] These are discrete rounded lesions that begin as dark red or purplish macules and progress to "bull's-eye" erythematous halos surrounding a central vesicle or ulcer. They have also been described in bacteremias with *Aeromonas* spp. and other gram-negative rods and fungi.[27] Sometimes biopsies or aspirations of a skin lesion with cultures and Gram stain may yield a diagnosis before blood cultures.

The most dramatic skin lesions occur with fulminant meningococcemia. These are diffuse petechial, purpuric, ecchymotic lesions that signal the presence of DIC. Petechiae may also be seen in infections with gram-positive organisms (e.g., in asplenic patients with pneumococcus infection) and in association with endocarditis. During the early phases of sepsis, the skin will be warm and flushed because of reduced peripheral vascular resistance. As the patient progresses to clinical shock, blood supply to the skin is reduced and the extremities become mottled, cyanotic, and cool.

Cardiovascular Manifestations

The hemodynamic picture of septic shock is complex and not static. It is often thought to begin with a hyperdynamic phase characterized by increased cardiac output and decreased systemic vascular resistance (warm shock).[28] This is considered a classic example of distributive shock, that is, a maldistribution of blood flow to different body compartments. As the various mediators of septic shock contribute to microvascular dysregulation, cardiac output becomes inadequate to maintain normal perfusion pressures and shock ensues.[6, 28–33] Swan-Ganz monitoring would then show decreased cardiac output and increased systemic vascular resistance (cold shock). As perfusion to tissues decreases, energy requirements are partially met by anaerobic metabolism, which leads to lactic acidemia. It is unclear whether the decreased perfusion and microvascular abnormalities are primary causes of organ failure in sepsis or just other associated events.[1]

TABLE 67–2 ■ Organisms Responsible for Sepsis in Relation to Host Factors

HOST FACTORS	ORGANISMS OF PARTICULAR IMPORTANCE
Asplenia	Encapsulated organisms: *Streptococcus pneumoniae, Haemophilus influenzae, Neisseria meningitidis, Capnocytophaga canimorsus, Babesia microti*
Cirrhosis	*Vibrio, Yersinia,* and *Salmonella* spp.; other gram-negative rods; encapsulated organisms
Alcoholism	*Klebsiella* spp., pneumococcus
Diabetes	*Mucor* and *Pseudomonas* spp. (malignant external otitis), *Escherichia coli, Staphylococcus aureus*
Steroids	*Mycobacterium tuberculosis,* fungi, herpesvirus
Neutropenia	Enteric gram-negative rods, *Pseudomonas, Aspergillus, Candida,* and *Mucor* spp.; *S. aureus*
T-cell abnormalities	*Listeria, Salmonella,* and fungal and mycobacterial spp.; herpesvirus group (herpes simplex virus, cytomegalovirus, varicella-zoster virus); parasites

Despite normal to high measurements of cardiac output, there is growing evidence of significant myocardial dysfunction in septic shock.[31, 32] A myocardial depressant factor is most likely responsible, although nothing definite has been isolated as yet.[1, 34] Tumor necrosis factor (TNF) has properties that inhibit myocyte contractility and may be one of several cytokines responsible for myocardial dysfunction in patients with sepsis.[35]

When measured serially, significant differences in cardiac indices and oxygen use were noted in survivors and nonsurvivors of septic shock 8 hours before the hypotensive crisis.[33] This suggests that a patient's outcome may be determined before any evidence of shock exists. Others have demonstrated the prognostic significance of heart rate and systemic vascular resistance in survivors of septic shock. Survivors are more likely to have heart rates below 106 beats per minute initially, then progressively slower heart rates and higher systemic vascular resistance during the first 24 hours.[28]

In late shock, tissue hypoperfusion leads to progressive acidosis as cardiac output falls, accompanied by refractory hypotension and inevitable death. Efforts to increase cardiac output with fluids and ionotropic agents often prove futile.[31] This has led some researchers to postulate that a metabolic block triggered by sepsis prevents tissues from the normal oxidative use of available substrate.[36, 37]

TABLE 67–3 ■ Factors Influencing Survival with Bacteremia

Severity of the underlying disease[2, 3, 5, 10, 11]
Appropriate antibiotic use[2, 4, 10–12]
Microorganism[3, 5, 7, 10, 11, 22]
Advanced age[10, 12]
Site of infection (respiratory > abdominal > urinary)[3, 10]
Nosocomial versus community-acquired infection[2, 3, 9]
Magnitude of bacteremia[2, 3]
Polymicrobial bacteremia[2, 4, 8]
Complications of sepsis (shock, hypothermia, anuria)[11, 12]

Pulmonary Manifestations

The earliest response to sepsis is tachypnea, which may be followed by a wide array of respiratory signs. These may range from hyperventilation and respiratory alkalosis to acute respiratory distress syndrome (ARDS) and, finally, failure of the respiratory muscles. The exact pathophysiologic mechanism of the lung damage is unclear; it probably involves numerous mediators activated by sepsis and a resultant increased alveolar capillary permeability. The increase in pulmonary edema is associated with a ventilation-perfusion mismatch, a widened alveolar-arterial oxygen gradient, and reduced lung compliance.[38, 39]

ARDS may complicate sepsis 10% to 40% of the time, increasing the mortality to 80% to 90%.[40–42] Establishing a diagnosis is arbitrary at times but usually includes arterial oxygen tension of less than 50 mm Hg despite a fraction of inspired oxygen greater than 50%, diffuse alveolar infiltrates without cardiomegaly or other signs of heart failure, and a pulmonary capillary wedge pressure below 15 mm Hg. Host factors do not seem to predispose patients to ARDS, but infections with gram-negative organisms are more often associated with ARDS.[40]

In the later stage of ARDS, as a preterminal event, oxygenation becomes impossible despite 100% inspired oxygen and high levels of positive end-expiratory pressure.

Hematologic Findings

Most patients with sepsis will exhibit a neutrophilic leukocytosis from both a stress-related demargination early and a release of less mature granulocytes from the marrow reserve later. Leukemoid reactions with leukocyte counts of 50,000/mm^3 or more are sometimes observed. Significant neutropenia is seen in infections with intracellular pathogens (*Brucella* spp., *Salmonella typhi, Listeria* spp., rickettsiae, viral infections) and overwhelming bacteremias. Alcoholic patients and the elderly are at greater risk for sepsis-related neutropenia, the presence of which is associated with a higher mortality.[4, 12]

A low platelet count and observance of toxic granulation, Döhle bodies, and vacuolization of the neutrophil on a complete blood count may be early clues to bacteremia.[43] DIC is characterized by fibrin deposition and thrombosis of the microvasculature. Hemorrhage results from consumption of platelets and clotting factors.[44] Elevated fibrin degradation products, prolonged prothrombin time, and decreased platelets, fibrinogen, and clotting factors are diagnostic of DIC. Hemolytic anemias may complicate infections with *Clostridium* and *Mycoplasma* spp. and may occur in association with DIC.

Renal and Gastrointestinal Manifestations

Renal insufficiency in sepsis is multifactorial. It depends to varying degrees on the host, the microbe, and the therapeutic interventions.[45] Glomerular lesions are seen with endocarditis (especially staphylococcal) and other unrelated infectious processes. Tubulointerstitial disease related to various bacteria and antibiotic therapy is well known. Most often, renal failure is attributed to acute tubular necrosis, which may be caused by hypotension, volume depletion, or any one of the numerous mediators of septic shock.

Sepsis is also associated with upper gastrointestinal tract bleeding[46] and is often seen in patients with coagulopathies and mechanical ventilation.[47] Liver dysfunction usually causes a cholestatic jaundice and may result from red blood cell lysis or hepatocellular dysfunction.[48] For unexplained reasons, sepsis with *Bacteroides* spp. is often accompanied by hyperbilirubinemia.[49] Precipitous rises in transaminase levels usually indicate shock liver from a hypotensive episode and generally fall rapidly as blood pressure is restored.

Hypoglycemia may complicate sepsis with a variety of bacteria and should be looked for in patients who have any change in mental status or seizures.[50] The pathogenesis is unclear, but patients with underlying liver disease are more likely to become hypoglycemic with sepsis.[51] Inhibition of gluconeogenesis and depletion of hepatic glycogen stores have been implicated.[52]

Multiorgan Dysfunction

When there is evidence of dysfunction in two or more systems (pulmonary, renal, gastrointestinal, central nervous, and hepatic), the diagnosis of multiorgan dysfunction syndrome can be made. Mortality rises in proportion to the number of organ systems involved.[53, 54] When four or more systems are involved, mortality is nearly 100%.

Mediators of the Inflammatory Response Syndrome

The systemic response to insult such as overwhelming infection or trauma involves a complicated cascade of biologic events culminating in hemodynamic compromise and organ damage. Triggering substances such as bacteria-derived endotoxin induce the production of endogenous mediators, which in turn act in an interdependent fashion to stimulate the reticuloendothelial, complement, and coagulation systems. It seems reasonable that the coordinated effect of localized inflammation is an attempt to physiologically contain and overcome offenses such as bacterial invasion. However, when the inflammatory response is no longer contained, and regulatory mechanisms are overwhelmed, systemic complications such as sepsis may occur (Fig. 67–2). Research in the last two decades has concentrated on characterizing and moderating these mediators of sepsis.

The events leading to sepsis typically involve the production and release of microbial toxins. In sepsis associated with gram-negative infection, the cell wall constituent known as endotoxin induces the release of proinflammatory mediators. Endotoxin, or lipopolysaccharide, consists of a three-part complex of species-specific O-antigens, core polysaccharide, and glucosamine-based phospholipid (lipid A). The core–lipid A portion is antigenically conserved among gram-negative species and possesses most of the complex's biologic activity. Endotoxin is known to be a potent stimulus for the production of TNF-α as well as of other cytokines and inflammatory cells. Endotoxin potency is augmented by lipopolysaccharide binding protein found in human serum. In addition to facilitating bacterial opsonization, the resulting endotoxin–lipopolysaccharide binding protein complexes bind readily to CD14 receptors on monocytes and macrophages.[55] Complement and coagulation cascades are affected by endotoxin through the activation of Hageman factor (factor XII).[56]

Toxin production is not restricted to gram-negative bacteria as is seen with the exotoxin produced by *Staphylococcus aureus* in toxic shock syndrome. Gram-positive bacterial, fungal, viral, and even parasitic organisms may elicit cell wall and other antigenic products that trigger the inflammatory response.[20]

Development of SIRS in the absence of gram-negative infection suggests other principal mediators unrelated to endotoxin. Of these, TNF-α has received the most attention. TNF-α is released early in SIRS by activated monocyte/macrophages and endothelial cells and stimulates the induction of secondary proinflammatory cytokines such as interleukin (IL)–1, IL-6, and platelet-activating factor.[57] Additional reactions include the induction of endothelial adhesion molecules, which promote neutrophil adherence to endothelium, and the enhancement of phagocytosis. Although TNF-α is considered pivotal in the production of the inflammatory cascade, the half-life of TNF-α is brief, and significant levels are not necessary to maintain the inflammatory response of sepsis.[58]

Cytokines may behave independently or in concert with other modulators to provoke the inflammatory cascade. IL-1 acts synergistically with TNF-α to promote fever, hypotension, and shock. Other actions include release of IL-6 and platelet-activating factor as well as endothelial cell activation and increased endothelial adhesion molecule expression.[55] Platelet-activating factor similarly functions to amplify the release of cytokines.[55] IL-6, on the other hand, while promoting neutrophil activation and accumulation, also acts in an antiinflammatory fashion by down-regulating TNF-α production and release. Similar antiinflammatory cytokines include IL-8, a potent chemoattractant for neutrophils but a substance that may also function to limit neutrophil-endothelial cell adherence; and IL-10, which decreases production of IL-1, IL-6, and TNF-α.[59]

Sepsis mediator activation results in damage to endovascular tissue with subsequent vascular disruption, hemodynamic compromise, and end-organ tissue damage. TNF-α and interleukin metabolism of arachidonic acid results in the manufacture of leukotrienes, thromboxane A_2, and prostaglandins, which increase vascular permeability and vasodilation. Endotoxin-induced nitric oxide production by macrophage and endothelial cells acts as a potent vasodilator.[60] TNF-α probably acts as a myocardial depressant substance.[35] Stimulated neutrophils release lysosomal enzymes and oxygen radicals, augmenting vascular and tissue compromise. Platelet aggregation and activation of the complement and coagulation cascades lead to thrombosis and hemorrhage and further impair tissue perfusion.[57]

Table 67–4 provides examples of the numerous mediators of sepsis and highlights steps that have been or are currently being investigated as targets for immunomodulation therapies.

Therapy

Patients in septic shock are probably best managed in an intensive care unit with Swan-Ganz and arterial catheters. Proof that invasive monitoring improves survival is from retrospective studies only.[61, 62] Measurements of right-sided heart pressures, pulmonary artery wedge pressures, and cardiac outputs are useful both in diagnosing sepsis (decreased systemic vascular resistance, increased cardiac output) and in following the response to volume replacement (avoiding pulmonary edema).[64, 65]

The essential therapies for septic shock include (1) antibiotics, (2) fluid replacement, (3) oxygen, and (4) vasopressors. Early antibiotic administration may dampen the inflammatory cascade, although studies have shown increased levels in serum endotoxin as a response to antimicrobial use.[63] Antibiotics should be chosen on the basis of potential sources of infection, epidemiologic concerns (community-acquired versus nosocomial infection), and underlying host factors (see Table 67–2). Broad-spectrum agents are recommended until culture results become available. In general, the use of combination therapy is advocated to (1) provide broad coverage for both gram-positive and gram-negative bacteremias, (2) prevent the selection of resistance, and (3) possibly afford the added benefit of synergy. Combination therapy may in-

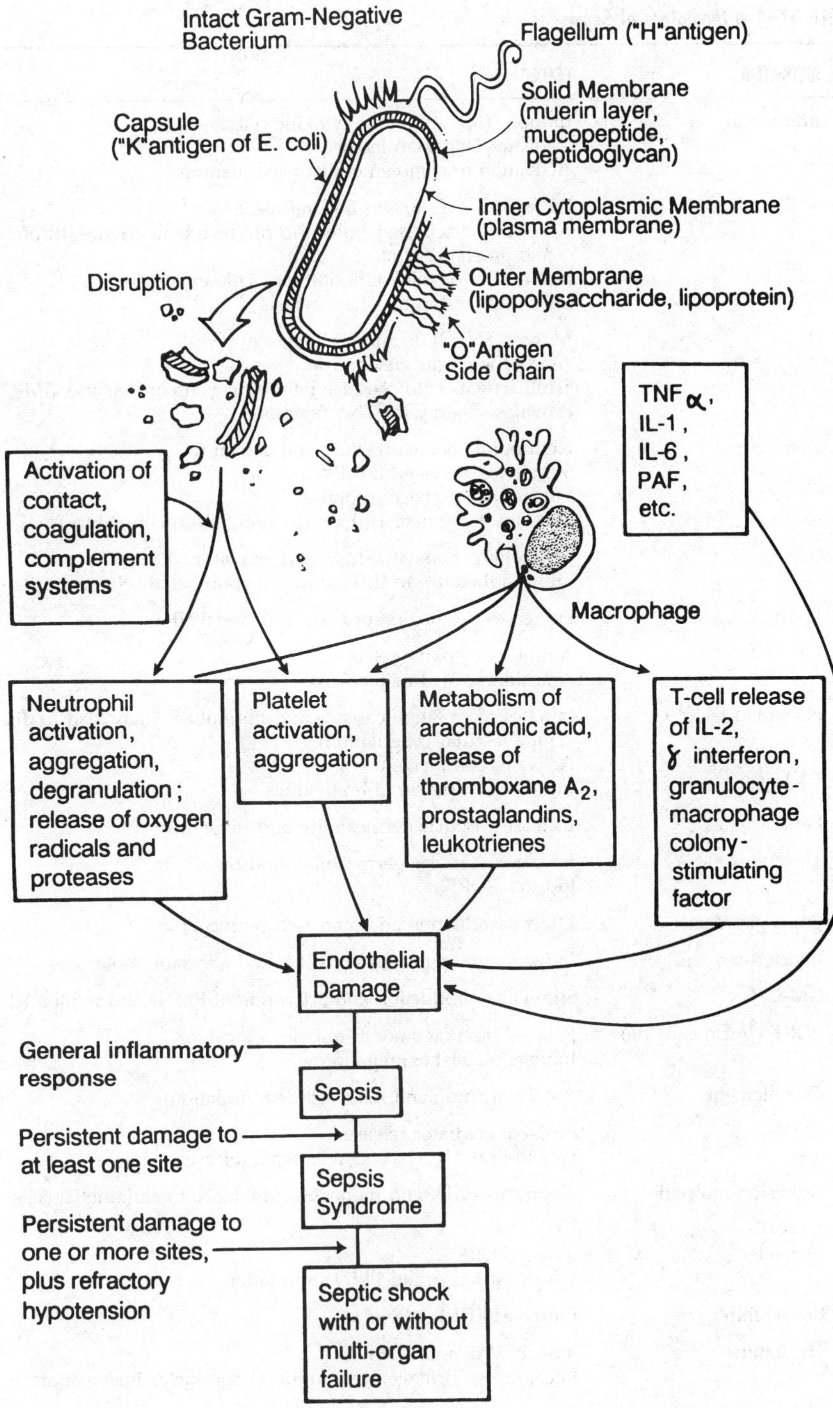

FIGURE 67–2 □ Mechanisms underlying gram-negative sepsis. This figure provides a framework for understanding how sepsis and systemic inflammatory response syndrome may occur. The pathways are not distinct, however, and effects may vary from individual to individual, depending on physiologic conditions. If general homeostasis is not restored, the systemic inflammatory response will produce clinical evidence of sepsis, and persistent endothelial damage at one site will ultimately result in organ dysfunction. GM-CSF, Granulocyte-macrophage colony-stimulating factor; IFN-γ, interferon-γ; IL, interleukin; PAF, platelet-activating factor; TNF-α, tumor necrosis factor-α. (Modified from Bone RC: The pathogenesis of sepsis. Ann Intern Med 115:457–469, 1991.)

clude an aminoglycoside (dosed to achieve high therapeutic levels with close monitoring to avoid associated toxic effects) along with a third-generation cephalosporin, or carbapenem for *Pseudomonas* and other resistant gram-negative rod coverage. Vancomycin should be considered when gram-positive organisms are likely (e.g., catheters, intravenous drug abuse). Once an organism is identified, therapy should be narrowed unless the patient's condition remains unstable.

Because of extensive capillary leakage and peripheral vasodilation, volume requirements may be enormous. Cardiac output in these patients may not respond to fluid challenges as expected,[31] so care must be taken with indiscriminate hydration. Pulmonary artery wedge pressures should be maintained between 12 and 15 mm Hg. Vasopressors are used when the blood pressure cannot be maintained with intravenous fluids. High-dose dopamine and norepinephrine (with low-dose dopamine to protect renal blood flow) are usually the first-line agents.[66, 67] Dobutamine and isoproterenol may be useful adjuncts.

Correcting hypoxemia may require mechanical ventilation and positive end-expiratory pressure. Because of concerns about barotrauma with high levels of positive end-expiratory pressure and oxygen toxicity with high prolonged fraction of inspired oxygen, a balance must be worked out to ensure adequate oxygen saturation with the least risk. Hyperbaric oxygenation and extracorporeal oxygenation have not proved to be superior to conventional therapy.

All other modalities in the treatment of septic shock are

TABLE 67–4 ■ Mediators of Sepsis

MEDIATOR*	EFFECT	POSSIBLE TREATMENT MODALITIES
Endotoxin	Induces TNF and other cytokine release Activates Hageman factor Activation of complement and coagulation	Polyclonal antisera Monoclonal antibodies
TNF-α	Induces IL-1, IL-6, and PAF release Arachidonic acid metabolism to produce leukotrienes, thromboxane A_2, and prostaglandins Induces endothelial adhesion molecule expression Enhances neutrophil phagocytosis	Monoclonal antibodies Recombinant TNF receptors
IL-1	Induces TNF, IL-6, and PAF release Arachidonic acid metabolism T-cell activation to produce interferon-γ, other ILs, and GM-CSF Provides synergy for TNF function	IL-1 receptor antagonists Soluble IL-1 receptors
IL-6	Neutrophil chemoattractant and activator Stimulates activated B cells Induces acute-phase response May down-regulate TNF production (antiinflammatory)	
IL-8	Neutrophil chemoattractant and activator Limits adherence to IL-1–activated endothelial cells (antiinflammatory)	
IL-10	Decreases production of IL-1, IL-6, and TNF	
PAF	Amplifies cytokine release Arachidonic acid metabolism	PAF antagonists
Hageman factor	Initiates coagulation cascade and fibrinolysis (may lead to disseminated intravascular coagulation) Activates complement Induces production of bradykinin	Monoclonal antibodies
Leukotrienes	Increase vascular permeability and resistance	
Thromboxane A_2	Increases vascular permeability and resistance Induces EDRF	Inhibitors or antagonists
Prostaglandins	Effect vasodilation and increased permeability	Inhibitors or antagonists
Interferon-γ	Induces and augments TNF, ILs, and adhesion molecules	
GM-CSF	Stimulates production and activation of PMNs and mononuclear cells	
EDRF (?nitrous oxide)	Relaxes vascular smooth muscle Inhibits platelet aggregation	
Complement	PMN activation and mast cell degranulation	
PMNs	Promote mediator release Free radical and lysosomal enzyme release	
Adhesion molecule	Augments PMN and monocyte adherence to endothelial cells	Monoclonal antibodies to adhesion molecules
Platelets	Induce EDRF Vasoconstriction and PMN stimulation	
Bradykinin	Promotes EDRF release	
Thrombin	Induces PAF and EDRF Encourages fibrinogen consumption and factor inactivation	
Myocardial depressant substance (? TNF)	Reversible myocardial depression, ventricular dilation, and decreased left ejection fraction	
Nitrous oxide	Potent vasodilator	

*EDRF, Endothelium-derived relaxing factor; GM-CSF, granulocyte-macrophage colony-stimulating factor; IL, interleukin; PAF, platelet-activating factor; PMN, polymorphonuclear leukocyte; TNF, tumor necrosis factor.

From Bone RC: The pathogenesis of sepsis. Ann Intern Med 115:457–469, 1991.

considered controversial. The use of high-dose corticosteroids is not indicated as adjunct therapy in the management of sepsis. Three large clinical trials failed to document improved mortality in corticosteroid-treated individuals with shock.[68–70]

New directions in the treatment of SIRS and sepsis involve attempting to modify the inflammatory cascade. By interfering with mediators of the inflammatory response, endothelial and parenchymal organ damage might be minimized or avoided. Support for this approach has come from numerous animal and several human studies. Initial work involving the use of polyclonal antisera to endotoxin in human gram-negative sepsis documented a protective effect with reduced mortality.[71] The problems of pooled immunoglobulin, such as variability in specific antibody concentrations and the risk for transmission of infectious agents, have encouraged research in the area of monoclonal antibody production. Two randomized, double-blind, and placebo-controlled multicenter trials attempted to evaluate the efficacy of murine monoclonal (E5)[72] and mouse-human hybridized monoclonal (HA-1A)[73] immunoglobulin M antibodies to endotoxin in the setting of gram-negative sepsis with and without shock. In both studies, overall mortality was not affected compared with placebo; however, subgroup analysis identified improved 30-day mortality and decreased end organ damage in the E5 study subgroup presenting with gram-negative bacteremia without shock. Likewise, significantly improved 30-day mortality was reported in the gram-negative bacteremic HA-1A study subgroup, regardless of the presence of shock. A second E5 trial designed to evaluate the specific subgroup of gram-negative bacteremic patients not in shock failed to show statistically significant improved mortality, although a trend toward improved survival was seen in those patients with major end organ damage.[74] Further U.S. Food and Drug Administration–directed work after the study showed that these agents are currently controversial.[75] Consequently, these agents have not been approved as adjunct therapy in the treatment of sepsis. The lack of conclusive findings in these trials is disappointing but not indicative of future inability to affect the inflammatory response by manipulation of endotoxin function.

Intervention at the level of common denominator mediators would allow the potential treatment of severe systemic inflammatory response regardless of gram-negative involvement. TNF-α neutralization by monoclonal antibody administration has been promising; passive and active immunization in animal models challenged with gram-negative and gram-positive organisms exhibited survival advantages over nontreated groups.[76–79] Published results of a multicenter prospective trial involving the use of mouse-human hybridized monoclonal antibody to TNF-α showed an early (day 3) significant reduction in mortality in septic shock patients receiving drug compared with placebo; however, this benefit was not sustained through day 28, when only a trend toward improved mortality was observed in patients in shock.[80] It remains to be seen whether timely TNF-α immunoregulation is feasible when the natural production of this cytokine is so early and transient.

Another approach to mediator blockade is the use of cytokine receptor antagonists and soluble receptor molecules. Naturally occurring serum inhibitors to IL-1 act by competitively binding to IL-1 cell surface receptors. A recombinant form of this inhibitor, recombinant IL-1 receptor antagonist, has been evaluated in clinical trials.[81] There was a trend toward a dose-related increase in survival in patients with a larger predicted risk of mortality and organ dysfunction.

The multitude of factors involved in SIRS and sepsis and their complicated proinflammatory and antiinflammatory effects suggest that adequate pharmacologic control may require intervention at several levels through an immunologic "cocktail" provided in addition to standard treatment modalities. Such an approach may involve antiproteases as well as prostaglandin, complement, and nitric oxide inhibitors. The contributory effect of these individual therapies awaits delineation through experimental research.

Until we know more about the physiologic basis of sepsis, the complex interactions of mediators on human tissue, and the effects of artificially modifying them, mortality is likely to remain high given the limitations of present therapies.

References

1. Parillo JE: Pathogenetic mechanisms of septic shock. N Engl J Med 328:1471, 1993.
2. Dupont HL, Spink WW: Infections due to gram-negative organisms: An analysis of 860 patients with bacteremia at the University of Minnesota Medical Center 1959–1966. Medicine (Baltimore) 48:307, 1969.
3. Kreger BE, Craven DE, Carling PC, McCabe WR: Gram-negative bacteremia. III. Reassessment of etiology, epidemiology and ecology in 612 patients. Am J Med 68:332, 1980.
4. Weinstein MP, Murphy JR, Reller LB, Lichtenstein KA: The clinical significance of positive blood cultures: A comprehensive analysis of 500 episodes of bacteremia and fungemia in adults. II. Clinical observations, with special reference to factors influencing prognosis. Rev Infect Dis 5:54, 1983.
5. McCabe WR, Jackson GG: Gram-negative bacteremia. II. Clinical, laboratory, and therapeutic observations. Arch Intern Med 110:856, 1962.
6. Parillo JE, moderator: Septic shock in humans: Advances in the understanding of pathogenesis, cardiovascular dysfunction, and therapy. Ann Intern Med 113:227, 1990.
7. McCabe WR, Treadwell TL, De Maria A: Pathophysiology of bacteremia. Am J Med 75:7018, 1983.
8. McCabe WR, Jackson GG: Gram-negative bacteremia. I. Etiology and ecology. Arch Intern Med 110:847, 1962.
9. McGowen JE, Barnes MW, Finland MW: Bacteremia at Boston City Hospital: Occurrence and mortality during 12 selected years (1935–1972) with special reference to hospital-acquired cases. J Infect Dis 132:316, 1975.
10. Bryan CS, Reynolds KL, Brenner ER: Analysis of 1,186 episodes of gram-negative bacteremia in non-university hospitals: The effects of antimicrobial therapy. Rev Infect Dis 5:629, 1983.
11. Bryant RE, Hood AF, Hood CE, Koening MG: Factors affecting mortality of gram-negative rod bacteremia. Arch Intern Med 127:120, 1971.
12. Kreger BE, Craven DE, McCabe WR: Gram-negative bacteremia. IV. Re-evaluation of clinical features and treatment in 612 patients. Am J Med 68:344, 1980.
13. Bone RC: Why new definitions of sepsis and organ failure are needed. Am J Med 95:348, 1993.
14. Bone RC, Balk RA, Cerra FB, et al: Definitions of sepsis and organ failure and guidelines for the use of innovative therapies in sepsis. Chest 101:1644, 1992.
15. Rangel-Frausto MS, Pittet D, Costigan M, et al: The natural history of the systemic inflammatory response syndrome (SIRS). JAMA 273:117, 1995.
16. Knaus WA, Wagner DP, Draper EA, et al: The APACHE III prognostic prediction of hospital mortality for critically ill hospitalized adults. Chest 100:1619, 1991.
17. Bannerjee SN, Emori TG, Culver DH, et al: Secular trends in nosocomial primary bloodstream infections in the United States, 1980–1989. Am J Med 91:865, 1991.
18. Schaberg DR, Culver DH, Gaynes RP: Major trends in the microbial etiology of nosocomial infection. Am J Med 91:725, 1991.
19. Bamberger DM, Gurley MB: Microbial etiology and clinical characteristics of distributive shock. Clin Infect Dis 18:726, 1994.
20. Bone RC: Gram-positive organisms and sepsis. Arch Intern Med 154:26, 1994.
21. Bone RC: The pathogenesis of sepsis. Ann Intern Med 115:457, 1991.
22. Miller PJ, Wenzel RP: Etiologic organisms as independent predictors of death and morbidity associated with bloodstream infections. J Infect Dis 156:471, 1987.
23. Washington JA: Blood cultures: Principles and techniques. Mayo Clin Proc 50:91, 1975.
24. Musher DM: Cutaneous and soft tissue manifestations of sepsis due to gram-negative enteric bacilli. Rev Infect Dis 2:854, 1980.
25. Greene SL, Su WP, Muller SA: Ecthyma gangrenosum: Report of clinical, histopathologic and bacteriologic aspects of eight cases. J Am Acad Dermatol 11:781, 1984.
26. Dorff GJ, Geimer NF, Rosenthal DR, et al: *Pseudomonas* septicemia: Illustrated evolution of its skin lesion. Arch Intern Med 128:591, 1971.
27. Shackelford PG, Ratzan SA, Shearer WT: Erythema gangrenosum produced by *Aeromonas hydrophila*. J Pediatr 83:100, 1973.
28. Parker MM, Shelhamer JH, Natanson C, et al: Serial cardiovascular variables in survivors and nonsurvivors of human septic shock: Heart rate as an early predictor of prognosis. Crit Care Med 15:923, 1987.

29. Weil MH, Nishijima H: Cardiac output in bacterial shock. Am J Med 64:920, 1978.
30. Parrillo JE: The cardiovascular pathophysiology of sepsis. Annu Rev Med 40:469, 1989.
31. Ognibene FP, Parker MM, Natanson C, et al: Depressed left ventricular performance: Response to volume infusion in patients with sepsis and septic shock. Chest 93:903, 1988.
32. Parker MM, Shelhamer JH, Bacharach SL, et al: Profound but reversible myocardial depression in patients with septic shock. Ann Intern Med 100:483, 1984.
33. Abraham E, Bland RD, Cobo JC, Shoemaker WC: Sequential cardiorespiratory patterns associated with outcome in septic shock. Chest 85:75, 1984.
34. Parrillo JE, Burch C, Shelhamer JH, et al: A circulating myocardial depressant substance in humans with septic shock. J Clin Invest 76:1539, 1985.
35. Cunnion RE: Myocardial depressant substance. Ann Intern Med 113:237, 1990.
36. Siegel JH, Cerra FB, Coleman B, et al: Physiological and metabolic correlations in human sepsis. Surgery 86:163, 1979.
37. Mizock B: Septic shock: A metabolic perspective. Arch Intern Med 144:579, 1984.
38. Dantzker DR, Brock CJ, De Hart P, et al: Ventilation perfusion distributions in the adult respiratory distress syndrome. Am Rev Respir Dis 120:1039, 1979.
39. Clowes G: Pulmonary abnormalities in sepsis. Surg Clin North Am 54:993, 1974.
40. Fein AM, Lippmann M, Holtzman H, et al: The risk factors, incidence, and prognosis of ARDS following septicemia. Chest 83:40, 1983.
41. Fowler AA, Hamman RI, Good JT, et al: Adult respiratory distress syndrome in gram-negative sepsis. Ann Intern Med 98:593, 1983.
42. Kaplan RL, Sahn SA, Petty TL: Incidence and outcome of the respiratory distress syndrome in gram-negative sepsis. Arch Intern Med 139:867, 1979.
43. Malcolm ID, Fogel KM, Katz M: Vacuolization of the neutrophil in bacteremia. Arch Intern Med 139:675, 1979.
44. Mant MJ, King EG: Severe, acute disseminated intravascular coagulation. Am J Med 67:557, 1979.
45. Spector DA, Millan J, Zauber N, et al: Glomerulonephritis and *Staphylococcus aureus* infections. Clin Nephrol 14:256, 1980.
46. Altemeier WA, Fullen WO, McDonough JJ: Sepsis and gastrointestinal bleeding. Ann Surg 175:759, 1972.
47. Schuster DP, Rowley H, Feinstein S, et al: Prospective evaluation of the risk of upper gastrointestinal bleeding after admission to a medical intensive care unit. Am J Med 76:623, 1984.
48. Zimmerman HJ, Fang M, Utili R, et al: Jaundice due to bacterial infection. Gastroenterology 77:362, 1979.
49. Chow AW, Guze LB: Bacteroidaceae bacteremia: A clinical experience with 112 patients. Medicine (Baltimore) 53:93, 1974.
50. Miller SR, Wallace RJ, Musher DM, et al: Hypoglycemia as a manifestation of sepsis. Am J Med 68:649, 1980.
51. Nouel O, Bernuau J, Rueff B, et al: Hypoglycemia: A common complication of septicemia in cirrhosis. Arch Intern Med 141:1477, 1981.
52. Filkins JP, Cornell RP: Depression of hepatic gluconeogenesis and the hypoglycemia of endotoxic shock. Am J Physiol 227:778, 1974.
53. Fry DE, Pearlstein L, Fulton RL, Polk HC: Multiple system organ failure. Arch Surg 115:136, 1980.
54. Bell RC, Coalson JJ, Smith JD, et al: Multiple organ system failure and infection in adult respiratory distress syndrome. Ann Intern Med 99:293, 1983.
55. Giroir BP: Mediators of septic shock: New approaches for interrupting the endogenous inflammatory cascade. Crit Care Med 21:780, 1993.
56. Kalter ES, Daha MR, ten Cate SW, et al: Activation and inhibition of Hageman factor–dependent pathways and the complement system in uncomplicated bacteremia or bacterial shock. J Infect Dis 151:1019, 1985.
57. Bone RC: The systemic inflammatory response syndrome: Does the new name mean new therapies? Clin Immunother 1:369, 1994.
58. St. John RC, Dorinsky PM: Immunologic therapy for ARDS, septic shock, and multiple-organ failure. Chest 103:932, 1993.
59. Glauser MP, Heumann D, Baumgartner JD, Cohen J: Pathogenesis and potential strategies for prevention and treatment of septic shock: An update. Clin Infect Dis 18:s205, 1994.
60. Lorente JA, Landin L, Renes E, et al: Role of nitric oxide in the hemodynamic changes of sepsis. Crit Care Med 21:759, 1993.
61. Li TCM, Phillips MC, Shaw L, et al: On site physician staffing in a community hospital intensive care unit: Impact on test and procedure use and on patient outcome. JAMA 252:2023, 1984.
62. Reynolds HN, Raupt MT, Thill-Baharozian, et al: Impact of critical care physician staffing on patients with septic shock in a university hospital medical intensive care unit. JAMA 260:3446, 1988.
63. Shenap JL, Flynn PM, Barrett FF, et al: Serial quantitation of endotoxemia and bacteremia during therapy for gram-negative bacterial sepsis. J Infect Dis 157:565, 1988.
64. Ognibene FP: Management of septic shock. Ann Intern Med 113:240, 1990.
65. Packman MI, Rackow C: Optimum left heart filling pressure during fluid resuscitation of patients with hypovolemic and septic shock. Crit Care Med 11:165, 1983.
66. Desjars P, Pinaud M, Potel G, et al: A reappraisal of norepinephrine therapy in human septic shock. Crit Care Med 15:134, 1987.
67. Meadows D, Edwards D, Wilkins RG, Nightingale P: Reversal of intractable septic shock with norepinephrine therapy. Crit Care Med 16:663, 1988.
68. Sprung CL, Caralis PV, Marcial E, et al: The effects of high-dose corticosteroids in patients with septic shock: A prospective, controlled study. N Engl J Med 311:1137, 1987.
69. Bone RC, Fisher CJ Jr, Clemmer TP, et al: A controlled clinical trial of high-dose methylprednisolone in the treatment of severe sepsis and septic shock. N Engl J Med 317:653, 1987.
70. Hinshaw L, Peduzzi P, Young E, et al: Effect of high-dose glucocorticoid therapy on mortality in patients with clinical signs of systemic sepsis. The Veterans Administration Systemic Sepsis Cooperative Study Group. N Engl J Med 317:659, 1987.
71. Zeigler EJ, McCutchan JA, Fierer J, et al: Treatment of gram-negative bacteremia and shock with human antiserum to a mutant *Escherichia coli*. N Engl J Med 307:1225, 1982.
72. Greenman RL, Schein RMH, Martin MA, et al: A controlled clinical trial of E5 murine monoclonal IgM antibody to endotoxin in the treatment of gram-negative sepsis. JAMA 266:1097, 1991.
73. Zeigler EJ, Fisher CJ Jr, Sprung CL, et al: Treatment of gram-negative bacteremia and septic shock with HA-1A human monoclonal antibody against endotoxin—A randomized, double-blind, placebo-controlled trial. N Engl J Med 324:429, 1991.
74. Wenzel R, Bone R, Fein A, et al: Results of a second double-blind, randomized, controlled trial of antiendotoxin antibody E5 in gram-negative sepsis. *In* Program and Abstracts of the 31st Interscience Conference on Antimicrobial Agents and Chemotherapy; September 29–October 2, 1991; Chicago, IL.
75. Warren HS, Danner RL, Munford RS: Anti-endotoxin monoclonal antibodies—A second look. N Engl J Med 326:1151, 1992.
76. Beutler B, Milsark IW, Cerami AC: Passive immunization against cachectin/tumor necrosis factor protects mice from lethal effect of endotoxin. Science 229:869, 1985.
77. Tracey KJ, Fong Y, Hesse DG, et al: Anti-cachectin/TNF monoclonal antibodies prevent septic shock during lethal bacteraemia. Nature 330:662, 1987.
78. Hinshaw LB, Tekamp-Olson P, Chang ACK, et al: Survival of primates in LD100 septic shock following therapy with antibody tumor necrosis factor (TNFα). Circ Shock 30:279, 1990.
79. Hinshaw LB, Emerson TE Jr, Taylor FB, et al: Lethal *Staphylococcus aureus*–induced shock in primates: Prevention of death with anti-TNF antibody. J Trauma 33:568, 1992.
80. Abraham E, Wunderink R, Silverman H, et al: Efficacy and safety of monoclonal antibody to human tumor necrosis factor-α in patients with sepsis syndrome. A randomized, controlled, double-blind, multicenter clinical trial. JAMA 273:934, 1995.
81. Fisher CJ, Dhainaut JFA, Opal SM, et al: Recombinant human interleukin-1 receptor antagonist in treatment of patients with sepsis syndrome: Results from a randomized, double-blind, placebo-controlled trial. JAMA 271:1836, 1994.

68

Endocarditis

Oksana M. Korzeniowski
Donald Kaye

The pathogenesis, clinical identification, and bacteriologic diagnosis of infective endocarditis were well recognized long before adequate therapy was available. Up to the 1940s, infective endocarditis was a progressively debilitating, incurable, fatal disease that usually affected young people.[1] The advent of antibiotics made it possible to eradicate infection in nearly all cases of infective endocarditis, provided that the diagnosis was made and treatment was begun sufficiently early. Fatalities occurred as a result of irreversible anatomic injury, such as heart failure or cerebral hemorrhage.[2]

In the last 50 years, the population susceptible to disease, the predisposing lesions, and the infective agents have changed[3, 4]; nevertheless, the incidence of the infection (about 20 cases per million population) has remained the same as in the preantibiotic era.[5]

Characteristics of the Disease

Infective endocarditis usually refers to bacterial or fungal infection within the heart. Extracardiac endothelium can also be colonized by microorganisms, and the infection (more properly called endarteritis) produces a clinical syndrome indistinguishable from infective endocarditis.[6] Endocarditis was initially classified as acute or subacute on the basis of the clinical course as observed before availability of antimicrobial therapy and in a population at risk that consisted mainly of patients with congenital or rheumatic heart disease (RHD).[7] Acute endocarditis denoted infection of a normal valve by a virulent organism such as *Staphylococcus aureus* or *Streptococcus pneumoniae,* which rapidly destroyed the heart valve and caused widespread metastatic foci. Death occurred in less than 6 weeks. Subacute endocarditis referred to infection of abnormal valves with relatively avirulent organisms, such as viridans streptococci. The course was indolent (up to 2 years), and metastatic foci were uncommon. Such classic presentations of infective endocarditis are now encountered less frequently. Currently, patients with prosthetic cardiac valves, users of illicit parenteral drugs, and persons with mitral valve prolapse, instead of patients with RHD, account for the majority of cases of endocarditis. The bacteriology in each population differs, and correlations between organism and course of disease are variable. Current useful classifications refer to underlying anatomy and infecting organism and serve as a basis for therapy and clinical prognosis.

Native Valve Endocarditis

Sixty percent to 80% of persons with native valve endocarditis who do not use parenteral drugs have an identifiable predisposing cardiac lesion.[8] In most recent series, mitral valve prolapse has been the underlying lesion in 30% to 50% of cases.[9, 10] Although the frequency of mitral valve prolapse is three times greater in women than in men, men with mitral valve prolapse and systolic murmur are at considerably higher risk for development of infective endocarditis. Men older than 45 years are particularly at risk.[11] RHD accounts for approximately 30% of the heart lesions in patients with endocarditis.[12–14] Most patients with RHD and endocarditis are middle-aged or older, reflecting the worldwide decline in the occurrence of rheumatic fever and carditis. This reservoir is likely to increase and become younger if the outbreaks of rheumatic fever with high frequency of valvulitis noted in the 1980s continue to occur.[15] In RHD, the mitral valve is most commonly involved, followed by the aortic valve. Both valves are infected simultaneously in less than 5%.[16] A tricuspid valve may occasionally be affected by RHD.[17] Congenital heart disease is the underlying lesion in 10% to 20% of patients. Routine closure of patent ductus arteriosus by medical or surgical means has considerably reduced the number of young people at risk. Other predisposing lesions include ventricular septal defects, subaortic and valvular aortic stenosis, tetralogy of Fallot, coarctation of the aorta, Marfan syndrome, and pulmonary stenosis but not uncomplicated atrial septal defects. Degenerative heart disease, particularly calcific aortic stenosis, is important in predisposing the elderly to infective endocarditis.[18] Syphilitic aortic valves are unusual as the underlying lesion.

Infective endocarditis on a native valve in a non–drug abuser remains predominantly a disease of men (observed male/female ratio, 3:1).[14]

CAUSES

Streptococci (50% to 70%), enterococci (10%), and staphylococci (25%) account for the majority of cases of endocarditis on native valves in non–drug abusers[14, 16, 19] (Table 68–1). Viridans streptococci, normal inhabitants of the oropharynx, account for more than half of all streptococcal infections.[13] This group includes a variety of *Streptococcus* species, including *S. sanguis, S. salivarius, S. mutans,* and *S. mitior,* most of which are highly susceptible to penicillin.[20, 21] With the recent emergence of occasional strains resistant to penicillin, determination of penicillin susceptibility of the infecting organism is advisable.[22] Infections caused by these organisms occur mainly on abnormal heart valves, and patients frequently report recently having undergone dental procedures.

Enterococci (formerly classified as streptococci and now reclassified as a separate genus) and other members of Lancefield group D are most commonly isolated from the remainder of patients with endocarditis. The genus *Enterococcus* contains at least 12 species including *E. faecalis, E. faecium, E. durans, E. avium,* and *E. gallinarum.*[23, 24] Infections are most commonly caused by *E. faecalis* and *E. faecium.* They are α-, β-, or γ-hemolytic and normally inhabit the gastrointestinal tract and the anterior urethra. Enterococci can attack normal or damaged heart valves. Most patients are men 60 years or older who frequently give a recent history of genitourinary manipulation, trauma, or disease (cystoscopy, urethral catheterization, or prostatectomy); less often, women younger than 40 years who have undergone abortion, pregnancy, or cesarean section are affected. Correct biochemical identification and in vitro susceptibility testing are critical because of the worldwide emergence and nosocomial spread of multidrug-resistant strains.[25] Classically, enterococci are not killed by penicillin alone because of intrinsic low-level resistance to β-lactams conferred by low-affinity penicillin binding proteins, so large doses of penicillin must be used and an aminoglycoside must be added to achieve a bactericidal effect on these organisms.[21, 26] Enterococci, particularly *E. faecium,* are capable of acquiring new resistance determinants from other species and of serving as a reservoir of resistance genes for other gram-positive organisms.[25] Resistance to β-lactams has been

TABLE 68–1 ■ Frequency of Microbial Pathogens in Infective Endocarditis

	NATIVE VALVE (%)		PROSTHETIC VALVE (%)	
ORGANISMS	Nonaddicts	Addicts	Early (<2 mo)	Late (>2 mo)
Streptococci	50–70	20	5–10	25–30
Enterococci	10	8	<1	5–10
Staphylococci	25	60	45–50	30–40
S. aureus	23	59	15–20	10–12
S. epidermidis	2	1	25–30	23–28
Gram-negative bacilli	<1	10	20	10–12
Fungi	<1	5	10–12	5–8
Diphtheroids	<1	2	5–10	4–5
Miscellaneous organisms	5–10	1–5	1–5	1–5
Multiple organisms	<1	5	8	8
Culture-negative results	5–10	10–20	5–10	5–10

acquired as the result of the transfer of a β-lactamase gene from staphylococci.[27, 28] Transfer of genes encoding aminoglycoside-modifying enzymes through plasmids and transposons has resulted in increasing prevalence of strains with high-level resistance to all aminoglycosides.[29, 30] Rapid simultaneous worldwide emergence of partial or total resistance to glycopeptide antibiotics (vancomycin, teicoplanin, and daptomycin) now presents the specter of lack of effective treatment for endocardial infection with multidrug-resistant enterococci.[31]

Streptococcus bovis and *Streptococcus equinus* are group D streptococci, but they differ biochemically from enterococci and are usually readily killed by penicillin alone.[32] *S. bovis* endocarditis occurs principally in persons older than 60 years and is frequently associated with the presence of colonic polyps (67% versus 21% of patients with enterococcal endocarditis) or colonic malignant neoplasm (18% versus 2% for enterococcal endocarditis).[33, 34] *S. bovis* accounts for about 10% of cases of endocarditis.

Other Lancefield group streptococci account for less than 5% of cases of endocarditis. Group A and group B streptococci can attack normal valves and produce distant metastases. Diabetic patients are particularly at risk for group B organisms. Susceptibility to penicillin G varies.[35]

Staphylococci cause 25% of cases of native valve endocarditis.[36, 37] Most are coagulase-positive *(S. aureus)*; coagulase-negative *(Staphylococcus epidermidis)* species account for less than 10% of isolates.[38, 39] The great majority of staphylococci, whether acquired in the hospital or in the community, are highly resistant to penicillin G owing to their ability to elaborate β-lactamase. In the past decade, an increasing prevalence of methicillin-resistant isolates of *S. aureus* and *S. epidermidis* in hospitals, nursing homes, and community settings has also been noted, rendering β-lactam agents ineffective in some geographic locales as empirical therapy before demonstration of susceptibility.[40] *S. aureus* endocarditis is usually fulminant with multiple metastatic abscesses. Normal or damaged valves can be affected and are rapidly destroyed. *S. epidermidis* causes an indolent infection of abnormal valves.

Almost all species of bacteria are occasionally identified as causes of native valve endocarditis. Most commonly encountered are *S. pneumoniae*,[41] *Neisseria gonorrhoeae*,[42] *Haemophilus* species, *Pseudomonas, Listeria*, and diphtheroids. The clinical course can be fulminant or indolent. Serum-susceptible gram-negative enteric organisms and anaerobic organisms are less capable of sustaining endocardial infection.[43] Spirochetes (e.g., *Spirillum minus*), cell wall–deficient bacteria, intracellular organisms *(Legionella)*, rickettsiae *(Coxiella burnetii)*, and chlamydiae are rare causes of endocarditis.

Fungi rarely cause native valve endocarditis in the absence of intravenous drug abuse. Factors that predispose to fungemia (i.e., intravenous catheters, severe underlying illness, corticosteroids, prolonged use of broad-spectrum antibiotics, cytotoxic agents) can result in endocarditis. *Candida, Torulopsis*, and *Aspergillus* species are usually implicated. The course is indolent but grave; large vegetations frequently embolize to major vessels in the lower extremities.[44]

Endocarditis in Intravenous Drug Abusers

The frequency of endocarditis in intravenous drug abusers (IVDAs) is difficult to estimate, although studies have documented that approximately 13% of febrile IVDAs presenting to urban emergency departments have infective endocarditis.[45, 46] In urban tertiary medical centers, patients who are IVDAs account for 20% to 50% of infective endocarditis cases. There appear to be differences in relative risk for infection based on the drugs used (i.e., cocaine versus heroin or amphetamines), the frequency of use, and the modes of drug preparation.[47] IVDAs with endocarditis are usually male (male/female ratio, 3:1), and their mean age is 30 years.[48] Approximately 20% have underlying cardiac disease, usually either congenital lesions or residua of previous endocarditis. Echocardiographic studies have demonstrated mild degrees of tricuspid valve insufficiency in previously normal valves of IVDAs, which may explain the predilection for right-sided infective endocarditis among drug users.[9] The tricuspid valve is infected in about 54%, the aortic valve in 25%, and the mitral valve in 20%. Mixed right- and left-sided endocarditis occurs in 6%.[48, 49] The skin is the most frequent source of the microorganisms responsible for endocarditis, although contamination of drugs and associated paraphernalia also contributes to bacteremia.[50]

S. aureus is isolated in approximately 60% of cases, various species of streptococci and enterococci from almost 20% to 30%, gram-negative bacilli (predominantly *Pseudomonas* and *Serratia* species) from 10%, and fungi (usually *Candida*) from 5%. More than one microorganism is isolated from the blood of 5% of addict patients. Multiple organisms either can cause the primary infection or can be acquired during the course of therapy. *S. aureus*, by far the most frequent organism isolated in tricuspid valve endocarditis, accounts for 80% of clinical isolates.[48–50] Similarly, in 70% to 80% of cases of *S. aureus* endocarditis in IVDAs, only the tricuspid valve is involved.

The majority (70% to 100%) of addicts with tricuspid valve endocarditis are noted to have pneumonia or multiple septic emboli, but the murmur of tricuspid valve insufficiency frequently is not present or may be misinterpreted as a functional or flow murmur.[51] Moreover, patients with a syndrome compatible with tricuspid valve endocarditis may actually have an extracardiac focus of endovascular infection (i.e., septic thrombophlebitis involving the subclavian or femoral venous system) rather than endocarditis.[52]

There do not appear to be clinical or pathophysiologic differences in endocarditis in IVDAs with concurrent human immunodeficiency virus infection.[46, 53, 54] Although infective endocarditis is usually reported in the early stages of human immunodeficiency virus infection, the clinical stage of human immunodeficiency virus infection does not appear to affect the outcome of treatment. Valve replacement surgery does not seem to accelerate human immunodeficiency virus–related immunodeficiency.[55, 56]

Prosthetic Valve Endocarditis

Patients with congenital, rheumatic, arteriosclerotic, and degenerative valve disease as well as patients with hemodynamic impairment secondary to infective endocarditis may receive a prosthetic valve. Prosthetic valve infections account for 10% to 20% of all cases of endocarditis. The overall frequency of endocarditis in patients with prosthetic valves is 1% to 4%.[57–59] By convention, prosthetic valve endocarditis (PVE) is termed early when symptoms appear within 60 days of valve insertion and late when they occur thereafter. The early and late groups differ in clinical features, microbial patterns, and mortality rates.

Early PVE generally reflects contamination arising in the perioperative period. Most contamination probably occurs intraoperatively through direct wound inoculation or contamination of the bypass machine. Postoperative sources include intravenous catheters (particularly central lines), arterial lines, urethral catheters, cardiac pacing wires, and endotracheal tubes. The attack rate for early PVE before 1969 was 2.5% of all patients undergoing valve replacement and has been 0.75% of all such patients subsequently. Despite use of prophylactic antibiotics, staphylococcal infection accounts for 45% to 50% of early PVE. *S. epidermidis* is the organism most often isolated (average frequency, 25% to 30%); *S. aureus* causes 15% to 20% of infections. The remainder of cases are caused by gram-negative aerobic organisms (approximately 20%), fungi (particularly *Candida* and *Aspergillus*, 10% to 12%),[60] streptococci and enterococci (5% to 10%), and diphtheroids (5% to 10%).

Late PVE occurs after valves have been endothelialized.[61] The incidence depends on the length of follow-up. It has been estimated to occur at an overall incidence of 0.2% to 0.5% per patient-year. The source of infection is presumed to be transient bacteremia seeding the valve. Thus, the bacteriology more closely resembles that of native valve endocarditis. Viridans streptococci are the organisms isolated most often (25% to 30%); median time to onset of PVE is 24 months after valve implantation. Other streptococci and enterococci account for 5% to 10%. Infections with staphylococci (*S. epidermidis*, 23% to 28%; *S. aureus*, 10% to 12%), gram-negative bacilli (10% to 12%), fungi (5% to 8%), and diphtheroids (4% to 5%) occur more frequently in the first 18 months after implantation of the valve. Infections other than those caused by streptococci, enterococci, and *S. aureus* often reflect delayed clinical appearance of infections acquired perioperatively.[62]

In contrast to native valve endocarditis, the aortic prosthetic valve is more prone to prosthetic valve infection. No definite pattern of infection occurs when both aortic and mitral prosthetic valves are present, but the frequency of infection after multiple valve implantation is higher than after replacement of either valve alone. There currently seems to be no significant difference in infectibility between mechanical and heterograft valves. The frequency of PVE after replacement of an infected native valve is approximately 4%, much higher than after replacement of an uninfected valve. However, it is usually not caused by the originally infecting organism. An increased occurrence of PVE has been associated with the black race, male sex, and longer cardiopulmonary bypass time.

Early PVE is often associated with valve dysfunction or dehiscence, a fulminant course, and a high mortality rate. Depending on the infecting organism, late PVE is commonly indistinguishable clinically from that in patients without a prosthesis, but it may also present with a fulminant course.

Pathogenesis

Three hemodynamic factors predispose patients to the development of infective endocarditis: a high-velocity jet stream, flow from a high- to a low-pressure chamber, and a comparatively narrow orifice separating the two chambers that creates a pressure gradient.[63, 64] The lesions of infective endocarditis tend to form just beyond the narrowed orifice through which the high-velocity jet stream passes (i.e., on the ventricular surfaces of the incompetent aortic valve, on the atrial surface of the incompetent mitral or tricuspid valve, and on the walls of the pulmonary artery at the orifice of the patent ductus arteriosus). Satellite lesions can also grow where the jet stream strikes the endocardium (e.g., the atrial wall opposite the mitral orifice in mitral regurgitation, the papillary muscle of the left ventricle in aortic regurgitation, and the surface of the pulmonary artery opposite the patent ductus arteriosus). The force of the jet stream against these sites presumably denudes the endothelium and promotes deposition of clumps of fibrin and platelets, which form sterile vegetations called nonbacterial thrombotic endocarditis. Sterile vegetations can also occur in patients with wasting disease, particularly malignant neoplasia (marantic endocarditis); in areas surrounding foreign bodies, such as intracardiac catheters; and at surgical sites, particularly vascular incisions and implants.[65] Infective endocarditis occurs when microorganisms are deposited onto the sterile vegetation during the course of bacteremia.[66, 67] Organisms that adhere well to platelets, fibrin, or fibronectin and are resistant to host defense mechanisms such as complement and other serum factors are most likely to colonize sterile vegetations and at lower inocula.[68, 69] Subsequent deposition of platelets and fibrin over the bacteria forms a "protected site" into which phagocytic cells penetrate poorly, allowing survival and proliferation of the microorganisms. Fresh vegetations of infective endocarditis are composed of clumps of microorganisms, platelets, fibrin, occasional red blood cells, and a few leukocytes attached to the surface of a valve leaflet, chorda, or ventricular endocardium.[70] Underlying valve destruction may coexist. The morphologic characteristics of vegetations can vary, depending on the nature of the infecting organism and the activity of the disease, from small, flat, granular lesions to large, pedunculated, friable masses. Unimpaired bacterial growth results in extremely high colony counts (10^9 to 10^{10} bacteria per gram of tissue). As vegetations heal during the process of bacteriologic cure, infiltration by polymorphonuclear leukocytes and fibroblasts leads to fibrosis, hyalinization, and sometimes calcification. Finally, the lesion is covered by endothelium.[71]

A disparity in clinical course and response to antimicrobial therapy between left-sided and right-sided infective endocarditis has long been noted in animal models of infective endocarditis and in patients. The exact mechanisms remain largely undefined, although increases in oxygen tensions resulting in increased intravegetation bacterial populations, higher rates of spontaneous emergence of antimicrobial-resistant strains, more frequent establishment of extracardiac foci of infection with resultant sustained bacteremia and valvular reseeding, reduced intralesional penetration of antibiotics, and attenuated penetration of vegetation by phagocytic cells may account for the increased severity of left-sided versus right-sided endocarditis.[72]

Organisms that possess little inherent pathogenicity, such as viridans streptococci, usually implant only on sites of preexisting nonbacterial thrombotic endocarditis; more virulent organisms, such as *S. aureus* or *S. pneumoniae*, may be able to infect apparently normal valves.

Conditions that predispose to bacteremia, particularly with the common causative organisms for infective endocarditis, have been examined extensively. Transient bacteremia occurs whenever an area heavily colonized with bacteria is traumatized. The degree of bacteremia is proportional to the number of organisms that inhabit the area. The number of organisms in blood usually does not exceed 10 per mL, and intravascular residence is transient, lasting no more than 15 to 30 minutes.[73] Transient bacteremias are most commonly associated with dental extraction; periodontal surgery; and invasive oropharyngeal, gastrointestinal, urologic, or gynecologic diagnostic or surgical procedures. Spontaneous bacteremia in the absence of trauma occurs with lung and skin infections and in patients with severe periodontal disease. Viridans streptococci are the bacteria most commonly isolated from blood, alone or mixed with other species, after trauma to tissues of the mouth. A wide variety of trivial events, such as chewing and tooth brushing, induce streptococcal bacteremia. This may explain why 85% of cases of endocarditis caused by mouth organisms cannot be related to dental procedures.[74, 75] Enterococcal and gram-negative bacillus bacteremias occur commonly after genitourinary or gastrointestinal surgery or instrumentation. Although about half of patients with enterococcal endocarditis report genitourinary tract manipulation before the onset of their disease, only six cases possibly related to gastrointestinal diagnostic procedures have been described.[74] An antecedent staphylococcal infection has been reported in 31% of patients with staphylococcal endocarditis.

Pathophysiology

The symptoms and signs of infective endocarditis are highly variable and depend on the organ system involved. Clinical features result from the local intracardiac infectious process and its attendant complications, bland or septic embolization of fragments of vegetations to virtually any organ, constant bacteremia with seeding of distant foci, and development of immune complex–associated disease.[64]

Intracardiac infection can lead to perforation of the valve leaflet or rupture of the chordae tendineae, interventricular septum, or papillary muscle. Infections, particularly with *S. aureus*, may result in valve ring abscesses and may extend into the myocardium to produce burrowing abscesses and purulent pericardial effusions. Conduction abnormalities, fistulae between chambers of the heart and pericardium or major vessels, and aneurysms of the sinus of Valsalva may result. Large vegetations such as those caused by fungi or *Haemophilus* species can occlude a valve orifice. Healing of the infection may cause scar formation and subsequent valvular stenosis or insufficiency. Myocarditis and myocardial infarction may be due to coronary artery emboli, myocardial abscesses, or immune complex vasculitis.

Embolic phenomena are common in infective endocarditis. Most often, the renal, splenic, coronary, and cerebral circulatory systems are involved. Pulmonary emboli occur in right-sided endocarditis, and large emboli suggest fungal infection. Infarcts or abscesses may result, depending on whether septic or bland embolization has occurred. Septic embolization to the vasa vasorum or direct bacterial invasion of the arterial wall produces mycotic aneurysms. The most commonly involved vessels include the cerebral arteries, aorta, and sinus of Valsalva; a ligated ductus arteriosus; and the superior mesenteric, splenic, coronary, and pulmonary arteries.[76, 77] Rupture of the weakened vessel may occur acutely or years later.

The persistent bacteremia of endocarditis stimulates both the humoral and cellular immune systems.[78, 79] Specific antibodies of the immunoglobulin M, G, or A class, having opsonic, agglutinating, and complement-fixing properties, as well as cryoglobulins and macroglobulins have been described in infective endocarditis. Nonspecific generalized hypergammaglobulinemia also develops as in many other chronic infections. Circulating immune complexes are found in virtually all patients. Immune complex deposition along the glomerular basement membrane results in the development of glomerulonephritis (focal, membranoproliferative, or diffuse).[80] Arthritis and peripheral manifestations of infective endocarditis, such as Osler nodes, have been attributed to immune complex deposition in joints and in mucocutaneous vessels. Effective treatment leads to disappearance of circulating immune complexes. Rheumatoid factor (anti–immunoglobulin G immunoglobulin M antibody) develops in about 50% of patients with subacute infective endocarditis. The titer correlates with the level of hypergammaglobulinemia and decreases in response to therapy.

Clinical Manifestations

Symptoms of endocarditis generally start within 2 weeks of the precipitating bacteremia.[64, 81] Nonspecific symptoms such as malaise, fatigue, night sweats, anorexia, and weight loss are common, particularly with organisms of low pathogenicity (e.g., viridans streptococci). The onset of infection with organisms of high pathogenicity (e.g., *S. aureus*) is usually explosive. Fever is present in almost all patients with endocarditis but may be absent in elderly persons; in persons who suffer severe debility, renal failure, or congestive heart failure; or in those treated previously with antibiotics. The fever is usually low grade (temperature less than 39°C) except with acute disease.

Heart murmurs are almost always present, except in acute infections and with right-sided or mural infection. The appearance of a new regurgitant murmur or true changes in a preexisting murmur (not changes in intensity due to changes in heart rate or cardiac output) are uncommon but when present suggest acute staphylococcal disease and correlate with development of congestive heart failure.

Splenomegaly (present in about 30% of cases), petechiae (20% to 40%), and clubbing of the fingers (10% to 20%) tend to occur in disease of long duration (greater than 6 weeks). Petechiae are most frequently found on the conjunctivae, palate, buccal mucosa, and extremities; they may be embolic or vasculitic. Splinter hemorrhages (subungual, linear, dark red streaks) are nonspecific. They are often related to trauma. Lesions located proximally in the nail bed are more suggestive of endocarditis than are distal lesions. Osler nodes (small, tender nodules, usually on the finger or toe pads, that persist for hours to days) occur in 10% to 25% of patients but are also a feature of other diseases. Immune complexes have been demonstrated in dermal vessels of Osler nodes. Janeway lesions are due to septic emboli and are most commonly seen in acute endocarditis. They are nontender hemorrhagic areas on the palms and soles. Roth spots (oval retinal hemorrhages with a pale center located near the optic disk) occur in less than 5% of patients with endocarditis and are also found in patients with connective tissue disease and hematologic disorders. Musculoskeletal complaints (arthralgia or arthritis) may mimic rheumatologic disorders. Systemic emboli may occur during or after therapy and are recognized in about a third of patients. Pulmonary emboli are common in addicts with tricuspid valve endocarditis (70% to 100% are noted to have pneumonia or septic pulmonary emboli)[48] and can also be seen in left-sided endocarditis with left-to-right cardiac shunts. Neurologic manifestations are present in about one third of patients with endocarditis.[82, 83] Major cerebral emboli to the middle cerebral artery system account for 25% and mycotic aneurysms for 2% to 10%, but brain abscesses and purulent meningitis, cerebral arteritis, intracerebral bleeding, and encephalomalacia have been documented. Mycotic aneurysms are usually silent; symptoms may be those of an expanding mass or a catastrophic hemorrhage. Congestive heart failure is the most common complication of infective endocarditis. Contributing factors include valve destruction, myocarditis, coronary artery emboli with infarction, and myocardial abscesses. Renal disease is present in most patients with endocarditis and is due to abscesses (uncommon), infarction (50%), or glomerulonephritis (up to 80%). Renal insufficiency may result.

Laboratory Features

A normochromic, normocytic anemia is present in 70% to 90% of cases of endocarditis and worsens with duration of illness. The white cell count is usually normal; the differential count may be shifted left slightly.[84] In acute endocarditis (particularly staphylococcal), leukocytosis and thrombocytopenia may be present, but not anemia. The erythrocyte sedimentation rate is almost always elevated, except with heart or kidney failure. Rheumatoid factor is present in 50% of patients with endocarditis for 3 to 6 weeks. Circulating immune complexes are present in virtually all patients, but hypergammaglobulinemia is detected in only one quarter. High serum titers of antibodies directed against teichoic acid constituents of the cell wall of staphylococci suggest endocarditis or other deep-seated infection.[85] Unfortunately, false-positive reactions and cross-reactions with other gram-positive bacteria limit their usefulness in diagnosis. Large mononuclear cells can occasionally be seen on peripheral blood smears, but the yield is greater (25%) if the first drop of blood obtained after earlobe massage and puncture is examined. Intraleukocytic bacteria can be seen in buffy coat preparations of blood in about 50% of patients.[86]

The urinalysis is usually abnormal, with proteinuria or microscopic hematuria in most patients. Reduction in serum complement parallels the occurrence of abnormal renal function, especially that due to diffuse glomerulonephritis.[87]

The bacteremia in endocarditis is continuous, so the blood culture is the critical diagnostic laboratory test. Blood cultures are positive in more than 95% of patients; if any culture is positive, all are likely to be positive. Because the magnitude of bacteremia is constant, timing of cultures based on temperature is not rational. In subacute disease, in the absence of previous therapy, three cultures should be obtained in a 3- to 6-hour period, after which therapy is initiated. Therapy for acute disease should not be delayed for more than 2 to 3 hours. Cultures should be obtained at least 30 minutes apart to prove that the bacteremia was continuous. Results of blood cultures may be negative in as many as 25% of patients who recently received outpatient antibiotic therapy,[88] and on the basis of clinical status, it may be necessary to delay treatment to maximize the chance of obtaining positive blood cultures. Only one culture should be obtained from each venipuncture using anaerobic as well as aerobic techniques. The yield of positive cultures is increased by observing them for 3 weeks and making periodic blind Gram stains and subcultures.[89] Hypertonic media may improve recovery of cell wall–deficient bacteria from previously treated patients.[90] Addition of pyridoxine hydrochloride to media will improve chances of isolating nutritionally deficient variant streptococci.[91] Arterial blood cultures or cultures of bone marrow offer no advantage over venipuncture.[92]

Results of blood cultures may be negative in infections with fastidious organisms such as *Haemophilus parainfluenzae, Brucella* species, or anaerobes.[93] Prolonged incubation, up to 4 weeks, may increase the recovery rate. Fifty percent of patients with *Candida* endocarditis and almost all with *Aspergillus, Histoplasma, C. burnetii,* or *Chlamydia psittaci* endocarditis have negative blood culture results.[94, 95] Because large peripheral emboli are common in fungal endocarditis, embolectomy with histologic examination and culture of the embolus may be diagnostic. Serologic procedures have not proved useful in the diagnosis of fungal endocarditis. Q fever *(C. burnetii)* and psittacosis *(C. psittaci)* endocarditis are diagnosed by serologic tests.[95]

Cardiac ultrasonography has assumed an increasingly important role in the assessment and management of patients with suspected infective endocarditis.[4, 70, 96, 97] Two-dimensional transthoracic echocardiography (TTE) combined with Doppler echocardiography has become widely accepted as the technique for identifying underlying valvular abnormalities and their hemodynamic consequences. Serial echocardiography findings can contribute to decisions for surgical intervention and intraoperatively guide the eventual cardiac repairs. Limitations include relative insensitivity to small vegetations, poor visibility of periannular complications, and inability to detect abnormalities on prosthetic valves as a result of acoustic shadowing and poor acoustic windows. Transesophageal echocardiography (TEE) uses a transducer on the end of a gastroscope and takes advantage of the close apposition of the esophagus to the heart to improve visibility of small vegetations, both atrial chambers, pulmonic valve, aortic valve anulus, proximal ascending aorta, and mechanical and bioprosthetic valves.[98–101] Mycotic aneurysms, intracardiac shunts, and valve ring abscesses are also better visualized. Compared with TTE, TEE is superior in delineating small (less than 5 mm) vegetations (sensitivity of 90% to 95% versus 70% to 75% for TTE), perivalvular abscesses (sensitivity of 87% versus 28% for TTE), and prosthetic valve abnormalities (sensitivity of 82% versus 36% for TTE). The negative predictive value for infective endocarditis of a single TEE is greater than 90%, depending on the clinical circumstances and the absence of a prosthetic valve. Repeated TEE should be performed when suspicion of infection remains high and the initial study is not diagnostic.

Diagnosis

The protean manifestations of infective endocarditis duplicate the clinical findings of atrial myxoma, acute rheumatic fever, marantic endocarditis, collagen-vascular diseases, and thrombotic thrombocytopenic purpura. Endocarditis should be suspected when a heart murmur and unexplained fever are present for at least 1 week, in febrile IVDAs, in young persons with a sudden neurologic event, and in patients with a prosthetic valve who have fever or valve dysfunction. A definite diagnosis must be based on positive blood cultures or positive cultures of surgical specimens (vegetations),[14] but overdiagnosis and underdiagnosis are common, particularly in patients with atypical presentations or negative blood cultures. Clinical case criteria first proposed by Pelletier and Petersdorf[17] in 1977 included predisposing valvular disease, bacteremia, embolic phenomena, and evidence of an active endocardial process. These were modified in 1981 by Von Reyn and colleagues[14] by including practical definitions for the individual elements (i.e., type of underlying heart disease, duration of persistently positive blood cultures). Additional modifications were proposed by Durack and coworkers[102] in 1994 using echocardiography, behavioral risk factors (IVDA), and microbial species as further refinements. In a study examining the criteria used by blinded experts to determine the probability of a patient's having infective endocarditis, the number of positive blood cultures and the type of infecting organism were the strongest predictors of classification of a patient as a case of infective endocarditis when risk factors were excluded from analysis.[103] When blood cultures were ambiguous, the presence of a vegetation on the echocardiogram most often served as supporting evidence.

In the absence of positive results of blood cultures, a search must be made for other causes of fever (e.g., another occult illness, drug-related fever, or postcardiotomy or postpump fever).

Treatment

Inside the vegetation, infecting organisms exist at high densities in a state of reduced metabolic activity, protected from host defenses.[104] Because cure requires eradication of all the organisms by antimicrobial agents, bactericidal rather than bacteriostatic agents must be used in high enough concentrations and for a long enough period to sterilize the vegetation.[105] Parenteral therapy is preferable because it achieves higher and more predictable serum antibiotic levels than does oral treatment. Central intravascular catheters should be avoided because they increase the risk for superinfection of a vegetation. The antimicrobial susceptibility of the infecting organism should be determined accurately; the organism should be saved for future testing of serum bactericidal activity, further antimicrobial susceptibility testing if a change in therapy is indicated, determination of synergistic combinations of antibiotics, or comparison with a relapse strain. A peak serum bactericidal titer (the highest dilution of the serum while the patient is receiving antibiotics that kills a standard inoculum of the infecting organism in vitro) of 1:8 or greater generally indicates adequate therapy.[106] Adequate therapeutic efficacy may be anticipated in streptococcal, enterococcal, and staphylococcal endocarditis with regimens containing penicillins, cephalosporins, or vancomycin, provided that the organisms are susceptible to these drugs. In these instances, routine assays of titer are unnecessary. Determination of the titer is most valuable when response to therapy is suboptimal, when endocarditis is due to an unusual organism, or when an unconventional treatment regimen is used.[26]

In the past several years, a trend toward outpatient management of patients with uncomplicated infective endocarditis has evolved. Parenteral regimens using permanent intravenous catheters and antibiotics with long therapeutic half-lives have given results comparable to treatment rendered in inpatient settings.[107, 108]

Blood cultures should be obtained soon after antimicrobial therapy is instituted to ensure that the bacteremia has been eradicated. Although anticoagulants inhibit vegetation formation and allow more rapid eradication of microorganisms on the valve, their use in endocarditis is contraindicated because of an increased risk for fatal intracranial hemorrhage.

Specific Antimicrobial Regimens

While culture results are awaited, empirical antimicrobial therapy should be directed at the organism or organisms most likely to cause infection in the presenting clinical setting. For patients with a native valve and a subacute clinical course, therapy should be directed against enterococci, which are more antibiotic resistant than streptococci; in those patients with an acute course, treatment should cover *S. aureus*. In IVDAs, therapy should be directed against *S. aureus* (including methicillin-resistant organisms in cities with high endemic rates of this organism among IVDAs) and gram-negative bacilli. Patients with prosthetic valves should receive empirical antibiotic coverage for methicillin-resistant *S. epidermidis* and gram-negative bacilli. When the organism has been identified, the antimicrobial coverage should be directed specifically. If cultures remain negative but endocarditis is likely and a clinical response has occurred, the empirical treatment is continued. Recommendations for the specific antimicrobial treatment of streptococcal, enterococcal, and staphylococcal endocarditis have been published.[26]

Streptococci

Regimens for streptococcal and enterococcal endocarditis are based principally on the minimal inhibitory concentration (MIC) of the isolate to penicillin G.[26]

Highly Penicillin Susceptible Viridans Streptococci (MIC no more than 0.1 μg/mL). These recommendations (Table 68–2) also apply to infection with *S. bovis*, a penicillin-sensitive nonenterococcal group D streptococcus. Penicillin G alone for 4 weeks (regimen A) gives cure rates of 99%. Addition of gentamicin (regimen B or C) produces synergistic killing and sterilizes cardiac vegetations more rapidly. Equivalent cure rates are obtained in 2 weeks. Regimen B is appropriate only for uncomplicated infections. Regimen A is preferred for patients who are likely to have side effects with aminoglycosides (those with renal insufficiency, with eighth nerve disease, or older than 65 years). Penicillin for 4 weeks with an aminoglycoside for the first 2 weeks (regimen C) is used to treat relapse or in the presence of complications such as shock and extracardiac foci of infection. A 6-week regimen of penicillin with an aminoglycoside for at least the first 2 weeks is recommended for patients with PVE. Regimen D can be used in the hospital or for home therapy. Alternative regimens for penicillin-allergic patients include regimen D for those with a history of penicillin rash and regimen E for those who experience anaphylaxis.

With nutritionally deficient variant strains, regimen F should be used.

Relatively Penicillin Resistant Streptococci (MIC between 0.1 and 0.5 μg/mL). Treatment with 18 million units daily of penicillin in combination with an aminoglycoside (regimen C) is recommended for strains of viridans streptococci and strains of *S. bovis* relatively resistant to penicillin.[109, 110] When penicillin cannot be used because of development of a rash, a cephalosporin can be substituted for the penicillin (regimen D); the aminoglycoside should be continued. For patients with immediate-type allergic reactions, vancomycin alone (regimen E) for 4 weeks is the substitute of choice.

Enterococci and Viridans Streptococci (MIC of at least 0.5 μg/mL). Enterococci are relatively resistant to penicillin G (median MIC, 2 μg/mL) and uniformly resistant to cephalosporins. Because penicillin, ampicillin, and vancomycin are not bactericidal for enterococci, treatment of enterococcal endocarditis requires the addition of an aminoglycoside (regimen F routinely, or regimen G for persons allergic to penicillin) for cure of approximately 75% of patients. Therapy usually lasts 4 weeks but should be extended to 6 weeks when symptoms have existed for more than 3 months, the course is complicated, or infection is present on a prosthetic valve.

The synergistic bactericidal effect of aminoglycosides on

TABLE 68–2 ■ Treatment of Infective Endocarditis

STREPTOCOCCI

Viridans streptococci and *Streptococcus bovis*

- Penicillin G susceptible (MIC* ≤ 0.1 μg/mL)
  - Regimen A: Penicillin G at 12–18 million units/d intravenously (IV) in divided doses q 4 h for 4 wk
  - Regimen B: Penicillin as in regimen A plus gentamicin 1 mg/kg IV q 8 h both for 2 wk
  - Regimen C: Penicillin plus gentamicin for 2 wk as in regimen B with penicillin continued 2 wk longer
  - †Regimen D: Ceftriaxone at 2 g IV or intramuscularly (IM) daily for 4 wk
  - †Regimen E: Vancomycin at 15 mg/kg IV q 12 h for 4 wk
- Relatively penicillin G resistant (MIC > 0.1 μg/mL but < 0.5 μg/mL)
  - Regimen C
  - †Regimen D or E

Enterococci and viridans streptococci (MIC ≥ 0.5 μg/mL)

- Regimen F: Penicillin G 18–30 million units/d or ampicillin at 12 g/d IV in divided doses q 4 h, plus gentamicin at 1 mg/kg IV q 8 h or streptomycin at 7.5 mg/kg IM q 12 h, both for 4–6 wk
- †Regimen G: Vancomycin at 15 mg/kg IV q 12 h plus gentamicin or streptomycin as in regimen F, both for 4–6 wk

Prosthetic valve (see text)

STAPHYLOCOCCI

Native valve

- Methicillin susceptible *(Staphylococcus epidermidis, Staphylococcus aureus)*
  - Regimen H: Nafcillin at 2 g IV q 4 h for 4–6 wk with or without gentamicin 1 mg/kg IV q 8 h for the first 3–5 d
  - †Regimen I: Cefazolin at 2 g IV q 8 h for 4–6 wk with or without gentamicin as in regimen H
  - †Regimen J: Vancomycin at 15 mg/kg IV q 12 h for 4–6 wk
- Methicillin resistant
  - Regimen J

Prosthetic valve

- Methicillin susceptible
  - Regimen H, I, or J: for 6–8 wk with gentamicin for the first 2 wk and rifampin at 300 mg orally q 8 h for 6–8 wk
- Methicillin resistant
  - Regimen J: for 6–8 wk with gentamicin for the first 2 wk and rifampin at 300 mg orally q 8 h for 6–8 wk

*MIC, Minimal inhibitory concentration.
†Regimens for patients allergic to penicillin.

enterococci occurs only when growth in vitro is inhibited by 2000 μg/mL of the aminoglycoside. The degree of resistance as well as the susceptibility to individual aminoglycosides is highly variable, so testing in vitro should be routine. Synergism is more likely with gentamicin than with streptomycin. Other aminoglycosides may lack activity against *E. faecium.* In many locales, enterococci resistant to 2000 μg/mL or more of gentamicin have become common.[111] Although some of these gentamicin-resistant strains are inhibited by streptomycin, most are resistant to all aminoglycosides. It is unlikely with strains resistant to all aminoglycosides that the addition of an aminoglycoside would be of benefit. For these organisms, aminoglycosides probably should be excluded from the regimen, and the duration of therapy should be prolonged to 8 to 12 weeks. Relapse is more likely in infections with these organisms. Patients infected with β-lactamase–producing enterococci should receive either ampicillin-sulbactam or vancomycin plus an aminoglycoside antibiotic if they do not demonstrate concurrent aminoglycoside resistance.[112–114] Nosocomially acquired enterococcal strains run a real possibility of being vancomycin resistant or of demonstrating resistance to penicillins and aminoglycosides, thus posing a major therapeutic dilemma.[115, 116] Antibiotic selection should be based on in vitro susceptibility and synergy by testing. If teicoplanin sensitivity is demonstrated in a vancomycin- and β-lactam–resistant strain, this agent should be used.[117] When organisms are resistant to β-lactam antibiotics, aminoglycosides, vancomycin, and teicoplanin, regimens incorporating ciprofloxacin, rifampin, tetracycline, chloramphenicol, and novobiocin may be tried. Such regimens have been tested in animal models and used in patients with enterococcal bacteremia with variable success.[118] Human cases of infective endocarditis caused by these resistant strains have so far been reported only rarely and with poor outcomes.[119, 120] Duration of therapy in these circumstances is undefined. Investigational agents such as Synercid (quinupristin plus dalfopristin) may be of some benefit.

Isolation of a highly penicillin resistant viridans streptococcus, an event still uncommon in the United States, may require substitution of a glycopeptide antibiotic for penicillin.[22, 121]

Staphylococci

Most staphylococci are resistant to penicillin G because they elaborate β-lactamase.[122, 123] Drugs of choice for the treatment of most patients with native valve staphylococcal endocarditis are semisynthetic penicillinase-resistant penicillins such as nafcillin (regimen H) or first-generation cephalosporins (regimen I). Patients who cannot tolerate penicillins or cephalosporins should receive intravenous vancomycin (regimen J). A large percentage of coagulase-negative staphylococci *(S. epidermidis)* and an increasing percentage of coagulase-positive strains *(S. aureus)* are methicillin resistant; these strains are resistant to all penicillins and cephalosporins, and intravenous vancomycin (regimen J) is the only option. Addition of an aminoglycoside to these regimens for the first 3 to 5 days hastens clearing of bacteremia, but evidence of improved outcome is lacking, and routine administration of an aminoglycoside is not recommended.[60, 124] Treatment for 4 weeks is standard; prolonged courses of 6 weeks or longer are indicated for patients with metastatic or intracardiac abscesses or otherwise complicated courses. As vancomycin use for the treatment of *S. aureus* infective endocarditis has increased, suboptimal clinical outcomes have been documented and concerns have been raised regarding the comparative efficacy of all glycopeptide antibiotics (i.e., vancomycin, teicoplanin, daptomycin) versus the β-lactam agents.[4] Delays in in vitro bacterial killing as well as prolonged fever and bacteremia in patients have been documented with vancomycin and teicoplanin even with uncomplicated right-sided endocarditis caused by methicillin-sensitive strains.[125] More disturbing have been reports of bacteriologic failures even when organisms are demonstrably vancomycin sensitive. Failures of the antibiotic have been variously attributed to high protein binding, poor penetration of drug into vegetations, inadequate killing of stationary-phase bacteria, and rapid renal clearance.[37]

Tricuspid valve infections in drug addicts are more susceptible to antimicrobial therapy, and relatively short courses of treatment (e.g., nafcillin plus tobramycin for 2 weeks) have been proposed.[126] Outcome depends on careful selection of patients without large vegetations, left-sided endocarditis, or extracardiac metastatic foci of infection. Because of unacceptably high failure rates, short-course therapy with a vancomycin-aminoglycoside combination is not recommended.[127, 128] There is also some advocacy for oral treatment of uncomplicated right-sided infective endocarditis. A regimen consisting of a fluoroquinolone and rifampin has shown promise in preliminary trials; however, bacteriologic and clinical failures have been documented.[129] The linkage of quinolone resistance with methicillin resistance further limits the widespread usefulness of these agents in IVDAs with staphylococcal infective endocarditis.

Staphylococcal Endocarditis in the Presence of Intracardiac Prosthetic Material. In the absence of contradictory evidence in vitro, all *S. epidermidis* organisms causing PVE should be assumed to be methicillin resistant. Optimal antibiotic therapy is provided by vancomycin plus rifampin for 6 to 8 weeks with an aminoglycoside added for the first 2 weeks of therapy. Rifampin resistance can develop during therapy.[130] If myocardial abscess or valve dysfunction is present, surgery is required. Combination therapy is also recommended for *S. aureus* PVE. Methicillin-sensitive strains should be treated with a penicillinase-resistant penicillin together with rifampin for 6 to 8 weeks and gentamicin for the first 2 weeks; when methicillin-resistant strains are present, vancomycin must be used.

Other Organisms

Endocarditis caused by gram-negative bacilli, anaerobes, and other uncommon pathogens should be treated with the regimen of bactericidal drugs that demonstrates the best activity in vitro.[131] If efficacy in vitro can be demonstrated, the best results are obtained by combining penicillins, cephalosporins, or vancomycin with an aminoglycoside and administering the drugs for 4 to 6 weeks. Because of the emergence of β-lactamase–producing strains of the HACEK group, coupled with the difficulty in performing their antimicrobial susceptibility testing, third-generation cephalosporins (regimen D) have replaced ampicillin as the recommended therapy.[26] Quinolone antibiotics, such as ciprofloxacin, have expanded treatment options for gram-negative bacillary endocarditis by allowing prolonged oral administration of these agents. As of yet, clinical experience is limited, but anecdotal reports indicate successful outcomes even in *Pseudomonas* endocarditis.[132] Serum bactericidal titers should be monitored. Valve replacement may be necessary in addition to antimicrobial therapy. Currently available antifungal agents do not cure fungal endocarditis, so a combined medical (amphotericin B, alone or with other antifungal agents) and surgical (excision of the vegetation or valve replacement) approach is advocated in the treatment of fungal endocarditis. Outcome is poor at best, and relapses are common after discontinuation of therapy. The availability of imidazole agents active against *Candida* and *Aspergillus* species provides feasible agents for long-term oral antifungal treatment and suppression. A report of fungal infective endocarditis on prosthetic valves has indicated a marked improvement in outcome when postoperative antifungal suppression is maintained indefinitely.[60]

Surgery in the Management of Endocarditis

The three principal indications for surgical intervention in infective endocarditis are congestive heart failure, uncontrolled infection, and prosthetic valve dysfunction.[133, 134] In patients with acute aortic regurgitation from endocarditis complicated by congestive heart failure, mortality exceeds 50%.[135, 136] Immediate valve replacement is essential. Valve replacement is also indicated for patients with persistently positive blood culture results despite appropriate antimicrobial therapy, when appropriate microbicidal therapy is not available (infections caused by organisms such as fungi or certain gram-negative bacilli), when recurrent relapse occurs despite appropriate antimicrobial therapy, or with prosthetic valve dysfunction or dehiscence.[137–139] Surgery often becomes necessary for PVE caused by organisms other than streptococci. Persistence of infection with the same organism has been uncommon after valve replacement.[140] Postoperative antimicrobial therapy should be continued long enough to eradicate metastatic foci of infection. Valvulectomy without valve implantation may suffice in right-sided endocarditis.[141, 142] Myocardial or valve ring abscesses must be drained surgically.[143] Myocardial invasion extending from the valve anulus is common in PVE.[144] Prompt surgical intervention may be lifesaving. Surgery should be considered when large vegetations are demonstrated by echocardiography and there are recurrent arterial emboli during therapy.[145] Several echocardiographic studies have now determined that the rate at which emboli occur during treatment is time dependent; a greater than threefold reduction of embolic events occurs between the first week and weeks 2 to 3 of effective antibiotic treatment, regardless of the size, shape, mobility, and location of the vegetations.[146, 147] Heart transplantation has been performed in a patient with intractable heart failure resulting from infective endocarditis.[148]

Prognosis

The fever of most patients subsides by 3 to 5 days after antimicrobial therapy is begun. Persistence or recurrence of fever may be due to associated myocardial or metastatic abscesses, recurrent emboli, superinfection of the vegetation, or, most often, febrile reactions to antimicrobial agents.[149] Development of petechiae, Osler nodes, emboli, rupture of mycotic aneurysms, and congestive heart failure may continue even after effective antimicrobial therapy. Blood cultures performed 2 to 4 weeks after completion of therapy detect the majority of relapses.

The factors that predispose to a poor prognosis in infective endocarditis are nonstreptococcal disease, development of heart failure, aortic valve involvement, presence of large vegetations, infection of a prosthetic valve, older age, and valve ring or myocardial abscesses.[150]

The cure rate for streptococcal endocarditis is about 90%. Failures are due to heart failure, embolic phenomena, rupture of mycotic aneurysms, complications of cardiac surgery, or renal failure.[26] For nonaddicts, mortality from *S. aureus* endocarditis ranges from 25% to 40%, whereas cure rates in drug addicts exceed 90%.[122] Death is more likely to occur during the initial 2 weeks of therapy as a consequence of congestive heart failure, rupture of mycotic aneurysms, or widespread metastatic infection. Results are poor in endocarditis caused by fungi and gram-negative bacilli. The overall mortality rate from PVE in the last 10 years averaged 54%.[57] The mortality for early disease (74%) is significantly higher than that for late disease (43%). More recent results using combination antimicrobial therapy and early surgery are more encouraging and show reductions in mortality to 25% to 40% regardless of microbial cause, high-risk subgroups, or severity of illness.[137–139] About 10% of patients will suffer additional episodes of endocarditis.

Prevention

Although there is no definite proof that antibiotic prophylaxis reduces the risk for endocarditis, indirect evidence that it should do so is generally accepted.[74, 75, 151–154] Furthermore, although the disease is uncommon (1 to 5 per 1000 hospital admissions[14]), the sequelae of infection, in terms of mortality and residual valve damage, are so severe that prophylaxis is

TABLE 68–3 ■ Recommendations for Prophylaxis Against Endocarditis

PROCEDURE	RISK FACTORS	PATIENT-RELATED FACTORS DETERMINING CHOICE OF REGIMEN	RECOMMENDED REGIMEN
Dental, oral or upper respiratory tract (viridans streptococci)	Standard regimen	Ability to take oral antibiotic and no allergy to penicillin	Amoxicillin at 3.0 g orally (PO) 1 h before procedure; then 1.5 g 6 h after initial dose
		Inability to take oral antibiotic and no allergy to penicillin	Ampicillin, intravenously (IV) or intramuscularly (IM), at 2.0 g 30 min before procedure; then ampicillin at 1.0 g IV or IM or amoxicillin at 1.5 g PO 6 h after initial dose
		Allergy to penicillin	Erythromycin ethylsuccinate at 800 mg or erythromycin stearate at 1.0 g PO 2 h before procedure; then half the dose *or* Clindamycin at 300 mg PO 1 h before procedure and 150 mg 6 h after initial dose
		Inability to take oral antibiotic and allergy to penicillin	Clindamycin at 300 mg IV 30 min before procedure and 150 mg PO or IV 6 h after initial dose
	Patient considered at extremely high risk and not a candidate for standard regimen	No penicillin allergy	Ampicillin at 2.0 g IV or IM plus gentamicin at 1.5 mg/kg IV or IM 30 min before procedure; followed by amoxicillin at 1.5 g PO 6 h after initial dose or by repeat of parenteral regimen 8 h after initial dose
		Allergy to penicillin	Vancomycin at 1.0 g IV in 1 h starting 1 h before procedure; no repeated dose necessary
Genitourinary or lower gastrointestinal tract (*Enterococcus*)	Standard regimen	No penicillin allergy	Ampicillin at 2.0 g IV or IM plus gentamicin at 1.5 mg/kg IV or IM 30 min before procedure; amoxicillin at 1.5 g PO 6 h after initial dose, or repeat parenteral regimen 8 h after initial dose
		Allergy to penicillin	Vancomycin at 1 g IV in 1 h plus gentamicin at 1.5 mg/kg IM or IV 1 h before; (optional) repeat 8–12 h later
	Minor procedures in low-risk patients	Oral regimen, no penicillin allergy	Amoxicillin at 3 g PO 1 h before; then 1.5 g PO 6 h later

recommended for patients with predisposing cardiac lesions who undergo procedures known to cause bacteremia. The conditions for which prophylaxis is recommended are valvular or congenital heart disease (except for uncomplicated atrial septal defects or surgically corrected cardiac lesions without prosthetic implants more than 6 months after operation), intracardiac prostheses (except pacemakers), asymmetric septal hypertrophy, and a previous episode of endocarditis. Mitral valve prolapse is common, and the risk for endocarditis is only moderately increased. Therefore, prophylaxis is recommended only for patients with insufficiency (i.e., significant murmur).[151] Recommendations for prophylaxis, as published by numerous authoritative groups,[152, 153, 155, 156] are summarized in Table 68–3.

Prophylaxis for dental and other traumatic procedures in the mouth, nose, throat, or esophagus that are likely to cause bleeding is aimed at the viridans streptococci. The regimens are tailored to the patient's ability to take oral medications, a history of allergy to penicillin, and the risk for developing endocarditis. Whenever possible, simple oral regimens increase the likelihood of compliance. Amoxicillin has become the preferred general regimen because it is well absorbed even in the presence of food, provides blood levels that are bactericidal for most viridans streptococci for many hours, and is more effective than penicillin in reducing bacteremia.[151] For genitourinary and lower gastrointestinal tract procedures that are likely to cause significant trauma (e.g., urethral catheterization, prosthetic surgery, vaginal hysterectomy, colonic or gallbladder surgery), prophylaxis is directed against enterococci. Combination parenteral regimens are recommended, except for minor repetitive procedures in persons not at high risk for endocarditis. Fiberoptic endoscopy even with biopsy carries such a low risk that prophylaxis is not justified except possibly in extremely high risk patients such as those with prosthetic valves.

Prophylaxis for cardiac surgery, including implantation of prosthetic devices, patches, and sutures, is directed against staphylococci.[156] The usual regimen is intravenous administration of cefazolin, 2 g, plus gentamicin, 1.5 mg/kg, at induction of anesthesia, followed by repeated doses 8 and 16 hours later. With the emergence of methicillin-resistant *S. epidermidis* (and, more recently, methicillin-resistant *S. aureus*) as an important nosocomial pathogen, substitution of intravenous vancomycin (15 mg/kg in 1 hour starting 1 hour before the procedure; 10 mg/kg after completion of bypass; then 7.5 mg/kg every 6 hours for three doses) for cefazolin may be prudent. Vancomycin is also used to treat patients who are hypersensitive to penicillin and cephalosporins.

References

1. Kelson SR, White PD: Notes on 250 cases of subacute bacterial streptococcal endocarditis studied and treated between 1927 and 1939. Ann Intern Med 22:40, 1940.
2. Christie RV: Penicillin in subacute bacterial endocarditis. Br Med J 1:4539, 1948.
3. McCartney AC: Changing trends in infective endocarditis. J Clin Pathol 45:945, 1992.
4. Bayer AS: Infective endocarditis. Clin Infect Dis 17:313, 1993.
5. Gray IR: Infective endocarditis 1937–1987. Br Heart J 57:211, 1987.
6. Parkhurst GF, Decker JP: Bacterial aortitis and mycotic aneurysms of the aorta: A report of 12 cases. Am J Pathol 31:821, 1955.
7. Kerr A Jr: Subacute Bacterial Endocarditis. Springfield, IL, Charles C Thomas, 1955, pp 3–343.
8. Weinberger I, Rotenberg Z, Zacharovitch D, et al: Native valve infective endocarditis in the 1970's versus the 1980's: Underlying cardiac lesions and infecting organisms. Clin Cardiol 13:94, 1990.
9. Naggar CZ, Forgacs P: Infective endocarditis: A challenging disease. Med Clin North Am 70:1279, 1986.
10. McKinsey DS, Ratts TE, Bisno AL: Underlying cardiac lesions in adults with infective endocarditis. Am J Med 82:681, 1987.
11. Frary CJ, Devereux RB, Kramer-Fox R, et al: Clinical and health care cost consequences of infective endocarditis in mitral valve prolapse. Am J Cardiol 73:263, 1993.
12. Moulsdale MT, Eykyn SJ, Phillips I: Infective endocarditis, 1970–1979. A study of culture-positive cases in St. Thomas' Hospital. Q J Med 49:315, 1980.
13. Venezio FR, Westenfelder GO, Cook VF, et al: Infective endocarditis in a community hospital. Arch Intern Med 142:789, 1982.
14. Von Reyn CF, Levy BS, Arbeit RD, et al: Infective endocarditis: An analysis based on strict case definitions. Ann Intern Med 94:505, 1981.
15. Denny FW Jr: A 45 year perspective on the streptococcus and rheumatic fever: The Edward H. Kass lecture in infectious disease history. Clin Infect Dis 19:1110, 1994.
16. DiNubile MJ, Calderwood SB, Steinhaus DM, Karchmer AW: Cardiac conduction abnormalities complicating native valve active infective endocarditis. Am J Cardiol 58:1213, 1986.
17. Pelletier LL, Petersdorf RG: Infective endocarditis: A review of 125 cases from the University of Washington Hospital, 1963–72. Medicine (Baltimore) 56:287, 1977.
18. Stekelberg JM, Melton LJ IV, Ilstrup DM, et al: Influence of referral bias on the apparent clinical spectrum of infective endocarditis. Am J Med 88:582, 1990.
19. Kaye D: Changing pattern of infective endocarditis. Am J Med 78(Suppl 6B):157, 1985.
20. Roberts RB, Kueger AG, Gross KC: The species of viridans streptococci associated with microbial endocarditis: Incidence and antimicrobial sensitivity. Trans Am Clin Climatol Assoc 89:36, 1977.
21. Tuazon CU, Gill V, Gill F: Streptococcal endocarditis: Single vs. combination antibiotic therapy and role of various species. Rev Infect Dis 8:54, 1986.
22. Guiot HF, Corel LJ, Vossen JM: Prevalence of penicillin-resistant viridans streptococci in healthy children and in patients with malignant hematological disorders. Eur J Clin Microbiol Infect Dis 13:645, 1994.
23. Musher DM: *Streptococcus faecalis* and other group D streptococci. *In* Mandell GL, Douglas RG, Bennet JE (eds): Principles and Practice of Infectious Diseases. New York, John Wiley & Sons, 1985, pp 1152–1155.
24. Rouff KL: Recent taxonomic changes in the genus *Enterococcus*. Eur J Clin Microbiol Infect Dis 9:75, 1990.
25. Low DE, Willey BM, Betschel S, Kreiswirth B: Enterococci: Pathogens of the 90's. Eur J Surg Suppl 573:19, 1994.
26. Wilson W, Karchmer AW, Dajani AS, et al: Antibiotic treatment of adults with infective endocarditis due to streptococci, enterococci, staphylococci, and HACEK microorganisms. JAMA 274:1706, 1995.
27. Murray BE, Singh KV, Markowitz SM, et al: Evidence for clonal spread of a single strain of β-lactamase producing *Enterococcus (Streptococcus) faecalis* to six hospitals in five states. J Infect Dis 163:780, 1991.
28. Patterson JE, Zervos MJ: Susceptibility and bacterial activity studies of four β-lactamase–producing enterococci. Antimicrob Agents Chemother 33:251, 1989.
29. Patterson JE, Masecar BL, Kauffman CA, et al: Gentamicin resistant plasmids of enterococci from diverse geographic areas are heterogeneous. J Infect Dis 158:212, 1988.
30. Eliopoulos GM: Aminoglycoside resistant enterococcal endocarditis. Infect Dis Clin North Am 7:117, 1993.
31. Shlaes DM, Elter L, Guttmann L: Synergistic killing of vancomycin-resistant enterococci of classes A, B, and C by combinations of vancomycin, penicillin and gentamicin. Antimicrob Agents Chemother 35:776, 1991.
32. Hoppes WL, Lerner PL: Nonenterococcal group-D endocarditis caused by *Streptococcus bovis*. Ann Intern Med 81:588, 1974.
33. Leport C, Bure A, Leport J, Vilde JL: Incidence of colonic lesions in *Streptococcus bovis* and enterococcal endocarditis. Lancet 1:748, 1987.
34. Emiliani VJ, Chodos JE, Comer GM, et al: *Streptococcus bovis* brain abscess associated with an occult colonic villous adenoma. Am J Gastroenterol 85:78, 1990.
35. Bayer AS, Chow AW, Anthony BF, Guze LB: Serious infections in adults due to group B streptococci. Clinical and serotypic characterization. Am J Med 61:498, 1976.
36. Bayer AS: Staphylococcal bacteremia and endocarditis: State of the art. Arch Intern Med 142:1169, 1982.
37. Mortara LA, Bayer AS: *Staphylococcus aureus* bacteremia and endocarditis—New diagnostic and therapeutic concepts. Infect Dis Clin North Am 7:53, 1993.
38. Whitener C, Caputo GM, Weitekamp MR, Karchmer AW: Endocarditis due to coagulase-negative staphylococci: Microbiologic, epidemiologic and clinical considerations. Infect Dis Clin North Am 7:81, 1993.
39. Caputo GM, Archer GL, Calderwood SB, et al: Native valve endocarditis due to coagulase-negative staphylococci: Clinical and microbiologic features. Am J Med 83:619, 1987.
40. Voss A, Milatovic D, Wallrauch-Schwarz C, et al: Methicillin-resistant *Staphylococcus aureus* in Europe. Eur J Clin Microbiol Infect Dis 13:50, 1994.
41. Bruyn GAW, Thompson J, Vandermeer JWM: Pneumococcal endocarditis in adult patients: A report of five cases and review of the literature. Q J Med 74:33, 1990.
42. Owens JE, Kelchak JA: Gonococcal endocarditis: Report of a case and review of the literature. J S C Med Assoc 86:93, 1990.
43. Yersin B, Glauser MP, Guze PA, et al: Experimental *Escherichia coli* endocarditis in rats: Roles of serum bactericidal activity and duration of catheter placement. Infect Immun 56:1273, 1988.
44. Rubinstein E, Noriega ER, Simberkoff MS, et al: Fungal endocarditis: Analysis of 24 cases and review of the literature. Medicine (Baltimore) 54:331, 1975.
45. Bayer AS, Ward JI, Ginzton LE, Shapiro SM: Evaluation of new clinical criteria for diagnosis of infective endocarditis. Am J Med 96:211, 1994.
46. Weisse AB, Heller DR, Schimenti RJ, et al: The febrile parenteral drug user: A prospective study in 121 patients. Am J Med 94:274, 1993.
47. Chambers HF, Morris DL, Tauber MG, Modin G: Cocaine use and the risk for endocarditis in intravenous drug users. Ann Intern Med 106:833, 1987.
48. Reisberg BE: Infective endocarditis in the narcotic addict. Prog Cardiovasc Dis 22:193, 1979.
49. Hecht SR, Berger M: Right-sided endocarditis in intravenous drug users. Prognostic features in 102 episodes. Ann Intern Med 117:560, 1992.
50. Vlahov D, Sullivan M, Astemborski J: Bacterial infections and skin cleaning prior to injection among intravenous drug users. Public Health Rep 107:595, 1992.
51. Chambers HF, Korzeniowski OM, Sande MA, the National Collaborative Endocarditis Study Group: *Staphylococcus aureus* endocarditis: Clinical manifestations in addicts and nonaddicts. Medicine (Baltimore) 62:170, 1983.
52. Murray HW: Infections in drug abusers. *In* Mandell GL, Douglas RG, Bennet JE (eds): Principles and Practice of Infectious Diseases. New York, John Wiley & Sons, 1985, p 1665.
53. Valencia ME, Guinea J, Soriano V, et al: Study of 164 episodes of infective endocarditis in drug addicts: Comparison of HIV positive and negative patients. Rev Clin Esp 194:535, 1994.

54. Carrel T, Schaffner A, Vogt P, et al: Endocarditis in intravenous drug addicts and HIV infected patients: Possibilities and limitations of surgical treatment. J Heart Valve Dis 2:140, 1993.
55. Lemma M, Vanelli P, Beretta L, et al: Cardiac surgery in HIV positive intravenous drug addicts: Influence of cardiopulmonary bypass on the progression to AIDS. Thorac Cardiovasc Surg 40:279, 1992.
56. Brau N, Esposito RA, Simberkoff MS: Cardiac valve replacement in patients infected with the human immunodeficiency virus. Ann Thorac Surg 54:552, 1992.
57. Cowgill LD, Addonizio VP, Hopeman AR, Harken AH: Prosthetic valve endocarditis. Curr Probl Cardiol 11:617, 1986.
58. Heimburger TS, Duma RJ: Infections of prosthetic heart valves and cardiac pacemakers. Infect Dis Clin North Am 3:221, 1989.
59. Grover FL, Cohen DJ, Oprian C, et al: Determinants of the occurrence of and survival from prosthetic valve endocarditis. Experience of the Veteran's Affair Cooperative Study on Valvular Heart Diseases. J Thorac Cardiovasc Surg 108:207, 1994.
60. Muehrcke DD: Fungal prosthetic valve endocarditis. Thorac Cardiovasc Surg 7:20, 1995.
61. Tornos P, Sanz E, Permanyar-Miralda G, et al: Late prosthetic valve endocarditis. Immediate and long term prognosis. Chest 101:37, 1992.
62. Bayer AS, Nelson RJ, Slama TG: Current concepts in prevention of prosthetic valve endocarditis. Chest 97:1203, 1990.
63. Rodbard S: Blood velocity and endocarditis. Circulation 27:18, 1963.
64. Weinstein L, Schlesinger JJ: Pathoanatomic, physiologic and clinical correlates in endocarditis. N Engl J Med 291:832, 1122, 1974.
65. Lopez JA, Ross RS, Fishbein MC, Siegel RJ: Nonbacterial thrombotic endocarditis: A review. Am Heart J 113:773, 1987.
66. Baddour LM, Christensen GD, Lowrance JH, Simpson WA: Pathogenesis of experimental endocarditis. Rev Infect Dis 11:452, 1989.
67. Baddour LM, Christensen GD, Lowrance JH, Simpson WA: Production and progress of the disease in rabbits. Br J Exp Pathol 54:142, 1973.
68. Bisno AL: Probing the pathogenesis of infective endocarditis. J Lab Clin Med 112:1, 1988.
69. Sullam PM, Drake TA, Sande MA: Pathogenesis of endocarditis. Am J Med 78(Suppl 6B):110, 1985.
70. Vegetations, valves, and echocardiography (Editorial). Lancet 2:1118, 1988.
71. Roberts WC, Buchbinder NA: Healed left-sided infective endocarditis: A clinicopathological study of 59 patients. Am J Cardiol 40:876, 1977.
72. Bayer AS, Norman DC: Valve site-specific pathogenic differences between right sided and left sided bacterial endocarditis. Chest 98:200, 1990.
73. Everett ED, Hirschmann JV: Transient bacteremia and endocarditis prophylaxis: A review. Medicine (Baltimore) 56:61, 1977.
74. Durack DT: Current issues in the prevention of infective endocarditis. Am J Med 78(Suppl 6B):149, 1985.
75. VanderMeer JTM, VanWijk W, Thompson J, et al: Efficacy of antibiotic prophylaxis for prevention of native valve endocarditis. Lancet 339:135, 1992.
76. Mansur AJ, Grinberg M, Leao PP, et al: Extracranial mycotic aneurysms in infective endocarditis. Clin Cardiol 9:65, 1986.
77. Brust JCM, Dickinson PCT, Hughes JEO: The diagnosis and treatment of cerebral mycotic aneurysms. Ann Neurol 27:238, 1990.
78. Phair JP, Clarke J: Immunology of infective endocarditis. Prog Cardiovasc Dis 22:137, 1979.
79. Bayer AS, Theofilopoulos AN: Immunopathogenetic aspects of infective endocarditis. Chest 97:204, 1990.
80. McKinsey DS, McMurray TL, Flynn JM: Immune complex glomerulonephritis associated with *Staphylococcus aureus* bacteremia: Response to corticosteroid therapy. Rev Infect Dis 12:125, 1990.
81. Lerner PL, Weinstein L: Infective endocarditis in the antibiotic era. N Engl J Med 274:388, 1966.
82. Salgado AV, Furlan AJ, Keys TF, et al: Neurologic complications of endocarditis: A 12-year experience. Neurology 39:173, 1989.
83. Tunkel AR, Kaye D: Neurologic complications of infective endocarditis. Neurol Clin 11:419, 1993.
84. Weinstein L, Rubin RH: Infective endocarditis—1973. Prog Cardiovasc Dis 26:239, 1973.
85. Bayer AS, Lam K, Ginzton L, et al: *Staphylococcus aureus* bacteremia: Clinical, serologic, and echocardiographic findings in patients with and without endocarditis. Arch Intern Med 147:457, 1987.
86. Powers DL, Mandell GL: Intraleukocytic bacteria in endocarditis patients. JAMA 227:312, 1974.
87. Gutman RA, Striker GE, Gilliland BC, et al: The immune complex glomerulonephritis of bacterial endocarditis. Medicine (Baltimore) 51:1, 1972.
88. Pazin GJ, Saul S, Thompson ME: Blood culture positivity: Suppression by outpatient antibiotic therapy in patients with bacterial endocarditis. Arch Intern Med 142:263, 1982.
89. Kaye D: Infecting Microorganisms in Infective Endocarditis. Baltimore, University Park Press, 1976.
90. Washington JA II: The role of the microbiology laboratory in the diagnosis and antimicrobial treatment of infective endocarditis. Mayo Clin Proc 57:22, 1982.
91. Carey RB, Gross KC, Roberts RB: Vitamin B6–dependent *Streptococcus mitior (mitis)* isolated from patients with systemic infections. J Infect Dis 131:722, 1975.
92. Beeson PB, Brannon ES, Warren JV: Observations on the sites of removal of bacteria from the blood in patients with bacterial endocarditis. J Exp Med 81:9, 1945.
93. Tunkel AR, Kaye D: Endocarditis with negative blood cultures. N Engl J Med 326:1215, 1992.
94. Rudd RM, Hill PR, Kopelman P, Parker DJ: Fungal endocarditis after homograft valve replacement: Difficulties in diagnosis and treatment. Thorax 35:686, 1980.
95. Fernandez-Guerrero ML: Zoonotic endocarditis. Infect Dis Clin North Am 7:135, 1993.
96. Schwinger ME, Tunick PA, Freedberg RS, et al: Vegetations on endocardial surface struck by regurgitant jets: Diagnosis by transesophageal echocardiography. Am Heart J 119:1212, 1990.
97. Jaffe WM, Morgan DE, Pearlman AS: Infective endocarditis, 1983–1988: Echocardiographic findings and factors influencing morbidity and mortality. J Am Coll Cardiol 15:1227, 1990.
98. Shapiro SM, Young E, DeGuzman S, et al: Transesophageal echocardiography in the diagnosis of infective endocarditis. Chest 105:377, 1994.
99. Grayburn PA: Southwestern Internal Medicine Conference: Clinical applications of transesophageal echocardiography. Am J Med Sci 307:151, 1994.
100. Daniel WG, Muggi A, Grote J, et al: Comparison of transthoracic and transesophageal echocardiography for detection of abnormalities of prosthetic and bioprosthetic valves in the mitral and aortic positions. Am J Cardiol 71:210, 1993.
101. Lowry RW, Zoghbi WA, Baker WB, et al: Clinical impact of transesophageal echocardiography in the diagnosis and management of infective endocarditis. Am J Cardiol 73:1089, 1994.
102. Durack DT, Lukes AS, Bright DK, et al: New criteria for diagnosis of infective endocarditis: Utilization of specific echocardiographic findings. Am J Med 96:200, 1994.
103. Berlin JA, Abrutyn E, Strom BL, et al: Assessing diagnostic criteria for active infective endocarditis. Am J Cardiol 73:887, 1994.
104. Durack DT, Beeson PB: Experimental bacterial endocarditis II. Survival of bacteria in endocardial vegetations. Br J Exp Pathol 53:50, 1972.
105. Bayer AS, Crowell D, Nast CC: Intravegetation antimicrobial distribution in aortic endocarditis analyzed by computer-generated model. Chest 97:611, 1990.
106. Wolfson JS, Swartz MN: Drug therapy: Serum bactericidal activity as a monitor of antibiotic therapy. N Engl J Med 312:968, 1985.
107. Francioli P, Etienne J, Hoigne R, et al: Treatment of streptococcal endocarditis with a single daily dose of ceftriaxone sodium for 4 weeks. Efficacy and outpatient treatment feasibility. JAMA 267:264, 1992.
108. Francioli PB: Ceftriaxone and outpatient treatment of infective endocarditis. Infect Dis Clin North Am 7:97, 1993.
109. Meeson J, McColm AA, Acred P: Differential response to benzylpenicillin in vivo of tolerant and non-tolerant variants of *Streptococcus sanguis*. II. J Antimicrob Chemother 25:103, 1990.
110. DiNubile MJ: Treatment of endocarditis caused by relatively

resistant nonenterococcal streptococci: Is penicillin enough? Rev Infect Dis 12:112, 1990.
111. Eliopoulos GM, Eliopoulos CT: Therapy of enterococcal infections. Eur J Clin Microbiol Infect Dis 9:118, 1990.
112. Ingerman M, Pitsakis PG, Rosenberg A, et al: β-Lactamase production in experimental endocarditis due to aminoglycoside resistant *Streptococcus faecalis*. J Infect Dis 155:1226, 1987.
113. Besnier JM, Leport C, Bure A, et al: Vancomycin-aminoglycoside combinations in therapy of endocarditis caused by *Enterococcus* species and *Streptococcus bovis*. Eur J Clin Microbiol Infect Dis 9:130, 1990.
114. Eliopoulos GM, Thauvin-Eliopoulos C, Moellering RC Jr: Contribution of animal models in the search for effective therapy for endocarditis due to enterococci with high-level resistance to gentamicin. Clin Infect Dis 15:58, 1992.
115. Jordens JZ, Bates J, Griffiths DT: Faecal carriage and nosocomial spread of vancomycin-resistant *Enterococcus faecium*. J Antimicrob Chemother 34:515, 1994.
116. Shlaes DM, Binczewski B, Rice LB: Emerging antimicrobial resistance and the immunocompromised host. Clin Infect Dis 17(Suppl 2):S527, 1993.
117. Leclerg R, Dutka-Malen S, Brisson-Noel A, et al: Resistance of enterococci to aminoglycosides and glycopeptides. Clin Infect Dis 15:495, 1992.
118. Whitman MS, Pitsakis PG, Zausner A, et al: Antibiotic treatment of experimental endocarditis due to vancomycin- and ampicillin-resistant *Enterococcus faecium*. Antimicrob Agents Chemother 37:2069, 1993.
119. Venditti M, Biavasco F, Varaldo PE, et al: Catheter-related endocarditis due to glycopeptide-resistant *Enterococcus faecalis* in a transplanted heart. Clin Infect Dis 17:524, 1993.
120. McDonald GR: Endocarditis after ciprofloxacin therapy for enterococcal pyelonephritis with bacteremia. J Tenn Med Assoc 86:527, 1993.
121. Martinez F, Martin-Luengo F, Garcia A, et al: Treatment of experimental endocarditis caused by penicillin-resistant *Streptococcus sanguis* with different doses of teicoplanin. Methods Find Exp Clin Pharmacol 16:247, 1994.
122. Karchmer AW: Staphylococcal endocarditis: Laboratory and clinical basis for antibiotic therapy. Am J Med 78(Suppl 6B):116, 1985.
123. Rouse MS, Walcox RM, Henry NK, et al: Ciprofloxacin therapy of experimental endocarditis caused by methicillin-resistant *Staphylococcus epidermidis*. Antimicrob Agents Chemother 34:273, 1990.
124. Korzeniowski O, Sande MA, the National Collaborative Endocarditis Study Group: *Staphylococcus aureus* endocarditis: Clinical manifestations in patients addicted to parenteral drugs and in nonaddicts. Ann Intern Med 97:496, 1982.
125. Levine DP, Fromm BS, Reddy BR: Slow response to vancomycin or vancomycin plus rifampin therapy among patients with methicillin-resistant *Staphylococcus aureus* endocarditis. Ann Intern Med 115:674, 1991.
126. Chambers HF, Miller RT, Newman MD: Right-sided *Staphylococcus aureus* endocarditis in intravenous drug abusers: Two week combination therapy. Ann Intern Med 109:619, 1988.
127. Chambers HF: Short-course combination and oral therapies of *Staphylococcus aureus* endocarditis. Infect Dis Clin North Am 7:69, 1993.
128. DiNubile MJ: Short-course antibiotic therapy for right-sided endocarditis caused by *Staphylococcus aureus* in injecting drug users. Ann Intern Med 121:873, 1994.
129. Chambers HF: Treatment of infection and colonization caused by methicillin-resistant *Staphylococcus aureus*. Infect Control Hosp Epidemiol 12:29, 1994.
130. Simon GL, Smith RH, Sande MA: Emergence of rifampin resistant strains of *Staphylococcus aureus* during combination therapy with vancomycin and rifampin: A report of two cases. Rev Infect Dis 5:5507, 1983.
131. Cohen PS, Maguire JH, Weinstein L: Infective endocarditis caused by gram-negative bacteria: A review of the literature 1945–1977. Prog Cardiovasc Dis 22:205, 1980.
132. Ugun O, Akalin HE, Unal S, et al: Long-term oral ciprofloxacin in the treatment of prosthetic valve endocarditis due to *Pseudomonas aeruginosa*. Scand J Infect Dis 24:797, 1992.
133. DiNubile MJ: Surgery in active endocarditis. Ann Intern Med 96:650, 1982.
134. Alsip SG, Blackstone EH, Kirklin JW, Cobbs CG: Indications for cardiac surgery in patients with active infective endocarditis. Am J Med 78:138, 1985.
135. Abdelnoor M, Nitter-Hauge S, Trettli S: Relative survival of patients after heart valve replacement. Eur Heart J 11:23, 1990.
136. Jones EL, Weintraub WS, Craver JM, et al: Ten-year experience with the porcine bioprosthetic valve: Interrelationship of valve survival and patient survival in 1,050 valve replacements. Ann Thorac Surg 49:370, 1990.
137. David TE: The surgical treatment of patients with prosthetic valve endocarditis. Semin Thorac Cardiovasc Surg 7:47, 1995.
138. Yu VL, Fand GD, Keys TF: Prosthetic valve endocarditis: Superiority of surgical valve replacement versus medical therapy only. Ann Thorac Surg 58:1073, 1994.
139. Grover FL, Cohen DJ, Oprian C, et al: Determinants of the occurrence of and survival from prosthetic valve endocarditis. J Thorac Cardiovasc Surg 108:207, 1994.
140. Tuna IC, Orszulak TA, Schaff HV, et al: Results of homograft aortic valve replacement for active endocarditis. Ann Thorac Surg 49:619, 1990.
141. Yee ES, Khonsari S: Right-sided infective endocarditis: Valvuloplasty, valvectomy or replacement? J Cardiovasc Surg 30:744, 1989.
142. Urbulu A, Holmes RJ, Asfaw I: Surgical treatment of intractable right-sided infective endocarditis: 25 years experience. J Heart Valve Dis 2:129, 1993.
143. D'Agostino RS, Miller DC, Stenson EB, et al: Valve replacements in patients with native valve endocarditis: What really determines operative outcome. Ann Thorac Surg 40:429, 1985.
144. Rocchiccioli C, Chastre J, Lecompte Y, et al: Prosthetic valve endocarditis: The case for prompt surgical management. J Thorac Cardiovasc Surg 92:784, 1986.
145. Buda AL, Zotz RL, LeMire MS, Bach DS: Prognostic significance of vegetations detected by two-dimensional echocardiography in infective endocarditis. Am Heart J 112:1291, 1986.
146. Steckelberg JM, Murphy JG, Ballard D, et al: Emboli in infective endocarditis: The prognostic value of echocardiography. Ann Intern Med 114:635, 1991.
147. Heinle S, Wilderman N, Harrison JK, et al: Value of transthoracic echocardiography in predicting embolic events in active infective endocarditis. Am J Cardiol 74:799, 1994.
148. DiSesa VJ, Sloss LJ, Cohn LH: Heart transplantation for intractable prosthetic valve endocarditis. J Heart Transplant 9:142, 1990.
149. Wilson WR, Guiliani ER, Danielson GK, Geraci LE: Management of complications of infective endocarditis. Mayo Clin Proc 57:162, 1982.
150. Verheul HA, Van den Brink RB, Van Vreeland T, et al: Effects of changes in management of active infective endocarditis on outcome in a 25 year period. Am J Cardiol 72:682, 1993.
151. Kaye D: Prophylaxis for infective endocarditis: An update. Ann Intern Med 104:419, 1986.
152. Lang S, Morris A: Infective endocarditis: Current recommendations for prophylaxis. Drugs 34:279, 1987.
153. Fekete T: Controversies in the prevention of infective endocarditis related to dental procedures. Dent Clin North Am 34:79, 1990.
154. Kaye D, Abrutyn E: Prevention of bacterial endocarditis: 1991. Ann Intern Med 114:803, 1991.
155. Dajani AS, Bisno AL, Chung KL, et al: Prevention of bacterial endocarditis. Recommendation by the American Heart Association. JAMA 264:2919, 1990.
156. Bayer AS, Nelson RJ, Slama TG: Current concepts in prevention of prosthetic valve endocarditis. Chest 97:1203, 1990.

69

Vascular Graft Infections

Thomas F. O'Donnell, Jr.
Harold J. Welch
Richard A. Nitzberg

Vascular infections are fortunately rather rare, averaging about 2% in most series. Although improvements in surgical techniques and perioperative management have led to decreased mortality and amputation rates (Table 69–1), graft infections always present a formidable challenge to both the vascular surgeon and the infectious disease consultant. Vascular infections can be divided into (1) those that involve the native vessel primarily, without a previous vascular reconstruction; and (2) those that are associated with the insertion of a synthetic graft or with a vascular reconstructive procedure. Although the most frequent causes of primary vascular infections in the 1970s and 1980s were organisms such as salmonellae, which are hematogenously spread from an initial enteric portal of entry, this cause is now rare. Now, direct inoculation of bacteria into the vessels, associated with drug abuse, is much more common in primary arterial infection. This chapter focuses on those infections related to vascular surgery.

Incidence

The incidence of graft infection varies with the site of the graft. With intraabdominal aortic level procedures, the infection rate is approximately 1%; with infrainguinal reconstructions, the rate is 2% to 4%. The primary culprit in these cases is groin dissection, as seen in the higher rates of aortofemoral grafts versus intraabdominal aortic procedures. For a variety of reasons, the rate of graft infections is higher with emergency operations, such as those performed for ruptured aneurysms, than with elective procedures. Mortality rates also vary with the anatomic location of the graft and are highest at the aortic level. In contrast, limb loss may be higher with infrainguinal vascular infections, perhaps because alternative routes of revascularization are limited. The data in Table 69–1 underline the fact that graft infections, although rare, are a lethal problem confronting both the surgeon and the infectious disease consultant.

Etiology

Although the bacterium responsible for most graft infections is usually identified, the origin of the infection often remains unclear. Two probable mechanisms of graft infection are bacteremic seeding and direct contamination at the time of surgery (Table 69–2). Bacteremic seeding of grafts, such as has been described with *Pseudomonas* infections of autogenous vein grafts after *Pseudomonas* urinary tract infections,[1] and with aortic infections after angiograms,[2] supports the theory of hematogenous seeding of vascular prostheses. Reports of aortic graft sepsis from *Pasteurella multocida* after a dog bite confirm bacteremic seeding as a mechanism of late graft infection.[3]

The timing of hematogenous bacterial contamination appears to be critical to infectivity. In experimental studies, all dogs challenged with an intravenous bolus infusion of *Staphylococcus aureus* immediately after graft implantation developed graft infection,[4] whereas only 30% developed sepsis when the same bacterial challenge was given at 1 year. Obviously, the degree of graft endothelialization in such experimental models determines infectibility because an intact luminal surface provides a barrier against infection. Studies with endothelium-seeded prosthetic graft show that these grafts are more resistant to infection than are their nonseeded counterparts.[5] In humans, the lack of complete endothelialization of a prosthesis and the presence of defects in the pseudointima probably account for instances of late graft infection via a hematogenous route that occur 4 to 5 years after implantation. Certainly, in the perioperative period,

TABLE 69–1 ■ Graft Infections*

AUTHOR	NUMBER	TYPE OF INFECTION	TIME TO INFECTION (mo)	TREATMENT	MORTALITY (%)	AMPUTATION (%)
Aortic Level						
Kuestner et al (1995)[21]	33	AEF	73.2	IGR/EAB	27.3	9.1
Sharp et al (1994)[55]	27	18 PGI/9 AEF	62.5	IGR/EAB ISR, PGE	3.7	0
Kieffer et al (1993)[15]	43	34 PGI/9 AEF	63.6	ISAGR	12	0
Bacourt and Koskas (1992)[56]	98	PGI/AEF	37	IGR/EAB	24	10
McCarthy et al (1992)[57]	17	PGI	—	IGR/EAB	18	0
Ricotta et al (1991)[58]	32	24 PGI/8 AEF	34	PGE ± EAB IGR ± EAB	25	13
Quiniones-Baldrich et al (1991)[59]	45	PGI/AEF	40.3	PGE ± EAB	24	11
Reilly et al (1984)[60]	92	59 PGI	25	IGR ± EAB	10	25
		33 AEF	33	IGR/EAB	21	24
Infrainguinal Level						
Calligaro et al (1991)[52]	35	PGI/VGI	—	IGR ± EAB, PGE, GP	2.8	7
Cherry et al (1992)[14]	39	PGI	2	IGR + EAB; GP	7.6	28
Mertens et al (1995)[61]	67	PGI	3	GP; IGR; PGE	18	40

*AEF, Aortoenteric fistula; IGR, infected graft removal; EAB, extraanatomic bypass; PGI, prosthetic graft infection; ISR, in situ replacement; PGE, partial graft excision; ISAGR, in situ allograft replacement; VGI, vein graft infection; GP, graft preservation.

when the pseudointima consists of a variety of proteins and cellular elements from the blood that afford only a weak barrier against bacterial invasion, numerous opportunities exist for hematogenous contamination, such as from central venous and arterial lines or from urinary catheters.

Another mechanism for prosthetic graft infection, bacterial colonization of grafts by direct contamination, is probably the most common cause. This conclusion is supported by studies such as those of Schwartz and coworkers,[6] who demonstrated that, when cultured, more than 10% of abdominal aortic aneurysms grew bacteria—a potential source of graft contamination. The relationship between positive bacterial culturing from aortic aneurysm walls and subsequent graft infection was first emphasized by Ernst and associates,[7] who cultured bacteria from the aneurysm wall in 12 of 78 patients. One patient subsequently developed graft sepsis. Ernst observed that those patients with ruptured aneurysms had a fourfold higher positive culture rate (38%) than did those who underwent elective surgery for aneurysms (10%). The clinical studies of Malone and associates[8] revealed that the incidence of graft infections rose with the number of "redo" vascular operations; that is, reoperative surgery for failed grafts carries with it a greater risk of vascular infections. Later studies by Durham and coworkers[9] showed that patients with negative arterial wall cultures failed to develop graft infections, whereas a significant number of patients with positive arterial wall cultures went on to develop graft infections. Like Malone and coworkers, Durham and coworkers demonstrated that patients undergoing reoperative vascular surgery had a significant increase in the incidence of graft infection, especially if the arterial wall culture was positive. On the basis of these studies, these investigators recommended that intraoperative cultures be done for all patients undergoing vascular *reoperation*. If arterial wall cultures are positive, long-term antibiotics may be indicated. This recommendation is supported by the work of Bergamini,[10] who found a 24% positive culture rate in patients undergoing reoperation for anastomotic aneurysms without signs of suppuration or frank sepsis. Of 18 patients with positive cultures in Bandyk's study,[11] 12 represented reoperations and the predominant bacterium was *Staphylococcus epidermidis*.

Direct contamination of vascular prostheses usually occurs at the time of implantation, which implies a break in surgical technique. In vitro models of bacterial adherence demonstrate that microorganisms readily adhere to prosthetic grafts. Knitted Dacron exhibited the greatest degree of adherence.[12] Direct graft contamination can occur at the time of implantation by contact with skin flora, especially in inguinal incisions. Alternatively, this contamination may occur after contact of the graft, surgeon's hands, or instruments with the patient's skin for a prolonged period.

Known or occult enteric injury also can directly contaminate grafts, whereas inadequate sterilization can, rarely, cause graft infection. The lymphatic system appears to play an important role in preventing graft infection, especially in patients with ischemic limbs. In a study utilizing a canine model, femoral polytetrafluoroethylene (PTFE) interposition grafts were implanted after procedures that produced unilateral limb ischemia.[13] Ipsilateral inoculation of both *Escherichia coli* and *S. aureus* into the ischemic limb produced graft infections in those animals that had their lymphatics transected or preserved. By contrast, there was a significant reduction in positive graft cultures in the group of animals that had either excision or ligation of the lymphatics in the ischemic limb. These findings suggest that the lymphatics may contribute to graft infection, possibly by absorbing and then transporting bacteria to the site of graft implantation. The clinical implications of this work are important and dictate that careful isolation, transection, and ligation of groin lymphatics may reduce the incidence of graft infections.

Finally, direct extension of superficial wound infections can cause graft infection. This is the most common mechanism in the groin, where either excessive moisture or poor technique or both in wound closure, particularly in obese patients, will result in wound breakdown. This mechanism is also seen in grafts tunnelled subcutaneously, such as femoropopliteal, axillofemoral, and axilloaxillary bypasses. Direct extension is also the mechanism for aortoenteric fistula formation. Adherence of bowel, most commonly the duodenum, to aortic grafts results in erosion of the bowel wall, allowing the luminal bacteria to infect the graft.

TABLE 69–2 ■ Causes of Graft Infection

BACTEREMIC SEEDING

Source: urinary tract, arteriographic puncture site, or other distant inoculation site

DIRECT CONTAMINATION

Source: aortic wall, e.g., aneurysm, break in surgical technique
- Surgeon's hands or instruments
- Graft contact with skin
- Entertomy—planned or inadvertent
- Lymphatic disruption
- Direct extension from septic site
- Aortoenteric fistula
- Wound breakdown that exposes graft

Bacteriology

The time interval from surgery to graft infection may be as little as 2 days[14] to as long as 18 years.[15] Early graft infections are caused by virulent strains, particularly *S. aureus* and gram-negative bacteria such as *Pseudomonas, Klebsiella, Proteus,* and *Enterobacter. S. aureus* has been the most common organism causing graft infections, which has been isolated in one third to one half of cases.[16, 17] The common skin contaminant *S. epidermidis* now accounts for a greater number of infections. Although *E. coli* and other gram-negative organisms are more commonly found in classic late graft infections (Table 69–3), Bandyk and associates[18] found *S. epidermidis* to be the responsible organism in more than 50% of their cases of late graft infections. They related this increase in frequency to the unique protective mechanism of this bacterium. *S. epidermidis* can produce a biofilm of mucin "slime" that surrounds the organism as a protective barrier. The organism remains dormant and is usually associated with late infections months to years after graft implantation. The infection commonly presents as an anastomotic aneurysm that is often accompanied by a mucinous perigraft cavity. These organisms induce a complex host-organism response that causes weakening at the graft-to-host artery anastomosis.

The role of anaerobic bacteria, especially in aortofemoral graft infections, has been elucidated by Brook.[19] In a 10-year review of aortofemoral graft infections, anaerobes were cultured from 13 of 16 specimens (82%). Predisposing conditions, which included leg ulcers, gangrene, reoperation, and diabetes, existed in more than 50% of these patients.

Culture results show mixed flora in many instances. Calligaro and coworkers[20] grew both gram-positive and gram-negative organisms from 16 of 42 wounds, whereas many other cultures were positive for several species of gram-positive or gram-negative bacteria. Keustner and colleagues[21] grew multiple organisms in 44% of cultures from secondary aortoenteric fistulas.

Adhesion of bacteria to vascular grafts varies among types

TABLE 69–3 ■ Bacteriology of Graft Infection

	TYPES OF BACTERIA IN CULTURE (%)						
ORGANISM	Szilagy et al (1972)[25] (n = 48)	Liekweig and Greenfield (1977)[17] (n = 22)	Bunt (1983)[41] (n = 205)	Bandyk et al (1984)[11] (n = 30)	Calligaro et al (1990)[20] (n = 30)	Quinones-Baldrich et al (1991)[59] (n = 45)	Cherry et al (1992)[14] (n = 39)
Staphylococcus (coagulase-positive)	33	41	43	8	24	13	31
Staphylococcus (coagulase-negative)	15	—	—	42	24	21	10
Streptococcus (nonhemolytic)	5	—	—	6	51	5	18
Escherichia coli	23	9	17	11	10	18	(28% gram-negative)
Proteus	6	1	8	—	20	5	
Pseudomonas	2	14	10	3	33	21	8
Mixed						39	20
Negative culture						21	10

of grafts and bacteria. Schmidt and associates[12] examined the adherence of four strains of bacteria to three types of graft materials. All strains had a higher affinity for velour knitted Dacron than for expanded PTFE, and both *S. aureus* and *E. coli* had a higher affinity for velour knitted Dacron than for woven Dacron. When a mucin-producing strain of *S. epidermidis* was compared with a non–mucin-producing strain, the former had a much higher adherance to both expanded PTFE and knitted Dacron. The authors also showed that longer incubation allowed greater adhesion for the mucin-producing strain. In addition, the mucin-producing strain of *S. epidermidis* adhered to the graft wall in clusters, whereas the non–mucin-producing strain of *S. epidermidis, S. aureus,* and *E. coli* primarily adhered as single organisms.

Despite clinically obvious graft infections, cultures are sometimes negative, or intraoperative culture results may not agree with preoperative culture results. Perioperative antibiotics may be responsible for negative postoperative cultures. Goldstone and Effeney,[22] who noted negative cultures in 40% of proven graft infections, urged that the graft material itself be submitted for culture. Padberg and colleagues[23] used the techniques of ultrasonic bath treatment, direct ultrasonic disruption, and Vortex mixing to quantitatively culture bacteria from seeded Dacron grafts. They found the 5-minute ultrasonic bath treatment to be consistently better than the other two methods.

Fungal infections of vascular prosthetics are rare and are usually associated with disseminated infection. Graft infections with *Candida, Coccidioides, Aspergillus,* and other fungi may be the presenting manifestation of more widespread involvement.

Prophylactic Antibiotics

Antibiotics are routinely given before vascular surgery for two reasons: (1) the synthetic graft acts as a foreign body; and (2) there is a high risk of mortality or limb loss from graft infections. Usually, a first-generation cephalosporin such as cefazolin (Kefzol) is infused 1 to 2 hours before the skin incision is made and is continued for 24 to 48 hours after the vascular procedure. In a prospective randomized study of more than 450 patients, Kaiser and associates[24] showed that such a regimen reduced wound infections from 6.8% in a placebo-treated group to 0.9% in a cefazolin-treated group (Table 69–4). Although graft infections were also reduced in the antibiotic-treated group, this finding only *approached* statistical significance—all four graft infections occurred in the placebo group. Before this report, retrospective studies by Szilagyi and coworkers[25] and Fry and Lindenauer[26] noted a low incidence of graft infections in patients not treated with prophylactic antibiotics, 1.2% and 1.34%, respectively. These authors thought that a low rate of graft infections in the absence of routine prophylaxis argued against the use of prophylactic antibiotics. To the contrary, in their retrospective studies, Goldstone and Moore[27] found a threefold decrease in graft sepsis with the use of antibiotics. Edwards and coworkers,[16] in a review of 2614 arterial prosthetic graft procedures carried out for an 11-year period, observed that prophylactic antibiotics had been given in 22 of 24 cases of graft infection. In only 7 of the 22, however, had antibiotics been given according to the usual and appropriate protocol.

What has not yet been settled is how long to administer the prophylactic antibiotics. Edwards and colleagues[16] noted that more than 50% of surgical wound infections had a distant site of infection, of which 30% were related to urinary tract infections and 25% to respiratory tract sepsis. Despite routine administration of antibiotics, May and associates[28] found that 14% of their patients had positive Foley catheter cultures and that 16% had positive sputum cultures. Certainly, such findings would argue for both prompt removal of Foley catheters and antibiotic protection until their removal.

Prevention

Recognized risk factors for graft infections include reoperation, septic complications, and inadvertent or planned entry into the gastrointestinal tract at the time of graft placement. Obviously, reoperation cannot be avoided, but avoidance of gastrointestinal tract mishaps helps prevent graft infections.

TABLE 69–4 ■ Prospective Evaluation of the Role of Prophylactic Antibiotics in Vascular Surgery

AUTHOR	ANTIBIOTIC	NUMBER IN TRIAL	INCIDENCE OF INFECTION (%) Placebo	Treated
Kaiser et al (1978)[24]	Cefazolin	462	6.8	0.9
Pitt et al (1980)[34]	Cephradine	231	22.6	2.6

Placement of autogenous grafts, when possible, as opposed to synthetic grafts, can also reduce the incidence of vascular infections. It is well known that graft infections occur more frequently when a synthetic graft is used.[29] As noted earlier, careful division and ligation of groin lymphatics are helpful in preventing graft infections.[13] Attention to detail in excluding the graft from contact with the bowel postoperatively is imperative. This involves covering the graft with aneurysm sac (when appropriate), careful closure of the retroperitoneum, and use of omental patches where necessary. Earnshaw and colleagues[30] showed that although pathogenic organisms could be isolated from the skin preoperatively in 35% of patients studied, none of these organisms could be cultured from inguinal lymph nodes. Other studies have shown no benefit from the use of prophylactic closed suction drainage of inguinal wounds in patients undergoing vascular reconstruction.[31] Despite the occurrence of hematomas, seromas, and lymphoceles, closed suction drainage demonstrated no advantage over primary wound closure. The benefit of topical antibiotic wound irrigation has been shown. The retrospective studies of Lord and coworkers[32] showed a 0.23% incidence of wound infections in 434 patients who had topical wound irrigation, whereas Halasz[33] showed equal efficacy between topical and systemic antibiotics. In one of the few prospective trials to examine this issue, Pitt and associates[34] demonstrated a beneficial effect of wound irrigation, but the higher than usual wound infection rate in the control group weakened the impact of the study.

Further attempts to reduce graft infections have focused on either bonding or saturating prosthetic grafts with antibiotics, including rifampin, gentamicin, and ciprofloxacin. The risk of graft infection is probably greatest in the perioperative period; one study demonstrated that when antibiotics were added to the blood used for preclotting Dacron grafts, the frequency of graft sepsis was lowered.[35] Greco and colleagues[36] and others[37, 38] showed that antibiotic bonding to prosthetic grafts may be useful when a new graft must be placed in the setting of an infection. Torsello and coworkers[39] had no early (6-month) infections in rifampin-soaked aortic grafts placed in situ. Further work on the binding process is necessary because antibiotics can be leached out quickly with flowing blood.[40]

General measures that surgical staff can follow, such as showering with antiseptic soap 24 to 48 hours before surgery, not shaving the operative area until the patient is in the operating room, and using iodine- and povidone-impregnated drapes, help reduce wound and graft infection when coupled with meticulous surgical technique. Prophylactic antibiotics are beneficial but probably do not need to be given beyond 48 hours.

Classification

Graft infection is classified in the following ways: (1) level of septic involvement, (2) distal or proximal site, (3) type of bacteria, and (4) type of graft (Table 69–5). A type 1 infection involves the skin only and type 2 the subcutaneous tissue and skin. Type 3 is considered a true graft infection, in which the shaft with or without the anastomosis is involved. In his extensive clinical review, Bunt[41] suggested that vascular graft infection should be classified as (1) graft infection, (2) graft enteric erosion, (3) graft enteric fistula, or (4) aortic stump sepsis. He observed that the incidences of graft infection and graft enteric fistula were comparable, whereas the incidences of graft enteric erosion and aortic stump sepsis were much less, approximately 10% of the former. It is clear that the clinical diagnosis and subsequent management are related to the type of infection; therefore, they are discussed separately.

TABLE 69–5 ■ Classification of Graft Infections

Level of involvement:	Type 1—Skin only Type 2—Skin and subcutaneous tissue Type 3—Graft involvement: shaft alone or shaft and anastomosis
Site: Proximal (aortic) or distal (infrainguinal)	
Type of bacteria	
Type of graft:	Synthetic or autogenous; proximal and distal anastomotic locations
Bunt classification:	Graft infection Graft—enteric erosion Graft—enteric fistula Aortic stump infections

Clinical Presentation

The incidence of graft infection has not changed significantly over the past 20 years, although there has been a slight decline. More than three fourths of graft infections occur in the groin.[25, 27] Although earlier studies showed that a significant portion of graft infections occurred early, most later studies show infection developing an average of 4 to 6 years after implantation. The type of graft also influences the onset of graft sepsis. Infections associated with aortofemoral grafts tend to present earlier than aortoiliac grafts, probably owing to the superficial location of the femoral limb. With grafts located in the femoral region, patients usually exhibit localized signs of sepsis—an inguinal mass accompanied or unaccompanied by redness, pain, and fever (Table 69–6). The mass frequently progresses to frank drainage so that a sinus tract develops. A false aneurysm may be a sign of graft infection in approximately 10% of patients, whereas a smaller number present with evidence of hemorrhage, graft occlusion, or septic emboli. For infections involving grafts that are contained entirely within the abdomen, such as a tube or an aortoiliac graft, localized signs are unusual. Generally, the patient complains of recurrent febrile episodes, malaise, and weight loss—typical signs of occult sepsis. Blood cultures may be positive.

Graft enteric fistulae usually present with bleeding from the gastrointestinal tract (Table 69–7). The degree of bleeding depends on the site of the fistula. Massive acute bleeding is characteristic of fistulae that involve the graft-to-aorta anastomosis (Fig. 69–1), whereas fistulae involving the shaft of the graft more commonly bleed in low volume. In these situations, the bleeding is usually from the mucosa of the gastroin-

TABLE 69–6 ■ Clinical Diagnosis of Graft Infections (Average from Literature)

TYPE OF INFECTION	%
General	
Localized cellulitis or abscess	50
Fever	37
Systemic infection	25
Leukocytosis	26
Draining sinus	20
False aneurysm	16
Anastomotic bleeding	12
Graft occlusion	8
Septic emboli	6
Aortic Level	
Herald bleeding	76
Acute gastrointestinal bleeding	56
Chronic gastrointestinal bleeding	40

TABLE 69–7 ■ Aortoenteric Fistula: New England Medical Center and University of California, San Francisco Experiences*

	NEMC	UCSF
Number of patients	13	33
Original procedure		
Aneurysm	7	15
Occlusive	6	17
Both		1
Occurrence after implantation (y)	5.5	6.1
Site of AEF		
Duodenum	9	23
Jejunum	4	6
Other		5
Presenting symptoms		
Gastrointestinal bleeding	8	22
Shock	0	8
Fever	7	22
Sinus tract	0	5
Septic emboli	0	9
Positive blood culture results	8	11 (n = 15)
Diagnosis (diagnostic for AEF)		
Upper gastrointestinal tract series	2/7	1/8
Arteriography	0/9	0/30
Endoscopy	4/10	2/17
Computed tomography		8/24

*AEF, Aortoenteric fistula; NEMC, New England Medical Center; UCSF, University of California, San Francisco.

testinal tract, which has become irritated by the prosthetic graft.[42, 43] Patients in these cases may be febrile, but if blood cultures are positive, the prognosis is less good.[44]

Diagnosis

The diagnosis of graft infection may leave the surgeon with the uneasy sense of a suspected rather than a confirmed infection at a time when a major procedure associated with potentially high mortality and morbidity rates must be undertaken. Some clues can be derived from the physical examination. An erythematous, tender, pulsatile mass in the inguinal region or elsewhere suggests graft sepsis (see Table 69–6). A draining sinus in the area of a graft is clear-cut evidence of graft infection (Fig. 69–2). Nonspecific studies include laboratory measurements of white cell count, erythrocyte sedimentation rate, and blood cultures. The yield of specific diagnostic studies depends on the site and the type of infection. Radiologic techniques for detailing infections can be divided into those that detect anatomic abnormalities and those that reveal sites of inflammation. In patients with suspected graft infection, we have found that anatomic definition by computed tomography is the most helpful diagnostic study because it examines both the retroperitoneum and the perigraft tissue.[45] Computed tomography may reveal a collection of fluid around the main body of the graft or its limbs, blurring of the usual tissue planes in the retroperitoneum, or air collections around the graft (Fig. 69–3). False aneurysms may be detected (Fig. 69–4). With an aortoenteric fistula, oral contrast medium may sometimes be seen delineating the contour of the graft (Fig. 69–5). Another attractive feature of computed tomography is that it may delineate other possible sites of infection unrelated to the graft.

Magnetic resonance imaging is also useful, particularly in identifying perigraft fluid. However, fluid persists in up to 22% of patients at 12 weeks and may not be completely resolved for up to 24 weeks. Combined use of axial spin echo and short-tau inversion recovery (STIR) imaging has been shown to be highly accurate for diagnosing graft infections.[46]

Ultrasonography has also been used. However, other than

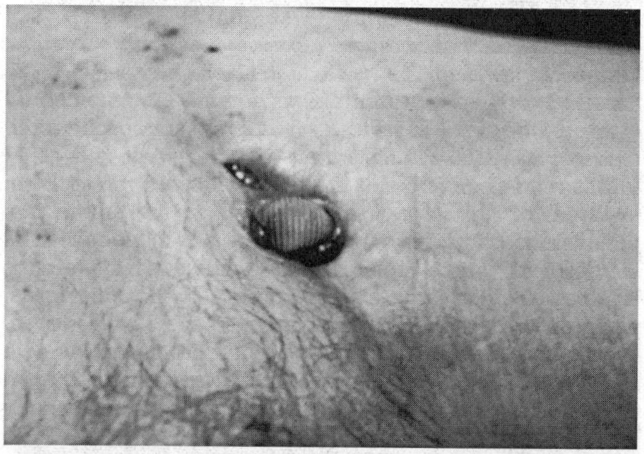

FIGURE 69–2 □ Obvious extrusion of graft through inguinal wound in a patient with a draining sinus and graft infection. This patient had had an aortofemoral bypass graft several years ago and was referred for management of this infection.

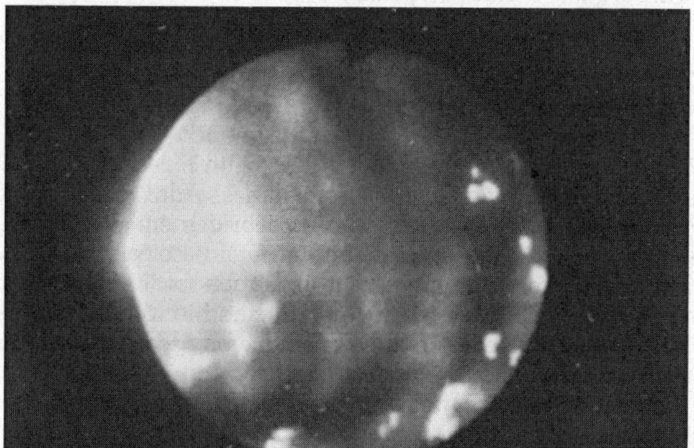

FIGURE 69–1 □ Endoscopic view of an aortoenteric fistula. Whitish, highly reflective material at the left (at 9 o'clock position) represents graft fabric; mucosa with hemorrhage is seen to fill the remainder of the circle.

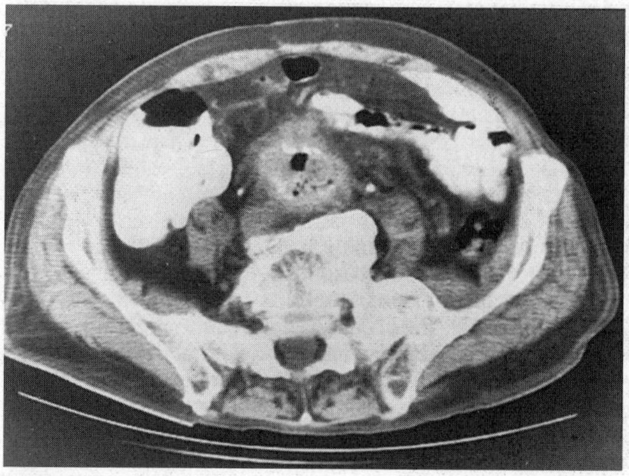

FIGURE 69–3 □ Computed tomographic scan of a patient with a graft infection. Blurring of the usual tissue planes in the retroperitoneum as well as air is observed around the shaft of the aortic graft.

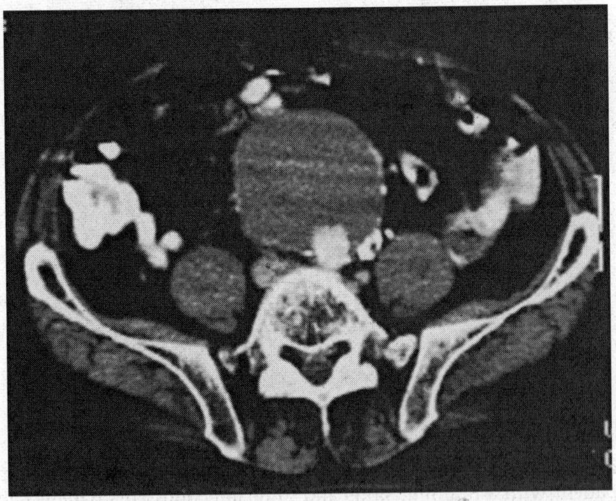

FIGURE 69–4 ▫ Computed tomographic scan of a false aneurysm in a patient with an aortoenteric fistula. The presence of the aortic anastomotic aneurysm was inferential evidence of a suspected aortoenteric fistula. This view is above the graft anastamosis and reveals the false aneurysm and overlying bowel.

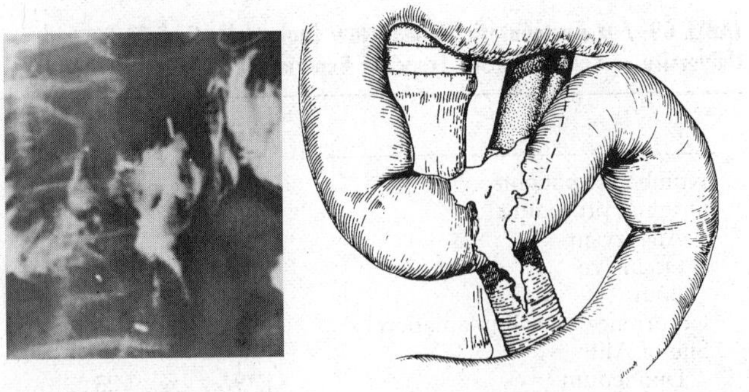

FIGURE 69–6 ▫ Upper gastrointestinal tract series in a patient with an aortoenteric fistula. The schematic drawing on the right illustrates the barium study on the left. The ulcer appeared in the fourth portion of the duodenum overlying the aortic anastomosis.

confirming the presence of a false aneurysm, ultrasound techniques have been disappointing in the evaluation of graft sepsis.

Contrast studies (Fig. 69–6) may also be helpful not only in diagnosing the presence of infection but also in planning the operative approach and the procedure. A patient with a clearly evident draining sinus should undergo sinography to define the level of wound infection as superficial or deep, the latter with graft involvement. In addition to demonstrating the runoff, arteriography may reveal an unsuspected false aneurysm, which provides suggestive evidence of graft sepsis (Fig. 69–7).

Radionuclide scans enjoyed an initial rush of enthusiasm, but this enthusiasm has been tempered by their overall lower than expected sensitivity. Because of normal postoperative inflammation, these scans are not useful in the first 3 to 5 months after graft implantation. Labeling leukocytes with indium 111 or technetium Tc 99m–HMPAO has produced a diagnostic accuracy of 80% to 100%.[47, 48] Polyclonal human immunoglobulin G scans and gallium scans are other options, each with its own advantages and disadvantages.[49]

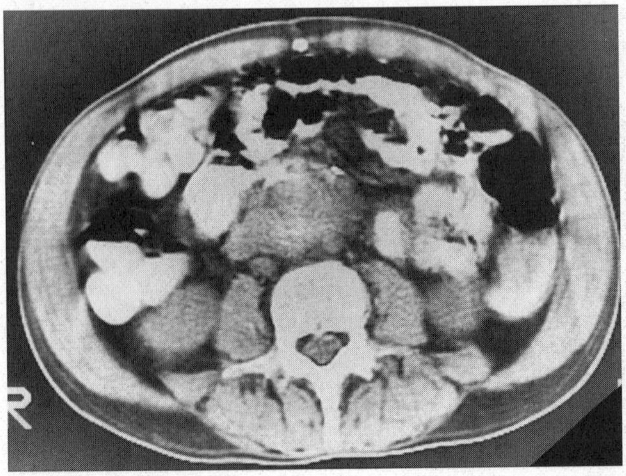

FIGURE 69–5 ▫ Computed tomographic scan of an aortoenteric fistula with oral contrast medium from the duodenum delineating the aortic graft (11 o'clock position of the graft).

Radionuclide studies should be combined with other imaging techniques, such as computed tomography or magnetic resonance imaging, to increase diagnostic accuracy.

Endoscopy is extremely useful in stable patients suspected of having an aortoenteric fistula. Gastroduodenoscopy must be carried out to the fourth portion of the duodenum. Occasionally, the graft material itself will be visualized (see Fig. 69–1), but any mucosal abnormality must be viewed with suspicion. Endoscopy must exclude other sources of bleeding, such as varices and ulcers; however, normal examination results do not necessarily exclude an aortoenteric fistula. Stable patients with lower gastrointestinal tract bleeding or guaiac-positive stools, and normal upper gastrointestinal tract endoscopic results, should undergo flexible sigmoidoscopy to evaluate a possible graft-sigmoid fistula.

If the diagnosis of graft sepsis is made preoperatively, attempts to determine the extent of infection (e.g., an entire graft or just one limb of an aortobifemoral graft) should be made. This may aid in planning the scope of the graft removal surgery. Unfortunately, a diagnosis of graft infection may be suspected but not confirmed despite multiple tests, and the patient must undergo exploration in the operating room. The major finding at surgery determining graft infection is how well the graft itself is incorporated, or healed, in the perigraft tissue. Findings of perigraft mucin or slime, bile staining, and easy dissection of perigraft tissue indicate graft infection. Padberg and associates,[50] using culture techniques described earlier, compared graft incorporation and graft culture results. They found that graft disincorporation correlated with the presence of bacteria in 71% of cases and that graft incorporation excluded bacteria in 97%.

Therapy

The "gold standard" for treating an infected vascular prosthetic is complete removal of the graft with revascularization through clean, noninfected tissue planes. Additional tenets include (1) complete resection and débridement of infected perigraft tissue, with special care to obtain a clean proximal arterial stump; (2) drainage or irrigation of the perigraft infection; (3) appropriate perioperative and long-term antibiotics; and (4) use of monofilament (vice-braided) sutures for arterial closure (Fig. 69–8).

Unfortunately, the gold standard of therapy carries the greatest risks of morbidity and mortality to the patient. As a result, clinicians have challenged the gold standard with a variety of treatments aimed at decreasing these risks. Even the gold standard has variations in management, particularly for infected aortic grafts.[51] Removal of the infected graft and revascularization can be performed in a staged manner, in

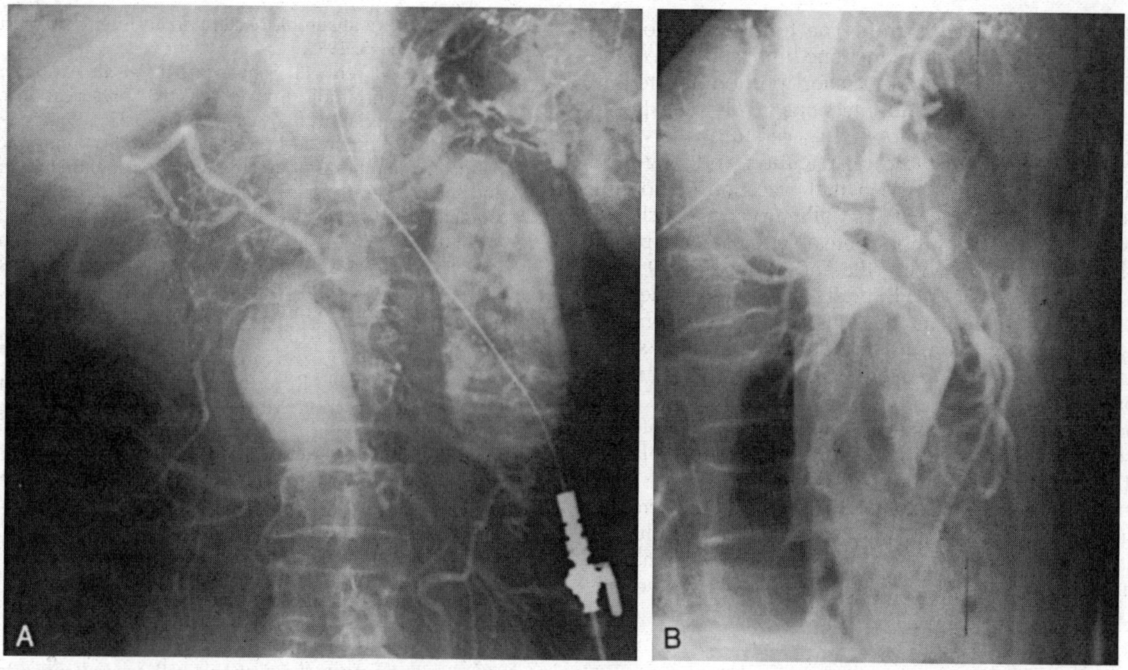

FIGURE 69–7 □ Anteroposterior *(A)* and lateral *(B)* arteriograms of a patient with an aortic false aneurysm and gastrointestinal bleeding. Subsequent exploration revealed an aortoenteric fistula that was treated by graft excision and extraanatomic bypass by axillofemoral bypass.

which the extraanatomic bypass is done followed by graft removal a few days later. Although the theoretical risk for infecting the new extraanatomic bypass exists, in practice the risk is quite low. This approach allows the patient to have two shorter, less stressful procedures. Alternatively, the procedures may be done in a sequential approach, in which the lower extremities are perfused via an extraanatomic bypass, immediately followed by total aortic graft excision. Another option is the synchronous approach, which includes graft resection either before or after an in-line reconstruction. All these approaches include total resection of the infected graft.

Less extensive options include partial graft resection and

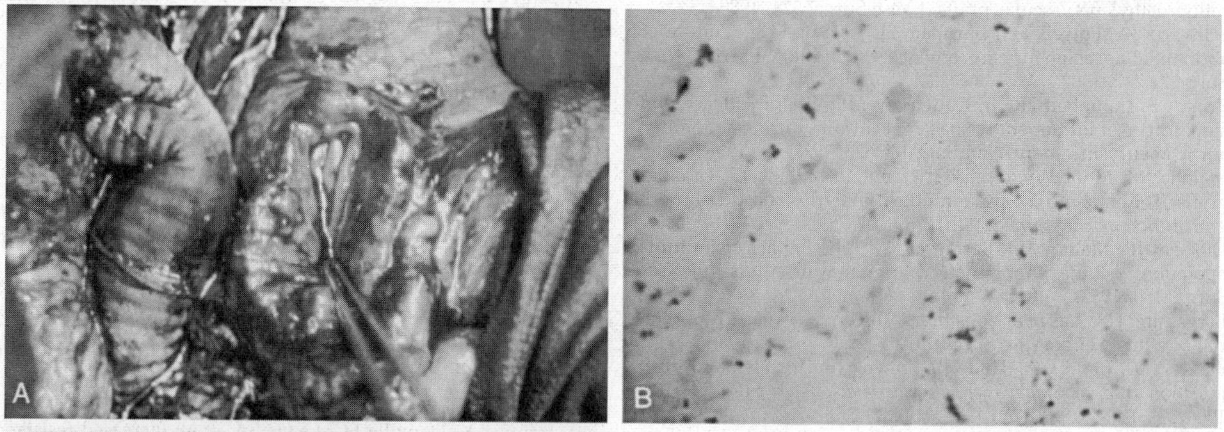

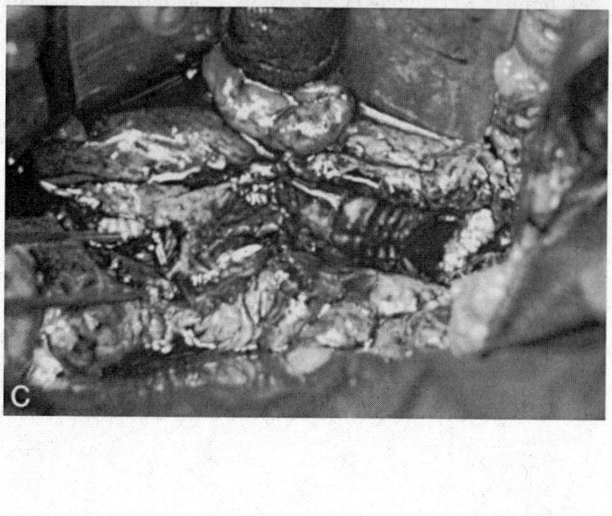

FIGURE 69–8 □ *A*, Bile-stained aortofemoral graft secondary to an aortoenteric fistula. Forceps point to the duodenum, which was densely adherent to the shaft of the aortic limb. *B*, Immediate Gram stain of periaortic tissue shows multiple gram-positive organisms. *C*, Completed aortic stump closure and fistula. Forceps point to open bowel, which was subsequently closed.

nonresection of the infected graft. The former is an option for aortobifemoral grafts when only one limb is involved and for infrainguinal grafts with only a short portion infected. In patients with superficial wound infections involving exposed grafts, several authors have reported successful preservation of the graft using local wound care, irrigation, and long-term antibiotics. One dictum has been that infections involving anastomoses require graft excision. Calligaro and associates[52] examined this issue. The authors were able to preserve patent grafts with infections involving the anastomosis in 10 of 11 patients having vein or PTFE grafts. They recommended graft excision if (1) there was bleeding from the anastomosis, (2) the graft was occluded, (3) the patient was in a septic condition from the graft infection, or (4) the graft was made of Dacron.[52]

Another alternative to the gold standard includes infected graft resection and regrafting in situ (i.e., simply replacing the graft). The new graft should be autogenous tissue (vein or endarterectomized artery), PTFE, or antibiotic-treated graft. The virulence of the primary pathogen will influence this decision. Cryopreserved aortic allografts have been used as in situ replacements with good success,[15] as have venous allografts.[53, 54]

References

1. Campbell OR, Bartlett FF: Postoperative *Pseudomonas* urinary tract infections as a source of bacterial contamination of an autogenous vein graft. J Vasc Surg 5:492, 1987.
2. Cullen PJ, Leahy AL, McBride KD, et al: Angiographically induced infection of the aorta. Ann Vasc Surg 1:386, 1986.
3. Sannella NA, Tavano P, McGoldrick DM, et al: Aortic graft sepsis caused by *Pasteurella* multocida. J Vasc Surg 5:887, 1987.
4. White JV, Freda J, Kozar R, et al: Does bacteremia pose a threat to synthetic vascular graft? Surgery 102:498, 1987.
5. Keller JD, Falk J, Bjornson HS, et al: Bacterial infectability of chemically implanted endothelial cell–seeded expanded polytetrafluoroethylene vascular grafts. J Vasc Surg 7:524, 1988.
6. Schwartz JA, Powell TW, Burnham SJ, Johnson G Jr: Culture of abdominal aortic aneurysm contents. An additional series. Arch Surg 122:777, 1987.
7. Ernst CB, Campbell HC Jr, Daugherty ME, et al: Incidence and significance of intraoperative bacterial cultures during abdominal aortic aneurysmectomy. Ann Surg 185:626, 1977.
8. Malone JM, Moor WS, et al: Bacteremic infectibility of vascular grafts: The influence of pseudointimal integrity and duration of graft function. Surgery 78:211, 1975.
9. Durham JR, Malone JM, Bernhard VM: The impact of multiple operations on the importance of arterial wall cultures. J Vasc Surg 5:160, 1987.
10. Bergamini TM: Vascular prostheses: Infections caused by bacterial biofilms. Semin Vasc Surg 3:101, 1990.
11. Bandyk DF, Berni GA, Thide BL, Towne JB: Aortofemoral graft infection due to *Staphylococcus epidermidis.* Arch Surg 119:102, 1984.
12. Schmitt DD, Bandyk DF, Pequet AJ, Towne JB: Bacterial adherence to vascular prostheses. A determinant of graft infectivity. J Vasc Surg 3:732, 1986.
13. Rubin JR, Malone JM, Goldstone J: The role of the lymphatic system in acute arterial prosthetic graft infections. J Vasc Surg 2:92, 1985.
14. Cherry KJ, Roland CF, Pairolero PC, et al: Infected femorodistal bypass: Is graft removal mandatory? J Vasc Surg 15:295, 1992.
15. Kieffer E, Bahini A, Koskas F, et al: In situ allograft replacement of infected infrarenal aortic prosthetic grafts: Results in forty-three patients. J Vasc Surg 17:349, 1993.
16. Edwards WH Jr, Martin RS 3rd, Jenkins JM, et al: Primary graft infections. J Vasc Surg 6:235, 1987.
17. Liekwig WJ Jr, Greenfield LJ: Vascular prosthetic infections: Collected experience and results of treatment. Surgery 81:335, 1977.
18. Bandyk DF, Beramini TM, Kinney EV, et al: In situ replacement of vascular prostheses infected by bacterial biofilms. J Vasc Surg 13:575, 1991.
19. Brook I: Role of anaerobic bacteria in aortofemoral graft infection. Surgery 104:843, 1988.
20. Calligaro KD, Veith FJ, Schwartz ML, et al: Are gram-negative bacteria a contraindication to selective preservation of infected prosthetic arterial grafts? J Vasc Surg 16:337, 1992.
21. Keustner LM, Reilly LM, Jicha DL, et al: Secondary aortoenteric fistula: Contemporary outcome with use of extraanatomic bypass and infected graft excision. J Vasc Surg 21:184, 1995.
22. Goldstone J, Effeney DJ: Prevention of arterial graft infections. *In* Bernhard VM, Towne JB (eds): Complications in Vascular Surgery, ed 2. New York, Grune & Stratton, 1985, pp 487–498.
23. Padberg FT, Smith SM, Eng RH: Optimal method for culturing vascular prosthetic grafts. J Surg Res 53:384, 1992.
24. Kaiser AB, Clayson RR, Mulherin JL, et al: Antibiotic prophylaxis in vascular surgery. Ann Surg 188:283, 1978.
25. Szilagyi DE, Smith RF, Elliott JP, Vrandecic MP: Infection in arterial reconstruction with synthetic grafts. Ann Surg 176:321, 1972.
26. Fry WJ, Lindenauer SM: Infection complicating the use of plastic arterial implants. Arch Surg 94:600, 1967.
27. Goldstone J, Moore WS: Infection in vascular prostheses: Clinical manifestations and surgical management. Am J Surg 128:225, 1974.
28. May AL, Darling RC, Brewster DC, et al: A comparison of the use of cephalothin and oxacillin in vascular surgery. Arch Surg 115:56, 1980.
29. Keller JD, Falk J, Bjorston HS, et al: Bacterial infectability of chemically implanted endothelial cell–seeded expanded polytetrafluoroethylene vascular grafts. J Vasc Surg 7:524, 1988.
30. Earnshaw JJ, Berridge DC, Slack RC, et al: Do preoperative chlorhexidine baths reduce the risk of infection after vascular reconstruction? Eur J Vasc Surg 3:323, 1989.
31. Healy DA, Keyser J 3rd, Holcomb GW 3rd, et al: Prophylactic closed suction drainage of femoral wounds in patients undergoing vascular reconstruction. J Vasc Surg 10:166, 1989.
32. Lord JM, Rossi G, Daliawa M: Intraoperative antibiotic wound lavage: An attempt to eliminate postoperative infections in arterial and clean procedures. Ann Surg 185:634, 1977.
33. Halasz NA: Wound infection and topical antibiotics: The surgeon's dilemma. Arch Surg 112:1240, 1977.
34. Pitt HA, Postier RG, MacGowan WA, et al: Prophylactic antibiotics in vascular surgery: Topical, systemic or both? Ann Surg 192:356, 1980.
35. White JV, Benvenisty AI, Reemtsma K, et al: Simple methods for direct antibiotic protection of synthetic vascular grafts. J Vasc Surg 1:372, 1984.
36. Greco RS, Trooskin SZ, Donetz AP, Harvey RA: The application of antibiotic bonding to the treatment of established vascular prosthetic infection. Arch Surg 120:71, 1985.
37. Modak SM, Sampath L, Fox CL, et al: A new method for the direct incorporation of antibiotics in prosthetic vascular grafts. Surg Gynecol Obstet 164:143, 1987.
38. Sheh PM, Modak S, Fox CL, et al: PTFE graft treated with silver noflaxacin (AGNF): Drug retention and resistance to bacterial challenge. J Surg Res 42:298, 1987.
39. Torsello G, Sandmann W, Gehrt A, Jungblut RM: In situ replacement of infected vascular prostheses with rifampin-soaked vascular grafts: Early results. J Vasc Surg 17:768, 1993.
40. Birinyi LK, Douville EC, Lewis SA, et al: Increased resistance to bacteremic graft infection after endothelial cell–seeding. J Vasc Surg 5:193, 1987.
41. Bunt TJ: Synthetic vascular graft infections. I. Graft infections. Surgery 93:733, 1983.
42. Champion MC, Sullivan SN, Coles JC, et al: Aortoenteric fistula. Incidence, presentation, recognition, management. Ann Surg 195:314, 1982.
43. Bunt TJ: Synthetic vascular graft infections. II. Graft-enteric erosion and graft-enteric fistulas. Surgery 94:1, 1983.
44. O'Donnell TF, Scott G, Shepard A, et al: Improvements in the diagnosis and management of aortoenteric fistula. Am J Surg 149:481, 1985.
45. Qvarfordt PG, Reilly LM, Mark AS, et al: Computerized tomographic assessment of graft incorporation after aortic reconstruction. Am J Surg 150:227, 1985.
46. Hansen ME, Yucel EK, Waltman AC: STIR imaging of synthetic vascular graft infection. Cardiovasc Intervent Radiol 16:30, 1993.

47. LaMurglia GM, Fischman AJ, Strauss HW, et al: Utility of indium 111–labeled human immunoglobulin G scan for the detection of focal vascular graft infection. J Vasc Surg 10:20, 1989.
48. Prats E, Banzo J, Abos MD, et al: Diagnosis of prosthetic vascular graft infection by technetium-99m-HMPAO-labeled leukocytes. J Nucl Med 35:1303, 1994.
49. Wakefield TW: Diagnosis of aortic graft infection. *In* Ernst CB, Stanley JC (eds): Current Therapy of Vascular Surgery. Philadelphia, BC Decker, 1991.
50. Padberg FT, Smith SM, Eng RH: Accuracy of disincorporation for identification of vascular graft infection. Arch Surg 130:183, 1995.
51. Reilly LM, Stoney RJ, Goldstone J, Ehrenfeld WK: Improved management of aortic graft infection: The influence of operation sequence and staging. J Vasc Surg 5:412, 1987.
52. Calligaro KD, Westcott CJ, Buckley RM, et al: Infrainguinal anastomotic arterial graft infections treated by selective graft preservation. Ann Surg 216:74, 1992.
53. Fujitani RM, Bassiouny HS, Gewertz BL, et al: Cryopreserved saphenous vein allogenic homografts: An alternative conduit in lower extremity arterial reconstruction in infected fields. J Vasc Surg 15:519, 1992.
54. Snyder SO, Wheeler JR, Gregory RT, et al: Freshly harvested cadaveric venous homografts as arterial conduits in infected fields. Surgery 101:283, 1987.
55. Sharp WJ, Hoballah JJ, Moran CR, et al: The management of the infected aortic prosthesis: A current decade of experience. J Vasc Surg 19:844, 1994.
56. Bacourt F, Koskas F: Axillobifemoral bypass and aortic exclusion for vascular septic lesions: A multicenter retrospective study of 98 cases. Ann Vasc Surg 6:119, 1992.
57. McCarthy WJ, McGee GS, Lin WW, et al: Axillary-popliteal bypass provides successful limb salvage after removal of infected aortofemoral grafts. Arch Surg 127:974, 1992.
58. Ricotta JJ, Faggioli GL, Stella A, et al: Total excision and extra-anatomic bypass for aortic graft infection. Am J Surg 162:145, 1991.
59. Quinones-Baldrich WJ, Hernandez JJ, Moore WS: Long-term results following surgical management of aortic graft infection. Arch Surg 126:507, 1991.
60. Reilly LM, Ahmay H, Lusby RJ, et al: Late results following surgical management of vascular graft infection. J Vasc Surg 1:36, 1984.
61. Mertens RA, O'Hara PJ, Hertzer NR, et al: Surgical management of infrainguinal arterial prosthetic graft infections: Review of a thirty-five year experience. J Vasc Surg 21:782, 1995.

70

Pericarditis and Myocarditis

Darryl See
Jeremiah Tilles

Because the myocardium, or muscular layer of the heart, is in anatomic proximity to the pericardial sac that surrounds the heart, many diseases that affect one structure also involve the other. However, the etiology and pathophysiology of inflammatory diseases that affect the myocardium or pericardium are usually distinct, and when both are involved the pathology of one usually predominates. Furthermore, there are marked differences in the clinical presentation, course, and prognosis of diseases of one tissue versus the other. For these reasons, the inflammatory disorders that affect the two structures are discussed separately in this chapter.

Pericarditis

Because pericarditis, or inflammation of the pericardium, may present clinically as acute pericarditis, recurrent acute pericarditis, or constrictive pericarditis, these overlapping clinical entities are discussed sequentially. The presentation of acute pericarditis is rapid and usually self-limited. Only a small proportion of affected patients develop either fulminant disease or one of the chronic forms of the disease.[1] Recurrent, or acute relapsing, pericarditis is a subset of acute pericarditis that is characterized by periodic episodes similar in clinical presentation to those seen with the acute syndrome.[2] Another chronic form of the illness, constrictive pericarditis, presents with signs and symptoms of restricted cardiac filling and is characterized by a fibrotic pericardium.[3] Each of the three syndromes may manifest pericardial effusion and may be accompanied by cardiac tamponade.

The pericardium is composed of two mesothelial surfaces. The visceral pericardium is firmly adherent to the epicardial surface of the heart; the parietal pericardium has attachments to the sternum, the great vessels, and the diaphragm. There is usually 10 to 50 mL of clear fluid between the two layers. Drainage occurs into the thoracic and the right lymphatic ducts, maintaining a homeostatic condition. However, inflammation of either surface may cause elaboration of substances such as fibrin, fluid, blood, and cells, which can overwhelm the drainage mechanisms.[4] Thus, excess fluid accumulates in the pericardial sac. The exudate may be serous, serofibrinous, fibrinous, suppurative, or hemorrhagic.

Cardiac tamponade results when the imposition of the accumulated fluid is sufficient to restrict ventricular filling during diastole. The outcome is a reduction in cardiac output and an increase in both systemic and pulmonary venous pressures.[5]

Acute Pericarditis

ETIOLOGY

The causes of acute pericarditis are multiple, including many infectious and noninfectious etiologies (Table 70–1). The most common recognized causes are viral, especially the group B coxsackieviruses.[6] Other common viral pathogens include group A coxsackieviruses, echoviruses, adenoviruses, mumps virus, hepatitis B virus, and influenza virus. Myocarditis is frequently present. Many cases are idiopathic and thought to be most likely secondary to unrecognized viral infections. Bacterial infections of the pericardium have become relatively rare in the antibiotic age.[7] Most infections now occur in elderly patients, infants, and individuals with either underlying immunosuppression or chronic illness. The bacterial infections that do occur may be a consequence of (1) direct extension of infection from local structures, such as the lungs, the endocardium, or the mediastinum[8]; (2) direct inoculation of organisms into the pericardium from penetrating injuries to the chest wall or cardiac surgery[9]; or, rarely, (3) direct seeding of the pericardium by bacteria in the blood stream. The bacterial spectrum involved has shifted. Thus, *Streptococcus pneumoniae*, which was the predominant etiologic agent in the past, is now uncommon.[10] In its place, *Staphylococcus aureus* has become the most prevalent bacterial pathogen isolated, and when present is associated with high morbidity and mortality.[11] The incidence of infections caused by gram-negative rods is rising; these cases are usually nosocomially acquired cases in immunocompromised hosts.[12]

Because tuberculous pericarditis complicates about 1% to 2% of cases of untreated pulmonary tuberculosis, there is still a high incidence of tuberculous pericarditis in some underdeveloped countries.[13] Many cases are clinically inapparent until the late hemodynamic consequences of constrictive pericarditis occur. Tuberculosis is now an uncommon cause of pericarditis in developed countries. Fungal pericarditis with *Candida* species, *Aspergillus* species, *Coccidioides immitis*, or *Cryptococcus neoformans* may occur as a consequence of disseminated infection in immunocompromised patients.[14] Parasitic infections of the pericardium are rare but may accompany primary infection at other sites with *Toxoplasma gondii, Entamoeba histolytica*, or *Schistosoma* species. Among the noninfectious etiologies of pericarditis, uremia, postmyocardial infarction syndrome, and collagen-vascular diseases are most frequently reported in the United States.

CLINICAL PRESENTATION

The most common symptom of acute idiopathic, or viral, pericarditis is chest pain (Table 70–2). Typically, the pain is sharp, precordial, and often worse with inspiration or coughing.[15] The pain is usually alleviated by leaning forward and is exacerbated by lying down. In addition to pain, fever and constitutional symptoms such as fatigue, myalgia, and arthralgia are usually reported by patients. Dry cough is also a common symptom, and dyspnea is usually present in patients with tamponade.

TABLE 70–1 ■ Causes of Acute Pericarditis

INFECTIOUS	NONINFECTIOUS
Viruses	**Diseases and Injuries**
Coxsackieviruses A and B	Acute myocardial infarction
Echovirus	Post–irradiation injury
Adenovirus	Post–cardiac surgery
Influenza virus	Collagen-vascular diseases
Epstein-Barr virus	Systemic lupus erythematosus
Varicella-zoster virus	Scleroderma
Cytomegalovirus	Wegener granulomatosis
Herpes simplex virus	Acute rheumatic fever
Mumps virus	Scleroderma
Hepatitis B virus	Dermatomyositis
	Familial Mediterranean fever
Fungi	Sarcoidosis
Histoplasma capsulatum	Neoplasm
Aspergillus spp.	Hypothyroidism
Candida spp.	Dissecting aortic aneurism
Blastomyces dermatitidis	Uremia
Coccidioides immitis	
Cryptococcus neoformans	**Drugs**
	Procainamide
Bacteria	Hydralazine
Streptococcus aureus	Methysergide
Streptococcus pneumoniae	Minoxidil
Enteric gram-negative rods	Phenytoin
Actinomyces spp.	Heparin
Legionella pneumophila	
Neisseria meningitidis	
Haemophilus influenzae	
Campylobacter jejuni	
Borrelia burgdorferi	
Mycoplasma pneumoniae	
Brucella spp.	
Salmonella spp.	
Anaerobic streptococci	
Nocardia asteroides	
Mycobacterium tuberculosis	
Mycobacterium avium complex	
Parasites	
Toxoplasma gondii	
Schistosoma spp.	
Entamoeba histolytica	
Trypanosoma cruzi	
Trichinella spiralis	

TABLE 70–2 ■ Clinical and Laboratory Features of Acute Pericarditis

SYMPTOMS	SIGNS
Chest pain	Three-part friction rub
Dry cough	Evidence of tamponade
Fatigue	Muffled heart sounds
Myalgias	Pulsus paradoxus
Arthralgias	Tachycardia
Dyspnea	Hypotension
	Jugular venous distention
	Peripheral edema
LABORATORY ABNORMALITIES	
Elevated erythrocyte sedimentation rate	
Leukocytosis	
ELECTROCARDIOGRAPHIC CHANGES	
ST segment elevation in most leads	
ST segment depression in aVR and V_1	
T wave inversions	
PR segment depression	
IMAGING STUDIES	
Pericardial thickening by computed tomography or magnetic resonance imaging	
Enlarged heart silhouette on chest radiograph (if effusion present)	
Pericardial effusion on echocardiogram	

The most frequent physical finding associated with pericarditis is a friction rub.[16] Auscultation classically reveals a three-part rub, reflecting contact of the inflamed pericardial tissue with the myocardium during ventricular and atrial systole and during rapid ventricular filling in early diastole. The finding of the characteristic three-part rub is pathognomonic for pericarditis, but the lack of a rub does not exclude the diagnosis. In one large series, a 50% incidence of a friction rub was reported in patients with acute pericarditis.[17] The pericardial rub may be obscured by cardiac murmurs, wheezing, rhonchi, rales, or a pleural friction rub. It may be confused with the Hamman crunch, which is associated with air in the mediastinum. When tamponade is present, physical findings frequently include hypotension, distended neck veins, muffled heart sounds, tachycardia, and paradoxical arterial pulse (defined as a decline of systolic arterial pressure greater than 10 mm Hg during inspiration).

Laboratory abnormalities frequently encountered in patients with acute pericarditis include an elevated erythrocyte sedimentation rate and leukocytosis early in the disease.[18,19] Cardiac isoenzyme levels are elevated when myocarditis is also present.

Electrocardiographic changes are present in 50% to 90% of patients with acute pericarditis.[20] Characteristic findings include ST segment elevation in most leads, ST segment depression in aVR and V_1, PR segment depression, and widespread T wave inversion. QRS voltage decreases only if there is considerable pericardial effusion, and patients usually maintain sinus rhythm unless underlying heart disease is present. Chest radiographs may show enlargement of the cardiac silhouette in the presence of pericardial effusion. Computed tomography and magnetic resonance imaging can be used to quantitate effusion or to demonstrate pericardial thickening or masses.[21, 22] Pericardial effusion can also be quantitated by echocardiography.[23]

SPECIFIC DIAGNOSIS

The etiologic diagnosis of acute pericarditis is usually presumptive in patients found to have concomitant conditions known to be associated with pericardial involvement, such as uremia, acute myocardial infarction, metastatic neoplasia, post–irradiation or post–cardiac surgery, myxedema, or collagen-vascular disease.[24] Similarly, documentation of adjacent purulent infection, bacteremia, or systemic disease with tuberculosis or fungus can give a presumptive diagnosis. Presumptive diagnosis of a viral etiology can be made either by isolation of a virus from throat or stool culture or by serologic demonstration of recent infection with a specific virus (e.g., by documentation of a fourfold rise in specific antibody titers between acute and convalescent serum samples or by identification of the presence of specific immunoglobulin M antibody). However, such diagnostic attempts are often unfruitful. This may be due in part to incomplete testing because the large number of potential viral pathogens require exhaustive numbers of testing conditions. Definitive diagnosis of a virus etiology is possible if the virus is isolated from aspirated pericardial fluid. However, owing to the risks of complications, pericardiocentesis is usually not recommended in an otherwise healthy individual with suspected viral or idiopathic pericarditis. Diagnostic pericardiocentesis is indicated in certain clinical situations (Table 70–3), including cases involving patients with suspected purulent effusion, immunocompromised individuals, patients with cardiac tamponade, and individuals with a prolonged, unexplained pericarditis.[25]

TREATMENT

Nonspecific Therapy

All patients with acute pericarditis require pain management, bed rest, and hemodynamic monitoring.[19] Emergency needle pericardiocentesis is required for patients with cardiac tamponade and unstable hemodynamic status.[26] In stable patients with tamponade, surgical drainage is preferred. Pericardial biopsy should be performed during the procedure if the diagnosis is unclear. Recurrent tamponade is an indication for a pericardial window or pericardial resection.[27]

Specific Therapy

Idiopathic (Viral) Pericarditis. Nonsteroidal antiinflammatory agent therapy is indicated for viral pericarditis.[19] Most authorities believe that steroids should be avoided because of the associated risk of enhancing viral replication, especially if the myocardium is involved. For patients with a documented infection with a treatable virus, appropriate antiviral agents can be considered on an experimental basis because, to date, the rarity of the syndrome has precluded demonstration of clinical efficacy. Thus, acyclovir can be considered for patients with a documented herpes simplex or varicella-zoster virus infection; amantadine or rimantadine can be considered for patients with confirmed or suspected influenza A virus infection; and intravenous ganciclovir or foscarnet can be considered in immunocompromised patients with cytomegalovirus infection. In each case, approval of the local Human Studies Institutional Review Board would be required because the U.S. Food and Drug Administration has not been able to approve the drug specifically for use in pericarditis.

Bacterial Pericarditis. A prolonged course of an appropriate intravenous antibiotic must be used for a patient with bacterial involvement of the pericardium. For example, *S. aureus* should be treated for 4 to 6 weeks with high doses of intravenous nafcillin. Alternatively, intravenous vancomycin can be used for a patient allergic to penicillin or infected with a methicillin-resistant strain. In most cases, surgical drainage of the pericardial fluid is required, and for recurrent purulent effusion, pericardiectomy may be necessary.[28]

Tuberculous Pericarditis. A patient with tuberculous pericarditis must be treated with three or four appropriate agents for 9 months.[29] In addition, adrenal corticosteroids are recommended to reduce inflammation and prevent the development of constrictive pericarditis.[30] Pericardiectomy is required for those patients with progressive pericardial thickening.[31]

TABLE 70–3 ■ Indications for Pericardiocentesis in Acute Pericarditis

Suspected purulent effusion (high fevers, positive bacterial culture at other sites)
Immunocompromised patient
Cardiac tamponade
Suspected malignancy
Prolonged course without a clear diagnosis

Acute Relapsing Pericarditis

Some patients with acute pericarditis develop recurrent episodes. Several prospective studies have suggested a recurrence rate of 9% to 32% for patients with idiopathic acute pericarditis.[32–34] The incidence in postinfarction and posttraumatic cases appears to be higher.[35]

Acute relapsing pericarditis is defined as pericarditis occurring at least 3 months after a well-documented, resolved episode of acute pericarditis in a patient who has no evidence of active systemic disease.[36] The symptoms, signs, and laboratory abnormalities are similar to those of acute pericarditis. Recurrent episodes tend to be less severe than the original presentation, and deaths are rare. The duration, frequency, and number of relapses are extremely variable. Some patients have only one relapse, whereas others continue to have lifelong recurrences. The overall incidence of cardiac tamponade or constrictive pericarditis or both appears to be less than 10%, regardless of the frequency or the severity of the recurrences.[37]

The pathophysiology of recurrent pericarditis is unknown. Although the mechanism is thought to be autoimmune, systemic immunologic studies are usually unremarkable.[36] The theory remains unproven, with histopathologic examination revealing only chronic inflammatory changes. Fortunately, the majority of cases respond to nonsteroidal antiinflammatory agents. Although most patients can be treated with an intermittent course, a few individuals require prolonged therapy. Attacks that are unresponsive to nonsteroidal antiinflammatory agents and extremely severe attacks are best managed with corticosteroid therapy.[37] The role of pericardiectomy is controversial. Although one study showed benefit in a majority of cases,[38] most experts recommend the procedure only for patients with extremely severe or frequent episodes that are unresponsive to steroids, and for those rare patients with constrictive pericarditis. Cardiac tamponade should be managed as with acute pericarditis and tends not to recur after drainage and therapy.

Constrictive Pericarditis

Acute pericarditis due to almost any cause may be followed by constrictive pericarditis. Untreated bacterial infections, tuberculosis, and connective tissue diseases appear to be the most common etiologies.[39] Both the visceral and the parietal pericardia become fibrotic, obliterating the pericardial space, reducing expansion of the heart during filling, and diminishing both venous return and cardiac output. The condition is usually insidious in onset, with patients eventually presenting with dyspnea, orthopnea, dry cough, malaise, and abdominal swelling.[40] Abnormal physical findings include elevated venous pressure, ascites, hepatomegaly, peripheral edema, pleural effusion, and pulsus paradoxus.[40] The hemodynamic findings are characterized by equal elevation of right and left ventricular filling pressures. Although patients with restrictive cardiomyopathy may present with similar clinical findings, patients with constrictive pericarditis will be differentiated when pericardial thickening is demonstrated by computed tomography or magnetic resonance imaging.[41] Furthermore, in patients with restrictive cardiomyopathy, hypertrophic myocardium can be demonstrated by echocardiography.[42] Although mild cases of constrictive pericarditis may be managed with diuretics and inotropic agents, the treatment for most cases is pericardiectomy.[43] Steroid therapy is not beneficial.

Myocarditis

The myocardium constitutes the bulk of the heart, with respect to both weight and volume. The predominant tissue is a system of myocardial fibrils, composed of individual myocytes. Other cellular elements include vascular structures, autonomic nerves, and dendritic cells. Although clinical and histopathologic evidence of myocarditis, or inflammation of the myocardium, has been described since the mid-19th century,[44, 45] the etiology of most current cases eludes diagnostic efforts; the pathogenesis of myocardial damage remains incompletely explained; and effective treatment is still a challenge. The pathogenesis of initial myocardial damage involves several mechanisms, including direct cytolytic effects on myocytes from toxins or microorganisms, indirect cellular damage from the initial host response to the inciting factor, and immune phenomena. In some patients, a prolonged secondary host response supervenes. Although the pathogenesis of this process has been poorly worked out in humans, murine models suggest a mononuclear cell–mediated autoimmune process.[46] The spectrum of clinical disease in humans varies from asymptomatic disease, which appears to be have a high incidence in the general population,[47] to minimally symptomatic disease, and ultimately to a progressively more severe syndrome that includes constitutional symptoms, chest pain, arrhythmias, heart failure, or a combination of some of or all these signs, which can occasionally lead to sudden death.[48] In some patients with myocardial inflammation, regardless of the severity at the onset, persistent myocarditis develops and may lead to progressive heart failure and dilated cardiomyopathy.

ETIOLOGY

Although myocarditis usually occurs in conjunction with a more general disease process, isolated myocarditis is also seen. Numerous infectious and noninfectious causes have been associated with myocardial involvement (Table 70–4). Among otherwise healthy individuals, viruses are the most frequent causes of myocarditis, especially the group B coxsackieviruses.[49] In one serologic study, 49% of cases of acute myocarditis were associated with elevated immunoglobulin M titers and attributed to one of the six coxsackievirus B serotypes.[50] Other reports have suggested that up to 5% of cases of coxsackievirus B infection are associated with myocardial involvement.[51] It has been estimated that in the United States 2 to 10 million coxsackievirus B infections occur annually; thus, the incidence of coxsackievirus B–associated myocarditis appears to be extremely high.[47] In the majority of these cases, myocardial involvement is not clinically apparent. Coxsackievirus B infections are more common in children than in adults, especially among those from lower socioeconomic groups.[52] One autopsy study of children who died from a variety of causes showed that 24% had coxsackievirus B antigen–positive myocarditis that had been clinically inapparent.[53] Other enteroviruses (i.e., echovirus and group A coxsackieviruses) have also been associated with myocarditis. Furthermore, studies using polymerase chain reaction amplification for the detection of viral nucleic acid have suggested that adenoviruses may also be a frequent cause of viral myocarditis.[54]

TABLE 70–4 ■ Causes of Myocarditis

CAUSES IN IMMUNOCOMPETENT PATIENTS	
Infectious	**Noninfectious**
Viruses	***Diseases and Injuries***
Coxsackieviruses A and B	Giant cell myocarditis
Echovirus	Sarcoidosis
Lymphocytic choriomeningitis virus	Acute necrotizing eosinophilic myocarditis
Influenza viruses A and B	Kawasaki disease
Varicella-zoster virus	Peripartum cardiomyopthy
Epstein-Barr virus	Post–irradiation injury
Mumps virus	Endocrine diseases
Measles virus	Phenochromocytoma
Rubella virus	Hyperthyroidism
Adenovirus	Hypothyroidism
Rabies virus	***Drugs***
Yellow fever virus	Alcohol
Dengue virus	Dobutamine
Chikungunya virus	Cocaine
Poliomyelitis virus	Emetine
Arbovirus	Doxorubicin
Bacteria	Cyclophosphamide
Streptococcus pyogenes	Daunorubicin
Actinomyces spp.	Methyldopa
Legionella pneumophilia	Opiates
Chlamydia trachomatis	Tetracycline
Clostridium perfringens	Sulfonamides
Neisseria meningitidis	Interferons
Salmonella spp.	Interleukin-2
Rickettsia spp.	***Autoimmune Diseases***
Brucella spp.	Still disease
Staphylococcus aureus	Dermatomyositis
Borrelia burgdorferi	Rheumatoid arthritis
Treponema pallidum	Systemic lupus erythematosus
Mycoplasma pneumoniae	***Toxins and Poisons***
Chlamydia psittaci	Arsenic
Corynebacterium diphtheriae	Lead
Fungi	Carbon monoxide
Blastocystis hominis	Scorpion stings
Parasites	Rheumatic fever
Trichinella spiralis	Scleroderma
Entamoeba histolytica	
Trypanosoma cruzi	
Trypanosoma brucei gambiense	
Trypanosoma brucei rhodesiens	
CAUSES IN IMMUNOCOMPROMISED PATIENTS	
Infectious	**Noninfectious**
Viruses	Metastatic Kaposi's sarcoma
Herpes simplex virus	Lymphoma
Cytomegalovirus	
Human immunodeficiency virus	
Fungi	
Aspergillus spp.	
Candida spp.	
Cryptococcus neoformans	
Coccidioides immitis	
Parasites	
Toxoplasma gondii	

The incidence of the diverse nonviral etiologies of infectious myocarditis is low in the United States. Myocarditis with bacterial pathogens continues to occur when infectious foci are established in the myocardium of bacteremic patients. In addition, contiguous myocardial involvement may accompany bacterial pericarditis, and perivalvular abscesses may complicate some cases of bacterial endocarditis. Parasitic infections of the myocardium are encountered primarily in underdeveloped countries. Thus, *Trypanosoma cruzi*, acquired through the bite of the reduviid bug, is a common cause of acute myocarditis in South and Central America.[55] Chronic myocarditis, thought to be autoimmune, occurs in approximately 20% to 40% of individuals infected with *T. cruzi*.[56] A similar course can be observed in persons infected with one of the African species *Trypanosoma brucei gambiense* or *Trypanosoma brucei rhodesiense*. Ironically, it is particularly in the most highly developed countries that infection with *Trichinella spiralis* tends to occur and be manifest by involvement of both the skeletal and myocardial striated muscle.[57]

Immunocompromised patients may have myocardial involvement in association with disseminated infections by opportunistic organisms. Many of these infections are clinically silent. Several autopsy studies of patients who died of acquired immunodeficiency syndrome have revealed unsuspected pathologic changes in the heart in more than 50% of cases.[58–60] Viral pathogens commonly involving the myocardium in patients with diminished cellular immunity include cytomegalovirus and herpes simplex virus. The human immunodeficiency virus itself has been shown to infect myocytes.[61] Furthermore, in patients with acquired immunodeficiency syndrome both *C. neoformans* and *T. gondii* are increasingly being recognized as causes of myocarditis.[62, 63] It is of interest that in neutropenic patients either *Aspergillus* or *Candida* species can occasionally infect the heart.

INCIDENCE

It is apparent from the preceding discussion that the available evidence indicates that myocarditis is common in the general population, although most cases are asymptomatic and therefore never diagnosed clinically. One study showed a prevalence of electrocardiographic changes consistent with myocarditis in 1% of military recruits with a variety of acute infections.[64] Various autopsy series have indicated a prevalence of clinically inapparent myocarditis of 1% to 14%,[65, 66] and it is estimated that 5% to 15% of sudden deaths in healthy young persons are caused by previously unrecognized myocarditis.[67] The rate may be much higher in infants and small children. One study showed histologic evidence of myocarditis in 48% of infants who had died from a variety of causes.[53]

PATHOGENESIS

A variety of mechanisms of tissue damage have been identified in infectious myocarditis. An etiologic agent may infect and kill myocytes directly,[68] or alternatively, extracellular toxins such as those elaborated by *Clostridium perfringens*, *Streptococcus pyogenes*, and *Corynebacterium diphtheriae* may attack the myocardium.[69] Furthermore, elements in the early host inflammatory response to infection may also directly damage myocytes. Thus, perforin, a product of cytotoxic lymphocytes, has been shown to mediate myonecrosis, and there is suspicion that proinflammatory cytokines such as interleukin-1 and tumor necrosis factor may also damage myocytes.[70] In addition, severe inflammation can induce in myocytes the rapid formation of intracellular calcium deposits, which ultimately may lead to death of these cells.[71] Intracoronary vasculitis and ischemia can be caused by rickettsial infections[72] and the etiologic agent of Kawasaki disease, which is thought to be infectious in etiology, although this has not been proved.[73] Even enteroviral infections in mice have been shown to be capable of causing narrowing of coronary vessel lumina and tissue ischemia.[74]

The pathogenesis of persistent viral myocarditis in humans has not been fully characterized. However, murine models have suggested that the process is autoimmune. During the first several days of infection, cardiotropic viruses replicate in the myocardium; then they are cleared by early immune mechanisms.[46] In some strains of mice, infection with the virus stimulates autoantibody production against myosin heavy chain.[75] There appear to be shared epitopes between some coxsackievirus strains and the mouse cardiac α-myosin heavy chain.[76] Furthermore, myosin is normally an intracellular protein but can be found in the extracellular milieu in virus-infected myocardium. This process appears to stimulate the production of antimyosin autoantibodies. Administration of myosin heavy chain to susceptible, uninfected mice results in myocarditis.[77] The role of autoantibodies in the autoimmune process is unclear, however, because passive transfer of high-titer myosin autoantibodies fails to induce myocarditis in healthy mice.[78] The myosin is processed by antigen-presenting cells and stimulates type 1 helper T cells to produce interferon-γ and other cytokines. Macrophages are recruited and stimulated; they produce interleukin-1 and tumor necrosis factor, which may mediate myocyte destruction.[79] Studies have shown that the administration of anti–interleukin-1[80] or anti–tumor necrosis factor[81] antibodies abrogates the immune destruction of myocytes. Finally, because it has been demonstrated that cytotoxic lymphocytes kill myocardial cells that express autoantigens,[82] it may well be that cellular autoimmunity is the critical factor in murine myocarditis. Studies with mice have shown that viral nucleic acid is still present in the myocardium weeks after replicating virus is no longer demonstrable.[83] Whether viral antigens are still present is unclear because the current tests for protein are less sensitive than those for nucleic acids. The mechanism by which the persistent presence of a virus could contribute to the autoimmune process is also unknown.

CLINICAL PRESENTATION

As noted previously, the available evidence indicates that most cases of myocarditis are asymptomatic. Clinically apparent acute viral myocarditis in adults usually occurs several days after a nonspecific influenza-like or respiratory illness. In infants, immunocompromised individuals, and patients with nonviral infectious etiologies, there is usually no prodrome. In these patients, myocardial involvement is believed to occur in phase with the initial involvement of other tissues.[68] Similarly, there is typically no prodrome in patients with a noninfectious etiology. In both immunocompetent and immunocompromised patients, chest pain is a common complaint; it may be pleuritic or may be described as a pressure-type pain similar to coronary ischemic pain.[84] Palpitation, fever, dyspnea, malaise, and arthralgia are also common symptoms. Symptoms of heart failure may accompany severe cases. Abnormal physical findings in patients with myocarditis include fever, tachycardia, tachypnea, arrhythmias, gallop rhythm, murmer of mitral or triscuspid regurgitation, and signs of heart failure. Cardiac isoenzyme levels are frequently elevated.[85] Electrocardiographic abnormalities include nonspecific ST segment and T wave changes.[84] Echocardiograms may reveal variable degrees of cardiac dysfunction or myocardial thickening or both.[86] Gallium scans[87] and indium 111–labeled antimyosin antibody[88] tests are frequently positive.

DIAGNOSIS

Definitive diagnosis of myocarditis is based on endomyocardial biopsy. However, correlation of histologic evidence of myocardial inflammation with clinical manifestations of myocarditis is highly variable. Sampling error probably accounts for much of this variability, but lack of uniformity in interpreting the biopsy specimens is also important. The Dallas criteria were devised by a panel of experts to minimize this problem.[89] Thus, endomyocardial biopsy specimens are classified into one of three categories: (1) active myocarditis (leukocyte infiltration and myocardial necrosis without evidence of ischemia), (2) borderline myocarditis (presence of leukocytes without necrosis), and (3) no myocarditis (absence of both leukocytes and necrosis).

The etiologic diagnosis of viral myocarditis is usually presumptive in otherwise normal adults. A positive immunoglobulin M titer for a specific virus, a fourfold rise in titer of specific viral antibody between acute and convalescent serum samples, or isolation of a virus from cerebrospinal fluid, throat, or stool provides both direct evidence of recent viral infection and, in the presence of myocarditis, indirect evidence of myocardial infection with the same organism. Unfortunately, in otherwise healthy adult patients, viruses cannot usually be isolated from endomyocardial biopsy specimens. However, identification of the viral nucleic acid in a myocardial biopsy specimen by, alternatively, in situ hybridization or polymerase chain reaction techniques has been demonstrated and holds promise for the future.[90, 91]

Viral agents are more readily isolated from the myocardium of children and immunocompromised adult patients. Thus, biopsies with cell culture for viruses and histopathologic examination for inclusion bodies and giant cells (characteristic of members of the herpesvirus group) should be considered in such patients, especially in those with fulminant disease.

In patients with suspected nonviral causes of infectious myocarditis, endomyocardial biopsy with appropriate stains for parasites—as well as both stains and cultures for fungi, bacteria, and mycobacteria—should be performed as indicated. For the noninfectious etiologies, a careful evaluation of the entire clinical picture is essential and should be supplemented with specific laboratory tests if available and myocardial biopsy.

TREATMENT

Because a majority of clinically recognized cases of myocarditis are either of unknown etiology or caused by viruses for which specific antiviral agents are not currently available, supportive therapy is the mainstay of treatment. Bed rest is recommended and is supported by studies demonstrating an adverse outcome for animals exercised during acute myocarditis.[92, 93] Supplemental oxygen is considered important adjuvant therapy. Patients should be monitored for arrhythmias and treated with appropriate antiarrhythmic agents if needed. Heart failure should be treated with diuretics, inotropic agents, afterload reduction, or a combination of these therapeutic options. Severe cases may require temporary cardiac support by intraaortic balloon pumps or ventricular assist devices.[94] For some of the uncommon etiologies of viral myocarditis, specific antiviral agents have been approved for other conditions. A prolonged course of a particular agent given in a high dose could be considered on an experimental basis (with approval of the Human Studies Institutional Review Committee). Thus, a prolonged course of acyclovir could be considered for patients with documented infection with herpes simplex virus or varicella-zoster virus; intravenous ganciclovir or foscarnet could be considered for cytomegalovirus myocarditis; and azidothymidine and/or other antiretroviral agents should be considered for myocarditis in patients with the human immunodeficiency virus. Agents of the WIN class have been effective in treating enteroviral myocarditis in mice but are not available for human use.[95] Patients with mycobacterial, bacterial, fungal, or parasitic myocarditis should receive the appropriate specific chemotherapy. Myocardial abscesses associated with endocarditis also require surgical drainage.

Studies with children[96] and mice[97] have suggested a beneficial role for intravenous immunoglobulin G in cases of severe, acute myocarditis. Although interferon had also demonstrated efficacy in several studies of murine viral myocarditis when given soon after inoculation of the virus,[98, 99] it is not currently recommended for use in humans because of the potential for exacerbating any early autoimmune process. Administration of either corticosteroids[100] or nonsteroidal antiinflammatory agents[101] during acute myocarditis in animal models has had deleterious effects. Similarly, the use of metoprolol, a β-blocker, was associated with increased mortality in a murine model of viral myocarditis.[102]

The treatment of persistent myocarditis is controversial. Because this disease is considered autoimmune in origin, many trials of immunosuppressive agents have been reported, but unfortunately the studies have been found to be inadequately controlled. Studies using corticosteroids, cyclosporine, cyclophosphamide, and azathioprine have yielded conflicting information,[103–106] and use of these agents is not currently recommended. The use of antithymocyte serum has proved beneficial in murine viral myocarditis,[107] but its efficacy in humans is not known. It is postulated that severe, persistent myocarditis may eventually result in dilated cardiomyopathy.[108] At that stage, transplantation should be considered.

References

1. Fowler N, Manitas G: Infectious pericarditis. Prog Cardiovasc Dis 16:323, 1973.
2. Levy R, Patterson M: Acute serofibrinous pericarditis of undetermined cause. Am J Med 8:34, 1950.
3. Dalton J, Pearson R, White P: Constrictive pericarditis: A review and long-term follow-up of 78 cases. Ann Intern Med 45:445, 1956.
4. Roberts W, Spray T: Clinical and morphologic spectrum of pericardial heart disease. Curr Probl Cardiol 2:1, 1977.
5. Engel P, Hon H, Fowler N, et al: Echocardiographic study of right ventricular wall motion in cardiac tamponade. Am J Cardiol 50:1021, 1982.
6. Brodie H, Marchessault V: Acute benign pericarditis caused by coxsackie group B. N Engl J Med 262:1278, 1960.
7. Hall I: Purulent pericarditis. Postgrad Med J 65:444, 1989.
8. Buchbinder N, Roberts W: Left-sided valvular active infective endocarditis: A study of 45 necropsy patients. Am J Med 53:20, 1972.
9. Bulkley BH, Klacsmann PG, Hutchins GM: A clinicopathological study of post-thoracotomy purulent pericarditis. A continuing problem of diagnosis and therapy. J Thorac Cardiovasc Surg 73:408, 1977.
10. Kauffman C, Watanakumnakorn C, Phair J: Purulent pneumococcal pericarditis. Am J Med 54:743, 1973.
11. Rubin R, Moellering R: Clinical, microbiologic and therapeutic aspects of purulent pericarditis. Am J Med 59:68, 1975.
12. Gould K, Barnett J, Sanfors J: Purulent pericarditis in the antibiotic era. Arch Intern Med 134:923, 1974.
13. Larrieu A, Tyers G, Williams E, et al: Recent experience with tuberculous pericarditis. Ann Thorac Surg 29:464, 1980.
14. Acierno L: Cardiac complications in acquired immunodeficiency syndrome (AIDS): A review. J Am Coll Cardiol 13:1144, 1989.
15. Smith W: Coxsackie B myopericarditis in adults. Am Heart J 80:34, 1970.
16. Spodnick D: Acoustic phenomena in pericardial disease. Am Heart J 81:114, 1971.
17. Spodick D: Pericardial rub: Prospective multiple observer inves-

tigation of pericardial friction rub in 100 patients. Am J Cardiol 35:357, 1975.
18. Shabetai R: Acute pericarditis. Cardiol Clin 8:639, 1990.
19. Houghton J: Pericarditis and myocarditis: Which is benign and which isn't? Postgrad Med J 91:273, 1992.
20. Spodick D: Electrocardiogram in acute pericarditis. Distributions of morphologic and axial changes by stages. Am J Cardiol 33:470, 1974.
21. Stark D, Higgens C, Lanzer P: Magnetic resonance imaging of the pericardium: Normal and pathologic findings. Radiology 150:469, 1984.
22. Isner J, Carter B, Bankoff M, et al: Computed tomography in the diagnosis of pericardial heart disease. Ann Intern Med 97:473, 1982.
23. Horowitz M, Schultz C, Stinson E, et al: Sensitivity and specificity of echocardiographic diagnosis of pericardial effusion. Circulation 50:239, 1974.
24. Spodick D: Pericarditis in systemic diseases. Cardiol Clin 8:709, 1990.
25. Permanyer-Miralda G, Sagrista-Sauleda J, Soler-Soler J: Primary acute pericardial disease: A prospective series of 231 consecutive patients. Am J Cardiol 56:623, 1985.
26. Maisch B: Pericardial diseases, with a focus on etiology, pathogenesis, pathophysiology, new diagnostic imaging methods, and treatment. Curr Opin Cardiol 9:379, 1994.
27. Piehler J, Pluth J, Schaff H, et al: Surgical management of effusive pericardial disease. Thorac Cardiovasc Surg 90:506, 1985.
28. Morgan R, Stephenson LW, Woolf PK, et al: Surgical treatment of purulent pericarditis in children. J Thorac Cardiovasc Surg 85:527, 1983.
29. Dutt A, Moers D, Stead W: Short-course chemotherapy for extrapulmonary tuberculosis: Nine years' experience. Ann Intern Med 104:7, 1986.
30. Strang J, Kakaza H, Gibson D, et al: Controlled clinical trial of complete open surgical drainage and of prednisone in treatment of tuberculous pericardial effusion in Transkei. Lancet 2:759, 1988.
31. Fowler N: Tuberculous pericarditis. JAMA 266:99, 1991.
32. Evans E: Acute nonspecific benign pericarditis. JAMA 143:954, 1950.
33. Connolly D, Burchell H: Pericarditis: A ten year survey. Am J Cardiol 7:7, 1961.
34. Carmichael D, Sprague H, Wyman S, et al: Acute nonspecific pericarditis. Circulation 3:321, 1951.
35. Dressler W: The post–myocardial-infarction syndrome: A report on forty-four cases. Arch Intern Med 103:28, 1959.
36. Fowler N: Recurrent pericarditis. Cardiol Clin 8:621, 1990.
37. Fowler N, Harbin A: Recurrent acute pericarditis: Follow-up study of 31 patients. J Am Coll Cardiol 7:300, 1986.
38. Hatcher C, Logue R, Logan W, et al: Pericardiectomy for recurrent pericarditis. J Thorac Cardiovasc Surg 62:371, 1971.
39. Cameron J, Oesterle S, Baldwin J, et al: The etiologic spectrum of constrictive pericarditis. Am Heart J 113:354, 1987.
40. Paul O, Castlemen B, White P: Chronic constrictive pericarditis: A study of 53 cases. Am J Med Sci 216:361, 1948.
41. Sutton F, Whitley N, Applefield M: The role of echocardiography and computed tomography in the evaluation of constrictive pericarditis. Am Heart J 109:350, 1985.
42. Vaitkus P, Kussmaul W: Constrictive pericarditis versus restrictive cardiomyopathy: A reappraisal and update of diagnostic criteria. Am Heart J 122:1431, 1991.
43. Tuna I, Danielson G: Surgical management of pericardial diseases. Cardiol Clin 8:683, 1990.
44. Woodruff JF: Viral myocarditis—A review. Am J Pathol 101: 427, 1980.
45. Bengtsson E, Orndahl G: Complications of mumps with special reference to the incidence of myocarditis. Acta Med Scand 149:381, 1954.
46. Reyes M, Lerner A: Coxsackievirus myocarditis—With special reference to acute and chronic effects. Prog Cardiovasc Dis 27:373, 1985.
47. Pallansch M: Epidemiology of group B coxsackieviruses. *In* Bendinelli M, Friedman H (eds): Coxsackieviruses—A General Update. New York, Plenum Publishing, 1988, p 399.
48. See D, Tilles J: Viral myocarditis. Rev Infect Dis 13:951, 1991.
49. Hirschman S, Hammer G: Coxsackievirus myopericarditis. Am J Cardiol 34:224, 1974.
50. Frisk G, Torfason E, Diderholm H: Reverse immunoassays of IgM and IgG antibodies to coxsackie B viruses in patients with acute myopericarditis. J Med Virol 14:191, 1984.
51. Bell E, Grist N: Coxsackievirus infections in patients with acute cardiac disease and chest pain. Scott Med J 13:47, 1968.
52. Melnick J: Enteroviruses: Polioviruses, coxsackieviruses, echoviruses, and newer enteroviruses. *In* Fields BN, Knipe DM, Chanock RM, et al (eds): Virology. New York, Raven Press, 1985, pp 739–751.
53. Burch G, Shih-Chien S, Kang-Chu C, et al: Interstitial and coxsackievirus B myocarditis in infants and children. JAMA 203:55, 1968.
54. Martin A, Webber S, Fricker F: Acute myocarditis: Rapid diagnosis by PCR in children. Circulation 90:330, 1994.
55. Rosenbaum M: Chagasic myocardiopathy. Prog Cardiovasc Dis 7:199, 1964.
56. Mott K, Hagstrom J: The pathologic lesions of the cardiac autonomic nervous system in chronic Chagas' myocarditis. Circulation 31:273, 1965.
57. Grey D, Morse B, Philips W: Trichinosis with neurologic and cardiac involvement. Review of the literature and report of three cases. Ann Intern Med 57:230, 1962.
58. Anderson D, Virmani R, Reilly J, et al: Prevalent myocarditis at necropsy in the acquired immunodeficiency syndrome. J Am Coll Cardiol 11:792, 1988.
59. Lewis W: AIDS: Cardiac findings from 115 autopsies. Prog Cardiovasc Dis 32:207, 1989.
60. Fink L, Reichek N, Sutton MG: Cardiac abnormalities in acquired immunodeficiency syndrome. Am J Cardiol 54:1161, 1984.
61. Grody W, Cheng L, Lewis W: Infection of the heart by the human immunodeficiency virus. Am J Cardiol 66:203, 1990.
62. Lewis W, Lipsick J, Cammarosano C: Cryptococcal myocarditis in acquired immunodeficiency syndrome. Am J Cardiol 9:1240, 1985.
63. Hofman P, Drici MD, Gibelin P, et al: Prevalence of toxoplasma myocarditis in patients with the acquired immunodeficiency syndrome. Br Heart J 70:376, 1993.
64. Sahi T, Karjalainen J, Viitasalo M, et al: Myocarditis in connection with viral infection in Finnish conscripts. Med Ann Finn Mil 57:198, 1982.
65. Saphir O: Myocarditis: A general review with an analysis of 240 cases. Arch Pathol 33:88, 1942.
66. Kline T, Saphir O: Myocarditis in senescence. Am Heart J 65:446, 1963.
67. Kramer MR, Drori Y, Lev B: Sudden death in young soldiers. High incidence of syncope prior to death. Chest 93:345, 1988.
68. Lerner A, Wilson F: Virus cardiomyopathy. Prog Med Virol 15:63, 1973.
69. Gore I: Myocardial changes in fatal diphtheria: Summary of observations in 221 cases. Am J Med Sci 215:257, 1948.
70. Young L, Joag S, Zheng L, et al: Perforin-mediated myocardial damage in acute myocarditis. Lancet 336:1019, 1990.
71. Stallion A, Rafferty J, Warner B, et al: Myocardial calcification: A predictor of poor outcome for myocarditis treated with extracorporeal life support. J Pediatr Surg 29:492, 1994.
72. Marin-Garcia J, Mirvis D: Myocardial disease in Rocky Mountain spotted fever: Clinical, functional, and pathologic findings. Pediatr Cardiol 5:149, 1984.
73. Newburger J, Sanders S, Burns J, et al: Left ventricular contractility and function in Kawasaki syndrome: Effect of intravenous gamma globulin. Circulation 79:1237, 1989.
74. Silver M, Kowalczyk D: Coronary microvascular narrowing in acute murine coxsackie B3 myocarditis. Am Heart J 118:173, 1989.
75. Alvarez FL, Neu N, Rose NR, et al: Heart-specific autoantibodies induced by coxsackievirus B3: Identification of heart autoantigens. Clin Immunol Immunopathol 43:129, 1987.
76. Beisel K, Srinivasappa, Prabhakar B: Identification of a putative shared epitope between coxsackie B4 and alpha cardiac myosin heavy chain. Clin Exp Immunol 86:49, 1991.
77. Neu N, Rose N, Beisel K, et al: Cardiac myosin induces myocarditis in genetically predisposed mice. J Immunol 139:3630, 1987.
78. Neu N, Plocer B, Ofner C, et al: Cardiac myosin-induced

myocarditis—Heart autoantibodies are not involved in the induction of the disease. J Immunol 145:4094, 1990.
79. Lane J, Neumann D, Lafond-Walker A, et al: Role of IL-1 and tumor necrosis factor in coxsackie virus–induced autimmune myocarditis. J Immunol 151:1682, 1993.
80. Neumann D, Lane J, Allen G, et al: Viral myocarditis leading to cardiomyopathy: Do cytokines contribute to pathogenesis? Clin Immunol Immunopathol 68:181, 1993.
81. Henke A, Mohr C, Sprenger H, et al: Coxsackievirus B3–induced production of tumor necrosis factor—alpha, IL-1 beta, and IL-6 in human myocytes. J Immunol 148:2270, 1992.
82. Huber S, Simpson K, Weller A, et al: Immunopathogenic mechanisms in experimental myocarditis: Evidence for autoimmunity to the viral receptor and antigenic mimicry between the virus and myocyte. *In* Schultheiss HP (ed): New Concepts in Viral Heart Disease. Berlin, Springer-Verlag, 1988, pp 179–188.
83. Wee L, Liu P, Penn L: Persistence of viral genome into late stages of murine myocarditis detected by polymerase chain reaction. Circulation 86:1605, 1992.
84. Heikkila J, Karjalainen J: Evaluation of mild acute infectious myocarditis. Br Heart J 47:381, 1982.
85. Karjalainen J, Heikkila J: "Acute pericarditis:" Myocardial enzyme release as evidence for myocarditis. Am Heart J 111:546, 1986.
86. Nieminen M, Heikkila J, Karjalainen J: Echocardiography in acute infectious myocarditis: Relation to clinical and electrocardiographic findings. Am J Cardiol 53:1331, 1984.
87. Alpert LI, Welch P, Fisher N: Gallium-positive Lyme disease myocarditis. Clin Nucl Med 9:617, 1985.
88. Yasuda T, Palacios I, Dec G, et al: Indium 111–monoclonal antimyosin antibody imaging in the diagnosis of acute myocarditis. Circulation 76:306, 1987.
89. Aretz H, Billingham M, Edwards W, et al: Myocarditis: A histopathologic definition and classification. Am J Cardiovasc Pathol 1:3, 1986.
90. Lozinski G, Davis G, Krous H, et al: Adenovirus myocarditis: Retrospective diagnosis by gene amplification from formalin-fixed, paraffin-embedded tissues. Hum Pathol 25:733, 1994.
91. Petitjean J, Kopecka H, Freymuth F, et al: Detection of enteroviruses in endomyocardial biopsy by molecular approach. J Med Virol 37:76, 1992.
92. Kiel R, Smith F, Chason J, et al: Coxsackievirus B3 myocarditis in C3H/Hej mice: Description of an inbred model and the effect of exercise on virulence. Eur J Epidemiol 5:348, 1989.
93. Tilles J, Elson S, Shaka J, et al: Effects of exercise on coxsackie A9 myocarditis in adult mice. Proc Soc Exp Biol Med 117:777, 1964.
94. Kesler K, Pruitt A, Turrentine M, et al: Temporary left-sided mechanical cardiac support during acute myocarditis. J Heart Lung Transplant 13:268, 1994.
95. See DM, Tilles JG: Treatment of coxsackievirus A9 myocarditis in mice with WIN 54954. Antimicrob Agents Chemother 36:425, 1992.
96. Drucker N, Colan S, Lewis A, et al: Gamma globulin treatment of acute myocarditis in the pediatric population. Circulation 89:252, 1994.
97. Weller A, Hall M, Huber S: Polyclonal immunoglobulin therapy protects against cardiac damage in experimental coxsackievirus-induced myocarditis. Eur Heart J 13:115, 1992.
98. Lutton C, Guantt C: Ameliorating effects of interferon beta and anti-interferon beta on coxsackievirus B3–induced myocarditis in mice. J Interferon Res 5:137, 1985.
99. Matsumori A, Tomioka N, Kawai C: Protective effect of recombinant alpha interferon on coxsackievirus B3 myocarditis in mice. Am Heart J 115:1229, 1988.
100. Tomioka N, Kishimoto C, Matsumari A, et al: Effects of prednisolone on acute viral myocarditis in mice. J Am Coll Cardiol 7:868, 1986.
101. Rezkalla S, Khatib G, Khatib R: Coxsackievirus B3 murine myocarditis: Deleterious effects of non-steroidal anti-inflammatory agents. J Lab Clin Med 107:393, 1986.
102. Rezkalla S, Kloner R, Khatib G, et al: Effect of metoprolol on the acute phase of coxsackievirus B3 murine myocarditis. J Am Coll Cardiol 12:412, 1988.
103. O'Connell J, Mason J: Diagnosing and treating active myocarditis. West J Med 150:458, 1989.
104. Hosenpud J, McAnulty J, Miles N: Lack of objective improvement in ventricular systolic function in patients with myocarditis treated with azathioprine and prednisone. J Am Coll Cardiol 6:797, 1985.
105. Vignola P, Aonuma K, Swaye P, et al: Lymphocytic myocarditis presenting as unexplained ventricular arrhythmias: Diagnosis with endomyocardial biopsy and response to immunosuppression. J Am Coll Cardiol 4:812, 1984.
106. Mortensen S, Baandrup U, Buch J, et al: Immunosuppressive therapy of biopsy-proven myocarditis: Experiences with corticosteroids and cyclosporine. Int J Immunother 1:35, 1985.
107. Kishimoto C, Abelmann W: Monoclonal antibody therapy for prevention of acute coxsackievirus B3 myocarditis in mice. Circulation 79:1300, 1989.
108. Matsumori A, Kawai C: An animal model of congestive (dilated) cardiomyopathy: Dilatation and hypertrophy of the heart in the chronic stage in DBA/2 mice with myocarditis caused by encephalomyocarditis virus. Circulation 66:355, 1982.

GASTROINTESTINAL TRACT

71

Approach to the Patient with Diarrhea

Juan C. Bandres
Herbert L. DuPont

Diarrhea is a difficult term to define, but it always implies a change in bowel habits. In general, mild diarrhea can be defined as the production of three or fewer loose stools per day without abdominal or systemic symptoms and no required change in activities. Moderate or severe diarrhea can be defined as the production of four or more loose stools per day, or a total of 200 g or more of feces per day, usually associated with local symptoms (abdominal cramps, nausea, vomiting, tenesmus) or systemic symptoms (fever, malaise, dehydration) with a forced modification of activities (moderate diarrhea) or temporary incapacitation (severe diarrhea).

Epidemiology, Etiology, and Clinical Features

In approaching a patient with diarrhea, the physician should understand that the questions that may uncover the cause are those related to the individual risk factors and the symptoms.

Risk Factors

Physicians seeking the cause of diarrhea should inquire about certain risk factors and predisposing events:

- Is the diarrhea associated with recent travel to a developing country? Bacterial enteropathogens most often cause traveler's diarrhea.
- Is the patient taking a drug known to be associated with diarrhea? The most commonly implicated drugs include antimicrobial agents, laxatives, antacids, alcohol, and antineoplastic drugs. Others can cause diarrhea in some patients, and a temporal relationship between drug ingestion and symptoms should raise a strong suspicion that the drug is the causative agent.
- Is the patient a homosexual male, or does the patient have acquired immunodeficiency syndrome or another immunosuppressive disease? The mode of organism acquisition (fecal-oral or rectal) and the state of immunodepression determine the type of illness that results.
- Have other members of the same household or other confined group experienced diarrhea at approximately the same time? In common-source outbreaks, an incubation period can often be established. This information, coupled with the clinical picture, often leads to the proper diagnosis.

Symptoms

Although diarrheal illness may not show important specific differences according to the causative agent, a number of enteric disease syndromes suggest a cause or category of causal agents (Table 71–1):

- Are the patient's stools soft (semiformed) or watery? Soft stools can be produced by motility abnormalities such as irritable bowel syndrome or increased dietary fiber, whereas watery stools are usually a sign of a potentially important diarrheal disease. The stool volume and their numbers may suggest disease of small bowel (large volume, small number) or colon origin (small volume, larger number).
- Do the stools contain blood or mucus? Small amounts of mucus in the stools should raise the question of irritable bowel syndrome; large amounts, invasive bacterial diarrhea or idiopathic inflammatory bowel disease. Blood in the stool (dysentery) should lead to the diagnosis of inflammatory mucosal disease of the colon—acute infection with invasion of the mucosa, ischemia, radiation injury, diverticulitis, or idiopathic ulcerative colitis.
- Has the patient had local symptoms, including incontinence, abdominal cramps, urgency, or tenesmus? These symptoms are usually related to an acute inflammatory disease, and localizing them may give clues to the specific organ involved. For example, severe crampy pain in the lower left side quadrant in an older patient with diarrhea suggests diverticulitis, whereas crampy periumbilical pain in a patient with previous gastric surgery suggests small bowel disease.
- Has the patient had systemic symptoms, such as fever, nausea, vomiting, anorexia, or weight loss? The answer to this question can be useful in differentiating between chronic and acute processes and mild and severe ones. A patient who has diarrhea with high fever, nausea, and vomiting is most likely to have an infectious process; a patient with chronic diarrhea, weight loss, and few other systemic symptoms is most likely to have a malabsorption process. When vomiting is the predominant symptom, vi-

TABLE 71–1 ■ Clinical Features of Acute Diarrhea

CLINICAL OBSERVATION	ANATOMIC CONSIDERATION	PATHOGENS TO CONSIDER
Passage of few, voluminous stools	Diarrhea of small bowel origin	*Vibrio cholerae*, enterotoxigenic *Escherichia coli*, *Shigella* strains early in the infection, *Giardia*
Passage of many small-volume stools	Diarrhea of large bowel origin	*Shigella, Salmonella, Campylobacter, Entamoeba histolytica*
Tenesmus, fecal urgency, dysentery	Colitis	*Shigella, Salmonella, Campylobacter, E. histolytica*
Vomiting as the predominant symptom	Gastroenteritis	Viral agents (rotavirus, Norwalk virus) or intoxication *(Staphylococcus aureus, Bacillus cereus)*
Fever as the predominant finding	Mucosal invasion	*Shigella, Salmonella, Campylobacter,* viral agents (rotavirus, Norwalk virus)

ral gastroenteritis or a food-borne intoxication is suggested. A febrile illness suggests a mucosally invasive pathogen or an inflammatory process.

The answers to these questions should enable the physician to further define the type of general process that is causing the diarrhea. At this point it should be possible to decide whether the patient requires admission to the hospital. In general, patients who need to be in the hospital are those with excessive fluid and electrolyte losses through stool or vomitus, those whose intractable nausea and vomiting prevent oral rehydration, infants or elderly patients whose condition appears toxic and who have high fever, and those with severe diarrhea who have an underlying immunosuppressive disease.

Specific Settings

Traveler's Diarrhea

Traveler's diarrhea characteristically strikes persons from developed countries who travel in Latin America, southern Asia, Africa, or any region where diarrhea is hyperendemic. The illness usually has its onset during the first 1 to 2 weeks of the stay in the new country, but onset can occur any time, depending on when the traveler consumes contaminated food. The signs and symptoms may vary according to the organism, although the vast majority of cases show no characteristic clinical picture. The causative agents are varied, but bacterial enteropathogens are responsible for more than two thirds of cases. Enterotoxigenic *Escherichia coli* is responsible for nearly half the cases.

Drug-Related Diarrhea

Diarrhea often follows the use of an antimicrobial agent. Sometimes an alteration in the bowel flora produces limited and mild consequences. At other times the cause is the proliferation of an enteropathogen, *Clostridium difficile*, that is usually inhibited by the intestinal flora. Once *C. difficile* is allowed to proliferate, it produces a toxin that causes characteristic mucosal damage consisting of pseudomembranous or plaquelike lesions, usually in the distal colon. Patients typically present with a watery, bloody diarrhea—and occasionally systemic symptoms such as fever. The diagnosis is suggested by the history of ingestion of the medication and a positive result on fecal leukocyte examination and is confirmed by identification of *C. difficile* toxin in stool specimens.

Other agents that often cause diarrhea are magnesium antacids, laxatives, and high-fiber foods. Oral contraceptives and other drugs can cause allergic vasculitis and production of bloody diarrhea due to hemorrhagic colitis.

Diarrhea in a Homosexual Male or an Immunocompromised Patient

Diarrhea and acute proctitis are common problems for homosexual males. The reasons include (1) the higher frequency of fecal-oral transmission of organisms (illness can be caused by any enteric pathogen in this setting; multiple agents often are present); (2) direct inoculation of *Neisseria gonorrhoeae*, herpes simplex virus, *Chlamydia trachomatis*, or *Treponema pallidum* into the rectum during receptive anal intercourse; and (3) the immunosuppression of some patients who have the acquired immunodeficiency syndrome (*Cryptosporidium, Isospora*, cytomegalovirus, *Salmonella, Mycobacterium avium-intracellulare*, herpes simplex virus).

Diarrhea Associated with Ingestion of Contaminated Food or Water

These cases usually affect two or more persons who ingest a common meal or beverage. In general, the characteristics of the disease are similar in all affected persons, although individual susceptibility accounts for minor differences in symptoms. Often this process is caused by a bacterium or a virus, by toxic chemicals, or, more rarely, by parasites (Table 71–2). As a general rule, syndromes that appear within minutes after the ingestion of contaminated food or water are due to chemical poisons; onset during the first 6 hours implicates preformed enterotoxins, as elaborated by *Staphylococcus aureus* or *Bacillus cereus*; onset between 6 and 12 hours suggests *Clostridium perfringens* toxin; and appearance of symptoms more than 12 hours later is usually due to viruses (Norwalk virus) or bacterial agents (*Shigella, Salmonella, Campylobacter*, or diarrheogenic *E. coli*).

Diagnosis

Many tests can help pinpoint the cause of diarrhea. The history and physical examination (including examination of the stool) are important, but certain laboratory tests should

TABLE 71–2 ■ Characteristics of Diarrhea Associated with Ingestion of Contaminated Food or Water*

INCUBATION PERIOD (h)	VOMITING	ABDOMINAL CRAMPS	FEVER	CAUSATIVE AGENT	DIAGNOSTIC TESTS
1–6	+ +	–	–	*Staphylococcus aureus, Bacillus cereus* enterotoxin (preformed)	Detection of toxin in food (usually clinical diagnosis)
8–16	±	+	–	*Clostridium perfringens, B. cereus* enterotoxin (produced in vivo)	Isolation of organisms from food or stools
12–72	±	+	±	*Shigella, Salmonella, Campylobacter jejuni, Vibrio parahaemolyticus, Yersinia enterocolitica*, enteroinvasive *Escherichia coli*, enterotoxigenic *E. coli, Vibrio cholerae*	Isolation of organisms from food or stools
12–72	+ +	+	±	Norwalk virus	Serum titers, identification of organisms in stool by electron immunomicroscopy or antigen by enzyme-linked immunosorbent assay (research laboratory only)

*–, Absent; ±, mild; +, moderate; + +, severe.

be considered in the general approach to patients with diarrhea.

Fecal Leukocyte Examination

A specimen of fresh stool (mucus is preferred and often can be obtained by applicator stick) is mixed with two drops of dilute Loeffler methylene blue and is examined under the microscope. The possible findings include few white blood cells (negative result), many (positive), or none. The presence of a few white blood cells is usually considered an indeterminate result and does not help clarify the diagnosis. A positive test usually indicates the presence of diffuse colonic mucosal inflammation that is caused by either an invasive bacterium or an idiopathic inflammatory disease. A negative result indicates preformed toxin; an infection by a virus, a parasite, or a toxigenic bacterium; or a small bowel process.

Examination for Parasites

Examination of feces for parasites is indicated for patients with a history of persistent diarrhea (2 weeks or longer) or of travel to mountainous areas or to Russia, those who have been in contact with daycare centers, and homosexual males. Sometimes this examination should include duodenal aspirate and specimens from duodenal biopsy. The most important parasitic causes of diarrhea are *Giardia lamblia, Entamoeba hystolytica*, and *Cryptosporidium*. At least three different specimens should be examined carefully if parasites are strongly suspected because these organisms are not always detectable when present. Different techniques can be used to concentrate the specimens and improve the sensitivity of the test.

Stool Culture

Material for stool cultures should be taken from every patient with severe diarrhea who requires hospitalization, from those with temperature higher than 102°F, those with a positive test for fecal leukocytes, and those with persistent diarrhea. Most laboratories can identify the common bacterial pathogens—*Salmonella, Shigella, Campylobacter*, and *Yersinia*—but every effort should be made to direct the laboratory to the likely pathogen in the case, based on the characteristics of the disease. In cases in which *Vibrio parahaemolyticus* or *Vibrio cholerae* is suspected (after ingestion of contaminated seafood or a visit to an area endemic for cholera), the stool specimens should be plated on special media that are not used routinely. If the diarrhea occurs after ingestion of hamburger or if it is associated with the hemolytic-uremic syndrome, the stool culture should be screened for *E. coli* O157:H7 or Shiga toxin–producing *E. coli*.

Virus Detection

Rotavirus and enteric adenovirus can be identified in stool specimens with a commercial kit. Norwalk virus can be detected only by research laboratories.

Proctosigmoidoscopy

The indications for proctosigmoidoscopy for diarrhea are limited to homosexual males, to patients with moderate to severe diarrhea that runs a chronic course, to those whose signs and symptoms suggest idiopathic inflammatory disease, and to those in whom the diagnosis of *E. histolytica* or colitis associated with antimicrobial therapy cannot be confirmed by other, simpler methods.

Treatment

There are three forms of therapy for patients with acute diarrhea: (1) fluids and electrolytes; (2) nonspecific antidiarrheal therapy; and (3) antimicrobial therapy. Each has a role in certain cases. All patients with significant vomiting

TABLE 71–3 ■ Antimicrobial Agents and Recommended Therapy in Infectious Diarrheal Diseases

		DOSAGE*	
DIAGNOSIS	DRUG	Adults	Children
Shigellosis	Trimethoprim-sulfamethoxazole	160 mg trimethoprim/800 mg sulfamethoxazole bid for 3 d	10 mg trimethoprim/50 mg sulfamethoxazole/kg/d in two doses for 3 d
	Norfloxacin	400 mg bid for 3 d	Not appropriate
	Ciprofloxacin	500 mg bid for 3 d	Not appropriate
	Ofloxacin	300 mg bid for 3 d	Not appropriate
	Fleroxacin	400 mg qd for 3 d	Not appropriate
Campylobacter jejuni enterocolitis	Norfloxacin	400 mg bid for 5 d	Not appropriate
	Ciprofloxacin	500 mg bid for 5 d	Not appropriate
	Ofloxacin	300 mg bid for 5 d	Not appropriate
	Fleroxacin	400 mg qd for 5 d	Not appropriate
	Erythromycin	500 mg qid for 5 d	50 mg/kg/d in four doses for 5 d
Traveler's diarrhea	As for shigellosis		
Giardiasis	Metronidazole	250 mg tid for 10 d	20 mg/kg d in four doses/d for 10 d
	Furazolidone	100 mg tid for 7 d	5 mg/kg/d in four doses/d for 7 d
Amebiasis	Metronidazole	750 mg tid for 5 d	50 mg/kg/d in three doses/d for 10 d
	plus Iodoquinol	650 mg tid for 21 d	40 mg/kg/d in three doses/d for 21 d

*bid, Twice daily; qd, each day; qid, four times daily; tid, three times daily.

or diarrhea—particularly very young and elderly patients—should be encouraged to drink fluids and to consume salt (e.g., from saltine crackers). More aggressive treatment, including potassium replacement, is indicated for those with dehydration. The two most successful types of nonspecific drugs are the antisecretory agents (bismuth subsalicylate) and antimotility preparations (loperamide, diphenoxylate). Bismuth subsalicylate, 30 mL every 30 minutes for eight doses for 2 days in adult patients, reduces diarrhea symptoms by about 50%. No other salicylate products should be taken because of the potential for salicylate intoxication. Loperamide-like drugs are even more effective. The customary initial dose of loperamide is 4 mg, followed by 2 mg after each loose bowel movement, not to exceed 8 to 16 mg/d. These drugs should not be taken by patients who have fever or bloody stools because they could potentiate invasive bacterial disease. Antimicrobial drugs are restricted for use in shigellosis (trimethoprim-sulfamethoxazole), *Campylobacter jejuni* enterocolitis (erythromycin or quinolone for adults, erythromycin for children), traveler's diarrhea (quinolone for adults, trimethoprim-sulfamethoxazole plus erythromycin for children), giardiasis (furazolidone for young children, for others metronidazole or quinacrine), and amebiasis (metronidazole plus iodoquinol) (Table 71–3).

Prophylaxis and Prevention

General Measures

Prevention of infectious diarrhea is usually based on avoiding contaminated food or water when traveling in endemic areas. Only food or water heated to 60°C (a temperature that is considered too hot to touch) can be considered safe to consume.

Prophylaxis

Different regimens have been used for prophylaxis of diarrhea for travelers in endemic areas. Both antimicrobial drugs (trimethoprim-sulfamethoxazole, norfloxacin, and doxycycline) and nonantimicrobial agents (bismuth subsalicylate) have been proved effective, although travelers should not be encouraged to use chemoprophylaxis without proper education.

Bibliography

- Blacklow NR, Greenberg HB: Viral gastroenteritis. N Engl J Med 325:252, 1991.
- DuPont HL: Gastrointestinal Infections. *In* Stein JH (ed): Internal Medicine, ed 4. St. Louis, Mosby–Year Book, 1994, p 1915.
- DuPont HL, Ericsson CD: Prevention and treatment of traveler's diarrhea. N Engl J Med 328:1821, 1993.
- Gorbach SL (ed): Infectious Diarrhea. Boston, Blackwell Scientific Publications, 1986.
- Guerrant RL, Bobak DA: Bacterial and protozoal gastroenteritis. N Engl J Med 325:327, 1991.

72

Shigellosis

Gerald T. Keusch

Shigella causes acute inflammatory colitis and bloody diarrhea, which in its most characteristic clinical presentation is manifested by the dysentery syndrome, a clinical triad consisting of cramps, painful straining to pass stools (tenesmus), and a frequent, small-volume, bloody mucoid discharge[1] (Fig. 72–1). In the United States and other highly industrialized societies, *Shigella sonnei* is the most common isolate, whereas *Shigella flexneri* predominates in developing countries.[2, 3] Since the late 1960s, after an absence of half a century, epidemics caused by *Shigella dysenteriae* type 1 have occurred in Latin America, Africa, and Asia and have been associated with high morbidity and, in infants and young children and elderly patients, high mortality rates.[4]

Epidemiology

Transmission of *Shigella* infection is primarily from person to person, facilitated by the ability of as few as a few hundred organisms to cause infection and illness.[5] Thus, it is relatively easy to transfer an infectious inoculum by the fingers, by food or water (which may lead to common-source epidemics), and even by contaminated fomites. The genus is highly adapted to the human host, and only a few higher primates appear to become naturally infected.[4]

Shigellosis is primarily a pediatric disease, presumably because of the lack of preexisting immunity and the greater likelihood that children will transfer the organism by the fecal-oral route.[1–4] In the United States, the majority of *S. sonnei* cases are found in patients younger than 10 years, with most infections occurring in children younger than 5 years.[2, 4] In contrast, the average age of patients in the United States with *S. flexneri* infection has steadily risen, particularly among young adult men.[6] It is presumed that this is the consequence of sexually transmitted infection among young male homosexuals. Shigellosis remains a problem among developmentally delayed and mentally retarded individuals,[7] and it has become a particular problem in daycare settings.[8] The rates of bacteriologically documented infections, as reported to the Centers for Disease Control and Prevention, have averaged approximately 6 per 100,000 population, increasing in some years to more than 9 per 100,000, primarily as the result of large outbreaks of *S. sonnei*.[9] Infections in young children accounted for the majority of these cases. The incidence in children younger than 4 years was 27 per 100,000, compared with approximately 2 per 100,000 in adults older than 20 years. Infections were also most commonly reported from urban regions with large populations of low-income minority groups and from Native American reservations. However, because most cases in the United States are not bacteriologically documented and, indeed, may be so mild that medical attention is not sought or obtained, these data represent gross underestimates.

The aforementioned rates should be compared with those documented in prospective cohort studies in a typical rural village in Guatemala, where the isolation rate for *Shigella* was 9800 per 100,000 children younger than 4 years with diarrheal

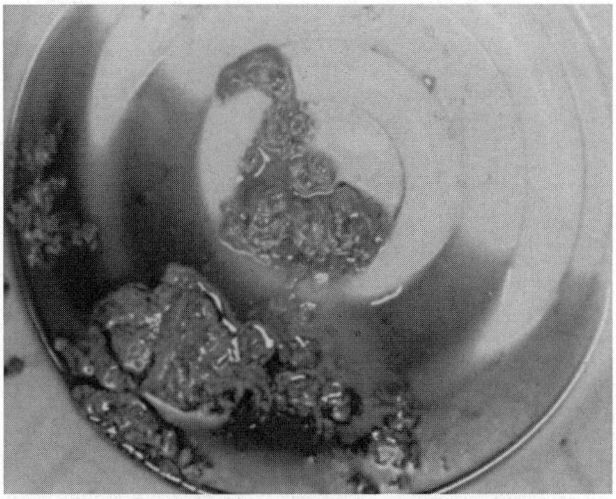

FIGURE 72–1 ▫ A characteristic stool of shigellosis, with mucoid stool mixed with a small amount of bloody fluid. The typical dysenteric stool, consisting of a small amount of grossly bloody mucus, is actually uncommon. (From Keusch GT, Formal SB, Bennish ML: Shigellosis. *In* Warren KS, Mahmoud AAF [eds]: Tropical and Geographical Medicine, Vol 2. New York, McGraw-Hill, 1990, pp 762–776.)

illness.[10] More than 50% of the children had more than one documented *Shigella* infection, yielding an overall incidence rate of approximately 125,000 per 100,000 children per year. Similar isolation rates of 9700 per 100,000 children with diarrhea have been reported from Bangladesh.[3]

Because of the small inoculum needed, the infection is readily transmitted in families.[11] The index case is usually a preschool child; secondary attack rates average approximately 20% and may be as high as 40%, with young children generally developing symptomatic infection and adults having asymptomatic disease. Mild infection is self-limited, with a typical duration of 5 to 7 days. Prolonged carriage beyond 2 months in convalescence is uncommon unless there is evidence of protein-energy malnutrition.

Clinical Manifestations

Although commonly described as bacillary dysentery, implying a bloody dysenteric presentation, most clinical shigellosis caused by *S. sonnei* in the United States is a watery diarrhea quite indistinguishable from other bacterial and viral causes of mild to moderate diarrhea. More severe inflammatory manifestations occur when *S. flexneri* is isolated and are especially common when *S. dysenteriae* type 1 is the causative agent.[1] The initial symptom is usually fever, followed by the onset of watery diarrhea that contains numerous leukocytes that are detectable by light microscopy. In a few hours to a few days, depending on the species of the infecting organism and perhaps on host resistance, the diarrhea may turn bloody (see Fig. 72–1), with or without the other signs and symptoms of dysentery.[12] The initial symptoms of clinical illness in children may be respiratory or central nervous system findings, but cultures of airway secretions and cerebrospinal fluid in these patients are negative, and the true diagnosis becomes apparent when the diarrhea begins and the stools are cultured. However, such extraintestinal presentations are quite rare, although the initial manifestation of infection in young children may be a seizure associated with rapidly rising fever.[13] The episode is generally a single seizure, and, except for affecting somewhat older children, it is otherwise clinically similar to a febrile seizure. Neurologic findings, such as altered consciousness, may be due to either electrolyte abnormalities or hypoglycemia (discussed further on). Occasionally, patients present with encephalopathic manifestations, most commonly in *S. flexneri* infection, with bizarre posturing and unresponsiveness[14] (Fig. 72–2).

Either local or systemic manifestations may complicate the illness. The most severe colonic complication, toxic megacolon (Fig. 72–3), occurs primarily during *S. dysenteriae* type 1 infection and is related to the severity of the colitis.[15] Perforation of the colon can also occur, with a significant increase in the case-fatality rate. In some young children, continued straining at stool and poorly developed ligamentous support of the terminal colon and the rectum results in rectal prolapse. The prolapse usually reduces spontaneously and does not require intervention except to keep the mucosa moist. Protein-losing enteropathy of varying severity occurs in most patients with colonic inflammation, but in children in developing countries it is a major factor in the later development of protein-energy malnutrition.[16]

Systemic complications include bacteremia with the infecting strain or other Enterobacteriaceae originating from the stool, occurring especially in young, malnourished, weaned infants and occasionally resulting in disseminated intravascular coagulopathy,[17] leukemoid reactions, and the hemolytic-uremic syndrome, with the last two complications seen almost exclusively in *S. dysenteriae* type 1 infection.[18] In addition, reactive arthritis and even full-blown Reiter syndrome, both of which are strongly associated with *S. flexneri* infection, particularly in patients with human leukocyte antigen B27,[19] and profound metabolic abnormalities such as hyponatremia[20] and hypoglycemia[21] can be significant problems.

Pathogenesis

In humans, the major pathologic findings are in the colon, where *Shigella* invades the mucosa and results in an inflammatory colitis of varying severity.[22] Lesions are more common and profound in the distal colon and become progressively less severe in the transverse colon and ascending colon.[23] Histologic findings include mucosal edema and hemorrhage, crypt hyperplasia, goblet-cell discharge, a marked inflammatory infiltrate in the lamina propria, epithelial cell damage and death, superficial ulcerations, and an inflammatory exu-

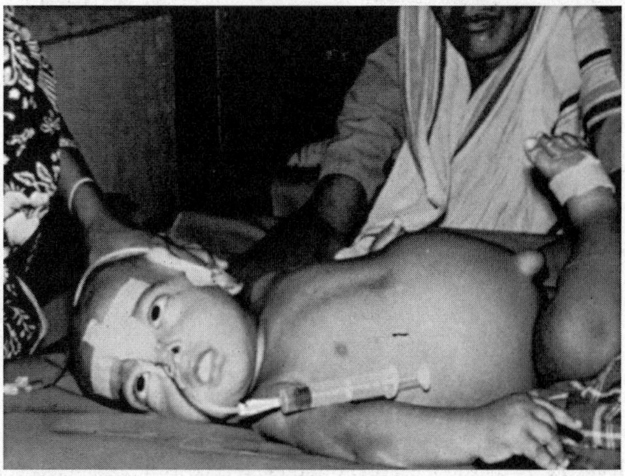

FIGURE 72–2 ▫ Encephalopathic manifestations of *S. flexneri* infection. Posturing, staring, and unresponsiveness can be appreciated in this Bangladeshi child. (Courtesy of Dr. Michael L. Bennish, New England Medical Center, Boston, MA.)

date in the lumen and the stool (Fig. 72–4). The invasive process is quite complex, requires the contribution of multiple genetic loci in the organism, both chromosomal and plasmid, and is essential for virulence.[24] The nature of the initial contact between the nonmotile organism and the target host cell is not understood; however, contact of the pathogen with the surface of the colonic cell triggers ingestion within membrane-bounded vesicles as the organism induces the polymerization of actin fibrils in a process analogous to that of phagocytosis.[25] This process is followed by rapid lysis of the phagocytic vacuole with release of the invading organism into the cytoplasm, where it is able to multiply. Actin polymerization then occurs at one pole of the organism, resulting in a propulsive force dubbed the "actin motor," which drives the bacteria to the plasma membrane of the host cell, using energy derived from hydrolysis of adenosine triphosphate resulting from a bacterial adenosine triphosphatase.[26] This force is enough to propel the bacterium, still within the host cell and bounded by the host cell membrane, to protrude into adjacent cells.[27] Subsequent fusion of the host cell membranes results in transfer of *Shigella* organisms from one cell to the next without ever exiting the intracellular milieu.[28] In this manner, foci of infection develop, leading to local cell injury, death, and sloughing and the production of the characteristic ulcerations of the intestinal mucosa associated with dysentery.

Various data suggest the importance of the induced inflammatory response early in the course of mucosal infection to pathogenesis. In in vitro studies in cultured human intestinal cell monolayers, addition of bacteria to the apical surface of the cells and of human neutrophils to the basal surface results in considerably increased transfer of bacteria across the monolayer, occurring primarily at intracellular tight junctions.[29] Invasion of *Shigella* in vivo in the ligated rabbit ileal loop model also supports this role of the host cell neutrophilic response because the number of invading bacteria increases dramatically when neutrophilic infiltration occurs. Introduction of antibody to the neutrophil surface antigen, CD18, can reduce the extent of the neutrophilic response.[30] Perfusion of animals with the cytokine antagonist interleukin-1 receptor antagonist before infection of ileal loops with *S. flexneri* significantly reduces bacterial invasion, the extent of mucosal inflammation, and tissue destruction.[31]

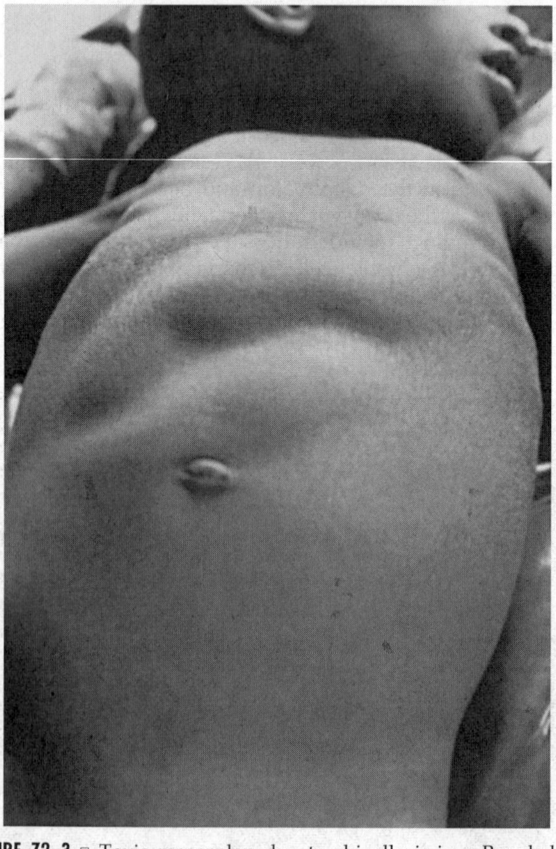

FIGURE 72–3 ▫ Toxic megacolon due to shigellosis in a Bangladeshi infant. The dilated bowel is easily seen. (From Keusch GT, Formal SB, Bennish ML: Shigellosis. *In* Warren KS, Mahmoud AAF [eds]: Tropical and Geographical Medicine, Vol 2. New York, McGraw-Hill, 1990, pp 762–776.)

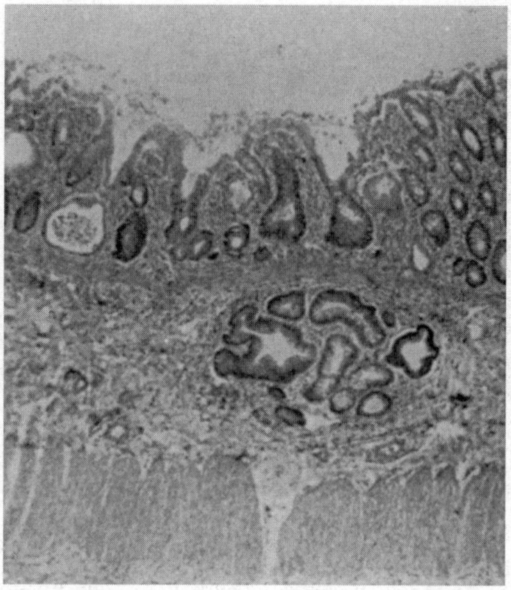

FIGURE 72–4 ▫ Section of colon from a fatal *S. flexneri* infection in a 1-year-old Bangladeshi infant with a 1-month history of dysentery, presenting with rectal prolapse and acute kwashiorkor. There are disruption and sloughing of the epithelial cell layer, an inflammatory exudate in the lamina propria, a crypt abscess on the left, and an extension of glands into the submucosa on the right. (From Butler T, Dunn D, Dahms B, Islam M: Causes of death and the histopathologic findings in fatal shigellosis. Pediatr Infect Dis J 8:767–772, 1989.)

The cellular inflammatory response is accompanied by the production of inflammatory cytokines, which are detectable in both serum and stool.[32] An increase in all cytokine-producing cells in the rectal mucosa has been demonstrated in humans with dysentery.[33] This increase persists for several weeks, perhaps explaining why anorexia and the metabolic consequences of shigellosis are so severe in these cases[34] and why malnutrition is a major associated factor in morbidity.[18]

In addition to effecting invasion, *S. dysenteriae* type 1 produces the cytotoxin protein Shiga toxin. In an experimental primate model of shigellosis, an isogenic toxin-negative *S. dysenteriae* type 1 strain caused much milder illness, with much less inflammation and bleeding, compared with that caused by the parental wild-type toxin-positive strain.[35] Shiga toxin binds to host cells expressing the blood group–active glycolipid Gb3 (globotriaosylceramide), specifically to its terminal galactose-α1→4-galactose disaccharide.[36] Tissue culture and rabbit intestinal cells that express this determinant are able to bind toxin. When toxin is translocated to the cytoplasm by a receptor-mediated endocytosis, the RNA glycohydrolase enzymatic activity of the A subunit cleaves a specific residue in the 28S ribosomal RNA of the 60S ribosomal subunit, irreversibly inhibiting protein synthesis and leading to cell death.[1] Biologic effects are determined in large part by selectivity in toxin binding. In the rabbit small bowel, for example, only villus cells express the principal glycolipid toxin receptor (Gb3), bind toxin, and are inhibited in protein synthesis.[37] These findings are associated with depressed sodium absorption, which is a major function of the villus cell. Because the crypt cell is not affected, basal fluid secretion continues. The combination of diminished absorption and normal secretion results in the net accumulation of fluid within the lumen. Although no studies have documented a small bowel phase in human shigellosis, this mechanism could explain the observed "net secretory" state described in monkey jejunum in the course of experimental *S. flexneri* type 2a infection,[38] and the early watery diarrhea phase in human shigellosis.[1]

Because the genes for Shiga toxin are restricted to *S. dysenteriae* type 1 strains, this mechanism would not account for watery diarrhea due to other *Shigella* species. Two new enterotoxins, designated ShET1 and ShET2, have been described in *Shigella*.[39, 40] Both alter electrolyte transport in rabbit small bowel mucosa in vitro and result in fluid accumulation in ligated ileal loops in vivo. ShET1 is encoded by a chromosomal gene in *S. flexneri* type 2 but not other serotypes or *Shigella* species.[41] ShET2 is plasmid encoded and is significantly homologous to a previously described enterotoxin of enteroinvasive *Escherichia coli*.[42] Humans develop neutralizing antibody to the ShET toxins, indicating that these substances are produced during infection. Their role, however, remains speculative, intriguing, and unproven.

It is likely that Shiga toxin directly contributes to the pathogenesis of hemolytic-uremic syndrome associated with *S. dysenteriae* type 1 infection, because the same complication occurs after infection with Shiga toxin–producing serotypes of *E. coli,* such as O157:H7, but not with non–toxin-producing serotypes.[43] Although the mechanism is not known with certainty, it is postulated to be related to the ability of Shiga toxin to bind to and damage endothelial cells, initiating the microangiopathic hemolysis and glomerular lesions of hemolytic-uremic syndrome.

Hyponatremia in shigellosis is common in children in developing countries and is likely a consequence of inappropriate antidiuretic hormone secretion.[18, 20] If this is true, the mechanism by which excess antidiuretic hormone is released remains to be determined. Hypoglycemia also occurs frequently and appears to be due in large part to inadequate gluconeogenic responses.[21] Other metabolic responses generally associated with inflammatory bowel diseases, such as muscle catabolism and protein-losing enteropathy, may be manifestations of the release of metabolically active cytokines such as interleukin-6 and tumor necrosis factor or other similar mediator peptides in the inflamed bowel so characteristic of the infection.[44]

Therapy

Because the fluid losses in shigellosis are not great, dehydration is not typically an important problem, even when the insensible losses secondary to fever and rapid respiration are included. If dehydration occurs, it is readily managed in most patients by oral rehydration therapy.[45]

The keystone to specific management is the use of effective antimicrobial agents, which lower mortality and reduce the duration of illness.[1] The major problem is to select antimicrobial drugs to which the organism remains sensitive.[46] It should be remembered that the phenomenon of transferable multiple drug resistance was described for the first time among patients with *Shigella* infections in Japan in the mid-1950s, and multidrug resistance remains a problem.[47] In addition to their common resistance to the penicillins and to the extended-spectrum, second-generation penicillins—streptomycin, tetracycline, and chloramphenicol—many strains are now also resistant to trimethoprim-sulfamethoxazole, especially those originating in developing countries. In the United States, documented drug resistance can be overcome by use of a third-generation cephalosporin or, in adults, a 4-fluoroquinolone.[47] The quinolones are not currently approved for use in patients younger than 17 years because of the possibility of associated cartilage damage similar to that reported in young rodents receiving long-term high doses of these drugs. Although the risk to humans appears remote, only when there are sufficient clinical data on the safety of quinolones in young children from controlled clinical trials will we be able to determine when and in whom they can be safely used.

In developing countries, the high frequency of multidrug resistance now often necessitates the use of nalidixic acid (although it is not licensed in the United States for this indication) because other effective drugs either are not available or are too expensive. Five days of therapy with an effective drug is the usual regimen, but it is likely that shorter and less expensive courses will also be effective, an idea that is currently being evaluated.[48] It is not certain that early and appropriate treatment will reduce the prevalence of complications such as hemolytic-uremic syndrome, and indeed some authors have suggested that antibiotic therapy increases the risk of some of these complications.[49]

Severe shigellosis in children in Bangladesh is frequently accompanied by clinically significant hyponatremia, with serum sodium levels lower than 120 mmol/L.[20] Infusion of 3% saline has been advocated by some (12 mL/kg in 2 hours, which is sufficient to produce an increase in serum sodium levels of approximately 10 mmol/L), and rapid reversal of the associated central nervous system depression has been observed.[18] Once there is a response, free access to water should be restricted because hyponatremia recurs if patients are allowed to drink as much as they want. Because severe hyponatremia occurs primarily with infection caused by *S. dysenteriae* type 1 and *S. flexneri*, particularly in young, poorly nourished infants and children, it is only rarely observed in the United States.

Hypoglycemia in shigellosis is most frequently associated with *S. flexneri* and may be seen in both developed and developing countries, especially in young children.[21] Pathogenesis appears to be an inadequate gluconeogenic response, and a blood glucose level lower than 1 mmol/L requires rapid infusion of glucose—for example, 5.6 mmol (1 g) of dextrose per kilogram of body weight in 5 to 10 minutes—followed by intravenous fluids containing 278 mmol (50 g) of dextrose per liter at a rate determined by the patient's fluid needs. Ultimately, management depends on control of infection per se, which restores glucose metabolism to normal.

In poorly nourished infants and children, special attention should be given to continuing nutritional rehabilitation because the catabolic stress of shigellosis is known to continue well into the convalescent period. Malnourished patients may require months of special nutritional therapy to replete body stores of protein, energy, and minerals.[50]

The typical febrile seizure of shigellosis usually does not require more than appropriate measures to reduce body temperature, including use of antipyretics.[13] Only uncommonly is it necessary to administer barbiturates or other anticonvulsive medication.

References

1. Acheson DWK, Keusch GT: *Shigella* and enteroinvasive *Escherichia coli. In* Blaser MJ, Smith PD, Ravdin JI, et al (eds): Infections of the Gastrointestinal Tract. New York, Raven Press, 1995, pp 763–784.

2. Laboratory Confirmed *Shigella* Surveillance Annual Summary, 1991–1992. Atlanta, Centers for Disease Control and Prevention, Foodborne and Diarrheal Diseases Branch, 1995.
3. Zaman K, Yunus M, Baqui AH, Hossain KM: Surveillance of shigellosis in rural Bangladesh: A 10 year review. J Pakistan Med Assoc 41:75–78, 1991.
4. Keusch GT, Bennish ML: Shigellosis. *In* Evans AS, Brachman P (eds): Bacterial Infections of Humans, ed 3. New York, Plenum Publishing (in press).
5. DuPont HL, Levine MM, Hornick RB, Formal SB: Inoculum size in shigellosis and implications for expected mode of transmission. J Infect Dis 159:1126–1128, 1989.
6. Tauxe RV: The persistence of *Shigella flexneri* in the United States: The increased role of the adult male. Am J Public Health 78:1432–1435, 1988.
7. Coles FB, Kondracki SF, Gallo RJ, et al: Shigellosis outbreaks at summer camps for the mentally retarded in New York State. Am J Epidemiol 130:966–975, 1989.
8. Bartlett AV, Moore M, Gary GW, et al: Diarrheal illness among infants and toddlers in day care centers. I. Epidemiology and pathogens. J Pediatr 107:495–502, 1985.
9. Lee LA, Shapiro CN, Hargrett-Bean N, Tauxe RV: Hyperendemic shigellosis in the United States: A review of surveillance data for 1967–1988. J Infect Dis 164:894–900, 1991.
10. Cruz JR, Cano F, Bartlett AV, Mendez H: Infection, diarrhea and dysentery caused by *Shigella* species and *Campylobacter jejuni* among Guatemalan rural children. Pediatr Infect Dis J 13:216–223, 1994.
11. Wilson R, Feldman RA, Davis J, LaVenture M: Family illness associated with *Shigella* infection: The interrelationship of age of the index patient and the age of the household members in acquisition of illness. J Infect Dis 143:130–132, 1981.
12. DuPont HL, Hornick RB, Dawkins A, et al: The response of man to virulent *Shigella flexneri* 2a. J Infect Dis 119:296–299, 1969.
13. Askenazi S, Dinari G, Zenulunov A, Nitzan M: Convulsions in shigellosis: Evaluation of possible risk factors. Am J Dis Child 141:208–210, 1987.
14. Goren A, Freier S, Passwell JH: Lethal toxic encephalopathy due to childhood shigellosis in a developed country. Pediatrics 89:1189–1193, 1992.
15. Bennish ML, Azad KA, Yousefzadeh D: Intestinal obstruction during shigellosis: Incidence, clinical features, risk factors, and outcome. Gastroenterology 101:626–634, 1991.
16. Bennish ML, Salam MA, Wahed MA: Enteric protein loss during shigellosis. Am J Gastroenterol 88:53–57, 1993.
17. Struelens MJ, Patte D, Kabir I, et al: *Shigella* septicemia: Prevalence, presentation, risk factors and outcome. J Infect Dis 152:784–790, 1985.
18. Bennish ML, Harris JR, Wojtyniak BJ, Struelens M: Death in shigellosis: Incidence and risk factors in hospitalized patients. J Infect Dis 161:500–506, 1990.
19. Stieglitz H, Lipsky P: Association between reactive arthritis and antecedent infection with *Shigella flexneri* carrying a 2-Md plasmid and encoding an HLA-B27 mimetic epitope. Arthritis Rheum 36:1387–1391, 1993.
20. Samadi AR, Wahed MA, Islam MR, Ahmed SM: Consequences of hyponatraemia and hypernatraemia in children with acute diarrhoea in Bangladesh. Br Med J 286:671–673, 1983.
21. Bennish ML, Azad AK, Rahman O, Phillips RE: Hypoglycemia during diarrhea in childhood. Prevalence, pathophysiology, and outcome. N Engl J Med 3222:1357–1363, 1990.
22. Islam MM, Azad K, Bardhan PK, et al: Pathology of shigellosis and its complications. Histopathology 24:65–71, 1994.
23. Speelman P, Kabir I, Islam M: Distribution and spread of colonic lesions in shigellosis: A colonoscopic study. J Infect Dis 150:899–903, 1984.
24. Parsot C: *Shigella flexneri*: Genetics of entry and intercellular dissemination in epithelial cells. Curr Top Microbiol Immunol 192:217–241, 1994.
25. Goldberg MB, Sansonetti PJ: *Shigella* subversion of the cellular cytoskeleton: A strategy for epithelial colonization. Infect Immun 61:4941–4946, 1993.
26. Zychlinsky A, Perdomo JJ, Sansonetti PJ: Molecular and cellular mechanisms of tissue invasion by *Shigella flexneri*. Ann N Y Acad Sci 730:197–208, 1994.
27. Bernardini ML, Mounier J, d'Hauteville H, et al: Identification of icsA, a plasmid locus of *Shigella flexneri* that governs bacterial intra- and intercellular spread through interactions with F-actin. Proc Natl Acad Sci USA 86:3867–3871, 1989.
28. Allaoui A, Mounier J, Prevost MC, et al: *icsB*: A *Shigella flexneri* virulence gene necessary for the lysis of protrusions during intercellular spread. Mol Microbiol 6:1605–1616, 1992.
29. Perdomo JJ, Gounon P, Sansonetti PJ: Polymorphonuclear leukocyte transmigration promotes invasion of colonic epithelial monolayer by *Shigella flexneri*. J Clin Invest 93:633–643, 1994.
30. Perdomo OJ, Cavaillon JM, Huerre M, et al: Acute inflammation causes epithelial invasion and mucosal destruction in experimental shigellosis. J Exp Med 180:1307–1319, 1994.
31. Sansonetti PJ, Arondel J, Cavaillon J-M, Huerre M: Role of interleukin-1 in the pathogenesis of experimental shigellosis. J Clin Invest 96:884–892, 1995.
32. Raqib R, Wretlind B, Andersson J, Lindberg AA: Cytokine secretion in acute shigellosis is correlated to disease activity and directed more to stool than to plasma. J Infect Dis 171:376–384, 1995.
33. Raqib R, Lindberg AA, Wretlind B, et al: Persistence of local cytokine production in shigellosis in acute and convalescent stages. Infect Immun 63:289–296, 1995.
34. Rahman MM, Kabir I, Mahalanabis D, Malek MA: Decreased food intake in children with severe dysentery due to *Shigella dysenteriae* 1 infection. Eur J Clin Nutr 46:833–838, 1992.
35. Fontaine A, Arondel J, Sansonetti PJ: Role of Shiga toxin in the pathogenesis of bacillary dysentery, studied by using a *Tox*⁻ mutant of *Shigella dysenteriae* 1. Infect Immun 56:3099–3109, 1988.
36. Jacewicz M, Clausen H, Nudelman E, et al: Pathogenesis of shigella diarrhea. XI. Isolation of a shigella toxin–binding glycolipid from rabbit jejunum and HeLa cells and its identification as globotriaosylceramide. J Exp Med 163:1391–1404, 1986.
37. Kandel G, Donohue-Rolfe A, Donowitz A, Keusch GT: Pathogenesis of *Shigella* diarrhea. XVI. Selective targeting of Shiga toxin to villus cells of rabbit jejunum explains the effect of the toxin on intestinal electrolyte transport. J Clin Invest 84:1509–1517, 1989.
38. Rout WR, Formal SB, Giannella RA, Dammin GJ: Pathophysiology of *Shigella* diarrhea in the rhesus monkey: Intestinal transport, morphological, and bacteriological studies. Gastroenterology 68:270–278, 1975.
39. Fasano A, Noriega FR, Maneval DR Jr, et al: *Shigella* enterotoxin 1: An enterotoxin of *Shigella flexneri* 2a active in rabbit small intestine in vivo and in vitro. J Clin Invest 95:2853–2861, 1995.
40. Nataro JP, Seriwatana J, Fasano A, et al: Cloning and sequencing of a new plasmid-encoded enterotoxin in enteroinvasive *E. coli* and *Shigella*. Presented at the 29th Joint Conference on Cholera and Related Diseases. Bethesda, MD, National Institutes of Health, 1993, pp 144–147.
41. Noriega FR, Liao FM, Formal SB, et al: Prevalence of *Shigella* enterotoxin 1 (ShET1) among *Shigella* clinical isolates of diverse serotypes. J Infect Dis 172:1408–1411, 1995.
42. Fasano A, Kay BA, Russell RG, et al: Enterotoxin and cytotoxin production by enteroinvasive *Escherichia coli*. Infect Immun 58:3717–3723, 1990.
43. Hofmann SL: Southwestern Internal Medicine Conference: Shiga-like toxins in hemolytic-uremic syndrome and thrombotic thrombocytopenic purpura. Am J Med Sci 306:398–406, 1993.
44. de Silva DG, Mendis LN, Sheron N, et al: Concentrations of interleukin 6 and tumour necrosis factor in serum and stools of children with *Shigella dysenteriae* 1 infection. Gut 34:194–198, 1993.
45. Varavithya W, Sunthornkachit R, Eampokalap B: Oral rehydration therapy for invasive diarrhea. Rev Infect Dis 13(Suppl 4):325–331, 1991.
46. Bennish ML, Salam MA: Rethinking options for the treatment of shigellosis. J Antimicrob Chemother 30:243–247, 1992.
47. Bennish ML, Levy SB: Antimicrobial resistance of enteric pathogens. *In* Blaser MJ, Smith PD, Ravdin JI, et al (eds): Infections of the Gastrointestinal Tract. New York, Raven Press, 1995, pp 1499–1523.
48. Bennish ML, Salam MA, Khan WA, Khan AM: Treatment of shigellosis. III. Comparison of one- or two-dose ciprofloxacin with standard 5-day therapy. Ann Intern Med 117:727–734, 1992.
49. Butler T, Islam MR, Azad MAK, Jones PK: Risk factors for development of hemolytic-uremic syndrome during shigellosis. J Pediatr 110:894–897, 1987.
50. Keusch GT, Scrimshaw NS: Selective primary health care: Strategies for control of disease in the developing world. XXIII. Control of infection to reduce the prevalence of infantile and childhood malnutrition. Rev Infect Dis 8:273–287, 1986.

73

Salmonella Infections

Kalpana D. Shere
Marcia B. Goldberg
Robert H. Rubin

The genus *Salmonella* includes more than 2500 serovars, which are capable of infecting a wide array of hosts, ranging from humans and domestic animals to reptiles, birds, and insects. With the important exception of *Salmonella typhi* and *Salmonella paratyphi*, for which there are no zoonotic reservoirs, the various salmonellae are almost ubiquitous as both commensals and pathogens in the animal kingdom. Those that are pathogens cause a variety of clinical syndromes in both animals and humans.[1]

Salmonellae are facultative anaerobic gram-negative rods, usually motile by peritrichous flagella, that are members of the family Enterobacteriaceae.[2] The genus *Salmonella* was named in honor of D. E. Salmon, an American veterinarian who first isolated *Salmonella choleraesuis* from pigs with hog cholera in 1884.[3] *S. typhi*, the causative agent of typhoid fever, was discovered in the mesenteric nodes and spleens of persons dying of typhoid fever in 1880 by Eberth and was first cultured in 1884 by Gaffky.[4]

Over the years, the taxonomy and the nomenclature of the genus *Salmonella* have been gradually restructured. Currently, all the *Salmonella* serovars belong to two species: *S. bongor* and *S. choleraesuis*. *S. bongor* contains fewer than 10 extremely rare serovars. The remaining serovars (more than 2500) are included within *S. choleraesuis*, which is subdivided into six subspecies: *S. arizonae*, *S. choleraesuis*, *S. gallinarum*, *S. paratyphi* A, *S. pullorum*, and *S. typhi*. All the serovars in subspecies *S. choleraesuis* are named, whereas serovars in other subspecies are not.[2] Strictly, the name *S. typhi* should be written *Salmonella* subspecies *choleraesuis* serovar *typhi*. To avoid confusion, in this chapter we refer to the various *Salmonella* serovars by the conventional, albeit less stringent, system currently used in the literature. For a more detailed discussion of the taxonomy, microbiology, and molecular pathogenesis of this important group of organisms, the reader is directed to Chapter 205. The scope of this chapter includes the epidemiology, the clinical syndromes, the diagnosis, and the management of both nontyphoidal and typhoidal *Salmonella* infection.

Epidemiology

Typhoid Fever

Improvements in sanitation, water supplies, and food hygiene since the 1920s have dramatically decreased the prevalence of typhoid fever in the United States (Fig. 73–1). In 1920, there were 35,994 cases of typhoid fever reported. Since 1965, the number of cases per year has rarely exceeded 500.[5] Between 1982 and 1991, there were on average 456 cases per year and one death per year attributable to typhoid fever.[6] This trend holds in other developed countries as well. It was originally hoped that, as carriers slowly died from natural causes and fewer individuals became carriers because of the low prevalence, the incidence of typhoid fever would continue to decrease and the illness would eventually be eradicated. However, since 1965, the number of reported cases of typhoid has remained fairly constant, largely owing to the importation of the disease by returning tourists, immigrants, and migrant laborers.[5]

Because there is no zoonotic reservoir of *S. typhi*, the two main sources for transmission are patients with acute disease and, more commonly, chronic carriers. Patients with acute disease and chronic carriers excrete large numbers of organisms, approximately 1 to 10 billion organisms per gram of stool.[1] Carriers are defined as persons who have recovered from the acute illness and continue to shed *S. typhi* for longer than 1 year. In endemic areas, contaminated water is the usual vehicle for transmission. In nonendemic areas, food contaminated by a carrier is the most frequent source.

In endemic areas, the highest attack rates occur in children. In contrast, in the United States, typhoid fever is most prevalent in age groups most likely to travel to endemic areas. Large-scale outbreaks related to contamination of food or water with *S. typhi* have become rare in the United States; a large proportion of cases continue to be imported. A review of 2666 cases of acute typhoid fever between 1975 and 1984 revealed that 62% (70% between 1983 and 1984) were acquired through foreign travel. From 1982 to 1984, the countries that contributed the most travel-associated cases were Peru, India, Pakistan, Chile, and Haiti.[5] A review of cases of typhoid fever in New York City from 1980 through 1990 revealed a similar trend, with 66% of cases related to foreign travel[7] (Fig. 73–2). Infrequently, microbiology technicians, nurses, nurses' aides, and physicians acquire *S. typhi* through occupational exposure, presumably related to lack of attention to both barrier isolation techniques and proper hand washing. Direct person-to-person transmission is rare, but anal-oral transmission has been demonstrated in homosexual males.[8] Owing to the relatively low incidence of typhoid fever in the United States, there is a paucity of information on the incidence of typhoid fever among patients with acquired immunodeficiency syndrome (AIDS). In Lima, Peru, where typhoid fever is endemic, the reported rate of *S. typhi* and *S. paratyphi* for individuals infected with human immunodeficiency virus (HIV) was estimated to be approximately 60 times that of the general population.[9]

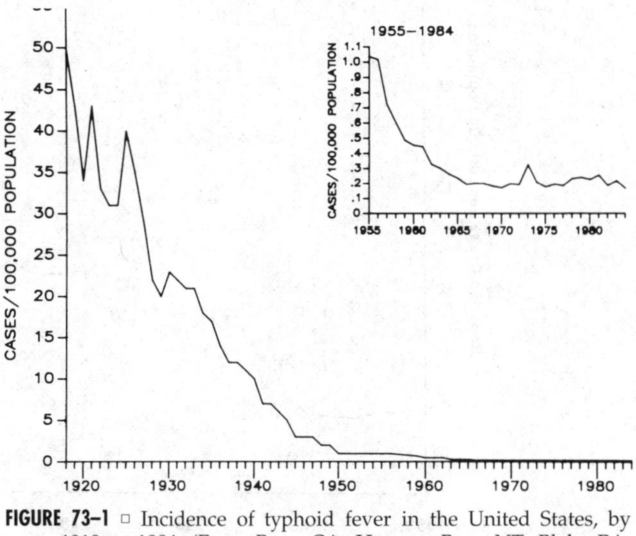

FIGURE 73–1 □ Incidence of typhoid fever in the United States, by year, 1918 to 1984. (From Ryan CA, Hargrett-Bean NT, Blake PA: *Salmonella typhi* infections in the United States, 1975–1984: Increasing role of foreign travel. Rev Infect Dis 11:1–8, 1989. © University of Chicago, Publisher.)

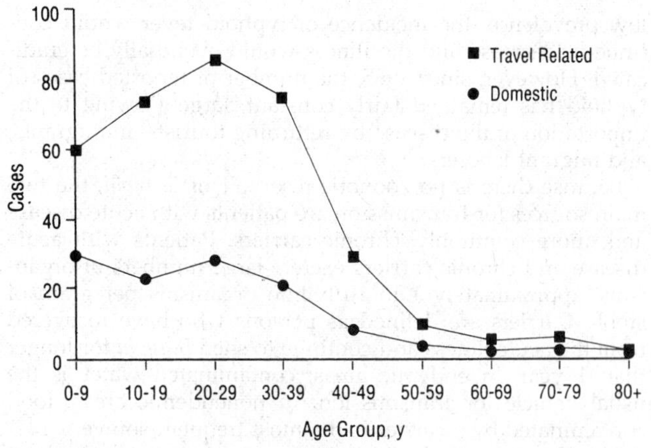

FIGURE 73–2 □ Typhoid fever in New York City. Distribution is given by age group, 1980 through 1990. (From Mathieu JJ, Henning KJ, Bell E, Frieden TR: Typhoid fever in New York City, 1980 through 1990. Arch Intern Med 154:1713–1718, 1994. © University of Chicago, Publisher.)

Nontyphoidal Salmonellosis

The incidence of human nontyphoidal salmonellosis in the United States steadily increased from 1955 to 1985. Since then, with the exception of 1985, when the largest food-borne outbreak ever reported to the Centers for Disease Control and Prevention (CDC) occurred, the reported incidence of nontyphoidal salmonellosis has remained fairly constant, with an average of 47,121 cases per year[6] (Fig. 73–3). These reported cases, which are tabulated primarily in outbreak investigations, are thought to represent only 1% of the actual number of nontyphoidal *Salmonella* infections each year; the total number is estimated to be between 1 and 4 million.[10] The average number of deaths attributed to nontyphoidal salmonellosis from 1982 to 1991 was 88 per year. The overwhelming majority of reported cases for which race was specified in 1993 occurred in Caucasians.[6]

There is a marked seasonal variation in the occurrence of nontyphoidal *Salmonella* infections; peak incidences in summer and fall are due to many small outbreaks of food poisoning. The highest rates of nontyphoidal *Salmonella* infections are observed in children younger than 5 years, particularly infants; rates in persons 20 to 40 years old and in persons older than 70 years are also slightly higher than in the general population[6, 11] (Fig. 73–4).

In contrast to *S. typhi* disease, the nontyphoidal *Salmonella* infections are widely distributed among different animal species. A wide variety of agricultural products, processed foods, and domestic animals have been vectors in *Salmonella* outbreaks. Chicken, egg products, beef, turkey, and pork are responsible for the largest proportion of salmonellosis with an identified origin.[12] The most common isolates in human infections closely resemble those isolated from these animal sources[13] (Table 73–1). In addition to eggs, poultry, and dairy products, items such as chocolate, fruit, rattlesnake meat, kangaroo meat, and marijuana have been implicated in *Salmonella* outbreaks.[14–18] Contact with infected pets such as turtles, iguanas, lizards, ducklings, and snakes causes a small percentage of outbreaks.[19–23]

It is not surprising that of the 2397 outbreaks of food-borne illness reported to the CDC from 1983 to 1987, *Salmonella* accounted for 57% of those attributed to bacteria and was the most frequently reported bacterial pathogen in each year. For each of the 5 years, the most commonly reported food preparation practice that contributed to food-borne disease was improper storage or holding temperature. The second most commonly reported practice was poor personal hygiene. For the majority of *Salmonella* outbreaks during time period, delicatessens, cafeterias, and restaurants were the places in which contaminated food was eaten.[24]

Since the mid-1980s, egg-borne *Salmonella* infections have become a major health problem in the United States, largely due to *Salmonella enteritidis*. From 1976 through 1989, the

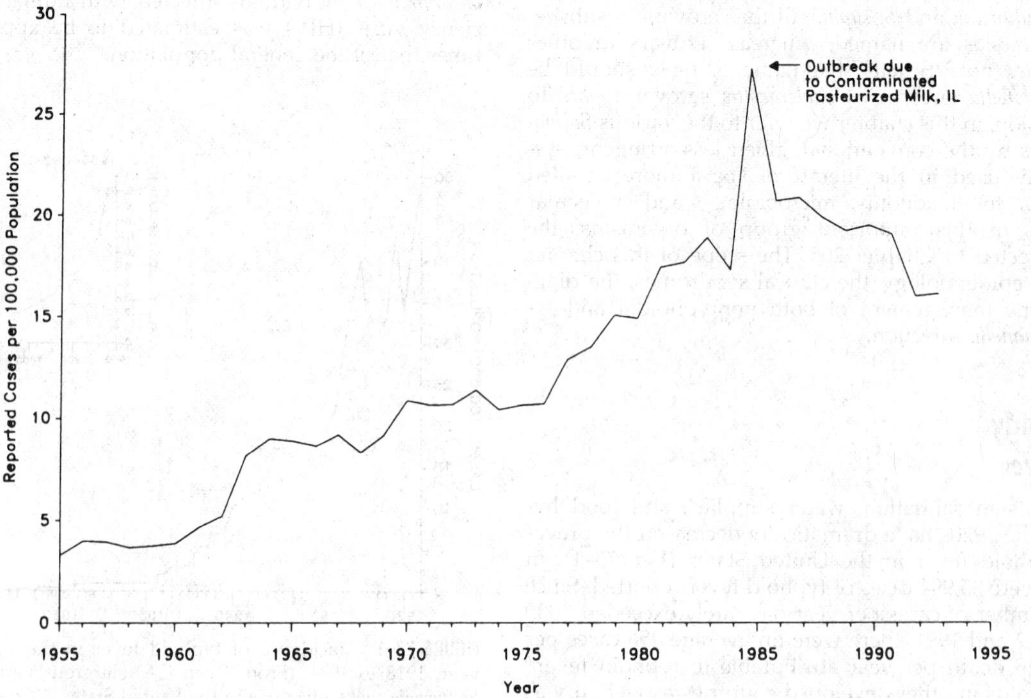

FIGURE 73–3 □ Salmonellosis (excluding typhoid fever) in the United States, by year, 1955 to 1993. (From Centers for Disease Control and Prevention: Summary of notifiable diseases, United States—1993. MMWR Morbid Mortal Wkly Rep 42:50, 1994.)

isolation rate of *S. enteritidis* increased such that in 1990, it was the most frequent isolate in the United States. *S. enteritidis* outbreaks initially reported in the New England states have spread to include Mid-Atlantic and South Atlantic states (Fig. 73–5). Of the 380 outbreaks of *S. enteritidis* infection occurring in the United States from 1985 to 1991, grade A shell eggs were implicated in 82%.[25] In the past, egg-borne salmonellosis was caused by cracked or dirty eggs, but more recent outbreaks have involved intact grade A shell eggs. Approximately 1 per 10,000 shell eggs contains *S. enteriditis*.[26] The organism is known to infect and localize in the ovaries of laying hens; transovarian transmission may be one mode of contamination. *Salmonella* species can penetrate and enter an egg through an intact as well as a cracked shell. Similarly, both transovarian and horizontal transmissions can sustain infection in flocks being raised for meat. *Salmonella* bacteria are present on a small number of broiler chickens at the time of slaughter, and unsanitary conditions in slaughterhouses allow spread of these bacteria among carcasses.[12, 27] Strategies to alter feeds with additives such as propionic acid and lactose, γ-ray irradiation, quarantine of contaminated birds, and development of vaccines for chickens are being explored.[12, 28, 29] Reported multistate outbreaks of food contaminated with *S. enteritidis* illustrate the persistence of this problem.[30]

The mass production and wide geographic distribution of foodstuffs can greatly increase the scope and the extent of an outbreak of salmonellosis. In particular, contamination of processing equipment, conveyor belts, and other machinery associated with mass processing of foodstuffs can greatly amplify the extent of *Salmonella* contamination.[1] A prime example of this phenomenon is a 1985 *Salmonella typhimurium* epidemic that affected more than 16,000 persons in a six-state area of the midwestern United States. In this epidemic, contamination of valves through which huge volumes of raw milk passed resulted in secondary infection of previously sterile milk with the epidemic strain. Because this dairy supplied the contaminated milk to large population centers throughout the Midwest, a major epidemic ensued.[31]

Because the source of most nontyphoidal *Salmonella* infection in humans is animals being raised for food, animal husbandry practices have a significant effect on human disease. For example, feeding domestic animals *Salmonella*-con-

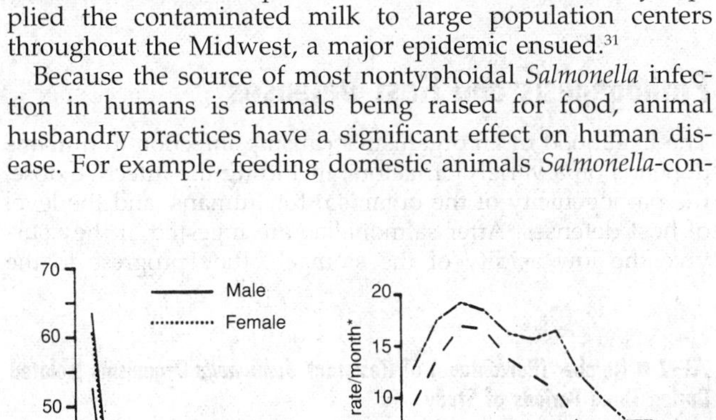

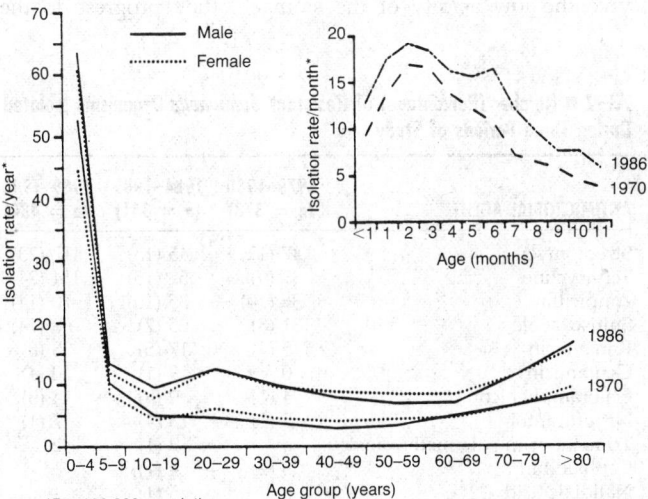

FIGURE 73–4 □ *Salmonella* isolation rates in the United States, by age and sex of patient and year, 1970 and 1986. (From Harrett-Bean NT, Pavia AT, Tauxe RV: *Salmonella* isolates from humans in the United States, 1984–1986. MMWR CDC Surveill Summ 2:25–31, 1988.)

TABLE 73–1 ■ Most Common Human *Salmonella* Isolates in the United States, 1992

SEROTYPES	ISOLATES No.	ISOLATES %
S. typhimurium	7894	22.9
S. enteritidis	6547	19.0
S. heidelberg	2519	7.3
S. hadar	1526	4.4
S. newport	1478	4.3
S. agona	748	2.2
S. thompson	689	2.0
S. javiana	646	1.9
S. oranienberg	595	1.7
S. montevideo	558	1.6
Other	11,320	32.7
Total	34,520	100.0

From the Enteric Diseases Branch, Bacterial and Mycotic Diseases Division, Centers for Disease Control and Prevention, Atlanta, 1992 (unpublished).

taminated fishmeal or other contaminated feeds has resulted in widespread infection both in domestic animals and in the humans who came into contact with these animals.[32, 33] In addition, the use of subtherapeutic concentrations of antibiotics as nonspecific growth factors in the feed has been shown to foster development of antibiotic-resistant strains of *Salmonella* that can ultimately cause human disease.[34] When such agricultural practices are combined with the selective pressures of antibiotic use in humans and the propensity of salmonellae to acquire plasmids that carry genes that mediate antibiotic resistance, it is not surprising that antibiotic resistance is common among these bacteria. Since the mid-1980s, there has been a significant increase in the frequency of antimicrobial-resistant *Salmonella* infections in the United States (Fig. 73–6). Moreover, organisms isolated from patients have been resistant to a wide range of antimicrobial agents[35] (Table 73–2). Outbreaks of salmonellosis in nursing homes and hospitals pose a particular threat because the case-fatality rate for salmonellosis is much higher in these settings. Of all food-borne disease outbreaks in nursing homes from 1975 to 1987, *Salmonella* was the most frequently reported pathogen, accounting for 52% of outbreaks and 81% of deaths.[36] Of the 380 outbreaks of *S. enteritidis* from 1985 to 1991, 59 of those that occurred in nursing homes or hospitals resulted in 90% of all deaths. The case-fatality rate was estimated to be 70 times greater than that in other settings.[25]

Because of the frequent presence of salmonellae in our food sources, it is important to emphasize that despite at times heroic public health measures, the major defense against human infection is appropriate food handling and cooking practices. Cooking food to temperatures greater than 70°C for longer than 12 minutes decreases the risk of salmonellosis. Because salmonellae have been shown to survive in boiled, fried, and scrambled eggs, particularly if some of the yolk remains liquid, the use of pasteurized eggs has been advocated for individuals in nursing homes and hospitals and for patients with immunodeficiencies.[36–38] Food safety measures for eggs and egg-containing foods, as outlined by the World Health Organization, are listed in Table 73–3.[39]

Several case series have demonstrated that nontyphoidal salmonellosis tends to be more prolonged, severe, and recurrent in patients with AIDS.[40–43] One review reported a 20-fold increase in the annual incidence of *Salmonella* infections in men with AIDS compared with men without AIDS.[44] The proportion of *Salmonella* blood isolates among 25- to 49-year-old men in states with a high incidence of AIDS increased

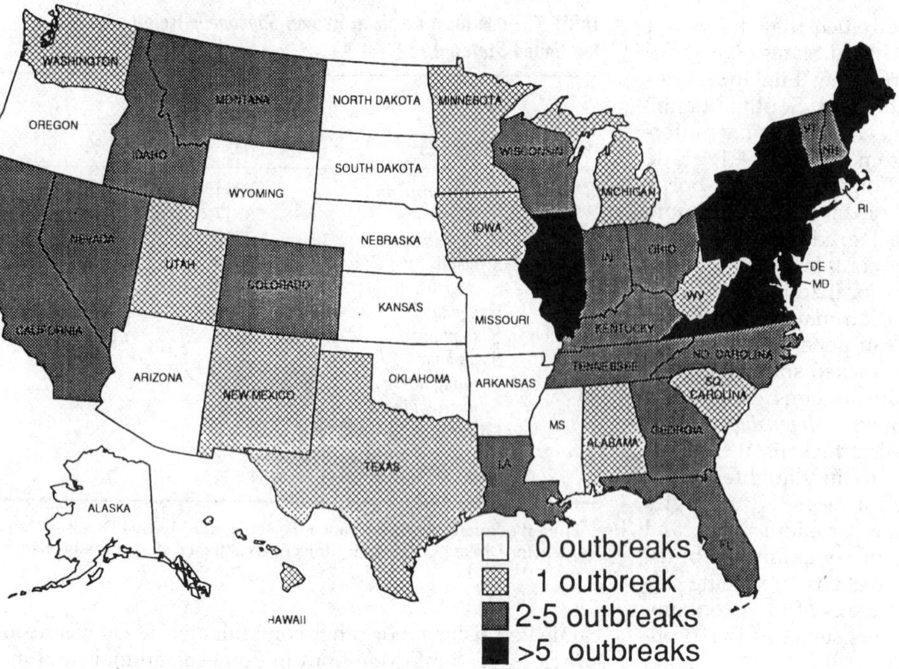

FIGURE 73–5 □ Number of states reporting outbreaks of *S. enteritidis* infection between 1985 and 1991. (From Mishu B, Koehler J, Lee L, et al: Outbreaks of *Salmonella enteritidis* infections in the United States, 1985–1991. J Infect Dis 169:547–552, 1994. © University of Chicago, Publisher.)

by about fourfold from 1978 to 1987.[45] The increased incidence and severity of salmonellosis in AIDS patients underline the importance of food counseling and safe food-handling procedures in this population.[46]

From both clinical and public health perspectives, a great deal of emphasis is placed on the full identification of a particular *Salmonella* isolate. Clinically, this information is useful in predicting what clinical events are apt to occur because different *Salmonella* serotypes are more or less likely to produce a particular syndrome. From the public health standpoint, identification of the organism is the primary tool for delineating and tracing epidemics. Such identification includes serotyping and, when an outbreak is suspected, the use of such molecular epidemiologic techniques as plasmid profiles, restriction endonuclease digestion of plasmid and chromosomal DNA, nucleic acid hybridization, and phage typing. Outbreak detection depends on the full identification of isolates because the major clues to the presence of an outbreak are clustering of cases of a rare serotype, an unusually large number of isolations of a particular serotype from a defined area, and changes in the normal geographic distribution of a particular serotype. Molecular techniques can then be applied to prove that different isolates of the same serotype are indeed identical and thus likely to emanate from the same source.[47–50]

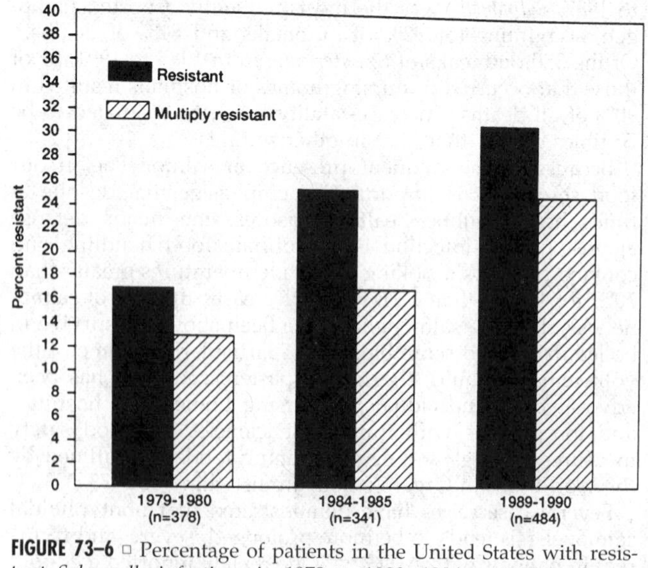

FIGURE 73–6 □ Percentage of patients in the United States with resistant *Salmonella* infections in 1979 to 1980, 1984 to 1985, and 1989 to 1990. (From Lee LA, Puhr ND. Maloney EK, et al: Increase in antimicrobial-resistant *Salmonella* infections in the United States, 1989–1990. J Infect Dis 170:128–134, 1994. © University of Chicago, Publisher.)

Pathogenesis and Host Defenses

The likelihood of an organism's causing infection in humans depends on a variety of factors, including the infective dose, the pathogenicity of the organism for humans, and the level of host defenses. After salmonallae are ingested, if they survive the low acidity of the stomach, they progress to the

73–2 ■ Number (Percentage) of Resistant *Salmonella* Organisms Isolated During Three Periods of Study

ANTIMICROBIAL AGENT	1979–1980 (*n* = 378)	1984–1985 (*n* = 341)	1989–1990 (*n* = 484)
Streptomycin	47 (12)	45 (13)	112 (23)
Tetracycline	33 (9)	52 (15)	114 (24)
Ampicillin	36 (10)	35 (10)	70 (14)
Sulfisoxazole	31 (8)	25 (7)	68 (14)
Kanamycin	15 (4)	17 (5)	38 (8)
Gentamicin	0	3 (1)	20 (4)
Chloramphenicol	4 (1)	9 (3)	14 (3)
Nitrofurantoin	5 (1)	13 (4)	7 (1)
Trimethoprim-sulfamethoxazole	0	2 (1)	2
Cephalothin	6 (2)	4 (1)	1
Nalidixic acid	0	5 (1)	1
Colistin	0	2 (1)	0

From Lee LA, Puhr ND, Maloney EK, et al: Increase in antimicrobial-resistant *Salmonella* infections in the United States, 1989–1990. J Infect Dis 170:128–134, 1994. © University of Chicago, Publisher.

TABLE 73–3 ■ Food Safety Measures for Eggs and Foods Containing Eggs

- Shell eggs should be refrigerated (<10°C) during storage.
- If available, eggs already processed for safety (i.e., pasteurized eggs) should be used. Dried egg powder presents a lesser risk of contamination, provided that it is handled properly during storage as well as after reconstitution.
- Eggs that have not been processed for safety should be cooked until all parts reach a minimal temperature of 70°C, at which point both the yolk and the white have become firm. Scrambled eggs need to be cooked in small batches until they are firm (not runny) throughout. Boiled eggs, depending on their initial size and temperature, may require a minimal boiling period of 7–9 min so that the yolk becomes firm. Similarly, dishes made with raw eggs should be well cooked.
- Leftovers and foods prepared in advance should be refrigerated (<10°C). Stored food must be reheated thoroughly before eating so that all parts of the food again reach a minimal temperature of 70°C.
- Food handlers should wash their hands thoroughly before preparing food, after handling foods likely to be contaminated, including shell eggs, and after every interruption in food preparation, particularly after using the toilet.
- Shell eggs should not be washed. If they are soiled with fecal matter, blood, or some other substance, they may be washed and should be used without delay.
- Cracked eggs are more likely to be contaminated and present a higher health risk.

From World Health Organization: Food safety measures for eggs and foods containing eggs. World Health Forum 14:437–438, 1993.

distal small bowel, where they penetrate the epithelial barrier. Ileal M cells are a type of intestinal epithelial cell found overlying Peyer patches, which are known to internalize organisms and small particles from the intestinal lumen and transfer them to underlying macrophages and leukocytes. These cells may be the primary site of entry. In enteric fever, salmonellae are then transported in vacuoles to the basal-cell membrane and exocytosed into the lamina propria and the lymphatic system, where they gain access to the blood stream, the spleen, the liver, and other parts of the reticuloendothelial system. Some organisms may reach the liver through the portal circulation. *Salmonella* species that cause gastroenteritis remain localized in the mucosa.[1, 51, 52] The molecular basis for *Salmonella* virulence is detailed in Chapter 205.

The minimal infective dose in humans is not clear. On the basis of results of studies involving volunteers from 1950 through the 1970s, it was long widely believed that a large inoculum of salmonellae was necessary to produce infection. However, few of the volunteer studies assessed the minimal infective dose. As few as 25 organisms caused disease in one human volunteer. In one review of 12 outbreaks of typhoid fever, the estimated number ingested ranged from 17 organisms to 100 billion organisms, and in more than 50% of the outbreaks, fewer than 1000 organisms were estimated to be ingested. In addition to the dose of organisms ingested, the serotype of the organism is important. For example, *S. pullorum,* which is adapted to chickens, produces infection in humans rarely and only when a large number of organisms (more than 1 billion) are ingested. In contrast, *S. typhimurium* and *S. enteritidis* may cause infection in humans with a relatively small number of organisms.[53]

Human host resistance to infection from salmonellae can be divided into two general categories: nonspecific host defenses, which are well delineated, and specific host defenses, which are at present poorly understood. Three nonspecific host defense mechanisms have been identified as protective against *Salmonella* infection: gastric acidity, normal gastric motility, and normal intestinal flora. Abnormalities in one or more of these mechanisms will result in an increased incidence and severity of clinical disease due to *Salmonella* infection[54, 55] (Table 73–4). Salmonellae will generally be killed instantly at a pH less than 2 and more slowly at a pH between 2 and 3.[56] Thus, impairment of gastric acid secretion due to achlorhydria, administration of antacids or histamine H_2 blockers, gastric resection, or vagotomy allows salmonellae to escape the bactericidal environment of the stomach. Age has been shown to be an important factor in *Salmonella* infections. Because infants produce little hydrochloric acid and the incidence of achlorhydria is greater for persons older than 60 years, these may be additional factors that place these age groups at higher risk for infection.[53] Rapid gastric emptying may allow bacteria to escape from the stomach into the duodenum. Medication-dependent diabetics have been shown to be at increased risk for *Salmonella* infection, possibly because of abnormalities of gastric acid secretion and motility seen in these patients.[57] Finally, abrogation of resistance conferred by normal gastrointestional flora as a result of broad-spectrum antibiotics, purgatives, or bowel surgery predisposes patients to infection.[54] Prior antimicrobial exposure appears to increase the risk of infection with both antimicrobial-sensitive and -resistant salmonellae, presumably by changing the gastrointestinal flora.[58] In experimental infections with *S. typhi*, treatment with streptomycin before exposure to bacteria reduced the number of organisms necessary to cause disease in both mice and humans.[59, 60] In this last category, a not uncommon clinical scenario is the transformation of the asymptomatic *Salmonella* carrier state into symptomatic disease after either administration of antibiotics or abdominal surgery.

Specific host defenses against salmonellae are incompletely understood. Clinical observations suggest that intracellular killing of these organisms by activated macrophages is of critical importance. Thus, patients with defects of macrophage function, such as those with AIDS or chronic granulomatous disease, are less able to eradicate these organisms. Moreover, illnesses such as sickle cell anemia and other hemoglobinopathies, malaria, bartonellosis, louse-borne relapsing fever, disseminated histoplasmosis, and certain forms of malignancy, in which "blockade" of macrophage function occurs, are associated with an increased incidence and severity of *Salmonella* infection.[61–63] Less information is available about the impact of T-lymphocyte deficiency and antibody deficiency syndromes on the course of salmonellosis, although severe infections in transplant patients and in those with antibody deficiency syndromes have been reported. In normal hosts, the correlation between protection against *S. typhi* and the levels of specific antibodies to different *Salmonella* antigens is poor. Protection from reinfection after the

TABLE 73–4 ■ Conditions That Predispose to *Salmonella* Infection

Decreased gastric acidity (e.g., secondary to antacids, H_2 blockers, H^+,K^+-ATPase inhibitors, or gastric resection)
Decreased gastrointestinal motility (e.g., secondary to opiates)
Alterations of normal intestinal flora (e.g., secondary to broad-spectrum antibiotics, purgatives, or bowel surgery)
Acquired immunodeficiency syndrome
Lymphoproliferative disease
Conditions associated with "macrophage blockade" (hemolysis, bartonellosis, malaria, histoplasmosis)
Inflammatory bowel disease (possible predisposing condition)
Schistosomiasis
Diabetes mellitus

occurrence of natural infection has been shown to be partial at best.[1, 48]

Clinical Manifestations

The clinical manifestations of *Salmonella* infection can be divided into four different syndromes, each of which requires a different diagnostic and therapeutic approach: (1) gastroenteritis, (2) enteric fever, (3) bacteremia with or without metastatic infection, and (4) the asymptomatic carrier state. In addition, there are specific populations, particularly the immunocompromised host, for whom the effects of *Salmonella* infection require special attention. Theoretically, any *Salmonella* serotype can cause any of the clinical syndromes. In fact, certain serotypes are especially associated with a certain constellation of clinical manifestations; for example, *S. newport* and *S. anatum* commonly cause gastroenteritis; *S. typhi* and *S. paratyphi* A, *S. schottmuelleri*, and *S. hirschfeldii* (the last three are the paratyphoid strains and were formerly known as *S. paratyphi* A, B, and C, respectively) are the principal causes of enteric fever; and *S. choleraesuis*, although it enters the host through a gastrointestinal portal, rarely causes gastrointestinal manifestations but commonly causes bacteremia or metastatic infection. One organism, *S. typhimurium*, stands out for its propensity for causing the full array of clinical syndromes. In the United States, *S. typhimurium* is the most common cause of gastroenteritis, bacteremia, and the asymptomatic carrier state[1, 48] (Table 73–5).

Gastroenteritis

The most commonly recognized clinical syndrome caused by *Salmonella* is gastroenteritis, which can be caused by any of the serotypes. Typically, the symptoms of nausea and vomiting begin 8 to 48 hours after exposure to the organism and subside within a few hours. Very soon thereafter, diarrhea and colicky abdominal pain develop, primarily in the periumbilical area and the right lower quadrant. The extent of the diarrhea is quite variable, ranging from a few loose stools to a cholera-like, profuse, watery diarrhea, to a dysentery-like syndrome with bloody, slimy stools and associated symptoms of rectal urgency and tenesmus. Similarly, abdominal findings on physical examination can range from the very mild to an extreme that suggests acute appendicitis, cholecystitis, or a ruptured viscus. In particular, *Salmonella* gastroenteritis (like bacterial gastroenteritis due to *Campylobacter jejuni* and *Yersinia enterocolitica*) is an important cause of "pseudoappendicitis," a clinical syndrome that usually occurs in the first two decades of life and closely mimics typical appendicitis. A moderate elevation in temperature (<39°C) may be present in 50% of patients and usually returns to normal within 1 or 2 days. Patients may sometimes complain of chills as well. Transient bacteremias probably occur in 1% to 4% of patients. In most situations, it is trivial, but in patients with certain underlying conditions (see following discussion), it is a major concern because of the possibility of metastatic seeding.[1, 48, 64]

TABLE 73–5 ■ Summary of Clinical Syndromes of *Salmonella* Infection

SYNDROME	MOST COMMON CAUSATIVE SEROTYPES	SYMPTOMS AND FINDINGS
Gastroenteritis	*S. typhimurium* *S. enteritidis* *S. newport* *S. anatum*	Moderate fever, nausea, vomiting, diarrhea, variable abdominal discomfort
Enteric fever	*S. typhi* *S. paratyphi A* *S. schottmuelleri* *S. hirschfeldii*	Prolonged fever, headache, myalgias, nausea, constipation or diarrhea, hypertrophy of reticuloendothelial system, possible metastatic infection, possible immune complex deposition
Bacteremia, with or without metastatic disease	*S. typhimurium* *S. choleraesuis* *S. heidelberg*	Fever, possible nausea, vomiting, possible diarrhea, abdominal discomfort, possible cardiovascular infection, possible metastatic infection
Chronic carrier state	*S. typhimurium*	Asymptomatic

Certain underlying conditions are associated with more severe gastroenteritis syndromes, with malnutrition, AIDS, achlorhydria, and inflammatory bowel disease being the most notable. Each of these conditions is associated with more severe and prolonged diarrhea and a higher rate of blood stream invasion with its potential consequences.[48]

The diagnosis of *Salmonella* gastroenteritis is based on the history and the stool culture. The diagnosis should be suspected in any patient who presents with a febrile gastroenteritis syndrome, particularly if there is an epidemiologic history that includes eating at a fast-food establishment, the possibility of having ingested inadequately cooked chicken or eggs, or a history of contact with persons with similar clinical syndromes. Stools of patients with *Salmonella* gastroenteritis are usually not bloody, but they may contain occult blood and a moderate number of polymorphonuclear leukocytes. Mild leukocytosis may be present, but the white cell count is most often normal.[48] Stool cultures are preferable to rectal swabs, and enrichment broth and media are important for isolation of the organisms.[65, 66]

Enteric Fever

Enteric fever is a multiorgan process that is caused by *Salmonella* and is characterized by (1) prolonged fever; (2) sustained blood stream infection without endothelial or endocardial seeding; (3) profound hypertrophy and activation of the reticulendothelial system, particularly the intestinal and the mesenteric lymphoid tissue, the liver, and the spleen; and (4) metastatic infection and immunologic complications such as immune complex deposition, leading to multiorgan dysfunction.[1, 48]

In theory, any *Salmonella* serotype is capable of producing an enteric fever syndrome. In fact, the majority of cases of enteric fever are caused by *S. typhi* and the paratyphoid strains (*S. paratyphi* A, *S. schottmuelleri*, and *S. hirschfeldii*). Regardless of the serotype involved, the clinical manifestations of enteric fever are qualitatively identical. However, the disease's severity, mortality rate, relapse rate, duration, and associated incidence of complications are greater in patients infected with *S. typhi*.[1, 48]

The incubation period of enteric fever depends on the size of the inoculum. It may be as short as 3 days or as long as 60 days; typically, the incubation period is 1 to 2 weeks. Approximately 10% of patients experience diarrhea during the first week after exposure. Many asymptomatic individuals have transiently positive stool cultures during this period. Fever is usually the earliest indication of disease, rising in a stepwise fashion in 2 to 3 days up to 39°C to 40°C. Appropriate antibiotic therapy eliminates fever during 3 to 5 days.[60] Signs and symptoms associated with enteric fever include

TABLE 73–6 ■ Symptoms in Typhoid Fever During Three Periods of Study (Percentage)

SYMPTOMS	1939–1944* (*n* = 360)	1964† (*n* = 507)	1973 (*n* = 105)
Fever	100	75	93
Headache	90	78	59
Diarrhea	43	37	57
Anorexia	91	NA‡	39
Abdominal pain	19	35	39
Chills	37	16	37
Vomiting	54	24	35
Cough	86	37	28
Nausea	54	NA	23
Muscle pains	91	25	12
Constipation	79	38	10
Weakness	87	NA	10
Dysuria	3	NA	7
Sore throat	84	NA	6
Dizziness	25	NA	3
Seizures	0	0	1

*See Stuart and Pullen.[68]
†See Walker.[118]
‡NA, Not available.
Reprinted by permission of the publisher from Hoffman TA, Ruiz CJ, Counts GW, et al: Waterborne typhoid fever in Dade County, Florida. Clinical and therapeutic evaluation of 105 bacteremic patients. Am J Med 59:481–487, 1975. Copyright 1975 by Excerpta Medica Inc.

fever, chilly sensation, myalgias, abdominal pain, headache, rose spots, cough, and sore throat. Comparison of signs and symptoms noted in three large outbreaks of typhoid fever shows that although fever is almost always present, the other findings may be quite variable (Table 73–6). Interestingly, symptoms such as sore throat, weakness, myalgias, constipation, and anorexia were apparently more common in patients with typhoid fever in the preantibiotic era study conducted by Stuart and Pullen.[68] Physical examination of the abdomen may reveal some tenderness, distention, hepatomegaly, and splenomegaly. Although relative bradycardia and rose spots are classically associated with enteric fever, they may be absent in the majority of patients.[67, 68]

The clinical syndrome caused by *S. typhi* in infants and young children is often different from that seen in adults. In its more severe form, it may appear as sepsis, especially in children younger than 2 years. However, one large study of 648 infants during the typhoid season (January to March 1983) in Chile revealed that *S. typhi* and *S. paratyphi* can cause a mild, self-limited bacteremic illness that was previously often misdiagnosed as a respiratory illness or a viral syndrome. In addition, diarrhea is seen more commonly than constipation in young children.[69, 70]

The major complications of enteric fever are perforations of the terminal ileum or proximal colon and hemorrhage from ulcerations in the same area. These complications occur in patients whose disease has been progressing for 2 weeks or more. They remain the leading causes of death in patients with typhoid fever. Other complications include psychosis, hepatitis, cholecystitis, pneumonitis, pericarditis, and meningitis. With prompt specific therapy, complications are rare. Relapses occur in up to 10% to 15% of patients treated with ampicillin, chloramphenicol, or trimethroprim-sulfamethoxazole, usually 2 weeks after cessation of therapy. Frequently, the relapse is a self-limited febrile illness, but a few patients may need another short course of an antibiotic.[60]

The role of endotoxin in the production of the signs and symptoms of typhoid fever has been studied extensively. Circulating endotoxin has been demonstrated only in patients infected with *S. typhi* who present with septic shock. In all infected patients, it has been postulated that local concentrations of endotoxin are responsible for cytotoxic and ischemic damage. These reactions may result in intestinal hemorrhage and perforation. Many signs and symptoms can be related to the known toxic and pyrogenic effects of endotoxin.[71]

Laboratory data in patients with enteric fever may reveal leukopenia or leukocytosis, but the leukocyte count is usually normal. Elevations in liver function tests, specifically of aspartate transaminase, alanine transaminase, alkaline phosphatase, and lactate dehydrogenase, may be seen. Examination of the stool frequently reveals a moderate number of polymorphonuclear leukocytes.[1, 48]

The definitive diagnosis depends on the isolation of the organism from the patient. Cultures of bone marrow aspirate, blood, urine, feces, bile, and rose spots yield varying results (Table 73–7). Cultures of bone marrow aspirates are the most sensitive (positive in 90% of cases). They are usually positive more quickly than are cultures of other specimens, and, unlike with blood cultures, the prior use of antibiotics does not diminish their yield. Blood cultures are positive in approximately 50% to 70% of patients with enteric fever. Stool cultures yield the organism in approximately 90% of cases if

TABLE 73–7 ■ Yield of Cultures from Various Sites During the Course of Untreated Typhoid Fever

TIME COURSE	Incubation Period *Ingestion* ↓	Stage of Active Invasion *Wk #1*	*Wk #2*	Established Disease *Wk #3*	*Wk #4*	Convalescent Period *Wk #5*	Period of Late Focal Complications *Indefinite*
BLOOD CULTURES	Negative	←—— 80%–90% ——→		Negative unless continued disease or relapse occurs			
STOOL CULTURES	Transiently positive	Negative	←—— 80% Positive ——→		←—— 50% Positive →		Decreasing incidence of positive cultures with time: 20% at 2 mo 10% at 3 mo 3% at 1 y
URINE CULTURES	Negative	Negative	←—— 25% Positive ——→		←—— 10% Positive →		Decreasing incidence of positive cultures
ANCILLARY CULTURES (bone marrow, rose spot)	Negative	Negative	←—— 80%–90% Positive ——→ / ←—— 60% Positive ——→		Decreasing incidence of positive cultures		
WIDAL TEST	Negative	←—— 20% Positive ——→		←—— 50% Positive ——→	←—— 80% Positive ——→		

numerous attempts are made. The duodenal string test yields the organism in about 70% of cases but is probably no more reliable than blood cultures. A combination of two or more cultures from different sites is the most sensitive diagnostic approach.[72–74]

Several serologic methods have been developed for the detection of *S. typhi* antigens and antibodies. The classic Widal test, a serum agglutination test for *Salmonella* O and H antigens, is still widely used in developing countries. Limitations of the test include difficulty in its interpretation in areas where *S. typhi* infection is endemic and baseline antibody titers of the population are unknown and poor standardization of the antigens.[75, 76] In addition, vaccine administration, other systemic inflammatory processes, and infection with nontyphoidal strains of *Salmonella* can cause elevations in these antibody levels.[1] Other serologic tests include enzyme-linked immunosorbent assay for immunoglobulins M and G antibodies against *S. typhi* lipopolysaccharide, the coagglutination test, counterimmunoelectrophoresis, and radioimmunoassay.[74, 77, 78] None of these tests is widely used owing to cost or lack of sensitivity, specificity, or rapidity.

Bacteremia and Metastatic Infection

Invasion of the blood stream by *Salmonella* organisms, whether part of the transient bacteremia that can occur in the setting of the gastroenteritis syndrome or part of the more sustained bacteremia of enteric fever, carries the potential for metastatic infection. Salmonellae have a unique capacity to metastasize, particularly to sites of preexisting structural abnormality. Major sites of concern are cardiovascular lesions, skeletal lesions, malignancies, and the meninges (spread to the meninges is particularly common in infants); however, almost any organ in the body may be affected. The serotype that most typically produces both sustained bacteremia and metastatic infection is *S. choleraesuis*, and this organism continues to be responsible for the highest incidence of such events per episode of human infection. Because of major improvements in the pork industry, however, human infection with this particular serotype has become much less common, and *S. typhimurium*, *S. enteritidis*, and *S. heidelberg* are now the *Salmonella* serotypes most likely to cause this array of clinical problems.[1, 48, 79]

CARDIOVASCULAR INFECTIONS

The critical information in a case of *Salmonella* bacteremia is the degree of bacteremia. High-grade bacteremia (greater than 50% of three or more cultures of blood drawn over several hours grow the organism) is suggestive of focal intracardiac or intravascular infection. Salmonellae have a unique propensity to localize on abnormal cardiovascular surfaces, particularly atherosclerotic aneurysms, plaques of the aorta and ileofemoral vessels, and abnormal surfaces of the endocardium.[64, 82, 83] *Salmonella* vascular infections have been reported in the thoracic and the abdominal portions of the aorta, the coronary arteries, the peripheral arteries, the arteriovenous fistulae, and a Dacron bypass graft. Abdominal aortic infections are most common, followed by infections of the femoral arteries, the thoracic aorta, and the iliac arteries. In *Salmonella* infections of abdominal aortic aneursyms, *S. typhimurium* is most commonly isolated, followed by *S. choleraesuis* and *S. enteritidis*. Complications include psoas abscesses and lumbar vertebral osteomyelitis.[82] Because the presentation is usually subacute and may be subtle, Rubin and Weinstein[1] have identified a set of suggestive presentations that may be useful: (1) a prolonged fever after an episode of gastroenteritis; (2) pain in the back, abdomen, or chest accompanied by *Salmonella* bacteremia; (3) recurrence of *Salmonella* bacteremia during or after adequate therapy; (4) vertebral osteomyelitis or paravertebral masses associated with *Salmonella* bacteremia; and (5) *Salmonella* bacteremia in patients with prosthetic vascular grafts. The mortality rate associated with *Salmonella* vascular infections is quite high, and both early surgical intervention and early medical therapy are necessary. Under the coverage of antibiotic therapy, surgical excision of the infected sites and reconstruction along clean tissue planes should be performed. Surgery should not be delayed in an attempt to eradicate the infection with antibiotics alone because the mortality rate associated with medical therapy alone has been reported to be as high as 100%. Most infected patients require 6 weeks of antibiotic therapy, but patients who are immunosuppressed or at high risk for reinfection may require longer courses of therapy.[82, 83]

Endocarditis due to salmonellae is rare. The majority of patients reported with *Salmonella* endocarditis have preexisting heart disease. Most cases involve the mitral or the aortic valve. The high incidence of isolated mural endocarditis with *Salmonella* underscores the organism's propensity for seeding abnormal surfaces of the endocardium. *S. choleraesuis*, *S. typhimurium*, and *S. enteritidis* are the most frequent serotypes seen. Complications include valve perforation, valve ring abscess, atrial septal abscess, atrioventricular wall perforation, and rupture of the cusps. In addition, *Salmonella* has been reported to cause myocarditis, pericarditis, coronary arteritis, and pacemaker infections.[82]

Because of the high incidence of underlying cardiovascular disease in persons older than 50 years, endothelial and endocardial infection with *Salmonella* is predominantly a disease of the elderly: as many as 25% of patients older than 50 years who have documented *Salmonella* bacteremia develop cardiovascular infection.[84] These data suggest that, although antibiotics may prolong fecal excretion of salmonellae, they may be justified for *Salmonella* gastroenteritis in the subset of patients with underlying cardiovascular disease.

BONE AND JOINT INFECTIONS

Although any skeletal site can become infected, *Salmonella* infections of bone typically involve the long bones, the chondrosternal junctions, and the spine. Skeletal infection is particularly common at sites of skeletal injury or abnormality, at sites of trauma, in areas that have been injured in the setting of sickle cell disease, and with skeletal prostheses. Most patients have involvement of one bone, but many patients with sickle cell disease may have two or more sites affected. Predisposing conditions include diabetes mellitus, corticosteroid therapy, systemic lupus erythematosus, sickle cell anemia, and age younger than 5 years. The overall prognosis is good with 2 to 4 weeks of antibiotic therapy.[1, 48, 82]

Suppurative arthritis may occur as an extension from a contiguous site of osteomyelitis or as a separate site of metastatic infection. Young age, immunosuppression, corticosteroids, and sickle cell anemia are predisposing conditions. The most commonly involved areas are the knee, the shoulder, the hip, and the sacroiliac joints. *S. typhimurium* is the most common causative serotype. The high incidence of positive blood cultures in both *Salmonella* osteomyelitis and septic arthritis suggests that the majority of cases are hematogenous in origin. Antibiotic therapy for 4 weeks with repeated arthrocentesis generally produces favorable results.[1, 48, 82]

Salmonella gastroenteritis may be complicated with reactive arthritis, which is usually a migratory polyarthritis occurring on the average of 10 days after the gastrointestinal episode. Knees, ankles, and wrist joints are most frequently affected. In one review, human leukocyte antigen B27 was present in 90% of patients with *Salmonella* reactive arthritis. Associated complications such as conjunctivitis and urethritis usually occur before or at the onset of arthritis. Approximately 25% of patients have the triad of arthritis, conjunctivitis, and urethritis associated with Reiter syndrome. The average duration of symptoms is 5.5 months. Cultures of blood, urine, and urethral and joint fluid are negative. The pathogenesis is unclear, but *Salmonella*-specific antibodies (particularly immunoglobulin A) have been identified in the serum and the synovial fluid of patients with this syndrome. In addition, there is direct evidence that *Salmonella* antigens and lipopolysaccharide are present in the joint space in these individuals. Antiinflammatory agents are the mainstay of therapy.[82, 85, 86]

CENTRAL NERVOUS SYSTEM INFECTIONS

Meningitis due to *Salmonella* is primarily a disease of young children: more than 50% of cases occur in newborns, and in these infants it tends to have a fulminant course. In those patients who survive, there is a high rate of neurologic sequelae, including residual seizures, hydrocephalus, ventriculitis, abscess formation, subdural empyema, and permanent disability. Four weeks of intravenous antibiotic therapy is usually necessary.[88] Because of the long-term sequelae associated with *Salmonella* meningitis, even with optimal therapy, it is recommended that physicians attempt to prevent this condition by administering antibiotics to all children younger than 1 year with *Salmonella* gastroenteritis.

Focal intracranial *Salmonella* infections such as brain abscesses, subdural empyemas, and epidural abscesses are rare. Unlike meningitis, focal intracranial infections tend to occur in adults as well as in children. Brain abscesses occur more often in adults, and subdural empyemas are seen more often in children. Predisposing factors include meningitis, trauma, and intracranial hematoma. Surgical drainage with antibiotic therapy is generally associated with a good prognosis.[88]

ABDOMINAL INFECTIONS

Intraabdominal *Salmonella* infection usually involves the hepatobiliary system and the spleen. Cholecystitis is the most frequently observed intraabdominal infection. Liver abscesses usually occur in patients with preexisting liver disease, and splenic abscess are associated with sickle cell disease. Other intraabdominal infections reported include pancreatic abscesses, subphrenic abscesses, adrenal abscesses, and peritonitis.[82]

PULMONARY INFECTIONS

Pleuropulmonary infecton due to *Salmonella* is rare and generally occurs in patients with either abnormalities of the pulmonary parenchyma or pleura or underlying disease. Typically, these patients present with an acute onset of symptoms and lobar infiltrates. Blood and stool cultures are positive in 50% of these patients. Complications develop frequently and include abscesses, empyemas, hemoptysis, pleural effusions, and bronchopleural fistulae. The majority of patients with uncomplicated pneumonia do well with a 2-week course of antiobiotic therapy. Complicated pneumonias often require surgical intervention as well as prolonged antibiotic therapy.[89]

GENITOURINARY INFECTIONS

Salmonella genitourinary infections generally occur in patients with preexisting genitourinary structural abnormalities (e.g., obstruction, reflux, calculous disease, or abnormalities secondary to tuberculosis or schistosomiasis), malignancy, and immunosuppression. In addition to antibiotic therapy, correction of the structural abnormalities is often necessary for cure. Owing to the high rate of relapse, cultivation of surveillance urine cultures during follow-up is recommended.[90, 91]

Genital infections due to *Salmonella* are rare but have been reported in testicular and ovarian abscesses, epididymitis, prostatitis, and septic abortion.[82]

SOFT TISSUE INFECTIONS

Burns, trauma, sickle cell disease, diabetes mellitus, and immunosuppression predispose patients to soft tissue infections with *Salmonella*. Mastitis, endophthalmitis, parotid abscess, thyroiditis, and thyroid abscess due to *Salmonella* have been reported. However, the skin is the most frequent site of *Salmonella* soft tissue infection. Skin infections due to *S. dublin* may be seen in veterinarians and farmers exposed to birthing cattle.[82]

Chronic Carrier State

The chronic carrier state refers to the persistence of salmonellae in stool or urine for periods of a year or longer. It develops in less than 1% of persons who have had nontyphoidal salmonellosis and approximately 2% to 3% of patients who have had typhoid fever. The biliary tree is the principal site in the gastrointestinal tract where these organisms are harbored; there is an excellent correlation between difficulty in eradicating the carrier state and the presence of gallstones or biliary scarring. The urinary carrier state has been reported in 0.2% to 3.3% of patients with typhoid fever. The urinary carrier state is strongly associated with obstructive uropathy from stones, strictures, tumors, tuberculosis, or schistosomiasis. Chronic urinary carriage is uncommon, except in areas of endemic schistosomiasis, where it may reach 5%.[1, 48, 90, 91]

A transient, asymptomatic carrier state that persists for less than 1 year is probably the most common outcome of ingesting salmonellae. In one review of 32 studies of nontyphoidal salmonellae excretion, patients younger than 5 years were found to have a median duration of excretion of 7 weeks, and 40% were culture-negative at 20 weeks. In older children and adults, the median duration of excretion was 3 to 4 weeks, and 90% were culture-negative at 9 weeks.[92] After *S. typhi* infection, organisms can be recovered from 50% of cases after 1 month, in 20% after 2 months, and in 10% after 3 months. Although children are more likely to have prolonged convalescent carriage, they usually do not develop the carrier state. Women are three times as likely as men to develop the carrier state after infection with *S. typhi*.[1, 48] In addition to stool cultures, a simple passive hemagglutination test based on highly purified Vi antigen can be used to identify chronic *S. typhi* carriers.[74]

Infection in Special Clinical Settings

Salmonella *and Human Immunodeficiency Virus Infections*

Since the first reports of *Salmonella* infections in AIDS patients in 1983, it has become clear that patients with HIV infection are more susceptible than the normal host to infection with *Salmonella*. These patients are more prone to bacteremic events, prolonged infections, complications, and relapses after adequate antimicrobial therapy. The incidence of *Salmonella* bacteremia in AIDS patients has been calculated to be 20 to 100 times that of the general population.[44, 93] This group of patients is also at risk for recurrent *Salmonella* bacteremia, which is now a criterion for the CDC classification of AIDS.

Often *Salmonella* infections in patients with HIV disease may occur before other manifestations of HIV infection. *Salmonella* bacteremia in a patient at risk for HIV infection should suggest the diagnosis of AIDS. The serotypes most commonly isolated from the blood stream of AIDS patients are *S. typhimurium* and *S. enteritidis*. Characteristic gastrointestinal symptoms are often absent. Complications such as meningitis, pulmonary abscess, subcutaneous abscess, peritonitis, brain abscesses, and septic arthritis have been reported. Aside from defects in cell-mediated immunity, factors such as frequent prior use of antibiotics and hematologic abnormalities may contribute to the increased susceptibility seen in these patients.[93–95]

Treatment of *Salmonella* infections in HIV-infected patients poses a particular problem because the rate of relapse is high. Although there is no consensus on the duration of therapy for *Salmonella* infection in these patients, appropriate intravenous therapy followed by 1 to several months of suppressive therapy seems reasonable.[40–43] Some authors have reported success with 1 to 8 months of ciprofloxacin therapy.[96] In addition, some preliminary data suggest that zidovudine alone may prevent relapses of *Salmonella* infection.[97] Relapse is not uncommon despite prolonged suppressive therapy, and some patients may require lifelong suppression.

Salmonella *and Malignancy*

Bacteremia occurs in 35% to 49% of *Salmonella* infections in patients with neoplastic disease. Focal infections are seen frequently, particularly pleuropulmonary disease. Patients with lymphoproliferative disease are at particular risk for disseminated salmonellosis. Predisposing factors in this group of patients includes antineoplastic therapy, chemotherapy, antacid use, corticosteroids, granulocytopenia, and surgery. Despite appropriate and prolonged therapy, the rates of mortality and relapse are relatively high.[98, 99]

Salmonella *and Renal Transplant Recipients*

Like other patients with immunosuppression, renal transplant recipients have extremely high rates of bacteremia (60%) and extraintestinal complications (35%) when infected with *Salmonella*. Unusual sites of focal infections reported include the maxillary sinus, axillary vein thrombosis, hemodialysis fistula, and testes. Asymptomatic bacteriuria is frequently present and may be prolonged (longer than 3 months). Many renal transplant patients present with a gastroenteritis prodrome followed by bacteremia and metastatic infection. Antimicrobial therapy of febrile gastroenteritis syndromes in this group of patients is warranted, with such therapy directed against nontyphoidal *Salmonella* and *Listeria*.[100, 101]

Salmonella *and Inflammatory Bowel Disease*

The relationship between *Salmonella* infection and idiopathic inflammatory bowel disease, particularly ulcerative colitis, is complex and, at present, incompletely understood. At least three different clinical scenarios have been noted. (1) Acute *Salmonella* gastroenteritis can mimic acute idiopathic disease, clinically, radiographically, endoscopically, and pathologically, but the process resolves completely with recovery from the infection. (2) Patients with a history of inflammatory bowel disease who acquire *Salmonella* infection have a much more severe clinical syndrome than the usual gastroenteritis, involving a high rate of bowel invasion with bacteremia, toxic megacolon, systemic toxicity, and even death. (3) Uncommonly, a patient with no previous history of inflammatory bowel disease who presents with *Salmonella* gastroenteritis develops chronic inflammatory bowel disease, suggesting that the infection triggered this disease diathesis.[48]

Salmonella *and Schistosomiasis*

Patients with schistosomiasis are at risk for the development of a chronic, systemic *Salmonella* syndrome. The bacteria infect the schistosomes and appear to be sequestered therein, protected from the effects of antimicrobial therapy. The clinical syndrome that ensues is characterized by chronic *Salmonella* bacteremia that can persist for years, marked hypertrophy of the reticuloendothelial system (most profoundly demonstrated by massive hepatosplenomegaly), wasting, and hyperglobulinemia. The clinical presentation may mimic kala-azar or lymphoma. Eradication of this condition requires effective treatment of both the schistosomiasis and the salmonellosis.[102–104]

Clinical Management

Although each of the clinical syndromes caused by *Salmonella* requires a different series of management decisions (Table 73–8), three general principles underlie antimicrobial management of all forms of salmonellosis: (1) *Salmonella* exhibits a high rate of plasmid-mediated resistance, particularly to such traditionally used drugs as ampicillin. (2) There is incomplete correlation between results of antimicrobial susceptibility testing in vitro and the possible clinical efficacy of a particular antibiotic. (3) Although in vitro resistance does correlate with clinical failure, in vitro sensitivity does not necessarily correlate with clinical benefit. At present, effective anti-*Salmonella* drugs (if in vitro testing reveals sensitivity) include the traditional drugs chloramphenicol, ampicillin, amoxicillin, and trimethroprim-sulfamethoxazole as well as third-generation cephalosporins, such as ceftriaxone and cefoperazone, and the fluoroquinolones.[48]

Gastroenteritis

The primary approach to *Salmonella* gastroenteritis includes fluid and electrolyte replacement, control of nausea and vomiting, and, under certain circumstances, antibiotic prophylaxis. The use of agents that alter bowel motility is discouraged, as such therapy can increase the incidence and the extent of bacteremia. Antibiotic treatment of gastroenteritis per se does not alter the course of this infection in normal hosts. In addition, antibiotic therapy has been associated with an increased duration and frequency of the intestinal carrier state. Although the quinolones have a favorable pharmacokinetic profile against *Salmonella*, ciprofloxacin was shown in one randomized, placebo-controlled, double-blind trial to have a high bacteriologic relapse rate in patients with salmonellosis and to be associated with prolonged fecal carriage.[105] At present, therapy with antibiotics for patients with *Salmonella* gastroenteritis should be viewed principally as a prophylactic effort aimed at persons for whom even transient bacteremia could have catastrophic consequences. When they do or might have *Salmonella* gastroenteritis, the following groups of patients should be considered for such prophylaxis: (1) newborn infants because of the high risk of meningitis; (2) patients older than 50 years because of the high risk of infecting atherosclerotic plaques or an aneurysm; (3) those who have lymphoproliferative disorders; (4) those who have suspected or known anatomic cardiovascular disease; (5) those who have significant bone or joint disease, including the presence of prostheses or other foreign bodies; (6) those with sickle cell disease or other forms of chronic hemolysis; (7) those with transplants; and (8) those with HIV infection.[48]

TABLE 73–8 ■ Management of *Salmonella* Infections

CLINICAL SYNDROME	TREATMENT	ANTIBIOTICS OF CHOICE
Gastroenteritis		
Normal host	No antibiotics	
Newborn infants Persons older than 50 y Lymphoproliferative disease Anatomic cardiovascular disease Bone or joint disease, especially in patients with prostheses Sickle cell disease or other chronic hemolysis Transplant recipients HIV infection	Antibiotic prophylaxis until patient is afebrile for 24 h	Ciprofloxacin by mouth (PO), trimethoprim-sulfamethoxazole PO, amoxicillin PO, cefriaxone intravenously (IV), cefoperazone IV, ciprofloxacin IV, trimethoprim-sulfamethoxazole IV, ampicillin IV
Enteric fever	Antibiotic therapy for 10–14 d	Ciprofloxacin PO/IV, ceftriaxone IV, cefoperazone IV, chloramphenicol PO/IV, ampicillin IV, trimethroprim-sulfamethoxazole IV
Bacteremia		
Without metastatic infection	Antibiotic therapy for 7–14 d	Chloramphenicol IV, ampicillin IV, trimethoprim-sulfamethoxazole IV/PO, ciprofloxacin IV/PO, cefriaxone IV, cefoperazone IV
With extraintestinal nonvascular metastatic infection	Antibiotic therapy for 2–4 wk and drainage of focal infection, where appropriate	
Vascular metastatic infection	Antibiotic therapy for 4–6 wk and excision of infected sites where possible	
Chronic carrier state		
Normal biliary tract	Antibiotic therapy for 4–6 wk	Ampicillin PO, amoxicillin PO, trimethoprim-sulfamethoxazole PO, ciprofloxacin PO
Biliary tract disease	Parenteral antibiotics for 10–14 d and cholecystectomy	Chloramphenicol IV, ampicillin IV, trimethoprim-sulfamethoxazole IV/PO, ciprofloxacin IV/PO, ceftriaxone IV, cefoperazone

The best antimicrobial regimen for bacteremia prophylaxis is not known. When oral therapy is feasible, our own preference is ciprofloxacin, 500 mg two times per day; trimethroprim-sulfamethoxazole, two double-strength tablets two times per day; or amoxicillin, 500 mg three times per day. If parenteral therapy is necessary, intravenous ceftriaxone, ciprofloxacin, trimethoprim-sulfamethoxazole, or ampicillin in full doses is prescribed. Therapy is continued until the patient has been afebrile for more than 24 hours.

Enteric Fever

Unlike the situation with *Salmonella* gastroenteritis, antimicrobial therapy is clearly efficacious in the treatment of enteric fever. Chloramphenicol was first used to treat *S. typhi* infections in 1948. It became the drug of choice because there was a uniform response pattern: the temperature returned to normal in 3.5 to 5 days, and patients felt better within 24 to 48 hours and recovered completely in 10 to 14 days. Mortality rates were reduced from 15% to 20% to 1.0% to 1.5%. Chloramphenicol, ampicillin, and trimethoprim-sulfamethoxazole have been the mainstays of therapy. The emergence of chloramphenicol-resistant strains and fear of the infrequent but severe bone marrow toxicity of chloramphenicol have curtailed use of this drug in some countries. However, because of its low cost and excellent oral bioavailabity, chloramphenicol is still widely used in developing countries.[106, 107]

The fluoroquinolones (e.g., ciprofloxacin, 500 mg two times per day for 10 to 14 days) have been shown to be effective in the treatment of enteric fever. They have emerged as the drugs of choice in the treatment of enteric fever for several reasons. Multidrug-resistant organisms have been reported in areas such as Latin America, the Indian subcontinent, and the Middle East. Currently, the incidence of antimicrobial resistance against the fluoroquinolones is lower than that seen against the traditional agents used against typhoid fever. The fluoroquinolones achieve high concentrations in bile, bowel, and urinary tract. In addition, they reach high concentrations within macrophages, where they exhibit a bactericidal effect.[108–111]

The third-generation cephalosporins cefotaxime, ceftriaxone, and cefoperazone are effective against *S. typhi*, with overall cure rates of approximately 90% and relapse rates of approximately 5%. Second-generation cephalosporins, despite in vitro susceptibility, have an unacceptably low cure rate and are not recommended. Similarly, aminoglycoside antibiotics are effective in vitro but do not effect clinical cure. Aztreonam is not recommended for similar reasons.[112, 113]

High-dose dexamethasone therapy in conjunction with chloramphenicol therapy was shown to reduce the case-fatality rate of severe enteric fever from 55.6% to 10% in one study involving 38 patients. Patients included in the study had severe disease with either abnormal state of consciousness (delirium, obtundation, stupor, or coma) or shock. There was no significant difference in the incidence of complications among the survivors in either group. The use of high-dose glucocorticoid therapy seems justified in the small subset of patients with severe enteric fever.[114]

Bacteremia with or Without Metastatic Infection

Bacteremic *Salmonella* infection merits antimicrobial therapy once sufficient blood cultures have been drawn to delineate the level of bacteremia. When sustained bacteremia is present, an effort should be made to rule out a cardiovascular site of infection. Transient bacteremia with extraintestinal nonvascular infection requires 2 to 4 weeks of antibiotic therapy and, when appropriate, surgical drainage of the focal infection. Transient bacteremia without metastatic infection should be treated for 7 to 14 days, preferably with a bactericidal drug. If relapse occurs, an aggressive search for a metastatic focus, particularly of the cardiovascular system, should be undertaken, and a 4- to 6-week course of treatment initiated, coupled with surgical intervention.[1, 48]

Chronic Carrier State

Success of antimicrobial therapy of the chronic carrier state depends on whether anatomic abnormalities of the biliary tract are present. In the absence of biliary tract disease, a 4- to 6-week course of ampicillin or amoxicillin at doses of 2 to 4 g/d or trimethoprim-sulfamethoxazole at doses of one to two double-strength tablets two times per day is effective in more than 80% of cases. For chronic carriers with gallbladder disease, the rate of failure with ampicillin is approximately 75%. In some small studies, ciprofloxacin in doses of 500 to 750 mg two times per day for 4 weeks has been shown to be successful in eradicating the carrier state.[48, 115–117]

When biliary tract disease is present, medical therapy fails in the majority of cases. Cholecystectomy without concomitant antibacterial therapy results in a 70% to 80% cure rate, but with significant morbidity and mortality, secondary to dissemination of the salmonellae at the time of surgery. The best results are obtained with the combination of cholecystectomy and a 10- to 14-day course of parenteral antibiotics initiated before surgery. The level of serum antibodies to the Vi antigen serves as a useful marker of the success of the treatment of chronic carriers because carriers will usually revert to being seronegative after successful treatment.[7, 48]

Prevention

Recommendations for typhoid vaccination are discussed in Chapter 205.

References

1. Rubin RH, Weinstein L: Salmonellosis: Microbiologic, Pathologic, and Clinical Features. New York, Stratton International, 1977.
2. Holt JG, Kreig NR, Sneath PHA, et al (eds): Bergey's Manual of Determinative Bacteriology, ed 9. Baltimore, Williams & Wilkins, 1994.
3. Foster WD: A History of Medical Bacteriology and Immunology. London, Cox and Wyman, 1970.
4. Burrows W. Textbook of Microbiology. Philadelphia, WB Saunders, 1985.
5. Ryan CA, Hargrett-Bean NT, Blake PA: *Salmonella typhi* infections in the United States, 1975–1984: Increasing role of foreign travel. Rev Infect Dis 11:1, 1989.
6. Centers for Disease Control and Prevention: Summary of notifiable diseases, United States, 1993. MMWR Morbid Mortal Wkly Rep 42:50, 1994.
7. Mathieu JJ, Henning KJ, Bell E, Frieden TR: Typhoid fever in New York City, 1980 through 1990. Arch Intern Med 154:1713, 1994.
8. Dritz SK, Braff EH: Sexually transmitted typhoid fever. N Engl J Med 296:1359, 1977.
9. Gotuzzo E, Frisancho O, Sanchez J, et al: Association between the acquired immunodeficiency syndrome and infection with *Salmonella typhi* or *Salmonella paratyphi* in an endemic typhoid area. Arch Intern Med 151:381, 1991.
10. Chalker RB, Blaser MJ: A review of human salmonellosis: III. Magnitude of *Salmonella* infection in the United States. Rev Infect Dis 10:111, 1988.
11. Hargrett-Bean NT, Pavia AT, Tauxe RV: *Salmonella* isolates from humans in the United States, 1984–1986. MMWR CDC Surveill Summ 2:25, 1988.
12. Hui YH, Gorham JR, Murrell KD, Cliver DO (eds): Foodborne Disease Handbook, Diseases Caused by Bacteria, Vol 1. New York, Marcel Dekker, 1994.
13. Centers for Disease Control and Prevention, Enteric Diseases Branch, Bacterial and Mycotic Diseases Divison. Atlanta, Centers for Disease Control and Prevention, 1995.
14. Gill ON, Sockett PN, Bartlett CL, et al: Outbreak of *Salmonella napoli* infection caused by contaminated chocolate bars. Lancet 1:547, 1983.
15. Centers for Disease Control and Prevention: Multistate outbreak of *Salmonella poona* infections—United States and Canada, 1991. MMWR Morbid Mortal Wkly Rep 40:549, 1991.
16. Babu K, Sonnenberg M, Kathpalia S, et al: Isolation of salmonellae from dried rattlesnake preparations. J Clin Microbiol 28:361, 1990.
17. Bensink JC, Ekaputra I, Taliotis C: The isolation of *Salmonella* from kangaroos and feral pigs processed for human consumption. Aust Vet J 68:106, 1991.
18. Taylor DN, Wachsmuth IK, Shangkuan Y, et al: Salmonellosis associated with marijuana. N Engl J Med 306:1249, 1982.
19. Cohen ML, Potter M, Pollard R, et al: Turtle-associated salmonellosis in the United States. JAMA 243:1247, 1980.
20. Centers for Disease Control and Prevention: Iguana-associated salmonellosis—Indiana. MMWR Morbid Mortal Wkly Rep 41:38, 1992.
21. Centers for Disease Control and Prevention: Lizard-associated salmonellosis—Utah. MMWR Morbid Mortal Wkly Rep 41: 610, 1992.
22. Centers for Disease Control and Prevention: *Salmonella* hadar associated with pet ducklings—Connecticut, Maryland, and Pennsylvania 1991. MMWR Morbid Mortal Wkly Rep 41:185, 1992.
23. Fonseca RJ, Dubey LM: *Salmonella montevideo* sepsis from a pet snake. Pediatr Infect Dis J 13:550, 1994.
24. Bean NH, Griffin PM, Goulding JS, Ivey CB: Foodborne disease outbreaks, 5-year summary, 1983–1987. MMWR CDC Surveill Summ 39:15, 1990.
25. Mishu B, Koehler J, Lee L, et al: Outbreaks of *Salmonella enteritidis* infections in the United States, 1985–1991. J Infect Dis 169:547, 1994.
26. Centers for Disease Control and Prevention: Update: *Salmonella enteritidis* infections and shell eggs—United States, 1990. MMWR Morbid Mortal Wkly Rep 39:909, 1990.
27. Cox NA, Bailey JS, Mauldin JM, et al: Extent of salmonellae contamination in breeder hatcheries. Poult Sci 70:416, 1991.
28. Clavero MR, Monk JD, Beuchat LR: Inactivation of *Escherichia coli* O157:H7, salmonellae, and *Campylobacter jejuni* in raw ground beef by gamma irradiation. Appl Environ Microbiol 60:2069, 1994.
29. Cooper GI, Venables LM, Woodbard MJ, et al: Vaccination of chickens with strain CVL30, a genetically defined *Salmonella enteritidis* aroA live oral vaccine candidate. Infect Immun 62:4747, 1994.
30. Centers for Disease Control and Prevention: Outbreak of *Salmonella enteritidis* associated with nationally distributed ice cream products—Minnesota, South Dakota, and Wisconsin, 1994. MMWR Morbid Mortal Wkly Rep 43:740, 1994.
31. Ryan CA, Nickels MK, Hargrett-Bean NT, et al: Massive outbreak of antimicrobial resistant salmonellosis traced to pasteurized milk. JAMA 258:3269, 1987.
32. Clark GM, Kaufmann AF, Gangarosa EJ, Thompson MA: Epidemiology of an international outbreak of *Salmonella agona*. Lancet 2:490, 1973.
33. Gangarosa EJ, Barker WH, Barne WB, et al: Man vs. animal feeds as the source of human salmonellosis. Lancet 1:878, 1973.
34. Holmberg SD, Osterholm MT, Senger KA, et al: Drug-resistant *Salmonella* from animals fed antimicrobials. N Engl J Med 311:617, 1984.
35. Lee LA, Puhr ND, Maloney EK, et al: Increase in antimicrobial-resistant *Salmonella* infections in the United States, 1989–1990. J Infect Dis 170:128, 1994.
36. Levine WC, Smart JF, Archer DL, et al: Foodborne disease outbreaks in nursing homes, 1975 through 1987. JAMA 266:2105, 1991.
37. Humphrey TJ, Greenwood M, Gilbert RJ, et al: The survival of salmonellas in shell eggs cooked under simulated domestic conditions. Epidemiol Infect 103:35, 1989.

38. Altekruse S, Hyman F, Klontz K, et al: Foodborne bacterial infectons in individuals with the human immunodeficiency virus. South Med J 87:170, 1994.
39. World Health Organization: Food safety measures for eggs and foods containing eggs. World Health Forum 14:437, 1993.
40. Nadelman RB, Mathur-Wagh U, Yancovitz, Mildvan D: *Salmonella* bacteremia associated with the acquired immunodeficiency syndrome (AIDS). Arch Intern Med 145:1968, 1985.
41. Smith PD, Macher AM, Bookman MA, et al: *Salmonella typhimurium* enteritis and bacteremia in the acquired immunodeficiency syndrome. Ann Intern Med 102:207, 1985.
42. Jacobs JL, Gold JW, Murray HW, et al: *Salmonella* infections in patients with the acquired immnunodeficiency syndrome. Ann Intern Med 102:186, 1985.
43. Glaser JB, Morton-Kute L, Berger SR: Recurrent *Salmonella typhimurium* bacteremia associated with the acquired immunodeficiency syndrome. Ann Intern Med 102:189, 1985.
44. Cecum CL, Chaissson RE, Rutherford GW, et al: Incidence of salmonellosis in patients with AIDS. J Infect Dis 156:998, 1987.
45. Levine WC, Buehler JW, Bean NH, Tauxe RV: Epidemiology of nontyphoidal *Salmonella* bacteremia during the human immunodeficiency virus epidemic. J Infect Dis 164:81, 1991.
46. Griffin PM, Tauxe RV: Food counseling for patients with AIDS (Letter). J Infect Dis 158:668, 1988.
47. O'Brien TF, Hopkins JD, Gilleece ES, et al: Molecular epidemiology of antibiotic resistance in *Salmonella* from animals and human beings in the United States. N Engl J Med 307:1, 1982.
48. Goldberg MB, Rubin RH: The spectrum of *Salmonella* infection. Infect Dis Clin North Am 2:571, 1988.
49. Gershman M: Single phage-typing set for differentiating salmonellae. J Clin Microbiol 5:302, 1977.
50. Wachsmuth IK, Kiehlbauch JA, Bopp DN, et al: The use of plasmid profiles and nucleic acid probes in epidemiologic investigations of foodborne, diarrheal diseases. Int J Food Microbiol 12:77, 1991.
51. Formal SB, Hale TL, Sansonetti PJ: Invasive enteric pathogens. Rev Infect Dis 5:702, 1983.
52. Finlay BB, Falkow S: Common themes in microbial pathogenicity. Microbiol Rev 53:210, 1989.
53. Blaser MJ, Newman LS: A review of human salmonellosis: I. Infective dose. Rev Infect Dis 4:1096, 1982.
54. Hook EW: Salmonellosis: Certain factors influencing the interaction of *Salmonella* and the human host. Bull N Y Acad Med 37:499, 1961.
55. Giannella RA, Broitman SA, Zamcheck N: *Salmonella* enteritis. I. Role of reduced gastric secretion in pathogenesis. Am J Dig Dis 16:1000, 1971.
56. Gorden J, Small PLC: Acid resistance in enteric bacteria. Infect Immun 61:364, 1993.
57. Telzak EE, Greenberg MS, Budnick LD: Diabetes mellitus—A new described risk factor for infecton from *Salmonella enteritidis*. J Infect Dis 164:538, 1991.
58. Pavia AT, Shipman LD, Wells JG: Epidemiologic evidence that prior antimicrobial exposure decreases resistance to infection by antimicrobial-sensitive *Salmonella*. J Infect Dis 161:255, 1990.
59. Miller CP, Bohnhoff M: Changes in the mouse's enteric microflora associated with enhanced susceptibility to *Salmonella* infection following streptomycin treatment. J Infect Dis 113:59, 1963.
60. Hornick RB, Greisman SE, Woodward TE, et al: Typhoid fever: Pathogenesis and immunologic control. N Engl J Med. 283:686, 1970.
61. Kaye D, Gill FA, Hook EW: Factors influencing host resistance to *Salmonella* infections: The effects of hemolysis and erythrophagocytosis. Am J Med Sci 254:205, 1967.
62. Gill FA, Kaye D, Hook EW: The influence of erythrophagocytosis on the interaction of macrophages and *salmonella* in vitro. J Exp Med 124:173, 1966.
63. Wheat LJ, Rubin RH, Harris NL, et al: Systemic salmonellosis in patients with disseminated histoplasmosis. Arch Intern Med 147:561, 1987.
64. Saphra I, Winter JW: Clinical manifestations of salmonellosis in man: An evaluation of 7779 human infections identified at the New York *Salmonella* Center. N Engl J Med 256:1128, 1957.
65. McCall CE, Martin WT, Boring JR: Efficiency of cultures of rectal swabs and faecal specimens in detecting *Salmonella* carriers: Correlation with numbers of salmonellae excreted. J Hyg (Lond) 64:261, 1966.
66. Chattopadhyay B, Pilfold JN: The effect of prolonged incubation of Selenite F broth on the rate of isolation of *Salmonella* from faeces. Med Lab Sci 33:191, 1976.
67. Hoffman TA, Ruiz CJ, Counts GW: Waterborne typhoid fever in Dade County, Florida: Clinical and therapeutic evaluation of 105 bacteremic patients. Am J Med 59:481, 1975.
68. Stuart BM, Pullen RL: Typhoid fever: Clinical analysis of 360 cases. Arch Intern Med 78:629, 1946.
69. Ferreccio C, Levine MM, Manterola A, et al: Benign bacteremia caused by *Salmonella typhi* and *paratyphi* in children younger than two years. J Pediatr 104:899, 1984.
70. Mahle WT, Levine MM: *Salmonella typhi* infection in children younger than five years of age. Pediatr Infect Dis 12:627, 1993.
71. Hornick RB, Greisman SE, Woodward TE: Typhoid fever: Pathogenesis and immunologic control. N Engl J Med 283:739, 1970.
72. Gilman RH, Terminel M, Levine MM, et al: Relative efficacy of blood, urine, rectal swab, bone marrow, and rose-spot cultures for recovery of *Salmonella typhi* in typhoid fever. Lancet 1:1211, 1975.
73. Hoffman SL, Punjabi NH, Rockhill RC: Duodenal string-capsule culture compard with bone-marrow, blood and rectal-swab cultures for diagnosing typhoid and paratyphoid fever. J Infect Dis 149:157, 1984.
74. Edelman R, Levine MM: Summary of an international workshop on typhoid fever. Rev Infect Dis 8:329, 1986.
75. Schroeder SA: Interpretation of serologic test for typhoid fever. JAMA 206:839, 1968.
76. Pang V, Puthucheary SD: Significance and value of the Widal test in the diagnosis of typhoid fever in an endemic area. J Clin Pathol 36:471, 1983.
77. Nardiello S, Pizzella T, Russo M, Bruno G: Serodiagnosis of typhoid fever by enzyme-linked immunosorbent assay determination of anti-*Salmonella typhi* lipopolysaccharide antibodies. J Clin Microbiol 20:718, 1984.
78. Shetty NP, Srinivasa H, Bhat P: Coagglutination and counter immunoelectrophoresis in the rapid diagnosis of typhoid fever. Am J Clin Pathol 84:80, 1985.
79. Cherubin CE, Neu HC, Imperatol PJ, et al: Septicemia with nontyphoid salmonella. Medicine (Baltimore) 53:365, 1974.
80. Black PH, Kunz LJ, Swartz MN: Salmonellosis—A review of some unusual aspects. N Engl J Med 262:864, 1960.
81. Saphra I, Wasserman M: *Salmonella choleraesuis:* A clinical and epidemiologic evaluation of 329 infections identified between 1940 and 1954 in the New York *Salmonella* Center. Am J Med Sci 228:525, 1954.
82. Cohen JI, Bartlett JA, Corey GR: Extra-intestinal manifestations of *Salmonella* infections. Medicine (Baltimore) 66:349, 1987.
83. Oskoui R, Davis WA, Gomes MN: *Salmonella aortitis:* A report of a successfully treated case with a comprehensive review of the literature. Arch Intern Med 153:517, 1993.
84. Cohen PS, O'Brien TF, Schoenbaum S, et al: The risk of endothelial infection in adults with *Salmonella* bacteremia. Ann Intern Med 89:931, 1978.
85. Maki-Ikola O, Yli-Kerttula U, Saario R, et al: *Salmonella* specific antibodies in serum and synovial fluid in patients with reactive arthritis. Br J Rheumatol 31:25, 1992.
86. Granfors K, Jalkanen S, Lindberg A: *Salmonella* lipopolysaccharide in synovial cells form patients with reactive arthritis. Lancet 335:685, 1990.
87. Rabinowitz SG, MacLeod NR: *Salmonella* meningitis. A report of three cases and a review of the literature. Am J Dis Child 123:259, 1972.
88. Rodriguez RE, Valero V, Watanakunakorn C: *Salmonella* focal intracranial infections: Review of the world literature (1884–1984) and report of an unusual case. Rev Infect Dis 8:31, 1986.
89. Aguado JM, Obeso G, Cabanillas JJ, et al: Pleuropulmonary infections due to nontyphoidal strains of *Salmonella*. Arch Intern Med 150:54, 1990.
90. Scott MB, Cosgrove MD: *Salmonella* infection and the genitourinary system. J Urol 118:64, 1977.
91. Melzer M, Altmann G, Rakowszcyk M, et al: *Salmonella* infections of the kidney. J Urol 94:23, 1965.
92. Buchwald DS, Blaser MJ: A review of human salmonellosis: II. Duration of excretion following infection with nontyphi *Salmonella*. Rev Infect Dis 6:345, 1984.

93. Sperber SJ, Schleupner CJ: Salmonellosis during infection with human immunodeficiency virus. Rev Infect Dis 9:925, 1987.
94. Satue JA, Aguado JM, Ramon Costa J, et al: Pulmonary abscess due to non-*typhi Salmonella* in a patient with AIDS (Letter). Clin Infect Dis 19:555, 1994.
95. Olive AT, Tena X: *Salmonella* septic arthritis in patients with human immunodeficiency virus. J Rheumatol 21:1172, 1994.
96. Jacobson MA, Hahn SM, Gerberding JL, et al: Ciprofloxacin for *Salmonella* bacteremia in the acquired immunodeficiency syndrome. Ann Intern Med 110:1027, 1989.
97. Salmon D, Detruchis P, Leport C: Efficacy of zidovudine in preventing relapses of *Salmonella* bacteremia in AIDS. J Infect Dis 163:415, 1991.
98. Wolfe MS, Louria DB, Armstrong D, Blevins A: Salmonellosis in patients with neoplastic disease. A review of 100 episodes at Memorial Cancer Center over a 13-year period. Arch Intern Med 128:546, 1971.
99. Noriega LM, Van der Auwera P, Daneau D, et al: *Salmonella* infections in cancer center. Support Care Cancer 2:116, 1994.
100. Samra Y, Shaked Y, Maier MK: Nontyphoid salmonellosis in renal transplant recipients: Report of five cases and review of the literature. Rev Infect Dis 8:431, 1986.
101. Rubin RH, Young LS: Clinical Approach to Infection in the Compromised Host, ed 3. New York, Plenum Publishing, 1994.
102. Neves J, Raso P, Marinko PP: Prolonged septicemic salmonellosis intercurrent with *Schistosoma mansoni* infection. J Trop Med Hyg 74:9, 1971.
103. Rocha H, Kirk JW, Hearey CD Jr: Prolonged *Salmonella* bacteremia in patients with *Shistosoma mansoni* infection. Arch Intern Med 128:254, 1971.
104. Young SW, Higashi G, Kamel R, et al: Interactions of salmonellae and schistosomes in host-parasite relations. Trans R Soc Trop Med Hyg 67:797, 1973.
105. Neill MA, Opal SM, Heelan J, et al: Failure of ciprofloxacin to eradicate convalescent fecal excretion after acute salmonellosis: Experience during an outbreak in health care workers. Ann Intern Med 114:195, 1991.
106. Vazquez V, Calderon E, Rodriquez R: Chloramphenicol-resistant strains of *Salmonella typhosa*. N Engl J Med 286:1220, 1972.
107. Gilman RH, Terminel M, Levine MM, et al: Comparison of trimethoprim-sulfamethoxazole and amoxicillin in therapy chloramphenicol-resistant and chloramphenicol-sensitive typhoid fever. J Infect Dis 132:630, 1975.
108. Asperilla MO, Smego RA Jr, Scott LK: Quinolone antibiotics in the treatment of *Salmonella* infections. Rev Infect Dis 12:873, 1990.
109. Lewin CS: Treatment of multiresistant *Salmonella* infection. Lancet 337:47, 1991.
110. Reid TMS: The treatment of non-typhic salmonellosis. J Antimicrob Chemother 29:4, 1992.
111. Blaser MJ, Smith PD, Ravdin JI, et al (eds): Infections of the Gastrointestinal Tract. New York, Raven Press, 1995.
112. Soe GB, Overturf GD: Treatment of typhoid fever and other systemic salmonelloses with cefotaxime, ceftriaxone, cefoperazone, and other newer cephalosporins. Rev Infect Dis 9:719, 1987.
113. Choo KE, Ariffin WA, Ong KH, et al: Aztreonam failure in typhoid fever. Lancet 337:498, 1991.
114. Hoffman SL, Punjabi NH, Kumala S, et al: Reduction of mortality in chloramphenicol-treated severe typhoid fever by high-dose dexamethasone. N Engl J Med 310:82, 1984.
115. Dinbar A, Altman G, Tulcinsky DB: The treatment of chronic biliary *Salmonella* carriers. Am J Med 47:236, 1969.
116. Diridl G, Pichler H, Wolf D: Treatment of chronic *Salmonella* carriers with ciprofloxacin. Eur J Clin Microbiol 5:260, 1986.
117. Cherubin CE, Kowalski J: Nontyphoidal *Salmonella* carrier state treated with norfloxacin. Ann Intern Med 85:100, 1990.
118. Walker W: The Aberdeen typhoid outbreak of 1964. Scot Med J 10:466, 1965.

74

Escherichia coli Infections

R. Bradley Sack

History

Escherichia coli species are well known as the most common facultative bacterial species in the large bowel flora. Although their concentrations are approximately 100 times smaller than those of the anaerobes that occupy this same ecologic niche, *E. coli* strains are the most common organisms that the diagnostic laboratory encounters on routine enteric isolation plates. Until approximately the last 25 years, they were considered (outside of an epidemic situation in a hospital nursery) normal flora, and their importance lay in their being differentiated from known enteric pathogens such as *Salmonella* and *Shigella*.

In the mid-1960s, veterinary workers[1] first described certain strains of *E. coli* in young animals that produced enterotoxins; in the late 1960s,[2] similar strains were found in India in humans who had a disease resembling cholera. Epidemiologic and clinical studies then went on to show that these were indeed important diarrheal pathogens worldwide—and probably the most common bacterial diarrheal pathogens of all! Other subtypes of *E. coli* have since been described, and the older nursery outbreak strains (so-called enteropathogenic serotypes) have been characterized more fully.[3] We can now differentiate at least six different categories of *E. coli* that are known to be or suspected of being diarrheogenic: enterotoxigenic, enteropathogenic, enteroinvasive, enterohemorrhagic, enteroaggregative, and diffusely adherent. It is also likely that additional diarrheogenic strains of *E. coli* have yet to be differentiated. In this chapter, I discuss the known pathogenic categories of diarrheogenic *E. coli*.

Characteristics of the Pathogen

All of the diarrheogenic *E. coli* share the basic properties of the species. They all have cell walls that contain lipopolysaccharides, and they can be serogrouped according to their O antigens. Most have flagella, although many strains are nonmotile. Approximately 173 O antigens and 56 flagellar antigens have been differentiated in *E. coli*, a diversity of antigens that has proved useful in the broad characterization of the species. They can also be differentiated by their outer membrane proteins, phage types, plasmid profiles, structural pili, secretory products, and genetic elements.

Enterotoxigenic E. coli

Enterotoxigenic *E. coli* strains (ETEC) are defined primarily by one or both of the enterotoxins they produce. One is commonly called LT, for heat-labile enterotoxin, and the other ST, for heat-stable enterotoxin. Both enterotoxins have been completely purified and their amino acid compositions defined; in addition, LT has been partially synthesized and ST completely synthesized. The genes controlling the production of these enterotoxins, which reside on transferable plasmids, have also been completely cloned and sequenced. The bio-

TABLE 74–1 ■ Properties of *Escherichia coli* Enterotoxins*

TOXIN	PRODUCED BY	MOLECULAR WEIGHT	SUBUNIT STRUCTURE	GENETIC CONTROL	MECHANISM OF ACTION
LT	ETEC	86,000	1α + 5β	Plasmid	Adenylate cyclase activation
ST	ETEC	~2,000	Single peptide, 18–19 amino acids	Plasmid	Guanylate cyclase activation
SLT-1	EHEC	70,000	1α + 5β	Bacteriophage	Inhibits protein synthesis, binds to 60S ribosome
SLT-2†	EHEC	68,000	1α + 5β	Bacteriophage	Inhibits protein synthesis, binds to 60S ribosome
EAST1	EAggEC	4,100	Single peptide	Plasmid	Guanylate cyclase activation

*All have been purified; genes have been cloned and sequenced. LT, Heat-labile enterotoxin; ST, heat-stable enterotoxin; SLT, Shiga-like toxin; ETEC, enterotoxigenic *E. coli;* EHEC, enterohemorrhagic *E. coli;* EAggEC, enteroaggregative *E. coli.*
†Presumed ratio of A and B subunits.

chemical and antigenic properties of the two enterotoxins are summarized in Table 74–1.

ETEC are also characterized by the structural pili they produce. Whereas almost all *E. coli* strains produce common type 1 mannose-sensitive pili, only ETEC produce specific types of mannose-resistant pili; these are important in facilitating colonization of the mucosal surfaces of the small bowel (Fig. 74–1). Not all ETEC have been shown to produce these pili, however, and there may be other nonstructural colonization factors, such as lectins and hemagglutinins, that are also important in these strains. All ETEC must possess some mechanism for initiating and maintaining colonization of the small intestine, because noncolonizing strains are not diarrheogenic. The genes controlling pili production are also located on plasmids, which may be the same ones that carry the genes for enterotoxin production. To date, at least nine known colonization factors have been described, and within some of these groups are several antigenic subtypes.[4]

Many strains of ETEC can also be differentiated by their characteristic serotypes. Of the large possible numbers of serotypes available into which the plasmids for enterotoxin and pilus production could be inserted, there seem to be only a limited number that can stably carry these plasmids and thus remain virulent. The flagellar antigens do not appear to be specific virulence antigens, although they are important in the recognition of ETEC strains. There seems to be a geographic distribution of some of these stable ETEC serotypes. Those found commonly in Kenya, for instance, are different from those found in Peru, but other ETEC serotypes are distributed worldwide, such as O6:H16. Because production of enterotoxin and pili is also highly correlated with serotype, geographic differences in enterotoxin production are also found. For example, strain O78:H11 invariably produces LT, ST, and colonization factor I and is found primarily in Southeast Asia. Table 74–2 lists the common ETEC serotypes.

ETEC may be further differentiated by common biotype patterns. A series of biochemical tests has been devised that differentiates ETEC into identifiable biotypes.[5] No single biochemical test, however, accurately predicts whether an *E. coli* strain is enterotoxigenic, so no simple surrogate markers for ETEC are available. Identification must come from the recognition of the enterotoxin produced or the appropriate enterotoxin genes carried by the organism (see later).

Enteropathogenic E. coli

Enteropathogenic serotypes of *E. coli* (EPEC) have traditionally been identified by their specific O and H antigens (see Table 74–2). Such identification was developed in the 1940s as a way of recognizing epidemic *E. coli* strains during nursery outbreaks.[6] This antedated any knowledge of the mechanism whereby these strains were causing diarrhea. Only relatively recently have other virulence properties been recognized that make these strains easier to identify. An adhesion assay has been developed in tissue culture cells, which is useful in

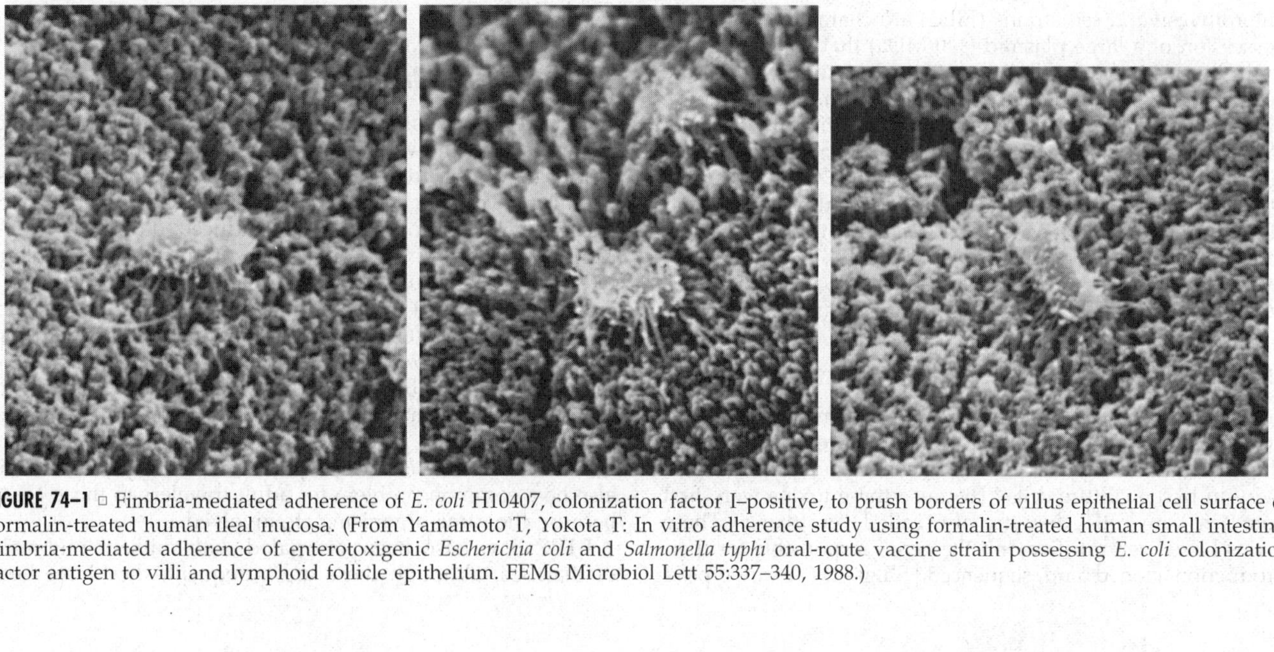

FIGURE 74–1 □ Fimbria-mediated adherence of *E. coli* H10407, colonization factor I–positive, to brush borders of villus epithelial cell surface of formalin-treated human ileal mucosa. (From Yamamoto T, Yokota T: In vitro adherence study using formalin-treated human small intestine: Fimbria-mediated adherence of enterotoxigenic *Escherichia coli* and *Salmonella typhi* oral-route vaccine strain possessing *E. coli* colonization factor antigen to villi and lymphoid follicle epithelium. FEMS Microbiol Lett 55:337–340, 1988.)

TABLE 74–2 ■ Most Commonly Recognized Serogroups (Serotypes) of Diarrheogenic *Escherichia coli**

ETEC†	EPEC‡	EIEC‡	EHEC
O6:H16	O26:H–,11	O28ac	O157:H7
O8:H9	O55:H–,6,7	O29	O26:H11
O15:H11	O86:H–,2,34	O112	O111:H–,8
O25:H42	O111:H–,2,12,21	O124	O113:H21
O27:H7,20	O114:H12	O136	O121:H19
O63:H12,30	O119:H6	O143	O145:H–
O78:H11,12	O125ac:H21	O144	
O128:H7	O126:H27	O152	
O149:H10	O127:H–,6,9,21	O164	
O159:H4,34	O128ab:H2		
	O142:H6		
	O158:H23		

*ETEC, Enterotoxigenic *E. coli;* EPEC, enteropathogenic *E. coli;* EIEC, enteroinvasive *E. coli;* EHEC, enterohemorrhagic *E coli.*
†More than 100 serotypes have been identified as ETEC.
‡List may vary, according to different laboratories.

identifying EPEC. These particular strains adhere in a focal manner[7] to HEp-2 cells in a way that can easily be recognized under the microscope (Fig. 74–2). This assay seems to be a marker for a virulence property in vivo that allows EPEC strains to adhere to and efface the brush border of the small intestinal mucosal cells, but without damaging the cells further (Fig. 74–3). These EPEC strains are not known to produce any recognized enterotoxins. Large concentrations of actin can be demonstrated immediately beneath the areas of bacterial attachment, indicating disruption of the endothelial cytoskeleton, and studies have indicated that some invasion of tissue culture cells occurs.

Although it is not known how EPEC actually produce diarrhea, they share many common properties that appear to be important virulence factors.[8] These include a large EPEC adherence factor (EAF) plasmid that carries genetic material controlling the localized adherence phenomenon, genes *(bfp)* for bundle-forming pili that are thought to mediate attachment to intestinal epithelial cells, and chromosomal genes *eae* that are responsible for the attaching and effacing lesion in intestinal mucosa. These genes are readily identified by DNA probes and can be used for diagnostic purposes.

Enteroinvasive E. coli

Enteroinvasive *E. coli* strains (EIEC) are characterized by the possession of a large plasmid (140 MDa) that contains genes controlling the production of invasion proteins, which are necessary for the virulence of the organism. The virulence properties of EIEC are thought to be identical to those of *Shigella* organisms, and indeed these organisms are more closely related taxonomically to *Shigella* than to other *E. coli.* Often they share the properties of not fermenting lactose and of agglutinating in antisera directed against the lipopolysaccharide of *Shigella.*

EIEC also possess a relatively small array of O antigens, which can be used to identify the organisms (see Table 74–2).

Enterohemorrhagic E. coli

Enterohemorrhagic *E. coli* strains (EHEC) are characterized by their ability to produce large amounts of one or more Shiga-like toxins, which are identified by their cytotoxic activity in tissue culture cells.[9] (Because these toxins were first noted in Vero cells, they are also called verotoxins.) These toxins have been purified and the genes responsible for their production cloned and sequenced. Shiga-like toxin type 1 is almost identical to the Shiga toxin produced by *Shigella dysenteriae* type 1 (there is a single amino acid difference) and is immunologically identical to Shiga toxin. A second toxin, called Shiga-like toxin type 2, has similar biologic activity but is immunologically and structurally distinct. Variants of Shiga-like toxin type 2 have also been described, which differ in their physiologic and immunologic characteristics. Table 74–1 also summarizes the known Shiga-like toxins and their properties.

The genes for the production of these toxins are located not on plasmids but on bacteriophages that have infected the bacterial cells. EHEC belong to only a relatively few serotypes. The classic serotype is O157:H7, which has been responsible for almost all outbreaks in the United States; other serotypes have been identified as causing outbreaks in Canada and Europe (see Table 74–2).

Enteroaggregative E. coli

Enteroaggregative *E. coli* strains (EAggEC) are identified by their typical aggregative, building block adherence to HEp-2 tissue culture cells[10] (see Fig. 74–2). Many strains possess a large plasmid that carries genes mediating this type of adherence as well as the production of a small heat-stable enterotoxin (EAST1) that is similar to STa produced by ETEC.[11] Most strains also produce bundle-forming pili, which are thought to mediate adherence. There seems to be some degree of heterogeneity within EAggEC as evidenced by differences in virulence.

Diffusely Adherent E. coli

Diffusely adherent *E. coli* strains (DAEC) are also identified by their adherence pattern to HEp-2 cells; bacteria are dispersed singly over the epithelial cells without clumps (see Fig. 74–2). Both chromosomal and plasmid genes have been identified that control this type of adherence, through fimbria and nonfimbrial adhesion.

Epidemiology

All of the diarrheogenic *E. coli* strains are transmitted by the fecal-oral route, in the manner of all other bacterial enteric pathogens. They do have distinctly different epidemiologic patterns of disease, each of which is discussed separately (Table 74–3).

Enterotoxigenic Strains

ETEC are the most commonly isolated bacterial cause of acute diarrhea the world over.[12] Throughout the developing world, they most frequently produce acute diarrheal disease in children younger than 2 years. Each child probably experiences several episodes of ETEC-induced diarrheal disease during this period. ETEC may also produce severe cholera-like diarrhea in adults living in areas where the organism is common, such as in India and Bangladesh. ETEC are perhaps best known to Western physicians, because they are responsible for approximately 40% to 70% of episodes of traveler's diarrhea. It is possible to generally predict the seriousness of the problem of traveler's diarrhea from the frequency of diarrheal episodes in children who live in the area to be visited. If diarrhea is a major problem in the children, it will also be a common problem for adult travelers to those areas, because the same organisms are involved.

ETEC have also been associated with nursery outbreaks of diarrhea, although these are infrequent; they have been

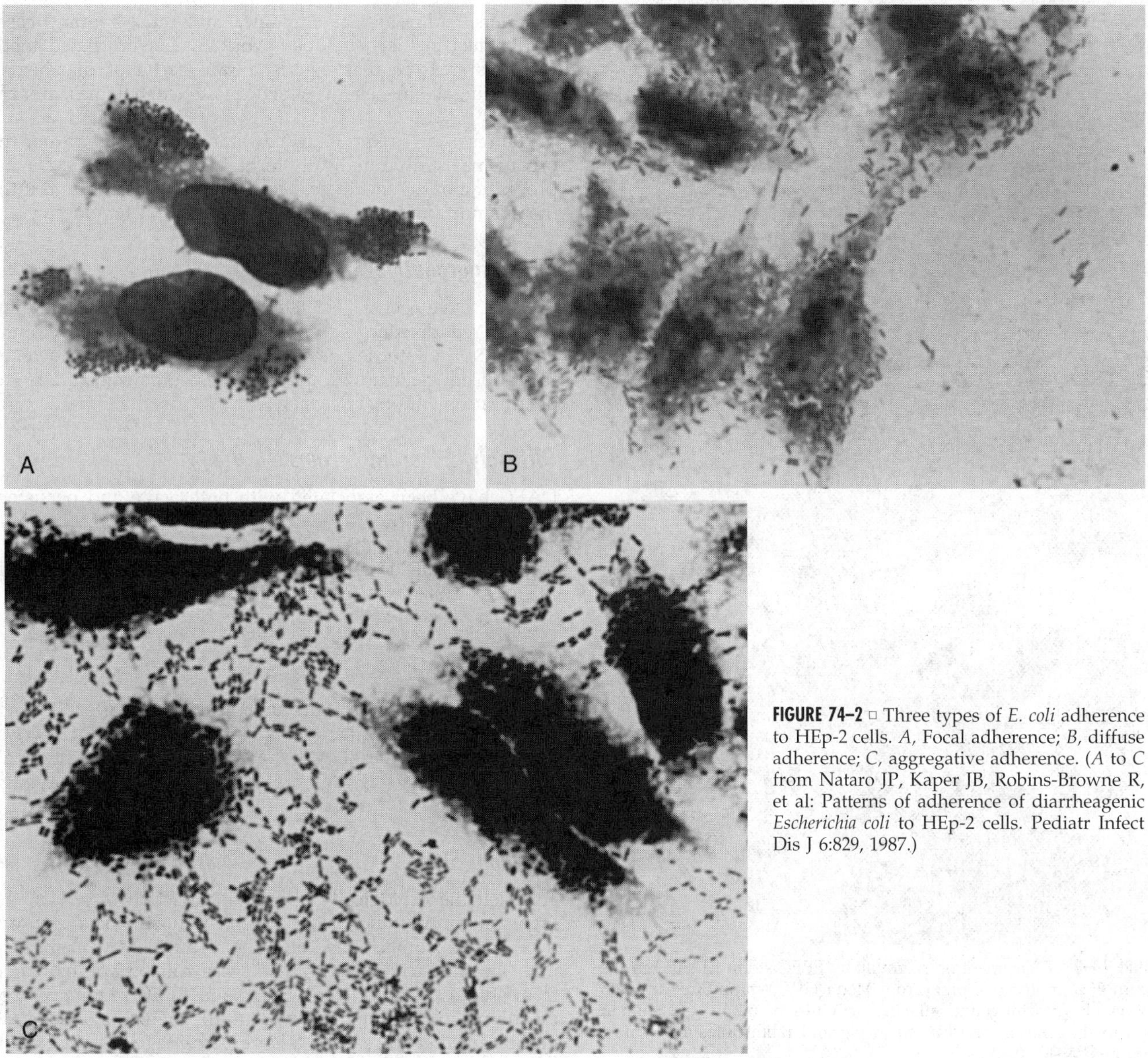

FIGURE 74–2 □ Three types of *E. coli* adherence to HEp-2 cells. *A,* Focal adherence; *B,* diffuse adherence; *C,* aggregative adherence. (*A* to *C* from Nataro JP, Kaper JB, Robins-Browne R, et al: Patterns of adherence of diarrheagenic *Escherichia coli* to HEp-2 cells. Pediatr Infect Dis J 6:829, 1987.)

associated with common-source outbreaks of diarrheal disease secondary to sewage contamination of water supplies.[13]

The common vehicle of transmission is usually fecally contaminated food. This is particularly a problem in the warm areas of the world where refrigeration of food is less than optimal.

There are no known nonhuman hosts for human ETEC. There are animal strains of ETEC that are important causes of diarrhea in animals such as piglets and calves, but these strains do not naturally cause diarrhea in humans. Likewise, human ETEC strains do not cause diarrhea in animals under natural conditions, although animal models can be infected experimentally. Presumably their virulence factors, particularly their colonization factors, are species specific.

Humans may carry the organisms asymptomatically, and such persons are probably the most important reservoir. ETEC are presumably carried in the large bowel rather than in the small bowel and so cause no illness in this location.

Enteropathogenic Strains

EPEC have been known historically by their ability to produce highly virulent disease in young children, particularly in hospital nursery settings. These outbreaks have now all but disappeared in the developed world, but they may still occur in hospitals in developing countries, where sanitation may be less than ideal. EPEC also cause sporadic illness in young children throughout the developing world, but usually less frequently than ETEC. They have also been implicated as a cause of persistent diarrhea in young children.[14] It is not known exactly why older children or adults do not seem to develop illness from these organisms; adult volunteers infected experimentally do develop acute diarrheal illness.[15]

Enteroinvasive Strains

EIEC have been associated principally with diarrhea outbreaks secondary to contaminated food items, such as soft cheeses.[16] Although they have been described as agents in sporadic disease in children and in travelers, illnesses that they cause seem to be generally infrequent.

Enterohemorrhagic Strains

EHEC are the most important of the diarrheogenic *E. coli* in the United States and the rest of the developed world. They

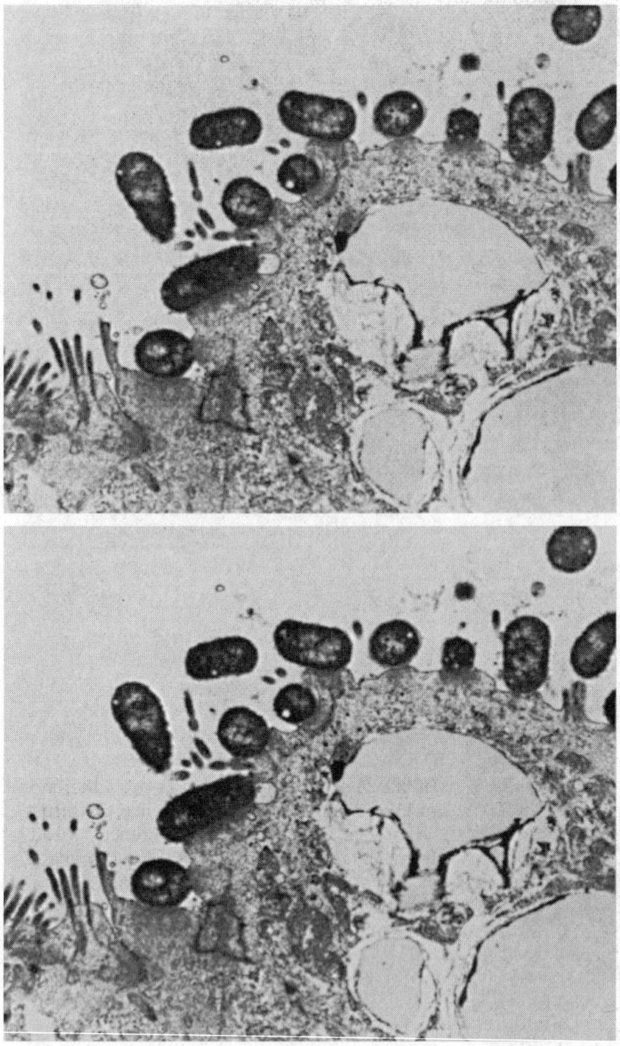

FIGURE 74–3 ▫ Effacement of microvilli by EPEC strain E128012 in the cecum of a gnotobiotic pig. (From Moon HW, Whipp SC, Argenzio RA, et al: Attaching and effacing activities of rabbit and human enteropathogenic *Escherichia coli* in pig and rabbit intestines. Infect Immun 41:1340, 1983.)

are transmitted primarily through processed foods and are thus important organisms because they signify economic "development." This organism was first described as a cause of diarrhea (hemorrhagic colitis) during outbreaks traced to the ingestion of undercooked hamburgers at fast-food restaurants.[17] Other outbreaks have been seen in nursing homes where processed foods were served to large numbers of residents.[18] Although the organism may cause sporadic cases of diarrhea in the developed world where processed foods are consumed regularly, it is a rare cause of diarrhea in developing countries in which these technologies are not used.

The reservoir is known to be cattle, which may harbor the organisms asymptomatically in their intestinal tracts. During processing of the meat, fecal contamination occurs, and if the meat is not thoroughly cooked, transmission may occur.

Enteroaggregative Strains

EAggEC have been associated primarily with persistent diarrhea in children in several studies from the developing world. Not all studies have shown an association, however. It is still not clear how important these organisms are in the overall problem of diarrhea.

Diffusely Adherent Strains

DAEC have been associated with both acute and persistent diarrhea in children from the developing world in some studies, although most findings of such studies have been negative. Of all the categories of *E. coli* discussed, this one is the least secure in terms of its association with diarrhea.

Pathogenesis

All these organisms produce diarrheal disease after the colonization of specific areas of the gastrointestinal tract. ETEC, EPEC, EAggEC, and DAEC specifically colonize the small bowel; EIEC and EHEC preferentially colonize the large bowel.

Inoculum Size

To reach the ecologically appropriate section of bowel, the organisms must first pass through the hostile acid environment of the stomach. The numbers of viable organisms that must be ingested to produce disease can be approximated from studies of volunteers. ETEC and EPEC require a large inoculum, in the neighborhood of 10^8 to 10^{10} organisms, to induce diarrheal disease in a large percentage of young adult male volunteers. The infectious dose is probably considerably smaller in naturally acquired infection, because the infection rate is clearly much lower. Persons with decreased gastric acid secretion are at higher risk, because a smaller inoculum is needed to cause infection. Volunteers fed EIEC required a similarly large inoculum; this is in contrast to the small inoculum (10^3 or less) of *Shigella* often needed to produce disease. This suggests that EIEC lack some of the virulence factors inherent to *Shigella*, in spite of their many similarities.

Although volunteers have not been fed EHEC, one can

TABLE 74–3 ■ Epidemiologic Features of Diarrheogenic *Escherichia coli* Infection*

E. COLI STRAIN†	INOCULUM SIZE‡	SPORADIC CASES	NURSERY OUTBREAKS	FOOD-BORNE OUTBREAKS	WATER-BORNE OUTBREAKS	CAUSE OF TRAVELER'S DIARRHEA
ETEC	10^8–10^{10}	Usual	Rare	No	Yes	Most common
EPEC	10^8–10^{10}	Usual	Rare (except in developing countries)	No	No	No
EIEC	10^8–10^{10}	Uncommon	No	Yes	No	Uncommon
EHEC	$\leq 10^3$	Uncommon	No	Yes	No	No

*All are spread by fecally contaminated food and water.
†ETEC, Enterotoxigenic *E. coli;* EPEC, enteropathogenic *E. coli;* EIEC, enteroinvasive *E. coli;* EHEC, enterohemorrhagic *E. coli.*
‡Inoculum size as determined in volunteers, except for EHEC.

extrapolate this information from known outbreaks of disease. Transmission has been clearly described in some outbreaks as going from person to person, after the ingestion of a common contaminated food source, suggesting that a small inoculum (perhaps similar to that for *Shigella*) is sufficient to cause infection.

No information is available on the inoculum size necessary to cause disease for EAggEC and DAEC. Volunteers have been challenged with large doses of these two categories without consistent results.

Colonization

The pili of ETEC are known to be important for colonization of the small bowel. These pili recognize receptors (not well characterized as yet) on the surface of the small bowel mucosal cells to which they attach, anchoring the organisms to the small bowel surface where they then continue to multiply to large numbers. Because the normal resident flora of the small bowel is scarce (no more than about 10^3 organisms per gram of tissue), no displacement of normal flora needs to occur. The rapidly growing ETEC reach concentrations of 10^6 to 10^8 per gram of small bowel mucosa, and these large numbers of rapidly dividing organisms produce the enterotoxins that are responsible for the outpouring of fluid from mucosal cells.

EPEC also colonize the small bowel to large concentrations by way of bundle-forming pili. Colonization by these organisms results in characteristic effacement of the brush border cells (see Fig. 74–3).

Little is known of the details of colonization of the large bowel by EIEC and EHEC. They must compete with the normal abundant resident microbial flora in this location, which is on the order of 10^9 to 9^{11} organisms per gram of feces. EHEC are known to possess a fimbrial adhesion, which promotes large bowel mucosal adherence and may be an important virulence factor.

EAggEC and DAEC have had fimbria and adhesions identified, but little is known of the actual colonization process.

Enterotoxin Production

ETEC produce enterotoxins, either LT or ST, that are directly responsible for the diarrheal illness. The biochemical and enzymatic pathways whereby these enterotoxins cause fluid loss have been studied extensively. LT is known to be closely related both structurally and antigenically to cholera enterotoxin and produces fluid loss by the same mechanisms.

After attachment of the B subunit of LT to the ganglioside G_{M1}, the A subunit enters the membrane and activates adenylate cyclase, which results in an increase in cyclic adenosine monophosphate in the cell. The increased amounts of cyclic adenosine monophosphate increase chloride secretion by the crypt cells and inhibit neutral sodium chloride absorption by villus cells. These secretory and absorptive defects lead to the accumulation of fluid in the small bowel, which overwhelms the absorptive capacity of the large bowel, resulting in diarrhea. The binding of the enterotoxin to the mucosal cells is irreversible, and the physiologic effects of the toxin continue throughout the cells' normal life span, which is usually 2 or 3 days in this part of the intestine.

ST also binds to small bowel mucosal cells but in a reversible fashion; the receptors involved have not yet been clearly defined. The toxin stimulates guanylate cyclase, leading to the production of cyclic guanosine monophosphate, which then brings about changes in the cells' secretory and absorptive functions similar to those produced by LT.

EHEC produce their characteristic disease through the production of their Shiga-like toxins, which lead to inhibition of protein synthesis and cell death through attachment of their A subunits to the 60S ribosome of the cells. Not only does the toxin kill mucosal cells; evidence suggests that it may be absorbed intact into the blood stream and also result in death of endothelial cells, thus initiating the hemolytic-uremic syndrome, which is frequently a sequela of infection by these organisms.

No enterotoxins have been identified in EPEC, EIEC, and DAEC. Some strains of EAggEC produce a small heat-stable enterotoxin (EAST1), which resembles the STa of ETEC, but it is not known whether this is important in the pathogenesis of diarrhea.

Invasiveness

EIEC possess invasive properties for the mucosal cells of the large bowel similar to those of *Shigella*. Some of the outer membrane invasion proteins are identical to those of *Shigella*; the genes coding for them, which reside on the large plasmid that these strains invariably carry, are homologous to those of *Shigella*.

Histopathology

ETEC colonize the small bowel and induce fluid secretion as a result of enterotoxin release without causing histologic damage to the mucosal cells. The only differences from normal mucosa are the discharge of mucus from the goblet cells and some minimal inflammation and edema of the lamina propria.

EPEC result in effacement of the brush border microvilli (seen in Fig. 74–3) of the small intestine but without evidence of invasion of the cells or inducement of an inflammatory response.

EIEC invade large bowel mucosal cells in a way similar to *Shigella* and produce a marked inflammatory lesion in the mucosa.

EHEC produce an adherence-effacing lesion in large bowel mucosal cells, similar to the lesions produced by EPEC in the small bowel. No invasion of the mucosa is seen, and no inflammatory response is produced. Cell destruction and death are presumably direct effects of the Shiga-like toxins.

No information is available on the histopathologic changes of the intestine in infection with EAggEC or DAEC.

Clinical Manifestations

All diarrheogenic *E. coli* strains produce acute diarrheal syndromes that reflect the pathogenic mechanisms involved. All illnesses, with the exception of some of the EPEC infections, usually last only a few days and are self-limited, presumably owing to the appearance of secretory antibodies in the intestinal tract that limit the colonization process. A summary of some of the salient features of the diarrheal illnesses is given in Table 74–4.

Diarrhea due to ETEC is characteristically voluminous, watery, and without inflammatory cells in the fluid. Large fluid losses result in dehydration, the most serious clinical consequence. The fluid loss may occasionally be so marked that the syndrome of clinical cholera may be produced. The patient usually does not have fever or severe abdominal cramps. The disease is usually relatively short, lasting approximately 2 to 4 days, although it can persist for 7 to 10 days.

Diarrhea due to EPEC is similar to the description given before, but the volume of the diarrhea is usually less. Children may also experience fever, but there are no inflammatory cells in the diarrhea fluid. The infection may occasionally

TABLE 74–4 ■ Clinical and Pathologic Features of Diarrheogenic *Escherichia coli* Infection*

E. COLI STRAIN	CLINICAL SYNDROME	SITE OF INFECTION	HISTOPATHOLOGIC CHANGE
ETEC	Watery diarrhea	Small bowel	None
EPEC	Watery diarrhea	Small bowel	Effacement of brush border
EIEC	Dysentery	Large bowel	Invasive, inflammatory
EHEC	Hemorrhagic colitis, hemolytic-uremic syndrome	Large bowel	Effacement of brush border, not inflammatory

*ETEC, Enterotoxigenic *E. coli;* EPEC, enteropathogenic *E. coli;* EIEC, enteroinvasive *E. coli;* EHEC, enterohemorrhagic *E. coli.* Information is not available for enteroaggregative *E. coli* and diffusely adherent *E. coli.*

be persistent and, if not treated adequately, may last longer than 2 weeks. In the majority of cases, however, the disease is also relatively short-lived, like ETEC-induced disease.

Disease caused by EIEC is identical to shigellosis, with fever, abdominal cramping and tenesmus, and frequent stools that contain inflammatory cells and sometimes blood as well. The disease is usually more protracted than that of other *E. coli* diarrheas and may last an average of 5 to 7 days.

EHEC cause a unique clinical syndrome of hemorrhagic colitis.[19] The illness begins as watery diarrhea that may last a day or so. This is followed by grossly bloody, watery stool without inflammatory cells in the fluid, and without fever, which usually lasts another 2 to 4 days. In approximately 10% of patients, a hemolytic-uremic syndrome develops during the recovery period or within a few days afterward, which is characterized by hemolysis, thrombocytopenia, and uremia and may require dialysis. Both young and older patients with this infection seem particularly susceptible to these severe complications, which may be lethal.

Clinical illness produced by EAggEC and DAEC is not well characterized. EAggEC and DAEC have been associated with persistent diarrhea in small children but have a lesser association with acute diarrhea, which is difficult to explain. Volunteer studies have not been particularly helpful; challenge with some EAggEC has produced diarrhea in only a few volunteers, whereas other strains have not produced diarrhea. Results of challenge with DAEC have been uniformly negative.

Diagnosis

The causal organism can be suspected on the basis of the clinical presentation and the characteristics of the stool. Watery stools without inflammatory cells suggest ETEC, EPEC, EAggEC, or DAEC; dysentery-type stools suggest EIEC; and hemorrhagic stools suggest EHEC. The final diagnosis rests on the identification of the causal agent in the stool (Table 74–5). Unfortunately, with the exception of EHEC, there are no easy tests to identify most of these organisms, and routine clinical diagnostic laboratories are not able to make the identification. The diagnostic tests described here are primarily research tools that have been used in epidemiologic studies[3] (see Table 74–5).

ETEC are recognized by the enterotoxins they produce or by the genes that control enterotoxin production. Enterotoxins can be identified in the laboratory by use of animal models, tissue culture assays, or immunologic assays. DNA probes and polymerase chain reaction are used for genetic recognition. Today, DNA probes are widely used for identification, but these are largely research tools.

EPEC may be recognized by serotyping; assays of adherence, such as the HEp-2 cell tissue culture assay; and DNA probes. Unfortunately, serotyping is difficult to perform and to interpret. Only antisera that recognize O antigens are available commercially, and serogrouping alone is not adequate to identify the organism. Virulence properties correlate with the O:H serotype rather than with the O serogroup alone. Moreover, some serogroups have been identified, such as O114 and O128, in which several of the diarrheogenic subtypes of *E. coli* can be found. Serotyping is done routinely only in diarrhea outbreak situations and by a few laboratories, such as those of the Centers for Disease Control and Prevention, which have the capability to perform the tests adequately.

EIEC can be identified by animal tests of invasion, such as the Sereny test; they can be identified presumptively by serogrouping; and they can also be identified by DNA probes and polymerase chain reaction.

EHEC can be identified by looking specifically for the major serotype known to be involved, O157:H7. A medium has been devised, by the addition of sorbitol to MacConkey agar base, that allows the laboratory to screen for sorbitol-negative *E. coli,* which can then be serotyped with O157:H7 antisera. Both the O and H types must be determined, because not all O157 strains are enterohemorrhagic. In the past, only stools that contained blood were examined for this organism; it is now recommended that all diarrheal stools sent to a clinical diagnostic laboratory be cultured on sorbitol–MacConkey agar. Strains are also identified by their production of Shiga-like toxins in tissue culture cells or by immunologic assays, DNA probes, and polymerase chain reaction.

EAggEC can be suspected on the basis of their clumping on the surface of liquid media[20]; they are positively identified by their characteristic adherence pattern on tissue culture cells or by DNA probes, which recognize a large virulence plasmid that codes for fimbria and the EAST1 toxin. These organisms do not fall into clear serotype patterns.

DAEC are best recognized by their adherence pattern on tissue culture cells, although DNA probes have been developed against genes controlling for fimbria and an outer membrane protein. Serotyping is not useful in their recognition.

Retrospective serologic diagnosis is usually not helpful in these diseases; high titers of serum antibodies are not regularly produced. In the case of EHEC, however, it is possible to demonstrate antibodies against Shiga-like toxins and O157 lipopolysaccharide in convalescents' sera. Antibodies to LT and pilus antigens can also be detected in convalescent patients with ETEC diarrhea, although such tests are not usually run.

The differential diagnosis for diarrheal diseases includes the entire list of bacterial, viral, and parasitic enteric pathogens. Diarrheal diseases due to ETEC, EPEC, EAggEC, and DAEC may be difficult to distinguish clinically one from another and from those due to *Vibrio cholerae* and rotavirus. EIEC infections are identical clinically to those due to *Shigella* and *Campylobacter.* EHEC infections may be confused clinically with shigellosis or with enterocolitis caused by *Clostridium difficile.*

Therapy

The basic therapy for all diarrheal diseases in which clinical dehydration is a feature is fluid replacement with solutions

TABLE 74–5 ■ Methods for Detecting Diarrheogenic *Escherichia coli* Infection*

E. COLI STRAIN	DIFFERENTIAL ENTERIC MEDIA USEFUL	USUAL ANIMAL MODELS	TISSUE CULTURE ASSAYS†	IMMUNOASSAYS†	DNA PROBES	POLYMERASE CHAIN REACTION	SEROTYPING USEFUL	SERUM ANTIBODIES
ETEC								
LT	No	Ileal loop RITARD	Y1 adrenal cells	LT/fimbria	LT/fimbria	LT	Yes	Anti-LT, antifimbria
ST	No	Infant mouse	None	ST/fimbria	ST/fimbria	None	Yes	No
EPEC	No	None	HEp-2 cells (adherence)	None	EAF *eae* *bfp*	None	Yes	No
EIEC	May be lactose-negative on MacConkey agar	Sereny test	HeLa cells (invasion)	None	Invasion proteins	Invasion proteins	Yes	No
EHEC	Sorbitol-negative on sorbitol–MacConkey agar	Infant rabbit	Vero cells; endothelial cells	SLT-1 SLT-2	SLT-1 SLT-2 *eae*	SLT-1 SLT-2	Yes	Antitoxin, anti-LPS
EAggEC	No	None	HEp-2 cells (adherence)	None	Virulence plasmid	Portion of virulence plasmid	No	No
DAEC	No	None	HEp-2 cells (adherence)	None	Fimbria	None	No	No

*ETEC, Enterotoxigenic *E. coli;* LT, heat-labile enterotoxin; ST, heat-stable enterotoxin; EPEC, enteropathogenic *E. coli;* EIEC, enteroinvasive *E. coli;* EHEC, enterohemorrhagic *E. coli;* EAggEC, enteroaggregative *E. coli;* DAEC, diffusely adherent *E. coli;* EAF, EPEC adherence factor; SLT, Shiga-like toxin; LPS, lipopolysaccharide.

†Free toxin can often be detected in stools of patients with ETEC (LT and ST) and EHEC as well as in colony isolates.

of appropriate electrolytes. In most cases, this can be done by the oral route, using solutions similar to those suggested by the World Health Organization. These fluids will not shorten the duration of the diarrhea or decrease the stool volume, but they will correct and maintain hydration for the duration of the illness.

Specific antimicrobial therapy is known to be effective only in selected circumstances. Because the laboratory identification of these diarrheogenic *E. coli* will not be immediately forthcoming, treatment may have to be presumptive. The best example of this is the use of antimicrobials in the treatment of traveler's diarrhea[21] (see Chapter 81). Any of four drugs has been shown to be clinically useful in the treatment of traveler's diarrhea: doxycycline, trimethoprim-sulfamethoxazole, norfloxacin, and ciprofloxacin. (Many diarrheogenic organisms are now resistant to tetracyclines, so these are no longer used for this purpose.) These drugs, which are active against most strains of ETEC as well as *Shigella,* shorten the course of diarrhea to about 24 to 36 hours. Because ETEC infections are difficult to diagnose presumptively in any other setting, only a few clinical trials have been done other than in travelers; antibiotics are not thought to be indicated.

In patients with known acute or persistent diarrhea caused by EPEC, antibiotics have been shown to be effective in terminating the illness. The antibiotics used depend on the sensitivities of the *E. coli* isolated; many strains are resistant to multiple antibiotics.

Antibiotics are useful for patients with dysentery symptoms in which *Shigella* are involved. Although no clinical trials have been done for antibiotics in EIEC disease owing to the infrequency of this infection, the results should be similar to those achieved in treating shigellosis.

Antibiotic therapy has not been shown to be useful in treating hemorrhagic colitis due to EHEC. In fact, there is some evidence that the use of antibiotics in this illness may actually predispose to the development of the hemolytic-uremic syndrome, although the mechanisms involved are not known.

There is no information on the use of antibiotics for treatment of diarrhea thought to be due to EAggEC or DAEC.

Other agents that may be used in selected cases include antimotility drugs such as loperamide and bismuth subsalicylate. Antimotility agents are contraindicated in small children and in patients with invasive pathogens such as EIEC or *Shigella.*

Early feeding is an important part of therapy for children in the developing world. Because diarrheal illness is one of the major contributing factors to malnutrition, food should not be withheld during a diarrheal illness. Food can be given immediately after the short initial period of rehydration.

Prevention

All diarrheal diseases can be prevented to a large extent by improving water purity and sanitation, which will prevent transmission of the infectious agents. Education in personal hygiene measures such as hand washing will help break the cycle of direct fecal-oral transmission. Improved food-processing procedures and food handling and preparation will also interrupt the spread of these fecal pathogens. Improvement in methods for meat processing is of primary importance in interrupting the spread of EHEC in developed countries.

One specific diarrheal syndrome caused mainly by ETEC can be prevented with a short course of antibiotics. A number of studies have indicated that prophylactic antibiotics (the same ones used for treatment) will decrease the attack rate of traveler's diarrhea by about 80% to 90% when given for periods of up to 3 weeks to travelers to the developing world[22] (see Chapter 81). This is presumably due to their effect on ETEC and other sensitive bacteria that are important agents of this disease. Because all these agents have a low rate of undesirable side effects, they should not be used uniformly for all travelers. They can, however, be prescribed for selected travelers for whom the risks and benefits of the prophylaxis can be well defined and accepted.

The oral administration of cow's milk with high titers of antibodies against ETEC has been shown to give volunteers a high degree of protection against challenge with ETEC.[23] Whether this type of passive immunization will be useful for travelers or children remains to be determined.

Prevention of *E. coli*–induced diarrheal disease by vaccines is only a theoretical possibility at this time. Because the numbers of serotypes, colonization factors, and enterotoxins are multiple, it may never be possible to have a single broad-spectrum vaccine against all diarrheogenic *E. coli.* The most promising vaccine, from a public health viewpoint and based on the theoretical possibilities for development, is that against ETEC. Results of field studies have already demonstrated that an oral cholera vaccine containing the B subunit will give short-term protection against diarrhea caused by LT-producing *E. coli.*[24] Laboratory studies in progress may eventually lead to an even more effective oral vaccine that will induce protective secretory antibodies against not only LT but also the other major virulence antigens of these organisms.

References

1. Smith HW, Halls S: Studies of *Escherichia coli* enterotoxin. J Pathol Bacteriol 93:531, 1967.
2. Sack RB, Gorbach SL, Banwell JG, et al: Enterotoxigenic *Escherichia coli* isolated from patients with severe cholera-like disease. J Infect Dis 123:378, 1971.
3. Jerse AE, Kopecko DJ: Molecular approaches to bacterial detection and species/subspecies characterization: The diarrheagenic *Escherichia coli* groups. Curr Opin Gastroenterol 11:89, 1995.
4. McConnell MM, Hibberd ML, Penny ME: Surveys of human enterotoxigenic *Escherichia coli* from three different geographical areas for possible colonization factors. Epidemiol Infect 106:477, 1991.
5. Orskov I, Orskov F: Special O:K:H serotypes among enterotoxigenic *Escherichia coli* strains from diarrhea in adults and children. Med Microbiol Immunol 163:99, 1977.
6. Bray J: Isolation of antigenically homogeneous strains of *Bact. coli neapolitanum* from summer diarrhoea of infants. J Pathol 57:239, 1945.
7. Cravioto A, Gross RJ, Scotland SM, et al: An adhesive factor found in strains of *Escherichia coli* belonging to the traditional infantile enteropathogenic serotypes. Curr Microbiol 3:95, 1979.
8. Donnenberg MS, Kaper JB: Enteropathogenic *Escherichia coli.* Infect Immun 60:3953, 1992.
9. O'Brien AD, Holmes RK: Shiga and Shiga-like toxins. Microbiol Rev 51:206, 1987.
10. Vial PA, Robins-Browne R, Lior H, et al: Characterization of enteroadherent-aggregative *Escherichia coli,* a putative agent of diarrheal disease. J Infect Dis 158:70, 1988.
11. Savarino SJ: Diarrhoeal disease: Current concepts and future challenges. Enteroadherent *Escherichia coli*: A heterogeneous group of *E. coli* implicated as diarrhoeal pathogens (Review). Trans R Soc Trop Med Hyg 87(Suppl 3):49, 1993.
12. Huilan S, Zhen LG, Mathan MM, et al: Etiology of acute diarrhoea among children in developing countries: A multicentre study in five countries. Bull World Health Organ 69:549, 1991.
13. Rosenberg ML, Koplan JP, Wachsmuth IK, et al: Epidemic diarrhea at Crater Lake from enterotoxigenic *Escherichia coli.* Ann Intern Med 86:714, 1977.
14. Rothbaum R, McAdams AJ, Giannella R, et al: A clinicopathologic study of enterocyte adherent *Escherichia coli*: A cause of protracted diarrhea in infants. Gastroenterology 83:441, 1982.

15. Levine MM, Bergquist EJ, Nalin DR, et al: *Escherichia coli* strains that cause diarrhoea but do not produce heat-labile or heat-stable enterotoxins and are noninvasive. Lancet 1:1119, 1978.
16. Tulloch EF, Ryan KJ, Formal SB, et al: Invasive enteropathogenic *Escherichia coli* dysentery. Ann Intern Med 79:13, 1973.
17. Riley LW, Remis RS, Helgerson SD, et al: Hemorrhagic colitis associated with a rare *Escherichia coli* serotype. N Engl J Med 308:681, 1983.
18. Carter AO, Borczyk AA, Carlson JAK, et al: A severe outbreak of *Escherichia coli* O157:H7–associated hemorrhagic colitis in a nursing home. N Engl J Med 317:1496, 1987.
19. Riley LW: The epidemiologic, clinical, and microbiological features of hemorrhagic colitis. Annu Rev Microbiol 41:383, 1987.
20. Albert MJ, Qadri F, Haque MA, Bhuiyan NA: Bacterial clump formation at the surface of liquid culture as a rapid test for identification of enteroaggregative *Escherichia coli.* J Clin Microbiol 31:1397, 1993.
21. Sack RB: Treatment and prevention of travelers' diarrhea. *In* Holmgren J, Lindberg A, Mollby R (eds): Development of Vaccines and Drugs Against Diarrhea. 11th Nobel Conference, Stockholm 1985. Lund, Sweden, Studentlitteratur, 1986.
22. Sack RB: Antimicrobial prophylaxis of travelers' diarrhea: A selected summary. Rev Infect Dis 8:S160, 1986.
23. Tacket CO, Losonsky G, Link H, et al: Protection by milk immunoglobulin concentrate against oral challenge with enterotoxigenic *Escherichia coli.* N Engl J Med 318:1240, 1988.
24. Clemens JD, Sack DA, Harris JR, et al: Cross-protection by B subunit–whole cell cholera vaccine against diarrhea associated with heat-labile toxin-producing enterotoxigenic *Escherichia coli*: Results of a large-scale field trial. J Infect Dis 158:372, 1988.

75

Escherichia coli O157:H7 and Other Shiga Toxin–Producing *E. coli*

Thomas G. Boyce
David L. Swerdlow
Patricia M. Griffin

Shiga toxin–producing *Escherichia coli* strains are so named because they elaborate either or both of two phage-encoded toxins that are similar to the cytotoxin produced by *Shigella dysenteriae* type 1.[1, 2, 2a] These toxins are also called verocytotoxins because of their toxicity to Vero tissue culture cells. *E. coli* O157:H7, designated by its somatic (O) and flagellar (H) antigens, is the most commonly identified of the Shiga toxin–producing *E. coli.* Since it was first linked to human illness in 1982,[3] *E. coli* O157:H7 has emerged as a major cause of both outbreak-associated and sporadic diarrhea in North America. The initial report described two outbreaks of gastrointestinal illness that were associated with eating undercooked ground beef from the same fast-food restaurant chain. Shortly after that report, investigators in Canada demonstrated the association of infection with *E. coli* O157:H7 and development of the hemolytic-uremic syndrome (HUS).[1] Several studies have since demonstrated that infection with *E. coli* O157:H7 is responsible for the vast majority of cases of HUS, a major cause of acute renal failure in children.[1, 4–10] A national consensus conference convened in 1994 concluded that *E. coli* O157:H7 infection is a serious national problem in terms of severity of illness, medical costs, lost productivity, and epidemic potential.[11]

Escherichia coli O157:H7

Epidemiology

E. coli O157:H7 has been isolated in many parts of the world, including Europe, Asia, Australia, Africa, and South America.[12] However, its prevalence in these areas is unknown. Cases have most commonly been reported from Canada and the United States.[13] In the United States, sporadic cases and outbreaks are more frequently reported from states in the northern part of the country. Whether this indicates the true distribution of the organism or is a result of more thorough screening and reporting has not been determined. *E. coli* O157:H7 infections are more common in warmer months, with a peak occurrence from June through September.[14, 15] This seasonal variation may reflect the natural ecology of the organism, increased ground beef consumption, or some other factor.

Because many laboratories in the United States do not routinely culture stools for *E. coli* O157:H7,[16, 17] the true incidence of infections is unknown. A prospective, population-based study done in the Seattle area in 1985 to 1986 reported an incidence of eight infections per 100,000 persons per year.[18] On the basis of this figure, *E. coli* O157:H7 is estimated to cause 21,000 infections in the United States annually. In U.S. and Canadian studies comparing the isolation rate of *E. coli* O157:H7 with that of other bacterial enteric pathogens, *E. coli* O157:H7 has commonly been isolated more frequently than *Shigella*.[15, 18–22] *E. coli* O157:H7 is isolated at a particularly high rate if the diarrhea is bloody. In Canada, studies of bloody stool specimens have demonstrated isolation rates of 15% to 39%.[23–26]

E. coli O157:H7 is probably a relatively new pathogen. The organism was first identified in the 1982 outbreaks by serotyping methods that had been in use for several years, and retrospective analysis of *E. coli* collections found no *E. coli* O157:H7 isolates in the United States before 1975.[3] The frequency of infections with *E. coli* O157:H7 has probably been increasing slowly since the middle of this century. This may be inferred from data on the incidence of HUS, a sentinel disease for *E. coli* O157:H7 infection. HUS was first described in 1955,[27] and a global review of all reported pediatric cases up to 1965 concluded that an increase in incidence had occurred in the previous decade.[28] Studies of 10-year periods in Minnesota and Washington have shown that independent of ascertainment bias, the incidence of HUS increased between the early 1970s and late 1980s.[29, 30] However, a study of HUS from 1971 to 1990 in Utah found no significant increase in cases during the study period.[9]

The number of outbreaks of *E. coli* O157:H7 infection reported to the Centers for Disease Control and Prevention increased dramatically between 1992 and 1994 (Fig. 75–1). Part of this rise may be attributed to increased reporting and increased screening for *E. coli* O157:H7 by laboratories. The number of states requiring *E. coli* O157:H7 infections to be reported increased from 2 in 1987 to 32 by January 1, 1995[31] (see Fig. 75–1). To strengthen national surveillance and aid in detection of outbreaks, *E. coli* O157:H7 infection should be made reportable in all states. However, unless clinical laboratories routinely screen stool specimens for *E. coli*

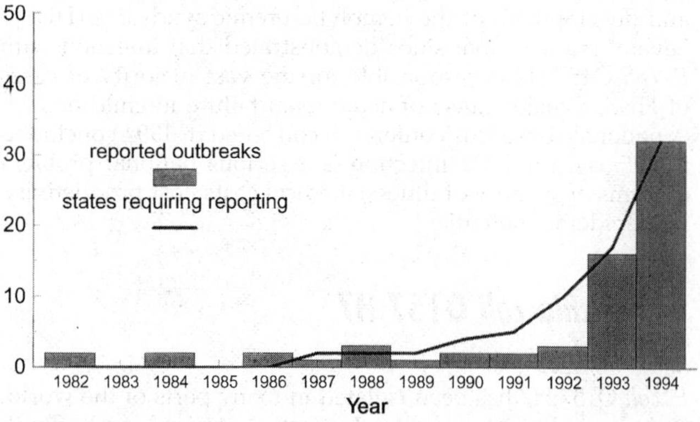

FIGURE 75–1 □ Number of outbreaks of *E. coli* O157:H7 infection reported to the Centers for Disease Control and Prevention and the number of states requiring reporting of *E. coli* O157:H7 infections, 1982 to 1994.

O157:H7, outbreaks are likely to go undetected, even in states in which it is a reportable disease.[16]

The majority of *E. coli* O157:H7 outbreaks have been the result of transmission through foods of bovine origin.[13] The most common vehicle is undercooked ground beef, although roast beef,[32] dry-cured salami,[31] and unpasteurized milk[33] have also been implicated. The largest reported U.S. outbreak affected more than 700 persons (including 4 who died) in four western states and was traced to undercooked hamburgers from a fast-food chain.[34, 35] Most other outbreaks have been caused by foods or beverages that were probably cross-contaminated by beef products or by cow manure. These include an outbreak traced to manured vegetables[36] and one from unpasteurized cider made from apples that had fallen to the ground.[37]

Other modes of transmission have also been documented, including water-borne transmission associated with an unchlorinated municipal water supply,[38] transmission to persons swimming in a fecally contaminated lake,[39] and transmission from person to person in child-care centers and institutional settings.[34, 40–42] Nosocomial spread[43] and laboratory-acquired infection have also been reported.[44, 45] The ease with which the organism is spread from person to person suggests that as with *Shigella*, the infectious dose is low.

The duration of excretion of *E. coli* O157:H7 is longer in young children and in those patients who develop HUS. In one study of sporadic cases, stool cultures from 53% of children 4 years of age and younger still yielded *E. coli* O157:H7 3 weeks after onset of diarrhea, compared with 8% of those from older children and adults.[15] Another study reported a median duration of fecal shedding of 13 days (range, 2 to 62 days) among children with diarrhea or hemorrhagic colitis and 21 days (range, 5 to 124 days) among patients who developed HUS.[46] Although asymptomatic infection and prolonged carriage may occasionally occur, *E. coli* O157:H7 is not part of the normal human bowel flora.[12]

Pathogenesis

The mechanisms by which *E. coli* O157:H7 causes diarrhea and HUS are incompletely understood. Virulence factors include the organism's adherence to mucosal surfaces and its production of one or more Shiga toxins. Adherence of *E. coli* O157:H7 to animal and tissue culture cells is described as attaching-effacing adherence and is characterized by dissolution of the brush border at the site of attachment.[47] Attachment to mucosal surfaces prevents loss of bacteria into the environment and permits the delivery of toxin to the cell surface in a concentrated manner.[48]

Most strains of *E. coli* O157:H7 produce Shiga toxin-2 with or without Shiga toxin-1. Shiga toxins are composed of a single A subunit and five B subunits.[49] The B subunits bind the toxin to cells by interaction with a membrane glycolipid called globotriosylceramide. The A subunit is an *N*-glycosidase that inactivates the 60S ribosomal subunit and thus blocks peptide elongation.[50] The exact role of Shiga toxin in diarrheal illness is unknown; it may act both locally and systemically on the gut mucosa. The histologic pattern of human colonic injury caused by *E. coli* O157:H7 infection is similar to that of *Clostridium difficile* colitis, which is caused by a locally acting toxin.[51] This similarity suggests that Shiga toxin may also play a role in colonic injury.

Colonic vascular damage by Shiga toxin may provide access for additional Shiga toxin, lipopolysaccharide, and other inflammatory mediators to the circulation, thus initiating HUS. This possibility is supported by the finding that among persons with *E. coli* O157:H7 infection, those with bloody diarrhea appear more likely than those with nonbloody stools to develop HUS.[52]

The increased rate of infection and complications in children younger than 5 years and the elderly suggests some role for immunity. However, whether circulating antibody to O157 lipopolysaccharide or to Shiga toxin decreases the likelihood of infection is unknown. Protective immunity has not been demonstrated in humans; children without known immunologic abnormalities have been infected twice.[53, 54]

Clinical Manifestations

The spectrum of clinical manifestations of *E. coli* O157:H7 infection is broad, often making the diagnosis difficult. The organism causes asymptomatic infection, nonbloody diarrhea, bloody diarrhea (hemorrhagic colitis), HUS, thrombotic thrombocytopenic purpura (TTP), and death.[55] In reported U.S. outbreaks, 23% of patients were hospitalized, 6% developed HUS or TTP, and 1.2% died.[12] On the basis of this death rate, *E. coli* O157:H7 may cause as many as 250 U.S. deaths each year.

The typical incubation period is 3 to 4 days, although incubation periods as short as 1 day and as long as 8 days have been reported.[12] Incubation periods longer than 8 days may represent secondary spread.[56, 57] Illness typically begins with severe abdominal cramps and nonbloody diarrhea, which may become grossly bloody by the second or third day of illness. About half of patients have nausea and vomiting. Other infectious causes of diarrhea are often considered (Table 75–1). However, unlike most bacterial enteric infections, fever is usually low grade or absent.[55] This may lead clinicians to suspect noninfectious causes, such as inflammatory bowel disease, ischemic colitis, or, in children, intussusception (see Table 75–1). Because the abdominal pain and tenderness may be severe, appendicitis or another acute sur-

TABLE 75–1 ■ Differential Diagnosis of Colitis Caused by *Escherichia coli* O157:H7

INFECTIOUS CAUSES	NONINFECTIOUS CAUSES
Shigella	Ulcerative colitis
Salmonella	Crohn disease
Campylobacter	Intussusception
Yersinia enterocolitica	Ischemic colitis
Clostridium difficile	Diverticulosis
Entamoeba histolytica	Appendicitis

From Boyce TG, Swerdlow DL, Griffin PM: *Escherichia coli* O157:H7 and the hemolytic-uremic syndrome. N Engl J Med 333:364–368, 1995.

gical condition may be the initial diagnosis, leading to exploratory laparotomy.[55, 58] Early reports suggested that the presence of fecal leukocytes was uncommon in patients infected with *E. coli* O157:H7.[55] However, a later report suggested that compared with stools of patients infected with *Salmonella*, *Shigella*, or *Campylobacter*, stools of patients infected with *E. coli* O157:H7 were nearly twice as likely to contain fecal leukocytes.[59]

Patients with *E. coli* O157:H7 infection may have profuse, bloody stools, mimicking gastrointestinal hemorrhage. Alternatively, the diarrhea may be minimally blood streaked or remain nonbloody. In reported outbreaks, the percentage of patients with *E. coli* O157:H7 infection who develop bloody diarrhea has varied widely, from 35%[38] to 90%.[34] Thus, although bloody stools are common with *E. coli* O157:H7 infection, the diagnosis must be considered for patients with nonbloody diarrhea as well.

Edema and submucosal hemorrhage in the ascending and transverse colon may be demonstrated on barium enema examination by a thumbprinting pattern.[3] At endoscopy, the colonic mucosa appears edematous and hyperemic, sometimes with superficial ulcerations.[51] Pathologic findings include infectious or ischemic patterns of colonic injury, usually in a patchy distribution, and sometimes with fibrin microthrombi.[51] Pseudomembranes may be present, making the distinction between *C. difficile* pseudomembranous colitis and infection with *E. coli* O157:H7 difficult.[51, 60]

Symptoms of infection with *E. coli* O157:H7 usually subside in about a week with no obvious sequelae. However, approximately 6% of patients develop HUS,[12] which is usually diagnosed about 6 days (range, 2 to 14 days) after the onset of diarrhea.[1] Probably the most common cause of acute renal failure in children, HUS is characterized by microangiopathic hemolytic anemia, thrombocytopenia, and renal failure, often accompanied by central nervous system manifestations.[61] Young children and the elderly are at the greatest risk for developing this syndrome.[13] Among persons infected with *E. coli* O157:H7, early predictors for progression to HUS include bloody diarrhea, fever, an elevated leukocyte count, and treatment with antimotility agents.[42, 52, 62]

TTP includes all the clinical features of HUS, although the renal injury is typically less severe and neurologic involvement is often more prominent; it is usually diagnosed in adults.[63] Few cases are preceded by a diarrheal prodrome[13]; however, postdiarrheal TTP is probably the same disorder as HUS.[13, 63, 64]

Among patients with HUS, predictors of severity include an elevated white cell count,[8, 9, 65] a severe gastrointestinal prodrome,[66] early-onset anuria,[9] and age younger than 2 years.[9] One quarter of patients develop neurologic impairment, including seizures in 20%, coma or obtundation in 15%, and stroke in 4%.[9, 67, 68] Approximately one half of patients with HUS require dialysis, and three quarters receive red blood cell transfusions.[9, 29, 30] HUS is a multisystem disease; relatively common extrarenal manifestations include pancreatitis in 20% of patients, diabetes mellitus in 8%, and hepatomegaly or elevated liver enzyme levels in 40%.[68] The mortality rate of HUS is 3% to 5%,[9, 29, 30] and 5% of surviving patients have severe sequelae, such as end-stage renal disease or permanent neurologic injury.[9]

Not all deaths of patients with *E. coli* O157:H7 infection are due to HUS. In published U.S. outbreaks in which at least 1 death was reported, 7 of 19 deaths occurred among patients who did not have HUS or TTP[34, 36, 38, 42, 57, 58]; all seven of those persons were elderly.

Diagnosis

E. coli O157:H7 infection should be suspected in any patient with bloody stools or HUS. The diagnosis should also be considered for persons with nonbloody diarrhea who have a suggestive exposure history, such as consumption of undercooked ground beef or unpasteurized milk. During an outbreak, clinical suspicion should be raised to detect milder cases. If only bloody stools are cultured for *E. coli* O157:H7, some infections will be missed.

Routine stool cultures will not detect the organism; however, a simple and inexpensive screening method is available to all laboratories. Unlike 80% to 90% of human fecal flora, *E. coli* O157:H7 does not ferment sorbitol rapidly, enabling laboratories to screen for it using sorbitol-MacConkey agar.[23] The colorless, sorbitol-negative colonies are selected and assayed for the O157 antigen with use of commercially available antiserum.[69] Sorbitol-negative *E. coli* organisms that agglutinate in O157 antisera may be presumptively identified as *E. coli* O157:H7, pending the determination of H type in a reference laboratory.

Recommendations from a national consensus conference regarding laboratory screening for *E. coli* O157:H7 have been published.[11] It is recommended that all stools submitted for examination for bacterial enteric pathogens also be cultured for *E. coli* O157:H7. In particular, the consensus conference emphasized that *E. coli* O157:H7 may be the most common enteropathogen isolated from stools with visible blood; therefore, at least all bloody stools should be cultured on sorbitol-MacConkey medium. As of January 1995, however, only about half of all clinical laboratories in the United States routinely screened all bloody stools for *E. coli* O157:H7.[17] Thus, when the diagnosis is suspected, physicians should specifically request that the laboratory culture for *E. coli* O157:H7. Because the recovery rate of the organism may decline rapidly after the first 6 days of illness,[10] stool cultures should be obtained as early as possible.

Serologic diagnosis using detection of antibodies to O157 lipopolysaccharide is performed in research laboratories only.[70] Tests for rapid detection of *E. coli* O157[71] and of Shiga toxin in stool are currently being developed. Such tests would be helpful in conducting treatment trials and in selecting patients for close monitoring.

Treatment

There is no proven specific therapy for patients with *E. coli* O157:H7 infection. Some retrospective studies have suggested that patients who were treated with an antimicrobial agent such as trimethoprim-sulfamethoxazole were more likely to develop HUS,[42] but one study reported the opposite result.[62] Only one prospective study of antimicrobial therapy has been reported.[72] In that study, trimethoprim-sulfamethoxazole had no significant effect on the course of gastrointestinal symptoms, duration of excretion, or progression to HUS. However, patients in that study began treatment a mean of 7 days after onset of diarrhea. There is a theoretical concern regarding the use of antibiotics for patients with *E. coli* O157:H7 infection. Subinhibitory concentrations of trimethoprim-sulfamethoxazole and ciprofloxacin have been shown to increase production of Shiga toxin in vitro.[73, 74] A multicenter trial of early antibiotic therapy is greatly needed, but until then, antimicrobial drugs should probably be avoided. Promising future therapies for *E. coli* O157:H7 infection include orally administered toxin-binding resins[75] and antitoxin given intravenously.

Antimotility agents are contraindicated in patients with bloody diarrhea. One retrospective study of patients with *E. coli* O157:H7 infection receiving antimotility drugs showed an increased risk for development of HUS,[62] and another study demonstrated increased severity of neurologic manifestations in those with HUS.[67]

During the week after onset of diarrhea, patients with

documented infection should be monitored for signs and symptoms of HUS, such as pallor and oliguria. For high-risk patients (such as those younger than 5 years and the elderly), monitoring of peripheral blood count, blood smear, and urinalysis during this period is prudent. The management of patients with HUS is supportive and includes meticulous attention to fluid and electrolyte balance; dialysis is often necessary.[76] Investigational therapies include the use of fresh-frozen plasma, plasmapheresis, and intravenous immune globulin.[76]

Prevention

The dose of *E. coli* O157:H7 that leads to infection is likely to be low; for this reason, patients infected with the organism should be considered highly contagious.[77] Person-to-person spread is especially common in daycare centers, where children may not wash their hands thoroughly after defecating and where there are many possibilites for close contact with other children. One study found a secondary attack rate of 22% within daycare centers.[40] Data from another study suggested that person-to-person spread may be a more important risk factor for childhood HUS than direct exposure to ground beef.[78] Exclusion of infected children from daycare until two consecutive stool cultures are negative has been shown to prevent ongoing transmission.[40] However, if this policy is to be successful, parents must be persuaded not to take an infected child to a different daycare center, which could result in more widespread transmission. A single negative stool culture during convalescence should not engender false confidence, because excretion of *E. coli* O157:H7 may be intermittent.[46, 77] The most important preventive measure for child-care centers is supervised hand washing for all children.

Once a presumptive *E. coli* O157:H7 is isolated, the local health department should be notified immediately. This is especially important if the patient is a nursing home resident or attends a daycare center, so that personnel in these settings can heighten surveillance for diarrheal illness. Cases of HUS and clusters of bloody diarrhea should also be reported, even if infection with *E. coli* O157:H7 has not been proved.[77] In the large January 1993 outbreak affecting persons in the western United States, early detection and reporting of *E. coli* O157:H7 infections and HUS enabled a rapid recall of contaminated ground beef and prevented an estimated 800 infections.[34]

The publicity of such large outbreaks has led to the perception that *E. coli* O157:H7 infection is most likely to be acquired by eating a hamburger in a fast-food restaurant. However, most cases of *E. coli* O157:H7 infection are probably sporadic, and ingestion of undercooked ground beef prepared in the home may be just as great a risk factor for infection.[79, 80] Patients should be counseled about the need to cook ground beef until the interior is no longer pink and juices run clear.

Because therapy for infection with *E. coli* O157:H7 is limited to supportive care, prevention of infection is paramount. Control measures on farms and in slaughtering and processing plants are greatly needed, as are better education strategies to promote safe food-handling practices.[11]

Other Shiga Toxin–Producing *Escherichia coli*

Although more than 100 Shiga toxin–producing serotypes of *E. coli* have been isolated from humans,[12] not all such serotypes have been shown to cause diarrhea or HUS. Those Shiga toxin–producing *E. coli* serotypes that cause bloody diarrhea are sometimes referred to as enterohemorrhagic *E. coli*. However, non-O157 Shiga toxin–producing *E. coli* serotypes appear less likely than *E. coli* O157:H7 to cause bloody diarrhea.[15, 19] It is possible that some non-O157 Shiga toxin–producing *E. coli* serotypes tend to cause bloody diarrhea, others cause nonbloody diarrhea, and others are not human pathogens. Some of the non-O157 Shiga toxin–producing *E. coli* serotypes most frequently isolated from persons with diarrhea are O26:H11 and O111:NM (nonmotile).[13] An outbreak of bloody diarrhea and HUS in South Australia was traced to dry sausage contaminated with *E. coli* O111:NM.[81] In 1994, the first reported outbreak of gastroenteritis in the United States attributable to a non-O157 Shiga toxin–producing *E. coli*, *E. coli* O104:H21, occurred in Montana. Illness was associated with drinking improperly pasteurized milk from a local dairy.[82]

Unlike screening for *E. coli* O157:H7, which is easily accomplished using sorbitol-MacConkey medium, techniques to identify other Shiga toxin–producing *E. coli* are not available in most laboratories.[12] Thus, if a cluster of patients with bloody diarrhea or HUS is detected and stool cultures do not yield *E. coli* O157:H7, the clinician should request that the state public health laboratory examine specimens for other Shiga toxin–producing *E. coli*.

Conclusions

Of the Shiga toxin–producing *E. coli*, *E. coli* O157:H7 is the most important serotype from both clinical and public health standpoints. In addition to causing bloody and nonbloody diarrhea, it is responsible for most cases of HUS in North America. Our knowledge about the pathophysiology, spectrum of illness, and modes of transmission for this organism has increased dramatically in recent years. However, it is still unknown whether antimicrobial, antitoxin, or other therapy can ameliorate the diarrheal illness or prevent HUS. As more laboratories begin to culture for *E. coli* O157:H7, the number of recognized infections will continue to increase. Until laboratory screening for this organism becomes routine, however, clinicians should ask their laboratories to culture stools for *E. coli* O157:H7 when the diagnosis is suspected.

References

1. Karmali MA, Petric M, Lim C, et al: The association between idiopathic hemolytic uremic syndrome and infection by verotoxin-producing *Escherichia coli*. J Infect Dis 151:775, 1985.
2. Strockbine NA, Marques LRM, Newland JW, et al: Two toxin-converting phages from *Escherichia coli* O157:H7 strain 933 encode antigenically distinct toxins with similar biologic activities. Infect Immun 53:135, 1986.

2a. Calderwood SB, Acheson DWK, Keusch GT, et al: Proposed new nomenclature for Shiga-like toxin (verotoxin) family. ASM News 62:118, 1996.

3. Riley LW, Remis RS, Helgerson SD, et al: Hemorrhagic colitis associated with a rare *Escherichia coli* serotype. N Engl J Med 308:681, 1983.
4. Bitzan M, Moebius E, Ludwig K, et al: High incidence of serum antibodies to *Escherichia coli* O157 lipopolysaccharide in children with hemolytic-uremic syndrome. J Pediatr 119:380, 1991.
5. Bitzan M, Ludwig K, Klemt M, et al: The role of *Escherichia coli* O157 infections in the classical (enteropathic) haemolytic uraemic syndrome: Results of a Central European, multicentre study. Epidemiol Infect 110:183, 1993.
6. Neill MA, Tarr PI, Clausen CR, et al: *Escherichia coli* O157:H7 as the predominant pathogen associated with the hemolytic uremic syndrome: A prospective study in the Pacific Northwest. Pediatrics 80:37, 1987.
7. Rowe PC, Orrbine E, Lior H, et al: A prospective study of exposure to verotoxin-producing *Escherichia coli* among Canadian

children with haemolytic uraemic syndrome. Epidemiol Infect 110:1, 1993.
8. Rowe PC, Orrbine E, Wells GA, et al: Epidemiology of hemolytic-uremic syndrome in Canadian children from 1986 to 1988. J Pediatr 119:218, 1991.
9. Siegler RL, Pavia AT, Christofferson RD, Milligan MK: A 20-year population-based study of postdiarrheal hemolytic uremic syndrome in Utah. Pediatrics 94:35, 1994.
10. Tarr PI, Neill MA, Clausen CR, et al: *Escherichia coli* O157:H7 and the hemolytic uremic syndrome: Importance of early cultures in establishing the etiology. J Infect Dis 162:553, 1990.
11. Brotman M, Giannella RA, Alm PF, et al: Consensus conference statement: *Escherichia coli* O157:H7 infections—An emerging national health crisis, July 11–13, 1994. Gastroenterology 108:1923, 1995.
12. Griffin PM: *Escherichia coli* O157:H7 and other enterohemorrhagic *Escherichia coli*. *In* Blaser MJ, Smith PD, Ravdin JI, et al: Infections of the Gastrointestinal Tract. New York, Raven Press, 1995, pp 739–761.
13. Griffin PM, Tauxe RV: The epidemiology of infections caused by *Escherichia coli* O157:H7, other enterohemorrhagic *E. coli*, and the associated hemolytic uremic syndrome. Epidemiol Rev 13:60, 1991.
14. Ostroff SM, Kobayashi JM, Lewis JH: Infections with *Escherichia coli* O157:H7 in Washington state: The first year of statewide disease surveillance. JAMA 262:355, 1989.
15. Pai CH, Ahmed N, Lior H, et al: Epidemiology of sporadic diarrhea due to verocytotoxin-producing *Escherichia coli*: A two-year prospective study. J Infect Dis 157:1054, 1988.
16. Centers for Disease Control and Prevention: Laboratory screening for *Escherichia coli* O157:H7—Connecticut, 1993. MMWR Morbid Mortal Wkly Rep 43:192, 1994.
17. Boyce TG, Pemberton AG, Wells JG, Griffin PM: Screening for *Escherichia coli* O157:H7: A nationwide survey of clinical laboratories. J Clin Microbiol 33:3275, 1995.
18. MacDonald KL, O'Leary MJ, Cohen ML, et al: *Escherichia coli* O157:H7, an emerging gastrointestinal pathogen: Results of a one-year, prospective, population-based study. JAMA 259:3567, 1988.
19. Bokete TN, O'Callahan CM, Clausen CR, et al: Shiga-like toxin–producing *Escherichia coli* in Seattle children: A prospective study. Gastroenterology 105:1724, 1993.
20. Cahoon FE, Thompson JS: Frequency of *Escherichia coli* O157:H7 isolation from stool specimens. J Infect Dis 33:914, 1987.
21. Gransden WR, Damm MA, Anderson JD, et al: Further evidence associating hemolytic uremic syndrome with infection by verotoxin-producing *Escherichia coli* O157:H7. J Infect Dis 154:522, 1986.
22. Marshall WF, McLimans CA, Van Scoy RE, Anhalt JP: Results of a 6-month survey of stool cultures for *Escherichia coli* O157:H7. Mayo Clin Proc 65:787, 1990.
23. March SB, Ratnam S: Sorbitol-MacConkey medium for detection of *Escherichia coli* O157:H7 associated with hemorrhagic colitis. J Clin Microbiol 23:869, 1986.
24. Pai CH, Gordon R, Sims HV, Bryan LE: Sporadic cases of hemorrhagic colitis associated with *Escherichia coli* O157:H7: Clinical, epidemiologic, and bacteriologic features. Ann Intern Med 101:738, 1984.
25. Bryant HE, Athar MA, Pai CH: Risk factors for *Escherichia coli* O157:H7 infection in an urban community. J Infect Dis 160:858, 1989.
26. Ratnam S, March SB: Sporadic occurrence of hemorrhagic colitis associated with *Escherichia coli* O157:H7 in Newfoundland. Can Med Assoc J 134:43, 1986.
27. Gasser C, Gautier E, Steck A: Hämolytisch-urämische Syndrome: Bilaterale Nierenrindennekrosen bei akuten erworbenen hämolytischen Anämien. Schweiz Med Wochenschr 85:205, 1955.
28. Piel CF, Phibbs RH: The hemolytic-uremic syndrome. Pediatr Clin North Am 13:295, 1966.
29. Martin DL, MacDonald KL, White KE, et al: The epidemiology and clinical aspects of the hemolytic uremic syndrome in Minnesota. N Engl J Med 323:1161, 1990.
30. Tarr PI, Neill MA, Allen J, et al: The increasing incidence of the hemolytic-uremic syndrome in King County, Washington: Lack of evidence for ascertainment bias. Am J Epidemiol 129:582, 1989.
31. Centers for Disease Control and Prevention: *Escherichia coli* O157:H7 outbreak linked to commercially distributed dry-cured salami—Washington and California, 1994. MMWR Morbid Mortal Wkly Rep 44:157, 1995.
32. Centers for Disease Control: Foodborne outbreak of gastroenteritis caused by *Escherichia coli* O157:H7—North Dakota, 1990. MMWR Morbid Mortal Wkly Rep 40:265, 1991.
33. Oregon Health Division: *Escherichia coli* O157:H7 outbreak traced to raw milk. Commun Dis Summ 42:1, 1993.
34. Bell BP, Goldoft M, Griffin PM, et al: A multistate outbreak of *Escherichia coli* O157:H7–associated bloody diarrhea and hemolytic uremic syndrome from hamburgers: The Washington experience. JAMA 272:1349, 1994.
35. Griffin PM, Bell BP, Cieslak PR, et al: Large outbreak of *Escherichia coli* O157:H7 infections in the western United States: The big picture. *In* Karmali MA, Goglio AG (eds): Recent Advances in Verocytotoxin-Producing *Escherichia coli* Infections: Proceedings of the 2nd International Symposium and Workshop on Verocytotoxin (Shiga-Like Toxin)–Producing *Escherichia coli* Infections, Bergamo, Italy, 27–30 June 1994. Amsterdam, Elsevier Science Publishing, 1994, pp 7–12.
36. Cieslak PR, Barrett TJ, Griffin PM: *Escherichia coli* O157:H7 infection from a manured garden. Lancet 342:367, 1993.
37. Besser RE, Lett SM, Weber JT, et al: An outbreak of diarrhea and hemolytic uremic syndrome from *Escherichia coli* O157:H7 in fresh-pressed apple cider. JAMA 269:2217, 1993.
38. Swerdlow DL, Woodruff BA, Brady RC, et al: A waterborne outbreak in Missouri of *Escherichia coli* O157:H7 associated with bloody diarrhea and death. Ann Intern Med 117:812, 1992.
39. Keene WE, McAnulty JM, Hoesly FC, et al: A swimming-associated outbreak of hemorrhagic colitis caused by *Escherichia coli* O157:H7 and *Shigella sonnei*. N Engl J Med 331:579, 1994.
40. Belongia EA, Osterholm MT, Soler JT, et al: Transmission of *Escherichia coli* O157:H7 infection in Minnesota child day-care facilities. JAMA 269:883, 1993.
41. Spika JS, Parsons JE, Nordenberg D, et al: Hemolytic uremic syndrome and diarrhea associated with *Escherichia coli* O157:H7 in a day care center. J Pediatr 109:287, 1986.
42. Pavia AT, Nichols CR, Green DP, et al: Hemolytic-uremic syndrome during an outbreak of *Escherichia coli* O157:H7 infections in institutions for mentally retarded persons: Clinical and epidemiologic observations. J Pediatr 116:544, 1990.
43. Karmali MA, Arbus GS, Petric M, et al: Hospital-acquired *Escherichia coli* O157:H7 associated haemolytic uraemic syndrome in a nurse (Letter). Lancet 1:526, 1988.
44. Booth L, Rowe B: Possible occupational acquisition of *Escherichia coli* O157 infection. Lancet 342:1298, 1993.
45. Burnens AP, Zbinden R, Kaempf L, et al: A case of laboratory acquired infection with *Escherichia coli* O157:H7. Zentralbl Bakteriol 279:512, 1993.
46. Karch H, Russman H, Schmidt H, et al: Long-term shedding and clonal turnover of enterohemorrhagic *Escherichia coli* O157 in diarrheal diseases. J Clin Microbiol 33:1602, 1995.
47. Moon HW, Whipp SC, Argenzio RA, et al: Attaching and effacing activities of rabbit and human enteropathogenic *Escherichia coli* in pig and rabbit intestines. Infect Immun 41:1340, 1983.
48. Zafriri D, Oron Y, Eisenstein BI, Ofek I: Growth advantage and enhanced toxicity of *Escherichia coli* adherent to tissue culture cells due to restricted diffusion of products secreted by the cells. J Clin Invest 79:1210, 1987.
49. Karmali MA: Infection by verocytotoxin-producing *Escherichia coli*. Clin Microbiol Rev 2:15, 1989.
50. Tesh VL, O'Brien AD: The pathogenic mechanisms of Shiga toxin and the Shiga-like toxins. Mol Microbiol 5:1817, 1991.
51. Griffin PM, Olmstead LC, Petras RE: *Escherichia coli* O157:H7–associated colitis: A clinical and histological study of 11 cases. Gastroenterology 99:142, 1990.
52. Carter AO, Borczyk AA, Carlson JAK, et al: A severe outbreak of *Escherichia coli* O157:H7–associated hemorrhagic colitis in a nursing home. N Engl J Med 317:1496, 1987.
53. Siegler RL, Griffin PM, Barrett TJ, Strockbine NA: Recurrent hemolytic uremic syndrome secondary to *Escherichia coli* O157:H7 infection. Pediatrics 91:666, 1993.
54. Robson WLM, Leung AK, Miller-Hughes, DJ: Recurrent hemorrhagic colitis caused by *Escherichia coli* O157:H7. Pediatr Infect Dis J 12:699, 1993.
55. Griffin PM, Ostroff SM, Tauxe RV, et al: Illnesses associated with

Escherichia coli O157:H7 infections: A broad clinical spectrum. Ann Intern Med 109:705, 1988.
56. Salmon RL, Farrell ID, Hutchison JG, et al: A christening party outbreak of haemorrhagic colitis and haemolytic uraemic syndrome associated with *Escherichia coli* O157:H7. Epidemiol Infect 103:249, 1989.
57. Ryan CA, Tauxe RV, Hosek GW, et al: *Escherichia coli* O157:H7 diarrhea in a nursing home: Clinical, epidemiological, and pathological findings. J Infect Dis 154:631, 1986.
58. Ostroff SM, Griffin PM, Tauxe RV, et al: A statewide outbreak of *Escherichia coli* O157:H7 infections in Washington state. Am J Epidemiol 132:239, 1990.
59. Slutsker L, Ries A, Maloney K, Griffin P, the *Escherichia coli* O157:H7 Study Group: Clinical features of *Escherichia coli* O157:H7 infection: How wise is conventional wisdom? *In* Program and Abstracts of the 35th Interscience Conference on Antimicrobial Agents and Chemotherapy; September 20, 1995; San Francisco. American Society for Microbiology, 1995, Washington, DC, p 314.
60. Case records of the Massachusetts General Hospital. Weekly clinicopathological exercises. Case 25-1994. N Engl J Med 330:1811, 1994.
61. Pickering LK, Obrig TG, Stapleton FB: Hemolytic-uremic syndrome and enterohemorrhagic *Escherichia coli*. Pediatr Infect Dis J 13:459, 1994.
62. Cimolai N, Carter JE, Morrison BJ, Anderson JD: Risk factors for the progression of *Escherichia coli* O157:H7 enteritis to hemolytic-uremic syndrome. J Pediatr 116:589, 1990.
63. Ruggenenti P, Remuzzi G: Thrombotic thrombocytopenic purpura and related disorders. Hematol Oncol Clin North Am 4:219, 1990.
64. Ashkenazi S: Role of bacterial cytotoxins in hemolytic uremic syndrome and thrombotic thrombocytopenic purpura. Annu Rev Med 44:11, 1993.
65. Robson WL, Fick GH, Wilson PC: Prognostic factors in typical postdiarrhea hemolytic-uremic syndrome. Child Nephrol Urol 9:203, 1988.
66. Lopez EL, Devoto S, Fayad A, et al: Association between severity of gastrointestinal prodrome and long-term prognosis in classic hemolytic-uremic syndrome. J Pediatr 120:210, 1992.
67. Cimolai N, Morrison BJ, Carter JE: Risk factors for the central nervous system manifestations of gastroenteritis-associated hemolytic-uremic syndrome. Pediatrics 90:616, 1992.
68. Siegler RL: Spectrum of extrarenal involvement in postdiarrheal hemolytic-uremic syndrome. J Pediatr 125:511, 1994.
69. March SB, Ratnam S: Latex agglutination test for detection of *Escherichia coli* serotype O157. J Clin Microbiol 27:1675, 1989.
70. Barrett TJ, Green JH, Griffin PM, et al: Enzyme-linked immunosorbent assays for detecting antibodies to Shiga-like toxin I, Shiga-like toxin II, and *Escherichia coli* O157:H7 lipopolysaccharide in human serum. Curr Microbiol 23:189, 1991.
71. Park CH, Hixon DL, Morrison WL, Cook CB: Rapid diagnosis of enterohemorrhagic *Escherichia coli* O157:H7 directly from fecal specimens using immunofluorescence stain. Am J Clin Pathol 101:91, 1994.
72. Proulx F, Turgeon JP, Delage G, et al: Randomized, controlled trial of antibiotic therapy for *Escherichia coli* O157:H7 enteritis. J Pediatr 121:299, 1992.
73. Karch H, Strockbine NA, O'Brien AD: Growth of *Escherichia coli* in the presence of trimethoprim-sulfamethoxazole facilitates detection of Shiga-like toxin producing strains by colony blot assay. FEMS Microbiol Lett 35:141, 1986.
74. Walterspiel JN, Ashkenazi S, Morrow AL, Cleary TG: Effect of subinhibitory concentrations of antibiotics on extracellular Shiga-like toxin I. Infection 20:25, 1992.
75. Armstrong GD, Rowe PC, Goodyer P, et al: A phase I study of chemically synthesized verotoxin (Shiga-like toxin) Pk-trisaccharide receptors attached to chromosorb for preventing hemolytic-uremic syndrome. J Infect Dis 171:1042, 1995.
76. Siegler RL: Management of hemolytic-uremic syndrome. J Pediatr 112:1014, 1988.
77. Tarr PI: *Escherichia coli* O157:H7: Clinical, diagnostic, and epidemiological aspects of human infection. Clin Infect Dis 20:1, 1995.
78. Rowe PC, Orrbine E, Lior H, et al: Diarrhoea in close contacts as a risk factor for childhood haemolytic uraemic syndrome. The CPKDRC co-investigators. Epidemiol Infect 110:9, 1993.
79. LeSaux N, Spika JS, Friesen B, et al: Ground beef consumption in noncommercial settings is a risk factor for sporadic *Escherichia coli* O157:H7 infection in Canada. J Infect Dis 167:500, 1993.
80. Centers for Disease Control and Prevention: *Escherichia coli* O157:H7 outbreak linked to home-cooked hamburger—California, July 1993. MMWR Morbid Mortal Wkly Rep 43:213, 1994.
81. Centers for Disease Control and Prevention: Community outbreak of hemolytic uremic syndrome attributable to *Escherichia coli* O111:NM—South Australia 1995. MMWR Morbid Mortal Wkly Rep 44:550, 1995.
82. Centers for Disease Control and Prevention: Outbreak of acute gastroenteritis attributable to *Escherichia coli* serotype O104:H21—Helena, Montana, 1994. MMWR Morbid Mortal Wkly Rep 44:501, 1995.

76

Campylobacter Infections

Ban Mishu Allos

Campylobacter species are an important cause of gastrointestinal infections in both the developing and the developed world. These previously underrecognized microorganisms are now known to be one of the most common causes of bacterial diarrhea worldwide. In the United States, more than 99% of reported *Campylobacter* isolates are *Campylobacter jejuni*.[1] The clinical features of this organism as well as its microbiology and epidemiology are contained in Chapter 207.

Because the selective media commonly used to detect *C. jejuni* may not permit growth of other *Campylobacter* species, these "atypical" isolates may not be detected despite their presence in stools. In parts of the world where *Campylobacter* isolation procedures are used that permit growth of atypical species (other than *C. jejuni* or *Campylobacter coli*), only 44% of strains are *C. jejuni*.[2] Indeed, worldwide, only 80% of identified *Campylobacter* strains are *C. jejuni*.[3] This chapter highlights the microbiology, epidemiology, and clinical characteristics of *Campylobacter* and *Campylobacter*-like organisms other than *C. jejuni* and *C. coli*.

Campylobacter fetus

C. fetus, formerly *Vibrio fetus* and *Campylobacter fetus* subsp. *fetus*, was first recognized as a cause of abortion in sheep and cattle in the early 20th century.[4] The organism was later recognized as a human pathogen causing bacteremia and other extraintestinal illness in immunocompromised persons.

Prolonged incubation of blood cultures is required for detection of *C. fetus* bacteremia because 3 to 25 days may be required for primary isolation from blood. The organisms grow better in aerobic bottles. Isolation of *C. fetus* from stools presents additional difficulties. Because most *C. fetus* strains are susceptible to cephalothin, use of cephalothin-containing media (commonly used to isolate *C. jejuni* from stools) will not permit the growth of *C. fetus* or other atypical *Campylobacter* strains. Therefore, an alternative detection method is needed. Because *Campylobacter* organisms are quite small (0.3 to 0.6 μm in diameter), stools may be filtered through a

0.45- to 0.65-μm filter onto an antibiotic-free medium. This filtration technique is now considered the optimal method for isolation of *Campylobacter* species from stools.

Like other *Campylobacter* species, *C. fetus* is microaerophilic, requiring 3% to 5% oxygen for growth. The organism does not ferment carbohydrates; most strains are nitrate-, catalase-, and oxidase-positive. *C. fetus* grows well at 25°C and 37°C, but unlike most *C. jejuni* strains, it does not grow at 42°C. (However, exceptional *C. fetus* strains are able to grow at this higher temperature.[5]) *C. fetus* is resistant to nalidixic acid, is susceptible to cephalothin, and lacks pyrazinamidase activity—features that help distinguish it from *C. jejuni* (Table 76–1).

C. fetus infections remain rare; only 265 isolates were reported to the Centers for Disease Control and Prevention *Campylobacter* Surveillance System between 1982 and 1989.[6] Most *C. fetus* infections are extraintestinal and occur in immunocompromised persons (Table 76–2); 75% of infected persons have underlying malignant disease, diabetes, alcoholism, cirrhosis or other liver disease, or acquired immunodeficiency syndrome or are receiving immunosuppressive therapy.[7, 8] Among adults with *C. fetus* infection, men outnumber women 3 to 1.[7]

Because *C. fetus* has a tropism for vascular tissue, any patient with *C. fetus* infection should be carefully evaluated for septic thrombophlebitis. Infections may also be associated with endocarditis or mycotic aneurysms.[9, 10] In pregnant animals, intestinal infection with *C. fetus* may lead to hematogenous spread followed by placental and fetal infection and death.[11] Similarly, in pregnant women, gastrointestinal *C. fetus* infection (with or without symptoms) may be followed by placental infection[12]; 80% of fetuses and neonates die even when maternal infection is mild and appropriate antibiotics are given.[13, 14] *C. fetus* infections may also cause salpingitis, septic arthritis, cellulitis, abscesses, meningitis, peritonitis, osteomyelitis, urinary tract infections, or cholecystitis.[15–20] Occasionally, *C. fetus* may produce uncomplicated enteritis in healthy persons.[5, 7, 21]

The most likely route of human infection with *C. fetus* is through the gastrointestinal tract. The organism is rarely isolated from stools; however, 40% of patients with *C. fetus* bacteremia report diarrhea.[22] Perhaps normal hosts are able to contain infection within the gut, whereas immunocompromised hosts cannot. Although only one third of patients with *C. fetus* bacteremia report contact with farm animals, it is likely that humans acquire infection from animals. *C. fetus* is isolated from sheep, cattle, poultry, reptiles, and swine[23] (Table 76–3). Human consumption of food or water contaminated with intestinal contents of infected animals probably results in transmission of infection.[24] Outbreaks of *C. fetus* infection have resulted from consumption of unpasteurized milk[5, 25] and raw liver.[26, 27]

The resistance of *C. fetus* to the bactericidal activity of normal human serum could account for the high proportion of *C. fetus* infections that result in bacteremias.[28, 29] Human *C. fetus* isolates are covered by a surface (S) layer protein forming a paracrystalline surface array that functions as a capsule and strongly inhibits binding of C3b.[30] Disruption of C3b binding explains both serum and phagocytosis resistance that has been observed; S^+ strains are not recognized by the alternative pathway of complement.

Serious *C. fetus* infections may be treated with ampicillin or third-generation cephalosporins.[19] An aminoglycoside may be added to the regimen in treating endocarditis; the duration of therapy should be at least 4 weeks. Two to 3 weeks of therapy is needed to treat *C. fetus* infections of the central nervous system. Erythromycin is usually not effective in the treatment of *C. fetus* infections.

The prognosis of patients with *C. fetus* infections depends largely on their general state of health. Immunocompetent patients with uncomplicated enteritis do well without antibiotic therapy. Immunocompromised persons with systemic infections require parenteral antibiotics but may still have a poor outcome. The overall mortality associated with *C. fetus* infections is 20%.[31, 32]

Campylobacter upsaliensis

C. upsaliensis is a thermotolerant *Campylobacter* that can cause gastroenteritis and bacteremia in humans. It was first identified in the stools of dogs[33] but in 1985 was recognized as a human pathogen.[34] The name *C. upsaliensis* was validated in 1991.[35]

C. upsaliensis is distinguished from other *Campylobacter* species by its susceptibility to nalidixic acid and cephalothin[36] (see Table 76–1). Like *C. fetus, C. upsaliensis* cannot grow on commonly used *Campylobacter*-selective media containing antibiotics; stools suspected of harboring this organism must be filtered onto an antibiotic-free medium.[2] Other microbiologic characteristics of most *C. upsaliensis* strains include a negative hippurate hydrolysis test result, positive nitrate reduction and indole acetate test results, and a negative or weakly positive catalase test result.[37]

Like many other *Campylobacter* species, *C. upsaliensis* is principally a gastrointestinal pathogen; typical illness is characterized by watery diarrhea, abdominal cramps, and low-grade fever (see Table 76–2). Onset of symptoms is usually abrupt, and illness is usually self-limited; prolonged or relapsing illness occasionally occurs.[38–40] Few patients have bloody stools or fecal leukocytes. *C. upsaliensis* may cause bacteremia, usually in persons with other chronic underlying illness.[36, 39, 41] The gastrointestinal tract is likely to be the source of these systemic infections.

Humans acquire *C. upsaliensis* infections through contact with dogs and cats[33, 39, 42] (see Table 76–3). The occurrence appears to increase during the fall.[40] Although the frequency of *C. upsaliensis* infections is not known with certainty, when filtration methods (i.e., antibiotic-free media) are used to culture stools, 12% to 22% of isolated *Campylobacter* strains are *C. upsaliensis*.[43–45] When other methods are used for culture, less than 1% of isolated strains are identified as *C. upsaliensis*.[46, 47] Fluoroquinolones are the drug of choice for treatment of *C. upsaliensis* infections.[48] Erythromycin resistance is encountered in 4% to 18% of *C. upsaliensis* isolates.[39, 44, 49]

Campylobacter hyointestinalis

C. hyointestinalis is principally known as a cause of enteritis in swine (see Table 76–3), but this organism may also cause diarrhea in immunocompromised persons and homosexual men. The organism is catalase- and nitrate reductase–positive, which helps distinguish it from other *Campylobacter* species (see Table 76–1). *C. hyointestinalis* is thermotolerant in that it survives at 42°C but grows most abundantly at 37°C.[50] Some *C. hyointestinalis* strains require a hydrogen-enhanced atmosphere for growth.[51]

Several published studies report the isolation of *C. hyointestinalis* from stools of patients with watery diarrhea; however, the organism has also been isolated from stools of asymptomatic persons.[51–53] Symptomatic *C. hyointestinalis* infections usually occur in homosexual men and immunocompromised or elderly persons[3] (see Table 76–2). The organism is also found in the stools of young or malnourished children with diarrhea.[2] *C. hyointestinalis* has been cultured from the blood of one patient after bone marrow transplantation.[3] All clinical

TABLE 76–1 ■ Biochemical Characteristics of *Campylobacter* and Related Species*

ORGANISM	CAT	NIT RED	IND ACE	ARYLSULF	PYRAZIN	HIPP	NAL	CEPH	H_2S Rapid†	H_2S Lead Ace	TSI	GROWTH AT 25°C	GROWTH AT 37°C	GROWTH AT 42°C	H_2 REQUIRED
C. jejuni bio. 1‡	+	+	+	−	+	+	S	R	−	++	−	−	+	+	−
C. jejuni bio. 2‡	+	+	+	+	+	+	S	R	+	++	−	−	+	+	−
C. coli	+	+	+	−	+	−	S	R	−	++	−	−	+	+	−
C. fetus	+	+	−	−	−	−	R	S	−	+	−	+	+	−	−
C. upsaliensis	(+)	+	+	−	+	−	S	S	−	(+)	−	−	+	(+)	d
C. lari	+	+	−	−	+	−	R	R	+	+	−	−	+	+	−
C. hyointestinalis	+	+	−	−	−	−	R	S	−	5+	3+	(+)	+	+	d
Helicobacter fennelliae§‖	+	−	+	+	−	−	S	(S)	−	+	−	−	+	−	−
Helicobacter cinaedi§	+	+	−	−	−	−	S	(S)	−	(+)	−	−	+	−	−
C. jejuni subsp. *doylei*	(+)	−	+	−	+	(+)	S	(S)	−	−	−	−	+	(+)	d
Arcobacter cryaerophilus¶	+	+	+	−	−	−	S	(R)	−	−	−	+	+	−	−
Arcobacter butzleri¶	(+)	+	+	−	−	−	S	(R)	−	−	−	−	+	(+)	−
C. sputorum bio. *sputorum*	−	+	−	+	+	−	R	S	+	5+	3+	−	+	+	−
C. sputorum bio. *bubulus*	−	+	−	+	−	−	R	S	+	5+	3+	−	+	(+)	−
C. sputorum bio. *faecalis*	+	+	−	+	+	−	R	S	+	5+	3+	−	+	+	−
C. concisus	−	+	−	+	+	−	(R)	S	−	3+	(+)	−	+	(−)	+
C. mucosalis	−	+	−	−	−	−	R	S	−	5+	+	(−)	+	(−)	+
C. curvus	−	+	+	+	+	−	R	S	−	5+	+	−	+	+	+
C. rectus	−	+	+	+	+	−	S	R	−	3+	+	−	+	+	+

*CAT, Catalase; NIT RED, nitrate reduction; IND ACE, indole acetate; ARYLSULF, arylsulfatase; PYRAZIN, pyrazinamidase; HIPP, hippurate hydrolysis; NAL, nalidixic acid resistance; CEPH, cephalothin resistance; Lead Ace, lead acetate; TSI, triple sugar iron; +, positive; (+), most strains positive; −, negative; (−), most strains negative; R, resistant; (R), most strains resistant; S, susceptible; (S), most strains suceptible; d, some isolates grow much better in hydrogen-enhanced growth conditions.

† Rapid H_2S method of Skirrow and Benjamin (Skirrow MB, Benjamin J: Differentiation of enteropathogenic *Campylobacter* [Letter]. J Clin Pathol 33:1122, 1980).

‡ *C. jejuni* subsp. *jejuni* biotypes 1 and 2 refer to Skirrow's scheme. Susceptibilities are based on 30-μg disks.

§ Spreading, noncolonial growth.

‖ Hypochlorite odor.

¶ Aerobic growth occurs at 30°C.

TABLE 76–2 ■ Clinical Features Associated with *Campylobacter* and Related Species Implicated as Causes of Human Illness

SPECIES	COMMONLY ENCOUNTERED CLINICAL FEATURES	LESS COMMONLY ENCOUNTERED CLINICAL FEATURES
C. jejuni	Fever, diarrhea, abdominal pain	Bacteremia
C. coli	Fever, diarrhea, abdominal pain	Bacteremia
C. fetus	Bacteremia, sepsis, meningitis, vascular infections	Diarrhea, relapsing fevers
C. upsaliensis	Watery diarrhea, low-grade fever, abdominal pain	Bacteremia, abscesses
C. lari	Gastroenteritis, abdominal pain, diarrhea	Colitis, appendicitis
C. hyointestinalis	Watery or bloody diarrhea, vomiting, abdominal pain	Bacteremia
Helicobacter fennelliae	Chronic, mild diarrhea; abdominal cramps; proctitis	Bacteremia in persons infected with human immunodeficiency virus and in children
Helicobacter cinaedi	Chronic, mild diarrhea; abdominal cramps; proctitis	Bacteremia in persons infected with human immunodeficiency virus and in children
C. jejuni subsp. *doylei*	Gastroenteritis	Chronic gastritis, bacteremia in children
Arcobacter cryaerophilus	Gastroenteritis	Bacteremia
Arcobacter butzleri	Fever, diarrhea, abdominal pain, nausea	Bacteremia, appendicitis
C. sputorum	Lung, perianal, groin, axillary abscesses	
Hydrogen-requiring *Campylobacter* species*	Periodontitis	Diarrhea, osteomyelitis, bacteremia in children

*Includes *C. rectus, C. curvus,* and *C. concisus.*

C. hyointestinalis isolates tested have been susceptible to erythromycin.

Campylobacter lari

C. lari, formerly *C. laridis,* is a nalidixic acid–resistant *Campylobacter* that may cause acute diarrheal illness in normal hosts and bacteremia in immunocompromised persons. Few microbiologic features distinguish *C. lari* from other *Campylobacter* species. Most *C. lari* strains are oxidase- and catalase-negative; the hippurate hydrolysis test result is negative[54] (see Table 76–1). Unlike *C. jejuni, C. lari* strains do not hydrolyze indole acetate.[55]

C. lari is isolated with high frequency from seagulls, kittiwakes, and crows[54, 56–58] (see Table 76–3), which may be a source of transmission to humans; the organism is infrequently found in poultry.[59] Rivers and other surface waters may also be a source of *C. lari* infection.[22, 60] A water-borne outbreak of gastroenteritis caused by *C. lari* infection occurred in Ontario after drinking water became contaminated by surface waters frequented by seagulls.[61]

Several reports document the presence of *C. lari* in stools of immunocompetent and immunocompromised persons with diarrhea.[62–64] *C. lari* bacteremia occurs in immunocompromised persons[47, 65–67] (see Table 76–2). Patients with uncomplicated diarrheal disease due to *C. lari* may not require treatment with antibiotics. For patients with more severe disease, antibiotics are indicated; the organism is susceptible to erythromycin, clindamycin, chloramphenicol, aminoglycosides, and imipenem.[62, 64, 65] In addition to nalidixic acid resistance, most *C. lari* isolates are resistant to penicillin, vancomycin, all cephalosporins, and trimethoprim.[62, 64] Quinolone-resistant strains have been reported in persons infected with human immunodeficiency virus.[62]

TABLE 76–3 ■ Animal Reservoirs for Atypical *Campylobacter* Species

SPECIES	RESERVOIR
C. fetus	Cattle, sheep
C. upsaliensis	Dogs, cats
C. hyointestinalis	Pigs, cattle, hamsters
C. lari	Seagulls, crows, kittiwakes, poultry, monkeys, seals
Helicobacter cinaedi and *Helicobacter fennelliae*	Hamsters, dogs
Arcobacter cryaerophilus and *Arcobacter butzleri*	Pigs, primates, ostrich, cattle
C. jejuni subsp. *doylei*	None known
Hydrogen-requiring *Campylobacter* species	Lambs, pigs
C. sputorum and subspecies	Cattle, sheep

Helicobacter cinaedi and *Helicobacter fennelliae*

H. cinaedi and *H. fennelliae* were first called *Campylobacter*-like organisms and later *Campylobacter cinaedi* and *Campylobacter fennelliae;* in 1991, they were recognized as members of the *Helicobacter* genus.[68] These microorganisms cause enteritis and proctocolitis in homosexual men; they may also cause bacteremia.

H. cinaedi and *H. fennelliae* grow best at 37°C and not at all at 42°C or 25°C[23, 69] (see Table 76–1). *H. fennelliae* colonies have an odor similar to that of household chlorine bleach. *H. cinaedi* and *H. fennelliae* may be distinguished by serologic tests,[70] sodium dodecyl sulfate–polyacrylamide gel electrophoresis,[71] and arylsulfatase activity.[21]

Campylobacter-like organisms were first identified in the stools of homosexual men with gastrointestinal symptoms.[72, 73] Up to 8% of homosexual men's stools contained *Campylobacter*-like organisms,[74] whereas stools from women and heterosexual men did not.[73] The source of human infection with *H. cinaedi* and *H. fennelliae* is not known; however, the organisms have been isolated from dogs and hamsters[75, 76] (see Table 76–3), suggesting possible animal-to-human transmission.

Infections with *H. cinaedi* and *H. fennelliae* may produce illness that is mild and consists only of a few loose stools per day.[77] However, they may produce illness similar to *C. jejuni* gastroenteritis with fever, diarrhea, and abdominal cramps. These infections may also be associated with anal discharge and pain, tenesmus, and hematochezia[73] (see Table 76–2). Blood and leukocytes may be found in stools. Sigmoidoscopic examination may show ulceration and mucosal bleeding; on histopathologic examination, crypt abscesses and polymorphonuclear leukocytes are found scattered through the lamina propria.[73]

Numerous reports document *H. cinaedi* bacteremia in patients with human immunodeficiency virus infection or acquired immunodeficiency syndrome[78, 79]; there are fewer reports of *H. fennelliae* bacteremia.[79, 80] Bacteremia due to these organisms may present only with low-grade fevers, malaise, and lethargy, but some patients report a preceding gastrointestinal illness. Hypotension and other signs of sepsis are not usually present. No fatal outcomes resulting from *H. cinaedi* and *H. fennelliae* have been described.

Reports from South Africa suggest that *H. cinaedi* and *H. fennelliae* infections may also cause gastroenteritis in heterosexual men and in women and children.[2, 75, 77, 81, 82] One report documented the presence of *H. cinaedi* in the cerebrospinal fluid of a neonate whose mother reported one third-trimester diarrheal illness.[83]

All *H. cinaedi* and *H. fennelliae* isolates are resistant to trimethoprim; most are also resistant to metronidazole. Thirteen percent of isolates from pediatric patients are resistant to erythromycin[2]; 28% of isolates from adult men are erythromycin and clindamycin resistant.[84] Oral fluoroquinolones (ciprofloxacin, 500 mg orally every 12 hours, or ofloxacin, 200 to 400 mg orally every 12 hours) are the treatment of choice for persistent *H. cinaedi* and *H. fennelliae* infections.[85, 86] Other antimicrobial agents that have documented in vitro activity against these organisms include ampicillin, gentamicin, tetracycline, doxycycline, ceftriaxone, rifampin, streptomycin, nalidixic acid, and chloramphenicol.[84]

Arcobacter cryaerophilus and *Arcobacter butzleri*

A. cryaerophilus and *A. butzleri* (formerly *Campylobacter cryaerophila* and *Campylobacter butzleri*) are aerobic organisms that may cause bacteremia and gastroenteritis. The organisms were removed from the genus *Campylobacter* to *Arcobacter* in 1991.[68] *A. butzleri* is frequently isolated from nonhuman primates[87, 88] (see Table 76–3). *A. cryaerophilus* is frequently isolated from urban sewage, especially near swine slaughter houses,[89] and from pig fetuses.[90, 91] The route of transmission of these organisms to humans is not known. Only three *A. cryaerophilus* human isolates have been confirmed, two from blood and one from stool.[92] Human *A. butzleri* infection occurs more commonly; among 631 Thai children with diarrhea, *A. butzleri* was the most frequent atypical "*Campylobacter*" isolated from stools.[46] Of 43 patients with *A. butzleri* isolated from their stools, more than 50% had abdominal pain and nausea; many also had fever, chills, vomiting, and malaise.[92] Abdominal cramps may be the predominant symptom associated with *A. butzleri* infection. In an outbreak of *A. butzleri* infection at an Italian elementary school, all 10 affected children had recurrent attacks of abdominal cramps, two to three times per day for about 10 days; none had diarrhea.[93]

Campylobacter jejuni Subspecies *doylei*

This subspecies of *C. jejuni* is only recently being recognized for its pathogenic potential in humans. During a 30-month study in South Africa, *C. jejuni* subsp. *doylei* composed more than 10% of *Campylobacter* strains isolated from children with gastroenteritis. Of the 142 *C. jejuni* subsp. *doylei*–infected children, 81% had diarrhea, 14% had bloody stools, and 20% had fecal leukocytes.[2] Eleven patients were bacteremic (see Table 76–2). Studies in other parts of the world have not shown as high a frequency of infection with *C. jejuni* subsp. *doylei;* however, even in these studies, infection with the organism was associated with diarrhea in children.[2, 43, 44, 46, 94] *C. jejuni* subsp. *doylei* may be distinguished from other *Campylobacter* species by its ability to reduce nitrate to nitrite[95] (see Table 76–1). The organism is susceptible to both cephalothin and nalidixic acid.[96]

Hydrogen-Requiring *Campylobacter* Species

Four species of *Campylobacter*—*C. concisus, C. mucosalis* (formerly *C. sputorum* subsp. *mucosalis*), *C. rectus* (formerly *Wolinella recta*), and *C. curvus* (formerly *Wolinella curva*)—are known to require hydrogen for growth. A strong association exists between *C. concisus* and human periodontal disease.[97–99] Most recently, *C. concisus* has been associated with gastrointestinal illness. Studies in South Africa[2, 100] and Belgium[101, 102] have detected *C. concisus* in 2.4% to 12.3% of adults and children with gastroenteritis. *C. rectus* is also associated with periodontal disease and is isolated from 80% of adults and children with this condition.[103] *C. rectus* has not been associated with gastrointestinal illness. The role of *C. curvus* in causing human disease is not yet known, but this organism may also be associated with periodontal disease[104] and gastroenteritis.[89, 102] *C. mucosalis* is an important veterinary pathogen causing proliferative enteritis in lambs and pigs.[105, 106] Only three human isolates (two from stool, one from blood) have been reported.[66, 107]

Campylobacter sputorum

C. sputorum and its subspecies have occasionally been associated with human disease,[108–110] but a causal role has not been established.

Conclusions

As detection methods for *Campylobacter* and related organisms improve, other new species may be identified as human pathogens and the isolation rate of atypical species may rise. Increasing understanding of the source of infection and pathogenesis of these infections will enhance the ability to both prevent and treat these illnesses.

References

1. Tauxe RV, Hargrett-Bean N, Patton CM, Wachsmuth IK: *Campylobacter* isolates in the United States, 1982–1986. MMWR CDC Surveill Summ 37:1–13, 1988.
2. Lastovica AJ, Le Roux E: Prevalence and distribution of *Campylobacter* spp. in the diarrhoeic stools and blood cultures of pediatric patients. Acta Gastroenterol Belg 56(Suppl):34, 1993.
3. Allos BM, Lastovica A, Blaser MJ: Atypical campylobacters and related organisms. *In* Blaser MJ, Smith PD, Ravdin JI, et al (eds): Infections of the Gastrointestinal Tract. New York, Raven Press, 1995, pp 849–866.
4. McFadyean J, Stockman S: Report of the department of committee appointed by the Board of Agriculture and Fisheries to inquire into epizootic abortions. Appendix to part III Abortion in sheep. London, His Majesty's Stationery Office, 1913, pp 1–29.
5. Klein BS, Vergeront JM, Blaser MJ, et al: *Campylobacter* infection associated with raw milk: An outbreak of gastroenteritis due to *Campylobacter jejuni* and thermotolerant *Campylobacter fetus* subsp. *fetus*. JAMA 255:361–364, 1986.
6. Mishu B, Patton C, Tauxe RV: Clinical and epidemiologic features of non-*jejuni* campylobacters. *In* Nachamkin I, Blaser MJ, Tompkins LS (eds): *Campylobacter jejuni*: Current Status and

Future Trends. Washington, DC, American Society for Microbiology, 1992, pp 31–41.
7. Guerrant RL, Lahita RG, Winn EC Jr, Roberts RB: Campylobacteriosis in man: Pathogenic mechanisms and review of 91 bloodstream infections. Am J Med 65:484–592, 1978.
8. Francioli P, Herztein J, Grob JP, et al: *Campylobacter fetus* subspecies *fetus* bacteremia. Arch Intern Med 145:289–292, 1985.
9. Anolik JR, Mildvan D, Winter JW, et al: Mycotic aortic aneurysm: A complication of *Campylobacter fetus* septicemia. Arch Intern Med 143:609–610, 1983.
10. Morrison VA, Lloyd BK, Chia JKS, Tuazon CU: Cardiovascular and bacteremic manifestations of *Campylobacter fetus* infection: Case report and review. Rev Infect Dis 12:387–392, 1990.
11. Miller VA, Jenson R, Gilroy JJ: Bacteremia in pregnant sheep following oral administration of *Vibrio fetus.* Am J Vet Res 20:677–679, 1959.
12. Lowrie DB, Pearce JH: The placental localisation of *Vibrio fetus.* J Med Microbiol 3:607–614, 1970.
13. Eden AH: Perinatal mortality caused by *Vibrio fetus.* Review and analysis. J Pediatr 68:297–304, 1966.
14. Simor AE, Karmali MA, Jadavji T, Roscoe M: Abortion and perinatal sepsis associated with *Campylobacter* infection. Rev Infect Dis 8:397–402, 1986.
15. Franklin B, Ulmer DD: Human infection with *Vibrio fetus.* West J Med 120:200–204, 1974.
16. Kilo C, Hagemann PO, Maryi J: Septic arthritis and bacteremia due to *Vibrio fetus* (Letter). Am J Med 38:962, 1965.
17. Brown WJ, Sautter R: *Campylobacter fetus* septicemia with concurrent salpingitis. J Clin Microbiol 6:72–75, 1977.
18. Wens R, Dratwa M, Potvliege C, et al: *Campylobacter fetus* peritonitis followed by septicaemia in a patient on continuous ambulatory peritoneal dialysis. J Infect 10:249–251, 1985.
19. Neuzil K, Wang E, Haas D, Blaser MJ: Persistence of *Campylobacter fetus* bacteremia associated with absence of opsonizing antibodies. J Clin Microbiol 32:1718–1720, 1994.
20. Yao JDC, Ng HMC, Campbell I: Prosthetic hip joint infection due to *Campylobacter fetus.* J Clin Microbiol 31:3323–3324, 1993.
21. Burnens AP, Nicolet J: Three supplementary diagnostic tests for *Campylobacter* species and related organisms. J Clin Microbiol 31:708–710, 1993.
22. Brennhound O, Kapperud G, Langeland G: Survey of thermotolerant *Campylobacter* spp. and *Yersinia* spp. in three surface water sources in Norway. Int J Food Microbiol 15:327–338, 1992.
23. Smibert RM: Genus *Campylobacter.* Sebald and Véron 1963, 907[AL]. *In* Krieg NR, Holt HG (eds): Bergey's Manual of Systematic Bacteriology, Vol 1. Baltimore, Williams & Wilkins, 1984, pp 111–118.
24. Blaser MJ, Taylor DN, Feldman RA: Epidemiology of *Campylobacter jejuni* infections. Epidemiol Rev 5:157–176, 1983.
25. Taylor PR, Weinstein WM, Bryner JH: *Campylobacter fetus* infection in human subjects: Association with raw milk. Am J Med 66:779–783, 1979.
26. Centers for Disease Control: *Campylobacter* sepsis associated with "nutritional therapy"—California. MMWR Morbid Mortal Wkly Rep 30:294–295, 1981.
27. Centers for Disease Control: Premature labor and neonatal sepsis caused by *Campylobacter fetus,* subsp. *fetus*—Ontario. MMWR Morbid Mortal Wkly Rep 33:483–489, 1984.
28. Blaser MJ, Smith PF, Kohler PA: Susceptibility of *Campylobacter* isolates to the bactericidal activity in human serum. J Infect Dis 151:227–235, 1985.
29. Blaser MJ, Smith PF, Hopkins JA, et al: Pathogenesis of *Campylobacter fetus* infections. Serum-resistance associated with high molecular weight surface proteins. J Infect Dis 155:696–706, 1987.
30. Blaser MJ, Smith PF, Repine JE, Joiner KA: Pathogenesis of *Campylobacter fetus* infections. Failure of C3b to bind explains serum and phagocytosis resistance. J Clin Invest 81:1434–1444, 1988.
31. Dickgiesser N, Kasper G, Kihm W: *Campylobacter fetus* ssp. *fetus* bacteremia: A patient with liver cirrhosis (Letter). Infection 11:288, 1983.
32. Rao GG, Karim QN, Maddocks A, et al: *Campylobacter fetus* infections in two patients with AIDS. J Infect 20:170–172, 1990.
33. Sandstedt K, Ursing J, Walder M: Thermotolerant *Campylobacter* with no or weak catalase activity isolated from dogs. Curr Microbiol 8:209–213, 1983.
34. Steele TW, Sangster N, Lanser JA: DNA relatedness and biochemical features of *Campylobacter* spp. isolated in Central and South Australia. J Clin Microbiol 22:71–74, 1985.
35. International Union of Microbiological Societies: Validation of the publication of new names and new combinations previously effectively published outside the IJSB. Int J Syst Bacteriol 41:580–581, 1991.
36. Lastovica AJ, Le Roux E, Penner JL: *"Campylobacter upsaliensis"* isolated from blood cultures of pediatric patients. J Clin Microbiol 27:657–659, 1989.
37. Sandstedt K, Ursing J: Description of *Campylobacter upsaliensis* sp. nov. previously known as the CNW group. Syst Appl Microbiol 14:39–48, 1991.
38. Megraud F, Bonnet F: Unusual campylobacters in human feces. J Infect 12:275–276, 1986.
39. Patton CM, Shaffer N, Edmonds P, et al: Human disease associated with *"Campylobacter upsaliensis"* (catalase-negative or weakly positive *Campylobacter* species) in the United States. J Clin Microbiol 27:66–73, 1989.
40. Walmsley SL, Karmali MA: Direct isolation of thermophilic *Campylobacter* species from human feces on selective agar medium. J Clin Microbiol 27:668–670, 1989.
41. Chusid MJ, Wortmann DW, Dunne WM: *"Campylobacter upsaliensis"* sepsis in a boy with acquired hypogammaglobulinemia. Diagn Microbiol Infect Dis 13:367–369, 1990.
42. Owen RJ, Hernandez J: Occurrence of plasmids in *"Campylobacter upsaliensis"* (catalase negative or weak group) from geographically diverse patients with gastroenteritis or bacteremia. Eur J Epidemiol 6:111–117, 1990.
43. Albert MJ, Tee W, Leach A, et al: Comparison of a blood-free medium and a filtration technique for the isolation of *Campylobacter* spp. from diarrhoeal stools of hospitalized patients in central Australia. J Med Microbiol 37:176–179, 1992.
44. Goossens H, Vlaes L, De Boeck M, et al: Is *"Campylobacter upsaliensis"* an unrecognised cause of human diarrhoea? Lancet 336:584–586, 1990.
45. Goossens H, Pot B, Vlaes L, et al: Characterization and description of *Campylobacter upsaliensis* isolated from human feces. J Clin Microbiol 28:1039–1046, 1990.
46. Taylor DN, Diehlbauch JA, Tee W, et al: Isolation of group 2 aerotolerant *Campylobacter* species from Thai children with diarrhea. J Infect Dis 163:1062–1067, 1991.
47. Skirrow MB, Jones DM, Sutcliffe E, Benjamin J: *Campylobacter* bacteremia in England and Wales, 1981–91. Epidemiol Infect 110:567–573, 1993.
48. Preston MA, Simor AE, Walmsley SL, et al: In vitro susceptibility of *"Campylobacter upsaliensis"* to twenty-four antimicrobial agents. Eur J Clin Microbiol Infect Dis 9:822–824, 1990.
49. da Silva-Tatley FM, Lastovica AJ, Steyn LM: Plasmid profiles of *"Campylobacter upsaliensis"* isolated from blood cultures and stools of pediatric patients. J Med Microbiol 37:8–14, 1992.
50. Edmonds P, Patton CM, Griffin PM, et al: *Campylobacter hyointestinalis* associated with human gastrointestinal disease in the United States. J Clin Microbiol 25:685–691, 1987.
51. Vandamme P, De Ley J: Proposal for a new family, Campylobacteraceae. Int J Syst Bacteriol 41:451–455, 1991.
52. Salana SM, Tabor H, Richter M, Taylor DE: Pulsed-field gel electrophoresis for epidemiologic studies of *Campylobacter hyointestinalis* isolates. J Clin Microbiol 30:1982–1984, 1992.
53. Minet J, Growbois B, Megraud F: *Campylobacter hyointestinalis:* An opportunistic enteropathogen? J Clin Microbiol 26:2659–2660, 1988.
54. Von Graevgenitz A: A revised nomenclature of *Campylobacter laridis, Enterobacter intermedium,* and *"Flavobacterium branchophilia."* Int J Syst Bacteriol 40:211, 1990.
55. Popovic-Uroic T, Patton CM, Nicholson MA, Kiehlbauch JA: Evaluation of indoxylacetate hydrolysis test for rapid differentiation of *Campylobacter, Helicobacter,* and *Wolinella* species. J Clin Microbiol 28:2335–2339, 1990.
56. Glunder G, Petermann S: The occurrence and characterization of *Campylobacter* spp. in silver gulls *(Larus argentatus),* three-toed gulls *(Rissa tridactyla),* and house sparrows *(Passer domesticus).* Zentralbl Veterinarmed B 36:123–130, 1989.
57. Kakkar M, Dogra SC: Prevalence of *Campylobacter* infections in animals and children in Haryana, India. J Diarrhoeal Dis Res 8:34–36, 1990.

58. Maruyama S, Tanaka T, Katsube Y, et al: Prevalence of thermophilic campylobacters in crows *(Corvus lavaillantii, Corvus corne)* and serogroups of the isolates. Jpn J Vet Sci 52:1237–1244, 1990.
59. Kazawala RR, Jiwa SF, Nkya AE: The role of management systems in the epidemiology of thermophilic campylobacters among poultry in eastern zone of Tanzania. Epidemiol Infect 110:273–278, 1993.
60. Bolton FJ, Coates D, Hutchinson DN, Godfree AF: A study of thermophilic *Campylobacter* in a river system. J Appl Bacteriol 62:167–176, 1987.
61. Borczyk A, Thompson S, Smith D, Lior H: Water-borne outbreak of *Campylobacter laridis*–associated gastroenteritis. Lancet 1:164–165, 1987.
62. Evans TG, Riley D: *Campylobacter laridis* colitis in a human immunodeficiency virus–positive patient treated with a quinolone. Clin Infect Dis 15:172–173, 1992.
63. Tauxe RV, Patton CM, Edmonds P, et al: Illness associated with *Campylobacter laridis,* a newly recognized *Campylobacter* species. J Clin Microbiol 21:222–225, 1985.
64. Simor AE, Wilcox L: Enteritis associated with *Campylobacter laridis.* J Clin Microbiol 25:10–12, 1987.
65. Nachamkin I, Stowell C, Skalina D, et al: *Campylobacter laridis* causing bacteremia in an immunosuppressed patient. Ann Intern Med 101:55–57, 1984.
66. Soderstrom C, Schalen C, Walder M: Septicaemia caused by unusual *Campylobacter* species (*C. laridis* and *C. mucosalis*). Scand J Infect Dis 23:369–371, 1991.
67. Vargas J, Carzo JE, Perez MJ, et al: Enfermedades infecciosas. Microbiol Clin 10:155–157, 1992.
68. Vandamme P, Falsen E, Rossau R, et al: Revision of *Campylobacter, Helicobacter,* and *Wolinella* taxonomy: Emendation of generic descriptions and proposal of *Arcobacter* gen. nov. Int J Syst Bacteriol 41:88–103, 1991.
69. Griffiths PL, Moreno GS, Park RW: Differentiation between thermophilic *Campylobacter* species by species-specific antibodies. J Appl Bacteriol 72:467–472, 1992.
70. Flores BM, Fennell CL, Stamm WE: Characterization of *Campylobacter cinaedi* and *C. fennelliae* antigens and analysis of human immune response. J Infect Dis 159:635–640, 1989.
71. On SLW, Owen RJ, Lastovica A, et al: Taxonomic study of *Helicobacter (Campylobacter) fennelliae* from clinical material by numerical analysis of one-dimensional electrophoretic protein patterns. Microbial Ecol Health Dis 4:S103, 1991.
72. Quinn TC, Stamm WE, Goodell SE, et al: The polymicrobial origin of intestinal infections in homosexual man. N Engl J Med 309:76–82, 1983.
73. Quinn TC, Goodell SE, Fennell CL, et al: Infections with *Campylobacter jejuni* and *Campylobacter*-like organisms in homosexual men. Ann Intern Med 101:187–192, 1984.
74. Laughon BE, Vernon AA, Druckman DA, et al: Recovery of *Campylobacter* species from homosexual men. J Infect Dis 158:464–467, 1988.
75. Burnens AP, Angeloy-Wick B, Nicolet J: Comparison of *Campylobacter* carriage rates in diarrheic and healthy pet animals. J Vet Med Ser B 39:175–180, 1992.
76. Gebhart CJ, Fennell CL, Murtaugh MP, Stamm WE: *Campylobacter cinaedi* is the normal intestinal flora in hamsters. J Clin Microbiol 27:1692–1694, 1989.
77. Grayson ML, Tee W, Dwyer B: Gastroenteritis associated with *Campylobacter cinaedi.* Med J Aust 150:214–215, 1989.
78. Burman WJ, Cohn DL, Reves RR, Wilson ML: Multifocal cellulitis and monoarticular arthritis as manifestations of *Helicobacter cinaedi* bacteremia. Clin Infect Dis 20:564–571, 1995.
79. Ng VL, Hadley WK, Fennell CL, et al: Successive bacteremias with *Campylobacter cinaedi* and *Campylobacter fennelliae* in a bisexual male. J Clin Microbiol 25:2008–2009, 1987.
80. Kemper CA, Mickelson P, Morton A, et al: *Helicobacter (Campylobacter) fennelliae*–like organisms as an important but occult cause of bacteremia in a patient with AIDS. J Infect 26:97–101, 1993.
81. Wilcox CM, Byford BA, Forsmark CE, et al: *Campylobacter*-like organisms are uncommon pathogens in patients infected with the human immunodeficiency virus. J Clin Microbiol 28:2370–2371, 1990.
82. Burnens AP, Stanley J, Schaad VB, Nicolet J: Novel *Campylobacter*-like organism resembling *Helicobacter fennelliae* isolated from a boy with gastroenteritis and from dogs. J Clin Microbiol 31:1916–1917, 1993.
83. Orlicek SL, Welch DF, Kuhls TL: Septicemia and meningitis caused by *Helicobacter cinaedi* in neonate. J Clin Microbiol 31:569–571, 1993.
84. Flores BM, Fennell CL, Holmes KK, Stamm WE: In vitro susceptibility of *Campylobacter*-like organisms to twenty antimicrobial agents. Antimicrob Agents Chemother 28:188–191, 1985.
85. Sacks LV, Labriola AM, Gill VJ, Gordin FM: Use of ciprofloxacin for successful eradication of bacteremia due to *Campylobacter cinaedi* in a human immunodeficiency virus–infected patient. Rev Infect Dis 13:1066–1068, 1993.
86. Decker CF, Martin GJ, Barham WB, Paparello SF: Bacteremia due to *Campylobacter cinaedi* in a patient infected with human immunodeficiency virus. Clin Infect Dis 15:178–179, 1992.
87. Anderson KF, Kiehlbauch JA, Anderson DC, et al: *Arcobacter (Campylobacter) butzleri*–associated diarrheal illness in a nonhuman primate population. Infect Immun 61:2220–2223, 1993.
88. Russell RG, Kiehlbauch JA, Gebhart CJ, DeTolla LJ: Uncommon *Campylobacter* species in infant *Macaca nemestrina* monkeys housed in a nursery. J Clin Microbiol 30:3024–3027, 1992.
89. Stamp S, Varoli O, Zanetti F, DeLuca G: *Arcobacter cryaerophilus* and thermophilic campylobacters in a sewage treatment plant in Italy: Two secondary treatments compared. Epidemiol Infect 110:633–639, 1993.
90. Neill SD, Ellis WA, Obrien JJ: The biochemical characteristics of *Campylobacter*-like organisms from cattle and pigs. Res Vet Sci 25:368–372, 1978.
91. Boudreau M, Higgins R, Mittal KR: Biochemical and serological characterization of *Campylobacter cryaerophilia.* J Clin Microbiol 29:54–58, 1991.
92. Kiehlbauch JA, Brenner DJ, Nicholson MA, et al: *Campylobacter butzleri* sp. nov. isolated from humans and animals with diarrheal illness. J Clin Microbiol 29:376–385, 1991.
93. Vandamme P, Pigina P, Benzi G, et al: Outbreak of recurrent abdominal cramps associated with *Arcobacter butzleri* in Italian school. J Clin Microbiol 30:2335–2337, 1992.
94. Lastovica AJ, Kirby R, Ambrosio RE: Clinical isolates of thermophilic *Campylobacter* spp. with no or weak catalase activity (Abstr). *In* Pearson AD, Skirrow MB, Lior H, Rowe B (eds): *Campylobacter* III. London, Public Health Laboratory Service, 1985, p 201.
95. Steele TW, Owen RJ: *Campylobacter jejuni* subspecies *doylei* (subsp. nov.), a subspecies of nitrate-negative campylobacters isolated from human clinical specimens. Int J Syst Bacteriol 38:316–318, 1988.
96. Firehammer BD: The isolation of vibrios from ovine feces. Cornell Vet 55:482–494, 1965.
97. Tanner ACR, Badger S, Lai CH, et al: *Wolinella* gen. nov., *Wolinella succinogenes (Vibrio succinogenes* Wolin et al.) comb. nov., and description of *Bacteroides gracilis* sp. nov., *Wolinella recta* sp. nov., *Campylobacter concisus* sp. nov., and *Eikenella corrodens* from humans with periodontal disease. Int J Syst Bacteriol 31:432–435, 1981.
98. Tanner ACR, Dzink JL, Ebersole JL, Socransky SS: *Wolinella recta, Campylobacter concisus, Bacteroides gracilis,* and *Eikenella corrodens* from periodontal lesions. J Periodont Res 22:327–330, 1987.
99. Badger SJ, Tanner ACR: Serological studies of *Bacteroides gracilis, Campylobacter concisus, Wolinella recta,* and *Eikenella corrodens,* all from humans with periodontal disease. Int J Syst Bacteriol 31:446–451, 1981.
100. Lastovica AJ, Le Roux E, Warren R, Klump H: Clinical isolates of *Campylobacter mucosalis.* J Clin Microbiol 31:2835–2836, 1993.
101. Vandamme P, Falsen E, Pot B, et al: Identification of EF group 22 campylobacters from gastroenteritis cases as *Campylobacter concisus.* J Clin Microbiol 27:1775–1781, 1989.
102. Lauwers S, Kevreker T, Van Etterijck R, et al: Isolation of *Campylobacter concisus* from human feces. Microbial Ecol Health Dis 4:S91, 1991.
103. Rams TE, Feik D, Slots J: *Campylobacter rectus* in human periodontitis. Oral Microbiol Immunol 8:230–235, 1993.
104. Tanner ACR, Listgarten MA, Ebersole JL: *Wolinella curva* sp. nov.: *"Vibrio succinogenes"* of human origin. Int J Syst Bacteriol 34:275–282, 1984.
105. Lawson GHK, Rowland AC: *Campylobacter sputorum* subsp. *mucosalis. In* Butzler JP (ed): *Campylobacter* Infection in Man and Animals. Boca Raton, FL, CRC Press, 1984, pp 207–225.

106. Megraud F, Elharrif Z: Isolation of *Campylobacter* species by filtration. Eur J Clin Microbiol 4:437–438, 1985.
107. Figura N, Guglielmetti P, Zanchi A, et al: Two cases of *Campylobacter mucosalis* enteritis in children. J Clin Microbiol 31:727–728, 1993.
108. Raffi F, Derriennic M, Michault A, et al: Infections humaines a *Campylobacter sputorum:* A propos de deux observations. Med Mal Infect 65–68, 1985.
109. Borczyk A, Lior H, McKeown A, Svendsen H: Isolations of *Campylobacter sputorum* associated with human infection (Abstr 211). *In* Kaijser B, Falsen E (eds): *Campylobacter* IV. Götenborg, Sweden, University of Götenborg, 1987, p 166.
110. On SL, Ridgewell F, Cryan B, Azadian BS: Isolation of *Campylobacter sputorum* biovar *sputorum* from an axillary abscess. J Infect 24:175–179, 1992.

77

Yersinia enterocolitica Infections

Edward J. Bottone

Yersinia enterocolitica, a gram-negative coccobacillus, was first isolated in the United States in 1934 by McIver and Pike[1] from a 53-year-old farm dweller with two facial abscesses. Although it was not fully characterized as *Y. enterocolitica* by these authors, retrospective examination of the isolate (which was on deposit at the New York State Department of Health) by Schleifstein and Coleman,[2] along with three additional isolates from enteric contents, led these investigators to propose the name *Bacterium enterocoliticum* for these previously unidentified microorganisms.[3] Interestingly, while the major emphasis in studying the basic microbiology and clinical manifestations of *Y. enterocolitica* and *Yersinia pseudotuberculosis* was taking place in European countries,[4] heightened awareness of *Y. enterocolitica* in the United States was propelled in 1976 by the food-borne outbreak of *Y. enterocolitica* gastrointestinal infection involving 222 subjects in upstate (Holland Patent) New York.[5]

The genus *Yersinia* is composed of 10 species, of which three, *Yersinia pestis* (plague bacillus), *Y. enterocolitica,* and *Y. pseudotuberculosis,* are well-recognized human pathogens. Whereas isolates of *Y. pestis* and *Y. pseudotuberculosis* are inherently pathogenic, virulence among *Y. enterocolitica* isolates is a function of biotype and serotype (see later).

Many of the basic microbiologic attributes of *Y. enterocolitica* are influenced by growth temperature. For instance, *Y. enterocolitica* is nonmotile at 37°C but motile at 25°C; acetylmethylcarbinol (Voges-Proskauer test) is produced at 25°C but not at 37°C; plasmid-encoded virulence factors are expressed at 37°C and lost at 25°C. Therefore, full characterization of an isolate as *Y. enterocolitica* should include tests determined at two incubation temperatures.[4]

Y. enterocolitica grows on a variety of bacteriologic media including enteric media used for the isolation of other enteric bacterial species. On these media, however, *Y. enterocolitica* produces pinpoint colonies after 24 hours of incubation and may be overlooked in clinical specimens (e.g., feces) containing a multiplicity of bacterial species. Thus, awareness of growth patterns on widely used enteric isolation media will aid recognition and recovery (Table 77–1). Although routine enteric media such as MacConkey agar support the growth of *Y. enterocolitica,* the use of cefsulodin-irgasan-novobiocin agar[5] greatly aids recovery when *Y. enterocolitica* is strongly suspected (see Table 77–1).

The stools of patients with acute gastroenteritis due to classic *Y. enterocolitica* serotypes (O3, O5,27, O8, O9) are productive of numerous colonies of *Y. enterocolitica* on routine isolation media.[6] However, in those instances when *Y. enterocolitica* is sought during convalescence from acute enteritis or for surveillance during an "outbreak," cold (4°C) enrichment of stool specimens in phosphate-buffered saline for up to 4 weeks with periodic subculture may enhance recovery.[7] *Y. enterocolitica* isolates recovered after prolonged cold enrichment should be biotyped and serotyped before clinical significance is ascribed to the isolate. In many instances, such isolates are of an environmental origin (biotype 1A) and lack virulence attributes.[6, 7]

Compared with *Y. pestis* and *Y. pseudotuberculosis, Y. enterocolitica* strains are biochemically heterogeneous, a characteristic that is linked to ecologic distribution, virulence potential, and serogroup designation. Biochemical characteristics distinguishing *Y. enterocolitica* from *Y. pseudotuberculosis* and *Y. pestis* and from closely related species are noted in Table 77–2. Biotyping schemas based on 12 biochemical reactions have been developed for *Y. enterocolitica* and revised by Wauters and colleagues[8] (Table 77–3). On the basis of these 12 reactions, six biogroups have been established that also correlate with human pathogenic potential (Table 77–4). In the United States, biotype 4, serotype O3 has emerged as the most frequently isolated serotype, exceeding serotype O8.[9] This trend was first noted in New York in the 1980s.[9–11] Wauters and coworkers[8] proposed six biogroups of *Y. enterocolitica,* with biogroup 6 being composed of strains designated biogroups 3A and 3B by Bercovier and colleagues.[12] Characterization of strains in biogroups 3A and 3B has led to species ascription as *Yersinia bercovieri* and *Yersinia mollaretii*[13] (see Table 77–2).

Y. enterocolitica isolates may be serologically typed by slide agglutination with rabbit antisomatic O antisera into 57 serotypes,[14] which, as noted before, correlate with human pathogenic strains and their ecologic distribution. Because cross-reactions may occur with other *Yersinia* species, and because some *Yersinia* isolates showing specific antigens were later reclassified as separate species, serotyping is useful in conjunction with biotyping as an index of the clinical significance of a *Y. enterocolitica* isolate. Further assessment of the

TABLE 77–1 ■ Colony Characteristics of *Yersinia enterocolitica* on Commonly Used Isolation Media

MEDIUM	GROWTH PATTERN
MacConkey agar	Pinpoint, colorless (pink), 24 h; 0.5–1.0 mm, 48 h
Hektoen enteric agar	Pinpoint, salmon colored due to sucrose fermentation; mimics "coliform" colonies
Xylose-lysine-deoxycholate agar	Pinpoint, yellow colonies due to xylose fermentation; mimics coliform colonies
Eosin–methylene blue agar	Pinpoint, lavender colonies with metallic sheen (48 h) due to sucrose fermentation; mimics colonies of *Escherichia coli*
Cefsulodin-irgasan-novobiocin agar	Red colonies with a transparent border 0.5–1.0 mm after 24 h at 25°C

TABLE 77–2 ■ Select Biochemical Tests Differentiating *Yersinia enterocolitica* from Closely Related Species*

	Yersinia							
TEST	***enterocolitica†***	***pseudotuberculosis***	***pestis***	***frederiksenii***	***intermedia***	***kristensenii***	***mollaretii***	***bercovieri***
Fermentation								
Glucose	+	+	+	+	+	+	+	+
Sucrose	+	0	0	+	+	0	+	+
Rhamnose	0	+	0	+	+	0	0	0
Raffinose	0	0	0	0	+	0	0	0
Melibiose	0	+	v	0	+	0	0	0
Cellobiose	+	0	0	+	+	+	+	+
Sorbose	v	0	0	+	+	+	+	0
Ornithine decarboxylase	+	0	0	+	+	+	+	+
Voges-Proskauer	+ (25°C)	0	0	+	+	0	0	0
Indole	v	0	0	+	+	v	0	0
Urease production	+	+	0	+	+	+	+	+
Motility (25°C)	+	+	0	+	+	+	+	+

*+, Positive; 0, negative; v, variable.
†Biotype 5 strains may vary in some reactions. See Table 77–3.

pathogenicity and epidemiology of a given *Y. enterocolitica* isolate may be achieved through bacteriophage typing, which also relates biotypes and serotypes to secondary autoimmune sequelae and epidemiologic distribution (Table 77–5).

Epidemiologically, until the late 1970s, most reports of *Y. enterocolitica* infections originated from Europe, with incipient reports appearing from South Africa,[17] Japan,[18] and the United States.[5] Today, however, as a consequence of heightened awareness by clinicians and microbiologists, *Y. enterocolitica* infections have been documented almost globally.[19] Whereas a cooler seasonal prevalence has long been recognized in European countries, such a correlation with cases has not been found in the United States or other countries.[19] It has been speculated that the frequency of infection is correlated with the porcine reservoir of pathogenic serotypes (O3, O5,27, O8, O9)[19a] and consumption of undercooked or raw pork products[20] or even their preparation.[21] Most sporadic infections with *Y. enterocolitica* cannot be traced to a specific vehicle, although ingestion of contaminated milk or other foods, contact with sick animals or index cases (?), and transfusion of contaminated blood seem to be the main routes of transmission and acquisition of this bacterial pathogen. At present, in the United States, most sporadic cases have been associated with serogroup O3 isolates[9, 11, 19]; five of seven common-source outbreaks have been caused by serogroup O8, and one each by serogroup O13a,13b and O3.[19, 21] Reasons accounting for serogroup O8 involvement in the majority of food-borne outbreaks in the United States may center on its innate virulence, which is analogous to that of *Salmonella typhi* among salmonellae.

Pathogenesis

The most common clinical manifestation of *Y. enterocolitica* infection ensues subsequent to ingestion of a pathogenic strain of the bacterium. Once ingested, virulent *Y. enterocolitica* traverse the host lumen through M cells,[22] which are especially abundant over Peyer patches in the terminal ileum, to gain access to the lamina propria. Studies in animal mod-

TABLE 77–3 ■ Biochemical Characteristics Used to Determine Biogroups of *Yersinia enterocolitica**

	BIOGROUP					
CHARACTERISTIC	**1A**	**1B†**	**2**	**3**	**4**	**5**
Lipase activity	+	+	0	0	0	0
Salicin (acid 24 h)	+	0	0	0	0	0
Esculin hydrolysis (24 h)	+/0	0	0	0	0	0
Xylose (acid production)	+	+	+	+	0	v
Trehalose (acid production)	+	+	+	+	+	0
Indole production	+	+	0	0	0	0
Ornithine decarboxylase	+	+	+	+	+	+(+)
Voges-Proskauer test	+	+	+	+	+	+(+)
Pyrazinamidase activity	+	0	0	0	0	0
Sorbose (acid production)	+	+	+	+	+	0
Inositol (acid production)	+	+	+	+	+	+
Nitrate reduction	+	+	+	+	+	0

*+, Positive; 0, negative; (+), delayed positive; v, variable.
†Biogroup 1B is composed mainly of strains isolated in the United States.
Modified from Wauters G, Kandolo K, Janssens M: Revised biogrouping scheme of *Yersinia enterocolitica*. Contrib Microbiol Immunol 9:14–21, 1987. S Karger, Basel, publisher.

TABLE 77–4 ■ Correlation of Pathogenic Potential of *Yersinia enterocolitica* with Biogroup, Serogroup, and Ecologic Distribution

ASSOCIATED WITH HUMAN INFECTIONS	BIOGROUP	SEROGROUPS	ECOLOGIC DISTRIBUTION
Yes	1B	O8; O4; O13a,13b; O18; O20; O21	Environment? Pig (O8) Mainly in the United States
	2	O9; O5,27	Pigs
	3	O1,2,3; O5,27	Chinchilla
	4	O3	Pigs
	5	O2,3	Hare
No*	1A	O5; O6,30; O7,8; numerous	Environment Food, water Animal and human feces

Y. enterocolitica isolates comprising biogroup 1A may be recovered from asymptomatic humans as commensals. These strains, however, may be opportunistic pathogens in patients with underlying disorders.

els with *Y. enterocolitica* serogroups O3 and O8 have established that the initial site of involvement is Peyer patches of the distal ileum, which results in the formation of microabscesses, ulceration of the overlying epithelium, and an inflammatory reaction.[23, 24] Infection subsequently spreads to the mesenteric lymph nodes, which may lead to abscesses in the medullary region and pain in the lower quadrant mimicking appendicitis. Acute enteritis with inflammatory cells and occasionally bloody, watery stools characterize infection in children. Furthermore, concomitant *Y. enterocolitica* bacteremia may be present in infants with enteritis.[11] In young adults, acute terminal ileitis and mesenteric adenitis are the more common presentations[25] (Table 77–6). Extensive ulceration of the intestinal tract and death have occurred in the course of *Y. enterocolitica* serotype O8 infection.[26, 27] *Y. enterocolitica* also produces a heat-stable enterotoxin, but its role in diarrheal disease is disputed because it is maximally produced below 30°C in late log-phase broth cultures.[28]

Although *Y. enterocolitica* is primarily a gastrointestinal tract pathogen, extraintestinal spread is a function of host

TABLE 77–5 ■ Correlation Between Serogroup, Biogroup, and Phage Type of Pathogenic *Yersinia enterocolitica* with Geographic Distribution and Secondary Sequelae of Infection*

GEOGRAPHIC DISTRIBUTION	SEROGROUP	BIOGROUP	PHAGE TYPE	SECONDARY SEQUELAE
United States	O8	1B	10†	No
	O3	4	9B	No
Canada	O3	4	9B	No
Europe	O3	4	8	Yes
	O9	2	10	Yes
Japan	O3	4	8	Rare[18]
South Africa	O3	4	9A	?‡

*Secondary sequelae are arthritis and erythema nodosum.
†New bacteriophage typing system developed.[15]
‡Probable but not definitive.[16]

TABLE 77–6 ■ Spectrum of *Yersinia enterocolitica* Infections

Gastrointestinal infections
- Enterocolitis, especially in young children; concomitant bacteremia may also be present
- Pseudoappendicitis syndrome (children older than 5 y; adults)
  - Acute mesenteric lymphadenitis
  - Terminal ileitis

Septicemia
- Especially in immunosuppressed individuals and those with iron overload or being treated with desferrioxamine
- Transfusion related

Metastatic infections after septicemia
- Focal abscesses: liver, kidney, spleen, lung
- Cutaneous manifestations: cellulitis, pyomyositis, pustules and bullous lesions
- Pneumonia, cavitary pneumonia
- Meningitis
- Panophthalmitis
- Endocarditis, infected mycotic aneurysm
- Osteomyelitis

Postinfection sequelae; associated with human leukocyte antigen B27
- Arthritis
- Myocarditis
- Glomerulonephritis
- Erythema nodosum

Pharyngitis

status and the pathogenic potential of the infecting strain. For instance, *Y. enterocolitica* serogroup O8 septicemia in a previously healthy 75-year-old individual mimicked typhoid fever in its presentation.[29] Secondary manifestations of bacteremia may involve every organ of the body including the central nervous system[30, 31] and may even lead to cutaneous lesions[30, 32] (see Table 77–6).

Peculiar to *Y. enterocolitica* is the increased occurrence of bacteremia in patients with iron overload or in those being administered desferrioxamine B, an iron-chelating agent.[33] *Y. enterocolitica* serotypes O3, O5,27, and O9, which are regarded as low-virulence species, require iron overload to cause septicemia or show animal lethality.[33] By way of contrast, highly virulent serotype O8 *Y. enterocolitica* does not require exogenous iron to cause septicemia or lethality in animals. The difference between these serotypes resides in the production under conditions of iron starvation of an iron-complexing siderophore and an outer membrane receptor for chelated iron by the highly pathogenic O8 serotype.[34] The gene coding for the iron-regulated synthesis of the outer membrane protein is absent in low-pathogenicity strains (e.g., O3),[34] necessitating their need for exogenous free or chelated iron.[33] Although it is not conclusive, the nonanimal lethal group of *Y. enterocolitica* has been shown to express an outer membrane protein of 82,000 daltons that cross-reacts serologically with the O8 siderophore and may serve a similar function in iron transport.[35]

Bacteremia with *Y. enterocolitica* may also occur by direct inoculation of *Y. enterocolitica* through contaminated blood for transfusion. Twenty-six cases of transfusion-associated *Y. enterocolitica* bacteremia have been documented since the first report in 1975[36] (personal review). The cases were predominantly associated with transfusion of packed red blood cells even of autologous origin[37] and resulted in shock in all and death in 14 of the 26 patients transfused. The source of *Y. enterocolitica* contamination was blood donors with asymptomatic bacteremia subsequent to an antecedent diarrheal episode.

Secondary nonsuppurative sequelae of *Y. enterocolitica* infection include polyarticular arthritis and erythema nodosum reported mainly among northern Europeans.[38–40] Polyarthritis onset is acute and is preceded by a history of fever and gastrointestinal disturbance. Symptoms of polyarthritis are manifested predominantly in weight-bearing joints (e.g., knees, ankles, and fingers). Joint involvement with pain and swelling occurs in rapid succession during a 2-week course. Synovial fluid may show a polymorphonuclear response, but although cultures are sterile, yersinial antigen may be present. Symptoms may persist for up to 4 months with a tendency toward chronicity in the absence of rheumatoid factor.[40] Predisposing factors for reactive arthropathy, but not erythema nodosum, include the presence of human leukocyte antigen B27 (in 80% of individuals).[41] In these patients, joint symptoms were more severe. Reiter syndrome,[41] myocarditis,[42] and glomerulonephritis[43] have also been reported as late sequelae in *Y. enterocolitica* infection. In glomerulonephritis, patients presented with proteinuria and hematuria, and *Yersinia* antigen complexed with immunoglobulin G and complement could be demonstrated in basement membranes by immunofluorescence.[44]

In Europe and northern European (Scandinavian) countries, *Y. enterocolitica* serotype O3, phage type 8, and serotype O9 are the common causes of yersiniosis. Phage type 8 isolates of serotype O3 are unique to Europe where the majority, if not all, secondary postinfectious sequelae occur, in contrast to Canada and South Africa, for example, where *Y. enterocolitica* serotype O3, phage types 9B and 9A, respectively, predominate but cases of reactive arthritis or other secondary sequelae have not been definitively documented.[4, 16]

Through serologic studies, *Y. enterocolitica* has also been associated with various thyroid disorders, including Graves disease, nontoxic goiter, and Hashimoto thyroiditis.[45] Antibody titers to serotype O3 *Y. enterocolitica* have been detected in up to 52% of patients with thyroid disorders in the United States[46] and Israel.[47] At the time of these studies, however, serotype O3 *Y. enterocolitica* had not yet emerged as a significant pathogen in the United States and was rarely encountered in Israel. These data suggest nonspecific serologic cross-reactions between *Y. enterocolitica* O3 or cross-reactivity with human thyrotropin receptor rather than a causal role for *Y. enterocolitica* in thyroid disorders.[48]

Virulence Factors

In concert with the plague bacillus *(Y. pestis)* and *Y. pseudotuberculosis,* human pathogenic strains of *Y. enterocolitica* possess a variety of plasmid- and chromosome-encoded virulence determinants. Those specified by a 70- to 75-kb plasmid are under exquisite temperature control, being expressed mainly at 37°C and in reduced copy number at 25°C.[49] Thus, with acquisition of the bacterium from an inanimate reservoir (e.g., food or water), adaptation to host temperature (37°C) results in synthesis of several virulence determinants that confer resistance to phagocytosis by polymorphonuclear leukocytes[50] and intracellular killing by macrophages[51] and resistance to serum bactericidal activity.[52] Also shared with *Y. pestis* and *Y. pseudotuberculosis* are plasmid-encoded V and W surface antigens, which may also provide antiphagocytic activity.[53]

Chromosomally encoded determinants include production of an outer membrane protein named invasin. When the gene *(inv)* encoding this surface component is introduced into a noninvasive *Escherichia coli,* invasiveness for several cultured epithelial cell lines is confered on the recipient.[54] The binding sites for invasin on host cells is a group of β_1 integrins.[55] Binding of *Y. enterocolitica* to these integrins results in cytoskeletal alteration of the host cell and internalization of the bacterium (parasite-mediated endocytosis).[55] Functional invasin is absent from *Y. pestis,* which gains access to host tissue by direct inoculation through a flea bite or by inhalation. Of significance is that invasin is maximally produced at 25°C, which may aid initial colonization of host tissues when the bacterium is obtained from an environmental source. Subsequent adaptation to 37°C triggers the plasmid-encoded virulence attributes and another chromosomally encoded outer membrane protein necessary to establish an infectious nidus in the human host. The latter surface component, which also confers invasiveness on *Y. enterocolitica,*[56] is coded by a specified chromosomal locus termed *ail* for the attachment/invasion locus. Presence of the *ail* gene also allows yersiniae to resist serum bactericidal activity.[57]

In contrast to *inv, ail* is expressed at 37°C and may therefore augment the initial invasive attribute contributed by *inv,* while the bacterium undergoes a thermal transition from ambient or refrigerated temperatures to host (37°C) temperature. The *ail* locus is commonly found among *Y. enterocolitica* serotypes associated with human infections and is absent from "environmental" isolates.[58]

Treatment

Surveys have shown that isolates of *Y. enterocolitica* are susceptible in vitro to trimethoprim-sulfamethoxazole, third-generation cephalosporins (ceftriaxone, cefotaxime, ceftizoxime, cefmenoxime, ceftazidime), aminoglycosides, imipenem, aztreonam, and quinolones.[59, 60] *Y. enterocolitica* isolates comprising serotypes O3 and O9 produce two distinct chromosomally encoded β-lactamases (A and B)[61] that inactivate a wide variety of penicillins and first-generation cephalosporins. Strains comprising serotype O5,27 produce only β-lactamase B, whereas serotype O8 isolates show resistance to ampicillin and cephalothin but to a lesser degree.[60] Despite antibiotic susceptibility to common agents (e.g., trimethoprim-sulfamethoxazole), there is still controversy over the need to treat uncomplicated *Y. enterocolitica* enteritis.[19, 25, 59] The mean duration of symptoms in untreated enteritis in children is 14 days.[62] In a placebo-controlled double-blind study of trimethoprim-sulfamethoxazole in *Y. enterocolitica* enteritis in children, Pai and coworkers[63] not only failed to show earlier resolution of symptoms but also showed prolongation (relapse) of bacteriologic cure as well. These investigators, however, began therapy late (11th or 12th day) in the course of enteritis of the 19 children studied. As they noted, treatment begun at the outset of symptoms might have had a different outcome. Worthy of consideration, however, is the concomitant *Yersinia* bacteremia that may occur in infants with enteritis.[11, 64]

Extraintestinal infection such as bacteremia in compromised hosts or in those with iron overload merits antiyersinial therapy. A retrospective analysis of 43 cases of bacteremia showed that third-generation cephalosporins in combination with other antibiotics resulted in a successful outcome in 85% of cases.[65] In this series, fluoroquinolones alone or in combination with an aminoglycoside or a third-generation cephalosporin were shown to be highly effective in 15 of 43 patients treated. Resolution of symptoms and of bacteremia ensued within 1 to 4 days. Older β-lactams failed in 18 cases; when used alone, amoxicillin-clavulanate failed in all of 6 cases. These authors concluded that all antibiotics active against aerobic gram-negative bacilli can be used for the treatment of *Y. enterocolitica* septicemia and that fluoroquinolones (pefloxacin, ofloxacin, ciprofloxacin) constitute the best treatment. Focal extraintestinal disease of liver, bones, joints, and central nervous system may require prolonged (3 weeks or more) therapy.

Prevention

Y. enterocolitica is widely distributed in terrestrial and freshwater ecosystems; it has been recovered from the intestinal tract of numerous mammalian species and from birds, insects, frogs, crabs, and oysters. In many instances, yersinial isolates recovered from these reservoirs are nonpathogenic members of biotype 1A. In terms of pathogenic serotypes, the pig is the only animal source clearly associated with serotypes O3, O5,27, and O9, especially in regions where the frequency of *Y. enterocolitica* infection is particularly elevated. To date, a clear-cut reservoir for the highly pathogenic serotype O8 strain has not been identified. Prevention of food-borne outbreaks requires adherence to known preventive measures (e.g., pasteurization, maintenance of sanitation policies for food-processing equipment, establishment of programs for minimizing contamination of finished products) as have been instituted for another food-borne pathogen, *Listeria monocytogenes*.[66] Avoiding contact with animal excreta in household or environmental settings may also reduce transmission.

References

1. McIver MA, Pike RM: Chronic glanders-like infection of face caused by an organism resembling *Flavobacterium pseudomallei.* Whitmore. *In* Clinical Miscellany, Mary Imogene Bassett Hospital, Cooperstown, New York, 1934, pp 16–20.
2. Schleifstein J, Coleman MB: An unidentified microorganism resembling *A. lignieri* and *Past. pseudotuberculosis* and pathogenic for man. N Y State J Med 39:1749, 1939.
3. Schleifstein J, Coleman MB: *Bacterium enterocoliticum.* Annual Report of Division of Laboratories and Research. Albany, NY, New York State Department of Health, 1943, p 56.
4. Bottone EJ: *Yersinia enterocolitica:* A panoramic view of a charismatic microorganism. Crit Rev Microbiol 5:211, 1977.
5. Black RE, Jackson RJ, Tsai T, et al: Epidemic *Yersinia enterocolitica* infection due to contaminated chocolate milk. N Engl J Med 298:76, 1978.
6. Van Noyen R, Vandepitte J, Wauters G: Nonvalue of cold enrichment of stools for isolation of *Yersinia enterocolitica* serotype 3 and 9 from patients. J Clin Microbiol 11:127, 1980.
7. Pai CH, Sorger S, Lafleur L, et al: Efficacy of cold enrichment techniques for recovery of *Yersinia enterocolitica* from human stools. J Clin Microbiol 9:70, 1979.
8. Wauters G, Kandolo K, Janssens M: Revised biogrouping scheme of *Yersinia enterocolitica*. Contrib Microbiol Immunol 9:14, 1987.
9. Bottone EJ: Current trends of *Yersinia enterocolitica* isolates in the New York City area. J Clin Microbiol 17:63, 1983.
10. Shayegani M, DeForge I, McGlynn DM, Root T: Characteristics of *Yersinia enterocolitica* and related species isolated from human, animal and environmental sources. J Clin Microbiol 14:304, 1981.
11. Bottone EJ, Gullans CR, Sierra MF: Disease spectrum of *Yersinia enterocolitica* serogroup 0:3, the predominant cause of human infection in New York City. Contrib Microbiol Immunol 9:56, 1987.
12. Bercovier H, Brault J, Barre N, et al: Biochemical, serological and phage types characteristics of 459 *Yersinia* strains isolated from a terrestrial ecosystem. Curr Microbiol 1:353, 1978.
13. Wauters GM, Janssens M, Steigerwalt AG, et al: *Yersinia mollaretii* sp. nov. and *Yersinia bercovieri* sp. nov., formerly called *Yersinia enterocolitica* biogroups 3A and 3B. Int J Syst Bacteriol 38:424, 1988.
14. Wauters G: Antigens of *Yersinia enterocolitica. In* Bottone EJ (ed): *Yersinia enterocolitica.* Boca Raton, FL, CRC Press, 1981, p 41.
15. Baker PM, Farmer JJ III: New bacteriophage typing system for *Yersinia enterocolitica, Yersinia kristensenii, Yersinia frederiksenii,* and *Yersinia intermedia:* Correlation with serotyping, biotyping and antibiotic susceptibility. J Clin Microbiol 15:491, 1982.
16. Robins-Browne RM, Rabson AR, Koornhoff HJ: *Yersinia enterocolitica* in South Africa. *In* Bottone EJ (ed): *Yersinia enterocolitca.* Boca Raton, FL, CRC Press, 1981, pp 193–203.
17. Rabson AR, Hallett AF, Koornhoff HJ: Generalized *Yersinia enterocolitica* infection. J Infect Dis 131:447, 1975.
18. Zen-Yoji H: Epidemiologic aspects of yersiniosis in Japan. *In* Bottone EJ (ed): *Yersinia enterocolitica.* Boca Raton, FL, CRC Press, 1981, pp 206–216.
19. Cover TL, Aber RC: *Yersinia enterocolitica.* N Engl J Med 321:16, 1989.

19a. Doyle MP, Hugdahl MB, Taylor SL: Isolation of virulent *Yersinia enterocolitica* from porcine tongues. Appl Environ Microbiol 42:661, 1981.

20. Tauxe RV, Vandepitte J, Wauters G, et al: *Yersinia enterocolitica* infections and pork: The missing link. Lancet 1:1129, 1987.
21. Lee LA, Gerber AR, Lonsway DR, et al: *Yersinia enterocolitica* infections in infants and children associated with the household preparation of chitterlings. N Engl J Med 322:984, 1990.
22. Grützkau A, Hanski C, Naumann M: Comparative study of histopathological alterations during intestinal infection of mice with pathogenic and non-pathogenic strains of *Yersinia enterocolitica* serotype O:8. Virchows Arch A Pathol Anat Histopathol 423:97, 1993.
23. Carter PB: Human *Yersinia enterocolitica* infection: Laboratory models. *In* Bottone EJ (ed): *Yersinia enterocolitica.* Boca Raton, FL, CRC Press, 1981, pp 74–81.
24. Robins-Browne RM, Tzopori S, Gonis G, et al: The pathogenesis of *Yersinia enterocolitica* infection in gnotobiotic piglets. J Med Microbiol 19:297, 1985.
25. Wormser GP, Keusch GT: *Yersinia enterocolitica:* Clinical observations. *In* Bottone EJ (ed): *Yersinia enterocolitica.* Boca Raton, FL, CRC Press, 1981, pp 83–93.
26. Gutman LT, Ottesen EA, Quan TJ, et al: An interfamilial outbreak of *Yersinia enterocolitica* enteritis. N Engl J Med 288:1372, 1973.
27. Bradford WD, Noce PS, Gutman LT: Pathologic features of enteric infection with *Yersinia enterocolitica.* Arch Pathol 98:17, 1974.
28. Boyce JM, Evans EJ Jr, Evans DG, DuPont HL: Production of heat-stable, methanol-soluble enterotoxin by *Yersinia enterocolitica.* Infect Immun 25:532, 1979.
29. Keet EE: *Yersinia enterocolitica* septicemia. Source of infection and incubation period identified. N Y State J Med 74:2226, 1974.
30. Sonnenwirth AC: Bacteremia with and without meningitis due to *Yersinia enterocolitica, Edwardsiella tarda, Commamonas terrigena,* and *Pseudomonas maltophilia.* Ann N Y Acad Sci 174:488, 1970.
31. Mary RS, Johnson JE III: *Yersinia enterocolitica* meningitis with septicemia and spontaneous peritonitis. N C Med J 40:691, 1979.
32. Olbrych TG, Zarconi J, File TM Jr, et al: Bullous skin lesions associated with *Yersinia enterocolitica* septicemia. Am J Med Sci 287:38, 1984.
33. Robins-Browne RM, Prpic JK: Effects of iron and desferrioxamine on infections with *Yersinia enterocolitica.* Infect Immun 43:108, 1985.
34. Carniel E, Mercereau-Puijalon O, Bonnefoy S: The gene coding for the 190,000 dalton iron-regulated protein of *Yersinia* species is present only in highly pathogenic strains. Infect Immun 57:1211, 1989.
35. Heesemann J, Hantke K, Vocke T, et al: Virulence of *Yersinia enterocolitica* is closely associated with siderophore production expression of an iron-repressible outer membrane polypeptide of 65,000 Da and pesticin sensitivity. Mol Microbiol 8:397, 1993.
36. Bruining A, DeWilde-Beekhuizen CCM: A case of contamination of donor blood by *Yersinia enterocolitica* type 9. Medilon 4:30, 1975.
37. Haditsch M, Binder C, Gabriel C, et al: *Yersinia enterocolitica* septicemia in autologous blood transfusion. Transfusion 34:907, 1994.
38. Ahvonen P, Sievers K, Aho K: Arthritis associated with *Yersinia enterocolitica* infection. Acta Rheumatol Scand 15:232, 1969.
39. Laitenen O, Tuuhea J, Ahvonen P: Polyarthritis associated with *Yersinia enterocolitica* infection. Clinical features and laboratory findings in nine cases with severe joint symptoms. Ann Rheum Dis 31:34, 1972.
40. Winblad S: Arthritis associated with *Yersinia enterocolitica* infections. Scand J Infect Dis 7:191, 1975.
41. Laitinen O, Leirisalo M, Skylv G: Relation between HLA-B27 and clinical features in patients with *yersinia* arthritis. Arthritis Rheum 20:1121, 1977.
42. Agner E, Larsen JH, Leth A: *Yersinia enterocolitica* carditis as a differential diagnosis—And the prognosis of this disease. Scand J Rheumatol 7:26, 1979.

43. Denneberg T, Friedberg M, Samuelsson T, Winblad S: Glomerulonephritis in infections with *Yersinia enterocolitica* O–serotype 3. I. Evidence for glomerular involvement in acute cases of yersiniosis. Acta Med Scand 209:97, 1981.
44. Friedberg M, Denneberg T, Brun C, et al: Glomerulonephritis in infections with *Yersinia enterocolitica* O–serotype 3. II. The incidence and immunological features of *Yersinia* infection in a consecutive glomerulonephritis population. Acta Med Scand 209:103, 1981.
45. Bech K, Nerup J, Larsen JH: *Yersinia enterocolitica* infection and thyroid diseases. Acta Endocrinol 84:87, 1977.
46. Shenkman L, Bottone EJ: Antibodies to *Yersinia enterocolitica* in thyroid disease. Ann Intern Med 85:735, 1976.
47. Weiss M, Rubinstein E, Bottone EJ, et al: *Yersinia enterocolitica* antibodies in thyroid disorders. Isr J Med Sci 15:553, 1979.
48. Toivanen P, Toivanen A: Does *Yersinia* induce autoimmunity? Int Arch Allergy Immunol 104:107, 1994.
49. Straley SC, Skrzypek E, Plano GV, Bliska JB: Yops of *Yersinia* spp. pathogenic for humans. Infect Immun 61:3105, 1993.
50. Lian C, Hwang WS, Pai CH: Plasmid-mediated resistance to phagocytosis in *Yersinia enterocolitica.* Infect Immun 55:1176, 1987.
51. Une T: Studies on the pathogenicity of *Yersinia enterocolitica.* II. Interaction with cultured cells in vitro. Microbiol Immunol 21:365, 1977.
52. Pai CH, DeStephano L: Serum resistance associated with virulence in *Yersinia enterocolitica.* Infect Immun 35:605, 1982.
53. Perry RD, Brubaker RR: Vwa^{+} phenotype of *Yersinia enterocolitica.* Infect Immun 40:166, 1983.
54. Isberg RR, Falkow S: A single genetic locus encoded by *Yersinia pseudotuberculosis* permits invasion of cultured animal cells by *Escherichia coli* K-12. Nature 317:262, 1985.
55. Isberg RR, Leong JM: Multiple β_1 chain integrins and receptors for invasin, a protein that promotes bacterial penetration into mammalian cells. Cell 60:861, 1990.
56. Miller VL, Falkow S: Evidence for two genetic loci from *Yersinia enterocolitica* that can promote invasion of epithelial cells. Infect Immun 56:1242, 1988.
57. Brett SJ, Mazorov AV, Charles IG, et al: Bacterial resistance to complement killing mediated by the Ail protein of *Yersinia enterocolitica.* Proc Natl Acad Sci USA 89:3561, 1992.
58. Miller VL, Farmer JJ III, Hill WE, et al: The *ail* locus is found uniquely in *Yersinia enterocolitica* serotypes commonly associated with disease. Infect Immun 57:121, 1989.
59. Hoogkamp-Korstanje JA: Antibiotics in *Yersinia enterocolitica* infections. J Antimicrob Chemother 20:123, 1987.
60. Hornstein MJ, Jupeau AM, Scavizzi MR, et al: In vitro susceptibilities of 126 clinical isolates of *Yersinia enterocolitica* to 21 beta-lactam antibiotics. Antimicrob Agents Chemother 27:807, 1985.
61. Cornelis G: Distribution of beta-lactamases A and B in some groups of *Yersinia enterocolitica* and their role in resistance. J Gen Microbiol 91:391, 1975.
62. Marks MI, Pai CH, Lafleur L, et al: *Yersinia enterocolitica* gastroenteritis: A prospective study of clinical, bacteriologic, and epidemiologic features. J Pediatr 96:26, 1980.
63. Pai CH, Gillis F, Tuomanen E, et al: Placebo-controlled double-blind evaluation of trimethoprim-sulfamethoxazole treatment of *Yersinia enterocolitica* gastroenteritis. J Pediatr 104:308, 1984.
64. Shapiro ED: *Yersinia enterocolitica* septicemia in normal infants. Am J Dis Child 135:477, 1981.
65. Gayraud M, Scavizzi MR, Mollaret HH, et al: Antibiotic treatment of *Yersinia enterocolitica* septicemia: A retrospective review of 43 cases. Clin Infect Dis 17:405, 1993.
66. Tappero JW, Schuchat A, Deaver RA, et al: Reduction in the incidence of human listeriosis in the United States. Effectiveness of prevention efforts? JAMA 273:1118, 1995.

78

Cholera and Related Illnesses Caused by *Vibrio* Species and *Aeromonas*

David A. Sack

Cholera is an acute diarrheal disease that, in severe cases, can lead to such massive fluid loss that normal, healthy people die of dehydration and shock within a few hours. In developing countries, epidemics can occur in massive outbreaks, leading to thousands of cases and deaths in a few days or weeks. Thus, cholera has earned respect as one of the great epidemic diseases. Cholera is caused by enterotoxigenic strains of *Vibrio cholerae* belonging to serogroup O1 or O139. These strains are members of the Vibrionaceae family, along with other serogroups of *V. cholerae* and other species of *Vibrio*, as well as *Aeromonas* spp. and *Plesiomonas shigelloides.* The pathogenic species of *Vibrio* include *V. mimicus, V. vulnificus, V. fluvialis, V. parahaemolyticus, V. hollisae, V. furnissii, V. alginolyticus, V. metschnikovii, V. damsela,* and *V. cincinnatiensis.* Formerly, the vibrios were simply classified as either *V. cholerae* O1, with epidemic potential, or nonagglutinating vibrios, which were unlikely to spark an epidemic. Now it is clear that many of the vibrio strains have characteristic pathogenic patterns and need to be speciated beyond simply carrying out agglutination tests with the O1 antiserum.

The vibrios share several common features. They are all motile, gram-negative, rod-shaped organisms with a single polar flagellum. Their natural habitat is environmental waters, and their spread and epidemic patterns are highly linked to the ecologic changes of the water in which they persist. Thus, in temperate climates, they are more common during the warmer summer months, when they can be isolated from water, plankton, and shellfish. Most infections in humans occur during this time. In tropical areas, their seasonality is more complex, as transmission may occur throughout the year. Halophilic (salt-loving) species require salt for growth and are generally isolated from saltwater sources. As with the illness caused by *V. cholerae* O1, most of the illnesses caused by the vibrios are diarrheal; however, certain species, especially *V. vulnificus,* may cause bacteremia and wound infections. The pathogenicity of *Aeromonas* spp. and *P. shigelloides* is less certain, but these bacteria probably cause diarrheal illness in some cases and rarely also lead to systemic infections.

Vibrio cholerae O1 and O139

History

Cholera has been endemic to the Indian subcontinent and other parts of the world for centuries. It was inadvertently introduced into Europe in 1817 during the age of colonial expansion. Subsequently, it spread around the world in successive pandemics and reached U.S. port cities in the mid-1800s. Cholera even followed pioneers across the American

West, contaminating the drinking water of the wagon trains. The current seventh pandemic, involving *V. cholerae* biotype el tor, serogroup O1, began in Indonesia in 1961 and is continuing in Asia and Africa. A focus of infection continues on the Gulf Coast of the United States even without environmental contamination with sewage.[1] In most years, a few persons who eat undercooked seafood from the Gulf Coast in August develop cholera.[2]

There have been two more recent landmarks in the history of cholera. First, Latin America had remained free of cholera for 100 years until 1991, when cholera appeared in Peru and subsequently spread to nearly all other Latin American countries.[3] After initial epidemics, the number of Latin American cases has dropped. By 1997, cholera had not spread to any of the Caribbean islands.

Second, in 1992, a new serogroup of epidemic cholera—*V. cholerae* O139—appeared in Bangladesh and India along the Bay of Bengal.[4] Previously, all epidemic strains of cholera belonged to serogroup O1, but this new strain caused epidemics like previous epidemics with serogroup O1. Because of its association with the Bay of Bengal, it was given the name *V. cholerae* O139 (synonym Bengal). Scientists are monitoring this new strain to determine whether it will continue its expansion outside Asia, invade other regions, and become the eighth pandemic strain.[5, 6]

Because of its high case-fatality rates, physicians throughout history desperately attempted to develop effective treatments. Unfortunately, these treatments had more to do with the popular medical philosophy of the day than with a reasonable approach to the disease. In the 19th century, cholera was treated with bleeding, laxatives, enemas, and a variety of herbs, and the therapy undoubtedly contributed to high case-fatality rates. Even Osler's textbook advocated injections of morphine, ice by mouth, brandy, and tannic acid enemas. A few physicians, however, realized that the key event of cholera was loss of fluids and attempted to replace them with intravenous fluids. For example, Latta[7] used intravenous saline as early as 1831[8] and a few of his patients survived, but sterile fluids and supplies were not available then, and case-fatality rates remained high, with many deaths caused by sepsis.

By the early 1900s, Rogers,[8a] working in Calcutta, began using improved intravenous fluids to treat cholera and gradually the case-fatality rates began to decrease. Still, the case-fatality rates did not reach their current low level of less than 1% until the 1960s, when physicians learned to use isotonic intravenous fluids that approximated the electrolyte composition of the diarrhea stool being lost. The development of rational intravenous fluids saved patients who were able to get this treatment,[9, 10] but the important public health breakthrough came with the development of oral rehydration fluids in the late 1960s in Calcutta and Dhaka.[11, 12]

In terms of etiology, Snow[13] in 1855 first described the relation between risk of cholera and the use of contaminated water and hypothesized the presence of a toxin that was being spread by way of water. Koch is generally credited with discovering the bacterium in 1884, although Pacini may have found the *Vibrio* as early as 1854. Regardless of this earlier claim, Koch's discovery quickly led to an appreciation of the infectious nature of the disease. Within a year, scientists developed a killed, whole-cell injectable vaccine, variations of which were widely used for many decades and which is still available—even though its use is discouraged.

Epidemiology

Cholera is spread by eating or drinking contaminated food or water. In common-source outbreaks, a specific food[14] or water supply can often be identified; however, the two sources usually overlap, because market food is often washed with contaminated water or leftover food is mixed with water. Because the environmental reservoir for *Vibrio* is water and shellfish, seafood has often been implicated, especially in the United States, where other vehicles are not present.[15] In endemic areas, many foods and water sources can spread the bacterium.

The risk of cholera in the United States and other industrialized countries is small. A few cases have resulted from contaminated seafood from the Gulf Coast,[15] and a few cases have resulted from imported food.[16, 17] Thus, cholera is primarily a disease of developing countries in areas where water and hygiene are substandard. Internationally, cholera is a reportable disease; however, the true global disease burden from cholera remains uncertain. On the basis of sample reporting, there are an estimated 6 million cases of cholera per year, associated with about 600,000 hospitalizations and about 120,000 deaths in the world.[18] Unfortunately, the national stigma associated with cholera and the fear of economic reprisals lead many countries in Asia and Africa to avoid reporting cases, so it has not been possible to detect trends in cholera epidemiology outside the Americas. Figure 78–1 shows the spread of *V. cholerae* O139 in Asia (*A*) and O1 in Latin America (*B*).

Cholera can be divided, somewhat arbitrarily, into endemic cholera and epidemic cholera. In areas with endemic cholera, such as the Ganges delta, cholera occurs regularly, with most cases appearing during cholera seasons. In some areas, two seasons are seen each year, whereas in other regions a single peak season is observed. In Asia, the highest rate of cholera occurs in childhood; naturally acquired immunity protects older individuals from the high illness rates seen in childhood.[19] Still, most cases are seen in older children and adults because they represent a much larger segment of the population.[20, 21] In Latin America, case rates have remained highest in adult men, perhaps because of increased exposure, even though cholera has become endemic.

Epidemic cholera occurs among populations who have had no previous exposure to cholera but become exposed suddenly. The explosive outbreaks of cholera in Africa caused by contaminated water sources, especially in refugee camps, are examples of epidemic cholera.[22, 23] Incidence rates and fatality rates in these epidemics are generally high because the population has little immunity and facilities for case management are not developed.

Certain factors have been identified that increase the risk of cholera infection and, in those who become infected, increase the disease's severity. Because vibrios are acid sensitive, hypochlorhydria, antacids, and gastric resection increase the risk of developing cholera.[24–28] For reasons that are not understood, persons with blood group O are at higher risk for el tor cholera (but not classic cholera) than persons with other blood groups.[29–31] Breast-feeding has a strong protective effect, and cholera is rare in infants who are nursing. Although nursing infants have less exposure to pathogens, the breast milk itself is protective.[32, 33]

Pathogenesis

Cholera occurs when the bacterium is ingested in sufficient numbers to pass through the gastric acid barrier and enter the small intestine, where they colonize the upper small intestine. Colonization is facilitated by colonization pili, of which two types have been described: toxin-coregulated pilus[34] and mannose-sensitive hemagglutinin pilus[35, 36] (Fig. 78–2).

When they have colonized the intestine, the bacteria secrete cholera toxin, a protein (molecular weight 84,000) with a central active (A) subunit surrounded by five binding (B)

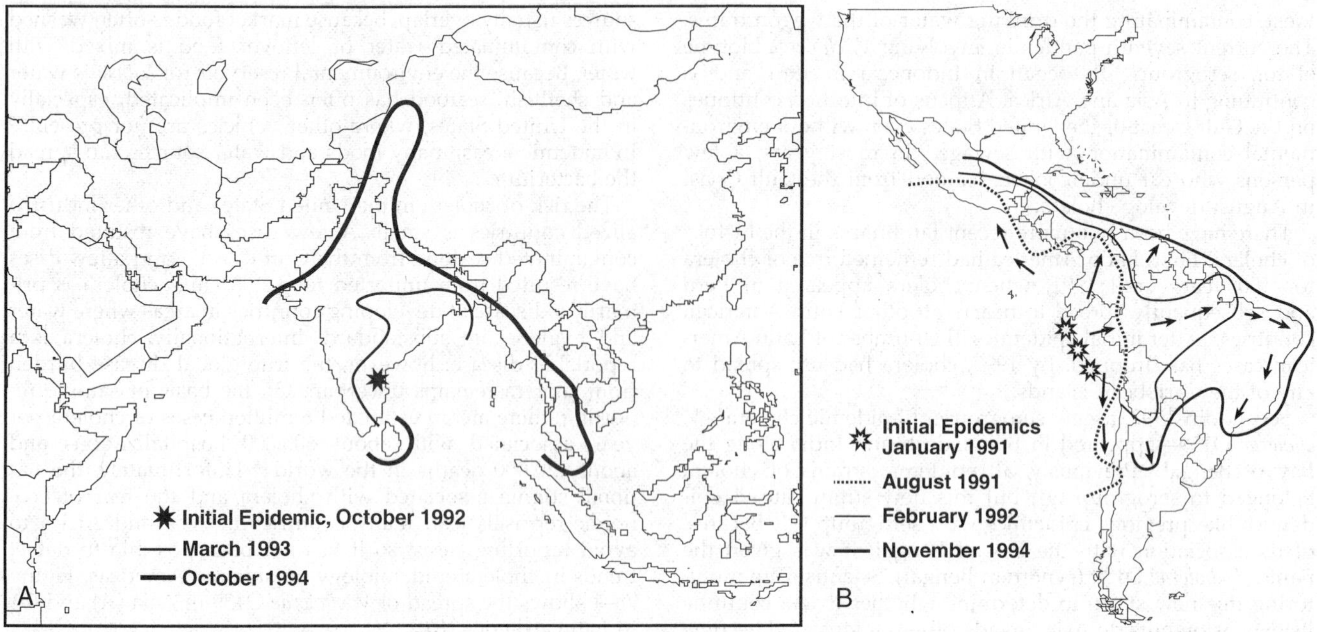

FIGURE 78–1 □ Map of the spread of *V. cholerae* O139 (synonym Bengal) through Asia *(A)* and of *V. cholerae* biotype el tor through South America *(B)*. (Data provided by the Centers for Disease Control and Prevention, Atlanta.)

subunits (Figs. 78–3 and 78–4). The B subunit attaches irreversibly to its mucosal cell receptor, G_{M1} ganglioside, which makes up part of all mammalian cell membranes. The A subunit is injected into the cell, and in a process involving stimulation of adenylate cyclase, it leads to the secretion of chloride and water.[37–39] The rate of fluid secretion overwhelms the reabsorptive capacity of the small and large intestines and the net secretions pass out as watery diarrhea. Although the functions of the mucosal cells are disturbed by the biochemical changes, the mucosa is not inflamed and there is no cytotoxic effect. Cholera toxin is similar in structure and function to a toxin of *Escherichia coli* called heat-labile toxin, and antibodies to cholera toxin also neutralize heat-labile toxin.

The volume and biochemical characteristics of the diarrhea fluid are important to the pathogenesis of cholera and its complications, because all of the signs and symptoms of cholera are explained by the loss of this fluid. The diarrhea fluid is an isotonic filtrate of serum that is modified only by exchange mechanisms that can take place before the fluid is excreted; in severe cases the transit time is so short that there is little time for exchange of electrolytes. Thus, the cholera stool contains a high concentration of sodium and bicarbonate and a low concentration of potassium, similar to serum.[40] Because the mucosa is not inflamed, the stool contains little protein. Thus, the effect of the toxin is to induce the rapid loss of an isotonic, alkaline fluid, and because the loss occurs rapidly, the fluid comes from the circulating and extracellular spaces. This results in dehydration, hypovolemia, hemoconcentration, potassium deficiency, and metabolic acidosis.[9, 41]

Clinical Manifestations

The spectrum of severity in cholera varies tremendously. Some individuals infected with this bacterium may experience no symptoms and some have mild diarrhea, whereas others develop severe, dehydrating watery diarrhea and excrete large volumes of nonbloody rice-water stool. The latter

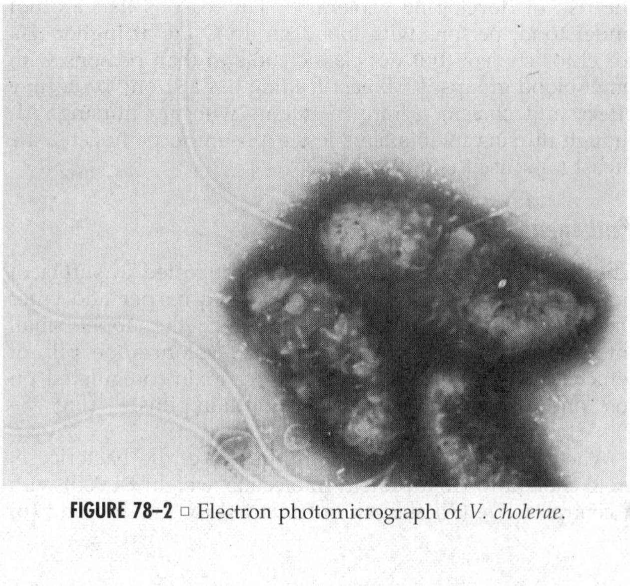

FIGURE 78–2 □ Electron photomicrograph of *V. cholerae.*

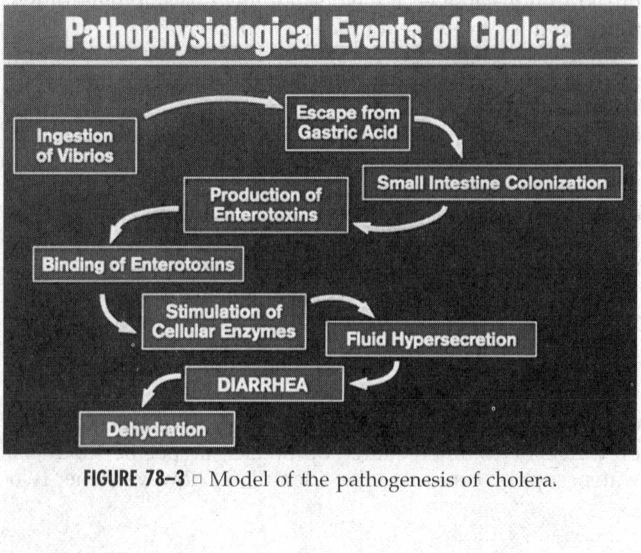

FIGURE 78–3 □ Model of the pathogenesis of cholera.

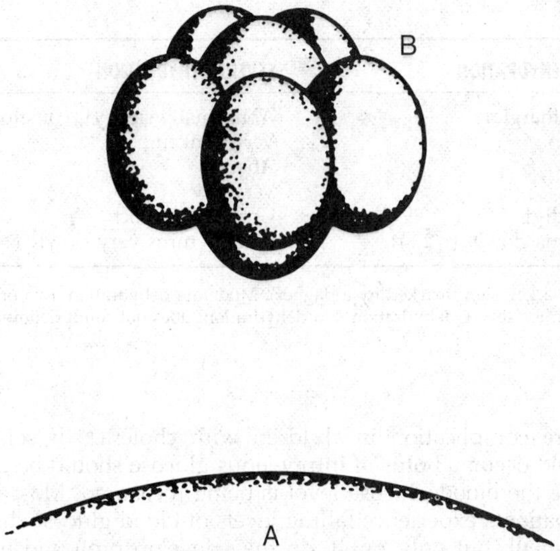

FIGURE 78–4 □ Model of cholera toxin showing the five binding (B) subunits surrounding a single active (A) subunit.

syndrome, often called cholera gravis, is a life-threatening condition in which perfectly healthy persons can become moribund and die within a few hours.[42, 43] These severely affected patients generally have associated symptoms of nausea, vomiting, and muscle cramps and signs of shock. Volumes of stools may exceed 1 L/h in adults or more than 10 mL/kg per hour in children. As the fluid loss continues, dehydration progresses, the radial pulse becomes weak, the blood pressure drops to undetectable levels, the mental status becomes depressed, and coma ensues. Gasping hyperventilation frequently occurs because of metabolic acidosis. If cholera gravis is left untreated, at least 50% of patients with it die, yet almost all of these patients survive if given effective rehydration therapy.

Diagnosis

Cholera should be suspected in persons with severe watery diarrhea, especially if they live in a cholera endemic area, have just returned from a cholera endemic area, or have eaten high-risk foods during the warm months. Except for travelers returning from cholera endemic areas[44] and a few exceptional cases resulting from imported contaminated foods,[16, 45] all U.S. cases occur in the summer (usually August) after consumption of shellfish from the Gulf of Mexico. In the United States, fecal specimens from all suspected cases should be cultured for vibrios, generally using thiosulfate citrate bile salts sucrose (TCBS) agar.[46] Positive isolates should be reported immediately to the state health department and the isolate should be sent for confirmation. Highly sensitive and specific rapid diagnostic kits* that detect vibrio cell wall antigen directly in stool are now available.[47, 48]

In cholera endemic areas, the diagnosis of new cases in the region should be confirmed with stool cultures, and a sample surveillance system is advisable to confirm a proportion of cases. During epidemics, most patients who have cholera symptoms do in fact have cholera, and culture confirmation of every case is not necessary. Cultures from a systematic sample of cases are useful for monitoring antibiotic sensitivity patterns, which can change during an epidemic season.

Patients with cholera develop a serologic response. If confirmation of the diagnosis is needed, acute serum and convalescent serum samples show a fourfold increase in vibriocidal antibodies.[46]

**V. cholerae* SMART kits, New Horizons Diagnostics, Columbia, Maryland.

Treatment

Treatment of cholera consists of rehydration therapy and antibiotics. Of these, rehydration is by far the more important because even severely affected patients survive without antibiotics but not without rehydration. To rehydrate appropriately, the hydration status of the patient is first assessed and a determination of the degree of dehydration is made.[49] The stage of dehydration is generally categorized as not dehydrated, some dehydration, or severely dehydrated. For severely dehydrated patients, intravenous fluids with Ringer lactate (or another suitable polyelectrolyte solution) are given to rapidly (e.g., in 2 to 4 hours) correct the fluid deficit.[9, 10, 50] This requires a large-bore needle and may require more than one infusion at a time. Severely dehydrated patients are assumed to have lost 10% of their body weight and this volume needs to be replaced. Thus, a 50-kg patient needs 5 L of Ringer lactate. Moderately dehydrated patients can generally be rehydrated with oral rehydration solution (ORS) and are assumed to have lost 7.5% of their body weight.[49] Those without signs of dehydration are not critically ill, but signs of dehydration do not appear until more than 5% of the body weight has been lost. Thus, those who have watery stools and are suspected of having cholera should be rehydrated with ORS, with volumes to approximate 5% of the body weight.

Clinical criteria (Table 78–1) are used to determine the state of dehydration, but laboratory tests can be used to confirm the patient's condition. The laboratory changes include a raised plasma protein level and raised hematocrit (resulting from hemoconcentration) and a lowered serum bicarbonate value (resulting from the metabolic acidosis). The potassium concentration generally remains in the normal range, but it falls as acidosis is corrected during rehydration unless potassium is included in the rehydration fluids.

While the patient is being rehydrated, continuing stool losses are noted, and equivalent volumes of ORS are provided to replace these ongoing losses.[49] If possible, a cholera cot (a camping cot with a hole cut beneath the buttock area to allow stool to pass into a bucket underneath) is used to facilitate the monitoring of these ongoing losses. The patient's hydration status must be monitored especially carefully during the critical first 24 hours, and occasional passing of urine is a helpful sign of hydration. Table 78–2 shows the composition of cholera stool and of rehydration solutions.

ORS is generally prepared from packets, although some prepare it from locally available ingredients. The composition of ORS is shown in Table 78–2. ORS that contains 40 to 80 g of rice in place of 20 g of glucose per liter is superior for cholera patients, in that the purging rate and duration of diarrhea are lessened by about 30% to 40%.[51, 52] Commercial preparations of rice ORS* are now available.

Oral antibiotics are given to kill the *Vibrio* and thus to decrease the duration of the illness.[49, 53–55] They should be given as early in the illness as possible, although a few hours delay may be needed to rehydrate and to allow vomiting to cease. A single dose of doxycycline, 300 mg, is effective against sensitive strains. Resistant strains also frequently cause epidemics, and alternative antibiotics (e.g., ciprofloxacin, as a 1-g single dose[55a]) may be needed.[56–59] These are shown in Table 78–3.

*CeraLyte, Cera Products, Columbia, Maryland.

TABLE 78–1 ■ Signs and Symptoms of Dehydration in Patients with Acute Diarrhea*

SIGN OR SYMPTOM	NO DEHYDRATION	MODERATE DEHYDRATION	SEVERE DEHYDRATION
Level of consciousness	Normal alert	Irritable, lethargic†	Abnormally sleepy†, comatose†
Eyes	Normal	Sunken	Very sunken
Tears (in children)	Present	Absent	Absent
Mucous membranes	Moist	Dry	Very dry
Thirst (tested)	Normal	Drinks avidly†	Unable to drink†
Skin pinch	Normal	Pinch returns slowly (<2 s)†	Pinch returns very slowly (>2 s)†

*Severe dehydration: two or more signs in the fourth column, at least one of which is a key sign (marked by a dagger). Moderate dehydration: two or more signs in the third column (including one with a dagger) but does not fulfill the definition for severe dehydration. No dehydration: does not fulfill definition for moderate or severe; no signs of dehydration.

Complications

ORS Failure. After initial rehydration, a few patients with severe cholera again become dehydrated even while being given ORS. This is generally due to severe vomiting and severe purging in excess of oral intake. For example, if the purging rate exceeds 10 mL/kg per hour, it is difficult to administer sufficient ORS to maintain hydration.[60] Likewise, vomiting in some patients prevents efficient oral replacement. In these cases, the patients should be rehydrated again with intravenous fluids.

Renal Failure. Acute tubular necrosis can occur if rehydration is insufficient (e.g., if fluid replacement prevents death but does not correct the shock). These patients need to be rehydrated to reestablish the circulating volume, but their potassium levels need to be monitored to avoid hyperkalemia. Occasionally, dialysis may be needed, but usually the renal failure is reversible.

Cholera Sicca. Signs of dehydration and shock can occur in the absence of severe purging when fluid collects in the intestine without being expelled. The abdominal swelling and shock can be mistaken for an acute surgical emergency. Treatment is the same as with other severe cases: replacement of fluids.

Hypokalemia. Hypokalemia may occur if potassium is not adequately replaced. Symptoms include abdominal distention and ileus, urinary retention, and cardiac arrhythmias.

Pulmonary Edema. This may result from overhydration with intravenous fluids. It is more likely if saline rather than Ringer lactate is used, because the acidosis is not corrected.

Hypoglycemia. Hypoglycemia, manifested by seizures, is a rare complication in children with cholera.[60] If seizures should occur, a bolus of intravenous glucose should be given while the blood glucose level is being measured. Most cholera patients experience falling levels of blood glucose during treatment, but only rarely do they develop profound hypoglycemia.

Abortion and Premature Delivery. Pregnant women with cholera frequently abort or deliver prematurely, apparently because of placental circulatory insufficiency.[61] Rapid rehydration decreases the likelihood of this complication. Centers that see many cases of cholera need to make provisions for delivering premature infants.

Fever and Chills. These are not a part of the cholera syndrome, but if they occur, pyrogens in the intravenous fluid or an intravenous line infection is the most likely cause.

Prevention

Improvements in water quality and sanitation are the long-term strategies for prevention. As these goals cannot be realized quickly, persons traveling in cholera areas should use boiled or bottled water and avoid high-risk foods and drinks (e.g., raw seafood, foods from street vendors, and drinks with ice).

Oral vaccines are becoming available in Europe and may be available soon in other parts of the world, and they will be recommended for persons traveling to cholera endemic areas. Two types of vaccines have been developed[62]: a killed oral vaccine[21, 63–65] and a live attenuated vaccine.[66, 67] Both are safe and effective and provide significant protection for several years. The currently available killed injectable vaccine is

TABLE 78–2 ■ Electrolyte Composition of Cholera Stool in Adults and Children and of Solutions Used to Rehydrate Cholera Patients

	CONCENTRATION (mmol/L)					
MATERIAL	Na^+	K^+	Cl^-	HCO_3^-	Citrate	Carbohydrate
Cholera stool						
Adults	135	15	100	45		—
Children	105	25	90	30		—
Rehydration fluid						
Cereal ORS (for oral use)*	90	20	80		10†	20–50
Glucose ORS (for oral use)*	90	20	80		10	111
Ringer lactate (for IV‡ use)	131	4	111		29	—
Dhaka solution (for IV use)	133	13	98		48	—
Normal saline (for IV use)§	154	—	154		—	—

*Glucose oral rehydration solution (ORS) contains (per liter) NaCl, 3.5 g; KCl, 1.5 g; trisodium citrate, 2.9 g; and glucose, 20 g. This has a total osmolality of 311 mOsm. The electrolytes in cereal ORS are the same, but the glucose is replaced by a cereal (e.g., rice) 40–80 g/L. Cereal ORS has a total osmolality of about 220–250.

†Either sodium bicarbonate, 2.5 g (which provides 30 mmol of bicarbonate), or trisodium citrate, 2.9 g (which provides 10 mmol of citrate), can be used as the base. The World Health Organization prefers citrate.

‡IV, Intravenous.

§Use normal saline only for patients in shock when Ringer solution or another polyelectrolyte solution is not available. Immediately start ORS to replace potassium and base, which are not included in saline.

TABLE 78–3 ■ Antimicrobial Agents Used in the Treatment of Cholera*

ANTIBIOTIC	ADULT DOSE	PEDIATRIC DOSE
Doxycycline	300 mg single dose† or 100 mg bid for 3 d	
Tetracycline	500 mg qid for 3 d	12.5 mg/kg qid for 3 d‡
Furazolidone	100 mg qid for 3 d§	1.25 mg/kg qid for 3 d
TMP-SMX	TMP at 160 mg + SMX at 800 mg bid for 3 d	TMP at 5 mg/kg + SMX at 25 mg/kg bid for 3 d‖
Ciprofloxacin¶	250 mg bid for 3 d	Not approved for children

*bid, Twice daily; qid, four times daily; TMP-SMX, trimethoprim-sulfamethoxazole.
†The drug of choice for most situations because a single dose can be used.
‡Be aware of policies against using tetracycline for children in whom teeth staining can occur.
§Furazolidone is the drug of choice for pregnant women.
‖TMP-SMX is the preferred drug for children.
¶Reserve for strains resistant to all other antibiotics.

not recommended because of local inflammatory reactions, short duration of protection (6 months), and low level of protection (50%).

Prophylactic antibiotics are sometimes used during cholera outbreaks when the strain is tetracycline sensitive. If used, a single dose of doxycycline, 300 mg, can be given to members of the immediate household but not to others in the neighborhood or community. Wide-scale use of prophylactic antibiotics quickly leads to the development of resistant strains.[68, 69]

Other Vibrios Generally Associated with Diarrhea

Non-O1 Vibrio cholerae

Strains of *V. cholerae* that do not agglutinate with antiserum O1 or O139 are termed non-O1 *V. cholerae*. They may still induce severe diarrhea, even though they do not cause epidemics, and thus they do not present the same public health risk as serotypes O1 and O139.

EPIDEMIOLOGY

The ecologic niche of the non-O1 *V. cholerae* is similar to that of cholera. These strains are associated with contaminated water or with shellfish, especially raw oysters and crabs. Non-O1 *V. cholerae* strains are, however, more widely distributed than O1 *V. cholerae* and are frequently isolated in the estuaries and bays of the United States, as well as in developing countries.[70–73] In developing countries, these organisms are usually not distinguished from the many bacterial pathogens causing diarrhea; hence, less is known about their transmission. In the United States or Mexico, however, patients with non-O1 *V. cholerae* infection have generally eaten raw or undercooked shellfish. In temperate climates, nearly all cases occur during the summer months.

PATHOGENESIS

Many of the non-O1 *V. cholerae* strains have been found to produce an enterotoxin nearly identical to cholera toxin, and a few other strains produce a heat-stable toxin closely related to the heat-stable enterotoxin of *E. coli*.[74, 75] However, the presence of these toxins has not altogether explained the mechanism of illness, as some strains have been associated with diarrhea yet produced neither of these two toxins.[76] Also, some episodes have been associated with significant fevers, a feature not seen in O1 cholera. Thus, multiple virulence factors are likely responsible for illnesses.

Non-O1 *V. cholerae* strains occasionally cause wound infection and sepsis,[77] especially in patients with predisposing illnesses, such as liver cirrhosis or immunosuppression.

CLINICAL MANIFESTATIONS

Diarrhea is the most common presentation for non-O1 *V. cholerae* infections, and these illnesses cannot be distinguished clinically from watery diarrhea caused by other organisms. Although individual patients can have a severe cholera-like illness with severe dehydration, diarrhea caused by non-O1 *V. cholerae* tends to be less severe than that in cholera. Fever and severe abdominal cramps may be seen and occasionally blood is present in the stool. The illness is self-limited with diarrhea lasting a few days.[72]

Wound infections and sepsis present in a manner similar to those seen with *V. vulnificus* (see later).

DIAGNOSIS

Persons with acute diarrhea should have a stool culture for vibrios with TCBS medium,[46] especially if there is a recent history of eating shellfish. Suspected colonies should be confirmed, and if there is doubt about their identity they should be referred to the state health department.

TREATMENT

Treatment for diarrhea caused by non-O1 *V. cholerae* is the same as the treatment in cholera, following principles of rehydration therapy according to the degree of dehydration using intravenous and/or oral rehydration fluids. The benefit of antibiotics has not been shown, but in severe cholera-like cases, doxycycline, a 300-mg single dose, or ciprofloxacin, 250 to 500 mg twice a day for 3 days, can be used. (Note: There have been no clinical trials for non-O1 *V. cholerae* infections; hence, these doses are based on treatment of O1 *V. cholerae*.) Those with milder cases need no antibiotics. Systemic infections require antibiotics according to sensitivity patterns. Tetracycline is generally used but others may also be effective, according to sensitivity patterns.

PREVENTION

There are no vaccines for non-O1 *V. cholerae* and the illness is sufficiently rare that one is not needed. Persons traveling to areas where there is a risk of ingesting vibrios should use boiled or bottled water and should avoid high-risk seafood, especially during the warmer months.

Vibrio mimicus

Diarrhea caused by *V. mimicus* is similar to that caused by *V. cholerae* except that it does not occur in epidemics. The pathogenesis involving the cholera toxin is the same, although additional toxins may also play a role. Like other vibrios, *V. mimicus* is associated with seafood consumption. Treatment, according to the degree of dehydration, is the same as that for cholera.[78–82] Rarely, *V. mimicus* may cause systemic infections.[83, 84]

Vibrio parahaemolyticus

V. parahaemolyticus is a halophilic vibrio that generally causes diarrhea but may rarely cause wound and systemic infections as well.[85, 86] Like the other vibrios, *V. parahaemolyticus* is associated with saltwater and seafood, and many of the U.S. cases result from eating raw oysters.[87] Cases are reported from all continents, but this infection is especially common in Japan, where it accounts for a majority of bacterial gastroenteritis cases. The popularity of raw fish in Japan probably accounts for the high number of cases there.

Most cases of diarrhea associated with *V. parahaemolyticus* cannot be distinguished from watery diarrhea caused by other agents, but in some cases the stool becomes bloody and patients may have fever. Virulence of *V. parahaemolyticus* is thought to be related to a hemolysin that is found in most clinical isolates and can be detected using Wagatsuma agar or molecular methods.[88–91] Treatment follows the same guidelines for rehydration as described for cholera. Antibiotics have not been shown to be helpful.

Although *V. parahaemolyticus* usually infects persons with normal immune systems, studies have shown increased risk for persons immunosuppressed because of human immunodeficiency virus infection or immunosuppressive drugs. Persons with these conditions should avoid raw seafood, especially during the warmer months.

Vibrio fluvialis

V. fluvialis (formerly called group EF-6 and group F *Vibrio*) is closely related biochemically to *Aeromonas*. It is ubiquitous in brackish waters and, like other vibrios, can infect persons by way of seafood. Patients infected with *V. fluvialis* have had diarrhea symptoms often with vomiting, abdominal pain, and fever. The fluid loss can lead to severe dehydration, similar to that in cholera. Treatment is similar to that for cholera with regard to fluid replacement, depending on the degree of dehydration. A major outbreak of *V. fluvialis* infection occurred in Bangladesh in 1977, but similar large-scale outbreaks have not been reported since then.[92, 93]

Vibrio furnissii

As with other vibrios, transmission of *V. furnissii* is associated with seafood and has been linked to diarrhea.[94, 95] Rehydration therapy for this illness uses the strategy described for cholera.

Vibrio hollisae

V. hollisae has been associated with diarrhea caused by eating seafood. Few cases have been reported, but the bacterium grows poorly on TCBS agar; hence, little is known of its true incidence. Rehydration, using guidelines as for cholera, is needed for patients with severe dehydration.[95–98] Rarely it may also cause septicemia[99, 100] in a manner similar to *V. vulnificus*.

Vibrios Generally Associated with Wound and Systemic Infections

Several *Vibrio* species lead primarily to wound infections and spontaneous septicemia, in patients with predisposing risk factors. These include *V. vulnificus, V. alginolyticus, V. damsela,* and possibly *V. cincinnatiensis.* Rarely, these species may cause diarrhea.

Vibrio vulnificus

V. vulnificus is primarily an extraintestinal pathogen, causing severe illness characterized by sepsis and wound infections, especially in persons with certain underlying diseases, including cirrhosis[101–104] (related to alcohol, hepatitis B, hepatitis C, or other causes), hemochromatosis (or other conditions with an excess of iron),[105, 106] thalassemia,[107] acquired immunodeficiency syndrome,[102] and diabetes. Although this is a rare infection for normal hosts in the United States, it is a major risk for persons with these conditions who become exposed, and because of its high case-fatality rate, it is the leading cause of death among the vibrio-caused illnesses in the United States and in many other countries.[108–114] Risk of exposure is highly related to seawater temperature, as the organism prospers in warmer waters (>15°C). Oysters are an especially high-risk food during warm months because the bacteria can multiply in mollusks. They also are found in high concentrations in intestines of certain fishes; hence, cleaning fish can also be risky.[115, 116]

Vibrio sepsis, which generally occurs within a day or two after eating undercooked seafood, is a nonspecific acute fever that progresses rapidly to hypotension and septic shock. Case-fatality rates for this syndrome have exceeded 50%, and patients require immediate supportive care and antibiotics, especially tetracycline or ciprofloxacin.

Wound infections occur after trauma with contamination by seawater, especially during the warmer months. Typical injuries have been cuts sustained while cleaning fish or shelling crabs. During the next 1 to 2 days, the wound becomes inflamed and may be associated with bullous skin lesions. The case-fatality rate for this infection is also substantial, about 25%, and aggressive treatment is needed with antibiotics and possibly wound débridement.

Other more unusual presentations for *V. vulnificus* infections include peritonitis,[117] corneal ulcer,[118] epiglottitis,[119] meningitis,[107] endometritis,[120] and osteomyelitis.[121]

Virulence of *V. vulnificus* is thought to be due to a bacterial capsular polysaccharide that makes the organism resistant to serum. A high proportion of the isolates from infections produce this capsule, but most environmental isolates do not; thus, the presence of the capsule appears to be a marker of pathogenicity.[122–127] This species is also able to utilize iron from the host tissue and from heme to promote growth and production of toxins.[128–131] Several toxins and extracellular enzymes have been identified that contribute to its pathogenicity.[132–135]

Because case-fatality rates are so high, persons at high risk must be warned of the dangers of exposure to undercooked seafood and of wounds sustained while in saltwater, especially during summer months.

Vibrio alginolyticus

V. alginolyticus is rarely isolated from humans but, like other vibrios, is associated with marine environments. Most infections have been associated with wounds sustained while in saltwater, and some of these infections have been severe. It has also been associated with ear infections. As with other vibrio wound infections, immunocompromised persons are at higher risk.[136–146]

Other Vibrios

V. metschnikovii, a common bacterium in marine environments, was isolated from the blood of a patient with gallbladder disease, but its role in the person's illness was not clear.[147]

V. damsela, previously known as EF-5, a pathogen for damselfish, has infected wounds of persons exposed to seawater and caused severe necrotizing infections.[95, 148–150]

V. cincinnatiensis was reported to cause meningitis and sepsis in a single case report of a patient with no marine exposure.[151]

Aeromonas Species

Aeromonas species are gram-negative, oxidase-positive, motile rods that are part of the normal flora of surface waters. On the basis of biochemical characteristics, three species have been designated: *Aeromonas hydrophila, Aeromonas sobria,* and *Aeromonas caviae*. Initially, it was thought that speciation would help identify clinically relevant features, but this has not yet become clear. They are considered to be causes of diarrhea by some, but their etiologic role in diarrhea is not yet clear because case-control studies have found similar rates of isolation in cases and control subjects, depending on the method of isolation,[152] and their rate of isolation is probably a marker for surface water consumption in the population. If *Aeromonas* species are enteropathogens, probably only some strains are pathogens. Markers of pathogenicity have been proposed, such as exotoxin production, but the correlation of these with virulence is not yet clear.[153, 154] Syndromes of diarrhea that have been seen in patients from whom *Aeromonas* species were isolated have included acute watery diarrhea, bloody diarrhea, and persistent diarrhea; hence, a typical clinical syndrome has not emerged.[155] Some patients with *Aeromonas*-associated diarrhea have responded to trimethoprim-sulfamethoxazole or tetracycline, but *Aeromonas* is generally resistant to ampicillin.

Two unique features of *Aeromonas* species are their ability to multiply in cold conditions and relative resistance to chlorine. Thus, refrigerated foods are more likely to become contaminated, and water from municipal systems with lower levels of chlorine is more likely to contain *Aeromonas* species.

Although their etiologic role in diarrhea remains undefined, they are occasional causes of systemic infection including wound infection, bacteremia, and meningitis.[156]

Plesiomonas shigelloides

P. shigelloides is a motile gram-negative, oxidase-positive rod that also lives in surface waters. It is also considered a potential enteropathogen, but its true relation to diarrhea is not clear. A few cases of diarrhea have been ascribed to this agent, but clinical studies have shown little difference between the rates of isolation in case and control subjects, and volunteers who were challenged with *P. shigelloides* have not developed illness,[157] nor have travelers with this infection developed serologic responses. Cases that have been described were related to oysters or other seafood or were related to travel to developing countries.[152, 158] Tests for specific virulence factors, such as invasiveness or enterotoxins, have generally been negative.

Among the 43 serogroups of *P. shigelloides,* the most common serotype, type 17, has a cell wall identical to that of *Shigella sonnei*. It is speculated that repeated exposure to this serotype by drinking surface water may stimulate a local intestinal immune response and protect people in developing countries from infection with *S. sonnei.*[159]

P. shigelloides is a rare cause of systemic infection and sepsis, usually in immunocompromised hosts.

References

1. Blake PA, Allegra DT, Snyder JD, et al: Cholera—A possible endemic focus in the United States. N Engl J Med 302:305–309, 1980.
2. Blake PA: Epidemiology of cholera in the Americas. Gastroenterol Clin North Am 22:639–660, 1993.
3. From the Centers for Disease Control. Update: Cholera—Western Hemisphere, and recommendations for treatment of cholera. JAMA 266:1186, 1189, 1991.
4. Large epidemic of cholera-like disease in Bangladesh caused by *Vibrio cholerae* O139 synonym Bengal. Cholera Working Group, International Centre for Diarrhoeal Diseases Research, Bangladesh. Lancet 342:387–390, 1993.
5. Bodhidatta L, Echeverria P, Hoge CW, et al: *Vibrio cholerae* O139 in Thailand in 1994. Epidemiol Infect 114:71–73, 1995.
6. Siddique AK, Zaman K, Akram K, et al: Emergence of a new epidemic strain of *Vibrio cholerae* in Bangladesh. An epidemiological study. Trop Geogr Med 46:147–150, 1994.
7. Latta T: Letter from Dr. Latta to the Secretary of the Central Board of Health, London, affording a view of the rationale and results of his practice in the treatment of cholera by aqueous and saline solutions. Lancet 2:274–277, 1831.
8. O'Shaughnessy WB: Proposal of a new method of treating blue epidemic cholera by the injection of highly oxygenated salts into the venous system. Lancet 1:366–371, 1831.

8a. Rogers LE: Bowel Diseases in the Tropics. London, Froude, Hodder, and Stoughton, 1921.

9. Carpenter CC, Mondal A, Sack RB: Clinical studies in Asiatic cholera II: Development of 2:1 saline lactate regimen. Comparison of this regimen with traditional modes of treatment. Bull Johns Hopkins Hosp 118:174–196, 1966.
10. Cash RA, Toha KMM, Nalin DR: Acetate in the correction of acidosis secondary to diarrhoea. Lancet 2:302–303, 1969.
11. Pierce NF, Banwell JG, Mitra RC: Effect of intragastric glucose-electrolyte infusion upon water and electrolyte balance in Asiatic cholera. Gastroenterology 55:333–343, 1968.
12. Hirschhorn N, Kinzie JL, Sachar DB, et al: Decrease in net stool output in cholera during intestinal perfusion with glucose-containing solutions. N Engl J Med 279:176–188, 1968.
13. Snow J: On the Mode of Communication of Cholera, ed 2. London, John Churchill, 1855.
14. St. Louis ME, Porter JD, Helal A, et al: Epidemic cholera in West Africa: The role of food handling and high-risk foods. Am J Epidemiol 131:719–728, 1990.
15. Weber JT, Levine WC, Hopkins DP, Tauxe RV: Cholera in the United States, 1965–1991. Risks at home and abroad. Arch Intern Med 154:551–556, 1994.
16. Taylor JL, Tuttle J, Pramukul T, et al: An outbreak of cholera in Maryland associated with imported commercial frozen fresh coconut milk. J Infect Dis 167:1330–1335, 1993.
17. From the Centers for Disease Control. Cholera associated with imported coconut milk. JAMA 267:1320, 1323, 1992.
18. Institute of Medicine: New Vaccine Development, Establishing Priorities, Vol II. Diseases of Importance in Developing Countries. Washington, DC, Institute of Medicine, 1986, pp 378–389.
19. Glass RI, Becker S, Huq MI, et al: Endemic cholera in rural Bangladesh, 1966–1980. Am J Epidemiol 116:959–970, 1982.
20. Siddique AK, Zaman K, Baqui AH, et al: Cholera epidemics in Bangladesh: 1985–1991. J Diarrhoeal Dis Res 10:79–86, 1992.
21. Clemens JD, Sack DA, Harris JR, et al: Field trial of oral cholera vaccines in Bangladesh: Results from three-year follow-up. Lancet 335:270–273, 1990.
22. Siddique AK, Salam A, Islam MS, et al: Why treatment centres failed to prevent cholera deaths among Rwandan refugees in Goma, Zaire. Lancet 345:359–361, 1995.
23. Public health impact of Rwandan refugee crisis: What happened in Goma, Zaire, in July, 1994? Goma Epidemiology Group. Lancet 345:339–344, 1995.
24. van Loon FP, Clemens JD, Shahrier M, et al: Low gastric acid

as a risk factor for cholera transmission: Application of a new non-invasive gastric acid field test. J Clin Epidemiol 43:1361–1367, 1990.
25. Nalin DR, Levine RJ, Levine MM, et al: Cholera, non-vibrio cholera, and stomach acid. Lancet 2:856–859, 1978.
26. Cash RA, Alam J, Toaha KM: Gastric acid in cholera patients. Lancet 2:1192, 1970.
27. Giannella RA, Broitman SA, Zamcheck N: The gastric acid barrier to enteric infection in man: In vivo and in vitro studies. Gut 13:251–256, 1972.
28. Sack FH, Pierce NF, Hennessey KN, et al: Gastric acid in cholera and non-cholera diarrhea. Bull WHO 47:31–36, 1972.
29. Barua D, Paguio AS: ABO blood groups and cholera. Ann Hum Biol 4:489–492, 1977.
30. Clemens JD, Sack DA, Harris JR, et al: ABO blood groups and cholera: New observations on specificity of risk and modification of vaccine efficacy. J Infect Dis 159:770–773, 1989.
31. Glass RI, Holmgren J, Haley CE, et al: Predisposition for cholera of individuals with O blood group. Possible evolutionary significance. Am J Epidemiol 121:791–796, 1985.
32. Clemens JD, Sack DA, Chakraborty J, et al: Field trial of oral cholera vaccines in Bangladesh: Evaluation of anti-bacterial and anti-toxic breast-milk immunity in response to ingestion of the vaccines. Vaccine 8:469–472, 1990.
33. Glass RI, Stoll BJ: The protective effect of human milk against diarrhea. A review of studies from Bangladesh. Acta Paediatr Scand [Suppl] 351:131–136, 1989.
34. Herrington DA, Hall RH, Losonsky G, et al: Toxin, toxin-coregulated pili, and the *toxR* regulon are essential for *Vibrio cholerae* pathogenesis in humans. J Exp Med 168:1487–1492, 1988.
35. Osek J, Svennerholm AM, Holmgren J: Protection against *Vibrio cholerae* El Tor infection by specific antibodies against mannose-binding hemagglutinin pili. Infect Immun 60:4961–4964, 1992.
36. Osek J, Jonson G, Svennerholm AM, Holmgren J: Role of antibodies against biotype-specific *Vibrio cholerae* pili in protection against experimental classical and El Tor cholera. Infect Immun 62:2901–2907, 1994.
37. Field M: Role of cyclic nucleotides in enterotoxic diarrhea. Adv Cyclic Nucleotide Res 12:267–277, 1980.
38. Holmgren J: Actions of cholera toxin and the prevention and treatment of cholera. Nature 292:413–417, 1981.
39. Holmgren J, Lonnroth I, Mansson J, Svennerholm L: Interaction of cholera toxin and membrane G_{M1} ganglioside of small intestine. Proc Natl Acad Sci USA 72:2520–2524, 1975.
40. Molla AM, Rahman M, Sarker SA, et al: Stool electrolyte content and purging rates in diarrhea caused by rotavirus, enterotoxigenic *E. coli*, and *V. cholerae* in children. J Pediatr 98:835–838, 1981.
41. Carpenter CC, Mitra PP, Sack RB: Clinical studies in Asiatic cholera I. Preliminary observations. Bull Johns Hopkins Hosp 118:165–173, 1966.
42. Quick RE, Vargas R, Moreno D, et al: Epidemic cholera in the Amazon: The challenge of preventing death. Am J Trop Med Hyg 48:597–602, 1993.
43. Siddique AK, Akram K, Islam Q: Why cholera still takes lives in rural Bangladesh. Study of an epidemic. Trop Doct 18:40–42, 1988.
44. Besser RE, Feikin DR, Eberhart-Phillips JE, et al: Diagnosis and treatment of cholera in the United States. Are we prepared? JAMA 272:1203–1205, 1994.
45. Finelli L, Swerdlow D, Mertz K, et al: Outbreak of cholera associated with crab brought from an area with epidemic disease. J Infect Dis 166:1433–1435, 1992.
46. Centers for Disease Control and Prevention: Laboratory Methods for the Diagnosis of *Vibrio cholerae*. Atlanta, Centers for Disease Control and Prevention, 1994.
47. Hasan JA, Huq A, Tamplin ML, et al: A novel kit for rapid detection of *Vibrio cholerae* O1. J Clin Microbiol 32:249–252, 1994.
48. Rahman M, Sack DA, Mahmood S, Hossain A: Rapid diagnosis of cholera by coagglutination test using 4-h fecal enrichment cultures. J Clin Microbiol 25:2204–2206, 1987.
49. World Health Organization: Management of the Patient with Cholera. Geneva, World Health Organization, 1991. WHO/CDD/SER/91.5.
50. Rahaman MM, Majid MA, Monsur KA: Evaluation of two intravenous rehydration solutions in cholera and non-cholera diarrhoea. Bull WHO 57:977–981, 1979.
51. Gore SM, Fontaine O, Pierce NF: Impact of rice based oral rehydration solution on stool output and duration of diarrhoea: Meta-analysis of 13 clinical trials. BMJ 304:287–291, 1992.
52. Molla AM, Ahmed SM, Greenough WB 3d: Rice-based oral rehydration solution decreases the stool volume in acute diarrhoea. Bull WHO 63:751–756, 1985.
53. Alam AN, Alam NH, Ahmed T, Sack DA: Randomised double blind trial of single dose doxycycline for treating cholera in adults. BMJ 300:1619–1621, 1990.
54. Sack DA, Islam S, Rabbani H, Islam A: Single-dose doxycycline for cholera. Antimicrob Agents Chemother 14:462–464, 1978.
55. De S, Chaudhuri A, Dutta P, et al: Doxycycline in the treatment of cholera. Bull WHO 54:177–179, 1976.
55a. Khan WA, Bennish ML, Seas C, et al: Randomised controlled comparison of single dose ciprofloxacin and doxycyclin for cholera caused by *Vibrio cholerae* O1 or O139. Lancet 348:296–300, 1996.
56. Pastore G, Rizzo G, Fera G, Schiraldi O: Trimethoprim-sulphamethoxazole in the treatment of cholera. Comparison with tetracycline and chloramphenicol. Chemotherapy 23:121–128, 1977.
57. Uylangco C, Santiago L, Pescante M, et al: Pivmecillinam, cotrimoxazole and oral mecillinam in gastroenteritis due to *Vibrio* spp. J Antimicrob Chemother 13:171–175, 1984.
58. Khan WA, Begum M, Salam MA, et al: Comparative trial of five antimicrobial compounds in the treatment of cholera in adults. Trans R Soc Trop Med Hyg 89:103–106, 1995.
59. Burans JP, Podgore J, Mansour MM, et al: Comparative trial of erythromycin and sulphatrimethoprim in the treatment of tetracycline-resistant *Vibrio cholerae* O1. Trans R Soc Trop Med Hyg 83:836–838, 1989.
60. Sack DA, Islam S, Brown KH, et al: Oral therapy in children with cholera: A comparison of sucrose and glucose electrolyte solutions. J Pediatr 96:20–25, 1980.
61. Ayangade O: The significance of cholera outbreak in the prognosis of pregnancy. Int J Gynaecol Obstet 19:403–407, 1981.
62. Development of vaccines against cholera and diarrhoea due to enterotoxigenic *Escherichia coli*: Memorandum from a WHO meeting. Bull WHO 68:303–312, 1990.
63. Clemens JD, Sack DA, Harris JR, et al: Field trial of oral cholera vaccines in Bangladesh. Lancet 2:124–127, 1986.
64. Holmgren J, Svennerholm AM, Jertborn M, et al: An oral B subunit: Whole cell vaccine against cholera. Vaccine 10:911–914, 1992.
65. Sanchez JL, Vasquez B, Begue RE, et al: Protective efficacy of oral whole-cell/recombinant-B-subunit cholera vaccine in Peruvian military recruits. Lancet 344:1273–1276, 1994.
66. Levine MM, Kaper JB: Live oral vaccines against cholera: An update. Vaccine 11:207–212, 1993.
67. Levine MM, Kaper JB, Herrington D, et al: Safety, immunogenicity, and efficacy of recombinant live oral cholera vaccines, CVD 103 and CVD 103-HgR. Lancet 2:467–470, 1988.
68. Khan MU: Efficacy of short course antibiotic prophylaxis in controlling cholera in contacts during epidemic. J Trop Med Hyg 85:27–29, 1982.
69. Sack RB: Prophylactic antibiotics? The individual versus the community. N Engl J Med 300:1107–1108, 1979.
70. Morris JG Jr, Black RE: Cholera and other vibrioses in the United States. N Engl J Med 312:343–350, 1985.
71. Finch MJ, Valdespino JL, Wells JG, et al: Non-O1 *Vibrio cholerae* infections in Cancun, Mexico. Am J Trop Med Hyg 36:393–397, 1987.
72. Morris JG Jr, Wilson R, Davis BR, et al: Non-O group 1 *Vibrio cholerae* gastroenteritis in the United States: Clinical, epidemiologic, and laboratory characteristics of sporadic cases. Ann Intern Med 94:656–658, 1981.
73. Oo KN, Myint T, Nwe YY, Aye T: *Vibrio* spp. isolated from natural waters of the city of Yangon, Myanmar. J Diarrhoeal Dis Res 11:105–107, 1993.
74. Yamamoto K, Takeda Y, Miwatani T, Craig JP: Evidence that a non-O1 *Vibrio cholerae* produces enterotoxin that is similar but not identical to cholera enterotoxin. Infect Immun 41:896–901, 1983.
75. Arita M, Takeda T, Honda T, Miwatani T: Purification and characterization of *Vibrio cholerae* non-O1 heat-stable enterotoxin. Infect Immun 52:45–49, 1986.
76. Morris JG Jr, Picardi JL, Lieb S, et al: Isolation of nontoxigenic

Vibrio cholerae O group 1 from a patient with severe gastrointestinal disease. J Clin Microbiol 19:296–297, 1984.

77. Pitrak DL, Gindorf JD: Bacteremic cellulitis caused by non-serogroup O1 *Vibrio cholerae* acquired in a freshwater inland lake. J Clin Microbiol 27:2874–2876, 1989.
78. Arita M, Honda T, Miwatani T, et al: Purification and characterization of a heat-stable enterotoxin of *Vibrio mimicus*. FEMS Microbiol Lett 63:105–110, 1991.
79. Kaper JB, Nataro JP, Roberts NC, et al: Molecular epidemiology of non-O1 *Vibrio cholerae* and *Vibrio mimicus* in the U.S. Gulf Coast region. J Clin Microbiol 23:652–654, 1986.
80. Spira WM, Fedorka-Cray PJ: Purification of enterotoxins from *Vibrio mimicus* that appear to be identical to cholera toxin. Infect Immun 45:679–684, 1984.
81. Shandera WX, Johnston JM, Davis BR, Blake PA: Disease from infection with *Vibrio mimicus*, a newly recognized *Vibrio* species. Clinical characteristics and epidemiology. Ann Intern Med 99:169–171, 1983.
82. Davis BR, Fanning GR, Madden JM, et al: Characterization of biochemically atypical *Vibrio cholerae* strains and designation of a new pathogenic species, *Vibrio mimicus*. J Clin Microbiol 14:631–639, 1981.
83. Albert MJ, Kabir I, Neogi PK, Kibriya AK: *Vibrio mimicus* bacteraemia in a child. J Diarrhoeal Dis Res 10:39–40, 1992.
84. Klontz KC, Cover DE, Hyman FN, Mullen RC: Fatal gastroenteritis due to *Vibrio fluvialis* and nonfatal bacteremia due to *Vibrio mimicus*: Unusual vibrio infections in two patients. Clin Infect Dis 19:541–542, 1994.
85. Blake PA, Weaver RE, Hollis DG: Diseases of humans (other than cholera) caused by vibrios. Annu Rev Microbiol 34:341–367, 1980.
86. Klontz KC: Fatalities associated with *Vibrio parahaemolyticus* and *Vibrio cholerae* non-O1 infections in Florida (1981 to 1988). South Med J 83:500–502, 1990.
87. Haddock RL, Cabanero AF: The origin of non-outbreak *Vibrio parahaemolyticus* infections on Guam. Trop Geogr Med 46:42–43, 1994.
88. Joseph SW, Colwell RR, Kaper JB: *Vibrio parahaemolyticus* and related halophilic vibrios. Crit Rev Microbiol 10:77–124, 1982.
89. Shirai H, Ito H, Hirayama T, et al: Molecular epidemiologic evidence for association of thermostable direct hemolysin (TDH) and TDH-related hemolysin of *Vibrio parahaemolyticus* with gastroenteritis. Infect Immun 58:3568–3573, 1990.
90. Honda T, Sornchai C, Takeda Y, Miwatani T: Immunological detection of the Kanagawa phenomenon of *Vibrio parahaemolyticus* on modified selective media. J Clin Microbiol 16:734–736, 1982.
91. Tada J, Ohashi T, Nishimura N, et al: Detection of the thermostable direct hemolysin gene *(tdh)* and the thermostable direct hemolysin–related hemolysin gene *(trh)* of *Vibrio parahaemolyticus* by polymerase chain reaction. Mol Cell Probes 6:477–487, 1992.
92. Klontz KC, Desenclos JC: Clinical and epidemiological features of sporadic infections with *Vibrio fluvialis* in Florida, USA. J Diarrhoeal Dis Res 8:24–26, 1990.
93. Tacket CO, Hickman F, Pierce GV, Mendoza LF: Diarrhea associated with *Vibrio fluvialis* in the United States. J Clin Microbiol 16:991–992, 1982.
94. Brenner DJ, Hickman-Brenner FW, Lee JV, et al: *Vibrio furnissii* (formerly aerogenic biogroup of *Vibrio fluvialis*), a new species isolated from human feces and the environment. J Clin Microbiol 18:816–824, 1983.
95. Morris JG Jr, Miller HG, Wilson R, et al: Illness caused by *Vibrio damsela* and *Vibrio hollisae*. Lancet 1:1294–1297, 1982.
96. Carnahan AM, Harding J, Watsky D, Hansman S: Identification of *Vibrio hollisae* associated with severe gastroenteritis after consumption of raw oysters. J Clin Microbiol 32:1805–1806, 1994.
97. Abbott SL, Janda JM: Severe gastroenteritis associated with *Vibrio hollisae* infection: Report of two cases and review. Clin Infect Dis 18:310–312, 1994.
98. Kothary MH, Richardson SH: Fluid accumulation in infant mice caused by *Vibrio hollisae* and its extracellular enterotoxin. Infect Immun 55:626–630, 1987.
99. Rank EL, Smith IB, Langer M: Bacteremia caused by *Vibrio hollisae*. J Clin Microbiol 26:375–376, 1988.
100. Lowry PW, McFarland LM, Threefoot HK: *Vibro hollisae* septicemia after consumption of catfish (Letter). J Infect Dis 154:730–731, 1986.
101. Arnold M, Woo ML, French GL: *Vibrio vulnificus* septicaemia presenting as spontaneous necrotising cellulitis in a woman with hepatic cirrhosis. Scand J Infect Dis 21:727–731, 1989.
102. Chin KP, Lowe MA, Tong MJ, Koehler AL: *Vibrio vulnificus* infection after raw oyster ingestion in a patient with liver disease and acquired immune deficiency syndrome–related complex. Gastroenterology 92:796–799, 1987.
103. Wongpaitoon V, Sathapatayavongs B, Prachaktam R, et al: Spontaneous *Vibrio vulnificus* peritonitis and primary sepsis in two patients with alcoholic cirrhosis. Am J Gastroenterol 80:706–708, 1985.
104. *Vibrio vulnificus* and patients with liver disease. FDA Drug Bull 15:5–6, 1985.
105. Brennaman B, Soucy D, Howard RJ: Effect of iron and liver injury on the pathogenesis of *Vibrio vulnificus*. J Surg Res 43:527–531, 1987.
106. Wright AC, Simpson LM, Oliver JD: Role of iron in the pathogenesis of *Vibrio vulnificus* infections. Infect Immun 34:503–507, 1981.
107. Katz BZ: *Vibrio vulnificus* meningitis in a boy with thalassemia after eating raw oysters. Pediatrics 82:784–786, 1988.
108. Hlady WG, Mullen RC, Hopkin RS: *Vibrio vulnificus* from raw oysters. Leading cause of reported deaths from foodborne illness in Florida. J Fla Med Assoc 80:536–538, 1993.
109. Warnock EW 3d, MacMath TL: Primary *Vibrio vulnificus* septicemia. J Emerg Med 11:153–156, 1993.
110. *Vibrio vulnificus* infections associated with raw oyster consumption—Florida, 1981–1992. MMWR Morbid Mortal Wkly Rep 42:405–407, 1993.
111. Chuang YC, Yuan CY, Liu CY, et al: *Vibrio vulnificus* infection in Taiwan: Report of 28 cases and review of clinical manifestations and treatment. Clin Infect Dis 15:271–276, 1992.
112. Park SD, Shon HS, Joh NJ: *Vibrio vulnificus* septicemia in Korea: Clinical and epidemiologic findings in seventy patients. J Am Acad Dermatol 24:397–403, 1991.
113. Morris JG Jr: *Vibrio vulnificus*—A new monster of the deep? Ann Intern Med 109:261–263, 1988.
114. Klontz KC, Lieb S, Schreiber M, et al: Syndromes of *Vibrio vulnificus* infections. Clinical and epidemiologic features in Florida cases, 1981–1987. Ann Intern Med 109:318–323, 1988.
115. DePaola A, Capers GM, Alexander D: Densities of *Vibrio vulnificus* in the intestines of fish from the U.S. Gulf Coast. Appl Environ Microbiol 60:984–988, 1994.
116. Cook DW: Effect of time and temperature on multiplication of *Vibrio vulnificus* in postharvest Gulf Coast shellstock oysters. Appl Environ Microbiol 60:3483–3484, 1994.
117. Holcombe DJ: *Vibrio vulnificus* peritonitis. A unique case. J La State Med Soc 143:27–28, 1991.
118. DiGaetano M, Ball SF, Straus JG: *Vibrio vulnificus* corneal ulcer. Case reports. Arch Ophthalmol 107:323–324, 1989.
119. Mehtar S, Bangham L, Kalmanovitch D, Wren M: Adult epiglottitis due to *Vibrio vulnificus*. Br Med J (Clin Res) 296:827–828, 1988.
120. Tison DL, Kelly MT: *Vibrio vulnificus* endometritis. J Clin Microbiol 20:185–186, 1984.
121. Vartian CV, Septimus EJ: Osteomyelitis caused by *Vibrio vulnificus* (Letter). J Infect Dis 161:363, 1990.
122. Reddy GP, Hayat U, Bush CA, Morris JG Jr: Capsular polysaccharide structure of a clinical isolate of *Vibrio vulnificus* strain BO62316 determined by heteronuclear NMR spectroscopy and high-performance anion-exchange chromatography. Anal Biochem 214:106–115, 1993.
123. Hayat U, Reddy GP, Bush CA, et al: Capsular types of *Vibrio vulnificus*: An analysis of strains from clinical and environmental sources. J Infect Dis 168:758–762, 1993.
124. Reddy GP, Hayat U, Abeygunawardana C, et al: Purification and determination of the structure of capsular polysaccharide of *Vibrio vulnificus* M06-24. J Bacteriol 174:2620–2630, 1992.
125. Yoshida S, Ogawa M, Mizuguchi Y: Relation of capsular materials and colony opacity to virulence of *Vibrio vulnificus*. Infect Immun 47:446–451, 1985.
126. Shinoda S, Kobayashi M, Yamada H, et al: Inhibitory effect of capsular antigen of *Vibrio vulnificus* on bactericidal activity of human serum. Microbiol Immunol 31:393–401, 1987.

127. Amako K, Okada K, Miake S: Evidence for the presence of a capsule in *Vibrio vulnificus*. J Gen Microbiol 130:2741–2743, 1984.
128. Amaro C, Biosca EG, Fouz B, et al: Role of iron, capsule, and toxins in the pathogenicity of *Vibrio vulnificus* biotype 2 for mice. Infect Immun 62:759–763, 1994.
129. Zakaria-Meehan Z, Massad G, Simpson LM, et al: Ability of *Vibrio vulnificus* to obtain iron from hemoglobin-haptoglobin complexes. Infect Immun 56:275–277, 1988.
130. Simpson LM, Oliver JD: Siderophore production by *Vibrio vulnificus*. Infect Immun 41:644–649, 1983.
131. Testa J, Daniel LW, Kreger AS: Extracellular phospholipase A_2 and lysophospholipase produced by *Vibrio vulnificus*. Infect Immun 45:458–463, 1984.
132. Miyoshi S, Hirata Y, Tomochika K, Shinoda S: *Vibrio vulnificus* may produce a metalloprotease causing an edematous skin lesion in vivo. FEMS Microbiol Lett 121:321–325, 1994.
133. Wright AC, Morris JG Jr: The extracellular cytolysin of *Vibrio vulnificus*: Inactivation and relationship to virulence in mice. Infect Immun 59:192–197, 1991.
134. Nishina Y, Miyoshi S, Nagase A, Shinoda S: Significant role of an exocellular protease in utilization of heme by *Vibrio vulnificus*. Infect Immun 60:2128–2132, 1992.
135. Kreger A, Lockwood D: Detection of extracellular toxin(s) produced by *Vibrio vulnificus*. Infect Immun 33:583–590, 1981.
136. Patterson TF, Bell SR, Bia FJ: *Vibrio alginolyticus* cellulitis following coral injury. Yale J Biol Med 61:507–512, 1988.
137. Janda JM, Brenden R, DeBenedetti JA, et al: *Vibrio alginolyticus* bacteremia in an immunocompromised patient. Diagn Microbiol Infect Dis 5:337–340, 1986.
138. Hasyn JJ, Mauer TP, Warner R, Von Hake C: Isolation of *Vibrio alginolyticus* from a patient with chronic otitis media: Report of case and review of biochemical activity. J Am Osteopath Assoc 87:560–562, 1987.
139. Opal SM, Saxon JR: Intracranial infection by *Vibrio alginolyticus* following injury in salt water. J Clin Microbiol 23:373–374, 1986.
140. Lessner AM, Webb RM, Rabin B: *Vibrio alginolyticus* conjunctivitis. First reported case. Arch Ophthalmol 103:229–230, 1985.
141. Taylor R, McDonald M, Russ G, et al: *Vibrio alginolyticus* peritonitis associated with ambulatory peritoneal dialysis. Br Med J (Clin Res) 283:275, 1981.
142. Schmidt U, Chmel H, Cobbs C: *Vibrio alginolyticus* infections in humans. J Clin Microbiol 10:666–668, 1979.
143. English VL, Lindberg RB: Isolation of *Vibrio alginolyticus* from wounds and blood of a burn patient. Am J Med Technol 43:989–993, 1977.
144. Ciufecu C, Nacescu N, Florescu D: Middle ear infection due to *Vibrio alginolyticus*. Bacteriological characterization. Acta Microbiol Acad Sci Hung 26:95–98, 1979.
145. Pezzlo M, Valter PJ, Burns MJ: Wound infection associated with *Vibrio alginolyticus*. Am J Clin Pathol 71:476–478, 1979.
146. Pien F, Lee K, Higa H: *Vibrio alginolyticus* infections in Hawaii. J Clin Microbiol 5:670–672, 1977.
147. Jean-Jacques W, Rajashekaraiah KR, Farmer JJ 3rd: *Vibrio metschnikovii* bacteremia in a patient with cholecystitis. J Clin Microbiol 14:711–712, 1981.
148. Yuen KY, Ma L, Wong SS, Ng WF: Fatal necrotizing fasciitis due to *Vibrio damsela*. Scand J Infect Dis 25:659–661, 1993.
149. Perez-Tirse J, Levine JF, Mecca M: *Vibrio damsela*. A cause of fulminant septicemia. Arch Intern Med 153:1838–1840, 1993.
150. Coffey JA Jr, Harris RL, Rutledge ML, et al: *Vibrio damsela*: Another potentially virulent marine vibrio. J Infect Dis 153:800–802, 1986.
151. Bode RB, Brayton PR, Colwell RR, et al: A new *Vibrio* species, *Vibrio cincinnatiensis*, causing meningitis: Successful treatment in an adult. Ann Intern Med 104:55–56, 1986.
152. Sack DA, Chowdhury KA, Huq A, et al: Epidemiology of *Aeromonas* and *Plesiomonas diarrhoea*. J Diarrhoeal Dis Res 6:107–112, 1988.
153. Wadstrom T, Ljungh A: *Aeromonas* and *Plesiomonas* as food and waterborne pathogens. Int J Food Microbiol 12:303–311, 1991.
154. Janda JM: Recent advances in the study of the taxonomy, pathogenicity, and infectious syndromes associated with the genus *Aeromonas*. Clin Microbiol Rev 4:397–410, 1991.
155. Agger WA, McCormick JD, Gurwith MJ: Clinical and microbiological features of *Aeromonas hydrophila*–associated diarrhea. J Clin Microbiol 21:909–913, 1985.
156. Janda JM, Guthertz LS, Kokka RP, Shimada T: *Aeromonas* species in septicemia: Laboratory characteristics and clinical observations. Clin Infect Dis 19:77–83, 1994.
157. Herrington DA, Tzipori S, Robins-Browne RM, et al: In vitro and in vivo pathogenicity of *Plesiomonas shigelloides*. Infect Immun 55:979–985, 1987.
158. Holmberg SD, Farmer JJ 3d: *Aeromonas hydrophila* and *Plesiomonas shigelloides* as causes of intestinal infections. Rev Infect Dis 6:633–639, 1984.
159. Sack DA, Hoque AT, Huq A, Etheridge M: Is protection against shigellosis induced by natural infection with *Plesiomonas shigelloides*? Lancet 343:1413–1415, 1994.

79

Clostridium difficile–Associated Diarrhea and Colitis

John G. Bartlett

Clostridium difficile, the major recognized agent of antibiotic-associated diarrhea and colitis, was originally reported as an agent of enteric disease in 1977.[1] This organism produces a spectrum of disease, ranging from simple and self-limited diarrhea to its most advanced and characteristic form, pseudomembranous colitis (PMC). *C. difficile* produces at least two toxins, toxin A and toxin B, which are responsible for clinical expression and pathologic changes.[2] An unusual feature of *C. difficile* is that it causes disease almost exclusively in the presence of antibiotic exposure.

Historical Perspective

A retrospective review of *C. difficile*–induced enteric disease shows three quite different lines of investigation: studies of the anatomy of PMC, studies of *C. difficile,* and studies of antibiotic-associated cecitis in rodent models.[2]

The anatomic studies began with the initial report of pseudomembranous lesions of the intestinal tract by Finney in 1893.[3] The case involved a 22-year-old patient of William Osler who underwent gastric surgery and postoperatively developed severe diarrhea that proved to be a lethal complication. Autopsy showed lesions that appeared as "diphtheritic membranes" in the small bowel. Pseudomembranous enterocolitis remained a relatively rare condition until the introduction of antibiotics. In the early 1950s, pseudomembranous enterocolitis became a relatively common complication of antibiotic therapy, especially with tetracycline and chloramphenicol. *Staphylococcus aureus* was the major nosocomial pathogen at the time, and it was implicated as the agent of this disease by virtue of recovery from stool.[4] A retrospective review of the data did not provide persuasive evidence for a causal role for *S. aureus* because the majority of the patients receiving antimicrobial agents harbored the organism; however, the role of *S. aureus* as the agent of antibiotic-associated colitis was not seriously challenged until there was renewed interest in the disease during the 1970s. The most important study was of a condition that became known as clindamycin colitis, conducted by Tedesco and coworkers[5] at Barnes Hospital in 1974. This was a prospective evaluation of 200 patients treated with clindamycin; 42 (21%) developed diarrhea and 20 (10%) had PMC at endoscopy. Stool cultures from these patients failed to grow *S. aureus* despite the relative ease of detecting this organism with selective media. A retrospective review of the Barnes Hospital experience indicates that the extraordinary frequency of this complication presumably reflects an epidemic of *C. difficile,* an impression supported by analysis of stored stool specimens from that epidemic, which revealed *C. difficile* toxin after the tissue culture assay was described 5 years later.[2]

The second series of relevant experiments in the history of *C. difficile* concerns the rodent model of antibiotic-associated colitis. Hambra and coworkers[6] reported in 1943 that attempts to determine the potential utility of penicillin for the treatment of gas gangrene in a guinea pig model were complicated by lethality that was ascribed to penicillin per se. Necropsy examinations showed large ceca filled with hemorrhagic fluid, and subsequent work showed that nearly all antibiotics may be lethal to guinea pigs and that hamsters are equally susceptible. A particularly important contribution was reported by Green[7] in 1974, who noted that stools and tissues of affected animals showed cytotoxic changes in cultured cells. No virus could be propagated, but he concluded that a latent virus was responsible. A similar observation was made in 1977 by Larson and colleagues,[8] who used stool specimens from patients with PMC.

Studies of *C. difficile* itself began with the demonstration of *C. difficile* as a component of the normal intestinal flora of newborn infants by Hall and O'Toole[9] in 1935. These investigators noted that this organism produced a "neurotoxin"; they observed that the cell-free supernatant of broth cultures was lethal when injected into experimental animals. In spite of this finding, the clinical significance of *C. difficile* remained enigmatic. The most comprehensive report on the organism before that time was the doctoral thesis of Hafiz[10] at the University of Leeds under the supervision of Professor Oakley, a noted authority on *Clostridium* organisms. Hafiz noted that the organism was widespread and could be recovered from stools of various animals. He also observed that most strains produced the lethal toxin, although in varying quantities, in vitro.

The three landmark studies were all reported in 1974.[3, 7, 10] Nevertheless, there was no way at that time to realize that the organism described in detail by Hafiz produced the cytotoxin noted by Green that caused the lesions described by Tedesco.

What subsequently brought these three lines of investigation together were studies utilizing the hamster model of antibiotic-associated colitis. This work showed that cecal contents contained a filterable protein toxin that was cytopathic in cell culture and would reproduce typical lesions when injected intracecally into healthy recipient animals.[1] Both the organism and its cytopathic toxin could be detected in all hamsters with antibiotic-induced disease and in nearly all patients with antibiotic-associated PMC.[11]

Pathophysiology

Factors contributing to the pathogenesis of *C. difficile*–associated diarrhea and colitis include (1) a source of the organism, presumably the host's normal flora or an environmental source (the latter is especially important in epidemics); (2) an altered intestinal flora that results from antibiotic exposure; (3) toxin production, reflecting rapid growth of toxigenic strains at the time the competing flora is suppressed; and (4) a poorly understood, age-related susceptibility.

Colonization Rates

C. difficile may be detected in stool with the use of selective media, such as the media containing cycloserine and cefoxitin, as originally described by George and colleagues.[12] The recovery rate for healthy adults is usually 2% to 3%[12–14] (Table 79–1); for patients who recently received antimicrobial agents and do not have diarrhea, it is 5% to 15%[14]; and for hospitalized patients the range is 10% to 25% whether or not they were exposed to an antibiotic.[15] The isolation rate in healthy infants is highly variable, ranging from 5% to 70%.[9, 14, 16, 17] Variable but often high carrier rates persist during the first 8 months of life, until the "normal adult flora" becomes established and the isolation rate subsequently approximates the 2% to 3% rate noted in healthy adults.[14, 16, 17]

Antibiotic Exposure

A striking feature of *C. difficile* is that it appears to cause enteric disease almost exclusively in the presence of antibiotic exposure. Virtually all drugs with an antibacterial spectrum of activity have been implicated, most frequently those that have a pronounced impact on the colon flora, primarily cephalosporins, ampicillin or amoxicillin, and clindamycin.[18–20] The most frequent inducing agents in more recent years have been cephalosporins, especially in nosocomial cases.[21–23] Less frequently implicated are penicillins other than ampicillin, erythromycin, quinolones, and trimethoprim-sulfamethoxazole. Rare inducing agents include fluoroquinolones, rifampin, parenteral aminoglycosides, sulfonamides, metronidazole, and tetracycline. For most drugs, the dose, the route of administration, and the duration of treatment seem to have little effect on the frequency or the severity of this complication. In addition, activity in vitro against *C. difficile* bears little apparent relevance. For example, the minimal inhibitory concentrations (MICs) of vancomycin and ampicillin are nearly identical, despite the fact that the former is highly effective therapy and the latter is one of the most common offending agents.[24]

Toxins

There are two toxins, designated A and B; both are produced by *C. difficile* during log-phase growth of vegetative forms.[25–27] Most strains are toxigenic, and virtually all toxigenic strains produce both toxins under identical culture

TABLE 79–1 ■ Clinical Experience with Tissue Culture Assay for *Clostridium difficile* Toxin and Culture for *C. difficile*

PATIENT'S CATEGORY	ISOLATION OF *C. DIFFICILE* (%)	*C. DIFFICILE* TOXIN ASSAY (%)
Antibiotic-associated diarrhea/colitis		
Antibiotic-associated diarrhea without colitis	15–30	15–25
Pseudomembranous colitis	90–100	90–100
Antibiotic exposure without diarrhea	10–20	2–8
Gastrointestinal diseases unrelated to antibiotics	2–3	0–1
Healthy adults	2–3	0–0.5
Healthy neonates	30–70	5–60

conditions, although there are strain variations in the amount of toxin produced and there are differences between the toxins in biologic activity.[25–30] Toxin B is a 270- to 279-kDa protein that is a potent cytotoxin causing nonlethal disruption of actin microfilaments of the cytoskeleton.[25, 26, 31, 32] Toxin A is a 308-kDa protein that causes similar cytotoxic changes but is about 1000 times less potent in tissue culture assays. Toxin A induces neutrophilic infiltration, increased myoelectric activity, and severe mucosal damage in loop assays of small bowel or colon of guinea pigs, hamsters, rats, mice, and rabbits.[25–27, 33] Toxin B has no activity in these loop assays using rodent models, suggesting that toxin B is responsible for tissue culture changes and toxin A is responsible for enteric disease. Studies with human intestinal cells (T84) in Ussing chambers showed that toxin B was about 10 times more potent in permeability and morphologic changes.[34] The implication is that both toxins may be important in clinical expression in patients.

Age-Related Risk

Numerous studies have shown high carriage rates of both *C. difficile* and its toxin among healthy neonates.[14, 16, 17] This is the only population in which the toxin is found in the stool at high frequency in the absence of clinical expression. One suggested explanation is that the infant gut simply is not susceptible.[35] In addition, population-based studies in Sweden have shown that the incidence of *C. difficile* toxin–positive stools is 20 to 100 times greater for persons older than 60 years than for those 10 to 20 years old.[13] Serologic assays indicate that most healthy persons older than 5 to 10 years have circulating antibody to toxin A, toxin B, or both, but this apparently does not confer protection.[36] These data suggest that the aging process is associated with increasing susceptibility to colonization, toxin production, and disease caused by *C. difficile*, although the mechanism is not known.

Clinical Features

Signs and Symptoms

The single symptom that is found in nearly all patients with PMC is diarrhea. Only 10% to 25% of all patients with antibiotic-associated diarrhea have positive toxin assays for *C. difficile*.[2, 20] The majority of the toxin-negative cases are enigmatic. Clinical features that specifically suggest *C. difficile*–associated enteric disease in the patient with antibiotic-associated diarrhea are as follows: severity of diarrhea based on gut symptoms and systemic response; evidence for colitis with cramps, fever, leukocytosis, or fecal leukocytes; lack of a dose relationship; and epidemic or endemic disease with nosocomial cases. Some antimicrobial agents cause high rates of diarrhea but are not disproportionately represented in *C. difficile*–associated disease. These include cefixime, amoxicillin-clavulanate, and cefoperazone.[37]

C. difficile most often causes mild or moderate diarrhea that resolves when the implicated agent is simply discontinued. Other features in more seriously ill patients[38–44] include fever, which is usually low grade but the temperature may reach 105°F; leukocytosis that averages 15,000 cells per mm^3 but may reach leukemoid levels of 50,000 cells per mm^3 or higher; and loose stools that may reach 15 to 30/d. Because this is a protein-losing enteropathy, hypoalbuminemia is common and pedal edema or anasarca is a late complication in advanced cases.[45] Stool examinations for fecal leukocytes are positive by direct methylene blue stain in 40% to 50% of cases and by stool lactoferrin in 60% to 80%.[22, 46, 47]

Serious complications in patients with *C. difficile*–induced diarrhea or colitis include severe dehydration, electrolyte imbalance, hypotension, hypoalbuminemia with anasarca, toxic megacolon, and colonic perforation. Extraintestinal symptoms are infrequent, except for the complications noted that are ascribed largely to severe colitis and diarrhea, although occasional patients have polyarthritis.[48–50] Three findings that appear to be somewhat unique to *C. difficile* diarrhea (compared with that caused by other bacterial agents) include its propensity to be prolonged or chronic, the characteristic anatomic feature of PMC, and hypoalbuminemia.

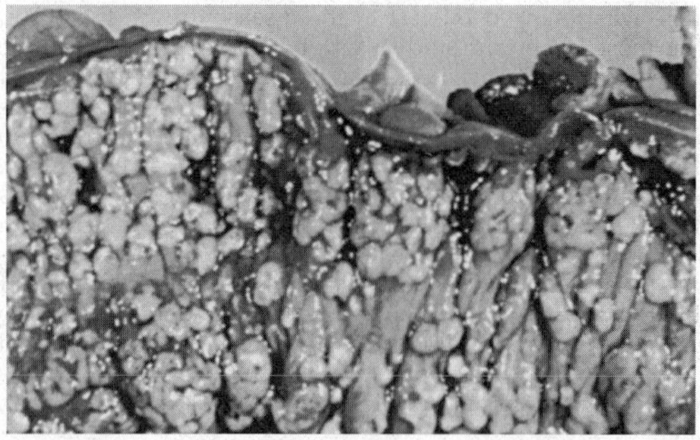

FIGURE 79–1 □ Resected colon showing pseudomembranous colitis.

Pathologic Changes

Endoscopy in patients with antibiotic-associated diarrhea shows a spectrum of changes on gross inspection, including an entirely normal mucosa, erythema, edema, severe inflammation, or, the most characteristic feature, pseudomembranous lesions. With PMC, gross inspection shows multiple, elevated, yellowish white plaques that vary in size from a few millimeters to 5 to 10 mm[5, 51, 52] (Fig. 79–1). Early lesions are punctate, but with advanced disease the pseudomembranes may coalesce and eventually slough to leave large denuded areas.

Histologic studies indicate that the pseudomembrane typically arises from a point of superficial ulceration and is accompanied by acute or chronic inflammatory changes in the lamina propria.[40, 41] The pseudomembrane is composed of fibrin, mucin, inflammatory cells, and sloughed mucosal epithelial cells (Fig. 79–2). There is no evidence of bacterial

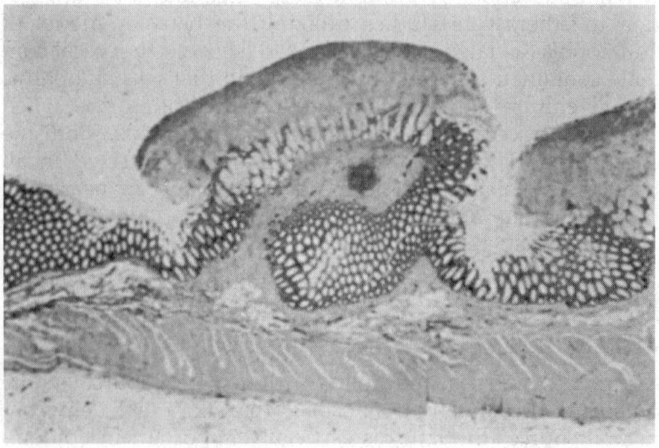

FIGURE 79–2 □ Histopathology of the lesion in Figure 79–1 showing the pseudomembrane.

invasion of the bowel mucosa, and no typical organisms are found within the pseudomembrane.

Diagnostic Studies

Diagnostic studies in patients with antibiotic-associated diarrhea or colitis are separated into those used to define anatomic changes and those used to detect the agent of disease. For anatomic studies, radiographs are usually nonspecific, although plain films of the abdomen in patients with colitis may show a markedly edematous colon with distention and distorted haustral markings.[53, 54] Contrast studies may show rounded filling defects that outline plaques, but most patients have nondiagnostic findings, owing to excessive mucus secretion, underpenetration of barium, or minimal involvement. The diagnostic yield is improved with air contrast studies, but these must be performed with caution because of the potential complication of colon perforation. Characteristic findings with computed tomography are changes restricted to the colon without small bowel involvement, colonic thickening that averages 10 to 15 mm, and ascites fluid[55, 56] (Fig. 79–3). Changes in the colon may be focal or pancolonic. Only approximately 50% of patients with positive toxin assays show changes on the computed tomographic scan.

The preferred method for determining anatomic changes is endoscopy. In most patients the distal colon is involved, so sigmoidoscopy is often adequate; however, as many as one third of the patients have lesions restricted to the right colon, necessitating colonoscopy.[57] The typical changes are those noted previously—punctate lesions that stud the colonic mucosa with an intervening mucosa that is normal or erythematous (Fig. 79–4). The role of endoscopy in these patients is often controversial. Because the procedure is unpleasant, because it is expensive, and because therapeutic decisions are usually based on the severity of clinical symptoms, the *C. difficile* toxin assay is the preferred diagnostic test.

Methods to detect *C. difficile* and its toxins are summarized in Table 79–2. Most authorities consider the tissue culture assay to be the "gold standard."[41–43] This requires the demonstration of a cytopathic toxin that is neutralized by *C. difficile* or *Clostridium sordellii* antitoxin.[58–59] Results with this assay in various populations are summarized in Table 79–1. The major disadvantages of the test are that many laboratories do not offer tissue culture technology and there is a 24- to 48-hour delay for results. The major technical error made in processing is the routine use of excessive dilutions of the

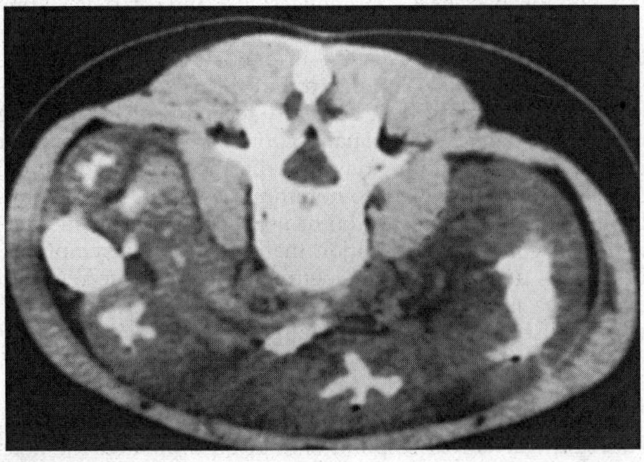

FIGURE 79–3 □ Computed tomographic scan of abdomen showing colitis due to *C. difficile,* with thickened colonic mucosa.

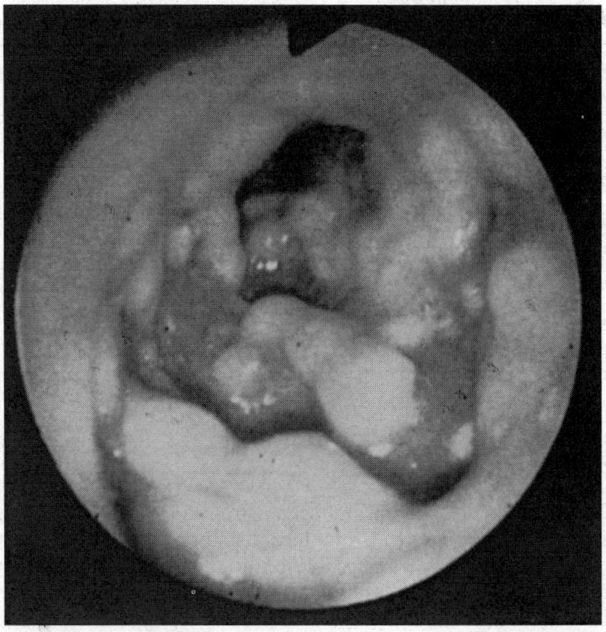

FIGURE 79–4 □ Pseudomembranous plaques seen with colonoscopy in a patient with *C. difficile*–associated PMC.

specimens; 10% to 20% of positive assays show a titer of 1:10 or less with undiluted specimens or only a 1:4 dilution.[60] The toxin titer may be evaluated using serial dilutions of stool, but there appears to be little correlation between the severity of disease and toxin titers. False-negative results are unusual, provided the specimen is processed by a competent laboratory using a sufficiently low dilution of the specimen. False-positive assays are so frequent in children younger than 1 year that the test is virtually useless in this population. Among adults, false-positive results are occasionally encountered in patients who are receiving antibiotics but do not have diarrhea. In addition, the toxin assays may remain positive long after symptoms have resolved. These observations indicate that the test is useful for initial diagnosis but it is not a reliable method to monitor response to therapy.

The first commercially available alternative to the tissue culture assay was the latex agglutination assay, introduced in the early 1980s. This assay was intended to detect toxin A of *C. difficile,* but subsequent work showed that it detected a nontoxic protein produced not only by *C. difficile* but also by other clostridial species.[61] The preferred test in most laboratories in the 1990s is the enzyme immunoassay. Reagents are now available from multiple suppliers for detection of toxin A or toxins A and B. Major advantages of these assays compared with tissue culture assays are the ease of technical performance and the speed with which results are completed, usually 2 to 3 hours. Also, sensitivity and specificity rates of these assays (63% to 89% and 95% to 100%, respectively) are higher than rates reported with tissue cultures.[60, 62–65] Other techniques for toxin detection that are being developed are a dot immunoblot[66] and polymerase chain reaction to amplify gene fragments that encode for toxin A or B.[67, 68] Some authorities advocate stool cultures to supplement toxin assays.[69–71] Advantages are that sensitivity is good when experienced technicians perform the assay, and this permits strain identity in epidemics. Disadvantages are the technical expertise required, the 48- to 72-hour delay for results, and the relative nonspecificity of results due to high rates of carriage in the population of greatest interest: hospitalized patients and patients receiving antibiotics (see Table 79–1).

TABLE 79–2 ■ Diagnostic Tests for Detection of *Clostridium difficile*–Associated Diarrhea

VARIABLE	TISSUE CULTURE ASSAY	LATEX PARTICLE AGGLUTINATION	ENZYME IMMUNOASSAY	DOT IMMUNOBLOT	POLYMERASE CHAIN REACTION	CULTURE
Source	Commercial microtiter wells	Commercially available	Four suppliers	Commercially available	Experimental	Cycloserine-cefoxitin-fructose agar, others
Product detected	Toxin B	Glutamate dehydrogenase	Toxin A or toxin A plus toxin B	Toxin A	Toxin B gene, toxin A gene, or both	Organism ± toxigenic potential in vitro
Time required	28–48 h	30 min	2–4 h	30 min	2–4 h	24–72 h
Clinical correlations	Best sensitivity with proper dilutions; good specificity	Least sensitive and specific; some use as screening test only	Good specificity; fair sensitivity; may require two or three tests	Initial studies promising	Good sensitivity; fair specificity	Good sensitivity; poor specificity due to high carriage rates in hospitalized patients and antibiotic recipients

Epidemiology

C. difficile is a sporulating organism that survives well in nature and appears to be widely distributed in the environment.[10] It is also a transferable pathogen that poses a threat to patients in hospitals and in chronic care facilities, where there is nosocomial exposure and a large population of susceptible hosts, owing to the frequency of antibiotic use.[5, 15, 39–44, 72–81] Within such institutions, *C. difficile* may be endemic or epidemic in selected areas. Several investigators have found environmental sources of *C. difficile*, primarily in case-associated areas.[76, 77, 81] For example, Kim and associates[76] isolated the organism in environmental samplings from 37 of 114 (32%) case-associated areas but in only 6 of 445 (1.3%) controlled sites.[75] The primary sources for positive cultures in such studies have been toilets, bed pans, floors, and the hands of personnel. The hospital environment may pose considerable risk for acquisition of *C. difficile*, even in the absence of an epidemic of clinically apparent disease. McFarland and coworkers[15] sampled rectal swab material sequentially from 428 hospitalized patients and found that 112 (26%) harbored *C. difficile* at some time during their hospital course; of these 112, 6 (6%) were apparently colonized before hospitalization, 23 (21%) had been in a nursing home before their hospitalization, and 83 (74%) acquired the organism during hospitalization. Most of the patients had no symptoms. Risks identified for both increased rates of carriage and increased rates of diarrhea include advanced age, severe underlying disease, and exposure to selected antibiotics, especially clindamycin and cephalosporins.[5, 22, 23, 41–44, 78]

Epidemiologic studies often include methods to type strains to monitor epidemiology and to correlate strain types with virulence according to clinical correlations and in vivo toxin production. Strain-typing methods include plasmid fingerprinting, protein analysis, immunoblotting, polyacrylamide gel electrophoresis, serotyping, restriction endonuclease analysis, polymerase chain reaction, ribotyping, bacteriocin typing, and restriction fragment length polymorphism.[73, 74, 82–89] There is no consensus on the optimal test,[89] and most hospital laboratories do not offer these assays.

Treatment

Treatment of *C. difficile*–associated diarrhea or colitis includes discontinuation of the implicated agent, implementation of supportive measures, and, in selected cases, oral administration of metronidazole or vancomycin. Antiperistaltic agents should be avoided.[90] Some patients require continued antibiotic treatment of the underlying condition; in these cases, it is advised to give oral metronidazole or vancomycin and change the suspected inducing agent to an alternative agent that infrequently causes this complication, such as fluoroquinolone, doxycycline, parenteral aminoglycoside, trimethoprim-sulfamethoxazole, sulfonamide, parenteral vancomycin, or metronidazole.

Antimicrobial Treatment

Many patients respond when the implicated agent is simply discontinued and do not require antibiotic treatment of the antibiotic-induced complication.[91] The major advantage is avoidance of the risk of relapsing *C. difficile*–associated diarrhea or colitis. Indications for antibiotic treatment are arbitrary and include severe diarrhea, diarrhea accompanied by systemic signs or evidence of colitis, ileus, and persistent symptoms after antibiotics have been discontinued. The drug usually administered in these cases is oral vancomycin or oral metronidazole.[41–43, 91–93] Some patients cannot take oral drugs owing to recent surgery, ileus, intolerance of an agent, or other gastrointestinal complications. The experience with parenteral vancomycin or metronidazole in such cases is anecdotal and inconsistent.[94]

Metronidazole is generally regarded as the preferred treatment based on cost, demonstrated efficacy, and the opportunity to avoid vancomycin, which may promote vancomycin-resistant *Enterococcus faecium* in nosocomial cases.[40–42, 93, 95, 96] A theoretical disadvantage of metronidazole is nearly complete absorption so that levels in the colonic lumen are nil. This is a toxin-mediated disease, with *C. difficile* retained entirely in the colonic lumen without invasion, meaning that drug in the colonic lumen is the assumed goal of therapy.

Vancomycin is considered the gold standard based on extensive experience with highly impressive results from 1978 to 1985, when many of the patients had serious disease with established PMC, systemic signs, and/or devastating diarrhea.[40–43, 91] My experience with 100 patients with established PMC showed that 97% responded.[93] The initial dose used in early trials was 2 mg/d, but this is substantial overkill and the standard dose currently recommended is 125 mg four times daily.[42] The usual response is impressive; fever usually resolves within 1 day, and diarrhea resolves in 4 to 5 days.[42, 91–93] Patients who do not improve within several days usually have toxic megacolon or ileus, or they have an alternative or concurrent condition that accounts for symptoms. Responses are similar with metronidazole, but the reported experience is generally restricted to patients with less advanced disease.[96]

Treatment Failure

Patients who fail to respond should be evaluated for ileus and alternative diagnoses with various studies, including computed tomography or endoscopy or both. Oral vancomycin is the preferred agent for patients who are seriously ill or unresponsive to alternative treatment. Options in patients with ileus are parenteral administration of metronidazole and enteric administration of vancomycin by mouth or intubation. In my colleagues' and my experience, approximately 0.4% of patients fail to respond and are candidates for surgery.[97] The usual indications for surgery are persistent or progressive signs of systemic toxicity, persistent diarrhea, signs of peritonitis (although perforation is rare), and progressive colonic disease as seen on sequential computed tomographic scans. In these cases, the procedure of choice is a total colectomy.

Relapse

The major complication with either oral metronidazole or vancomycin is relapse. This occurs only with antimicrobial treatment; it is found with equal frequency after treatment with vancomycin, bacitracin, and metronidazole, and the frequency is reported at 5% to 50%,[91, 93, 96, 98] with a rate of 24% in the largest series.[93] Most patients respond well to a second course of antibiotics, but approximately 2% to 5% have multiple relapses, defined as four or more relapses after antimicrobial treatment.[91, 93] The clinical features of relapses are quite stereotyped: the patient responds to standard treatment, but 2 to 28 days (usually 3 to 7 days) after antimicrobial treatment is discontinued, he or she reports that the same symptoms have recurred. Stool assays for toxin at that time will be positive, and cultures yield *C. difficile* that is usually the same strain as the original isolate. Nevertheless, stool assays for *C. difficile* toxin are often positive after treatment in patients who do not have relapses, indicating that the toxin assay should not be used to define relapse. Similarly, stool cultures are usually positive at the termination of treatment, and these isolates show continued susceptibility to the agent used for therapy.[91–99] Vancomycin fails to eradicate *C. difficile* from the colon, despite levels that are usually several hundred times higher than the MIC. (Levels achieved in the colonic lumen with standard doses are 350 to 500 μg/g, and the highest MIC ever measured for a strain of *C. difficile* is 16 μg/mL.[98, 100]) This persistence presumably reflects sporulation, and the assumption is that these strains revert to vegetative forms that replicate and produce toxin when vancomycin (or metronidazole) is discontinued.[101]

There are several methods that can be used to manage the patients with multiple relapses; all work some of the time and none works all of the time (Table 79–3). The method we prefer is a 10- 14-day course of vancomycin or metronidazole, followed by a second stage of treatment consisting of "pulse dose" vancomycin, 125 mg given orally every second day for 4 weeks.[91] An alternative method for the second phase of treatment is administration of cholestyramine, 4-g packet three times per day, plus *Lactobacillus* (e.g., Lactinex), 1 g four times per day, for 4 weeks. The theory used to justify these tactics is that the first phase is given to gain control of the disease and the second phase is an attempt to inhibit *C. difficile* until the normal flora becomes reestablished. Other methods used to manage relapses are administration of tapering doses of vancomycin,[102] vancomycin plus rifampin,[103] or intravenous immunoglobulin[104, 105] and attempts to manip-

TABLE 79–3 ■ Treatment of *Clostridium difficile*–Induced Diarrhea and Colitis

I. Nonspecific treatment
  A. Discontinuation of implicated antimicrobial agent (i.e., discontinuation of treatment or change to an alternative regimen unlikely to cause this complication)
  B. Implementation of supportive measures: correction of fluid losses and electrolyte imbalances essential; parenteral hyperalimentation rarely indicated; role of corticosteroids in seriously ill patients not established
  C. Avoidance of antiperistaltic agents
  D. Observance of enteric isolation precautions for hospitalized patients
II. Specific treatment and dosages*
  A. Antimicrobial agents (advocated only if symptoms are severe or persist)
    1. Oral agent (preferred)
      (a) Vancomycin: 125 mg PO qid, 7–14 d (efficacy is established)
      (b) Metronidazole: 250 mg PO tid, 7–14 d (efficacy is established)
      (c) Alternative: bacitracin, 25,000 units PO qid, 7–14 d (efficacy is established)
    2. Oral treatment precluded by NPO status, ileus, intolerance of medicines
      (a) Parenteral agents: metronidazole: 500 mg IV q 6 h (experience is anecdotal and variable; oral treatment should be given whenever feasible)
      (b) Vancomycin (0.5–2 g/d) via long tube in small bowel or via endoscopy or rectal tube in colon
  B. Alternative treatments
    1. Anion exchange resins
      (a) Cholestyramine, 4-g packet PO tid, 5–14 d (efficacy is established)
      (b) Cholestipol, 5-g packet PO tid, 5–10 d
    2. Alteration of fecal flora: Lactinex (or alternative *Lactobacillus* preparation) 1-g packet PO qid, 7–14 d
III. Multiple relapses
  A. Vancomycin or metronidazole PO 10–14 d, followed by
    1. Cholestyramine 4-g packet PO tid plus *Lactobacillus* 1 g PO qid, 3–4 wk
    2. Vancomycin, 125 mg PO qod, 3 wk
  B. Vancomycin plus rifampin, 7–14 d[103]
  C. Experimental agents
    1. *Saccharomyces boulardii*: vancomycin 125 mg PO qid or metronidazole 250 mg PO tid ≥4 d with addition of *S. boulardii* as two 250-mg capsules bid, 4 wk[105, 106]
    2. *Lactobacillus* GG: 1 tab (10^{10}organisms) bid × 3 wk after course of vancomycin or metronidazole[107]
    3. Intravenous immunoglobulin: 400 mg/kg q 3 wk (reported primarily in pediatric patients and in an adult with immunoglobulin A deficiency)[104]
    4. Rectal instillation of feces: 50 g fresh stool from healthy donor in 500 mL saline delivered by enema[108]
    5. Rectal instillation of broth cultures of bacterial isolates from healthy donors: strains selected based on in vitro inhibition of *C. difficile*, cultured to 10^9/mL, 2 mL of each mixed in anaerobic glovebox with 180 mL saline and given by enema[109]

*PO, By mouth; qid, four times daily; tid, three times daily; qod, every other day; bid, twice daily; tab, tablet; NPO, nothing by mouth; IV, intravenously.

ulate the fecal flora with oral administration of *Saccharomyces boulardii*,[106] oral administration of *Lactobacillus* GG,[107] rectal instillations of stool from healthy donors,[108] and rectal instillations of broth cultures of stool isolates.[109]

Infection Control

C. difficile–induced enteric disease may be endemic or epidemic in acute care hospitals, chronic care facilities, and daycare centers, all settings where there is clustering of people rendered vulnerable by high rates of antibiotic use.[40–43, 70, 72–81, 110] Patients in acute and chronic care facilities should preferably be in private rooms with bathroom facilities until diarrhea resolves. There should be enteric precautions, with careful attention to hand washing and use of gloves.[20, 73, 74, 111, 112] In epidemics it may be necessary to institute controls on use of major inducing agents, primarily clindamycin and cephalosporins.[78]

Evaluation of epidemics includes identification of cases with increased use of toxin assays and a surveillance log book to determine epidemiologic patterns. Some authorities recommend stool cultures and strain typing of isolates from cases and carriers.[82–89] However, most laboratories do not offer either stool cultures for *C. difficile* or strain typing of isolates. Interventions in epidemics include sequestering patients, assiduous attention to enteric precautions, cleansing environmental sources with sporicidal germicides, and antibiotic control to limit use of clindamycin or cephalosporins or both. Some physicians favor treatment of carriers with vancomycin or metronidazole, although, as noted earlier, this does not eradicate the carrier state and may actually cause this complication.

References

1. Bartlett JG, Onderdonk AB, Cisneros AB, et al: Clindamycin-associated colitis due to toxin-producing species of *Clostridium* in hamsters. J Infect Dis 136:701, 1977.
2. Bartlett JG: *Clostridium difficile:* Clinical considerations. Rev Infect Dis 12:S243, 1990.
3. Finney JMT: Gastroenterostomy for cicatrizing ulcer of pylorus. Bull Johns Hopkins Hosp 4:53, 1893.
4. Hummel RO, Altemeier WA, Hill EO: Iatrogenic staphylococcal enterocolitis. Ann Surg 160:551, 1964.
5. Tedesco FJ, Barton RW, Alpers DH: Clindamycin-associated colitis: A prospective study. Ann Intern Med 81:429, 1974.
6. Hambra DM, Rake G, McKeet CM, et al: The toxicity of penicillin as prepared for clinical use. Am J Med Sci 206:642, 1943.
7. Green RH: The association of viral activation with penicillin toxicity in guinea pigs and hamsters. Yale J Biol Med 47:166, 1974.
8. Larson HE, Parry JV, Price AB, et al: Undescribed toxin in pseudomembranous colitis. Br Med J 1:1246, 1977.
9. Hall IC, O'Toole E: Intestinal flora in newborn infants with a description of a new pathogenic anaerobe, *Bacillus difficiles.* Am J Dis Child 49:380, 1935.
10. Hafiz S: *Clostridium difficile* and Its Toxins. Leeds, England, University of Leeds, 1974. PhD dissertation.
11. Bartlett JG, Chang TW, Gurwit M, et al: Antibiotic-associated pseudomembranous colitis due to toxin-producing clostridia. N Engl J Med 298:531, 1978.
12. George WL, Sutter VL, Citron D, et al: Selective and differential medium for isolation of *Clostridium difficile.* J Clin Microbiol 9:214, 1979.
13. Aronsson B, Mollby R, Nord CE: Antimicrobial agents and *Clostridium difficile* in acute enteric disease: Epidemiological data from Sweden, 1980–1982. J Infect Dis 151:476, 1985.
14. Viscidi R, Willey S, Bartlett JG: Isolation rates and toxigenic potential for *Clostridium difficile* isolates from various patient populations. Gastroenterology 81:5, 1981.
15. McFarland LV, Mulligan ME, Kwok RYY, et al: Nosocomial acquisition of *Clostridium difficile* infection. N Engl J Med 320:204, 1989.
16. Larson HE, Barclay FE, Honour P, et al: Epidemiology of *Clostridium difficile* in infants. J Infect Dis 146:727, 1982.
17. Holst E, Helin I, Mardh P: A recovery of *Clostridium difficile* in children. Scand J Infect Dis 13:41, 1981.
18. Bartlett JG: Antimicrobial agents implicated in *Clostridium difficile* toxin–associated diarrhea or colitis. Johns Hopkins Med J 149:6, 1981.
19. George WL, Rolfe RD, Finegold SM: *Clostridium difficile* and its cytotoxin in feces of patients with antimicrobial agent–associated diarrhea and miscellaneous conditions. J Clin Microbiol 15:1049, 1982.
20. Wilcox MH: Cleaning up *Clostridium difficile* infection. Lancet 348:767, 1996.
21. Golledge CL, McKenzie T, Riley TV: Extended spectrum cephalosporins and *Clostridium difficile.* J Antimicrob Chemother 23:929, 1989.
22. Manabe YC, Vinetz JM, Moore RD, et al: *Clostridium difficile* colitis: An efficient clinical approach to diagnosis. Ann Intern Med 123:835, 1995.
23. Anand A, Bashey B, Mir T, Glatt AE: Epidemiology, clinical manifestation, and outcome of *Clostridium difficile*–associated diarrhea. Am J Gastroenterol 89:519, 1994.
24. Dzink JA, Bartlett JG: In vitro susceptibility of *Clostridium difficile* isolates from patients with antibiotic-associated diarrhea or colitis. Antimicrob Agents Chemother 17:695, 1980.
25. Taylor NS, Thorne G, Bartlett JG: Comparison of two toxins produced by *Clostridium difficile.* Infect Immun 34:1036, 1981.
26. Sullivan NM, Pettett S, Wilkins TD: Purification and characterization of toxins A and B of *Clostridium difficile.* Infect Immun 35:1032, 1982.
27. Lima AM, Lyerly DM, Wilkins TD, et al: Effects of *Clostridium difficile* toxins A and B in rabbit small and large intestine in vivo and cultured cells in vitro. Infect Immun 56:582, 1988.
28. Fluit AC, Wolfhagen MJHM, Verdonk GPHT, et al: Nontoxigenic strains of *Clostridium difficile* lack the genes for both toxin A and toxin B. J Clin Microbiol 29:2666, 1991.
29. Borriello SP, Wren BW, Hyde S, et al: Molecular, immunological, and biological characterization of a toxin A–negative, toxin B–positive strain of *Clostridium difficile.* Infect Immun 60:4192, 1992.
30. Johnson S, Sypura WD, Gerding DN, et al: Selective neutralization of a bacterial enterotoxin by serum immunoglobulin A in response to mucosal disease. Infect Immun 63:3166, 1995.
31. Fiorentini C, Malorni W, Paradisi S, et al: Interaction of *Clostridium difficile* toxin A with cultured cells: Cytoskeletal changes and nuclear polarization. Infect Immun 58:2329, 1990.
32. Just I, Selzer J, Wilm M, et al: Glucosylation of Rho proteins by *Clostridium difficile* toxin B. Nature 375:500, 1995.
33. Burakoff R, Zhao L, Celifarco AJ, et al: Effects of purified *Clostridium difficile* toxin A on rabbit distal colon. Gastroenterology 190:348, 1995.
34. Riegler M, Sedivy R, Pothoulakis C, et al: *Clostridium difficile* toxin B is more potent than toxin A in damaging human colonic epithelium in vitro. J Clin Invest 95:2004, 1995.
35. Eglow R, Pothoulakis C, Itzkowitz S, et al: Diminished *Clostridium difficile* toxin A sensitivity in newborn rabbit ileum is associated with decreased toxin A receptor. J Clin Invest 90:822, 1992.
36. Viscidi R, Laughon BE, Yolken R, et al: Serum antibody response to toxins A and B of *Clostridium difficile.* J Infect Dis 148:93, 1983.
37. Gilbert DN: Aspects of the safety profile of oral antimicrobial agents. Infect Dis Clin Pract 4(Suppl 2):103, 1995.
38. George WL, Rolfe RD, Finegold SM: *Clostridium difficile* and its cytotoxin in feces of patients with antimicrobial agent–associated diarrhea and miscellaneous conditions. J Clin Microbiol 15:1049, 1982.
39. Bartlett JG, Taylor NW, Chang TW, Dzink JA: Clinical and laboratory observations in *Clostridium difficile* colitis. Am J Clin Nutr 33:2521, 1981.
40. Mogg GM, Keighley M, Burdon D, et al: Antibiotic-associated colitis—A review of 66 cases. Br J Surg 66:738, 1979.
41. Bartlett JG: Antibiotic-associated diarrhea. Clin Infect Dis 15:573, 1992.
42. Fekety R, Shah AB: Diagnosis and treatment of *Clostridium difficile* colitis. JAMA 269:71, 1993.

43. Kelly C, Pothoulakis C, LaMont JT: *Clostridium difficile* colitis. N Engl J Med 330:257, 1994.
44. Gerding DN: Disease associated with *Clostridium difficile* infection. Ann Intern Med 110:255, 1989.
45. Rybolt AH, Laughon BE, Greenough WB, et al: Protein-losing enteropathy associated with *Clostridium difficile* infection. Lancet 1:1353, 1989.
46. Yong WH, Mattia AR, Ferraro MJ: Comparison of fecal lactoferrin latex agglutination assay and methylene blue microscopy for detection of fecal leukocytes in *Clostridium difficile*–associated disease. J Clin Microbiol 32:1360, 1994.
47. Schleupner MA, Garner DC, Sosnowski KM, et al: Concurrence of *Clostridium difficile* toxin A enzyme–linked immunosorbent assay, fecal lactoferrin assay, and clinical criteria with *C. difficile* cytotoxin titer in two patient cohorts. J Clin Microbiol 33:1755, 1995.
48. Putterman C, Rubinow A: Reactive arthritis associated with *Clostridium difficile* pseudomembranous colitis. Semin Arthritis Rheum 22:420, 1993.
49. Mermel LA, Osborn TG: *Clostridium difficile*–associated reactive arthritis in an HLA-B27 positive female: Report and literature review. J Rheumatol 16:133, 1989.
50. Rollins DE, Moeller D: Polyarthritis associated with clindamycin-induced colitis. JAMA 231:1228, 1975.
51. Price AB, Davies DR: Pseudomembranous colitis. J Clin Pathol 30:1, 1977.
52. Summer HW, Tedesco FJ: Rectal biopsy in clindamycin-associated colitis. Arch Pathol 99:237, 1975.
53. Stanley RJ, Melson GL, Tedesco FJ: The spectrum of radiographic findings in antibiotic-related pseudomembranous colitis. Radiology 111:519, 1974.
54. Stanley RJ, Melson GL, Tedesco FJ, et al: Plain-film findings in severe pseudomembranous colitis. Radiology 118:7, 1976.
55. Fishman E, Kavuru M, Kulzlman JE, et al: CT of pseudomembranous colitis: Radiologic, clinical and pathologic correlation. Radiology 180:57, 1991.
56. Boland GW, Lee MJ, Cats AM, et al: Antibiotic-induced diarrhea: Specificity of abdominal CT for the diagnosis of *Clostridium difficile* disease. Radiology 191:103, 1994.
57. Tedesco FJ, Corless JK, Brownstein RE: Rectal sparing in antibiotic-associated pseudomembranous colitis: A prospective study. Gastroenterology 83:1259, 1982.
58. Chang TW, Lauermann M, Bartlett JG: Cytotoxicity assay in antibiotic-associated colitis. J Infect Dis 140:765, 1979.
59. Bartlett JG: Laboratory diagnosis of antibiotic-associated colitis. Lab Med 12:347, 1981.
60. Laughon BE, Viscidi RP, Gdovin SL, et al: Enzyme immunoassays for detection of *Clostridium difficile* toxins A and B in fecal specimens. J Infect Dis 149:781, 1984.
61. Lyerly DM, Barroso LA, Wilkins TD: Identification of the latex test–reactive protein of *Clostridium difficile* as glutamate dehydrogenase. J Clin Microbiol 29:2639, 1991.
62. Walker RC, Ruane PJ, Rosenblatt JE, et al: Comparison of culture, cytotoxicity assays, and linked immunosorbent assay for toxin A and toxin B in the diagnosis of *Clostridium difficile*–related enteric disease. Diagn Microbiol Infect Dis 5:61, 1986.
63. DiPersio JP, Varga FJ, Conwell DL, et al: Development of a rapid enzyme immunoassay for *Clostridium difficile* toxin A and its use in the diagnosis of *C. difficile*–associated disease. J Clin Microbiol 29:2724, 1991.
64. Barbut F, Kajzer C, Planas N, Petit J-C: Comparison of three enzyme immunoassays, a cytotoxicity assay, and toxigenic culture for diagnosis of *Clostridium difficile*–associated diarrhea. J Clin Microbiol 31:963, 1993.
65. Merz CS, Kramer C, Forman M, et al: Comparison of four commercially available rapid enzyme immunoassays with cytotoxin assay for detection of *Clostridium difficile* toxins(s) from stool specimens. J Clin Microbiol 32:1142, 1994.
66. Kurzynski TA: Evaluation of *C. difficile* CUBE test for detection of *Clostridium difficile*–associated diarrhea. Diagn Microbiol Infect Dis 15:493, 1992.
67. Kato N, Ou C-Y, Kato H, et al: Detection of toxigenic *Clostridium difficile* in stool specimens by the polymerase chain reaction. J Infect Dis 167:455, 1993.
68. Kuhl SJ, Tang YJ, Navarro L, et al: Diagnosis and monitoring of *Clostridium difficile* infections with the polymerase chain reaction. Clin Infect Dis 16(Suppl 4):234, 1993.
69. Bond F, Payne G, Borriello SP, Humphreys H: Usefulness of culture in the diagnosis of *Clostridium difficile* infection. Eur J Clin Microbiol Infect Dis 14:223, 1995.
70. Gerding DN, Johnson S, Peterson LR, et al: *Clostridium difficile*–associated diarrhea and colitis. Infect Control Hosp Epidemiol 16:459, 1995.
71. Riley TV, Cooper M, Bell B, Golledge CL: Community-acquired *Clostridium difficile*–associated diarrhea. Clin Infect Dis 20(Suppl 2):263, 1995.
72. McFarland LV, Surawicz CM, Stamm EW: Risk factors for *Clostridium difficile* carriage and *C. difficile*–associated diarrhea in a cohort of hospitalized patients. J Infect Dis 162:678, 1990.
73. Samore MH, DeGirolami PC, Tlucko A, et al: *Clostridium difficile* colonization and diarrhea at a tertiary care hospital. Clin Infect Dis 18:181, 1994.
74. Samore MH, Venkataraman L, DeGirolami PC, et al: Clinical and molecular epidemiology of sporadic and clustered cases of nosocomial *Clostridium difficile* diarrhea. Am J Med 100:32, 1996.
75. Simor AE, Yake SL, Tsimidis K: Infection due to *Clostridium difficile* among elderly residents of a long-term care facility. Clin Infect Dis 17:672, 1993.
76. Kim KH, Fekety R, Botts DH, Brown D: Isolation of *Clostridium difficile* from the environment and contacts of patients with antibiotic-associated colitis. J Infect Dis 143:42, 1981.
77. Mulligan ME, George WL, Rolfe RD, et al: Epidemiological aspects of *Clostridium difficile*–induced diarrhea and colitis. Am J Clin Nutr 33:2533, 1981.
78. Pear SM, Williamson TH, Bettin KM, et al: Decrease in nosocomial *Clostridium difficile*–associated diarrhea by restricting clindamycin use. Ann Intern Med 120:272, 1994.
79. Gerding DN, Olson M, Peterson R, et al: *Clostridium difficile*–associated diarrhea and colitis in adults. A prospective case controlled epidemiologic study. Arch Intern Med 146:95, 1986.
80. Bender BS, Laughon BE, Gaydos C, et al: Is *Clostridium difficile* endemic in chronic care facilities? Lancet 2:11, 1986.
81. Johnson S, Clabots CR, Linn FV, et al: Nosocomial *Clostridium difficile* colonisation and disease. Lancet 336:97, 1990.
82. Clabots CR, Peterson LR, Gerding DN: Characterization of a nosocomial *Clostridium difficile* outbreak by using plasmid profile typing and clindamycin susceptibility testing. J Infect Dis 158:731, 1988.
83. Pantosti A, Cerquetti M, Gianfrilli PM: Electrophoretic characterization of *Clostridium difficile* strains isolated from antibiotic-associated colitis and other conditions. J Clin Microbiol 26:540, 1988.
84. Mulligan ME, Halebian S, Kwok RYY, et al: Bacterial agglutination and polyacrylamide gel electrophoresis for typing *Clostridium difficile*. J Infect Dis 153:267, 1986.
85. Tabaqchali S, O'Farrell S, Holland D, Silman R: Typing scheme for *Clostridium difficile*: Its application in clinical and epidemiological studies. Lancet 1:935, 1984.
86. Kuijper EJ, Oudbier JH, Stuifbergen WNHM, et al: Application of whole-cell DNA restriction endonuclease profiles to the epidemiology of *Clostridium difficile*–induced diarrhea. J Clin Microbiol 25:751, 1987.
87. McFarland LV, Elmer GW, Stamm WE, Mulligan ME: Correlation of immunoblot type, enterotoxin production, and cytotoxin production with clinical manifestations of *Clostridium difficile* infection in a cohort of hospitalized patients. Infect Immun 59:2456, 1991.
88. Clabots CR, Johnson S, Bettin KM, et al: Development of a rapid and efficient restriction endonuclease analysis typing system for *Clostridium difficile* and correlation with other typing systems. J Clin Microbiol 31:1870, 1993.
89. Brazier JS: An international study on the unification of nomenclature for typing *Clostridium difficile*. Clin Infect Dis 20(Suppl 2):325, 1995.
90. Novak E, Lee JE, Seckman CE, et al: Unfavorable effect of atropine-diphenoxylate (Lomotil) therapy in lincomycin-caused diarrhea. JAMA 235:1451, 1976.
91. Bartlett JG: Treatment of *Clostridium difficile* colitis. Gastroenterology 89:1192, 1985.
92. Fekety R, Silva J, Armstrong J, et al: Treatment of antibiotic-associated colitis with vancomycin. Rev Infect Dis 3:S273, 1981.
93. Bartlett JG: Treatment of antibiotic-associated pseudomembranous colitis. Rev Infect Dis 6:S235, 1984.

94. Guzman R, Kirkpatrick J, Forward K, Lim F: Failure of parenteral metronidazole in the treatment of pseudomembranous colitis (Letter). J Infect Dis 158:1146, 1988.
95. Centers for Disease Control and Prevention: Recommendation for preventing the spread of vancomycin resistance. MMWR Morb Mort Weekly Rep 44(RR-12):1, 1995.
96. Teasley DG, Gerding DN, Olson MM, et al: Prospective randomised trial of metronidazole versus vancomycin for *Clostridium difficile*–associated diarrhoea and colitis. Lancet 2:1043, 1983.
97. Lipsett PA, Samantaray DK, Tam ML, et al: Pseudomembranous colitis: A surgical disease? Surgery 116:491, 1994.
98. Young GP, Ward PB, Bayley M: Antibiotic-associated colitis due to *Clostridium difficile*: Double-blind comparison of vancomycin with bacitracin. Gastroenterology 89:1038, 1985.
99. Walters BA, Roberts R, Stafford R, et al: Relapse of antibiotic-associated colitis: Endogenous persistence of *Clostridium difficile* during vancomycin therapy. Gut 24:206, 1983.
100. Burdon DW, Brown JD, Youngs D, et al: Antibiotic susceptibility of *Clostridium difficile*. J Antimicrob Chemother 5:307, 1979.
101. Onderdonk AB, Cisneros RL, Bartlett JG: *Clostridium difficile* in gnotobiotic mice. Infect Immun 28:277, 1980.
102. Tedesco FJ: Treatment of recurrent antibiotic-associated pseudomembranous colitis. Am J Gastroenterol 77:330, 1982.
103. Buggy BP, Fekety R, Silva J: Therapy of relapsing *Clostridium difficile*–associated diarrhea and colitis with the combination of vancomycin and rifampin. J Clin Gastroenterol 9:155, 1987.
104. Leung DY, Kelly CP, Boguniewicz M, et al: Treatment with intravenously administered gamma globulin of chronic relapsing colitis induced by *Clostridium difficile* toxin. J Pediatr 118:633, 1991.
105. Hassett J, Meyers S, McFarland L, Mulligan ME: Recurrent *Clostridium difficile* infection in a patients with selective IgG1 deficiency treated with intravenous immune globulin and *Saccharomyces boulardii*. Clin Infect Dis 20(Suppl 2):266, 1995.
106. McFarland LV, Surawicz CM, Greenberg RN, et al: A randomized placebo-controlled trial of *Saccharomyces boulardii* in combination with standard antibiotics for *Clostridium difficile* disease. JAMA 271:1913, 1994.
107. Gorbach S, Chang T-W, Goldin B: Successful treatment of relapsing *C. difficile* colitis with *Lactobacillus* GG. Lancet 2:1519, 1987.
108. Schwan A, Sjolin S, Trottestam U, et al: Relapsing *Clostridium difficile* enterocolitis cured by rectal infusion of normal feces. Scand J Infect Dis 16:211, 1984.
109. Tvede M, Rask-Madsen J: Bacteriotherapy for chronic relapsing *Clostridium difficile* diarrhoea in six patients. Lancet 6:1156, 1989.
110. Costas M, Holmes B, On SL, et al: Investigation of an outbreak of *Clostridium difficile* infection in a general hospital by numerical analysis of protein patterns by sodium dodecyl sulfate-polyacrylamide gel electrophoresis. J Clin Microbiol 32:759, 1994.
111. Silva J, Lezzi C: *Clostridium difficile* as a nosocomial pathogen. J Hosp Infect 2(Suppl A):378, 1988.
112. Kaatz GW, Gitlin SD, Schaberg DR, et al: Acquisition of *Clostridium difficile* from the hospital environment. Am J Epidemiol 127:1289, 1988.

80

Viral Gastroenteritis

Neil R. Blacklow

Viral gastroenteritis is an extremely common illness that affects all age groups worldwide. Both epidemic and endemic patterns of infection occur. In a comprehensive 10-year study of illnesses among American families, viral gastroenteritis was found to be second in frequency only to the common cold.[1] It is responsible for a considerable loss of time from work and school,[2] aside from the distress it produces in those afflicted. In the United States, viral gastroenteritis is a relatively benign and self-limited illness, although it can be severe, and even lethal, in infants and in elderly or debilitated patients.[3]

History

The agents responsible for this common illness were not defined until the 1970s and 1980s. This is in marked contrast to the viruses of acute respiratory tract disease and common childhood febrile and exanthematous illnesses, which were defined in the 1950s and 1960s. The reason for the delay was the inability to cultivate the responsible organisms from diarrheal stools in cell cultures and laboratory animals. Controlled epidemiologic studies in the 1950s and 1960s had shown that known cultivatable enteric viruses such as echovirus and coxsackievirus were not important causes of gastroenteritis.[4] Studies performed during the 1940s and 1950s established that the disease syndrome could be induced and serially propagated in volunteers by oral administration of bacteria-free filtrates of diarrheal stool, but these infectious materials failed to yield cultivatable agents.[5] The causative viruses were discovered only when electron microscopy and advanced laboratory techniques that could identify agents without in vitro cultivation were available. The result was the discovery in the 1970s of two major medically important causes of viral gastroenteritis, rotavirus and Norwalk virus.[6, 7] It is interesting that the various viral gastroenteritis agents known today still are not cultivatable or replicate inefficiently in vitro. Thus, antigen detection techniques and electron microscopy are the mainstays for detecting viral gastroenteritis agents.

Etiologic Agents

Several different viruses are associated with gastroenteritis (Table 80–1). Detailed discussion of the characteristics of each of these viruses is provided in Part VIII of this text. There are four agents for which an important role in diarrhea is well established, namely, rotavirus, calicivirus (for which Norwalk virus is the prototype), astrovirus, and enteric adenovirus types 40 and 41.[8–11] Non–group A rotavirus definitely causes gastroenteritis, but the extent to which and frequency with which this occurs are unclear.[12, 13] Coronavirus-like particles have been detected in feces in some studies, but a clearcut disease association has been difficult to establish.[14] Not noted in Table 80–1 is pestivirus, the antigens of which have been found in preliminary studies of the stools of some infants with gastroenteritis[15]; however, viral particles have yet to be detected and the medical significance of these findings is unclear.

The agents of viral gastroenteritis belong to diverse virologic groupings (see Table 80–1). Some are larger agents (rotavirus, enteric adenovirus, non–group A rotavirus, and enteric coronavirus), whereas others are small round viral particles (calicivirus and astrovirus, which are discussed together in Chapter 271). Most of the viral gastroenteritis agents (except enteric adenovirus) contain RNA. Only rotavirus, enteric adenovirus, and astrovirus have replicated in and been adapted to cell culture, and, for each of these viruses, the efficiency of viral isolation from human stools is low. Thus, cell culture is not used for clinical diagnosis of viral gastroenteritis.

The individual viral gastroenteritis agents have unique

TABLE 80–1 ■ Agents of Viral Gastroenteritis*

VIRUS	VIRION DIAMETER (nm)	NUCLEIC ACID TYPE	REPLICATION IN CELL CULTURE	MEDICAL IMPORTANCE DEMONSTRATED	LABORATORY DIAGNOSTIC TESTS
Rotavirus	70–75	dsRNA	Yes	Yes	ELISA, EM, NAA
Calicivirus (e.g., Norwalk virus)	27–40	ssRNA	No	Yes	ELISA, NAA, IEM in research laboratories
Enteric adenovirus	70–80	dsDNA	Yes	Yes	ELISA, EM, NAA
Astrovirus	27–32	ssRNA	Yes	Yes	EM; ELISA in research laboratories
Non–group A rotavirus	70–75	dsRNA	No	Partially	EM plus NAA; ELISA in research laboratories
Enteric coronavirus	100–150	ssRNA	No	No	EM

*ss, Single stranded; ds, double stranded; ELISA, enzyme-linked immunosorbent assay; EM, electron microscopy; IEM, immunoelectron microscopy; NAA, viral nucleic acid analysis.

characteristics. Rotavirus possesses 11 segments of double-stranded RNA, and four serotypes are medically important causes of diarrhea; Norwalk virus is the prototype 27-nm virus for the calicivirus group, sometimes also called small round-structured viruses (e.g., Snow Mountain, Hawaii); enteric adenovirus types 40 and 41 are specific serotypes that are quite fastidious in their requirements for cultivation in vitro, in contrast to the other conventional adenoviruses; astrovirus has a star shape contained within a sphere; non–group A rotavirus lacks a common group antigen shared by conventional rotaviruses and therefore possesses a different genomic pattern even though it appears morphologically indistinguishable; enteric coronavirus-like particles are often difficult to distinguish from artifacts on electron microscopic examination of diarrheal stool specimens.

Despite our knowledge of viral gastroenteritis agents, a specific agent has not been identified for approximately one third to one half of all suspected cases of viral gastroenteritis when all available research diagnostic techniques are employed. Presumably, additional agents remain to be discovered.

Epidemiology

Viral gastroenteritis occurs primarily in two epidemiologically distinct clinical forms.[16] One entity develops predominantly in infants and young children and is usually sporadic and occasionally epidemic. This form of illness is typified by rotavirus, a major human pathogen that produces severe diarrhea that lasts for 3 to 9 days and is usually accompanied by vomiting and fever.[17] Disease typically occurs during the winter months in temperate climates.[18] The incubation period is short (1 to 3 days) and spread is by the fecal-oral route. Infants and children 4 to 24 months old, who are affected most often,[18] are usually symptomatic and may develop severe diarrhea and dehydration requiring oral, or even parenteral, fluid replacement. Adult contacts of ill infants usually develop asymptomatic infections, and only rarely severe clinical disease.[19, 20] Nosocomial rotaviral outbreaks are well described. Rotavirus accounts for 30% to 50% of pediatric cases of gastroenteritis that necessitate hospitalization and probably a similar proportion of outpatient diarrhea in this age group. It is estimated that between 25,000 and 80,000 children are hospitalized with rotaviral diarrhea in the United States each year and about 150 die.[21] Enteric adenovirus types 40 and 41 are agents of pediatric diarrhea in temperate climates; they are reported to produce 3% to 10% of cases.[10, 22] Some calicivirus strains also cause this syndrome and in one study were responsible for 3% of diarrhea cases in daycare settings.[23–25] Astrovirus causes about 2% to 10% of endemic pediatric diarrhea, worldwide, and is an important pathogen in daycare center diarrhea.[11, 26, 27]

The second clinical entity is characteristically epidemic and consists of family and community-wide outbreaks of gastroenteritis among school-age children, family contacts, and adults. This form of illness is typified by the prototype calicivirus strain, Norwalk virus. In contrast to the first clinical entity, infants and young children are typically spared. Outbreaks occur throughout the year without a seasonal predilection.[9] The incubation period is quite short (12 to 48 hours), and spread is by the fecal-oral route.[28] Because of the short incubation period and explosive disease onset, a respiratory route of spread is hypothesized and some limited epidemiologic evidence exists to back this theory.[29] Vomiting, or diarrhea, or both develop rapidly and typically last only 1 to 2 days.[28] A variety of descriptive labels have been applied to this clinical entity, such as winter vomiting disease, epidemic collapse, epidemic diarrhea and vomiting, and acute infectious nonbacterial gastroenteritis.[5] Approximately 40% of viral gastroenteritis outbreaks in the United States are associated with Norwalk virus.[9] Epidemiologic settings often involve contaminated drinking or swimming water, ingestion of raw or inadequately cooked shellfish, recreational camps, military populations, cruise ships, nursing homes, schools, and community or family locations. Calicivirus strains other than Norwalk virus (e.g., Snow Mountain, Hawaii, Taunton, Otofuke, and Sapporo) are all derived from epidemic outbreaks, similar to Norwalk virus itself, and their epidemiologic settings appear to be similar to those of Norwalk virus.[30–32]

Non–group A rotavirus has been described as producing medically important disease only in China, where severe outbreaks of diarrheal disease with a water-borne route of spread have affected many adults as well as children.[13] Because this association with disease in adults is unusual for rotavirus, this agent has also been called adult diarrhea rotavirus.[33] Enteric coronavirus remains a controversial potential pathogen; some reports associate it with severe necrotizing diarrhea in newborns.[34] Its pathogenic potential is obscured by its presence in the stools of both ill and well persons, particularly in developing countries.[14]

Pathogenesis

The pathogenesis of viral gastroenteritis is similar for each agent. The most comprehensive data available are derived from studies of human volunteers infected experimentally by oral administration of Norwalk virus. At the time of disease onset, a mucosal lesion develops in the proximal small intestine, which has been examined in biopsy specimens taken at the duodenojejunal junction.[35] This lesion (Fig. 80–1) has also been found in volunteers infected with another calicivirus, Hawaii virus.[36] Villi are blunted, and there is an intense inflammation of the lamina propria with ingress of mononuclear cells and polymorphonuclear leukocytes. The crypts of the villi are hypertrophic, and although the intestinal mucosal surface epithelial cells are grossly intact, they are clearly damaged, as evidenced by their vacuolization. Electron microscopic examination of these epithelial cells reveals damage to their microvillous architectural substructure. The virus and its antigens have not been detected within involved mucosal cells by electron microscopy or immunofluorescence, probably because of the virus' small size and patchy distribution. These histopathologic changes seen with the Norwalk or Hawaii strain of calicivirus persist for up to 2 weeks, long after clinical recovery has taken place.

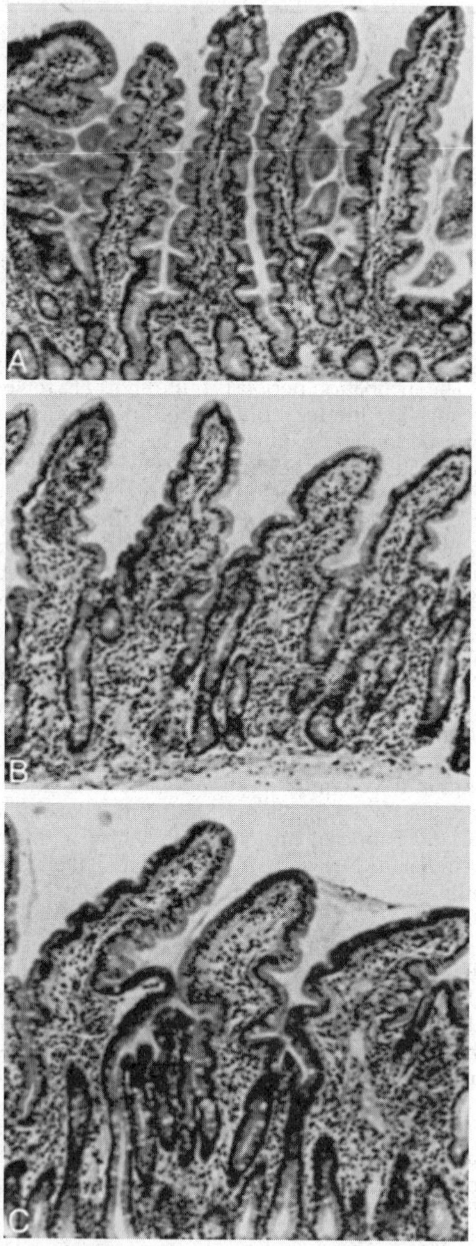

FIGURE 80–1 □ Biopsy specimens of the small intestine before and after oral ingestion of Norwalk agent (hematoxylin-eosin, × 100). *A*, Before ingestion, villi are tall, and the cellularity of the lamina propria is normal. *B*, Two days after ingestion, the villi are shortened, the crypts are hypertrophied and contain increased numbers of mitoses, and the cellularity of the lamina propria is increased. *C*, Six days after ingestion, shortened villi, hypertrophied crypts, and increased mitoses persist. (From Schreiber DS, Blacklow NR, Trier JS: The mucosal lesion of the proximal small intestine in acute infectious non-bacterial gastroenteritis. N Engl J Med 288:1319, 1973.)

Accompanying this small intestinal lesion is bowel dysfunction manifested by malabsorption of fat and xylose.[4, 5, 35] Malabsorption has been found for at least 1 week after disease onset. Decreased levels of intestinal brush border enzymes occur during disease, whereas adenylate cyclase levels remain normal within epithelial cells of the small intestine.

In contrast to the small intestine, the gastric mucosa remains histologically normal during Norwalk virus illness, as does its secretions of acid, pepsin, and intrinsic factor[37]; however, gastric emptying is markedly delayed, as evidenced by physiologic studies that indicate altered gastric motor function.[38] This may explain the frequency of nausea and vomiting seen with Norwalk virus illness. Thus, use of the term gastroenteritis, rather than just enteritis, seems justified for this infection. The colonic mucosa remains normal, a finding that is consistent with the usual absence of fecal leukocytes in this syndrome.

The pathogenesis of human rotavirus infection has been studied in naturally infected children, and the findings resemble those seen with Norwalk virus–infected volunteers.[39] In contrast to Norwalk virus, however, rotavirus and its antigens have been detected within the mucosal epithelial cells of the small intestine,[40] and in rare fatal cases the involvement of the virus may extend from its usual duodenal and jejunal location to the large bowel.[41] The major pathophysiologic mechanism for rotaviral diarrhea seems to be decreased absorption of salt and water because of selective infection of the absorptive intestinal villus cells, resulting in net fluid secretion, isotonic dehydration, and compensated metabolic acidosis.[42] Dehydration occurs frequently but is normally less than 5%, except in severe cases, the most extreme of which require hospitalization.

Clinical Manifestations

Viral gastroenteritis can vary widely in its clinical features, ranging from asymptomatic or mild illness to complete prostration, dehydration, and circulatory collapse. Diarrhea is typical for a noninflammatory form of gastroenteritis, with watery stools lacking fecal leukocytes and blood. The clinical characteristics of rotavirus and calicivirus (e.g., Norwalk virus) illnesses are often indistinguishable, but there can be differences.

Rotavirus illness usually has a sudden onset of fever and vomiting in infants and young children, and watery diarrhea often develops later.[17] Although fever is typically low grade, it can be high in some dehydrated patients. Diarrhea normally lasts from 3 to 9 days and is self-limited, although relapses occasionally occur. Chronic or prolonged diarrhea can occur in patients who are immunosuppressed (e.g., for bone marrow transplantation) or have primary immunodeficiency diseases. Findings referable to the respiratory tract may occur, such as pharyngeal or tympanic membrane erythema,[43] but the virus has not been detected in the respiratory tract of patients with gastroenteritis. Severe dehydration is more common with rotavirus disease than with other enteric viral, bacterial, or parasitic pathogens. There are numerous reports of rotavirus in association with a variety of syndromes such as intussusception, Kawasaki syndrome, Reye's syndrome, and inflammatory bowel disease; however, the relationships are probably not causal. A disease association seems strongest for some cases of neonatal necrotizing enterocolitis.[34]

Calicivirus (e.g., Norwalk virus) illness develops abruptly. Some patients experience primarily vomiting, others diarrhea, and still others both.[28] Affected persons often also have abdominal cramps, myalgia, low-grade fever, headache, or malaise. The illness typically renders the patient prostrate and unable to work; however, it is short-lived, usually resolving spontaneously 24 to 48 hours after the onset of symptoms. Some patients have developed a transient leukocytosis, but the white cell count remains normal in most. Fatalities are extremely rare and are limited to elderly and debilitated persons.[3]

Diagnosis

Clinical and epidemiologic features of an acute diarrheal illness may suggest viral gastroenteritis, but usually the findings are not distinctive enough to confirm the diagnosis. Some nonviral pathogens commonly produce a noninflammatory diarrhea with watery stools lacking fecal leukocytes—a clinical picture that is indistinguishable from viral gastroenteritis. Thus, to diagnose viral diarrhea with certainty, the specific causal agent must be detected. The primary diagnostic tests are immunoassays, principally enzyme-linked immunosorbent assay (ELISA), and electron microscopy, which can detect the presence of the virus or its antigens in stool specimens (see Table 80–1).

Rotavirus infection can be diagnosed in stool specimens rapidly in many hospital diagnostic laboratories with the use of commercially available ELISA test kits. More sensitive than rotavirus latex agglutination tests, ELISAs permit a specific diagnosis within 4 hours. Tests that utilize monoclonal antibodies against rotavirus seem to be more specific and sensitive than those that employ polyclonal sera.[44] Rotavirus in feces usually correlates with acute diarrhea caused by this pathogen.

Infection with enteric adenovirus types 40 and 41 can be diagnosed rapidly in stool specimens using commercially available ELISA test kits. The diagnosis of the other agents of viral gastroenteritis requires either an electron microscope or access to one of a few research laboratories that specialize in this field. Electron microscopy, specifically immunoelectron microscopy, is available as a diagnostic tool in only a limited number of medical centers, and furthermore, considerable technical experience is necessary with the use of an electron microscope specifically for the diagnosis of the pathogens of viral gastroenteritis. ELISA and viral nucleic acid detection tests are available for the diagnosis of several agents such as the Norwalk, Snow Mountain, and Hawaii strains of calicivirus as well as astrovirus,[45–49] but these assays are currently restricted to a few research laboratories.

Treatment

Specific antiviral therapy is not available for any of the agents of viral gastroenteritis, so therapy is directed at fluid replacement. Most patients can be managed with oral rehydration solutions that are commercially available and contain glucose or sucrose plus electrolytes[50, 51] (see Chapter 83). Severely dehydrated patients, usually those who are elderly, debilitated, or infant, may require parenteral fluid and electrolyte replacement.[50] Immunodeficient children with chronic rotavirus infection have responded to therapy with human milk containing rotavirus antibody, but normal children have failed to show improvement with this treatment. In experimentally infected volunteers, bismuth subsalicylate reduced the severity and duration of abdominal cramping caused by Norwalk virus.

Prevention

Considerable effort is being directed at the development of a live attenuated oral vaccine to prevent rotavirus infection by the four medically important serotypes.[52] No vaccine is licensed, although vaccine candidates are currently undergoing clinical trials (see Chapter 263). Immunity to Norwalk virus is short-lived (see Chapter 271) and the rationale for development of a vaccine appears uncertain.

Standard infection control measures for enteric infections, emphasizing hand washing, are required for prevention of nosocomial viral gastroenteritis in hospital and nursing home units as well as in homes and daycare centers. Cohorting of infected patients and staff can control disease transmission in hospitals, nursing homes, and daycare centers. Use of proper food preparation and water purification practices can prevent Norwalk virus and other calicivirus disease outbreaks.

Controversy exists over whether some infants may derive protection against severe rotavirus diarrhea from breast-feeding,[53] but if this protection exists it clearly is not complete, nor is it seen in all infants. Oral administration of human serum globulin possessing rotaviral antibodies provides significant protection against illness for low-birth-weight infants[54]; however, there is currently little interest in measures for passive immunization, and most attention is being directed toward developing a vaccine.

References

1. Dingle JH, Badger GF, Feller AE, et al: A study of illness in a group of Cleveland families. I. Plan of study and certain general observations. Am J Hyg 58:16, 1953.
2. National Center for Health Statistics: Current Estimates from the Health Interview Survey, United States. Rockville, MD, National Center of Health Statistics, 1973. U.S. Dept. of Health, Education, and Welfare publication (HRA) 74-1512.
3. Gangarosa RE, Glass RI, Lew JF, Boring JR: Hospitalizations involving gastroenteritis in the United States, 1985: The special burden of the disease among the elderly. Am J Epidemiol 135:281, 1992.
4. Schreiber DS, Trier JS, Blacklow NR: Recent advances in viral gastroenteritis. Gastroenterology 73:174, 1977.
5. Blacklow NR, Dolin R, Fedson DS, et al: Acute infectious nonbacterial gastroenteritis: Etiology and pathogenesis. Ann Intern Med 76:993, 1972.
6. Kapikian AZ, Wyatt RG, Dolin R, et al: Visualization by immune electron microscopy of a 27-nm particle associated with acute infectious nonbacterial gastroenteritis. J Virol 10:1075, 1972.
7. Bishop RF, Davidson GP, Holmes IH, Ruck BH: Detection of a new virus by electron microscopy of faecal extracts from children with acute gastroenteritis. Lancet 1:149, 1974.
8. Brandt CD, Kim HW, Yolken RH, et al: Comparative epidemiology of two rotavirus serotypes and other viral agents associated with pediatric gastroenteritis. Am J Epidemiol 110:243, 1979.
9. Kaplan JE, Gary GW, Baron RC, et al: Epidemiology of Norwalk gastroenteritis and the role of Norwalk virus in outbreaks of acute nonbacterial gastroenteritis. Ann Intern Med 96:756, 1982.
10. Kotloff KL, Losonsky GA, Morris JG, et al: Enteric adenovirus infection and childhood diarrhea: An epidemiological study in three clinical settings. Pediatrics 84:219, 1989.
11. Herrmann JE, Taylor DN, Echeverria P, Blacklow NR: Astroviruses as a cause of gastroenteritis in children. N Engl J Med 324:1757, 1991.
12. Dolin R, Treanor JJ, Madore HP: Novel agents of viral enteritis in humans. J Infect Dis 155:365, 1987.
13. Hung T, Chen G, Wang C, et al: Waterborne outbreak of rotavirus diarrhoea in adults in China caused by a novel rotavirus. Lancet 2:1139, 1984.
14. Ashley C, Caul EO: Human enteric coronavirus. *In* Farthing MJG (ed): Viruses and the Gut. London, Swan Press, 1989, pp 91–95.
15. Yolken R, Leister F, Almeido-Hill J, et al: Infantile gastroenteritis

associated with excretion of pestivirus antigens. Lancet 1:517, 1989.
16. Blacklow NR, Greenberg HB: Viral gastroenteritis. N Engl J Med 325:252, 1991.
17. Rodriguez WJ, Kim HW, Arrobio JO, et al: Clinical features of acute gastroenteritis associated with human reovirus-like agent in infants and young children. J Pediatr 91:188, 1977.
18. Kapikian AZ, Kim HW, Wyatt RG, et al: Human retrovirus-like agent as the major pathogen associated with winter gastroenteritis in hospitalized infants and young children. N Engl J Med 294:965, 1976.
19. Wenman WM, Hinde D, Feltham S, Gurwith M: Rotavirus infection in adults: Results of a prospective family study. N Engl J Med 301:303, 1979.
20. Echeverria P, Blacklow NR, Cukor G, et al: Rotavirus as a cause of severe gastroenteritis in adults. J Clin Microbiol 18:663, 1983.
21. Prospects for immunizing against rotavirus. *In* New Vaccine Development: Establishing Priorities, Vol I. Diseases of Importance in the United States. Washington, DC, National Academy Press, 1985, pp 410–423.
22. Uhnoo I, Goran W, Lennart S, Johansson ME: Importance of enteric adenoviruses 40 and 41 in acute gastroenteritis in infants and young children. J Clin Microbiol 20:365, 1984.
23. Matson DO, Estes MK, Glass RI, et al: Human calicivirus-associated diarrhea in children attending day care centers. J Infect Dis 159:71, 1989.
24. Cubitt WD: The candidate caliciviruses. Ciba Found Symp 128:126, 1987.
25. Riepenhoff-Talty M, Saif LJ, Barrett HJ, et al: Potential spectrum of etiological agents of viral enteritis in hospitalized infants. J Clin Microbiol 17:352, 1983.
26. Lew JF, Moe CL, Monroe SS, et al: Astrovirus and adenovirus associated with diarrhea in children in day care settings. J Infect Dis 164:673, 1991.
27. Blacklow NR, Herrmann JE: Astrovirus gastroenteritis. Trans Am Clin Climatol Assoc 106:58, 1994.
28. Dolin R, Blacklow NR, DuPont H, et al: Transmission of acute infectious nonbacterial gastroenteritis to volunteers by oral administration of stool filtrates. J Infect Dis 123:307, 1971.
29. Sawyer LA, Murphy JJ, Kaplan JE, et al: 25- to 30-nm virus particle associated with a hospital outbreak of acute gastroenteritis with evidence for airborne transmission. Am J Epidemiol 127:1261, 1988.
30. Ando T, Monroe SS, Gentsch JR, et al: Detection and differentiation of antigenically distinct small round-structured viruses (Norwalk-like viruses) by reverse transcription–PCR and Southern hybridization. J Clin Microbiol 33:64, 1995.
31. Lew JF, Kapikian AZ, Valdesuso J, Green KY: Molecular characterization of Hawaii virus and other Norwalk-like viruses: Evidence for genetic polymorphism among human caliciviruses. J Infect Dis 170:535, 1994.
32. Wang J, Jiang X, Madore HP, et al: Sequence diversity of small, round-structured viruses in the Norwalk virus group. J Virol 68:5982, 1994.
33. Penaranda ME, Ho MS, Fang ZY, et al: Seroepidemiology of adult diarrhea rotavirus in China, 1977 to 1987. J Clin Microbiol 27:2180, 1989.
34. Vaucher YE, Ray CG, Minnich LL, et al: Pleomorphic, enveloped, virus-like particles associated with gastrointestinal illness in neonates. J Infect Dis 145:27, 1982.
35. Schreiber DS, Blacklow NR, Trier JS: The mucosal lesion of the proximal small intestine in acute infectious non-bacterial gastroenteritis. N Engl J Med 288:1318, 1973.
36. Schreiber DS, Blacklow NR, Trier JS: The small intestinal lesion induced by Hawaii agent acute infectious nonbacterial gastroenteritis. J Infect Dis 129:705, 1974.
37. Widerlite L, Trier JS, Blacklow NR, Schreiber DS: Structure of the gastric mucosa in acute infectious nonbacterial gastroenteritis. Gastroenterology 68:425, 1975.
38. Meeroff JC, Schreiber DS, Trier JS, Blacklow NR: Abnormal gastric motor function in viral gastroenteritis. Ann Intern Med 92:370, 1980.
39. Davidson GP, Barnes GL: Structural and functional abnormalities of the small intestine in infants and young children with rotavirus enteritis. Acta Paediatr Scand 68:181, 1979.
40. Bishop RF, Davidson GP, Holmes IH, Ruck BJ: Virus particles in epithelial cells of duodenal mucosa from children with acute nonbacterial gastroenteritis. Lancet 2:1281, 1973.
41. Carolson JAK, Middleton PJ, Szymanski MT, et al: Fatal rotavirus gastroenteritis: An analysis of 21 cases. Am J Dis Child 132:477, 1978.
42. Tallett S, MacKenzie C, Middleton P, et al: Clinical laboratory and epidemiological features of viral gastroenteritis in infants and children. Pediatrics 60:217, 1977.
43. Lewis HM, Parry JV, Davies HA, et al: A year's experience of the rotavirus syndrome and its association with respiratory illness. Arch Dis Child 54:339, 1979.
44. Dennehy PH, Gauntlet DR, Tente WE: Comparison of nine commercial immunoassays for the detection of rotavirus in fecal specimens. J Clin Microbiol 26:1630, 1988.
45. Herrmann JE, Nowak NA, Blacklow NR: Detection of Norwalk virus in stools by enzyme immunoassay. J Med Virol 17:127, 1985.
46. Treanor JJ, Madore HP, Dolin R: Development of an enzyme immunoassay for the Hawaii agent of viral gastroenteritis. J Virol Methods 22:207, 1988.
47. Jiang X, Wang J, Graham DY, Estes MK: Detection of Norwalk virus in stool by polymerase chain reaction. J Clin Microbiol 30:2529, 1992.
48. DeLeon R, Matsui SM, Baric RS, et al: Detection of Norwalk virus in stool specimens by reverse transcriptase–polymerase chain reaction and nonradioactive oligoprobes. J Clin Microbiol 30:3151, 1992.
49. Herrmann JE, Nowalk NA, Perron-Henry DM, et al: Diagnosis of astrovirus gastroenteritis by antigen detection with monoclonal antibodies. J Infect Dis 161:226, 1990.
50. Santosham M, Daun RS, Dillman L, et al: Oral rehydration therapy of infantile diarrhea. A controlled study of well-nourished children hospitalized in the United States and Panama. N Engl J Med 306:159, 1985.
51. Santosham M, Burns B, Nadkarni V, et al: Oral rehydration therapy for acute diarrhea in ambulatory children in the United States: A double-blind comparison of four different solutions. Pediatrics 76:159, 1985.
52. Bernstein DI, Glass RI, Rodgers G, et al: Evaluation of rhesus rotavirus monovalent and tetravalent reassortant vaccines in US children. JAMA 273:1191, 1995.
53. Cushing AH, Anderson L: Diarrhea in breast-fed and non–breast-fed infants. Pediatrics 70:921, 1982.
54. Barnes GL, Doyle IW, Hewson PH, et al: A randomised trial of oral gammaglobulin in low-birth-weight infants infected with rotavirus. Lancet 1:1371, 1982.

81

Traveler's Diarrhea

Sherwood L. Gorbach

On the scale of life's tribulations, traveler's diarrhea (TD) is neither the most perilous nor the most debilitating illness, but an episode of intestinal agonies during a trip abroad can certainly rank among the more memorable events of a lifetime. Diarrheal disease has plagued travelers for centuries. Whether the trip is for business or pleasure, military conquest or amusement, TD has infiltrated all ranks, given rise to numerous theories of causation, and achieved worldwide fame by its various euphemisms, some of which are lilting, others scatologic. Among the approximately 300 million travelers who cross their national borders each year, about 16 million travel from industrialized countries to developing countries. In view of an incidence of diarrhea in the range of

30% to 50%, it can be said, at least for these hapless travelers, that travel broadens their minds as it loosens their bowels.

Diarrheal disorders have been noted in hippocratic writings and in the Bible. Travelers throughout the ages have referred discreetly in their journals to episodes of intestinal indisposition. But the credit for scientific study of TD belongs to Kean, who undertook a classic series of investigations in the 1950s of students traveling to Europe and Mexico.[1, 2] Besides describing the clinical and epidemiologic features, he made the seminal observation, in a well-designed, placebo-controlled trial, that antimicrobial drugs can provide protection against the illness, thereby implicating bacterial pathogens as the cause.[3] In his final contribution to this subject, Kean participated in the team effort that led to the discovery of enterotoxigenic *Escherichia coli* (ETEC) as the major culprit in this illness.[4]

Characteristics of the Pathogen

Traditional folklore of TD has spawned such etiologic theories as change in the water, too much noonday sun, spicy foods, and the general vicissitudes of travel. As improved laboratory methods became available, particularly testing for ETEC,[4, 5] it became apparent that TD is caused in the main by infectious microorganisms that are acquired in food and drink.[6–9] Several studies have isolated specific microbial pathogens from the feces of sick tourists. The causal link between infection and clinical disease has been solidified by field trials that have demonstrated the efficacy of antibacterial drugs in preventing and treating TD[8, 10–13]; indeed, prevention rates of 80% or more, achieved with a variety of antimicrobial drugs, strongly implicate bacterial pathogens, and probably gram-negative enteric organisms, as the cause of most TD cases.

Etiologic studies of TD have been carried out in many parts of the world. Travelers to Mexico have undergone the most intensive scrutiny: 19 reports have been published since 1974.[4, 5, 14–30] There have also been seven investigations of TD in other parts of Latin America,[31–37] as well as nine investigations of travelers to Asia[38–46] and four studies of travelers to Africa.[37, 47–49] An array of pathogens have been found, but it is apparent that the leading culprits are various forms of *E. coli*, particularly ETEC (Table 81–1). Some geographic differences have become apparent in the isolation rates of ETEC in travelers. In Latin America, for example, the median isolation rate of ETEC in TD cases has been 42% (range 26% to 72%), compared with a median of 16% in Asia (range 0% to 37%).[9] Enteroadherent *E. coli* organisms, which are characterized by their ability to adhere to HEp-2 cells in tissue culture, have been recovered from approximately 15% of travelers with diarrhea in Mexico[27] and from Mexican children who have diarrhea.[50] Three patterns of adherence have been described in cases of diarrhea: local, aggregative, and diffuse. Whereas the first two types have been implicated convincingly in field trials and volunteer studies, the pathogenicity of *E. coli* with diffuse adherence is somewhat doubtful as a result of failure of two such strains to induce diarrhea in a volunteer challenge study.[51] In travelers, fecal colonization with enteroaggregative *E. coli* increased 10-fold during their journey, but there was no evidence that such colonization was associated with diarrhea.[52] Enteroinvasive strains of *E. coli* similar to *Shigella* account for 5% of TD cases in Mexico, according to one study.[53]

TABLE 81–1 ■ Microbial Pathogens in Traveler's Diarrhea

	FREQUENCY	
PATHOGEN	Average (%)	Range (%)
Enterotoxigenic *Escherichia coli*	40–60	0–72
Enteroadherent *E. coli*	15	—
Invasive *E. coli*	<5	0–5
Shigella	10	0–30
Salmonella	<5	0–15
Campylobacter	<5	0–15
Vibrio	<5	0–30
Aeromonas	<5	0–30
Rotavirus	5	0–36
Giardia lamblia	<5	0–6
Entamoeba histolytica	<5	0–6
Cryptosporidium	<5	—
No pathogen identified	40	22–83

The serotypes of ETEC strains have been quite variable.[8] With the exception of O128:H7, none of these ETEC serotypes shares an antigen with the familiar serotypes of enteropathogenic *E. coli*.[54] Certain serotypes, such as O6:H16, are found worldwide, whereas others are peculiar to certain countries.[8]

Shigella species have been encountered in approximately 10% of TD cases, although the rate of isolation varies from 0% to more than 20%.[15, 22, 24, 25] The disease caused by *Shigella* tends to be more severe than the usual form of TD. In a report from Cancun, Mexico, *Shigella dysenteriae* type 1 was isolated from tourists.[55] This is the most virulent strain of *Shigella*, and in some of these cases the disease was associated with the hemolytic-uremic syndrome. In addition, many of these strains were resistant to trimethoprim-sulfamethoxazole (TMP-SMX).

Salmonella organisms are found in less than 5% of TD cases, although the incidence is higher among travelers to Asia, particularly in the more developed areas of Asia, than in travelers to Latin America or Africa.[6, 7, 9] There is also a geographic difference in isolation rates of *Campylobacter jejuni*, which accounts for 15% to 20% of TD cases in Thailand and Bangladesh,[45, 56] compared with less than 5% in Mexico[27] and elsewhere. Vibrios, particularly *Vibrio parahaemolyticus*, and *Aeromonas* species have also been isolated more often in travelers to Asia and North Africa than to Latin America or Africa.[6, 7, 9, 40, 41, 43–45, 57, 58]

Among the parasites, *Giardia lamblia* is a hazard to travelers in Leningrad,[59] but not necessarily in Latin America and Asia.[4, 13, 14, 45, 56] Amebiasis, which has been characterized by Elsdon Dew as the "refuge of the diagnostically destitute," is relatively uncommon in Mexico[4, 14] and Asia.[40, 45, 56] *Cryptosporidium* has been isolated only sporadically in travelers.[60–62] A newly described protozoan organism belonging to the coccidian genus *Cyclospora* (formerly known as cyanobacterium-like bodies) has been identified in the stools of both travelers in Nepal and local people in Peru.[63, 64] In the travelers, *Cyclospora* was associated with chronic diarrhea.

Viral diarrhea is generally thought to be more common in children than in adults, but rotavirus has been isolated from adult travelers in Mexico[14, 18, 20, 25, 65] and Honduras,[32, 33] as well as Asia.[38, 39, 45] In a study of viral pathogens in the stools of U.S. military personnel with diarrhea who were deployed in South America and West Africa, rotavirus was found in 11% and Norwalk virus in 10%.[37]

Several studies have reported more than one pathogen in TD cases, up to 15% in Mexico[14, 29] and 33% in Thailand.[45] To confuse the issue further, no pathogens have been identified, despite careful laboratory study, in more than 40% of cases, from all parts of the world.* The high incidence of mixed infections, along with the inability to isolate pathogens in

*References 4, 5, 12–15, 19, 21, 22, 25–27, 31–39, 43–45, 47, 66.

many cases, casts some doubt on the veracity of etiologic studies altogether. Nevertheless, the striking efficacy of prophylaxis and treatment directed against bacterial pathogens suggests that TD is indeed a bacterial infection in most cases.

Epidemiology

TD is a syndrome consisting of a twofold or greater increase in the frequency of bowel movements, usually unformed, and commonly associated with other symptoms such as abdominal cramps, nausea, bloating, and urgency. Travelers at risk are defined as persons from industrialized countries visiting for a period of up to 1 month a region or country where there is increased risk of the disease.

The major determinant of risk is the destination. According to studies of nearly 20,000 European tourists to various locations, it has been possible to define three zones of risk. High-risk destinations, where the incidence of TD ranges from 20% to 50%, include Latin America, Africa, the Middle East, and Asia. Intermediate-risk destinations, with a 10% to 20% incidence of TD, include southern European countries, Israel, and a few Caribbean islands. Low-risk areas, where the incidence is less than 8%, include Canada, the United States, Northern Europe, Australia, New Zealand, and a number of the Caribbean islands.[67] These estimates, however, are based on questionnaires filled out by returning travelers. In summarizing the experience from 34 prospective studies, a somewhat greater TD risk emerges: median TD rates of 53% (21% to 100%) in Latin America, 54% (21% to 57%) in Asia, and 54% (36% to 62%) in Africa.[9]

The national origin of the traveler is another important factor in TD liability. At an international conference in Teheran held in 1968, participants from the United States and Northern Europe had a 36% attack rate, compared with only 8% for colleagues from developing countries and 2% for local Iranians.[68] Similar findings were noted in an international congress in Mexico.[69] Longer residence in the tropical country also leads to increased resistance to TD,[16] but previous short-term travel to areas of high risk does not necessarily produce protection.[4, 40]

The purpose of travel and eating style both play significant roles in risk of developing this illness. The greatest frequency of diarrhea occurs in people traveling as students or itinerant tourists, the lowest risk in those visiting relatives, and intermediate risk in business travelers.[67, 70] Most diarrhea occurs in people who eat in restaurants and school cafeterias, and the risk is particularly high, as might be imagined, for those who succumb to the wares of street vendors. The safest place to eat is in a private home.[67, 70] Younger travelers, particularly those 20 to 29 years of age, have the highest risk, and the lowest TD rates are noted in those older than 55 years.[2, 70] In accordance with the general susceptibility of younger travelers, it appears that small children are even more vulnerable. In a retrospective Swiss survey of children and adolescents, most with a destination in Latin America or Africa, TD occurred within 2 weeks in 40%, 9%, 22%, and 36% in the age groups 0 to 2 years, 3 to 6 years, 7 to 14 years, and 15 to 20 years, respectively. Thereafter the incidence declined to 23% at the age of 70 years or more.[71] Whether this apparent respect for advancing age is due to immunity gained after frequent attacks or to less adventuresome eating habits is a source of speculation.

TD is acquired through ingestion of fecally contaminated food or beverages.[19, 67, 70, 72, 73] In one study, foods in Mexico were more likely to contain fecal coliforms and enteric pathogens than similar foods from Houston, Texas.[73] Especially risky foods include uncooked vegetables, meat, and seafood. Tap water, ice, unpasteurized milk and dairy products, and unpeeled fruits are also associated with increased risk. High-level contamination with enteric bacteria is found in food from school cafeterias, restaurants, and street vendors; the highest counts are found in dairy products, although some contamination is found even in cooked foods.[19, 72, 74] Bottled carbonated beverages (especially flavored beverages), beer, wine, hot coffee or tea, and water boiled or appropriately treated with chlorine are relatively safe. Some studies, however, show that drinking bottled uncarbonated mineral water increased the risk of water-borne infection.[75–77] Enteropathogens can be killed in water hotter than 65°C, which is too hot to touch when it comes from a faucet; in one study only 1 of 14 hotels in Mexico had hot tap water that was hotter than 65°C.[78] Dietary indiscretion is penalized by an increased risk of TD. Yet, even the most conscientious travelers were unable to resist such temptations, and 98% of Swiss travelers consumed unsafe food and beverages during the first 3 days of an overseas journey: 71% consumed salads or uncooked vegetables, and 53% accepted ice cubes in drinks.[79] Hence, dietary advice, although universally recognized as important and of proven efficacy, is rarely heeded by even the most informed, responsible travelers.

Clinical Features

The definition of TD has varied according to investigator.[4, 11, 14, 40, 67] Most studies define TD as the passage of three or more loose stools in a 24-hour period in association with at least one of the following symptoms or signs of enteric disease: nausea, vomiting, abdominal cramps, fever, fecal urgency, tenesmus, or the passage of bloody or mucoid stools.[80] This definition has been modified to require either four or more loose stools in a 24-hour period or three or more loose stools in an 8-hour period with at least one of these additional symptoms or signs.[81, 82] As a working definition, however, any bowel movement that fits the shape of the container is considered diarrhea. The disease does not begin immediately after the traveler's arrival but generally 2 to 3 days later.[4, 67, 70] Although most people have 3 to 5 loose stools per day, about 20% can have 6 to 15 watery motions.[4, 14] The average duration of illness in untreated subjects is 3 to 5 days, but a few unfortunate ones have persistent diarrhea throughout their stay.[4, 67, 70]

Watery, loose stools are the most common complaint, along with an array of associated symptoms (Table 81–2). Approximately 2% to 10% have fever, bloody stools, or both, and they are more likely to have shigellosis.[83] In general, persons with a milder clinical presentation, regardless of the patho-

TABLE 81–2 ■ Associated Symptoms in Traveler's Diarrhea

SYMPTOM	% OF SUBJECTS
Gas	79
Fatigue	74
Cramps	68
Nausea	61
Fever	56
Abdominal pain	53
Anorexia	53
Headache	39
Chills	38
Back pain	35
Dizziness	34
Vomiting	29
Malaise	24
Arthralgia	23

gen, experience more rapid resolution of disease than those with more severe symptoms, but even mild disease can produce an illness that lasts 4 to 5 days. Travelers with identifiable pathogens in their stools had a longer duration of diarrhea and more symptoms than those with culture-negative stools; invasive bacteria, especially *Campylobacter,* produced the most severe disease.[84] Despite the impressive list of symptoms, less than 1% of travelers are admitted to a local hospital, and no reports of death caused by diarrhea have been recorded among several hundred thousand insured travelers from Switzerland.[67, 70]

Treatment

Treatment of all forms of diarrhea entails two modalities: fluid replacement and appropriate drugs. In TD cases, severe dehydration is encountered rarely, so fluid losses can be repaired generally with soft drinks, fruit juices, and some clear fluids. Drug treatment is directed at suppressing the pathogen, as with antibiotics, or at reducing fluid and electrolyte losses with antisecretory agents. Not all patients require drug treatment, however, as shown by an analysis of U.S. adult travelers to Guadalajara, Mexico.[80] If diarrhea was mild, defined as one or two loose stools per 24 hours with only one symptom of enteric disease, 60% of affected persons did well by the second day and only 22% continued to have mild diarrhea. As the etiology was essentially the same in patients with mild or severe TD, the results suggest that travelers with mild TD be advised to wait before instituting antimicrobial therapy until at least three unformed stools are passed during 24 hours.

Several antibiotics have been used successfully in treatment of TD (Table 81–3). TMP-SMX or TMP alone reduced duration of diarrhea from 93 hours to approximately 30 hours.[21] Ciprofloxacin was as effective as TMP-SMX.[29] Fleroxacin,[85] norfloxacin,[86] and aztreonam[87] have also been used successfully for treatment of TD. Studies have shown that a single dose of ciprofloxacin[88] or fleroxacin[85] is effective, although one study found that a 3-day regimen of ciprofloxacin was more effective than a single dose.[89] On the other hand, furazolidone and ampicillin were disappointing as therapeutic measures.[90]

Antimotility drugs have enjoyed considerable support among tourists for providing relief from the intestinal indignities of travel, and their approbation is supported by good scientific studies.[36, 91, 92] Loperamide induces rapid improvement demonstrable even on the first day of therapy, when the results were significantly better than those obtained with either placebo or bismuth subsalicylate (BSS).[36] The concern about potentially exacerbating a case of dysentery with an antimotility drug[93] has largely been dispelled by clinical experience; patients with shigellosis, even infection with *S. dysenteriae* type 1, have been treated inadvertently with loperamide as the only drug, and they had a normal resolution without evidence of prolonged illness or delayed expulsion of the pathogen.[36, 91, 92]

The most effective relief from symptoms of TD has been provided by a combination of an antimicrobial drug and an antimotility drug. In a study of travelers to Mexico, the combined use of loperamide and TMP-SMX curtailed diarrhea in 1 hour, compared with 30 hours with either drug alone or 59 hours with placebo.[94] Even in the severest forms of TD, those with fecal leukocytes or blood-tinged stool, the

TABLE 81–3 ■ Antimicrobial Treatments for Traveler's Diarrhea

TREATMENT REGIMEN*		DURATION OF DIARRHEA (h)	REFERENCE
TMP-SMX	1 DS tablet bid × 5 d	29†	22
TMP	200 mg bid × 5 d	31†	
Placebo		93	
Furazolidone	100 mg qid × 5 d	57	90
Ampicillin	500 mg qid × 5 d	72	
Bicozamycin	500 mg qid × 3 d	28†	25
Placebo		64	
Ciprofloxacin	500 mg bid × 5 d	29†	29
TMP-SMX	1 DS tablet bid × 5 d	20†	
Placebo		81	
TMP-SMX	2 DS tablets × 1 dose	28†	94
Loperamide	4 mg; then 2 mg × 3 d	33	
TMP-SMX + loperamide		1†	
Placebo		59	
Ciprofloxacin	500 mg × 1 dose	25†	88
Placebo		54	
Ciprofloxacin	750 mg × 1 dose	36	89
Ciprofloxacin + loperamide	750 mg × 1 dose 4 mg; then 2 mg qid	34	
Ciprofloxacin + loperamide	750 mg bid × 3 d 4 mg; then 2 mg qid	44	
Aztreonam	100 mg PO tid × 5 d	33†	87
Placebo		68	

*DS, Double strength; bid, twice daily; qid, four times daily; PO, orally.
†Significantly shorter than with placebo.

median duration of illness was 4.5 hours, a remarkable result in this setting. Other investigators, however, have not seen any benefit in adding loperamide to an effective antibiotic such as ciprofloxacin in treating TD.[89]

BSS has been effective in treating mild to moderate TD. BSS is an insoluble complex of trivalent bismuth and salicylate. The drug possesses antimicrobial activity on the basis of the bismuth and antisecretory properties related to the salicylate moiety.[95] In the four therapeutic trials conducted in Mexico or West Africa, BSS reduced frequency of diarrhea significantly over placebo, but results were generally better when the higher dose (4.2 g/d) was used.[36, 96–99] These studies demonstrate that BSS has modest efficacy in ameliorating symptoms and reducing fluid losses in TD when higher doses are used and a low incidence of side effects.[96]

The current recommendations for treating TD are somewhat different from those made by the National Institutes of Health Consensus Conference.[100, 101] For mild to moderate diarrhea, generally less than four bowel movements per day, without blood or fever, either loperamide or BSS can be used effectively. For more severe forms of diarrhea, the optimal therapy at present seems to be a combination of an antimotility drug and an effective antimicrobial drug.[13, 94]

Prevention

It is certainly beneficial to prevent an attack of diarrhea, especially one that can interfere with an overseas journey. Having stated the obvious, such prevention is not easy to accomplish, unless one travels with sterile, hermetically sealed containers of food and drink. Four approaches to preventing TD can be conceived: avoiding unsafe foods and beverages, use of antiinfective drugs, use of other medications, and immunization.

Certain precautions about eating habits should be observed, to prevent not only diarrhea but other food- and water-borne diseases as well. An association between consumption of salads with raw vegetables and TD risk has been found,[14] but not in all studies.[69] High risk of TD has also been associated with eating raw meat and fish and dairy products.[72–74, 102, 103] Although there is a direct relationship between dietary indiscretions and the incidence of TD,[83] other studies have failed to show any benefit from dietary restriction, probably because this advice is followed more in theory than in practice.[70, 72, 104–106] Bottled beverages are generally safe, although some reported epidemics have been associated with contaminated bottled drinks.[75–77, 107] Carbonated beverages are safer than noncarbonated ones, owing to the low pH, generally 4.0 to 5.0, which has antibacterial properties.[74, 108] Tea or coffee prepared with boiling water is generally safe when consumed while it is still hot. Because the venue of food consumption determines the risk of TD, travelers are advised not to eat food from street vendors. Despite these recommendations it is apparent that most travelers are unable to maintain perfect vigilance during a pleasure trip; so this approach, although universally recommended, does not in reality provide complete protection.[79]

Antimicrobial drugs have been used extensively for prevention of TD. Since the classic study by Kean and colleagues in 1962,[3] 16 placebo-controlled trials have been conducted* (Table 81–4). Significant protection compared with placebo was noted in all but three studies, two of which involved neomycin[3, 109] and the third doxycycline in twice-weekly doses rather than the usual daily doses.[33] Protection rates have varied from 28% to 100%; the lower rates have been seen with what would now be recognized as poorly effective antimicrobial drugs, such as sulfonamides and streptomycin,[3, 109] or when a high level of resistance to the drug is found in ETEC isolated in the area.[34, 44] In studies employing TMP-SMX, protection rates have ranged from 71% to 95%[21, 24]; with norfloxacin or ciprofloxacin the protection rates are 68% to 94%.[26, 111–113]

The incidence of side effects has also varied considerably, depending in part on how carefully the subjects are followed. The lowest rates are recorded in studies in which retrospective questionnaires are used to tabulate side effects. On the other hand, when the research team is on site, making frequent data collections, a higher incidence of untoward effects is observed.[11] With TMP-SMX, 14% of subjects reported a rash with the higher dose[21] and 2% to 3% with the lower dose.[24] In the doxycycline trials, nausea and vomiting were the most common complaints (4% to 12% of subjects).[10] In one of the studies involving norfloxacin,[25] 2% of subjects developed a rash related to the study drug.

Antimicrobial resistance can develop in the intestinal flora of subjects taking antibiotic prophylaxis.[44, 48, 114, 115] In addition, travelers tend to acquire the microflora of their new environment,[115] and in developing countries the general enteric flora has many resistant organisms.[34, 44, 48, 116] For this reason travel to Mexico, even without taking antibiotics, can lead to acquisition of an antibiotic-resistant enteric flora.[117] The enteric pathogens, especially *Shigella*[46, 54, 116, 118] and ETEC,[34, 44, 48, 116] have a high degree of resistance to several antimicrobial agents in many developing countries. Resistance has been increasing to TMP-SMX[37, 118] and tetracycline,[118] which are widely used for TD, yet resistance to quinolones was not observed in strains isolated from TD in two studies.[37, 118] If these trends continue, as they undoubtedly will, the criteria and the drug choice for treating TD will need to be revised.

When considering the use of antimicrobial prophylaxis, it is necessary to balance the benefits of widespread prophylactic use in several million travelers each year with the potential drawbacks. The known risks include allergy and adverse effects such as rashes, photosensitivity of the skin, blood disorders, Stevens-Johnson syndrome, staining of children's teeth, and induction of other infections by the antimicrobial drug, for example, antibiotic-associated colitis, *Candida* vaginitis, and possibly salmonellosis. In addition, excessive use of these agents would apply pressure to select for bacterial resistance to antimicrobial drugs in general, which is a problem that exists already in many developing countries.[116]

Antimicrobial agents are not recommended for universal use by travelers.[13, 100, 101, 119, 120] This position is justified by the excellent results of early and aggressive treatment of TD, which, as outlined earlier, can reduce the duration of diarrhea to an average of 1 hour if a combination of antimicrobial and antimotility drugs is used.[94] By avoiding prophylactic antimicrobial agents, only people traveling to high-risk areas who actually develop moderate to severe TD (less than 30% of travelers at risk) are exposed to the side effects of antimicrobial agents, and this exposure is restricted to a period of 1 to 3 days.

BSS has been used for prevention of TD because of its antimicrobial and antisecretory activities.[95] The bismuth moiety has been shown to suppress several bacterial pathogens in vitro[121, 122] at concentrations that can be achieved in the intestinal tract. Indeed, the isolation of bacterial pathogens from the stools of patients with infectious diarrhea is markedly reduced in BSS-treated patients compared with placebo-treated control subjects.[97, 123, 124] In clinical prevention trials, the larger dose of 4.2 g/d (60 mL four times a day [qid]) in the liquid form, or 2.1 g/d (two tablets qid) in the tablet form, produced protection rates of 62% and 65%, respectively[20, 30]; the lower dose of 1.05 g/d (one tablet qid) gave protection of only 35% to 40%.[30, 124] A severe form of TD

*References 3, 10, 21, 24, 26, 28, 33, 34, 44, 48, 109–113.

TABLE 81–4 ■ Antimicrobial Prophylaxis of Traveler's Diarrhea

YEAR (REFERENCE)	COUNTRY	ANTIMICROBIAL AGENT	DOSAGE*	TD (%)	PROTECTION (%)
1962 (3)	Mexico	Neomycin	500 mg bid	16	24
		Phthalylsulfathiazole	1000 mg bid	12	51†
		Placebo		24	—
1967 (109)	Various	Streptotriad	1 tablet bid	13	28†
		Neomycin-sulfa	1 tablet bid	17	0
		Placebo		17	—
1976 (48)	Kenya	Doxycycline	100 mg qid	6	86†
		Placebo		43	—
1977 (49)	Morocco	Doxycycline	100 mg qid	8	83†
		Placebo		46	—
1978 (33)	Honduras	Doxycycline	100 mg twice weekly	33	27
		Placebo		45	—
1980 (34)	Honduras	Doxycycline	100 mg qid	32	68‡
		Placebo		100	—
1980 (44)	Thailand	Doxycycline	100 mg qid	10	59‡
		Placebo		24	—
1981 (110)	Mexico	Doxycycline	100 mg qid	4	81†
		Placebo		21	—
1983 (40)	Egypt and Far East	Mecillinam	200 mg qid	13	75†
		Placebo		53	—
1982 (21)	Mexico	TMP-SMX	1 DS tablet bid	16	71†
		Placebo		55	—
1983 (24)	Mexico	TMP-SMX	1 DS tablet qid	2	95†
		TMP	200 mg qid	14	59†
		Placebo		33	—
1985 (28)	Mexico	Bicozamycin	500 mg qid	0	100†
		Placebo		53	—
1986 (26)	Mexico	Norfloxacin	400 mg qid	7	88†
		Placebo		60	—
1987 (111)	Various	Norfloxacin	200 mg bid	11	68†
		Placebo		34	—
1990 (112)	Egypt	Norfloxacin	400 mg qid	2	92†
		Placebo		26	—
1989 (113)	Tunisia	Ciprofloxacin	500 mg qid	4	94†
		Placebo		64	—

*bid, Twice daily; qid, four times daily; DS, double strength.
†Significantly different from placebo.
‡High incidence (~50%) of doxycycline-resistant ETEC.

was studied in a laboratory setting in which ETEC was administered to volunteers, and the efficacy of BSS as a prophylactic agent was convincingly established.[123] It appears that BSS provides modest protection against TD but only when the traveler is conscientious about taking the higher dose.

Among drugs other than antimicrobials, halogenated hydroxyquinolines have enjoyed popular use. In a review of field trials, some studies have shown benefit and others have failed to find any salutary effect.[125] Notwithstanding its questionable efficacy for prophylaxis of TD, this class of drug should not be used by travelers, nor in other situations either, because of the reported association with subacute myelooptic neuropathy.[126, 127]

Various commercial preparations of *Lactobacillus* and *Streptococcus faecium* (SF 68) have been used prophylactically for TD, and the effects have generally been negative.[17, 96, 128] A study in animals has shown that lactobacilli that have the ability to adhere to the intestinal mucosa can prevent colonization with *E. coli*.[129] This concept was incorporated in a preparation known as *Lactobacillus* GG, which was shown to reduce TD by 40% in one of two hotels studied in Turkey.[130]

Various starches, talcs, chalks, and absorbent compounds have been prescribed for diarrheal diseases for as long as recorded history. Kaolin and pectin, for example, are included in several proprietary formulations, yet there is no substantive evidence that these products can alter the volume or electrolyte content of diarrhea stool,[131–133] and they are not recommended for use in TD.[134]

Although several avenues appear promising, there is no current vaccine or immunologic intervention that can be recommended for preventing TD. Most work is focused on controlling ETEC, because it is the major pathogen.[37, 135, 136] Another approach employs cholera vaccine or the toxin B subunit, which induces protection against ETEC.[137] These various approaches are being pursued vigorously in several laboratories, and active vaccine or passive antibodies may become available in the future for use in TD as well as the important problem of diarrhea in developing countries.

References

1. Kean BH, Waters SR: The diarrhea of travelers. N Engl J Med 216:71, 1959.
2. Kean BH: The diarrhea of travelers to Mexico: Summary of five-year study. Ann Intern Med 59:605, 1963.
3. Kean BH, Schaffner W, Brennan RW, Waters SR: The diarrhea of travelers. V. Prophylaxis with phthalylsulfathiazole and neomycin sulphate. JAMA 180:367, 1962.
4. Gorbach SL, Kean BH, Evans DG, et al: Travelers' diarrhea and toxigenic *Escherichia coli*. N Engl J Med 292:933, 1975.
5. Shore EG, Dean AG, Holik KJ, Davis BR: Enterotoxin-producing *Escherichia coli* and diarrheal disease in adult travelers: A prospective study. J Infect Dis 129:577, 1974.

6. Black RE: Pathogens that cause travelers' diarrhea in Latin America and Africa. Rev Infect Dis 12(Suppl 1):S131, 1990.
7. Taylor DN, Echeverria P: Etiology and epidemiology of travelers' diarrhea in Asia. Rev Infect Dis 12(Suppl 1):S136, 1990.
8. Sack RB: Travelers' diarrhea: Microbiologic bases for prevention and treatment. Rev Infect Dis 12(Suppl 1):S59, 1990.
9. Black RE: Epidemiology of traveler's diarrhea and relative importance of various pathogens. Rev Infect Dis 12(Suppl 1):S73, 1990.
10. Sack RB: Antimicrobial prophylaxis of travelers' diarrhea: A selected summary. Rev Infect Dis 8(Suppl 2):S160, 1986.
11. DuPont HL, Ericsson CD, Johnson PC, Cabada FJ: Antimicrobial agents in the prevention of travelers' diarrhea. Rev Infect Dis 8(Suppl 2):S167, 1986.
12. DuPont HL, Ericcson CD, Reves RR, Galindo E: Antimicrobial therapy for travelers' diarrhea. Rev Infect Dis 8(Suppl 2):S217, 1986.
13. DuPont HL: Travellers' diarrhoea. Which antimicrobial? Drugs 45:910, 1993.
14. Merson MH, Morris GK, Sack DA, et al: Travelers' diarrhea in Mexico: A prospective study of physicians and family members attending a congress. N Engl J Med 294:1299, 1976.
15. DuPont HL, Olarte J, Evans DG, et al: Comparative susceptibility of Latin America and United States students to enteric pathogens. N Engl J Med 295:1520, 1976.
16. DuPont HL, Haynes GA, Pickering LK, et al: Diarrhea of travelers to Mexico: Relative susceptibility of United States and Latin American students attending a Mexican university. Am J Epidemiol 105:37, 1977.
17. Pozo-Olano J de D, Warram JH Jr, Gómez RG, Cavazos MG: Effect of a lactobacilli preparation on travelers' diarrhea: A randomized double-blind clinical trial. Gastroenterology 74:829, 1978.
18. Vollett JJ, Ericsson CD, Gibson G, et al: Human rotavirus in an adult population with travelers' diarrhea and its relationship to the location of food consumption. J Med Virol 4:81, 1979.
19. Ericsson CD, Pickering LK, Sullivan P, DuPont HL: The role of location of food consumption in the prevention of travelers' diarrhea in Mexico. Gastroenterology 79:812, 1980.
20. DuPont HL, Sullivan P, Evans DG, et al: Prevention of travelers' diarrhea (emporiatric enteritis): Prophylactic administration of subsalicylate bismuth. JAMA 243:237, 1980.
21. DuPont HL, Evans DG, Rios N, et al: Prevention of travelers' diarrhea with trimethoprim-sulfamethoxazole. Rev Infect Dis 4:533, 1982.
22. DuPont HL, Reves RR, Galindo E, et al: Treatment of travelers' diarrhea with trimethoprim-sulfamethoxazole alone. N Engl J Med 307:841, 1982.
23. Freeman LD, Hooper DR, Lathen DF, et al: Brief prophylaxis with doxycycline for the prevention of travelers' diarrhea. Gastroenterology 84:276, 1983.
24. DuPont HL, Galindo E, Evans DG, et al: Prevention of travelers' diarrhea with trimethoprim-sulfamethoxazole and trimethoprim alone. Gastroenterology 84:75, 1983.
25. Ericsson CD, DuPont HL, Sullivan P, et al: Bicozamycin, a poorly absorbable antibiotic, effectively treats travelers' diarrhea. Ann Intern Med 98:20, 1983.
26. Johnson PC, Ericsson CD, Morgan DR, DuPont HL: Prophylactic norfloxacin for acute travelers' diarrhea. Clin Res 32:870A, 1984.
27. Mathewson JJ, Johnson PC, DuPont HL, et al: A newly recognized cause of travelers' diarrhea: Enteroadherent *Escherichia coli*. J Infect Dis 151:471, 1985.
28. Ericsson CD, DuPont HL, Galindo E, et al: Efficacy of bicozamycin in preventing travelers' diarrhea. Gastroenterology 88:473, 1985.
29. Ericsson CD, Johnson PC, DuPont HL, et al: Ciprofloxacin or trimethoprim-sulfamethoxazole as initial therapy for travelers' diarrhea. Ann Intern Med 106:216, 1987.
30. DuPont HL, Ericsson CD, Johnson PC, et al: Prevention of travelers' diarrhea by the tablet formulation of bismuth subsalicylate. JAMA 257:1347, 1987.
31. Guerrant RL, Rouse JD, Hughes JM, Rowe B: Turista among members of the Yale Glee Club in Latin America. Am J Trop Med Hyg 29:895, 1980.
32. Sheridan JF, Aurelian L, Barbour G, et al: Travelers' diarrhea associated with rotavirus infection: Analysis of virus-specific immunoglobulin classes. Infect Immun 31:419, 1981.
33. Santosham M, Sack RB, Froehlich J, et al: Biweekly prophylactic doxycycline for travelers' diarrhea. J Infect Dis 143:598, 1981.
34. Sack RB, Santosham M, Froehlich JL, et al: Doxycycline prophylaxis of travelers' diarrhea in Honduras, an area where resistance to doxycycline is common among enterotoxigenic *Escherichia coli*. Am J Trop Med Hyg 33:460, 1984.
35. Sack RB, Froehlich JL, Orskov F, Orskov I: Doxycycline is an effective treatment for travellers' diarrhoea. J Diarrhoeal Dis Res 3:144, 1986.
36. Johnson PC, Ericsson CD, DuPont HL, et al: Comparison of loperamide with bismuth subsalicylate for the treatment of acute travelers' diarrhea. JAMA 255:757, 1986.
37. Bourgeois AL, Gardiner CH, Thornton SA, et al: Etiology of acute diarrhea among United States military personnel deployed to South America and west Africa. Am J Trop Med Hyg 48:243, 1993.
38. Escheverria P, Hodge FA, Blacklow NR, et al: Travelers' diarrhea among United States Marines in South Korea. Am J Epidemiol 108:68, 1978.
39. Escheverria P, Ramirez G, Blacklow NR, et al: Travelers' diarrhea among US Army troops in South Korea. J Infect Dis 139:215, 1979.
40. Escheverria P, Blacklow NR, Sanford LB, Cukor GG: Travelers' diarrhea among American Peace Corps volunteers in rural Thailand. J Infect Dis 143:767, 1981.
41. Black FR, Gaarslev K, Orskov F, et al: Mecillinam, a new prophylactic for travellers' diarrhoea: A prospective double-blind study in tourists travelling to Egypt and the Far East. Scand J Infect Dis 15:189, 1983.
42. Kudoh Y: Imported bacterial diarrheal disease in Tokyo (in Japanese). Medico 15:6392, 1984.
43. Abe H, Ichiki S, Hashimoto S, et al: Isolation and characterization of enterotoxigenic *Escherichia coli* from patients with travellers' diarrhoea in Osaka. J Diarrhoeal Dis Res 2:83, 1984.
44. Echeverria P, Sack RB, Blacklow NR, et al: Prophylactic doxycycline for travelers' diarrhea in Thailand. Further supportive evidence of *Aeromonas hydrophila* as an enteric pathogen. Am J Epidemiol 120:912, 1984.
45. Taylor DN, Echeverria P, Blaser MK, et al: Polymicrobial aetiology of travellers' diarrhoea. Lancet 1:381, 1985.
46. Taylor DN, Houston R, Shum DR, et al: Etiology of diarrhea among travelers and foreign residents in Nepal. JAMA 260:1245, 1988.
47. Sack DA, Kaminsky DC, Sack RB, et al: Enterotoxigenic *Escherichia coli* diarrhea of travelers: A prospective study of American Peace Corps volunteers. Johns Hopkins Med J 141:63, 1977.
48. Sack DA, Kaminsky DC, Sack RB, et al: Prophylactic doxycycline for travelers' diarrhea: Results of a prospective double-blind study of Peace Corps volunteers in Kenya. N Engl J Med 298:758, 1978.
49. Sack RB, Froehlich JL, Zulich AW, et al: Prophylactic doxycycline for travelers' diarrhea: Results of a prospective double-blind study of Peace Corps volunteers in Morocco. Gastroenterology 76:1368, 1979.
50. Mathewson JJ, Oberhelman RA, DuPont HL, et al: Enteroadherent *Escherichia coli* as a cause of diarrhea among children in Mexico. J Clin Microbiol 25:1917, 1987.
51. Tacket CO, Moseley SL, Kay B, et al: Challenge studies in volunteers using *Escherichia coli* strains with diffuse adherence to HEp-2 cells. J Infect Dis 162:550, 1990.
52. Cohen MB, Hawkins JA, Weckbach LS, et al: Colonization by enteroaggregative *Escherichia coli* in travelers with and without diarrhea. J Clin Microbiol 31:351, 1993.
53. Wanger AR, Murray BE, Echeverria P, et al: Enteroinvasive *Escherichia coli* in travelers with diarrhea. J Infect Dis 158:640, 1988.
54. Orskov I, Orskov F: Significance of surface antigens in relation to enterotoxigenicity of *E. coli*. *In* Ouchterlony O, Holmgren J (eds): Cholera and Related Diarrheas. New York, S Karger, 1980, pp 134–141.
55. Parsonnet J, Greene KD, Gerber AR, et al: *Shigella dysenteriae* type I infections in US travelers to Mexico 1988. Lancet 2:543, 1989.
56. Speelman P, Struelens MJ, Sanyal SC, Glass RI: Detection of

Campylobacter jejuni and other potential pathogens in travelers' diarrhoea in Bangladesh. Scand J Gastroenterol 84(Suppl):19, 1983.
57. Spiratanaban A, Reinprayoon S: *Vibrio parahaemolyticus*: A major cause of travelers' diarrhea in Bangkok. Am J Trop Med Hyg 31:128, 1982.
58. Hanninen ML, Salmi S, Mattila L, et al: Association of *Aeromonas* spp. with travellers' diarrhoea in Finland. J Med Microbiol 42:26, 1995.
59. Jokipii L, Jokipii AMM: Giardiasis in travelers: A prospective study. J Infect Dis 130:295, 1974.
60. Jokipii L, Pohjola S, Jokipii AMM: *Cryptosporidium*: A frequent finding in patients with gastrointestinal symptoms. Lancet 2:358, 1983.
61. Sterling CR, Seegar K, Sinclair NA: *Cryptosporidium* as a causative agent of travelers' diarrhea (Letter). J Infect Dis 153:380, 1986.
62. Soave R, Ma P: Cryptosporidiosis: Travelers' diarrhea in two families. Arch Intern Med 145:70, 1985.
63. Hoge CW, Shlim DR, Rajah R, et al: Epidemiology of diarrhoeal illness associated with coccidian-like organism among travellers and foreign residents in Nepal. Lancet 341:1175, 1993.
64. Ortega YR, Sterling CR, Gilman RH, et al: *Cyclospora* species—A new protozoan pathogen of humans. N Engl J Med 328:1308, 1993.
65. Bolivar R, Conklin RH, Vollett JJ, et al: Rotavirus in travelers' diarrhea: Study of an adult student population in Mexico. J Infect Dis 137:324, 1978.
66. Luscher D, Altwegg M: Detection of shigellae, enteroinvasive and enterotoxigenic *Escherichia coli* using the polymerase chain reaction (PCR) in patients returning from tropical countries. Mol Cell Probes 8:285, 1994.
67. Steffen R: Epidemiologic studies of travelers' diarrhea, severe gastrointestinal infections, and cholera. Rev Infect Dis 8(Suppl 2):S122, 1986.
68. Kean BH: Turista in Teheran: Travellers' diarrhoea at the Eighth International Congresses of Tropical Medicine and Malaria. Lancet 2:583, 1969.
69. Lowenstein MS, Balows A, Gangarosa EJ: Turista at an international congress in Mexico. Lancet 1:529, 1973.
70. Steffen R, van der Linde F, Gyr K, Schar M: Epidemiology of diarrhea in travelers. JAMA 249:1176, 1983.
71. Pitzinger B, Steffen R, Tschopp A: Incidence and clinical features of traveler's diarrhea in infants and children. Pediatr Infect Dis J 10:719, 1991.
72. Tjoa WS, DuPont HL, Sullivan P, et al: Location of food consumption and travelers' diarrhea. Am J Epidemiol 106:61, 1977.
73. Wood LV, Ferguson LE, Hogan P, et al: Incidence of bacterial enteropathogens in foods from Mexico. Appl Environ Microbiol 46:328, 1983.
74. Blaser MJ: Environmental interventions for the prevention of travelers' diarrhea. Rev Infect Dis 8(Suppl 2):S142, 1986.
75. Blake PA, Rosenberg ML, Florencia J, et al: Cholera in Portugal, 1974. II. Transmission by bottled mineral water. Am J Epidemiol 105:344, 1977.
76. Harris JR: Are bottled beverages safe for travelers? (Editorial). Am J Public Health 72:787, 1982.
77. Communicable Diseases (Scotland) Unit: Outbreak of illness associated with holiday in Soviet central Asia. Commun Dis Scotl Wkly Rep 19:7, 1984.
78. Bandres JC, Mathewson JJ, DuPont HL: Heat susceptibility of bacterial enteropathogens. Implications for the prevention of travelers' diarrhea. Arch Intern Med 148:2261, 1988.
79. Kozicki M, Steffen R, Schar M: "Boil it, cook it, peel it, or forget it": Does this rule prevent travelers' diarrhoea? Int J Epidemiol 14:169, 1985.
80. Ericsson CD, DuPont HL: Travelers' diarrhea: Approaches to prevention and treatment. Clin Infect Dis 16:616, 1993.
81. Hyams KC, Bourgeois AL, Merrell BR, et al: Diarrheal disease during Operation Desert Shield. N Engl J Med 325:1423, 1991.
82. Turner AC: Travellers diarrhoea. Ann Soc Belg Med Trop 59:109, 1979.
83. Ericsson CD, Patterson TF, DuPont HL: Clinical presentation as a guide to therapy for travelers' diarrhea. Am J Med Sci 294:91, 1987.
84. Mattila L: Clinical features and duration of traveler's diarrhea in relation to its etiology. Clin Infect Dis 19:728, 1994.
85. Steffen R, Jori R, DuPont HL, et al: Efficacy and toxicity of fleroxacin in the treatment of travelers' diarrhea. Am J Med 94:182S, 1993.
86. Mattila L, Peltola H, Siitonen A, et al: Short-term treatment of traveler's diarrhea with norfloxacin: A double-blind, placebo-controlled study during two seasons. Clin Infect Dis 17:779, 1993.
87. DuPont HL, Ericsson CD, Mathewson JJ, et al: Oral aztreonam, a poorly absorbed yet effective therapy for bacterial diarrhea in US travelers to Mexico. JAMA 267:1932, 1992.
88. Salam I, Katelaris P, Leigh-Smith S, Farthing MJ: Randomised trial of single-dose ciprofloxacin for travellers' diarrhoea. Lancet 344:1537, 1994.
89. Petruccelli BP, Murphy GS, Sanchez JL, et al: Treatment of traveler's diarrhea with ciprofloxacin and loperamide. J Infect Dis 165:557, 1992.
90. DuPont HL, Ericsson CD, Galindo E, et al: Furazolidone versus ampicillin in the treatment of travelers' diarrhea. Antimicrob Agents Chemother 26:160, 1984.
91. Schiller LR, Santa Ana CA, Morawksi SG, Fordtran JS: Mechanism of the antidiarrheal effect of loperamide. Gastroenterology 86:1475, 1984.
92. Van Loon FPL, Bennish ML, Speelman P, Butler C: Double-blind trial of loperamide for treating acute watery diarrhoea in expatriates in Bangladesh. Gut 30:492, 1989.
93. DuPont HL, Hornick RB: Adverse effect of Lomotil therapy in shigellosis. JAMA 226:1525, 1973.
94. Ericsson CD, DuPont HL, Mathewson JJ, et al: Treatment of traveler's diarrhea with sulfamethoxazole and trimethoprim and loperamide. JAMA 263:257, 1990.
95. Gorbach SL: Bismuth therapy in gastrointestinal diseases. Gastroenterology 99:863, 1990.
96. Steffen R: Worldwide efficacy of bismuth subsalicylate in the treatment of travelers' diarrhea. Rev Infect Dis 12(Suppl 1):S80, 1990.
97. DuPont HL, Sullivan P, Pickering LK, et al: Symptomatic treatment of diarrhea with bismuth subsalicylate among students attending a Mexican university. Gastroenterology 73:715, 1977.
98. Steffen R, Mathewson JJ, Ericsson CD, et al: Travelers' diarrhea in West Africa and in Mexico: Fecal transport systems and liquid bismuth subsalicylate for self-therapy. J Infect Dis 57:1008, 1988.
99. Steffen R, Heusser R, Tschopp A, DuPont HL: Efficacy and side effects of six agents in the self-treatment of travelers' diarrhoea. Travel Med Int 6:153, 1988.
100. Gorbach SL, Edelman R (eds): Travelers' diarrhea: National Institutes of Health Consensus Development Conference. Rev Infect Dis 8:109, 1986.
101. Consensus Conference: Travelers' diarrhea. JAMA 253:2700, 1985.
102. Kendrick MA: Summary of study on illness among Americans visiting Europe, March 31, 1969–March 30, 1970. J Infect Dis 126:685, 1972.
103. Gangarosa EJ, Kendrick MA, Loewenstein MS, et al: Global travel and travelers' health. Aviat Space Environ Med 51:265, 1980.
104. Turner AC: Travellers diarrhoea. Trans Med Soc Lond 92–93:64, 1975–77.
105. Chang T-W: Traveler's diarrhea (Letter). Ann Intern Med 89:428, 1978.
106. Ryder RW, Oquist CA, Greenberg H, et al: Travelers' diarrhea in Panamanian tourists in Mexico. J Infect Dis 144:442, 1981.
107. Gonzales-Cortes A, Gangarosa EJ, Parrilla C, et al: Bottled beverages and typhoid fever: The Mexican epidemic of 1972–73. Am J Public Health 72:844, 1982.
108. Koser SA, Skinner WW: Viability of the colon typhoid group in carbonated water and carbonated beverages. J Bacteriol 7:111, 1922.
109. Turner AC: Traveler's diarrhoea: A survey of symptoms, occurrence, and possible prophylaxis. Br Med J 4:453, 1967.
110. Freeman LD, Hooper DR, Lathen DF, et al: Brief prophylaxis with doxycycline for the prevention of travelers' diarrhea. Gastroenterology 84:276, 1983.
111. Wistrom J, Norrby SR, Burman LG, et al: Norfloxacin versus placebo for prophylaxis against travellers' diarrhoea. J Antimicrob Chemother 20:563, 1987.

112. Scott DA, Haberberger RL, Thornton SA, Hyams KC: Norfloxacin for the prophylaxis of travelers' diarrhea in US military personnel. Am J Trop Med Hyg 42:160, 1990.
113. Rademaker CM, Hoepelman IM, Wolfhagen MJ, et al: Results of a double-blind placebo-controlled study using ciprofloxacin for prevention of travelers' diarrhea. Eur J Clin Microbiol Infect Dis 8:690, 1989.
114. Murray BE, Rensimer ER, DuPont HL: Emergence of high-level trimethoprim resistance in fecal *Escherichia coli* during oral administration of trimethoprim or trimethoprim-sulfamethoxazole. N Engl J Med 306:130, 1982.
115. Stenderup J, Orskov I, Orskov F: Changes in serotype and resistance pattern of the intestinal *Escherichia coli* flora during travel. Results from a trial of mecillinam as a prophylactic against travellers' diarrhoea. Scand J Infect Dis 15:367, 1983.
116. Murray BE: Resistance of *Shigella, Salmonella*, and other selected enteric pathogens to antimicrobial agents. Rev Infect Dis 8(Suppl 2):S172, 1986.
117. Murray BE, Mathewson JJ, DuPont HL, et al: Emergence of resistant fecal *Escherichia coli* in travelers not taking prophylactic antimicrobial agents. Antimicrob Agents Chemother 34:515, 1990.
118. Vila J, Gascon J, Abdalla S, et al: Antimicrobial resistance of *Shigella* isolates causing traveler's diarrhea. Antimicrob Agents Chemother 38:2668, 1994.
119. Preventing travellers' diarrhoea (Editorial). Lancet 2:144, 1988.
120. Steffen R, Boppart I: Travellers' diarrhoea. Baillieres Clin Gastroenterol 1:361, 1987.
121. Cornick NA, Silva M, Gorbach SL: In vitro antibacterial activity of bismuth subsalicylate. Rev Infect Dis 12(Suppl 1):S9, 1990.
122. Manhart MD: In vitro antimicrobial activity of bismuth subsalicylate and other bismuth salts. Rev Infect Dis 12(Suppl 1):S11, 1990.
123. Graham DY, Estes MK, Gentry LO: Double-blind comparison of bismuth subsalicylate and placebo in the prevention and treatment of enterotoxigenic *Escherichia coli*–induced diarrhea in volunteers. Gastroenterology 85:1017, 1983.
124. Steffen R, DuPont HL, Heusser R, et al: Prevention of travelers' diarrhea by the tablet form of bismuth subsalicylate. Antimicrob Agents Chemother 29:625, 1986.
125. Steffen R, Heusser R, DuPont HL: Prevention of travelers' diarrhea by nonantibiotic drugs. Rev Infect Dis 8(Suppl 2):S151, 1986.
126. Tsubaki T, Honma Y, Hoshi M: Neurologic syndrome associated with clioquinol. Lancet 1:696, 1971.
127. Baumgartner G, Gawel MJ, Kaeser HE, et al: Neurotoxicity of halogenated hydroxyquinolines: Clinical analysis of cases reported outside Japan. J Neurol Neurosurg Psychiatry 42:1073, 1979.
128. Clemens ML, Levine MM, Black RE, et al: *Lactobacillus* prophylaxis for diarrhea due to enterotoxigenic *Escherichia coli*. Antimicrob Agents Chemother 20:104, 1981.
129. Itoh K, Freter R: Control of *Escherichia coli* populations by a combination of indigenous clostridia and lactobacilli in gnotobiotic mice and continuous-flow cultures. Infect Immun 57:559, 1989.
130. Oksanen PJ, Salminen S, Saxelin M, et al: Prevention of travellers' diarrhoea by *Lactobacillus* GG. Ann Med 22:53, 1990.
131. Durrington PN, Manning AP, Bolton CH, Hartog M: Effect of pectin on serum lipids and lipoproteins, whole-gut transit time, and stool weight. Lancet 2:394, 1976.
132. Cummings JH, Southgate DAT, Branch WJ, Wiggins HS: The digestion of pectin in the human gut and its effect on calcium absorption and large bowel function. Br J Nutr 41:477, 1979.
133. Portnoy BL, DuPont HL, Pruitt D, et al: Antidiarrheal agents in the treatment of acute diarrhea in children. JAMA 236:844, 1976.
134. Donowitz M, Wicks J, Sharp GWG: Drug therapy for diarrheal diseases: A look ahead. Rev Infect Dis 8(Suppl 2):S188, 1986.
135. Sack RB, Kline RL, Spira WM: Oral immunization of rabbits with enterotoxigenic *Escherichia coli* protects against intraintestinal challenge. Infect Immun 56:387, 1988.
136. Svennerholm A-M, Vidal YL, Holmgren J, et al: Role of PCF8775 antigen and its coli surface subcomponents for colonization, disease, and protective immunogenicity of enterotoxigenic *Escherichia coli* in rabbits. Infect Immun 56:523, 1988.
137. Clemens JD, Sack DA, Harris JR, et al: Cross-protection by B subunit–whole cell cholera vaccine against diarrhea associated with heat-labile toxin-producing enterotoxigenic *Escherichia coli*: Results of a large-scale field trial. J Infect Dis 158:372, 1988.

82

Food Poisoning

David R. Snydman

Food-borne illness is a significant public health problem. It is a major cause of morbidity and an infrequent cause of mortality in the United States.[1] From 1988 to 1991, 2000 outbreaks were reported to the Centers for Disease Control and Prevention (CDC) from virtually all 50 states. The number of ill individuals in these outbreaks exceeded 60,000 and there were 64 deaths. Surveillance suggests that these outbreaks are grossly underreported; the true scope of disease related to food is probably 10 to 100 times more frequent. Estimates of 6 million to 99 million cases at a cost of $5 billion to $23 billion have been made.[2]

For most public health authorities, a food-borne disease outbreak is defined by two criteria: (1) two or more persons experience a similar illness, usually gastrointestinal, after ingestion of a common food, and (2) epidemiologic analysis implicates food as the source of the illness. There are certain exceptions to this definition. For example, one case of botulism or chemical poisoning constitutes an outbreak for epidemiologic investigation and control purposes.

Reported food-borne outbreaks are generally divided into two categories: (1) laboratory confirmed, that is, outbreaks in which evidence of a specific etiologic agent is obtained and specific laboratory criteria are met, and (2) undetermined, that is, outbreaks in which epidemiologic evidence implicates a food source but adequate laboratory confirmation is not obtained.

Food poisoning is defined as an illness caused by the consumption of food contaminated with pathogenic microorganisms, their toxins, or chemicals.[3] Food poisoning can be related to bacteria, bacterial toxins, parasites (e.g., trichinosis), viruses (e.g., hepatitis), and chemicals (e.g., in mushrooms). Food poisoning caused by bacteria constitutes approximately two thirds of the recognized food-borne outbreaks in the United States for which an etiology can be determined. However, it should be noted that only about 40 such outbreaks fulfill the criteria for a confirmed etiology[1] (Table 82–1).

The major recognized etiologies of bacterial food poisoning are generally limited to about a dozen bacteria, namely *Salmonella, Staphylococcus aureus, Clostridium perfringens, Shigella*, toxigenic or enteropathogenic *Escherichia coli, Bacillus cereus, Clostridium botulinum*, vibrios including *Vibrio cholerae, Campylobacter, Yersinia, Aeromonas*, and *Listeria*. Other agents such as streptococci and *Arizona* species have also infrequently been implicated as agents in food-borne illness in the United States.

Salmonella outbreaks predominate among the confirmed outbreaks and constitute almost a third of all reported cases of food-borne illness. This may be due in part to ease of recognition and to the awareness of physicians and the public. Among other bacterial causes of food-borne outbreaks, *C.*

TABLE 82–1 ■ Confirmed Food-Borne Disease Outbreaks, Cases, and Deaths, 1988 to 1991, United States, as Reported to the Centers for Disease Control and Prevention

	1988		1989		1990		1991		TOTAL		DISTRIBUTION		TOTAL DEATHS
	Outbreak	Cases	Outbreak	Cases	Outbreak	Cases	Outbreak	Cases	Outbreak	Cases	Outbreak	Cases	
Bacterial													
Bacillus cereus	5	51	3	61	5	43	5	253	18	408	0.9	0.7	0
Campylobacter	4	134	8	295	3	72	6	93	21	594	1.0	1.0	0
Clostridium botulinum	20	49	13	24	12	22	11	25	56	120	2.8	0.2	10
Clostridium perfringens	0	0	7	436	11	1,240	10	1,213	28	2,889	1.4	4.7	1
Escherichia coli	2	109	1	3	2	80	3	33	8	225	0.4	0.4	0
Listeria monocytogenes	0	0	1	2	0	0	0	0	1	2	0.05	0.003	0
Salmonella	94	2,987	117	4,920	136	6,290	122	4,146	469	18,343	23.2	29.9	34
Shigella	6	3,581	6	257	8	834	4	112	24	4,784	1.2	7.8	0
Staphylococcus aureus	8	245	14	524	13	372	9	331	44	1,472	2.2	2.4	0
Streptococcus group A	0	0	1	35	1	12	1	100	3	137	0.1	0.2	0
Vibrio cholerae	0	0	0	0	1	26	2	6	3	32	0.1	0.05	1
Vibrio parahaemolyticus	0	0	0	0	4	21	0	0	4	21	0.2	0.03	0
Vibrio vulnificus	0	0	0	0	1	2	0	0	1	2	0.05	0.003	1
Chemical													
Ciguatoxin	4	8	19	66	11	44	7	50	41	168	2.0	2.7	0
Heavy metals	2	19	1	7	0	0	0	0	3	26	0.1	0.04	0
Mushroom	2	9	0	0	1	5	2	4	5	18	2.5	0.03	0
Scombrotoxin	16	65	17	80	11	194	17	40	61	379	3.0	0.6	1
Paralytic shellfish	1	6	0	0	2	24	2	35	5	65	2.5	0.1	2
Other chemical	4	32	0	0	2	3	3	30	9	65	4.5	0.1	0
Parasitic													
Giardia	0	0	1	21	3	129	2	32	6	182	3.0	0.3	0
Trichinella spiralis	3	34	4	15	2	105	1	41	10	195	5.0	0.3	0
Viral													
Hepatitis A	12	795	7	329	9	452	7	114	35	1,885	1.7	3.1	6
Norwalk virus	0	0	1	42	0	0	0	0	1	42	0.05	0.07	0
Confirmed	183	8,124	221	7,117	237	4,958	214	6,658	855	26,857	42.4	43.7	60
Unknown etiology	268	7,608	284	8,750	295	9,925	315	8,239	1162	34,552	57.6	56.3	4
Total	451	15,732	505	15,867	532	19,883	529	14,897	2017	61,409	100	100	64

From Bean NH, Goulding JS, Lao C, Angulo FJ: Surveillance for foodborne-disease outbreaks—United States, 1988–1992. MMWR CDC Surveill Summ 45(5):1–66, 1996.

botulinum, followed by *S. aureus* and *Shigella,* have been among the most commonly recognized. However, two chemical causes, ciguatoxin and scombrotoxin, have increasingly been recognized as among the more common causes of food-borne outbreak.[1]

Etiologic patterns may vary throughout the world. These patterns are dependent on many factors, such as food preferences, physician and public awareness, and laboratory capabilities. For example, in the United States *Salmonella* and *S. aureus* are among the agents most commonly involved in food-borne outbreaks, being present in more than 50% of these outbreaks.[1, 3] In contrast, *Salmonella* is implicated in more than 90% of the recognized food-borne illness in England and Wales.[4] Japan, on the other hand, has different etiologic patterns, probably related to many of the aforementioned factors. *Vibrio parahaemolyticus* gastroenteritis was first described in that country; *V. parahaemolyticus* is the dominant pathogen in food-borne outbreaks and is present in more than 50% of the reported outbreaks.[5]

In the past decade in the United States, there has been a marked change in the epidemiology of food-borne disease.[6] The decline in food-borne outbreaks caused by *S. aureus* and *C. perfringens* has been accompanied by increasing rates of salmonellosis and the recognition of major new food-borne pathogens, such as *E. coli* O157:H7 and *Listeria monocytogenes*.[7, 8] Furthermore, a greater appreciation for *Campylobacter jejuni* and Norwalk virus, described in the 1970s as agents of food-borne disease, has emerged.[9, 10]

Some of these changes may be due to a shift in dietary habits with a marked increase in per capita consumption of fresh vegetables, fresh fruit, cheese, and poultry.[6] Furthermore, importation of exotic fruits and vegetables, especially from Mexico and South America, has grown. There has also been a trend toward increased consumption of food from commercial service establishments, leading to the potential for outbreaks caused by infected food handlers.

In addition to exotic foods and changing practices, unusual outbreaks such as thyrotoxicosis related to consumption of bovine thyroid glands in ground beef[11] and eosinophilic myalgia syndrome related to contaminated L-tryptophan[12] point not only to the impact widespread food distribution may have in multistate outbreaks but also to unusual clinical manifestations that may occur as a result of food poisoning.

This chapter focuses primarily on the major toxin-mediated, short-incubation food poisoning syndromes. For a complete discussion of individual pathogens the reader is referred to the respective chapters.

Bacterial Causes of Food-Borne Illness

Many microorganisms are associated with food-borne disease. Table 82–2 lists the major bacterial causes, some epidemiologic and clinical features, and diagnostic media. For a more complete discussion of each bacterial pathogen, the reader is referred to individual chapters in the text.

Staphylococcus aureus

Dack and coworkers[13] were the first to prove that staphylococcal food poisoning was due to toxin production by *S. aureus*. They performed classic experiments with human volunteers, demonstrating that culture filtrates of staphylococci isolated from a cream-filled sponge cake, which had been the implicated vehicle in a food-borne outbreak, could cause gastroenteritis.[14] After these reports appeared, staphylococcal food poisoning became widely appreciated, and today staphylococci are among the most common agents implicated in food-borne disease.

PATHOPHYSIOLOGY

The microbiologic distinguishing characteristics of *S. aureus* are outlined in Chapter 191. Six immunologically distinct *S. aureus* enterotoxins have been described, termed A, B, C, D, E, and F.[15, 16] These enterotoxins are heat-resistant, single-polypeptide chains that contain large quantities of lysine, aspartic and glutamic acids, and tyrosine. They range in molecular weight from 28,366 to 34,700. The precise mechanism of action is not yet known; however, when they were tested in a rat intestinal loop model, net transport of water and solute occurred.[17] These toxins were emetic when administered to monkeys and cats.[17] The toxic shock–producing toxin, enterotoxin F, has not been associated with food-borne disease.[18]

Enterotoxins A, B, C, D, and E have all been implicated in outbreaks of staphylococcal food poisoning in the United States and United Kingdom. Most implicated strains produce A or A and D. Surprisingly, from 1979 to 1981 all the reported staphylococcal food-borne outbreaks were due to enterotoxin A.[19]

There are three requisites for staphylococcal food poisoning to occur: (1) contamination of a food with enterotoxin-producing staphylococci, (2) a food that has suitable growth requirements for the organisms, and (3) an allotment of time and temperature at which the organism can multiply.

EPIDEMIOLOGY

S. aureus was the third most common bacterial agent implicated in bacterial food poisoning from 1988 to 1991.[1] Outbreaks are characterized by explosive onset between 1 and 6 hours after consumption of a contaminated vehicle (median 3 hours). Attack rates are usually quite high because small quantities of enterotoxin can cause illness. Secondary cases are not of concern in this type of food poisoning.

Outbreaks related to staphylococci can occur at all times of the year, but most outbreaks are reported during the warm weather months.

Many different foods have been implicated in staphylococcal food poisoning. However, some foods are frequently implicated: ham, canned beef, pork, or any salted meat and cream-filled cakes or pastries such as cream puffs. Potato and macaroni salads are occasionally involved. Foods that have a high salt content (ham) or sugar content (custard) selectively favor the growth of staphylococci.

CLINICAL FEATURES

The symptoms of staphylococcal food poisoning are primarily profuse vomiting, nausea, and abdominal cramps, often followed by diarrhea. In severe cases, blood may be observed in the vomitus or stool. Rarely, hypotension and marked prostration occur. Fatalities are unusual and recovery is complete in 24 to 48 hours. Fever is not a common accompaniment but may be present if dehydration is severe.

DIAGNOSIS

Staphylococcal food poisoning should be considered in anyone who presents with severe vomiting, nausea, cramps, and some diarrhea. A history of ingesting meats of high salt or protein content may be helpful. Usually, the best epidemiologic clue is the short incubation period (1 to 7 hours). Of the agents of bacterial food-borne diseases, only *B. cereus* has a similar incubation period with a marked vomiting syndrome.[20] Because the *B. cereus* vomiting syndrome is so closely associated with fried rice, an easy epidemiologic distinction can usually be made.[21]

TABLE 82–2 ■ Characteristics of Bacterial Food Poisoning

ORGANISM	COMMON VEHICLES	MEDIAN INCUBATION PERIOD (h)	TOXIN, PRIMARY IN PATHOGENESIS	CLINICAL FEATURES*	MEDIAN DURATION (d)†	SECONDARY ATTACK RATES (%)	SOURCES OF DIAGNOSTIC MATERIAL	LABORATORY DIAGNOSIS‡
Bacillus cereus	Fried rice, vanilla sauce, cream	2 (1–16)	Heat stable	V, C, D, (33%)	0.4 (0.2–0.5)	—	Vomitus, stool, or food	$>10^5$ colonies on peptone–beef extract egg yolk agar; need controls for stool analysis (may be normal flora), serotyping
	Vanilla sauce, meatballs, boiled beef, barbecued chicken	9 (6–14)	Heat labile	D, C, V	1 (1–2)	—		
Campylobacter jejuni	Milk, chicken, pet animals, beef	48 (24–240)	?	D, F, C, B, H, M, N, V	7 (2–30)	25	Stool or rectal swab	Brucella agar base with vancomycin, polymyxin, and trimethoprim grown in reduced oxygen
Clostridium perfringens	Beef, turkey, chicken	12 (8–22)	Heat labile	D, C (N, V, F rare)	1 (0.3–3)	—	Stool or rectal swab; food, food contact surfaces	Egg yolk–free tryptose-sulfite-cycloserine agar; Hobbs or bacteriocin typing
Escherichia coli	Salads, beef	24 (8–44)	Heat labile	D, C, N, H, F, M	3 (1–4)	0	Stool or rectal swab	MacConkey medium; *E. coli* must be tested for toxin production (see Chapter 74)
	Salami							
	Apple cider		Heat stable	F, M, D, C				
		72 (24–112)	Verotoxin	B, C, F, hemolytic-uremic syndrome	5 (?)	20	Stool or rectal swab, serum	Sorbital MacConkey medium, serotyping, ELISA, PCR, antibody
Listeria monocytogenes	Milk, raw vegetables, coleslaw, dairy products, poultry, beef	?	?	D, F, C, N, V, blood	?	10	Stool or rectal swab	Cold enrichment, nutrient broth potassium thiocyanate and nalidixic acid
Staphylococcus aureus	Ham, pork, canned beef, cream-filled pastry	3 (1–6)	Heat stable	V, N, C, D, F (rare)	1 (0.3–1.5)	—	Stool, vomitus; food or food contact surfaces; nasal, hand, purulent lesion from food preparer	Egg yolk–tellurite-glycine-pyruvate agar or mannitol salt; phage type isolates; enterotoxin testing
Salmonella	Eggs, meat, poultry, tomatoes, cantaloupe	24 (5–72)	—	D, C, N, V, F, H, B (rare), enteric fever	3 (0.5–14)	30–50	Stool or rectal swab from patients and food preparation workers; raw food	*Salmonella-Shigella,* deoxycholate-citrate, Hektoen enteric, or xylose-lysine-deoxycholate; phage typing for *Salmonella* typhimurium
Shigella	Milk, salads (potato, tuna, turkey)	24 (7–168)	—	C, F, D, B, H, N, V	3 (0.5–14)	40–60	Stool or rectal swab from patients or food preparation workers; food	Same media as above; colicin typing
Vibrio parahaemolyticus	Seafood, rarely salt water or salted vegetables	12 (2–48)	?	D, C, N, V, H, F (25%), B (rare)	3 (2–10)	—	Stool or rectal swab; food, food contact surfaces; seawater	Thiosulfate citrate bile salts agar; test for Kanagawa phenomenon (see text), serotyping
Yersinia enterocolitica	Chocolate or raw milk, pork	?72 (2–144)	Heat stable (see text)	F, C, D, V, pharyngitis, arthritis, mesenteric adenitis, rashes	7 (2–30)	20	Stool from food preparer	Cold enrichment; serotyping, serology

*B, Bloody diarrhea; C, crampy abdominal pain; D, diarrhea; F, fever; H, headache; M, myalgias; N, nausea; V, vomiting.
†Ranges are given in parentheses.
‡ELISA, enzyme-linked immunosorbent assay; PCR, polymerase chain reaction.

The diagnosis can be confirmed by culturing the epidemiologically incriminated food, the skin or nose of the food handler, or occasionally the vomitus or stools of affected individuals. Any *S. aureus* recovered can be typed using phage or molecular methods such as pulsed-field gel electrophoresis to prove that the isolated strains are identical.

Several methods have been developed for detection of staphylococcal enterotoxin, including immunofluorescence, hemagglutination, radioimmunoassay, and enzyme-linked immunoassay, which can detect nanogram quantities of enterotoxin.[22] These should be considered research tools.

Bacillus cereus

The classic description of the illness caused by *B. cereus* was that of Hauge,[23] who described four Norwegian outbreaks involving 600 people in 1955. Interestingly, the vehicle in all four outbreaks appeared to be a vanilla sauce. Samples of sauce in each instance contained *B. cereus* in concentrations greater than 10^6 per mL. The patients suffered from diarrhea that was profuse and watery, associated with abdominal pain and nausea but rarely with vomiting. Fever was distinctly uncommon, and all symptoms usually abated within 12 hours. The incubation period in these outbreaks was about 10 hours.

Hauge[23] demonstrated in himself that vanilla sauce inoculated with a strain of *B. cereus* isolated from an outbreak of gastrointestinal illness and allowed to incubate for 24 hours would cause severe abdominal pain and diarrhea 13 hours after consumption. He was able to culture *B. cereus* from his stool as well.

The first well-documented outbreak of gastrointestinal disease in the United States was reported by Midura and coworkers in 1970.[24] In 1974 a vomiting syndrome caused by *B. cereus* that involved fried rice was recognized.[25] This report heralded the realization that this organism may be responsible for two distinct food-borne syndromes.

MICROBIOLOGY AND PATHOPHYSIOLOGY

B. cereus is a gram-positive, catalase-positive, aerobic spore-forming rod. Most strains are β-hemolytic. Several extracellular toxins are produced by strains of *B. cereus* and may contribute to their virulence.[26] An enterotoxin has been described that produces fluid accumulation in rabbit ileal loops, alters vascular permeability in the skin of rabbits, kills mice when injected intravenously, and stimulates the adenylate cyclase–cyclic AMP system in intestinal epithelial cells.[27]

A second heat-stable toxin of molecular weight 5000 has been isolated from a strain of *B. cereus* implicated in an outbreak of vomiting-type illness that produced vomiting when fed to rhesus monkeys.[27]

EPIDEMIOLOGY

Eighteen outbreaks of *B. cereus* gastroenteritis affecting 408 persons were reported to the CDC from 1988 to 1991. Most reported outbreaks have attack rates of 50% to 75%. In the reported vomiting-type outbreaks, virtually all individuals who consumed contaminated fried rice became ill. There is no risk of secondary cases.

The median incubation period for the diarrheal outbreaks reported in the United States was 9 hours (range 6 to 14 hours). The median incubation period for the outbreaks of emetic illness has been 2 hours (range 2 to 3 hours).

The reports of most outbreaks of the vomiting syndrome in the United States and of outbreaks in Great Britain implicated fried rice as the vehicle. The diarrheal illness, however, has been related to a variety of vehicles including boiled beef, sausage, chicken soup, vanilla sauce, and puddings.

Illness characterized by vomiting as the major finding can be attributed to the common practice in Chinese restaurants of allowing large portions of boiled rice to drain unrefrigerated to avoid clumping. The flash frying in the final preparation of the fried rice does not produce enough heat to destroy the preformed heat-stable toxin.[28]

CLINICAL FEATURES

The diarrheal, long-incubation illness is characterized by diarrhea (96%), abdominal cramps (75%), and vomiting (23%). Fever is uncommon. The duration of illness has ranged from 20 to 36 hours, with a median of 24 hours.

The emetic form of the illness has the predominant symptoms of vomiting (100%) and abdominal cramps (100%). Diarrhea is present in only one third of affected individuals. The duration of this illness has ranged from 8 to 10 hours (median 9 hours). In both types of illness the disease is usually mild and self-limited.

DIAGNOSIS

The diagnosis of *B. cereus* food poisoning should be considered in any individual who has diarrhea without fever in association with lower abdominal cramps. The disease caused by *C. perfringens* is so similar to that of *B. cereus* that they cannot be differentiated clinically or epidemiologically; culture methods are required.

The vomiting syndrome must be differentiated from *S. aureus* food poisoning. The association with fried rice is useful in differentiating the two organisms.

The diagnosis can be made by the isolation of 10^5 or more *B. cereus* organisms per gram from the incriminated food item. *B. cereus* can sometimes be found in the stools of healthy persons; therefore, isolation of the organism from feces may not be suitable confirmation unless negative stool cultures are obtained from an appropriate control group.

Clostridium perfringens

C. perfringens was first recognized and confirmed in the United States as a food-borne pathogen in 1945 by McClung,[29] who studied four outbreaks of diarrhea related to the consumption of chickens steamed 24 hours before consumption. *C. perfringens* was isolated from the cooked chickens.

Shortly after McClung's discovery, filtrates from strains of *C. perfringens* were administered by mouth to human subjects.[30] Cramps and diarrhea occurred in some individuals but the incubation period was short, 45 to 80 minutes. Living cultures induced cramps and bloating in 4 hours and diarrhea several hours thereafter. Hobbs and colleagues[30] elegantly confirmed these results and outlined the epidemiologic features of the disease in Great Britain in 1953.

Another discovery in the late 1940s was the outbreak of a severe and often lethal intestinal condition termed enteritis necroticans or Darmbrand that affected more than 400 people in Germany.[31] This outbreak was similar to others described later in New Guinea and termed pig-bel.[32] Both conditions were due to *C. perfringens.*

MICROBIOLOGY

Clostridia are gram-positive, spore-forming obligate anaerobes. The microbiologic features are outlined in Chapter 222. Although all species grow better under anaerobic conditions,

C. perfringens is remarkably aerotolerant and may survive exposure to oxygen for as long as 72 hours.

PATHOPHYSIOLOGY

C. perfringens is known to produce 12 toxins that are active in tissues, as well as several enterotoxins. Diarrheal disease is caused by a heat-labile, protein enterotoxin with a molecular weight of approximately 34,000.[33] This toxin is nondialyzable, precipitated by ammonium sulfate, antigenic, and inactivated by pronase but not by trypsin, lipase, or amylase.[34] Duncan and colleagues[34–37] have shown that the toxin is a structural component of the spore coat and is formed during sporulation. The toxin can be shown to cause fluid accumulation in the rabbit ileal loop model[35, 36] (the toxin is described in greater detail in Chapter 222).

An enterotoxin has been isolated from strains of *C. perfringens* type C implicated in the pig-bel syndrome in New Guinea in the 1950s. This enterotoxin seems to be quite similar if not identical to the one described for type A strains.[37]

EPIDEMIOLOGY

C. perfringens food poisoning is the sixth most common food-borne disease in the United States. Epidemics of *C. perfringens* illness are usually characterized by high attack rates with a large number of affected individuals; the average number of affected individuals per outbreak has been more than 100 from 1988 to 1991. There is no risk of secondary transmission. The incubation period in most outbreaks varies between 8 and 14 hours (median of 12 hours) but can be as long as 72 hours.

More cases of *C. perfringens* food poisoning are reported in the fall and winter months, presumably because stews and turkey are more likely to be consumed in winter.

Virtually every outbreak has roast, boiled, stewed, or steamed meats or poultry as the vehicle of infection. The organism is ubiquitous, usually found in the gastrointestinal tract or in soil. The implicated food invariably undergoes a period of inadequate cooling during which the redox potential of the food is in a reduced state that allows the spores to germinate. This usually happens below 50°C.

CLINICAL FEATURES

C. perfringens food poisoning is characterized by watery diarrhea and severe, crampy abdominal pain, usually without vomiting, beginning 8 to 24 hours after the incriminated meal. Fever, chills, headache, or other signs of infection are usually not present.

The illness is of short duration, 24 hours or less. Rare fatalities have been recorded in debilitated or hospitalized patients who are victims of clostridial food poisoning.

Enteritis necroticans or pig-bel is a much more severe, necrotizing disease of the small intestine with high mortality. After a 24-hour incubation period, illness ensues with intense abdominal pain, blood diarrhea, vomiting, and shock. The mortality rate in this illness is about 40%, and death is usually due to intestinal perforation. Outbreaks of pig-bel in New Guinea have been clearly related to orgiastic consumption of pig in large native feasts. The pig is improperly cooked and large quantities are consumed during 3 to 4 days.

DIAGNOSIS

The diagnosis of *C. perfringens* food poisoning should be considered in any diarrheal illness characterized by abdominal pain and moderate to severe diarrhea, unaccompanied by fever or chills. Many other individuals are usually involved in the outbreak, and the suspect food is beef or chicken that has been stewed, roasted, or boiled earlier and then allowed to sit without proper refrigeration.

The major laboratory criterion for diagnosis is the isolation of the same organism from epidemiologically incriminated food and from the stools of ill individuals. If no food specimens are available, the isolation of organisms with the same serotype in stools of most ill individuals, and not in the stools of suitable control subjects, would suffice for the diagnosis. In the absence of either of these findings, a culture of the incriminated food containing 10^5 organisms per gram or more is suggestive. Studies have demonstrated *C. perfringens* toxin in the stools of affected individuals.[38] Serologic diagnosis is difficult because a high proportion of healthy individuals have antibody to *C. perfringens*.

Clostridium botulinum

The growth of *C. botulinum* in food is associated with the production of a potent neurotoxin. Ingestion of this toxin causes botulism, a neuroparalytic disease that may be fatal.[39] Outbreaks and sporadic cases have been associated with meat, fish, and vegetables that are contaminated and improperly processed. From 1988 to 1991, there were 56 outbreaks of botulism in the United States associated with 120 cases and 10 fatalities.

The toxins produced after germination of *C. botulinum* spores in inadequately processed foods may lead to the development of an acute gastrointestinal illness usually within 18 to 24 hours after ingestion of the toxin. When neurologic disease occurs, constipation is most common, but nausea, vomiting, and even diarrhea may occur before the onset of paralysis. This disease is caused by one of three distinct heat-labile neurotoxins designated A, B, and E.[40] The syndrome of infant botulism is thought to result from ingestion of spores with toxin production in vivo.[41] A more complete discussion of this illness may be found in Chapter 221. Botulism outbreaks have been generally associated with ingestion of low-acidity home-canned vegetables, fruits, or fish.[42] Outbreaks have been associated with ingestion of sauteed onions, chopped garlic, and baked potatoes.[43, 44] Botulism may be confirmed by the demonstration of toxin in the serum or stool of ill people and in the incriminated food or by the isolation of *C. botulinum* from feces of ill people. Therapy is discussed in Chapter 221.

Escherichia coli

In the past 10 years, the emergence of verotoxin-producing *E. coli* of serotype O157:H7 (along with other serotypes) as a major food-borne pathogen has been remarkable.[7, 45] Furthermore, these verotoxin-producing strains have been associated with the development of the hemolytic-uremic syndrome.

The significance of this pathogen as a cause of food-borne disease is not evident from examination of the CDC surveillance data from 1988 to 1991 (see Table 82–1). However, from 1991 to 1994 the number of outbreaks reported to the CDC increased from 4 to 30.[46] Some of this increase can be attributed to increased screening for the organism and reporting to public health authorities. In the past 2 years, multistate outbreaks with hundreds of cases and a number of deaths, especially among children, have been linked to contaminated, undercooked beef.[45, 47] Furthermore, these outbreaks have resulted in clusters of cases of hemolytic-uremic syndrome. Additional vehicles of transmission such as cold pressed apple cider[47] and dry cured salami have been recognized.[48]

E. coli O157:H7 is present in the intestines of approximately 1% of healthy cattle.[45] The process of slaughter and grinding presumably leads to contamination of beef, which, if the beef is undercooked, may lead to subsequent transmission. It should be noted that there are many other verotoxin-producing *E. coli* serotypes that may cause diarrheal illness; therefore, screening for the O157:H7 serotype clearly under-represents the frequency of such infections.[49]

The spectrum of disease may vary from nonbloody to bloody diarrhea, even frank hemorrhagic colitis, the hemolytic-uremic syndrome, thrombocytopenic purpura, and death. In the outbreaks with *E. coli* O157:H7, about 25% of the patients have required hospitalization, about 5% developed hemolytic-uremic syndrome, and about 1% died.[50]

The secondary attack rate in outbreaks in nursing homes and daycare centers has been reported to be as high as 20%, perhaps reflecting a low inoculum necessary for transmission.[51] For a more complete discussion of this pathogen the reader is referred to Chapter 75.

Listeria monocytogenes

This organism is also becoming increasingly recognized as a food-borne pathogen.[52] *Listeria* is a gram-positive, motile rod that is relatively heat resistant. *Listeria* is widely distributed in nature, found in the intestinal tracts of various animals and humans and in sewage, soil, and water.[52]

There is now sufficient evidence that *Listeria* is causally related to food-borne illness from investigations of a number of epidemics. Contaminated coleslaw, raw vegetables, raw and pasteurized milk, and Mexican-style soft cheeses have been implicated as vehicles for epidemic listeriosis.[53–56] The sources of sporadic *Listeria* infection are less well understood, although one can culture the organism from a high proportion of raw poultry or beef or ready-to-eat meat products.[54]

The syndromes one usually associates with *Listeria* include meningitis, bacteremia, and focal metastatic disease. It has frequently been noted that gastrointestinal symptoms, such as diarrhea, precede the recognized onset of bacteremic disease. The organism has a propensity to affect adults who are either immunosuppressed or pregnant. As a reflection of this host susceptibility, the most common cause of mortality associated with food-borne illness from 1983 to 1987 was epidemic listeriosis, which accounted for 70 deaths.[57]

The exact rate of food-borne transmission in sporadic cases of listeriosis is not known. Stool carriage among humans has been documented.[54] Because the incubation period to disease onset may be more than a week, it may be difficult to pinpoint the food exposures that occurred before case recognition. However, a commercial food monitoring program initiated by the U.S. Food and Drug Administration detected *L. monocytogenes* in 2% to 3% of all processed diary products that were tested, reflecting the widespread distribution of this organism in nature.[58] There has been a reduction in the incidence of human listeriosis in the United States, perhaps as a result of industry, regulatory, and educational efforts.[59] Surveillance estimates suggest about a 45% reduction in illness and death related to *L. monocytogenes*.

This organism is discussed in greater detail in Chapter 199.

Salmonella

Salmonella is the most commonly documented cause of food poisoning. In the United States alone there were 469 recorded outbreaks and 18,343 cases resulting in 34 fatalities.[1] Given estimates that as few as 10% of cases are actually reported, this pathogen is even more common. Furthermore, there was a doubling of reports to the CDC from 1975 until 1985. The marked increase in salmonellosis has in part been attributed to increasing contamination of poultry and grade A eggs.[60] Certain serotypes have been epidemiologically linked to particular animal species, *Salmonella hadar* with turkey products[60] and *Salmonella dublin* with raw cow's milk.[61] Details regarding *Salmonella* pathogenesis and therapy are provided in Chapters 73 and 205.

Vibrio parahaemolyticus

V. parahaemolyticus was first recognized as a potential food-borne pathogen by Fujino and coworkers[62, 63] when it was isolated from autopsy materials collected in relation to a food-poisoning outbreak. During the next decade, many other outbreaks in Japan were associated with a pleomorphic, halophilic, hemolytic gram-negative organism similar to the one described by Fujino and coworkers and variously named *Pasteurella parahaemolytica*, *Pseudomonas enteritis*, and *Oceanomonas parahaemolytica*.[63] The vehicles in these outbreaks were usually raw fish, shellfish, and cucumbers in brine. Extensive taxonomic studies by Sakazaki and colleagues[64] and Fujino[63] revealed that the organisms in question belonged to the genus *Vibrio*, and the new species designation *V. parahaemolyticus* was officially adopted.

Volunteer feeding experiments in Japan in the 1960s supplied further evidence of the pathogenicity of this organism.[65] Kato and coworkers[65] made the next major advance when they observed that strains isolated from ill humans caused hemolysis on Wagatsuma blood agar, whereas strains obtained from routine food samples lacked this characteristic. It was suggested that this trait correlated with pathogenicity. Indeed, this was borne out in volunteer studies, because only hemolytic strains were pathogenic in humans. This has been termed the Kanagawa phenomenon.[65]

Japanese workers, using various culture media with a high salt content, showed that *V. parahaemolyticus* accounts for between 50% and 70% of reported food-borne disease in Japan during the summer months.[5] This organism has also been implicated in outbreaks described in the United States and Great Britain.

MICROBIOLOGY AND PATHOPHYSIOLOGY

V. parahaemolyticus is a gram-negative, straight or curved rod, that is pleomorphic, halophilic, and facultatively anaerobic. This organism is part of the genus *Vibrio*, which includes *V. cholerae*, *V. alginolyticus*, *V. vulnificus*, and other species (see Chapter 208).

Several investigators have demonstrated an invasive ability of *V. parahaemolyticus*. Calia's laboratory demonstrated blood stream invasion of suckling rabbits after oral challenge with *V. parahaemolyticus*.[66] Histologic studies of rabbit ileal loop tissue after exposure to broth cultures have shown evidence of bacterial invasion of the mucosa accompanied by severe inflammation.[67, 68]

EPIDEMIOLOGY

It is difficult to assess the real incidence of food poisoning caused by *V. parahaemolyticus* in the United States. There were only four outbreaks from 1988 to 1991 affecting 21 individuals. In Japan, *V. parahaemolyticus* food poisoning accounts for as many as 60% of all individuals with bacterial food poisoning.

The attack rates in epidemics reported in the United States have varied from 24% to 86% of exposed individuals and the number of affected individuals from 6 to 600. No secondary cases have been reported in either the United States or Japan, although two individuals with long incubation periods (96 hours) may have been secondary cases in one outbreak. The median incubation period for most outbreaks has been 13 to 23 hours; the range has been quite variable, from 4 to 48 hours.

There has been a striking association of *V. parahaemolyticus* infection in the United States with coastal states as well as cruise ships. Most outbreaks have occurred in Maryland, but Massachusetts, Louisiana, New Jersey, Texas, and Washington have all reported outbreaks. In addition, there have been several epidemics on cruise ships. The majority of reported cases have occurred during the warm months (June to October).

Although most outbreaks of *V. parahaemolyticus* gastroenteritis have been recorded in Japan, many other countries in Southeast Asia, as well as Australia and Great Britain, have documented this infection. The organism itself is ubiquitous in marine waters and can be found on the U.S. coastline, in Canada, Great Britain, the Netherlands, and virtually all of Southeast Asia. In the United States, outbreaks have been related to crabs (both steamed and processed), shrimp (both cooked and uncooked), and oysters.

CLINICAL FEATURES

Explosive watery diarrhea is the cardinal manifestation of more than 90% of cases. Abdominal cramps, nausea, vomiting, and headache are common. Fever and chills occurred in approximately 25% of cases. Clinically, this illness resembles that produced by nontyphoidal salmonellosis. However, in one epidemic case in the United States, a bloody dysenteric syndrome was observed with fecal leukocytes and superficial ulcerations on sigmoidoscopic examination; a small percentage of cases in a cruise ship outbreak also reported bloody diarrhea.

The illness has generally been mild, with a median duration of 3 days (range 2 hours to 10 days). There have been no deaths in the 1000 cases reported in the United States. This has generally been the experience in Japan, although in the first outbreak reported by Fujino,[62] 20 of 272 ill individuals died.

The diarrhea is usually not profuse like that of *V. cholerae*. Yet, in one outbreak in Great Britain, hypotension and shock occurred in three of five cases. The spectrum of disease is apparently quite varied.

V. parahaemolyticus can occasionally cause wound infections. Most cases in the United States have been related to trauma associated with a marine environment.

DIAGNOSIS

V. parahaemolyticus should be considered in any outbreak of diarrheal illness related to seafood occurring in the warm months. The occurrence of mild but explosive watery diarrhea with or without dysentery (bloody, mucoid stools) in association with abdominal cramps, nausea, vomiting, and headache is most characteristic.

Rectal swabs or stool specimens should be streaked onto thiosulfate citrate bile salts agar or bromothymol blue–Teepol agar plates and incubated at 35°C to 37°C for 18 to 24 hours. Studies have shown mannitol salt agar to be an acceptable alternative medium.

Other Organisms

A number of other bacteria have been implicated in food-borne diarrheal illness. Many reports are unconvincing or unconfirmed.

ARIZONA

The organism *Arizona* is a motile gram-negative rod closely related to *Salmonella*.[69] It has been implicated in outbreaks of gastroenteritis and enteric fever. Various vehicles have included eggs or poultry as the contaminated product.[70] Because of the similarities to *Salmonella*, contaminated animal products should be considered the usual vehicle.

The syndromes caused by *Arizona* are also similar to salmonellosis. Gastroenteritis, enteric fever, bacteremia, and localized infection have been described. The incubation period is similar to that of *Salmonella*. Usually 24 to 48 hours after ingestion of contaminated food, symptoms develop. Fever, headache, nausea, vomiting, abdominal pain, and watery diarrhea may occur. Marked prostration may occur. Symptoms may persist for several days. Therapy and prevention are also similar to the methods employed for salmonellosis.

PLESIOMONAS AND AEROMONAS

Plesiomonas shigelloides is a gram-negative rod from the family Vibrionaceae. The organism has been associated with diarrheal illness.[71] At least two outbreaks have been reported, one related to ingestion of raw oysters.[72] Individuals who have become ill did so 48 hours after ingesting raw oysters. It is thought that the organism is enteroinvasive on the basis of lack of discernible toxins and the presence of blood and fecal polymorphonuclear leukocytes in stools of individuals with diarrhea.[72]

The role of *Aeromonas* species as food-borne pathogens is unclear.[73, 74] The organisms can be isolated from a number of environmental sources, including water and eggs. Enterotoxins have been described in *Aeromonas hydrophila*.[75] Case-control studies in some series have implicated these organisms as a cause of diarrhea.[76]

Chronic Diarrhea

A chronic diarrheal syndrome has been described in individuals drinking raw milk. It was described originally in Brainerd, Minnesota, where individuals developed acute watery diarrhea that persisted for an average of 2 years.[77] The etiologic agent has not been identified. Diarrhea began approximately 2 weeks after ingestion of the product. In addition, there has been a second outbreak of a similar illness associated with a restaurant, suggesting that a food vehicle other than raw milk may be involved.[78]

Viruses

The two most common viral causes of food poisoning are hepatitis A virus and Norwalk virus.[1] Viral gastroenteritis is one of the most common causes of food-borne illness in Minnesota.[6] Hepatitis A infection associated with food has been linked to raw shellfish, but efficient transmission from infected food handlers can also occur.[79] Norwalk virus has also become an important food poisoning pathogen.[6] Humans are the only known reservoir for both viruses. Norwalk virus food poisoning is marked by high attack rates, presumably because of the low inoculum necessary to transmit infection.[80–82] Transmission can occur from contaminated salads, frosting, and raw oysters.[83–84] For a complete discussion of hepatitis A and Norwalk virus the reader is referred to Chapters 260 and 271, respectively.

Parasitic Disease

A number of parasites have been implicated in food-borne disease, including *Trichinella spiralis, Entamoeba histolytica, Giardia lamblia, Ascaris lumbricoides, Taenia saginata, Taenia solium,*

Anisakis, and *Diphyllobothrium latum*. From 1988 to 1991, only *G. lamblia* was reported to the CDC.[1] Outbreaks associated with these parasites are uncommon. However, in one investigation the inoculum of *G. lamblia* necessary to cause disease was quite low.[7] Water-borne outbreaks caused by *Cryptosporidium* have reached national prominence.[85] In addition, there has been one reported outbreak related to fresh pressed apple cider.[86] The life cycles, modes of transmission, and discussions of these parasites can be found in their respective chapters.

Syndromes Related to Chemicals

In addition to bacterial food poisoning, which primarily causes diarrheal syndromes with abdominal cramps and fever, there are a number of food-borne diseases related to chemicals, many of which are not due to microbial pathogens. Individuals who develop nausea and vomiting with or without abdominal cramps within an hour of food consumption usually have disease primarily related to heavy metal poisoning. Copper, zinc, tin, and cadmium have generally caused such outbreaks.[87, 88] The time from consumption to onset of disease is generally 5 to 15 minutes. Nausea, vomiting, and cramps usually occur and resolve several hours after removal of the offending agent by vomiting.

Several syndromes are characterized by paresthesias occurring within one to several hours after ingestion of the toxin. The major ones include fish poisoning, Chinese restaurant syndrome, and niacin poisoning.[89–91] The Chinese restaurant syndrome has been characterized by a burning sensation in the neck, abdomen, and arms along with chest tightness. Headache, flushing, weakness, nausea, and abdominal cramps have also been described. Symptoms are thought to be caused primarily by excessive amounts of monosodium L-glutamate, although not all the substances that cause this syndrome have been well defined.[91] Usually illness is treated symptomatically and resolves within hours. Another syndrome that is associated with burning or facial flushing is niacin poisoning, which can occur within less than an hour of ingestion and generally resolves rapidly.[92]

The fish and shellfish poisoning syndromes are outlined in Table 82–3. Four major syndromes are described, namely scombroid, ciguatera, paralytic shellfish, and neurotoxic shellfish poisoning.[89] Most of these syndromes occur within hours of ingestion. Scombroid poisoning is characterized by symptoms that are typical of a histamine reaction.[93] Burning of the mouth and throat, flushing, and headache frequently occur. In many cases urticaria and bronchospasm can also be present. Symptoms are thought to be the result of histamine and inhibitors of histamine that are produced by enzymatic decarboxylation of histamine by marine-associated bacteria.[94] Histamine, cadaverine, and putrescine have been detected in samples from one outbreak that was associated with a nonscombroid fish, a bluefish.[95] The patients can be treated with an antihistamine, and symptoms usually resolve without serious consequences. Infusion of cimetidine has also been reported to be beneficial.[96]

There are several types of shellfish poisoning, classified as paralytic and neurotoxic.[97] The toxins associated with these two distinct syndromes are saxitoxins. Symptoms in paralytic shellfish poisoning include paresthesias, shortness of breath, muscle weakness or paralysis, and respiratory insufficiency.[89, 96–98] Neurotoxic shellfish poisoning tends to be milder, and respiratory paralysis has not been reported. The duration of illness generally ranges from a few hours to a few days for either paralytic or neurotoxic shellfish poisoning. The saxitoxin found in both neurotoxic and paralytic shellfish poisoning is formed by dinoflagellates.[98, 99] Saxitoxin is heat stable and blocks nerve and muscle action potential by interfering with sodium permeability. Many patients with paralytic or neurotoxic shellfish poisoning develop the onset of symptoms within several hours of ingestion. The same is true for neurotoxic shellfish poisoning. These syndromes are generally confined to coastal areas of the world. Neurotoxic shellfish poisoning has been reported primarily from the Gulf and Atlantic coasts of Florida and occurs in spring and fall. Paralytic shellfish poisoning generally occurs between May and November. Cases have been reported from the Pacific and Atlantic coasts of North America, Japan, the western coast of continental Europe, South Africa, South America, and New Zealand.

Ciguatera fish poisoning should be distinguished from paralytic shellfish poisoning by symptoms characterized by a more abdominal component, including abdominal cramps, nausea, vomiting, and diarrhea.[100, 101] Although patients may have numbness and paresthesia of the lips and tongue, dry mouth, myalgias, blurred vision, photophobia, transient blindness, and a sharp shooting pain in the legs have also been reported. In addition, there may be a sensation of looseness and pain in the teeth and a reversal of cold and hot sensation. Respiratory paralysis may occur. Ciguatoxin has been demonstrated to be similar to the toxins described in paralytic shellfish poisoning.[102] The duration of ciguatoxin poisoning tends to be longer than that seen with the neurotoxic or paralytic shellfish poisonings.[103] Acute illness may range for days to months, and pain has been reported to occur for years after an episode.[103] The species of fish consumed include barracuda, snapper, and grouper. The toxin is found in reef-dwelling shellfish that are ingested by bottom-dwelling fish. The Caribbean and Pacific islands are the areas predominantly affected. The treatment is supportive, including respiratory support.

Mushroom Poisoning Syndromes

A number of clinical syndromes associated with the ingestion of toxic mushrooms have been described (Table 82–4). A syndrome with a short incubation period in which patients develop confusion, restlessness, visual disturbances, and lethargy has been described.[104] Several *Amanita* species of mushrooms that contain ibotenic acid or muscimol are responsible for this syndrome. Another species of mushroom causes an illness in which parasympathetic hyperactivity is pronounced with salivation, blurred vision, sweating, and diarrhea. In addition, patients may develop bradycardia or bronchospasm. Symptoms usually resolve in 24 hours. This syndrome is caused by the chemical muscarine found in *Inocybe* and *Clitocybe* species.[105] An acute psychotic reaction caused by toxins found in several species of mushrooms has been described. Mushroom intoxication can also cause a disulfiram-like reaction if alcohol is consumed. A number of mushrooms can cause a gastroenteritis. The toxins have not been well characterized.

By far the most lethal mushroom poisoning syndromes are due to the amatoxins and phallotoxins found in the species *Amanita phalloides*, *Amanita virosa*, *Amanita verna*, *Galerina autumnalis*, *Galerina marginata*, or *Galerina venenata*. After ingestion the syndrome is heralded by abdominal cramps and diarrhea; however, after apparent improvement in symptoms, patients develop both liver and renal failure.[106] A mortality of at least 50% has been reported. A similar syndrome without renal failure has been described after ingestion of *Gyromitra*. The toxin associated with this species does not appear to cause acute renal failure; however, significant hepatic failure has been described.

TABLE 82–3 ■ Fish and Shellfish Poisoning Syndromes

SYNDROME	FISH	INCUBATION PERIOD	SYMPTOMS	DURATION	GEOGRAPHIC LOCATION	TOXIN
Scombroid	Tuna, mackeral, bonito, skipjack, mahi-mahi	5 min–1 h	Histamine reaction, burning, flushing urticaria, nausea vomiting, bronchospasm	Hours	Coast (Hawaii, California)	Histamine and saurine
Ciguatera	Barracuda, snapper, grouper, amberjack	1–6 h	Nausea, vomiting, diarrhea, blurred vision, photophobia, shooting pains, hot-cold temperature reversal, hypotension, respiratory paralysis	Days, months	35° north–35° south latitude (Hawaii, Florida)	Ciguatoxin
Paralytic shellfish	Shellfish, *Gonyaulax catenella, Gonyaulax tamarensis*	5 min–4 h	Paresthesias, dysphagia, paralysis	Hours–days	>30° north and <30° south New England, West Coast	Saxitoxin
Neurotoxic shellfish	Shellfish, dinoflagellates, *Gymnodinium breve*	5 min–4 h	Paresthesias	Hours–days	Gulf Coast, Atlantic Coast (Florida)	Saxitoxin

Adapted from references 90–101.

TABLE 82–4 ■ Mushroom Poisoning Syndromes

SYNDROME	INCUBATION PERIOD (h)	SPECIES	TOXIN
Confusion, restlessness, visual disturbances lethargy	2	*Amanita muscaria* *Amanita pantherina*	Ibotenic acid, muscimol
Parasympathetic activity	2	*Inocybe* sp. *Clitocybe* sp.	Muscarine
Hallucinations	2	*Psilocybe* sp. *Panaeolus* sp.	Psilocybin Psilocin
Disulfiram	2	*Coprinus atramentarius*	Disulfiram-like substances
Gastroenteritis	2	Many	Unknown
Hepatorenal failure	6–24	*Amanita phalloides* *Amanita virosa* *Amanita verna* *Galerina autumnalis* *Galerina marginata* *Galerina venenata*	Amatoxins Phallotoxins
Hepatic failure	6–24	*Gyromitra* sp.	Gyromitrin

Water-Borne Disease

Occasionally clusters of water-borne disease that may mimic a food-borne epidemic are reported. The most common cause of water-borne disease has been *G. lamblia* (see Chapter 286), which has been responsible for several large outbreaks associated with municipal water supplies. *Cryptosporidium* has been responsible for community-wide outbreaks.[85] Other water-borne outbreaks have been caused by *Shigella*, hepatitis A virus, nontyphoid *Salmonella*, *Salmonella typhi*, enterotoxigenic *E. coli*, *C. jejuni*, and viral agents, including Norwalk virus and others.

Control and Prevention

The common theme that ties all food-borne illnesses together is the presence of an improper food handling procedure before food consumption.

In a review of the factors responsible for food-borne outbreaks in the United States during a 15-year period, Bryan[106] has shown that inadequate refrigeration is the single factor most frequently implicated in food-borne outbreaks (Table 82–5). Usually more than one factor is associated with an outbreak, and inadequate refrigeration, advance preparation of food without adequate storage, and improper reheating or cooling are usually present to one degree or another.[106] To a lesser degree, contaminated equipment, cross-contamination, and food preparation personnel with poor personal hygiene may contribute to outbreaks. Contaminated raw ingredients are frequently part of the process as well. The ubiquity of *B. cereus* and *C. perfringens* makes it mandatory that food be cooked properly and, when stored, cooled properly. The failure to refrigerate food properly is the major problem in staphylococcal disease, the only difference being the contamination of the food by a carrier at some point before service. It becomes obvious that control must be based on inhibiting bacterial growth, preventing contamination after preparation, and killing potential pathogens with cooking. In general, foods should be heated to an internal temperature of 165°F, but lower temperatures for longer periods may be equally effective. Once cooked or processed, foods must be held at a temperature of 40°F or below.

Although these control measures are standard, many places where food preparation takes place do not abide by these guidelines. It is through diligent efforts by public health officials that reported outbreaks are investigated and food preparation techniques corrected. Therefore, recognition and reporting of food-borne illness are instrumental in the control of the problem. Education of the public, nurses, physicians, and eating establishments is crucial to the control of food-borne illness. Carriage of most of the organisms considered in this chapter is not a problem, with the exception of staphylococci and *Salmonella*. Because staphylococcal carriage is a necessary step in the development of staphylococcal food-borne illness, education of food handlers to watch for boils and pustules should be emphasized. Except for *S. typhi*, carriage of *Salmonella* is not the usual means of transmission of these organisms.

TABLE 82–5 ■ Factors That Contributed to Food-Borne Disease Outbreaks in the United States from 1961 to 1976

FACTOR	% IMPLICATED*
Inadequate refrigeration	47
Food prepared too far in advance of service	21
Infected person with poor personal hygiene	21
Inadequate cooking	16
Inadequate holding temperature	16
Inadequate reheating	12
Contaminated raw ingredients	11
Cross-contamination	7
Dirty equipment	7

*Values total more than 100% because more than one factor may contribute to food-borne outbreak.

From Bryan FL: Epidemiology of foodborne diseases. *In* Reimann H, Bryan FL (eds): Food-borne Infections and Intoxications, ed 2. New York, Academic Press, 1979, pp 3–69.

Treatment

For each of the pathogens enumerated here, treatment is beyond the scope of this chapter. In general, for the illnesses that are self-limited and mediated by toxins, antibiotics play little role in either therapy or prophylaxis. Invasive disease caused by *Salmonella* or *Campylobacter* may require antibiotic therapy. Disease caused by *Shigella* or *Listeria* requires antibiotic treatment, a discussion of which can be found in their respective chapters. Fluid replacement and supportive therapy are the major considerations in all of these illnesses.

Immunization

In general, immunization has not been attempted in these diseases. The immunogenicity of many of the toxins described has not been totally defined, and the populations at risk are so vast that immunization may not be practical. An interesting report on using a clostridial toxoid prepared from type C cultures in New Guinea suggests the prevention of pig-bel in children.[107]

References

1. Bean NH, Goulding JS, Lao C, Angulo FJ: Surveillance for foodborne disease outbreaks—United States. MMWR Morb Mortal Wkly Rep (in press).
2. Todd E: Epidemiology of foodborne illness: North America. Lancet 336:788–790, 1990.
3. Centers for Disease Control: Foodborne Disease Surveillance. Annual Summary 1981. Atlanta, Centers for Disease Control, 1983.
4. Bryan FL, Fanelli MJ, Reimann H: *Salmonella* infections. *In* Reimann H, Bryan FL (eds): Foodborne Infections and Intoxications, ed 2. New York, Academic Press, 1979, pp 73–130.
5. Sakazaki R: Halophilic vibrio infections. *In* Reimann H (ed): Foodborne Infections and Intoxications. New York, Academic Press, 1969, pp 115–119.
6. Hedberg CW, MacDonald KL, Osterholm MT: Changing epidemiology of food-borne disease: A Minnesota perspective. Clin Infect Dis 18:671–682, 1994.
7. MacDonald KL, O'Leary MJ, Cohen ML, et al: *Escherichia coli* 0157:H7, an emerging gastrointestinal pathogen. JAMA 259:3567–3570, 1988.
8. Lovett J: *Listeria monocytogenes*. *In* Doyle MP (ed): Foodborne Bacterial Pathogens. New York, Marcel Dekker, 1989, pp 283–310.
9. Skirrow MB: *Campylobacter* perspectives. Public Health Laboratory Service. Microbiol Diagn 6:113–117, 1989.
10. Morse DL, Guzewich JJ, Hanrahan JP, et al: Widespread outbreaks of clam- and oyster-associated gastroenteritis: Role of Norwalk virus. N Engl J Med 314:678–681, 1986.
11. Hedberg CW, Fishbein DB, Janssen RS, et al: An outbreak of thyrotoxicosis caused by consumption of bovine thyroid gland in ground beef. N Engl J Med 316:993–998, 1987.
12. Belongia EA, Hedberg CW, Gleich GJ, et al: An investigation of the cause of the eosinophilia-myalgia syndrome associated with tryptophan use. N Engl J Med 323:357–365, 1990.
13. Dack GM, Cary WE, Woolpert O, Wiggers H: An outbreak of food poisoning proved to be due to a yellow hemolytic *Staphylococcus*. J Prev Med 4:167–175, 1930.
14. Dack GM, Jordan EO, Woolpert O: Attempts to immunize human volunteers with *Staphylococcus* filtrates that are toxic to man when swallowed. J Prev Med 5:151–159, 1931.
15. Dack GM: *Staphylococcus* food poisoning. *In* Dack GM (ed): Food Poisoning. Chicago, University of Chicago Press, 1956, pp 109–158.
16. Sullivan R, Asano T: Effects of staphylococcal enterotoxin B on intestinal transport in the rat. Am J Physiol 222:1793–1799, 1971.
17. Minor TE, March EH: *Staphylococcus aureus* and staphylococcal food poisoning. J Milk Food Technol 34:21–29, 77–83, 227–241, 1972; 35:447–476, 1973.
18. Bergdoll MS, Crass BA, Reiser RF, et al: A new staphylococcal enterotoxin, enterotoxin F, associated with toxic-shock-syndrome *Staphylococcus aureus* isolates. Lancet 1:1017–1021, 1981.
19. Holmberg SD, Blake PA: Staphylococcal food poisoning in the United States. New facts and old misconceptions. JAMA 25:487–489, 1984.
20. Terranova W, Blake PA: *Bacillus cereus* food poisoning. N Engl J Med 298:143–144, 1978.
21. Mortimer PR, McCann G: Food-poisoning episodes associated with *Bacillus cereus* in fried rice. Lancet 1:1043–1045, 1974.
22. Saunders GC, Bartlett ML: Double-antibody solid-phase enzyme immunoassay for the detection of staphylococcal enterotoxin A. Appl Environ Microbiol 34:518–522, 1977.
23. Hauge S: Food poisoning caused by aerobic spore forming bacilli. J Appl Bacteriol 18:591–595, 1955.
24. Midura T, Gerber M, Wood R, Leonard AR: Outbreak of food poisoning cause by *Bacillus cereus*. Public Health Rep 85:45–48, 1970.
25. Portnoy BL, Goepfert JM, Harmon SM: An outbreak of *Bacillus cereus* food poisoning resulting from contaminated vegetable sprouts. Am J Epidemiol 103:589–594, 1976.
26. Turnbull PCB, Nottingham JF, Ghosh AC: A severe necrotic enterotoxin produced by certain food, food poisoning and other clinical isolates of *Bacillus cereus*. Br J Exp Pathol 58:273–280, 1977.
27. Turnbull PCB: Studies on the production of enterotoxins by *Bacillus cereus*. J Clin Pathol 29:941–948, 1976.
28. Lund BM. Foodborne disease due to *Bacillus* and *Clostridium* species. Lancet 336:982–986, 1990.
29. McClung LS: Human food poisoning due to growth of *Clostridium perfringens* (*Cl. welchii*) in freshly cooked chicken: A preliminary note. J Bacteriol 50:229–233, 1945.
30. Hobbs BC, Smith ME, Oakley CL, et al: *Clostridium welchii* food poisoning. J Hyg 51:75–101, 1953.
31. Zeissler J, Rassfeld-Sternberg L: Enteritis necroticans due to *Clostridium welchii* type F. Br Med J 1:267–270, 1949.
32. Murrell TGC, Egerton JR, Rampling A, et al: The ecology and epidemiology of the pig-bel syndrome in man in New Guinea. J Hyg 64:375–396, 1966.
33. Stark RL, Duncan CL: Biological characteristics of *Clostridium perfringens* type A enterotoxin. Infect Immun 4:89–96, 1971.
34. Duncan CL, Strong DH: *Clostridium perfringens* type A food poisoning. I. Response of the rabbit ileum as an indication of enteropathogenicity of strains of *Clostridium perfringens* in monkeys. Infect Immun 3:167–170, 1971.
35. Duncan CL: Time of enterotoxin formation and release during sporulation of *Clostridium perfringens* type A. J Bacteriol 113:932–936, 1973.
36. Skjelkvale R, Duncan CL: Enterotoxin formation by different toxigenic types of *Clostridium perfringens*. Infect Immun 11:563–575, 1975.
37. Skjelkvale R, Duncan CL: Characterization of enterotoxin purified from *Clostridium perfringens* type C. Infect Immun 11:1061–1068, 1975.
38. Bartholomew BA, Stringer MF, Watson GN, Gilbert RJ: Development and application of an enzyme linked immunosorbent assay for *Clostridium perfringens* type A enterotoxin. J Clin Pathol 38:222–228, 1985.
39. Horwitz MH, Hughes JM, Merson MH, et al: Food-borne botulism in the United States, 1970–75. J Infect Dis 136:153–157, 1977.
40. Arnon SS, Midura TF, Clay SA, et al: Infant botulism: Epidemiological, clinical and laboratory aspects. JAMA 237:1946–1952, 1977.
41. MacDonald KL, Cohen ML, Blake PA: The changing epidemiology of adult botulism in the United States. Am J Epidemiol 124:794–799, 1986.
42. MacDonald KL, Spengler RF, Hathaway CL, et al: Type A botulism from sauteed onions. JAMA 253:1275–1278, 1985.
43. St. Louis ME, Peck SHS, Bowering D, et al: Botulism from chopped garlic: Delayed recognition of a major outbreak. Ann Intern Med 108:363–368, 1988.
44. Griffin PM, Tauxe RV: The epidemiology of infections caused by *Escherichia coli* O157:H7, other enterohemorrhagic *E. coli*, and the associated hemolytic uremic syndrome. Epidemiol Rev 13:60–98, 1991.
45. Boyce TG, Swerdlow DL, Griffin PM: *Escherichia coli* O157:H7 and the hemolytic-uremic syndrome. N Engl J Med 333:364–368, 1995.
46. Bell BP, Goldoft M, Griffin PM, et al: A multistate outbreak of *Escherichia coli* O157:H7–associated bloody diarrhea and hemolytic uremic syndrome from hamburgers. The Washington experience. JAMA 272:1349–1353, 1994.
47. Besser RE, Lett SM, Weber TJ, et al: An outbreak of diarrhea and hemolytic uremic syndrome from *Escherichia coli* O157:H7 in fresh-pressed apple cider. JAMA 269:2217–2220, 1993.
48. Centers for Disease Control and Prevention: *Escherichia coli* O157:H7 outbreak linked to commercially distributed dry-cured salami—Washington and California, 1994. MMWR Morb Mortal Wkly Rep 44:157–160, 1995.
49. Interim guidelines for the control of infections with Vero cytotoxin producing *Escherichia coli* (VTEC). Subcommittee of the PHLS Working Group on Vero cytotoxin producing Escherichia coli (VTEC). Commun Dis Rep CDR Rev 5:R77–R81, 1995.
50. Griffin PM, Ostroff SM, Tauxe RV, et al: Illnesses associated

with *Escherichia coli* 0157:H7 infections. A broad clinical spectrum. Ann Intern Med 109:705–712, 1988.
51. Belongia EA, Osterholm MT, Soler JJ, et al: Transmission of *Escherichia coli* 0157:H7 infection in Minnesota child day-care facilities. JAMA 269:883–888, 1993.
52. Gellin GB, Broome CV: Listeriosis. JAMA 261:1313–1320, 1989.
53. Schlech WF III, Lavigne PM, Bortolussi RA, et al: Epidemic listeriosis—Evidence for transmission by food. N Engl J Med 308:203–206, 1983.
54. Fleming DW, Cochis L, MacDonald KL, et al: Pasteurized milk as a vehicle of infection in an outbreak of listeriosis. N Engl J Med 312:404–407, 1985.
55. Ho JL, Shands KN, Friedland G, et al: A multi-hospital outbreak of type 4b *Listeria monocytogenes* infections involving patients from eight Boston hospitals. Arch Intern Med 146:520–524, 1986.
56. Tappero JW, Schucart A, Deaver KA, et al: Reduction in the incidence of human listeriosis in the United States. Effectiveness of prevention efforts? JAMA 273:1118–1122, 1995.
57. Centers for Disease Control: Foodborne and Waterborne Disease Outbreaks. Five Year Summary, 1983–1987. Atlanta, Centers for Disease Control, 1990.
58. *Listeria* Contamination Seen Controlled by Normal Sanitation Procedures. Washington, DC, National Association of Federal Veterinarians, 1987, p 2.
59. St. Louis ME, Morse DL, Potter ME, et al: The emergence of grade A eggs as a major source of *Salmonella enteritis* infections. New implications for the control of salmonellosis. JAMA 259:2103–2107, 1988.
60. Fowler NG, Mead GC: *Salmonella* in poultry (Letter). Lancet 337:118–119, 1991.
61. Maguire H, Cowden J, Jacob M, et al: An outbreak of *Salmonella dublin* infection in England and Wales associated with soft unpasteurized cows' milk cheese. Epidemiol Infect 109:389–396, 1992.
62. Fujino T, Okuno Y, Nahada D, et al: On the bacteriological examination of shirasu-food poisoning. Med J Osaka Univ 4:299–304, 1953.
63. Fujino T, Sakazaki R, Tamura K: Designation of the type of strain of *Vibrio parahaemolyticus* and description of 200 strains of the species. Int J Syst Bacteriol 24:447–499, 1974.
64. Sakazaki R, Tamura K, Kato T, et al: Studies on the enteropathogenic facultatively halophilic bacteria, *Vibrio parahaemolyticus*. III. Enteropathogenicity. Jpn J Med Sci Biol 21:325–331, 1968.
65. Kato T, Obara Y, Ichinose H, et al: Hemolytic activity and toxicity of *Vibrio parahaemolyticus*. Jpn J Bacteriol 21:442–443, 1966.
66. Calia FM, Johnson DE: Bacteremia in suckling rabbits after oral challenge with *Vibrio parahaemolyticus*. Infect Immun 11:1222–1225, 1975.
67. Yahagi H: Early features of infection in ligated loops of the rabbit small intestine inoculated with *Shigella flexneri* 3a, enteropathogenic *E. coli, Escherichia coli* and *Vibrio parahaemolyticus*, the second report: Gross appearance and histologic findings of ligated loops after inoculation. Keio J Med 16:133–145, 1967.
68. Yahagi H, Ghoda A, Sasaki S: Early features of infection in ligated loops of the rabbit small intestine inoculated with *Shigella flexneri* 3a, enteropathogenic *E. coli, Escherichia coli* and *Vibrio parahaemolyticus*, the third report: Study of bacterial invasiveness with the fluorescent antibody technique. Keio J Med 16:119–131, 1967.
69. Johnson RH, Lutwick LI, Huntley GA, Vosti KL: *Arizona hinshawii* infections. New cases, antimicrobial sensitivities, and literature review. Ann Intern Med 85:587–592, 1976.
70. Kumar MC, Nivas SC, Bahl AK, et al: Studies on natural infection and egg transmission of *Arizona hinshawii* 7:1, 7, 8 in turkeys. Avian Dis 18:416–426, 1974.
71. Holmberg SD, Wachsmuth IK, Hickman-Brenner FW, et al: *Plesiomonas* enteric infections in the United States. Ann Intern Med 105:690–694, 1986.
72. Rutala WA, Sarubi FA Jr, Finch CS, et al: Oyster-associated outbreak of diarrhoeal disease possibly caused by *Plesiomonas shigelloides* (Letter). Lancet 1:739, 1982.
73. Holmberg SD, Farmer JJ III: *Aeromonas hydrophila* and *Plesiomonas shigelloides* as causes of intestinal infections. Rev Infect Dis 6:633–639, 1982.
74. Singh DV, Sanyal SC: Enterotoxicity of clinical and environmental isolates of *Aeromonas* spp. J Med Microbiol 36:269–272, 1992.
75. Agger WA, McCormick JD, Gurwith MJ: Clinical and microbiologic features of *Aeromonas hydrophila*–associated diarrhea. J Clin Microbiol 21:909–913, 1985.
76. Namdari H, Bottone EJ: Microbiologic and clinical evidence supporting the role of *Aeromonas caviae* as a pediatric enteric pathogen. J Clin Microbiol 28:837–840, 1990.
77. Osterholm MT, MacDonald KL, White KE, et al: An outbreak of a newly recognized chronic diarrhea syndrome associated with raw milk consumption. JAMA 256:484–490, 1986.
78. Martin DL, Hoberman LJ: A point source outbreak of chronic diarrhea in Texas. No known exposure to raw milk (Letter). JAMA 256:469, 1986.
79. Snydman DR, Dienstag JL, Stedt BL, et al: Use of IgM–hepatitis A antibody testing to investigate a common-source, food-borne outbreak. JAMA 245:827–830, 1981.
80. Blacklow NR, Greenberg HB: Viral gastroenteritis. N Engl J Med 325:252–264, 1991.
81. Morse DL, Guzewich JJ, Hanrahan JP, et al: Widespread outbreaks of clam- and oyster-associated gastroenteritis. Role of Norwalk virus. N Engl J Med 314:678–681, 1986.
82. Kaplan JE, Schonberger LB, Varano G, et al: An outbreak of acute nonbacterial gastroenteritis in a nursing home: Demonstration of person-to-person transmission by temporal clustering of cases. Am J Epidemiol 116:940–948, 1982.
83. Kuritsky JN, Osterholm MT, Greenberg HB, et al: Norwalk gastroenteritis: A community outbreak associated with bakery product consumption. Ann Intern Med 100:519–521, 1984.
84. Kohn MA, Farley TA, Ando T, et al: An outbreak of Norwalk virus gastroenteritis associated with eating raw oysters. Implications for maintaining safe oyster beds. JAMA 273:466–471, 1995.
85. MacKenzie WR, Hoxie NJ, Proctor ME, et al: A massive outbreak in Milwaukee of cryptosporidium infection transmitted through the public water supply. N Engl J Med 331:161–167, 1994.
86. Millard PS, Gensheimer KF, Addiss DG, et al: An outbreak of cryptosporidiosis from fresh pressed apple cider. JAMA 272:1592–1596, 1994.
87. Semple AB, Parry WH, Phillips DE: Acute copper poisoning: An outbreak traced to contaminated water from a corroded geyser. Lancet 2:700, 1960.
88. Brown MA, Thom JV, Orth GL, et al: Food poisoning involving zinc contamination. Arch Environ Health 8:657–661, 1964.
89. Mills AR, Passmore R: Pelagic paralysis. Lancet 1:161–163, 1988.
90. Schaumburg HH, Byck B, Gerstl R, Mashman JH: Monosodium L-glutamate: Its pharmacology and role in the Chinese restaurant syndrome. Science 163:826–828, 1969.
91. Hudson PJ, Vogt RL: A foodborne outbreak traced to niacin overenrichment. J Food Prot 48:249–251, 1985.
92. Merson MH, Baine WB, Gangarosa EJ, et al: Scombroid fish poisoning: Outbreak traced to commercially canned tuna fish. JAMA 228:1268–1269, 1974.
93. Foo LY. Scombroid poisoning—Recapitulation on the role of histamine. N Z Med J 85:425–427, 1977.
94. Etkind P, Wilson ME, Gallagher K, et al: Bluefish-associated scombroid poisoning. An example of the expanding spectrum of food poisoning from seafood. JAMA 258:3409–3410, 1987.
95. Blakesley ML: Scombroid poisoning: Prompt resolution of symptoms with cimetidine. Ann Emerg Med 12:104–106, 1983.
96. Hughes JM, Merson MH: Fish and shellfish poisoning. N Engl J Med 295:1117–1120, 1976.
97. Porkiss MEE, Horstman DA, Harpur D: Paralytic shellfish poisoning. A report of 17 cases in Cape Town. S Afr Med J 55:1017–1021, 1979.
98. Ghazarossian VE, Schantz EJ, Schnoes HK, et al: Identification of poison in toxic scallops from a *Gonyaulax tamarensis* red tide. Biochem Biophys Res Commun 59:1219–1224, 1974.
99. Schantz EJ, Ghazarossian VE, Schnoes HK, et al: The structure of saxitoxin. J Am Chem Soc 97:1238–1246, 1975.
100. Engleberg NC, Morris JG Jr, Lewis J, et al: Ciguatera fish poisoning: A major common-source outbreak in the U.S. Virgin Islands. Ann Intern Med 98:336–337, 1983.
101. Bagnis R, Kuberski T, Laugier S: Clinical observations on 3,009 cases of ciguatera fish poisoning in the south pacific. Am J Trop Med Hyg 28:1067–1073, 1979.
102. Bidard JN, Vijverberg HPM, Frelin C, et al: Ciguatoxin is a novel type of Na^+ channel toxin. J Biol Chem 259:8353–8357, 1984.

103. Morris JG Jr, Lewin P, Hargrett NT, et al: Clinical features of ciguatera fish poisoning. A study of disease in the US Virgin Islands. Arch Intern Med 142:1090–1092, 1982.
104. Lampe KF: Toxic fungi. Annu Rev Pharmacol Toxicol 19:85–102, 1979.
105. Paaso B, Harrison DL: A new look at an old problem. Mushroom poisoning. Am J Med 58:505–507, 1975.
106. Bryan FL: Epidemiology of foodborne diseases. *In* Reimann H, Bryan FL (eds): Foodborne Infections and Intoxications, ed 2. New York, Academic Press, 1979, pp 3–69.
107. Lawrence G, Shann F, Freestone DS, Walker PD: Prevention of necrotising enteritis in Papua New Guinea by active immunisation. Lancet 1:227–230, 1979.

83

Specific and Nonspecific Treatment of Diarrhea

Stephen J. Savarino
Myron M. Levine

The worldwide burden of diarrheal diseases remains high, particularly in settings where potable water and sanitation are unavailable and personal hygiene practices are primitive. In the first half of this century, the treatment of diarrheal diseases was still generally guided by empiricism; however, this has changed in the past several decades. New agents that cause diarrhea have been identified. Major virulence properties of enteric pathogens have been revealed. Increased understanding of gut physiology has led to improved rehydration therapy. Antibiotics have become available to treat specific enteric infections. In this chapter, we describe the benefits and risks offered by various specific and nonspecific interventions in an effort to foster a rational approach to treatment of the patient with infectious diarrhea.

Fluid Therapy

The most common complication of diarrheal illness is dehydration; if severe, dehydration can lead to hypovolemia, acidosis, shock, and death. Young and old persons and those with underlying diseases are most vulnerable. Cholera at any age and diarrhea caused by enterotoxigenic *Escherichia coli* (ETEC) or rotavirus in infants can result in frequent, voluminous stools. The cornerstone of therapy for all diarrheal diseases is rehydration designed to correct fluid and electrolyte deficits and replace ongoing losses.

Early rehydration initiated at the onset of diarrhea can prevent dehydration. If the patient presents with clinically evident dehydration, rehydration must be instituted promptly. Intravenous fluid therapy is necessary for only a small proportion of patients, including those with severe dehydration and shock (for whom intravenous fluid therapy may be lifesaving), diminished mental status, symptomatic electrolyte disturbances, paralytic ileus, excessively high purging rate, or intractable vomiting. Rapid infusion of an appropriate solution such as Ringer lactate to vigorously expand the intravascular volume is followed by the administration of additional rehydration fluids (preferably by the oral route) to replace the remaining deficit and to provide for ongoing losses and maintenance requirements. Intravenous fluid therapy is employed fairly frequently in industrialized countries, where it is often a route of convenience rather than the superior method.

The majority of patients with diarrhea in all settings can be effectively treated with oral rehydration. This therapy is simple to administer, inexpensive, and highly efficacious.[1, 2] Glucose-based oral rehydration therapy rests on the observation that active transport of glucose is coupled with sodium transport in the small intestine,[3] a process that is preserved during diarrheal illness. Other solutes, such as amino acids and dipeptides, are also actively and independently cotransported with sodium. These observations have led to the concept of a "supersolution," which would contain multiple actively transported substrates and be so potent in stimulating absorption as to actually diminish diarrheal losses while achieving rehydration. Regrettably, so far no solution has consistently achieved such results in clinical studies.[4–6]

Throughout the developing world, the World Health Organization (WHO) recommends the use of a single oral rehydration solution (WHO-ORS) with a sodium concentration of 90 mEq/L for diarrheal illness of all causes in all ages.[7] By concurrently offering appropriate amounts of low-solute fluids, WHO-ORS can be used to prevent dehydration as well as to replace deficits of body water and electrolytes.[8–11] The reader is referred to a review article for a more detailed discussion of its use.[12] WHO-ORS oral rehydration therapy is as efficacious as intravenous fluid therapy in treating hyponatremic and isotonic dehydration; its use in hypernatremic dehydration results in a lower frequency of seizures.[13, 14]

Some physicians in industrialized countries have been reluctant to use WHO-ORS owing to its relatively high sodium content. As an alternative, a two-solution approach has become popular; a rehydration solution (sodium concentration 60 to 75 mEq/L) is used for replacement of deficits, and a second solution (sodium concentration 45 to 50 mEq/L) is used to replace ongoing losses.

Although glucose-based oral rehydration therapy effectively replaces diarrheal losses, it does not abate stool output. Rice powder–electrolyte solutions, which deliver higher densities of glucose to the small intestine in the form of complex starches along with amino acids and small peptides, offer potential advantages over glucose-electrolyte solutions. Compared with WHO-ORS in a number of studies, rice powder–electrolyte solution proved superior in treating dehydration due to cholera and noncholera diarrhea. Oral intake requirement, stool output, and duration of diarrhea were all significantly reduced in the group treated with the rice powder–electrolyte solution, particularly in patients with more severe dehydration.[15–17]

Antimicrobial Therapy

In general, antimicrobial agents are prescribed too liberally for treatment of diarrheal diseases. In fact, most illness is mild and self-limited and can be treated with fluid therapy alone. The widespread use of antibiotics in some areas has provided selective pressures leading to antibiotic resistance among enteropathogens, complicating the treatment of patients who warrant antibiotics. For many bacterial diarrheas, controlled studies to establish the efficacy of specific antibiotics either have not been done or have shown no benefits; viral diarrheas obviously do not respond to such treatment. Nevertheless, antibiotics have proven efficacy in the treatment of certain bacterial and protozoan enteric infections and may be warranted for treating others when the illness is complicated or severe (Table 83–1).

Shigellosis

Shigella is the most common cause of dysentery. One serotype, *Shigella dysenteriae* type 1, causes particularly fulminant illness and is associated with a high case-fatality rate. In controlled clinical trials, several antibiotics have been shown to shorten the illness and duration of *Shigella* excretion. Information from such trials is critical because in vitro susceptibility does not necessarily correlate with efficacy in vivo. Several antibiotics, including cephalexin[18] and cefaclor,[19] are of little value clinically despite favorable activity in vitro. In addition, as effective antibiotics have achieved broad use, widespread resistance has developed. From the 1940s through the mid-1970s, sulfa drugs, tetracycline, and ampicillin were successively the drugs of choice for treating shigellosis, until resistant strains became highly prevalent. The utility of trimethoprim-sulfamethoxazole (TMP-SMX), the drug of choice in many areas in the 1980s, is being eroded worldwide by increasing levels of resistance.[20–23] TMP-SMX resistance genes are often found on plasmids that encode multiple other antibiotic resistances.

Nalidixic acid and the newer quinolone derivatives have been employed to treat infections caused by *Shigella* strains that are resistant to other antibiotics. In South Asia, rapid emergence of *S. dysenteriae* resistance to nalidixic acid has occurred, limiting the utility of this agent.[24] These findings argue for judicious use of antibiotics in treating moderate to severe shigellosis, guided by susceptibility testing and epidemiologic surveillance, and the continued search for effective new agents.

For sensitive strains, a 5-day course of tetracycline, ampicillin, or TMP-SMX to treat shigellosis has been shown to shorten the illness and the duration of pathogen excretion (Table 83–2). A single large dose (stosstherapy) of tetracycline has efficacy comparable to a 5-day regimen.[25] One study showed that tetracycline stosstherapy may be effective even against strains that demonstrate tetracycline resistance in vitro.[26] However, this observation has not been corroborated, and it is prudent to use antimicrobial agents to which *Shigella* strains are likely to be sensitive. Tetracycline is contraindicated in pregnancy and in children younger than 7 years because of its associated tooth discoloration; the safety of stosstherapy has not been evaluated in these groups. Although clinical response to stosstherapy with ampicillin compares favorably with that to a 5-day regimen, it was associated with significantly higher rates of bacteriologic failure in a study from Bangladesh.[27] Amoxicillin is ineffective in the treatment of shigellosis for reasons that are ill understood.[28] TMP-SMX continues to be a drug of choice in many areas where resistant strains remain uncommon. In parts of Asia and Africa, where TMP-SMX–resistant *Shigella* strains have become common,[23, 24, 29] nalidixic acid has been shown to be effective for treatment of shigellosis.[20]

Several clinical trials have demonstrated the effectiveness of ciprofloxacin and norfloxacin in the treatment of shigellosis.[29–32] Limited experience has shown that single-dose therapy with ciprofloxacin is effective treatment against disease caused by all *Shigella* spp. except *S. dysenteriae*, for which a 5-day course of therapy is superior.[33] In areas where resistance has eroded the utility of other available antibiotics, the fluoroquinolones, particularly ciprofloxacin, represent the drug of choice. Several of the quinolones have been associated with arthropathies in young animals,[34] and case reports of ciprofloxacin-associated arthropathy in children have appeared.[35] For this reason, the quinolones, except nalidixic acid, were not approved in the past for use in children and pregnant or nursing women. However, evidence is accumulating to support cautious use of the fluoroquinolones for treatment of severe, multidrug-resistant *Shigella* infections in children when effective alternatives are unavailable.[36, 37] Pivmecillinam is currently the only oral antibiotic alternative to nalidixic acid for treatment of children with resistant shigellosis.[24] Ceftriaxone, administered parenterally once daily for 2 to 5 days, is an alternative that has utility in developed countries.[38]

Salmonella *Gastroenteritis*

The effect of antibiotic treatment on uncomplicated nontyphoidal *Salmonella* gastroenteritis has been studied in several randomized placebo-controlled trials. Variously employing chloramphenicol,[39] neomycin,[40] TMP-SMX,[41] and ampicillin and amoxicillin,[42, 43] these studies failed to show any benefit over placebo in terms of diminishing duration or severity of diarrheal illness or duration of pathogen excretion. One study found that children treated with either oral amoxicillin or ampicillin had a significantly higher frequency of bacteriologic relapse, not infrequently associated with recurrence of diarrhea.[43] Whereas the fluoroquinolones show excellent in vitro activity against salmonellae, a randomized, placebo-controlled, double-blind trial found that no significant clinical or bacteriologic benefit was conferred by treatment with ciprofloxacin.[44] On the basis of these studies, antibiotics are not recommended for treatment of uncomplicated *Salmonella* gastroenteritis in adults, children, or infants 12 weeks of age or older.

Infants younger than 12 weeks, patients with hemoglobinopathies, and individuals with acquired immunodeficiency syndrome who develop *Salmonella* gastroenteritis are at increased risk for developing bacteremia and metastatic complications such as meningitis, septic arthritis, and osteomyelitis.[45] It is recommended that these high-risk groups be treated with antibiotics. Some authorities extend this recommendation to include patients with malignant neoplasms and other immunosuppressive conditions,[46] although data are lacking.

TABLE 83–1 ■ Relative Indications for Use of Antimicrobial Agents in Diarrheal Disease Caused by Specific Etiologic Agents in Immunocompetent Hosts

CLEARLY INDICATED	SOMETIMES INDICATED	NOT INDICATED
Shigellosis	Nontyphoidal salmonellosis (in infants <12 wk of age)	Rotavirus
Cholera	Enteropathogenic *E. coli* (nursery outbreaks or persistent infection)	Other viral agents
Enterotoxigenic *Escherichia coli* traveler's diarrhea*	Enteroinvasive *E. coli*	Nontyphoidal salmonellosis
Amebiasis	*Campylobacter* (early treatment of dysentery)	Cryptosporidiosis
Giardiasis	*Clostridium difficile* colitis	
	Non–*Vibrio cholerae* vibrios	
	Enteroaggregative *E. coli* (persistent diarrhea)	

*Enterotoxigenic *E. coli* is the most common cause of acute traveler's diarrhea, and certain antibiotics are highly effective.

TABLE 83–2 ■ Recommended Antibiotic Dosage Regimens for the Treatment of Shigellosis

	DOSE AND DURATION	
ANTIBIOTIC	Infants and Children	Adults and Adolescents
Oral		
TMP-SMX*	10 mg/kg/d of TMP and 50 mg/kg/d of SMX in 4 divided doses for 5 d	160 mg of TMP and 800 mg of SMX q 12 h for 5 d
Ampicillin	100 mg/kg/d in 4 divided doses for 5 d	500 mg q 6 h for 5 d
Norfloxacin		400 mg q 12 h for 5 d Stosstherapy: 100 mg/kg in 1 dose
Tetracycline		500 mg q 6 h for 5 d Stosstherapy: 2.5 g in 1 dose
Ciprofloxacin		500 mg q 12 h for 5 d
Nalidixic acid	55 mg/kg/d in 4 divided doses for 5–7 d	1 g q 6 h for 5–7 d
Parenteral		
Ceftriaxone	50 mg/kg single daily dose for 5 d	

*TMP-SMX, Trimethoprim-sulfamethoxazole.

Usually ampicillin or amoxicillin (200 mg/kg per day for infants, 2 to 3 g/d for adults) or chloramphenicol (75 mg/kg per day for children, 2 to 3 g/d for adults) for 7 to 10 days is appropriate, although susceptibility patterns in vitro should guide the choice. Except for use in infants and children, fluoroquinolones are an excellent choice for treatment of severe or invasive nontyphoidal *Salmonella* infections when isolates are likely to be resistant to other antibiotics.[47, 48]

Campylobacter jejuni *Enteritis*

In the past 15 years, *Campylobacter* enteritis has become recognized as a common diarrheal disease worldwide, with a spectrum of illness ranging from watery diarrhea to frank dysentery. Several placebo-controlled trials of erythromycin in children and adults have demonstrated significant curtailment of pathogen excretion in treated groups.[49–51] However, only one study, in which infants with dysentery were treated with erythromycin (50 mg/kg per day for 5 days) early in their illness, has demonstrated significant amelioration of diarrheal illness.[52] A study from Bangkok noted a high proportion of erythromycin-resistant *Campylobacter* isolates,[53] although similar findings have generally not been reported elsewhere.

Several studies have been conducted using fluoroquinolones for treatment of campylobacteriosis in adults. In three randomized double-blind trials in which a 3- to 5-day course of either norfloxacin (400 mg twice daily) or ciprofloxacin (500 mg twice daily) was compared with placebo, a modest reduction in the duration of diarrhea was observed.[54–56] Emergence of fluoroquinolone-resistant *Campylobacter* isolates in several areas has been documented, which may limit the utility of these agents in this disease.[55, 57, 58] Azithromycin is a new oral macrolide antibiotic that attains high tissue concentrations and shows good in vitro activity against *Campylobacter* spp.[59] In one trial, azithromycin was shown to be as efficacious as ciprofloxacin in treating adults with *Campylobacter* enteritis.[58]

On the basis of data currently available, it is reasonable that patients presenting early with moderate to severe enteritis be treated with erythromycin if *Campylobacter* infection is suspected. Further studies with azithromycin and the fluoroquinolones are necessary before their use can be recommended.

Enterotoxigenic Escherichia coli *Infections*

ETEC, which produces a toxin-mediated secretory diarrhea, is a frequent cause of diarrhea in travelers to developing areas and is also endemic among children in such areas. In a placebo-controlled trial among Bangladeshi adults with ETEC-induced diarrhea, tetracycline significantly shortened pathogen excretion, although only limited clinical benefits were noted.[60] TMP-SMX treatment has demonstrated clinical and bacteriologic efficacy compared with placebo in ETEC-induced diarrhea in three separate studies involving American volunteers,[61] adult travelers in Mexico,[62] and young Mexican children.[63] As high rates of resistance to tetracycline, ampicillin, and TMP-SMX have emerged in some areas,[64, 65] the fluoroquinolones, which are highly active against ETEC in vitro,[66] have been shown to be useful. A short course of ciprofloxacin, norfloxacin, or ofloxacin shortens the duration of ETEC-associated diarrhea compared with placebo.[56, 67, 68]

In areas where ETEC is prevalent, it is recommended that adult traveler's diarrhea be treated promptly with TMP-SMX (160 mg of TMP and 800 mg of SMX twice daily for 5 days). In areas with a high prevalence of TMP-SMX resistance, ciprofloxacin (500 mg twice daily for 3 to 5 days) or norfloxacin (300 mg twice daily) is the considered drug of choice. Although definitive data are not available, pediatric travelers should also be treated early in their course of diarrheal illness with TMP-SMX (TMP at 4 mg/kg and SMX at 20 mg/kg twice daily for 5 days). Antibiotics are not routinely recommended for suspected ETEC-induced diarrhea in persons indigenous to areas where ETEC is endemic. A vast amount of clinical experience from oral rehydration studies in which the causative agents were identified supports this contention. In persons from endemic areas, degrees of background immunity tend to make ETEC infections self-limited and amenable to oral rehydration therapy alone.

Enteropathogenic Escherichia coli *Infections*

Enteropathogenic *E. coli* (EPEC) is an important cause of diarrhea in infants younger than 6 months of age in many developing areas of the world; occasional nursery and community outbreaks still occur in industrialized countries. In the 1960s, oral neomycin was sometimes used to treat EPEC-induced diarrhea,[69] but its use is now discouraged because neomycin commonly causes intestinal malabsorption and diarrhea as adverse effects. In an Ethiopian trial, EPEC-infected infants receiving either mecillinam or TMP-SMX for 5 days had significantly better clinical and bacteriologic cure rates compared with an untreated control group.[70] Two studies of EPEC-infected infants and children employing ampicillin had different outcomes; one showed a favorable clinical and bacteriologic response[71] and the other no difference[42] compared with placebo. Given the paucity of data, a reasonable approach is to employ an antibiotic such as TMP-SMX when EPEC is implicated as the cause of severe or persistent diarrhea in a young infant or in a nursery outbreak situation.

Enteroinvasive and Enterohemorrhagic Escherichia coli *Infections*

Enteroinvasive *E. coli* (EIEC) has many similarities to *Shigella* in its virulence properties and pathogenesis. Like *Shigella*, EIEC can cause dysentery. EIEC infections are thought to be responsive to the same agents as are used to treat shigellosis, although there have been no controlled trials to support this, and few published antibiotic susceptibility data are available.

Enterohemorrhagic *E. coli* (EHEC) causes hemorrhagic colitis and is also associated with hemolytic-uremic syndrome and thrombotic thrombocytopenic purpura. In the only controlled trial to date, no benefit was afforded to patients with O157:H7 EHEC-associated enteritis who received TMP-SMX.[72] Although not definitive, some retrospective analyses suggest that the use of antibiotics in EHEC diarrhea constitutes a risk factor for progression to hemolytic-uremic syndrome.[73, 74] Pending further study, routine antibiotic therapy for EHEC-associated diarrhea or colitis is not recommended.

Yersinia enterocolitica *Enteritis*

Y. enterocolitica is a common cause of enteritis and dysentery in young children, particularly in certain cooler regions such as northern Europe. Infected adolescents frequently present with mesenteric lymphadenitis; extraintestinal infections, including septicemia, have been reported (albeit infrequently) in patients with certain underlying conditions, most notably iron overload states. In general, isolates are susceptible in vitro to aminoglycosides, tetracycline, chloramphenicol, TMP-SMX, third-generation cephalosporins, and quinolones,[75] but data are lacking to support their use in uncomplicated diarrhea. In the only placebo-controlled trial, in which children with *Yersinia* enteritis were treated on average 12 days into their illness, TMP-SMX offered no beneficial clinical or bacteriologic effect.[76] On the basis of available information, it is recommended that antibiotic therapy be limited to patients with particularly severe or chronic *Y. enterocolitica* enteritis and to those with focal extraintestinal or systemic infections, the choice of antibiotics being guided by susceptibility testing in vitro.

Cholera

Vibrio cholerae O1 and O139 strains cause a secretory diarrhea characterized by voluminous purging. As an adjunct to fluid therapy, antibiotics are of proven benefit. Tetracycline, the drug of choice, markedly diminishes the volume and duration of diarrhea and fluid replacement requirements and curtails the excretion of the pathogen.[77, 78] Adults may be given 500 mg four times daily or 2 g once daily for 2 days, with equivalent results. Because duration of therapy is short, it is considered safe for use in children (125 mg four times daily for 2 to 4 days). Although they are inferior to tetracycline, other antibiotics such as doxycycline,[79] chloramphenicol,[77] and furazolidone[80] have proven efficacy in treating cholera. In one small study, norfloxacin (400 mg twice daily for 5 days) was shown to be effective in treatment of severe cholera in adults.[81] Furazolidone may be used as an alternative treatment for children and pregnant women. Reported outbreaks associated with tetracycline-resistant strains in Africa and Asia[82, 83] underscore the importance of alternatives to tetracycline. Preliminary data suggest that antibiotics used to treat *V. cholerae* O1, including tetracycline, are also effective therapy for *V. cholerae* O139 (Bengal).[84] Whereas *V. cholerae* O1 strains are typically sensitive to TMP-SMX, *V. cholerae* O139 strains isolated so far have been resistant.[85]

Clostridium difficile *Diarrhea and Colitis*

C. difficile is the most common agent of antibiotic-associated pseudomembranous colitis and is less frequently implicated in antibiotic-associated diarrhea without colitis. Antimicrobial therapy is warranted for patients with *C. difficile*–induced colitis or diarrhea that does not respond to discontinuation of the offending antibiotic.[86] Multiple studies have documented the efficacy and safety of oral vancomycin,[87] which is considered the drug of choice. A dosage of 125 mg, four times daily for 7 to 14 days, is generally adequate, although some patients may require up to 2 g daily. Because of its high cost and the frequency of clinical relapse (6% to 39%), other agents have been sought. Both oral metronidazole, 250 mg four times daily,[88] and bacitracin, 20,000 units four times daily,[89] appear to be comparable clinically to vancomycin. Metronidazole has, in fact, become the first-line agent in many institutions because it is considerably less expensive than vancomycin. Its use is contraindicated in pregnant and nursing women because of the theoretical potential for human teratogenesis, and concurrent alcohol consumption is proscribed because of a disulfiram-like effect.

Cases of multiple relapses and relapse associated with adynamic ileus are especially problematic. For multiple relapses, uncontrolled studies have shown a favorable response to an extended course of cholestyramine in tandem with oral vancomycin as well as to bacteriotherapy (see later), although what is the optimal therapy has not been established. In patients who are unable to tolerate oral therapy, limited anecdotal experience using parenteral metronidazole and vancomycin has met with both success and failure with each agent.[90] Demonstrable achievement of therapeutic intracolonic metronidazole levels after parenteral dosing[91] favors its use, although more controlled studies with these agents and a search for other therapies need to be pursued.

Amebiasis, Giardiasis, Cryptosporidiosis, and Isosporiasis

Amebiasis, giardiasis, cryptosporidiosis, and isosporiasis are discussed in Part XII of this text.

Clinical Approach to Treatment of Infectious Diarrhea

The clinician faces a series of therapeutic decisions when a patient presents with infectious diarrhea. The foremost concern should be the patient's state of hydration. After this is assessed and appropriate fluid therapy instituted, the indication for antimicrobial therapy must be determined. This hinges on whether the likely offending pathogen is amenable to such therapy. It is helpful to categorize the patient's disease into one of six clinical types (Table 83–3). Depending on the geographic setting, which pathogen most frequently causes each type of diarrhea varies somewhat.

The majority of patients present with simple diarrhea, characterized by watery stools without blood, low-grade fever, abdominal cramps, malaise, and occasional vomiting. Viral pathogens, mainly rotavirus, are the most frequent etiologic agents of pediatric diarrhea in many settings and clearly do not warrant antibiotic therapy. In developing areas, bacterial pathogens including ETEC and EPEC are more frequent

TABLE 83–3 ■ Clinical Presentations and Likely Agents of Acute Diarrheal Disease

CLINICAL TYPE	PATIENTS (APPROXIMATE %)	LIKELY AGENT*	
		Industrialized Countries	Developing Countries
Simple diarrhea	90	Rotavirus, other viruses, *Salmonella*, *Campylobacter jejuni*	Rotavirus, ETEC, *C. jejuni*
Dysentery	5–10	*Shigella*, *C. jejuni*, EIEC, *Yersinia*	*Shigella*, *C. jejuni*, *Entamoeba histolytica*, EIEC
Persistent diarrhea (>14 d)	3–4	*Giardia*, *Salmonella*, *Yersinia*	EPEC, *Giardia*, EAggEC
Severe purging of rice-water stools	1†	Rotavirus, *Salmonella*	*Vibrio cholerae*, ETEC
Hemorrhagic colitis	<1	EHEC	EHEC, *Shigella dysenteriae* type 1
Repeated vomiting without diarrhea	1–2		
Acute	1	Norwalk virus, other viruses	Viruses, *Giardia*
Persistent	<0.5	*Giardia*	*Giardia*, *Strongyloides*

*ETEC, Enterotoxigenic *E. coli;* EIEC, enteroinvasive *E. coli;* EPEC, enteropathogenic *E. coli;* EHEC, enterohemorrhagic *E. coli;* EAggEC, enteroaggregative *E. coli.*
†More common in cholera endemic areas.

offenders, so adult travelers to such areas who have moderate to severe watery diarrhea are likely to respond to early institution of TMP-SMX or a fluoroquinolone, which are active against ETEC.

In any setting, when the patient presents with dysentery, the physician must consider the invasive bacterial pathogens, such as *Shigella*, *Campylobacter*, and EIEC. In many areas, *Shigella* is the most common agent, and empirical therapy with TMP-SMX is generally indicated (ciprofloxacin or nalidixic acid in areas with widespread TMP-SMX resistance). It may be reasonable to include erythromycin along with TMP-SMX for *Campylobacter* coverage in patients who present early with dysentery. One clue to the presumptive diagnosis of *C. jejuni* enteritis is the notation of characteristic darting motility of vibrio-shaped organisms on examination of a wet preparation of stool.[92] Because the fluoroquinolones are active against both *Shigella* and *Campylobacter*, they appear to represent reasonable monotherapy for dysentery in adults, although the emergence of *Campylobacter* resistance to the quinolones may disturb this approach. In developing areas where *Entamoeba histolytica* is endemic, stool examination for amoebae must be performed to determine whether antiprotozoal therapy is warranted. In the appropriate setting (e.g., the hospitalized patient receiving antibiotics), *C. difficile* must be considered another potentially treatable cause of bloody diarrhea.

Tetracycline therapy is warranted for patients in endemic cholera areas who present with voluminous rice-water purging. Patients with persistent diarrhea may suffer profound nutritional losses, and detailed evaluation for an infectious agent may uncover a treatable cause, such as giardiasis.

Nonspecific Therapies

A plethora of nonantibiotic antidiarrheal agents are used in the hope of achieving symptomatic relief of diarrheal illness. Few are both innocuous and effective. Kaolin-pectin preparations are innocuous but essentially ineffective. They serve to increase the consistency of the diarrheal stool, but the water and electrolyte content of the stools is unchanged.[93] Kaolin-pectin preparations may be regarded as placebos and prescribed accordingly, if the clinician desires.

Bacteriotherapy, enteral administration of nonpathogenic microorganisms to inhibit growth of enteropathogens, is another innocuous modality without a clear indication. *Lactobacillus acidophilus* is commonly prescribed for treatment of acute diarrhea, although there is little evidence from controlled studies that such preparations can prevent or ameliorate infectious diarrheas.[94, 95] *Lactobacillus casei* strain GG has shown more promise. In two randomized placebo-controlled studies, oral administration of 10^{10-11} colony-forming units twice daily for 2 days was well tolerated and hastened recovery from acute watery diarrhea in children.[96, 97] An uncontrolled study described the successful use of rectal instillation of a mixture of 10 different bacteria in the treatment of chronic relapsing *C. difficile*–associated diarrhea. Administration of this preparation led to recolonization with *Bacteroides* species (absent in all patients before treatment) and elimination of *C. difficile*, associated with cessation of diarrhea.[98]

Chlorpromazine inhibits the secretory effect of cholera toxin and *E. coli* heat-labile toxin in vitro.[99] Clinical trials in cholera patients have shown that chlorpromazine can significantly diminish the voluminous diarrhea,[100] but the doses required to achieve a therapeutic effect may induce somnolence and thereby interfere with a patient's ability to ingest oral rehydration solutions. For this reason, chlorpromazine has not been approved for this use.

Opioids, including paregoric and codeine, have long been employed to relieve diarrhea. Synthetic opioids such as diphenoxylate and loperamide have been licensed more recently, and loperamide is now available over-the-counter. One of their most prominent effects is to decrease intestinal motility. The synthetic opioids may also have antisecretory effects. The advisability of using antimotility agents is the subject of considerable debate among physicians experienced in the treatment of diarrheal diseases. Some evidence from animal models and clinical studies speaks against the use of antimotility agents in patients with invasive bacterial infections such as shigellosis. For example, guinea pigs are normally resistant to *Shigella*, but if they are pretreated with paregoric, fatal enteritis follows oral inoculation with *Shigella*.[101] Moreover, volunteers experimentally challenged with *Shigella* who were treated with diphenoxylate after developing clinical illness exhibited higher fever and prolonged excretion of *Shigella* compared with untreated infected volunteers.[102] In contrast, a study found that treatment of *Shigella* dysentery with ciprofloxacin and loperamide hastened the resolution of diarrhea in comparison to antibiotic alone, and no deleterious effects were observed.[103]

We advocate a reasoned, conservative approach to the use of opioids in patients with infectious diarrheas. These drugs should not be used in the treatment of diarrheal disease in children or adults living in developing countries, because invasive bacterial diarrheas are common in such areas; therapy must be as economical as possible; and any diversion from an emphasis on oral rehydration is considered ill-advised. Loperamide, apparently the safest of the opioids, may be used as an adjunct to therapy in adults or older children with nonbloody diarrhea in industrialized countries, as long as appropriate precautions are taken (e.g., examination for fecal leukocytes) to ascertain that it is unlikely that the diarrhea is due to an invasive bacterial enteropathogen such as *Shigella*. Some physicians prescribe loperamide for adult travelers with mild to moderate watery diarrhea, particularly when abdominal cramps are prominent. We advocate a conservative approach that limits use of such agents to a single dose at the outset of antibiotic therapy.[104, 105]

Bismuth subsalicylate (BSS) has been widely studied as an antidiarrheal agent. Its effects are probably mediated by the salicylate component, although studies with ETEC-induced diarrhea suggest that the bismuth compound may act to inhibit intraluminal attachment or growth.[106] Field studies in adults with traveler's diarrhea have shown the liquid suspension of BSS to provide moderate relief of symptoms,[107] although this formulation has not been shown to diminish the water content or total weight of stools more than placebo does.[108] Because of the inconvenient dosing regimen with the liquid formulation, BSS in tablet form has been studied. BSS tablets reduce the occurrence of traveler's diarrhea for up to 3 weeks when used prophylactically but have not been efficacious in relieving established diarrhea.[106, 109] The salicylate component of BSS is readily absorbed, and serum levels in the range of 70 to 80 fg/mL have been recorded after multiple doses in adults. Therefore, patients taking aspirin, those with aspirin hypersensitivity or bleeding diathesis, and young children should avoid its use.

In two of three small inpatient studies using moderate (25 mg/kg per day) doses of aspirin to treat acute diarrhea in infants and children in developing countries, it was shown to diminish intestinal fluid losses.[110, 111] In the one study in which no beneficial effect was demonstrated, EPEC was the most commonly identified pathogen.[112] Despite promising animal data,[113] the few studies of indomethacin as an antidiarrheal agent either were poorly controlled[114] or demonstrated no efficacy.[115] Until more safety and efficacy data are available, the use of aspirin or indomethacin in the symptomatic treatment of diarrhea cannot be advocated.

Cholestyramine, a nonabsorbable exchange resin, has been studied in a number of settings. It significantly shortened the duration of acute diarrhea in infants, among whom rotavirus was the most common pathogen.[116] A few small uncontrolled studies suggested that cholestyramine may have a beneficial effect in treating persistent diarrhea in infants in developing countries and antibiotic-associated diarrhea and colitis, particularly in those patients who suffer multiple relapses after oral vancomycin therapy.[117, 118] Potential adverse effects include development of hyperchloremic acidosis in young children and in persons with renal insufficiency and interference with absorption of other drugs.

Octreotide is a somatostatin analog that has been approved for use in treating diarrhea that results from certain hormone-secreting tumors. Several case reports provide anecdotal evidence of a dramatic antidiarrheal effect when it is used in patients with acquired immunodeficiency syndrome who have severe secretory diarrhea associated with *Cryptosporidium*.[119, 120]

References

1. Santosham M, Daum RS, Dillman L, et al: Oral rehydration therapy of infantile diarrhea: A controlled study of well-nourished children hospitalized in the United States and Panama. N Engl J Med 306:1070, 1982.
2. Tamer AM, Friedman LB, Maxwell SRW, et al: Oral rehydration of infants in a large urban U.S. medical center. J Pediatr 107:14, 1985.
3. Schedl HP, Clifton JA: Solute and water absorption by human small intestine. Nature 199:1264, 1963.
4. Nalin DR, Cash RA: Oral or nasogastric maintenance therapy for diarrhoea of unknown aetiology resembling cholera. Trans R Soc Trop Med Hyg 64:769, 1970.
5. Santosham M, Burns BA, Reid R, et al: Glycine-based oral rehydration solution: Reassessment of safety and efficacy. J Pediatr 109:795, 1986.
6. Patra FC, Sack DA, Islam A, et al: Oral rehydration formula containing alanine and glucose for treatment of diarrhoea: A controlled trial. BMJ 298:1353, 1989.
7. World Health Organization: The Treatment and Prevention of Acute Diarrhoea: Practical Guidelines, ed 2. Geneva, World Health Organization, 1989, p 39.
8. Ahmed SM, Islam MR, Butler T, et al: Effective treatment of diarrhoeal dehydration with an oral rehydration solution containing citrate. Scand J Infect Dis 18:65, 1986.
9. Sack DA, Islam S, Brown KH, et al: Oral therapy in children with cholera: A comparison of sucrose and glucose electrolyte solutions. J Pediatr 96:20, 1980.
10. Nalin DR, Levine MM, Mata L, et al: Oral rehydration and maintenance of children with rotavirus and bacterial diarrhoeas. Bull World Health Organ 57:453, 1979.
11. Cutting WAM, Belton NR, Gray JA, et al: Safety and efficacy of three oral rehydration solutions for children with diarrhoea (Edinburgh 1984–85). Acta Pediatr Scand 78:253, 1989.
12. Levine MM, Pizarro D: Advances in therapy of diarrheal dehydration: Oral rehydration. Adv Pediatr 31:207, 1984.
13. Pizarro D, Posada G, Villavicencio N, et al: Oral rehydration in hypernatremic and hyponatremic diarrheal dehydration: Treatment with oral glucose/electrolyte solution. Am J Dis Child 137:730, 1983.
14. Pizarro D, Posada G, Levine MM, et al: Hypernatremic diarrheal dehydration treated with "slow" (12-hour) oral rehydration therapy: A preliminary report. J Pediatr 104:316, 1984.
15. Gore SM, Fontaine O, Pierce NF: Impact of rice-based oral rehydration solution on stool output and duration of diarrhoea: Meta-analysis of 13 clinical trials. BMJ 304:287, 1992.
16. Lebenthal E, Khin-Maung-U, Rolston DDK, et al: Thermophilic amylase-digested rice-electrolyte solution in the treatment of acute diarrhea in children. Pediatrics 95:198, 1995.
17. Molina S, Vettorazzi C, Peerson JM, et al: Clinical trial of glucose–oral rehydration solution (ORS), rice dextrin–ORS, and rice flour–ORS for the management of children with acute diarrhea and mild or moderate dehydration. Pediatrics 95:191, 1995.
18. Nelson JD, Haltalin KC: Comparative efficacy of cephalexin and ampicillin for shigellosis and other types of acute diarrhea in infants and children. Antimicrob Agents Chemother 7:415, 1975.
19. Ostrower VG: Comparison of cefaclor and ampicillin in the treatment of shigellosis. Postgrad Med J 55(Suppl):82, 1979.
20. Salam MA, Bennish ML: Therapy for shigellosis. I. Randomized, double-blind trial of nalidixic acid in childhood shigellosis. J Pediatr 113:901, 1988.
21. Griffin PM, Tauxe RV, Redd SC, et al: Emergence of highly trimethoprim-sulfamethoxazole–resistant *Shigella* in a native American population: An epidemiologic sudy. Am J Epidemiol 129:1042, 1989.
22. Tiemens KM, Shipley PL, Correia RA, et al: Sulfamethoxazole-trimethoprim–resistant *Shigella flexneri* in northeastern Brazil. Antimicrob Agents Chemother 25:653, 1984.
23. Tuttle J, Ries AA, Chimba RM, et al: Antimicrobial-resistant epidemic *Shigella dysenteriae* type 1 in Zambia: Modes of transmission. J Infect Dis 171:371, 1995.
24. Bennish ML, Salam MA, Hossain MA, et al: Antimicrobial resistance of *Shigella* isolates in Bangladesh, 1983–1990: Increasing frequency of strains multiply resistant to ampicillin, trimethoprim-sulfamethoxazole, and nalidixic acid. Clin Infect Dis 14:1055, 1992.
25. Lionel NDW, Abeyasekera FJB, Samarasinghe HG, et al: A comparison of a single dose and a five day course of tetracycline therapy in bacillary dysentery. J Trop Med Hyg 72:170, 1969.
26. Pickering LK, DuPont HL, Olarte J, et al: Single-dose tetracycline therapy for shigellosis in adults. JAMA 239:853, 1978.
27. Gilman RH, Spira W, Rabbani H, et al: Single-dose ampicillin therapy for severe shigellosis in Bangladesh. J Infect Dis 143:164, 1981.
28. Nelson JD, Haltalin KC: Amoxicillin less effective than ampicillin against *Shigella* in vitro and in vivo: Relationship of efficacy to activity in serum. J Infect Dis 129(Suppl):S222, 1974.

29. Lolekha S, Vibulbandhitkit S, Poonyarit P: Response to antimicrobial therapy for shigellosis in Thailand. Rev Infect Dis 13(Suppl 4):S342, 1991.
30. Bennish ML, Salam MA, Haider R, et al: Therapy for shigellosis: II. Randomized, double-blind comparison of ciprofloxacin and ampicillin. J Infect Dis 162:711, 1990.
31. Gotuzzo E, Oberhelman RA, Maguina C, et al: Comparison of single-dose treatment with norfloxacin and standard 5-day treatment with trimethoprim-sulfamethoxazole for acute shigellosis in adults. Antimicrob Agents Chemother 33:1101, 1989.
32. Bhattacharya SK, Bhattacharya MK, Dutta P, et al: Randomized clinical trial of norfloxacin for shigellosis. Am J Trop Med Hyg 45:683, 1991.
33. Bennish ML, Salam MA, Khan WA, Khan AM: Treatment of shigellosis: III. Comparison of one- or two-dose ciprofloxacin with standard 5-day therapy. A randomized, blinded trial. Ann Intern Med 117:727, 1992.
34. Schluter G: Ciprofloxacin: Review of potential toxicologic effects. Am J Med 82(Suppl 4A):91, 1987.
35. Alfaham M, Holt ME, Goodchild MC: Arthropathy in a patient with cystic fibrosis taking ciprofloxacin. Br Med J 295:699, 1987.
36. Fontaine O: Antibiotics in the management of shigellosis in children: What role for the quinolones? Rev Infect Dis 11(Suppl 5):S1145, 1989.
37. Shaad UB, Salam MA, Aujard Y, et al: Use of fluoroquinolones in pediatrics: Consensus report of an International Society of Chemotherapy commission. Pediatr Infect Dis J 14:1, 1995.
38. Eidlitz-Marcus T, Cohen YH, Nussinovitch M, et al: Comparative efficacy of two- and five-day courses of ceftriaxone for treatment of severe shigellosis in children. J Pediatr 123:822, 1993.
39. MacDonald WB, Friday F, McEacharn M, et al: The effect of chloramphenicol in *Salmonella* enteritis of infancy. Arch Dis Child 29:238, 1954.
40. Joint Project by Members of the Association for the Study of Infectious Disease: Effect of neomycin in noninvasive *Salmonella* infections of the gastrointestinal tract. Lancet 2:1159, 1970.
41. Kazemi M, Gumpert TG, Marks MI, et al: A controlled trial comparing sulfamethoxazole-trimethoprim, ampicillin, and no therapy in the treatment of *Salmonella* gastroenteritis in children. J Pediatr 83:646, 1973.
42. de Olarte DG, Trujillo H, Agudelo N, et al: Treatment of diarrhea in malnourished infants and children: A double-blind study comparing ampicillin and placebo. Am J Dis Child 127:379, 1974.
43. Nelson JD, Kusmiesz H, Jackson LH, et al: Treatment of *Salmonella* gastroenteritis with ampicillin, amoxicillin, or placebo. Pediatrics 65:1125, 1980.
44. Sanchez C, Garcia-Restoy E, Garau J, et al: Ciprofloxacin and trimethoprim-sulfamethoxazole versus placebo in acute uncomplicated *Salmonella* enteritis: A double-blind trial. J Infect Dis 168:1304, 1993.
45. Torrey S, Fleisher G, Jaffe, D: Incidence of *Salmonella* bacteremia in infants with *Salmonella* gastroenteritis. J Pediatr 108:718, 1986.
46. Committee on Infectious Diseases, American Academy of Pediatrics: 1994 Red Book: Report of the Committee on Infectious Diseases, ed 23. Elk Grove Village, IL, American Academy of Pediatrics, 1994, p 414.
47. Wessalowski R, Thomas L, Kivit J, et al: Multiple brain abscesses caused by *Salmonella enteritidis* in a neonate: Successful treatment with ciprofloxacin. Pediatr Infect Dis J 12:683, 1993.
48. Gendrel D, Raymond J, Legall MA, et al: Use of pefloxacin after failure of initial antibiotic treatment in children with severe salmonellosis. Eur J Clin Microbiol Infect Dis 12:209, 1993.
49. Anders BJ, Lauer BA, Paisley JW, et al: Double-blind placebo-controlled trial of erythromycin for treatment of *Campylobacter* enteritis. Lancet 1:131, 1982.
50. Pitkanen T, Petterson T, Ponka A: Effect of erythromycin on the fecal excretion of *Campylobacter fetus* subspecies *jejuni.* J Infect Dis 145:128, 1982.
51. Pai CH, Gillis F, Tuomanen E, et al: Erythromycin in treatment of *Campylobacter* enteritis in children. Am J Dis Child 137:286, 1983.
52. Salazar-Lindo E, Sack RB, Chea-Woo E, et al: Early treatment with erythromycin of *Campylobacter jejuni*–associated dysentery in children. J Pediatr 109:355, 1986.
53. Taylor DN, Blaser MJ, Echeverria P, et al: Erythromycin-resistant *Campylobacter* infections in Thailand. Antimicrob Agents Chemother 31:438, 1987.
54. Pichler HET, Diridl G, Stickler K, et al: Clinical efficacy of ciprofloxacin compared with placebo in bacterial diarrhea. Am J Med 82(Suppl 4A):329, 1987.
55. Wistrom J, Jertborn M, Ekwall E, et al: Empiric treatment of acute diarrheal disease with norfloxacin: A randomized, placebo-controlled study. Ann Intern Med 117:202, 1992.
56. Mattila L, Peltola H, Siitonen A, et al: Short-term treatment of traveler's diarrhea with norfloxacin: A double-blind, placebo-controlled study during two seasons. Clin Infect Dis 17:779, 1993.
57. Endtz HP, Ruijs GJ, van Khageren B, et al: Quinolone resistance in campylobacter isolated from man and poultry following the introduction of fluoroquinolones in veterinary medicine. J Antimicrob Chemother 27:199, 1991.
58. Kuschner RA, Trofa AF, Thomas RJ, et al: Use of azithromycin for the treatment of *Campylobacter* enteritis in travelers to Thailand, an area where ciprofloxacin resistance is prevalent. Clin Infect Dis 21:536, 1995.
59. Gordillo ME, Singh KV, Murray BE: In vitro activity of azithromycin against bacterial enteric pathogens. Antimicrob Agents Chemother 37:1203, 1993.
60. Merson M, Sack RB, Islam S, et al: Disease due to enterotoxigenic *Escherichia coli* in Bangladeshi adults: Clinical aspects and a controlled trial of tetracycline. J Infect Dis 141:702, 1980.
61. Black RE, Levine MM, Clements ML, et al: Treatment of experimentally induced enterotoxigenic *Escherichia coli* diarrhea with trimethoprim, trimethoprim-sulfamethoxazole, or placebo. Rev Infect Dis 4:540, 1982.
62. DuPont HL, Reves RR, Galindo E, et al: Treatment of traveler's diarrhea with trimethoprim-sulfamethoxazole and with trimethoprim alone. N Engl J Med 307:841, 1982.
63. Oberhelman RA, de la Cabada J, Garibay EV, et al: Efficacy of trimethoprim-sulfamethoxazole in treatment of acute diarrhea in a Mexican pediatric population. J Pediatr 110:960, 1987.
64. Echeverria P, Verhaert L, Ulyangco CV, et al: Antimicrobial resistance and enterotoxin production among isolates of *Escherichia coli* in the Far East. Lancet 2:589, 1978.
65. Sack RB, Santosham M, Froehlich JL, et al: Doxycycline prophylaxis of traveler's diarrhea in Honduras, an area where resistance to doxycycline is common among enterotoxigenic *Escherichia coli.* Am J Trop Med Hyg 33:460, 1984.
66. Goossens H, Mol PD, Coignau J, et al: Comparative in vitro activities of aztreonam, ciprofloxacin, norfloxacin, ofloxacin, HR 810 (a new cephalosporin), RU28965 (a new macrolide), and other agents against enteropathogens. Antimicrob Agents Chemother 27:388, 1985.
67. Ericsson CD, Johnson PC, DuPont HL, et al: Ciprofloxacin or trimethoprim-sulfamethoxazole as initial therapy for travelers' diarrhea. Ann Intern Med 106:216, 1987.
68. DuPont HL, Ericsson CD, Mathewson JJ, et al: Five versus three days of ofloxacin therapy for traveler's diarrhea: A placebo-controlled study. Antimicrob Agents Chemother 36:87, 1992.
69. Nelson JD: Duration of neomycin therapy for enteropathogenic *Escherichia coli* diarrheal disease: A comparative study of 113 cases. Pediatrics 48:248, 1971.
70. Thoren A, Wolde-Mariam T, Stintzing G, et al: Antibiotics in the treatment of gastroenteritis caused by enteropathogenic *Escherichia coli.* J Infect Dis 141:27, 1980.
71. Haltalin KC, Kusmiesz HT, Hinton LV, et al: Treatment of acute diarrhea in outpatients: Double-blind study comparing ampicillin and placebo. Am J Dis Child 124:554, 1972.
72. Proulx R, Turgeon JP, Delage G, et al: Randomized, controlled trial of antibiotic therapy for *Escherichia coli* O157:H7 enteritis. J Pediatr 121:299, 1992.
73. Ostroff SM, Kobayashi JM, Lewis JH: Infections with *Escherichia coli* O157:H7 in Washington State: The first year of statewide disease surveillance. JAMA 262:355, 1989.
74. Martin DL, MacDonald KL, White KE, et al: The epidemiology and clinical aspects of the hemolytic uremic syndrome in Minnesota. N Engl J Med 323:1161, 1990.
75. Hoogkampe-Korstanje JA: Antibiotics in *Yersinia enterocolitica* infections. J Antimicrob Chemother 20:123, 1987.
76. Pai CH, Gillis F, Tuomanen E, et al: Placebo-controlled double-

blind evaluation of trimethoprim-sulfamethoxazole treatment of *Yersinia enterocolitica* gastroenteritis. J Pediatr 104:308, 1984.
77. Lindenbaum J, Greenough WB, Islam MR: Antibiotic therapy of cholera in children. Bull World Health Organ 37:529, 1967.
78. Wallace CK, Anderson PN, Brown TC, et al: Optimal antibiotic therapy in cholera. Bull World Health Organ 39:239, 1968.
79. Rahaman MM, Majid MA, Alam AKMJ, et al: Effects of doxycycline in actively purging cholera patients: A double-blind clinical trial. Antimicrob Agents Chemother 10:610, 1976.
80. Pierce NF, Banwell JG, Mitra RC, et al: Controlled comparison of tetracycline and furazolidone in cholera. Br Med J 3:277, 1968.
81. Bhattacharya SK, Bhattacharya MK, Dutta P, et al: Double-blind, randomized, controlled clinical trial of norfloxacin for cholera. Antimicrob Agents Chemother 34:939, 1990.
82. World Health Organization: Cholera surveillance. Multiply antibiotic-resistant O-group 1 *Vibrio cholerae*. Week Epidemiol Rec 38:292, 1980.
83. Maimone F, Coppo A, Pazzani C, et al: Clonal spread of multiply resistant strains of *Vibrio cholerae* O1 in Somalia. J Infect Dis 153:802, 1986.
84. Khan WA, Dhar U, Begum M, et al: Antimicrobial treatment of cholera in adults due to *Vibrio cholerae* O139 (Bengal) infection. Presented at the Fifth International Symposium on New Quinolones; 1994; Singapore. Abstract 96.
85. Swerdlow DL, Ries AA: *Vibrio cholerae* non-O1—The eighth pandemic? Lancet 342:382, 1993.
86. Gerding DN: Epidemiology and management of *Clostridium difficile* infection. Contemp Intern Med 2:55, 1990.
87. Bartlett JG: Treatment of antibiotic-associated pseudomembranous colitis. Rev Infect Dis 6(Suppl 1):S235, 1984.
88. Teasley DG, Gerding DN, Olson MM, et al: Prospective randomised trial of metronidazole versus vancomycin for *Clostridium difficile*–associated diarrhoea and colitis. Lancet 2:1043, 1983.
89. Young GP, Ward PB, Bayley N, et al: Antibiotic-associated colitis due to *Clostridium difficile*: Double-blind comparison of vancomycin with bacitracin. Gastroenterology 89:1038, 1985.
90. Oliva SL, Guglielmo BJ, Jacobs R, et al: Failure of intravenous vancomycin and intravenous metronidazole to prevent or treat antibiotic-associated pseudomembranous colitis. J Infect Dis 159:1154, 1989.
91. Bolton RP, Culshaw MA: Faecal metronidazole concentrations during oral and intravenous therapy for antibiotic-associated colitis due to *Clostridium difficile*. Gut 27:1169, 1986.
92. Paisley JW, Mirretts S, Laver BA, et al: Darkfield microscopy of human feces for presumptive diagnosis of *Campylobacter fetus* subsp. *jejuni* enteritis. J Clin Microbiol 15:61, 1982.
93. Portnoy BL, DuPont HL, Pruitt D, et al: Antidiarrheal agents in the treatment of acute diarrhea in children. JAMA 236:844, 1976.
94. Pozo-Olano JD, Warram JHJ, Gomez RG, et al: Effect of lactobacilli preparation on traveler's diarrhea: A randomized double-blind clinical trial. Gastroenterology 74:829, 1978.
95. Zoppi G, Balsamo V, Deganello A, et al: Oral bacteriotherapy in clinical practice. II. The use of different preparations in the treatment of acute diarrhoea. Eur J Pediatr 139:22, 1982.
96. Isolauri E, Juntunen M, Rautanen T, et al: *Lactobacillus* strain (*Lactobacillus casei* sp. strain GG) promotes recovery from acute diarrhea in children. Pediatrics 88:90, 1991.
97. Raza S, Graham SM, Allen SJ, et al: *Lactobacillus* GG promotes recovery from acute nonbloody diarrhea in Pakistan. Pediatr Infect Dis J 14:107, 1995.
98. Tvede M, Rask-Madsen J: Bacteriotherapy for chronic relapsing *Clostridium difficile* diarrhoea in six patients. Lancet 1:1156, 1989.
99. Holmgren J, Lange S, Lonnroth I: Reversal of cyclic AMP–mediated intestinal secretion in mice by chlorpromazine. Gastroenterology 75:1103, 1978.
100. Rabbani GH, Greenough WB, Holmgren J, et al: Chlorpromazine reduces fluid loss in cholera. Lancet 1:410, 1979.
101. Formal SB, Abrams GD, Schneider H, et al: Experimental *Shigella* infections: VI. Role of the small intestine in an experimental infection in guinea pigs. J Bacteriol 85:119, 1963.
102. DuPont HL, Hornick RB: Adverse effect of Lomotil therapy in shigellosis. JAMA 226:1525, 1973.
103. Murphy GS, Bodhidatta L, Echeverria P, et al: Ciprofloxacin and loperamide in the treatment of bacillary dysentery. Ann Intern Med 118:582, 1993.
104. Van Loon FPL, Bennish ML, Speelman P, et al: Double-blind trial of loperamide for treating acute watery diarrhoea in expatriates in Bangladesh. Gut 30:492, 1989.
105. Ericsson CD, DuPont HL, Mathewson JJ, et al: Treatment of traveler's diarrhea with sulfamethoxazole and trimethoprim and loperamide. JAMA 263:257, 1990.
106. Graham DY, Estes MK, Gentry LO: Double-blind comparison of bismuth subsalicylate and placebo in the prevention and treatment of enterotoxigenic *Escherichia coli*–induced diarrhea in volunteers. Gastroenterology 85:1017, 1983.
107. Steffen R, Mathewson JJ, Ericsson CD, et al: Travelers' diarrhea in West Africa and Mexico: Fecal transport systems and liquid bismuth subsalicylate for self-therapy. J Infect Dis 157:1008, 1988.
108. DuPont HL, Sullivan P, Pickering LD, et al: Symptomatic treatment of diarrhea with bismuth subsalicylate among students attending a Mexican university. Gastroenterology 73:715, 1977.
109. DuPont HL, Ericsson CD, Johnson PC, et al: Prevention of travelers' diarrhea by the tablet formulation of bismuth subsalicylate. JAMA 257:1347, 1987.
110. Burke V, Gracey M, Suharyono N, et al: Reduction by aspirin of intestinal fluid loss in acute childhood gastroenteritis. Lancet 1:1329, 1980.
111. Gracey M, Phadke MA, Burke V, et al: Aspirin in acute gastroenteritis: A clinical and microbiological study. J Pediatr Gastroenterol Nutr 3:692, 1984.
112. Mohan M, Daral TS, Singh HP, et al: Aspirin in childhood gastroenteritis. J Diarrhoeal Dis Res 3:215, 1985.
113. Wald A, Gotterer GS, Rajendra GR, et al: Effect of indomethacin on cholera-induced fluid movement, unidirectional sodium fluxes, and intestinal cAMP. Gastroenterology 72:106, 1977.
114. Neumann SZ: Childhood diarrhoea and its treatment with indomethacin in Libya. Trop Doct 10:24, 1980.
115. Rabbani GH, Butler T: Indomethacin and chloroquine fail to inhibit fluid loss in cholera. Gastroenterology 89:1035, 1985.
116. Isolauri E, Vesikari T: Oral rehydration, rapid feeding, and cholestyramine for treatment of acute diarrhea. J Pediatr Gastroenterol Nutr 4:366, 1985.
117. Kreutzer EW, Milligan FD: Treatment of antibiotic-associated pseudomembranous colitis with cholestyramine resin. Johns Hopkins Med J 143:67, 1978.
118. Pruksananonda P, Powell KR: Multiple relapses of *Clostridium difficile*–associated diarrhea responding to an extended course of cholestyramine. Pediatr Infect Dis J 8:175, 1989.
119. Cook DJ, Kelton JG, Stanisz AM, et al: Somatostatin treatment for cryptosporidial diarrhea in a patient with the acquired immunodeficiency syndrome (AIDS). Ann Intern Med 108:708, 1988.
120. Katz MD, Erstad BL, Rose C: Treatment of severe *Cryptosporidium*-related diarrhea with octreotide in a patient with AIDS. Drug Intell Clin Pharm 22:134, 1988.

84

Whipple's Disease

Patrick I. Okolo, III
Theodore M. Bayless

Whipple's disease is a rare systemic disorder caused by an actinobacterium known as *Tropheryma whippelii*.[1] The periodic acid–Schiff (PAS)–positive microorganism and the characteristic macrophage response can be identified in almost all organ systems. Small intestinal involvement is characteristic. Several studies have implicated an impaired cellular immune response in patients with Whipple's disease.[2-5] This host susceptibility may be inherited because Whipple's disease almost exclusively affects white males in Europe and North America.[6]

In the early phase of the disease, the clinical features are multisystemic, with relapsing arthralgias, polyserositis, and lymphadenopathy. Diarrhea with or without malabsorption, weight loss, hyperpigmentation, endocarditis, and central nervous system (CNS) abnormalities are prominent findings in the later stages of the disease.

Before the use of antibiotics to treat this disease, its course was unrelenting and ultimately fatal. Intestinal biopsy provided a method of diagnosis, and treatment with antibiotics has greatly improved outcome. The response to antibiotics is usually rapid and sometimes complete. Relapses can be seen with inadequate therapy and less commonly with adequate therapy. Cardiac and CNS involvement may become predominant in the setting of relapse and can make treatment difficult.

History

Initial Description

In 1907, George Hoyt Whipple, who later became the 1934 Nobel laureate in physiology, provided a thorough account of a 36-year-old physician's chronic illness.[7] Diarrhea, weight loss, arthritis, and cough were prominent features. Whipple gave an extremely detailed and accurate description of the histologic findings in the small bowel and mesenteric lymph nodes. He described large frothy cells crowding the lamina propria with a tendency to alteration of the villous architecture. Whipple named the illness "intestinal lipodystrophy" despite the fact that he clearly recognized bacteria in one lymph node. The gland had been stained with a silver stain and demonstrated great numbers of "peculiar rod shaped organisms," measuring 2 μm or less. As with many diseases, earlier reports of what seem to be the same disease are later discovered. Dobbins,[6] in his extensive review of the literature, credited Allchin and Hebb with first reporting a patient with this disorder in 1895. In 1961, Yardley and Fleming[8] at Johns Hopkins Hospital obtained preserved tissue from Whipple's original 1907 case and showed the presence of many PAS-positive macrophages in the intestinal lymph nodes. This provided the confirmation that the original patient did indeed have Whipple's disease. Because of Whipple's accurate description and his recognition of a possible role of bacteria in the pathogenesis of the disorder, it seems reasonable and still proper to call it Whipple's disease.

Multisystem Involvement and Distinguishing Macrophage Stains

Before the use of antibiotics, the disease was almost invariably fatal and the diagnosis was made at autopsy. The first antemortem diagnosis was made in 1947 on the basis of examination of a lymph node removed at laparotomy.[9] By 1948, it was established that the characteristic macrophages in Whipple's disease contained glycoprotein mucopolysaccharide, because they stained with PAS.[10] The systemic nature of the illness was proved by the demonstration of typical macrophages in peripheral lymph nodes, adrenal glands, liver, heart valves, CNS, and many other nonintestinal tissues.[11] In 1950, it was shown that the malabsorption was secondary to injury of intestinal epithelial cells as a result of lymphatic obstruction.[12] In 1961, Yardley and Hendrix[13] demonstrated bacterial invasion of intestinal epithelial cells.

ANTIBIOTIC RESPONSE

In 1952, Pauley[14] reported "the apparent success of chloramphenicol in promoting a remission" in a patient with well-documented Whipple's disease. The patient's physician, Dr. G. Andr, had decided to try the antibiotic. This opened up the possibility of antibiotic treatment of Whipple's disease.

BACTERIAL ORIGIN CONFIRMED

Yardley and Hendrix[13] at Johns Hopkins Hospital and Chears and Ashworth[15] in Texas almost simultaneously reported in 1961 that a bacterial organism was demonstrable by electron microscopy in infected tissues. The organism measured 1.0 μm in length and 0.2 μm in width. The bacterium could be visualized at light microscopy with Giemsa stains. Both groups suggested that the intracellular material in the macrophages was derived from the bacteria, and they thought that the disease was most certainly an unusual infection. During the same period, a number of groups were reporting dramatic responses of patients with Whipple's disease after treatment with various antibiotics, and thus a previously undiagnosable, invariably fatal illness became a readily diagnosable and curable disease.

SINGLE ORGANISM INVOLVED

Keren and colleagues[16] at Johns Hopkins Hospital used an indirect immunofluorescence technique in 1976 to demonstrate a uniform pattern of immunofluorescent staining of various bacterial antigens within foamy macrophages from three patients with Whipple's disease. Utilizing molecular techniques, Relman and colleagues[1] in 1992 were able to identify the previously unidentified causative organism of Whipple's disease and named it *T. whippelii*.

Epidemiology

Demography

Dobbins[6] provided an excellent analysis of demographic data in a study of 664 patients, including 574 males and 90 females. In male patients, the median age at diagnosis was 49.1 years; that for female patients was 51 years. The age at diagnosis was maximal in the fifth decade for men but in the seventh decade for women. Only 9 of the 664 patients were younger than 31 years at diagnosis. The racial distribution of the disease was almost exclusively white. Only 10 of the patients were black, of whom 8 were male and 2 were female. Of the patients analyzed by Dobbins, only 15 were nonwhite.

Occupations

There have been suggestions that this illness occurs more commonly in rural situations. Dobbins[6] was able to confirm this in his review of the occupations of 191 patients. Farmers accounted for 23% of the total. The frequency in farm workers is three times that expected from the total number of farmers in the United States work force. Combining those who work in farming and construction and those who work as machinists and who might therefore be expected to have major contact with soil or animals, one can account for two thirds of the total known occupations of affected persons.

Clustering

There are three reports of siblings with the illness, including one family with possible multigenerational involvement.[17] There have been some reports of clustering, including three patients from a French village and four patients from an Italian village.[18] In a U.S. report, 7 of 19 patients from the state of North Carolina lived within a 20-mile radius of Fayetteville.[19]

Causes of Death

In the review by Dobbins,[6] 179 of the 664 analyzed patients died of Whipple's disease itself. Sixty-eight of these patients lived in the postantibiotic era. The major cause of death was disease too advanced to be treated effectively. In some patients, a delay in diagnosis allowed the disease to enter the terminal stage. In others, irreversible disease occurred as a result of CNS or cardiovascular relapses caused by inadequate treatment. The importance of keeping a reasonable index of suspicion for this disease cannot be overemphasized. In the Dobbins review, 16 deaths occurred as recently as between 1980 and 1986.

Immunology and Pathology

Patients with Whipple's disease clearly manifest an inadequate immune response to the causative organism. They are unable to clear the organism from intracellular residues. Several small studies have suggested a defect of cellular immunity. Demonstrable abnormalities include decreased lymphocyte mitogenicity to concavalin A and phytohemagglutinin.[3] Skin testing for recall antigens is also abnormal.[4, 20] In one study, the serum of patients with Whipple's disease manifested inhibitory properties during active disease.[5] Proliferation assays clearly showed higher proliferation rates of peripheral blood mononuclear cells among all groups of patients when cells were mixed with control serum; more important, there was decreased proliferation of control mononuclear cells when they were mixed with patients' serum.[5] In the same study, patients with the disease manifested a persistent reduction in peripheral blood mononuclear cell CD11b expression (complement receptor 3α-chain). Abnormalities of CD11b have been implicated previously in congenital leukocyte adhesion deficiency.[21]

Complement receptor 3α activity has been implicated in macrophage accumulation and cellular adhesion.[22, 23] Thus, defective CD11b expression in patients with Whipple's disease may be one of the major contributory factors in the inadequate immune response to the causative organism and may play a role in determining susceptibility to the disease.

There are also demonstrable abnormalities of mucosal immunity in Whipple's disease. Ectors and colleagues[24] found decreased phagocytic potential, decreased CD4/CD8 ratio, and increased numbers of intraepithelial lymphocytes in a study of small bowel mucosa from 16 Belgian patients with Whipple's disease.

The immune deficiency may be genetically determined. In the review by Dobbins,[6] 14 of 53 patients (26%) were positive for human leukocyte antigen (HLA) B27. The expression of HLA-B27 in ethnic groups prone to develop Whipple's disease ranges from 0.3% to 6.9%, so the 26% HLA-B27 positivity suggests that this antigen is increased in patients with Whipple's disease. It has been hypothesized that this genetic association may play a role in determining the presence of cellular immune deficiency.

In terms of immunopathology, a granulomatous inflammatory reaction may occur in Whipple's disease. The polyvisceral granulomata resemble those in sarcoidosis. Nine percent of the cases reviewed by Dobbins[6] contained evidence of granulomatous changes, especially in the liver, mesentery, and peripheral lymph nodes as well as intestine, brain, and lung. Other sites of granulomata reported in the literature include synovium and kidneys.[25, 26] PAS staining of lymph nodes containing granulomata has sometimes led to a conclusive diagnosis of Whipple's disease in patients with an otherwise elusive diagnosis.

Etiology, Pathogenesis, and Diagnosis

Even though it was clear for many years that the etiologic agent in Whipple's disease was a single, gram-positive organism found just below the basal epithelial layer, identification of this organism was not possible because of difficulties in culturing it. Relman and colleagues[1] were able to identify the previously unculturable organism using molecular techniques on tissue from 5 patients with histopathologically confirmed Whipple's disease and 10 control patients. The 16S bacterial ribosomal RNA was amplified by the polymerase chain reaction (PCR) with a sequential combination of broad and then specific primers as described by Chen and coworkers.[27] The diagnostic PCR concept is based on the highly conserved sequences that are shared by all bacterial organisms on the 16S ribosomal RNA. These sequences are interspersed with variable regions that are distinct for different bacteria. The PCR first uses broad primers that bind to the highly conserved sequence. The nucleotide sequence is then analyzed, and specific primers for the variable regions are used for a second-stage PCR. The nucleotide sequence of the amplicon provides a specific diagnostic PCR product (Fig. 84–1).

With this strategy, Relman and colleagues[1] identified a specific PCR product in a patient with Whipple's disease and then used the specific primers on five other patients who all had positive tests. The control patients did not have a single false-positive result. The phylogenetic position of this bacterium was determined by computer-aided analysis and found to be the actinobacteria. The etiologic agent of Whipple's disease, thus positively identified, was named *T. whippelii.*

The utility of this method in the diagnosis of Whipple's

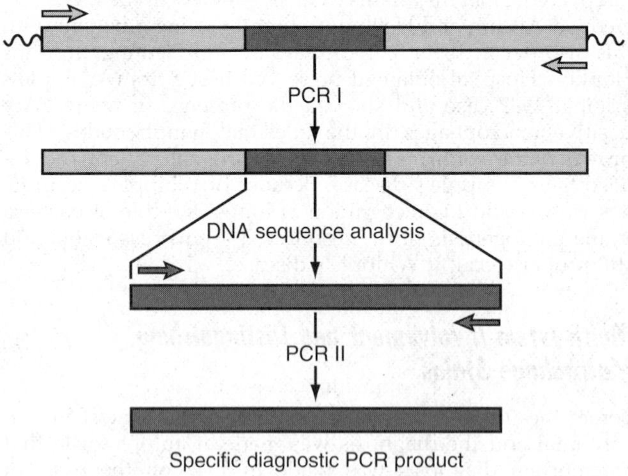

FIGURE 84–1 □ Strategy for the development of a specific PCR assay for Whipple's disease. A segment from the 16S ribosomal RNA gene, encompassing conserved sequences *(light shading)* and variable regions *(dark shading)* is amplified using primers that bind to the conserved sequences (*light shaded arrows,* PCR I). The nucleotide sequence of a variable region is determined and specific primers *(dark shaded arrows)* are designed on the basis of the new sequence information. These primers are used to selectively amplify a Whipple's disease–specific DNA fragment (PCR II). (Adapted from von Weizsacker F, Blum E: Impact of molecular biology in gastroenterology. Digestion 54:125–129, 1993. By permission of S Karger, Basel.)

disease has been examined further. Lowsky and coworkers[28] described two patients for whom the diagnosis was made by molecular analysis of peripheral blood. With whole-blood DNA, PCR yielded an amplicon and subsequent sequence analysis demonstrated 100% homology of an examined variable portion to *T. whippelii*. Rickman and colleagues[29] reported a patient with chronic uveitis and little clinical evidence of Whipple's disease in whom the diagnosis of ocular Whipple's disease was made by PCR of vitreous fluid. The described patient also had molecular evidence of duodenal infection without clinical symptoms.

These reports suggest that PCR may yet be the most sensitive and accurate method of diagnosing Whipple's disease, especially in the context of previously treated disease.

Treatment and Prognosis

Before the observation of the effectiveness of antibiotics in 1952, Whipple's disease was invariably fatal; it continued to be so until the early 1960s. The immediate response to antibiotics is often described as spectacular. Treatment, usually lasting 1 to 2 years, has been given to more than 400 patients. Responses have occurred to a variety of antibiotics, thus depriving us of a specific antibiotic probe to identify the organism. More than 200 patients have received tetracycline, although the next largest group, more than 50 patients, received penicillin, streptomycin, and tetracycline. Other patients have received tetracycline combinations, penicillin, or ampicillin alone. There are 15 documented responses to trimethoprim-sulfamethoxazole (TMP-SMX) combinations, and seven patients responded to TMP-SMX alone, chloramphenicol alone, or erythromycin alone.[6]

The condition of the surface epithelium in the intestine improves within 1 week, whereas free bacteria may exist in the lamina propria for up to 9 weeks during therapy. The PAS-positive macrophages, however, clear at a much lower rate, so that 6 months or even 12 months after beginning therapy, prominent macrophages may still be present. The membranous materials of the macrophages, which presumably represent bacterial cell walls, are eventually replaced by granular material. In his most recent review, Dobbins[6] did not think that the presence of the PAS-positive macrophages is significant, and he advised against intestinal biopsy for routine follow-up of patients who are doing well clinically after institution of therapy. We had previously utilized disappearance of the membranous material within the PAS-positive macrophages as a sign that therapy had been adequate, but we have no data to support this view. Antibiotic treatment should be given for a long period, probably at least 1 year, although there is some evidence that 3 months of therapy may be sufficient for a few patients.

Relapses after presumably inadequate therapy are much more common than had been appreciated originally. In the largest review, by Keinath and colleagues,[30] there were 31 relapses among 88 treated patients. The relapses may be manifested by recurrence of the patient's original symptoms or may be characterized by development of new symptoms, particularly in the CNS. Only 1 of 11 patients who suffered CNS manifestations and relapse of symptoms responded to new courses of antibiotics, whereas 19 of 20 patients with intestinal symptoms responded to reinstitution of therapy.[30] Knox and coworkers[31] had emphasized the phenomenon of CNS relapses after inadequate antibiotic therapy. In the review by Keinath's group,[30] 13 of the 31 patients who suffered a relapse had a CNS relapse. The prominent symptoms were dementia, ataxia, hypothalamic signs, and ophthalmoplegia. It is probably reasonable to assume that all patients with Whipple's disease have a degree of CNS invasion at some point. At the time of Knox and colleagues' report[31] in 1976, they recommended using antibiotics in the initial therapy that could be expected to cross the blood-brain barrier.

Treatment of Whipple's disease with tetracycline or penicillin would not be expected to effectively eradicate the subclinical involvement of the CNS, because these two antibiotics do not adequately penetrate uninflamed meninges.[32] TMP-SMX does penetrate uninflamed meninges, reaches receptors on leukocytes, is effective after oral administration, and can be administered safely for long periods. It may be necessary to add folinic acid at 3 mg/d, especially to a malnourished patient, if long-term TMP-SMX therapy is to be used.

TMP-SMX was compared with oral tetracycline in a nonrandomized, partially retrospective study of 30 patients. In this study,[33] TMP-SMX was clearly superior to oral tetracycline in inducing clinical remission as well as in the treatment of CNS disease. TMP-SMX did not prevent CNS manifestations in all patients, however. One patient of eight treated with TMP-SMX developed aqueductal stenosis with consequent hydrocephalus. The authors concluded that TMP-SMX was a clearly superior regimen to oral tetracycline but suggested that a highly active bactericidal compound with good CNS penetration should be used for the treatment of CNS Whipple's disease. Cooper and colleagues[32] reported the case of a patient who presented with evidence of CNS Whipple's disease 14 months after initiation of therapy with TMP-SMX. He was treated with cefixime, an oral third-generation cephalosporin, resulting in resolution of his symptoms and regression of white matter abnormalities previously noted at magnetic resonance imaging.[32] In another report, treatment with a quinolone, pefloxacin, resulted in successful treatment of a patient who presented with CNS symptoms and no other manifestations of Whipple's disease.[34]

The current recommendations by Dobbins,[6] based on extensive review of the literature, include parenteral penicillin G, 1.2 million units, plus streptomycin at 1.0 g daily for 10 to 14 days, followed by one double-strength tablet of sulfamethoxazole given twice daily for 1 year. If the patient is severely ill, the double-strength tablet could be given three times a day for 2 weeks and then twice daily for 1 year, with administration of folinic acid, 3 mg/d, to prevent folic acid deficiency. Because CNS relapses have not occurred in patients who have been treated with parenteral penicillin and streptomycin, it might be reasonable to use these two agents followed by oral penicillin, such as penicillin VK, 250 mg four times a day for 1 year, if the patient is unable to tolerate sulfonamides.

There is also one report of the use of 20 million units of penicillin intravenously per 24 hours for the initial 30 days of treatment when there was a suspicion of subclinical cerebral involvement of Whipple's disease. Long-term therapy of all patients with Whipple's disease is important. If all symptoms disappear and there is a complete remission, there is probably no need for routine follow-up with intestinal biopsy; however, intestinal biopsy should be done at the time of any symptomatic relapse, regardless of the system involved, to try to demonstrate whether the intestinal phase has been reactivated. If possible, efforts should be made to search for the presence of free bacilli by electron microscopy in any tissues that might be involved—intestine or brain—or by examining cerebrospinal fluid. The presence of free bacilli seen by electron microscopy is currently accepted as a clear establishment of relapse.

When the CNS has not been involved, early repeated treatment of relapses has been effective no matter what antibiotic was chosen; however, only 1 of 11 patients with CNS relapses is known to have responded, and this patient responded to oral TMP-SMX after failing to respond to a variety of other antibiotics, including chloramphenicol. A Jarisch-Herxheimer reaction has been reported on four occasions during initial treatment with oral or intravenous penicillin. A systemic reaction developed within 12 to 24 hours, including temperature elevations, chills, headache, hypertension, and, in two patients, severe abdominal pain and chest pain.[35] Adrenocorticosteroids were given for 1 week to one patient to control a presumed Jarisch-Herxheimer reaction.[36] This reaction is similar to that seen 42 hours after the initial treatment of syphilis with penicillin. Presumably, endotoxin or some other product released from the bacteria causes this reaction. Other possible explanations are depletion of endogenous opioids and activation of the complement system.[36]

Summary

Whipple's disease is a rare infectious disease that seems to occur in a specific population of middle-aged white men who have significant exposure to soil and/or to a rural environment. There is evidence that there are subtle immune defects in these patients; the predominance of HLA-B27 suggests a genetic predisposition.

The etiologic agent is *T. whippelii*, a gram-positive actinomycete that stains positively with PAS. The organism multiplies in the lamina propria of the intestinal mucosa and in other organs without exciting a vigorous immune response. The bacterium is sensitive to a variety of antibiotics; however, eradication and cure require prolonged antibiotic therapy. CNS involvement portends relative resistance to antibiotic therapy.

It is recommended that therapy include the use of antibiotics to which the organism is sensitive as well as antibiotics that cross the blood-brain barrier to help eliminate the subclinical CNS invasion. Current recommendations include penicillin and streptomycin for 2 weeks, followed by 1 year of TMP-SMX therapy.

Relapses, especially in the CNS, can be extremely resistant to therapy; however, there are some reports that fluoroquinolones may help in this setting. Deaths from Whipple's disease continue to occur, largely because of late recognition of the illness or because of CNS and cardiac involvement.

The ability to recognize and treat this disease should continue to improve with the identification of the causative organism and the description of newer molecular techniques of detection in tissues and body fluids.

References

1. Relman DA, Schmidt TM, MacDermott RP, Falkow S: Identification of the uncultured bacillus of Whipple's disease. N Engl J Med 327:293–301, 1992.
2. Martin F, Vilseck J, Dobbins WO, et al: Immunological alterations in patients with treated Whipple's disease. Gastroenterology 63:6–18, 1972.
3. Maxwell JD, Ferguson A, McKay AM, et al: Lymphocytes in Whipple's disease. Lancet 1:887–889, 1968.
4. Groll A, Volberg LS, Simon JB, et al: Immunological defects in Whipple's disease. Gastroenterology 63:943–950, 1972.
5. Marth T, Roux M, von Herbay AV, et al: Persistent reduction of complement receptor 3 alpha-chain expressing mononuclear blood cells and transient inhibitory serum factors in Whipple's disease. Clin Immunol Immunopathol 72:217–226, 1994.
6. Dobbins WO III: Whipple's Disease. Springfield, IL, Charles C Thomas, 1987.
7. Whipple GH: A hitherto undescribed disease characterized anatomically by deposits of fat and fatty acids in the intestinal and mesenteric lymphatic tissue. Bull Johns Hopkins Hosp 18:381–391, 1907.
8. Yardley JH, Fleming WH 2d: Whipple's disease: A note regarding PAS-positive granules in the original case. Bull Johns Hopkins Hosp 109:76–79, 1961.
9. Oliver Pascual E, Galan J, Oliver Pascual A, Castillo E: Un caso de lipodistrofica intestinal con lesions gangliones mesentericas de granulomatosis lipofagica (enfermed de Whipple). Rev Esp Enferm Apar Dig 6:213–226, 1947.
10. Black-Schaffer B: Tinctorial demonstration of glycoprotein in Whipple's disease. Proc Soc Exp Biol Med 72:225–227, 1949.
11. Sieracki JC: Whipple's disease: Observation on systemic involvement. Arch Pathol 66:464–467, 1958.
12. Hendrix JP, Black-Shaffer B, Withers RW, Handler P: Whipple's intestinal lipodystrophy: Report of 4 cases. Arch Intern Med 85:91–131, 1950. [See addendum in Arch Intern Med 85:131, 1950.]
13. Yardley JH, Hendrix TR: Combined electron and light microscopy in Whipple's disease. Bull Johns Hopkins Hosp 109:80–87, 1961.
14. Pauley JW: A case of Whipple's disease (intestinal lipodystrophy). Gastroenterology 22:128–133, 1952.
15. Chears WC Jr, Ashworth CT: Electron microscopic study of the intestinal mucosa in Whipple's disease. Demonstration of encapsulated bacilliform bodies in the lesion. Gastroenterology 41:129–138, 1961.
16. Keren DF, Weisburger WR, Yardley JH, et al: Whipple's disease: Demonstration by immunofluorescence of similar bacterial antigens in macrophages from three cases. Johns Hopkins Med J 139:51–59, 1976.
17. Clancy RL, Tomkins WAF, Muckle TJ, et al: Isolation and characterization of an aetiological agent in Whipple's disease. Br Med J 3:568–570, 1975.
18. Puite RH, Tesluk H: Whipple's disease. Am J Med 19:383–400, 1955.
19. Capron JP, Thevenin A, Delamarre J, et al: Whipple's disease: Study of 3 cases and epidemiological and radiological remarks. Lille Med 20:842–845, 1975.
20. Feurle GE, Dorken B, Schopf E, Lenhard V: HLA B27 and defects in the T-cell system in Whipple's disease. Eur J Clin Invest 9:385–389, 1979.
21. Patarroyo M, Makgoba MW: Leucocyte adhesion to cells. Molecular basis, physiological relevance, and abnormalities. Scand J Immunol 32:129–164, 1989.
22. Tuomanen EI, Saukkonen K, Sande S, et al: Reduction of inflammation, tissue damage, and mortality in bacterial meningitis in rabbits treated with monoclonal antibodies against adhesion-promoting receptors of leukocytes. J Exp Med 170:959–969, 1989.
23. Ding A, Wright SD, Nathan C: Activation of mouse peritoneal macrophages by monoclonal antibody to Mac-1 (complement receptor type 3). J Exp Med 165:733–749, 1987.
24. Ectors N, Geboes K, De Vos R, et al: Whipple's disease: A histological, immunocytochemical and electronmicroscopic study of the immune response in the small intestinal mucosa. Histopathology 21:1–12, 1992.
25. Dhib M, Heron F, Francois A, et al: Kidney granuloma in Whipple's disease. BMJ 307:1067–1068, 1993.
26. Rouillon A, Menkes CJ, Gerster JC, et al: Sarcoid-like forms of Whipple's disease. Report of 2 cases. J Rheumatol 20:1070–1072, 1993.
27. Chen K, Neimark H, Rumore P, Steinman CR: Broad range DNA probes for detecting and amplifying eubacterial nucleic acids. FEMS Microbiol Left 48:19–24, 1989.
28. Lowsky R, Archer GL, Fyles G, et al: Diagnosis of Whipple's disease by molecular analysis of peripheral blood. N Engl J Med 331:1343–1346, 1994.
29. Rickman LS, Freeman W, Green R, et al: Brief report: Uveitis caused by *Tropheryma whippelii* (Whipple's bacillus). N Engl J Med 332:363–366, 1995.
30. Keinath RD, Merrell DE, Vlietstra R, Dobbins WO III: Antibiotic treatment and relapse in Whipple's disease: Long-term follow-up of 88 patients. Gastroenterology 88:1867–1873, 1985.
31. Knox DL, Bayless TM, Pittman FE: Neurologic disease in patients with treated Whipple's disease. Medicine (Baltimore) 55:467–476, 1976.
32. Cooper GS, Blades EW, Remler BF, et al: Central nervous system Whipple's disease: Relapse during therapy with trimethoprim-sulfamethoxazole and remission with cefixime. Gastroenterology 106:782–786, 1994.

33. Feurle GE, Marth T: An evaluation of antimicrobial treatment for Whipple's disease. Tetracycline versus trimethoprim-sulfamethoxazole. Dig Dis Sci 39:1642–1648, 1994.
34. Amarenco P, Roullet E, Hannoun L, Marteau R: Progressive supranuclear palsy as the sole manifestation of systemic Whipple's disease treated with pefloxacine (Letter). J Neurol Neurosurg Psychiatry 54:1121–1122, 1991.
35. Reed JI, Sipe JD, Wohlgethan JR, et al: Response of the acute-phase reactants, C-reactive protein and serum amyloid A protein, to antibiotic treatment of Whipple's disease. Arthritis Rheum 28:352–355, 1985.
36. Vellar ID, Niall JF, Davis NA, Hope R: Whipple's disease: A report of two cases. Med J Aust 1:661–663, 1974.

85

Intraabdominal Infections

Robert E. Condon
Dietmar H. Wittmann

The approach to patients suffering from intraabdominal infections is governed by the limitation of time available to establish proper treatment. An exact diagnosis, although the ultimate goal, may not be made before treatment is initiated. Some authors discuss this entity under the term acute abdomen, meaning the presence of abnormal abdominal signs and symptoms that require an immediate work-up to explain them so that appropriate action can be taken. In this context, early diagnosis and treatment of potentially life-threatening disease result in a better outcome and—*cum granum sale*—any delay correlates exponentially with mortality.

The most valuable information is obtained from the patient's description of the circumstances of the presenting symptoms. The specific time of onset and the duration of complaints are of utmost importance. The diagnosis of intraabdominal infection is purely clinical. There is seldom a role for sophisticated technology or time-consuming laboratory tests and similar nonessential diagnostic procedures.

The accepted classification of intraabdominal infection is a division into primary and secondary peritonitis (Table 85–1). This arcane classification has little clinical utility; clinicians referring to suppurative intraabdominal infection use the term peritonitis without qualification. Some authors discuss tertiary peritonitis as a new entity seen in patients recovering from secondary peritonitis and experiencing an ongoing failure of host defenses without any further true infectious challenge.[1–3]

Definition

Intraabdominal infection and peritonitis are not synonymous, although both terms are used clinically to describe a suppurative intraabdominal process. Peritonitis means inflammation of the peritoneum or of a part of it. The peritoneum is formed by a single layer of mesothelial cells together with underlying loose connective tissue[4] and comprises a total area of approximately 1.8 m^2. It covers all of the intestinal organs and the abdominal wall, the diaphragm, the retroperitoneum, and the pelvis. In older textbooks, the area of the peritoneum is described as approximately equal to the area of the skin, drawing an analogy of the systemic responses in intraabdominal infection with those of burn injuries to the skin.

Intraabdominal infection implies the presence in the peritoneal cavity of an infectious disease process due to an identifiable causative infecting microorganism. The body's response to intraabdominal infection is similar to that described for peritonitis. Peritonitis can be regarded as a general class of which a specific entity is intraabdominal infection.

The leviathan response of the peritoneum to inflammation influences all of the varieties of clinical presentation of intraabdominal infection. Inflammatory edema resulting in thickening of the peritoneum by only 1 mm would require shifting 8 L of fluid into the peritoneum from the extracellular space, leading to hypovolemia and deleterious effects on systemic tissue perfusion. Consequently, intraabdominal infections are not solely a local disease but affect the entire body, resulting in early signs of organ dysfunction that may be detected at the initial work-up.[5]

Host Response

The inflammatory reaction of secondary peritonitis that occurs in intraabdominal infection is triggered by influx into the abdominal cavity of bacteria-laden gastrointestinal contents or chemical irritants. In primary peritonitis, with a low initial bacterial inoculum, this reaction is not as fulminant. Bacteria and their toxins ultimately play a key role in all forms of intraabdominal infection. Immediately after the initial influx of bacteria into the free peritoneal cavity, the bacteria multiply at a rate that depends on their adaptability to the new environment.[6] The damage caused by these events takes the following course.

Histamine and other vasoactive substances are released owing to mast cell degranulation after cell damage to the

TABLE 85–1 ■ Classification of Intraabdominal Infection

PRIMARY PERITONITIS
Spontaneous peritonitis of childhood
Spontaneous peritonitis of adult
Peritonitis in patients with continuous ambulatory peritoneal dialysis
Tuberculosis peritonitis
SECONDARY PERITONITIS
Spontaneous peritonitis (spontaneous acute)
Gastrointestinal tract perforation
Bowel wall necrosis
Pelvic peritonitis
Peritonitis after translocation of bacteria
Postoperative peritonitis
Leak of an anastomosis
Leak of a suture line
Stump insufficiency
Other iatrogenic leaks
Posttraumatic peritonitis
Peritonitis after blunt abdominal trauma
Peritonitis after penetrating abdominal trauma
TERTIARY PERITONITIS
Peritonitis without pathogens
Peritonitis with fungi
Peritonitis with low-grade pathogenic bacteria
INTRAABDOMINAL ABSCESS
Intraabdominal abscess with secondary peritonitis
Intraabdominal abscess with tertiary peritonitis

peritoneum (Fig. 85–1). The complement system is activated, and chemotaxis is induced. Vasoactive substances increase the permeability of vessels. In combination with chemotaxis, this promotes an influx of polymorphonuclear granulocytes. Both in-migrating and local macrophages phagocytose bacteria as well as detritus and foreign bodies. This process is supported by the activated complement system, which promotes opsonization. Finally, phagocytosed bacteria are destroyed and the dead bacteria and phagocytic cells are carried away, primarily through the lymphatic stomata and channels in the diaphragm.

Owing to increased vascular permeability, plasma exudes into the free peritoneal cavity, leading to fibrin formation. Necrotic, bacteria-containing detritus is delimited, leading to abscess formation (Fig. 85–2). In the developing abscess, bacteria continue to divide, producing toxins and enzymes that together with the proteolytic enzymes of macrophages liquefy the abscess content, creating high osmotic pressure. Because oxygen and nutrients cannot easily cross the abscess membrane, anaerobic glycolysis is promoted within the abscess, which finally results in an anaerobic environment of high pressure in which growth of obligate anaerobic bacteria is promoted. Rupture of such an abscess into the peritoneal cavity may reinitiate the process of diffuse bacterial peritonitis, but with a different primary causative microorganism.

Absorption of exudate and pus through diaphragmatic lymphatic channels represents an important defense mechanism of the peritoneal cavity. This defense reaction is enhanced by respiratory motion in connection with the diaphragmatic lymphatic "valves." Eight tenths of the exudate and toxins generated in most intraabdominal infections is eventually absorbed through the diaphragmatic-thoracic lymphatic channels into the central venous circulation. Intraabdominal infection thus affects the entire organism at an early stage. Rapid intraabdominal clearance of considerable amounts of bacteria and noxious material can lead to damage in all organ systems.[7–11] In effect, a local-regional infection

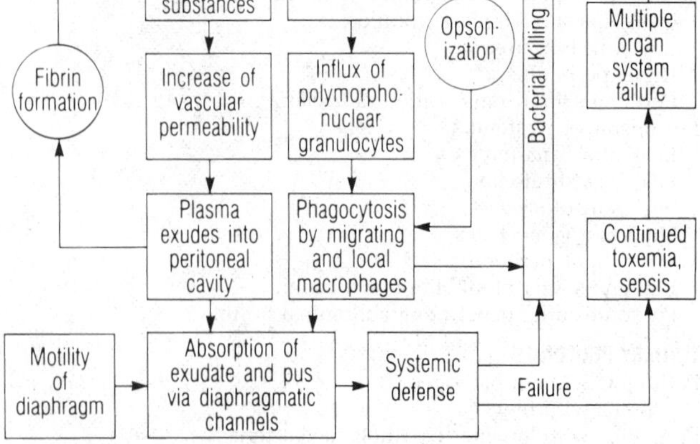

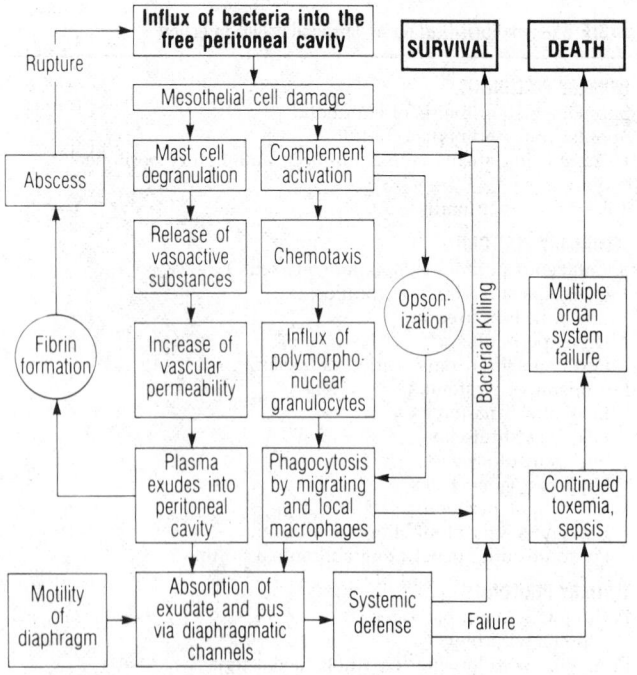

FIGURE 85–1 ▫ The evolution of intraabdominal infection. Bacterial contamination of the peritoneal cavity initiates a sequence of local and systemic responses that culminate in the survival or death of the patient.

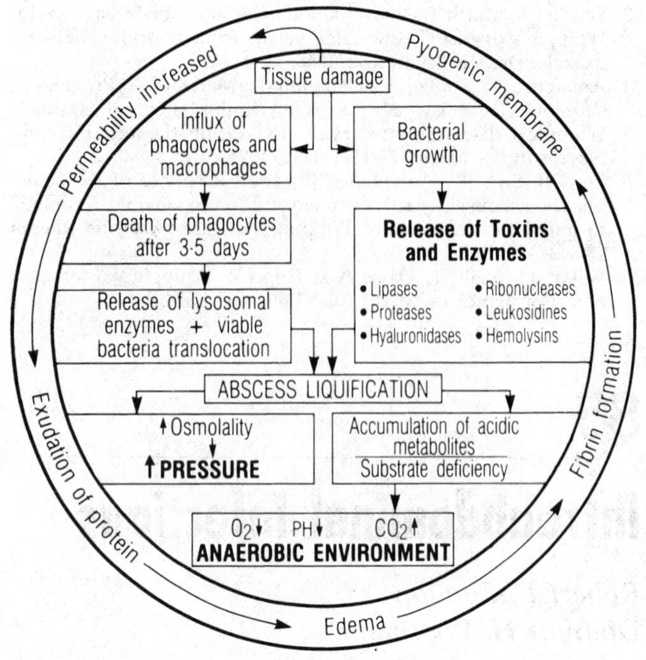

FIGURE 85–2 ▫ Pathophysiologic processes during formation of an abscess.

turns into a severe systemic infection mediated by cytokines, autacoids, eicosanoids, nitric oxide, and other inflammatory mediators.[12]

The inflammatory reaction of the peritoneum produces significant sequestration of fluid in the peritoneal cavity. The inflammatory edema expanding the peritoneum may result in a relatively acute fluid loss of 5 to 8 L from the circulation. This leads initially to hypovolemic shock, followed by dehydration and, finally, death in connection with toxin-induced shock. The signs and symptoms of sepsis are mainly due to the products of bacterial breakdown. Hypoxia forms the turnstile of all the involved pathophysiologic mechanisms (Fig. 85–3). Hypoxia results from the inability of cells to use oxygen for energy-generating processes.

A hyperdynamic cardiovascular response occurs that attempts to compensate for what is perceived by the body as a cellular oxygen deficit. Clinically, high cardiac output and low systemic vascular resistance are seen, coupled with deficient cellular oxygen use so that highly oxygenated blood returns to the venous system. Compounding factors may be toxic respiratory insufficiency with reduced pulmonary oxygen transport, thus further reducing oxygen delivery to the tissues. This process contributes to cell death and aggravates the endotoxin–macrophage–nitric oxide inhibition of adenosine triphosphate synthesis in the mitochondria. Gradual cell death of organs leads to sequential organ system failure.[12]

Pathophysiologic Changes That Lead to Vital Organ Damage

Heart: dehydration, tachycardia, hypotension, reduction of cardiac output and venous return with decreased peripheral resistance (blood pooling), hypoxia, shock. Progressive peripheral cell death eventually leads to a hypodynamic circulation and the low cardiac output of the failing or dying heart.

Lung: decreased ventilatory space due to inflammatory edema and increased abdominal pressure, disturbance

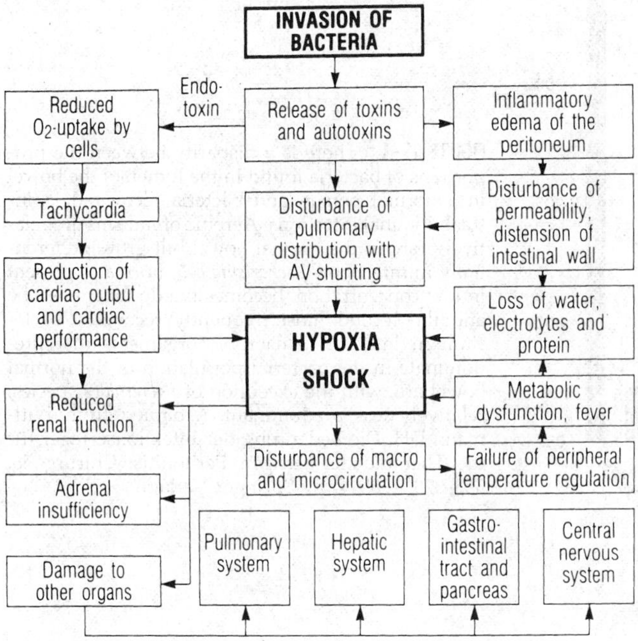

FIGURE 85–3 □ The systemic pathophysiologic responses in intraabdominal infection are largely mediated through disturbed oxygen-dependent processes.

of pulmonary ventilation-perfusion with atrial venous shunting, increased pulmonary resistance, nitric oxide–induced alveolar cell destruction, increased oxygen transfer distance, pulmonary insufficiency (acute respiratory distress syndrome), hypoxia.

Kidney: reduced perfusion secondary to hypovolemia and increased intraabdominal pressure, retention of toxic metabolites, hypoxic and toxic damage to renal epithelia, increase in urea nitrogen and creatinine, renal insufficiency.

Intestine: local hypoxia, increased sympathetic activity, disproportional bacterial growth, bowel distention, increased intraabdominal pressure, abdominal compartment syndrome.

Liver: hypoxic cell damage, reduced protein synthesis, impaired Kupffer cell function, reduced metabolic detoxification, reduced perfusion due to increased intraabdominal pressure.

Bacteriology

Normal Bowel Flora

Bacterial counts in the gastrointestinal tract vary greatly, from nearly sterile in the fasting, normal, low-pH stomach to high concentrations of bacteria approaching 10^{12} per mL feces in the distal colon. Of the more than 400 different species of intestinal bacteria, most are symbiotic saprophytes, and only a few are capable of survival outside the bowel.[6, 13–15]

Esophagus and Stomach. Normally, there are fewer than 1000 organisms per milliliter of fluid in the esophagus and stomach. There are no obligate anaerobes; the flora is composed chiefly of α-hemolytic streptococci, lactobacilli, yeasts, and some swallowed oral bacteria. There is a direct correlation between the pH of the stomach (normally between 2 and 3) and the bacterial concentration. In achlorhydria, the count ranges from 100,000 to 10 million per mL. Anesthesia reduces gastric acid secretion and thus permits an increase in the microbial count. Higher bacterial concentrations in the stomach are also associated with the administration of histamine H_2-receptor antagonists; this needs to be considered when upper gastrointestinal tract perforation occurs in patients receiving such drugs, especially patients who are being treated in the intensive care unit for other reasons. Studies of stomach bacteria after resection or vagotomy consistently show an increased bacterial count.[16]

Duodenum and Jejunum. In the duodenum and jejunum, there are 100 to 10,000 bacteria per milliliter, primarily hemolytic streptococci, lactobacilli, transitory oral flora, and in rare cases, *Enterobacter* species and some types of *Bacteroides*. Duodenal diverticula and biliary calculous disease contribute to higher bacterial counts, as does previous gastrectomy with a blind duodenal stump or ileus of any cause.

Ileum. With decreasing distance from the ileocecal valve, the bacterial count increases, reaching values of 1 to 10 million per mL in the distal ileum.[15] Lactobacilli and streptococci are most frequent; *Bacteroides* and *Enterobacter* species are found in equal concentrations in the terminal ileum. High counts are found in any pathologic bowel state, such as ileus, obstruction, or chronic inflammatory disease.

Colon. Two thirds of dry fecal matter consists of bacteria. Less than 0.3% of these bacteria are Enterobacteriaceae. Moore and Holdeman[6] identified 400 to 500 different bacterial species in the large bowel. The ratio of anaerobic to aerobic organisms is 3000:1 to 10,000:1. The total bacterial count is 3.8×10^{12} per mg dry stool (Table 85–2).

Pathogens and Virulence Selection

The pathogens that cause intraabdominal infections come primarily from the intestine and associated hollow organs. Knowledge of the types and frequency of pathogenic bacteria usually resident in various segments of the bowel provides the basis for a presumptive diagnosis of the most likely pathogens before culture and sensitivity findings are available. The intestinal flora, however, is dependent on other factors—age, race, diet, previous operations, malnutrition, gastric acidity, bile salt excretion, gut motility, immune mechanisms, and prior administration of antibiotics.[6, 17] These factors alter the spectrum of possible target bacteria for therapy. In addition, the qualitative distribution of bacteria within their normal environment may be altered by various virulence factors outside the gastrointestinal tract.[18–22]

Once outside the intestines, only those bacteria that can withstand the host defense system survive for any length of time.[18] The consequence is a selection of virulent species after viscus perforation and other forms of intraabdominal infection (Fig. 85–4). Information about the pathogenicity of individual bacterial species is particularly important in the mixed infections usually seen with intraabdominal infection, because there are multiple possibilities of synergistic interactions and there may also be antagonistic ones.

Current microbiologic identification and sensitivity testing

TABLE 85–2 ■ Mean Concentration* of Selected Intraluminal Bacteria

BACTERIA	CONCENTRATION
Streptococci	$10^{6.5}$
Bacillus species	$10^{7.0}$
Enterococci	$10^{7.5}$
Escherichia coli	$10^{8.0}$
Bifidobacteria	$10^{8.3}$
Anaerobic cocci	10^{10}
Eubacteria	$10^{10.5}$
Clostridia	$10^{10.5}$
Bacteroides species	10^{11}

*Per milligram of dried feces.

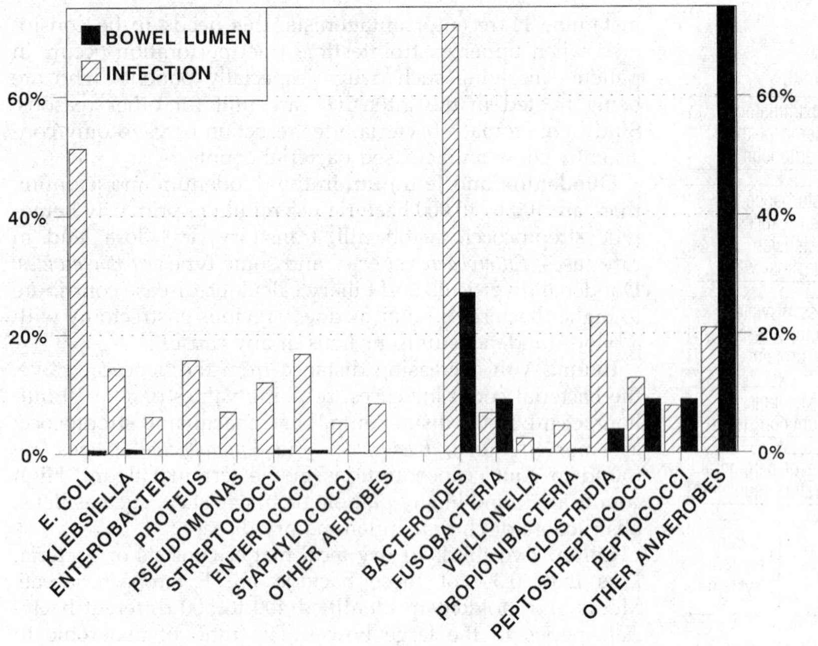

FIGURE 85–4 □ There is a disparity between the proportions of bacteria found in the lumen of the bowel in a normal person and bacteria recovered in intraabdominal infections. Aerobic organisms are relatively rare in the normal bowel but grow preferentially in infections. *Escherichia coli,* normally present in low concentration, becomes the dominant aerobe and the second most frequently recovered bacterium in infection. Anaerobic organisms that predominate in the bacterial population of the normal bowel are, with the exception of *Bacteroides* species, relatively less predominant. (Adapted from Wittmann DH: Die Bedeutung der Infektionserreger für die Therapie der eitrigen Peritonitis. Chirurg 56: 363–370, 1985. © by Springer-Verlag.)

methods available in hospitals do not meet the optimal requirements for management of antibacterial chemotherapy.[23] Results need to be available within a short time after the cultures are taken if the physician is to be able to institute selective antibiotic therapy without risking increased mortality and morbidity due to delay in starting that therapy. The desired time frame is in the range of minutes and will probably never be achieved. Therefore, presumptive antimicrobial therapy should be started as soon as an intraabdominal infection is diagnosed.

The initial therapy may be modified when specific sensitivity data are available, but changing antibiotics is not absolutely indicated unless the initial regimen is failing. Often, results of the initial bacteriologic assessment may be impaired because of inadequate specimen sampling or inappropriate transport time, especially in patients who have their laparotomy outside of the regular working hours of the laboratory. Antibiotic choice should not be based on such potentially flawed bacteriologic reports, which usually show predominance of transport-resistant bacteria such as enterococci that are of little pathogenic importance.

Isolation of Pathogens

The isolation of pathogens poses many problems for the usual hospital clinical laboratory. Almost any bacterium known to be pathogenic for humans may be seen on a Gram stain (see Fig. 85–4) obtained from the usual patient with peritonitis. Except to confirm that a mixed bacterial flora is present, the Gram stain is of little help. Many pathogens die off rapidly after the initial sampling and cannot be cultured easily by the hospital bacteriologist. Subsequent antibiotic therapy may fail if it is based on bacteriologic test results gained under suboptimal conditions. It is surprising, however, how similar are the results concerning distribution and frequency of pathogens from different studies using the best available techniques[23, 24] (Table 85–3).

The data of Table 85–3 record the important pathogens that should be considered target bacteria for therapy. *Escherichia coli* is the most commonly isolated pathogen. Its relative frequency in abdominal infections exceeds its intraluminal frequency by about 300 times, indicating that *E. coli* has a better chance of survival outside its natural environment, thus confirming its pathogenicity. The second most commonly isolated bacteria in intraabdominal infections are gram-negative obligate anaerobes, particularly *Bacteroides fragilis.* These organisms, in combination with other nonobligate anaerobes, are responsible for abscess formation. Other important organisms to be covered by initial chemotherapy are clostridia and gram-positive anaerobic cocci. Staphylococci and pseudomonads are unimportant as initial patho-

TABLE 85–3 ■ Pathogens of 900 Intraabdominal Infections Isolated in Six Independent Studies

	ISOLATES	
PATHOGEN	**Number**	**%**
AEROBES		
Escherichia coli	462	38
Klebsiella species	129	10
Enterobacter species	56	5
Proteus species	141	11
Pseudomonas aeruginosa	63	5
Staphylococcus aureus	46	4
Enterococcus faecalis	150	12
Other streptococci	107	9
Other aerobes	75	6
Total	1229	48
ANAEROBES		
Bacteroides fragilis	329	24
Other *Bacteroides* species	318	24
Fusobacteria	61	5
Veillonella	22	2
Peptococci	71	5
Peptostreptococci	113	8
Clostridia	205	15
Propionibacteria	41	3
Other	189	14
Total	1349	52
Grand total	2578	

Data from Wittmann DH: Treatment of Peritonitis: Antibiotic Concentration Dynamics at the Site of Infection as Criterion of Antimicrobial Chemotherapy. Habilitation. Hamburg, Medizinische Fakultät der Universität, 1985. Thesis.

gens in peritonitis. Enterococci are frequently isolated, but their pathogenic role is not yet defined; these organisms may act as a cofactor in the development of abscesses induced by obligate anaerobes.

Sepsis

Patients with intraabdominal infections die of the deleterious effects of their own immune response to infection, a process defined as sepsis and septic shock, and best measured by the Acute Physiology and Chronic Health Evaluation II (APACHE II) score (Fig. 85–5). Sepsis is most commonly induced by endotoxin released from dying facultative bacteria such as *E. coli*.[25] The term sepsis has been used to denote systemic response to infection and its pathophysiologic changes. Sepsis is the most common cause of death in the intensive care unit and is the 13th most common cause of death in the United States; 400,000 patients develop sepsis annually, in 200,000 it progresses to septic shock, and 100,000 patients die annually.[26] Microorganisms (such as *E. coli*) therefore constitute the major target for antibiotic therapy if the threat of mortality and organ failure is to be reduced.

Clinical Features of Intraabdominal Infection

Every case of intraabdominal infection, of whatever cause, initiates a sequence of responses involving the peritoneum, the bowel, and the body fluid compartments, which then produces secondary endocrine, cardiac, respiratory, renal, and metabolic responses (see Figs. 85–1 and 85–3). In certain forms of peritonitis, notably acute suppurative peritonitis, additional responses due to the presence of infection also occur. These pathophysiologic responses form the basis of schemes to stratify mortality risk among patients with peritonitis.[25, 26]

Abdominal pain is almost always the predominant symptom, unless its perception is masked by the administration of analgesics or the presence of a fresh surgical wound. The pain may have been sudden in onset, associated with rupture of a viscus, or more insidious. When fully developed, pain is steady, unrelenting, burning, and aggravated by any motion. Pain is usually most intense in the region of most advanced peritoneal inflammation. Decreasing intensity and extent of pain with time suggest localization of the inflammatory process, whereas increasing intensity and extent imply the presence of spreading peritonitis.

Anorexia is almost always present. Nausea is frequent and may be accompanied by vomiting. The patient usually complains of thirst and of feeling feverish, often with intermittent chills. Temperature usually ranges between 38°C and 40°C; the fever is more spiking in character in younger and healthier patients, whereas older or debilitated patients may exhibit only a modest febrile response. Tachycardia and a diminished palpable peripheral pulse volume are indicative of hypovolemia. As hypovolemia progresses, compensatory initial vasoconstrictive responses may be overwhelmed with the rapid appearance of hypovolemic shock. Respirations are typically rapid and shallow: rapid because of greater tissue demands for oxygen and the need to correct developing acidosis, and shallow because deep respiration intensifies the perception of abdominal pain.

The abdomen is distended, quiet to auscultation, and tender to palpation. Tenderness is present over the entire extent of the peritoneum involved in the inflammatory process and is maximal usually in the region of the organ in which the process originated. In some cases, maximal tenderness is found over the advancing edge of peritoneal inflammation. Direct, percussive, and referred rebound tenderness confirms the presence of peritoneal irritation. Percussion tenderness sometimes is more accurate than direct palpation in locating the point of maximal tenderness and in delineating the extent of peritoneal irritation.

Rigidity of the abdominal muscles is produced—initially by voluntary guarding—after involvement of the parietal peritoneum by inflammation but also by reflex muscle spasm. Reflex spasm may become so severe that boardlike abdominal rigidity is produced. Hyperresonance due to accumulating gas in the paralyzed, distended intestines can usually be demonstrated easily by percussion.

Some bowel sounds may be audible on auscultation early in intraabdominal infection, but as inflammation spreads, the nearly silent abdomen of adynamic ileus ("atonia") supervenes. Rectal and vaginal examinations are essential steps to locate the extent of tenderness and the possible presence of a pelvic mass. Vaginal examination of the cervix may provide clues to the origin of the inflammatory process.

Leukocytosis is common in acute intraabdominal infection, but the total white cell count, taken alone without a differential count, can be misleading. Massive peritoneal inflammation may mobilize sufficient numbers of leukocytes into the diseased area to produce peripheral leukopenia. Leukocytosis of more than 25,000 and leukopenia of less than 4000 white cells per mm^3 are both associated with higher mortality. The differential count provides the essential evidence of the presence of acute inflammation by showing a moderate to marked leftward shift even if the total white cell count is normal.

The radiologic picture in an acute intraabdominal infection is of paralytic ileus. Inflammatory exudate and edema of the intestinal wall may produce widening of the spaces between adjacent bowel loops noted on a flat film of the abdomen.

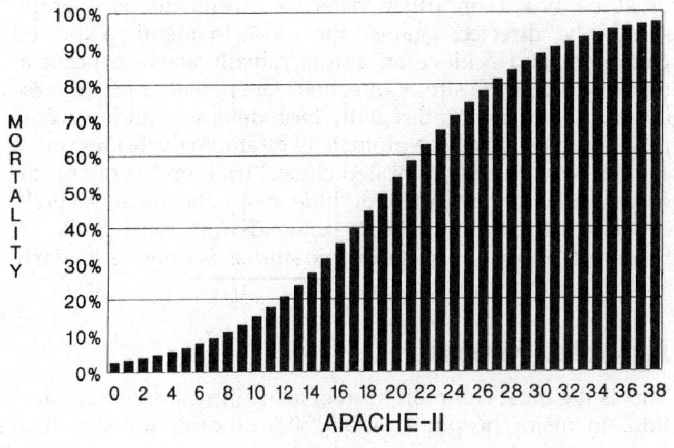

FIGURE 85–5 □ Relation between APACHE II score and predicted mortality for patients with intraabdominal infection. (From Wittmann DH, Condon RE, Walker AP: Peritonitis and intraabdominal infection. *In* Schwartz S [ed]: Principles of Surgery, ed 6. New York, McGraw-Hill, 1993, pp 1449–1483. Reproduced with permission of The McGraw-Hill Companies.)

Peritoneal flank fat lines and the retroperitoneal psoas shadows may be obliterated. Free air may be visible on an upright abdominal or lateral decubitus film if a ruptured hollow viscus is the cause of peritonitis or if peritonitis is well established and due to gas-forming bacteria such as *E. coli.* Air beneath the diaphragm may also be noted on radiographs of the chest, especially if the patient remains in an upright position for 5 minutes before the film is made.

Therapy

The therapeutic goal is reduction of mortality. The mortality of intraabdominal infection was about 90% at the turn of the 19th century, when management was mainly nonoperative and supportive. Through the application of the following surgical principles of early, definitive treatment, mortality in the worst cases has been reduced by more than 50%[27, 28]:

- Closure, resection, or exteriorization to control the source of infection
- Elimination or reduction of the concentration of bacteria, toxins, and necrotic material in the peritoneal cavity
- Treatment of residual bacteria with antimicrobial drugs
- Decompression of abdominal compartment syndrome
- Restoration of organ function

After its initial introduction into medical practice, antibiotic therapy did not reduce the mortality of intraabdominal infection, although it was successful in treating many other surgical infections. Poor isolation techniques that obscured the participation of anaerobes in peritonitis and limited activity of the drugs initially available against the endotoxin-producing Enterobacteriaceae were major factors responsible for the initial failure of antibiotic therapy in peritonitis.

During the last two decades, however, the mortality risk of peritonitis has diminished. Reliable studies of advanced peritonitis have been published that report mortality rates of 30% and less.[29–31] The improvement can be attributed to a better understanding of the true pathogens of intraabdominal infections and to antimicrobial therapy targeted at these microorganisms. Improved surgical technique is another important factor.[1] Some authors have reported better survival rates in a subset of high-risk patients with intraabdominal infection treated more aggressively by planned repeated laparotomy.[28–30, 32] The relaparotomy program should start as early as possible after diagnosis but not before the operative reduction of the bacterial inoculum, which helps to reduce the threat of endotoxemia.[23, 25, 33–36]

Antibiotic therapy should be started as early as possible after diagnosis as it also helps to reduce endotoxemia. Specific, directed treatment is not possible, however, because the infecting microorganisms and their sensitivities are not precisely known. Consequently, the choice of antimicrobial must be based on other criteria.[32] Antimicrobial therapy should be directed against the most frequently expected pathogens and achieve an antimicrobially active concentration of drug at the site of infection. The potential for adverse interaction of antibiotics with host defenses, and possible toxic effects such as the ototoxicity of aminoglycosides, must also be considered. Controlled clinical trial reports of antimicrobial efficacy are often of little help; the most severely diseased patients have been excluded from most trials.[37, 38] Sampling of pus for bacteriologic studies is done as an early step in operative treatment.

Perforation Peritonitis

This is the most common form of acute intraabdominal infection. In major hospitals, about 80% of cases are due to a variety of primary necrotic lesions of the gastrointestinal tract or of other intraabdominal organs; 10% to 20% of perforations are seen in patients after abdominal operations (postoperative peritonitis). In 58% of patients, frank perforation of the gastrointestinal tract due to peptic ulcer disease, diverticulitis, appendicitis, or a malignant lesion leads to the infection (Table 85–4). Bowel wall necrosis, either after strangulation caused by incarcerated hernia or due directly to impaired vascular flow, is the cause of infection in 20% of cases.

TABLE 85–4 ■ Causes of Peritonitis

CAUSES OF PERITONITIS	ALL PATIENTS		PATIENTS WHO DIED	
	Number	%	Number	%
Perforation	331	58	58	18
Bowel wall necrosis	116	20	42	36
Trauma	10	2	2	20
Postoperative leak	80	14	23	29
Abscess	26	5	5	19
Not specified	4	1	2	
Total	567	100	132	23

Infection After Perforation of Stomach and Duodenum

Infection after peptic ulcer perforation presents acutely; the patient is usually able to identify the exact time at which the perforation occurred. This form of peritonitis is initially chemical in nature but with the passage of a short time becomes infected through bacterial translocation. The patient most often seeks help early owing to severe pain, and operative repair is often possible before systemic dissemination of infection and organ failure occur. The proper management is simple closure. Some authors recommend additional definitive treatment of the peptic ulcer disease if the perforation is less than 12 hours old.

The high mortality rate of anastomotic leakage or suture line breakdown after gastroduodenal operations is explained by the fact that the duodenum is retroperitoneally fixed and cannot be exteriorized, and the source of infection often cannot be adequately controlled or closed. Consequently, infective material and proteolytic enzymes are delivered continuously into the peritoneal cavity, sustaining the infection.

Infection After Pancreatitis

Translocation of bacteria is probably the mechanism of the progression from chemical inflammation to intraabdominal infection. The combination of tissue necrosis due to proteolytic and lipolytic pancreatic juice and the presence of intestinal bacteria is the reason for the high mortality. The diagnosis of pancreatitis is not difficult; a history of midepigastric pain radiating to the back in combination with elevated levels of amylase and lipase in serum and urine suggests the correct diagnosis. The transition from pancreatitis to diffuse peritonitis is more difficult to diagnose, and thus antimicrobial therapy is often started late, when deterioration and multiorgan system failure have already occurred. In this type of advanced disease, multiple planned reoperations may be necessary.[36, 39]

Infection After Small Bowel Perforation

Symptoms of intraabdominal infection after small bowel perforation fall into two major categories:

1. Ileus precedes peritonitis. Colic and other features of bowel obstruction are the leading signs and symptoms initially, gradually changing to those of localized or diffuse peritonitis with fever and leukocytosis.

2. Bowel wall necrosis due to inadequate vascular supply or inflammation leads to perforation. Peritonitis may be diagnosed at a late stage owing to a lack of initial symptoms. Often these patients are operated on late in the evolution of their peritonitis, and the mortality rate is more than 50%. This contributes to the mortality figure of 36% in patients who had peritonitis after bowel wall necrosis (see Table 85–4).

Infection and Appendicitis

In formal usage, appendicitis meets the criteria of a local peritonitis, but this disease is not usually included under secondary suppurative peritonitis because of the strictly localized inflammation and the extremely low mortality in typical cases. If the appendix has perforated, however, the disease may become life threatening, especially when the omentum is not able to contain the infection and then diffuse suppurative peritonitis results. The symptoms of appendicitis are outlined in Chapter 88. When peritonitis develops, there is usually a sudden deterioration in the clinical status. Treatment is more likely to be successful once the appendix is removed and the source of infection is thus controlled. This explains the lower mortality rate of 13% in the series recorded in Table 85–5.

Disseminated intraabdominal infection from appendicitis is not seen as often today as in the first decades of this century, when vital statistics showed that appendicitis was the major cause of peritonitis seen in hospitals.[28] Because the human life span has increased, other organ origins of peritonitis are now seen more often, and diseases of aged persons, cancer and diverticulitis, for example, are more frequently the cause of intraabdominal infections.

Infection After Colon Perforation

Colon perforation due to diverticulitis or cancer is a common cause of diffuse, suppurative peritonitis. Postoperative peritonitis due to a disrupted anastomosis is seen most frequently after a colon operation. A myriad of bacteria gain access to the peritoneal cavity through the perforated colon. This factor, together with the many associated diseases in the population of elderly patients with colon disease, contributes to the high mortality rate of 37% (see Table 85–5). This group of patients particularly benefits from planned relaparotomy for which the overall mortality rate is only 23%. The basis for successful treatment (i.e., the elimination of the infectious source) is accomplished through colostomy or exteriorization and resection of the diseased colon.

TABLE 85–5 ■ Organ Source of Origin of Peritonitis

	ALL PATIENTS		THOSE WHO DIED	
ORIGIN OF PERITONITIS	**Number**	**%**	**Number**	**%**
Stomach and duodenum	175	31	38	22
Biliary tract	50	9	8	16
Pancreas	11	2	4	36
Small bowel	71	13	27	38
Appendix	125	22	16	13
Colon	117	21	43	37
Genitourinary system	14	2	3	21
Other	4	1	1	25
Total	567	100	140	25

Infection After Perforation of the Genitourinary Tract

A variety of conditions may cause peritonitis originating from the genitourinary tract. Ruptured perinephric abscess and ruptured chronic cystitis after radiation therapy for female reproductive tract cancer are examples. Pelvic peritonitis due to sexually transmitted infection is seen in young women; usually there is acute, severe abdominal pain. The condition is easily diagnosed by Gram stain if it is suspected. Treatment is only with antimicrobials in nearly all cases.

Postoperative Peritonitis

Postoperative peritonitis is usually due to a leak from a suture line and is discovered only after some delay, as a rule between the fifth and seventh postoperative days. Delay contributes to the high mortality rate.[37] A suture line leak is easier to repair if it is observed in the colon, small bowel, or stomach compared with leaks of the duodenum or esophagus. Upper gastrointestinal tract disease after an operation allows only a limited therapeutic correction, because these organs are fixed or closely attached to the retroperitoneum and the infectious source cannot be totally excluded or controlled under most circumstances. Resection of the anastomosis or of the diseased bowel segment is better than repair. Staged abdominal repair using a temporary abdominal closure device may be of particular benefit to this subset of patients with intraabdominal infections; we were able to reduce mortality to 24%.[28, 29, 33, 36]

Posttraumatic Peritonitis

Peritonitis may develop in patients with injuries after blunt trauma who have unrecognized intraabdominal disease, such as ruptured mesentery with obliteration of the vascular supply to the small or large bowel or a frank bowel perforation. This type of intraabdominal infection is usually severe because it is masked by other injuries. Treatment does not differ from that of intraabdominal infection generally.

Contamination of the abdominal cavity seen after penetrating abdominal trauma is usually not considered an intraabdominal infection. Only one third of patients with penetrating trauma to the colon actually sustain documented contamination of the peritoneal cavity, although many trials testing the efficacy of antimicrobials erroneously use this subset of patients as being representative of peritonitis.[40]

Tertiary Peritonitis

Patients who are unable to contain an infection, whether because of inadequate host defense mechanisms or overwhelming infection, may go on to develop persistent diffuse peritonitis, which Rotstein and Meakins[41] have called tertiary peritonitis. The clinical picture is one of occult sepsis manifested by hyperdynamic cardiovascular findings, low-grade fever, and a general hypermetabolic state. These patients have the clinical picture of sepsis without the presence of a well-defined focus of infection and are often subjected to laparotomies in the hope of improving drainage of recurrent or residual collections of infected fluid. These infected fluid collections are different from true abscesses, because they are not delimited by an inflammatory membrane or capsule. These patients frequently die with multiple organ system failure as the result of cellular asphyxia. Bacteria of low pathogenic potential, usually selected by antimicrobial therapy, are isolated from these patients. The bacterial isolates include multiresistant, coagulase-negative staphylococci, enterococci, and species of pseudomonads and fungi. These microorganisms do not seem to be readily affected by antimicrobial treatment, which suggests a generalized failure of host defenses.

References

1. Wittmann DH: Symposium of intra-abdominal infections: Introduction. World J Surg 14:145, 1990.
2. Dellinger EP, Wertz MJ, Meakins JL, et al: Surgical infection stratification system for intra-abdominal infection. Arch Surg 120:21, 1985.
3. Nyström PO, Bax R, Dellinger EP, et al: Proposed definitions for diagnosis, severity scoring, stratification, and outcome for trials on intraabdominal infection. World J Surg 14:148, 1990.
4. Lierse W: Das Peritoneum. Anatomische Grundlagen. Chirurg 56:357, 1985.
5. Hau T, Ahrenholz DH, Simmons RL: Secondary bacterial peritonitis: The biologic basis of treatment. *In* Ravitch MM, Steinchen FM (eds): Current Problems in Surgery. Chicago, Year Book Medical Publishers, 1979.
6. Moore WEC, Holdeman LV: Human fecal flora: The normal fecal flora of 20 Japanese-Hawaiians. Appl Microbiol 27:961, 1974.
7. Baue AE: Multiple, progressive, or sequential systems failure. A syndrome of the 1970's. Arch Surg 110:779, 1975.
8. Fry DE, Pearlstein L, Fulton RL, et al: Multiple system organ failure: The role of uncontrolled infection. Arch Surg 115:136, 1981.
9. Stahl TJ, Cerra FB: Hemodynamic and metabolic response to infection. *In* Simmons RL, Howard RJ (eds): Surgical Infectious Disease. Norwalk, CT, Appleton & Lange, 1988, pp 209–232.
10. Goris RJA: Pathophysiology of multiple organ failure with "sepsis." Med Link 82:546, 1987.
11. Tighe D, Moss R, Boghossian S, et al: Multi-organ damage resulting from experimental faecal peritonitis. Clin Sci 76:269, 1989.
12. Wittman DH: Peritonitis—Intra-abdominal Infection—Intra-abdominal Abscess. Austin, TX, RG Landes, 1995.
13. Drasar BS, Hill MJ: Human Intestinal Flora. London, Academic Press, 1974.
14. Finegold SM: Microflora of the gastrointestinal tract. *In* Wilson SE, Finegold SM, Williams RA (eds): Intra-abdominal Infection. New York, McGraw-Hill, 1982, pp 1–22.
15. Bentley DW, Nichols RL, Condon RE, et al: The microflora of the human ileum and intra-abdominal colon: Results of direct needle aspiration at surgery and evaluation of technique. J Lab Clin Med 79:421, 1972.
16. Clark JS, Bartlett JG, Finegold SM: Bacteriology of the gut and its clinical implications. West J Med 121:359, 1976.
17. Greenlee HB, Gelbart SM, DeOrio AJ: The influence of gastric surgery on intestinal flora. Am J Clin Nutr 30:1826, 1977.
18. Collee JG: Factors contributing to loss of anaerobic bacteria in transit from the patient to laboratory. Infection 8:145, 1980.
19. Meleney FL, Ollp J, Harvey HD, et al: Peritonitis: II. Synergism of bacteria commonly found in peritoneal exudates. Arch Surg 25:709, 1932.
20. Bartlett JG, Onderdonk AB, Louie TJ, et al: A review. Lesson from an animal model of intra-abdominal sepsis. Arch Surg 113:853, 1978.
21. Onderdonk AB, Weinstein W, Sullivan NM, et al: Experimental intraabdominal abscesses in rats: Quantitative bacteriology of infected animals. Infect Immun 10:1256, 1974.
22. Hagen CJ, Wood WS, Hashimoto T: In vitro stimulation of *Bacteroides fragilis* growth by *Escherichia coli.* Eur J Clin Microbiol 1:338, 1982.
23. Wittmann DH, Syrrakos B, Wittmann MM: Advances in the diagnosis and treatment of intra-abdominal infection. *In* Nyhus L, Nichols RL (eds): Problems in General Surgery: Surgical Sepsis, 1992 and Beyond. Philadelphia, JB Lippincott, 1993, pp 604–627.
24. Wittmann DH: Treatment of Peritonitis: Antibiotic Concentration Dynamics at the Site of Infection as Criterion of Antimicrobial Chemotherapy. Habilitation. Hamburg, Medizinische Fakultät der Universität, 1984. Thesis.
25. Prins JM, van Deventer SJH, Kuijper EJ, Speelman P: Clinical relevance of antibiotic-induced endotoxin release. Antimicrob Agents Chemother 38:121, 1995.
26. Parrillo JE: Pathogenic mechanisms of septic shock. N Engl J Med 328:1471, 1993.
27. Kirschner M: Die Behandlung der akuten eitrigen freien Bauchfellentzundung. Langenbecks Arch Chir 142:53, 1926.
28. Wittmann DH, Bansal N, Bergstein JM, et al: Staged abdominal repair compares favorably when adjusting for prognostic factors with a logistic model. Theor Surg 9:201, 1994.
29. Aprahamian C, Wittmann DH: Operative management of intraabdominal infection. Infection 19:453, 1991.
30. Schein M, Hirshberg A, Hashmonai M: The surgical management of severe intra-abdominal infection. Surgery 112:489, 1992.
31. Ohmann C, Wittmann DH, Wacha H: Prospective evaluation of prognostic scoring systems in peritonitis. Eur J Surg 159:167, 1994.
32. Wittmann DH, Bergstein JM, Frantzides CT: Calculated empiric antimicrobial therapy for mixed surgical infections. Infection 19(Suppl 6):345, 1991.
33. Wittmann DH, Aprahamian C, Bergstein JM: Etappenlavage, advanced diffuse peritonitis managed by planned multiple laparotomies utilizing zippers, slide fastener, and Velcro analogue for temporary abdominal closure. World J Surg 14:218, 1990.
34. Hurley JC: Antibiotic-induced release of endotoxin: A reappraisal. Clin Infect Dis 15:840, 1992.
35. Shenep JL: Antibiotic-induced bacterial cell lysis: A therapeutic dilemma. Eur J Clin Microbiol 5:11, 1986.
36. Wittmann DH: Intra-abdominal Infections: Pathophysiology and Treatment. New York, Marcel Dekker, 1991.
37. Solomkin JS, Meakins JL Jr, Allo MD, et al: Antibiotic trials in intra-abdominal infections. A critical evaluation of study design and outcome reporting. Ann Surg 200:29, 1984.
38. Wittmann DH: Standard cephalosporin for surgical infections. Diagn Microbiol Infect Dis 22:173, 1995.
39. Stone HH, Strom PR, Mullins RJ: Pancreatic abscess management by subtotal resection and packing. World J Surg 8:340, 1984.
40. Bohnen JMA, Solomkin JS, Dellinger EP, et al: Guidelines for clinical care: Anti-infective agents for intra-abdominal infection: A Surgical Infection Society policy statement. Arch Surg 127:83, 1992.
41. Rotstein OD, Meakins JL: Diagnostic and therapeutic challenges of intra-abdominal infections. World J Surg 14:159, 1990.

86

Peritonitis

Ronald Lee Nichols
James W. C. Holmes
Jeffrey W. Smith

Although many types of intraabdominal infections are reported in the surgical literature, peritonitis, which secondarily follows the interruption of the continuity of the gastrointestinal tract by trauma, intrinsic disease, or surgery, is most common. The degree of dissemination of the infection within the peritoneal cavity depends primarily on five factors: (1) the location and size of the primary leak, (2) the nature of the underlying injury or disease, (3) the presence of peritoneal adhesions from previous disease states or operations, (4) the duration of the present illness, and (5) the efficiency of the local and systemic host defense mechanisms.

The Peritoneal Membrane

The adult peritoneal membrane, made up of a single layer of mesothelial cells, measures approximately 1.7 m^2, which closely approximates the total cutaneous surface area. This membrane lines the peritoneal cavity and viscera within this space, forming the largest preformed extravascular space in the body. The space is normally lubricated with about 20 to 50 mL of clear yellow fluid transudate, which has been reported to possess some intrinsic antibacterial activity.[1, 2] This peritoneal fluid normally contains less than 300 cells per mm^3, mostly macrophages and lymphocytes; however, when inflammation or infection is present, rapid increases of the total fluid volume and cell counts occur, with a shift in cell type to neutrophils predominantly.

The ability of the peritoneal membrane to participate in fluid exchange and absorption is well documented. The hyperosmolar nature of the peritoneal fluid in bacterial peritonitis can result in a rapid inflow of 300 to 500 mL of fluid per hour into the peritoneal space, which can lead to a hypovolemic condition unless therapy is initiated promptly. Some have likened the hemodynamic effect of acute generalized peritonitis to that of burns covering 50% or more of the body surface.[1]

Although the entire peritoneal membrane participates in fluid and solute exchange, the diaphragmatic lymphatics specifically absorb particulate matter.[3] It is only in this region that lymphatic collecting vessels (lacunae) form small pores (stomata) that penetrate the mesothelial basement membrane and open directly into the peritoneal cavity. Peritoneal fluid flows through the stomata into the lacunae during relaxation of the diaphragm while contraction empties the lymphatics into efferent ducts. Flow is aided by one-way valves in the thoracic lymphatics that prevent reversal of these dynamics. Because each stoma ranges from 8 to 12 μm in size and most bacteria are 0.5 to 2 μm in diameter, the bacteria are cleared rapidly from the peritoneal cavity by this mechanism. This clearance has been shown to be delayed when the patient is in the upright position and increased by the bent-down position. During peritonitis, it has been observed that intraabdominal fibrin formation is enhanced, whereas fibrinolytic activity is reduced. The fibrin clots within the peritoneum can trap bacteria and reduce clearance, increase abscess formation, and protect bacteria caught in the fibrin from antimicrobial agents and immunologic defense mechanisms. Fibrin alone is readily lysed by the fibrinolytic enzymes present in the healthy peritoneal cavity.[4] The use of heparin has been shown to be of benefit in experimental peritonitis by preventing the additional apposition of fibrin and therefore improving the clearing mechanisms.[5]

The effect of recombinant tissue plasminogen activator was studied in a rat model of generalized *Escherichia coli* and *Bacteroides fragilis* peritonitis by van Goor and coworkers.[6] The tissue plasminogen activator was shown to reduce abscess formation but also resulted in early bacteremia and increased mortality. Abscesses that formed consisted of *E. coli* and other species of intestinal origination, thus showing bacterial translocation. It is apparent that further studies should be performed to ascertain whether this treatment modality would be of clinical benefit.

Experimental investigations have shown that the peritoneal mesothelium sloughs readily even after only brief exposure to air or saline solution; rapid regeneration begins within hours of these exposures and is completed within a week of the injury.[7] Whether this healing occurs from differentiations of local macrophages into mesothelium or from the mesothelial cells from the opposing peritoneal surfaces is unclear.

Experimental Intraperitoneal Infections

Experimental studies of intraperitoneal sepsis have contributed much to our understanding of the pathophysiologic and microbiologic events as well as the therapeutic considerations significant in clinical infection. Weinstein and coworkers[8] studied antimicrobial agents in the treatment of experimentally induced intraperitoneal sepsis in rats. In their experimental model, pooled colonic contents from the rats were placed into gelatin capsules and then surgically positioned within the peritoneal cavity.[9] They used a constant inoculum and observed that a two-stage disease developed in untreated rats. Initially, death caused by acute peritonitis was observed in 37% of the rats, whereas all of the survivors developed late intraabdominal abscesses. In the antibiotic-treated rats, gentamicin alone (aerobic coverage) reduced the acute mortality to 4%, but 98% of the survivors later developed abscesses. Clindamycin therapy alone (anaerobic coverage) was associated with an acute mortality rate of 35%, but the frequency of late intraabdominal abscesses in survivors was only 5%. A combination of gentamicin and clindamycin produced the salutary effects of each agent—an acute mortality rate of 7% and a frequency of late abscess formation of 6% in the survivors. These studies, which were done with appropriate microbiologic manipulations, suggested that coliform organisms caused the early deaths due to peritonitis and that anaerobes were principally responsible for the late complications of intraabdominal abscess formation.

Subsequent experimental studies by Onderdonk and colleagues[10] stressed the importance of *E. coli* in acute mortality in experimental peritonitis. Their results also suggested that intraabdominal abscesses are formed by a synergistic relationship between anaerobic and facultative bacteria. They were unable to cause early septicemic death or late abscess formation when only *B. fragilis* was used as the inoculum. They also found that implanting 5 × 10^7 enterococci alone in the capsule placed in the peritoneal cavity caused neither early septicemic mortality nor late abscess formation, whereas the placement of a mixed inoculum of *E. coli* plus enterococci failed to result in abscess formation. However, when combinations of *B. fragilis* or *Fusobacterium* organisms with enterococci were used, a high rate of intraperitoneal abscess was observed. These investigators thought that the pathogenicity of the enterococcus rested in its ability to act synergistically with the anaerobes in the formation of abscesses.

Further experimental studies,[11, 12] however, identified a polysaccharide capsule external to the outer membrane in some strains of the *B. fragilis* group. On the basis of slight differences in biochemical reactions, it has been determined that of the many different subspecies of *B. fragilis,* only *B. fragilis* subspecies *fragilis* has this capsule. This subspecies is more frequently isolated from clinical infections, despite its relatively low numbers in human stool, than are the other subspecies.[13]

Our laboratory[14, 15] modified these techniques and thereby widened the spectrum of experimental intraabdominal sepsis so that a disease more similar to that observed in humans could be induced. We found that in the rats studied the mortality rate due to acute peritonitis increased with increasing doses of human stool inoculum.[14] The results of this study revealed that only the broad-spectrum antibiotic agents with aerobic and anaerobic coverage significantly decreased the early mortality rate due to peritonitis in the large-inoculum group compared with the control group, whereas all the tested agents singly or in combination significantly decreased the mortality rate in the middle-inoculum group compared with the control group.

The activity of gentamicin has been noted to be decreased in acidic environments such as the interior of abscesses and the peritoneum during peritonitis. Sawyer and coworkers[16] showed that the minimal inhibitory concentration of gentamicin against an *E. coli* strain increased eightfold, whereas the minimal inhibitory concentration to aztreonam only doubled. They further compared the effectiveness of gentamicin with that of aztreonam for aerobic antibacterial coverage in a murine model of intraperitoneal abscess formation due to *E. coli* and *B. fragilis*. Each was combined with clindamycin for anaerobic coverage. They were able to show that aztreonam plus clindamycin was superior to gentamicin plus clindamycin in preventing abscess formation (33% versus 0%) and in eliminating *E. coli* from those abscesses that did form (100% versus 61%).

Other experimental studies have disclosed the adjuvant action that hemoglobin plays in peritonitis.[17] Although the exact mechanism of this action is unproved, most authors agree that it is based on the ability of hemoglobin to delay the clearance of the bacteria from the peritoneal cavity.[18] Hall and associates[19] have presented evidence that this mechanism may rest on the ability of hemoglobin to inhibit the chemotactic response of the polymorphonuclear neutrophils by interfering with the effective interaction of the cytotoxin to the receptor on the cell well.

The value of intraperitoneal irrigation with both antibiotic solutions and povidone-iodine has also been studied in experimental fecal peritonitis.[20] In this study, lethal fecal peritonitis was prevented in 5 of 17 (29%) animals after 0.1% kanamycin peritoneal irrigation; all other groups treated by irrigation with saline solution or varying concentrations of povidone-iodine (and no parenteral antibiotics) had no survivors. When appropriate systemic antibiotics have been administered before peritoneal irrigation to animals with fecal peritonitis, the results indicated no better survival or less abscess formation after lavage with aminoglycoside than with saline alone.[21] Similar findings were observed even when the lavage solution used antibiotics with both aerobic and anaerobic activity[22]; intraperitoneal lavage with a dilute solution of hydrogen peroxide appeared to have a significantly greater toxic effect than benefit compared with a control group treated with saline solution.[23]

Despite aggressive surgical intervention and antibiotic therapy, morbidity and mortality can remain high in patients with diffuse peritonitis. A possible explanation is that the immune system is adversely affected by the infectious process causing an immunosuppression. This suppression may be mediated by the increased release of cytokines such as interleukin-1 or tumor necrosis factor (TNF) or by a decreased ability of immune system cells to identify and destroy infecting bacteria.[24, 25]

Brown and coinvestigators[26] have shown an improved survival rate when the immunomodulator muramyl dipeptide was given 24 hours before the onset of experimental peritonitis, whereas no protection has been observed when this or another immunostimulant was given at the time of bacteria inoculation.[27–29] Dunn and coworkers[29] showed a clearly defined additive effect of muramyl dipeptide pretreatment given with a prophylactic dose of cefoxitin in a human fecal peritonitis rat model.

Sawyer and associates[30] studied the effects of pretreatment with cefoxitin and anti-TNF antibody on mortality and serum TNF levels in a murine model of mixed *E. coli* and *B. fragilis* peritonitis. At low- and intermediate-inocula levels, only the cefoxitin prevented death, and all groups demonstrated low serum TNF levels. At the high-inoculum level, mortality was uniform in all groups except the cefoxitin and anti-TNF antibody group. This group and the anti-TNF antibody group both showed significantly reduced levels of serum TNF at 6 hours. They concluded that the cytokine response was dependent on both the nature of the insult (inocula level) and the therapeutic intervention.

McMasters and Cheadle[31] pretreated experimental peritonitis in mice with the immunomodulator compounds muramyl dipeptide or monophosphoryl lipid A. Neither agent altered the expression of TNF-α during peritonitis. They concluded that peritonitis is associated with an early increase in peritoneal macrophage TNF-α. Tissues remote from the infection demonstrated less marked changes, indicating that the immunosuppression is related to the proximity to the infectious process.

Experimental work has suggested that biomaterials in the peritoneal cavity may influence intraabdominal infection. One study showed increased bacterial translocation and serum levels of TNF and interleukin-6 in rats implanted with *E. coli* and rubber drain pieces compared with *E. coli* or rubber alone.[32] Histologic examination also revealed a more pronounced inflammatory response as well in this group. The authors thus concluded that the presence of a biomaterial (rubber drain) aggravates intraabdominal sepsis.

Secondary Bacterial Peritonitis

Secondary bacterial peritonitis is a frequently encountered clinical condition that usually arises after gastrointestinal tract leakage within the peritoneal cavity. This leakage may follow perforation of diseased viscera or blunt or penetrating trauma to the abdomen.

Characteristics of the Pathogen

Altemeier,[33] in 1938, was the first to stress the polymicrobial aerobic and anaerobic nature of the bacterial flora of peritonitis resulting from acute appendiceal perforation. In 1942, he reported on the pathogenicity of the aerobic and anaerobic bacteria isolated from the peritoneal exudate of these 100 cases of acute perforated appendicitis in experimental animals.[34] The primary conclusions of this study were as follows: (1) the great majority of the bacteria did not produce fatal peritonitis when injected in pure culture; (2) many avirulent strains of bacteria, particularly *E. coli*, became highly virulent in the presence of dead sterile tissue within the peritoneal cavity; (3) in mixed culture, these bacteria show a synergistic action producing a high degree of pathogenicity; and (4) acute perforated appendicitis peritonitis appears to be an infection resulting from the synergistic activities of the various bacterial symbionts present in a given case. These important studies were not elaborated on for nearly three decades, until modern techniques for the isolation and growth of anaerobic bacteria allowed better classification in both normal flora and postoperative infection studies.[35–37]

INTESTINAL MICROFLORA

The numbers and types of microorganisms increase progressively down the gastrointestinal tract. In normal humans, the stomach and proximal small intestine support a sparse bacterial flora of both aerobes and anaerobes (less than 10^4 colony-forming units [CFU]/mL).[38] Acidity and motility appear to be the major factors that inhibit the growth of bacteria in the stomach. Diseases of the stomach and duodenum may compromise these factors. Thus, in cases of bleeding or obstructing duodenal ulcer, gastric ulcer, or carcinoma, the microflora of the stomach usually increases, being composed principally of anaerobes from the oral cavity and aerobic coliforms.

The microflora of the distal small bowel represents a transitional zone between the microfloras of the upper and lower gastrointestinal tract; modest numbers of aerobic and anaerobic microorganisms (up to 10^8 CFU/mL) are usually present.[39, 40] The largest concentrations of anaerobes are in the colon, where up to 10^{11} CFU per gram of stool or milliliter of intestinal aspirate can be identified.[41] Coliforms are also present in the colon in concentrations of 10^8 CFU/g.

This anatomic location of microorganisms within the gastrointestinal tract in part accounts for the differences in septic complications associated with injuries to the upper and lower tract. Sepsis that occurs after upper intestinal leaks is generally less severe and associated with less morbidity and mortality than is sepsis due to leaks that follow colon injuries.

Microbiology of Intraperitoneal Sepsis

The numbers of aerobic and anaerobic bacteria isolated from sites of intraabdominal sepsis depend on the nature of the microflora of the diseased or traumatized organ. A complex polymicrobial flora results from contamination from the gastrointestinal tract. The polymicrobial nature of the pathogens in patients with intraabdominal infection is evident from several reports,[42–45] which, when combined, showed that the average number of strains of bacteria isolated from the infected sites ranged from 2.5 to 5.0. These figures included an average of 1.4 to 2.0 aerobes and 2.4 to 3.0 anaerobes per infection. One or more anaerobic species was isolated from 65% to 94% of the patients (Table 86–1).

The commonly isolated aerobes in all of the studies included *E. coli* and *Klebsiella, Streptococcus, Proteus,* and *Enterobacter* species; the anaerobes isolated most frequently were *Bacteroides, Peptostreptococcus,* and *Clostridium* species. *B. fragilis* was the anaerobe most often isolated. Along with other species of *Bacteroides, B. fragilis* accounted for 30% to 60% of all the anaerobic isolates in these studies. Purely anaerobic intraabdominal sepsis was usually reported in less than 15% of the cases, whereas purely aerobic infections were noted in about 10%. Both aerobes and anaerobes were involved in more than 75% of the cases of intraabdominal infections.

In addition, highly antibiotic resistant strains, such as *Pseudomonas aeruginosa, Serratia marcescens,* and *Acinetobacter* or *Providencia* species, are frequently isolated from patients who have an intraabdominal septic event within the hospital setting.[46] The microbiology of persistent peritonitis in patients with long hospitalizations, repeated courses of antibiotics, multiple operations, or admissions to the intensive care unit favors the growth of breakthrough microorganisms such as *Staphylococcus epidermidis* or *Enterococcus* and *Candida* species.[47, 48] Other rarer organisms have infrequently been recovered from patients with peritonitis, especially after continuous ambulatory peritoneal dialysis (CAPD). These include *Nocardia, Lactobacillus, Listeria, Streptococcus pneumoniae, Aeromonas, Campylobacter, Mycobacterium,* and *Brevibacterium.*[49–56] The origin of these organisms has been shown to include both internal and external sources.

An early work suggested that exposure to atmospheric oxygen during the course of an operation was the dominant factor controlling the recovery of anaerobic bacteria from the peritoneum.[57] The investigators based this idea on their empirical observations that they were able to recover anaerobic bacteria in nearly all instances of traumatic colon injury or perforated appendicitis immediately after opening the peritoneum. However, in only 10% of the cases were they able to recover the organisms after 1 to 2 hours of operative time. We studied this concept in clinical peritonitis by taking aerobic and anaerobic cultures during surgery.[58] The findings suggested that a selective suppression of anaerobic bacteria by atmospheric oxygen does not exist. Species of both aerobic and anaerobic bacteria may increase or decrease during the course of an operation, which probably relates to the degree of initial contamination as well as the degree of mechanical débridement and irrigation performed. Additional studies showed reliable aerobic and anaerobic bacterial recovery from experimental peritoneal exudates collected on transfer swabs and exposed to room air for up to 24 hours. These studies suggested that clinically implicated aerobic bacterial strains appear to be relatively aerotolerant.

Clinical Features

Secondary bacterial peritonitis occurs after the leakage of endogenous microorganisms from a diseased or traumatized intraperitoneal hollow viscus. The extent of dissemination of the infections within the peritoneal cavity depends primarily on many local factors, including the presence of adhesions from previous operations, the presence of a well-functioning omentum, and the size and location of the primary site of leakage. Localization of the spread usually results in the formation of intraperitoneal, retroperitoneal, or visceral abscesses, whereas generalized peritonitis is most commonly seen after penetrating or blunt abdominal trauma and rarely after organ perforation when the spread of infection is not localized.

Abdominal pain is present in all cases of peritonitis; when it is localized to one region of the abdomen, it is associated with rebound tenderness and muscle guarding in the area of organ perforation. In generalized peritonitis, the pain and tenderness are found over the entire abdomen and are aggravated by any movement, including coughing or jarring the hospital bed. Associated muscle rigidity is present, which in extreme cases may result in the so-called boardlike abdomen. Patients with peritonitis also have fever and a progressive tachycardia that occurs secondary to the third-space loss within the peritoneal cavity. If treatment is delayed, hypovolemia develops rapidly and shock follows. Early shock is usually due to hypovolemia alone, whereas later it is due to both hypovolemia and sepsis. Abdominal distention is due to the accumulation of fluid and debris in the peritoneal cavity as well as to increases in the intraluminal bowel gas and liquid due to the associated paralytic ileus (Fig. 86–1).

TABLE 86–1 ■ Microorganisms Isolated from Patients with Intraabdominal Infections

SERIES (YEAR)	NUMBER OF CASES STUDIED	AVERAGE NUMBER OF MICROORGANISMS PER INFECTION	AVERAGE NUMBER OF AEROBES PER INFECTION	AVERAGE NUMBER OF ANAEROBES PER INFECTION	NUMBER OF CASES WITH ANAEROBES/NUMBER STUDIED (%)
Altemeier et al[42] (1973)	501	2.5	Not available	Not available	Not available (65)
Gorbach et al[44] (1974)	46	5.0	2.0	3.0	40/60 (87)
Swenson et al[43] (1974)	64	3.8	1.4	2.4	52/64 (81)
Gorbach et al[45] (1975)	67	4.8	1.9	2.9	63/67 (94)

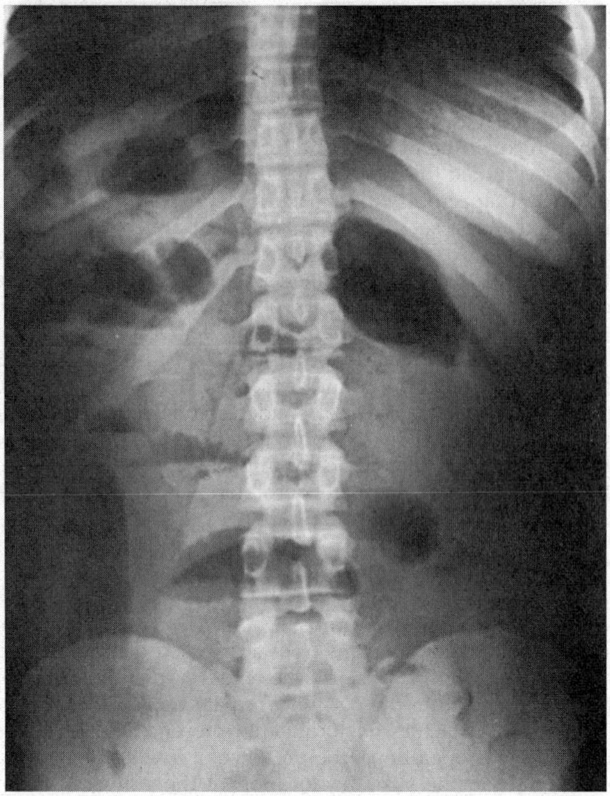

FIGURE 86–1 □ Upright radiograph of the abdomen demonstrates the presence of small intestinal air-fluid levels in addition to the free peritoneal fluid.

Bowel sounds are usually diminished early in the course of disease and become absent as time passes.

Diagnosis

The diagnosis of diffuse peritonitis is usually based on the clinical history and typical physical findings. Associated increases of the peripheral leukocyte counts are frequently observed, most often exceeding 15,000/mm^3 with a shift to the left. Basic radiographic examination may be helpful in showing evidence of free air below the diaphragm on chest films (Fig. 86–2) or the finding of mild distention of the small and large intestine associated with an intraperitoneal fluid collection between the bowel loops. Specialized radiographic procedures are most helpful in searching for localized intraabdominal collections and are rarely necessary to make the diagnosis. Paracentesis may be required to confirm the diagnosis. If gross pus, intestinal contents, or feces is aspirated, the diagnosis is confirmed. A Gram stain of the aspirated fluid offers immediate insights concerning the cause of the peritonitis. Bacterial cultures should always be performed so that further therapy can be based on knowledge of the pathogens and their antibiotic susceptibility patterns.

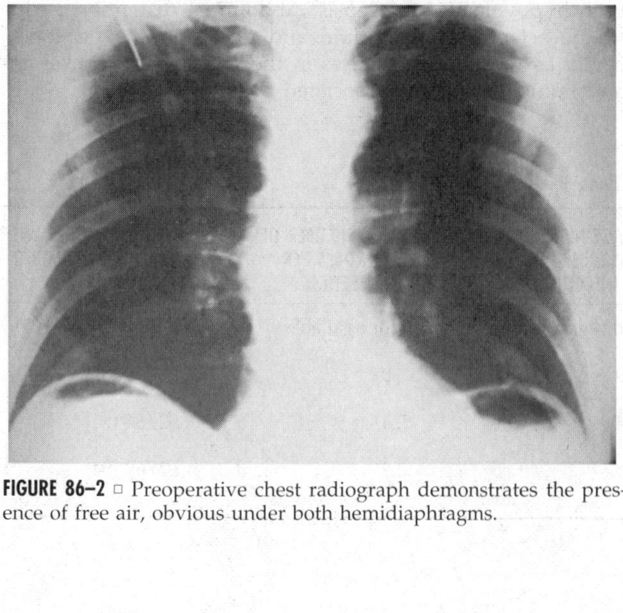

FIGURE 86–2 □ Preoperative chest radiograph demonstrates the presence of free air, obvious under both hemidiaphragms.

Attempts have been made to evaluate the severity of peritonitis by use of a variety of scoring systems. These include the Acute Physiology and Chronic Health Evaluation II (APACHE II), the Mannheim Peritonitis Index, and the Peritonitis Index Altona II. Although they have limited value in clinical trials to define risk, compare treatments, and define inclusion criteria, they have not been shown to be of diagnostic value in individual patients to predict outcomes.[59]

Treatment

The most critical aspect of the treatment of secondary bacterial peritonitis is early diagnosis and prompt surgical intervention. Preoperative care requires rapid monitoring of arterial and venous pressures as well as of urinary output. Frequent monitoring allows better fluid resuscitation during the perioperative course. Optimal preoperative care includes oxygenation of the tissues aided by the use of nasal cannula, administration of blood products in anemic patients, and use of vasoactive or inotropic agents as indicated. Intubation and respiratory assistance initiated at the time of operation are continued for varying periods during the postoperative period to prevent hypoxia. Preoperative placement of a nasogastric tube helps to decompress the accumulated gastrointestinal gas and fluid contents, which reduces pressure on the diaphragm and improves pulmonary ventilation. It appears that early bowel decompression also facilitates early return of intestinal motility during the postoperative course. The use of sedatives, analgesics, and antibiotics should be initiated only after the diagnosis of peritonitis has been made and the surgical procedure planned.

The nutritional requirements of these septic patients can be enormous, depending on the severity of the infection and the patient's prior health. Parenteral alimentation or enteral feedings delivered by a jejunostomy tube placed at the time of surgery are routinely recommended in severely septic patients or those with preoperative malnutrition.

Despite advances in the understanding of the pathophysiologic events that occur in patients with intraabdominal infection, the mortality and morbidity remain significant. Some investigators believe that improvement in these rates may be possible if study design and outcome reporting become standardized. This will allow better comparison of different treatment regimens in equivalent populations of patients, steps that may help to detect small differences.[60, 61] In addition to the general aspects of perioperative care just addressed, the true mainstays of treatment for peritonitis remain antibiotic selection and operative therapy.

ANTIBIOTIC SELECTION

Unlike superficial wound abscesses, for which surgical drainage alone usually suffices, intraabdominal sepsis is best managed by a combination of surgical repair, diversion, or drainage plus appropriate parenterally administered antibiotic agents. The antibiotic therapy should be initiated a soon as the diagnosis is made during the preoperative course and continued during the operative procedure and into the postoperative period. The choice of the ideal agent or agents and the necessary length of the therapeutic course remain controversial and unproven; however, the spectrum of activity of the chosen antibiotics based on early experimental[8, 15] and clinical[46, 62] studies must have activity against both the colonic aerobes and anaerobes including *B. fragilis*.

Instead of a list of the countless antibiotic studies that report equal efficacy in intraabdominal sepsis, a list of agents commonly used singly or in combination is offered (Table 86–2). Gorbach[63] has reviewed this subject and listed the agents that should be expected to be effective in this clinical setting.

The importance of using antibiotic agents that are effective against both aerobic and anaerobic gastrointestinal bacteria was demonstrated in a prospective study of 100 abdominal trauma patients reported in 1973.[62] This study revealed a significantly increased rate of anaerobic septicemia and intraabdominal infections in the group of patients treated with cephalothin-kanamycin (aerobic coverage) compared with those treated with clindamycin-kanamycin (aerobic and anaerobic coverage). The authors appropriately stated on the basis of these results that anaerobic bacteria appear to be a significant cause of infection in abdominal trauma.

Hofstetter and coinvestigators[64] in 1984 reported on their prospective study of 119 abdominal trauma patients. Results of this heterogeneous group appeared to indicate that a short-term course with a single drug, cefoxitin, was as safe and effective as the use of a triple-drug regimen of aminoglycoside, ampicillin, and clindamycin. The authors also suggested that it might be prudent to consider leaving the skin and subcutaneous tissues open in patients who had hollow viscus injury because of the high rate of localized wound infection in this clinical setting. Prospective randomized studies of purely penetrating abdominal trauma carried out during the same period reached similar conclusions in regard to the efficacy of antibiotic therapy.[65–67] Results of cefoxitin alone were found to be equal to those of combination therapy,[65–67] whereas cefoxitin alone was superior to cefamandole alone.[65, 67] These differences in efficacy of single cephalosporin agents were attributed to the varying activity of these agents against the anaerobe *B. fragilis*. The antibiotic agents used in these studies generally lacked efficacy against the enterococci, which were frequently isolated from infected sites in mixed culture. Despite their isolation, rarely was it necessary to alter the original antibiotic therapy to have a successful outcome; however, a similar study has stressed the ability of certain broad-spectrum cephalosporins to result in enterococcal overgrowth in this clinical setting.[68]

A trend has developed during the past several years to reduce the duration of antibiotic therapy after penetrating abdominal trauma with gastrointestinal contamination. Dellinger and colleagues[69] compared 12-hour and 5-day therapy in patients with colon injuries and saw no significant differences. Low numbers of patients may have resulted in a low statistical power to find a true difference. Fabian and coworkers[70] showed no differences in infectious outcome between 1- and 5-day therapy. They did not consider the severity of injuries in assigning therapy duration. When the abdominal trauma index was compared with infection, it was noted that those with more severe injuries did have increased infection rates. A study by Nichols and colleagues[71] allocated patients who had sustained penetrating abdominal trauma to either 2 or 5 days of antibiotics on the basis of the severity of their injuries and predicted infection risk. The patients predicted to have a low probability of infection who received 2 days of treatment showed the same rates of infection (10% major, 12% minor) as historical control patients who had received 5 days of treatment (9% major, 14% minor). Results of this study indicate that risk factors can be used to identify low-risk patients who require only short-term antibiotic therapy. Other patients are at greater risk for infection despite prolonged antibiotics and delayed wound closure. The use of the initial peritoneal culture in penetrating abdominal trauma and in other clinical settings in which there is no established intraabdominal infection has been reported to have no predictive value for the development of postoperative infection or for the pathogen identified from such infections when they occurred.[66, 72]

Because of the increasing frequency of β-lactamase–producing bacteria implicated in intraabdominal sepsis,[73] several studies have been conducted with use of antibiotic regimens containing β-lactamase inhibitors. Walker and colleagues[74] compared ampicillin-sulbactam with cefoxitin in patients with culture-positive peritoneal infections. Clinical success was found to be similar in the two groups, as were the rates of adverse events. Piperacillin-tazobactam was compared with either clindamycin plus gentamicin or imipenem-cilastatin in three trials of patients with severe intraabdominal infections.[75–77] The results indicated that the β-lactamase inhibitor–containing therapy was equivalent to the comparator regimen in two studies[75, 77] and superior in one.[76] The usefulness of therapy with β-lactamase inhibitors has been shown to be at least the same as that of standard treatment, and it might prove to be beneficial in cases of infection with β-lactamase–producing organisms.

The Surgical Infection Society in 1992 issued guidelines for the use of antiinfective agents in intraabdominal infections.[78] The guidelines were restricted to infections derived from the gastrointestinal tract and took into account various factors, including results from experimental and clinical studies and the pharmacokinetics, mechanisms of action, resistance, and safety of antibiotics. They stressed that antimicrobial coverage must provide a sufficient spectrum of activity against both facultative (aerobic) gram-negative bacilli and obligate anaerobic gram-negative bacilli. Regimens with little or no activity against these organisms are not acceptable. Their recommendations include the following: single-agent therapy with cefoxitin, cefotetan, cefmetazole, or ticarcillin-clavulanate for community-acquired infections of mild to moderate

TABLE 86–2 ■ Parenteral Antibiotic Agents Used for Coverage of Aerobic and Anaerobic Components of the Human Colonic Microflora

COMBINATION THERAPY

Aerobic coverage—to be combined with a drug having anaerobic activity
- Amikacin
- Aztreonam
- Ceftriaxone
- Ciprofloxacin
- Gentamicin
- Tobramycin

Anaerobic coverage—to be combined with a drug having aerobic activity
- Chloramphenicol
- Clindamycin
- Metronidazole

SINGLE-DRUG THERAPY

Aerobic-anaerobic coverage—single agent
- Ampicillin-sulbactam
- Cefoxitin
- Ceftizoxime
- Imipenem-cilastatin*
- Meropenem*
- Piperacillin-tazobactam
- Ticarcillin-clavulanate

*If selected, should be used for the treatment of hospital-acquired infection.

severity; single-agent therapy with imipenem-cilastatin or combination therapy with either a third-generation cephalosporin, aztreonam, or an aminoglycoside plus clindamycin or metronidazole for more severe infections.

Finally, the choice of individual antibiotic agents or combinations must be influenced by many factors, including efficacy, toxicity, local hospital microbial sensitivity patterns, and price.[63, 68, 79–81]

SURGICAL TECHNIQUES

The type of surgical procedure to be performed depends on what intraperitoneal disease is identified. The goal of the procedure should be to arrest peritoneal contamination and to débride necrotic tissue, remove debris and foreign bodies, and drain all localized purulent collections. Many mechanical techniques designed to reduce the bacterial burden within the peritoneal cavity have been advocated in addition to the primary surgical procedure[82] (Table 86–3).

The first of these techniques, intraoperative peritoneal irrigation, is used almost universally to treat secondary bacterial peritonitis. The irrigation is carried out at the end of the operative procedure either with a pour-in technique or with a jet lavage device using 2 or 3 L of irrigant. The evidence indicates that this technique does reduce the number of bacteria present, especially when it is done before fibrin has been deposited within the peritoneal cavity.[83]

The use of antibiotic irrigation of the peritoneal cavity in the face of peritonitis became popular in the mid-1960s.[84, 85] A review of 29 investigators' descriptions of the use of various antibiotic solutions in intraperitoneal irrigations for peritonitis has failed to prove the efficacy of the technique.[86] Until definite evidence of clinical efficacy is available, physicians must exercise caution before routinely using this technique, which may result in significant toxic effects because of peritoneal absorption,[87] increased expense, and increased deposition of peritoneal adhesions.[88] The use of varying concentrations of povidone-iodine irrigations in the bacterially contaminated abdomen was first recommended by Sindelar and Mason[89] in 1979. In their study, which did not completely standardize the use of systemic antimicrobial administration, the frequency of postoperative intraabdominal abscesses was reduced from 9 of 88 patients (10.2%) by the saline irrigation to 1 of 80 patients (1.3%) by irrigation with 0.1% iodine. Despite initial clinical enthusiasm, experimental studies of peritonitis have demonstrated that this technique can actually increase the mortality rate in peritonitis, presumably by damaging host defense mechanisms.[20, 90] In contrast, wound irrigation alone with local antibiotics or antiseptics continues to be a safe, commonly used technique, especially when primary wound closure is done.

In 1987, Leiboff and Soroff[91] published their critical review of 39 studies concerning the use of closed postoperative catheter peritoneal lavage in generalized peritonitis. Three of four prospective randomized studies showed unfavorable results with this technique, whereas 25 of 27 noncomparative studies showed favorable results. The authors concluded that the therapeutic value of this procedure remains unknown and that there remains a need for a large-scale, prospective, randomized study to evaluate the efficacy of closed postoperative catheter peritoneal lavage in the treatment of generalized peritonitis. As yet, this has not been done.

TABLE 86–3 ■ Intraoperative Mechanical Techniques Used in Intraabdominal Sepsis

Irrigation of the peritoneal cavity (pour-in or jet lavage)
- Saline solution
- Antibiotic solutions
- Povidone-iodine

Closed peritoneal catheter lavage
Radical surgical débridement
Leaving the peritoneal cavity open
Reoperation
- Use of surgical zipper or other temporary closure techniques
- Classic techniques

Radical surgical débridement was advocated by Hudspeth[92] in 1975. To date, no clinical study has confirmed the remarkable results of this study, and one prospective randomized study has shown no advantages of the radical over the conservative approach.[93]

Another technique recommended by Steinberg[94] in 1979 for acute generalized suppurative peritonitis was leaving the peritoneal cavity open. Twelve of 14 patients so treated had successful postoperative courses with no recurrent infections and no major complications such as evisceration of the abdominal contents.

Reoperation for intraabdominal sepsis, based on clinical judgment, has been recommended on the basis of a retrospective study of 50 patients.[95] The authors found that laboratory tests were not helpful in predicting the presence of infections on reexploration, but if reoperation was performed before the development of organ failure, the authors believed that the risk associated with a negative exploration is worth taking.

Teichmann and colleagues[96] were among the first to report a prospective study of a new concept of scheduled multiple laparotomies with abdominal lavage in 61 patients for the treatment of diffuse peritonitis. This process, which they named etappenlavage, consists of scheduled reoperations of the abdominal cavity to ensure exclusion of the infected source, promote maximal elimination of necrotic material, and allow prompt recognition of complications to effect immediate repair. They modified the technique for the last 31 patients in that reoperation was facilitated by closing the abdomen with a zipper. This technique was revised and further studied by Wittmann and coworkers[97] in a series of 117 patients with severe advanced suppurative peritonitis. They compared the technique using retention sutures, simple zippers, slide fasteners, and a Velcro analog (artificial bur). The patients required an average of 6.1 reoperations and showed a reduction of 34% to 93% predicted mortality (APACHE II or Surgical Infection Society Modified APACHE II scoring) to 24%. More complications were seen with retention sutures, and decompression of the abdomen was not allowed by retention sutures or the simple zipper. The Velcro analog was seen to be the most practical method of temporary abdominal closure. An additional study by this group further showed the usefulness and safety of this artificial bur.[98] There is some thought among surgeons that operations after multiple scheduled reoperations and lavage might prove difficult because of increased amounts of adhesions and a generally "hostile" abdomen. This, however, was not seen in a series of 12 patients requiring later operations to restore bowel continuity or for abdominal wall reconstruction.[99]

I (RLN) favor the technique of scheduled reoperations for high-risk patients with diffuse peritonitis and think that daily unzipping should be accomplished in the operating room until evidence of continued peritoneal sepsis is absent. Other investigators have recommended reoperation only when clinical findings or laboratory tests indicate continued intraabdominal infection.[100, 101]

In summary, the treatment of secondary bacterial peritonitis requires prompt initial diagnosis followed by adequate surgery and efficacious parenteral antibiotics. For high-risk patients, I (RLN) recommend that the abdomen be closed with a surgical zipper to allow daily reoperation until the evidence of continued sepsis is absent.

Primary Peritonitis

Less than 1% of the cases of bacterial peritonitis occur spontaneously, without evidence of intraabdominal organ perforation, and are referred to as primary peritonitis. Presumably, in most cases, the bacterial offenders reach the peritoneal cavity by hematogenous spread. Although this syndrome is seen more frequently in infants and children, it appears to be decreasing. Primary peritonitis has been diagnosed most frequently in the following groups: normal infants and children, patients with cirrhosis, and children with nephrotic syndrome. Even more rarely, it has been diagnosed in patients with systemic lupus erythematosus or Fitz-Hugh–Curtis syndrome.

The occurrence of primary peritonitis in normal infants and children accounts for more than 10% of cases of diffuse peritonitis.[102] In infants, the peak occurrence is before age 2 months, predominantly in girls; in children, it usually occurs between 5 and 9 years of age with equal frequency in boys and girls. In children with the nephrotic syndrome, boys predominate and the mean age of presentation of the primary peritonitis is about 4 years.[103] In this group, the most important pathogens are streptococci, particularly pneumococci, followed by coliforms such as *E. coli*.

The first cases of this disease in patients with cirrhosis were observed about 40 years ago. The frequency of primary peritonitis in cirrhosis patients appears to be about 6%.[104]

The causative bacterial flora in primary peritonitis associated with cirrhosis is a single microorganism in more than 90% of cases.[104] Although pneumococci were the most frequently isolated pathogen earlier in this century, the rate has decreased in more recent times. Today, the coliforms, especially *E. coli*, are most commonly implicated, followed by streptococci. Anaerobic bacteria are rarely found in primary peritonitis and if isolated would suggest secondary bacterial peritonitis. With the perihepatitis of the Fitz-Hugh–Curtis syndrome, the organisms isolated would generally be a gonococcus or *Chlamydia* species.[105]

The four most frequently implicated routes of bacterial contamination in primary peritonitis are hematogenous, direct from the female genital tract, contagious spread of infection from the retroperitoneal or supradiaphragmatic region, and migration of endogenous intestinal bacteria.

In a patient with cirrhosis or nephrosis, the presence of ascites is of great importance in the pathogenesis of primary peritonitis because it provides a nutritious and protective environment for the invading bacteria.

The symptoms and finding of primary peritonitis are generally less acute and develop slowly compared with those of secondary bacterial peritonitis. Nevertheless, they can mimic both early appendicitis and a catastrophic abdominal illness.[106] Fever associated with abdominal pain and tenderness and muscle guarding or rigidity with rebound are common. Leukocytosis is characteristic, and abdominal radiographs rarely provide any clues to the presence of intraabdominal disease, including masses or free air.

If primary peritonitis is suspected, it can be diagnosed by paracentesis, with or without peritoneal lavage. Infected fluid contains at least 300 white cells per mm^3, and usually more than 500.[107] Gram stain of the peritoneal fluid usually provides insights to the offending microorganism, and culture provides definitive identification. The finding on Gram stain of mixed flora of gram-positive and gram-negative microorganisms is highly suggestive of secondary bacterial peritonitis.

The mortality rate associated with primary peritonitis in children early in this century approached 100%, with or without operation. Since the advent of effective antibiotics and vaccines, the rate has fallen below 10% for children and below 50% for neonates.[102] The development of primary peritonitis in cirrhosis is associated with a high mortality rate, approaching 90% to 95%, owing principally to the complications of cirrhosis, including hepatic decompensation.

The treatment of primary peritonitis most frequently includes an exploratory laparotomy to rule out surgically correctable lesions that cause secondary bacterial peritonitis. In high-risk patients who have suggestive findings clinically and on peritoneal tap, appropriate empirical antibiotic therapy may be successful. This treatment regimen can be modified when culture and sensitivity results are available for organisms in the peritoneal fluid.

Other Atypical Forms of Infective Peritonitis

Barium Peritonitis

Perforation of the gastrointestinal tract during the course of a radiographic procedure that uses barium sulfate is a dreaded complication. Experimental models have indicated that the combination of barium and intestinal contents produces a more virulent peritonitis than either does alone.[13, 14] It is thought that the water-insoluble barium tenaciously binds to intestinal bacteria. This lethal mixture, which is difficult if not impossible to remove surgically, results in multiple foci of intraabdominal infection. The best chance for survival occurs when the disease is localized. The best treatment is prevention! Several recommendations have been offered to decrease the risk of this occurrence.[108] Once the diagnosis is made, successful therapy depends largely on the general health of the patient before this event; on appropriate choice of parenteral antibiotics aimed at the intestinal flora; and on multiple surgical procedures designed to divert, débride, and drain the affected areas.

Peritonitis Associated with Intraperitoneal Prosthesis

Peritonitis may occur in patients who have indwelling synthetic catheters for peritoneal dialysis or peritoneal venous or ventriculoperitoneal shunts. This complication is most common in CAPD patients owing to the relatively large numbers of these procedures; however, the frequency has decreased with general improvements in catheter design.[109] The repeated connecting and disconnecting of the administration sets to the indwelling catheter and any breakdown of aseptic technique are the major causes of CAPD peritonitis. The average rate of peritonitis is reported to be 1.3 to 1.4 episodes per patient-year.[110] The most frequently isolated organisms, usually originating from the skin flora, are coagulase-negative staphylococci (30% to 45%).[111, 112] A lesser number of cases are due to *Staphylococcus aureus* (10% to 20%), streptococci (10% to 15%), and gram-negative organisms (20% to 35%). Peritonitis in CAPD patients may result from decreased host phagocytic efficiency with depressed phagocytosis and bactericidal capacity of peritoneal macrophages. Diagnosis is usually made when a cloudy effluent is seen, with or without clinical signs or symptoms such as abdominal pain or tenderness, fever, nausea, vomiting, chills, or increased dialysate white cell count. The intraperitoneal route for antibiotic administration allows most patients with uncomplicated peritonitis to be treated as outpatients. A large number of antibiotics including cephalosporins, aminoglycosides, and penicillins have been used to treat CAPD peritonitis.[110] Vancomycin (intravenously or intraperitoneally) is the

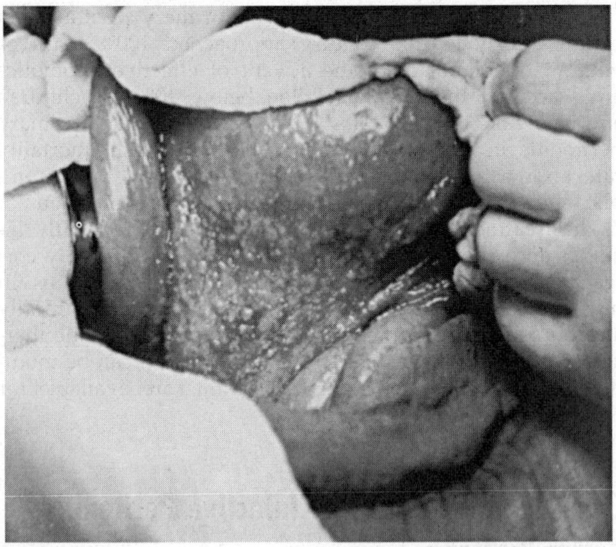

FIGURE 86–3 ▫ Operative picture of a patient with tuberculous peritonitis. The multiple tubercles can be seen on the intestinal serosa and on the root of the mesentery.

most commonly used antibiotic for gram-positive bacteria; aminoglycosides (intravenously or intraperitoneally) are commonly used for gram-negative infections. Although there have been several reports of successful therapy with oral quinolones such as ciprofloxacin and ofloxacin, their efficacy has not been proved conclusively.[113, 114]

Successful treatment mandates large doses of specific systemic antimicrobials, and frequently it is necessary to remove and subsequently replace the affected foreign body; however, peritoneal dialysis catheters rarely need to be removed unless there is associated infection of the subcutaneous tunnel. In this setting, continuous dialysis is instituted to prevent fluid loculation and adhesion formation until the patient is asymptomatic.

Tuberculous Peritonitis

Tuberculous peritonitis is today a rare disease.[115] In most cases, a primary pulmonary focus is present, which allows the spread of *Mycobacterium tuberculosis* hematogenously to the peritoneal cavity. Abdominal pain, progressively increasing abdominal girth, fever, weight loss, night sweats, and ascites are common. Paracentesis rarely is helpful, but laparoscopy or exploratory surgery discloses multiple tubercles scattered throughout the peritoneal cavity (Fig. 86–3). Treatment with triple antituberculosis drugs is most often successful.

References

1. Ahrenholz DH, Simmons RL: Peritonitis and other intraabdominal infections. *In* Howard RJ, Simmons RL (eds): Surgical Infectious Diseases, ed 2. Norwalk, CT: Appleton & Lange, 1988, pp 605–646.
2. Bercovici B, Michel J, Miller J, et al: Antimicrobial activity of human peritoneal fluid. Surg Gynecol Obstet 141:885, 1975.
3. Tsilibary EC, Wissig SL: Absorption from the peritoneal cavity: SEM study of the mesothelium covering the peritoneal surface of the muscular portion of the diaphragm. Am J Anat 149:127, 1977.
4. Dunn DL, Rotstein OD, Simmons RL: Fibrin in peritonitis. Arch Surg 119:139, 1984.
5. Hau T, Simmons RL: Heparin in the treatment of experimental peritonitis. Ann Surg 187:294, 1978.
6. van Goor H, de Graaf JS, Kooi K, et al: Effect of recombinant tissue plasminogen activator on intra-abdominal abscess formation in rats with generalized peritonitis. J Am Coll Surg 179:407, 1994.
7. Watters WB, Buck RC: Scanning election microscopy of mesothelial regeneration in the rat. Lab Invest 26:604, 1972.
8. Weinstein WM, Onderdonk AB, Bartlett JG, et al: Antimicrobial therapy of experimental intraabdominal sepsis. J Infect Dis 132:282, 1975.
9. Weinstein WM, Onderdonk AB, Bartlett JG, et al: Experimental intraabdominal abscesses in rats: Development of an experimental model. Infect Immun 10:1250, 1974.
10. Onderdonk AB, Bartlett JG, Louie T, et al: Microbial synergy in experimental intraabdominal abscess. Infect Immun 13:22, 1976.
11. Kasper DL: The polysaccharide capsule of *Bacteroides fragilis* subspecies *fragilis*: Immunochemical and morphologic definition. J Infect Dis 133:79, 1976.
12. Onderdonk AB, Kasper DL, Cisneros RL, et al: The capsular polysaccharide of *Bacteroides fragilis* as a virulence factor; comparison of the pathogenic potential of encapsulated and unencapsulated strains. J Infect Dis 136:82, 1977.
13. Bartlett JG, Onderdonk AB, Louie T, et al: A review: Lessons from an animal model of intraabdominal sepsis. Arch Surg 113:853, 1978.
14. Nichols RL, Smith JW, Balthazar ER: Peritonitis and intraabdominal abscess: An experimental model for the evaluation of human disease. J Surg Res 25:129, 1978.
15. Nichols RL, Smith JW, Fossedal EN, et al: Efficacy of parenteral antibiotics in the treatment of experimentally induced intraabdominal sepsis. Rev Infect Dis 1:302, 1979.
16. Sawyer RG, Adams RB, Pruett TL: Aztreonam vs. gentamicin in experimental peritonitis and intra-abdominal abscess formation. Am Surg 60:849, 1994.
17. Davis JH, Hull AB: A possible toxic factor in abdominal injury. J Trauma 2:291, 1962.
18. Filler RM, Sleeman HK: Pathogenesis of peritonitis I. The effect of *Escherichia coli* and hemoglobin on peritoneal absorption. Surgery 61:385, 1967.
19. Hall T, Nelson RD, Fiegel VD, et al: Mechanisms of the adjuvant action of hemoglobin in experimental peritonitis. 2. Influence of hemoglobin on human leukocyte chemotaxis in vitro. J Surg Res 22:174, 1977.
20. Lally KP, Nichols RL: Various intraperitoneal irrigation solutions in treating experimental fecal peritonitis. South Med J 74:789, 1981.
21. Lally KP, Shorr LD, Nichols RL: Adjunctive aminoglycoside lavage: Lack of efficacy in experimental fecal peritonitis. J Pediatr Surg 20:541, 1985.
22. Lally KP, Tretten JC, Torma MJ: Adjunctive antibiotic lavage in experimental peritonitis. Surg Gynecol Obstet 156:605, 1983.
23. Lawson KJ, Lavery I: Hydrogen peroxide vs normal saline lavage in experimental fecal peritonitis. Cleve Clin J Med 54:279, 1987.
24. Brown JM, Grosso MA, Harken AH: Cytokines, sepsis and the surgeon. Surg Gynecol Obstet 169:568, 1988.
25. Ertel W, Morrison MH, Wang P, et al: The complex pattern of cytokines in sepsis. Ann Surg 214:141, 1991.
26. Brown GL, Foshee H, Pietsch J, et al: Muramyl dipeptide enhances survival from experimental peritonitis. Arch Surg 121:47, 1986.
27. Almdahl SM, Bogwald J, Hoffman J, et al: Protection by aminated glucan in experimental endogenous peritonitis. Eur Surg Res 19:79, 1987.
28. Browder W, Williams D, Sherwood E, et al: Synergistic effect of nonspecific immunostimulation and antibiotics in experimental peritonitis. Surgery 102:206, 1987.
29. Dunn CW, Horton JW, Walker PB: Additive effect of an immunomodulator and broad-spectrum antibiotic in fecal peritonitis. Am J Surg 157:548, 1989.
30. Sawyer RG, Adams RB, May AK, et al: Anti–tumor necrosis factor antibody reduces mortality in the presence of antibiotic-induced tumor necrosis factor release. Arch Surg 128:73, 1993.
31. McMasters KM, Cheadle WG: Regulation of macrophage TNFα, IL-1β, and Ia (I-Aα) mRNA expression during peritonitis is site dependent. J Surg Res 54:426, 1993.
32. Guo W, Soltesz V, Ding JW, et al: Abdominal rubber drain piece

aggravates intra-abdominal sepsis in the rat. Eur J Clin Invest 24:540, 1994.
33. Altemeier WA: The bacterial flora of acute perforated appendicitis with peritonitis: A bacteriologic study based upon one hundred cases. Ann Surg 107:517, 1938.
34. Altemeier WA: The pathogenicity of the bacteria of appendicitis peritonitis: An experimental study. Surgery 11:374, 1942.
35. Nichols RL, Smith JW: Modern approach to the diagnosis of anaerobic sepsis. Surg Clin North Am 55:21, 1975.
36. Bentley DN, Nichols RL, Condon RE, et al: The microflora of the human ileum and intraabdominal colon: Results of direct needle aspiration at surgery and evaluation of the techniques. J Lab Clin Med 79:421, 1972.
37. Nichols RL: Intraabdominal sepsis: Characterization and treatment. J Infect Dis 135(Suppl):S54, 1977.
38. Nichols RL, Smith JW: Intragastric microbial colonization in common disease states of the stomach and duodenum. Ann Surg 182:557, 1975.
39. Gorbach SL, Bartlett JG: Anaerobic infections. N Engl J Med 290:1177, 1974.
40. Nichols RL, Condon RE, Bentley DW, et al: Ileal microflora in surgical patients. J Urol 105:351, 1971.
41. Nichols RL, Condon RE, Gorbach SL, et al: Efficacy of preoperative antimicrobial preparation of the bowel. Ann Surg 176:227, 1972.
42. Altemeier WA, Culbertson WR, Fullen WD, et al: Intraabdominal abscesses. Am J Surg 125:701, 1973.
43. Swenson RM, Lorber B, Michaelson TC, et al: The bacteriology of intraabdominal infections. Arch Surg 109:398, 1974.
44. Gorbach SL, Thadepalli H, Norsen J: Anaerobic microorganisms in intraabdominal infections. *In* Balows A, DeHaan RM, Dowell VR Jr, Guze LB (eds): Anaerobic Bacteria: Role in Disease. Springfield, IL, Charles C Thomas, 1974, pp 399–407.
45. Gorbach SL: Anaerobic infections: Treatment of intraabdominal sepsis. Ann Intern Med 83:377, 1975.
46. Tally FP, McGowan K, Kellum JM, et al: A randomized comparison of cefoxitin with or without amikacin and clindamycin plus amikacin in surgical sepsis. Ann Surg 193:318, 1981.
47. Rotstein DD, Pruett TL, Simmons RL: Microbiologic features and treatment of persistent peritonitis in patients in the intensive care unit. Can J Surg 29:247, 1986.
48. Nichols RL, Musik AC: Enterococcal infections in surgery—The mystery continues! Clin Infect Dis 15:72, 1992.
49. Lopes JO, Alves SH, Benevenga JP, et al: *Nocardia asteroides* peritonitis during continuous ambulatory peritoneal dialysis. Rev Inst Med Trop Sao Paulo 35:377, 1993.
50. Sanyal D, Bhandari S: CAPD peritonitis caused by *Lactobacillus rhamnosus.* J Hosp Infect 22:325, 1992.
51. Kent SJ, Van Scoy MS, Skerrett S: *Listeria monocytogenes* peritonitis with review of the literature. Aust N Z J Med 24:405, 1994.
52. Schoenmakers EAJM, Brummer RM, van Tiel FH: Spontaneous bacterial peritonitis due to *Streptococcus pneumoniae* in a male who did not have another concurrent infection. Clin Infect Dis 19:551, 1994.
53. Muñoz P, Fernández-Baca V, Peláez T, et al: *Aeromonas* peritonitis. Clin Infect Dis 18:32, 1994.
54. Perkins DJ, Newstead GL: *Campylobacter jejuni* enterocolitis causing peritonitis, ileitis and intestinal obstruction. Aust N Z J Surg 64:55, 1994.
55. Gruner E, Pfyffer GE, von Graevenitz A: Characterization of *Brevibacterium* ssp. from clinical specimens. J Clin Microbiol 31:1408, 1993.
56. Giladi M, Lee BE, Berlin OG, Panosian CB: Peritonitis caused by *Mycobacterium kansasii* in a patient undergoing continuous ambulatory peritoneal dialysis. Am J Kidney Dis 19:597, 1992.
57. Stone HH, Kolb LD, Geheber CE: Incidence and significance of intraperitoneal anaerobic bacteria. Ann Surg 181:705, 1975.
58. Hardin WD, Aran AJ, Smith JW, et al: Aerotolerance of commonly encountered anaerobic bacteria—Fact or fancy? South Med J 75:1051, 1982.
59. Ohmann C, Wittmann DH, Wacha H, and the Peritonitis Study Group: Prospective evaluation of prognostic scoring systems in peritonitis. Eur J Surg 159:267, 1993.
60. Dellinger EP, Wertz MJ, Meakins JL, et al: Surgical infection stratification system for intraabdominal infection. Arch Surg 120:21, 1985.
61. Solomkin JS, Meakins JL, Allo MD, et al: Antibiotic trials in intraabdominal infections: A critical evaluation of study design and outcome reporting. Ann Surg 200:29, 1984.
62. Thadepalli H, Gorbach SL, Broido PW, et al: Abdominal trauma, anaerobes and antibiotics. Surg Gynecol Obstet 173:270, 1973.
63. Gorbach SL: Treatment of intraabdominal infection. Am J Med 7(Suppl):107, 1984.
64. Hofstetter SR, Pachter HL, Bailey AA, et al: A prospective comparison of two regimens of prophylactic antibiotics in abdominal trauma: Cefoxitin versus triple drug. J Trauma 24:307, 1984.
65. Gentry LO, Feliciano DV, Lea AS, et al: Perioperative antibiotic therapy for penetrating injuries of the abdomen. Ann Surg 200:561, 1984.
66. Nichols RL, Smith JW, Klein DB, et al: Risk of infection after penetrating abdominal trauma. N Engl J Med 311:1065, 1984.
67. Jones RC, Thal ER, Johnson NA, et al: Evaluation of antibiotic therapy following penetrating abdominal trauma. Ann Surg 201:576, 1985.
68. Feliciano DV, Gentry LO, Bitondo CG, et al: Single agent cephalosporin prophylaxis for penetrating abdominal trauma—Results and comment on the emergence of the enterococcus. Am J Surg 152:674, 1986.
69. Dellinger EP, Wertz MJ, Lennard ES, Oreskovich MR: Efficacy of short-course antibiotic prophylaxis after penetrating abdominal injury: A prospective randomized trial. Arch Surg 121:23, 1986.
70. Fabian TC, Croce MA, Payne LW, Kudsk KA: Duration of antibiotic therapy for penetrating abdominal trauma: A prospective trial. Surgery 112:788, 1992.
71. Nichols RL, Smith JW, Robertson GD, et al: Prospective alterations in therapy for penetrating abdominal trauma. Arch Surg 128:55, 1993.
72. Browder W, Smith JW, Vivoda LM, et al: Nonperforative appendicitis: A continuing surgical dilemma. J Infect Dis 159:1088, 1989.
73. Aldridge KE: Anaerobes in polymicrobial surgical infections: Incidence, pathogenicity, and antimicrobial resistance. Eur J Surg Suppl 573:31, 1994.
74. Walker AP, Nichols RL, Wilson RF, et al: Efficacy of a β-lactamase inhibitor combination for serious intra-abdominal infections. Ann Surg 217:115, 1993.
75. Niinikoski J, Havia T, Alhava E, et al: Piperacillin/tazobactam versus imipenem/cilastatin in the treatment of intra-abdominal infections. Surg Gynecol Obstet 176:255, 1993.
76. Eklund AE, Nord CE, and Swedish Study Group: A randomized multicenter trial of piperacillin/tazobactam versus imipenem/cilastatin in the treatment of severe intra-abdominal infections. J Antimicrob Chemother 31(Suppl A):79, 1993.
77. Polk HC, Fink MP, Laverdiere M, et al: Prospective randomized study of piperacillin/tazobactam therapy of surgically treated intra-abdominal infection. Am Surg 59:598, 1993.
78. Bohnen JMA, Solomkin JS, Dellinger AP, et al: Guidelines for clinical care: Anti-infective agents for intra-abdominal infection, a Surgical Infection Society policy statement. Arch Surg 127:83, 1992.
79. Nichols RL, Wikler MA, McDevitt JT, et al: Coagulopathy associated with extended-spectrum cephalosporins in patients with serous infection. Antimicrob Agents Chemother 31:281, 1987.
80. DiPiro JT, Mansberger JA, Davis JB Jr: Current concepts in clinical therapeutics: Intra-abdominal infections. Clin Pharm 5:34, 1986.
81. Ho JL, Barza M: Role of aminoglycoside antibiotics in the treatment of intraabdominal infection. Antimicrob Agents Chemother 31:485, 1987.
82. Nichols RL: The treatment of intraabdominal infections in surgery. Diagn Microbiol Infect Dis 12:195(S), 1989.
83. Schumer W, Lee DK, Jones B: Peritoneal lavage in postoperative therapy of late peritoneal sepsis. Preliminary report. Surgery 55:841, 1964.
84. DiVincenti FC, Cohn I Jr: Intraperitoneal kanamycin in advanced peritonitis. A preliminary report. Am J Surg 3:147, 1966.
85. Noon GP, Beall AC Jr, Jordan GL Jr, et al: Clinical evaluation of peritoneal irrigation with antibiotic solution. Surgery 62:73, 1967.
86. Roth RM, Gleckman RA, Gantz NM, et al: Antibiotic irrigations—A plea for controlled clinical trials. Pharmacotherapy 5:222, 1985.

87. Pissiotis CA, Nichols RL, Condon RE: Absorption and excretion of intraperitoneally administered kanamycin sulfate. Surg Gynecol Obstet 134:995, 1972.
88. Rappaport WD, Holcomb M, Valente J, et al: Antibiotic irrigation and the formation of intraabdominal adhesions. Am J Surg 158:435, 1989.
89. Sindelar WF, Mason GR: Intraperitoneal irrigation with povidone-iodine solution for the prevention of intraabdominal abscesses in the bacterially contaminated abdomen. Surg Gynecol Obstet 148:409, 1979.
90. Ahrenholz DH, Simmons RL: Povidone-iodine in peritonitis. I. Adverse effects of local instillation in experimental *E. coli* peritonitis. J Surg Res 26:458, 1979.
91. Leiboff AR, Soroff HS: The treatment of generalized peritonitis by closed postoperative peritoneal lavage. Arch Surg 122:1005, 1987.
92. Hudspeth AS: Radical surgical debridement in the treatment of advanced generalized bacterial peritonitis. Arch Surg 110:1233, 1975.
93. Polk HC, Fry DE: Radical peritoneal débridement for established peritonitis: The results of a prospective randomized clinical trial. Ann Surg 192:350, 1980.
94. Steinberg D: On leaving the peritoneal cavity open in acute generalized suppurative peritonitis. Am J Surg 137:216, 1979.
95. Machiedo GW, Tikellis J, Suval W, et al: Reoperation for sepsis. Am Surg 51:149, 1985.
96. Teichmann W, Wittmann DH, Andreone PA: Scheduled reoperations *(Etappenlavage)* for diffuse peritonitis. Arch Surg 121:147, 1986.
97. Wittmann DH, Aprahamian C, Bergstein JM: Etappenlavage: Advanced diffuse peritonitis managed by planned multiple laparotomies utilizing zippers, slide fastener, and Velcro analogue for temporary abdominal closure. World J Surg 14:218, 1990.
98. Wittmann DH, Aprahamian C, Bergstein JM, et al: A burr-like device to facilitate temporary abdominal closure in planned multiple laparotomies. Eur J Surg 159:75, 1993.
99. Sleeman D, Sosa JL, Gonzalez A, et al: Reclosure of the open abdomen. J Am Coll Surg 180:200, 1995.
100. Andrus C, Doering M, Herrmann VM, et al: Planned reoperation for generalized intraabdominal infection. Am J Surg 152:682, 1986.
101. Butler JA, Huang J, Wilson SE: Repeated laparotomy for postoperative intraabdominal sepsis. Arch Surg 122:702, 1987.
102. McDougal WS, Izant RJ Jr, Zollinger RM Jr: Primary peritonitis in infancy and childhood. Ann Surg 181:310, 1975.
103. Speck WT, Dresdale SS, McMillan RW: Primary peritonitis and the nephrotic syndrome. Am J Surg 127:267, 1974.
104. Correra JP, Conn HO: Spontaneous bacterial peritonitis in cirrhosis: Endemic or epidemic? Med Clin North Am 59:963, 1975.
105. Wilner-Hanssen P, Westrom L, Mardh PA: Chlamydial perihepatitis. Scand J Infect Dis 32(Suppl):77, 1982.
106. Golden GT, Shaw A: Primary peritonitis. Surg Gynecol Obstet 135:513, 1972.
107. Conn HO: Spontaneous bacterial peritonitis: Multiple revisitations. Gastroenterology 70:455, 1976.
108. Grobmyer AJ III, Kerlan RA, Peterson CM, et al: Barium peritonitis. Am Surg 2:116, 1984.
109. Rubin J, Ray R, Barnes T, et al: Peritonitis in continuous ambulatory peritoneal dialysis patients. Am J Kidney Dis 2:602, 1983.
110. Balaie GR, Eisele G: Continuous ambulatory peritoneal dialysis: A review of its mechanics, advantages, complications, and areas of controversy. Ann Pharmacother 26:1409, 1992.
111. von Graevenitz A, Amsterdam D: Microbiological aspects of peritonitis associated with continuous ambulatory peritoneal dialysis. Clin Microbiol Rev 5:36, 1992.
112. Saklayen MG: CAPD peritonitis. Incidence, pathogens, diagnosis and management. Med Clin North Am 74:997, 1990.
113. Smith JA: Treatment of intra-abdominal infections with quinolones. Eur J Clin Microbiol Infect Dis 10:330, 1991.
114. Janknegt R: CAPD peritonitis and fluoroquinolones: A review. Perit Dial Int 11:53, 1991.
115. Dineen P, Homan WP, Grafe WR: Tuberculous peritonitis: 43 years' experience in diagnosis and treatment. Ann Surg 184:717, 1976.

87

Intraabdominal Abscesses

Avery B. Nathens
Ori D. Rotstein

Intraabdominal abscesses are localized collections of purulent material that are walled off from the rest of the peritoneal cavity by inflammatory adhesions, loops of intestine and their mesentery, the greater omentum, and other viscera. The development of an abscess reflects the successful prevention of disseminated infection by local host defense mechanisms in the peritoneal cavity. However, complete resolution of infection is thwarted by the inability of immune cells to function within the microenvironment of the abscess cavity.

Abscesses may occur in the peritoneal cavity, either within or outside the abdominal viscera, or in the retroperitoneum. Nonvisceral abscesses within the peritoneal cavity represent a consequence of a disruption of the gastrointestinal tract, whether it occurs spontaneously or posttraumatically. Visceral abscesses most commonly occur from hematogenous or lymphatic spread of bacteria to the particular organ. Retroperitoneal abscesses originate through one of several mechanisms, including perforation of the gastrointestinal tract into the retroperitoneal space or hematogenous or lymphatic spread of bacteria to the retroperitoneal organs, particularly into the inflamed pancreas. Visceral abscesses refer to abscesses originating in the liver or spleen. These as well as retroperitoneal abscesses related to the pancreas and kidney are discussed elsewhere in this book. The present discussion focuses on the pathogenesis, diagnosis, and management of nonvisceral abscesses of the peritoneal cavity.

Etiology

Intraabdominal abscesses arise in three general settings: (1) after perforation of the gastrointestinal tract with resolution of diffuse peritonitis in which a loculated area of infection persists and evolves into an abscess, (2) after a spontaneous or traumatic perforation of the gastrointestinal tract, and (3) in the postoperative period after anastomotic disruption. The formation of abscesses in each of these settings depends on the normal function of peritoneal defense mechanisms that serve to sequester and wall off infection.

The etiology and location of abscesses have changed in time owing to advances in antibiotic therapy and improved surgical technique. Altemeier and colleagues[1] reviewed a series of 540 abscesses in 501 patients during an 11-year period spanning 1961 to 1972. Nonvisceral intraperitoneal abscesses constituted approximately 36% of all cases reviewed. Most of these were located in the right lower quadrant (44%), and appendicitis was deemed to be the underlying pathologic process in 50%. Later series have documented that more than 80% of intraabdominal abscesses occur in the postoperative period, with the majority following pancreaticobiliary or colorectal surgery[2, 3] (Table 87–1). This may be a reflection of the technically difficult anastomoses in the former and the large bacterial load in the latter. More than 30% of abscesses are associated with clear evidence of an anastomotic leak.[3, 4] By contrast, intraabdominal abscesses unassociated with

TABLE 87–1 ■ Frequency of Postoperative Abscess Formation in Relation to Site of Initial Operation

SITE OF INITIAL OPERATION	FREQUENCY OF POSTOPERATIVE ABSCESS (%)
Pancreas and biliary tract	20
Colon	15
Stomach	9
Retroperitoneum	9
Trauma	9
Duodenum	8
Appendix	6
Kidney and adrenal gland	5
Small intestine	4
Spleen	4
Liver	4
Vascular	2
Uterus and ovary	1
Others	11

From Levison MA, Zeigler D: Correlation of APACHE II score, drainage technique and outcome in postoperative intra-abdominal abscess. Surg Gynecol Obstet 172:89–94, 1991. By permission of Surgery, Gynecology & Obstetrics, now known as the Journal of the American College of Surgeons.

prior operation are most commonly due to inflammatory processes with a small, localized perforation as in appendicitis, diverticulitis, and Crohn disease.[3, 5]

The spectrum of organisms inoculating the peritoneum after violation of the gastrointestinal tract is remarkably diverse. The distal small bowel and colon contain more than 500 species of bacteria at a concentration of 10^{12} organisms per gram of luminal contents with an anaerobe/aerobe ratio of 1000:1.[6, 7] Whereas large numbers of bacteria may contaminate the peritoneal cavity, early events involved in abscess formation result in both a marked simplification and a change in the rank order of their prevalence from that found in the gastrointestinal tract (Table 87–2). Cultures obtained from abscesses under optimal conditions usually reveal mixed aerobic and anaerobic species, with *Escherichia coli, Enterococcus*, and *Bacteroides fragilis* predominating. The process of simplification provides evidence for the existence of interactions among bacterial species and between bacteria and host defense mechanisms that allow an ideal environment for abscess formation. The central role of *B. fragilis* in abscess formation has been delineated in a series of experiments in which known quantities of *E. coli, B. fragilis, Fusobacterium varium*, or enterococcus within gelatin capsules were inoculated in the peritoneal cavity. Neither *E. coli* nor enterococci produced intraabdominal abscesses, nor did combinations of the two aerobes or the two anaerobes. By contrast, a mixed anaerobe-aerobe inoculum consistently produced intraperitoneal abscesses. Subsequent work has provided evidence that the capsular polysaccharide complex derived from *B. fragilis* is the primary virulence determinant necessary for abscess formation.[8, 9] Intraperitoneal administration of this complex without live organisms results in bacteriologically sterile abscesses, yet they are histologically identical to those formed in response to viable bacteria.

TABLE 87–2 ■ Comparison of Common Bacterial Isolates from Normal Colonic Flora and from Intraabdominal Abscesses

COLONIC ISOLATES*		ABSCESS ISOLATES†	
Rank	**Organism**	**Rank**	**Organism**
1	*Bacteroides vulgatus*	1	*Escherichia coli*
2	*Fusobacterium prausnitzii*	2	*Enterococcus*
3	*Bifidobacterium adolescentis*	3	*Klebsiella*
4	*Eubacterium aerofaciens*	4	*Bacteroides fragilis*
5	*Peptostreptococcus productus II*	5	*Pseudomonas*
6	*Bacteroides thetaiotaomicron*	6	*Staphylococcus*
7	*Eubacterium eligens*	7	*Candida*
8	*Peptostreptococcus productus I*	8	*Enterobacter*
9	*Eubacterium biforme*	9	*Clostridium*
10	*Eubacterium aerofaciens III*	10	*Proteus*
11	*Bacteroides distasonis*	11	*Serratia*
28	*Bacteroides ovatus*		
29	*Bacteroides fragilis*		
59–75	*Enterococcus*		
76–113	*Escherichia coli, Klebsiella*		

*Adapted from Moore WEC, Holdeman LV: Human fecal flora: The normal flora of 20 Japanese-Hawaiians. Appl Microbiol 27:961–979, 1974. © by Springer-Verlag.

†Adapted from Olson MM, Allen MO: Nosocomial abscess. Results of an eight-year prospective study of 32,284 operations. Arch Surg 124:356–361, 1989; and Olak J, Christou NV, Stein LA, et al: Operative vs percutaneous drainage of intra-abdominal abscesses. Comparison of morbidity and mortality. Arch Surg 121:141–146, 1986.

In the postoperative patient, resistant gram-negative organisms or yeast may be isolated as a result of extensive use of empirical broad-spectrum antibiotics in the preoperative setting. In addition, such organisms may develop when antibiotics are used empirically for postoperative febrile episodes in an attempt to "treat the fever" rather than drain the abscess.

Pathogenesis of Abscess Formation

Bacterial contamination of the peritoneal cavity initiates a complex series of events that ultimately result in abscess formation. After peritoneal soiling, massive bacterial contamination is limited by mechanical clearance through the diaphragmatic lymphatics such that more than 60% of organisms are cleared within the first 60 minutes of contamination.[10] Locally, peritoneal macrophages and mesothelial cells elaborate proinflammatory mediators in response to lipopolysaccharide derived from gram-negative bacteria, leading to hyperemia, exudation of protein-rich fluid containing fibrinogen, and a massive influx of phagocytic cells.[11, 12] This phagocytic phase lasts approximately 48 to 72 hours, during which time the majority of organisms are ingested either by neutrophils during the early inflammatory response or by peritoneal macrophages at later time points.

The early events set the stage for the localization phase in which residual bacteria and inflammatory cells are localized within fibrinous exudates, loops of bowel, and omentum. Fibrin deposition is mediated by the procoagulant effect of activated macrophages and damaged peritoneal mesothelial cells through the cellular expression of tissue factor, which initiates the coagulation cascade.[13, 14] Further, fibrin deposition is facilitated through a reduction in peritoneal fibrinolytic activity mediated by a marked increase in peritoneal fluid plasminogen activator inhibitor.[15] The initiation of coagulation in response to bacterial infection is recognized as a mechanism that is both protective and potentially harmful. During the early phases of peritonitis, fibrin matrices serve to sequester bacteria within the peritoneal cavity and further localize the contamination by causing loops of intestine to adhere to both each other and the omentum, thereby preventing disseminated infection and bacteremia. The protective role of fibrin is demonstrated by studies in which fibrin deposition is prevented through the administration of tissue plasminogen activator[16] or systemic fibrinogen depletion.[17] Both interventions significantly increase bacteremia and mortality in a rodent model of intraabdominal infection.

By virtue of its ability to effectively wall off and contain infection locally, peritoneal fibrin deposition plays an important role in abscess formation. The ability of fibrin to enmesh microorganisms appears to protect the bacteria from normal host clearance mechanisms, thereby permitting unopposed proliferation and ultimately the establishment of an abscess.[18, 19] That fibrin deposition is a necessary component of abscess formation has been outlined in a series of experiments in which aerosolized fibrinogen administered into the contaminated peritoneum augments formation of abscesses,[20] whereas fibrinolytic agents almost completely abrogate their development.[16]

The contribution of the specific and the nonspecific cellular immune responses to the localization phase of abscess formation remains poorly defined. Classically, phagocytic cells have been considered to constitute the major cellular defense against intraabdominal infection. As described before, peritoneal macrophages appear to be important in abscess development through induction of procoagulant activity on exposure to bacterial lipopolysaccharide.[21] However, evidence suggests that the ability of the capsular polysaccharide complex of *B. fragilis* to induce the formation of abscesses is dependent on the presence of nonimmune $CD4^+/CD8^+$ T cells.[22] Furthermore, rodent studies have demonstrated that abscess formation can be prevented by preimmunization with capsular polysaccharide complex, an effect dependent on specific $CD8^+$ T lymphocytes.[22, 23] Adoptive transfer with these cells prevented abscess formation in naive mice, as did the passive transfer of a soluble cell lysate derived from these immune T cells.[24] By contrast, systemic[25] or peritoneal[26] exposure to a combination of live *E. coli* and *B. fragilis* increased the number of intraabdominal abscesses in a murine intraabdominal abscess model. Although contradictory, these findings represent novel concepts implicating specific cell-mediated immunity in the pathogenesis of intraabdominal abscesses.

The subsequent processes involved in abscess formation and persistence are important to consider. A mature abscess consists of a central core containing necrotic debris, dead cells, and bacteria; a surrounding ring of neutrophils and macrophages; and a peripheral ring consisting of smooth muscle cells and fibroblasts within a collagen capsule.[27] The evolution from an infected phlegmonous mass to a well-defined abscess suggests a process by which bacteria are able to sequester themselves within a milieu where they are protected from the host's attempts to effect ultimate resolution of the infection. The chemical, bacterial, and physical microenvironment of an abscess leads to microbial persistence. Table 87–3 summarizes the potential mechanisms whereby bacterial clearance is frustrated, leading to persistent localized infection.

Clinical Manifestations

In contrast to patients with diffuse generalized peritonitis in whom the symptoms and physical findings are obvious, patients with intraabdominal abscesses frequently have less conspicuous findings. The local symptoms and signs vary with the source and location of the abscess and with the underlying status of the patient. Enteroparietal abscesses produce pain, tenderness, and a palpable, diffuse abdominal mass. Interloop, intramesenteric, and subphrenic abscesses are more cryptic because the visceral peritoneum is innervated by splanchnic rather than somatic pain fibers, and no mass can be palpated. Patients with subphrenic abscesses may additionally have hiccups, cough, tachypnea, or jaundice.[49] Nonspecific thoracic manifestations include pleural effusions, elevation of the diaphragm, and decreased basilar breath sounds.[50, 51] Retroperitoneal abscesses may produce only lumbar or ileopsoas muscle spasm or referred pain to the hip, groin, or knee.[52] Chronic psoas abscesses may present with an irritable hip and back pain with a flexion deformity of the hip and wasting of the quadriceps femoris.[53] Pelvic abscesses can be palpated on rectal examination but usually give few symptoms. Intractable diarrhea may occur as the presenting feature in as many as 20% of patients owing to irritability of the sigmoid colon as a result of the adjacent inflammatory process.[54]

The most common systemic sign of an intraabdominal abscess is a low-grade fever. This is frequently associated with anorexia, general malaise, and weakness. Systemic evidence of inflammation is often reflected in the peripheral leukocyte count, as noted by a leukocytosis or a left shift toward immature forms. Additional laboratory investigation adds little to confirm the diagnosis.

TABLE 87–3 ■ Local Factors in Abscesses That Favor Microbial Persistence

FACTOR	EFFECT	REFERENCE
Microenvironmental		
Hypoxia	Impairs neutrophil migration and killing	28–30
Low pH	Impairs neutrophil migration, phagocytosis, and killing	28, 31–33
Hyperosmolarity	Impairs neutrophil phagocytosis, cell degranulation, and killing	34, 35
Hypercapnia	Reduced phagocytic cell cytoplasmic pH leads to cell dysfunction	36
Microbiologic		
Bacterial synergy	Optimizes microenvironment for bacterial growth, provision of nutrients between bacterial partners	37, 38
High concentrations of bacterial by-products/cell wall components/proteases	Impaired phagocytic function, local tissue damage, complement depletion	39
Adjuvant Materials		
Necrotic debris	Complement depletion, neutrophil deactivation	40, 41
Blood, hemoglobin, fibrin	Impaired phagocytic cell function, reduced access of cell to bacteria	19, 42
Barium sulfate	Reduced access of cells to bacteria	43
Bile salts	Toxic to neutrophils	44
Hemostatic agents	Impaired neutrophil function	45
Foreign body	Premature activation of neutrophils	46, 47
Unknown	Impaired macrophage antigen-presenting capacity	48

In the postoperative patient, the abdominal symptoms are masked by incisional pain and postoperative analgesics. Physical examination is notoriously unreliable in this period—in most patients the abdomen is distended and tender. In addition, the clinical findings associated with an intraabdominal abscess may be masked by the administration of antibiotics to the patient. The median time from initial operation to clinical presentation in a series of 114 abscesses was 8 days.[4] In this series, the median time from presentation of abscess symptoms to drainage was 4 days. The systemic response to antibiotic therapy in the period after surgery for peritonitis may also provide a clue to the presence of residual intraabdominal infection. Studies have suggested that antibiotics may be discontinued in this setting with low probability of subsequent infection (less than 1%) if the patient is afebrile, has a normal leukocyte count, and has a band count less than 3%.[55, 56] This normalization usually occurs within 5 to 10 days. Extension beyond this period indicates persistent infection and should direct the physician to more intensive radiologic investigation.[55, 56] At times, the first sign of postoperative abscess formation may be progressive organ dysfunction leading to multiple organ failure.[57] Similarly, immunocompromised patients may present with shock as the only indication of ongoing intraabdominal infection. Occasionally, the reporting of an unexpected positive blood culture, particularly if it is polymicrobial or contains an anaerobe, will provide the first evidence of an intraabdominal abscess.[58, 59]

Diagnosis

Diagnosis is based on clinical suspicion of an abscess and radiologic confirmation. Conventional plain film radiographs of the abdomen may reveal loculated extraluminal gas collections or mottled soft tissue masses, either of which is indicative of abscess formation. More subtle signs include the presence of a localized ileus or obliteration of the psoas shadow or flank stripes. Chest radiographs may document the presence of a pleural effusion or atelectasis, features that may indicate the presence of a subphrenic collection.[60] A limited contrast-enhanced examination may be useful to investigate the integrity of an anastomosis in the postoperative period or to differentiate the stomach from an extraluminal mass noted on a plain film. At best, conventional radiographic techniques offer indirect evidence of an abscess. Suspicion of an abscess based on the clinical picture should direct the physician to the use of imaging techniques to confirm the diagnosis and anatomically define the abscess.

Advances in ultrasonography and computed tomography (CT) have allowed the accurate and expeditious diagnosis of intraabdominal abscess in almost all patients. These techniques have largely replaced conventional radiography and nuclear scintigraphy; new techniques, such as magnetic resonance imaging, have yet to achieve a significant role.

Ultrasonography is a sensitive tool for the detection and localization of fluid collections in the abdomen and pelvis. It is rapid and noninvasive, and it does not expose the patient to additional radiation. It has real-time capabilities that can visualize bowel peristalsis, thereby enhancing differentiation between fluid-filled bowel and abscesses. The availability of mobile machines permits bedside examination, allowing safe examination of critically ill patients in the intensive care unit without the added risk of transporting them to the radiology department. Sensitivity and specificity of ultrasonography in the detection of abscesses are in the range of 80% to 90%, depending on the site of the abscess and skill of the operator.[61, 62] The right upper quadrant, pelvis, and left upper quadrant (when the spleen is present) are best visualized by ultrasonography, and it is therefore most appropriate to limit its use to these regions.[63] In addition, the use of endoluminal probes allows transvaginal or transrectal visualization and drainage of deep pelvic abscesses, an advantage not offered by other techniques.[64, 65]

The principal disadvantages of ultrasound examination are related to its technical limitations and lack of specificity in the postoperative setting. Intestinal gas reflects transmitted sound waves and prevents imaging of large areas of the abdomen, pelvis, and retroperitoneum. This may be a particular problem in the postoperative setting in patients with an ileus when multiple distended air-filled bowel loops make examination difficult. Patients with open wounds, extensive dressings, drains, or stomas are poorly suited for ultrasound examination because of the lack of acoustic windows.

CT has several advantages over the use of ultrasonography and proves to be the most accurate technique available for the diagnosis of intraabdominal abscesses.[61, 66] Sensitivity and specificity are in the range of 97.5% and 85%, respectively.[61] Its advantages include higher resolution, operator independence, and an ability to see deep to bone and gas-filled structures without the need for an intact abdominal wall. It has proved excellent in visualizing the retroperitoneum, with a sensitivity approaching 100%, in contrast to a sensitivity of 67% for ultrasonography.[52] Optimal detection by CT depends on the administration of intravenous contrast material and gastrointestinal contrast to opacify bowel. Gastrointestinal contrast enhancement improves the differentiation of fluid-filled bowel from an abscess. Criteria for the identification of an abscess by CT include identification of an area of low attenuation in an extraluminal location. The CT attenuation of material within an abscess cavity falls between that of water and soft tissue (0 to 40 Hounsfield units). Intracavitary gas, thick or irregular walls, contrast enhancement of the wall, heterogeneous internal debris, and displacement of surrounding viscera or edema of the adjacent tissue planes are additional useful features.[63] A long air-fluid level within an abscess suggests a fistulous connection to the bowel.[67]

The major disadvantages of CT are the requirement for a cooperative patient who will remain immobile and the lack of portability of the unit. In addition, the expense of the machine limits its widespread availability. The accuracy of the scan is reduced in patients in whom the gastrointestinal tract is not opacified with contrast material. In this setting, the scans are limited in their ability to distinguish fluid-filled bowel loops from an abscess. Interloop abscesses, which represent 4% of all abscesses, are also poorly visualized with CT.[68] Finally, artifacts related to the presence of surgical clips or residual barium in the gastrointestinal tract may limit the accuracy of this technique.

Whereas both ultrasonography and CT demonstrate a high degree of accuracy with respect to anatomic localization of fluid collections, both are somewhat limited in their ability to discern the origin of the collection. Fluid-filled collections simulating abscesses include hematomas, bilomas, lymphoceles, seromas, and urinomas. In two prospective studies, 19% to 23% of asymptomatic patients had evidence of fluid collections on the fourth or fifth postoperative day.[69, 70] Most of these were crescent shaped and conformed to the peritoneal recesses. Only 6% of patients still demonstrated fluid on the eighth postoperative day, suggesting that most were sterile collections relating to the surgical procedure rather than early abscesses.[70] In those patients in whom diagnosis is in doubt, ultrasound- or CT-guided diagnostic aspiration can contribute to an accurate diagnosis by providing fluid for Gram stain and culture. Percutaneous needle aspiration of intraabdominal collections for the purpose of diagnosis therefore represents an important adjuvant technique to scanning.[71] This technique will help guide the physician with respect to further surgery, therapeutic percutaneous drainage, or conservative management.

Studies comparing ultrasonography with CT generally demonstrate CT to be the superior modality with respect to accuracy.[72, 73] However, the advantages and disadvantages of each technique (summarized in Table 87–4) must be considered in the particular clinical setting and with consideration of the resources and expertise available.

Nuclear scintigraphy using either gallium citrate Ga 67 or indium In 111 has a limited role in the diagnosis of intraabdominal abscesses. Gallium has an affinity for iron-binding proteins present on leukocytes and on bacterial surfaces and is thus concentrated at sites of infection.[74] The detection of an abscess is based on increased uptake outside of expected sites. However, gallium is excreted in the colon and accumulates in the stool. An enema is necessary to clear radiolabeled stool and allow interpretation of the study. Other disadvantages of this technique include the false-positive imaging of neoplasms and the 24- to 72-hour delay required between injection of the radionuclide and the scanning procedure.

In a white blood cell scan, ^{111}In in the form of the chelate with oxyquinoline is used to label leukocytes drawn from the patient.[61, 75] After labeling, the cells are reinjected into the patient, and the patient is scanned with a gamma camera. Although conceptually attractive, this technique has several shortcomings. Labeling of granulocytes with ^{111}In requires a highly skilled technician. In addition, because this technique depends on delivery of neutrophils to a site of acute inflammation, it may be associated with a significant number of false-negative test results in patients with chronic infection.[61] Neither ^{111}In nor gallium scans are effective in the early postoperative period. Peritoneal inflammation at this time will attract the isotopes, and all sites at which dissection has occurred will show isotope localization. There may be some benefit from these scanning techniques in the later postoperative period (greater than 2 weeks), once inflammation has quiesced.[76] Finally, these tests do not provide sufficiently accurate localization of the collection to permit diagnostic needle aspiration or insertion of a percutaneous drainage catheter. In general, these two techniques do not add much to the diagnostic armamentarium of intraabdominal infection. They may be useful as an initial screening examination in patients who are not critically ill and do not have a localizing site of infection. If uptake is noted in the abdomen, subsequent CT or ultrasound scanning may be used to better define the lesion.

The role of magnetic resonance imaging in the diagnosis of intraabdominal abscesses requires further definition. Initial studies have suggested potential advantages.[77] Surgical clips do not interfere with imaging, and intravenous contrast enhancement is not necessary to outline the abscess or distinguish it from adjacent structures. In addition, sagittal section may be useful in the pelvis to provide improved anatomic definition. The extended time required for imaging and the excellent sensitivity and specificity of CT and ultrasonography suggest only a minor role for magnetic resonance imaging in the diagnosis of intraabdominal infection. The use of spectroscopy to evaluate parameters such as tissue pH may ultimately be helpful in differentiating among various fluid collections, an ability presently lacking with ultrasonography and CT.

Management

Three basic principles guide the management of intraabdominal abscesses. These include (1) supportive care of the patient; (2) antibiotic administration; and (3) drainage of the abscess, either percutaneously or operatively.

Supportive Management

Patients with intraabdominal abscess show a spectrum of clinical presentations ranging from a low-grade fever to frank septic shock. In general, these patients have intravascular volume depletion that calls for fluid resuscitation and monitoring. The intensity of resuscitation and monitoring depends on the status of the patient. Hourly monitoring of vital signs, urine output, and mental status may be necessary. In the critically ill individual, Swan-Ganz catheterization and invasive arterial monitoring are essential to direct initial resuscitation, particularly if administration of inotropic agents is necessary. Hypoxemia may be present for several reasons. Atelectasis, basilar pneumonia, and pleural effusions may exist secondary to abdominal distention and elevation of the diaphragm or a subdiaphragmatic inflammatory process. Intraabdominal infection is intimately associated with the development of a host-derived systemic inflammatory response mediated by several proinflammatory mediators, perhaps the most important of which are tumor necrosis factor, interleukin-1, and interleukin-6.[78, 79] If the process is advanced, early signs of organ dysfunction may develop, resulting in hemodynamic instability, the adult respiratory distress syndrome, and renal dysfunction. Adjunctive mediator-directed therapy using antibodies directed against endotoxin[80] or tumor necrosis factor[81] has not demonstrated any significant benefit. An attempt to modulate the inflammatory response with the use of corticosteroids[82] has been demonstrated to be deleterious in patients with documented infection. Subset

TABLE 87–4 ■ Role of Ultrasonography and Computed Tomography in the Diagnosis of Intraabdominal Abscesses

	ULTRASONOGRAPHY	COMPUTED TOMOGRAPHY
Advantages	Rapid	Higher resolution
	Portable	Superior imaging of the retroperitoneum
	No ionizing radiation	Operator independent
	Visualizes bowel peristalsis—may allow differentiation of bowel from abscess	
	Greatest sensitivity in right upper quadrant, pelvis	
Disadvantages	Limited sensitivity in obese patients due to signal attenuation	Requires transport of the patient—difficult in the critically ill patient
	Limited sensitivity in patients with gaseous abdominal distention (e.g., ileus)	Barium sulfate, metallic clips may cause image distortion
	Operator dependent	Not available in all centers
	Technically difficult in presence of open abdominal wounds, stomas, or bulky abdominal dressings	Expensive

analysis in two large clinical trials using antagonists directed against platelet-activating factor[83] or the interleukin-1 receptor[84] has demonstrated marginal efficacy in patients with sepsis at greatest risk for mortality. Although it is conceptually attractive, the role of mediator-directed therapy remains to be defined, and its use is limited to carefully controlled clinical trials.

Nutritional support is important to prevent further debilitation. Patients in whom abscesses develop in the postoperative period are already at a nutritional disadvantage because they have usually spent 7 to 10 days without adequate calorie intake. The marked catabolic response associated with sepsis further aggravates this problem. Historically, total parenteral nutrition has been preferred in patients with intraabdominal infection. However, evidence suggests that nutritional supplementation by the enteral route may reduce the frequency of infectious complications and improve the immune status of critically ill patients.[85–87] Furthermore, enteral feeding within 24 hours of laparotomy appears to be well tolerated in the majority of patients. Similarly, patients with enterocutaneous fistulae may be managed by use of this approach as long as adequate drainage prevents further contamination of the peritoneal cavity.[88]

Antimicrobial Therapy

Empirical antibiotic therapy should be initiated once the diagnosis of intraabdominal abscess is suspected. Antimicrobial therapy should include an agent or agents with activity against both aerobic and anaerobic organisms. Previously, dual-agent therapy with an aminoglycoside and an antianaerobe agent such as metronidazole was considered the "gold standard." The development of second- and third-generation cephalosporins, carbapenems, monobactam agents, and acylureidopenicillins (in combination with a β-lactamase inhibitor) has resulted in the availability of several single-agent or combination regimens of equal or improved efficacy[89] (Table 87–5).

Newer quinolone agents such as ciprofloxacin in combination with metronidazole or clindamycin show particular promise in facilitating the management of intraabdominal abscess formation. The availability of both intravenous and oral preparations allows initial intravenous therapy followed by a course of oral therapy.[89a] This may significantly reduce costs related to both the antimicrobial agents and the hospital stay without compromising efficacy.

The decision regarding a particular regimen is based on consideration of both the efficacy and toxicity profile in each patient. Abscess isolates do not usually demonstrate significant antimicrobial resistance—a second-generation cephalosporin with anaerobic activity or ticarcillin in combination with a β-lactamase inhibitor is usually satisfactory. Debilitated, immunocompromised, or critically ill patients are at risk for resistant organisms and thus require special consideration. In these patients, the use of imipenem-cilastatin is of documented efficacy.[90, 91]

Supportive care and antimicrobial therapy serve primarily as adjuncts to drainage of the abscess cavity. Antibiotics alone are unlikely to be effective for numerous reasons. These include poor penetration of antibiotics into the abscess center; inactivation of antibiotics in the low pH, hypoxic suppurative environment; and inactivity of the drug against a large bacterial inoculum.[92, 93] Drainage of an abscess reverses these adverse conditions and increases the efficacy of the antibiotics.

TABLE 87–5 ■ Antibiotic Therapy for Intraabdominal Abscesses

MONOTHERAPY	COMBINATION THERAPY
Mild to Moderate Infections	
Cefoxitin	Antianaerobe plus aminoglycoside
Cefotetan	Antianaerobe plus third-generation cephalosporin
Cefmetazole	
Piperacillin-tazobactam	Antianaerobe plus ciprofloxacin (oral or intravenous regimen)
Ticarcillin-clavulanate	
	Clindamycin plus aztreonam
Severe Infections	
Imipenem-cilastatin	

From Bohnen JMA, Solomkin JS, Dellinger EP, et al: Guidelines for clinical care: Anti-infective agents for intraabdominal infection. Arch Surg 127:83–89, 1992. Copyright 1992, American Medical Association.

Drainage

Percutaneous abscess drainage (PAD) has become the interventional approach of choice for the management of intraabdominal abscesses, having superseded operative drainage as the first line of therapy. In early studies, attempts at PAD were limited to simple abscesses—well-defined, unilocular collections without evidence of enteral communication and no significant tissue necrosis. Multiple or multiloculated abscesses, those that form a fistula to adjacent organs or bowel, and abscesses containing viscous fluid, debris, or necrotic material were defined as complex and were formerly considered contraindications to PAD. However, extensive experience in the last decade has demonstrated that percutaneous management of complex abscesses is feasible and represents a reasonable approach in almost all cases.

The care of patients undergoing PAD is similar to that of those undergoing operative drainage. Intravenous antibiotic therapy should be administered before the procedure. Either ultrasonography or CT is used to image the abscess and provide guidance for abscess drainage. The choice of technique depends largely on the size and location of the abscess, operator preference, and status of the patient. For example, portable ultrasound examination and PAD may be performed at the bedside in critically ill unstable patients, a distinct advantage over CT. Once the abscess is visualized, percutaneous drainage is achieved with use of a modified Seldinger technique. A fine needle (20 or 22 gauge) is guided into the collection both for localization and aspiration of a sample of fluid. A guide wire is placed through the needle into the cavity, and then an 8.3 F to 14 F catheter is placed into the cavity over the guide wire, followed by removal of the guide wire. Larger bore tubes do not necessarily lead to more effective drainage. The principal determinant of drain efficacy is the presence of multiple large side holes that prevent catheter occlusion with abscess contents. Complex abscesses including those with multiple septa, hematoma, or thick purulent fluid within the abscess pose particularly difficult management problems because of catheter occlusion and ineffective drainage. Preliminary experimental[94] and clinical[95] studies suggest a potential role for intracavitary urokinase in reducing abscess fluid viscosity through its fibrinolytic effect. Intracavitary urokinase appears to be safe, without adverse effects on systemic coagulation. However, its value remains to be demonstrated in controlled clinical studies.

Close monitoring of both the patient and the percutaneous drain is as vital to outcome for the patient as is postoperative care after operative drainage. Catheters are placed to gravity drainage or low suction. Daily irrigation with 10 to 15 mL of saline should be performed to maintain catheter patency. Repeated CT or ultrasound examination and sinograms are necessary to ensure a progressive reduction in cavity size and to discern whether any enteral communication exists. Criteria for removal of the percutaneous catheter include (1) clinical resolution of septic parameters as judged by the patient's well-being, normal temperature, and normal leukocyte count; (2) minimal serous drainage from the catheter; and (3) radiologic evidence of abscess resolution as judged by sinogram or abdominal imaging. Some authors have recommended gradual removal of the catheter during 1 to 2 days,[96] although this is not our preference. The overall duration of drainage varies widely from 7 to 47 days.[97] In general, the prolonged drainage periods are due to the presence of an enteric communication. Major complications of percutaneous drainage occur in 0% to 5% of patients and include hemorrhage, intestinal perforation and enteric fistulae, and empyemas resulting from inadvertent transpleural passage of the catheter.[98–100]

A clinical response to drainage should be observed within 48 to 72 hours of drainage. The development or persistence of fever and leukocytosis within 72 hours of drainage is worrisome and suggests a definite need for reevaluation.[101] Possible reasons for failure include ineffective drainage because of inadequate catheter size or position, an undrained area of contiguous abscess, a large enteric communication, or the presence of a second unrecognized abscess. A repeated CT scan with or without a sinogram will elucidate the cause of persistent infection. Residual abscesses can then be percutaneously drained or the catheter repositioned if necessary (Fig. 87–1). If residual infections exist that cannot be adequately drained, or if no residual collections are seen, a formal laparotomy should be performed.

Outcome after percutaneous drainage is stratified as a curative success, palliative success, or failure.[102, 103] A curative success provides complete cure without the need for additional percutaneous or operative intervention. Palliative success implies the use of percutaneous drainage when cure is impossible, such as an unresectable, infected tumor mass. More frequently, palliative success refers to the ability of percutaneous drainage to act as a temporizing measure providing for stabilization of the patient before definitive operative management. This is particularly important in the management of diverticular abscesses. Before the use of PAD, patients presenting with a diverticular abscess required a two- or three-stage procedure including abscess drainage, proximal diverting colostomy, sigmoid colectomy and anastomosis, and reversal of colostomy. However, in more than two thirds of patients, local control of the abscess with PAD allows single-stage sigmoid colectomy and primary anastomosis in an elective setting.[97, 100] Similarly, patients presenting with spontaneous abscesses as a result of a perforated viscus may be treated with initial percutaneous drainage. Operative intervention may then be postponed or deemed unnecessary, depending on the nature of the underlying disease.[104] Most spontaneous and postoperative abscesses occur as a result of perforation of a viscus or anastomotic leak. The enteral communication often presents as a sudden increase in drainage of gastrointestinal contents from the catheter. Many of these fistulae may be managed conservatively, provided that the intraabdominal infection is controlled. Various factors including local conditions and site of origin of the fistula influence the likelihood of spontaneous closure (Table 87–6). These warrant consideration in the clinical decision-making process.

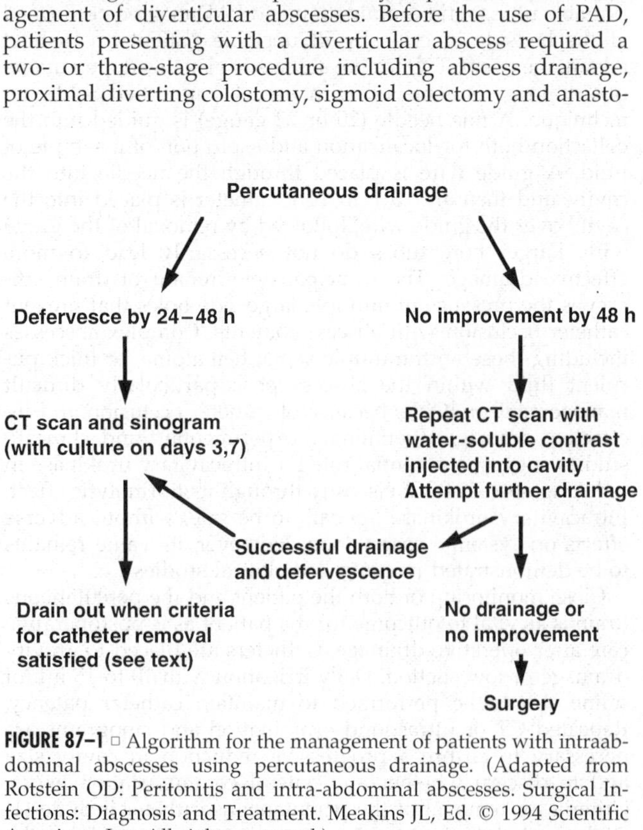

FIGURE 87–1 Algorithm for the management of patients with intraabdominal abscesses using percutaneous drainage. (Adapted from Rotstein OD: Peritonitis and intra-abdominal abscesses. Surgical Infections: Diagnosis and Treatment. Meakins JL, Ed. © 1994 Scientific American, Inc. All rights reserved.)

TABLE 87–6 ■ Probability of Fistula Closure in Relation to Underlying Disease and Location

DISEASE AND LOCATION	SPONTANEOUS CLOSURE RATE (%)
Local Factor	
Local infection/abscess	Virtually 0
Complete anastomotic dehiscence	Virtually 0
Retained foreign body	Virtually 0
Epithelialization of tract	Virtually 0
Distal obstruction	Virtually 0
Crohn disease	8
Irradiation of small bowel	14
Tract <2 cm	17
Malignant neoplasm	26
Closure rate with none of these factors	32
Origin of Fistula	
Esophagus	82
Stomach	43
Duodenum (end)	50
Duodenum (lateral)	27
Jejunum	21
Ilium	19
Pancreas	67
External biliary tree	60
Cecum/appendix	44
Colon	30
Rectum	30

Adapted from Reber HA, Roberts C, Way LW, Dunphy JE: Management of external gastrointestinal fistulas. Ann Surg 188:460–467, 1978.

An overall success rate of 81% to 89% has been reported for PAD.[105–109] The type, location, and cause of the abscess have a significant influence on outcome. Simple abscesses are successfully drained in 82% to 95% of cases, whereas complex collections are associated with a 45% to 69% success rate. Equivalent rates of success have been documented with use of PAD or operative drainage for simple abscesses, whereas complex abscesses may be treated successfully more often by operation,[110] although it is probably reasonable to attempt PAD as a first-line approach. In certain situations, operative management should be resorted to without primary PAD. Clearly, when the abscess is inaccessible or ill-defined, or CT demonstrates multiple small abscesses or an infected phlegmon, an operative approach is necessary to ensure adequate drainage. With accurate CT localization, a direct (often extraserous) approach to abscesses in the subphrenic, subhepatic, or pelvic regions can be taken. A general laparotomy under these circumstances is unnecessary and may lead to complications such as enteric fistulae and bleeding. On the other hand, laparotomy is usually necessary when abscesses are in the lesser sac or when multiple abscesses are present. In addition, fluid collections developing in the early postoperative period (less than 72 hours) are usually not amenable to percutaneous drainage, because the collection is rarely localized. This frequently represents an anastomotic dehiscence, which requires a laparotomy to deal with both the anastomosis and peritoneal contamination.

In most patients, normal host defense mechanisms localize the infectious process as an abscess, allowing relatively straightforward management by either percutaneous or operative drainage. There is a subset of critically ill patients at risk for intraabdominal abscesses who manifest a systemic inflammatory response yet demonstrate no evidence of intraabdominal abscesses on imaging studies. At laparotomy, only poorly defined, serosanguineous collections are found, rather than discrete purulent abscesses.[111, 112] Peritoneal cultures yield organisms that are traditionally considered to be of low virulence, including *Enterococcus, Candida,* coagulase-negative staphylococcus, and *Pseudomonas aeruginosa.*[111–113] Associated organ dysfunction is common. This triad of organ dysfunction, poorly localized intraabdominal infection, and atypical pathogens constitutes a syndrome coined tertiary peritonitis.[111] It is believed that the imparied host defense mechanisms of critical illness render the localization process and subsequent abscess formation ineffective. The significance of these organisms is unclear. Their presence may be related to selection by antibiotic pressures or may be an indication of impaired systemic immunity. Management is complex and usually involves multiple laparotomies and intensive supportive therapy. Despite this, mortality is as high as 64%.[112]

Prevention

Intraabdominal abscesses most frequently occur after surgery on the gastrointestinal tract as a result of anastomotic leak. In this setting, prevention of postoperative sepsis is dependent on meticulous surgical technique. Anastomoses should be performed between ends of bowel that are free from tension and are well vascularized. Meticulous hemostasis should be achieved and foreign bodies avoided.

Abscesses after surgery for secondary peritonitis usually represent foci of residual infection. Prevention of abscess formation involves (1) elimination of the source of contamination, (2) reduction of bacterial contamination, and (3) specific measures geared toward the prevention of recurrent infection. The source of contamination is controlled by closing, excluding, or resecting the perforated viscus. Primary anastomoses are at increased risk for dehiscence when they are performed in the setting of acute inflammation or in the immunocompromised patient.[114] Bowel exteriorization should be performed to circumvent the potential dangers of anastomotic breakdown. This is necessary in almost all cases, although in the setting of acute diverticulitis requiring operation, an intracolonic bypass tube has been used to protect the anastomoses. The device consists of a soft, pliable tube anastomosed to the submucosa of the proximal colon, which is expelled 10 to 14 days postoperatively. Two clinical trials using this technique have demonstrated the efficacy of this technique after colonic perforations of various causes.[115, 116] Although these preliminary reports are promising, further studies are required to define those patients most likely to benefit.

After secondary peritonitis, normal host defense mechanisms are overwhelmed by massive bacterial contamination. Techniques aimed at controlling bacterial contamination are geared toward reducing the bacterial inoculum to a level at which normal host defense mechanisms can eliminate the few remaining organisms. At operation, gross purulent exudates are aspirated, and loculations are gently opened and débrided. Particulate debris, such as fecal matter or other gross intestinal contents, is removed to optimize bacterial clearance. Intraoperative peritoneal lavage using saline or saline-antibiotic combinations has been attempted with variable success. A prospective study by Schein and coworkers[117] did not demonstrate any improvement in mortality or postoperative abscess formation in patients receiving saline lavage or saline lavage with chloramphenicol. Peritoneal lavage may have deleterious effects on endogenous clearance mechanisms. Saline lavage may impair phagocytosis and leukocyte migration.[118] Antibiotics or antiseptics in the lavage fluid may impair neutrophil chemotaxis[119] and microbial killing[120] and may potentiate adhesion formation.[121] These data suggest a limited or potentially deleterious impact of intraoperative lavage. As a result, reduction of bacterial contamination should be limited to thorough cleansing with suction and moist swabs.[122]

In the setting of diffuse peritonitis, a variety of adjuvant surgical techniques have been advocated to prevent residual infection and abscess formation. On the basis of theoretical arguments that fibrin deposited within the peritoneal cavity in response to bacterial contamination served as a nidus for abscess formation, Hudspeth[123] advocated the use of radical peritoneal débridement in patients with fibrinopurulent peritonitis. This technique involved the meticulous débridement of fibrinous exudates off the peritoneal surface. The sole randomized study in which this technique was compared with standard techniques demonstrated no advantage to its use and in fact suggested a potentially deleterious effect due to the induction of hemorrhage.[124]

Postoperative peritoneal lavage represents another measure designed to limit recurrent infection. At the time of operation for secondary peritonitis, drains are left in situ, and lavage using saline with or without antibiotics is started in the immediate postoperative period. Numerous studies have evaluated the role of postoperative peritoneal lavage in the treatment of general peritonitis.[125] However, most are limited by severe flaws in study design. Nonrandomized comparative studies have generally shown improved outcome with postoperative peritoneal lavage. However, those using a prospective randomized study design were unable to confirm these encouraging results.[117] The technique is extremely labor-intensive, requires intensive care unit monitoring, and is potentially complicated by the development of an enteric fistula due to catheter erosion. As a result, there appears to be no strong justification for its use at present. Randomized prospective studies using well-defined populations of high-risk patients are necessary to further define its role.

In critically ill patients with significant peritoneal contamination, two additional operative approaches designed to limit recurrent intraabdominal infection have been suggested. Scheduled or planned relaparotomy is the practice of performing repeated operations at fixed intervals (24 to 72 hours) regardless of the patient's clinical condition. Difficulties encountered with this approach center on the need for repeated, forceful closure of the abdominal wall in the presence of significant visceral edema. Abdominal closures under tension are at risk for dehiscence and may compromise perfusion of the abdominal wall, viscera, and kidneys as well as limit ventilation.[126, 127] As a result, an open abdomen approach has been proposed to obviate the need for abdominal closure—in effect treating the entire abdominal cavity as an abscess. Complications of this technique include evisceration, massive fluid losses, spontaneous fistulae, and contamination of the open wound. In addition, sedation of the patient and

TABLE 87–7 ■ Components of the APACHE II Severity of Illness Scoring System

I ACUTE PHYSIOLOGY PARAMETERS:
0 (normal) to 4 points (markedly abnormal)
Temperature
Mean blood pressure
Heart rate
Respiratory rate
Oxygenation
Arterial pH
Serum sodium level
Serum potassium level
Hematocrit
Glasgow Coma Scale score
White cell count
Serum creatinine value

II AGE POINTS

Age (y)	Points
<44	0
45–54	2
55–64	3
65–74	5
>75	6

III CHRONIC HEALTH POINTS
If the patient has a history of severe organ system insufficiency or is immunocompromised, points are assigned as follows:
Nonoperative or emergency postoperative patients: 5
Elective postoperative patients: 2

APACHE II score = I + II + III

Data from Knaus WA, Draper EA, Wagner DP, Zimmerman JE: Apache II: A severity of disease classification system. Crit Care Med 13:818–829, 1985.

mechanical ventilation are required and necessitate management in an intensive care setting.

As a result of difficulties encountered with scheduled relaparotomy and the open abdomen approach, a compromise has been reached by using various means of temporary abdominal closure. Retention meshes, polyurethane foam, gauze packing, and Marlex mesh with or without an insewn zipper have all been used, with the last becoming increasingly popular. Closure with Marlex mesh reduces the requirement for mechanical ventilation, prevents evisceration, and may lower the rate of iatrogenic fistula. Independent of the technique used, the entire abdomen should be explored manually, breaking down adhesions between loops and débriding fibrinous exudates, fluid, and necrotic debris. Frequent explorations allow early recognition of enteric fistula, a problem that may significantly complicate management in these patients. Repeated explorations are continued until clinical sepsis has subsided and the abdominal cavity appears clean as judged by the presence of healthy granulation tissue and adhesion formation. Nonabsorbable mesh (Marlex) may be removed at 7 to 9 days, once adhesions eliminate the possibility of evisceration. One major technical problem with this technique relates to an inability to explore the entire abdomen once the peritoneal surface starts to granulate and loops of bowel become adherent to each other and the abdominal wall. This problem has been circumvented by performing sequential CT scans in these patients. Inaccessible collections (usually in the subphrenic spaces) may be managed by percutaneous drainage.

A major difficulty in interpreting the efficacy of these approaches is the heterogeneous nature of intraabdominal infection. This is compounded by the lack of adequate prospective studies comparing these treatment modalities. Despite these concerns, early reports evaluating the outcome of this approach were optimistic. A report by Walsh and colleagues[128] examined the use of the Marlex mesh technique in the treatment of diffuse nonlocalizing peritonitis in patients stratified by use of the Acute Physiology and Chronic Health Evaluation II (APACHE II) severity of illness scoring system[129] (Table 87–7). With postoperative peritonitis, patients receiving a mesh at the time of reoperation had a mortality rate that was one third that expected on the basis of APACHE II scoring. The greatest benefit occurred in those patients with midrange APACHE II scores, a finding confirmed in studies by Garcia-Sabrido and coworkers.[130] In a prospective evaluation of 239 patients with severe peritonitis, there was no difference in mortality whether patients were treated with conventional abdominal closure, a mesh-zipper, or open gauze packing.[131] On the basis of a compilation of 642 patients from 22 series, Schein and colleagues[122] concluded that there was insufficient evidence to recommend either open management or scheduled relaparotomy in patients with severe peritonitis. In addition, the use of mesh is not without complications. In excess of 10% of patients develop fistulae as a result of small bowel perforations directly attributable to the presence of the mesh.[132]

Prognosis

Intraabdominal abscesses are associated with rates of mortality in the range of 7% to 29%.[2, 105, 130, 133, 134] This broad range reflects the heterogeneity of the populations of patients described in the literature. The principal determinant of outcome relates to the severity of illness at abscess presentation, a measure easily quantitated by APACHE II scores. The risk for mortality correlates with the APACHE II score at abscess presentation[2, 105, 134] (Fig. 87–2). In 1980, Fry and coworkers[135] reported a mortality rate of 32% in patients with intraabdominal abscesses. Organ failure, bacteremia, recurrent or multiple abscesses, and subphrenic or lesser sac abscesses were predictive of mortality. In most cases, deaths were attributed to inadequate drainage. Olson and Allen[4] demonstrated per-

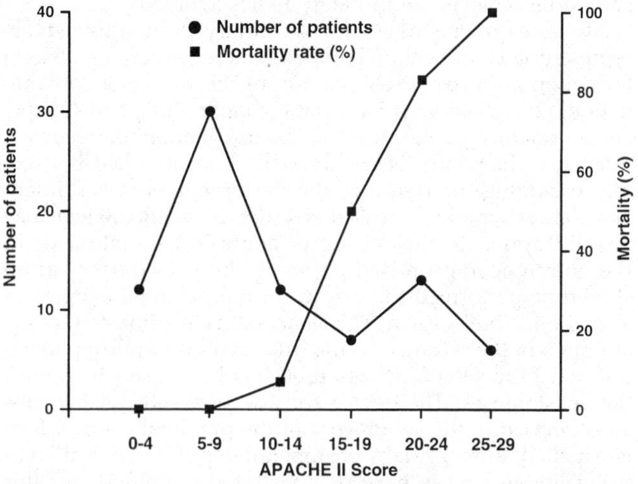

FIGURE 87–2 □ Distribution of patients and mortality with respect to APACHE II scores. Although the majority of patients with intraabdominal abscesses have relatively low APACHE II scores, the mortality arises from the 10% to 20% of patients with APACHE II scores higher than 15. (Adapted from Levison MA, Zeigler D: Correlation of APACHE II score, drainage technique and outcome in postoperative intra-abdominal abscess. Surg Gynecol Obstet 172:89–94, 1991. By permission of Surgery, Gynecology & Obstetrics, now known as the Journal of the American College of Surgeons.)

sistent abscesses in 41% of patients at autopsy, again implicating inadequate drainage as a factor contributing to mortality.

Several nonrandomized, retrospective studies have compared the outcomes of percutaneous and operative drainage in patients stratified by severity of illness. All demonstrate equivalent mortality rates.[2, 105, 134] There may be a slight benefit to operative drainage in patients with APACHE II scores greater than 15, although the small number of patients in this particular study precludes any definitive conclusion.[2] Deveney and colleagues[136] compared the mortality rate of patients with intraabdominal abscesses treated between 1973 and 1978 before the use of CT, ultrasonography, and percutaneous drainage with that of patients treated between 1981 and 1986, when these modalities were available. Mortality dropped from 39% to 21% during this period. This reduction in mortality was accompanied by a greater proportion of patients with predrainage localization, successful initial drainage, and a decreased frequency of predrainage organ failure. There was no difference in mortality in patients in the later group treated with PAD or operation, suggesting that the reduction in mortality was due to earlier and more precise abscess localization rather than the particular drainage technique used. Duration of drainage appears to be longer in patients treated percutaneously,[2, 134] but this does not appear to have an impact on the length of hospital stay.[105] Most patients may be discharged from the hospital with the drainage tube in place, once evidence of systemic sepsis has abated.

Summary

Intraabdominal abscesses may occur after diffuse peritonitis, after spontaneous or traumatic perforation of the gastrointestinal tract, or in the postoperative period as a result of anastomotic disruption. Abscess formation occurs as a result of the unique suppurative environment leading to bacterial proliferation and frustration of local host defenses. Diagnosis is made by abdominal imaging with either CT or ultrasonography. Drainage remains the most important intervention in facilitating abscess resolution. Percutaneous drainage is highly successful and may be carried out with either curative or palliative intent. Antimicrobial therapy is of secondary importance and should be directed against aerobic and anaerobic organisms, most commonly *E. coli* and *B. fragilis*. Intraabdominal abscesses are associated with a mortality of 7% to 29%, with the most important outcome predictor being the severity of illness at the time of abscess drainage.

References

1. Altemeier WA, Culbertson WR, Fullen WD, et al: Intra-abdominal abscesses. Am J Surg 125:70, 1973.
2. Levison MA, Zeigler D: Correlation of APACHE II score, drainage technique and outcome in postoperative intra-abdominal abscess. Surg Gynecol Obstet 172:89, 1991.
3. Lambiase RE, Deyoe L, Cronan JJ, et al: Percutaneous drainage of 335 consecutive abscesses: Results of primary drainage with 1-year follow-up. Radiology 184:167, 1992.
4. Olson MM, Allen MO: Nosocomial abscess. Results of an eight-year prospective study of 32,284 operations. Arch Surg 124:356, 1989.
5. Field TC, Pickleman J: Intraabdominal abscess unassociated with prior operation. Arch Surg 120:821, 1985.
6. Stone HH, Kolb LD, Geheber CE: Incidence and significance of intraperitoneal anaerobic bacteria. Ann Surg 181:705, 1975.
7. Moore WEC, Holdeman LV: Human fecal flora: The normal flora of 20 Japanese-Hawaiians. Appl Microbiol 27:961, 1974.
8. Tzianabos AO, Onderdonk AB, Zaleznik DF, et al: Structural characteristics of polysaccharides that induce protection against intra-abdominal abscess formation. Infect Immun 62:4881, 1994.
9. Tzianabos AO, Onderdonk AB, Rosner B, et al: Structural features of polysaccharides that induce intra-abdominal abscesses. Science 262:4116, 1993.
10. Steinberg B: Infections of the Peritoneum. New York, Hoeber, 1944.
11. Lanfrancone L, Boraschi D, Ghiara P, et al: Human peritoneal mesothelial cells produce many cytokines (granulocyte colony-stimulating factor [CSF], granulocyte-monocyte-CSF, macrophage-CSF, interleukin-1 [IL-1], and IL-6) and are activated and stimulated to grow by IL-1. Blood 80:2835, 1992.
12. Dunn DL, Barke RA, Ewald DC, et al: Macrophages and translymphatic absorption represent the first line of defense in the peritoneal cavity. Arch Surg 122:105, 1987.
13. Hau T, Simmons RL: Secondary bacterial peritonitis: The biologic basis of treatment. Curr Probl Surg 16:1, 1979.
14. Rosenthal GA, Levy G, Rotstein OD: Induction of macrophage procoagulant activity by *Bacteroides fragilis*. Infect Immun 57:338, 1989.
15. van Goor H, de Graaf JS, Sluiter WJ, et al: Fibrinolytic activity in the abdominal cavity of rats with faecal peritonitis. Br J Surg 81:1046, 1994.
16. van Goor H, de Graaf JS, Kooi K, et al: Effect of recombinant tissue plasminogen activator on intra-abdominal abscess formation in rats with generalized peritonitis. J Am Coll Surg 179:407, 1994.
17. McRitchie DI, Girotti MJ, Glynn MF, et al: Effect of systemic fibrinogen depletion on intraabdominal abscess formation. J Lab Clin Med 118:48, 1991.
18. Ciano PS, Colvin RB, Dvorak AM, et al: Macrophage migration in fibrin gel matrices. Lab Invest 54:62, 1986.
19. Rotstein OD, Pruett TL, Simmons RL: Fibrin in peritonitis V. Fibrin inhibits phagocytic killing of *E. coli* by human polymorphonuclear leukocytes. Ann Surg 203:413, 1986.
20. Dubrow T, Schwartz RJ, McKissock J, et al: Effect of aerosolized fibrin solution on intraperitoneal contamination. Arch Surg 126:80, 1991.
21. Chapman HA, Zdenek V, Hibbs JB: Coordinate expression of macrophage procoagulant activity and fibrinolytic activity in vitro and in vivo. J Immunol 130:261, 1983.
22. Shapiro ME, Kasper DL, Zaleznik DF, et al: Cellular control of abscess formation: Role of T cells in the regulation of abscesses formed in response to *Bacteroides fragilis*. J Immunol 137:341, 1986.
23. Shapiro ME, Onderdonk AB, Kasper DL, et al: Cellular immunity to *Bacteroides fragilis* capsular polysaccharide. J Exp Med 154:1188, 1982.
24. Zaleznik DF, Finberg RW, Shapiro ME, et al: A soluble suppressor T cell factor protects against experimental intraabdominal abscesses. J Clin Invest 75:1023, 1985.
25. Sawyer RG, Adams RB, Spengler MD, et al: Transient and distant infections after later intraperitoneal abscess formation. Arch Surg 126:164, 1991.
26. Sawyer RG, Adams RB, Spengler MD, et al: Preexposure of the peritoneum to live bacteria increases later mixed intraabdominal abscess formation and delays mortality. J Infect Dis 163:664, 1991.
27. Joiner KA, Onderdonk AB, Gelfand JA, et al: A quantitative model for subcutaneous abscess formation in mice. Br J Exp Pathol 61:97, 1980.
28. Rotstein OD, Feigel VD, Simmons RL, et al: The deleterious effect of reduced pH and hypoxia on neutrophil migration in vitro. J Surg Res 45:298, 1988.
29. Mandell GL: Bactericidal activity of aerobic and anaerobic polymorphonuclear neutrophils. Infect Immun 9:337, 1974.
30. Knighton DR, Halliday B, Hunt TK: Oxygen as an antibiotic. The effect of inspired oxygen on infection. Arch Surg 119:199, 1984.
31. Simchowitz L: Intracellular pH modulates the generation of superoxide radicals by human neutrophils. J Clin Invest 76:1079, 1985.
32. Liberek T, Topley N, Jorres A, et al: Peritoneal dialysis fluid inhibition of polymorphonuclear leukocyte respiratory burst activation is related to the lowering of intracellular pH. Nephron 65:260, 1993.

33. Tonetti M, Cavellero A, Botta GA, et al: Intracellular pH regulates the production of different oxygen metabolites in neutrophils: Effects of organic acids produced by anaerobic bacteria. J Leukoc Biol 49:180, 1991.
34. Hampton MB, Chambers ST, Vissers MC, et al: Bacterial killing by neutrophils in hypertonic environments. J Infect Dis 169:839, 1994.
35. Kazilek CJ, Merkle CJ, Chandler DE: Hyperosmotic inhibition of calcium signals and exocytosis in rabbit neutrophils. Am J Physiol 23:C709, 1988.
36. Simchowitz L, Cragoe EJ: Regulation of human neutrophil chemotaxis by intracellular pH. J Biol Chem 261:6492, 1986.
37. Rotstein OD, Pruett TL, Simmons RL: Mechanisms of microbial synergy in polymicrobial surgical infections. Rev Infect Dis 7:151, 1985.
38. Sawyer RG, Spengler MD, Adams RB, et al: The peritoneal environment during infection: The effect of monomicrobial and polymicrobial bacteria on pO_2 and pH. Ann Surg 213:253, 1991.
39. Howard RJ: Microbes and their pathogenicity. *In* Howard RJ, Simmons RL (eds): Surgical Infectious Diseases, ed 2. Norwalk, CT, Appleton & Lange, 1988, pp 1–13.
40. Finlay-Jones JJ, Kenny PA, Nulsen MF, et al: Pathogenesis of intraabdominal abscess formation: Abscess-potentiating agents and inhibition of complement-dependent opsonization of abscess-inducing bacteria. J Infect Dis 164:1173, 1991.
41. Yamada Y, Hefter K, Burke JA, et al: An in vitro model of the wound microenvironment: Local phagocytic cell abnormalities associated with in situ complement activation. J Infect Dis 155:998, 1987.
42. Pruett TL, Rotstein OD, Fiegel VD, et al: Mechanism of the adjuvant effect of hemoglobin in experimental peritonitis: VIII. A leukotoxin is produced by *Escherichia coli* metabolism in hemoglobin. Surgery 96:375, 1984.
43. Yamamura M, Nishi M, Furubayashi H, et al: Barium peritonitis. Report of a case and review of the literature. Dis Colon Rectum 28:347, 1985.
44. Cho J, Rotstein OD, Pruett TL: The adjuvant effect of bile salts in experimental peritonitis. Surg Forum 35:231, 1984.
45. Hill GB: Enhancement of experimental anaerobic infections by blood, hemoglobin, and hemostatic agents. Infect Immun 1984:443, 1978.
46. Zimmerli W, Waldvogel FA, Vaudaus P, et al: Pathogenesis of foreign body infection: Description and characteristics of an animal model. J Infect Dis 146:487, 1982.
47. Zimmerli W, Lew PD, Waldvogel FA: Pathogenesis of foreign body infection: Evidence for a local granulocyte defect. J Clin Invest 73:1191, 1984.
48. Gallinaro RN, Naziri W, McMasters KM, et al: Alteration of mononuclear cell immune-associated antigen expression, interleukin-1 expression, and antigen presentation during intraabdominal infection. Shock 1:1330, 1994.
49. Sherman NJ, Davis JR, Jesseph JE: Subphrenic abscess. A continuing hazard. Am J Surg 117:117, 1969.
50. Carter R, Brewer LA: Subphrenic abscess: A thoracoabdominal clinical complex. Am J Surg 108:165, 1964.
51. Boyd DP: The intrathoracic complications of subphrenic abscess. J Thorac Cardiovasc Surg 38:771, 1959.
52. Crepps JT, Welch JP, Orlando R: Management and outcome of retroperitoneal abscesses. Ann Surg 205:276, 1987.
53. Durning P, Schofield PF: Diagnosis and management of psoas abscess in Crohn's disease. J R Soc Med 77:33, 1984.
54. Longo WE, Milsom JW, Lavery IC, et al: Pelvic abscess after colon and rectal surgery—What is optimal management? Dis Colon Rectum 36:936, 1993.
55. Stone HH, Bourneuf AA, Stinson LD: Reliability of criteria for predicting persistent or recurrent sepsis. Arch Surg 120:17, 1985.
56. Lennard ES, Dellinger EP, Wertz MJ: Implications of leukocytosis and fever at conclusion of antibiotic therapy for intraabdominal sepsis. Ann Surg 195:19, 1982.
57. Polk HC, Shields CL: Remote organ failure: A valid sign of occult intraabdominal infection. Surgery 81:310, 1977.
58. Ing AF, Mclean APH, Meakins JL: Multiple-organism bacteremia in the surgical intensive care unit: A sign of intraperitoneal sepsis. Surgery 90:779, 1981.
59. Fry DE, Garrison RN, Polk HCJ: Clinical implications in *Bacteroides* bacteremia. Surg Gynecol Obstet 149:189, 1979.
60. DeCosse JJ, Poulin TL, Fox PS, et al: Subphrenic abscess. Surg Gynecol Obstet 138:841, 1974.
61. Knochel JO, Koehler PR, Lee TG: Diagnosis of abdominal abscesses with computed tomography, ultrasound, and In-111 leukocyte scans. Radiology 137:427, 1980.
62. Taylor KJW, Wasson JFM, De Graaf C, et al: Accuracy of greyscale ultrasound diagnosis of abdominal and pelvic abscesses in 220 patients. Lancet 1:83, 1978.
63. Gazelle GS, Mueller PR: Abdominal abscesses: Imaging and intervention. Radiol Clin North Am 32:913, 1994.
64. vanSonnenberg E, D'Agostino HB, Casola G, et al: US-guided transvaginal drainage of pelvic abscesses and fluid collections. Radiology 181:53, 1991.
65. Bennett JD, Kozak RI, Taylor BM, et al: Deep pelvic abscesses: Transrectal drainage with radiologic guidance. Radiology 185:825, 1992.
66. Dobrin PB, Gully PH, Greenlee HB, et al: Radiologic diagnosis of an intraabdominal abscess. Do multiple tests help? Arch Surg 121:41, 1986.
67. Jaques P, Mauro M, Yankaskas B, et al: CT features of intraabdominal abscesses: Prediction of successful percutaneous drainage. AJR 146:1041, 1986.
68. Baker ME, Blinder RA, Rice RP: Diagnostic imaging of abdominal fluid collections and abscesses. Crit Rev Diagn Imaging 25:233, 1986.
69. Aveline B, Guimaraes R, Bely N, et al: Intraabdominal serous fluid collections after appendectomy: A normal sonographic finding. AJR 161:71, 1993.
70. Neff CC, Simeone JF, Ferrucci JTJ, et al: The occurrence of fluid collections following routine abdominal surgical procedures: Sonographic study in asymptomatic post operative patients. Radiology 146:463, 1983.
71. Haaga JR, Weinstein AJ: CT-guided percutaneous aspiration and drainage of abscesses. AJR 135:1187, 1980.
72. Korobkin M, Callun PW, Filly RA, et al: Comparison of computed tomography, ultrasonography, and gallium-67 scanning in the evaluation of suspected abdominal abscesses. Radiology 129:89, 1978.
73. Moir C, Robins RE: Role of ultrasonography, gallium scanning and computerized tomography in the diagnosis of intraabdominal abscess. Am J Surg 143:582, 1982.
74. Hoffer P: Gallium mechanisms. J Nucl Med 21:282, 1980.
75. Dutcher JP, Schiffer CA, Johnston GS: Rapid migration of 111-indium labelled granulocytes to sites of infection. N Engl J Med 304:586, 1981.
76. Fry DE, Clevenger FW: Reoperation for intra-abdominal abscess. Surg Clin North Am 71:159, 1991.
77. Wall SD, Fisher MR, Amparo EG, et al: Magnetic resonance imaging in the evaluation of abscesses. AJR 144:1217, 1985.
78. Casey LC, Balk RA, Bone RC: Plasma cytokine and endotoxin levels correlate with survival in patients with the sepsis syndrome. Ann Intern Med 119:771, 1993.
79. Bellomo R: The cytokine network in the critically ill. Anaesth Intensive Care 20:288, 1992.
80. Ziegler EJ, Fisher CJ, Sprung CL, et al: Treatment of gram-negative bacteremia and septic shock with HA-1A human monoclonal antibody against endotoxin. N Engl J Med 324:429, 1991.
81. Abraham E, Wunderdink R, Silverman H, et al: Efficacy and safety of monoclonal antibody to human tumor necrosis factor alpha in patients with sepsis syndrome. JAMA 273:934, 1995.
82. Bone RC, Fisher CJ, Clemmer TP, et al: A controlled clinical trial of high-dose methylprednisone in the treatment of severe sepsis and septic shock. N Engl J Med 317:653, 1987.
83. Dhainaut J-FA, Tenaillon A, Le Tulzo Y, et al: Platelet activating factor receptor antagonist BN 52021 in the treatment of severe sepsis: A randomized, double blind, placebo controlled, multicenter, clinical trial. Crit Care Med 22:1720, 1994.
84. Fisher CJ, Dhainaut J-FA, Opal SM, et al: Recombinant human interleukin-1 receptor antagonist in the treatment of patients with sepsis syndrome. JAMA 271:1836, 1995.
85. Moore F, Feliciano D, Andrassy R, et al: Early enteral feeding, compared with parenteral, reduces postoperative septic complications: The results of a meta-analysis. Ann Surg 216:172, 1992.
86. Moore FA, Moore EE, Jones TN, et al: TEN versus TPN following major abdominal trauma—Reduced septic morbidity. J Trauma 29:916, 1989.

87. Cerra F: Nutrient modulation of inflammatory and immune function. Am J Surg 161:230, 1991.
88. Levy E, Frileux P, Cugnenc PH, et al: High-output external fistulae of the small bowel: Management with continuous enteral nutrition. Br J Surg 76:676, 1989.
89. Bohnen JMA, Solomkin JS, dellinger EP, et al: Guidelines for clinical care: Anti-infective agents for intraabdominal infection. Arch Surg 127:83, 1992.
89a. Solomkin JJ, Reinhart HH, Dellinger EP, et al: Results of a randomized trial comparing sequential intravenous/oral treatment with ciprofloxacin plus metronidazole to imipenem/cilastatin for intra-abdominal infections. Ann Surg 223:303, 1996.
90. Hackford AW, Tally FP, Reinhold RB, et al: Prospective study comparing imipenem-cilastatin with clindamycin and gentamicin for the treatment of serious surgical infections. Arch Surg 123:322, 1988.
91. Solomkin JS, Dellinger EP, Christou NV, et al: Results of a multicenter trial comparing imipenem/cilastatin to tobramycin/clindamycin for intraabdominal infections. Ann Surg 212:581, 1990.
92. Galandiuk S, Lamos J, Montgomery W, et al: Antibiotic penetration of experimental intra-abdominal abscesses. Am Surg 61:521, 1995.
93. Bryant RE: Effect of the suppurative environment on antibiotic activity. *In* Root RK, Sande MA (eds): New Dimensions in Antimicrobial Therapy. New York, Churchill Livingstone, 1984, pp 313–337.
94. Park JK, Kraus FC, Haaga JR: Fluid flow during percutaneous drainage procedures: An in vitro study of the effects of fluid viscosity, catheter size, and adjunctive urokinase. AJR 160:165, 1993.
95. Lahorra JM, Haaga JR, Stellato T, et al: Safety of intracavitary urokinase with percutaneous abscess drainage. AJR 160:171, 1993.
96. van Sonnenberg E, Ferrucci JT, Mueller PR, et al: Percutaneous drainage of abscesses and fluid collections: Techniques, results, and applications. Radiology 142:1, 1982.
97. Stabile BE, Puccio E, van Sonnenberg E, et al: Preoperative percutaneous drainage of diverticular abscesses. Am J Surg 159:99, 1990.
98. Samelson SL, Ferguson MK: Empyema following percutaneous drainage of upper abdominal abscesses. Chest 102:1612, 1992.
99. Stylianos S, Martin EC, Starker PM, et al: Percutaneous drainage of intra-abdominal abscesses following abdominal trauma. J Trauma 29:584, 1989.
100. Schecter S, Eisenstat TE, Oliver GC, et al: Computerized tomographic scan–guided drainage of intra-abdominal abscesses. Dis Colon Rectum 37:984, 1994.
101. Brolin RE, Flancbaum L, Ercoli FR, et al: Limitations of percutaneous catheter drainage of abdominal abscesses. Surg Gynecol Obstet 173:203, 1991.
102. Rotstein OD: Peritonitis and intra-abdominal abscesses. *In* Wilmore DW, Brennan MF, Harken AH, et al (eds): Scientific American: Care of the Surgical Patient. New York, Scientific American, 1992, pp 1–24.
103. Pruett TL, Rotstein OD, Crass J, et al: Percutaneous aspiration and drainage for suspected intra-abdominal infection. Surgery 96:731, 1984.
104. Flancbaum L, Nosher JL, Brolin RE: Percutaneous catheter drainage of abdominal abscesses associated with perforated viscus. Am Surg 56:52, 1990.
105. Hemming A, Davis NL, Robins RE: Surgical versus percutaneous drainage of intra-abdominal abscesses. Am J Surg 161:593, 1991.
106. Haaga JR: Imaging intraabdominal abscesses and nonoperative drainage procedures. World J Surg 14:204, 1990.
107. Gerzof SG, Johnson WC, Robbins AH, Nabseth DC: Expanded criteria for percutaneous abscess drainage. Arch Surg 120:227, 1985.
108. Brolin RE, Nosher JL, Leiman S: Percutaneous catheter versus open surgical drainage in the treatment of abdominal abscesses. Am Surg 150:102, 1984.
109. Goletti O, Lippolis PV, Chiarugi M, et al: Percutaneous ultrasound-guided drainage of intra-abdominal abscesses. Br J Surg 80:336, 1993.
110. Malangoni MA, Shumate CR, Thomas HA, et al: Factors influencing the treatment of intra-abdominal abscesses. Am J Surg 159:167, 1990.
111. Rotstein OD, Pruett TL, Simmons RL: Microbiologic features and treatment of persistent peritonitis in patients in the intensive care unit. Can J Surg 29:247, 1986.
112. Nathens AB, Rotstein OD, Marshall JC: Tertiary peritonitis: Clinical features of a complex nosocomial infection. Crit Care Med 21(Suppl):S129, 1993.
113. Sawyer RG, Rosenlof LK, Adams RB, et al: Peritonitis into the 1990's: Changing pathogens and changing strategies in the critically ill. Am Surg 58:82, 1992.
114. Schrock TR, Deveney CW, Dunphy JE: Factors contributing to leakage of colonic anastomoses. Ann Surg 197:513, 1973.
115. Ravo B, Mishrick A, Addei K, et al: The treatment of perforated diverticulitis by one stage intracolonic bypass procedure. Surgery 102:771, 1987.
116. Rosati C, Smith L, Deitel M, et al: Primary colorectal anastomosis with the intracolonic bypass tube. Surgery 112:618, 1992.
117. Schein M, Gecelter G, Freinkel W, et al: Peritoneal lavage in abdominal sepsis. A controlled clinical study. Arch Surg 125:1132, 1990.
118. Dunn DL, Barke RA, Ahrenholz DH, et al: The adjuvant effect of peritoneal fluid in experimental peritonitis: Mechanism and clinical implications. Ann Surg 199:37, 1984.
119. Majeski JA, McClellan MA, Alexander JW: Evaluation of leukocyte chemotactic response in the presence of antibiotics. Surg Forum 16:83, 1975.
120. Hansbrough JF, Zapata-Sirvent RL, Cooper ML: Effects of topical antimicrobial agents on the human neutrophil respiratory burst. Arch Surg 126:603, 1991.
121. Rappaport WD, Holcomb M, Valente J, et al: Antibiotic irrigation and the formation of intraabdominal adhesions. Am J Surg 158:435, 1989.
122. Schein M, Hirshberg A, Hashmonai M: Current surgical management of severe intraabdominal infection. Surgery 112:489, 1992.
123. Hudspeth AS: Radical debridement in the treatment of advanced generalized bacterial peritonitis. Arch Surg 110:1233, 1975.
124. Polk HC, Fry DE: Radical peritoneal debridement for established peritonitis: The result of a prospective randomized clinical trial. Ann Surg 192:350, 1980.
125. Leiboff AR, Soroff HS: The treatment of generalized peritonitis by closed postoperative peritoneal lavage: A critical review of the literature. Arch Surg 122:1005, 1987.
126. Richards WO, Scovill W: Acute renal failure associated with increased intra-abdominal pressure. Ann Surg 197:183, 1983.
127. Richardson JD, Trinkle JK: Hemodynamic and respiratory alteration with increased intraabdominal pressure. J Surg Res 20:401, 1976.
128. Walsh GL, Chiasson P, Hedderich G: The open abdomen. The Marlex mesh and zipper technique: A method of managing intraabdominal infection. Surg Clin North Am 68:25, 1988.
129. Knaus WA, Draper EA, Wagner DP, et al: Apache II: A severity of disease classification system. Crit Care Med 13:818, 1985.
130. Garcia-Sabrido JL, Tallado JM, Christou NV, et al: Treatment of severe intra-abdominal sepsis and/or necrotic foci by an "open-abdomen" approach. Arch Surg 123:152, 1988.
131. Christou NV, Barie PS, Dellinger EP, et al: Surgical Infection Society intra-abdominal infection study. Prospective evaluation of management techniques and outcome. Arch Surg 128:193, 1993.
132. Mastboom WJB, Kuypers HHC, Schoots FJ, et al: Small bowel perforations complicating the open treatment of generalized peritonitis. Arch Surg 124:689, 1989.
133. Mughal MM, Bancewicz J, Irving MH: Laparostomy: A technique for the management of intractable intraabdominal sepsis. Br J Surg 73:253, 1986.
134. Olak J, Christou NV, Stein LA, et al: Operative vs percutaneous drainage of intra-abdominal abscesses. Comparison of morbidity and mortality. Arch Surg 121:141, 1986.
135. Fry DE, Garrison N, Heitsch RC, et al: Determinants of death in patients with intraabdominal abscess. Surgery 88:517, 1980.
136. Deveney CW, Lurie K, Deveney KE: Improved treatment of intra-abdominal abscess. Arch Surg 123:1126, 1988.

88

Appendicitis

Gordon L. Telford
Robert E. Condon

Appendicitis can occur at any age; it accounts for approximately 1% of all surgical operations.[1] Although rare in infants, appendicitis becomes increasingly common throughout childhood, reaching its maximal frequency between the ages of 10 and 30 years.

Pathophysiology

Obstruction followed by infection is the most likely pathogenesis of appendicitis.[2, 3] The appendiceal lumen first becomes obstructed by hyperplasia of submucosal lymphoid follicles, fecalith, foreign body, stricture, tumor, pinworms *(Enterobius vermicularis)*, or other pathologic state. Once it is obstructed, mucus accumulates within the lumen of the appendix, and intraluminal pressure increases. The accumulated mucus is converted into pus by luminal bacteria, continued secretion combined with the relative inelasticity of the serosa leads to a further increase in pressure in the lumen. Lymphatic obstruction ensues, leading to edema, diapedesis of bacteria, and mucosal ulceration. Continued secretion results in a further rise in intraluminal pressure, leading to venous obstruction, increasing edema, and ischemia of the appendix, and acute suppurative appendicitis ensues.

Progression of this pathologic process results in venous and arterial thromboses in the wall of the appendix and gangrenous appendicitis. The final stage in the progression of acute appendicitis is perforation through a gangrenous infarct and spilling of accumulated pus.

Microbiology

The flora of the lumen of the appendix is that of the lumen of the colon, a mixture of aerobic and anaerobic organisms.[4] The flora cultured from infections resulting from acute appendicitis is representative of the flora of the lumen of the appendix (Table 88–1). More than 90% of wound infections resulting from an episode of acute appendicitis are polymicrobial; most commonly, five different species of bacteria are cultured. In order of prevalence, bacterial isolates include *Bacteroides, Escherichia coli*, other gram-negative aerobes, and anaerobic and aerobic streptococci.

TABLE 88–1 ■ Relative Prevalence of Bacterial Flora of the Appendix

AEROBES	%	ANAEROBES	%
Escherichia coli	80	*Bacteroides fragilis* group	89
Klebsiella-Enterobacter	57	Other *Bacteroides* spp.	25
Enterococcus faecalis group	26	Streptococci	64
Other gram-positive cocci	8	Clostridia	13
Other aerobes	43	Other anaerobes	41
No growth	1	No growth	4

Data from the Surgical Microbiology Research Laboratory, Medical College of Wisconsin, Milwaukee, Wisconsin, 1990.

Symptoms

Although the symptom history varies, the cardinal symptoms of acute appendicitis are usually present.[1, 5] The symptoms usually begin with epigastric or periumbilical abdominal pain, followed by anorexia and nausea. Vomiting, if it occurs, appears next. After a variable time, usually about 8 hours, the pain becomes localized to the right side and usually into the right lower quadrant.

Pain

Acute appendicitis typically begins with diffuse, central, minimally severe visceral pain. This is followed in 8 hours by somatic pain that is more severe and usually well localized to the right lower quadrant. Atypical pain that does not follow the classic visceral-somatic sequence is common in acute appendicitis, however, occurring in up to 45% of patients. Atypical pain, while it is localized to the right lower quadrant, may remain visceral. Conversely, the pain may never become localized. Atypical pain is found more frequently in older patients.

Patients with high retrocecal appendicitis may present with only diffuse pain in the right flank. Similarly, patients whose entire appendix is within the true pelvis may never develop somatic pain and, instead, may have tenesmus and vague discomfort in the suprapubic area.

Anorexia, Nausea, and Vomiting

Anorexia and nausea are present in almost all cases of acute appendicitis. The presence or absence of vomiting should not be a criterion for the diagnosis of appendicitis. When vomiting does occur, it is not persistent and begins after the onset of pain with such regularity that if it antedates pain, the diagnosis of appendicitis should be questioned. If vomiting is persistent, the diagnosis should also be questioned.

Constipation and Diarrhea

A history of constipation or diarrhea of recent onset is not exceptionally helpful in the diagnosis of appendicitis.

Physical Examination

Typical physical signs of acute appendicitis include localized tenderness, muscle guarding, and rebound tenderness. Cutaneous hyperesthesia, right-sided pelvic tenderness on rectal examination, and the presence of a psoas or obturator sign are less common and tend to be dependent on the examiner. Although a normal temperature is often present, temperature up to 38°C occurs, but in the typical case of appendicitis, high fever is uncommon.

If the appendix ruptures, the physical findings change. If the infection is contained, the patient often develops a soft, tender mass in the right lower quadrant, and the area of tenderness now encompasses the entire right lower quadrant. Involuntary guarding becomes evident and rebound tenderness more marked. The patient's temperature is more like that seen with abscess formation and may rise to 39°C and be associated with tachycardia.

If appendiceal rupture fails to localize, the patient develops the signs and symptoms of diffuse peritonitis. Tenderness and guarding become generalized, the temperature remains above 38°C and spikes to 40°C, and the pulse rises above 100 beats per minute.

Tenderness and Muscle Guarding

On routine abdominal examination, an area of maximal tenderness is often elicited in the area of the McBurney point. In high retrocecal appendicitis, tenderness may occur over a large area, and there may be no signs of muscle spasm. In pelvic appendicitis, neither sign may be present. Both signs are often absent or minimal in aged persons.

Signs of peritoneal inflammation or irritation in the right lower quadrant are also helpful in the diagnosis. Coughing or bouncing on the heels produces this type of pain. Rebound tenderness and muscle guarding can usually be elicited. Rovsing sign, pain elicited in the right lower quadrant by palpation pressure in the left lower quadrant, is another type of rebound tenderness and can be present in acute appendicitis.

Abdominal Mass

As the disease process progresses, it may be possible to palpate a tender mass in the right lower quadrant. Although the mass may be due to an abscess, it can also result from adherence of the omentum and loops of intestine to an inflamed appendix.

Rectal Examination

Rectal examination, although essential for all patients suspected of having appendicitis, is helpful only in those few whose appendix lies almost wholly within the pelvis. In these patients, a thorough rectal examination may be the only way to elicit tenderness.

Laboratory Tests

Laboratory tests have little value in the early diagnosis of acute appendicitis. Up to one third of patients, particularly older ones,[6] have a normal total leukocyte count with acute appendicitis.[1,7] The differential white cell count often reveals a shift to the left with an increase in the percentage of polymorphonuclear neutrophils.[7] In considering the diagnosis of appendicitis, clinical findings take precedence over the white cell count or other laboratory observations when they are at variance.

The urinalysis is helpful in the differential diagnosis of patients with lower abdominal pain only when it reveals that a urinary tract lesion is causing the symptoms. Patients with advanced appendicitis and abscess formation or generalized peritonitis may have abnormal results of liver function tests.

Radiologic Examination

Abdominal radiographs are seldom helpful in the diagnosis of acute appendicitis, except when they demonstrate a fecalith or exclude other diagnoses such as acute cholecystitis, perforated duodenal ulcer, perforated colon cancer, and acute diverticulitis. Cecal distention or a sentinel loop of distended small intestine in the right lower quadrant is frequently present in appendicitis.

A mass can often be demonstrated extrinsic to the cecum late in the course of appendicitis. There may be scoliosis to the right, absence of the right psoas shadow, and signs of edema of the abdominal wall. With late appendicitis and generalized peritonitis, there will be an ileus pattern with generalized gas throughout the small and large intestines.

Barium enema examination, although not indicated in cases in which the diagnosis of acute appendicitis is evident on clinical grounds, can be helpful in some situations.[8,9] It can be helpful in young women, in whom the diagnosis is still in question after observation and in whom the negative laparotomy rate is high. It can also be helpful in patients with a debilitating systemic disease such as leukemia, for whom the operative risk is markedly increased. Findings of significance on barium enema examination are nonfilling or partial filling of the appendix and an extrinsic defect on the cecum (the reversed three sign).[9,10]

An experienced radiologist is able to diagnose acute appendicitis using ultrasonography with an accuracy greater than 90%.[11–13] Appendicitis is diagnosed if the maximal cross-sectional diameter of the appendix exceeds 6 mm, if the appendix is noncompressible, if an appendicolith is present, or if a complex mass is demonstrated. Other criteria that are not universally agreed on include rigidity and nonmobility. Nonvisualization of the appendix is not a criterion for appendicitis. More prospective studies are necessary to identify the most appropriate criteria for the ultrasound diagnosis of acute appendicitis. Ultrasonography is also useful in the diagnosis of perforated appendicitis with abscess formation.

Although more expensive, computed tomography (CT) has been demonstrated to be effective in the diagnosis of acute appendicitis with an accuracy greater than 90%.[14,15] The cost can be reduced by performing a limited, unenhanced CT scan with no significant loss in diagnostic accuracy.[14] Appendicitis is diagnosed when the appendix is thickened with a diameter greater than 6 mm and there are inflammatory changes in the periappendiceal fat (streaking and poorly defined increased attenuation).[14–16] Both the presence of pericecal inflammation without an inflamed appendix and an appendicolith without the presence of periappendiceal inflammation are insufficient to diagnose acute appendicitis. As with ultrasonography, the specific criteria for the CT diagnosis of acute appendicitis are not universally agreed on, and further prospective studies are necessary to identify the most appropriate criteria.

Acute Appendicitis in Infants and Young Children

The diagnosis of acute appendicitis can be difficult in this age group. The patient is usually unable to give an accurate history. Appendicitis is uncommon and acute nonspecific abdominal pain is common in infants and children. Because of such factors, diagnosis and treatment are delayed, and complications develop.[17] The suspicion of appendicitis is often not aroused until the appendix has ruptured and the child is obviously ill.[18] Two thirds of young children with appendicitis have symptoms for more than 3 days before appendectomy.[17] Vomiting, fever, irritability, flexing of the thighs, and diarrhea are likely early signs. Abdominal distention is the most consistent physical finding. As in adults, the total leukocyte count is not a reliable test.

The frequency of perforation in infants younger than 1 year is almost 100%, and although it decreases with age, it is still 50% at age 5 years. The mortality rate in this age group remains as high as 5% because of the aforementioned factors.

Appendicitis in Young Women

Whereas the overall frequency of "negative laparotomy" in patients suspected of having appendicitis is as high as 20%, the frequency in women younger than 30 years is as high as 45%. The majority of the misdiagnoses are accounted for by pain associated with ovulation; diseases of the ovaries, tubes, and uterus; and urinary tract infections (cystitis). If a young woman has atypical pain, muscle guarding in the right lower quadrant is absent, and there is no fever, leukocystosis, or leftward shift in the differential white cell count, then it is best to observe the patient and to perform frequent reexaminations. If the patient's signs and symptoms remain stable after several hours, it is appropriate to perform a barium enema examination or a CT scan.

Appendicitis During Pregnancy

The risk of appendicitis during pregnancy is the same as in nonpregnant women of the same age; the frequency is 1 in every 2000 pregnancies. Appendicitis occurs more often during the first two trimesters, during which period the symptoms are similar to those seen in nonpregnant women.[13] Surgery should be performed during pregnancy when appendicitis is suspected just as it would be in a nonpregnant woman. As in nonpregnant patients, the effects of a negative laparotomy are minor, whereas the effects of ruptured appendicitis can be catastrophic. If peritonitis and sepsis ensue, the infant mortality rate—due both to prematurity and to the effects of sepsis—increases.

The mortality rate for appendicitis during pregnancy is due mainly to delay in diagnosis. In the final analysis, early appendectomy is the appropriate therapy in suspected appendicitis during all stages of pregnancy.[19]

Appendicitis in Elderly Persons

Appendicitis has a much greater mortality rate among elderly than among young adults. The increased risk appears to be due both to delay in seeking medical care and to delay in making the diagnosis.[20, 21] Elderly persons have the classic symptoms, but they are often less pronounced. Right lower quadrant pain localizes later and may be milder. On initial physical examination, the findings are often minimal, although right lower quadrant tenderness eventually develops.[22] Distention of the abdomen and a clinical picture suggestive of small bowel obstruction are commonly seen. More than 30% of elderly patients have a ruptured appendix at the time of operation.[22]

Differential Diagnosis

When the classic symptoms of appendicitis are present, the diagnosis is usually made easily and is seldom missed. It is most important to rule out diseases that do not require operative therapy and can be made worse by operation, for example, pancreatitis, myocardial infarction, and basilar pneumonia.

The diseases in young children that are most frequently mistaken for acute appendicitis are gastroenteritis, *Yersinia enterocolitica* enterocolitis and associated mesenteric lymphadenitis, Meckel's diverticulitis, pyelitis, small intestinal intussusception, enteric duplication, and basilar pneumonia.

In teenagers and young adults, the differential diagnosis is different for men and women. In young women, it includes diseases of the ovaries and tubes, such as ruptured ectopic pregnancy, mittelschmerz, endometriosis, and salpingitis[23]; chronic constipation also needs to be considered. In young men, the differential diagnosis is smaller and includes the acute onset of regional enteritis, right-sided renal or ureteral calculus, torsion of the testes, and acute epididymitis. In both young men and young women, *Y. enterocolitica* enterocolitis and associated mesenteric lymphadenitis should be considered.

In older persons, the differential diagnosis of acute appendicitis includes diverticulitis, perforated peptic ulcer, acute cholecystitis, acute pancreatitis, intestinal obstruction, perforated cecal carcinoma, mesenteric vascular occlusion, rupturing aortic aneurysm, and the disease entities mentioned before for young adults. Although rare, amebic infection of the cecum with cecal dilatation can mimic appendicitis. Because it can cause leukocytosis, fever, nausea, vomiting, and abdominal cramps, *Salmonella* infection can also mimic appendicitis and must be considered in patients with diarrhea who report that other family members or friends have gastroenteritis.

Treatment

Preoperative Preparation

It is not necessary to rush a patient with a presumed diagnosis of acute appendicitis directly to the operating room. All patients, especially those with a presumed diagnosis of peritonitis, should be adequately prepared and then taken to the operating room. Patients with a palpable right lower quadrant mass may be managed initially without operation.[24]

Intravenous fluid replacement should be initiated and the patient resuscitated. Once urine output reaches acceptable levels (more than 30 mL/h), it can be assumed that resuscitation is complete. Nasogastric suction is helpful for patients with peritonitis and a profound ileus. If the patient's body temperature is greater than 39°C, measures should be taken to reduce fever before beginning an operation.

Antibiotic Therapy

Before antibiotics were available, the mortality rate for acute appendicitis was in the range of 8% to 15%. Today, it is less than 1%. Although other factors are involved, antibiotic therapy is a major factor in improving the mortality rate.

The risk of an infectious complication becomes greater as the state of the appendix worsens. The frequency of wound infection after removal of a normal appendix or an appendix in the early stages of appendicitis is in the range of 5% to 10%. The risk increases by threefold or fourfold with gangrene and to one of every two patients with perforation.

More than 100 clinical trials have now been conducted at a number of institutions to measure the efficacy of antibiotics in appendicitis. The results of these studies clearly indicate that antibiotics decrease infectious complications for all stages of appendicitis so that a preoperative "single shot" of an efficacious antibiotic regimen is indicated in every patient having an operation for suspected appendicitis. The same cannot be said for the use of antimicrobial and antiseptic solutions to irrigate the abdominal cavity and the wound. Few studies in which irrigants were used have demonstrated reduction of the infection rate.

Infections resulting from acute appendicitis are polymicrobial, and aerobe-anaerobe synergy plays a pathogenic role. An antibiotic that is active against both aerobes and anaerobes is needed. A large number of antibiotics and antibiotic combinations have been demonstrated to be effective. These include second-generation cephalosporins (cefoxitin, cefotetan), third-generation cephalosporins (ceftazidime, ceftizoxime) combined with an antianaerobe agent (metronidazole, clindamycin), the expanded-spectrum penicillins combined with β-lactamase inhibitors (ampicillin-sulbactam, ticarcillin-clavulanate), aztreonam plus clindamycin, and doxycycline as well as the traditional but now outmoded aminoglycoside-antianaerobe and "triple-antibiotic" combinations. Our current preference is to use a broad-spectrum antibiotic, such as cefoxitin, 1 to 2 g intravenously in adults, in patients with suspected appendicitis. If, at the time of operation, the appendicitis is uncomplicated, administration of antibiotics is stopped.

Antibiotics should be continued postoperatively as the clinical condition indicates in patients who have a gangrenous or ruptured appendix and localized or generalized peritonitis. This often entails treatment for a week or so. More important is the selection of an end point for therapy; we stop giving antibiotics when the white cell count is normal with a normal differential count, the temperature has not been elevated for 24 hours, and the patient is taking food without problems. If these conditions have not been achieved by the 10th postoperative day, CT for an abdominal or pelvic abscess may be appropriate. Antibiotic therapy should be changed or stopped, depending on the clinical circumstances.

Examination Under Anesthesia

After the induction of anesthesia, the patient's abdomen should be palpated systematically. Such an examination may, on occasion, demonstrate other disease to be the cause of the patient's symptoms, such as acute cholecystitis. It may also be possible to palpate an appendiceal mass that will confirm the suspected diagnosis.

Uncomplicated Appendicitis Without a Palpable Mass

When the diagnosis of uncomplicated acute appendicitis has been made, appendectomy should be performed as an emergency procedure. The earlier the diagnosis is made and the sooner the appendectomy is performed, the better is the prognosis. Uncomplicated appendectomy should have a surgical mortality rate of less than 0.1%. In contrast, the mortality rate for ruptured appendicitis can be as high as 10%.

The recommended incision for a routine appendectomy is a transverse incision (Rockey-Davis, Fowler-Weir-Mitchell; Fig. 88–1). Exposure of the appendix through this incision is much better than that obtained through the classic McBurney incision, particularly in patients who have a retrocecal appendix or are obese.

The gridiron, or muscle-splitting, incision (McBurney incision) is the one most widely used for uncomplicated appendicitis, largely because of surgical tradition rather than its particular utility. The exposure through a McBurney incision can be awkward, especially for a retrocecal appendix, unless the appendix lies immediately below the incision. If necessary, the incision can be extended medially, partially transecting the rectus sheath, but this maneuver is usually helpful only for a pelvic appendix.

If the diagnosis of acute appendicitis is in doubt and exploratory laparotomy is indicated, a vertical midline incision is appropriate. If an appendiceal mass is encountered, the midline incision can be closed and a more direct approach to the lesion made through a right lower quadrant incision.

After the peritoneum is opened, the appendix is identified by following the anterior cecal taenia to the base of the appendix. The inflamed appendix is coaxed into the wound by gentle traction. If the appendix is retrocecal or retroperitoneal, or if the local inflammation and edema are intense, exposure is improved by dividing the lateral peritoneal reflection of the cecum. At the end of the maneuver, the cecum should lie within the wound, and the appendix should be at the level of the anterior abdominal wall (see Fig. 88–1).

Once the appendix has been freed, the mesoappendix is

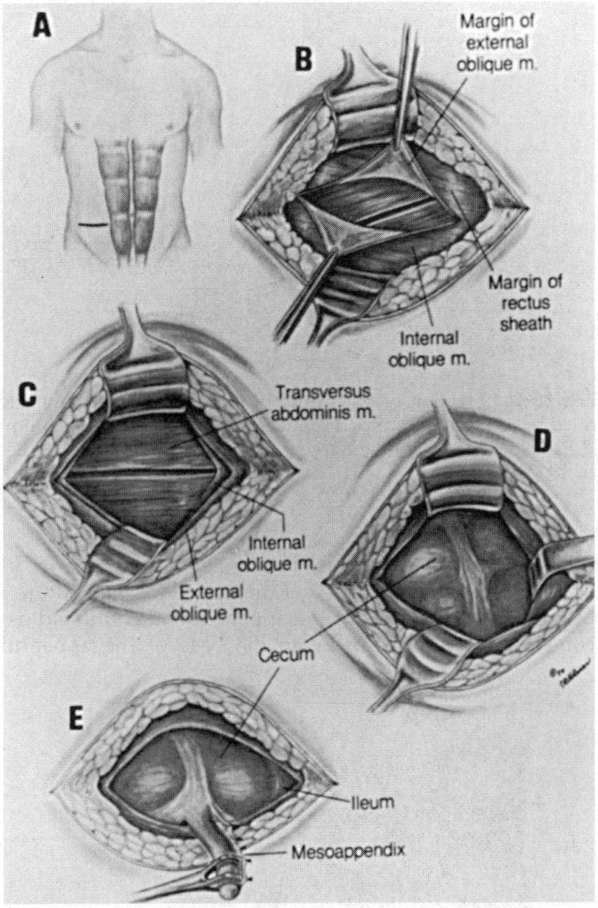

FIGURE 88–1 □ Steps in performing an appendectomy through a transverse incision. *A*, Placement of the skin incision. *B* and *C*, External and internal oblique and transversus abdominis muscles are divided in the direction of their fibers. *D*, After incision of the peritoneum, the cecum is exposed and the appendix is located by following the anterior cecal taenia inferiorly. *E*, The cecum is mobilized into the wound by incising its lateral peritoneal reflections. (From Condon RE: Appendicitis. *In* Moody FG, Carey LC, Jones RS, et al [eds]: Surgical Treatment of Digestive Diseases. Chicago, Year Book Medical Publishers, 1986.)

transected, beginning at its free border by taking small bites of the mesoappendix between pairs of hemostats placed approximately 1 cm from and parallel to the appendix. This process is repeated until the base of the appendix is reached.

There are three ways to handle the appendiceal stump: simple ligation, inversion, and a combination of the two. Either simple ligation or inversion is acceptable, and both have comparable rates of complications. The combination of ligation and inversion is not recommended because it does not reduce the risk of septic complications[25] but does create conditions conducive to development of an intramural abscess or a mucocele. Also, the ligated and inverted appendiceal stump can appear later as a cecal "tumor," a source of diagnostic difficulties in the future.[26]

Simple ligature of the appendiceal stump is accomplished by crushing the appendix at its base with a hemostat, then removing the hemostat and replacing it on the appendix just distal to the crushed line. A ligature of monofilament suture is placed in the groove produced by the crushing clamp and is tied tightly (Fig. 88–2). The appendix is transected just proximal to the hemostat and removed. Inversion of an unligated stump using a Z stitch (Fig. 88–3), rather than the more conventional purse-string suture, is preferred. The upper

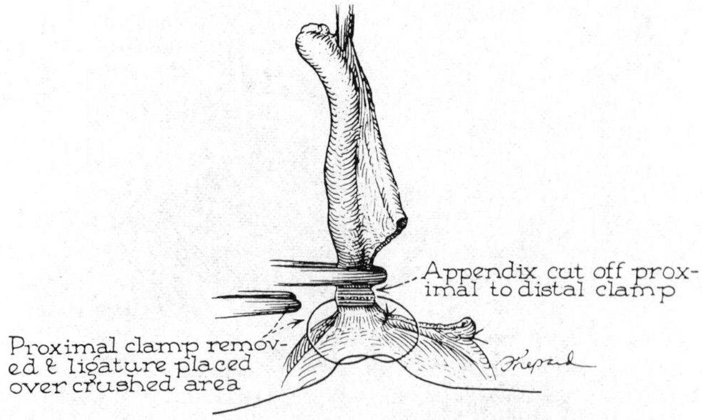

FIGURE 88–2 □ Ligation of the stump of the appendix in the groove formed by a crushing clamp. (From Partipilo AV: Surgical Technique and Principles of Operative Surgery, ed 6. Philadelphia, Lea & Febiger, 1957.)

level of the Z stitch is placed as a Lembert suture in the cecum, just distal to the base of the appendix. The suture is brought around the base of the appendix and continued as a second Lembert suture beneath the base of the appendix.

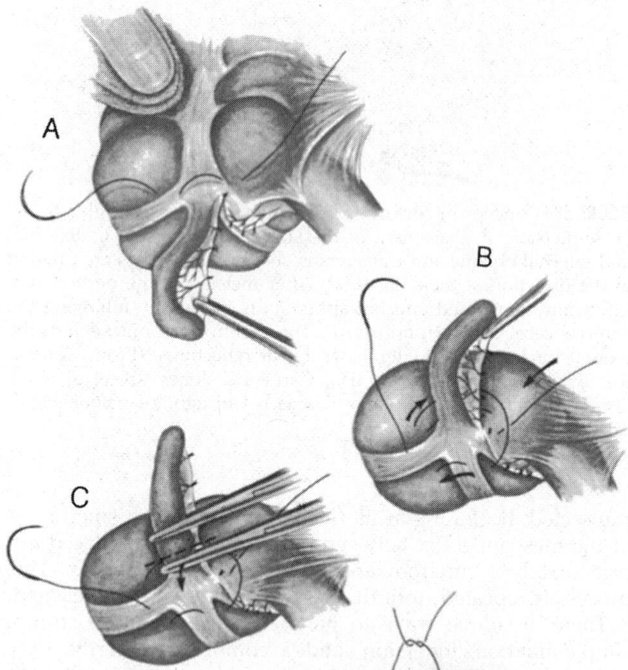

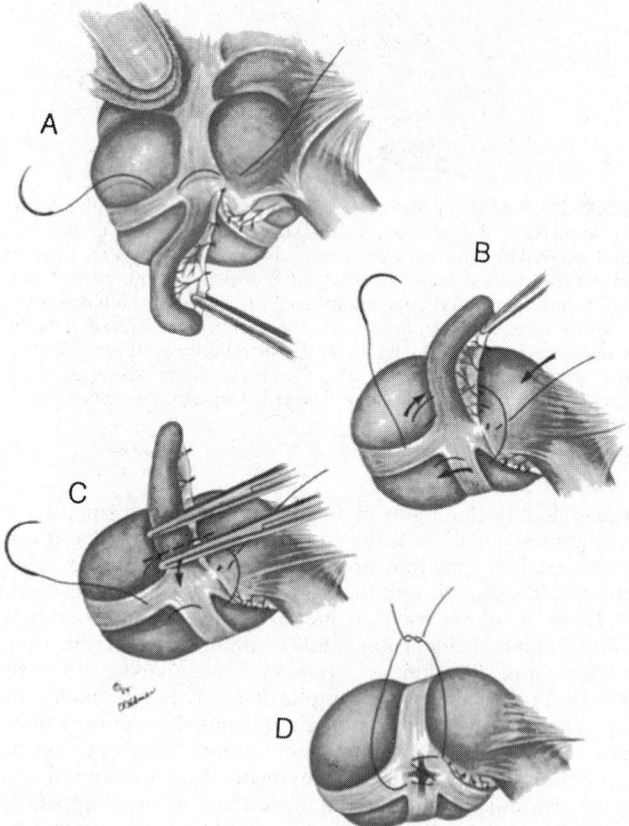

FIGURE 88–3 □ Use of a Z stitch to invert the unligated appendiceal stump. *A*, Two bites of the suture are placed in the cecum 1 cm distal to the base of the appendix. *B*, The suture is then brought around the appendix medially, and two additional bites are placed beneath the base of the appendix. *C*, The appendix is then transected. *D*, The stump of the appendix is inverted into the cecum and the clamp is removed as the suture is tightened. (From Adams JT: Z-stitch suture for inversion of the appendiceal stump. Surg Gynecol Obstet 127:1321, 1968. By permission of Surgery, Gynecology & Obstetrics, now known as the Journal of the American College of Surgeons.)

The appendix is transected between clamps; the stump is inverted into the cecum; the proximal clamp is removed; and the ends of the Z stitch are tied over the stump of the appendix, which is not ligated. If the appendiceal stump is unsuitable for inversion because of edema, it should be simply ligated and not inverted.

Laparoscopy has gained acceptance in the diagnosis and treatment of acute appendicitis.[27] If uncomplicated appendicitis is encountered at the time of laparoscopy, an appendectomy can be performed with relative ease. If a normal appendix is encountered, the abdomen can be examined with the laparoscope, thus avoiding a large abdominal incision.

Perforated or Gangrenous Appendicitis with a Periappendiceal Mass

When a mass is detected by examination under anesthesia that was not appreciated preoperatively, a transverse incision is made over the most prominent portion of the mass. The muscles and aponeuroses are split along their lines of cleavage in gridiron fashion. If the peritoneal cavity is entered, the wound should be packed immediately to prevent contamination of the abdominal cavity. Any fluid or pus is aspirated, and a specimen is sent for culture and sensitivity studies. A finger should be used to break up any loculations. As mentioned earlier, the mass may be made up of omentum and loops of small intestine that are adherent to the inflamed appendix, and an abscess may not be present. If feasible, appendectomy is then performed; it is usually not possible to invert the stump, so simple ligation is preferred.

In a patient with a gangrenous appendix and little or no periappendiceal pus, it is not necessary to place a subfascial drain. If there is a periappendiceal abscess and the tissues are so fixed as to create a dead space, the cavity should be drained with one or more closed suction drains brought out through a separate stab incision.

Before fascial closure, the right iliac fossa and the wound should be liberally irrigated. Muscles and aponeuroses should be closed with interrupted sutures. Whether the skin should be closed is a matter of controversy. Studies in children indicate that primary closure is a safe practice[28, 29]; experience in adults indicates that the skin should be left open, to be closed with adhesive paper tapes on the fifth or sixth postoperative day. Parenteral antibiotics should be given for 5 days after operation or until clinical signs indicate absence of infection and the white cell count and differential count are normal. Rectal examination for a pelvic abscess is performed daily. The patient should be discharged from the hospital only after discontinuing antibiotics for 24 hours without developing a fever.

Perforated Appendicitis with Localized Abscess Formation

If, at the time of initial physical examination, a well-localized periappendiceal mass is found and the patient's symptoms are improving, it is acceptable in healthy adults to initiate parenteral antibiotic treatment and to observe the patient expectantly. This form of therapy is not appropriate for children, pregnant women, or elderly patients. For two thirds of cases, expectant treatment of an appendix mass succeeds and interval appendectomy can be performed later. If the patient's symptoms do not subside, an emergency operation should be performed with the diagnosis of localized abscess.

The skin incision for drainage of a periappendiceal abscess is made just medial to the crest of the ileum at the level of the abscess. With use of a muscle-splitting technique, the lateral edge of the peritoneum is exposed and pushed medially so that the abscess is approached from its lateral aspect. Once it is entered, a finger should be used to break up the loculations. Any fluid or pus is sent for culture and sensitivity study. If the appendix can be freed without breaking down adhesions, appendectomy should be performed. If an appendectomy is not performed, an interval appendectomy should be done 6 to 8 weeks after the abscess has ceased to drain and the wound is completely healed.

After the wound has been thoroughly irrigated with normal saline, a closed suction drain should be inserted into the abscess cavity and brought out through a separate stab wound in the flank. The muscles and aponeuroses are closed with interrupted nonabsorbable sutures, and the skin and subcutaneous tissues are packed open with saline-soaked gauze. The drain should be left in place until it is draining less than 50 mL/d; then it is advanced progressively until it is removed.

Systemic antibiotics should be continued for 5 days postoperatively or until signs of sepsis have cleared and the white cell count and differential count are normal. A daily rectal examination should be done to detect pelvic abscess. The patient should be discharged from the hospital only after having discontinued antibiotics for 48 hours without developing a fever.

Perforated Appendicitis with Diffuse Peritonitis

The major cause of mortality from appendicitis is generalized peritonitis, so for a patient with a diagnosis of acute appendicitis whose physical signs are consistent with diffuse peritonitis, immediate exploration is indicated. If a perforated appendix and diffuse peritonitis are documented at operation, an appendectomy should be performed and the abdomen thoroughly irrigated. The use of drains in diffuse peritonitis is not recommended unless there are localized abscesses that require drainage.[30] The wound and postoperative care should be handled as described in a patient with a periappendiceal abscess.

Normal Appendix When Appendicitis Is Suspected

Whenever a patient undergoes exploratory laparotomy, especially through a right lower quadrant incision, for the diagnosis of acute appendicitis and a normal appendix is found, a careful search for other disease should be made and an appendectomy should be performed. The cause of the symptoms should be identified and treated, or the surgeon should be sure that no lesion requiring treatment is present. The normal appendix is removed to avoid diagnostic confusion in the future.

If the history and physical examination findings are appropriate for the diagnosis of acute appendicitis, it is not an error to perform an exploratory laparotomy and remove what appears to be a normal appendix. A policy of early surgical intervention on the basis of clinical suspicion has been demonstrated overall to reduce both the morbidity and mortality of acute appendicitis.

Complications

Postoperative complications occur in 5% of patients with an unperforated appendix but in more than 30% of those with a gangrenous or perforated appendix. The most frequent complications after appendectomy are wound infection, intraabdominal abscess, fecal fistula, pylephlebitis, and intestinal obstruction.

Subcutaneous tissue infection is the most common complication after appendectomy. The organisms most frequently cultured are anaerobic *Bacteroides* species and the aerobes *Klebsiella, Enterobacter,* and *E. coli.*[31] When early signs of wound infection (undue pain and edema) are present, the skin and subcutaneous tissue should be opened. The wound should be packed with saline-soaked gauze and reclosed with Steri-Strips in 4 to 5 days.

Pelvic, subphrenic, or other intraabdominal abscesses occur in up to 20% of patients with a gangrenous or perforated appendix. Such abscesses are accompanied by recurrent fever, malaise, and anorexia. CT is a great help in making the diagnosis of intraabdominal abscess. When abscesses are diagnosed, they should be drained either operatively or percutaneously under CT or ultrasound guidance.

Some fecal fistulae close spontaneously, provided that there is no anatomic reason for the fistula to remain open. Obviously, those that do not close spontaneously require operation. Pylephlebitis, or portal pyemia, is characterized by jaundice, chills, and high fever. It is a serious illness that frequently leads to multiple liver abscesses. The infecting organism is usually *E. coli.* This complication has become rare with the routine use of antibiotics in complicated appendicitis. Although not frequent, true mechanical bowel obstruction may occur as a complication of acute appendicitis. As for any other mechanical small bowel obstruction, operative therapy is indicated.

References

1. Lewis FR, Holcroft JW, Boey J, Dunphy JE: Appendicitis: A critical review of diagnosis and treatment in 1,000 cases. Arch Surg 110:677, 1975.
2. Wangensteen OH, Dennis C: Experimental proof of obstructive origin of appendicitis in man. Ann Surg 110:629, 1939.
3. Dennis C: Physiologic behavior of the human appendix and the problem of appendicitis: Reaction of the appendix to drugs. Arch Surg 43:1021, 1941.
4. Altemeier WA: The bacterial flora of acute perforated appendicitis with peritonitis: A bacteriologic study based upon one hundred cases. Ann Surg 107:517, 1938.
5. Pieper R, Kager L, Nasman P: Acute appendicitis: A clinical study of 1018 cases of emergency appendectomy. Acta Chir Scand 148:51, 1982.
6. Hubbell DS, Barton WK, Soloman OD: Leukocytosis in appendicitis in older patients. JAMA 175:139, 1961.
7. Bolton JP, Craven ER, Croft RJ, Menzies-Gow N: An assessment of the value of the white cell count in the management of suspected acute appendicitis. Br J Surg 62:906, 1975.
8. Rajagopalan AE, Mason JH, Kennedy M, Pawlikowski J: The value of the barium enema in the diagnosis of acute appendicitis. Arch Surg 112:531, 1977.
9. Jona JZ, Belin RP, Selke AC: Barium enema as a diagnostic aid in children with abdominal pain. Surg Gynecol Obstet 144:351, 1977.
10. Smith DE, Kirchmer NA, Stewart DR: Use of the barium enema in the diagnosis of acute appendicitis and its complications. Am J Surg 138:829, 1979.
11. Hayden CK, Kuchelmeister J, Lipscomb TS: Sonography of acute appendicitis in childhood: Perforation versus nonperforation. J Ultrasound Med 11:209, 1992.
12. Sivit CJ, Newman KD, Boenning DA, et al: Appendicitis: Usefulness of US in diagnosis in a pediatric population. Radiology 185:549, 1992.
13. Rioux M: Sonographic detection of the normal and abnormal appendix. AJR 158:773, 1992.
14. Malone AJ, Wolf CR, Malmed AS, Melliere BF: Diagnosis of acute appendicitis: Value of unenhanced CT. AJR 160:763, 1993.
15. Balthazar EJ, Megiban AJ, Siegel SE, Birnbaum BA: Appendicitis: Prospective evaluation with high-resolution CT. Radiology 180:21, 1991.
16. Shapiro MP, Gale ME, Gerzof SG: CT of appendicitis: Diagnosis and treatment. Radiol Clin North Am 27:753, 1989.
17. Stone HH, Sanders SL, Martin JD: Perforated appendicitis in children. Surgery 69:673, 1971.

18. Graham JM, Pokorny WJ, Harberg FJ: Acute appendicitis in preschool age children. Am J Surg 139:247, 1980.
19. Gomez A, Wood M: Acute appendicitis during pregnancy. Am J Surg 137:180, 1979.
20. Owens BJ III, Hamit HF: Appendicitis in the elderly. Ann Surg 187:392, 1978.
21. Thorbjarnarson B, Loehr WJ: Acute appendicitis in patients over the age of sixty. Surg Gynecol Obstet 125:1277, 1967.
22. Burns RP, Cochran JL, Russell WL, Bard RM: Appendicitis in mature patients. Ann Surg 201:695, 1985.
23. Bongard F, Landers DV, Lewis F: Differential diagnosis of appendicitis and pelvic inflammatory disease. A prospective analysis. Am J Surg 150:90, 1985.
24. Hoffman J, Lindhard A, Jensen H-E: Appendix mass: Conservative management without interval appendectomy. Am J Surg 1248:379, 1984.
25. Kingsley DPE: Some observations on appendectomy with particular reference to technique. Br J Surg 56:491, 1969.
26. Myllariemi H, Perttala Y, Peltokallio P: Tumor-like lesions of the cecum following inversion of the appendix. Dig Dis 19:547, 1974.
27. Gotz F, Pier A, Badier C: Modified laparoscopic appendectomy in surgery: A report of 388 operations. Surg Endosc 4:6, 1990.
28. Neilson IR, Laberge JM, Nguyen LT, et al: Appendicitis in children: Current therapeutic recommendations. J Pediatr Surg 25: 1113, 1990.
29. Burnweit C, Bilik R, Shandling B: Primary closure of contaminated wounds in perforated appendicitis. J Pediatr Surg 26: 1362, 1991.
30. Haller JA, Shaker IJ, Donahoo JS, et al: Peritoneal drainage versus nondrainage for generalized peritonitis from ruptured appendicitis in children. Ann Surg 177:595, 1973.
31. Leigh DA, Simmons K, Normal E: Bacteria flora of the appendix fossa in appendicitis and postoperative wound infection. J Clin Pathol 27:997, 1974.

89

Diverticulitis

Dietmar H. Wittmann
Moshe Schein
Constantine T. Frantzides

Acute diverticulitis is the inflammation of congenital or acquired colonic diverticula. The terms diverticulosis and diverticulitis must not be confused. The former indicates the presence of symptomatic or silent diverticular disease; the latter signifies an infectious process developing in the former. The incidence of the disease increases with age. Most often it occurs as a complication of acquired diverticulosis of the sigmoid colon.[1, 2] In the Western world, the sigmoid colon is the segment affected in 90% of the cases of diverticulitis,[3] whereas in Asian countries, such as Japan, right-sided disease is more common.[4, 5] It is estimated that the annual risk for acute diverticulitis in the population with diverticulosis of the colon is 1% to 3%.[6] Diverticulosis affects 30 million Americans annually, bringing 200,000 to the hospital and incurring health care costs exceeding a third of a billion dollars.[6] Several studies strongly suggest that symptomatic diverticulosis in younger patients (i.e., younger than 40 to 50 years) is prone to severe complications and would usually require, at some stage, surgical treatment.[7, 8]

Pathogenesis

The pathophysiologic mechanism of colonic diverticulum formation is multifactorial. It must involve spaces of high intracolonic pressure and areas of relative weakness in the colon wall. In manometric and cinematographic studies, high-pressure waves coincide with bandlike contractions that occlude short segments, leading to herniation of the mucosa.[9] This mechanism is not uniformly accepted and other theories have been proposed. The tensile strength and elasticity of the colon decline with age and are more marked in the left colon, which is the narrowest and thickest part, suggesting that the mechanical properties of the bowel wall are main etiologic factors. Because tensile strength is a probable factor in the firmness of colon wall and the process of aging is associated with an increase in type I collagen and a decrease in type III collagen[10] in some tissues, this could explain the increased incidence of diverticulosis with age.

The striking differences in the incidence of diverticulosis, so common in the Western world and almost nonexistent in African populations, must be emphasized. Probably, inequalities in nutritional habits are responsible: high-residue diets of Africans produce bulkier feces and as a result a thinner and more elastic colon wall. Conversely, the end result of the low-residue Western dietary habits is the narrow, contracted, divericulum-prone colon.[11] Acute diverticulitis usually originates in a narrow-necked diverticulum with impacted fecal material. A reactive inflammatory edema obstructs the neck and prevents intraluminal drainage of the fecal material, which contains up to 400 different species of bacteria in large numbers.[12] This leads to the development of diverticular microempyema, an accumulation of pus in the preformed diverticulum. Increased pressure in the diverticulum leads to microperforation of the mucosa, promoting the leakage of intraluminal bacteria into adjacent sterile tissues or the free abdominal cavity. The patient's host defense mechanisms respond with the formation of a peridiverticular infiltrate, consisting of omentum and adjacent structures, to prevent fecal contamination of the peritoneal cavity.

A wide variety of disease processes may follow, ranging in severity from acute inflammation without pus formation to acute fecal peritonitis, with abscess formation representing the middle of the spectrum (Table 89–1). The end result of the initial process depends on the size of the perforation and the magnitude of the bacterial challenge versus the local host response. An abscess develops when bacterial toxins and the host's proteolytic enzymes liquefy the central oxygen- and nutrient-depleted necrotic areas—an ideal condition for further growth of anaerobic bacteria. The abscess might perforate into the free peritoneal cavity or into adjacent organs, most commonly the urinary bladder. Occasionally, it spreads along retroperitoneal tissue planes into the skin, especially in the left groin. The prevalence of fistula formation among patients with colonic diverticular disease is reported to be 12%.[13, 14]

The free perforation via the bowel wall (Fig. 89–1) releases

TABLE 89–1 ■ The Spectrum of Perforative Diverticular Disease

Acute simple diverticulitis (acute inflammation without pus formation)
Localized purulent process
Local peritonitis (peridiverticular infiltrate)
Abscess
Fistula (vagina, bladder, bowel, skin)
Diffuse fecal peritonitis
After perforation of a diverticulum
After perforation of a peridiverticular abscess

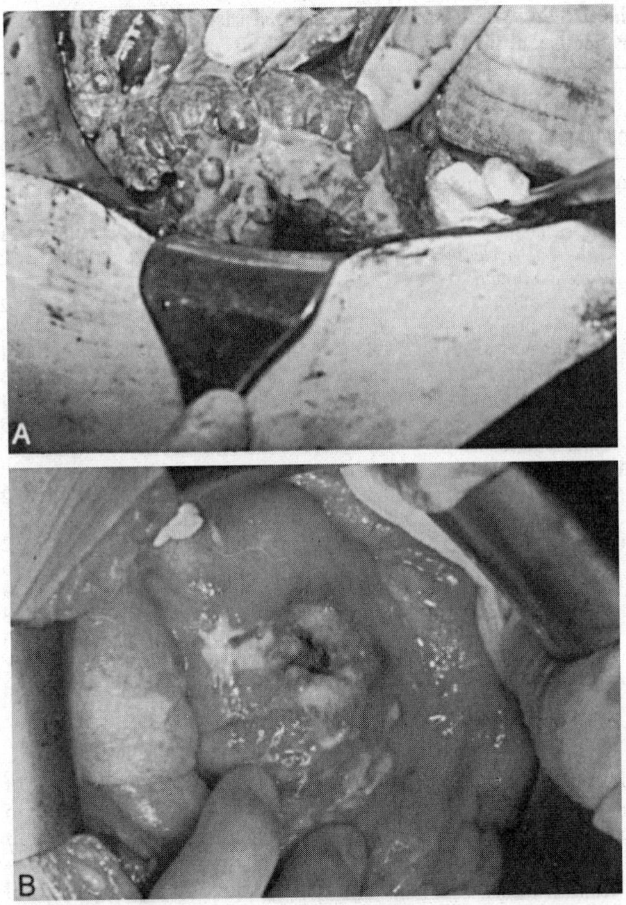

FIGURE 89–1 □ Peritonitis caused by perforated diverticulum. *A*, Peritonitis with fibrinous exudate and diverticula of the sigmoid colon. *B*, Inflammation of the peritoneum caused by a perforated diverticulum of the sigmoid colon.

high inocula of proliferating bacteria into the peritoneal cavity and results in a generalized peritonitis that is associated with a high mortality rate. It is well recognized that nonsteroidal antiinflammatory drugs interfere with local "walling-off" mechanisms. Hence, severe perforative complications of acute diverticulitis are significantly more common in patients who ingest these drugs.[15]

Clinical Manifestations

The clinical scenario may be labeled a "left-sided appendicitis." The most prominent symptom is steady, deep-seated, left lower quadrant pain, which may at times be crampy and intermittent. Because the sigmoid colon is mobile, the symptoms and signs may refer to other quadrants of the abdomen. Changes in bowel function may occur: usually constipation but sometimes diarrhea or alternating diarrhea and constipation. Low-grade or spiking fever with chills is usually present if the disease is severe. Nausea and vomiting are not common unless there is perforation, peritonitis, or bowel obstruction. Urinary symptoms such as frequency, urgency, and dysuria may be present when the inflammation extends to the bladder. Dysuria and urinary frequency associated with pneumaturia and fecaluria are diagnostic of colovesical fistula.

The physical examination usually reveals left lower quadrant abdominal tenderness with muscle guarding. Occasionally on deep palpation a tender, fixed mass may be felt, which is indicative of suppurative pericolitis. When severe inflammation is present, abdominal muscle guarding makes the palpation of such a mass impossible. At times, the mass can be felt on rectal digital examination. Blood and mucus may be seen on the examining finger, but profuse hemorrhage is uncommon. In cases with free perforation into the peritoneal cavity, the symptoms and signs of generalized peritonitis prevail.

Diagnosis

Chest and abdominal radiographs should be obtained at the time of admission to the hospital to rule out free perforation or bowel obstruction. Contrast-enhanced studies, if indicated, should always be performed with low pressure and water-soluble contrast media, and sigmoidoscopy should never be done with insufflation of air. We believe that there is little, if any, indication for these diagnostic procedures during the acute phase of the disease, although they may be of great value when performed after the symptoms have subsided, to exclude inflammatory bowel disease or neoplasia. Colonoscopy in patients with symptomatic sigmoid diverticular disease has revealed an associated carcinoma in 7 patients and adenomatous polyps in 29. Barium enema examination has been inaccurate.[16] Studies suggest that computed tomography may be helpful not only in the diagnosis of diverticulitis and its complications[17] but also in selecting the therapeutic regimen.[18–20] The visualization of a triad consisting of a diverticulum, a segmentally thickened colon, and extraluminal fluid collection, with or without associated gas, correctly identifies an abscess. The combination of diverticulum, thickened colon, and an adjacent, gas-containing edematous bladder points to a colovesical fistula.[21] Computed tomography combined with diatrizoate meglumine (Gastrografin) enema has been used prospectively to assess the severity of the acute attack. Mild diverticulitis has been defined as localized colon wall thickening of less than 5 mm with inflammation of pericolic fat. The same findings associated with an abscess, extraluminal air, or extraluminal Gastrografin suggested a severe attack of diverticulitis. Most patients classified as having a mild disease responded to conservative treatment, whereas those considered to have a severe attack required an urgent operation or an interval procedure after nonoperative treatment.[8] Because a pericolic phlegmon should be managed differently than a pericolic abscess, the differentiation of these conditions may obviate undue delay or undue rush in the management of diverticulitis. Although laboratory and radiologic findings can at times be valuable in the evaluation of acute diverticulitis, we believe that the diagnosis should be based principally on the clinical evaluation. Computed tomography should be performed selectively for patients in whom abscess or fistulization is suspected after they fail to improve rapidly with conservative therapy.

Treatment

General Considerations

Treatment of acute sigmoid diverticulitis is best considered under the following headings: (1) medical (nonoperative) management, (2) operative management of infectious complications, and (3) medical and surgical prevention of recurrent episodes.

Generally, our practical therapeutic approach (Table 89–2) is based on the extent of the process (see Table 89–1). Acute inflammation without pus formation is managed conservatively, localized suppuration requires an immediate or de-

TABLE 89–2 ■ Management of Acute Diverticulitis: Authors' Recommendations

DISEASE PROCESS	MANAGEMENT
Acute simple diverticulitis	Nonoperative treatment
Diverticular abscess	Percutaneous drainage plus delayed elective sigmoid resection
Diverticular fistula	Resection of fistula and sigmoid colon Colocutaneous fistula may heal spontaneously
Diffuse peritonitis	Sigmoid resection and primary anastomosis plus planned reoperations; Hartmann procedure in desperate situations

layed operation, and the diffuse process is treated by an emergency laparotomy. About 80% of patients admitted to the hospital for diverticular disease are managed medically with antibiotics and a low-residue diet. Only 10% to 20% require an emergency operation, and at operation generalized or fecal peritonitis is found in 20% to 60% of these.[22]

Medical (Nonoperative) Treatment

An attack of mild, noncomplicated, acute phlegmonous diverticulitis usually responds to conservative therapy. The colon is "rested" with a low-residue diet. If ileus develops the patient is given nothing by mouth. If analgesics are required, the agent of choice appears to be pentazocine, which has been shown to reduce the motility of the sigmoid in patients with diverticulitis.[23] Meperidine may be preferred because it is less likely to produce disorientation.

Antibiotic therapy is initiated. It is required on the assumption that pathogenic bacteria within the stool flora are responsible for the acute infectious process. Antimicrobials should suppress growth of both endotoxin-producing facultative aerobes and obligate anaerobes, even if blood cultures grow only a single species. The microbial pathogenicity of the disease process favors the development of synergistic infection by organisms that include *Escherichia coli*, *Bacteroides fragilis*, and other *Bacteroides* species, clostridia, and anaerobic streptococci. Therefore, "blind" or even empirical antimicrobial chemotherapy is antiquated and should be discarded in favor of calculated antibiotic therapy[24] (Table 89–3).

Because it is impossible to investigate pathogens directly in infected diverticula, pathogens isolated in peritonitis after perforation of the colon most closely delineate the target bacteria[24, 25] (Table 89–4). The antibiotic concentration at the site of infection should surpass the minimal inhibitory concentration (MIC) for the targeted bacteria. Antimicrobial concentrations measured in peritoneal fluid have been shown to be more representative of drug levels at the infectious site

TABLE 89–3 ■ Essentials of Calculated Antimicrobial Therapy

Consideration of typical spectrum of infecting bacteria
Consideration of pathogenicity of different bacteria and synergistic or antagonistic interactions
Consideration of the antibiotic concentration sustained at the infectious site after a given dose
Consideration of toxicity of antibiotics under the specific circumstances
Consideration of antibiotic interaction with host defense
Consideration of results of controlled clinical trials

TABLE 89–4 ■ Bacteria Isolated in Intraabdominal Infections After Perforation of the Large Bowel in 48 Patients

ORGANISM	ISOLATES Number	%
Aerobes (facultative anaerobes)		
Escherichia coli	39	81
Klebsiella sp.	10	21
Enterobacter cloacae	1	2
Proteus mirabilis	7	15
Proteus vulgaris	1	2
Streptococci group A	3	6
Streptococci groups C + D	2	4
Enterococcus faecalis	16	33
Pseudomonas aeruginosa	2	4
Other aerobes	7	15
Total aerobes	88	
Anaerobes (obligate anaerobes)		
Bacteroides fragilis	25	52
Other *Bacteroides*	22	46
Fusobacterium	1	2
Peptostreptococci	7	15
Clostridium perfringens	9	19
Other clostridia	4	8
Other anaerobes	6	13
Total anaerobes	74	

than the serum concentration. After a dose of 500 mg of metronidazole, a concentration of 2 to 4 mg/L is present in peritoneal fluid for about 12 hours, a concentration sufficient for most anaerobic bacteria. *B. fragilis* generally cannot survive at this concentration of metronidazole. A dose interval of 12 hours is sufficient. Because its bioavailability is greater than 90% after oral or rectal administration, the route of administration does not significantly influence the concentration at the infectious site.

The antimicrobial choice should include activity against *E. coli* and other less common gram-negative enteric organisms. In 104 studies, 10,413 strains of *E. coli* were tested using standardized techniques (test inoculum 6.0 log_{10} colony-forming units per milliliter) against cefotaxime, ceftazidime, and moxalactam and other β-lactam antibiotics. No strain had an MIC higher than the concentrations achieved in peritoneal fluid for 2 g of cefotaxime, ceftazidime, and moxalactam. Of the *E. coli* strains, 26%, 19%, and 13% had MICs higher than the antibiotic concentrations achieved at the infectious site for 2 g of cefoxitin, 1.5 g of cefuroxime, and 2 g of cefoperazone, respectively. More than 35% of the *E. coli* strains had MICs that were greater than the peritoneal fluid concentrations for 5 g of mezlocillin and piperacillin at 50 mg/kg given intravenously.[26] No properly conducted prospective randomized antibiotic trials have dealt with diverticulitis only. Other trials of antibiotics for so-called intraabdominal infections provided insufficient information to help in choosing the right antibiotic because they excluded the most seriously ill patients from being enrolled in the studies.[27] Furthermore, many patients in these studies were described as having intraabdominal infections and had just simple abdominal contamination resulting from penetrating bowel injury. Therefore, the choice of antibiotic is better based on the pharmacodynamics mentioned earlier.

The antibiotic of choice should therefore include cefotaxime, ceftazidime, or similar third-generation cephalosporins in combination with 500 mg of metronidazole (Table 89–5) or clindamycin for coverage of the pathogenic anaerobes. Clindamycin, 1200 mg every 12 hours intravenously (or the traditional but not so good 600 mg every 6 hours), may be

TABLE 89–5 ■ Recommendations for Antimicrobial Therapy for Diverticulitis

AGENT	DOSE (mg)	ADMINISTRATION*
Fixed combinations		
Imipenem-cilastatin	1000	q 8 h IV
Ampicillin-sulbactam	3000	q 6 h IV
Ticarcillin–clavulanate	3100	q 8 h IV
Piperacillin-tazobactam	4500	q 8 h IV
Amoxicillin–clavulanate	500/125	q 8 h PO
Combinations of antianaerobic drugs with cephalosporins and monobactams		
Metronidazole	500	q 12 h IV, or PO or rectally
	or	
Clindamycin	1200	q 12 h IV or 600 mg q 8 h PO
	in combination with	
Cefotaxime	2000	q 8–12 h IV
	or	
Ceftizoxime	2000	q 12 h IV
	or	
Ceftriaxone	2000	q 12 h IV
Alternative combinations		
Clindamycin	1200	q 12 h IV
	in combination with	
Aztreonam	2000	q 8 h IV

* IV, Intravenously; PO, orally.

combined with 2000 mg of aztreonam for effective treatment. Ceftazidime should not be used for diverticulitis (it should be reserved for *Pseudomonas aeruginosa* infections). Monotherapy with an intravenous drug such as moxalactam, 2 g every 12 hours; cefotetan, 2 g every 12 hours; or imipenem, 1000 mg every 8 hours, may have the same effect as combinations owing to their excellent activity against *E. coli* and obligate anaerobes. Fixed combinations such as imipenem-cilastatin, 1000 mg every 8 hours, and the newly approved penicillin–β-lactamase inhibitor combinations are alternative choices. Combinations with metronidazole and quinolones seem attractive because both drugs can be given orally. Valid clinical experience, however, is pending.

Today the value of aminoglycosides seems to be limited to certain classes of patients who may be infected by bacteria that are resistant to the third-generation cephalosporins. In such patients who have in previous weeks been exposed to antibiotics or to a hospital environment, the additive effect of aminoglycosides plus β-lactams on certain strains of multidrug-resistant bacteria may be utilized.

The classic combination of an aminoglycoside plus clindamycin has been widely used. At present, this regimen may be used under specific circumstances when potentially less toxic alternatives cannot be administered. When diverticulitis progresses to peritonitis, renal function may be impaired as a result of the systemic repercussions of the infectious process. The nephrotoxic potential of aminoglycosides may be clinically relevant even if serum levels are monitored.

Because there have been few randomized controlled clinical studies of diverticulitis, one may be tempted to base patients' management on the results of numerous antibiotic trials for intraabdominal infection of gut origin, but the value of these trials is limited by the excessively restrictive criteria for selection of patients.[27]

Patients with milder symptoms of acute diverticulitis, such as low-grade fever and minimal signs of peritoneal irritation, might be given oral antibiotics to avoid hospitalization. Among the drugs suggested have been oral ciprofloxacin in combination with clindamycin or metronidazole. Another possibility is amoxicillin–clavulanate potassium (Augmentin), which gives broad aerobic and anaerobic coverage.

Surgical Treatment

OPERATIVE TREATMENT OF INFECTIOUS COMPLICATIONS

The perforation of a diverticulum allows a direct communication between the lumen of the colon and adjacent sterile tissues or the free abdominal cavity, resulting in a spectrum of conditions (see Table 89–1) that require selective therapy. The choice of the specific surgical technique has been controversial for many decades.[22] Previously, the surgical management of complicated diverticulitis has been based on guidelines suggested by Mayo,[28] Lockhart-Mummary,[29] and Smithwick.[30] During the past 50 years, surgeons have relied on a diverting colostomy or multiple-stage procedures that involve high risk for mortality and morbidity. There is currently a trend that favors a single-stage repair with resection of the sigmoid colon without protective colostomy.[31–36] The existence of several published studies that report unfavorable results for staged repair, the availability of potent antibiotics, and better surgical intensive care are probably reasons for this rapid change. Some authors believe that primary anastomosis can be performed even in the presence of obstruction or perforation.[37–40] This can be accomplished with[41] or without[42] an intraoperative colonic preparation.

A collective review of the literature[22] outlined the superiority of the one-stage resection over all other more "conservative" procedures. ("Secure suture of a perforation has never really been possible."[43]) Poor outcome seen with suture closure and drainage plus colostomy confirms this statement. Nevertheless, one might reason that multiple-stage procedures are usually performed on the most severely ill patients and represent a negative selection. In 1981, Sakai and colleagues[44] published a report of multiple-stage series with no associated mortality in this high-risk group of patients. In it, primary resection was performed and the abdomen was left open to allow repeated débridement and control of the healing of the anastomosis. Furthermore, the authors of most studies of multiple-stage operation fail to report the cumulative morbidity and mortality for all stages.

Staged abdominal repair (e.g., planned abdominal reexplorations) (Fig. 89–2) may be the best treatment option for a high-risk group.[45] If the patient's physiologic derangement predicts a high risk of death on the basis of the Acute Physiology and Chronic Health Evaluation II (APACHE II) score[46] and if débridement cannot be accomplished in a single procedure, staged abdominal repair should be considered. In this procedure the infected abdominal cavity is treated like an open wound that is closed temporarily. This allows daily reexploration and débridement until the septic focus is under control and anastomotic healing is ensured. Temporary abdominal closure can be accomplished by using Marlex mesh with a zipper, Ethizip, or a Velcro-like artificial bur.[45] In one series, planned, staged abdominal reexplorations were performed in 10 consecutive patients suffering from diffuse fecal peritonitis. There was no mortality, attesting to the importance of aggressive, repeated peritoneal "toilet" when fecal contamination is massive.[47]

Occasionally, the invading bacteria and adjuvants of infection are confined in a localized abscess, which may be demonstrable at the time of diagnosis. Computed tomography–guided percutaneous drainage may be a good treatment option.[48, 49] The bacterial inoculum is reduced considerably, allowing optimal effectiveness of antimicrobials. The resection of the diseased colon could be delayed and subsequently performed electively. If clinical resolution is not seen within 48 hours, an urgent operation should be performed. It must

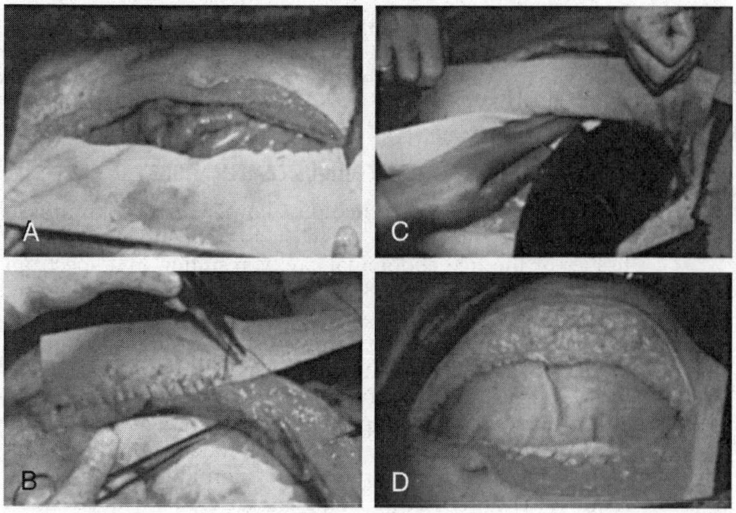

FIGURE 89–2 □ Abdominal wound with artificial bur adhesive sheets (Velcro) sutured to the abdominal fasciae to ease temporary abdominal closure between planned repeated laparotomies every 24 hours (staged abdominal repair). *A,* The looped sheet of the artificial bur is sutured to the abdominal fascia on one side of the abdominal wound. *B,* The hooked sheet of the artificial bur is sutured to the opposite abdominal fascia. *C,* The looped sheet is pushed underneath the hooked sheet covering the intestines. *D,* The hooked sheet adheres to the looped sheet and the abdominal wound is closed, leaving a gap between the fascia to decompress the abdominal compartment syndrome that is often seen in diffuse peritonitis after diverticular perforation.

be hoped that in the future there will be more controlled trials to determine the best treatment options. Our current therapeutic recommendations are summarized in Table 89–2.

MEDICAL AND SURGICAL PREVENTION OF RECURRENT EPISODES

After the successful conservative management of the acute episode, a high-fiber diet to relieve pain and bowel dysfunction is recommended. The role of the high-fiber diet, which reduces the pressure in the diseased colon segment, is generally accepted for uncomplicated diverticular disease. Clinical trials, however, have not presented suitable control groups for comparison,[50] and evidence demonstrating a reduction in the recurrence rate is not available. Adequate fiber intake may be furnished by five slices (150 g) of whole wheat bread or by varying amounts of widely marketed cereals.[51]

Prevention of recurrences by primary resection of the diseased colon segment has been advocated for recurrent disease, which is seen in 50% of the cases. The risk of life-threatening complications is the basis for indicating interval sigmoid resection after conclusion of acute inflammatory symptoms.[52] Currently, the interval sigmoid colon resection is advocated by most surgeons,[52] although it is not uniformly agreed upon whether it should follow the first or the second acute episode.[53] Common indications for delayed elective sigmoidectomy after the first attack include

1. Young patients (40 to 50 years old) who are prone to complicated recurrences
2. Suspicion of an underlying carcinoma
3. Demonstrable complications such as fistulae, residual abscess, or colonic stenosis

Certainly, a recurrent episode of acute diverticulitis is an indication for a sigmoidectomy. If appropriate, elective surgical resection should be performed 8 to 10 weeks after the acute episode. This time interval permits resolution of the inflammatory reaction. The operation of choice is primary resection of the sigmoid colon without colostomy. The entire distal sigmoid colon needs to be resected and anastomosed to the upper rectum to avoid recurrent diverticulitis.[54] More proximal diverticula-bearing colon segments should be left alone, as the risk of symptomatic disease originating proximal to the resected sigmoid is minimal.[55] It is difficult to assess the overall benefit of this management. In one study, 7% of patients who had resection for diverticular disease suffered recurrent disease.[55] In a separate series, long-term follow-up (3 to 15 years) demonstrated that half of the patients had only one repeated episode of acute diverticulitis.[52]

Acute Diverticulitis in a Solitary Cecal Diverticulum

This rare condition is encountered during 1 of 500 emergency laparotomy procedures or, when compared with acute appendicitis, had a ratio of 1:220. Thus, even busy surgeons would not treat more than a few such cases during their lifetime. The condition usually develops in an age group intermediate to those of patients with acute appendicitis and sigmoid diverticulitis. The clinical presentation mimics that of acute appendicitis but is perhaps less dramatic. In the majority of patients, a diagnosis of acute appendicitis is made, leading to an operation. Occasionally, a correct initial diagnosis is established, with the help of a contrast study or computed tomographic examination, ordered because of atypical symptoms or the history of a previous appendectomy.

When a definitive diagnosis of cecal diverticulitis is established, nonoperative treatment, along lines similar to those described for sigmoid diverticulitis, should be attempted and in most cases is successful. Most patients, however, undergo laparotomy, during which the typical finding consists of a cecal mass (phlegmon). Differentiation from carcinoma or Crohn disease may be extremely difficult. When the possibility of cecal diverticulitis is entertained, a correct intraoperative diagnosis can be made by palpation (a fecalith within the diverticulum) or through a colotomy. In such a situation the procedure should consist of local excision of the diverticulum followed by primary closure of the colonic defect. When accurate diagnosis is in doubt, most authors agree that an immediate right hemicolectomy with an ileocolic anastomosis is the safest option.[56]

References

1. Boles RS Jr, Jordan SM: The clinical significance of diverticulosis. Gastroenterology 35:579, 1958.
2. Horner JL: Natural history of diverticulosis of the colon. Am J Dig Dis 3:343, 1958.
3. Rodkey GV, Welch CE: Changing patterns in the surgical treatment of diverticular disease. Ann Surg 200:466, 1984.
4. Kovalcik PJ, Surstarsic DL: Cecal diverticulitis. Ann Surg 47:72, 1981.
5. Schuler JG, Bayley J: Diverticulitis of the cecum. Surg Gynecol Obstet 156:743, 1983.
6. Griffin HE, Mendeloff AI: Epidemiology of digestive disease. Washington, DC, US Government Printing Office, 1978. US De-

partment of Health, Education, and Welfare publication NIH 79-1887:11–33.
7. Quriel K, Schwartz SI: Diverticular disease in the young patient. Surg Gynecol Obstet 156:1, 1983.
8. Ambrosetti P, Robert J, Witzig JA, et al: Prognostic factors from computed tomography in acute left colonic diverticulitis. Br J Surg 79:117, 1992.
9. Painter NS, Truelove SC, Ardran GM, Tuckey M: Segmentation and the localization of intraluminal pressures in the human colon, with special reference to the pathogenesis of colonic diverticula. Gastroenterology 49:169, 1965.
10. Bornstein P: Disorders of connective tissue function and the aging process: A synthesis and review of current concepts and findings. Mech Ageing Dev 5:305, 1976.
11. Watters DAK, Smith AN: Strength of the colon wall in diverticular disease. Br J Surg 77:257, 1990.
12. Bentley DW, Nichols RL, Condon RE, Gorbach SL: The microflora of the human ileum and intra-abdominal colon: Results of direct needle aspiration at surgery and evaluation of technique. J Lab Clin Med 79:421, 1972.
13. Fazio WV, Church MJ, Jagelman GD, Wearley LF: Colocutaneous fistulas complicating diverticulitis. Dis Colon Rectum 30:89, 1987.
14. Woods JR, Lavery CI, Fazio WV, et al: Internal fistulas in diverticular disease. Dis Colon Rectum 31:591, 1988.
15. Campbell K, Steele RJ: Non-steroidal anti-inflammatory drug and complicated diverticular disease: A case-control study. Br J Surg 78:190, 1991.
16. Boulous PB, Cowen AP, Karamanolis DG, Clark GC: Diverticula, neoplasia, or both? Early detection of carcinoma in sigmoid diverticular disease. Ann Surg 202:607, 1985.
17. Morris J, Stellato TA, Lieberman J, Haaga JR: The utility of computed tomography in colonic diverticulitis. Ann Surg 104:128, 1986.
18. Lieberman JM, Haagar JR: Computed tomography of diverticulitis. J Comput Assist Tomogr 7:431, 1983.
19. Goldman SM, Fishman EK, Gatewood OMB, et al: Demonstration of colovesical fistulae secondary to diverticulitis. J Comput Assist Tomogr 8:462, 1984.
20. Raval B, Lamki N, St. Ville E: Role of computed tomography in diverticulitis. J Comput Tomogr 11:144, 1987.
21. Labs JD, Sarr MG, Fishman EK, et al: Complications of acute diverticulitis of the colon: Improved diagnosis with computerized tomography. Am J Surg 155:331, 1988.
22. Krukowski ZH, Matheson NA: Emergency surgery for diverticular disease complicated by generalized and faecal peritonitis: A review. Br J Surg 71:921, 1984.
23. Stanciu C, Bennett JR: Colonic response to pentazocine. Br J Med 1:312, 1974.
24. Wittmann DH, Bergstein JM, Frantizdes C: Calculated empiric antimicrobial therapy for mixed surgical infections. Infection 19(Suppl):345, 1991.
25. Onderdonk AB, Kaspar DL, Mansheim BJ, et al: Experimental animal models for anaerobic infections. Rev Infect Dis 1:291, 1979.
26. Wittmann DH: Treatment of Peritonitis: Antibiotic Concentration Dynamics at the Site of Infection as Criterion of Antimicrobial Chemotherapy. Hamburg University Medical School, Hamburg, Germany, 1984. Thesis.
27. Solomkin JS, Meakins JL Jr: Antibiotic trials in intra-abdominal infections: A critical evaluation of study design and outcome reporting. Ann Surg 201:29, 1984.
28. Mayo WJ: Acquired diverticulitis of the large intestine. Surg Gynecol Obstet 5:8, 1907.
29. Lockhart-Mummary JP: Late results in diverticulitis. Lancet 2:1041, 1938.
30. Smithwick RH: Experiences with the surgical management of diverticulitis of the sigmoid. Ann Surg 115:969, 1942.
31. Eng K, Ranson JHC, Locaslio SA: Resection of the perforated segment: A significant advance in treatment of diverticulitis with free perforation or abscess. Am J Surg 133:67, 1977.
32. Grief JM, Fried G, McSherry CK: Surgical treatment of perforated diverticulitis of the sigmoid colon. Dis Colon Rectum 23:483, 1980.
33. Eisenstat TE, Rubin RJ, Salrari EP: Surgical management of diverticulitis: The role of the Hartmann procedure. Dis Colon Rectum 26:429, 1983.
34. Auguste L, Borrero E, Wise L: Surgical management of perforated colonic diverticulitis. Arch Surg 120:450, 1985.
35. Lambert ME, Knox RA, Schofield RF, et al: Management of the septic complications of diverticular disease. Br J Surg 73:576, 1986.
36. Silvis R, Keeman JN: Complicated diverticulitis in acute surgery. Neth J Surg 40:117, 1988.
37. Dandekar NV, McCann WJ: Primary resection and anastomosis in the management of perforation of diverticulitis of the sigmoid flexure and diffuse peritonitis. Dis Colon Rectum 12:172, 1969.
38. Farkouh E, Hellon G, Allard M, et al: Resection and primary anastomosis for diverticulitis with perforation and peritonitis. Can J Surg 25:314, 1982.
39. Madden JL: Primary resection in the treatment of acute perforations of the colon with abscess or diffuse peritonitis. *In* Delaney JP, Varco RL (eds): Controversies in Surgery II. Philadelphia, WB Saunders, 1983, p 349.
40. Wittmann DH, Kellinghusen C, Frommelt L: Peritonitis after perforations of sigma diverticula. *In* Wittmann DH (ed): Intra-Abdominal Infections. Munich, Futuramed Verlag, 1983, pp 535–542.
41. Saadia R, Schein M: Intra-operative colonic lavage. Dis Colon Rectum 32:78, 1988.
42. Mealy K, Salman A, Arthur G: Definitive one-stage emergency large bowel surgery. Br J Surg 75:1216, 1988.
43. Condon RE: Management of the acute complications of diverticular disease: Peritonitis and septicemia. Dis Colon Rectum 19:296, 1976.
44. Sakai L, Daake J, Kaminski DL: Acute perforation of sigmoid diverticuli. Am J Surg 142:12, 1981.
45. Wittmann DH, Aprahamian C, Bergstein J: Etappenlavage: Advanced diffuse peritonitis managed by planned multiple laparotomies utilizing zippers, slide fastener, and Velcro for temporary abdominal closure. World J Surg 14:218, 1990.
46. Wittmann DH, Nyström PO: Multicenter validation of APACHE II score for intraabdominal infection. Surg Res Commun 8(Suppl):27, 1990.
47. Schein M, Decker GAG: The Hartmann procedure. Extended indications in severe intra-abdominal infection. Dis Colon Rectum 31:126, 1988.
48. Neff CC, van Sonnenberg E, Casola G, et al: Diverticular abscesses: Percutaneous drainage. Radiology 163:15, 1987.
49. Saini S, Mueller PR, Wittenberg J, et al: Percutaneous drainage of diverticular abscess. Arch Surg 121:475, 1986.
50. Almy TP, Howell DA. Diverticular disease of the colon. N Engl J Med 302:324, 1980.
51. The high-fiber diet: Its effect on the bowel. Med Lett 17:93, 1975.
52. Chappuis CW, Cohn I Jr: Acute colonic diverticulitis. Surg Clin North Am 68:301, 1988.
53. Manousos ON: Diverticular disease of the colon. Dig Dis 7:86, 1989.
54. Benn PL, Wolff BG, Ilstrup DM: Level of anastomosis and recurrent colonic diverticulitis. Am J Surg 151:269, 1986.
55. Wolff BG, Ready RL, MacCarty RL, et al: Influence of sigmoid resection on progression of diverticular disease of the colon. Dis Colon Rectum 27;645, 1984.
56. Schmit PJ, Bennion RS, Thompson JE: Cecal diverticulitis: A continuing diagnostic dilemma. World J Surg 15:367, 1991.

LIVER AND BILIARY TRACT

90

Approach to the Patient with Infection of the Liver

H. Franklin Herlong

Liver function may be adversely affected by infectious diseases because of direct invasion of the liver or by the effects of bacteremia and sepsis. Clinical manifestations are varied and depend on the infectious organism, the host's immune response, and the effects of therapeutic agents. The number of different infectious agents causing hepatic abnormalities is large, and the clinical syndromes are broad. In other chapters, specific diseases such as viral hepatitis are discussed. This chapter focuses on the differential diagnosis of several clinical scenarios involving the liver in which infectious diseases may be important.

Patients with Abnormal Hepatic Biochemical Test Results

The detection of abnormal hepatic biochemical test results is often the first evidence of liver disease. These abnormalities are increasingly noted in asymptomatic individuals who donate blood, as a part of routine blood testing during annual physical examinations, or in the investigation of other diseases. Elevations in aspartate aminotransferase (AST) and alanine aminotransferase (ALT) values are sensitive indicators of hepatocellular injury. ALT is located primarily in the cytosol of the hepatocyte and is more specific for liver disease. AST is located primarily in the mitochondrion of the hepatocyte and is also found in skeletal muscle, leukocytes, erythrocytes, brain, and kidney.[1] Isolated AST elevation may accompany myocardial or cerebral ischemia, muscle injury, heavy exercise, or hemolysis. Spuriously low aminotransferase levels have been reported in uremia.[2] The degree of aminotransferase elevation does not correlate with the severity of liver injury and is of little prognostic value. However, the height of elevation may help determine the cause of the liver injury.[3] The highest aminotransferase elevations (greater than 5000 IU/L) are seen with ischemic liver injury, drug-induced liver disease from direct hepatotoxins such as acetaminophen, and viral hepatitis. In diseases like hemochromatosis, α_1-antitrypsin deficiency, and nonalcoholic steatohepatitis, the aminotransferase levels are frequently less than five times the upper limit of normal. Occasionally, acute obstruction of the biliary tract from a common duct stone can cause markedly elevated aminotransferase values.[4] Alcoholic liver disease causes a characteristic aminotransferase pattern. The AST/ALT ratio is greater than 2:1, and the ALT value is frequently normal or minimally elevated. The decrease in ALT activity results from an alcohol-induced reduction in the conversion of pyridoxine to pyridoxal phosphate, a cofactor necessary for ALT activity.[5]

Serum alkaline phosphatase is most useful in detecting disorders of the biliary tract. Elevation in serum alkaline phosphatase may result from abnormalities of the extrahepatic biliary tree (calculi, stricture, or tumor), the main hepatic ducts (cholangiocarcinoma, sclerosing cholangitis), the septal and interlobular bile ducts (primary biliary cirrhosis, granulomata), or the hepatocyte-canalicular membrane (oral contraceptives, anabolic steroids, rifampin).[6] The height of serum alkaline phosphatase elevation is not useful in differentiating extrahepatic from intrahepatic cholestasis. Elevated serum alkaline phosphatase levels in the absence of hepatic involvement have been detected in patients with hypernephroma or Hodgkin's disease.[7] Certain tumors such as bronchogenic carcinoma may produce an alkaline phosphatase with an isoenzyme pattern distinct from that of liver and bone. Serum alkaline phosphatase levels tend to rise with age and may be outside reported normal ranges in older people without evidence of liver disease.[3]

The serum γ-glutamyl transpeptidase concentration is a sensitive indicator of hepatobiliary disease, but a lack of specificity limits its usefulness.[8] Many drugs including alcohol can induce γ-glutamyl transpeptidase activity in the absence of liver disease.[9, 10] Serum γ-glutamyl transpeptidase is used to confirm the hepatic origin of an elevated alkaline phosphatase value. Because alcohol induces γ-glutamyl transpeptidase activity, it has sometimes been used as a surrogate marker of alcohol consumption.[11]

The height of serum bilirubin elevation is of little prognostic value in acute liver disease but correlates with mortality in chronic cholestatic liver diseases such as primary biliary cirrhosis and sclerosing cholangitis.[12] The mean serum bilirubin concentration is normally slightly higher in men than in women.[1] Isolated indirect (unconjugated) hyperbilirubinemia is associated with hemolysis or Gilbert syndrome. In these disorders, the bilirubin level is rarely greater than 4 mg/dL.[1] Even with biliary tract obstruction, the bilirubin levels rarely exceed 30 mg/dL because extrahepatic clearance, largely through urinary excretion, balances bilirubin production.[1] Extreme elevations in serum bilirubin are seen when hemolysis complicates parenchymal liver disease, such as viral hepatitis in a patient with sickle cell disease.

Clinical signs and symptoms are also useful in establishing the cause of liver disease.[13] Pruritus in a middle-aged woman with an elevated alkaline phosphatase level suggests primary biliary cirrhosis. Urticaria may be seen during the prodromal stage of acute hepatitis B.[14] Postadolescent acne in a young woman suggests autoimmune liver disease; porphyria cutanea tarda is found in a significant number of patients with hepatitis C.[15]

Autoimmune phenomena such as immune thrombocytopenic purpura, renal tubular acidosis, or thyroiditis may be associated with autoimmune liver diseases such as chronic hepatitis, primary biliary cirrhosis, or sclerosing cholangitis. Arthralgias and arthritis have been reported in up to 20% of patients during the preicteric phase of viral hepatitis. Syndromes associated with hepatitis B include polyarteritis nodosa and glomerulonephritis.[14] Concurrent hepatitis C is seen in many patients with cryoglobulinemia.[16]

Abnormalities in hepatic biochemical tests are common in systemic infections and result either from direct parenchymal or biliary tract involvement or as a manifestation of the effects of inflammatory mediators on liver function.[17–20] Multisystemic dysfunction is common in patients with sepsis and has been labeled the sepsis syndrome.[21, 22] A mild degree of aminotransferase and alkaline phosphatase elevation with varying degrees of hyperbilirubinemia is typical.[23] Jaundice in the absence of abnormalities of other hepatic tests probably results from an isolated defect in the excretion of conjugated bilirubin.[24] Endotoxemia occurring in the setting of gram-negative infections causes a decrease in bile flow with a concomitant reduction in excretion of bilirubin and other organic ions. The effects of endotoxin probably account for many of the cases of jaundice seen in serious infections.[25] Hepatic blood flow is also depressed in sepsis.[26, 27] Coincidental hepatic dysfunction may occur in a septic patient because of hepatotoxic medications, the effects of parenteral nutrition, or concomitant biliary tract obstruction. Abnormalities in liver function usually resolve promptly after treatment of sepsis with appropriate antibiotics.

Certain organisms can cause characteristic hepatopathies. Toxic shock syndrome, a multisystemic disorder, is caused by colonization or infection with a strain of *Staphylococcus aureus* producing toxic shock syndrome toxin 1.[28] Although hypotension is common in toxic shock syndrome, the degree of AST elevation is less than that seen in patients with similar degrees of hypotension from other causes. Typically, hepatic histology shows steatosis with inflammation of the septal and interlobular bile ducts.[29] Occasionally, bile duct rupture is seen with infiltration of the portal areas with neutrophils, lymphocytes, and eosinophils.[30]

A mild nonspecific reactive hepatitis, on histologic examination of the liver, similar to that seen in viral hepatitis, may accompany Legionnaires' disease, listeriosis, *Yersinia* bacteremia, or Lyme disease.[31–34]

Neisseria gonorrhoeae and *Chlamydia trachomatis* cause a perihepatitis resulting from direct spread of the organism from the genital tract to the liver by the fallopian tubes.[35, 36] *Chlamydia* has been isolated from the ascitic fluid in such patients.[37] Inoculation also occurs through the blood or lymphatics because this condition has been described in men. Localized peritonitis causes formation of adhesions between the visceral and parietal peritoneum overlying the liver. Table 90–1 summarizes laboratory and pathologic findings in a variety of systemic infections.[17]

Adverse reactions to therapeutic agents may cause hepatic biochemical abnormalities in patients with infectious diseases. Hepatotoxic reactions may cause hepatocellular necrosis or cholestasis; many adverse reactions cause some degree of both. Hepatotoxicity may be related to the route of administration as with tetracycline, which causes microvesicular fat accumulation when high doses are given intravenously but has no effect when it is administered orally.[38] Toxicity may be dose related with acetaminophen or idiosyncratic with drugs like oxacillin.[39] Combinations of certain drugs may affect hepatotoxicity. Rifampin-isoniazid combinations lead to a higher frequency of hepatic injury than does either

TABLE 90–1 ■ Hepatic Biochemical Abnormalities in Infectious Diseases*

INFECTION OR BACTERIA	AST, ALT	ALKALINE PHOSPHATASE	BILIRUBIN	PATHOLOGIC CHANGE
Sepsis syndrome	+	+	+	Intrahepatic cholestasis, focal necrosis, mild portal inflammation
Pneumococcal pneumonia	+	+	+	Focal necrosis
Toxic shock syndrome	+ + +	+	+	Centrilobular necrosis and cholestasis; vasculitis, steatosis, cholangitis
Listeriosis	+ +	+ +	+ +	Microabscesses, granulomata, cholestasis
Legionnaires' disease	+ +	+ +	+	Mild portal mononuclear infiltrate; neutrophils in sinusoids; cholestasis; microabscesses
Brucellosis	+	+ +	+	Granulomata; portal inflammation
Neisseria gonorrhoeae	NL	NL	NL	Fibrinous adhesions of the liver capsule (Fitz-Hugh–Curtis syndrome)
Yersinia	+	+ +	+ +	Preexisting iron overload; granulomata; cholestasis; abscesses
Salmonellosis	+	+	+	Hyperplasia of Kupffer cells, which aggregate into "typhoid nodules"
Nocardiosis	+	+ +	+	Granulomata with acid-fast organisms
Spirochete				
Treponema pallidum				
Congenital	+ +	+	+ +	Mild focal necrosis
Secondary	+	+ +	+ +	Focal necrosis, granulomata; portal inflammation
Tertiary	+	+ +	+	Granulomata with central necrosis; rare vasculitis; gummata, hepar lobatum
Borrelia burgdorferi (Lyme disease)	+ +	+	+	Moderate portal inflammation, Kupffer cell hyperplasia
Leptospirosis	+ +	+ +	+ + + +	Centrilobular necrosis, cholestasis; portal inflammation
Other				
Coxiella burnetii (Q fever)	+ + +	+	+	Doughnut granulomata
Rickettsia rickettsii (Rocky Mountain spotted fever)	+	+	+	Mild focal necrosis
Chlamydia trachomatis	NL	NL	NL	Fibrous pericapsular adhesions (Fitz-Hugh–Curtis syndrome)
Chlamydia psittaci	+	+	+	Mild focal necrosis

*AST, Aspartate aminotransferase; ALT, alanine aminotransferase; NL, normal; +, less than twice normal; + +, 2–4 times normal; + + +, 5–10 times normal; + + + +, greater than 10 times normal.

drug alone.[40] Drug formulation may affect the prevalence of adverse hepatic reactions. Erythromycin estolate has a much greater rate of hepatotoxicity than does erythromycin propionate or ethylsuccinate.[41] Some drugs affect only an isolated component of liver function. Rifampin interferes with the uptake of bilirubin by a direct effect on receptor proteins within the hepatocyte, leading to elevated serum levels of unconjugated bilirubin.[42]

Systemic infections develop frequently in patients with chronic liver disease. Fortunately, in most patients, these infections can be treated with antibiotics that have little toxicity. When possible, aminoglycosides should be avoided in patients with chronic liver disease because of the increased risk of nephrotoxicity.[43] The β-lactam group of antibiotics is effectively cleared in patients with chronic liver disease, making them especially useful in this group of patients. However, cephalosporins that contain a methyltetrazole thiol group (cefamandole, cefoperazone) inhibit the synthesis of vitamin K–dependent clotting factors and should not be used in patients with chronic liver disease.[44]

Patients with Focal Hepatic Lesions

The widespread availability of hepatic imaging studies has resulted in the early recognition of focal hepatic lesions in both symptomatic and asymptomatic individuals. Hepatic masses may be cystic or solid (Table 90–2). Cystic defects may be caused by benign simple cysts, infections (pyogenic abscess, amebic abscess, echinococcal cyst), or rarely neoplasms (cystadenoma, cystadenocarcinoma). Most solid lesions are caused by tumors that are benign (hepatic adenoma, focal nodular hyperplasia, hemangioma) or malignant (hepatocellular carcinoma, metastasis, cholangiocarcinoma, angiosarcoma).

Cystic Lesions

Simple cysts of the liver are the most common cause of focal hepatic defects. They are seen sporadically or less commonly in association with adult polycystic disease.[45] Intrahepatic cystic lesions can communicate with the biliary tract (Caroli disease).[46] Most benign simple cysts are asymptomatic, but they can become large enough to cause right upper quadrant pain. Simple cysts arise from an aberration in the development of intrahepatic bile ducts.[47] The biliary epithelium secretes fluid that gradually accumulates and forms cysts. The cysts enlarge in time because they lack effective drainage. Complications of simple cysts are rare but include infection, bleeding, and obstruction of the biliary tract.[48]

Fever, chills, right upper quadrant pain, leukocytosis, and positive blood culture results suggest pyogenic liver abscess.[49] Patients occasionally have only nonspecific malaise and dull abdominal pain. Diaphragmatic irritation with referred pain to the right shoulder is common. In elderly debilitated patients, signs of pyogenic liver abscess can be minimal, causing delays in diagnosis. Liver abscesses in recipients of liver transplants can present a diagnostic dilemma because hepatic denervation prevents the pain of hepatic enlargement. Laboratory test abnormalities are unimpressive with a modest elevation in alkaline phosphatase and aminotransferase values.[50] Jaundice is rare unless the abscess compresses the biliary tract. Pyogenic liver abscesses may be single or multiple and are detected in either lobe of the liver. Pyogenic liver abscesses result from three routes of infection: biliary tract, hematogenous, or extension of contiguous infection.[51] Most pyogenic liver abscesses are caused by cholangitis associated with obstruction of the biliary tract by tumor, stricture, or calculi. These abscesses are often multiple and affect both lobes of the liver. Less often, pyogenic liver abscesses result from pylephlebitis caused by portal bacteremia from diverticular disease, appendicitis, intraabdominal abscesses, or in-

TABLE 90–2 ■ Focal Hepatic Lesions

LESION	RISK FACTORS	RADIOGRAPHIC FINDINGS
Cystic		
Simple cyst	Genetic predisposition (polycystic disease)	Smooth cystic border with low-density contents
Pyogenic abscess	Biliary tract, intraabdominal infection; penetrating wounds or trauma	Low-density lesion containing echogenic material
Amebic abscess	Residence in or travel to endemic area; homosexual men	Elevated hemidiaphragm pleural effusion, irregular cystic edge
Hydatid cyst	Travel to or residence in endemic regions	Elevated hemidiaphragm, cyst wall calcification, daughter cysts with detached membranes
Cystadenocarcinoma	Congenital cyst	Thick irregular cyst wall
Solid		
Benign tumors		
Adenoma	Oral contraceptives	Vascular hypodense lesions; no ^{99m}Tc uptake
Focal nodular hyperplasia	—	^{99m}Tc uptake; hypodense avascular lesions
Hemangioma	—	^{99m}Tc-tagged red blood cell study
Malignant		
Hepatocellular carcinoma	Hepatitis B or C, cirrhosis, mycotoxins	Hypodense lesion with nonhomogeneous contrast enhancement
Cholangiocarcinoma	*Clonorchis*, sclerosing cholangitis; polycystic disease; choledochal cyst; Thorotrast	Hypodense lesion; dilated intrahepatic ducts
Angiosarcoma	Vinyl chloride, anabolic steroids, Thorotrast	Hypodense vascular lesion
Metastasis	Primary tumor risk	Hypodense lesions; locality dependent or primary

flammatory bowel disease.[52] Liver abscesses predominate in the right lobe because the mesenteric veins, which drain the region of the body responsible for the majority of hepatic abscesses, supply the greater proportion of the blood supply to the right lobe.[53] Abscesses may also result from extension of contiguous infection from subhepatic abscesses, cholecystitis, or pancreatitis.[54] In about one quarter of cases, pyogenic liver abscesses are cryptogenic.[52] Liver abscesses associated with cholangitis or intraabdominal infections are caused by multiple organisms including enteric gram-negative bacilli and anaerobes. Abscesses caused by a single organism such as *S. aureus* or streptococci are usually caused by hematogenous spread.[55] Patients with diabetes mellitus or underlying liver disease, particularly hemochromatosis, are susceptible to liver abscesses caused by *Yersinia enterocolitica*.[56] Fungal abscesses are less common and are frequently found simultaneously in the liver and spleen.

Amebic liver abscess should be considered in patients who have recently traveled to endemic areas such as Mexico or South America. For unknown reasons, most patients with amebic abscesses are males and are younger than patients with bacterial liver abscesses.[57] Amebic abscesses are seen with increased frequency in homosexual men.[58]

Amebic abscesses occur most commonly in the right lobe of the liver, often near the diaphragm. Amebic abscesses are indistinguishable radiographically from pyogenic abscess.[59] Fever and right upper quadrant pain with tender hepatomegaly are common. Clinical signs or symptoms of colonic amebiasis are often absent in patients with amebic liver abscesses. Most patients have a leukocytosis, but eosinophilia is rare. In many patients, amebic trophozoites or cysts are not detected in the stool.

The diagnosis is made when imaging tests show a focal hepatic defect in an appropriate clinical setting. Hemagglutination test results are usually positive; a negative result makes the diagnosis unlikely. Ultrasonographically guided aspiration can confirm the diagnosis but is usually unnecessary. Rarely, secondary bacterial infection can convert an amebic abscess to a pyogenic abscess.[60] Metronidazole is the treatment of choice for amebic abscesses.[59]

Hydatid disease of the liver is caused by the tapeworm *Echinococcus granulosus*, and develops in areas of the world where sheep are plentiful, such as South America and the Middle East. In the United States, the disease appears solely in immigrants or travelers. Because the hydatid cyst grows so slowly, most patients are unaware of the infection until the cyst reaches a large size. Right upper quadrant pain and hepatomegaly are the most common presenting symptoms and usually develop only when the cyst dies and a pericystitis from leakage of the fluid produces pain and low-grade fever. Secondary bacterial infection causes symptoms identical with pyogenic abscess. The cyst may rarely rupture into the peritoneum or bile ducts. If the cyst adheres to the diaphragm, rupture into the pleural space is possible.[61]

The physical examination is often unimpressive except for hepatomegaly, and laboratory tests show minimal abnormalities.[62] Serologic tests are useful in making the diagnosis of hydatid disease. The indirect hemagglutination test is used most commonly for screening. Because it becomes negative after cure, it can be used to assess efficacy of treatment. However, this test is not particularly sensitive; false-negative responses occur in about 20% of patients. The immunoelectrophoretogram is the most specific test available.[63]

Open surgical evacuation of hydatid cysts with obliteration of the cystic cavity remains the treatment of choice for symptomatic hydatid disease.[64] In patients with recurrent disease or when surgery is contraindicated, systemic administration of anthelmintic drugs is another possibility.

Solid Lesions

Benign tumors of the liver include hepatic adenoma and focal nodular hyperplasia. Most hepatic adenomas are associated with the use of estrogens and less commonly anabolic steroid use, glycogen storage diseases, and tyrosinemia.[65, 66] Patients with hepatic adenomas may present with vague right upper quadrant pain, a palpable liver mass, an acute abdomen due to intraabdominal hemorrhage, or an incidental abnormality discovered on hepatic imaging for other reasons.[67] Most hepatic adenomas are solitary and develop in the right lobe of the liver. Hepatic adenomas caused by oral contraceptives often regress with discontinuation of estrogens.[68] On rare occasions, malignant degeneration has been reported in patients with hepatic adenomas.[69–71] Focal nodular hyperplasia is more common than hepatic adenomas, but evidence for an association between focal nodular hyperplasia and oral contraceptive use is weak.[72] Most likely, focal nodular hyperplasia is caused by developmental vascular abnormalities with secondary hyperplasia. Most patients with focal nodular hyperplasia are asymptomatic but may develop pain if there has been hemorrhage into the lesion. The majority of focal nodular hyperplasia lesions are solitary and frequently subcapsular. A central fibrous scar caused by fibrosepta radiating from the center of the lesion is considered diagnostic.[73]

Hemangiomas are common benign hepatic lesions that are often asymptomatic. Cavernous hemangiomas (greater than 5 cm) may cause pain. Large hemangiomas of the liver may produce differential diagnostic problems for the clinician and radiologist, particularly in patients with known malignant disease or risk factors for malignant hepatic tumors.

Malignant tumors of the liver include hepatocellular carcinoma, cholangiocarcinoma, and angiosarcoma. Risk factors for hepatocellular carcinoma include underlying cirrhosis, hepatitis B and C, exposure to aflatoxin or vinyl chloride, and hereditary tyrosinemia. Less well defined risk factors for hepatocellular carcinoma include anabolic steroid use, hemochromatosis without cirrhosis, and Wilson disease.[74–76] Hepatocellular carcinoma may be discovered incidentally in patients with cirrhosis but most often is diagnosed when a known cirrhotic patient develops worsening fatigue, weight loss, or right upper quadrant pain.

Risk factors for cholangiocarcinoma include congenital biliary tract diseases such as Caroli disease or choledochal cysts, sclerosing cholangitis, and certain biliary tract parasites *(Clonorchis sinensis)*.[77, 78] It is difficult to recognize the development of a cholangiocarcinoma in a patient with preexisting biliary tract disease such as sclerosing cholangitis.

Malignant tumors often metastasize to the liver and are more common than primary malignant hepatic tumors. Tumors metastasizing to the liver most commonly include those with portal venous drainage (stomach and intestine). Lung tumors are next highest; pancreatic tumors account for only 4% of metastatic hepatic lesions.

Patients with Granulomatous Liver Disease

Hepatic granulomata develop when the reticuloendothelial system of the liver is exposed to certain foreign antigens that may be infectious (tuberculosis, cytomegalovirus infection, brucellosis) or noninfectious (beryllium, allopurinol).[79] The antigen may never be identified, as is the case with sarcoidosis or Hodgkin's disease[80, 81] (Table 90–3).

The clinical presentation depends on the cause of the granulomatous inflammation. Granulomata may be seen on a liver biopsy specimen obtained as a part of the evaluation of a fever of undetermined origin or in the evaluation of hepatic

TABLE 90–3 ■ Causes of Hepatic Granulomata

INFECTION	Rickettsial
Bacterial	Q fever
Tuberculosis	Viral
Atypical mycobacteria (acquired immunodeficiency syndrome)	Cytomegalovirus
Leprosy	Epstein-Barr virus
Brucellosis	**DRUGS AND OTHER AGENTS**
Tularemia	Allopurinol
Listeriosis	Sulfonamides
Fungal	Quinidine
Histoplasmosis	Beryllium
Coccidioidomycosis	Talc
Candidiasis	**MISCELLANEOUS CAUSES**
Parasitic	Sarcoid
Schistosomiasis	Primary biliary cirrhosis
Toxocariasis	Crohn disease
Spirochetal	Hodgkin's disease
Syphilis	Hypogammaglobulinemia

biochemical abnormalities.[82] Whereas many patients with hepatic granulomata are asymptomatic, others are febrile and complain of vague right upper quadrant pain, weight loss, and occasional night sweats. The hepatic biochemical profile in hepatic granulomatous disease is characterized by a moderate elevation of alkaline phosphatase with minimal aminotransferase elevation. Jaundice is unusual, and synthetic function as measured by serum albumin concentration and prothrombin time is usually preserved. Histologic examination of the liver is often helpful in patients with suspected granulomatous disease.[83] In addition, the liver biopsy specimen may be cultured or stained for specific infectious agents.

Hepatic granulomata are found in virtually all patients with military tuberculosis and may also be seen in patients in whom the clinical evidence of tuberculosis is limited to the lung or other organs.[84] Certain infections produce characteristic histologic abnormalities. Caseous necrosis suggests tuberculosis; well-developed epithelioid granulomata with giant cells, asteroid bodies, and Schaumann inclusions are seen in sarcoidosis.[83] Clusters of histiocytes without well-defined epithelioid granulomata are typical of cytomegalovirus infection and brucellosis.[85] Granulomata with central clearing (doughnut granulomata) suggest Q fever.[86] Examination of the liver biopsy specimen with polarized light may show talc within granulomata.

The cause of granulomatous liver disease varies regionally and with the population studied. Granulomata are commonly seen in patients with acquired immunodeficiency syndrome and are frequently caused by a variety of infectious agents.[87] Patients living in the desert Southwest would have a higher prevalence of coccidioidomycosis; in developing countries, tuberculosis would be more common.[88]

Simon and Wolff[89] described a group of patients with prolonged unexplained fever and granulomatous inflammation in the liver in whom no infectious agent could be identified. They observed a favorable response to therapy with corticosteroids. Subsequently, this disorder has been called idiopathic granulomatous hepatitis. Patients suspected of having this syndrome should receive corticosteroids only after attempts to prove an infectious cause have been unsuccessful. Some patients who have failed to respond to corticosteroid therapy or have unacceptable side effects have responded to methotrexate.[90]

Management of Patients with Ascites

Cirrhosis is the most common cause of ascites, but extrahepatic disorders may cause fluid accumulation in the peritoneal cavity. Pancreatitis, tuberculosis, malignant tumors, serositis, and hypothyroidism can cause ascites in the absence of liver disease. The development of ascites in a patient with cirrhosis implies a poor prognosis; less than half of patients are alive 2 years later.

A diagnostic paracentesis is helpful when ascites is first detected or when there is unexplained deterioration in the status of a previously compensated cirrhotic patient. Useful tests in the differential diagnosis of ascites include cell count with differential, total protein and albumin concentrations, lactate dehydrogenase activity, and culture for aerobic bacteria.[91] Anaerobic cultures are included if secondary peritonitis is suspected.[92] If there is clinical evidence of pancreatic ascites, tuberculosis, or tumor, then measurement of ascitic fluid amylase, culture for acid-fast bacilli, and cytopathologic examination should be included.

The serum–ascitic fluid albumin gradient can help establish the cause of ascites.[93] A gradient between the serum and ascitic fluid albumin concentration greater than 1.1 g/dL suggests portal hypertension. Smaller gradients are seen in nonhepatic causes, such as peritoneal malignant neoplasms, tuberculosis, pancreatic ascites, or the nephrotic syndrome when the portal pressure is normal.[94] In patients with cirrhosis and portal hypertension, the serum–ascitic fluid albumin gradient may remain high even when there is peritoneal infection (Table 90–4).

Bacterial infection of ascitic fluid is a common complication of cirrhosis.[95] The infection is designated secondary peritonitis when it results from perforation of the bowel or when bacteria enter the ascitic fluid from localized infections, such as perinephric or subhepatic abscesses. In most patients with

TABLE 90–4 ■ Ascitic Fluid Analysis*

ETIOLOGY	PROTEIN (g/dL)	S-A ALBUMIN GRADIENT	CELL COUNT (/mm³)	PREDOMINANCE	OTHER LABORATORY TESTS
Cirrhosis	<2.0	>1.1	<200	Mononuclear	↑ WHVP
Cardiogenic	>2.5	>1.1	<250	Mononuclear	↑ CVP, normal WHVP
Pancreatic	>2.5	<1.1	>500	PMN/mononuclear	↑ Fluid amylase
Myxedema	>2.5	>1.1	>200	Mononuclear	↑ TSH
Spontaneous bacterial peritonitis	>2.0	<1.1	>250	PMN	+ Culture
Chylous	>2.5	<1.1	>200	Mononuclear	↑ Fluid triglycerides
Tuberculosis	>2.5	<1.1	>500	Mononuclear	+ Biopsy
Chlamydial	>4.0	<1.1	>500	Mononuclear	+ Fluid culture
Malignant neoplasms	>2.5	<1.1	<200	Tumor	↑ Fluid LDH

*S-A, Serum–ascitic fluid; PMN, polymorphonuclear leukocyte; WHVP, wedged hepatic vein pressure; CVP, central venous pressure; TSH, thyroid-stimulating hormone; LDH, lactate dehydrogenase.

cirrhosis, the infection occurs with no obvious sight of inoculation and is designated spontaneous bacterial peritonitis (SBP).[96] In many of these patients, no signs or symptoms of infection are detected.[97] Secondary peritonitis cannot be differentiated from SBP on the basis of clinical symptoms or signs. Ascitic fluid analysis is necessary to diagnose bacterial infection and determine whether it is primary or secondary.[98]

Empirical antibiotic therapy is indicated with an ascitic fluid polymorphonuclear leukocyte count greater than 250/mm^3.[99] Direct inoculation of the ascitic fluid into blood culture bottles at the bedside can increase the yield of positive cultures.[100] Gram stain of the fluid is positive in only 10% of infected specimens.[101] As a result, the choice of empirical antibody coverage is based on the epidemiology of SBP infection. A single gram-negative bacillus is most often encountered, followed by streptococci and staphylococci.[102] Anaerobic organisms are cultured from the fluid in less than 1% of cases of SBP.[103]

A third-generation cephalosporin such as cefotaxime covers most of the organisms frequently isolated in SBP, except for enterococci.[104] Aminoglycosides should be avoided unless organism sensitivity mandates these agents because of the high rate of nephrotoxicity in patients with cirrhosis.[43] Occasionally, a positive ascitic fluid culture will be obtained when the polymorphonuclear leukocyte count is less than 250/mm^3 in the fluid.[105] In these patients, a repeated paracentesis with culture and cell count is indicated. If the repeated culture is negative and the cell count remains low, no treatment is necessary.[106]

Culture-negative neutrocytic ascites is diagnosed when the ascitic fluid culture shows no growth and the polymorphonuclear leukocyte count is greater than 250/mm^3. The clinical signs, symptoms, course, and mortality of patients with culture-negative neutrocytic ascites are not different from those of patients with SBP.[107]

A rare variant of ascitic fluid infection is polymicrobial bacterascites, in which multiple organisms are cultured from the ascitic fluid but the polymorphonuclear leukocyte count is less than 250/mm^3. This is virtually diagnostic of inadvertent bowel puncture by the paracentesis needle.[108]

It is important to distinguish SBP from secondary peritonitis because secondary peritonitis usually requires surgical intervention. Secondary peritonitis should be suspected in the following setting: ascitic fluid protein concentration greater than 1 g/dL, glucose level less than 50 mg/dL, or multiple organisms cultured from the fluid.[98, 99] If preliminary data suggest secondary peritonitis, metronidazole is added for initial empirical coverage. An aggressive search is then instituted for evidence of colonic or biliary tract perforation or loculated infections such as subhepatic or perinephric abscesses.

The pathogenesis of SBP has not been established, but it presumably results from colonization of the ascitic fluid from bacteria entering the systemic circulation.[106] Patients whose ascitic fluid contains less than 1 g/dL of protein are at risk for recurrent episodes of bacterial peritonitis.[109] This increased susceptibility to infection is related to a reduction in ascitic fluid opsonic activity from reduced levels of ascitic fluid complement.[110] The value of prophylactic administration of antibiotics to prevent recurrent SBP has not been established.[111, 112] SBP implies a poor prognosis in patients with cirrhosis and is often used as a criterion for liver transplantation.[113]

Whereas bacterial infection accounts for the majority of cases of peritonitis, nonbacterial infections do occur most commonly from mycobacteria and chlamydiae. In chlamydial peritonitis, the serum–ascitic fluid albumin gradient is low, there is a mononuclear leukocytosis of the fluid, and fluid protein levels are often high.[37, 114] Tuberculous peritonitis usually causes a high fluid protein level and low serum–ascitic fluid albumin gradient with a mononuclear predominance in the fluid. Fluid culture for acid-fast bacilli is often negative, and the diagnosis is established by peritoneoscopy when white plaques are seen on the liver surface and peritoneum. Histologic and culture data obtained from peritoneal biopsy confirm the diagnosis.[115]

References

1. McIntyre N, Rosalki S: Biochemical investigation of liver disease. *In* McIntyre N, Benhamou J, Bircher J, et al (eds): Oxford Textbook of Clinical Hepatology. Oxford, UK, Oxford University Press, 1991, p 294.
2. Cohen G, Goffinet J, Donabedian K: Observations on decreased serum glutamate oxaloacetic transaminase (SGOT) in azotemic patients. Ann Intern Med 84:275, 1976.
3. Baker A: Liver chemistry tests. *In* Kaplowitz N (ed): Liver and Biliary Disease. Baltimore, Williams & Wilkins; 1992, p 182.
4. Ginsburg A: Very high levels of SGOT and LDH in patients with extrahepatic biliary tract obstruction. Am J Gastroenterol 15:803, 1970.
5. Diehl AM, Potter J, Boitnott J, et al: Relationship between pyridoxal 5′-phosphate deficiency and aminotransferase levels in alcoholic hepatitis. Gastroenterology 86:632, 1984.
6. Kaplan M: Alkaline phosphatase. Gastroenterology 62:452, 1972.
7. Kaplan M, Brensilver H: Significance of elevated liver alkaline phosphatase in serum. Gastroenterology 68:221A, 1975.
8. Zein M, Discombe G: Serum gamma glutamyl transpeptidase activity as a diagnostic aid. Lancet 2:748, 1970.
9. Henny J, Siest G, Schiele F, et al: Use of the reference state concept for interpretation of laboratory tests; drug effect on gamma-glutamyl transferase. Adv Biochem Pharmacol 3:209, 1982.
10. Rosalki S, Rau D: Serum gamma-glutamyl transpeptidase activity in alcoholism. Clin Chim Acta 39:41, 1972.
11. Moussavian S, Becker R, Piepmeyer J: Serum gammaglutamyl transpeptidase and chronic alcoholism. Dig Dis Sci 30:211, 1985.
12. Muraca M, Fevery J, Blanckaert N: Analytic aspects and clinical interpretation of serum bilirubin. Semin Liver Dis 8:137, 1988.
13. McIntyre N: Symptoms and signs of liver disease. *In* McIntyre N, Benhamou J, Bircher J, et al (eds): Oxford Textbook of Clinical Hepatology. Oxford, UK, Oxford University Press, 1991, p 273.
14. Seefe LB, Koff RS: Evolving concepts of the clinical and serologic consequences of hepatitis B virus infection. Semin Liver Dis 6:11, 1986.
15. Navas S, Bosch O, Castillo I, et al: Porphyria cutanea tarda and hepatitis C and B virus infection: A retrospective study. Hepatology 21:279, 1995.
16. Sansonno D, Cornacchiulo V, Iacobelli AR, et al: Localization of hepatitis C virus antigens in liver and skin tissues of chronic hepatitis C virus–infected patients with mixed cryoglobulinemia. Hepatology 21:305, 1995.
17. Kibbler C: Bacterial infection and the liver. *In* McIntyre N, Benhamou J, Bircher J, et al (eds): Oxford Textbook of Clinical Hepatology. Oxford, UK, Oxford University Press, 1991, p 656.
18. Jaundice due to bacterial infection. Gastroenterology 77:362, 1979.
19. Eley A, Hargreaves T, Lambert HP: Jaundice in severe infections. Br Med J 2:75, 1965.
20. Rayner BL, Willcox PA: Community-acquired bacteraemia; a prospective survey of 239 cases. Q J Med 69:907, 1988.
21. Gimson AES: Hepatic dysfunction during bacterial sepsis. Intensive Care Med 13:162, 1987.
22. Bank JG, Foulis AK, Ledingham I, et al: Liver function in septic shock. J Clin Pathol 35:1249, 1982.
23. Carvana J, Montes M, Camara D, et al: Functional and histopathologic changes in the liver during sepsis. Surg Gynecol Obstet 154:653, 1982.
24. Utili R, Abernathy C, Zimmerman H: Inhibition of Na^+/K^+-ATPase by endotoxin; a possible mechanism for endotoxin induced cholestasis. J Infect Dis 136:583, 1977.
25. Utili R, Abernathy C, Zimmerman H: Studies on the effects of *E. coli* endotoxin on canalicular bile formation in the isolated perfused rat liver. J Lab Clin Med 89:471, 1977.

26. Lang C, Bagby GJ, Ferguson JL, et al: Cardiac output and redistribution of organ blood flow in hypermetabolic sepsis. Am J Physiol 246:R331, 1984.
27. Gottlieb M, Sarfeh I, Stratton H: Hepatic perfusion and splanchnic oxygen consumption in patients post surgery. J Trauma 23:836, 1983.
28. Davis J, Chesney P, Wand P: Toxic-shock syndrome: Epidemiologic features, recurrence, risk factors and prevention. N Engl J Med 303:1429, 1980.
29. Gourley G, Chesney P, Davis J, et al: Acute cholestasis in patients with toxic-shock syndrome. Gastroenterology 81:928, 1981.
30. Ishak K, Rogers W: Cryptogenic acute cholangitis—Association with toxic shock syndrome. Am J Clin Pathol 76:619, 1981.
31. Kirby B, Snyder K, Meyer R, et al: Legionnaires disease: Report of sixty-five nosocomially acquired cases and review of the literature. Medicine (Baltimore) 59:188, 1980.
32. Yu V, Miller W, Wing E, et al: Disseminated listeriosis presenting as acute hepatitis. Am J Med 73:773, 1982.
33. Rabson A, Hallett A, Koornhof H: Generalized *Yersinia enterocolitica* infection. J Infect Dis 131:447, 1975.
34. Goellner M, Agger W, Burgess J, et al: Hepatitis due to recurrent Lyme disease. Ann Intern Med 108:707, 1988.
35. Cano A, Fernandez C, Scapa M, et al: Gonococcal perihepatitis: Diagnostic and therapeutic value of laparoscopy. Am J Gastroenterol 79:280, 1984.
36. Muller-Schoop J, Wang S, Munzinger J, et al: *Chlamydia trachomatis* as possible cause of peritonitis and perihepatitis in young women. Br Med J 1:1022, 1978.
37. Haight J, Ockner S: *Chlamydia trachomatis* perihepatitis with ascites. Am J Gastroenterol 83:323, 1988.
38. Briggs R: Tetracycline and the liver. N Engl J Med 269:1386, 1963.
39. Dismukes W: Oxacillin-induced hepatic dysfunction. JAMA 226:861, 1973.
40. Zimmerman H: Agents employed in the treatment of infectious and parasitic diseases. *In* Zimmerman H (ed): Hepatotoxicity. New York, Appleton-Century-Crofts, 1978, p 468.
41. Bachman B, Boyd W, Brady P: Erythromycin ethylsuccinate–induced cholestasis. Am J Gastroenterol 77:397, 1982.
42. Capelle P, Dhumeaux D, Mora M, et al: Effect of rifampicin on liver function. Gut 13:366, 1972.
43. Moore R, Smith C, Lietman P: Increased risk of renal dysfunction due to interaction of liver disease and aminoglycosides. Am J Med 80:1093, 1986.
44. Raiford D, Mitchell M: Disorders of drug disposition. *In* Rector W (ed): Complications of Chronic Liver Disease. St. Louis, Mosby–Year Book, 1992, p 238.
45. Summerfield J, Nagafuchi Y, Sherlock S, et al: Hepatobiliary fibropolycystic disease. A clinical and histological review of 51 patients. J Hepatol 2:141, 1986.
46. Caroli J, Corcos V: La dilatation congenitale des voies biliaries intrahepatiques. Rev Mediochir Mal Foie 39:1, 1964.
47. Desmet V: Intrahepatic bile ducts under the lens. J Hepatol 1:545, 1985.
48. Williams A, Wild S, Palmer K: Adult hepatic fibropolycystic disease presenting as obstructive jaundice. Gut 31:1082, 1990.
49. Miedema B, DiNeen P: The diagnosis and treatment of pyogenic liver abscesses. Ann Surg 200:328, 1984.
50. Perera M, Kirk A, Noone P: Presentation, diagnosis and management of liver abscess. Lancet 2:629, 1980.
51. Lee K-T, Sheen P, Chen J, et al: Pyogenic liver abscess: Multivariate analysis of risk factors. World J Surg 15:372, 1991.
52. Branum G, Tyson G, Branum M, et al: Hepatic abscess. Changes in etiology, diagnosis and management. Ann Surg 212:655, 1990.
53. Eisenberg P, Mueller P, Rattner D: Hepatic abscesses. *In* Pitt HA, Carr-Locke DL, Ferrucci JT (eds): Hepatobiliary and Pancreatic Disease: The Team Approach to Management. Boston, Little, Brown, 1995, p 81.
54. Reddy K, Jeffers L, Livingstone A, et al: Pyogenic liver abscess complicating common bile duct stenosis secondary to chronic calcific pancreatitis. Gastroenterology 86:953, 1984.
55. Moore-Gillon J, Eykyn S, Phillips I: Microbiology of pyogenic liver abscess. Br Med J 283:819, 1981.
56. Khanna R, Levendoghu H: Liver abscess due to *Yersinia enterocolitica*: Case report and review of the literature. Dig Dis Sci 34:636, 1989.
57. Katzenstein D, Rickerson V, Braude A: New concepts of amoebic liver abscess derived from hepatic imaging, serodiagnosis and hepatic enzymes in 67 cases in San Diego. Medicine (Baltimore) 61:237, 1982.
58. Goldmeier D, Sargeaunt PG, Price AB, et al: Is *Entamoeba histolytica* in homosexual men a pathogen? Lancet 1:641, 1986.
59. Barnes P, DeCork K, Reynolds T, et al: A comparison of amoebic and pyogenic abscess of the liver. Medicine (Baltimore) 66:472, 1987.
60. Greenstein A, Sachar D: Pyogenic and amoebic abscesses of the liver. Semin Liver Dis 8:210, 1988.
61. Schaefer J, Khan M: Echinococcosis (hydatid disease): Lessons from experience with 59 patients. Rev Infect Dis 13:243, 1991.
62. Langer J, Rose O, Keystone J, et al: Diagnosis and management of hydatid disease of the liver. Ann Surg 199:412, 1984.
63. Miguet J, Bresson-Hadni S: Alveolar echinococcosis of the liver. J Hepatol 8:373, 1989.
64. Magistrelli P, Masetti R, Coppola K, et al: Surgical treatment of hydatid disease of the liver. A 20 year experience. Arch Surg 126:518, 1991.
65. Grange J, Guechot J, Legendre C, et al: Liver adenoma and focal nodular hyperplasia in a man with high endogenous sex steroids. Gastroenterology 93:1409, 1987.
66. Neuberger J, Nunnerley H, Davis M, et al: Oral-contraceptive–associated liver tumours: Occurrence of malignancy and difficulties in diagnosis. Lancet 1:273, 1980.
67. Leese T, Olivier F, Bismuth H: Liver cell adenomas. A 12-year surgical experience from a specialist hepato-biliary unit. Ann Surg 208:558, 1988.
68. Knowles D, Casarella W, Johnson P, et al: The clinical, radiologic, and pathologic characterization of benign hepatic neoplasm. Medicine (Baltimore) 57:223, 1978.
69. Foster J, Berman M: The malignant transformation of liver cell adenomas. Arch Surg 129:712, 1994.
70. Liang-Che T: Oral contraceptive–associated liver cell adenoma and hepatocellular carcinoma. Cancer 68:341, 1991.
71. Ferrell L: Hepatocellular carcinoma arising in a focus of multilobular adenoma. Am J Surg Pathol 17:525, 1993.
72. Shortell C, Schwartz S: Hepatic adenoma and focal nodular hyperplasia. Surg Gynecol Obstet 173:426, 1991.
73. Welch T, Sheedy P, Johnson C, et al: Focal nodular hyperplasia and hepatic adenoma: Comparison of angiography, CT, US, and scintigraphy. Radiology 156:593, 1985.
74. Overly W, Dankoff J, Wang B, et al: Androgens and hepatocellular carcinoma in an athlete. Ann Intern Med 100:158, 1984.
75. Wilkinson M, Portmann B, Williams K: Wilson's disease and hepatocellular carcinoma. Possible protective role of copper. Gut 24:767, 1983.
76. Di Bisceglie A, Rustgi V, Hoofnagle J, et al: Hepatocellular carcinoma. Ann Intern Med 108:390, 1988.
77. Ona F, Dytoc J: *Clonorchis* associated cholangiocarcinoma. Gastroenterology 101:831, 1991.
78. Tompkins R, Saunders K, Boslyn J, et al: Changing patterns in diagnosis and management of bile duct cancer. Ann Surg 211:164, 1990.
79. Adams D: THe granulomatous inflammatory response. A review. Am J Pathol 84:164, 1976.
80. Kadin M, Donaldson S, Dorfman K: Isolated granuloma in Hodgkin's disease. N Engl J Med 283:859, 1970.
81. Guckian J, Perry J: Granulomatous hepatitis. An analysis of 63 cases and review of the literature. Ann Intern Med 65:1081, 1965.
82. Guckian J, Perry J: Granulomatous hepatitis of unknown etiology. An etiologic and functional evaluation. Am J Med 44:207, 1968.
83. Klatskin G, Yesner R: Hepatic manifestations of sarcoidosis and other granulomatous diseases. A study based on histological examination of tissue obtained by needle biopsy of the liver. Yale J Biol Med 23:207, 1950.
84. Korn R, Kellow W, Heller P, et al: Hepatic involvement in extrapulmonary tuberculosis. Histologic and functional characteristics. Am J Med 27:60, 1959.
85. Cervantes F, Bruguera M, Carbonell J, et al: Liver diseases in brucellosis. A clinical and pathological study of 40 cases. Postgrad Med J 58:346, 1982.
86. Bernstein M, Edmondson H, Barbour B: The liver lesion in Q

fever. Clinical and pathologic features. Arch Intern Med 16:491, 1965.
87. Gordon S, Reddy K, Gould E, et al: The spectrum of liver disease in the acquired immunodeficiency syndrome. J Hepatol 2:475, 1986.
88. Forbus W, Bestebreurtje A: Coccidioidomycosis: A study of 95 cases of the disseminated type with special reference to the pathogenesis of the disease. Surgeon 99:653, 1946.
89. Simon HB, Wolff SM: Granulomatous hepatitis and prolonged fever of unknown origin: A study of 13 patients. Medicine (Baltimore) 52:1, 1973.
90. Knox T, Kaplan M, Gelfand J, et al: Methotrexate treatment of idiopathic granulomatous hepatitis. Ann Intern Med 122:592, 1995.
91. Rector W: Sodium retention and ascites formation. *In* Rector W (ed): Complications of Chronic Liver Disease. St. Louis, Mosby–Year Book, 1992, p 68.
92. Targan S, Chow A, Guze L: Role of anaerobic bacteria in spontaneous peritonitis of cirrhosis. Am J Med 62:397, 1977.
93. Rector W, Reynolds T: The serum-ascites albumin gradient is superior to the ascites total protein concentration in the separation of "transudative" and "exudative" ascites. Am J Med 77:83, 1986.
94. Mauer K, Manzione N: Usefulness of the serum-ascites albumin difference in separating transudative from exudative ascites. Dig Dis Sci 33:1208, 1988.
95. Conn H: Spontaneous peritonitis and bacteremia in Laennec's cirrhosis caused by enteric organisms: A relatively common but rarely recognized syndrome. Ann Intern Med 60:568, 1964.
96. Conn H, Fessel J: Spontaneous bacterial peritonitis in cirrhosis: Variations on a theme. Medicine (Baltimore) 50:161, 1971.
97. Pinzello G, Simonetti RG, Craxi A, et al: Spontaneous bacterial peritonitis: A prospective investigation in predominantly nonalcoholic cirrhotic patients. Hepatology 3:545, 1983.
98. Runyon BA, Hoefs JC: Ascitic fluid analysis in the differentiation of spontaneous bacterial peritonitis from gastrointestinal tract perforation into ascitic fluid. Hepatology 4:447, 1984.
99. Akriviadis E, Runyon B: The value of an algorithm in differentiating spontaneous from secondary bacterial peritonitis. Gastroenterology 98:127, 1990.
100. Runyon B, Umland E, Merlin T: Inoculation of blood culture bottle with ascitic fluid: Improved detection of spontaneous bacterial peritonitis. Arch Intern Med 147:73, 1987.
101. Runyon B, Canawati H, Akriviadis E: Optimization of ascitic fluid culture technique. Gastroenterology 95:1351, 1988.
102. Hoefs J, Runyon B: Spontaneous bacterial peritonitis. Dis Mon 31:1, 1985.
103. Sheckman P, Onderdonk A, Bartlett J: Anaerobes in spontaneous peritonitis. Lancet 2:1223, 1977.
104. Remola A, Navasa M, Arroyo V: Experience with cefotaxime in the treatment of spontaneous bacterial peritonitis in cirrhosis. Diagn Microbiol Infect Dis 22:141, 1995.
105. Runyon B: Monomicrobial bacterascites: A potentially lethal variant of spontaneous bacterial peritonitis (Abstr). Hepatology 6:1140, 1986.
106. Runyon B: Spontaneous bacterial peritonitis. *In* Rector W (ed): Complications of Chronic Liver Disease. St. Louis, Mosby–Year Book, 1992, p 85.
107. Runyon B, Hoefs J: Culture-negative neutrocytic ascites: A variant of spontaneous bacterial peritonitis. Hepatology 4:1209, 1984.
108. Runyon B, Canawati H, Hoefs J: Polymicrobial bacterascites: A unique entity in the spectrum of infected ascitic fluid. Arch Intern Med 146:2173, 1986.
109. Runyon B: Low-protein-concentration ascitic fluid is predisposed to spontaneous bacterial peritonitis. Gastroenterology 91:1343, 1986.
110. Runyon B, Morrissey R, Hoefs J, et al: Opsonic activity of human ascitic fluid: A potentially important protective mechanism against spontaneous bacterial peritonitis. Hepatology 5:634, 1985.
111. Singh N, Gayowski T, Yu V, et al: Trimethoprim-sulfamethoxazole for the prevention of spontaneous bacterial peritonitis in cirrhosis: A randomized trial. Ann Intern Med 122:595, 1995.
112. Rolachon A, Cordier L, Bacq Y, et al: Ciprofloxacin and long-term prevention of spontaneous bacterial peritonitis: Results of a prospective controlled trial. Hepatology 22:1171, 1995.
113. Ukah F, Merhav H, Kramer D, et al: Early outcome of liver transplantation: Patients with a history of spontaneous bacterial peritonitis. Transplant Proc 25:1113, 1993.
114. Korula J: Ascites: Pathogenesis, characteristics, complications and treatment. *In* Kaplowitz N (ed): Liver and Biliary Diseases. Baltimore, Williams & Wilkins, 1992, p 529.
115. Burack W, Hollister R: Tuberculous peritonitis. A study of forty-seven proved cases encountered by a General Medical Unit in twenty-five years. Am J Med 28:510, 1960.

91

Type A Viral Hepatitis

Stanley M. Lemon

Type A viral hepatitis occurs as a result of infection with a hepatotropic picornavirus, hepatitis A virus (HAV). Signs and symptoms reflect acute infection of the hepatocyte with HAV and its subsequent clearance by several different immune mechanisms. The disease itself is probably largely immunopathologic in nature. Among the multiple viral agents now recognized to cause acute hepatitis in humans, HAV and hepatitis E virus share a unique potential for epidemic spread. Both viruses lack lipid envelopes and are transmitted predominantly by the fecal-oral route. Chronic viral hepatitis is not associated with either HAV or hepatitis E virus, and, unlike the viruses responsible for hepatitis B, hepatitis D, and hepatitis C, there is no evidence for long-term persistence of these viruses after acute infection.

Virology

The biology of HAV is considered in greater detail in Chapter 260; only selected aspects relevant to the clinical picture of hepatitis A are considered here. HAV is currently classified within the genus *Hepatovirus* of the family Picornaviridae.[1, 2] It is distantly related to enteroviruses and the human rhinoviruses, causative agents of the common cold, but has little nucleotide sequence relatedness with these viruses.[3, 4] The HAV particle is 27 nm in diameter, has no envelope, and consists of a 7.5-kb, positive-sense single-stranded RNA genome tightly encapsidated within a protein shell composed of 60 copies each of three (perhaps four) different structural proteins[3, 5] (see Fig. 260–1). There is no antigenic cross-relatedness between HAV and other picornaviruses or other viruses that cause acute hepatitis in humans. HAV replication occurs in the cytoplasm of hepatocytes and appears to follow a general scheme resembling that of poliovirus, the best studied member of the picornavirus family.

Like the enteroviruses, HAV is stable at low pH (indicating its ability to survive gastric acidity), but the thermal stability of the HAV virion is significantly greater than that of poliovirus and other picornaviruses.[6–8] In suspension, the infectivity of HAV is not appreciably affected by incubation for several minutes at temperatures up to 60°C. It is likely that the stability of the virus under adverse conditions of temperature and pH promotes its spread in the environment and its propensity for causing epidemics. Because of the absence of a lipid envelope, the virus is resistant to lipid solvents and is not inactivated by solvent-detergent treatments commonly used to ensure virus safety of blood products.[9]

The nucleotide sequences of human HAV isolates generally differ from each other by less than 20%; even greater conservation (>95%) is evident in the amino acid sequences of the capsid proteins.[4] Thus, HAV displays significantly less genetic variability than that observed among diverse poliovirus strains. However, analysis of a large number of HAV strains indicates the existence of at least seven distinct HAV genotypes that differ from each other at more than 15% of nucleotide positions within regions of the genome encoding the structural proteins[10, 11] (see Chapter 260). HAV strains recovered from humans constitute four of these genotypes (genotypes I, II, III, and VII); viruses in the remaining three genotypes (IV, V, and VI) are simian strains that have subtle antigenic differences and have thus far been recovered only from naturally infected nonhuman primates (cynomolgus monkeys and African green monkeys). The high level of antigenic conservation that is evident at the molecular level is associated with absence of significant antigenic variability among human HAV strains, and even the simian viruses can be considered members of the same single HAV serotype.[12, 13]

HAV is the only human hepatitis virus that has been reliably propagated in conventional cell cultures.[14–16] This has allowed development of conventional vaccines for prevention of hepatitis A that contain inactivated virus grown in cell culture (discussed later). Although the virus replicates in several different types of primate cell cultures in vitro, it does so slowly and less efficiently than does poliovirus. HAV does not induce a shutdown of host cell macromolecular synthesis, and replication in vitro is usually not associated with a cytopathic effect. It seems likely that replication in vivo resembles that which is generally seen in vitro, and these features of the HAV replication cycle probably contribute to the lengthy incubation period of hepatitis A, which averages about 4 weeks. Virus that has been adapted to more efficient growth in cell culture over a number of passages has often been shown to be attenuated when used to challenge otherwise susceptible nonhuman primates (chimpanzees, owl monkeys, tamarins).[17, 18] Such viruses have been evaluated as candidate attenuated vaccine strains in humans[19, 20] (see Chapter 260). Several highly cell culture–adapted variants of HAV are cytopathic in cell culture and form plaques.[8] Although the pathogenicity of such viruses has not been tested in animal models, these viruses are likely to be highly attenuated in vivo.

In general, inoculation of cultures of permissive cells with HAV results in the establishment of persistent infection. Despite this, there are no existing clinical or virologic data supporting long-term persistence of HAV infection in humans. A possible exception may be infected premature infants, in whom epidemiologic evidence supports occasionally prolonged fecal shedding of the virus.[21] Presumably, this reflects the immaturity of the host's immune system. In addition, relapses have been reported up to 4 months after the acute illness in adults[22, 23] (discussed later). Although virus has been found in clinical samples during such relapses, such patients have provided no conclusive evidence of long-term persistence of virus. The failure of the virus to establish persistent infection in humans suggests that immune responses to HAV are usually quite effective, even in severely immunocompromised individuals such as those with advanced human immunodeficiency virus infection. These immune clearance mechanisms include the development of antibodies capable of neutralizing HAV[24]; the proliferation of virus-specific, human leukocyte antigen–restricted cytotoxic T cells[25–27]; and the induction of interferons.[28]

Epidemiology

Virus Transmission

Hepatitis A has a worldwide distribution, but it is particularly common in developing countries with poor public health sanitation. Transmission of HAV almost always occurs by the fecal-oral route.[29] Spread of the virus is facilitated by the exceptional stability of the viral capsid, and HAV may be transmitted through contaminated ground water or contaminated food.[30, 31] Common-source outbreaks are often related to infected food handlers who are involved in the preparation of uncooked foods, particularly salads. However, a large number of vehicles have been incriminated in transmission of the virus. Remarkably, in several outbreaks it seems likely that lettuce or other produce may have been contaminated at its source or in the wholesale distribution chain. Despite the impressive nature of such common-source outbreaks, the majority of hepatitis A cases occur in a sporadic and endemic fashion (Table 91–1).

Occasional transmission of HAV by blood or blood products is well documented, although it is rare.[32, 33] For transmission to be related to blood transfusion, the donor must give blood during the early stages of the infection when viremic but not yet ill (discussed later). The transmission of HAV to hemophilic patients in Europe by some lots of high-purity, solvent-detergent–inactivated factor VIII preparations can be attributed to use of large donor plasma pools containing commercially procured plasma; the high purity of the final product, which contains low quantities of potentially protective immunoglobulins; and the absence of a virus inactivation process effective against HAV.[9, 33] Blood-borne transmission of HAV may occur more commonly among needle-sharing users of illicit drugs.[34, 35] All forms of blood-borne transmission of HAV reflect the fact that viremia persists for several weeks during acute infection (Fig. 91–1).

Incidence and Prevalence

Seroprevalence surveys have shown that the prevalence of previous infection (ascertained by the presence of antibody to the virus, anti-HAV) is directly related to age, socioeconomic status, and the general level of public health sanitation.[36, 37] Infection is common early in life in many developing countries and generally quite rare among the well-developed economies of northern Europe. Thus, the prevalence of HAV varies widely among different geographic regions, largely reflecting existing sanitation practices. The United States has an intermediate level of endemicity of this virus.[37] Although 24,238 clinical cases of hepatitis A were reported to the Centers for Disease Control and Prevention in the United States during 1993, a much greater number of cases probably go unreported. Hepatitis A is most prevalent in the southwestern part of the country and is generally less common in the northeast.[37] Native Americans living on reservations are at increased risk.[38, 39] Many cases of hepatitis A are acquired as part of extended, community-based outbreaks that do not have readily apparent sources.

TABLE 91–1 ■ Reported Risk Factors for Hepatitis A by Mutually Exclusive Groups

RISK FACTOR	PATIENTS WITH ACUTE HEPATITIS A (%)
Personal contact with hepatitis case	24.0
Daycare association	15.1
Foreign travel	5.5
Outbreak associated	4.7
Male homosexual	3.8
Illicit parenteral drug use	2.4
Unknown	44.5

Data from the Viral Hepatitis and Surveillance Program, Centers for Disease Control and Prevention, 1992 (n = 9886).[37]

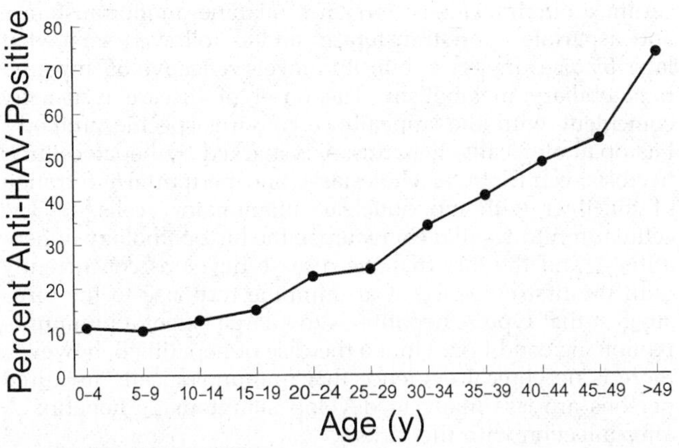

FIGURE 91–1 □ Prevalence of antibody to HAV in residents of the United States, by age group. Data are from the National Health and Nutrition Examination Survey, with subjects studied between 1976 and 1980. (From Lemon SM, Shapiro CN: The value of immunization against hepatitis A. Infect Agents Dis 3:38–49, 1994.)

In studies carried out in the late 1970s, approximately one half of Americans had serologic evidence of prior infection by 50 years of age[37] (see Fig. 91–1). To a large extent, this probably reflects a higher national incidence of HAV infection earlier in this century. The majority of adult Americans younger than age 50 are susceptible to infection with this virus, explaining why foreign travel to developing countries with poor public health sanitation remains an important risk factor for acquisition of hepatitis A. Long-term fluctuations in the rates of infectious hepatitis (presumed to be largely hepatitis A) have been reported over periods spanning decades in several developed regions, including the United States. However, within the United States, this cyclic variation in incidence seems to have disappeared.

There are no apparent differences in the virulence of HAV strains circulating in different regions of the world, although the typical age at which infection occurs varies widely and influences the incidence of accompanying disease (discussed later).

Risk Factors for Acquisition

Risk factors that have been associated with hepatitis A within the United States are shown in Table 91–1.[37] Close personal contact with infected persons remains the most commonly reported risk factor. This usually entails living in the same household with such individuals. Less intense contact, such as being in the same classroom or work environment, most often does not lead to transmission.

Contact with young children attending group daycare also represents an important factor in acquisition of hepatitis A.[40–43] Group daycare centers are frequently a locus for spread of the infection. The risk of secondary transmission is greatest from infected children younger than the age of 2 to 3 years who are not yet toilet trained, especially because infection in these young children is often clinically silent. The risk of disease is substantially greater in older siblings and caregivers, who are much more likely to develop signs and symptoms of hepatitis A than the infants who serve as silent "vectors" for amplification of the virus.[41] In some communities, group daycare centers may contribute substantially to community-wide occurrence rates of hepatitis A and may be the focus of extended, community-wide outbreaks of disease.[40, 41, 44] Perhaps for similar reasons, a number of hospital-based outbreaks of hepatitis A have been reported in pediatric units, especially neonatal intensive care units.[21, 45–48] Clinical evidence of hepatitis is generally confined to the staff of such units, although infection has been documented in patients.

Homosexually active males with multiple partners are also at increased risk for hepatitis A, as they are for other enterically transmitted pathogens.[49–51] Transmission of virus is facilitated by oral-anal contact. In this setting, hepatitis A typically presents as urban outbreaks of disease in which a significant proportion of reported cases occur among gay males. Because of the absence of a chronic carrier state, the risk of HAV infection among homosexually active men is likely to be episodic and dependent on the presence of HAV in the community and its entry into the gay male population in particular.

It has been suggested that sanitation workers and hospital housekeeping personnel may be at increased risk of acquiring hepatitis A, but there are few data in support of these contentions.

With the exception of illicit drug use, all of the risk factors shown in Table 91–1 are easily related to an increased probability of fecal-oral transmission. The nature of the relationship between drug abuse and hepatitis A is complicated and remains unclear.[34, 35] To some extent, infection of drug users may reflect poor sanitation and living conditions. However, as suggested earlier, it is likely that many cases associated with drug use are due to parenteral transmission of HAV via contaminated needles. The strongest piece of evidence in support of this conclusion is that the frequency of drug use as a risk factor for hepatitis A in the United States peaked in the late 1980s and since then has declined substantially. This parallels precisely changes in the rates of parenterally transmitted hepatitis B and C associated with illicit drug use. Reductions in the occurrence of hepatitis in drug users are possibly related to education about the acquired immunodeficiency syndrome and needle exchange programs. The risk of infection in hemophilic patients receiving high-purity, solvent-detergent–inactivated factor VIII preparations[33] is likely to have been eliminated by changes in virus inactivation procedures.

Pathogenesis

Virologic Events

Present understanding of the pathogenesis of hepatitis A derives from studies of naturally and experimentally infected humans[52–56] and nonhuman primates (chimpanzees, marmosets, and owl monkeys).[57–60] HAV antigen has been described in intestinal cells of infected tamarins,[61] a finding confirmed in orally challenged owl monkeys. In addition, small amounts of virus have been found in saliva during acute hepatitis A, suggesting that replication might occur in the oropharynx.[62] Despite these findings, the mechanism by which virus first reaches the liver remains unclear. Virus is present in the liver within a week of oral inoculation of nonhuman primates.

The dominant site of virus replication in vivo is the hepatocyte, although small amounts of viral antigen have been found in lymph nodes and spleen and along the glomerular basement membrane in infected primates.[63] Virus replicated in the liver is shed into the bile, from which it reaches the intestines and exits via the stool.[57, 64] Considerable replication and shedding of virus occur in completely asymptomatic individuals during the incubation phase of the disease (Fig. 91–2), suggesting that virus replication is by itself noncytopathic.[65] The clinical findings thus correlate well with the characteristically slow, noncytopathic replication of wild-type HAV in cell culture. Studies of experimentally infected owl

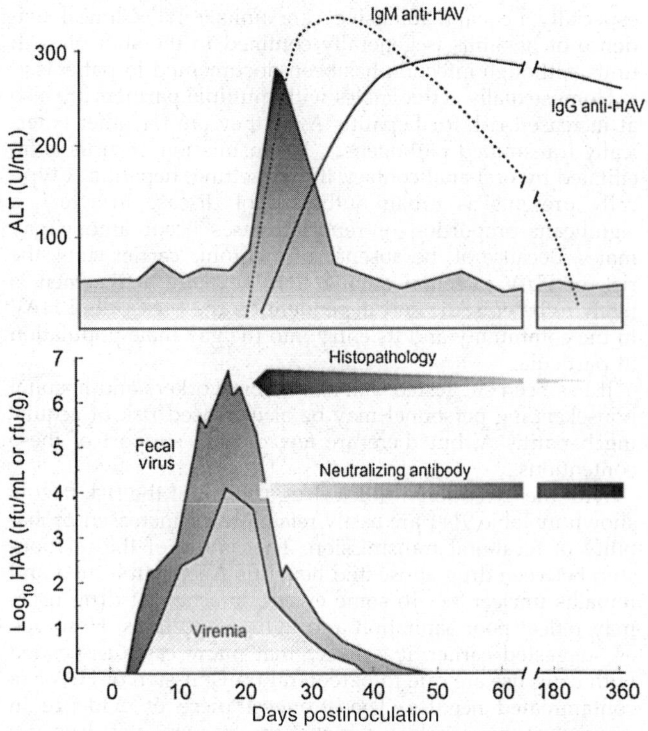

FIGURE 91–2 □ Virologic events accompanying HAV infection in an experimentally inoculated owl monkey. The events mimic hepatitis A in humans, although the disease is generally milder in nonhuman primates. The top panel depicts serum alanine aminotransferase (ALT) activity *(shaded area)* and the serum IgG *(solid line)* and IgM *(dashed line)* antibody responses to the virus. The bottom panel depicts the recovery of infectious virus from feces and serum (as measured by radioimmunofocus assay) and the presence of serum neutralizing antibody and liver histopathologic changes. (From Lemon SM, Binn LN, Marchwicki R, et al: In vivo replication and reversion to wild type of a neutralization-resistant variant of hepatitis A virus. J Infect Dis 161:7–13, 1990. © by The University of Chicago Press.)

monkeys indicate that infectious virus first appears in the stool within the first week after oral or intravenous inoculation. The quantity of virus shed in feces increases during a period of 2 to 3 weeks, reaching a maximum just before the onset of clinical symptoms.[66]

Lesser amounts of virus are found in the blood[62, 66] (see Fig. 91–2). At any point in time, the titer of virus found in serum of experimentally infected primates is approximately 1000-fold less than the titer of virus in feces. However, the temporal course of viremia follows fecal shedding closely, indicating that it also derives from the liver.[66] Viremia typically persists for up to 3 weeks, occasionally longer. Small quantities of infectious virus continue to be present in serum for a week or more after the appearance of symptoms and the development of neutralizing antibody. During experimental HAV infections in owl monkeys, up to 10^4 to 10^5 infectious virus particles have been found per milliliter of serum.[66] Maximal viremia titers may be even higher in humans. Thus, there is a brief window in which parenteral transmission may easily occur with sharing of needles among drug users. During this period, still higher titers of virus are generally found in liver tissue.

The symptoms of hepatitis A usually have their onset about 4 weeks after exposure, but this timing may range from 2 to 6 weeks. In experimentally infected primates, higher dose inocula lead to shorter incubation periods. Acute liver cell injury is marked chemically by elevations of the serum aminotransferase enzymes (alanine aminotransferase and aspartate aminotransferase) and is followed somewhat later by rises in serum bilirubin levels reflective of impaired hepatobiliary metabolism. The onset of disease is usually coincident with the appearance of virus-specific antibody. Histopathologically, hepatitis A is marked by hepatocellular necrosis, centrilobular cholestasis, and periportal infiltration of the liver with mononuclear inflammatory cells.[67–69] The cellular infiltrates that characterize the histopathology of hepatitis A and the fact that the disease develops concurrently with the first evidence of an immune response to the virus suggest that type A hepatitis is to a large extent an immunopathologic condition. Unlike the case of hepatitis B, however, there is no clinical evidence that immunologically impaired persons are less likely to develop symptomatic hepatitis A after infection with the virus.

Immune Response to Hepatitis A Virus Infection

Total serum immunoglobulins are often nonspecifically elevated during hepatitis A, and rheumatoid factor (immunoglobulin [Ig] M antibodies to IgG) is often present. Virus-specific antibodies of all three major isotypes, IgM, IgG, and IgA, appear early in the course of the illness.[29, 56, 70] IgM antibody is the most useful diagnostic marker for acute hepatitis A, because the duration of the IgM response is generally limited to less than 6 months after infection. On the other hand, IgG antibody to HAV persists for many years, perhaps lifelong in most patients. Tests for these antibodies are described in Chapter 260. Both IgG and IgM antibodies have been shown to have virus-neutralizing activity.

Antibody-antigen complexes have been described in patients with acute type A hepatitis.[71] These contain antiviral IgM antibody and viral capsid proteins. However, circulating immune complexes and antiviral antibody probably do not contribute significantly to disease development. It is more likely that liver injury is mediated by virus-specific, cytotoxic $CD8^+$ T cells that are present in the liver[25–27] and less specific natural killer cells.[72] The virus-specific cellular target for cytotoxic T cells is not known. As proposed for hepatitis B, the elaboration of interferon-γ by virus-specific $CD8^+$ cells probably results in the recruitment of nonspecific inflammatory cells to the site of virus replication.[28] These inflammatory cells play an important role in the production of the disease. Virus replication is sensitive to interferon, and interferons probably contribute to elimination of the virus in acutely infected persons.

Lifelong immunity is afforded by persisting levels of serum neutralizing antibody, but there is limited evidence that asymptomatic reinfection may occur in older individuals living in areas of high HAV endemicity.[56, 73] In such cases, primary infection presumably occurred at an early age and was followed by a loss of detectable serum antibody later in life. Reinfection may occur in the setting of household exposure to HAV and is marked by reappearance of serum antibody (IgG without an IgM response) in the absence of clinically evident disease.

Surprisingly, secretory immunity appears not to play a major role in defense against hepatitis A.[74] Although virus-specific IgA has been detected in fecal extracts by immunoassays, virus-neutralizing activity has not been reproducibly found in saliva or fecal extracts.[74, 75] This lack of a significant secretory IgA response may reflect low levels of virus replication in intestinal tissues but remains somewhat perplexing. It has important implications for vaccine-induced immunity (discussed later). Because the presence of serum antibodies prevents infection of the liver (which is the source of most virus shed in feces), such antibodies should limit the extent to which an exposed person can transmit the virus to others.

Thus, unlike the case of inactivated poliovirus vaccine, serum neutralizing antibodies produced by an inactivated HAV vaccine should be effective in preventing transmission of virus within an immunized population.

Clinical Manifestations

Acute Hepatitis A

The clinical manifestations accompanying infection with HAV[29, 76, 77] are listed in Table 91–2. These differ between adults and young children, as most children younger than 2 years experience asymptomatic infection or an infection marked with symptoms other than those suggestive of hepatic inflammation.[29, 41] On the other hand, the majority of adults older than 18 years develop clinical evidence of hepatitis in association with HAV infection, and up to two thirds may become clinically icteric.[78] The most common symptoms are nausea, dark urine, and light stools. Fever may be impressive by history but is most often not present by the time the patient seeks medical attention. Diarrhea is reported more often by children (or their parents) than by adults, although the reason for this difference remains uncertain. Other evidence of extrahepatic involvement is uncommon, although meningoencephalitis and renal failure have been reported in association with hepatitis A.[79, 79a]

The acute illness associated with HAV infection lasts from 1 to 3 weeks but may be followed by a period of prolonged convalescence. Serum liver-specific enzyme elevations may persist for a number of weeks but are always normal on long-term follow-up (1 year). There is no evidence for progression to chronic viral hepatitis, although it has been suggested that acute hepatitis A may trigger the onset of chronic autoimmune hepatitis in certain genetically predisposed individuals.[80] If so, this must be a rare event.

Cholestatic Hepatitis A

In some patients, there may be a prolonged period of jaundice (more than 12 weeks) after an episode of acute hepatitis A and the subsidence of serum alanine aminotransferase and aspartate aminotransferase levels toward normal.[81] In addition to pruritus associated with cholestasis, patients with this condition (which has been termed cholestatic hepatitis A) may complain of diarrhea and weight loss. Eventually, the serum bilirubin level returns to normal over a period of weeks with complete resolution of the illness. The challenge to the clinician is to avoid inappropriate surgical maneuvers in such patients. The pathogenic basis for prolonged cholestasis is not known, but the fact that it may improve after a brief course of corticosteroid therapy suggests an immune-mediated process.[81] Patients with this condition are probably not infectious.

Relapsing Hepatitis A

Occasional cases of relapsing hepatitis A occur after otherwise typical acute hepatitis A.[22, 23] These cases have been marked by recrudescent clinical signs and symptoms and worsening of biochemical indices of liver inflammation after a period of apparent convalescence lasting from 1 to 4 months. Several reported cases have developed simultaneous increases in titer of total serum antibodies against HAV, and in most cases there is persistence of IgM anti-HAV. It is not clear, however, whether IgM anti-HAV persists in such patients for longer periods than in most uncomplicated cases of acute hepatitis A. In one report, HAV was shed in feces during clinical relapse, and in another viral RNA was reportedly found in serum by a reverse transcription–polymerase chain reaction assay.[22, 23] Although supervening infections with other hepatitis agents have not been excluded in all cases, reports of relapsing hepatitis A have occurred with sufficient frequency to suggest that the phenomenon is real. Such relapses are not well explained by existing concepts of the pathogenesis of hepatitis A. Even in cases of relapsing hepatitis A, however, complete recovery is the rule. Occasional patients may complain of fatigue persisting beyond 12 months, but it is difficult to relate these symptoms specifically to previous infection with HAV.

Fulminant Hepatitis A

Fulminant hepatitis is marked by clinical failure of hepatic synthetic functions with associated bleeding diathesis and coma. HAV accounts for approximately 10% to 20% of all cases of fulminant viral hepatitis.[82, 83] Risk factors for development of fulminant disease include an age older than 50 years and preexisting chronic liver disease of other viral or nonviral

TABLE 91–2 ■ Symptoms Associated with Hepatitis A, B, and Non-A, Non-B in Adults*

	PREVALENCE OF SYMPTOMS (%)		
FINDING	Hepatitis A (18 Patients)	Hepatitis B (214 Patients)	Hepatitis Non-A, Non-B (68 Patients)
Jaundice	88	83	82
Dark urine	68	79	89
Fatigue	63	74	77
Light-colored stools	58	48	37
Loss of appetite	42	56	62
Distaste for cigarettes (smokers only)	45	57	63
Nausea or vomiting	26	46	56
Abdominal pain	37	51	51
Fever or chills	32	25	25
Headache	26	26	25
Muscle pain	26	21	17
Diarrhea	16	30	15
Constipation	16	17	19
Joint pain	11	30	21
Sore throat	0	12	14

*Findings in U.S. Army personnel admitted to the hospital with a serologically proven hepatitis virus infection. Most cases of hepatitis non-A, non-B were probably due to hepatitis C virus infection.

Data from references 29, 76.

causes.[84, 85] Fulminant hepatitis A is often fatal, although survival rates are higher than with fulminant hepatitis B or non-A, non-B, non-C disease. Approximately 70 fatal infections are reported annually in United States. Liver transplantation has been successful in a number of cases.

Diagnosis

The clinical signs and symptoms of hepatitis A do not allow its differentiation from hepatitis B or other forms of viral hepatitis in individual cases (see Table 91–2). A specific diagnosis may be suggested by unusual epidemiologic circumstances (such as involvement in a common-source epidemic or recent return from overseas travel), but serologic confirmation is always required. The diagnosis of acute hepatitis A thus rests on the specific detection of IgM anti-HAV[70, 86] (see Chapter 260). This serum marker is usually indicative of HAV infection having occurred within the preceding 6 months, although IgM persistence has been described for up to 12 months in some patients. Total serum antibody to HAV may also be measured as an index of previous infection (and immunity) to the virus. However, commercially available non–isotype-specific tests for anti-HAV antibodies are relatively insensitive and have a detection threshold of about 100 mIU/mL based on use of a World Health Organization reference reagent. Such tests often do not detect protective levels of antibody present after administration of immune globulin (IG) or a single dose of inactivated hepatitis A vaccine (discussed later).

Treatment

There are no available antiviral agents with activity against HAV, so management of acute hepatitis A is directed at control of symptoms and has at best a limited impact on the course of the disease. Hospitalization is usually not recommended for the typical patient with acute hepatitis A, although it may be indicated for patients who are severely ill or elderly patients who are less able to weather the illness. Certainly, evidence of confusion or prolongation of the prothrombin time should prompt early hospitalization. Bed rest has never been shown to have any effect other than improving the patient's comfort. Patients may be returned to full activity as soon as symptoms subside. A brief course of corticosteroid therapy has been suggested for patients with persistent jaundice and high serum bilirubin levels (cholestatic hepatitis)[81] but should be used with caution even in this special circumstance. No specific therapy has been shown to be of benefit in patients with fulminant hepatitis A. General medical support, including vitamin K for bleeding diathesis and measures to reduce cerebral edema, should be aggressively pursued. Orthotopic liver transplantation may be lifesaving.

Prevention

Immune Globulin

The use of pooled human IG for prevention of symptomatic hepatitis A in exposed individuals dates back to World War II, when it was shown to be approximately 80% effective in preventing infectious hepatitis among U.S. soldiers overseas.[87] When given after exposure, IG probably limits viremia and secondary intrahepatic spread of the virus. This would have the effect of reducing the number of hepatocytes that are ultimately infected, explaining the ability of IG to limit symptoms even though allowing development of normal immunity (so-called passive-active immunization).[88] IG (0.02 mL/kg) is considered effective up to 2 weeks after exposure,[89] although it may have some beneficial effects even later in the course of the infection. Administration of IG at this dosage leads to low but protective levels of serum antibody, on the order of 20 to 40 mIU/mL. These levels are generally not detectable in commercially available assays for anti-HAV.[90] When given before exposure (0.02 to 0.06 mL/kg every 3 to 6 months), IG may completely prevent infection. Postexposure prophylaxis is generally recommended after household exposure to hepatitis A or other close personal exposures considered likely to result in transmission, whereas preexposure prophylaxis is usually confined to travelers to highly endemic regions (Table 91–3). However, inactivated HAV vaccine has become available and may be preferable to IG for preexposure prophylaxis in many circumstances

TABLE 91–3 ■ Prevention of Hepatitis A with Immune Globulin and Inactivated Vaccine

GROUP AT RISK	IMMUNE GLOBULIN		HAV VACCINE
	Postexposure*	Preexposure†	
Known high risk of hepatitis A: prophylaxis is indicated			
Household or close personal contact with hepatitis A patient	√		
Travel to highly endemic regions		√	√‡
Male homosexual with multiple partners			√
High risk of severe disease if infected: strongly consider prophylaxis			
Chronic liver disease of viral or nonviral causes			√
Possibly increased risk of hepatitis A: consider prophylaxis			
Users of illicit parenteral drugs			√
Staff of group daycare centers			√
Handlers of nonhuman primates			√
Residents of institutions for the developmentally disabled, prisons, and so forth			√
Staff of neonatal intensive care units			√
Sanitation workers			√
Increased risk of transmitting HAV if infected: consider prophylaxis			
Children (<3 y) in group daycare			√
Food handlers			√

*0.02 mL/kg.
†0.02–0.06 mL/kg depending on duration of travel or protection indicated.
‡Vaccine is preferable if the traveler can be immunized 2–4 wk before departure and if multiple trips are anticipated. IG can be given with vaccine for immediate protection.

(discussed later). A detailed discussion of recommendations for use of IG may be found elsewhere.[91]

IG administration has few side effects. Patients who are IgA deficient, however, are subject to allergic reactions after administration of IG, especially with recurrent doses.

Inactivated Hepatitis A Vaccine

Inactivated hepatitis A vaccines have been developed by several commercial vaccine manufacturers, and two of these vaccines (Havrix, SmithKline Beecham; Vaqta, Merck & Co.) have been approved for sale in the United States.[37, 92–95] These vaccines are prepared by formaldehyde inactivation of HAV particles produced in infected human diploid cells. The inactivated viral antigen is subsequently adsorbed to aluminum hydroxide for its adjuvant effect. The purity of these vaccines varies considerably between manufacturers, but this has not been shown to correlate with differences in safety or efficacy. These vaccines appear to be exceptionally safe, with only minor local and systemic side effects that are similar in frequency and severity to those seen with the recombinant hepatitis B vaccine. After licensure of Havrix in Europe and the distribution of millions of doses, more serious adverse events have been reported (anaphylaxis, Guillain-Barré syndrome) but at extraordinarily low frequencies. Some reported instances of anaphylaxis may be related to the vaccine or its vehicle, but equally rare neurologic adverse events have an uncertain association with administration of the vaccine.

In general, a single dose of inactivated hepatitis A vaccine is sufficient to induce levels of antibodies to HAV that, although relatively low, are greater than those present after a single 0.02 mL/kg dose of IG.[95–98] These levels of antibody protect against clinical hepatitis A but may or may not lead to seroconversion in commercially available assays for anti-HAV. There is no added risk to immunizing an individual who is already seropositive for anti-HAV. The decision to check antibody before immunization should be based on cost-effectiveness and should reflect the probability of seropositivity, cost of the antibody test, and cost of the vaccine. Screening for antibody generally would not be cost-effective in younger American adults (see Fig. 91–1).

The currently recommended adult immunization schedule for Havrix specifies a single dose of 1440 enzyme-linked immunosorbent assay (ELISA) antigen units given by intramuscular injection. Although some evidence supports the presence of antibody within 2 weeks of administration of a single dose of Havrix, it is much preferred to immunize travelers at least 4 weeks before departure. IG can be given simultaneously with the vaccine (at different injection sites), affording travelers immediate protection with only a small negative effect on vaccine immunogenicity.[99] A booster dose of vaccine given 6 to 12 months after the first dose leads to marked increases in antibody titer and extends the duration of protection. Pediatric recommendations are for three doses of Havrix (360 ELISA antigen units each) on a 0-, 1-, and 6- to 12-month schedule or two doses of 720 ELISA antigen units given 6 to 12 months apart. Vaqta is administered as a two-dose regimen, with doses separated by 6 to 12 months (25 antigen units per dose for children, and 50 antigen units per dose for adults). These recommended dosages and schedules are confusing because of the absence of an internationally recognized HAV antigen standard. Protection should last more than 5 years, based on the results of antibody levels obtained in early studies. There are as yet no recommendations for late booster doses and generally no reason to check serum antibody levels after vaccination.

Two prospective clinical trials have confirmed a high level of clinical efficacy of inactivated hepatitis A vaccines in prevention of hepatitis A in immunized children. In one study, protection against clinical disease was 100% within 3 weeks after administration of a single dose of Vaqta.[100] One month after this immunization, the median level of serum anti-HAV antibody approximated that present after a protective dose of IG. Detailed analysis indicated that this early vaccine-induced antibody, although highly protective, differs qualitatively from the antibody that is present in IG. The early antibody probably has lower affinity for the virus than anti-HAV in IG. This makes it difficult to quantitate and compare serologic responses to different vaccines, as the existing antibody standard is an IG preparation. In a second clinical trial, Havrix was shown to be equivalently protective in immunized Thai schoolchildren.[101] In this study, however, surveillance for hepatitis A cases did not commence until after a second dose of vaccine had been given, preventing an analysis of the efficacy of a single vaccine dose.[102] Although clinical studies of efficacy in adults are lacking, these vaccines are likely to be highly protective on the basis of a comparison of the induced antibody levels with those present after administration of IG.

Suggested recommendations for use of inactivated HAV vaccine[37] are summarized in Table 91–3, although formal recommendations had not yet been published by the U.S. Public Health Service at the time of preparation of this chapter. In general, immunization should be considered for those at increased risk of acquiring hepatitis A, those at increased risk for severe or fulminant disease should they become infected, and those who may be at increased risk of transmitting the infection to others (see Table 91–3). Inactivated HAV vaccines are capable of providing effective control of community-wide outbreaks of hepatitis A.[100, 103]

Whereas IG remains the preventive modality of choice for postexposure prophylaxis of close personal contacts of hepatitis A cases, vaccine is generally preferable to IG for most preexposure indications. However, a good case for the use of IG could be made for persons who anticipate only a single overseas trip of limited duration to a hepatitis A endemic region. Inactivated hepatitis A vaccine is expensive, and its cost will affect the decision-making process. Although the price may be reduced by competition with the entry of new products into the market, inactivated HAV vaccine is unlikely to receive wide enough use to reduce the overall incidence of hepatitis A in the United States or other countries with moderate or high rates of hepatitis A.[37] Effective control of hepatitis A would require universal immunization of children, especially those in group daycare. This will probably require the development of equally safe and effective vaccines that are less expensive to manufacture and administer. Candidate attenuated vaccines have been tested in limited clinical trials[19, 20] but have not proved sufficiently immunogenic to warrant further development (see Chapter 260). Immunization of food handlers would be likely to prevent many food-borne outbreaks of hepatitis A, but the cost-effectiveness of this strategy is uncertain.

Acknowledgment

This work was supported in part by grant AI-32599 from the U.S. Public Health Service.

References

1. Lemon SM, Robertson BH: Current perspectives in the virology and molecular biology of hepatitis A virus. Semin Virol 4:285, 1993.
2. Lemon SM: Hepatitis A virus: Current concepts of the molecular virology, immunobiology, and approaches to vaccine development. Rev Med Virol 2:73, 1992.

3. Cohen JI, Ticehurst JR, Purcell RH, et al: Complete nucleotide sequence of wild-type hepatitis A virus: Comparison with different strains of hepatitis A virus and other picornaviruses. J Virol 61:50, 1987.
4. Ticehurst JR, Cohen JI, Feinstone SM, et al: Replication of hepatitis A virus: New ideas from studies with cloned cDNA. *In* Semler BL, Ehrenfeld E (eds): Molecular Aspects of Picornavirus Infection and Detection. Washington, DC, American Society for Microbiology, 1989, p 27.
5. Feinstone SM, Kapikian AZ, Purcell RH: Hepatitis A: Detection by immune electron microscopy of a viruslike antigen associated with acute illness. Science 182:1026, 1973.
6. Siegl G, Weitz M, Kronauer G: Stability of hepatitis A virus. Intervirology 22:218, 1984.
7. Scholz E, Heinricy U, Flehmig B: Acid stability of hepatitis A virus. J Gen Virol 70:2481, 1989.
8. Lemon SM, Murphy PC, Shields PA, et al: Antigenic and genetic variation in cytopathic hepatitis A virus variants arising during persistent infection: Evidence for genetic recombination. J Virol 65:2056, 1991.
9. Lemon SM, Murphy PC, Smith A, et al: Removal/neutralization of hepatitis A virus during manufacture of high purity, solvent/detergent factor VIII concentrate. J Med Virol 43:44, 1994.
10. Jansen RW, Siegl G, Lemon SM: Molecular epidemiology of human hepatitis A virus defined by an antigen-capture polymerase chain reaction method. Proc Natl Acad Sci USA 87:2867, 1990.
11. Robertson BH, Jansen RW, Khanna B, et al: Genetic relatedness of hepatitis A virus strains recovered from different geographic regions. J Gen Virol 73:1365, 1992.
12. Ping L-H, Lemon SM: Antigenic structure of human hepatitis A virus defined by analysis of escape mutants selected against murine monoclonal antibodies. J Virol 66:2208, 1992.
13. Lemon SM, Jansen RW, Brown EA: Genetic, antigenic, and biologic differences between strains of hepatitis A virus. Vaccine 10(Suppl 1):S40, 1992.
14. Provost PJ, Hilleman MR: Propagation of human hepatitis A virus in cell culture in vitro. Proc Soc Exp Biol Med 160:213, 1979.
15. Daemer RJ, Feinstone SM, Gust ID, Purcell RH: Propagation of human hepatitis A virus in African green monkey kidney cell culture: Primary isolation and serial passage. Infect Immun 32:388, 1981.
16. Binn LN, Lemon SM, Marchwicki RH, et al: Primary isolation and serial passage of hepatitis A virus strains in primate cell cultures. J Clin Microbiol 20:28, 1984.
17. Provost PJ, Bishop RP, Gerety RJ, et al: New findings in live, attenuated hepatitis A vaccine development. J Med Virol 20:165, 1986.
18. Taylor KL, Murphy PC, Asher LVS, et al: Attenuation phenotype of a cell culture–adapted variant of hepatitis A virus (HM175/p16) in susceptible New World owl monkeys. J Infect Dis 168:592, 1993.
19. Midthun K, Ellerbeck E, Gershman K, et al: Safety and immunogenicity of a live attenuated hepatitis A virus vaccine in seronegative volunteers. J Infect Dis 163:735, 1991.
20. Sjogren MH, Purcell RH, McKee K, et al: Clinical and laboratory observations following oral or intramuscular administration of a live, attenuated hepatitis A vaccine candidate. Vaccine 10(Suppl 1):S135, 1992.
21. Rosenblum LS, Villarino ME, Nainan OV, et al: Hepatitis A outbreak in a neonatal intensive care unit: Risk factors for transmission and evidence of prolonged viral excretion among preterm infants. J Infect Dis 164:476, 1991.
22. Sjogren MH, Tanno H, Fay O, et al: Hepatitis A virus in stool during clinical relapse. Ann Intern Med 106:221, 1987.
23. Glikson M, Galun E, Oren R, et al: Relapsing hepatitis A. Review of 14 cases and literature survey. Medicine (Baltimore) 71:14, 1992.
24. Lemon SM, Binn LN: Serum neutralizing antibody response to hepatitis A virus. J Infect Dis 148:1033, 1983.
25. Vallbracht A, Gabriel P, Maier K, et al: Cell-mediated cytotoxicity in hepatitis A virus infection. Hepatology 6:1308, 1986.
26. Vallbracht A, Maier K, Stierhof Y-D, et al: Liver-derived cytotoxic T cells in hepatitis A virus infection. J Infect Dis 160:209, 1989.
27. Fleischer B, Fleischer S, Maier K, et al: Clonal analysis of infiltrating T lymphocytes in liver tissue in viral hepatitis A. Immunology 69:14, 1990.
28. Maier K, Gabriel P, Koscielniak E, et al: Human gamma interferon production by cytotoxic T lymphocytes sensitized during hepatitis A virus infection. J Virol 62:3756, 1988.
29. Lemon SM: Type A viral hepatitis: New developments in an old disease. N Engl J Med 313:1059, 1985.
30. Hooper RR, Juels CW, Routenberg JA, et al: Outbreak of type A viral hepatitis at the Naval Training Center, San Diego: Epidemiologic evaluation. Am J Epidemiol 105:148, 1977.
31. Bergeisen GH, Hinds MW, Skaggs JW: A waterborne outbreak of hepatitis A in Meade County, Kentucky. Am J Public Health 75:161, 1985.
32. Weisfuse IB, Graham DJ, Will M, et al: An outbreak of hepatitis A among cancer patients treated with interleukin-2 and lymphokine activated killer cells. J Infect Dis 161:647, 1990.
33. Mannucci PM, Gdovin S, Gringeri A, et al: Transmission of hepatitis A to patients with hemophilia by factor VIII concentrates treated with organic solvent and detergent to inactivate viruses. Ann Intern Med 120:1, 1994.
34. Widell A, Hansson BG, Moestrup T, Nordenfelt E: Increased occurrence of hepatitis A with cyclic outbreaks among drug addicts in a Swedish community. Infection 11:198, 1983.
35. Centers for Disease Control: Hepatitis A among drug abusers. MMWR Morb Mortal Wkly Rep 37:297, 1988.
36. Dienstag JL, Szmuness W, Stevens CE, Purcell RH: Hepatitis A virus infection: New insights from seroepidemiologic studies. J Infect Dis 137:328, 1978.
37. Lemon SM, Shapiro CN: The value of immunization against hepatitis A. Infect Agents Dis 3:38, 1994.
38. Gildon B, Makintubee S, Istre GR: Community-wide outbreak of hepatitis A among an Indian population in Oklahoma. South Med J 85: 9, 1992.
39. Bulkow LR, Wainwright RB, McMahon BJ, et al: Secular trends in hepatitis A virus infection among Alaska natives. J Infect Dis 168:1017, 1993.
40. Benenson MW, Takafuji ET, Bancroft WH, et al: A military community outbreak of hepatitis type A related to transmission in a child care facility. Am J Epidemiol 112:471, 1980.
41. Hadler SC, Webster HM, Erben JJ, et al: Hepatitis A in day-care centers: A community-wide assessment. N Engl J Med 302:1222, 1980.
42. Gingrich GA, Hadler SC, Elder HA, Ash KO: Serologic investigation of an outbreak of hepatitis A in a rural day-care center. Am J Public Health 73:1190, 1983.
43. Hadler SC, McFarland L: Hepatitis in day care centers: Epidemiology and prevention. Rev Infect Dis 8:548, 1986.
44. Hadler SC, Erben JJ, Matthews R, et al: Effect of immunoglobulin on hepatitis A in day-care centers. JAMA 249:48, 1983.
45. Noble RC, Kane MA, Reeves SA, Roeckel I: Posttransfusion hepatitis A in a neonatal intensive care unit. JAMA 252:2711, 1984.
46. Krober MS, Bass JW, Brown JD, et al: Hospital outbreak of hepatitis A: Risk factors for spread. Pediatr Infect Dis 3:296, 1984.
47. Orenstein WA, Wu E, Wilkins J, et al: Hospital-acquired hepatitis A: Report of an outbreak. Pediatrics 67:494, 1981.
48. Watson JC, Fleming DW, Borella AJ, et al: Vertical transmission of hepatitis A resulting in an outbreak in a neonatal intensive care unit. J Infect Dis 167:567, 1993.
49. Corey L, Holmes KK: Sexual transmission of hepatitis A in homosexual men: Incidence and mechanism. N Engl J Med 302:435, 1980.
50. Christenson B, Brostrom C, Bottiger M, et al: An epidemic outbreak of hepatitis A among homosexual men in Stockholm: Hepatitis A, a special hazard for the male homosexual subpopulation in Sweden. Am J Epidemiol 116:599, 1982.
51. Stewart T, Crofts N: An outbreak of hepatitis A among homosexual men in Melbourne. Med J Aust 158:519, 1993.
52. Ward R, Krugman S, Giles JP, et al: Infectious hepatitis: Studies of its natural history and prevention. N Engl J Med 258:407, 1958.
53. Krugman S, Ward R, Giles JP: The natural history of infectious hepatitis. Am J Med 32:717, 1962.
54. Krugman S, Ward R, Giles JP, et al: Infectious hepatitis: Detec-

tion of virus during the incubation period and in clinically inapparent infection. N Engl J Med 261:729, 1959.
55. Boggs JD, Melnick JL, Conrad ME, Felsher BF: Viral hepatitis: Clinical and tissue culture studies. JAMA 214:1041, 1970.
56. Decker RH, Overby LR, Ling C-M, et al: Serologic studies of transmission of hepatitis A in humans. J Infect Dis 139:74, 1979.
57. Schulman AN, Dienstag JL, Jackson DR, et al: Hepatitis A antigen particles in liver, bile, and stool of chimpanzees. J Infect Dis 134:80, 1976.
58. Dienstag JL, Feinstone SM, Purcell RH, et al: Experimental infection of chimpanzees with hepatitis A virus. J Infect Dis 132:532, 1975.
59. Holmes AW, Deinhardt F, Wolfe L, et al: Specific neutralization of human hepatitis type A in marmoset monkeys. Nature 243:419, 1973.
60. LeDuc JW, Lemon SM, Keenan CM, et al: Experimental infection of the New World owl monkey *(Aotus trivirgatus)* with hepatitis A virus. Infect Immun 40:766, 1983.
61. Karayiannis P, Jowett T, Enticott M, et al: Hepatitis A virus replication in tamarins and host immune response in relation to pathogenesis of liver cell damage. J Med Virol 18:261, 1986.
62. Cohen JI, Feinstone S, Purcell RH: Hepatitis A virus infection in a chimpanzee: Duration of viremia and detection of virus in saliva and throat swabs. J Infect Dis 160:887, 1989.
63. Mathiesen LR, Drucker J, Lorenz D, et al: Localization of hepatitis A antigen in marmoset organs during acute infection with hepatitis A virus. J Infect Dis 138:369, 1978.
64. Coulepis AG, Locarnini SA, Lehmann NI, Gust ID: Detection of hepatitis A virus in the feces of patients with naturally acquired infections. J Infect Dis 141:151, 1980.
65. Dienstag JL, Feinstone SM, Kapikian AZ, et al: Faecal shedding of hepatitis-A antigen. Lancet 1:765, 1975.
66. Lemon SM, Binn LN, Marchwicki R, et al: In vivo replication and reversion to wild type of a neutralization-resistant variant of hepatitis A virus. J Infect Dis 161:7, 1990.
67. Dienstag JL, Popper H, Purcell RH: The pathology of viral hepatitis types A and B in chimpanzees. Am J Pathol 85:131, 1976.
68. Teixera MR Jr, Weller IVD, Murray A, et al: The pathology of hepatitis A in man. Liver 2:53, 1982.
69. Keenan CM, Lemon SM, LeDuc JW, et al: Pathology of hepatitis A infection in the owl monkey *(Aotus trivirgatus)*. Am J Pathol 115:1, 1984.
70. Lemon SM, Brown CD, Brooks DS, et al: Specific immunoglobulin M response to hepatitis A virus determined by solid-phase radioimmunoassay. Infect Immun 28:927, 1980.
71. Margolis HS, Nainan OV, Krawczynski K, et al: Appearance of immune complexes during experimental hepatitis A infection in chimpanzees. J Med Virol 26:315, 1988.
72. Kurane I, Binn LN, Bancroft WH, Ennis FA: Human lymphocyte responses to hepatitis A virus–infected cells: Interferon production and lysis of infected cells. J Immunol 135:2140, 1985.
73. Villarejos VM, Serra CJ, Anderson-Visona K, Mosley JW: Hepatitis A virus infection in households. Am J Epidemiol 115:577, 1982.
74. Stapleton JT, Lange DK, LeDuc JW, et al: The role of secretory immunity in hepatitis A virus infection. J Infect Dis 163:7, 1991.
75. Locarnini SA, Coulepis AG, Kaldor J, Gust ID: Coproantibodies in hepatitis A: Detection by enzyme-linked immunosorbent assay and immune electron microscopy. J Clin Microbiol 11: 710, 1980.
76. Lemon SM, Lednar WM, Bancroft WH, et al: Etiology of viral hepatitis in American soldiers. Am J Epidemiol 116:438, 1982.
77. Tong MJ, El-Farra NS, Grew MI: Clinical manifestations of hepatitis A: Recent experience in a community teaching hospital. J Infect Dis 171(Suppl 1):S15, 1995.
78. Lednar WM, Lemon SM, Kirkpatrick JW, et al: Frequency of illness associated with epidemic hepatitis A virus infections in adults. Am J Epidemiol 122:226, 1985.
79. Bromberg K, Newhall DN, Peter G: Hepatitis A and meningoencephalitis. JAMA 247:815, 1982.
79a. Nachbaur K, König H, Rumpelt HJ, et al: Acute renal failure complicating non-fulminant hepatitis A. Clin Nephrol 45:398, 1996.
80. Vento S, Garofano T, di Perri G, et al: Identification of hepatitis A virus as a trigger for autoimmune chronic hepatitis type 1 in susceptible individuals. Lancet 337:1183, 1991.
81. Gordon SC, Reddy KR, Schiff L, Schiff ER: Prolonged intrahepatic cholestasis secondary to acute hepatitis A. Ann Intern Med 101:635, 1984.
82. Mathiesen LR, Skinhoj P, Nielsen JO, et al: Hepatitis type A, B, and non-A non-B in fulminant hepatitis. Gut 21:72, 1980.
83. Rakela J, Redeker AG, Edwards VM, et al: Hepatitis A virus infection in fulminant hepatitis and chronic active hepatitis. Gastroenterology 74:879, 1978.
84. Hadler SC: Global impact of hepatitis A virus infection: Changing patterns. *In* Hollinger FB, Lemon SM, Margolis HS (eds): Viral Hepatitis and Liver Disease. Baltimore, Williams & Wilkins, 1991, p 14.
85. Forbes A, Williams R: Changing epidemiology and clinical aspects of hepatitis A. Br Med Bull 46:303, 1990.
86. Decker RH, Kosakowski SM, Vanderbilt AS, et al: Diagnosis of acute hepatitis A by HAVAB-M, a direct radioimmunoassay for IgM anti-HAV. Am J Clin Pathol 76:140, 1981.
87. Gellis SS, Stokes J Jr, Brother GM, et al: The use of human immune serum globulin (gamma globulin) in infectious (epidemic) hepatitis in the Mediterranean theater of operations. I. Studies on prophylaxis in two epidemics of infectious hepatitis. JAMA 128: 1062, 1945.
88. Krugman S, Ward R, Giles JP, Jacobs AM: Infectious hepatitis: Studies on the effect of gamma globulin and on the incidence of inapparent infection. JAMA 174:323, 1960.
89. Winokur PL, Stapleton JT: Immunoglobulin prophylaxis for hepatitis A. Clin Infect Dis 14:580, 1992.
90. Stapleton JT, Jansen RW, Lemon SM: Neutralizing antibody to hepatitis A virus in immune serum globulin and in the sera of human recipients of immune serum globulin. Gastroenterology 89:637, 1985.
91. Protection against viral hepatitis. Recommendations of the Immunization Practices Advisory Committee (ACIP). MMWR Morb Mortal Wkly Rep 39(RR-2):1, 1990.
92. Lewis JA, Armstrong ME, Larson VM, et al: Use of a live attenuated hepatitis A vaccine to prepare a highly purified, formalin-inactivated hepatitis A vaccine. *In* Hollinger FB, Lemon SM, Margolis HS (eds): Viral Hepatitis and Liver Disease. Baltimore, Williams & Wilkins, 1991, p 94.
93. Andre FE, Hepburn A, D'Hondt E: Inactivated candidate vaccines for hepatitis A. Prog Med Virol 37:72, 1990.
94. Clemens R, Safary A, Hepburn A, et al: Clinical experience with an inactivated hepatitis A vaccine. J Infect Dis 171(Suppl 1):S44, 1995.
95. Green MS, Cohen D, Lerman Y, et al: A trial of the reactogenicity and immunogenicity of an inactivated hepatitis A vaccine. Isr J Med Sci 30:485, 1994.
96. Ellerbeck EF, Lewis JA, Nalin D, et al: Safety profile and immunogenicity of an inactivated vaccine derived from an attenuated strain of hepatitis A virus. Vaccine 10:668, 1992.
97. Newcomer W, Rivin B, Reid R, et al: Immunogenicity, safety and tolerability of varying doses and regimens of inactivated hepatitis A virus vaccine in Navajo children. Pediatr Infect Dis J 13:640, 1994.
98. DeFraites RF, Feighner BH, Binn LN, et al: Immunization of US soldiers with a two-dose primary series of inactivated hepatitis A vaccine: Early immune response, persistence of antibody, and response to a third dose at 1 year. J Infect Dis 171(Suppl 1):S61, 1995.
99. Green MS, Cohen D, Lerman Y, et al: Depression of the immune response to an inactivated hepatitis A vaccine administered concomitantly with immune globulin. J Infect Dis 168:740, 1993.
100. Werzberger A, Mensch B, Kuter B, et al: A controlled trial of a formalin-inactivated hepatitis A vaccine in healthy children. N Engl J Med 327:453, 1992.
101. Innis BL, Snitbhan R, Kunasol P, et al: Protection against hepatitis A by an inactivated vaccine. JAMA 271:1328, 1994.
102. Lemon SM: Inactivated hepatitis A vaccines. JAMA 271:1363, 1994.
103. Príkazsky V, Oleár V, Cernoch A, et al: Interruption of an outbreak of hepatitis A in two villages by vaccination. J Med Virol 44:457, 1994.

92

Hepatitis B and Hepatitis D

Raymond S. Koff

HEPATITIS B

Epidemiology

Incubation Period

The incubation period of hepatitis B, defined as the interval between exposure to hepatitis B virus (HBV) and elevation of the serum aminotransferase levels, has a broad peak of between 60 and 90 days, with a range of 30 to 180 days. The incubation period, if taken as the period between exposure to HBV and the initial appearance of the hepatitis B surface antigen (HBsAg) in serum, the earliest marker of infection routinely detected, may be as short as 1 to 2 weeks. Biochemical evidence of hepatitis is usually present within a month or two after HBsAg is identified.

Epidemiologic Patterns

HBV infection occurs throughout the world with a highly variable prevalence. HBV transmission is not dependent on serial propagation; a human reservoir, currently estimated to be approximately 300 million persistently infected individuals, is present in nearly all communities of the world (Fig. 92–1). HBV infection has been identified in highly endemic zones in geographically remote and culturally isolated populations (e.g., South Pacific Islanders and Alaskan Natives) as well as in large, densely populated regions (e.g., sub-Saharan Africa and Asia). Approximately 1.2 million North Americans are HBV carriers. HBV infection occurs early in life in most high-prevalence areas. As a consequence of maternal-neonatal transmission and horizontal spread between young children, markers of prior HBV infection may be found in most children by 10 to 15 years of age in these endemic regions.[1]

In contrast, in moderate-prevalence populations, the rate of infection peaks later; a substantial proportion of the population may have markers of HBV infection by age 25 years. Sexual activity plays an important role in this pattern. In the United States, as in many low-prevalence areas, markers of HBV infection are found in less than 4% of the general population. They are found more frequently in Asian Americans and in black persons than in white persons. In general, in low-prevalence populations, such as in the United States, sexual activity, injection drug use, occupationally acquired infection, nonsexual household or intrafamilial spread, and dialysis and use of multiple blood products are the principal identified mechanisms of HBV transmission (Fig. 92–2). Imported cases in immigrants and travelers returning from high-prevalence countries are of minor importance. In about 25% to 30% of cases, no risk factor can be identified; unrecognized or inapparent permucosal or percutaneous spread is responsible. Although transfusion-associated hepatitis B has become a rare event in the United States since the introduction of serologic screening of blood donors, recipients of multiple blood products, such as patients with hemophilia A, have had a substantial risk for HBV infection.[2]

In the United States, the risk of HBV transmission among young children appears to be low.[3] Peak attack rates of HBV are seen in the 15- to 39-year-old age group. These infections represent nearly 75% of all reported cases and support the concept of HBV infection as a sexually transmitted disease. A progressive decline in the frequency of acute hepatitis B is anticipated as a consequence of universal vaccination of infants and young adolescents.

Modes of Transmission

Contact Transmission. Horizontal transfer of HBV-contaminated body secretions, including semen, cervicovaginal secretions, blood, and saliva, is involved in contact transmission between sexual partners and between some household members not engaging in sexual activity. HBV DNA may be present in spermatozoa and leukocytes in semen and in the leukocytes present in the saliva of acutely and persistently infected individuals. Transfer of contaminated body fluids to nonsexual household and family contacts is most likely to

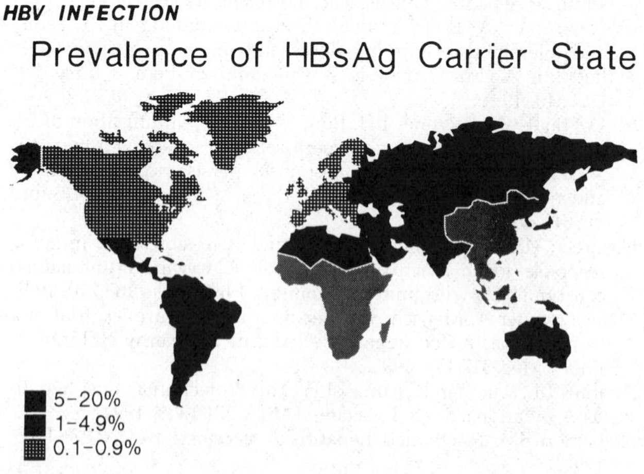

FIGURE 92–1 □ The global prevalence of the HBV carrier state. High-endemicity zones, in which the HBsAg carrier rate approaches or occasionally exceeds 20%, are found in Southeast Asia and in sub-Saharan Africa. (Courtesy of the Clinical Teaching Project, American Gastroenterological Association.)

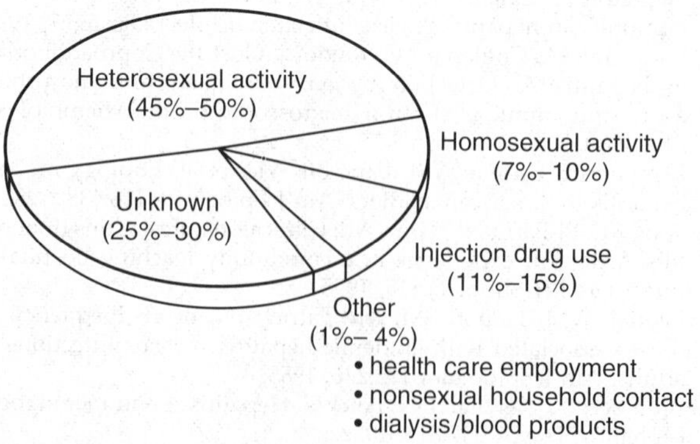

FIGURE 92–2 □ Major risk factors for the acquisition of HBV infection in the United States. (Adapted from McQuillan G, Alter MJ, Everhart JE: Viral hepatitis. *In* Everhart JE [ed]: Digestive Diseases in the United States. Washington, DC, US Government Printing Office, 1994, pp 127–156. NIH publication 94–1447.)

occur by child-to-child transmission and may involve such diverse mechanisms as shared eating utensils, teething rings, toys, and toothbrushes. Transmission may be efficient when the infected individual is developmentally disadvantaged and institutionalized.[4] The infectivity of body fluids and the contagiousness of persistently infected individuals appear to decrease with increasing age, concomitantly with loss of serum markers of viral replication (e.g., HBV DNA).[5]

Maternal-Neonatal Transmission. No more than 5% to 10% of neonatal HBV infections appear to result from in utero infection.[6] The presumed mechanism of maternal-neonatal infection is transplacental leakage of HBV-contaminated maternal blood resulting from uterine contractions and disruption of placental barriers during labor and delivery. The majority of neonatal HBV infections are a consequence of exposure of the newborn to HBV during labor, delivery, or the early postpartum period. HBV DNA has been identified by polymerase chain reaction amplification in colostral specimens.[7] However, breast-feeding does not increase the risk of transmission in infants of infected mothers provided that they are immunized shortly after birth with hepatitis B immune globulin (HBIG) and hepatitis B vaccine. Data on the efficacy of delivery by cesarean section in reducing the risk of infection are conflicting.

Maternal-neonatal HBV transmission occurs most frequently when the mother is an HBV carrier who is hepatitis B e antigen (HBeAg)–positive or when she develops HBV infection during the third trimester or early postpartum period. Nearly 90% of the infants of HBeAg-positive carrier women will be infected; about 10% to 15% of the infants of HBeAg-negative women will be infected[8] (Fig. 92–3). In the infants of the HBeAg-positive mothers, most infections will be persistent (i.e., the infant becomes an HBV carrier). In contrast, most infections in the infants of HBeAg-negative mothers are transient infections. The strongest independent predictor of the risk of persistent infection in the infant is the maternal HBV DNA level.[8] The risk increases with increasing maternal HBV load.

Percutaneous Transmission. Percutaneous inoculation appears to be an efficient mode of HBV transfer. HBV infection is exceedingly common in injecting drug users who share needles and other inoculation equipment, in those who inject frequently, and in those who attend "shooting galleries."[9] It was also common among health care workers exposed through accidental needlesticks with contaminated equipment in the era before widespread use of HBV vaccines in this occupational group. Unfortunately, among the unvaccinated, HBV transmission still occurs. In one study of health care workers, the seroprevalence of HBV in the unvaccinated was 22%, and the incidence density rate, expressed as new infections per 100 person-years, was 3.05 for HBV.[10]

Tissue penetrations with any form of contaminated instruments (e.g., acupuncture needles, tattoo needles, and ear-piercing equipment) may be responsible for sporadic cases as well as for mini-outbreaks of infection. Communal use of water for bathing has been implicated in the development of outbreaks of HBV among track-finders with multiple cuts and scratches. An extreme example of percutaneous transmission, HBV infection after transplantation of HBV-contaminated organs, has become uncommon since donor screening has been implemented. In the medical office, in the hospital laboratory, or at the bedside, permucosal transfer may result from splashing accidents when mucosal surfaces are exposed to contaminated biomaterials, such as blood or other body fluids.

Unestablished Routes of Spread. Respiratory or airborne transmission and food- and water-borne spread are not accepted epidemiologic entities. The role of biting insects remains speculative.

Pathogenesis and Pathology

The principal hepatic histologic lesions of acute HBV infection are foci of hepatocyte necrosis, with loss of cells (dropout), ballooning degeneration, and acidophilic (Councilman-like) bodies, which are mummified, necrotic hepatocytes. Necrosis and inflammation may be most prominent in the centrilobular zones; an endophlebitis may be present. Whereas the lobular architecture is intact, a diffuse mononuclear cell infiltrate may be prominent within the lobule and within expanded portal tracts, which may demonstrate segmental ero-

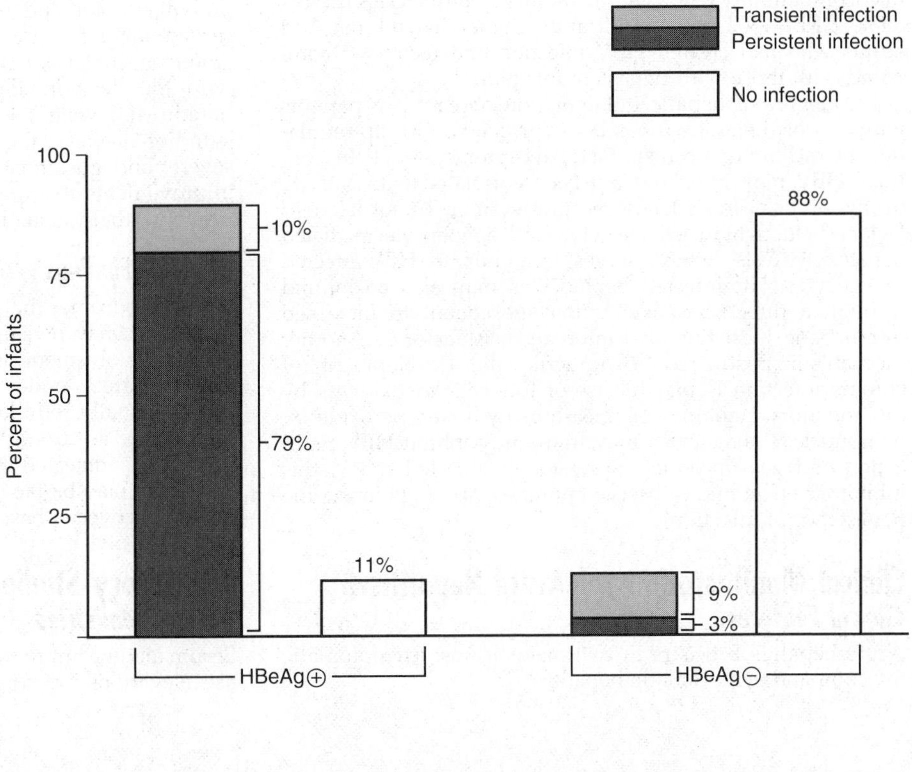

FIGURE 92–3 □ Infant HBV infection rates and the HBeAg status of the HBsAg-positive carrier mother. As shown here, most infections in the infants of HBeAg-positive mothers are persistent. (Adapted from Burk RD, Hwang L-Y, Ho GYF, et al: Outcome of perinatal hepatitis B virus exposure is dependent on maternal virus load. J Infect Dis 170:1418–1423, 1994.)

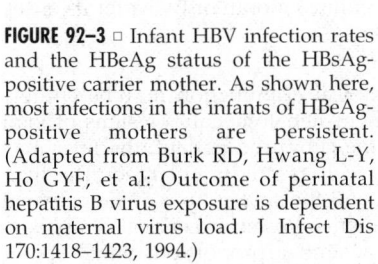

sion of the limiting plate. The $CD8^+$ cytotoxic lymphocyte appears to be the predominant mononuclear cell in the liver of the patient with HBV infection; it is closely associated with infected hepatocytes. Natural killer lymphocytes are also prominent. The mononuclear macrophages of the liver, the Kupffer cells, appear enlarged and hyperplastic.

In general, hepatocyte injury in HBV infection does not appear to be due to a direct cytopathic effect of the virus. The production of HBV and its gene products by the hepatocytes of HBV carriers in whom liver histology and function may be entirely normal suggests that liver injury is likely to be mediated by mechanisms other than direct HBV-induced cytotoxicity. Nonetheless, in some instances (e.g., after liver transplantation for end-stage chronic hepatitis B with active viral replication), the rapid onset of HBV reinfection of the graft and the development of severe hepatitis in the immunosuppressed recipient suggest a direct role for the virus. Whether specific gene products, such as the hepatitis B core antigen (HBcAg), are directly cytotoxic remains speculative despite the early observation that cultured cells expressing this material may develop cytopathic alterations.[11]

Cell-mediated immune mechanisms are thought to be key in the pathogenesis of liver injury in hepatitis B. The precise mechanisms are still poorly understood. Major histocompatibility complex–restricted cytotoxic T-lymphocyte activity, antibody-dependent cell-mediated cytotoxicity, and natural killer cell activity have been postulated to be involved. Activation of cytotoxic (cytolytic) T lymphocytes directed against specific target viral antigens (e.g., HBcAg) expressed on the hepatocyte membrane has received considerable attention. Viral antigen-independent activation of cytotoxic T lymphocytes may also play a role. T-lymphocyte recognition of HBV-infected hepatocytes may require display of HBcAg or other viral antigens on the surface of the hepatocyte membrane and display of human leukocyte antigen (HLA) class I antigens before immunocytolysis can be effected.[12]

The mechanisms responsible for the development of chronic HBV infection also remain incompletely understood. The high frequency of chronic infection in those infected early in life and in the immunocompromised suggests that immunologic tolerance may play a key role. Genetically determined host factors also appear to play a role in HBV persistence. In a study of the polymorphism of the major histocompatibility complex, the frequency of the class II HLA allele DRB1*1302 was significantly higher in children and adults who had cleared HBV infection and recovered compared with those with persistent infection.[13]

The degree of hepatic inflammation observed in patients with chronic hepatitis B has been correlated with up-regulation of the tumor necrosis factor receptor system.[14] In contrast, HBV replication has not been correlated with activity of the tumor necrosis factor receptor system. Tumor necrosis factor-α is thought to activate cytotoxic T-lymphocyte–mediated hepatocyte lysis, which serves to eliminate HBV-infected hepatocytes. Noninfected hepatocytes may also be injured through a direct cytotoxic action subsequent to increased intrahepatic induction of tumor necrosis factor-α. Another mechanism postulated to underlie the development of chronic infection is that release of intracellular oxidants by inflammatory cytokines or release of hydrogen peroxide by mononuclear phagocytes may transiently inhibit HBV replication and gene product expression in infected cells[15]; this inhibitory effect may subserve immune evasion, favoring the persistence of infection.

Clinical Manifestations of Acute Hepatitis B

Clinical Features

Acute hepatitis B occurs in two major forms: asymptomatic infection and symptomatic hepatitis.

Asymptomatic Hepatitis. Asymptomatic HBV infection can be either subclinical or inapparent. In subclinical infection, abnormal blood test results reflecting hepatic injury (i.e., elevated serum aminotransferase levels) are present, but jaundice and symptoms are absent. In inapparent infection, symptoms and biochemical abnormalities are not detected; inapparent infections are identified by serologic studies. In neonates and young children with HBV infection, asymptomatic infection is typical. The ratio of subclinical and inapparent infection remains ill-defined. In contrast to experience in children, symptomatic disease is more frequently encountered in adolescents and adults.

Symptomatic Hepatitis. In symptomatic disease in adults, about one in four patients will have jaundice. Symptomatic hepatitis without jaundice is termed anicteric hepatitis. The clinical features of anicteric hepatitis are identical, save for the absence of jaundice, to those of icteric hepatitis, but they are milder and often abbreviated. Gastrointestinal symptoms, either alone or in combination with influenza-like symptoms, including mild fever, may be the predominant clinical features of anicteric hepatitis. Malaise, fatigue, weakness, and anorexia may or may not be present.

Preicteric (Prodromal) Features. The onset of symptoms in hepatitis B is usually insidious. In a few patients, no symptoms occur before the onset of jaundice. However, more typically, a set of constitutional, gastrointestinal, and to a lesser extent respiratory symptoms may be seen during a preicteric prodromal phase that may last for several weeks. In about 25% of patients, the preicteric phase may be less than 1 week long. Lassitude, fatigue, myalgias and arthralgias, anorexia, and nausea and vomiting may be the most prominent complaints. In less than 10% of patients, an immune complex–mediated, extrahepatic serum sickness–like syndrome may be the initial or major preicteric feature. In affected patients, combinations of polyarthritis, angioedema, urticaria, maculopapular eruptions, and more rarely hematuria and proteinuria reflecting glomerular involvement or cutaneous or systemic vasculitis are observed (Fig. 92–4). The polyarthritis is typically symmetric, involves chiefly the distal joints (e.g., the proximal interphalangeal joints and, to a lesser extent, the larger axial and appendicular joints), and usually subsides with the development of jaundice.

Icteric and Recovery Phases. Darkening of the urine to a brownish color and lightening of stool color are often observed for a few days before the appearance of jaundice. Anorexia, malaise, nausea, and vomiting transiently worsen with the development of jaundice, and pruritus may be noted. Mild weight loss may occur. Within a few days, as jaundice deepens, the constitutional symptoms become less severe, and gustatory and olfactory acuity returns with an improvement in appetite. Jaundice peaks and then disappears gradually, usually within a month or two after its onset.

Physical Findings

In the prodrome, the physical examination may be entirely normal or may reveal slight hepatomegaly or signs of joint or skin involvement. In the jaundiced patient, the liver may be moderately tender as well as mildly enlarged. The liver edge is usually rounded, and the spleen tip may be palpated in as many as 20% of patients. Posterior cervical lymphadenopathy is detected in a similar proportion. Small spider angiomas may be recognized. These findings disappear during the recovery phase.

Laboratory Studies

Blood Chemistries

Serum alanine aminotransferase and aspartate aminotransferase elevations are found in the late prodromal phase and

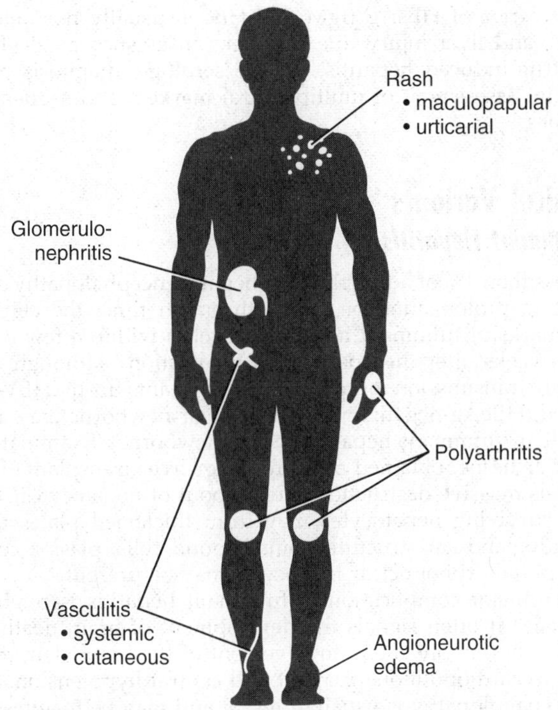

FIGURE 92–4 □ Extrahepatic manifestations of the HBV-associated, immune complex–mediated, serum sickness–like syndrome seen in the prodrome of acute hepatitis B. (Courtesy of the Clinical Teaching Project, American Gastroenterological Association.)

reach peak levels, usually 10 to 100 times the upper limits of normal, during the early icteric phase. Serum bilirubin levels peak 1 to 8 days after peak aminotransferase levels. In most icteric patients, maximal serum bilirubin levels are below 10 mg/dL. Higher levels suggest severe disease or a cholestatic element to the hepatitis. In the convalescent phase, both serum aminotransferase and bilirubin levels decline toward normal; minor elevations of the aminotransferases may persist for a few months even after serum bilirubin levels are normal. Typically, serum alkaline phosphatase levels are normal or only mildly elevated, and only minimal alterations in hepatic synthetic function (prothrombin time and serum albumin levels) are found.

Serologic Tests

Hepatitis B Surface Antigen. The first readily identifiable serologic marker of acute HBV infection is the HBsAg (Fig. 92–5). It appears before the development of elevated levels of alanine aminotransferase. In patients in whom the HBV-associated prodromal serum sickness–like syndrome is recognized, HBsAg may be the only marker present in serum samples. In most HBV-infected patients, HBsAg becomes serologically undetectable, by conventional polyclonal radioimmunoassay or enzyme-linked immunosorbent assay, within a few weeks to a few months after its appearance. In about 10% of patients, HBsAg has disappeared by the time symptoms develop. In contrast, persistence of HBsAg beyond 6 months suggests the development of the HBV carrier state. Pre-S proteins (pre-S1 and pre-S2) have been identified in the sera of HBV-infected patients during the period in which HBsAg is present and HBV replication is active. Pre-S2 protein disappears earlier than pre-S1 protein; both disappear while HBsAg is still present.[16] The corresponding anti–pre-S antibodies, immunoglobulin (Ig) M and IgG, develop shortly thereafter and may persist for some time or may disappear with the development of circulating anti-HBs.[17–19] Assays for pre-S proteins and antibodies are not commercially available.

Hepatitis B e Antigen. This derivative of the HBcAg is usually detected within a few days to a few weeks after the appearance of HBsAg in acute HBV infection. The HBcAg is not generally detected in serum. HBeAg is a marker of active HBV replication because its presence is correlated, imperfectly, with the presence of HBV particles and HBV DNA in serum. However, mutations in the precore (pre-C) region of HBV DNA result in HBV infections in which HBeAg is not produced but active viral replication may be present. In uncomplicated acute HBV infection, HBeAg disappears before HBsAg disappears. Shortly after the disappearance of HBeAg, its corresponding antibody, anti-HBe, becomes detectable. This marker may persist for prolonged periods.

Hepatitis B Virus DNA. Circulating HBV DNA can be detected during the early phase of acute HBV infection; during this period, it is the single best marker of active HBV replication. Several weeks later, it as well as HBeAg is generally undetectable when measured by slot blot hybridization techniques.[20] In most patients, HBeAg clearance occurs before clearance of HBV DNA.[21] However, in self-limited acute hepatitis B, HBV DNA may be detected by the more sensitive technique of polymerase chain reaction amplification in serum and peripheral blood mononuclear cells for as long as several years after clinical, biochemical, and apparent serologic remission.[22] The HBV DNA in mononuclear cells appears to be transcriptionally active. Whether persistent detection of HBV DNA indicates continuing replication in the liver remains uncertain, as does the potential infectivity of blood containing minute quantities of HBV DNA.

In contrast, the prolonged presence of HBV DNA, detected by the less sensitive hybridization techniques, usually indicates persistent infection with continuing viral replication and continued infectivity. Whereas HBV DNA has been identified in an extrachromosomal site in the hepatocytes of patients with active HBV replication, it seems likely that integration of HBV DNA into the DNA of the hepatocyte may occur randomly throughout the infectious process. The detection of HBV DNA in peripheral mononuclear cells of blood (i.e., T cells, B cells, monocytes), in bone marrow stem cells,[23] and in other extrahepatic tissues suggests that replication of HBV may not be limited to the liver.

Antibody to the Hepatitis B Core Antigen (Anti-HBc). Anti-HBc is detected shortly after HBsAg is detected and before the appearance of anti-HBs. Initially, the predominant immunoglobulin class of anti-HBc is IgM. Peak levels of IgM

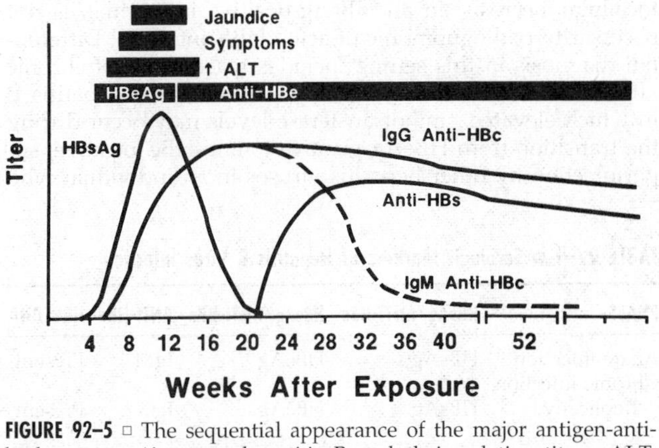

FIGURE 92–5 □ The sequential appearance of the major antigen-antibody systems in acute hepatitis B and their relative titers. ALT, Alanine aminotransferase. (From Koff RS: Acute and chronic hepatitis B. *In* Seeff LB, Lewis JH [eds]: Current Perspectives in Hepatology. New York, Plenum Publishing, 1989, pp 23–33.)

anti-HBc are reached within several weeks of the onset of infection; IgM anti-HBc persists considerably longer than HBsAg. A positive test response for IgM anti-HBc is the most sensitive test for the identification of acute HBV infection. IgM anti-HBc will be detected in the 10% of patients who have lost HBsAg by the time of first testing. After reaching peak levels, IgM anti-HBc diminishes in titer and disappears in most patients with acute HBV infection by 4 to 8 months after its appearance.[24] Test results for total anti-HBc remain positive nonetheless. The predominant form of anti-HBc found during late convalescence and thereafter for years to decades after acute HBV infection is IgG anti-HBc. Levels of anti-HBc decline slowly during a prolonged period.

Antibody to the Hepatitis B Surface Antigen (Anti-HBs). As the titer of HBsAg declines with time in acute HBV infection, anti-HBs, its corresponding antibody, becomes detectable and reaches peak levels within a few months. This antibody is believed to be the neutralizing, protective antibody. During the late convalescent phase of acute HBV infection, anti-HBs titers begin to decrease. The rate of decline is slow; anti-HBs remains detectable for many years to decades. In some patients, a distinct minority, anti-HBs may eventually become undetectable. In a small proportion of patients, anti-HBs is lost early or never becomes detectable.

Diagnosis

The diagnosis of HBV infection requires identification of serologic markers. Through use of these markers, it is possible to identify acute HBV infection, the replicative and nonreplicative phases of chronic HBV infection, and the recovery phase (Table 92–1).

Specific Serologic Diagnosis of Acute Hepatitis B

The serologic diagnosis of acute HBV infection is based on the presence of HBsAg and IgM anti-HBc. Although nearly all patients with acute infection are HBsAg-positive for some time, HBsAg will have disappeared by the time illness is recognized and serologic testing is undertaken in about 10%. Testing for IgM anti-HBc identifies all acutely infected patients, regardless of whether HBsAg is still present. HBeAg and HBV DNA are typically present during the acute phase of illness, but because their identification adds little useful information, they are not routinely measured.

Differential Diagnosis

Acute hepatitis, as defined by symptoms and signs and the presence of typical laboratory abnormalities indicating hepatocellular necrosis, in an HBsAg-positive individual, is not necessarily pathognomonic of acute HBV infection. Differential diagnosis in this setting includes reactivation of chronic HBV infection, a seroconversion flare in chronic hepatitis B in which elevated aminotransferase levels may occur during the transition from HBeAg-positive to anti-HBe–positive, superinfection by other hepatitis viruses in an individual who is a carrier of HBsAg (IgM anti-HBc is usually not detectable), and liver injury due to other causes such as alcohol- or drug-induced hepatitis. Precise serologic diagnosis may require assessment of multiple viral markers and sequential studies.

TABLE 92–1 ■ Serologic Markers of Hepatitis B Virus Infection

PHASE	HBsAg/ANTI-HBs	HBeAg/ANTI-HBe	ANTI-HBc	HBV DNA
Acute infection	HBsAg	HBeAg	IgM	Present
Chronic infection				
Replicative phase	HBsAg	HBeAg	IgG	Present
Nonreplicative phase	HBsAg	Anti-HBe	IgG	Absent
Recovery	Anti-HBs	Anti-HBe	IgG	Absent

Clinical Variants

Fulminant Hepatitis

In less than 1% of adult patients, hepatic encephalopathy and striking prolongation of the prothrombin time, the clinical hallmarks of fulminant hepatitis, develop within a few days to 8 weeks after the onset of HBV infection. Although unusual, transmission of pre-C HBV mutants from HBV-infected, HBeAg-negative mothers to their newborns may also result in fulminant hepatitis in the newborn.[25] Examination of liver tissue, obtained at necropsy or liver transplantation, reveals massive destruction and dropout of hepatocytes. The few surviving hepatocytes may form thickened plates and pseudoglandular structures. Small round cells, plasma cells, and polymorphonuclear leukocytes may be present.

The major complication of fulminant hepatitis is cerebral edema.[26] It often signals the development of brain death or brain stem involvement. Involvement of the brain stem may lead to cardiopulmonary arrest and central hypotension. Severe coagulopathy is usually present and may be manifested by gastrointestinal bleeding. Sepsis may be prominent; in some patients, severe, life-threatening hypoglycemia or insulin-resistant nonketotic hyperglycemia may dominate the clinical findings. In addition to hepatic failure, other organ systems eventually fail, reducing the likelihood of recovery. Fatality rates in patients with severe disease often exceed 75%. Emergency liver replacement for patients near death from fulminant hepatitis, by means of orthotopic liver transplantation, is associated with a survival rate of about 60%.[27]

Cholestatic Hepatitis

In rare patients with clinically mild acute HBV infection, jaundice is prolonged and total serum bilirubin levels may exceed 10 mg/dL. Pruritus and weight loss may be present, but these patients usually feel reasonably well. The disorder is so rare that one should strongly consider the coexistence of another disease (e.g., drug-induced cholestasis).

Relapsing Hepatitis

In exceedingly rare instances, patients who have recovered from HBV infection may once again develop symptoms and elevations in serum aminotransferase values. Other causes, including reactivation of chronic hepatitis B or HBeAg to anti-HBe seroconversion flares, should be considered because they are considerably more common. Whereas relapsing hepatitis may lead to prolonged illness, resolution may be anticipated if persistent infection does not supervene.

Chronic Hepatitis B Virus Infection

Chronic HBV infection is defined operationally as the persistence of HBsAg for at least 6 months. The highest risk for HBV persistence is found in neonates born to HBV carrier women who are HBeAg-positive and have high levels of HBV DNA.[8] Of these neonates, 80% to 90% progress to chronic infection.[28] In contrast, 30% of children infected before 6 years of age develop chronicity. Among adults infected by HBV, more than 95% recover completely. In about 1% to 5%, persistent infection may be associated with chronic hepatitis or an asymptomatic carrier state. In general, persistent infection occurs with a higher frequency in males than in females and among individuals with impaired immunity. Among adults with acute HBV infection, high serum levels of HBsAg, HBeAg, and HBV DNA during the first few weeks of infection appear to predict progression to chronic infection.[29]

Natural History

Asymptomatic Carriers. Persistently HBsAg-positive patients with normal serum aminotransferase levels, as well as other normal liver chemistries, are termed asymptomatic or healthy carriers. Most of these individuals are HBeAg-negative, and most have normal or minimally abnormal results of liver biopsy on initial evaluation. Follow-up studies, during a period of more than a decade, indicate that recurrent HBV replication, hepatitis D or C virus superinfection, and histologic progression are not seen in these carriers, even in those few patients who developed mild or transient serum aminotransferase elevations on sequential study.[30] A few patients with sustained serum aminotransferase elevations may experience HBV reactivation and histologic progression to chronic hepatitis. Although no carriers developed hepatocellular carcinoma during follow-up,[30] whether this will remain so on further follow-up remains uncertain. A few patients may spontaneously lose HBsAg positivity on follow-up. HBsAg clearance in asymptomatic HBsAg carriers appears to occur at an annual rate of about 0.8%. In contrast, HBsAg clearance in patients with chronic hepatitis B is slightly lower at a rate of about 0.5% annually.[31] The cumulative probability of clearing HBsAg is greater in asymptomatic carriers than in those with chronic hepatitis B.

Chronic Hepatitis B. The natural history of chronic hepatitis B is variable. There is a large body of data indicating that continuing viral replication is highly correlated with progression of disease and reduced life expectancy. It is estimated that approximately 10% of patients with chronic hepatitis B spontaneously cease to have detectable viral replication, as reflected in loss of HBeAg or HBV DNA, during the first year after identification and each year thereafter. Unless these patients experience relapse, hepatic inflammation and hepatocyte necrosis are diminished, and the likelihood of developing cirrhosis, liver failure, and premature death are reduced. Relapses, often called reactivation, are recognized by the reappearance of HBeAg or HBV DNA and occur in about 7% of those who have lost HBeAg in the first year and in about 3% per year thereafter. Among patients with chronic hepatitis B in whom viral replication continues, the annual probability of developing cirrhosis has been estimated to be 12%, and the annual probability that liver failure will ensue in those with cirrhosis is estimated to be close to 6%.[32]

The development of hepatocellular carcinoma, an extraordinarily prevalent malignant neoplasm in many parts of the world, has been etiologically linked with chronic HBV infection. In regions in which the HBV carrier state is high, hepatocellular carcinoma is a leading cause of cancer-related death. The precise oncogenic mechanism remains ill-defined.[33] Patients with chronic hepatitis B associated with cirrhosis have an annual incidence of hepatocellular carcinoma estimated to be close to 2.5%.[32] Hepatocellular carcinoma is also seen in some patients with chronic hepatitis B in the absence of cirrhosis. However, more than 90% of HBV-associated hepatocellular carcinoma occurs in individuals with cirrhosis.

The natural history of chronic hepatitis B associated with the pre-C HBV mutant remains incompletely understood. In individuals with chronic HBV infection in whom the pre-C mutant had emerged, either an asymptomatic carrier state with normal alanine aminotransferase levels or a more severe and progressive liver disease may be predominant.[34]

Pathology

Examination of liver biopsy specimens reveals portal and periportal inflammation with small round cells, hepatocyte degeneration and necrosis that may be confluent (bridging necrosis), and the formation of fibrous septa. The predominant inflammatory cell is the cytotoxic T lymphocyte; plasma cells are also present. The inflammatory infiltrate may spill over and erode the limiting plate of the portal triad, producing the lesion termed piecemeal necrosis. During active phases of disease and during relapses, lobular inflammation may be similar to that seen in acute hepatitis B, with scattered acidophilic bodies. In most patients with chronic hepatitis B, HBsAg may be demonstrated in hepatocyte cytoplasm with immunostaining or routine orcein staining. Occasional hepatocytes may have a ground-glass appearance.

Clinical Manifestations

Patients with chronic hepatitis B may be asymptomatic, may experience fatigue, or may have symptoms of end-stage liver disease. During active phases of the disease, malaise and weakness may be striking. Elevated serum aminotransferase levels are usually found; levels may be increased from 2- to 20-fold. In patients with elevated serum bilirubin levels, prolonged prothrombin times, and reduced serum albumin levels, severe disease should be anticipated. The development of edema, ascites, splenomegaly and hypersplenism, or esophageal varices strongly suggests the presence of cirrhosis and portal hypertension. In no more than 1% to 3% of patients with chronic hepatitis B, extrahepatic manifestations resembling the immune complex–mediated serum sickness–like syndrome seen in the prodrome of acute hepatitis B may be striking. These include cryoglobulinemia, arthritis, membranous or membranoproliferative glomerulonephritis, and generalized vasculitis.

Specific Serologic Diagnosis of Chronic Hepatitis B

HBsAg and anti-HBc (IgG) are present in nearly all patients with chronic hepatitis B (Fig. 92–6). HBeAg and HBV DNA are detected in those with active viral replication (see Table 92–1) with the notable exception that HBeAg may be absent in patients with the pre-C HBV variant. Surprisingly, a small proportion of patients may have low-titer, low-affinity heterotypic anti-HBs. In this circumstance, the presence of anti-HBs has no clinical importance. In patients in whom HBV

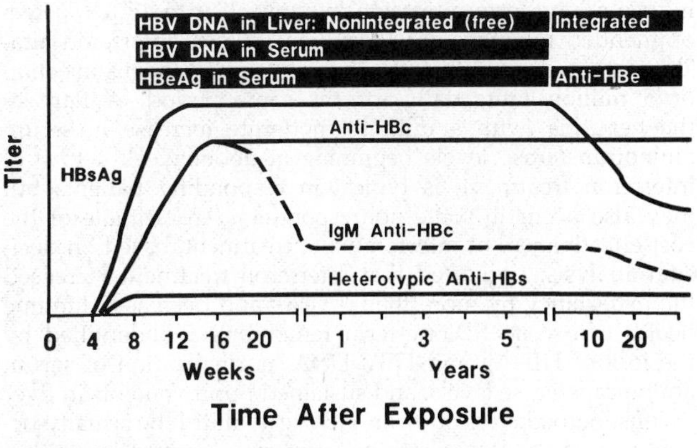

FIGURE 92–6 □ The sequential serologic appearance of the major antigen-antibody systems and HBV DNA (in serum and liver) in chronic hepatitis B. (From Koff RS: Acute and chronic hepatitis B. *In* Seeff LB, Lewis JH [eds]: Current Perspectives in Hepatology. New York, Plenum Publishing, 1989, pp 23–33.)

reactivation occurs, HBV DNA and HBeAg usually reappear in serum concurrently with elevation of serum aminotransferases.

Although distinctly uncommon, HBV DNA has been detected in asymptomatic healthy blood donors without conventional serologic markers of HBV infection or elevated serum alanine aminotransferase levels.[35] The natural history of these curious chronic HBV infections remains ill-defined. Similarly, HBV DNA has also been detected in as many as 3% of HBsAg-negative patients with presumed alcoholic liver disease.[36] Whether HBV exerts a synergistic or additive effect on the liver injury in this setting is uncertain.

Treatment

Acute Hepatitis B

Treatment of acute HBV infection is unsatisfactory. Only supportive and symptomatic measures are currently available. Physical activity restrictions are best determined by the patient and should be based on the patient's view of his or her sense of well-being. Dietary restrictions are usually unnecessary as long as a well-balanced diet can be consumed. Specific antiviral pharmacologic therapy is under development. Early treatment with interferon, with the goal of reducing the risk of progression to chronic HBV infection, is theoretically possible, but because 95% of adult infections are self-limited, this approach is impractical. Other potential approaches include the development of drugs that inhibit the attachment of HBV to target cells, prevent the uncoating of HBV, inhibit HBV DNA polymerase and reverse transcriptase activity, impair nucleocapsid production, and prevent the coating of the nucleocapsid with HBsAg. If successful, each of these approaches may lead to impaired synthesis of intact virions and may reduce the frequency of persistent infection. Corticosteroids should not be used, regardless of the severity of the clinical disease.

Asymptomatic Carriers

No effective treatment of asymptomatic, healthy HBsAg carriers is currently available. Treatment with interferon is not recommended. Repeated administration of HBV vaccine has no influence on the carrier state.

Chronic Hepatitis B

A large number of prospective, controlled studies have shown that treatment with interferon alfa of patients with chronic hepatitis B in whom HBV replication is active will induce a long-term remission in about 35% to 45%.[32, 37] Recommended regimens are 10 million units of interferon alfa-2b three times a week for 16 weeks by subcutaneous injection or 5 million units daily for the same period. A flare in the hepatitis, with a mild to moderate increase in serum aminotransferase levels beginning at about week 4 to 8 of interferon treatment, is typical in responding patients but may also occur in some nonresponders. An estimate of the cost-effectiveness of interferon alfa treatment, based on decision analysis, suggested that interferon treatment increased life expectancy by more than 3 years and decreased lifetime health care costs.[32] Long-term remissions are identified by the loss of HBeAg and HBV DNA, normalization of serum aminotransferase levels, and sustained improvements in liver lesions. Seroconversion from HBeAg to anti-HBe usually occurs during the last month of interferon treatment or within 3 months of treatment in chronic hepatitis B.[38] Interferon treatment may also induce remissions in patients with extrahepatic disorders (e.g., glomerulonephritis) associated with chronic HBV infection.

Among patients with chronic hepatitis B treated with interferon, missense mutations were significantly more common in the precore-core gene of nonresponders or relapsed patients than in long-term responders.[39] These observations suggest that responsiveness to interferon in chronic hepatitis B may be related to HBV genomic variability.

For patients nonresponsive to interferon, several drugs are currently under evaluation in the laboratory or in clinical trials. These include the nucleoside analogs lamivudine and famciclovir, foscarnet, thymosin, antisense oligonucleotides, ribozymes, triple-helix oligomers, and inhibitors of oligosaccharide trimming.[40–42] Unexpected and unacceptable toxic effects associated with the use of fialuridine, a nucleoside analog, ended clinical trials with this potent inhibitor of mitochondrial function.

In patients with advanced disease, in whom clinical evidence of decompensation is present (e.g., jaundice, ascites, encephalopathy, or previous esophageal variceal bleeding), treatment with interferon is less likely to be beneficial and may lead to severe acute flares of disease and life-threatening side effects.[43] Whether the drugs just described will prove effective in these patients is also uncertain.

End-Stage Chronic Hepatitis B with Cirrhosis

For patients with advanced, life-threatening disease, liver transplantation has had some success.[44] Enthusiasm for this approach has been dampened, however, by a high frequency of recurrent infection in the graft, largely attributed to the existence of extrahepatic reservoirs of infection in patients with active viral replication, that may lead to rapidly progressive disease, the need for retransplantation, and early demise. Studies suggest that this sequence can be interrupted by the administration of HBIG during the operative procedure and routinely thereafter.[45] Route of administration and dosing schedules are currently under study. The utility of other drugs (e.g., lamivudine) is also under study in the transplantation setting.

Hepatocellular Carcinoma

Management remains difficult because the prognosis is exceedingly poor in most patients. Although screening of patients with chronic hepatitis B and cirrhosis for hepatocellular carcinoma by serial measurement of serum α-fetoprotein and ultrasound examination of the liver has been advocated, the benefits of screening remain controversial, and many of the lesions detected have not been resectable.[46] Resection of small tumors is more effective than chemotherapy or radiotherapy, but multifocal lesions are not uncommon, and relatively few patients are cured by hepatic resection. Orthotopic liver transplantation for pretransplantation-identified or incidentally discovered large HBV-related hepatocellular carcinomas is associated with a poor outcome and cannot be recommended.[44] The role of percutaneous ethanol injection and chemoembolization in the treatment of unresectable disease remains under study.

Prevention

General Measures

Limiting the exchange of secretions occurring during sexual activity and practicing "safe" sex as well as avoiding percutaneous exposures are desirable goals for the prevention of HBV transmission. Unfortunately, educational resources and efforts in this direction are limited, and modification of such behaviors in many individuals is exceedingly difficult. Even if behavior can be changed, a reduction in HBV transmission cannot be guaranteed because in as many as 25% to 30% of patients with acute HBV infection, the specific route of infection and likely source remain uncertain. The key to control of HBV infection is immunoprophylaxis.

Immunization

Anti-HBs is the protective, neutralizing antibody responsible for immunity to HBV infection. Passive immunization, the administration of exogenous, preformed anti-HBs in the form of HBIG prepared from donors who have recovered from HBV infection, is rarely used alone. Active immunization, through the use of HBV vaccine, and combined active-passive immunization (HBV vaccine and HBIG) are the preferred approaches. HBsAg is the active immunogenic material in the yeast-recombinant HBV vaccines (Recombivax HB and Engerix-B) commercially available in the United States. These vaccines contain HBsAg particles but lack HBV DNA, HBcAg, HBeAg, or pre-S sequences. They are safe, immunogenic, effective, and expensive. Although the vaccines are rendered impotent by freezing, heating for 1 week at 45°C or for 1 month at 37°C has not affected immunogenicity.[47] Plasma-derived HBV vaccines, also containing HBsAg particles, are relatively inexpensive, compose 80% of total world HBV vaccine production, and are widely used abroad. They are no longer available in the United States.

The immune response to active immunization by vaccination is limited to anti-HBs alone; the response to natural infection with HBV involves induction of both anti-HBc and anti-HBs[48] (Fig. 92–7). Titers of anti-HBs after vaccination are usually lower than those found after natural infection. Breakthrough infections in vaccinated individuals can be attributed to hyporesponsiveness or nonresponsiveness to HBV vaccine (see later) or, rarely, to infection by the HBV escape mutant in which the "a" determinant of HBsAg cannot be neutralized by vaccine-induced anti-HBs.[49] The HBV vaccine–induced escape mutant has been identified in Italy, Singapore, Japan, Africa, and infrequently in the United States.

Anti-HBs titers after vaccination diminish with time. Whereas anti-HBs levels also fall after natural infection, the duration of protection is lifelong in nearly all instances of natural infection. The duration of protection after vaccine-induced immunity remains uncertain (see later). A specific, critical threshold value of anti-HBs above which immunity is solid and below which immunity is uncertain has yet to be unequivocally established. Nonetheless, a threshold level of greater than 10 mIU/mL has been considered indicative of seroprotection. The duration of anti-HBs persistence is highly correlated with the peak titer after the third or fourth dose.[50]

Although the available recombinant, yeast-derived vaccines contain different amounts of HBsAg protein, postvaccination anti-HBs levels in young, healthy recipients are probably similar, and it is assumed that they offer similar early protective efficacy. Whether long-term protection will differ remains to be established. Even at 10 years after initial vaccination, when the titer of anti-HBs may have fallen below 10 mIU/mL in as many as 40% or is undetectable, continued protection against clinical hepatitis and persistent HBV infection has been demonstrated.[51] The timing of and necessity for booster doses more than 10 years after successful vaccination remain uncertain. However, boosters are recommended in immunosuppressed populations such as patients undergoing maintenance hemodialysis if, on annual testing, anti-HBs levels fall below 10 mIU/mL.

The major host factors affecting vaccine immunogenicity are age and immunocompetency. Smoking and obesity may also be linked to a diminished responsiveness.[52] Neonates and children respond superbly, with the development of anti-HBs in more than 95% of vaccinees. Adults older than 40 years respond less well.[53] In older individuals and in immunosuppressed populations, there may be some advantage in using Engerix-B, the recombinant product with higher concentrations of HBsAg protein.[54] Severely immunosuppressed individuals may not respond to HBV vaccination and are unlikely to respond after a second vaccination series.

Route, Dose, and Vaccine Schedule. HBV vaccines are given intramuscularly into the deltoid muscle in children and adults and into the anterolateral muscle of the thigh in infants in a three-dose schedule (0, 1, and 6 months) or a four-dose schedule (0, 1, 2, and 12 months). Other schedules (e.g., first dose at 2 months of age, second at 4 months, and third at 12 months) may also be used in infants. Anti-HBs levels peak at 1 to 3 months after the third dose. In adults, the conventional dose (given three times in the standard schedule) is 10 or 20 μg of HBsAg protein. Infants may be vaccinated with lower doses. Because the long-term efficacy of low-dose, intradermal regimens remains to be established, they are not recommended. Accelerated dose schedules in which the interval between vaccine doses is shortened may provide more rapid induction of protective levels, but long-term protection with such schedules has not yet been studied.

Adverse Effects of Immunization. The major side effect of HBIG and HBV vaccine is transient pain at the injection site. Neither human immunodeficiency virus nor HBV and other hepatitis viruses have been transmitted by HBIG and HBV vaccines prepared in the United States.

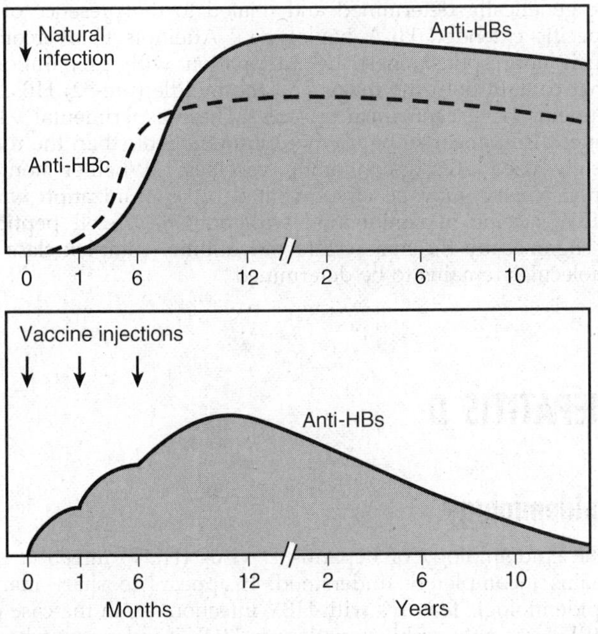

FIGURE 92–7 □ The immune response to natural infection with HBV *(top)* involves induction of both anti-HBc and high-titer anti-HBs. In contrast, the response to HBV vaccine *(bottom)* is limited to anti-HBs.

Candidates for Immunoprophylaxis

Preexposure Prophylaxis. Shortly after the introduction of HBV vaccines, only high-risk groups were targeted for immunization. That policy had no impact on the overall infection rate. The current strategy for HBV control in the United States is screening of pregnant women for HBsAg and administration of HBIG and HBV vaccine to their neonates, combined with universal vaccination of all other infants, "catch-up" vaccination of preteenagers or early adolescents, and continuing vaccination of high-risk populations. The cost-effectiveness of these recommendations has been studied by use of the tools of decision analysis.[55] Universal infant immunization was first recommended in late 1991 in the United States, and vaccination of preteenagers was recommended in 1995. Because catch-up HBV vaccination of older children and adolescents is unlikely to occur through typical health care visits, which are infrequent in this age group, other settings may be required to deliver vaccine. School-based HBV vaccination programs in San Francisco, Baton Rouge, and Oregon have completed the three-dose vaccine program in 65% to 78% of targeted school populations.[56] School-based programs, in Framingham and Natick, Massachusetts, have delivered three doses of vaccine to 98% of eligible 10- and 11-year-old children.

Universal infant immunization programs had been initiated in more than 75 countries by the end of 1996, and many other countries are attempting to develop programs. Effective control in many parts of the developing world has been hindered by imperfect existing immunization infrastructure and the absence of funding for new vaccination programs.

Preexposure prophylaxis with the HBV vaccine is recommended for individuals in high-risk categories, for example, household contacts of HBsAg-positive individuals; homosexual or bisexual men; individuals with a history of episodes of sexually transmitted diseases; health care workers regularly exposed to blood or blood-contaminated secretions (such as surgeons and pathologists; medical technicians and blood bank technologists; dialysis staff; operating room, intensive care, and emergency room nurses; and dentists and dental professionals); first responders (e.g., police, firefighters); parenteral drug users; workers and residents in institutions for the mentally retarded; recurrent recipients of high-risk blood products; and inmates of prisons in which parenteral drug use or homosexual behavior may continue. Immunization at an early age, for example, for health care students and other trainees, is more likely to be effective than later immunization.[57]

Travelers to HBV endemic regions who are likely to require medical assistance or in whom intimate contact with the local population is anticipated are also candidates for preexposure vaccination. Other high-risk groups appropriately considered for universal immunization include Alaskan Natives and Pacific Islanders. Refugees or adopted children from countries at high risk for HBV infection (Southeast Asia, sub-Saharan Africa, eastern Europe, and the former Soviet Union) should probably be screened for HBV infection; if the carrier state or chronic hepatitis B is identified, susceptible household contacts should be vaccinated.

Postexposure Prophylaxis. For susceptible health care workers who have not been vaccinated but are inadvertently exposed to HBV through needlesticks, lacerations, or splashing accidents, combined passive-active immunization with HBIG and HBV vaccine has been recommended. HBIG is given intramuscularly in a dose of 0.06 mL/kg body weight as early as possible after exposure, and the first of three doses of HBV vaccine is given at another site in the deltoid muscle at the same time or within several days. The second and third vaccine doses are given 1 and 6 months later. Earlier administration of the second and third vaccine doses, in an accelerated schedule, with or without prior HBIG is under study.

Sexual contacts of patients with acute HBV infection should receive a single dose of 0.06 mL of HBIG per kilogram of body weight within 14 days of exposure; there is no current evidence that vaccination of contacts of acutely infected individuals is necessary. However, for susceptible male homosexuals or promiscuous heterosexuals, HBV vaccine should be initiated at the same time.

HBV vaccine alone has been recommended for susceptible intimate and household contacts of index cases with chronic HBV infection. Immunoprophylaxis is not recommended for the casual contacts of HBsAg-positive persons, whether they are acutely or chronically infected.

Prevention of maternal-neonatal transmission of HBV requires screening of all pregnant women to determine carrier status. For neonates of HBsAg-positive women, a dose of 0.5 mL of HBIG should be given within a few hours of birth into the anterolateral muscle of the thigh of the neonate; HBV vaccine is given in the contralateral thigh within a week of birth and repeated at 1 and 6 months. Some data suggest that an accelerated vaccine schedule using higher vaccine dosages without HBIG may be as effective as combined passive-active immunization.[58] The protective efficacy of the combined program approaches 90% to 95%.[58] Immunized infants should be tested for HBV markers at about 12 months of age. The presence of HBsAg indicates treatment failure; the presence of both anti-HBs and anti-HBc suggests that infection occurred but was modified by immunoprophylaxis; the presence of anti-HBs alone suggests vaccine-induced immunity. A number of studies suggest that immunity has persisted for at least 8 to 12 years after vaccination of infants and that boosters are not needed during this period.[59, 60]

Remaining Issues

New HBV vaccines are on the drawing boards. Combination vaccines incorporating HBV vaccine with other pediatric vaccines into one formulation are likely to become available in the near future. Another approach to immunization, currently under study in the laboratory, is the direct injection of HBV DNA encoding HBsAg into muscle tissue. This gene transfer approach has led to the production of anti-HBs in inoculated animals.[61] Incorporation of the variant antigens of the escape HBV mutant into the next generation of vaccine may be necessary if the prevalence of the escape mutant, now rare, increases.

A small number of otherwise healthy, immunocompetent individuals may be hyporesponsive (anti-HBs levels of less than 10 mIU/mL) after three doses of the current HBV vaccines. An additional two or three doses may produce somewhat more vigorous responses in about half.[62] In contrast, an even smaller number of patients appear to be absolutely nonresponsive. Nonresponsiveness in this setting appears to be genetically determined and related to the presence of a specific extended HLA haplotype.[63] Attempts to overcome such nonresponsiveness by vaccination with preparations that contain both the major and the middle (pre-S2) HBsAg proteins have been unsuccessful.[64] These experimental vaccines also appear to be no more immunogenic than the routinely used HBsAg-containing vaccines.[53] Whether nonresponsiveness may be circumvented by immunization with HBV vaccine in conjunction with a helper T-cell peptide recognized by the major histocompatibility complex class II molecules remains to be determined.[65]

HEPATITIS D

Epidemiology

The epidemiology of hepatitis D virus (HDV) infection remains incompletely understood. It appears to share many epidemiologic features with HBV infection. As in the case of HBV, large geographic variations in HDV infection rates have been identified. Somewhat surprisingly, given the close biologic interrelationship of HDV with HBV, the prevalence of

HDV infection among HBV-infected patients with chronic liver disease is highly variable. In some areas, such as Southeast Asia, HDV infections are uncommon; in others, such as the Amazon region of South America, HDV infection appears to by hyperendemic. Among the 300 million worldwide HBsAg carriers, it is estimated that as many as 15 million (5%) are infected by HDV.[66]

Incubation Period

The incubation period of HDV infection appears to have a range of a few weeks to several weeks or months, based on limited observations in transfusion-associated cases and experimental transmission studies in chimpanzees.[67, 68] The length of the incubation period, measured from HDV exposure to the development of serum alanine aminotransferase elevations, was related to the size of the HDV inoculum in infected chimpanzees; it varied from 24 days when an undiluted inoculum was given to 51 days in the animal given the highest dilution inoculum.

Epidemiologic Patterns

Modes of transmission are similar to those associated with HBV infection. HDV infections can be either acute or persistent. Persistent HDV infections may induce chronic liver disease and are believed to facilitate the spread of HDV among individuals infected by HBV. HDV may spread rapidly in susceptible populations and may spill over into other populations within communities. HDV infection has been identified in nearly all parts of the world, but prevalence rates vary widely. Two different epidemiologic patterns are recognized: one that appears to be endemic, and the other nonendemic.[69] The endemic pattern has been seen in the countries of the Mediterranean littoral, in the Balkans, in European regions of the former Soviet Union, in parts of Africa and the Middle East, and in the Amazon basin of South America. Outbreaks in these areas may result from the introduction of HDV-infected individuals into susceptible (HBV carrier) populations. HDV is spread in endemic regions chiefly by person-to-person direct contact between HDV-infected individuals and HBV carriers; intrafamilial and sexual routes of spread are common.

HDV infection is infrequent in the general population of nonendemic regions such as North America and northern Europe. In these areas, HDV infections occur with moderate frequency in HBsAg-positive persons at risk for percutaneous exposure (i.e., injecting drug users and hemophiliacs). Outbreaks of HDV infection have been noted in such individuals and in their intimate contacts. A high prevalence of HDV infections has been identified in prisoners. In this case, HDV infection is assumed to result from the increased frequency of injecting drug use among those incarcerated. These data suggest that in nonendemic regions, HDV infection is largely confined to that narrow segment of the population who are exposed by direct percutaneous inoculation.

Modes of Transmission

HDV is a blood-borne pathogen. Few studies have evaluated the presence of HDV or HDV RNA in body fluids other than blood. Percutaneous spread, as among injecting drug users, is clearly a major mode of transmission. Posttransfusion acquisition of HDV infection has also been recognized, particularly among hemophiliac patients who have received large quantities of clotting factors. In one study of American patients with hemophilia A, 75% had a serologic marker of previous HBV infection, and 13% of these had antibodies to HDV.[70] Other modes of transmission include person-to-person contact spread through intimate or inapparent transmission through open skin lesions or spread through household contamination. These observations suggest that HDV may be present in the same body fluids as HBV is. Contact transmission of HDV is believed to involve the same mechanisms as in contact transmission of HBV but is likely to be far less efficient. Promiscuous sexual behavior remains a major risk factor for acquisition of HDV among HBV carriers. For example, among HBsAg-positive prostitutes, HDV infection rates are considerably higher than those seen in the general population of HBsAg-positive individuals. HDV infection rates in homosexual or bisexual men have been independently associated with injecting drug use, the number of sexual partners, and rectal trauma. Maternal-neonatal spread may also occur, but its epidemiologic importance seems minor. Persistence of active HDV and HBV infections provides a reservoir of HDV and HBV carriers who may serve as sources of infection in some populations.

Immunopathogenesis and Pathology

The immunopathogenesis of HDV infection is poorly understood. The relative contributions of a direct cytopathic effect versus an immunologic mechanism remain to be determined. Morphologic features suggestive of a direct cytopathic effect on the hepatocyte include the presence of microvesicular steatosis, vacuolization, and focal necrosis, with a paucity of parenchymal mononuclear inflammatory cells.[71] However, studies of transgenic mice in which both HDV antigen isoforms are expressed revealed no evidence of hepatocyte injury.[72] These observations suggest that HDV gene products are not directly cytopathic. No relationship between the severity of the initial lesions of acute hepatitis D and the development of HDV-associated chronic hepatitis has been recognized. In contrast, a significant positive relationship was observed between the expression of HDV antigens and the presence of inflammation in the liver in chronic hepatitis D, suggesting the importance of immune mechanisms in perpetuating injury. Furthermore, in the patient with HDV and HBV infection in whom liver transplantation is undertaken, HDV can be demonstrated immunohistochemically within 1 week in the transplanted graft, but hepatocellular injury is delayed until HBV reinfection ensues, usually more than 3 months after transplantation.[73] These observations support the notion that HDV requires HBV for its pathogenicity. The nature of the mechanisms responsible for the induction of hepatocyte injury requires further investigation.

Serologic Diagnosis

Serologic diagnosis of HDV infection should be sought only in patients shown to be HBsAg-positive or in those in whom HBsAg-negative acute hepatitis B is recognized by demonstration of IgM anti-HBc and in whom coinfection with HDV is considered. In all other settings, HDV infection in persons who are HBsAg-negative must be exceedingly rare. Whereas immunohistochemical demonstration of intrahepatic HDV antigen appears to be a sensitive marker of active HDV infection, this approach is impractical because it requires liver biopsy. Detection of HDV RNA in serum by polymerase chain reaction also appears to be highly sensitive and specific for ongoing viral replication in chronic hepatitis D,[74] but approved assays are not yet available.

Coinfection

A variety of serologic responses indicative of HDV infection have been identified in patients with acute, self-limited HDV coinfection with HBV (Fig. 92–8). Circulating HDV antigen and serum HDV RNA (detected by dot blot analysis or polymerase chain reaction) appear during the late incubation period and early acute phase of illness concurrently with the detection of HBsAg but are present transiently.[75] Commercial assays for HDV antigen are not yet approved for use in the United States. Research radioimmunoassays and enzyme-linked immunosorbent assays indicate that HDV antigen disappears early from serum, before or concurrently with the clearance of HBsAg and coincident with the development of the corresponding antibodies to HDV antigen (anti-HDV). Although viremia is usually short-lived, HDV RNA may persist in some instances for prolonged periods even when HDV antigen and anti-HDV are undetectable.[76] Unfortunately, assays for serum HDV antigen and HDV RNA remain research tools, not widely available. As a consequence, antibody markers of HDV infection are the principal widely available tools used for serologic diagnosis.

Seroconversion to IgM anti-HDV, as determined by either radioimmunoassay or enzyme-linked immunosorbent assay, usually occurs within several days to a few weeks after the onset of illness. IgM anti-HDV is seldom detectable for longer than 2 to 8 weeks. It is usually followed by IgG anti-HDV, which may also disappear in a number of weeks, or it may persist for as long as 6 months in low titers or occasionally for as long as 1 to 2 years.[77, 78] One or more of these markers may be absent in a typical case of acute HDV infection or, curiously, may appear during the convalescent phase.

Hepatitis D Virus Superinfection

In HDV superinfection of HBsAg-positive HBV carriers, HDV antigen and HDV RNA are detectable in serum and HDV antigen is identifiable in the liver.[79, 80] Simultaneously, a reduction in HBV replication and a consequent decrease in the titer of circulating HBsAg may ensue. Rarely, this HDV inhibition of HBV replication results in the termination of the HBsAg carrier state. As shown in Figure 92–9, IgM anti-HDV appears during the superinfection and may be followed or accompanied by the brisk and *sustained* production of IgG anti-HDV in high titers. In a large proportion of superinfected patients, HDV infection becomes persistent, and HDV antigen and HDV RNA may remain detectable in serum; large quantities of HDV antigen can also be detected in hepatocytes by immunofluorescent techniques. High titers of IgG anti-HDV, variable titers of IgM anti-HDV, and serum HDV RNA positivity by polymerase chain reaction are maintained in persistent HDV infection.

Clinical Spectrum

In HDV and HBV coinfections, the acute illness resembles uncomplicated hepatitis B in the majority of instances (Fig. 92–10). In a small proportion, less than 15%, the disease may be severe, as reflected by the development of a prolonged prothrombin time or hepatic encephalopathy, and fatalities may occur in a few cases as a consequence of fulminant disease with massive hepatic necrosis. In some outbreaks, a striking frequency of fatal disease may be seen. For example, in a major outbreak of virulent HDV infection in the city of Worcester, Massachusetts, among injecting drug users, in which serologic analysis revealed that most cases represented coinfection with both HBV and HDV, a case-fatality rate of 8% was observed.[81] Because most HBV infections acquired as an adult are short-lived, and because HDV infection cannot persist after recovery from HBV, the majority of coinfections are self-limited and chronic HDV infection is distinctly uncommon.

In HDV superinfection of HBV carriers (see Fig. 92–10), the acute disease is more likely to be severe, and chronic, progressive hepatitis is more frequent than in HDV and HBV coinfections. Furthermore, cirrhosis or hepatic failure is a common sequela of chronic hepatitis D because of persistent HDV infection.[82] In a prospective study of Yucpa Indian HBV carriers in Venezuela in whom the consequences of HDV

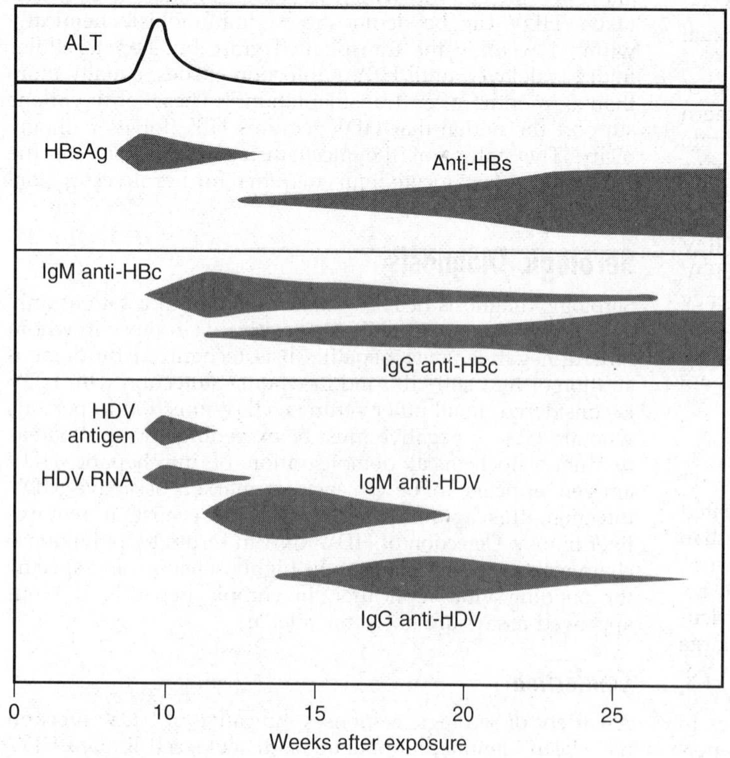

FIGURE 92–8 ▫ Schematic illustration of the sequence of biochemical and serologic events seen in self-limited HDV and HBV coinfection. ALT, Alanine aminotransferase.

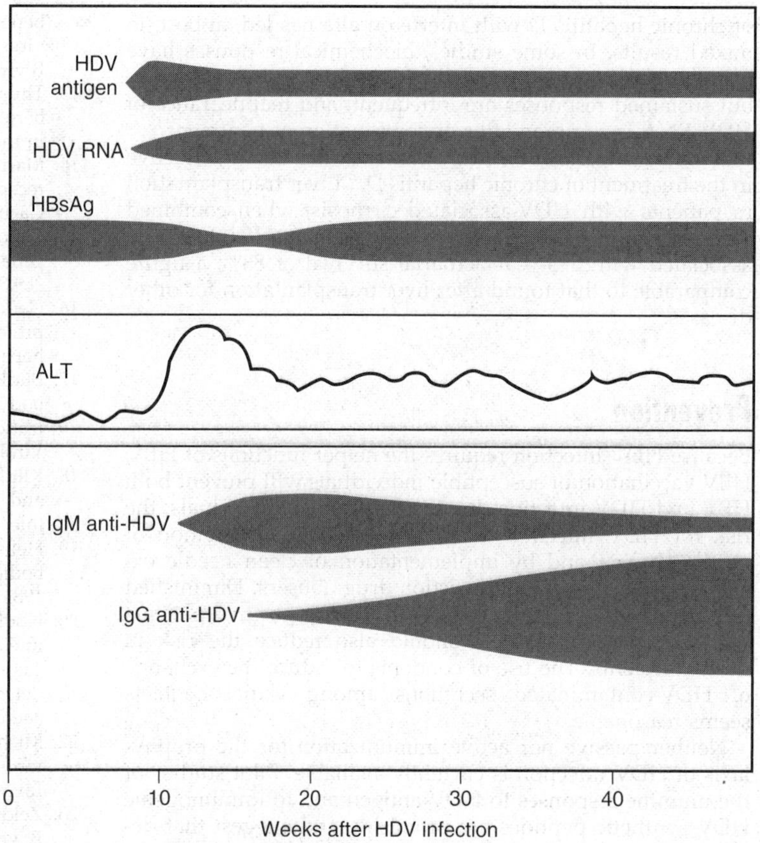

FIGURE 92–9 ▫ Schematic illustration of the sequence of serological and biochemical events in HDV superinfection of HBV carriers. ALT, Alanine aminotransferase.

superinfection were evaluated, more than half of HDV-infected persons had moderate to severe chronic liver disease compared with none of the non–HDV-infected individuals.[82] Mortality rates in HDV-infected individuals varied from 7% to 9% per year; most deaths were due to rapidly progressive chronic liver disease or the development of fulminant hepatitis.

The risk for progression from chronic hepatitis D to cirrhosis appears to be greater than for patients with chronic hepatitis B alone, and the rate of progression may be striking. In one study, progression to cirrhosis was observed in more than 50% of patients with chronic hepatitis D after a little more than 2 years of follow-up.[83] The role of HDV superinfection in the development of hepatocellular carcinoma in HBsAg-positive patients is still uncertain. Although a direct role remains to be established, the expression of the c-*myc* protooncogene in the hepatocyte nuclei of patients with chronic hepatitis D has been reported,[84] and there is support for the notion that HDV infection enhances the risk for malignant transformation in the younger patient.

The preceding notwithstanding, the morbidity and mortality associated with HDV infection may have been overestimated in early studies of the natural history of HDV infection. Increasingly, as more data are collected, evidence of less severe infections has accumulated, indicating that the spectrum of disease severity associated with HDV is considerably broader than initially believed and that HDV infections may not invariably be highly pathogenic.

Treatment

No specific therapy has yet been shown to alter the natural history of either acute or chronic HDV infections. Treatment

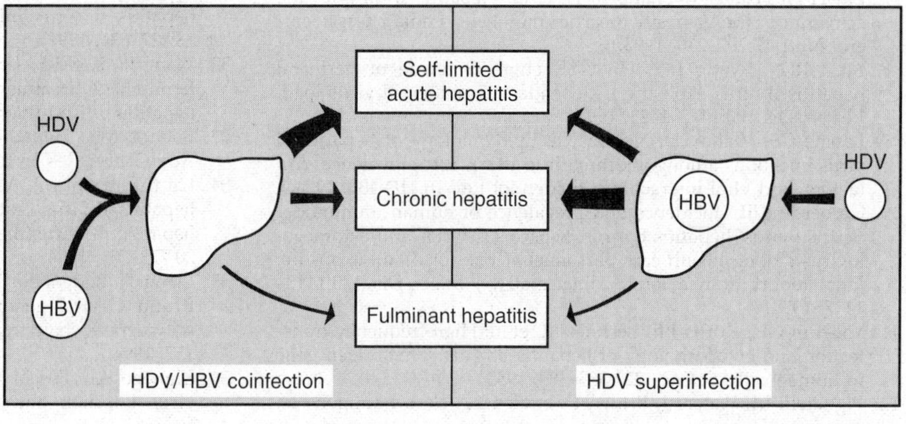

FIGURE 92–10 ▫ Schematic illustration of the sequelae of HDV and HBV coinfection *(left)* and HDV superinfection of HBV carriers *(right)*.

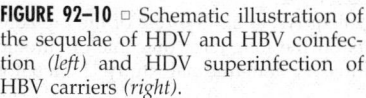

of chronic hepatitis D with interferon alfa has led, at best, to mixed results. In some studies, biochemical responses have been observed in those treated with high doses of interferon, but sustained responses are infrequent, and reappearance of HDV RNA is common after discontinuation of treatment.[85, 86] In a small, uncontrolled study, ribavirin has been ineffective in the treatment of chronic hepatitis D.[87] Liver transplantation in patients with HDV-associated cirrhosis, when combined with long-term passive administration of anti-HBs, has been associated with a 5-year actuarial survival of 88%, a figure comparable to that found after liver transplantation for other diseases.[88]

Prevention

Because HDV infection requires the helper functions of HBV, HBV vaccination of susceptible individuals will prevent both HBV and HDV infection. In HBsAg-positive individuals, the risk for HDV infection may be reduced by prohibition of needle sharing and by implementation of clean needle exchange programs among injection drug abusers. Diminished use of untreated blood products in HBsAg-positive patients with hemostatic disorders should also reduce the risk in these recipients. The use of condoms to reduce the exchange of HDV-contaminated secretions among sexual contacts seems reasonable.

Neither passive nor active immunization for the prophylaxis of HDV infection is currently available. Pilot studies of the immune responses to HDV antigen and to immunogenic HDV synthetic peptides are promising and suggest that development of an effective vaccine is a feasible goal.[89]

References

1. Margolis HS, Alter MJ, Hadler SC: Hepatitis B: Evolving epidemiology and implications for control. Semin Liver Dis 11:84–92, 1991.
2. Kumar A, Kulkarni R, Murray DL, et al: Serologic markers of viral hepatitis A, B, C, and D in patients with hemophilia. J Med Virol 41:205–209, 1993.
3. McQuillan G, Alter MJ, Everhart JE: Viral hepatitis. *In* Everhart JE (ed): Digestive Diseases in the United States. Washington, DC, US Government Printing Office, 1994, pp 127–156. NIH publication 94-1447.
4. Van Damme P, Cramm M, Van der Auwera J-C, et al: Horizontal transmission of hepatitis B virus. Lancet 345:27–29, 1995.
5. Whittle HC, Maine N, Pilkington J, et al: Long-term efficacy of continuing hepatitis B vaccination in infancy in two Gambian villages. Lancet 345:1089–1092, 1995.
6. Stevens CE, Toy PT, Tong MJ, et al: Perinatal hepatitis B virus transmission in the United States. Prevention by passive-active immunization. JAMA 253:1740–1745, 1985.
7. Lin H-H, Hsu H-Y, Chang M-H, et al: Hepatitis B virus in the colostra of HBeAg-positive carrier mothers. J Pediatr Gastroenterol Nutr 17:207–210, 1993.
8. Burk RD, Hwang L-Y, Ho GYF, et al: Outcome of perinatal hepatitis B virus exposure is dependent on maternal virus load. J Infect Dis 170:1418–1423, 1994.
9. Levine OS, Vlahov D, Nelson KE: Epidemiology of hepatitis B virus infections among injecting drug users: Seroprevalence, risk factors, and viral interactions. Epidemiol Rev 16:418–436, 1994.
10. Gerberding JL: Incidence and prevalence of human immunodeficiency virus, hepatitis B virus, hepatitis C virus, and cytomegalovirus among health care personnel at risk for blood exposure: Final report from a longitudinal study. J Infect Dis 170:1410–1417, 1994.
11. Yoakum GH, Korba BE, Lechner JR, et al: High-frequency transfection and cytopathology of hepatitis B virus core antigen gene in human cells. Science 222:385–389, 1983.
12. Pignatelli M, Waters J, Brown D, et al: HLA class I antigens on hepatocyte membrane during recovery from acute hepatitis B virus infection and during interferon therapy in chronic hepatitis B virus infection. Hepatology 6:349–353, 1986.
13. Thursz MR, Kwiatkowski D, Allsopp CEM, et al: Association between an MHC class II allele and clearance of hepatitis B virus in the Gambia. N Engl J Med 332:1065–1069, 1995.
14. Marinos G, Naoumov NV, Rossol S, et al: Tumor necrosis factor receptors in patients with chronic hepatitis B virus infection. Gastroenterology 108:1453–1463, 1995.
15. Zheng Y-W, Yen TSB: Negative regulation of hepatitis B virus gene expression and replication by oxidant stress. J Biol Chem 269:8857–8862, 1994.
16. Gerken G, Manns M, Gerlich WH, et al: Pre-S encoded surface proteins in relation to the major viral surface antigen in acute hepatitis B virus infection. Gastroenterology 92:1864–1868, 1987.
17. Budkowska A, Riottot M-M, Dubreuil P, et al: Monoclonal antibody recognizing pre-S(2) epitope of hepatitis B virus: Characterization of pre-S(2) epitope and anti–pre-S(2) antibody. J Med Virol 20:111–125, 1986.
18. Klinkert M-Q, Theilmann L, Pfaff E, Schaller H: Pre-S1 antigens and antibodies early in the course of acute hepatitis B virus infection. J Virol 58:522–525, 1986.
19. Hellstrom U, Sylvan S, Kuhns M, et al: Absence of pre-S2 antibodies in natural hepatitis B virus infection. Lancet 2:889–893, 1986.
20. Hoofnagle JH, Schafer DF: Serologic markers of hepatitis B virus infection. Semin Liver Dis 6:1–10, 1986.
21. Tassopoulos NC, Kuhns MC, Koutelou MG, et al: Quantitative detection of hepatitis B virus DNA in sera from patients with acute hepatitis B. Dig Dis Sci 38:2156–2162, 1993.
22. Michalak TI, Pasquinelli C, Guilhot S, Chisari FV: Hepatitis B virus persistence after recovery from acute viral hepatitis. J Clin Invest 93:230–239, 1994.
23. Zeldis JB, Mugishima H, Steinberg HN, et al: In vitro hepatitis B virus infection of human bone marrow cells. J Clin Invest 78:411–417, 1986.
24. Chernesky M, Mahony J, Castriciano S, et al: Diagnostic significance of anti-HBc IgM prevalence related to symptoms in Canadian patients acutely or chronically infected with hepatitis B virus. J Med Virol 20:269–277, 1986.
25. Hawkins AE, Gilson RJC, Beath SV, et al: Novel application of a point mutation assay: Evidence for transmission of hepatitis B viruses with precore mutations and their detection in infants with fulminant hepatitis B. J Med Virol 44:13–21, 1994.
26. Fingerote RJ, Bain VG: Fulminant hepatic failure. Am J Gastroenterol 88:1000–1010, 1993.
27. Wall WJ, Adams PC: Liver transplantation for fulminant hepatic failure: North American experience. Liver Transplant Surg 1:178–182, 1995.
28. Hyams KC: Risks of chronicity following acute hepatitis B virus infection: A review. Clin Infect Dis 20:992–1000, 1995.
29. Fong T-L, Di Bisceglie AM, Biswas R, et al: High levels of viral replication during acute hepatitis B infection predict progression to chronicity. J Med Virol 43:155–158, 1994.
30. de Franchis R, Meucci G, Vecchi M, et al: The natural history of asymptomatic hepatitis B surface antigen carriers. Ann Intern Med 118:191–194, 1993.
31. Liaw Y-F, Sheen I-S, Chen T-J, et al: Incidence, determinants and significance of delayed clearance of serum HBsAg in chronic hepatitis B virus infection: A prospective study. Hepatology 13:627–631, 1991.
32. Wong JB, Koff RS, Tine F, Panker SG: Cost-effectiveness of interferon-alfa 2b treatment for hepatitis B e antigen–positive chronic hepatitis B. Ann Intern Med 122:664–675, 1995.
33. Buenda MA: Hepatitis B viruses and hepatocellular carcinoma. Adv Cancer Res 59:167–226, 1992.
34. Lai ME, Solinas A, Mazzoleni AP, et al: The role of the pre-core hepatitis B virus mutants on the long-term outcome of chronic hepatitis B virus hepatitis. A longitudinal study. J Hepatol 20:773–781, 1994.
35. Liang TJ, Bodenheimer HC, Yankee R, et al: Presence of hepatitis B and C viral genomes in US blood donors as detected by polymerase chain reaction amplification. J Med Virol 42:151–157, 1994.
36. Zignego AL, Foschi M, Laffi G, et al: "Inapparent" hepatitis B virus infection and hepatitis C virus replication in alcoholic

subjects with and without liver disease. Hepatology 19:577–582, 1994.
37. Wong DKH, Cheung AM, O'Rourke K, et al: Effect of alpha-interferon treatment in patients with hepatitis B e antigen–positive chronic hepatitis B. Ann Intern Med 119:312–323, 1993.
38. Perrillo R, Mimms L, Schechtman K, et al: Monitoring of antiviral therapy with quantitative evaluation of HBeAg: A comparison with HBV DNA testing. Hepatology 18:1306–1312, 1993.
39. Naoumov NV, Thomas MG, Mason AL, et al: Genomic variations in the hepatitis B core gene: A possible factor influencing response to interferon alfa treatment. Gastroenterology 108:505–514, 1995.
40. Schalm SW, de Man RA, Heijtink RA, et al: New nucleoside analogues for chronic hepatitis B. J Hepatol 22(Suppl 1):52–56, 1995.
41. Block TM, Lu X, Platt FM, et al: Secretion of human hepatitis B virus is inhibited by the imino sugar *N*-butyldeoxynojirimycin. Proc Natl Acad Sci USA 91:2235–2239, 1994.
42. Offensperger W-B, Blum HE, Gerok W: Molecular therapeutic strategies in hepatitis B virus infection. Clin Invest 72:737–741, 1994.
43. Hoofnagle JH, Di Bisceglie, Waggoner JG, Park Y: Interferon alfa for patients with clinically apparent cirrhosis due to chronic hepatitis B. Gastroenterology 104:1116–1121, 1993.
44. Eason JD, Freeman RB Jr, Rohrer RJ, et al: Should liver transplantation be performed for patients with hepatitis B? Transplantation 57:1588–1593, 1994.
45. Samuel D, Muller R, Alexander G, et al: Liver transplantation in European patients with the hepatitis B surface antigen. N Engl J Med 329:1842–1847, 1993.
46. Colombo M, De Franchis R, Del Ninno E, et al: Hepatocellular carcinoma in Italian patients with cirrhosis. N Engl J Med 325:675–680, 1991.
47. Van Damme P, Cramm M, Safary A, et al: Heat stability of a recombinant DNA hepatitis B vaccine. Vaccine 10:366–367, 1992.
48. Stevens CE, Taylor PE: Hepatitis B vaccine: Issues, recommendations, and new developments. Semin Liver Dis 6:23–27, 1986.
49. Fortuin M, Karthigesu V, Allison L, et al: Breakthrough infections and identification of a viral variant in Gambian children immunized with hepatitis B vaccine. J Infect Dis 169:1374–1376, 1994.
50. Gesemann M, Scheiermann N: Quantification of hepatitis B vaccine–induced antibodies as a predictor of anti-HBs persistence. Vaccine 13:443–447, 1995.
51. Hadler SC, Francis DP, Maynard JE, et al: Long-term immunogenicity and efficacy of hepatitis B vaccine in homosexual men. N Engl J Med 315:209–214, 1986.
52. Winter AP, Follett AC, McIntyre J, et al: Influence of smoking on immunological responses to hepatitis B vaccine. Vaccine 12:771–772, 1994.
53. Clements ML, Miskovsky E, Davidson M, et al: Effect of age on the immunogenicity of yeast recombinant hepatitis B vaccines containing surface antigen (S) or preS2+S antigens. J Infect Dis 170:510–516, 1994.
54. Treadwell TL, Keeffe EB, Lake J, et al: Immunogenicity of two recombinant hepatitis B vaccines in older individuals. Am J Med 95:584–588, 1993.
55. Bloom BS, Hillman AL, Fendrick M, Schwartz JS: A reappraisal of hepatitis B virus vaccination strategies using cost-effectiveness analysis. Ann Intern Med 118:298–306, 1993.
56. Centers for Disease Control and Prevention: Hepatitis B vaccination of adolescents—California, Louisiana, and Oregon, 1992–1994. MMWR Morbid Mortal Wkly Rep 43:605–609, 1994.
57. Margolis HS, Presson AC: Host factors related to poor immunogenicity of hepatitis B vaccine in adults. Another reason to immunize early. JAMA 270:2971–2972, 1993.
58. Andre FE, Zuckerman AJ: Review: Protective efficacy of hepatitis B vaccines in neonates. J Med Virol 44:144–151, 1994.
59. Coursaget P, Leboulleux D, Soumare M, et al: Twelve-year follow-up study of hepatitis B immunization of Senegalese infants. J Hepatol 21:250–254, 1994.
60. Marion SA, Pastore MT, Pi DW, Mathias RG: Long-term follow-up of hepatitis B vaccine in infants of carrier mothers. Am J Epidemiol 140:734–746, 1994.
61. Davis HL, Michel M-L, Mancini M, et al: Direct gene transfer in skeletal muscle: Plasmid DNA-based immunization against the hepatitis B virus surface antigen. Vaccine 12:1503–1509, 1994.
62. Stuve J, Aronsson B, Frenning B, et al: Seroconversion after additional vaccine doses to non-responders to three doses of intradermally or intramuscularly administered recombinant hepatitis B vaccine. Scand J Infect Dis 26:468–470, 1994.
63. Alper CA, Kruskall MS, Marcus-Bagley BS, et al: Genetic prediction of nonresponse to hepatitis B vaccine. N Engl J Med 321:708–712, 1989.
64. Pillot J, Poynard T, Elias A, et al: Weak immunogenicity of the preS2 sequence and lack of circumventing effect on the unresponsiveness to the hepatitis B virus vaccine. Vaccine 13:289–294, 1995.
65. Hervas-Stubbs S, Berasain C, Golvano JJ, et al: Overcoming class II–linked non-responsiveness to hepatitis B vaccine. Vaccine 12:867–871, 1994.
66. Rizzetto M, Ponzetto A, Forzani I: Epidemiology of hepatitis delta virus: Overview. Prog Clin Biol Res 364:1–20, 1991.
67. Rizzetto M, Canese MG, Gerin JL, et al: Transmission of the hepatitis B virus–associated delta antigen to chimpanzees. J Infect Dis 141:590–602, 1980.
68. Ponzetto A, Hoyer BH, Popper H, et al: Titration of the infectivity of hepatitis D virus in chimpanzees. J Infect Dis 155:72–78, 1987.
69. Polish LB, Gallagher M, Fields HA, Hadler SC: Delta hepatitis: Molecular biology and clinical and epidemiological features. Clin Microbiol Rev 6:211–229, 1993.
70. Kumar A, Kulkarni R, Murray DL, et al: Serologic markers of viral hepatitis A, B, C, and D in patients with hemophilia. J Med Virol 41:205–209, 1993.
71. Lefkowitch JH, Goldstein H, Yatto R, et al: Cytopathic liver injury in acute delta virus hepatitis. Gastroenterology 92:1262–1266, 1987.
72. Guilhot S, Huang S-N, Xia YP, et al: Expression of the hepatitis delta virus large and small antigens in transgenic mice. J Virol 68:1052–1058, 1994.
73. Davies S, Lau JY, O'Grady JG, et al: Evidence that hepatitis D virus needs hepatitis B virus to cause hepatocellular damage. Am J Clin Pathol 98:554–558, 1992.
74. Simpson LH, Battegay M, Hoofnagle JH, et al: Hepatitis delta virus RNA in serum of patients with chronic delta hepatitis. Dig Dis Sci 39:2650–2655, 1994.
75. Gupta S, Govindarajan S, Cassidy WM, et al: Acute delta hepatitis: Serological diagnosis with particular reference to hepatitis delta virus RNA. Am J Gastroenterol 86:1227–1231, 1991.
76. Negro F, Bergmann KF, Baroudy BM, et al: Chronic hepatitis D virus (HDV) infection in hepatitis B virus carrier chimpanzees experimentally superinfected with HDV. J Infect Dis 158:151–159, 1988.
77. Hoofnagle JH: Type D (delta) hepatitis. JAMA 261:1321–1325, 1989.
78. Shattock AG, Morris M, Kinane K, et al: The serology of delta hepatitis and the detection of IgM anti-HD by EIA using serum derived delta antigen. J Virol Methods 23:233–240, 1989.
79. Buti M, Esteban R, Jardi R, et al: Chronic delta hepatitis: Detection of hepatitis delta virus antigen in serum by immunoblot and correlation with other markers of delta viral replication. Hepatology 10:907–910, 1989.
80. Govindarajan S, Gupta S, Valinluck B, et al: Correlation of IgM anti–hepatitis D virus (HDV) to HDV RNA in sera of chronic HDV. Hepatology 10:34–35, 1989.
81. Lettau LA, McCarthy JG, Smith MH, et al: Outbreak of severe hepatitis due to delta and hepatitis B viruses in parenteral drug abusers and their contacts. N Engl J Med 317:1256–1262, 1987.
82. Hadler SC, de Monzon MA, Rivero D, et al: Epidemiology and long-term consequences of hepatitis delta virus infection in the Yucpa Indians of Venezuela. Am J Epidemiol 136:1507–1516, 1992.
83. Buti M, Mas A, Sanchez-Tapias JM, et al: Chronic hepatitis D in intravenous drug addicts and non-addicts. A comparative clinico-pathological study. J Hepatol 7:169–174, 1988.
84. Tappero G, Natoli G, Anfossi G, et al: C-myc expression in cells infected with hepatitis delta virus. *In* Hadziyannis SJ, Taylor JM, Bonino F (eds): Hepatitis Delta Virus. Molecular Biology, Pathogenesis, and Clinical Aspects. New York, Wiley-Liss, 1993, pp 175–179.
85. Farci P, Mandas A, Coiana A, et al: Treatment of chronic hepatitis D with interferon alfa-2a. N Engl J Med 330:88–94, 1994.
86. Rosina F, Cozzolongo R: Interferon in HDV infection. Antiviral Res 24:165–174, 1994.

87. Garripoli A, Di Marco V, Cozzolongo R, et al: Ribavirin treatment for chronic hepatitis D: A pilot study. Liver 14:154–157, 1994.
88. Samuel D, Zignego A-L, Reynes M, et al: Long-term clinical and virological outcome after liver transplantation for cirrhosis caused by chronic delta hepatitis. Hepatology 21:333–339, 1995.
89. Gerin JL, Casey JL, Bergmann KF: The molecular biology of hepatitis delta virus: Recent advances. *In* Nishioka K, Suzuki H, Mishiro S, Oda T (eds): Viral Hepatitis and Liver Disease. Tokyo, Springer-Verlag, 1994, pp 38–41.

93

Hepatitis C

Raymond S. Koff

Epidemiology

Incubation Period

The incubation period of hepatitis C varies widely between 2 and 20 weeks, with a mean of about 7 to 10 weeks.[1] Short incubation periods, of less than 4 weeks, have occasionally been reported in recipients of contaminated factor VIII concentrates and in nosocomial outbreaks, but serologic confirmation of hepatitis C virus (HCV) infection was not available at the time. Viremia occurs during the incubation period and may precede the initial serum alanine aminotransferase (ALT) elevation by at least 12 days in experimentally infected chimpanzees.[2] HCV RNA has been detected in a serum sample 2 weeks after transfusion in a patient who developed antibodies to HCV (anti-HCV) at the 16th week.[3]

Epidemiologic Patterns

HCV infections are widely distributed throughout the world; most are chronic.[4] In fact, it is currently believed that no more than 15% to 20% of acutely infected patients recover completely, losing HCV RNA, normalizing serum ALT levels, and eventually losing anti-HCV.[5] As shown in Table 93–1, high seroprevalence rates of HCV infection have been reported from geographically diverse regions; infection rates approach 15% in some areas, whereas infection rates in neighboring areas are no higher than 1% to 2%. Although not completely understood, high rates may be a consequence of iatrogenic transmission through the reuse of contaminated needles, syringes, or other instruments used purposefully for scarification or non–health care–related tissue penetrations.[6] Although genotypes 1a and 1b are the predominant HCV infections in the United States, genotype patterns vary widely, as shown in Figure 93–1.

Hepatitis C appears to account for about 15% of the acute viral hepatitis reported in the United States during the past decade. Most acute HCV infections occur in young adults, although all age groups are affected. The Centers for Disease Control and Prevention has estimated that an average of 150,000 HCV infections occurred annually in the United States during the 1980s. However, on the basis of data from the Centers for Disease Control and Prevention's four-sentinel county study and adjustments for underreporting, a decline of more than 75% in HCV incidence has occurred since 1989. This decline is thought to reflect a decrease in blood-borne transmission[7]—injection drug use– and transfusion-associated hepatitis C. Despite the decline, studies suggest the presence of a large reservoir of HCV infection in the United States. Currently, about 1.8% of the population, or roughly 4 million individuals, have evidence of past or present HCV infection based on detection of anti-HCV. Seroprevalence rates are higher in black than in white persons and peak in the 30- to 39-year-old age group. HCV-infected individuals constitute a large potential reservoir of infection, and many have chronic liver disease. It is estimated that as many as 8000 to 10,000 deaths annually can be attributed to chronic hepatitis C.

Modes of Transmission

Percutaneous Transmission. As soon as serologic testing for HCV infection became available, it was recognized that hepatitis C was the major complication of transfusion of blood and blood products. Approximately 90% of cases could be attributed to HCV.[8] By the mid-1990s, as a consequence of changes in the donor population resulting from self-exclusion of individuals with risk factors for human immunodeficiency virus (HIV) infection, from the introduction of surrogate testing of blood donors (serum ALT and anti–hepatitis B core antigen), and from markedly improved anti-HCV screening techniques (second-generation assays), transfusion-associated HCV infection became a rarity with no more than one case per 3000 to 6000 transfused units. However, the potential infectivity of blood products was highlighted by the occurrence of an outbreak of acute HCV infection between October 1993 and June 1994 among recipients of a commercial intravenous immune globulin product subsequently removed from the worldwide market.[9] Although intramuscular immune globulin products prepared in the United States may contain HCV RNA, these have a remarkable historical record of safety.[10] The precise mechanism responsible for the failure of these products to transmit HCV remains uncertain.

Organ transplantation from anti-HCV–positive donors has been another recognized mode of transmission and has been shown to increase the risk for development of liver disease in recipients.[11] However, short-term follow-up studies of infected recipients failed to reveal an adverse influence on survival of either the graft or the patient. Screening of donors

TABLE 93–1 ■ Global Endemicity Rates of Hepatitis C Virus Based on Anti-HCV Seroprevalence Data (First- or Second-Generation Assays) from the General Population or Blood Donors in Selected Countries

ENDEMICITY PATTERN	COUNTRY	SEROPREVALENCE (%)
Low endemicity (0%–2.5%)	Hong Kong	0.5
	Sweden	0.7
	Australia	0.8
	South Africa	0.9
	United States	1.8
	Ethiopia	2.0
	Taiwan	2.5
Moderate endemicity (>2.5%–5%)	Yemen	2.6
	South Sudan	3
	Peru	3
	Japan	4
	Senegal/Tunisia/Burundi	4
	Kiribati	5
High endemicity (>5%)	Philippines	5
	Zaire	6
	Libya	8
	Egypt	14
	Cameroon	15

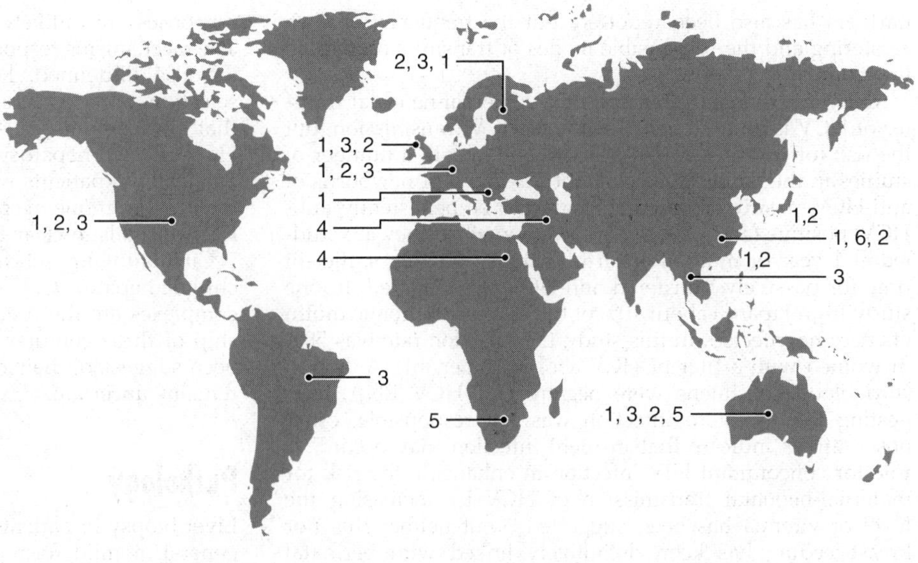

FIGURE 93–1 □ Global distribution of HCV genotypes in blood donors. Order reflects decreasing prevalence of genotype. (Adapted from van der Poel CL, Cuypers HT, Reesink HW: Hepatitis C virus six years on. Lancet 344[8935]:1475–1479, 1994. © by The Lancet Ltd. 1994.)

for anti-HCV has become standard practice and should reduce the risk for infection. Transplantation of HCV-positive organs into HCV-positive recipients is undertaken in some transplantation centers.[12]

Hepatitis C was also commonly identified in injecting drug users who shared injection equipment. Risk factors associated with acquisition of HCV infection have been identified in the Centers for Disease Control and Prevention's four–sentinel county study (Table 93–2). By 1992, more than one third of reported cases could be linked with blood-borne transmission; just below 30% of acute HCV infections were associated with injection drug use, and 6% were associated with blood transfusion, hemodialysis, or health care employment.[7] Recognized or inapparent percutaneous inoculations, through needlestick accidents or contamination of minor lacerations or other breaks in the integrity of the skin, appear to be responsible for occupationally acquired HCV infections among health care workers. A limited number of studies indicate that the infection rate after accidental needlesticks with HCV-contaminated equipment among health care workers varies between 6% and 10%. However, in studies of health care personnel at risk for blood exposure, the seroprevalence of HCV was similar to that reported in the general population or in blood donors,[13, 14] and incidence density rate, expressed as new infections per 100 person-years, was relatively low at 0.08.[13] In contrast, as a consequence of blood transfusion and possibly nosocomial spread by dialysis machines and intraunit spread, as many as 10% to 45% of hemodialysis patients are HCV infected.

Acupuncture performed without sterilization between patients and the use of nonsterilized needles, syringes, and knives by practitioners of folk medicine may be responsible for some episodes of community-acquired HCV infection.[15]

TABLE 93–2 ■ Risk Factors Associated with Hepatitis C Virus Infection in the Centers for Disease Control and Prevention's Four–Sentinel County Study (1992)

RISK FACTOR	%
Injection drug use	29
Heterosexual activity	8
Household contact	4
Transfusion	4
Health care employment	2
Low socioeconomic status or high-risk behavior or contacts*	45
Unknown	8

*Behavior or contacts more than 6 mo before onset of illness.

Contact Transmission. Person-to-person spread seems likely to be responsible for the transmission of HCV from acutely or chronically infected individuals to their intimate, sexual contacts, but the frequency of contact transmission remains controversial. The risk for transmission is thought to be correlated with the frequency of sexual exposure and duration of exposure. As might be anticipated, anti-HCV prevalence rates in female prostitutes are increased and may vary between 1% and 12%; anti-HCV positivity has also been found in nearly 10% of sexually active homosexual men,[16] although reported seroprevalence rates have varied widely between 0% and 50%.[17] Injection drug use by homosexual men has been found to confound the association with HCV infection in some studies; however, even after controlling for percutaneous exposures, the number of lifetime sexual partners and the number of oral- or anal-receptive partners were weakly associated with HCV seroprevalence.[17] In the Centers for Disease Control and Prevention's four–sentinel county study (see Table 93–2), about 12% of identified cases could be linked with either heterosexual activity or household contact, which included exposure to a sexual partner or a household member with hepatitis or exposure to multiple sexual partners. In my experience, about 10% of cohabitating sexual partners of anti-HCV–positive patients are found to be anti-HCV–positive, excluding those partners with other risk factors for infection, and seroconversions have been identified on follow-up in a small number of susceptible spouses. In other studies in the United States, about 5% of the sexual partners of HCV-infected individuals are found to be anti-HCV–positive. However, sexual transmission of HCV from women infected in the 1970s with contaminated anti–D immunoglobulin has not been documented; none of their husbands developed markers of HCV infection.[18] In contrast, in one study from Japan,[19] 27% of spouses of patients with chronic hepatitis C were found to be anti-HCV–positive, and HCV RNA was detected in 16%. In that study, HCV infection rates in spouses increased with duration of cohabitation; rates were 9% if they were married less than 30 years, and 24% if they were married more than 30 years. Although the precise mechanisms remain unknown, HCV transmission from men to women seems to be more efficient than transmission from women to men.[20] Intrafamilial clustering of HCV infection among household members other than sexual partners has also been reported, but the frequency of such clustering and the responsible modes of transmission remain uncertain.[21]

Maternal-Neonatal Transmission. Maternal-neonatal transfer of HCV is an established mode of HCV transmission, but the risk for transmission appears to be low.[18] In a number of studies in the United States, about 3% to 5% of newborns of anti-HCV–positive women are found to be persistently anti-HCV–positive (and HCV RNA–positive) when they are studied at 1 year or more after birth, thereby allowing sufficient time for passively transfered anti-HCV to be cleared. In one study from Japan,[22] about 10% of the infants of viremic mothers became infected. In this study, the infection rate was 50% in women with a titer of HCV above 10^6 per mL. Although cord blood specimens were negative for HCV RNA, suggesting that in utero infection was not responsible, other observations indicate that in utero infection may occur.[23] A role for concomitant HIV infection in enhancing the risk for maternal-neonatal transmission of HCV by increasing the level of viremia has been suggested,[24] but neither this nor breast-feeding has been definitively linked with perinatal transmission.[25]

Unestablished Routes of Spread. Although a variable proportion of HCV-infected patients do not admit to a specific risk factor associated with transmission, a large number of such individuals come from low socioeconomic levels. Others admit to high-risk behaviors, but not in the 6 months preceding the onset of illness (see Table 93–2). There are no data supporting respiratory or airborne transmission of HCV. Similarly, food-borne spread and water-borne spread are unlikely modes of transmission. The role of arthropod vectors in transmission is unknown. HCV RNA has been detected in cell-free samples of tears and aqueous humor of patients with anti-HCV.[26] Whether tears or corneal transplants can transmit infection remains uncertain.

Pathogenesis

The pathogenesis of liver disease in HCV infection remains somewhat obscure. HCV antigens, including core, envelope, NS3, NS4, and NS5, have been demonstrated by in situ hybridization or through immunohistochemical staining in hepatocytes and occasional bile duct epithelium,[27] but not in hepatocyte nuclei, in Kupffer or sinusoidal lining cells, or in blood vessels.[28] HCV is not believed to be directly cytopathic. However, at high levels of viremia (e.g., in the immunosuppressed transplant recipient), a direct cytopathic effect is possible but not proved. The occurrence of persistent viremia in the absence of liver disease in some patients with HCV infection suggests that there may be nonvirulent strains, immunologic tolerance to HCV, or extrahepatic replication. The precise mechanisms remain to be defined. Both $CD4^+$ and $CD8^+$ cells have been identified in the livers of infected individuals with chronic hepatitis C; it seems likely that damage to the hepatocyte is mediated by cellular mechanisms. The $CD4^+$ cell response is probably directed against all of the putative HCV antigens. The $CD8^+$ cytotoxic response also appears to be polyclonal; epitopes on the HCV antigens are recognized by $CD8^+$ cells in peripheral blood and within the liver.[29] However, although immunostaining has identified fairly homogeneously distributed HCV core antigen within hepatocyte cytoplasm, its expression does not correspond to either hepatocellular necrosis or lymphocytic inflammation.[30] These observations suggest that the HCV core antigen is not a major target of the immune response. The nature of the critical target antigens remains ill-defined.

The occurrence of severe chronic hepatitis C in patients with agammaglobulinemia indicates that humoral immune responses are unlikely to be responsible for hepatic injury.[9] The mechanisms responsible for persistence of HCV infection are also ill-defined. Persistence may be a consequence of selection of virus strains that produce inhibitory peptides that interfere with cell-mediated mechanisms for eliminating HCV-infected hepatocytes. Proof of this hypothesis is not yet available. In patients with chronic hepatitis C, it seems likely that the immune response maintains inflammation in the liver but fails to clear HCV.

Circulating immune complexes are present in patients with chronic hepatitis C. Conglutinin-binding circulating immune complexes are the predominant form.[31] Although a relationship of these complexes with more severe liver disease has been suggested, their role in the pathogenesis of liver injury remains uncertain.

Pathology

Liver biopsy in patients with acute HCV infection reveals, in general, a mild form of hepatitis with portal lymphocytic inflammation, parenchymal inflammation, and focal hepatocyte necrosis in the form of ballooning or acidophilic bodies.

Histopathologic analysis of liver specimens from patients with chronic hepatitis C has revealed four histologic lesions useful in distinguishing hepatitis C from B: bile duct damage; lymphoid follicles or aggregates, occasionally with germinal centers; large-droplet fat; and periportal Mallory body–like material.[32] Bile duct injury includes cytoplasmic swelling, vacuolation, acidophilia, nuclear pleomorphism, and loss of nuclear polarity without loss of ducts.[33] Although unusual, multiple granulomata and multinucleated giant cells may be found in about 10% of livers obtained from patients undergoing transplantation for chronic hepatitis C with cirrhosis.[34] Progression of chronic hepatitis C to cirrhosis may be seen in as few as 2% to as many as 20% of patients after 20 years of infection, and an important proportion of patients with cirrhosis may later develop hepatocellular carcinoma (HCC) (see later). In retrospective studies, the mean period from onset of infection (1) to diagnosis of chronic hepatitis C has been about 10 years; (2) to diagnosis of cirrhosis, about 20 years; and (3) to development and diagnosis of HCC, about 30 years. These intervals are shorter, 6, 10, and 15 years, respectively, in patients who acquire infection after age 50 years.[35]

The detection of markers of HCV infection in as many as one quarter to one third of patients with alcoholic liver disease has suggested a role for both HCV and alcohol in the pathogenesis of liver disease in these patients.[36] The mechanism responsible for this apparently synergistic effect remains to be defined. Similarly, the finding of a high prevalence of anti-HCV and the detection of HCV RNA in serum and liver in patients with porphyria cutanea tarda suggest an important role for HCV in the liver injury observed in affected patients.[37]

Concurrent hepatitis B virus, hepatitis D virus, and HIV infections are not uncommon among HCV-infected individuals, particularly in those who have acquired HCV through injecting drug use or receipt of multiple blood products (e.g., hemophilic patients). The spectrum of hepatitis severity in affected patients is broad; in some but not all studies, enhanced morbidity and excessive mortality have been found in patients with concurrent HCV and HIV infections. Further study is required to define the clinical impact of these coinfections, the mechanism of altered pathogenicity, and the response to therapy. Similarly, the natural history of dual infection by HCV and hepatitis B virus remains poorly understood. Alternating dominance in replication, presumably due to in vivo interference between the two agents, has been reported,[38] but its impact on disease progression or severity is uncertain.

Clinical Manifestations

Clinical Features

Many infections are presumed to be inapparent or subclinical. Symptomatic hepatitis is found in a minority of cases, and jaundice is seen in less than one quarter of symptomatic patients. Prodromal features may be absent or so abbreviated that they fail to be recognized or may last as long as 2 weeks. A prodrome with a serum sickness–like syndrome, arthralgias, and pruritic or nonpruritic papular or papulovesicular eruptions on the trunk or anterior surfaces of the arms has been described but is rare. Fever is uncommon, and hepatomegaly is present in less than one third of patients.

Cryoglobulinemia may be present in one third to one half of patients with chronic hepatitis C,[39] and HCV RNA has been detected by polymerase chain reaction (PCR) both in serum and in the isolated cryoglobulins of affected patients. However, only 1% to 2% of patients with HCV-associated cryoglobulinemia have symptomatic disease manifested as purpura, vasculitis, or peripheral neuropathy. Membranoproliferative glomerulonephritis, usually linked with HCV-associated cryoglobulinemia, is also unusual; glomerular deposition of immune complexes of HCV and anti-HCV appears responsible.[40] HCV antigens have also been identified in normal-appearing blood vessels in anti-HCV–positive, HCV RNA–positive patients with mixed cryoglobulinemia.[41] This observation suggests that deposition of HCV antigens precedes vascular damage.

Blood Chemistries

Peak serum levels of the aminotransferases tend to be lower than in hepatitis A or B virus infections, but there is considerable overlap when groups of patients are compared. Nonetheless, serum ALT levels infrequently exceed 2000 IU/mL and are less than 800 IU in about 50% of patients.[42] Episodic fluctuations in the serum levels of ALT and aspartate aminotransferase are a frequent but not invariable feature of acute or chronic hepatitis C. This biphasic or multiphasic pattern is thought to reflect recurrent waves of hepatocyte necrosis, presumably a consequence of complex alterations in the interaction of the immune system with HCV-infected hepatocytes and the possible emergence of HCV neutralization escape mutants. Hematologic studies are usually unremarkable during the course of uncomplicated acute hepatitis C; rarely, aplastic anemia has been seen in the convalescent phase of clinically recognized infection. Autoimmune serologic markers (e.g., rheumatoid factor, antinuclear and anti–smooth muscle antibodies) are common in chronic hepatitis C[39] and may also be present in acute HCV infection.

Extrahepatic Diseases

In addition to HCV-associated mixed cryoglobulinemia and its associated complications, a number of extrahepatic disorders have been linked with chronic HCV infection. These include sialadenitis, resembling Sjögren syndrome; membranoproliferative glomerulonephritis; non-Hodgkin's lymphoma; lichen planus; and Mooren corneal ulcer, an extremely rare form of chronic ulcerative keratitis.[36]

Serologic Studies and Diagnosis

Acute Hepatitis C

The first identifiable marker of acute HCV infection is the appearance in serum of HCV RNA, which may be detected by PCR amplification within a few weeks of exposure[3] (Fig. 93–2). However, PCR amplification to detect HCV RNA remains an expensive investigational tool, and although commercial assays are available for HCV RNA detection, none has received approval from the U.S. Food and Drug Administration. In addition to PCR assays, a less sensitive branched DNA signal amplification assay has been widely used to quantitate HCV RNA levels.[43] Serologic diagnosis of acute HCV infection rests on the detection of antibodies to recombinant HCV antigens. These antigens have included C22-3 from the core region, C33c from NS3, C100-3 and 5-1-1 from NS4, and NS5 from the NS5 region.[44] The first-generation immunoassays, measuring antibody to the C100-3 nonstructural antigen of HCV, were imperfect, in part because antibodies developed slowly and in part because of false-positive reactions. False-positive test results were commonly found in low-prevalence populations such as blood donors, although this did not negate the value of the assay in preventing transfusion-associated hepatitis C.[45] Second- and third-generation enzyme immunoassays and recombinant immunoblot assays that employ multiple antigens from both structural and nonstructural regions of the HCV genome have increased sensitivity and specificity. As shown in Figure 93–2, antibodies to C22-3 and C33c may be the first anti-HCV antibodies to appear in HCV infection. Anti-NS5 appears somewhat later; anti–C100-3 appears to be the last antibody to be detected in acute, self-limited infection.

Antibodies to HCV antigens may be detected in more than 60% of patients during the acute phase of illness; seroconversion occurs weeks to months later in another 35%. In perhaps 5% of infected patients, current assays for anti-HCV may remain persistently negative, although the presence of circulating HCV RNA indicates the presence of infection. Although HIV infection has been associated with an impaired anti-HCV response,[46] HIV infection probably accounts for only a small proportion of HCV-infected individuals without anti-HCV. Attempts to develop an assay for immunoglobulin antibodies to the HCV envelope proteins appear promising; prototype assays have been studied, but only few data are available. Third-generation immunoassays, with increased sensitivity, are widely used; these may further shorten the

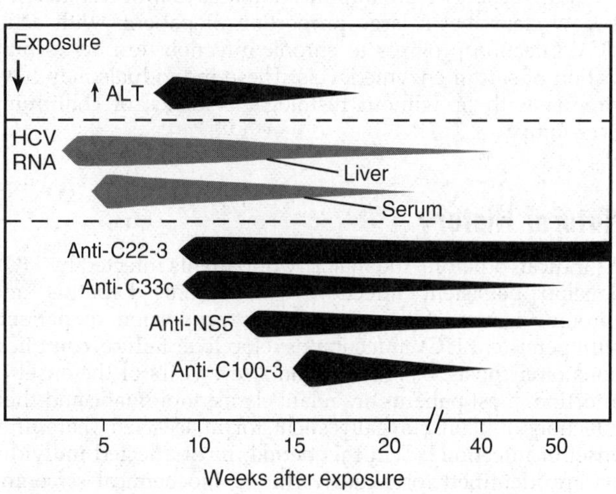

FIGURE 93–2 □ Sequence of serum alanine aminotransferase (ALT) elevation and appearance and clearance of serologic markers of HCV infection in self-limited acute hepatitis C.

window for the development of anti-HCV in acute hepatitis C. Antibodies to the E2 glycoprotein have been identified in 50% of patients with acute hepatitis C and may be present early in the course of infection.[47]

Anti-HCV generally persists for prolonged periods after acute infection. Limited data suggest that the titers of anti-C33c, anti-NS5, and anti–C100-3 may decline while levels of anti–C22-3 may be maintained for considerably longer (see Fig. 93–2). In apparent self-limited HCV infection (at most 10% to 20% of infections), in which serum enzyme levels return to normal and HCV RNA is consistently absent from serum at follow-up, anti-HCV may be lost within a 10-year period. Unfortunately, even in patients in whom biochemical resolution of the disease appears to have occurred, HCV RNA may persist in serum for prolonged periods, and chronic liver disease may be present. In patients in whom biochemical evidence of chronic HCV infection follows the acute infection, nearly all remain anti-HCV–positive when tested by second-generation assays, and all continue to have circulating HCV RNA.

Chronic Hepatitis C

In chronic hepatitis associated with HCV, HCV RNA is detected consistently throughout the course of infection, and viral load appears to increase in time. Viremia may be lifelong. In patients with chronic HCV infection, clearance of HCV RNA may rarely be temporary, with reappearance of viremia at follow-up.[48] HCV replication may be increased in advanced liver disease and may play a role in progression of disease.[49] In general, patients with chronic hepatitis C, if defined by persistence of elevated serum aminotransferase levels for more than 6 months, have anti-HCV detected by second-generation assays and circulating HCV RNA by PCR amplification. However, in a few individuals (e.g., blood donors) with detectable HCV RNA with or without elevated serum ALT levels, the second-generation immunoassays for anti-HCV remain negative.[50] It seems likely that the absence of anti-HCV may be correlated with the presence of low levels of HCV RNA[51] and may be related in part to specific HCV genotypes. It has been reported that serologic reactivity to the C100-3 and 5-1-1 proteins, measured with the four-antigen, second-generation recombinant immunoblot assay, was reduced in genotypes 2b and 3a compared with HCV genotypes 1a and 1b.[52] However, with a third-generation recombinant immunoblot assay, the prevalence of measured antibodies did not differ among different HCV genotypes.[53]

On the basis of PCR amplification assays for HCV RNA, it is now clear that a large proportion of patients with acute HCV infection progress to chronic infection despite normalization of serum enzyme levels. These individuals may have viremia with or without histologic evidence of continuing liver injury.

Natural History

As indicated before, the majority of patients infected by HCV develop persistent infection with chronic hepatitis and chronic viremia. Although a minor proportion of patients with persistent HCV infection develop liver failure, complications of cirrhosis, or HCC within a few years of the onset of infection, most patients are relatively asymptomatic and their infections remain clinically silent for at least 20 years after onset of infection.[54, 55] In this period, most affected individuals are identified fortuitously during biochemical screening or blood donor screening. In an important proportion (about 30%) of these patients with biochemically defined chronic hepatitis C, overt chronic liver disease is recognized as a consequence of infection 20 years earlier.[55] End-stage liver disease with manifestations of liver failure may develop thereafter, leading to symptoms, a reduced survival rate, and referral for lifesaving liver transplantation. In fact, by the middle of the 1990s, chronic hepatitis C had become the single most common form of liver disease for which liver transplantation was undertaken in the United States. A number of potential predictors of rapid disease progression have been identified in some but not all studies; these include high levels of HCV RNA in serum, HCV genotype 1b, concomitant alcohol-induced liver disease, older age at the time of HCV acquisition, agammaglobulinemia, and increased hepatic iron concentration.

Clinical Variants

Fulminant Hepatitis

In the United States, HCV is a rare cause of fulminant hepatitis.[56] However, in some countries of the world (e.g., Taiwan), HCV infection has been identified in nearly one half of patients with fulminant non-A, non-B hepatitis.[57] Because anti-HCV appearance may be delayed, sequential studies or detection of HCV RNA may be necessary for diagnosis.

Hepatocellular Carcinoma

HCC in chronic HCV infection appears to develop predominantly through evolution from cirrhosis.[58] In a rare patient with HCC, cirrhosis may be absent, and a more direct carcinogenic effect of HCV has been postulated. The mechanism of that action is unknown. Positive and negative HCV RNA strands have been detected in both tumor and nontumor liver tissue in affected patients, suggesting that the tumor supports HCV replication.[59] Progression of HCV-induced liver disease to HCC was observed in 27% of patients with HCV-related cirrhosis after 15 years of follow-up in Japan,[60] an area in which HCV is a major cause of HCC. In fact, the cumulative risk for development of HCC in a 50-year-old HCV-positive Japanese blood donor has also been estimated to be 28% within the following 15 years.[61]

Treatment

Acute Hepatitis C

Treatment of HCV infection has been focused predominantly on patients with chronic hepatitis C. Relatively few studies of patients with acute HCV infection are currently available; those limited studies that have been published, largely from outside the United States, suggest that treatment of acute hepatitis C with interferon may reduce the risk of chronicity and increase the likelihood of a sustained loss of HCV RNA. However, treatment of acute hepatitis C with interferon is not approved in the United States and should be considered experimental. Candidates for interferon treatment may be those patients in whom HCV RNA is found more than 1 month after the onset of illness.[62]

Chronic Hepatitis C

The goals of treatment of chronic hepatitis C have been to relieve symptoms; to eradicate HCV, thereby eliminating infectivity and decreasing ongoing HCV-induced liver injury; and to prevent progression of hepatitis to end-stage liver disease—cirrhosis and HCC. At present, the therapy of choice appears to be interferon. Interferon alfa-2a and alfa-2b, the only approved treatment for chronic hepatitis C in the United

States, when given in a dose of 3 million units three times a week for 6 months, produce a biochemical response (normalization of serum ALT levels) in about 50% of patients at completion of treatment. Histologic improvement in the necroinflammatory liver lesions may be seen, and levels of HCV viremia are often reduced in patients with this biochemical response. Complete eradication of HCV RNA from serum, peripheral blood mononuclear cells, and liver has been reported but is uncommon.[63] Unfortunately, as many as 70% to 80% of the responding patients may relapse, within a few months to a year after the discontinuation of treatment, with elevation of serum ALT levels and a return of circulating HCV RNA. Treatment with interferon may change the spectrum of HCV quasi species identically in serum and in liver, because the same quasi species appear to be present in serum and liver,[64] but reversion to the original pattern may occur after relapse. Hence, with the standard 6-month drug regimen, no more than 10% to 20% of treated patients will have a sustained response lasting at least 3 years.

Initial response rates have been highest among younger patients and those of lower body weight; in women, those with shorter disease duration, and nondrinkers of alcohol; and with low serum HCV RNA levels, HCV genotypes other than type 1, absence of cirrhosis, and low hepatic iron concentrations.[65–68] Sustained response rates appear to be higher in patients in whom serum HCV RNA is absent at the end of treatment. However, absence of HCV RNA in liver may be a better predictor of a sustained response. In fact, patients with detectable hepatic levels of HCV RNA have a significantly higher rate of relapse than do patients with absent HCV RNA in liver biopsy specimens.[69] An increasing number of studies suggest that initial treatment periods of at least 12 to 18 months may increase the sustained response rate, as measured by histologic improvement, clearance or reduction of HCV RNA, and normalization of serum ALT levels,[70, 71] and may be more effective than repeated shorter regimens. Lower dose regimens appear unlikely to be beneficial, even if given for prolonged periods.[71]

For patients who do not respond to interferon treatment, dose escalation may be attempted but is successful in only a small proportion.[72] Unfortunately, no clearly effective treatment is currently available for the majority of nonresponders. The nucleoside analog ribavirin may induce a biochemical remission but has no influence on HCV viremia. Combination therapies (e.g., interferon plus ribavirin or ursodeoxycholic acid or nonsteroidal antiinflammatory agents, or *N*-acetylcysteine) have produced equivocal results in small trials.[73, 74] Inhibitors of the serine protease of HCV are under development.[75] Corticosteroids may reduce serum ALT levels in some patients but, in general, increase levels of viremia, an undesirable effect.[76]

Liver Transplantation. Patients with end-stage liver disease associated with HCV infection are candidates for liver transplantation. Recurrence of HCV appears to be almost invariable on follow-up of transplant recipients, but damage to the allograft may be present in less than half of those with posttransplantation HCV infection.[77] In contrast to hepatitis B virus infection, posttransplantation HCV infection is generally mild and often clinically silent; progressive disease leading to hepatic failure is uncommon. Short-term survival of patients with posttransplantation HCV infection may be comparable to or slightly lower than survival in patients with other liver diseases. Large-scale long-term follow-up studies are not yet available.

Treatment of HCV-Related Hepatocellular Carcinoma. Management of affected patients remains a problem. Five-year survival rates generally do not exceed 10%, and median survival is often measured in months rather than years. Treatment of early or small HCC includes hepatic resection and orthotopic liver transplantation (most successful when the cancer is an incidental finding at surgery). For more advanced, unresectable disease, percutaneous ethanol injection, chemoembolization, and chemotherapy have been used; their benefits remain uncertain.

Treatment of Extrahepatic Disorders Linked with HCV. Interferon treatment of patients with cryoglobulinemia associated with hepatitis C may result in improvement in cutaneous vasculitis and a reduction of cryoglobulin levels, immunoglobulin levels, rheumatoid factor and anti-HCV titers, and serum creatinine levels, particularly in patients in whom HCV RNA levels are suppressed during therapy.[78] Among patients with HCV-associated glomerulonephritis, proteinuria may decrease during treatment with interferon, but renal function appears unlikely to improve.[79] Unfortunately, after cessation of interferon treatment, recurrence of viremia, cryoglobulinemia, and proteinuria is common. Experiences with treatment of the other extrahepatic disorders is limited.

Prevention

General Measures

Continued screening of blood donors for anti-HCV, screening of blood products such as immune globulin products for HCV RNA, and implementation of universal precautions in health care settings may further reduce the frequency of blood-borne HCV infection. Safe sex practices may reduce the risk for transmission among sexual partners.

Passive Immunization

Experimental studies of HCV infection in chimpanzees have indicated that in vivo infection with HCV can elicit a neutralizing antibody, but it is a restricted response, isolate specific.[80] There is no convincing evidence that conventional immune globulin provides any protection against HCV infection; it is not recommended for HCV prophylaxis in any setting. Whether a high-titer hepatitis C immune globulin can provide protection remains to be demonstrated.

Active Immunization

The heterogeneity of HCV and the identification of multiple HCV genotypes have important implications with regard to the development of an HCV vaccine. Superinfection by another genotype of a patient chronically infected with one HCV genotype has been observed[81]; a protective vaccine may require antigenic material from a multitude of HCV genotypes. Of even greater concern are the observations indicating that primary infection with HCV may not induce protective immunity in the chimpanzee model of infection.[82] Nonetheless, an attempt to develop a prototype vaccine has been reported.[83] Envelope glycoproteins from one strain of HCV were used to immunize chimpanzees. Five of seven animals challenged with low doses of the same strain, at the peak of the antibody response, appeared to be protected.[83] Confirmation of this work with use of higher doses of the challenging virus and challenges at nonpeak antibody periods will be necessary. Other approaches, such as adoptive immunotherapy and the development of a T-lymphocyte–based HCV vaccine, are on the drawing boards and hold considerable research interest.

References

1. Aach RD, Stevens CE, Hollinger FB, et al: Hepatitis C virus infection in post-transfusion hepatitis—An analysis with first- and second-generation assays. N Engl J Med 325:1325–1329, 1991.

2. Hollinger FB, Gitnick GL, Aach RD, et al: Non-A, non-B hepatitis transmission in chimpanzees: A project of the transfusion-transmitted viruses study group. Intervirology 10:60–68, 1978.
3. Kato N, Yokosuka O, Hosoda K, et al: Detection of hepatitis C virus RNA in acute non-A, non-B hepatitis as an early diagnostic tool. Biochem Biophys Res Commun 192:800–807, 1993.
4. Alter MJ, Margolis HS, Krawczynski K, et al: The natural history of community-acquired hepatitis C in the United States. N Engl J Med 327:1899–1905, 1992.
5. Mauser-Bunschoten EP, Bresters D, van Drimmelen AAJ, et al: Hepatitis C infection and viremia in Dutch hemophilia patients. J Med Virol 45:241–246, 1995.
6. Hayashi J, Kishihara Y, Yamaji K, et al: Transmission of hepatitis C virus by health care workers in a rural area of Japan. Am J Gastroenterol 90:794–799, 1995.
7. McQuillan G, Alter MJ, Everhart JE: Viral hepatitis. *In* Everhart JE (ed): Digestive Diseases in the United States. Washington, DC, US Government Printing Office, 1994, pp 127–156. NIH publication 94-1447.
8. Donahue JG, Munoz A, Ness PM, et al: The declining risk of post-transfusion hepatitis C virus infection. N Engl J Med 327: 369–373, 1992.
9. Centers for Disease Control and Prevention: Outbreak of hepatitis C associated with intravenous immunoglobulin administration—United States, October 1993–June 1994. MMWR Morbid Mortal Wkly Rep 43:505–509, 1994.
10. Yu MYW, Mason BL, Tankersley DL: Detection and characterization of hepatitis C virus RNA in immune globulin. Transfusion 34:596–602, 1994.
11. Pereira BJG, Wright TL, Schmid CH, et al: A controlled study of hepatitis C transmission by organ transplantation. Lancet 345: 484–487, 1995.
12. Mulligan DC, Goldstein RM, Crippin JS, et al: Use of anti-hepatitis C virus seropositive organs in liver transplantation. Transplant Proc 27:1204–1205, 1995.
13. Gerberding JL: Incidence and prevalence of human immunodeficiency virus, hepatitis B virus, hepatitis C virus, and cytomegalovirus among health care personnel at risk for blood exposure: Final report from a longitudinal study. J Infect Dis 170:1410–1417, 1994.
14. Zuckerman J, Clewley G, Griffiths P, Cockcroft A: Prevalence of hepatitis C antibodies in clinical health-care workers. Lancet 343:1618–1620, 1994.
15. Kiyosawa K, Tanaka E, Sodeyama T, et al: Transmission of hepatitis C in an isolated area in Japan: Community-acquired infection. Gastroenterology 106:1596–1602, 1994.
16. Buchbinder SP, Katz MH, Hessol NA, et al: Hepatitis C virus infection in sexually active homosexual men. J Infect 29:263–269, 1994.
17. Osmond DH, Charlebois E, Sheppard HW, et al: Comparison of risk factors for hepatitis C and hepatitis B virus infection in homosexual men. J Infect Dis 167:66–71, 1993.
18. Meisel H, Reip A, Faltus B, et al: Transmission of hepatitis C virus to children and husbands by women infected with contaminated anti–D immunoglobulin. Lancet 345:1209–1211, 1995.
19. Akahane Y, Kojima M, Sugai Y, et al: Hepatitis C virus infection in spouses of patients with type C chronic liver disease. Ann Intern Med 120:748–752, 1994.
20. Thomas DL, Zenilman JM, Alter HJ, et al: Sexual transmission of hepatitis C virus among patients attending sexually transmitted diseases clinics in Baltimore—An analysis of 309 sex partnerships. J Infect Dis 171:768–775, 1995.
21. Takahashi M, Yamada G, Doi T, et al: Intrafamilial clustering of genotypes of hepatitis C virus RNA. Acta Med Okayama 48:293–297, 1994.
22. Ohto H, Terazawa S, Sasaki N, et al: Transmission of hepatitis C virus from mothers to infants. N Engl J Med 330:744–750, 1994.
23. Weiner AJ, Thaler MM, Crawford K, et al: A unique, predominant hepatitis C virus variant found in an infant born to a mother with multiple variants. J Virol 67:4365–4368, 1993.
24. Zanetti AR, Tanzi E, Paccagnini S, et al: Mother-to-infant transmission of hepatitis C virus. Lancet 345:289–291, 1995.
25. Manzini P, Saracco G, Cerchier A, et al: Human immunodeficiency virus infection as risk factor for mother-to-child hepatitis C virus transmission; persistence of anti–hepatitis C virus in children is associated with the mother's anti–hepatitis C virus immunoblotting pattern. Hepatology 21:328–332, 1995.
26. Shimazaki J, Tsubota K, Fukushima Y, Honda M: Detection of hepatitis C virus RNA in tears and aqueous humor (Letter). Am J Ophthalmol 118:524–525, 1994.
27. Marrogi AJ, Cheles MK, Gerber MA: Chronic hepatitis C: Analysis of host immune response by immunohistochemistry. Arch Pathol Lab Med 119:232–234, 1995.
28. Krawczynski K, Beach MJ, Bradley DW, et al: Hepatitis C virus antigen in hepatocytes: Immunomorphologic detection and identification. Gastroenterology 103:622–629, 1992.
29. Cerny A, Chisari FV: Immunological aspects of HCV infection. Intervirology 37:119–125, 1994.
30. Uchida T: Pathology of hepatitis C. Intervirology 37:126–132, 1994.
31. Tsai J-F, Margolis HS, Jeng J-E, et al: Circulating immune complexes in chronic hepatitis related to hepatitis C and B viruses infection. Clin Immunol Immunopathol 75:39–44, 1995.
32. Lefkowitch JH, Schiff ER, Davis GL, et al: Pathological diagnosis of chronic hepatitis C: A multicenter comparative study with chronic hepatitis B. Gastroenterology 104:595–603, 1993.
33. Kaji K, Nakanuma Y, Sasaki M, et al: Hepatic bile duct injuries in chronic hepatitis C: Histopathologic and immunohistochemical studies. Mod Pathol 7:937–945, 1994.
34. Emile JF, Sebagh M, Feray C, et al: The presence of epithelioid granulomas in hepatitis C virus–related cirrhosis. Hum Pathol 24:1095–1097, 1993.
35. Tong MJ, El-Farra NS, Reikes AR, et al: Clinical outcomes after transfusion-associated hepatitis C. N Engl J Med 332:1463–1466, 1995.
36. Koff RS, Dienstag JL: Extrahepatic manifestations of hepatitis C and the association with alcoholic liver disease. Semin Liver Dis 15:101–109, 1995.
37. Navas S, Bosch O, Castillo I, et al: Porphyria cutanea tarda and hepatitis C and B viruses infection: A retrospective study. Hepatology 21:279–284, 1995.
38. Koike K, Yasuda K, Yotsuyanagi H, et al: Dominant replication of either virus in dual infection with hepatitis viruses B and C. J Med Virol 45:236–239, 1995.
39. Pawlotsky J-M, Roudot-Thoraval F, Simmonds P, et al: Extrahepatic immunologic manifestations in chronic hepatitis C and hepatitis C virus serotypes. Ann Intern Med 122:169–173, 1995.
40. Johnson RJ, Gretch DR, Yamabe H, et al: Membrano-proliferative glomerulonephritis associated with hepatitis C virus infection. N Engl J Med 328:465–470, 1993.
41. Sansonno D, Cornacchiulo V, Iacobellii AR, et al: Localization of hepatitis C virus antigens in liver and skin tissues of chronic hepatitis C virus–infected patients with mixed cryoglobulinemia. Hepatology 21:305–312, 1995.
42. Bhandari BN, Wright TL: Hepatitis C: An overview. Annu Rev Med 46:309–317, 1995.
43. Martinot-Peignoux M, Marcellin P, Gournay J, et al: Detection and quantitation of serum HCV-RNA by branched DNA amplification in anti-HCV positive blood donors. J Hepatol 20:676–678, 1994.
44. Garson JA, Tedder RS: The detection of hepatitis C infection. Rev Med Virol 3:75–83, 1993.
45. Donahue JG, Munoz A, Ness PM, et al: The declining risk of post-transfusion hepatitis C virus infection. N Engl J Med 327:369–373, 1992.
46. Marcellin P, Martinot-Peignoux M, Elias A, et al: Hepatitis C virus (HCV) viremia in human immunodeficiency virus–seronegative and -seropositive patients with indeterminate HCV recombinant immunoblot assay. J Infect Dis 170:433–435, 1994.
47. Lesniewski R, Okasinski G, Carrick R, et al: Antibody to hepatitis C virus second envelope (HCV-E2) glycoprotein: A new marker of HCV infection closely associated with viremia. J Med Virol 45:415–422, 1995.
48. Wang JT, Wang T-H, Sheu J-C, et al: Posttransfusion hepatitis revisited by hepatitis C antibody assays and polymerase chain reaction. Gastroenterology 103:609–616, 1992.
49. Hagiwara H, Hayashi N, Mita E, et al: Quantitation of hepatitis C virus RNA in serum of asymptomatic blood donors and patients with type C chronic liver disease. Hepatology 17:545–550, 1993.
50. Sugitani M, Inchauspe G, Shindo M, Prince AM: Sensitivity of serological assays to identify blood donors with hepatitis C viraemia. Lancet 339:1018–1019, 1992.

51. Yuki N, Hayashi N, Kasahara A, et al: Hepatitis C virus replication and antibody responses toward specific hepatitis C virus proteins. Hepatology 19:1360–1365, 1994.
52. Zein NN, Rakela J, Persing DH: Genotype-dependent serologic reactivities in patients infected with hepatitis C virus in the United States. Mayo Clin Proc 70:449–452, 1995.
53. Pawlotsky J-M, Roudot-Thoraval F, Pellet C, et al: Influence of hepatitis C virus (HCV) genotypes on HCV recombinant immunoblot assay patterns. J Clin Microbiol 33:1357–1359, 1995.
54. Seeff LB, Buskell-Bales Z, Wright EC, et al: Long-term mortality after transfusion-associated non-A, non-B hepatitis. N Engl J Med 327:1906–1911, 1993.
55. Seeff LB: Natural history of viral hepatitis, type C. Semin Gastrointest Dis 6:20–27, 1995.
56. Gordon FD, Anastopoulos H, Khettry U, et al: Hepatitis C infection: A rare cause of fulminant hepatic failure. Am J Gastroenterol 90:117–120, 1995.
57. Chu C-M, Sheen I-S, Liaw Y-F: The role of hepatitis C virus in fulminant viral hepatitis in an area with endemic hepatitis A or B. Gastroenterology 107:189–195, 1994.
58. Resnick RH, Koff RS: Hepatitis C–related hepatocellular carcinoma. Arch Intern Med 153:1672–1677, 1993.
59. Gerber MA, Shieh YSC, Shim K-S, et al: Detection of replicative hepatitis C virus sequences in hepatocellular carcinoma. Am J Pathol 141:1271–1277, 1992.
60. Ikeda K, Saitoh S, Koida I, et al: A multivariate analysis of risk factors for hepatocellular carcinogenesis: A prospective observation of 795 patients with viral and alcoholic cirrhosis. Hepatology 18:47–53, 1993.
61. Tanaka H, Hiyama T, Tsukuma H, et al: Cumulative risk of hepatocellular carcinoma in hepatitis C virus carriers: Statistical estimations from cross-sectional data. Jpn J Cancer Res 85:485–490, 1994.
62. Fried MW, Hoofnagle JH: Therapy of hepatitis C. Semin Liver Dis 15:82–91, 1995.
63. Romeo R, Pol S, Berthelot P, Brechot C: Eradication of hepatitis C virus RNA after alpha-interferon therapy. Ann Intern Med 121:276–277, 1994.
64. Sakamoto N, Enomoto N, Kurosaki M, et al: Comparison of the hypervariable region of hepatitis C virus genomes in plasma and liver. J Med Virol 46:7–11, 1995.
65. Nousbaum J-P, Pol S, Nalpas B, et al: Hepatitis C virus type 1b (II) infection in France and Italy. Ann Intern Med 122:161–168, 1995.
66. Okazaki T, Yoshihara H, Suzuki K, et al: Efficacy of interferon therapy in patients with chronic hepatitis C. Comparison between non-drinkers and drinkers. Scand J Gastroenterol 29:1039–1043, 1994.
67. Hayashi J, Ohmiya M, Kishihara Y, et al: A statistical analysis of predictive factors of response to human lymphoblastoid interferon in patients with chronic hepatitis C. Am J Gastroenterol 89:2151–2156, 1994.
68. Olynk JK, Reddy KR, Di Bisceglie AM, et al: Hepatic iron concentration as a predictor of response to interferon alfa therapy in chronic hepatitis C. Gastroenterology 108:1104–1109, 1995.
69. Shindo M, Arai K, Sokawa Y, Okuno T: Hepatic hepatitis C virus RNA as a predictor of a long-term response to interferon-alpha therapy. Ann Intern Med 122:586–591, 1995.
70. Kasahara A, Hayashi N, Hiramatsu N, et al: Ability of prolonged interferon treatment to suppress relapse after cessation of therapy in patients with chronic hepatitis C: A multicenter randomized controlled trial. Hepatology 21:291–297, 1995.
71. Poynard T, Bedossa P, Chevallier M, et al: A comparison of three interferon alfa-2b regimens for the long-term treatment of chronic non-A, non-B hepatitis. N Engl J Med 332:1457–1462, 1995.
72. Marcellin P, Pouteau M, Martinot-Peignoux M, et al: Lack of benefit of escalating dosage of interferon alfa in patients with chronic hepatitis C. Gastroenterology 109:156–165, 1995.
73. Boucher E, Jouanolle H, Andre P, et al: Interferon and ursodeoxycholic acid combined therapy in the treatment of chronic viral C hepatitis: Results from a controlled randomized trial in 80 patients. Hepatology 21:322–327, 1995.
74. Schvarcz R, Yun ZB, Sonnerborg A, et al: Combined treatment with interferon alpha-2b and ribavirin for chronic hepatitis C in patients with a previous non-response or non-sustained response to interferon alone. J Med Virol 46:43–47, 1995.
75. Pizzi E, Tramontano A, Tomei L, et al: Molecular model of the specificity pocket of the hepatitis C virus protease: Implications for substrate recognition. Proc Natl Acad Sci USA 91:888–892, 1994.
76. Magrin S, Craxi A, Fabiano C, et al: Hepatitis C viremia in chronic liver disease: Relationship to interferon-alpha or corticosteroid treatment. Hepatology 19:273–279, 1994.
77. Poterucha JJ, Gross JB Jr: Hepatitis C after liver transplantation. Gastroenterology 108:1314–1317, 1995.
78. Misiani R, Bellavita P, Fenili D, et al: Interferon alfa-2a therapy in cryoglobulinemia associated with hepatitis C virus. N Engl J Med 330:751–756, 1994.
79. Johnson RJ, Gretch DR, Couser WG, et al: Hepatitis C virus–associated glomerulonephritis. Effect of alpha-interferon therapy. Kidney Int 46:1700–1704, 1994.
80. Farci P, Alter HJ, Wong DC, et al: Prevention of hepatitis C virus infection in chimpanzees after antibody-mediated in vitro neutralization. Proc Natl Acad Sci USA 91:7792–7796, 1994.
81. Kao J-H, Chen P-J, Lai M-Y, Chen D-S: Superinfection of heterologous hepatitis C virus in a patient with chronic type C hepatitis. Gastroenterology 105:583–587, 1993.
82. Farci P, Alter HJ, Govindarajan S, et al: Lack of protective immunity against reinfection with hepatitis C virus. Science 258:135–140, 1992.
83. Choo QL, Kuo G, Ralston R, et al: Vaccination of chimpanzees against infection by the hepatitis C virus. Proc Natl Acad Sci USA 91:1294–1298, 1994.

94

Hepatitis E

Raymond S. Koff

Epidemiology

Incubation Period and Virus Shedding

The incubation period of hepatitis E is variable, with a reported range of 15 to 65 days in most water-borne outbreaks and a mean of about 40 days. The hepatitis E virus (HEV) is shed in the stools of infected patients. It seems likely, on the basis of studies of HEV in the bile and feces of experimentally infected cynomolgus macaques, that the virus is shed in the feces after transport of HEV from the liver into bile and then into the duodenal contents. Whether replication occurs in the intestine remains uncertain. The duration of fecal shedding is 4 to 11 weeks in the macaque, and the titer of HEV RNA is higher in feces than in serum in these animals.[1] The demonstration of HEV in extrahepatic tissues and other body fluids has yet to be reported. The precise duration of fecal shedding of HEV, the duration of viremia, and the titer of circulating HEV during the viremic period have yet to be established in infected human subjects but are generally believed to be short-lived (Fig. 94–1). However, in one study, viremia was identified between as early as 1 week and as late as 4 months after the onset of jaundice, and protracted viremia was present in 15% of patients.[2] In one patient, fecal shedding of HEV RNA continued up to the 52nd day after onset of icterus. Despite these provocative findings, neither an intestinal carrier state nor persistent viremia has been established.

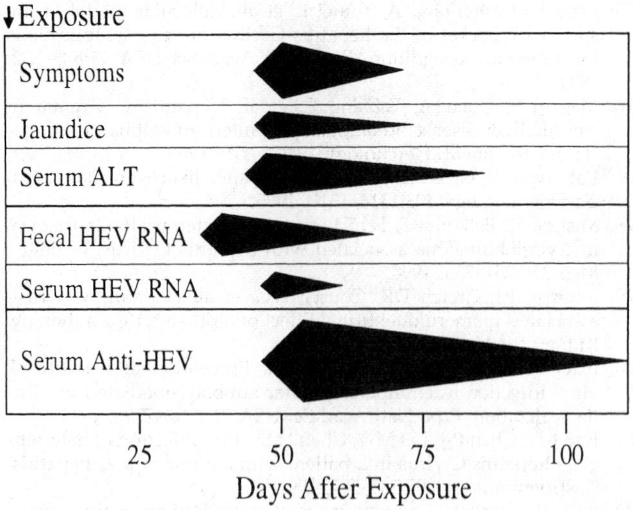

FIGURE 94–1 □ Proposed scheme of clinical, biochemical, virologic, and serologic events in acute hepatitis E infection. ALT, Alanine aminotransferase.

Epidemiologic Patterns

HEV has been linked with epidemic and endemic disease in developing countries, particularly in the Indian subcontinent, Asia, and Africa. Limited seroprevalence data suggest that less than 3% of the population of developed countries have detectable antibody to HEV (Table 94–1); in contrast, higher seroprevalence rates have been identified in developing countries. The specificity of anti-HEV detection in developed nations, in the absence of known epidemic or endemic disease, remains to be established. Outbreaks of HEV infection have been recognized in Mexico[3] and may be present elsewhere in the Americas. In fact, as shown in Table 94–1, there is serologic evidence that the virus has circulated among rural populations and rural Amerindians in Venezuela.[4] However, there is little evidence that HEV is highly endemic in the New World. Acute hepatitis E is seen in developed nations throughout the world, but in these instances, the infection is imported by travelers and immigrants from the developing world; endemic foci have yet to be identified and secondary transmission has yet to be reported in developed nations. Sporadic cases of HEV infection in the developing world may serve as a reservoir of infection during periods between outbreaks.

TABLE 94–1 ■ Seroprevalence of Anti-HEV in Selected Countries and Regions

COUNTRY OR REGION	ANTI-HEV PREVALENCE (%)	
Taiwan	0	(healthy subjects)
United States	0.5	
Ukraine	0.5	
South Africa	<2	
Europe	<2	
Italy	0.74	(healthy subjects)
	0.9	(blood donors)
Thailand	2	
Venezuela	1.6	(pregnant women, Caracas)
	4	(rural population)
	5	(rural Amerindians)
Tajikistan	8.5	
Saudi Arabia	9.5	(blood donors)
Egypt	24.5	(blood donors)

Although the epidemiology of HEV infection resembles that of hepatitis A, there are distinct differences. HEV infection is thought to be the most common form of clinically apparent sporadic hepatitis in the young adult population of developing countries; hepatitis A may be the most common form of subclinical or inapparent infection in children in these same areas. Whereas hepatitis A is generally mild, even during pregnancy, hepatitis E is often a severe disorder in pregnancy with high case-fatality rates (see later).

Modes of Transmission

Outbreaks of hepatitis E have been repeatedly linked to fecal contamination of water supplies. Some endemic infections also appear to result from fecal-oral transmission due to continuing contamination of water and breakdown in purification techniques. Intrafamilial person-to-person transmission occurs but plays a minor role in the spread of infection.[5] Maternal-neonatal transmission has been documented; intrauterine infection may be responsible.[6] A high frequency of abortions and intrauterine deaths results from such infections. Affected surviving infants may have clinical and biochemical evidence of HEV infection.

Limited serologic studies suggest that the seroprevalence of anti-HEV increases with age. This may represent either a cohort effect, with a decreasing incidence of infection in the recent past, or an accumulation of infections or reinfections over time. The weight of available evidence suggests that immunity to HEV infection does develop and that most infections are primary infections rather than reinfections. In one study of an outbreak of hepatitis E,[7] the presence of immunoglobulin (Ig) G anti-HEV appeared to protect contacts of patients. Evidence of resistance to reinfection has also been documented in experimental studies in nonhuman primates.[8]

Pathogenesis and Pathology

The pathogenesis of HEV infection is poorly understood. Although direct HEV-induced cytopathogenic actions remain possible and are favored by the finding of relatively fewer intrahepatic lymphocytes than in other forms of viral hepatitis, the importance of this circumstantial observation is uncertain. Immunologically mediated mechanisms of hepatocyte injury have not been excluded. In fact, small round cells (predominantly T lymphocytes) are the predominant cell component of the inflammatory infiltrates seen on examination of liver tissue from infected cynomolgus monkeys. Infiltration of both lymphocytes and monocytes in areas of hepatocyte loss and direct contact between lymphocytes and hepatocytes may be prominent features.[9] In liver biopsy specimens of some patients, regenerating liver cells arrange themselves in a ductlike pattern known as pseudoglandular transformation; this lesion is common in hepatitis E but is nonspecific.

Experimental transmission of HEV to cynomolgus macaques by intravenous inoculation resulted in increases in serum alanine aminotransferase levels at days 10 to 19 and hepatic histologic changes at days 12 to 14; HEV antigen could be detected in liver and bile at days 14 to 22.[10] Histopathologic changes became most prominent at days 18 to 25; serum anti-HEV was first detected at days 27 to 39, before or at the time of the peak alanine aminotransferase level. By day 39, hepatic HEV antigen was no longer detectable but histologic lesions persisted. These observations suggested the possibility of two phases of HEV infection. In the first, HEV might replicate in the liver, and a mild hepatitis may be seen as a consequence of a viral or immune-mediated effect. The second phase might begin with the development of a humoral immune response that results in clearing of HEV but worsening of the hepatic histologic changes. Further studies will be needed to confirm this notion of biphasic infection.

Clinical Manifestations

In typical outbreaks, highest attack rates of clinically apparent disease are usually found in individuals between 15 and 40 years of age. In children, most infections are anicteric. In most adult patients with hepatitis E, the disease is clinically indistinguishable from other forms of viral hepatitis. Serum enzyme elevations are usually monophasic. Jaundice may last for 2 to 3 weeks; serum bilirubin and serum alanine aminotransferase levels return to normal within 2 months (see Fig. 94–1). Cholestasis may be a prominent feature. In one study of hepatitis E in a predominantly adult population,[11] cholestasis was evident, as identified by the presence of pruritus and clay-colored stools, in 25%. About 5% of patients may develop generalized lymphadenopathy during the course of the illness. Overall case-fatality rates due to fulminant hepatitis E are usually in the range of 0.5% to 3%.

Serologic Studies and Diagnosis

IgM antibody to HEV (IgM anti-HEV) has been detected regularly and early in hepatitis E and may persist for at least 6 weeks after the peak of the illness.[7] IgG anti-HEV is also present early, peaks about 2 weeks or more after the onset of clinical disease, and remains detectable at lower levels for at least 20 months.[7] Serum HEV RNA may be present in nearly three quarters of IgM anti-HEV–positive patients during the acute phase.[2] In some patients, HEV RNA may be present alone; in others, IgM anti-HEV may be present alone. For uncertain reasons, the appearance of IgG anti-HEV may be delayed in some patients.[11] The presence of IgG anti-HEV in low-prevalence populations without evidence of endemic or epidemic disease may reflect false-positive test results because of cross-reactivity with another agent or nonspecificity of these assays.

No immunoassay for diagnosis of hepatitis E has been approved for use in the United States. A fluorescent antibody–blocking assay, developed at the Centers for Disease Control and Prevention, has been the most reliable assay but continues to be a research tool. Enzyme immunoassays and Western blot assays based on the detection of antibody to synthetic HEV peptides and polymerase chain reaction assays for HEV RNA are under development and may become commercially available in the near future.

Clinical Variants and Sequelae

The acute hepatitis associated with HEV infection has been shown to be self-limiting, except in the few patients in whom fulminant hepatitis ensues. To date, no form of chronic liver disease (chronic hepatitis, cirrhosis, or hepatocellular carcinoma) has been linked to infection by HEV. In pregnant women, particularly in the third trimester, a surprisingly high proportion (10% to 20%) of HEV infections result in fulminant hepatitis with a high risk for maternal and intrauterine fetal or neonatal mortality. The mechanism underlying the enhanced virulence of HEV in the third trimester of pregnancy remains to be determined. HEV-like particles have been identified in the liver of a pregnant woman who died of fulminant HEV infection.[12]

Treatment

No specific treatment of hepatitis E is available. Although pregnant women with fulminant hepatitis E should be considered candidates for liver transplantation, experience remains limited.

Prevention

Passive Immunization

Passive immunization of cynomolgus monkeys with anti-HEV–titered convalescent serum from experimentally infected animals did not protect against challenge with live HEV.[1] Conventional immune globulin manufactured in the United States is unlikely to contain anti-HEV and is not likely to be useful in the prophylaxis of this infection. Unfortunately, immune globulin prepared in developing countries where the disease is endemic also appears to have insufficient anti-HEV levels to prevent infection. Unless a high-titered, hyperimmune preparation can be developed from convalescent sera, passive immunization is unlikely to be of value.

Active Immunization

Immunization of cynomolgus monkeys with a 55-kDa recombinant HEV fusion protein from the second open reading frame of HEV protected against challenge with live HEV.[1] These promising studies suggest that it should be possible to develop a vaccine to protect against outbreaks and sporadic cases within endemic areas and to protect travelers to these developing countries.

References

1. Tsarev SA, Tsareva TS, Emerson SU, et al: Successful passive and active immunization of cynomolgus monkeys against hepatitis E. Proc Natl Acad Sci USA 91:10198–10202, 1994.
2. Nanda SK, Ansari IH, Acharya SK, et al: Protracted viremia during acute sporadic hepatitis E virus infection. Gastroenterology 108:225–230, 1995.
3. Velazquez O, Stetler HC, Avila C, et al: Epidemic transmission of enterically transmitted non-A, non-B hepatitis in Mexico, 1986–1987. JAMA 263:3281–3285, 1990.
4. Pujol FH, Favorov MO, Marcano T, et al: Prevalence of antibodies against hepatitis E virus among urban and rural populations in Venezuela. J Med Virol 42:234–236, 1994.
5. Aggarwal R, Naik SR: Hepatitis E: Intrafamilial transmission versus waterborne spread. J Hepatol 21:718–723, 1994.
6. Khuroo MS, Kamili S, Jameel S: Vertical transmission of hepatitis E virus. Lancet 345:1025–1026, 1995.
7. Bryan JP, Tsarev SA, Iqbal M, et al: Epidemic hepatitis E in Pakistan: Patterns of serologic response and evidence that antibody to hepatitis E virus protects against disease. J Infect Dis 170:517–521, 1994.
8. Arankalle VA, Favorov MO, Chadha MS, et al: Rhesus monkeys infected with hepatitis E virus (HEV) from the former USSR are immune to subsequent challenge with an Indian strain of HEV. Acta Virol 37:515–518, 1993.
9. Soe S, Uchida T, Suzuki K, et al: Enterically transmitted non-A, non-B hepatitis in cynomolgus monkeys: Morphology and probable mechanism of hepatocellular necrosis. Liver 9:135–145, 1989.
10. Longer CF, Denny SL, Caudill JD, et al: Experimental hepatitis E: Pathogenesis in cynomolgus macaques *(Macaca fascicularis)*. J Infect Dis 168:602–609, 1993.
11. Khuroo MS, Rustgi VK, Dawson GJ, et al: Spectrum of hepatitis E virus infection in India. J Med Virol 42:281–286, 1994.
12. Asher LV, Innis BL, Shrestha MP, et al: Virus-like particles in the liver of a patient with fulminant hepatitis and antibody to hepatitis E virus. J Med Virol 31:229–233, 1990.

95

Pyogenic Liver Abscess

John G. Bartlett

Because the liver is exposed to bacteria in both the systemic and the portal circulations, it would seem relatively vulnerable to bacterial infections. Nevertheless, the extensive network of reticuloendothelial cells that lines the sinusoids seems highly protective, and this appears to be one of the most effective sites of bacterial clearance.[1] The most common bacterial infection is pyogenic abscess. Even this is relatively rare, but when it occurs it often represents a life-threatening infection that may be difficult to detect and controversial with respect to management strategies.

History

Hepatic abscesses were originally described in 1836 by John Bright.[2] Ochsner[3] published his classic review in 1938, which included 575 cases culled from the literature: 35% were amebic and 34% occurred in association with appendicitis. The mortality rate at that time was 80%, and it remained in the 65% to 80% range until the mid-1960s. During the past 30 years, there have been three important changes in our understanding and management of pyogenic liver abscesses: (1) imaging techniques were developed that remarkably facilitated detection; (2) refinements in the microbiology showed that anaerobic bacteria were major pathogens; and (3) percutaneous drainage methods were introduced as an alternative to surgery. Pyogenic liver abscess continues to be a somewhat elusive clinical condition, but the aforementioned developments have driven mortality rates down to the 10% to 20% range.

Incidence

Hepatic abscesses accounted for 0.04% to 0.007% of all hospitalizations in the preantibiotic era.[4, 5] A review of 18,300 autopsies in 1932 by Collins[5] showed 111 cases for an autopsy incidence of 0.6%. Since that time the incidence has declined, possibly owing to the availability of antibiotic therapy. A review of nine cases from the Henry Ford Hospital from 1950 to 1960 indicated that these accounted for 0.005% of all hospital admissions, and another review published in 1973 indicated an incidence of 0.007%.[6, 7] Another review at Duke showed 58 patients with this diagnosis during the period 1968 to 1982, representing 15 cases per 100,000 admissions.[8]

Pathophysiology

Pyogenic abscesses usually are secondary to another condition, although 15% to 30% are considered "cryptogenic." The most common associated conditions are biliary tract disease, hepatic neoplasms, infections of the portal system, infections at distant anatomic sites, and trauma.[8–36] The distribution of associated conditions is reviewed in Table 95–1, which presents data from a review of 885 cases reported in the literature from 1954 to 1979 by McDonald and Howard[9] and a review of 55 cases at Duke from 1968 to 1982 by McDonald and coworkers.[8]

TABLE 95–1 ■ Associated Conditions in Liver Abscess

SOURCE	McDONALD AND HOWARD[9] Literature Review	McDONALD ET AL[8] Duke University Hospital
Cases	885	55
Period	1954–1979	1968–1982
Associated conditions (%)		
Biliary tract disease	33	36
Neoplastic disease	10	22
Portal system infection	12	12
Other infection	13	15
Trauma	3	4
Unknown	21	15

Data from McDonald AP, Howard RJ: Pyogenic liver abscess. World J Surg 4:369, 1980; and McDonald MI, Corey GR, Gallis HA, Durack DT: Single and multiple pyogenic liver abscesses: Natural history, diagnosis and treatment, with emphasis on percutaneous damage. Medicine (Baltimore) 63:291, 1984.

The most common associated condition at present is ascending cholangitis secondary to biliary obstruction or manipulation secondary to calculus, stricture, or malignancy. This accounted for only 14% of hepatic abscesses in the prechemotherapy era, according to the review of 575 cases by Ochsner,[3] but it now accounts for approximately 30%.[8, 13–19, 22, 24–33]

Hematogenous infection of the liver may occur via the hepatic artery or, more frequently, the portal vein. In the report by Ochsner and colleagues,[3] 34% were associated with appendicitis, but these now account for less than 1%. Other associated infections that may reach the liver via the portal circulation include inflammatory diseases of the small and large bowel, diverticulitis, pancreatic infections, splenic infections, peritonitis, intraabdominal abscesses, and omphalitis. The most common of these at present are infections involving the colon. There has been increasing recognition of hepatic abscesses in patients with Crohn disease, an incidence reported at 0.5% to 3%.[37–39] Hematogenous infection of the liver may occur from primary foci at extraabdominal sites through the hepatic artery. These include diverse conditions, may occur in association with hepatic trauma, and often involve a relatively unusual bacterium, such as *Staphylococcus aureus*. A distinctive variant of this pattern is jugular septic thrombophlebitis with bacteremia almost invariably due to *Fusobacterium necrophorum* and multiple hepatic abscesses.

Infections that may reach the liver parenchyma by direct extension include penetrating tumors of the gastrointestinal tract, cholecystitis, pancreatitis, perihepatic abscess, and penetrating duodenal or gastric ulcer.

Miscellaneous conditions of the liver that may be complicated by pyogenic abscesses include trauma, tumors (hepatomas or metastatic cancer), infected cysts, and foreign bodies. Malignancies were second only to biliary tract disease in the Duke series,[8] but most were extrahepatic tumors involving the biliary tract or pancreas accompanied by biliary tract obstruction. Nevertheless, Robertson and colleagues[10] reported that 16% of all hepatic abscesses reported during a 25-year interval represented secondary infections of neoplastic lesions of the liver.

Hepatic abscess is being recognized more often in immunosuppressed hosts, including those with defective B-cell function,[40, 41] chronic granulomatous disease,[42] diabetes,[43] sickle cell disease,[44] or defective cell-mediated immunity,[45–47] including recipients of liver transplants[48] and patients with acquired immunodeficiency syndrome.[49] As expected, those associated with defective cell-mediated immunity usually involve opportunistic fungi.

Approximately 20% of pyogenic liver abscesses have no associated underlying condition and are referred to as cryptogenic. Cryptogenic liver abscesses are usually solitary.[8, 14, 25]

Microbiology

The review of 575 reported cases of hepatic abscess by Ochsner[3] in 1938 indicated that approximately one third were due to amebiasis and the balance were "pyogenic." Since that time, the relative incidence of amebic liver abscesses in industrialized countries has declined. In the United States they now account for only about 10% of all liver abscesses, although there may be great interhospital differences according to the population served. In U.S. hospitals serving a large population of Hispanic immigrants, amebic abscesses may account for the majority of cases,[50] and in developing countries these clearly constitute the majority.[51–54]

Microbiologic studies of pyogenic abscesses in the preantibiotic era implicated *Escherichia coli* in 30%, *Streptococcus* in 27%, and *Staphylococcus* in 26%; cultures for the remaining 30% were sterile.[3] The literature review by McDonald and Howard[9] showed that the major isolates in 604 patients reported from 1954 to 1979 included *E. coli* (37%), *S. aureus* (23%), *Proteus* (13%), *Klebsiella* or *Enterobacter* species (12%), and *Streptococcus* (17%). Anaerobic bacteria accounted for 6% in this review, and 7% of patients had sterile lesions. A major revision of the bacteriology of pyogenic liver abscess followed the 1972 report by Sabbaj and associates,[11] which showed anaerobes in 25 of 47 cases (45%; Table 95–2). A subsequent review by Finegold[12] summarized the anaerobic bacteriology in 310 reported patients with liver abscesses ascribed to anaerobic bacteria reported before 1976. The most common of the 379 strains reported were microaerophilic and anaerobic streptococci (96 isolates), *F. necrophorum* (47), *Bacteroides fragilis* (33), *Clostridium* (38), *Actinomyces* (32), and unspeciated strains of *Bacteroides* (39) and of *Fusobacterium* (34). The reports by Finegold[12] and Sabbaj[11] both include a substantial number of "microaerophilic streptococci." Many of these are now properly classified as *Streptococcus intermedius* or *Streptococcus milleri,* which appear to be especially common in cryptogenic liver abscesses and hepatic abscess associated with Crohn disease.[55, 56]

Most studies show that 30% to 50% of blood cultures of patients with pyogenic abscesses are positive and that cultures of liver aspirates usually show a polymicrobial flora. Many of these infections are due to mixtures of aerobic and anaerobic bacteria. The most common isolates from blood or aspirates are coliforms, various streptococci (aerobic, microaerophilic, and anaerobic), and anaerobic gram-negative bacilli, principally *Fusobacterium* and *Bacteroides* species.

Less common causes of pyogenic liver abscess include *Listeria monocytogenes,*[57] *Yersinia enterocolytica* (especially in patients who have hemachromatosis or who receive iron therapy),[58–60] *Pasteurella multocida* (with animal exposure),[61] *Actinomyces* (usually cryptogenic),[62–64] *Pseudomonas pseudomallei* (which causes the majority of pyogenic abscesses in countries where melioidosis is endemic),[65] and tuberculosis.[49, 66] In children, the major pathogen is *S. aureus,*[67–71] although some find the mixed flora with anaerobes to predominate.[72] A distinctive syndrome of hepatic candidiasis with multiple microabscesses is recognized with increasing frequency in immunocompromised hosts, especially patients with acute granulocytic leukemia.[73–75]

TABLE 95–2 ■ Bacteriology of Liver Abscess: 25 Cases Involving Anaerobic Bacteria

BACTERIA	NUMBER OF LIVER ISOLATES	NUMBER OF BLOOD ISOLATES
Anaerobes	30	14
Peptostreptococci	6	2
Microaerophilic streptococci	7	7
Fusobacteria	5	1
Bacteroides fragilis	5	2
Other *Bacteroides* sp.	5	2
Aerobes	7	6
Streptococci	4	3
Escherichia coli	2	2
Proteus	1	0

From Sabbaj J, Sutter VL, Finegold SM: Anaerobic pyogenic liver abscess. Ann Intern Med 77:629, 1972.

Clinical Features

Age

In the preantibiotic era the predominant age group consisted of 30- to 40-year-old individuals, but the reduction in cases associated with appendicitis has been accompanied by a shift in age prevalence, so that most more recent series show a predominance of patients in the sixth and seventh decades of life. Nevertheless, a relatively large number of cases are reported in children.[68–72]

Symptoms

The usual systemic signs of infection include fever, chills, malaise, and anorexia. Most patients appear severely ill and have spiking fever, although the fever pattern is quite varied and may be continuous or intermittent. Most patients also complain of right side upper quadrant pain that may radiate to the right shoulder. In some instances, the infection persists for long periods and is associated with signs of chronic infection, such as weight loss and anemia. This was noted in 30% to 50% of cases in the extensive literature review by McDonald and Howard.[9]

Physical Examination

Approximately two thirds of patients with pyogenic liver abscesses have a large, tender liver. Perhaps the most useful specific finding is a localized point of tenderness, which must be carefully sought by a fingertip march over the intercostal spaces of the right upper quadrant. Before scanning technology was available, this technique was used to identify the site for needle aspiration, in an effort to confirm the diagnosis, and the relatively low yield may be one of the reasons that these lesions were often detected only at autopsy. Jaundice is unusual and often reflects extrahepatic biliary disease rather than involvement of the liver itself. Breath sounds may be reduced or absent at the right base, owing to an overlying pleural effusion or splinting.

Laboratory Tests

The typical findings are those of systemic infection and impaired hepatic function (Table 95–3). Most patients have leukocytosis with a leftward shift and anemia. Indicators of hepatic dysfunction commonly include slight elevation in the bilirubin value, elevated alkaline phosphatase and hepatic aminotransferase levels, and hypoalbuminemia. Especially

TABLE 95–3 ■ Laboratory Findings in Liver Abscess

PARAMETER	NO. ABNORMAL/ NO. TESTED (%)
Leukocytosis	
White cells >10,000/mm^3	316/445 (71)
Anemia	
Hemoglobin <12 g/dL	165/349 (47)
Elevated bilirubin level	
>2 mg/dL	117/299 (39)
Hypoalbuminemia	
<2 g/dL	130/238 (55)
Elevated alkaline phosphatase level	139/300 (46)
Abnormal chest radiograph	181/344 (53)

Adapted from McDonald AP, Howard RJ: Pyogenic liver abscess. World J Surg 4:369, 1980.

characteristic are elevated alkaline phosphatase and low serum albumin values. Chest radiographs show abnormalities in at least half the cases, but the findings are nonspecific. Typical features include an elevation of the right diaphragm, a right side pleural effusion, and atelectasis of the right lower lobe. Gas in the liver parenchyma on plain films of the abdomen is considered virtually diagnostic, but it is present infrequently.[76] Also, it may be difficult to distinguish gas collections in the biliary tract, the portal vein, or the bowel. A right side lateral view or contrast studies may be helpful in making this distinction.

Hepatic Scans

The availability of scanning techniques is probably the most important development in management guidelines for suspected liver abscesses and is largely credited with the substantial reduction in mortality rate in more recent series. There are now numerous scanning techniques from which to choose, and the selection depends on the clinical setting and availability (Fig. 95–1 and Table 95–4).

The liver scan using technetium Tc 99m sulfur colloid shows a localized area of reduced uptake at the site of infection. Numerous studies have shown positive results in 70% to 98% of cases.[8, 77, 78] The major causes of false-negative

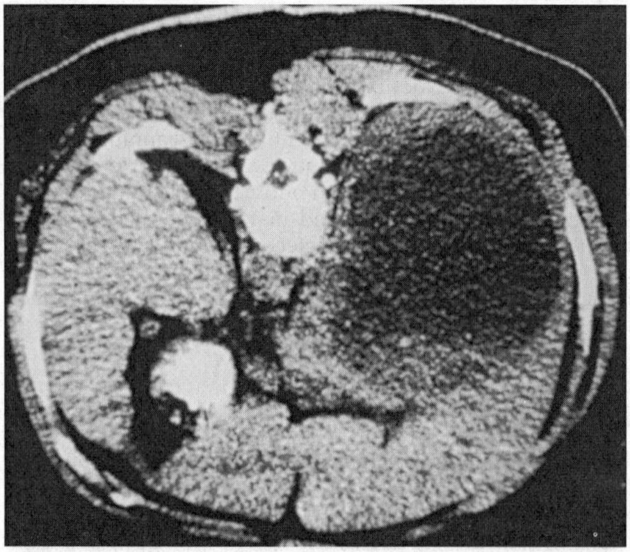

FIGURE 95–1 □ Magnetic resonance image showing a large hepatic abscess.

readings are microscopic abscesses (smaller than 2 cm) and occasionally poor uptake due to hepatic failure. A disadvantage of these scans is that they do not distinguish abscesses from tumors, cysts, hemangiomas, and other intrahepatic lesions.

Ultrasonography demonstrates areas of echogenicity that may be quite variable. Most lesions are round with irregular walls; they may be cystic, multiloculated, or septate, or they may show internal echoes indicating debris. The sensitivity of the test is somewhat technician dependent, but most report that it is 70% to 90%.[77–86] False-negative results are ascribed to suboptimal technique, failure to detect small abscesses, difficult interpretation confounded by overlying bowel gas, and misinterpretation of subcapsular collections as ascites. Advantages of ultrasonography are the ability to perform the test at the bedside, which is a notable advantage for seriously ill patients. Sonograms complement the technetium scan in distinguishing solid from cystic lesions, and they may also be used to guide drainage.

Gallium citrate scans show a sensitivity of 90% to 95% but do not distinguish inflammatory lesions from neoplasms.[77, 78, 85, 87, 88] Another problem is the time required to perform the test—24 to 72 hours. Indium 111–labeled white blood cell scans offer advantages in that the label tracks only to inflammatory lesions, it is not excreted in the bowel, and the test may be done after several hours rather than days. Despite these advantages, the largely anecdotal published experience with indium scans includes both false-negative[89] and false-positive[90] results.

Computed tomography is generally regarded as the most sensitive and specific method of detecting pyogenic abscesses of the liver. Typical lesions are sharply demarcated low-density masses of 20 to 30 Hounsfield units. Gas is detected within the abscess in 20% to 30% of patients, presumably produced by gas-forming organisms, primarily anaerobic bacteria, or occasionally coliforms such as *E. coli* or *Klebsiella.* The use of intravenous contrast medium increases the sensitivity of the test, which is usually reported to be 90% to 100%.[77, 78, 84–86, 91–95] Advantages of computed tomography include the potential for guided aspiration, the ability to detect smaller lesions (resolution limit 0.5 cm), the utility of the test in defining other sites of intraabdominal pathology, and the ability to distinguish tumors, cysts, and hematomas as causes of the focal defects. Nevertheless, such distinctions are not always easy, and occasional false-negative readings have been reported. Relative merits of magnetic resonance imaging compared with computed tomography are unclear.[85]

It should be noted that all scanning techniques are considered unreliable early in the course of hepatic candidiasis in the neutropenic host.[73–75, 96] With resolution of neutropenia, ultrasonography or computed tomography will usually demonstrate typical lesions.[74]

Etiologic Diagnosis

The major diagnostic challenge in many cases is the differentiation of pyogenic and amebic abscesses because this distinction dictates therapeutic decisions. With pyogenic abscesses, blood culture results are often positive, and the presence of common associated diseases (e.g., biliary tract disease, inflammation involving the bed of portal circulation, hemochromatosis, and Crohn disease) facilitates the identification of pyogenic abscess. Amebic abscesses are most common in immigrants from or travelers to endemic areas, and these persons are usually young, previously healthy adults. Most do not have concurrent amebic colitis, although a stool examination will sometimes yield the parasite. The most reliable diagnostic test is serology using enzyme-linked immunosorbent assays, which are almost invariably positive with inva-

TABLE 95–4 ■ Diagnostic Imaging of Hepatic Abscess

IMAGING METHOD	SENSITIVITY (%)	COMMENT
Technetium scintigraphy	80–90	Lesions <2 cm not detected; nonspecific: does not distinguish abscesses, hematomas, tumors, or cysts
Gallium citrate scanning	90–95	Fails to distinguish neoplastic and inflammatory conditions; requires ≥24 h
Sonography	70–90	Many false-negative results; complements technetium scintiscan; distinguishes solid vs. cystic lesions; may be used to guide percutaneous drainage; avoids radiation exposure; may be performed at bedside
Computed tomography	90–100	Detects lesions as small as 0.5 cm; detects extrahepatic abdominal lesions; sensitivity improves with contrast; often helpful in distinguishing abscesses, tumors, cysts, and hematomas; may be used to guide percutaneous drainage

sive disease.[97, 98] Aspirates from patients who have needle aspiration should have stains and culture for acid-fast bacteria, aerobic and anaerobic bacteria, and fungi; the sniff test indicating putrid discharge is considered diagnostic of anaerobic infection. Hepatic candidiasis in the neutropenic host may be extremely elusive because scans are often negative, as are cultures of blood and liver.[73–75]

Treatment

The treatment of amebic liver abscess is antibiotic therapy, usually using metronidazole followed by diloxanide furoate, iodoquinol, or paromomycin. About 10% of patients require surgery owing to extrahepatic complications, rupture, or failure to respond.[51–54] Some patients undergo a diagnostic aspiration, which appears to hasten the initial response but provides no clear advantage with long-term follow-up in uncomplicated amebic abscesses.[99] Some authorities think that there is an advantage with routine percutaneous aspiration for amebic abscesses, especially those that exceed 6 cm in diameter.[99, 100]

Pyogenic abscesses sometimes respond to antimicrobial treatment alone,[101, 102] but most authorities advocate drainage. The major issue is the method of drainage, with three options: surgery, percutaneous drainage with insertion of a drain, or percutaneous aspiration. Each approach is accompanied by antibiotic treatment.

Surgical Drainage

The two operative approaches are extraserous drainage and transperitoneal drainage. Extraserous drainage was previously preferred because it avoids contamination of the peritoneal cavity. The extraserous approach involves a subcostal incision for anterior abscesses or a transpleural approach for a more posterior abscess. The problems are the limited ability to explore the liver (which increases the likelihood that adjacent or accessory abscesses will be overlooked) and the inability to identify sites of intraabdominal disease that may represent underlying lesions. With progress in surgical sepsis control, most surgeons now favor the transperitoneal approach using appropriate antibiotic coverage and peritoneal toilet. This affords the surgeon the opportunity to palpate the liver, aspirate suspicious lesions, and detect associated conditions in the abdominal cavity. The postoperative complication rate is generally reported at 30% to 40%, and the principal problems are recurrence of abscesses, intraabdominal abscesses, and wound infections.

Percutaneous Drainage

Percutaneous drainage was developed in the mid-1970s as an alternative to surgical drainage. Potential advantages are reduced cost, no need for general anesthesia, avoidance of postoperative complications, and apparently shorter recovery period. Potential disadvantages are that the liver cannot be explored and that sites of intraabdominal pathology may go undetected. The drain may be placed by trocar insertion or over a guide wire (Seldinger technique). Principles of drain management are analogous to those for drains placed at surgery. Gerzof and coworkers[94, 107] emphasized that dependent drainage is not mandatory, that drains should be left in place for at least 2 to 3 weeks, that instillation of contrast material is contraindicated, and that instillation of antibiotics is not necessary. Multiple drains may be placed for patients with multiple hepatic abscesses, and as many as eight discrete abscesses have been drained in this fashion in a single patient (Gerzof S, personal communication). The published experience shows morbidity and mortality rates that are as low or lower than those achieved with surgery.[32, 84–86, 103–113] Although surgical treatment of hepatic abscesses is still controversial, most authorities now conclude that it should be reserved for cases that fail to respond to percutaneous drainage.

Antibiotic Treatment

McFadzean and colleagues[101] reported the successful treatment of 14 patients with solitary liver abscesses using both parenteral and percutaneous instillation of antibiotics in 1953. At that time prompt surgical drainage was considered the mainstay of therapy. Although authors occasionally reported successful antibiotic management of anecdotal cases, this impression that surgery was required prevailed until the late 1970s. In 1979, Maher and colleagues[102] from the Los Angeles County–University of Southern California Medical Center reported successful medical management of six patients. Since then, other reports have supported the impression that antibiotic treatment alone is satisfactory[114–116] (Table 95–5). In many of these cases, percutaneous aspiration was used to determine the microbiology to facilitate antibiotic selection, and this assisted drainage as well. Others have been less successful with this approach.[117] In some instances, patients have been treated empirically with metronidazole for suspected amebic abscess; subsequent serology excluded this

TABLE 95–5 ■ Medical Management of Hepatic Abscess

SOURCE	MANAGEMENT	CURE RATE
Berger and Osborne[114]	Antibiotics + aspiration	15/15 (100%)
Herbert et al[115]	Antibiotics ± aspiration	9/10 (90%)
Reynolds[116]	Antibiotics ± aspiration	13/15 (87%)
McCorkell and Niles[117]	Antibiotics ± aspiration	1/14 (7%)

diagnosis, although the prompt clinical response implicated anaerobic infection and the possibility of avoiding a drainage procedure.

ANTIBIOTIC SELECTION

Most hepatic abscesses contain pathogens similar to those in intraabdominal sepsis—coliforms and anaerobic bacteria. Thus, the regimens commonly used to treat intraabdominal sepsis are often advocated for empirical use in pyogenic liver abscesses. This decision is obviously simplified if the bacterial population of the lesion is defined, as by aspiration of the abscess, although the clinical experience has taught that bacteriologic patterns are largely predictable. Problematic organisms that may not be addressed with commonly used regimens include *Pseudomonas aeruginosa,* enterococci, and *S. aureus.* Metronidazole is often included in the initial regimen owing to the possibility of amebiasis as well as optimal activity versus anaerobes. The use of an aminoglycoside with metronidazole is ill-advised, owing to the apparent importance of aerobic and microaerophilic streptococci, especially *S. milleri.* Commonly recommended regimens include a third-generation cephalosporin combined with metronidazole or clindamycin, an aminoglycoside with metronidazole and ampicillin, or some other regimen that is commonly used in intraabdominal sepsis.

Prognosis

The mortality rate reported by Ochsner for his series in the preantibiotic era was 80%.[3] During the early antibiotic era, numerous reports indicated a persistently high mortality rate, in the range of 65% to 80%. More recent reports have shown decreased mortality rates of 10% to 25%, presumably owing to more accurate and earlier diagnosis. The major factor that now influences outcome is the number of abscesses.[8] Most studies show that, regardless of the type of therapy or the period of review, substantially higher mortality rates are associated with multiple abscesses than with single abscesses. In the series by Ochsner,[3] the difference was 37% versus 90%; in the Duke series representing the modern experience, the difference was 15% versus 41%.[8] Mortality also seems to correlate directly with age and with associated diseases.[118]

References

1. Beeson PB, Brannon ES, Warren JV: Observations on the sites of removal of bacteria from the blood in patients with bacterial endocarditis. J Exp Med 81:9, 1945.
2. Bright J: Observations on jaundice: More particularly on that form of the disease which accompanies diffused inflammation of the liver. Guys Hosp Rep 1:630, 1836.
3. Ochsner A, Debakey M, Murray S: Pyogenic abscesses of the liver. II. An analysis of forty-seven cases with review of the literature. Am J Surg 40:292, 1938.
4. Norris GW, Farley DC: Abscess of the liver. Med Clin North Am 10:17, 1926.
5. Collins AN: Abscess of the liver. Minn Med 15:756, 1932.
6. Knowles R, Rinaldo JA: Pyogenic hepatic abscess secondary to sigmoid diverticulitis. Gastroenterology 38:262, 1960.
7. Ribaudo JM, Ochsner A: Intrahepatic abscesses: Amebic and pyogenic. Am J Surg 125:570, 1973.
8. McDonald MI, Corey GR, Gallis HA, Durack DT: Single and multiple pyogenic liver abscesses: Natural history, diagnosis and treatment, with emphasis on percutaneous drainage. Medicine (Baltimore) 63:291, 1984.
9. McDonald AP, Howard RJ: Pyogenic liver abscess. World J Surg 4:369, 1980.
10. Robertson RD, Foster JH, Peterson CG: Pyogenic liver abscess studies by cholangiography: Case report and 25 year review. Ann Surg 32:521, 1966.
11. Sabbaj J, Sutter VL, Finegold SM: Anaerobic pyogenic liver abscess. Ann Intern Med 77:629, 1972.
12. Finegold SM: Anaerobic Bacteria in Human Disease. New York, Harcourt, 1977.
13. de la Maza LM, Naeim F, Berman L: The changing etiology of liver abscess. JAMA 227:161, 1974.
14. Heymann AD: Clinical aspects of grave pyogenic abscess of the liver. Surg Gynecol Obstet 149:209, 1979.
15. McFadzean AJS, Chang KPS, Wong CC: Colitary pyogenic abscess of the liver treated by closed aspiration and antibiotics. Br J Surg 41:141, 1953.
16. Pitt HA, Zuidema GD: Factors influencing mortality in the treatment of pyogenic hepatic abscess. Surg Gynecol Obstet 140:228, 1975.
17. Pyrtek LJ, Bartus SA: Hepatic pyemia. N Engl J Med 272:551, 1965.
18. Rubin RH, Swartz MN, Malt R: Hepatic abscess: Changes in clinical, bacteriologic and therapeutic aspects. Am J Med 57:601, 1974.
19. Warren KW, Hardy KJ: Pyogenic hepatic abscess. Arch Surg 97:40, 1968.
20. Altemeier WA: Pyogenic liver abscess. *In* Schiff L, Schiff ER (eds): Diseases of the Liver. Philadelphia, JB Lippincott, 1983.
21. Balasegaram M: Management of hepatic abscess. Curr Prob Surg 18:285, 1981.
22. Chattopadhyay B: Pyogenic liver abscess. J Infect 6:5, 1983.
23. DeBakey ME, Jordan GL: Hepatic abscesses, both intra- and extra-hepatic. Surg Clin North Am 57:325, 1977.
24. Pyogenic liver abscess (Editorial). Br Med J 280:1155, 1980.
25. Lee JF, Block GE: The changing clinical pattern of hepatic abscesses. Arch Surg 104:465, 1972.
26. Brodine WN, Schwartz SI: Pyogenic liver abscess. Br J Hosp Med 26:47, 1981.
27. Neoptolemos JP, Macpherson DS: Pyogenic liver abscess. Br J Hosp Med 26:47, 1981.
28. Dietrich RB: Experience with liver abscess. Am J Surg 147:288, 1984.
29. Perera MR, Kirk A, Noone P: Presentation, diagnosis and management of liver abscess. Lancet 2:629, 1980.
30. Price JE, Joseph WL, Mulder DG: Diagnosis and treatment of intra-hepatic abscess. Am Surg 33:820, 1967.
31. Wintch RW, Reines HD, Rambo WM: Liver abscess: A changing entity. Am Surg 48:11, 1982.
32. Yinnon AM, Hadas-Halpern I, Shapiro M, et al: The changing clinical spectrum of liver abscess: The Jerusalem experience. Postgrad Med J 70:436, 1994.
33. Georges RN, Deitch EA: Pyogenic hepatic abscess. South Med J 86:1233, 1993.
34. Teh LB, Ng HS, Kwok KC, et al: Liver abscess—A clinical study. Ann Acad Med Singapore 15:176, 1986.
35. Mehta RB, Parija SC, Chetty DV, Smile RR: Management of 240 cases of liver abscess. Int Surg 71:91, 1986.
36. Levitt MD, Quinlan MF, Sheiner HJ: Liver abscess in Western Australia (1974–1983). Aust N Z J Surg 56:341, 1986.
37. Mir-Madjlessi SH, McHenry MC, Farmer RG: Liver abscess in Crohn's disease. Report of four cases and review of the literature. Gastroenterology 91:987, 1986.
38. Vakil N, Hayne G, Sharma A, et al: Liver abscess in Crohn's disease. Am J Gastroenterol 89:1090, 1994.
39. Greenstein AJ, Sachar DB, Lowenthal D, et al: Pyogenic liver abscess in Crohn's disease. Q J Med 56:505, 1985.
40. Tweedy CR, White WB: Multiple *Fusobacterium nucleatum* liver abscesses. Association with a persistent abnormality in humoral immune function. J Clin Gastroenterol 9:194, 1987.
41. Francis IR, Glazer GM, Amendola MA, Trenkner SW: Hepatic abscesses in the immunocompromised patient: Role of CT in detection, diagnosis, management, and follow-up. Gastrointest Radiol 11:257, 1986.
42. Skibber JM, Lotze MT, Garra B, Fauci A: Successful management of hepatic abscesses by percutaneous catheter drainage in chronic granulomatous disease. Surgery 99:626, 1986.
43. Chew SK, Lim HS, Mah PK, et al: Pyogenic hepatic abscess and diabetes mellitus—A probable association. Ann Acad Med Singapore 14:261, 1985.

44. Shulman ST, Beem MO: A unique presentation of sickle cell disease. Pyogenic hepatic abscess. Pediatrics 47:1019, 1971.
45. Shirkhoda A, Lopez-Berestein G, Holbert JM, Luna MA: Hepatosplenic fungal infection: CT and pathologic evaluation after treatment with liposomal amphotericin B. Radiology 159:349, 1986.
46. Shenep JL, Kalwinsky DK, Feldman S, Pearson TA: Mycotic cervical lymphadenitis following oral mucositis in children with leukemia. J Pediatr 106:243, 1985.
47. DeVoe PW, Buckley RH, Shirley LR, et al: Successful immune reconstitution in severe combined immunodeficiency despite Epstein-Barr virus and cytomegalovirus infections. Clin Immunol Immunopathol 34:48, 1985.
48. Kusne S, Dummer JS, Singh N, et al: Infections after liver transplantation. An analysis of 101 consecutive cases. Medicine (Baltimore) 57:132, 1988.
49. Pottipati AR, Dave PB, Gumaste V, et al: Tuberculosis abscess of the liver in acquired immunodeficiency syndrome. J Clin Gastroenterol 13:549, 1991.
50. Nordestgaard AG, Stapleford L, Worthen N, et al: Contemporary management of amebic liver abscess. Am Surg 58:315, 1992.
51. Ahmed M, McAdam KP, Sturm AW, et al: Systemic manifestations of invasive amebiasis. Clin Infect Dis 15:974, 1992.
52. Chuah SK, Chang-Chien CS, Sheen IS, et al: The prognostic factors of severe amebic liver abscess: A retrospective study of 125 cases. Am J Trop Med Hyg 46:398, 1992.
53. Meng XY, Wu JX: Perforated amebic liver abscess: Clinical analysis of 110 cases. South Med J 87:985, 1994.
54. Hai AA, Singh A, Mittal VL, et al: Amoebic liver abscess. Review of 220 cases. Int Surg 76:81, 1991.
55. Moore-Gillon JC, Eykyn SJ, Phillips I: Microbiology of pyogenic liver abscess. Br Med J 283:819, 1981.
56. Chua D, Reihart HH, Sobel JD: Liver abscess caused by *Streptococcus milleri*. Rev Infect Dis 11:197, 1989.
57. Braun TI, Travis D, Dee RR, et al: Liver abscess due to *Listeria monocytogenes:* Case report and review. Clin Infect Dis 17:267, 1993.
58. Vadillo M, Corbella X, Pac V, et al: Multiple liver abscesses due to *Yersinia enterocolitica* discloses primary hemochromatosis: Three case reports and review. Clin Infect Dis 18:938, 1994.
59. Leighton PM, MacSween HM: *Yersinia* hepatic abscesses subsequent to long-term iron therapy. JAMA 257:964, 1987.
60. Hopewood AH, Riddle BW: *Yersinia enterocolitica* hepatic abscesses. J Ky Med Assoc 84:13, 1986.
61. Cortez JC, Shapiro M, Awe RJ: *Pasteurella multocida* liver abscess. Am J Med Sci 292:107, 1986.
62. Mongiardo N, De Rienzo B, Zanchetta G, et al: Primary hepatic actinomycosis. J Infect 12:65, 1986.
63. Roesler PJ Jr, Willis JS: Hepatic actinomycosis: CT features. J Comput Assist Tomogr 10:335, 1986.
64. Miyamoto MI, Fang FC: Pyogenic liver abscess involving *Actinomyces:* Case report and review. Clin Infect Dis 16:303, 1993.
65. Vatcharapreechasakul T, Suputtamongkol Y, Dance DA, et al: *Pseudomonas pseudomallei* liver abscesses: A clinical, laboratory, and ultrasonographic study. Clin Infect Dis 14:412, 1992.
66. Kubota H, Ageta M, Kubo H, et al: Tuberculous liver abscess treated by percutaneous infusion of antituberculous agents. Intern Med 33:351, 1994.
67. Moore SW, Millar AJ, Cywes S: Conservative initial treatment of liver abscesses in children. Br J Surg 81:872, 1994.
68. Vachon L, Diament MJ, Stanley P: Percutaneous drainage of hepatic abscesses in children. J Pediatr Surg 21:366, 1986.
69. Bilfinger TV, Hayden CK, Oldham KT, Lobe TE: Pyogenic liver abscesses in nonimmunocompromised children. South Med J 79:37, 1986.
70. Diament MJ, Stanley P, Kangarloo H, Donaldson JS: Percutaneous aspiration and catheter drainage of abscesses. J Pediatr 108:204, 1986.
71. Karrar ZA, Abdullah MA: Pyogenic liver abscess in children: A report of three patients and review of the literature. Ann Trop Paediatr 5:97, 1985.
72. Brook I, Fraizer EH: Role of anaerobic bacteria in liver abscesses in children. Pediatr Infect Dis J 12:743, 1993.
73. Haron E, Feld R, Tuffnell P, et al: Hepatitis candidiasis: An increasing problem in immunocompromised patients. Am J Med 83:17, 1987.
74. Thaler M, Pastakia B, Shawker T, et al: Hepatic candidiasis in cancer patients: The evolving picture of the syndrome. Ann Intern Med 108:88, 1988.
75. Flannery MT, Simmons DB, Saba H, et al: Fluconazole in the treatment of hepatosplenic candidiasis. Arch Intern Med 152:406, 1992.
76. Lee TY, Wan TY, Tsai CC: Gas-containing liver abscess: Radiological findings and clinical significance. Abdom Imaging 19:47, 1994.
77. Rubinson HA, Isikoff MB, Hill MC: Diagnostic imaging of hepatic abscesses: A retrospective analysis. AJR 135:735, 1980.
78. Kemeny MM, Sugarbaker PH, Smith TJ, et al: A prospective analysis of laboratory tests and imaging studies to detect hepatic lesions. Ann Surg 195:163, 1982.
79. Conter RL, Pitt HA, Tompkins RK, et al: Differentiation of pyogenic from amebic hepatic abscesses. Surg Gynecol Obstet 162:114, 1986.
80. Kandel G, Marcon NE: Pyogenic liver abscess: New concepts of an old disease. Am J Gastroenterol 79:65, 1984.
81. Rubin RH, Swartz MN, Malt R: Hepatic abscess: Changes in clinical, bacteriological and therapeutic aspects. Am J Med 57:601, 1974.
82. Kuligowska E, Noble J: Sonography of hepatic abscesses. Semin Ultrasound 4:102, 1983.
83. Newlin N, Silver TM, Stuck KJ, et al: Ultrasonic features of pyogenic liver abscess. Radiology 139:155, 1981.
84. Donovan AJ, Yellin AE, Ralls PW: Hepatic abscess. World J Surg 15:162, 1991.
85. Barreda R, Ros PR: Diagnostic imaging of liver abscess. Crit Rev Diagn Imaging 33:29, 1992.
86. Philips RL: Computed tomography and ultrasound in the diagnosis and treatment of liver abscesses. Australas Radiol 38:165, 1994.
87. Fawcett HD, Lantieri RL, Frankel A, McDougall IR: Differentiating hepatic abscess from tumor. AJR 135:53, 1980.
88. Shih WJ, Domstad PA, DeLand FH: "Hot" and "cold" lesions detected by gallium-67 scintigraphy in a pyogenic liver abscess. Eur J Nucl Med 10:123, 1985.
89. Haentjens M, Piepsz A, Schell-Frederick E, et al: Limitations in the use of indium-111-oxine–labeled leukocytes for the diagnosis of occult infection in children. Pediatr Radiol 17:139, 1987.
90. Lomena F, Abello R, Garcia A, et al: False-positive early indium-111 leukocyte scan. Clin Nucl Med 12:391, 1987.
91. Buchman TG, Zuideman GD: The role of computerized tomographic scanning in the surgical management of pyogenic hepatic abscess. Surg Gynecol Obstet 153:1, 1981.
92. Callen PW: Computed tomographic evaluation of abdominal and pelvic abscesses. Radiology 131:171, 1979.
93. Haaga JR, Weinstein AJ: CT-guided percutaneous aspiration and drainage of abscesses. AJR 135:1187, 1980.
94. Gerzof SG, Robbins AH, Johnson WC, et al: Percutaneous catheter drainage of abdominal abscesses: A five-year experience. N Engl J Med 305:653, 1981.
95. Mathiew D, Vasile N, Fagniez PL, et al: Dynamic CT features of hepatic abscesses. Radiology 154:749, 1985.
96. Vasquez TE, Evans DG, Schiffman H, Ashburn WL: Fungal splenic abscesses in the immunocompromised patient. Correlation of imaging modalities. Clin Nucl Med 12:36, 1987.
97. Abd-Alla MD, Jackson TF, Gathiram V, et al: Differentiation of pathogenic *Entamoeba histolytica* infections from nonpathogenic infections by detection of galactose-inhibitable adherence protein antigen in sera and feces. J Clin Microbiol 31:2845, 1993.
98. Flores BM, Reed SL, Ravdin JI, et al: Serologic reactivity to purified recombinant and native 29-kilodalton peripheral membrane protein of pathogenic *Entamoeba histolytica.* J Clin Microbiol 31:1403, 1993.
99. Ramini A, Ramani R, Kumar MS, et al: Ultrasound-guided needle aspiration of amoebic liver abscess. Postgrad Med J 69:38, 1993.
100. Adams EB, MacLeod IN: Invasive amebiasis. II. Amebic liver abscess and its complications. Medicine 56:325, 1977.
101. McFadzean AJR, Chang KPS, Wong CC: Solitary abscess of the liver treated by closed aspiration and antibiotics: Fourteen cases with recovery. Br J Surg 41:141, 1953.
102. Maher JA, Reynolds TB, Yellin AE: Successful medical treatment of pyogenic liver abscess. Gastroenterology 77:618, 1979.

103. Kraulis JE, Bird BL, Colapinto ND: Percutaneous catheter drainage of liver abscess: An alternative to open drainage. Br J Surg 67:400, 1980.
104. Attar B, Levendoglu H, Cuasay NS: CT-guided percutaneous aspiration and catheter drainage of pyogenic liver abscesses. Am J Gastroenterol 81:550, 1986.
105. Bertel CK, van Heerden JA, Sheedy PF: Treatment of pyogenic hepatic abscesses. Surgical vs. percutaneous drainage. Arch Surg 121:554, 1986.
106. Porter JA, Loughry CW, Cook AJ: Use of the computerized tomographic scan in the diagnosis and treatment of abscesses. Am J Surg 150:257, 1985.
107. Gerzof SG, Johnson WC, Robbins AH, Nabseth DC: Intrahepatic pyogenic abscesses: Treatment by percutaneous drainage. Am J Surg 149:487, 1985.
108. Moulds-Merritt C, Frazee RC: Therapeutic approach to hepatic abscesses. South Med J 87:884, 1994.
109. Chou FF, Sheen-Chen SM, Chen YS: Prognostic factors for pyogenic abscess of the liver. J Am Coll Surg 179:727, 1994.
110. Stain SC, Yellin AE, Donovan AJ, et al: Pyogenic liver abscess. Modern treatment. Arch Surg 126:991, 1991.
111. Vary TC, Kimball SR: Regulation of hepatic protein synthesis in chronic inflammation and sepsis. Am J Physiol 262:445, 1992.
112. Hansen N, Vargish T: Pyogenic hepatic abscess: A case for open drainage. Am Surg 59:219, 1993.
113. Nosher JL, Giudici M, Needell GS, et al: Elective one-stage abdominal operations after percutaneous catheter drainage of pyogenic liver abscess. Am Surg 59:658, 1993.
114. Berger LA, Osborne DR: Treatment of pyogenic liver abscesses by percutaneous needle aspiration. Lancet 1:132, 1982.
115. Herbert DA, Rothman J, Fogel DA, et al: Pyogenic liver abscesses: Successful non-surgical therapy. Lancet 1:134, 1982.
116. Reynolds TB: Medical treatment of pyogenic liver abscess. Ann Intern Med 96:373, 1982.
117. McCorkell SJ, Niles NL: Pyogenic liver abscesses: Another look at medical management. Lancet 1:803, 1985.
118. Land MA, Moinuddin M, Bisno AL: Pyogenic liver abscess: Changing epidemiology and prognosis. South Med J 78:1426, 1985.

96

Amebic Liver Abscess

J. Joseph Marr

History

Amebiasis is an intestinal disease that occasionally spreads to involve the liver or, rarely, to pass beyond the liver and enter the systemic circulation. It is one of the best known of the diarrheal illnesses. The pathogenic organism *Entamoeba histolytica* is a cause of substantial morbidity in developing countries and is one of the most important intestinal diseases to which travelers are exposed.

Experiments that demonstrated that amoebae are pathogenic were first performed approximately a century ago by Losch, in St. Petersburg, Russia, when lesions were induced in a dog with dysenteric stool.[1] In 1891, Councilman and Lafleur demonstrated the distinction between bacillary and amebic dysentery, as reported by Kean and coworkers.[2] Although the disease is endemic in most developing countries, some of the best studied epidemics have been in the United States. One of the best known occurred at the Chicago Century of Progress Exposition in 1933, the result of a cross-connection between sewage and water lines.[3] The organism is widespread in the developing world and can be found in approximately 5% of persons in many areas of temperate climate. For this reason, contamination of drinking water not uncommonly results in epidemic spread of the disease.

Characteristics of the Pathogen

E. histolytica is an anaerobic protozoan classified in the subphylum Sarcodina. There are several species in the genus *Entamoeba* but only *E. histolytica* is believed to produce disease in humans. Other members of this genus that may be confused with *E. histolytica* are *Entamoeba coli, Entamoeba gingivalis, Entamoeba hartmanni*, and *Entamoeba polecki*. The organism is distinct from members of the genera *Naegleria* and *Acanthamoeba*, which are free-living.

E. histolytica has two forms: the trophozoite, which is the vegetative form, and the cyst. The cyst is highly tolerant of environmental extremes; it also resists destruction by mildly corrosive agents. It is ideally suited to protect the organism outside its host. When the cyst is ingested, it undergoes a nuclear division to form eight nuclei, which is characteristic of this organism and helps distinguish it from the similar looking *E. coli*. The organism excysts to form eight trophozoites. The excystation occurs in the large bowel because it requires the presence of anaerobic flora to maintain the necessary low redox potential. The trophozoites continue to divide in the large bowel and, depending on the infecting dose, may produce no symptoms, mild symptoms, or severe invasive disease. During the course of the infection, some of the trophozoites encyst again and are shed into the environment to complete the life cycle.

Epidemiology

Amebiasis is spread by fecal-oral transmission. In developing countries, where sanitary measures may be less stringent, transmission of the organism is relatively common. In the United States, persons at greatest risk for acquiring the disease are those in institutions for the mentally retarded and travelers to the developing world. It has become evident that homosexual and bisexual males are also at increased risk of acquiring amebiasis and other diarrheal illnesses. This increased incidence of diarrheal disease among homosexuals was originally given the name "gay bowel syndrome" and is now known to be a manifestation of superinfection in persons infected with the human immunodeficiency virus.

Pathogenesis

The major pathologic feature of intestinal amebiasis is local ulcerative destruction of the wall of the large intestine (Fig. 96–1). Cytolysis requires intact amebic microfilament function and calcium flux.[4, 5] Cytotoxic amebic proteins have been described. Amebic proteolytic enzymes may be responsible for the initial destruction of epithelial barriers, but these activities do not correlate with virulence in vivo.[6] The organisms also have collagenase activity, which is associated with the membrane of the trophozoite and correlates with strain virulence.[7] For a more complete review of the specifics of importance of amebic strain variation and certain host factors, see Ravdin and coworkers.[5]

The mechanism of tissue lysis (hence the name *E. histolytica*) is not clear. It is known that lysis requires direct contact with the tissue and is calcium dependent. The ulcers are found only in the large bowel, presumably because of the

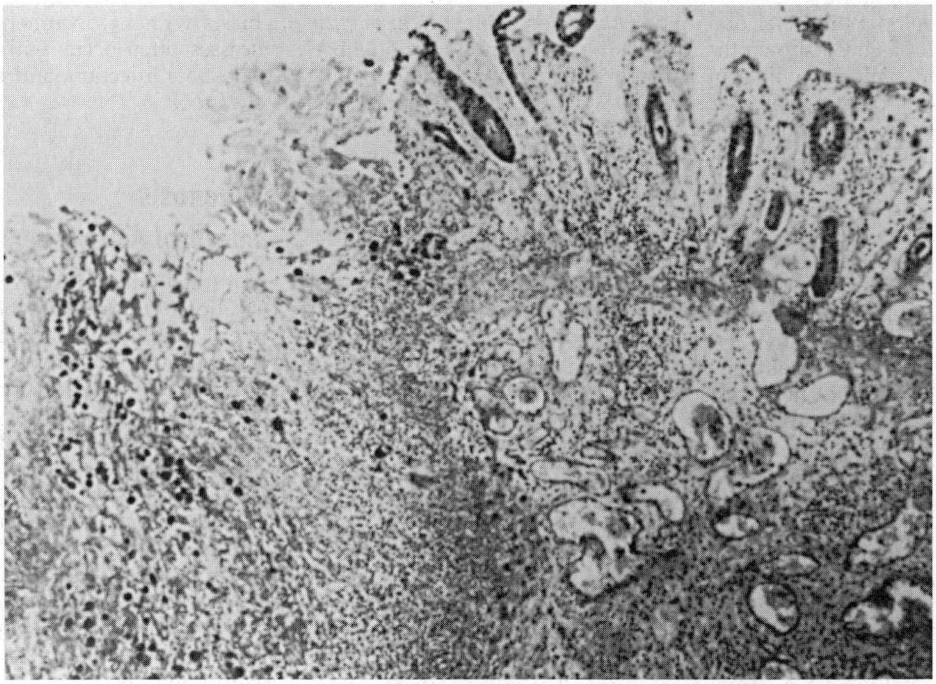

FIGURE 96–1 □ Light micrograph demonstrates a flask-shaped ulcer in a pathologic specimen from a patient with severe colonic amebiasis (periodic acid–Schiff stain, × 16). (From Ravdin JI, Guerrant RL: A review of the parasite cellular mechanisms involved in the pathogenesis of amebiasis. Rev Infect Dis 4:1185–1207, 1982. © by The University of Chicago Press.)

anaerobic nature of this protozoan, which requires a low redox potential for growth and development. Once the organism begins to destroy the tissue, liquefactive necrosis and the organism's ability to destroy leukocytes[8] sustain the anaerobic environment even in the absence of accompanying fecal bacteria. Severe amebiasis results in necrotic ulcerations, which may perforate to the peritoneum, although this complication is unusual. Dissemination from the large bowel to the liver occurs by way of the portal venous system. Because the portal blood tends to be shunted into the right lobe of the liver by the admixture of blood from the splenic vein, hepatic amebic abscesses tend to be located in that lobe (Fig. 96–2). Occasionally, the organisms enter the inferior mesenteric venous system and bypass the liver to cause pulmonary infection or pass into the systemic circulation to produce infection in accordance with the distribution of the cardiac output. Severe hepatic amebic abscesses can enter the hepatic venous system and thereby pass into the systemic circulation as well. Extension of extraintestinal amebiasis beyond the liver is unusual, however.

The destructive potential of these protozoans is significant, and the architecture of the invaded tissue generally is lost. There is liquefactive necrosis in the intestinal ulcers and complete destruction of the liver parenchyma in areas where abscesses form (see Fig. 96–2). The organisms themselves are found not in the central portions of the abscesses but at the margins. For this reason, the nature of the lesion should be confirmed by biopsy of the edge of the ulcer or the margin of the hepatic abscess rather than the central necrotic material.

When there is extraintestinal disease, infected humans de-

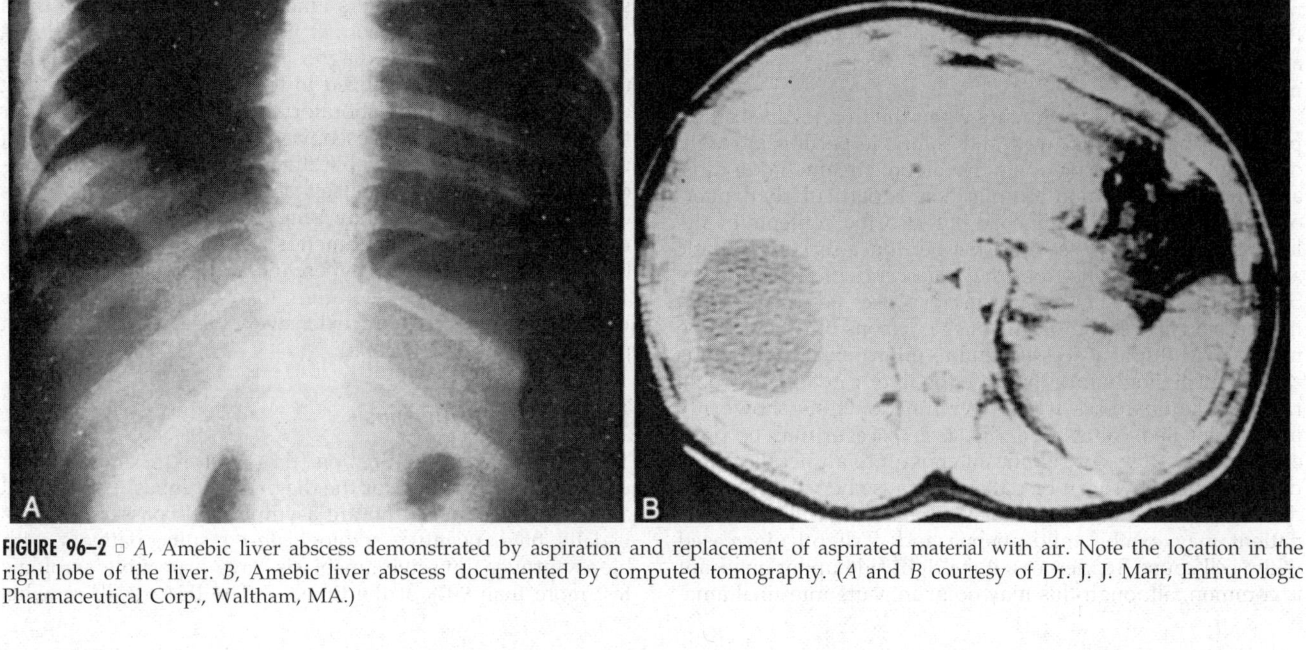

FIGURE 96–2 □ *A*, Amebic liver abscess demonstrated by aspiration and replacement of aspirated material with air. Note the location in the right lobe of the liver. *B*, Amebic liver abscess documented by computed tomography. (*A* and *B* courtesy of Dr. J. J. Marr, Immunologic Pharmaceutical Corp., Waltham, MA.)

velop a high titer of antibodies directed against *E. histolytica.* It has been shown that there is no rise in immunoglobulin G in patients with acute amebic dysentery or asymptomatic cyst passers; however, persons with active hepatic amebiasis have significant increases. This is a measure of extraintestinal invasion and is the basis for the enzyme-linked immunosorbent assay, which is always positive in persons with liver abscess (see later). This same study demonstrated that persons with active amebic dysentery had increases in immunoglobulin M but asymptomatic cyst passers did not. This is additional evidence of the benign nature of the latter form of amebiasis.[9] Humoral immunity is associated with activation of the alternative complement pathway,[10] but recurrent colonic and hepatic amebiasis is well documented despite the presence of high antibody titers.[11, 12] However, some clinical data indicate that the recurrence of invasive colitis or liver abscess is rare in areas of high endemicity.[13] Thus, there may be value to continued exposure to the organism.[14] This is supported experimentally by studies with SCID (severe combined immunodeficient) mice, which showed that, when challenged intrahepatically, these mice uniformly developed abscesses.[15] Transfer of polyclonal antiserum protected about 50% of the mice from hepatic infection. This suggests that both humoral immunity and lymphocyte mediated immunity are important in protection against amebic liver abscess.

Like most eukaryotic organisms that invade tissue, amoebae provoke a cell-mediated immune response. Evidence for the role of cell-mediated immunity in the prevention of invasive amebic disease is accumulating.[5] Amoebae destroy neutrophils, monocytes, and peripheral blood mononuclear cells; however, human monocyte–derived macrophages can kill virulent amebic trophozoites after suitable activation.[16]

Clinical Manifestations

Clinical manifestations of amebiasis can be classified as follows: (1) asymptomatic infection, (2) intestinal amebiasis, and (3) extraintestinal amebiasis. Most persons infected with this organism have no symptoms. The organism may be eliminated spontaneously, or it may persist silently. There is little correlation between symptoms of intestinal disease and the presence of the organism in stool samples.

The clinical manifestations probably depend on the dose of organisms ingested. Symptomatic intestinal amebiasis may present as mild lower abdominal discomfort, lower abdominal pain with diarrhea, or severe colitis with bloody diarrhea. Because tissue is invaded, the person often is febrile. There are blood and leukocytes in the stool, and abdominal pain may be significant.

Extraintestinal disease occurs when the trophozoites either perforate the intestinal wall and enter the peritoneal cavity or progress to the liver via the blood stream. Peritonitis, although an uncommon complication, is particularly dangerous because not only amoebae but also the contents of the large bowel are released into the peritoneal cavity. Hepatic abscess usually results from the coalescence of areas of amebic hepatitis as the liquefactive necrosis becomes the predominant lesion. These are usually single lesions but they can be multiple. Multiple abscesses tend to interconnect. Symptoms can be surprisingly mild because the liver can accommodate rather large abscesses while liver function tests show only mildly elevated values (see Fig. 96–2*A*). Fever may be present, but it is often not significant enough to attract the attention of either physician or patient. Because hepatic abscesses due to amoebae are often subacute or chronic lesions, the patient may exhibit mild anemia and a slightly increased white cell count. Tenderness of the right side upper quadrant is common, although this may occur in acute intestinal amebiasis without documented hepatic involvement. Liver abscesses often occur without clinical evidence of preexisting intestinal infection, and the organism may not be present in the stool.

Diagnosis

Intestinal Amebiasis

Intestinal infection with *E. histolytica* is diagnosed by demonstration of the cysts or the trophozoites in stool specimens. In the United States, the demonstration of either is considered diagnostic of infection; in developing countries, where infection is common, such persons may be considered asymptomatic carriers. The success of identifying amoebae depends on the techniques for identification of trophozoites, which is, in turn, a function of the frequency with which the disease exists in the community and the average specimen load for the laboratory. The best methods for identification are given here.

Direct Examination. A fresh stool specimen or a specimen obtained during endoscopy can be examined directly for the presence of motile, erythrocyte-containing amoebae. The specimen should be mixed with saline and examined on a warm microscope stage. The characteristic motility is directed, linear movement. Endoscopy specimens have the greatest yield when the edge of the ulcer is scraped or a biopsy of the margin is taken.

Fixed Specimens. Identification of the hematophagous trophozoites can be accomplished by fixing the stool specimen in polyvinyl alcohol after it is smeared on a microscope slide. These can be stained with trichrome or iron hematoxylin. The most difficult differential diagnosis is between *E. histolytica* and *E. coli.* The former can be differentiated by the central position of nucleolus and the fine peripheral chromatin pattern.

Stool Centrifugation. If the stool specimen is to be concentrated, it can be suspended in 6% formalin solution for fixation and centrifuged. It is then resuspended in formol-ether (5:1). After centrifugation, a drop of the sediment can be examined with a drop of dilute iodine solution (1% to 2%) for the presence of cysts.

Fresh Stool Culture. *E. histolytica* can be cultured from fresh stool, but this method is somewhat cumbersome and generally is done only in specialized laboratories. A single stool examination discovers amebiasis only about one third of the time. For this reason, at least three specimens should be submitted before the diagnosis is excluded.[17, 18] Occasionally, disease may be localized to the cecum or the ascending colon, and the yield on laboratory examination is low. Under these circumstances, endoscopy with biopsy or scraping of the lesion may be a valuable diagnostic technique. The disease generally manifests itself as small hemorrhagic areas or small ulcers, which may range in diameter from a few millimeters to a few centimeters. In ulcerative colitis, the bowel is more generally hyperemic and bleeds more easily. The erythema is diffuse rather than punctate. Shigellosis is characterized by more extensively diseased bowel with purulent, ulcerative lesions.

Extraintestinal Amebiasis

The indirect hemagglutination (IHA) test is the most widely used serologic method for the diagnosis of invasive intestinal amebiasis.[19] Persons who are asymptomatic passers of cysts usually have negative serologic test results; patients with biopsy-proven invasive amebiasis have a positive serologic test more than 90% of the time.[19, 20] The IHA result remains elevated (at least 1:128) for many years after the invasive disease. This test is useful in the diagnosis of invasive or extraintestinal amebiasis; it is also useful for persons who have nonamebic inflammatory bowel disease because the result is rarely false-positive.[21] The aforementioned enzyme-linked immunosorbent assay appears to be as good as the IHA test but has not yet received sufficient clinical testing to recommend it.

The best methods for demonstrating an amebic liver abscess are computed tomography and ultrasonography (see Fig. 96–2*B*). Radionuclide scanning, used frequently in the past, has been replaced by these two modalities. Gallium scans may be helpful in differentiating bacterial and amebic abscesses because the amebic abscess has a "cold" central area. The isotope is taken up at the border, where leukocytes are present.[22, 23] The result of the IHA test is almost always positive when an amebic liver abscess is present. In this situation there may be no trophozoites or cysts in the stool; however, a stool examination should be performed because the finding of amoebae assists in the diagnosis of the liver mass. In the past, diagnostic aspiration was frequently used (see Fig. 96–2*A*). The characteristic material obtained is an odorless brown liquid that generally does not contain amoebae. As with the intestinal lesion, these organisms are more commonly found in the wall of the abscess. In the presence of a positive IHA result, a therapeutic trial with metronidazole is indicated rather than aspiration. The symptoms resolve rapidly in response to this therapy. If they do not, diagnostic aspiration is indicated to differentiate the lesion from a pyogenic abscess or neoplasm.

Treatment

From a therapeutic viewpoint, amebiasis may be considered according to whether it is asymptomatic or symptomatic. There is complete agreement that persons with symptomatic disease, whether intestinal or extraintestinal, should be treated. The question of whether to treat asymptomatic cyst passers is not resolved. Asymptomatic persons who have little or no chance of becoming reinfected should be treated. However, persons who are likely to become reinfected because they reside in a highly endemic area and homosexual men and others who exhibit promiscuous behavior will derive little benefit from therapy, and for them, emphasis should be placed on reducing the risk of reinfection. An exception to this rule is an acute outbreak of disease in an institution, such as a psychiatric facility, where a number of asymptomatic infections will exist. Under these circumstances it is beneficial to attempt to eliminate the infection from the institution.

Patients with extraintestinal amebiasis or symptomatic intestinal disease should be treated. Drug treatment varies with the site of infection: the lumen of the bowel, the wall of the intestine, extraintestinal sites. In general, metronidazole is the drug of choice for both intestinal and extraintestinal disease and is associated with a cure rate of greater than 90%. It is given as 750 mg three times per day for 5 to 10 days. Metronidazole has few serious side effects, but it is known to produce a disulfiram-like effect, and patients should be cautioned not to drink alcohol while taking the drug. It may also potentiate the anticoagulant effect of coumarin. A metallic taste is a not uncommon side effect, and there may be some epigastric discomfort as well. The urine of some patients may become red or brown owing to metabolic products of the drug.

Patients who do not respond to metronidazole are rare, but they may be treated with dihydroemetine (available from the Centers for Disease Control and Prevention) or, in the case of liver abscess, with the addition of chloroquine. The dose of dihydroemetine is 1 to 1.5 mg/kg per day for 5 days (maximal dose is 90 mg/d). The chloroquine dose is 600 mg of the base per day for 2 days, then 300 mg of base per day for 2 to 3 weeks.

Asymptomatic intestinal infections are treated with iodoquinol at a dose of 650 mg three times per day for 20 days. The second choice is diloxanide furoate at a dose of 500 mg three times per day for 10 days; it is available from the Centers for Disease Control and Prevention. Both are more effective than metronidazole for asymptomatic infection.

Dihydroemetine is prepared from ipecac and its toxic effects are many. The most common are gastrointestinal—diarrhea, nausea, and vomiting in one third of patients. The diarrhea is due to a direct action of the drug on the intestinal smooth muscle; the nausea and the vomiting are probably central in origin. Cardiovascular toxicity is the most important side effect. Symptoms include hypotension, precordial pain, arrhythmias, tachycardia, and dyspnea. These manifestations may mimic myocardial infarction. About half of patients exhibit electrocardiographic changes. Iodoquinol is poorly absorbed and for this reason is only a luminal agent. Like other iodine compounds, it may interfere with the results of thyroid function tests and can cause iodine dermatitis. Diloxanide furoate has few serious side effects. More detailed discussions of the pharmacology and toxicity of these antiparasitic agents may be found in Chapter 35.

The role of invasive procedures in the treatment of amebic abscess is no longer an area of debate. Needle aspiration is unnecessary for most patients for relief of symptoms or for therapy.[23] Approximately 10% to 15% of patients may require reduction in the size of the abscess before a therapeutic response is observed, and for them, needle aspiration may be useful. Surgical drainage is rarely necessary and should be avoided unless the abscess is inaccessible to needle drainage and response to therapy has not occurred within 5 or 6 days. Surgical procedures for drainage were relatively common in the past, but the advent of metronidazole has all but eliminated them. Similarly, there is rarely any need to correct amebic bowel perforation or peritonitis surgically.[24]

Prevention

No immunization is available for amebic infections, and prevention consists of efforts to eradicate fecal contamination of food and water. The most commonly contaminated items are fresh vegetables and water. The nonspecific antiseptics, such as low doses of chlorine or iodine, do not kill amoebae. Only boiling is absolutely effective. The most important factors in elimination of the infection are effective waste disposal and water purification. The avoidance by homosexual males and others of sexual practices that expose them to fecal contact will prevent infection in this population. Preventing infection in institutionalized persons, especially those who are mentally retarded, is difficult and generally resolves itself into close supervision of personal hygiene.

References

1. Losch FA: Massive development of amebas in the large intestine. Am J Trop Med Hyg 24:383, 1875.
2. Kean BH, Mott KE, Russel AJ: Tropical medicine and parasitology: Classic investigations. Ithaca, NY, Cornell University Press, 1978, p 79.
3. Select Committee: Amebiasis outbreak in Chicago: Report of a special committee. JAMA 102:369, 1934.
4. Ravdin JI, Kroft BY, Guerrant RL: Cytopathogenic mechanisms of *Entamoeba histolytica*. J Exp Med 152:377, 1980.

5. Ravdin JI, Sperelakis N, Guerrant RL: Effect of ion channel inhibitors on the cytopathogenecity of *Entamoeba histolytica.* J Infect Dis 146:335, 1982.
6. Jarumilinta R, Maegraith BG: Enzymes of *Entamoeba histolytica.* Bull WHO 41:269, 1969.
7. Gadasi H, Kessler E: Correlation of virulence and collagenolytic activity in *Entamoeba histolytica.* Infect Immun 39:528, 1983.
8. Jarumilinta R, Kradolfer F: The toxic effect of *Entamoeba histolytica* on leucocytes. Ann Trop Med Parasitol 58:375, 1964.
9. el-Ganayni GA, Attia RA, el-Naggar HM: Some immunological studies on amoebiasis. J Egypt Soc Parasitol 24:357, 1994.
10. Kapin R, Kapin NR, Carmona M, Ortiz-Ortiz L: Effect of complement depletion on the induction of amebic liver abscess in the hamster. Arch Invest Med (Mex) 11(Suppl 1):173, 1980.
11. Krupp IM, Powell SJ: Comparative study of the antibody response in amebiasis. Am J Trop Med Hyg 20:421, 1971.
12. Jenkinson SG, Hargrove MD, Jr: Recurrent amebic abscess of the liver. JAMA 232:277, 1975.
13. Sepulveda B, Martinez-Palomo A: Immunology of amoebiasis *Entamoeba histolytica. In* Cohen S, Warren VS (eds): Immunology of Parasitic Disease, ed 2. Oxford, UK, Blackwell Scientific Publications, 1982, p 170.
14. Tissl D: Immunology of *Entamoeba histolytica* in human and animal hosts. Rev Infect Dis 4:1154, 1982.
15. Cieslak PR, Virgin HW 4th, Stanley SL Jr: A severe combined immunodeficient (SCID) mouse model for infection with *Entamoeba histolytica.* J Exp Med 176:1605, 1992.
16. Salata RA, Pearson RD, Murphy CF, Ravdin JI: The interaction of *Entamoeba histolytica* with human white blood cells: Killing of virulent amebae by the activated macrophage. J Clin Invest 76:491, 1985.
17. Thacker SB, Simpson S, Gordon TJ, et al: Parasitic disease control in a residential facility for the mentally retarded. Am J Public Health 69:1279, 1979.
18. Mathur TN, Kaur J: The frequency of excretion of cysts of *Entamoeba histolytica* in known cases of nondysenteric amoebic colitis based on twelve stool examinations. Indian J Med Res 61:330, 1973.
19. Patterson M, Healy GR, Shabot JM: Serologic testing for amoebiasis. Gastroenterology 78:136, 1980.
20. Wolfe MS: Nondysenteric intestinal amebiasis: Treatment with diloxanide furoate. JAMA 224:1601, 1973.
21. Healy GR, Sumner CK: The indirect hemoglutination test for amebiasis in patients with inflammatory bowel disease. Am J Dig Dis 17:97, 1972.
22. Shabot JM, Patterson M: Amebic liver abscess 1966–1976. Dig Dis 23:110, 1978.
23. Katzenstein D, Rickerson B, Braude A: New concepts of amebic liver abscess derived from hepatic imaging, serodiagnosis, and hepatic enzymes in sixty-seven consecutive cases in San Diego. Medicine (Baltimore) 61:237, 1982.
24. Kapoor OP, Joshi BR: Multiple amoebic liver abscesses. A study of fifty-six cases. J Trop Med Hyg 75:4, 1972.

97

Cholecystitis and Cholangitis

Russell A. Williams
Samuel E. Wilson

Acute Calculous Cholecystitis

Gallstone disease is one of the most common afflictions of developed countries, and operations on the biliary tree are the most frequently performed abdominal procedures. Up to 500,000 cases are reported annually in the United States. Acute cholecystitis is associated with gallstones in 95% of cases, and only 5% are acalculous.

Epidemiology

PREVALENCE

The prevalence of gallstones is difficult to estimate accurately because figures based on autopsy series are not necessarily representative of those in living populations. Rates reported from oral cholecystographic or ultrasonographic studies also highlight symptomatic patients, and the larger, asymptomatic population is often not assessed by these investigations. At autopsy, the frequency of gallstones varies with age, race, and sex and ranges from 14% to 39% (Table 97–1).

NATURAL HISTORY

Autopsy studies show that approximately 75% of patients have asymptomatic gallstones.[1] The proportion of these asymptomatic patients who subsequently develop symptoms or complications has been estimated to be 15% at 10 years and 18% at 15 and 20 years.[2] Of patients who already have symptoms, 35% to 39% continue to have biliary pain or develop complications.[3, 4]

At Henry Ford Hospital 11.6% of 19,277 patients with benign biliary disease had acute cholecystitis; at Massachusetts General Hospital 20.8% of 2835 operations for cholecystitis were performed for acute disease.

TABLE 97–1 ■ Factors Associated with Incidence of Gallstones

FACTOR	EFFECT ON INCIDENCE
Ethnicity	Marked increase in Pima Indians, Mexicans, and Swedes
Geography	High incidence in United States, Great Britain, and Australia
Age	Increases with age
Sex	More common in females than in males
Pregnancy	Increases with parity
Obesity	
Clofibrate therapy	
Ileal disease or resection[33]	
Cirrhosis	Increases two- to threefold[34]
Total parenteral nutrition	Increases with prolonged therapy[35]
Hemolysis	

TABLE 97–2 ■ Microorganisms in Bile in Acute Cholecystitis: Classification of 199 Organisms

AEROBES—174 (87%)			
Gram-negative—132 (66%)		Gram-positive—42 (21%)	
Escherichia coli	77	*Enterococcus faecalis*	30
Klebsiella	22	β-Hemolytic streptococci	4
Proteus	13	*Staphylococcus epidermidis*	4
Enterobacter	8	*Streptococcus viridans*	1
Pseudomonas	4		
ANAEROBES—25 (13%)			
Gram-negative—1%		Gram-positive—23 (12%)	
Bacteroides sp.	2	*Clostridium perfringens*	16
		Peptostreptococcus	7

From Keighley MRB: Micro-organisms in the bile. A preventable cause of sepsis after biliary surgery. Ann R Coll Surg Engl 59:328, 1977.

The incidence of acute cholecystitis increases with the age of the population of patients, and this may reflect the presence of preexisting chronic cholecystitis with obliterative changes of the cystic artery.

Sex distribution is equal in childhood, but among adults, women are affected more frequently than men. Multiple pregnancies appear to be associated with increased frequency of acute cholecystitis.

Many patients give a history of episodes of biliary colic or acute cholecystitis. The rate of early recurrence varies from 5.3% to 23% but increases to 59% after 6 years.[5–7]

Pathogenesis

In the majority of patients, the cystic duct is obstructed by a gallstone and the hydrostatic pressure in the gallbladder lumen is markedly elevated. Bile salts and phospholipases (which transform phospholipids to cytotoxic lyso compounds) cause an initial chemical cholecystitis. Prostaglandin production increases in the inflamed gallbladder and stimulates secretion of fluid by the epithelium and contraction of the gallbladder wall. The fluid secretion results in increased hydrostatic pressure, which impairs the microcirculation and decreases both the viability of the gallbladder wall and the clearance rate of noxious intraluminal agents.

Bacteriology

Infection of the gallbladder appears to be a secondary phenomenon, with up to 60% of patients' gallbladder bile cultures being positive and the percentage increasing with the duration of cholecystitis.[8] Aerobic gram-negative rods predominate (55%), followed by streptococci (30%) and anaerobes (15%) (Table 97–2). Single species are found in 30% of patients, but the majority have multiple organisms.[9] In most patients, cultures from the gallbladder wall and gallbladder bile grow the same organisms.

The incidence of infection with anaerobes is increased in older patients and in patients with current choledocholithiasis.[10] Invasion of ischemic or necrotic gallbladder wall by gas-forming bacteria (especially *Clostridium*) is most common in elderly male diabetic patients; the result is emphysematous cholecystitis.

The biliary tract of healthy persons usually does not harbor bacteria.[11] Contamination from the duodenum may occur via the bile ducts. Supportive evidence is that the incidence of infected bile is lower when tumors completely obstruct the biliary tree than when stones or iatrogenic strictures produce partial obstruction. Bile may also be contaminated by portal venous bacteremia or via the lymphatics.

Pathology

The gallbladder becomes tense and edematous, and the surface is a lusterless gray-red color. As the serosal inflammation progresses, adhesions form to adjacent structures (gastrohepatic omentum, duodenum, porta hepatis, colon). If the obstruction is not relieved, the tension causes ischemia and gangrene, particularly in the fundus, where the blood supply is poorest. Most cases do not progress beyond the initial chemical phase, with resolution leading to changes of chronic cholecystitis. In 15% of cases, complications may occur, with gangrene and perforation.

Histologic examination of gallbladder tissue shows hemorrhage and edema with an inflammatory infiltrate consisting mostly of monocytes with relatively few neutrophils and bacteria (Fig. 97–1).

Clinical Manifestations

Acute cholecystitis usually follows an attack of biliary colic that persists longer than 6 hours. Initially the pain may be epigastric, but later it becomes localized to the right side upper quadrant and radiates to the right subscapular region. Severe and constant, it is often associated with nausea and vomiting. Fever develops in most patients, but rigors are unusual unless there are associated bile duct stones and cholangitis. Mild jaundice occurs in some patients, but deeper jaundice usually indicates choledocholithiasis.

The main findings on physical examination are tenderness and guarding in the right side upper quadrant; in some patients a mass may be palpable. Generalized peritoneal tenderness is found in patients with free perforation, but clinical signs do not always correlate with severity of the disease, especially in older patients.

ACUTE CHOLECYSTITIS DURING PREGNANCY

The incidence of acute cholecystitis increases with multiple pregnancies, and it is not uncommon for this to be the initial presentation of biliary disease in women. Medical therapy is recommended during the first trimester, but surgical treatment during the second trimester is safer, is associated with a low rate of fetal loss, and is recommended for patients who present during this stage of the pregnancy. Others recommend postpartum cholecystectomy as the safest option,[12] and this certainly applies when cholecystitis begins during the third trimester.

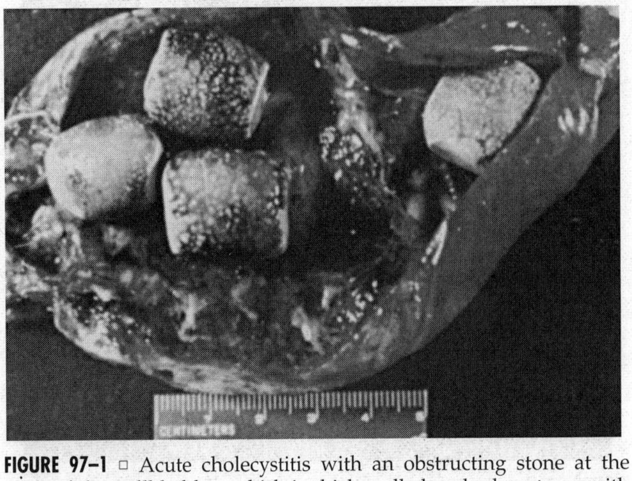

FIGURE 97–1 □ Acute cholecystitis with an obstructing stone at the neck of the gallbladder, which is thick walled and edematous, with serosal inflammation.

CHOLECYSTITIS IN ELDERLY PERSONS

Acute cholecystitis in patients older than 65 years is a serious condition associated with a high incidence of complications and a significantly greater mortality rate. Often the diagnosis is made late because of minimal or masked signs,[13] and early surgery is recommended unless there are serious medical contraindications. The increased incidence of complications (gangrene, perforation, and empyema) and the frequently associated cardiovascular and pulmonary disorders in these patients account for a 9% mortality rate, as opposed to 1.6% in younger persons.

Diagnosis

There is usually mild leukocytosis with minor biochemical abnormalities (elevated transaminase and alkaline phosphatase values). Slightly elevated serum amylase values are common, but marked elevation is associated with biliary pancreatitis. At Harbor–UCLA Medical Center, the mean serum amylase level in patients with biliary pancreatitis was 2465 mU/mL (normal was 20 to 110 mU/mL).

The plain radiograph of the abdomen is rarely helpful in establishing the diagnosis (calcified stones in 10% of patients and gas in the gallbladder with emphysematous cholecystitis), but it is valuable for excluding other disease. Oral cholecystography is not useful in the acute phase, and intravenous cholangiography is now essentially of historical interest.

Ultrasonography with real-time scanning has become the most widely used screening test for acute cholecystitis. At the same examination, other intraabdominal sites (pancreas, liver, and appendix) can be screened. Its accuracy in detecting gallstones is 90% to 95%,[14] but the interpretation of the criteria for diagnosing acute cholecystitis, which include stone impaction, focal gallbladder tenderness, pericholecystic fluid collections, and changes in the gallbladder wall, in many cases depends on the experience of the technician (Fig. 97–2).

Radionuclide imaging with technetium Tc 99m–labeled agents (lidofenin [hepatoiminodiacetic acid], iminodiacetic acid, PIPIDA [*p*-isopropyliminodiacetic acid, iprofenin]) has enabled clinicians to diagnose or exclude acute cholecystitis with great accuracy. It is noninvasive, easy to read, applicable even in jaundiced patients, and it provides good images of the intra- and extrahepatic ducts. It is sensitive for determining patency of the cystic duct, and visualization of the gallbladder effectively excludes the diagnosis of acute cholecystitis (Figs. 97–3 and 97–4). False-positive results (failure to visualize a gallbladder not involved by acute cholecystitis) are encountered in patients who are receiving parenteral nutrition, have severe intercurrent illness, are alcoholic, or have gallstone pancreatitis.

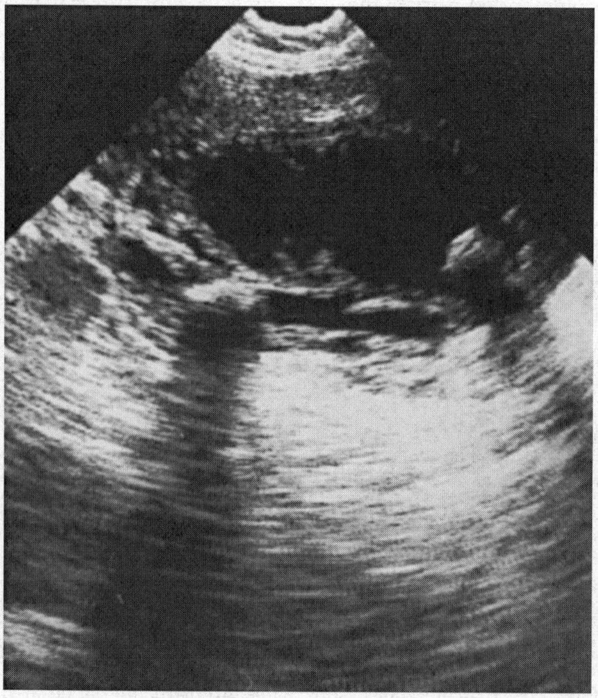

FIGURE 97–2 □ Ultrasonographic examination shows a distended gallbladder with a calculus causing acoustic shadowing.

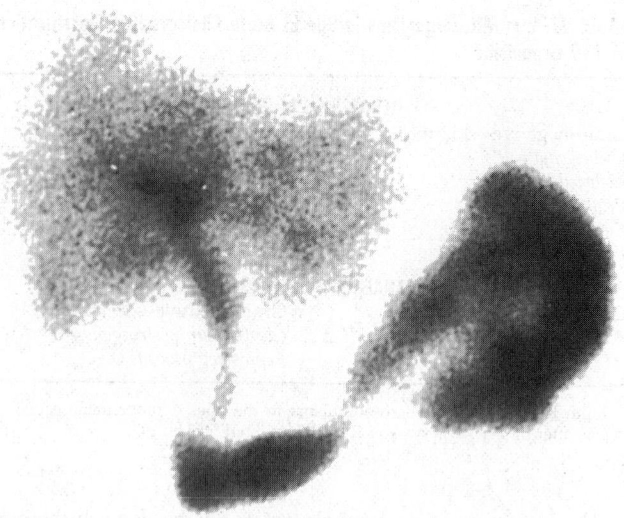

FIGURE 97–3 □ Lidofenin scan in acute cholecystitis shows absence of gallbladder filling and normal free-draining bile duct.

Initially ultrasonography should be used to screen for gallstones and signs of acute cholecystitis. If no stones are present on ultrasonograms, the physician then performs radionuclide studies in search of acute acalculous cholecystitis. Many conditions simulate acute cholecystitis: acute pancreatitis, perforated peptic ulcer, retrocecal appendicitis, liver abscess, hepatitis, pyelonephritis, myocardial infarction, and right side lowerlobe pneumonia.

Complications

GANGRENE AND PERFORATION

Patchy gangrene affecting the fundus of the gallbladder is found in 8% of patients, and perforation affects a like number. Perforation of the gallbladder may be acute (with generalized peritonitis), subacute (with a pericholecystic abscess), or chronic (with fistulous communication involving another viscus).

Perforation is more common in older patients and in those who have diabetes or acalculous or emphysematous cholecystitis. The reported incidence varies widely between series, ranging from 12% in a collected series[15] to 1%.[16] An incidence of approximately 5.4% to 6% is close to the experience of most surgeons who perform operations in the acute phase of the disease.[17, 18]

The mechanism of perforation is probably related to vascular congestion and subsequent ischemia and necrosis. The signs and symptoms are not distinctive; many cases are diagnosed late or are missed, which accounts for the 30% to 50% mortality rate for patients with free perforation.

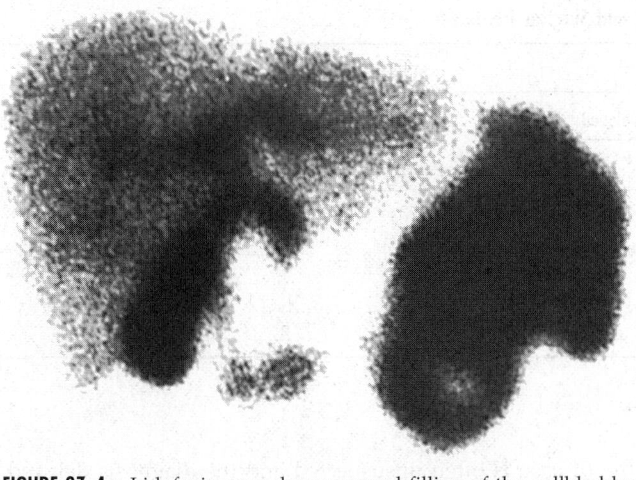

FIGURE 97–4 □ Lidofenin scan shows normal filling of the gallbladder and biliary tree with free flow into the duodenum and proximal bowel.

EMPYEMA

The reported frequency of empyema varies from 1% to 9%, but the higher figures may overestimate the incidence because milky contents of the acutely inflamed gallbladder may present precipitate of calcium carbonate and cholesterol rather than true pus (Fig. 97–5). It usually affects older patients, and fever, leukocytosis, and a tender mass are typical, but as with perforation, minimal disturbance with few signs is not uncommon in debilitated, elderly patients. As many as 15% of older patients may have liver abscess or subphrenic abscess.[13]

PANCREATITIS

The incidence of pancreatitis associated with acute cholecystitis varies widely, depending on whether the diagnosis is established with serum amylase value, imaging technique, or operative findings. It is interesting to note how infrequently acute pancreatitis is reported in patients who undergo surgery for acute cholecystitis immediately or early in the disease. For patients who undergo surgery during their hospitalization for gallstone pancreatitis the incidence of acute cholecystitis ranges from 13% to 14%.[19, 20] In our series of 46 patients who had early surgery for gallstone pancreatitis at Harbor–UCLA Medical Center, only 6 (13%) had acute cholecystitis by histologic criteria. The pancreatitis is usually the edematous interstitial type. Other rare complications include hemobilia and hemoperitoneum. Cholangitis is unusual unless there are also stones in the bile duct, a condition that occurs in about 15% of patients.[21] Cholangitis and jaundice may occasionally be caused by obstruction of the common hepatic duct by a large cystic duct stone.[22] Rarely, biliary peritonitis may occur without perforation of the gallbladder.

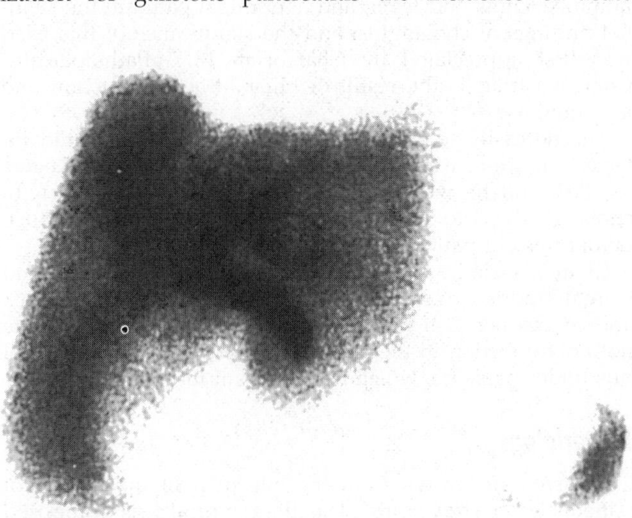

FIGURE 97–5 □ Lidofenin scan shows free flow of tracer in the bile duct and proximal bowel but absence of gallbladder filling and a large defect in the inferior aspect of the liver due to a gallbladder empyema.

Treatment

Treatment options for acute cholecystitis include medical therapy and surgery.[7, 23–27] The two approaches are compared in Table 97–3.

Medical Therapy. Initial management for all patients is medical—intravenous fluids, analgesia, nasogastric suction if vomiting occurs, and antibiotics. Antibiotics probably do not influence the progression of the disease and have not been shown to decrease the incidence of local complications such as empyema and pericholecystic collections. When used preoperatively, they do, however, decrease the incidence of septicemia and wound infection.

Antibiotics effective against gram-negative rods should be used. Second- and third-generation cephalosporins (cefotetan, moxalactam, and cefotaxime), ureidopenicillins (mezlocillin and piperacillin), ampicillin, aminoglycosides, and trimethoprim have been shown to be effective against the usual forms of acute cholecystitis. The antibiotic regimen may need to be refined for patients who are found at operation to have extensive sepsis, for patients with emphysematous cholecystitis or cholangitis, and for those whose clinical status deteriorates in response to the aforementioned regimens. Additional coverage for gram-positive aerobes and anaerobes may have to be provided in such situations.

Urgent Surgical Treatment. Most patients are managed by the medical regimen, and only a few require urgent intervention, for reasons such as follows: (1) failure of medical therapy with clinical deterioration, (2) generalized peritonitis, (3) emphysematous or acalculous cholecystitis, (4) empyema, and (5) diagnostic uncertainty, when other intraabdominal conditions cannot be excluded. Many patients who require urgent intervention are old and infirm, and for those who are unduly compromised, cholecystostomy may be performed under local anesthesia, provided extensive gangrene, perforation, or associated bile duct stones and cholangitis are not present. However, percutaneous cholecystostomy has been performed successfully in unfit patients.[28]

Cholecystostomy is rarely performed today, which may reflect improvements in anesthesia and resuscitation and the broader training of residents in elective biliary surgery. Nevertheless, cholecystostomy should be viewed not as a therapeutic failure but as a sign of mature judgment and experience in cases in which the anatomy is obscured by inflammation and persistent prolonged attempts to perform cholecystostomy are not in the patient's best interest.

Planned cholecystectomy is usually performed after cholecystostomy, and the procedure has not been associated with greater morbidity or mortality than elective cholecystectomy, but in many elderly patients no further treatment or dissolution therapy may be appropriate.

Emphysematous Cholecystitis

Emphysematous cholecystitis, an uncommon variant of acute cholecystitis, is associated with gallbladder infection by gas-

TABLE 97–3 ■ Mortality in Acute Cholecystitis: Comparison of Medical Therapy and Surgical Treatment

	MEDICAL THERAPY		SURGICAL THERAPY					
			Delayed		Early		Urgent	
AUTHOR	Patients	Deaths	Patients	Deaths	Patients	Deaths	Patients	Deaths
Payne[23]	265	0	265	7	133	0		
Essenhigh[24]	312	20	137	*	22	1	95	12
Kune and Birks[25]			73	0	162	1	27	5
Reiss et al[26]					182	1		
Van der Linden and Edlund[27]	185	4	141	7			10	3
Rosi and Midel[7]	107	5	173	9	234	5	31	6

*Deaths were not reported.

forming organisms (most commonly *Clostridium perfringens*, often with *Escherichia coli* and anaerobic streptococci as co-pathogens). It is associated with gallstones in 72% of cases and has a predilection for older male diabetic patients.

The presentation varies from a mild illness simulating the more usual form of acute cholecystitis to a serious fulminant disease associated with rapid clinical deterioration. The diagnosis may be confirmed by use of a radiograph that shows gas in the gallbladder lumen or wall. Gangrene and perforation occur with greater frequency than in ordinary forms of cholecystitis and may be related to obliterative vascular changes in the cystic artery, particularly in diabetic patients. The treatment recommended is immediate cholecystectomy and aggressive antibiotic therapy with anaerobic coverage (penicillin and metronidazole). The mortality rate in reported series averages 15%.

Acute Acalculous Cholecystitis

Acute acalculous cholecystitis, another variant of acute cholecystitis, accounts for 5% of cases of acute cholecystitis and has been described in a variety of settings. Half of all cases of acute cholecystitis in children are acalculous disease.[12] Clinical cholecystitis is a well-known complication of infusion chemotherapy and of primary systemic diseases such as typhoid fever, brucellosis, and miliary tuberculosis and *Campylobacter*, cytomegalovirus, *Cryptosporidium*, and *Candida albicans* infections.

The more usual settings in which acalculous cholecystitis occurs are in association with critical illness, parenteral nutrition, trauma, and thermal injury. It may develop after intra- or extraabdominal procedures.

Pathophysiology

Numerous factors have been implicated in the pathogenesis of acalculous cholecystitis, including (1) bile stasis after massive transfusions, prolonged fasting, or dehydration, leading to cystic duct obstruction; (2) functional obstruction of the ampulla of Vater by opiates; and (3) ischemic mucosal injury in low-flow states and multisystem failure. Anatomic variants that cause cystic duct obstruction (adhesions, enlarged cystic duct node, and tortuous cystic artery) rarely cause cholecystitis.

Clinical Aspects

Acute acalculous cholecystitis demonstrates a male predominance, higher incidences of gangrene and perforation, and a higher mortality rate than ordinary acute cholecystitis. The clinical settings in which it occurs account for the fact that the disease is often unsuspected and the diagnosis delayed. The symptoms and signs are often subtle and not characteristic, particularly in patients who are recovering from an abdominal procedure or are critically ill.

A mass may be palpable in up to 40% of patients, but the most useful investigation is ultrasonography, which may show a large gallbladder with a thickened wall and a pericholecystic collection. Computed tomography has proved to be a valuable alternative, but radionuclide studies are unreliable because in many of the clinical settings associated with acalculous cholecystitis these studies yield false-positive results.

Treatment

Cholecystectomy should be performed as soon as possible because progression to gangrene (52%) or perforation (11%) is likely to be fatal if diagnosis and treatment are delayed until cholecystostomy is no longer possible. Aggressive management of critically ill patients including prophylactic cholecystectomy in patients with total parenteral nutrition–induced gallbladder disease and in those receiving perfusion chemotherapy, may decrease the incidence of this serious complication.

Ascending and Suppurative Cholangitis

Jaundice, chills and fever, and abdominal pain are the sentinel findings of cholangitis, and the significance of this triad was first appreciated by Charcot in 1877. Pathologically, Charcot's triad is the result of biliary tract obstruction and infection.

The necessity for surgical drainage of the obstructed infected bile duct was suggested by Captain Leonard Rogers in 1803, and he was inspired to operate on a patient with cholangitis and to insert a glass tube to drain the bile duct. Before this, all patients died of suppurative cholangitis.

Charcot's triad was expanded in 1959, when Reynolds and Dargan[29] added two more signs of severe cholangitis: shock and central nervous system depression. These signs indicate not only infection in the biliary tree but also the presence of pus under pressure, which needs urgent intervention.

Bacteriology

Organisms are grown from the bile duct of up to 90% of patients with cholangitis. The flora typically is composed of multiple organisms, the majority of which are aerobic, predominantly *E. coli* and *Klebsiella* and *Streptococcus* species. These same organisms are isolated from the gallbladder of patients with cholecystitis; however, in cholangitis, particularly in patients who had previous bile duct surgery that has been complicated by stricture formation, anaerobic organisms are more common. The anaerobic organisms are *Bacteroides fragilis* and *C. perfringens*.

Animal experiments have shown that particles of a size comparable to gram-negative bacteria translocate rapidly from within the hepatic duct to the blood stream in response to only modest pressure gradients across the biliary system wall.[30] Similarly, infection itself generates elevated pressure, leading to unremitting bacteremia and septic shock if the bile duct is not decompressed by drainage.[31]

Epidemiology

Most often, cholangitis develops as a complication of stones in the biliary tree. Although stone disease of the biliary tract is among the most common surgical diseases in the United States and choledocholithiasis is common, cholangitis is a rare complication of gallstones. It accounted for 2 of every 1000 hospital admissions and 17 of 955 patients with biliary disease in one series seen by a gastroenterologist.[31]

In surgical series, approximately 10% of patients with a prior diagnosis of biliary disease develop suppurative cholangitis, and one third of all patients who have a common duct operation have had cholangitis. About half the patients who develop cholangitis are elderly, often older than 70 years.

Pathogenesis

The clinical presentations of the two forms of cholangitis, ascending and suppurative, have overlapping features. The difference between the two is in the degree of biliary obstruction: with partial obstruction and bacterial multiplication in the bile ducts pressure does not increase dramatically. Bacteria are showered intermittently into the blood stream, producing the characteristic remitting and relapsing clinical course of ascending cholangitis.

Suppurative cholangitis develops in a completely obstructed biliary system. Pressure rises rapidly as the infection evolves into frank purulence within the biliary system, and there is unremitting translocation of bacteria into the blood stream. The clinical course in suppurative cholangitis is toward rapidly progressive septic shock and death.

Ascending cholangitis can evolve into suppurative cholangitis, as complete bile duct occlusion develops secondary to inflammatory thickening of the duct wall and production of tenacious mucopurulent material and "biliary mud" within the bile ducts.

Multiple abscesses often develop in the liver, which may be the source of persistent sepsis even though bile duct obstruction is relieved. The bile ducts dilate and become thick walled; at times they may even resemble the small bowel. With continued unrelenting obstruction, biliary cirrhosis may supervene.

Bactibilia, the presence of bacteria in the bile, occurs with varying frequency, depending on the patient's age and other conditions in the biliary tract. It is more likely to be found in elderly persons who have stones in the duct and obstructive jaundice, particularly if they have previously had surgery in the biliary area. Asymptomatic bactibilia evolves to symptomatic, clinical disease with increasing biliary obstruction.

The ducts are most often obstructed by stones. In some cases there are stones in the gallbladder as well. In other cases they were missed during a previous operation, particularly cholecystectomy, or they since formed. Cholangitis may be the first indication of the presence of a stone in the patient's bile duct.

Clinical Manifestations

The majority of patients have Charcot's triad. The fever develops suddenly and can be associated with paroxysmal shaking; mild jaundice often follows; and pain develops in the right side upper quadrant that radiates to the back and is associated with deep tenderness.

Many patients experience this triad of signs and symptoms intermittently over a protracted period, even years, but some patients present with the triad plus shock and nervous system depression, indicating severe suppuration in the biliary tree.

Diagnosis

Charcot's triad is not exclusively a manifestation of cholangitis; it occurs also in other inflammatory diseases of the gallbladder and pancreas and with hepatitis. The constellation may not always be complete, and at times, a patient with cholangitis may present with septicemia or fever of undetermined origin. A positive blood culture, particularly one that grows one or more of the organisms that are characteristic of the biliary flora, should prompt the physician to consider cholangitis.

The most common biochemical abnormality among liver function tests is a modest elevation in bilirubin level. Accompanying this, the serum alkaline phosphatase value is often elevated, indicating bile duct obstruction.

Plain radiographs of the abdomen rarely show gas in the bile ducts (produced by gas-forming pathogens such as *Clostridium*). Radiopaque stones in the gallbladder or along the course of the bile duct are rare findings and serve as sentinels to direct attention to the biliary system.

If cholangitis is suspected, imaging of the biliary system is done expeditiously. If cholangitis is present, this demonstrates a dilated thick-walled duct, typically containing stones, and often indicates the level of obstruction, usually in the larger, more distal bile duct, but sometimes in the more proximal ducts, including either the right or left hepatic duct system. The most likely cause of obstruction is gallstones, but if no stones are found, other causes, such as previous bile duct injury leading to stricture or carcinoma in the biliary system, must be considered.

As part of the ultrasonographic investigation of suspected cholangitis, the liver is examined for the presence of abscesses and the gallbladder for accompanying disease, particularly gallstones. Usually ultrasonographic examination of the biliary system is sufficient to confirm the diagnosis of cholangitis. Computed tomography is less efficient for showing stones in the biliary system but does show duct lesions and abscesses in the liver.

Studies performed to outline the biliary tract, such as transhepatic cholangiography and endoscopic retrograde cholangiopancreatography, are invasive and demand special equipment and personnel. Each elevates the pressure in the biliary tree and produces bacteremia and an exacerbation of the patient's clinical condition, so at times, in the examination study room or after returning to the ward from the examination suite, the patient develops florid septic shock. This should be anticipated, and patients undergoing these examinations need pretreatment with intravenous fluids and antibiotics well before the study is performed. These studies not only outline the biliary tree but also define the specific obstructive lesion.

Such invasive studies are not obtained routinely but are considered if the cause of the biliary obstruction is unusual (e.g., traumatic stricture, which needs good definition to plan for surgery) or if the patient is unfit for surgery and it is thought that endoscopic sphincterotomy or transhepatic biliary drainage is the safest means of decompression and, at times, particularly with choledocholithiasis, of curing the obstruction.

Treatment

Most patients with cholangitis respond well to antimicrobial therapy against the biliary flora and fluid administration to expand intravascular volume. Some patients respond well initially to this regimen then relapse into shock soon thereafter. Rarely, the treatment is ineffective because the septic shock is profound. Both situations are life threatening and require urgent decompression of the biliary system. This may be accomplished by endoscopic sphincterotomy and insertion of a drainage tube into the bile duct via the endoscope, or, less satisfactory, drainage can be achieved percutaneously. The latter technique often aggravates sepsis and leads to biliary cutaneous fistulae.

Surgery has been the usual means of treating cholangitis. At operation it is usually possible to effect permanent relief of the obstruction, either by removing stones from the bile duct or by draining a bile duct obstructed by fibrous stricture or malignant disease into adjacent bowel. The simplest means for draining the bile duct operatively is to insert a large T tube.

The choice of surgical procedure depends on the severity of the patient's illness at the time. If the patient is in shock or has responded poorly to fluids and antimicrobial therapy, the simplest procedure (e.g., insertion of a T tube) may secure survival. If the patient is in remission after an episode of ascending cholangitis, a complete, more extensive surgical procedure to alleviate biliary obstruction and permanently reestablish drainage is indicated. Patients treated with simple T-tube drainage undergo definitive surgery once recovered fully from shock.

References

1. Sato T, Matsushiro T: Surgical indications in patients with silent gallstones. Am J Surg 128:368, 1974.
2. Gracie WA, Ransohoff DF: The natural history of silent gallstones. The innocent gallstone is not a myth. N Engl J Med 307:798, 1982.
3. Wenckert A, Robertson B: The natural history of gallstone disease: Eleven-year review of 781 unoperated cases. Gastroenterology 50:376, 1966.
4. Watts JMcK, Bradley BM, Whiting MJ: Studies on the outcome of untreated gallstone disease. Southeast Asian J Surg 7:8, 1984.
5. Burnett W: The management of acute cholecystitis. Aust N Z J Surg 41:25, 1971.
6. Newman HF, Northup JD, Rosenblum M, Abrams H: Complications of cholelithiasis. Am J Gastroenterol 50:476, 1968.
7. Rosi PA, Midel AI: Acute cholecystitis. An analysis of current treatment. Surg Clin North Am 47:147, 1967.
8. Claesson BEB, Holmlund DEW, Matzsch TW: Microflora of the gallbladder related to duration of acute cholecystitis. Surg Obstet Gynecol 162:531, 1986.
9. Keighley MRB: Microorganisms in the bile. A preventable cause of sepsis after biliary surgery. Ann R Coll Surg Engl 59:329, 1977.
10. Shimada K, Inamatsu T, Yamashiro M: Anaerobic bacteria in biliary disease in elderly patients. J Infect Dis 135:850, 1977.
11. Csendes A, Fernandez M, Uribe P: Bacteriology of the gallbladder bile in normal subjects. Am J Surg 129:629, 1975.
12. Hiatt JR, Hiatt JCG, Williams RA: Biliary disease in pregnancy: Strategy for surgical management. Am J Surg 150:263, 1986.
13. Morrow DJ, Thompson J, Wilson SE: Acute cholecystitis in the elderly: A surgical emergency. Arch Surg 118:1149, 1978.
14. Cooperberg PL, Burhenne HJ: Real-time ultrasonography. Diagnostic technique of choice in calculous gallbladder disease. N Engl J Med 302:1277, 1980.
15. Diffenbaugh WG, Sarver FE, Strohl EL: Gangrenous perforation of the gallbladder. Arch Surg 59:742, 1949.
16. Lee AE: The management of acute cholecystitis. Br J Surg 45:523, 1958.
17. Essenhigh DM: Perforation of the gall-bladder. Br J Surg 55:175, 1968.
18. Pines B, Rabinovitch J: Perforation of the gallbladder in acute cholecystitis. Ann Surg 140:170, 1954.
19. Stone HH, Fabian TS, Dunlop WE: Gallstone pancreatitis. Biliary tract pathology in relation to timing of operation. Ann Surg 194:305, 1981.
20. Frei GJ, Frei VT, Thirlby RC, McClelland RN: Biliary pancreatitis: Clinical presentation and surgical management. Am J Surg 151:170, 1986.
21. Coelho JC, Buffara M, Pozzoban CE, et al: Incidence of common bile duct stones in patients with acute and chronic cholecystitis. Surg Obstet Gynecol 158:76, 1984.
22. Koehler RE, Melson GL, Lee JKT, Long L: Common hepatic duct obstruction by cystic duct stone: Mirizzi syndrome. Am J Roentgenol 132:1007, 1977.
23. Payne RA: Evaluation of the management of acute cholecystitis. Br J Surg 56:200, 1969.
24. Essenhigh DM: Management of acute cholecystitis. Br J Surg 53:1032, 1966.
25. Kune GA, Birks D: Acute cholecystitis. An appraisal of current methods of treatment. Med J Aust 2:218, 1970.
26. Reiss R, Pikelnie S, Engelberg M: The value of early surgery and routine operative cholangiography in the management of acute cholecystitis. World J Surg 3:107, 1979.
27. Van der Linden W, Edlund G: Early versus delayed cholecystectomy: The effect of a change in management. Br J Surg 68:753, 1981.
28. Klimberg S, Hawkins I, Vogel SB: Percutaneous cholecystostomy for acute cholecystitis in high-risk patients. Am J Surg 153:125, 1987.
29. Reynolds BM, Dargan EL: Acute obstructive cholangitis. Ann Surg 150:299, 1959.
30. Huang T, Bass JA, Williams RD: The significance of biliary pressure in cholangitis. Arch Surg 98:629, 1969.
31. Andrew DJ, Johnson SE: Acute suppurative cholangitis, a medical and surgical emergency: A review of ten years' experience emphasizing early recognition. Am J Gastroenterol 54:141, 1970.
33. Cohen S, Kaplan M, Gottlieb L, Patterson J: Liver disease and gallstones in regional enteritis. Gastroenterology 60:237, 1971.
34. Bouchier IAD: Postmortem study of the frequency of gallstones in patients with cirrhosis of the liver. Gut 10:705, 1969.
35. Roslyn JJ, Pitt HA, Mann L, et al: Parenteral nutrition–induced gallbladder disease: A reason for early cholecystectomy. Am J Surg 148:58, 1984.

PANCREAS AND SPLEEN

98

Infection After Acute Pancreatitis

Ernst Klar
Andrew L. Warshaw

Classification

Acute pancreatitis is generally a self-limited disease that subsides uneventfully. In perhaps 15% of cases, the inflammatory process becomes complicated, usually with the generation of necrotic tissue such that there is a basis for secondary infection.[1] Although several variations on this theme exist, with overlapping signs and symptoms, the term pancreatic abscess has been widely used to encompass the varieties.[2] Emphasis has been placed on separating pancreatic abscesses into the components of the spectrum,[3] but it is likely that most of the morphologic differences to be described are reflections of the point in the development of the process at which it becomes evident, rather than of uniquely different pathogeneses.[4]

Pancreatic Phlegmon

The term phlegmon, as applied in acute pancreatitis, was suggested by Kune and King[5] and Warshaw[6] to describe the ligneous pancreatic and peripancreatic tissue swelling and inflammation that may persist for weeks or even months after the attack. The process may resolve spontaneously or may evolve to necrosis of the affected areas, either in small (even microscopic) patches or over large, confluent areas (regional necrosis). The latter are at particular risk of becoming infected,[7] but infection may occur even without grossly apparent necrosis.[8] Some writers dislike the term phlegmon because it does not describe a clearly defined entity, but it is precisely that element of uncertainty and potential for evolution and change that makes the phlegmon an important concept in our eyes.[4]

Acute Pseudocyst

A pancreatic pseudocyst is a pool of pancreatic secretions within a nonepithelialized cavity. In chronic pancreatitis, pseudocysts are thought to develop behind an obstructed duct, and they rarely become clinically infected[9] unless bacteria are introduced iatrogenically, usually by pancreatography. In acute pancreatitis, glandular destruction creates a soup of escaped secretions, blood, and necrotic tissue that becomes walled off by adjacent structures and eventually encapsulated by granulation tissue. Bacterial infection of this debris, although relatively uncommon, converts the collection to an infected pseudocyst.[10] The feature that distinguishes this entity from the other forms of infection is the well-formed capsule of the pseudocyst.

Pancreatic Abscess

Pancreatic abscess is the easiest of the pancreatic infections to envision, a collection of pus. As such, it is probably the end result of tissue destruction, liquefaction, and infection. Morphologically it may be similar in its late stages to other forms of intraabdominal abscess. Earlier in its evolution, as with the infected pseudocyst, there is usually considerable semisolid debris—chunks of necrotic tissue in the cavity.

Infected Pancreatic Necrosis

Infected necrosis is the term favored when the content of the infected areas is mainly solid rather than liquid pus. This was previously included with pancreatic abscesses, but Beger and colleagues[1] have argued that the clinical characteristics and fulminance of infected necrosis are sufficiently different to warrant a distinctive label.

Pathogenesis

Pancreatic infection occurs in 1% to 9% of cases of acute pancreatitis.[2, 11–19] There is no apparent relation to the antecedent cause of pancreatitis (gallstone, alcoholism). Although some have found little relation between the severity of the initial presentation and the likelihood of developing an abscess,[19–21] others do report a correlation between the number of Ranson prognostic signs and subsequent infection,[13, 17] probably reflecting the amount of tissue injury that serves as the bacterial culture medium. For this reason it has been noted that so-called extended pancreatic necrosis, in which retroperitoneal tissues outside the pancreas proper are involved in the necrotizing process, are even more likely to become infected.[22] Most patients who die from acute pancreatitis, if they have survived the initial circulatory deficits, have infection in the area of injury.[23]

Healthy pancreas is highly resistant to infection, even by injection of bacteria directly into the gland. Strong circumstantial evidence suggests that devitalized tissues are the necessary prerequisite for successful establishment of bacterial infection in the pancreas.[24] Using percutaneous needle sampling of tissues in acute pancreatitis, Gerzof and coworkers[8] found extremely low rates of infection in peripancreatic fluid, intermediate rates in phlegmons, and high rates in necrotic tissues. Beger and colleagues[1] found the prevalence of infection in necrotic pancreatic tissues to be about 40%, with the earliest infections occurring within 7 days and reaching a maximal prevalence (71%) by 3 weeks. In Beger and colleagues'[1] large experience, pancreatic and peripancreatic necrosis appears to be a prerequisite for infection. In fact, the more extensive the necrosis, especially if it extends well beyond the pancreas into the retroperitoneal surroundings, the more likely is the chance of infection.

The mechanisms that contribute to this injury probably include both enzymatic digestion and ischemia. Activation of proteases and cathepsins in the pancreatic cell is believed to contribute to cell death. It has been proposed that in patients who develop widespread tissue injury, the endogenous protease control mechanisms that utilize α_1-antiprotease and α_2-macroglobulin to bind, inactivate, and transport the escaped proteases have been overwhelmed.[18]

Ischemic injury would appear to be added to the enzymatic component and may be the critical extra factor in converting edematous to necrotizing pancreatitis.[18, 25] In experimental necrotizing pancreatitis, blood flow to the pancreas is reduced,[26, 27] and interference with pancreatic perfusion by injection of micropheres[28] or ligation of pancreatic arteries[29] converts an edematous process to a necrotizing one. Similarly, pharmacologic reduction of pancreatic perfusion by vasoconstrictor drugs increases the severity of experimental pancreatitis.[30]

The precise route by which microorganisms reach the pancreas is not fully established but may comprise direct transmural spread of bacteria from the colon[6] across the peritoneal cavity as well as lymphatic[21] or hematogenous[31] seeding, especially in the presence of impaired function of the hepatic reticuloendothelial system.[32–36] The biliary tract may be an important source of infection in that subgroup of patients whose pancreatitis is caused by a common duct stone and who may therefore have associated cholangitis.

Increased intestinal permeability with translocation of bacteria from the gut lumen is generally considered to be the most likely initial step of pancreatic infection. Disruption of normal enteric mucosal barrier[37] has been defined as the basic mechanism of bacterial translocation in conditions of bowel ischemia or inflammation and in shock, regardless of the underlying disease entity.[38–40] Further insight into the pathogenesis of septic complications during acute pancreatitis was gained by application of different antibiotic regimens in a rodent model of acute necrotizing pancreatitis.[41] Because early pancreatic infection could be reduced by either gut decontamination or a systemic antibiotic that is concentrated by the pancreas (e.g., imipenem), direct bacterial spread from the gut and hematogenous seeding appear to interplay in initiation of infection. In contrast, extrapancreatic infection in distant sites such as the kidney could be prevented only by systemic antibiotic therapy, a finding consistent with the dominant role of bacteremic and hematogenous spread.

Although infection is not important in the early lethality of pancreatitis,[42] bacterial contamination of the pancreas and other sites has been shown to occur early in experimental pancreatitis.[41, 43] Indirect evidence for bacteremia and invasive infection during the early stages of human pancreatitis comes from the finding of measurable endotoxin levels in peripheral blood of patients with severe pancreatitis before any other sign of local infection.[44]

The typical organisms found in pancreatic infections are coliforms and other enteric species[1, 2, 8 13, 19, 21] (Table 98–1). Multiple organisms, rather than a single species, are common. Anaerobes such as *Bacteroides* are occasionally found in pancreatic infections, but they are not common.[21] This absence is not explained simply by inadequate culture techniques, for they are found no more often when special efforts are made. *Candida albicans* is a rare primary agent in pancreatic abscesses[45, 46] but is being recovered more frequently as a superinfecting organism in patients treated with prolonged courses of antibiotics. A primary tuberculous abscess of the pancreas has been reported.[47]

TABLE 98–1 ■ Microorganisms Found in 45 Pancreatic Infections*

ORGANISM	NO. OF SPECIMENS
Escherichia	22
Enterococcus	17
Staphylococcus	16
Klebsiella	6
Proteus	4
Candida albicans	3
Pseudomonas	3
Streptococcus	2
Torulopsis glabrata	1
Haemophilus parainfluenzae	1
Diphtheroids	1
Serratia marcescens	1
Negative culture (positive Gram stain for organisms on smear)	5

*More than one organism was propagated from 20 specimens.

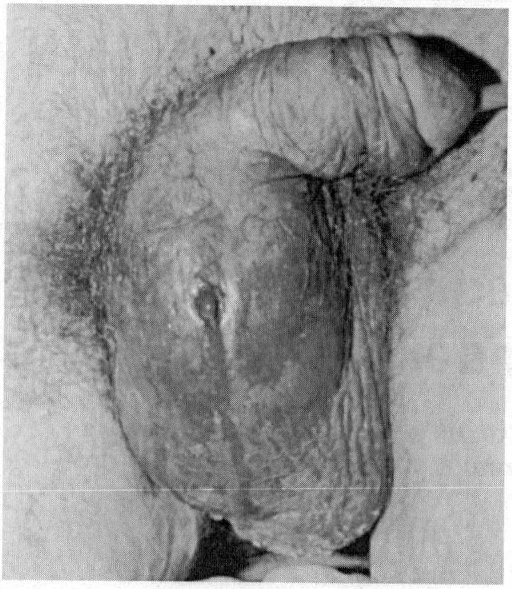

FIGURE 98–1 □ Retroperitoneal extension of a pancreatic abscess with necessitation out through the scrotum.

Pancreatic infections frequently spread out from the pancreas. They usually follow retroperitoneal tissue planes, most often down the paracolic gutters or out between the leaves of the mesenteries of the large and small intestines. It is believed that these extensions are facilitated by the activated pancreatic proteolytic enzymes, which are admixed in the abscess contents and which potentiate the erosion of tissues along the advancing front. Pancreatic abscesses have been known to reach and necessitate out the scrotum[6] (Fig. 98–1) or to travel up the mediastinum to the neck. Along the way they can perforate into the peritoneal cavity, into an intraabdominal hollow viscus, into the pleural space, or even into a bronchus.[48] Their aggressive behavior is not matched by other forms of intraabdominal abscess.

Clinical Manifestations

The presentations of pancreatic infection are those of sepsis. They range over a spectrum of severity from inapparent to fulminant, but two relatively distinct patterns can be distinguished in the continuum.[3, 19, 21] In the first, the patient seems to recover from the acute attack, may seem to be well for 1 to 5 weeks (latent period), and then develops a fever, leukocytosis, and perhaps other signs of intraabdominal infection.[13, 17, 19, 20, 24] These patients usually have distinct, well-demarcated pancreatic abscesses, as described before. The second pattern is that of the patient who never recovers from the presenting inflammatory episode but continues to be acutely ill with clinical signs of fluid sequestration, hyperdynamic cardiac function, circulatory instability, and fever. Patients in this second group appear to be sicker and more toxic. The tempo of their illness tends to force recognition of the complication by 10 to 14 days after onset, an average of 2 weeks earlier than the first group.[19, 21] When examined by computed tomography (CT) or at operation, the infected tissues have not yet fully liquefied but have the same appearance as sterile (not yet infected) necrosis.[7, 8, 49] We believe that these two groups of patients do not represent different processes but only different points in the temporal course

TABLE 98–2 ■ Presenting Symptoms and Signs of Pancreatic Infections in 45 Patients

SIGN OR SYMPTOM	NO.	%
Fever	39	87
Abdominal pain	37	82
Abdominal tenderness	28	62
Palpable mass	22	50
Nausea or vomiting	21	47
Distention	12	27
Jaundice	7	16
Systemic sepsis	3	7
Pulmonary failure	2	4
Gastrointestinal bleeding	1	2

of pancreatic necrosis and infection. In the first group, the subsiding of pancreatitis allows the process to advance to liquefaction. In the second, the ongoing necrotizing pancreatitis forces earlier intervention at a time before liquefaction and conversion to a pocket of pus can occur. Pancreatic abscess and infected necrosis in this view should not be considered as mutually exclusive but rather as closely related and complementary.[4]

The symptoms and signs of pancreatic infection are not specific, whether present or absent.[17, 19, 20] Table 98–2, drawn from our own experience, illustrates the more common findings, but equally important it shows that any or all may be absent. Even fever was missing in 13% of cases. However, all the features may also be produced by sterile necrosis. To wit, the local and systemic effects of pancreatic necrosis may mimic almost exactly those of an infected process, even including the hyperdynamic, high-output cardiocirculatory dysfunction.[50] Thus, the clinical picture cannot be relied on to make the diagnosis of pancreatic infection.[20, 24]

Diagnosis

Infection in acute pancreatitis should be considered in any patient who is febrile after the first several days or who becomes febrile after a period of quiescence. However, patients' clinical profiles after infection may be indistinguishable from those of uninfected edema and necrosis. High-spiking fevers are suggestive but not specific. Routine laboratory indices are helpful but not specifically diagnostic. Clearly, other sources of infection, such as the lungs, the urinary tract, and intravenous lines, must be evaluated, but pancreatic sepsis must be suspected even in the absence of abdominal signs or palpable masses.

Table 98–3 shows data from 45 patients with proven pancreatic abscess. In many of these cases the findings are not striking, and in some they are even normal. The white cell count usually did not exceed 15,000/mm^3, and 13% of the patients had results in the normal range. The serum amylase value was increased in less than half of the patients. These findings have been confirmed in several studies[3, 19, 20] and emphasize the difficulties in separating patients with infected necrosis from those with a still sterile process by routine tests.[13, 24]

TABLE 98–3 ■ Routine Laboratory Findings in 45 Pancreatic Infections

FINDING	NO.
White cell count (/mm^3) >20,000	6
15,000–20,000	7
10,000–15,000	26
<10,000	6
Serum amylase >25 Russell units	19
Alkaline phosphatase >40 IU	18
Serum aspartate aminotransferase >40 units	23
Bilirubin >1.2 mg/dL	17
Calcium <8.5 mg/dL	25
Albumin <3 g/dL	20

Radiographic abnormalities are common, but most are also insensitive and nonspecific. The classic soap bubble sign (mottled lucencies that are a combination of necrotic tissues and gas bubbles[13, 17] in the retroperitoneal tissues; Fig. 98–2) occurs infrequently (4 of 45 patients in our series).[19] Contrast studies of the upper gastrointestinal tract yield only indirect evidence of visceral displacement, stenosis, or obstruction, albeit commonly (40 of 45). Seventy-one percent of our patients had an abnormal chest radiograph that showed pleural effusions, atelectasis, or pneumonitis.

Of the imaging techniques, CT has proved to be much superior to ultrasonography in its ability to show areas of liquefaction within and around pancreatic inflammatory masses.[19, 21, 51] Also, in 30% of patients the ultrasonographic examination is technically unsatisfactory because of excess bowel gas. At least 75% of abscesses can be demonstrated with CT,[12, 13, 19, 21, 52] and many more can be suspected.[19] Although gas in the fluid collection is widely accepted as proof of infection[53, 54] (Fig. 98–3), it is missing in the majority of patients with confirmed abscesses[55, 56] and rarely may be present in the pancreas without an abscess,[57] presumably indicating a pancreatic-enteric fistula.

As already noted, certain groups of patients are at higher risk: those who have had a fulminant presentation with multiple clinical and laboratory signs of severity[13, 17, 58, 59]; those with laboratory suggestions of necrosis, including elevated serum levels of C-reactive protein[59–62] and phospholipase[62]; and those with CT evidence of necrosis.[49, 51]

There has been a particular attempt to use CT to identify patients at increased risk of developing an abscess. Clavien and associates[55] found that the majority of patients with extensive phlegmonous extrapancreatic spread shown within 36 hours of admission develop a pancreatic abscess. Balthazar and Ranson and their colleagues[22, 63] developed a grading system that utilized the extent of the inflammatory process and the number of collections in and around the pancreas to estimate the probability of subsequent infection. The inci-

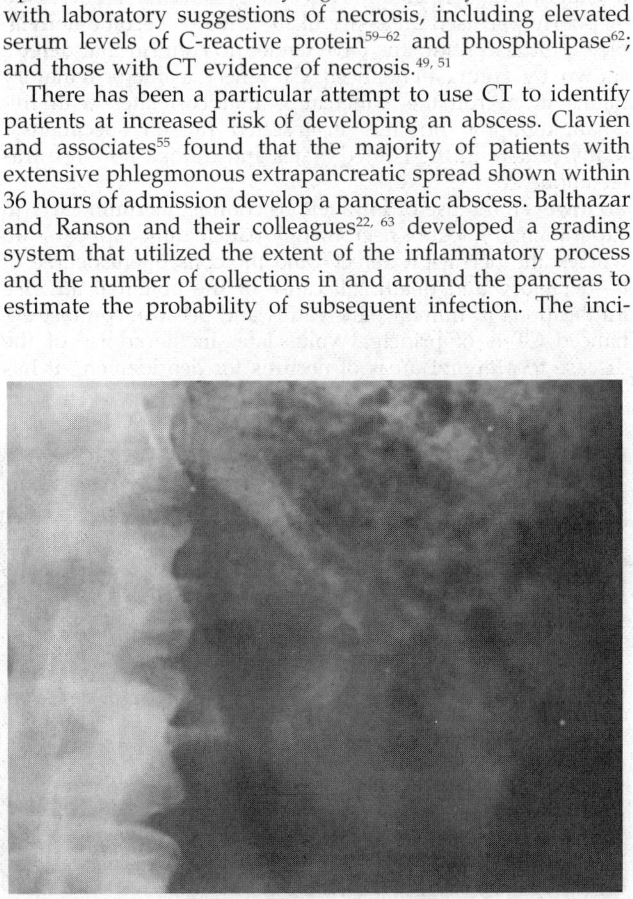

FIGURE 98–2 □ Abdominal radiograph showing the classic soap bubble sign of a pancreatic abscess.

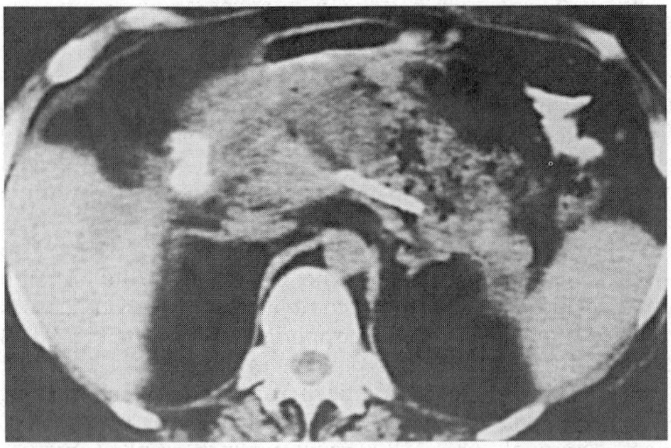

FIGURE 98–3 □ Computed tomographic scan of a pancreatic abscess showing gas bubbles in a large volume of regional necrosis.

dence of abscesses in patients whom they graded as having the most severe disease was 60% to 80%. In a comparable population of patients, these results were not reproduced by means of a similar scoring system that emphasized more the retroperitoneal changes and associated ascites and pleural effusions.[64]

Of greatest current interest is so-called dynamic angio-CT, CT performed during rapid injection of a large volume of intravenous contrast medium. The principle of this technique is that the CT image of well-perfused pancreatic parenchyma will be enhanced by the contrast medium,[65] whereas nonperfused areas will be readily distinguished[66] (Fig. 98–4). Studies in experimental pancreatitis have suggested that nonperfused or poorly perfused areas are likely to be or become nonviable.[67] Studies in humans have tended to confirm that defects shown by contrast-enhanced CT reflect a microcirculatory injury in necrotizing pancreatitis that correlates with microangiographic findings in resected human specimens.[68] Many centers in the United States and Europe now use this technique.[44, 51, 55, 69–71]

However, the use of intravenous contrast medium early in experimental acute necrotizing pancreatitis appears to worsen the perfusion defect[72] and the consequent degree of tissue injury and death.[73] Because of the potential adverse implications in human pancreatitis and because contrast-enhanced CT is of principal value later in the course of the disease to pinpoint areas of necrosis for débridement, it has been suggested that the use of intravenous contrast material be avoided in the first few days of acute pancreatitis.[73]

It is clear that pancreatic infection may be suspected in appropriate clinical situations that turn out to be sterile and that unsuspected infection may be present. The latter circumstance suggests that bacteria may enter and proliferate in the damaged tissues in an occult fashion for a considerable time before generating clinical manifestations. The only diagnostic test that can reliably distinguish a sterile from an infected pancreatic inflammatory process is a culture of those tissues. Even blood cultures are positive in only a minority of pancreatic abscesses,[13, 17, 21] and they do not pinpoint the origin of the septicemia. Patients with positive blood cultures may be more likely to die.[21]

Studies have now proved that it is safe to sample pancreatic inflammatory masses and collections by percutaneous thin-needle aspiration under CT guidance.[8, 74] They have shown remarkable accuracy in both proving and disproving infection. Gerzof's group showed that about 60% of patients who were suspected of harboring infection were infected.[8] Peripancreatic fluid collections were not commonly infected (15%), whereas phlegmons or acute pseudocysts and necrotic areas frequently were (more than 50%). They had no false-positive cultures, no false-negatives, and no contamination caused by the needle aspiration (testimony to the excellence of their technique). In their patients, 22% of the infections were found within 7 days after the onset of the attack and 55% within 14 days, confirming the observations of Beger's group, who obtained cultures during surgical débridement for necrotizing pancreatitis.[1] Heretofore it was thought that pancreatic infection occurred later, usually after 2 or 3 weeks, when clinical signs became evident. These new data emphasize that infection may get an early start and be present for an indeterminate time before it causes systemic effects. Percutaneous needle aspiration under CT guidance has rapidly become the undisputed technique of choice for exposing infection of pancreatic inflammatory masses, and it appears to be virtually as good for confirming contemporaneous sterility of the process.

Treatment

There is no firm evidence that pancreatic abscesses can be prevented. Even timely fluid therapy is not known to forestall pancreatic necrosis.[27] Although prophylactic antibiotics are often given, they have not been shown to reduce the

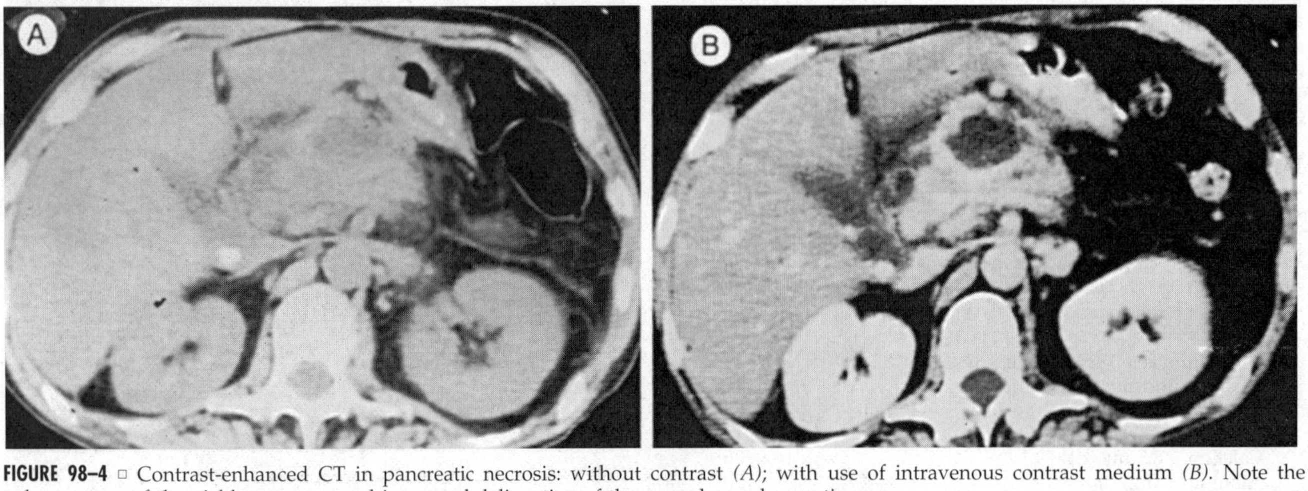

FIGURE 98–4 □ Contrast-enhanced CT in pancreatic necrosis: without contrast *(A)*; with use of intravenous contrast medium *(B)*. Note the enhancement of the viable pancreas and improved delineation of the nonenhanced necrotic area.

incidence of infection.[75–79] Premature feeding is said to increase the chance of abscess formation,[17] but this theory has not been appropriately tested. Nonetheless, it is common practice to use parenteral broad-spectrum antibiotics directed primarily at colon flora in patients with severe pancreatitis who are considered to be at excessive risk of secondary infection. It has been proposed that it would be desirable to choose antibiotics that are secreted by the pancreas or otherwise reach concentrations in the pancreatic juices that are effective in vitro against the common pathogens[80]; however, the assumption that antibiotic levels in the pancreatic secretions are of any importance is unproved, and it seems more probable that penetration into the parenchyma and peripancreatic tissues is of greater importance.

Once an abscess is present, antibiotics alone cannot cure it. It is likely that a pancreatic abscess will be uniformly lethal unless it is adequately evacuated and drained. Percutaneous catheter drainage of pancreatic abscesses has a limited role. Whereas percutaneous drainage of other kinds of intraabdominal abscesses has been highly successful (up to 90%),[81–83] the technique has been less successful with pancreatic abscesses[81, 84, 85] mainly because of the loculations and the solid and semisolid necrotic debris, which do not readily pass through the catheters.[85] In spite of these difficulties, percutaneous catheterization may have a valid place in selected cases: as a preliminary means of decompressing and stabilizing a critically ill septic patient; when surgical access to the abscess is particularly difficult or dangerous; and for drainage of small recurrent or satellite abscesses, especially after multiple surgical drainage procedures.[19, 84, 86]

In general, surgical drainage and débridement should be considered the definitive therapy for pancreatic abscesses.* Although some have advocated formal subtotal[89] or even total[90] pancreatectomy, mortality rates up to 60% for resection in this situation seem excessive.

In our opinion, an upper midline incision represents the best access, allowing wide exposure for thorough exploration of the entire abdomen in search of multiple loculations, which are present in up to 30% of patients.[6, 21] Others have favored upper abdominal transverse incisions.[87] Especially for the first drainage operation, small lateral or flank incisions have the disadvantage of limiting the débridement and hampering the control of possible hemorrhage.

The transmesocolic approach to the pancreas (Fig. 98–5) is often most expeditious and safest in avoiding damage to the transverse colon and the stomach when they are densely adherent to the pancreas. This route is particularly valuable when surgeons are reoperating on patients who have had prior gastric surgery, who have a gastrostomy tube anchoring the stomach, or who have recurrent abscess after drainage through a different approach. After the abscess cavity is emptied of pus, special attention must be directed toward the evacuation of necrotic tissue. Blunt digital dissection is most discriminating between debris and viable tissue, including major vascular structures, which often line the walls or traverse abscess cavities. External drainage should be carefully implemented in all extensions of the cavity and is best accomplished with multiple soft suction drains and stuffed rubber drains brought out through several separate stab wounds[19, 21] (Fig. 98–6). This technique has the advantage of providing both packing and large paths for slough and drainage of devitalized tissues and yet minimizes the risk of incisional hernia. The stuffed drains should be left in place for at least 1 week and subsequently be removed one at a time to allow the cavity to contract around the remaining drains. The suction drains should remain in place until the volume of drainage is small and any fistulae have closed. Using this technique, we have observed a striking decrease in mortality rate for pancreatic abscesses and infected necrosis, from 38% to 5% between 1973 and 1983.[19] This parallels a trend seen elsewhere as well.[21, 36, 87, 88] We attribute the improvement to better ability to detect the lesions with CT and to a more aggressive stance toward early and adequate débridement.

For the subgroup with much remaining necrotic tissue and not just a loculation of pus, Beger's group has advocated the use of an extended period of irrigation of the cavity, whether or not the necrosis is infected.[44] The concept is that local lavage is more effective than drains alone in facilitating the egress of sloughed material. They continue to irrigate the cavity with saline for up to several weeks (median 25 days), usually until the returns no longer contain debris or increased quantities of pancreatic enzymes. The results are excellent, and the mortality rate is 8.4%.

There has been renewed interest in open packing of infected necrosis.[87, 90, 91] The concept is based on the tendency

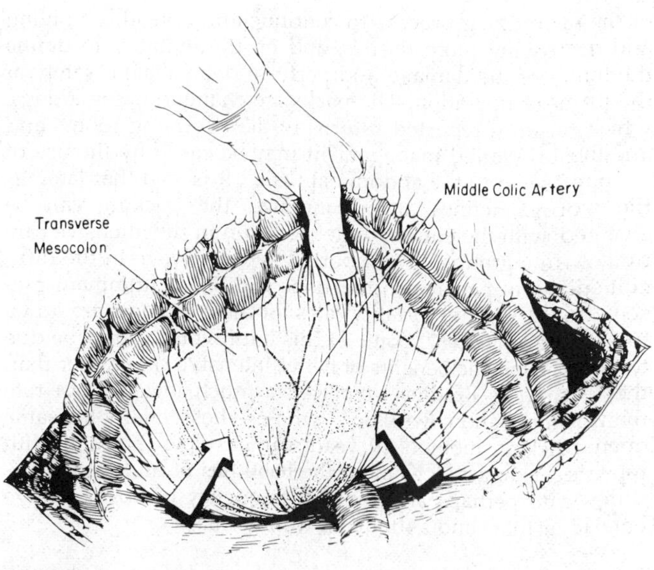

FIGURE 98–5 □ Transmesocolic approach to drainage and débridement of the pancreas.

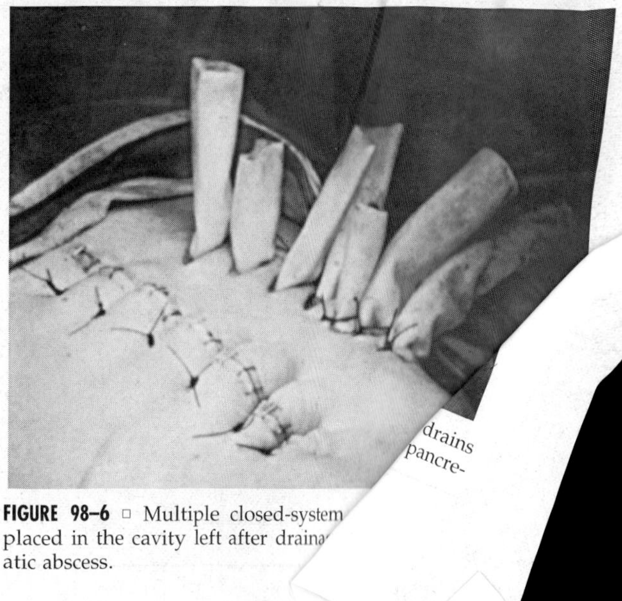

FIGURE 98–6 □ Multiple closed-system drains placed in the cavity left after draina- pancreatic abscess.

*References 13, 14, 17, 19, 21, 36, 44, 87, 88.

of the necrotizing process to continue and spread, involving and destroying more tissues, and on the inability to define the limits of the damage and perform débridement safely at the primary operation. The packs are changed every 2 days, which requires repeated returns to the operating rooms and anesthesia. Wound management may be eased by the use of a zipper sewn to the abdominal wall.[91] It is said that later, as the wound defines and granulates, the packing can be changed with the patient under sedation in the intensive care unit. A few groups have reported better salvage in the difficult subset of pancreatic infections with early fulminant presentation. Current mortality rates for these patients are down to 9% to 22%.[21, 87, 88, 91] Some of this improvement may be due to the nonspecific benefits of better intensive care rather than the technique: Bradley[87] reported a much lower death rate than Bolooki and coworkers,[14] who used essentially the same open packing method 19 years earlier. Open packing with repeated changes does incur the liabilities of multiple procedures and perhaps an increased frequency of postoperative enteric fistulae and abdominal wall hernias.[87]

Complications

Although the number of complications has declined, they still occur in up to three fourths of patients[13, 19, 21, 88, 89] (Table 98–4). The causes of death from pancreatic abscess are principally a combination of the ongoing necrotizing process, uncontrolled sepsis, hemorrhage, and multiple organ failure.[19, 21]

Recurrent abscesses, which, in some cases, may instead be additional abscesses missed in the first drainage procedure, have been described in 30% to 40% in earlier series.[2, 11, 12, 92]

We have found that a technique of thorough abdominal exploration and maximal débridement at the first operation reduces the incidence of complications to 16%.[19] Although the principal tactics should still consist of surgical drainage, percutaneous catheter drainage can be beneficial under these circumstances as an adjunct therapeutic tool if directed toward small additional abscesses to which surgical access is hazardous owing to previous operations.[19, 84, 86]

Hemorrhage from the abscess cavity is second only to progressive sepsis as the cause of death from pancreatic abscesses. Intraoperative bleeding most likely results from decompression of necrotic vessels or vascular trauma by the débridement and is best controlled by packing if direct ligation proves difficult.[88] Serious problems can arise from hemorrhage at later stages owing to difficulties in surgical access and localization of the bleeding source. Transcatheter arterial embolization[19, 93] or balloon occlusion[93] has proved to be beneficial with regard to the temporary control of hemorrhage and allows reexploration, débridement, and repacking under more favorable conditions.

Fistulae occurring after drainage and débridement of a pancreatic abscess are common[13, 19, 87–89, 94–96] (see Table 98–4) because of necrosis of organs, presumably a combined effect of local ischemia due to small-vessel thrombosis and of enzymatic digestion.[95] Of course, direct injury by the surgeon or the drains is also a possibility. Pancreatic fistulae occur in about 30% of patients.[19, 88, 94] Spontaneous closure within weeks or months is common,[12, 19, 94] but persistence of fistulae may indicate an isolated pancreatic segment, usually the tail, which later requires resection or closure with a Roux-en-Y loop of jejunum.[94, 96]

The incidence of enteric fistulae varies from 10% to 31%.[88] Although some may heal spontaneously if well channelled and the hole is small, colocutaneous fistula often requires a proximal colostomy to help control sepsis, subsequent segmental resection of the damaged colon, and later reanastomosis.[97, 98]

Healing of lesser colon injuries may lead to symptomatic stenosis that requires resection.[99] Duodenal fistulae do not often heal spontaneously and may require internal drainage into a Roux-en-Y jejunal loop or even pancreatoduodenectomy. Gastric fistulae have additional potential for major hemorrhage, perhaps because of digestion by the high-volume acid output.[95] Some gastric fistulae close, but it has been suggested that gastric resection and reconstruction be undertaken after 4 weeks' unsuccessful waiting.[95]

Prevention

Measures to reduce the chances of developing a pancreatic abscess should probably be directed toward limitation of necrosis as a precursor in the earlier stages of acute pancreatitis. Because pancreatic ischemia has been shown to play

TABLE 98–4 ■ Complications After Drainage of 45 Cases of Pancreatic Abscess and Infected Necrosis

	PERIOD 1 (1974–1978)		PERIOD 2 (1979–1983)		PERIODS 1 AND 2		
COMPLICATIONS	No.	%	No.	%	No.	%	NO. DIED
Hemorrhage	9	35	1	5	10	22	7
Pancreatic fistula	8	31	6	32	14	31	1
Colonic necrosis	1	4	1	5	2	4	1
Colonic fistula	1	4	1	5	2	4	0
Duodenal fistula	1	4	1	5	2	4	1
Gastric fistula	1	4	0	0	1	2	0
Systemic sepsis	7	27	1	5	8	18	8
Recurrent abscess	4	15	3	16	7	16	1
Renal failure	3	12	1	5	4	9	4
Respiratory failure	3	12	0	0	3	7	3
Pulmonary emboli	1	4	0	0	1	2	1
Pneumonia	6	23	3	16	9	20	0
Wound infection	5	19	1	5	6	13	0
...manent diabetes	2	8	1	5	3	7	0
...ic vein thrombosis	1	4	0	0	1	2	0
...nal hernia	0		1	5	1	2	0
...f patients with complications	24	92	14	74	38	84	
...aths	10	38	1	5	11	24	26

a key role in the pathogenesis of experimental necrotizing pancreatitis,[26, 27, 29, 97, 100] stabilization of the pancreatic microcirculation may be paramount. There is no evidence that ischemic injury to the pancreas and peripancreatic tissues is prevented. In experimental animals the use of dextran solutions may be promising.[26] Short-term peritoneal lavage effectively reverses early circulatory dysfunction of acute pancreatitis but does not prevent later abscesses.[50, 101] Prolonged peritoneal lavage may have some prophylactic benefit.[102] Neither suppression of pancreatic secretion by atropine, glucagon, calcitonin, or somatostatin nor inhibition of pancreatic enzymes by aprotinin or any other agent has been successful.[103, 104]

Once regional necrosis has appeared, choosing the right time for operative intervention to forestall invasive sepsis is problematic. Experts agree that nonoperative observation suffices if the areas of necrosis demonstrated by contrast-enhanced CT are small and if the patient's condition is clinically stable. These limited areas of injury can, and often do, heal without infection or other complications. Larger areas of regional necrosis are less likely to resolve and may evolve by a process of liquefaction into a pseudocyst or become infected. Inasmuch as the extent of the necrosis generally correlates with the likelihood of bacterial contamination,[1] which in turn is associated with higher rates of morbidity and mortality, preemptive surgical débridement has been advocated for patients whose necrosis seems to represent more than 50% of the pancreas, regardless of whether superinfection has already taken place.[44]

In severe human pancreatitis, the contamination rate ranges between 40% and 50% during the first week of the disease.[1, 105] Historically, only one retrospective study has shown that the prophylactic use of antibiotics in acute pancreatitis decreased the incidence of pancreatic infection.[106] Subsequent retrospective[75, 76] and randomized prospective[77–79] studies were unable to confirm these results. However, the broad-spectrum penicillins used in those studies are now recognized to provide insufficient coverage for the typical spectrum of bacteria found in pancreatic infection. These antibiotics have also been shown to be unable to penetrate into pancreatic tissues sufficiently to achieve effective bactericidal levels. It has been suggested that a blood-pancreas barrier may limit drug uptake into the pancreas.[105, 107–110] In an experimental model in rats, early treatment with imipenem and ciprofloxacin, which have good pancreatic tissue penetration,[107, 108] resulted in significant reduction of pancreatic infection, of late septic complications, and of mortality.[111] In the only clinical study of imipenem, a controlled multicenter trial evaluated the effect of this agent in 74 patients with necrotizing pancreatitis. Patients receiving imipenem as prophylactic therapy were compared with patients in whom the antibiotic was administered only if pancreatic infection was confirmed by fine-needle aspiration. Although prophylaxis with imipenem resulted in a reduction in the incidence of infection in necrotic and peripancreatic tissues, there was no difference in the necessity for operative intervention or in mortality.[105] In our opinion, prophylactic antibiotic therapy with imipenem or a quinolone can nonetheless be justified in severe necrotizing pancreatitis on the basis of the unequivocal results in the animal studies.[111] Further clinical trials seeking to prove similar benefits in humans will undoubtedly be forthcoming.

Because the gut is considered the main source of bacterial contamination in acute pancreatitis, selective decontamination of the digestive tract offers a logical therapeutic tool in eliminating the gram-negative bacteria that are the principal pathogens.[112, 113] Nonetheless, data on selective decontamination of the gut in acute pancreatitis are almost nonexistent. In one study, nine patients with severe acute pancreatitis and respiratory failure who were treated by selective gut decontamination were compared with a historical control group of six patients treated in the same department before the concept of selective decontamination of the gut was introduced. After selective decontamination was introduced, it was said to have resulted in a reduced rate of infection, but survival was not improved.[114] One controlled multicenter clinical trial of selective decontamination found a significant reduction of mobidity and mortality by reduction of gram-negative colonization of the digestive tract and subsequent pancreatic infection rate.[115, 116]

References

1. Beger HG, Bittner R, Block S, et al: Bacterial contamination of pancreatic necrosis. A prospective clinical study. Gastroenterology 91:433, 1986.
2. Warshaw AL: Pancreatic abscesses. N Engl J Med 287:1234, 1972.
3. Bittner R, Block S, Buechler M, et al: Pancreatic abscess and infected pancreatic necrosis. Different local septic complications in acute pancreatitis. Dig Dis Sci 32:1082, 1987.
4. Warshaw AL: Lowering the level of uncertainty in late pancreatitis. Gastroenterology 93:1434, 1987.
5. Kune GA, King R: The late complications of acute pancreatitis: Pancreatic swelling, cyst and abscess. Med J Aust 1:1241, 1973.
6. Warshaw AL: Inflammatory masses following acute pancreatitis. Phlegmon, pseudocyst, and abscess. Surg Clin North Am 54:621, 1974.
7. Sostre CF, Flournoy JG, Bova JG, et al: Pancreatic phlegmon. Clinical features and course. Dig Dis Sci 30:918, 1985.
8. Gerzof SG, Banks PA, Robbins AH, et al: Early diagnosis of pancreatic infection by computed tomography–guided aspiration. Gastroenterology 93:1315, 1987.
9. Colhoun E, Murphy JJ, MacEarlean DP: Percutaneous drainage of pancreatic pseudocysts. Br J Surg 71:131, 1984.
10. Glazer G, Dudley HAF: Pancreatic abscess: An incomplete descriptive phrase. Br J Surg 71:401, 1984.
11. Altemeier WA, Alexander JW: Pancreatic abscess: A study of 32 cases. Arch Surg 87:80, 1963.
12. Aranha GV, Prinz RA, Greenlee HB: Pancreatic abscess: An unresolved surgical problem. Am J Surg 144:534, 1982.
13. Becker JM, Pemberton JH, DiMagno EP, et al: Prognostic factors in pancreatic abscess. Surgery 96:455, 1984.
14. Bolooki H, Jaffe B, Gliedman ML: Pancreatic abscesses and lesser omental sac collections. Surg Gynecol Obstet 126:1301, 1968.
15. Donohue PE, Nyhus LM, Baker RJ: Pancreatic abscess after alcoholic pancreatitis. Arch Surg 115:905, 1980.
16. Farringer JL, Robbins LB, Pickens DR: Abscess of the pancreas. Surgery 60:964, 1966.
17. Ranson JHC, Spencer FC: Prevention, diagnosis, and treatment of pancreatic abscess. Surgery 82:99, 1977.
18. Warshaw AL: Problems of pancreatitis. Jpn J Surg 16:385, 1986.
19. Warshaw AL, Jin G: Improved survival in 45 patients with pancreatic abscess. Ann Surg 202:408, 1985.
20. Fink AS, Hiatt JR, Pitt HA, et al: Indolent presentation of pancreatic abscess. Experience with 100 cases. Arch Surg 123:1067, 1988.
21. Malangoni MA, Shallcross JC, Seiler JG, et al: Factors contributing to fatal outcome after treatment of pancreatic abscess. Ann Surg 203:605, 1986.
22. Balthazar EJ, Ranson JHC, Naidich DP, et al: Acute pancreatitis: Prognostic value of CT. Radiology 156:767, 1985.
23. Renner IG, Savage WT III, Pantoja JL, et al: Death due to acute pancreatitis. A retrospective analysis of 405 autopsy cases. Dig Dis Sci 30:1005, 1985.
24. Block S, Buchler M, Bittner R, et al: Sepsis indicators in acute pancreatitis. Pancreas 2:499, 1987.
25. Warshaw AL, O'Hara PJ: Susceptibility of the pancreas to ischemic injury in shock. Ann Surg 188:593, 1978.
26. Klar E, Herfarth CH, Messmer K: Therapeutic effect of isovolemic hemodilution with dextran 60 on the impairment of pancreatic microcirculation in acute biliary pancreatitis. Ann Surg 211:346, 1990.

27. Klar E, Messmer K, Warshaw AL, Herfarth C: Pancreatic ischaemia in experimental acute pancreatitis: Mechanism, significance and therapy. Br J Surg 77:1205, 1990.
28. Pfeffer RB, Lazzarini-Robertson A, Safadi D, et al: Gradations of pancreatitis, edematous through hemorrhagic, experimentally produced by controlled injection of microspheres into blood vessels in dogs. Surgery 51:764, 1962.
29. Popper HL, Necheles H, Russel KC: Transition of pancreatic edema into pancreatic necrosis. Surg Gynecol Obstet 87:79, 1948.
30. Klar E, Rattner DW, Compton C, et al: Adverse effect of therapeutic vasoconstrictors in experimental acute pancreatitis. Ann Surg 214:168, 1991.
31. Webster MW, Pasculle AW, Myerowitz RL, et al: Postinduction bacteremia in experimental acute pancreatitis. Am J Surg 138:418, 1979.
32. Medich DS, Lee TK, Mehlehm MF, et al: Pathogenesis of pancreatic sepsis. Am J Surg 165:46, 1993.
33. Tarpila E, Nystrom PO, Frinzen L, et al: Bacterial translocation during acute pancreatitis in rats. Eur J Surg 159:109, 1993.
34. Widdison AL, Karanija ND, Alvarez C, et al: Sources of pancreatic pathogens in acute necrotizing pancreatitis. Gastroenterology 100:A304, 1991.
35. Edmiston CE, Condon RE: Bacterial translocation. Surg Gynecol Obstet 173:73, 1991.
36. Runkel NS, Moody FG, Smith GS, et al: The role of the gut in the development of sepsis in acute pancreatitis. J Surg Res 51:18, 1991.
37. Ryan CM, Schmidt J, Lewandrowski K, et al: Gut macromolecular permeability in pancreatitis correlates with severity of disease in rats. Gastroenterology 104:890, 1993.
38. O'Dwyer ST, Michie HR, Ziegler TR, et al: A single dose of endotoxin increases intestinal permeability in healthy humans. Arch Surg 123:1459, 1988.
39. Maejima K, Deitch EA, Berg RD: Bacterial translocation from the gastrointestinal tracts of rats receiving thermal injury. Infect Immun 43:6, 1984.
40. Baker JW, Deitch EA, Berg RD, et al: Hemorrhagic shock induces bacterial translocation from the gut. J Trauma 28:896, 1988.
41. Foitzik TH, Fernández–del Castillo C, Ferraro MJ, et al: Pathogenesis and prevention of early pancreatic infection in experimental acute necrotizing pancreatitis. Ann Surg 222:179, 1995.
42. Rattner DW, Napolitano LM, Corsetti J, et al: Bacterial infection is not necessary for lethal necrotizing pancreatitis in mice. Int J Pancreatol 5:99, 1989.
43. Foitzik TH, Mithöfer K, Ferraro MJ, et al: Time course of bacterial infection of the pancreas and its relation to disease severity in a rodent model of acute necrotizing pancreatitis. Ann Surg 220:193, 1994.
44. Beger HG, Buchler M, Bittner R, et al: Necrosectomy and postoperative local lavage in necrotizing pancreatitis. Br J Surg 75:207, 1988.
45. Richter JM, Jacoby GA, Schapiro RH, et al: Pancreatic abscess due to *Candida albicans.* Ann Intern Med 97:221, 1982.
46. Howard JM, Bieluch VB: Pancreatic abscess secondary to *Candida albicans.* Pancreas 4:120, 1989.
47. Stambler JB, Kilbaner MI, Bliss CM, et al: Tuberculous abscess of the pancreas. Gastroenterology 83:922, 1982.
48. Iglehart JD, Mansback C, Postlethewait R, et al: Pancreatico–bronchial fistula: Case report and review of the literature. Gastroenterology 90:759, 1986.
49. White EM, Wittenberg J, Mueller PR, et al: Pancreatic necrosis: CT manifestations. Radiology 158:343, 1986.
50. Beger HG, Bittner R, Buchler M, et al: Hemodynamic data pattern in patients with acute pancreatitis. Gastroenterology 90:74, 1986.
51. Block S, Maier W, Bittner R, et al: Identification of pancreas necrosis in severe acute pancreatitis: Imaging procedures versus clinical staging. Gut 27:1035, 1986.
52. Saxon A, Reynolds JT, Doolas A: Management of pancreatic abscesses. Ann Surg 194:545, 1981.
53. Jeffrey RB, Federle MP, Cello JP, et al: Early computed tomography in severe acute pancreatitis. Surg Gynecol Obstet 154:170, 1982.
54. Siegelman SS, Copeland BE, Saba GP, et al: CT of fluid collections associated with pancreatitis. AJR 134:1121, 1980.
55. Clavien PA, Hauser H, Meyer P, et al: Value of contrast-enhanced computerized tomography in the early diagnosis and prognosis of acute pancreatitis. A prospective study of 202 patients. Am J Surg 155:457, 1988.
56. Federle MP, Jeffrey RB, Cross RA, et al: Computed tomography of pancreatic abscesses. AJR 136:879, 1981.
57. White M, Simeone JF, Wittenberg J: Air within a pancreatic inflammatory mass: Not necessarily a sign of abscess. J Clin Gastroenterol 5:173, 1983.
58. Ranson JHC, Rifkind KM, Turner JW: Prognostic signs and nonoperative peritoneal lavage in acute pancreatitis. Surg Gynecol Obstet 143:209, 1976.
59. Wilson C, Heads A, Shenkin A, et al: C-reactive protein, antiproteases and complement factors as objective markers of severity in acute pancreatitis. Br J Surg 76:177, 1989.
60. Buchler M, Malfertheiner P, Schoetensack C, et al: Sensitivity of antiproteases, complement factors and C-reactive protein in detecting pancreatic necrosis. Results of a prospective clinical study. Int J Pancreatol 1:227, 1986.
61. Mayer AD, McMahon MJ, Bowen M, et al: C-reactive protein: An aid to assessment and monitoring of acute pancreatitis. J Clin Pathol 37:207, 1984.
62. Puolakkainen P, Valtonen V, Paananen A, et al: C-reactive protein (CRP) and serum phospholipase A2 in the assessment of the severity of acute pancreatitis. Gut 28:764, 1987.
63. Ranson JHC, Balthazar E, Caccavale R, et al: Computed tomography and the prediction of pancreatic abscess in acute pancreatitis. Ann Surg 201:656, 1985.
64. Vernacchia FS, Jeffrey RB, Federle MP, et al: Pancreatic abscess: Predictive value of early abdominal CT. Radiology 162:435, 1987.
65. Nuutinen P: Contrast-enhanced computed tomography in acute oedematous pancreatitis. Surg Res Commun 1:251, 1987.
66. Schroder T, Kivisaari L, Standertskjold-Nordenstam CG, et al: The clinical significance of contrast-enhanced computed tomography in acute pancreatitis. Ann Chir Gynaecol 73:268, 1984.
67. Kivisaari L, Somer K, Standertskjold-Nordenstam CG, et al: A new method for the diagnosis of acute hemorrhagic-necrotizing pancreatitis using contrast-enhanced CT. Gastrointest Radiol 9:27, 1984.
68. Nuutinen P, Kivisaari L, Schroder T: Contrast-enhanced computed tomography and microangiography of the pancreas in acute human hemorrhagic/necrotizing pancreatitis. Pancreas 3:53, 1988.
69. London NJM, Neoptolemos JP, Lavelle J, et al: Contrast-enhanced abdominal computed tomography scanning and prediction of severity of acute pancreatitis: A prospective study. Br J Surg 76:266, 1989.
70. Bradley EL, Murphy F, Ferguson C: Prediction of pancreatic necrosis by dynamic pancreatography. Ann Surg 210:495, 1989.
71. Larvin M, Chalmers AG, Robinson PJ, et al: Débridement and closed cavity irrigation for the treatment of pancreatic necrosis. Br J Surg 76:465, 1989.
72. Foitzik TH, Bassi DG, Fernández–del Castillo C, et al: Intravenous contrast medium impairs oxygenation of the pancreas in acute necrotizing pancreatitis in the rat. Arch Surg 129:706, 1994.
73. Foitzik TH, Bassi DG, Schmidt J, et al: Intravenous contrast medium accentuates the severity of acute necrotizing pancreatitis in the rat. Gastroenterology 106:207, 1994.
74. Hiatt JR, Fink AS, King W III, et al: Percutaneous aspiration of peripancreatic fluid collections: A safe method to detect infection. Surgery 101:523, 1987.
75. Cogbill CL, Song KT: Acute pancreatitis. Arch Surg 100:673, 1970.
76. Kodesch R, Dupont HL: Infectious complications of acute pancreatitis. Surg Gynecol Obstet 136:763, 1973.
77. Howes R, Zuidema GD, Cameron JL: Evaluation of prophylactic antibiotics in acute pancreatitis. J Surg Res 18:197, 1975.
78. Finch WT, Sawyers JL, Schenker SA: A prospective study to determine the efficacy of antibiotics in acute pancreatitis. Ann Surg 183:667, 1976.
79. Craig RM, Dordal E, Myles L: The use of ampicillin in acute pancreatitis. Ann Intern Med 83:831, 1975.
80. Bradley EL: Antibiotics in acute pancreatitis. Current status and future directions. Am J Surg 158:472, 1989.
81. Gerzof SG, Robbins AH, Johnson WC, et al: Percutaneous cathe-

ter drainage of abdominal abscesses: A five-year experience. N Engl J Med 305:653, 1981.
82. Gerzof SG, Johnson WC, Robbins AH, Nabseth DC: Expanded criteria for percutaneous abscess drainage. Arch Surg 120:227, 1985.
83. Gerzof SG, Johnson WC, Robbins AH, et al: Percutaneous drainage of infected pancreatic pseudocysts. Arch Surg 119:888, 1984.
84. Pickelman J, Moncada R: The role of percutaneous drainage of pancreatic abscess. Am Surg 8:451, 1987.
85. Steiner E, Mueller PR, Hahn PF, et al: Complicated pancreatic abscesses: Problems in interventional management. Radiology 167:443, 1988.
86. Walters R, Herman CM, Neff R, et al: Percutaneous drainage of abscesses in the postoperative abdomen that is difficult to explore. Am J Surg 149:623, 1985.
87. Bradley EL: Management of infected pancreatic necrosis by open drainage. Ann Surg 206:542, 1987.
88. Pemberton JH, Becker JM, Dozois RR, et al: Controlled open lesser sac drainage for pancreatic abscess. Ann Surg 203:600, 1986.
89. Stone HH, Strom PR, Mullins RJ: Pancreatic abscess management by subtotal resection and packing. World J Surg 8:340, 1984.
90. Alexandre JF, Guerrari MT: Role of total pancreatectomy in the treatment of necrotizing pancreatitis. World J Surg 5:369, 1981.
91. Garcia-Sabrido JL, Tallado JM, Christou NV, et al: Treatment of severe intraabdominal sepsis and/or necrotic foci by an "open-abdomen" approach. Zipper and zipper-mesh techniques. Arch Surg 123:152, 1988.
92. Holden JL, Berne TV, Rossoff L: Pancreatic abscess following acute pancreatitis. Arch Surg 111:858, 1976.
93. Waltman AC, Luers PR, Athanasoulis CA, et al: Massive arterial hemorrhage in patients with pancreatitis. Complementary role of surgery and transcatheter occlusive techniques. Arch Surg 121:439, 1986.
94. Fielding GA, McLatchie GR, Wilson C, et al: Acute pancreatitis and pancreatic fistula formation. Br J Surg 76:1126, 1989.
95. Warshaw AL, Moncure AC, Rattner DW: Gastrocutaneous fistulas associated with pancreatic abscesses. An aggressive entity. Ann Surg 210:603, 1989.
96. Schmidt J, Warshaw AL: Surgical treatment of pancreatic fistulas: Rationale, timing and technique. *In* Bassi C, Vesentini S (eds): Topics on Pancreatic Fistulas. Berlin, Springer-Verlag, 1993, pp 176–194.
97. Russell JC, Welch JP, Clark DG: Colonic complications of acute pancreatitis and pancreatic abscess. Am J Surg 146:558, 1983.
98. Bouillot JL, Alexandre JH, Vuong NP: Colonic involvement in acute necrotizing pancreatitis: Results of surgical treatment. World J Surg 13:84, 1967.
99. Bradley EL: Enteropathies. *In* Bradley EL (ed): Complications of Pancreatitis. Philadelphia, WB Saunders, 1982, pp 265–292.
100. Becker H, Vinten-Johansen J, Buckberg GD, et al: Correlation of pancreatic blood flow and high-energy phosphates during experimental pancreatitis. Eur Surg Res 14:203, 1982.
101. Mayer AD, McMahon MJ, Corfield AP, et al: Controlled clinical trial of peritoneal lavage for the treatment of severe acute pancreatitis. N Engl J Med 312:399, 1985.
102. Ranson JHC, Berman RS: Long peritoneal lavage decreases pancreatic sepsis in severe acute pancreatitis. Ann Surg 211:708, 1990.
103. Steinberg WM, Schlesselman SE: Treatment of acute pancreatitis. Gastroenterology 93:1420, 1987.
104. Crist DW, Cameron JL: The current management of acute pancreatitis. Adv Surg 20:69, 1987.
105. Pederzoli P, Bassi C, Vesentini S, et al: A randomized multicenter clinical trial of antibiotic prophylaxis of septic complications in acute necrotizing pancreatitis with imipenem. Surg Gynecol Obstet 176:480, 1993.
106. Evans FC: Pancreatic abscesses. Am J Surg 117:537, 1969.
107. Bassi C, Pederzoli P, Vesentini S: Behavior of antibiotics during human necrotizing pancreatitis. Antimicrob Agents Chemother 38:830, 1994.
108. Büchler M, Malfertheiner P, Friess H: Human pancreatic tissue concentration of bactericidal antibiotics. Gastroenterology 103:1902, 1992.
109. Burns GP, Stein TA, Kabnick LS: Blood-pancreatic juice barrier to antibiotic excretion. Am J Surg 151:205, 1986.
110. Trudel JL, Wittnich C, Brown RA: Antibiotics bioavailability in acute experimental pancreatitis. J Am Coll Surg 178:475, 1994.
111. Mithöfer K, Fernández–del Castillo C, Ferraro MJ, et al: Antibiotic treatment improves survival in experimental acute necrotizing pancreatitis. Gastroenterology 110:232, 1996.
112. Van der Waaij D, Manson WL, Arends JP, et al: Clinical use of selective decontamination: The concept. Intensive Care Med 16:212, 1990.
113. Wells CL, Jechorek RP, Maddau MA, et al: Effects of clindamycin and metronidazole on intestinal colonization and translocation of *Enterococcus* in mice. Antimicrob Agents Chemother 32:1769, 1988.
114. McClelland P, Van Saene HKF, Murray A, et al: Prevention of bacterial infection and sepsis in acute severe pancreatitis. Ann R Coll Surg Engl 74:329, 1992.
115. Luiten EJT, Hop WCJ, Lange JF, et al: Controlled clinical trial of selective decontamination for the treatment of severe acute pancreatitis. Ann Surg 222:57, 1995.
116. Schmidt J, Hotz HG, Foitzik TH, et al: Intravenous contrast medium aggravates the impairment of pancreatic microcirculation in necrotizing pancreatitis in the rat. Ann Surg 221:257, 1995.

99

Splenic Abscess

Pamela A. Lipsett
Thomas R. Gadacz

Splenic abscess is an unusual source of intraabdominal sepsis. However, in several series, the incidence of splenic abscess appears to be increasing.[1–4] In population-based autopsy series, its reported incidence is between 0.2% and 0.7%.[5, 6] In this chapter the classification, causes, diagnosis, treatment, and outcome of splenic abscess are discussed.

Classification and Etiology

Splenic abscess can be classified in many ways. The most common method is based on the organisms cultured from the abscess. In recent times, the microbiology has changed. Table 99–1 shows the organisms and their incidence from a review of 227 patients.[1] Aerobic bacteria accounted for 44% of pathogens, with *Streptococcus* and *Staphylococcus* being the most common organisms. Anaerobic bacteria accounted for 12%, with mixed organisms, *Bacteroides*, and *Propionibacterium* predominating. Reports of fungal organisms in splenic abscesses are increasing in frequency. One case, which was reported before 1978, accounted for 2% of all organisms; however, fungal organisms are responsible for 26% of the reported cases today. The most common fungal organism is *Candida*.[7] In intravenous drug abusers, *Staphylococcus aureus* is present in 45% of the reported cases of splenic abscess.[1] Acquired immunodeficiency syndrome–related splenic abscesses have been seen with several organisms, including *Salmonella*,[8] disseminated *Mycobacterium avium-intracellulare*,[9] and fungi. In all series, about one fourth of patients with a splenic abscess will not have an organism cultured from the abscess cavity or from blood.

Splenic abscesses can also be classified as solitary or multi-

TABLE 99–1 ■ Microbiology of Splenic Abscess

BACTERIAL FINDINGS	%*
Aerobic Bacteria	59.4
Streptococcus	16.0
Staphylococcus	14.7
Salmonella	7.3
Other Gram-Negative Bacteria	21.4
Escherichia coli	36.0
Proteus	20.0
Shigella	18.0
Klebsiella	2.0
Unspecified coliforms	6.0
Pseudomonas	2.0
Anaerobes	12.1
Mixed organisms	32.0
Bacteroides	25.0
Propionibacterium	21.0
Clostridium	14.0
Streptococcus	11.0
Fusobacterium	4.0
Fungi	2.4
Sterile Cultures	26.6

*N = 230.

TABLE 99–2 ■ Predisposing Conditions in 227 Patients with a Splenic Abscess

RISK FACTOR	%
Infectious Etiology	68.80
Endocarditis	15.30
Urinary tract infection/surgery	8.10
Otitis media	3.30
Appendicitis	2.80
Pneumonia	2.80
Brucellosis	2.30
Lung abscess	2.30
Malaria	1.90
Diverticulitis	1.90
Amebiasis	0.95
Miscellaneous	11.90
Sepsis syndrome	11.90
Noninfectious Etiology	31.20
Trauma	16.70
Hemoglobinopathy	11.90
Contiguous diseases	23.00

ple[10] (Fig. 99–1). Solitary splenic abscesses are usually detected at an early stage. These abscesses have a better prognosis and are usually not associated with multiorgan sepsis. Multiple splenic abscesses are clinically covert, have a high mortality rate, and are part of multiorgan sepsis. In several reports, multiple splenic abscesses have accounted for increasing numbers of cases. These multiple cases are also associated with immunosuppressed states.

Another method of classification is based on the source of infection or the underlying disease.[10] In general, major risk factors are metastatic infection, trauma, contiguous infection, hematologic disorders, and immunodeficiency states. Specific risk factors for these disease categories and the incidence of these factors in 227 patients are shown in Table 99–1. Infection, especially endocarditis, is the most common cause. Trauma is a cause in 17% and hemoglobinopathies in 12%. Twenty percent of abscesses are discovered at autopsy.

Pathogenesis

The pathogenesis of a splenic abscess is divided into three categories: (1) pyogenic infection that may produce a bacteremia or septic embolization to the spleen, (2) splenic infarction due to ischemia secondary to hemoglobinopathy or nonpenetrating trauma, or (3) a contiguous process that may extend into the spleen. Table 99–2 lists the frequency of disease processes that contribute to splenic abscess.[11] Sepsis is by far the most common underlying condition, with endocarditis being the most common septic process. Of those without infection as a predisposing cause, trauma was present in 16% and hemoglobinopathy was present in 11.9%. Contiguous extension from diverticulitis, perforated neoplasm, perforated peptic disease, or pancreatic infection is common. In 17.9% of patients, there were associated diseases

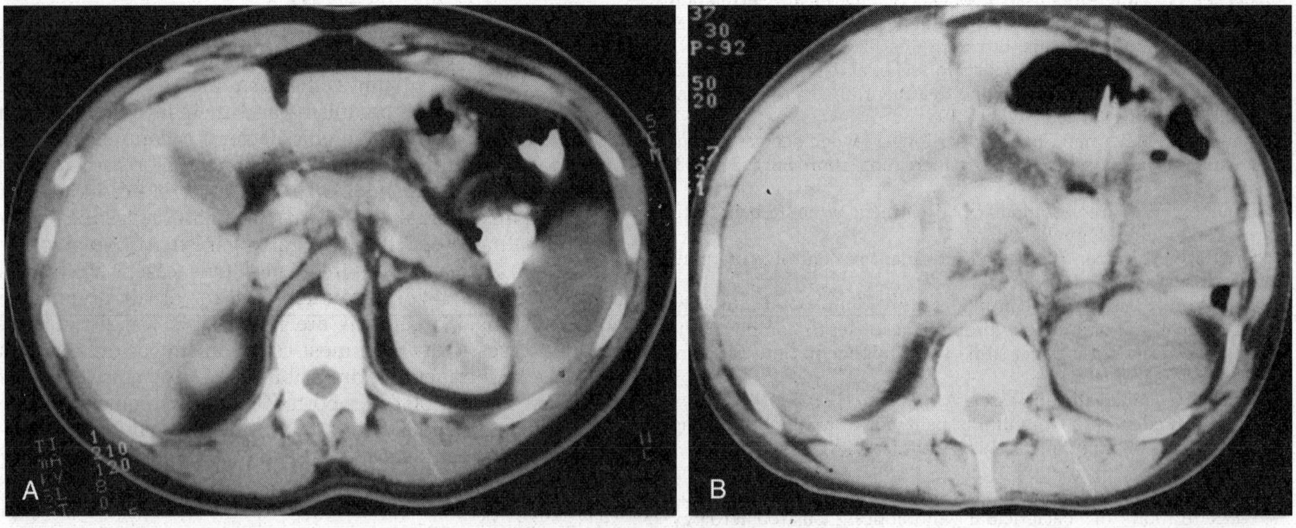

FIGURE 99–1 □ *A*, Unilocular hypodense splenic abscess secondary to endocarditis. The infecting organism was *Staphylococcus*. The patient was treated successfully with a splenectomy. *B*, A hypodense spleen with an air bubble seen on a computed tomographic scan. The contiguous colonic and pancreatic process mandated a splenectomy. Multiple enteric organisms were cultured.

such as chemotherapeutic immunosuppression, drug abuse, diabetes, alcoholism, or primary splenic disorders (e.g. amyloidosis and Felty syndrome).

Diagnosis

History and Physical Examination

The signs and symptoms of a splenic abscess are often not specific and are frequently related to the underlying disease (i.e., endocarditis). Table 99–3 characterizes the clinical findings in 227 patients.[1] Fever is present in 92.5% of patients with splenic abscess. Abdominal pain is present in 60% of patients, and pain specifically in the left upper quadrant is present in 39% of patients. Abscesses in the upper pole of the spleen may cause pain in the left shoulder owing to diaphragmatic irritation, whereas deep-seated infections may be asymptomatic. Signs and symptoms in the left side of the chest may occur, with a decrease in breath sounds in the left lower chest due either to lung parenchymal consolidation or to pleural effusion. Splenomegaly is present in slightly more than half of these patients. A splenic rub is rare.

Laboratory Findings

Leukocytosis is present in 70% to 88% of patients but is a variable finding. In one large series, the while cell count varied between 2400 and 41,000/mm^3.[11] In general, other serum laboratory studies were not helpful.

Radiographic Findings

Radiographic findings are nonspecific in up to 80% of cases of splenic abscess.[11, 12] In 33% of cases, an elevated left hemidiaphragm was found; in 28%, a left pleural effusion was found.[11] Abdominal x-ray films in 45 patients showed an abnormal soft tissue mass in 35.6% and air-fluid levels in the left upper quadrant in 11.1%. Barium studies may show a medial displacement of the stomach, but this finding is nonspecific. Other more definitive studies such as ultrasonography or, more specifically, computed tomography (CT) are indicated.

Radioisotopic Scanning

Technetium Tc 99m and gallium citrate Ga 67 scans have reported accuracy rates of 80% to 90%. Abscesses larger than 2 cm are frequently demonstrated, but 80% to 90% of the smaller abscesses are not well seen, and false-negative results are frequently noted. Although the sensitivity of radionuclide scans is not different from that of ultrasonography, the delay between injection and visualization make ultrasonography a better alternative when CT is unavailable. Thus, radionuclide scans are not recommended for the evaluation of patients with a suspected splenic abscess.[13]

TABLE 99–3 ■ Presenting Signs of Splenic Abscess

CLINICAL FEATURE	%
Fever	92.5
Abdominal pain	57.5
Left upper quadrant pain	39.2
Pleuritic pain	15.8
Toxic syndrome	15.4
Vomiting	14.0
Abdominal tenderness	60.1
Left upper quadrant tenderness	38.2
Splenomegaly	56.0

Ultrasonography

A splenic abscess usually presents as an echogenic pattern at ultrasonograpy. Often multiple septa and variable internal echo patterns are seen. When compared with CT scans, ultrasound investigations of the spleen are slightly less effective in establishing a diagnosis of a splenic abscess.[13] False-negative studies are more often seen,[12, 14, 15] and technical difficulties may be caused by overlying ribs or bowel gas.

Computed Tomography

CT is a useful adjunct in localizing an intraabdominal source of infection, especially when enhanced with intravenous contrast material. CT attenuation of the spleen is typically homogenous on noncontrast scans. An intravenous bolus injection with dynamic CT enhances the ability to visualize abnormal heterogeneous areas of the spleen.[16] With CT, a bacterial splenic abscess is frequently seen as a low-density center of fluid or necrotic tissue, unless a capsule has developed, in which case mild enhancement may be seen. Air within an intrasplenic collection is diagnostic of an abscess, although most abscesses do not contain air.[16] In patients with fungal microabscesses, typically lesions are smaller than 2 cm, are multiple, and are hypodense. Occasionally, a central focus of higher attenuation or wheel-within-a wheel pattern may be seen.[17] Granulomatous infections of the spleen are often seen as multiple irregular hypodense lesions in patients with mild splenomegaly. This population of patients may also have abdominal lymphadenopathy, high-attenuation ascites, nodular peritoneal thickening, and hepatomegaly.[18] The advantage of CT in establishing the diagnosis lies in its superior sensitivity compared with ultrasonography or scintigraphy, especially in cases of multilocular abscesses and fungal abscesses and in patients younger than 40 years.[7, 10, 12, 13, 19] CT is the imaging technique of choice for detection and characterization of splenic abscesses.

Treatment

The "gold standard" treatment of a splenic abscess is still splenectomy and intravenous antibiotics.[6, 10, 12] Percutaneous drainage of a splenic abscess may be used if the patient has a unilocular abscess, is in unstable condition from a recent operation, has had multiple previous operations, or has significant risks of standard surgical drainage.[14, 20] In patients with human immunodeficiency virus disease, splenectomy may improve the CD4$^+$ cell count and may also clear a continuing source of recurrent infection.

Percutaneous abscess drainage of the spleen can be safely employed only when a drainage window that avoids adjacent thoracic, gastrointestinal, and vascular structures is present.[6] In general, anterior approaches on the abdominal wall should be avoided, and the posterior abdominal wall offers better dependent drainage and safety. The catheter should be placed at the most dependent portion of the cavity, and a Gram stain and culture for aerobes, anaerobes, fungi and mycobacteria should be done routinely. At the time of catheter placement, the catheter should be irrigated copiously when the cavity has been evacuated so as to remove necrotic debris.

While the catheter remains in place, irrigation with 10 to 25 mL of saline should be done routinely. The catheter can be removed when the drainage is scant and the cavity has decreased in size as evidenced by a sinogram, ultrasound scan, or CT scan. In children, the possibility of an infected splenic cyst exists, and failure of the cavity to resolve invariably requires splenectomy or splenotomy. If the patient does not improve, splenectomy is advised. Percutaneous drainage is most likely to succeed when the abscess collection is unilocular and has a discrete wall and no internal septation. Abscesses containing thick, tenacious necrotic debris are less likely to be successfully drained percutaneously, as are phlegmons, poorly defined cavities, microabscesses, multiple abscesses, and abscesses originating from a contigous process. Percutaneous drainage of a multiloculated abscess is almost uniformly unsuccessful; however, for a single loculation, percutaneous drainage has been reported to be effective 75% to 90% of the time.[14, 19] In one series by Faught and associates,[2] 3 of 10 patients were treated successfully with percutaneous drainage. Another four patients retrospectively could have been candidates for percutaneous drainage. However, these 4 patients had additional intraabdominal disease, and 3 of 10 patients presented with peritonitis or hemorrhage and required immediate surgical intervention.[2] All morbidity (3 in 10) and mortality (1 in 10) occurred in the splenectomy group. Nonetheless, splenectomy remains the standard treatment for most patients.

For most patients undergoing surgical treatment, a midline operative approach allows examination of the entire abdomen if other areas of sepsis are suspected; otherwise, a subcostal incision is acceptable. In the presence of previous trauma or an enlarged spleen, vascular control of the splenic artery is obtained at the celiac axis. The splenic attachments are incised, and short gastric vessels are ligated and divided. The hilar vessels are identified and ligated, and the spleen is removed. After copious irrigation, the splenic bed is drained.

A splenotomy is occasionally indicated, and care is taken not to enter the pleural cavity or the rest of the abdominal cavity. Percutaneous or extraserosal drainage is indicated in high-risk patients when the spleen and abscess have adhered to the abdominal wall. This treatment option is exceptionally rare.

Broad-spectrum antibiotics should be initiated when a splenic abscess is diagnosed. This therapy should include agents effective against staphylococcal, streptococcal, and gram-negative bacteria. A semisynthetic penicillin or a cephalosporin plus an aminoglycoside is appropriate. If a contiguous abdominal process is suspected, an anaerobic agent should be added, and usually three antibiotics such as ampicillin, gentamicin, and metronidazole are given until the bacteria are identified and the sensitivities are known. In immunosuppressed patients, antifungal coverage should be initiated early in the disease process.

Outcome

In a review of the outcome of splenic abscesses, all untreated cases had a fatal outcome (Table 99–4). With antibiotics alone there is a 50% mortality rate in patients who have a pyogenic abscess, and the mortality rate is 6.2% in patients with a fungal abscess when treated only with antifungal agents (usually amphotericin). One hundred two patients were treated with splenectomy. The mortality rate was 7.81% and the morbidity rate was 11%. Thirty-three patients with unilocular abscesses were treated with a splenotomy or with percutaneous drainage without mortality; however, the morbidity rate was 12% and the failure rate was 30%.[12] Two thirds of all splenic abscesses in adults are solitary, and one third are multiple. In children, however, the exact opposite is true.[21–24] Solitary abscesses are generally easier to diagnose and treat and are usually caused by streptococci, staphylococci, hemoglobinopathies, or *Salmonella*. Multiple abscesses tend to be caused by *Candida*. The prognosis is clearly related to multisystem organ failure, age, and associated diseases. With early diagnosis and treatment, the mortality can be as low as 7%.[11, 12] A solitary abscess has a favorable prognosis with a mortality rate of 14%, whereas with multiple abscesses the mortality rate is 87%.[14]

The best treatment of an established fungal abscess is unclear because individual experiences are small in number. Most patients are cured by a combination of antifungal agents and splenectomy. One report has confirmed that 12 of 16 patients with a fungal abscess were cured with antifungal agents alone, and the mortality rate did not differ from that of an immediate splenectomy. These data suggest that confirmed fungal abscesses in the spleen may be treated with prolonged antifungal agents alone provided that complete resolution is confirmed by CT. However, a large fungal abscess may be better treated by percutaneous abscess drainage or by splenectomy, and a failing patient can be treated successfully by splenectomy.

TABLE 99–4 ■ Success and Mortality Rates for Treatment Options for a Splenic Abscess

TREATMENT	*n*	SUCCESS (%)	MORTALITY (%)
Splenectomy			
Bacterial	81	94	6
Fungal	21	86	14
Combined	102	92	8
Drainage Procedures			
Splenotomy	11	73	0
Percutaneous	22	68	0
Combined	33	70	0
Antibiotics Alone			
Bacterial	6	50	50
Fungal	16	75	6
No Treatment	11	0	100

References

1. Alsono-Cohen MA, Galera MJ, Ruiz M, et al: Splenic abscess. World J Surg 14:513–517, 1990.
2. Faught WE, Gilbertson JJ, Nelson EW: Splenic abscess: Presentation treatment options and results. Am J Surg 158:612–614, 1989.
3. Tikkakoski T, Siniluoto T, Päiväsalo M, et al: Splenic abscess: Imaging and intervention. Acta Radiol 33:561–565, 1992.
4. Paris S, Weiss SM, Ayers WH, et al: Splenic abscess. Am Surg 60:358–361, 1994.
5. Chulay JD, Lankerani MR: Splenic abscess. Am J Med 61:513–522, 1976.
6. Sarr MG, Zuidema GD: Splenic abscess—Presentation, diagnosis, and treatment. Surgery 92:480–485, 1982.
7. Helton WS, Carrico CJ, Zaveruha PA, Schaller R: Diagnosis and treatment of splenic fungal abscesses in the immune-suppressed patient. Am Surg 121:580–586, 1986.
8. Torres JR, Casas JR, Balda E, Cebrian J: Multifocal *Salmonella* splenic abscess in a HIV-infected patient. Trop Geogr Med 44:66–68, 1992.
9. Agarwala S, Bhatnagar V, Mitra DK, et al: Primary tubercular abscess of the spleen. J Pediatr Surg 27:1580–1581, 1992.
10. Gadacz TR: Splenic abscess. World J Surg 9:410–415, 1985.
11. Chun CH, Raff MJ, Contreras L, et al: Splenic abscess. Medicine (Baltimore) 59:50–65, 1980.
12. Nelken N, Ignatius J, Skinner M, Christensen N: Changing clinical spectrum of splenic abscess. A multicenter study and review of the literature. Am J Surg 154:27–34, 1987.
13. Grant E, Mertens MA, Mascatello VJ: Splenic abscess: Comparison of four imaging methods. AJR 132:465–466, 1979.

14. Gleich S, Wolin DA, Herbsman H: A review of percutaneous drainage in splenic abscess. Surg Gynecol Obstet 167:211–216, 1988.
15. Van Sonneberg E, Ferrucci JT, Muellar PR, et al: Percutaneous drainage of abscesses and fluid collections. Technique, results and applications. Radiology 142:1–10, 1982.
16. Rabushka LS, Kawashima A, Fishman ER: Imaging of the spleen: CT with supplemental MR examination. Radiographics 14:307–332, 1994.
17. Coslowitz PL, Labs JD, Fishman EK, et al: The changing spectrum of splenic abscess. Clin Imaging 13:201–207, 1989.
18. Choi BI, Im JC, Han MC, et al: Hepatosplenic tuberculosis with hypersplenism: CT evaluation. Gastrointest Radiol 14:265–267, 1989.
19. Van der Laan RT, Verbeeten B Jr, Smits NJ, et al: Computed tomography in the diagnosis and treatment of solitary splenic abscesses. J Comput Assist Tomogr 13:71–74, 1989.
20. Quinn SF, van Sonnenberg E, Casola G, et al: Interventional radiology in the spleen. Radiology 161:289–291, 1986.
21. Keidl CM, Chusid MJ: Splenic abscesses in childhood. Pediatr Infect Dis J 8:368–373, 1989.
22. Smith MD Jr, Masaki N, Camel JE, et al: Management of splenic abscess in immunocompromised children. J Pediatr Surg 28:823–826, 1993.
23. Akoh JA, Auld CD: Splenic abscess: Is conservation applicable? Br J Clin Pract 46:274–275, 1992.
24. Thorne MT, Chwals WJ: Treatment of complicated congenital splenic cysts. J Pediatr Surg 28:1635–1636, 1993.

OTHER SURGICAL INFECTIONS

100

Approach to the Patient with Postoperative Fever

E. Patchen Dellinger

Postoperative fever is not unusual and is always a source of concern to the physician and the patient. Most physicians and patients associate fever with infection, and the empirical prescription of antibiotics is a common response. To put these concerns into perspective and to analyze the best approach to this common phenomenon, I will consider the definition of fever, the correlation between postoperative fever and postoperative infection, and other possible causes of postoperative fever.

Definitions and Incidence

Fever can be defined as any temperature higher than 37°C, but the normal variability of temperature among individuals and the even greater variability of temperature in the postoperative period render this definition too nonspecific to be useful clinically. Dykes[1] found that 82% of 162 nonobstetric postoperative patients had a recorded temperature higher than 37°C in the first postoperative week. Figure 100–1 illustrates the range of unexplained fevers observed after four different representative surgical procedures. Other definitions of postoperative fever use 38°C as the lower limit, but the duration criterion varies: within 3 days of operation,[2] while in the hospital,[3] within 10 days of operation,[4] during the first 7 days,[5] for 2 consecutive days,[6] for 48 hours,[7] and for 8 hours during the first 6 days.[8] These reports record the incidence of postoperative fever to be between 14% and 89%. In the same reports, the prevalence of infection varied from 2% to 13% for all patients and between 5% and 62% for febrile patients. The proportion of febrile patients who are infected appears to increase as the definition of fever becomes more rigorous[1–13] (Table 100–1). However, as the definition of postoperative fever becomes more rigorous, a greater proportion of infected patients no longer meet the definition of fever. The result is that the overall accuracy of fever as an index of infection changes little, if at all (Dellinger EP, personal observations).[5, 14–16] Triulzi and associates[17] reported on 109 patients having spinal fusion procedures with an infection rate of 7%. The average duration of fever in infected patients was 4 days compared with 3 days in patients without infection.[17] The mean day for diagnosis of infection was day 8 with a median of day 14. Clearly, the great majority of febrile postoperative patients are not infected, and indeed, as many as 50% of infected patients may not be febrile,[7, 13] depending on the definition of postoperative fever.

Because fever is common in the absence of infection, it is important to consider causes of postoperative fever other than infection. Atelectasis without infection is commonly cited as a cause of postoperative fever, although the mechanism is not known. Some work has suggested that the fever

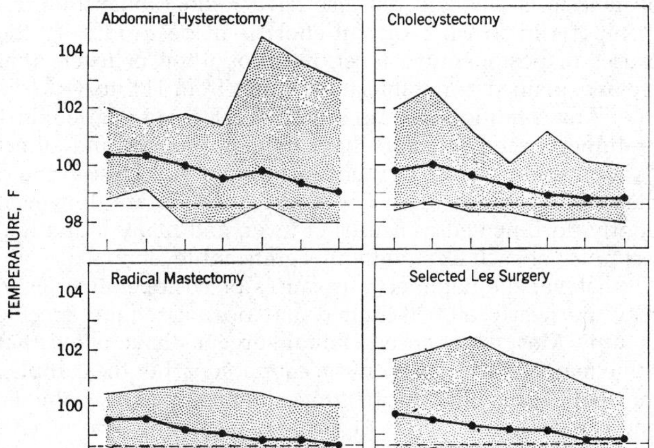

FIGURE 100–1 □ Mean, maximal, and minimal daily temperatures in four groups of 20 consecutive patients with unexplained fevers. (From Dykes MHM: Unexplained postoperative fever. Its value as a sign of halothane sensitization. JAMA 216:641–644, 1971.)

TABLE 100–1 ■ Postoperative Fever Definitions and Incidence of Fever and Infection

INVESTIGATOR	PATIENTS/OPERATION	FEVER CRITERION (°C)	DURATION	PATIENTS: NUMBER	PATIENTS: No. Febrile (% of Total)	PATIENTS: No. Infected (% of Total)	PATIENTS: Febrile and Infected (%)
Dykes[1]	Nonobstetric	>37	Any, days 1–7	133	104 (78)	31* (23)	30*
Yeung et al[2]	Pediatric	≥38	Any, days 1–3	256	73 (29)	4 (2)	5
Miholic et al[3]	Open heart	≥38	Any	115	102 (89)	7 (6)	7
Pien et al[4]	Coronary bypass	≥38	Any, days 1–9	263	174† (66)	24 (9)	14
Mellors et al[5]	Abdominal operations	≥38.1	Any, days 1–7	434	163 (38)	26 (6)	16
Garibaldi et al[6]	General surgical	≥38	2 consecutive days	871	194 (22)	113 (13)	58
Galicier and Richet[7]	General surgical	≥38	Persists 48 h in hospital	570	78 (14)	48 (8)	62
Freischlag and Busuttil[8]	Abdominal operations	≥38.5	Twice in 8 h, days 1–6	464	71 (15)	19 (4)	27
Le Gall et al[9]	Intensive care unit patients/abdominal operations	≥39	Any, days 3–10	Only febrile patients	100 (100)	89 (89)	89
Rantala et al[10]	Abdominal operations	>38.5	>24 h postoperatively	Only febrile patients	107 (100)	48 (45)	45
Engoren[11]	Open heart	≥38	Days 0–2	100	37 (37)	0	0
		≥38.5	Days 0–2	100	14 (14)	0	0
Petrelli et al[12]	Colorectal operations	>38	Any, days 1–7	77	37 (48)	0	0
Giangobbe et al[13]	Cholecystectomy	≥38.4 or ≥38	Any time in hospital twice, 4 h apart	176	28 (16)	10 (6)	7

*Includes both infected patients and patients with diagnosed noninfectious causes of fever (atelectasis and hematoma).
†Number projected from the incidence in a subset of uninfected patients.

that often accompanies atelectasis may be caused by the production of interleukin-1 and tumor necrosis factor by pulmonary macrophages[18]; however, although atelectasis may be responsible for some postoperative fevers, many patients who have a postoperative fever show no physical or radiographic signs of atelectasis, and many patients with radiographic evidence of atelectasis are not febrile.[11, 16] Roberts and associates[16] found that 37 of 109 febrile patients did not have radiographic evidence of atelectasis, whereas 82 of 154 patients with atelectasis did not have fever. Similarly, in patients who had no preexisting cardiac or pulmonary disease, Ejlertsen and associates[19] found a large group with atelectasis but no fever after upper abdominal operations. Dykes[1] found no patients with distinctive physical findings of atelectasis who did not also have radiographic findings. In reports in which a careful effort is made to identify the causes of postoperative fever, the proportion of fevers that are unexplained or noninfectious varies from 11% to 84%.[1, 5, 6, 9, 15, 16] Any condition that can cause the release of interleukin-1 or tumor necrosis factor—hematoma formation and direct tissue trauma, pulmonary embolism, and atelectasis—could theoretically cause fever. These explanations are, however, poorly documented as causes of fever, and many individual examples of each exist without significant fever.

Whatever the noninfectious causes of postoperative fever, they are nearly all self-limited and do not require specific therapy. Most experienced clinical surgeons have noted that some temperature elevation is a common part of the complex metabolic response to major surgical injury. In many patients, one can observe a series of changes beginning 3 to 6 days after the operation. Within a 24-hour period, temperature normalizes, the pulse rate falls to preoperative levels, bowel function returns, fluid balance sheets show diuresis of the interstitial (third space) fluid accumulated during the procedure, and the patient begins to smile spontaneously and take an interest in his or her personal appearance again (positive lipstick sign). Two exceptions to this self-limited course include major pulmonary collapse, which should be treated by physical measures for reexpansion, and pulmonary embolism, which is treated with anticoagulation or other specific measures. The clinician's primary approach to a postoperative fever, therefore, is appropriately focused on the possibility of infection, although in most cases none is found. Although the surgical incision is the natural area of concern, it is not the location of the majority of postoperative infections and, in fact, often is not even the most common.[2, 5, 7, 8, 20, 21] The two most common sites of infection are wounds and the urinary tract. Following these sites are respiratory tract infections and then a number of much less common ones, including intravenous catheter–associated infections, other blood stream infections, sinusitis, and infections entirely unrelated to the operative procedure.

Importance of Timing

The approach to a patient with postoperative fever must account for the relative likelihood that different causes will produce fever at different times after operation and the importance or urgency of diagnosis of the different causes. Garibaldi and associates[6] found that 38% of all postoperative fevers occurred within 48 hours after an operation, but the great majority (73%) of these early fevers were noninfectious in origin (Fig. 100–2). Of fevers originating on the first day, 80% were noninfectious, whereas most of the remaining 20% were respiratory in origin. On the second and third days, new fevers were still 55% to 65% noninfectious. Only on the fifth postoperative day was a new fever as likely to represent a surgical site infection as to be noninfectious.[6] Of all fevers that began 5 days or longer after operation, 42% were caused by wound infections, 29% by urinary tract infections, 12% by respiratory tract infections, and only 10% were noninfectious. Galicier and Richet[7] found that most fevers due to infection began on the third postoperative day or later, whereas almost 95% of fevers without an infectious origin began within 4 days of the operation. Pien and coworkers[4] found that less

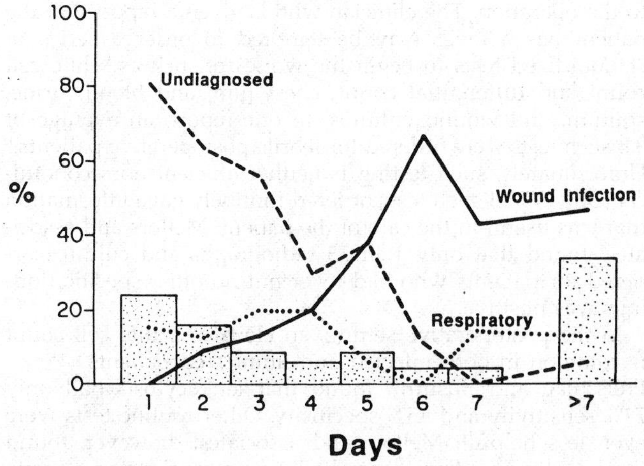

FIGURE 100–2 ▫ Vertical bars indicate the percentage of all fevers that appear each respective day. Lines indicate the percentage of new fevers on each day that are due to wound infection (———) or respiratory infection (··········) or are unexplained (– – – –) (Data from Garibaldi RA, Brodine S, Matsumiya S, Coleman M: Evidence for the non-infectious etiology of early postoperative fever. Infect Control 6:273–277, 1985.)

than 10% of patients with noninfectious fevers after coronary artery bypass operations were febrile after the fourth postoperative day, whereas 25% of fevers that were still present or began after the fourth day were due to infections. Data also do not support the commonly held belief that the intensity of the fever (higher than 39°C or 40°C) during the first 5 to 7 postoperative days is more likely to distinguish infected from uninfected patients or severe from minor infections[5, 6, 14, 15] (Figs. 100–3 and 100–4).

Urgent Causes of Early Fever

These data influence the approach to early (within 48 hours) postoperative fever. The great majority of these fevers are noninfectious and self-limited. This does not mean that such fevers can be ignored, but it does mean that an extensive laboratory or radiographic work-up is not indicated. Two rare but lethal infections should be considered when high fever presents in the first 24 to 48 hours after an operation. Both should be detected by physical examination, and each febrile postoperative patient should be examined to rule out these infections.

After an abdominal operation, an unnoticed injury to the bowel or a leaking anastomosis that causes peritoneal soiling with intestinal contents usually results in an early, high fever. It also causes striking cardiovascular disturbances, marked fluid sequestration, and specific physical findings. An abdominal examination and a review of the clinical setting should suffice to discover this problem, although the abdominal examination is made more difficult by the proximity of a recent incision. This potential complication is best evaluated by the operating surgeon, who is aware of the details of the operative procedure, including any unusual or untoward events.

Most wound infections are not evident on physical examination before the fourth postoperative day; in fact, most infections are discovered considerably later. However, an invasive soft tissue infection due to one or two organisms can manifest during the first 48 hours and represents a major threat to the patient. These organisms are the β-hemolytic streptococci and the histotoxic *Clostridium* species. Infections caused by these organisms are discussed in detail in other chapters. Diagnosis is made by inspection of the wound and by a Gram stain of any fluid in the wound.

An even rarer cause of fever in the first 48 hours after operation is toxic shock syndrome associated with a *Staphylococcus aureus* wound infection. During an 18-month period in 1980 and 1981, the Centers for Disease Control and Prevention confirmed 13 such cases among 16 suspected cases.[22] This finding represented less than 1% of all cases of toxic shock syndrome reported to the Centers for Disease Control and Prevention during that interval. Seven of the 13 cases had their onset within 48 hours after operation. Fever, diarrhea, and vomiting were the earliest signs. The most characteristic presentation was fever, profuse watery diarrhea, erythroderma, and hypotension. Local signs of wound infection were often absent initially. The best treatment is not known, but drainage and irrigation of the wound in combination with a systemic antistaphylococcal antibiotic seem reasonable.[23]

Antibiotic-associated enterocolitis due to *Clostridium difficile* is another potential cause of postoperative fever. It can occur within 1 or 2 days after operation and antibiotic administration but is often delayed and can occur several weeks later. It should be considered in any hospitalized patient who has received antibiotics and who has diarrhea. Cases have been reported after a single short course of prophylactic antibiotics.[24, 25] In one report, 55% of all cases of *C. difficile*

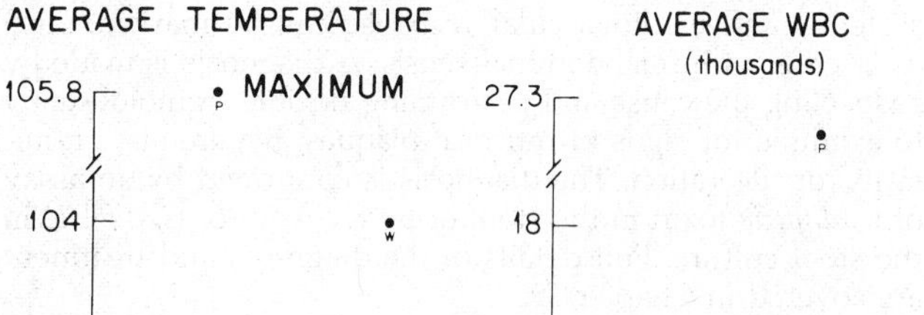

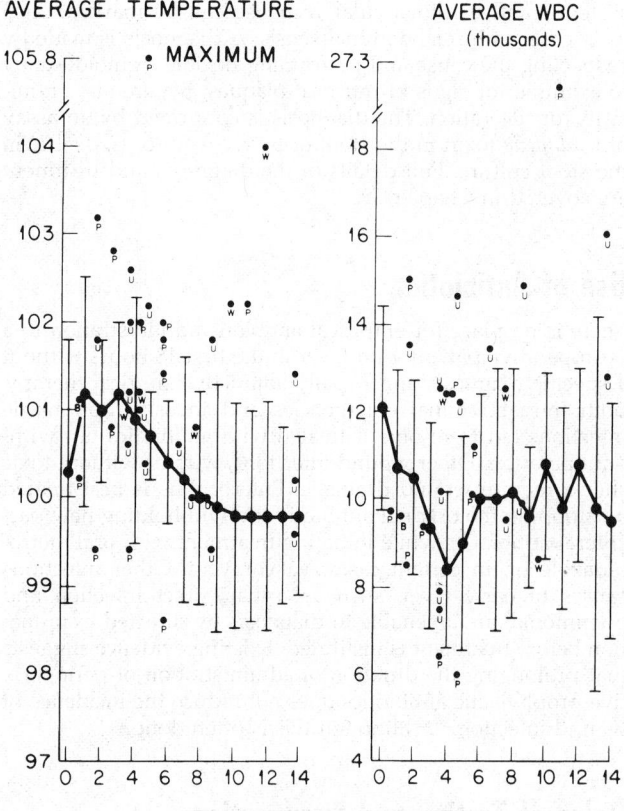

FIGURE 100–3 ▫ Curves represent mean values ±1 SD for daily maximal temperature and white cell count for 154 patients without infection. Individual points represent values for the 35 patients with infection on the day infection was documented. P, Pneumonia; W, wound infection; U, urinary tract infection; B, bacteremia. (From Bell DM, Goldmann DA, Hopkins CC, et al: Unreliability of fever and leukocytosis in the diagnosis of infection after cardiac valve surgery. J Thorac Cardiovasc Surg 75:87–90, 1978.)

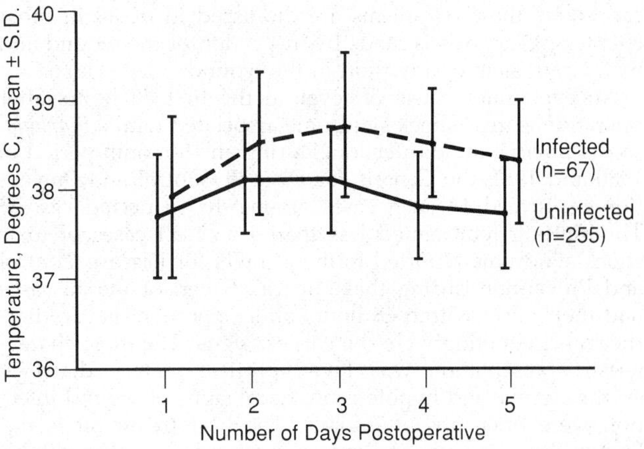

FIGURE 100–4 □ Mean daily maximal temperature ±1 SD for 67 patients with (- - - -) and 255 patients without (———) postoperative infection after celiotomy for penetrating abdominal injury.

colitis in a 10-year period occurred on the surgical service. Perioperative prophylaxis was the most common indication for preceding antibiotics and accounted for 25% of all cases.[24] Many, but not all, patients have fever, and abdominal cramps and leukocytosis are also common.[26, 27] White blood cells are present in the stool smear in approximately half of the cases and, if present, suggest colitis rather than toxic shock. The systemic and cardiovascular response can be marked, such as in cases of intraabdominal sepsis. A diagnosis is made by suspecting the cause and performing flexible sigmoidoscopy to examine for signs of mucosal plaques, hyperemia, granularity, or ulceration. The diagnosis is confirmed by an assay of *C. difficile* toxin in the stool or by recovery of *C. difficile* in the stool culture. Full details of the diagnosis and treatment are covered in Chapter 79.

Use of Antibiotics

There is no place for empirical antibiotic administration to a postoperative patient with fever in the first 48 hours without a specific diagnosis and usually adjunctive surgical therapy. Both intraabdominal emergencies and invasive soft tissue infections fail to resolve if treated with antibiotics but without operation. Other wound infections, with or without toxic shock, require wound drainage. Enterocolitis is best treated by stopping the original antibiotic and withholding new parenteral antibiotics while initiating treatment with oral metronidazole or, in certain cases, vancomycin. Other infectious causes of early fever, such as urinary tract infection and pneumonia, are amenable to diagnosis by directed examination before treatment is instituted. Existing evidence suggests that prolonging the duration of administration of perioperative prophylactic antibiotics does not reduce the incidence of wound infection,[28–32] although this is often done.[33–35]

Roles of Testing and Examination

After the third or fourth postoperative day, the likelihood that a new or persistent fever is infectious in origin is greater and begins to exceed the probability that a noninfectious cause is responsible (see Fig. 100–2). A variety of diagnoses should be considered in decreasing order of likelihood: surgical site infection (in either the incision or a deeper operative site), urinary tract infection, respiratory tract infection, intravascular catheter–associated infection, and others unrelated to the operation. The clinician who is given a report that the patient has a fever may be tempted to order a series of standardized tests to begin the work-up, such as white cell count and differential count, chest film, and blood, urine, sputum, and wound cultures. In one report, an average of 3.8 such tests were ordered for febrile postoperative patients.[8] Unfortunately, such testing is neither efficient nor economical. Only 7% of such tests ordered routinely gave information that was useful in the care of the patient. Mellors and associates[5] found that only 1 in 73 radiographs and cultures ordered for patients who had fever but no other specific findings was positive.

In the postoperative setting, an elevated white cell count is common in both infected and uninfected patients.[8, 14, 15, 36] Freischlag and Busuttil[8] found that leukocytosis had only 74% sensitivity and 45% specificity. Other routine tests were even less helpful. Mellors and associates,[5] however, found that greater specificity was obtained by considering a white cell count that was either greater than 10,000/mm^3 or less than 5000/mm^3, compared with a count simply greater than a specific level.

A physical examination done by a physician with knowledge of the recent history and details of the operative procedure is most helpful for diagnosing postoperative infections. Tests suggested by this examination are likely to confirm a clinical diagnosis. A wound infection is diagnosed by inspecting the wound. Urinary tract infections are rare in postoperative patients who have not been catheterized and have no history of prior urinary tract infections or acute symptoms. Urinalysis and a Gram smear of an unspun drop of urine give valuable information about the likelihood of a urinary tract infection a day before culture results are available. Ordering a sputum culture for a patient who does not have a productive cough and thoracic findings on physical examination is unrewarding and merely produces information regarding the bacterial content of the oropharynx. Intravascular catheters that have been in position for 3 days or more should be changed at the onset of a new fever, and cultures of the catheter should be obtained.

Blood cultures should be part of the evaluation of any fever that occurs after the fourth postoperative day in a patient with a permanent intravascular device such as a cardiac valve or vascular graft. Blood cultures obtained from postoperative patients with fever whose course is otherwise routine rarely grow organisms. They are indicated for patients who are clinically septic, but only as an adjunct, and even then they are most often negative in postoperative patients, even those with documented bacterial infection.[9] In a study of the utility of blood cultures for diagnosis in febrile postoperative patients, Theuer and associates[37] reported on 364 cultures obtained during 108 febrile events in 72 patients. All patients had temperatures above 38.6°C, and the average temperature was 38.9°C in patients both with and without positive blood cultures. Among the 364 cultures obtained, there were 5 positive cultures, 4 contaminated cultures, and 355 cultures without growth. None of the 85 cultures obtained on the first 3 days after operation were positive. Of cultures obtained on days 4 through 10, 8% were positive.[37]

A postoperative patient with signs of systemic sepsis must be assumed to have a life-threatening infection at the operative site unless it is proved otherwise, and this nearly always demands direct diagnostic procedures and finally operative intervention. In none of these settings does a patient benefit from empirical administration of antibiotics before a presumptive clinical diagnosis is made and an appropriate operative intervention is instituted. Antibiotic administration without diagnosis and indicated operative intervention may temporarily suppress clinical evidence of infection, such as fever, cause a delay in making a diagnosis, and increase the risk of secondary complications such as the multiple organ failure syndrome.

Intraabdominal Infections

A deep intraabdominal infection is a less common but more serious complication of abdominal surgery than wound infection, urinary tract infection, respiratory tract infection, or infection of intravascular devices. Approximately 4% of all abdominal operations are followed by an urgent reoperation within the next month, and about half of these are required for a deep infectious complication[38–41] (Table 100–2). However, a patient with high fever and systemic sepsis who qualifies for admission to an intensive care unit after an abdominal operation is much more likely to have an intraabdominal infection.[9] Intraabdominal infection has a mortality rate in the range of 15% to 50%, depending on the population of patients and other risk factors.[42–45] A delay in diagnosis is common and increases mortality, especially in the immediate postoperative period.[45]

The seriousness of a postoperative intraabdominal infection is the stimulus for a great deal of testing in patients with postoperative fever. As discussed earlier for other potential postoperative infections, blind reliance on blood tests and radiographs is not an effective strategy. Only about 11% to 29% of patients with documented intraabdominal infection have positive blood cultures.[9, 43, 44] Specialized radiographic tests are needed for diagnosis in the minority of cases.[46] In the specific circumstance of septic intensive care unit patients, computed tomography used as the primary study often fails to yield information that is helpful in determining the treatment of the patient.[47] The most sensitive instrument for suspecting infection and determining its most likely location continues to be a conscientious physician utilizing the time-honored skills of history and physical examination. Computed tomography can be extremely useful, however, for confirming a suspicion and planning the best therapeutic approach.[48]

Less Common Causes of Fever

If the work-up outlined here does not produce a diagnosis, less common causes of postoperative fever must be considered. Fever caused by a drug must be considered in any febrile patient, but it is a diagnosis of exclusion. A patient who has in place devices such as a nasogastric or nasotracheal tube may develop purulent sinusitis due to nosocomial organisms.[49] Purulent nasal drainage implies the diagnosis, but it may not be present. In one study of trauma patients, serous or purulent otitis media was a sensitive and specific indicator of paranasal sinusitis.[50] Sinus mucosal thickening or fluid, with or without an air-fluid level, may be detected by plain films or by computed tomography, but computed tomography is more sensitive, especially in the presence of tubes, bandages, and fractures. A sinus puncture for a Gram smear and culture, the definitive diagnostic test, also provides information about pathogens and sensitivity.

Gout can be triggered by surgical stress, which may unmask previously undiagnosed disease. In a 10-year experience at the Jackson Veterans Affairs Hospital, 295 patients with the preoperative diagnosis of gout had surgical procedures, and 45 (15%) developed postoperative gout. Another seven patients had their first diagnosed gout attack during the postoperative period during this same 10-year interval. The average temperature of these 52 patients was 38.2°C, and the attacks occurred between 1 and 17 days postoperatively with a mean of 4 days. Eighty-five percent occurred in the lower extremity, whereas 87% were monoarticular, but only 15% had classic podagra.[51]

Any patient can develop parotitis, but elderly and dehydrated patients and those with poor oral hygiene are at higher risk. It is marked by local pain and swelling and sometimes by edema overlying the gland. In some cases, pus can be expressed from the duct. Parotitis is treated with antistaphylococcal antibiotics and sometimes by incision of the gland.

Transfusion-associated viral infection should be considered when a fever develops 3 weeks or longer after a procedure in which blood transfusions were used. The most common cause has been hepatitis C, followed by hepatitis B.[52–55] The availability of a serologic test for hepatitis C should reduce this occurrence, but modern prospective series recording the incidence of hepatitis after transfusion have not been published since the availability of this test. After transfusion, cytomegalovirus can also cause a mononucleosis-like syndrome. This is commonly associated with cardiac surgery that requires cardiopulmonary bypass, but it has also been reported after noncardiac surgery.[56] It may be more common in patients who have undergone splenectomy. When a directed examination of the operative site, urinary tract, lungs, and intravascular devices does not reveal the source of fever, the approach is a meticulous complete physical examination and detailed history, just as for other patients with fever.

Summary

Postoperative fever is common, both with and without postoperative infectious complications. In the first 2 to 4 days after operation, most fevers are noninfectious in origin and resolve without specific therapy. It is important, however, to rule out a peritoneal leak of enteric contents and invasive soft tissue infection with directed physical examination. The clinician should also be aware of the remote possibility of toxic shock syndrome associated with staphylococcal wound infection. After the fourth postoperative day, a new or persis-

TABLE 100–2 ■ Repeated Laparotomy for Infection

INVESTIGATOR	PRIMARY LAPAROTOMIES (NO.)	REPEATED LAPAROTOMY		REPEATED LAPAROTOMY FOR INFECTION	
		No.	%	No.	%
Hinsdale and Jaffe[41]	5,532	119	2	77	65
Harbrecht et al[40]	1,633	133	7	60	53
Zer et al[39]	3,679	95	3	33	35
Bunt[38]	2,657	192	7	93	48
Total	13,501	519	3.8	263	51

tent fever is more likely to represent an infectious complication, although many self-limited, noninfectious fevers can still occur. The most effective diagnostic approach is a review of the operative and preoperative history and a physical examination. Laboratory tests and radiographic examinations are best directed by the results of the physical examination rather than being ordered routinely in response to a fever. Neither prolongation of perioperative prophylactic antibiotics nor the initiation of empirical therapeutic antibiotics is indicated without a presumptive clinical diagnosis and a plan for operative intervention when indicated.

References

1. Dykes M: Unexplained postoperative fever: Its value as a sign of halothane sensitization. JAMA 216:641, 1971.
2. Yeung RS, Buck JR, Filler RM: The significance of fever following operations in children. J Pediatr Surg 17:347, 1982.
3. Miholic J, Hiertz H, Hudec M, et al: Fever, leucocytosis and infection after open heart surgery. A log-linear regression analysis of 115 cases. Thorac Cardiovasc Surg 32:45, 1984.
4. Pien FD, Ho PWL, Fergusson DJG: Fever and infection after cardiac operation. Ann Thorac Surg 33:382, 1982.
5. Mellors JW, Kelly JJ, Gusberg RJ, et al: A simple index to estimate the likelihood of bacterial infection in patients developing fever after abdominal surgery. Am Surg 54:558, 1988.
6. Garibaldi RA, Brodine S, Matsumiya S, Coleman M: Evidence for the noninfectious etiology of early postoperative fever. Infect Control 6:273, 1985.
7. Galicier C, Richet H: A prospective study of postoperative fever in a general surgery department. Infect Control 6:487, 1985.
8. Freischlag JB, Busuttil RW: The value of postoperative fever evaluation. Surgery 94:358, 1983.
9. Le Gall JR, Fagniez PL, Meakins J, et al: Diagnostic features of early high post-laparotomy fever: A prospective study of 100 patients. Br J Surg 69:452, 1982.
10. Rantala A, Niinikoski J, Lehtonen O-P: Early *Candida* isolations in febrile patients after abdominal surgery. Scand J Infect Dis 25:479, 1993.
11. Engoren M: Lack of association between atelectasis and fever. Chest 107:81, 1995.
12. Petrelli NJ, Stulc JP, Rodriguez-Bigas M, et al: Nasogastric decompression following elective colorectal surgery: A prospective randomized study. Am Surg 59:632, 1993.
13. Giangobbe MJ, Rappaport WD, Stein B: The significance of fever following cholecystectomy. J Fam Pract 34:437, 1992.
14. Bell DM, Goldmann DA, Hopkins CC, et al: Unreliability of fever and leukocytosis in the diagnosis of infection after cardiac valve surgery. J Thorac Cardiovasc Surg 75:87, 1978.
15. Dellinger EP, Wertz MJ, Oreskovich MR, et al: Specificity of fever and leukocytosis after laparotomy for penetrating abdominal trauma. J Trauma 23:633, 1983.
16. Roberts J, Barnes W, Pennock M, et al: Diagnostic accuracy of fever as a measure of postoperative pulmonary complications. Heart Lung 17:166, 1988.
17. Triulzi DJ, Vanek K, Ryan DH, et al: A clinical and immunologic study of blood transfusion and postoperative bacterial infection in spinal surgery. Transfusion 32:517, 1992.
18. Kisala JM, Ayala A, Stephan RN, et al: A model of pulmonary atelectasis in rats: Activation of alveolar macrophage and cytokine release. Am J Physiol 264:R610, 1993.
19. Ejlertsen T, Nielsen PH, Jepsen S, Olsen A: Early diagnosis of postoperative pneumonia following upper abdominal surgery. A study in patients without cardiopulmonary disorder at operation. Acta Chir Scand 155:93, 1989.
20. Horan TC, White JW, Jarvis WR, et al: Nosocomial infection surveillance, 1984. MMWR CDC Surveill Summ 35:17SS, 1986.
21. Dellinger E, Oreskovich M, Wertz M, et al: Risk of infection following laparotomy for penetrating abdominal injury. Arch Surg 119:20, 1984.
22. Bartlett P, Reingold AL, Graham DR, et al: Toxic shock syndrome associated with surgical wound infections. JAMA 247:1448, 1982.
23. Goodpasture HC, Voth DW: Toxic shock syndrome—Additional perspectives. JAMA 247:1464, 1982.
24. Jobe BA, Grasley A, Deveney KE, et al: *Clostridium difficile* colitis: An increasing hospital-acquired illness. Am J Surg 169:480, 1995.
25. Yee J, Dixon CM, McLean AP, et al: *Clostridium difficile* disease in a department of surgery. The significance of prophylactic antibiotics. Arch Surg 126:241, 1991.
26. George WL: Antimicrobial agent-associated colitis and diarrhea: Historical background and clinical aspects. Rev Infect Dis 6:S208, 1984.
27. Bartlett JG: Antibiotic-associated colitis. Dis Mon 30:6, 1984.
28. Dellinger E, Wertz M, Lennard E, et al: Efficacy of short-course antibiotic prophylaxis after penetrating intestinal injury. Arch Surg 121:23, 1986.
29. Dellinger E, Caplan E, Weaver L, et al: Duration of preventive antibiotic administration for open extremity fractures. Arch Surg 123:333, 1988.
30. Dellinger E, Miller S, Wertz M, et al: Risk of infection after open fracture of the arm or leg. Arch Surg 123:1320, 1988.
31. Strachan C, Black J, Powis S, et al: Prophylactic use of cephazolin against wound sepsis after cholecystectomy. Br Med J 1:1254, 1977.
32. Mendelson J, Portnoy J, De Saint Victor JR, Gelfand MM: Effect of single and multidose cephradine prophylaxis on infectious morbidity of vaginal hysterectomy. Obstet Gynecol 53:31, 1979.
33. Shapiro M, Townsend TR, Rosner B, et al: Use of antimicrobial drugs in general hospitals: Patterns of prophylaxis. N Engl J Med 301:351, 1979.
34. Classen DC, Evans RS, Pestotnik SL, et al: The timing of prophylactic administration of antibiotics and the risk of surgical wound infection. N Engl J Med 326:281, 1992.
35. Currier JS, Campbell H, Platt R, et al: Perioperative antimicrobial prophylaxis in middle Tennessee, 1989–90. Rev Infect Dis 12:S874, 1991.
36. Goodman JS, Shaffner W, Collins HA, et al: Infection after cardiovascular surgery: Clinical study including examination of antimicrobial prophylaxis. N Engl J Med 278:117, 1968.
37. Theuer CP, Bongard FS, Klein SR: Are blood cultures effective in the evaluation of fever in perioperative patients? Am J Surg 162:615, 1991.
38. Bunt TJ: Urgent relaparotomy: The high-risk, no-choice operation. Surgery 98:555, 1985.
39. Zer M, Dix S, Dintsman M: The timing of relaparotomy and its influence on prognosis. Am J Surg 139:338, 1980.
40. Harbrecht PJ, Garrison RN, Fry DE: Early urgent relaparotomy. Arch Surg 119:369, 1984.
41. Hinsdale JG, Jaffe BM: Re-operation for intraabdominal sepsis: Indications and results in modern critical care setting. Ann Surg 199:31, 1984.
42. Hau T, Ahrenholz DH, Simmons RL: Secondary bacterial peritonitis: The biologic basis of treatment. Curr Probl Surg 16:1, 1979.
43. Lennard ES, Minshew BH, Dellinger EP, et al: Stratified outcome comparison of clindamycin-gentamicin vs chloramphenicol-gentamicin for treatment of intra-abdominal sepsis. Arch Surg 120:889, 1985.
44. Dellinger E, Wertz M, Meakins L, et al: Surgical infection stratification system for intra-abdominal infection. Arch Surg 120:21, 1985.
45. Bohnen J, Boulanger M, Meakins JL, et al: Prognosis in generalized peritonitis: Relation to cause and risk factors. Arch Surg 118:285, 1983.
46. Wright HK, Dunn E, MacArthur JD, et al: Specific but limited role of new imaging techniques in decision making about intraabdominal abscesses. Am J Surg 143:456, 1982.
47. Norwood SH, Civetta JM: Abdominal CT scanning in critically ill surgical patients. Ann Surg 202:166, 1985.
48. Hoogewoud H-M, Rubli E, Terrier F, et al: The role of computerized tomography in fever, septicemia and multiple system organ failure after laparotomy. Surg Gynecol Obstet 162:539, 1986.
49. Deutschman C, Wilton P, Sinow J, et al: Paranasal sinusitis associated with nasotracheal intubation: A frequently unrecognized and treatable source of sepsis. Crit Care Med 14:111, 1986.
50. Christensen L, Schaffer S, Ross SE: Otitis media in adult trauma patients: Incidence and clinical significance. J Trauma 31:1543, 1991.
51. Craig MH, Poole GV, Hauser CJ: Postsurgical gout. Am Surg 61:56, 1995.
52. Aach RD, Kahn RA: Posttransfusion hepatitis: Current perspective. Ann Intern Med 92:539, 1980.

53. Kahn RA, Barrios SDP: Diseases transmitted by blood transfusion. *In* Rutman RC, Miller WV (eds): Transfusion Therapy: Principles and Procedures. Rockville, MD, Aspen Publishers, 1985, p 311.
54. Kahn RA: Diseases transmitted by blood transfusion. Hum Pathol 14:241, 1983.
55. Aach RD, Stevens CE, Hollinger FB, et al: Hepatitis C virus infection in post-transfusion hepatitis: An analysis with first- and second-generation assays. N Engl J Med 325:1325, 1991.
56. Drew WL, Miner RC: Transfusion-related cytomegalovirus infection following noncardiac surgery. JAMA 247:2389, 1982.

101

Surgical Wound Infection

Ronald Lee Nichols

Wound infections remain a major source of postoperative morbidity, accounting for about a quarter of the total number of nosocomial infections.[1, 2] Today, many of these infections are first recognized in the outpatient clinic or in the patient's home because of the large number of operations done in the outpatient setting.[2] This leads to errors in establishing the true frequency of their occurrence but undoubtedly decreases the overall real cost and prolongation of hospital stay. The pathogens implicated in the development of wound infections remain largely the microorganisms from the exogenous environment and the endogenous organ microflora. Many perioperative factors have been identified that increase the frequency of the development of postoperative wound infection. Avoidance of these factors as well as the appropriate use of perioperative antibiotic prophylaxis has decreased the incidence of wound infection.

The rate of wound infection varies from surgeon to surgeon, from hospital to hospital, and from one surgical procedure to another and most important from one patient to another (Table 101–1). One of the earliest comprehensive reviews showed that the overall postoperative infection rate was approximately 7.4%.[3] In 1976, wound infections accounted for approximately 24% of the total number of nosocomial infections.[4] This figure represented more than 500,000 wound infections or about 2.8 per 100 operations performed. Previous published data have shown that the average hospital stay was noted to double and the cost of hospitalizations was correspondingly increased when postoperative wound infection developed after six commonly performed operations during the mid-1970s.[5] These figures of real cost and length of hospital stay are undoubtedly lower today for most surgical procedures that are done as outpatient procedures or those that require only a short postoperative stay. In these cases, most of the wound infections are diagnosed and treated in the outpatient clinic or in the patient's home. However, major complications such as deep sternal wound infections continue to have a grave impact, increasing the duration of hospitalization as much as 20-fold and the cost of hospitalization 5-fold.[6] The development of any surgical wound infection after open heart surgery has also been shown to result in a significant net loss of reimbursement to the hospital compared with uninfected cases, a factor that should serve as a potent incentive to hospitals to minimize the occurrence of postoperative wound infections.[7]

TABLE 101–1 ■ Overall Rate of Wound Infections After Surgical Procedures

REFERENCE	REPORTED RATE (%)	COMMENTS
National Academy of Sciences,[3] 1964	7.4	5-hospital 2.5-y survey (15,613 operations)
Cruse,[44] 1981	4.7	10-y single-hospital study, standardized definitions, 28-d follow-up (62,939 operations)
Haley et al,[4] 1985	2.8	1-y (1975–1976) nationwide survey (18,271,858 operations)
Olson and Lee,[45] 1990	2.5	10-y review at a single medical center (40,915 operations)

During the 1980s, many significant observations were reported from data collected by the ongoing Study on the Efficacy of Nosocomial Infection Control (SENIC) project.[8] In addition to the benefits from well-organized infection surveillance and control program improvements, significant advances have occurred in the appropriate use of prophylactic antibiotics in the surgical patient and in the accurate identification of those patients who are at greatest risk for the development of surgical wound sepsis in the various surgical procedures. The identification of high-risk patients in each specific surgical procedure will allow prospective alteration in therapy studies, which will be conducted and reported during the 1990s.[2]

Description of Clinical Wound Infections

To carry out surveillance, prevention, and control of surgical wound infections, it is necessary to use a commonly employed set of definitions. The Hospital Infections Program, Center for Infectious Diseases of the Centers for Disease Control and Prevention (CDC), previously developed a set of definitions to be used for the surveillance of nosocomial infections in the hospitals participating in the National Nosocomial Infections Surveillance System.[9] These definitions were modified in 1992 to include specific sites of deep organ or space surgical site infections and to replace the term wound infections with surgical site infections.[10] The wound infections are divided into incisional and deep and are considered to be nosocomial (hospital acquired) only if there is no evidence that the infection was present or incubating at the time of hospital admission. The definitions for superficial and deep incisional surgical site infections are presented in Table 101–2.

Most superficial surgical site infections are diagnosed sometime between the fourth and eighth postoperative day (late). When infection occurs during the first 48 hours after operation (early), it is characteristically a rapidly moving gangrenous infection caused by a single type of microorganism, either a *Clostridium* species or β-hemolytic *Streptococcus*.[2] In these rare cases, the dramatic clinical presentation may include profound systemic toxic effects and rapid local advance of the infection, often involving all layers of the body wall.

Traditional Wound Classification: A Time for Reassessment

Classification of the surgical wound in the operating room by surgeons and nurses is a time-honored routine that has

TABLE 101–2 ■ Definiitons of Surgical Site (Surgical Wound) Infections

SUPERFICIAL INCISIONAL SURGICAL SITE INFECTIONS

Occurs within 30 d of operative procedure

Involves skin, subcutaneous tissue, or muscle above fascia

Includes at least one of the following:
- Purulent drainage from the incision or drain located above the fascia
- Organisms isolated from culture of fluid or tissue from incision closed primarily
- Signs or symptoms of infection, such as pain or tenderness, local swelling, redness, or heat
- Incision is deliberately opened by surgeon, unless culture-negative
- Diagnosis of infection by surgeon or attending physician

Does not include stitch abscess, episiotomy or newborn circumcision site infections, infected burn wounds, or infections extending into fascia or muscle

DEEP INCISIONAL SURGICAL SITE INFECTIONS

Occurs within 30 d of operative procedure if no implant* is left in place or within 1 y if an implant is in place

Appears related to the operative procedure

Involves deep soft tissues or spaces at or beneath the fascial layer

Includes at least one of the following:
- Purulent drainage from the deep incision or drain located above the fascia but not the organ space component of the surgical site
- A deep incision that spontaneously dehisces or is deliberately opened by a surgeon when the patient has at least one of the following signs or symptoms:
  - Fever (temperature >38°C)
  - Localized pain or tenderness unless the incision is culture-negative
- An abscess or other evidence of infection seen on direct examination, during surgery, or by histopathologic examination
- Diagnosis of a deep incisional infection by a surgeon or attending physician

*Nonhuman-derived implantable foreign body (e.g., prosthetic heart valve, nonhuman vascular graft, mechanical heart, or hip prosthesis) that is permanently placed in a patient during surgery.

been practiced for at least 30 years, since the study by the National Academy of Sciences National Research Council on the influence of ultraviolet irradiation on surgical wound infection.[3] This traditional method uses four classes of wounds based on the risk level and type of contamination expected or observed at operation.[2] Clean surgical wounds (class I) are those in which only exogenous (airborne) contamination is expected or observed; the predicted rate of wound infection, largely due to gram-positive microorganisms such as *Staphylococcus aureus*, is approximately 2%. Clean-contaminated (class II) wounds are those in which generally both exogenous and endogenous (aerobic-anaerobic) bacterial contamination occurs during elective operations; the infection rate in this category is estimated at 5% to 15% and is usually due to the polymicrobial endogenous flora. Contaminated wounds (class III) are those with early endogenous leakage or delayed exogenous contamination in the absence of established clinical infection; they carry a greater than 15% infection rate. In dirty-infected wounds (class IV), in which active infection is encountered during operation, a postoperative infection rate of greater than 30% is anticipated.

During the last decade, problems have been identified with the use of this traditional wound classification system and the accuracy of the predicted infection rates in each category. The major limitation lies in the lack of attention to the varying risk for infection among subjects in each class of wound. Haley and coworkers[11] at the CDC were among the first to describe the importance of identifying the varying individual risks for infection among patients in each of the traditional four categories of wounds. This and other timely studies on risk factors for surgical wound infection have been stressed in Chapter 44. From this analysis, we understand today that the risk for infection in each traditional category of surgical procedures varies greatly, depending on the individual patient's risk factors. The infection rate in clean surgical procedures cannot be assumed to be low.[12] Haley and colleagues[11] created a simplified index of the risk for infection that consists of the total number of the following risk factors: abdominal operation, operation longer than 2 hours, contaminated or dirty-infected operation, and three or more diagnoses. They compared this risk index with the traditional wound classifications (Table 101–3) and found a great range of infection rates among each of the traditional classes, from

TABLE 101–3 ■ Comparision of Rates of Surgical Wound Infections Using Either the Traditional Classification System or the Simplified Risk Index for 58,498 Patients Undergoing Surgical Procedures at 338 SENIC Hospitals in 1970

	INFECTION RATE (%) FOR A SIMPLIFIED RISK INDEX* OF					
TRADITIONAL WOUND CLASS	0	1	2	3	4	All
Class I: Clean	1.1	3.9	8.4	15.8	—	2.9
Class II: Clean-contaminated	0.6	2.8	8.4	17.7	—	3.9
Class III: Contaminated	—	4.5	8.3	11.0	23.9	8.5
Class IV: Dirty-infected	—	6.7	10.9	18.8	27.4	12.6
All	1.0	3.6	8.9	17.2	27.0	4.1

*Total number of the following risk factors: abdominal operation; operation longer than 2 h; contaminated or dirty-infected operation; three or more diagnoses.
Data from Haley RW, Culver DH, Morgan WM, et al: Identifying patients at high risk of surgical wound infection. Am J Epidemiol 121:206, 1985.

1% to 16% for clean surgery to 7% to 27% in dirty-contaminated cases. Realization of the presence of the patient's risk factors in each surgical procedure will result in more accurate assessment of the initial risk for wound infection and will allow prophylactic or therapeutic interventions, which may ideally lead to an overall decrease in the occurrence of wound infection.

A reported 13-year study of the development of postoperative wound infection in a large group of patients undergoing clean surgery has also stressed the great variation in the rate of infection for different patients with varying risks.[13] High wound infection rates similar to those reported in contaminated surgery were found in patients having splenectomy in the presence of schistosomiasis (21.2%) and for abdominal incisional hernia repair (14.7%).

In conclusion, the traditional four-class system of estimating risk for postoperative wound infection is largely dependent on the nature and extent of perioperative contamination, reflecting little focus on the individual patient's risk factors.[14] In addition, the classification levels overlap. Although this system has served well, the data presented indicate that a simplified two-tiered system could be more effective. The risk for postoperative wound infection depends largely on the combined effects of the nature and extent of perioperative contamination as well as the individual patient's risk factors. More attention should now be focused on delineating the general risk factors, including specific disease or operative factors, for infection in the surgical patient.

Pathogens Implicated in Surgical Wound Infections

The pathogens that are isolated from surgical wound infections vary, primarily on the basis of the type of surgical procedure undertaken[15, 16] (Table 101–4). In clean surgical procedures in which the gastrointestinal, gynecologic, and respiratory tracts have not been entered, *S. aureus* from the exogenous environment or the patient's skin flora is the usual cause of infection. In the other categories of surgical procedures including clean-contaminated, contaminated, and dirty-infected, the polymicrobial aerobic-anaerobic flora closely resembling the normal endogenous microflora of the surgically resected organ constitutes the most frequently isolated pathogens.[17]

The importance of thoughtfully carried out epidemiologic and microbiologic investigations of the changing patterns of nosocomial pathogens both in outbreak investigations and in national surveillance data has been stressed since the early 1960s.[18] Evidence reported from the SENIC project and the National Nosocomial Infections Surveillance System has shown that the rate of nosocomial infections caused by different pathogens continues to change.[19] The number of nosocomial infections caused by gram-positive cocci, which had been declining, is again increasing, with the emergence of coagulase-negative staphylococci as important nosocomial pathogens.[20, 21] Edmiston and colleagues[21] have observed that the majority of prosthetic vascular graft infections are now caused by mucin-producing strains of *Staphylococcus epidermidis*, which express varying degrees of adherence to the synthetic substrates.

Antibiotic-resistant strains of both gram-positive and gram-negative microorganisms are being increasingly isolated from infections in postoperative patients and from the hospital environment.[22, 23] Rapidly growing mycobacteria, *Rhodococcus bronchialis*, and *Candida tropicalis* have been implicated in outbreaks of both deep and superficial wound infections after open heart surgery.[24–26] In the case of the mycobacterial infections, about 80% of the cardiac isolates were from the southern coastal states, and the heterogeneity of the isolates suggests that most are unrelated but are derived from local environmental sources rather than from contaminated commercial surgical materials or devices.[24] This finding of heterogeneity among the isolates of rapidly growing mycobacteria has also been reported in wound infections after augmentation mammaplasty despite case clustering in Texas and other southern coastal states.[27] The outbreaks of wound infection due to both *R. bronchialis* and *C. tropicalis* were identified to be common-source cluster epidemics; the removal of the sources from the cardiac team terminated the outbreaks.[25, 26]

The importance of the strict enforcement of infection control policies within the operating room has been the subject of two reports.[28, 29] An outbreak of infection due to *Serratia marcescens* was reported in eight patients who had undergone cardiovascular surgery in one hospital.[28] Two of the patients became bacteremic, and one died. The epidemiologic investigation identified the cause of the outbreak to be contaminated skin cream used by a scrub nurse. This nurse also wore artificial nails, which are known to increase the carriage rate of gram-negative bacteria. The outbreak stopped after the use of the cream was discontinued. In the other study, a relatively new intravenous anesthetic, propofol, was implicated in a large number of postoperative wound and other infections.[29] This drug has a unique lipid base that can support microbial growth if it is contaminated. Sixty-two patients at seven hospitals developed infections after adminis-

TABLE 101–4 ■ Common Potential Pathogens Causing Surgical Wound Infections

TYPE OF SURGICAL PROCEDURE	POTENTIAL PATHOGENS
Clean	
Cardiac, vascular, orthopedic	*Staphylococcus aureus, Staphylococcus epidermidis,* enteric gram-negative bacilli
Clean-Contaminated or Contaminated	
Gastroduodenal	Aerobic and anaerobic streptococci, enteric gram-negative bacilli, *Bacteroides* sp. not *fragilis*
Biliary	Enteric gram-negative bacilli, enterococci, clostridia
Colorectal (elective)	Enteric gram-negative bacilli, *B. fragilis,* peptostreptococci, clostridia
Small intestine	Enteric gram-negative bacilli, *B. fragilis,* peptostreptococci
Appendectomy	Enteric gram-negative bacilli, *B. fragilis,* peptostreptococci, enterococci
Vaginal or abdominal hysterectomy; cesarean section; abortion	Enteric gram-negative bacilli, *B. fragilis,* enterococci, clostridia, group B streptococci
Dirty-Infected	
Penetrating abdominal trauma	Enteric gram-negative bacilli, *B. fragilis,* peptostreptococci, clostridia, enterococci
Other traumatic wounds	*S. aureus,* clostridia, group A streptococci

tration of propofol. These infections, at first, were attributed to the surgeon or procedure performed. Subsequently, it was found that extrinsic contamination of the drug had resulted from numerous breaks in infection control technique by the anesthesia personnel.[29, 30] Contaminated drug was then administered to the patients, resulting in the infections.

Factors That Relate to Surgical Wound Infection and the Patient's Risk Factors

Many factors including length of preoperative hospital stay, use of antibiotic prophylaxis, preoperative cleansing and shaving techniques, use of prophylactic drains, and elective operation done in the presence of an active remote infection have been proved to influence the development of postoperative wound infections.[2] Many other factors have been considered, without convincing evidence, to influence postoperative wound infection, including preoperative scrub technique, surgical glove damage, barrier materials, and laminar flow air-handling systems in the operating room.[2] Anecdotal experience and commercial interests rather than scientific studies usually account for these associations. A thoughtful review by Sebben[31] offered recommendations that are thought to be essential elements of infection control for office-based surgical practice, including modern concepts of instrument sterilization, skin cleansing, and insights into the use of prophylactic antibiotics.

These factors as well as general risk factors related to the patient are described in Chapter 44 and therefore are not reviewed again here.

Risk Factors for Infection in Specific Operative Procedures

Many clinical studies of risk factors for infection in specific operative procedures have been published during the 1980s. Knowledge of the presence or absence of these risk factors in the perioperative period may allow alterations of infection control techniques in the studies conducted in the future (Table 101–5).

TABLE 101–5 ■ Risk Factors Implicated* in Increased Surgical Wound Infection Rates After Specific Operative Procedures

PROCEDURE	RISK FACTORS
Penetrating abdominal trauma	Increased age Left colon injury requiring colostomy Increased transfusions at surgery Increased number of injured organs or associated injuries Increased colon injury score Significant intraperitoneal contamination
Elective colonic resection	Duration of operation Location of resection
Nonperforative appendicitis	Nonuse of perioperative antibiotics Surgeon's determination of gangrenous appendix
Abdominal or vaginal hysterectomy	Increased operative time
Cardiac surgery	Obesity Diabetes Prolonged hospitalization Prolonged stay in intensive care unit Prolonged mechanical ventilation Preexisting chronic pulmonary disease or postoperative pneumonia Increased age Prolonged use of Foley catheter Reexploration Postoperative weight gain Placement of intraaortic balloon pump Postoperative blood products Male sex
Vascular surgery for lower limb arterial ischemia	Rest pain Skin necrosis Increased age
Gastroduodenal surgery	Low gastric acidity Reduced gastrointestinal motility
Biliary surgery	Age >70 y Previous biliary tract surgery Jaundice, acute cholecystitis, or common duct stones

*One or more controlled clinical studies.

Shapiro and coinvestigators[32] in 1982 were the first to use logistic regression analysis to identify the risk factors for operative site infections in abdominal or vaginal hysterectomy. They observed that an increasing duration of operative time was associated with a decreasing effect of antibiotic prophylaxis in preventing operative site infection. The statistically significant benefit of antibiotic prophylaxis in procedures lasting 1 hour or less was lost in operations lasting more than 3.3 hours. Using a similar logistic regression analysis of the risks for infection after penetrating abdominal trauma, we showed that a statistically higher risk for infection was associated with the increasing age of the patient, an injury to the left colon necessitating colostomy, a large number of transfusions at surgery, and a large number of injured organs identified at operation.[33] The presence of shock on arrival to the hospital, which was found to increase the risk for infection when this factor was analyzed individually, did not add predictive power. We then conducted a double-blind, randomized study of 170 patients with traumatic perforation of the gastrointestinal tract who were administered an advanced-generation cephalosporin.[34] At surgical closure, patients were divided into infection risk groups (below 40%, low; 40% to 70%, middle; and above 70%, high) by use of the logistic regression formula based on four proven risk factors—age, blood replacement, ostomy, and number of organs injured. Patients in the low-risk group received 2 days of antibiotic therapy; those in the middle- and high-risk groups received 5 days of antibiotic therapy. Those patients in the low- and middle-risk groups had primary wound closure; those in the high-risk group had their wounds packed open and closed later. Most of the patients (144 [85%]) were in the low-risk group. Their major and minor infection rates (10% and 12%, respectively) were not significantly different from 145 historical control subjects receiving 5 days of antibiotic therapy (9% major, 14% minor).[33] Patients in the middle- and high-risk groups showed a greater rate of major infections (46%) but a similar rate of minor infections (12%). The results indicated that risk factors can be used to identify low-risk patients who require only short-term antibiotic therapy and primary wound closure. The remaining patients were shown to be at greater risk for infection despite prolonged antibiotic therapy and delayed wound closure.

In a published large single-hospital study of wound infections after cesarean section, significantly higher rates of infections were observed in clinic patients (15.8%) compared with private patients (6.0%).[35] All significant individual risk factors for infection including emergency versus elective operation, number of vaginal examinations before operation, duration of operation, vertical skin incision, and category of surgeon were overrepresented in the group of clinic patients. There was no difference in the wound infection rate among potentially infected patients whether or not prophylactic antibiotics were used.

A prospective study of nonperforated appendicitis, using a logistic regression analysis of risk factors, has shown that the risk for postoperative wound infection related only to the failure to use perioperative antibiotics and the surgeon's determination of the appendix as gangrenous.[36] The highest infection probability (77%) was predicted in those patients receiving placebo and having a gangrenous appendix, the lowest (2%) in those receiving an antibiotic perioperatively and not having a gangrenous appendix at surgery. Perioperative antibiotic prophylaxis had a beneficial effect in decreasing hospital stay.

Kaiser and associates,[37] studying elective colon resection and different approaches to preoperative antibiotic prophylaxis, have shown a direct correlation between the duration of operation and the postoperative infection rate. In operations lasting less than 3 hours, no infections were identified when the antibiotic prophylaxis was with a parenteral agent alone or a combination of oral and parenteral agents. However, in operations lasting more than 4 hours, a significant reduction of infection was observed in those patients receiving the combination prophylactic regimen. Coppa and Eng,[38] in a similar study of elective colon resection, have stressed that postoperative wound infections are associated with the length of operation and location of the colonic resection (intraperitoneal colon resection versus rectal resection). These authors showed that the wound infection rate in high-risk patients with long operations (longer than 215 minutes) and rectal resection could be reduced significantly by the use of a combination of oral and parenteral prophylactic antibiotics. Whether to repair the injured colon primarily or to do a colostomy has been the subject of a prospective study of colonic injuries after penetrating abdominal trauma.[39] Using logistic regression analysis, the authors have identified that transfusion of four or more units, more than two associated injuries, significant intraperitoneal contamination, and increasing colon injury severity scores significantly correlate with increased frequencies of postoperative wound and intraabdominal infections. The authors concluded that nearly all penetrating colon wounds can be repaired primarily regardless of risk factors.

Many current studies have been published concerning the risk factors for wound and deep sternal infections after median sternotomy for cardiac surgical procedures.[2] Knowledge of these risk factors is required to aid surgeons and patients in making judgments about the relative benefits of surgery and to alert nursing personnel to be particularly aware of early signs of infection in patients at high risk.[40] This may also be helpful in planning additional prophylactic measures for high-risk patients. There are a large number of individual risk factors identified in this population of patients[2] (see Table 101–5). The use of bilateral internal mammary arterial grafting in coronary revascularization procedures has been shown to be a risk factor for infection in some studies.[2]

The risk factors for wound infection after vascular surgery have been reported after a study of 100 consecutive patients with lower limb arterial ischemia.[41] The authors found a significant number of patients harboring pathogenic organisms on their skin preoperatively in those with rest pain and skin necrosis. Another risk factor was increasing age of the patient, whereas claudication or the presence of an aneurysm was not.

Undoubtedly, risk factor studies accomplished in the next decade, for other operative procedures, will aid in our discovery of the high-risk patient, which will allow prospective alterations in preventive techniques in this group.

Surveillance of the Surgical Wound

Traditional surveillance of the surgical wound, which was practiced widely into the 1970s, depended primarily on infection control personnel's searching for positive cultures from the microbiology laboratory. The finding of a positive culture of wound drainage or exudate triggered a review of the patient's chart and of the patient if he or she was still hospitalized. Errors in this approach were due to inadequate and widely varying definitions of surgical wound infection in addition to the missing of clinical infection when cultures were not done for infected patients or when the culture result was negative in infected patients.

With use of a representative sample of U.S. general hospitals (SENIC project), the efficacy of infection surveillance and control on the prevention of nosocomial infections was established by the CDC in 1985.[42] A 32% reduction in nosocomial infections was noted from 1970 to the period from 1975 to 1976 in the participating hospitals where the essential components of the intensive infection surveillance and control programs were practiced. These effective programs included conducting organized concurrent surveillance and control activities and having a trained effectual infection control physician, an infection control nurse per 250 beds, and a system for reporting infection rates to practicing surgeons. It was estimated that because only a few hospitals had these programs, only 6% of the nation's approximately 2 million nosocomial infections were actually being prevented by the mid-1970s, leaving another 26% to be prevented by universal adoption of these programs. Among hospitals without effective programs, the overall infection rate increased by 18% from 1970 to 1976. In an update of the SENIC project[43] using information collected in 1983 from a random sample of hospitals, it was found that the intensity of infection surveillance and control activities had greatly increased from 1976. The number of hospitals with an infection control nurse per 250 beds increased from 22% to 57%, although the number with a physician trained in infection control remained low (15%). There was an increase in the number of hospitals having effective programs to prevent urinary tract infections, bacteremias, and pneumonias, but this was not the case for surgical wound infection. Also noted was that the percentage of hospitals doing surgical wound infection surveillance had decreased (from 90% to 79%), and those reporting surgeon-specific infection rates to surgeons had decreased (from 19% to 13%). At this point, it is estimated that 9% of the nosocomial infections were being prevented, whereas 32% could be prevented if all hospitals adopted the most effective programs.

The first comprehensive, single-hospital, 10-year prospective study of wound infection surveillance was reported in 1981[44] (see Table 101–1). In this study, all wounds were inspected by a single surgical nurse. Definitions of wound infections were standardized, and surveillance was continued by telephone up to 28 days, when a final report on each wound was made. An overall infection rate of 4.7% was identified. Each surgeon received an annual report showing the surgeon's individual rate of infection in clean wounds as well as the average clean wound infection rate of the patients of the other surgeons in corresponding surgical divisions. A monthly computer report of the infection rates, especially stressing the clean wound, was discussed at the division of surgery and the infection control committee meetings. The bottom line of this report was a reduction of almost 50% in the overall wound infection rate as well as of the clean infection rate within 6 months after institution of this surveillance program.

In a later 10-year wound infection surveillance program, procedure-specific rates rather than surgeon-specific rates were calculated annually.[45] The results of this study (see Table 101–1) showed a significant reduction in wound infection rates in the last 9 years of surveillance in every class of surgical wound compared with the index year rates. Estimated savings in hospital room costs alone reached $3 million during the 10 years.

The improvement in wound infection rates in all of these studies was the direct result of periodic clinical interventions based on the surveillance data, which have already been described in the section dealing with the factors that prevent surgical wound infections. The use of computer surveillance to improve the use of antibiotic administration in both the prevention and the treatment of nosocomial infections, including wound infections, has also been stressed.[46, 47] Many different computer-based programs have been developed for the monitoring of surgical wound infections and the identification of risk factors for the development of infection.[48, 49]

Shorter lengths of hospitalization and the increasing numbers of outpatient operations have heightened our awareness of the importance of posthospital surveillance to accurately document the presence of surgical wound infection. Follow-up of patients for at least 30 days after operation is generally required to rule out the presence of a superficial wound infection. Large studies have shown that at present, about 50% of all infections can be identified after hospital discharge if adequate surveillance is carried out.[50, 51] In addition to the data obtained from clinic visits, questionnaires for the physician and patient sent out approximately 30 days after discharge from the hospital have appeared to offer the best efficacy in determining the true rate of surgical wound infection.[50]

Most studies concerning the collection and confidential distribution of surgeon-specific wound infection rates, especially in clean surgical procedures, have shown a reduction of surgical wound infection after the use of this approach.[52, 53] However, an editorial has stressed that to prove the validity of surgeon-specific wound infection rates, it is required to adjust for surgical procedure as well as for the severity of the patient's illness.[54]

A standardized effective surveillance program to detect and control surgical wound infection has proved to be of benefit in reducing the frequency of these infections. It is urged that all hospitals implement these programs.[55]

Implications for the Future

The number of patients admitted to hospitals for inpatient surgery will continue to decrease while the numbers of outpatient surgical procedures will continue to increase. The severity of the patient's illness and the risk for postoperative wound infection and other septic events in hospitalized patients will increase. These trends will require effective infection surveillance in both the hospital and the outpatient setting for collection of meaningful data. Continued advances in computer technology will improve the collection and integration of pertinent clinical, laboratory, and surgical information and will greatly facilitate surveillance, analysis, and control of infections in the surgical wound.

Specific patient-related risk factors for each operative procedure will be reported, and these risk factors will be used to plan prospective alterations in therapy studies with the intention of doing less for the low-risk patient and increasing the preventive and therapeutic modalities in the high-risk patient.

Further progress in the area of chemotherapeutic development will occur, with the emphasis being placed on the use of oral or local regimens. The use of antibiotic prophylaxis before operative procedures will continue to be streamlined, largely on the basis of further pharmacokinetic data that will influence administration techniques and limit the total dosage. Operative procedures that use foreign body implants may be done with implants that have been commercially bonded or prepared with antibiotics or antiseptics. Immunomodulators will be used to help prevent infectious complications in the immunosuppressed host. Infection control committees will ideally pay more attention to proper surveillance of the surgical wound than to the discussion of the relative merits of sacred cows.

References

1. Nichols RL: Postoperative wound infection. N Engl J Med 307:1701, 1982.
2. Nichols RL: Surgical wound infection. Am J Med 91(Suppl 3B):54, 1991.
3. National Academy of Sciences, National Research Council: Postoperative wound infections: The influence of ultraviolet irradiation of the operating room and of various other factors. Ann Surg 160(Suppl 2):1, 1964.
4. Haley RW, Culver DH, White JW, et al: The nationwide nosocomial infection rate: A new need for vital statistics. Am J Epidemiol 121:159, 1985.
5. Green JW, Wenzel RP: Postoperative wound infection: A controlled study of the increased duration of hospital stay and direct cost of hospitalization. Ann Surg 185:264, 1977.
6. Taylor GJ, Mikell FL, Moses HW, et al: Determinants of hospital charges for coronary artery bypass surgery: The economic consequences of postoperative complications. Am J Cardiol 65:309, 1990.
7. Boyce JM, Potter-Bynoe G, Dziobek L: Hospital reimbursement patterns among patients with surgical wound infections following open heart surgery. Infect Control Hosp Epidemiol 11:89, 1990.
8. Haley RW, Quade D, Freeman HE, Bennett JV: The SENIC Project. Study on the efficacy of nosocomial infection control (SENIC Project). Summary of study design. Am J Epidemiol 111:472, 1980.
9. Garner JS, Jarvis WR, Emori TG, et al: CDC definitions for nosocomial infections, 1988. Am J Infect Control 16:128, 1988.
10. Horan TC, Gaynes RP, Martone WJ, et al: CDC definitions of nosocomial surgical site infections, 1992: A modification of CDC definitions of surgical wound infections. Am J Infect Control 20:271, 1992.
11. Haley RW, Culver DH, Morgan WM, et al: Identifying patients at high risk of surgical wound infection. Am J Epidemiol 121:206, 1985.
12. Nichols RL: Wound infection rates following clean operative procedures: Can we assume them to be low? Infect Control Hosp Epidemiol 13:455, 1992.
13. Ferraz EM, Bacelar TS, Aguiar JL, et al: Wound infection rates in clean surgery: A potentially misleading risk classification. Infect Control Hosp Epidemiol 13:457, 1992.
14. Nichols RL: Classification of the surgical wound: A time for reassessment and simplification. Infect Control Hosp Epidemiol 14:253, 1993.
15. Abramowicz M: Antimicrobial prophylaxis in surgery. Med Lett 37:79, 1995.
16. American Medical Association: Antimicrobial chemoprophylaxis for surgical patients. Drug Evaluations Annual. Chicago, American Medical Association, 1995, pp 1369–1376.
17. Nichols RL: Prevention of infection in high risk gastrointestinal surgery. Am J Med 76:111, 1984.
18. Kundsin RB, Walter CW, Morin P: *Staphylococcus aureus* UC-18: Agent of nosocomial infections. Science 145:1322, 1964.
19. Hughes JM: Study on the efficacy of nosocomial infection control (SENIC Project): Results and implications for the future. Chemotherapy 34:553, 1988.

20. Large M, Stubbs E, Benn R, et al: A study of coagulase-negative staphylococci isolated from clinically significant infections at an Australian teaching hospital. Pathology 21:19, 1989.
21. Edmiston CE Jr, Schmitt DD, Seabrook GR: Coagulase-negative staphylococcal infections in vascular surgery: Epidemiology and pathogenesis. Infect Control Hosp Epidemiol 10:111, 1989.
22. Andersen BM, Sorlie D, Hotvedt R, et al: Multiply beta-lactam resistant *Enterobacter cloacae* infections linked to the environmental flora in a unit for cardiothoracic and vascular surgery. Scand J Infect Dis 21:181, 1989.
23. The Hospital Infection Control Practices Advisory Committee (HICPAC): Recommendations for preventing the spread of vancomycin resistance—Special communication. Am J Infect Control 23:87, 1995.
24. Wallace RJ Jr, Musser JM, Hull SI, et al: Diversity and sources of rapidly growing mycobacteria associated with infections following cardiac surgery. J Infect Dis 159:708, 1989.
25. Isenberg HD, Tucci V, Cintron F, et al: Single-source outbreak of *Candida tropicalis* complicating coronary bypass surgery. J Clin Microbiol 27:2426, 1989.
26. Richet HM, Craven PC, Brown JM, et al: *Rhodococcus bronchialis* sternal wound infections following coronary artery bypass graft surgery. N Engl J Med 324:104, 1991.
27. Wallace RJ Jr, Steele LC, Labidi A, et al: Heterogeneity among isolates of rapidly growing mycobacteria responsible for infections following augmentation mammoplasty despite case clustering in Texas and other southern coastal states. J Infect Dis 160:281, 1989.
28. Centers for Disease Control and Prevention: Sleuths track nosocomial outbreak to skin cream. Hosp Infect Control 22:65, 1995.
29. Bennett SN, McNeil MM, Bland LA, et al: Postoperative infections traced to contamination of an intravenous anesthetic, propofol. N Engl J Med 333:147, 1995.
30. Nichols RL, Smith JW: Bacterial contamination of an anesthetic agent. N Engl J Med 333:184, 1995.
31. Sebben JE: Sterile technique and the prevention of wound infection in office surgery—Part II. J Dermatol Surg Oncol 15:38, 1989.
32. Shapiro M, Munoz A, Tager IB, et al: Risk factors for infection at the operative site after abdominal or vaginal hysterectomy. N Engl J Med 307:1661, 1982.
33. Nichols RL, Smith JW, Klein DB, et al: Risk of infection after penetrating abdominal trauma. N Engl J Med 311:1065, 1984.
34. Nichols RL, Smith JW, Robertson GD, et al: Prospective alterations in therapy for penetrating abdominal trauma. Arch Surg 128:55, 1993.
35. Webster J: Post-caesarean wound infection: A review of the risk factors. Aust N Z J Obstet Gynaecol 28:201, 1988.
36. Browder W, Smith JW, Vivoda LM, et al: Nonperforative appendicitis: A continuing surgical dilemma. J Infect Dis 159:1088, 1989.
37. Kaiser AB, Herrington JL Jr, Jacobs JK, et al: Cefoxitin versus erythromycin, neomycin, and cefazolin in colorectal operations. Ann Surg 198:525, 1983.
38. Coppa GF, Eng K: Factors involved in antibiotic selection in elective colon and rectal surgery. Surgery 104:853, 1988.
39. George SM Jr, Fabian TC, Voeller GR, et al: Primary repair of colon wounds: A prospective trial in nonselected patients. Ann Surg 209:728, 1989.
40. Lillienfeld DE, Vlahov D, Tenney JH, et al: Obesity and diabetes as risk factors for postoperative wound infections after cardiac surgery. Am J Infect Control 16:3, 1988.
41. Earnshaw JJ, Slack RCB, Hopkinson BR, et al: Risk factors in vascular surgical sepsis. Ann R Coll Surg Engl 70:139, 1988.
42. Haley RW, Culver DH, White JW, et al: The efficacy of infection surveillance and control programs in preventing nosocomial infections in US hospitals. Am J Epidemiol 121:182, 1985.
43. Haley RW, Morgan WM, Culver DH, et al: Update from the SENIC project: Hospital infection control: Recent progress and opportunities under prospective payment. Am J Infect Control 13:97, 1985.
44. Cruse P: Wound infection surveillance. Rev Infect Dis 3:734, 1981.
45. Olson MM, Lee JT Jr: Continuous, 10-year wound infection surveillance: Results, advantages, and unanswered questions. Arch Surg 125:794, 1990.
46. Evans RS, Larsen RA, Burke JP, et al: Computer surveillance of hospital-acquired infections and antibiotic use. JAMA 256:1007, 1986.
47. Larsen RA, Evans RS, Burke JP, et al: Improved perioperative antibiotic use and reduced surgical wound infection through use of computer decision analysis. Infect Control Hosp Epidemiol 10:316, 1989.
48. Bremmelgaard A, Raahave D, Beier-Holgersen R, et al: Computer-aided surveillance of surgical infections and identification of risk factors. J Hosp Infect 13:1, 1989.
49. Kjaeldgaard P, Cordtz T, Sejberg D, et al: The DANOP-DATA system: A low cost personal computer based program for monitoring of wound infections in surgical ward. J Hosp Infect 13:273, 1989.
50. Brown RB, Bradley S, Opitz E, et al: Surgical wound infections documented after hospital discharge. Am J Infect Control 15:54, 1987.
51. Krukowski ZH, Matheson NA: Ten-year computerized audit of infection after abdominal surgery. Br J Surg 75:857, 1988.
52. Condon RE, Schulte WJ, Malangoni MA, et al: Effectiveness of a surgical wound surveillance program. Arch Surg 118:303, 1983.
53. Mead PB, Pories SE, Hall P: Decreasing the incidence of surgical wound infection. Arch Surg 121:458, 1986.
54. Scheckler WE: Surgeon-specific wound infection rates—A potentially dangerous and misleading strategy. Infect Control Hosp Epidemiol 9:145, 1988.
55. Nichols RL: Surveillance of the surgical wound. Infect Control Hosp Epidemiol 11:513, 1990.

102

Gas Gangrene and Other Clostridial Skin and Soft Tissue Infections

Sherwood L. Gorbach

Clostridial species are associated with a variety of skin and soft tissue infections. The clinical presentation may be acute and dramatic, with tissue destruction and gangrene that progresses over a few hours to an inexorably lethal outcome, or these organisms can coexist in apparent symbiosis with other bacteria in a chronic, suppurative infection, such as diabetic foot ulcer, which can persist for months and even years. The most important distinction in classifying clostridial infections is clinical evidence of toxin production, which causes local effects on muscle, with destruction and gangrene, and systemic effects such as hypotension, renal failure, and hemolysis. In a classic paper, MacLennan[1] described what he termed "the histotoxic clostridial infections," a classification based mostly on his experiences with clostridial infections in wartime. This simple approach has become somewhat outdated since other forms of toxigenic clostridial infections have been described in civilian practice. Beside the typical traumatic injuries described by MacLennan, whether associated with war wounds, civilian violence, or major trauma, serious, nontraumatic cases have been recognized, some of which occur with classic myonecrosis and others with spreading cellulitis and overwhelming toxinosis but without direct involvement of muscle (Table 102–1).

Gas gangrene is a necrotizing, gas-forming process of muscle associated with systemic signs of toxemia.[1–10] The appearance of affected muscle is distinctive, and the diagnosis of

TABLE 102–1 ■ Classification of Clostridial Skin and Soft Tissue Infections

TOXIGENIC INFECTIONS
Traumatic gas gangrene
Wounds of violence—gunshot, projectile missiles, stabbings, anal impalement
War wounds
Civilian violence
Major traumatic injuries
Motor vehicle and motorcycle accidents
Industrial accidents
Open fractures
Minor trauma
Puncture wounds
Insect bites
Intramuscular injections
Subcutaneous injections, especially epinephrine
Postoperative gas gangrene
Gastrointestinal operations
Gallbladder operations
Uterine gas gangrene
Post partum
Septic abortion
Nonpregnant women
Spontaneous (nontraumatic) myonecrosis
Local (contiguous spread from a focus)
Colon cancer
Intraabdominal abscess
Distant (metastatic) spread
Colon cancer, various other types
Neutropenia (leukemia, cyclic neutropenia)
Crepitant cellulitis or fasciitis, with systemic toxinosis
NONTOXIGENIC INFECTIONS
Crepitant cellulitis or fasciitis, localized
Suppurative skin and soft tissue infections
Diabetic foot ulcer and stump infections
Decubitus ulcers
Suppurative myositis
Intravenous drug abuse
Intramuscular injection

gas gangrene can be made on direct inspection of the open wound. Histologically, there is gelatinous necrosis of muscle cells, with early loss of striations and nuclei, in the absence of acute inflammation or infiltration of polymorphonuclear leukocytes.

Microbiology

Clostridium perfringens type A is the leading cause of gas gangrene, reported in about 80% of such cases (range from 50% to 100%).[4, 8, 10] *Clostridium novyi* or *Clostridium septicum* is the pathogen in most of the remaining cases. Some reports have implicated *Clostridium histolyticum, Clostridium bifermantans, Clostridium sporogenes*, and *Clostridium fallax*, although the evidence for their role is rather tenuous.[4, 10–12] The incriminated pathogen is isolated in pure culture in about half of cases, and in the remainder an assortment of aerobic and anaerobic organisms coexist in the contaminated wound.[10]

Pathophysiology

Among the 12 toxins elaborated by *C. perfringens*, the α-toxin, a phospholipase C (lecithinase), is the major, and probably the only, toxin responsible for the local (myonecrosis) and systemic (shock, hemolysis) effects (see Chapter 222). Minute amounts of α-toxin are lethal to mice; in rabbits, it causes bradycardia, hypotension, and a dose-dependent reduction in myocardial function.[13] Guinea pigs immunized with α-toxin are protected against challenge by the organism itself or the purified toxin. The availability of purified α-toxin and knowledge of the genetics of the toxin have brought additional data confirming the central role of this toxin in the clinical presentation of gas gangrene. By using genetic manipulation techniques it was possible to produce a vaccine that contained fragments of α-toxin possessing both phospholipase C and hemolytic activity. This vaccine provided protection in a mouse model against lethal effects of a challenge by 10 LD_{100} (10 times the lethal dose) of *C. perfringens* type A organisms.[14] The role of α-toxin was also examined by a genetic approach that used "knockout" mutants of *C. perfringens* type A. The mutant strain that failed to produce α-toxin could not cause gas gangrene in a mouse myonecrosis model, whereas the parent strain with intact α-toxin production had full virulence in this model.[15] An oxygen-labile hemolysin, θ-toxin, is also lethal to mice, and it depresses myocardial function in rabbits, not directly as α-toxin, but indirectly, perhaps through release of an endogenous mediator such as platelet activating factor.[16] However, θ-toxin is considerably less potent than α-toxin, and it requires cysteine for activation. Although θ-toxin, and others elaborated by *C. perfringens*, may play some role, it is still believed that α-toxin is the major effector of gas gangrene.

The physiologic state of the wound site is critical to allowing the organism to germinate and produce its toxins. The proper conditions are a low oxidation-reduction potential, anoxia, and the availability of various peptides and amino acids.[7] Calcium ion is also needed because α-toxin requires this ion for interaction with substrate.[17] Because α-toxin has a high affinity for lipids, it is bound locally to tissue and circulating toxin is not generally found.[16, 18, 19] In animal experiments, the minimal infecting dose of the organism is 1000 times greater for normal muscle tissue than for devitalized muscle. The infecting dose can be reduced by 10^6 when devitalized tissue is contaminated with sterile dirt.[20] Many of these promoting factors are found in traumatic wounds.

Epidemiology

Estimates of the annual number of cases of gas gangrene in the United States range from 1000 to 3000.[6, 10] In Great Britain, a case of gas gangrene was seen in a general hospital every 2 years,[21] a figure not unlike that reported in Cincinnati, Ohio.[4] Referral centers admit approximately 10 cases per year.[10] Throughout history, gas gangrene has been tied intimately to the battlefield.[1, 7] Because of improved treatment in combat zones, there has been a gratifying reduction in the incidence of gas gangrene associated with war wounds: 5% in World War I, 0.7% in World War II, 0.2% in the Korean War, and 0.02% in the Vietnam War.[1–3, 22, 23] *C. perfringens* is often present in war wounds: MacLennan[1] reported that 20% to 30% of wounds were contaminated by the organism, but only 0.32% of them developed gas gangrene. A review of 187,936 open traumatic wounds showed a contamination rate with clostridia of 3.8% to 39%, but less than 2% of patients actually developed gas gangrene.[3, 4]

In peacetime practice, traumatic injuries account for half of the cases of gas gangrene, the remainder being divided between postoperative complications (30%) and spontaneous (nontraumatic) gas gangrene (20%).[6, 8–10, 24–26] Among the trauma cases, major trauma is responsible for more than 70%; the most common causes are motor vehicle accidents, particularly those involving motorcycles, followed by crush injuries, industrial accidents, gunshot wounds, and burns. Minor injury is noted in 30% of the trauma category—puncture wounds, insect bites, simple lacerations, intramuscular injections, and subcutaneous injections, especially with epinephrine.[27] Postoperative gas gangrene, which accounts for 30% of cases, is related to the following operative sites, in order of frequency: appendix, biliary tract, colon, small intestine, and upper gastrointestinal tract.[28] Those in the spontaneous gas gangrene group have diverse underlying diagnoses, including colon cancer, diabetes, vascular disease, neutropenia, and intraabdominal infection.

Gas gangrene is two to three times more common in males than females. The average age is 35 to 40 years, but children and elders are also affected. The location of gas gangrene is important in terms of management and overall survival. In 80% of traumatic cases the disease originates in an extremity, and in the head or trunk area in 20%, whereas in postoperative cases the figures are reversed. In spontaneous cases, the head and trunk are the favored sites.[10]

Because clostridia are distributed so widely in nature—they can be cultured from virtually all soil samples[7] as well as from multiple environmental sites in a hospital, including air and dust (even in the operating room)—it is difficult to know where the infecting strain originated.[29, 30] Nevertheless, it is believed that most infections, particularly those involving trauma or surgery, are associated with endogenous strains from the patient's own flora, although outbreaks within a hospital have been recognized.[29, 30] In battlefield conditions, a soldier's uniform is covered with a patina of excrement that harbors large numbers of clostridial spores; a penetrating wound is liable to be contaminated with pieces of this soiled clothing, as well as dirt and other particulate matter. Not all clostridial strains are equally capable of causing gas gangrene. In animal challenge experiments, those strains isolated from feces or from infected wounds are considerably more virulent than are strains obtained from soil samples.[7, 20]

Clinical Features

Gas Gangrene

Although gas gangrene is relatively rare, its dramatic presentation and often devastating outcome make each case a memorable event in the personal experience of a physician. Local destruction of muscle and soft tissues and systemic signs of toxemia and hypotension dominate the clinical picture. The onset generally comes 1 to 4 days after the initiating event, although it can start as early as 8 hours or as late as 3 weeks. The initial symptom is gnawing pain in the wound that persists after surgical repair, increasing in severity and extending somewhat beyond the original borders over the next few hours. The skin becomes intensely edematous. It changes from an initial pallor to a magenta hue, often accompanied by large, hemorrhagic bullae. A thin, watery discharge appears early in the course. The discharge has an unpleasant, foul-sweet odor. Microscopic examination reveals abundant gram-positive rods and a remarkable paucity of inflammatory cells. Tachycardia, which cannot be explained by the degree of fever or circulatory changes, is an early finding. Profuse sweating is a constant feature. The temperature can be elevated or even normal. Later, hypotension that is unresponsive to fluid administration and renal failure ensue.

In gas gangrene, the appearance of the involved muscles is characteristic and quite unlike that of any other surgical infection. It must be viewed by direct operative exposure, because many of the changes are not apparent on inspection through the edges of a traumatic wound. Initially, the muscle is pale and edematous, looking like a piece of steak that has been seared over a charcoal fire. The muscle does not contract when stimulated. Further dissection reveals beefy, red, nonviable muscle tissue. A brownish, watery discharge with bubbles of gas seeps through the wound. As the disease progresses, the muscle becomes frankly gangrenous, black, and extremely friable, but by this time the patient is near death. It is important to establish the diagnosis of myonecrosis as early as possible, so that all devitalized, necrotic muscle can be resected. Gas production is often a late finding, and although highly suggestive of gas gangrene, it should not be used as a pathognomonic sign, nor should its absence be allowed to disparage the diagnosis (see Chapter 222 for additional discussion of gas production).[31, 32]

The mental status of a patient with gas gangrene is an extraordinary feature of the disease process. Despite profound hypotension, renal failure, and advancing crepitation, these patients may be remarkably alert and extremely sensitive to their surroundings. They are aware of their impending doom, and a sense of terror can be read in their furtive gaze. This intense mental awareness is mercifully suspended just before death, when the patient lapses into toxic delirium and eventually into a coma.

Minor trauma may precipitate a severe, even lethal, case of gas gangrene. Insect bites, puncture wounds, and superficial lacerations have been incriminated.[10] Intramuscular injections have been the predisposing cause in a number of patients, particularly those with diabetes.[27, 33, 34] Epinephrine and other vasoconstrictors are most dangerous in this regard;[35] other drugs have included insulin, barbiturate, potassium chloride, and pentazocine.[33] Diabetes patients appear to be at increased risk of developing gas gangrene, not only from injections but also from injuries in the lower extremity.[36, 37]

Gas gangrene of the eye and orbit usually follows traumatic panophthalmitis.[38–42] A penetrating wound of the globe is the portal of entry. The ensuing infection destroys vision, and it is usually necessary to enucleate the eye or eviscerate the orbit. Surprisingly, the postoperative course is uneventful, and these patients are not at the high risk of death that those are who have other forms of gas gangrene. There are also mild cases of clostridial conjunctivitis.[39, 43] A laboratory report of the organism in a conjunctival discharge is greeted with considerable skepticism owing to the benign clinical course.

Uterine Gas Gangrene. Clostridial invasion of the myometrium can produce an overwhelming infection that starts 2 to 3 days after the inciting event.[44–48] Before abortion was legalized in the United States and in many European countries, septic abortion was the major cause of uterine gas gangrene. This complication occurred in 0.5% to 10% of septic abortions. In the United States, gas gangrene was a leading cause of maternal death, a situation that still prevails in countries where unsanitary abortions are carried out.[44, 49] Although rare, uterine gas gangrene can complicate normal delivery,[49, 50] cesarean section,[49, 51] and amniocentesis.[52] Both mother and newborn are endangered by the infection. Nonpregnant women can develop uterine gas gangrene in association with uterine cancer, leiomyoma, and curettage for choriocarcinoma.[53, 54]

Uterine gas gangrene is heralded by the dramatic onset of fever, rapid pulse, and severe toxemia. Hypotension is a regular feature of the syndrome, and for some patients unexplained hypotension is the initiating event. Renal output is invariably reduced, accompanied in the early stages by "port wine" urine secondary to hemoglobinuria; it usually progresses to anuria and acute cortical necrosis, which necessitates renal dialysis. Jaundice may progress with extraordinary rapidity, owing to massive intravascular hemolysis caused by the α-toxin (lecithinase).[55] As a result, the patient's skin and sclerae assume a deep, mahogany discoloration in a matter of hours. Peripheral blood smears show crinkled and shaggy erythrocytes. Pelvic findings may be minimal even at this point, although an x-ray film can demonstrate the presence of gas in the midline, related to the uterine wall but distinct from the intestine, as well as in surrounding pelvic structures. Computed tomography can demonstrate gas bubbles in the uterine wall even when the standard radiograph and ultrasonogram do not.

Two forms of pathologic process are recognized. A milder form consists of a superficial decidual infection limited to the uterine contents. This infection can liberate large amounts of toxin so that the clinical features are fully expressed with only minimal local disease. Simple curettage is usually sufficient to remove the necrotic tissue at the site of infection. The second—and more serious—form of gas gangrene involves invasion of uterine muscle and gelatinous necrosis of tissue. As in the disease associated with skeletal muscle, there are remarkably few inflammatory cells associated with this process. The infection can spread beyond the uterus itself into the structures of the pelvis. Mortality rates up to 70% have been reported for uterine gas gangrene, but total hysterectomy, when performed early for the more severe form of invasive disease, can reduce the mortality rate to less than 10%.[45]

Clostridium sordellii has been associated with fatal postpartum infection.[56, 57] In each of the reported cases, the postpartum infection occurred in a rather limited, inconspicuous site, such as a retained vaginal sponge or cesarean section operative site, or associated with endometritis. A galloping, downhill course with hypotension and shock was observed in each of these women. Cases of soft tissue infections and bacteremia have also been reported with *C. sordellii* with a better outcome than in the postpartum cases.[58] Neither uterine myonecrosis nor gas formation was present. *C. sordellii* elaborates a factor known as β-toxin, which when injected in animals causes necrosis, edema, hemorrhage, and death.[59, 60] This lethal toxin may actually consist of two toxins, which seem to be similar to toxin A and toxin B of *Clostridium difficile*.[61, 62] The gene of the cytotoxin of *C. sordellii*, known as L, shares homologies with the C-terminal of the *C. difficile* cytotoxin gene, although there are clear structural differences.[63] There are also immunologic and cytotoxic effects that are different among the two toxins of *C. difficile* and toxin L of *C. sordellii*.[64]

Spontaneous (Nontraumatic) Myonecrosis

A variant of the classic picture of gas gangrene is one that arises spontaneously, without an apparent source, at least at onset. Three clinical forms are recognized (see Table 102–1). The *local* form is associated with an intraabdominal or pelvic focus of infection from which clostridia spread into surrounding muscle. The usual setting is "silent" colon cancer or occasionally a diverticular abscess. The disease is characterized by the presence of gas in the flank or thigh muscles, along with hypotension and renal failure.[10, 33, 65] The initiating event may also be perforation of a viscus during bladder catheterization or barium enema.[66, 67]

The second form of spontaneous gas gangrene is *distant* "metastatic" spread of the infection, which originates in a colon cancer or in neutropenic enterocolitis but presents as a gas-forming, necrotizing infection of an extremity or, less commonly, the abdominal wall.[33, 65, 68–71] The unique features of this form of gas gangrene are the absence of trauma, the isolation of *Clostridium* as the sole pathogen, and an abbreviated course, with spreading crepitation and rapid clinical deterioration. The crepitation advances relentlessly during a period of hours, until the entire limb, and even the trunk, is involved. Unlike classic gas gangrene, which tends to be a more localized process, the organism spreads rapidly in these cases through tissue planes, producing massive volumes of gas and advancing far beyond the border of necrotic muscle. Renal failure, hemolytic anemia, and hypotension are usually present, and the patient succumbs 1 to 3 days after onset.[68, 69] More than 90% of these cases are associated with colon cancer, which is occult in nearly half the patients.[68]

The third form of spontaneous gas gangrene is a related, and perhaps earlier, stage of this metastatic process: *crepitant cellulitis* and *fasciitis* with overwhelming toxinosis in the absence of direct muscle invasion.[65, 68, 72, 73] The disease manifests with dramatic abruptness, spreading through fascial planes with widespread gas formation, moving in a virtually visual fashion. Physical examination reveals diffuse crepitation but relatively little pain over the muscles. The process usually begins in an extremity and spreads rapidly to the trunk. Systemic signs of overwhelming clostridial toxemia are present, often leading rapidly to death less than 24 hours from onset.[69, 72] It can be said of this infection, as it was said of cholera in the past, that it is a disease that begins where other diseases end—with death. Pathologic examination fails to show the muscle necrosis characteristic of gas gangrene, although an inflammatory reaction can be seen in the muscle groups adjacent to the affected fascial planes. (A condition analogous to crepitant cellulitis caused by *C. sordellii* occurs in the uterus as noted earlier.)

In spontaneous gas gangrene, the pathogen has been *C. perfringens* in two thirds of cases and *C. septicum* in the remainder,[65, 68, 69] although *C. septicum* may be the more common pathogen in the variety associated with crepitant cellulitis and fasciitis.[69] Colon cancer,[74] leukemia, and various forms of neutropenia, including cyclic neutropenia and neutropenic enterocolitis,[75] have been the underlying cause. Overall mortality in the cases associated with malignancy is 70%, and the highest mortality rates are noted in patients with *C. septicum* infection who have a short incubation period and a rapid course. (See Chapter 222 for discussion of *C. septicum* bacteremia.)

Nontoxigenic Clostridial Infections

Clostridial cellulitis, without signs of systemic toxinosis, is a localized suppurative process that tracks along fascial planes with abundant gas formation yet lacks the systemic signs of clostridia toxin activity. It has a rather leisurely progression—an incubation period of 3 to 5 days and a slower course than that of gas gangrene.[1, 4] Clostridial cellulitis, along with anaerobic streptococcal cellulitis, was reported frequently during World War II, but both conditions are rather rare in more recent times, probably because of more aggressive treatment of traumatic wounds and large-dose antibiotic therapy.

Suppurative skin and soft tissue infections may involve clostridia, usually along with other organisms. About one third of foot ulcers in diabetic patients harbor clostridia[76, 77]; careful bacteriologic studies reveal several different species, most commonly *C. perfringens*.[78, 79] Gas formation is a frequent finding in diabetic foot ulcer, but most cases are caused by gram-negative enteric bacilli and streptococci rather than by clostridia.[31] Gas gangrene is rare in diabetic foot ulcers, although crepitant cellulitis has been described arising from the ulcer or an infected stump amputation. Decubitus ulcer is another site of infection with clostridia, which can even invade the blood stream.[80–82]

Clostridia cause a form of suppurative myositis. This condition differs from gas gangrene because it lacks systemic findings, has a relatively benign course, and produces less muscle destruction. The infection is localized in a single muscle, and it can be managed with simple drainage, leaving a functional muscle group.[83] In intravenous drug abusers, clostridial suppurative myositis manifests with local pain and tenderness, eventually developing into a discrete area of fluctuance that requires surgical drainage. The main sites are the thigh and the forearm. The pathologic findings include subcutaneous abscess in the muscle with an intense inflammatory response that may involve adjacent soft tissues and fascia. A similar condition has been associated with injections of various therapeutic drugs, particularly in diabetic patients.[34] These clinical forms resemble tropical myositis, although the tropical disease is usually caused by *Staphylococcus aureus*.

Diagnosis

In its severe forms, gas gangrene produces an unmistakable clinical picture—myonecrosis, shock, and renal failure. By the time gas gangrene is clinically evident, however, the patient is usually doomed. Thus, it is important to make the diagnosis at the earliest moment to halt the progression of the disease and avoid dire complications that might require mutilating surgery. Initial suspicion should be aroused when the patient complains of unrelenting pain in a wound site even after it has been surgically repaired. Tight, bulging retention sutures or a tight cast over a compound fracture should be warning signs. A rapid pulse in an afebrile patient who has sustained trauma is another ominous sign. The diagnosis of myonecrosis is established by direct examination of the incriminated muscle. The typical appearance, along with failure of the muscle to respond to stimuli and poor blood supply, indicates its nonviable nature. The watery, brownish, foul-smelling discharge shows under the microscope an abundance of gram-positive rods and no inflammatory cells. Culture, which usually propagates the organism within 24 hours, shows *C. perfringens* in most cases. Gas, when present, is useful in diagnosis, but it also can be misleading. Crepitation can be found in nontoxigenic clostridial infections as well as in streptococcal infections. It can also be seen with infections caused by coliforms. These conditions can be excluded by careful examination of the muscle and Gram stain examination of the discharge. Patients with spontaneous gas gangrene present with crepitant cellulitis and severe systemic signs, often before direct muscle invasion occurs. Material from the fascial plane is obtained by needle aspiration, and a Gram stain examination can establish the diagnosis. Radiography, ultrasonography, and computed tomography may be useful to indicate the presence of incipient gas and to delineate the margins of infection. Such examinations are particularly valuable when the muscle is relatively inaccessible, as in the flank or pelvis.

Treatment

The most important therapeutic modality in gas gangrene is adequate *surgical débridement*. All necrotic muscle must be removed because it provides a nidus for proliferation of the organism and toxin production. This may involve amputation of an involved limb, wide resection of limb muscles, removal of abdominal musculature, or hysterectomy. In the absence of adequate resection, antibiotics do not quell this infection.[4, 10–12, 28, 84–86]

Antibiotic therapy is an important adjunct to surgical management. It is generally agreed that penicillin is the drug of choice.[4, 10, 86–88] For experimental clostridial infections, several drugs, including penicillin, chloramphenicol, and tetracycline, are effective as prophylaxis or therapy.[3, 89–93] Antibiotics that inhibit protein synthesis, such as clindamycin, tetracycline, and chloramphenicol, are superior to cell wall–active agents such as penicillin, probably owing to suppression of toxin production by the former group of drugs.[94, 95] The combination of penicillin and clindamycin produces better results than either drug alone in some animal experiments.[96] Because resistance to penicillin among clostridia is still rather uncommon (see Chapter 222) and the clinical experience with this drug remains favorable, the drug regimen for treatment of gas gangrene should include penicillin. At least 50% of these wounds are contaminated by other aerobic and anaerobic bacteria,[10] and additional drugs are often needed. Clindamycin would be a reasonable choice for anaerobic bacteria and to add synergistic activity to penicillin against clostridia[96]; another drug, such as an aminoglycoside or a third-generation cephalosporin, should be employed for gram-negative organisms. Because there has never been a controlled trial of antibiotic therapy for gas gangrene, such recommendations are based on clinical experience, supported by data from studies in vitro and from animal experiments.

Antitoxin had been recommended in earlier times, based primarily on the excellent results published from the wartime experiences.[1, 8, 9] The antiserum was raised in horses against five clostridial species. Severe allergic reactions were reported, and several authorities[24, 86, 97] including Altemeier,[3, 4] who had not used the antitoxin since 1943, recommended against using it. This view was endorsed by the National Research Council and the U.S. Department of Defense,[4] and the production of antitoxin has been discontinued; all current supplies are outdated.

Hyperbaric oxygen (HBO), a procedure used for treating gas gangrene during the past 35 years,[98] is still highly controversial, mostly because its adherents are so convinced of its efficacy that they have not conducted a randomized clinical trial. In vitro, oxygen at 3.0 atmospheres is bactericidal to many strains of clostridia[99] and inhibits production of α-toxin.[100] In a dog model of clostridial infection, neither surgery nor HBO therapy produced survivors; antibiotic treatment alone was associated with a 50% rate of survival, the addition of surgery resulted in 70% survival, and the use of HBO along with surgery and antibiotics produced 95% survival.[101] HBO also reduced morbidity and mortality in a mouse model of clostridial infection.[25, 102] Clearly, animals treated with surgery alone fare worse than those treated with surgery and HBO.[103] When antibiotics are added to the equation, which simulates the clinical situation, the results are less convincing for HBO. In one study either clindamycin or metronidazole improved survival in challenge experiments, but HBO did not have an additive effect,[104] and in the other study the best results were seen with clindamycin compared with metronidazole, penicillin, or HBO, and its superior efficacy was not further enhanced by HBO.[105] Several groups have reported good experiences with HBO in clinical cases of gas gangrene,[10, 37, 73, 86, 106–109] the overall mortality rate being 25%.[10] It is difficult to judge its value from reading the literature, but this author can aver from limited personal experience that the effect of HBO therapy for gas gangrene can be quite dramatic. Having stated this, there are certain problems with such a therapeutic modality, not the least of which is the logistic challenge of moving desperately ill patients to appropriately equipped centers. In addition, HBO has certain untoward effects, including oxygen toxicity, barotrauma, decompression sickness, lung damage, and fire hazard,[10, 110, 111] but these complications are infrequent.[10, 112–115] During the acute period, HBO is administered at 2.0 to 2.5 atmospheres, three times a day, and this regimen has not caused a chamber-related death in more than 20,000 compressions.[10] It would be reasonable to conclude that patients with gas gangrene should be treated with HBO when a facility is

TABLE 102–2 ■ Features of Gas Gangrene Associated with Poor Outcome

Shock
Long incubation period (>30 h)
Spontaneous or postoperative cause
Location in trunk
Older age
Male sex
Underlying disease (cancer, diabetes)
Leukopenia
Renal failure
Hemolysis

Adapted from Hart GB, Lamb RC, Strauss MB: Gas gangrene. J Trauma 23:991–1000, 1983.

readily available. To be sure, some centers without an HBO chamber have reported excellent results; for example, Altemeier and Fullen[4] had a 15% mortality rate in their cases, one of the best records in the literature.

Prognosis

Survival from gas gangrene is related to several factors (Table 102–2). The best results (90% survival or better) are seen in younger patients with traumatic myonecrosis involving a single extremity.[10] At the other extreme, only 20% of patients with spontaneous gas gangrene, particularly those with leukemia or *C. septicum* infection, survive.[4, 33, 68, 73, 97] Treatment also influences survival. During the world wars, before antibiotic and HBO treatments, mortality rates of 30% were common.[2] When the full range of treatment options—surgery, antibiotics, and HBO—is applied in experienced centers, cases of traumatic gas gangrene have less than 10% mortality, and the overall mortality rate for all cases is 25%.[10, 116] Amputations are required in 15% to 20% of patients with gas gangrene, most often in those with traumatic or spontaneous myonecrosis in an extremity.[10] Risk factors associated with a poor outcome are evidence of shock on admission, incubation period longer than 30 hours, and cancer or leukemia as an underlying disease.[10, 68]

Prevention

The best prevention of gas gangrene in trauma cases is good surgical management at the earliest moment, because antibiotics by themselves cannot prevent the disease. The basic principles were articulated more than 70 years ago by Wilensky: "The opening up completely of the entire wound including all pockets; the removal of all dirt and the mechanical cleansing of the wound; the removal of all foreign bodies; the eradication of all hematomata, small and large; the removal of all muscle tissue which is in any way compromised; complete hemostasis. It is imperative to institute wide and abundant drainage."[10, 117]

References

1. MacLennan JD: The histotoxic clostridial infections of man. Bacteriol Rev 26:177, 1962.
2. MacLennan JD: Anaerobic infections of war wounds in the Middle East. Lancet 2:94, 1943.
3. Finegold SM: Anaerobic Bacteria in Human Disease. New York, Academic, 1977, pp 418–428.
4. Altemeier, WA, Fullen WD: Prevention and treatment of gas gangrene. JAMA 217:806, 1971.
5. Weinstein L, Barza M: Gas gangrene. N Engl J Med 289:1129, 1973.
6. Hitchcock CR, Demello FJ, Haglin JJ: Gangrene infection: New approaches to an old disease. Surg Clin North Am 55:1403, 1975.
7. Smith LDS: The Pathogenic Anaerobic Bacteria, ed 2. Springfield, IL, Charles C Thomas, 1975, pp 115–324.
8. Caplan ES, Kluge RM: Gas gangrene: Review of 34 cases. Arch Intern Med 136:788, 1976.
9. Cameron HU, Ford M: Gas gangrene—Need it occur? Can Med Assoc J 119:1207, 1978.
10. Hart GB, Lamb RC, Strauss MB: Gas gangrene. J Trauma 23:991, 1983.
11. DeHaven KE, Evarts CM: The continuing problem of gas gangrene: A review and report of illustrative cases. J Trauma 11:983, 1971.
12. Hitchcock CR, Haglin JJ, Arnar O: Treatment of clostridial infection with hyperbaric oxygen. Surgery 62:759, 1967.
13. Alouf JE, Jolivet-Reynaud C: Purification and characterization of *Clostridium perfringens* δ toxin. Infect Immun 31:536, 1981.
14. Williamson ED, Titball RW: A genetically engineered vaccine against the alpha-toxin of *Clostridium perfringens* protects mice against experimental gas gangrene. Vaccine 11:1253, 1993.
15. Awad MM, Bryant AE, Stevens DL, Rood JI: Virulence studies on chromosomal alpha-toxin and theta-toxin mutants constructed by allelic exchange provide genetic evidence for the essential role of alpha-toxin in *Clostridium perfringens*-mediated gas gangrene. Mol Microbiol 15:191, 1995.
16. Stevens DL, Troyer BE, Merrick DT et al: Lethal effects and cardiovascular effects of purified α and θ toxins from *Clostridium perfringens*. Infect Dis 157:272, 1988.
17. Jolivet-Reynaud C, Moreau H, Alouf JE: Purification of α toxin from *Clostridium perfringens*. Methods Enzymol 165:91, 1988.
18. Ellner PD: Fate of partially purified ^{14}C-labeled toxin of *Clostridium perfringens*. J Bacteriol 82:275, 1961.
19. Bullen JJ: Role of toxins in host-parasite relationships. *In* Montie TC, Kadis S, Aji SJ (eds): Microbial Toxins, Vol 2. London, Academic Press, 1972, pp 109–158.
20. Altemeier WA, Furste WL: Studies in virulence of *Clostridium welchii*. Surgery 25:12, 1949.
21. Parker MT: Postoperative clostridial infections in Britain. Br Med J 3:671, 1969.
22. Simeone F: Clostridial myositis. *In* Symposium on Military Medicine in the Far East Command. Surg Circ Lett Med Sect (Suppl) September 1951.
23. Brown PW, Kinman PB: Gas gangrene in a metropolitan community. J Bone Joint Surg Am 56:1445, 1974.
24. Eraklis AJ, Filler RM, Pappas AM, et al: Evaluation of hyperbaric oxygen as an adjunct in the treatment of anaerobic infections. Am J Surg 117:485, 1969.
25. Holland JA, Hill GB, Wolfe WG, et al: Experimental and clinical experience with hyperbaric oxygen in the treatment of clostridial myonecrosis. Surgery 77:75, 1975.
26. Skiles MS, Covert GK, Fletcher HS: Gas-producing clostridial and nonclostridial infections. Surg Gynecol Obstet 147:65, 1978.
27. Hallagan LF, Scott JL, Horowitz BC, Feied CF: Clostridial myonecrosis resulting from subcutaneous epinephrine suspension injection. Ann Emerg Med 21:434, 1992.
28. Fromm D, Siles W: Postoperative clostridial sepsis of the abdominal wall. Am J Surg 118:517, 1969.
29. Lowbury EJL, Lilly HA: The sources of hospital infection of wound with *Clostridium welchii*. J Hyg 56:169, 1958.
30. Eickhoff TC: An outbreak of surgical wound infections due to *Clostridium perfringens*. Surg Gynecol Obstet 114:102, 1962.
31. Bessman AN, Wagner W: Nonclostridial gas gangrene: Report of 48 cases and review of the literature. JAMA 233:958, 1975.
32. Nichols RL, Smith JW: Gas in the wound: What does it mean? Surg Clin North Am 55:1289, 1975.
33. Nordkild P, Crone P: Spontaneous clostridial myonecrosis: A collective review and report of a case. Ann Chir Gynaecol 75:274, 1986.
34. Kershaw CJ, Bulstrode CJK: Gas gangrene in a diabetic after intramuscular injection. Postgrad Med J 64:812, 1988.
35. Harvey PW, Purnell GV: Fatal case of gas gangrene associated with intramuscular injection. Br Med J 1:744, 1968.
36. Kahn O: The incidence and significance of gas gangrene in a diabetic population. Angiology 25:462, 1974.

37. Kofoed H, Riegels-Nielsen P: Myonecrotic gas gangrene of the extremities. Acta Orthop Scand 54:220, 1983.
38. Walker S: Prognosis of *Bacillus welchii* panophthalmitis. Arch Ophthalmol 19:406, 1938.
39. Henkind P, Fedukowicz H: *Clostridium welchii* conjunctivitis. Arch Ophthalmol 70:791, 1963.
40. Leavitt JM, Stam J: *Clostridium perfringens* panophthalmitis. Arch Ophthalmol 84:227, 1970.
41. Duke-Elder S: System of Ophthalmology. London, Kimpton, 1872, pp 405–410.
42. Crock GW, Heriot WJ, Janakiraman P, Weiner JM: Gas gangrene infection of the eyes and orbits. Br J Ophthalmol 69:143, 1985.
43. Walsh T: Clostridial ocular infection. Case report of gas gangrene panophthalmitis. Br J Ophthalmol 49:472, 1965.
44. Ragan WD: Gas gangrene complicating term pregnancy. Obstet Gynecol 15:332, 1960.
45. Decker WH, Hall W: Treatment of abortions infected with *Clostridium welchii*. Am J Obstet Gynecol 19:545, 1966.
46. Pritchard JA, Whaley PJ: Abortion complicated by *Clostridium perfringens* infection. Am J Obstet Gynecol 111:484, 1971.
47. Smith LP, McLean AP, Maughan GB: *Clostridium welchii* septicotoxemia: A review and report of 3 cases. Am J Obstet Gynecol 110:135, 1971.
48. Patchell RD: Gas gangrene complicating term pregnancy. Obstet Gynecol 28:64, 1966.
49. Dylewski J, Wisenfeld H, Latour A: Postpartum uterine infection with *Clostridium perfringens*. Rev Infect Dis 2:470, 1989.
50. Kirkpatrick CJ, Werdehausen K, Jaeger J, Braining H: Fatal *Clostridium perfringens* infection after normal term pregnancy. Arch Gynecol 231:167, 1982.
51. Browne JT, Van Derhor AH, McConnell TS, Wiggins JW: *Clostridium perfringens* myometritis complicating cesarean section: Report of 2 cases. Obstet Gynecol 28:64, 1966.
52. Fray RE, Davis TP, Brown EA: *Clostridium welchii* infection after amniocentesis. Br Med J 288:901, 1984.
53. Lacey CG, Futoran R, Murrow CP: *Clostridium perfringens* infection complicating chemotherapy for choriocarcinoma. Obstet Gynecol 47:337, 1976.
54. Braverman J, Adachi A, Lev-Gur M, et al: Spontaneous clostridia gas gangrene of uterus associated with endometrial malignancy. Am J Obstet Gynecol 156:1205, 1987.
55. Becker RC, Giuliani M, Savage RA, Weick JK: Massive hemolysis in *Clostridium perfringens* infections. J Surg Oncol 35:13, 1987.
56. Soper DD: Clostridial myonecrosis arising from an episiotomy. Obstet Gynecol 68:265, 1986.
57. McGregor JA, Soper DE, Lovell G, Todd JK: Maternal deaths associated with *Clostridium sordellii* infection. Am J Obstet Gynecol 161:987, 1989.
58. Spera RV Jr, Kaplan MH, Allen SL: *Clostridium sordellii* bacteremia: Case report and review. Clin Infect Dis 15:950, 1992.
59. Willis AT: Clostridia of Wound Infection. London, Butterworth, 1969.
60. Nakamura SN, Tanabe K, Yamakawa K, Nishida S: Cytotoxin production by *Clostridium sordelli* strains. Microbiol Immunol 27:495, 1983.
61. Popoff MR: Purification and characterization of *Clostridium sordellii* lethal toxin and cross-reactivity with *Clostridium difficile* cytotoxin. Infect Immun 55:35, 1987.
62. Martinez RD, Wilkins TD: Purification and characterization of *Clostridium sordellii* hemorrhagic toxin and cross-reactivity with *Clostridium difficile* toxin A (enterotoxin). Infect Immun 56:1215, 1988.
63. Green GA, Schue V, Monteil H: Cloning and characterization of the cytotoxin L-encoding gene of *Clostridium sordellii*: Homology with *Clostridium difficile* cytotoxin B. Gene 161:57, 1995.
64. Baldacini O, Girardot R, Green GA, et al: Comparative study of immunological properties and cytotoxic effects of *Clostridium difficile* toxin B and *Clostridium sordellii* toxin L. Toxicon 30:129, 1992.
65. Jendrzejewski JW, Jones S, Newcombe R, Gilbert DN: Nontraumatic clostridial myonecrosis. Am J Med 65:542, 1978.
66. Amar AD, Ratiff RK: Gas gangrene of the urinary bladder and abdominal wall following catheterization. J Urol 80:130, 1958.
67. Reckman LS, Short WF, Cooper WM: Barium enema septicemia—Occurrence in a patient with leukemia. JAMA 226:62, 1973.
68. Kornbluth AA, Danzig JB, Bernstein LH: *Clostridium septicum* infection and associated malignancy: Report of 2 cases and review of the literature. Medicine (Baltimore) 68:30, 1989.
69. Stevens DL, Musher DM, Watson DA, et al: Spontaneous, nontraumatic gangrene due to *Clostridium septicum*. Rev Infect Dis 12:286, 1990.
70. Buckley D, Kudsk K: Occult gastrointestinal carcinoma causing metastatic clostridial soft-tissue infection: Report of two cases. Dis Colon Rectum 31:306, 1988.
71. Bretzke ML, Bubrick MP, Hitchcock CR: Diffuse spreading *Clostridium septicum* infection, malignant disease and immune suppression. Surg Gynecol Obstet 166:197, 1988.
72. Gorbach SL: Case records of the Massachusetts General Hospital, case 49—1979. N Engl J Med 301:1276, 1979.
73. Hitchcock CF, Bubrick MP: Gas gangrene infections of the small intestine, colon and rectum. Dis Colon Rectum 19:112, 1976.
74. Lorimer JW, Eidus LB: Invasive *Clostridium septicum* infection in association with colorectal carcinoma. Can J Surg 37:245, 1994.
75. Lev R, Sweeney KG: Neutropenic enterocolitis: Two unusual cases with review of the literature. Arch Pathol Lab Med 117:524, 1993.
76. Manson MH: Pathogenic gas-producing anaerobic bacilli in chronic ulcers. Arch Surg 24:752, 1932.
77. Louie TJ, Bartlett JG, Tally FP, Gorbach SL: Aerobic and anaerobic bacteria in diabetic foot ulcers. Ann Intern Med 85:461, 1976.
78. Sapico FL, Canawati HN, Witte JL, et al: Quantitative aerobic and anaerobic bacteriology of infected diabetic feet. J Clin Microbiol 12:413, 1980.
79. Sapico FL, Witte JL, Canawati HN, et al: The infected foot of the diabetic patient: Quantative microbiology and analysis of clinical features. Rev Infect Dis 6:S171, 1984.
80. Wilson WR, Martin WJ, Wilkowske CJ, Washington JA II: Anaerobic bacteremia. Mayo Clin Proc 47:639, 1972.
81. Rissing JP, Crowder JG, Dunfee T, White A: *Bacteroides* bacteremia from decubitus ulcers. South Med J 67:1179, 1974.
82. Chow AW, Galpin JE, Guze LB: Clindamycin for treatment of sepsis caused by decubitus ulcers. J Infect Dis 135:S65, 1977.
83. Gorbach SL, Thadepalli H: Isolation of *Clostridium* in human infections: Evaluation of 114 cases. J Infect Dis 131:S81, 1975.
84. Duff JH, McLean APH, MacLean LD: Treatment of severe anaerobic infections. Arch Surg 101:314, 1970.
85. Klein RS, Berger SA, Yekutiel P: Wound infection during the Yom Kippur war: Observations concerning antibiotic prophylaxis and therapy. Ann Surg 182:15, 1975.
86. Darke SG, King AM, Slack WK: Gas gangrene and related infection: Classification, clinical features and aetiology, management and mortality: A report of 88 cases. Br J Surg 64:104, 1977.
87. Knight RJ: Reception and resuscitation of casualties in South Vietnam. Experience at the First Australian Field Hospital. Lancet 2:29, 1972.
88. Finegold SM, George WL, Mulligan ME: Anaerobic infections. Part II. Dis Mon 31:1, 1985.
89. Hac LR: Experimental *Clostridium welchii* infection. IV. Penicillin therapy. J Infect Dis 71:164, 1944.
90. Altemeier WA, McMurrin JA, Alt LP: Chloromycetin and aureomycin in experimental gas gangrene. Surgery 28:621, 1950.
91. Freeman WA, McFadzean JA, Whelan JPF: Activity of metronidazole against experimental tetanus and gas gangrene. J Appl Bacteriol 31:443, 1968.
92. Irvin TT, Moir ERS, Smith G: Treatment of *Clostridium welchii* infection with hyperbaric oxygen. Surg Gynecol Obstet 127:1058, 1968.
93. Owen-Smith MS, Matheson JM: Successful prophylaxis of gas gangrene of the high-velocity missile wound in sheep. Br J Surg 55:36, 1968.
94. Stevens DL, Maier KA, Laine BM, Mitten JE: Comparison of clindamycin, rifampin, tetracycline, metronidazole, and penicillin for efficacy in prevention of experimental gas gangrene due to *Clostridium perfringens*. J Infect Dis 155:220, 1987.
95. Stevens DL, Maier KA, Mitten JE: Effect of antibiotics on toxin production and viability of *Clostridium perfringens*. Antimicrob Agents Chemother 31:213, 1987.
96. Stevens DL, Laine BM, Mitten JE: Comparison of single and combination antimicrobial agents for prevention of experimental gas gangrene caused by *Clostridium perfringens*. Antimicrob Agents Chemother 31:312, 1987.

97. Roding B, Groeneveld PHA, Boerema I: Ten years of experience in the treatment of gas gangrene with hyperbaric oxygen. Surg Gynecol Obstet 134:579, 1972.
98. Brummelkamp WH, Hogendjik J, Boerema I: Treatment of anaerobic infections (clostridial myositis) by drenching the tissues with oxygen under high atmospheric pressure. Surgery 49:299, 1961.
99. Hill GB, Osterhout S: Experimental effects of hyperbaric oxygen on selected clostridial species: I. In-vivo studies. J Infect Dis 125:17, 1972.
100. Van Unnik AJM: Inhibition of toxin production in *Clostridium perfringens* in vitro by hyperbaric oxygen. Antonie van Leeuwenhoek 31:181, 1965.
101. Demello FJ, Haglin JJ, Hitchcock CR: Comparative study of experimental *Clostridium perfringens* infection in dogs treated with antibiotics, surgery, and hyperbaric oxygen. Surgery 73:936, 1973.
102. Hill GB, Osterhout S: Experimental effects of hyperbaric oxygen on selected clostridial species: II. In vivo studies in mice. J Infect Dis 125:26, 1972.
103. Hirn M: Hyperbaric oxygen in the treatment of gas gangrene and perineal necrotizing fasciitis: A clinical and experimental study. Eur J Surg Suppl (570):1, 1993.
104. Muhvich KH, Anderson LH, Mehm WJ: Evaluation of antimicrobials combined with hyperbaric oxygen in a mouse model of clostridial myonecrosis. J Trauma 36:7, 1994.
105. Stevens DL, Bryant AE, Adams K, Mader JT: Evaluation of therapy with hyperbaric oxygen for experimental infection with *Clostridium perfringens* [see comments]. Clin Infect Dis 17:231, 1993.
106. Unsworth IP, Sharo PA: Gas gangrene. An 11-year review of 73 cases managed with hyperbaric oxygen. Med J Aust 140:256, 1984.
107. Gibson A, Davis FM: Hyperbaric oxygen therapy in the management of *Clostridium perfringens* infections. N Z Med J 99:617, 1986.
108. Hirn M, Niinikoski J: Hyperbaric oxygen in the treatment of clostridial gas gangrene. Ann Chir Gynaecol 77:37, 1988.
109. Grim PS, Gottlieb LJ, Boddie A, Batson E: Hyperbaric oxygen therapy. JAMA 263:2216, 1990.
110. Brummelkamp WH, Boerema I, Hogendijk L: Treatment of clostridial infections with hyperbaric oxygen drenching. A report on 26 cases. Lancet 1:235, 1963.
111. Slack WK, Hanson GC, Chew HER: Hyperbaric oxygen in the treatment of gas gangrene and clostridial infections. A report of 40 patients treated in a single-person hyperbaric oxygen chamber. Br J Surg 56:505, 1969.
112. Bernhard WF, Filler RM: Hyperbaric oxygenation: Current concepts. Am J Surg 115:661, 1968.
113. DeHaven KE, Evarts CM: The continuing problem of gas gangrene: A review and report of illustrative cases. J Trauma 11:983, 1971.
114. Davis JC, Dunn JM, Hagood CO, et al: Hyperbaric medicine in the US Air Force. JAMA 224:205, 1973.
115. Johnson JT, Gillespie TE, Cole JR, et al: Hyperbaric oxygen therapy for gas gangrene in war wounds. Am J Surg 118:839, 1969.
116. Heimbach RD: Gas gangrene: Review and update. HBO Rev 1:41, 1980.
117. Wilensky AO: Gas gangrene. Surg Gynecol Obstet 27:187, 1918.

103

Necrotizing Skin and Soft Tissue Infections

Sherwood L. Gorbach

The severe skin and soft tissue infections differ from the milder, superficial infections by clinical presentation, coexisting systemic manifestations, and treatment strategies.[1–3] They are often "deep and devastating": deep because they involve the fascial and muscle compartments, and devastating because they cause major destruction of tissue and can lead to a fatal outcome. It is important to recognize such infections because appropriate interventions can reduce loss of vital structures and reduce mortality (Table 103–1). These conditions are usually "secondary" infections in that they develop from an initial break in the skin related to trauma or surgery. They can be monomicrobial, usually streptococcal or staphylococcal, or polymicrobial, involving a mixed aerobe-anaerobe bacterial flora.

Five clinical features suggest the presence of a deep and severe infection of the skin and its deeper structures:

1. Severe pain, which is constantly present.
2. Bullous lesions, related to occlusion of deep blood vessels that traverse the fascia or muscle compartments. Bullae are not diagnostic of deep infections because they can also be found in association with superficial infections (erysipelas, cellulitis, toxic shock syndrome, disseminated intravascular coagulation, purpura fulminans), some toxins (e.g., from brown recluse spider bites), and primary dermatologic conditions (e.g., pyoderma gangrenosum).
3. Gas in the soft tissues, which is detected by palpation, radiography, or scanning. The gases are produced by metabolic activity of the aerobic or anaerobic bacteria. When anaerobes are present, there is also a distinctive odor of putrefaction.
4. Systemic toxicity manifested by fever, leukocytosis, delirium, and renal failure.
5. Rapid spread centrally along fascial planes.

Another distinction from the milder skin infections is that these necrotizing deep infections usually require surgical intervention along with antimicrobial drugs for cure. The choice of drugs is based on the specific organisms present, and there may be a monomicrobial flora or a polymicrobial flora (Table 103–2). Whereas preservation of as much viable tissue as possible is attempted, it is necessary to perform bold resection of all necrotic material and incise the fascial planes until the full extent of purulence is realized.

Necrotizing Fasciitis

Necrotizing fasciitis is a relatively rare infection involving subcutaneous tissues with extensive undermining and tracking along fascial planes.[4, 5] Although it was originally associated with group A *Streptococcus pyogenes*, it is apparent that the disease can be caused by other microorganisms, including anaerobic streptococci, *Staphylococcus aureus*, *Bacteroides*, and a mixed anaerobic-aerobic flora.[6]

TABLE 103–1 ■ Necrotizing Soft Tissue Infections

PARAMETER	GAS-FORMING CELLULITIS	SYNERGISTIC NECROTIZING CELLULITIS	GAS GANGRENE	"STREPTOCOCCAL" MYONECROSIS	NECROTIZING FASCIITIS	INFECTED VASCULAR GANGRENE	STREPTOCOCCAL INFECTION
Predisposing conditions	Traumatic	Diabetes, prior local lesions, perirectal lesions	Traumatic or surgical wound	Trauma, surgery	Diabetes, trauma, surgery, perineal infection	Arterial insufficiency	Traumatic or surgical wound
Incubation period	>3 d	3–14 d	1–4 d	3–4 d	1–4 d	>5 d	6 h–2 d
Etiologic organisms	Clostridia, others	Mixed aerobic-anaerobic flora	Clostridia, especially *Clostridium perfringens*	Anaerobic streptococci	Mixed aerobic-anaerobic flora	Mixed aerobic-anaerobic flora	*Streptococcus pyogenes*
Systemic toxicity	Minimal	Moderate to severe	Severe	Minimal until late in course	Moderate to severe	Minimal	Severe
Course	Gradual	Acute	Acute	Subacute	Acute to subacute	Subacute	Acute
Wound findings							
Local pain	Minimal	Moderate to severe	Severe	Late only	Minimal to moderate	Variable	Severe
Skin appearance	Swollen, minimal discoloration	Erythematous or gangrene	Tense and blanched, yellow-bronze, necrosis with hemorrhagic bullae	Erythema or yellow-bronze	Blanched, erythema, necrosis with hemorrhagic bullae	Erythema or necrosis	Erythema, necrosis
Gas	Abundant	Variable	Usually present	Variable	Variable	Variable	No
Muscle involvement	No	Variable	Myonecrosis	Myonecrosis	No	Myonecrosis limited to area of vascular insufficiency	No
Discharge	Thin, dark, sweetish or foul odor	Dark pus or "dishwater," putrid	Serosanguineous, sweet or foul odor	Seropurulent	Seropurulent or dishwater, putrid	Minimal	None or sero-sanguineous
Gram stain	PMNs, gram-positive bacilli	PMNs, mixed flora	Sparse PMNs, gram-positive bacilli	PMNs, gram-positive cocci	PMNs, mixed flora	PMNs, mixed flora	PMNs, gram-positive cocci in chains
Surgical therapy	Débridement	Wide filleting incisions	Extensive excision, amputation	Excision of necrotic muscle	Wide filleting incisions	Amputation	Débridement of necrotic tissue

*PMNs, Polymorphonuclear leukocytes.

From Bartlett JG: Clostridial myonecrosis and other clostridial diseases. *In* Wyngaarden JB, Smith LH Jr, Bennett JC (eds): Cecil Textbook of Medicine, ed 19. Philadelphia, WB Saunders, 1992, p 1679.

Clinical Features

Extension from a skin lesion is seen in 80% of cases. The initial lesion is often trivial, such as a minor abrasion, insect bite, injection site (in the case of heroin addicts), or boil. Rare cases have arisen in a Bartholin gland abscess or perianal abscess, from which the infection spreads to fascial planes of the perineum, thigh, groin, and abdomen. The remaining 20% of patients have no visible skin lesion. The initial presentation is that of cellulitis, which advances slowly. During the next 2 to 4 days, however, there is systemic toxicity with high temperatures. The patient is disoriented and lethargic. The local site shows the following features: cellulitis (90%); edema (80%); skin discoloration or gangrene (70%); and anesthesia of involved skin (frequent, but the true incidence is unknown).

The most distinguishing clinical feature is the wooden-hard feel of the subcutaneous tissues. In cellulitis or erysipelas, the subcutaneous tissues can be palpated and are yielding, but in fasciitis the underlying tissues are firm, and the fascial planes and muscle groups cannot be discerned by palpation. It is often possible to observe a broad erythematous track in the skin, along the route of the fascial plane, as the infection advances cephalad in an extremity. If there is an open wound, probing the edges with a blunt instrument permits ready dissection of the superficial fascial planes well beyond the wound margins. There is remarkably little pain associated with this procedure.

Bacteriology

Monomicrobial Form. Pathogens in this form are group A β-hemolytic *S. pyogenes*, *S. aureus*, and anaerobic streptococci (*Peptostreptococcus*). Staphylococci and hemolytic streptococci occur with about equal frequency, and approximately one third of patients will have both pathogens simultaneously. Most patients acquire their infection outside the hospital. The majority of these infections present in the extremities, approximately two thirds in the lower extremity. There is often an underlying cause, such as diabetes, arteriosclerotic vascular disease, or venous insufficiency with edema. In some instances, a chronic vascular ulcer changes into a more acute process. The mortality in this group is high, approaching 50% in patients with severe vascular disease.

Polymicrobial Form. An array of anaerobic and aerobic organisms can be cultured from the involved fascial plane: from 1 to 15 types of bacteria, with an average of 5 in each wound. Most of the organisms originate from the bowel flora (e.g., coliforms and anaerobic bacteria). The polymicrobial infection is associated with four clinical settings:

1. Surgical procedures, especially bowel resections and penetrating trauma, can be complicated by cellulitis, leading to a superficial fascial dissection.

2. An infection proceeding from a decubitus ulcer, minor trauma, or perianal abscess can involve the buttocks and perineum. Owing to the proximity of the anus, contamination by fecal bacteria is universally present.

TABLE 103–2 ■ Pharmacologic Treatment of Necrotizing Infections of the Skin, Fascia, and Muscle

FIRST-LINE TREATMENT	SECOND-LINE TREATMENT OR PENICILLIN-ALLERGIC PATIENTS
Mixed infections	
Imipenem-cilastatin Ticarcillin-clavulanate Ampicillin-sulbactam Piperacillin-tazobactam	Cefoxitin, clindamycin, or metronidazole and an aminoglycoside
Streptococcal infections	
Penicillin (and clindamycin, for toxic shock or necrotizing fasciitis)	Cefazolin Vancomycin
Staphylococcus aureus infections	
Nafcillin Cloxacillin Vancomycin (for resistant strains)	Cefazolin Vancomycin

3. In intravenous drug users, the upper extremities are frequently involved at the site of injection. Because the needles and "works" are contaminated, unusual organisms such as *Pseudomonas* and *Citrobacter* can be isolated, sometimes in association with anaerobes.

4. The lesion can spread from a Bartholin abscess or a minor vulvovaginal infection. Some cases have been associated with pudendal block anesthesia during delivery. Whereas mixed infections are usually noted in this setting, some cases are caused by a single pathogen, particularly anaerobic *Streptococcus.*

Diagnosis

It may not be possible to diagnose fasciitis on first seeing the patient. Overlying cellulitis is a frequent accompaniment. That the process involves the deeper fascial planes is suggested by the following features:

1. Failure to respond to initial antibiotic therapy. Cellulitis usually improves, with lowering of fever and reduction in local signs, within 24 to 48 hours. Fasciitis is a more stubborn infection and shows little improvement in the initial few days.
2. Hard, wooden feel of the subcutaneous tissue, extending beyond the area of apparent skin involvement.
3. Systemic toxicity, often with altered mental status.

A computed tomographic scan or magnetic resonance image may show exudate extending along the fascial plane. The most important diagnostic feature of necrotizing fasciitis is the appearance of the fascial planes at surgery. On direct inspection, the fascia is swollen and dull gray in appearance, with stringy areas of necrosis. A thin, brownish exudate emerges from the wound. Even on deep dissection, there is no true pus. Extensive undermining of surrounding tissues is present, and the fascial planes can be dissected with a gloved finger or a blunt instrument. A Gram stain of the exudate demonstrates the pathogens and provides an early clue to therapy. Gram-positive cocci in chains suggest *Streptococcus* (either group A or anaerobic). Large gram-positive cocci in clumps suggest *S. aureus.* A mixed flora suggests polymicrobial infection. Cultures are best obtained from the deep tissues. If the infection has emanated from a contaminated skin wound, such as a vascular ulcer, the bacteriology of the superficial wound is not necessarily indicative of the deep tissue infection. An array of coliforms, staphylococci, and various streptococci can be isolated from the ulcer, but the fascia may yield a pure culture or single organism, such as anaerobic streptococci or *S. aureus.* Direct needle aspiration of the advancing edge has been advocated as a means of obtaining material for culture, but this technique is nearly always unproductive. A definitive bacteriologic diagnosis can be established only by culture of the fascia at operation or by positive blood culture.

Treatment

Surgical intervention is the major therapeutic modality in cases of necrotizing fasciitis. However, some patients can be treated with large doses of appropriate antibiotics and thereby avoid potentially mutilating surgery. The decision to undertake aggressive surgery should be based on the following:

1. Failure to respond to antibiotics after a reasonable trial is the most common index. A response to antibiotics should be judged by reduction in fever and toxic effects and lack of advancement of fasciitis.
2. Profound toxic response, fever, hypotension, or advancement of the skin and soft tissue infection during antibiotic therapy is an indication for surgical intervention.
3. When the local wound shows extensive necrosis with easy dissection along the fascia by a blunt instrument, more complete incision and drainage are required.

The patient should be well hydrated and adequately transfused before the surgical procedure is begun. With the patient under general anesthesia, the skin is incised or the wound is widened down to the fascial plane for complete inspection. Finger dissection along the fascial plane determines the extent of the linear incision. Multiple incisions or "fillets" are usually required to delineate adequately the extent of involvement. Loose gauze dressings are packed into the wound and changed every 6 hours or as required. Wet-to-dry dressings are used to facilitate mechanical débridement. As the dressings are removed, the depth of the wound should be inspected by a gloved finger to determine any extension that requires further incision. The first procedure is almost never sufficient to determine the extent of involvement. As further tracks are discovered, the patient is returned to the operating room for additional incision and débridement. Although no discrete pus is encountered, these wounds can discharge copious amounts of tissue fluid. For this reason, aggressive fluid and colloid therapy is a necessary adjunct.

Antimicrobial therapy, when administered appropriately, can minimize the extent of, and even avert, surgical intervention, especially in those cases in which the distinction between cellulitis and fasciitis is difficult. The antimicrobial must be directed at the pathogens and used in high doses for a prolonged time, usually 2 to 3 weeks.

The overall mortality in necrotizing fasciitis is 20% to 30%. Adverse risk factors include diabetes, advanced arteriosclerotic disease, and lesions that involve an extremity and that then progress into the buttocks or back muscles or onto the chest wall.

Anaerobic Streptococcal Myositis

Myositis is a more indolent process than the other streptococcal infections. Involvement of the muscle and fascial planes is usually associated with trauma or a surgical procedure. There may be severe local pain. The overlying skin appears as a gangrenous wound that emits a foul, watery, brown discharge. Bleb formation is common. Crepitus may be apparent in the surrounding tissue. The gas formation can be extensive, with tracking into the adjacent healthy tissues. Inspection of the muscle reveals redness and edema with some local destruction. There is no myonecrosis, however, and the muscle contracts under the scalpel. Although there is generalized toxicity and fever and even organ failure, the patient is usually not as ill as someone with gas gangrene.

The initial approach to a crepitant skin infection is to obtain a sample of exudate for Gram stain and open the wound for inspection of muscle and soft tissue. The major distinctions between the disease caused by anaerobic streptococci and clostridia are as follows. Systemic effects are less prominent with the streptococcal form. This infection does not cause hypotension and renal failure, as does the clostridial disease. On inspection, the involved muscle remains viable in the streptococcal disease, although there may be inflammatory reaction and edema. True myonecrosis is not found. The anaerobic streptococcal form can produce considerable gas, which occurs early in the course, whereas clostridial infections tend to have less gas and usually as a late development. The discharge from the wound is a thin, brown ooze that shows gram-positive cocci and multiple polymorphonuclear leukocytes on the Gram stain slide. By contrast, the discharge in gas gangrene shows gram-positive rods but few polymorphonuclear leukocytes.

For treatment, incision and drainage of the infected wound are critical. The necrotic tissue and debris are resected, but the inflamed muscle should not be removed because it can heal and become functionally useful. The incision should be packed with moist dressings.

Antibiotic treatment is highly effective. These organisms are all sensitive to penicillin or ampicillin, which should be administered in high doses.

Streptococcal Gangrene (Meleney Streptococcal Gangrene, β-Streptococcal Gangrene)

Streptococcal infection can progress to cause severe destruction of the superficial layers of skin. This form of gangrene most frequently occurs in the extremities, associated with minor trauma, puncture wound, or surgical incision, but it can occur in postoperative abdominal incisions. The initial event is erysipelas, with the typical findings of pain, erythema, edema, and advancing border. Within 1 to 2 days, the center of the lesion becomes dark red, then blue-black, with formation of bullae and gangrene of the skin and subcutaneous tissues. The surrounding tissue is fiery red, raised, and edematous. Deeper fascia and muscle may also be involved. Surgical management involves débridement of the gangrenous skin and incision and drainage of the surrounding tissues and fascial planes. Because it is important to release the pressure on the skin and subcutaneous tissues, the incisions should be extended beyond the areas of gangrene and far enough into the superficial fascia to establish good drainage. The limb should be elevated to promote drainage and dressed with moist packs for superficial débridement. Although no discrete pockets of pus are to be found, there is significant oozing of tissue fluid, which must be made up by appropriate intravenous administration of fluid and colloids. High-dose penicillin or ampicillin is also given.

Progressive Bacterial Synergistic Gangrene (Meleney Gangrene)

Meleney synergistic gangrene is an indolent process characterized by poor wound healing with elevation and erythema of the surrounding skin. This is a postoperative infection that typically occurs in the vicinity of retention suture or in a drain site after an abdominal operation. It occasionally occurs in other areas, such as an incision of the chest wall. The diagnosis is recognized 1 to 2 weeks after operation, when the lesion has extended circumferentially with three zones of involvement: a central area of necrosis; a middle zone of violaceous, tender, edematous tissue; and an outer zone of bright erythema. Local pain and tenderness are nearly always present. However, fever and systemic toxicity are usually absent.

This condition is caused by synergistic (cooperative) association between *S. aureus* and a microaerophilic or anaerobic *Streptococcus*. These organisms can be isolated from the outer zone of infection; sampling the central zone of necrosis, however, yields a mixed flora of coliforms that does not reflect the essential pathologic process. Synergy has also been demonstrated in mixed infections of *S. aureus* and β-hemolytic *S. pyogenes* and of aerobes and anaerobes.[7]

In the preantibiotic era, Meleney advocated extensive resection of all nonviable tissue as well as extension of the incision beyond the area of induration and necrosis to include some healthy tissue. The availability of antibiotics has eliminated the requirement for such radical excision. It is now recommended that all necrotic tissue be removed, with inspection of subcutaneous structures for burrowing tracks. Wet-to-dry dressings should then be employed. Daily inspection should reveal any extension of the process that requires additional débridement. A heterograft or homograft may be necessary to cover the wound. Antimicrobial therapy should be directed at the two major pathogens, *S. aureus* and the anaerobic *Streptococcus*. A semisynthetic penicillin (nafcillin or oxacillin) or a cephalosporin can be used.

Pyomyositis

Pyomyositis refers to a discrete abscess within an individual muscle group caused in the main by *S. aureus*. On occasion, *Streptococcus pneumoniae* or a gram-negative enteric rod is the responsible pathogen. Because of its geographic distribution, this condition is often referred to as tropical pyomyositis,[8] but cases are increasingly recognized in temperate climates, especially in patients with human immunodeficiency virus infection or diabetic patients.[9, 10] The presenting findings are localized pain in a single muscle group, muscle spasm, and fever. The disease occurs most often in an extremity, but any muscle group can be involved, including the psoas or muscles of the trunk. Initially, it may not be possible to palpate a discrete abscess because the infection is localized deep within the muscle, but the area has a firm, woody feel on palpation, along with pain and tenderness. In the early stages, an ultrasound or computed tomographic scan is needed to make the diagnosis, which can be confused with deep vein thrombosis, but in more advanced cases, a bulging abscess is apparent. Blood cultures are positive in 5% to 30% of cases. Surgical incision and drainage are required, along with appropriate antibiotics.

Synergistic Necrotizing Cellulitis

This is a highly lethal polymicrobial infection that produces extensive necrosis of skin and soft tissues with progressive undermining along fascial planes.[11] The process may be indolent at first, presenting after 7 to 10 days of mild symptoms. Patients are often afebrile or have only low-grade fever and lack systemic toxicity in the early stages. The initial lesion in the skin is a small area of necrosis or reddish brown bleb with extreme local tenderness. However, the superficial appearance belies the widespread destruction of the deeper tissues. By direct inspection through skin incisions, there is extensive gangrene of the superficial tissues and fat, with gelatinous necrosis of fascia and muscle. The discharge is brown, rather thin and watery, with a foul odor; such exudate has been labeled dishwater pus. Gram stain reveals a mixed flora with abundant polymorphonuclear leukocytes. Gas can be palpated in the tissues in 25% of patients.

The most common site of involvement is the perineum, seen in one half of patients. The major predisposing causes are perirectal abscess and ischiorectal abscess; these conditions track to the deeper structures of the pelvis, leading to a severe form of the disease. A more superficial form involves the buttocks without extension to deeper muscles. Approximately 40% of patients have involvement of the thigh and leg. Some infections arise in the adductor compartment of the thigh, often extending from an infected amputation stump or diabetic gangrene. Lesions in the lower leg are usually associated with vascular disease or diabetic foot ulcers. The remaining 10% of cases occur in the upper extremities or in the neck, most frequently in patients with vascular disease or diabetes.

Seventy-five percent of patients have diabetes mellitus, which may be relatively mild and discovered only at the time of admission. Some patients present with ketoacidosis. Cardiovascular or renal disease is seen in 50% of patients. Obesity is common, found in more than 50% of patients.

This is a mixed aerobic-anaerobic infection, consisting of organisms that have their origin in the intestinal tract.[11, 12] Of the aerobes, coliforms, such as *Escherichia coli, Klebsiella,* and *Proteus,* are most common. The anaerobes include *Bacteroides, Peptostreptococcus, Clostridium,* and *Fusobacterium.* Approximately one third of patients have positive blood cultures, usually a coliform, *Bacteroides,* or *Peptostreptococcus.*

Surgical management of synergistic necrotizing cellulitis involves radical débridement of involved tissues, followed by wet-to-dry dressing and mechanical débridement. When the lower extremity is involved, as in diabetes, an amputation is usually required. In the perineum, infection that is confined to the buttocks can be managed with complete surgical excision; however, deeper infection in the pelvis, extending from perirectal disease, is difficult to approach by complete resection and may require repeated sessions of débridement in the operating room to achieve adequate drainage. Antibiotic therapy involves a spectrum broad enough to cover both aerobes and anaerobes.

There is a 50% mortality in this disease. The patient usually succumbs to septic shock and circulatory collapse. Adverse risk factors include diabetes, especially ketoacidosis; severe renal disease; and involvement of deep tissues of the pelvis and perineum.

Nonclostridial Crepitant Cellulitis

Gas-forming organisms can involve the skin, either primarily or as an extension from deeper structures. The origin of infection may be an abdominal wound, perianal disease, or operative incisions that have become secondarily infected. Tracking of gas-forming organisms from deeper sites of infection may also present as crepitant cellulitis without a break in the skin. This can be noted in the perineal area, associated with ischiorectal abscess, or in the flank, communicating with perinephric abscess. Among the bacteria isolated are anaerobic organisms such as *Bacteroides* or anaerobic streptococci *(Peptostreptococcus)* and coliform bacteria, especially *E. coli* and *Klebsiella*. Diabetic patients are more likely to acquire such infections, especially in the lower extremities. These emphysematous infections are generally not as serious as those associated with clostridia, because the nonclostridial pathogens do not liberate systemic toxins.

The surgical approach should be aggressive but tailored specifically to the underlying cause of infection. Extensive resection is usually not required; the gas is not an index of underlying necrosis but rather reflects tracking of the infection along the fascial or lymphatic planes. Antibiotic therapy is directed at a mixed aerobic-anaerobic flora until culture reports are available.

Noninfectious processes can be associated with gas in subcutaneous tissues:

1. On the chest wall, at the site of thoracocentesis, chest tube insertion, or a thoracic procedure, there may be subcutaneous emphysema that tracks extensively along subcutaneous tissues.
2. A tracheotomy provides a portal for air to track along the tissues of the neck, even to the anterior chest wall. Transtracheal aspiration by a needle produces local emphysema in approximately 10% of cases.
3. On rare occasion, a thin column of gas is palpated or seen by x-ray examination along the course of an intravenous catheter in the arm. This is most likely caused by a central venous pressure line or a Swan-Ganz catheter. This is a benign condition, not associated with infection in the lines or the surrounding veins.

Fournier Gangrene

This is a variant of synergistic gangrene that involves the scrotum and penis and has an explosive onset.[13, 14] The average age at onset is 50 to 60 years. Most men have significant underlying disease, particularly diabetes. It can also occur in healthy men, without other illnesses. One third of patients have no preceding cause; the remaining individuals have one of the following conditions: ischiorectal abscess; perianal fistula; erysipelas of the perineum; bowel disease (rectal carcinoma, diverticulitis); scrotal traumas; or prior urogenital surgery, especially involving the periurethral glands. In recent times, this disease has been observed in alcoholic men who develop pressure sores of the scrotum and perineum by sitting in the same position in a drunken stupor. Dissection of pancreatic juice through the retroperitoneum has on rare occasion presented as scrotal gangrene.

The infection can begin insidiously with a discrete area of necrosis on the scrotum, which can then move with advancing skin necrosis rapidly in 1 to 2 days. The route of infection is thought to be through Buck fascia, spreading along the planes of the dartos fascia of the scrotum and penis. The infection may then extend to Colles fascia of the perineum and even to Scarpa fascia of the abdominal wall. At the outset, it tends to be superficial gangrene, limited to skin and subcutaneous tissue, extending to the base of the scrotum. The testes, glans penis, and spermatic cord are usually spared because they have a separate blood supply. There may be extension to the perineum and the anterior abdominal wall through the fascial planes.

Most cases are caused by a mixed flora of aerobic and anaerobic bacteria, similar to those noted in synergistic necrotizing cellulitis. Staphylococci are frequently present, usually in mixed culture but occasionally as a single pathogen. *Pseudomonas* is another common organism in the mixed culture.

Prompt and aggressive surgical débridement should be instituted with removal of all necrotic tissue, sparing the deeper structures when possible. It is often necessary to return to the operating room on several occasions for the necessary resection of necrotic tissue. Diversion of the fecal or urinary stream is necessary in some but not all cases.

Antibiotic therapy should cover the range of organisms in the mixed culture. Special attention is paid to staphylococci and pseudomonads. Even with optimal surgical and medical therapy, mortality ranges from 10% to 40% in various series.

References

1. Ahrenholz DH: Necrotizing soft-tissue infections. Surg Clin North Am 68:199–214, 1988.
2. Lewis RT: Necrotizing soft-tissue infections. Infect Dis Clin North Am 6:693–703, 1992.
3. File TM Jr, Tan JS: Treatment of skin and soft-tissue infections. Am J Surg 169:27s–33s, 1995.
4. Giuliano A, Lewis F Jr, Hadley K, Blaisdell FW: Bacteriology of necrotizing fasciitis. Am J Surg 134:52–57, 1977.
5. Howard RJ, Pessa ME, Brennaman BH, Ramphal R: Necrotizing soft-tissue infections caused by marine vibrios. Surgery 98:126–130, 1985.
6. Rea WJ, Wyrick WJ Jr: Necrotizing fasciitis. Ann Surg 172:957–964, 1970.
7. Kingston D, Seal DV: Current hypotheses on synergistic microbial gangrene. Br J Surg 77:260–264, 1990.
8. Sissolak D, Weir WR: Tropical pyomyositis. J Infect 29:121–127, 1994.
9. Belsky DS, Teates CD, Hartman ML: Case report: Diabetes mellitus as a predisposing factor in the development of pyomyositis. Am J Med Sci 308:251–254, 1994.
10. Walling DM, Kaelin WG Jr: Pyomyositis in patients with diabetes mellitus. Rev Infect Dis 13:797–802, 1991.
11. Stone HH, Martin JD Jr: Synergistic necrotizing cellulitis. Ann Surg 175:702–711, 1972.
12. Brook I, Frazier EH: Clinical features and aerobic and anaerobic microbiological characteristics of cellulitis. Arch Surg 130:786–792, 1995.
13. Salvino C, Harford FJ, Dobrin PB: Necrotizing infections of the perineum. South Med J 86:908–911, 1993.
14. Laucks SS 2nd: Fournier's gangrene. Surg Clin North Am 74:1339–1352, 1994.

104

Surgical Infections in Trauma

Ronald C. Jones

Trauma is the fourth most common cause of death, after diseases of the heart, malignant neoplasms, and cerebrovascular diseases.[1] It is the leading cause of death in persons aged 1 through 37 years.[2] After hemorrhage and closed head injury, sepsis is the next most common cause of death in patients who sustain abdominal trauma, and it is a leading cause of postoperative morbidity.[3, 4] As many as 24% of trauma patients admitted to hospitals develop a nosocomial infection, and patients requiring 5 days or more in the intensive care unit have an infection rate of 60%.[5]

The source of a nosocomial infection is either exogenous or endogenous. Infection after penetrating abdominal trauma usually results from endogenous organisms introduced by perforation of the gastrointestinal tract. The bacterial population of the large bowel is 10^{11} to 10^{12} bacteria per gram of stool, and anerobes outnumber aerobes by 1000 to 10,000.[6] The most common aerobe is *Escherichia coli*, and the most common anaerobe is *Bacteroides*.[7] The large intestine provides an ideal anaerobic environment and a low oxidation-reduction potential. A less common cause of infection is exogenous bacteria, which may be carried into the wound on pieces of clothing, dirt, or foreign bodies by a knife or bullet. Gram-positive infections due to staphylococcal, streptococcal, or clostridial infections may result. During the immediate resuscitation, contamination may result from breach in sterile technique while intravenous and urinary catheters are inserted or arterial lines or during arteriography.

Local and Systemic Factors

Many factors are responsible for infection after trauma—the number and virulence of organisms, blood supply or viability of tissue, host resistance, shock, adequacy of surgical débridement, tissue tension, dead space, hemostasis, age, and associated diseases.[8] Normal tissue has remarkable resistance to microorganisms, whereas devitalized tissue has a limited capacity for resistance.[9–11] Clinical experience has long shown that there is an inverse relationship between the vascularity of an area and its susceptibility to infection. Débridement remains the most important adjunct in the prevention of infection.

Host Defense Mechanisms

As the severity of injury increases, there are progressively more abnormalities in host defense mechanisms.[12, 13] Host defense mechanisms include humoral (antibody) responses, complement, phagocytic cells, the cell-mediated system, and barrier defense of the gastrointestinal tract. There are numerous humoral mediators of acute-phase responses, including interleukin-1 and prostaglandins. Delayed hypersensitivity skin testing has proved to be a reliable method of identifying anergic patients who are at increased risk of developing postoperative sepsis.[14] Within 2 hours of sustaining severe injuries, patients have alterations in host defense mechanisms that activate the complement cascade. Chemotaxis and phagocytosis are impaired.[15, 16] Treatment of the patient with impaired host defense mechanisms is by parenteral nutrition, restoration of blood volume, adequate oxygenation, débridement, good hemostasis, and evaluation for a possible source of infection.[17]

Prophylactic Antibiotics

Sepsis is related to the length of the interval between bacterial contamination of the traumatic wound and the initiation of treatment designed to prevent sepsis. The effectiveness of preventive antibiotics in surgical wounds has been shown to be no more than 3 hours.[18] Antibiotics should be started as soon as possible after injury for which such drugs are indicated.

In 1965, more than 400 patients who sustained penetrating abdominal trauma were reviewed to determine the preventive benefit of penicillin and tetracycline. Approximately half of the patients received antibiotics before or during their operation and the other half, in the recovery room, when infection developed, or never (i.e., therapeutic group).[19] Gunshot wounds were associated with four times more cases of sepsis than were stab wounds (Table 104–1). Patients in shock had twice as many septic complications as did normotensive patients (24% versus 11%). The overall infection rate was

TABLE 104–1 ■ Effects of Preventive Antibiotics in Penetrating Abdominal Trauma

	PREOPERATIVE OR INTRAOPERATIVE TREATMENT			POSTOPERATIVE OR THERAPEUTIC			TOTALS		
	Patients Treated	Patients with Infection		Patients Treated	Patients with Infection		Patients Treated	Patients with Infection	
TYPE OF TRAUMA	*N*	*N*	%	*N*	*N*	%	*N*	*N*	%
Stab wounds	77	0	0	111	5	4.5	188	5	2.6
Gunshot wounds	113	8	7	102	15	15	215	23	10.7

reduced from 9% to 4.5% with the early use of antibiotics. Based on the biphasic animal model experiments, a second study was initiated, which included 122 patients who sustained penetrating abdominal trauma (Jones RC, personal communication, 1980). The patients were randomized into three groups that received clindamycin plus tobramycin, no antibiotics, or cefoxitin. The infection rate for combination therapy was 16%, for no antibiotics 44%, and for the single agent 10%. Antibiotic therapy did prevent sepsis in a clinical setting, but there was no difference between single-agent and combination therapy (Jones RC, personal communication, 1980).

Another study compared cephalothin plus kanamycin with clindamycin plus kanamycin in patients with gastrointestinal tract trauma.[20] Anaerobes were frequently isolated from infections in the patients receiving cephalothin-kanamycin, whereas clindamycin-kanamycin almost eliminated them. O'Donnell and colleagues[21] subsequently demonstrated that single-agent carbenicillin was comparable to the combination of clindamycin-gentamicin; thus, routine use of an aminoglycoside was shown to be unnecessary for abdominal trauma.

Jones and colleagues[22] evaluated 257 patients to determine whether single-agent therapy was comparable to combination therapy and whether anaerobes played a role in infection after trauma. Patients were randomized to receive combination therapy (clindamycin-tobramycin); cefamandole, which is not active against *Bacteroides fragilis*; or cefoxitin, which is active against aerobes and anaerobes. The overall infection rate with clindamycin-tobramycin was 20%; with cefamandole, 29% and with cefoxitin, 13%. Among patients who sustained colon or small bowel injuries the infection rates rose to 29%, 45%, and 15%, respectively (Table 104–2). This study demonstrated that single-agent antimicrobial therapy was as effective as combination therapy and that antibiotics active against *B. fragilis* and other anaerobes are necessary in the preoperative treatment of the trauma patient. In the absence of colon injury, there was no difference in infection rate, regardless of what antibiotic was given.[22]

TABLE 104–2 ■ Penetrating Abdominal Trauma: Colon and/or Small Bowel Injuries at Parkland Memorial Hospital, December 1980 to June 1983

ANTIBIOTIC	NUMBER OF PATIENTS	NUMBER OF INFECTIONS (%)	BACTEREMIA, ABDOMINAL ABSCESS, OPERATIVE SOFT TISSUE
Cleocin/tobramycin	51	15 (29%)	7 (14%)
Mandol	44	20 (45%)	11 (26%)
Cefoxitin	52	8 (15%)	5 (10%)
I versus III		$P = .086$	$P = .515$
II versus I and III		$P = .006$	$P = .048$

Several studies have confirmed that results of single-agent therapy are comparable to those of combination therapy.[23, 24] Fabian demonstrated that single-agent therapy with ticarcillin-clavulanate (Timentin) was comparable to combination therapy with clindamycin-gentamicin for treating penetrating abdominal trauma.[23] Nichols and associates[25] demonstrated an overall infection rate of 20% using cefoxitin, versus 23% with clindamycin-gentamicin. Risk factors for development of infection after trauma include older age, injury to the left side of the colon, massive transfusion, and multiple injured organs. Gentry and colleagues[27] evaluated cefamandole, cefoxitin, and ticarcillin-tobramycin for penetrating abdominal trauma. The intraabdominal abscess rates were identical (6%) for cefoxitin and combination therapy and were half that for cefamandole (Table 104–3) (12%).[26] Thus, preventive antibiotics, either a single agent or a combination, are beneficial when given before operation to patients with abdominal trauma.

The appropriate duration of preventive antibiotic treatment is unknown. Various studies have included recommendations ranging from 12 hours to 5 days.[22–28] For gastrointestinal injury, between 1 and 3 days' therapy is adequate.[28a, 28b] Patients without gastrointestinal injury and without massive tissue destruction can probably stop taking antibiotics within 24 hours.

Bacteremia in Trauma

Bacteremia often follows gunshot wounds to the colon, and gram-negative organisms account for 70% of the isolates; anaerobes are isolated from 20% of patients.[29] The overall mortality rate for patients with bacteremia after trauma is approximately 40%. Of a group of patients with bacteremia, two thirds had sustained colon injuries and 75% gunshot wounds. This supports a study by Gibson and colleagues,[31] who noted that 75% of patients who developed intraabdominal abscess had previously sustained a gunshot wound. *Enterococcus* may be the only organism isolated from blood cultures and appears to be a significant pathogen. Isolation of an *Enterococcus* species is rare immediately after trauma; more often these organisms are present after multiple complications. The most common gram-negative aerobes isolated were *Klebsiella pneumoniae* and *E. coli*, followed by *Enterobacter, Pseudomonas*, and *Serratia* species. It was unusual to isolate anaerobes after blunt trauma, but the rate was 28% after penetrating trauma. Resistant organisms, such as *Pseudomonas aeruginosa, Serratia marcescens*, and *Enterobacter cloacae*, were uncommon isolates in patients who had not undergone surgery. Antibiotic coverage may not have to be as broad for hospital patients who have penetrating or blunt abdominal trauma; nevertheless, several antibiotic choices are available (Table 104–4). In another group of patients who sustained pancreatic trauma, 15% developed bacteremia and half of them had an associated colon injury. Patients with colon

TABLE 104–3 ■ Single-Agent Therapy for Penetrating Abdominal Trauma*

INVESTIGATOR	PATIENTS (N)		INFECTIONS (%)		ABDOMINAL ABSCESS (%)	
Jones et al[22]	Cef	CT	Cef	CT	Cef	CT
	94	85	13	20	5	4
Gentry et al[26]	Cef	TT	Cef	TT	Cef	TT
	50	51	6	10	6	6
Nichols et al[25]	Cef	CG	Cef	CG	Cef	CG
	70	75	20	23	4	7

*Cef, Cefoxitin; TT, ticarcillin-tobramycin; CG, clindamycin-gentamicin; CT, clindamycin-tobramycin.

injury usually require antibiotic treatment for 2 to 5 days, depending on the severity.[32] Depending also on the severity of illness, single-agent therapy or combination therapy is indicated, especially for *Pseudomonas* organisms. Broad-spectrum coverage is used until culture results are available. Alternatives to aminoglycoside antibiotics are aztreonam and third-generation cephalosporins such as ceftazidime.

Intraoperative Management of Fecal Contamination

Peritonitis is usually accompanied by sequestration of extracellular fluid, which requires liberal administration of a balanced salt solution. It is mandatory that the source of fecal contamination be eliminated, and this is best accomplished by a proximal colostomy or colon repair. Once peritonitis is diagnosed, antibiotic therapy is initiated, the choice of drug being based on the site of infection and the suspected pathogens. Anaerobic organisms including *B. fragilis*, *Clostridium*, and *Peptostreptococcus* species are common in both generalized peritonitis and postoperative intraabdominal abscess. Many antibiotic combinations and single agents are capable of producing clinical improvement or cure of peritonitis. Dawes and colleagues[33] have demonstrated that the risk of infection after colon injury is related to the patient's age, number of associated injuries, number of blood transfusions, and injury to the spleen. In the absence of these risk factors, the likelihood of infection after colon injury and primary repair or resection is low. If these four risk factors are present, a colostomy is usually indicated.[22, 33]

Thompson and Moore[34] evaluated right- and left-sided colon injuries that were managed by either primary repair or resection and found no difference in wound infection rates (7%) or abscess formation rates (14%). Some physicians have thought that the left-sided colon may not heal as well as the right-sided colon; however, Schrock and Christiansen[35] found no difference in leakage of ileocolic and left colon anastomoses in elective operations.

TABLE 104–4 ■ Antibiotics for Penetrating Abdominal Trauma

ANTIBIOTIC	DOSE	TREATMENT DAYS
Cefoxitin	1 g q 4 h[22]	2
	2 g q 6 h[26]	2
	2 g q 6 h[27]	3
	2 g q 6 h[25]	5
Clindamycin	600 mg q 6 h[25]	
Gentamicin	1.7 mg/kg q 8 h	2–5
Ticarcillin	3 g q 4 h[26]	2
Tobramycin	1.5 mg/kg q 8 h	
Timentin	3 g q 4 h[23]	1
Mezlocillin	4 g q 6 h[70]	2–5

Peritonitis

The organisms that usually cause infections after abdominal trauma are Enterobacteriaceae and anaerobic bacteria.[36] *B. fragilis* species are the predominant anaerobes isolated, along with *Peptostreptococcus* organisms. Weinstein and colleagues[37, 38] developed an experimental model in rats and subsequently described two phases of peritonitis. Onderdonk and coworkers[39] described synergy between anaerobes and facultative bacteria as the mechanism for intraabdominal abscess formation. Early death of the animal was usually due to *E. coli* infection, but almost 100% of those that survived developed intraabdominal abscess from which *B. fragilis* was isolated. More than 100 patients with peritonitis were evaluated, and the most common gram-positive organisms were as follows: *Streptococcus* and *Enterococcus* species[29]; gram-negative aerobes, *E. coli* and *Klebsiella*; anaerobes, *Peptostreptococcus* and *B. fragilis* or *Bacteroides* species.

Imipenem (Primaxin), a carbapenem, has the broadest antimicrobial activity of any antibiotic developed, is relatively nontoxic, and is active against both aerobes and anaerobes, including *B. fragilis*. It is a useful antibiotic for empirical treatment of moderate to severe intraabdominal infections, for resistant organisms, and for severe pulmonary infections in patients in a step-down intensive care unit.[40] For established *Pseudomonas* sepsis, imipenem is combined with an aminoglycoside. Imipenem is not recommended for prophylaxis and is not to be used to treat mild infections. Other single agents for mild to moderate peritonitis include cefoxitin and cefotetan. Agents such as clindamycin or metronidazole combined with an aminoglycoside or metronidazole-ceftazidime or clindamycin-aztreonam have been used without risk of aminoglycoside toxicity.

Intraperitoneal Antibiotic Irrigation

The incidence of infection is lower after antibiotic irrigation than if no antibiotic therapy is given, but it is unclear whether intraperitoneal antibiotic irrigation adds anything to the effects of systemic antibiotic therapy. Intraperitoneal antibiotic irrigation produces measurable levels of antibiotic in serum; however, they are not as high as those achieved by intravenous administration of drug. Aminoglycoside peritoneal irrigation can rapidly produce antibiotic serum levels in the toxic range.[41]

Intraabdominal Abscess After Surgery for Trauma

In one series, 86% of the abscesses followed gunshot wounds of the abdomen, and 60% of patients sustained a colon

TABLE 104–5 ■ Prevalence of Intraabdominal Abscess After Surgery for Trauma in 50 Patients*

INFECTION SITE	PREVALENCE (%)
Colon	60
Small bowel only	12
Bacteremia	36
Mortality rate	22

*Injury: gunshot wounds, 86%; SGW, 6%; stab wounds, 8%.

injury[29] (Table 104–5). Thus, colon injury is a predictor of increased incidence of complications. The most common gram-positive aerobe isolated was *Enterococcus*, present in approximately 60% of the abscesses but almost always in association with other organisms. *Staphylococcus* species were present in approximately 15% of patients. The most common gram-negative aerobe was *E. coli*, whereas *Enterobacter* species were present in 20% of cases. *B. fragilis* or other *Bacteroides* species were isolated from approximately 25% of patients, and *Clostridium perfringens* or other clostridia from 22% (Table 104–6). As in bacteremia, *Pseudomonas* is not often associated with the first intraabdominal complication of trauma.[29] Of the patients with intraabdominal abscess, more than a third had associated bacteremia. Clinical findings before drainage of the abscess frequently include temperature elevations to 102°F to 105°F and white cell counts of 20,000 to 50,000/mm^3. The mortality rate for intraabdominal abscess is approximately 20%.[30]

Computed tomography is specific for diagnosing intraabdominal abscess. Sonography is often fruitless owing to overlying gas from ileus.[42] It is usually possible to predict on which side a subphrenic abscess will develop, depending on whether there has been an associated liver or spleen injury.[32, 43] At the time of surgical or percutaneous drainage, a needle is inserted in the abscess and pus is withdrawn in a syringe and sent to the laboratory for aerobic and anaerobic culture. Percutaneous drainage of an intraabdominal abscess is successful in approximately 80% of patients.[44]

Major drain tract infections—and possibly intraabdominal abscess formation—are more often associated with the use of Penrose and sump drains.[32] More recently, closed suction drainage is being used to drain solid organs. Early drainage of an intraabdominal abscess is the most important aspect of management with adjuvant antibiotic therapy. Early surgical drainage or percutaneous drainage of an intraabdominal abscess reduces the risk of death. Antibiotic therapy is directed to both aerobes and anaerobes. Until culture results are available, single-antibiotic therapy is usually adequate. Antibiotics that are known to be effective for treatment of intraabdominal abscess include imipenem (Primaxin), ticarcillin-clavulanate, ampicillin-sulbactam (Unasyn), piperacillin, cefoxitin, and cefotetan.

Closed Chest Drainage

The use of prophylactic antibiotics in the management of trauma patients with chest tubes remains controversial. Some have demonstrated a significant decrease in the incidence of empyema using cefoxitin or clindamycin during the interval when the chest tube is in place,[45, 46] whereas others have failed to demonstrate any difference in rate of infection using tetracycline.[47] The majority of patients who require closed chest tube drainage have associated injuries and, therefore, other indications for antibiotic prophylaxis.

Pulmonary Infections in the Intensive Care Unit

One of the most difficult problems is to determine whether to treat an intubated patient in the intensive care unit with antibiotics. Most of these patients have abnormal chest x-ray findings, are semiconscious, and tend to aspirate. They may develop gram-negative pneumonia, because gram-negative organisms colonize the trachea within 3 or 4 days of admission to the intensive care unit. To culture oropharyngeal secretions is probably not productive because of the colonization of the pharynx. If the patient is not intubated, transtracheal aspiration may be performed. Cultures of specimens obtained from bronchoscopy are valuable in identifying the pathogen. Pneumonia may be treated by single-agent therapy, but if *Pseudomonas aeruginosa* is suspected, combination therapy with an aminoglycoside is preferable.[48] For suspected *Staphylococcus* infection, vancomycin is administered. A third-generation cephalosporin combined with an aminoglycoside is active against *Pseudomonas* species. The treatment for established empyema is rib resection.[49]

Postsplenectomy Infection

Since the recognition of postsplenectomy sepsis (commonly due to the pneumococcus) attempts have been made to repair the spleen or perform partial splenectomy. In addition to pneumococcal organisms, overwhelming infection may also be due to *E. coli, Haemophilus influenzae*, or *Meningococcus, Staphylococcus*, or *Streptococcus* species.[50] Pneumovax and prophylactic penicillin are frequently recommended to treat children who have undergone splenectomy. The duration of effectiveness of Pneumovax for adults is unclear.[51] Malangoni and associates[51] reviewed 245 adults who underwent splenectomy for trauma; only 3 developed serious late infection (2 to 15 years after splenectomy), 2 caused by *Streptococcus pneumoniae*. None of the patients died.

TABLE 104–6 ■ Bacteriology of 50 Intraabdominal Abscesses After Trauma

AEROBES (90%)	NUMBER OF PATIENTS	ANAEROBES (48%)	NUMBER OF PATIENTS
Enterococcus	29	*Peptococcus*	10
Staphylococcus aureus	2 (2 MR)*	*Peptostreptococcus*	4
Streptococcus	3	*Bacteroides*	14
Escherichia coli	26	*Clostridium*	11
Enterobacter	10	*Fusobacterium*	2
Pseudomonas	5	*Eubacterium*	2
Klebsiella	4		
Proteus	4		

*MR, Methicillin resistant.

Multisystem Organ Failure

In multisystem organ failure, there is sequential instead of simultaneous organ failure, usually starting with the lungs and followed by liver, gastrointestinal tract, and kidneys. Pulmonary failure is first manifested by acute respiratory distress syndrome.[52] Sepsis and organ failure can be produced by activating the inflammatory response: bacteria, endotoxin, and ischemic tissue can all activate this response. More than half of the patients with acute respiratory distress syndrome develop the sepsis syndrome, which is followed by multisystem organ failure. Although sepsis may initiate multisystem organ failure, in approximately half the patients the source of infection cannot be found.[53] To prevent multisystem organ failure it is important that the source of infection be identified and treated with appropriate antibiotics.

It is becoming apparent that bacterial translocation from the bowel lumen to mesenteric lymph nodes and the portal circulation follows trauma and shock. Phagocytes ingest intestinal bacteria, transporting them outside the intestine, but fail to accomplish intracellular killing, which results in liberation of bacteria outside the intestine.[54, 55] The mortality rate after failure of two or three organs is 50% to 75%. Early enteral feeding, which may keep the gut barrier intact, may decrease multisystem organ failure.[56]

Orthopedic Trauma

Cephalothin or nafcillin can produce a significant reduction in infections that follow open fractures and hip fractures.[58–60] Stroth and associates[61] reviewed patients with open and closed fractures and found that posttraumatic osteomyelitis continues to be a major problem, occurring in almost half of the patients who develop an infection. Although *Staphylococcus* species are often isolated, as many or more gram-negative organisms are isolated, necessitating a broad spectrum of preventive antibiotic coverage.[61] Success or failure in preventing infection after open fracture depends on the adequacy of débridement, blood supply, presence of foreign bodies, and whether primary skin closure can be accomplished. One series reviewed antibiotic prophylaxis for open fractures and suggested that when fracture wounds were less than 1 cm long and not associated with extensive soft tissue damage antibiotics be administered for only 24 hours. For patients with extensive soft tissue damage and arterial injury that requires repair, a minimum of 48 hours' antibiotic prophylaxis is recommended.[62] Appropriate antibiotics for both gram-positive and gram-negative aerobic coverage include cefamandole and cefotaxime.[63] The third-generation cephalosporins are not recommended because of their decreased antistaphylococcal activity. Patients with higher bacterial counts at the time of closure have a higher incidence of postoperative sepsis, which is not related to the type of irrigation (mechanical or syringe) or to whether antibiotic irrigation was used.[64] Patients treated with antibiotics for more than 2 days may have a higher incidence of infection compared with patients treated on a short-term basis. Antibiotic prophylaxis may include a penicillinase-resistant synthetic penicillin or vancomycin combined with a third-generation cephalosporin.

Neurosurgical Trauma

Cerebrospinal fluid rhinorrhea is a sequela of only 2% or 3% of acute head injuries.[65, 66] Experts disagree about whether prophylactic antibiotics should be administered to patients with cerebrospinal fluid rhinorrhea. For antibiotics to be effective they must cross the blood-brain barrier. Those that do so most effectively are the penicillins and chloramphenicol (Chloromycetin). Klastersky and associates[67] found that penicillin reduced the incidence of bacterial meningitis in patients with rhinorrhea or otorrhea. Brawley and Kelly[65] noted only one case of meningitis during a 15-year period among patients treated with prophylactic antibiotics. MacGee and associates[68] were unable to demonstrate a statistically significant difference in the incidence of meningitis in patients who received prophylactic antibiotics after cerebrospinal fluid rhinorrhea. Gilbert and associates[69] reported the successful treatment of six patients, noting cessation of cerebrospinal fluid leaks and conversion to sterile cerebrospinal fluid within 72 hours.

Summary

Trauma patients appear to be at increased risk for wound infection, bacteremia, and intraabdominal abscess formation following gunshot wounds and colon injury. Initial fluid, resuscitation, blood replacement, and débridement of damaged tissue are more important than is antibiotic administration. Gram-negative aerobes appear to predominate in patients who develop bacteremia after abdominal trauma. Anaerobic isolates are common in patients with intraabdominal abscess. Knowledge of the hospital's antibiotic sensitivity pattern is important for appropriate antibiotic selection for an established infection.

References

1. National Center for Health Statistics: US Department of Health and Human Services: Monthly Vital Statistics Report. Advance Report of Final Mortality Statistics 1983. 34(Suppl 2):6, 1985.
2. Mullen JT: The magnitude of the problem of trauma. J Trauma 24:1070, 1974.
3. Caplan ES, Hoyt N: Infection surveillance and control in the severely traumatized patient. Am J Med 70:638, 1981.
4. Jones RC: Management of pancreatic trauma. Ann Surg 187:555, 1978.
5. Schimpff SC, Miller RM, Polakavetz S, et al: Infection in the severely traumatized patient. Ann Surg 179:353, 1974.
6. Bartlett JG: The normal flora. *In* Condon RE, Gorbach SL (eds): Surgical Infections, Selective Antibiotic Therapy. Baltimore, Williams & Wilkins, 1981, pp 4–5.
7. Gorbach SL, Nahas L, Lerner PI, Weinstein I: Studies of intestinal microflora. I: Effects of diet, age, and periodic sampling on numbers of fecal microorganisms in man. Gastroenterology 53:845, 1967.
8. Hunt PK, Jawetz E, Hutchinson JGP, Dunphy JE: A new model for the study of wound infection. J Trauma 7:298, 1967.
9. Elek FD, Conen PE: The virulence of staphylococcal pryogenes for man. A study of the problems of wound infection. Br J Exp Pathol 38:573, 1957.
10. Altemeier WA, Wilsin J: Antimicrobial therapy in injured patients. JAMA 173:527, 1960.
11. Evans BG: The enhancement of bacterial infections by adrenalin. Br J Exp Pathol 19:20, 1948.
12. Meakins JL, MacLean APH, Kelly R, et al: Delayed hypersensitivity and neutrophil chemotaxis. Effect of trauma. J Trauma 8:240, 1978.
13. Schneider RP, Christou NV, Meakins JL, Nohn C: Humoral immunity in surgical patients with and without trauma. Arch Surg 126:143, 1991.
14. Pietsch JB, Meakins JL: Predicting infection in surgical patients. Surg Clin North Am 59:185, 1979.
15. MacLean LD: Host resistance in surgical patients. J Trauma 19:297, 1979.
16. MacLean LD, Meakins JL, Taguchi K, et al: Host resistance in sepsis and trauma. Ann Surg 182:207, 1975.

17. Pruett TL, Rothstein OD, et al: Mechanisms of the adjunct effect of hemoglobin in experimental peritonitis. Surgery 96:375, 1984.
18. Burke JF: The effective period of preventive antibiotic action in experimental incisions and dermal lesions. Surgery 50:161, 1961.
19. Jones RC: Antibiotics in trauma. *In* Condon RE, Gorbach SL (eds): Surgical Infections. Baltimore, Williams & Wilkins, 1981.
20. Thadepalli H, Gorbach SL, Broido PW, et al: Abdominal trauma, anaerobes and antibiotics. Surg Gynecol Obstet 137:270, 1973.
21. O'Donnell V, Mandal AK, Lou MA, Thadepalli H: Evaluation of carbenicillin and a comparison of clindamycin and gentamicin combined therapy in penetrating abdominal trauma. Surg Gynecol Obstet 147:525, 1978.
22. Jones RC, Thal ER, Johnson NA: Evaluation of antibiotic therapy following penetrating abdominal trauma. Ann Surg 201:576, 1985.
23. Fabian TC, Boldreghini SJ: Antibiotics in penetrating abdominal trauma: Comparison of ticarcillin plus clavulanic acid with gentamicin plus clindamycin. Am J Med 79(Suppl 5B):157, 1985.
24. Hofstetter SR: A prospective comparison of two regimens of prophylactic antibiotics in abdominal trauma: Cefoxitin versus triple drug. J Trauma 24:307, 1984.
25. Nichols RL, Smith JW, Klein DB, et al: Risk of infection after penetrating abdominal trauma. N Engl J Med 311:1065, 1984.
26. Gentry LO, Feliciano DV, Scott L, et al: Perioperative antibiotic therapy for penetrating injuries of the abdomen. Ann Surg 200:561, 1984.
27. Heseltine PNR, Berne RV, Yellin AE, et al: The efficacy of cefoxitin versus clindamycin-gentamicin in surgically treated stab wounds of the bowel. J Trauma 26:241, 1986.
28. Dellinger EP, Wert MJ, Lennard ES, et al: Efficacy of short-course antibiotic prophylaxis after penetrating intestinal injury: A prospective randomized trial. Arch Surg 121:23, 1986.
28a. Fabian TC, Croce MA, Payne LW, et al: Duration of antibiotic therapy for penetrating abdominal trauma: A prospective trial. Surgery 112:788, 1992.
28b. Weigelt JA, Easley SM, Thal ER, et al: Abdominal surgical wound infection is lowered with improved perioperative enterococcus and bacteroides therapy. J Trauma 34:579, 1993.
29. Jones RC: New Directions in Antimicrobial Therapy, Infections in Trauma—A Symposium. St. James, Barbados, Stuart Pharmaceuticals, 1983, p 17.
30. Goins WA, Rodriguez A, Joshi M, Jacobs D: Intra-abdominal abscess after blunt abdominal trauma. Ann Surg 212:60, 1990.
31. Gibson DM, Feliciano DV, Mattox KL: Intraabdominal abscess after penetrating abdominal trauma. Am J Surg 142:699, 1981.
32. Jones RC: Management of pancreatic trauma. Am J Surg 150:698, 1985.
33. Dawes LG, Aprahamian MD, Condon RE, et al: The risk of infection after colon injury. Surgery 100:796, 1986.
34. Thompson JS, Moore EE: Comparison of penetrating injuries of the right and left colon. Ann Surg 193:414, 1981.
35. Schrock TR, Christiansen N: Management of penetrating injuries of the colon. Surg Gynecol Obstet 135:65, 1972.
36. Swenson RM, Lorber BM, Michaelson TC, et al: The bacteriology of intraabdominal infections. Arch Surg 109:398, 1974.
37. Weinstein WM, Onderdonk AB, Bartlett JG, Gorbach SL: Experimental intraabdominal abscesses in rats: Development of an experimental model. Infect Immun 10:1250, 1974.
38. Weinstein WM, Onderdonk AB, Bartlett JG, et al: Antimicrobial therapy of experimental intraabdominal sepsis. J Infect Dis 132:282, 1975.
39. Onderdonk AB, Bartlett JG, Louiet T, et al: Microbial synergy in experimental intraabdominal abscess. Infect Immun 13:22, 1976.
40. Solomkin JS, Dellinger EP, Christou NV, Busuttil RW: Results of a multicenter trial comparing imipenem/cilastatin to tobramycin/clindamycin for intra-abdominal infections. Ann Surg 212:581, 1990.
41. Duke J: Clinical pharmacology of intravenous and intraperitoneal aminoglycoside antibiotics in the prevention of wound infections. Ann Surg 188:66, 1978.
42. Saini S, Kellum JM, O'Leary MP, et al: Improved localization and survival in patients with intraabdominal abscesses. Am J Surg 145:136, 1983.
43. Norwood SH, Civetta JM: Abdominal CT scanning in critically ill surgical patients. Ann Surg 202:166, 1985.
44. Gerzof S, Robbins AH, Johnson WC, et al: Percutaneous catheter drainage of abdominal abscesses: A five year experience. N Engl J Med 305:653, 1981.
45. LoCurto JJ, Tischler CD, Swan KG, et al: Tube thoracostomy and trauma—antibiotics or not? J Trauma 26:1067, 1986.
46. Grover FL, Richardson JD, Fewel JG, et al: Prophylactic antibiotics in the treatment of penetrating chest wounds. J Thorac Cardiovasc Surg 74:538, 1977.
47. Mandel AK: Prophylactic antibiotics and no antibiotics compared in penetrating chest trauma. J Trauma 25:639, 1985.
48. Hoyt NJ, Kaplan ES: Identification and prevention of infections in the critically ill population. Crit Care Q 6:17, 1983.
49. Lemmer JH, Botham MJ, Oringer MB: Modern management of adult thoracic empyema. J Thorac Cardiovasc Surg 90:849, 1985.
50. Francke EL, Neu HC: Postsplenectomy infection. Surg Clin North Am 61:135, 1981.
51. Malangoni MA, Dillon LD, Klamar TW, et al: Factors influencing the risk of early and late serious infections in adults after splenectomy for trauma. Surgery 96:775, 1984.
52. Baue AE: Multiple, progressive or sequential systems failure: A syndrome of the 1970s. Arch Surg 110:779, 1975.
53. Carrico CJ, Meakins JL, Marshall JC, et al: Multiple organ failure syndrome. Arch Surg 121:196, 1986.
54. Wells CL, Maddaus MA, Simmons RL: Proposed mechanisms for the translocation of intestinal bacteria. Rev Infect Dis 10:958, 1988.
55. Deitch E, Winterlon J, Li M, et al: The gut as a portal of entry for bacteremia. Ann Surg 205:681, 1987.
56. Serra FB, Shronts EP, Konstantinides NN, et al: Enteral feeding in sepsis: A prospective, randomized, double-blind trial. Surgery 98:632, 1985.
57. Stoutenbeek CP, Van Saene HK, Miranda DR, Zandstra DF: The effect of selective decontamination of the digestive tract on colonization and infection rate in multiple trauma patients. Intensive Care Med 10:185, 1984.
58. Boyd JJ, Burke JF, Colton T: A double-blind clinical trial of prophylactic antibiotics in hip fractures. J Bone Joint Surg Am 55:6, 1973.
59. Burnett JW, Gustilo RB, Williams DN, et al: Prophylactic antibiotics in hip fractures, a double-blind prospective study. J Bone Joint Surg Am 62:457, 1980.
60. Tengve B, Kjellander J: Antibiotic prophylaxis in operations on trochanteric femoral fractures. J Bone Joint Surg Am 60:97, 1978.
61. Stroth AI, Fry DE, Polk HC: Infections morbidity in extremity fractures. J Trauma 26:757, 1986.
62. Antrum RM, Solomkin JS: A review of antibiotic prophylaxis for open fractures. Orthop Rev 16:246, 1987.
63. Gatell JM, Riba J, Lozano ML, et al: Prophylactic cefamandole in orthopaedic surgery. J Bone Joint Surg Am 66:1219, 1984.
64. Merritt K: Factors increasing the risk of infection in patients with open fractures. J Trauma 28:823, 1988.
65. Brawley BW, Kelly WA: Treatment of basal skull fractures with and without cerebrospinal fluid fistulae. J Neurosurg 26:57, 1967.
66. Raaf J: Posttraumatic cerebrospinal fluid leaks. Arch Surg 95:648, 1967.
67. Klastersky J, Sadeghi M, Brihaye J: Antimicrobial prophylaxis in patients with rhinorrhea or otorrhea: A double-blind study. Surg Neurol 6:111, 1976.
68. MacGee EE, et al: Meningitis following an acute traumatic cerebrospinal fluid fistula. J Neurosurg 33:312, 1970.
69. Gilbert VE, Beals JD Jr, Natelson SE, Tyler WA: Treatment of cerebrospinal fluid leaks and gram-negative bacillary meningitis with large doses of intrathecal amikacin and systemic antibiotics. Neurol Surg 18:402, 1986.
70. Lou MA, Thadepalli H, Mandal AK: Safety and efficacy of mezlocillin: A single-drug therapy for penetrating abdominal trauma. J Trauma 28:1541, 1988.

105

Burns

Basil A. Pruitt, Jr.
Albert T. McManus
Seung H. Kim

Burn injury destroys the cutaneous mechanical barrier to microorganisms; coagulates the proteinaceous components of the damaged tissue, which renders the burn wound avascular; and impairs both the humoral and cellular limbs of the immune system. These effects of the burn injury make the burn patient particularly susceptible to infection in remote sites as well as the burn wound per se. Before 1964, the burn wound was the most common site of life-threatening infection; however, the use of effective topical antimicrobial chemotherapy since that time has significantly reduced the incidence of invasive burn wound infection. That decrease in burn wound infection has been associated with improved survival of patients with burns of up to 80% of the total body surface.[1]

Burn Wound Care

Topical antimicrobial chemotherapy is initiated as soon as the patient is hemodynamically stable and the burn wounds have been cleansed and débrided. Such therapy limits proliferation and invasion by the bacteria that initially colonize the surface of the burn wound. There are three topical agents of documented effectiveness in controlling the microbial density in the burn wound: mafenide acetate burn cream, 0.5% silver nitrate soaks, and silver sulfadiazine burn cream[2] (Table 105–1). The physical characteristics of the latter two agents are such that they act principally on the surface of the wound and are most effective when application is begun within the first 24 to 48 hours after injury, before microbial penetration of the eschar has occurred. Mafenide acetate burn cream has similar antimicrobial activity on the wound surface, but the solubility of mafenide acetate permits it to penetrate into the burned tissue, where it exerts its antimicrobial action and controls proliferation of microorganisms both within the eschar and at the viable-nonviable tissue interface.

Excision of the burn wound is commonly begun as soon as possible after resuscitation is complete (usually the third to fifth postburn day). Early excision with immediate grafting in patients with available donor sites effects wound closure and reduces the length of time that the wound is at risk for infection. There are other patients with associated injuries or other complicating conditions who are not able to undergo excision, usually because of respiratory failure, cardiac failure, or sepsis-related coagulopathy.[3] In those patients and patients in whom the extent of burn prevents excision of all burn wounds at a single sitting, topical chemotherapy must be continued until resolution of organ failure occurs or excision of the burn wound can be completed. Because the protection provided by topical antimicrobial agents is imperfect, some burn patients, most commonly those with burns of more than 30% of the total body surface, may develop invasive burn wound infection.[4]

Burn Wound Infection

The diagnosis of infection in burn patients is confounded by the fact that most of the systemic and many of the laboratory

TABLE 105–1 ■ Effective Topical Burn Wound Antimicrobial Agents

PARAMETER	MAFENIDE ACETATE BURN CREAM	0.5% SILVER NITRATE SOAKS	SILVER SULFADIAZINE BURN CREAM
Spectrum of antimicrobial activity	Gram-negative bacteria—selectively good activity Gram-positive bacteria—good activity Yeasts—minimal activity	Gram-negative bacteria—good activity Gram-positive bacteria—good activity Yeasts—good activity	Gram-negative bacteria—selectively good activity Gram-positive bacteria—good activity Yeasts—good activity
Method of wound care	Exposure: applied after daily cleansing and renewed 12 h later	Occlusive dressings changed two or three times per day	Exposure or light dressing impregnated with agent: applied after daily cleansing and renewed 12 h later if exposure method used
Advantages	Easily applied Penetrates eschar Wound appearance readily monitored No resistance of *Pseudomonas* Joint motion unrestricted	Painless No hypersensitivity reactions Dressings reduce evaporative heat loss No gram-negative resistance Effective against yeasts	Easily applied Painless Wound appearance readily monitored when exposure method used Effective against yeasts
Disadvantages	Painful on partial-thickness burns Inhibition of carbonic anhydrase results in self-limited acidosis Cutaneous hypersensitivity reactions in 7% of patients	Causes deficits of sodium, potassium, calcium and chloride No eschar penetration Limitation of joint motion by dressings Methemoglobinemia—rare Argyria—rare Staining of environment and equipment	Limited eschar penetration Neutropenia—usually transient Hypersensitivity—infrequent Resistance of clostridia and certain gram-negative bacteria Rapid appearance of plasmid-mediated resistance to sulfonamides and multiple other antibiotics

signs of infection are mimicked by the physiologic response to severe injury.[5] Because clinical and laboratory signs are not reliable in making the diagnosis of infection in severely burned patients, reliance must be placed on daily examination of the entire burn wound to identify changes indicative of infection before systemic spread has occurred. The examination of the wound is best carried out at the time of daily cleansing when all dressings and topical applications have been removed. Focal dark red, brown, or black discoloration of the burn wound is the most common tinctorial change associated with burn wound infection, but the reliability of this sign may be compromised by hemorrhage into the burn wound caused by local trauma, which can produce similar changes.[6] Conversion of an area of partial-thickness injury to full-thickness necrosis is the most reliable sign of burn wound infection.[7] As noted in Table 105–2, there are other clinical signs typically associated with infections caused by specific organisms; ecthyma gangrenosa and green discoloration of the subcutaneous fat are characteristic of *Pseudomonas* infections, and saponification of the subcutaneous fat, unexpectedly rapid spontaneous separation of the eschar, and rapidly expanding ischemic necrosis are typical of fungal infections. The appearance of vesicular lesions in the nasolabial area of healing burn wounds is typical of herpes simplex virus infections. The identification of any of these local signs necessitates more precise assessment of the microbial status of the burn wound.

Cultures of the burn wound surface are useful in only an epidemiologic sense, and even quantitative cultures merely identify the density of colonizing organisms on or in nonviable tissue. Studies by McManus and colleagues[8] have documented that low quantitative culture counts in tissue obtained from a burn wound biopsy sample correlate well with the absence of invasive infection but that high counts are unreliable as an indication of the presence of infection. These investigators found that less than 50% of the biopsy specimens having quantitative culture counts of 10^5 or more organisms per gram of tissue were associated with histologic evidence of invasive infection. The histologic examination of a burn wound biopsy specimen is the most reliable and rapid way of making the critical differentiation between the colonization of nonviable tissue and the invasion of viable tissue.

Whenever any of the clinical signs of burn wound infection are identified, a burn wound biopsy specimen should be obtained from the area of the wound showing the most pronounced changes. A 500-mg lenticular tissue sample (the specimen must include viable subcutaneous tissue underlying the burn eschar) is obtained using a scalpel (Fig. 105–1*A* and *B*). If local anesthesia is necessary, the anesthetic agent should be injected at the periphery of the intended biopsy site to avoid distorting the morphologic characteristics of the biopsy specimen. One half of the bisected specimen is cultured to identify the organisms present and their antibiotic sensitivities. The other half of the specimen is processed for histologic examination by the pathologist using either a rapid-section technique requiring 4 hours for section preparation or a frozen-section technique requiring approximately 30 minutes for section preparation.[9, 10] Because the frozen-section technique is associated with a 4% falsely negative diagnosis rate, a specimen initially processed by that technique should be subsequently processed by regular-section technique. The histologic identification of microorganisms in unburned viable tissue confirms the diagnosis of invasive burn wound infection. The other histologic findings listed in Table 105–3 are not diagnostic of invasive burn wound infection but should heighten the pathologist's index of suspicion and prompt a meticulous search for microorganisms in the unburned tissue included in the specimen.

The microbial status of a biopsy sample can be staged according to the scheme detailed in Table 105–4. If the histologic examination reveals only colonization, no change in wound care is required. If serial biopsy examinations reveal progression from stage IA to stage IC, such evidence of microbial proliferation and eschar penetration justifies alteration of wound care. A histologic diagnosis of stage II necessitates alteration of wound care including urgent burn wound excision as well as systemic antimicrobial therapy. A biopsy diagnosis of stage IIC, indicating involvement of the microvasculature and lymphatics, portends hematogenous spread to remote tissues and organs and mandates close monitoring of the lungs and heart—common sites of metastatic spread (Fig. 105–2).

The burn wound biopsy histologic findings must always be evaluated with respect to the patient's clinical condition. A stage I histologic diagnosis or negative biopsy report for a septic burn patient in whom no other source of infection exists necessitates immediate biopsy of another area of the burn wound that shows changes typical of infection. If histologic examination of that biopsy specimen also fails to confirm invasive infection, wound monitoring is continued and new or expanding areas of wound changes are subjected to biopsy as they appear.

A diagnosis of invasive burn wound infection should prompt immediate therapeutic intervention. If a nonabsorbable topical agent is being used, it should be discontinued and twice-daily application of mafenide acetate burn cream instituted. Supportive measures should be employed to correct and maintain organ function and to prevent initiation of the cascade of multiple sequential organ failure. Systemic administration of an antibiotic active against the infecting

TABLE 105–2 ■ Clinical Signs of Burn Wound Infection

I. Systemic
   A. Temperature change*
      Hyperthermia: early sign
      Hypothermia: late sign of severe infection
   B. Tachycardia*
   C. Hyperventilation*
   D. Pain: may be obscured by burn wound sensitivity
   E. Ileus*
   F. Disorientation and obtundation*
   G. Glucose intolerance*
II. Local
   A. Conversion of partial-thickness injury to full-thickness necrosis
   B. Color change of wound: focal dark red, brown, or black eschar discoloration
   C. Hemorrhagic discoloration of subeschar tissues
   D. Degeneration of granulation tissue and formation of neoeschar
   E. Edema of unburned skin at margins of wound
   F. Erythematous or violaceous discoloration of unburned skin at margins of wound
   G. Green pigment visible in subcutaneous fat†
      Pale gray or yellow cheesy-appearing fat necrosis (soap formation)‡
   H. Nodular necrotic lesions (ecthyma gangrenosum) in unburned skin†
   I. Unexpectedly rapid separation of eschar‡
   J. Rapid centrifugal expansion of ischemic necrotic lesion with surrounding edema‡
   K. Vesicular lesions in healed or healing partial-thickness burns§
   L. Crusted serrated margins of partial-thickness facial burns§

*Produced by extensive burn injury per se.
†Characteristic of *Pseudomonas* infections.
‡Characteristic of fungal infections.
§Characteristic of herpes simplex virus type 1 infections.

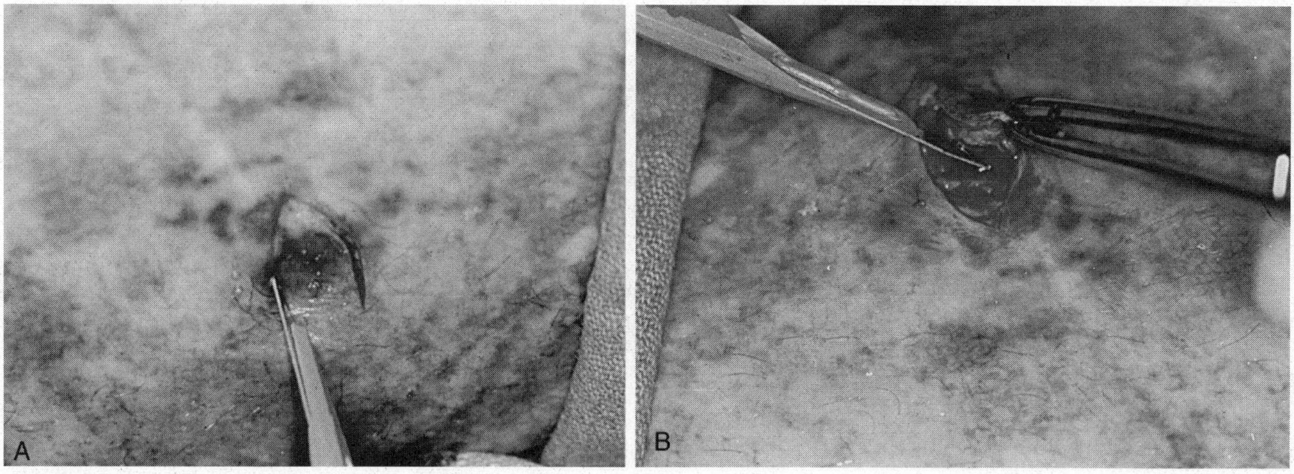

FIGURE 105–1 □ *A,* A scalpel is used to obtain a burn wound biopsy specimen from an area of the burn wound showing focal dark red and black discoloration typical of invasive infection. *B,* Elevation of the biopsy specimen demonstrates that unburned subcutaneous tissue is included in the sample. Note that bleeding into the biopsy wound also confirms viability of the tissue at the line of excision.

organism should be started. If no prior cultures have been taken of the burn wound, the selection of antibacterial agents should be based on the Gram stain characteristics of the organisms identified in the biopsy sections. Ideally, prior microbial surveillance data from the patient's wounds or from a prior biopsy can be used to guide antibiotic selection. If such information is not available, the results of the unit's microbial surveillance program should be used to determine the antibiotics most likely to be effective. The potential cost savings of a culture-based selection of an appropriate and less expensive agent further justifies the use of a prospective microbial surveillance system.[11]

The hypermetabolism and hyperdynamic circulation of the burn patient alter both the metabolism and excretion rate of antibiotic agents, necessitating careful monitoring of peak and trough levels to ensure adequacy of therapy. The increased effective renal blood flow characteristic of burn patients can markedly decrease the effective half-life of antibiotics that are excreted primarily by the renal route.[12, 13]

Even though the overall incidence of invasive burn wound infection has decreased markedly, *Pseudomonas aeruginosa* remains the most common causative bacterium, and it is typically sensitive to high concentrations of broad-spectrum penicillins. Accordingly, one half of the daily dose of a broad-spectrum penicillin, such as piperacillin, suspended in 1000 mL of normal saline should be immediately infused into the subeschar tissues beneath all infected areas of the wound using a No. 20 spinal needle to minimize the number of injection sites. The patient should then be scheduled for excision of the infected tissue within the next 12 hours and a second subeschar antibiotic infusion performed immediately before that procedure to minimize hematogenous dissemination of viable bacteria during the excision.

Excision of the infected tissue is carried out with the patient under general anesthesia by using a scalpel to remove all tissue superficial to the investing fascia. If the infection involves the investing fascia or subfascial tissues, those should be excised as well. Once one is certain that the excision has removed all infected tissue, the wound should be covered with a biologic dressing or skin substitute to prevent desiccation of the wound bed. If the adequacy of the excision is uncertain, 5% mafenide acetate or 0.5% silver nitrate soak dressings should be applied. In either case, the patient should be returned to the operating room 24 to 48 hours later for examination of the wound after removal of the wound dressings. If there is no evidence of residual infection, the wounds can be closed by skin grafting. However, if there is residual wound infection, repeated débridement should be carried out, the wounds dressed as before, and the patient returned to the operating room 24 to 48 hours later for examination of the wounds.

The development of generalized invasive burn wound infection can be forestalled and the high mortality associated with it reduced by scheduled wound surveillance and the use of wound biopsies to identify infection at an early stage.

TABLE 105–3 ■ Histologic Signs of Burn Wound Infection

Microorganisms present in unburned tissue
Exaggerated inflammatory reaction in unburned tissue
Hemorrhage into viable subeschar tissue
Small vessel thrombosis and ischemic necrosis of unburned tissue
Intracellular viral inclusions
Type A Cowdry bodies: light microscopy
Virions: electron microscopy
Dense microbial growth*
Surrounding hair follicles and sweat glands
Marked proliferation in subeschar space
Dense mononuclear cell infiltration with multinucleated giant cells containing fungal spores
Epithelioid granuloma formation with fungal hyphae in soft tissue

*Typical of deep colonization.

TABLE 105–4 ■ Classification of Microbial Status of Burn Wounds

Stage I.	Colonization of nonviable tissue
	A. Superficial colonization: microorganisms present on burn wound surface
	B. Microbial penetration: microorganisms present in variable thickness of eschar
	C. Subeschar proliferation: multiplication of microorganisms in the subeschar space or neocolonization in which microorganisms are present on desiccated tissue exposed by prior escharectomy
Stage II.	Invasion of variable tissue
	A. Microinvasion: microscopic foci of microorganisms in unburned viable tissue immediately beneath eschar
	B. Generalized invasion: multifocal or diffuse penetration of microorganisms into viable subcutaneous tissue
	C. Microvascular invasion: microorganisms present in unburned small blood vessels and lymphatics

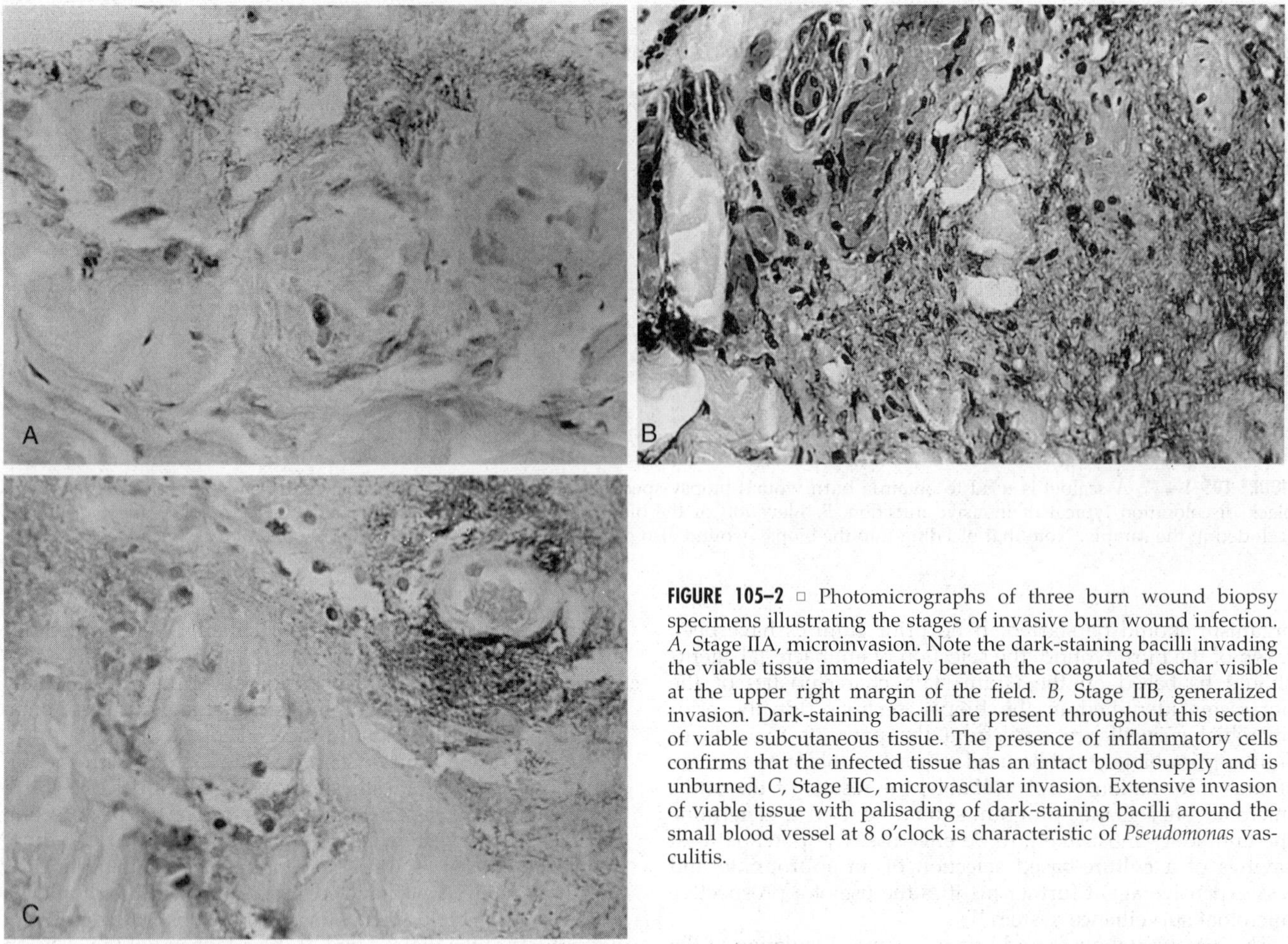

FIGURE 105–2 □ Photomicrographs of three burn wound biopsy specimens illustrating the stages of invasive burn wound infection. *A,* Stage IIA, microinvasion. Note the dark-staining bacilli invading the viable tissue immediately beneath the coagulated eschar visible at the upper right margin of the field. *B,* Stage IIB, generalized invasion. Dark-staining bacilli are present throughout this section of viable subcutaneous tissue. The presence of inflammatory cells confirms that the infected tissue has an intact blood supply and is unburned. *C,* Stage IIC, microvascular invasion. Extensive invasion of viable tissue with palisading of dark-staining bacilli around the small blood vessel at 8 o'clock is characteristic of *Pseudomonas* vasculitis.

The effectiveness of this protocol has been documented by the results obtained in a group of 19 extensively burned patients with histologically verified invasive *Pseudomonas* burn wound infection treated by subeschar antibiotic infusion and, when the patient's condition permitted, surgical excision of the infected tissue.[14] Although 9 of the 19 patients died with uncontrolled infection, the wound infection was controlled in 10 patients, of whom 5 later died from other causes. In the five patients who survived both the episode of invasive infection and their burn injury, no positive blood cultures were obtained before excision of the infected tissue, confirming that the infectious process had been identified and controlled before bacterial spread through the microvasculature to the general circulation.

Burn wound infections caused by gram-positive cocci, chief among which are the staphylococci, tend to be localized, although the initially present microabscesses may slowly expand with time. Removal of the burned tissue overlying a solitary staphylococcal abscess may be sufficient treatment, but the presence of multiple microabscesses may necessitate excision of extensive areas of the eschar utilizing a variant of tangential excision. A disproportionate systemic response in a patient with a staphylococcal infection should alert one to the possibility that the infecting strain is causing systemic toxicity by production of exotoxins such as toxic shock syndrome toxin 1. Such patients should be treated by systemic administration of vancomycin.

The usually mild and self-limiting cellulitis that frequently involves only a few centimeters of skin immediately adjacent to the burn wound in the first week after burn is considered to represent the inflammatory reaction to tissue degradation products diffusing from the wound. Antibiotic treatment is not required for this nonmicrobial form of cellulitis. The rarity of β-hemolytic streptococcal cellulitis has led most surgeons to abandon the use of prophylactic penicillin in the immediate postburn period.[15] However, if cellulitic changes characterized by bright red, rapidly spreading erythema with or without lymphangititis develop, a presumptive diagnosis of β-hemolytic streptococcal cellulitis should be made, cultures taken, and penicillin therapy initiated.

Staphylococcal pustular eruptions with patchy epidermal sloughing in areas of healed partial-thickness wounds (Fig. 105–3) or healed grafts may be treated with topical application of mupirocin. This agent, which is derived from *Pseudomonas fluorescens,* has rapid action against most strains of staphylococci, and clinical use of this agent at the U.S. Army Institute of Surgical Research (U.S. Army Burn Center) has not been associated with the development of resistance or opportunistic overgrowth.

Candidal Infections

The overall incidence of bacterial burn wound infection has significantly decreased and that related to *P. aeruginosa* has precipitously receded during the past 25 years, during which time the incidence of nonbacterial burn wound infections has increased.[11] *Candida* species are the most common nonbacterial colonizers of burn wounds. An example of such colonization by *Candida albicans* of nonviable eschar (biopsy stage IA) is presented in Figure 105–4. This situation typically remains confined to burned tissue without invasion and thus requires

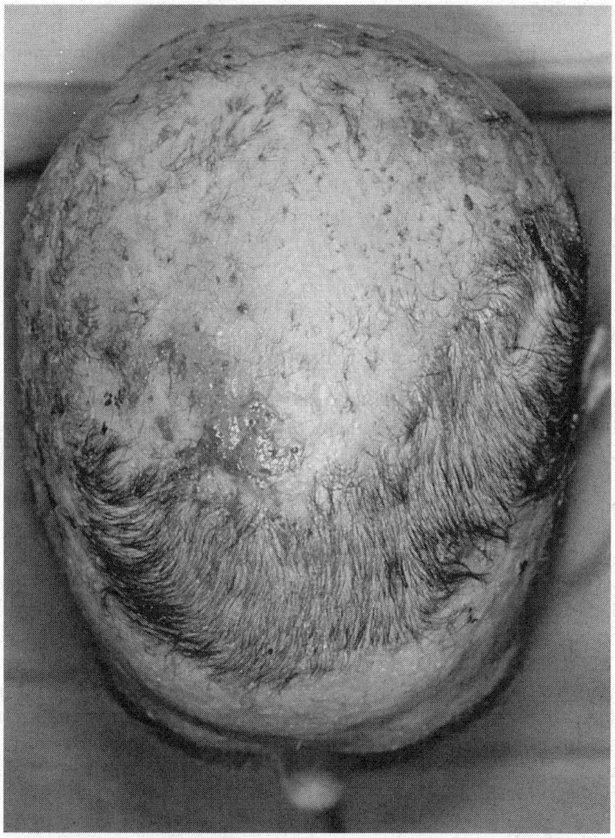

FIGURE 105–3 □ Superficial staphylococcal infection with patchy epidermal loss surrounding hair follicles in a previously healed partial-thickness scalp burn (45th postburn day).

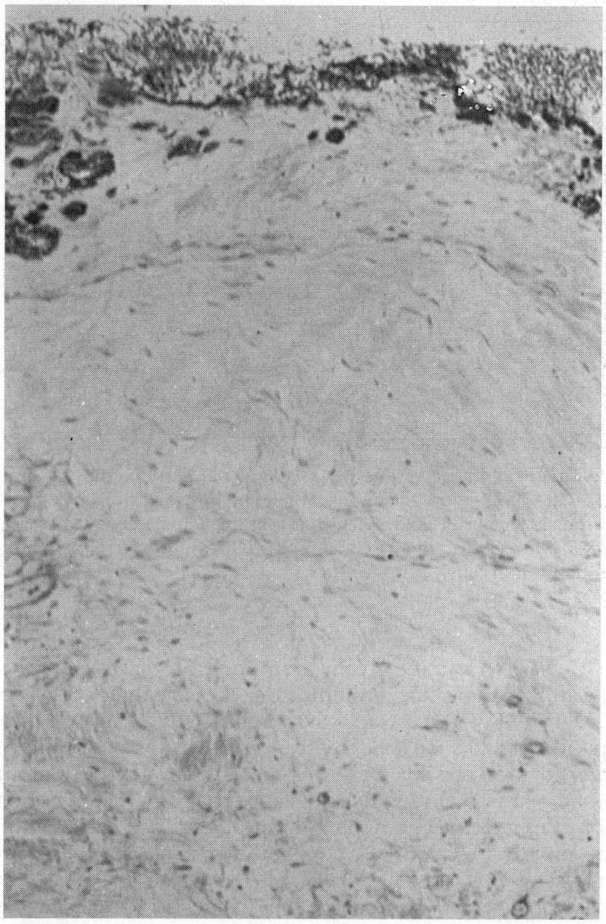

FIGURE 105–4 □ Colonization of nonviable eschar with *Candida albicans* (stage IA).

no specific treatment.[16] Candidal infection of a previously excised burn wound exposed in the interstices of a mesh graft or an excised burn wound exposed by loss of skin grafts requires treatment by twice-daily application of a topical antifungal agent such as clotrimazole cream or ciclopirox olamine cream. Excision of the infected tissue may be necessary if such treatment is ineffective in preventing extension of the disease process. In patients requiring excision of foci of candidal infection, systemic administration of amphotericin B should be instituted.

During the period 1985 to 1994, 150 candidal infections were documented in 2213 burn patients treated at the U.S. Army Burn Center (Table 105–5). Those infections included 93 of the urinary tract, 40 of the blood, and only 6 of the burn wound. Infection with this nonbacterial opportunist commonly occurred in patients with extensive burns, many of whom had received broad-spectrum antibiotics perioperatively at the time of burn wound excisions and for the treatment of other infections. The average times of candidal colonization of the burn wound (35th postburn day), of candidal urinary tract infection (40th postburn day), and of other candidal infections (47th postburn day) are all consistent with that possibility. Irrigation of the bladder with amphotericin B solution (50 mg per 1000 mL of sterile water per day for 7 days) is recommended for the treatment of *Candida* cystitis, but the urine may not clear until the urethral catheter is removed. Candidemia requires a full course of systemic amphotericin B therapy (0.5 to 0.7 mg/kg per day for 7 to 10 days).

Fungal Infections

Filamentous fungi are much more apt to cause invasive burn wound infection than are candidal organisms. Between January 1, 1985, and December 31, 1994, at the U.S. Army Burn Center, 45 burn wound invasions caused by filamentous (true) fungi were observed. These infections occurred at an average of 22 days after the burn in a group of severely burned patients who had burns involving an average of 66% of the total body surface. The infections occurred earlier than the candidal wound infections noted before. *Aspergillus* species, the most common filamentous fungi that caused burn wound infections, typically remained confined to the subcutaneous tissue and rarely traversed tissue planes.[17] As with invasive bacterial burn wound infection, the diagnosis of invasive fungal infection is best made by the histologic examination of a burn wound biopsy specimen (Fig. 105–5). Treatment of such infections consists of twice-daily topical application of an antifungal agent such as clotrimazole cream

TABLE 105–5 ■ ***Candida* Infection in Burn Patients, 1985 to 1994**

SITE OF INFECTION	NUMBER OF INFECTIONS
Urinary tract	93
Blood	40
Burn wound	6
Respiratory tract	3
Pneumonia—2	
Tracheitis—1	
Eye	3
Vagina	3
Vein	2

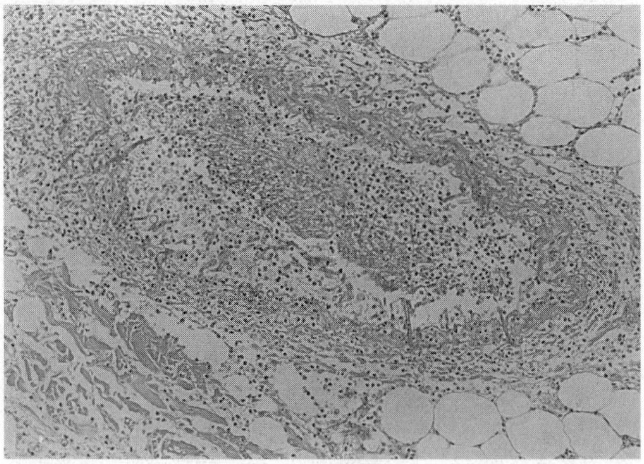

FIGURE 105–5 □ Invasive fungal (*Aspergillus* sp.) burn wound infection, stage IIC. Note hyphal penetration into the lumen of the small vessel in the center of the field. Such microvascular involvement increases the likelihood of hematogenous spread of the infection to remote tissues and organs.

or ciclopirox olamine cream, institution of systemic amphotericin B therapy, and prompt excision of the infected tissue.

Members of the group Phycomycetes, particularly *Mucor* species, are the most aggressive of the filamentous fungi.[18] Infections caused by these organisms spread rapidly along tissue planes and readily cross fascial barriers. The predilection of phycomycotic hyphae to invade vessels accounts for the rapidly expanding ischemic necrosis and the frequency of distant metastases characteristic of infections caused by these organisms (Fig. 105–6). The diagnosis is best made by the identification of broad nonseptate hyphae in unburned tissue. All forms of topical therapy appear to be ineffective in controlling phycomycotic infections and immediate surgical intervention is required. The extent of surgical excision required is often defined by a rim of edema at the outermost limit of the disease process. What has been termed radical débridement is carried out to ensure removal of all infected tissue and reduce the risk of further local extension and

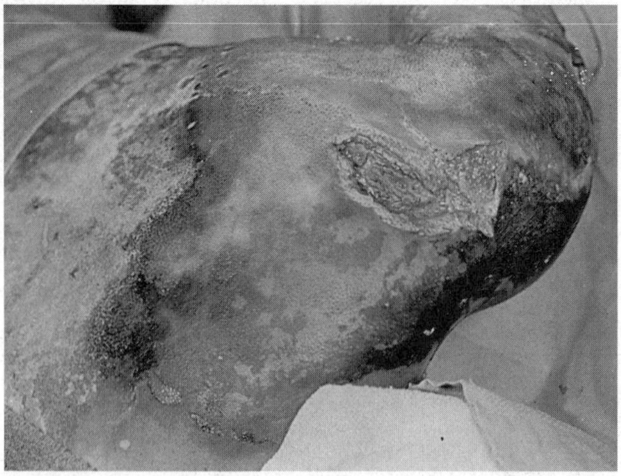

FIGURE 105–6 □ Invasive mucormycosis of the burn wound of the left shoulder of this patient necessitated a forequarter amputation. Note the black ischemic discoloration over the top of the shoulder and at the margin of the expanding infection near the midline of the upper back and at the lower margin of the scapula inferiorly. Involvement of the unburned underlying muscles was confirmed by biopsy of the ischemic muscle exposed at the upper margin of the scapula.

hematogenous dissemination to remote tissues. If a phycomycotic infection in a limb has traversed the investing fascia and involves significant amounts of underlying muscle, amputation may be necessary to control the infectious process, as was the case in 26 (35%) of 75 patients with phycomycotic burn wound infections treated between 1954 and 1983.[19] A full course of parenteral amphotericin B should be administered to all patients with invasive phycomycotic wound infections.

Viral Infections

Viral infections in burn patients are relatively uncommon, as indicated by the occurrence of only seven herpes simplex virus type 1 infections in the 2213 patients treated at the U.S. Army Burn Center in the period 1985 to 1994. Herpetic infections occur most commonly in healing or recently healed partial-thickness burns, particularly those in the nasolabial area (Fig. 105–7*A*). The diagnosis of herpetic burn wound infection is most reliably made by the histologic examination of a biopsy specimen or scrapings from the cutaneous lesions. Because the vesicles are easily ruptured and readily colonized by bacteria from the surrounding skin, the light microscopic characteristics of herpes simplex virus 1 infections, that is, type A Cowdry bodies (Fig. 105–7*B*), may be obscured. In this case, electron microscopy can be used to identify intracellular virions[20] (Fig. 105–7*C*). Topical application of acyclovir (Zovirax), which may inactivate the virus and prevent further development of cutaneous lesions, is most effective when done early in the course of lesion development.

Although herpetic infections occur most commonly in healing partial-thickness burns and remain localized, such infections may occur in other tissues as documented by autopsy evidence of herpetic involvement of the airway in three patients during the period 1985 to 1994. Occasionally, systemic herpesvirus infections involving multiple organs such as the liver, lung, spleen, adrenal, and bone marrow occur.[20] Unexplained hypotension or other signs of systemic sepsis in a burn patient with no other source of infection and rapidly spreading cutaneous herpetic lesions should alert one to the possibility of a systemic herpes simplex virus infection. If the patient has an intact coagulation system, a percutaneous hepatic biopsy may confirm hepatic involvement and justify the institution of systemic antiviral therapy with acyclovir, 10 mg/kg three times daily for 10 days.[21]

Cytomegalovirus is the other virus most commonly recovered from burn patients.[22, 23] The majority of cytomegalovirus infections have involved the aerodigestive tract, as documented by autopsy findings in four patients with airway involvement during the period 1985 to 1994. Systemic cytomegalovirus infection may produce varying degrees of jaundice associated with the clinical signs of low-grade infection. In such patients, documentation of rising cytomegalovirus titers in successive serum samples enables one to avoid the potentially deleterious effects of inappropriate broad-spectrum antibiotic administration. Ganciclovir is the antiviral agent of choice for the treatment of cytomegalovirus infection (7.5 to 10 mg/kg per day for up to 20 days).

Other Infections

That infection remains the most frequent cause of morbidity and mortality in burn patients indicates the pervasive effect of the global immunosuppression that is induced in direct proportion to the extent of burn injury. During the 10-year period 1985 to 1994, infection was considered the primary cause of death in 102 (48%) of 211 fatal burns (Table 105–6).

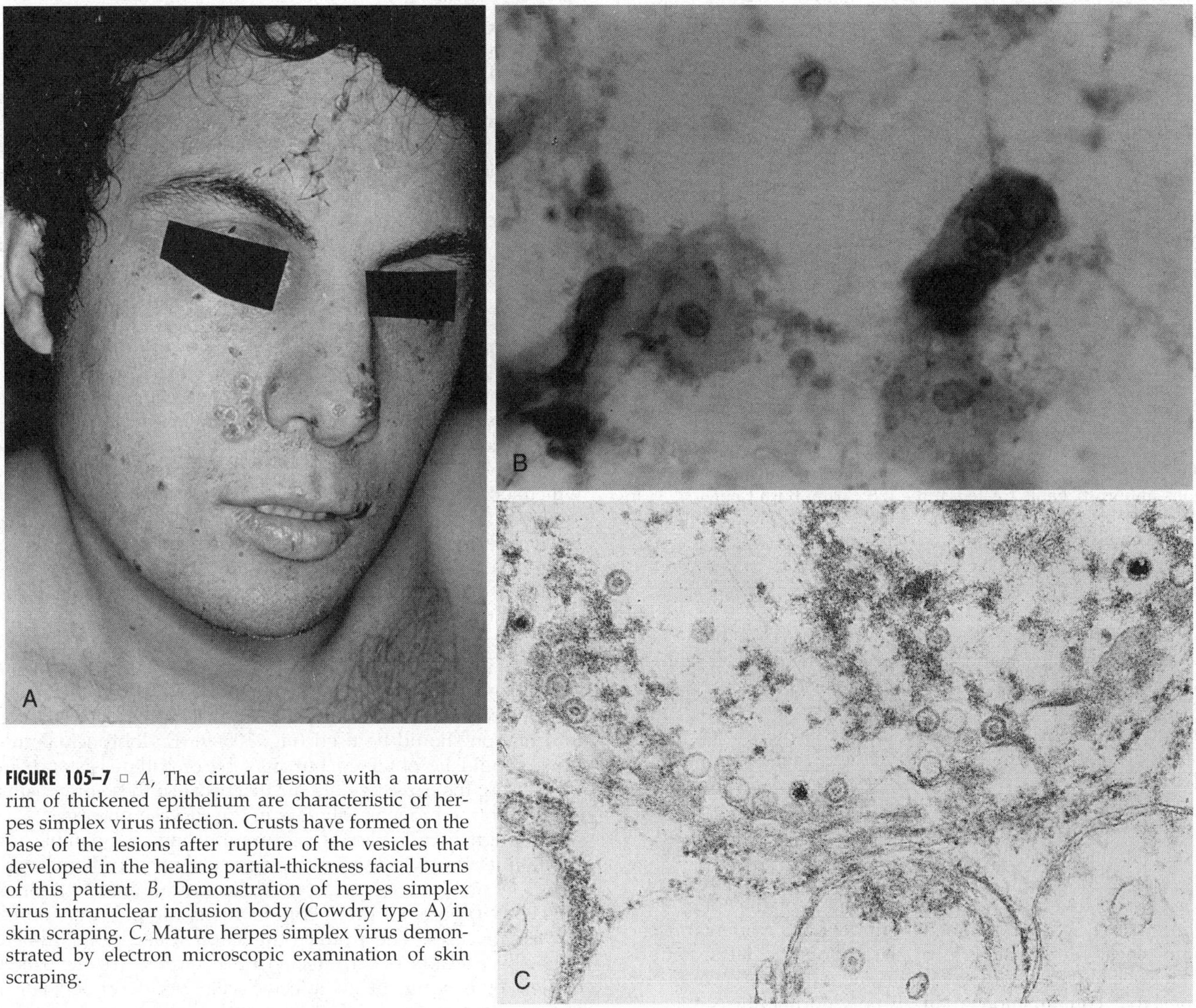

FIGURE 105–7 □ *A,* The circular lesions with a narrow rim of thickened epithelium are characteristic of herpes simplex virus infection. Crusts have formed on the base of the lesions after rupture of the vesicles that developed in the healing partial-thickness facial burns of this patient. *B,* Demonstration of herpes simplex virus intranuclear inclusion body (Cowdry type A) in skin scraping. *C,* Mature herpes simplex virus demonstrated by electron microscopic examination of skin scraping.

The effectiveness of topical chemotherapy and current wound care techniques is attested to by the fact that invasive burn wound infection was considered to be the primary cause of death in only 7 patients, whereas pneumonia was present in 80 (38%) of the 211 fatal burns. During the past two decades, the predominant organisms causing infections in burn patients have also changed dramatically.[6, 24, 25] Gram-negative opportunistic organisms have receded in importance, and *Staphylococcus aureus,* the most frequent infecting organism, has been recovered from 33% of all infections in patients treated at the U.S. Army Burn Center (Fig. 105–8).

TABLE 105–6 ■ Infections as Cause of Death in Fatal Burns, 1985 to 1994

Number of fatal burns: 211		
Pneumonia	80	
Invasive burn wound infection	7	
Sepsis	4	
Abscess	3	
Bacterial endocarditis	2	
Enterocolitis	2	
Staphylococcal scalded skin syndrome	1	
Cytomegalovirus infection	1	
Peritonitis	1	
Gastrointestinal infection	1	
Total	102	(48.3%)

Control of the microbial population of the burn wound has altered the predominant site of infection in burn patients, the types of organisms causing pneumonia, and the predominant form of pneumonia that occurs in those patients. Before the development of topical antimicrobial burn wound therapy, hematogenous pneumonia occurred with twice the frequency of airborne pneumonia (or bronchopneumonia), but since that time the incidence of airborne pneumonia has greatly exceeded that of hematogenous pneumonia and at present it represents only 10% of pulmonary infections. The frequency of pneumonia necessitates close clinical and radiographic monitoring to make a timely diagnosis of pneumonia and differentiate between the two forms of pulmonary infection.

Bronchopneumonia

Airborne pneumonia, or bronchopneumonia, usually begins as a tracheobronchitis that causes necrosis of the airway mucosa and subsequently extends distally to involve the alveoli.[26] The infectious process then spreads to involve a variable volume of pulmonary parenchyma. This disease process is nonrandom in distribution, involves mainly dependent areas of the lung, and is a frequent complication in

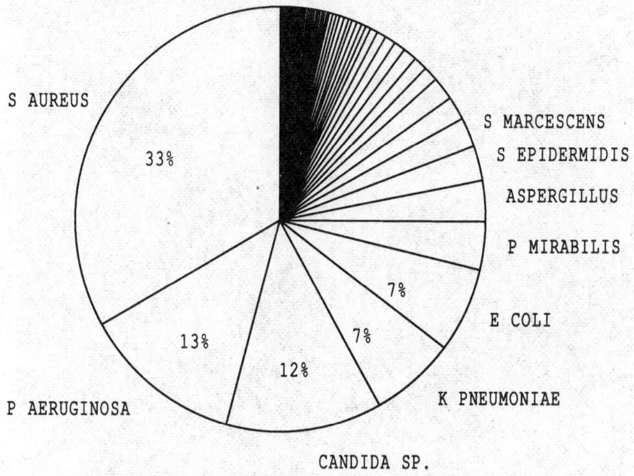

FIGURE 105–8 □ Frequency of recovery of microorganisms from infections in burn patients treated at the U.S. Army Burn Center, 1985 to 1994. Unlabeled segments represent organisms causing less than 4% of infections.

patients with inhalation injury.[27] The incidence of brochopneumonia in burn patients with moderate or severe inhalation injury was 38.4%, as compared with 9.1% for patients without inhalation injury.[28] This form of pneumonia is fatal in only approximately one third of patients but is the primary cause of death in 80% of burn patients who expire with the disease.[26]

The initial radiographic changes characteristic of bronchopneumonia occur in the lower lobes and take the form of irregular linear infiltrates resembling those of atelectasis. If the disease process is uncontrolled, the infiltrates spread and coalesce to involve ever greater portions of the lung, even entire lobes. Whenever such infiltrates are evident on the daily chest film, a sample of the endobronchial secretions should be obtained for Gram stain and culture. Airway secretions that contain more than 25 polymorphonuclear leukocytes and fewer than 25 squamous cells per high-power field are considered representative of endobronchial secretions and correlate well with the presence of respiratory tract infection.[29] Although the use of protected biopsy brushes and even endoscopically directed bronchoalveolar lavage has been recommended to improve the accuracy of bacteriologic assessment of the lower respiratory tract in mechanically ventilated patients,[30–32] in our experience the culture results of endoscopically guided bronchoalveolar lavage in burn patients have been no different from those of blind endobronchial aspiration.

Aspirate findings consistent with respiratory tract infection in the presence of radiographic changes and/or clinical findings compatible with that diagnosis warrant the institution of antibiotic therapy. With improvements in burn wound management and in isolation of patients, *S. aureus* has replaced *P. aeruginosa* and other gram-negative opportunists as the most common causative organism of bronchopneumonia in burn patients.[11, 33, 34] Consequently, the initial selection of antibiotics should be based on the results of the microscopic examination of bronchial secretions and the current results of the patient's surveillance cultures. The presence of resistance to the penicillinase-resistant penicillins such as methicillin proscribes the use of all β-lactam antibiotics. To avoid the selection of cross-resistant strains by such agents and ensure effectiveness of treatment, vancomycin is always used for the treatment of staphylococcal infections at the U.S. Army Burn Center. No pathogens resistant to this agent have been observed since the initiation of this policy in 1978, a 17-year period. The initial antibiotic therapy may subsequently be altered, if necessary, on the basis of the patient's endobronchial culture and sensitivity results.

In a patient with clinical signs of infection but no radiographically evident infiltrates or other source of infection, an endobronchial aspirate indicative of respiratory tract infection is consistent with the diagnosis of tracheobronchitis. That process should be treated with antibiotics selected on the basis of the microscopic examination of the aspirate and the predominant nosocomial flora.

Hematogenous Pneumonia

Hematogenous pneumonia begins as a necrotizing capillaritis caused by blood-borne bacteria. The infection then spreads to adjacent alveoli, forming a nodular lesion, which may ultimately erode into bronchi. This form of pneumonia, which occurs in a random distribution depending on the location of the vessels in which bacteria lodge, presents relatively late in the postburn course with the average time of diagnosis being the 17th postburn day.[26] The sudden appearance of a dense rounded infiltrate on the chest radiograph is consistent with a diagnosis of hematogenous pneumonia and should prompt a search for the primary site of infection and the initiation of systemic antibiotic therapy based on surveillance cultures from the patient. If culture data for the patient are not available, the institution's current surveillance information should be used (Fig. 105–9). Endobronchial cultures should be obtained but may be of little assistance in identifying the causative organisms, because these organisms erode into the bronchi only late in the disease process.

Although occult visceral perforation and inapparent soft tissue infections may serve as primary sources of hematogenous pneumonia, an invasive burn wound infection or a focus of suppurative thrombophlebitis is the primary source in 98% of cases. The primary infection must be controlled either by excision of an infected burn wound (as described earlier) or excision of an infected vein (as described later) to prevent continued pulmonary and systemic seeding. The mortality associated with hematogenous pneumonia exceeds 90%, but as a reflection of its being secondary to a remote infection, it is infrequently the primary cause of death.[26]

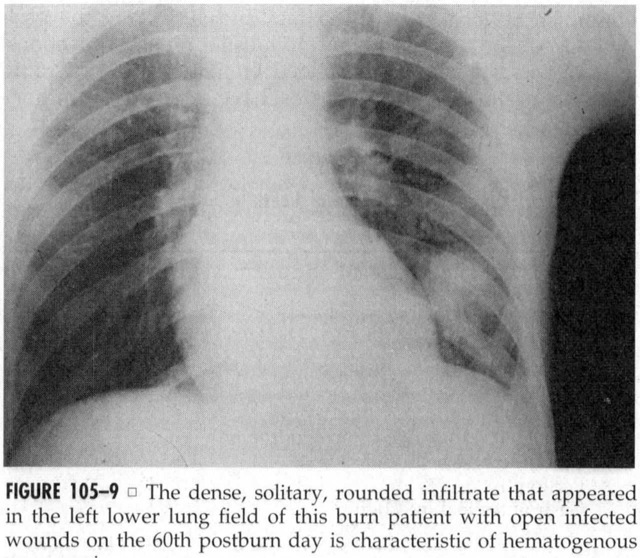

FIGURE 105–9 □ The dense, solitary, rounded infiltrate that appeared in the left lower lung field of this burn patient with open infected wounds on the 60th postburn day is characteristic of hematogenous pneumonia.

Suppurative Thrombophlebitis

Intraluminal suppuration can occur in any previously cannulated vein. Cannula composition, the characteristics of the infused fluids, the duration of cannulation, microbial seeding of the infusion system, and lodgment of blood-borne bacteria on the fibrin sleeve that forms around the cannula can all serve as contributory factors in the development of suppurative thrombophlebitis.[35] The risk of microbial seeding of the fibrin sleeve on the intravascular cannula is particularly high in burn patients, in whom bacteremia occurs in association with 21% of all wound débridement procedures, with the incidence of positive blood cultures related directly to the extent of the burn and the magnitude of wound manipulation.[36] Since 1979, strict limitation of venous cannulation duration to no more than 72 hours has reduced the incidence of this infection. In the period 1982 to 1990, the incidence was 0.71%, compared with 6.9% before the initiation of this policy.[6]

Suppurative thrombophlebitis typically begins at the site of cannula tip placement and can extend for surprisingly long distances both proximally and distally from the site. The diagnosis of suppurative thrombophlebitis should be considered for any burn patient with a pulmonary infiltrate characteristic of hematogenous pneumonia and no other apparent source of infection. Local signs of infection are present in less than 30% of the burn patients who develop this disease.[37] Consequently, all previously cannulated veins, beginning with the most recently cannulated vessel and progressing to the most remotely cannulated vessel, may have to be explored to locate the infection. The site of cannula tip residence should be surgically exposed and the vein excised. The diagnosis of suppurative thrombophlebitis is confirmed if intraluminal pus is identified. If a nonsuppurative intraluminal clot is present, however, that section of vein should be excised and both the vein and the clot cultured and subjected to histologic examination. A positive culture or the presence of microorganisms in the clot or the vein wall confirms the diagnosis of suppurative thrombophlebitis (Fig. 105–10).

Suppurative thrombophlebitis is treated by excision of the infected vein and the systemic administration of antibiotics active against the infecting organism. Because multiple areas of intraluminal infection may be present proximal to the relatively normal-appearing "skip" areas, the excision should continue to the point at which the vein becomes a tributary of the next higher order of veins or to the point at which the vein wall is unequivocally normal and brisk retrograde flow of unaltered blood is noted. After excision of the infected vein and any grossly involved tributaries, the venectomy wounds should be loosely packed and covered with an occlusive dressing. Skin grafting or secondary closure is carried out after resolution of the infection and the local inflammatory changes.

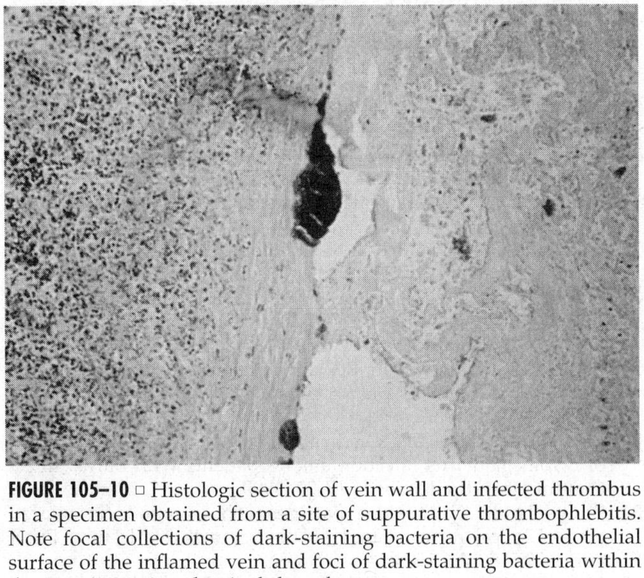

FIGURE 105–10 □ Histologic section of vein wall and infected thrombus in a specimen obtained from a site of suppurative thrombophlebitis. Note focal collections of dark-staining bacteria on the endothelial surface of the inflamed vein and foci of dark-staining bacteria within the organizing intraluminal thrombus.

Suppuration may occur even in high-flow central veins that cannot be readily excised. Central vein suppuration should be treated by a full maximum-dose course of antibiotic therapy with addition of heparin anticoagulation if pulmonary emboli develop. Balloon catheter extraction of an infected thrombus from a central vein has been reported, but rethrombosis at the site of vein wall inflammation limits the effectiveness of such intervention.[38]

Persistence of the septic state after excision of a focus of suppurative thrombophlebitis may be due to residual infection proximal to the level of excision, requiring proximal extension of the prior level of excision. Alternatively, it may be due to suppuration within another vein, requiring identification and excision of the other infected vein. Hematogenous pneumonia or acute bacterial endocarditis secondary to dissemination of the infection before excision of the involved vein may also cause persistence of the septic state, necessitating specific therapy as described for those processes.

Acute Endocarditis

The prolonged need for intravenous infusions, the high incidence of suppurative thrombophlebitis, and the previously noted frequency of bacteremia related to burn wound manipulation have all been incriminated in the relatively high incidence of acute endocarditis in burn patients. During the period 1969 to 1974, 1.3% (22 of 1699) of patients treated at the U.S. Army Burn Center developed acute bacterial endocarditis; in the past two decades, however, only five cases have occurred. The incidence has decreased in concert with the declining incidence of invasive burn wound infections.[39] In burn patients, acute endocarditis is slightly more common on the right side of the heart, although either or both sides may be involved. The identification of murmurs characteristic of this disease is difficult in the presence of the markedly hyperdynamic circulation of the burn patient.

The diagnosis of acute bacterial endocarditis should be entertained if the same organism, particularly coagulase-positive *S. aureus*, is recovered from two or more blood cultures in a burn patient with sepsis and no other apparent infection. Two-dimensional echocardiographic examination can be used to identify valvular lesions, but small foci of infection may go undetected. If no other source of infection is identified, systemic antibiotic therapy should be initiated and treatment continued for at least 3 weeks or until the blood cultures clear. Cardiac catheterization should be performed if antibiotic therapy fails to clear the septicemia or if valvular insufficiency occurs along with other signs of infection. Treatment can be delayed and repeated blood cultures done when a positive blood culture is obtained for a patient whose general condition is inconsistent with sepsis. If exogenous contamination can be excluded, systemic antibiotic therapy should be initiated if the same organism is recovered from two successive blood cultures, even if the patient is not clinically septic. Falsely negative culture results can be minimized if the blood for cultures is drawn as the patient's temperature is rising or, in a patient already receiving antibiotic therapy, immediately before a scheduled antibiotic dose, when circulating levels of the antibiotic are lowest.

Recovery of multiple organisms from a single blood culture or different organisms from successive blood cultures in critically ill burn patients with life-threatening complications is indicative of loss of effective host resistance and should not be discounted as a consequence of technical error. Maximum doses of an antibiotic or antibiotics active against all of the recovered organisms should be administered to such patients, and the septic focus from which the microorganisms arose should be identified and controlled.

The organism recovered from the blood determines the impact of septicemia on the burn patient. A review spanning 25 years has demonstrated that gram-negative septicemia and candidemia significantly increased the mortality associated with the extent of burn, whereas gram-positive septicemia had no demonstrable effect on expected mortality.[40] Improvements in wound care and general care have resulted in a reduction of the comorbid effect of gram-negative septicemia.

Infection Control

The types of organisms that cause infections in burn patients can be influenced by manipulating the patients' environment.[41, 42] During a 10-year period at the U.S. Army Burn Center, improvement in isolation of patients was associated with significant reductions in both the frequency and the associated added mortality of infection. The changes observed were related to the use of single-bed isolation of seriously burned patients and reduction of between-patient contact. Assignment of nursing personnel to specific patients, regulating other staff traffic to flow from new patients to convalescent patients, and prevention of contact with convalescent patients who serve as a reservoir for multiply resistant organisms were effective in reducing interpatient transfer of organisms and prevented the establishment of endemic burn center strains. Environmental control measures included strict enforcement of hand-washing, gowning, and gloving policies.

The quality assurance of isolation of patients and infection control were based on a microbial surveillance program. Cultures were obtained from the wound surface, upper respiratory system (sputum), and urinary tract at admission and then three times per week throughout each patient's hospital course. Antibiotic sensitivity testing was done on *S. aureus* and *P. aeruginosa* or the principal gram-negative species isolated at each site. Patients with multiply resistant organisms acquired in other hospitals before burn center admission or detected during hospitalization were assigned to a patient-specific care team.[15]

The high incidence of infectious complications in burn patients mandates that every burn center establish its own infection control committee and a microbial surveillance program. The surveillance database can document the organism types and antimicrobial sensitivity patterns for the individual patient's flora from time of admission throughout the hospital course. This permits temporal documentation of colonization and the early identification of specific microorganisms when clinical signs of infection develop. The availability of antibiotic sensitivity data also permits selection of pathogen-specific agents, which reduces the high costs associated with empirical use of newer broad-spectrum agents.

Each burn center should establish an infection control committee that can use clinically relevant and appropriate definitions of infections that occur in burn patients to monitor the results of the microbial surveillance program and thus to identify temporal changes in the endemic flora, clusters of infection, changes in the types of infections that occur, and the predominant causative organisms.[6] The committee should also assess the appropriateness of antibiotic use. Lastly, outcome analyses must be conducted to identify organism-related effects on morbidity and mortality and thereby identify needed modifications of procedures for care of patients and environmental control.

References

1. Pruitt BA Jr, Mason AD Jr: Epidemiological, demographic and outcome characteristic of burn injury. *In* Herndon DN (ed): Total Burn Care. London, WB Saunders, 1996.
2. Pruitt BA Jr: The burn patient: II. Later care and complications of thermal injury. Curr Probl Surg 16:6–10, 1979.
3. McManus WF, Mason AD Jr, Pruitt BA Jr: Excision of the burn wound in patients with large burns. Arch Surg 124:718–720, 1989.
4. Goodwin CW, Pruitt BA Jr: Management of surgical infections: Pathogenesis, diagnosis, and treatment. *In* Davis JH, Sheldon GF (eds): Clinical Surgery. St. Louis, CV Mosby, 1995, pp 355–412.
5. Pruitt BA Jr: Infection: Cause or effect of pathophysiologic change in burn and trauma patients. *In* Paubert-Braquet M (ed): Lipid Mediators in the Immunology of Shock. New York, Plenum Publishing, 1987, pp 31–42.
6. Pruitt BA Jr, McManus AT: The changing epidemiology of infection in burn patients. World J Surg 16:57–67,1992.
7. Pruitt BA Jr, McManus AT, Kim SH, et al: Use of burn wound biopsy in the diagnosis and treatment of burn wound infection. *In* Lorenz S, Zellner PR (eds): Die Infektion beim Brandverletzten. Darmstadt, Germany, Steinkopf Verlag, 1993, pp 55–63.
8. McManus AT, Kim SH, McManus WF, et al: Comparison of quantitative microbiology and histopathology in divided burn wound biopsy specimens. Arch Surg 122:74–76, 1987.
9. Kim SH, Hubbard GB, Worley BL, et al: A rapid section technique for burn wound biopsy. J Burn Care Rehabil 6:433–435, 1985.
10. Kim SH, Hubbard GB, McManus WF, et al: Frozen section technique to evaluate early burn wound biopsy: A comparison with the rapid section technique. J Trauma 25:1134–1137, 1985.
11. McManus AT, Mason AD Jr, McManus WF, et al: Control of *Pseudomonas aeruginosa* infection in burned patients. Surg Res Commun 12:61–67, 1992.
12. Aulick LH, Goodwin CW Jr, Becker BA, et al: Visceral blood flow following thermal injury. Ann Surg 193:112–116, 1981.
13. Zaske DE, Sawchuk RJ, Gerding DN, et al: Increased dosage requirements of gentamicin in burn patients. J Trauma 16:824–828, 1976.
14. McManus WF, Goodwin CW Jr, Pruitt BA Jr: Subeschar treatment of burn-wound infection. Arch Surg 118:291–294, 1983.
15. McManus AT, McManus WF, Mason AD Jr, et al: Beta-hemolytic streptococcal burn wound infections are too infrequent to justify penicillin prophylaxis (Letter). Plast Reconstr Surg 93:650, 1994.
16. Bruck HM, Nash G, Stein JM, et al: Studies on the occurrence and significance of yeast and fungi in the burn wound. Ann Surg 176:108–110, 1972.
17. Becker WK, Cioffi WG, McManus AT, et al: Fungal burn wound infection: A 10 year experience. Arch Surg 126:44–48, 1991.
18. Majeski JA, MacMillan BG: Fatal systemic mycotic infections in the burned child. J Trauma 17:320–322, 1977.
19. Pruitt BA Jr: Phycomycotic infections. Probl Gen Surg 1:664–678, 1984.
20. Foley FD, Greenawald KA, Nash G, et al: Herpesvirus infection in burned patients. N Engl J Med 282:652–656, 1970.
21. Brandt SJ, Tribble CG, Lakeman AD, et al: Herpes simplex burn wound infections: Epidemiology of a case cluster and responses to acyclovir therapy. Surgery 98:338–343, 1985.
22. Deepe GS Jr, MacMillan BG, Linnemann CC Jr: Unexplained fever in burn patients due to cytomegalovirus infection. JAMA 248:2299–2301, 1982.
23. Bale JF Jr, Kealey GP, Massanari RM, et al: The epidemiology of cytomegalovirus infection among patients with burns. Infect Control Hosp Epidemiol 11:17–22, 1990.
24. Pruitt BA Jr: Cadaverous particles and infections in injured man—Clinical review based on the Semmelweis lecture. Eur J Surg 159:515–520, 1993.
25. McManus AT, Mason AD Jr, McManus WF, et al: A decade of

reduced gram-negative infections and mortality associated with improved isolation of burned patients. Arch Surg 129:1306–1309, 1994.
26. Pruitt BA Jr, DiVincenti FC, Mason AD Jr, et al: The occurrence and significance of pneumonia and other pulmonary complications in burned patients: Comparison of conventional and topical treatments. J Trauma 10:519–531, 1970.
27. Shirani KZ, Pruitt BA Jr, Mason AD Jr: The influence of inhalation injury and pneumonia on burn mortality. Ann Surg 205:82–87, 1987.
28. Rue LW, Cioffi WG, Mason AD, et al: Improved survival of burned patients with inhalation injury. Arch Surg 128:772–780, 1993.
29. Bartlett JG, Brewer NS, Ryan KJ: Laboratory diagnosis of lower respiratory tract infections. Washington JA II (ed): Cumitech 7: Laboratory Diagnosis of Lower Respiratory Tract Infections. Washington, DC, American Society for Microbiology, 1978, pp 4–7.
30. Gong H Jr, Soffer MJ, Ertle AR, et al: Diagnostic efficacy of a nasotracheal protected specimen brush in patients with suspected bacterial pneumonia. Diagn Microbiol Infect Dis 11:87–100, 1988.
31. Papazian L, Martin C, Albanese J, et al: Comparison of two methods of bacteriologic sampling of the lower respiratory tract: A study in ventilated patients with nosocomial bronchopneumonia. Crit Care Med 17:461–464, 1989.
32. Stover DE, Zaman MB, Hajdu SI, et al: Bronchoalveolar lavage in the diagnosis of diffuse pulmonary infiltrates in the immunosuppressed host. Ann Intern Med 101:1–7, 1984.
33. Taylor GD, Kibsey P, Kirkland T, et al: Predominance of staphylococcal organisms in infections occurring in a burns intensive care unit. Burns 18:332–335, 1992.
34. Frame JD, Kangesu L, Malik WM: Changing flora in burn and trauma units: Experience in the United Kingdom. J Burn Care Rehabil 13:281–286, 1992.
35. Pruitt BA Jr, McManus WF, Kim SH, et al: Diagnosis and treatment of cannula related intravenous sepsis in burn patients. Arch Surg 191:546–554, 1980.
36. Sasaki TM, Welch GW, Herndon DN, et al: Burn wound manipulation–induced bacteremia. J Trauma 19:46–48, 1979.
37. Pruitt BA Jr, Stein JM, Foley FD, et al: Intravenous therapy in burn patients: Suppurative thrombophlebitis and other life threatening complications. Arch Surg 100:399–404, 1970.
38. Stein JM: In discussion: Pruitt BA Jr, Stein JM, Foley FD, et al: Intravenous therapy in burn patients: Suppurative thrombophlebitis and other life threatening complications. Arch Surg 100:399–404, 1970.
39. Baskin TW, Rosenthall A, Pruitt BA Jr: Acute bacterial endocarditis: A silent source of sepsis in the burn patient. Ann Surg 184:618–621, 1976.
40. Mason AD Jr, McManus AT, Pruitt BA Jr: Association of burn mortality and bacteremia: A twenty-five year review. Arch Surg 121:1027–1031, 1986.
41. McManus AT, McManus WF, Mason AD Jr, et al: Microbial colonization in a new intensive care burn unit: A prospective cohort study. Arch Surg 120:217–223, 1985.
42. Shirani KZ, McManus AT, Vaughan GM, et al: Effects of environment on infection in burn patients. Arch Surg 121:31–36, 1986.

URINARY TRACT

106

Approach to the Patient with Urinary Tract Infection

Walter E. Stamm
Ann E. Stapleton

The term urinary tract infection (UTI) is applied to a wide variety of clinical conditions, ranging from asymptomatic bacteriuria on the one hand to acute pyelonephritis with gram-negative septicemia on the other. Many designations have been used to subdivide UTIs: symptomatic and asymptomatic, complicated and uncomplicated, upper tract and lower tract infection, among others. These schemes frequently overlap and do not correspond well to epidemiologically related groups of patients recognized by clinicians. In this chapter, symptomatic UTI in adults is subdivided into three groups: acute uncomplicated cystitis in women; acute uncomplicated pyelonephritis in women; and complicated UTIs in men or women. Most acute symptomatic UTIs in adults fall into one of these categories. Asymptomatic bacteriuria is discussed separately; it may be associated with any of the three groups. Being able to place a patient's complaint in one of the groups allows the physician to predict the likely infecting organisms and to choose an agent for empirical therapy.

Causative Pathogens

More than 95% of UTIs are caused by a single bacterial species. *Escherichia coli* is the agent of more than 80% of uncomplicated cystitis and pyelonephritis (Table 106–1). Interestingly, relatively few O serogroups produce the majority of these uncomplicated infections (O2, O4, O8, O18ab, O75, O150); they are known collectively as uropathogenic *E. coli* clones.[1] The proportion of cases of recurrent UTIs due to other organisms (usually *Klebsiella, Proteus,* or *Enterobacter* species or enterococci) is greater, as is the likelihood of isolating an organism with increased antibiotic resistance. From hospital-acquired UTIs a much wider range of organisms other than *E. coli* are isolated (see Table 106–1). Antibiotic-resistant isolates are common in nosocomial UTIs, particularly if the patient received prior courses of antimicrobial treatment.

Coagulase-negative staphylococci are often considered urinary contaminants, but studies have clearly demonstrated a pathogenic role for *Staphylococcus saprophyticus*.[2, 3] In urine specimens, this species can be reliably identified as a coagulase-negative staphylococcus that is resistant to novobiocin.[4] The vast majority of *S. saprophyticus* infections occur in young women, most commonly in the spring and summer. In northern Europe,[5, 6] *S. saprophyticus* has accounted for up to one third of acute uncomplicated UTIs in young women, whereas in the United States *S. saprophyticus* has usually accounted for 5% to 15% of acute cystitis episodes.[7]

Anaerobic bacteria, lactobacilli, corynebacteria, streptococci (other than enterococci), and *Staphylococcus epidermidis* are the predominant organisms isolated from the normal flora of

TABLE 106–1 ■ Microbial Species Most Often Associated with Specific Types of Urinary Tract Infections

MICROBE	ACUTE UNCOMPLICATED CYSTITIS (%)	ACUTE UNCOMPLICATED PYELONEPHRITIS (%)	COMPLICATED UTI (%)	CATHETER-ASSOCIATED UTI (%)
Escherichia coli	79	89	32	24
Staphylococcus saprophyticus	11	0	1	0
Proteus	2	4	4	6
Klebsiella	3	4	5	8
Enterococci	2	0	22	7
Pseudomonas	0	0	20	9
Mixed	3	5	10	11
Other	0	2	5	10
Yeast	0	0	1	28
S. epidermidis	0	0	15	8

Data in columns one and two are from 607 episodes of cystitis and 84 episodes of pyelonephritis in Seattle; data from columns 3 and 4 from Platt R, Polk BF, Murdock B, Rosner B: Risk factors for nosocomial urinary tract infection. Am J Epidemiol 124:977, 1986, and Gasser TC, et al: Treatment of complicated UTIs with ciprofloxacin. Am J Med 82(Suppl 4):278, 1987.

the perineum and distal urethra, but they seldom cause UTI.[8] These organisms are among the most common urinary contaminants.

Staphylococcus aureus bacteriuria often indicates metastatic infection of the kidney following bacteremia; ascending cystitis or pyelonephritis due to *S. aureus* is extremely unusual in patients who have not undergone instrumentation.[9] Adenoviruses (especially type 11) cause epidemic hemorrhagic cystitis in children, particularly boys,[10] and may be underestimated as an endemic cause of cystitis.

The role of other organisms in urinary infection remains unclear. Using special media, Maskell and colleagues[11] have isolated fastidious microaerophilic organisms from many women with the acute dysuria–frequency syndrome, but the causal role of these organisms is disputed by others.[12] *Gardnerella vaginalis* can be isolated from the urine of women with and without urinary tract symptoms, but its pathogenic role is likewise often uncertain.[13] *Ureaplasma urealyticum* and *Mycoplasma hominis* probably account for some cases of acute pyelonephritis, and perhaps some cases of cystourethritis.[14, 15] *Haemophilus influenzae* may, on occasion, cause community-acquired UTI.

Epidemiology

Table 106–2 summarizes the prevalence of UTI, the male/female ratio, and major risk factors for patients by age group. Prevalence of bacteriuria in the neonatal period is approximately 1%,[16] and infections during this period are often associated with bacteremia. Many are associated with functional or anatomic abnormalities of the urinary tract. In the first year of life, the frequency of UTI is higher in males than in females.[17] Between ages 1 and 5 years, the prevalence of bacteriuria in girls rises to 4.5%, whereas in boys it falls to 0.5%.[18] Infections in young boys are often associated with congenital anomalies of the urinary tract. More recently, an intact foreskin has been identified as an important risk factor for UTIs in this group.[19] Between one third and one half of UTIs in girls in the first 5 years of life are associated with vesicoureteral reflux, and this appears to be a critical period in determining whether renal scarring will occur.[20, 21]

The prevalence of bacteriuria in schoolgirls in the United States is approximately 1%; 5% of girls experience bacteriuria at some time. Most such episodes are not associated with renal abnormalities.[22, 23] Bacteriuria is rare in elementary school–age boys.

During late adolescence, the occurrence of UTI increases strikingly in young women. Approximately 20% of young women have at least one episode of acute dysuria each year, most due to bacterial infections.[24] An estimated 6 million cases of acute cystitis occur in young women each year, making these among the most frequent infections in this age group.[25] This figure probably understates the true incidence of these infections, because at least half of all UTIs resolve without coming to medical attention. During this period of life, UTIs are 50 times more common in women than in men. Major risk factors in women of this age group appear to be sexual intercourse and diaphragm and spermicide use (see later). Among young men who develop an uncomplicated UTI, homosexuality (perhaps due to exposure of the urethra to *E. coli* during insertive rectal intercourse), lack of circumcision, and human immunodeficiency virus infection appear to be important risk factors.[26, 27]

TABLE 106–2 ■ Overview of the Epidemiology of Urinary Tract Infections by Age Group

	FEMALES		MALES	
AGE GROUP (Y)	Prevalence (%)	Risk Factors	Prevalence (%)	Risk Factors
<1	1	Anatomic or functional urologic abnormalities	1	Anatomic or functional urologic abnormalities
1–5	4–5	Congenital abnormalities, vesicoureteral reflex	0.5	Congenital abnormalities, uncircumcised penis
6–15	4–5	Vesicoureteral reflux	0.5	None
16–35	20	Sexual intercourse, spermicide use, diaphragm use	0.5	Homosexuality, uncircumcised, human immunodeficiency virus infection
36–65	35	Gynecologic surgery, bladder prolapse, postmenopausal estrogen deficiency	20	Prostatic hypertrophy, obstruction, catheterization, surgery
>65	40	As for those age 36–65, plus incontinence, chronic catheterization	35	As for those age 36–65, plus incontinence, long-term catheterization

In the later years of life, the incidence of UTI increases sharply in both sexes and the female/male ratio declines. Many of these infections occur in the setting of catheterization, instrumentation, and bladder outlet obstruction due to prostatic hypertrophy.[28]

Pathogenesis

Community-acquired UTIs usually result from entry into the bladder of bacteria that colonize the anterior urethra or the vaginal introitus.[28, 29] Blood-borne or lymphatic spread of pathogens from distant sites of infection occurs occasionally. Relapsing infection from unresolved foci in the prostate, kidney, or calculi may seed other parts of the urinary tract. Rarely, bacteria spread from the bowel to the bladder via a fistulous communication, as in Crohn disease or malignancy. Characteristically, polymicrobial infection and pneumaturia result in such cases.

The pathogenesis of community-acquired UTI has been studied most carefully in young women, because they have the most infections.[30] The short female urethra allows bacteria colonizing the distal urethra to enter the bladder after urethral massage, which in part explains the association of UTIs and bacteriuria with sexual activity.[31] In addition, the proximity of the urethral meatus to the rectum in women facilitates colonization of the periurethral area with coliform bacteria.

In prospective studies, it has been repeatedly observed that the organisms that eventually cause UTIs usually colonize the vagina and the periurethral area beforehand.[32] Factors that promote colonization of the vaginal introitus are poorly understood. Both colonization of the vaginal introitus and bacteriuria due to *E. coli* have been strongly associated with diaphragm and spermicide use,[33] which may account for the apparently increased risk of UTI associated with sexual activity.[34] Although the mechanism of this association is not yet clear, it is probably at least partly a perturbation of the vaginal flora caused by spermicides. Certain antibiotics, especially β-lactams, also promote introital colonization with *E. coli*.[35]

Bacterial adherence to vaginal and uroepithelial cells represents the initial step in colonization of the lower urinary tract.[36] An important unresolved question is the extent to which epithelial cells vary in their susceptibility to bacterial attachment, either from person to person or in one person at different times. Several studies have demonstrated that uroepithelial cells from women prone to recurrent UTI bind larger numbers of bacteria than do cells from women with no history of UTI.[37, 38] This observation suggests that some women may be genetically predisposed to UTI, a hypothesis that is further supported by the fact that nonsecretors of blood group antigens have an increased risk of recurrent UTI and their uroepithelial cells bind *E. coli* in greater numbers than do cells from secretors.[39, 40] The biochemical basis for these observations may lie in the fact that vaginal epithelial cells from nonsecretors contain unique uropathogenic *E. coli*–binding glycosphingolipids that are not present in cells from secretors.[41] Alternatively, other factors such as estrogenic hormones appear to influence bacterial binding to epithelial cells and may alter the risk of UTI.[42] Spermicide use could also influence the likelihood of bacterial attachment to uroepithelial cells, either by directly altering the epithelial cell surface or by eliminating the normal vaginal flora.

Bacterial Virulence Factors

In comparison with "nonuropathogeneic" *E. coli* from the normal fecal flora, uropathogenic *E. coli* strains appear to belong to several distinct clones that exhibit specific virulence factors, including increased adherence to vaginal[43] and uroepithelial cells,[44] resistance to the bactericidal activity of human serum,[45] production of hemolysin[46] and of cytotoxic necrotizing factor-1,[47] carboxylesterase B electrophoretic pattern,[48] presence of chromosomal aerobactin,[49] and increased amounts of K capsular antigen.[50] These organisms belong to a limited number of O, K, and H serogroups. Their adhesive properties are important determinants, not only of infectivity but also in some cases of a propensity to develop upper tract infections. Adhesion is mediated by specific bacterial ligands, which attach as lectins to host cell wall carbohydrate residues that serve as receptors.[51] These ligands are usually small proteins located at the tips of bacterial fimbriae.[51, 52] Most *E. coli* strains (and many other Enterobacteriaciae) possess type 1 fimbriae, which bind mannoside residues on vaginal epithelial and uroepithelial cells.[53] Binding can be competitively inhibited by α-methyl mannoside and is said to be mannose sensitive. Although type 1 pili appear to be important in animal models of UTI, their pathogenic role in humans has not been clearly demonstrated. *E. coli* strains that cause upper UTIs usually express other adhesins that cannot be inhibited by an α-methyl mannoside and were thus originally called mannose-resistant adhesins. Eighty percent to 90% of uropathogenic *E. coli* strains that express mannose-resistant adhesins recognize a specific glycolipid receptor found on human erythrocytes and uroepithelial cells.[54, 55] The minimal recognition structure for this adhesin is a disaccharide moiety, α-D-galactopyranosyl-(1→4)-β-galactopyranoside, which is present on the globoseries glycosphingolipid on epithelial and erythrocyte membranes.[56] For this reason, these fimbriae have been called gal-gal fimbriae by some workers. Because this structure also constitutes a major part of the P blood group antigen on erythrocytes,[57] it has been named the P fimbria. Other mannose-resistant adhesins that do not recognize this disaccharide moiety are termed X adhesins[58]; the specific recognition sites for several X adhesins have been determined.[58]

Considerable evidence supports the importance of specific bacterial virulence factors in the pathogenesis of UTI. The importance of adhesion in uropathogenicity, for example, is demonstrated in experiments in which *E. coli* colonization of the mouse bladder can be prevented by mannose (i.e., competitive blockade of the mannose-sensitive adhesin).[59] Antibodies directed against P fimbriae block adherence to epithelial cells in vitro and prevent upper tract infection in a mouse model of pyelonephritis.[60] An *E. coli* vaccine utilizing gal-gal pili has been developed that prevents pyelonephritis in the same model.[61] Adhesion, often fimbria mediated, probably also plays a central role in the uropathogenicity of other bacterial species, such as *S. saprophyticus* and *Klebsiella*, but has been less studied.

Once attachment to uroepithelial cells occurs, bacterial virulence factors other than adhesins become important.[62] Most uropathogenic strains produce hemolysin, which may be important in initiating tissue invasion and cell damage or in making iron available to invading *E. coli*. Siderophores, such as aerobactin, are iron-scavenging proteins that are found with increased frequency in uropathogenic strains. The presence of K antigen protects bacteria from phagocytosis by leukocytes. Endotoxin derived from the *E. coli* cell wall is an important initiator of the inflammatory process in the kidney. Many or all of these virulence factors characteristically are found in *E. coli* strains isolated from infections, especially those involving the kidney, in urologically normal patients. Thus, these factors appear necessary for such strains to infect the intact host; however, they are less important in patients with structural or functional abnormalities of the urinary tract. *E. coli* strains infecting the upper tracts of children with vesicoureteral reflux or adults with urologic abnormalities, for example, do not exhibit the typical virulence factors found in the uropathogenic *E. coli* strains infecting nonimpaired hosts.[62]

Host Defense Mechanisms in the Urinary Tract

Small numbers of bacteria presumably enter the female bladder frequently, but established infection rarely ensues. A variety of host factors act in concert to protect against infection.[63] The flushing and diluting effects of urine accumulation and voiding help to clear infection. The acidity, high urea concentration, and extremes of osmolality in urine make it a poor culture medium for many anaerobic and fastidious bacteria[64] and inhibit growth of many other organisms. Bacteria grow less avidly in urine collected from men than from women, probably because of the inhibitory activity of prostatic secretions.[65] Tamm-Horsfall protein may act as a barrier to infection with Enterobacteriaceae, because it contains large numbers of mannose residues, which bind the mannose-sensitive adhesins on these bacteria and competitively inhibit attachment to epithelial cells.[66] Taken together, these factors often successfully defend the bladder against small bacterial inocula, but they may be overcome by larger inocula or by more virulent bacteria. Foreign bodies such as stones and structural abnormalities provide such good refuge for bacteria that they may be extremely difficult or impossible to eradicate with antimicrobial agents.

Once infection is established, a local inflammatory response develops, with an influx of polymorphonuclear leukocytes and macrophages that ingest and destroy bacteria.[67] Interleukin-6 and interleukin-8 appear in the urine in patients with lower tract UTI and often in both the urine and serum of patients with acute pyelonephritis.[68, 69] Urine inhibits the phagocytic functions of polymorphonuclear leukocytes, including migration, aggregation, and killing. The inflammatory response itself is in part responsible for the symptoms of cystitis. In contrast to pyelonephritis,[70] cystitis is seldom associated with a marked systemic or local antibody response to the infecting organism,[71] and reinfection with the same strain may occur.

Overview of Clinical Manifestations

The symptoms of UTI in young children are notoriously nonspecific; often the major manifestations are fever, poor feeding, and vomiting.[72] Abdominal discomfort may be present. UTI must always be excluded when a child has unexplained fever. After early childhood, the classic symptoms of dysuria, urgency, and frequency are more common. Adult women with cystitis generally void frequently and urgently, usually in small volumes,[73] and they often experience a sensation of lower abdominal heaviness or lower back pain. The urine may be turbid, and it is frankly bloody in one third of cases. Onset of symptoms is usually abrupt. Most cases respond rapidly to antimicrobial treatment, and many resolve even without therapy. If untreated, some patients progress over several days to develop signs and symptoms of upper tract involvement—fever, rigors, vomiting, flank pain. Studies that compared clinical signs and symptoms with the localization of bacteria to the upper or lower urinary tract by laboratory techniques have demonstrated a poor correlation between clinical manifestations and site of infection.[74, 75]

In elderly persons, UTIs often produce no symptoms, and, as in childhood, when symptoms and signs are present they are frequently nonspecific. In addition, frequency, urgency, nocturia, and incontinence may have multiple causes in this age group. Physicians should not hesitate to collect urine for culture when an elderly patient has unexplained fever, increased urinary frequency, incontinence, or lower abdominal discomfort. Patients with neurogenic bladders or an indwelling catheter usually have few or no symptoms referable to the bladder when they develop a UTI; signs and symptoms of pyelonephritis and unexplained fever or septicemia are more common.

Acute Uncomplicated Cystitis

Acute uncomplicated cystitis generally occurs in young women, but it may also be seen in older men and women and in children. Typical symptoms include dysuria, urinary frequency, urgency, voiding of small volumes, incontinence, and suprapubic or pelvic pain. Suprapubic tenderness is present in about 10% of patients with cystitis, and gross hematuria in about 30%, but both are relatively specific findings for cystitis in this group of patients.[76]

Acute cystitis must be differentiated from other conditions in which dysuria may be a prominent symptom, especially vaginitis and urethral infections caused by sexually transmitted pathogens. Table 106–3 summarizes the characteristic features that are useful in assigning a patient with dysuria to one of these diagnostic categories.[77]

About 10% to 35% of patients with characteristic symptoms of acute uncomplicated cystitis are discovered also to have unrecognized infection of the upper urinary tract (occult renal infection) when localization studies such as the bladder washout test, selective ureteral catheterization, or antibody-coated bacteria tests are run.[78–80] The likelihood of occult renal infection in a patient presumed to have acute cystitis appears to be greater for women whose symptoms have persisted at least 7 days or who have a history of recent UTI and for those in lower socioeconomic groups.

Acute Pyelonephritis

Patients with acute pyelonephritis characteristically present with the symptoms of localized flank, low back, or abdominal pain and systemic symptoms such as fever, rigors, sweats, headache, nausea, vomiting, malaise, and prostration.[81] Antecedent or concomitant symptoms of cystitis may or may not be present. Fever and flank pain are relatively specific indicators of acute renal infection.

TABLE 106–3 ■ Factors That Distinguish Acute Cystitis from Vaginitis and Urethritis

FACTOR	ACUTE CYSTITIS	ACUTE URETHRITIS	VULVOVAGINITIS
Pathogen	*Escherichia coli, Staphylococcus saprophyticus*	*Chlamydia trachomatis, Neisseria gonorrhoeae*, herpes simplex virus	*Candida, Trichomonas*
Symptoms	Internal dysuria, frequency, urgency, hematuria	Internal dysuria, frequency, urgency, vaginal discharge	External dysuria, vaginal discharge, vaginal odor
Onset	Abrupt; symptoms severe	Gradual; symptoms mild	Gradual; symptoms mild
History	Prior UTI, diaphragm use	New sexual partner	Dyspareunia
Physical findings	Suprapubic tenderness	Cervicitis	Vulvovaginitis

A wide spectrum of illness is encountered among patients with acute pyelonephritis, ranging from mild disease to full-blown gram-negative sepsis. Volume contraction from recurrent vomiting may necessitate intravenous administration of fluids and antimicrobial agents. A minority of patients with acute pyelonephritis develop complications such as necrotizing intrarenal and perinephric abscesses[82] or gram-negative sepsis.[83] These severe manifestations occur primarily in patients with associated urinary tract obstruction, diabetes, or other immunosuppressive conditions[84, 85] and often necessitate aggressive diagnostic and therapeutic efforts, including emergency ultrasonography or computed tomography, and in some cases, hemodynamic monitoring, pressors, assisted ventilation, or urologic surgical procedures.

Complicated Urinary Tract Infections

In addition to being classified by the presumed anatomic site of infection, UTIs are often categorized as complicated or uncomplicated, depending on the presence or absence of host conditions known to promote infection, account for persistence of infection, or lead to a recurrence[85, 86] (Table 106–4). Generally, uncomplicated cystitis and uncomplicated pyelonephritis occur in young women who lack evidence of structural or functional urologic abnormalities; thus, among females, complicated infections primarily affect premenarchal girls and postmenopausal women. All UTIs in males should be considered complicated until proved otherwise. As indicated earlier, the clinical manifestations that accompany complicated UTI are more often atypical and nonspecific. When complicating host factors are present, antimicrobial resistance is more common, response to therapy is often disappointing (even with agents active against the patient's pathogen),[85] and severe complications of infection are more frequent. Antimicrobial and adjunctive therapies may require modification in the presence of complicating factors (see later).

Diagnosis

Confirmation of a UTI requires documentation of bacteriuria by culture. Suprapubic aspiration avoids potential contamination of the urine during collection but is rarely used in practice, except in children and certain other patients. Urethral catheterization can also be used to collect a specimen for urine culture; contamination of specimens collected by in-and-out catheterization is infrequent compared with that of voided specimens, but the procedure is uncomfortable for the patient, time-consuming, and thus rarely used. If a patient has an indwelling catheter, specimens for culture should be obtained from the specimen collection port on the catheter.

Urine Culture

In clinical practice, urine for culture is usually voided unless a catheter is in place, so specimens are often contaminated with perineal bacteria. Quantitative cultures and specific identification of the organisms in urine are used to distinguish culture contaminants (usually in small numbers and usually nonpathogenic species, often several of them) from true infective agents (usually larger numbers of typical uropathogens only).[87] The urine bacterial concentration is usually determined by inoculating a culture dish with a known volume of urine (10^{-2} or 10^{-3} mL), or it can be estimated using a dip-culture method.[88] The finding of more than 10^5 bacteria per milliliter of voided urine was shown by Kass, Sanford, and others to differentiate infected from contaminated urine of women with asymptomatic bacteriuria or acute pyelonephritis.[87–89] Since these studies were published, many physicians have considered at least 10^5 colony-forming units (CFU) per milliliter to be a necessary criterion for the diagnosis of any urinary infection; however, about one third of women with acute cystitis caused by *E. coli, S. saprophyticus*, and *Proteus* species have colony counts in midstream urine between 10^2 and 10^4 CFU/mL.[90, 91] Similarly, acute pyelonephritis has been reported in association with low bacterial counts in voided urine.[92] Thus, in acutely symptomatic women, a more appropriate threshold value for defining "significant bacteriuria" is more than 10^2 CFU/mL of a known uropathogen.[90, 91] Failure to use this criterion for such patients seriously compromises the sensitivity of the urine culture. Many microbiology laboratories use culture techniques that accurately detect 10^3 but not 10^2 CFU/mL, so a 10^3 CFU/mL criterion may be more practical for many clinicians and laboratorians. Clinicians should encourage their clinical laboratory to utilize techniques that detect 10^3 CFU/mL and to report the results of cultures that grow 10^3 to 10^5 CFU/mL of a uropathogen.

As alternatives to standard culture methods, several more rapid methods for the detection of bacteriuria have been developed and are reviewed in detail elsewhere.[93] These methods detect bacterial growth by using photometry or bioluminescence and can provide results in as little as 2 hours. In general, these methods achieve a sensitivity of 95% to 98% and better than 99% negative predictive value compared with conventional cultures when bacteriuria is defined as at least 10^5 CFU/mL. Thus, they are excellent for screening out negative cultures by this definition of bacteriuria. Unfortunately, the sensitivity of these tests falls to unsatisfactory levels when they are asked to detect bacteriuria between 10^2 and 10^4 CFU/mL, which is necessary in patients with symptoms of acute disease.

TABLE 106–4 ■ Complicating Factors in Urinary Tract Infection

Male sex
Pregnancy
Diabetes
Immunosuppression
Hospital-acquired UTI
Recent antibiotic use
Catheterization or instrumentation of the urinary tract
Stone or urinary tract structural abnormality

Rapid Noncultural Diagnostic Tests

Rapid tests for detecting urinary leukocytes, erythrocytes, and bacteria permit presumptive confirmation of UTI at the time of initial evaluation without the expense and delays associated with urine culture. Among women with acute uncomplicated infection, when pyuria in voided urine specimens is carefully assessed using the hemocytometer method and when UTI is defined as more than 10^2 CFU/mL of a uropathogen plus acute urinary tract symptoms, pyuria is a highly sensitive indicator of UTI.[93] In fact, its absence should call into question the diagnosis of UTI in this group of patients. Unfortunately, assessment of pyuria using the centrifuged urine sediment method that is employed in many laboratories is far less accurate and reproducible than counting leukocytes in uncentrifuged urine using a chamber method. The former method should be discouraged. The leukocyte esterase dipstick method is somewhat less sensitive in identifying pyuria than the hemocytometer method,[94] but it can serve as an alternative approach when microscopy is not available. Pyuria is a less sensitive and specific indicator of complicated or catheter-associated UTI than of uncomplicated infection, but assessment of pyuria should be undertaken in such patients suspected of having a UTI.

Microscopic hematuria is found in 40% to 60% of cases of acute cystitis and is uncommon in other dysuric syndromes of young women; therefore, for this group, hematuria is a highly specific indicator of cystitis. In elderly persons, urinary calculi or tumors must be considered when hematuria is observed. Microscopic bacteriuria, which is most conveniently assessed using gram-stained, uncentrifuged urine, is found in more than 90% of UTIs in which colony counts are at least 10^5 CFU/mL and is a highly specific finding.[95] Bacteria are not readily detected microscopically with infections of lower colony counts (10^2 to 10^4 CFU/mL). Thus, microscopic hematuria and bacteriuria lack sensitivity but are reasonably specific for UTI in most groups of patients. Failure to detect them in a patient whose symptoms are consistent with UTI should not be interpreted as evidence against the diagnosis. At the same time, the presence of bacteriuria or hematuria in a patient with acute dysuria is strong evidence of bacterial UTI.

Selection of Laboratory Tests

Many authorities recommend that urine culture and antimicrobial susceptibility testing be performed whenever a UTI is suspected. However, the spectrum of infecting bacterial species and their antimicrobial susceptibility profiles are highly predictable in patients with acute cystitis. Further, treatment decisions are usually made, and therapy is often completed, before culture results are known in such patients. Thus, it may be more cost-effective to manage patients who have symptoms and urinalysis findings characteristic of acute, uncomplicated cystitis without an initial urine culture. In a study of women with uncomplicated infection, pretreatment urine cultures were not predictive of the therapeutic outcome and were considered unnecessary.[96] Another study[97] estimated that the routine use of pretherapy urine cultures in acute cystitis increased costs by 40% but decreased the overall duration of symptoms by only 10%.

In view of these data, when patients have symptoms and signs suggestive of acute cystitis but no complicating factors, one approach that is increasingly used is to provide empirical antimicrobial therapy and do no laboratory testing unless the patient fails to improve. Alternatively, a urinalysis or a leukocyte esterase dipstick test can be performed.[98] If results indicate pyuria or bacteriuria, these tests provide sufficient documentation of UTI, and urine culture and susceptibility testing can be omitted. Urine culture should be performed, however, when symptoms and urine examination findings leave the diagnosis of cystitis in question. Pretreatment culture and susceptibility tests are also essential to the management of patients with suspected upper tract infections and those who have complicating factors, because in these situations a variety of pathogens may be present and antibiotic therapy is best tailored to the individual organism.[99]

Treatment

General Principles

All symptomatic UTIs should be treated with antimicrobial drugs. Ideally, the least toxic, least expensive drug should be prescribed for a period long enough to eradicate the infection. The antibacterial spectrum of the drug should cover the likely infecting organisms but should minimally disrupt the normal gut and perineal flora. Successful treatment of uncomplicated lower UTIs correlates with the inhibitory concentration of antimicrobial agent achieved in the urine, not in plasma or tissue.[79] Some antimicrobial agents that are used successfully to treat cystitis (e.g., nitrofurantoin[79]) do not achieve microbicidal blood or tissue levels but are excreted in high concentrations in the urine. Urinary concentrations of many antibiotics are much higher than corresponding levels in other body fluids and may even exceed the minimal inhibitory concentration of some resistant organisms. This probably accounts for the clinical observation that some patients with cystitis are cured by antibiotics to which the infecting organism was apparently resistant. Urinary pH is an important determinant of antibacterial activity in vitro of some antimicrobials, such as erythromycin and the aminoglycosides, but it is rarely important clinically.

A variety of nonspecific adjunctive measures are recommended to supplement antimicrobial treatment of UTIs.[100] Patients with UTIs are usually advised to drink as much water as they can. The diluting and flushing out of nonadherent bacteria from the bladder may rapidly reduce the bacteria count in the urine and provide temporary symptomatic relief. In some cases, a large fluid load may be sufficient to clear the infection, but often as urine flow diminishes, bacterial counts rise again and symptoms appear. Other effects of "forcing fluids" may not be beneficial: urinary acidification is reduced, antibacterial substances in the urine are diluted, and obstruction or reflux may be exacerbated. Nonspecific treatment to reduce bladder discomfort and dysuria such as potassium citrate and phenazopyridine have little place in the management of bacterial cystitis. Phenazopyridine is occasionally helpful in women with recurrent dysuria, who have no documented infection.

Acute Cystitis

The traditional approach to treating acute cystitis was 7 to 10 days' therapy with an oral antibiotic; however, single-dose therapy (SDT) is effective in treating most women with acute cystitis, is less costly, and is associated with significantly fewer side effects than longer therapy.[101, 102] However, in controlled trials in which the sample size was adequate to allow detection of 15% to 20% differences in efficacy, SDT has been less effective than 7- to 10-day therapy.[103, 104] In addition, high-risk patients such as pregnant women; those with diabetes, immunosuppressive conditions, or urinary tract anomalies; and those who experienced symptoms for at least 7 days before therapy started are more likely to have occult upper tract infection and to not be cured by SDT or to develop complications if the infection is not eradicated.[103, 104]

Cure rates with SDT are in part related to the drug used. Higher cure rates have generally been observed with trimethoprim, trimethoprim-sulfamethoxazole, and fluoroquinolones, whereas lower cure rates have been observed with ampicillin, amoxicillin, and other β-lactam agents. This probably results mainly from the rapid urinary excretion of the latter compounds and the prolonged urinary excretion of the former. In addition, trimethoprim is concentrated in renal tissues to a greater extent than is ampicillin.[105] The high incidence of resistance to ampicillin among pathogens from community-acquired UTIs (Table 106–5) also contributes substantially to the decreased efficacy of ampicillin and amoxicillin in antibody-coated bacteria–positive infections.

SDT may also be less effective because it does not eradicate vaginal *E. coli* as effectively as 10-day therapy. Perhaps the majority of "relapses" after SDT actually represent failure of such therapy to eliminate *E. coli* from the vaginal reservoir, followed rapidly by ascending reinfection.

Studies have evaluated the use of a 3-day course of therapy for treatment of cystitis. On theoretical grounds, 3-day therapy can be expected to be more effective than SDT, especially in patients with unrecognized complicating factors, and may

TABLE 106–5 ■ Susceptibility of Urinary Tract Infection Pathogens to Commonly Used Antibiotics in Selected Situations*

ANTIBIOTIC	CYSTITIS (%)	ACUTE PYELONEPHRITIS (%)	COMPLICATED UTI (%)
Ampicillin	72	57	30
First-generation cephalosporin	91	60	51
Third-generation cephalosporin	N/A	95	95
Gentamicin	N/A	95	81
Nitrofurantoin	96	N/A	N/A
Trimethoprim-sulfamethoxazole	89	70	63
Fluoroquinolone	99	98	95

*Author's unpublished data. N/A indicates not available.
Modified from Johnson JR, Stamm WE: Diagnosis and treatment of acute urinary tract infections. Infect Dis Clin North Am 1:773–791, 1987.

be more effective than SDT in eradicating *E. coli* from the vaginal reservoir. Three-day regimens of trimethoprim, trimethoprim-sulfamethoxazole, fluoroquinolones, or doxycycline have been associated with an incidence of adverse effects as low as that seen with SDT, and with cure rates that appear comparable to those achieved with longer courses of therapy.[106, 107] Thus, 3-day therapy may be the preferred short-course regimen for treating acute uncomplicated lower UTI, although further studies are needed. Short-course therapy (Table 106–6; see Table 106–5) should be reserved for patients presumed to have acute cystitis and no known complicating factors. When complicating factors are present in such patients, therapy should be continued for at least 7 days.

Acute Pyelonephritis

Patients with acute pyelonephritis can be subdivided into three groups: (1) those with mild acute pyelonephritis that can be managed in an outpatient setting; (2) those with acute uncomplicated pyelonephritis who are sufficiently ill to require hospitalization for parenteral therapy; and (3) those with complicated infection occurring in the setting of prior catheterization, hospitalization, urologic surgery, or known urologic abnormalities. The first group, who represent a minority of patients with acute pyelonephritis, can be treated successfully as outpatients with oral antibiotics, provided adequate compliance and follow-up can be ensured.[108] A cost analysis showed that outpatient therapy for acute pyelonephritis was considerably less expensive than inpatient therapy.[109]

Therapy for the second group, the majority of patients with acute pyelonephritis, necessitates hospital admission, intravenous fluids, and parenteral antibiotics because of the patient's extreme debility and inability to take oral medications. The combination of ampicillin and an aminoglycoside has traditionally been recommended as empirical therapy for patients hospitalized with uncomplicated acute pyelonephritis, ampicillin being continued alone if the infecting organism proves to be susceptible. However, because of the increasing frequency of resistance to ampicillin, even among community-acquired *E. coli* strains (see Table 106–5), its attractiveness as part of a regimen for empirical therapy of gram-negative infections is much diminished. A major advantage of the traditional ampicillin-gentamicin regimen is its effectiveness against both *Enterococcus* and *Pseudomonas* organisms, in addition to other gram-negative bacilli, but for uncomplicated acute pyelonephritis such coverage is usually unnecessary. Given the availability of a number of alternative intravenous antibiotics that are active against most Enterobacteriaceae and the capability of excluding enterococcal infection with the urine Gram stain, it may be preferable to initiate therapy for acute uncomplicated pyelonephritis due to gram-negative bacilli with a single intravenous agent such as trimethoprim-sulfamethoxazole, a fluoroquinolone, a third-generation cephalosporin, or an aminoglycoside alone while awaiting culture results. The choice of which of these drugs to use depends on cost considerations and on local antimicrobial sensitivity patterns. Therapy can be modified after 24 to 48 hours, when susceptibility testing results are available. Parenteral therapy should be used until symptoms improve, fever disappears, and the patient is able to take fluids by mouth.

We find that the duration of therapy for acute pyelonephritis in women need not be longer than 14 days.[110] Shorter courses of therapy are curative for some cases of acute pyelonephritis, as reflected in reports of success with as little as 5 days' therapy[111, 112]; however, in one controlled trial, 1 week of therapy using the combination of pivampicillin and pivmecillinam resulted in significantly more bacteriologic recurrences than 3 weeks of therapy.[113] Thus, routine use of less than 14 days' therapy is not supported by currently available comparative clinical trials.

As in lower UTIs, the presence of complicating factors in patients with upper UTI argues for more aggressive management, closer follow-up, and a longer course of therapy. Reference to recent urine culture reports or to the Gram stain examination of the initial urine specimen may be used to broaden the spectrum of empirical antimicrobial coverage but should not be relied on to narrow it. Consideration should be given to making urologic consultation part of the initial management of such patients. Similarly, patients with suspected pyelonephritis who have symptoms of renal colic or a stone on their admission abdominal x-ray film or who fail to improve after 3 days' appropriate antibiotic therapy should be suspected of harboring a stone or of having an underlying anatomic abnormality, urinary tract obstruction, or an acquired complication of infection such as intrarenal abscess. In such cases, ultrasonography, computed tomography, or excretory urography should be performed and urologic consultation obtained if indicated.

Asymptomatic Bacteriuria

Generally, children with asymptomatic bacteriuria should be treated. Bacteriuria in pregnancy is associated with a high risk of developing acute pyelonephritis and may jeopardize the pregnancy.[114] Women should thus be screened for bacteriuria during pregnancy and treated promptly (see later). For adults who are not pregnant, there is little convincing evidence that treating asymptomatic bacteriuria is beneficial.[115, 116] Exceptions may include selected high-risk patients such as those with neutropenia or a renal transplant. At present, there is no reason to treat asymptomatic bacteriuria in elderly patients. Although the mortality rate for hospitalized patients with bacteriuria has been higher than that for patients without bacteriuria,[117] this probably relates to the frequency with which seriously ill patients are catheterized and the mortality associated with bacteremic catheter-associ-

TABLE 106–6 ■ Empirical Treatment Regimens for Selected Clinical Situations

CLINICAL SITUATION	EXPECTED PATHOGENS	ANTIBIOTIC THERAPY*	EXPECTED OUTCOME	COMMENTS
Acute uncomplicated cystitis	*Escherichia coli* (>90%) *Staphylococcus saprophyticus*	Therapy for 3 d with TMP-SMX, TMP, norfloxacin, ofloxacin, ciprofloxacin, sulfa; or nitrofurantoin for 7 d	Cure > 95%, relapse rare; subsequent reinfection possible	Therapy is extended to 7 d for following situations: unreliable patient, recent infection, 7 d of symptoms, diabetes, pregnancy, age <12 or >65 y
Acute pyelonephritis, no clinical evidence of stones or urologic disease, no evidence of sepsis, mild illness	*E. coli* (>90%)	14-d course of ofloxacin, ciprofloxacin, or TMP-SMX given orally to outpatient	Cure > 90%; ~10% reinfection; relapse rare	With relapse, calculi or urologic disease is ruled out; then 2–6 wk with appropriate drug treatment eradicates focus
Acute pyelonephritis, with suspected gram-negative sepsis or severe illness	*E. coli* (>90%) *Klebsiella, Proteus*	14-d course of therapy; start with initial IV gentamicin or third-generation cephalosporin or fluoroquinolone for 3 d followed by PO therapy	Cure > 80%; may relapse as described above	Hospitalization, parenteral antibiotics, other measures to manage shock; obstruction relieved if present
Infection with calculi or urologic abnormality	*E. coli, Proteus, Klebsiella, Pseudomonas;* occasionally *Staphylococcus* or *Enterococcus*	At least 14-d course directed by culture results and sensitivities; begin with ampicillin plus gentamicin	Dependent on relief of underlying condition	Therapy before culture results are known depends on degree of illness and local sensitivity patterns (see text)
Nosocomial infection in catheterized patient; no clinical evidence of pyelonephritis or sepsis	*E. coli, Proteus, Klebsiella, Pseudomonas, Serratia, Enterococcus*	Often none if catheter can be withdrawn and patient is asymptomatic; if catheter cannot be withdrawn, treat symptomatic patients and selected asymptomatic patients, immunosuppressed patients (especially renal transplant recipients), and those at high risk of sepsis (old age, severe underlying disease)	Usually eradicated if catheter is withdrawn; treatment usually fails otherwise	Therapy based on culture results and sensitivities
Asymptomatic bacteriuria	*E. coli* (>90%) in young women; diverse spectrum in elderly	Treatment not always needed (see text); pregnant women and men about to undergo urologic surgery are treated as for acute uncomplicated cystitis	Cure 70%	Two cultures should be positive before treatment is undertaken

*TMP-SMX, Trimethoprim-sulfamethoxazole; IV, intravenous; PO, oral.

ated UTI. Therefore, asymptomatic bacteriuria should not be treated in most cases of catheter-associated UTI.

Prophylaxis of Recurrent Infection in Women

Many women have occasional episodes of cystitis, but in a minority, recurrent episodes occur with such frequency (three or more per year) that antimicrobial prophylaxis is justified. These patients can be divided into two groups: (1) those with structural or functional abnormalities of the urinary tract (and an associated tendency to develop pyelonephritis or relapsing infection), and (2) the great majority, who have a normal picture at intravenous pyelography, infections confined to the lower urinary tract, and repeated reinfections. In some of these women, infections can be temporally related to sexual intercourse or diaphragm use, but in the majority no predisposing factor is apparent. The recurrent infections tend to cluster in time[118]; that is, the likelihood of a subsequent infection is greatest at the end of the treatment course and then diminishes progressively the longer that the woman is infection free.

Simple measures such as voiding immediately after sexual intercourse or substituting an alternative form of contraception for a diaphragm may be effective for women for whom these factors are related to recurrent infection. Three antimicrobial strategies can be employed: (1) continuous low-dose prophylaxis[119]; (2) self-administered single-dose treatment[120]; and (3) postcoital single-dose prophylaxis.[121]

For continuous low-dose prophylaxis, trimethoprim (with or without sulfamethoxazole), nitrofurantoin, and norfloxacin have been evaluated extensively and are highly effective.[119] Most experience has been gained with trimethoprim-sulfamethoxazole; it is tolerated well and produces an excellent therapeutic index when used long term. Side effects are rare but usually develop in the first few weeks of therapy. Emergence of resistant strains is unusual with these drugs, and their efficacy does not appear to diminish with extended use. Other drugs have been used for long-term prophylaxis, but experience with them is more limited, and in general results have not been as good.

The choice of management strategy depends on the factors that predispose to recurrent infection, the numbers of infections per year, and the preference of the patient.[122] In general, continuous prophylaxis is preferred for women who experience three infections or more per year. Patient-administered SDT or 3-day therapy should be reserved for women who have two or three infections per year, and postcoital prophylaxis for women who relate their infections to sexual activity. The costs of prophylaxis and patient-administered SDT with trimethoprim-sulfamethoxazole are approximately the same.[120] There are no clear guidelines as to when to stop prophylaxis, but most often it is given for at least 6 months. Most women's infections return at the preprophylaxis rate when the drug is withdrawn.[123]

Among postmenopausal women, estrogen deficiency is associated with an increased risk of recurrent UTI[124] and with alterations of the vaginal flora favoring colonization with uropathogens.[125] In a double-blind, placebo-controlled trial, treatment with topical intravaginal estradiol cream was shown to ameliorate these derangements of the vaginal flora and to dramatically reduce the risk of recurrent UTI among these women.[126]

Urinary Tract Infection in Pregnancy

Asymptomatic bacteriuria occurs in 4% to 7% of pregnancies,[127] the risk increasing with parity, lower socioeconomic status, and age. Several physiologic changes account for this predisposition to infection in pregnancy, including estrogen-induced and progesterone-induced dilation of the uterus, bladder, and renal pelvis; increased bladder capacity; hydroureter and decreased ureteral peristalsis; and vesicoureteral reflux. Approximately one third of untreated pregnant women with bacteriuria develop upper tract infections, usually in the third trimester, in contrast with a rate of less than 1% in patients without bacteriuria in early pregnancy.[128] The incidence of pyelonephritis in bacteriuric women can be reduced to less than 5% by appropriate therapy. Thus, more than 75% of cases of acute pyelonephritis in pregnancy can be prevented by screening for and treating asymptomatic bacteriuria early in pregnancy. Prevention of pyelonephritis in pregnancy also prevents associated fetal morbidity (principally prematurity).

Women should be screened for bacteriuria at their first antenatal clinical visit. Sulfonamides, nitrofurantoin, ampicillin, cephalexin, and nalidixic acid are all considered safe to use early in pregnancy. Sulfonamides should not be used near term, owing to the theoretical risk that kernicterus may be induced in the newborn by sulfonamide displacement of bilirubin from plasma albumin binding sites. Trimethoprim, a dihydrofolate reductase inhibitor, is not generally recommended in pregnancy, because there is some evidence of fetal toxicity with high doses in experimental animals; however, in pregnant humans there is no evidence of teratogenicity or other adverse effects. Tetracyclines and fluoroquinolones are contraindicated in pregnancy.

At present, a 7-day course of antimicrobial agent would seem a reasonable treatment of choice for asymptomatic bacteriuria or uncomplicated lower UTI during pregnancy if careful follow-up is possible.[129] Patients should be followed up 2 weeks after completing therapy and then at monthly intervals. The aim of follow-up is to detect and treat asymptomatic bacteriuria as promptly as possible and therefore to prevent the development of acute pyelonephritis.

Catheter-Associated Infections

Catheter-associated UTIs constitute 35% to 40% of all hospital-acquired infections.[130] The majority of these infections are asymptomatic, but some produce the clinical manifestations of cystitis described earlier. More important, catheter-associated bacteriuria is the most common source of gram-negative bacteremia in hospitalized patients[131] and has been associated with a threefold increase in mortality,[132] prolonged hospital stay, and increased hospital costs.

Bacteria gain entry to the catheterized bladder in three ways: they may be introduced during catheterization, they may enter on the external surface of the catheter in the urethral mucus sheath (periurethral route),[133] or they may enter the drainage system by contamination of the collecting bag or disconnection of the junction between the catheter and collecting tube and ascend through the lumen of the catheter (intraluminal route).[133] The importance of the intraluminal route is illustrated by the marked reduction in the incidence of catheter-associated UTI since the introduction of sterile, closed drainage systems. Presently, in hospitals where closed, sterile drainage is used, the periurethral route of infection appears to be the most frequent route of bacterial entry, especially in women. Antecedent rectal and periurethral colonization plays an important role in the subsequent development of catheter-associated bacteriuria, as it does in women with cystitis.[133] In one study, urethral colonization preceded the development of catheter-associated UTI in 67% of women and 29% of men.[133]

The overall risk of infection increases with the time that the catheter is in place. About 50% of men and women catheterized for 2 weeks develop bacteriuria, and all patients with permanent indwelling catheters eventually become infected. Risk of catheter-associated UTI is greater in women, in patients whose sterile, closed drainage system is disconnected, and in patients who are not receiving systemic antibiotics.

Prevention of Infection

Closed, sterile drainage systems significantly reduce the incidence of catheter-associated infection. Provided that the system is not breached, bacteriuria can be prevented in the majority of patients for up to 10 days with modern collecting systems and catheters. In general, antibiotic ointments and creams applied to the urethral meatus have not been protective; however, one study showed that twice-daily application of a polyantimicrobial cream to the urethral meatus significantly reduced infection in women with periurethral colonization at the time of catheterization.[134] Silver-impregnated catheters may prevent bacteriuria, especially in patients catheterized long term.[135, 136] Systemic antibiotic treatment has a definite short-term effect in reducing the prevalence of UTIs in catheterized patients, but in the long term it predisposes to infection by resistant strains. This approach may be appropriate for short-term coverage of high-risk patients, but it is unwise for periods of catheterization longer than 1 week.

Treatment

In general, catheter-associated bacteriuria should be treated only in patients with symptomatic infection. When treatment is to be started, it is preferable to remove the catheter, start appropriate therapy, and then reintroduce a new catheter and drainage system if indwelling catheterization is still necessary. Concretions on the internal surface of the catheter often serve as a reservoir for bacteria, where they may be protected from antimicrobial drugs much as they are in urinary calculi. If such "infected" catheters are left in place, relapsing infection will occur when antimicrobial therapy is stopped. If fever and flank pain are present, parenteral treatment should be started immediately. Evidence is insufficient to cite an optimal duration of treatment for catheter-associated UTI; 7 days' therapy is usual. Resistant bacteria and fungi (usually *Candida*) are often isolated in catheterized patients receiving multiple courses of broad-spectrum antimicrobials. Symptomatic bacterial infections should be treated on the basis of antimicrobial sensitivities. Yeast isolation does not necessarily require treatment, because many episodes clear without treatment, but repeated isolations or symptomatic infections should be treated with oral fluconazole or amphotericin B irrigations.[137, 138]

References

1. Ørskov F, Ørskov I: Summary of a workshop on the clone concept in the epidemiology, taxonomy and evolution of the Enterobacteriaceae and other bacteria. J Infect Dis 148:346, 1983.
2. Latham RH, Running K, Stamm WE: Urinary tract infections in young women caused by *Staphylococcus saprophyticus*. JAMA 250:3063, 1983.
3. Mabeck CD: Significance of coagulase-negative staphylococcal bacteriuria. Lancet 2:1150, 1969.
4. Pereira AT: Coagulase-negative strains of staphylococcus possessing antigen 51 as agents of urinary infection. J Clin Pathol 15:252, 1962.
5. Hovelius B, Mardh P-A: *Staphylococcus saprophyticus* as a common cause of urinary tract infections. Rev Infect Dis 6:328, 1984.
6. Wallmark G, Arremark I, Telander B: *Staphylococcus saprophyticus*: A frequent cause of urinary tract infection among female outpatients. J Infect Dis 138:791, 1978.
7. Jordan PA, Irvani A, Richard GA, et al: Urinary tract infection caused by *Staphylococcus saprophyticus*. J Infect Dis 142:510, 1980.
8. Marrie TJ, Swantee CA, Hartlen M: Aerobic and anaerobic urethral flora of healthy females in various physiological age groups and females with urinary tract infections. J Clin Microbiol 11:654, 1980.
9. Demuth PJ, Gerding DN, Crossley K: *Staphylococcus aureus* bacteriuria. Arch Intern Med 139:78, 1979.
10. Manalo D, Mufson MA, Zollar IM, Mandad VN: Adenovirus infection in acute hemorrhagic cystitis: A study in 25 children. Am J Dis Child 121:281, 1971.
11. Maskell R, Pead L, Sanderson RA: Fastidious bacteria and the urethral syndrome. Lancet 2:1277, 1983.
12. Gargan RA, Brumfitt W, Hamilton-Miller JMT: Do anaerobes cause urinary infection? Lancet 1:37, 1980.
13. Fairley KF, Birch DF: Unconventional bacteria in urinary tract disease: *Gardnerella vaginalis*. Kidney Int 23:862, 1983.
14. Stamm WE, Running K, Hale J, Holmes KK: Etiologic role of *M. hominis* and *U. urealyticum* in women with the acute urethral syndrome. Sex Transm Dis 10:318S, 1983.
15. Thomsen AC: Mycoplasmas in human pyelonephritis: Demonstration of antibodies in serum and urine. J Clin Microbiol 8:197, 1978.
16. Bran JL, Levison ME, Kaye D: Entrance of bacteria into the female urinary bladder. N Engl J Med 259:626, 1972.
17. Abbott GD: Neonatal bacteriuria: A prospective study in 1460 infants. Br Med J 1:267, 1972.
18. Randolph MF, Greenfield M: The incidence of asymptomatic bacteriuria and pyuria in infancy. A study of 400 infants in private practice. J Pediatr 65:57, 1964.
19. Herzog LW: Urinary tract infections and circumcision. Am J Dis Child 143:348, 1989.
20. Smellie JM, Normand ICS: Bacteriuria, reflux and renal scarring. Arch Dis Child 50:581, 1975.
21. Editorial: Bacteriuria—When does it matter? Lancet 2:1155, 1979.
22. Kunin CM: The natural history of recurrent bacteriuria in school girls. N Engl J Med 282:1443, 1970.
23. Gillenwater JY, Harrison RB, Kunin CM: Natural history of bacteriuria in schoolgirls: A long-term case-control study. N Engl J Med 301:369, 1979.
24. Sanford JP: Urinary tract symptoms and infections. Annu Rev Med 26:485, 1975.
25. National Center for Health Statistics: Ambulatory medical care rendered in physicians' offices—United States—1975. Adv Data 12:1, 1977.
26. Barnes RC, Daifuku R, Roddy RE, Stamm WE: Urinary tract infection in sexually active homosexual men. Lancet 2:171, 1986.
27. Spach DH, Stapleton AE, Stamm WE: Lack of circumcision increases the risk of urinary tract infection in young men. JAMA 267:679, 1992.
28. Lipsky BA: Urinary tract infections in men. Epidemiology, pathophysiology, diagnosis, and treatment. Ann Intern Med 110:138, 1989.
29. Stamey TA, Timothy M, Millar M, Mikhara G: Recurrent urinary tract infections in adult women. The role of introital enterobacteria. Calif Med 115:1, 1971.
30. Svanborg-Eden C, Hausson S, Jodal U, et al: Host-parasite interaction in the urinary tract. J Infect Dis 157:421, 1988.
31. Nicolle LE, Harding GKM, Preiksaitis J, Ronald AR: The association of urinary tract infections with sexual intercourse. J Infect Dis 146:579, 1982.
32. Stamey TA: Pathogenesis and Treatment of Urinary Tract Infections. Baltimore, Williams & Wilkins, 1972.
33. Hooton TM, Hillier S, Johnson C, et al: *Escherichia coli* bacteriuria and contraceptive method. JAMA 265:64, 1991.
34. Strom BL, Collins M, West SL, et al: Sexual activity, contraceptive use, and other risk factors for symptomatic and asymptomatic bacteriuria: A case-control study. Ann Intern Med 107:816, 1987.
35. Herthelius BM, Hedström KG, Möllby R, et al: Pathogenesis of urinary tract infections—Amoxicillin induces genital *E. coli* colonization. Infection 5:263, 1988.
36. Reid G, Sobel JD: Bacterial adherence in the pathogenesis of urinary tract infection: A review. Rev Infect Dis 9:470, 1987.
37. Svanborg-Eden C, Jodal U: Attachment of *E. coli* to urinary sediment epithelial cells from urinary tract infection–prone and healthy children. Infect Immun 26:837, 1979.
38. Schaeffer AJ, Jones JM, Dunn JK: Association of in vitro *E. coli* adherence to vaginal and buccal epithelial cells with susceptibility of women to recurrent urinary tract infections. N Engl J Med 304:1062, 1981.
39. Kinane DF, Blackwell CC, Brettle RP, et al: ABO blood group, secretor state, and susceptibility to recurrent urinary tract infection in women. Br Med J 285:7, 1982.
40. Lomberg H, Cedergren B, Leffler H, et al: Influence of blood group on the availability of receptors for attachment of uropathogenic *E. coli*. Infect Immun 51:919, 1986.
41. Stapleton A, Nudelman E, Clausen H, et al: Binding of uropathogenic *Escherichia coli* R45 to glycolipids extracted from vaginal epithelial cells is dependent on the histo–blood group secretor status. J Clin Invest 90:965, 1992.
42. Reid G, Brooks HJK, Bacon DF: In vitro attachment of *E. coli* to human epithelial cells: Variation in receptivity during the menstrual cycle and pregnancy. J Infect Dis 148:412, 1983.
43. Schaefer AJ, Jones JM, Falkowski WS, et al: Variable adherence of uropathogenic *Escherichia coli* to epithelial cells from women with recurrent urinary tract infection. J Urol 128:1227, 1982.
44. Svanborg-Edén C, Hanson LÅ, Jodal U, et al: Variable adherence to normal urinary tract epithelial cells of *Escherichia coli* strains associated with various forms of urinary tract infections. Lancet 2:490, 1976.
45. Bjorksten B, Kaijser B: Interaction of human serum and neutrophils with *Escherichia coli* strains: Difference between strains isolated from urine of patients with pyelonephritis or asymptomatic bacteriuria. Infect Immun 22:308, 1978.
46. Hughs C, Hacker J, Roberts A, Boegel A: Hemolysin production as a virulence marker in symptomatic and asymptomatic urinary tract infections caused by *Escherichia coli*. Infect Immun 39:546, 1983.
47. Blanco J, Blanco M, Alonso MP, et al: Characteristics of haemolytic *Escherichia coli* with particular reference to production of cytotoxic necrotizing factor type 1 (CNF1). Res Microbiol 143:869, 1992.

48. Johnson JR, Goullet P, Picard B, et al: Association of carboxylesterase B electrophoretic pattern with expression of urovirulence factor determinants and antimicrobial resistance among strains of *Escherichia coli* that cause urosepsis. Infect Immun 59:2311, 1991.
49. Johnson JR, Moseley SL, Roberts PL, Stamm WE: Aerobactin and other virulence genes among strains of *E. coli* causing urosepsis: Association with patient characteristics. Infect Immun 56:405, 1988.
50. Roberts AP, Phillips R: Bacteria causing symptomatic urinary tract infection or bacteriuria. J Clin Pathol 32:492, 1979.
51. Reid G, Sobel JD: Bacterial adherence in the pathogenesis of urinary tract infection—A review. Rev Infect Dis 9:470, 1987.
52. Korhonen TK, Leffler H, Svanborg-Eden C: Binding specificity of piliated strains of *Escherichia coli* and *Salmonella typhimurium* to epithelial cells, *Saccharomyces cerevisiae* cells and erythrocytes. Infect Immun 32:796, 1981.
53. Ofek I, Mirelman D, Sharon N: Adherence of *Escherichia coli* to human mucosal cells mediated by mannose receptors. Nature 265:623, 1977.
54. Väisänen V, Tallgren LG, Mäkelä PH, et al: Mannose resistant haemagglutination and P antigen recognition are characteristic of *Escherichia coli* causing primary pyelonephritis. Lancet 2:1366, 1981.
55. Leffler H, Svanborg-Eden C: Glycolipid receptors for uropathogenic *E. coli* on human erythrocytes and uroepithelial cells. Infect Immun 34:920, 1981.
56. Källenius G, Möllby R, Svenson SB, et al: Identification of a carbohydrate receptor recognized by uropathogenic *Escherichia coli*. Infection 8(Suppl 3):5288, 1980.
57. Källenius G, Svenson SB, Hultberg H, et al: Occurrence of P-fimbriated *Escherichia coli* in urinary tract infections. Lancet 2:1369, 1981.
58. Nowicki B, Moulds J, Hull R, Hull S: A hemagglutinin of uropathogenic *E. coli* recognizes the Dr blood group antigen. Infect Immun 56:1057, 1988.
59. Aronson M, Medalia O, Schori L, et al: Prevention of colonization of the urinary tract of mice with *Escherichia coli* by blocking of bacterial adherence with methyl-α-D-mannopryanoside. J Infect Dis 139:329, 1979.
60. O'Hanley PD, Lark D, Falkow S, Schoolnik G: A globoside binding *E. coli* pilus vaccine prevents pyelonephritis (Abstr). Clin Res 31:372, 1983.
61. O'Hanley P, Lark D, Falkow S, Schoolnik G: Molecular basis of *Escherichia coli* colonization of the upper urinary tract in BALB/c mice: Gal-Gal pili immunization prevents *Escherichia coli* pyelonephritis in the BALB/c mouse model of human pyelonephritis. J Clin Invest 75:347, 1985.
62. Stamm WE, Hooton TM, Johnson JR, et al: Urinary tract infections: From pathogenesis to treatment. J Infect Dis 159:635, 1989.
63. Sobel JD: Pathogenesis of urinary tract infections. Host defenses. Infect Dis Clin North Am 1:855, 1987.
64. Kaye D: Antibacterial activity of human urine. J Clin Invest 47:237, 1968.
65. Stamey TA, Fair WR, Timothy MM: Antibacterial nature of prostatic fluid. Nature 218:444, 1968.
66. Ørskov S, Ferencz A, Ørskov F: Tamm-Horsfall protein or uromucoid in the normal urinary slime that traps type 1 fimbriated *Escherichia coli*. Lancet 1:887, 1980.
67. Mulholland SG: Lower urinary tract antibacterial defense mechanisms. Invest Urol 17:93, 1979.
68. Ko YC, Mukaida N, Ishiyama S, et al: Elevated interleukin-8 levels in the urine of patients with urinary tract infections. Infect Immun 61:1307, 1993.
69. De Man P, Jodal U, Van Kooten C, Svanborg C: Bacterial adherence as a virulence factor in urinary tract infection. APMIS 98:1053, 1990.
70. Rene P, Silverblatt FJ: Serological response to *Escherichia coli* pili in pyelonephritis. Infect Immun 37:749, 1982.
71. Rene P, Dinolfo M, Silverblatt FJ: Serum and urogenital antibody response to *Escherichia coli* pili in cystitis. Infect Immun 38:542, 1982.
72. Bran JL, Levison ME, Kaye D: Entrance of bacteria into the female urinary bladder. N Engl J Med 259:626, 1972.
73. Komaroff AL: Acute dysuria in women. N Engl J Med 310:368, 1984.
74. Jones SR, Smith JW, Sanford JP: Localization of urinary tract infection by detection of antibody-coated bacteria in urine sediment. N Engl J Med 290:591, 1974.
75. Latham RH, Stamm WE: Role of fimbriated *Escherichia coli* in urinary tract infection in adult women: Correlation with localization studies. J Infect Dis 149:835, 1984.
76. Wong ES, Fennell CL, Stamm WE: Urinary tract infection among women attending a clinic for sexually transmitted diseases. Sex Transm Dis 11:18, 1984.
77. Johnson JR, Stamm WE: Diagnosis and treatment of acute urinary tract infections. Infect Dis Clin North Am 1:773, 1987.
78. Fairley KF, Carson NE, Gutch RC, et al: Site of infection in acute urinary tract infection in general practice. Lancet 2:615, 1971.
79. Stamey TA, Govan DE, Palmer JM: The localization and treatment of urinary tract infections: The role of bactericidal urine levels as opposed to serum levels. Medicine (Baltimore) 44:1, 1965.
80. Thomas V, Shelokov A, Forland M: Antibody-coated bacteria in the urine and the site of urinary tract infection. N Engl J Med 290:588, 1974.
81. Johnson JR, Lyons MF 2d, Pearce W, et al: Therapy for women hospitalized with acute pyelonephritis: A randomized trial of ampicillin versus trimethoprim-sulfamethoxazole for 14 days. J Infect Dis 103:325, 1991.
82. Ahlering TE, Boyd SD, Hamilton CL, et al: Emphysematous pyelonephritis: A 5-year experience with 13 patients. J Urol 134:1086, 1985.
83. Bahnson RR: Urosepsis. Urol Clin North Am 13:627, 1986.
84. Cattell WR: Urinary tract infections in adults—1985. Postgrad Med J 61:907, 1985.
85. Anderson RU: Urinary tract infections in compromised hosts. Urol Clin North Am 13:727, 1986.
86. Preheim LC: Complicated urinary tract infections. Am J Med 79:62, 1985.
87. Sobel JD, Kaye D: Urinary tract infections. *In* Mandell GL, Douglas RG Jr, Bennett JE (eds): Principles and Practice of Infectious Diseases, ed 2. New York, John Wiley & Sons, 1985.
88. Cohen SN, Kass EH: A simple method for quantitative urine culture. N Engl J Med 277:176, 1967.
89. Stamm WE: Recent developments in the diagnosis and treatment of urinary tract infections. West J Med 137:213, 1982.
90. Stamm WE, Counts GW, Running KR, et al: Diagnosis of coliform infection in acutely dysuric women. N Engl J Med 307:463, 1982.
91. Stamm WE: Quantitative urine cultures revisited (Editorial). Eur J Clin Microbiol 3:279, 1984.
92. Bollgren I, Engström CF, Hammarlind M, et al: Low urinary counts of P-fimbriated *Escherichia coli* in presumed acute pyelonephritis. Arch Dis Child 59:102, 1984.
93. Pappas PG: Laboratory in the diagnosis and management of urinary tract infections. J Gen Intern Med 75:313, 1991.
94. Carroll KC, Hale DC, Von Boerum DH, et al: Laboratory evaluation of urinary tract infections in an ambulatory clinic. Am J Clin Pathol 101:100, 1994.
95. Jenkins RD, Fenn JP, Matsen JM: Review of urine microscopy for bacteriuria. JAMA 255:3397, 1986.
96. Schultz HJ, McCaffrey LA, Keys TF, Nobrega FT: Acute cystitis: A prospective study of laboratory tests and duration of therapy. Mayo Clin Proc 59:391, 1984.
97. Carlson KJ, Mulley AG: Management of acute dysuria: A decision-analysis model of alternative strategies. Ann Intern Med 102:244, 1985.
98. Stamm WE, Hooton TM: Management of urinary tract infections in adults. N Engl J Med 329:1328, 1993.
99. Stamm WE: When should we use urine cultures? Infect Control 7:431, 1986.
100. Kunin CM: Detection, Prevention and Management of Urinary Tract Infections, ed 4. Philadelphia, Lea & Febiger, 1987.
101. Bailey RR: Single-dose therapy for uncomplicated urinary tract infections. N Z Med J 98:327, 1985.
102. Sheehan G, Harding GKM, Ronald AR: Advances in the treatment of urinary tract infection. Am J Med 76:141, 1984.
103. Fihn SD: Single-dose antimicrobial therapy for urinary tract infections: "Less is more"? or "Reductio ad absurdum"? (Editorial). J Gen Intern Med 1:62, 1986.
104. Philbrick JT, Bracikowski JP: Single-dose antibiotic treatment

for uncomplicated urinary tract infections. Arch Intern Med 145:1672, 1985.
105. Glauser MP, Lyons JM, Braude AI: Prevention of pyelonephritis due to *Escherichia coli* in rats with gentamicin stored in kidney tissue. J Infect Dis 139:172, 1979.
106. Charlton CAC, Crowther A, Davies JG, et al: Three-day and ten-day chemotherapy for urinary tract infections in general practice. Br Med J 1:124, 1976.
107. McCue JD: Urinary tract infection and dysuria. Cost-conscious evaluation and antibiotic therapy. Postgrad Med 80:133, 1986.
108. Stamm WE, McKevitt M, Counts GW: Acute renal infection in women: Treatment with trimethoprim-sulfamethoxazole or ampicillin for two or six weeks. A randomized trial. Ann Intern Med 106:341, 1987.
109. Patton JP, Nash DB, Abrutyn E: Urinary tract infections: Cost considerations. Med Clin North Am 75:495, 1991.
110. Ronald AR: Optimal duration of treatment for kidney infection (Editorial). Ann Intern Med 106:467, 1987.
111. Stamey TA: Recurrent urinary tract infections in female patients: An overview of management and treatment. Rev Infect Dis 9(Suppl 2):S195, 1987.
112. Bailey RR, Peddie BA: Treatment of acute urinary tract infection in women (Letter). Ann Intern Med 107:430, 1987.
113. Jernelius H, Zbornik J, Bauer C: One or three week treatment of acute pyelonephritis. A double-blind comparison using a fixed combination of pivampicillin plus pivmecillinam. Acta Med Scand 223:469, 1988.
114. Kaitz AL, Hodder EW: Bacteriuria and pyelonephritis of pregnancy: A prospective study of 616 women. N Engl J Med 265:667, 1961.
115. Nicolle LE, Mayhew WJ, Bryan C: Prospective randomized comparison of therapy and no therapy for asymptomatic bacteriuria in elderly institutionalized women. Am J Med 83:27, 1987.
116. Wong EW, Stamm WE: Urethral infections in men and women. Annu Rev Med 34:337, 1983.
117. Dontas AS, Kasviki-Charvati P, Papanayiotou PC: Bacteriuria and survival in old age. N Engl J Med 304:939, 1981.
118. Kraft JK, Stamey TA: The natural history of symptomatic recurrent bacteriuria in women. Medicine (Baltimore) 56:55, 1947.
119. Stamm WE, Counts GW, Wagner KF, et al: Antimicrobial prophylaxis of recurrent urinary tract infection. Ann Intern Med 92:770, 1980.
120. Wong ES, McKevitt M, Running K, et al: Management of recurrent urinary tract infections with patient-administered single-dose therapy. Ann Intern Med 102:302, 1985.
121. Stapleton A, Latham R, Johnson C, Stamm WE: Post-coital antimicrobial prophylaxis for recurrent urinary tract infection: A randomized, double-blind, placebo-controlled trial. JAMA 264:703, 1990.
122. Stamm WE: Prevention of urinary tract infections. Am J Med 76(Suppl 5A):148, 1984.
123. Stamm WE, Counts GW, McKevitt M, et al: Urinary prophylaxis with trimethoprim and trimethoprim-sulfamethoxazole—Efficacy, influence on the natural history of recurrent bacteriuria, and cost control. Rev Infect Dis 4:450, 1982.
124. Romano JM, Kaye D: UTI in the elderly: Common yet atypical. Geriatrics 36:113, 1981.
125. Stamey TA, Sexton CC: The role of vaginal colonization with Enterobacteriaceae in recurrent urinary tract infections. J Urol 113:214, 1975.
126. Raz R, Stamm WE: A controlled trial of intravaginal estrogen in postmenopausal women with recurrent urinary tract infection. N Engl J Med 329:753, 1993.
127. Norden CW, Kass EH: Bacteriuria of pregnancy: A critical appraisal. Annu Rev Med 19:431, 1968.
128. Kincaid-Smith P: Bacteriuria in pregnancy. Lancet 1:395, 1965.
129. Vercaigne LM, Zhanel GG: Recommended treatment for urinary tract infection in pregnancy. Ann Pharmacother 28:248, 1994.
130. Stamm WE, Martin SM, Bennett JV: Epidemiology of nosocomial infections due to gram-negative bacilli: Aspects relevant to the use of vaccines. J Infect Dis 136(Suppl):S151, 1977.
131. Kreger BE, Craven DE, Carling PC, McCabe WR: Gram-negative bacteriuria. III: Reassessment of aetiology, epidemiology, and ecology in 612 patients. Am J Med 68:332, 1980.
132. Platt R, Polk BF, Murdock B, Rosner B: Mortality associated with nosocomial urinary tract infection. N Engl J Med 307:637, 1982.
133. Stamm WE: Catheter-associated urinary tract infections: Epidemiology, pathogenesis, and prevention. Am J Med 91(Suppl 3B):3B-65S, 1991.
134. Butler HK, Kunin CM: Evaluation of polymyxin catheter lubricant and impregnated catheter. J Urol 100:560, 1968.
135. Schaeffer AJ, Story KO, Johnson SM: Effect of silver oxide/trichlorolsoganuric acid antimicrobial drainage system on catheter-associated bacteriuria. J Urol 139:69, 1988.
136. Johnson JR, Roberts PR, Olsen RJ, et al: Prevention of catheter-associated urinary tract infection with a silver oxide-coated urinary catheter: Clinical and microbiological correlates. J Infect Dis 162:1145, 1990.
137. Wong-Beringer A, Jacobs RA, Guglielmo BJ: Treatment of funguria. JAMA 267:2780, 1992.
138. Sanford JP: The enigma of candiduria: Evolution of bladder irrigation with amphotericin B for management—from anecdote to dogma and a lesson from Machiavelli. Clin Infect Dis 16:145, 1993.

107

Urethritis, Prostatitis, Epididymitis, and Orchitis

Edwin M. Meares, Jr.

Urethritis

Inflammations and infections of the urethra are exceedingly common in male and female patients and arise from a wide range of inciting causes. In male patients, urethritis most commonly is caused by sexually transmitted organisms: *Neisseria gonorrhoeae, Chlamydia trachomatis*, and *Ureaplasma urealyticum*. In female patients, urethritis most often presents as the acute urethral syndrome, or urethrocystitis, caused by infections with coliforms and *Staphylococcus saprophyticus*, and less often with *C. trachomatis* and *N. gonorrhoeae*.

Gonococcal Urethritis in Male Patients

Urethritis, the most common clinical manifestation of gonorrhea in men, typically occurs after an incubation period of 2 to 7 days. Most patients present with dysuria and a purulent urethral discharge, singly or in combination. About 20% to 30% of heterosexual men with symptomatic gonococcal urethritis are also infected with *C. trachomatis*.[1] Unless therapy is given concurrently for this organism, these men develop postgonococcal urethritis after single-dose, gonococcus-specific therapy. An estimated 1% to 5% of men with gonococcal urethritis are asymptomatic, do not seek medical attention, and serve as a reservoir, transmitting disease to uninfected sexual partners.[1] Acute epididymitis and urethral strictures are the most common genitourinary tract complications of gonococcal urethritis.

The diagnosis of gonococcal urethritis in symptomatic men is confirmed with about 95% sensitivity and specificity when Gram-stained smears of urethral discharge disclose gram-negative diplococci within polymorphonuclear leukocytes.[1] Absolute confirmation is made by culture of urethral specimens on selective media (e.g., Thayer-Martin medium), incubation in a moist environment in 5% carbon dioxide atmosphere at 34°C to 36°C, and identification of *N. gonorrhoeae* organisms. Antimicrobial susceptibility tests are desirable if available.

A summary of key papers presented at a symposium held at the Centers for Disease Control and Prevention in Atlanta outlined background issues that led to its 1993 Sexually Transmitted Disease Treatment Guidelines. Moran and Levine[3] concluded: "Many single-dose antimicrobial regimens are effective against uncomplicated urogenital and rectal gonorrhea. Of those available in the United States, ceftriaxone, 125 mg IM [intramuscularly], cefixime, 400 mg orally, ciprofloxacin, 500 mg orally, and ofloxacin, 400 mg orally, appear to offer the best balance of proven efficacy and safety." Ceftriaxone and cefixime appear to be effective against incubating syphilis; cefixime is questionably effective; and neither ciprofloxacin nor ofloxacin is effective against *Treponema pallidum*.[3] Currently, spectinomycin, 2 g intramuscularly, is recommended for treatment of gonorrhea only in persons who cannot tolerate cephalosporins or quinolones.

Weber and Johnson[4] have reviewed new treatments for *C. trachomatis* and concluded that azithromycin and ofloxacin are the most important agents. Although there are many acceptable ways to treat simultaneous infections with *N. gonorrhoeae* and *C. trachomatis*, the following appear to be most efficacious and safe: ceftriaxone, 125 mg intramuscularly, plus doxycycline, 100 mg orally twice daily for 7 days; ceftriaxone, 125 mg intramuscularly, plus azithromycin, 1 g orally once; ofloxacin, 400 mg orally twice daily for 7 days.

Nongonococcal Urethritis in Male Patients

Nongonococcal urethritis (NGU), caused mainly by *C. trachomatis* and occasionally by *U. urealyticum*, is the most common form of male urethritis in the United States.[1, 2] The incubation period is typically 7 to 21 days. The clinical manifestation is dysuria or urethral discharge, or both. The dysuria is variable, often absent, and sometimes associated with urethral itching; the discharge is typically mucoid to watery and is less pronounced and purulent than that of gonorrhea. An estimated 10% of men with NGU are asymptomatic.[1] The diagnosis of NGU is usually established by failure to demonstrate gonococci on Gram stain examination and on culture in a male patient who has four or more polymorphonuclear leukocytes per high-power field at microscopy of a urethral smear or sediment from a 10-mL sample of first-voided urine. Infection caused by *C. trachomatis* can be confirmed by direct immunofluorescence with monoclonal antibodies when this test is available; otherwise, infection caused by *C. trachomatis* or *U. urealyticum* is confirmed only by means of special tissue culture techniques. Potential genitourinary tract complications of NGU include epididymitis and urethral strictures; however, the most serious consequence is the potential transmission of *C. trachomatis* to a female sexual partner, who may develop ascending infection and serious sequelae.

The recommended treatment of NGU is doxycycline, 100 mg by mouth twice daily for 7 days, or ofloxacin, 400 mg orally twice daily for 7 days, or azithromycin, 1 g orally once. Whenever possible, sexual partners should be treated simultaneously.

Acute Urethral Syndrome in Female Patients

The acute urethral syndrome consists of dysuria and frequency (plus variable other lower tract symptoms) in women whose bladder urine on culture shows no growth or low bacteria counts. Stamm and coworkers[5] observed that the bladder urine of women with acute lower urinary tract symptoms often contains significantly fewer bacterial colony-forming units (CFUs) than the traditional diagnostic criterion of at least 100,000 per mL midstream urine. Indeed, only 51% of women with symptomatic urinary tract infection (UTI) caused by coliform bacteria were identified by using the diagnostic criterion of at least 100,000 CFU/mL. Moreover, these investigators showed that a count of at least 100 CFU/mL in the clean-voided urine of a symptomatic woman with acute dysuria was a sensitive and specific indicator of true coliform infection (as defined by culture of a catheterized or suprapubic aspirate specimen). Fihn and Stamm[6] have categorized acutely dysuric women into groups for whom there are specific therapeutic implications:

1. Vaginitis (32%)
2. Typical cystitis, with growth of at least 100,000 CFU/mL midstream urine (32%)
3. Acute urethral syndrome (36%)
   a. Pyuria
      Bladder bacteriuria less than 100,000 CFU/mL (15%)
      C. trachomatis infection (7%)
   b. No pyuria, sterile urine (12%)
   c. Other pathogens, including herpes simplex virus and *N. gonorrhoeae* (2%)

To properly treat the acute urethral syndrome, the clinician must recognize the underlying cause. Many women with pyuria and "low-count" bacteriuria actually have bacterial urethrocystitis and should be treated with pathogen-specific antimicrobial therapy. In a second group, cultures are positive for organisms that may be transmitted sexually. These women and their sexual partners should be treated with an appropriate regimen: doxycycline, ofloxacin, or azithromycin for *C. trachomatis* infection; ceftriaxone plus doxycycline or azithromycin, or ofloxacin alone for gonorrhea (for routes of administration and dosing see under urethritis in male patients earlier). In a third group, no causative agent is identified, but, curiously, the dysuria still responds to antimicrobial therapy (e.g., doxycycline, 100 mg by mouth twice daily for 10 days). A small group of women with no pyuria and no apparent pathogen respond poorly to antimicrobial therapy. Some of them apparently have a functional voiding abnormality and respond to therapy with an α-adrenergic blocking agent, such as prazosin, 1 or 2 mg by mouth twice daily.[7] Still others' symptoms improve during therapy with an anticholinergic agent (e.g., oxybutynin chloride, 5 mg by mouth three times daily) or diazepam (2 to 5 mg by mouth three times daily).

Excretory urography is seldom warranted in evaluation; however, in cases of recurrent acute urethral syndrome, cystoscopy helps to rule out specific urethral abnormalities such as diverticula. Bladder biopsy may be necessary to rule out interstitial cystitis or mucosal dysplasia. Videourodynamic testing may demonstrate a primary voiding dysfunction in women who have sterile cultures and no pyuria and who respond poorly to empirical antimicrobial therapy.[7] Women prone to recurrent bouts of acute urethral syndrome caused by recurrent bacterial infection are best managed by use of long-term, low-dose, preventive antibacterial therapy.

Prostatitis

Inflammatory disorders of the prostate gland are common but confusing because they occur in distinct forms—prostatitis syndromes. Therapeutic outcomes therefore vary with the clinician's ability to recognize and properly treat specific types of prostatitis. Common, uncommon, and suspected but not proved types of prostatitis are shown in Table 107–1. The most common varieties—acute bacterial prostatitis (ABP), chronic bacterial prostatitis (CBP), nonbacterial prostatitis

TABLE 107–1 ■ Classification of Prostatitis

Common types	
	Acute bacterial prostatitis
	Chronic bacterial prostatitis
	Chronic bacterial prostatitis with infected calculi
	Nonbacterial prostatitis
	Prostatodynia
Uncommon types	
	Gonococcal prostatitis
	Tuberculous prostatitis
	Parasitic prostatitis
	Mycotic prostatitis
	Nonspecific granulomatous prostatitis
	Noneosinophilic variety
	Eosinophilic variety
Suspected but unproven types	
	Prostatitis due to *Ureaplasma* species (*Mycoplasma* species)
	Prostatitis due to *Chlamydia trachomatis*
	Prostatitis due to viruses

(NBP), and prostatodynia (PD)—have many similar features and certain distinctive ones.

Bacterial prostatitis is associated with UTI, positive cultures localizing the pathogen to the prostatic secretions, and excessive inflammatory cells (leukocytes and macrophages containing fat particles) in the expressed prostatic secretions (EPS). ABP is an abrupt, febrile illness with marked constitutional and genitourinary tract signs and symptoms; CBP is a less dramatic disorder featuring relapsing recurrent UTI caused by persistence of the pathogen in the prostatic secretory system despite courses of antibacterial therapy. Patients with NBP, in contrast, have excessive numbers of inflammatory cells in their EPS despite a typically negative history of documented UTI and negative results of urinary and prostatic fluid cultures. This syndrome is called NBP because no infectious organism can be found. Patients with PD have symptoms that suggest prostatitis but have no history of UTI and normal EPS by microscopy and culture.

Etiology and Pathogenesis

The pathogens in bacterial prostatitis are similar in type and distribution to those that cause UTIs: strains of *Escherichia coli* predominate; however, infections caused by other Enterobacteriaceae and *Pseudomonas* species also occur.[8]

Among my patients who have documented CBP, about 82% are infected with a single pathogen and the remainder by two or more pathogens.[8] The role of gram-positive bacteria as agents of prostatitis is controversial. Enterococci do cause bacterial prostatitis and associated recurrent enterococcal bacteriuria. Likewise, hospital-acquired, catheter-associated prostatitis caused by *Staphylococcus aureus* is found occasionally.[8] The causative role in prostatitis of other gram-positive bacteria (e.g., coagulase-negative staphylococci, micrococci, non–group D streptococci, diphtheroids) is doubtful. These organisms are not reproducibly localized to the prostate and do not cause relapsing recurrent UTI as do gram-negative pathogens and enterococci.[8]

Possible routes of bacterial infection of the prostate include (1) ascending urethral infection, (2) reflux of infected urine into prostatic ducts that empty into the posterior urethra, (3) invasion by rectal bacteria by direct extension or lymphatic spread, and (4) hematogenous infection.

Blacklock[9] and Stamey[10] independently studied men with CBP and their female sexual partners and concluded that some men probably develop bacterial prostatitis as a consequence of ascending urethral infection resulting from urethral inoculation during sexual relations. Because they are frequently associated with urethral colonization by pathogenic bacteria and ascending UTI, both urethral catheter and condom catheter drainage systems can produce bacterial prostatitis.[8] In addition, bacterial prostatitis is known to develop after transurethral prostatectomy in men who have infected urine.

Studies have shown that urine commonly refluxes into prostatic ducts and that intraprostatic urinary reflux probably is the most important route for introducing bacteria into the prostate.[8] Moreover, high-grade intraprostatic urinary reflux with sterile urine may be the cause of nonbacterial, "chemical" forms of prostatitis.[11]

Diagnosis

GENERAL LABORATORY FINDINGS

Prostatic massage for microscopy and culture of the EPS is important in the diagnosis of prostatitis syndromes; however, accurate interpretation is impossible unless the first-voided 10 mL of urine (urethral specimen) and a midstream urine sample (bladder specimen) obtained immediately before prostatic massage are also evaluated. Inflammatory cells and bacteria of nonprostatic origin can easily contaminate the EPS and lead to erroneous conclusions.[8, 12] The same concerns apply to isolated microscopy and culture of semen. When urethral and midstream urine specimens show insignificant pyuria, the finding of at least 15 white blood cells per high-power field denotes prostatic inflammation.[8, 12] Another important sign of prostatitis is large numbers of macrophages containing fat droplets in the prostatic secretions.[8, 12] Whereas an excessive number of inflammatory cells in the prostatic secretions denotes prostatic inflammation, it does not distinguish bacterial prostatitis from nonbacterial forms.

Bacterial prostatitis, and to a lesser extent NBP, is associated with secretory dysfunction of the prostate gland.[8, 12] Although most of the physical and chemical characteristics of the prostatic secretions are altered, the most important changes are increased alkalinity of the secretions and depressed levels of zinc. This secretory dysfunction, especially increased alkalinity of the secretions, affects pharmacokinetics, and the depressed zinc level may increase the susceptibility of the prostate to bacterial infection.[8, 13] (Zinc serves as a potent antibacterial factor against bacterial prostatitis and ascending UTI in men.[14]) The specificity of these markers in the differential diagnosis of prostatitis syndromes, however, remains undefined.

Bacterial prostatitis quickly leads to the elaboration of pathogen-specific antibody in the serum and especially in the prostatic fluid of patients.[15] This immune response is an important investigative tool for confirming bacterial prostatitis and following the response to treatment.[16]

In patients with ABP that is cured by antimicrobial therapy, antigen-specific immunoglobulin (Ig) G in both serum and prostatic fluid is elevated at the onset of the infection but declines slowly in the ensuing 6 to 12 months. On the other hand, the level of antigen-specific IgA in prostatic fluid rises significantly at the onset of infection and begins to decline only after 12 months, whereas an initial elevation of IgA in the serum disappears after only 1 month.

In patients with CBP that is cured by antimicrobial therapy, levels of antigen-specific IgA and IgG in prostatic fluid are elevated at the onset of treatment but begin to decline slowly to normal levels—IgG after about 6 months and IgA not until about 24 months. Patients with CBP that is not cured by antimicrobial therapy have persistently elevated levels of antigen-specific IgG and IgA in prostatic fluid.

BACTERIOLOGIC LOCALIZATION CULTURES

The clinician can easily and accurately confirm the diagnosis of bacterial prostatitis, especially CBP, by performing bacterial localization cultures. This method, first introduced in 1968 by Meares and Stamey,[17] is reliable when carried out properly. Culture of prostatic fluid from a man with CBP often grows small numbers of bacteria. Because CBP is usually a focal tissue infection, no absolute count of bacterial colonies on culture is diagnostic. Instead, the bacterial counts in specimens of urethral and midstream bladder urine and of EPS—all obtained at the same time—must be compared. Both careful collection of segmented specimens and immediate culturing after collection (Fig. 107–1, Table 107–2) and the application of microbiologic techniques capable of quantifying small numbers of bacteria are essential for proper diagnosis.

If the bladder urine is sterile or nearly so, urethral colonization or infection is indicated by a much higher count in the first 10 mL of urine that is passed (VB_1) than in either the EPS or the first 10 mL of urine voided after prostatic massage (VB_3). With bacterial prostatitis, the reverse is true. If culture of bladder urine (VB_2) shows heavy bacteriuria, 2 or 3 days' treatment with an antimicrobial agent that is active in urine but not in prostatic tissue (e.g., 500 mg penicillin G by mouth every 6 hours or 100 mg nitrofurantoin by mouth every 8 hours) should be given before segmented specimens are collected. The diagnosis of CBP is best confirmed when the numbers of pathogenic bacteria in the prostatic specimens exceed by at least 10-fold those in the VB_1 and VB_2 specimens.

Acute Bacterial Prostatitis

ABP is an acute infection of the prostate typically caused by enteric bacteria, mainly coliforms (especially *E. coli*) and *Pseudomonas aeruginosa*.[8, 16] Because the clinical presentation of ABP is well defined, the clinician usually makes the diagnosis without difficulty, although the nonurologist may mistakenly think the patient has acute pyelonephritis. The typical clinical picture is sudden onset of chills, fever, perineal and low back pain, and symptoms of both irritative and obstructive voiding dysfunction. On examination, the prostate is tender, swollen, indurated, and warm. These findings alone are usually sufficient for a presumptive diagnosis of ABP. Some patients develop acute bacterial epididymitis; some experience transient bacteremia. Other findings are generalized malaise and prostration, arthralgia, myalgia, and acute urinary retention.

Prostatic secretions are typically abnormal: at microscopy numerous leukocytes and macrophages packed with fat droplets are seen; culture shows heavy growth of the bacterial pathogen. Prostatic massage is not recommended, however, because it is painful for the patient and may lead to bacteremia. Because bacteriuria usually accompanies ABP, the causative agent can usually be identified by culture of voided urine.

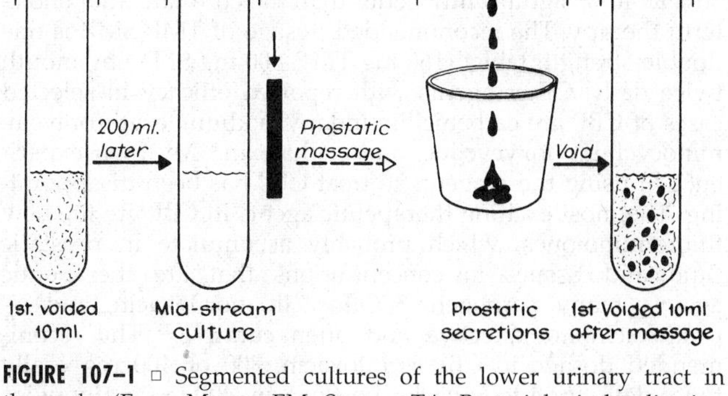

FIGURE 107–1 □ Segmented cultures of the lower urinary tract in the male. (From Meares EM, Stamey TA: Bacteriologic localization patterns in bacterial prostatitis and urethritis. Invest Urol 5:492–518, 1968.)

Patients with ABP usually respond promptly to pathogen-specific therapy, even with antimicrobial agents that normally diffuse poorly into prostatic secretions. The intense inflammation of ABP appears to allow drugs that are normally excluded to accumulate at therapeutic levels in the prostatic secretory system, interstitium, and stroma. Hospitalization may be necessary for patients who develop acute urinary retention or who need parenteral antimicrobial therapy.

Pathogen-specific antimicrobial therapy should be administered when the infecting organism can be identified by culture and sensitivity tests. While these results are pending, empirical therapy is indicated. For oral therapy, four excellent alternatives are trimethoprim-sulfamethoxazole (TMP-SMX), 160 mg TMP and 800 mg SMX; ofloxacin, 300 or 400 mg; norfloxacin, 400 mg; and ciprofloxacin, 500 mg; for each, the dosage is twice daily by mouth. For parenteral therapy, excellent choices are TMP-SMX, 8 to 10 mg/kg body weight (based on the TMP component) in two to four divided doses every 6, 8, or 12 hours intravenously, or gentamicin plus ampicillin (1 mg/kg gentamicin intravenously every 8 hours; 2 g ampicillin intravenously every 6 hours). If the clinical response and results of susceptibility tests are favorable, therapy should be continued at full dosage for a minimum of 30 days to prevent the development of CBP. Patients receiving parenteral therapy can usually be switched to a suitable oral agent within 1 week or as early as 48 hours after the fever subsides. Adjunctive therapy includes adequate hydration, analgesics, antipyretics, and stool softeners. Acute urinary retention is best managed by placing a punch suprapubic catheter under local anesthesia. Transurethral catheterization or instrumentation should be avoided.

With proper management, most patients with ABP are cured. Careful follow-up is indicated, however, because persistent infection of the prostate may develop. Another potential complication of ABP is prostatic abscess. Because prostatic abscess is seldom cured by antimicrobial therapy alone, a suspected abscess should be confirmed by means of transrectal ultrasonography or pelvic computed tomography. In addition to antimicrobial therapy, surgical or percutaneous drainage of the abscess is usually necessary.[18]

Chronic Bacterial Prostatitis

CBP has variable clinical features. Many patients have no histories of a preceding bout of ABP. Some men are asymptomatic and are found to have CBP only when bacteriuria is discovered incidentally. Most patients, however, complain of mild to moderate symptoms of irritative voiding dysfunction: urinary urgency, frequency, nocturia, and dysuria. Many patients complain of pain and discomfort in the low back and in the perineal, suprapubic, penile, scrotal, or groin areas. Some patients have hemospermia and postejaculatory discomfort, but chills and fever are unusual unless ABP evolves. Single or recurrent bouts of bacterial epididymitis occasionally develop. Rectal palpation of the prostate reveals nothing specific: the prostate may feel normal, variably indurated, tender, or boggy. The most characteristic feature of CBP is its unique role in causing relapsing, recurrent UTIs.[8, 12, 16] Because in patients with CBP most antimicrobial agents accumulate poorly in the prostatic secretory system (where the bacteria reside), these bacteria persist unaltered within the prostate during treatment. Therapy may sterilize the urine and resolve

TABLE 107–2 ▪ Segmented Cultures of 15 Men with Chronic Bacterial Prostatitis

		COLONIES PER MILLILITER				
PATIENT	**ANTIBIOTIC**	**VB_1***	**VB_2***	**EPS***	**VB_3***	**ORGANISM**
1	Yes	90	0	800	20	*Escherichia coli*
	No	10	0	1,000	20	*E. coli*
2	Yes	0	0	1,000	0	*Enterococcus*
	Yes	20	0	4,000	10	*Enterococcus*
3	Yes	50	0	165	150	*E. coli*
		0	0	50	20	*Enterobacter aerogenes*
		0	0	560	50	*Proteus mirabilis*
		0	0	140	0	*Proteus morganii*
	Yes	0	0	660	190	*E. coli*
		10	0	400	40	*E. aerogenes*
		0	0	500	20	*P. mirabilis*
		0	0	200	0	*P. morganii*
4	Yes	20	0	5,000	50	*Klebsiella*
	Yes	50	0	100,000	1,000	*Klebsiella*
5	No	60	0	1,000	20	*E. coli*
	No	640	40	100,000	220	*E. coli*
6	Yes	0	0	5,000	100	*E. coli*
	Yes	50	10	10,000	1,500	*E. coli*
7	Yes	120	0	3,600	370	*E. coli*
	No	2,000	200	100,000	4,000	*E. coli*
8	Yes	250	20	5,000	330	*Klebsiella*
	No	0	0	50	0	*Klebsiella*
	No	20	0	10,000	2,000	*Klebsiella*
9	Yes	10,000	150	100,000	10,000	*E. coli*
	Yes	110	0	1,500	810	*E. coli*
10	No	2,000	60	4,000	250	*Enterococcus*
	No	600	60	4,000	2,000	*Enterococcus*
	No	260	20	7,200	90	*Enterococcus*
	Yes	20	20	500	30	*Enterococcus*
11	Yes	30	0	10,000	—	*E. coli*
	Yes	0	0	3,600	—	*E. coli*
12	Yes	800	20	—	5,000	*E. coli*
	Yes	10,000	800	100,000	10,000	*E. coli*
13	No	0	0	10,000	600	*E. coli*
	Yes	0	0	7,000	10	*E. coli*
	Yes	0	0	4,000	120	*E. coli*
14	Yes	0	0	700	200	*P. mirabilis*
	Yes	30	0	1,000	10	*P. mirabilis*
15	Yes	2,500	300	20,000	10,000	*Pseudomonas*
	Yes	110	70	30,000	750	*Pseudomonas*

*VB_1, First 10 mL of urine voided (urethral culture); VB_2, midstream aliquot (bladder culture); EPS, expressed prostatic secretions from prostatic massage (prostatic culture), VB_3, first 10 mL of urine voided immediately after prostatic massage (prostatic culture).

From Meares EM Jr: Prostatitis and related disorders. *In* Walsh PC, Retik AB, Stamey TA, Vaughan ED Jr (eds): Campbell's Urology, ed 6. Philadelphia, WB Saunders, 1986, pp 807–822.

the symptoms, but after the patient stops the medication, the prostatic pathogen typically reinfects the urine and the symptoms of CBP recur.[8, 12, 16]

Prostatic calculi develop in postpubertal men with astonishing frequency. Transrectal ultrasonography indicates that prostatic stones are detected in about 75% of middle-aged men and in about 100% of elderly men.[19] Furthermore, ultrasonography demonstrates prostatic stones in about 70% of men who have no other radiographic signs of prostatic stones. Calculi within the prostate typically are not infected and cause no symptoms or harm, provided they remain confined to the prostate. In certain men with prostatic stones and relapsing, recurrent UTIs, however, the stones have proved to be infected and are the source of the relapsing UTIs.[20, 21] The condition is similar to infected renal calculi: the infection associated with infected prostatic calculi cannot be cured unless the stones are surgically removed. Because prostatic calculi are common and can become infected primarily or secondarily, infected calculi may play the most important role in the failure of antimicrobial therapy to cure CBP.

Several antimicrobial agents are said to be effective in the treatment of CBP, but TMP-SMX has the best cure rates confirmed in reported prospective studies.[8, 16] Among patients who received TMP-SMX at full dosage for 4 to 16 weeks, the rate of cure in various studies has been about 30% to 40%, significantly better than the cure rate after short-term therapy. The recommended dosage of TMP-SMX is one double-strength tablet (160 mg TMP, 800 mg SMX) by mouth twice daily. Other agents with reported efficacy in selected cases of CBP are carbenicillin indanyl sodium, erythromycin, minocycline, doxycycline, and cephalexin.[8] My own experience in using these agents to treat CBP has been disappointing. The most exciting therapeutic agents in CBP are the new fluoroquinolones, which probably accumulate in prostatic fluid and tissues in concentrations that are therapeutic against many pathogens.[22] Ofloxacin, norfloxacin, and ciprofloxacin are effective and often curative.[23] The recommended dosage in CBP is ofloxacin, 300 or 400 mg orally twice daily for 4 to 6 weeks, norfloxacin, 400 mg orally twice daily for 30 days, or ciprofloxacin, 500 mg orally twice daily for 30 days.

Patients who are not cured by medical therapy generally can be managed satisfactorily with long-term suppressive therapy using low-dose medication.[8, 12, 16] Two preferred regimens are TMP-SMX, one single-strength tablet (80 mg TMP, 400 mg SMX) by mouth daily, and nitrofurantoin, 100 mg once or twice daily by mouth. Patients who cannot be managed satisfactorily by medical therapy should be considered for surgical therapy. Appropriate antimicrobial therapy combined with thorough transurethral prostatectomy can be curative, provided all foci or infected tissue and calculi are removed.[24]

Nonbacterial Prostatitis and Prostatodynia

NBP is an inflammation of the prostate of inderminate cause. PD has been described as a special type of NBP in which patients have symptoms of NBP, especially those of a "pelvic pain syndrome," but no history of UTI and normal EPS at microscopy and culture.[25] Brunner and coworkers[26] studied approximately 600 men attending a special prostatitis clinic and found that 64% had NBP and 31% had PD. My experience and that of others.,[27] however, indicate that the term PD should probably be dropped. Indeed, patients with PD at times do show excessive numbers of white blood cells in their prostatic expressates.[16] Patients with PD and NBP have the same abnormalities on videourodynamic studies, and treatment of the two conditions is essentially the same.

The patient with NBP/PD typically is a man 20 to 45 years old who has variable symptoms of irritative and obstructive voiding dysfunction but has no history of UTI and has negative culture results. The person's EPS may or may not show excessive numbers of leukocytes. A predominant complaint is pain: perineal, suprapubic, scrotal, low back, or urethral, especially pain referred to the tip of the urethra. Although some patients have "tight" anal sphincters and tender prostates or paraprostatic tissues on digital rectal examination, physical examination discloses no specific abnormalities.

Studies by Kirby and coworkers[11] indicate that NBP/PD is a chemical prostatitis caused by the intraprostatic reflux of urine. Investigations of the cause of NBP/PD by several researchers generally have excluded as causative agents gram-positive bacteria (other than *Enterococcus* and *S. aureus*), fungi, obligate anaerobic bacteria, trichomonads, and viruses.[8, 16] The possible role of *Mycoplasma* species, *Ureaplasma* species, and *C. trachomatis* remains controversial,[8] but studies using cultures and immunologic tests in men with NBP/PD indicate these organisms are not agents of NBP/PD.[28–31]

Videourodynamic studies of patients with NBP/PD demonstrate that most have a spastic dysfunction of the bladder neck and prostatic urethra.[32–34] The postulated basis of symptoms in these patients is as follows: smooth muscle spasm of the bladder neck and prostatic urethra, resulting in intraprostatic and ejaculatory duct urinary reflux, which leads to a chemical prostatitis, seminal vesiculitis, and even epididymitis. Some patients with NBP/PD appear to suffer mainly from tension myalgia of the pelvic floor.[34] Symptoms in these patients are thought to arise from habitual contraction and spasm of the pelvic floor skeletal muscles. Still other patients with NBP/PD seem to have stress as a primary cause.

The bladder neck and prostate are rich in α-adrenergic receptors; therefore, α-adrenergic blocking agents can reduce or eliminate the smooth muscle spasm that leads to the clinical symptoms in NBP/PD. The use of α-blockade is therefore the most important method of treating patients who have NBP/PD. New α-blockers, terazosin and doxazosin, are preferred over the older α-blockers, prazosin and phenoxybenzamine, because of once-daily dosing and fewer adverse side effects. To avoid adverse side effects, these drugs must be given initially at a low dosage. The dosage is then increased slowly until the desired relief of symptoms is achieved. In my experience, most patients need 10 to 15 mg of terazosin or 4 to 8 mg of doxazosin, each taken daily at bedtime. Patients with tension myalgia of the pelvic floor respond best to treatment using diazepam, 5 mg orally three times daily, alone or in combination with an α-blocker. When stress seems a major factor, the patient should be referred to a psychiatrist or a psychologist.

Epididymitis

Etiology and Pathogenesis

Inflammation of the epididymis is sometimes the result of trauma or chemical irritation associated with reflux of sterile urine from the urethra through the vas deferens. Most cases of acute epididymitis, however, are infections that can be divided into (1) a sexually transmitted type associated with urethritis and usually caused by *C. trachomatis*, *N. gonorrhoeae*, or both, and (2) an essentially non–sexually transmitted type associated with UTI and prostatitis caused mainly by Enterobacteriaceae or *Pseudomonas* species.[35, 36]

Ascending infection from the urethra, prostate, or bladder urine appears to cause most cases of infectious epididymitis. Infected urine or secretions are thought to enter the ejaculatory ducts by reflux or direct extension and ascend the vas deferens to colonize and infect the epididymis.[35] A congenital abnormality, especially an ectopic ureter draining into the ipsilateral seminal vesicle, should be suspected in cases of recurrent epididymitis in a young boy. Bacteriuric males who undergo genitourinary tract instrumentation, catheterization, or surgery are at high risk for developing epididymitis.

Clinical Manifestations

Painful swelling of the affected side of the scrotum is the basic manifestation. At the onset, an enlarged, indurated, and tender epididymis can usually be distinguished from the testis; however, within a few hours, the epididymis and testis may seem to become one tender mass. Acute epididymitis is typically a unilateral, febrile illness that is variably associated with a urethral discharge or signs and symptoms of prostatitis or UTI. Rectal examination may suggest an underlying ABP. Scrotal ultrasonography helps distinguish acute epididymitis from other conditions such as torsion or neoplasia, especially when an acute reactive hydrocele evolves. Urethral swabs and voided urethral (VB_1) and midstream (VB_2) specimens should be subjected to a Gram stain and culture for proper diagnosis before treatment is initiated. When sexually transmitted acute epididymitis is suspected, stain and culture for *N. gonorrhoeae* should always be performed. Likewise, attempts should be made to test for *Chlamydia* as the pathogen.

Non–Sexually Transmitted Acute Epididymitis

Nonvenereal acute epididymitis occurs mainly in middle-aged and older men and is usually caused by coliform bacteria or *Pseudomonas* organisms.[35, 36] When the infecting organism can be identified, prompt initiation of pathogen-specific antimicrobial therapy is indicated. Severe cases may require hospitalization and the administration of parenteral antibiotics (e.g., an aminoglycoside plus ampicillin or a cephalosporin); less severe cases may be treated at home with oral antimicrobial agents. Especially when an underlying bacterial prostatitis is suspected, my preference is to prescribe TMP-

SMX, one double-strength tablet (160 mg TMP, 800 mg SMX) twice daily for 4 weeks, or ofloxacin, 400 mg twice daily by mouth for 4 weeks, or ciprofloxacin, 500 mg twice daily by mouth for 4 weeks. When parenteral therapy is used initially, after about 1 week, a suitable oral agent should be given instead and continued for 3 weeks. Some clinicians recommend short courses of therapy (about 10 days); however, like bacterial prostatitis, acute epididymitis is a tissue infection that is likely to relapse if the duration of therapy is insufficient.

Sexually Transmitted Acute Epididymitis

Sexually transmitted acute epididymitis usually occurs before age 35 years, in association with urethritis in men who have no underlying genitourinary tract abnormalities.[35, 36] Absence of gram-negative rods on a Gram stain or culture of urethral and urinary specimens is typical. Smears positive for gram-negative intracellular diplococci or positive cultures are diagnostic for infection by *N. gonorrhoeae*. When available, urethral cultures or immunologic tests should be used to identify *C. trachomatis*; otherwise, chlamydial infection is assumed by exclusion.

Preferred therapy consists of ofloxacin, 400 mg by mouth four times daily for 21 days, or doxycycline, 100 mg by mouth twice daily for 21 days. For gonococcal urethritis and epididymitis, an alternative may be ciprofloxacin, 500 mg orally four times daily for 21 days, or a 10-day course of a parenteral second- or third-generation cephalosporin.

Orchitis

Orchitis, a relatively uncommon inflammation of the testicle, is usually the result of a blood-borne viral infection. The leading cause of viral orchitis is mumps, which rarely causes orchitis in prepubertal males but involves one or both testes in 20% to 30% of postpubertal males.[35, 37, 38] Orchitis, unilateral in about two thirds of cases, usually follows the onset of the parotitis by a few days. The clinical course varies considerably. Some patients have only slight testicular swelling and tenderness and minimal constitutional signs; others experience severe testicular swelling and pain with high fever and marked constitutional signs. The illness may last only 4 to 5 days in mild cases but up to 4 weeks in severe cases. Postinfectious atrophy occurs in about 50% of involved testes; patients with marked bilateral atrophy may become infertile.[35, 38] Because no antiviral agent is currently available to treat the mumps virus specifically, only supportive therapy can be given.

Pyogenic orchitis is usually a result of contiguous spread of a bacterial infection originating in the ipsilateral epididymis, but it may also result from rickettsial or parasitic infections.[38] The responsible pathogens are usually coliforms or *Pseudomonas*, although strains of staphylococci or streptococci are occasionally involved. Affected patients usually have fever and marked pain and swelling of the affected testes. Parenteral antimicrobial therapy, specific for the pathogen when possible, should be administered. Orchiectomy may be needed if an abscess or testicular infarction develops.

Granulomatous orchitis is rare but is sometimes seen in patients who have actinomycosis or a systemic fungal disease, such as blastomycosis, histoplasmosis, and coccidioidomycosis. Tuberculous orchitis and syphilitic orchitis are seldom seen today. Antiinfective agents that are appropriate for the underlying disease are indicated in therapy.

Testicular trauma or torsion of the spermatic cord may lead to marked swelling and progressive ischemia of the testis with resultant noninfectious orchitis. Scrotal ultrasonography, isotope scans, and Doppler blood flow studies may assist in diagnosis, but surgical exploration is often necessary.

References

1. Dallabetta G, Hook EW III: Gonococcal infections. Infect Dis Clin North Am 1:25, 1987.
2. Hooton TM, Barnes RC: Urethritis in men. Infect Dis Clin North Am 1:165, 1987.
3. Moran JS, Levine WC: Drugs of choice for the treatment of uncomplicated gonococcal infections. Clin Infect Dis 20(Suppl 1):S47, 1995.
4. Weber JT, Johnson RE: New treatments for *Chlamydia trachomatis* genital infection. Clin Infect Dis 20(Suppl 1):S66, 1995.
5. Stamm WE, Counts GW, Running KR, et al: Diagnosis of coliform infection in acutely dysuric women. N Engl J Med 307:463, 1982.
6. Fihn SD, Stamm WE: The urethral syndrome. Semin Urol 1:121, 1983.
7. Barbalias GA, Meares EM Jr: Female urethral syndrome: Clinical and urodynamic perspectives. Urology 23:208, 1984.
8. Meares EM Jr: Acute and chronic prostatitis: Diagnosis and treatment. Infect Dis Clin North Am 1:855, 1987.
9. Blacklock NJ: Anatomical factors in prostatitis. Br J Urol 46:47, 1974.
10. Stamey TA: Pathogenesis and Treatment of Urinary Tract Infections. Baltimore, Williams & Wilkins, 1980.
11. Kirby RS, Lowe D, Bultitude MI, et al: Intraprostatic urinary reflux: An aetiological factor in abacterial prostatitis. Br J Urol 54:729, 1982.
12. Meares EM Jr: Prostatitis syndromes: New perspectives about woes. J Urol 123:141, 1980.
13. Meares EM Jr: Prostatitis: Review of pharmacokinetics and therapy. Rev Infect Dis 4:475, 1982.
14. Fair WR, Couch J, Wehner N: Prostatic antibacterial factor: Identity and significance. Urology 7:169, 1976.
15. Shortliffe LMD, Wehner N, Stamey TA: The defection of a local prostatic immunologic response to bacterial prostatitis. J Urol 125:509, 1981.
16. Meares EM Jr: Prostatitis and related disorders. *In* Walsh PC, Gittes RF, Perlmutter AD, Stamey TA (eds): Campbell's Urology, ed 5. Philadelphia, WB Saunders, 1986, pp 868–887.
17. Meares EM, Stamey TA: Bacteriologic localization patterns in bacterial prostatitis and urethritis. Invest Urol 5:492, 1968.
18. Meares EM Jr: Prostatic abscess (Editorial). J Urol 136:1281, 1986.
19. Peeling WB, Griffiths GJ: Imaging of the prostate by ultrasound. J Urol 132:217, 1984.
20. Meares EM Jr: Infection stones of the prostate gland. Laboratory diagnosis and clinical management. Urology 4:560, 1974.
21. Eykyn S, Bultitude MI, Mayo ME, et al: Prostatic calculi as a source of recurrent bacteriuria in the male. Br J Urol 46:527, 1974.
22. Larsen EH, Gasser TC, Dorflinger T, et al: The concentration of various quinolone derivatives in the human prostate. *In* Weidner W, Brunner H, Krause W, Rothauge CF (eds): Therapy of Prostatitis. Munich, W Zuckschwerdt Verlag, 1986, pp 35–39.
23. Naber KG: Use of quinolones in urinary tract infection and prostatitis. Rev Infect Dis 11(Suppl 5):S1321, 1989.
24. Meares EM Jr: Chronic bacterial prostatitis: Role of transurethral prostatectomy (TURP) in therapy. *In* Weidner W, Brunner H, Krause W, Rothauge CF (eds): Therapy of Prostatitis. Munich, W Zuckschwerdt Verlag, 1986, pp 193–197.
25. Drach GW, Fair WR, Meares EM Jr, et al: Classification of benign diseases associated with prostatic pain: Prostatitis or prostatodynia. J Urol 120:266, 1978.
26. Brunner H, Weidner W, Schiefer H-G: Studies of the role of *Ureaplasma urealyticum* and *Mycoplasma hominis* in prostatitis. J Infect Dis 147:807, 1983.
27. Neal DE Jr, Moon TD: Use of terazosin in prostatodynia and validation of a symptom score questionnaire. Urology 43:460, 1994.
28. Berger RE, Krieger JN, Kessler D, et al: Case-control study of men with suspected chronic idiopathic prostatitis. J Urol 141:328, 1989.
29. Mardh P-A, Ripa KT, Colleen S, et al: Role of *Chlamydia trachomatis* in nonacute prostatitis. Br J Vener Dis 54:330, 1978.
30. Doble A, Thomas BJ, Walker MM, et al: The role of *Chlamydia*

trachomatis in chronic abacterial prostatitis: A study using ultrasound-guided biopsy. J Urol 141:332, 1989.
31. Shortliffe LMD, Elliott KM, Sellers RG, et al: Measurement of chlamydial and ureaplasmal antibodies in serum and prostatic fluid of men with nonbacterial prostatitis (Abstr). J Urol 133:276A, 1985.
32. Meares EM Jr, Barbalias GA: Prostatitis: Bacterial, nonbacterial and prostatodynia. Semin Urol 1:146, 1983.
33. Barbalias GA, Meares EM Jr, Sant GR: Prostatodynia: Clinical and urodynamic characteristics. J Urol 130:514, 1983.
34. Meares EM Jr: Prostatodynia: Clinical findings and rationale for treatment. *In* Weidner W, Brunner H, Krause W, Rothauge CF (eds): Therapy of Prostatitis. Munich, W Zuckschwerdt Verlag, 1986, pp 207–212.
35. Meares EM Jr: Nonspecific infections of the genitourinary tract. *In* Tanagho EA, McAninch JW (eds): Smith's General Urology, ed 12. Norwalk, CT, Appleton & Lange, 1988, pp 196–245.
36. Berger RE: Urethritis and epididymitis. Semin Urol 1:138, 1983.
37. Beard CM, Benson RC, Kelalis PP, et al: The incidence and outcome of mumps orchitis in Rochester, Minnesota, 1935 to 1974. Mayo Clin Proc 52:3, 1977.
38. Krieger JN: Epididymitis, orchitis, and related conditions. Sex Transm Dis 11:173, 1984.

108

Renal Abscess

Edwin M. Meares, Jr.

Intrarenal Abscess

Renal Cortical Abscess

ETIOLOGY AND PATHOGENESIS

Most renal cortical abscesses, or renal carbuncles, develop from hematogenous spread of *Staphylococcus aureus* (90% of cases) infection at distant sites, most often skin lesions.[1] Intravenous (IV) drug abuse, diabetes mellitus, and hemodialysis are predisposing factors.[2, 3] In contrast to other intrarenal abscesses, renal cortical abscesses rarely result from ascending infection.[2, 3] Initially microabscesses develop, and they enlarge and coalesce to form a fluid-filled mass with a thick wall. This cortical abscess can eventually rupture through the renal capsule to form a perinephric abscess. Most renal carbuncles are unilateral (97%) solitary lesions (77%), and 63% affect the right kidney.[2, 3]

CLINICAL FEATURES

Patients in the second through fourth decades of life most often develop renal carbuncles; men are affected three times more than women.[2, 3] Chills, fever, and localized costovertebral angle tenderness are the typical clinical features. Early in the course, when the abscess does not communicate with the collecting system, there are no urinary symptoms. Physical examination may disclose a flank mass or loin bulge with loss of lumbar lordosis.

The hemogram typically shows moderate to marked leukocytosis, mainly neutrophils and many bands. When there is no communication between cortical abscesses and the collecting system, the results of urinalysis are normal and urine culture grows no pathogens. Blood cultures are often negative.

DIAGNOSIS

Imaging studies are essential for identifying the renal cortical abscess and for a differential diagnosis. Results of excretory urography are nonspecific and seldom contribute to diagnosis. Radionuclide scanning using gallium citrate Ga 67 and indium 111–labeled white blood cells may assist in diagnosis, but certain conditions—renal cell carcinoma, ureteral obstruction, severe nonsuppurative pyelonephritis—can produce false-positive findings.[2–5] Ultrasonography (US) can readily confirm a renal abscess, especially after the microabscesses coalesce to form a fluid-filled, thick-walled mass. Unfortunately, the US appearance of a renal abscess in its early stages may be mistaken for a renal neoplasm.[5, 6] Renal arteriography often fails to differentiate a renal abscess from a hypovascular or cystic renal neoplasm. Computed tomography (CT), with or without use of contrast agents, is the most accurate diagnostic imaging modality for identifying renal abscess[5–7] (Fig. 108–1). Aspiration of the abscess under US or CT guidance not only assists in diagnosis and identification of the causative agent but also may establish therapeutic drainage.

TREATMENT

The traditional mainstays of therapy have been the administration of appropriate antimicrobial agents and surgical drainage.[1–3] However, renal cortical abscesses, particularly those caused by *S. aureus,* have been treated successfully with antimicrobial agents alone.[2, 3] Recommended antistaphylococcal agents are oxacillin and nafcillin; either drug is given in IV doses of 100 to 200 mg/kg per day every 4 hours. Alternative therapy might be vancomycin, 1 g IV every 12 hours; cefazolin, 2 g IV every 8 hours; or cephalothin, 2 g IV every 4 hours. Parenteral therapy is continued for 10 to 14 days and followed by oral antistaphylococcal therapy for another 14 to 28 days. If no favorable clinical response (relief of pain, reduction of fever) is evident after 48 hours' therapy, the clinician should suspect a resistant pathogen or complicating factors, such as a perinephric abscess. In such cases, an attempt at aspiration and drainage by placing an appropriate percutaneous catheter under US or CT control is indicated.[3, 5, 6, 8] If this proves unsuccessful, open surgical drainage is necessary.

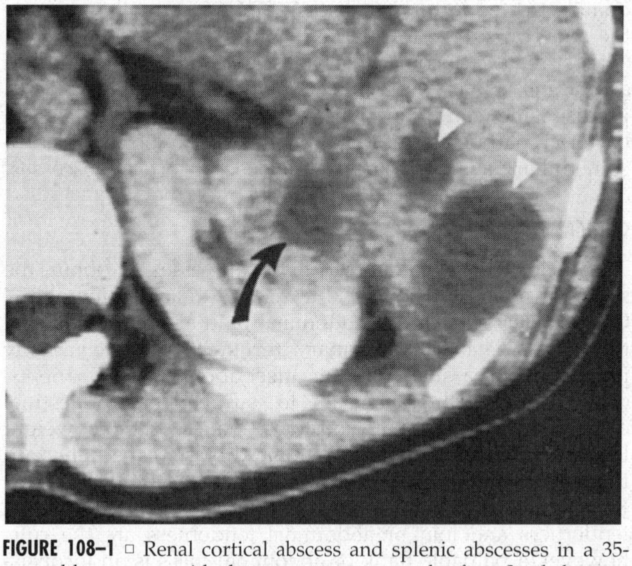

FIGURE 108–1 □ Renal cortical abscess and splenic abscesses in a 35-year-old woman with hematogenous spread of a *Staphylococcus aureus* skin infection. Computed tomography after intravenous injection of contrast material shows a cystic lesion in the left kidney with a low-density center and enhancing thick wall *(curved arrow)* and two similar lesions in the spleen *(arrowheads).*

Renal Corticomedullary Abscess

ETIOLOGY AND PATHOGENESIS

Renal corticomedullary abscesses generally evolve from an underlying urinary tract abnormality, such as an obstruction or a vesicoureteral reflux.[2, 3, 9] Whereas staphylococcal infections most often are responsible for renal carbuncles, coliform bacteria, especially strains of *Escherichia coli, Klebsiella,* and *Proteus,* most often are the agents of corticomedullary abscesses.[1, 2]

Several types of severe acute and chronic infectious processes are related to or associated with corticomedullary abscesses. Acute focal bacterial nephritis, also called acute lobar nephronia or focal pyelonephritis, is a severe acute parenchymal infection without liquefaction that occurs in one or more renal lobes.[3, 5, 10] The infection is thought to be limited to the lobes affected by intrarenal reflux. That this solid inflammatory mass, if untreated, may eventually liquefy and become a corticomedullary abscess is an interesting postulate.

Xanthogranulomatous pyelonephritis, a rare but important severe renal inflammatory disease, is often associated with intrarenal corticomedullary abscesses complicating a chronic urinary tract infection (usually coliform bacteria), renal calculi, and obstructive nephropathy.[1, 3, 5] The inflammatory process may involve part or all of the kidney (stage I), extend beyond the renal capsule to involve the perirenal fat within Gerota fascia (stage II), or involve the retroperitoneum and adjacent structures more extensively (stage III).[11] The typical histologic changes of xanthogranulomatous pyelonephritis include severe acute and chronic inflammation plus characteristic xanthoma cells, which are macrophages containing phagacytosed cholesterol and lipid materials.[1, 2, 11]

In adults, most corticomedullary abscesses are associated with renal calculi, obstructive uropathy, and damaged kidneys; in children, corticomedullary abscesses are generally associated only with vesicoureteral reflux.[2, 9] Another important predisposing condition, especially in adults, is diabetes mellitus.[1, 2] Aerobic, gram-negative bacilli are the usual pathogens in all age groups.[1–3] An initial infection of the renal medulla, subsequent liquefaction, and eventual involvement of the renal cortex apparently constitute the pathogenic process of a corticomedullary abscess. Inadequately treated intrarenal abscesses may eventually perforate the renal capsule to form a perinephric abscess.

Most renal corticomedullary abscesses occur as a result of ascending urinary tract infection in patients who have a predisposing condition, which explains the differences in bacterial pathogens and anatomic location between corticomedullary abscesses and staphylococcal cortical abscesses.

CLINICAL FEATURES

The incidence of corticomedullary abscesses is about the same for males and females but rises with advancing age.[2, 3] Chills, fever, and loin or abdominal pain are prominent features. Dysuria and other urinary tract symptoms are variably present. Nausea and vomiting affect about 65% of patients, often causing the clinician to suspect gastrointestinal disease.[2, 3] Constitutional symptoms (malaise, fatigue, weight loss) occur in patients with chronic disease, especially xanthogranulomatous pyelonephritis and associated abscesses. Physical findings are often nonspecific. Costovertebral angle tenderness and loin or abdominal tenderness are the rule; however, a palpable flank or abdominal mass is an inconsistent finding.[2, 3]

Because corticomedullary abscesses usually communicate with the collecting system, the findings of urinalysis typically are abnormal and the infecting pathogens (mainly coliforms, less often *Pseudomonas* species, *S. aureus,* and others) generally grow readily in urine culture.[1–3] Compared with patients who have renal cortical abscesses, patients with corticomedullary abscesses more often have positive blood cultures. Other laboratory abnormalities include anemia (75%), hypoalbuminemia (60%), and hypergammaglobulinemia (α_1- and α_2-globulin, 79%).[2, 3]

DIAGNOSIS

Because the medical history, physical findings, and results of routine laboratory tests are nonspecific, imaging studies, especially US and CT, are imperative for making the diagnosis of corticomedullary abscess. In acute focal bacterial nephritis, the renal US image may appear normal or show a solid hypoechoic mass that is poorly demarcated from adjacent normal parenchyma but deforms the renal contour and obliterates corticomedullary definition.[5] Noncontrast CT usually fails to demonstrate the lesion. Postcontrast CT, however, usually demonstrates a poorly defined, wedge-shaped, hypodense area without liquefaction[5] (Fig. 108–2). The inflammatory mass may involve one or several renal lobes. The varied radiographic characteristics of xanthogranulomatous pyelonephritis were reviewed in detail by Piccirillo and coworkers.[5] An obstructed, poorly functioning or nonfunctioning kidney containing calculi is a characteristic finding (Fig. 108–3).

The sonographic appearance of intrarenal abscesses, whether cortical or corticomedullary, is variable: they may lack internal echoes (mimicking cysts or calyceal diverticula), appear highly reflective (simulating neoplasms), or may contain sparse, low-density echoes.[5, 6] CT, with or without the use of IV contrast material, is the most definitive imaging technique for diagnosing intrarenal abscesses. CT shows a low-attenuation (0 to 20 Hounsfield units), distinctly marginated parenchymal lesion that fails to enhance after IV administration of contrast medium.[5, 6]

TREATMENT

Experience shows that, like cortical abscesses caused by staphylococci, corticomedullary abscesses caused by coli-

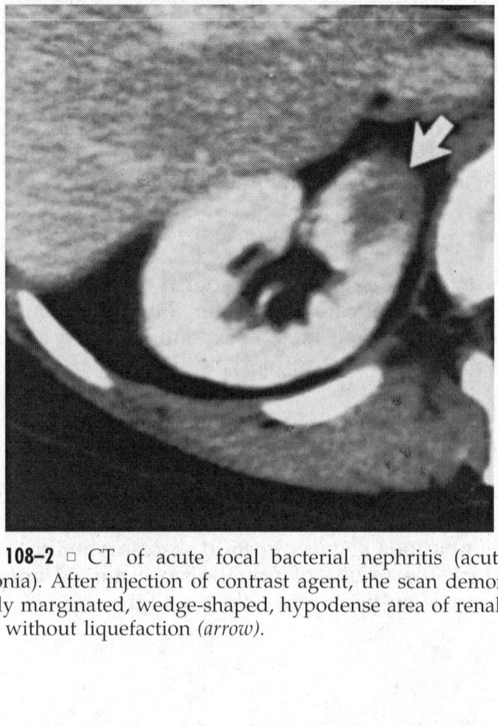

FIGURE 108–2 □ CT of acute focal bacterial nephritis (acute lobar nephronia). After injection of contrast agent, the scan demonstrates a poorly marginated, wedge-shaped, hypodense area of renal parenchyma without liquefaction *(arrow).*

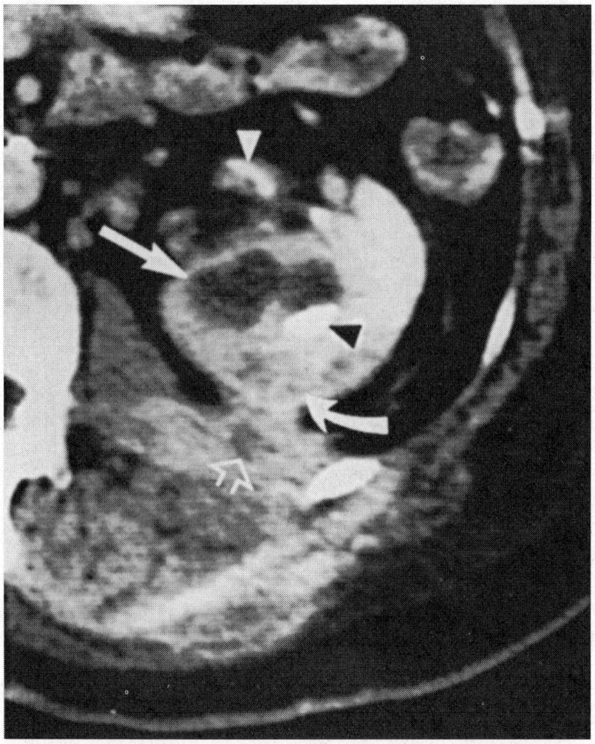

FIGURE 108–3 □ Xanthogranulomatous pyelonephritis with suppurative process extending into the perinephric space in a 51-year-old woman. CT of the left kidney after IV injection of contrast material shows calculi *(arrowheads)*, hydronephrosis *(straight white arrow)*, parenchymal suppuration with liquefaction *(curved white arrow)*, and extension of the process through the renal capsule into the perinephric space (perinephric abscess, *short open arrow*).

forms can sometimes be treated with antimicrobial agents alone without drainage.[2, 3] This is especially true for acute focal bacterial nephritis and often for small lesions with minimal liquefaction that are confined to the renal parenchyma. In addition to intensive antimicrobial therapy, moderate to large unilocular abscesses must usually be drained, preferably by insertion of a percutaneous catheter.[6] Multilocular abscesses frequently must be drained by open surgical incision. Patients with xanthogranulomatous pyelonephritis and poorly functioning kidneys usually require nephrectomy.

Initial antibacterial therapy should include a combination of ampicillin, 1 g every 4 to 6 hours, or cefazolin, 1 g every 8 hours, IV, plus an aminoglycoside—gentamicin or tobramycin, 1 mg/kg every 8 hours, IV, adjusting the dose appropriately for decreased renal function. A fluoroquinolone, such as ciprofloxacin or ofloxacin, is a good choice for infection caused by gram-negative bacteria; the drug can be given IV at first, followed by the oral form.[12, 16] Depending on the clinical response and results of culture and sensitivity tests, combination therapy is continued or adjusted appropriately. Parenteral therapy is continued until symptoms abate, fever has resolved for at least 48 hours, and repeated imaging demonstrates a favorable response. A suitable oral antimicrobial agent is eventually given for 2 to 4 weeks, until clinical and radiologic examinations demonstrate complete resolution of the process. Early diagnosis and proper therapy usually ensure a favorable outcome.

Perinephric Abscess

Etiology and Pathogenesis

Perinephric abscesses form mainly as a result of rupture of an intrarenal abscess into the perinephric space, so the agents are the same as those of intrarenal abscesses: *S. aureus* (cortical abscess) and aerobic, gram-negative bacteria, mainly strains of *E. coli, Proteus,* and *Klebsiella* (corticomedullary abscess). Other coliforms, *Pseudomonas* species, gram-positive bacteria, and obligate anaerobic bacteria are occasionally involved.[1, 2, 4, 14, 15] Fungi, especially *Candida* species, and *Mycobacterium tuberculosis* at times are responsible. Abscess cultures grow multiple microbes in about 25% of cases.[2] The abscess is usually confined by Gerota fascia to the perinephric space but may extend throughout the retroperitoneum to affect surrounding structures. Predisposing factors are the same as those involved with intrarenal abscesses.

Clinical Features

The often insidious nature and confusing clinical presentation of a perinephric abscess make early recognition difficult. Data from reported series indicate that most patients with a perinephric abscess have symptoms for 2 to 3 weeks before they consult a physician.[2, 4] Depending on the clinical acumen of the physician the patient consults, the diagnosis of perinephric abscess may be delayed several days longer. Fever, the only universal sign, may early on be considered of unknown origin. Pain in the affected flank eventually develops in most patients. Costovertebral angle tenderness and flank tenderness, with or without a palpable loin or abdominal mass, are the most prominent findings at physical examination. The diaphragm on the affected side may be elevated and fixed, with or without an associated ipsilateral pleural effusion. The patient may complain of pleuritic chest pain secondary to the diaphragmatic irritation from cephalad extension of the suppuration. Scoliosis (concavity to the affected side) commonly develops from spasm of the psoas muscle, which may also cause pain on bending away from the affected side, active flexion of the ipsilateral thigh against resistance, or extension of the thigh during ambulation. Likewise, irritation of the psoas muscle or iliohypogastric, ilioinguinal, genitofemoral, or femorocutaneous nerves may refer pain to the ipsilateral hip area. Abdominal tenderness and guarding, suggestive of intraperitoneal disease, sometimes confound the diagnosis. A painful bulge in the loin with overlying erythema and edema of the tissues is a late sign but is suggestive of perinephric abscess.

Routine laboratory test results are variably altered. Blood tests usually show only mild leukocytosis with neutrophilia, an elevated erythrocyte sedimentation rate, and variable anemia. Azotemia is uncommon unless bilateral renal disease is present. Pyuria and proteinuria are often found, but hematuria is not. About 30% of patients have a normal urinalysis result, and about 40% have sterile urine cultures.[1, 2, 4] Blood cultures are positive in only 40% of cases.[2]

Diagnosis

That a perinephric abscess has an insidious onset and clinical course with highly variable features, often making early recognition difficult, must be emphasized. The most important aspect of early diagnosis is a high index of suspicion on the part of the clinician, coupled with the performance of appropriate radiographic imaging studies.

CHEST AND ABDOMINAL RADIOGRAPHY

Chest films are helpful if they show an elevated or fixed hemidiaphragm, pleural effusion, empyema, lung abscess, lower lobe infiltrate or atelectasis, or apical scarring, especially in patients with tuberculous abscesses. Abdominal radiography may demonstrate thoracolumbar scoliosis (concavity toward the affected side), mass effect, renal calculi, poorly visualized or effaced renal outline, poorly visualized or effaced psoas shadows, gas in the renal or perirenal area, and Mathe sign of renal fixation.[4] It must be emphasized, however, that none of these findings is specifically diagnostic of a perinephric abscess.

EXCRETORY UROGRAPHY

Excretory urography with tomography demonstrates an abnormality on the affected side in 80% to 85% of cases.[4] Findings include variable abnormalities: poor or no visualization of the affected kidney; mass effect; displacement of the kidney, renal pelvis, or ureter; calculi; calicectasis; and obstruction (with or without a calculus). None of these findings is specifically diagnostic of a perinephric abscess.

RADIONUCLIDE IMAGING AND RENAL ARTERIOGRAPHY

Radionuclide scanning with ^{67}Ga- or ^{111}In-labeled white blood cells may assist in diagnosis but plays a minor role. These scans take 2 to 3 days for interpretation and do not differentiate perinephric abscesses from several other renal diseases.[2, 4] Renal arteriography, a highly invasive study, often fails to differentiate inflammatory masses from neoplasia and is seldom indicated because US and CT scans yield better results.

ULTRASONOGRAPHY AND COMPUTED TOMOGRAPHY

Both US and CT are useful in the diagnosis of perinephric abscess, but CT best demonstrates the full extent of involvement.[6, 7] Piccirillo and coworkers[5] provided an excellent detailed review of specific US and CT findings in perinephric abscess. CT abnormalities include a soft tissue mass of low central attenuation (0 to 20 Hounsfield units), an inflammatory wall with slightly higher attenuation on noncontrast views, the rind sign (a rim of increased density in the abscess wall after IV injection of contrast medium), obliteration of surrounding tissue planes, ipsilateral enlargement of the kidney or psoas muscle, thickening of Gerota fascia, and gas or air-fluid level in the lesion[4–6] (see Fig. 108–3). Absolute confirmation and identification of the causative agent or agents are made by percutaneous aspiration of the abscess under US or CT control.

Treatment

Early, thorough surgical drainage plus proper antimicrobial therapy is always indicated; antimicrobial therapy alone is inadequate for management of a perinephric abscess. Traditional surgical drainage has been open incision, irrigation, débridement, and placement of drains exiting the retroperitoneum, or immediate nephrectomy when necessary. More recently, however, drainage by placement of a percutaneous catheter under US or CT control has proved effective in selected cases.[3, 4, 6, 8, 16] Open surgical drainage or nephrectomy should be performed expeditiously if percutaneous drainage proves inadequate.

Parenteral antimicrobial therapy is initially directed against staphylococci and coliforms, the most likely pathogens, until culture and sensitivity test results are available. The same agents and dosage outlined for treatment of intrarenal abscesses are recommended. Depending on the clinical response and culture and sensitivity results, appropriate changes can be made as indicated. Parenteral, and ultimately oral, antimicrobial therapy is given until clinical and repeated imaging findings indicate resolution of the infectious process.

In the past, owing to errors and delays in diagnosis, the mortality rates for patients with perinephric abscess have ranged from 20% to 57%; up to 34% were diagnosed only at autopsy.[2, 4, 14, 15] It is encouraging that Sheinfeld and coworkers[4] reported a series of 15 patients with perinephric abscess, treated at their institution between 1979 and 1983, who had excellent outcomes and no deaths. Fowler and Perkins[7] cured all 57 patients who were diagnosed and underwent drainage; in 4 patients the abscess escaped detection, contributing to their death. This emphasizes what can be accomplished by early recognition by means of modern imaging techniques and prompt drainage combined with proper antimicrobial therapy.

References

1. Meares EM Jr: Nonspecific infections of the genitourinary tract. *In* Tanagho EA, McAninch JW (eds): Smith's General Urology, ed 12. Norwalk, CT, Appleton & Lange, 1988, pp 196–245.
2. Patterson JE, Andriole VT: Renal and perirenal abscesses. Infect Dis Clin North Am 1:907, 1987.
3. Andriole VT: Renal and perirenal abscess. *In* Schrier RW, Gottschalk CW (eds): Diseases of the Kidney, ed 4. Boston, Little, Brown, 1987, pp 1049–1064.
4. Sheinfeld J, Erturk E, Spataro RD, et al: Perinephric abscess: Current concepts. J Urol 137:191, 1987.
5. Piccirillo M, Rigsby C, Rosenfield AT: Contemporary imaging of renal inflammatory disease. Infect Dis Clin North Am 1:927, 1987.
6. Gerzof SG, Gale ME: Computed tomography and ultrasonography for diagnosis and treatment of renal and retroperitoneal abscesses. Urol Clin North Am 9:185, 1982.
7. Fowler JE Jr, Perkins T: Presentation, diagnosis and treatment of renal abscesses: 1972–1988. J Urol 151:847, 1994.
8. Gerzof SC, Robbins AH, Johnson WC, et al: Percutaneous catheter drainage of abdominal abscesses. A five-year experience. N Engl J Med 305:653, 1981.
9. Timmons JW, Perlmutter AD: Renal abscess: A changing concept. J Urol 115:229, 1976.
10. Nosher JL, Tamminen JL, Amorosa JK, et al: Acute focal bacterial nephritis. Am J Kidney Dis 11:36, 1988.
11. Malek RS, Elder JS: Xanthogranulomatous pyelonephritis. A critical analysis of 26 cases and of the literature. J Urol 119:589, 1978.
12. Andriole VT: Use of quinolones in treatment of prostatitis and lower urinary tract infections. Eur J Clin Microbiol Infect Dis 10:342, 1991.
13. Rubenstein E, Keller N: Fluoroquinolones: Present uses. Infect Dis Clin Pract 3(Suppl 3):S195, 1994.
14. Salvatierra O Jr, Bucklew WB, Morrow JW: Perinephric abscess: A report of 71 cases. J Urol 98:296, 1967.
15. Thorley JD, Jones SR, Sanford JP: Perinephric abscess. Medicine (Baltimore) 53:41, 1974.
16. Siegel JF, Smith A, Moldwin R: Minimally invasive treatment of renal abscess. J Urol 155:52, 1996.

SEXUALLY TRANSMITTED DISEASES

109

Approach to the Patient with Sexually Transmitted Disease

H. Hunter Handsfield

In few areas of infectious diseases have changes in epidemiology and in our understanding of the clinical manifestations been as profound as in the field of sexually transmitted diseases (STDs) in the past two decades. All facets of "emerging infections" are reflected in recent STD trends, including the appearance or recognition of new pathogens and syndromes, evolution of antimicrobial resistance in formerly susceptible pathogens, increasing importance of viral pathogens, and rapid worldwide spread fostered by international travel and trade. The recognized spectrum of STDs includes at least 50 distinct clinical syndromes caused by more than 25 pathogenic organisms and viruses. Table 109–1 lists the predominant syndromes and complications of STDs, in the approximate order of their importance to human health, and the pathogens associated with them. In each instance, sexual contact is an important mode of transmission if not the only one. This chapter presents some general principles for clinicians who care for patients who have or are at risk for STDs.

The major STDs are more serious for women than for men. Many are transmitted more efficiently from male to female than the reverse, probably because the vagina serves as a reservoir that prolongs the exposure of susceptible mucous membranes to infectious secretions. Women are more likely than men to have asymptomatic or minimally symptomatic infections early in the clinical course, fostering delays in seeking health care. Diagnosis of STDs is more difficult in women, because the clinical findings are less specific and many microbiologic tests are less sensitive than in men. Finally, infected women are at greater risk than are men for severe or permanent sequelae, such as infertility, ectopic pregnancy, cancer, and serious consequences for the fetus and newborn. Thus, prevention, treatment, and control of STDs is important primarily to protect and preserve the health of women.

The expansion of the perceived spectrum of STDs in the past two decades has largely involved recognition of the importance of the viral STD pathogens, such as the human immunodeficiency viruses (HIVs), type 2 herpes simplex virus (HSV), hepatitis B virus, the human papillomaviruses, and cytomegalovirus. The rising case rates of the viral STDs probably reflect both enhanced recognition and true increases in incidence and prevalence. The viral STDs have a greater potential than those caused by bacteria for sustained transmission outside the traditional high-risk groups, because prolonged infection permits sustained transmission in populations with low rates of sexual partner change. Partly for the same reason, health care behaviors have less influence on disease occurrence and complications of viral than of bacterial STDs. As a result, primary prevention of new infections through behavioral intervention is the primary control measure currently available for the viral STDs, pending development of new vaccines or curative therapy.

Most STDs, including but not limited to those that cause overt genital ulceration, enhance the efficiency of HIV transmission.[1] This probably occurs from increased HIV production by inflammatory cells that accumulate at sites of infection, resulting in an elevated potential for transmission, and from the enhanced susceptibility of such cells to HIV, so that persons with STDs are more likely to acquire HIV if they are exposed. The importance of these theoretical considerations was confirmed in a community-based study in Tanzania, where institution of STD clinical services, without specific HIV prevention efforts, resulted in a reduced rate of HIV seroconversion compared with control communities where STD services were not offered.[2] Variations in the frequency of heterosexually transmitted HIV infection are largely due to differences in the prevalence of other STDs. In many settings, preventing the traditional STDs is probably one of the most cost-effective approaches to preventing HIV infection.[1–3]

Epidemiologic Principles

Despite substantial improvements in diagnosis and treatment in the past several decades, STDs are endemic or epidemic in virtually all societies, and they are a prime example of the influence that behavioral and demographic factors can have on an infectious disease despite the availability of effective therapy and other technologic advances.

Risk Factors and Risk Markers

The principal risk factor for acquisition and transmission of STDs is sexual behavior, including the number and selection of partners and specific sexual practices, which in turn predict exposure to sexually transmitted infections and may affect the efficiency of transmission of some pathogens. Secondary risk factors include coinfection with other STDs; male (and perhaps female) circumcision; contraceptive practices; and certain health care behaviors, such as the decision to cease sexual activity and promptly seek medical attention for genital symptoms. These causal factors should be distinguished from risk markers, which are indirect indicators of sexual behavior.[4] Risk markers are primarily demographic and social characteristics, such as race, ethnicity, marital status, sexual orientation, socioeconomic level, residence (e.g., urban or rural), and substance abuse. Some predictors function as both risk factors and risk markers. Examples include gender and age, which influence both behavior and susceptibility to infection.[4]

Core Populations

All STDs are transmitted with less than 100% efficiency, so that a minimal frequency of sexual partner change is necessary to propagate an STD in a population. Population subgroups in which sexual behavior is sufficient to sustain the epidemic are defined as core groups. The core transmission hypothesis was developed for gonorrhea,[5] and studies have

TABLE 109–1 ■ Sexually Transmitted Pathogens, Copathogens, and Clinical Syndromes*

SYNDROME	PRIMARY PATHOGENS	SECONDARY PATHOGENS AND COPATHOGENS
Acquired immunodeficiency syndrome and related disorders	HIV (types 1 and 2)	Numerous opportunistic pathogens
Acute pelvic inflammatory disease and its primary complications, female infertility, ectopic pregnancy, chronic pelvic pain	*Neisseria gonorrhoeae, Chlamydia trachomatis*	*Mycoplasma hominis, Prevotella* sp., *Peptococcus* sp., *Bacteroides* sp., coliform bacteria, other vaginal flora
Neonatal or perinatal complications (premature delivery, chorioamnionitis, TORCHES syndrome, pneumonia, conjunctivitis, cognitive impairment, immunodeficiency)	*N. gonorrhoeae, C. trachomatis,* CMV, HSV (types 1 and 2), *Treponema pallidum,* group B streptococcus, HIV	*Ureaplasma urealyticum, M. hominis,* vaginal anaerobes
Neoplasia (squamous cell cancer of cervix, anus, vulva, penis; Kaposi's sarcoma; lymphoma; hepatocellular carcinoma)	Human papillomavirus (types 16, 18, 34, 45, others), HIV, hepatitis B virus, Kaposi's sarcoma virus	
Lower genital tract infections in women		
Mucopurulent cervicitis and urethritis	*C. trachomatis, N. gonorrhoeae,* HSV	*Trichomonas vaginalis*
Vaginitis, vulvovaginitis	*Trichomonas vaginalis, Candida* sp.	Anaerobic vaginal flora, other yeasts
Bacterial vaginosis	Primary pathogen(s) unknown	*Gardnerella vaginalis, M. hominis, Mobiluncus* sp., anaerobic vaginal flora
Anogenital warts	Human papillomaviruses (especially types 6 and 11)	
Viral hepatitis	Hepatitis viruses (A, B, C, D)	
Male urethritis	*N. gonorrhoeae, C. trachomatis, U. urealyticum* (?), *Mycoplasma genitalium* (?)	*T. vaginalis,* HSV-1 and HSV-2
Genital ulcer–lymphadenopathy syndromes	*T. pallidum,* HSV-1, HSV-2, *Haemophilus ducreyi, C. trachomatis* (LGV strains), *Calymmatobacterium granulomatis*	Pyogenic bacteria, *Candida* sp., other fungi
Arthritis	*N. gonorrhoeae, C. trachomatis,* hepatitis B virus, HIV (?)	*U. urealyticum, M. hominis*
Epididymitis	*C. trachomatis, N. gonorrhoeae*	Genitourinary pathogens
Tertiary syphilis	*T. pallidum*	
Proctitis, proctocolitis	Same as for urethritis, cervicitis	
Enteric infections, enterocolitis	*Shigella* sp., *Giardia lamblia, Entamoeba histolytica, Campylobacter* sp., HIV (?)	
Mononucleosis	CMV, human herpesvirus type 6 (?), Epstein-Barr virus, HIV (?)	
Ectoparasite infestation	*Sarcoptes scabiei* (scabies mite), *Phthirus pubis* (crab louse)	Pyogenic bacteria
Molluscum contagiosum	Molluscum contagiosum virus	

*Listed in approximate order of importance to human health. TORCHES, Toxoplasmosis, rubella, cytomegalovirus, herpes, syphilis; HIV, human immunodeficiency virus; CMV, cytomegalovirus; HSV, herpes simplex virus; LGV, lymphogranuloma venereum.

provided empirical support for the central role of core transmission in the epidemiology of this infection.[6, 7] The same concept applies to all STDs.

These concepts have been described mathematically according to the formula $R_0 = \beta cD$.[5, 8, 9] R_0 is the reproductive rate of an infection, defined as the number of additional cases generated by each infection introduced into a population; thus, when R_0 is 1.0, the prevalence remains stable, and values below 1.0 and above 1.0 are associated with declining or rising prevalences, respectively. As shown by the formula, the reproductive rate is determined by the product of three factors. β represents infectivity, the likelihood of transmission during a single sexual encounter between an infected person and a susceptible one. (Barrier contraceptives are effective in prevention because they reduce β.) The symbol c represents the frequency with which infected and susceptible persons encounter one another; simplistically, this is the rate at which members of the population change sexual partners. (Education to promote monogamy or reduced numbers of partners is an effort to limit the value of c in the population.) The symbol D represents the mean duration of infection from acquisition to treatment, spontaneous resolution, or, for HIV infection, death. (For the bacterial STDs, D is reduced by case finding and early antimicrobial therapy.)

The value of β, the efficiency of transmission, is relatively constant for most STDs, averaging about 20% to 50% for heterosexual vaginal intercourse. Accordingly, differences in the epidemiology of gonorrhea and genital herpes, for example, can be explained by their differences in the rate of partner change *(c)* and the mean duration of infection *(D)*. For gonorrhea, D varies from days to a few weeks, because early symptoms lead promptly to treatment, many infections resolve spontaneously, and efforts are made to notify and treat partners. The formula dictates that if D is low, a high rate of partner change *(c)* is required to sustain R_0 at a level of 1.0 or greater. Therefore, gonorrhea is concentrated in relatively small core groups that are characterized by extremely high rates of partner change. By contrast, the duration of genital herpes is measured in years and perhaps for the life of the infected person; as a result, the prevalence of infection can be maintained despite low rates of partner change, and genital herpes is therefore common in the entire population. Chlamydial infection occupies an intermediate position; the mean duration of infection is longer than that of the other bacterial STDs but substantially shorter than that of herpes or human papillomavirus infection. Thus, *Chlamydia trachomatis* core groups are characterized by intermediate rates of partner change, so the infection is common in a broader segment of the population than gonorrhea but in a narrower one than the viral STDs. For heterosexual transmission of HIV, β is probably less than 1% (i.e., less than one transmission for each 100 sexual encounters). Thus, despite the prolonged duration *(D)* of HIV infection, sustaining HIV prevalence in a population requires either high rates of partner change *(c)* or enhancement of transmission efficiency (β), for example, by other STDs or traumatic sexual practices, such as anal intercourse. Of course, for all STDs, the actual situation is much more complex than described here. For example, β is not constant during the course of infection and varies with specific sexual practices, and the variability of *c* in a population has influence in addition to the mean rate of partner change.[8, 9]

Asymptomatic Carriers

Most persons with genital symptoms cease sexual activity and seek health care. It follows that infected persons who transmit STDs to their sexual partners are likely to have no symptoms or to have mild symptoms that they ignore. Those with asymptomatic infections continue sexual activity and accumulate in the population.[10] Other persons, perhaps especially in socioeconomically disadvantaged populations or where health care is not readily available, continue sexual activity despite overt symptoms.[11] These observations explain the importance of taking active steps to ensure that sexual partners of infected persons are notified and treated. More often than not, the partner who transmitted an STD to a newly infected person will not spontaneously seek medical attention.[10, 11]

Clinical and Public Health Considerations

Several unique aspects of STDs and the populations at risk affect clinical management. The Centers for Disease Control and Prevention periodically issues guidelines for management of patients with STDs, including recommendations for clinical assessment, prevention, and control.[12]

Clinical Evaluation and Risk Assessment

In addition to routine clinical care, the management of patients with STDs or at risk entails measures to assess risk, reduce the likelihood of future infections and complications, and protect the health of the patients' sexual partners and the public at large.

Assessment of risk requires an accurate social and sexual history, including appraisal of factors that influence sexuality, such as substance abuse. Although taking such a history is daunting to some clinicians, a forthright and sensitive approach usually produces accurate information and need not be time-consuming. This sets the stage for counseling and education that can maximize compliance with treatment and follow-up and reduce the risk of future STD episodes. Risk reduction counseling should usually emphasize monogamy or the judicious selection of sexual partners, use of condoms, and for those with ongoing risk, periodic screening examinations. Patients should be advised about the protective value of sexual abstinence until a permanent, mutually monogamous relationship is established, but this is an impractical ideal for many persons at risk.

Clinicians who provide STD care should have immediate access to tests for HIV infection; syphilis serology; specific tests for *Neisseria gonorrhoeae*, *C. trachomatis*, and HSV; microscopy for examination of Gram-stained smears and wet mounts of vaginal secretions; and Papanicolaou smears, which should be routinely obtained for women at risk for STDs. Type-specific serologic tests for HSV antibody are clinically useful, but most commercially offered assays do not accurately distinguish HSV-1 from HSV-2 antibody, despite some laboratories' claims to the contrary. Providers who serve populations with high prevalences of syphilis should have access to darkfield microscopy for detection of *Treponema pallidum*.

Ideally, a specific diagnosis should be made and treatment and counseling guided accordingly. In some instances, an etiologic diagnosis is known before treatment is given, such as when a positive result is received for a screening test for *C. trachomatis* or a Gram-stained smear is diagnostic of gonorrhea. More often, however, an empirical management decision must be made before the etiologic diagnosis is known, as when a patient presents with mucopurulent cervicitis, pelvic inflammatory disease, or a genital ulcer. Acute symptoms usually require immediate therapy, and some patients may not defer sexual activity while awaiting test results. Accordingly, clinicians must be cognizant of the usual causes of the common STD syndromes in the populations they serve, recognizing that the causes vary geographically and fluctuate over time. However, even when initial care must be based on clinical grounds ("syndromic management"), it is good practice to obtain specific diagnostic tests whenever practical, even when the results will not be known until after treatment is started.[12]

Principles of Treatment

Historically, STD patients have been considered unlikely to comply with prolonged treatment, resulting in an emphasis on single-dose therapy. In fact, persons with STDs may be no less reliable than other patients, but an STD carries implications for continued transmission that magnify the importance of therapeutic compliance. Directly observed, single-dose treatment should therefore be used whenever practical; it is indicated for almost all cases of uncomplicated gonorrhea, chlamydial infection, primary or secondary syphilis, and many cases of nongonococcal urethritis and chancroid. If multiple-dose treatment must be given, the clinician should make a special effort to counsel the patient about the necessity of compliance. When practical, even multiple-dose drugs should be given directly to the patient in the office and the first dose should be observed, rather than giving a prescription to be filled, especially when the patient must pay for therapy. In a study of women with acute pelvic inflammatory disease diagnosed in an urban emergency department, 30% failed to fill their prescriptions for doxycycline.[13]

Management of sexual partners is an integral part of treating patients with STDs. Failure to ensure treatment of the partner is often tantamount to not treating the index case, because of the risk for reinfection. The physician should take specific steps to examine partners personally or to make specific referrals elsewhere; vague advice to "make sure your partner gets checked" is often not heeded.

The traditional recommendation is that all partners of infected patients should be examined and that it is inappropriate to provide "blind" treatment without examination or referral. Compliance with treatment may be poor among partners who are not directly counseled, and they are unlikely to fully understand the nature of the infection. Coinfections that were not apparent in the index case are often discovered in the partner. Without examination, the opportunity is missed to bring still other partners to treatment. Blind treatment may also entail medicolegal risk, for example, if therapy causes a serious side effect.

Nevertheless, for the bacterial STDs, the overriding goal is to ensure that patients' partners are treated. Anecdotal experience in STD clinics suggests that referral of partners by either index patients or trained counselors results in treatment of 40% or less of the male partners of women with chlamydial infection or gonorrhea. In an uncontrolled study in Sweden, reinfection with *C. trachomatis* was substantially less frequent in women given antibiotics to treat their partners than in women whose partners were referred for therapy.[14] Although the clinician should always attempt to arrange for examination and diagnostic testing of the partner, blind treatment may be appropriate if the traditional approach is unsuccessful or impractical.

Clinical and Prevention Services for Sexually Transmitted Diseases in a Managed Care Environment

The rapid evolution of managed care as a paradigm for delivery of health care services and capitation as a mechanism for funding them raises numerous questions about STD management. Will screening for common pathogens be funded and routinely provided? Will there be fiscal and operational pressures toward syndromic management without definitive diagnosis? Will providers and health maintenance organizations be willing and able to offer same-day care for patients with "epidemiologic" urgency, such as when a patient has trivial (or no) symptoms but may transmit infection to others if not treated promptly? How can effective risk reduction counseling be integrated into highly efficient delivery of services in a busy clinic? How will sexual partners be managed when they do not participate in the patients' managed care plans? A controlled study showed that screening sexually active women for chlamydial infection in a large health maintenance organization reduced the frequency of pelvic inflammatory disease by 60%, clearly a cost-effective outcome.[15] Other studies have also demonstrated the cost-effectiveness of screening women for *C. trachomatis*.[16] For many prevention strategies, however, few objective data are available to document similar outcomes, notwithstanding the beliefs and recommendations of many public health authorities. Until more controlled studies are available, clinicians and managed care organizations will be required to make pragmatic decisions and integrate the following procedures into their practices whenever possible.

Education and Counseling

Counseling and education are important not only for patients who currently have an STD or are at risk but also for all young people in primary health care settings for primary prevention. When practical, such counseling should begin before the patient becomes sexually active. The clinician should emphasize sexual safety. Providers should tell patients that abstinence and permanent, mutual monogamy are certain prevention strategies. In most cases, however, the emphasis will be on reducing the number of sexual partners, selectivity in choosing partners, and consistent use of condoms. Other educational messages should address the recognition of and response to symptoms of STDs and the links between STDs and substance abuse. In general, education and counseling based on pragmatic rationales are more readily accepted by persons at risk than is advice justified on moral or religious grounds.[17]

Screening

The occurrence of an STD is a "sentinel event" that reflects unprotected sexual activity, and diagnosis of any STD often should include screening for additional ones. Other criteria for screening depend on the epidemiology of STDs in the local population and a balance among cost, test performance, anticipated yield, potential impact of case detection on public health, and frequency of complications. Screening has a central role in the control of gonorrhea, syphilis, chlamydial infection, and HIV infection. Screening has been proposed in various settings for HSV infection, human papillomavirus infection, and other STDs, but its value in preventing these infections has not been determined.

A difficult dilemma is that screening yields that are high on a population basis may not be sufficient to sustain a clinician's resolve to continue testing his or her patients at risk. For example, a 5% prevalence of chlamydial infection in sexually active young women demands routine testing, but a yield of only one infection in 20 patients screened may tempt a clinician to restrict testing to patients who seem to be at particular risk—a strategy that almost always fails to detect most infections in the population.[16] The development of urine-based testing for *C. trachomatis* and *N. gonorrhoeae* will simplify screening decisions and procedures for these infections.[18]

Partner Notification

Notification and referral of the sexual partners of infected persons are traditional components of programs for prevention and control of syphilis and gonorrhea, and these measures clearly apply as well to chlamydial infection. The importance of partner referral for the control of HIV infection and other viral STDs has been controversial, principally because medical interventions have not been documented to affect transmission, except for immunization against hepatitis B. However, notification is also important to ensure that the partners receive appropriate treatment and behavioral counseling.

All partner notification is necessarily voluntary, because if a patient refuses to divulge a partner's name and the partner is unknown to the clinician, notification is impossible. To be effective, partner notification programs must be undertaken with the highest regard for the privacy of the affected persons. Ideally, the index patient should personally inform the partners, but that person often cannot or will not do so. In most states, the local or state health department is available to assist in partner notification for patients with selected STDs, especially syphilis, and frequently for those with gonorrhea, chlamydial infection, or HIV infection.

Reporting

Documentation of STD morbidity locally and nationally is integral to control. Prevention programs can be rationally designed only when such data are available, and resources can be targeted to the core populations only if their occurrence, location, and demographic characteristics are known. Health care providers should report all cases of designated STDs to health authorities according to local regulations; failure to do so contributes to the continued spread of STDs.

References

1. Wasserheit JN: Epidemiological synergy: Interrelationships between human immunodeficiency virus infection and other sexually transmitted diseases. Sex Transm Dis 19:61, 1992.
2. Grosskurth H, Mosha F, Todd J, et al: Impact of improved treatment of sexually transmitted diseases on HIV infection in rural Tanzania: Randomised controlled trial. Lancet 346:530, 1995.
3. Roseberry W: AIDS prevention and mitigation in sub-Saharan Africa: An updated World Bank strategy. Geneva, Switzerland, The World Bank, 1996. Report 15569-AFR.
4. Aral SO, Holmes KK: Epidemiology of sexual behavior and sexually transmitted diseases. *In* Holmes KK, et al (eds): Sexually Transmitted Diseases, ed 2. New York, McGraw-Hill, 1990, pp 19–36.

5. Yorke JA, Hethcote HW, Nold A: Dynamics and control of the transmission of gonorrhea. Sex Transm Dis 5:51, 1978.
6. Rice RJ, Roberts PL, Handsfield HH, Holmes KK: Sociodemographic distribution of gonorrhea incidence: Implications for prevention and behavioral research. Am J Public Health 81:1252, 1991.
7. Rothenberg RB, Potterat JJ: Temporal and social aspects of gonorrhea transmission: The force of infectivity. Sex Transm Dis 15:88, 1988.
8. May RM, Anderson RM: Transmission dynamics of HIV infection. Nature 326:137, 1987.
9. Brunham RC, Nagelkerke NJ, Plummer FA, Moses S: Estimating the basic reproductive rates of *Neisseria gonorrhoeae* and *Chlamydia trachomatis*: The implications of acquired immunity. Sex Transm Dis 21:353, 1994.
10. Handsfield HH, Lipman TO, Harnisch JP, et al: Asymptomatic gonorrhea in men. Diagnosis, natural course, prevalence and significance. N Engl J Med 290:117, 1973.
11. Hook EW III, Brady WE, Reichart CA, et al: Determinants of emergence of antibiotic-resistant *Neisseria gonorrhoeae*. J Infect Dis 159:1900, 1987.
12. Centers for Disease Control and Prevention: 1993 Sexually transmitted diseases treatment guidelines. MMWR Morbid Mortal Wkly Rep 42(RR-14):1, 1993.
13. Brookoff D: Compliance with doxycycline therapy for outpatient treatment of pelvic inflammatory disease. South Med J 87:1088, 1994.
14. Ramstedt K, Forssman L, Johannisson G: Contact tracing in the control of genital *Chlamydia trachomatis* infection. Int J STD AIDS 2:116, 1991.
15. Scholes D, Stergachis A, Heidrich FE, et al: Prevention of pelvic inflammatory disease by screening for cervical chlamydial infection. N Engl J Med 334:1362, 1996.
16. Marrazzo JM, Celum CL, Hillis SD, et al: Performance and cost-effectiveness of selective screening criteria for *Chlamydia trachomatis* infection in women: Implications for a national chlamydia control strategy. Sex Transm Dis (in press).
17. Brandt AM: No Magic Bullet: A Social History of Venereal Disease in the United States Since 1890, ed 2. New York, Oxford University Press, 1987.
18. Lee HH, Chernesky MA, Schachter J, et al: Diagnosis of *Chlamydia trachomatis* genitourinary infection in women by ligase chain reaction assay of urine. Lancet 345:213, 1995.

110

Gonorrhea

Edward W. Hook
Jonathan M. Zenilman

To most nonmedical personnel, the term gonorrhea elicits the image of a sexually transmitted disease (STD) uniformly manifested as urethral discharge and dysuria among men or vaginal discharge in women. All too often, this widely held but overly simplistic concept is an impediment to accurate diagnosis and management of gonorrhea. Whereas these widely appreciated symptoms are present in many patients with gonorrhea, a substantial proportion are asymptomatic or present with other signs or symptoms. Misconceptions regarding clinical presentations of gonorrhea sometimes lead clinicians to fail to consider gonorrhea screening or diagnosis in patients at risk. Likewise, the same misconceptions that sometimes lead clinicians to miss gonorrhea diagnosis also occasionally make it difficult to convince patients of their risk for gonococcal infection or that gonorrhea screening might be appropriate despite the absence of clinically apparent findings. *Neisseria gonorrhoeae* is a gram-negative diplococcus that infects only humans, causing a spectrum of clinical syndromes (Table 110–1). Proper diagnosis and management require an appreciation of the epidemiology of *N. gonorrhoeae,* an awareness of the entire spectrum of possible clinical presentations, and an understanding of current recommendations for gonorrhea therapy.

Epidemiology

Despite declines, gonorrhea remains one of the most common reportable bacterial infections in the United States. In 1995, 392,848 cases of gonorrhea were reported to the Centers for Disease Control and Prevention (CDC).[1] This figure, however, underrepresents the magnitude of the problem; it has been estimated that as many as half of all gonorrhea cases are not reported owing to either poor compliance with reporting requirements or treatment of patients on the basis of clinical (e.g., signs and symptoms or Gram stain examination) or epidemiologic (e.g., history of sexual exposure to a partner with gonorrhea) criteria without culture confirmation.

In 1978, the number of gonorrhea cases reported to the CDC peaked at 1,013,436 and then began to decline—gradually at first, then at an accelerating pace in the era of human immunodeficiency virus and acquired immunodeficiency syndrome.[1–3] The observed declines have not been uniform throughout the population. Gonorrhea has declined most dramatically among homosexually active men and among whites of both sexes, whereas smaller declines have been observed among the minority (primarily African-American and Hispanic) inner-city populations in whom gonorrhea has always been most common. For example in 1995, rates of reported gonorrhea were 37 times higher for African-Americans than for whites. Whereas part of this disparity reflects increased care from public clinics where reporting is generally better, the infection is also more common in African-Americans. Similarly, changes in gonorrhea rates have been most dramatic among older persons and have changed little for adolescents, the group at highest risk for infection[2]

TABLE 110–1 ■ Clinical Presentations of Gonorrhea

NEONATES
Asymptomatic mucosal infection
Conjunctivitis
Disseminated gonococcal infection
MEN
Asymptomatic mucosal infection
Urethritis
Proctitis
Pharyngitis
Epididymitis
Disseminated gonococcal infection
WOMEN
Asymptomatic mucosal infection
Cervicitis
Urethritis
Proctitis
Pharyngitis
Skene or Bartholin gland infection
Pelvic inflammatory disease (endometritis, salpingitis, peritonitis)
Disseminated gonococcal infection

(see later). Another factor likely to have contributed indirectly to changing gonorrhea rates is the widespread changes in preferred contraceptive measures. Condoms and spermicidal preparations containing nonoxynol 9 reduce the risk for gonorrhea acquisition.[3] In contrast, use of oral contraceptive pills may make the risk for acquiring gonorrhea greater for women than when no contraceptive measure at all is used.[4]

Gonorrhea epidemiology is also closely related to age, and gonorrhea is a disease of youth.[1, 2] In 1995, 77% of gonorrhea cases reported to the CDC occurred in individuals 15 to 29 years of age.[1] Although this age effect is present in both sexes, it is more pronounced in female patients. Gonorrhea rates in women are uniformly highest in young women. Except in neonates, gonococcal infections are nearly always the consequence of sexual transmission, and risk for gonorrhea acquisition is influenced by a number of covariates related to individual susceptibility, sexual partners, and practices. The high gonorrhea rates for young women probably reflect not only relatively rapid accrual of sexual partners soon after young persons become sexually active but possibly also a biologically based increase in susceptibility among young women compared with older women. This increased susceptibility appears to be related to the presence of larger areas of cervical ectropion (columnar epithelial cells on the surface of the ectocervix) in younger women, which affords a larger area of susceptible target cells for inoculation of gonococcal infection.[5] Certain behaviors are likewise associated with increased risk for gonorrhea. Persons who have multiple sexual partners and prostitutes and their clients have long been considered to be at increased risk for gonorrhea.[6, 7] Studies have demonstrated that sexual activity associated with illicit drug use (parenteral or nonparenteral) and sex with new partners are also risk factors. Likewise, regardless of numbers of partners, persons in relationships they characterize as casual, as opposed to serious, are at increased risk for gonorrhea.[6]

Thus, epidemiologic considerations are sometimes useful as a guide in making decisions regarding whom to screen for gonorrhea. In a given population, for instance, the yield of routine gonorrhea screening is usually highest among younger persons, those who have recently had sex with new partners, and those who use illicit drugs. Geographic variation in gonorrhea rates also affects the yield of routine gonorrhea screening; rates are higher among lower socioeconomic class, minority, inner-city populations than in nearby suburban middle- or upper-class populations.

Diagnostic Considerations

Gram stain examination and culture isolation remain the favored methods for detection of *N. gonorrhoeae*; however, available nonculture methods are improving and becoming more widely used. The frequent absence or nonspecificity of symptoms, the potential complications of untreated infection, and the proven benefit of routine screening of populations at risk make the time and cost for gonorrhea detection important considerations in choosing methods for diagnosis. A number of other rapid, nonculture methods for detecting *N. gonorrhoeae* have become available.

Specimen Collection

Proper specimen collection is important to ensure optimal yield of most gonorrhea tests. In men with detectable urethral discharge, expressed urethral exudate may be used for Gram staining or culture.[8, 9] Proper specimen collection from asymptomatic men or men with symptoms who lack expressible discharge involves insertion 1.5 to 2 cm into the urethra of a wire-shafted swab tipped with calcium alginate or synthetic fibers by a rotatory motion. For diagnosis of urogenital tract gonorrhea in women, specimens should always be collected from the uterine endocervix. If the endocervical specimen is to be evaluated by Gram stain, adherent cervicovaginal secretions should be removed from the cervical os with use of large cotton-tipped swabs before the specimen is obtained. Specimens obtained for Gram stain should be rolled, rather than rubbed, onto a glass microscope slide, lest the morphologic features of inflammatory cells be distorted. Specimens collected for culture from any site should always use calcium alginate or synthetic fiber–tipped swabs. Substances contained in wooden-shafted, cotton-tipped swabs may be toxic for *N. gonorrhoeae*, particularly if the swab is to be placed in transport medium for transfer to the laboratory rather than plated directly onto culture media.[8]

Gram Stain

For detection of gonococcal urethritis or cervicitis in persons who have symptoms or are at high risk, Gram stain examination rapidly provides accurate diagnostic information. The examination can be performed in minutes; the reagents cost pennies per test; and, if positive, the results are highly specific.[9] The result of a Gram stain preparation is considered positive if gram-negative diplococci are seen within polymorphonuclear leukocytes. If gram-negative diplococci are seen extracellularly in the presence of polymorphonuclear leukocytes, the Gram stain is termed equivocal for gonorrhea, and in most instances this is sufficient indication to warrant initiation of treatment. The presence of gram-negative diplococci without associated polymorphonuclear leukocytes is difficult to interpret and does not necessarily indicate the presence of gonococcal infection.

For symptomatic men with gonococcal urethritis, the sensitivity of Gram stain is approximately 95% to 98%, and the specificity is in excess of 95%. For women with gonococcal cervicitis, sensitivity is somewhat less (40% to 60%); however, specificity again exceeds 95%. For asymptomatic men, Gram stain of urethral specimens has a sensitivity similar to that for cervical specimens (e.g., 40% to 60%), and although specificity is slightly lower than that for other sites, it still exceeds 90%. Gram stain of rectal specimens is sometimes complicated by the presence of nongonococcal, gram-negative diplococci, which may be mistaken for *N. gonorrhoeae*; nonetheless, it is sometimes useful for evaluation of symptomatic proctitis in persons who practice receptive rectal intercourse. In contrast, owing to the high prevalence of nongonococcal *Neisseria* species and other gram-negative cocci in the pharynx, Gram stain examination is not a recommended means for diagnosis of pharyngeal gonorrhea.

Culture Diagnosis

For optimal recovery of *N. gonorrhoeae*, mucosal specimens obtained for culture should be inoculated directly onto selective media and placed into a 35°C to 37°C incubator containing a 5% to 7% carbon dioxide atmosphere. Many effective transport media are available that sustain the viability of *N. gonorrhoeae* for several hours, permitting specimens to be transported to the laboratory from areas where it is not possible to stock culture media. In general, these transport media sustain gonococcal viability for periods in excess of 6 to 12 hours.

Selective media for isolation of *N. gonorrhoeae* from mucosal specimens usually contain antimicrobial substances to suppress growth of other microorganisms (bacteria and fungi) that might overgrow and obscure the presence of the relatively small colonies characteristic of *N. gonorrhoeae*.[10]

Comparative studies have shown that although antimicrobial agents contained in selective media may inhibit growth of a small proportion of gonococcal isolates, that proportion is no larger than the proportion that go undetected as the result of overgrowth in specimens plated on nonselective media.[10–12] The gonococcal strains that are most likely to cause disseminated gonococcal infection (DGI) are more fastidious. As a result, specimens from patients with possible DGI should routinely be cultured onto nonselective chocolate agar to optimize culture isolation rates. The selective media most widely used for *N. gonorrhoeae* culture from mucosal sites include modified Thayer-Martin, Martin-Lewis, and New York City medium. Any of these provides suitably efficient isolation of *N. gonorrhoeae,* and all are, by and large, comparable with regard to their potential usefulness.

Methods Other Than Culture and Gram Stain for Gonorrhea Detection

Many nonculture diagnostic tests have become available that detect gonococcal antigens, gonococcal enzyme activity, or gonococcal genetic material.[13, 14] In 1994, more than one third of tests for gonorrhea performed in the United States were nonculture tests. The majority of these tests used a single-stranded DNA probe that detected gonococcal ribosomal RNA in test specimens and has a specificity of 99% and a sensitivity close to that of culture on selective media for detection of *N. gonorrhoeae*.

In 1996, the first amplified nucleic acid detection test for gonorrhea diagnosis was approved in the United States. This test, a ligase chain reaction assay, is as sensitive and specific as culture for gonorrhea diagnosis but has the advantage of performing equally well with use of swab or voided urine specimens in both men and women. The simplified specimen collection procedures for amplified nucleic acid detection tests using assays such as ligase chain reaction and polymerase chain reaction may greatly simplify screening for gonorrhea and other STDs.[15]

Clinical Presentation

Asymptomatic Mucosal Infection

Asymptomatic infections may occur at any potential mucosal site of gonococcal infection (urethra, cervix, rectum, pharynx, conjunctiva) and are usually detected by screening or culture evaluation of patients who report recent exposure to sexual partners with gonorrhea. Asymptomatic urethral and cervical infections are present in approximately 10% and 40% to 50%, respectively, of men and women who report exposure to sexual partners with gonorrhea. The prevalence of asymptomatic urethral gonorrhea in military recruits and other otherwise unselected populations of sexually active men has been 0.5% to 2%. More often than not, pharyngeal and rectal gonococcal infections are asymptomatic.[16, 17] Asymptomatic mucosal infections are also disproportionately common among patients with DGI.[18, 19] It is not known whether this represents a risk factor for dissemination in patients with asymptomatic (and therefore untreated) mucosal gonorrhea or is a reflection of the propensity of the distinctive strains that most often cause disseminated infection also to cause asymptomatic mucosal infection. Detection of asymptomatic infection through screening of populations identified as high risk on the basis of sociodemographic characteristics, age, or history is an important facet of efforts to control gonorrhea. Because persons with asymptomatic infection are less likely to abstain from sexual activity than are those who develop symptoms, they probably contribute disproportionately to gonococcal infection rates within communities.

Local Gonococcal Infections in Men

Symptomatic urethritis is the most common presentation of gonorrhea in men. Urethral discharge and dysuria usually develop 2 to 5 days after exposure to an infected sexual partner. The majority of men with symptomatic gonococcal urethritis have a purulent urethral discharge, which often becomes copious if it is untreated. Dysuria may be the sole symptom of gonococcal infection and tends to be mild to moderate in severity.

The most common local complication of gonococcal infection in men is acute epididymitis, which usually presents as gradually increasing unilateral scrotal pain. Examination of patients with epididymitis may yield heretofore unnoticed urethral discharge as well as tenderness or swelling of the epididymis. Acute epididymitis must be expeditiously differentiated from testicular torsion, which tends to be more acute in onset and usually is not associated with urethral discharge. In cases in which clinical differentiation is difficult, a urologist should be consulted immediately to preserve testicular viability in the event of torsion. For patients younger than 40 years, treatment of epididymitis targets *N. gonorrhoeae* and *Chlamydia trachomatis* as well, because coinfection is common. In men older than 40 years, as structural abnormalities of the urinary tract become more common, epididymitis may be caused by gram-negative rods and other urinary tract pathogens as well as STD pathogens.

Rarely, men with gonococcal urethritis present with other complications of infection, such as gonococcal cellulitis, penile lymphangitis, or periurethral abscess. In such patients, routine treatment for gonorrhea usually results in rapid resolution of these findings.

Local Gonococcal Infections in Women

The uterine cervix is the primary site of infection in women with acute uncomplicated gonorrhea. Whereas gonococcal cervicitis in women is often asymptomatic, women with local gonococcal infections may complain of increased vaginal discharge, genital itch, or dysuria. Because the same symptoms may also result from urinary tract infections, vaginal infections, or cervicitis due to other causes, evaluation of such complaints in sexually active women should include urinalysis (and culture when indicated); evaluation of vaginal secretions for candidiasis, trichomoniasis, and bacterial vaginosis; and tests for *N. gonorrhoeae* and *C. trachomatis*. Urethral cultures propagate the pathogen for 40% to 60% of women with gonococcal cervicitis, and the presence of urethral infection may help to explain dysuria as a common symptom of gonorrhea in women. In hysterectomized women, the primary site of infection is the urethra, because vaginal epithelium is relatively resistant to gonococcal infection. Women with local gonococcal infection may also present with local complications resulting from infection of Skene or Bartholin glands. In either case, these complications present with local pain and swelling.

Pelvic inflammatory disease (PID) is the most important complication of gonococcal infections.[20–22] PID is a generic designation that may refer to endometritis, salpingitis, peritonitis, or a combination of these findings. Gonococcal PID usually results from ascension of *N. gonorrhoeae* from the site of primary infection (the cervix) into the upper genital tract. Symptoms of PID may include unilateral or bilateral lower abdominal cramps, dyspareunia, and intramenstrual bleeding. These symptoms may be severe or so mild that women with PID do not mention them; in such cases, the signs of PID are detected at the time of physical examination. Clinical signs associated with PID on bimanual pelvic examination include fundal or adnexal (usually bilateral) tenderness, signs of peritonitis, and occasionally adnexal masses or fullness. On speculum examination, as in gonococcal cervicitis, a grossly purulent cervical discharge may be present, although frequently it is not. PID is most often a polymicrobial illness, and women with gonococcal PID are likely to have concurrent infection with *C. trachomatis* or an array of vaginal flora, including gram-negative rods, gram-positive cocci, and anaerobic bacteria.[20, 21] The tubal abnormalities and scarring that may result from PID or associated tuboovarian abscess are major causes of infertility, and ectopic pregnancy represents the major source of PID-associated morbidity. After a single episode of symptomatic PID, approximately 10% of women have bilateral tubal occlusion and resultant infertility, and women who do not have tubal obstruction have an approximately 10-fold greater risk for ectopic pregnancy.

Anorectal Gonorrhea

Anorectal gonorrhea is unusual in heterosexual men. Asymptomatic anorectal gonococcal infection occurs in approximately 30% to 50% of women with cervical gonorrhea and is thought most often to arise from local contamination by cervicovaginal secretions. Obviously, however, women and homosexually active men who participate in receptive anal intercourse with infected sexual partners are also at risk for developing anorectal gonorrhea. Although most men with anorectal gonorrhea are asymptomatic, some develop signs of acute proctitis (rectal discharge, pain, tenesmus). Among homosexually active men with symptomatic proctitis, coinfection with a variety of pathogens is common.[17] As a result, homosexually active men who present for evaluation of symptomatic proctitis should also be thoroughly evaluated for a wide variety of other potential pathogens. The pathogens, differential diagnosis, and diagnostic approach to homosexually active men with proctitis are reviewed in Chapter 120.

Disseminated Gonococcal Infections

Approximately 1% to 2% of patients with untreated gonorrhea progress to DGI, a bacteremic illness that most often presents with myalgia, arthralgia, asymmetric polyarthritis, or a characteristic dermatitis.[18, 19] Although DGI is a bacteremic illness, patients with this syndrome often are not clinically toxic. Not infrequently, the illness is characterized as influenza-like; the mean temperature of patients with DGI is 37.9°C at time of presentation, and the mean peripheral leukocyte count is 10,550/mm^3.[19] Whereas *N. gonorrhoeae* mucosal infection is present in most cases of DGI, it is frequently asymptomatic. Therefore, all potential mucosal sites of infection (urethra or cervix, pharynx, rectum) should be sampled for *N. gonorrhoeae* when the differential diagnosis includes DGI.

The two most common presentations of DGI are acute asymmetric polyarthritis and dermatitis, which sometimes may be present with painful tenosynovitis of the extremities.[18, 19] The arthritis of DGI tends to be asymmetric, most often involving joints of the hands, wrists, ankles, or knees, although nearly any joint may be affected. In patients with arthritis, the joint fluid polymorphonuclear leukocyte concentration may range from a few hundred cells to more than 20,000/mm^3. The likelihood of isolating *N. gonorrhoeae* appears to correlate relatively well with the magnitude of synovial fluid leukocyte concentration; higher isolation rates occur in patients with higher cell counts.[19] Overall, 20% to 30% of DGI patients' synovial fluid cultures propagate the pathogen.

The dermatitis of DGI is characteristically composed of a small number of skin lesions (usually fewer than 30) that are located predominantly on the extremities. Extremities are more often involved distally than proximally, and the natural history of the lesions is that they begin as tender papules, which then go on to become necrotic pustules and to ulcerate. Many patients with such lesions characterize them as insect bites. The classic skin lesion of DGI is a necrotic pustule on an erythematous base, and lesions in different stages of evolution are often present concurrently. The lesions are often somewhat tender to the touch. Attempts at culture isolation of DGI skin lesions is rarely productive. On occasion, DGI may be complicated when seeding of heart valves or the meninges results in gonococcal endocarditis or meningitis.[23–25] Either complication is potentially life threatening and should be treated aggressively and vigorously.

Therapeutic Considerations

Uncomplicated Gonorrhea

In the 1990s, therapy for infections due to *N. gonorrhoeae* has become complicated by appreciation of the increasing prevalence of diverse forms of gonococcal antimicrobial resistance (Table 110–2). For nearly 50 years, a penicillin was the choice for gonorrhea therapy worldwide; however, by 1989, penicillin resistance had become widespread, severely compromising its usefulness as treatment of choice for gonorrhea.[26, 27] Antimicrobial resistance of *N. gonorrhoeae* may be due to plasmid-mediated β-lactamase production; to plasmid-mediated resistance to tetracycline; or to chromosomally mediated resistance to a wide variety of antibiotics, including penicillin, tetracycline, and spectinomycin[26, 28–33] (see Table 110–2 and Chapter 201). In addition to antimicrobial resistance, other important considerations in choosing therapeutic agents for gonococcal infections include their utility against coinfecting pathogens (principally *C. trachomatis*), their ease of administration (single-dose therapy enhances compliance), and their cost (given the fact that many patients with gonorrhea have limited financial resources and so are dependent on the services of publicly funded STD clinics for therapy).[27]

TABLE 110–2 ▪ Mechanisms for *Neisseria gonorrhoeae* Antimicrobial Resistance

	β-LACTAMASE PRODUCTION	PLASMID-MEDIATED TETRACYCLINES	CHROMOSOMAL
Acronym*	PPNG	TRNG	CRMNG
Acquisition	Single-step plasmid acquisition	Single-step plasmid acquisition	Cumulative effect of multiple chromosome mutations
Mechanism	β-Lactamase production	Unknown; Tet(M)–mediated	Multiple, different mechanisms
Antimicrobials affected	β-Lactams (penicillins)	Tetracyclines	β-Lactams, tetracyclines, quinolones, erythromycins, spectinomycin
Laboratory detection	Rapid, single step	Nonspecific screening; disk sensitivity screening useful	Minimal inhibitory concentration determination is time-consuming

*PPNG, Penicillinase-producing *N. gonorrhoeae* (NG); TRNG, tetracycline-resistant NG; CRMNG, NG with chromosomal resistance to penicillin.

Persons at risk for one STD are often at increased risk for others as well. For patients with gonorrhea, the two most common coinfecting pathogens are *C. trachomatis* and, in women, *Trichomonas vaginalis*. It is estimated that at least 10% to 20% of men and 30% to 40% of women with uncomplicated gonorrhea have concurrent *Chlamydia* infections. No inexpensive single-dose therapy currently recommended for gonorrhea reliably eradicates *Chlamydia* organisms, and the currently recommended anti-*Chlamydia* treatment regimens are not reliable for gonorrhea. Therefore, it is recommended that patients treated for gonorrhea also be treated routinely for possible *Chlamydia* infection at the time of gonorrhea therapy. Because *Chlamydia* testing is relatively costly and usually requires several days for results, the cotreatment approach is thought to be more cost-effective and efficient.[34]

In women, coexisting infection with *T. vaginalis* can often be detected by microscopic examination of saline preparations of vaginal fluid. In some women, however, the presence of trichomoniasis may become apparent only after treatment of gonorrhea. Thus, for women with persistent or new complaints of vaginal discharge or discomfort, repeated examination is necessary to differentiate failure of gonorrhea treatment from trichomoniasis or vaginal candidiasis complicating therapy.

In the past, it was recommended that repeated attempts at culture isolation be performed 4 to 7 days after completion of therapy for patients with uncomplicated gonorrhea to ensure that they had been cured (test-of-cure cultures). Since the 1989 revision of the CDC STD treatment guidelines, this recommendation was dropped for patients treated with recommended regimens in favor of the suggestion that rescreening (as opposed to test-of-cure evaluation) be conducted 1 to 2 months subsequent to therapy.[27] The current recommendation is based on the assumption that reacquisition of gonorrhea or acquisition of another STD is more common than asymptomatic treatment failure. For patients treated with any of the alternative regimens listed in Table 110–3, test-of-cure evaluation continues to be suggested as a result of the limited experience to date with those regimens.

Complicated Gonococcal Infections

In the 1970s and early 1980s, isolates from patients with DGI were found to be more sensitive to penicillin than were isolates from patients with uncomplicated gonorrhea; however as the prevalence of gonococcal antimicrobial resistance has increased, β-lactamase–producing *N. gonorrhoeae* and gonococci with clinically significant penicillin resistance have been isolated from a number of patients with disseminated infection.[24, 35] Therefore, penicillin is no longer recommended

TABLE 110–3 ■ Therapy for Gonococcal Infections

UNCOMPLICATED GONORRHEA

Preferred Regimen

Ceftriaxone, 125 mg intramuscularly (IM)
or
Cefixime, 400 mg orally (PO)
or
Ciprofloxacin, 500 mg PO
or
Ofloxacin, 400 mg PO
plus
A regimen effective against *Chlamydia trachomatis*, such as
Doxycycline,*† 100 mg PO twice daily (bid) × 7 d
or
Azithromycin, 1.0 g PO as a single dose

Alternative Regimens

Spectinomycin, 2 g IM
or
Ceftizoxime, 500 mg IM
or
Cefotaxime, 500 mg IM
or
Cefoxitin, 2 g IM
or
Cefuroxime axetil, 1 g PO
or
Cefpodoxime proxetil, 200 mg PO
or
Enoxacin, 400 mg PO
or
Lomefloxacin, 400 PO
or
Norfloxacin, 800 mg PO

EPIDIDYMITIS

Ceftriaxone, 250 mg IM
plus
Doxycycline,*† 100 mg PO bid × 7 d

PELVIC INFLAMMATORY DISEASE

Inpatient Management

Cefoxitin, 2 g intravenously (IV) q 6 h
or
Cefotetan, 2 g IV q 12 h
plus
Doxycycline, 100 mg PO or IV q 12 h until improved, *then*
Doxycycline, 100 mg PO bid to complete 10–14 d course
or
Clindamycin, 900 mg IV q 8 h
plus
Gentamicin, 2 mg/kg (maintenance dose) IM or IV q 8 h until improved, *then*
Doxycycline, 100 mg PO bid to complete 10- to 14-d course

Outpatient Management

Cefoxitin, 2 g IM
plus
Probenecid, 1.0 g PO
or
Ceftriaxone, 250 mg IM
or
Equivalent cephalosporin
plus
Doxycycline,* 100 mg PO bid for 10–14 d

DISSEMINATED GONOCOCCAL INFECTION

(unless *C. trachomatis* coinfection is ruled out, therapy should be given with or followed by doxycycline,* 100 mg PO bid × 7 d)
Ceftriaxone, 1 g IM or IV q 24 hr
or
Ceftizoxime, 1 g IV q 8 h
or
Cefotaxime, 1 g IV q 8 h until symptoms resolve, *then* complete 7–d course with
Cefuroxime axetil, 500 mg PO bid
or
Amoxicillin, 500 mg with clavulanate three times daily
or
Ciprofloxacin,† 500 mg PO bid

*Tetracycline, 500 mg PO four times daily, or erythromycin, 500 mg PO four times daily, may be substituted for the preferred doxycycline, as needed.
†Quinolone and tetracycline antibiotics are contraindicated in pregnancy.

as initial therapy for patients with suspected DGI.[27] Because the differential diagnosis of DGI also includes other serious infections such as endocarditis or meningococcemia, initial hospitalization is recommended to confirm the diagnosis and to ensure that patients are responding to therapy. After therapeutic response, patients with DGI may be discharged to complete therapy as outpatients with oral medications such as cefuroxime, ciprofloxacin, or amoxicillin-clavulanate.

Although the gonococcus is one of the pathogens most frequently isolated from patients with PID, the syndrome is often polymicrobial and clinical findings are not useful for determining likely pathogens. As a result, therapeutic regimens for PID should be effective not only for *N. gonorrhoeae* but also for chlamydiae, gram-negative vaginal organisms, group B streptococci, and anaerobes. In the currently recommended regimens for PID therapy, the agents with acceptable utility against the gonococcus include cefoxitin, cefotetan, gentamicin, and ceftriaxone.

Evaluation of Sexual Partners

The most common cause of treatment failure in patients treated for gonorrhea is repeated exposure to untreated sexual partners. Because asymptomatic partners of persons with uncomplicated or complicated gonococcal infections are at substantially increased risk for asymptomatic infection, treatment of all partners within the preceding 30 days is recommended, regardless of the presence or absence of signs or symptoms of infection. This accomplishes the dual purpose of providing therapy for asymptomatically infected persons who may have infected the initial patient (source contacts) and treating partners who may have acquired infection as the result of exposure to the initial patient after his or her acquisition of infection (spread contacts), who may be asymptomatic or still incubating the infection.

References

1. Division of STD Prevention: Sexually Transmitted Disease Surveillance, 1995. US Department of Health and Human Services, Public Health Service. Atlanta, Centers for Disease Control and Prevention, September 1996.
2. Rice RJ, Aral SO, Blount JH, Zaidi AA: Gonorrhea in the United States 1975–1984: Is the giant only sleeping? Sex Transm Dis 14:83, 1987.
3. Declining rates of rectal and pharyngeal gonorrhea among males—New York City. MMWR Morbid Mortal Wkly Rep 33:295, 1984.
4. Austin H, Louv W, Alexander J: A case-control study of spermicides and gonorrhea. JAMA 251:2822, 1984.
5. Louv WC, Austin H, Perlman J, Alexander WJ: Oral contraceptive use and the risk of chlamydial and gonococcal infections. Am J Obstet Gynecol 160:396, 1989.
6. Upchurch DM, Brady WE, Reichart CA, Hook EW III: Behavioral contributions to acquisition of gonorrhea in patients attending an inner city sexually transmitted disease clinic. J Infect Dis 161:938, 1990.
7. Hook EW, Brady WE, Reichart CA, et al: Determinants of emergence of antibiotic-resistant *Neisseria gonorrhoeae*. J Infect Dis 159:900, 1989.
8. Goodhart ME, Ogden J, Zaidi AA, Kraus S: Factors affecting the performance of smear and culture tests for the detection of *Neisseria gonorrhoeae*. Sex Transm Dis 9:63, 1982.
9. Lossick JG, Smeltzer MP, Curran JW: The value of the cervical Gram stain in the diagnosis and treatment of gonorrhea in women in a veneral disease clinic. Sex Transm Dis 9:124, 1982.
10. Mirrett S, Reller LB, Knapp JS: *Neisseria gonorrhoeae* strains inhibited by vancomycin in selective media and correlation with auxotype. J Clin Microbiol 14:94, 1981.
11. Bonin P, Tanino TT, Handsfield HH: Isolation of *Neisseria gonorrhoeae* on selective and nonselective media in a sexually transmitted disease clinic. J Clin Microbiol 19:218, 1984.
12. Reichart CA, Rupkey LM, Brady WE, Hook EW III: Comparison of GC-lect and modified Thayer-Martin media for isolation of *Neisseria gonorrhoeae*. J Clin Microbiol 27:808, 1989.
13. Jaffe HW, Kraus SJ, Edwards TA, et al: Diagnosis of gonorrhea using a genetic transformation test on mailed clinical specimens. J Infect Dis 146:275, 1982.
14. Ulsen JV, Michel MF, van Strik R, et al: Experience with a modified solid-phase enzyme immunoassay for detection of gonorrhea in prostitutes. Sex Transm Dis 13:1, 1986.
15. Smith KR, Ching S, Lee H, et al: Evaluation of ligase chain reaction for use with urine for identification of *Neisseria gonorrhoeae* in females attending a sexually transmitted disease clinic. J Clin Microbiol 33:455, 1995.
16. Wiesner PJ, Tronca E, Bonin P, et al: Clinical spectrum of pharyngeal gonococcal infection. N Engl J Med 288:181, 1973.
17. Quinn TC, Stamm WE, Goodell SE, et al: The polymicrobial origin of intestinal infections in homosexual men. N Engl J Med 309:576, 1983.
18. Holmes KK, Counts GW, Beaty HN: Disseminated gonococcal infection. Ann Intern Med 74:979, 1971.
19. Handsfield HH, Wiesner PJ, Holmes KK: Treatment of the gonococcal arthritis-dermatitis syndrome. Ann Intern Med 84:661, 1976.
20. Eschenbach DA, Buchanan TM, Pollock HM, et al: Polymicrobial etiology of acute pelvic inflammatory disease. N Engl J Med 293:166, 1975.
21. Wasserheit JN, Bell TA, Kiviat NB, et al: Microbial causes of proven pelvic inflammatory disease and efficacy of clindamycin and tobramycin. Ann Intern Med 104:187, 1986.
22. Wolner-Hanssen P, Paavonen J, Kiviat N, et al: Outpatient treatment of pelvic inflammatory disease with cefoxitin and doxycycline. Obstet Gynecol 71:595, 1988.
23. Disseminated gonorrhea caused by penicillinase-producing *Neisseria gonorrhoeae*—Wisconsin, Pennsylvania. MMWR Morbid Mortal Wkly Rep 36:161, 1987.
24. Black JR, Brint M, Reichart CA: Successful treatment of gonococcal endocarditis with ceftriaxone. J Infect Dis 157:1281, 1988.
25. Disseminated gonococcal infections and meninigitis—Pennsylvania. MMWR Morbid Mortal Wkly Rep 33:158, 1984.
26. Schwarcz SK, Zenilman JM, Schnell D, et al: National surveillance for antimicrobial resistance in *Neisseria gonorrhoeae*. JAMA 264:1413, 1990.
27. Centers for Disease Control and Prevention: 1993 sexually transmitted diseases guidelines. MMWR Morbid Mortal Wkly Rep 42(RR-14):57, 1993.
28. Plasmid-mediated antimicrobial resistance in *Neisseria gonorrhoeae*—United States, 1988 and 1989. MMWR Morbid Mortal Wkly Rep 284:293, 1990.
29. Knapp JS, Biddle JW, DeWitt WE, Johnson SR: Frequency and distribution in the United States of strains of *Neisseria gonorrhoeae* with plasmid-mediated, high-level resistance to tetracycline. J Infect Dis 155:819, 1987.
30. Morse SA, Johnson SR, Biddle JW, Roberts MC: High-level tetracycline resistance in *Neisseria gonorrhoeae* is result of acquisition of streptococcal tetM determinant. Antimicrob Agents Chemother 30:664, 1986.
31. Handsfield HH, Sandstrom EG, Knapp JS, et al: Epidemiology of penicillinase-producing *Neisseria gonorrhoeae* infections. N Engl J Med 306:950, 1982.
32. Boslego JW, Tramont EC, Takafuji ET, et al: Effect of spectinomycin use on the prevalence of spectinomycin-resistant and of penicillinase-producing *Neisseria gonorrhoeae*. N Engl J Med 317:272, 1987.
33. Faruki H, Kohmescher RN, McKinney WP, Sparling PF: A community-based outbreak of infection with penicillin-resistant *Neisseria gonorrhoeae* not producing penicillinase (chromosomally mediated resistance). N Engl J Med 313:607, 1985.
34. Washington AE, Browner WS, Korenbrot CC: Cost-effectiveness of combined treatment for endocervical gonorrhea. JAMA 257:2056, 1987.
35. Buch LM, Boscia JA: Disseminated multiple antibiotic-resistant gonococcal infection: Needed changes in antimicrobial therapy. Ann Intern Med 107:692, 1987.

111

Chlamydial Infections

Julius Schachter

History

The human diseases caused by *Chlamydia trachomatis* have been recognized since antiquity.[1] Trachoma is described in Egyptian papyruses. Lymphogranuloma venereum was described by John Hunter in the 18th century. The genital tract infections, such as nongonococcal urethritis (NGU) and neonatal ophthalmia caused by *C. trachomatis*, were recognized after the identification of the gonococcus. With the introduction of ocular (Credé) prophylaxis with silver nitrate drops to prevent ophthalmia neonatorum and of methods to diagnose gonococcal infections, it became apparent that conjunctivitis in infants and urethritis in adult men had nongonococcal forms. Chlamydial inclusions were seen in specimens from such cases in the first decade of this century. A breakthrough in chlamydial research was the introduction in 1965 of a cell culture isolation method. With use of this test, several groups published studies finding that one third to one half of men with NGU had chlamydial infections.[1, 2] Since then, the clinical syndromes associated with these infections have rapidly expanded.[3]

Characteristics of the Pathogen

C. trachomatis is an obligate intracellular bacterium. It is one of four species within the genus *Chlamydia*.[4–6] Two others, *Chlamydia psittaci* and *Chlamydia pneumoniae*, are also human pathogens. Chlamydiae are separated from other bacteria on the basis of a unique life cycle. *C. trachomatis* is differentiated from the other species on the basis of sulfonamide sensitivity and production of inclusions that contain glycogen.

Chlamydiae have evolved a specialized outer membrane structure that is adapted to the requirements of the life cycle. The infectious elementary body is a small (approximately 350 nm) rigid form that is not metabolically active. Structural rigidity is maintained by cross-linked cysteine-rich proteins, not by muramic acid. Inside a susceptible host cell, reduction of the disulfide bonds results in a more flexible and permeable membrane. The larger (approximately 1000 nm) intracellular form, called the reticulate body, is metabolically active and divides by binary fission. It is not stable in the extracellular environment. Toward the end of the cycle, the reticulate bodies change to elementary bodies that are released when the cell lyses.

Chlamydiae are antigenically complex. They possess a genus-specific lipopolysaccharide antigen. Antigens of species and serotype specificity are found in the major outer membrane protein.[7] This is a cysteine-rich protein composing 60% of the weight of the outer membrane.[8]

A more detailed description of biologic properties of the organism can be found in Chapter 232.

Epidemiology

C. trachomatis is considered our most common sexually transmitted bacterial pathogen.[9] Current estimates are that more than 4 million infections occur annually in the United States. These infections are worldwide in distribution. Infants can acquire the infection when they pass through the infected birth canal. Sporadic cases of conjunctivitis occur when infective genital discharges are inoculated into the eye. Prospective studies have shown that at least 60% to 70% of perinatally exposed infants are infected.[10] Approximately one in six exposed infants develops pneumonia, and approximately one in three develops conjunctivitis.[11]

Because of the long (approximately 48 to 72 hours) growth cycle of the bacterium, the incubation periods for chlamydial infections are relatively long, typically 1 to 3 weeks. The efficiency of sexual transmission of chlamydiae is not known. Contact tracing studies reveal infection rates of 85% for female source contacts of men with chlamydial urethritis.[12] Inapparent infections are common. In screening settings, up to 70% of the women with chlamydial infection have neither signs nor symptoms of the infection.[13] If untreated, chlamydial infections can persist for years.

Individuals with lower genital tract infection are at risk for upper genital tract disease.[14] The rates at which these occur are not known. Approximately 1 in 10 young women with cervical chlamydial infection will develop clinically evident pelvic inflammatory disease. However, perhaps an even larger proportion may develop asymptomatic upper genital tract infections. These can lead to tubal factor infertility and ectopic pregnancy.[15]

A number of risk factors for chlamydial infection can be identified. Age is the most important one. The highest infection rates are found in sexually active adolescents. Among teenagers, approximately 15% of sexually active girls and 5% to 10% of sexually active boys have chlamydial infections.[2, 16–18] Other risk factors include recent change in partner, failure to use barrier methods of contraception, low socioeconomic status, and use of oral contraceptives.[2, 13, 19] One important risk factor is the diagnosis of gonorrhea.[2] Approximately 20% of men and 40% of women with gonorrhea have concomitant chlamydial infection.

The proportions cited reflect data from studies performed before the introduction of *Chlamydia* control programs. It has become obvious in a number of settings that the prevalence of *C. trachomatis* infections can drop dramatically with the introduction of broad-based screening and treatment programs. In cities where *Chlamydia* prevalence is dropping, the chlamydial contribution to various disease states is changing as well.

Pathogenesis

Pathogenic mechanisms for chlamydial diseases are not clear. Chlamydial infection can induce local lymphoproliferation in the form of lymphoid follicles.[1] The trachoma biotype of *C. trachomatis*, the common sexually transmitted pathogen, grows only in squamocolumnar cells. There is suggestive but not conclusive evidence that much of the pathologic process is mediated by immune responses and that second infections are more damaging. Sensitizing antigens have been identified from animal studies.[20] The leading candidate for a sensitizing antigen has been characterized as a member of the 60-kDa heat shock protein (HSP 60) family.[21] This antigen has been shown to be capable of inducing inflammation in previously sensitized animals. The soluble antigen is loosely bound to the elementary body and is excreted by infected cells and may be produced by cells when infection has been suppressed by the action of lymphokines.[22] Women suffering from tubal factor infertility or ectopic pregnancy may have high levels of antibodies to HSP 60.[23–24]

Clinical Manifestations

Genital Tract Disease

The most common manifestation of sexually transmitted infections is NGU in men[2, 25] (Table 111–1). This syndrome is defined by exclusion, that is, the failure to find *Neisseria gonorrhoeae* organisms in urethral specimens from a man with urethritis. NGU is more common than gonococcal urethritis. The age distribution is similar for NGU and gonococcal urethritis. Most cases occur in the 15- to 25-year-old group. NGU is more common than gonococcal urethritis in men of higher socioeconomic class and in heterosexual men.

NGU is characterized by pyuria. There is usually a mucoid to mucopurulent discharge. It is less purulent than the typical discharge of gonococcal urethritis. However, the clinical findings in NGU and gonococcal urethritis have sufficient overlap to render diagnosis purely on clinical grounds inaccurate. Men without overt discharge can have NGU. A common method of diagnosing NGU is to demonstrate a "significant" number of polymorphonuclear leukocytes (PMNs) in either a first-catch urine specimen or a smear prepared from a urethral swab. If a Gram stain of discharge shows many PMNs but no intracellular diplococci, a presumptive diagnosis of NGU is made. There is no unanimity as to the significant number of PMNs. For resuspension of the centrifuged sediment of a 10- to 15-mL sample of first-catch urine, the usual criterion is 15 or more PMNs per × 400 high-power field; for a smear obtained by urethral swabbing, the cutoff is 5 or more PMNs per × 1000 field.[26]

Postgonococcal urethritis is a special subset of NGU. It is seen in men who have been successfully treated for gonococcal infection and either develop symptoms shortly after therapy or remain symptomatic.[27] *C. trachomatis* is the leading cause of this condition, being responsible for 70% to 90% of cases. β-Lactam drugs in dosages used to treat gonorrhea are largely ineffective against chlamydiae. Because of the high (more than 20%) double infection rate, the Centers for Disease Control and Prevention has recommended that all cases of gonorrhea in heterosexual men be treated presumptively for chlamydial infection.[28]

Although NGU was long considered to be a trivial condition, it is now recognized that serious complications can result. Ascending infections can occur, resulting in epididymitis.[29] *C. trachomatis* is the leading cause of epididymitis in sexually active young men. Rectal infections are not uncommon. Screening studies in gay men attending venereal disease clinics found that approximately 6% of asymptomatic men yielded *Chlamydia* from rectal swabs, compared with a 12% recovery rate from men with proctitis.[30] *C. trachomatis* can be recovered from the pharynx of sexually active adults at risk for genital tract infection.

In the woman, the most commonly affected site is the cervix, where the organism can cause a mucopurulent endocervicitis.[2] This condition is characterized by a mucopurulent endocervical discharge, often accompanied by easily induced bleeding and edema within a zone of ectopy.[31] Asymptomatic and inapparent infections are often found during screening of women having routine pelvic examinations for cervical cytology or birth control advice. Approximately 70% of the infections detected during screening were not associated with any abnormal clinical findings.[13]

Because women with gonorrhea often have chlamydial infection, the same rationale as discussed before for men has been applied to treatment of women with gonorrhea. It is even more important to treat women with gonorrhea for chlamydial infection. Women have double infection rates approximately twice as high as those observed in men (35% to 45% of women with gonorrhea have concomitant chlamydial infection). Eradication of the chlamydiae will reduce the subsequent development of salpingitis.[2, 32]

Efforts have been made to establish clinical criteria for diagnosing chlamydial cervicitis. Swab tests can be used to demonstrate a purulent discharge (a white swab inserted in the endocervical canal will be colored yellow in the presence of a purulent discharge) or easily induced bleeding (a swab rubbed against the endocervical wall will be reddened by bleeding caused by pressure if the cervix is edematous and inflamed).[31] These tests have a predictive value of 30% to 50% for *C. trachomatis* infection in different populations and have been used as a guideline for presumptive therapy[2, 9, 28] (Table 111–2).

Some common features can be associated with chlamydial infection among symptomatic women. *C. trachomatis* is a parasite of columnar epithelium; as yet, it has not been found to be capable of growth in squamous cells. Thus, the organism does not cause vaginitis. The major susceptible sites within the lower genital tract would be in the endocervix, within the squamocolumnar junction, and in the urethra when chlamydial infection has been associated with sterile pyuria in some populations of women.[33] The association of chlamydiae with the urethral syndrome was shown in college-age women. It is unwise to generalize those findings to other populations of women.

Evidence suggesting a chlamydial etiology for some cases of bartholinitis has been developed.[34] What proportion of cases may be attributed to chlamydiae is uncertain, because most had both chlamydial and gonococcal infections.

Ascending genital infection is common. Acute salpingitis is the most important complication of sexually transmitted chlamydial infection.[14] *C. trachomatis* is found in the endometrium or fallopian tubes of approximately 25% of women with acute salpingitis in the United States and at higher rates in western Europe.[35–37] As expected, younger women are at higher risk.[14] Chlamydial salpingitis tends to be clinically milder than salpingitis associated with gonococcal or mixed anaerobic infections. *Chlamydia*-infected women usually have a longer prodrome before being admitted to the hospital.[38] *C. trachomatis* is also associated with complications of salpingitis, such as the Fitz-Hugh–Curtis syndrome (perihepatitis).[39]

TABLE 111–1 ■ Proportion of Common Genital Tract Disease Attributed to *Chlamydia trachomatis*

CONDITION	PERCENTAGE DUE TO *CHLAMYDIA*
Nongonococcal urethritis	35–50
Postgonococcal urethritis	>70
Epididymitis, young men	>60
Mucopurulent endocervicitis	30–50
Acute salpingitis	25–50

TABLE 111–2 ■ Clinical Conditions Calling for Presumptive Therapy for *Chlamydia trachomatis* Infection

POPULATION	CONDITIONS
Men	Nongonococcal urethritis
	Postgonococcal urethritis
	Epididymitis
	Gonorrhea
	Female partner with conditions listed below
Women	Mucopurulent endocervicitis
	Acute salpingitis
	Gonorrhea
	Male partner with conditions listed above

Chlamydiae are important causes of tubal factor infertility and ectopic pregnancy as a result of tubal damage after salpingitis.[15, 35, 40] Unfortunately, because chlamydial salpingitis can be clinically mild, or even inapparent, evidence of chlamydial infection is often first obtained retrospectively by serologic tests performed during evaluation for infertility.

The endometrium may be involved in women with generalized pelvic inflammation.[41] It is uncertain whether endometrial chlamydial infection occurs as part of a pathway involving spread from cervix to oviduct (as is likely to be the case for women with salpingitis) or whether there is a discrete self-limited chlamydial endometritis.[42] Other studies have reported recovery of chlamydiae from the endometrium of asymptomatic nonpregnant women.[43] It seems likely that chlamydial endometritis exists as a distinct entity, although it is obviously impossible to tell whether it is part of the spectrum of a progressive disease process.

Women who are *Chlamydia*-positive in the first trimester of their pregnancies may develop postpartum endometritis after a vaginal delivery.[44] The role of *C. trachomatis* in other complications of pregnancy is controversial. Some studies have found an association between chlamydial infection and fetal wastage and prematurity.[45, 46] Other studies have not confirmed these findings or have shown that only a small subset of women with chlamydial infection (those with immunoglobulin M antibody) had an excess prematurity rate.[47, 48]

Neonatal Disease

Approximately 5 to 21 days after birth, the infant develops a mucopurulent conjunctivitis.[1] Hyperemia and discharge are the most prominent findings. Follicles are not seen unless the condition persists for longer than a month. Conjunctivitis is usually self-limiting and resolves in a few months without treatment. It is not considered to be a sight-threatening condition. Corneal damage is minimal, although some keratitis and micropannus can develop. Conjunctival scarring is relatively uncommon, although sheet scarring may follow the disease in infants who develop pseudomembranes. These scars do not result in lid deformity. Occasional cases persist, and severe disease, which may threaten vision, can rarely develop.[49]

The incubation period for chlamydial pneumonia of infants is usually between 2 and 12 weeks.[50, 51] The infants will often have a prodrome of rhinitis, and many will have had conjunctivitis. Affected infants are usually afebrile, are markedly tachypneic and occasionally apneic, and have a staccato cough. They are hypergammaglobulinemic, particularly in the immunoglobulin M class. A relative eosinophilia occurs in approximately one third of affected infants. Radiographs usually show hyperinflation.

The spectrum of chlamydial respiratory involvement in infants is broad. Nasopharyngeal infections are common.[50] Some infants develop a severe rhinitis, without lower respiratory tract involvement, that can occasionally interfere with respiration.[52] The pathogenesis of chlamydial pneumonia probably reflects descending infection, and bronchiolitis can occur. Infants with chlamydial pneumonia typically fall into the category of infants with failure to thrive and often have only mild respiratory distress, with tachypnea being the prominent finding.[50] The infants occasionally have severe respiratory problems and may become apneic and require respiratory assistance, but more often they can be managed on an outpatient basis. Most infants with chlamydial pneumonia develop asthma or obstructive airway disease,[53] even after successful treatment of the acute disease.

Conjunctivitis in Adults

Inclusion conjunctivitis in adults is an acute follicular conjunctivitis that must be differentiated from adenoviral keratoconjunctivitis by microbiologic tests. The condition has an incubation period of approximately 1 to 3 weeks. It is typically seen in sexually active young adults and results from exposure to infected genital discharges. It is similar in presentation to early trachoma, although it is not considered to be a sight-threatening condition. It can become chronic, although most cases clear spontaneously after several months if they are not treated.

Diagnosis

It has long been considered that isolation in a cell culture system is the most efficient way of diagnosing *C. trachomatis* infection.[54] Although this procedure is usually only 80% to 90% sensitive in expert laboratories, it has still been more sensitive than the antigen detection methods. The major variable in diagnosis has been adequate specimen collection because appropriate samples of involved epithelial cells must be collected, and it is important that specimens be processed relatively quickly and that a cold chain be maintained. Cycloheximide-treated McCoy cells are the most commonly used system. The nonculture methods that are more widely available include direct fluorescent antibody test, enzyme immunoassay, and direct DNA probes.[55–57]

Under good conditions (expert specimen collectors, well-trained microscopists), the direct fluorescent antibody tests have a sensitivity of approximately 80% (compared with culture) and a specificity of 97% to 98% for detecting chlamydial infection of the cervix.[58] This is slightly better performance than is obtained with most enzyme immunoassays or the direct DNA probes.

Amplified DNA probe technology, such as polymerase chain reaction or ligase chain reaction, is much more sensitive.[59–61] There have been some concerns about the possible importance of inhibitors in the early versions of the commercially available polymerase chain reaction tests.[62] When inhibitors have not been a problem, this procedure has actually been more sensitive than culture. Multicenter clinical trials have found ligase chain reaction to be far more sensitive than culture, and this test has been found efficient in detecting chlamydial infection with use of urine samples from men and women.[60, 63]

Infant conjunctivitis may be diagnosed readily by any of the cytologic tests. Giemsa stain is adequate in diagnosing severe cases of conjunctivitis, whereas the antigen detection techniques are sensitive. The agent may be easily isolated.

A specific diagnosis for pneumonia may be more difficult because of sampling problems, but the organism can often be isolated from the nasopharynx or tracheobronchial aspirates.[50] Serologic testing may be the method of choice for diagnosing chlamydial pneumonia because of the sampling problems. Infants with chlamydial pneumonia almost always develop high immunoglobulin M antibody levels, and because of their defined exposure (at birth), the diagnosis may be readily established on the basis of a single point titer of specific antichlamydial immunoglobulin M antibodies above 1:32 in the microimmunofluorescence test.[64]

Serologic tests do not play a role in diagnosing uncomplicated lower genital tract infections.[65] A major problem is a high prevalence of antibodies to *C. trachomatis* in high-risk populations. The complement fixation test is relatively insensitive for diagnosing infections with the trachoma biotype. The microimmunofluorescence test is the serologic test of choice.[66] Because of the high titers seen in upper genital tract disease, serology can play a supportive role in establishing a diagnosis of chlamydial salpingitis or epididymitis.

On clinical grounds, the spectrum of chlamydial genital tract disease is similar to that of gonococcal infection, and patients should be tested for both.

TABLE 111–3 ■ Treatment of Chlamydial Infections

	FIRST CHOICE		SECOND CHOICE	
ORGANISM AND CONDITION	Drug	Dose*	Drug	Dose*
C. psittaci				
Psittacosis†	Tetracycline	250 mg qid × 3 wk	Erythromycin	250 mg qid × 3 wk
C. trachomatis				
Genital tract infections (e.g., urethritis, cervicitis)	Doxycycline	100 mg bid × 1 wk	Azithromycin	1 g orally, single dose
Pregnant women	Erythromycin	250 mg qid × 2 wk	Amoxicillin	500 mg tid × 1 wk
Infant pneumonia	Erythromycin	10 mg/kg qid × 2 wk	Sulfisoxazole	37.5 mg/kg qid × 2 wk
Inclusion conjunctivitis (infants)	Erythromycin	10 mg/kg qid × 2 wk	Sulfisoxazole	37.5 mg/kg qid × 2 wk
Inclusion conjunctivitis (adults)	Tetracycline	250 mg qid × 3 wk	Erythromycin	250 mg qid × 3 wk

*qid, Four times daily; tid, three times daily; bid, twice daily.
†Similar regimens are probably effective for *C. pneumoniae* (TWAR) infection.

Treatment

One gram of oral azithromycin given in a single dose is now considered the treatment of choice for uncomplicated lower genital tract infections with *C. trachomatis*.[9, 28] This is as effective as a week-long course of oral doxycycline.[67] The currently recommended guidelines for treating these infections are shown in Table 111–3. Chlamydial infection in the infant calls for oral therapy with erythromycin. Conjunctivitis usually responds to 7 to 10 days of therapy; pneumonia should be treated for 14 to 21 days.[9, 28] Topical therapy is not recommended for conjunctivitis because of relatively high failure rates and because systemic therapy will prevent subsequent development of pneumonia. Treatment of pelvic inflammatory disease should always include antimicrobials effective against *C. trachomatis* (see Chapter 117).

Prevention

Guidelines for a *Chlamydia* control program have been developed, but no such control program is currently in effect because of economic constraints.[9] Recommended methods for these infections include the relatively nonspecific measures used for other sexually transmitted diseases. These include screening of high-risk populations and examination and treatment of contacts. No vaccines are available, although this is currently an area of intensive research efforts.

It is clear that programs involving screening of high-risk populations may identify many infected individuals. Unfortunately, such programs are not in wide use. Where programs are present, they focus only on women, because women have routine pelvic examinations. With the current potential for screening high-risk populations by testing first-catch urine specimens, there is a real possibility for successful broad-based *Chlamydia* control programs. Where active screening and treatment programs have been in effect for a long time (these programs have mostly involved family planning clinics), dramatic reductions in prevalence of infection have been noted.

There is one instance in which effective control measures are currently available. Perinatal chlamydial infections can be prevented by a program of screening pregnant women and treating those found to be infected with erythromycin.[68] Because attack rates have been fairly consistent in most studies, the prevalence of chlamydial infection in pregnant women will determine the cost-benefit relationship of this stratagem. A number of studies have found that more than 20% of pregnant women have chlamydial infection. Such prenatal clinics would clearly be appropriate sites for screening and treatment.

References

1. Schachter J, Dawson CR (eds): Human Chlamydial Infections. Littleton, MA, PSG Publishing, 1978.
2. Stamm WE, Holmes KK: *Chlamydia trachomatis* infections of the adult. *In* Holmes KK, Mardh P-A, Sparling PF, et al (eds): Sexually Transmitted Diseases. New York, McGraw-Hill, 1990, pp 181–193.
3. Schachter J: Chlamydial infections. N Engl J Med 298:428, 490, 540, 1978.
4. Moulder JW, Hatch TP, Kuo CC, et al: Order II. Chlamydiales Storz and Page 1971. *In* Krieg NR, Holt JG (eds): Bergey's Manual of Systematic Bacteriology, Vol 1. Baltimore, Williams & Wilkins, 1984, pp 729–739.
5. Grayston JT, Kuo C-C, Campbell LA: *Chlamydia pneumoniae* sp. nov. for *Chlamydia* strain TWAR. J Syst Bacteriol 39:88, 1989.
6. Fukushi H, Hirai K: *Chlamydia pecorum*—The fourth species of genus *Chlamydia*. Microbiol Immunol 37:516, 1993.
7. Caldwell HD, Schachter J: Antigenic analysis of the major outer membrane protein of *Chlamydia* spp. Infect Immun 35:1024, 1982.
8. Caldwell HD, Kromhout J, Schachter J: Purification and partial characterization of the major outer membrane protein of *Chlamydia trachomatis*. Infect Immun 31:1161, 1981.
9. Centers for Disease Control and Prevention: Recommendations for the prevention and management of *Chlamydia trachomatis* infections, 1993. MMWR 42(RR-12):5, 1993.
10. Schachter J, Grossman M, Sweet RL: Prospective study of perinatal transmission of *Chlamydia trachomatis*. JAMA 255:3374, 1986.
11. Alexander ER, Harrison HR: Role of *Chlamydia trachomatis* in perinatal infection. Rev Infect Dis 5:713, 1983.
12. Oriel JD, Ridgway GL: Studies of the epidemiology of chlamydial infection of the human genital tract. *In* Mardh P-A, Holmes KK, Oriel JD, et al (eds): Chlamydial Infections: Proceedings, 5th International Symposium, Lund, Sweden, June 15–19, 1982. Amsterdam, Elsevier, 1982, pp 425–428.
13. Schachter J, Stoner E, Moncada J: Screening for chlamydial infections in women attending family planning clinics: Evaluations of presumptive indicators for therapy. West J Med 138:375, 1983.
14. Mardh P-A, Oriel D: Genital chlamydial infections. *In* Bowie WR, Caldwell HD, Jones RP, et al (eds): Chlamydial Infections: Proceedings of the Seventh International Symposium on Human Chlamydial Infections. New York, Cambridge University Press, 1990, pp 293–302.
15. Cates W Jr: Sexually transmitted organisms and infertility: The proof of the pudding. Sex Transm Dis 11:113, 1984.

16. Shafer MA, Blain B, Beck A: *Chlamydia trachomatis*: Important relationships to race, contraception, lower genital tract infection, and Papanicolaou smears. J Pediatr 104:141, 1984.
17. Podgore JK, Holmes KK, Alexander ER: Asymptomatic urethral infections due to *Chlamydia trachomatis* in male US military personnel. J Infect Dis 146:828, 1982.
18. Shafer MA, Prager V, Shalwitz J: Prevalence of urethral *Chlamydia trachomatis* and *Neisseria gonorrhoeae* among asymptomatic, sexually active adolescent boys. J Infect Dis 156:223, 1987.
19. Handsfield HH, Jasman LL, Roberts PL: Criteria for selective screening for *Chlamydia trachomatis* infection in women attending family planning clinics. JAMA 255:1730, 1986.
20. Watkins NG, Hadlow WJ, Moos AB, et al: Ocular delayed hypersensitivity: A pathogenic mechanism of chlamydial conjunctivitis in guinea pigs. Proc Natl Acad Sci USA 83:7480, 1986.
21. Morrison RP, Belland RJ, Lyng K, Caldwell HD: Chlamydial disease pathogenesis. The 57-kD chlamydial hypersensitivity antigen is a stress response protein. J Exp Med 170:1271, 1989.
22. Beatty WL, Byrne GI, Morrison RP: Morphologic and antigenic characterization of interferon gamma–mediated persistent *Chlamydia trachomatis* infection in vitro. Proc Natl Acad Sci USA 90:3998, 1993.
23. Wagar EA, Schachter J, Bavoil P, Stephens RS: Differential human serologic response to two 60,000 molecular weight *Chlamydia trachomatis* antigens. J Infect Dis 162:922, 1990.
24. Toye B, Laferriere C, Claman P, et al: Association between antibody to the chlamydial heat-shock protein and tubal infertility. J Infect Dis 168:1236, 1993.
25. Holmes KK, Handsfield HH, Wang S-P, et al: Etiology of nongonococcal urethritis. N Engl J Med 292:1199, 1975.
26. Bowie WR: Comparison of Gram stain and first-voided urine sediment in the diagnosis of urethritis. Sex Transm Dis 5:39, 1978.
27. Oriel JD, Ridgway GL, Reeve P: The lack of effect of ampicillin plus probenecid given for genital infections with *Neisseria gonorrhoeae* on associated infection with *Chlamydia trachomatis*. J Infect Dis 133:568, 1976.
28. Centers for Disease Control and Prevention: 1993 Sexually transmitted diseases treatment guidelines. MMWR 42(RR-14):51, 1993.
29. Berger RE, Alexander ER, Monda GE, et al: *Chlamydia trachomatis* as a cause of acute "idiopathic" epididymitis. N Engl J Med 298:301, 1978.
30. Quinn TC, Goodell SE, Mkrtichian E, et al: *Chlamydia trachomatis* proctitis. N Engl J Med 305:195, 1981.
31. Brunham RC, Paavonen J, Stevens CE, et al: Mucopurulent cervicitis—The ignored counterpart in women of urethritis in men. N Engl J Med 311:1, 1984.
32. Stamm WE, Guinan ME, Johnson C, et al: Effect of treatment for *Neisseria gonorrhoeae* on simultaneous infection with *Chlamydia trachomatis*. N Engl J Med 310:545, 1984.
33. Stamm WE, Wagner KF, Amsel R, et al: Causes of the acute urethral syndrome in women. N Engl J Med 303:409, 1980.
34. Davies JA, Rees E, Hobson D, et al: Isolation of *Chlamydia trachomatis* from Bartholin's ducts. Br J Vener Dis 54:409, 1978.
35. Mardh P-A, Ripa T, Svensson L, et al: *Chlamydia trachomatis* infection in patients with acute salpingitis. N Engl J Med 296:1377, 1977.
36. Wasserheit JN, Bell TA, Kiviat NB, et al: Microbial causes of proven pelvic inflammatory disease and efficacy of clindamycin and tobramycin. Ann Intern Med 104:187, 1986.
37. Sweet RL, Schachter J, Robbie M: Failure of beta lactam antibiotics to eradicate *Chlamydia trachomatis* in the endometrium despite apparent clinical cure of acute salpingitis. JAMA 250:2641, 1983.
38. Swenson CE, Donegan E, Schachter J: *Chlamydia trachomatis* induced salpingitis in mice. J Infect Dis 148:1101, 1983.
39. Muller-Schoop JW, Wang S-P, Munzinger J, et al: *Chlamydia trachomatis* as possible cause of peritonitis and perihepatitis in young women. Br Med J 1:1022, 1978.
40. Chow JM, Yonekura ML, Richwald GA, et al: The association between *Chlamydia trachomatis* and ectopic pregnancy. A matched-pair, case-control study. JAMA 263:3164, 1990.
41. Kiviat NB, Wolner-Hanssen P, Peterson M, et al: Localization of *Chlamydia trachomatis* infection by direct immunofluorescence and culture in pelvic inflammatory disease. Am J Obstet Gynecol 154:865, 1986.
42. Mardh P-A, Moller BR, Ingerselv HJ, et al: Endometritis caused by *Chlamydia trachomatis*. Br J Vener Dis 57:191, 1981.
43. Cleary RE, Jones RB: Recovery of *Chlamydia trachomatis* from the endometrium of infertile women with serum antichlamydial antibodies. Fertil Steril 44:233, 1985.
44. Wager GP, Martin DH, Koutsky L, et al: Puerperal infectious morbidity: Relationship to route of delivery and to antepartum *Chlamydia trachomatis* infection. Am J Obstet Gynecol 138:1028, 1980.
45. Martin DH, Koutsky L, Eschenbach DA, et al: Prematurity and perinatal mortality in pregnancies complicated by maternal *Chlamydia trachomatis* infections. JAMA 247:1585, 1982.
46. Gravett MG, Nelson HP, DeRouen T, et al: Independent associations of bacterial vaginosis and *Chlamydia trachomatis* infection with adverse pregnancy outcome. JAMA 256:1899, 1986.
47. Harrison HR, Alexander ER, Weinstein L, et al: Cervical *Chlamydia trachomatis* and mycoplasmal infections in pregnancy: Epidemiology and outcomes. JAMA 250:1721, 1983.
48. Sweet RL, Landers DV, Walker C, et al: *Chlamydia trachomatis* infection and pregnancy outcome. Am J Obstet Gynecol 156:824, 1987.
49. Mordhorst CH, Wang S-P, Grayston JT: Childhood trachoma in a nonendemic area. JAMA 239:1765, 1978.
50. Beem MO, Saxon EM: Respiratory tract colonization and a distinctive pneumonia syndrome in infants infected with *Chlamydia trachomatis*. N Engl J Med 296:306, 1977.
51. Harrison HR, English MG, Lee CK, et al: *Chlamydia trachomatis* infant pneumonitis: Comparison with matched controls and other infant pneumonitis. N Engl J Med 298:702, 1978.
52. Cohen SD, Azimi PH, Schachter J: *Chlamydia trachomatis* associated with severe rhinitis and apneic episodes in a one-month-old infant. Clin Pediatr 21:498, 1982.
53. Weiss SG, Newcomb RW, Beem MO: Pulmonary assessment of children after chlamydial pneumonia of infancy. J Pediatr 108:659, 1986.
54. Schachter J: Chlamydiae. *In* Balows A, Hausler WJ Jr, Hermann KL, et al (eds): Manual of Clinical Microbiology, ed 5. Washington, DC, American Society for Microbiology, 1991, pp 1045–1053.
55. Schachter J: Immunodiagnosis of sexually transmitted disease. Yale J Biol Med 58:443, 1985.
56. Tam MR, Stamm WE, Handsfield HH, et al: Culture-independent diagnosis of *Chlamydia trachomatis* using monoclonal antibodies. N Engl J Med 310:1146, 1984.
57. Howard LV, Coleman PF, England BJ, et al: Evaluation of Chlamydiazyme for the detection of genital infections caused by *Chlamydia trachomatis*. J Clin Microbiol 23:329, 1986.
58. Stamm WE: Diagnosis of *Chlamydia trachomatis* genitourinary infections. Ann Intern Med 108:710, 1988.
59. Bobo L, Coutlee F, Yolken RH, et al: Diagnosis of *Chlamydia trachomatis* cervical infection by amplified DNA with an enzyme immunoassay. J Clin Microbiol 28:1968, 1990.
60. Chernesky MA, Lee H, Schachter J, et al: Diagnosis of *Chlamydia trachomatis* urethral infection in symptomatic and asymptomatic men by testing first-void urine in a ligase chain reaction assay. J Infect Dis 170:1308, 1994.
61. Schachter J, Stamm WE, Quinn TC, et al: Ligase chain reaction to detect *Chlamydia trachomatis* infection of the cervix. J Clin Microbiol 32:2540, 1994.
62. Bauwens JE, Clark AM, Stamm WE: Diagnosis of *Chlamydia trachomatis* endocervical infections by a commercial polymerase chain reaction assay. J Clin Microbiol 31:3023, 1993.
63. Lee HH, Chernesky MA, Schachter J, et al: Diagnosis of *Chlamydia trachomatis* genitourinary infection in women by ligase chain reaction assay of urine. Lancet 345:213, 1995.
64. Schachter J, Grossman M, Azimi PH: Serology of *Chlamydia trachomatis* in infants. J Infect Dis 146:530, 1982.
65. Schachter J: Chlamydiae. *In* Rose NR, Conway de Macario E, Fahey JL, et al (eds): Manual of Clinical Laboratory Immunology, ed 4. Washington, DC, American Society for Microbiology, 1992, pp 661–666.
66. Wang S-P, Grayston JT, Alexander ER, Holmes KK: A simplified microimmunofluorescence test with trachoma–lymphogranuloma venereum (*Chlamydia trachomatis*) antigens for use as a screening test for antibody. J Clin Microbiol 1:250, 1975.
67. Martin D, Mroczkowski T, Dalu AZ, et al: A controlled trial of a single dose of azithromycin for the treatment of chlamydial urethritis and cervicitis. N Engl J Med 327:921, 1992.
68. Schachter J, Sweet RL, Grossman M, et al: Experience with the routine use of erythromycin for chlamydial infections in pregnancy. N Engl J Med 314:276, 1986.

112

Syphilis

Daniel M. Musher
Robert E. Baughn

Treponema pallidum is a natural pathogen only for humans. Infection is spread from infected to uninfected individuals by sexual contact; by transplacental passage, leading to congenital syphilis; or rarely by laboratory accident or blood transfusion. The infecting organism enters the body through inapparent breaks in abraded areas of the skin; older theories that the corkscrew motion of *T. pallidum* enables penetration through unbroken epithelium are no longer accepted today. Within the tissues, local replication and dissemination via lymphatics occur simultaneously, thus setting the stage for secondary (disseminated) syphilis. Secondary syphilis resolves spontaneously, leading to a latent stage. Primary syphilis and secondary syphilis together with the first year of latency constitute early syphilis. Except for the now-unusual relapse to secondary syphilis, reappearance of disease after a latent period has been called tertiary syphilis. Human immunodeficiency virus (HIV) infection has had a major impact on the natural evolution of this disease; neurologic disease that appears after a much shorter delay is called neurosyphilis but is not designated as tertiary infection. The clinical manifestations of each stage of syphilis are listed in Table 112–1.

Pathogenesis and Clinical Manifestations

Primary Syphilis

Fourteen to 21 days after inoculation of *T. pallidum* into a dermal site, a red, painless papule 0.5 to 2 cm in diameter appears at the site of inoculation. Within a few days the papule ulcerates, producing the typical chancre of primary syphilis, an ulcerated area sometimes covered by a slight yellowish or grayish exudate and surrounded by a slightly indurated margin (Fig. 112–1). The chancre usually does not cause the patient pain, but it may be somewhat tender on examination. Chancres are generally round, although they may be elongated, following tissue lines. Modest enlargement of inguinal lymph nodes, frequently bilaterally, is observed in the majority of patients who have genital lesions. Although solitary lesions were once said to be characteristic, multiple lesions frequently occur.[1]

Because of their venereal origin, primary syphilitic chancres most frequently occur in the genital, perineal, anal, or oral area; however, any part of the body may be affected. Most chancres are found on the penis of men and on the labia, fourchette, or cervix of women. Chancres in the anus or rectum are particularly common in homosexual men. When these lesions cause pain on defecation or rectal bleeding, they can be confused with hemorrhoids or even a neoplasm,[2] but they often go unnoticed, as do those on the labia and cervix. In most instances, active syphilis in women and in homosexual men is usually not diagnosed until the secondary stage. If untreated, syphilitic chancres heal spontaneously within 3 to 8 weeks. The mechanism for healing is obscure; some kind of local immunity is responsible, because secondary lesions appear during or after the regression of the primary ones. Differentiating a syphilitic chancre from chancroid, the soft chancre caused by infection with *Haemophilus ducreyi*, may be impossible on clinical grounds, although a great degree of tenderness, a yellow exudate over the lesion, or striking inguinal lymphadenopathy with thin and shiny overlying skin is suggestive of chancroid. Simple trauma, especially to the penis, or a fixed drug eruption may cause lesions resembling chancre. Lesions of herpes simplex virus infection usually are not a problem of differential diagnosis, but coinfection by both organisms may occur.

Secondary (Disseminated) Syphilis

Lesions of secondary syphilis result from the hematogenous dissemination of treponemes from syphilitic chancres, and the term disseminated syphilis might be more appropriate.[3] More than 3 weeks elapse between the deposition of *T. pallidum* in the dermis and emergence of these lesions; this delay in development and the failure of the involved sites to develop into lesions that resemble primary chancres reflect a degree of humoral and/or cellular immunity that modifies the evolution of infection. Thus, secondary syphilis appears 4 to 10 weeks after the initial appearance of primary lesions, although in some patients who present with disseminated lesions there is an overlap, and a careful examination discloses a primary chancre. Cases of "malignant" syphilis (lues maligna), in which disseminated lesions resemble primary

TABLE 112–1 ■ Clinical Manifestations of Syphilis by Stages*

PRIMARY	SECONDARY	TERTIARY
Chancre on penis, labia, vagina, cervix, anus, rectum, lips, mouth, nipple, navel, finger Inguinal lymphadenopathy Condyloma latum†	Rash Condyloma latum Lymphadenopathy Hepatitis (subclinical) Systemic: fever, malaise, weight loss Neurologic: headache, meningismus, meningitis, cranial nerve disorders (optic neuritis, deafness, otitis), cerebrovascular accident Periostitis Uveitis, iritis Glomerulonephritis Arthritis	Benign late syphilis (gummata) of skin, subcutaneous tissues, bones, testis, liver Aortitis, aortic aneurysm Neurosyphilis: tabes dorsalis, paresis, psychosis, dementia, meningitis, cerebrovascular accident, spinal cord disease

*Early neurosyphilis, as seen in HIV-infected persons, is specifically not included in this table (see text).
†Most commonly extension from a primary lesion, this condition may precede the onset of secondary (disseminated) syphilis, in which case it represents a stage intermediate between primary and secondary disease. Less frequently, condyloma latum appears in intertriginous areas during secondary (disseminated) infection.

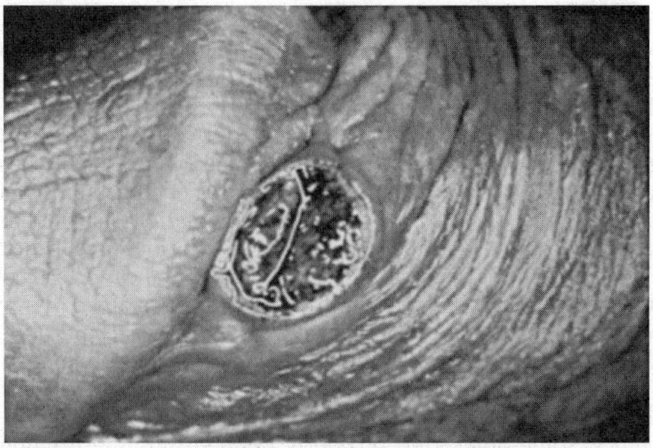

FIGURE 112–1 □ Typical syphilitic chancre with clearly demarcated, slightly indurated margin and nonpurulent base.

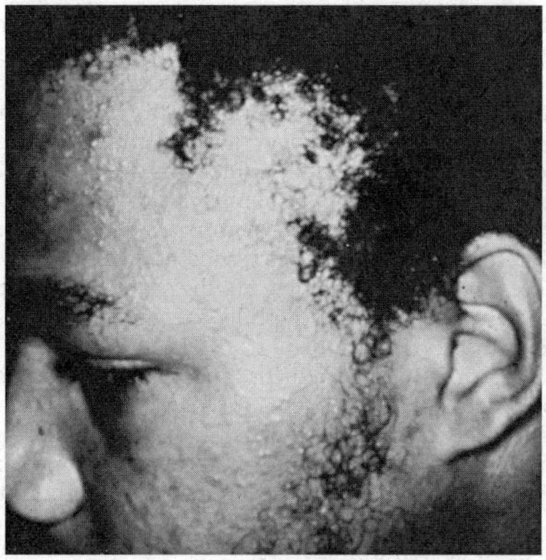

FIGURE 112–3 □ Alopecia associated with secondary syphilis. (Slide provided by the late Dr. John Knox.)

chancres, are rare; host factors that permit this unusual manifestation of syphilis have not been identified. The clinical picture of lues maligna resembles that seen after intravenous injection of a large inoculum of *T. pallidum* into rabbits; because there has been no immune response during a primary stage of infection, multiple skin chancres appear all over the body.

The initial finding in disseminated syphilis is said to be an evanescent macular rash that is usually overlooked by the patient and not observed by the physician. A few days later a symmetric papular eruption appears, involving the entire trunk and the extremities, including palms of the hands and soles of the feet. The papules are red or reddish brown, discrete, and usually 0.5 to 2 cm in diameter (Fig. 112–2). They are generally scaly, although they may be smooth, follicular, or, rarely, pustular. Except for the involvement of palms and soles, syphilis may be difficult to distinguish from pityriasis rosea or psoriasis. Vesicles are said not to occur, although vesiculopustular lesions are seen on rare occasions and are common on the palms or soles. Circular (anular) lesions occur on the face of dark-skinned persons.[4] Hypo- or hyperpigmentation may be seen. Alopecia (Fig. 112–3) occurs in some cases. Mucosal lesions, either small, superficial, ulcerated areas with grayish borders that resemble painless aphthous ulcers or larger gray plaques, are also common. Erosive gastritis has been documented in rare instances.

Condyloma latum refers to one or more large, raised, whitish or gray lesions found in warm, moist areas. These lesions were originally described as a manifestation of secondary

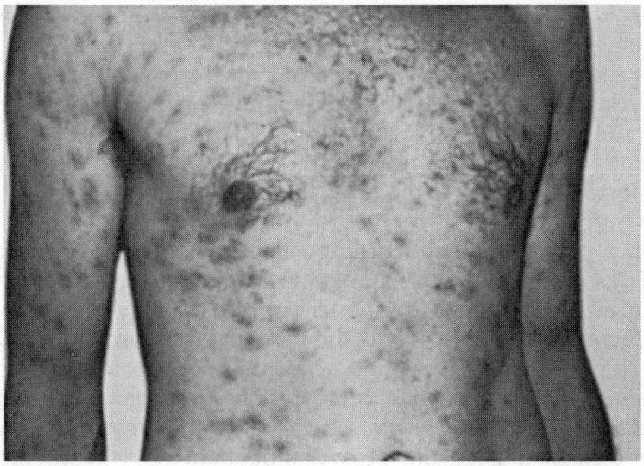

FIGURE 112–2 □ Typical generalized rash of secondary syphilis.

syphilis, reflecting local breakdown of secondary lesions with extension of infection in areas of tissue trauma; most frequently, the axilla and groin were involved.[5] Today, it is far more common to observe condylomata in an area adjacent to a primary chancre, generally in the perineum or around the anus, resulting from extension from the primary lesion. These lesions appear before or soon after the generalized lesions. In this situation the local spread of treponemes from a primary lesion in a favorable environment is responsible; the condyloma represents an intermediate stage of infection, because, strictly speaking, it does not reflect dissemination.

Secondary syphilis is a systemic disease, and interest in the dermatologic manifestations should not blind the physician to the presence of other symptoms, such as malaise, sore throat, headache, weight loss, low-grade fever, or muscle aches.[6] The presence of pruritus has received emphasis in the modern era, and it may be severe. Lymph node enlargement is present in the great majority of patients. In one prospective study, 75% of infected persons had palpable inguinal nodes, and 38% had palpable axillary, 28% posterior cervical, 18% femoral, and 17% epitrochlear nodes.[6] Periosteal inflammation was said to be clinically apparent in one fourth of cases in the prepenicillin era, skull, tibia, sternum, and ribs being involved most often; at present, symptomatic involvement occurs only rarely. Subclinical hepatitis can be detected by laboratory studies in 10% of cases and is supported by histologic findings.[7] Occasionally, symptomatic hepatitis results.

Neurologic manifestations that appear in early syphilis have received increased attention, especially because of the relation with concurrent HIV infection, which is discussed in detail later. Before the occurrence of HIV infection, abnormalities in the cerebrospinal fluid (CSF)—increased white blood cells, elevated protein level, a positive Veneral Disease Research Laboratory (VDRL) test, or the presence of viable *T. pallidum* organisms—were detected in up to 40% of cases of secondary syphilis in the absence of neurologic abnormalities.[8, 9] However, no more than 1% to 2% of patients with secondary syphilis were found to have symptoms or signs of central nervous system involvement, including meningismus, meningitis, headaches, and mental changes; cranial nerve abnormalities such as ocular palsy, deafness, or nystagmus, and internuclear ophthalmoplegia; cerebrovascular accidents; or signs of spinal cord or nerve root involvement such as tingling, weakness, and hyporeflexia. These findings are sometimes called early neurosyphilis. Before the penicillin era, they were included under the term neurorecurrence because they nearly always occurred in subjects who had received inadequate therapy for syphilis.[10] There may be some degree of overlap between these neurologic manifestations of early, secondary syphilis and some of the classic manifestations of late or tertiary neurosyphilis. It is important to note, however, that at this stage the symptoms are reversible with treatment. Progression to late neurosyphilis was uncommon, even in the prepenicillin era, if treatment was continued until the CSF returned to normal. As discussed later and reviewed elsewhere,[10] both the frequency and the severity of neurologic involvement in secondary syphilis are greatly increased in persons with HIV infection.

Iritis, anterior uveitis, arthritis, and glomerulonephritis or nephrotic syndrome also occur in secondary syphilis. Circulating immune complexes that contain treponemal antigen and human fibronectin together with antibody and complement are present in this stage of infection,[11] and their deposition in relevant organs is thought to play a role in the pathogenesis of these syndromes.

Latent Syphilis

The natural history of untreated secondary syphilis is marked by spontaneous resolution after a period of 3 to 12 weeks, leaving the patient free of lesions and of symptoms. If treatment has not been given, this naturally attained asymptomatic state is called latency. In the pretreatment era, 25% of patients whose infection had become latent had a recrudescence of active, secondary syphilis.[12] Because these relapses usually occurred within 1 year of the onset of latency, this period was called early latency. Relapses after this time were rare, so after 1 year without recurrence of disease and before the onset of tertiary syphilis untreated persons were said to have entered the late latent period. Patients with late latent syphilis are immune to reinfection with *T. pallidum*.[13]

At present, patients are diagnosed as having latent syphilis if they have a reactive serologic test for syphilis (STS) that measures antibody to cardiolipin (see the later section on laboratory diagnosis) in the absence of any apparent signs of disease and if a test for specific antitreponemal antibody (*T. pallidum* hemagglutination assay) is positive. Strictly speaking, the diagnosis is proved only if an entirely normal CSF excludes the possibility of neurosyphilis. These persons probably represent a heterogeneous group in regard to their syphilitic infection. Some may have an unrecognized chancre. Others may have had an unrecognized chancre that healed and have not yet developed disseminated disease. Some subjects may still have a reactive test after having been given antibiotic treatment for some unrelated condition, syphilis not having been thought to be present. Others may retain reactive STS despite being cured of the infection (a "serofast" state). The majority of patients with positive STS and *T. pallidum* hemagglutination assay results but without signs of active syphilitic infection probably do not have true latent infection, although from a public health point of view they are generally regarded as if they do.

Tertiary Syphilis

Clinical manifestations of tertiary syphilis[14] develop after a highly variable latent period, usually longer than 2 years. The incidence varies greatly, depending on how careful a search is made for the manifestations. Among a large group of untreated patients who were observed for many years, benign late syphilis became clinically apparent in 15%, cardiovascular syphilis in 10%, and neurosyphilis in 7%.[12] However, some authorities have stated that the longer patients are observed without treatment, the greater the percentage who develop cardiovascular syphilis,[15] and, in one study, some cardiovascular abnormalities attributable to syphilis were said to be present at autopsy in up to 80% of untreated subjects.[16] At present, in the United States, all these syndromes of tertiary syphilis are extremely rare.

Benign late syphilis is characterized by the presence of gummata—true granulomas with epithelioid and giant cells and central necrosis in nonvital structures such as skin, soft tissue, bones, and cartilage and parenchymal organs such as liver or testes. The pathogenesis of these lesions is obscure. Early reports that claimed to identify treponemes in tertiary lesions were based on examination of silver-stained tissue sections, which tended to produce false-positive results. One study used fluorescent staining to demonstrate treponemes,[17] but the lesion itself was not so clearly a tertiary one. Rather than a response to the presence of large numbers of treponemes, some other kind of poorly defined immune reaction is thought to be responsible. The nature of the immune reaction is further obscured by the fact that there is no relation between the location of primary or disseminated lesions and the eventual site of gummata.

Benign late syphilis usually presents with isolated lesions of the skin and subcutaneous tissues over the face and neck and at sites on the extremities that are exposed to minor trauma such as the elbows.[18] Indurated, nodular, or ulcerated lesions that describe an arc or an irregular full circle are characteristic. Tissue destruction and scarring may result. Peripheral hyperpigmentation is seen, with central scarring. Untreated, these lesions may persist for several years. Late syphilis of bone affects the tibia, fibula, clavicle, and skull, although any bone (or bones) may be involved.[14] Pain and swelling are consistent with the periosteal location of the granulomatous reaction. Destruction of cartilage also plays an important part in determining the clinical appearance of lesions. Large visceral gummata may be asymptomatic or may cause symptoms referable to the involved organ.

Syphilitic aortitis results from involvement of the vasa vasorum of the aorta and resulting medial necrosis. The majority of patients are asymptomatic. Clinical syndromes that used to be observed relatively frequently and that still occur occasionally include aneurysm of the ascending aorta, rarely with erosion into the bones of the thorax, aortic insufficiency, left ventricular hypertrophy, and congestive heart failure.[19] Involvement of the ostia of the coronary arteries may cause symptoms of ischemic heart disease. Syphilis of the aorta is recognized radiographically by calcifications or aneurysm in the ascending aorta. This complication may become manifest years after active disease of the aorta has subsided, probably resulting from continued mechanical stress in an already damaged vital area. The VDRL reaction is negative in one third of patients at the time when syphilitic disease of the aorta is diagnosed.

Late neurosyphilis may cause any of a number of syndromes, including tabes dorsalis, manic-depressive behavior, psychosis, dementia, paresis, and death. Syndromes that overlap those of early neurosyphilis include meningitis, cerebrovascular accident, and myelitis. A mixed picture may result.[20] Although typical examples of "classic" cases are reported,[21] the usual picture appears to be more varied.[22–25] Proving a diagnosis of neurosyphilis, or, for that matter, being certain that the existing literature on the subject includes only proven cases, may be exceedingly difficult. The clinical picture is nonspecific, STS in the CSF may be negative in up to 25% of cases, and the CSF may be entirely normal in 10% to 15% of patients who are thought to have the disease.[22–24] Because the fluorescent treponemal absorption antibody test of CSF gives a false-positive reaction in an appreciable percentage of syphilitic patients who are not thought to have neurosyphilis, it should not be used.

Relation Between Syphilis and HIV Infection

There is little to suggest that the dermatologic manifestations of syphilis are more striking in HIV-infected persons, nor has an increase in syphilitic hepatitis, arthritis, or osteitis been specifically documented. This may not be surprising, as the lesions of secondary syphilis may be immunologically mediated, owing to deposition of circulating immune complexes.[26] In contrast, concurrent HIV infection appears to have a profound impact on neurologic involvement in syphilis.[10, 27, 28] Neurosyphilis has been seen both more often and in younger patients in the past few years than ever before. Many cases have been described in the context of therapeutic failure with conventional doses of penicillin (see the later treatment section); their importance in terms of our understanding the pathogenesis of syphilis in these subjects is just as great. Numerous individual case reports have documented the rapid progression of early syphilis to neurosyphilis, manifested in meningitis, optic neuritis, deafness, or the symptoms of nervous system disorders.[10, 29–35] Cranial nerve defects appear with or without meningitis, and vasculitis with appropriate radiographic documentation has also been described, causing cerebrovascular accidents.

The term quaternary neurosyphilis has been revived to describe necrotizing encephalitis in an HIV-infected patient.[34] Most important, cases of early neurosyphilis, which were nearly unheard of before 1980, have become commonplace. Patients with this kind of disease may have acquired immunodeficiency syndrome or only serologic evidence of HIV infection. In many cases, the concurrent HIV infection has been documented for the first time when neurologic complications of syphilis were recognized.

Laboratory Diagnosis

The most specific and sensitive method for verifying the diagnosis of primary syphilis is the finding of treponemes with characteristic appearance by dark-field microscopic examination of fluid obtained from the surface of the chancre. This test result is nearly always positive if a good specimen can be obtained. If no exudate is present, abrading the chancre and adding a drop or two of saline yields an adequate specimen. Secondary lesions can also be examined in this fashion, although greater technical facility may be required.

The darkfield examination is actually the only test that is required specifically to establish the diagnosis of primary syphilis. Anticardiolipin antibody, as measured by an STS such as the VDRL or the rapid plasma reagin (RPR), is present, generally at a relatively low level, in about 80% of patients at the time they come to medical attention for primary syphilis. Tests that measure antibody to surface proteins of *T. pallidum* by a hemagglutination assay (*T. pallidum* hemagglutination assay or microhemagglutination assay–*T. pallidum* [MHA-TP]) are positive in about 90% of such cases. Thus, a negative result does not exclude the diagnosis, nor, for that matter, does a positive one establish it, because antibody may be present as a result of some earlier infection. Nevertheless, STSs are generally requested to provide a baseline for follow-up after therapy. In contrast, once antibody to surface proteins appears, causing a positive MHA-TP, it persists for life; this greatly limits the usefulness of this test for any purpose other than excluding a diagnosis of syphilis, if negative.

In secondary syphilis, STS results are always positive, nearly always at a high dilution (at least 1:32). Thus a truly negative RPR result in a patient with a disseminated rash that is thought to be syphilitic actually excludes the diagnosis. However, most laboratories do not perform serum dilutions unless the physician indicates that the diagnosis of syphilis is suspected clinically and/or requests that dilution be done; in this situation, the prozone phenomenon, in which a high concentration of antibody is present but is not detected in undiluted serum, may obscure a positive reading. HIV-infected subjects tend to have a positive STS result with unusually high titers. Isolated case reports of secondary syphilis with a negative RPR result in an HIV-infected patient[36] may well be the exceptions that prove the rule. The RPR MHA-TP result is always positive in secondary disease.

In latent syphilis the RPR result may be positive, but the level generally subsides with time. Gummatous tertiary syphilis also has high-level RPR reactivity, presumably reflecting a continuing immune response, as the histologic picture suggests. In the case of aortitis, the decline of the VDRL titer may reflect subsidence of active inflammation, although progressive damage of the aorta results from continued mechanical stress.

The diagnosis of neurosyphilis can be exceedingly problematic. The clinical picture is nonspecific, being consistent with a wide range of neurologic or neuropsychiatric syndromes. The serum RPR is reactive, usually at a low dilution (e.g., up to 1:4), but it may be weakly reactive or even nonreactive. A negative MHA-TP test excludes the diagnosis of late syphilis, but a positive one clearly does not establish a diagnosis. The CSF may show a modest pleocytosis with a predominance of lymphocytes, an elevated protein value, and a positive VDRL result. The CSF MHA-TP result is often false-positive and cannot be used unless immunoglobulin M reactive with *T. pallidum* antigens is measured specifically or immunoglobulin G is titrated for comparison of CSF and serum levels,[37] procedures that are not generally available in the United States. CSF is said by some authorities to be entirely normal in up to 25% of cases of neurosyphilis,[22–24] although others[38] do not necessarily agree. Thus, because neurosyphilis may cause any of a variety of neurologic or psychiatric findings and all laboratory studies may be normal except the serum MHA-TP, it is not possible to fully exclude this diagnosis in any older person who has ever had syphilis and who has symptoms or signs of neuropsychiatric disease. This becomes a major, unsolved, and seemingly insoluble problem for physicians who have a hospital-based practice with elderly patients who have not been under their personal care for many years.

To summarize, even though the MHA-TP test is highly sensitive and specific for *T. pallidum* infection, clinically, it is not useful for establishing a diagnosis of syphilis in most situations because a positive result may always reflect an earlier infection. The principal usefulness of the MHA-TP test is to obtain a negative result, which excludes any diagnosis of syphilis other than early primary disesae. STSs, on the other hand, are neither specific nor highly sensitive, although positivity in high titer (1:16 or greater) generally signifies active infection with *T. pallidum.* Detecting treponemes by darkfield examination remains the surest way that the laboratory can support a clinical diagnosis of syphilis. As a good general principle, consideration of one veneral disease should lead to consideration of another; for example, any person with syphilis should be studied for antibody to HIV, hepatitis B virus, and others, and vice versa.

Treatment

Treatment schedules for syphilis are listed in standard textbooks as well as in brochures available from the Centers for Disease Control and Prevention and from state and city departments of public health. Especially with the advent of HIV infection, the subject is vastly more complicated than might have been imagined, and recommendations are being reformulated. Eventually, it may be best to evaluate each case individually, as is the custom for other diseases, using official recommendations only as guidelines. The time course for untreated syphilis is given in Figure 112–4.

Early Syphilis, No HIV Infection

After treatment with 2.4 million units of benzathine penicillin, more than 95% of all patients with primary syphilis are apparently cured of their disease. The VDRL result returns to negative in 1 to 2 years in nearly all cases. Treatment of secondary syphilis with 2.4 million units of benzathine penicillin also seems to cure the vast majority of patients, but some authorities have recorded a serologic failure rate as high as 25%.[39] Fiumara[40] has claimed that two such treatments 7 days apart cause the VDRL result to return to negative in every instance. A small proportion of patients who are cured of their secondary syphilis retain low-grade VDRL reactivity throughout life (the so-called serofast state).[41] These treatments probably do not produce a biologic cure; treponemes persist in lymph nodes and the central nervous system of treated patients and experimental animals,[42, 43] a fact that becomes important in considering treatment of HIV-infected subjects.

Even in the era before the acquired immunodeficiency syndrome, isolated case reports showed that 2.4 million units of benzathine penicillin may arrest all but the neurologic manifestations of secondary syphilis.[44] This finding is consistent with the miniscule levels of penicillin that are present in the central nervous system after benzathine penicillin therapy.[45] The rarity of neurosyphilis before 1980 argues that, in practice, recommended doses of penicillin were remarkably successful in curing syphilis. In the absence of neurologic abnormalities and in subjects who do not have HIV infection it seems reasonable to treat secondary syphilis with two treatments each of 2.4 million units benzathine penicillin.

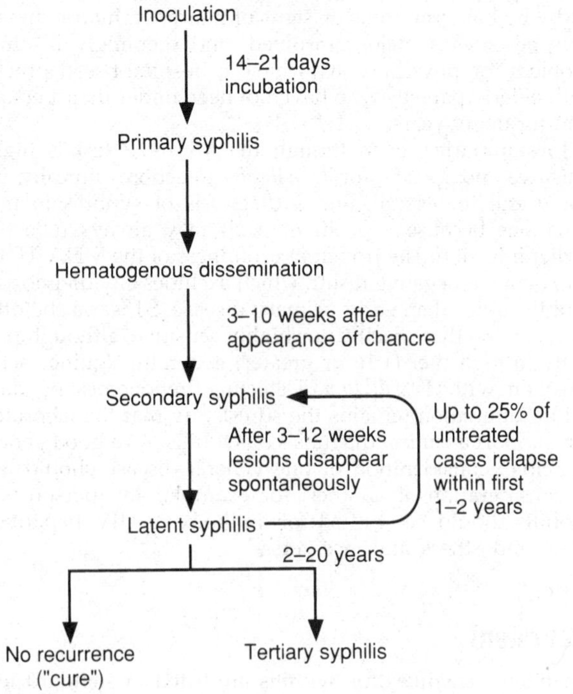

FIGURE 112–4 □ Time course of untreated syphilis. Treatment at any stage with accepted doses of penicillin nearly always eliminates disease (exceptions are late manifestations of tertiary syphilis and immunologic compromise caused by HIV infection).

Latent and Late Syphilis, No HIV Infection

Latent syphilis presents a problem. As noted earlier, the diagnosis is based on a reactive RPR test in an asymptomatic subject. In the majority of instances in the United States today, this serologic result reflects previously treated rather than active infection. Nevertheless, the official recommendation—that two treatments of 2.4 million units benzathine penicillin be given at weekly intervals unless neurosyphilis is also present—is reasonable. Although many of these subjects may not require treatment, it is not possible to identify them, so all are treated as a public health measure. A problem arises from the guidelines of the Centers for Disease Control and Prevention, which consider it "desirable" to perform lumbar puncture in every patient with latent syphilis, to exclude asymptomatic neurosyphilis. Some factors help to extenuate this recommendation: (1) The vast majority of latent infections have been arrested or cured (i.e., no later appearance of tertiary syphilis) by two or three doses, each of 2.4 million units benzathine penicillin. (2) For all the concern about treating proven neurosyphilis with benzathine penicillin, there are few well-documented case reports of therapeutic failure. (3) The character of the CSF may be within normal limits in neurosyphilis, so the lumbar puncture does not rule out the diagnosis. Some authorities[46] have concluded that the likelihood of serious complications resulting from lumbar puncture, as uncommon as they might be, still outweighs the potential benefits. It may be reasonable and certainly more practical to treat with three doses of benzathine penicillin at weekly intervals and do no spinal tap unless symptoms of neurologic disease are present.

Although benzathine penicillin (three doses of 2.4 million units at weekly intervals) yields barely detectable or undetectable CSF levels of penicillin, this regimen appears to have arrested neurosyphilis in the vast majority of cases. Nevertheless, the World Health Organization[47] has recommended against its use. It is probably preferable to treat late neurosyphilis with 2 weeks of daily procaine penicillin. Some authorities (including the first choice of the Centers for Disease Control and Prevention) prefer larger doses of penicillin (e.g., 10 to 24 million units per day intravenously for 10 days) in the absence of any data suggesting that this dosage will lead to a better outcome. Syphilologists generally talk of arrest of neurosyphilis rather than cure, because in most cases return to a normal state is not expected. Those who advocate routine use of higher doses of penicillin have not advanced any data to support higher rates of cure, and enormous doses of penicillin may not eradicate *T. pallidum* from experimental animals or humans.[43]

Treatment of Syphilis in HIV-Infected Patients

All of the foregoing considerations set the stage for discussion of this difficult subject.[10] If *T. pallidum* travels to seemingly privileged areas, such as the lymph nodes and central nervous system, where it escapes the normally lethal effects of penicillin, what might be expected in the presence of severe immunosuppression? Although one early report[48] suggested that HIV-infected patients with early syphilis respond slowly to 2.4 million units of benzathine penicillin, two subsequent studies[49, 50] have suggested that the response of early syphilis to therapy is not altered by HIV infection. What is impressive is the number of cases in which treatment with benzathine penicillin is followed by rapid progression to neurosyphilis,[10, 51–53] a clinical finding that has been supported by documentation of persisting treponemes in the CSF of HIV-infected patients.[54] These problems have been recognized, but, as yet, there is no consensus about the recommended therapeutic approach. In the opinion of this author, minimal therapy for early syphilis (primary or secondary infection without neurologic involvement) in HIV-infected patients appears to be two doses each of 2.4 million units of benzathine penicillin at weekly intervals; three such doses would be preferable. A less practical alternative is injection of 1.2 million units of procaine penicillin daily or of 1 g of ceftriaxone on alternate days for 10 to 15 days. Erythromycin or tetracycline cannot be recommended because of failure to produce adequate levels in the central nervous system. If either is used in a case in which desensitization to penicillin would be necessary but cannot be achieved, both physician and patient should be fully aware of the need for close monitoring and the concern over failure to cure neurologic disease. For syphilis with neurologic (including ophthalmologic or otologic) involvement, 10 days of intravenous penicillin, 24 million units per day, is recommended. Alternative therapy, including ceftriaxone, 1 g/d, is probably equally effective. Both of these regimens are associated with rates of failure plus relapse that approach 30%.[35, 55] It is entirely possible that daily procaine penicillin for 10 to 14 days would be as effective. Clearly, with any treatment regimen, careful attention needs to be given both to clinical response and to the subsequent serum VDRL reaction.

References

1. Chapel TA: The variability of syphilitic chancres. Sex Transm Dis 5:68, 1978.
2. Drusin LM, Singer C, Valenti AJ, Armstrong D: Infectious syphilis mimicking neoplastic disease. Arch Intern Med 137:156, 1977.
3. Musher DM, Knox JM: Syphilis and yaws. *In* Schell RF, Musher DM (eds): Pathogenesis and Immunology of Treponemal Infections. New York, Marcel Dekker, 1983, pp 101–120.
4. Friedman PS, Wright DJ: Observations on syphilis in Addis Ababa. 2. Prevalence and natural history. Br J Vener Dis 53:276, 1977.
5. Shrivastava SN, Singh G: Extensive condyloma lata. Br J Vener Dis 53:23, 1977.
6. Chapel TA: The signs and symptoms of secondary syphilis. Sex Transm Dis 7:161, 1980.
7. Jozsa L, Timmer M, Somogyi T, Feher J: Hepatitis syphilitica: A clinico-pathological study of 25 cases. Acta Hepatogastroenterol 24:344, 1977.
8. Mills CH: Routine examination of cerebrospinal fluid in syphilis: Its value in regard to more accurate knowledge, prognosis and treatment. Br Med J 2:527, 1936.
9. Bauer TJ, Price EV, Cutler JC: Spinal fluid examinations among patients with primary or secondary syphilis. Am J Syph 36:309, 1952.
10. Musher DM, Hamill RJ, Baughn RE: Effect of human immunodeficiency virus (HIV) infection on the course of syphilis and on the response to treatment. Ann Intern Med 113:872, 1990.
11. Baughn RE, McNeely MC, Jorizzo JL, Musher DM: Characterization of the antigenic determinants and host components in immune complexes from patients with secondary syphilis. J Immunol 136:1406, 1986.
12. Clark EG, Danbolt N: The Oslo study of the natural course of untreated syphilis: An epidemiologic investigation based on a re-study of the Boeck-Bruusgaard material. Med Clin North Am 48:613, 1964.
13. Magnuson HJ, Thomas EW, Olansky S, et al: Inoculation syphilis in human volunteers. Medicine (Baltimore) 35:33, 1956.
14. Kampmeier RH: The late manifestations of syphilis: Skeletal, visceral and cardiovascular. Med Clin North Am 48:667, 1964.
15. Kemp JE, Cochems KD: Studies in cardiovascular syphilis: Influence of treatment of early syphilis upon incidence of cardiovascular syphilis. Am J Syph Gonorrhea Vener Dis 21:625, 1937.
16. Heggtveit HA: Syphilitic aortitis: A clinicopathologic autopsy study of 100 cases, 1950 to 1960. Circulation 29:346, 1964.
17. Handsfield HH, Lukehart SA, Sell S, et al: Demonstration of *Treponema pallidum* in a cutaneous gumma by indirect immunofluorescence. Arch Dermatol 719:677, 1983.
18. Olansky S: Late benign syphilis (gumma). Med Clin North Am 48:653, 1964.
19. Grabau W, Emanuel R, Ross D, et al: Syphilitic aortic regurgitation: An appraisal of surgical treatment. Br J Vener Dis 52:366, 1976.
20. Perdrup A, Jorgensen BB, Pedersen NS: The profile of neurosyphilis in Denmark: A clinical and serological study of all patients in Denmark with neurosyphilis disclosed in the years 1971–1979 incl. by Wassermann reaction (CWRM) in the cerebrospinal fluid. Acta Derm Venereol Suppl (Stockh) 96:1, 1981.
21. Talbot MD, Morton RS: Neurosyphilis: The most common things are most common. Genitourin Med 61:95, 1985.
22. Hooshmand H, Escobar MR, Kopf SW: Neurosyphilis: A study of 241 patients. JAMA 219:726, 1972.
23. Catterall RD: Neurosyphilis. Br J Hosp Med 17:585, 1977.
24. Luxon L, Greenwood RJ, Lees AJ: Neurosyphilis today. Lancet 1:90, 1979.
25. Binder RL, Dickman WA: Psychiatric manifestations of neurosyphilis in middle-aged patients. Am J Psychiatry 137:6, 1980.
26. Jorizzo JL, McNeely MC, Baughn RE, et al: Role of circulating immune complexes in human secondary syphilis. J Infect Dis 153:1014, 1986.
27. Holtom PD, Larsen RA, Leal ME, Leedom JM: Prevalence of neurosyphilis in human immunodeficiency virus–infected patients with latent syphilis. Am J Med 93:9, 1992.
28. Katz DA, Berger JA, Duncan RC: Neurosyphilis: A comparative study of the effects of infection with human immunodeficiency virus. Arch Neurol 50:243, 1993.
29. Folk JC, Weingeist TA, Corbett JJ, et al: Syphilitic neuroretinitis. Am J Ophthalmol 95:480, 1983.
30. Harris RL, Rutecki PA, Donovan DT, et al: Fever, headache and hearing loss in a young homosexual man. Hosp Pract 20:167, 170, 1985.
31. Zaidman GW: Neurosyphilis and retrobulbar neuritis in a patient with AIDS. Ann Ophthalmol 18:260, 1986.
32. Zambrano W, Perez GM, Smith JL: Acute syphilitic blindness in AIDS. J Clin Neurol Ophthalmol 7:1, 1987.
33. Johns DR, Tierney M, Felsenstein D: Alteration in the natural history of neurosyphilis by concurrent infection with the human immunodeficiency virus. N Engl J Med 316:1569, 1987.
34. Morgello S, Laufer H: Quaternary neurosyphilis. N Engl J Med 319:1549, 1989.
35. Gordon SM, Eaton ME, George R, et al: The response of symptomatic neurosyphilis to high-dose intravenous penicillin G in patients with human immunodeficiency virus infection. N Engl J Med 331:1469, 1994.
36. Hicks CB, Benson PM, Lupton GP, Tramont EC: Seronegative secondary syphilis in a patient infected with the human immunodeficiency virus (HIV) with Kaposi sarcoma. Ann Intern Med 107:492, 1987.
37. Prange HW, Moskophidis M, Schipper HI, Muller F: Relationship between neurological features and intrathecal synthesis of IgG antibodies to *Treponema pallidum* in untreated and treated human neurosyphilis. J Neurol 230:241, 1983.
38. Swartz M: Neurosyphilis. *In* Holmes KK, Mardh P-A, Sparling PF, Wiesner PJ (eds): Sexually Transmitted Diseases. New York, McGraw-Hill, 1984, pp 313–334.
39. Leslie N: Treatment of early infectious syphilis with benzathine penicillin G. *In* Proceedings of World Forum on Syphilis and Other Treponematoses, September 4–8, 1962, Washington, DC. Washington, DC, US Public Health Service, 1964. USPHS publication 997.
40. Fiumara NJ: Treatment of primary and secondary syphilis. Serological response. JAMA 243:2500, 1980.
41. Schroeter AL, Lucas JB, Price EV, Falcon VH: Treatment of early syphilis and reactivity of serological tests. JAMA 221:471, 1972.
42. Collart P, Borel L-J, Durel P: Significance of spiral organisms found, after treatment, in late human and experimental syphilis. Br J Vener Dis 40:81, 1964.
43. Yobs AR, Clark JW Jr, Mothershed SE, et al: Further observations on the persistence of *Treponema pallidum* after treatment in rabbits and humans. Br J Vener Dis 44:116, 1968.
44. Tramont EC: Persistence of *Treponema pallidum* following penicilling G therapy. A report of two cases. JAMA 236:2206, 1976.
45. Goh BT, Smith GW, Samarasinghe L, et al: Penicillin concentrations in serum and cerebrospinal fluid after intramuscular

injection of aqueous procaine penicillin 0.6 MU with and without probenecid. Br J Vener Dis 60:371, 1984.
46. Wiesel J, Rose DN, Silver AL, et al: Lumbar puncture in asymptomatic neurosyphilis. Arch Intern Med 145:465, 1985.
47. Treponemal infections. World Health Org Tech Rep Ser 674:1, 1982.
48. Frederick WR, Delapenha R, Barnes S, et al: Secondary syphilis and HIV infection (Abstr 1175). Abstracts of the 28th Interscience Conference. Antimicrob Agents Chemother 320, 1988.
49. Gourevitch MN, Selwyn PA, Davenny K, et al: Effect of HIV infection on the serologic manifestations and response to treatment of syphilis in intravenous drug users. Ann Intern Med 118:350, 1993.
50. Hutchinson CM, Hook EW III, Shepherd M: Altered clinical presentation of early syphilis in patients with human immunodeficiency virus infection. Ann Intern Med 121:94, 1994.
51. Bayne LL, Schmidley JW, Goodin DS: Acute syphilitic meningitis. Its occurrence after clinical and serologic cure of secondary syphilis with penicillin G. Arch Neurol 43:137, 1986.
52. Jorgensen J, Tikjob G, Weisman K: Neurosyphilis after treatment of latent syphilis with benzathine penicillin. Genitourin Med 62:129, 1986.
53. Berry CD, Hooton TM, Collier AC, Lukehart SA: Neurologic relapse after benzathine penicillin therapy for secondary syphilis in a patient with HIV infection. N Engl J Med 316:1587, 1987.
54. Lukehart SA, Hood EW III, Baker-Zander SA, et al: Invasion of the central nervous system by *Treponema pallidum:* Implications for diagnosis and treatment. Ann Intern Med 109:855, 1988.
55. Dowell ME, Ross PG, Musher DM, et al: Response of latent syphilis or neurosyphilis to ceftriaxone in persons infected with human immunodeficiency virus. Am J Med 93:481, 1992.

113

Genital Herpes

Michael N. Oxman

Genital herpes (herpes genitalis) is an acute inflammatory herpes simplex virus (HSV) infection of the male or female genital tract that may result from either an initial (primary or nonprimary) or a recurrent HSV infection. Initial episodes of genital herpes are sexually transmitted exogenous infections. They may be caused by HSV type 1 (HSV-1) or HSV type 2 (HSV-2), but the latter predominates. Although self-limited, an initial episode of genital herpes results in a lifelong latent infection of sacral sensory neurons that innervate the initially infected skin and mucous membranes. Periodically thereafter, latent virus reactivates and travels within sensory axons back to the site of infection. This may result in another episode of disease (i.e., recurrent genital herpes) or in asymptomatic HSV shedding. Little noted three decades ago, genital herpes is now a major concern of sexually active adults and their physicians. This reflects the increasing frequency and recognition of HSV infections of the genital tract; the realization, during a period of increased sexual permissiveness, that genital herpes is a sexually transmitted disease (STD); and the introduction of effective chemotherapy. It also reflects the realization that genital herpes is currently incurable and, because of its tendency to recur, endows infected individuals with a lifelong potential to transmit the disease to others.

History

Although herpes labialis (herpes febrilis, "fever blisters," cold sores) was well described as early as the first century AD, it was not until the 18th century that a clear description of genital herpes (herpes genitalis, herpes progenitalis) appeared.[1] This was published in 1736 by Jean Astruc,[2] physician to the King of France, in his treatise on venereal diseases. Astruc did not give the disease a name, but he vividly described the lesions of genital herpes in men and women, as well as those of rectal herpes in recipients of anal intercourse.

Genital herpes was well recognized by 19th century venereologists, who published excellent descriptions of the disease and called attention to its generally benign nature, its tendency to recur in the same anatomic area, and its association with a previous history of a recognized STD such as gonorrhea, syphilis, or chancroid.[3, 4] Unna,[5] a German venereologist, described genital herpes as a "vocational disease" of prostitutes, reporting its occurrence in 4% to 9% of prostitutes admitted to the Hamburg General Hospital from 1878 through 1881. He reemphasized earlier observations of the frequent occurrence of genital herpes in persons with a prior history of a recognized STD, as well as its frequent recurrence in men after coitus and in women at the time of menstruation. Unna[6] also provided the first description of the histopathology of the genital lesions.

Despite the association of genital herpes with recognized STDs, the preponderance of recurrent (endogenous) infections tended to obscure its contagious nature. It was not until the early part of this century that Grüter,[7] Lipschütz,[8] and other European investigators established the infectious etiology of herpes labialis and genital herpes by transmitting infection to experimental animals. Lipschütz[8] called attention to the transmission of genital herpes by sexual contact and demonstrated that the viruses responsible for herpes labialis and genital herpes were biologically and antigenically different. However, this work appears to have been ignored. In 1946, Slavin and Gavett[9] isolated HSV from lesions of the vulva, demonstrated that "herpetic vulvovaginitis" was a manifestation of primary HSV infection, and described the conjugal transmission of genital herpes from a husband with penile herpes to his wife. Despite these observations, genital herpes was still not widely accepted as an STD until the rediscovery of the two HSV serotypes in the late 1960s, and the development of assays to distinguish between them permitted the different epidemiologies of HSV-1 and HSV-2 to be delineated.[10–12]

Investigators during the past three decades have greatly expanded our knowledge of the epidemiology, natural history, and spectrum of diseases caused by HSV-1 and HSV-2; the structure of the virion and of the genomes of the two HSV serotypes; the mechanisms of gene expression and virus replication; and the identity and biologic function of individual viral gene products.[13–15] These advances have led to the development of new techniques of molecular epidemiology and rapid viral diagnosis, type-specific serologic assays, and effective antiviral therapy. They have also yielded new insights into the HSV-host interaction, especially the mechanisms of HSV latency and reactivation, and laid the foundation for the development of HSV vaccines. These points are discussed in detail in Chapter 240.

Microbiology

HSV-1 and HSV-2 are closely related members of the Herpesviridae, a large and successful family of viruses that includes six other human representatives: varicella-zoster virus (VZV); human cytomegalovirus; Epstein-Barr virus; and three recently discovered viruses—human herpesviruses 6, 7, and 8 (HHV-6, HHV-7, and HHV-8). The reader is referred to Chapter 240 for a detailed discussion of the microbiology of HSV-1 and HSV-2, including their classification, structure, biologic properties, replication, and antigenic characteristics. These subjects are reviewed only briefly here.

HSV-1 and HSV-2 are morphologically indistinguishable from each other and from other members of the Herpesviridae. The HSV virion consists of a central core containing the viral genome enclosed within an icosahedral protein shell, or capsid, approximately 100 nm in diameter and composed of 162 identical protein subunits (capsomers). The resulting structure, the HSV nucleocapsid, is surrounded by an amorphous layer of viral protein (the tegument) and, finally, by a lipoprotein envelope derived from the nuclear membrane of the infected host cell. The complete virion is roughly spherical with a diameter of 150 to 200 nm. Embedded in the lipid bilayer of the virus envelope and visible as radially oriented spikes in electron micrographs (see Fig. 240–1) are viral glycoproteins that interact with the surface of susceptible host cells to mediate virus attachment and enable the nucleocapsid to penetrate into the cell cytoplasm. Because of the essential role of these envelope glycoproteins in initiating HSV infection, only intact enveloped virions are fully infectious. This accounts for the lability of HSV; infectivity is rapidly destroyed by organic solvents, detergents, proteolytic enzymes, heat, drying, and extremes of pH. The envelope glycoproteins are antigenic and elicit neutralizing antibodies and cell-mediated immunity. Several also interact with host defense mechanisms to protect virions and infected cells from immune recognition and lysis.

The HSV genome is a linear double-stranded molecule of DNA of approximately 150 kb (molecular weight of about 100×10^6), with a guanine plus cytosine content of 68% (HSV-1) or 69% (HSV-2). The genomes of HSV-1 and HSV-2 share about half their nucleotide sequences and have colinear genetic maps.[14] Each HSV-1 gene appears to have a functionally interchangeable HSV-2 homolog with which it shares at least some nucleotide sequences and that occupies the same relative position in the HSV-2 genome. Consequently, intertypic recombinants are viable, and most of the 70 or more HSV-1–encoded proteins are antigenically related to their HSV-2 homologs (see Chapter 240). Because of their antigenic relatedness, most of the structural and nonstructural proteins of HSV-1 and HSV-2 elicit cross-reactive immune responses.[10–13, 15–20] This provides a degree of heterotypic immunity when individuals infected with one HSV serotype are subsequently exposed to the other (see later), but it has complicated serodiagnosis and seroepidemiologic investigations (see Chapter 240). Fortunately, two of the HSV envelope glycoproteins, gC and gG, elicit mainly type-specific immune responses, and this has permitted the development of type-specific immunologic assays for identification of HSV isolates, serologic diagnosis of infection, and seroepidemiologic investigations.[15, 16, 18–25]

Despite these similarities, many homologous coding and noncoding regions of the two HSV serotypes differ in length because of type-specific insertions and deletions of genetic information. This results in type-specific differences in restriction endonuclease cleavage sites and in the sizes of viral proteins, which form the basis of laboratory techniques to differentiate HSV-1 from HSV-2.[26–32] Strains belonging to a single HSV serotype also exhibit genetic variation but of a much smaller magnitude than that observed between HSV-1 and HSV-2. This results in restriction endonuclease polymorphisms that are easily detected among epidemiologically unrelated strains of HSV-1 and HSV-2 and serve as useful markers for epidemiologic investigations.[33–37] Epidemiologically related HSV isolates (e.g., the strain of HSV-2 isolated from a case of primary genital herpes and the strain of HSV-2 isolated from a recurrence of genital herpes in the sexual partner from whom the infection was acquired) have identical restriction endonuclease "fingerprints," whereas unrelated strains of the same HSV serotype do not.[35–37] Although their similarities are much greater than their differences, HSV-1 and HSV-2 can also be distinguished by a number of antigenic, biologic, and biochemical differences (see Table 240–1).

HSV differs from all other human herpesviruses in having a broad host range. HSV-1 and HSV-2 can infect many experimental animals, including rats, mice, hamsters, guinea pigs, rabbits, nonhuman primates, and chick embryos, as well as a wide variety of cell cultures derived from human and animal tissues. This makes it relatively easy to isolate HSV in the laboratory if the appropriate clinical specimens are obtained and handled properly to prevent this relatively labile virus from losing infectivity.

Epidemiology

Genital herpes may be caused by HSV-1 or HSV-2, although HSV-2 predominates. Both viruses are transmitted by close personal contact, which results in the direct transfer of virus by infected secretions or from an infected mucocutaneous surface to the recipient's mucous membrane or skin. Because the intact stratum corneum is resistant to infection, transmission to cutaneous sites generally requires some disruption of this barrier, either by trauma or by disease. Furthermore, HSV is labile. Thus, despite experimental evidence that it can survive for hours on a variety of contaminated surfaces, there is no documented transmission from inanimate objects such as toilet seats or from swimming pools or hot tubs, and there is no evidence of natural transmission by aerosols.[15, 18, 38–42]

HSV-1 and HSV-2 are both distributed throughout the world. Humans are the only natural reservoir, and no vectors are involved in transmission. The capacity of both viruses to establish lifelong latent infections with periodic reactivation and virus shedding ensures their survival in populations too small and isolated to support the continuous circulation of viruses causing such epidemic diseases as measles and influenza. Consequently, both HSV-1 and HSV-2 are endemic in virtually every human society.[43, 44] Whereas the genomic DNA of isolates of HSV-1 and HSV-2 from different geographic locations and even of epidemiologically unrelated isolates from the same location have distinct restriction endonuclease fingerprints, no consistent biologic differences have been documented.[29, 33–36, 45, 46] There is no clear evidence of different racial susceptibility to HSV-1 or HSV-2, and there is no significant seasonal variation in the occurrence of overt disease. However, sexual transmission is more efficient from men to women than from women to men,[47, 48] and the prevalence of antibody to HSV-2 is higher in women than in men, even after controlling for other risk factors.[23–25, 49, 50] In addition, when symptomatic, genital herpes is usually more severe in women than in men (see later).

Studies to ascertain the prevalence of HSV-1 and HSV-2 infection have been complicated by two characteristics of HSV. (1) Most initial HSV-1 and HSV-2 infections (i.e., at least two thirds) are asymptomatic or unrecognized, and reactivation of latent infection results in asymptomatic virus shedding far more often than in overt disease.[13, 15, 17, 18, 23–25, 38, 41, 42, 47–82] Thus, at any given time, persons shedding HSV asymptomatically (most of whom are unaware of ever having been infected) outnumber those with clinical disease. Consequently, clinical surveys greatly underestimate the incidence and prevalence of HSV infection. (2) The immune response to HSV is largely to cross-reacting antigenic determinants, making it difficult to discriminate between antibodies to one HSV serotype in persons who were previously infected with the other.* This problem has been solved by the development of Western blot and enzyme immunoassays that employ as antigens the gG envelope glycoproteins of HSV-1 and HSV-2, which elicit primarily type-specific immune responses.[21–25, 84, 85]

The prevalence of HSV-1 and HSV-2 infection is best assessed by serologic surveys that identify previously infected (i.e., seropositive) individuals, most or all of whom shed HSV intermittently and thus constitute the source of virus responsible for most new infections. The only infected persons not detected by such surveys are those who are newly infected and are tested before their antibody response has exceeded the threshold of the assay, and the rare individuals who fail to mount a detectable immune response to the particular HSV antigen employed.

Since their putative anatomic divergence and separate evolution some 8 to 10 million years ago[86] (see Chapter 240), HSV-1 and HSV-2 have differed in their mode of transmission and thus in their epidemiology. HSV-1, which generally causes infections of the oropharynx and eye (see Table 240–1), is transmitted primarily by contact with infected oral secretions or lesions. This is favored by crowding and poor hygiene, and consequently the incidence and prevalence of HSV-1 infection are inversely related to socioeconomic status.[42, 51, 52, 87, 88] Until the middle of this century, almost everyone was infected with HSV-1 before puberty and thus had acquired a degree of heterologous immunity to HSV-2. However, the age-specific prevalence of antibodies to HSV-1 has been decreasing in the past 40 years in Western industrialized countries, especially in middle-class populations, as the standard of living improved.[15, 18, 23–25, 42, 52, 87–92]

The prevalence of antibodies to HSV-1 in white adults in the United States has decreased from nearly 100% to 40% to 60%, but it is only 25% in white 14-year-olds and 25% to 30% in white college students; the figures remain much higher in black persons (70% in 14-year-olds and 50% to 60% in college students), undoubtedly reflecting lower socioeconomic status and crowded living conditions during childhood.[15, 18, 23–25, 42, 51, 52, 82, 91, 92] The increasing proportion of the white middle-class population now reaching puberty without having been infected with HSV-1, which induces partial immunity to subsequent HSV-2 infection, is an important factor underlying the current epidemic of symptomatic genital herpes and helps explain the increasing frequency with which HSV-1 is being isolated from patients with initial episodes of genital herpes. It may also help explain why black persons, despite having a much higher prevalence of antibodies to HSV-2 than do white persons, appear to have a lower prevalence of symptomatic genital herpes.[23, 24, 50]

HSV-2 is transmitted sexually by contact with infected genital secretions or mucocutaneous surfaces. Thus, HSV-2 infection is rare before puberty, and its acquisition thereafter is related to sexual activity. The rate of infection is highest between the ages of 15 and 35 years, with more than 80% of all initial HSV-2 infections occurring in this age group. The prevalence of antibodies to HSV-2 varies from essentially zero in children younger than 14 years and celibate adults to more than 80% in prostitutes.† Once a rare disease among members of the white middle class, symptomatic genital herpes has increased dramatically in prevalence in the United States and Europe since the mid-1960s.[13, 15, 18, 41, 50, 63, 92, 94, 96–102] In the United States, visits to physicians for initial episodes of symptomatic genital herpes now exceed 1 per 1000 persons per year,[96, 98] and symptomatic genital herpes accounts for 1% to 8% of visits to STD clinics, 0.1% to 1% of visits to general gynecology offices, and 0.6% to 4% of visits to university health services.[15, 18, 41, 103–105] Contributing factors include the increasing sexual activity of white middle-class adolescents,[106] the decreased use of barrier contraceptives, and the reduced proportion of white middle-class adolescents with partial immunity to HSV induced by earlier HSV-1 infection.[18, 23, 24, 42, 50, 92, 96–99]

Seroepidemiologic studies employing type-specific assays have demonstrated HSV-2 antibody prevalence rates of less than 1% in a group of South Carolina first-year college students, 20% to 22% in pregnant women in California and in women attending family planning clinics in western Pennsylvania, more than 30% in middle-class women receiving care in an Atlanta health maintenance organization and in a Seattle family practice clinic, and 16% in a representative cross-section of men and women aged 15 to 74 years in the United States sampled between 1976 and 1980.[15, 23–25, 50, 71, 81, 92, 94, 102] Sixty percent to 80% of these seropositive individuals have no history of symptomatic genital herpes. Antibody prevalence is substantially higher in men and women attending STD clinics and in sexually active homosexuals than in the general population.[50, 80, 85, 92, 94, 101, 103] Prospective serologic studies have shown that the incidence of initial HSV-2 infection is about 1% to 2% per year in college students, 2% per year in middle-class women of childbearing age, 5% to 10% per year in multipartnered heterosexual STD clinic patients, and 5% per year in sexually active homosexual men.[15, 18, 25, 50, 71, 92, 94, 96, 97]

Risk factors for HSV-2 infection include multiple sexual partners, early age at first intercourse, years of sexual activity, history of other STDs, low family income, race, and gender; the age-specific prevalence of antibodies to HSV-2 is two to three times higher in black than in white persons, and consistently higher in women than in men, even after controlling for other risk factors.[15, 18, 23–25, 49, 50, 92, 94, 96, 100–103] In heterosexual women in the United States, the probability of being infected with HSV-2 increases markedly with the number of sexual partners. It is less than 10% in women with 1 lifetime sexual partner and increases to 40% with 2 to 10, 60% with 11 to 50, and more than 80% with more than 50 lifetime sexual partners.[92] The corresponding probabilities of HSV-2 infection in heterosexual men are less than 1%, 20%, 35%, and 70%.[92] The higher infection rates in women may be explained, at least in part, by the observation that men with genital HSV-2 infection have more recurrences than do women.[107] As in the case of HSV-1, latency and asymptomatic virus shedding play a critical role in maintaining HSV-2 in human populations, and the majority of new HSV-2 infections are acquired from a sexual partner shedding virus in the absence of recognized disease.[24, 47, 48, 50, 73, 74, 76, 80–82, 85] All seropositive individuals are latently infected and probably experience reactivation at least occasionally. In otherwise healthy men and women, the incidence of asymptomatic virus shedding from the genital tract is approximately 1% to 2% on any given day, but it is substantially higher in persons with frequent symptomatic recurrences, in the first several months after the initial episode of infection, and in the days immediately before and after a symptomatic recurrence.* The data outlined before indicate that there are now between 40 and 60 million people in the United States (16% to 22%) infected with HSV-2 and that more than 1 million new infections occur each year.

Although HSV-1 and HSV-2 appear to be adapted to different anatomic sites (see discussion in Chapter 240 and Table 240–1), the decreasing prevalence of HSV-1 infections before puberty in affluent populations and the increasing popularity

*References 10–13, 15, 18, 21, 22, 41, 42, 50, 52, 70, 83–85.

†References 12, 13, 15, 17, 18, 23–25, 38, 41, 42, 50, 52, 63, 71, 92–103.

*References 13, 15, 18, 41, 53–69, 71–75, 77–80, 94, 97, 107, 108.

of oral-genital sexual practices are changing the epidemiology of HSV-1 and HSV-2 infections. HSV-1 is now causing disease in territory formerly inhabited exclusively by HSV-2 (e.g., below the waist) and vice versa. For example, 10% to 40% of initial episodes of genital herpes are now caused by HSV-1.* Although primary genital herpes caused by HSV-1 is clinically indistinguishable from primary genital herpes caused by HSV-2, the rate of subsequent recurrences, both symptomatic and asymptomatic, is 5- to 10-fold lower when disease is caused by HSV-1 than by HSV-2.[13, 77, 78, 107, 109, 110]

Neonatal HSV infections, two thirds of which are caused by HSV-2, are usually acquired during passage through the infected birth canal of a mother with asymptomatic genital herpes.† Intrauterine infection is responsible for a small minority of cases. Infection may also be acquired postnatally from the mother or another adult with nongenital HSV infection or by nosocomial transmission in the nursery. The risk for infection is much higher in infants born to mothers with initial (primary or nonprimary) rather than recurrent genital HSV infections. The incidence of neonatal HSV infection in the United States is estimated to be between 1 in 3000 and 1 in 5000 live births, and it may be on the rise because of the increasing incidence of genital herpes and the decreasing prevalence of prior HSV-1 infection, which probably reduces the risk for transmission from mother to infant.[15, 18, 38, 42, 50, 71, 75, 94, 115–117]

Prior infection with HSV-2 increases the risk for acquiring human immunodeficiency virus infection, presumably because of the capacity of HSV-2 to produce genital ulcers.[92, 118]

Pathology and Pathogenesis

The pathologic changes of genital herpes are the result of cytopathic effects induced by HSV in infected cells plus local inflammatory responses. At the level of the cell, HSV infection is ultimately cytolytic, but before lysis infected cells undergo a series of characteristic cytopathic changes, including the formation of eosinophilic intranuclear inclusion bodies and fusion with adjacent infected and uninfected cells, that give the lesions a distinctive and diagnostically significant histopathologic appearance. Although influenced by the anatomic site and extent of infection and by the nature of the host response, the histopathology of HSV infection is similar at all sites. Moreover, the skin and mucous membrane lesions caused by HSV-1 and HSV-2 are histopathologically indistinguishable from each other and from lesions caused by VZV, and there are no discernible histopathologic differences between the lesions of primary and recurrent genital herpes.

HSV is introduced into the genital mucosa or abraded skin by genital-genital or oral-genital sexual contact with a partner who has a symptomatic or, more typically, an asymptomatic genital or oropharyngeal HSV infection. Virus can also be introduced by a finger moistened with HSV-1–containing saliva or bearing a herpetic whitlow. The HSV replicates in cells of the stratum spinosum, producing characteristic cytopathic effects that include cell swelling ("ballooning degeneration"), loss of intercellular bridges, development of Cowdry type A eosinophilic intranuclear inclusion bodies, and membrane changes that cause infected cells to fuse with adjacent infected and uninfected cells to form multinucleated giant cells. The involved cells are soon separated by intercellular edema that, together with inflammation and capillary dilatation in the underlying lamina propria, results in the formation of an erythematous papule. The infection and degeneration of additional epithelial cells and the continuing influx of edema fluid eventually elevate the uninvolved stratum corneum to form a delicate, clear, intraepidermal vesicle that contains fibrin, degenerating epithelial cells, multinucleated giant cells, and large amounts of infectious virus (see Fig. 240–6). Adjacent vesicles may coalesce to form small bullae. Capillary dilatation and infiltration by inflammatory cells are pronounced in the underlying dermis or lamina propria, but necrosis is absent. Inflammatory cells invade from below and the fluid becomes cloudy, transforming the vesicle into a pustule. The fluid is soon absorbed, leaving an adherent crust that dries and hardens. The crust is eventually shed when the underlying epithelium has regenerated from uninfected cells in the germinal layer, and the lesions heal without scarring.

*References 15, 18, 50, 63, 75, 77–80, 92–99, 104–108.
†References 13, 15, 18, 38, 50, 52, 71–75, 94, 111–116.

In moist areas, such as the cervix, vagina, and labia minora in women and under the foreskin in uncircumcised men, the vesicles are macerated and quickly rupture, liberating infectious virus and leaving tender, painful, shallow ulcers. Virus liberated from ruptured vesicles spreads the infection locally to the cervix, vagina, vulva, and, often, the surrounding skin. Nongenital sites, including the anal canal, buttocks, and thighs, are often also involved.[50, 63, 78–80, 119] These may be sites of initial infection or may be infected by autoinoculation or by retrograde neural ("zosteriform") spread of HSV from newly infected sacral ganglia.[120, 121] In most infected individuals, virus replication and cell destruction are rapidly terminated at the site of inoculation, and the infection remains asymptomatic or unrecognized. In some cases, however, virus replication and cell destruction are more extensive, resulting in clinically manifest disease (i.e., symptomatic primary or nonprimary first episodes of genital herpes) with lesions at the portal of entry, spread of virus to regional lymph nodes, and some degree of viremia.[15, 38, 63, 94, 122–125] In the normal host, nonspecific and specific defense mechanisms combine to localize infection, terminate virus replication, and eventually eliminate infectious virus from tissues at the portal of entry and from any sites of viremic spread (see later).

Early in the course of both symptomatic and asymptomatic infections, HSV invades local sensory or autonomic nerve endings. Viral nucleocapsids are transported within axons to regional sensory[126–128] or autonomic[129] ganglia, where lifelong latent infections are established in neurons (see Chapter 240). Thereafter, despite the host's immunity, this latent virus is periodically reactivated, either spontaneously or induced by various stimuli, which may include trauma to the ganglion or nerve root, fever, menstruation, ultraviolet light, sexual intercourse, and emotional stress.[15, 38, 87, 130–137] The reactivated virus travels within the axon back to the periphery and reinfects epithelial cells in the genital skin or mucous membranes. There, virus replication and cell-to-cell spread may produce intraepidermal vesicles like those produced during the initial infection. When reactivation of latent HSV results in clinically manifest disease, it is called a recurrence or an episode of recurrent genital herpes. In the normal host, immune mechanisms rapidly limit local virus replication and spread, so that recurrent genital herpes is generally less severe, less extensive, and of shorter duration than initial episodes of genital herpes (Fig. 113–1). In fact, in most instances, the local infection is so circumscribed that no recognized lesions are produced, and reactivation results only in asymptomatic virus shedding.

Immune Responses and Other Host Defenses

In the normal host, an array of overlapping local and systemic defense mechanisms limit HSV replication and spread, destroy HSV-infected cells, and eventually eliminate infectious virus. These defenses fall into two categories, nonspecific and specific, which are most clearly differentiated during

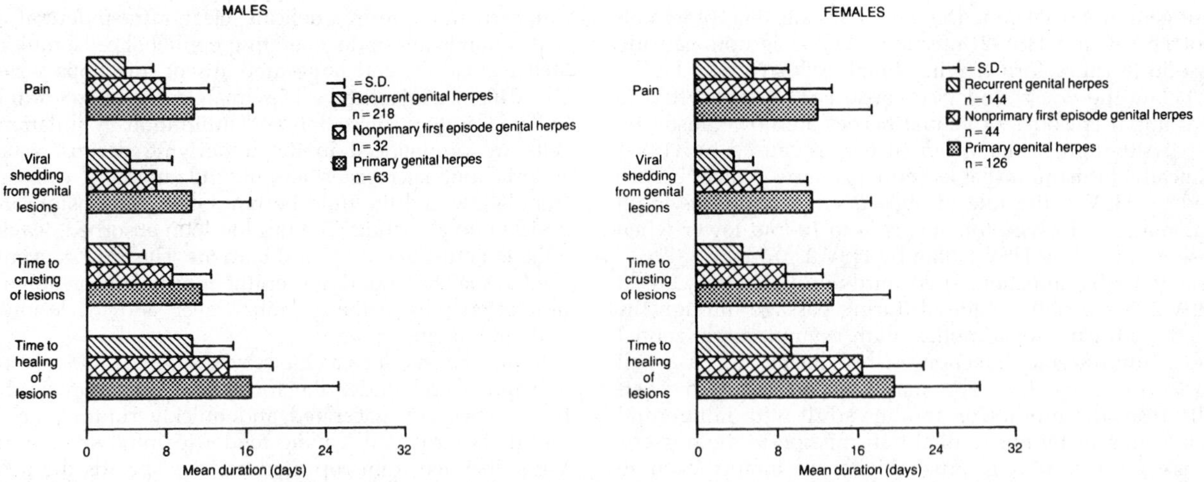

FIGURE 113–1 ▫ The duration of symptoms and signs of primary, nonprimary first-episode, and recurrent genital herpes in men and women. SD, Standard deviation. (From Corey L, Adams HG, Brown ZA, Holmes KK: Genital herpes simplex virus infections: Clinical manifestations, course, and complications. Ann Intern Med 98:958–972, 1983.)

primary HSV infections. Only nonspecific defenses are operative during the first several days of primary infection, that is, until specific immune responses develop, yet these are sufficient to prevent the development of clinically manifest disease in the majority of infected individuals. Specific (immune) and nonspecific host defenses are discussed in detail in the corresponding section of Chapter 240.

The normal cornified epithelium is an important nonspecific barrier to the initiation and spread of HSV infection. When it is defective (e.g., in patients with atopic eczema or burns), HSV infections are frequently severe, widespread, and occasionally disseminated. The female genital tract includes a much greater area of mucous membrane and moist, minimally cornified epithelium than does the male counterpart, and this may account for the greater severity of primary genital herpes in women as well as their more frequent development of complications related to local extension and to spread of virus to extragenital sites. It may also contribute to the greater risk for transmission of genital herpes from men to women than from women to men.

Once primary HSV infection is initiated in the skin or mucous membranes, a number of nonspecific defense mechanisms are mobilized, producing a local inflammatory response. These include complement activation; production of interferons and other lymphokines; and the activity of neutrophils, monocytes, macrophages, and natural killer cells. Together, they slow HSV replication and limit its spread.[138]

Antibodies to HSV are first detected several days after the onset of infection; they are elicited by epitopes on most of the HSV-encoded proteins, but those that are protective are directed primarily at the envelope glycoproteins, which are exposed on the surface of virions and virus-infected cells.[16, 138–145] They include complement-dependent and complement-independent neutralizing antibodies, antibodies that mediate the complement-dependent lysis of HSV-infected cells, and antibodies that mediate antibody-dependent cellular cytotoxicity (ADCC), that is, the lysis of HSV-infected cells by Fc receptor–bearing effector cells. These specific immune responses, especially ADCC, further inhibit virus replication at the portal of entry and at any sites of viremic spread, and they prevent further virus dissemination.[138, 145] Somewhat later, during the second week of infection, HSV immune T lymphocytes can be detected. These include lymphocytes, which proliferate and produce interferon-γ and other lymphokines in response to HSV antigens, and cytotoxic T lymphocytes, which are able to destroy HSV-infected cells early in the virus replication cycle before any progeny virus is produced.[138, 146–154] Acquired immunity to HSV involves T-cell recognition of type-specific and cross-reactive epitopes, prominant Th1 responses, and discordant Th2 responses with substantial production of interleukin-10 but little interleukin-4.[146]

Because of the multiplicity and overlap of these host defenses, it is difficult to determine the exact role and relative importance of each. Nevertheless, clinical and experimental observations (discussed in Chapter 240) indicate that the natural resistance of the normal epithelium and the virucidal and cytolytic capacities of macrophages and natural killer cells play a crucial role in localizing infection at the portal of entry and slowing virus replication during the first few days, before specific immune responses have developed. When these defenses are deficient, as they are in patients with eczema or extensive burns and in the newborn, there is risk for early virus dissemination and overwhelming systemic infection.[75, 138, 155–166] ADCC, the appearance of which coincides with resolution of the systemic symptoms of primary HSV infections, also has an important role in limiting virus replication at the portal of entry and preventing visceral dissemination. For example, deficiencies in ADCC, due primarily to numerical or functional deficiencies in effector cells, are associated with a markedly increased risk for severe disseminated HSV infection in the newborn and in certain patients with leukemia; and the presence of antibodies mediating ADCC is predictive of better outcome in neonatal HSV infections.[71, 72, 75, 143, 145, 162–169] Finally, HSV-reactive T lymphocytes appear to be required for the eventual eradication of infectious virus from mucocutaneous sites of infection.[138, 141, 146–150] Patients with deficient T-lymphocyte function, such as those with acquired immunodeficiency syndrome (AIDS), develop severe, persistent, locally progressive, mucocutaneous HSV infections but rarely have hematogenous dissemination.[138, 148, 170] Although patients with deficient cell-mediated immunity are subject to more frequent and more severe HSV recurrences, no specific defect has been consistently identified in otherwise normal individuals who suffer frequent episodes of recurrent genital herpes.[15, 18, 38, 41, 94, 138, 148, 161]

Clinical Manifestations

The clinical manifestations of genital herpes are influenced by the prior experience of the host with HSV, the serotype and amount of virus initiating infection, local conditions (e.g., trauma) at the site of infection, and host factors such as immunocompetence and gender. Because of the existence of two antigenically cross-reactive HSV serotypes, and the prevalence of asymptomatic infections, the characterization of HSV infections as primary (i.e., the initial HSV infection of a host with no immunity to either HSV-1 or HSV-2) or recurrent (i.e., symptomatic HSV infection caused by reactivation of latent [endogenous] HSV) does not reflect the complexity of the situation. Immunity to HSV is incomplete, as evidenced by the frequent recurrence of disease (e.g., recurrent genital herpes) in the presence of homologous humoral and cell-mediated immunity and by the ability to induce symptomatic infection in seropositive individuals by inoculating their skin with homologous virus.[171] Nevertheless, the clinical efficacy of homologous immunity is considerable, as indicated by the reduced extent and severity of recurrent as compared with primary infections and by the presence of substantial, although incomplete, resistance to exogenous reinfection by the same HSV serotype.[35–37]

Because of their extensive cross-reactivity, HSV-1 and HSV-2 both induce heterologous humoral and cell-mediated immune responses. Consequently, infection with one HSV serotype reduces susceptibility to infection by the other and moderates the severity of those infections that do occur. This has been demonstrated in seroepidemiologic studies showing that the prevalence of antibodies to HSV-2 is lower in women with antibodies to HSV-1 than in HSV-1–seronegative women, indicating that HSV-1 infection, presumably acquired in childhood, provides partial protection from subsequent HSV-2 infection.[24, 92, 101, 172] These studies also showed that women with antibodies only to HSV-2 were more likely to have a history of symptomatic genital herpes than were women with antibodies to both viruses, indicating that preexisting immunity to HSV-1 reduces the severity of those HSV-2 infections that do occur, so that a higher proportion are subclinical. The protective effect of prior HSV-1 infection has been confirmed by prospective transmission studies in couples discordant for antibodies to HSV-2.[47, 48] The risk for acquiring HSV-2 infection was three to four times greater in women who lacked antibodies to HSV-1 and HSV-2 than in women with previously acquired antibodies to HSV-1.

The effect of heterologous immunity has also been demonstrated by prospective clinical studies showing that initial episodes of genital herpes caused by HSV-2 are less severe in patients with serologic evidence of prior HSV-1 infection than in those with no preexisting antibodies to HSV-1 or HSV-2.[15, 38, 63, 76, 94, 107] In addition, initial episodes of genital herpes caused by HSV-1 are extremely rare in patients with preexisting antibodies to HSV-1, indicating that previous (presumably oropharyngeal) HSV-1 infection protects against genital herpes caused by the same HSV serotype. Finally, because most primary and nonprimary first-episode infections are asymptomatic but still result in the establishment of latent infections that are subject to periodic reactivation, many people experiencing their first recognized episode of symptomatic genital herpes are not, as they believe, experiencing an initial episode of exogenous infection. Instead, they are suffering their first symptomatic recurrence caused by reactivation of a latent infection established in the course of an earlier asymptomatic or unrecognized primary infection.[15, 38, 50, 63, 70, 94] Such episodes frequently result in confusion and consternation, especially when they occur in one member of a monogamous couple, neither of whom has any history of recognized genital herpes. In this situation, a clear understanding that the source of the virus responsible for the episode may be endogenous rather than exogenous is often more therapeutic than antiviral therapy.

These considerations, important in counseling patients and in evaluating any forms of treatment or prophylaxis, lead us to classify an initial episode of clinically manifest genital herpes as a primary first episode if it occurs in a person with no previous HSV infection at any site, as evidenced by the absence of antibodies to HSV-1 and HSV-2; a nonprimary first episode if it occurs in a person with preexisting antibodies to the heterologous HSV serotype (e.g., a first episode of symptomatic genital herpes caused by HSV-2 in a person with preexisting antibodies to HSV-1); and a recurrent episode if it occurs in a person with preexisting antibodies to the same HSV serotype (recognizing that the earlier homotypic infection could have been at a different anatomic site) (Table 113–1). The average duration and severity of clinical disease are greater in primary than in nonprimary first episodes of genital herpes, and episodes of recurrent genital herpes are usually the shortest and least severe (see Fig. 113–1). However, there is sufficient overlap that distinctions are often difficult to make on clinical grounds in any individual patient.

Primary and Initial Nonprimary Genital Herpes

The incubation period after sexual contact is usually 3 to 7 days, with a range of 1 day to more than 2 weeks.[38, 53, 54, 63, 94, 173] Most infections in both sexes are asymptomatic, but symptomatic primary genital herpes is more severe in women than in men. Women have a larger total area of lesions, more intense and prolonged local symptoms, more frequent constitutional symptoms, more extragenital lesions, and more complications. They have a higher frequency than men of dysuria (83% versus 44%), urethritis (85% versus 27%), meningitis (36% versus 13%), and pharyngitis (13% versus 7%).[63, 174–183] Primary genital herpes in women (i.e.,

TABLE 113–1 ■ Classification of Genital Herpes Simplex Virus Infections

CLINICAL PRESENTATION	HERPES SIMPLEX VIRUS ISOLATED	ANTIBODIES TO HERPES SIMPLEX VIRUS IN ACUTE SERUM	CLASSIFICATION	SOURCE OF VIRUS
First (recognized) episode	HSV-2	None	Primary HSV-2	Exogenous
	HSV-1	None	Primary HSV-1	Exogenous
	HSV-2	HSV-1	Initial nonprimary HSV-2	Exogenous
	HSV-1	HSV-2	Initial nonprimary HSV-1*	Exogenous
	HSV-2	HSV-2 ± HSV-1	Recurrent HSV-2†	Endogenous‡
	HSV-1	HSV-1 ± HSV-2	Recurrent HSV-1†	Endogenous‡
Recurrence	HSV-2	HSV-2 ± HSV-1	Recurrent HSV-2	Endogenous‡
	HSV-1	HSV-1 ± HSV-2	Recurrent HSV-1	Endogenous‡

*Rarely observed.
†First recognized reactivation of latent HSV in an individual whose initial (primary or nonprimary) infection was asymptomatic or unrecognized.
‡Reactivation of endogenous latent HSV infection.

primary herpetic vulvovaginitis) often begins with the appearance of herpetic vesicles, but this may be preceded by a short period of local burning, tenderness, and erythema of the labia minora and vaginal introitus. Typical herpetic vesicles first appear on the external genitalia, usually involving the labia majora, labia minora, vaginal vestibule, and introitus. New lesions continue to appear bilaterally in the same areas, and the eruption often extends to the mons pubis, clitoris, urethral orifice, perianal skin, buttocks, and thighs. In most areas within the labia minora, vesicles quickly rupture, leaving shallow, exquisitely tender ulcers covered with a yellowish gray exudate and surrounded by a red areola (Fig. 113–2). In drier areas, such as the outer surface of the labia majora and the adjacent skin, vesicles may remain intact, evolve into pustules, and then crust in several days.

New lesions continue to appear for a week or more. They are often extensive and may coalesce, forming bullae and large areas of ulceration that resembles a second-degree burn. The vaginal mucosa and vulva are inflamed and edematous. The cervix is almost always involved, and there is usually a profuse watery vaginal discharge. Examination typically reveals diffuse friability of the cervical epithelium; sometimes there is extensive ulceration and, occasionally, severe necrotic cervicitis.[180] Herpetic cervicitis is sometimes the only clinical manifestation of primary genital herpes. Most patients have severe vulvar pain, exquisite tenderness of the affected tissues, and dysuria, which is sometimes severe enough to cause urinary retention. Dysuria is nearly always associated with urethritis and the presence of HSV in the urine. HSV appears to be present in the urine in a higher proportion of patients with primary genital herpes caused by HSV-1 than by HSV-2.[80]

The majority of infected women have constitutional symptoms, including fever, headache, malaise, and myalgias, which usually peak during the first 3 to 4 days and disappear by the end of the first week. Most also develop bilateral painful inguinal and pelvic lymphadenopathy. The local symptoms generally worsen during the first week, reach a peak between days 8 and 10, and then gradually subside. Even when severe, primary genital herpes is normally self-limited. Virus replication is maximal during the first 3 to 4 days and declines thereafter; the mean duration of virus shedding is 11 to 12 days, although a few patients may shed virus for several weeks. Pain usually remits in 10 to 14 days, and healing occurs without scarring in 2 to 4 weeks. Mucosal lesions heal without crusting. The cervix, which is involved in 90% or more of women with symptomatic primary genital herpes, appears to be the source of virus that may be shed for weeks after visible lesions have healed and symptoms have disappeared.[15, 18, 38, 56, 58, 71, 94, 173, 180–183]

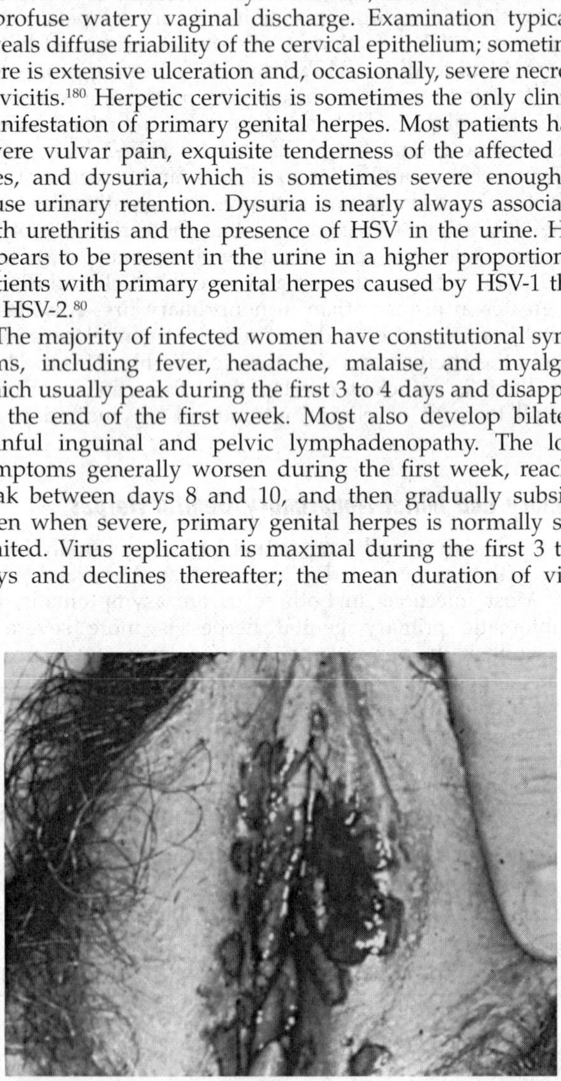

FIGURE 113–2 □ Primary genital herpes in the female patient. This young woman with primary herpetic vulvovaginitis has shallow, exquisitely tender ulcers on the inner surface of the labia majora, the labia minora, and the vaginal mucosa. The ulcers are covered with a yellowish gray exudate and surrounded by a narrow zone of erythema. Further examination also reveals herpetic cervicitis. (From Oxman MN: Genital herpes. *In* Braude AI, Davis CE, Fierer J [eds]: Infectious Diseases and Medical Microbiology, ed 2. Philadelphia, WB Saunders, 1986, pp 1041–1054.)

In men, the lesions of primary genital herpes usually appear bilaterally on the glans penis, the prepuce, and the shaft of the penis and less often on the scrotum, thighs, and buttocks. Their evolution is similar to that in women. In dry skin (e.g., on the shaft of the penis), they progress from papule to vesicle to pustule to crust and then heal, usually by the middle of the third week. In moist areas (e.g., under the prepuce), the vesicles are quickly macerated and evolve into ulcers identical to those described in women. New lesions continue to appear for a week or more, and there is local pain, tenderness, inflammation, and edema. Dysuria, usually associated with herpetic urethritis and accompanied by a small amount of clear mucoid urethral discharge, occurs in 30% to 40% of men with primary genital herpes. It is generally more painful than the dysuria of gonococcal or nongonococcal urethritis, and HSV can usually be isolated from urethral swabs. There is bilateral tender inguinal and pelvic lymphadenopathy, but this is less severe and of shorter duration than in women. Less than half of men with primary genital herpes have significant constitutional symptoms. Virus is present in large amounts during the first 3 to 5 days, and the mean duration of virus shedding is 10 to 11 days. Pain usually resolves during the second week, and healing occurs without scarring in 2 to 3 weeks.

The clinical manifestations and course of primary genital herpes caused by HSV-1 and HSV-2 are indistinguishable. However, the frequency of subsequent recurrences is lower after primary genital herpes caused by HSV-1 (see later).

The clinical manifestations of nonprimary first-episode genital herpes are similar to those of true primary genital herpes, but the disease is less severe and of shorter duration (see Fig. 113–1). There is a marked reduction in the frequency of constitutional symptoms, extragenital lesions, and complications, and a smaller proportion of women shed HSV from the cervix.[38, 41, 63, 75, 77, 94, 107, 176–179]

Recurrent Genital Herpes

Sixty percent to 90% of individuals with symptomatic primary or nonprimary first-episode genital herpes experience one or more episodes of recurrent genital herpes during the subsequent year. The recurrence rate is lower for HSV-1 than for HSV-2.[63, 77, 78, 107, 109, 110] The mean monthly rate of recurrence for genital herpes caused by HSV-1 is 0.08, compared with 0.34 for genital herpes caused by HSV-2, and approximately 40% of HSV-2–infected patients will have six or more recurrences per year.[107] This may explain why HSV-1 is isolated from 10% to 40% or more of patients with primary genital herpes but from only 1% to 5% of patients with recurrent disease. Interestingly, a study of patients with concurrent genital and oropharyngeal infections with the same HSV serotype showed that the oropharyngeal recurrence rate is higher for HSV-1 (0.12 per month) than for HSV-2 (0.001 per month). These differences in site-specific recurrence rates may reflect the adaptation of HSV-1 and HSV-2 to different anatomic niches[86] (see also Chapter 240). The rate of symptomatic recurrence is approximately 20% higher in men than in women.[107]

Recurrent genital herpes is usually less severe and of shorter duration than either primary or nonprimary first-episode infection (see Fig. 113–1). Although the same sites tend to be affected, there are fewer lesions, the area involved is more circumscribed, and the lesions are usually unilateral.[63, 94, 184, 185] Most patients have a prodrome of tenderness, pain, burning, tingling, or itching at the site of the impending eruption, beginning from a few hours to 1 or 2 days before the appearance of lesions. Some have a prodrome of ipsilateral sacral neuralgia, with severe burning, aching, or lancinating pain in the leg, buttock, or genital area. The lesions of recurrent genital herpes begin as clusters of tiny erythematous papules, which quickly develop into clusters of tiny vesicles on an erythematous base (Fig. 113–3). They sometimes coalesce, and they evolve in the same manner as in primary genital herpes but more rapidly. There is also less pain, fewer days of new lesion formation, and a much smaller total area of lesions.

The clinical manifestations of recurrent genital herpes are more severe in women than in men.[38, 41, 63, 94, 107, 173, 181–185] In women, the lesions are almost always painful. They are most often located on the labia minora, labia majora, or perineum but may also occur on the mons pubis, perianal skin, or buttocks.[119] Some women have linear ulcerations in the fourchette, which resemble inflamed excoriations and often are not recognized as herpetic by patients or their physicians.[38, 41, 63, 94, 173, 182–185] Lymphadenopathy may be present, but fever and constitutional symptoms are uncommon, and only about a quarter of women with recurrent genital herpes have dysuria. Virus is present in much smaller amounts in recurrent than in primary herpetic lesions (mean peak titers of 10^3 plaque-forming units or less per swab versus 10^5 plaque-forming units or more per swab); virus is shed for an average of 5 days, and its recovery after the seventh day is uncommon. Pain also disappears during the first week, and the lesions generally heal within 8 to 10 days. The frequency of positive cervical cultures (5% to 10%) is much lower during recurrent than during primary genital herpes. Furthermore, there are no visible cervical lesions, and the amount of virus present is at least 1000-fold less than the amount present during primary infections.[38, 41, 56, 58, 94, 173, 182, 183]

In men, recurrent genital herpes most often presents with one or more patches of grouped vesicles (see Fig. 113–3) on the shaft of the penis, prepuce, or glans. Lesions, which are usually unilateral, begin as papules and, on dry skin, evolve into vesicles, pustules, and crusts in the same manner as the lesions of herpes labialis.[38, 63, 94, 173, 181, 184, 185] Under the prepuce, vesicles are quickly macerated, forming shallow painful ulcers. There may be mild inguinal lymphadenopathy, but constitutional symptoms are rare and urethritis is uncommon. Urethral cultures are positive for HSV in less than 5% of men with recurrent genital herpes. The titer of virus is lower in recurrent than in primary lesions, and HSV can rarely be recovered after 4 or 5 days. Pain is present in about 60% of men with recurrent genital herpes. It is usually mild and disappears with the virus. Lesions heal in 7 to 10 days.

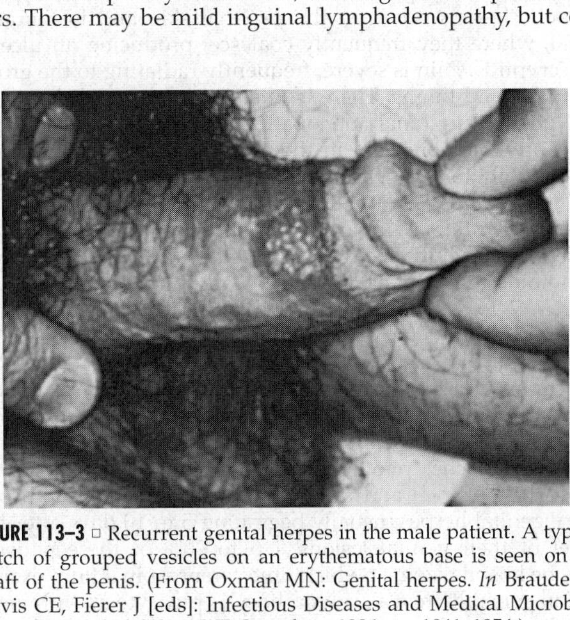

FIGURE 113–3 □ Recurrent genital herpes in the male patient. A typical patch of grouped vesicles on an erythematous base is seen on the shaft of the penis. (From Oxman MN: Genital herpes. *In* Braude AI, Davis CE, Fierer J [eds]: Infectious Diseases and Medical Microbiology, ed 2. Philadelphia, WB Saunders, 1986, pp 1041–1054.)

In approximately 5% of patients, recurrent herpes genitalis may present with a single, large, shallow, minimally tender ulcer, up to 1 cm in diameter, that has a clean, granular base and a sharply demarcated border. This lesion, which has been called a herpetic chancre,[183] may be mistaken for a syphilitic chancre. Because both herpes genitalis and syphilis may coexist in the same patient,[186, 187] laboratory diagnosis is essential.

Symptomatic genital HSV infections are only the tip of an iceberg.* The majority of primary genital HSV infections are asymptomatic or unrecognized, and 70% to 80% of people with antibodies to HSV-2 have no history of symptomatic genital herpes. Nevertheless, these seropositive individuals are latently infected and experience periodic virus reactivation, as evidenced by virus shedding. However, the majority of these reactivations are also asymptomatic or unrecognized. Consequently, episodes of asymptomatic virus shedding are far more frequent than episodes of symptomatic recurrent genital herpes.* The rate of asymptomatic virus shedding is generally 1% to 2% in immunocompetent persons with antibody to HSV-2, but it is substantially higher (e.g., 6% or more) in the first few months after initial HSV-2 infection, in the days immediately before and after a symptomatic recurrence, and in individuals with a high rate of symptomatic recurrence.[50, 77–80, 188, 189] HSV DNA can be detected by polymerase chain reaction (PCR) at a rate approximately eight times higher than that reported for infectious virus,[188, 189] but the biologic significance of low levels of HSV DNA in the absence of infectious virus remains to be determined. Asymptomatic shedding appears to be at least as common from the usual lesion site on the vulva as from the cervix, and anal shedding is also frequently documented.[61–66, 77–80, 94, 108] The epidemiologic importance of asymptomatic genital HSV infection is underlined by the observation that the majority of the mothers of infants with neonatal herpes have had no signs or symptoms of genital herpes during pregnancy and no history of prior symptomatic genital herpes.[15, 71, 72, 75, 111–115, 118]

Complications of Genital Herpes

Although often physically and mentally distressing, genital herpes in the normal host is almost always self-limited and usually resolves spontaneously without major complications or sequelae. Those complications that do occur may be divided into three categories: (1) bacterial or fungal superinfection; (2) extragenital infection or aberrant behavior by the virus in an apparently normal person; and (3) HSV infections in compromised hosts.

Bacterial and fungal superinfections are surprisingly uncommon. Rarely, balanoposthitis occurs in an uncircumcised man as a result of bacterial superinfection of herpes ulcers on the prepuce, and candidal balanitis is seen occasionally. Ulcerative lesions in moist skin areas may also become superinfected. *Candida* vaginitis occurs in about 10% of women with primary genital herpes and is more frequent in patients with diabetes. These complications usually respond to local therapy and rarely require systemic antibiotics.

Most complications of genital herpes result from infection

*References 18, 23–25, 38, 41, 50, 63, 68, 69, 71–82, 94, 108, 117, 188, 189.

of extragenital sites. Virus may reach these sites by direct extension, autoinoculation, viremia, or neural spread. Extragenital sites may also be infected exogenously at the time of genital infection, for example, concurrent oral and genital HSV-1 infection as a result of exposure to infected saliva.[190] These complications are much more frequent in primary than in nonprimary infections, and they are more common and generally more severe in women than in men. Once established, these extragenital HSV infections may recur, but they are rarely initiated during episodes of recurrent genital herpes.[63, 94, 119, 191]

Infection of the cervix occurs in almost every woman with symptomatic primary genital herpes and probably causes much of the profuse watery vaginal discharge that usually begins shortly after the onset of the disease.[63, 94] In addition, the cervix appears to be the site of infection in many asymptomatic cases of genital herpes, which actually constitute the majority of genital HSV-2 infections. On occasion, the cervical infection may be extremely severe, producing necrotic cervicitis.[180] Symptoms include profuse vaginal discharge; dysuria; abdominal, pelvic, or genital pain; and constitutional symptoms. The cervix is extremely tender, bleeds easily, and exhibits extensive superficial necrosis with sloughing of necrotic epithelium. Healing occurs spontaneously in 2 to 3 weeks. Herpetic cervicitis may occur in the absence of other genital lesions. Rarely, extensive herpetic infection of the glans penis can produce necrotizing balanitis. Misdiagnosis and inappropriate therapy are common.[192, 193]

Herpetic urethritis frequently accompanies primary genital herpes, occurring in 30% to 40% of men and more than 80% of women.[38, 63, 94, 174–179] Typical herpetic lesions may be visible near the urethral meatus, or they may be intraurethral. There is usually severe burning pain on micturition but minimal discharge. Typical intranuclear inclusion bodies and multinucleated giant cells may be demonstrated in urethral smears. The urethritis may recur, with or without recurrent genital lesions, and herpetic urethritis may be the only clinical manifestation of primary genital herpes. Herpetic cystitis has also been observed in patients with primary genital herpes and may account for some instances of dysuria and urinary retention.[194] In many cases, virus may reach the bladder by direct extension from the urethra or by neural transmission from infected sacral ganglia. The occurrence of cystitis caused by HSV-1 in adults with oropharyngeal HSV infection suggests that the bladder may also be infected as a result of viremia.

Ten percent to 30% of patients with primary genital herpes caused by HSV-1 or HSV-2 develop symptomatic herpetic pharyngotonsillitis, often as their first manifestation of HSV infection.[38, 63, 94, 110] In most cases, virus is probably introduced directly by oral-oral or oral-genital contact, but it may also reach the pharynx by viremia. Clinical manifestations range from mild erythema to severe exudative pharyngotonsillitis, which may even result in pharyngeal obstruction.[195] Most patients have constitutional symptoms and anterior cervical lymphadenopathy. Many are misdiagnosed as having streptococcal pharyngitis or infectious mononucleosis, especially if genital signs and symptoms are absent or ignored.

During primary genital herpes, cutaneous lesions frequently appear on the buttocks, thighs, or other areas of skin below the waist. They may result from contiguous spread, zosteriform neural transmission from newly infected sacral ganglia, or autoinoculation. When these lesions recur (typically in the absence of any genital lesions), they may resemble herpes zoster and are often associated with a prodrome of deep neuralgic pain. However, frequent recurrence distinguishes this syndrome of "zosteriform herpes simplex" from true herpes zoster caused by VZV, which rarely recurs in the same dermatome.[38, 51, 119, 196]

Autoinoculation of the finger during primary genital herpes may result in a herpetic whitlow that is indistinguishable from the whitlows that occur in hospital personnel as a result of contact with HSV-1 in saliva and respiratory secretions (Chapter 240). Most herpetic whitlows in adults (other than in dental and hospital personnel) are associated with primary genital herpes and are caused by HSV-2.[197, 198] These troublesome lesions occur primarily in women and tend to recur. Autoinoculation occasionally results in skin lesions at other sites and appears to be responsible for herpetic keratoconjunctivitis, which may be seen in as many as 1% of patients with primary genital herpes.[63, 94]

Severe disseminated HSV infections are common in immunosuppressed children and adults (see later). Yet, although viremia probably occurs during most cases of primary genital herpes in the normal host, it is seldom clinically manifest and virtually never documented. Rarely, apparently healthy young adults with primary genital herpes develop disseminated infection. This generally involves the skin, rather than internal organs, and produces a disease that is virtually indistinguishable from varicella.[38, 51, 199, 200] The illness is self-limited and usually resolves in 12 to 15 days. However, skin lesions commonly recur at sites of primary cutaneous infection. Very rarely there is severe, often fatal, visceral dissemination that may or may not be accompanied by vesicular lesions in the skin. Multiple organs are involved, but fulminant HSV hepatitis is usually predominant clinically and is generally accompanied by leukopenia, thrombocytopenia, and disseminated intravascular coagulation. This syndrome, fatal in the majority of untreated cases, occurs with greatest frequency in pregnant women, usually during the third trimester. Some cases have been associated with primary oropharyngeal HSV-1 infections, but most have accompanied primary genital herpes caused by either HSV serotype.[15, 38, 51, 71, 94, 201–215] The disease in these pregnant women resembles that observed in renal transplant recipients and other immunosuppressed patients and in the neonate (see later). HSV-specific cellular immunity is depressed during the third trimester of pregnancy,[216] and this may explain the susceptibility of pregnant women to disseminated HSV infection.

Anorectal herpes and herpetic proctitis may occur as complications of genital herpes in women, the virus spreading from the vulva to the perineum, anus, and anal canal directly or by zosteriform spread from infected sacral ganglia. However, most cases result from anal intercourse, and the disease is seen most frequently in homosexual men.[217–219] Typical herpetic lesions occur on the perianal skin and in the anal canal, where they frequently coalesce, producing an ulcerative cryptitis. Pain is severe, frequently radiating to the groin, buttocks, and thighs. There is often a serous rectal discharge and bilateral inguinal adenopathy, and constitutional symptoms are common. Pain in the anal canal usually results in reflex inhibition of defecation and sometimes tenesmus. Sacral ganglionitis and autonomic dysfunction frequently result in sacral neuralgia, urinary retention, and impotence.[217–220] In spite of its severity, the disease is self-limited; the neurologic symptoms resolve, and healing usually occurs without scarring in 2 to 4 weeks. Recurrent attacks of anal herpes are common after primary infection.

Neurons play a crucial role in the pathogenesis of HSV infections, and thus it is not surprising that many complications of genital herpes involve the central and peripheral nervous systems. Symptoms of meningitis, including fever, severe headache, photophobia, and stiff neck, develop in about 10% of men and more than 30% of women with primary genital herpes, usually beginning 5 to 10 days after the onset of their genital lesions. Up to 20% of these patients may be hospitalized, at which time cerebrospinal fluid examination generally reveals a lymphocytic pleocytosis with moderately elevated protein concentration and normal glucose concentration.[94, 221–228] Nearly all cases are caused by HSV-2, which can be isolated from the cerebrospinal fluid. Concurrent isolation of HSV from the blood is uncommon, and the frequent association of meningitis with signs and symptoms of lumbosacral ganglionitis and radiculomyelitis, including urinary retention, abdominal and lower extremity muscle weakness, and paresthesia and anesthesia over sacral dermatomes, suggests that virus reaches the central nervous system by neural spread rather than by viremia.[94, 221–228] The meningitis usually follows a brief and benign course, but the associated lumbosacral ganglionitis and radiculomyelitis may not resolve for several months.[220, 221, 226] Ascending myelitis is a rare complication.[221, 229] Aseptic meningitis recurs in 20% to 30% of patients, usually in association with episodes of recurrent genital herpes. The recurrences are usually milder than the initial episode. The detection of HSV-2 DNA in the cerebrospinal fluid of 10 of 13 patients with benign recurrent lymphocytic (Mollaret) meningitis suggests that this syndrome is usually a complication of genital herpes.[230] Only 3 of the 10 patients had a history of genital herpes, emphasizing the clinical importance of asymptomatic and unrecognized HSV infections.

Recurrent genital herpes and recurrent zosteriform herpes involving the skin below the waist may be associated with severe local neuralgia, usually in an L5-S1 dermatome distribution. When the recurrent herpetic lesions and neuralgia involve the extremities, there may also be local edema and lymphangitis. The neuralgia may precede the eruption by several days and usually resolves along with the cutaneous lesions.[38, 226, 231–233] Although resolution is generally complete and multiple recurrences occur without permanent residua, repeated attacks during a period of years may sometimes result in chronic pain and permanent sensory and motor deficits. A similar syndrome is occasionally seen with recurrent herpetic whitlow. Primary genital or anal herpes is sometimes complicated by urinary retention, and this may be accompanied by neuralgic pain and blunting of sensation over the sacral dermatomes. Patients with this syndrome have hypotonic bladders and cerebrospinal fluid pleocytosis, indicating that the urinary retention reflects acute herpetic ganglionitis or lumbosacral radiculomyelitis.[38, 220, 234–236] This complication of genital herpes normally resolves spontaneously without residua in 7 to 10 days; the only report of prolonged dysfunction was in a patient treated with corticosteroids.[223]

Recurrent genital herpes may be associated with recurrent episodes of erythema multiforme or Stevens-Johnson syndrome. As is the case with HSV-1, this complication appears to be an allergic response to circulating HSV antigens or antigen-antibody complexes. The lesions are not the direct result of replications of HSV-2 in the skin or mucous membranes (see Chapter 240).

Persons with compromised host defenses are at increased risk for severe, even fatal, HSV infections. Those at greatest risk appear to have abnormal cellular immunity, eczema, or burns. The risk to the compromised patient and the nature of the pathologic process appear to be the same with HSV-1 and HSV-2. Most episodes of genital herpes in these patients are recurrent infections, and they often evolve normally and resolve without complications. Sometimes, however, the local lesions do not resolve but slowly progress to form a deep, gradually enlarging ulcer with a sharp erythematous border and a necrotic base covered with purulent exudate; there are often satellite lesions in adjacent areas of skin. These chronic progressive herpetic ulcers are usually exquisitely tender. They contain large amounts of HSV and may persist for months. They occur most frequently in patients with severely depressed cell-mediated immunity, and they often heal spontaneously when cellular immunity improves on induced remission of lymphoreticular malignant neoplasms or reduction in iatrogenic immunosuppression in organ allograft recipients.

Male homosexuals with AIDS often have chronic progressive perianal herpetic ulcers.[170, 237] In spite of their severity, these lesions are rarely associated with constitutional symptoms or hematogenous dissemination of HSV. Genital herpes sometimes disseminates in immunocompromised patients, producing widespread cutaneous lesions or fatal involvement of multiple visceral organs, especially the liver. This highly lethal complication of genital herpes, seen most often in organ allograft recipients in the first month after transplantation, is usually a consequence of reactivation of latent endogenous HSV infection, although it may also result from exogenous infection introduced by the transplanted organ.[238–240] It may be prevented by the use of acyclovir prophylaxis.[240]

Asymptomatic shedding of HSV-2 is markedly increased in immunocompromised patients. In one study, the prevalence of asymptomatic shedding by HSV-2–seropositive women was found to be four times greater in human immunodeficiency virus–infected women than in uninfected control subjects, and it was greatest in those with the lowest $CD4^+$ cell counts.[241]

Neonatal Herpes Simplex Virus Infection

One of the most serious complications of genital herpes occurs when infection in a pregnant woman is transmitted to her newborn infant.[15, 38, 71, 75, 113–115] The infant is usually infected perinatally during passage through the birth canal of a mother with asymptomatic genital herpes. In some cases, ascending infection occurs shortly before birth, usually in a woman with prolonged rupture of membranes. Ascending infection can also be iatrogenic, introduced by a fetal monitor.[242] The risk for neonatal infection is estimated to be as high as 30% for infants born to mothers shedding virus at delivery as a result of an initial primary or nonprimary infection, compared with 2% to 3% (and probably substantially lower) when virus shedding at term results from a recurrent infection.[75, 115–117] In addition, asymptomatic shedding of HSV at the onset of labor due to recently acquired primary infection is associated with preterm delivery, whereas shedding due to an asymptomatic recurrence of genital herpes acquired before pregnancy is not.[243] Congenital infection, a consequence of primary maternal HSV infection occurring earlier in pregnancy, is responsible for 3% to 5% of infected neonates.[75, 244–246] Some infants acquire infection postnatally from the mother, other family members, or nursery personnel with nongenital HSV infections or by nosocomial transmission from another infected infant.[75, 247–250] The observation that one third of neonatal HSV infections are now caused by HSV-1 indicates the potential importance of these sources of infection. The overall rate of occurrence of neonatal HSV infection in the United States is estimated to be between 1 in 3000 and 1 in 5000 live births.[75, 115]

In contrast to other forms of HSV infection, infection of the newborn is virtually never asymptomatic. Its clinical presentation reflects the site and extent of virus replication. The initial clinical manifestations of neonatal herpes usually appear during the first or second week of life, but they may be present at birth or delayed until the infant is 1 month of age. Congenital (intrauterine) infection presents at birth with a triad of skin vesicles or scarring; eye disease, including chorioretinitis and often herpetic keratoconjunctivitis; and microcephaly or hydranencephaly. Mortality is high, and survivors have severe sequelae. Prepartum intrauterine (ascending) infection results in the appearance of skin lesions at birth or within 24 hours thereafter but no evidence of prepartum infection of other organs. These infants respond well to antiviral therapy. Infants infected during delivery or postnatally present with one of three patterns of disease: (1) disease localized to the portal of entry, that is, the skin, eyes, or mouth; (2) encephalitis with or without skin, eye, or mouth disease; or (3) disseminated infection involving multiple organs, including the brain, lungs, liver, heart, adrenals, and skin.[15, 75, 111–114]

Infants in whom infection appears to remain localized to the skin, eyes, or mouth generally present at 10 to 11 days of life. Herpetic skin vesicles are present in about 90%, often on the presenting part, but they may be few in number. Most of these infants survive without treatment, but some develop disseminated disease or encephalitis, and 30% to 40% develop significant neurologic or ocular sequelae. Treatment has reduced the frequency of sequelae to about 10%, but even treated newborns suffer repeated recurrences during infancy.

Infants with encephalitis present later, at about 16 to 17 days of life, with a clinical picture resembling bacterial meningitis. Only about 60% have skin vesicles to aid diagnosis. Mortality without treatment is approximately 50%, and most survivors have severe neurologic and ocular sequelae.

Infants with disseminated neonatal HSV infections develop initial manifestations late in the first week of life. These are relatively nonspecific, consisting of lethargy, fever or hypothermia, vomiting, and poor feeding. Jaundice, purpuric rash, apneic spells, respiratory distress, and cyanosis may also appear. The clinical picture often resembles bacterial sepsis. Many of these infants have clinical evidence of central nervous system involvement, and seizures are common. The disease progresses rapidly, with the frequent development of pneumonia, shock, and disseminated intravascular coagulation. About 90% of these infants die, usually in the second week of life, and most survivors have severe neurologic sequelae. Herpetic skin lesions fail to develop in nearly one quarter of these infants. Antiviral therapy has reduced the mortality to 55% in infants with disseminated infection and to 15% in infants with encephalitis, and it has increased the proportion of survivors who function normally at 1 year of age.[112] Moreover, the availability of experimental treatment protocols has led to earlier diagnosis, increasing the proportion of infants recognized with localized infection of the skin, eyes, or mouth, many of whom would develop disseminated or central nervous system infection if untreated.[114] The natural history and clinical manifestations of neonatal HSV infection are discussed in detail by Whitley[15] and Whitley and Arvin.[75]

Diagnosis

The diagnosis of genital herpes is often clinically apparent, especially when there are typical grouped vesicles and a history of recurrent episodes. However, a number of other diseases can cause ulcerative genital lesions that may be confused with those of genital herpes, and lesions caused by HSV are often atypical, especially in immunocompromised patients. Moreover, the rate of dual infections is higher than random.[99, 186, 187, 191, 251] Thus, laboratory diagnosis is often required, and it is always desirable. The availability of specific antiviral agents now places a high premium on early and reliable diagnosis. The diagnosis of HSV infection is discussed in detail in Chapter 240.

Virus isolation in cell culture is the "gold standard" for the diagnosis of HSV infections. It offers high sensitivity and specificity when specimens are obtained early in the course of HSV infection (i.e., at the vesicular stage) and handled properly to avoid loss of infectivity (see Chapter 240). It also yields virus for subsequent studies, such as measurement of sensitivity to antiviral drugs and restriction endonuclease fingerprinting, and it may detect pathogens other than HSV. However, even with culture enhancement techniques,[252–255] results are not available for at least 24 hours and often longer. Because many therapeutic decisions require diagnostic information in minutes to hours, much effort has been devoted to developing methods for rapid diagnosis.[19, 255–264]

The simplest technique for rapid diagnosis of HSV infection is the examination of cells scraped from the base of a vesicle or ulcer (Tzanck smear) or scraped from the surface of the cervix or the vaginal mucosa (Papanicolaou smear) and stained by the Papanicolaou or Paragon multiple stain technique, as described in Chapter 240. Multinucleated giant cells with eosinophilic intranuclear inclusion bodies indicate HSV or VZV infection. Virus antigen detection and identification (e.g., by immunofluorescent or immunoenzyme staining) using monoclonal antibodies to HSV-1, HSV-2, and VZV can increase sensitivity and provide a specific diagnosis, distinguishing HSV from VZV and HSV-1 from HSV-2.[19, 255–259] A punch biopsy specimen taken at the edge of a lesion provides better tissue for cytologic and immunologic diagnosis, especially in atypical ulcerative lesions, such as those observed in immunocompromised patients.[170]

Rapid direct detection and identification of HSV antigens and nucleic acids in clinical specimens are now a reality. These techniques are specific and sensitive when applied to herpetic lesions and can even detect viral proteins and nucleic acids late in the course of infection, when infectious virus may no longer be recovered.[15, 255–261] However, they lack the sensitivity required to detect the small amounts of virus shed during asymptomatic recurrences of genital herpes,[255, 260, 261] which appear to be responsible for about half of all neonatal HSV infections[71, 72, 75, 115] as well as for the majority of new genital HSV infections.[41, 47–50, 73, 74] The application of PCR to detection of HSV DNA sequences in clinical specimens provides a solution to this problem.[188, 189, 230, 255, 261–264] Use of primers from HSV DNA sequences that are common to HSV-1 and HSV-2 (e.g., gB, DNA polymerase) permits detection of either HSV serotype, whereas primers from type-specific DNA sequences can be used to identify the HSV serotype involved.[15, 75, 255, 261–263] The increased sensitivity of this technique has led to the recognition that benign recurrent lymphocytic meningitis is usually a complication of recurrent genital herpes, although most cases occur in HSV-2–seropositive individuals with asymptomatic or unrecognized infections.[230] PCR has also proved to be substantially more sensitive than virus isolation for detection of symptomatic and asymptomatic virus shedding in patients with genital herpes.[188, 189, 255, 261, 264] Its clinical application has led to a three- to eightfold increase in the estimated frequency of HSV shedding by HSV-2–seropositive women.[188, 189, 264] Not surprisingly, culture-positive specimens contain much larger quantities of HSV DNA than do culture-negative specimens. The clinical significance of small quantities of HSV DNA in the absence of infectious virus remains to be determined.

Type-specific serologic assays have been developed in which serum samples are reacted with HSV proteins that have predominantly type-specific epitopes (e.g., gG1 or gC1 from HSV-1 and gG2 from HSV-2) in solid-phase enzyme immunoassays or with electrophoretically separated HSV-1 and HSV-2 proteins in Western blot assays.[21–25, 85, 92, 255, 261] The enzyme immunoassays are accurate and simple to perform on large numbers of serum samples, but antibodies to gG2 may not develop until 6 to 8 weeks after initial HSV-2 infections and remain undetectable in some patients, especially immunosuppressed patients (e.g., AIDS patients) with culture-proven recurrent HSV-2 infections.[22, 255] Western blot assays are more cumbersome, but they can detect early seroconversion, identify HSV-2 infections even when antibodies to gG2 are not detectable, and detect seroconversion to HSV-2 in patients with prior HSV-1 infections despite their early anamnestic response to type-common epitopes. They are also useful for distinguishing primary and nonprimary first episodes of HSV infection and for determining previous infection with HSV-1 or HSV-2, or both (e.g., for screening organ donors and recipients, pregnant women and their sexual partners, and potential vaccine recipients). The clinical application of these type-specific assays has revolutionized the serologic diagnosis of genital herpes and led to a clear delineation of the epidemiology of HSV-1 and HSV-2 infections.[21–25, 50, 85, 92, 255] Unfortunately, these assays are generally available only in research laboratories. Commercially available enzyme immunoassays do not reliably discriminate between HSV-1 and HSV-2 infections despite claims to the contrary.[84] These assays are useful only for confirming a diagnosis of primary HSV infection by documenting the absence of antibodies to HSV in the acute-phase serum and their development during convalescence, and for identifying persons not infected with either HSV serotype. Because recurrent genital herpes only rarely induces a significant increase in the titer of antibodies to HSV, serologic assays are not helpful in confirming that diagnosis.

The diseases to be considered in the differential diagnosis of herpes genitalis are syphilis, chancroid, lymphogranuloma venereum, granuloma inguinale, vaccinia, herpes zoster, erythema multiforme, Behçet syndrome, mucocutaneous manifestations of inflammatory bowel disease, contact dermatitis, candidiasis, and impetigo.[251] Multinucleated giant cells and eosinophilic Cowdry type A intranuclear inclusion bodies indicate the presence of either HSV or VSV; direct detection and identification of HSV antigens or nucleic acids or virus isolation can give the specific diagnosis. Because patients are often simultaneously infected by more than one agent, it is important to rule out at least some of the other possibilities even if an HSV infection is documented.[186, 187]

Syphilis is the most important of these diseases.[186, 187] The chancre of syphilis may mimic the ulcerative lesions of genital herpes, although it tends to be more indurated, indolent, and painless. The mucous patches of secondary syphilis may also resemble the ulcerated lesions of genital herpes, but they are usually accompanied by a generalized rash or other secondary manifestations. The diagnosis should be attempted by darkfield examination and serology. Serologic follow-up is essential.

The ulcers of chancroid are soft and painful with ragged undermined margins, and there is prominent painful, often fluctuant, inguinal adenopathy. The demonstration of *Haemophilus ducreyi,* a small gram-negative rod, in smears of the ulcer or by culture can help establish the diagnosis. The diagnosis of lymphogranuloma venereum and granuloma inguinale is discussed in Chapter 114. Vaccinia, which should rarely be seen now that routine smallpox vaccination has been abandoned, can be differentiated from HSV and VZV infections by the presence of cytoplasmic inclusion bodies and the absence of intranuclear inclusion bodies and multinucleated giant cells. The histopathologic appearance of erythema multiforme and Behçet syndrome is different from that of genital herpes, and both are accompanied by characteristic lesions outside the genital area. However, erythema multiforme is induced by genital herpes in some patients, and the lesions may therefore coexist. Bacterial and candidal infections may be diagnosed by Gram-stained smears and cultures.

With the advent of effective chemotherapy, it has become essential to establish the diagnosis early in the course of life-threatening HSV infections, such as neonatal HSV infections and disseminated HSV infections in immunocompromised children and adults.[202–214, 238–240, 265] Because the majority of infected infants are born to mothers without signs or symptoms or even a history of genital herpes, and because obvious external sources of infection are lacking in most infected children and adults, this requires a high index of suspicion. Any skin lesion should be examined by Tzanck smear, one or more HSV antigen detection methods (e.g., immunoperoxidase staining), and viral culture, and blood should be cultured for HSV. Lesions should be sought in the mouth, and the eyes should be examined for herpetic conjunctivitis. Any infant with signs of sepsis or meningitis, but with negative bacterial cultures or a poor response to appropriate antibiotics, is suspect. Mouth, conjunctivae, urine, stool, blood, and cerebrospinal fluid should be cultured for HSV; the mother should also be examined and cultures performed. HSV DNA should be sought in these specimens by use of PCR techniques.[255, 261] Disseminated enterovirus infection can resemble neonatal herpes, and the two infections may rarely coexist.

Treatment

No treatment is presently available that can eradicate latent HSV infections or prevent the establishment of HSV latency. Nevertheless, antiviral chemotherapy is effective in shortening the course and reducing the severity of primary, first-episode nonprimary, and recurrent genital HSV infections in immunocompetent and immunocompromised patients. Moreover, suppressive therapy can markedly reduce the frequency of symptomatic recurrences and asymptomatic virus shedding. Acyclovir (9-[2-hydroxyethoxymethyl]guanine) has been proved effective for the treatment of genital herpes and has been the mainstay of therapy for the past 15 years.[266–269] Acyclovir is a guanosine analog that is selectively phosphorylated by HSV deoxypyrimidine kinase (thymidine kinase) and thus concentrated in HSV-infected cells. Cellular enzymes then convert the resulting acyclovir monophosphate to acyclovir triphosphate, which is a selective inhibitor of HSV DNA polymerase. In addition, any acyclovir triphosphate that is incorporated into DNA causes chain termination.[270] As a consequence of these properties, acyclovir is a highly effective and nontoxic inhibitor of HSV replication. Strains of HSV-1 are generally more sensitive to acyclovir than are strains of HSV-2, but current dosages employed (see later) produce concentrations in serum and body fluids well in excess of those required to inhibit the replication of HSV-2 in vitro. Two licensed prodrugs, famciclovir and valacyclovir, provide much greater oral bioavailability than does acyclovir. This permits less frequent dosing and results in blood levels of antiviral activity heretofore achievable only with intravenous acyclovir.[271–275]

A number of randomized placebo-controlled double-blind studies have demonstrated the therapeutic efficacy of intravenous, oral, and topical acyclovir in immunologically normal persons with first-episode genital herpes. In patients with first episodes severe enough to warrant hospitalization, intravenous acyclovir (5 mg/kg every 8 hours for 5 days) begun within 7 days of onset markedly reduced the duration of virus shedding (more than 75%) and of local and constitutional symptoms (more than 50%). Healing time was reduced by more than 50%, and the development of new lesions and complications was prevented.[174–176] Oral acyclovir (200 mg five times daily for 10 days) begun within 6 days of onset has also reduced virus shedding and new lesion formation (more than 70%), shortened the duration of local and constitutional symptoms, and shortened the times to crusting and healing of lesions in patients with primary first-episode genital herpes.[177–179]

In patients with nonprimary first-episode genital herpes,

oral acyclovir markedly reduced the duration of virus shedding but did not have a significant effect on the clinical course of the disease, presumably because of the late initiation of therapy relative to the shorter normal duration of nonprimary first-episode disease.[177–179, 268, 269]

Topical acyclovir (5% in polyethylene glycol ointment applied four times daily for 7 days) reduced the duration of virus shedding in patients with primary and nonprimary first-episode genital herpes and shortened the clinical course of local disease in patients with primary infections, but it was significantly less effective than oral or intravenous acyclovir.[276, 277] Moreover, in contrast to oral and intravenous acyclovir, topical acyclovir did not decrease new lesion formation or reduce the duration of dysuria, vaginal discharge, or constitutional symptoms.[276, 277] Thus, topical acyclovir is not recommended for treatment of first-episode genital herpes. No form of therapy appears to prevent the establishment of neuronal latency, and in no group of treated patients has any reduction in the frequency or severity of subsequent recurrences been demonstrated.[63, 107, 174–179, 266–269] Nevertheless, the observation that patients with prolonged primary HSV-2 infections (duration of 35 days or longer) have more frequent episodes of recurrent genital herpes than do patients with shorter primary infections[107] suggests that early treatment of first-episode genital herpes (which would be expected to shorten the course of the disease) might reduce the frequency of subsequent recurrences.

In patients with recurrent genital herpes, oral acyclovir (200 mg five times daily for 5 days) begun within 48 hours of onset reduced the duration of virus shedding and new lesion formation and modestly shortened the times to crusting and healing of lesions.[177, 184] When therapy was initiated at the onset of symptoms, the clinical effects of acyclovir were greater, but they were still far smaller than those observed in first episodes of genital herpes. Topical acyclovir had no clinically significant effect on the course of disease.[185] Treatment of recurrent genital herpes with acyclovir did not reduce the frequency or severity of subsequent episodes. The treatment of initial and recurrent genital herpes is reviewed in detail in references 266 to 269.

A number of well-designed clinical trials have demonstrated that oral and intravenous dosing acyclovir is extremely effective for the treatment (and prophylaxis) of severe mucocutaneous HSV infections in immunocompromised patients.[278–283] Excellent results have been obtained with oral dosages of 200 mg or 400 mg four or five times daily and intravenous dosages or 5 mg/kg or 250 mg/m^2 every 8 to 12 hours. When infection is disseminated or involves internal organs such as the liver, early initiation of treatment with acyclovir (e.g., before the diagnosis has been confirmed) may be lifesaving.[240] Treatment of herpetic proctitis with oral acyclovir, 400 mg five times daily for 10 days, markedly decreases virus shedding and speeds resolution of the disease. The higher dose of acyclovir is preferred because herpetic proctitis often occurs in homosexual men who may be immunocompromised because of human immunodeficiency virus infections.[284] No significant hematologic, renal, or hepatic toxicity has been observed in patients with normal renal function treated with oral acyclovir for genital herpes, although reversible neurotoxicity has been reported in patients with renal failure and in bone marrow transplant recipients treated with intravenous acyclovir.[285] Acyclovir dosage adjustment is required in patients with diminished renal function. Immunosuppressive therapy should be reduced, if possible, in immunocompromised patients with HSV infection.

Patients with primary or nonprimary initial episodes of genital herpes benefit significantly from treatment with oral acyclovir. The regimen approved by the U.S. Food and Drug Administration, 200 mg five times daily for 10 days, is widely used, but 400 mg three times daily (i.e., every 8 hours) for 10 days is equally effective and much more convenient.[286] This regimen is recommended (Table 113–2). Higher doses (800 mg five times daily) offer no additional clinical benefit but are associated with gastrointestinal side effects.[287] Intravenous acyclovir is appropriate for initial use in patients hospitalized with severe first-episode genital herpes or for complications such as aseptic meningitis or sacral ganglionitis. When the patient improves, the course may be completed with oral acyclovir. In contrast, the normal course of recurrent genital herpes is often so circumscribed that many patients perceive relatively little benefit from treatment, even when it is initiated during the prodrome. The standard treatment regimen for recurrent genital herpes has been 200 mg five times daily for 5 days, but the equally effective and more convenient regimen of 400 mg three times daily (i.e., every 8 hours) is now recommended[286] (see Table 113–2). Many patients with a history of more prolonged and severe recurrences who do appear to benefit from therapy find that they can reduce the dose of acyclovir after the first day or two (e.g., to 200 mg three times daily) or even eliminate the fourth and fifth days of treatment without perceiving any loss of efficacy. Thus, in individuals with recurrent genital herpes, decisions to employ therapy, reduce dosage, use prophylactic (suppressive) therapy (see later), or simply let nature take its course are best left to the patient, with the physician's guidance. In this regard, it is often useful for the patient to keep a daily calendar to record the nature and durations of recurrences, prodromal symptoms, and therapy.

Treatment of neonatal HSV infections with intravenous acyclovir or vidarabine for 10 days has significantly reduced mortality and increased the proportion of infants who appear to function normally at 1 year of age. The two drugs appear comparable in efficacy. However, considerable morbidity and mortality still exist among treated infants, and there is evidence of relapse and of progressive neurologic deterioration after cessation of therapy.[15, 75, 111–114, 288, 289] In this regard, long-term suppressive therapy with oral acyclovir has been shown to markedly reduce cutaneous recurrences in infants with virologically confirmed neonatal herpes with disease confined to the skin, eyes, and mouth.[290] However, the effect on neurologic outcome remains to be determined. Whereas intravenous acyclovir (10 mg/kg or 500 mg/m^2 every 8 hours for 10 days) is currently recommended for treatment of neonatal HSV infection, studies are continuing in an attempt to develop more effective diagnostic and therapeutic strategies. See references 15, 75, 112–114, 288, 289, and 290.

Prevention

Prevention of HSV infection and disease is a particularly complicated problem because of the unique characteristics of the HSV-host interaction. For example, the high rate of asymptomatic initial and recurrent infections, the frequent development of symptomatic recurrent disease in individuals whose initial infection was asymptomatic, and the dominant role of asymptomatic virus shedding in transmission all emphasize the need to distinguish between preventing infection and preventing disease. These problems as well as potential goals and strategies for the prevention of HSV infection and disease are discussed in the section on prevention and treatment in Chapter 240.

Prevention of Genital Herpes Simplex Virus Infection

Prevention of exposure is, at present, the only proven means of preventing genital HSV infection. Because men with symp-

TABLE 113–2 ■ Treatment and Suppression of Genital Herpes in Immunocompetent Persons

DRUG	ROUTE	DOSE	FREQUENCY	DURATION
Initial Episode (Primary and Nonprimary)				
Recommended				
Acyclovir	Oral	400 mg	q 8 h	10 d*
Acyclovir	Intravenous	5 mg/kg	q 8 h	7–10 d*†
Alternatives				
Acyclovir	Oral	200 mg	5 times daily	10 d*
Famciclovir	Oral	250 mg	q 12 h	10 d*
Valacyclovir	Oral	1.0 g	q 12 h	10 d*
Recurrent Genital Herpes (Episodic Treatment)				
Recommended				
Acyclovir	Oral	400 mg	q 8 h	5 d
Alternatives				
Acyclovir	Oral	200 mg	5 times daily	5 d
Famciclovir	Oral	125 mg	q 12 h	5 d
Valacyclovir	Oral	500 mg	q 12 h	5 d
Suppression of Frequently Recurring Genital Herpes				
Recommended				
Acyclovir	Oral	400 mg	q 12 h	Daily
Alternative				
Acyclovir	Oral	200 mg	3 or 4 times daily	Daily
Investigational				
Famciclovir	Oral	250 mg	q 12 h	Daily
Valacyclovir	Oral	500 mg	q 12 h	Daily

*Or until lesions resolve.
†In patients requiring hospitalization or with complications such as aseptic meningitis.

tomatic genital herpes appear to transmit infection to 75% or more of susceptible consorts, men with prodromal symptoms or active genital herpes should refrain from sexual intercourse. Women with prodromal symptoms, symptomatic genital herpes, or visible but asymptomatic genital lesions should also refrain from sexual intercourse. Oral-genital contact can transmit infection in either direction. Thus, individuals with herpes labialis should refrain from oral-genital sexual activity. Unfortunately, this approach will be only modestly successful because of the role of asymptomatic virus shedding in transmission. Despite that the concentration of virus and the duration of shedding are less during asymptomatic than during symptomatic recurrences, the majority of initial genital HSV infections are acquired from a sexual partner with no history of genital herpes who is shedding virus without recognizing any signs or symptoms of infection.[47–50, 73, 74] The risk for infection under these circumstances can probably be reduced by using condoms, and perhaps also diaphragms and spermicidal foams containing surfactants that can inactivate extracellular HSV. Patients should also be educated to recognize symptoms and signs of mild recurrences so that they can avoid exposing partners.

Because infants born by vaginal delivery to mothers with active genital herpes at term are at significant risk for developing neonatal herpes, it is generally advised that women with active genital herpes at term have a cesarean section.[15, 71, 75, 115] However, the efficacy of this procedure has not been proved. Prepartum ascending infections occur, and a number of infants born by cesarean section to mothers with intact membranes have developed neonatal HSV infection.[75, 114, 115] This difficult problem is detailed elsewhere.[75, 115] Suffice it to say that prevention of neonatal HSV infection is complicated by the fact that the majority of infected infants are born to mothers with no signs or symptoms of genital herpes, no history of previous episodes of genital herpes, and no history of genital herpes in their sexual partners. The relatively low frequency of neonatal infection and the low risk for transmission from women with asymptomatic recurrences make any strategy involving the screening of pregnant women at term for asymptomatic virus shedding (e.g., by PCR) extremely expensive.[64, 66–68, 71, 72, 75, 115, 168, 188] Because asymptomatic primary genital HSV infections near term appear to account for about half of all neonatal HSV infections,[71, 75, 115, 168] every effort should be made, perhaps even including abstinence, to avoid initial genital HSV infections during the last month of pregnancy. Serologic testing of pregnant women and their sexual partners could be used to identify susceptible pregnant women at risk for genital or orogenital exposure from seropositive partners.[81]

Immediate postexposure administration of acyclovir or of antibodies to HSV can reduce the frequency of HSV infection and latency in experimental animals (see Chapter 240). Clinical trials are under way to assess this approach in infants exposed to HSV during delivery. Acyclovir suppression during pregnancy in an attempt to reduce virus shedding at delivery has not been assessed. However, acyclovir, 400 mg three times daily from 36 weeks' gestation, has been administered to pregnant women experiencing their first episode of symptomatic genital herpes during pregnancy in an attempt to reduce the need for cesarean section. None of 21 treated patients had clinical evidence of recurrent genital herpes at delivery, compared with 9 of 25 placebo recipients (all of whom underwent cesarean section).[291] Although asymptomatic virus shedding would be expected to have been reduced as well,[79, 189] this was not assessed, and the effect of this strategy on the risk for neonatal HSV infection remains to be determined. Also remaining to be determined is whether immediate postexposure prophylaxis with acyclovir can lower the frequency of genital herpes in seronegative adults.

Prophylaxis (Suppression) of Frequently Recurring Genital Herpes

Long-term prophylaxis with oral acyclovir has been shown to markedly reduce the rate and severity of recurrent genital herpes in individuals with frequent recurrences (six or more per year). However, whereas the rate of recurrence is reduced by 75% to more than 90%, about half of treated patients still experience one or more recurrences per year. Moreover, treatment does not prevent asymptomatic HSV shedding or abolish latency, even when it is continued for more than 5 years; recurrences resume when suppressive therapy is stopped.[79, 266–269, 292–303] Both dose and frequency of dosing affect the efficacy of suppression. Dosage schedules tested have included doses of 200 mg to 800 mg administered as often as four times daily. Daily treatment is more effective than intermittent treatment, and at least two doses per day are required for effective suppression. Although recurrence rates were reported to be somewhat lower with 200 mg four times daily than with 400 mg twice daily,[302] greatly increased convenience favors 400 mg twice daily, the most extensively tested and widely recommended regimen. Patients who respond poorly to a given regimen often show improved response to higher or more frequent dosing. Thus, dosage schedules must be individualized. It seems reasonable to begin with 400 mg twice daily. Apparently compliant patients who continue to report frequent recurrences despite continuous therapy at a dose of 400 mg of acyclovir two or three times daily should be examined and cultured during one or two recurrences. It is far more common to mistake other genital signs and symptoms for recurrent genital herpes than to fail suppressive therapy. A trial of suppressive therapy with famciclovir or valacyclovir should be considered because these prodrugs have much greater oral bioavailability than acyclovir.[269, 271–275] Virus isolates should also be tested for acyclovir sensitivity. Because of the tendency of recurrences to decrease in frequency in time (measured in years) in the absence of therapy, patients receiving prophylactic acyclovir should have treatment stopped periodically (e.g., after 12 to 18 months of suppression) to reevaluate the need for its continuation.

Suppression with prophylactic oral acyclovir also appears to be beneficial for patients with frequent recurrences that are associated with severe complications, such as recurrent meningitis, herpetic whitlow, erythema multiforme, and severe neuralgia. However, controlled studies are lacking in these patients.

Reduction in symptomatic recurrences and in asymptomatic shedding have not been proved to reduce transmission. Nevertheless, in view of the 94% reduction in asymptomatic shedding reported when recently infected women were given 400 mg of acyclovir twice daily,[79, 189] suppressive therapy with acyclovir should be offered to all patients with frequent recurrences as well as to those with a history of recent or severe initial infections.

Treatment and Prophylaxis of Recurrent Genital Herpes in Immunocompromised Patients

Recurrent HSV infections are a major cause of illness in patients undergoing organ and bone marrow transplantation as well as remission-induction chemotherapy for acute leukemia; 60% to 90% of seropositive patients develop mucocutaneous HSV infections during the early posttransplant period, when immunosuppression is greatest (see Chapter 240). A number of placebo-controlled studies have shown that acyclovir (250 mg/m^2 or 5 mg/kg intravenously every 8 to 12 hours, or 200 mg to 400 mg orally three to five times per day) provides effective prophylaxis, reducing the frequency of recurrences by 90% or more.[268, 269, 281–283, 304–308] The frequency of life-threatening disseminated HSV infections and HSV hepatitis in organ allograft recipients underscores the benefits of posttransplantation acyclovir prophylaxis in such severely immunosuppressed patients.

Prophylaxis of recurrent genital herpes in patients with AIDS is also effective, although higher doses may be required.[267–269, 308] In addition, the development of acyclovir resistance is an increasingly troublesome problem in profoundly immunosuppressed patients, especially those with AIDS receiving acyclovir, both for prophylaxis and for therapy. Selection of acyclovir-resistant HSV may be a greater problem in immunosuppressed patients receiving episodic rather than suppressive therapy, presumably because virus replication is more extensive in those receiving episodic therapy.[309, 310] It is important to employ adequate doses of acyclovir (400 mg at least three times daily) and ensure compliance. Although nearly all clinically significant acyclovir-resistant mutants of HSV have been isolated from immunocompromised patients, it is only a matter of time before the widespread use of acyclovir leads to the selection and transmission of resistant virus among immunocompetent patients as well.[311] This crucial problem is discussed in Chapter 240 as well as in references 312 to 317.

The most effective method for the prevention of infection by a ubiquitous virus, especially when most exposures are unrecognized, is immunization. The problem in the case of HSV is complicated by the phenomenon of latency and by the incomplete immunity provided by natural infection. Nevertheless, there are reasons for optimism. These include the significant reduction in the rate and severity of HSV-2 infections in persons with prior HSV-1 infections, the rarity of superinfection with different strains of the same HSV serotype in immunocompetent persons, and the antigenic stability of both HSV-1 and HSV-2. This optimism has been reinforced by a number of studies in animal models, which demonstrated significant protection from exogenous HSV-1 and HSV-2 infections by immunization with inactivated, attenuated, and replication-incompetent whole-virus vaccines, by purified and recombinant envelope glycoprotein vaccines, and by viral DNA vaccines.[318–327] Several experimental vaccines have entered clinical trials; preliminary data suggest that with appropriate adjuvants, recombinant glycoprotein vaccines induce good levels of humoral and cell-mediated immunity in seronegative individuals. Placebo-controlled efficacy studies are currently under way.

Therapeutic immunization to reduce the frequency of recurrent HSV infections has a long and colorful history.[327] A completed placebo-controlled study employing a recombinant HSV-2 glycoprotein D vaccine showed a small but statistically significant reduction in recurrences.[328] Further studies with combinations of glycoproteins and improved adjuvants are currently under way.

Summary

Enormous progress has been made during the past three decades in our understanding of HSV infections in general and of genital herpes in particular. Physicians are now able to offer their patients effective treatment for symptomatic genital herpes as well as advice that should help reduce its transmission. Many life-threatening infections can be prevented or, if diagnosed early, effectively treated. Unfortunately, however, it seems unlikely that we will be successful in eradicating latent HSV infections or eliminating genital herpes from the human population, as we have smallpox. Nevertheless, HSV vaccines now being developed and evaluated, new methods for rapid diagnosis, new antiviral agents, and a clearer understanding of the natural history and epidemiology of HSV infection by patients and their physicians can be expected to markedly reduce the morbidity and mortality of genital HSV infections in the future.

References

1. Hutfield DC: History of herpes genitalis. Br J Vener Dis 42:263, 1966.
2. Astruc J: De Morbis Venereis, Libri Sex. Paris, Cavelier, 1736, pp 254–255.
3. Bateman TA: A Practical Synopsis of Cutaneous Diseases. London, Longman, 1813.
4. Greenough FB: Herpes progenitalis. Arch Dermatol 7:1, 1881.
5. Unna PG: On herpes progenitalis, especially in women. J Cutan Vener Dis 1:321, 1883.
6. Unna PG: The Histopathology of the Diseases of the Skin. Edinburgh, Clay, 1896, p 145.
7. Grüter W: Experimentelle und Klinische Untersuchungen über den sogenanneten Herpes cornea. Berl Versamm Ophthalmol Ges 42:162, 1920.
8. Lipschütz B: Untersuchungen über die Aetiologie der Krankheiten der Herpesgruppe (Herpes zoster, Herpes genitalis, Herpes febrilis). Arch Dermatol Syph 136:428, 1921.
9. Slavin HB, Gavett E: Primary herpetic vulvovaginitis. Proc Soc Exp Biol Med 63:343, 1946.
10. Schneweis KE: Serologische Untersuchungen zur Typendifferenzierung des Herpesvirus hominis. Z Immunitaetsforsch Exp Ther 124:24, 1962.
11. Plummer G: Serological comparison of the herpesviruses. Br J Exp Pathol 45:135, 1964.
12. Nahmias AJ, Dowdle WR: Antigenic and biologic differences in herpesvirus hominis. Prog Med Virol 10:110, 1968.
13. Corey L, Spear PG: Infections with herpes simplex viruses. N Engl J Med 314:686, 749, 1986.
14. Roizman B, Sears AE: Herpes simplex viruses and their replication. *In* Fields BN, Knipe DM, Howley PM (eds): Fields Virology, ed 3. Philadelphia, Lippincott-Raven, 1996, pp 2231–2295.
15. Whitley RJ: Herpes simplex viruses. *In* Fields BN, Knipe DM, Howley PM (eds): Fields Virology, ed 3. Philadelphia, Lippincott-Raven, 1996, pp 2297–2342.
16. Spear PG: Glycoproteins specified by herpes simplex viruses. *In* Roizman B (ed): The Herpesviruses, Vol 3. New York, Plenum Publishing, 1985, pp 309–373.
17. Rawls WE: Herpes simplex virus types 1 and 2 and *Herpesvirus simiae*. *In* Lennette EH, Schmidt NJ (eds): Diagnostic Procedures for Viral, Rickettsial and Chlamydial Infections. Washington, DC, American Public Health Association, 1979, pp 309–373.
18. Nahmias AJ, Keyserling H, Lee FK: Herpes simplex viruses 1 and 2. *In* Evans AS (ed): Viral Infections of Humans: Epidemiology and Control, ed 3. New York, Plenum Publishing, 1989, pp 393–417.
19. Pereira L, Dondero DV, Gallo D, et al: Serological analysis of herpes simplex virus types 1 and 2 with monoclonal antibodies. Infect Immun 35:363, 1982.
20. Carmack MA, Yasukawa LL, Chang SY, et al: T cell recognition and cytokine production elicited by common and type-specific glycoproteins of herpes simplex virus type 1 and type 2. J Infect Dis 174:899, 1996.
21. Lee FK, Coleman RM, Pereira L, et al: Detection of herpes simplex virus type-2 specific antibody with glycoprotein G. J Clin Microbiol 22:641, 1985.
22. Ashley RL, Militoni J, Lee F, et al: Comparison of western blot (immunoblot) and glycoprotein G–specific immunodot enzyme assay for detecting antibodies to herpes simplex virus type 1 and 2 in human sera. J Clin Microbiol 26:662, 1988.
23. Johnson RE, Nahmias AJ, Magder LS, et al: A seroepidemiologic survey of the prevalence of herpes simplex virus type 2 infection in the United States. N Engl J Med 321:7, 1989.
24. Breinig MK, Kingsley LA, Armstrong JA, et al: Epidemiology of genital herpes in Pittsburgh: Serologic, sexual, and racial correlates of apparent and inapparent herpes simplex infections. J Infect Dis 162:299, 1990.
25. Gibson JJ, Hornung CA, Alexander GR, et al: A cross-sectional study of herpes simplex virus types 1 and 2 in college students: Occurrence and determinants of infection. J Infect Dis 162:306, 1990.
26. Honess RW, Watson DH: Unity and diversity in the herpesviruses. J Gen Virol 37:15, 1977.
27. Morse LS, Pereira L, Roizman B, Schaffer PA: Anatomy of HSV DNA. XI. Mapping of viral genes by analysis of polypeptides and functions specified by HSV-1 × HSV-2 recombinants. J Virol 26:389, 1978.
28. Preston VG, Davison AJ, Marsden HS, et al: Recombinants between herpes simplex virus types 1 and 2: Analyses of genome structures and expression of immediate-early polypeptides. J Virol 28:499, 1978.
29. Hayward GS, Frenkel N, Roizman B: The anatomy of herpes simplex virus DNA: Strain differences and heterogeneity in the locations of restriction endonuclease cleavage sites. Proc Natl Acad Sci USA 72:1768, 1975.
30. Lonsdale DM: A rapid technique for distinguishing herpes simplex virus type 1 and type 2 by restriction enzyme technology. Lancet 1:849, 1979.
31. Cassai EN, Sarmiento M, Spear PG: Comparison of the virion proteins specified by herpes simplex virus types 1 and 2. J Virol 16:1327, 1975.
32. Marsden HS, Stow ND, Preston VG, et al: Physical mapping of herpes simplex virus induced polypeptides. J Virol 28:624, 1978.
33. Buchman TG, Simpson T, Nosal C, et al: The structure of herpes simplex virus DNA and its application to molecular epidemiology. Ann N Y Acad Sci 354:279, 1980.
34. Buchman TG, Roizman B, Adams G, Stover BH: Restriction endonuclease fingerprinting of herpes simplex virus DNA: A novel epidemiologic tool applied to a nosocomial outbreak. J Infect Dis 138:488, 1978.
35. Buchman TG, Roizman B, Nahmias AJ: Demonstration of exogenous reinfection with herpes simplex virus type-2 by restriction endonuclease fingerprinting of viral DNA. J Infect Dis 140:295, 1979.
36. Schmidt OW, Fife KH, Corey L: Reinfection is an uncommon occurrence in patients with symptomatic recurrent genital herpes. J Infect Dis 149:645, 1984.
37. Lakeman FD, Nahmias AJ, Whitley RJ: Analysis of DNA from recurrent genital herpes simplex virus isolates by restriction endonuclease digestion. J Sex Transm Dis 13:61, 1986.
38. Oxman MN: Genital herpes. *In* Braude AI, Davis CE, Fierer J (eds): Infectious Diseases and Medical Microbiology, ed 2. Philadelphia, WB Saunders, 1986, pp 1041–1054.
39. Nerurkar LS, West F, May M, et al: Survival of herpes simplex virus in water specimens collected from hot tubs in spa facilities and on plastic surfaces. JAMA 250:3081, 1983.
40. Douglas JM, Corey L: Fomites and herpes simplex viruses: A case for nonvenereal transmission? JAMA 250:3093, 1983.
41. Guinan ME, Wolinsky SN, Reichman RC: Epidemiology of genital herpes simplex virus infection. Epidemiol Rev 7:127, 1985.
42. Rawls WE, Campione-Piccardo J: Epidemiology of herpes simplex virus type 1 and 2. *In* Nahmais A, Dowdle W, Schinazi R (eds): The Human Herpesviruses: An Interdisciplinary Perspective. Amsterdam, Elsevier North Holland, 1981, pp 137–152.
43. Black FL, Hierholzer WJ, Pinheiro F, et al: Evidence for persistence of infectious agents in isolated human populations. Am J Epidemiol 100:230, 1974.
44. Black FL: Infectious diseases in primitive societies. Science 187:515, 1975.
45. Hammer SM, Buchman TG, D'Angelo LJ, et al: Temporal cluster of herpes simplex encephalitis: Investigation by restriction endonuclease cleavage of viral DNA. J Infect Dis 141:436, 1980.
46. Whitley RJ, Lakeman AD, Nahmias AJ, Roizman B: DNA restriction enzyme analysis of herpes simplex virus isolates obtained from patients with encephalitis. N Engl J Med 307:1060, 1982.
47. Mertz GJ, Benedetti J, Ashley R, et al: Risk factors for the sexual transmission of genital herpes. Ann Intern Med 116:197, 1992.
48. Bryson YJ, Dillon M, Bernstein DI, et al: Risk of acquisition of

genital herpes simplex virus type 2 in sex partners of persons with genital herpes: A prospective couple study. J Infect Dis 167:942, 1993.
49. Cowan FM, Johnson AM, Ashley R, et al: Antibody to herpes simplex virus type 2 as serological marker of sexual lifestyle in populations. BMJ 309:1325, 1994.
50. Mertz GJ: Epidemiology of genital herpes infections. Infect Dis Clin North Am 7:825, 1993.
51. Oxman MN: Herpes stomatitis. *In* Braude AI, Davis CE, Fierer J (eds): Infectious Diseases and Medical Microbiology, ed 2. Philadelphia, WB Saunders, 1986, pp 752–772.
52. Whitley RJ: Epidemiology of herpes simplex viruses. *In* Roizman B (ed): The Herpesviruses, Vol 3. New York, Plenum Publishing, 1985, pp 1–44.
53. Ng ABP, Reagin JW, Yen SS: Herpes genitalis—Clinical and cytopathologic experience with 256 patients. Obstet Gynecol 36:645, 1970.
54. Poste G, Hawkins DF, Thomlinson J: Herpesvirus hominis infection of the female genital tract. Obstet Gynecol 40:871, 1972.
55. Bolognese RJ, Corson SL, Fuccilo DA: Herpes virus hominis type II infections in asymptomatic pregnant women. Obstet Gynecol 48:507, 1976.
56. Adam E, Kaufman RH, Mirkovic RR, Melnick JL: Persistence of virus shedding in asymptomatic women after recovery from herpes genitalis. Obstet Gynecol 54:171, 1979.
57. Rattray MC, Corey L, Reeves WC, et al: Recurrent genital herpes among women: Symptomatic versus asymptomatic viral shedding. Br J Vener Dis 54:252, 1978.
58. Ekwo E, Wong YW, Myers M: Asymptomatic cervicovaginal shedding of herpes simplex virus. Am J Obstet Gynecol 134:102, 1979.
59. Tejani N, Klein SW, Kaplan M: Subclinical herpes simplex genitalis infections in the perinatal period. Am J Obstet Gynecol 135:547, 1979.
60. Adam E, Dreesman GE, Kaufman RH, Melnick JL: Asymptomatic virus shedding after herpes genitalis. Am J Obstet Gynecol 137:827, 1980.
61. Scher J, Bottone E, Desmond E, Simons W: The incidence and outcome of asymptomatic herpes simplex genitalis in an obstetric population. Am J Obstet Gynecol 144:906, 1982.
62. Vontver LA, Hickok DE, Brown Z, et al: Recurrent herpes simplex virus infection in pregnancy: Infant outcome and frequency of asymptomatic recurrences. Am J Obstet Gynecol 142:75, 1982.
63. Corey L, Adams HG, Brown ZA, Holmes KK: Genital herpes simplex virus infections: Clinical manifestations, course, and complications. Ann Intern Med 98:958, 1983.
64. Harger JH, Pazin GJ, Armstrong JA, et al: Characteristics and management of pregnancy in women with genital herpes simplex virus infection. Am J Obstet Gynecol 145:784, 1983.
65. Hankins GDV, Cunningham FG, Luby JP, et al: Asymptomatic genital excretion of herpes simplex virus during early labor. Am J Obstet Gynecol 150:100, 1984.
66. Wittek AE, Yeager AS, Au DS, Hensleigh PA: Asymptomatic shedding of herpes simplex virus from the cervix and lesion site during pregnancy. Am J Dis Child 138:439, 1984.
67. Arvin AM, Hensleigh PA, Prober CG, et al: Failure of antepartum maternal cultures to predict the infant's risk of exposure to herpes simplex virus at delivery. N Engl J Med 315:796, 1986.
68. Prober CG, Hensleigh PA, Boucher FD, et al: Use of routine viral cultures at delivery to identify neonates exposed to herpes simplex virus. N Engl J Med 318:887, 1988.
69. Simkovich JW, Soper DE: Asymptomatic shedding of herpesvirus during labor. Am J Obstet Gynecol 158:588, 1988.
70. Sullender WM, Yasukawa LL, Schwartz M, et al: Type-specific antibodies to herpes simplex virus type 2 (HSV-2) glycoprotein G in pregnant women, infants exposed to maternal HSV-2 infection at delivery, and infants with neonatal herpes. J Infect Dis 157:164, 1988.
71. Prober CG, Arvin AM: Genital herpes and the pregnant woman. Curr Clin Top Infect Dis 10:1, 1989.
72. Yeager AS, Arvin AM: Reasons for the absence of a history of recurrent genital herpes infections in mothers of neonates infected with herpes simplex virus. Pediatrics 73:188, 1984.
73. Mertz GJ, Schmidt O, Jourden JL, et al: Frequency of acquisition of first-episode genital infection with herpes simplex virus from symptomatic and asymptomatic source contacts. Sex Transm Dis 12:33, 1985.
74. Rooney JF, Felser JM, Ostrove JM, Straus SE: Acquisition of genital herpes from an asymptomatic sexual partner. N Engl J Med 314:1561, 1986.
75. Whitley RJ, Arvin A: Herpes simplex virus infections. *In* Remington JS, Klein JO (eds): Infectious Diseases of the Fetus and Newborn Infant, ed 4. Philadelphia, WB Saunders, 1995, pp 354–376.
76. Cowan FM, Johnson AM, Ashley R, et al: Relationship between antibodies to herpes simplex virus (HSV) and symptoms of HSV infection. J Infect Dis 174:470, 1996.
77. Koelle DM, Benedetti J, Langenberg A, Corey L: Asymptomatic reactivation of herpes simplex virus in women after the first episode of genital herpes. Ann Intern Med 116:433, 1992.
78. Wald A, Zeh J, Selke S, et al: Virologic characteristics of subclinical and symptomatic genital herpes infections. N Engl J Med 333:770, 1995.
79. Wald A, Zeh J, Barnum G, et al: Suppression of subclinical shedding of herpes simplex virus type 2 with acyclovir. Ann Intern Med 124:8, 1996.
80. Koutsky LA, Stevens CE, Holmes KK, et al: Underdiagnosis of genital herpes by current clinical and viral-isolation procedures. N Engl J Med 326:1533, 1992.
81. Kulhanjian JA, Soroush V, Au DS, et al: Identification of women at unsuspected risk of primary infection with herpes simplex virus type 2 during pregnancy. N Engl J Med 326:916, 1992.
82. Brown ZA, Benedetti JK, Watts DH, et al: A comparison between detailed and simple histories in the diagnosis of genital herpes complicating pregnancy. Am J Obstet Gynecol 172:1299, 1995.
83. McClung H, Seth P, Rawls WE: Relative concentrations in human sera of antibodies to cross-reacting and specific antigens of herpes simplex virus types 1 and 2. Am J Epidemiol 104:192, 1976.
84. Ashley R, Cent A, Maggs V, et al: Inability of enzyme immunoassays to discriminate between infections with herpes simplex virus types 1 and 2. Ann Intern Med 115:520, 1991.
85. Safrin S, Arvin A, Mills J, Ashley R: Comparison of the Western immunoblot assay and a glycoprotein G enzyme immunoassay for detection of serum antibodies to herpes simplex virus type 2 in patients with AIDS. J Clin Microbiol 30:1312, 1992.
86. Gentry GA, Lowe M, Alford G, Nevins R: Sequence analysis of herpesviral enzymes suggests an ancient origin for human sexual behavior. Proc Soc Natl Acad Sci USA 65:2658, 1988.
87. Juel-Jensen BE, MacCallum FO: Herpes Simplex, Varicella and Zoster: Clinical Manifestations and Treatment. Philadelphia, JB Lippincott, 1972.
88. Burnet FM, Williams SW: Herpes simplex: A new point of view. Med J Aust 1:637, 1939.
89. Smith IW, Peutherer JF, MacCallum FO: The incidence of *Herpesvirus hominis* antibody in the population. J Hyg (Camb) 65:395, 1967.
90. Wentworth BB, Alexander ER: Seroepidemiology of infections due to members of the herpesvirus group. Am J Epidemiol 94:496, 1971.
91. Glezen WP, Fernald GW, Lohr JA: Acute respiratory disease of university students with special reference to the etiologic role of herpesvirus hominis. Am J Epidemiol 101:111, 1975.
92. Nahmias AJ, Lee FK, Bechman-Nahmias S: Sero-epidemiological and -sociological patterns of herpes simplex virus infection in the world. Scand J Infect Dis 69:19, 1990.
93. Hatherley LI, Hayes K, Jack I: Herpesvirus in an obstetric hospital. Prevalence of antibodies in patients and staff. Med J Aust 2:325, 1980.
94. Corey L: Genital herpes. *In* Holmes KK (ed): Sexually Transmitted Diseases, ed 2. New York, McGraw-Hill, 1990, pp 391–413.
95. Duenas A, Adam E, Melnick JL, Rawls WE: Herpes virus type-2 in a prostitute population. Am J Epidemiol 95:483, 1972.
96. Chuang T-Y, Su WP, Perry HO, et al: Incidence and trend of herpes progenitalis. A 15-year population study. Mayo Clin Proc 58:436, 1983.
97. Becker TM, Stone KM, Cates W Jr: Epidemiology of genital herpes infections in the United States: The current situation. J Reprod Med 31:359, 1986.
98. Centers for Disease Control: Genital herpes infections—United States, 1966–1984. MMWR Morbid Mortal Wkly Rep 35:402, 1986.

99. Catterall RD: Biological effects of sexual freedom. Lancet 1:315, 1981.
100. Christenson B, Bottiger M, Svensson A, Jeansson S: A 15-year surveillance study of antibodies to herpes simplex virus types 1 and 2 in a cohort of young girls. J Infect 25:147, 1992.
101. Cunningham AL, Lee FK, Ho DWT, et al: Herpes simplex virus type 2 antibody in patients attending antenatal or STD clinics. Med J Aust 158:525, 1993.
102. Oliver L, Wald A, Kim M, et al: Seroprevalence of herpes simplex virus infections in a family medicine clinic. Arch Fam Med 4:228, 1995.
103. Siegle D, Golden E, Washington AE, et al: Prevalence and correlates of herpes simplex infections: The population-based AIDS in multiethnic neighborhoods study. JAMA 268:1702, 1992.
104. Sumaya CV, Marx J, Ullis K: Genital infections with herpes simplex virus in a university student population. Sex Transm Dis 7:16, 1980.
105. Kalinyak JE, Fleagle G, Docherty JJ: Incidence and distribution of herpes simplex virus types 1 and 2 from genital lesions in college women. J Med Virol 1:173, 1977.
106. Centers for Disease Control: Premarital sexual experience among adolescent women—United States, 1970–1988. MMWR Morbid Mortal Wkly Rep 39:929, 1991.
107. Benedetti JK, Corey L, Ashley R: Recurrence rates in genital herpes after symptomatic first-episode infection. Ann Intern Med 121:847, 1994.
108. Brock BV, Selke S, Benedetti J, et al: Frequency of asymptomatic shedding of herpes simplex virus in women with genital herpes. JAMA 263:418, 1990.
109. Reeves WC, Corey L, Adams HG, et al: Risk of recurrence after first episodes of genital herpes: Relation to HSV type and antibody response. N Engl J Med 304:315, 1981.
110. Lafferty WE, Coombs RW, Benedetti J, et al: Recurrences after oral and genital herpes simplex virus infection. Influence of site of infection and viral type. N Engl J Med 316:1444, 1987.
111. Whitley RJ, Nahmias AJ, Soong S-J, et al: Vidarabine therapy of neonatal herpes simplex virus infection. Pediatrics 60:495, 1980.
112. Whitley R, Arvin A, Prober C, et al: A controlled trial comparing vidarabine with acyclovir in neonatal herpes simplex virus infection. N Engl J Med 324:444, 1991.
113. Whitley R, Arvin A, Prober C, et al: Predictors of morbidity and mortality in neonates with herpes simplex virus infections. N Engl J Med 324:450, 1991.
114. Whitley RJ, Corey L, Arvin A, et al: Changing presentation of herpes simplex virus infection in neonates. J Infect Dis 158:109, 1988.
115. Prober CG, Corey L, Brown ZA, et al: The management of pregnancies complicated by genital infections with herpes simplex virus. Clin Infect Dis 15:1031, 1992.
116. Prober CG, Sullender WM, Yasukawa LL, et al: Low risk of herpes simplex virus infections in neonates exposed to the virus at the time of vaginal delivery to mothers with recurrent genital herpes simplex virus infections. N Engl J Med 316:240, 1987.
117. Brown ZA, Benedetti J, Ashley R, et al: Neonatal herpes simplex virus infection in relation to asymptomatic maternal infection at the time of labor. N Engl J Med 324:1247, 1991.
118. Greenblatt RM, Lukehart SA, Plummer FA, et al: Genital ulceration as a risk factor for human immunodeficiency virus infection. AIDS 2:47, 1988.
119. Benedetti JK, Zeh J, Selke S, Corey L: Frequency and reactivation of nongenital lesions among patients with genital herpes simplex virus. Am J Med 98:237, 1995.
120. Stanberry LR, Kern ER, Richard JT, et al: Genital herpes in guinea pigs: Pathogenesis of the primary infection and description of recurrent disease. J Infect Dis 146:397, 1982.
121. Blyth WA, Harbour DA, Hill JT: Pathogenesis of zosteriform spread of herpes simplex virus in the mouse. J Gen Virol 65:1477, 1984.
122. Kipping R, Downie A: Generalised infection with herpes simplex. Br Med J 10:247, 1948.
123. Ruchman J, Dodd K: Recovery of herpes simplex virus from the blood of a patient with herpetic rhinitis. J Lab Clin Med 35:434, 1950.
124. Becker WB, Kipps A, McKenzie D: Disseminated herpes simplex virus infection: Its pathogenesis based on virological and pathological studies in 33 cases. Am J Dis Child 115:1, 1968.
125. Craig CP, Nahmias AJ: Different patterns of neurologic involvement with herpes simplex virus types 1 and 2: Isolation of herpes simplex virus type 2 from the buffy coat of two adults with meningitis. J Infect Dis 127:365, 1973.
126. Bastian FO, Rabson AS, Yee CL, Tralka TS: Herpesvirus hominis: Isolation from human trigeminal ganglion. Science 178:306, 1972.
127. Baringer JR, Swoveland P: Recovery of herpes simplex virus from human trigeminal ganglia. N Engl J Med 288:648, 1973.
128. Baringer JR: Recovery of herpes simplex virus from human sacral ganglions. N Engl J Med 291:828, 1974.
129. Warren KG, Brown SM, Wrobelwska Z, et al: Isolation of latent herpes simplex virus from the superior cervical and vagus ganglions of human beings. N Engl J Med 298:1068, 1978.
130. Cushing H: The surgical aspects of major neuralgia of the trigeminal nerve. A report of 20 cases of operation upon the gasserian ganglion with anatomic and physiologic notes on the consequence of its removal. JAMA 44:773, 860, 920, 1002, 1088, 1905.
131. Baringer JR: Herpes simplex virus infection of nervous tissue in animals and man. Prog Med Virol 20:1, 1975.
132. Stevens JG: Latent herpes simplex virus and the nervous system. Curr Top Microbiol Immunol 70:31, 1975.
133. Warren SL, Carpenter CM, Boak RA: Symptomatic herpes, a sequela of artificially 'induced' fever: Incidence and clinical aspects; recovery of virus from herpetic vesicles and comparison with a known strain of herpes virus. J Exp Med 71:155, 1940.
134. Greenberg MS, Brightman VJ, Ship II: Clinical and laboratory differentiation of recurrent intraoral herpes simplex virus infections following fever. J Dent Res 48:385, 1969.
135. Carton CA, Kilbourne ED: Activation of latent herpes by trigeminal sensory-root section. N Engl J Med 246:172, 1952.
136. Pazin GJ, Ho M, Jannetta PJ: Reactivation of herpes simplex virus after decompression of the trigeminal nerve root. J Infect Dis 138:405, 1978.
137. Segal AL, Katcher AH, Brightman VG, Miller MF: Recurrent herpes labialis, recurrent aphthous ulcers and the menstrual cycles. J Dent Res 53:797, 1974.
138. Lopez C, Arvin AM, Ashley R: Immunity to herpesvirus infections in humans. *In* Roizman B, Whitley RJ, Lopez C (eds): The Human Herpesviruses. Philadelphia, Lippincott-Raven, 1993, p 397.
139. Kohl S, Adam E, Matson DO, et al: Kinetics of human antibody responses to primary genital herpes simplex virus infection. Intervirology 18:164, 1982.
140. Oh SH, Douglas JM, Corey L, Kohl S: Kinetics of humoral immune response measured by antibody-dependent cell-mediated cytotoxicity and neutralization assays in genital herpes virus infections. J Infect Dis 159:328, 1989.
141. Blacklaws BA, Nash AA: Immunologic memory to herpes simplex virus type 1 glycoproteins B and D in mice. J Gen Virol 71:863, 1990.
142. Balachandran N, Bachetti S, Rawls WE: Protection against lethal challenge of BalB/C mice by passive transfer of monoclonal antibodies to five glycoproteins of herpes simplex virus type 2. Infect Immun 37:1132, 1982.
143. Kohl S, Strynadka NCJ, Hodges RS, Periera LA: Analysis of the role of antibody-dependent cellular cytotoxic antibody activity in murine neonatal herpes simplex virus with antibodies to synthetic peptides of glycoprotein D and monoclonal antibodies to glycoprotein B. J Clin Invest 86:273, 1990.
144. Mester JC, Glorioso JC, Rouse BT: Protection against zosteriform spread of herpes simplex virus by monoclonal antibodies. J Infect Dis 163:263, 1991.
145. Kohl S: Role of antibody-dependent cellular cytotoxicity in defense against herpes simplex virus infections. Rev Infect Dis 13:108, 1991.
146. Carmack MA, Yasukawa LL, Chang SY, et al: T cell recognition and cytokine production elicited by common and type-specific glycoproteins of herpes simplex virus type 1 and type 2. J Infect Dis 174:899, 1996.
147. Kirchner H: Immunobiology of infection with herpes simplex virus. Monogr Virol 13:1, 1982.
148. Hirsch MS: Herpes group virus infections in the compromised host. *In* Rubin RH, Young LS (eds): Clinical Approach to Infection in the Immunocompromised Host, ed 2. New York, Plenum Publishing, 1988, p 347.

149. Kohl S: Herpes simplex virus immunology: Problems, progress and promises. J Infect Dis 152:435, 1985.
150. Nash AA, Leung KN, Wildy P: The T-cell mediated immune response of mice to herpes simplex virus. *In* Roizman B, Lopez C (eds): The Herpesviruses, Vol 4. New York, Plenum Publishing, 1985, pp 87–102.
151. Glorioso JC, Kees U, Kumel G, et al: Identification of herpes simplex virus type 1 (HSV-1) glycoprotein gC as the immunodominant antigen for HSV-1 specific memory cytotoxic T lymphocytes. J Immunol 135:575, 1985.
152. Martin S, Cantin E, Rouse BT: Evaluation of antiviral immunity using vaccinia virus recombinants expressing cloned genes for herpes simplex virus type 1 glycoproteins. J Gen Virol 70:1359, 1989.
153. Witmer LA, Rosenthal KL, Graham FL, et al: Cytotoxic T lymphocytes specific for herpes simplex virus (HSV) studied using adenovirus vectors expressing HSV glycoproteins. J Gen Virol 71:387, 1990.
154. Martin S, Zhu X, Silverstein SJ, et al: Murine cytotoxic T lymphocytes specific for herpes simplex virus type 1 recognize the immediate early protein ICP4 but not ICPO. J Gen Virol 71:2391, 1990.
155. Wenner HA: Complications of infantile eczema caused by the virus of herpes simplex: Description of the clinical characteristics of an unusual eruption and identification of an associated filterable virus. Am J Dis Child 67:247, 1944.
156. Ruchman I, Welsh AL, Dodd K: Kaposi's varicelliform eruption: Isolation of the virus of herpes simplex from cutaneous lesions of three adults and one infant. Arch Dermatol Syph 56:846, 1947.
157. Wheeler CE Jr, Abele DC: Eczma herpeticum, primary and recurrent. Arch Dermatol 93:162, 1966.
158. Foley FD, Greenwald KA, Nash G, Pruitt BA: Herpesvirus infection in burned patients. N Engl J Med 282:652, 1970.
159. Hayden FG, Himel HN, Heggers JP: Herpesvirus infections in burn patients. Chest 106:15S, 1994.
160. Hirsch MS, Zisman B, Allison AC: Macrophages and age-dependent resistance to herpes simplex virus in mice. J Immunol 104:1160, 1970.
161. Wilson CB: Developmental immunology and role of host defenses in neonatal susceptibility. *In* Remington JS, Klein JO (eds): Infectious Diseases of the Fetus and Newborn Infant, ed 3. Philadelphia, WB Saunders, 1990, pp 17–67.
162. Whitley R, Arvin A, Prober C, et al: Predictors of morbidity and mortality in neonates with herpes simplex virus infections. N Engl J Med 324:450, 1991.
163. Kohl S, West MS, Prober CG, et al: Neonatal antibody-dependent cellular cytotoxicity antibody levels are associated with the clinical presentation of neonatal herpes simplex virus infection. J Infect Dis 160:770, 1989.
164. Kohl S: Protection against murine neonatal herpes simplex infections by lymphokine-treated human leukocytes. J Immunol 144:307, 1990.
165. Taylor S, Bryson YJ: Impaired production of γ-interferon by newborn cells in vitro due to a functionally immature macrophage. J Immunol 134:1493, 1985.
166. Wilson CB, Westall J, Johnston L, et al: Decreased production of interferon-gamma by human neonatal cells. J Clin Invest 77:860, 1986.
167. Yeager AS, Arvin AM, Urbani L, Kemp JA: Relationship of antibody to outcome in neonatal herpes simplex virus infections. Infect Immun 29:532, 1980.
168. Prober CG, Sullender WM, Yasukawa LL, et al: Low risk of herpes simplex virus infections in neonates exposed to the virus at the time of vaginal delivery to mothers with recurrent genital herpes simplex virus infections. N Engl J Med 316:240, 1987.
169. Ashley RL, Dalessio J, Burchett S, et al: Herpes simplex virus-2 (HSV-2) type-specific antibody correlates of protection in infants exposed to HSV-2 at birth. J Clin Invest 90:511, 1992.
170. Siegal FP, Lopez C, Hammer GS, et al: Severe acquired immunodeficiency in male homosexuals, manifested by chronic perianal ulcerative herpes simplex lesions. N Engl J Med 305:1039, 1981.
171. Lazar MP: Vaccination for recurrent herpes simplex infection: Initiation of a new disease site following use of unmodified material containing the live virus. Arch Dermatol 73:70, 1956.
172. Oberle MW, Rosero-Bixby L, Lee FK, et al: Herpes simplex virus type 2 antibodies: High prevalence in monogamous women in Costa Rica. Am J Trop Med Hyg 41:224, 1989.
173. Brown ZA, Kern ER, Spruance SL, Overall JC: Clinical and virologic course of herpes simplex genitalis. West J Med 130:414, 1979.
174. Mindel A, Adler MW, Sutherland S, Fiddian AP: Intravenous acyclovir treatment for primary genital herpes. Lancet 1:697, 1982.
175. Corey L, Fife KH, Benedetti JK, et al: Intravenous acyclovir for the treatment of primary genital herpes. Ann Intern Med 98:914, 1983.
176. Peacock JE Jr, Kaplowitz LG, Sparling PF, et al: Intravenous acyclovir therapy of first episodes of genital herpes: A multicenter double-blind, placebo-controlled trial. Am J Med 85:301, 1988.
177. Nilsen AE, Aasen T, Halsos AM, et al: Efficacy of oral acyclovir in the treatment of initial and recurrent genital herpes. Lancet 2:571, 1982.
178. Bryson YJ, Dillon M, Lovett M, et al: Treatment of first episodes of genital herpes simplex virus infection with oral acyclovir: A randomized double-blind controlled trial in normal subjects. N Engl J Med 308:916, 1983.
179. Mertz GJ, Critchlow CW, Benedetti J, et al: Double-blind placebo-controlled trial of oral acyclovir in first-episode genital herpes simplex virus infection. JAMA 252:1147, 1984.
180. Wilcox RR: Necrotic cervicitis due to primary infection with virus of herpes simplex. Br Med J 1:610, 1968.
181. Adams HG, Renson EA, Alexander ER, et al: Genital herpetic infection in men and women: Clinical course and effect of topical application of adenine arabinoside. J Infect Dis 133(Suppl):A151, 1976.
182. Guinan ME, MacCalman J, Kern ER: The course of untreated recurrent genital herpes simplex infection in 27 women. N Engl J Med 304:759, 1981.
183. Chang TW, Fiumara NJ, Weinstein L: Genital herpes: Some clinical and laboratory observations. JAMA 229:544, 1974.
184. Reichman RC, Badger GJ, Mertz GJ, et al: Treatment of recurrent genital herpes simplex infections with oral acyclovir: A controlled trial. JAMA 251:2103, 1984.
185. Reichman RC, Badger GJ, Guinan ME, et al: Topically administered acyclovir in the treatment of recurrent herpes simplex genitalis: A controlled trial. J Infect Dis 147:336, 1983.
186. Chapel TA, Jeffries CD, Brown WJ: Simultaneous infection with *Treponema pallidum* and herpes simplex virus. Cutis 24:191, 1979.
187. Fiumara NJ, Schmidt-Ulrick B, Comite H: Primary herpes simplex and primary syphilis: A description of seven cases. Sex Transm Dis 7:130, 1980.
188. Cone RW, Hobson AC, Brown Z, et al: Frequent detection of genital herpes simplex virus DNA by polymerase chain reaction among pregnant women. JAMA 272:792, 1994.
189. Wald A, Corey L, Cone R, et al: Frequent genital herpes simplex virus 2 shedding in immunocompetent women. J Clin Invest 99:1092, 1997.
190. Embil JA, Manuel FR, McFarlane ES: Concurrent oral and genital infection with an identical strain of herpes simplex virus type 1. Sex Transm Dis 8:70, 1981.
191. Hutfield DC: Herpes genitalis. Br J Vener Dis 44:241, 1968.
192. Pertherer JF, Smith IW, Robertson DHH: Necrotising balanitis due to a generalized primary infection with herpes simplex virus type 2. Br J Vener Dis 55:48, 1979.
193. Powers RD, Rein MF, Hayden FG: Nectrotizing balanitis due to herpes simplex type 1. JAMA 248:215, 1982.
194. Person DA, Kaufman RH, Gardner HL, Rawls WE: Herpesvirus type 2 genitourinary tract infections. Am J Obstet Gynecol 116:993, 1973.
195. Tustin AW, Kaiser AB: Life-threatening pharyngitis caused by herpes simplex virus, type 2. Sex Transm Dis 6:23, 1979.
196. Slavin HB, Ferguson JJ: Zoster-like eruptions caused by the virus herpes simplex. Am J Med 8:456, 1950.
197. Glogau R, Hanna L, Jawetz E: Herpetic whitlow as part of genital virus infection. J Infect Dis 136:689, 1977.
198. Gill MJ, Arlette J, Buchan K: Herpes simplex virus infection of the hand. Am J Med 84:89, 1988.
199. Long JC, Wheeler CE, Briggaman RA: Varicella-like infection due to herpes simplex, Arch Dermatol 114:406, 1978.
200. Naraqi W, Jackson GG, Jonasson OM: Viremia with herpes simplex type 1 in adults: Four nonfatal cases, one with features of chickenpox. Ann Intern Med 85:165, 1976.

201. Connor RW, Lorts G, Gilbert DN: Lethal herpes simplex virus type 1 hepatitis in a normal adult. Gastroenterology 76:590, 1979.
202. Gelven PL, Gruber KK, Swiger FK, et al: Fatal disseminated herpes simplex in pregnancy with maternal and neonatal death. South Med J 89:732, 1996.
203. Flewett TH, Parker RGF, Philip WM: Acute hepatitis due to herpes simplex virus in an adult. J Clin Pathol 22:60, 1969.
204. Eron L, Kosinski K, Hirsch MS: Hepatitis in an adult caused by herpes simplex virus type 1. Gastroenterology 71:500, 1976.
205. Joseph TJ, Vogt PJ: Disseminated herpes with hepatoadrenal necrosis in an adult. Am J Med 56:735, 1974.
206. Whorton CM, Thomas DM, Denham SW: Fatal systemic herpes simplex virus type 2 infection in a healthy young woman. South Med J 76:81, 1983.
207. Francis TJ, Osuntokum BO, Kemp GE: Fulminant hepatitis due to herpes hominis in an adult human. Am J Gastroenterol 57:329, 1972.
208. Goyette RE, Donowho EM, Hieger LR, Plunkett G: Fulminant herpesvirus hominis hepatitis during pregnancy. Obstet Gynecol 43:191, 1974.
209. Young EJ, Chafizadeh E, Oliveira VL, Genta RM: Disseminated herpesvirus infection during pregnancy. Clin Infect Dis 22:51, 1996.
210. Hensleigh PA, Glover DB, Cannon M: Systemic herpesvirus hominis in pregnancy. J Reprod Med 22:171, 1979.
211. Kobbermann T, Clark L, Griffin WT: Maternal death secondary to disseminated herpesvirus hominis. Am J Obstet Gynecol 6:742, 1980.
212. Peacock JE Jr, Sarubbi FA: Disseminated herpes simplex virus infection during pregnancy. Obstet Gynecol 61:13s, 1983.
213. Chase RA, Pottage JC Jr, Haber MH, et al: Herpes simplex virus hepatitis in adults: Two case reports and review of the literature. Rev Infect Dis 9:329, 1987.
214. Lagrew DC, Furlow TG, Hager D, Yarrish YL: Disseminated herpes simplex virus infection in pregnancy. Successful treatment with acyclovir. JAMA 252:2058, 1984.
215. Whittaker JA, Hardson MD: Severe thrombocytopenia after generalized HSV-2 infection. South Med J 72:864, 1978.
216. Kumar A, Madden DL, Nankervis GA: Humoral and cell-mediated immune responses to herpesvirus antigens during pregnancy—A longitudinal study. J Clin Immunol 4:12, 1984.
217. Jacobs E: Anal infections caused by herpes simplex virus. Dis Colon Rectum 19:151, 1976.
218. Goodell SE, Quinn RC, Mkrtichian E, et al: Herpes simplex virus proctitis in homosexual men. Clinical, sigmodoscopic, and histopathological features. N Engl J Med 308:868, 1983.
219. Oates JK, Greenhouse PRDH: Retention of urine in anogenital herpetic infection. Lancet 1:691, 1979.
220. Goldmeier D: Herpetic proctitis and sacral radiculomyelopathy in homosexual men. Br Med J 2:549, 1979.
221. Oxman MN: Herpes simplex encephalitis and meningitis. *In* Braude AI, Davis CE, Fierer J (eds): Infectious Diseases and Medical Microbiology, ed 2. Philadelphia, WB Saunders, 1986, pp 1114–1131.
222. Terni M, Caccialanza P, Cassai E, Kieff E: Aseptic meningitis in association with herpes progenitalis. N Engl J Med 285:503, 1971.
223. Craig CP, Nahmias AJ: Different patterns of neurologic involvement with herpes simplex virus type 1 and 2: Isolation of herpes simplex virus 2 from the buffy coat of two adults with meningitis. J Infect Dis 127:365, 1973.
224. Stalder H, Oxman MN, Dawson DM, Levin MJ: Herpes simplex meningitis: Isolation of herpes simplex virus type 2 from cerebrospinal fluid. N Engl J Med 289:1296, 1973.
225. Skoldenberg B, Jeansson S, Wolontis S: Herpes simplex virus type 2 and acute aseptic meningitis: Atypical features of cases with isolation of herpes simplex virus from cerebrospinal fluids. Scand J Infect Dis 7:227, 1975.
226. Bergström T, Vahlne A, Alestig K, et al: Primary and recurrent herpes simplex virus type 2–induced meningitis. J Infect Dis 162:322, 1990.
227. Sawanobori S, Onishi S, Matsuyama S, Irie H: HSV-1 and acute aseptic meningitis. Lancet 1:756, 1974.
228. Harford CG, Wellinghoff W, Weinstein RA: Isolation of herpes simplex virus from the cerebrospinal fluid in viral meningitis. Neurology 25:198, 1975.
229. Klastersky J, Cappel R, Snoeck JM, et al: Ascending myelitis in association with herpes-simplex virus. N Engl J Med 287:182, 1972.
230. Tedder DG, Ashley R, Tyler KL, Levin MJ: Herpes simplex virus infection as a cause of benign recurrent lymphocytic meningitis. Ann Intern Med 121:334, 1994.
231. Hinthorn DR, Baker LH, Romig DA, Liu C: Recurrent conjugal neuralgia caused by herpesvirus hominis type 2. JAMA 236:587, 1976.
232. Krohel GB, Richardson JR, Farrell DF: Herpes simplex neuropathy. Neurology 26:596, 1976.
233. Layzer RB, Conant MA: Neuralgia in recurrent herpes simplex. Arch Neurol 31:233, 1974.
234. Caplan LR, Kleeman FJ, Berg S: Urinary retention probably secondary to herpes genitalis. N Engl J Med 297:918, 1977.
235. Chang T-W: Transient neurogenic bladder in genital herpes. J Infect 1:375, 1979.
236. Gerber SI, Cromie WJ: Herpes simplex virus type 2 infection associated with urinary retention in the absence of genital lesions. J Pediatr 128:250, 1996.
237. Safrin S, Ashley R, Houlihan C, et al: Clinical and serologic features of herpes simplex virus infections in patients with AIDS. AIDS 5:1107, 1991.
238. Taylor RJ, Saul SH, Dowling JN, et al: Primary disseminated herpes simplex infection with fulminant hepatitis following renal transplantation. Arch Intern Med 141:1519, 1981.
239. Elliott WC, Houghton DC, Bryant RE, et al: Herpes simplex type 1 hepatitis in renal transplantation. Arch Intern Med 140:1656, 1980.
240. Kusne S, Schwartz M, Breinig MK, et al: Herpes simplex virus hepatitis after solid organ transplantation in adults. J Infect Dis 163:1001, 1991.
241. Augenbraun M, Feldman J, Chirgwin K, et al: Increased genital shedding of herpes simplex virus type 2 in HIV-seropositive women. Ann Intern Med 123:845, 1995.
242. Kaye EM, Dooling EC: Neonatal herpes simplex meningoencephalitis associated with fetal monitor scalp electrodes. Neurology 31:1045, 1981.
243. Brown ZA, Benedetti J, Selke S, et al: Asymptomatic maternal shedding of herpes simplex virus at the onset of labor: Relationship to preterm labor. Obstet Gynecol 87:483, 1996.
244. Florman AL, Gershon AA, Blackett RP, Nahmias AJ: Intrauterine infection with herpes simplex virus: Resultant congenital malformation. JAMA 225:129, 1973.
245. Hutto C, Arvin A, Jacobs R, et al: Intrauterine herpes simplex virus infections. J Pediatr 110:97, 1987.
246. Baldwin S, Whitely RJ: Intrauterine herpes simplex virus infection. Teratology 39:1, 1989.
247. Light IJ: Postnatal acquisition of herpes simplex virus by the newborn infant. A review of the literature. Pediatrics 63:480, 1979.
248. Adams G, Stover BH, Keenlyside RA, et al: Nosocomial herpetic infections in a pediatric intensive care unit. Am J Epidemiol 113:126, 1981.
249. Linnemann CC Jr, Buchman TG, Light IJ, et al: Transmission of herpes simplex virus type-1 in a nursery for the newborn: Identification of viral species isolated by DNA fingerprinting. Lancet 1:964, 1978.
250. Sullivan-Bolyai JZ, Fife KH, Jacobs RF, et al: Disseminated neonatal herpes simplex virus type 1 from a maternal breast lesion. Pediatrics 71:455, 1983.
251. Corey L, Holmes KK: Genital herpes simplex virus infections: Current concepts in diagnosis, therapy and prevention. Ann Intern Med 98:973, 1983.
252. Cleaves CA, Wilson DJ, Wold AD, Smith TF: Detection and serotyping of herpes simplex virus in MRC-5 cells by use of centrifugation and monoclonal antibodies 16 h post inoculation. J Clin Microbiol 21:29, 1985.
253. Michalski FJ, Shaikh M, Sahraie F, et al: Enzyme-linked immunosorbent assay spin amplification technique for herpes simplex virus. J Clin Microbiol 19:548, 1986.
254. Warford AL, Chung JW, Drill AE, Steinberg E: Amplification techniques for detection of herpes virus in neonatal and maternal genital specimens obtained at delivery. J Clin Microbiol 27:1324, 1989.
255. Ashley R: Laboratory techniques in the diagnosis of herpes simplex infection. Genitourin Med 69:174, 1993.

256. Goldstein LC, Corey L, McDougall JK, et al: Monoclonal antibodies to herpes simplex viruses: Use in antigenic typing and rapid diagnosis. J Infect Dis 147:829, 1983.
257. Richman DD, Cleveland PH, Redfield DC, et al: Rapid viral diagnosis. J Infect Dis 149:298, 1984.
258. Corey L: Laboratory diagnosis of herpes simplex virus infections. Principles guiding the development of rapid diagnostic tests. Diagn Microbiol Infect Dis 4:1115, 1986.
259. Fife KH, Corey L: Herpes simplex virus. *In* Holmes KK (ed): Sexually Transmitted Diseases, ed 2. New York, McGraw-Hill, 1990, pp 941–952.
260. Verano L, Michalski FJ: Herpes simplex virus antigen direct detection in standard transport medium by DuPont Herpchek enzyme-linked immunosorbent assay. J Clin Microbiol 28:2555, 1990.
261. Ashley R: Current concepts in laboratory diagnosis of herpes simplex infections. *In* Sacks SL, Strauss SE, Whitley RJ, Griffiths PD (eds): Clinical Management of Herpes Viruses. New York, IOS Press, 1995, pp 137–174.
262. Hardy DA, Arvin AM, Yasukawa LL, et al: Use of polymerase chain reaction for successful identification of asymptomatic genital infections with herpes simplex virus in pregnant women at delivery. J Infect Dis 162:1031, 1990.
263. Aurelius E, Johansson B, Skoldenberg B, Forsgren M: Encephalitis in immunocompetent patients due to herpes simplex virus type 1 or 2 as determined by type-specific polymerase chain reaction and antibody assays of cerebrospinal fluid. J Med Virol 39:179, 1993.
264. Cone RW, Hobson AC, Palmer J, et al: Extended duration of herpes simplex virus DNA in genital lesions detected by the polymerase chain reaction. J Infect Dis 164:757, 1991.
265. Stanberry LR, Floyd-Reising SA, Connelly BL, et al: Herpes simplex viremia: Report of eight pediatric cases and review of the literature. Clin Infect Dis 18:401, 1994.
266. Guinan ME: Oral acyclovir for treatment and suppression of genital herpes simplex virus infection: A review. JAMA 255:1747, 1986.
267. Stone KM, Whittington WL: Treatment of genital herpes. Rev Infect Dis 12(Suppl 6):610, 1990.
268. Whitley RJ, Gnann JW Jr: Acyclovir: A decade later. N Engl J Med 327:782, 1992.
269. Mertz GJ: Management of genital herpes. Adv Exp Med Biol 394:1, 1996.
270. Elion GB: Acyclovir: Discovery, mechanism of action, and selectivity. J Med Virol Suppl 1:2, 1993.
271. Vere Hodge RA: Famciclovir and penciclovir. The mode of action of famciclovir including its conversion to penciclovir. Antiviral Chem Chemother 4:67, 1993.
272. Sacks SL: Use of penciclovir and famciclovir in the management of genital herpes. Curr Probl Dermatol 24:219, 1996.
273. Sacks SL, Aoki FY, Diaz-Mitoma F, et al: Patient-initiated, twice-daily oral famciclovir for early recurrent genital herpes: A randomized, double-blind multicenter trial. JAMA 276:44, 1996.
274. Weller S, Blum MR, Doucette M, et al: Pharmacokinetics of the acyclovir pro-drug valaciclovir after escalating single- and multiple-dose administration to normal volunteers. Clin Pharmacol Ther 54:595, 1993.
275. Spruance SL, Tyring SK, DeGregorio B, et al: A large-scale placebo-controlled dose-ranging trial of peroral valaciclovir for episodic treatment of recurrent herpes. Arch Intern Med 156:1729, 1996.
276. Corey L, Nahmias AJ, Guinan ME, et al: A trial of topical acyclovir in genital herpes simplex virus infections. N Engl J Med 306:1313, 1982.
277. Corey L, Benedetti J, Critchlow C, et al: Treatment of primary first episode genital herpes simplex virus infections with acyclovir: Results of topical, intravenous, and oral therapy. J Antimicrob Chemother 12:79, 1983.
278. Wade JC, Newton B, McLaren C, et al: Intravenous acyclovir to treat mucocutaneous herpes simplex virus infection after marrow transplantation: Double-blind trial. Ann Intern Med 96:265, 1982.
279. Meyers JD, Wade JC, Mitchell CD, et al: Multicenter collaborative trial of intravenous acyclovir for treatment of mucocutaneous herpes simplex virus infection in immunocompromised host. Am J Med 73:229, 1982.
280. Shepp DH, Newton BA, Dandliker PS, et al: Oral acyclovir therapy for mucocutaneous herpes simplex virus infections in immunocompromised marrow transplant recipients. Ann Intern Med 102:783, 1985.
281. Saral R, Burns WH, Laskin OL, et al: Acyclovir prophylaxis of herpes simplex virus infections: A randomized, double-blind, controlled trial in bone-marrow-transplant recipients. N Engl J Med 305:63, 1981.
282. Wade JC, Newton B, Flournoy N: Acyclovir for prevention of herpes simplex virus reactivation after marrow transplantation. Ann Intern Med 100:823, 1984.
283. Shepp DH, Dandliker PS, Flournoy N, Meyers JD: Sequential intravenous and twice-daily oral acyclovir for extended prophylaxis of herpes simplex virus infection in marrow transplant patients. Transplantation 43:654, 1987.
284. Rompalo AM, Mertz GJ, Davis LG, et al: Oral acyclovir for treatment of first-episode herpes simplex virus proctitis. JAMA 259:2879, 1988.
285. Wade JC, Meyers JD: Neurologic symptoms associated with parenteral acyclovir treatment after marrow transplantation. Ann Intern Med 98:921, 1983.
286. Drugs for non-HIV viral infections. Med Lett Drugs Ther 36:27, 1994.
287. Wald A, Benedetti J, Davis G, et al: A randomized, double-blind, comparative trial comparing high- and standard-dose oral acyclovir for first-episode genital herpes. Antimicrob Agents Chemother 38:174, 1994.
288. Gutman LT, Wilfert CM, Eppes S: Herpes simplex virus encephalitis in children: Analysis of cerebrospinal fluid and progressive neurodevelopmental deterioration. J Infect Dis 154:415, 1986.
289. Sullivan-Bolyai JZ, Hull H, Wilson C, et al: Presentation of neonatal herpes simplex virus infections: Implications for a change in therapeutic strategy. Pediatr Infect Dis J 5:309, 1986.
290. Kimberlin D, Powell D, Gruber W, et al: Administration of oral acyclovir suppressive therapy after neonatal herpes simplex virus disease limited to the skin, eyes and mouth: Results of a Phase I/II trial. Pediatr Infect Dis J 15:247, 1996.
291. Scott LL, Sanchez PJ, Jackson GL, et al: Acyclovir suppression to prevent cesarean delivery after first-episode genital herpes. Obstet Gynecol 87:69, 1996.
292. Straus SE, Takiff HE, Seidlin M, et al: Suppression of frequently recurring genital herpes: A placebo-controlled double-blind trial of oral acyclovir. N Engl J Med 310:1545, 1984.
293. Douglas JM, Critchlow C, Benedetti J, et al: A double-blind study of oral acyclovir for suppression of recurrences of genital herpes simplex virus infection. N Engl J Med 310:1551, 1984.
294. Straus SE, Croen KD, Sawyer MH, et al: Acyclovir suppression of frequently recurring genital herpes: Efficacy and diminishing need during successive years of treatment. JAMA 260:2227, 1988.
295. Mertz GJ, Jones CC, Mills J, et al: Acyclovir Study Group. Long-term acyclovir suppression of frequently recurring genital herpes simplex virus infection. A multicenter double-blind trial. JAMA 260:201, 1988.
296. Gold D, Corey L: Acyclovir prophylaxis for herpes simplex virus infection. Antimicrob Agents Chemother 31:361, 1987.
297. Mattison HR, Reichman RC, Benedetti J, et al: Double-blind placebo-controlled trial comparing long-term oral acyclovir therapy for management of recurrent genital herpes. Am J Med 85(2A):20, 1988.
298. Kinghorn GR: Long-term suppression with oral acyclovir of recurrent herpes simplex virus infections in otherwise healthy patients. Am J Med 85(2A):26, 1988.
299. Mostow SR, Mayfield JL, Marr JJ, Drucker JL: Suppression of recurrent genital herpes by single daily dosages of acyclovir. Am J Med 85(2A):30, 1988.
300. Straus SE, Seidlin M, Takiff HE, et al: Effect of oral acyclovir treatment on symptomatic and asymptomatic virus shedding in recurrent genital herpes. Sex Transm Dis 16:107, 1989.
301. Mindel A, Faherty A, Carney O, et al: Dosage and safety of long-term suppressive acyclovir therapy for recurrent genital herpes. Lancet 1:926, 1988.
302. Kroon S, Petersen CC, Andersen LP, et al: Long term suppression of severe recurrent genital herpes simplex infections with oral acyclovir: A dose titration study. Genitourin Med 66:101, 1990.
303. Goldberg LH, Kaufman R, Kurtz TO, et al: Long-term suppres-

sion of recurrent genital herpes with acyclovir. A 5-year benchmark. Acyclovir Study Group. Arch Dermatol 129:582, 1993.
304. Saral R, Ambinder RF, Burns WH: Acyclovir prophylaxis against herpes simplex virus infection in patients with leukemia. A randomized double-blind placebo-controlled study. Ann Intern Med 99:773, 1983.
305. Saral R: Management of mucocutaneous herpes simplex virus infections in immunocompromised patients. Am J Med 85:57, 1988.
306. Hann IM, Prentice HF, Blacklock HA, et al: Acyclovir prophylaxis against herpes virus infections in severely immunocompromised patients: Randomised double blind trial. Br Med J 287:384, 1983.
307. Gluckman E, Devergie A, Melo R, et al: Prophylaxis of herpes infections after bone-marrow transplantation by oral acyclovir. Lancet 2:706, 1983.
308. Conant MA: Prophylactic and suppressive treatment with acyclovir and the management of herpes in patients with acquired immunodeficiency syndrome. J Am Acad Dermatol 18:186, 1988.
309. Ljungman P, Ellis MN, Hackman RC, et al: Acyclovir-resistant herpes simplex virus causing pneumonia after marrow transplantation. J Infect Dis 162:244, 1990.
310. Wade JC, McLaren C, Meyers JD: Frequency and significance of acyclovir-resistant herpes simplex virus isolated from marrow transplant patients receiving multiple courses of treatment with acyclovir. J Infect Dis 148:1077, 1983.
311. Kost RG, Hill EL, Tigges M, Straus SE: Brief report: Recurrent acyclovir-resistant genital herpes in an immunocompetent patient. N Engl J Med 329:1777, 1993.
312. Chatis PA, Crumpacker CS: Resistance of herpesviruses to antiviral drugs. Antimicrob Agents Chemother 36:1589, 1992.
313. Coen DM: Acyclovir-resistant, pathogenic herpesviruses. Trends Microbiol 2:481, 1994.
314. Coen DM: Antiviral drug resistance in herpes simplex virus. *In* Mills J, Volberding PA, Corey L (eds): Antiviral Chemotherapy 4. New York, Plenum Publishing, 1996, pp 49–57.
315. Englund JA, Zimmerman ME, Swierkosz EM, et al: Herpes simplex virus resistant to acyclovir. Ann Intern Med 112:416, 1990.
316. Safrin S: Treatment of acyclovir-resistant herpes simplex and varicella zoster virus infections. Adv Expt Med Biol 394:59, 1996.
317. Balfour HH, Benson C, Braun J, et al: Management of acyclovir-resistant herpes simplex and varicella-zoster virus infections. J Acquir Immune Defic Syndr 7:254, 1994.
318. Burke RL: Current status of HSV vaccine development. *In* Roizman B, Whitley RJ, Lopez C (eds): The Human Herpesviruses. Philadelphia, Lippincott-Raven, 1993, p 367.
319. Whitley RJ, Meignier B: Herpes simplex vaccines. *In* Ellis RW (ed): Vaccines: New Approaches to Immunological Problems. Boston, Butterworth, 1991, p 223.
320. Burke RL: Development of a herpes simplex virus subunit glycoprotein vaccine for prophylactic and therapeutic use. Rev Infect Dis 13:S906, 1991.
321. Stanberry LR: Herpes simplex virus vaccines as immunotherapeutic agents. Trends Microbiol 3:244, 1995.
322. Morrison LLA, Knipe DM: Immunization with replication-defective mutants of herpes simplex virus type 1: Sites of immune intervention in pathogenesis of challenge virus infection. J Virol 68:689, 1994.
323. Morrison LA, Knipe DM: Mechanisms of immunization with a replication-defective mutant of herpes simplex virus 1. Virology 220:402, 1996.
324. Langenberg AG, Burke RL, Adair SF, et al: A recombinant glycoprotein vaccine for herpes simplex virus type 2: Safety and immunogenicity [corrected] [published erratum appears in Ann Intern Med 123:395, 1995]. Ann Intern Med 122:889, 1995.
325. Bourne N, Stanberry LR, Bernstein DI, Lew D: DNA immunization against experimental genital herpes simplex virus infection. J Infect Dis 173:800, 1996.
326. Boursnell MEG, Entwisle C, Blakeley D, et al: A genetically inactivated herpes simplex virus type 2 (HSV2) vaccine provides effective protection against primary and recurrent HSV2 disease. J Infect Dis 175:16, 1997.
327. McKenzie R, Straus SE: Therapeutic immunization for recurrent herpes simplex virus infections. *In* Mills J, Volberding PA, Corey L (eds): Antiviral Chemotherapy 4. New York, Plenum Publishing, 1996, pp 67–83.
328. Straus SE, Corey L, Burke RL, et al: Placebo-controlled trial of vaccination with recombinant glycoprotein D of herpes simplex virus type 2 for immunotherapy of genital herpes [see comments]. Lancet 343:1460, 1994.

114

Chancroid, Lymphogranuloma Venereum, and Granuloma Inguinale

Allan Ross Ronald
Michelle J. Alfa

Genital ulceration is a common presentation to health care providers who treat patients with sexually transmitted infections. In the United States, England, and Sweden, about 3% of patients present with ulcers. In clinics for sexually transmitted diseases in East Africa, Southeast Asia, and India, the prevalence of genital ulceration is 20% to 50%. Genital herpes and primary syphilis are the first and second most common cause of genital ulcers in Western societies; chancroid accounts for most ulcers in the developing world. Regardless of the cause, genital ulcers are often associated with regional lymphadenopathy. Etiologic identification requires laboratory investigation owing to the nonspecificity of clinical features.

Granuloma inguinale (GI) is rarely diagnosed in Western countries but is endemic in Papua New Guinea and in parts of India. Lymphogranuloma venereum (LGV) occurs only sporadically in the industrialized countries but is common in many developing countries.

Genital ulcers have assumed increasing importance owing to their epidemiologic association with the human immunodeficiency virus type 1 (HIV-1).[1] The association between "crack" cocaine use and chancroid[2] raises concern about outbreaks in North America and the resultant impact on transmission of HIV in this population. Indeed, Schulte and colleagues[3] indicated that chancroid is underreported in the United States. The need for a rapid, reliable, inexpensive diagnostic test for chancroid has been identified as a priority. Studies are under way to define the role of the various genital ulcerating agents as cofactors for retrovirus dissemination.

Chancroid and *Haemophilus ducreyi* Infection

History

In 1889, Ducrey[4] at the University of Naples published his discovery of the cause of soft chancre.[5] He inoculated three patients with pus from their own genital ulcers and at weekly intervals reinoculated a new site with material from the most recent ulcer. In each, he found a single microorganism in the ulcer exudate that he described as a "short, compact streptobacillary rod with rounded ends" that was observed within and outside neutrophils. He was unable to grow the organism in culture.

Earlier investigators, including Ricord in France, had clearly differentiated the primary hard chancre of syphilis from the soft chancre, or ulcus mole, of chancroid.[5] In France in 1852, Bassereau[6] further differentiated these two venereal ulcers by demonstrating that only patients with soft chancre could be reinfected at another skin site by autoinoculation of ulcer exudate.[5]

During the first two decades after Ducrey's discovery, a score of microbiologists and clinicians studied both the organism and the disease. *H. ducreyi* was cultured, and some of its growth requirements were characterized.

For the next six decades, there was a dearth of interest in *H. ducreyi* and chancroid—and fewer than 15 major publications. Only rarely was *H. ducreyi* cultured from patients with genital ulcers. Some public health authorities doubted that *H. ducreyi* was responsible for genital ulcerations, and some suggested that chancroid was an atypical presentation of herpes simplex virus. In 1938, Hanschell[7] described the efficacy of sulfonamides for the treatment of chancroid. The incidence declined dramatically, until in 1977 only 455 cases were reported in the United States.

During the past 20 years, outbreaks of chancroid in Canada, Greenland, and the United States provided opportunities to study *H. ducreyi* and to control outbreaks of chancroid.[8] In addition, the association between genital ulcer disease and HIV transmission has emphasized the need to improve diagnostic procedures because the inaccuracy of clinical diagnosis of genital ulcer disease has been well described.[9, 10] There has been an exponential growth of research interest and at least a dozen groups are actively investigating *H. ducreyi* and chancroid. These studies were critically reviewed by Trees and Morse.[11]

Biology of Haemophilus ducreyi

H. ducreyi is a small, gram-negative, bipolar-staining organism. In tissue sections, and occasionally in broth cultures, the characteristic spatial features were initially described as a "school of fish" arrangement or as streptobacillary, with long parallel chains or "railway tracks." *H. ducreyi* stains poorly with both safranin and crystal violet and can readily be overlooked with Gram stain. The colonies of *H. ducreyi* are yellow-gray and 0.5 to 1.0 mm in diameter (Fig. 114–1). Colonies are nonmucoid, are compact, and can be pushed intact across the surface of solid media when nudged by the inoculating loop. On first impression, the culture appears to be mixed because of the variable size and opacity of colonies. A clear medium using catalase as the source of heme has been described[12]; however, no completely defined medium has been described that permits growth of most strains of *H. ducreyi*. The organism requires a hemin level between 25 and 50 mg/L, serum, and the amino acids glutamine and cysteine. *H. ducreyi* grows well in both aerobic and anaerobic environments. Growth is enhanced in a water-saturated environment in 5% carbon dioxide.

The taxonomic placement of *H. ducreyi* within the genus *Haemophilus* has been controversial. Although *H. ducreyi* has a guanine plus cytosine content in the lower range of the genus *Haemophilus* and requires hemin as do other members of the genus, Albritton and coworkers[13] found that the related DNA homology with other members of the genus was only 0.18. Using the S1 nuclease method, Kasin and colleagues[14] found that 17 type strains of *Haemophilus* were no more than 6% related to *H. ducreyi*, and Carlone and associates[15] noted that *H. ducreyi* possesses isoprenoid structure types quite different from those of other *Haemophilus* species. These findings suggest that *H. ducreyi* should have a new taxonomic assignment, perhaps with the genus *Pasteurella*.

At present, *H. ducreyi* has no known unique immunologic or biochemical characteristics. It does reduce nitrate and produces alkaline phosphatase. It is also cytochrome oxidase–positive if the test is performed with tetraethyl-*p*-phenylenediamine. The organism is asaccharolytic in routine sugar fermentation tests and is also unable to metabolize polysaccharides but possesses a wide range of immunopeptidase and esterase activity.[16] Hemolytic activity is most readily detected by using horse erythrocytes.[17] The hemolysin is heat labile and protease sensitive.

Characterization of the structure and function of *H. ducreyi*

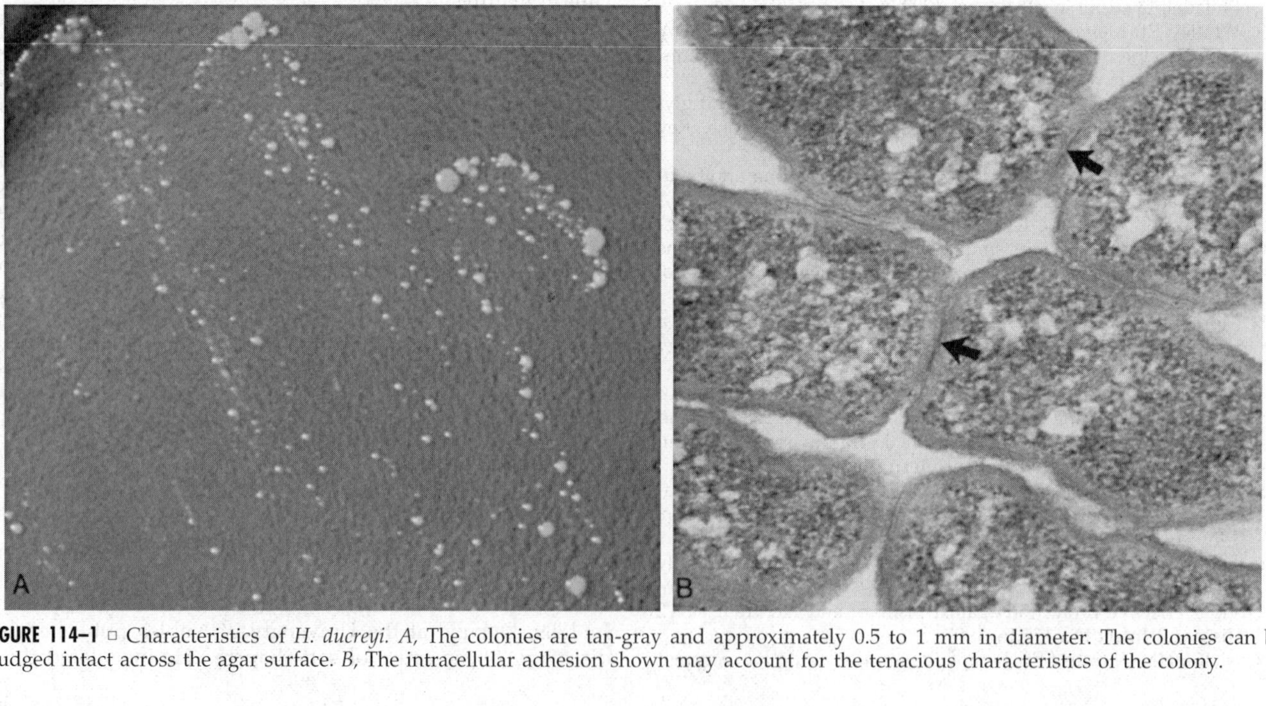

FIGURE 114–1 □ Characteristics of *H. ducreyi*. *A*, The colonies are tan-gray and approximately 0.5 to 1 mm in diameter. The colonies can be nudged intact across the agar surface. *B*, The intracellular adhesion shown may account for the tenacious characteristics of the colony.

antigens is well under way. Outer membrane proteins have been analyzed by sodium dodecyl sulfate–polyacrylamide gel electrophoresis, and seven polypeptide band patterns have been described.[18] A major outer membrane protein with a molecular mass of about 40,000 daltons is present in all strains and is reported to be a member of the OmpA family of proteins.[19] *H. ducreyi* infection elicits an antibody response.[20–22] This has been used in preliminary studies as a serologic test for the diagnosis of chancroid.[23] The lipopolysaccharide has been characterized as a rough type, similar to that of *Haemophilus* and *Neisseria* spp.[24] Parsons and colleagues[25] have described GroEL, a 57.8-kDa polypeptide, as the predominant protein produced by *H. ducreyi* grown at 33°C. The *groE* heat shock operon has a high degree of homology with the *groE* genes in other bacteria.[25]

The pathogenesis of *H. ducreyi* infections and its virulence determinants are still not well understood. Invasive strains seem to be resistant to the bactericidal activity of normal human serum and also resistant to phagocytosis and killing by neutrophils.[26] In preliminary studies, this appears to be due to phenotypic alterations in the lipopolysaccharide. A number of model systems have been developed including in vitro cell culture models,[27–29] a primate model,[30] a temperature-dependent rabbit model,[31] and human inoculation.[32] These models have indicated that *H. ducreyi* is able to attach to keratinocytes[29] and human epithelial cells.[28] The organism is able to invade epithelial cells by being taken up by vesicles and subsequent escape into the cytoplasm. Once it invades the subcutaneous tissues, it attaches to but does not invade human fibroblasts.[33] Human volunteer studies indicate that 2 weeks of infection with *H. ducreyi* stimulates a delayed-type hypersensitivity response. These volunteers when subsequently challenged were not immune.[32] Melaugh and coworkers[34] have shown that the terminal glycan structures on *H. ducreyi* lipooligosaccharide resemble those of paragloboside, a glycosphingolipid precursor of human blood group antigen and of some human cell gangliosides. Humans with chancroid develop antibodies against a 58.5-kDa heat shock protein[35] as well as antibodies to lipooligosaccharide of *H. ducreyi*,[21] but the significance of this has not been identified. Although animal models are promising,[36] human vaccines have not been developed, perhaps reflecting our inadequate understanding of the pathogenesis of chancroid.[37]

Epidemiology

The reservoir for *H. ducreyi* is controversial. In Kenya almost all prostitutes infected with *H. ducreyi* had genital ulceration, and the few asymptomatic women did not appear to have persistent carriage of *H. ducreyi*.[38] Women who were either source contacts or secondary contacts of men with chancroid were found to have genital ulcers. Epidemics of chancroid have been readily controlled in numerous outbreaks in Western countries by intensive follow-up of female contacts, particularly prostitutes, and treatment of persons who have ulcers. The male/female ratio in most studies averages about 8:1; presumably owing to the role of prostitutes in most outbreaks, small numbers of women infect many men. Men with foreskins have about three times the risk of circumcised men of acquiring *H. ducreyi* infection after similar exposure.[39] In North America, chancroid has occurred principally among Native Americans, blacks, and Hispanics. Although Kinghorn and coworkers[40] reported isolation of *H. ducreyi* from herpetic ulcers and from normal genital mucosa, these findings have not been confirmed by other investigators. Martin and DiCarlo[2] reported that an association between crack cocaine use in the United States and chancroid correlated with prostitutes who exchange sex for drugs. As discussed by Schulte and colleagues,[3] interpretation of surveillance information about chancroid is difficult, because diagnostic and confirmatory tests are inadequate. This is further compounded by the inaccuracy of clinical diagnosis of genital ulcer disease.[9]

Interaction of *Haemophilus ducreyi* and Human Immunodeficiency Virus

Epidemiologic studies in Nairobi and elsewhere in Africa consistently showed that men infected with HIV-1 are three times as likely as seronegative men to have a recent history of genital ulcers.[41] Subsequent studies have confirmed this finding.[42–44] In a prospective study of seronegative men, those who presented with chancroid had a fivefold greater risk of seroconversion during a mean follow-up period of 14 weeks than men who presented with urethritis.[45] The increased risk of seroconversion among men who acquired chancroid was further increased threefold in men who were not circumcised.[45] Uncircumcised men who presented with chancroid had a 48% risk of acquiring HIV from a sexual liaison.[45] More than 95% of HIV seroconversions among men with sexually transmitted diseases could be attributable to either recent acquisition of chancroid or the presence of a foreskin.[45]

Both cross-sectional and prospective studies have demonstrated that prostitutes with genital ulcers are at greater risk of acquiring HIV-1 than are prostitutes with no episodes of genital ulcer disease.[46] Overall, we estimate that among prostitutes in Nairobi, ulcers increase the risk of acquiring HIV-1 more than fivefold.

We conclude from these studies that genital ulcers are portals of HIV-1 entry and exit. Presumably, the immune response to *H. ducreyi* recruits and activates macrophages and T helper lymphocytes,[47] which dramatically increase the susceptibility of women to HIV-1 infection. Viral excretion into the vagina is increased in women with latent HIV-1 infection who develop *H. ducreyi* ulcers.[48]

Results of studies also suggest that women infected with HIV-1 are more susceptible to *H. ducreyi* genital ulceration: the prevalence of genital ulcers is twice that among HIV-1–seronegative women.[49]

It is apparent that HIV-1 and *H. ducreyi* interact in several ways to increase heterosexual transmission.[37, 42] Chancroid increases women's susceptibility to infection with HIV-1 and also markedly increases the likelihood of transmitting HIV-1 to sexual partners, doubling the prevalence of genital ulcer disease in women, and increasing the risk for men who have a foreskin of acquiring HIV-1 and *H. ducreyi* from their sexual partners (Fig. 114–2). This interactive process acts as an amplification cycle for HIV-1 and chancroid. Control of chan-

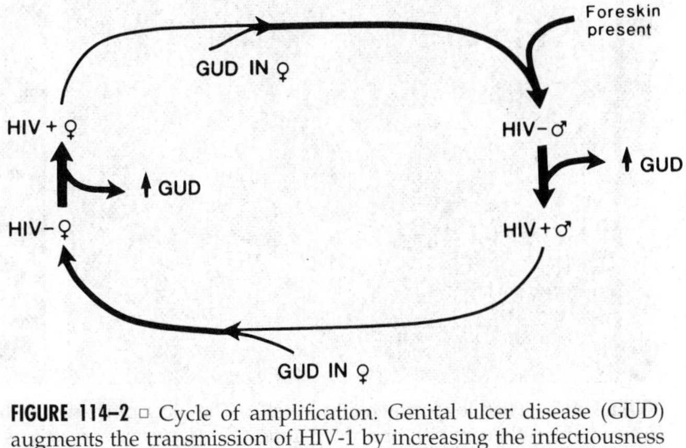

FIGURE 114–2 □ Cycle of amplification. Genital ulcer disease (GUD) augments the transmission of HIV-1 by increasing the infectiousness of women for their sexual partners and making them more susceptible to the virus.

croid is a critical strategy for slowing the epidemic of heterosexual HIV infection.

Histologic Features

Freinkel[50] has described three histologic zones in the fully developed chancroid ulcer: a narrow superficial zone of necrotic tissue, red blood cells, fibrin, and degenerate neutrophils; a broad middle zone of edematous inflammatory tissue with numerous small dilated vessels and strands of endothelial cells infiltrated with neutrophils; and a deep zone characterized by a dense infiltrate of plasma cells, lymphocytes, and macrophages (Fig. 114–3). *H. ducreyi* organisms are most readily seen in the superficial zone. In experimental human studies, Spinola and coworkers[32] found that 3 days after inoculation the dermis was infiltrated with T cells and macrophages. The keratinocytes and T cells had human leukocyte antigen DR expression consistent with a delayed-type hypersensitivity response. Crowson and colleagues[47] studied the histopathology of penile biopsy specimens and described psoriasiform hyperplasia and spongiosis in the epidermis. Exocytosis of mononuclear cells in the epidermis was noted in most biopsies and there was no cytolysis of keratinocytes. In the dermal area, a perivascular and interstitial mononuclear cell infiltrate was observed. Immunoperoxidase studies showed that the predominant mononuclear cell types were histiocytes and $CD4^+$ T lymphocytes. The histiocytes were mainly of Langerhans cell lineage ($UCHL1^+$, $S100^+$, $lysozyme^-$). Vasculitic changes were observed in the dermis. Granulomatis vasculitis was further evidence of a cell-mediated immune response.

Laboratory Diagnosis

Culture of *H. ducreyi* on agar medium has supplanted older methods of culture in blood or serum as the definitive technique for the diagnosis of chancroid. Gonococcal fetal calf serum agar, Mueller-Hinton horse blood agar, and rabbit heart infusion blood agar, each with added vancomycin, 3 mg/L, to inhibit overgrowth of gram-positive bacteria, are optimal culture media (isolation rates 50% to 80%). Studies have indicated that charcoal is an effective replacement for the fetal calf serum supplementation of media for the isolation of *H. ducreyi* from clinical samples.[51]

Specimens for culture should be obtained from the purulent ulcer base without extensive cleaning. Either cotton or Dacron swabs are adequate to collect the exudate. Transport systems have not been extensively studied for *H. ducreyi,* and swabs should be plated directly or within an hour of obtaining the specimen. However, newly formulated thioglycollate-hemin–based transport media containing either selenium dioxide, glutamine, and albumin or glutamine and albumin have been shown to facilitate enrichment of *H. ducreyi* when held at 4°C for 4 days.[52]

The exudate is streaked for isolation and the plate is incubated at 33°C to 34°C in an environment with 5% carbon dioxide and maximal humidity. A candle extinction jar with a moist paper towel is quite adequate. Growth is usually apparent only after 48 hours' incubation, and cultures should be held 5 days before being discarded as negative.

The positive predictive value of a culture that grows *H. ducreyi* is 100% (i.e., a positive culture defines an abnormal state). The sensitivity of culture for chancroid is about 80% in males who have clinical chancroid. All genital ulcers require careful dark-field microscopy and serology for syphilis, to exclude concomitant infection with *Treponema pallidum.*

H. ducreyi is further identified by its ability to reduce nitrate, a positive oxidase test, and a requirement for X factor.[5] Advances in using DNA probes and polymerase chain reaction for diagnosis[53–56] and serology for epidemiologic studies[21, 22, 57] appear promising.

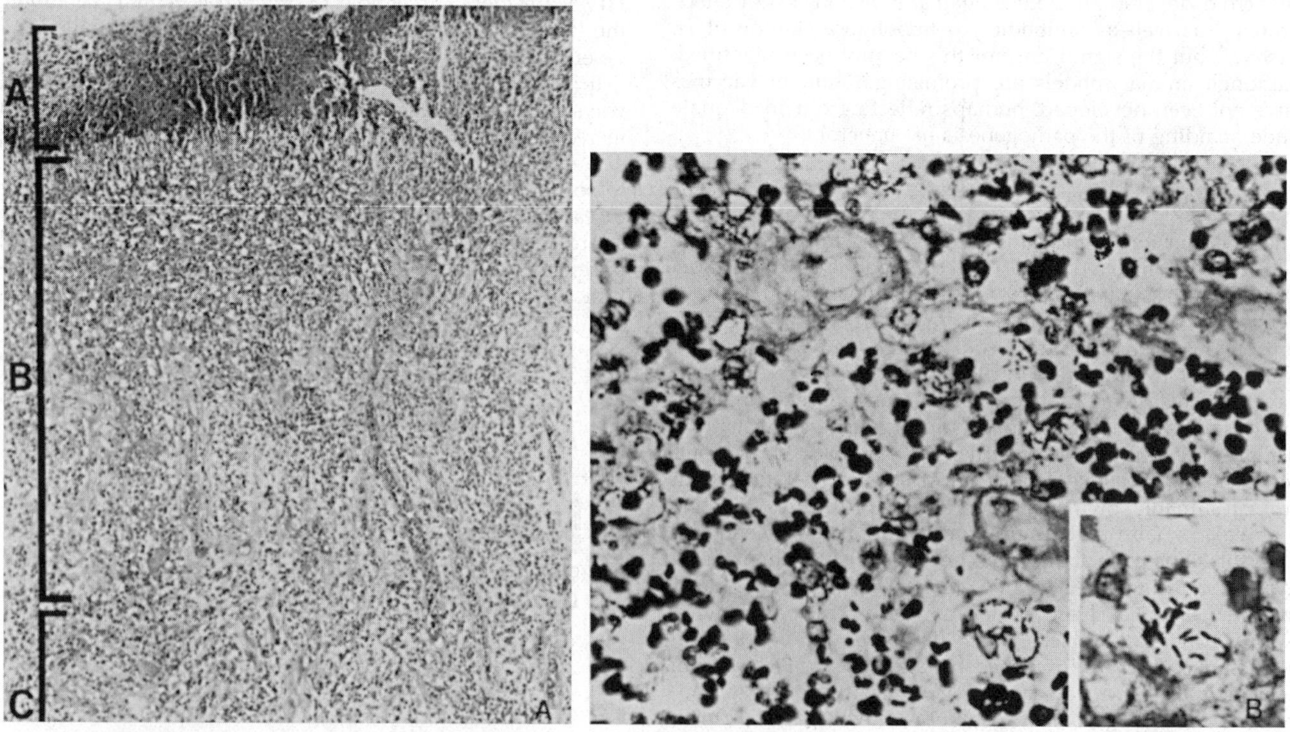

FIGURE 114–3 □ Histology of genital ulcers. *A,* The ulcer of chancroid has three distinct zones: narrow superficial zone (A); broad, middle zone with vascular chancre (B); and deep zone (C). *H. ducreyi* organisms are usually seen in the superficial zone (H&E, × 130). *B,* Granuloma inguinale shows Donovan bodies *(inset),* intracellular bipolar-staining, rod-shaped organisms (Warthin-Starry stain, × 796). (*A* and *B* from Freinkel AL: Histological aspects of sexually transmitted genital lesions. Histopathology 11:819–831, 1987.)

Clinical Presentation

H. ducreyi gains access through a break in the epithelium of the genital mucosa or skin. The inoculum necessary for infection is not known. After an incubation period of 3 to 10 days, an inflammatory papule develops, which rapidly ulcerates. Classically, chancroid ulcers bleed readily from an irregular granulomatous base of variable depth (Fig. 114–4). The ulcer is often filled with a grayish, necrotic purulent exudate. The ulcers are usually painful, although the skin surrounding the ulcer is not much inflamed. About half of chancroid ulcers have typical features, but this common presentation can be mimicked by other pathogens.

Gaisin and Heaton[58] described a number of different presentations, including giant ulcers formed when several smaller ones merge; a follicular type limited to hairy regions that resembles a pyogenic infection; dwarf chancroid with tiny shallow, round ulcers that resemble herpes; transient chancroid that is associated with acute regional lymphadenitis and resembles LGV; and painless single ulcers that resemble primary syphilis. About 10% of patients present with lesions that would be classified clinically as primary syphilis. Kraus and colleagues[59] described two patients with proliferative, raised, indurated, "beefy" lesions on the prepuce characteristic of GI, yet *H. ducreyi* was cultured from both patients.

The sensitivity and specificity of the clinical diagnosis are dependent on the relative proportion of genital ulcers that are due to *H. ducreyi.* In one study from Atlanta, more than 80% of typical chancroid lesions were due to herpes simplex virus.[60] In Kenya, the majority of ulcers of both sexes that clinically resemble herpes were due to chancroid.[61]

Certain sites on the genitalia are favored by *H. ducreyi.* In uncircumcised men, half the lesions occur on the prepuce and are about equally divided between the external and internal surface. Almost 10% of presentations occur as a septic sore, usually in the prepuce but occasionally on the shaft of the penis. Several milliliters of pus can be trapped in the skin when there is no obvious ulcer. Lesions occur on the glans, in the urethra, on the penile shaft, and on the scrotum and skin of the perineum. "Kissing" lesions are common on adjacent cutaneous surfaces. Circumferential ulcers on the coronal sulcus are a common presentation. In women, lesions occur, in order of decreasing frequency, on the fourchette, labia, perianal area, and medial aspect of the thighs. Cervical ulcers are uncommon, and vaginal wall ulcers are rare. Paronychial lesions are not uncommon.

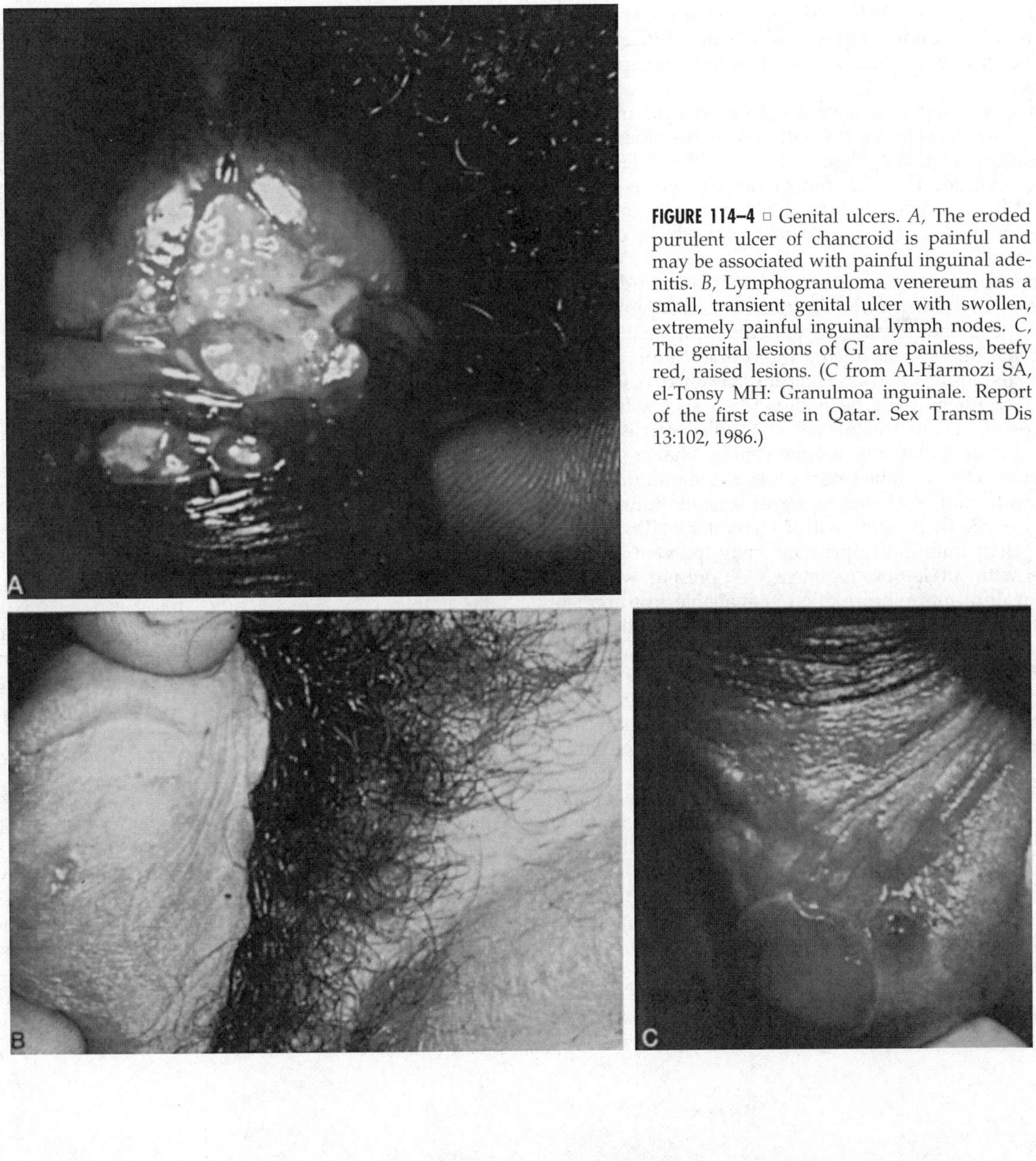

FIGURE 114–4 □ Genital ulcers. *A,* The eroded purulent ulcer of chancroid is painful and may be associated with painful inguinal adenitis. *B,* Lymphogranuloma venereum has a small, transient genital ulcer with swollen, extremely painful inguinal lymph nodes. *C,* The genital lesions of GI are painless, beefy red, raised lesions. (C from Al-Harmozi SA, el-Tonsy MH: Granulmoa inguinale. Report of the first case in Qatar. Sex Transm Dis 13:102, 1986.)

Painful inguinal adenitis occurs in about 40% of patients. It is unilateral in about half of them. Adenitis progresses to suppuration in most patients and a painful inguinal abscess or bubo develops. The overlying skin is stretched and erythematous. Aspiration is necessary to prevent rupture. Purulent urethritis and mucopurulent cervicitis are uncommon presentations of *H. ducreyi*.[62]

Patients with concomitant HIV-1 infection appear to have more extensive ulcers.

Dual infections of *H. ducreyi* plus either *T. pallidum* or herpes simplex virus occur in 2% to 3% of patients. In these cases, clinical features can be confusing and can usually be sorted out only with careful diagnostic investigation.

Human reinoculation studies indicated that infection does not provide immunity,[32] confirming earlier observations by Ducrey[4] and Bassereau[6] that infections recur. The duration of infection and relationship to development of immunity need clarification.

Antimicrobial Susceptibility and Treatment Regimens

Antimicrobial susceptibility tests should be performed with the agar dilution technique. Susceptibility varies markedly from one geographic area to another, and periodic surveys are necessary to make specific recommendations on optimal therapeutic regimens. Antimicrobial resistance has been reported to sulfonamides, tetracyclines, ampicillin and other penicillins, trimethoprim, chloramphenicol, streptomycin, and kanamycin.[63]

Plasmid-mediated resistance is responsible for most antibacterial resistance. During the outbreak in Winnipeg in 1976, Brunton and coworkers[64] described a 5.7-MDa β-lactamase–encoding plasmid. This plasmid carries the entire sequence of the 3.2 MDa gonococcal plasmid. Subsequently, three additional β-lactamase–encoding plasmids have been described in *H. ducreyi*.[63]

Treatment of chancroid has been evaluated in studies originating from both Africa and Southeast Asia. Optimal treatment regimens should cure all patients with genital ulcers and inguinal buboes, producing rapid eradication of *H. ducreyi* from the lesions and no clinical recurrence. A variety of treatment regimens have been prescribed successfully as a single-dose or 1-day treatment.[65, 66] Studies carried out in Kenya suggested that any regimen cures chancroid if the antibacterial activity in the serum exceeds the minimal inhibitory concentration of *H. ducreyi* for at least 48 hours[67]; however, experience in patients with concomitant HIV infection suggests that immunosuppression may prevent effective treatment with single-dose regimens.[68] At present, we recommend that until more information is available from patients with concomitant chancroid and HIV-1 infection, all patients be treated for at least 5 to 7 days. Several studies have shown that erythromycin, 500 mg four times a day for 7 days, is predictably effective. Two studies have shown that a single intramuscular dose of 250 mg of ceftriaxone predictably cures chancroid.[69, 70] However, a study of HIV-infected individuals found a much higher failure rate. Trimethoprim, alone or together with sulfonamides, is no longer effective in most areas of the world.[67] Amoxicillin combined with clavulanic acid prescribed thrice daily for 7 days is an effective regimen.[71] Of the fluoroquinolones, ciprofloxacin in a 3-day course of 500 mg twice daily is effective.[72] Other treatment regimens, including thiamphenicol, kanamycin, spectinomycin, enoxacin, and trimethoprim combined with rifampin have all been effective,[73] but many studies have had a limited number of patients and require confirmation. The sexually transmitted disease treatment guidelines recommend azithromycin as effective therapy for chancroid in patients who do not have HIV infection.[74, 75] When HIV infection is also present, the 7-day erythromycin treatment is preferred.[74]

Fluctuant buboes should be aspirated. Local ulcer treatment may relieve symptoms and facilitate removal of necrotic debris.

Prevention and Control

Chancroid control and eradication are becoming an urgent priority in light of the increasing evidence linking it to the explosive heterosexual spread of HIV-1. Studies in industrialized societies have shown that the disease can be eradicated with traditional principles of sexually transmitted disease control. This includes identification and treatment of contacts, examination and treatment of prostitutes, and effective treatment programs. In developing countries, education linking genital ulcer disease to acquired immunodeficiency syndrome and HIV together with effective programs to provide condoms to persons who continue to take risks may be effective in reducing the ongoing epidemic of chancroid. Targeted programs that focus on prostitutes and their clients may be particularly effective. Demonstration programs are urgently needed. The link between chancroid and the exchange of sex for drugs[2] is concerning.

Lymphogranuloma Venereum and *Chlamydia trachomatis* Serovars L1, L2, and L3

History

LGV was initially described by Wallace in 1833 and definitively characterized by Durand, Nicholas, and Favre in 1913. Rake and coworkers grew *C. trachomatis* from patients with LGV in 1940. LGV has been known as lymphopathia venerea, tropical bubo, and lymphogranuloma inguinale.

Biology of Lymphogranuloma Venereum Serovars of Chlamydia trachomatis

C. trachomatis serovars L1, L2, and L3 are the agents of LGV. Details of *C. trachomatis* biology are presented in Chapter 232. The serovars L1, L2, and L3 differ from other chlamydial serovars in that they are more invasive in the mouse model and have a tropism for lymphatic tissue.[76] Although the genus *Chlamydia* has been the subject of intense investigation in the past three decades, characterization of the LGV strain and the pathogenesis of this unique presentation of *C. trachomatis* have not kept pace, presumably owing to the infrequency of LGV infections in the industrialized world. Studies reveal that LGV biovars of *C. trachomatis* share the same glycosaminoglycan-dependent mechanisms for eukaryotic cell infection as the trachoma strains.[77] In addition, naturally occurring recombination of the major outer membrane protein of LGV has been described.[78]

Epidemiology

LGV is a rare disease in Europe and North America: fewer than 600 cases are reported annually in the United States. In Gambia and Swaziland, it accounted for 1% and 12% of genital ulcers, respectively. Clinically evident infection is 6 to 10 times more common in men than in women. LGV chlamydiae are transmitted by sexual contact, but the incidence after exposure is not known. Men are probably infectious until the primary ulcerative lesion heals, whereas women may have asymptomatic cervical infection that persists for months and serves as a reservoir for this pathogen. The incubation period varies from 5 to 21 days.

Laboratory Diagnosis

DIRECT EXAMINATION

The earliest diagnostic test for LGV was examination of the specimen by Giemsa stain for characteristic intracellular inclusions of *Chlamydia*.[79] This test is specific but insensitive and is usually positive in 50% of patients or less. Newer techniques that use antigen capture with methods incorporating immunofluorescence or enzyme-linked immunoassays have been used to detect *C. trachomatis,* but these tests are not specific for LGV serovars.

ISOLATION OF THE AGENT

Culture of *C. trachomatis* from an appropriate specimen and identification of the unique serovar is the definitive diagnostic test. The positive predictive value is 100% if the agent is isolated from the appropriate specimen, such as a suppurative lymph node or inflamed rectum in a symptomatic patient. Specimens for isolation of *C. trachomatis* should be collected as described in Chapter 232. To reduce cytotoxicity, bubo exudates should be diluted 1:10 before inoculating the cell culture. Typically, LGV strains can be inoculated directly onto the eukaryotic cells (HeLa 229 or McCoy) and do not need to be centrifuged onto them. The LGV serovars have a shorter growth cycle and the cell culture should be fixed and stained within 48 hours. Philip and coworkers[80] successfully isolated *C. trachomatis* from four of eight patients with classic LGV and one of eight patients with possible LGV. Unfortunately, cell culture as a diagnostic tool is severely limited by the sophistication of the technique. Also, the culture technology is substantially less sensitive in patients with more advanced disease.

SEROLOGIC TESTS

Since the description of the complement fixation test, serology has been the mainstay for the diagnosis of LGV.[81] The antigen is an acid polysaccharide common to all *Chlamydia* organisms, and cross-reactions occur with antibodies to non-trachomatis *Chlamydia* species. Although 20% to 30% of a general population of a sexually transmitted disease clinic have low titers of complement fixation antibody, patients with LGV usually have a titer of 1:64 or greater. The sensitivity of this test for the diagnosis of LGV is 80%. A fourfold rise or fall in titer further supports this diagnosis. In the context of the appropriate syndrome, a positive result of the complement fixation test is strongly predictive of LGV, whereas a low titer of 1:16 or less reliably excludes the diagnosis.

Microimmunofluorescence tests for the detection of *C. trachomatis* serovars L1, L2, and L3 now make possible serologic diagnosis of a specific serovar. The test utilizes as antigens yolk sac–grown serovar-specific elementary bodies.[82] The antibody titer is usually in excess of 1:512. Unfortunately, like all fluorescence tests, LGV microimmunofluorescence is subject to observer bias and it is not widely available.

THE FREI TEST

The Frei test is an intradermal test of delayed hypersensitivity to bubo pus or egg yolk *C. trachomatis* antigens. It is neither sensitive nor specific for LGV and is no longer recommended.

Clinical Features

LGV is a chronic disease with three stages, not unlike syphilis. The primary lesion is an inconspicuous, usually painless transient ulcer, most commonly on the coronal sulcus, that heals without scarring and is recalled by no more than 20% of patients (see Fig. 114–4). Cervicitis is the common primary lesion in women. LGV chlamydiae are carried by the macrophages to the regional nodes, which become exquisitely tender masses at the secondary stage. This may be associated with a nonspecific illness, with fever, chills, malaise, headache, and weight loss and a variety of systemic features, including meningoencephalitis, pneumonia, polyarthritis, and erythema nodosum. Lymphadenopathy is bilateral in about 30% of patients and may be so extensive that the inguinal mass of nodes is cleaved by the inguinal ligament, the pathognomonic groove sign. Over a course of 2 to 8 weeks, in the absence of treatment, the overlying skin becomes brawny and wrinkled with a characteristic violaceous hue, and the abscesses within the nodes coalesce and drain from one or more sinus tracts. In women, the sacral lymphatics as well as the iliac lymphatics are often involved with ongoing obstruction of lymph drainage from the rectum and uterus. Fibrosis of lymph nodes leads to lymphedema of the vulva and perineum with chronic pelvic pain.

An anorectal syndrome may be the presenting feature in women and homosexual men. A hemorrhagic proctitis progresses to a third stage, consisting of perirectal abscesses, rectal strictures, and fistulae. Rectal stricture associated with LGV is etiologically linked to rectal cancer.[83]

Antimicrobial Susceptibility and Treatment Regimens

The antimicrobial susceptibility of LGV strains is similar to that of other serovars of *C. trachomatis.* The organisms are routinely susceptible to tetracyclines, erythromycin, and sulfonamides. The prognosis of LGV is extremely variable and unpredictable. Many LGV patients have other sexually transmitted diseases, and the contribution of LGV to the total disease process is indeterminate. About 5% of patients who develop the inguinal lymph node syndrome develop either fistular lesions or a rectal stricture. Few controlled trials of antimicrobial therapy have been published. Although treatment has not been proved to influence the healing of the primary ulcer or the secondary lymphadenitis, most authorities recommend a 3-week course of treatment with either tetracycline or erythromycin, 500 mg four times daily.[84] Fluctuant lymph nodes should be aspirated as necessary to forestall rupture, but surgical incision should be avoided.

Control and Prevention

The value of strategies to reduce the transmission of LGV chlamydiae is unknown. Sexual partners without apparent disease should be treated with a 2-week course of either tetracycline or erythromycin.

Granuloma Inguinale

History

Granuloma tropicalis was first described in southern India in 1882 by McLeod. In 1905, Donovan described the intracellular "protozoan-like" inclusions.[85] The bacterial nature of the Donovan body was established in 1943, when bacteria from an ulcer were cultured in the yolk sac of embryonated eggs.

Biology of *Calymmatobacterium granulomatis*

Limited investigation has been conducted of the presumed agent, *C. granulomatis,* or of the disease itself. *C. granulomatis* is a gram-negative rod with a prominent capsule. In tissue smears, the bacteria are found in large histiocytic cells. They appear to reproduce in multiple foci in the cytoplasm until each vacuole contains hundreds of organisms, which are liberated on cell rupture. Although *C. granulomatis* has antigenic features that resemble those of the genus *Klebsiella,* it has not been grown consistently on artificial media and no cultures of the organism are known to exist. No biochemical or immunologic characteristics are known, and the organism is currently classified as an unassigned genus associated with the family Enterobacteriaceae.

Epidemiology

GI is endemic in southern India, Papua New Guinea, central Australia, and certain islands in the Caribbean. Although transmission is presumed to be sexual, other modes of infection are likely. For example, GI is common in children in regions of the world in which the disease is epidemic. The male/female ratio varies from 2:1 to 10:1.[85] Studies of sexual partners report infection in about 20% of individuals.

In the United States, fewer than 100 cases are reported annually, and some are presumably chancroid misdiagnosed as GI. The disease is thought to be only moderately contagious, and repeated exposure may be necessary. The incubation period is unknown but seems to vary from days to months. Rectal lesions have been described in homosexual patients.

Laboratory Diagnosis

The ulcerative lesion is scraped and the granulation tissue is spread on the slide, air dried, and stained with a Wright or Giemsa stain.[85] The classic findings are intracellular bacterial organisms, which appear as bipolar, black clusters of bacteria in the cytoplasm of large histiocytes. Performed correctly, this test is sensitive and specific for the diagnosis of GI. Donovan bodies can also be seen in tissue sections. Cultural techniques are not useful, as *C. granulomatis* cannot be cultured on artificial media and egg yolk inoculation is not a proven diagnostic procedure. No serologic test is available for the diagnosis of GI.

Clinical Features

The primary lesion is an indurated papule, generally at the portal of entry. These ulcerate but remain "clean, with a red cobblestone base," without purulence, the so-called exuberant beefy appearance (see Fig. 114–4). The lesions enlarge slowly over months, and even years, and may reach a diameter of 5 to 20 cm. The lesion is surprisingly painless. Secondary infection may result in necrosis and increased purulence. Local extension, healing, and fibrosis all occur simultaneously. Although systemic manifestations are uncommon, metastatic hematogenous spread to bones, joints, and the liver has occasionally been described. Regional lymphadenitis is rare, but the ulcerating lesion often extends onto the inguinal skin and produces pseudobuboes. O'Farrell and colleagues[9] reported that the clinical diagnosis of genital ulcers of GI was more accurate than that of other genital ulcers because the ulcers caused by *C. granulomatis* bled, were larger, and were not usually associated with inguinal lymphadenopathy, making their clinical presentation more clear-cut.

Lesions occur commonly on the prepuce of males and on the labia of females. About 5% of patients have cutaneous sites remote from the genitalia. Anal lesions are often verrucous. Scarring may lead to phimosis. A suspected epidemiologic association with genital neoplasms has not been confirmed. Spontaneous healing is rare, and recurrences are frequent after a successful course of therapy. GI is frequently misdiagnosed as carcinoma, and tissue biopsy should be carried out early when the presentation is atypical. Secondary syphilis that fails to respond to penicillin is also a frequent initial diagnosis.

Antimicrobial Susceptibility and Therapeutic Regimens

No susceptibility tests have been carried out in vitro so treatment regimens are empirical. Trimethoprim-sulfamethoxazole, one double-strength tablet (160 mg/800 mg) twice daily, has been effective in Zimbabwe.[86] Tetracycline and erythromycin, 500 mg four times a day, have also been effective. Chloramphenicol, streptomycin, and gentamicin have all been used successfully. Ampicillin is ineffective. Pregnant patients should be treated with trimethoprim-sulfamethoxazole or erythromycin. After initiation of antibacterial treatment, a clinical response is usually evident within 7 to 10 days. Therapy should be continued for 3 weeks. Relapse occurs in 10% to 20% of patients and requires more prolonged treatment. Clinical resistance to a number of agents, including tetracycline, has been reported. Treatment regimens should be altered after 2 weeks if significant improvement has not occurred. Studies indicate that ceftriaxone treatment with 7 to 26 g given by daily intramuscular injections consisting of 1 g of ceftriaxone in 2 mL of 1% lidocaine is optimal.[87] Despite a mean duration of infection of 3 years and multiple previously unsuccessful antibiotic treatments, all 12 patients studied showed significant clinical improvement and 4 patients had complete healing with no recurrence.

Prevention and Control

No useful information is available on primary prevention. Early diagnosis and treatment are effective in preventing the serious sequelae that can occur if treatment is delayed. Presumably, effective treatment of patients with lesions would reduce the prevalence in the population.

References

1. Simonsen JN, Cameron DW, Gakinya MN, et al: Human immunodeficiency virus infection in men with sexually transmitted diseases. N Engl J Med 319:274, 1988.
2. Martin DH, DiCarlo RP: Recent changes in the epidemiology of genital ulcer disease in the United States. The crack cocaine connection. Sex Transm Dis 21(2 Suppl):S76, 1994.
3. Schulte JM, Martich FA, Schmid GP, et al: Chancroid in the United States, 1981–1990: Evidence for underreporting of cases. MMWR CDC Surveill Summ 41:57, 1992.
4. Ducrey A: Experimental Untersuchungen über den Ansteckungsstoff des weichen Schankers und über die Bubonen. Monatsh Prakt Dermatol 9:387, 1889.
5. Kampmeier RH: The recognition of *Haemophilus ducreyi* as the cause of soft chancre. Sex Transm Dis 9:212, 1982.
6. Bassereau PI: Traite de affections de la peau symptomatiques de la syphilis. Paris, JB Bailliere, 1852.
7. Hanschell HM: Sulfonamide in the treatment of chancroid. Lancet 1:886, 1938.
8. Schmid GP, Sanders LL Jr, Blount JH, Alexander ER: Chancroid in the United States. Reestablishment of an old disease. JAMA 258:3265, 1987.
9. O'Farrell N, Hoosen AA, Coetzee KD, van den Ende J: Genital ulcer disease: Accuracy of clinical diagnosis and strategies to improve control in Durban, South Africa. Genitourin Med 70:7, 1994.
10. Ndinya-Achola JO, Kihara AN, Fisher LD, et al: Presumptive specific clinical diagnosis of genital ulcer disease (GUD) in a primary health care setting in Nairobi. Int J STD AIDS 7:201, 1996.

11. Trees DL, Morse SA: Chancroid and *Haemophilus ducreyi:* An update. Clin Microbiol Rev 8:357, 1995.
12. Totten PA, Stamm WE: Clear broth and plate media for culture of *Haemophilus ducreyi.* J Clin Microbiol 32:2019, 1994.
13. Albritton WL, Setlow JK, Thomas M, et al: Heterospecific transformation in the genus *Haemophilus.* Mol Gen Genet 193:358, 1984.
14. Kasin I, Grimont F, Grimont PAD, Sanson-Le Pors M-J: Lack of deoxyribonucleic acid relatedness between *Haemophilus ducreyi* and other *Haemophilus* species. Int J Syst Bacteriol 35:23, 1985.
15. Carlone GM, Schalla WO, Moss CW, et al: *Haemophilus ducreyi* isoprenoid quinone content and structure determination. Int J Syst Bacteriol 38:249, 1988.
16. Van Dyck E, Piot P: Enzyme profile of *Haemophilus ducreyi* strains isolated on different continents. Eur J Clin Microbiol 6:40, 1987.
17. Palmer KL, Grass S, Munson RS Jr: Identification of a hemolytic activity elaborated by *Haemophilus ducreyi.* Infect Immun 62:3041, 1994.
18. Odumeru JA, Ronald AR, Albritton WL: Characterization of cell proteins of *Haemophilus ducreyi* by polyacrylamide gel electrophoresis. J Infect Dis 148:710, 1983.
19. Spinola SM, Griffiths GE, Shanks KL, Blake MS: The major outer membrane protein of *Haemophilus ducreyi* is a member of the OmpA family of proteins. Infect Immun 61:1346, 1993.
20. Alfa MJ, Olson N, DeGagne P, et al: Use of an adsorption enzyme immunoassay to evaluate the *Haemophilus ducreyi* specific and cross-reactive humoral immune response of humans. Sex Transm Dis 19:309, 1992.
21. Alfa MJ, Olson N, DeGagne P, et al: Humoral immune response of humans to lipooligosaccharide and outer membrane proteins of *Haemophilus ducreyi.* J Infect Dis 167:1206, 1993.
22. Roggen EL, Hoofd G, Van-Dyck E, Piot P: Enzyme immunoassays (EIAs) for the detection of anti–*Haemophilus ducreyi* serum IgA, IgG, and IgM antibodies. Sex Transm Dis 21:36, 1994.
23. Museyi K, Van Dyck E, Vervoort T, et al: Use of an enzyme immunoassay to detect serum IgG antibodies to *Haemophilus ducreyi.* J Infect Dis 157:1039, 1988.
24. Odumeru JA, Wiseman GM, Ronald AR: Role of lipopolysaccharide and complement in susceptibility of *Haemophilus ducreyi* to human serum. Infec Immun 50:495, 1985.
25. Parsons LM, Waring AL, Shayegani M: Molecular analysis of the *Haemophilus ducreyi groE* heat shock operon. Infect Immun 60:4111, 1992.
26. Odumeru JA, Wiseman GM, Ronald AR: Relationship between lipopolysaccharide composition and virulence of *Haemophilus ducreyi.* J Med Microbiol 23:155, 1987.
27. Alfa MJ: Cytopathic effect of *Haemophilus ducreyi* for human foreskin cell culture. J Med Microbiol 37:43, 1992.
28. Totten PA, Lara JC, Norn DV, Stamm WE: *Haemophilus ducreyi* attaches to and invades human epithelial cells in vitro. Infect Immun 62:5632, 1994.
29. Brentjens RJ, Spinola SM, Campagnari AA: *Haemophilus ducreyi* adheres to human keratinocytes. Microb Pathog 16:243, 1994.
30. Totten PA, Morton WR, Knitter GH, et al: A primate model for chancroid. J Infect Dis 169:1284, 1994.
31. Purcell BK, Richardson JA, Radolf JD, Hansen EJ: A temperature-dependent rabbit model for production of dermal lesions by *Haemophilus ducreyi.* J Infect Dis 164:359, 1991.
32. Spinola SM, Wild LM, Apicella MA, et al: Experimental human infection with *Haemophilus ducreyi.* J Infect Dis 169:1146, 1994.
33. Alfa MJ, DeGagne P, Hollyer T: *Haemophilus ducreyi* adheres to but does not invade cultured human foreskin cells. Infect Immun 61:1735, 1993.
34. Melaugh W, Phillips NJ, Campagnari AA, et al: Structure of the major oligosaccharide from the lipooligosaccharide of *Haemophilus ducreyi* strain 35000 and evidence for additional glycoforms. Biochemistry 33:13070, 1994.
35. Brown TJ, Jardine J, Ison CA: Antibodies directed against *Haemophilus ducreyi* heat shock proteins. Microb Pathog 15:131, 1993.
36. Hansen EJ, Lumbley SR, Richardson JA, et al: Induction of protective immunity to *Haemophilus ducreyi* in the temperature-dependent rabbit model of experimental chancroid. J Immunol 152:184, 1994.
37. Sparling PF, Elkins C, Wyrick PB, Cohen MS: Vaccines for bacterial sexually transmitted infections: A realistic goal? Proc Natl Acad Sci USA 91:2456, 1994.
38. Plummer FA, D'Costa LJ, Nsanze H, et al: Epidemiology of chancroid and *Haemophilus ducreyi* in Nairobi, Kenya. Lancet 2:1293, 1983.
39. Hart G: Venereal disease in a war environment: Incidence and management. Med J Aust 1:808, 1985.
40. Kinghorn GR, Hafiz S, McEntegart MG: Pathogenic microbial flora of genital ulcers in Sheffield with particular reference to herpes simplex virus and *Haemophilus ducreyi.* Br J Vener Dis 58:377, 1982.
41. Greenblatt RM, Lukehart SA, Plummer FA, et al: Genital ulceration as a risk factor for human immunodeficiency virus. AIDS 2:47, 1988.
42. Telzak EE, Chiasson MA, Bevier PJ, et al: HIV seroconversion in patients with and without genital ulcer disease. A prospective study. Ann Intern Med 119:1181, 1993.
43. Augenbraun MH, McCormack WM: Sexually transmitted diseases in HIV-infected persons. Infect Dis Clin North Am 8:439, 1994.
44. Pepin J, Dunn D, Gaye I, et al: HIV-2 infection among prostitutes working in The Gambia: Association with serological evidence of genital ulcer diseases and with generalized lymphadenopathy. AIDS 5:69, 1991.
45. Cameron DW, Simonsen JN, D'Costa LJ, et al: Female to male transmission of human immunodeficiency virus type 1: Risk factors for seroconversion in men. Lancet 2:403, 1989.
46. Plummer FA, Simonsen JN, Cameron DW, et al: Co-factors in male-female sexual transmission of HIV. J Infect Dis 163:233, 1991.
47. Crowson AN, Magro CM, Alfa M, et al: A comparison histopathological, immunophenotypic, and ultrastructural study of penile chancroid lesions in HIV^+ and HIV^- African males. Lab Invest 70:45A, 1994.
48. Kreiss JK, Coombs R, Plummer F, et al: Isolation of human immunodeficiency virus from genital ulcers in Nairobi prostitutes. J Infect Dis 160:380, 1989.
49. Jessamine PG, Plummer FA, Ndinya-Achola JO, et al: Human immunodeficiency virus, genital ulcers and the male foreskin synergism in HIV-1 transmission. Scand J Infect Dis S61:181, 1990.
50. Freinkel AL: Histological aspects of sexually transmitted genital lesions. Histopathology 11:819, 1987.
51. Lockett AE, Dance DAB, Mabey DCW, Drasar BS: Serum-free media for isolation of *Haemophilus ducreyi.* Lancet 338:326, 1991.
52. Dangor Y, Radebe F, Ballard RC: Transport media for *Haemophilus ducreyi.* Sex Transm Dis 20:5, 1993.
53. Rossau R, Duhamel M, Jannes G, et al: The development of specific rRNA-derived oligonucleotide probes for *Haemophilus ducreyi,* the causative agent of chancroid. J Gen Microbiol 137:277, 1991.
54. Parsons LM, Shayegani M, Waring AL, Bopp LH: DNA probes for the identification of *Haemophilus ducreyi.* J Clin Microbiol 27:1441, 1989.
55. Johnson SR, Martin DH, Cammarata C, Morse SA: Alterations in sample preparation increase sensitivity of PCR assay for diagnosis of chancroid. J Clin Microbiol 33:1036, 1995.
56. Chui L, Albritton W, Paster B, et al: Development of the polymerase chain reaction for diagnosis of chancroid. J Clin Microbiol 31:659, 1993.
57. Thomas DL, Quinn TC: Serologic testing for sexually transmitted diseases. Infect Dis Clin North Am 7:793, 1993.
58. Gaisin A, Heaton CL: Chancroid: Alias the soft chancre. Int J Dermatol 3:188, 1975.
59. Kraus SJ, Werman BS, Biddle JW, et al: Pseudogranuloma inguinale caused by *Haemophilus ducreyi.* Arch Dermatol 118:494, 1982.
60. Salzman RS, Kraus SJ, Miller RG, et al: Chancroidal ulcers that are not chancroid. Cause and epidemiology. Arch Dermatol 120:636, 1984.
61. Nsanze H, Fast MV, D'Costa LJ, et al: Genital ulcers in Kenya. Clinical and laboratory study. Br J Vener Dis 57:378, 1981.
62. Kunimoto DY, Plummer FA, Namaara W, et al: Urethral infection with *Haemophilus ducreyi* in men. Sex Transm Dis 15:37, 1988.
63. McNicol PJ, Ronald AR: The plasmids of *Haemophilus ducreyi.* J Antimicrob Chemother 14:561, 1984.
64. Brunton J, Neier M, Erhman N, et al: Origin of small β-lactamase–specifying plasmids in *Haemophilus* species and *Neisseria gonorrhoeae.* J Bacteriol 168:374, 1986.

65. Plummer FA, Nsanze H, D'Costa LJ, et al: Single-dose therapy of chancroid with trimethoprim-sulfametrole. N Engl J Med 309:67, 1983.
66. Tyndall MW, Agoki E, Plummer FA, et al: Single dose azithromycin for the treatment of chancroid: A randomized comparison with erythromycin. Sex Transm Dis 21:231, 1994.
67. Dylewski J, D'Costa LJ, Nsanze H, Ronald AR: Single-dose therapy with trimethoprim-sulfametrole for chancroid in females. Sex Transm Dis 13:166, 1986.
68. MacDonald KS, Cameron WD, D'Costa LJ, et al: Evaluation of fleroxacin (Ro23-6240) as single oral dose therapy of culture-proven chancroid in Nairobi, Kenya. Antimicrob Agents Chemother 33:612, 1989.
69. Taylor DN, Pitarangsi C, Escheverria P, et al: Comparative study of ceftriaxone and trimethoprim-sulfamethoxazole for the treatment of chancroid in Thailand. J Infect Dis 152:1002, 1985.
70. Bowmer MI, Nsanze N, D'Costa LJ, et al: Single-dose ceftriaxone for chancroid. Antimicrob Agents Chemother 31:67, 1987.
71. Fast MV, Nsanze H, D'Costa LJ, et al: Treatment of chancroid by clavulanic acid with amoxicillin in patients with β-lactamase–positive *Haemophilus ducreyi* infection. Lancet 2:509, 1982.
72. Naamara W, Plummer FA, Greenblatt R, et al: Treatment of chancroid with ciprofloxacin: A prospective randomized clinical trial. Am J Med 82(Suppl 4A):317, 1987.
73. Schmid GP: The treatment of chancroid. JAMA 255:1757, 1986.
74. Levine WC, Berg AO, Johnson RE, et al: Development of sexually transmitted diseases treatment guidelines, 1993. New methods, recommendations, and research priorities. STD Treatment Guidelines Project Team and Consultants. Sex Transm Dis 21(2 Suppl):S96, 1994.
75. Centers for Disease Control and Prevention: 1993 sexually transmitted diseases treatment guidelines. MMWR Morb Mortal Wkly Rep 42(RR-14):1, 1993.
76. Brunham RC, Kuo C-C, Chen WJ: Systemic *Chlamydia trachomatis* infection in the mouse: A comparison of lymphogranuloma venereum and trachoma biovars. Infect Immun 48:78, 1985.
77. Chen JC, Stephens RS: Trachoma and LGV biovars of *Chlamydia trachomatis* share the same glycosaminoglycan-dependent mechanism for infection of eukaryotic cells. Mol Microbiol 11:501, 1994.
78. Hayes LJ, Yearsley P, Treharne JD, et al: Evidence for naturally occurring recombination in the gene encoding the major outer membrane protein of lymphogranuloma venereum isolates of *Chlamydia trachomatis*. Infect Immun 62:5659, 1994.
79. Joseph AK, Rosen T: Laboratory techniques used in the diagnosis of chancroid, granuloma inguinale, and lymphogranuloma venereum. Dermatol Clin 12:1, 1994.
80. Philip RN, Hill DA, Greaves AB, et al: Study of chlamydiae in patients with lymphogranuloma venereum and urethritis attending a venereal disease clinic. Br J Vener Dis 47:114, 1971.
81. Schachter J: Lymphogranuloma venereum and other nonocular *Chlamydia trachomatis* infections. *In* Hobson D, Holmes KK (eds): Nongonococcal Urethritis and Related Infections. Washington, DC, American Society for Microbiology, 1977, pp 91–97.
82. Wang SP, et al: A simplified method for immunological typing of trachoma–inclusion conjunctivitis–lymphogranuloma venereum organisms. Infect Immun 7:356, 1973.
83. Chopda NM, Desai DC, Sawant PD, et al: Rectal lymphogranuloma venereum in association with rectal adenocarcinoma. Indian J Gastroenterol 13:103, 1994.
84. Perine PL, Osoba AO: Lymphogranuloma venereum. *In* Holmes KK, Mardh P-A, Sparling PF, Wiesner PJ (eds): Sexually Transmitted Diseases, ed 2. New York, McGraw-Hill, 1990, pp 195–204.
85. Kuberski T: Granuloma inguinale (donovanosis). Sex Transm Dis 1:29, 1980.
86. Latif AS, Mason PR, Paraiwa E: The treatment of donovanosis (granuloma inguinale). Sex Transm Dis 1:27, 1988.
87. Merianos A, Gilles M, Chuah J: Ceftriaxone in the treatment of chronic donovanosis in central Australia. Genitourin Med 70:84, 1994.

115

Human Papillomaviruses and Anogenital Disease

Lawrence J. Eron

Human papillomaviruses (HPVs) produce squamous epithelial tumors. Certain types of HPV cause the common wart of the fingers, and others cause condylomata acuminata in the anogenital region (genital warts), some of which can become severely dysplastic and progress to invasive carcinoma. Genital HPV infection is responsible for 1 million new office consultations each year in the United States, making it the second most common sexually transmitted disease.[1]

Characteristics of Papillomaviruses

Taxonomy

Although originally classified with polyomavirus and simian virus 40, HPVs are a distinct group of viruses with their own biologic and genetic characteristics.[2, 3] They contain a double-stranded circular DNA genome larger than that of polyomaviruses (8000 base pairs versus 5000) and are larger in capsid diameter (55 versus 40 nm). Unlike the other papovaviruses, they are not easily propagated in tissue culture, so the various events of virus DNA replication, protein synthesis, and maturation are not well known.

Virulence Factors

It has not been possible to distinguish between HPVs by serologic methods. Rather, they are classified by DNA hybridization into 73 different types.[4] Viruses that possess more than 50% DNA homology with a test probe are assigned to that particular type. Some of these and their clinical syndromes are listed in Table 115–1. Types 6, 11, 42, 43, and 44 have been associated with benign, exophytic condylomata acuminata of the anogenital region, as well as low-grade dysplasias (cervical intraepithelial neoplasia [CIN], also

TABLE 115–1 ■ Types of Human Papillomaviruses

TYPE	SOURCE
HPV-1, -4	Plantar warts
HPV-2, -27, -29	Verruca vulgaris
HPV-3, -10, -26, -28	Flat warts
HPV-5, -8, -9, -12, -14, -15, -17, -19 to -25	Epidermodysplasia verruciformis
HPV-6, -11, -42, -43, -44	Genital warts and laryngeal papillomas
HPV-7	Butcher's warts
HPV-13, -32	Oral focal epithelial hyperplasia
HPV-16, -18, -30, -31, -33, -35, -39, -45, -51, -52, -56	Cervical dysplasia and carcinoma, bowenoid papulosis
HPV-30, -40	Laryngeal carcinoma

known as squamous intraepithelial lesions, grade 1), which are less likely to progress to more severe dysplasia and carcinoma.[5] Types 16, 18, 31, 33, 35, 39, 45, 51, 52, and 56 have frequently been associated with flat warts that may progress to more severe dysplasias, such as CIN grades 2 (moderate dysplasia) and 3 (severe dysplasia), and to invasive carcinomas of the cervix, vagina, and vulva.

Epidemiology

The HPV that causes clinical infection in the anogenital region is transmitted sexually; its incidence in the United States is 1 million new cases of genital warts per year.[1] It is relatively easily transmitted during intercourse, because fully 73% of sexual partners of persons with clinically evident genital HPV infection show evidence of HPV infection at their initial examination.[6] It may also be transmitted to the neonate as laryngeal papillomatosis, presumably during passage through an infected birth canal. Three percent of Papanicolaou smears (a relatively insensitive technique) of sexually active women show evidence of HPV infection,[7] whereas 10% to 30% of randomly selected normal persons show evidence of HPV infection by DNA probing of exfoliated cells.[8, 9] Of those attending a sexually transmitted disease clinic, 48% tested positive for HPV (mainly type 16) by DNA probing.[10]

Pathogenesis

At the Molecular Level

The HPV genome is organized into three distinct regions: an "early" region that encodes viral proteins necessary for DNA replication, transcription, and cell transformation; a "late" region that encodes the viral capsid proteins; and a control region known as the upstream regulatory region. Many of the proteins of these genes have been identified in bovine papillomavirus, and it is likely that the HPV genes encode proteins with similar functions.[4] The genes of the early region are designated *E1* to *E7* and those of the late region, *L1* to *L2* (Table 115–2). Despite its location in the early region, *E4* encodes a late protein that is synthesized only in productive infection.[11]

In productive infection, messenger RNA transcription from the early and late regions of the viral genome allows viral DNA replication and viral capsid synthesis, respectively. Virus assembly occurs and infectious virions are produced. In nonproductive infection, transcription of messenger RNA is from the early region only. Restriction of expression of the late region in nonproductive infection is thought to occur at the level of transcription initiation and termination.[12] Viral capsid synthesis and viral assembly do not occur, but early functions may transform the cell.

TABLE 115–2 ▪ Papillomavirus Gene Functions

GENE	FUNCTION
E1	Extrachromosomal DNA replication down- and up-regulation
E2	Transcription regulator against cell transformation
E3	Unknown
E4	Viral maturation
E5	Cellular transformation in bovine papillomavirus, control of plasmid numbers
E6	Cellular transformation, control of plasmid numbers
E7	Cellular immortalization, transcriptional transactivation
E8	DNA replication in bovine papillomavirus
L1	Major capsid protein (54,000 daltons)
L2	Minor capsid protein (76,000 daltons)

In benign condylomata caused by HPV-6 or HPV-11, productive infection produces many copies of HPV DNA per cell as extrachromosomal plasmids. In carcinomas of the genital tract from which HPV-16 or -18 DNA has been isolated, the HPV DNA genome integrates into one or more sites on the host chromosome, often in tandem arrays.[13] Integration of the virus into the host cell DNA usually occurs with disruption of the circular viral genome at a characteristic location within the *E1* and *E2* genes.[14] With loss of these two gene functions, E6 and E7 are deregulated and the cell is transformed.[15, 16]

The role of *E6* and *E7* as oncogenes is now firmly established.[17] Both viral proteins interfere with the p53 protein and the retinoblastoma tumor suppressor gene product, pRB, host proteins that normally control cell growth and differentiation. The role of these genes in HPV oncogenesis was predicted by three epidemiologic observations that suggested that infection by HPVs, although necessary, was not sufficient for malignant conversion.[18] First, there is a long latency period between HPV infection and the development of cancer of the cervix. Second, there is a low incidence of cervical cancer in those infected with "highly oncogenic" HPV types. Third, certain cofactors such as smoking and type 2 herpes simplex viral infection promote the development of cervical cancer. Indeed, progression of an HPV-transformed or immortalized cell clone to invasive growth as a cancer involves modification of host cell growth control genes.

Cell fusion studies have demonstrated at least four such host cell genes.[19] Some of these genes suppress viral oncogene expression posttranscriptionally, and others prevent transcription via activated macrophages.[20] One example is the p53-induced *p21* gene (also known as *Cip-1* or *Waf-1*), whose function interferes with cyclin-dependent kinases, thereby blocking phosphorylation of pRB.[21] Phosphorylation of pRB inactivates this protein, leading to deregulation of cell growth.

At the Cellular and Tissue Levels

To cause an infection, HPV must penetrate through gaps in the epithelium to gain access to the basal layer. Although there is no direct proof that the basal cells are the principal site of infection, they are the only dividing cells of the epithelium that could act as a reservoir to yield HPV in mature keratinocytes. Expression of the viral DNA in the basal layer is thought to be responsible for the proliferation of keratinocytes and blood vessels that results in a wart.

The clinical features, histologic appearance, and natural history of HPV infections are determined largely by the type of HPV DNA found within the lesions (Table 115–3). After an incubation period as long as 9 months, HPV-6 and -11 generally induce exophytic condylomata affecting anogenital skin and the lower vagina, although they may also produce flat condylomata.[22, 23] On histologic examination, these lesions display koilocytosis (cytoplasmic vacuolization). Occasionally, they may form huge condylomatous masses called verrucous carcinomas (Buschke-Löwenstein tumors), which are locally invasive but rarely metastatic.[24] Whereas HPV-6 and -11 cause exophytic condylomata on all genital areas, HPV-16, -18, -31, -33, and -35 show a predilection for the cervix and frequently progress to higher grades of CIN than are associated with HPV-6 and -11[1] (Table 115–4). Nuclear atypia and abnormal mitotic figures are seen and koilocytosis is frequently absent. These high-risk HPV types (especially type

TABLE 115–3 ■ Anogenital Lesions and Human Papillomavirus Infection

LESION	HPV TYPE
Condylomata acuminata	6, 11
Cervical intraepithelial neoplasia (grades 1, 2, and 3)	16, 18, 31, 33, 35, 39, 42, 43, 44, 45, 51, 52, 56
Bowenoid papulosis	16, 34, 37, 42
Buschke-Löwenstein tumors	6, 11
Invasive cervical carcinomas	16, 18, 31, 33, 35, 39, 45, 51, 52, 56
Vulvar carcinomas	16 (rarely 6, 11)
Penile carcinomas	16, 18

16) are detectable in 80% to 90% of grade 3 CIN lesions[25] and cervical cancers.[1, 22, 26]

Through the use of colposcopy it is now known that most cervical HPV infections are expressed as subclinical flat lesions, becoming visible only after the application of acetic acid.[10] Subclinical infection may represent an early phase of cervical infection in evolution to CIN.[27] In one study,[28] 16% of subclinical infection progressed to CIN 2 or 3 within a 12-month period.

The likelihood of developing cervical cancer may be forecast by the type of CIN. In one study,[29] 12% of CIN 1 lesions evolved into cancer, 20% CIN 2, and 75% of CIN 3. Because of the long lag time between initial infection and eventual malignant conversion, estimated to be 5 to 20 years,[30] and because not all HPV-16–infected women develop cervical cancer, other cofactors are probably responsible for malignant conversion. Other risk factors may include tobacco use[31, 32] and infection by other agents,[33, 34] including herpes simplex virus, which has been thought to be a cofactor,[35] perhaps acting by amplifying oncogenes or inducing mutations or recombinations. Immunosuppression may also function as a cofactor in tumor development.

HPV-16 and the more malignant HPV types also infect the vagina, vulva, and penis, where they may cause the same phenomena as in the cervix—subclinical infection, condylomata, and vulvar and vaginal intraepithelial neoplasia. As in the cervix, HPV-16 is most frequently associated with subclinical infection of the vagina, vulva, and penis, but the neoplastic potential at these sites is less well understood.[27] HPV-16 DNA has also been detected in such premalignant conditions as bowenoid papulosis and Bowen disease (see Table 115–3). Whereas HPV-16 is the most prevalent type in squamous cell carcinomas of the cervix, HPV-18 is preferentially associated with cervical adenocarcinomas.[36, 37] Penile cancers may harbor HPV-16 and -18.[38, 39]

HPV may also infect the perianal and intraanal regions, occasionally above the dentate line of the distal rectum. The presence of perianal condylomata, in either males or females, need not imply a history of anal intercourse, as condylomata on the vulva extend into the anal region in 18% of patients (who deny anal intercourse).[40]

HPV types 6 and 11 may cause oral lesions and laryngeal papillomatosis, which are believed to be transmitted by oral-genital sexual contact. Laryngeal papillomatosis may be transmitted to infants by intrapartum contact from an infected birth canal. Cesarean section as a measure to prevent intrapartum spread is controversial and at this time is not thought to be indicated.

TABLE 115–4 ■ Relation of Human Papillomavirus Type to Clinical Disease in the Cervix

	NO. OF ISOLATES FOR HPV TYPE				
DISEASE	6	11	16	18	31
Condyloma	15	7	1	1	0
CIN 1	5	1	3	1	2
CIN 2	6	0	15	1	5
CIN 3	1	0	16	1	3
Cervical cancer	0	0	5	3	1

Adapted from Reid R, Greenberg M, Jenson AB, et al: Sexually transmitted papillomaviral infections. I. The anatomic distribution and pathologic grade of neoplastic lesions associated with different viral types. Am J Obstet 156:212–222, 1987.

Immune Responses

Because persons who are immunoincompetent often develop more numerous warts that are refractory to therapy,[41] it is clear that the immune response is important in controlling HPV infection. Defects of humoral immunity do not influence the natural history of HPV infection.[42] Although regression of warts in some cases correlates temporally with the development of immunoglobulin G antibodies,[10] resolution may occur in their absence and reinfection may occur in their presence.

Cell-mediated immunity is more important in determining the progression or regression of HPV infection.[43] Regression of warts after therapy is frequently accompanied by enhanced responses in vitro and in vivo to tests for cell-mediated immunity to viral antigens.[44]

If immunity to HPV infection is similar to that for other viral infections, helper and cytotoxic T lymphocytes ought to recognize HPV antigens displayed on the cell surface in association with glycoproteins encoded by the major histocompatibility complex. The HPV antigen that is recognized is not likely to be the major capsid antigen that is shared by all HPV types. In patients with regressing flat warts, plantar and common warts may persist, suggesting that immunity may be type specific.[44]

Patients with refractory genital warts should be screened for antibody to human immunodeficiency virus, as refractoriness of genital warts to therapy may be a marker for human immunodeficiency virus infection and for decreased response to interferon.[45] Immunocompetent persons may have warts that are unresponsive to therapy because of a deficiency of local host response, thought to be a disorder of lymphokines.[44] This theory supports the case for lymphokines such as interferon for the therapy of refractory warts (see Treatment).

Animals whose warts have regressed are resistant to reinfection by HPV, suggesting a role for vaccine in increasing host resistance to HPV.[46] Injecting rabbits with papilloma extracts increases the rate and frequency of papilloma regression.[47] The immune response may also play a role in preventing regrowth after physical ablation of existing warts. Ablative therapies may alter HPV antigens in some way to render them more antigenic, thus recruiting the immune response to prevent relapse of treated warts despite the fact that the viral reservoir may remain after ablation.

Clinical Manifestations

HPV infection of the anogenital tract is usually asymptomatic but may occasionally cause pruritus and burning. It may occur subclinically as a flat wart, identified by "acetowhitening" (70% of cases), or it may occur as a papillary projection above the skin with a rich capillary bed (30% of cases; Fig. 115–1). The flat warts may be stable lesions that

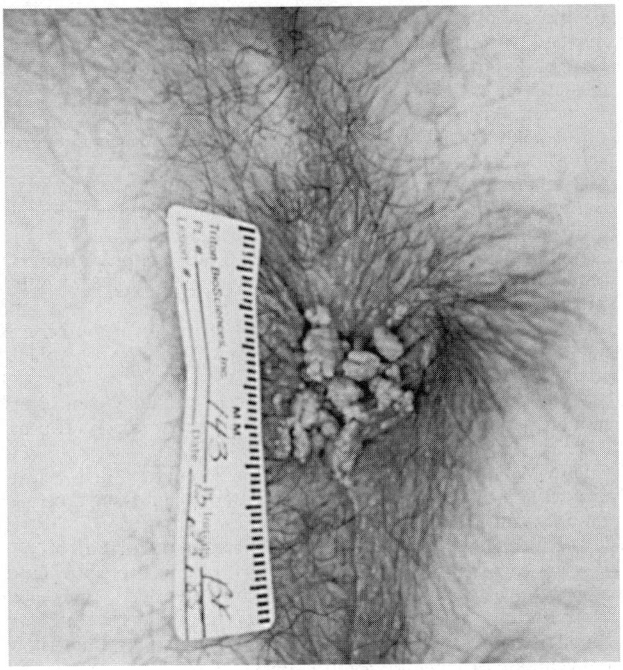

FIGURE 115–1 □ Genital warts involving the perianal region.

do not evolve into exophytic projections, or they may become increasingly dysplastic and progress to carcinoma in situ.[10]

In women, the exophytic types of warts are located most frequently in the posterior introitus, followed by the labia, clitoris, vaginal vestibule, and perianal region (Fig. 115–2). They may also occur on the cervix. When warts are present on the vulva, more than one third of patients have vaginal or cervical infection as well.[48, 49]

In uncircumcised men, the prepuce is most frequently affected, followed by the penile shaft, scrotum, and perianal area. The urethral meatus may be affected in asymptomatic men, but the proximal urethra rarely is,[6] although it may be in immunosuppressed persons and those with Buschke-Löwenstein tumors.[50]

Diagnosis

Condylomata acuminata must be differentiated from other growths in the genital area, including molluscum contagiosum, condylomata lata, keratoses, moles, and skin tags. The last entity may be especially difficult to distinguish in the vaginal area.

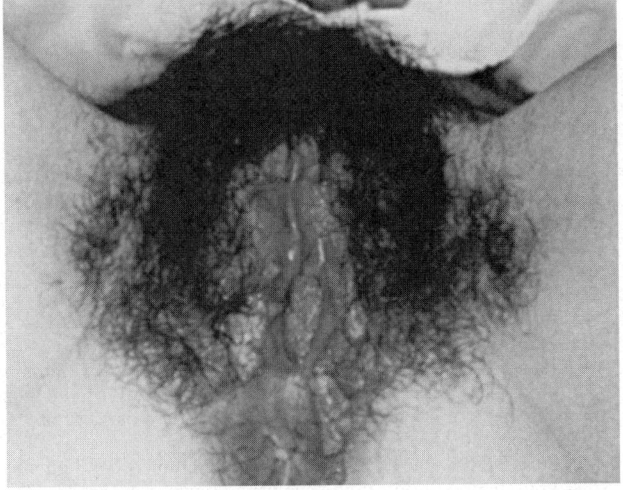

FIGURE 115–2 □ Genital warts involving the labia.

Because HPV cannot be grown in tissue culture, identification of HPV infection must be made on the basis of gross appearance: exophytic projections of skin containing a capillary loop within or flat areas that stain acetowhite on application of acetic acid. In the case of flat acetowhite areas, HPV infection should be confirmed by biopsy and examination for the typical changes of koilocytosis. Koilocytosis can also be identified on Papanicolaou smears of the cervix, as a general screen. DNA hybridization tests are useful for identifying the type of HPV but cannot yet be advocated for screening purposes.[51]

Treatment

Genital warts are often chronic HPV infections, and clinical cures frequently represent reversion to latency rather than disappearance of viral DNA from the treated area. HPV DNA is present in the normal epithelium adjacent to lesions. Relapse after therapy can be predicted by demonstration of HPV DNA sequences in biopsy specimens of adjacent tissue.[52] The most popular form of therapy in previous years, topical application of 25% podophyllin (washed off 6 hours later) weekly for 5 weeks, is ineffective, especially on dry areas of the penis (shaft and scrotum) and on the labia majora. Even in wet areas such as the prepuce or the labia minora, less than 50% efficacy rates are often reported,[53] as well as frequent recurrences.[54] In addition, podophyllin is not a standardized compound, and the proportion of active ingredient, podophyllotoxin, may vary from batch to batch. Podophyllotoxin has replaced podophyllin, although it is no more effective. Its use is contraindicated in pregnant women.

Another chemical method, topical application of 50% to 80% trichloroacetic acid or bichloroacetic acid, has less potential systemic toxicity and can be used by pregnant women. It produces a white slough that peels in a few days and it can be reapplied twice daily 3 days per week, up to 4 weeks; however, efficacy rates may not exceed those of podophyllin.[53, 54] It, too, is essentially ineffective on warts on keratinized epithelium.

A third topical drug, 5-fluorouracil, can produce impressive clearance (82%) of warts when used nightly for 1 week,[6] but this regimen may be intensely irritating.[55] Its efficacy, which relies on a differential degree of toxicity to normal and condylomatous epithelium, varies with the degree of dermatitis. Many persons may tolerate only one or two applications in a week.[55] After laser therapy, 5-fluorouracil has also been applied once or twice weekly to prevent relapse.[56, 57] Like other caustic therapies, it is not as effective on the labia majora as on the inside of the labia minora.[55]

A variety of ablative physical procedures have been utilized. Cryotherapy—two 1-minute freeze-thaw cycles induced by a probe or by liquid nitrogen—is the least painful because it does not require local anesthesia. It is more effective than podophyllin: the cure rate is 60% to 70% after approximately three to six weekly treatments.[58] Recurrences are common.

Electrocoagulation using a battery-powered instrument may yield a slightly higher clearance rate (70%) than cryosurgery,[59] but again, there are recurrences. Scarring may result, and a painful local injection of lidocaine for anesthesia is required.

Laser ablation is the treatment of choice for cervical lesions. It offers the advantage of precise control of depth, but again there are recurrences and morbidity may be high.[49, 56, 60] It requires local or general anesthesia. Because therapeutic laser equipment is quite expensive to purchase, it is not surprising that laser treatment is more expensive than any other modality, even when general anesthesia is not used.

Interferons and interferon inducers, such as imiquimod,[60a] offer the potential advantage of eradicating the HPV reservoir, owing to their antiviral and immune stimulating properties in addition to their antiproliferative effects. Interferon-α (leukocyte) is effective when injected into the lesion[61–63] and into muscle.[64] Interferon-β (fibroblast) has been shown to be effective,[65] and interferon-γ (immune) holds great promise.[66] All the interferons have toxic side effects (influenza-like symptoms) and relapses may still occur. The potential benefit of combining them with ablative therapies is being tested.

Certain types of condylomata are better suited for certain therapies. Exophytic vaginal condylomata may respond better to 5-fluorouracil than to laser, whereas flat cervical condylomata are better treated by laser.[56] Patients whose warts clear should be monitored for relapse monthly for 2 months after therapy and thereafter every 6 months. Large warts and warts older than 6 months are more likely to be resistant to therapy and to relapse after apparent clearance.

Prevention

Because approximately 70% of sexual partners of those with clinical genital HPV disease develop HPV infection, prevention is important. Theoretically, the use of condoms, nonoxynol 9 (an ingredient in vaginal contraceptive foams, gels, and sponges), or both ought to prevent spread of HPV during sexual intercourse, but no clinical trials have yet proved this. Efforts to develop a vaccine have been frustrated by our inability to grow HPV in tissue culture. Animal models of the rabbit[3] and the cow[67] have demonstrated the efficacy of an animal vaccine, but no vaccine has yet been developed for human testing. Should a vaccine become available, its potential for the control of HPV infection and cancer of the cervix would be vast indeed.

References

1. Reid R, Greenberg M, Jenson AB, et al: Sexually transmitted papillomaviral infections. I. The anatomic distribution and pathologic grade of neoplastic lesions associated with different viral types. Am J Obstet 156:212, 1987.
2. Howley PM, Broker TR (eds): Papillomaviruses: Molecular and Clinical Aspects. New York, Alan R Liss, 1985.
3. Syrjanen K, Gissmann L, Koss LG (eds): Papillomaviruses and Human Disease. Heidelberg, Springer-Verlag, 1987.
4. Howley PM, Schlegel R: The human papillomaviruses: An overview. Am J Med 85:155, 1988.
5. Campion MJ, McCance DJ, Cuzick J, et al: Progressive potential of mild cervical atypia: Prospective cytological, colposcopic, and virological study. Lancet 2:237, 1986.
6. Rosemberg SK, Greenberg MD, Reid R: Sexually transmitted papillomaviral infection in men. Obstet Gynecol Clin North Am 14:495, 1987.
7. Grubb GS: Human papillomavirus and cervical neoplasia. Epidemiological considerations. Int J Epidemiol 15:1, 1986.
8. Gissmann L, Schwarz E: Persistence and expression of human papillomavirus DNA in genital cancer. *In* Evered D, Chard C (eds): Papillomaviruses. Chichester, UK, John Wiley & Sons, 1986, pp 190–197.
9. Howley PM: On human papillomaviruses. N Engl J Med 315:1089, 1986.
10. Reid R, Laverty CR, Coppleson M, et al: Noncondylomatous wart virus infection of the cervix. Obstet Gynecol 55:476, 1980.
11. Doorbar J, Campbell D, Grand RJA, et al: Identification of the human papillomavirus-1a *E4* gene products. EMBO J 5:355, 1986.
12. Baker CC, Howley PM: Differential promoter utilization by the bovine papillomavirus in transformed cells and productively infected wart tissues. EMBO J 6:1027, 1987.
13. Broker TR: Structure and genetic expression of papillomaviruses. Obstet Gynecol Clin North Am 14:329, 1987.
14. Baker CC, Phelps WC, Lindgren V, et al: Structural and transcriptional analysis of human papillomavirus type 16 sequences in cervical carcinoma cell lines. J Virol 61:962, 1987.
15. Matlashewski G, Schneider J, Banks L, et al: Human papillomavirus type 16 DNA cooperates with activated *ras* in transforming primary cells. EMBO J 6:1741, 1987.
16. Bedell MA, Jones KH, Laimins LA: The E6-E7 region of human papillomavirus type 18 is sufficient for transformation of NIH 3T3 and rat-1 cells. J Virol 61:3635, 1987.
17. zur Hausen H: Molecular pathogenesis of cancer of the cervix and its causation by specific HPV types. Curr Top Microbiol Immunol 186:131, 1994.
18. zur Hausen H: Disrupted dichotomous intracellular control of human papillomavirus infection in cancer of the cervix. Lancet 343:955, 1994.
19. Chen TM, Pecoraro G, Defendi V: Genetic analysis of in vitro progression of human papillomavirus–transfected human cervical cells. Cancer Res 53:1167, 1993.
20. Rösl F, Lengert M, Albrecht J, et al: Differential regulation of the *JE* gene encoding the monocyte chemoattractant protein (MCP-I) in cervical carcinoma cells and derived hybrids. J Virol 68: 2142, 1994.
21. Xiong Y, Hannon GJ, Zhang H, et al: p21 is a universal inhibitor of cyclin kinases. Nature 366:701, 1993.
22. Pfister H: Relationship of papillomaviruses to anogenital cancer. Obstet Gynecol Clin North Am 14:349, 1987.
23. Gissmann L, Wolnik L, Ikenberg H, et al: Human papillomavirus types 6 and 11 DNA sequences in genital and laryngeal papillomas and in some cervical cancers. Proc Natl Acad Sci USA 80:560, 1983.
24. Buschke A, Lowenstein L: Uber carcinomahnliche Condylomata acuminata des Penis. Arch Dermatol Syphilol 163:30, 1931.
25. Lorincz AT, Temple GF, Patterson JA, et al: Correlation of cellular atypia and human papillomavirus deoxyribonucleic acid sequences in exfoliated cells of the uterine cervix. Obstet Gynecol 68:508, 1986.
26. Lorincz AT, Temple GF, Kurman RJ, et al: Oncogenic association of specific human papillomavirus types with cervical neoplasia. J Natl Cancer Inst 79:671, 1987.
27. Campion MJ: Clinical manifestations of HPV infection. Obstet Gynecol Clin North Am 14:363, 1987.
28. Evans AS, Monaghan JM: Spontaneous resolution of cervical warty dysplasia: The relevance of clinical and nuclear DNA features, a prospective study. Br J Obstet Gynaecol 92:165, 1985.
29. Felmar E, Payton C, Smietanka M: Human papillomavirus as a risk factor for cervical cancer. Prim Care Cancer 8:11, 1988.
30. Schreier AA, Allen WP, Laughlin C, et al: Prospects for human papillomavirus vaccine and immunotherapies. J Natl Cancer Inst 80:896, 1988.
31. Sasson IM, Haley NJ, Wylander EL, et al: Cigarette smoking and neoplasia of the uterine cervix: Smoke constituents in cervical mucus. N Engl J Med 312:315, 1985.
32. Holly EA, Petrakis NL, Friend NF, et al: Mutagenic mucus in the cervix of smokers. J Natl Cancer Inst 76:983, 1986.
33. Allerding TJ, Jordan SW, Boardman RE: Association of human papillomavirus and *Chlamydia* infections with incidence of cervical neoplasia. Acta Cytol 29:653, 1985.
34. Syrjanen K, Mantyjarvi R, Vayrynen M, et al: *Chlamydia* cervicitis in women followed up for human papillomavirus (HPV) lesions of the uterine cervix. Acta Obstet Gynecol Scand 64:467, 1985.
35. zur Hausen H: Herpes simplex virus in human genital cancer. Int Rev Exp Pathol 25:307, 1983.
36. Smotkin D, Berek JS, Fu YS, et al: Human papillomavirus deoxyribonucleic acid in adenocarcinoma and adenosquamous carcinoma of the uterine cervix. Obstet Gynecol 68:241, 1986.
37. Yoshikawa H, Matsukura T, Yamamoto E: Occurrence of human papillomavirus types 16 and 18 DNA in cervical carcinomas from Japan: Age of patients and histological type of carcinomas. Jpn J Cancer Res 76:667, 1985.
38. McCance DJ, Kalache A, Ashdown K, et al: Human papillomavirus types 16 and 18 in carcinomas of the penis from Brazil. Int J Cancer 37:55, 1986.

39. Villa LL, Lopes A: Human papillomavirus DNA sequences in penile carcinomas in Brazil. Int J Cancer 37:853, 1986.
40. Oriel JD: Epidemiology of human papillomaviruses. *In* De Palo G, Rilke F, zur Hausen H (eds): Herpes and Papillomaviruses. New York, Raven Press, 1986, pp 55–61.
41. Barnett N, Mak H, Winkelstein JA: Extensive verrucosis in primary immunodeficiency diseases. Arch Dermatol 119:5, 1983.
42. Kienzler JL: Humoral immunity to human papillomaviruses. Clin Dermatol 3:144, 1985.
43. Iwatsuki K, Tagami H, Takigawa M, et al: Plane warts under spontaneous regression: Immunopathologic study of cellular constituents leading to inflammatory reaction. Arch Dermatol 122:655, 1986.
44. Jenson AB, Kurman RJ, Lancaster WB: Tissue effects of and host response to human papillomavirus infection. Obstet Gynecol Clin North Am 14:397, 1987.
45. Douglas JM, Rogers M, Judson FN: The effect of asymptomatic infection with HTLV-III on the response of the anogenital warts to intralesional treatment with recombinant α_2-interferon. J Infect Dis 154:331, 1986.
46. Evans CA, Ito Y: Antitumor immunity in the Shope papilloma-carcinoma complex III. Responses to reinfection with viral nucleic acid. J Natl Cancer Inst 36:1161, 1966.
47. Evans CA, Gorman LR, Ito Y, et al: Antitumor immunity in the Shope papilloma-carcinoma complex of rabbits. I. Papilloma regression induced by homologous and autologous tissue vaccines. J Natl Cancer Inst 29:277, 1962.
48. Walker PG, Colley NV, Grubb C, et al: Abnormalities of the uterine cervix in women with vulvar warts. Br J Vener Dis 59:120, 1983.
49. Reid R: Superficial laser vulvectomy I. The efficacy of extended superficial ablation for refractory and very extensive condylomas. J Obstet Gynecol 151:1047, 1985.
50. Ray B: Condyloma acuminatum of the bladder. J Urol 117:739, 1977.
51. Lorincz AT: Detection of human papillomavirus infection by nucleic acid hybridization. Obstet Gynecol Clin North Am 14:451, 1987.
52. Ferenczy A, Mitao M, Nagai N, et al: Latent papillomavirus and recurrent genital warts. N Engl J Med 313:784, 1985.
53. von Krogh G: Condylomata acuminata 1983: An updated review. Semin Dermatol 2:109, 1983.
54. Jenson SL: Comparison of podophyllin applications with simple surgical excision in clearance and recurrence of perianal condylomata acuminata. Lancet 2:1146, 1985.
55. Krebs HB: The use of topical 5-fluorouracil in the treatment of genital condylomas. Obstet Gynecol Clin North Am 14:537, 1987.
56. Ferenczy A: Comparison of 5-fluorouracil and CO_2 laser for treatment of vaginal condylomata. Obstet Gynecol 64:773, 1985.
57. Sillman FH, Sedlis A: Anogenital papillomavirus infections and neoplasia in immunodeficient women. Obstet Gynecol Clin North Am 14:537, 1987.
58. Bashi SA: Cryotherapy versus podophyllin in the treatment of genital warts. Int J Dermatol 24:535, 1985.
59. Simmons PD, Langlet F, Thin RNT: Cryotherapy versus electrocautery in the treatment of genital warts. Br J Vener Dis 57:273, 1981.
60. Billingham RP, Lewis FG: Laser versus electrical cautery in the treatment of condylomata acuminata of the anus. Surg Gynecol Obstet 155:865, 1982.
60a. Eron LJ, Edwards L, Ferenezy A, et al: Treatment of genital warts with imiquimod cream. Clin Infect Dis 21:783, 1995.
61. Eron LJ, Judson F, Tucker S, et al: Interferon therapy for condylomata acuminata. N Engl J Med 315:1059, 1986.
62. Vance JC, Bart BJ, Hansen RC, et al: International recombinant α_2-interferon for the treatment of patients with condyloma acuminatum or verruca plantaris. Arch Dermatol 122:272, 1986.
63. Friedman-Kien AE, Eron LJ, Conant M, et al: Natural interferon-α for treatment of condylomata acuminata. JAMA 259:533, 1988.
64. Gall SA, Hughes CE, Trofatter K: Interferon for the therapy of condyloma acuminatum. Am J Obstet Gynecol 153:157, 1985.
65. Schonfeld A, Schattner A, Crespi M, et al: Intramuscular human interferon-β injections in treatment of condylomata acuminata. Lancet 1:1038, 1984.
66. Kirby PK, Kiviat N, Beckman A, et al: Tolerance and efficacy of recombinant human interferon-γ in the treatment of refractory genital warts. Am J Med 85:183, 1988.
67. Pilacinski WP, Glass DL, Glassman KF, et al: Development of a recombinant DNA vaccine against bovine papillomavirus infection in cattle. *In* Howley PM, Broker TR (eds): Papillomaviruses: Molecular and Clinical Aspects. New York, Alan R Liss, 1985, pp 247–272.

GYNECOLOGY AND OBSTETRICS

116

Approach to the Patient with Infection of the Pelvis

William J. Ledger

The toughest aspect of a physician's care of a woman with a pelvic infection is making a diagnosis, because signs and symptoms are vague and the cause is usually not obvious. Diagnosis is not automatic[1] (Table 116–1). For example, less than half of women whose acute salpingitis is confirmed by laparoscopy are febrile,[1] so the traditional logic that equates fever with this bacterial infection does not apply in women with pelvic inflammatory disease. In addition, the problems of diagnosis do not end with physical signs and symptoms. To aid in the diagnosis of pelvic infections, the laboratory

TABLE 116–1 ■ Classic Signs and Laboratory Findings of Salpingitis Observed in Women with a Laparoscopic Diagnosis of Salpingitis Compared with Women with Normal Pelvic Findings

CLINICAL AND LABORATORY FINDINGS	% WITH SALPINGITIS	% WITH NORMAL FINDINGS	STATISTICALLY SIGNIFICANT
Acute pelvic pain	94	94	No
Fever (temperature higher than 38°C)	32.9	14.1	Yes
Tender adnexal swelling or mass	49.5	24.5	Yes
Elevated erythrocyte sedimentation rate	75.9	52.7	Yes

From Jacobson L, Westrom L: Objectivized diagnosis of acute pelvic inflammatory disease. Diagnostic and prognostic value of routine laparoscopy. Am J Obstet Gynecol 105:1088–1098, 1969.

testing ordered by the physician must be selective.[2] This varies from the common mode of care in the United States before the economic restrictions brought about by such practice trends as diagnosis-related groups and health maintenance organizations. The old mode, in which a physician orders a battery of tests for comprehensive screening of a patient, is no longer acceptable economically. Medically, this is the case as well. A plethora of tests for a suspected pelvic infection may not be helpful; in fact, improper interpretation of standard microbiologic test results often confounds the diagnosis. Thus, accurate diagnosis of pelvic infections requires careful evaluation of the patient and the use of a limited number of relevant laboratory tests, results of which are most accurate when they are performed immediately by the physician.

An accurate initial diagnosis is the best basis for appropriate therapy. It is also important because once empirical antibiotic therapy begins, signs and symptoms are modified and the site of infection is rendered much more obscure.[3]

History

To obtain a relevant history from a patient suspected of having a pelvic infection, the physician's attitude must be friendly and open to put the patient at ease. A woman whose symptoms are important enough for her to seek medical care will be alert to the physician's body language or to a dismissive tone of voice. These women deserve the same consideration and attention to the detail of care as a patient with chest pain receives.

The patient should be permitted the freedom to describe her problem in her own words. The physician should not be in a hurry to arrive at a diagnosis. Questioning should progress at the patient's own pace and without interruption (Table 116–2). The physician can begin the interview by asking, Why are you here? Subsequently, questions can be employed to expand the patient's response in a nonjudgmental manner, for example, When did the problem begin? How does it bother you? Sometimes the patient recalls a specific event that will be helpful to the diagnosis. The patient can be prompted to expand her description, if it is necessary to clarify the problem. If the patient's problem is a discharge, is she aware of an odor? Is this what is bothering her? If so, what is she doing about it? If symptoms are related to her menstrual cycle, it can be a hint to the physician of some forms of vaginitis or salpingitis.

Most pelvic infections occur in sexually active women. Information about sexual activity must be sought without implying that any type of sexual activity is bad and that infection is a just punishment for the patient's transgressions. For a woman to be ill is not a crime. The questioning should be matter-of-fact and open, for example, Are you involved with anyone? An affirmative reply allows the physician to explore methods of contraception, which can help delineate some types of infection.

The end point of the initial interview occurs when the physician fully understands the reasons for the patient's visit. The entire interview process should be the patient's unrestricted exposé of problems and not the physician's checklist to fit the patient into a preordained diagnostic category.

TABLE 116–2 ■ Key Discussion Points in the Initial Patient Interview

Why are you here?
When did the problem begin?
How does it bother you?
Are you involved with anyone?

Physical Examination

All women should receive a general examination. Assessment of vital signs is important. In most women who have a pelvic infection, vital signs are usually normal, although some who have salpingitis have fever, and low blood pressure may indicate a seriously ill patient with septic shock. The remainder of the general examination is important because another pathologic process can be present that is not related to the symptoms that prompted the visit to the physician. Obstetrician-gynecologists can find breast lumps, a thyroid nodule, or a heart murmur that may be asymptomatic but nevertheless will require medical evaluation.

The focus of any physician's evaluation for pelvic infection is the pelvic examination. Anything less than this in an initial work-up is inadequate care for the patient. An adequate examination requires a table with stirrups, proper lighting, working equipment, and an assistant to aid the physician in the examination. The array of equipment needed is neither extensive nor expensive. It includes, at the least, a magnifying glass to evaluate lesions; 4% acetic acid to stain the vulva to delineate areas for biopsy; local anesthesia solution (1% lidocaine); a 25-gauge needle syringe; forceps; fine scissors for the biopsy; Monsel solution for hemostasis of the biopsy sites; slides and a microscope; saline solution; 10% potassium hydroxide; a strip of pH paper; and appropriate culture media for herpesvirus, *Chlamydia trachomatis*, *Neisseria gonorrhoeae*, and *Candida albicans*. More intricate equipment that will be helpful in some cases includes a colposcope and a vaginal ultrasound probe.

The pelvic examination should be unhurried and directed by the patient's history. The goal should be a complete evaluation without causing the patient discomfort. The key is to inform the patient of every step of the examination. The assistant should drape the sheets in such a way that the patient can see the physician, if she desires.

Examination of the vulva is guided by symptoms. If the patient has a "sore," the location should be pinpointed by the physician. If there is a painful lesion, material is obtained for culture for herpesvirus. Blood antibody studies for herpesvirus are sometimes not immediately helpful in the evaluation of a patient with a lesion; results can be negative in a patient with primary genital herpes or positive in a patient who does not have genital herpes but has had cold sores in her mouth in the past. A positive culture for herpesvirus confirms the diagnosis. However, one study showed that antibody testing is more sensitive than the culture in diagnosing genital herpes.[4] There are other diagnostic problems. Some women have what appear to be condylomata acuminata; biopsy of these should be done to confirm the diagnosis. If a woman complains of point tenderness at the introitus with sexual penetration or the insertion of a tampon, the site of discomfort should be sought with a cotton swab. Vestibular adenitis is manifested by a focal tenderness. Pressure with a swab produces excruciating pain.

The examination of the vagina begins with an unlubricated speculum; this prevents difficulties if pH evaluation or cultures are necessary. Tap water can be alkaline, and lubricants have antibacterial substances present. If the complaint is vaginal discharge, the extent and the quality of the discharge can usually be noted by the physician. Most gynecologic textbooks characterize the vaginal discharges associated with *C. albicans* vulvovaginitis and *Trichomonas vaginalis* vaginitis. These clinical entities are seldom that specific, and first impressions are often wrong. To avoid diagnostic errors, the clinician must do a number of quick diagnostic tests, each of which is accomplished in seconds, the results of which can point to the diagnosis.

The test for vaginal pH is important; the sample should be

from the side walls of the vagina, not from the endocervix, which is usually alkaline. The vaginal pH is normally less than 4.5 with *Candida* vaginitis, whereas it is usually higher in *T. vaginalis* vaginitis and bacterial vaginosis. The physician should smell the potassium hydroxide slide when vaginal secretions are added. An unpleasant fishy amine odor is common with bacterial vaginosis or *Trichomonas* vaginitis. The hanging drop preparation of saline and 10% potassium hydroxide should be examined microscopically. Trichomonads can usually be easily identified in the saline preparation; they are motile, and the beating flagella can be seen under high-power magnification. Clue cells have a characteristic appearance, with a speckled cytoplasm of the squamous epithelial cells and a serrated cell surface. To confirm the diagnosis of bacterial vaginosis, they should be present in large numbers and white blood cells should be virtually absent from the field.

The microscopic examination to confirm the diagnosis of *Candida* vaginitis is the most difficult, because the yeast elements are often not seen. This is the one common disorder of the vagina for which culture is helpful. Culture will propagate *Candida* organisms far more often than they can be detected by scanning hanging drop preparations for hyphae and mycelia.[5] This is especially important in patients with a chronic vaginal problem. Patients should not be subjected to long-term treatment for *Candida* infection unless the organisms are grown in culture. This does not meet their therapeutic needs, and too often women will develop a vaginal reaction caused by local sensitivity to the propylene glycol present in most vaginal creams and suppositories.

A number of diagnostic hints can be helpful in some patients with vaginitis. Because the presenting sign for salpingitis can be an abnormal vaginal discharge, cervical culture for *C. trachomatis* and *N. gonorrhoeae* is appropriate when the physician suspects this possibility; however, all vaginal cultures should propagate bacteria, because the vagina has a diverse bacterial flora, similar in variety to that of the lower bowel, with much smaller numbers of bacteria.[6] A positive bacterial culture should not automatically be equated with disease. The most harmful therapeutic interventions that I have seen over the years involve antibiotic treatment of patients because cultures of vaginal material grew an organism, for example, *Escherichia coli*. Treating a nonexistent entity, *E. coli* vaginitis, often results in antibiotic-induced *Candida* vaginitis and, in some cases, an allergic reaction to the antibiotics. Vaginitis must not be treated with antibiotics if the pathogen is not known. The patient will not get better, and the physician can cause harm.

Finally, if the patient complains of persistent vaginal burning with no definitive findings on pH, microscopic, or culture studies, consideration should be given to the possibility of allergic vaginitis[7] or vaginal flat warts due to papillomavirus.[8] Allergic vaginitis can be suspected if the patient can relate her vaginal symptoms to specific exposures, such as vaginal antifungal cream, vaginal spermicidal agents, or male ejaculate.[7] Witkin and colleagues[9] demonstrated the presence of immunoglobulin E antibodies and an increased number of eosinophils in the vaginal fluid of such women. If flat warts are suspected, colposcopic examination with acetic acid staining and biopsy with histologic preparation and DNA probes can be employed to make the diagnosis. I like the use of DNA probes, because there is often no agreement among pathologists about the microscopic diagnosis of condyloma. A positive finding with a DNA probe confirms the impression. A negative finding with a DNA probe does not rule out the possibility of a human papillomavirus infection, because the currently available probe tests only for a minority of the human papillomavirus strains.

For patients with a chronic vaginal problem, a Gram stain examination of vaginal secretions is useful. It provides a permanent record of the initial cytologic findings and a standard for comparison during follow-up. In addition, culture for *T. vaginalis* is in order when there is persistent vaginal discharge but microscopic and culture findings are normal. Small numbers of trichomonads may not be seen by a hanging drop microscopic examination but can be detected by culture.[2]

The cervix is the next site of evaluation. The gross visual evaluation of the cervix can be subject to misinterpretation. A large area of columnar epithelium on the surface can look inflamed and can bleed easily when a Papanicolaou smear specimen is obtained, a picture that many physicians equate with cervicitis. The best diagnostic aid is a cotton-tipped applicator gently rotated in the endocervical canal and then examined against a white background. Mucopus will be grossly evident, which confirms the clinical diagnosis of cervicitis.[10] It is especially important to perform this examination of the cervix when many white blood cells are seen in the vaginal smear. For example, large numbers of white blood cells should not be present on the vaginal smear of a patient with bacterial vaginosis. When they are, the physician should remember that it is possible for a patient to have two concurrent conditions, bacterial vaginosis and cervicitis. A cotton swab examination confirms the clinical diagnosis of cervicitis. In patients with cervicitis, endocervical cultures for *N. gonorrhoeae* and *C. trachomatis* should be done. To confirm *Chlamydia*, the "gold standard" in the past has been propagation of organisms in a tissue culture system. Most clinical laboratories have neither the facilities nor the personnel to do this. An alternative is the antigen detection system. Fluorescein-tagged species-specific monoclonal antibodies determine elementary bodies in the cellular material, or *Chlamydia* antigen can be detected in an eluted sample from a swab by using an enzyme immunoassay. The advantage of these tests is that they are easy to perform. Given the choice, all laboratory directors will pick this type of testing over tissue culture. The disadvantage is that they are not as sensitive or specific as a tissue culture. This means that some women with a *C. trachomatis* infection will not be diagnosed, and some women will be test-positive who are not infected. Newer, more sensitive tests are now available. The polymerase chain reaction is more sensitive than tissue culture for it can detect the presence of a small number of organisms that would not be detected by culture.[11] There are other tests being used in scientific studies. The persistence of *C. trachomatis* DNA has been verified by in situ hybridization or immunoperoxidase stain tests in women who have received what is considered to be an adequate antibiotic treatment regimen for *C. trachomatis* infection.[12] The significance of this observation will be the subject of many subsequent clinical studies.

The pelvic examination is difficult in a postoperative patient. There is a great deal of pelvic induration after pelvic surgery and usually no purulent discharge. This examination begins with the speculum. If the uterus is present, as it is after vaginal delivery or cesarean section, pregnancy termination, or myomectomy, the cervical os should be evaluated for the presence of purulent discharge or tissue. A ring forceps should be placed in the endocervical canal to determine the presence of and to remove retained placental tissue or membranes; a double-lumen culture device is employed for culture of facultative and anaerobic organisms.[13] The double-lumen technique is used to minimize the chances of endocervical contamination. Vaginal probe ultrasonography is being increasingly employed to determine the presence of retained tissue in the uterus. In the posthysterectomy patient, the vaginal cuff should be probed for purulent material. Some authors have described tortuous pelvic veins in a patient with septic pelvic thrombophlebitis, but I have never been impressed with my ability to do this clinically.[14] For me, this has been a diagnosis of exclusion in a patient who remains febrile after antibiotic treatment and has no evidence of a pelvic abscess. It is difficult by clinical examination to determine the presence or the site of a postoperative pelvic abscess because of the pelvic induration and tenderness present in all postoperative patients. Again, ultrasound examination is an excellent screening method because it can demonstrate the presence of fluid-filled masses. Better delineation of pelvic disease can be achieved with magnetic resonance imaging or computed tomography.

When salpingitis is suspected, the evaluation can be extremely important in making the diagnosis. The key to any evaluation is gentleness. Forceful pressure at the time of pelvic examination can cause pain and even more so when the pelvic viscera are inflamed because of infection. The physician's focus should be to determine whether there is adnexal tenderness or a mass. If pain is elicited and there is no pelvic mass, more forceful pressure to palpate the ovaries simply causes more pain without gaining any additional diagnostic information. Other important diagnostic studies should be obtained for these women. The least invasive and probably the most helpful is microscopic examination of a vaginal smear. Westrom[15] has stated that he has never found salpingitis confirmed by laparoscopy when there was not a large number of white blood cells on the vaginal smear. Clearly, white blood cells can be present in a patient with cervicitis, but this simple noninvasive test is especially helpful for confirming the diagnosis. If white blood cells are absent, causes other than infection should be searched for to determine the diagnosis. Culture material should be obtained from the endocervix for *N. gonorrhoeae* and *C. trachomatis*. Polymerase chain reaction should be used as the screen for *C. trachomatis*. Either simple culture or a DNA probe can be used for *N. gonorrhoeae*. Culdocentesis is a potentially valuable diagnostic technique. White blood cells and bacteria are not normally present in peritoneal fluid; when they are, they indicate peritoneal inflammation and infection. Monif[16] used this test as part of his ESP (endometritis, salpingitis, peritonitis) classification scheme of pelvic infection. Peritonitis was diagnosed when purulent material was recovered by culdocentesis. The biggest problem is the pain associated with the procedure. I have never had a patient on whom I performed culdocentesis allow me to do another one. Because of this, I try to be selective with this diagnostic approach. For the afebrile patient with minimal pelvic pain, white blood cells in a vaginal smear, and cervicitis, culdocentesis can be helpful in pinpointing the diagnosis. This should be performed after a gentle preliminary examination confirms an anteflexed uterus and no cul-de-sac masses. This invasive technique should be done without using a tenaculum, and the physician is limited to one attempt at needle insertion to limit pain. The widespread use of vaginal probe ultrasonography and needle guidance to obtain ova will probably spill over into gynecologic practice in the next decade and become a part of this diagnostic intervention. Ultrasonography has the advantage of confirming the presence of cul-de-sac fluid before a decision is made to insert the needle. Any fluid obtained should be examined under the microscope. White blood cells and bacteria are not normally present in these smears. Imaging techniques can be helpful in some patients. For patients who have a great deal of pain, a screening ultrasound examination can demonstrate a fluid-filled mass that cannot be detected by the pelvic examination. In many patients with pelvic pain, an adnexal pregnancy sac can be detected. Obviously, an ectopic pregnancy should not be treated with antibiotics. If the physician elicits a history of intravenous drug use by this patient or her sexual partner, blood should be drawn to screen for hepatitis B virus. If the patient agrees, blood should also be drawn to test for human immunodeficiency virus antibody.

This is an outline of the general approach to the patient with a pelvic infection. It emphasizes a hands-on evaluation because this skill yields the most accurate diagnosis.

References

1. Jacobson L, Westrom L: Objectivized diagnosis of acute pelvic inflammatory disease. Am J Obstet Gynecol 105:1088, 1969.
2. Eschenbach DA, Hillier SL: Advances in diagnostic testing for vaginitis and cervicitis. J Reprod Med 34:555, 1989.
3. Galask RP, Ohm MJ: Bacterial flora and mycotic infection of the vagina and cervix in posthysterectomy patients. Mykosen Suppl 1:236, 1978.
4. Koutsky LA, Stevens CE, Holmes KK, et al: Underdiagnosis of genital herpes by current clinical and viral-isolation procedures. N Engl J Med 326:1533, 1992.
5. McCormack WM, Starke KM, Zinner SH: Symptoms associated with vaginal colonization with yeast. Am J Obstet Gynecol 158:31, 1988.
6. Bartlett JG, Onderdonk AB, Drude E, et al: Quantitative bacteriology of the vaginal flora. J Infect Dis 136:271, 1977.
7. Witkin SS: Immunology of recurrent vaginitis. Am J Reprod Immunol Microbiol 15:34, 1987.
8. Spitzer M, Krumholz BA, Seltzer VL: The multicentric nature of disease related to human papillomavirus of the female lower genital tract. Obstet Gynecol 73:303, 1989.
9. Witkin SS, Jeremias J, Ledger WJ: Vaginal eosinophils and IgE antibodies to *Candida albicans* in women with recurrent vaginitis. J Med Vet Mycol 27:57, 1989.
10. Branham RC, Paavonen J, Stevens CE, et al: Mucopurulent cervicitis: The ignored counterpart in women of urethritis in men. N Engl J Med 311:1, 1984.
11. Witkin SS, Jeremias J, Toth M, Ledger WJ: Detection of *Chlamydia trachomatis* by the polymerase chain reaction in the cervices of women with acute salpingitis. Am J Obstet Gynecol 168:1438, 1993.
12. Patton DL, Askienazy-Elbhar M, Henry-Suchet J, et al: Detection of *Chlamydia trachomatis* in fallopian tube tissue in women with post-infectious tubal infertility. Am J Obstet Gynecol 171:95, 1994.
13. Eschenbach DA, Rosene K, Tompkins LS, et al: Endometrial cultures obtained by a triple-lumen method from afebrile postpartum women. J Infect Dis 153:1038, 1986.
14. Ledger WJ, Peterson EP: The use of heparin in the management of pelvic thrombophlebitis. Surg Gynecol Obstet 131:1115, 1970.
15. Westrom L: Clinical manifestation and diagnosis of pelvic inflammatory disease. J Reprod Med 28:703, 1983.
16. Monif GRG: Clinical staging of acute bacterial salpingitis and its therapeutic ramifications. Am J Obstet Gynecol 143:489, 1982.

117

Pelvic Inflammatory Disease and Tuboovarian Abscess

Richard L. Sweet

PELVIC INFLAMMATORY DISEASE

Among women, pelvic inflammatory disease (PID) is a major public health concern and the most common serious complication of the current epidemic of sexually transmitted diseases. It is estimated that 1 million women receive treatment for PID annually in the United States,[1–4] some 250,000 to 300,000 of whom are hospitalized.[5] However, from 1979 to 1988, hospitalization rates for PID decreased 36% from 3.5 to 2.2 hospitalizations per 1000 women.[6] The economic costs of PID and PID-associated ectopic pregnancy and infertility in the United States are estimated to be more than $4.2 billion in 1990 and more than $9 billion by 2000.[7]

Of more concern than the infection itself is that at least one of every four women who develop PID suffers serious long-term sequelae—infertility, ectopic pregnancy, tuboovarian abscess (TOA), pyosalpinx, chronic pelvic pain, or pelvic adhesive disease.[8] Approximately 20% are rendered infertile, and their risk for ectopic pregnancy increases 7- to 10-fold. Both risks increase with recurrences. TOA, the major early complication of acute PID, is diagnosed in 10% to 15% of patients hospitalized for treatment of acute PID. Last, nearly 20% of affected women develop symptoms of chronic pelvic adhesive disease.

To reduce these debilitating medical and economic consequences, we must improve our methods of prevention, detection, and treatment. Efforts to this end have been hindered by several factors. First, the clinical criteria of PID are imprecise; a lack of consensus among experts leaves clinicians with a diagnostic dilemma. Second, the major site of infection, the fallopian tube, is relatively inaccessible to culture, so the agent may not be identifiable. Finally, the polymicrobial nature of the infection confounds determination of the sequence of events and relative contributions of various organisms, including *Neisseria gonorrhoeae*, *Chlamydia trachomatis*, bacterial vaginosis–associated organisms, anaerobic and facultative bacteria, and other pathogens such as the genital mycoplasmas. Even some viruses, such as herpes simplex virus and cytomegalovirus, could play a role in PID.

Epidemiology

Considerable effort has been invested in research on predisposing factors for acute salpingitis. Women who have a history of acute salpingitis or PID are at increased risk for recurrences of PID. Westrom[9] noted that nearly one in four women with PID suffers a subsequent episode. A strong association exists between sexually transmitted pathogens, especially *N. gonorrhoeae* and *C. trachomatis*, and acute PID; women with a history of these sexually transmitted diseases are at increased risk for PID. Women with multiple sexual partners were found to be nearly five times more likely to develop PID than were monogamous women.[10] Jossens and colleagues[11] have reported that women with two or more sexual partners in the previous 30 to 60 days were at significantly increased risk for PID. In contradistinction, these authors noted that having multiple lifetime partners was not a risk factor for acute PID.[11]

Young age has also been associated with an increased frequency of PID. Westrom[9] reported that nearly 70% of women with acute salpingitis were 25 years of age or younger and that 33% had their first infection before age 19 years. Sexually active adolescents are three times more likely to develop PID than are 25- to 29-year-old women.[12] Indeed, among the group aged 13 to 15 years, this risk is increased 10-fold. It is thought that this dramatic risk is due to the high prevalence of sexually transmitted diseases among adolescents; to multiple sexual partners; and to failure to use contraceptives, several of which (condom, diaphragm, oral contraceptives) protect against PID. The intrauterine device (IUD) is an additional risk factor in the development of acute salpingitis. Initially, it was estimated that IUD users have a threefold to fivefold greater risk for developing PID.[12–16] Later studies have lowered this risk to a twofold to threefold increase compared with women who use no contraception. A syndrome of progressive endometritis has been associated with IUD use; menorrhagia, metrorrhagia, and leukorrhea were noted and were followed by progressive endometritis, parametritis, peritonitis, and pelvic abscess formation.[17] The IUD tail has been implicated as a potential mechanism by which bacteria ascend from lower to upper genital tract.[18] Animal studies have noted that the multifilament tails, especially ones that were frayed, are associated with higher bacterial counts in the endometrial cavity than is the monofilament tail.[19] The IUD itself interferes with host defense mechanisms (much as other foreign bodies do) within the uterine cavity to allow establishment of an upper genital tract infection. Oral contraceptives appear not only to protect against the development of PID but also to ameliorate the disease when it occurs, and patients who develop PID while taking them have a better prognosis for future fertility than do those using any other type of contraception or none.[20]

Bacterial vaginosis, a perturbation in which the lactobacilli-predominant normal vaginal microflora is replaced by high concentrations of *Gardnerella vaginalis*, anaerobic bacteria, and *Mycoplasma hominis*, has been shown to be a risk factor for acute PID.[21–25] The anaerobic organisms associated with bacterial vaginosis include *Prevotella* species, *Mobiluncus*, and peptostreptococci. Interestingly, Amsel and coworkers[25] demonstrated an association between IUD use and bacterial vaginosis, which may explain the role of IUD use as a risk factor for PID.

Etiology

Although research in the last 20 years has provided many insights into the causation of acute PID, the exact involvement and spread of organisms and the interaction between different organisms remain unknown.

Neisseria gonorrhoeae Infection

Salpingitis was traditionally categorized as gonococcal or nongonococcal, but this distinction has become outdated.

Initial work that employed cervical cultures to identify the pathogen revealed *N. gonorrhoeae* in a significant proportion of women with PID. Studies that used endocervical cultures identified *N. gonorrhoeae* in 33% to 81% of women with PID.[10, 26–30] Except for the presence of *N. gonorrhoeae* or *C. trachomatis*, cervical flora of women with acute salpingitis is not appreciably different from that of normal women.[31] That comparisons of organisms obtained by culdocentesis or laparoscopy with endocervical canal specimens have shown poor correlation suggests that cervical flora is not representative of the tubal flora of PID.[27–34]

Culdocentesis, laparoscopy, and sophisticated methods of anaerobe isolation have enabled investigators to identify a variety of aerobic and anaerobic bacteria from the peritoneal cavity of women with PID.[27, 29–33] The majority of these patients had a positive result on endocervical culture for *N. gonorrhoeae*. Interestingly, approximately one third had only *N. gonorrhoeae* in the abdominal cavity; another third had *N. gonorrhoeae* plus aerobes and anaerobes; and the remaining third had only aerobes and anaerobes (Table 117–1).

These studies confirmed the polymicrobial nature of PID. Still, the site of optimal organism retrieval was not known. Sweet and coworkers[32] compared cultures of specimens from culdocentesis and fallopian tube and found that the former frequently appeared to be contaminated by vaginal flora and so were unreliable. Results of subsequent comparisons of cultures of cul-de-sac fluid and tubal material were similar, lending further credence to the idea that retrieving culture specimens by the transvaginal route was unsatisfactory.[32] The unreliability of culdocentesis has been confirmed by Soper and colleagues.[35]

Two theories emerged to explain the pathogenesis of PID. The first proposed that either *N. gonorrhoeae* or *C. trachomatis* organisms initiate the process by producing tissue damage and changing the normal environment, allowing superinfection by aerobes and anaerobes from the cervix and vagina.[30, 31, 33] The second hypothesis is that PID must be a polymicrobial infection from the outset.[10, 32] Support for this hypothesis comes from studies that demonstrate the presence of aerobes and anaerobes in the fallopian tubes of women with salpingitis despite the absence of *N. gonorrhoeae* and *C. trachomatis*, even in the endocervix.[34]

To solve this problem, Sweet and coworkers[34] determined the chronologic variation in organisms involved in PID. *N. gonorrhoeae* organisms were recovered from the endocervix of 50% of PID patients and from the fallopian tubes of only 23%. Anaerobes were the organisms most commonly isolated from fallopian tube cultures. When these data were broken down into length of time from symptom onset, a pattern was suggested. *N. gonorrhoeae* organisms were isolated from the fallopian tubes of 70% of women whose cultures were inoculated within the first 24 hours of clinical infection, and the percentage steadily decreased as time progressed. Only 19% of cultures started after 48 hours propagated *N. gonorrhoeae*. The percentage of anaerobes was inversely proportional to that of *N. gonorrhoeae*.

The most widely held theory for the pathogenesis of *N. gonorrhoeae* in PID is that the pathogen gains access to the upper genital tract at or near the end of menses through the breakdown of local host defense mechanisms at the level of the cervix and can then spread directly to the adnexae. Between 66% and 75% of women with PID develop symptoms at the end of or just after menstruation.[36] Similarly, Sweet and coworkers[37] demonstrated that PID associated with *C. trachomatis* occurs at the end of or shortly after the menstrual period, with no cases of chlamydial PID noted after day 14 of the menstrual cycle.

Certain subsets of *N. gonorrhoeae* are thought to be more aggressive and have been found frequently to be associated with upper genital tract infections. Certain auxotypes (varied nutritional requirements), phenotypes, and serotypes have been incriminated and studied in great detail.[38–42] It has also been postulated that *N. gonorrhoeae* produces a lipopolysaccharide that causes a local toxic effect on the tubal epithelium, resulting in loss of cilia.[43]

Chlamydia trachomatis *Infection*

C. trachomatis infection is the most common sexually transmitted disease in the United States. Initially, it appeared to be more common in Scandinavia, where the organism was recovered from cervical cultures in 20% to 50% of patients with acute salpingitis[44–47] and from fallopian tube cultures in 30%.[44, 45, 47] Initial studies in the United States failed to identify *C. trachomatis* as a major putative agent in acute PID.[26, 27, 29, 32] However, serologic studies in Seattle and San Francisco demonstrated a fourfold rise in serum antibody titer in 20% to 23% of PID patients,[27, 32] suggesting that the organism was important in the United States as well. One possible reason for this discrepancy is that patients in the Scandinavian studies included many with milder forms of infection who might have been treated as outpatients in the United States, whereas the U.S. studies included only hospitalized patients. Patients with chlamydial salpingitis often have a milder clinical presentation, despite a higher erythrocyte sedimentation rate and more inflammation, resulting in more tubal damage.[48] More U.S. investigations have clearly demonstrated that *C. trachomatis* is a principal agent in acute PID and can be recovered from the upper genital tract of roughly 20% to 40% of patients with acute disease.[49, 50] Moreover, as Sweet's group noted, failure to provide antimicrobial coverage for chlamydiae results in persistent chlamydial infection in the upper genital tract despite supposed clinical cure.[49]

Additional evidence that *C. trachomatis* plays a role in acute salpingitis is indirect. Evaluation of infertile patients by hysterosalpingogram revealed that 91% of those whose

TABLE 117–1 ■ Isolation of *Neisseria gonorrhoeae* and Anaerobic and Facultative Bacteria from Patients with Acute Salpingitis

			CULDOCENTESIS		
STUDY	NUMBER OF PATIENTS	ENDOCERVICAL *N. GONORRHOEAE* (%)	*N. GONORRHOEAE* ONLY (%)	*N. gonorrhoeae* Plus Anaerobes/Facultatives (%)	Anaerobes/Facultatives Only (%)
Sweet et al[32]	26	50	31	31	31
Eschenbach et al[27]	54	39	28	5	24
Thompson et al[29]	30	80	21	21	58
Cunningham et al[30]	104	54	22	32	46
Chow et al[31]	20	65	0	5	90
Monif et al[33]	17	94	31	31	38

findings were abnormal also had a positive result on serologic tests for chlamydiae, compared with only 50% of women with normal radiographic findings.[51] Henry-Suchet and coworkers[52] noted that 50% of infertility patients undergoing surgery for repair of tubal obstruction tested positive for chlamydiae, but only 18% of control subjects did. Serologic studies have revealed that tubal factor infertility patients were two to three times more likely to have antichlamydia immunoglobulin G antibody than were control patients.[53, 54] Similarly, women with ruptured ectopic pregnancies have been shown to be significantly more likely to have serologic evidence of prior chlamydial infection than are matched intrauterine pregnancy control subjects.[55–64] Thus, the two major sequelae of acute PID have been associated with previous chlamydial infection.

Animal studies have also demonstrated the effect of chlamydial infection in producing tubal damage.[65–68] Swenson and coworkers[68] infected mouse fallopian tubes with *C. trachomatis*, recovered organisms from infected tissue for 3 weeks, noted that approximately 50% developed hydrosalpinges, and documented a high rate of subsequent infertility.

Mycoplasma hominis Infection

M. hominis has also been postulated to be a potential pathogen in PID, although the data are soft. Whereas a large percentage of women with acute salpingitis have antibodies against *M. hominis*, the organism is infrequently recovered from tubal and peritoneal fluid cultures from these women with PID.[69] Experimentation using tubal organ cultures has recorded decreased cilial activity after infection with this agent, but no cytopathic effect has yet been demonstrated.[70] Work has demonstrated that *M. hominis* is present in association with bacterial vaginosis.[25] Thus, any role that *M. hominis* might have in the etiology of acute PID is probably related to its presence in the microflora of bacterial vaginosis.

Infection with Anaerobic and Facultative Bacteria

Facultative and anaerobic bacteria are often isolated from fallopian tube and cul-de-sac cultures of women with PID.[26, 33, 49, 50] Those most often recovered are *Peptostreptococcus*, *Prevotella* (formerly *Bacteroides*) species, *Escherichia coli*, *G. vaginalis*, and facultative streptococci (Table 117–2). These organisms are commonly found in the lower genital tract, so whether they function initially as direct pathogens or whether they require the presence of an initiating organism such as *N. gonorrhoeae* or *C. trachomatis* remains controversial. Studies reporting the results of cultures obtained from the upper genital tract of patients with acute PID are summarized in Table 117–3. In these studies, mixed anaerobic and aerobic bacteria were the most commonly recovered group of organisms.[71–73] In a report, Jossens and colleagues[11] noted that in nearly one third of acute PID cases, only anaerobic and/or aerobic bacteria were recovered from the upper genital tract. In addition, among the 65% of acute PID patients with *N. gonorrhoeae* or *C. trachomatis* present, half also had anaerobic or aerobic bacteria recovered.[11] The anaerobes are worrisome in that the *Prevotella* group produce β-lactamase enzymes and are thus resistant to many antibiotics, including penicillin, ampicillin, and first-generation cephalosporins. In human fallopian tube organ cultures, *Bacteroides fragilis* has proved more destructive to tubal epithelium than has *N. gonorrhoeae*; extensive damage is generated within 4 days of infection.[74] These bacteria have also been implicated in the development of TOA in both humans and animal models.[75]

TABLE 117–2 ■ Bacteria Frequently Recovered from the Upper Genital Tract of Women with Acute Salpingitis

ANAEROBES	AEROBES
Prevotella bivia	*Gardnerella vaginalis*
Prevotella species	*Escherichia coli*
Peptostreptococcus species	Nonhemolytic streptococci
	Group B streptococci

TABLE 117–3 ■ Recovery of Microorganisms from the Upper Genital Tract of Women with Acute Pelvic Inflammatory Disease

	NUMBER (%) OF POSITIVE CULTURES		
INVESTIGATION	*Chlamydia trachomatis*	*Neisseria gonorrhoea*	Anaerobes and Facultatives
Brunham et al[71]	21 (40%)	8 (16%)	10 (20%)
Heinonen et al[72]	7 (19%)	15 (42%)	28 (78%)
Paavonen et al[21]	12 (34%)	4 (11%)	24 (69%)
Sweet[73]	45 (24%)	54 (39%)	129 (68%)
Wasserheit et al[50]	11 (44%)	8 (35%)	11 (44%)

Diagnosis

The timely diagnosis of PID has suffered from a lack of testing accuracy and standardization. Jacobson and Westrom,[76] studying women with the clinical diagnosis of PID by laparoscopy, were able to confirm the diagnosis in only 65%. On the other hand, a significant number of patients admitted with another diagnosis, such as acute appendicitis, ectopic pregnancy, ruptured ovarian cyst, or endometriosis, were found to have acute PID. Chaparro and coworkers[77] then studied women whose laparoscopic findings were consistent with PID and found that 64% had a clinical course suggestive of PID. These studies suggested that a large number of patients were either treated needlessly with antibiotics or inappropriately left untreated and subjected to the sequelae and complications of untreated salpingitis. The most common symptoms and physical findings in patients with laparoscopically confirmed acute salpingitis are listed in Table 117–4.[76] Among the presenting symptoms, only a history of fever or chills was significantly more common in the group with verified PID than in the control group whose pelvic findings at laparoscopy were normal. Whereas a documented fever, adnexal tenderness, elevated erythrocyte sedimentation

TABLE 117–4 ■ Frequency of Symptoms and Findings in 623 Cases of Surgically Documented Acute Pelvic Inflammatory Disease

	PATIENTS	
SYMPTOM OR FINDING	No.	%
Lower abdominal pain	585	94
Increased vaginal discharge	340	55
Fever or chills	257	41
Irregular bleeding	221	36
Urinary symptoms	116	19
Gastrointestinal symptoms	64	10
Fever on admission	205	33
Adnexal tenderness	573	92
Increased erythrocyte sedimentation rate	473	76
Abnormal vaginal discharge	394	63

TABLE 117–5 ■ Criteria for Diagnosis of Pelvic Inflammatory Disease

ALL THREE MUST BE PRESENT

History of low abdominal pain and presence of low abdominal tenderness, with or without evidence of rebound

Cervical motion tenderness

Adnexal tenderness

plus

ONE OF THESE MUST BE PRESENT

Temperature of at least 38°C

Leukocytosis with white cell count above 10,000/mm^3

A culdocentesis that yields peritoneal fluid containing white blood cells and bacteria

Presence of an inflammatory mass noted on pelvic examination or sonography

Elevated erythrocyte sedimentation rate

Evidence of *N. gonorrhoeae* or *C. trachomatis* in the endocervix

- A Gram stain from the endocervix revealing gram-negative intracellular diplococci suggestive of *N. gonorrhoeae*
- A monoclonal antibody–directed smear from endocervical secretions revealing *C. trachomatis*
- Mucopurulent endocervicitis

Presence of >10 white blood cells per oil-immersion field on Gram stain of endocervical discharge

rate, and abnormal vaginal discharge were statistically significantly more frequent among verified cases of acute PID, the differences were indistinct clinically.

To improve the accuracy of clinical diagnosis, Hager and coworkers[78] studied clinical and laboratory information from women found to have PID by laparoscopy and formulated standardized criteria for clinical diagnosis and for grading the severity of laparoscopically confirmed salpingitis. The criteria have since been revised and are listed in Table 117–5. Kahn and coworkers[79] reviewed studies addressing the diagnosis of acute PID in which laparoscopy was considered the diagnostic "gold standard." These authors noted that the history and physical findings were reasonably sensitive but nonspecific. The only factors that had both high sensitivity and specificity were elevated erythrocyte sedimentation rate or C-reactive protein and findings on endometrial biopsy positive for plasma cell endometritis.

Laparoscopy is the definitive technique for diagnosing PID. It is relatively safe, with a low complication rate, and permits both visualization of the pelvis and access to the fallopian tubes for direct culture. Method and coworkers[80] studied selected patients for a period of 4 years and found that no significant additional expense would have been incurred if all women admitted with a clinical diagnosis of PID had had the diagnosis verified by laparoscopy. Many clinicians advocate its routine use for suspected PID. It is extremely helpful when the diagnosis is in question, particularly for distinguishing PID from other surgical conditions such as appendicitis, ectopic pregnancy, and ruptured endometrioma. Paavomen and colleagues[81] demonstrated a close association between biopsy-proven plasma cell endometritis and visually confirmed acute salpingitis. This finding has been confirmed by Wasserheit,[50] Kiviat,[82] Sellors,[83] and Soper[24] and associates. The delay in diagnosis by endometrial biopsy limits its clinical usefulness.

Treatment of Uncomplicated Pelvic Inflammatory Disease

The goals in the management of acute PID are to preserve fertility, prevent ectopic pregnancy, and reduce long-term inflammatory sequelae. Optimal treatment of acute PID requires early diagnosis and prompt institution of antimicrobial therapy effective against the major pathogens known to be involved in the disease process. Studies using hysterosalpingographic and laparoscopic evaluation of tubal status have demonstrated that women treated early in the course of infection have a better chance of retaining tubal patency.[84] Hillis and colleagues[85] reported that women treated after 3 days or more of symptoms had a significantly greater infertility rate (19.7%) compared with those treated with less than 3 days of symptoms (8.3%). Although the advent of antibiotics has reportedly decreased sequelae of salpingitis such as abscess formation, infertility, and the need for operative intervention, major complications and sequelae still occur in a large portion of treated women.[8, 9, 86, 87] Investigation of PID in an animal model suggests that early antibiotic treatment may prevent infertility.[88]

Initially, single-agent antimicrobial therapy focused on eradication of *N. gonorrhoeae*. Most often, these drugs failed to eradicate both *C. trachomatis* and mixed aerobic-anaerobic bacteria important in the pathogenesis of PID,[89] and even the newer broad-spectrum cephalosporins do not always eliminate *C. trachomatis* from the endometrial cavity.[49]

In September 1993, the Centers for Disease Control and Prevention published new recommendations for the treatment of acute PID.[90] The guidelines for outpatient therapy of acute PID are provided in Table 117–6.

TABLE 117–6 ■ Treatment Guidelines for Acute Pelvic Inflammatory Disease

INPATIENT TREATMENT

Regimen A*

Cefoxitin, 2 g intravenously (IV) q 6 h, or cefotetan, 2 g IV q 12 h

plus

Doxycycline, 100 mg IV or orally q 12 h

Regimen B†

Clindamycin, 900 mg IV q 8 h

plus

Gentamicin loading dose (2 mg/kg) IV or intramuscularly (IM) followed by a maintenance dose (1.5 mg/kg) q 8 h

OUTPATIENT TREATMENT

Regimen A

Cefoxitin, 2 g IM, plus probenecid, 1 g orally in a single dose concurrently, or ceftriaxone, 250 mg IM, or other parenteral third-generation cephalosporin‡

plus

Doxycycline, 100 mg orally twice a day for 14 d

Regimen B

Ofloxacin, 400 mg orally twice a day for 14 d

plus

Either clindamycin, 450 mg orally 4 times a day, or metronidazole, 500 mg orally twice a day for 14 d

*Continued for at least 48 h after the patient demonstrates substantial clinical improvement, after which doxycycline 100 mg orally twice a day should be continued for a total of 14 d.

†Continued for at least 48 h after the patient demonstrates substantial clinical improvement, then followed with doxycycline 100 mg orally twice a day or clindamycin 450 mg orally 4 times a day to complete a total of 14 days of treatment.

‡Ceftizoxime or cefotaxime.

From Centers for Disease Control and Prevention: 1993 Sexually transmitted diseases treatment guidelines. MMWR Morbid Mortal Wkly Rep 42(RR-14):1, 1993.

Outpatient Antibiotic Therapy

Most of the studies on outpatient treatment are flawed by poor study design. Results of "unblinded," noncomparative studies have demonstrated good clinical responses in patients treated with a number of regimens prospectively comparing ampicillin with tetracycline[91, 92]; however, in a six-hospital collaborative study of ambulatory regimens, outpatient treatment resulted in clinical failure in 17% of patients.[93] Improved study designs employing pretreatment and post-treatment data have demonstrated the persistence of multiple strains of bacteria and have widened our definition of treatment success to include microbial eradication from the upper genital tract. Outpatient treatment is further complicated by poor compliance and by the lack of an oral drug preparation that can attain therapeutic concentrations in serum.

It is not clear whether either ambulatory treatment or parenteral antibiotic therapy prevents complications and long-term sequelae. Objective data must be generated to resolve this question. Owing to the high rate of ambulatory treatment failures, the considerable morbidity caused by PID, and the impression of improved outcome with early and effective parenteral therapy, the criteria for hospitalization of patients with PID have been broadened (Table 117–7). Indeed, some authorities recommend that all women with acute PID be hospitalized for combination parenteral antibiotic therapy.

Inpatient Antibiotic Therapy

A number of properly designed studies have been reported that compare inpatient treatment regimens. Two early studies reported equal initial clinical efficacy for the treatment regimens approved by the Centers for Disease Control and Prevention, (1) cefoxitin-doxycycline and (2) clindamycin-tobramycin or clindamycin-gentamicin.[50, 94] These combinations have become the standards against which new regimens are generally tested. Walker and coworkers[95] reported a metaanalysis of clinical trials for the treatment of acute PID. Of the 34 treatment trials published between 1966 and 1992, they accepted 21 as meeting their inclusion criteria. These studies addressed only initial clinical and microbiologic outcome; they did not assess the effect of treatment on sequelae such as infertility or ectopic pregnancy. The pooled clinical cure rates ranged from 75% to 94%, and the pooled microbiologic cure rates ranged from 71% to 100% (Tables 117–8 and 117–9). Other than the metronidazole plus doxycycline regimen, all other treatment regimens had excellent short-term clinical and microbiologic efficacy.

In general, combination regimens of either clindamycin plus an aminoglycoside or an extended-spectrum cephalosporin plus doxycycline have produced excellent initial clinical responses. Treatment with fluoroquinolone alone resulted in a high rate of posttreatment persistence of anaerobic bacteria in the endometrial cavity. Randomized, prospective studies with meticulous clinical or laparoscopic grading, microbial analysis, and long-term follow-up are desperately needed to assess how effective these regimens are in preventing subsequent episodes of PID and adverse reproductive sequelae.

TABLE 117–7 ■ Criteria for Hospitalization of Women with Acute Pelvic Inflammatory Disease

Possibly, all patients with suspected pelvic inflammatory disease
Presence of pelvic abscess or tuboovarian abscess
Concurrent pregnancy
Temperature > 38°C
Nausea and vomiting that preclude oral therapy
Adolescent patient
Intrauterine device in place
No response to outpatient therapy within 48 h
Failure to comply with oral regimen
Upper abdominal findings (e.g., rebound)

TABLE 117–8 ■ Pooled Cure Rates in the Treatment of Acute Pelvic Inflammatory Disease for Antibiotic Regimens with More Than One Study

DRUG REGIMEN	NUMBER OF STUDIES	NUMBER OF PATIENTS	CLINICAL CURE RATE (%)	MICROBIOLOGIC CURE RATE (%)*
Inpatient				
Clindamycin plus aminoglycoside	10	372	92	97
Cefoxitin plus doxycycline	7	338	93	98
Cefotetan plus doxycycline	2	86	94	100
Ciprofloxacin	4	90	94	96†
Metronidazole plus doxycycline	2	36	75	71
Outpatient				
Cefoxitin plus doxycycline	2	59	95	91

*Based on eradication of *N. gonorrhoeae* and *C. trachomatis.*
†High rate of persistent anaerobic bacteria.
Data from Walker CK, Kahn JG, Washington AE, et al: Pelvic inflammatory disease: Metaanalysis of antimicrobial regimen efficacy. J Infect Dis 168:969–978, 1993.

Adjunctive Therapy

Supportive Care. Many patients being treated for PID require supportive measures. Intravenous or oral hydration is usually needed to replace fluid losses secondary to fever or gastrointestinal tract distress. Bed rest, preferably in the semi-Fowler position, employs gravity to help localize the infection to the pelvis. Nonsteroidal antiinflammatory agents or narcotics are frequently needed for pain relief. Antipyretics may be used, especially during the first 24 hours of antibiotic treatment; thereafter, they should be discontinued to assess response to therapy. Finally, patients should abstain from sexual intercourse for 6 to 12 weeks after treatment.

Removal of Intrauterine Devices. Because IUDs work by altering host resistance, it is logical to remove them from patients with PID. Studies of resolution time demonstrate slower recovery when the IUD is left in place.[96, 97] No study has reported whether antibiotic therapy should be started before or after the IUD is removed. In theory, a therapeutic serum antibiotic level should lower the risk of introducing transient bacteremia by removing the IUD.

Treatment of Sexual Partners. To minimize reinfection, it is recommended that all partners of women with PID be screened for *N. gonorrhoeae* and *C. trachomatis*. Infected partners should be treated with a regimen that is effective against both organisms, usually a combination of ceftriaxone, 125 mg intramuscularly in a single dose, plus doxycycline, 100 mg orally twice daily for 7 days.

TABLE 117–9 ■ Reported Cure Rates in the Treatment of Acute Pelvic Inflammatory Disease for Antibiotic Regimens with Only a Single Study

DRUG REGIMEN	NUMBER OF PATIENTS	CLINICAL CURE RATE (%)	MICROBIOLOGIC CURE RATE (%)*
Inpatient			
Ceftizoxime plus tetracycline	18	88	100
Cefotaxime plus tetracycline	19	94	100
Sulbactam-ampicillin plus doxycycline	37	95	100
Outpatient			
Amoxicillin-clavulanate	35	100	100
Ofloxacin	37	95	100

*Based on eradication of *N. gonorrhoeae* and *C. trachomatis*.
Data from Walker CK, Kahn JG, Washington AE, et al: Pelvic inflammatory disease: Metaanalysis of antimicrobial regimen efficacy. J Infect Dis 168:969–978, 1993.

TUBOOVARIAN ABSCESS

A well-known early sequela of PID is TOA. Although most series report a 10% to 15% prevalence, it has been reported to occur in up to one third of patients hospitalized with PID.[98–105] Despite the clinical availability of many new and potent broad-spectrum antimicrobial agents for treatment of pelvic infections, pelvic abscess remains a major cause of morbidity and a diagnostic and therapeutic challenge for gynecologists.

Diagnosis

The most frequent presenting complaint (more than 90% of cases) of patients with TOA is abdominal or pelvic pain.[99, 100, 105–107] Most have fever and leukocytosis, but many patients who harbor a TOA have normal temperature and white cell count.[100] Temperature of at least 37.8°C has been reported in 60% to 80% of patients, and leukocytosis was reported in 66% to 80%.[98–100, 107–109] The findings of vaginal discharge, abnormal uterine bleeding, nausea, vomiting, diarrhea, dysuria, and frequency are inconsistent. Because the presenting signs and symptoms of uncomplicated PID and TOA are similar, diagnosis relies on identification of an inflammatory adnexal mass. Patients whose severe pain and tenderness preclude an adequate pelvic examination require further evaluation for a pelvic mass.

Various noninvasive imaging techniques facilitate the diagnosis of adnexal masses[110–120]: radionucleotide scanning, ultrasonography (US), computed tomography (CT), and magnetic resonance imaging. A newer additional technique is scintigraply with radiolabeled polyclonal immunoglobulin G, which has excellent sensitivity and specificity for detecting acute infection.[121, 122] Differentiation of a TOA from inflammatory masses with adherent bowel or omentum is appreciably improved with such techniques.

Gallium Ga 67–labeled and indium In 111–labeled white blood cell scans are sensitive in localizing intraabdominal abscesses.[112–115] The best results seem to be obtained with ^{111}In (reported accuracy 87%).[114] The diagnostic accuracy of radionucleotide scans for TOA has not been determined; thus, they are not generally used in these patients.

The most frequently used technique to confirm the diagnosis of TOA is US. Real-time US can be used to confirm the diagnosis of TOA and to measure response to therapy. The accuracy of US in the diagnosis of pelvic abscesses has been assessed in several retrospective studies.[110, 116–118, 123] Taylor and coworkers[116] described 220 patients with surgically proven abdominal or pelvic abscesses with the following results: 36 of 40 abdominal abscesses and 32 of 33 pelvic abscesses were correctly identified; 112 of 113 suspected abdominal abscesses and 33 of 34 suspected pelvic abscesses were correctly ruled out. Landers and Sweet[100] reported that 29 of 31 surgically confirmed TOAs were correctly diagnosed with US. TOAs were reported as complex adnexal masses or cyst-type masses with multiple internal echoes consistent with an abscess. The two false-positive results were simple cystic masses. A mass was correctly identified in all surgically confirmed TOAs and in 90% of the 67 patients with clinically diagnosed TOAs.[5] In a later report, Jasinsky and coworkers[123] compared the sensitivity of US and CT in the diagnosis of intraabdominal abscess. In this study, the sensitivity of US for pelvic abscesses was 42 of 56 (75%), and the sensitivity of CT was 14 of 15 (93%). The difference was attributed to the difficulty of imaging postoperative abscesses by US in oncology patients. In general, TOAs are visualized with a high degree of accuracy by use of standard US techniques, including vaginal probe studies.

CT has also been used extensively in both diagnosis and treatment of abdominal abscesses.[112–114] Despite its known sensitivity in the detection of abdominal abscesses, there is scant information on the accuracy of these scans for the diagnosis of TOA and other pelvic abscesses. One study on the accuracy of US, ^{67}Ga-enhanced scan, and CT in the diagnosis of abdominal abscesses reported the sensitivities as 82%, 96%, and 100%, respectively,[109] and the specificities as 91%, 65%, and 100%, respectively. Thus, CT appears to be accurate in detecting the presence of an abscess, at least in the abdomen. Because CT is significantly more expensive, the slightly higher degree of accuracy does not justify its use as a primary diagnostic tool. In general, our initial approach is to use US for the diagnosis of TOAs and to use CT as a backup. Virtually no data are available on the sensitivity and specificity of magnetic resonance imaging in evaluating pelvic abscess, but the technique is appealing because it discriminates between different tissue densities and fluid consistencies and does not employ ionizing radiation. Its expense precludes its use in the diagnosis of TOAs, except in unusual circumstances.

Organisms

The organisms isolated from TOAs are predominantly a mixed flora of anaerobes and facultative or aerobic organisms.[100, 124] When good anaerobic microbiologic methods are used, anaerobic bacteria are the most prevalent organisms isolated from TOAs. Anaerobic bacteria have been isolated from 63% to 100% of adnexal abscesses.[100, 125–129] In my experience, the predominant organisms isolated from TOA aspirates were *E. coli*, *B. fragilis*, a variety of *Prevotella* species, aerobic streptococci, and *Peptostreptococcus* species.[100]

It is rare to recover the gonococcus from a TOA. Landers and Sweet[100] recovered *N. gonorrhoeae* from only 3.8% of 53 TOA aspirates; the overall recovery rate of *N. gonorrhoeae* from the endocervix was 31% in their TOA population. It has been proposed that initial infection with the gonococcus leads to anaerobic invasion of the fallopian tubes.[31, 33] Subsequently, the facultative and anaerobic organisms may suppress the growth of *N. gonorrhoeae*, preventing its recovery.[130] Similarly, *C. trachomatis* has not been demonstrated to play a role in the causation of TOA. To date, I have been unable to recover *C. trachomatis* from the abscess content of the wall of TOAs.

Actinomycetes, most commonly *Actinomyces israelii*, a gram-positive anaerobe, has occasionally been found in association with PID and, more specifically, TOA. This organism has been reported in association with IUD use.[131–133] Burkman and coworkers[101] reported that 7 of 8 (88%) PID patients with actinomycetic infection had a TOA compared with 11 of 38 (29%) without. In other studies on TOA, actinomycetes have not been recovered. The exact role of these organisms in the pathogenesis of TOA is unclear. Their major role may be related to an association with IUD use and subsequent abscess formation.

Pathogenesis

A variety of factors that play a role in the pathogenesis of abscess formation have been identified: exotoxins with tissue-necrotizing potential; enzymes such as collagenase and heparinase; and virulence factors associated with the bacterial cell surface. The inflammatory response to antigenic stimuli has also been shown to play a role in this process. The exact mechanism of TOA formation has been difficult to establish.

Inflammatory damage to the endosalpinx results in a purulent exudate, which may spill from the fimbriated end of the fallopian tubes. In an attempt to localize and wall off the infection, the ovaries or other pelvic structures become involved in the inflammatory process. Organisms enter the ovary, presumably at an ovulation site, and subsequently invade tissue. Tissue planes are eventually lost, and the separation of tube and ovary is obscured as the abscess forms. It may remain localized, involving the tube and ovary alone, or it may involve other contiguous pelvic structures such as bowel, bladder, or the opposite adnexa. At any point in the progression, rupture may occur, exposing the peritoneal surface and other intraabdominal organs to a large amount of purulent material. This process can lead to overwhelming sepsis and further abscess formation. Fortunately, less than 1% or 2% of TOAs reach the stage when they rupture spontaneously, but a ruptured TOA is a true acute surgical emergency.

Association with Intrauterine Devices

The frequency of IUD use among patients who develop TOA has been reported in several studies to range from 20% to 54%.[100, 108, 109, 124, 134, 135] A strong correlation between IUD use and unilateral TOA was suggested by initial reports in the 1970s,[136, 137] but numerous subsequent investigations have noted that the frequency of unilateral abscesses ranged from 20% to 71%, and it was not significantly related to IUD use.[100, 108, 109, 135, 138]

Medical Therapy

Although it was long a clinical dictum that abscesses require surgical drainage or extirpation for cure, primary medical management with antibiotic therapy has become the initial approach to TOA in many centers as newer data have supported a conservative medical approach. Still, many patients continue to be managed primarily with surgery. Although highly effective, this approach is overzealous, because TOAs can be treated safely and effectively by conservative means. It has been suggested that even when a surgical approach is necessary, unilateral TOA can be treated with unilateral adnexectomy rather than total abdominal hysterectomy and bilateral salpingo-oophorectomy (TAH-BSO).

Numerous investigators have reported success with a conservative medical approach to the treatment of TOA* (Table 117–10). A favorable result can be expected in one half to two thirds of cases. A number of antimicrobial regimens were employed in these studies: Franklin's group[104] used mostly a penicillin and streptomycin combination; Gins-

*References 100, 102, 104, 108, 109, 135, 138–140.

TABLE 117–10 ■ Investigations of Treatment of Tuboovarian Abscess with Conservative Medical Therapy

STUDY	NUMBER OF CASES TREATED	INITIAL RESPONSE No.	INITIAL RESPONSE %	SUBSEQUENT PREGNANCY IN PATIENTS WITH FOLLOW-UP* No.	SUBSEQUENT PREGNANCY IN PATIENTS WITH FOLLOW-UP* %
Landers and Sweet[100]	217	175	81	8/58	13.8
Franklin et al[104]	120	110	90†	10/108	9.3
Ginsberg et al[108]	110	76	69	9/95	9.5
Edelman and Berger[109]	318	175	55	NS	NS
Scott[138]	33	24	73	NS	NS
Manara[135]	26	11	42	1/26	3.8
Hager[102]	32	5	16	4/8	50
Berkeley[5]	9	6	66	NS	NS
Hemsell et al[145]	41	39	95	6/41	14.6
Mercer et al[141]	20	12	60	NS	NS
Hemsell et al[139]	24	22	92	NS	NS
Reed et al[140]	119	90	70	NS	NS
Total	1069	745	69.7	38/336	11.3

*NS, Not stated.
†Includes some patients treated with colpotomy drainage.

berg's[108] used "broad-spectrum antibiotics"; Hager[102] and Manara[135] used parenteral penicillin or a first-generation cephalosporin in combination with an aminoglycoside. Mercer and coworkers[141] reported resolution of the TOA in 12 of 20 patients treated with various therapies, all of which included anaerobic coverage.

Because these abscesses contain significant concentrations of the resistant gram-negative anaerobes, such as *B. fragilis*, *Prevotella bivia*, and *Prevotella disiens*, better results should accrue from aggressive treatment with antibiotics that are effective against these organisms, such as clindamycin, metronidazole, the extended-spectrum penicillins, and the newer broad-spectrum second- and third-generation cephalosporins. In addition, broad-spectrum agents combined with β-lactamase inhibitors and the penems should prove efficacious as well, but further clinical trials are needed.

In Landers and Sweet's[100] series of 232 TOAs, response to therapy was determined on the basis of improvement in symptoms, absence of fever, reduction of pelvic tenderness, and shrinking of the mass (Table 117–11). Of 167 patients treated with antibiotics alone before discharge, reduction in mass size was observed in 25% of those who received penicillin alone, 49% who received penicillin and an aminoglycoside, and 68% who received regimens that included clindamycin ($P < .01$). Follow-up was available for 104 patients treated with antibiotic regimens that did not include clindamycin. Initial response was seen in 36.5%, compared with 68% of the 63 patients treated with regimens that included clindamycin. Surgical intervention was required for 42 patients during the initial hospitalization because of failure to respond to antimicrobial therapy alone. Of these, 64% had received drugs other than clindamycin and 36% received a regimen containing clindamycin. At follow-up 2 to 4 weeks after discharge, 46.4% of the former group and 86% of clindamycin-treated patients had further reduction or absence of adnexal masses.[100]

Reed and colleagues,[140] in a study comparing cefoxitin plus doxycycline with clindamycin plus gentamicin for treatment of TOA, reported that nearly 75% of TOAs responded to medical management alone with equivalent cure rates seen for both regimens. The studies by Landers and Sweet[100] and Reed and coworkers[140] clearly demonstrated the importance of antimicrobial therapy with an agent effective against *B. fragilis* and *Prevotella* species and the excellent results with such therapy in the management of TOA.

The factor most predictive of response to antimicrobial therapy alone is TOA size. Ginsberg and coworkers[108] reported that TOAs larger than 8 cm or that were bilateral were predictive of failure to respond to antimicrobial therapy alone. Similarly, Reed and coworkers[140] demonstrated that response to antimicrobial therapy was inversely proportional to abscess size.

Animal models have been developed to study the efficacy of various antimicrobial agents in the treatment of abscesses. Several studies have evaluated these drugs in treating experimental subcutaneous and intraperitoneal abscesses caused by *B. fragilis* or by mixed aerobic-anaerobic pathogens. Antibiotic levels and activity were measured in pus and serum, and abscess size response was assessed.[142–144] When the activity of 10 antimicrobial agents was measured in these subcutaneous abscesses by reduction in bacterial counts, it was found that the most active antimicrobials, in decreasing order of activity, were metronidazole, clindamycin, moxalactam, and cefoxitin.

Experience with cefoxitin, third-generation cephalosporins, or extended-spectrum penicillins in the management of TOAs is limited. In a clinical trial of 41 patients with TOA, 39 (95%) responded favorably to cefotaxime, a third-generation cephalosporin.[145] No patient required surgery at initial hospitalization, and two patients needed the addition of another antibiotic. Only six patients required further surgery for persistent mass. Six patients (15%) later became pregnant, and all had had abscesses larger than 7 cm, four of them bilateral. Other agents with similar activity should be tested for abscess in animal models and in comparative clinical trials.

TABLE 117–11 ■ Comparison of Regimens with and Without Clindamycin for Treatment of Tuboovarian Abscess

	REDUCTION OF SIZE AT HOSPITAL DISCHARGE		FURTHER REDUCTION OF SIZE AT 2–4 WK AFTER DISCHARGE	
ANTIBIOTIC REGIMEN	No. Responded	%	No. Treated	%
Antimicrobial regimens that included clindamycin	43/63	68.3	43/50	86.0
Antimicrobial regimens that excluded clindamycin	38/104	36.5	39/84	46.4

Adapted from Landers DV, Sweet RL: Tubo-ovarian abscess: Contemporary approach to management. Rev Infect Dis 5:876–884, 1983.

Treatment Rationale for Unruptured Tuboovarian Abscess

As described before, investigators have encouraged conservative management with antibiotics alone when possible.[100, 104, 108] I manage patients with TOAs conservatively, using the following guidelines. If a ruptured TOA is suspected, the patient's condition is stabilized, antibiotic therapy is instituted, and immediate surgical intervention is undertaken. If the diagnosis is in question or there is a reasonable likelihood of an alternative surgical condition, operative intervention is undertaken, with laparoscopy or laparotomy if necessary. Otherwise, the patient is given intravenous antibiotic therapy, usually clindamycin or metronidazole plus an aminoglycoside or cefoxitin, with broad-spectrum coverage that includes the resistant gram-negative anaerobes. The initial approach of antibiotics alone is appropriate for pyosalpinx, ovarian abscess, tuboovarian complex, and TOA. Because it is often difficult to distinguish which of these entities is present, a conservative initial approach eliminates the need to resolve the question.

If the patient does not respond to appropriate antibiotic therapy within 72 hours, surgical intervention should be considered. Patients are frequently slow to respond; it can take a full 3 days' treatment before clinical improvement becomes evident. Clinical judgment is crucial, and each case must be assessed according to the patient's needs and situation. The clinician must be aware also that the abscess may rupture and become a surgical emergency. If the patient's status suddenly deteriorates, surgery should be undertaken immediately.

Several factors have been identified that are predictive of antibiotic failure. Adnexal masses larger than 8 cm or bilateral adnexal involvement has been shown to be predictive of failure.[108, 140] Surprisingly, the presence of fever, degree of leukocytosis, and history of PID have no predictive value, but persistence of fever and rising white cell count in the face of ongoing antibiotic therapy strongly suggest that surgical intervention will be necessary.

Intraabdominal rupture is one of the most serious complications of TOA. It is a surgical emergency, and the mortality rate may be increased by unnecessary delay. With expectant conservative management, Pedowitz and Bloomfield[98] noted that all of the patients who had rupture of a TOA before 1947 died. After 1947, 127 cases were treated with a more aggressive surgical approach (TAH-BSO) combined with available medical adjuvants. The mortality rate dropped to 3.1%.[3] The physician's delay in establishing the diagnosis was cited as the most common preventable cause of death. Subsequent investigators have continued to show improved survival rates with aggressive surgical management of ruptured TOA.[106, 146] In 1977, Rivlin and Hunt[147] described 113 patients with ruptured TOA. The mortality rate was 7.1% in their series, but only 3% of the patients underwent hysterectomy. Unilateral adnexectomy, with preservation of hormonal and menstrual function, was accomplished in 73.5% of cases. Rivlin reported that only 17.5% of patients required further surgery later during the 1- to 5-year follow-up period. Landers and Sweet[100] described four patients with ruptured TOA who underwent unilateral adnexectomy; none required further surgery in the 2- to 10-year follow-up period, and one subsequently carried an intrauterine pregnancy to term. With modern antimicrobial agents and aggressive surgical intervention, ruptured unilateral TOA can be safely managed without removing the uterus and contralateral fallopian tube and ovary.

Surgical Approach to Unruptured Tuboovarian Abscess

A wide variety of surgical approaches to unruptured TOA have been employed through the years: extraperitoneal drainage, posterior colpotomy drainage, unilateral adnexectomy and TAH-BSO, and more recently, percutaneous and laparoscopic drainage. Abdominal extraperitoneal drainage of TOAs has been virtually replaced by other approaches. Posterior colpotomy, still used frequently by many clinicians, can be an effective mode of treatment when it is combined with antimicrobial therapy and restricted to patients with fluctuant abscesses in the midline that dissect the rectovaginal septum and are firmly attached to parietal peritoneum. These conditions severely limit the number of TOAs that can be safely drained by this procedure. The morbidity of this procedure can also be significant if these requirements are not met. Rubenstein and coworkers[148] reported in 1976 that of 65 patients with pelvic abscesses drained by colpotomy or rectal incision, nearly one third subsequently required a major operation because of residual pain or infection. In a 1982 combined series of 348 cases of colpotomy drainage reported by Rivlin and coworkers,[149] there were 23 cases of diffuse peritoneal sepsis (6.5%), resulting in six (26%) deaths. Rivlin and coworkers[150] also described their experience with colpotomy drainage in 59 patients, of whom 24 required further surgical intervention. Of greatest concern, 13 (54%) of these surgeries were performed as emergency procedures. Vaginal colpotomy drainage is seldom used on our service, for the following reasons: (1) there is a high rate of complications, and more definitive surgery is frequently required after colpotomy drainage[148–150]; (2) most TOAs do not meet the requirements for the vaginal approach (i.e., midline mass that adheres to pelvic peritoneum and dissects upper third of rectovaginal septum); and (3) with a conservative approach, many of these unilateral abscesses can be removed by the abdominal approach, offering a better chance for preservation of future fertility and hormone production.

Alternative Treatment Approaches

Percutaneous Drainage

Whereas percutaneous drainage is commonly employed in the treatment of intraabdominal abscesses, this technique has not often been applied to the treatment of TOA. US- or CT-guided drainage of intraabdominal abscesses has been reported to be successful in 75% to 89% of cases, obviating major surgery and minimizing the patient's discomfort, morbidity, and cost.[151–158] In addition, patients recover more rapidly and avoid the risk of general anesthesia and surgery. CT and US are also used to observe the response of these abscesses to the drainage technique. Repeated scans are generally performed within 48 hours after drainage to evaluate response. The drainage catheters can also be used to irrigate the abscess cavities and to inject contrast material to ensure reduction of cavity size on repeated scans. Several series have shown that percutaneous catheter drainage can be successfully used in treating pelvic abscesses. Van Sonnenberg and coworkers[152] reported a 78% success rate for 50 abscesses. Worthen and Gunning[153] used two methods of drainage for 35 patients with TOA: small abscesses were aspirated and large abscesses were drained with a catheter. Seven patients (20%) could not be treated by drainage or aspiration for technical reasons; for the remaining patients, the success rate was 94% (18 of 19) for aspiration drainage and 77% (7 of 9) for catheter drainage. Complications included a bowel laceration and an abscess rupture that required early intervention. Further trials of this approach against medical treatment are needed.

Laparoscopic Drainage

Laparoscopy has been suggested as a possible approach to the management of TOA.[159–162] It affords direct visualization of the abscess and confirms the diagnosis. The TOA is diagnosed under direct vision, adhesions are lysed, and purulent material is removed by suction; the peritoneal cavity can also be irrigated to remove necrotic tissue. In 1984, Henry-Suchet and coworkers[159] reported a series of 50 patients whose TOAs were managed laparoscopically. The reported overall clinical recovery rate was 90%, with almost complete disappearance of the adnexal mass and minimal adhesion formation after resolution of the acute infection. Reich and McGlynn[160] evaluated 25 women treated with this procedure. There was only one failure in the series; that woman required TAH-BSO 1 month after laparoscopic treatment. Minimal adhesions were found in five women who underwent second-look laparoscopy. Adducci[161] obtained similar results in seven cases and reported colpotomy drainage under laparoscopic control in nine patients with PID-associated pelvic abscesses. All nine responded well. Prospective studies are needed to compare the efficacy of antimicrobial therapy alone and antimicrobial therapy with drainage in resolving the abscess and preventing long-term sequelae.

Conservative Surgery Versus Total Hysterectomy with Bilateral Adnexectomy

The extent of surgery necessary to effect a cure when antibiotic therapy alone fails remains controversial. The approaches have ranged from simple drainage to complete removal of all reproductive organs by TAH-BSO.[98, 99, 156, 161] An alternative approach is a unilateral salpingo-oophorectomy for unilateral TOAs or a bilateral salpingo-oophorectomy for bilateral disease. Whereas a TAH-BSO is curative, the more conservative unilateral adnexectomy offers the potential for future fertility, maintenance of hormonal and menstrual function, and avoidance of the physiologic and psychologic effects of hysterectomy and gonadectomy.

Several investigators have reported results of conservative surgical management of patients with unilateral TOAs.[98, 99, 106, 108, 124, 135, 147] These data indicate that approximately 17% of patients treated with unilateral adnexectomy later require additional surgery. Rivlin and Hunt[147] combined conservative surgery with intraoperative and postoperative antibiotic peritoneal lavage for the treatment of 113 patients with ruptured TOA. They found that only four patients (3%) required hysterectomy during the initial hospitalization. Of the 83 patients treated with adnexal procedures (unilateral or bilateral) without removal of the uterus, 16 (19%) required further surgical intervention. An additional 19 patients reported by Landers and Sweet[100] were treated with unilateral adnexectomy; only 2 required subsequent surgery, and 3 subsequently became pregnant. Thus, it appears that although there is a risk that further surgery will be required, the conservative surgical approach does offer the TOA patient in whom initial antibiotic therapy fails another alternative to permanent sterilization and castration.

Another potential application of unilateral adnexectomy is in patients whose disease responds to initial antimicrobial therapy but whose mass persists. These patients may benefit from unilateral adnexectomy in terms of future fertility and recurrent disease. This approach needs to be evaluated in controlled trials. As in vitro fertilization techniques and donor embryo transplantation programs improve, the demand for a conservative surgical approach will increase.

Fertility After Tuboovarian Abscess

Fertility potential after a TOA has received little attention in the medical literature. Although several investigators have reported the frequency of subsequent pregnancy after lowing TOA, the follow-up data were limited, leaving it impossible to assess the number of patients attempting to conceive and their success rate.* The pregnancy rate has been reported to range from 9.5% to 13.8% after conservative medical management,[100, 104, 108, 145] 3.7% to 16% after unilateral adnexal procedures with preoperative antibiotics,[100, 108, 124] and 10% to 15% after antibiotics plus colpotomy drainage.[147, 149] Hager[102] published a series on 50 patients treated for TOA. A total of 11 of these patients had reproductive potential after treatment, but only 8 attempted to conceive. Four of the eight (50%) conceived a total of five intrauterine pregnancies. There were no ectopic pregnancies. In addition, he described five patients who underwent unilateral salpingo-oophorectomy and attempted to conceive; four were successful (80%). Although these rates of fertility are low, we may be dramatically underestimating reproduction potential after TOA unless we consider only the number of patients who attempt to conceive. Furthermore, few data have been published about vigorous treatment with antibiotics, such as clindamycin and metronidazole, that can penetrate abscesses. More investigation is also needed to determine the effects on fertility of newer antibiotics, laparoscopic drainage, and unilateral adnexectomy for unilateral TOA.

References

1. Curran JW: Economic consequences of pelvic inflammatory disease in the United States. Am J Obstet Gynecol 138:848, 1980.
2. Jones OG, Zaidi AA, St. John RK: Frequency and distribution of salpingitis and pelvic inflammatory disease in short-stay hospitals in the United States. Am J Obstet Gynecol 138:905, 1980.
3. St. John RK, Jones OG, Blount JH: The epidemiology and trend of pelvic inflammatory disease among hospitalized women. Sex Transm Dis 8:62, 1981.
4. Blount JH, Reynolds GH, Rice RJ: Pelvic inflammatory disease: Incidence and trends in private practice. MMWR CDC Surveill Summ 32:27SS, 1983.
5. Washington AE, Cates W, Zaidi AA: Hospitalizations for pelvic inflammatory disease: Epidemiology and trends in the United States, 1975 to 1982. JAMA 251:2529, 1984.
6. Rolfs RT, Galaid E, Zaidi AA: Epidemiology of pelvic inflammatory disease: Trends in hospitalizations and office visits, 1979–1988. *In* Joint Meeting of the CDC and NIH About Pelvic Inflammatory Disease, Prevention, Management and Research in the 1990s; September 4–5, 1990; Bethesda, MD.
7. Washington AE, Katz P: Cost of and payment source for pelvic inflammatory disease: Trends and projections 1983 through 2000. JAMA 266:2565, 1991.
8. Westrom L: Incidence, prevalence and trends of acute pelvic inflammatory disease and its consequences in industrialized countries. Am J Obstet Gynecol 38:880, 1980.
9. Westrom L: Effect of acute pelvic inflammatory disease on fertility. Am J Obstet Gynecol 122:707, 1975.
10. Eschenbach DA: Epidemiology and diagnosis of acute pelvic inflammatory disease. Obstet Gynecol 55:142S, 1980.
11. Jossens MOR, Schachter J, Sweet RL: Risk factors associated with pelvic inflammatory disease of differing microbial etiologies. Obstet Gynecol 83:989, 1994.
12. Bell TA, Holmes KK: Age-specific risks of syphilis, gonorrhea and hospitalized pelvic inflammatory disease in sexually experienced U.S. women. Sex Transm Dis 11:291, 1984.
13. Eschenbach DA, Harnisch JP, Holmes KK: Pathogenesis of acute pelvic inflammatory disease: Role of contraception and other risk factors. Am J Obstet Gynecol 128:838, 1977.
14. Ory HW: A review of the association between intrauterine devices and pelvic inflammatory disease. J Reprod Med 20:200, 1978.
15. Kaufman DW, Shapiro S, Rosenberg L, et al: Intrauterine contraceptive device use and pelvic inflammatory disease. Am J Obstet Gynecol 136:159, 1980.
16. Lee NC, Rubin GL, Ory HW, et al: Type of intrauterine device and the risk of pelvic inflammatory disease. Obstet Gynecol 62:1, 1983.
17. Burnhill MS: Syndrome of progressive endometritis associated with intrauterine contraceptive devices. Adv Planned Parenthood 8:144, 1973.
18. Sparks RA, Purrier BGA, Watt PJ, Ectein M: Bacterial colonization of uterine cavity: Role of tailed intrauterine contraceptive devices. Fertil Steril 282:1189, 1981.
19. Skangalis M, Mahoney CJ, O'Leary WM: Microbial presence in the uterine cavity as affected by varieties of intrauterine contraceptive devices. Fertil Steril 37:263, 1982.
20. Wolner-Hansen P, Svensson L, Mardh P-A, et al: Laparoscopic findings and contraceptive use in women with signs and symptoms suggestive of acute salpingitis. Obstet Gynecol 66:233, 1985.
21. Paavonen J, Teisala K, Heinonen PK, et al: Microbiological and histopathological findings in acute pelvic inflammatory disease. Br J Obstet Gynecol 94:454, 1987.
22. Eschenbach DA, Hillier S, Critchlow C, et al: Diagnosis and clinical manifestations of bacterial vaginosis. Am J Obstet Gynecol 158:819, 1988.
23. Hillier SL, Kiviat NB, Critchlow C, et al: Bacterial vaginosis associated bacteria as etiologic agents of pelvic inflammatory disease (Abstr). *In* Proceedings of the Annual Meeting of the Infectious Diseases Society of Obstetrics and Gynecology; August 6–8, 1992; San Diego, CA; p 12.
24. Soper D, Brockwell NJ, Dalton HP, Johnson D: Observations concerning the microbial etiology of acute salpingitis. Am J Obstet Gynecol 170:1008, 1994.
25. Amsel R, Totten PA, Spiegel CA, et al: Nonspecific vaginitis: Diagnostic criteria and microbiologic and epidemiologic associations. Am J Med 74:14, 1983.
26. Sweet RL, Mills J, Hadley KW, et al: Use of laparoscopy to determine the microbiologic etiology of acute salpingitis. Am J Obstet Gynecol 134:68, 1979.

*References 100, 102, 104, 124, 147, 149, 159, 160.

27. Eschenbach DA, Buchanan T, Pollock HM, et al: Polymicrobial etiology of acute pelvic inflammatory disease. N Engl J Med 293:166, 1975.
28. Lip J, Burgoyne X: Cervical and peritoneal bacterial flora associated with salpingitis. Obstet Gynecol 28:561, 1966.
29. Thompson SE, Hager WD, Wong KH, et al: The microbiology and therapy of acute pelvic inflammatory disease in hospitalized patients. Am J Obstet Gynecol 136:179, 1980.
30. Cunningham FG, Hauth JC, Gilstrap LC, et al: The bacterial pathogenesis of acute pelvic inflammatory disease. Obstet Gynecol 52:161, 1978.
31. Chow AW, Malkasian KL, Marshall JR, et al: The bacteriology of acute pelvic inflammatory disease. Am J Obstet Gynecol 122:876, 1975.
32. Sweet RL, Draper DL, Schachter J, et al: Microbiology and pathogenesis of acute salpingitis as determined by laparoscopy: What is the appropriate site to sample? Am J Obstet Gynecol 138:985, 1980.
33. Monif GRG, Welkos SL, Baer H, et al: Cul-de-sac isolates from patients with endometritis-salpingitis-peritonitis and gonococcal endocervicitis. Am J Obstet Gynecol 126:158, 1976.
34. Sweet RL, Draper D, Hadley WK: Etiology of acute salpingitis: Influence of episode number and duration of symptoms. Obstet Gynecol 58:62, 1981.
35. Soper DE, Brockwell NJ, Dalton HP: False-positive cultures of the cul-de-sac associated with culdocentesis in patients undergoing laparoscopy. Obstet Gynecol 77:134, 1991.
36. Eschenbach DA, Holmes KK: Acute pelvic inflammatory disease. Current concepts of pathogenesis, etiology and management. Clin Obstet Gynecol 18:35, 1975.
37. Sweet RL, Blankfort-Doyle M, Robbie MD, Schachter J: The occurrence of chlamydial and gonococcal salpingitis during the menstrual cycle. JAMA 255:2062, 1986.
38. Draper DL, James JF, Hadley WK, et al: Auxotypes and antibiotic susceptibilities of *Neisseria gonorrhoeae* from women with acute salpingitis. Sex Transm Dis 8:43, 1981.
39. Kellogg DS Jr, Peacock WL Jr, Deacon WE, et al: *Neisseria gonorrhoeae*. I. Virulence genetically linked to clonal variation. J Bacteriol 85:1274, 1963.
40. Kellogg DS Jr, Cohen IR, Norins LC, et al: *Neisseria gonorrhoeae*. II. Colonial variation and pathogenicity during 35 months in vitro. J Bacteriol 95:596, 1968.
41. Buchanan TM, Eschenbach DA, Knapp JS, et al: Gonococcal salpingitis is less likely to recur with *Neisseria gonorrhoeae* of the same principal outer membrane protein antigen type. Am J Obstet Gynecol 138:978, 1981.
42. McGee ZA, Johnson AP, Taylor-Robinson D: Pathogenic mechanisms of *Neisseria gonorrhoeae*: Observations on damage to human fallopian tubes in organ culture by gonococci of colony type I or colony type 4. J Infect Dis 143:413, 1981.
43. Melly MA, Gregg CR, McGee ZA: Studies of toxicity of *Neisseria gonorrhoeae* for human fallopian tube mucosa. J Infect Dis 143:423, 1981.
44. Mardh P-A, Ripa T, Swensson L, Westrom L: *Chlamydia trachomatis* infection in patients with acute salpingitis. N Engl J Med 298:1377, 1977.
45. Osser S, Persson K: Epidemiology and serodiagnostic aspects of chlamydia salpingitis. Obstet Gynecol 59:206, 1982.
46. Moller BR, Mardh P-A, Ahrons S, et al: Infections with *Chlamydia trachomatis*, *Mycoplasma hominis* and *Neisseria gonorrhoeae* in patients with acute pelvic inflammatory disease. Sex Transm Dis 8:198, 1981.
47. Gjonnaess H, Dalaker K, Anestad G, et al: Pelvic inflammatory disease: Etiologic studies with emphasis on chlamydial infection. Obstet Gynecol 59:550, 1982.
48. Swensson L, Westrom L, Ripa KT, et al: Differences in some clinical and laboratory parameters in acute salpingitis related to culture and serologic findings. Am J Obstet Gynecol 138:1017, 1980.
49. Sweet RL, Schachter J, Robbie M: Failure of β-lactam antibiotics to eradicate *Chlamydia trachomatis* from the endometrium in patients with acute salpingitis despite apparent clinical cure. JAMA 250:2641, 1983.
50. Wasserheit JN, Bell TA, Kiviat NB, et al: Microbial causes of proven pelvic inflammatory disease and efficacy of clindamycin and tobramycin. Ann Intern Med 104:187, 1986.
51. Punnonen R, Terho P, Nikkanen V, et al: Chlamydial serology in infertile women by immunofluorescence. Fertil Steril 31:656, 1979.
52. Henry-Suchet J, Catalan F, Loffredo V, et al: Microbiology of specimens obtained by laparoscopy from controls and from patients with pelvic inflammatory disease or infertility with tubal obstruction: *Chlamydia trachomatis*, *Ureaplasma urealyticum*. Am J Obstet Gynecol 138:1022, 1980.
53. Jones RB, Ardery BR, Hui S, et al: Correlation between serum antichlamydial antibodies and tubal factors as a cause of infertility. Fertil Steril 38:553, 1982.
54. Moore DE, Spadoni LR, Roy HM, et al: Increased frequency of serum antibodies to *Chlamydia trachomatis* in infertility due to distal tube disease. Lancet 2:574, 1982.
55. Gump DW, Gibson M, Ashikaga T: Evidence of prior pelvic inflammatory disease and its relationship to *C. trachomatis* antibody and intrauterine contraceptive device use in infertile women. Am J Obstet Gynecol 146:153, 1983.
56. Cevanini R, Possati G, LaPlaca M: *Chlamydia trachomatis* infection in infertile women. *In* Mardh P-A, Holmes KK, Oriel JD, et al (eds): Chlamydial Infections. Amsterdam, Elsevier Biomedical, 1982, pp 182–192.
57. Conway D, Caul EO, Hall MR: Chlamydial serology in fertile and infertile women. Lancet 1:191, 1984.
58. Kane JL, Woodland RM, Forsey T, et al: Evidence of chlamydial infection in infertile women with and without fallopian tube obstruction. Fertil Steril 42:6, 1984.
59. Sellors JW, Mahoney J, Chernesky M, et al: *Chlamydia trachomatis* in fertile and infertile Canadian women. *In* Chlamydia Infections. Sixth International Symposium Proceedings, June 1986. Cambridge, England, Cambridge University Press, 1986, p 233.
60. Brunham RS, MacLean IW, Binns B, et al: *Chlamydia trachomatis*: Its role in tubal infertility. J Infect Dis 152:1275, 1985.
61. Brunham RS, Binns B, McDowell J, et al: *Chlamydia trachomatis* infection in women with ectopic pregnancy. Obstet Gynecol 67:722, 1986.
62. Svensson L, Mardh P-A, Ahlgren M, et al: Ectopic pregnancy and antibiotics to *Chlamydia trachomatis*. Fertil Steril 44:313, 1985.
63. Hartford SL, Silva PD, diZerega GS, et al: Serologic evidence of prior chlamydial infection in patients with tubal ectopic pregnancy and contralateral tubal disease. Fertil Steril 47:118, 1987.
64. Chow JM, Yonekura L, Richard GA, et al: The association between *Chlamydia trachomatis* and ectopic pregnancy: A matched-pair, case-control study. JAMA 263:3164, 1990.
65. Patton DL, Halbert SA, Kuo C-C, et al: Host response to primary *Chlamydia trachomatis* infection of the fallopian tube in pig-tailed monkeys. Fertil Steril 40:829, 1983.
66. Ripa KT, Moller BR, Mardh P-A, et al: Experimental acute salpingitis in grivet monkeys provoked by *Chlamydia trachomatis*. Acta Pathol Microbiol Scand 87:65, 1979.
67. Sweet RL, Schachter J, Banks J, et al: Experimental chlamydial salpingitis in the guinea pig. Am J Obstet Gynecol 138:952, 1980.
68. Swenson CE, Donegan E, Schachter J: *Chlamydia trachomatis*–induced salpingitis in mice. J Infect Dis 148:1101, 1983.
69. Mardh P-A, Westrom L: Tubal and cervical cultures in acute salpingitis with special reference to *Mycoplasma hominis* and T-strain mycoplasma. Br J Vener Dis 46:179, 1970.
70. Mardh P-A, Westrom L, Ripa KT, et al: Pelvic inflammatory disease: Clinical, etiologic and pathophysiologic studies. *In* Holmes KK, Mardh P-A (eds): International Perspectives on Neglected Sexually Transmitted Diseases. New York, Hemisphere Publishing, 1983.
71. Brunham RL, Binns B, Guijon F, et al: Etiology and outcome of acute PID. J Infect Dis 158:510, 1988.
72. Heinonen PK, Teisala K, Punnoven R, et al: Anatomic sites of upper genital tract infection. Obstet Gynecol 66:384, 1985.
73. Sweet RL: Pelvic inflammatory disease and infertility in women. Infect Dis Clin North Am 1:199, 1987.
74. Hare MJ, Barnes CFJ: Fallopian tube culture in the investigation of *Bacteroides* as a cause of pelvic inflammatory disease. *In* Phillips I, Collier J (eds): Proceedings of the 2nd International Symposium on Metronidazole. London, Royal Society of Medicine, 1979.
75. Hammill HA, Owens WE, Ford LE, et al: A rat model of unilateral utero-tubo-ovarian abscess. Rev Infect Dis 6(Suppl 1):S96, 1984.

76. Jacobson L, Westrom L: Objectivized diagnosis of acute pelvic inflammatory disease: Diagnostic and prognostic value of routine laparoscopy. Am J Obstet Gynecol 105:1088, 1969.
77. Chaparro MV, Ghosh S, Nashed A, et al: Laparoscopy for the confirmation and prognostic evaluation of pelvic inflammatory disease. Int J Gynecol Obstet 15:307, 1978.
78. Hager WD, Eschenbach DA, Spence MR, Sweet RL: Criteria for diagnosis and grading of salpingitis. Obstet Gynecol 61:113, 1983.
79. Kahn JG, Walker CK, Washington AE, et al: Diagnosing pelvic inflammatory disease. A comprehensive analysis and considerations for developing a new model. JAMA 266:2594, 1991.
80. Method MW, Urnes PD, Neahring R, et al: Economic considerations in the use of laparoscopy for diagnosing pelvic inflammatory disease. J Reprod Med 32:759, 1987.
81. Paavonen J, Teisala K, Heinonen PK, et al: Endometritis and acute salpingitis associated with *Chlamydia trachomatis* and herpes simplex virus type two. Obstet Gynecol 65:288, 1985.
82. Kiviat NB, Wolner-Hanssen P, Eschenbach DA, et al: Endometrial histopathology in patients with culture-proved upper genital tract infection and laparoscopically diagnosed acute salpingitis. Am J Surg Pathol 14:167, 1990.
83. Sellors JW, Mahoney JB, Goldsmith C, et al: The diagnosis of pelvic inflammatory disease: The accuracy of clinical and laparoscopic findings. Am J Obstet Gynecol 164:113, 1991.
84. Viberg L: Acute inflammatory conditions of the uterine adnexa. Acta Obstet Gynecol Scand 43(Suppl 4):1, 1964.
85. Hillis SD, Joesoef R, Marchbanks PA, et al: Delayed care of pelvic inflammatory disease as a risk factor for impaired fertility. Am J Obstet Gynecol 168:1503, 1993.
86. Washington AE, Sweet RL, Shafer M-A: Pelvic inflammatory disease and its sequelae in adolescents. J Adolesc Health Care 6:298, 1985.
87. Sherris JD, Fox G: Infertility and sexually transmitted disease: A public health challenge. Popul Rep L 11:113, 1983.
88. Swensson CE, Sung ML, Schachter J: The effect of tetracycline treatment on chlamydial salpingitis and subsequent fertility in the mouse. Sex Transm Dis 13:40, 1986.
89. Thompson SE, Brooks CA, Eschenbach DA, et al: High failure rates in outpatient treatment of salpingitis with either tetracycline alone or penicillin-ampicillin combination. Am J Obstet Gynecol 152:635, 1985.
90. Centers for Disease Control and Prevention: 1993 Sexually transmitted diseases treatment guidelines. MMWR Morbid Mortal Wkly Rep 42(RR-14):1, 1993.
91. Wolner-Hanssen P, Paavonen J, Kiviat N, et al: Outpatient treatment of pelvic inflammatory disease with cefoxitin and doxycycline. Obstet Gynecol 71:595, 1988.
92. Wolner-Hanssen P, Paavonen J, Kiviat N, et al: Ambulatory treatment of suspected pelvic inflammatory disease with augmentin, with or without doxycycline. Am J Obstet Gynecol 158:577, 1988.
93. Thompson S, Holcomb G, Cheng S, et al: Antibiotic therapy of outpatient pelvic inflammatory disease (Abstr 671). *In* Program and Abstracts of the 20th Interscience Conference on Antimicrobial Agents and Chemotherapy. Washington, DC, American Society for Microbiology, 1980.
94. Sweet RL, Schachter J, Ohm-Smlith M, et al: Treatment of acute pelvic inflammatory disease: Cefoxitin and doxycycline vs clindamycin and tobramycin (Abstr 271). *In* Program and Abstracts of the 25th Interscience Conference on Antimicrobial Agents and Chemotherapy; September 29–October 2, 1985; Minneapolis, MN.
95. Walker CK, Kahn JG, Washington AE, et al: Pelvic inflammatory disease: Meta-analysis of antimicrobial regimen efficacy. J Infect Dis 168:969, 1993.
96. Thompson SE III, Hager WD, Wong K-H, et al: The microbiology and therapy of acute pelvic inflammatory disease in hospitalized patients. Am J Obstet Gynecol 136:179, 1980.
97. Brunham RC: Therapy for acute pelvic inflammatory disease: A critique of recent therapeutic trials. Am J Obstet Gynecol 148:235, 1984.
98. Pedowitz P, Bloomfield RD: Ruptured adnexal abscess with generalized peritonitis. Am J Obstet Gynecol 88:721, 1964.
99. Nebel WA, Lucas WE: Management of tuboovarian abscess. Obstet Gynecol 32:381, 1968.
100. Landers DV, Sweet RL: Tubo-ovarian abscess: Contemporary approach to management. Rev Infect Dis 5:876, 1983.
101. Burkman R, Schlesselman S, McCaffrey L, et al: The relationship of genital tract actinomycetes and the development of pelvic inflammatory disease. Am J Obstet Gynecol 143:585, 1982.
102. Hager WD: Follow-up of patients with tuboovarian abscess(es) in association with salpingitis. Obstet Gynecol 61:680, 1983.
103. Benigno BB: Medical and surgical management of the pelvic abscess. Clin Obstet Gynecol 224:1187, 1981.
104. Franklin EW, Hevron JE, Thompson JD: Management of the pelvic abscess. Clin Obstet Gynecol 16:66, 1973.
105. Brunham RC, Binns B, Guijon F, et al: Etiology and outcome of acute pelvic inflammatory disease. J Infect Dis 158:510, 1988.
106. Mickal A, Sellmann AH: Management of tuboovarian abscess. Clin Obstet Gynecol 12:252, 1969.
107. Clark JR, Moore-Hines S: A study of tubo-ovarian abscess at Howard University Hospital (1965 through 1975). J Natl Med Assoc 71:1109, 1979.
108. Ginsberg DS, Stern JL, Hamod KA, et al: Tubo-ovarian abscess: A retrospective review. Am J Obstet Gynecol 138:1055, 1980.
109. Edelman DA, Berger GS: Contraceptive practice and tubo-ovarian abscess. Am J Obstet Gynecol 138:541, 1980.
110. Filly RA: Detection of abdominal abscesses: A combined approach employing ultrasonography, computed tomography and gallium-67 scanning. J Assoc Can Radiol 30:202, 1979.
111. Norton L, Eule J, Burdick D: Accuracy of techniques to detect intraperitoneal abscess. Surgery 84:370, 1978.
112. Hopkins GB, Kan M, Mende CW: Gallium-67 scintigraphy and intraabdominal sepsis: Clinical experience in 140 patients with suspected intraabdominal abscess. West J Med 125:425, 1976.
113. Carroll B, Silverman PM, Goodwin DA, McDougall R: Ultrasonography and indium-111 white blood cell scanning for the detection of intraabdominal abscesses. Radiology 140:155, 1981.
114. Coleman RE, Black RE, Welch DM, et al: Indium-111–labeled leukocytes in the evaluation of suspected abdominal abscesses. Am J Surg 139:99, 1980.
115. Bicknell TA, Kohatsu S, Goodwin DA: Use of indium-111–labeled autologous leukocytes in differentiating pancreatic abscess from pseudocyst. Am J Surg 142:312, 1981.
116. Taylor KJK, DeGraaft MCI, Wasson JF, et al: Accuracy of greyscale ultrasound diagnosis of abdominal and pelvic abscesses in 220 patients. Lancet 1:83, 1978.
117. Spirtos NJ, Bernstine RL, Crawford WL, Rayle J: Sonography in acute pelvic inflammatory disease. J Reprod Med 27:312, 1982.
118. Uhrich PC, Sanders RC: Ultrasonic characteristics of pelvic inflammatory masses. J Clin Ultrasound 4:199, 1976.
119. Moir C, Robins RE: Role of ultrasound, gallium scanning and computed tomography in the diagnosis of intraabdominal abscess. Am J Surg 143:582, 1982.
120. Mitchell DG, Mintz MC, Spritzer CE, et al: Adnexal masses: MR imaging observations at 1.5T, with US and CT correlation. Radiology 162:319, 1987.
121. Fischman AJ, Rubin RH, Khaw BD, et al: Detection of acute inflammation with ^{111}In-labeled nonspecific polyclonal IgG. Semin Nucl Med 18:335, 1988.
122. Rubin RH, Fischman AG, Callahan RJ, et al: ^{111}In-labeled nonspecific immunoglobulin scanning in the detection of focal infection. N Engl J Med 321:935, 1989.
123. Jasinsky RW, Glazer GM, Francis IR, Harkness RL: CT and ultrasound in abscess detection at specific anatomic sites: A study of 198 patients. Comput Radiol 11:41, 1987.
124. Golde SH, Israel R, Ledger WJ: Unilateral tubo-ovarian abscess: A distinct entity. Am J Obstet Gynecol 127:807, 1977.
125. Svenson RM, Michaelson TC, Daly MJ, et al: Anaerobic bacterial infections of the female genital tract. Obstet Gynecol 42:538, 1973.
126. Thadepalli H, Gorbach SL, Keith L: Anaerobic infections of the female genital tract: Bacteriologic and therapeutic aspects. Am J Obstet Gynecol 117:1034, 1973.
127. Altemeier WA: The anaerobic streptococci in tubo-ovarian abscess. Am J Obstet Gynecol 39:1038, 1940.
128. Ledger WJ, Campbell C, Willson JR: Postoperative adnexal infections. Obstet Gynecol 31:83, 1968.
129. Pearson HE, Anderson GV: Genital bacteroidal abscesses in women. Am J Obstet Gynecol 107:1264, 1970.
130. Holmes KK, Eschenbach DA, Knapp JS: Salpingitis: Overview of etiology and epidemiology. Am J Obstet Gynecol 138:893, 1980.

131. Schiffer MA, Elguezabal A, Sultana M, Allen AC: Actinomycosis infections associated with intrauterine contraceptive devices. Obstet Gynecol 45:67, 1975.
132. Lomax CW, Harbert GM, Thornton WN: Actinomycosis of the female genital tract. Obstet Gynecol 48:341, 1976.
133. Gupta PK, Erozan YS, Frost JK: Actinomyces and the IUD: An update. Acta Cytol 22:281, 1978.
134. Golditch IM, Huston JE: Serious pelvic infections associated with intrauterine contraceptive devices. Int J Fertil 18:156, 1973.
135. Manara LR: Management of tubo-ovarian abscess. J Am Osteopath Assoc 81:476, 1982.
136. Taylor ES, McMillan JH, Green BE, et al: The intrauterine device. Obstet Gynecol 46:429, 1975.
137. Dawood MY, Birnbaum SJ: Unilateral tubo-ovarian abscess and an intrauterine contraceptive device. Obstet Gynecol 46:429, 1975.
138. Scott WC: Pelvic abscess in association with intrauterine contraceptive devices. Am J Obstet Gynecol 131:149, 1978.
139. Hemsell DL, Hemsell PG, Heard MC, Nobles BJ: Piperacillin and a combination of clindamycin and gentamicin for the treatment of hospital- and community-acquired acute pelvic infections including pelvic abscess. Surg Gynecol Obstet 165:223, 1987.
140. Reed SD, Landers DV, Sweet RL: Antibiotic treatment of tuboovarian abscess: Comparison or broad spectrum beta lactam agents versus clindamycin containing regimens. Am J Obstet Gynecol 164:1556, 1991.
141. Mercer LJ, Hajj SN, Ismail MA, Block BS: Use of C-reactive protein to predict the outcome of medical management of tuboovarian abscess. J Reprod Med 33:164, 1988.
142. Joiner KA, Lower BR, Dzink JL, Bartlett JG: Antibiotic levels in infected and sterile and sterile subcutaneous abscesses in mice. J Infect Dis 143:487, 1981.
143. Joiner K, Lowe B, Dzink J, Bartlett JG: Comparative efficacy of 10 antimicrobial agents in experimental infections with *Bacteroides fragilis*. J Infect Dis 145:561, 1982.
144. Bartlett JG, Marien GJ, Dezfulian M, Joiner KA: Relative efficacy of beta-lactam antimicrobial agents in two animal models of infections involving *Bacteroides fragilis*. Rev Infect Dis 5:S338, 1983.
145. Hemsell DL, Santos-Ramos R, Cunningham FG, et al: Cefotaxime treatment for women with community-acquired pelvic abscess. Am J Obstet Gynecol 151:771, 1985.
146. Collins CA, Jansen FW: Treatment of pelvic abscess. Clin Obstet Gynecol 2:512, 1959.
147. Rivlin ME, Hunt JA: Ruptured tubo-ovarian abscess: Is hysterectomy necessary? Obstet Gynecol 50:518, 1977.
148. Rubenstein PR, Mishell DR, Ledger WJ: Colpotomy drainage of pelvic abscess. Obstet Gynecol 48:142, 1976.
149. Rivlin ME, Golan A, Darling MR: Diffuse peritoneal sepsis associated with colpotomy drainage of pelvic abscess. J Reprod Med 27:406, 1982.
150. Rivlin ME: Clinical outcome following vaginal drainage of pelvic abscess. Obstet Gynecol 61:169, 1983.
151. Mandel SR, Body D, Jaques PF, et al: Drainage of hepatic, intraabdominal and mediastinal abscesses guided by computerized axial tomography. Am J Surg 145:120, 1983.
152. Van Sonnenberg E, Ferrucci JT, Mueller PR, et al: Percutaneous radiographically guided catheter drainage of abdominal abscesses. JAMA 247:190, 1982.
153. Worthen NJ, Gunning JE: Percutaneous drainage of pelvic abscess: Management of tuboovarian abscess. J Ultrasound Med 5:551, 1986.
154. Gerzof SG, Robbins AH, Johnson WC, et al: Percutaneous catheter drainage of abdominal abscesses. N Engl J Med 305:653, 1981.
155. Gronvall S, Gammelgaard J, Haubek A, Holm HH: Drainage of abdominal abscesses guided by sonography. Am J Radiol 138:527, 1982.
156. Van Sonnenberg E, Ferrucci JT, Mueller PR, et al: Percutaneous drainage of abscess and fluid collections. Techniques, results and applications. Radiology 142:1, 1982.
157. Kuligowska E, Conners SK, Shapiro JH: Liver abscess: Sonography in diagnosis and treatment. AJR 138:253, 1982.
158. Jeffrey RB Jr, Federle MP, Laing FC: Computed tomography of silent abdominal abscesses. J Comput Assist Tomogr 8:67, 1984.
159. Henry-Suchet J, Soler A, Loffredo V: Laparoscopic treatment of tuboovarian abscess. J Reprod Med 29:579, 1984.
160. Reich H, McGlynn F: Laparoscopic treatment of tuboovarian abscess and pelvic abscess. J Reprod Med 32:747, 1987.
161. Adducci JE: Laparoscopy in the diagnosis and treatment of pelvic inflammatory disease with abscess formation. Int Surg 66:359, 1981.
162. Kaplan AL, Jacobs WM, Ehresman JB: Aggressive management of pelvic abscess. Am J Obstet Gynecol 98:482, 1967.

118

Vaginitis, Cervicitis, and Endometritis

David A. Eschenbach

VAGINITIS

Complaint of an abnormal vaginal discharge is one of the most common reasons women visit primary care and specialist physicians. The discharge can be from a physiologic increase in fluid or from a vaginal or cervical infection. Vaginal infection results either from overgrowth of normal flora as in candidiasis and bacterial vaginosis (BV) or from sexual transmission as in trichomoniasis and cervicitis.

The Normal State of the Vagina

In menstruating women, the vagina is lined by a stratified squamous epithelium 40 cells thick during the proliferative phase and 20 cells thick during the secretory phase of the menstrual cycle.[1] Vaginal discharge fluid is a complex mixture of material in water. Most of the water is transudate from blood vessels just beneath the epithelial surface. Water egresses through intracellular channels between vaginal epithelial cells, which widen after ovulation.[2] Fluid is also derived from the cervix and endometrium. The remainder of vaginal discharge consists of water, sloughed epithelial cells, microorganisms, urea, protein (including enzymes), carbohydrates, fatty acids, and chemical by-products of microorganisms and the local cellular metabolism.[3] Vaginal fluid also contains T cells, immunoglobulins, cytokines, and probably a multitude of other components.[4]

Before puberty or at menopause, the vaginal epithelium is cuboid and the pH of vaginal discharge is 6 to 8. Under the influence of estrogen, the vaginal environment changes, glycogen collects in the vaginal epithelial cells, and the epithelium markedly thickens. The glycogen is metabolized by bacteria, particularly lactobacilli. The metabolism for both lactobacilli and vaginal epithelium produces high levels of lactic acid, which results in the low pH of vaginal fluid in menstruating women of 3.5 to 4.7.[5] The normal vaginal flora in women who are producing or taking estrogen is dominated by lactobacilli, which make up about 95% of the bacterial count.[6] Lactobacilli maintain their dominance over other vaginal microorganisms by producing lactic acid (and thus the low pH that inhibits most bacteria), hydrogen peroxide (which inhibits catalase-negative bacteria[7] and kills other bacteria), and other bactericidins. Other microorganisms that constitute vaginal flora include *Staphylococcus epidermidis*, diphtheroids, *Gardnerella vaginalis*, both aerobic and anaerobic streptococci, anaerobic *Prevotella* and *Bacteroides* species, and *Ureaplasma urealyticum*.[8, 9] About 15% of women carry *Escherichia coli*, group B streptococci, and *Candida* species. Lactobacilli concentration increases before menses, then decreases during menses.[10] The variation of other bacteria during the menstrual cycle is relatively small.[10] In premenarchal and postmenopausal patients, an increased number of anaerobic lactobacilli and other anaerobes occurs.

Examination of Cervical and Vaginal Discharges

A systematic examination of the discharge is required to accurately diagnose infection in symptomatic patients. Inspection is needed of the vagina for erythema and of the cervix for mucopus (yellow mucus on a cotton-tipped swab). Abnormal cervical discharge can be Gram stained to identify an excess of polymorphonuclear leukocytes (PMNs) of more than 30 per high-power field and determinations made for *Neisseria gonorrhoeae* and *Chlamydia trachomatis*. A pH of the vaginal discharge helps place patients in two general categories of vaginitis (Fig. 118–1). One drop of vaginal discharge is mixed with normal saline and covered with a coverslip, and another drop is mixed with 10% potassium hydroxide and smelled for the presence of amines before a coverslip is placed. In some cases, a smear for Gram stain or material for culture can be collected. An accurate diagnosis of vaginitis is highly dependent on microscopic findings. Therapy for vaginitis becomes relatively easy if the diagnosis is correct, and except for occasional recurrent infection, most therapeutic failures result from an incorrect diagnosis. Several specific elements should be actively sought by microscopy: long *Lactobacillus* morphotypes, small coccobacillary morphotypes, white blood cells, trichomonads, and clue cells in the saline slide and hyphae in the potassium hydroxide part of the slide (see Fig. 118–1).

Candidiasis

Candida species are present as commensals in about 15% of reproductive age women.[9, 10] Several predisposing factors for candidiases have been identified in the general population, including previous vaginal candidiases, frequency of coitus, oral and vaginal contraceptive use, and more than two episodes a week of passive oral-genital contact. Special factors that contribute to vaginal candidiases include antibiotic and corticosteroid use, diabetes, pregnancy, and acquired immunodeficiency syndrome.[11] In menstruating women, symptoms most commonly develop just before menses. Excessive warmth and moisture seem related to vulvovaginal candidiases. Rarely, men with genital candidiases will sexually transmit *Candida*. Tight clothing, tampon use, and douching are not related to vaginal candidiases.

Candida albicans is responsible for 85% to 90% of vaginal candidiases.[12] Other *Candida* species, such as *Candida glabrata*, *Candida krusei*, *Candida tropicalis*, and *Candida pseudotropicalis*, can also cause symptomatic infection. These non-*albicans* species are particularly common in patients with recurrent candidiases, and they have more resistance to azoles than *C.*

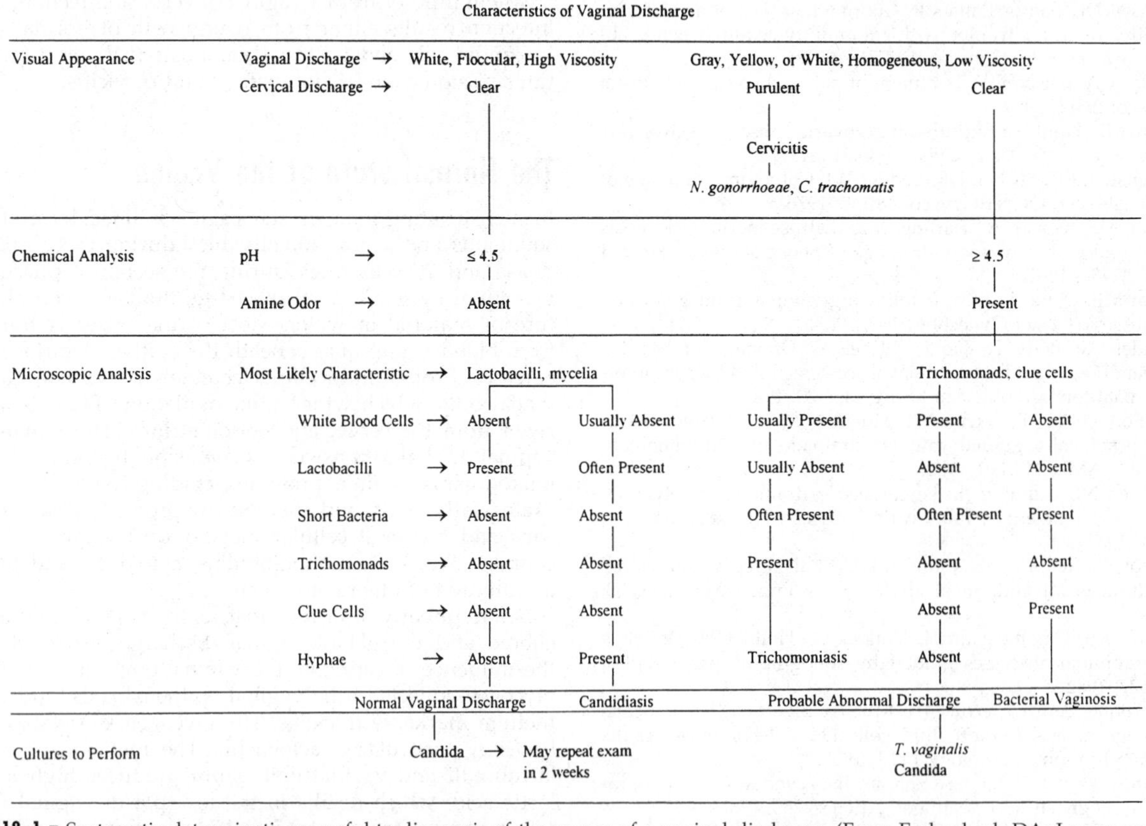
Characteristics of Vaginal Discharge
Visual Appearance
Vaginal Discharge →
White, Floccular, High Viscosity
Gray, Yellow, or White, Homogeneous, Low Viscosity
Cervical Discharge →
Clear
Purulent
Clear
Cervicitis
N. gonorrhoeae, C. trachomatis
Chemical Analysis
pH →
≤ 4.5
≥ 4.5
Amine Odor →
Absent
Present
Microscopic Analysis
Most Likely Characteristic →
Lactobacilli, mycelia
Trichomonads, clue cells
White Blood Cells →
Absent
Usually Absent
Usually Present
Present
Absent
Lactobacilli →
Present
Often Present
Usually Absent
Absent
Absent
Short Bacteria →
Absent
Absent
Often Present
Often Present
Present
Trichomonads →
Absent
Absent
Present
Absent
Absent
Clue Cells →
Absent
Absent
Absent
Present
Hyphae →
Absent
Present
Trichomoniasis
Absent
Normal Vaginal Discharge
Candidiasis
Probable Abnormal Discharge
Bacterial Vaginosis
Cultures to Perform
Candida →
May repeat exam in 2 weeks
T. vaginalis
Candida

FIGURE 118–1 □ Systematic determinations useful to diagnosis of the causes of a vaginal discharge. (From Eschenbach DA: Lower genital tract infections. *In* Galask RP, Larsen B [eds]: Infectious Diseases in the Female Patient. New York, Springer-Verlag, 1986, p 166.)

albicans does.[13] All species of *Candida* except *C. glabrata* exist in two forms, a blastospore and a germinated form with hyphae. The blastospore attaches to the epithelial cell and colonizes the surface. The germinated form is seen during infection in which *Candida* invades the superficial epithelium.[11]

Typical symptoms include vulvar pruritus, a burning sensation, superficial dysuria, and a white discharge. Vulvar erythema and at times a geographic rash can be present. The vagina is often erythematous; in about 25% of patients, a pathognomonic thick, dry, curdy vaginal discharge occurs. The vaginal pH is 4.7 or less, and hyphae are identified on wet mount or Gram-stained material at the low microscopic power. Among women with pruritus or other genital findings that could represent *Candida* infection, it is important to perform a culture for *Candida* when the microscopic examination result is negative. A culture identifies not only an increased number of symptomatic women with candidiasis compared with microscopy alone, and it excludes candidiasis in symptomatic women with an unclear diagnosis.[14]

Vaginal candidiasis is usually treated with one of the azoles, most commonly an intravaginal preparation. Intravaginal medication given for 3 to 7 days has better long-term efficacy than 1-day regimens do. Miconazole, clotrimazole, butoconazole, and terconazole are all available for intravaginal use[15] (Table 118–1). In the unusual situation when resistance occurs to one azole, resistance is present to all of the azoles. Oral fluconazole and itraconazole can be used to treat vaginal candidiases, but they offer little advantage over intravaginal preparations. Oral azole treatment is no more efficacious than local azole treatment, and for symptomatic patients, oral fluconazole may need to be repeated, increasing the cost.[16] Nystatin is no longer a first-line drug, but it can be useful when resistance develops to azoles. Boric acid (boric acid powder in gelatin capsules) is fungistatic, and intravaginal use can also be helpful for strains resistant to azoles.[17] Most patients rapidly become symptom free with any of the anti-*Candida* therapies. Allergy to the base in the vaginal preparation or other reasons for symptoms should be considered when patients receiving azoles have persistent or increasing symptoms. Rarely, patients with persistent symptoms have *Candida* resistant to azoles.

TABLE 118–1 ■ Treatment Regimens for Vaginal Candidiases

IMIDAZOLES	
Clotrimazole	200-mg vaginal tablet nightly for 3 d
	or
	100-mg vaginal tablet or 1% cream, 5 g intravaginally nightly for 7 d
Miconazole nitrate	250-mg vaginal suppository nightly for 3 d
	or
	100-mg vaginal suppository or 2% cream, 5 g intravaginally nightly for 7 d
Butoconazole	2% cream, 5 g intravaginally nightly for 3 d
Terconazole	80-mg vaginal suppository nightly for 3 d
	or
	0.4% cream, 5 g intravaginally nightly for 7 d
POLYENES	
Nystatin	100,000-unit vaginal tablet, 1 per vagina twice daily for 14 d
BORIC ACID	600 mg powder in gelatin capsules, 1 per vagina twice daily for 14 d

TREATMENT DURING PREGNANCY
Clotrimazole, miconazole, and terconazole may be used intravaginally for the treatment of symptomatic patients during pregnancy. It is suggested that use be deferred until the second trimester.

Recurrent Vaginal Candidiases

Candidiasis occurs in up to 75% of women at some time in their life, usually only one to three times. However, a small number of patients have frequent recurrences; those with four or more recurrences a year are considered to have frequent recurrent candidiasis.[18] Such patients should be examined or culture should be performed for *Candida* to ensure that recurrent symptoms are actually due to *Candida* and to rule out potentially resistant species. It is not clear whether these relapses occur with the same strain or are due to rapid recolonization from the skin or gastrointestinal tract.[19] Attempts to reduce *Candida* in the gastrointestinal tract only slightly influence recurrent infection,[20] although continued gastrointestinal tract suppression with 4 ounces of yogurt containing lactobacilli twice daily has reduced recurrence.[21] Sexual partner therapy is not useful, except for the treatment of men with symptomatic genital candidiasis.[22]

Patients with frequently recurrent candidiasis need to be scrutinized for risk factors, although few patients have risk factors. Patients with acquired immunodeficiency syndrome have an increased risk for vaginal candidiasis, but acquired immunodeficiency syndrome would rarely be diagnosed in this group of patients. Patients with frequent recurrences should receive 3 weeks of standard anti-*Candida* therapy with local or oral azoles followed by 6 to 12 months of suppressive therapy. Suppressive therapy with intravaginal azoles or boric acid given every third night and weekly fluconazole is most effective. Ketoconazole should no longer be used for candidiases because of hepatotoxic effects, but 100 mg (one-half tablet) of ketoconazole daily for 6 months reduced the recurrence rate from 75% in placebo-treated women to 25%.[18]

Trichomoniasis

Trichomonas vaginalis is a sexually transmitted protozoan. *T. vaginalis* can be recovered from the prostate gland of up to 70% of male sexual partners of women with trichomoniasis.[23] Symptoms of an uncomfortable or yellow vaginal discharge occur in about 40% to 50% of patients with *T. vaginalis* infection.[24, 25] Symptomatic women may have vulvar erythema and edema; about 60% have a purulent vaginal discharge, and 10% have a frothy vaginal discharge.[25] Pathognomonic punctate areas of red epithelium (strawberry lesions or colpitis macularis) were rarely observed with the naked eye but were observed by colposcopy in 44% of patients.[25] The vaginal pH is usually 4.7 or higher, and an elevated number of PMNs and the herky-jerky motion of the mobile trichomonad can be observed on saline wet mount. Fortunately, most symptomatic patients have trichomonads recognized by wet mount, but only about 50% of women with *T. vaginalis* recovered from the vagina have a high enough concentration of trichomonads to be found on wet mount. Modified Diamond media should be used for culture, although cultures are usually unnecessary.

T. vaginalis infection is treated with a 2-g single dose of metronidazole.[26] Seven-day metronidazole regimens can also be used (Table 118–2). Male partners require simultaneous treatment, which reduces failure rates from about 20% to 3%.[27, 28] Patients with recurrent infection should receive metronidazole for 7 days. Patients with severe symptoms in pregnancy should be treated with a 2-g single dose after

TABLE 118–2 ■ Treatment Regimens for Trichomoniasis

FOR INITIAL INFECTION
Metronidazole, 2 g orally as a single dose
Metronidazole, 500 mg orally twice daily for 7 d
Metronidazole, 250 mg orally 3 times daily for 7 d
FOR TREATMENT FAILURES
Re-treat with metronidazole, 500 mg twice daily for 7 d
FOR REPEATED TREATMENT FAILURES
Re-treat with metronidazole, 1 g orally twice daily plus 500 mg of intravaginal metronidazole twice daily for 7–10 d
TREATMENT DURING PREGNANCY
After the first trimester, metronidazole, 2 g orally as a single dose, for women with severe symptoms
The patient's sexual partner should be treated simultaneously.

the first trimester.[26] Although *T. vaginalis* infection has been associated with preterm birth, routine treatment in pregnancy is not presently recommended.[29]

Rarely, patients have strains of *T. vaginalis* that are relatively resistant to metronidazole, with levels of 100 μg or more of metronidazole needed for inhibition.[30] These patients fail to respond to 2 g of metronidazole daily for 2 to 10 days. They often require a 1-g oral dose of metronidazole twice daily plus an intravaginal dose of 500 mg of metronidazole twice daily (tablets crushed in a base at a concentration of 500 mg/5 mL, the volume of a vaginal applicator). This regimen causes considerable anorexia, nausea, and vomiting. Because serum metronidazole levels after an oral and an intravenous dose are nearly equal, there is no advantage to the use of intravenous metronidazole. Doses exceeding 3 g/d of metronidazole should be avoided because irreversible peripheral neuropathy can result.

Bacterial Vaginosis

BV is a syndrome in which the vaginal flora is no longer dominated by lactobacilli and there is an overgrowth of *G. vaginalis*, certain anaerobic bacteria, and *Mycoplasma hominis*.[6, 31] Facultative lactobacilli are found in only 20% to 25% of patients with BV, and most of these strains do not produce hydrogen peroxide. Anaerobic lactobacilli are found in 25% of patients with BV compared with 5% of those with normal vaginal flora.[7] Concomitant with the drop in the prevalence of facultative lactobacilli, an increase occurs in the prevalence and concentration of other microorganisms.

In a population-based study of pregnant women containing a cohort of both asymptomatic and symptomatic women with BV, a 10-fold increase occurred in the concentration of *G. vaginalis*, certain anaerobes, and *M. hominis* among patients with BV compared with those without vaginitis.[6] In a comparison of symptomatic patients with BV and control subjects without vaginitis, an increased concentration of 100-fold occurred for *G. vaginalis* and of 1000-fold for certain anaerobes in the BV group.[32] The anaerobes associated with BV include *Prevotella, Prevotella bivia, Bacteroides ureolyticus, Peptostreptococcus,* and *Mobiluncus*.[31–33] It is not clear which of the microorganisms are primary and which secondarily overgrow in BV. Amines including cadaverine, putrescine, and trimethylamine are metabolic products of this bacterial overgrowth that cause the fishy odor.[34, 35] These amines are bound to protein at a low pH, but alkalinization of vaginal fluid by semen during intercourse or by potassium hydroxide produces the fishy odor characteristic of BV. A variety of inorganic acids are also produced by the microorganisms in BV, including succinate, which is suspected of inhibiting PMN migration.[31]

Factors associated with BV include sexual activity, a new sexual partner, antibiotic use, *T. vaginalis*, and use of an intrauterine device. However, BV is not a classic sexually transmitted disease (STD) because no specific agents in the male partner have been found, and treatment of the man with metronidazole does not prevent recurrent BV.[36, 37]

About half of patients with BV are asymptomatic. Patients with BV complain of a fishy vaginal odor and increased vaginal discharge.[38] BV is present in about 15% to 20% of a general sexually active population, but the prevalence varies widely from 5% of asymptomatic college students to 30% to 45% of women attending STD clinics.[39, 40]

The clinical diagnosis of BV is based on the presence of three of the four following characteristics of vaginal discharge: (1) a pH above 4.5, (2) a thin (skim milk) appearance, (3) a fishy amine odor when 10% potassium hydroxide is placed on the discharge, and (4) clue cells.[39] Clue cells are vaginal epithelial cells that contain so many bacteria on their surface that the cell border is obscured. On wet mount, long *Lactobacillus* morphotypes are absent and numerous small coccobacillary forms are present. Gram stain criteria have been developed for BV. Gram stain diagnosis closely correlates with the diagnosis made by clinical criteria.[40–42] Gram stain criteria rely on a paucity of long gram-positive lactobacilli morphotypes and numerous small gram-negative and gram-positive *Gardnerella* and *Prevotella* rod morphotypes, gram-positive cocci, and gram-variable curved rod *Mobiluncus* morphotypes. Culture should not be used to diagnose BV because cultures for *G. vaginalis* are misleading and proper cultures for anaerobes are too expensive. Whereas virtually all women with BV have *G. vaginalis* isolated, so do half of women without vaginitis.[43] Therefore, the recovery of *G. vaginalis* is too nonspecific to be of any practical benefit to diagnose BV.

All symptomatic nonpregnant women, probably all pregnant women (see later), and nonpregnant women undergoing selected pelvic operations with BV should be treated. Asymptomatic nonpregnant women should not be treated. The reason for an expansion of the treatment group relates to data associating BV with upper genital tract infection and preterm delivery. Pregnant patients with BV have a 50% to 100% increased rate of preterm low-birth-weight delivery,[44] amniotic fluid infection,[45] and chorioamnion infection.[46] Treatment of BV reduces the preterm low-birth-weight rate to baseline levels.[47, 48] These data are convincing that BV needs to be routinely diagnosed and treated in pregnancy, although this is not yet routine.

The high concentration of potentially virulent bacteria in the vagina also appears related to other upper genital tract infections. Patients with BV who have a cesarean section have a sixfold increased rate of postpartum endometritis compared with control subjects.[49] Patients with BV undergoing therapeutic abortion have a threefold increased rate of pelvic inflammatory disease compared with control subjects, and metronidazole therapy reduces this rate to baseline levels.[50, 51] Patients with BV undergoing abdominal hysterectomy have a threefold to fourfold increased rate of vaginal cuff cellulitis compared with control subjects.[52, 53]

Two antimicrobials with high activity against anaerobic bacteria provide first-line therapy (Table 118–3). Both oral and intravaginal metronidazole and clindamycin regimens produce 80% to 90% cure rates.[26, 54–56] Single-dose metronidazole and 7-day amoxicillin-clavulanate regimens are also effective. Regimens with little or no activity against BV are still used but should be abandoned, including oral ampicillin, cephalosporins, quinolones, tetracycline, and erythromycin

TABLE 118–3 ■ Treatment Regimens for Bacterial Vaginosis

FOR INITIAL INFECTION IN SYMPTOMATIC PATIENTS	
Nonpregnant patients	
	Metronidazole, 500 mg orally twice daily for 7 d
	Metronidazole 0.75% gel intravaginally twice daily for 5 d
	Clindamycin, 300 mg orally 3 times daily for 7 d
	Clindamycin 2% cream intravaginally nightly for 7 d
Pregnant patients	
	Metronidazole, 500 mg twice daily for 7 d, *after the first trimester*
	Clindamycin, 300 mg orally 3 times daily for 7 d
FOR RECURRENT INFECTION IN SYMPTOMATIC PATIENTS	
Repeat treatment with vaginal metronidazole or clindamycin	
FOR ASYMPTOMATIC PATIENTS	
Antibiotic treatment should be given if the patient is at risk for upper genital tract infection from a surgical procedure	

and intravaginal triple sulfa cream and povidone-iodine (Betadine) gel. *Lactobacillus* given orally or intravaginally may be helpful in preventing recurrence, but no proof exists. As mentioned, metronidazole given to men has no effect on the recurrence of BV in their sexual partners.[36, 37]

CERVICITIS

Background

Terms such as cervical erosion, cervical ectopy, and cervical hypertrophy represent variances of the normal cervical anatomy rather than examples of cervical infection. Columnar epithelium lines the endocervical canal and secretes the mucus found in the endocervical canal. If columnar epithelium is located entirely inside the endocervical canal, it is not visible and the cervix has a "normal" appearance. However, columnar epithelium can often be present on the cervical portio, where it has a red appearance because columnar epithelium is only a few cells thick; the red color is from light reflecting off the blood in the superficial blood vessels. The extension of columnar epithelium onto the cervical portio is termed ectopy.[57] Ectopy is normal variation, and the amount of ectopic tissue visible on the cervical portio varies considerably from patient to patient. Most ectopy is unrelated to infectious agents; it appears rather to be related to female hormone levels. Ectopy commonly appears after menarche, and patients with a high level of hormones, such as those taking oral contraceptives, have an increased prevalence and areas of cervical ectopy.[58]

Mucopurulent cervicitis is the preferred and specific term for inflammation of cervical columnar epithelium. The presence of yellowish cervical mucus in the cervical canal or an abnormally increased number of PMNs on Gram-stained material from the endocervical canal is evidence of mucopurulent cervicitis.[59] A standard definition of cervicitis allows researchers to compare diseases regardless of what microorganism is recovered from the cervix. To date, microorganisms commonly correlated with the presence of mucopurulent cervicitis include *C. trachomatis*, *N. gonorrhoeae*, and herpes simplex virus (HSV).[58, 60] Follicular cervicitis and hypertrophic cervicitis are descriptive terms used for *C. trachomatis* cervical infection. The histologic appearance of *C. trachomatis* infection in the cervix is relatively well described, but less is known about histologic changes associated with the other two infections. Inflammatory cells are commonly found in the cervical epithelium and in the cervical stroma of patients without mucopurulent cervicitis who undergo biopsy to diagnose cervical dysplasia. The significance of PMNs in these patients with acute and chronic histologic cervicitis and their correlation with the microorganisms associated with mucopurulent cervicitis have not been determined, so the remainder of this chapter focuses on mucopurulent cervicitis.

Prevalence

The true prevalence of mucopurulent cervicitis has been underestimated in most clinical settings. The frequent failure to recognize mucopurulent cervicitis has been related to nonstandard definitions, to confusion with normal anatomy, and to inattention to physical signs. The prevalence of mucopus depends on the prevalence of these microorganisms in the population under study. In an STD clinic, the prevalence of mucopurulent cervicitis in women appears to be similar to the prevalence of both nongonococcal and gonococcal urethritis in men. Mucopurulent cervicitis has been reported in 24% to 40% of randomly selected female patients attending STD clinics and in 34% of consecutive women undergoing routine annual examinations at a university student health clinic.[59–61] Among patients with *C. trachomatis*, mucopurulent cervicitis was present in 64% to 95% of randomly sampled STD patients and in about one third of randomly sampled college students.[61]

Mucopurulent cervicitis was found in only 15% of STD patients with *N. gonorrhoeae*, and the frequency of mucopus among patients with *N. gonorrhoeae* but without *C. trachomatis* appears to be low.[61] Thus, *C. trachomatis* is more often associated with mucopus than is *N. gonorrhoeae*.

Importance

Uterine cervical infections are of considerable importance because they represent an important reservoir for the spread of sexually transmitted microorganisms. An important way to identify possible genital infection among women is by recognition and treatment of cervicitis, and it allows potentially infected men to be identified.

Cervicitis also provides a source of the intraluminal ascent of pathogenic organisms to the endometrium and endosalpinx. Cervical infections are central to the development of pelvic inflammatory disease. From 10% to 20% of women with cervical *N. gonorrhoeae* and at least 10% of patients with cervical *C. trachomatis* develop clinical manifestations of pelvic inflammatory disease.[62] It is well recognized that in 50% to 70% of patients, salpingitis is never recognized by the patient or her physician.[63, 64] Even when salpingitis is recognized promptly and treated, most of the acute tubal damage that later causes tubal infertility appears to have occurred before antibiotic therapy was instituted. Thus, the identification and treatment of cervicitis are key to reducing rates of infertility and ectopic pregnancy secondary to pelvic inflammatory disease.

A second important consequence of cervicitis is the possible ascent during pregnancy of infectious agents that produce chorioamnionitis, premature rupture of membranes, amniotic fluid infection, premature delivery, and puerperal and neonatal infections. Both *C. trachomatis* and *N. gonorrhoeae* have been related to these adverse perinatal outcomes.[65, 66]

Microorganisms

Three organisms have been related to mucopurulent cervicitis: *C. trachomatis*, *N. gonorrhoeae*, and HSV.[60] *C. trachomatis* has been more closely associated with the presence of mucopus than the other agents have. As mentioned earlier, a substantial proportion of patients with *C. trachomatis* have mucopus, and conversely, among patients with mucopus, 30% to 60% have *C. trachomatis*.[60] Overall, *C. trachomatis* is isolated from approximately 40% to 50% of patients with mucopus or an increased number of PMNs on Gram stain of cervical mucus. Many patients with *C. trachomatis* also have *N. gonorrhoeae*. The strong association between *C. trachomatis* and mucopus plus the weaker association between *N. gonorrhoeae* and mucopus is curious. Perhaps *C. trachomatis* infection is a more chronic process, with either no symptoms or chronic symptoms and signs, whereas *N. gonorrhoeae* infections need to be treated because of acute symptoms in the woman or her sexual contact. Acute primary HSV infection causes ulcerative lesions and an exudate covering the cervix, but neither mucopus nor ulcers are present with recurrent HSV infections.[67] Thus, whereas mucopurulent cervicitis from HSV appears to be a feature of only primary infection, inflammation is present on the Papanicolaou smear of patients with both primary and recurrent HSV infections.[67]

Other organisms, including *T. vaginalis* and *M. hominis*, and BV have not been consistently related to mucopurulent cervicitis or to the other cervical manifestations of infection when the presence of *C. trachomatis* is controlled. However, in one study, *U. urealyticum* remained associated with mucopurulent cervicitis after adjustment for the presence of *C. trachomatis*.[60] *U. urealyticum* has also been associated with nongonococcal urethritis in men, independently of *C. trachomatis*.

Clinical Diagnosis

Manifestations of mucopurulent cervicitis are difficult for either the patient or the physician to recognize. Organisms such as *C. trachomatis* can simultaneously infect the urethra, cervix, and rectum and thereby produce variable symptoms. Symptoms from cervical infection are often poorly localized, and they are frequently mistaken for vaginitis. Symptoms can include an increase in yellow vaginal discharge and, less commonly, postcoital spotting, vague lower abdominal pain, and mild discomfort with intercourse. However, cervical infections often produce no symptoms. In addition, cervical cultures for *C. trachomatis* and *N. gonorrhoeae* do not provide completely ideal information because results are positive in only about half of patients with mucopurulent cervicitis, and a large number of patients with mucopurulent cervicitis would not be detected by use of culture criteria alone. Further, in the past, physicians have not usually appreciated the clinical signs of cervical infection. Thus, compared with the recognition of nongonococcal urethritis in men, the recognition of cervicitis in women has been more of a problem.

Cervical mucus is normally clear and translucent. Yellow discharge observed on a white cotton swab best identifies cervical mucopus. However, vaginal discharge must be wiped from the face of the cervix so that vaginal discharge does not confuse this clinical test. Yellow mucopus is highly correlated with an increased number of PMNs on a Gram stain of cervical mucus from nonpregnant patients.[59] Opaque cervical mucus is common in pregnancy, and mucopus may be more difficult to distinguish from the normal secretion in pregnant patients.[68]

Easily produced bleeding of the columnar epithelium from the inflammation is the second most common manifestation of mucopurulent cervicitis after mucopus.[60] Bleeding occurs when the cervix is swabbed for Papanicolaou smears or cervical cultures. Other manifestations of mucopurulent cervicitis include the presence of erythema of the cervical ectopy.[60] In addition, edema or swelling of the columnar epithelium above the plane of the squamous epithelium has been noted in patients with cervicitis.[60, 61] The swelling is analogous to the follicular appearance of the conjunctiva among patients with *C. trachomatis* in the eye.

Laboratory Diagnosis

Endocervical mucus should be obtained on a swab to confirm the presence of mucopurulent cervicitis. Vaginal material must be wiped off the face of the cervix with a large cotton-tipped swab before cervical mucus is collected; otherwise, the Gram stain is likely to be uninterpretable because of vaginal bacteria or PMNs. A standard approach includes the reading of five representative fields under the high-power (× 1000) microscope objective.[59] An increased number of PMNs on the Gram stain is highly correlated with the presence of cervical pathogens. The exact number of PMNs needed to establish an abnormal number is population dependent. In earlier studies, a mean of 10 or more PMNs per × 1000 field was used to define cervicitis. A more liberal definition of a mean of 20 to 30 PMNs increases the specificity but lowers the sensitivity of the test.[59] Further evaluation of the mean number of PMNs to distinguish cervicitis is needed for pregnancy. Papanicolaou smears can also be used to detect the presence of an increased number of PMNs, and they aid in the diagnosis of cervicitis.[67] Papanicolaou smears cannot be used to specifically diagnose *C. trachomatis* infection.

Therapy

Therapy for mucopurulent cervicitis should cover *C. trachomatis* and *N. gonorrhoeae*. In a randomized comparison of oral tetracycline with oral amoxicillin, both agents unexpectedly treated *C. trachomatis* and cervicitis, and both were equally effective in eliminating mucopus and other cervical manifestations of cervicitis, including the PMN count in patients without *C. trachomatis* infection.[69] Only about half of the patients in this study had either *C. trachomatis* or *N. gonorrhoeae*, and the disappearance of mucopus among patients without these two bacteria suggests a bacterial infection even in the culture-negative patients with cervicitis. Despite the findings of this study, tetracycline is more active than amoxicillin against *C. trachomatis*, and tetracycline or doxycycline remains the preferable antibiotic to treat mucopurulent cervicitis, especially for patients with known *C. trachomatis* infection. Patients with penicillinase-producing *N. gonorrhoeae* do not usually respond to tetracycline, so ceftriaxone together with tetracycline would be preferable in these cases. Tetracycline should be administered in a dose of 500 mg four times a day, or doxycycline in a dose of 100 mg twice a day, for a total of 10 days.

ENDOMETRITIS

Background

Endometritis is an infection of the endometrial cavity, which is anatomically interposed between the cervix and fallopian tubes. Endometritis has not been well described in terms of pathologic and clinical manifestations. The endometrium of patients with endometritis may contain a large variety of inflammatory cells during menstrual sloughing, but the presence of plasma cells in the endometrium has been considered necessary to diagnose endometritis.[70] Leukocytes and lymphocytes are often present in large numbers in the endometrium of patients with plasma cells, but they are also normally present just before and during menses.

A high prevalence of plasma-cell endometritis has been found among patients with mucopurulent cervicitis. Fourteen (40%) of 35 women with cervical mucopus had plasma-cell endometritis.[71, 72] Endometritis is found in 80% to 90% of patients with salpingitis.[72] Plasma-cell endometritis appears to be infrequent among asymptomatic patients without mucopurulent cervicitis; it was found in 3% of 35 asymptomatic patients who underwent endometrial biopsy for evaluation of infertility.[71]

Microorganisms

Both *C. trachomatis* and, to a lesser extent, *N. gonorrhoeae* are associated with endometritis.[71, 72] The presence of BV has also been associated with plasma-cell endometritis.[73] *Chlamydia* inclusions can be identified in the endometrium by use of monoclonal antibodies. In fact, *C. trachomatis* was identified more frequently in endometrial tissue by monoclonal antibody than by cultures. In unusual circumstances, HSV has also been found in endometrium.[74]

Clinical Diagnosis

Endometritis has been associated with a history of intermenstrual vaginal bleeding and increased bleeding with menses. Up to half of the women of reproductive age who have an endometrial biopsy for abnormal uterine bleeding have had plasma-cell endometritis (unpublished data). The diagnosis of endometritis was not made clinically or by usual pathologic study in the majority of these women. Uterine tenderness has been recognized more frequently among patients with endometritis than among those without.[71] In addition, cervical motion tenderness and elevations of the erythrocyte sedimentation rate and the peripheral white cell count can be present with endometritis.

Careful bimanual examination may reveal mild uterine tenderness[71]; however, it is difficult to make the distinction between endometritis alone and endometritis with salpingitis on a clinical basis. Thus, in studies in which the diagnosis of salpingitis was not confirmed by laparoscopy, some patients with a clinical diagnosis of salpingitis in fact have had endometritis without salpingitis. This emphasizes the difficulties inherent in the clinical diagnosis of upper genital tract infection and the overlapping clinical findings between endometritis and salpingitis.

Laboratory Diagnosis

An endometrial biopsy appears to be the only reliable means to establish a diagnosis of endometritis. Endometrial biopsy is useful for establishing a diagnosis of endometritis or upper genital tract infection.[70] Patients with vague complaints for whom infection is not strongly suspected benefit from endometrial biopsy if the biopsy shows endometritis; however, an absence of plasma cells in the biopsy specimen does not rule out salpingitis because about 20% of patients with laparoscopically proven salpingitis have no evidence of plasma cells on endometrial biopsy.[72]

Therapy

Treatment of endometritis with ceftriaxone and azithromycin appears to eliminate plasma cells from the endometrium (unpublished data). It would seem reasonable to use the outpatient treatment of salpingitis to treat endometritis. A loading dose of antibiotic to treat gonorrhea should be followed by 14 days of antibiotics to inhibit *C. trachomatis*.[26] Treating endometritis is particularly important owing to the risk for infertility if salpingitis develops because patients are not treated or are undertreated.

Two special circumstances for endometritis exist. In at least one reported case, endometritis seemed related to reversible infertility. An asymptomatic infertile patient with plasma-cell endometritis and *C. trachomatis* noted on an endometrial biopsy sample became pregnant after therapy.[75] The second circumstance of endometritis exists after pregnancy. This has been most closely studied among patients who have had therapeutic abortion; about 20% of patients with *C. trachomatis* before the abortion develop laparoscopically confirmed salpingitis after the procedure.[76] The rate of postabortion salpingitis is five times greater among women with *C. trachomatis* than among those without. Manifestations often begin as low-grade abdominal pain and mild uterine tenderness indicative of endometritis. Symptoms and signs of endometritis have also been noted after term vaginal delivery; patients usually develop mild lower abdominal pain about 2 weeks after delivery. These patients are usually afebrile, and half have had *C. trachomatis*.[77]

Endometritis may be particularly important to identify and treat before tubal damage occurs. It has been well recognized in infertility literature that 50% to 70% of patients who are infertile because of occluded fallopian tubes have never had a recognized episode of salpingitis.[63, 64] Presumably, most of these patients had mild symptoms or atypical manifestations of upper genital tract infection. It is important that physicians identify and treat patients who present them with mild manifestations of pelvic infection.

References

1. Buros MH, Roig de Vargas-Linares CE: Ultrastructure of the vaginal mucosa. *In* Hafez ESE, Evans TN (eds): The Human Vagina. Amsterdam, Elsevier North Holland, 1978, pp 63–93.
2. Roig de Vargas-Linares CE: Vagina as a source of immunoglobulins. *In* Hafez ESE, Evans TN (eds): The Human Vagina. Amsterdam, Elsevier North Holland, 1978, p 42.
3. Huggins GR, Preti G: Vaginal odors and secretions. Clin Obstet Gynecol 24:355, 1981.
4. Moghissi KS: Vaginal fluid constituents. *In* Beller FK, Chumacher GFB (eds): The Biology of Fluids of the Female Genital Tract. Amsterdam, Elsevier North Holland, 1979.
5. Cohn L: Influence of pH on vaginal discharges. Br J Vener Dis 45:241, 1969.
6. Hillier SL, Krohn MA, Rabe LK, et al: The normal vaginal flora, H_2O_2-producing lactobacilli, and bacterial vaginosis in pregnant women. Clin Infect Dis 16(Suppl 4):S273, 1993.
7. Eschenbach DA, Davick PR, Williams BL, et al: Prevalence of hydrogen peroxide–producing *Lactobacillus* species in normal women and women with bacterial vaginosis. J Clin Microbiol 27:251, 1989.
8. Bartlett JG, Moon NE, Goldstein PR, et al: Cervical and vaginal bacterial flora: Ecologic niches in the female lower genital tract. Am J Obstet Gynecol 130:658, 1978.
9. Hill GB, Eschenbach DA, Holmes KK: Bacteriology of the vagina. Scand J Urol Nephrol Suppl 86:23, 1984.
10. Galask R, Brown WJ: Variation in vaginal bacterial flora. A preliminary report. Ann Intern Med 96(pt 2):931, 1982.
11. Sobel JD: Pathophysiology of vulvovaginal candidiasis. J Reprod Med 34(Suppl 8):572, 1989.
12. Morton RS, Raskid S: Candidal vaginitis: Natural history, predis-

posing factors and prevention. Proc R Soc Med 70(Suppl 4):3, 1977.
13. Spinillo A, Pizzoli G, Colonna L, et al: Epidemiologic characteristics of women with idiopathic recurrent vulvovaginal candidiasis. Obstet Gynecol 51:721, 1993.
14. Nyirjesy P, Seeney SM, Terry Grody MH, et al: Chronic fungal vaginitis: The value of cultures. Am J Obstet Gynecol 173:820, 1995.
15. Oral fluconazole for vaginal candidiasis. Med Lett 36:81, 1994.
16. Sobel JD, Brooker D, Stein E, et al: Single oral dose fluconazole compared with conventional clotrimazole topical therapy of *Candida* vaginitis. Am J Obstet Gynecol 172:1263, 1995.
17. Van Slyke KK, Michel VP, Rein MF: Treatment of vulvovaginal candidiasis with boric acid powder. Am J Obstet Gynecol 141:145, 1981.
18. Sobel JD: Recurrent vulvovaginal candidiasis: A prospective study of the efficacy of maintenance ketoconazole therapy. N Engl J Med 315:1455, 1986.
19. O'Connor MI, Sobel JD: Epidemiology of recurrent vulvovaginal candidiasis: Identification and strain differentiation of *Candida albicans*. J Infect Dis 154:358, 1986.
20. Nystatin Multicenter Study Group: Therapy of candidal vaginitis: The effect of eliminating intestinal *Candida*. Am J Obstet Gynecol 155:651, 1986.
21. Hilton E, Isenberg HD, Alperstein P, et al: Ingestion of yogurt containing *Lactobacillus acidophilus* as prophylaxis for candidal vaginitis. Ann Intern Med 116:418, 1992.
22. Buck A, Christenson ES: Treatment of vaginal candidosis with natamycin and effect of treating the partner at the same time. Acta Obstet Gynecol Scand 61:393, 1982.
23. Block E: Occurrence of trichomoniasis in sexual partners of women with trichomoniasis. Acta Obstet Gynecol Scand 35:398, 1959.
24. Krieger JN, Tam MR, Stevens CE, et al: Diagnosis of trichomoniasis. Comparison of conventional wet-mount examination with cytologic studies, cultures, and monoclonal antibody staining of direct specimens. JAMA 259:1223, 1988.
25. Wölner-Hanssen P, Krieger JN, Stevens CE, et al: Clinical manifestations of vaginal trichomoniasis. JAMA 261:571, 1989.
26. Centers for Disease Control and Prevention: 1993 Sexually transmitted diseases treatment guidelines. MMWR Morbid Mortal Wkly Rep 42:1, 1993.
27. Pereyra AJ, Lansing JD: Urogenital trichomoniasis: Treatment with metronidazole in 2002 incarcerated women. Obstet Gynecol 499, 1964.
28. Lossick JG: Single-dose metronidazole treatment for vaginal trichomoniasis. Obstet Gynecol 56:508, 1980.
29. Hardy PH, Hardy JV, Well EE, et al: Prevalence of six sexually transmitted agents among pregnant inter-city adolescents and pregnancy outcomes. Lancet 2:333, 1984.
30. Lossick JG, Muller M, Gorrell TE: In vitro drug susceptibility and doses of metronidazole required for cure in cases of refractory vaginal trichomoniasis. J Infect Dis 153:948, 1986.
31. Spiegel CA, Amsel R, Eschenbach DA, et al: Anaerobic bacteria in nonspecific vaginitis. N Engl J Med 303:601, 1980.
32. Holst E, Wathne B, Hovelius B, Mårdh P-A: Bacterial vaginosis: Microbiological and clinical findings. Eur J Clin Microbiol 6:536, 1987.
33. Martius J, Krohn MA, Hillier SL, et al: Relationship of vaginal *Lactobacillus* species, cervical *Chlamydia trachomatis*, and bacterial vaginosis to preterm birth. Obstet Gynecol 71:89, 1988.
34. Chen KCS, Amsel R, Eschenbach DA, Holmes KK: Biochemical diagnosis of vaginitis: Determination of diamines in vaginal fluid. J Infect Dis 145:337, 1982.
35. Brand JM, Galask RP: Trimethylamine: The substance mainly responsible for the fishy odor often associated with bacterial vaginosis. Obstet Gynecol 63:682, 1986.
36. Swedberg J, Steiner JF, Deiss F, et al: Comparison of single dose versus one week course of metronidazole on symptomatic bacterial vaginosis. JAMA 254:1046, 1985.
37. Vejtorp M, Bollerup AC, Vejtorp L, et al: Bacterial vaginosis: A double-blind randomized trial of the effect of treatment of the sexual partner. Br J Obstet Gynaecol 95:920, 1988.
38. Pheifer TA, Forsyth PA, Durfee MA, et al: Nonspecific vaginitis: Role of *Haemophilus vaginalis* and treatment with metronidazole. N Engl J Med 198:1429, 1978.
39. Amsel R, Totten PA, Spiegel CA, et al: Nonspecific vaginitis: Diagnostic criteria and microbial and epidemiologic associations. Am J Med 74:14, 1983.
40. Eschenbach DA, Hillier SL, Critchlow CW, et al: Diagnosis and clinical features associated with bacterial vaginosis. Am J Obstet Gynecol 158:819, 1988.
41. Spiegel CA, Amsel R, Holmes KK: Diagnosis of bacterial vaginosis by direct Gram stain of vaginal fluid. J Clin Microbiol 18:170, 1983.
42. Nugent RP, Krohn MA, Hillier SL: Reliability of diagnosing bacterial vaginosis is improved by a standardized method of Gram stain interpretation. J Clin Microbiol 29:297, 1991.
43. Totten PA, Amsel R, Hale J, et al: Selective differential human blood bilayer media for isolation of *Gardnerella (Haemophilus) vaginalis*. J Clin Microbiol 15:141, 1982.
44. Hillier SL, Nugent RP, Eschenbach DA, et al: The association of bacterial vaginosis *Bacteroides*, and *Mycoplasma hominis* with preterm low birth weight delivery. N Engl J Med 333:1737, 1995.
45. Gravett MG, Hummel D, Eschenbach DA, Holmes KK: Preterm labor associated with subclinical amniotic fluid infection and with bacterial vaginosis. Obstet Gynecol 67:229, 1986.
46. Hillier SL, Martius J, Krohn MA, et al: A case-control study of chorioamniotic infection and chorioamnionitis in prematurity. N Engl J Med 319:972, 1988.
47. Morales WJ, Schorr S, Albritton J: Effect of metronidazole in patients with preterm birth in preceding pregnancy and bacterial vaginosis: A placebo controlled double-blind study. Am J Obstet Gynecol 171:345, 1994.
48. Dennemark N, Meyer-Wilmes M, Schlüter R: Comparison of two treatments of bacterial vaginosis (BV) vs. non-treatment: Influence on incidence of premature birth (Abstr 35). Second European Congress of the European Society on Infectious Diseases of Obstetrics and Gynecology; October 29–November 5, 1995; Marbella, Spain.
49. Watts DH, Krohn MA, Hillier SL, Eschenbach DA: Bacterial vaginosis as a risk factor for postcesarean endometritis. Obstet Gynecol 75:52, 1990.
50. Larsson P, Bergman B, Forsum U, et al: *Mobiluncus* and clue cells as predictors of PID after first-trimester abortion. Acta Obstet Gynecol Scand 68:217, 1989.
51. Larsson P, Platz-Christensen J, Thejls H, et al: Incidence of pelvic inflammatory disease after first-trimester legal abortion in women with bacterial vaginosis after treatment with metronidazole: A double-blind, randomized study. Am J Obstet Gynecol 166:100, 1992.
52. Soper DE, Bump RC, Hurt WG: Bacterial vaginosis and trichomoniasis vaginitis are risk factors for cuff cellulitis after abdominal hysterectomy. Am J Obstet Gynecol 163:1016, 1990.
53. Larsson P, Platz-Christensen J, Forsum U, Påhlson C: Clue cells in predicting infections after abdominal hysterectomy. Obstet Gynecol 77:450, 1991.
54. Hillier SL, Lipinski CM, Briselden AM, Eschenbach DA: Efficacy of intravaginal 0.75% metronidazole gel for the treatment of bacterial vaginosis. Obstet Gynecol 81:963, 1993.
55. Fischbach F, Petersen EE, Weissenbacher ER, et al: Efficacy of clindamycin vaginal cream versus oral metronidazole in the treatment of bacterial vaginosis. Obstet Gynecol 82:405, 1993.
56. Greaves W, Chungafung J, Morris B, et al: Clindamycin versus metronidazole in the treatment of bacterial vaginosis. Obstet Gynecol 72:799, 1988.
57. Singer A, Jordan JA: The anatomy of the cervix. *In* Jordan JA, Singer A (eds): The Cervix. Philadelphia, WB Saunders, 1976, pp 13–36.
58. Critchlow CW, Wölner-Hanssen P, Eschenbach DA, et al: Determinants of cervical ectopia and of cervicitis: Age, oral contraception, specific cervical infection, smoking and drinking. Am J Obstet Gynecol 173:534, 1995.
59. Brunham RC, Paavonen JA, Stevens CE, et al: Mucopurulent cervicitis: The ignored counterpart in women of urethritis in men. N Engl J Med 311:1, 1984.
60. Paavonen JA, Stevens CE, Wölner-Hanssen P, et al: Colposcopic manifestations of cervical and vaginal infection. Obstet Gynecol Surv 43:373, 1988.
61. Paavonen JA, Critchlow CW, DeRouen T, et al: Etiology of cervical inflammation. Am J Obstet Gynecol 154:556, 1986.
62. Eschenbach DA, Holmes KK: Acute pelvic inflammatory disease:

Current concepts of pathogenesis, etiology and management. Clin Obstet Gynecol 18:35, 1975.
63. Moore DE, Spadoni LR, Foy HM, et al: Increased frequency of serum antibodies to *Chlamydia trachomatis* in women with distal tubal disease. Lancet 2:574, 1982.
64. Sellors JW, Mahoney JR, Chernesky MA, Rath DJ: Tubal factor infertility: An association with prior chlamydial infection and asymptomatic salpingitis. Fertil Steril 49:451, 1988.
65. Elliott B, Brunham RC, Laga M, et al: Maternal gonorrheal infection as a preventable risk for low birthweight. J Infect Dis 161:531, 1990.
66. Martin DH, Koutsky LA, Eschenbach DA, et al: Perinatal mortality and prematurity in pregnancies complicated by antepartum maternal *Chlamydia trachomatis* infection. JAMA 247:1585, 1982.
67. Eckert LO, Koutsky LA, Kiviat NB, et al: The inflammatory Pap smear: What does it mean? Obstet Gynecol 86:360, 1995.
68. Rapke JT, Berlin, Spence M, et al: Reproducibility of the diagnosis of cervicitis in pregnancy. Am J Perinatol 5:242, 1988.
69. Paavonen JA, Roberts PC, Stevens CE, et al: Treatment of mucopurulent cervicitis with doxycycline and amoxicillin. Am J Obstet Gynecol 161:128, 1989.
70. Kiviat NB, Wölner-Hanssen P, Eschenbach DA, et al: Endometrial histopathology in patients with culture-proved upper genital tract infections and laparoscopically diagnosed acute salpingitis. Am J Surg Pathol 14:167, 1990.
71. Paavonen JA, Kiviat NB, Brunham RC, et al: Prevalence and manifestation of endometritis among women with cervicitis. Am J Obstet Gynecol 152:280, 1985.
72. Wasserheit JN, Bell TA, Kiviat NB, et al: Microbial causes of proven pelvic inflammatory disease and efficacy of clindamycin and tobramycin. Ann Intern Med 104:187, 1986.
73. Korn AP, Bolang, Padian N, et al: Plasma cell endometritis in women with symptomatic bacterial vaginosis. Obstet Gynecol 85:387, 1995.
74. Sneider V, Behm FG, Mumaw VR: Ascending herpes endometritis. Obstet Gynecol 59:259, 1982.
75. Gump DW, Dickstein S, Gibson N: Endometritis related to *Chlamydia trachomatis* infection. Ann Intern Med 95:61, 1981.
76. Moller BR, Ahrons S, Laurin J, Mårdh P-A: Pelvic infection after elective abortion associated with *Chlamydia trachomatis*. Obstet Gynecol 59:210, 1982.
77. Hoyme UB, Kiviat NB, Eschenbach DA: Microbiology and treatment of late postpartum endometritis. Obstet Gynecol 68:226, 1986.

119

Infections Associated with Pregnancy, Delivery, and Abortion

Ronald S. Gibbs

Great advances have been made in our understanding of the pathophysiology, microbiology, treatment, and prevention of many genital tract infections associated with pregnancy. Controlled and randomized trials have provided a more reliable database for practice. In this chapter, developments in four areas are reviewed: intraamniotic infection, postpartum endometritis, wound and episiotomy infection, and prophylactic antibiotics.

Intraamniotic Infection

Clinically evident intrauterine infection occurs in approximately 1% to 4% of pregnancies and leads to increased maternal morbidity and excessive perinatal mortality and morbidity.[1] Many terms have been applied to this entity, including intraamniotic infection, amniotic fluid infection, clinical chorioamnionitis, amnionitis, and intrapartum infection. The condition is usually heralded by fever, maternal or fetal tachycardia, uterine tenderness, foul-smelling amniotic fluid, and maternal leukocytosis, especially in the presence of rupture of the membranes.

Pathophysiology and Microbiology

Intraamniotic infection usually occurs by an ascending route after the membranes have ruptured, but it may also occur with membranes intact in patients in labor, particularly in preterm gestations. Although infrequent, intraamniotic infection may be a complication of instrumentation of the intact uterus, as by amniocentesis, percutaneous umbilical blood sampling, or intrauterine transfusion. Several studies have described the microbiology of the amniotic fluid in cases of intraamniotic infection. Like many other pelvic infections, intraamniotic infection is usually polymicrobial, involving both aerobic and anaerobic bacteria. In a controlled study, Gibbs and colleagues[2] compared amniotic fluid microbes from 52 cases of intraamniotic infection with organisms from 52 matched control subjects. In 69% of the cases the amniotic fluid showed more than 10^2 colony-forming units (CFUs) of a high-virulence organism per milliliter of amniotic fluid. In comparison, only 7.7% of matched control amniotic fluid showed more than 10^2 CFUs/mL. In a study of 404 cases of intraamniotic infection, Sperling and colleagues[3] reported the results of amniotic fluid culture (Table 119–1). As shown, organisms commonly isolated included the genital mycoplasmas, anaerobes, *Gardnerella vaginalis,* and group B streptococci. Aerobic gram-negative rods and enterococci were isolated less often. Other findings confirm the wide array of organisms found in the amniotic fluid in intraamniotic infections. At present, evidence for the role of *Chlamydia trachomatis* in amniotic fluid infections is conflicting.

Diagnosis

Diagnosis of intramniotic infection often requires a high index of suspicion because early clinical criteria may be vague.

TABLE 119–1 ■ Selected Amniotic Fluid Isolates in 404 Cases of Intraamniotic Infection*

ISOLATE	NO. (%)
Ureaplasma urealyticum	190 (47)
Myeloplasma hominis	123 (30.4)
Bacteroides bovis	119 (29.4)
Gardnerella vaginalis	99 (24.5)
Group B streptococci	59 (14.6)
Peptostreptococci	38 (9.4)
Escherichia coli	33 (8.2)
Enterococci	22 (5.4)
Other aerobic gram-negative rods	21 (5.2)
Fusobacterium species	22 (5.4)
Bacteroides fragilis	14 (3.4)

*Organisms considered to have low virulence, such as lactobacilli and diphtheroids, are not shown. All specimens were collected by aspiration of an intrauterine pressure catheter after discarding the first 7 mL. Genital mycoplasmas were cultured qualitatively. For all other organisms shown, isolates were found in concentrations of at least 10^2 CFU/mL.

Adapted from Sperling RS, Newton E, Gibbs RS: Intraamniotic infection in low-birth-weight infants. J Infect Dis 157:113–117, 1988.

In addition, usual laboratory indicators of infection, such as positive stains of the amniotic fluid for organisms or leukocytes, are often found when there is no clinical evidence of infection.[4] The clinical diagnosis is usually based on maternal fever, maternal or fetal tachycardia, uterine tenderness, malodorous amniotic fluid, and leukocytosis.

Direct evaluation of amniotic fluid may provide important diagnostic information, with the specimen being obtained by either amniocentesis or aspiration of a transcervical pressure catheter. In specimens obtained by amniocentesis from symptomatic patients, there is a significant association between observing bacteria in a stain of uncentrifuged amniotic fluid and colony counts greater than 10^2 to 10^3 bacteria per milliliter.[2] However, when the specimen is collected via a transcervical pressure catheter, both leukocytes and bacteria may be present in women who do not develop clinical infection.[4] The determination of amniotic fluid glucose for diagnosing clinical chorioamnionitis has also been evaluated. Glucose levels greater than 20 to 25 mg/dL essentially exclude a positive culture in asymptomatic patients, whereas low values (less than 5 to 20 mg/dL) correlate well with both clinical evidence of chorioamnionitis and a positive amniotic fluid culture.[5] Blood and other fluids for culture, such as urine, should be obtained from the mother.

Treatment

It is generally agreed that delivery of the fetus is indicated, as well as antibiotic therapy. Findings have meaningfully advanced our knowledge of management. Timing of delivery has been an issue, but several studies have reported excellent maternal and neonatal outcomes without regard to arbitrary time limits.[6–8] Generally, cesarean section has been performed for obstetric indications such as prolonged labor or fetal distress and not for intraamniotic infection alone. No critical interval from time of diagnosis of amnionitis to delivery can be identified, provided management is not unduly delayed. Delivery is almost always fairly prompt: the mean interval from diagnosis of amnionitis to delivery is about 3 to 5 hours. Cesarean section rates are higher among patients with intraamniotic infection, generally about 40%. The reason is most likely that patients with intraamniotic infection often have an underlying abnormal labor to begin with, and they seem to be less sensitive to oxytocin. When abdominal delivery is necessary, excellent results are obtained with a transperitoneal low cervical cesarean section. Others in the past have advocated extraperitoneal cesarean section,[9] but this technique is not widely practiced and offers little objective advantage. Cesarean hysterectomy should be reserved for cases associated with prolonged hemorrhage or other concurrent indications for hysterectomy, such as placenta accreta.

Three studies have emphasized the importance of administering antibiotics during labor rather than in the puerperium. In 1987, we presented the results of a nonrandomized comparison of intrapartum and immediate postpartum administration of antibiotics (intravenous [IV] penicillin G plus gentamicin).[10] Of 257 women with clinically diagnosed intraamniotic infection, 82% had received antibiotics intrapartum whereas 18% (mainly those who delivered quickly) received the drugs immediately after delivery. There were no significant differences between these two groups in the distribution of low-birth-weight infants, maternal bacteremia, cesarean delivery, or organisms in the amniotic fluid. Infants of women who had received intrapartum treatment had significantly less neonatal sepsis (2.8% versus 19.6%, $P < .001$). Neonatal mortality caused by sepsis was also lower in infants whose mothers had been treated intrapartum (0.9% versus 4.3%), but this difference was not statistically significant. In 1988, Gilstrap and colleagues[11] reported that mothers who had received intrapartum antibiotic therapy were significantly less likely to have infants with group B streptococcal sepsis.

Because of the limitations of these retrospective studies, we thought that it was important to conduct a prospective, randomized clinical trial.[12] We used IV ampicillin plus gentamicin to treat mothers intrapartum and after delivery. All infants received the same regimen. When the neonate's workup was negative, antibiotics were discontinued after 72 hours. If sepsis or pneumonia was diagnosed, treatment was continued for 10 days. Results of this randomized trial are shown in Table 119–2.

From these studies we may conclude that intrapartum treatment reduces neonatal sepsis and that this benefit overshadows any theoretical objection (such as obscuring positive neonatal cultures) to intrapartum treatment of intraamniotic infection. An overall approach to patients who have intraamniotic infection is set forth in Table 119–3.

Postpartum Endometritis

Even with well-established principles for the use of prophylactic antibiotics, genital tract infections after delivery continue to be a common, and occasionally serious, threat to women after childbirth.

Pathogenesis

Most postpartum uterine infections are caused by vulvovaginal flora that ascend into the uterus. These organisms are

TABLE 119–2 ■ Maternal and Neonatal Outcomes in a Randomized Trial of Intrapartum Versus Immediate Postpartum Treatment of Women with Intraamniotic Infection

	TREATMENT GROUP		
CHARACTERISTICS	Intrapartum (N = 26)	Postpartum (N = 19)	P
Maternal			
Maximal temperature post partum (°F)*	99.8 ± 0.8	100.3 ± 1.1	.05
Hospital stay post partum (d)*	4.0 ± 1.0	5.0 ± 1.9	.05
Febrile days*	0.4 ± 0.7	1.5 ± 2.1	.05
Neonatal			
Early sepsis, no (%)	0	4 (21)	.03
Sepsis or pneumonia, no (%)	0	6 (32)	.003
Hospital stay (d)*	3.8 ± 11	5.7 ± 3.0	.02

*Mean ± SD.

Adapted from Gibbs RS, Dinsmoor MJ, Newton ER, Ramamurthy RS: A randomized trial of intrapartum versus immediate postpartum treatment of women with intra-amniotic infection. Obstet Gynecol 72:823–828, 1988.

TABLE 119–3 ■ Approach to the Patient with Intraamniotic Infection

Collect specimens for culture as indicated, including genital secretions and amniotic fluid if possible.
Begin antibiotic therapy as soon as cultures have been collected, even if delivery is anticipated shortly.
Cesarean delivery should be performed only for standard obstetric indications (such as abnormal labor, fetal distress), not for intraamniotic infection alone.

similar qualitatively to those obtained from infected amniotic fluid[13] (see Table 119–1). *C. trachomatis* may play a role in a relatively mild form of endometritis that follows vaginal delivery but does not appear to be a common pathogen in endometritis after cesarean delivery.

Risk factors for postpartum endometritis have been studied extensively. By far the leading risk factor is cesarean delivery, especially when performed during labor or after membrane rupture.[14] In addition to cesarean delivery itself, other risk factors are a group of covariables, including labor, rupture of the membranes and amniotic fluid colonization, vaginal examinations, and internal fetal monitoring. Women of low socioeconomic status, independent of race, appear to be at higher risk than women of middle socioeconomic status. Other variables sometimes reported to be independent risk factors for postpartum infection include postpartum anemia, obesity, type of anesthesia for cesarean section, duration of cesarean section, skill of the surgeon in cesarean section, and estimated blood loss during cesarean section.

Diagnosis

The diagnosis of uterine infection, referred to as endometritis or endomyometritis, is usually based on symptoms of fever, abdominal pain, malaise, and purulent or foul-smelling lochia; however, few patients exhibit all the signs and symptoms. Endomyometritis should be suspected when a patient has fever after delivery, especially when other risk factors are present. It is also important to recognize that patients who have a serious postpartum infection, such as that caused by group A or group B streptococci, may have high fever early in the puerperium but little in the way of localizing factors early. The diagnosis of uterine infection after delivery may be difficult because many patients have low-grade fever early in the puerperium. Such fever often resolves spontaneously after vaginal delivery but tends to persist after cesarean section.

Appropriate work-up of a patient with suspected endometritis includes a complete blood count, two sets of venous blood cultures, and a genital tract culture. No technique is commercially available to collect a uterine specimen that is not contaminated by organisms of the lower genital tract. For practical purposes, under most circumstances a swab culture of the lower uterine segment or cervix for aerobes usually suffices. Gram staining of the genital cultures may also be helpful when group A or group B streptococcal or clostridial infection is suspected.

Attention has been drawn to case series from Texas and Colorado describing fulminant, multiple organ system, puerperal infections with group A streptococci. Characteristics of these cases include bacteremia, shock, and end organ dysfunction. These cases have variable onset from 2 to 7 days after delivery and usually present with fever. Characteristically, the patients are free of underlying disease and commonly manifest disseminated intravascular coagulation, acute respiratory distress, renal insufficiency, and hepatic dysfunction. Gram stain and culture of the genital secretions may give an early diagnostic indication. Often there is a poor response to vigorous medical therapy, and hysterectomy may be needed to save the patient's life.[15]

Treatment

Using general supportive care and appropriate broad-spectrum antibiotic therapy, clinicians can expect the vast majority of patients with endomyometritis to improve within a few days. Well-controlled treatment trials have shown that antibiotic therapy with agents that are active against anaerobes was more successful than therapy with less active agents.[16] Most studies of therapy have addressed women who developed endomyometritis after cesarean section. A common standard for comparison is clindamycin plus gentamicin, a regimen that in the past yielded cure rates of 90% to 95%. Still, this combination is not without problems. In other trials the failure rate of clindamycin plus gentamicin has been reported to be as high as 20% to 25%.[17] Although the reasons are uncertain, it appears that part of the increase may be due to more widespread use of cephalosporins for prophylaxis. As a consequence, more enterococci are observed in endometrial cultures. We observed that enterococci are associated with an increased failure rate for clindamycin-gentamicin therapy.[18] Second, both clindamycin and gentamicin have serious, well-known side effects. Third, studies have revealed that it may be difficult to obtain a therapeutic level of aminoglycoside in obstetric patients, especially in the puerperium, because of rapid renal clearance.

We believe that routine determination of aminoglycoside levels in postpartum women is unnecessary and should be reserved for special circumstances, such as obese patients (for whom it may be difficult to estimate the proper dose), patients treated with drugs for more than a week, patients with renal compromise (who should probably receive alternative agents), and patients who are bacteremic or are not responding to therapy.

Many broad-spectrum penicillins, cephalosporins, and related antibiotics have become commercially available. Although no single agent is active against the entire array of organisms that cause postpartum endometritis, most have sufficient aerobic and anaerobic activity to merit consideration in obstetric infections. Small series of single-agent therapy with agents such as cefoxitin, cefotetan, cefoperazone, cefotaxime, piperacillin, ampicillin-sulbactam, and ticarcillin-clavulanate had high cure rates.

These new penicillins and cephalosporins are usually well tolerated and have few side effects. In addition, their pharmacokinetics in women after delivery are favorable. Administration of a single agent also demands less time and equipment, although the direct cost of these antibiotics is greater (Table 119–4).

Some studies have evaluated other combinations for therapy—metronidazole plus an aminoglycoside, clindamycin plus aztreonam. The former combination provides excellent anaerobic and gram-negative aerobic activity, but it does not provide optimal coverage of gram-positive aerobic organisms, in particular group B streptococci, so we do not recommend it primarily. Clindamycin plus aztreonam has the advantage of substituting the monobactam aztreonam for the aminoglycoside, and it performed as well as clindamycin plus aminoglycoside.

For patients who respond well to initial antibiotic therapy, studies have demonstrated that it is sufficient to continue the IV antibiotic therapy for 24 to 48 hours after the patient's fever disappears. The question of whether oral antibiotic therapy is needed as an adjunct to parenteral therapy by patients who have had a good response has been addressed in descriptive and comparative reports.[19–22] Results of these studies demonstrate that oral antibiotics are not necessary

TABLE 119–4 ■ Parenteral Regimens Used to Treat Endometritis

NO.	REGIMEN	"RESISTANT" ORGANISMS	COMMENTS
1	Penicillin-aminoglycoside	*Staphylococcus aureus*, many anaerobes	Inferior choice
2	Clindamycin-aminogycoside	Mainly enterococci	Often a standard for comparison
3	Clindamycin-aztreonam	Mainly enterococci	Alternative combination to clindamycin-gentamicin
4	Metronidazole-aminoglycoside	Group B streptococci, enterococci	Alternative combination to clindamycin-gentamicin
5	Cephalosporins: cefoxitin, cefotetan, cefotaxime, others	Enterococci, some anaerobes	Single drug alternative
6	Ureidopenicillins: piperacillin, mezlocillin, azlocillin	Some aerobic gram-negative rods, some *S. aureus*	Single drug alternative
7	Penicillin–β-lactamase inhibitors: ticarcillin-clavulanate; ampicillin-sulbactam	Some aerobic gram-negative rods	Single drug alternative
8	Carbapenems: imipenem-cilastatin	Some clostridia, some *S. aureus*	Reserve

because recurrence of endometritis or other genital tract infections is unusual (less than 4%).

We do employ oral antibiotic therapy in special circumstances, as when the course of infection is protracted and the response to parenteral antibiotics slow, and for *Staphylococcus aureus* bacteremia.

A patient whose infection does not respond to initial antibiotic therapy clearly presents a problem. It is appropriate to change therapy after 48 to 72 hours, unless the patient's condition is unstable, in which case changes may be needed more promptly. As Table 119–5 shows, diagnostic considerations include an infected mass in the pelvis or in the wound, a resistant organism, and an additional source of fever. It is also possible that the patient has been receiving appropriate antibiotics but in inadequate doses or by an inappropriate route. Under these circumstances, measurement of aminoglycoside may be helpful. Bedside examination and systematic review of the patient's course and cultures often reveal the source, and often changing antibiotics, as by adding penicillin to an aminoglycoside to cover enterococci, is effective even though the responsible organism is not identified. It is possible that these "failures" occur simply because sufficient time has not passed for the antibiotics to take effect.

In cases of poor response, diagnostic studies often identify a pelvic mass or a deep-seated wound infection. Ultrasonography of the abdomen and pelvis may reveal a mass. Acholonu and colleagues[23] reported using ultrasonography to guide percutaneous drainage of fluid collections in several women who developed fever after cesarean delivery. In most cases, this drainage and continued antibiotic therapy were followed by resolution of the fever. Computed tomography may also be useful in identifying a pelvic mass and pelvic thrombophlebitis. Because the usefulness of ultrasonography of the abdomen is limited in patients who have an open abdominal wound, computed tomography is particularly helpful in this situation.

TABLE 119–5 ■ Identified Causes of Poor Response to Antibiotic Therapy in Patients with Endometritis

CAUSE	APPROXIMATE PREVALENCE (%)
Infected mass, including abscess, hematoma, septic pelvic thrombophlebitis, pelvic cellulitis, retained placenta	40–50
Resistant organisms, commonly enterococci, in a patient receiving clindamycin-aminoglycoside or a cephalosporin	20
Additional cause, including catheter phlebitis, inadequate dose of antibiotics	10
No cause evident but response to empirical change in antibiotic therapy	20–30

Septic pelvic thrombophlebitis may occur in association with pelvic surgery, operative site infection after pelvic surgery, and pelvic inflammatory disease.[24] In studies conducted 2 years ago, pelvic thrombophlebitis was reported in 1% to 2% of patients with postoperative infection after cesarean delivery.[16, 25] In subsequent studies, broader spectrum agents have been used, and septic pelvic thrombophlebitis has been reported less frequently.

Pelvic vein thrombophlebitis appears to take two distinct clinical forms[25]—acute ovarian vein thrombosis and septic pelvic thrombophlebitis. Patients with the former condition usually have distinct clinical findings. Although not all of these patients are febrile, some have a moderately elevated temperature. The initial physical examination often suggests an acute process such as appendicitis or an insult to an ovarian cyst. This condition is often striking in its clinical appearance and prompts laparotomy, at which procedure the diagnosis is made.

The second presentation of septic pelvic thrombophlebitis is less distinctive and has been called enigmatic fever. Initially, patients may demonstrate many of the clinical signs of endometritis, but they usually experience definite improvement in all clinical parameters except persistent fever. Some may have a mass and tenderness. Usually, they do not appear critically ill and have no positive physical findings. The diagnosis usually is made by ruling out other causes of persistent fever with computed tomographic or ultrasonographic examination.

Several surgical and medical approaches have been utilized to treat pelvic vein thrombophlebitis. None of the trials has been randomized. Certain general principles for the management of patients with suspected pelvic vein thrombophlebitis have been established. In general, surgery should be reserved for patients who remain clinically ill despite adequate medical therapy or who present with acute abdomen. In this circumstance, several surgical procedures have been proposed as the operative technique of choice: bilateral ovarian vein ligation and inferior vena cava ligation; unilateral ovarian vein ligation, with or without vena cava ligation; excision of the infected vein, with or without ligation of the contralateral vein. The most reasonable approach seems to be ligation of the infected veins; concurrent ligation of the vena cava is indicated when the ovarian vein thrombus extends into this vessel.

Medical treatment for pelvic vein thrombophlebitis has traditionally consisted of antibiotic therapy with intravenous heparin in full therapeutic doses for 10 days. Most experts have not recommended continuing oral anticoagulation therapy after this interval, and late embolic phenomena are extremely rare. Although it is rarely necessary with modern antibiotic approaches, surgical intervention may be necessary to effect a cure. Indications for surgical therapy include control of overwhelming infection (such as in cases of group A streptococcal sepsis), drainage of a pelvic or subcutaneous abscess, removal of an infected thrombus, or exploration in an acutely ill patient who has not responded to appropriate medical therapy.

Wound and Episiotomy Infection

Abdominal wound infections are fairly common after cesarean section. In San Antonio, Texas, a prospective study of infections after cesarean section revealed that approximately 5% of 413 consecutive cases were complicated by wound infection.[26] Sweet and Ledger[26] and Moir-Bussy and colleagues[27] have reported a similar incidence of 6% after cesarean section. Additional series have found the rate of wound infection to vary between 5.4% and 9.4% of cesarean sections.[28–30]

Risk factors for wound abscess after cesarean delivery may be somewhat different from those for wound infection after other surgical procedures. First, patients undergoing cesarean delivery are young and their hospital stay is usually brief. Moreover, they rarely have serious underlying disease and the operation itself is relatively short. On the other hand, many cesarean sections are performed as emergency procedures, often in a field contaminated with large numbers of bacteria. It is most likely that organisms in contaminated amniotic fluid or other genital secretions produce the wound abscess. Risk factors reported in several studies of wound abscess after cesarean section include fever on admission, multiple vaginal examinations, prolonged surgical procedure, and significant blood loss during the procedure.[27] In a review of wound infection after cesarean section, Moir-Bussy and colleagues[27] from the United Kingdom reported that the use of drains was significantly associated with wound infections. In their study the most common organisms were *Streptococcus faecalis, Escherichia coli, Proteus* species, hemolytic streptococci, and *S. aureus*. In their study, anaerobes accounted for only 25 of 300 (8%) isolates, but this raises the question of whether microbiologic techniques were satisfactory.

Two studies have provided contemporary information regarding the microbiology of wound infection after a cesarean section. In 1988, investigators at the University of Washington noted that postoperative wound infections caused by cervical vaginal flora were associated with various obstetric factors (including prolonged labor, a longer duration of fetal monitoring, a larger number of vaginal examinations, and organisms isolated from the endometrium and cesarean section).[28] On the other hand, infections associated with *S. aureus* (accounting for approximately 25% of wound infections) were not associated with these features. It seemed that the former group of wound infections resulted from ascension of genital organisms, whereas the *S. aureus* infections had nosocomial sources. Roberts and colleagues[30] reported that the predominant isolates in wound infection were those commonly found in the lower genital tract, with the genital mycoplasmas being reported most often. Organisms usually associated with the skin were isolated less frequently, including coagulase-negative staphylococci in 32% of positive cultures and *S. aureus* in only 6%.

Abdominal wound infections after cesarean section are diagnosed and managed as are infections complicating other surgical procedures. Historically, the approach to the open wound after cesarean section has been closure by secondary intention including wound débridement, packing, and allowing the wound to close by granulation. There has been interest in secondary closure (en bloc closure techniques after the wound was granulating well). The hypothetic advantage of secondary closure is shortened time for healing and fewer hospital stays. Several randomized clinical trials have demonstrated that the secondary closure may be carried out easily—even without general anesthesia and without use of the operating room—resulting in benefits to the patients.[31–33]

Most of these infections are simple wound cellulitis or subcutaneous wound abscess. Life-threatening wound infections are extremely rare, but it is important to recognize the clinical features of necrotizing fasciitis, myonecrosis, and bacterial synergistic nonclostridial gangrene.

Although episiotomy and repair are performed with most vaginal deliveries, infection is a surprisingly infrequent complication. Simple episiotomy infection involves only the skin and subcutaneous tissue, including Scarpa fascia of the perineum adjacent to the episiotomy.[34] Common signs include local edema and erythema with exudate. It is important to recognize that more extensive findings should raise suspicion of a deeper or more serious infection. Treatment of simple episiotomy infection consists of opening, exploring, and debridement of the perineal wound. Drainage alone is usually satisfactory, but appropriate antibiotic therapy is indicated if there is marked cellulitis or isolation of group A streptococci. It is usually unnecessary to resuture a simple episiotomy infection, as most heal well by granulation. The exception is infections that have resulted in breakdown of the sphincter muscles or rectal mucosa. Such wounds are repaired when the field is free of infection. Studies have demonstrated that breakdown of fourth-degree episiotomies can be safely and effectively repaired early in the hospital course even if these breakdowns have been the result of infection. Success has been reported in approximately 90% of cases.[35–37] The technique includes initial débridement, intravenous antibiotics in nearly all cases, daily wound care, and then definitive repair after the patient has been afebrile for 24 to 48 hours and the wound is clean and covered with granulating tissue. Mechanical bowel preparation with an oral electrolyte solution (GoLYTELY) given as 1 gallon to be consumed until the patient has clear, watery stools is also common. Repairs have been performed using regional anesthesia and a layered closure with either chromic catgut or Vicryl.

One life-threatening episiotomy infection is necrotizing fasciitis, also known as superficial fascial necrosis.[38–40] Both layers of the superficial perineum (Camper and Colles fasciae) become necrotic, and infection spreads along fascial planes to the buttocks, thighs, pubis, and abdominal wall. Important features of this infection are noted in Table 119–6. In addition, patients may have marked hemoconcentration and hypocalcemia (because of saponification of fatty acids). Often this infection has been associated with group A streptococci, but other reports indicate that anaerobic bacteria may play important roles.

The essential part of therapy is adequate débridement in addition to appropriate broad-spectrum antibiotic therapy. Indications for surgical exploration of episiotomy infection include signs of edema or infection extending beyond the labia; asymmetric, particularly unilateral, edema with signs of infection; and signs of hypotension, toxicity, or deterioration. At surgery, necrotizing fasciitis may be recognized by the ease with which the skin is separated from the deep

TABLE 119–6 ■ Characteristics of Life-Threatening Episiotomy Infections

INFECTION	FEATURE
Superficial fascial necrosis (necrotizing fasciitis)	Edema and erythema, especially with unilateral edema or edema extending to abdomen, thighs, or buttocks. Edema may become brawny, and skin may become blue or black, with bullae or frank gangrene. Gray, watery discharge. Severe pain. Signs of toxicity or deterioration.
Myonecrosis	Severe pain, usually of sudden onset. Signs of toxicity. Early skin signs include mild local edema. In advanced cases, cutaneous gangrene, crepitus, and a bronzed appearance are evident in skin.

fascia, absence of bleeding along the incision lines, and a serosanguineous "dishwater" discharge. The potential role of frozen-section biopsy to determine the underlying diagnosis has been emphasized.[41] The débridement should be carried out until all necrotic tissue is removed.

Prophylactic Antibiotics

Since 1968, more than 25 randomized, placebo-controlled trials have reported benefits of prophylactic antibiotics in cesarean section.[42] In general, the risk of infection is 50% lower in patients who receive prophylactic antibiotics than in those who receive placebo. Prophylactic antibiotics decrease the incidence of endometritis, wound infection, and probably urinary tract infection. Adverse effects of prophylactic antibiotics include shifts in flora, pseudomembranous colitis, and direct toxic effects. Use of prophylaxis routinely (including use for low-risk patients) remains controversial. Several groups have argued for routine prophylaxis,[43, 44] whereas others have argued against such widespread use and for restriction to high-risk populations.[45, 46] Table 119–7 summarizes the author's recommendations.

Several studies have employed prophylactic antibiotics for either mothers or newborns in the presence of premature rupture of the membranes. Currently, the only standard recommendation would be to use selective intrapartum chemoprophylaxis (as with ampicillin) in group B streptococcus–positive patients who suffer preterm premature rupture of the membranes or prolonged (more than 12 to 18 hours) rupture of the membranes. The purpose of this selective prophylaxis, as demonstrated by Boyer and Gotoff,[47] is to reduce the risk of neonatal group B streptococcal sepsis.

The theory that subclinical infection may cause premature rupture of the membranes in the first place has prompted interest in prophylaxis. Although preliminary studies have demonstrated some benefit,[48] preventive therapy remains completely experimental.

Infected Abortion

Although septic abortion has decreased as a problem, life-threatening, infectious complications of abortion are occasionally a problem. Most complications of abortion in the United States today follow therapeutic abortion rather than illegal abortion, as the vast majority of pregnancy terminations are now performed in medical facilities. In the last 20 years, mortality rates from therapeutic abortion have decreased, and current data show a case-fatality rate of less than 1 per 100,000 therapeutic abortions. In comparison, the mortality rate associated with delivery at term is approximately 10 times greater than that after legal abortion.[49]

Predisposing factors to infection after abortion are incomplete abortion (failure to remove all products of conception) and uterine perforation. Principles of management of post-abortion infection have not changed substantially in the past 20 years. These include removal of remaining products of conception, broad-spectrum antibiotic therapy, and general supportive therapy as needed. In view of classic studies on the microbiology of infected abortion, broad-spectrum therapy is appropriate at the time of diagnosis and must include agents with optimal activity against anaerobes as well as common aerobic genital pathogens. In view of the disposition of a woman with infection after abortion to develop major complications, such as septic shock, empirical combination therapy with clindamycin plus gentamicin, for example, is appropriate. Alternative therapy with a single agent such as cefoxitin or a broad-spectrum cephalosporin or broad-spectrum penicillin may also be effective.

A number of studies have addressed prophylaxis for first-trimester abortion. In a double-blind study, Sonne-Holm and colleagues[50] noted that prophylaxis was effective only for patients who previously had a pelvic infection. Levallois and Rious[51] reduced the rate of pelvic infection in women with negative *Chlamydia* cultures from 3.0% to 0.4% ($P = .001$) by giving them 300 mg doxycycline instead of placebo. A benefit was seen in patients with positive *Chlamydia* cultures. Similarly, Darj and coworkers[52] found that single-dose doxycycline decreased postoperative infection from 6.2% in the placebo group to 2.1% in the treated group. In both of these studies, vomiting was a common side effect (18% in the study by Darj and 1.6% in the placebo group). Grimes and colleagues[53] argued for routine use of tetracycline in first-trimester abortion. Several studies have identified groups at high risk, such as patients with a history of gonorrhoea or pelvic infection and nulliparas who have multiple sexual partners. Adverse antibiotic effects are common, albeit minor,

TABLE 119–7 ■ Recommendations for Use of Prophylactic Antibiotics in Cesarean Section

Limit use of prophylactic antibiotics to women having cesarean at risk for postoperative infection.

When prophylaxis is used, a short-course regimen of one to three doses should be used. Considerable evidence now favors single-dose prophylaxis.

Antibiotics chosen for prophylaxis should be effective, safe, and inexpensive. Recommended agents include first-generation cephalosporins and ampicillin.

Newer, broader spectrum antibiotics have not been found to be more effective as prophylactic agents and should be reserved for therapy.

Administration of prophylaxis should be delayed until after cord is clamped to avoid potential consequences to the fetus.

Antibiotics are not more effective administered by irrigation than by IV injection.

When prophylaxis is used, patients who develop postprophylaxis fever or other signs of infections must be evaluated carefully. Appropriate cultures should be obtained, particularly because these patients are more likely to have resistant organisms.

When therapeutic antibiotics are necessary in these patients, initially use a broad-spectrum agent or a combination of broad-spectrum agents in view of the changes of flora brought about by even short-course prophylactic antibiotics.

complications, and widespread use of prophylaxis is likely to select out resistant organisms.

Patients undergoing therapeutic abortion who have positive tests for *Neisseria gonorrhoeae* or *C. trachomatis* should be treated with appropriate antibiotics with a minimum of delay. Even though the infection rate after abortion is low and most of these infections appear to be minor, most authorities also recommend routine use of doxycycline prophylaxis, for example, 200 mg before and 100 mg 12 hours after the procedure.[46]

References

1. Gibbs RS: Intraamniotic infections (intrauterine infections) in late pregnancy. *In* Sweet RL, Gibbs RS: Infectious Diseases of the Female Genital Tract, ed 3. Baltimore, Williams & Wilkins, 1985, pp 548–563.
2. Gibbs RS, Blanco JD, St Clair PJ, Castaneda YS: Quantitative bacteriology of amniotic fluid from patients with clinical intraamniotic infection at term. J Infect Dis 145:1, 1982.
3. Sperling RS, Newton E, Gibbs RS: Intraamniotic infection in low–birth weight infants. J Infect Dis 157:1, 1988.
4. Listwa HM, Dobek AS, Carpenter J, et al: The predictability of intrauterine infection by analysis of amniotic fluid. Obstet Gynecol 48:31, 1976.
5. Kiltz RJ, Burke MS, Porreco RP: Amniotic fluid glucose concentration as a marker for intra-amniotic infection. Obstet Gynecol 78:1, 1991.
6. Gibbs RS, Castillo MS, Rodgers PJ: Management of acute chorioamnionitis. Am J Obstet Gynecol 136:709, 1980.
7. Looff JD, Hager WD: Management of chorioamnionitis. Surg Gynecol Obstet 158:161, 1984.
8. Hauth JC, Gilstrap LC, Hankins GDV, et al: Term maternal and neonatal complications of acute chorioamnionitis. Obstet Gynecol 66:59, 1985.
9. Imig JR, Perkins RP: Extraperitoneal cesarean section: A new need for old skills. A preliminary report. Am J Obstet Gynecol 125:51, 1976.
10. Sperling RS, Ramamurthy RS, Gibbs RS: A comparison of intrapartum versus immediate postpartum treatment of intraamniotic infection. Obstet Gynecol 70:6, 1987.
11. Gilstrap LC III, Leveno KJ, Cox SM, et al: Intrapartum treatment of acute chorioamnionitis: Impact on neonatal sepsis. Am J Obstet Gynecol 159:579, 1988.
12. Gibbs RS, Dinsmoor MJ, Newton ER, Ramamurthy RS: A randomized trial of intrapartum versus immediate postpartum treatment of women with intraamniotic infection. Obstet Gynecol 72:6, 1988.
13. Rosene K, Eschenbach DA, Tompkins LS, et al: Polymicrobial early postpartum endometritis with facultative and anaerobic bacteria, genital mycoplasmas and *C. trachomatis:* Treatment with piperacillin or cefoxitin. J Infect Dis 153:1028, 1986.
14. Duff P: Pathophysiology and management of postcesarean endomyometritis. Obstet Gynecol 67:269, 1986.
15. Silver RM, Heddleston LN, McGregor JA, et al: Life-threatening puerperal infection due to group A streptococci. Obstet Gynecol 79:894, 1992.
16. di Zerega G, Yonekura L, Roy S, et al: A comparison of clindamycin-gentamicin and penicillin-gentamicin in the treatment of post-cesarean section endomyometritis. Am J Obstet Gynecol 134:238, 1979.
17. Herman G, Cohen AW, Talbot GH, et al: Cefoxitin versus clindamycin and gentamicin in the treatment of postcesarean section infections. Obstet Gynecol 67:371, 1986.
18. Walmer D, Walmer K, Gibbs RS: Enterococci in post-cesarean endometritis. Obstet Gynecol 71:159, 1988.
19. Cabbad M, Sijin O, Minkoff H: Short course of antibiotics for post–cesarean section endometritis. Am J Obstet Gynecol 157:908, 1987.
20. Soper DE, Kemmer CT, Conover WB: Abbreviated antibiotic therapy for the treatment of postpartum endometritis. Obstet Gynecol 69:127, 1987.
21. Dinsmoor MJ, Newton ER, Gibbs RS: Oral antibiotic therapy (POABTX) following intravenous antibiotic therapy (IVABTX) for postpartum endometritis (PPE) (Abstr). Quebec, Canada, Infectious Disease Society for Obstetrics and Gynecology, 1989.
22. Hager WD, Vernon M, Pascuzzi M: Efficacy of oral antibiotics following parenteral antibiotics for serious infections in obstetrics and gynecology (Abstr). Quebec, Canada, Infectious Disease Society for Obstetrics and Gynecology, 1989.
23. Acholonu F, Minkoff H, Delke I: Percutaneous draining of fluid collections in the bladder flap of febrile post–cesarean section patients: A report of seven cases. J Reprod Med 32:140, 1987.
24. Duff P, Gibbs RS: Pelvic vein thrombophlebitis: Diagnostic dilemma and therapeutic challenge. Obstet Gynecol Surv 38:365, 1983.
25. Gibbs RS, Jones PM, Wilder CJ: Antibiotic therapy of endometritis following cesarean section. Obstet Gynecol 52:31, 1978.
26. Sweet RL, Ledger WJ: Puerperal infections: A two year review. Am J Obstet Gynecol 117:1093, 1973.
27. Moir-Bussy BR, Hutton RM, Thompson JR: Wound infection after cesarean section. J Hosp Infect 5:359, 1984.
28. Emmons SL, Krohn M, Jackson M, et al: Development of wound infections among women undergoing cesarean section. Obstet Gynecol 72:559, 1988.
29. Webster J. Post-caesarean wound infection: A review of the risk factors. Aust N Z J Obstet Gynaecol 28:201, 1988.
30. Roberts S, Maccato M, Faro S, et al: The microbiology of post-cesarean wound morbidity. Obstet Gynecol 81:383, 1993.
31. Walters MD, Dombroski RA, Davidson SA, et al: Reclosure of disrupted abdominal incisions. Obstet Gynecol 76:597, 1990.
32. Dodson MK, Magann EF, Meeks GR: A randomized comparison of secondary closure and secondary intention in patients with superficial wound dehiscence. Obstet Gynecol 80:321, 1992.
33. Dodson MK, Magann EF, Sullivan DL, et al: Extrafascial wound dehiscence: Deep en bloc closure versus superficial skin closure. Obstet Gynecol 83:142, 1994.
34. Shy KK, Eschenbach DA: Fatal perineal cellulitis from an episiotomy site. Obstet Gynecol 54:292, 1979.
35. Ramin SM, Ramus RM, Little BB, et al: Early repair of episiotomy dehiscence associated with infection. Am J Obstet Gynecol 167:1104, 1992.
36. Hauth JC, Gilstrap LC, Ward SC, et al: Early repair of an external sphincter ani muscle and rectal mucosal dehiscence. Obstet Gynecol 67:806, 1986.
37. Hankins GDV, Hauth JC, Gilstrap LC, et al: Early repair of episiotomy dehiscence. Obstet Gynecol 75:48, 1990.
38. Golde S, Ledger WJ: Necrotizing fasciitis in postpartum patients: A report of four cases. Obstet Gynecol 50:670, 1977.
39. Meltzer RM: Necrotizing fasciitis and progressive bacterial synergistic gangrene of the vulva. Obstet Gynecol 61:757, 1983.
40. Ewing TL, Smale LE, Elliott FA: Maternal deaths associated with postpartum vulvar edema. Am J Obstet Gynecol 134:173, 1979.
41. Stamenkovic I, Lew PD: Early recognition of potentially fatal necrotizing fasciitis. The use of frozen-section biopsy. N Engl J Med 310:1689, 1984.
42. Gibbs RS: Antibiotic prophylaxis in obstetrics and gynecology. *In* Sweet RL, Gibbs RS: Infectious Diseases of the Female Genital Tract, ed 3. Baltimore, Williams & Wilkins, 1995, pp 729–745.
43. Mugford M, Kingston J, Chalmers I: Reducing the incidence of infection after caesarean section: Implications of prophylaxis with antibiotics for hospital resources. BMJ 299:1003, 1989.
44. Ehrenkranz NJ, Blackwelder WC, Pfaff SJ, et al: Infections complicating low-risk cesarean sections in community hospitals: Efficacy of antimicrobial prophylaxis. Am J Obstet Gynecol 162:337, 1990.
45. Howie PW, Davey PG: Prophylactic antibiotics and caesarean section. BMJ 300:2, 1990.
46. Hemsell DL: Prophylactic antibiotics in gynecologic and obstetric surgery. Rev Infect Dis 13(Suppl 10):S821, 1991.
47. Boyer KM, Gotoff SP: Prevention of early onset neonatal group B streptococcal disease with selective intrapartum chemoprophylaxis. N Engl J Med 314:1665, 1986.
48. Amon E, Lewis SV, Sibai BM, et al: Ampicillin prophylaxis in preterm premature rupture of the membranes: A prospective randomized study. Am J Obstet Gynecol 159:539, 1988.
49. Council on Scientific Affairs, American Medical Association: In-

duced termination of pregnancy before and after Roe v. Wade. Trends in mortality and morbidity of women. JAMA 268:3231, 1992.
50. Sonne-Holm S, Heisterbert L, Hebjorn S, et al: Prophylactic antibiotics in first trimester abortions: A clinical, controlled trial. Am J Obstet Gynecol 139:693, 1981.
51. Levallois P, Rious JE: Prophylactic antibiotics for suction curettage abortion: Results of a clinical controlled trial. Am J Obstet Gynecol 158:100, 1988.
52. Darj E, Stralin EB, Nilsson S: The prophylactic effect of doxycycline on postoperative infection rate after first-trimester abortion. Obstet Gynecol 70:755, 1987.
53. Grimes DA, Schulz KF, Cates W: Prophylactic antibiotics for curettage abortion. Am J Obstet Gynecol 150:689, 1984.

AIDS AND RELATED INFECTIONS

120

Approach to the Patient with Human Immunodeficiency Virus Infection: Clinical Features

Henry Masur

In the United States, about 650,000 to 900,000 people are infected with human immunodeficiency virus type 1 (HIV-1).[1, 2] Worldwide, many millions are infected,[3, 4] including males and females of all major ethnic groups and all age ranges from neonates to elders.[1–4] Health care providers in all disciplines can expect to deal with HIV-infected persons who need health care for problems unrelated to the HIV or who need diagnostic, therapeutic, or prophylactic services related to manifestations of HIV infection.[5] Health care providers can also anticipate continued concern and awareness on the part of uninfected persons who want information about the likelihood that they or their families will come into contact with or acquire HIV, either in the community or in health care facilities where they are receiving attention. Some persons become concerned that a wide variety of nonspecific symptoms and signs could indicate HIV disease even if they are not engaged in any high-risk behavior. Thus, every health care provider in the 1990s needs to be familiar with HIV. To an increasing degree, infectious disease practitioners are expected to be information resources in their medical facilities and to provide both consultations and primary care for infected persons. They are also expected to be information resources and leaders for their communities.

HIV produces a broad range of manifestations in humans, manifestations that originally were categorized into asymptomatic acquired immunodeficiency syndrome (AIDS)–related complex and AIDS.[6–9] Since then, it has been recognized that HIV can produce a range of manifestations that are not easy to fit accurately and usefully into a few categories. The range of manifestations includes an acute retroviral syndrome,[10–19] an asymptomatic period, and myriad clinical syndromes that can be mild to incidental[20–28] or severe and life threatening.[29–46] It is important to view HIV infection as a chronic, usually fatal process that is punctuated by manifestations that vary dramatically in type and severity from person to person. HIV disease progresses at an unpredictable rate.[47–61] The variations in rate of disease progression and specific manifestations are probably influenced by numerous factors, which may include route of HIV infection, size of HIV inoculum, sex, host genetic background, specific strain of infecting HIV, recent and past environmental exposures, and medical interventions. The variation in clinical course of HIV disease, much like the variation in clinical course of most infectious and noninfectious diseases, must be recognized by health practitioners so that an appropriate respect for the unpredictability of the disease can temper the real progress that is being made in understanding the course of this retroviral process, which is being increasingly better defined by techniques such as viral load monitoring.[52, 57, 60]

The clinical approach to a patient with HIV infection is predicated on the assumption that the patient is truly infected. As more serologic techniques become available to screen for HIV and then to confirm the presence of the retrovirus, it is essential to ascertain that the diagnosis has been unequivocally established (see Chapter 126). If the diagnosis is certain, the physician must initiate a series of assessments designed to evaluate where HIV disease is in its evolution, what processes currently present need to be diagnosed and treated, and what processes can be anticipated and either prevented or delayed. The physician must also initiate a process of education of the patient so that he or she can take an active role in the management of the retroviral infection, plan realistically for the future, and have the information necessary to minimize the likelihood of transmitting the virus to anyone else.

Natural History

Acute Retroviral Syndrome

One to 6 weeks after acquiring HIV infection, some patients experience a nonspecific febrile illness that is transient and self-limiting over several weeks.[10–19] The clinical features of this illness are variable but may include fever, malaise, fatigue, rash (maculopapular, urticarial, or roseola-like), arthralgias, myalgias, generalized adenopathy, pharyngitis, headache, photophobia, meningismus, diarrhea, peripheral neuropathy, and encephalitis. These manifestations are usually self-limiting during a few days to several weeks. There is nothing specific and diagnostic in the history and physical examination except a temporal relationship to a possible exposure. Because the symptoms and signs *are* nonspecific and most patients do not undergo a laboratory evaluation focused on HIV, it has been difficult to estimate what fraction of patients do develop this type of syndrome. One study reported an acute clinical syndrome in 41 of 46 individuals.[15] Another prospective study reported an acute syndrome in 55% of 22 seropositive patients, but 21% of 44 HIV-uninfected persons reported similar symptoms.[13] Many health care workers who have acquired HIV occupationally have reported acute illness.[11, 62]

The relationship of an acute syndrome to HIV infection can be established by laboratory tests. The erythrocyte sedimentation rate and transaminase levels may be elevated. Granulocytopenia and thrombocytopenia may be seen. Counts of total lymphocytes (including both $CD4^+$ and $CD8^+$ cells) characteristically fall, followed by transient increases in $CD8^+$ lymphocytes.[13, 14, 18, 63, 64] $CD4^+$ lymphocytes have been reported in one series to be 244 to 1055 cells per mm^3 within the first 4 weeks after acquisition of HIV.[15] $CD4^+$ lymphocytes may recover to preinfection numbers, but most patients demonstrate a fall of 100 to 200 cells in the first 6 months after seroconversion and an additional 100 cells in the next 6 months. In one review of 318 seroconverters, mean $CD4^+$ cell counts in the initial 12 months after seroconversion fell from 999 to 673/mm^3.[63] If a spinal tap is performed, cerebrospinal fluid pleocytosis with normal protein and glucose levels is often seen.[64]

HIV serologic studies sometimes show p24 antigen in the serum or cerebrospinal fluid within 2 weeks of exposure.[12, 64, 65] This p24 antigen often appears concurrently with acute symptoms and persists for 8 to 12 weeks until p24 antibody appears. Viremia can be detected during the period of clinical illness and disappears when p24 antibody becomes detectable.[13, 14, 19, 60] The magnitude of viremia and the duration of persistence correlate with prognosis. For almost all patients, the results of enzyme-linked immunosorbent assay and Western blot tests become positive within 2 to 4 months of HIV acquisition, although a few cases of persistent "seronegativity" with "culture positivity" have been reported.[66–69] Some of these cases of persistent seronegativity may represent flawed performance or interpretation of laboratory tests. Antibody to HIV proteins can be detected by Western blot somewhat before the enzyme-linked immunosorbent assay test becomes positive.[67]

It would thus appear that well over half of all persons who acquire HIV infection have a symptomatic syndrome. Many do not seek medical attention for this nonspecific syndrome, however. In addition, most health care providers would have no reason to initiate an HIV evaluation for this type of nonspecific disorder unless the patient drew attention to a history of potential HIV exposure. Preliminary studies suggest that early intervention with antiretroviral therapy can slow the decline of $CD4^+$ cells and reduce the number of clinical events during the initial several years of infection.[19] Whether a strategy of early intervention with antiretroviral therapy at the time an acute syndrome or seroconversion is recognized produces long-term benefit including prolonged survival remains to be adequately assessed.

Asymptomatic Stage

After acquisition of HIV infection and resolution of the acute retroviral syndrome, if one occurs, patients are free from life-threatening opportunistic infections or tumors for a median of about 8 years, although life-threatening processes have been documented as early as 2 years after seroconversion, and acute opportunistic infections occasionally occur as part of the acute retroviral syndrome.[27, 47, 56, 70–73] An increasing number of the 650,000 to 900,000 persons in the United States who have HIV infection are coming to medical attention before they develop an AIDS-defining illness or any HIV-related clinical manifestations.[6] They come voluntarily and involuntarily to medical attention because of increased awareness of HIV and its manifestations, both by health care practitioners and by the persons themselves who are at high risk. A distressingly large number of individuals, however, are still unaware that their behavior places them in a high-risk category for acquiring HIV infection, and a distressingly large number have HIV infection that is unknown to them until they develop a serious clinical manifestation.[72, 74]

When HIV infection is confirmed, it is important to assess the patient's prognosis. HIV causes disease by three basic mechanisms: (1) depletion of functional $CD4^+$ T lymphocytes, leading to susceptibility to opportunistic infections and tumors; (2) development of immune-mediated events caused, for instance, by antigen-antibody complexes to produce glomerulonephritis or thrombocytopenia; and (3) damage to specific organs such as heart, brain, or lungs by direct or indirect retroviral actions.

How rapidly these processes cause disease, or what the precise manifestations of disease are, is difficult to predict for any given patient. Most studies have assessed the rate of progression of HIV infection by measuring the time from seroconversion to the development of AIDS-related complex or AIDS or death or progression through standardized classification systems.[27, 47, 52, 70–73] The definition of AIDS by the Centers for Disease Control and Prevention[6, 9] is shown in Tables 120–1 and 120–2; the definition by the World Health Organization[7] is shown in Table 120–3; and the two most common classification systems, the Centers for Disease Control and Prevention system[9] and the Walter Reed system,[8, 75] are shown in Tables 120–2 and 120–4, respectively. These classification systems are useful for surveillance purposes and as objective staging systems for research protocols. For assessing the prognosis for an individual patient, however, they are not always ideally suited. For instance, a patient with Kaposi's sarcoma and a high $CD4^+$ cell count and a patient with cytomegalovirus (CMV) retinitis and a low $CD4^+$ cell count both meet the case definition of AIDS, although the two patients have vastly different prognoses. Similarly, some patients with persistent generalized adenopathy may have a low $CD4^+$ cell count and persistent fever and have a much worse prognosis than a patient with similar adenopathy but a normal $CD4^+$ cell count and normal temperature curve. Thus, the use of these staging systems in clinical practice may not provide the type of data most useful to the clinician.

The natural history of HIV infection has been dramatically altered by antiretroviral therapy, better prevention and therapy of opportunistic processes, and improved supportive care.[19, 27, 56, 57, 72, 74, 76–78] The likelihood of an initial AIDS-defining infection or tumor developing in an untreated person who is HIV seropositive probably averages about 4% to 10% per year after acquisition of HIV infection.[48–52, 55–57] The rate of transition from asymptomatic infection without AIDS to AIDS is relatively lower in the first few years after seroconversion. The incidence curve appears to be steeper thereafter. In a cohort study from San Francisco involving homosexual men who received little antiretroviral therapy or prophylaxis against opportunistic infection, the actuarial progression rate to AIDS during 9 years after seroconversion was 42%; an additional 32% had developed HIV-related disorders that did not meet the definition of AIDS over this period.[70] Similar results have been obtained in other studies involving homosexual men and hemophiliacs.[27, 48, 51, 52, 58, 59, 73] Rates of progression may differ in other populations of patients such as parenteral drug users or elderly transfusion recipients. In the era of increasingly potent antiretroviral therapies and increasingly effective chemoprophylaxis against opportunistic infections, rates of progression will be substantially altered.[72, 75]

TABLE 120–1 ■ Centers for Disease Control and Prevention Surveillance Case Definition for AIDS—1987

Diseases diagnosed definitively without confirmation of HIV infection in patients without other causes of immunodeficiency
- Candidiasis of the esophagus, trachea, bronchi, or lungs
- Cryptococcoses, extrapulmonary
- Cryptosporidiosis >1 mo duration
- Cytomegalovirus (CMV) infection of any organ except the liver, spleen, or lymph nodes in patients >1 mo old
- Herpes simplex, mucocutaneous (>1 mo duration), or of the bronchi, lungs, or esophagus of 1 mo duration
- Kaposi's sarcoma in patients <60 y old
- Primary central nervous system (CNS) lymphoma in patients <60 y old
- Lymphoid interstitial pneumonitis (LIP) and/or pulmonary lymphoid hyperplasia (PLH) in patients <13 y old
- *Mycobacterium avium* complex or *Mycobacterium kansasii* disseminated
- *Pneumocystis carinii* pneumonia
- Progressive multifocal leukoencephalopathy
- Toxoplasmosis of the brain in patients >1 mo old

Diseases diagnosed definitively with confirmation of HIV infection
- Multiple or recurrent pyogenic bacterial infections in patients <13 y old
- Coccidioidomycosis, disseminated
- Histoplasmosis, disseminated
- Isosporiasis >1 mo duration
- Kaposi's sarcoma, any age
- Primary CNS lymphoma, any age
- Non-Hodgkin's lymphoma (small, noncleaved lymphoma; Burkitt or non-Burkitt type; or immunoblastic sarcoma)
- Mycobacterial disease other than that caused by *Mycobacterium tuberculosis*, disseminated
- *M. tuberculosis* disease, extrapulmonary
- *Salmonella* septicemia, recurrent

Disease diagnosed presumptively with confirmation of HIV infection
- Candidiasis of the esophagus
- CMV retinitis
- Kaposi's sarcoma
- LIP/PLH in patients <13 y old
- Disseminated mycobacterial disease (not cultured)
- *P. carinii* pneumonia
- Toxoplasmosis of the brain in patients >1 mo old
- HIV encephalopathy
- HIV wasting syndrome

From Centers for Disease Control: Revision of the CDC surveillance case definition for acquired immunodeficiency syndrome. MMWR Morbid Mortal Wkly Rep 36(Suppl 1):1S–15S, 1987.

Some patients remain clinically well 10 to 20 years after they were first found to be seropositive. A few of these patients have normal or almost normal CD4$^+$ lymphocyte counts. These unusual patients, termed long-term nonprogressors, characteristically have preserved immune function and low viral burdens. Why they have been able to preserve immune function and what their ultimate outcome will be remain uncertain.[54, 61] Conversion of viral cultures or serology from positive to negative has been debated in one child with congenital HIV infection.[79] If this occurs in adults, it appears to be extraordinarily rare.

Clinical parameters can help to predict the likelihood of progression from an asymptomatic stage to a symptomatic or life-threatening manifestation of HIV (Table 120–5). Clinically, the presence of oral candidiasis in a seropositive patient who is not receiving corticosteroids or antibiotics and who does not have diabetes correlates with progression to AIDS,[21] as does the finding of oral hairy leukoplakia.[22, 26] These diagnoses must be arrived at by careful observation, and the inexperienced or hurried health care provider can often mistake saliva or products of poor oral hygiene for these entities.[80] Direct microscopic examination of mucosal scrapings for *Candida* organisms is helpful diagnostically; biopsy can also be diagnostic but is rarely necessary outside a research setting. Lymphadenopathy and dermatomal zoster correlate with HIV seropositivity but do not appear to correlate with likelihood of disease progression, although some data suggest that the site, extent, severity, or frequency of zoster may have some prognostic significance.[49–52, 81] Fever, night sweats, weight loss, and chronic diarrhea appear to correlate with likelihood of progression to AIDS.

Laboratory parameters, especially virologic assays, are receiving increasing attention.[57, 60, 82–107] The absolute peripheral CD4$^+$ lymphocyte count and the percentage of peripheral cells that are CD4$^+$ both correlate well with the likelihood of developing AIDS.[57, 60, 73, 82, 83] Retrospective and prospective studies show that the lower the absolute CD4$^+$ lymphocyte count or percentage, the more likely the patient is to develop life-threatening opportunistic infections.[57, 60, 73, 82–84, 108] For instance, CMV retinitis almost always occurs in patients with an absolute CD4$^+$ lymphocyte count less than 50/mm^3 or less than 5% CD4$^+$ cells.[77, 82, 103] *Pneumocystis carinii* pneumonia usually occurs in patients with a CD4$^+$ lymphocyte count below 100/mm^3 or less than 10%; *Pneumocystis* pneumonia occasionally develops in patients with CD4$^+$ counts of 100 to 250/mm^3 (10% to 25% CD4$^+$ cells) but rarely in patients with

TABLE 120–2 ■ 1993 Centers for Disease Control and Prevention AIDS Surveillance Case Definition and Staging System

CD4$^+$ CATEGORY		CLINICAL CATEGORIES		
Number of Cells	%	Asymptomatic or Acute HIV, PGL*	Symptomatic, not A or C	AIDS Indicator Conditions†
>499	>29	A1	B1	C1
200–499	14–28	A2	B2	C2
<200	<14	A3	B3	C3

*PGL, Persistent generalized lymphadenopathy.
†AIDS indicator conditions from 1987 are listed in Table 120–1; new AIDS indicator conditions are pulmonary tuberculosis, recurrent bacterial pneumonia, and invasive cervical cancer.
From Centers for Disease Control and Prevention: 1993 revised classification system for HIV infection and expanded surveillance case definition for AIDS among adolescents and adults. MMWR Morbid Mortal Wkly Rep 41(RR-17):1, 1992.

TABLE 120–3 ■ World Health Organization Adult Case Definition for AIDS

Major signs*
- >10% weight loss
- Diarrhea >1 mo duration
- Fever >1 mo duration

Minor signs*
- Cough >1 mo duration
- General pruritic dermatitis
- Recurrent herpes zoster
- Oropharyngeal candidiasis
- Progressive, disseminated herpes simplex
- Generalized lymphadenopathy

Diagnostic of AIDS
- Cryptococcal meningitis
- Disseminated Kaposi's sarcoma

*The presence of at least two major signs and one minor sign is diagnostic of AIDS.
From World Health Organization: Interim proposal for a WHO Staging System for HIV infection and diseases. Wkly Epidemiol Rec 65:221–224, 1990.

TABLE 120–4 ■ Walter Reed Staging Classification for HIV Infection in Adults

STAGE	HIV ANTIBODY OR VIRUS ISOLATION	CHRONIC LYMPHADENOPATHY	T HELPER CELLS/mm³	ANERGY	THRUSH	OPPORTUNISTIC INFECTION
0	–	–	>400	Normal	–	–
1	+	–	>400	Normal	–	–
2	+	+	>400	Normal	–	–
3	+	+/–	<400	Normal	–	–
4	+	+/–	<400	Partial	–	–
5	+	+/–	<400	Complete	+	–
6	+	+/–	<400	Complete	+	+

From Redfield RR, Wright DC, Tramont EC: The Walter Reed staging classification for HTLV-III/LAV infection. N Engl J Med 314:131–132, 1986.

more CD4⁺ cells than 250/mm³ (or more than 25%).[74, 82, 108] Some non–life-threatening opportunistic infections such as oral candidiasis and some serious opportunistic processes such as tuberculosis *(Mycobacterium tuberculosis)* may occur at somewhat higher CD4⁺ ranges than CMV retinitis or *Pneumocystis* pneumonia, but it seems clear that the lower a patient's CD4⁺ lymphocyte count or percentage, the more likely the patient is to develop an opportunistic infectious process. Whether protease inhibitors or immunomodulators such as interleukin-2 will modify this relationship is uncertain; to date there is no firm evidence that, after CD4⁺ cell count rises induced by these therapies, opportunistic infections will occur at unexpected CD4⁺ cell counts.

The percentage of peripheral mononuclear cells that are CD4⁺ is at least as useful as the absolute number of CD4⁺ cells for predicting the occurrence of opportunistic infections.[82, 83] The CD4⁺ cell percentage is a number measured directly by the fluorescent antibody cell sorter; the absolute number of CD4⁺ cells is derived by multiplying this percentage by the total lymphocyte count, which is itself the product of the white cell count and differential. The percentage usually fluctuates less than the absolute number, which is an advantage for monitoring, although clinicians are generally more accustomed to following absolute numbers. The CD4⁺/CD8⁺ ratio also correlates with susceptibility to infection and prognosis, but the correlation is not as strong as with the absolute number or percentage of CD4⁺ cells.[83]

The relationship of the CD4⁺ lymphocyte count to the development of opportunistic infectious complications of HIV infection is important in approaching the management of HIV infection. First, HIV infection implies that unless an effective therapeutic intervention is developed, immune function inexorably declines and infectious complications occur (antiretroviral therapy that is currently available may slow this decline but does not prevent it). Second, monitoring the immunologic decline provides the clinician with a means of anticipating certain complications. This anticipation should allow earlier diagnosis of these complications and reduction of the likelihood of certain complications if safe and effective prophylactic regimens can be instituted. Third, a rise in CD4⁺ lymphocyte number in response to some antiretroviral therapies, and perhaps to certain immunotherapies such as that with interleukin-2, predicts clinical, virologic, and immunologic benefit of therapeutic intervention.[56, 60, 86–88]

The presence of serum p24 antigen identifies patients who are more likely to develop an initial AIDS-defining illness during a defined follow-up period.[70–73] Conversely, high levels of anti-p24 antibody appear to be present in patients who are less likely to develop an initial AIDS-defining illness in a given period of follow-up.[89–93] Quantitative measurement of plasma viremia, currently performed by quantitative polymerase chain reaction tests or branched chain DNA assays, is becoming increasingly available.[56, 60] These assays provide information that is not only prognostically useful but also useful for demonstrating a response to antiretroviral therapy and subsequent prognosis in terms of fewer AIDS-defining illnesses and longer survival. These assays are likely to replace serology and p24 antigen assays as laboratory indicators of disease activity or prognosis.[56, 57, 60, 94–96]

When HIV infection is definitely diagnosed and the patient's prognosis is estimated, the health care provider must help the patient find resources to deal with the emotional, spiritual, psychologic, and financial aspects of the disease as well as the medical issues.[97] The patient needs to be encouraged to consider how HIV infection and its many ramifications affect family, friends, employment, living accommodations, and finances and to be made aware of issues such as health insurance, medical assistance, durable power of attorney, and wills. Referrals to psychologists, psychiatrists, social workers, support groups, or comprehensive assistance agencies may enhance the quality of the patient's subsequent existence as much as the medical help that is provided.

TABLE 120–5 ■ Parameters Predictive of Prognosis in HIV-Seropositive Persons

- Clinical
  - Oral thrush
  - Hairy leukoplakia
  - Persistent constitutional symptoms (including wasting)
  - Fever >2 wk duration
  - Chronic diarrhea
- Laboratory
  - Peripheral CD4⁺ lymphocyte (number, percentage, or ratio)
  - Plasma HIV RNA quantitation
  - HIV p24 antigen
  - Anti-HIV p24 antibody
  - Neopterin
  - Syncytium-inducing HIV-1 phenotype
  - Interferon-γ production
  - HIV resistance to antiretroviral drugs
  - β_2-Microglobulin
  - Hemoglobin

Symptomatic Stage

Symptomatic manifestations of HIV disease can occur at almost any juncture during the immunologic decline that HIV produces. As reviewed earlier, the manifestations that occur as the CD4⁺ cell count falls from 800 to 1200/mm³ (normal) to 200 to 250/mm³ are rarely life threatening, although tuberculosis, geographic fungal diseases, oropharyngeal candidiasis, lymphoma, and Kaposi's sarcoma can occur. At CD4⁺ cell counts below 200 to 250/mm³ the same manifestations can occur, but many life-threatening opportunistic pathogens (e.g., *P. carinii,* nontuberculous mycobacteria, CMV, cryptosporidia) become frequent causes of morbidity.[74, 82, 85, 109–114] Which manifestations an individual patient develops or when in the temporal evolution of HIV disease the first manifestation or subsequent ones occur is difficult to predict. For primary and secondary infectious manifestations, the patient's past and present microbial environments, in terms of person-to-person transmission, geographic location, and fortuitous events (e.g., exposure to contaminated food, waste, animals, or aerosols), are important determinants. *M. tuberculosis, Histoplasma capsulatum, Coccidioides immitis, Leishmania chagasi, Penicillium marneffei, Trypanosoma cruzi,* and *Isospora belli* are examples of pathogens with a strong geographic predisposition that could cause disease if the patient were exposed to the appropriate source, either early in life before acquiring HIV infection or subsequently, after HIV was well established. It has been assumed that most AIDS-related opportunistic infectious diseases are due to reactivation of latent pathogens. As organisms are characterized by more specific laboratory techniques, however, it is becoming clearer that at least some infectious complications are due to recent acquisition of primary infection or to reinfection with a newly acquired strain that is phenotypically or genotypically different from an infecting organism documented previously. Other factors that are not well understood also influence whether and when a patient develops certain manifestations. Chapters 122 through 125 provide details about the diagnosis and therapy of many HIV-related manifestations, and Tables 120–1 to 120–3 provide classification schemes for these manifestations. (The definition of AIDS made in 1984 was modified in 1985, 1987, and 1993.[6, 9]) As each manifestation occurs and appropriate diagnostic and therapeutic steps are taken, the health care provider needs to reconsider what the occurrence signifies prognostically: First, can the manifestation itself be successfully treated? Second, does therapy of the new manifestation interfere with current therapeutic, suppressive, or prophylactic regimens? Third, what does the occurrence of the manifestation indicate about the immunologic and virologic status of the patient and future clinical events? Appropriate communication with the patient about how these symptomatic episodes alter management and prognosis is in order.

Reduction of Complications

Once it is established that a patient definitely has HIV infection and where in the natural evolution of HIV disease the particular patient is, a major focus of management must be the prevention of complications of HIV disease. Either prevention or deferral of complications is likely to have a beneficial effect on the quality and duration of the patient's survival.

Management to reduce the number and frequency of complications and to prolong survival should include (1) antiretroviral therapy; (2) reduction of exposure to pathogens; (3) chemoprophylaxis and immunization; and (4) prompt and aggressive management of infections, tumors, and other complications when they do occur.

Antiretroviral and Immunomodulating Therapy

An expanding armamentarium of antiretroviral agents is available that can reduce the frequency of HIV-related complications and prolong survival. Zidovudine was the first drug that was definitively shown to reduce the number of HIV-related opportunistic infections and tumors and to prolong survival.[98–102] It has been clear that the clinical, virologic, and immunologic benefit of zidovudine is time limited largely by the development of retroviral resistance after months or years of therapy.[96] There was considerable controversy about the optimal time to initiate zidovudine to maximize the modest but important benefits that this drug can provide. Zidovudine can be associated with considerable toxicity and cost, issues that must be balanced against its potential benefit.

Since the development of zidovudine, evidence has accumulated that other regimens can provide more effective initial benefit, including didanosine alone or the combination regimen zidovudine plus didanosine, or zidovudine plus zalcitabine.[76] Thus, monotherapy with zidovudine is no longer considered a reasonable initial antiretroviral regimen.[114a, 114b] It is logical to assume that other potent regimens that provide more effective antiretroviral activity (as measured by reduction in plasma viremia) or more substantial immunologic effect (as measured by rise in $CD4^+$ cell count) would provide even more impressive clinical benefit.[56, 86, 87, 106, 107, 114a–114c] Trials using newer drugs such as the nucleoside reverse transcriptase inhibitors (e.g., lamivudine), nonnucleoside reverse transcriptase inhibitors (e.g., delaviridine or nevirapine), nucleotides (e.g., 9-(2-phosphonylmethoxyethyl)adenine [PMEA]), protease inhibitors (e.g., saquinavir, indinavir, ritonavir),[106, 107, 114a–114c] and other compounds need to be completed and analyzed to determine whether they do provide greater clinical benefit with acceptable safety, cost, and convenience. The issue of convenience can be an important issue if regimens involve an unpalatable quantity of pills, a burdensome drug schedule, or complicated drug interactions.[115] The optimal time to initiate these regimens, is controversial. Many clinicians now agree that antiretroviral therapy should be initiated for any symptomatic patient; for an asymptomatic patient with a $CD4^+$ cell count below 500/mm^3; for an asymptomatic patient with a $CD4^+$ cell count higher than 500/mm^3 and either a viral load greater than 30,000 to 50,000 copies per milliliter or a rapidly declining $CD4^+$ cell count.[114a]

Some clinicians would initiate therapy for an asymptomatic patient with a $CD4^+$ cell count higher than 500/mm^3 and only 5000 to 10,000 HIV RNA copies per milliliter.[114a]

Whatever initial regimen is initiated, the duration of benefit for a specific regimen is limited. It is currently unclear how best to determine when this benefit is waning, although it would obviously be desirable to change therapy before deterioration is extensive enough to permit occurrence of a clinical event such as an opportunistic infection. It is logical at least to follow $CD4^+$ cell counts and viral load and to change regimens when these surrogate markers change substantially.[55, 57] Many clinicians would advocate always adding at least two drugs to which the patient has never previously been exposed to minimize the likelihood that drug resistance will emerge rapidly. Such a strategic approach needs to be validated before it is accepted as the standard of care, even though it is logical, because it involves expensive laboratory monitoring. The use of these laboratory markers also requires considerable judgment: viral load, for instance, can increase temporarily as a result of immunization or concurrent events like herpes labialis or herpes genitalis.[109] Clinicians would not want to change therapeutic regimens because of occurrences that do not influence the clinical course or because of laboratory inconsistencies and errors.

More data about antiretroviral therapy are becoming available to help determine the best time to initiate therapy, the best time to switch therapy, the best agents to use, and the optimal doses. During this period of rapid change, health care professionals need to ascertain that the regimens they introduce into their practices represent documented improvements in management rather than fashionable concepts not warranted on the basis of reasonable data.

It is worth pointing out that early institution of antiretroviral therapy might help prevent some of the complications that appear to be closely linked to HIV in addition to preventing opportunistic infectious processes. Early institution of antiretroviral therapy may prevent or ameliorate HIV encephalopathy, myopathy, nonspecific pneumonitis, cardiomyopathy, or enteropathy. Similarly, some of the sequelae of immune complex disease, such as glomerulonephritis or thrombocytopenia, may be prevented or delayed by early antiretroviral intervention.

Most attention to treating the underlying, basic cause of HIV disease has focused on antiretroviral therapy. HIV is certainly an appropriate target for this focus, but most of the complications of HIV disease are caused by an insufficient number of appropriate CD4+ cells. Agents that improve immunologic function, such as interleukin-2, may also prove to provide considerable clinical benefit in conjunction with antiretroviral therapy.[88] This approach may be useful for maintaining CD4+ cells at normal numbers before they are diminished quantitatively or qualitatively. This approach may also be useful for patients whose immune function was comprised before antiretroviral therapy was initiated or despite aggressive antiretroviral efforts.[88]

Prophylaxis and Suppression of Specific Opportunistic Pathogens

REDUCTION OF EXPOSURE TO PATHOGENS

Patients with HIV infection, like all other humans, are constantly exposed to microorganisms in their environment.[74] Opportunistic pathogens are present in the air (e.g., *Pneumocystis, M. tuberculosis,* or *Streptococcus pneumoniae*), food (e.g., *Cryptosporidium* or *Salmonella*), and water (e.g., *Cryptosporidium*). Pathogens can also be acquired by specific activities such as sexual intercourse (e.g., CMV, *Treponema pallidum*), contact with children in daycare (e.g., CMV, *Cryptosporidium,* or *Salmonella*), contact with pets (e.g., *Salmonella, Cryptosporidium,* or *Bartonella* species), or working in prisons, shelters, or hospitals (e.g., *M. tuberculosis*). Patients with HIV infection cannot eliminate exposure to these pathogens, but they can consider whether they wish to modify their behavior to reduce exposure or at least be monitored carefully (e.g., by frequent tuberculin skin tests) to determine whether infection has taken place.[74] Even if patients already have serologic or skin test evidence of prior infection with a particular organism, it may be reasonable to reduce the potential for becoming infected with a different strain, a situation that is known to occur with tuberculosis[35, 36] and may occur with other pathogens.[115a]

Patients and their health care providers need to consider jointly whether the inconvenience of behavioral modification is warranted by the magnitude of likely benefit. An HIV-infected patient who is seronegative for CMV, for example, may wish to practice safe sex with an HIV-infected, CMV-seropositive sexual partner, even if the sexual relationship is monogamous. Conversely, if a patient lives in a city with a municipal water supply that conforms to accepted standards, it may not be worthwhile to use boiled or bottled water because the risk of acquiring cryptosporidiosis or other enteric pathogens is likely to be low.

CHEMOPROPHYLAXIS AND IMMUNIZATION OF SPECIFIC PATHOGENS

As long as antiretroviral therapy (and perhaps immunomodulating therapy) can prevent or slow the decline in CD4+ cell counts above 200/mm³, the number of serious infectious complications is substantially reduced. Antiretroviral and immunomodulatory strategies have not yet been devised that can prevent this decline indefinitely, however, and thus almost all patients eventually develop a level of immunodeficiency such that they would benefit from the addition of specific chemoprophylaxis or immunization to reduce the frequency of opportunistic infections.

In the last half of the 1990s, a wide and expanding array of drugs and immunizations are available that can reduce the frequency of specific opportunistic infections.[74, 77, 80, 105, 110–145] In addition, immunizations are available that it is logical to employ, even if their benefit is not proved. Using all the regimens that are available is impractical because of the number of pills required, their interactions, their toxicity, and their cost.[115] Thus, clinicians and patients need to consider the available options and give highest priority to the immunizations and drug regimens that are likely to prevent the most common and the most serious processes. For patients with different behavioral risk factors and for different geographic areas, those choices may differ. For instance, prophylaxis against *Pneumocystis* and *Mycobacterium avium* complex is more important in North America than in Brazil, where toxoplasmosis, tuberculosis, and fungal disease are more important.

For patients in the United States, the U.S. Public Health Service, in conjunction with the Infectious Disease Society of America, has issued guidelines suggesting prioritization of chemoprophylaxis and immunization.[74]

Pneumocystis pneumonia deserves particular attention because it is so frequent and so serious in North America. Before the era of antipneumocystis prophylaxis and antiretroviral therapy, 75% to 80% of patients with HIV infection eventually developed one or more episodes of *Pneumocystis* pneumonia.[108, 111, 112, 114] These were the most common causes of life-threatening opportunistic infection. Clinical studies have determined when in the natural course of HIV infection *Pneumocystis* pneumonia occurs and have defined highly effective, convenient, safe, and inexpensive prophylactic regimens.[81, 82, 111–114, 122–126] Several studies have convincingly shown a strong survival benefit for patients who receive antipneumocystis prophylaxis, independent of other factors such as antiretroviral regimen and CD4+ cell count.[74, 117–121] Thus, it is logical for *Pneumocystis* prophylaxis to be considered standard care and to be at the top of the priority list for chemoprophylactic options.

Antipneumocystis prophylaxis can be expected to reduce the frequency of *Pneumocystis* pneumonia, although no regimen is 100% effective. Convincing data demonstrate that if prophylaxis is initiated when the CD4+ cell count falls to 200/mm³ or (regardless of CD4+ cell count) when oral candidiasis, hairy leukoplakia, unexplained fever of 2 or more weeks in duration, or perhaps substantial weight loss occurs, most cases of *Pneumocystis* pneumonia can be prevented.[108, 113, 122–126] A few cases occur at higher CD4+ cell counts, before any indicator signs, but a larger number of patients would have to receive prophylaxis to prevent these relatively few cases.

A variety of regimens have been shown to have antipneumocystis activity.[113, 122–126] Trimethoprim-sulfamethoxazole is the regimen of choice because it is more effective than any other, is cheap and convenient, and has activity against other pathogens including *Toxoplasma gondii, S. pneumoniae,* and *Haemophilus influenzae*.[74, 113, 114] Dapsone alone is probably the second choice, although dapsone-pyrimethamine combinations are also effective. Aerosol pentamidine is also effective, as detailed in Chapter 122. The best regimen for an individual patient depends on a complex array of issues including the patient's ability to tolerate the various regimens, compliance issues, and cost.

Prevention of *M. tuberculosis* disease is also a high priority.[74, 127–131] It is well recognized that clinical disease is likely to occur if patients with HIV infection become infected with *M. tuberculosis*.[34–36, 127–129, 132–136] In addition, *M. tuberculosis* infection appears to stimulate enhanced retroviral activity. Not only does *M. tuberculosis* cause morbidity and mortality in the infected patient, but there is a sizable risk of transmission, especially because the patient is likely to habituate areas frequented by other highly susceptible individuals. Patients with no history of tuberculin reactivity should be retested at least annually and offered prophylaxis if their skin test becomes positive or if the test result is positive with no history of prophylaxis, as detailed in Chapter 166.[129, 130] It may be reasonable to offer tuberculosis prophylaxis to certain individuals at high risk regardless of tuberculin test status.[136] Isoniazid prophylaxis has been shown to provide survival benefit for tuberculin test–positive individuals.[136] Thus, it should be clear that chemoprophylaxis for tuberculosis, like that for *Pneumocystis*, should be standard care.

Prevention of bacterial infections is being recognized as a desirable goal to decrease the morbidity of these processes, as well as their potential to stimulate HIV replication. The use of immunization is controversial because efficacy has not been proved and because immunization could theoretically produce deleterious effects.[136] Some drugs, such as trimethoprim-sulfamethoxazole and macrolides, which are used for other purposes, appear to decrease the frequency of bacterial infections.[138] However, bacterial resistance to these drugs is likely to be an increasing problem.

Other opportunistic pathogens that cause serious complications can be prevented by chemoprophylaxis, including *M. avium* complex (rifabutin or azithromycin or clarithromycin),[79, 110, 137–139] CMV (oral ganciclovir),[140, 141] *Candida* and *Cryptococcus* (fluconazole),[80] and *Toxoplasma* (trimethoprim-sulfamethoxazole or dapsone-pyrimethamine).[124, 142–145] As other studies are completed, additional regimens will probably be shown to be capable of preventing opportunistic infections. Because each of these regimens is associated with toxicities and cost, several of them cause important drug interactions, and there is a limit to how many drugs an individual can take, a decision to add one or more of these regimens to antipneumocystis and antituberculosis chemoprophylaxis is difficult to standardize in any uniform manner for all patients. Some patients are able to tolerate and afford more pills than others, and they may be receiving other drugs that do not interact with the prophylactic agents. Another consideration, however, is that any of these chronic regimens may promote the development of resistant pathogens. That prospect may be sufficient to warrant declining a primary prophylactic regimen that has not proved to prolong survival or substantially improve quality of life compared with other strategies such as prompt therapy when disease is first recognized or when a surrogate marker such as an antigen or nucleic acid detection system indicates a high likelihood of clinical disease.

For opportunistic infections that are not life threatening, such as oral candidiasis or perirectal herpes simplex, primary prophylaxis is probably not as sensible as a strategy of waiting for the first episode of disease to occur, treating it, and then considering the desirability of chronic prevention. There are reports that reactivation of viruses such as herpes simplex virus may stimulate HIV replication, suggesting that suppression may be a desirable strategy to prevent immunologic decline. Until this concept is validated, however, there is no strong evidence on which to base recommendations for therapy.

Secondary prophylaxis needs to be considered after successful therapy for any opportunistic infection in a patient with HIV infection, regardless of whether the infection was merely annoying or life threatening. After therapy for any opportunistic pathogen in an HIV-infected patient, with the possible exception of *M. tuberculosis* and common bacterial pathogens, there is a great likelihood that another episode of the disease will occur within weeks or months, often in the same anatomic location as the original disease (e.g., the same locus in the brain for toxoplasmosis, the same locus in the retina for CMV retinitis).[74, 77] In some instances, the subsequent episode is almost certainly a relapse, because the original therapy suppressed but did not eradicate the original pathogen. This appears to be the situation with herpes simplex virus, varicella-zoster virus, CMV, *T. gondii*, and *Cryptococcus neoformans* infections, regardless of whether results of immediate posttherapy cultures and titers suggested active infection. Whether more aggressive therapy or more potent agents could eradicate all pathogens and obviate long-term therapy remains to be determined. In other instances, the subsequent episodes may represent relapse or reinfection with another strain; for *Pneumocystis* pneumonia and *Candida* infections it is not known which scenario occurs more commonly. In some situations secondary prophylaxis might represent long-term suppressive therapy; in other situations it might represent prevention of reinfection.

Regardless of terminology, a long-term regimen is indicated after acute therapy for most life-threatening opportunistic infections.[74, 77] These long-term regimens need to be convenient, inexpensive, effective, and compatible with other drugs taken for long periods, such as antiretroviral agents, if they are to gain widespread use.

For non–life-threatening infections, the desirability of secondary prophylaxis or long-term suppression depends on how severe and how frequent the relapses are. For perirectal herpes, for instance, chronic suppression with oral acyclovir might be desirable if relapses occurred predictably within a few weeks of terminating acute-phase therapy. In contrast, if relapses occurred only once or twice a year, it might be more convenient and cost-effective to treat each episode when it occurred, starting therapy promptly when symptoms or signs are first recognized.

Expeditious Treatment of Infections and Tumors

Prompt therapy of opportunistic infections and tumors is an important strategy if complications of host diseases are to be minimized. There is convincing evidence, for example, that early recognition and therapy of *Pneumocystis* pneumonia minimize the likelihood of respiratory failure or death.[146–149] It seems reasonable to assume that many of the chronic sequelae of *Pneumocystis* pneumonia, such as bronchopleural fistulae or severe pulmonary fibrosis, also occur less frequently if therapy is started earlier in the natural history of the infectious process. Similarly, early therapy of CMV colitis would be likely to reduce the frequency of bowel hemorrhage and perforation.[150] Early therapeutic intervention would also be a rational approach to minimizing acute and chronic sequelae of other life-threatening processes, such as toxoplasmosis, cryptococcosis, tuberculosis, histoplasmosis, central CMV retinitis, and salmonellosis. Therapy for many non–life-threatening processes—oral or vaginal candidiasis, perirectal or oral herpes simplex, painful cutaneous or disfiguring Kaposi's sarcoma lesions—is palliative. Because these infectious processes are usually symptomatic, prompt initiation of such therapy is appropriate. It must be recognized, however, that for certain non–life-threatening processes such as non-disfiguring, painless cutaneous Kaposi's sarcoma, early therapeutic intervention may be inconvenient and toxic without providing clear benefit to the patient. Thus, for some serious but not life-threatening processes prompt therapy may not be useful.

For prompt therapy of life-threatening processes to be initiated, both health care providers and patients need to be educated about which subtle signs and symptoms warrant immediate diagnostic evaluation. Both health care providers and patients need to recognize the enhanced urgency of evaluating subtle manifestations if the peripheral $CD4^+$ cell count is below 200 to 250/mm^3. The increasing availability of diagnostic studies that are noninvasive and inexpensive has enhanced the enthusiasm of health care providers and patients for initiating diagnosis early. Induced sputum examinations for *Pneumocystis*,[151] serum antigen tests for cryptococcal disease,[31] and lysis centrifugation or radiometric culture techniques for mycobacteria and fungi[152–156] are examples of sensitive and specific outpatient techniques that are less invasive and less costly than approaches used previously. Clinicians need to keep in mind, however, that when the index of suspicion is high for a life-threatening process and results of these screening tests are negative, more sensitive examinations such as bronchoscopy, lumbar puncture, computed tomography, percutaneous organ biopsy, and even surgical exploration and biopsy should in many instances be performed even if they are more expensive and more invasive and cause more morbidity.

Empirical Versus Specific Therapy

With any disease process, both health care providers and patients are often enthusiastic about treating a new manifestation empirically and thus avoiding the discomfort, inconvenience, cost, and morbidity of diagnostic procedures. There is a role for empirical therapy for certain complications of HIV disease, but the desirability of empirical therapy depends on four factors: how certain the identity of the pathogen is; how effective the empirical regimen is; how toxic and inconvenient the empirical regimen is; and how difficult it will be to establish the diagnosis later if the empirical regimen is not successful.[157]

When a patient with HIV infection develops pneumonia, for example, empirical therapy might be reasonable in certain circumstances. If hypoxemia is mild (e.g., room air partial pressure of oxygen greater than 70 to 80 torr or oxygen saturation greater than 95%), the process is not progressing rapidly, the $CD4^+$ cell count is below 200/mm^3, the chest radiograph is typical of *Pneumocystis* pneumonia, the patient is compliant and can tolerate an oral regimen, the patient has not been receiving trimethoprim-sulfamethoxazole prophylaxis, and diagnostic facilities are not readily available, then an empirical trial of trimethoprim-sulfamethoxazole might be reasonable. In this setting, the most likely treatable cause of pneumonia is *Pneumocystis*. If the patient becomes worse or fails to improve after 4 or 5 days, an induced sputum examination or bronchoalveolar lavage would be indicated.

Empirical therapy might also be appropriate for oral thrush, esophagitis, or a contrast-enhancing cerebral lesion. Because few processes mimic oral candidiasis, a clinical diagnosis of this entity can be made with a high degree of confidence by an experienced clinician and empirical antifungal therapy can be instituted. Most cases of esophagitis are caused by *Candida* species, and they respond within several days to topical, oral, or parenteral therapy. Topical nystatin, topical clotrimazole, or preferably oral fluconazole or itraconazole is generally tolerated well. Life-threatening complications of esophagitis caused by CMV, herpes simplex virus, or tumors are unusual. Thus, an empirical course of antifungal therapy for several days is reasonable in patients with clinical esophagitis. If the clinical response is not prompt and complete, the inconvenience, expense, and discomfort of a diagnostic procedure such as endoscopy are warranted.

For cerebral lesions that show contrast enhancement, empirical antitoxoplasma therapy is also appropriate. Although many infections and neoplastic processes can cause contrast-enhancing cerebral lesions in patients with HIV infection, almost all such masses are due to either *T. gondii* or lymphoma.[43, 45] If lesions represent *Toxoplasma,* there should be radiographic evidence of a response to pyrimethamine plus sulfadiazine within 2 weeks.[43, 45, 158, 159] If the lesions turn out to be due to lymphoma, little harm is likely to come to the patient, because cerebral lymphomas usually do not progress dramatically in such a short interval. Moreover, the success of therapy for lymphoma in this setting is modest, and waiting for 2 or 3 weeks is not likely to influence outcome adversely.

Thus, empirical therapy is warranted in certain clinical settings for patients with HIV infection. Given the cost, inconvenience, toxicity, and potential drug interactions associated with many therapies, however, empirical therapies need to be chosen judiciously.

Conclusion

Since AIDS was first recognized and described in 1981, dramatic progress has been made in understanding its etiology, pathogenesis, and natural history. New information on diagnosis, therapy, prophylaxis, and prognosis is rapidly becoming available. Clinicians need to assess these new approaches promptly but cautiously, so that those that provide clear benefit can be used and those that are not real improvements can be avoided or abandoned. The progress made in the 1980s provides clinicians in the 1990s with opportunities to improve the quality and duration of survival for the growing population of patients with HIV, an infectious process that is becoming increasingly chronic.

The second half of the 1990s is likely to see a changing array of clinical manifestations of HIV infection. First, the demographics of the HIV-infected populations are shifting, and more women and more drug abusers from lower socioeconomic strata are becoming infected. This shift should accentuate the reduction in frequency of Kaposi's sarcoma that is already occurring, because women and heterosexual intravenous drug abusers rarely develop it. In addition, less prosperous socioeconomic groups are more likely to have been exposed to *M. tuberculosis* and thus to develop tuberculosis when their immunity is suppressed. Other complications of poverty and drug abuse will be superimposed on manifestations of HIV in more and more patients. Members of lower socioeconomic groups are also less likely to obtain early medical intervention with antiretroviral therapy or evaluation of acute syndromes, so they are likely to come to medical attention with more florid, more advanced disease than was usually the case in the late 1980s. Second, antiretroviral therapy is slowing the progression of clinical disease and perhaps diminishing the severity of clinical complications. Patients will live longer and may ultimately manifest complications, such as cardiomyopathy, pneumonitis, or bowel dysfunction, that have been relatively uncommon so far. Third, the use of specific antiinfective prophylactic agents is having a considerable impact on clinical disease. Prophylaxis for *Pneumocystis* pneumonia, for instance, allows patients to live longer and ultimately provides an opportunity for more HIV-mediated processes such as cardiomyopathy, more neoplasms, and previously unrecognized opportunistic infections. Episodes of *Pneumocystis* pneumonia that do occur may be atypical in their pulmonary manifestations, may be extrapulmonary, and may be more difficult to diagnose and treat.[142–145] Thus, in the last half of the 1990s, clinicians caring for HIV-infected patients must remain alert to new and changing clinical manifestations, changes in sensitivity of various diagnostic approaches, and changes in the efficacy of therapeutic and prophylactic approaches.

As newer antiretroviral drugs are widely used and prophylactic antiinfective agents are used more widely and more chronically, drug resistance is likely to become a clinically important phenomenon that must be tested for and requires alterations in therapeutic regimens. Unless new drugs with novel mechanisms of action continue to be developed for HIV and for opportunistic pathogens, many of the gains of the 1980s and early 1990s may be eroded.

References

1. Karon JM, Rosenberg PS, McQuillan G, et al: Prevalence of HIV infection in the United States, 1984–1992. JAMA 276:126, 1996.
2. Karon JM, Buehler JW, Byers RH, et al: Projections of the number of persons diagnosed with AIDS and the number of immunosuppressed HIV-infected persons—United States, 1992–1994. MMWR Morbid Mortal Wkly Rep 41:1, 1992.
3. World Health Organization: AIDS, the current global situation of the HIV/AIDS pandemic. Wkly Epidemiol Rec 68:193, 1993.
4. World Health Organization: The HIV/AIDS Pandemic. 1993 Overview. Geneva, World Health Organization, 1993.
5. Northfelt DW, Hayward RA, Shapiro MF: The acquired immunodeficiency syndrome is a primary care disease. Ann Intern Med 109:773, 1988.
6. Centers for Disease Control: Revision of the CDC surveillance case definition for acquired immunodeficiency syndrome. MMWR Morbid Mortal Wkly Rep 36(Suppl 1):1S, 1987.
7. World Health Organization: Interim proposal for a WHO staging system for HIV infection and diseases. Wkly Epidemiol Rec 65:221, 1990.
8. Redfield RR, Wright DC, Tramont EC: The Walter Reed staging classification for HTLV-III/LAV infection. N Engl J Med 314:131, 1986.
9. Centers for Disease Control and Prevention: 1993 revised classification system for HIV infection and expanded surveillance case definition for AIDS among adolescents and adults. MMWR Morbid Mortal Wkly Rep 41(RR-17):1, 1992.
10. Cooper DA, Gold J, MacLean P, et al: Acute AIDS retrovirus infection. Definition of a clinical illness associated with seroconversion. Lancet 2:1376, 1984.
11. Daar ES, Mougdil T, Meyer RD, et al: Transient high level of viremia in patients with primary human immunodeficiency virus type 1 infection. N Engl J Med 324:961, 1991.
12. Kessler HA, Blauw B, Spear J, et al: Diagnosis of human immunodeficiency virus infection in seronegative homosexuals who present with an acute viral syndrome. JAMA 258:1196, 1987.
13. Niu MT, Stein DS, Schnittman SM: Primary human immunodeficiency virus type 1 infection: Review of pathogenesis and early treatment interventions in humans and animal retrovirus infections. J Infect Dis 168:1490, 1993.
14. Niu MT, Jermano JA, Reichelderfer P, et al: Summary of the National Institutes of Health workshop on primary human immunodeficiency virus type 1 infection. AIDS Res Hum Retroviruses 9:913, 1993.
15. Schacker T, Collier AC, Hughes J, et al: Clinical and epidemiologic features of primary HIV infection. Ann Intern Med 125:257, 1996.
16. Rustin MHA, Ridely CM, Smith MD, et al: The acute exanthem associated with seroconversion to human T-cell lymphotropic virus III in a homosexual man. J Infect Dis 12:161, 1986.
17. Denning DW, Anderson J, Rudge P, et al: Acute myelopathy associated with primary infection with human immunodeficiency virus. Br Med J 294:143, 1987.
18. Zaunders J, Carr A, McNally L, et al: Effect of primary HIV-1 infection on subsets of $CD4^+$ and $CD8^+$ T lymphocytes. AIDS 9:561, 1995.
19. Kinloch-DeLoes S, Hirschel BJ, Hoen B, et al: A controlled trial of zidovudine in primary human immunodeficiency virus infection. N Engl J Med 333:408, 1995.
20. Metroka CE, Cunningham-Rundles S, Pollack MS, et al: Persistent generalized lymphadenopathy in homosexual men. Ann Intern Med 99:585, 1983.
21. Klein RS, Harris CA, Small CB, et al: Oral candidiasis in high-risk patients as the initial manifestation of the acquired immunodeficiency syndrome. N Engl J Med 31:354, 1984.
22. Greenspan D, Greenspan JS, Hearst NG, et al: Relation of oral hairy leukoplakia to infection with the human immunodeficiency virus and the risk of developing AIDS. J Infect Dis 155:475, 1987.
23. Buchbinder SP, Katz MH, Hessol NA, et al: Herpes zoster and human immunodeficiency virus infection. J Infect Dis 166:1153, 1992.
24. Rowland RW, Escobar MR, Friedman RB, et al: Painful gingivitis may be an early sign of infection with the human immunodeficiency virus. Clin Infect Dis 16:233, 1993.
25. Feigal DW, Katz MH, Greenspan D, et al: The prevalence of oral lesions in HIV-infected homosexual and bisexual men: Three San Francisco epidemiological cohorts. AIDS 5:519, 1991.
26. Greenspan D, Greenspan JS: Oral manifestations of human immunodeficiency virus infection. Dent Clin North Am 37:21, 1993.
27. Saah AJ, Munoz A, Kuo V, et al: Predictors of the risk of development of acquired immunodeficiency syndrome within 24 months among gay men seropositive for human immunodeficiency virus type 1: A report from the Multicenter AIDS Cohort Study. Am J Epidemiol 135:1147, 1992.
28. Schafer A, Friedmann W, Mielke M, et al: The increased frequency of cervical dysplasia-neoplasia in women infected with the human immunodeficiency virus is related to the degree of immunosuppression. Am J Obstet Gynecol 164:593, 1991.
29. Kovacs JA, Hiemenz JW, Macher AM, et al: *Pneumocystis carinii* pneumonia: A comparison between patients with the acquired immunodeficiency syndrome and patients with other immunodeficiencies. Ann Intern Med 100:663, 1984.
30. Kalb RE, Grossman ME: Chronic perianal herpes simplex in immunocompromised hosts. Am J Med 80:486, 1986.
31. Kovacs JA, Kovacs AA, Polis M, et al: Cryptococcosis in the acquired immunodeficiency syndrome. Ann Intern Med 103:533, 1985.
32. Hawkins CC, Gold JWM, Whimbey E, et al: *Mycobacterium avium* complex infections in patients with the acquired immunodeficiency syndrome. Ann Intern Med 105:184, 1986.
33. DeHovitz JA, Pape JW, Boncy M, Johnson WD Jr: Clinical manifestations and therapy of *Isospora belli* infection in patients with acquired immunodeficiency syndrome. N Engl J Med 315:87, 1986.
34. Chaisson RE, Moore RD, Richman DD, et al: Incidence and natural history of *Mycobacterium avium*-complex infections in patients with advanced HIV disease treated with zidovudine. Am Rev Respir Dis 146:285, 1992.
35. Daley CL, Small PM, Schecter GF, et al: An outbreak of tuberculosis with accelerated progression among persons infected with the human immunodeficiency virus—An analysis using restriction-fragment length polymorphisms. N Engl J Med 326:231, 1992.
36. Edlin BR, Tokars JI, Grieco MH, et al: An outbreak of multidrug-resistant tuberculosis among hospitalized patients with the acquired immunodeficiency syndrome. N Engl J Med 326:1514, 1992.
37. NIH Conference: Gastrointestinal infections in AIDS. Ann Intern Med 116:63, 1992.
38. Grohmann GS, Glass RI, Pereira HG, et al: Enteric viruses and diarrhea in HIV-infected patients. N Engl J Med 329:14, 1993.
39. Hook EW, Marra CM: Acquired syphilis in adults. N Engl J Med 326:1060, 1992.
40. Ilortholary O, Meyohas MC, Dupont B, et al: Invasive aspergillosis in patients with acquired immunodeficiency syndrome: Report of 33 cases. Am J Med 95:177, 1993.
41. Janoof EN, Breiman RF, Daley CL, et al: Pneumococcal disease during HIV infection. Ann Intern Med 117:314, 1992.
42. Koehler JE, Quinn FD, Berger TG, et al: Isolation of *Rochalimaea* species from cutaneous and osseous lesions of bacillary angiomatosis. N Engl J Med 327:1625, 1992.
43. Luft BJ, Hafner R, Korzun AH, et al: Toxoplasmic encephalitis in patients with the acquired immunodeficiency syndrome. N Engl J Med 329:995, 1993.
44. McCutchan JA: Cytomegalovirus infections of the nervous system in patients with AIDS. Clin Infect Dis 20:747, 1995.

45. Porter SB, Sande MA: Toxoplasmosis of the central nervous system in acquired immunodeficiency syndrome. N Engl J Med 327:1643, 1992.
46. Reynolds P, Saunders LD, Layefsky ME, Lemp GF: The spectrum of acquired immunodeficiency syndrome (AIDS)–associated malignancies in San Francisco, 1980–1987. Am J Epidemiol 137:19, 1993.
47. Goedert JJ, Biggar RJ, Weiss SH, et al: Three year incidence of AIDS in five cohorts of HTLV-III–infected risk group members. Science 231:992, 1986.
48. Jaffe HW, Darrow WW, Echenberg DF, et al: The acquired immunodeficiency syndrome in a cohort of homosexual men: A six year follow-up study. Ann Intern Med 103:210, 1985.
49. Melbye M, Biggar JR, Ebbesen P, et al: Long-term HTLV-VIII seropositive homosexual men without AIDS develop measurable immunologic and clinical abnormalities: A longitudinal study. Ann Intern Med 104:496, 1986.
50. Moss AR, Bacchetti P, Osmond D, et al: Seropositivity for HIV and the development of AIDS or ARC. Three year follow-up of the San Francisco General Hospital cohort. Br Med J 296:745, 1988.
51. Goedert JJ, Kessler CM, Aledort LM, et al: A prospective study of human immunodeficiency virus type 1 infection and the development of AIDS in subjects with hemophilia. N Engl J Med 321:1141, 1989.
52. O'Brien TR, Blattner WA, Waters P, et al: Serum HIV-1 RNA levels and time to development of AIDS in the Multicenter Hemophilia Cohort Study. JAMA 276:105, 1996.
53. Samson M, Libert F, Doranz BJ, et al: Resistance to HIV-1 infection in caucasian individuals bearing mutant alleles of the CCR-5 chemokine receptor gene. Nature 382:722, 1996.
54. Cao Y, Qin L, Zhang L, et al: Virologic and immunologic characterization of long-term survivors of human immunodeficiency virus type 1 infection. N Engl J Med 332:201, 1995.
55. Graham NM, Zeger SL, Park LP, et al: The effects on survival of early treatment of human immunodeficiency virus infection. N Engl J Med 326:1037, 1992.
56. Katzenstein D, Hammer S, Hughes M, et al: The relation of virologic and immunologic markers to clinical outcomes after nucleoside therapy in HIV infected adults with 200 to 500 CD4 cells. N Engl J Med 335:1091, 1996.
57. Mellors JW, Rinaldo CR Jr, Gupta P, et al: Prognosis of HIV infection predicted by the quantity of virus in plasma. Science 272:1167, 1996.
58. Lemp GF, Payne SF, Temelso DN, et al: Survival trends for patients with AIDS. JAMA 263:402, 1990.
59. Munoz A, Vlahov D, Solomon L, et al: Prognostic indicators for development of AIDS among intravenous drug users. J Acquir Immune Defic Syndr 5:694, 1992.
60. Mellors JW, Kingsley LA, Rinaldo CR Jr, et al: Quantitation of HIV-1 RNA in plasma predicts outcome after seroconversion. Ann Intern Med 122:573, 1995.
61. Pantaleo G, Menzo S, Vaccarezza M, et al: Studies in subjects with long-term nonprogressive human immunodeficiency virus infection. N Engl J Med 332:209, 1995.
62. Stricof RL, Morse DL: HTLV-III/LAV seroconversion following a deep intramuscular needlestick injury. N Engl J Med 314:1115, 1986.
63. Stein DS, Korvick JA, Vermund SH: CD4+ lymphocyte cell enumeration for prediction of clinical course of human immunodeficiency virus disease: A review. J Infect Dis 165:352, 1992.
64. Goudsmit J, De Wolf F, Paul DA, et al: Expression of human immunodeficiency virus antigen (HIV-Ag) in serum and cerebrospinal fluid during acute and chronic infection. Lancet 2:177, 1986.
65. Cooper DA, Tindall B, Wilson E, et al: Characterization of T-lymphocyte responses during primary HIV infection. J Infect Dis 157:889, 1988.
66. Allain J-P, Laurian Y, Paul DA, et al: Serological markers in early stage of human immunodeficiency virus infection in hemophiliacs. Lancet 2:1233, 1986.
67. Gaines H, Sonnerborg A, Czaijkowski J, et al: Antibody response in primary human immunodeficiency virus infection. Lancet 1:1249, 1987.
68. Ranki A, Valle S-L, Krohn M, et al: Long latency period precedes overt seroconversion in sexually transmitted human immunodeficiency virus infection. Lancet 2:589, 1987.
69. Centers for Disease Control and Prevention: Persistent lack of detectable HIV-1 antibody in a person with HIV infection—Utah, 1995. MMWR Morbid Mortal Wkly Rep 45:181, 1996.
70. Lifson AR, Hessol NA, Rutherford GW: Progression and clinical outcome of infection due to human immunodeficiency virus. Clin Infect Dis 14:966, 1992.
71. Carne CA, Weller IVD, Loveday C, Adler MW: From persistent generalised lymphadenopathy to AIDS: Who will progress? Br Med J 294:868, 1987.
72. Hoover DR, Saah AJ, Bacellar H: Clinical manifestations of AIDS in the era of pneumocystis prophylaxis. N Engl J Med 329:1922, 1993.
73. Enger C, Graham M, Peng Y, et al: Survival from early, intermediate, and late stages of HIV infection. JAMA 275:1329, 1996.
74. Kaplan JE, Masur H, Holmes KK, et al: PHS/IDSA guidelines for the prevention of opportunistic infections in persons infected with human immunodeficiency virus: Introduction. Clin Infect Dis 21(Suppl 1):S1, 1995.
75. MacDonnell KB, Chmiel JS, Goldsmith J, et al: Prognostic usefulness of the Walter Reed staging classification for HIV infection. J Acquir Immune Defic Syndr 1:367, 1988.
76. Hammer S, Katzenstein D, Hughes M, et al: A trial comparing nucleoside monotherapy with combination therapy in HIV infected adults with CD4 counts from 200 to 500 per cubic millimeter. AIDS Clinical Trial Group Study Team. N Engl J Med 335:1081, 1996.
77. Gallant JE, Moore RD, Chaisson RE: Prophylaxis for opportunistic infections in patients with HIV infection. Ann Intern Med 120:932, 1994.
78. Montaner JSG, Schechter MT, Rachlis A, et al: Didanosine compared with continued zidovudine therapy for HIV-infected patients with 200 to 500 CD4 cells/mm^3. Ann Intern Med 123:561, 1995.
79. Bryson YJ, Pang S, Wei LS, et al: Clearance of HIV infection in a perinatally infected infant. N Engl J Med 332:833, 1995.
80. Powderly WG, Finkelstein DM, Feinberg J, et al: A randomized trial comparing fluconazole with clotrimazole troches for the prevention of fungal infections in patients with advanced human immunodeficiency virus infection. N Engl J Med 332:700, 1995.
81. Melbye M, Grossman RJ, Goedert JJ, et al: Risk of AIDS after herpes zoster. Lancet 1:728, 1987.
82. Masur H, Ognibene FP, Yarchoan R, et al: CD4 counts as predictors of opportunistic pneumonias in human immunodeficiency virus infected individuals. Ann Intern Med 111:223, 1989.
83. Taylor JMB, Fahey JL, Detels R, Giorgi JV: CD4 percentage, CD4 number, and CD4:CD8 ratio in HIV infection: Which to choose and how to use. J Acquir Immune Defic Syndr 2:114, 1989.
84. Hanson DL, Chu SY, Farizo KM, et al: Distribution of CD4+ T lymphocytes at diagnosis of acquired immunodeficiency syndrome–defining and other human immunodeficiency virus–related illnesses. Arch Intern Med 155:1537, 1995.
85. Donovan RM, Bush CE, Smereck SM, et al: Rapid decrease in unintegrated human immunodeficiency virus DNA after the initiation of nucleoside therapy. J Infect Dis 170:202, 1994.
86. Fiscus SA, DeGruttola V, Gupta P, et al: Human immunodeficiency virus type 1 quantitative cell microculture as a measure of antiviral efficacy in a multicenter clinical trial. J Infect Dis 171:305, 1995.
87. Graham NMH, Park LP, Piantadosi S, et al: Prognostic value of combined response markers among human immunodeficiency virus–infected persons: Possible aid in the decision to change zidovudine monotherapy. Clin Infect Dis 20:352, 1995.
88. Kovacs JA, Vogel S, Albert J, et al: Sustained increases in CD4 counts in HIV-infected patients treated with interleukin-2 during a randomized, controlled trial. N Engl J Med 335:1350, 1996.
89. Pan LZ, Cheng-Mayer C, Levy JA: Patterns of antibody response in individuals infected with the human immunodeficiency virus. J Infect Dis 155:626, 1987.
90. Goudsmit J, Lange JMA, Paul DA, Dawson GJ: Antigenemia and antibody titers to core and envelope antigens in AIDS, AIDS-related complex and subclinical human immunodeficiency virus infection. J Infect Dis 155:558, 1987.
91. Mayer KH, Falk LA, Paul DA, et al: Correlation of enzyme-linked immunosorbent assays for serum human immunodefi-

ciency virus antigen and antibodies to recombinant viral proteins with subsequent clinical outcomes in a cohort of asymptomatic homosexual men. Am J Med 83:208, 1987.

92. Weber JN, Clapham PR, Weiss RA, et al: Human immunodeficiency virus infection in two cohorts of homosexual men: Neutralising sera and association of anti-gag antibody with prognosis. Lancet 1:119, 1987.
93. Schupbach J, Haller O, Vogt M, et al: Antibodies to HTLV-III in Swiss patients with AIDS and pre-AIDS and in groups at risk for AIDS. N Engl J Med 312:265, 1985.
94. Ho DD, Moudgil T, Alam M: Quantitation of human immunodeficiency virus type 1 in the blood of infected persons. N Engl J Med 321:1621, 1989.
95. Coombs RW, Collier AC, Allain J-P, et al: Plasma viremia in human immunodeficiency virus infection. N Engl J Med 321:1626, 1989.
96. D'Aquila RT, Johnson VA, Welles SL, et al: Zidovudine resistance and HIV-1 disease progression during antiretroviral therapy. Ann Intern Med 122:401, 1995.
97. Drotman DD: Earlier diagnoses of human immunodeficiency virus (HIV) infection and more counseling. Ann Intern Med 110:680, 1989.
98. Fischl MA, Richman DD, Grieco MH, et al: The efficacy of azidothymidine (AZT) in the treatment of patients with AIDS and AIDS-related complex. N Engl J Med 317:185, 1987.
99. Fischl M, Richman DD, Causey AM, et al: Prolonged zidovudine therapy in patients with AIDS and advanced AIDS related complex. JAMA 262:2405, 1989.
100. Fischl MA, Parker CB, Pettinelli C, et al: A randomized controlled trial of a reduced daily dose of zidovudine in patients with the acquired immunodeficiency syndrome. N Engl J Med 323:1009, 1990.
101. Fischl MA, Richman DD, Hansen N, et al: The safety and efficacy of zidovudine (AZT) in the treatment of subjects with mildly symptomatic human immunodeficiency virus type 1 (HIV) infection—A double-blind placebo controlled trial. Ann Intern Med 112:727, 1990.
102. Volberding PA, Lagakos SW, Koch MA, et al: Zidovudine in asymptomatic human immunodeficiency virus infection—A controlled trial in persons with fewer than 500 CD4-positive cells per cubic millimeter. N Engl J Med 322:941, 1990.
103. Crowe SM, Carlin JB, Stewart KI, et al: Predictive value of CD4 lymphocyte numbers for the development of opportunistic infections and malignancies in HIV-infected persons. J Acquir Immune Defic Syndr 4:770, 1991.
104. Larder BA, Kemp SD, Harrigan R: Potential mechanism for sustained antiretroviral efficacy of AZT-3TC combination therapy. Science 269:696, 1995.
105. Pierce M, Crampton S, Henry D, et al: The effect of MAC and its prevention on survival in patients with advanced HIV infection. Presented at the 35th Annual Interscience Conference on Antimicrobial Agents and Chemotherapy Meeting; September 17–20, 1995; San Francisco; LB-18.
106. Collier AC, Coombs RW, Schoenfeld DA, et al: Treatment for human immunodeficiency virus infection with saquinavir, zidovudine, and zalcitabine. N Engl J Med 334:1011, 1996.
107. Massari F, Staszewski S, Berry P, et al: A double blind, randomized trial of indinavir (MK-639) alone or with zidovudine vs. zidovudine alone in zidovudine naive patients. Presented at the 35th Annual ICAAC Meeting; September 17–20, 1995; San Francisco; LB-6.
108. Phair J, Munoz A, Detels R, et al: The risk of *Pneumocystis carinii* among men infected with human immunodeficiency virus type 1. N Engl J Med 322:161, 1990.
109. O'Brien WA, Grovit-Ferbas K, Namazi A, et al: Human immunodeficiency virus–type 1 replication can be increased in peripheral blood seropositive patients after influenza vaccination. Blood 86:1082, 1995.
110. Centers for Disease Control and Prevention: Recommendations on prophylaxis and therapy for disseminated *Mycobacterium avium* complex for adults and adolescents infected with human immunodeficiency virus. MMWR Morb Mortal Wkly Rep 42(RR-9):14, 1993.
111. U.S. Public Health Service Task Force on Antipneumocystis Prophylaxis in Patients with Human Immunodeficiency Virus Infection: Recommendations for prophylaxis against *Pneumocystis carinii* pneumonia for persons infected with human immunodeficiency virus. J Acquir Immune Defic Syndr 6:46, 1993.
112. USPHS/IDSA Prevention of Opportunistic Infections Working Group: USPHS/IDSA guidelines for the prevention of opportunistic infections in persons infected with human immunodeficiency virus: A summary. MMWR Morb Mortal Wkly Rep 44(RR-8):1, 1995.
113. Bozzette SA, Finkelstein DM, Spector SA, et al: A randomized trial of three antipneumocystis agents in patients with advanced human immunodeficiency virus infection. N Engl J Med 332:693, 1995.
114. Masur H: Drug therapy: Prevention and treatment of *Pneumocystis* pneumonia. N Engl J Med 327:1853, 1992.
114a. Carpenter CCJ, Fischl MA, Hammer SM, et al: Antiretroviral therapy for HIV infection in 1996. Recommendations of an international panel. JAMA 276:146, 1996.
114b. Saag MS, Holodniy M, Kuritzkes DR, et al: HIV viral load markers in clinical practice. Nature Med 2:625, 1996.
114c. Markowitz M, Saag M, Powderly WG, et al: A preliminary study of ritonavir, an inhibitor of HIV-1 protease, to treat HIV-1 infection. N Engl J Med 333:1534, 1995.
115. Piscitelli SC, Flexner C, Minor JR, et al: Drug interactions in patients infected with human immunodeficiency virus. Clin Infect Dis 23:685, 1996.
115a. Tsolaki AG, Miller RF, Underwood AO, et al: Genetic diversity at the internal transcribed spacer region of the rRNA operon among isolates of *Pneumocystis carinii* from AIDS patients with recurrent pneumonia. J Infect Dis 174:141, 1996.
116. Centers for Disease Control and Prevention: 1995 revised guidelines for prophylaxis against *Pneumocystis carinii* pneumonia for children infected with or perinatally exposed to human immunodeficiency virus. MMWR Morb Mortal Wkly Rep 44(RR-4):1, 1995.
117. Osmond D, Charlebois E, Long W, et al: Changes in AIDS survival time in two San Francisco cohorts of homosexual men 1983–1993. JAMA 271:1083, 1994.
118. Lundgren JD, Barton SE, Katlama C, et al: *Pneumocystis carinii* pneumonia in European patients with AIDS. Multicenter Study Group on AIDS in Europe. Arch Intern Med 155:822, 1995.
119. Rutherford GW, Lifson AR, Hessol NA, et al: Course of HIV-1 infection in a cohort of homosexual and bisexual men: An 11 year follow-up study. Br Med J 301:1183, 1990.
120. Saah AJ, Hoover DR, He Y, et al: Factors influencing survival after AIDS: Report from the Multicenter AIDS Cohort Study (MACS). J Acquir Immune Defic Syndr 7:287, 1994.
121. Chaisson RE, Keruly J, Richman DD, Moore RD: *Pneumocystis* prophylaxis and survival in patients with advanced HIV infection treated with zidovudine. Arch Intern Med 152:2009, 1992.
122. Podzamczer D, Salazar A, Jimenez J, et al: Intermittent trimethoprim-sulfamethoxazole compared with dapsone-pyrimethamine for the simultaneous primary prophylaxis of *Pneumocystis* pneumonia and toxoplasmosis in patients infected with HIV. Ann Intern Med 122:755, 1995.
123. Schneider MME, Hoepelman AIM, Schattenkerk JKME, et al: A controlled trial of aerosolized pentamidine or trimethoprim-sulfamethoxazole as primary prophylaxis against *Pneumocystis carinii* pneumonia in patients with human immunodeficiency virus infection. N Engl J Med 327:1836, 1992.
124. Hardy WD, Feinberg J, Finkelstein DM, et al: A controlled trial of trimethoprim-sulfamethoxazole or aerosolized pentamidine for secondary prophylaxis of *Pneumocystis carinii* pneumonia in patients with acquired immunodeficiency syndrome. N Engl J Med 327:1842, 1992.
125. Girard PM, Landman R, Gaudebout C, et al: Dapsone-pyrimethamine compared with aerosolized pentamidine as primary prophylaxis against *Pneumocystis carinii* pneumonia and toxoplasmosis in HIV infection. N Engl J Med 328:1514, 1993.
126. Opravil M, Hirschel B, Lazzarin A, et al: Once-weekly administration of dapsone/pyrimethamine vs. aerosolized pentamidine as combined prophylaxis for *Pneumocystis carinii* pneumonia and toxoplasmic encephalitis in human immunodeficiency virus–infected patients. Clin Infect Dis 20:531, 1995.
127. Barnes PR, Bloch AB, Davidson PT, Snider DE Jr: Tuberculosis in patients with human immunodeficiency virus infection. N Engl J Med 324:1644, 1991.
128. Hopewell PC: Impact of human immunodeficiency virus infec-

tion on the epidemiology, clinical features, management, and control of tuberculosis. Clin Infect Dis 15:540, 1992.
129. American Thoracic Society, Centers for Disease Control and Prevention: Treatment of tuberculosis and tuberculosis infection in adults and children. Am J Respir Crit Care Med 149:1359, 1994.
130. Centers for Disease Control: Purified protein derivative (PPD)–tuberculin anergy and HIV infection: Guidelines for anergy testing and management of anergic persons at risk of tuberculosis. MMWR Morb Mortal Wkly Rep 40(RR-5):27, 1991.
131. Centers for Disease Control and Prevention: Guidelines for preventing the transmission of *Mycobacterium tuberculosis* in health-care facilities, 1994. MMWR Morb Mortal Wkly Rep 43(RR-13):1, 1994.
132. Beck-Sague C, Dooley SW, Hutton MD, et al: Hospital outbreak of multidrug-resistant *Mycobacterium tuberculosis* infections: Factors in transmission to staff and HIV-infected patients. JAMA 268:1280, 1992.
133. Dooley SW, Villarino ME, Lawrence M, et al: Nosocomial transmission of tuberculosis in a hospital unit for HIV-infected patients. JAMA 267:2632, 1992.
134. Fischl MA, Daikos GL, Uttamchandani RB, et al: Clinical presentation and outcome of patients with HIV infection and tuberculosis caused by multiple-drug-resistant bacilli. Ann Intern Med 117:184, 1992.
135. Pearson ML, Jereb JA, Frieden TR, et al: Nosocomial transmission of multidrug-resistant *Mycobacterium tuberculosis:* A risk to patients and health care workers. Ann Intern Med 117:191, 1992.
136. Pape JE, Jean SS, Ho JL, et al: Effect of isoniazid prophylaxis on incidence of active tuberculosis and progression of HIV infection. Lancet 342:268, 1993.
136a. Stanley SK, Ostrowski MA, Justement JS, et al: Effect of immunization with a common recall antigen on viral expression in patients infected with human immunodeficiency virus type 1. N Engl J Med 334:1222, 1996.
137. Nightingale SD, Cameron DW, Gordin FM, et al: Two controlled trials of rifabutin prophylaxis against *Mycobacterium avium* complex infection in AIDS. N Engl J Med 329:828, 1993.
138. Havlir DV, Dube MP, Sattler FR, et al: Prophylaxis against disseminated *Mycobacterium avium* complex with weekly azithromycin, daily rifabutin, or both. N Engl J Med 335:392, 1996.
139. Pierce M, Crampton S, Henry D, et al: A randomized trial of clarithromycin as prophylaxis against disseminated *Mycobacterium avium* complex infection in patients with advanced acquired immunodeficiency syndrome. N Engl J Med 335:384, 1996.
140. Brosgart CL, Craig C, Hillman D, et al: A randomized, placebo-controlled trial of the safety and efficacy of oral ganciclovir for prophylaxis of CMV retinal and gastrointestinal mucosal disease in HIV-infected individuals with severe immunosuppression. Presented at the 35th Annual Interscience Conference on Antimicrobial Agents and Chemotherapy Meeting; September 17–20, 1995; San Francisco; LB-10.
141. Spector SA, McKinley GF, Lalezari JP, et al: Oral ganciclovir for the prevention of cytomegalovirus disease in persons with AIDS. N Engl J Med 334:1491, 1996.
142. Mallolas J, Zamora L, Gatell JM, et al: Primary prophylaxis for *Pneumocystis carinii* pneumonia: A randomized trial comparing cotrimoxazole, aerosolized pentamidine and dapsone plus pyrimethamine. AIDS 7:59, 1993.
143. Luft BJ, Remington JS: Toxoplasmic encephalitis in AIDS. Clin Infect Dis 15:211, 1992.
144. Luft BJ, Hafner R, Korzun AH, et al: Toxoplasmic encephalitis in patients with the acquired immunodeficiency syndrome. N Engl J Med 329:995, 1993.
145. Carr A, Tindall B, Brew BJ, et al: Low-dose trimethoprim-sulfamethoxazole prophylaxis for toxoplasmic encephalitis in patients with AIDS. Ann Intern Med 117:106, 1992.
146. Brenner M, Ognibene FP, Lack E, et al: Prognostic factors and life expentancy of patients with acquired immunodeficiency syndrome and *Pneumocystis carinii* pneumonia. Am Rev Respir Dis 136:1199, 1987.
147. Bozzette SA, Sattler FR, Chiu J, et al: A controlled trial of early adjunctive treatment with corticosteroids for *Pneumocystis carinii* pneumonia in the acquired immunodeficiency syndrome. California Collaborative Treatment Group. N Engl J Med 323:1451, 1990.
148. Montaner JS, Lawson LM, Levitt N, et al: Corticosteroids prevent early deterioration in patients with moderately severe *Pneumocystis carinii* pneumonia and the acquired immunodeficiency syndrome (AIDS). Ann Intern Med 113:14, 1990.
149. Consensus statement on the use of corticosteroids as adjunctive therapy for pneumocystis pneumonia in acquired immune deficiency syndrome. N Engl J Med 323:1500, 1990.
150. Goodgame RW: Gastrointestinal cytomegalovirus disease. Ann Intern Med 119:924, 1993.
151. Kovacs JA, Ng V, Masur H, et al: Diagnosis of *Pneumocystis carinii* pneumonia: Improved detection in sputum using monoclonal antibodies. N Engl J Med 318:589, 1987.
152. Chuck SL, Sande MA: Infections with *Cryptococcus neoformans* with acquired immunodeficiency syndrome. N Engl J Med 321:794, 1989.
153. Truffot-Pernot C, Lecoeur HF, Maury L, et al: Results of blood cultures for detection of mycobacteria in AIDS patients. Tubercle 70:187, 1989.
154. Yagupsky P, Menegus M: Cumulative positivity rates of multiple blood cultures for *Mycobacterium avium-intracellulare* and *Cryptococcus neoformans* in patients with the acquired immunodeficiency syndrome. Arch Pathol Lab Med 114:923, 1990.
155. Havlir D, Kemper CA, Deresinski SC: Reproducibility of lysis-centrifugation cultures for quantification of *Mycobacterium avium* complex bacteremia. J Clin Microbiol 31:1794, 1993.
156. Stone BL, Cohn DL, Kane SM, et al: Utility of paired blood cultures and smears in diagnosis of disseminated *Mycobacterium avium* complex infections in AIDS patients. J Clin Microbiol 32:841, 1994.
157. Masur H, Shelhamer J: Empiric outpatient management of HIV-related pneumonia: Economical or unwise? Ann Intern Med 124:451, 1996.
158. Oksenhendler E, Charreau I, Tournerie C, et al: *Toxoplasma gondii* infection in advanced HIV infection. AIDS 8:483, 1994.
159. Leport C, Raffi F, Matherson S, et al: Treatment of central nervous system toxoplasmosis with pyrimethamine/sulfadiazine combination in 35 patients with the acquired immunodeficiency syndrome. Efficacy of long-term continuous therapy. Am J Med 84:94, 1988.

121

International Epidemiology of the Human Immunodeficiency Virus

Thomas C. Quinn
Richard E. Chaisson

Historical Perspective

In 1981, the first cases of the acquired immunodeficiency syndrome (AIDS) were recognized in previously healthy homosexual men residing in the United States.[1–4] During the next few years, additional cases were recognized in members of other high-risk groups, including injecting drug users (IDUs), hemophiliacs, and recipients of blood transfusions.[5] By 1984 it was evident that AIDS was already widespread throughout North America, the Caribbean, and parts of Central Africa, Europe, and Oceania.[6–10] By the end of the decade, it was clear that AIDS had become pandemic. By 1995 more than 1 million cases of AIDS from 192 countries had been officially reported[11] (Fig. 121–1). Allowing for underdiagnosis, incomplete reporting, and reporting delays, the World Health Organization (WHO) estimated that more than 4.5 million AIDS cases in adults and children have occurred worldwide and more than 2.5 million adults, children, and infants have died with AIDS[12] (see Fig. 121–1). Consequently, in the period of 1 to 15 years, AIDS had become recognized as the leading cause of death in major cities in the United States, Europe, and sub-Saharan Africa.[13–17]

After the recognition that the human immunodeficiency virus type 1 (HIV-1) was the etiologic agent of AIDS in 1984,[18, 19] it became evident that the clinical syndrome of AIDS and its associated mortality represented only a small portion of the greater epidemic of HIV-1 infection. From selected seroprevalence studies and mathematic models based on the natural history of HIV infection,[20–22] the WHO estimated that 18.5 million persons were infected with HIV-1 by 1995[12] (Fig. 121–2). These persons, distributed throughout most countries of the world, particularly Africa, Asia, the Americas, and Europe, represent the human reservoir of HIV infection from which continued transmission to other persons occurs. With an associated mortality rate greater than 90%[23] and with the current lack of a vaccine or curative drug, it is clear from these estimates that the HIV epidemic will continue to escalate worldwide and to have an enormous impact on public health in the next several decades.

Evolution of the Epidemic

Temporally, the HIV pandemic has undergone four major phases of evolution during the past three decades.[24] These phases can be characterized as emergence, dissemination, escalation, and stabilization. Before AIDS was ever recognized, HIV emerged from remote rural areas, where it might have been endemic at low levels, and disseminated to more populated, urban areas.[25] This resulted in rapid spread among high-risk populations such as female sex workers and their clients in developing countries and among homosexual men in industrialized countries.[7, 26] This first phase of emergence was followed by a phase of dissemination in which the virus quickly spread to various regions of the world primarily through population migration.[27] Although rural-to-urban migration and international travel played an important role in dissemination, another factor associated with migration was the enormous social disruption that occurred during this period of urbanization, particularly in sub-Saharan Africa.[28] This social disorganization and cultural change directly influenced vulnerability to HIV. During the next phase of escalation, which occurred in the 1980s, transmission of HIV was further amplified among high-risk populations, including IDUs and heterosexual partners of infected individuals.[26, 29] This resulted in further spread of HIV from restricted high-risk populations and segments of the general population in some regions. This phase of escalation is most dramatically illustrated in the densely populated regions of Southeast Asia, where it has been estimated that 3 million cumulative HIV infections have occurred within the past 5 years.[30–32]

A fourth phase of the HIV pandemic became evident as HIV prevalence and reported AIDS cases appeared to stabilize, particularly in the developed regions of Australia, North America, and Western Europe.[12, 33] Although such changes might represent a positive development from a prevention perspective, they may also indicate a transition from epidemic HIV to endemic HIV infection.[33] Stabilization of HIV prevalence in the United States, moreover, indicates that the number of deaths resulting from AIDS now equals the number of new HIV infections.[34, 35] Stabilization may also mask disproportionate increases in particular modes of transmission such as an increase in heterosexually transmitted HIV or disproportionate increase in new HIV infections among

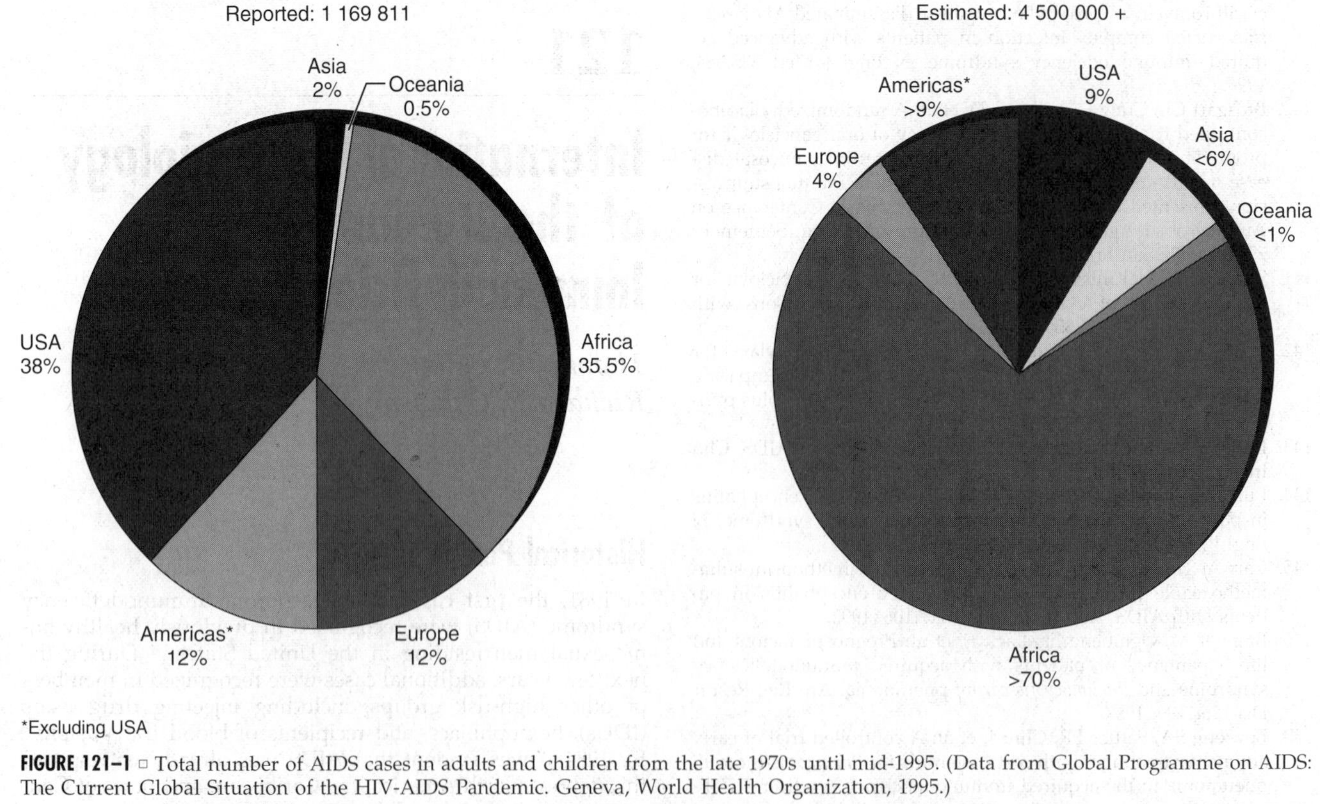

FIGURE 121–1 □ Total number of AIDS cases in adults and children from the late 1970s until mid-1995. (Data from Global Programme on AIDS: The Current Global Situation of the HIV-AIDS Pandemic. Geneva, World Health Organization, 1995.)

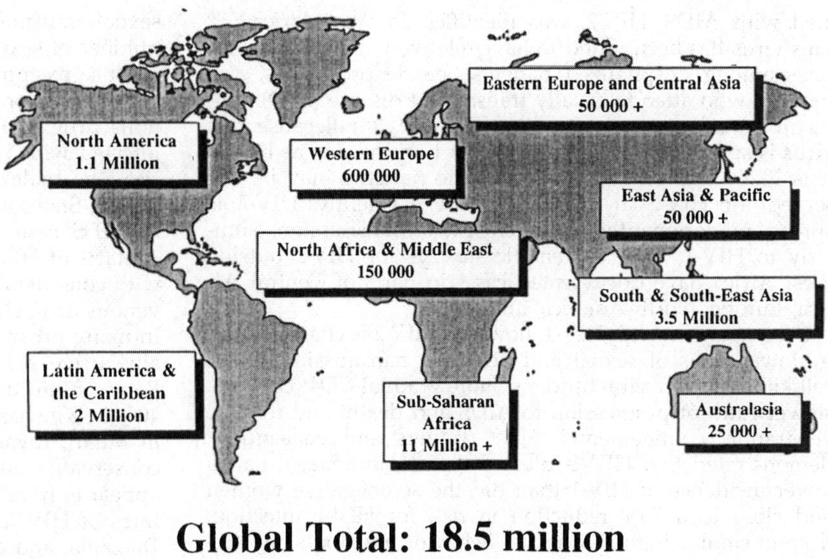

FIGURE 121–2 □ Estimated distribution of total adult HIV infections from late 1970s until mid-1995. (Data from Global Programme on AIDS: The Current Global Situation of the HIV-AIDS Pandemic. Geneva, World Health Organization, 1995.)

young people as evidenced in the United States and Europe.[12, 33, 36, 37] Stabilization of HIV prevalence and reported AIDS cases is simply one more facet of the evolving global nature of HIV infection. These trends of stabilization continue to occur in developed countries, and with escalation continuing in developing countries, it is evident that the major force of the epidemic will be in sub-Saharan Africa and Asia, where more than half of the world's population resides.[12, 32, 38]

The global pandemic of HIV infection consists of many different epidemics, each with its own dynamics, influenced by many factors such as the time of introduction, population density, and cultural and social factors that might increase vulnerability to HIV infection.[39] Figure 121–1 illustrates the incidence of HIV in various regions of the world. Even within some regions, the HIV epidemic consists of a multitude of smaller, ongoing epidemics, which, although related, pursue their own course with different velocities.[40] The spread of the epidemic has varied dramatically between the developed and developing countries, depending on the culture of the regions as well as many other social and behavioral patterns. Incidence rates have been highest in developing countries, where heterosexual transmission is most common, as in sub-Saharan Africa, the Caribbean, and Southeast Asia.[12, 27, 41] In addition to continued spread in already affected areas, HIV is spreading rapidly to communities and countries little affected during the 1980s. Nigeria, once considered an area of minimal HIV activity located between the West African and Central African epicenters, now estimates that it has at least 500,000 infected individuals.[12] Similarly, South Africa and Botswana estimate more than 500,000 and 100,000 HIV infections, respectively. In Southeast Asia, particularly India, Myanmar (Burma), and Thailand, the volatility of the pandemic is most dramatically seen.[38, 42] Because of the density of the population, there may be more HIV-infected individuals in the year 2000 in Southeast Asia than in any other regions of the world, including sub-Saharan Africa.[32, 38] With the continued escalation of HIV transmission in Asia and sub-Saharan Africa, it is estimated that nearly 90% of all HIV-infected people will reside in these developing countries by the year 2000.[12]

Molecular Epidemiology

The diversity of the global AIDS pandemic is also reflected in the heterogeneity of the viral subtypes, or clades, of HIV. On the basis of genetic sequence data, HIV-1 can be grouped into at least nine distinct genetic subtypes, A through H and subtype O.[43–45] In addition, there are at least five different subtypes of HIV-2, the predominant virus originally identified in West African countries.[46] A broad overview of the geographic distribution of HIV strains can be obtained from molecular epidemiologic studies, which can offer clues to how the virus spread between regions and continents.[47–49] Global diversity of HIV is most likely affected by the number of infected individuals and the overall rate of transmission. The pattern of global variation and distribution seems to have resulted from accidental trafficking (viral migration) than from diversification (viral mutation).[47] The uniform occurrence of the B subtype in the Americas and Europe represents a "founder" effect. Similarly, a subtype E virus recovered from Central Africa quickly emerged as the dominant form of the outbreak in female sex workers in Thailand and subtype B was found predominantly in IDUs in Thailand, providing evidence for two separate but concurrent epidemics.[50–52] Given the chance nature of HIV migrations, it is quite possible that one or more rare viral subtypes could be brought swiftly into ascendance: subtype F, a minor form in Brazil and Africa, has become a major form in Romania, and subtype G, found in Central Africa, appears to have been introduced into southern Russia.[53]

In some countries in Africa, which were either among the earliest centers of infection or had significant population migration and transmission, at least five viral subtypes are known to be present. Similarly, diversity is now being documented in India and in Brazil, where there is documentation of recombinants such as A-E and B-F.[47, 54–56] In some cases the degree of viral divergence within a given region may also reflect the duration of the epidemic. For example, in Africa there is already 20% to 30% genetic diversity within a genotype, whereas in Thailand this diversity is much more limited.[51] The immunologic importance of this genetic heterogeneity is not fully understood, but it is clear that any globally effective vaccine will have to induce protective immunity through a broad range of genetic and potentially antigenic subtypes. The low levels of genetic diversity seen in some regions of HIV-1 spread present rapidly closing windows of opportunity for vaccination against still relatively homologous viral challenge. The diversity in HIV subtypes may also have important biologic and immunologic implications. Intrinsic biologic properties of these viruses include infectivity and replication capacities that contribute to different epidemic curves.[50] In 1985 a second human retrovirus associated with AIDS, HIV-2, was identified in West Africa.[57, 58] This virus has been found to have relatively high prevalence rates among hospitalized patients, female prostitutes, and patients who attend sexually transmitted disease (STD) clinics in several countries of West Africa.[46, 59–61] Because this virus is spread by the same modes of transmission as HIV-1, it is likely that similar epidemiologic patterns may be observed for HIV-2 in the near future. Currently, HIV-2 is spread predominantly by heterosexual transmission, similarly to HIV-1.[46, 62, 63] Systematic surveys for HIV-2 outside West Africa have documented cases in parts of Central Africa, Europe, North America, and Brazil.

In comparison with HIV-1, however, HIV-2 is characterized by lower rates of sexual and perinatal transmission, lesser cell killing, lower viral burdens, more gradual $CD4^+$ cell loss, slower rates of progression to AIDS and death, and relative geographic confinement.[46, 62, 64–68] Travers and colleagues[69] demonstrated that HIV-2–infected women in Senegal had a lower incidence of HIV-1 than did the seronegative women and close to a 70% reduction in risk for HIV-1 infection, despite similar high-risk sexual behavior and the same frequency of STDs. These data suggested that the protection observed may be a result of cross-reactive immunity to epitopes conserved between HIV-1 and HIV-2. However, the study also demonstrated for the first time sequential infection with two different HIV subtypes, first with HIV-2 and then with HIV-1. Further studies are urgently needed to determine whether cross-reactive immunity can be induced to epitopes conserved between different strains of the virus.

Molecular techniques have also been utilized to investigate clusters of HIV infection. For example, in a Florida dental practice, molecular subtyping confirmed that a dentist's HIV-1 infection had been transmitted to several of his patients.[70–73] Although the study demonstrated that the patients were infected with the same HIV strain as the dentist, questions persist regarding how the infection occurred and whether new cases of this kind are likely to be encountered. Another case has been studied in southern Russia, where nearly 90 children became infected with the same strain.[53, 74] It is clear from this cluster and from a series in Australia in which four women were infected with a strain similar to one identified in a patient with AIDS that nosocomial transmission can and does occur, particularly with unsterilized instruments.[75]

With molecular typing it is possible to discern geographic differences in the proportion of cases acquired by one mode of transmission or another, but the three major modes of transmission, sexual, parenteral, and perinatal, still remain the major means of acquisition of either HIV-1 or HIV-2. Each of these modes of transmission is discussed in detail, with particular geographic references when appropriate.

Modes of Transmission

Sexual Transmission

Sexual transmission probably accounts for more than 80% of HIV-1 infection worldwide. In developed countries, homosexual transmission has been strongly associated with the number of sexual partners and the frequency at which they practice receptive anal intercourse.[76–78] As the prevalence of HIV-1 infection increased among bisexual men and intravenous drug abusers, an increasing number of women were infected with HIV-1 via heterosexual contact.[26, 33, 79–81] In Africa, the male/female ratio is 1:1.4,[7, 82, 83] and even in the United States and Europe the greatest proportional increase in AIDS cases has been documented among heterosexual contacts of HIV-1–infected persons.[26, 84, 85] Urban populations with consistently high rates of STDs, prostitution, and intravenous drug abuse have the highest rates of HIV-1 infection. In many urban centers of Central Africa, 5% to 20% of sexually active persons are already infected with HIV-1.[27, 83, 86] Rates of infection among some prostitute groups range from 40% in Kinshasa, Zaire, to 80% in Nairobi, Kenya, and 88% in Butari, Rwanda.[87–89] Rural areas that are culturally more conservative and where the incidence of STDs is much lower appear to have lower rates of HIV-1 infection, although rural rates of HIV infection are rising in some areas of Uganda, Tanzania, and other countries.[27] Certain risk factors, such as promiscuity, anal intercourse, sex with an infected person, prostitution, and other behavioral factors, appear to be responsible for increased risk of heterosexual transmission.

Although the relative efficiencies of bidirectional transmission have not been well documented, it is evident that most heterosexual transmission of HIV-1 among sexual partners occurs during vaginal intercourse and that receptive anal intercourse also increases the risk of infection for women (Table 121–1). Variable rates of heterosexual transmission of HIV-1 among sexual partners of infected persons have been documented in studies in the United States, Europe, and Africa.[36, 90] Reported rates of infection for sexual partners of an infected person range from 15% to 50% and are dependent on the presence or absence of other STDs, which may serve as cofactors for transmission, as well as on the relative infectivity of the infected individual. In studies by Goedert and coworkers,[91] the risk of transmission from one person to a sexual partner was greatest among those with $CD4^+$ cell counts of less than 200/mm^3 and those with p24 antigenemia.

An epidemiologic synergy has been demonstrated between HIV and STDs that is related to both behavioral and biologic factors[92] (Table 121–2). Epidemiologic studies from sub-Saharan Africa, Asia, Europe, and North America have suggested that there is approximately a fourfold greater risk of becoming HIV infected in the presence of a genital ulcer caused by syphilis and/or chancroid and a two- to threefold greater risk in the presence of other STDs such as gonorrhea, chlamydial infection, and trichomoniasis[92–97] (Fig. 121–3). In a WHO report the prevalence of four curable STDs, gonorrhea, chlamydial infection, syphilis, and trichomoniasis, was estimated to be 333 million individuals.[98] The greatest number of these STDs occur in Southeast Asia and sub-Saharan Africa, the two regions with the highest rates of HIV infection.[24]

With the strong association between STDs and HIV infection among heterosexuals, increased attention should be fo-

TABLE 121–1 ■ Geography and Human Immunodeficiency Virus Transmission Rates in 16 Serologic Studies of Heterosexual Couples

	NUMBER POSITIVE/TOTAL (%)*			
GEOGRAPHY	Female to Male	Male to Female	RELATIVE RISK†	*P* VALUE
United States	22/128 (17)	136/504 (27)	1.6	$P < .05$
Europe	57/427 (13)	308/1184 (26)	1.9	$P < .001$
Africa, Haiti	83/143 (58)	171/324 (53)	0.9	$P < .01$
Total	162/698 (23)	615/2012 (31)	1.3	$P < .01$

*Overall infection rate: 777/2710 (29%).
†Male-to-female versus female-to-male transmission rates.

TABLE 121–2 ■ Factors That Affect Infectiousness of or Susceptibility to Human Immunodeficiency Virus

INFECTIOUSNESS	SUSCEPTIBILITY
Acute primary HIV infection	Genital ulcerations
Advanced clinical stage of HIV	Other STDs
Genital ulcerations (chancroid, syphilis, herpes)	Lack of male circumcision
Cervical ectopy	Traumatic sex
Antiretroviral therapy (decreased infectiousness)	Lack of condom use
Consistent condom use (decreased infectiousness)	Anal intercourse
	Sex during menses

cused on integrated HIV-STD services.[99, 100] The development of programs with an integrated approach to inducing behavior change, promoting condom use, and controlling STDs would inevitably reduce the infectivity of HIV transmitters and the susceptibility of HIV-exposed persons. In Kinshasa, Zaire, investigators demonstrated that intensive STD diagnosis and treatment coupled with a condom distribution program for female sex workers successfully decreased both the incidence and the prevalence of both STDs and HIV.[99] In a national condom promotion campaign in Thailand, the prevalence of STDs declined nationwide with a subsequent decrease in HIV incidence[101] (Fig. 121–4). In another study, investigators demonstrated that a community-based syndromic approach to the treatment of symptomatic STDs led to a 42% decrease in HIV incidence compared with control villages in Mwanza, Tanzania.[102] In the Rakai district of Uganda, a community-based trial of mass treatment of STDs is being studied to determine whether a decline in the prevalence of STDs is also associated with a decline in HIV incidence.[103] Studies such as these are of particular importance because there is no clearly defined population of high-frequency transmitters, and in some regions the entire population is considered at risk.

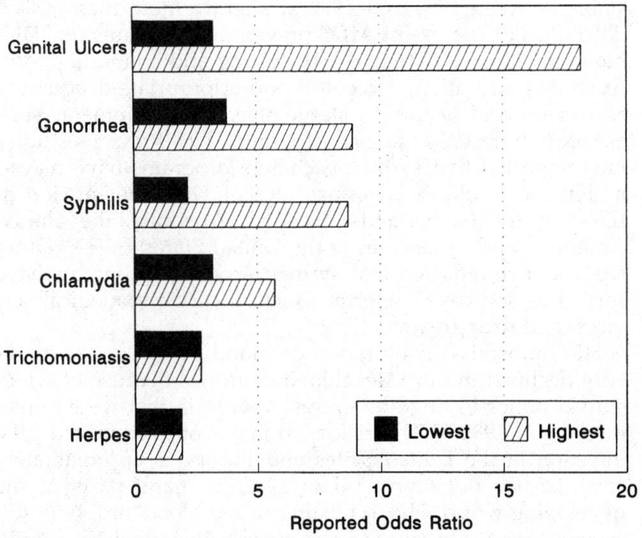

FIGURE 121–3 □ Relative risk of HIV infection by type of STD. Summary of risk estimates of STDs and HIV infection, drawn from prospective cross-sectional or case-controlled studies. All risks are expressed as odds ratios and indicate the highest and lowest reported risks of HIV infection in the presence of the STD compared with the risk for subjects without an STD. (Data from Wasserheit JN: Epidemiological synergy: Interrelationships between human immunodeficiency virus infection and other sexually transmitted diseases. Sex Transm Dis 19:61–77, 1992.)

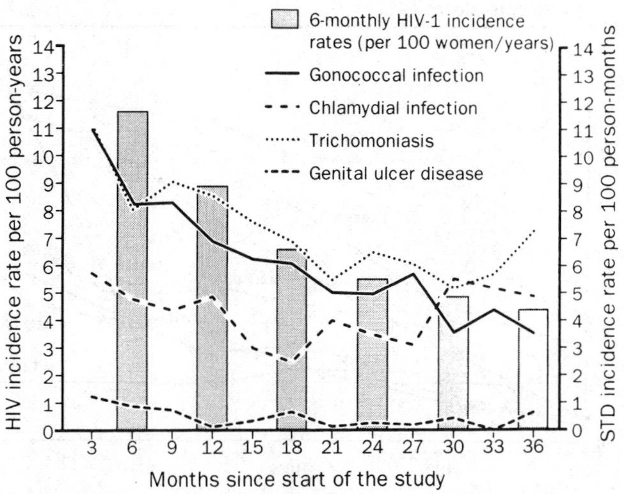

FIGURE 121–4 □ Time trends in incidence of HIV and other STDs among HIV-1–negative women followed up for a maximum of 36 months. (From Hanenberg RS, Rojanapithayakorn W, Kunasol P, Sokal DC: Impact of Thailand's HIV-control programme as indicated by the decline of sexually transmitted diseases. Lancet 344[8917]:243–245, 1994. © by The Lancet Ltd. 1994.)

Perinatal Transmission

With increasing evidence of HIV infection among women, perinatal transmission, which may occur in utero, during delivery, or postnatally via breast-feeding, continues to increase in areas where heterosexual transmission is most common (Fig. 121–5). Transmission rates have been highly variable in different regions, ranging from 13% to 52%[104, 105] (Table 121–3). Reanalysis of transmission on the basis of an international standard definition has shown that the rates of vertical transmission have much greater consistency within geographic areas than previously reported. Factors associated with increased perinatal transmission include advanced maternal stage of disease, increased viral titers, decreased maternal serum vitamin A levels, chorioamnionitis, maternal ane-

TABLE 121–3 ■ Presumptive Evidence of the Timing of Maternal-Infant Transmission of Human Immunodeficiency Virus

In utero
Identification of HIV in aborted fetal tissue from infected women
Presence of HIV in peripheral blood in about 50% of infected infants in the first week of life
Rapid progression of HIV disease in some infants
Peripartum
Higher transmission rates in first-born twins than in second-born twins
No detectable circulating virus in about 50% of infected infants in the first week of life
Decreased transmission with cesarean section
Lower transmission rates with administration of zidovudine to the mother in late pregnancy* and the peripartum period and to the infant in the neonatal period
Two distinct patterns of disease progression (rapid and less rapid) in infected infants
Absence of congenital malformations and symptoms and signs of HIV infection at birth

*In the AIDS Clinical Trial Group Protocol 076 trial, zidovudine therapy was started at a median of 26 wk of gestation.

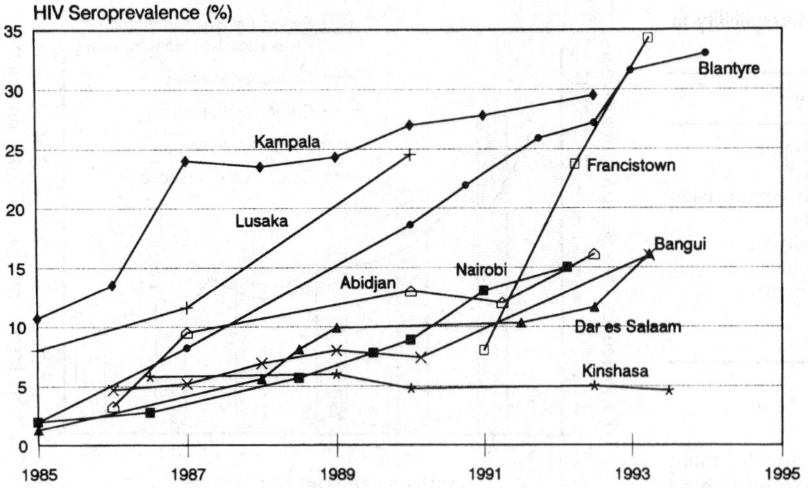

FIGURE 121–5 □ HIV seroprevalence for pregnant women in selected urban areas of Africa: 1985 to 1994. (Data from the U.S. Bureau of the Census: Trends and Patterns of HIV and AIDS Infection in Selected Developing Countries: Country Profiles: June 1994. Washington, DC, U.S. Bureau of the Census, 1994. Research Note 14.)

mia, low neutralizing titers to antibody, and titers to antibody to the V3 loop of glycoprotein gp120 of HIV[106–109] (see Table 121–3). The more common use of breast-feeding in developing countries may also contribute to increased perinatal transmission compared with that observed in developed countries. Data suggest that up to 15% of infants breast-fed by HIV-infected mothers may become infected through breast-feeding.[110] A metaanalysis of several prospective studies indicated that the risk attributable to breast-feeding ranged from 7% to 22%. Although bottle feeding is recommended for HIV-infected women in developed countries, this would not be appropriate in some countries with high rates of infectious diseases and poor sanitation.[111]

Strategies for reducing perinatally acquired HIV include preventing HIV infection among women in general and, for women infected with HIV, avoiding pregnancy or refraining from breast-feeding their infants[112] (Table 121–4). In addition, antiretroviral therapy with zidovudine has been shown to reduce significantly the risk for perinatal transmission from 25.5% to 8.3%, a 67.5% reduction.[113] In countries where zidovudine is available and affordable, these results have drawn attention to the importance of expanding prenatal HIV testing and of improving the care of infected women during pregnancy.[112] In countries where the cost is prohibitive, new trials are under way to examine modified timing and dosing of zidovudine for pregnant women to find the most cost-efficient method of reducing perinatal transmission. Other interventions being evaluated include passive immunization with hyperimmune sera to HIV, and a randomized trial of routine delivery versus cesarean section has been started in Europe.[114, 115] Interventions found to be successful, however, must be affordable and sustainable, particularly in developing countries, where the impact would be greatest.[116, 117]

TABLE 121–4 ■ Approaches to Reducing the Transmission of Human Immunodeficiency Virus from Mother to Child

Avoidance of breast-feeding
Antiretroviral therapy (for the mother during pregnancy and delivery and for the infant after birth)
Zidovudine
Other antiretroviral agents
Reduction in peripartum exposure
Cesarean section
Avoidance of intrapartum invasive procedures
Vaginal disinfection
Treatment of sexually transmitted diseases
Immunotherapy for the mother or infant (or both)
Passive therapy (monoclonal or polyclonal antibodies)
Active immunization

Parenteral Transmission

The third mode of infection is parenteral transmission, which includes blood transfusion and exposure to blood through reuse of needles or syringes among IDUs or in health care facilities where sterilization of instruments is inadequate. Transmission among IDUs is a major problem for developed countries and an increasing problem for countries such as those in Southeast Asia, Thailand, India, and Myanmar, as well as some countries of Latin America. Seroprevalence rates among IDUs vary widely but may be as high as 60% to 70% in some regions.[118] Although HIV incidence continues to rise among IDUs in some regions of the world, substantial HIV prevention programs targeting IDUs have resulted in stabilization of infection rates and in some cases a decline.[119] In a study in New York City, HIV seroprevalence remained stable between 1984 and 1992 at slightly more than 50%.[120] Attributes of successful AIDS prevention programs for IDUs have included confidential HIV testing and counseling, outreach and education, successful and appropriate drug abuse treatment, and access to sterile injecting equipment, such as through needle exchange programs.[121–125] Previous studies have reported that syringe exchange programs have played a significant role in lowering rates of HIV transmission in IDUs in the Netherlands, Sweden, Australia, the United Kingdom, and some cities of the United States.[122, 123, 126] Other studies have reported that syringe exchange programs have served as sources of referral to social services, medical services, and drug treatment.[119, 121–123, 126]

HIV transmission by blood or blood products has markedly declined in most developed countries because of widespread donor testing and exclusion criteria that were implemented in 1985.[127] The risk of transfusion-transmitted HIV infection in the United States and Europe is approximately 1 in 225,000 donations.[128] However, in many parts of the developing world, HIV screening of the blood supply is still severely limited because of cost factors. Nevertheless, a study in Zambia demonstrated in a cost-benefit analysis that screening of the blood supply cost three cents per person with a cost per case of HIV prevented calculated as $31.62.[129] An estimated 3625 undiscounted healthy years of life were saved, of which 69% were those of children younger than 6 years at a cost of $1.32 per year of life saved. In areas where universal screening of blood donations has not been implemented, progress toward a safer supply of blood and blood products can also be achieved through appropriate selection and retention of voluntary, nonremunerated, low-risk donors and through more rational use of blood aimed at decreasing the number of people receiving transfusions as well as using blood substitutes and plasma expanders whenever possible.

The risk of HIV transmission in a health care setting through accidental exposure to HIV-infected blood is estimated to be 0.3%, and the risk after mucocutaneous exposure is much less.[130, 131] However, the number of parenteral exposures of health care workers is thought to be considerable. In 1990, between 378,000 and 756,000 needlestick injuries were estimated to have occurred among health care workers in the United States. Of these, 1300 to 8300 probably involved patients known to be infected with HIV.[132] It is hoped that through the use of universal precautions, parenteral, mucous membrane, and nonintact skin exposure of health care workers to infectious blood has been limited.[131, 133, 134]

HIV transmission from an infected health care worker to a patient appears to be extremely rare. With the exception of the documented case of HIV transmission from an infected dentist to six patients, the probability of transmission from an HIV-infected surgeon to a patient is in the range of about 1 in 42,000 procedures to 1 in 20,000 procedures.[131, 135–137]

Other Modes of Transmission

Household transmission may occur when there is contact with blood or other body secretions or excretions from a person already known to be infected with HIV. Eight instances of HIV transmission in households through direct contact with blood or body secretions have now been reported.[138] Consequently, persons who provide nursing and care for HIV-infected persons in home settings should employ similar universal precautions to reduce exposure to blood and other body fluids. Because of the social, economic, and medical benefits of home care, the number of persons with HIV who receive health care outside hospitals is increasing.

Regional Epidemics

Sub-Saharan Africa

Although AIDS has had an enormous medical, cultural, and economic impact on all countries of the world, this disease has taken its greatest toll in the countries of sub-Saharan Africa. More than 12 million individuals—3% of the population of the subcontinent—have been infected with HIV.[12, 139, 140] More than half of these infected adults are women, and as many as 1 million African children are estimated to have been infected as a result of mother-to-infant transmission. In some geographic areas, specific population groups are disproportionately affected by the epidemic. Men and women between 20 and 40 years old, people with STDs, and people in certain occupational groups such as long-distance truck drivers, military personnel, and women employed in commercial sex usually have the highest prevalences of infection.[7, 27, 86] HIV prevalences higher than 80% have been reported for female sex workers in East Africa and Central Africa. In some areas, HIV infection has now been documented among members of the general population, as evidenced by the initially slow but accelerating spread among pregnant women. Seroprevalence of HIV among pregnant women ranges from 5% to 35%, with the highest rates in urban centers such as Blantyre, Kampala, Lusaka, Kinshasa, and Abidjan[104, 106, 141] (see Fig. 121–5). In some urban populations, more than 10% of the adults are infected and the annual incidence is estimated to be 3%.[142, 143]

Approximately 50% to 65% of HIV infections in Africa have been in East and Central Africa, an area that accounts for only 15% of the total population of sub-Saharan Africa. Serologic data indicate that the pandemic has continued to evolve, particularly in western and southern Africa.[12] In Nigeria, a country with more than 105 million inhabitants (20% of sub-Saharan Africa's population), HIV has been introduced and is rapidly spreading among female sex workers and their clients.[144, 145] Similarly, in southern Africa HIV prevalences of 20% to 30% have been documented among adults in major urban areas of Botswana.[12] South Africa witnessed a threefold increase in HIV prevalence between 1990 and 1992 in women attending antenatal clinics.[146]

AIDS has emerged as the leading cause of adult death in Abidjan, in Kinshasa, and in rural communities in Uganda and Tanzania.[13, 15, 16, 147] Excess deaths attributable to HIV are highest in 25- to 34-year-olds, usually a group with low mortality. Nearly 90% of deaths in this age group were in excess of background rates and were attributable to HIV. Because AIDS deaths are concentrated in childhood and young adult ages, their effects are substantial, reducing life expectancy by more than 20 years in several countries. Population growth will decline more rapidly than expected and the size of the African population in the year 2000 will be smaller than it would have been without AIDS. These additional HIV-AIDS cases will put an increasing strain on the health care systems, which are already overburdened, and on individual households, which are trying to manage with limited economic resources. Care and support for children orphaned by AIDS will be a growing concern throughout the region,[148] and the social, economic, and demographic impact of AIDS will be enormous. For a country with a current HIV prevalence of 8%, the expected increased demand for health care services ranges from 2.3% to 9.3% depending on the state of development of its health care sector.[139] The strong association of HIV with a burgeoning tuberculosis epidemic[149, 150] combined with the excess mortality associated with HIV infection underscores the critical importance of the HIV epidemic in Africa.

Asia

With more than half of the world's population, Asia is still in the early phases of an explosive HIV-AIDS epidemic. Although HIV was introduced much later in Asia than in the rest of the world, it is now estimated that more than 3.5 million people are infected with HIV.[12] Within the past year there has been an eightfold increase in the number of AIDS cases, from 30,000 to 250,000. By the year 2000 it is estimated that the HIV epidemic in Asia will surpass that already devastating sub-Saharan Africa. Furthermore, India will probably have the largest number of infected persons of any single country, with an estimated 5 million infected people.[30] With the population of India expected to reach 1 billion by the year 2000, the HIV epidemic has the potential to have a dramatic impact on that country. In addition to those in India, major HIV epidemics already exist in Thailand and Myanmar, and the epidemic has begun to emerge in Cambodia, Vietnam, Indonesia, China, Taiwan, Singapore, and the Philippines.[32, 38, 42]

The pattern of HIV spread in Asia appears to be different from that described in other regions. HIV was initially noted among IDUs in Thailand, Myanmar, and India. HIV seroprevalence increased dramatically between 1988 and 1991 from 1.2% to 45% in Thailand,[151–153] and in the northeastern state of Manipur, India, it rose from 55% to 80%.[30, 38, 154] In addition, the first evidence of HIV in Yunnan province of China, bordering Burma and Laos and considered part of the "golden triangle" of heroin exportation, demonstrated an alarming HIV prevalence of 43% to 82% in IDUs.[155, 156] Data from Malaysia and Vietnam show similar increases in HIV levels among IDUs.[12]

During this rise of HIV infection among IDUs, HIV infection was noted among female sex workers. Although highly variable by region, HIV prevalences of 30% to 65% have been reported among female sex workers in various cities of Thailand and India[30, 38, 41] (Fig. 121–6). Successive waves of heterosexual transmission from these sex workers to their male clients and subsequently to other sexual partners including spouses occurred, resulting in rapid spread of HIV to segments of the general population. Among military recruits in Thailand in 1993, HIV prevalence was 4% overall and 12.4% in recruits from the northern province of Chiang Mai.[157, 158] Among pregnant women, HIV prevalence rose to 8% in Chiang Mai and Chiang Rai in northern Thailand, and the overall prevalence for pregnant women in the country was estimated as 2%.[159] From these data, it was estimated that more than 840,000 persons in Thailand, or 1% of the Thai population, were HIV infected by 1994.[12] If this rate of HIV transmission continues, there will be 2 million to 4 million cumulative HIV infections in Thailand alone by the year 2000.

In urban centers in India, the rise in HIV seroprevalence among female sex workers and their sexual contacts has been equally dramatic (see Fig. 121–6). In a study of 2800 attendees of STD clinics in Pune, the overall HIV seroprevalence was 23.4%.[160] Among initially seronegative persons, the subsequent HIV incidence was 26.1 per 100 person-years of observation for female sex workers, 9.4 for men, and 8.4 for women who were not sex workers.[161] Recurrent genital ulcer disease and urethritis or cervicitis during the follow-up period were independently associated with an increased risk of seroconversion. Given the prevailing sexual practices, large population of HIV-infected female sex workers, low social status of women, male patronage of sex workers, high rates of STDs, low rates of condom use, and high frequency of IDU, a scenario similar to that described for India and Thailand is likely for many other populous countries of Asia.[32] For the more developed areas, such as Japan, South Korea, Taiwan, Singapore, and Hong Kong, HIV epidemics may not be as explosive, but there will probably be a slow and steady increase in HIV infections. Throughout Asia the HIV incidence could exceed 1 million new infections per year within the next few years.

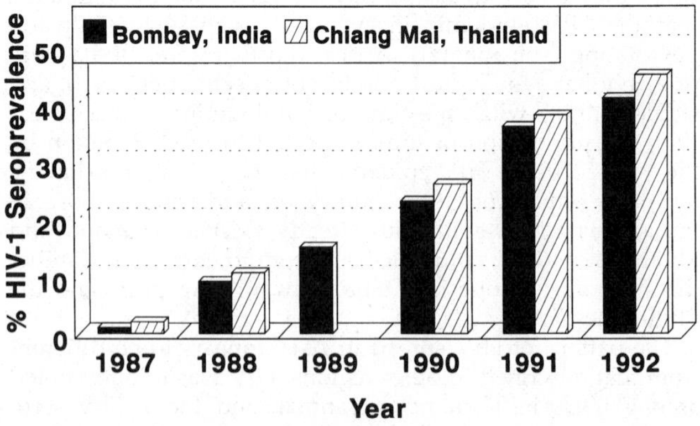

FIGURE 121–6 ▫ Seroprevalence rates for HIV infection among commercial sex workers in Thailand and India from 1986 through 1992. (Data from the U.S. Bureau of the Census: Trends and Patterns of HIV and AIDS Infection in Selected Developing Countries: Country Profiles: June 1994. Washington, DC, U.S. Bureau of the Census, 1994. Research Note 14.)

Oceania

Approximately 50,000 cumulative adult HIV infections have occurred in this region, with nearly half in Australia and New Zealand.[162] The annual reported number of HIV infections from these last two countries seems to have reached its peak, and since 1987 there has been a downward trend for both countries in the number of HIV infections reported each year. Most of the infections have occurred among homosexual men, and the male/female ratio among infected individuals is 7:1, indicating a lower degree of heterosexual transmission than that observed in other regions. The frequency of HIV infection among IDUs in Australia and New Zealand also remains lower than that in Western Europe or North America, probably because of the early availability of sterile injection equipment.

For most other countries of the Pacific region, the cumulative numbers of reported AIDS cases and HIV infections have been too few to allow meaningful analysis by time or mode of transmission. However, despite the low number of cases, there is a great potential for HIV to spread rapidly within this region. Epidemiologic and behavioral studies indicate generally high rates of injecting drug use, unprotected sexual activity including commercial sex, and a high prevalence of STDs. Moreover, many parts of Asia and the Pacific are undergoing rapid development. As trade, tourism, and migration increase, so may the opportunities for HIV dissemination.[162]

The Americas

Approximately 3 million cumulative HIV infections have occurred in the countries of the Americas, with more than 1 million in North America and 2 million in Latin America and the Caribbean.[12] Approximately 400,000 new HIV infections are estimated to occur each year, or 1000 new infections per day.[163]

The United States has had the highest number of reported AIDS cases in the world with more than 501,301 cases and 311,381 fatalities (62%) as of late 1995[33] (Fig. 121–7). During the early 1990s in the United States, HIV infection became the leading cause of death among men 25 to 44 years old and the fourth leading cause of death among women in the same age group, accounting for 19.9% and 7.3% of deaths, respectively[14] (Fig. 121–8). An evolving pattern in the epidemiology of HIV infection has become evident in the countries of the Americas. The AIDS surveillance case definition was substantially expanded in late 1987 and in 1993 to reflect increased knowledge of the natural history of HIV.[164, 165] Substantial differences in the distribution of cases were noted in 1995 compared with the early 1980s[33] (Fig. 121–9). For example, the proportion of cases among whites decreased from 60% to 43%, and the proportion among blacks and Hispanics increased from 25% to 38% and from 14% to 18%, respectively (Fig. 121–10*A*). The rates per 100,000 population for blacks and Hispanics (101 and 51, respectively) were substantially higher than rates for whites (17), Native Americans and Alaskan Natives (12), and Asians and Pacific Islanders (6). Substantial increases of cases were also noted among IDUs and heterosexuals. The proportion of cases among persons who reported injecting drug use increased from 17% to 27%, and the proportion of cases attributed to heterosexual transmission increased from 3% to 10% (Fig. 121–10*B*). As a result of increased heterosexual transmission, AIDS cases increased among women from 8% to 18%, and there was a proportional decrease in cases among homosexual men from 64% to 45%.

This increase in AIDS among women is also reflected in serosurveys of HIV infection in women. In a survey of infants

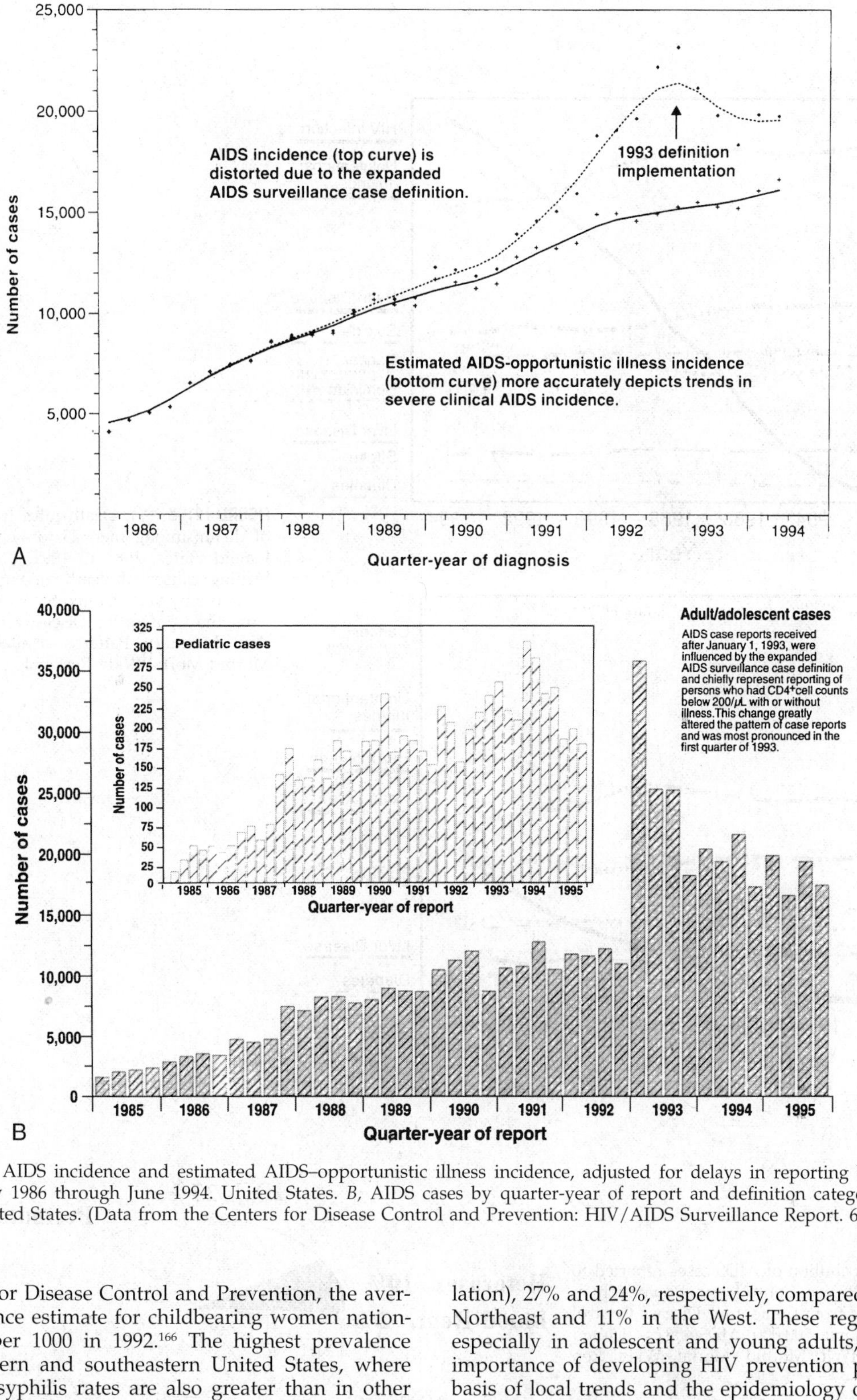

FIGURE 121–7 □ *A,* AIDS incidence and estimated AIDS–opportunistic illness incidence, adjusted for delays in reporting by quarter-year of diagnosis, January 1986 through June 1994. United States. *B,* AIDS cases by quarter-year of report and definition category, reported 1984 through 1994, United States. (Data from the Centers for Disease Control and Prevention: HIV/AIDS Surveillance Report. 6:1, 1994.)

by the Centers for Disease Control and Prevention, the average seroprevalence estimate for childbearing women nationwide was 1.7 per 1000 in 1992.[166] The highest prevalence was in the eastern and southeastern United States, where gonorrhea and syphilis rates are also greater than in other areas of the United States.[167] This association between STDs and increasing HIV infection rates among women suggests further heterosexual transmission.

Geographic patterns have also changed, as reflected by the largest proportion in increase of reported cases (31%) from the South.[33] The proportional increases in AIDS cases reported for the Midwest, Northeast, and West were 22%, 20% and 15%, respectively. Higher proportions of cases among adolescents and young adults (13 to 29 years old) also occurred in small metropolitan statistical areas (<500,000 population), 27% and 24%, respectively, compared with 9% in the Northeast and 11% in the West. These regional variations, especially in adolescent and young adults, underscore the importance of developing HIV prevention programs on the basis of local trends and the epidemiology of HIV transmission. In the South and Midwest, more detailed characterization of the epidemiologic patterns in small cities and rural areas is particularly important for developing effective, region-wide prevention programs.

The epidemic in children younger than 13 years of age is closely associated with the epidemic in women. By using findings from the HIV survey of childbearing women, an estimated 7000 HIV-infected women delivered infants in the United States during 1993. Assuming a perinatal transmission rate of 15% to 30%, approximately 1000 to 2000 infants

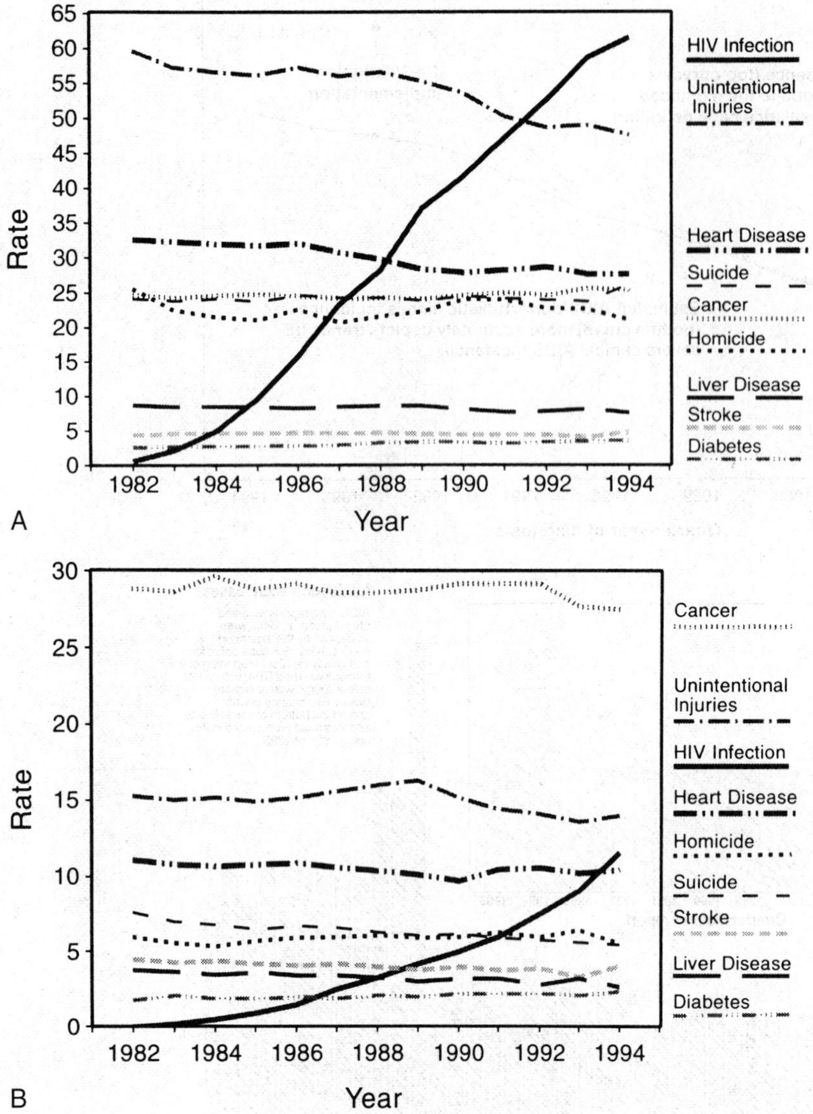

FIGURE 121–8 □ *A,* Death rates from leading causes of death among men 25 to 44 years old by year, United States, 1982 to 1994. *B,* Death rates from leading causes of death among women 25 to 44 years old by year, United States, 1982 to 1994. (Data from the Centers for Disease Control and Prevention: Mortality Patterns—United States. MMWR Morbid Mortal Wkly Rep 45:1, 1996.)

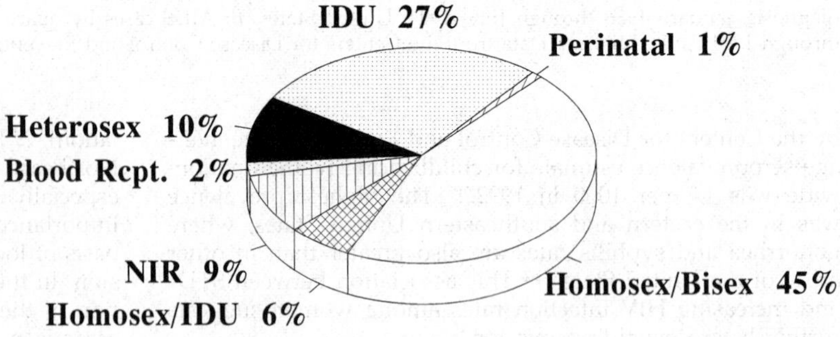

FIGURE 121–9 □ Distribution of AIDS cases reported to the Centers for Disease Control and Prevention in 1993 to 1995. (Data from Centers for Disease Control and Prevention: First 500,000 AIDS cases—United States, 1995. MMWR Morbid Mortal Wkly Rep 44:849–853, 1995.)

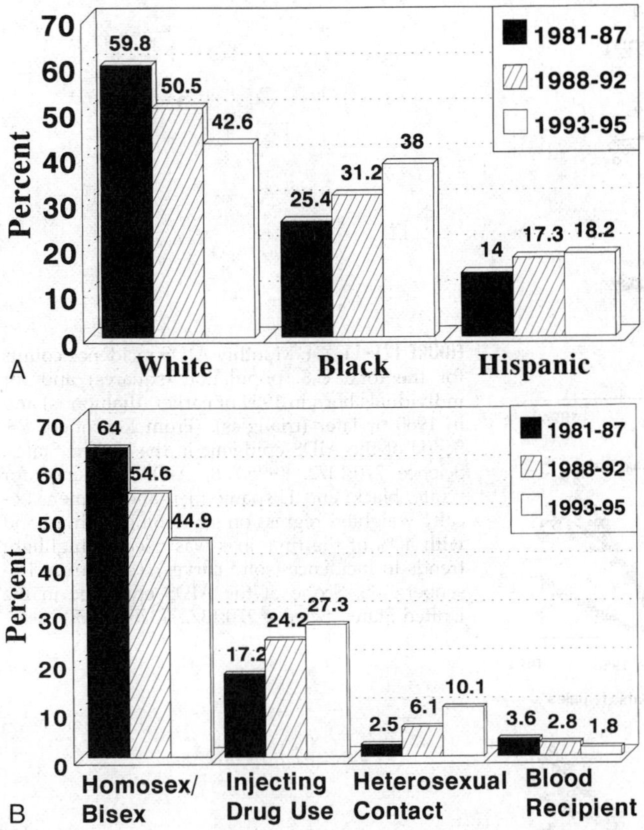

FIGURE 121–10 □ *A,* Percentage of persons with AIDS by race, ethnicity, and period of report in the United States from 1981 through 1995. *B,* Percentage of persons with AIDS by HIV exposure category and period of report in the United States from 1981 through 1995. (Data from Centers for Disease Control and Prevention: First 500,000 AIDS cases—United States, 1995. MMWR Morbid Mortal Wkly Rep 44:849–853, 1995.)

were perinatally infected with HIV infection in 1993.[112] HIV infection has become a leading cause of death for young children, currently ranked seventh for children 1 to 4 years old.[17] Further trends in AIDS incidence among children will be affected by the current recommendations of the U.S. Public Health Service for routine counseling and voluntary prenatal HIV testing for women and the use of zidovudine to prevent perinatal transmission.[112]

According to a mathematic model to reconstruct age-specific HIV infection rates in the United States from AIDS surveillance data, approximately 630,000 to 897,000 U.S. adults and adolescents were living with HIV infection in January 1993, including 107,000 to 150,000 women[168] (Table 121–5). The estimated incidence of HIV infection declined markedly over time among white males, especially those older than 30 years. In contrast, HIV incidence appeared to remain relatively constant among women and minorities (Fig. 121–11). In January 1993, HIV prevalence was highest among young adults in their late 20s and 30s and among minorities. An estimated 3% of black men and 1% of black women in their 30s were living with HIV infection as of that date. If infection rates remain at these levels, HIV can be considered endemic in the United States. Among white males, age-specific HIV prevalence peaked at about 1% among individuals in their early 30s. Prevalence rates were high among racial and ethnic minority men over a broad range of ages, 30 to 44 years. About 3% of black men and 1.5% of Hispanic men in this age range were living with HIV infection. The prevalence was about 1% for black women and 0.5% for Hispanic women in their late 20s and early 30s. The prevalence was lowest in white women. Thus, the highest national prevalence rates were seen among minorities and in particular among young black men. Approximately 1 of every 50 black men in the United States, 18 to 59 years old, may be infected with HIV.

To summarize the HIV-AIDS epidemic in the United States, the epidemic has evolved from a small outbreak among homosexual men in a few cities to a major killer of young adults. Moreover, the epidemic is continuing to evolve. Although there are encouraging reports of decreasing transmission among homosexual and bisexual men in general, data also indicate that new infections are occurring in this population, particularly among younger men. Heterosexual transmission is also becoming an increasingly important part of the U.S. epidemic, with certain groups at a disproportionately high risk. At greatest risk are the young, disadvantaged, and minority populations, particularly women living in the inner cities of the Northeast and in parts of the rural South. A major source of infection for these women has been male IDUs; transmission occurs particularly among women with multiple sexual partners and those who exchange sex for drugs or money. Transmission in these settings has also been facilitated by the presence of other STDs. Persons at highest risk for infection are often those who are the hardest to reach through conventional health education programs. Yet, these persons with their myriad social and economic problems are the individuals who need to be reached most urgently. Finally, the impact on the health care delivery system will be particularly dramatic. HIV seroprevalence in sentinel hospital patients ranged from 0.1% to 5.8%.[169] In one emergency department, the prevalence of HIV among unselected adults rose from 6% to 11.3% during a 4-year period.[170]

In Latin America and the Caribbean, the HIV pandemic is also continuing to evolve. Within the last 5 years there has been evidence of increasing heterosexual transmission, principally among bisexual men and their female sex partners and among female sex workers and their clients.[163, 171] In Brazil, the porportion of reported AIDS cases attributable to heterosexual transmission increased from 7.5% in 1987 to 26% in 1994.[12] HIV infections among IDUs are also a growing problem. For example, in Argentina the prevalence of HIV infection among IDUs ranges from 30% to 50%; in Brazil, from 20% to 60%.[12] Throughout the Caribbean, heterosexual transmission has been the predominant mode for at least a decade.[172] In Haiti, approximately 8% to 10% of the urban population and 5% of the rural population are infected, most

TABLE 121–5 ■ Estimated Number of Infected Persons and Prevalence of Human Immunodeficiency Virus Type 1 Infection in the United States as of January 1993 Estimated by Back-Calculation from AIDS Incidence Data

GROUP	NUMBER OF PERSONS ALIVE WITH HIV-1	SEROPREVALENCE OF HIV+ IN AGES 18–54 (%)
Men		
White	255,000	0.49
Black	184,000	2.29
Hispanic	97,000	1.44
Total	544,000	0.78
Women		
White	25,000	0.05
Black	67,000	0.74
Hispanic	24,000	0.34
Total	117,000	0.16
Grand total	660,000	0.47

Data from Rosenberg PS: Scope of the AIDS epidemic in the United States. Science 270:1372–1375, 1995.

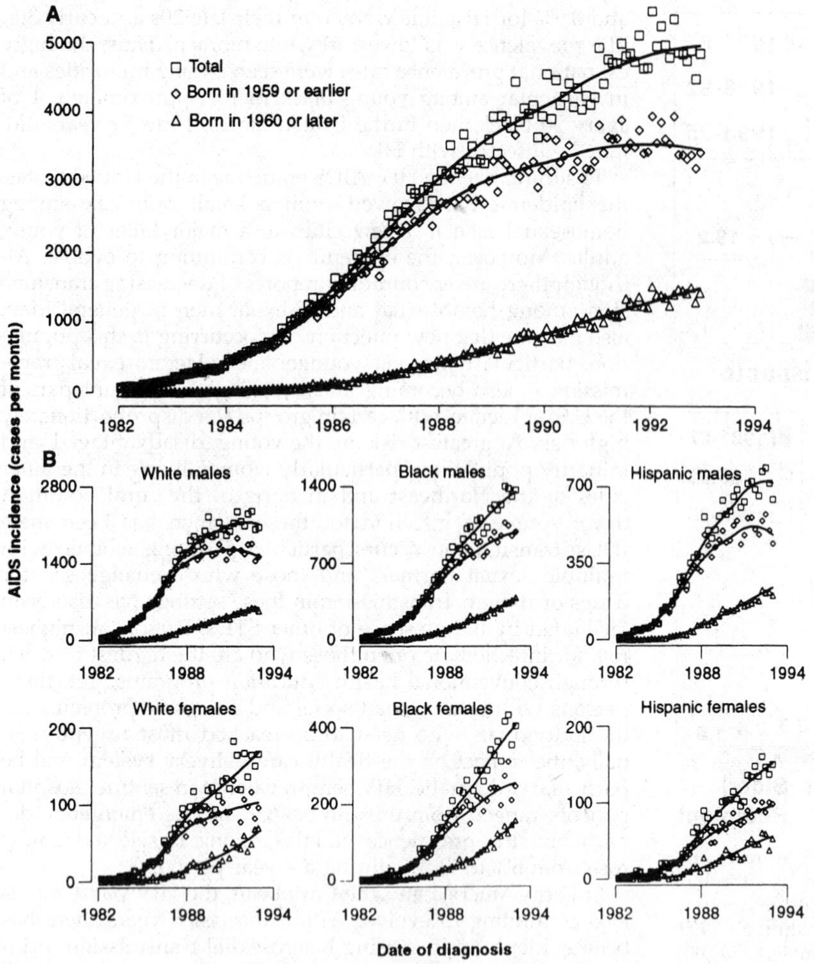

FIGURE 121-11 □ *A*, Monthly AIDS incidence counts for the total U.S. population (squares) and for individuals born in 1959 or earlier (diamonds) and in 1960 or later (triangles). (From Rosenberg PS: Scope of the AIDS epidemic in the United States. Science 270:1372, 1995.) *B*, AIDS incidence for white, black, and Hispanic men and women. Locally weighted regression smoothing with a band with 40% of the time axis was used to highlight trends in incidence (solid curves). (Data from Rosenberg PS: Scope of the AIDS epidemic in the United States. Science 270:1372–1375, 1995.)

through heterosexual contact.[8] It was estimated that 70% of new cases in the Caribbean will occur in young adults 20 to 45 years old and 12% in children under 15 years old.[173] Age-specific mortality will more than double in the 20- to 40-year age range. In terms of economic impact, it was estimated that the total annual cost of the epidemic will approach 2% to 5% of the gross domestic product in countries with limited resources. It is estimated that the direct cost of treating AIDS patients in Latin America and the Caribbean will amount to $2 billion by 1999, and indirect costs will be many times greater.[173]

Europe

Approximately a half-million individuals are estimated to be HIV infected in Western and Eastern Europe. Differences continue to exist in HIV transmission patterns between and even within individual countries. For example, the majority of AIDS cases in Scandinavia have occurred among heterosexual and bisexual men, whereas IDUs constitute two thirds or more of the cases reported in Italy and Spain. However, for all Europe the proportion of AIDS cases attributable to homosexual transmission fell from 62% to 36% between 1985 and 1992, whereas the proportion of transmission attributable to injecting drug use increased from 16% to 40%.[12] Transmission through heterosexual exposure has also increased, especially in urban populations with high rates of injecting drug use or STDs.[36, 81, 174] Between 14% and 18% of HIV-infected people in Europe may have acquired their infection heterosexually. Seroprevalence studies demonstrate increasing HIV incidence among patients attending STD clinics, female sex workers and their clients, and pregnant women. In countries such as Italy and Spain, where IDU transmission has been common, heterosexual transmission is rapidly increasing.

Data regarding the frequency and transmission of HIV infections in Eastern Europe are much more limited. Homosexual and heterosexual transmission appears to be a predominant route in some countries, although several localized outbreaks of nosocomial transmission have been reported among infants and young children.[12, 175, 176] In the Czech and Slovak republics, about two thirds of confirmed HIV infections are due to homosexual transmission. In Bulgaria, 75% are linked to heterosexual transmission. In Poland, 70% of HIV-infected people are IDUs and a seroprevalence survey demonstrated a prevalence of 10% in IDUs. In Eastern Europe, 2400 AIDS cases or two thirds of the total are children infected with HIV through unsafe medical practices.[12] In an outbreak in 1988 in the Kalmyk Republic of the Russian Federation, several hundred children were infected through injections of medicine using shared syringes that had been contaminated with HIV-infected blood.[176, 177] In a 1989 Romanian outbreak, it is believed that between 1000 and 2000 children were infected through transfusions of unscreened blood and possibly as a result of the use of unsterilized needles or syringes.[176] This variation in epidemiology probably reflects societal differences among the countries concerned. With westernization over the past few years there has been a marked increase in STDs such as gonorrhea and syphilis, and the incidence of hepatitis B is roughly 10 times that in the continent's western half. Consequently, Eastern

Europe has an explosive potential for HIV because all the transmission routes are present.

Natural History of Human Immunodeficiency Virus Type 1 Infection

Studies of the natural history of HIV-1 infection in homosexual men, hemophiliacs, and recipients of infected blood transfusions in developed countries have shown an annual progression rate of disease of approximately 2% to 5%.[178–182] Disease progression in HIV-1–infected African heterosexuals appears to be similar to the rate observed in white homosexual men and hemophiliacs. Among HIV-1–seropositive female prostitutes in Nairobi, 6% developed severe illness during a 12-months follow-up.[82] Among African men and women with lymphadenopathy syndrome or AIDS-related complex followed in Brussels, the annual progression rates to AIDS were 1.1% and 20.7%, respectively.[82] In Zaire, 6.3% of 56 persons who had become seropositive between 1984 and 1986 had developed AIDS-related conditions by the end of 1986, and 5% had developed AIDS.[183, 184] Among 91 already seropositive men and women who enrolled in the cohort in 1984, by 1986, a 2-year period, 16.3% had AIDS-related conditions, 3.3% had AIDS, and 11.9% had died with suspected AIDS.

Prognostic factors for disease progression were originally identified in cohort studies in Europe and the United States. A specific loss of immunoglobulin G antibodies against *gag* gene products of HIV-1 (p24) was identified with clinical progression of HIV-1 infection, whereas antibodies to viral *env* glycoproteins (gp41 and gp120/160) remained stable.[185–188] In these cohorts, an increase in *gag* viral antigen (p24) was also correlated with progression to AIDS, although p24 antigenemia was found less often in serum from African patients with AIDS than in serum from European or U.S. patients.[189, 190] These studies underscore the importance of viral RNA levels in predicting disease progression.

Whether microbial infections act as cofactors to enhance HIV-1 infection remains to be determined. Frequent exposure to a wide variety of infections in the developing world, such as malaria, mycobacterial infections, STDs, and infections with other viruses such as cytomegalovirus and herpes simplex virus, has been hypothesized to increase viral replication, thereby enhancing disease progression.[191] Coinfection with human T-cell lymphotropic virus type I, which occurs in many tropical areas, may also influence the natural history of HIV-1 infection, as cohort studies in Trinidad and Brazil demonstrated.[192, 193]

In addition to its association with STDs, HIV is associated with many other opportunistic infections. Most notable is its association with tuberculosis. Tuberculosis is already one of the leading causes of adult death in many developing countries, killing about 3 million people a year.[149, 194–197] An alarming increase in cases has been reported in parallel with the AIDS epidemic in many countries.[149, 198, 199] HIV infection is now the most potent biologic risk factor for the development of active tuberculosis.[150, 197, 200] People with latent tuberculosis may readily develop the disease when their immune system has been damaged by HIV. Of individuals who are dually infected, 5% to 10% may develop active tuberculosis each year.[201] Moreover, data from the United States indicate that some of the increase in active tuberculosis is attributable to new infections among those with HIV infection who have increased susceptibility to active tuberculosis.[202–206] About 30% to 50% of adults in most developing countries have latent tuberculosis infection.[149, 200]

Projections by the WHO suggest that the annual number of tuberculosis cases worldwide will reach 10.2 million by the year 2000.[194, 202] Even though several factors contribute to the increase, HIV infection plays a dominant role in many resource-poor countries. In some African countries heavily affected by the HIV epidemic, the number of tuberculosis cases annually has more than doubled, and the rates of HIV-associated tuberculosis are beginning to increase in parts of Asia. With these trends, tuberculosis control programs in many resource-poor countries are being overburdened. Potential solutions are allocating more resources for tuberculosis control, redistributing some activities to other parts of the health sector, and simplifying tuberculosis control activities so that more cases can be managed with the staff and resources available.[201] Underfunding is clearly a major obstacle to progress in the control of tuberculosis. DeCock and Wilkinson[207] have suggested an alternative approach to the treatment of tuberculosis similar to that described for STDs. The traditional etiologically based management of STDs failed at a public health level and is now being replaced by syndromic management aiming for compliance of patients with effective therapy without specific diagnostic confirmation. The new tuberculosis control strategy would incorporate reducing laboratory investigation, using one global regimen, providing all treatment on a directly observed basis, and integrating tuberculosis control program activities better into other health services provided at the district level.[207–209] This tuberculosis control strategy aims for maximal public health impact by ensuring adherence to effective therapy after diagnosis, delivered in a simple way, with minimal subsequent investigation. As the WHO has declared tuberculosis a global emergency, a uniform international response examining these strategies urgently needs to be evaluated.[202]

Future Projections

The long-term dimensions of the HIV pandemic cannot yet be forecast with confidence. However, on the basis of available data the WHO has projected that by the year 2000 there will be a cumulative total of more than 40 million infections in men, women, and children, of which more than 90% will be in developing countries.[12] The projected cumulative total of adult AIDS cases will be close to 10 million. By the year 2000 the cumulative number of HIV-related deaths in adults is predicted to rise from its current total of 2 million to more than 8 million individuals. Unless our interventions are more effective, between 15 million and 20 million new HIV infections will occur in the next 5 years. In addition, more than 5 million children younger than 10 years will be orphaned as a result of AIDS-related fatalities.[210, 211] The number of orphans will increase further in the early years of the next century as a result of the deaths of mothers who were infected with HIV in the 1990s. As the epidemic matures in some parts of the world, a large number of young people becoming sexually active will replenish the pool of susceptible people, especially in developing countries, where the base of the age pyramid is quite broad.[43] Evidence for a high incidence in young populations compared with older cohorts is already emerging for various countries. In the United States, the number of 13- to 21-year-olds who had become infected with HIV rose by 77% between 1991 and 1993. In sub-Saharan African countries the highest HIV seroprevalence rates are in women between 15 and 25 years old.[142]

Heterosexual spread of HIV is causing an epidemiologic shift of infection from high-risk populations such as homosexual men and IDUs to populations more reflective of the general population, especially adolescents and young women of childbearing age. As a consequence, the number of persons with AIDS will continue to increase, causing unprecedented personal suffering, high direct costs for medical care, reduced economic output, and a substantial indirect cost to society. The impact of HIV in many countries will be immense.

In conservative projections the annual number of new AIDS cases in North America and Western Europe during the next two decades is expected to remain fairly constant at close to 100,000. This is because HIV-infected persons will eventually develop AIDS and the annual HIV incidence in these regions, projected to be close to 100,000, will nearly equal the number of fatalities. In sub-Saharan Africa, the peak occurrence of AIDS, estimated at 750,000 cases per year, will not be reached until the middle of the next decade (Fig. 121–12). However, in Asia the annual number of AIDS cases will increase steadily in the next decade and will not begin to level off until 2010 at about 850,000 cases per year.[32] Although the absolute number of new HIV infections in Asia is equal to the high level found in Africa, the rate of new infections or new cases per year as a percentage of the adult population is still much lower in Asia than in sub-Saharan Africa. This is because the adult population of Asia is more than five times larger than the adult population of sub-Saharan Africa. If unchecked, the rising incidence in Asia will produce an unprecedented number of new cases in that region. On the basis of current data, cumulative HIV infections in Asia are conservatively projected to be more than 10 million (0.46% of the population) in the year 2000 and more than 18 million in 2010. In sub-Saharan Africa the cumulative number of HIV infections is projected to reach about 15 million in the year 2000 (3%) and about 20 million in 2010 (1.7%). In North America and Western Europe, conservative estimates are about 2 million cumulative HIV infections in the year 2000 (0.23%) and about 2.7 million infections in 2010 (0.17%).

Global Control of Human Immunodeficiency Virus Infection

Control of HIV infections has become a public health priority in most countries of the world. With no prospect for an effective vaccine or curative treatment in the near future, prevention is the only effective way to control HIV infection and AIDS. With an estimated 20 million HIV-infected people worldwide, the need for a global program to coordinate control activities was urgently needed. In 1986 the WHO created the Global Programme on AIDS, which developed three primary objectives: to prevent new HIV infections, to provide support and care to those already infected, and to link national and international efforts against AIDS.[82, 212] The basic tenets of control, including professional and public education on the modes of transmission, risk behavior reduction for persons at high risk, and screening of blood supplies to prevent further transmission by transfusions, are all attainable, but the obstacles to complete control are enormous.[213] Information alone is not sufficient motivation to change risk behaviors, and even intervention by screening blood donors has not been implemented in many developing countries owing to economic constraints and lack of adequate blood banking facilities and appropriate laboratory technology.

The modes of HIV transmission are common to all countries, but the relative importance and characteristics are variable in specific areas. For example, heterosexual transmission among prostitutes and their clients in certain cities in Africa and the Caribbean, homosexual transmission in North America and Europe, and HIV transmission by bisexual males in the Caribbean and South America are all forms of sexual transmission,[213] but curbing each requires different educational approaches and interventions. Although it is the most difficult objective in the control of AIDS, preventing HIV transmission by changing sexual behaviors, if successful, would have the greatest impact on the containment of AIDS. It is therefore important to direct educational efforts to persons who exhibit high-risk behavior and to adolescents. Whenever possible, AIDS education should be incorporated in existing health education programs. Reducing the risk of sexual transmission must be accomplished by limiting the number of sexual partners, especially anonymous partners, and increasing condom use. Spermicides containing nonoxynol 9 have been shown in the laboratory to inactivate HIV and may provide additional protection. With increasing evidence that HIV transmission is facilitated by genital ulcers and other STDs, programs to diagnose and treat these disease should be integrated into AIDS control efforts.[99, 101, 102]

The success of programs to prevent STDs depends on the delivery of messages to specific audiences and the provision of support services such as counseling and providing condoms to maximize compliance.[214] Because few data on sexual practices are available, surveys of knowledge, attitudes, and practices are needed to identify the culturally appropriate messages for various segments of the population in each country, such as prostitutes, adolescents, homosexual males, and bisexuals. Programs to prevent STDs have been undertaken before, and the success and failure of such programs should be examined so that mistakes made previously can be avoided in AIDS control programs.

Parenteral transmission of HIV remains a major problem,

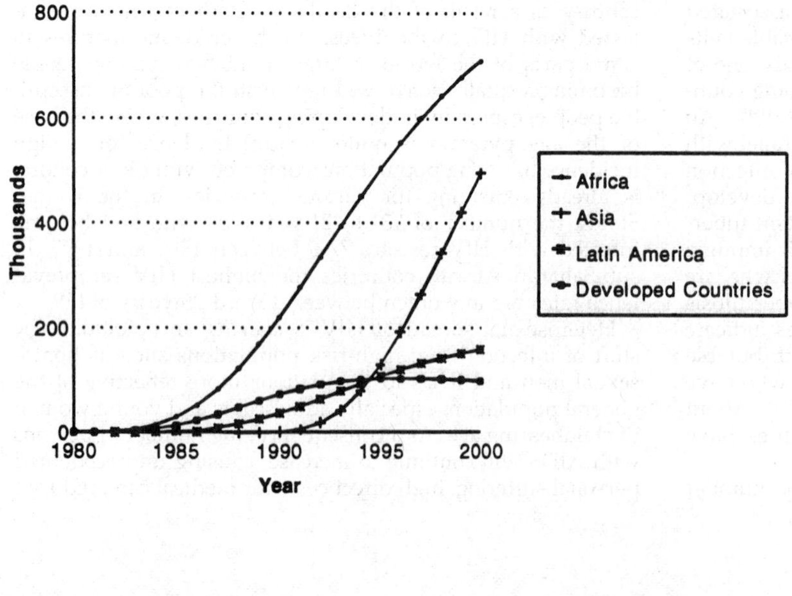

FIGURE 121–12 □ Estimated and projected annual adult AIDS incidences by macroregion, 1980 to 2000. (Data from Global Programme on AIDS: The Current Global Situation of the HIV-AIDS Pandemic. Geneva, World Health Organization, 1995.)

particularly among IDUs in developed countries and recipients of blood transfusions in developing countries where screening has not been implemented.[215] As with implementing changes in sexual behavior, the challenge of altering needle sharing habits among drug users is formidable. Advocating a change of behavior among drug users must be integrated into strategies at current treatment centers, which must be made more widely available.[216] Specific recommendations for the control of HIV-1 infection among IDUs include HIV antibody testing, which should be voluntary; free distribution of sterile needles and syringes; methadone maintenance and other drug treatment programs, which should be available on demand for all IDUs as a means of reducing the spread of HIV infection; and educational strategies to prevent persons from starting injecting drug use, which should be broad based and directed at all persons at high risk.[217] Among the target populations are IDUs who wish to enter drug treatment programs; current IDUs who do not want treatment for their drug abuse; persons who are not currently IDUs but who are at risk for becoming so; and all young people, especially those who live in areas with high rates of injecting drug use. In addition, sexual partners of staff and inmates of correctional facilities and all health care workers, counselors, and hospital personnel should be specifically educated about the potential risk of acquiring HIV infection through parenteral exposure to blood-contaminated needles and syringes and through sexual contact with an HIV-infected partner.[90]

Although transmission by blood transfusion is now rare in most industrialized countries, in some developing countries blood transfusions are probably the second most important route of HIV transmission, accounting for up to 10% of infections in adults and up to 30% in children. An HIV-free blood supply is an attainable goal with available technology and would have an immediate impact on the spread of AIDS. Major drawbacks have been logistic problems of setting up a blood bank screening infrastructure in developing countries. Donor deferral or screening of donors on the basis of clinical or epidemiologic criteria is unlikely to protect the blood supply and could drastically reduce the available donor pool; however, an intensive program to educate physicians about the risk of HIV transmission through transfusions and the development of stringent criteria for prescribing transfusions should dramatically decrease the number of blood transfusions.[218] Coupled with screening utilizing inexpensive, rapid diagnostic assays, these measures should help prevent further transmission of HIV by blood transfusion, even in remote rural areas.

In some developing countries such as those in Africa, the frequent exposure to blood-contaminated needles and syringes that are reused for medicinal purposes may result in a substantial number of HIV infections. The potential importance of HIV transmission by needle reflects several cultural factors that merit emphasis. Patients often express a strong preference for parenteral rather than oral therapy. Injections as well as scarifications may be administered in clinics or nonmedical sites by personnel inadequately trained in aseptic technique. Financial and other practical constraints also lead to reuse of disposable equipment and to inadequate sterilization of needles and instruments. In contrast, the lack of association between HIV seropositivity and childhood vaccination probably reflects the wider use of properly sterilized injection equipment and immunization programs.

Prevention of perinatal transmission of HIV depends primarily on the success of limiting the spread of HIV infection of women of childbearing age and use of antiretroviral drugs such as zidovudine for HIV-infected pregnant women. In the developed world, when a mother is HIV infected, the known and potential benefit of breast-feeding for the child should be compared with the incremental risk to the infant of becoming infected through breast-feeding. In developing countries, where safe and effective alternatives for breast-feeding are not generally available, breast-feeding by the biologic mother should continue to be the feeding method of choice, regardless of the mother's HIV infection status. The issues of childbearing, contraception, breast-feeding, and abortion are obviously complex and require different approaches depending on the cultural background of the population.

With the magnitude of the current AIDS epidemic and the continued escalation in spread of HIV infection, it is evident that control and prevention of AIDS will require a sustained long-term commitment. Research is still urgently needed to define the size of the problem in different geographic areas through serosurveys of representative samples of the population. Research is needed to clarify the dynamics of transmission and the possible role of intercurrent infections or other cofactors in increasing the risk of infection or of disease. Additional research is also urgently needed to develop effective control programs, which will rely on new studies of patterns of sexual behavior and the evaluation of the efficacy of health education interventions. The overall success of these national programs and the regional and global AIDS control efforts will depend on a unifying international political and societal commitment.

References

1. Gottlieb MS, Schroff R, Schanker HM, et al: *Pneumocystis carinii* pneumonia and mucosal candidiasis in previously healthy homosexual men: Evidence of a new acquired cellular immunodeficiency. N Engl J Med 305:1425, 1981.
2. Masur H, Michelis MA, Greene JB, et al: An outbreak of community-acquired *Pneumocystis carinii* pneumonia: Initial manifestation of cellular immune dysfunction. N Engl J Med 305:1431, 1981.
3. Siegal FP, Lopez C, Hammer GS, et al: Severe acquired immunodeficiency in male homosexuals, manifested by chronic perianal ulcerative herpes simplex lesions. N Engl J Med 305:1444, 1981.
4. Centers for Disease Control: Kaposi's sarcoma and *Pneumocystis* pneumonia among homosexual men—New York City and California. MMWR Morbid Mortal Wkly Rep 30:305, 1981.
5. Centers for Disease Control: Acquired immunodeficiency syndrome (AIDS) update—United States. MMWR Morbid Mortal Wkly Rep 32:309, 1983.
6. Mann JM, Chin J, Piot P, Quinn TC: The international epidemiology of AIDS. Sci Am 259(4):82, 1988.
7. Quinn TC, Mann JM, Curran JW, Piot P: AIDS in Africa: An epidemiologic paradigm. Science 234:955, 1986.
8. Pape J, Johnson WD Jr: AIDS in Haiti: 1982–1992. Clin Infect Dis 17(Suppl 2):S341, 1993.
9. Pape JW, Liautaud B, Thomas F, et al: Characteristics of the acquired immunodeficiency syndrome in a heterosexual population in Zaire. Lancet 2:65, 1984.
10. Piot P, Quinn TC, Taelman H, et al: Acquired immunodeficiency syndrome in a heterosexual population in Zaire. Lancet 2:65, 1984.
11. World Health Organization: AIDS—Global situation of the HIV/AIDS pandemic. Wkly Epidemiol Rec 70:193, 1995.
12. Global Programme on AIDS: The Current Global Situation of the HIV-AIDS Pandemic. Geneva, World Health Organization, 1995.
13. DeCock KM, Barrere B, Diaby L, et al: AIDS—The leading cause of adult death in the West African city of Abidjan, Ivory Coast. Science 249:793, 1990.
14. Selik RM, Chu SY, Buehler JW: HIV infection as leading cause of death among young adults in U.S. cities and states. JAMA 269:2991, 1993.
15. Mulder DW, Nunn AJ, Kamali A, et al: Two-year HIV-1–associated mortality in a Ugandan rural population. Lancet 343:1021, 1994.
16. Sewankambo NK, Wawer MJ, Gray RH, et al: Demographic

impact of HIV infection in rural Rakai district, Uganda: Results of a population-based cohort study. AIDS 8:1707, 1994.
17. National Center for Health Statistics: Annual Summary of Births, Marriages, Divorces, and Deaths: United States, 1993. Hyattsville, MD, U.S. Department of Health and Human Services, Public Health Service, 1994, pp 18–20.
18. Barre-Sinoussi F, Chermann JC, Rey F, et al: Isolation of a T-lymphotropic retrovirus from a patient at risk for acquired immune deficiency syndrome (AIDS). Science 220:868, 1983.
19. Gallo RC, Salahuddin SZ, Popovic M, et al: Frequent detection and isolation of cytopathic retroviruses (HTLV-III) from patients with AIDS and at risk for AIDS. Science 224:500, 1984.
20. Brookmeyer R: Reconstruction and future trends of the AIDS epidemic in the United States. Science 253:37, 1991.
21. Medley GF, Anderson RM, Cox DR, Billard L: Incubation period of AIDS in patients infected via blood transfusion. Nature 328:719, 1987.
22. Lui KJ, Darrow WW, Rutherford GW III: A model-based estimate of the mean incubation period for AIDS in homosexual men. Science 240:1333, 1988.
23. Rothenberg R, Woelfel M, Stoneburner R, et al: Survival with the acquired immunodeficiency syndrome. Experience with 5833 cases in New York City. N Engl J Med 317:1297, 1987.
24. Quinn TC: Global burden of the HIV pandemic. Lancet 348:99, 1996.
25. Nzilambi N, De Cock KM, Forthal DN, et al: The prevalence of infection with human immunodeficiency virus over a 10-year period in rural Zaire. N Engl J Med 318:276, 1988.
26. Curran JW, Jaffe HW, Hardy AM, et al: Epidemiology of HIV infection and AIDS in the United States. Science 239:610, 1988.
27. Quinn TC: Population migration and the spread of types 1 and 2 human immunodeficiency viruses. Proc Natl Acad Sci USA 91:2407, 1994.
28. Decosas J, Kane F, Anarfi JK, et al: Migration and AIDS. Lancet 346:826, 1995.
29. Piot P, Plummer FS, Mhalu JL, et al: AIDS: An international perspective. Science 239:573, 1988.
30. Bollinger RC, Tripathy SP, Quinn TC: The human immunodeficiency virus epidemic in India. Medicine (Baltimore) 74:97, 1995.
31. Mertens TE, Burton A, Stoneburner R, et al: Global estimates and epidemiology of HIV infections and AIDS. AIDS 8(Suppl 1):S361, 1994.
32. Chin J: Scenarios for the AIDS Epidemic in Asia. Asia-Pacific Population Research Reports, No 2, February 1995. Honolulu, HI.
33. Centers for Disease Control and Prevention: The first 500,000 AIDS cases—United States, 1995. MMWR Morbid Mortal Wkly Rep 44:849, 1995.
34. Anderson R: Mathematical models of the potential demographic impact of AIDS in Africa. AIDS 5(Suppl 1):S37, 1991.
35. Ades AE: Serial HIV seroprevalence surveys: Interpretation, design, and role in HIV/AIDS prediction. J Acquir Immune Defic Syndr Hum Retrovirol 9:490, 1995.
36. Haverkos HW, Quinn TC: The third wave: HIV infection among heterosexuals in the United States and Europe. Int J STD AIDS 6:227, 1995.
37. Centers for Disease Control and Prevention: Update: Acquired immunodeficiency syndrome—United States, 1994. MMWR Morbid Mortal Wkly Rep 44:64, 1995.
38. Kaldor JM, Sittitrai W, John TJ, Kitamura T: The emerging epidemic of HIV infection and AIDS in Asia and the Pacific. AIDS 8(Suppl 2):S165, 1994.
39. Mann J, Tarantola D: The state of the HIV/AIDS pandemic. *In* Mann J, Tarantola D, Netter J (eds): AIDS in the World, Vol II. London, Oxford University Press (in press).
40. Quinn TC, Zacarias FRK, St. John RK: HIV and HTLV-1 infections in the Americas: A regional perspective. Medicine (Baltimore) 68:189, 1989.
41. U.S. Bureau of the Census: HIV/AIDS in Asia. Washington, DC, U.S. Bureau of the Census, 1995. Research Note 18.
42. Brown T, Xenos P: AIDS in Asia: The gathering storm. *In* Asia-Pacific Issues, No 16. Honolulu, HI, East-West Center, 1994.
43. Myers G, Korber B, Wain-Hobson S, et al: Human Retroviruses and AIDS 1994. Los Alamos, NM, Los Alamos National Laboratory, 1994.
44. Kostrikis LG, Bagdades E, Cao Y, et al: Genetic analysis of human immunodeficiency virus type 1 strains from patients in Cyprus: Identification of a new subtype designated subtype I. J Virol 69:6122, 1995.
45. Gurtler LG, Hauser PH, Eberle J, et al: A new subtype of human immunodeficiency virus type 1 (MVP-5180) from Cameroon. J Virol 68:1581, 1994.
46. Marlink R: Biology and epidemiology of HIV-2. *In* Essex M, Kalengay M, Kanki P, et al (eds): AIDS in Africa. New York, Raven Press, 1994, pp 47–65.
47. Myers G: HIV: Between past and future. AIDS Res Hum Retroviruses 10:1317, 1994.
48. Artenstein AW, Coppola J, Brown AE, et al: Multiple introductions of HIV-1 subtype E into the Western Hemisphere. Lancet 346:1197, 1995.
49. Brodine SK, Mascola JR, Weiss PJ, et al: Detection of diverse HIV-1 genetic subtypes in the U.S.A. Lancet 346:1198, 1995.
50. Kunanusont C, Foy HM, Kreiss JK, et al: HIV-1 subtypes and male-to-female transmission in Thailand. Lancet 345:1078, 1995.
51. Weniger BG, Takebe Y, Ou C-Y, Yamazaki S: The molecular epidemiology of HIV in Asia. AIDS 8(Suppl 2):S13, 1994.
52. Ou C-Y, Takebe Y, Weiniger BG, et al: Independent introduction of two major HIV-1 genotypes into distinct high-risk populations in Thailand. Lancet 341:1171, 1993.
53. Bobkov A, Garaev MM, Rzhaninova A: Molecular epidemiology of HIV-1 in the former Soviet Union: Analysis of *env* V3 sequences and their correlation with epidemiologic data. AIDS 8:619, 1994.
54. Louwagie J, Delwart EL, Mullins JL, et al: Genetic analysis of HIV-1 isolates from Brazil reveals presence of two distinct genetic subtypes. AIDS Res Hum Retroviruses 10:561, 1994.
55. Morgado MG, Sabino EC, Shpaer EG, et al: V3 region polymorphisms in HIV-1 from Brazil: Prevalence of subtype B strains divergent from North American/European prototype and detection of subtype F. AIDS Res Hum Retroviruses 10:569, 1994.
56. Pieniazek D, Janini LM, Ramos A, et al: HIV-patients may harbor viruses of different phylogenetic subtypes: Implications for the evolution of the HIV/AIDS pandemic. Emerging Infect Dis 1:86, 1995.
57. Clavel F, Guetard D, Brun-Vezinet F, et al: Isolation of a new retrovirus from West African patients with AIDS. Science 233:343, 1986.
58. Kanki PJ, Barin F, M'Boup S, et al: New human T-lymphotropic retrovirus related to simian T-lymphotropic virus type III (STLV-IIIAGM). Science 232:238, 1986.
59. Clavel F, Mansinho K, Chamaret S, et al: Human immunodeficiency virus type 2 infection associated with AIDS in West Africa. N Engl J Med 316:1180, 1987.
60. Clavel F: HIV-2, the West African AIDS virus. AIDS 1:135, 1987.
61. De Cock KM, Adjorlolo G, Ekpini E, et al: Epidemiology and transmission of HIV-2. Why there is no HIV-2 pandemic. JAMA 270:2083, 1993.
62. Kanki P, M'Boup S, Marlink R, et al: Prevalence and risk determinants of human immunodeficiency virus type 2 (HIV-2) and human immunodeficiency virus type 1 (HIV-1) in West African female prostitutes. Am J Epidemiol 136:895, 1992.
63. Markovitz DM: Infection with the human immunodeficiency virus type 2. Ann Intern Med 118:211, 1993.
64. DeCock KM, Brun-Vezinet F: Epidemiology of HIV-2 infection. AIDS 3(Suppl 1):S89, 1989.
65. Kanki P: Biologic features of HIV-2. An update. AIDS Clin Rev 17, 1991.
66. Kanki PJ, Travers KU, M'Boup S, et al: Slower heterosexual spread of HIV-2 than HIV-1. Lancet 343:943, 1994.
67. Adjorlolo-Johnson G, De Cock KM, Ekpini E, et al: Prospective comparison of mother-to-child transmission of HIV-1 and HIV-2 in Abidjan, Ivory Coast. JAMA 272:462, 1994.
68. Kanki PJ, DeCock KM: Epidemiology and natural history of HIV-2. AIDS 8(Suppl 1):S85, 1994.
69. Travers K, Mboup S, Marlink R, et al: Natural protection against HIV-1 infection provided by HIV-2. Science 268:1612, 1995.
70. Ou C-Y, Ciesielski CA, Myers G, et al: Molecular epidemiology of HIV transmission in a dental practice. Science 256:1165, 1992.
71. Jaffe HW, McCurdy JM, Kalish ML, et al: Lack of HIV transmission in the practice of a dentist with AIDS. Ann Intern Med 121:855, 1994.
72. Ciesielski CA, Marianos DW, Schochetman G, et al: The 1990

Florida dental investigation: The press and the science. Ann Intern Med 121:886, 1994.
73. Ou CY, Ciesielski CA, Myers G, et al: Molecular epidemiology of HIV transmission in a dental practice. Science 256:1165, 1992.
74. Cheingsong-Popov R, Bobkov A, Garaev MM, et al: Identification of human immunodeficiency virus type 1 subtypes and their distribution in the Commonwealth of Independent States (former Soviet Union) by serologic V3 peptide-binding assays and V3 sequence analysis. J Infect Dis 168:292, 1993.
75. Chant K, Lowe D, Rubin G, et al: Patient-to-patient transmission of HIV in private surgical consulting rooms. Lancet 342:1548, 1993.
76. Kingsley LA, Zhou SYJ, Bacellar H, et al: Temporal trends in human immunodeficiency virus type 1 seroconversion 1984–1989. Am J Epidemiol 134:331, 1991.
77. Winkelstein W, Lyman DM, Padian N, et al: Sexual practices and risk of infection by the human immunodeficiency virus: The San Francisco Men's Health Study. JAMA 257:321, 1987.
78. Kingsley LA, Detels R, Kaslow R, et al: Risk factors for seroconversion to human immunodeficiency virus among male homosexuals. Lancet 1:345, 1987.
79. Padian NS: Heterosexual transmission of acquired immunodeficiency syndrome: International perspectives and national projections. Rev Infect Dis 9:947, 1987.
80. Centers for Disease Control and Prevention: Heterosexually acquired AIDS—United States, 1993. MMWR Morbid Mortal Wkly Rep 43:155, 1994.
81. Prevots DR, Ancelle-Park RA, Neal JJ, Remis RS: The epidemiology of heterosexually acquired HIV infection and AIDS in Western industrialized countries. AIDS 8(Suppl 1):S109, 1994.
82. Piot P, Plummer FA, Mhlau FS, et al: AIDS: An international perspective. Science 239:573, 1988.
83. Piot P, Goeman J, Laga M: The epidemiology of HIV and AIDS in Africa. *In* Essex M, Mboup S, Kanki P, Kalengayi M (eds): AIDS in Africa. New York, Raven Press, 1994, pp 157–172.
84. Piot P, Kreiss JK, Ndinya-Achola JO, et al: Heterosexual transmission of HIV. AIDS 2:1, 1988.
85. Quinn TC, Fauci AS: The changing demography of AIDS: Emergence of heterosexual transmission. *In* Isselbacher KJ, Braunwald E, Wilson JD, et al (eds): Harrison's Principles of Internal Medicine, Suppl 9. New York, McGraw-Hill, 1994, pp 1–9.
86. Piot P, Kapita BM, Were JBO, et al: AIDS in Africa: The first decade and challenges for the late 1990s. AIDS 5:S1, 1991.
87. Kreiss JK, Koech D, Plummer FA, et al: AIDS virus infection in Nairobi prostitutes. Spread of the epidemic to East Africa. N Engl J Med 314:414, 1986.
88. Mann JM, Nzilambi N, Piot P, et al: Human immunodeficiency viral infection and associated risk factors in female prostitutes in Kinshasa, Zaire. AIDS 2:255, 1988.
89. Piot P, Plummer FS, Rey MA, et al: Retrospective seroepidemiology of AIDS virus infection in Nairobi populations. J Infect Dis 155:1108, 1987.
90. Holmberg SD, Horsburgh CR, Ward JW, Jaffe HW: Biologic factors in the sexual transmission of human immunodeficiency viruses. J Infect Dis 160:116, 1989.
91. Goedert JJ, Eyster ME, Bigger RJ, et al: Heterosexual transmission of human immunodeficiency virus: Association with severe depletion of T-helper lymphocytes in men with hemophilia. AIDS Res Hum Retroviruses 4:355, 1987.
92. Wasserheit JN: Epidemiological synergy: Interrelationships between human immunodeficiency virus infection and other sexually transmitted diseases. Sex Transm Dis 19:61, 1992.
93. Otten M, Zaidi AA, Peterman TA, et al: High rate of HIV seroconversion among patients attending urban sexually transmitted disease clinics. AIDS 8:549, 1994.
94. Quinn TC, Glasser D, Cannon RO, et al: Human immunodeficiency virus infection among patients attending clinics for sexually transmitted diseases. N Engl J Med 318:197, 1988.
95. Latif AS, Katzenstein DA, Bassett MT, et al: Genital ulcers and transmission of HIV among couples in Zimbabwe. AIDS 3:519, 1989.
96. Laga M, Manoka A, Kivuvu M, et al: Non-ulcerative sexually transmitted diseases as risk factors for HIV-1 transmission in women: Results from a cohort study. AIDS 7:95, 1993.
97. Laga M, Diallo MO, Buve A: Inter-relationship of sexually transmitted diseases and HIV: Where are we now? AIDS 8(Suppl 1):S119, 1994.
98. World Health Organization: An Overview of Selected Curable Sexually Transmitted Diseases. Global Programme on AIDS. Geneva, World Health Organization, 1995.
99. Laga M, Alary M, Nzila N, et al: Condom promotion, sexually transmitted diseases treatment, and declining incidence of HIV-1 infection in female Zairian sex workers. Lancet 344:246, 1994.
100. Laga M: STD control for HIV prevention—It works. Lancet 346:518, 1995.
101. Hanenberg RS, Rojanapithayakorn W, Kunasol P, Sokal DC: Impact of Thailand's HIV-control programme as indicated by the decline of sexually transmitted diseases. Lancet 344:243, 1994.
102. Grosskurth H, Mosha F, Todd J, et al: Impact of improved treatment of sexually transmitted diseases on HIV infection in rural Tanzania: Randomised controlled trial. Lancet 346:530, 1995.
103. Wawer MJ: Community-based mass treatment of sexually transmitted diseases (Abstr). Presented at the International Society for Sexually Transmitted Diseases Research; August 27–31, 1995; New Orleans.
104. The Working Group on Mother-to-Child Transmission of HIV: Rates of mother-to-child transmission of HIV-1 in Africa, America, and Europe: Results from 13 perinatal studies. J Acquir Immune Defic Syndr Hum Retrovirol 8:506, 1995.
105. Peckham C, Gibb D: Mother-to-child transmission of the human immunodeficiency virus. N Engl J Med 333:298, 1995.
106. St. Louis M, Kamenga M, Brown C, et al: Risk for perinatal HIV-1 transmission according to maternal immunologic, virologic, and placental factors. JAMA 269:2853, 1993.
107. Burns DN, Landesman S, Muenz LR, et al: Cigarette smoking, premature rupture of membranes, and vertical transmission of HIV-1 among women with low $CD4^+$ levels. J Acquir Immune Defic Syndr 7:718, 1994.
108. Weisner B, Nachman S, Tropper P, et al: Quantitation of human immunodeficiency virus type 1 during pregnancy: Relationship of viral titer to mother-to-child transmission and stability of viral load. Proc Natl Acad Sci USA 91:8037, 1994.
109. Semba RLD, Miotti PG, Chiphangwi JD, et al: Maternal vitamin A deficiency and mother-to-child transmission of HIV-1. Lancet 343:1593, 1994.
110. Dunn DT, Newell ML, Ades AE, Peckham CS: Risk of human immunodeficiency virus type 1 transmission through breast-feeding. Lancet 340:585, 1992.
111. World Health Organization. Global Programme on AIDS. Consensus statement from the WHO/UNICEF consultation on HIV transmission and breast-feeding. Wkly Epidemiol Rec 67:177, 1992.
112. Centers for Disease Control and Prevention: U.S. Public Health Service recommendations for human immunodeficiency virus counseling and voluntary testing for pregnant women. MMWR Morbid Mortal Wkly Rep 44(RR-7):1, 1995.
113. Connor EM, Sperling RS, Gelber R, et al: Reduction of maternal-infant transmission of human immunodeficiency virus type 1 with zidovudine treatment. N Engl J Med 331:1173, 1994.
114. Strategies for prevention of perinatal transmission of HIV infection: Report of a consensus workshop, Siena, Italy, June 3–6, 1995. J AIDS Hum Virol 8:161, 1995.
115. European Collaborative Study: Caesarean section and risk of vertical transmission of HIV-1 infection. Lancet 343:1464, 1994.
116. Lallemant M, Le Coeur S, Tarantola D, et al: Antiretroviral prevention of HIV perinatal transmission (Letter). Lancet 343:1429, 1994.
117. Dabis F, Msellati P, Newell ML, et al: Methodology of intervention trials to reduce mother-to-child transmission of HIV with special attention to developing countries. AIDS 9(Suppl A):S67, 1995.
118. Des Jarlais DC, Friedman SR, Choopanya K, et al: International epidemiology of HIV and AIDS among injecting drug users. AIDS 6:1053, 1992.
119. Des Jarlais DC, Friedman SR, Friedmann P, et al: HIV/AIDS-related behavior change among injecting drug users in different national settings. AIDS 9:611, 1995.
120. Des Jarlais DC, Friedman SR, Sotheran JL, et al: Continuity and change within an HIV epidemic: Injecting drug users in New York City, 1984 through 1992. JAMA 271:121, 1994.
121. Waters JK, Estilio MJ, Clark GL, Corrick J: Syringes and needle

exchange as HIV/AIDS prevention for injection drug users. JAMA 271:115, 1994.
122. Lurie P, Reingold AC, Bowser B, et al: The Public Health Impact of Needle Exchange Programs in the United States and Abroad. Vol 1. Atlanta: Centers for Disease Control and Prevention, 1993.
123. Normand J, Vlahov D, Moses LE (eds): Preventing HIV Transmission: The Role of Sterile Needles and Bleach. Washington, DC, National Academy Press, 1995.
124. World Health Organization: Global Programme on AIDS. Geneva, World Health Organization, 1995. WHO/GPA/RID/PRS/95.1.
125. Centers for Disease Control and Prevention: Syringe exchange programs—United States, 1994–1995. MMWR Morbid Mortal Wkly Rep 44:684, 1995.
126. Des Jarlais DC, Hagan H, Friedman SR, et al: Maintaining low HIV seroprevalence in populations of injecting drug users. JAMA 274:1226, 1995.
127. Centers for Disease Control: Provisional Public Health Service interagency recommendations for screening donated blood and plasma for antibodies to the virus causing acquired immunodeficiency syndrome. MMWR Morbid Mortal Wkly Rep 34(1):1, 1985.
128. Ward JW, Holmberg SD, Allen JR: Transmission of human immunodeficiency virus (HIV) by blood transfusions screened as negative for HIV antibody. N Engl J Med 318:473, 1988.
129. Foster S, Buve A: Benefits of HIV screening of blood transfusions in Zambia. Lancet 346:225, 1995.
130. Centers for Disease Control: Recommendations for prevention of HIV transmission in health-care settings. MMWR Morbid Mortal Wkly Rep 36(Suppl 2):1S, 1986.
131. Gerberding JL: Management of occupational exposures to blood-borne viruses. N Engl J Med 332:444, 1995.
132. Centers for Disease Control: Public Health Service statement on management of occupational exposure to human immunodeficiency virus, including considerations regarding zidovudine postexposure use. MMWR Morbid Mortal Wkly Rep 39(RR-1):1, 1990.
133. Centers for Disease Control: Guidelines for prevention of transmission of human immunodeficiency virus and hepatitis B virus to health-care and public-safety workers. MMWR Morbid Mortal Wkly Rep 38(Suppl 6):1, 1989.
134. Centers for Disease Control: Update: Universal precautions for prevention of transmission of HIV, hepatitis B virus, and other bloodborne pathogens in health-care settings. MMWR Morbid Mortal Wkly Rep 37:377, 387, 1988.
135. Centers for Disease Control: Recommendations for preventing transmission of human immunodeficiency virus and hepatitis B virus to patients during exposure-prone invasive procedures. MMWR Morbid Mortal Wkly Rep 40(RR-8):1, 1991.
136. Centers for Disease Control: Update: Investigations of persons treated by HIV-infected health-care workers—United States. MMWR Morbid Mortal Wkly Rep 42:329, 1993.
137. Robert LM, Chamberland ME, Cleveland JL, et al: Investigations of patients of health care workers infected with HIV. Ann Intern Med 122:653, 1995.
138. Centers for Disease Control and Prevention: Human immunodeficiency virus transmission in household settings—United States. MMWR Morbid Mortal Wkly Rep 43:347, 1994.
139. Impact of HIV on delivery of health care in sub-Saharan Africa: A tale of secrecy and inertia (Editorial). Lancet 345:1315, 1995.
140. Stanford JL, Grange JM, Pozniak A: Is Africa lost? Lancet 338:557, 1991.
141. Miotti PG, Dallabetta G, Ndovi E, et al: HIV-1 and pregnant women: Associated factors, prevalence, estimate of incidence and role in fetal wastage in central Africa. AIDS 4:733, 1990.
142. Wawer M, Sewankambo N, Berkley S, et al: HIV incidence in a rural district of Uganda. BMJ 308:171, 1994.
143. U.S. Bureau of the Census: Trends and Patterns of HIV and AIDS Infection in Selected Developing Countries: Country Profiles: June 1994. Washington, DC, U.S. Bureau of the Census, 1994. Research Note 14.
144. Dada AJ, Oyewole F, Onofowokan R, et al: Demographic characteristics of retroviral infections (HIV-1, HIV-2, and HTLV-1) among female prostitutes in Lagos, Nigeria. J Acquir Immune Defic Syndr 269:2853, 1993.
145. Olaleye OD, Bernstein L, Ekweozor CC, et al: Prevalence of human immunodeficiency virus types 1 and 2 infections in Nigeria. J Infect Dis 167:710, 1993.
146. Swanevelder R: Fifth national HIV survey of women attending antenatal clinics, South Africa, October/November 1994. *In* Kustner H (ed): Epidemiological Comments, Vol 22, No 5. Washington, DC, U. S. Department of Health and Human Services, 1995, pp 90–100.
147. Dondero TJ, Curran JW: Excess deaths in Africa from HIV: Confirmed and quantified. Lancet 343:989, 1995.
148. Preble EA: Impact of HIV/AIDS on African children. Soc Sci Med 31:671, 1990.
149. Harries AD: Tuberculosis and human immunodeficiency virus infection in developing countries. Lancet 335:387, 1990.
150. DeCock KM, Soro B, Coulibaly I-M, Lucas SB: Tuberculosis and HIV infection in sub-Saharan Africa. JAMA 268:1581, 1992.
151. Weniger BG, Limpakarnjanarat K, Ungchusak K, et al: The epidemiology of HIV infection and AIDS in Thailand. AIDS 5(Suppl 2):S71, 1991.
152. Brown T, Sittirai W, Vanichseni S, Thisyakom U: The recent epidemiology of HIV and AIDS in Thailand. AIDS 8(Suppl 2):S131, 1994.
153. Kitayaporn D, Uneklabh C, Weniger BG, et al: HIV-1 incidence determined retrospectively among drug users in Bangkok, Thailand. AIDS 8:1443, 1994.
154. Naik TN, Sarkar S, Singh HL, et al: Intravenous drug users: A new high-risk group for HIV infection in India. AIDS 5:117, 1991.
155. Cheng H, Zhang J, Capizzi J, et al: Introduction of HIV-1 subtype E into Yunnan, China. Lancet 344:953, 1994.
156. Xia M, Kreiss JK, Holmes KK: Risk factors for HIV infection among drug users in Yunnan province, China: Association with intravenous drug use and protective effect of boiling reusable needles and syringes. AIDS 8:1701, 1994.
157. Nelson KE, Celentano DD, Supraset S, et al: Risk factors for HIV infection among young adult men in northern Thailand. JAMA 270:955, 1993.
158. Kitsiripornchai S: HIV-1 infection in young men entering the Royal Thai Army: Trends and demographic risk factors (Abstr). Presented at the Third International Conference on AIDS in Asia and the Pacific, Fifth National AIDS Seminar in Thailand; September 17–21, 1995; Chiang Mai, Thailand.
159. Brown T, Sittirai W: The HIV/AIDS epidemic in Thailand: Addressing the impact on children. *In* Asia-Pacific Population and Policy, No 35. Honolulu, HI, East-West Center Program on Population, 1995.
160. Rodrigues JJ, Mehendale SM, Shepherd ME, et al: Risk factors for HIV infection in people attending clinics for sexually transmitted diseases in India. BMJ 311:283, 1995.
161. Mehendale SM, Rodrigues JJ, Brookmeyer RS, et al: Incidence and predictors of human immunodeficiency virus type 1 seroconversion in patients attending sexually transmitted diseases clinics in India. J Infect Dis 172:1486, 1995.
162. World Health Organization: HIV and AIDS in the western Pacific region. *In* AIDS Surveillance Report: Western Pacific Region, No 5. Geneva, World Health Organization, 1995, pp 1–8.
163. Pan American Health Organization: AIDS Surveillance in the Americas. Quarterly Report. Washington, DC, Pan American Health Organization, 1995.
164. Centers for Disease Control and Prevention: Update: Impact of the expanded AIDS surveillance case definition. MMWR Morbid Mortal Wkly Rep 43:160, 1994.
165. Centers for Disease Control and Prevention: HIV/AIDS Surveillance Report. 6:1, 1994.
166. Gwinn M, Pappaioanou M, George JR, et al: Prevalence of HIV infection in childbearing women in the United States. Surveillance using newborn blood samples. JAMA 265:1704, 1991.
167. Rogers MF, Caldwell MB, Gwinn ML, Simonds RJ: Epidemiology of pediatric human immunodeficiency virus infection in the United States. Acta Paediatr Suppl 400:5, 1994.
168. Rosenberg PS: Scope of the AIDS epidemic in the United States. Science 270:1372, 1995.
169. Janssen RS, St. Louis ME, Satten G, et al: HIV infection among patients in U.S. acute-care hospitals: Strategies for the counseling and testing of hospital patients. N Engl J Med 327:445, 1992.
170. Kelen GD, Hexter DA, Hansen KN, et al: Trends in HIV infection among an inner-city emergency department patient popula-

tion: Implications for emergency department based HIV-screening programs. Clin Infect Dis 21:867, 1995.
171. Sawanpanyalert P, Ungchusak K, Thanprasertsuk S, Akarasewi P: HIV-1 seroconversion rates among female commercial sex workers, Chiang Mai, Thailand: A multi cross-sectional study. AIDS 8:825, 1994.
172. Wheeler VW, Radcliffe KW: HIV infection in the Caribbean. Int J STD AIDS 5:79, 1994.
173. Newton EAC, White FMM, Sokal DC, et al: Modeling the HIV/AIDS epidemic in the English-speaking Caribbean. Bull Pan Am Health Organ 28:239, 1994.
174. The European Study Group: European Community Concerted Action on HIV seroprevalence among sexually transmitted disease patients in 18 European sentinel networks. AIDS 7:393, 1993.
175. Kozlov AP, Volkova GV, Malykh AG, et al: Epidemiology of HIV infection in St. Petersburg, Russia. J Acquir Immune Defic Syndr 6:208, 1993.
176. Canosa CA: Epidemiology of HIV infection in children in Europe. Acta Paediatr Suppl 400:8, 1994.
177. Pokrovsky VV, Eramova IY, Arzamastsev VP, et al: Epidemiology of human immunodeficiency virus (HIV) infection in the USSR. Zh Mikrobiol Epidemiol Immunobiol 2:26, 1990.
178. Melnick SL, Sherer R, Louis TA, et al: Survival and disease progression according to gender of patients with HIV infection. JAMA 272:1915, 1994.
179. Hogg RS, Strathdee SA, Craib KJP, et al: Lower socioeconomic status and shorter survival following HIV infection. Lancet 344:1120, 1994.
180. Baltimore D: Lessons from people with nonprogressive HIV infection. N Engl J Med 332:259, 1995.
181. Osmond D, Charlebois E, Lang W, et al: Changes in AIDS survival time in two San Francisco cohorts of homosexual men, 1983 to 1993. JAMA 271:1083, 1994.
182. Schrager LK, Young JM, Fowler MG, et al: Long-term survivors of HIV-1 infection: Definitions and research challenges. AIDS 8(Suppl 1):S95, 1994.
183. Ngaly B, Ryder RW, Kapita B, et al: Human immunodeficiency virus infection among employees in an African hospital. N Engl J Med 319:1123, 1988.
184. Mann JM, Kapita B, Colebunders RL, et al: Natural history of HIV infection in Zaire. Lancet 2:707, 1986.
185. Polk BF, Fox R, Brookmeyer R, et al: Predictors of the acquired immunodeficiency syndrome developing in a cohort of seropositive homosexual men. N Engl J Med 317:1114, 1987.
186. Allain JP, Laurian Y, Paul DA, et al: Long-term evaluation of HIV antigen and antibodies to p24 and gp41 in patients with hemophilia: Potential clinical importance. N Engl J Med 317:1114, 1987.
187. Spira TJ, Kaplan JE, Feorino PM, et al: Human immunodeficiency virus viremia as a prognostic indicator in homosexual men with lymphadenopathy syndrome. N Engl J Med 317:1093, 1987.
188. Moss AR, Bacchetti P, Osmond D, et al: Seropositivity for HIV and the development of AIDS or AIDS-related condition: Three-year follow-up of the San Francisco General Hospital cohort. Br Med J 269:745, 1988.
189. Baillou A, Barin F, Allain JP, et al: Human immunodeficiency virus antigenemia in patients with AIDS and AIDS related disorders: A comparison between Europe and Central African populations. J Infect Dis 156:830, 1987.
190. Mellors JW, Kingsley LA, Rinaldo CR Jr, et al: Quantitation of HIV-1 RNA in plasma predicts outcome after seroconversion. Ann Intern Med 122:573, 1995.
191. Quinn TC, Piot P, McCormick JB, et al: Serologic and immunologic studies in patients with AIDS in North America and Africa. The potential of infectious agents as cofactors in human immunodeficiency virus infection. JAMA 257:2617, 1987.
192. Bartholomew C, Blattner W, Cleghorn F: Progression to AIDS in homosexual men co-infected with HIV and HTLV-1 in Trinidad (Letter). Lancet 2:1469, 1987.
193. Schechter M, Harrison LH, Halsey NA, et al: Coinfection with human T-cell lymphotropic virus type 1 and HIV in Brazil. JAMA 271:353, 1994.
194. Raviglione MC, Snider DE, Kochi A: Global epidemiology of tuberculosis. Morbididity and mortality of a worldwide epidemic. JAMA 273:220, 1995.
195. Perriens JH, Colebunders RL, Karahunga C, et al: Increased mortality and tuberculosis treatment failure rate among human immunodeficiency virus (HIV) seropositive compared with HIV seronegative patients with pulmonary tuberculosis treated with "standard" chemotherapy in Kinshasa, Zaire. Am Rev Respir Dis 144:750, 1991.
196. Ackah A, Coulibaly D, Digbeau H, et al: Response to therapy, mortality, and CD4+ lymphocyte counts in HIV-infected persons with tuberculosis in Abidjan, Côte d'Ivoire. Lancet 344:1323, 1994.
197. Espinal MA, Reingold AL, Koenig E, et al: Screening for active tuberculosis in HIV testing centre. Lancet 345:890, 1995.
198. Narian JP, Raviglione MC, Kochi A: HIV-associated tuberculosis in developing countries: Epidemiology and strategies for prevention. Tuber Lung Dis 73:311, 1992.
199. Garcia Garcia L, Valdespino Gomez JL, Garcia Sancho MC, et al: Epidemiology of AIDS and tuberculosis. Bull Pan Am Health Organ 29:37, 1995.
200. DeCock KM, Lucas SB, Lucas S, et al: Clinical research, prophylaxis, therapy, and care for HIV disease in Africa. Am J Public Health 83:1385, 1993.
201. DeCock KM: Screening for tuberculosis and HIV in resource-poor countries. Lancet 345:873, 1995.
202. World Health Organization: WHO Report on the Tuberculosis Epidemic, 1995. Geneva, World Health Organization, 1995. WHO/TB/95.183.
203. Small PM, Schecter GF, Goodman PC, et al: Treatment of tuberculosis in patients with advanced human immunodeficiency virus infection. N Engl J Med 324:289, 1991.
204. Centers for Disease Control: National action plan to combat multidrug-resistant tuberculosis. MMWR Morbid Mortal Wkly Rep 41(RR-11):1, 1992.
205. Centers for Disease Control and Prevention: Tuberculosis morbidity—United States, 1994. MMWR Morbid Mortal Wkly Rep 44:387, 1995.
206. Selwyn PA, Hartel D, Lewis VA, et al: A prospective study of the risk of tuberculosis among intravenous drug users with human immunodeficiency virus infections. N Engl J Med 320:545, 1989.
207. DeCock KM, Wilkinson D: Tuberculosis control in resource-poor countries: Alternative approaches in the era of HIV. Lancet 346:675, 1995.
208. Alwood K, Keruly J, Moore-Rice K, et al: Effectiveness of supervised, intermittent therapy for tuberculosis in HIV-infected patients. AIDS 8:1103, 1994.
209. Weis SE, Slocum PC, Blais FX, et al: The effect of directly observed therapy on the rates of drug resistance and relapse in tuberculosis. N Engl J Med 330:1179, 1994.
210. Chin J: Current and future dimensions of the HIV/AIDS pandemic in women and children. Lancet 336:221, 1990.
211. Preble EA: Impact of HIV/AIDS on African children. Soc Sci Med 31:671, 1990.
212. Mann JM, Chin J: AIDS: A global perspective. N Engl J Med 319:302, 1988.
213. Quinn TC, Zacarias FR, St. John RK: AIDS in the Americas: An emerging public health crisis (Editorial). N Engl J Med 320:1005, 1989.
214. Ngugi EN, Plummer FA, Simonsen JN, et al: Prevention of transmission of human immunodeficiency virus in Africa: Effectiveness of condom promotion and health education among prostitutes. Lancet 2:887, 1988.
215. Quinn TC, Kline R, Francis H, et al: Rapid latex agglutination assay using recombinant envelope polypeptide for the detection of antibody to the human immunodeficiency virus. JAMA 260:510, 1988.
216. Des Jarlais DC, Friedman SR, Stoneburner RL: HIV infection and intravenous drug use: Critical issues in transmission dynamics, infection, outcome and prevention. Rev Infect Dis 10:151, 1988.
217. Brickner PW, Torres RA, Barnes M, et al: Recommendations for control and prevention of human immunodeficiency virus infection in intravenous drug users. Ann Intern Med 110:833, 1989.
218. Greenberg AE, Nguyen-Dinh P, Mann JM, Kabote N: The association between malaria, blood transfusion, and HIV seropositivity in a pediatric population in Kinshasa, Zaire. JAMA 259:545, 1988.

122

Pulmonary Infections in Patients with Human Immunodeficiency Virus Infections

Philip C. Hopewell

The disorder that is now known as the acquired immunodeficiency syndrome (AIDS) was first identified when an unusual number of cases of *Pneumocystis carinii* pneumonia were recognized in homosexual men in California and New York.[1,2] Since the first reports of AIDS, the lungs have continued to be a frequent site of disease; *P. carinii* pneumonia, either alone or in combination with other opportunistic processes, has been the AIDS-defining diagnosis in up to 65% of reported cases, although this percentage has now decreased, presumably because of the widespread use of prophylaxis. Moreover, because reporting criteria have changed, most cases (85% in 1995) are defined by having less than 200 CD4⁺ T lymphocytes per mm³ of blood. In 1995, *P. carinii* pneumonia was the indicator diagnosis in 18% of the reported AIDS cases, still the largest single specific disease.[3] As experience with human immunodeficiency virus (HIV) infection has grown, so has the understanding of the broad array of both infectious and noninfectious disorders that occur in patients infected with HIV.[4–7]

In this chapter, I describe the pulmonary infections that occur in association with HIV infection and discuss how their management differs from management in patients not infected with HIV. In addition, a general approach to diagnosis of lung disease in the setting of HIV infection is presented. The reader is referred to the sections dealing with specific organisms for more detailed discussions of the diagnosis and general management of the disorders described in this chapter.

Natural History of Human Immunodeficiency Virus Infection

Knowledge of the natural history of HIV infection is useful in guiding the approach to evaluation of patients with lung disease. Awareness of the lung diseases that are likely to occur at the various stages of HIV infection makes possible application of appropriate diagnostic tests and empirical treatment until specific diagnoses can be established. Moreover, various preventive interventions are most effective at different stages of HIV infection.

Data from several studies describe indicators that predict the risk for progression to AIDS and thus are markers for the stage of HIV disease. In all studies, a lower number of circulating CD4⁺ lymphocytes (helper T cells) on enrollment correlated with an increased rate of developing AIDS. In addition, a progressive reduction in CD4⁺ cells was strongly associated with the risk for AIDS. The risk for AIDS has also been shown to be related directly to β_2-microglobulin concentration and HIV p24 antigenemia and inversely to level of HIV antibody, hemoglobin concentration, and platelet count.[8–14] Direct measurements of the amount of HIV in blood have been used to provide a more precise estimation of the activity of the process and to predict the progression to AIDS and survival.[15,16] In spite of the better precision and more direct inferences that can be drawn from HIV measurements, there is not sufficient information to relate these measurements to the likelihood of various pulmonary disorders. Clinical predictors of progression have also been identified—thrush (oral candidiasis), hairy leukoplakia, constitutional symptoms (unexplained fever and weight loss), and persistent unexplained diarrhea.

Particularly noteworthy was the finding by Moss and associates[13]; the men in their cohort who did not develop AIDS or other HIV-associated conditions nevertheless experienced a progressive reduction in the absolute number of CD4⁺ cells during the 3-year period of observation. The median CD4⁺ cell count in this subgroup fell from a baseline value of 626 to 428/mm³ at the end of 3 years, in consistent decrements of approximately 65 to 70 cells per year. This observation is indicative of the chronic, progressive nature of HIV disease during a time when it is subclinical.

The data provided by Moss and coworkers,[13] as well as those of other investigators, strongly suggest that the current most useful means of determining the stage of HIV disease in relation to the kinds of complications that can be anticipated is to measure the number of circulating CD4⁺ lymphocytes. Figure 122–1 presents a conceptualization of the effects of HIV infection on circulating CD4⁺ lymphocytes with time, showing the numbers of cells present in groups of patients with various HIV-associated diseases. Although the slope (rate of decline) of the terminal portion of the curve is not known, it is well established that the AIDS-defining opportunistic diseases generally do not occur until there is marked CD4⁺ cell depletion—usually less than 200 cells per mm³. It

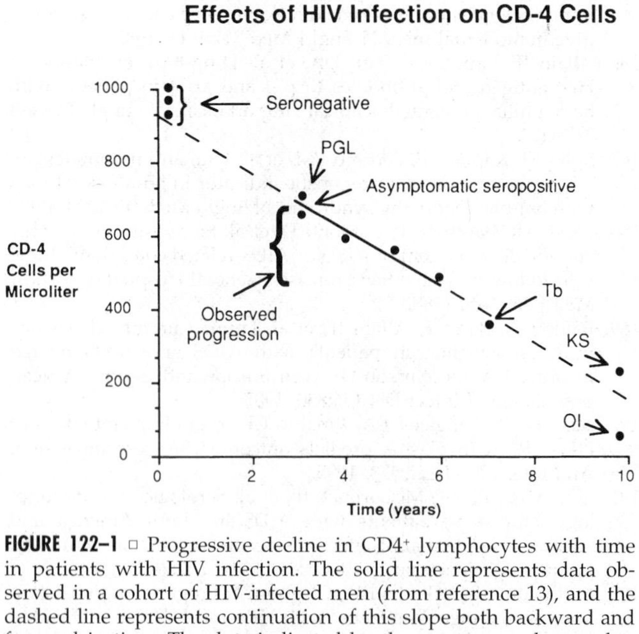

FIGURE 122–1 □ Progressive decline in CD4⁺ lymphocytes with time in patients with HIV infection. The solid line represents data observed in a cohort of HIV-infected men (from reference 13), and the dashed line represents continuation of this slope both backward and forward in time. The dots indicated by the arrows are the number of CD4⁺ lymphocytes found in seronegative persons and in persons with different HIV-related conditions. PGL, Progressive generalized lymphadenopathy; Tb, tuberculosis; KS, Kaposi's sarcoma; OI, opportunistic infection. (From Hopewell PC: Human immunodeficiency virus–associated lung disease: An overview. Semin Respir Infect 4:73–74, 1989.)

is also clear that other pulmonary infections, tuberculosis, for example, may occur with milder degrees of immune compromise.

Effects of Human Immunodeficiency Virus Infection on Lung Defenses

Because of the central role of the CD4+ lymphocyte in immune-mediated lung defenses, HIV infection has a progressive and ultimately profound effect on the ability of the lung to ward off or contain pathogenic organisms. As shown in Figure 122–2, the CD4+ cell is crucial to the functioning of alveolar macrophages and natural killer cells, and it conditions the response of B lymphocytes to specific antigens.[17] Moreover, HIV is known to infect macrophages and dendritic cells, perhaps interfering with their function; thus, HIV infection has a multifactorial effect on the ability of the lungs to respond to infectious agents.[17]

The most apparent HIV-induced abnormalities in host defenses involve cell-mediated immunity. Thus, the usual pathogens are those that induce a cell-mediated response. The suppression of this arm of the immune system is manifested clinically by reduction in reactivity to intradermally administered antigens such as tuberculin. The decrease in reactivity becomes more marked as the stage of HIV disease advances.[18] For example, in one study, 80% of patients with tuberculosis who were HIV infected but did not have AIDS had reactive tuberculin tests (at least 10 mm of induration), whereas in a second study, 49% of the patients with tuberculosis who subsequently developed AIDS and 25% of those who had AIDS when tuberculosis was diagnosed had reactive results.[19, 20]

Although the major HIV-induced abnormalities relate more to cell-mediated immunity than to humoral defenses, humoral immunity is nevertheless impaired. This is most clearly manifested by a diminished antibody response to specific antigens. Several studies have shown that increments in antibody concentrations produced by administration of pneumococcal or influenza vaccine are significantly smaller in subjects with more advanced HIV infection.[21, 22] Whether this observation is relevant to the increased frequency of pneumococcal pneumonia in HIV-infected persons is not clear.

Data from prospective cohort studies have shown that there is an increased frequency of lung disease throughout the course of HIV disease, or at least beginning well before the stage of advanced immunosuppression is reached. In early and midcourse HIV disease, acute bronchitis is the most frequent pulmonary disease encountered.[7] Pyogenic bacterial pneumonia and tuberculosis may occur at any point, early or late. *P. carinii* pneumonia and *Mycobacterium avium* complex disease occur only in patients with advanced immune suppression. The stage of HIV disease at which a given pathogen causes lung disease presumably relates to the virulence or pathogenicity of the organism. Thus, it is the interaction between host and parasite, or more precisely between the immune response and virulence factors of the organism, that determines when the organism will cause disease.

Pyogenic Bacterial Pneumonia

Although the frequency of pyogenic bacterial infections of the lung is not well quantified in HIV-infected patients, it is clear that the risk is greater than for persons without HIV infection.[6, 7, 23, 24] The organisms most often involved are *Streptococcus pneumoniae* and *Haemophilus influenzae,* both encapsulated organisms (although some strains of *H. influenzae* are not encapsulated).[24, 25] The clinical manifestations of pneumonia caused by these organisms in HIV-infected patients are not substantially different from the features of the diseases

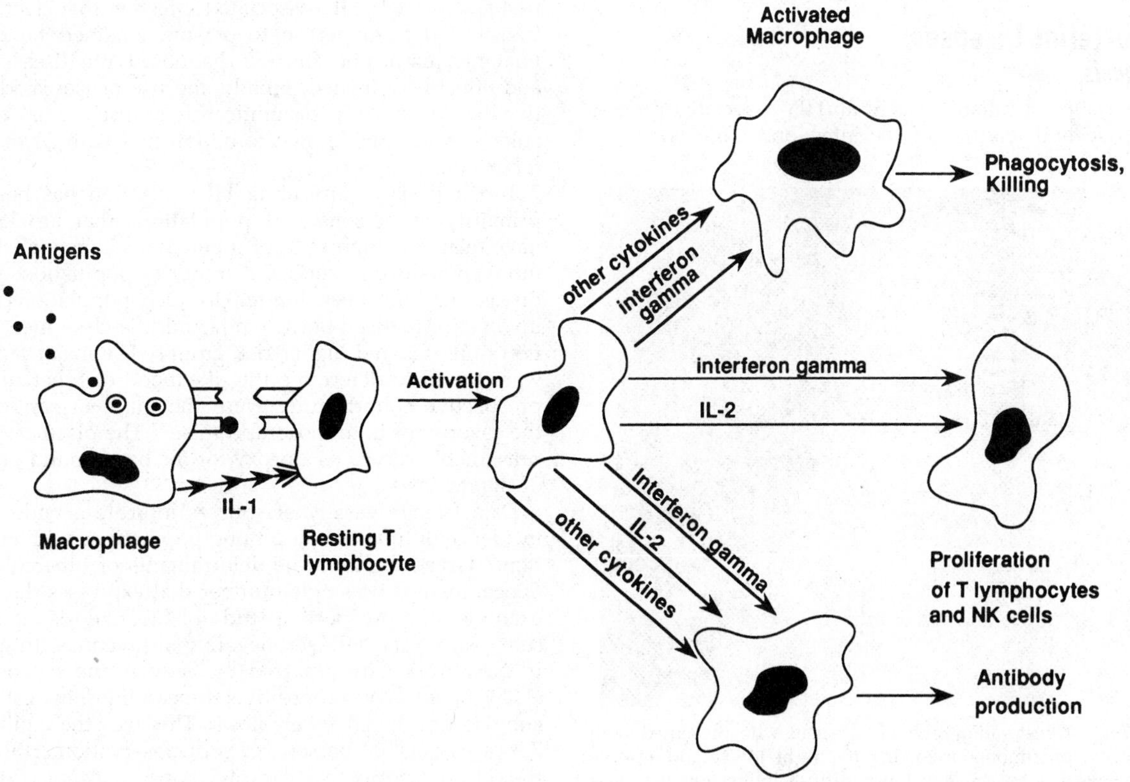

FIGURE 122–2 □ Interaction of CD4+ lymphocytes with other immune effector cells. IL-1, Interleukin-1; IL-2, interleukin-2; NK, natural killer.

in patients without HIV infection; however, multilobar involvement and bacteremia appear to be more common in the presence of HIV infection.

The approach to diagnosis is essentially the same as in an immunocompetent host. The diagnosis is usually suggested by the acuteness of the disease and the presence of a productive cough. Chest radiographs typically show focal consolidation, although diffuse infiltration may be seen occasionally and cavitation may occur, especially with type III *S. pneumoniae*. The diagnosis can be established by Gram stain and culture of the sputum; however, the results of sputum culture for *S. pneumoniae* may be falsely negative, and microscopic examination of Gram-stained sputum may be definitive. Blood cultures should also be obtained from any patient suspected of having pyogenic bacterial pneumonia. Other potentially diagnostic specimens, such as pleural or cerebrospinal fluid, should be obtained when the clinical situation indicates.

In spite of the greater frequency of bacteremia and multilobar involvement, the response to therapy of both pneumococcal and *H. influenzae* pneumonia tends to be good—or at least not worse than in the absence of HIV infection.[23, 25] Cefuroxime or another second-generation cephalosporin is reasonable empirical therapy until a specific diagnosis is established. Once an organism is identified, the spectrum of antimicrobial coverage can be narrowed. Failure to respond to what should be adequate therapy, or exacerbation after initial improvement, should suggest either that the diagnosis was wrong or that another disease has emerged, as in the patient whose chest films are shown in Figure 122–3.

Not all pyogenic bacterial pneumonias in patients with HIV infection are caused by *S. pneumoniae* or *H. influenzae*. The frequency of *Staphylococcus aureus* pneumonia may also be increased, and unusual pathogens are also found. The patient whose chest film is shown in Figure 122–4 had pneumonia and lung abscess caused by *Rhodococcus equi*. *Pseudomonas* and *Klebsiella* species have also been reported, as have *Legionella*.

Mycobacterial Diseases

Tuberculosis

The importance of tuberculosis as an HIV-associated process relates to several features of the infection.[26] First is its frequency, especially in populations that have a high prevalence of preexisting tuberculous infection. Second, tuberculosis is perhaps the only HIV-associated infection that clearly can be transmitted from person to person, whether the person is HIV infected or not. Third, if diagnosed, the disease is easily and effectively treated. Finally, the use of isoniazid preventive therapy is likely to significantly reduce the risk for tuberculosis in persons known to be infected with *Mycobacterium tuberculosis*.

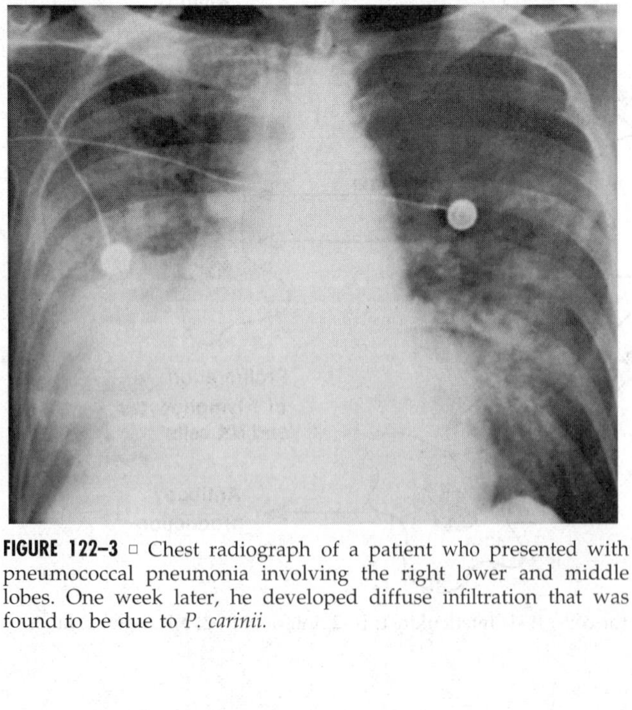

FIGURE 122–3 □ Chest radiograph of a patient who presented with pneumococcal pneumonia involving the right lower and middle lobes. One week later, he developed diffuse infiltration that was found to be due to *P. carinii*.

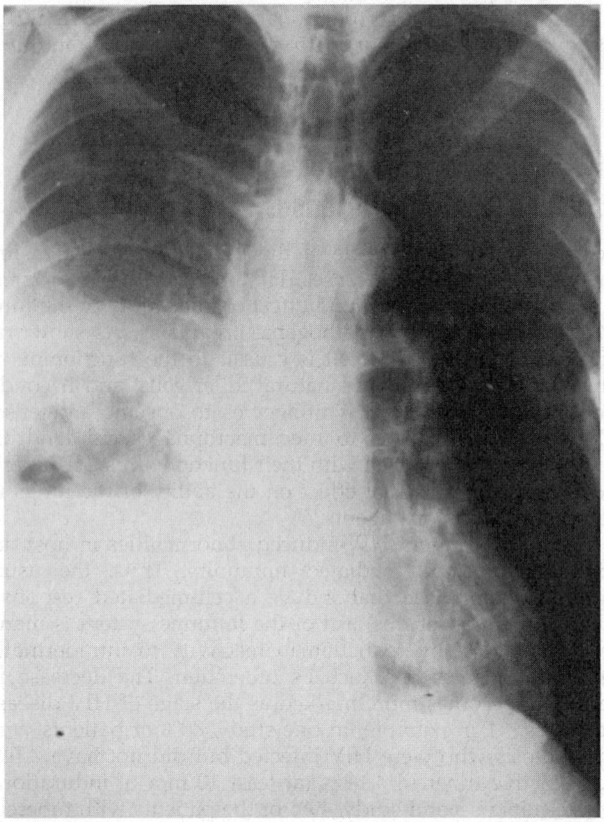

FIGURE 122–4 □ Chest radiograph of a patient showing a large lung abscess in the right lower hemithorax that was caused by *Rhodococcus equi*.

Tuberculosis complicating HIV infection has been noted primarily in persons and populations that are known to have relatively high rates of tuberculous infection—Haitians, intravenous drug users, and minority populations—but the disease has not been limited to such populations and has involved American-born, white, middle-class men in addition to recognized higher risk groups. The major factors that were found to determine the likelihood of tuberculosis in a prospective cohort study were the place of residence and the severity of immunocompromise.[27] The place of residence presumably served as a proxy for the background prevalence of tuberculosis.

Data from a variety of sources indicate a wide range of incidence of tuberculosis among populations with HIV infection.[26] Given the multiple determinants of tuberculosis incidence, there is no single number that expresses the risk. For example, in a prospective study of tuberculosis among HIV-seropositive and HIV-seronegative intravenous drug abusers in New York City reported by Selwyn and coworkers,[28] 7 (14%) of 49 HIV-seropositive, tuberculin skin test–positive subjects developed tuberculosis. This was the equivalent of 7.9 cases per 100 person-years of observation. However, in the cohort reported by Markowitz and colleagues,[27] the overall rate of tuberculosis was 0.76 per 100 person-years of observation. Within the cohort, the relative risk was 6.7 times greater among subjects from New York City and Newark compared with the subjects from Detroit, Chicago, Los Angeles, and San Francisco combined. Rates were significantly greater among persons with less than 200 CD4+ cells per mm^3 and among those with positive (5 mm or more) tuberculin reactions. Rates were not higher among anergic subjects.

The full impact of HIV infection on the epidemiology of tuberculosis has not been defined, either in the United States or in other countries. It is clear, however, that the influence is substantial. Assessment of the impact of HIV infection on the incidence of tuberculosis is hampered by there being few prospective studies that examine the prevalence of HIV among patients with tuberculosis. Data from Dade County, Florida, reported by Pitchenik and coworkers[29] showed that of 71 consecutive patients with tuberculosis, 22 (31%) had serologic evidence of HIV infection. Similar studies in San Francisco, which included only non–Asian-born adults, and in Seattle showed 29% and 23% rates of HIV seropositivity, respectively.[19, 30] In a longitudinal survey of the prevalence of HIV infection among patients in 13 tuberculosis clinics in the United States conducted by the Centers for Disease Control and Prevention, the seroprevalence rate increased from 13% in 1989 to 21% in 1991.[31] Data from other countries show much higher rates of HIV infection among persons with tuberculosis. As summarized by DeCock and associates,[32] various studies from Africa have reported the prevalence of HIV infection among patients with tuberculosis to range from 20% to 67%.

The clinical manifestations of tuberculosis in patients with HIV infection vary considerably, depending at what stage of HIV infection tuberculosis develops.[33] In most series, the majority of tuberculosis diagnoses have antedated the identification of nontuberculous, AIDS-defining disease. Apparently, the earlier tuberculosis develops, the more "usual" is its clinical presentation, whereas the later it occurs, the more atypical are its features.

Reports in the literature have emphasized that tuberculosis in persons with advanced HIV infection is frequently disseminated or involves extrapulmonary sites, has unusual radiographic manifestations, and commonly gives nonreactive tuberculin skin test results. Lymph node involvement, including intrathoracic adenopathy, was frequently described. In these series as well as in individual case reports, a variety of unusual manifestations have been noted—central nervous system involvement with brain abscesses, tuberculomas, and meningitis[30]; osteomyelitis[34]; pericarditis[34]; gastric tuberculosis[35]; tuberculous peritonitis[36]; and scrotal tuberculosis.[37] In addition, *M. tuberculosis* has been cultured from blood as well as from bone marrow.[38]

Despite the increased frequency of unusual forms of tuberculosis in persons with HIV infection, several reports have described a predominance of "standard" pulmonary disease.[19, 28] These reports presented series collected prospectively in which either tuberculosis patients had HIV antibody measured[19] or HIV-seropositive subjects were monitored for the development of tuberculosis.[28] Presumably, these patients' immunity was less profoundly compromised.

The atypical findings on chest radiographs of HIV-infected patients who have tuberculosis have received considerable emphasis. In retrospective studies, features that are not regarded as "typical" for pulmonary tuberculosis have been the norm.[26] Lower zone or diffuse lung infiltrations are often observed rather than the usual upper lobe involvement. Cavitation has been unusual, and intrathoracic adenopathy, an unusual finding in immunocompetent adults with tuberculosis, has been relatively frequent. Figure 122–5 shows a series of one patient's chest films made during a 17-day period. The initial finding was adenopathy (see Fig. 122–5*A*) that progressed to diffuse infiltration (see Fig. 122–5*B* and *C*) before a diagnosis of tuberculosis was established.

In the prospective study by Theuer and colleagues,[19] the radiographic findings in patients with HIV infection were indistinguishable from those in patients who were HIV-seronegative. The findings included typical upper lobe infiltration, often with cavitation.

Several additional radiographic features of tuberculosis in the setting of HIV infection are notable. Both in the cohort reported by Markowitz and colleagues[27] and in a retrospective analysis by Small and associates,[39] a substantial proportion (20% and 13.5%, respectively) had normal chest films. Small and coworkers[39] also described the evolution of radiographic findings with treatment of tuberculosis and noted that 10 of 13 (77%) patients who completed therapy and did not develop another pulmonary disease had complete resolution of the radiographic abnormalities.

As would be expected, persons with advanced HIV infection usually react minimally—or not at all—to the tuberculin skin test, but in earlier stages of the infection, reactivity may be sustained. The ability to respond to tuberculin is an indicator of the status of cell-mediated immunity, which in turn is an indicator of the stage of HIV infection. Most studies that describe the prevalence of reactive (at least 10 mm of induration) tuberculin tests indicate that approximately 40% of patients have positive reactions. In the study by Theuer and associates,[19] 80% of the HIV-seropositive patients with tuberculosis had positive tuberculin reactions. Because of the frequency of blunted skin test responses or anergy, it has been recommended that a reaction of at least 5 mm of induration to 5 tuberculin units of purified protein derivative be regarded as indicative of tuberculous infection in persons with HIV infection.[40]

Most reported series indicate that the prevalence of positive sputum smears and cultures in patients with pulmonary tuberculosis is the same among HIV-infected and noninfected persons.[27] In some instances, sputum induction or bronchoscopic procedures have been necessary to diagnose pulmonary tuberculosis. Specimens from any site of infection in patients who have or may have HIV infection should be examined for mycobacteria by smear and culture. Potential high-yield sources include lymph nodes, bone marrow, urine, and blood. Stool examinations that have been sensitive in detecting *M. avium* complex have not been useful for *M. tuberculosis*.

With a few notable exceptions, reported series of patients with tuberculosis and HIV infection demonstrate a good response to antituberculosis treatment,[26, 41] although in the series reported by Sunderam and coworkers,[34] there were three patients who had progressive disease and did not respond to the treatment. A case report from the same institution described a recurrence of tuberculosis in the scrotum after apparently successful treatment for pulmonary disease.[37] These reports have prompted concern about the adequacy of current standard 6-month therapy and subsequently recommendations that 9 months be the minimal duration of treatment for HIV-infected patients.[40, 42]

In a prospective study of treatment of tuberculosis in persons with HIV infection, Perriens and associates[43] showed that relapse rates were reduced by continuing therapy with isoniazid and rifampin for an additional 6 months for a total of 12 months of multidrug treatment. However, relapse rates in the HIV-infected group treated for 6 months were not different from the rate in the HIV-negative control group also treated for 6 months, and survival was not improved by the additional therapy.

Current recommendations indicate that for adult patients with HIV infection, treatment for tuberculosis should include

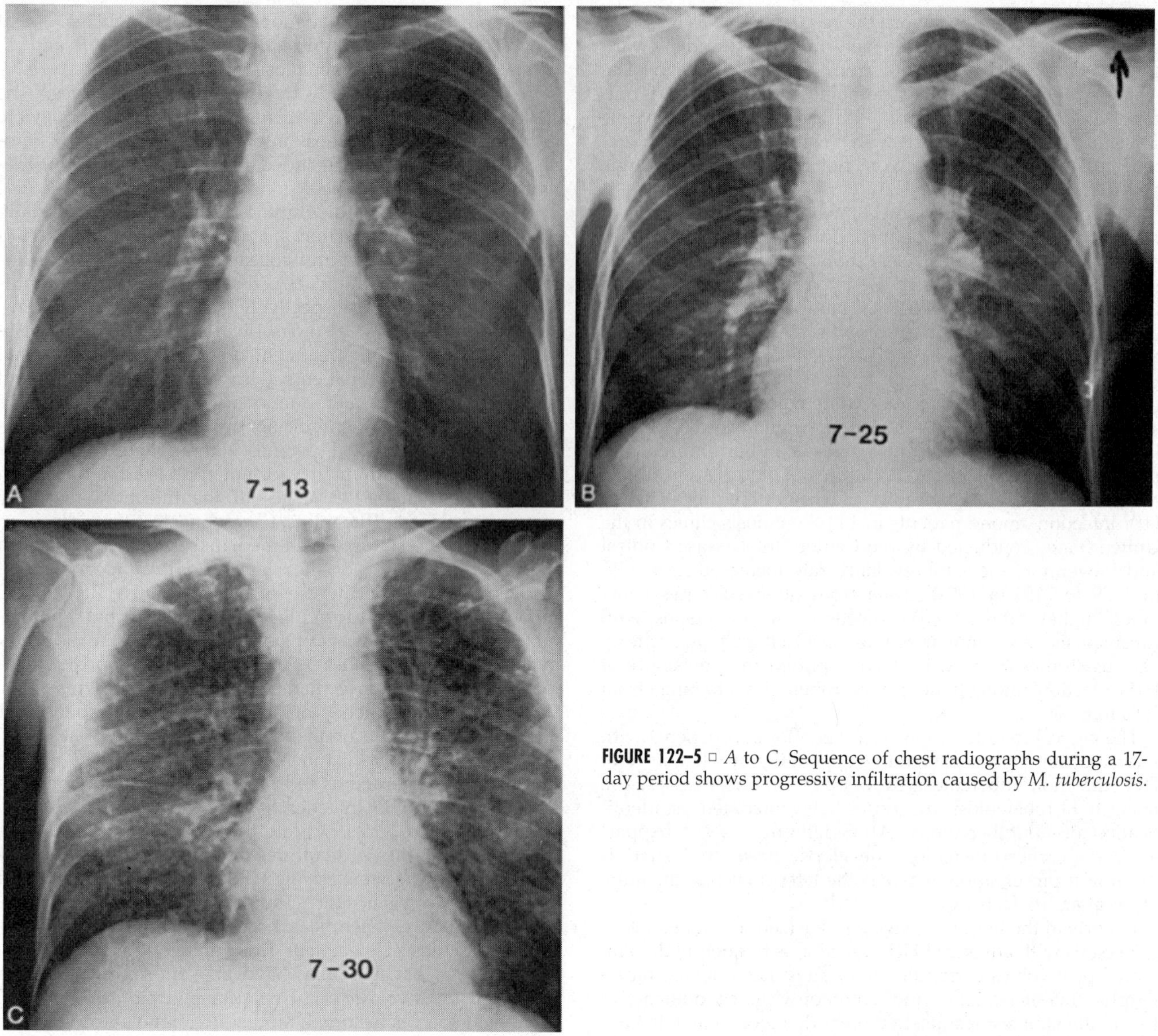

FIGURE 122–5 □ *A* to *C*, Sequence of chest radiographs during a 17-day period shows progressive infiltration caused by *M. tuberculosis*.

isoniazid at 300 mg/d, rifampin at 600 mg/d (450 mg for persons weighing less than 50 kg), ethambutol at 15 mg/kg per day, and pyrazinamide at 20 to 30 mg/kg per day during the first 2 months of therapy; isoniazid and rifampin should be continued for another 4 months, making the total duration of therapy 6 months.[44] Strong consideration should be given to administering therapy under direct observation to ensure adherence to the regimen. This can be facilitated by twice-weekly dosing after an initial phase of daily treatment.

Findings of at least one study suggested that persons with HIV infection have more adverse reactions to antituberculosis drugs,[20] so patients with HIV infection should be observed closely with appropriate laboratory and clinical monitoring.

Preventive therapy with isoniazid has been proved to be widely effective in preventing tuberculosis among various groups of persons with tuberculous infection, including persons infected with HIV.[45] For this reason, tuberculin testing should be a routine part of management of HIV infection. Patients who react with at least 5 mm of induration to 5 tuberculin units of purified protein derivative should be considered to have tuberculous infection and be offered preventive therapy. Although the usual recommended preventive therapy for persons with normal chest films is 6 months' treatment, 12 months' treatment is recommended for those who have HIV infection.[44]

Because tuberculosis is the only common HIV-associated infection that can be transmitted from person to person, including to persons who are not infected with HIV, it is extremely important that tuberculosis infection control measures be applied to persons with HIV infection. When patients are being evaluated because of respiratory symptoms or findings, respiratory precautions should be applied until tuberculosis is excluded. Sputum induction and bronchoscopy should be performed in areas with adequate ventilation and from which exhausted air is not recirculated to other parts of the building. Transmission of *M. tuberculosis* among persons with HIV infection has been documented in health care and residential facilities and has led to explosive outbreaks of tuberculosis.[46, 47]

Mycobacterium avium *Complex Disease*

Soon after the recognition of AIDS, it became apparent that a closely related group of nontuberculous mycobacteria, collectively named *M. avium* complex, was commonly isolated from multiple sites in patients with the syndrome.[48, 49] The occurrence of disseminated disease in patients without preexisting chronic lung disease who did not necessarily live in the southeastern United States, the major endemic focus of infection by *M. avium* complex, represented a major change in the epidemiology of the disease.

Because disseminated *M. avium* complex disease tends to occur late in the course of HIV infection, usually after another AIDS index diagnosis has been established, the true frequency is not known. It is clear, however, that among persons with HIV infection and less than 50 CD4+ lymphocytes per mm^3, disseminated *M. avium* complex disease is common if prophylactic therapy is not being given. In a study by Chin and coworkers,[50] 18% of a group of HIV-infected patients with CD4+ lymphocyte counts of 50/mm^3 or less who had not previously had disseminated *M. avium* complex disease and who were not receiving prophylaxis had the organism isolated from initial blood cultures obtained as part of an evaluation for symptoms. On continued follow-up of the patients who had negative initial cultures by Kaplan-Meier life table analysis, the cumulative probability of developing *M. avium* complex bacteremia was 32% after 6 months and 51% after 12 months.

Although in immunocompetent hosts the pathogenesis of *M. avium* complex disease involves recrudescence of latent infection, this does not appear to be the case in patients with HIV infection, for whom the epidemiologic patterns suggest progressive, recently acquired infection. How infection is acquired is not known, but the high frequency of gastrointestinal involvement suggests that the organism is ingested and the gut serves as the main portal of entry. However, in a study that attempted to identify environmental risk factors for acquisition of *M. avium* complex, Horsburgh and colleagues[51] were unable to find plausible environmental risks. Moreover, in a comprehensive environmental sampling, Yajko and associates[52] were able to isolate *M. avium* complex only from potting soil in house plant containers. Food and water, as well as other potential sources of oral acquisition, were not found to contain the organism.

In patients with advanced HIV infection, *M. avium* complex usually causes disseminated disease with involvement of bone marrow, lymph nodes, and multiple other organs. The organism can usually be isolated from blood. In the presence of dissemination, acid-fast bacilli may be seen in stool specimens and *M. avium* complex cultures; however, isolation from stool does not always indicate dissemination of the infection. Isolation of *M. avium* complex from either stool or respiratory tract specimens may precede subsequent disseminated disease.[53]

Much less commonly, *M. avium* complex may produce focal disease limited to the lung (Fig. 122–6). Endobronchial lesions may be seen at bronchoscopy, and these lesions contained granulomata in at least a few reports.[54] It has been speculated that this sort of involvement is more likely to occur in patients taking antiretroviral therapy who have had some restoration of immune function.

In most patients, *M. avium* involvement of tissues is characterized by large numbers of organisms and little or no inflammatory response. In spite of the widespread infiltration of organs and the large bacillary population, the disease is associated with surprisingly few clinical manifestations, presumably owing to the ablated host response produced by advanced HIV infection. The clinical features seen most often include fever, anemia, abdominal pain, and diarrhea.[55] Typically, intraabdominal lymph nodes are enlarged, sometimes markedly, and on computed tomographic scans have low-density, necrotic centers.[56] The diagnosis is usually established by isolating the organism from blood, bone marrow, lymph node (often by computed tomography–directed needle aspiration biopsy), or another organ.

Treatment of *M. avium* complex disease has improved dramatically, especially since the introduction of the new macrolide agents azithromycin and clarithromycin. Optimal regimens usually include a macrolide, rifabutin, and ethambutol. Several studies have indicated that a three-drug regimen, as before, is superior to two drugs.[57, 58]

For prevention of disseminated *M. avium* complex disease,

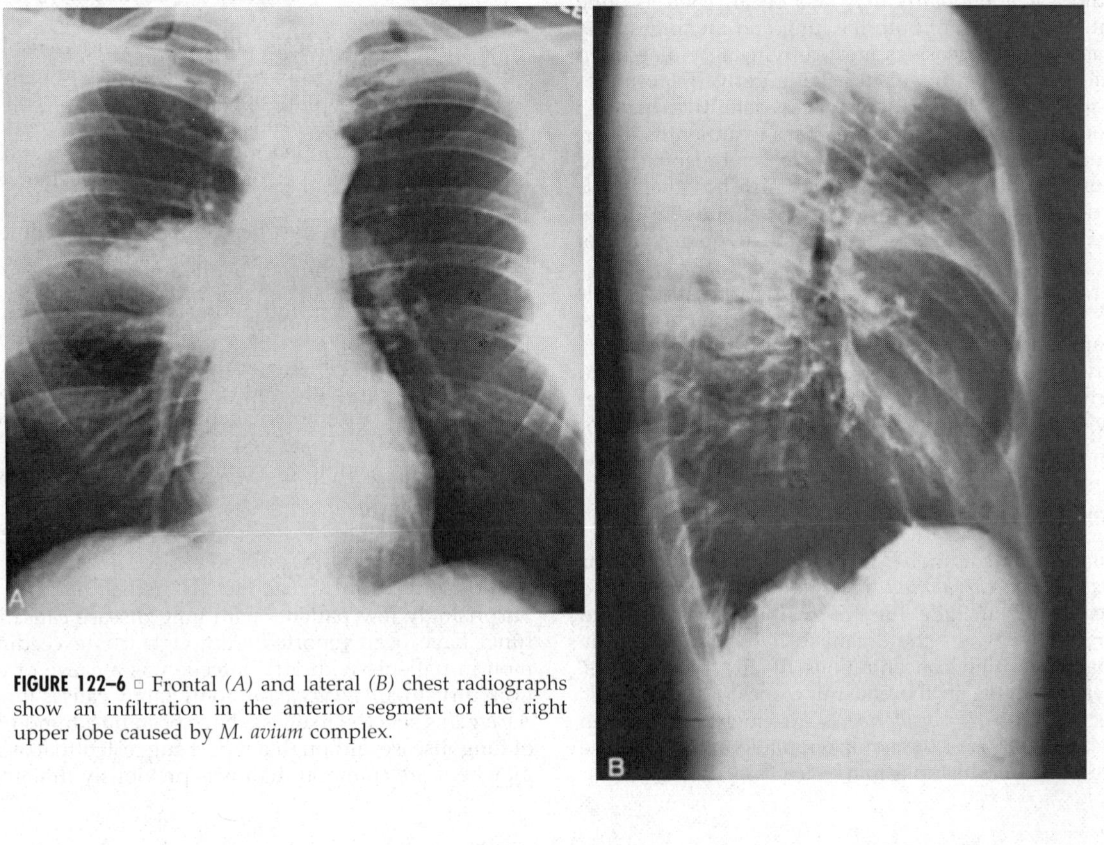

FIGURE 122–6 □ Frontal *(A)* and lateral *(B)* chest radiographs show an infiltration in the anterior segment of the right upper lobe caused by *M. avium* complex.

both clarithromycin and azithromycin have been shown to be effective and superior to rifabutin.[59, 60] Combinations of a macrolide with rifabutin have been somewhat more efficacious but have been associated with more side effects, particularly uveitis.

Infections with Other Nontuberculous Mycobacteria

Except for *M. avium* complex, infections with nontuberculous mycobacteria have been uncommon in patients with HIV infection. However, there are anecdotal suggestions that the frequency of disease caused by *Mycobacterium kansasii* is increasing. Through August 1987, only a total of 78 cases had been reported.[61] The *Mycobacterium* organisms that have been reported as index diagnoses or in isolated case reports include *M. kansasii, M. xenopi, M. scrofulaceum, M. szulgai, M. flavescens, M. gordonae, M. asiaticum,* and *M. malmoense.*[62]

Because of the infrequency of disease caused by these organisms, response to treatment and optimal regimens have not been described. *M. kansasii* would be expected to be responsive because of its susceptibility to standard antimycobacterial agents. The recommended regimen consists of isoniazid, rifampin, and ethambutol given for a minimum of 18 months.

Fungal Infections

Cryptococcosis

Disease caused by *Cryptococcus neoformans* is the most common fungal pulmonary infection in persons with AIDS, although the exact frequency is not known. The organism is thought to be widely distributed in the environment and to cause asymptomatic latent infections that later return, especially when immunosuppression occurs.

Cryptococcal pulmonary disease in HIV-infected patients takes several forms: focal consolidation, single or multiple nodular lesions, and interstitial infiltration.[67] Pleural effusions and intrathoracic adenopathy may also occur. There is often concurrent involvement of both the lung and meninges.[64]

Pulmonary cryptococcosis is most convincingly diagnosed by identification of the organism in lung-derived specimens from a patient with lung disease. Less definitive but still strong enough evidence on which to base treatment is detection of cryptococcal antigen in serum or cerebrospinal fluid in a patient who has lung disease for which no other cause has been demonstrated. Serum cryptococcal antigen test results can be false-negative, although the frequency is not known.

In general, AIDS patients with pulmonary cryptococcosis should be managed as if they have meningitis as well. A standard approach is to use amphotericin B, 0.7 to 0.8 mg/kg per day, for the initial phase (2 weeks) of therapy and then switch to oral fluconazole, 400 mg/d for the remainder of therapy (8 to 10 weeks).[65] Therapy is then maintained for the rest of the patient's life with fluconazole, 200 mg/d.

Histoplasmosis

Histoplasmosis is a common AIDS index diagnosis in areas where *Histoplasma capsulatum* is endemic. In the United States, these areas include the Mississippi, Missouri, and Ohio river valleys, where the organism lives predominantly in sites that have high concentrations of bird or bat feces. Among persons living in the endemic zones, asymptomatic latent infection with *H. capsulatum* is extremely common. In some areas, up to 80% of the adult population have positive skin test responses to histoplasmin.[66]

In persons with HIV infection, histoplasmosis may result from primary infection or recrudescence of latent infection. Because of the prevalence of primary infection in endemic zones and the potential for activation of latent infection, histoplasmosis may develop in persons who long ago moved from an endemic area and subsequently became immunocompromised. Thus, the disease should be considered in the differential diagnosis of lung disease in any patient with HIV infection, especially if the patient is known to have resided in an endemic area.

The clinical features of histoplasmosis in patients with HIV infection are nonspecific and include fever and weight loss and, when the lungs are involved, cough and dyspnea.[67] Lymphadenopathy, splenomegaly, and hepatomegaly are also common with disseminated disease, as is nearly always the case. Bone marrow involvement is extremely common and produces varying degrees of cytopenias.

The diagnosis of pulmonary histoplasmosis is established by identifying the organism in specimens obtained from the lungs. The organism may also be identified in blood, bone marrow, or other tissues and can be assumed to be the cause of lung disease if no other pathogen is found. The diagnosis can be strongly inferred from detection of *H. capsulatum* antigen in the blood or urine.[68] Standard serologic tests for antibodies are of little use in making a diagnosis.

Amphotericin B is the drug of choice for treating severe disseminated histoplasmosis in AIDS patients.[65] Itraconazole is probably as effective in less severe forms of the disease. Lifelong maintenance with itraconazole, 200 mg twice daily, has been shown to be successful in preventing relapse.[65]

Coccidioidomycosis

Like *H. capsulatum, Coccidioides immitis* has a limited endemic range in the United States, principally the southwestern states. The organism resides in soil and gains access to the body through the respiratory tract. The newly acquired infection may progress directly to disease or be contained and remain latent until, in the case of HIV infection, immunosuppression occurs.[69]

As with histoplasmosis, although the disease is much more prevalent in endemic areas, persons who acquire the infection in an endemic area may not develop the disease until much later, when they may reside elsewhere. Thus, coccidioidomycosis should be included in the differential diagnosis of pulmonary infection in persons with HIV infection, regardless of where they live.

Fever, cough, and dyspnea characterize the clinical presentation of coccidioidomycosis.[70] The radiographic features are nonspecific, bilateral nodules or reticulonodular infiltrates being most common. Intrathoracic adenopathy may also be present. The diagnosis requires histologic or cultural identification of *C. immitis* in specimens from the lungs. Intradermal tests and serologic studies are not useful in patients with HIV infection. Amphotericin B continues to be the drug of choice for AIDS-associated coccidioidomycosis.[65] Maintenance therapy should be continued with itraconazole or fluconazole.

Other Fungal Infections

Surprisingly few patients with lung disease caused by other fungi have been reported. Although it is exceedingly common in patients with HIV infection as a cause of oral infection (thrush), *Candida albicans* only rarely causes lung disease. *Aspergillus* species, likewise, have been uncommon as a cause of lung disease, although a report suggested that aspergillosis may be more common than was previously thought.[71]

Pneumocystis carinii Pneumonia

P. carinii pneumonia continues to be the most frequent cause of lung disease among persons with less than 200 $CD4^+$ lymphocytes per mm^3, in spite of wide use of effective prophylaxis.[7] As described previously, a major aspect of the natural history of HIV infection is progressive depletion of $CD4^+$ lymphocytes. Because *P. carinii* is not a particularly pathogenic organism, severe immune compromise, indicated by a marked reduction in $CD4^+$ lymphocytes, must be present for the organism to proliferate and cause disease. Masur and associates[72] have examined the circulating $CD4^+$ lymphocyte counts of HIV-infected patients and what related diseases were diagnosed at the time the counts were performed. Patients who were found to have *P. carinii* pneumonia had a median of 26 $CD4^+$ cells per mm^3 (interquartile range 12 to 62.5 cells per mm^3). In only 2 of 46 episodes of *P. carinii* pneumonia were the $CD4^+$ cell counts greater than 200 cells per mm^3. Similar results have been reported by Stansell and associates.[73]

The most common presenting symptoms of *P. carinii* pneumonia are fever, cough, and subsequently shortness of breath.[74] The shortness of breath usually progresses from being present only with exertion to being present at rest. Cough is generally nonproductive but may be associated with sputum in patients who smoke cigarettes or who have bacterial bronchitis or pneumonia as well as *P. carinii* pneumonia. At the time evaluation for *P. carinii* is undertaken, the respiratory symptoms may be prominent or relatively minor. Antiretroviral and antipneumocystis prophylaxis reduces the severity of *P. carinii* pneumonia if it does develop, so the presenting symptoms may be subtle. Conversely, patients who have not been under medical care and who do not readily seek medical attention may present with advanced pneumonia and marked symptoms.

For patients with *P. carinii* pneumonia, the physical examination is not particularly helpful; again, findings may be dominated by other HIV-associated diseases. Initial laboratory evaluation is also not especially helpful. Lymphopenia is common but not universal. As noted earlier, $CD4^+$ cell counts may be useful in identifying patients who have severe immune compromise and who, therefore, are at risk for having an opportunistic infection. A variety of other hematologic abnormalities, including anemia, leukopenia, and thrombocytopenia, may also occur.

On the chest radiograph, *P. carinii* most often causes diffuse interstitial infiltration involving all portions of the lungs equally.[75] Several variations of the basic pattern may be seen; the infiltration may be distributed somewhat unevenly throughout the lung or it may be more miliary in appearance (Figs. 122–7 and 122–8). Diffuse and focal airspace consolidation may also be caused by *P. carinii* pneumonia; this usually occurs as the disorder becomes more severe. Cystic changes or pneumatoceles have been noted, particularly during the healing process, as has cavitation within preexisting nodular lesions. Probably as an extension of the cystic or cavitary processes, spontaneous pneumothorax may occur (Fig. 122–9). Pleural effusions and intrathoracic adenopathy are uncommon.

There seems to be a general perception among clinicians caring for patients with *P. carinii* pneumonia that the frequency of unusual or "atypical" radiographic presentations is increasing. If true, it could be related simply to increasing experience with the disease, to the effects of antiviral therapy, or to the use of prophylaxis.

Arterial blood gas measurements are helpful in determining the severity of pulmonary involvement. Hypoxemia is frequent but not invariable, and hypocapnia may also be seen. An increase in the alveolar-to-arterial oxygen tension gradient, especially with exercise, has also been reported to be common in patients with *P. carinii* pneumonia.[76] Gallium-enhanced lung scanning has proved to be a sensitive although nonspecific test for the presence of *P. carinii* pneumonia, but because of the expense and time required for the study, it is not especially useful.

Although patients with *P. carinii* pneumonia often complain of cough, they rarely produce sputum that is suitable

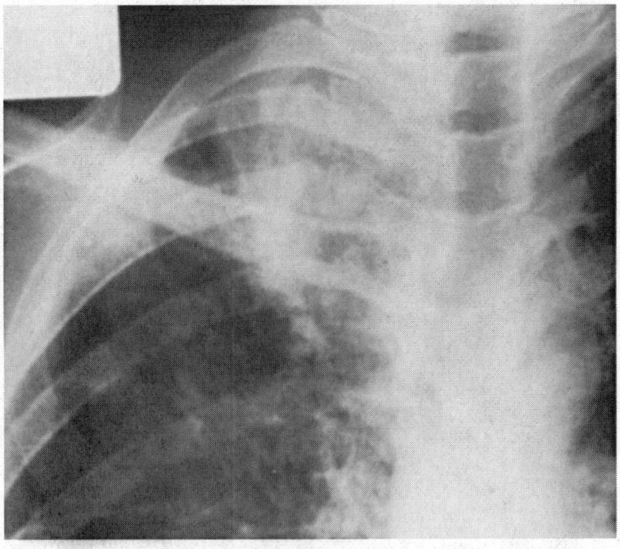

FIGURE 122–7 □ Detail of a frontal view chest radiograph shows a focal right upper lobe abnormality caused by *P. carinii.*

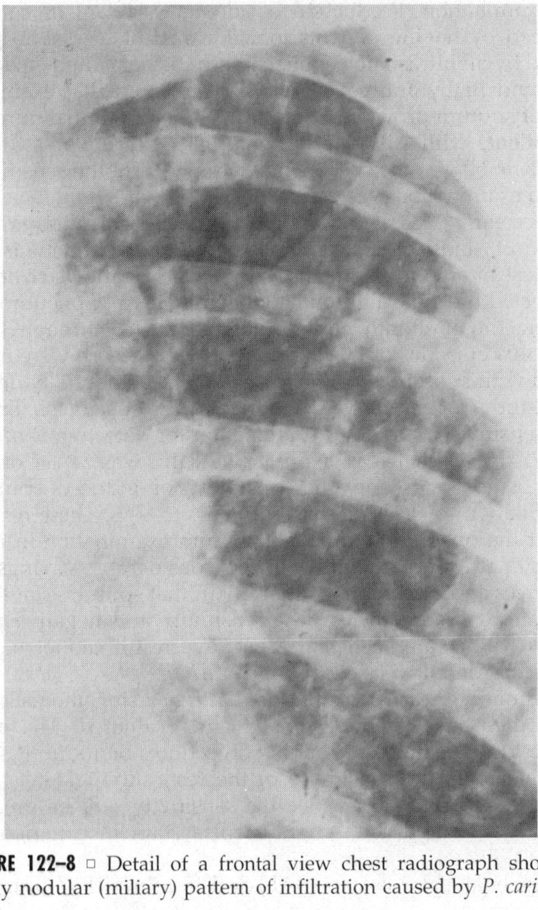

FIGURE 122–8 □ Detail of a frontal view chest radiograph shows a finely nodular (miliary) pattern of infiltration caused by *P. carinii.*

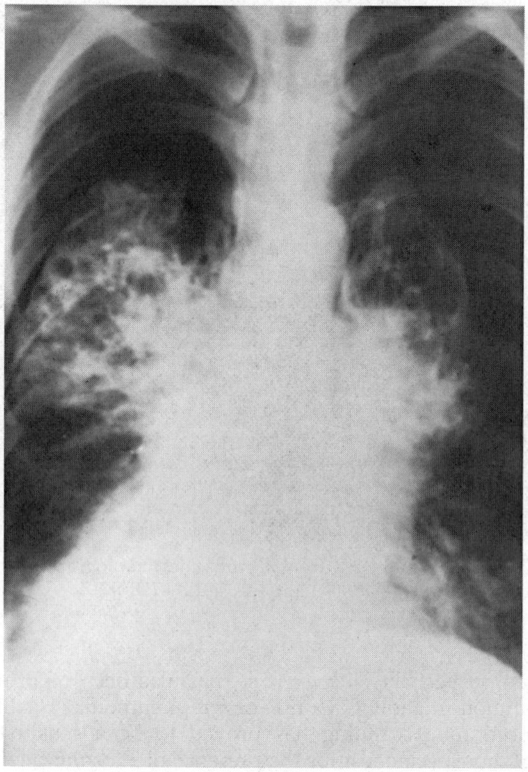

FIGURE 122–9 ▫ Chest radiograph showing bilateral spontaneous pneumothoraces and marked cystic changes in the lungs caused by *P. carinii.*

for examination. Production of adequate specimens can be induced by having patients inhale a mist of 3% saline produced by an ultrasonic nebulizer. Both Pitchenik and coworkers[77] and Bigby and colleagues[78] documented that examination of sputum provides a diagnosis for a substantial number of patients with AIDS. In both studies, *P. carinii* was found in 40% to 50% of the specimens examined, and the sensitivity of the examination was between 50% and 60%.

Since early 1986 at San Francisco General Hospital, examination of "induced sputum" has been used routinely as the first test in attempts to identify *P. carinii* in patients strongly suspected on clinical grounds of having *P. carinii* pneumonia. During the 10-month period September 1986 through June 1987, 404 episodes of HIV-associated lung disease were evaluated with sputum examination as the first potentially definitive study.[79] *P. carinii* was identified in 222 specimens (55%). The sensitivity of sputum examination for detecting *P. carinii* was 77%, and the negative predictive value was 64%. Consistently since that time, the sensitivity of induced sputum examination for *P. carinii* has been 75% to 80%. These results reflect the operational utility of sputum examination in routine practice and demonstrate the considerable savings of resources and discomfort to the patient that sputum examination affords. Nevertheless, the sensitivity and negative predictive values are such that a negative result cannot be regarded as definitively excluding *P. carinii.*

Immunofluorescent stains for *P. carinii* using monoclonal antibodies have been developed and evaluated. The data suggest that using these staining procedures on induced sputum increases the sensitivity of the test, although it is not clear that in routine practice the sensitivity will be greater than that of modified Wright-Giemsa stain in experienced hands.[80, 81]

Bronchoalveolar lavage (BAL) and transbronchial lung biopsy have proved sensitive in identifying pulmonary infections in AIDS patients. Stover and associates[82] reported the results of bronchoscopic procedures in 72 such patients. Both transbronchial biopsy and BAL had high yields (88% and 85%, respectively), and when they were used together, the yield was 94%. The yield was especially high for *P. carinii* (94%). Similar results were reported by Broaddus and coworkers,[83] who described the efficacy of BAL and transbronchial biopsy in detecting pulmonary pathogens in 276 fiberoptic bronchoscopic examinations performed on 171 patients known to have or suspected of having AIDS. Of 173 pathogens identified during the initial evaluation or in the subsequent month, the initial bronchoscopy detected 166 (96%). BAL and transbronchial biopsy had similar sensitivities of 86% (124 of 145) and 87% (133 of 153), respectively. For *P. carinii,* lavage had an 89% sensitivity and transbronchial biopsy was 97% sensitive. For patients who had both procedures performed, the sensitivity was 100%.

BAL alone has been reported by Golden and coworkers[84] to have a sensitivity for *P. carinii* of 97%. At the San Francisco General Hospital, we have reviewed our experience subsequent to the report by Broaddus and colleagues[83, 85] and found that only rarely was *P. carinii* identified in transbronchial biopsy specimens when it was not seen in BAL fluid. Thus, as a matter of course in patients known to have or suspected of having AIDS in whose sputum *P. carinii* is not found, we perform only BAL. If findings of that procedure are not diagnostic, the transbronchial biopsy is performed.

Empirical treatment remains controversial. On the negative side of the argument, another treatable process may be missed, and such an approach exposes the patient to the risks of therapy, perhaps without benefit. On the positive side, for patients who have classic clinical features, it has been demonstrated that a presumptive diagnosis can be established with a high degree of accuracy by experienced clinicians.[86] This approach may have some applicability for institutions that lack the capability of making diagnoses from induced sputum, but it does not seem to be justified when the majority of diagnoses can be established by this noninvasive and relatively inexpensive test.[85]

Treatment of *P. carinii* pneumonia in patients with AIDS is essentially the same as for patients with other forms of immunosuppression (see Chapter 292), but several points deserve mention. First, after therapy is instituted, patients with *P. carinii* pneumonia and AIDS tend to get sicker before they improve.[87] The response to a specific agent cannot be determined within the first 5 or 6 days of treatment. Second, adverse reactions to antipneumocystis agents are common in AIDS patients and tend to occur between days 5 and 15 of treatment. Third, patients with more severe forms of *P. carinii* pneumonia benefit from corticosteroid therapy. Several reports attest to the value of corticosteroid therapy in improving gas exchange in patients with severe *P. carinii* pneumonia.[88–91] There are several possible reasons that a corticosteroid might improve lung function in the setting of *P. carinii* pneumonia, so a benefit from this modality is plausible if the drug is given early in the course of disease.

Prophylaxis for *P. carinii* pneumonia has proved to be effective in and important for persons with HIV infection.[92, 93] Preventive therapy is indicated for patients who have any of the following: $CD4^+$ lymphocyte count less than 200/mm^3, unexplained and persistent fever, oral candidiasis, or prior *P. carinii* pneumonia. Trimethoprim-sulfamethoxazole is the prophylactic agent of choice. The superiority of trimethoprim-sulfamethoxazole has been convincingly demonstrated in prospective studies comparing the drug with aerosol pentamidine and with dapsone.[94, 95] The optimal regimen has not been clearly established. The best studied approach is one double-strength dose (160 mg of trimethoprim, 800 mg of sulfamethoxazole) daily, but twice- and thrice-weekly regimens may be equally effective. For persons who are intolerant of trimethoprim-sulfamethoxazole, dapsone at 50 mg daily, or aerosol pentamidine at 300 mg every month, is an effective substitute.[93, 96]

Viral Infections

Although a variety of viral pathogens have been isolated from the lungs of patients with HIV infection,[97] it is difficult to determine the frequency with which these agents actually cause pneumonitis. Members of the herpesvirus family, especially cytomegalovirus (CMV), are found commonly in lung-derived specimens. In general, however, it appears that CMV infection in patients with HIV infection does not impose additional morbidity or mortality.[98]

CMV infection generally occurs early in life and is easily contained by the normal host. It may be acquired later by sexual contact. Before the AIDS epidemic, CMV infection was demonstrated in nearly all sexually active homosexual men.[99] In patients with HIV infection, CMV may cause disease at multiple sites, including the retina, colon, and liver. Significant pulmonary involvement is uncommon, although some patients have definite CMV pneumonitis. Cytologic demonstration of typical cytopathic effect or isolation of the virus itself is not sufficient to establish a diagnosis; however, if compatible histologic findings and positive cultures occur in a person who has lung disease for which no other diagnosis can be identified, the diagnosis of CMV pneumonia may be inferred.

Treatment of CMV pneumonitis in patients with HIV has not proved to be particularly effective, although experience is limited. Ganciclovir has been useful in treating both retinitis and colitis, and foscarnet is probably equally effective; thus, either agent may be tried in patients with pneumonitis.

Other herpesvirus infections (herpes simplex, varicella-zoster, and Epstein-Barr virus infection) have also been implicated as causing lung disease in patients with HIV infection. Epstein-Barr virus (as well as HIV itself) has been suggested as the cause of lymphoid interstitial pneumonia on the basis of the finding of viral DNA in lung biopsy specimens.

Miscellaneous Infections

In determining the differential diagnosis of lung disease in a patient with HIV infection, one should keep in mind that the full spectrum of infections has not been described and that the data currently available may change in time and may be applicable only to specific groups or locales. Thus, infections that in this chapter are categorized as miscellaneous may in some groups or in some parts of the world be important. For example, infestation with *Strongyloides stercoralis* is extremely common in many parts of the world. With immune suppression, the hyperinfection may occur and produce multisystem disease, including pneumonia. This has not yet been described in patients with HIV infection, but it may be because the disease is most likely to occur in areas where diagnostic facilities are limited.

Toxoplasmosis in patients with HIV infection usually involves the central nervous system, although there are a few reports of pulmonary involvement that in several instances has caused respiratory failure and death.[100, 101] Diagnosis is based on finding tachyzoites in a lung-derived specimen. *Cryptosporidium* has also been identified as a cause of lung disease in patients with HIV infection.[102]

An Integrated Approach to Diagnosis

On the basis of the information contained in the foregoing discussion of the infectious pulmonary complications of HIV infection, a logical and systematic approach to diagnosis can be developed. The first question that must be answered is, Is the patient HIV infected? The answer may be known because HIV serologic tests have been conducted or the patient has previously had an HIV-related disease. If the HIV status is not known, the evaluation must usually proceed while the results of the test are pending.

The second question is, Is the disease HIV related? If the lung disease is thought to be infectious, the answer to this question is nearly always yes. However, not all respiratory symptoms of HIV-infected persons are caused by infection.

Third, the stage of HIV infection should be considered. This may be inferred from the presence or absence of conditions such as thrush or Kaposi's sarcoma or may be determined more directly by measurement of the $CD4^+$ cell count. In general, if the HIV infection is not advanced, organisms not usually considered to be opportunistic, such as pneumococci or *M. tuberculosis,* should be high on the list. With more advanced HIV disease, the whole spectrum of infection should be included.

The fourth consideration is the mode of presentation and the clinical features of the illness. For example, an acute illness with productive cough and evidence of lobar consolidation on the chest radiograph is much more likely to be pneumococcal pneumonia than *P. carinii* pneumonia and should be evaluated accordingly.

If the stage of HIV disease and the clinical features of the illness are suggestive of an opportunistic process, then the evaluation should be directed along these lines, with the goal of identifying a specific pathogen. In general, blood chemistry and antibody tests are not useful. *Cryptococcus* and *Histoplasma* antigen determinations may be diagnostic if positive.

The first step in attempting to identify a specific opportunistic organism is usually examination of sputum obtained by inhalation of hypertonic saline mist.[79, 103] Induced sputum specimens should be stained for *P. carinii.* If the organism is detected, the sputum should also be stained and cultured for *Mycobacterium.* Depending on the part of the country, fungal cultures may also be in order. If *P. carinii* is not found, processing the sputum for other organisms depends on the next steps to be taken. If bronchoscopy is to be performed for all patients with sputum examinations, for *P. carinii* negative processing sputum for mycobacteria and fungi is superfluous. If bronchoscopy is not planned, other pathogens should be sought in the sputum.

At the time of bronchoscopy, it must be decided whether only BAL is to be performed or whether transbronchial biopsy will be done as well. This decision depends in part on the degree of clinical suspicion of *P. carinii* pneumonia. As noted earlier, BAL is extremely sensitive for *P. carinii,* so transbronchial biopsy might not add to the yield but certainly adds to the rate of complications.

Lavage fluid and biopsy specimens (if obtained) should be examined for *P. carinii,* mycobacteria, and fungi. Routine viral culture of tissue or fluid has not been found to be useful. Likewise, routine culture of lavage fluid for pyogenic bacteria may not be useful because of upper airway contamination. If all studies, including transbronchial biopsy, are nondiagnostic, the next step must be individualized according to the clinical circumstances.

References

1. Gottlieb MS, Schroff R, Schanker HM, et al: *Pneumocystis carinii* pneumonia and mucosal candidiasis in previously healthy ho-

mosexual men. Evidence of a new acquired cellular immunodeficiency. N Engl J Med 305:1425, 1981.
2. Masur H, Michelis MA, Green JB, et al: An outbreak of community-acquired *Pneumocystis carinii* pneumonia. N Engl J Med 305:1431, 1981.
3. Centers for Disease Control and Prevention: HIV/AIDS Surveillance Report 7:18, 1995.
4. Murray JF, Felton CP, Garay S, et al: Pulmonary complications of the acquired immunodeficiency syndrome. Report of a National Heart, Lung, and Blood Institute Workshop. N Engl J Med 310:1682, 1984.
5. Murray JF, Garay SM, Hopewell PC, et al: Pulmonary complications of the acquired immunodeficiency syndrome: An update. Am Rev Respir Dis 135:504, 1987.
6. Wallace JM, Rao AV, Glassroth J, et al: Respiratory illness in persons with human immunodeficiency virus infection. Am Rev Respir Dis 148:523, 1993.
7. Wallace JM, Hansen NI, LaVange L, et al: Respiratory disease trends in the pulmonary complications of HIV infection study cohort. Am J Respir Crit Care Med (in press).
8. Goedert JJ, Biggar RJ, Weiss SH, et al: Three-year incidence of AIDS in five cohorts of HTLV-III infected risk group members. Science 231:992, 1986.
9. Polk BF, Fox R, Brookmeyer R, et al: Predictors of the acquired immunodeficiency syndrome developing in a cohort of seropositive homosexual men. N Engl J Med 310:61, 1987.
10. Eyster ME, Gail MH, Bollard JO, et al: Natural history of human immunodeficiency virus infections in hemophiliacs: Effects of T-cell subsets, platelet counts and age. Ann Intern Med 107:1, 1987.
11. Kaslow RA, Phair JP, Friedman HB, et al: Infection with the human immunodeficiency virus: Clinical manifestations and their relationship to immune deficiency. Ann Intern Med 107:474, 1987.
12. Goedert JJ, Biggar RJ, Melbye M, et al: Effect of T4 count and cofactors on the incidence of AIDS in homosexual men infected with human immunodeficiency virus. JAMA 257:331, 1987.
13. Moss AR, Bacchetti P, Osmond D, et al: Most men seropositive for HIV will progress to AIDS or ARC: Three year follow-up of the San Francisco General Hospital cohort. Br Med J 296:745, 1988.
14. Phair J, Muñoz A, Detels R, et al: Multicenter AIDS Cohort Study Group. The risk of *Pneumocystis carinii* pneumonia among men infected with human immunodeficiency virus type I. N Engl J Med 322:161, 1990.
15. O'Brien WA, Hartigan PM, Martin D, et al: Changes in plasma HIV-1 RNA and $CD4^+$ lymphocyte counts and the risk of progression to AIDS. N Engl J Med 334:426, 1996.
16. Mellors JW, Rinaldo CR Jr, Gupta P, et al: Prognosis in HIV-1 infection predicted by the quantity of virus in plasma. Science 272:1167, 1996.
17. Davis L, Beck JM, Shellito J: Update: HIV infection and pulmonary host defenses. Semin Respir Infect 8:75, 1993.
18. Markowitz N, Hansen NI, Wilcosky TC, et al: Tuberculin and anergy in HIV-seropositive and HIV-seronegative persons. Ann Intern Med 119:185, 1993.
19. Theuer CP, Hopewell PC, Elias D, et al: Human immunodeficiency virus infection in tuberculous patients. J Infect Dis 162:8, 1990.
20. Chaisson RE, Schecter GF, Theuer CP, et al: Tuberculosis in patients with the acquired immunodeficiency syndrome. Clinical features, response to therapy, and survival. Am Rev Respir Dis 136:570, 1987.
21. Huang BD, Ruben FL, Rinaldo CR, et al: Antibody response after influenza and pneumococcal immunization in HIV-infected homosexual men. JAMA 261:245, 1989.
22. Nelson KE, Clements ML, Miotti P, et al: The influence of human immunodeficiency virus (HIV) infection on antibody responses to influenza vaccines. Ann Intern Med 109:383, 1988.
23. Janoff E, Breiman R, Daley CL, Hopewell PC: Pneumococcal disease during HIV infection. Ann Intern Med 117:314, 1992.
24. Hirschtick RE, Glassroth J, Jordan MC, et al: Bacterial pneumonia in persons infected with the human immunodeficiency virus. N Engl J Med 333:845, 1995.
25. Witt DJ, Craven DE, McCabe WR: Bacterial infections in adult patients with the acquired immunodeficiency syndrome (AIDS) and AIDS-related complex. Am J Med 82:900, 1987.
26. Hopewell PC: Tuberculosis in persons with HIV infection. *In* Sande MA, Volberding PA (eds): The Medical Management of AIDS, ed 4. Philadelphia, WB Saunders, 1995, pp 416–436.
27. Markowitz N, Hansen NI, Hopewell PC, et al: Tuberculosis in a prospectively evaluated cohort of persons with HIV infection. Ann Intern Med (in press).
28. Selwyn PA, Hartel D, Lewis VA, et al: A prospective study of the risk of tuberculosis among intravenous drug users with human immunodeficiency virus infection. N Engl J Med 320:545, 1989.
29. Pitchenik AE, Burr J, Suarez M, et al: Human T cell–lymphotropic virus-III (HTLV-III) seropositivity and related disease among 71 consecutive patients in whom tuberculosis was diagnosed. Am Rev Respir Dis 135:875, 1987.
30. Nolan CM, Heckbert S, Elarth A, et al: Case-control study of the association between human immunodeficiency virus infection and tuberculosis (Abstr 4620). Presented at the Fourth International Conference on AIDS; 1988; San Francisco; p 1011.
31. Onorato J, McCombs S, Morgan WM, McCray E: HIV infection in persons in tuberculosis clinics, United States, 1988–1991 (Abstr WS-C 18-6). Presented at the Ninth International Conference on AIDS; 1993; Berlin; p 99.
32. DeCock KM, Soro B, Coulibali IM, Lucas SB: Tuberculosis and HIV infection in sub-Saharan Africa. JAMA 268:1581, 1992.
33. Jones BE, Young SMM, Antoniskis D, et al: Relationship of the manifestations of tuberculosis to CD4 cell counts in patients with human immunodeficiency virus infection. Am Rev Respir Dis 148:1292, 1993.
34. Sunderam G, McDonald RJ, Maniatis T, et al: Tuberculosis as a manifestation of the acquired immunodeficiency syndrome (AIDS). JAMA 256:362, 1986.
35. Brody JM, Muller DK, Zeman RK, et al: Gastric tuberculosis: A manifestation of acquired immunodeficiency syndrome. Radiology 159:347, 1986.
36. Barnes P, Leedon J, Radin DR, Chandrasoma P: An unusual case of tuberculous peritonitis in a man with AIDS. West J Med 144:467, 1986.
37. Sunderam G, Mangura BT, Lombardo JM, et al: Failure of optimal four-drug short-course tuberculosis chemotherapy in a compliant patient with human immunodeficiency virus infection. Am Rev Respir Dis 136:1475, 1987.
38. Saltzman BR, Motyl MR, Friedland GH, et al: *Mycobacterium tuberculosis* bacteremia in the acquired immunodeficiency syndrome. JAMA 256:390, 1986.
39. Small PM, Hopewell PC, Schecter GF, et al: Evolution of chest radiographs in treated patients with pulmonary tuberculosis and HIV infection. J Thorac Imaging 9:74, 1994.
40. Tuberculosis and human immunodeficiency virus infection: Recommendations of the Advisory Committee for the Elimination of Tuberculosis (ACET). MMWR Morbid Mortal Wkly Rep 39:236, 1989.
41. Small PM, Schecter GF, Goodman PC, et al: Treatment of tuberculosis, in patients with advanced human immunodeficiency virus infection. N Engl J Med 324:289, 1991.
42. Iseman MDR: Is standard chemotherapy adequate in tuberculosis patients infected with the HIV infection? Am Rev Respir Dis 176:1326, 1987.
43. Perriens JH, St. Louis ME, Mukadi JB, et al: Pulmonary tuberculosis in HIV-infected patients in Zaire. A controlled trial of treatment for either 6 or 12 months. N Engl J Med 332:779, 1995.
44. American Thoracic Society/Centers for Disease Control: Treatment and prevention of tuberculosis and tuberculosis infection in adults and children. Am J Respir Crit Care Med 149:1359, 1994.
45. Pape JW, Jean SS, Ho JL, et al: Effect of isoniazid prophylaxis on incidence of active tuberculosis and progression of HIV infection. Lancet 342:268, 1993.
46. Di Perri G, Cruciani M, Danzi MC, et al: Nosocomial epidemic of active tuberculosis among HIV-infected patients. Lancet 2:1502, 1989.
47. Daley CL, Small PM, Schecter GF, et al: An outbreak of tuberculosis with accelerated progression among persons infected with human immunodeficiency virus—An analysis using restriction-fragment–length polymorphisms. N Engl J Med 326:231, 1992.
48. Greene JB, Sidhu GS, Lewin S, et al: *Mycobacterium avium-intracellulare*: A cause of disseminated life-threatening infection in homosexuals and drug abusers. Ann Intern Med 97:539, 1982.

49. Horsburgh CR Jr, Selik RM: The epidemiology of disseminated nontuberculous mycobacterial infection in the acquired immunodeficiency syndrome (AIDS). Am Rev Respir Dis 139:4, 1989.
50. Chin DP, Reingold AL, Stone EN, et al: The impact of *Mycobacterium avium* complex bacteremia and its treatment on survival of AIDS patients—A prospective study. J Infect Dis 170:578, 1994.
51. Horsburgh CR Jr, Chin DP, Yajko DM, et al: Environmental risk factors for acquisition of *M. avium* complex in persons with human immunodeficiency virus infection. J Infect Dis 170:362, 1994.
52. Yajko DM, Chin DP, Gonzalez PC, et al: *Mycobacterium avium* complex in water, food and soil samples collected from the environment of HIV-infected individuals. J Acquir Immune Defic Syndr Hum Retrovirol 9:176, 1995.
53. Chin DP, Reingold AL, Horsburgh CR Jr, et al: Predicting *Mycobacterium avium* complex bacteremia in patients infected with human immunodeficiency virus: A prospectively validated model. Clin Infect Dis 19:668, 1994.
54. Packer SJ, Cesario T, Williams JH: *Mycobacterium tuberculosis* complex infection presenting as endobronchial lesions in immunocompromised patients. Ann Intern Med 109:389, 1988.
55. Hawkins CC, Gold JWM, Whimbey E, et al: *Mycobacterium avium* complex infections in patients with the acquired immunodeficiency syndrome. Ann Intern Med 105:184, 1986.
56. Nyberg DA, Federle MP, Jeffrey RB, et al: Abdominal CT findings of disseminated *Mycobacterium avium-intracellulare* in AIDS. AJR 145:297, 1985.
57. Shafran SD, and the Canadian MAC Study Group: The Canadian randomized open-label trial of combination therapy for MAC bacteremia: Final results. Presented at the 35th Interscience Conference on Antimicrobial Agents and Chemotherapy; September 17–20, 1995; San Francisco.
58. May T, and the CURAVIUM Group: A French randomized open trial of 2 clarithromycin combination therapies for MAC bacteremia: First results. Presented at the 35th Interscience Conference on Antimicrobial Agents and Chemotherapy; September 17–20, 1995; San Francisco.
59. Havlir DV, and the CCTG: A double-blind, randomized study of weekly azithromycin, daily rifabutin and combination azithromycin and rifabutin for the prevention of *Mycobacterium avium* complex (MAC) in AIDS patients. Presented at the Third Conference on Retroviruses and Opportunistic Infections; 1996; Washington, DC.
60. Benson CA, and the ACTG 196/CPCRA 009 Study Team: A phase III prospective, randomized, double-blind study of the safety and efficacy of clarithromycin (CLA) vs. rifabutin (RBT) vs. CLA + RBT prevention of *Mycobacterium avium* complex (MAC) disease in HIV^+ patients with CD4 counts <100 cells/mm^3. Presented at the Third Conference on Retroviruses and Opportunistic Infections; 1996; Washington, DC.
61. Horsburgh CR, Selik RM: The epidemiology of disseminated nontuberculous mycobacterial infection in the acquired immunodeficiency syndrome (AIDS). Am Rev Respir Dis 139:4, 1989.
62. Jacobson MA: Disseminated *Mycobacterium avium* complex and other bacterial infections. *In* Sande MA, Volberding PA (eds): Medical Management of AIDS, ed 4. Philadelphia, WB Saunders, 1995, pp 402–415.
63. Stansell JD: Pulmonary fungal infections in HIV-infected persons. Semin Respir Infect 8:116, 1993.
64. Chuck S, Sande MA: Infections with *Cryptococcus neoformans* in the acquired immunodeficiency syndrome. N Engl J Med 321:794, 1989.
65. Saag MS: Cryptococcosis and other fungal infections (histoplasmosis, coccidioidomycosis). *In* Sande MA, Volberding PA (eds): Medical Management of AIDS, ed 4. Philadelphia, WB Saunders, 1995, pp 437–459.
66. Edwards LD, Acquaviva FA, Livesay VT, et al: An atlas of sensitivity to tuberculin PPDB and histoplasmin in the United States. Am Rev Respir Dis 99(Suppl):1, 1969.
67. Johnson PC, Hamil RJ, Sarosi GA: Clinical review: Progressive disseminated histoplasmosis in the AIDS patient. Semin Respir Infect 4:139, 1989.
68. Wheat LJ, Connolly J, Springfield P, et al: *Histoplasma capsulatum* polysaccharide antigen detection in diagnosis and management of disseminated histoplasmosis in patients with AIDS. Am J Med 87:396, 1989.
69. Drutz DJ, Catanzaro A: State of the art: Coccidioidomycosis. Am Rev Respir Dis 117:559; 727, 1978.
70. Bronnimann DA, Adam RD, Galgiani JN, et al: Coccidioidomycosis in the acquired immunodeficiency syndrome. Ann Intern Med 106:372, 1987.
71. Denning DW, Follansbee SE, Scolaro M, et al: Pulmonary aspergillosis in the acquired immunodeficiency syndrome. N Engl J Med 324:654, 1991.
72. Masur H, Frederick P, Ognibene FP, et al: CD4 counts as predictors of opportunistic pneumonias in human immunodeficiency virus (HIV) infection. Ann Intern Med 111:223, 1989.
73. Stansell JD, Osmond DH, Charlebois E, et al: Predictors of *Pneumocystis carinii* pneumonia in HIV-infected persons. Am J Respir Crit Care Med (in press).
74. Kovacs JA, Hiemenz JW, Macher AM, et al: *Pneumocystis carinii* pneumonia: A comparison between patients with the acquired immunodeficiency syndrome and patients with other immunodeficiencies. Ann Intern Med 100:663, 1984.
75. Cohen BA, Pomeranz S, Rabinowitz JG, et al: Pulmonary complications of AIDS: Radiologic features. AJR 143:115, 1984.
76. Stover DE, White DA, Romano PA, et al: Spectrum of pulmonary disease associated with the acquired immune deficiency syndrome. Am J Med 78:429, 1985.
77. Pitchenik AE, Ganjei P, Torres A, et al: Sputum examination for the diagnosis of *Pneumocystis carinii* in the acquired immunodeficiency syndrome. Am Rev Respir Dis 133:226, 1986.
78. Bigby T, Margolskee D, Curtis J, et al: The usefulness of induced sputum in the diagnosis of *Pneumocystis carinii* pneumonia in patients with the acquired immunodeficiency syndrome. Am Rev Respir Dis 133:515, 1986.
79. Ng VL, Gartner I, Weymouth LA, et al: The use of mucolysed induced sputum for the identification of pulmonary pathogens associated with human immunodeficiency virus infection. Arch Pathol Lab Med 113:488, 1989.
80. Kovacs JA, Ng VL, Masur H, et al: Diagnosis of *Pneumocystis carinii* pneumonia: Improved detection in sputum with use of monoclonal antibodies. N Engl J Med 318:589, 1988.
81. Ng VL, Yajko DM, McPhaul LW, et al: Evaluation of an indirect fluorescent antibody stain for detection of *Pneumocystis carinii* in respiratory specimens. J Clin Microbiol 28:975, 1990.
82. Stover DE, White DA, Romano PA, Gellene RA: Diagnosis of pulmonary disease in the acquired immune deficiency syndrome: Roles of bronchoscopy and bronchoalveolar lavage. Am Rev Respir Dis 131:659, 1984.
83. Broaddus VC, Dake MD, Stulbarg MS, et al: Bronchoalveolar lavage and transbronchial biopsy for the diagnosis of pulmonary infections in patients with the acquired immunodeficiency syndrome. Ann Intern Med 102:747, 1985.
84. Golden JA, Hollander H, Stulbarg MS, Gamsu G: Bronchoalveolar lavage as the exclusive diagnostic modality for *Pneumocystis carinii* pneumonia. Chest 90:18, 1986.
85. Huang L, Hecht FM, Stansell JD, et al: Suspected *Pneumocystis carinii* pneumonia with a negative induced sputum examination: Is early bronchoscopy useful? Am J Respir Crit Care Med 151:1866, 1995.
86. Miller RF, Millar AB, Weller IVD, Semple JSG: Empirical treatment without bronchoscopy for *Pneumocystis carinii* pneumonia in the acquired immunodeficiency syndrome. Thorax 44:559, 1989.
87. Wharton JM, Coleman DL, Wofsy CB, et al: Trimethoprim-sulfamethoxazole or pentamidine for *Pneumocystis carinii* pneumonia in the acquired immunodeficiency syndrome. Ann Intern Med 105:37, 1985.
88. Montaner JSG, Lawson LM, Levitt N, et al: Corticosteroids prevent early deterioration in patients with moderately severe *Pneumocystis carinii* pneumonia and the acquired immunodeficiency syndrome (AIDS). Ann Intern Med 113:14, 1990.
89. Bozette SA, Sattler FR, Chiu J, et al: A controlled trial of early adjunctive treatment with corticosteroids for *Pneumocystis carinii* pneumonia in the acquired immunodeficiency syndrome. N Engl J Med 323:1451, 1990.
90. Gagnon S, Boota AM, Fischl MA, et al: Corticosteroids as adjunctive therapy for severe *Pneumocystis carinii* pneumonia in the acquired immunodeficiency syndrome. N Engl J Med 323:1444, 1990.
91. The National Institutes of Health—University of California Ex-

pert Panel for Corticosteroids as Adjunctive Therapy for *Pneumocystis* pneumonia: Consensus statement on the use of corticosteroids as adjunctive therapy for *Pneumocystis* pneumonia in the acquired immunodeficiency syndrome. N Engl J Med 323:1500, 1990.
92. Hopewell PC, Mazur H: *Pneumocystis carinii*: Current concepts. *In* Sande MA, Volberding PA (eds): Medical Management of AIDS, ed 4. Philadelphia, WB Saunders, 1995, pp 367–401.
93. Simonds RJ, Hughes WT, Feinberg J, Navin TR: Preventing *Pneumocystis carinii* pneumonia in persons infected with human immunodeficiency virus. Clin Infect Dis 21(Suppl):544, 1995.
94. Schneider MME, Hoepelman AIM, Eftnick-Schattenkirk JKM, et al: A controlled trial of aerosolized pentamidine or trimethoprim-sulfamethoxazole as primary prophylaxis against *Pneumocystis carinii* pneumonia in patients with human immunodeficiency virus infection. N Engl J Med 327:1836, 1992.
95. Bozzette SA, Finkelstein DM, Spector SA, et al: A randomized trial of three antipneumocystis agents in patients with advanced human immunodeficiency virus infection. N Engl J Med 332:693, 1995.
96. Leoung GS, Feigel DW Jr, Montgomery AB: Pentamidine for prophylaxis against *Pneumocystis carinii* pneumonia: The San Francisco community prophylaxis trial. N Engl J Med 323:769, 1990.
97. Wallace JM: Pulmonary infection in human immunodeficiency disease: Viral pulmonary infection. Semin Respir Infect 4:147, 1989.
98. Jacobson MA, Mills J, Rush J: Morbidity and mortality of patients with AIDS and first episode *Pneumocystis carinii* pneumonia is unaffected by concomitant pulmonary cytomegalovirus infection. Am Rev Respir Dis 144:6, 1991.
99. Mintz L, Drew WL, Miner RC, Braf EH: Cytomegalovirus infections in homosexual men: An epidemiologic study. Ann Intern Med 98:326, 1983.
100. Catterall JR, Hofflin JM, Remington JS: Pulmonary toxoplasmosis. Am Rev Respir Dis 133:704, 1986.
101. Schnapp LM, Geaghan SM, Campagna A, et al: *Toxoplasma gondii* pneumonitis in patients infected with the human immunodeficiency virus. Arch Intern Med 152:1073, 1992.
102. Brady EM, Margolis ML, Korzeniowski OM: Pulmonary cryptosporidiosis in acquired immunodeficiency syndrome. JAMA 252:89, 1984.
103. Ng V, Yajko D, Hadley WK: Update on laboratory tests for the diagnosis of pulmonary disease in HIV-1 infected individuals. Semin Respir Infect 8:86, 1993.

123

Gastrointestinal Complications of Human Immunodeficiency Virus Infection

John G. Bartlett

The gastrointestinal tract, from the mouth to the anus, is one of the most common sites for clinical expression of human immunodeficiency virus (HIV) infection. Most patients have oral candidiasis, and *Candida* esophagitis is second only to *Pneumocystis carinii* pneumonia as the initial opportunistic infection defining the acquired immunodeficiency syndrome (AIDS). Up to one third of patients develop perirectal lesions, primarily caused by herpes simplex virus (HSV); 30% to 80% experience chronic or intermittent diarrhea. Several gastrointestinal lesions appear to be somewhat uniquely associated with HIV infection, including visceral Kaposi's sarcoma, oral hairy leukoplakia, Whipple-like enteropathy caused by mycobacteria, chronic cryptosporidiosis, microsporidiosis, and cytomegalovirus (CMV) infections of the gut. Most of these complications occur relatively late in the course of HIV infection and represent opportunistic infections that reflect advanced immunosuppression. Many of these conditions contribute to wasting or protein-calorie malnutrition by reduction in nutritional intake or by excessive nutrient losses through malabsorption.

Types of Conditions

The Gay Bowel Syndrome

In the 1970s, there was increasing recognition of the gastrointestinal complications of homosexual men, including proctitis, proctocolitis, and enteritis.[1, 2] Pathogens encountered in these conditions include three groups: (1) enteric pathogens that are commonly recognized in other populations of patients, such as *Shigella*, *Entamoeba histolytica*, and *Giardia lamblia*; (2) sexually transmitted pathogens, including *Neisseria gonorrhoeae*, HSV, *Chlamydia trachomatis*, and *Treponema pallidum*; and (3) occasional enteric pathogens that may be idiosyncratic in this population of patients, such as *Campylobacter cinaedi* and *Campylobacter fennelliae*. The high prevalence of these pathogens in homosexual men presumably reflects promiscuity, sexual practices, and the high incidence of asymptomatic and untreated infections.[1, 2] Since the early 1980s, there has been a 10- to 20-fold decrease in rates of gonococcal proctitis and other sexually transmitted pathogens among gay men; this presumably reflects modified sexual practices that also resulted in a substantial reduction in transmission rates of HIV. The result is that the gay bowel syndrome is now relatively infrequent.

Oral Lesions (Table 123–1)

Oral lesions are common and often contribute to malnutrition. The most common include candidiasis (thrush), oral hairy leukoplakia, herpes simplex, aphthous ulcers, and various dental complications. Less common are Kaposi's sarcoma, CMV infections, and non-Hodgkin's lymphoma.

Thrush is occasionally seen in the acute HIV syndrome and in late-stage disease with low $CD4^+$ cell counts.[3] Early lesions are easily managed, but the late-stage disease can be problematic, especially with resistance complicating extensive exposure to azoles.[4] Many cases are asymptomatic; symptoms, when present, consist of mouth pain, taste perversion, and, with *Candida* esophagitis, odynophagia.[3–5] The diagnosis is usually made by clinical appearance. The most common presentation is that of characteristic pseudomembranous lesions, which are white, creamy plaques on an inflamed base located on the buccal mucosa, tongue, gingiva, and/or palate. The plaques are easily removed with scraping. The erythematous or "atrophic" form of thrush shows spotty or confluent red patches and is more elusive to identify.[3] The diagnosis may be established with a potassium hydroxide wet mount or Gram stain of an oral swab or scrapings to demonstrate typical yeast and pseudomycelia, but this is usually not necessary. Culture is not generally required except to detect resistant strains. Nearly all lesions found in early-stage disease are due to *Candida albicans*; late-stage dis-

TABLE 123–1 ■ Oral Lesions in Patients with Human Immunodeficiency Virus Infection

CONDITION	CLINICAL FEATURES	DIAGNOSIS	STAGE	TREATMENT	COMMENT
Candidiasis (thrush)	Pseudomembranous form: white, creamy plaques on inflamed base, buccal mucosa, tongue, gums, palate; scrapes off easily Erythematous form (atrophic): spotty or confluent red patches Hyperplastic form (*Candida* leukoplakia): white lesions that do not wipe off and respond to azole therapy *Symptoms*: Often asymptomatic; oral pain, taste perversion; odynophagia with esophagitis in late-stage disease	Clinical appearance Oral swab, scraping, or rinse specimen for (1) KOH preparation or Gram stain to show yeast and pseudomycelia and/or (2) culture, primarily to show azole susceptibility	$CD4^+$ cell count < 300/mm^3 Promote with antibiotic treatment More common and severe with late-stage disease	Local: clotrimazole troche, nystatin, amphotericin B Systemic: azoles—primarily fluconazole; intravenous (IV) amphotericin B occasionally required	Pseudomembranous lesions are most common; erythematous lesions are underdiagnosed. Colonization rates of *C. albicans* in mouth of healthy persons are 10%–40%. Risks for azole resistance are increased by prolonged exposure to azoles and late-stage disease.
Oral hairy leukoplakia	White fibrillar patches, usually on tongue, especially the lateral surface; do not scrape off (as in candidiasis) *Symptoms*: Often asymptomatic; pain, altered voice or taste	Clinical appearance Biopsy: epithelial hyperplasia with "hairs"	$CD4^+$ cell count < 300/mm^3	Usually not treated Symptomatic disease: oral acyclovir (high dose) or ganciclovir	Relapse is common when treatment is stopped. Epstein-Barr virus is implicated by electron microscopy, immunofluorescence, or Southern blot.
Herpes simplex	Small painful ulcers or vesicles on an erythematous base, usually on gingiva and palate *Symptoms*: Local pain	Clinical appearance Scraping: multinucleated giant cells with Tzanck preparation, culture or fluorescent antibody technique for HSV	Any stage: more common and severe with late-stage disease	Acyclovir by mouth or IV (valacyclovir and famciclovir also effective) Acyclovir resistance: foscarnet	Topical treatment (lidocaine, dyclonine [Dyclone], Benadryl, 5% cocaine) may be needed to permit oral feedings.
Aphthous ulcers	Small painful ulcers at any location in oral cavity *Symptoms*: Local pain, often severe ± voice change or dysphagia	Clinical appearance plus studies to exclude HSV	May occur at any stage; more severe in late-stage disease	Topical: fluocinonide, lidocaine, Dyclone, or dexamethasone Local injection: corticosteroids Systemic: corticosteroids or thalidomide	May be severe and debilitating.
Kaposi's sarcoma	Red or purple nodules, usually on palate or gingiva; most have cutaneous lesions also *Symptoms*: Usually asymptomatic; may be cosmetic concern or disruption of teeth	Clinical appearance Biopsy	$CD4^+$ cell count < 300/mm^3	Usually not treated Laser or intralesional vinblastine Large lesions: radiation	

ease with prolonged exposure to azoles often results in thrush involving *Candida tropicalis*, *Candida glabrata*, or other non-*albicans* strains or *C. albicans* resistant to azoles.[4, 6, 7] Topical treatment consists of orally administered clotrimazole troches, nystatin, or amphotericin. Refractory or recurrent disease is often managed with oral fluconazole or other azoles, but severe disease may require intravenous amphotericin B.

Oral hairy leukoplakia was first described in 1984[8] and is now reported in 10% to 25% of patients with HIV infection, usually at a relatively late stage of disease with $CD4^+$ cell counts less than 300/mm^3.[9] The typical lesion is a nonremovable patch on the tongue, especially the lateral surfaces that tend to show a corrugated texture; close inspection shows fibrillar projections, which account for the name. Electron microscopy and nucleic acid hybridization implicate Epstein-Barr virus,[10] and this expression of Epstein-Barr virus appears to be almost uniformly restricted to patients with immunosuppression. The major differential diagnosis is thrush; oral hairy leukoplakia can be distinguished by its anatomic location, difficulty in removing plaques with scraping (in contrast to thrush), a smear that fails to show *Candida* hyphae, lack of response to antimycotic treatment, or biopsy with histological characteristics of oral hairy leukoplakia.[11] Most patients are asymptomatic, and this lesion is commonly overlooked with routine inspection of the mouth.[12] The usual symptoms are pain, burning, and altered taste; symptoms and lesions resolve with acyclovir or ganciclovir but tend to recur when treatment is discontinued.[13]

Oral herpes is common in the general population, but in patients with advanced HIV infection the lesions are likely to be more extensive, more frequent, more likely to disseminate, and more refractory to treatment.[3] The usual appearance is painful vesicles or ulcers 1 to 3 mm in diameter on the lips and/or oral cavity. The major differential diagnosis is aphthous ulcers; features suggesting HSV include a prior history of typical oral herpetic lesions, positive Tzanck preparation (positive in about 75%), positive cultures for HSV (positive in about 80%), and response to treatment with acyclovir. These lesions may be quite painful and may be extensive with involvement of the mucous membranes and adjacent skin. The standard treatment is oral acyclovir in conventional doses, but high-dose oral acyclovir or intravenous acyclovir is sometimes required. Famciclovir and valacyclovir are also effective. Refractory cases suggest acyclovir resistance and may require foscarnet treatment for severe disease.

Aphthous ulcers may not be more common than in the general population, but they appear to be more severe and prolonged in patients with HIV infection. The lesions appear identical to HSV lesions and may be found any place in the oral cavity.[3] A biopsy, if done, shows nonspecific inflammation. Symptoms include pain, dysphagia, and altered speech. There are multiple treatments: topical treatment consists of fluocinonide (1:1 with orobase), dexamethasone elixir, and various combinations of lidocaine and steroids or intralesional steroids; severe or refractory cases often require systemic prednisone or thalidomide.[14] Other causes of vesicles or ulcers in the mouth include CMV, varicella-zoster virus, and molluscum contagiosum, but all of these are infrequent.

Periodontal disease is frequent in patients with HIV infection and may be severe. The most common form involves gingivitis and periodontitis as found in the general population, but these disorders are more common and more severe with advanced stages of HIV infection.[15] The usual presentation is a red gingival margin sometimes referred to as HIV gingivitis.[3] A less common but distinctive form of disease referred to as nectrotizing ulcerative periodontitis (formerly HIV-associated periodontitis) is characterized by local pain, spontaneous bleeding, intense erythema, edema, bone loss, and then tooth loss. Recommended treatment consists of débridement, scaling and root planing, and povidone-iodine irrigations, sometimes accompanied by topical chlorhexidine oral rinses and metronidazole.

Esophageal Disease (Table 123–2)

Esophageal disease is a leading gastrointestinal-related complication of HIV infection. The most frequent complaint is odynophagia, which may be an extremely debilitating symptom that contributes substantially to malnutrition. It is often seen relatively early in the course of HIV infection, and nearly all forms are treatable.[16, 17]

Candida is the most common cause of esophagitis, and Candida esophagitis is usually, but not always, accompanied by thrush. Distinctive features compared with other forms of esophagitis are that pain is diffuse, it is associated primarily with swallowing, and fever is unusual. Treatment is usually presumptive with endoscopy reserved for those who fail to respond or have an atypical presentation.[18, 19] The usual finding with endoscopy is pseudomembranous plaques that resemble the lesions found with thrush; brushings show yeast and pseudomycelia, and cultures may be done to detect azole-resistant strains. The usual treatment is oral azoles, either ketoconazole or fluconazole.[19] Most patients respond, but relapse rates are high and azole resistance is often problematic with late-stage disease and excessive azole exposure.[4, 20]

Esophageal ulcers are usually caused by CMV or are idiopathic (aphthous ulcers).[21] HSV as a cause is infrequent, is often associated with typical oral herpetic lesions, and is important to recognize because of the ease of effective treatment. All three forms of ulcerative esophagitis may cause severe odynophagia that is focal (rather than diffuse as seen with *Candida* infection) and causes chest pain (rather than pain precipitated only by swallowing). Endoscopy is necessary for detecting these forms of ulcerative esophagitis and is essential for distinguishing them from neoplastic processes. The treatment for CMV infection is intravenous ganciclovir and the short-term response is usually good, but the need for long-term maintenance treatment is controversial.[22, 23] Many of these patients have CMV retinitis, and concurrent esophagitis may influence decisions regarding management, for example, local or intraocular therapy versus intravenous treatment. The treatment of choice for idiopathic ulcers is prednisone, often with azoles for antifungal prophylaxis[24]; the alternative is thalidomide for refractory cases.[25]

Other diagnostic considerations in patients with dysphagia or odynophagia are drug-induced complications including those associated with dideoxycytidine or zidovudine[26] and selected unusual infections for this anatomic location such as *Mycobacterium avium* infection, tuberculosis, cryptosporidia infection, *P. carinii* infection, and histoplasmosis.[27] Tumors that may cause esophageal symptoms include Kaposi's sarcoma and non-Hodgkin's lymphoma. These require endoscopy for detection.

Recommended diagnostic tests depend on symptoms and stage of disease. With $CD4^+$ cell counts greater than 500/mm^3, the patient should be evaluated as in the absence of HIV infection. Essentially all of the HIV-associated complications that have been noted are seen with $CD4^+$ cell counts less than 300/mm^3, and most are seen with median $CD4^+$ cell counts of 20 to 50/mm^3. Barium studies are of limited value. Endoscopy is generally preferred to make the distinctions summarized earlier (see Table 123–2). Prior reports indicate that a likely diagnosis can be established by endoscopy in 70% to 95% of cases.[28]

TABLE 123–2 ■ Esophageal Disease in Patients with Acquired Immunodeficiency Syndrome*

CHARACTERISTIC	*CANDIDA* INFECTION	CYTOMEGALOVIRUS INFECTION	APHTHOUS ULCER	HERPES SIMPLEX
Frequency (as cause of esophageal symptoms)	50%–70%	10%–20%	10%–20%	2.5%
Clinical features				
Dysphagia	+ +	+	+	+
Odynophagia	+ +	+ + +	+ + +	+ + +
Oral lesions	Thrush—70%	None	None	HSV > 50%
Pain localization	Diffuse—esophageal	Focal—chest	Focal—chest	Focal—chest
Fever	None	Usually	None	Variable
Stage	$CD4^+$ cell count < 100/mm³	$CD4^+$ cell count < 50/mm³	$CD4^+$ cell count < 50/mm³	$CD4^+$ cell count < 150/mm³
Diagnosis				
Endoscopy	Usually treated empirically Pseudomembranous plaques	Ulcers—single or multiple discrete Biopsy—required to detect CMV	Ulcers—identical to those in CMV	Ulcers—shallow, small, confluent
Microbiology	Brush—yeast and pseudomycelia Culture for in vitro sensitivity test	Histopathology to show intranuclear inclusions; culture is inconclusive	Negative studies for alternative agents	Histopathology showing intracytoplasmic inclusions + multinucleated giant cells; HSV by fluorescent antibody stain or culture
Treatment				
Acute (2–3 wk)	Azoles; usually fluconazole Some require IV amphotericin	Ganciclovir Alternative is foscarnet	Systemic prednisone ± antifungal prophylaxis Thalidomide	Acyclovir by mouth or intravenously
Maintenance	Fluconazole or other azole only with repeated episodes	Arbitrary—some use only for recurrent disease	None	Arbitrary
Comment	Response to fluconazole: 85%	Should obtain ophthalmologic examination	May be severely debilitating	Relatively rare cause of esophageal ulcer Response to treatment is usually good

*+, Modest; + +, moderate; + + +, severe.

Enteric Infection

The frequency of diarrhea is usually reported as 30% to 60% of AIDS patients in developed countries and 60% to 90% in developing countries.[2, 29–40] However, the frequency in developed countries is not well studied in terms of well-accepted diagnostic criteria in large populations followed up for extended periods with appropriate control subjects. In general, diarrhea is defined on the basis of the number and duration of stools (≥ two to three a day for ≥ 2 or 3 days), character of stool (conforms to a container in which it is placed or water content exceeding 90%), or volume (more than 200 g/d in adults). Diarrhea is further defined as acute if present for less than 2 weeks, persistent if present more than 14 days, and chronic if the duration exceeds 30 days. Diarrhea constitutes an AIDS-defining diagnosis if it is present with at least two stools a day for more than 1 month accompanied by an otherwise unexplained weight loss exceeding 10%.

Management recommendations for diagnostic evaluation depend on clinical symptoms, stage of disease, and diagnostic resources. Acute diarrhea is usually caused by common bacterial or viral agents. Chronic diarrhea is usually caused by protozoan parasites (Microsporida, *Cryptosporidium*, *Isospora*, or *Cyclospora*), *M. avium*, or CMV. The relative frequency of these microbes is summarized in Table 123–3 on the basis of multiple studies from developed countries.[2, 34–42] Diagnostic probabilities depend to a large extent on the $CD4^+$ cell count and the distinction between acute and chronic diarrhea.

The usual diagnostic evaluation begins with the stool screen with culture for enteric pathogens (*Salmonella*, *Campylobacter jejuni*, *Shigella*, and, less frequently, *Yersinia*, *Aeromonas*, *Escherichia coli* O157:H7, and/or noncholera vibrios), stool for ova and parasites (preferably with acid-fast stain for detection of *Cryptosporidium*, *Isospora*, and *Cyclospora*), and a *Clostridium difficile* toxin assay (preferably with an enzyme immunoassay or tissue culture assay). A stool leukocyte examination, preferably using lactoferrin, is a good method for distinguishing inflammatory from secretory causes of diarrhea.[43] The common inflammatory causes of diarrhea in pa-

TABLE 123–3 ■ Prevalence of Enteric Pathogens in Patients with Acquired Immunodeficiency Syndrome with Diarrhea

PATHOGEN	MEAN (%)	RANGE (%)
Cryptosporidium	20	7–37
Microsporida	19	2–39
Cytomegalovirus	20	8–45
Mycobacterium avium	9	2–25
Giardia lamblia	5	2–12
Entamoeba histolytica	3	0–25
Campylobacter jejuni	3	0–11
Clostridium difficile	2	0–7
Salmonella sp.	2	0–25
Shigella	2	0–5
Isospora	1	0–4
Enteric viruses	4	2–10

tients with HIV infection include bacterial agents (especially *Salmonella, C. jejuni,* and *C. difficile*) and CMV. Protozoan parasites, viruses other than CMV, and *M. avium* are not commonly associated with fecal leukocytes and are consequently classified as agents of secretory diarrhea. Microsporida may be detected in stool using a special trichrome stain that is variable in terms of availability and technical expertise.[44]

Treatment of patients with acute diarrhea when *C. difficile* is unlikely or excluded may include a fluoroquinolone given empirically if symptoms are severe. Antiperistaltic agents are often advocated for empirical treatment of acute or chronic diarrhea. Patients with negative stool studies who are unresponsive to empirical therapy usually undergo endoscopy.[36–38] If the clinical presentation suggests colonic or inflammatory diarrhea (fever, cramps, fecal leukocytes), the usual initial anatomic study is lower endoscopy. If the symptoms suggest secretory diarrhea with malabsorption (large-volume stools, no fecal leukocytes, absence of fever, absence of cramps), there should be consideration of upper endoscopy, primarily for detection of microsporidiosis or *M. avium;* although *Cryptosporidium* is the most common cause of enteritis in late-stage HIV infection in many studies, the stool screening examination is sufficiently sensitive that endoscopy is infrequently required to establish this diagnosis.[38] If there is persistent or severe diarrhea combined with weight loss and a $CD4^+$ cell count less than 100/mm^3, many authorities recommend sigmoidoscopy or colonoscopy followed by upper endoscopy.[36, 45]

Previous experience indicates that approximately one third of HIV-infected patients with diarrhea that is sufficiently severe or prolonged to require a complete diagnostic evaluation as defined earlier have a negative evaluation for etiologic agents.[36–39] One study with long-term follow-up of such "pathogen-negative" HIV-infected patients with chronic diarrhea showed that most had low-volume diarrhea that resolved spontaneously or was easily controlled with antimotility agents.[45] It should be noted that small bowel biopsies of patients with advanced HIV infection show villus atrophy with crypt hyperplasia, but the consequences of these anatomic changes are unclear because the same histopathologic picture is seen as a manifestation of late-stage HIV infection whether diarrhea is present or absent.[37, 42]

Idiopathic diarrhea may be explained by multiple processes in late-stage HIV infection. One possibility is a previously undetected enteric pathogen such as enteroadherent *E. coli* as described later.[46, 47] Another possibility is that the anatomic changes noted earlier as characteristic features of AIDS enteropathy may also be a contributing factor, because these anatomic changes are associated with mild malabsorption of carbohydrates,[48] although the data on this point are inconsistent.[49] Another possible contributing factor is HIV infection of the gut as a direct effect. HIV has been found in the lamina propria of both the small bowel and the colon of HIV-infected patients, suggesting a possible role in clinical expression, although the virus is almost always within lymphocytes or macrophages and its presence and quantitation do not correlate with symptoms.[50, 51] Another possibility is that some of the gut symptoms are due to inflammatory mediators such as cytokines.[52] Bacterial overgrowth in the small bowel has been implicated in some studies, especially in association with hypochlorhydria, which is especially common in advanced HIV infection[53]; nevertheless, these patients show inconsistent responses to antibiotic treatment. Autonomic neuropathy is another potential explanation for some patients with enigmatic diarrhea.[54, 55]

Acute Diarrhea

DEFINITION

Acute diarrhea must be distinguished from chronic diarrhea on the basis of distinctions in terms of etiologic probabilities and management (Table 123–4). Many cases are mild and do not require diagnostic evaluation or treatment, many resemble irritable bowel syndrome,[45] and many result from medications including multiple antibiotics, enteral feedings, and anti-HIV agents such as zidovudine, dideoxyinosine, or ritonavir.

AGENTS

The most common infectious agents identified in patients with acute diarrhea are viruses and selected bacteria. Common viral agents are astroviruses, picobirnavirus, adenovirus, and small round viruses including calicivirus.[56–58] The most common bacterial pathogens are *Salmonella, C. difficile,* and possibly, enteroadherent *E. coli. Salmonella* is especially common[59–64] and may be seen with relatively high $CD4^+$ cell counts, reflecting the virulence of this organism even in immunocompetent patients.[59–63] Many present with symptoms of enteric fever without diarrhea, although gastroenteritis is another common presentation. The rate of salmonellosis in patients with HIV infection is estimated to be about 100-fold greater than that of those without HIV infection.[60, 61] In New York City, a crossing of reports of salmonellosis and the AIDS registry showed that the rate of *Salmonella* bacteremia per 100,000 populations was 457 for AIDS patients compared with 2.3 for those without AIDS, and the rate for *Salmonella* gastroenteritis per 100,000 was 393 in AIDS patients compared with 7.7 for those without AIDS.[61] The most frequent isolate appears to be *Salmonella typhimurium*.[60–63] Unusual features of salmonellosis in patients with HIV include the lack of an identifiable source of infection in most patients, high rates of bacteremia, and a propensity of infection to recur after discontinuation of antibiotic treatment.[60–63] Although most authorities do not recommend antibiotic treatment for *Salmonella* gastroenteritis, patients with advanced HIV infection should be treated, usually with a third-generation cephalosporin or a fluoroquinolone. The duration of treatment is arbitrary, but most continue for 4 to 6 weeks because of the frequency of recurrences. The frequency of salmonellosis is modified by the use of zidovudine, which has in vitro activity against this bacterium[64] and other Enterobacteriaceae, and prophylactic trimethoprim-sulfamethoxazole for *P. carinii*.

C. difficile is relatively common in patients with HIV infection, but most authorities believe that this simply reflects the frequency of antibiotic use in this population rather than any inherent HIV-associated risk.[65] Our studies of 200 HIV-infected patients with diarrhea showed that 25 (12.5%) had positive *C. difficile* toxin, assays, virtually all with positive toxin assays had recent exposure to antimicrobial agents, and the usual inducing antibiotics were those seen in the absence of HIV infection: cephalosporins, clindamycin, and ampicillin.[66] Occasional patients have unusual inducing agents such as trimethoprim-sulfamethoxazole, albendazole, or zidovudine.[67] It is not known whether the course of *C. difficile* infection is modified by the presence of HIV infection in terms of the severity of disease, response to therapy, or probability of relapse. The recommended treatment at present is the same as that advocated for patients without HIV infection, using metronidazole for patients with moderately severe disease or persistence of symptoms after withdrawal of the inducing agent; oral vancomycin is reserved for patients with severe disease or disease that fails to respond to metronidazole therapy.[66] Many authorities advocate avoidance of the inducing agent in the future, but this tactic does not have established validity.

Enteroadherent *E. coli* has been implicated as a possible cause of both acute and chronic diarrhea in patients with advanced HIV infection.[46, 47] This organism has been detected on histopathologic studies in the right colon or cecum, show-

TABLE 123–4 ■ Acute Infectious Diarrhea in Patients with Acquired Immunodeficiency Virus

AGENT	FREQUENCY* (%)	CLINICAL FEATURES	DIAGNOSIS	TREATMENT
Salmonella	5–15	Watery diarrhea; fever; fecal white blood cells (WBCs) variable: CD4$^+$ cell count variable; increased frequency with low CD4$^+$ cell count	Stool culture Blood culture	Ciprofloxacin (Cipro), 500–750 mg by mouth (PO) twice a day (bid) for 14 d Trimethoprim-sulfamethoxazole (TMP-SMX), 1–2 double-strength (DS) tablets PO bid for 14 d Ampicillin, 2 g/d PO or 6 g/d intravenously for 14 d (if sensitive) Third-generation cephalosporin or chloramphenicol Treatment may need to be extended in ≥4 wk
Shigella	1–3	Watery diarrhea or bloody flux; fever; fecal WBCs common; any CD4$^+$ cell count	Stool culture	Cipro, 500 mg PO bid for 3 d TMP-SMX, 1 DS tablet PO bid for 3 d
Campylobacter jejuni	4–8	Watery diarrhea or bloody flux; fever; fecal leukocytes variable; any CD4$^+$ cell count	Stool culture; most laboratories cannot detect *C. cinaedi, C. fennelli,* and others	Cipro, 500 mg PO bid for 3–5 d Erythromycin, 500 mg PO four times a day (qid) for 5 d
Clostridium difficile	10–15	Watery diarrhea; fecal WBCs variable; fever and leukocytosis common; antibacterial agent nearly always—especially clindamycin, ampicillin, and cephalosporins; any CD4$^+$ cell count	Endoscopy: pseudomembranous colitis, colitis, or normal Stool toxin assay: tissue culture of enzyme immunoassay preferred Computed tomographic scan: colitis with thickened mucosa	Metronidazole, 250–500 mg PO qid for 10–14 d Vancomycin, 125 mg PO qid for 10–14 d Antiperistaltic agents (diphenoxylate–atropine sulfate [Lomotil] or loperamide) contraindicated
Enteroadherent *Escherichia coli*	10–20	Watery diarrhea; acute, but may be chronic	Adherence to HEp-2 cells (research laboratories only)	Fluoroquinolone
Enteric viruses	15–30	Watery diarrhea; acute, but one third of cases become chronic; any CD4$^+$ cell count	Major agents: adenovirus, astrovirus, picobirnavirus, calicivirus,† clinical laboratories cannot detect these viruses	Supportive treatment: Lomotil or loperamide
Idiopathic	25–40	Variable Noninfectious causes—rule out medications, diet, irritable bowel syndrome; any CD4$^+$ cell count	Negative studies including culture, ova and parasites examination, and *C. difficile* toxin assay	Severe acute diarrhea: Cipro, 500 mg PO bid or ofloxacin, 200–300 mg PO bid for 5 d ± metronidazole‡

*Frequency among patients with acute diarrhea defined as three or more loose or watery stools for 3–10 d.
†Data from Grohmann et al.[58]
‡Data from Arch Intern Med 150:541, 1990; Ann Intern Med 117:202, 1992.

ing attachment to microvilli or aggregates at sites of damaged epithelium; it is identified by adherence to HEp-2 tissue culture cells,[47] but this technology is available only from research laboratories. Support for its role as an enteric pathogen is based on volunteer studies and prevalence in patients with diarrhea compared with control subjects. Enteroadherent *E. coli* has been found in up to 17% of patients with AIDS and diarrhea in the United States and 60% to 80% of HIV-infected patients in Zambia.[47] The suggested treatment is with a fluoroquinolone, but the experience is limited.

Chronic Diarrhea

The most common pathogens found in chronic diarrhea in nearly all reports are *Cryptosporidium*, Microsporida, *M. avium*, and CMV[29–44, 68–70] (Table 123–5). There is a long list of miscellaneous agents, including many of those described as agents of acute diarrhea, such as *Salmonella, C. difficile*, enteroadherent *E. coli*, and most of the enteric viral agents summarized earlier. The "big four" are discussed in the following.

Spore-forming protozoa that are associated with HIV infection include two that are common, *Cryptosporidium* and Microsporida, and two that are infrequent, *Isospora* and *Cyclospora*. Shared properties of these agents are the following: all have been identified as human pathogens, AIDS having increased awareness and recognition; they are intracellular pathogens found within enterocytes; spores or oocytes are shed in stool and represent the infecting source; malabsorption and morphologic changes are related to the organism load; they are most common in tropical areas and locations with poor sanitation; the source of acquisition is fecal-oral contamination or contaminated water or food; all may cause asymptomatic infection, self-limited diarrhea, or, in immunodeficient patients, chronic diarrhea; the diagnosis is based on microscopic examination of stool; and all are treatable, but results of treatment are quite variable[68] (Table 123–6). Pathologic changes are similar with all four and characterized by villus blunting and crypt hyperplasia analogous to changes summarized earlier for AIDS enteropathy. The life cycle starts with ingestion of the spore, followed by invasion of the enterocyte and replication with maturation to produce the infectious agent, the oocyst or spore, which is sloughed

TABLE 123–5 ■ Chronic Infectious Diarrhea in Patients with Acquired Immunodeficiency Syndrome

AGENT	FREQUENCY* (%)	CLINICAL FEATURES	DIAGNOSIS	TREATMENT
Microsporida *Enterocytozoon bieneusi* or *Septata intestinalis*	15–30	Enteritis; watery diarrhea; no fecal white blood cells (WBCs); fever uncommon; remitting disease over years; malabsorption; wasting; CD4+ cell count < 100/mm³	Special trichrome stain described† Biopsy—electron microscopy or Giemsa stain	Albendazole, 400–800 mg orally (PO) twice a day (bid) for 4 wk; larger doses may be required; efficacy is not established‡ (available only through Treatment IND) Metronidazole (anecdotal), 500 mg PO bid§
Cryptosporidium	10–30	Enteritis; watery diarrhea; no fecal WBCs; no fever; malabsorption; wasting; large stool volume with abdominal pain; remitting symptoms for months to years; CD4+ cell count < 200/mm³	Acid-fast bacillus smear of stool to show oocyst of 4–6 μm	Paromomycin, 500 mg PO four times a day (qid) for ≥4 wk Octreotide, 50–500 μg subcutaneously or intravenously (IV) three times a day (tid) (nonspecific) Azithromycin, 1200 mg PO bid for 1 d, then 1200 mg/d for 27 d, then 600 mg/d May require parenteral hyperalimentation
Cytomegalovirus	15–40	Colitis and/or enteritis; fecal WBCs and/or blood; cramps; fever; watery diarrhea ± blood; may cause perforation; hemorrhage, toxic megacolon, ulceration; CD4+ cell count < 50/mm³	Biopsy to show intranuclear inclusion bodies, preferably with inflammation, vasculitis Computed tomography (CT); segmental or pancolitis	Ganciclovir, 5 mg/kg IV bid Foscarnet, 40–60 mg/kg IV q 8 h Results of treatment variable‖; foscarnet and ganciclovir are equally effective¶
Mycobacterium avium	10–20	Enteritis; watery diarrhea; no fecal WBCs; fever and wasting common; diffuse abdominal pain in late stage; CD4+ cell count < 50/mm³	Positive blood cultures for *M. avium*; biopsy may show changes like Whipple's disease, but with acid-fast bacilli; CT may be supportive; hepatosplenomegaly, adenopathy, and thickened small bowel	Clarithromycin, 500 mg–1 g PO tid + ethambutol, 15 mg/kg/d; rifampin, 600 mg/d and/or clofazimine, 100 mg/d
Isospora	1–3	Enteritis; watery diarrhea; no fecal WBCs; no fever; wasting; malabsorption; CD4+ cell count < 100/mm³	Acid-fast bacillus smear of stool; oocytes 20–30 μm	Trimethoprim-sulfamethoxazole (TMP-SMX), 3–4 double-strength (DS) tablets/d Pyrimethamine, 50–75 mg/d PO
Entamoeba histolytica	1–3	Colitis; bloody stools; cramps; no fecal WBCs (bloody stools); most patients asymptomatic carriers; any CD4+ cell count	Stool ova and parasites (O&P) examination	Metronidazole, 500–750 mg PO or IV tid for 5–10 d, then iodoquinol, 650 mg PO tid for 21 d or paromomycin, 500 mg PO qid for 7 d
Giardia	1–3	Enteritis; watery diarrhea ± malabsorption, bloating; flatulence; any CD4+ cell count	Stool O&P examination	Quinacrine, 100 mg PO tid for 10 d or metronidazole, 250 mg PO tid for 10 d
Cyclospora cayetanensis	<1%	Enteritis; watery diarrhea; CD4+ cell count < 100/mm³	Stool acid-fast bacillus smear—resembles that of *Cryptosporidium*	TMP-SMX, 1 DS bid for 3 d
Small bowel overgrowth	Not known	Watery diarrhea; malabsorption; wasting; often associated with hypochlorhydria	Hydrogen breath test; quantitative culture of small bowel aspirate	Amoxicillin-clavulanate, 250–500 mg PO tid Doxycycline, 100 mg PO tid
Idiopathic	20–30	Watery diarrhea; malabsorption; no fecal WBCs	Biopsy shows villus atrophy, crypt hyperplasia + no identifiable cause despite endoscopy with biopsy and electron microscopy for Microsporida**	Supportive care: diphenoxylate–atropine sulfate (Lomotil) or loperamide Nutritional support

*Frequency among patients with advanced HIV infection and chronic diarrhea defined as more than two or three loose or watery stools a day for ≥21 d.
†Data from Weber et al.[104]
‡Data from Dieterich et al.[107]
§Schattenkerk JKME, van Gool T, van Ketel RJ, et al: Clinical significance of small-intestinal microsporidiosis in HIV infected individuals. Lancet 337:895, 1991.
‖Data from Dieterich et al[72] and Reed EC, Wolford JL, Kopecky KJ, et al: Ganciclovir for the treatment of cytomegalovirus gastroenteritis in bone marrow transplant recipients. Ann Intern Med 112:505, 1990.
¶Data from Blanshard et al.[81]
**Data from Bartlett et al.[38]

TABLE 123–6 ■ Comparison of Intestinal Spore-Forming Protozoa

CHARACTERISTIC	CRYPTOSPORIDIUM	MICROSPORIDA	ISOSPORA	CYCLOSPORA
Agents—human disease	*Cryptosporidium parvum*	*Enterocytozoon bieneusi* *Septata intestinalis*	*Isospora belli*	*Cyclospora cayetanensis*
Source of infection (suspected or established)	Humans, farm animals Food or water	Humans Food or water	Humans Food or water	Humans Food or water
Frequency in AIDS patients with diarrhea	10%–20%	6%–50% *E. bieneusi/S. intestinalis* = 7.1%	United States: 2% Developing countries: 10%–12%	United States: <1% Haiti: 11%
Clinical expression				
Immunocompetent persons	Self-limited diarrhea (3–25 d)	Nonpathogenic	Self-limited diarrhea	Self-limited diarrhea; may be chronic
AIDS patients	Most: transient or chronic diarrhea; may be devastating	Transient or chronic diarrhea	Transient or chronic diarrhea	Transient or chronic diarrhea
Extraintestinal disease	Biliary infection —	Biliary infection Disseminated disease	Biliary infection —	— —
Detection				
Modified acid-fast bacillus (AFB) stain	+	—	+	±
Size of oocyst	4–6 μm	1–2 μm	20–30 μm	8–10 μm
Diagnosis	AFB—stool	Trichrome or fluorescent antibody stain	AFB—stool	AFB—stool
Therapy	Paromomycin	*E. bieneusi*—none *S. intestinalis*—albendazole	Trimethoprim-sulfamethoxazole	Trimethoprim-sulfamethoxazole

Adapted from Goodgame RW: Understanding intestinal spore-forming protozoa: Cryptosporidia, microsporidia, isospora, and cyclospora. Ann Intern Med 124:429–441, 1996.

in the intestine. Detection is by acid-fast staining of stool with distinction based on morphology and the size of oocysts (see Table 123–6). The exception is Microsporida organisms, which are 1 to 2 μm and best seen with a modified trichrome or fluorescent stain.[44]

Specific Pathogens

Cytomegalovirus Infection

CMV gastrointestinal disease is found in about 20% of AIDS patients.[71] Nearly all have late-stage HIV infection with $CD4^+$ cell counts less than 100/mm^3, and the median $CD4^+$ cell count is 10 to 25/mm^3. Sites of involvement include virtually any level of the gastrointestinal tract, including the oral cavity, esophagus, stomach, small bowel, colon, and perirectal region. The accompanying clinical syndromes reflect the site: dysphagia and retrosternal pain are associated with esophageal involvement; ulcer symptoms that fail to respond to antacids or histamine H_2 blockers with gastroduodenitis; abdominal pain with malabsorption with steatorrhea when the small bowel is infected; and chronic diarrhea that may be watery, bloody, or associated with excessive mucus when the colon is involved. Most common is CMV colitis with inflammatory diarrhea with fecal leukocytes or blood, fever, and cramps.[72–76] Less common presentations include a solitary intestinal ulcer, toxic megacolon, intestinal perforation, or obstruction caused by mass lesions in the small bowel.[75] Typical findings of contrast studies include segmental colitis or pancolitis with mucosal granularity, thickened folds, spasticity, or superficial erosions.[77, 78] Colonic involvement may be diffuse, segmental, or restricted to the cecum. Computed tomography usually shows a thickened colonic mucosa with ulcerations, and endoscopy usually shows focal or diffuse inflammatory changes with hemorrhagic plaques and superficial ulcerations. Biopsy and histologic examination of typical lesions show CMV vasculitis with inflammation and hemorrhage in the lamina propria and typical intranuclear inclusions within endothelial cells.

The usual treatment is intravenous ganciclovir (5 mg/kg every 12 hours for 14 to 28 days). Response with esophagitis is usually good but is less impressive with colitis. A placebo-controlled trial in AIDS patients with CMV colitis showed that ganciclovir treatment reduced the number of cultures positive for CMV, improved colonoscopy scores, stabilized weight changes, and decreased the frequency of new extracolonic sites of CMV disease.[79] There was no significant change in diarrhea, abdominal pain, or fatigue. The role of maintenance therapy is variable depending on response and relapse after treatment is discontinued. Foscarnet is the alternative agent for patients who fail to respond to ganciclovir therapy.[80] A comparative trial of foscarnet versus ganciclovir showed that the two agents were equally effective.[81]

Cryptosporidiosis

Cryptosporidium parvum was originally described as an enteric pathogen of humans in 1976, and it has subsequently been implicated as a relatively common cause of infectious diarrhea in immunocompetent patients. In previously healthy persons, the disease is characterized by 3 to 25 days of diarrhea, abdominal pain, and malaise; a minority of patients have nausea, vomiting, or fever or require hospitalization.[68, 82] The disease is more common and more severe in patients with immunosuppression.[82–84] One study of 128 AIDS patients showed four patterns: asymptomatic carriage (4%); transient, self-limited disease (29%); chronic disease (60%); and fulminant disease (8%).[84] Clinical expression with severity and chronicity of symptoms depends largely on the $CD4^+$ cell count; patients with counts less than 50/mm^3 may have devastating diarrhea with fluid losses of 10 to 20 L/d and lifelong persistence of *Cryptosporidium*.[68, 83–85] Cryptosporidiosis is the initial AIDS-defining diagnosis in 2% to 4% of

AIDS patients, it is the most common cause of chronic diarrhea, and its frequency is higher in developing countries.[29–33, 86, 87] In the United States, *Cryptosporidium* organisms are found in stools of 10% to 20% of AIDS patients with diarrhea.[2, 36–38, 83–85] The usual method of detection is identification of typical oocysts utilizing modified Ziehl-Neelsen, modified Kinyoun acid-fast, auramine O fluorescent, or murine monoclonal antibody stains.[68, 83–90] Examination of small bowel biopsy specimens shows typical 4-μm circular organisms on the apical membrane of the enterocyte. Associated histologic changes include partial atrophy and distortion of the villi with a mononuclear infiltrate of the lamina propria, predominantly in the ileum and jejunum. Other sites of involvement of the gastrointestinal tract, including the esophagus and colon, have been reported. Biliary infections include a sclerosing cholangitis and acalculous cholecystitis.[68, 91–93] Patients with acalculous sclerosing cholangitis present with right upper quadrant pain and increasing alkaline phosphatase. This is a late-stage complication. With regard to therapy, extensive efforts have been made to treat cryptosporidial infections in immunocompromised hosts using a variety of therapeutic agents, but none has proved consistently effective.[94] The favored drug is paromomycin (500 mg three or four times daily), which has shown a modest benefit compared with placebo in terms of oocyte excretion and stool frequency.[95] Patients with biliary cryptosporidiosis do not respond to paromomycin[96]; uncontrolled studies show response to sphincterotomy, but results are variable and relief of pain is often temporary.[92, 93] The role of cholecystectomy is also unclear.[97] For patients with severe disease, the usual recommendation is elemental feedings, antiperistaltic agents, and possibly spiramycin or somatostatin.

Isosporosis

Isospora belli is also a protozoan parasite that invades microvilli of the small intestine, causing severe and protracted diarrhea in patients with AIDS. Histologic changes in the small bowel and diagnostic testing using small bowel biopsies or direct stool examination are analogous to those described for cryptosporidiosis.[68, 87, 98] On stool examination the organism is readily distinguished from *Cryptosporidium* on the basis of size[68, 99] (see Table 123–6). Data from the Centers for Disease Control and Prevention indicated that isosporosis is the initial AIDS-defining diagnosis for only about 0.2% of AIDS patients in the United States; however, the reported frequency of isosporidia among AIDS patients with chronic diarrhea from Zaire and Haiti has been as high as 19% and 15%, respectively.[29, 92] This organism is endemic in many parts of Africa, Asia and South America, but prevalence rates in AIDS patients in these locations are generally unknown.[68] Unlike *Cryptosporidium*, *I. belli* seems to respond well to trimethoprim-sulfamethoxazole, although the relapse rate is relatively high, suggesting the possible need for long-term maintenance therapy.[68, 98, 100, 101] Other treatment options include pyrimethamine and metronidazole.[100] Trimethoprim-sulfamethoxazole or sulfadoxine-pyrimethamine prevents recurrent disease.[100]

Microsporidiosis

Microsporida comprises monocellular parasites that have been recognized as human pathogens and are being recognized with escalating frequency among patients with AIDS and chronic diarrhea.[34, 36–38, 42, 101–103] Human infection has been reported almost exclusively in AIDS patients and usually in those with $CD4^+$ cell counts lower than 50/mm^3. Two species have been implicated as intestinal pathogens, *Enterocytozoon bieneusi* and *Septata intestinalis*. Both cause noninflammatory, usually intermittent, chronic diarrhea without fever; malabsorption studies show severe malabsorption of fat and D-xylose and low zinc levels.[34, 68] *E. bieneusi* is the more common species involved, *S. intestinalis* causes extraintestinal disease, and both species have been implicated in AIDS cholangiopathy. As the name implies, Microsporida organisms are small parasites that cannot be detected by routine microscopic studies of stool, and they are usually overlooked on small bowel biopsy examination as well. The usual method of recognition is by a modified trichrome stain of stool.[36, 68, 104–106] Small bowel biopsy appears to be more sensitive than stool examination. Stains advocated for detecting Microsporida in tissue include hematoxylin-eosin, Gram stain, toluidine blue, Warthin-Starry, and Giemsa stain.[68] Asymptomatic infection in the small bowel has been described.[105] With regard to therapy, albendazole (400 mg twice a day) is effective for *S. intestinalis*.[106] Albendazole is less effective for infections involving *E. bieneusi*, with only a modest reduction in stools and failure to eradicate the pathogen.[107]

Mycobacterium avium *Infection*

Prior studies indicated that 40% to 50% of late-stage AIDS patients develop disseminated *M. avium* infection, although this frequency is notably reduced with prophylaxis using rifabutin, clarithromycin, or azithromycin. Gastrointestinal involvement may be expressed clinically as diarrhea, malabsorption, weight loss, crampy abdominal pain, and fever. Pathologic changes noted with colonic involvement include edema, erythema, and friability, and biopsy specimens show typical acid-fast organisms within macrophages and free within the lamina propria.[108] With small bowel involvement, the typical pathologic changes are nearly identical to those of Whipple's disease, with foamy macrophages distended by vesicles containing periodic acid–Schiff–positive material in the lamina propria.[109] Nearly all patients have *M. avium* bacteremia.[110] The organism is commonly detected with acid-fast stains and cultures of stool,[111, 112] but this finding simply supports the diagnosis of disseminated infection and does not necessarily indicate invasion of the gut. The usual treatment is with combination antimicrobials, using clarithromycin plus ethambutol, sometimes with the addition of rifabutin or a fluoroquinolone. Relapses are common and are usually associated with resistance to clarithromycin.

Miscellaneous Infections

Patients with HIV infection are subject to the same types of enteric pathogens that are encountered in healthy hosts, although these infections may be unusually severe or prolonged in immunosuppressed persons. For example, AIDS patients with shigellosis often have *Shigella* bacteremia[113] or may have persistent infection[114]; infections with *Campylobacter* species may include bacteremia with opportunistic pathogens such as *Campylobacter fetus*, *C. jejuni*, or *C. cinaedi*.[115–117] Hemolytic-uremic syndrome and thrombotic thrombocytopenic purpura caused by verocytotoxin-producing *E. coli* have been reported in AIDS patients.[118, 119] *C. difficile* is presumably the most common bacterial pathogen. This appears to reflect the frequent exposure to antibacterial agents rather than a predisposition based on immunosuppression. The major agents implicated are cephalosporins, ampicillin, and clindamycin. Most patients respond to antibiotic withdrawal and treatment with metronidazole or oral vancomycin.[65, 66] The prominent role of protozoan parasites (*Cryptosporidium*, *Isospora*, and Microsporida) was summarized earlier. Other parasites are found occasionally but, excluding *E. histolytica* and *G. lamblia*, evidence to implicate them as agents of enteric disease is tenuous. Perhaps the most controversial is *Blasto-*

cystis hominis, which has been found in 5% to 15% of healthy persons and 35% to 50% of homosexual men and has occasionally been implicated as an agent of enteric disease in diverse hosts, including those with HIV infection.[120] When treatment is deemed appropriate, metronidazole is the preferred agent. There is no good evidence that *Endolimax nana, Entamoeba coli, Entamoeba hartmanni,* and other nonpathogenic parasites are peculiarly virulent in patients with HIV infection. The most common identified viral pathogens are CMV and HSV. Multiple enteric viruses have been found in AIDS patients with both acute and chronic diarrhea as summarized earlier.[56–58] These agents are not detectable with the usual laboratory resources and there is no specific treatment. Adenovirus is sometimes detected in the mucosa in intestinal biopsies, but its role in diarrhea is unclear.[56, 57] Adenovirus may be mistaken for Microsporida or CMV at light microscopy of intestinal specimens, and this mistake could have important therapeutic implications.[121] Fungi are uncommon causes of enteric infection, although there may be intestinal involvement with disseminated disease caused by histoplasmosis, aspergillosis, or cryptococcosis.[122–124] The most common is enteritis with disseminated *Histoplasma capsulatum.*[124]

Tumors

Tumors of the gastrointestinal tract associated with HIV infection include Kaposi's sarcoma, non-Hodgkin's lymphoma, cloacogenic carcinoma of the rectum, squamous cell carcinoma of the rectum and anus, squamous carcinoma of the tongue, and Burkitt lymphoma. The most common, Kaposi's sarcoma, may involve the gut in up to 40% to 50% of patients who have cutaneous lesions.[125, 126] Most are asymptomatic, although oral lesions may be painful, esophageal lesions may cause dysphagia, and lower gastrointestinal tract involvement may cause diarrhea, subacute intestinal obstruction, protein-losing enteropathy, or a rectal ulcer. Oral lesions are readily apparent on inspection, and endoscopy may show typical raised, red nodules, with or without central umbilication. Histologic confirmation is difficult owing to the depth of the lesions. In one study, only 7 of 30 lesions observed by endoscopy were confirmed with histologic examination.[126] The lymphomas associated with HIV infection are usually extranodal high-grade B-cell lymphomas. The gastrointestinal tract is involved in up to 20% of all HIV-infected patients with lymphomas, and there may be involvement of any site from the oral cavity to the rectum.

Wasting

The wasting syndrome is defined by the unintentional loss of 10% of body weight. The wasting syndrome is second only to *P. carinii* pneumonia as the most common cause of the initial AIDS-defining condition, accounting for 15% to 20% of cases. For many patients the weight loss is profound and is a factor contributing to death.[127] As with other chronic disease states, death occurs when the weight is 66% of ideal body weight.

There are multiple contributing factors to weight loss in patients with AIDS. Anorexia results from drug treatments, depression, oral or esophageal disease, or enteropathy.[128] Malabsorption may result in loss of nutrients. There is also derangement of intermediary metabolism with suppression of carbohydrate oxidation, increased triglyceride concentrations, and accelerated protein turnover.[129–132] The result is that ingested substrates are directed to fat rather than lean tissue. Energy balance is the product of energy intake and expenditure. A common thesis has been that increased resting energy expenditure is the cause of wasting in AIDS. Nevertheless, rapid weight loss during secondary infections appears to result from reduced energy intake rather than expenditure. The secondary infections are accompanied by fatigue that represents a compensatory mechanism to maintain weight and energy.[131–133]

A conclusion from these observations is that rapid weight loss usually indicates secondary infection and that weight gain accompanies recovery from infection. The implication is that rapid weight loss (more than 4 kg in ≤4 months) indicates secondary infection and that successful treatment of these complications is the optimal method for preventing devastating weight loss. A more gradual weight loss may indicate anorexia or malabsorption.

Nutritional support is considered a critical factor in disease management. The goal is to increase lean body mass rather than fat mass to improve fatigue and functional performance. Appetite stimulants such as dronabinol (Marinol) and megestrol (Megace) increase food intake and weight, although most of the weight gain is in fat. Anabolic agents such as growth hormone and anabolic steroids promote nitrogen retention with increase in fat-free mass. Thalidomide has been used for its potential benefit in suppressing tumor necrosis factor. Enteral and parenteral nutritional supports are used to increase energy intake and are useful primarily for patients with anorexia. Most studies have shown that drug therapy and supplemental feedings are associated with weight gains and improved quality of life, but the improvement is modest, the cost is often high, and there is no important effect on $CD4^+$ cell count.[134]

References

1. Quinn TC, Stamm WE, Goodell SE, et al: The polymicrobial origin of intestinal infections in homosexual men. N Engl J Med 309:576, 1983.
2. Laughon BE, Druckman DA, Vernon A, et al: Prevalence of enteric pathogens in homosexual men with and without AIDS. Gastroenterology 94:984, 1988.
3. Greenspan D, Greenspan JS: HIV-related oral disease. Lancet 348:729, 1996.
4. Maenza JR, Keruly JC, Moore RD, et al: Risk factors for fluconazole-resistant candidiasis in human immunodeficiency virus–infected patients. J Infect Dis 173:219, 1996.
5. Tavitian A, Raufman J-P, Rosenthal LE: Oral candidiasis as a marker for esophageal candidiasis in the acquired immunodeficiency syndrome. Ann Intern Med 104:54, 1986.
6. Greenspan D: Treatment of oral candidiasis in HIV infection. Oral Surg Oral Med Oral Pathol 78:211, 1994.
7. Baily GG, Perry FM, Denning DW, Mandal BK: Fluconazole-resistant candidosis in an HIV cohort. AIDS 8:787, 1994.
8. Greenspan D, Greenspan JS, Conant M, et al: Oral 'hairy' leukoplakia in male homosexuals: Evidence of association with both papillomavirus and a herpes-group virus. Lancet 2:831, 1984.
9. Greenspan JS, Greenspan D, Lennette ET, et al: Replication of Epstein-Barr virus within the epithelial cells of oral "hairy" leukoplakia, an AIDS-associated lesion. N Engl J Med 313:1564, 1985.
10. Greenspan D, Greenspan JS, Hearst NG, et al: Relation of oral hairy leukoplakia to infection with the human immunodeficiency virus and the risk of developing AIDS. J Infect Dis 155:475, 1987.
11. Aragues M, Sanchez Perez J, Fraga J, et al: Hairy leucoplakia: A clinical, histopathological and ultrastructural study in 33 patients. Clin Exp Dermatol 15:335, 1990.
12. Paauw DS, Wenrich MD, Curtis JR, et al: Ability of primary care physicians to recognize physical findings associated with HIV infection. JAMA 274:1380, 1995.
13. Resnick L, Herbst JS, Ablashi D, et al: Regression of oral hairy leukoplakia after orally administered acyclovir therapy. JAMA 259:384, 1988.
14. MacPhail LA, Greenspan D, Greenspan JS: Recurrent aphthous ulcers in association with HIV infection: Diagnosis and treatment. Oral Surg Oral Med Oral Pathol 73:283, 1992.

15. Winkler JR, Herrera C, Westenhouse J, et al: Periodontal disease in HIV-infected and uninfected homosexual and bisexual men. AIDS 6:1041, 1992.
16. Connolly GM, Hawkins D, Harcourt-Webster JN, et al: Oesophageal symptoms, their causes, treatment, and prognosis in patients with the acquired immunodeficiency syndrome. Gut 30:1033, 1989.
17. Laine L, Bobacini M: Esophageal disease in HIV infection. Arch Intern Med 154:1577, 1994.
18. Porro GB, Parente F, Cernuschi M: The diagnosis of esophageal candidiasis in patients with acquired immune deficiency syndrome: Is endoscopy always necessary? Am J Gastroenterol 84:143, 1989.
19. Rabeneck L, Laine L: Esophageal candidiasis in patients infected with HIV: A decision analysis to assess cost-effectiveness of alternative management strategies. Arch Intern Med 154:2705, 1994.
20. Laine L: The natural history of esophageal candidiasis after successful treatment in patients with AIDS. Gastroenterology 107:744, 1994.
21. Wilcox CM, Straub RF, Clark WS: Prospective evaluation of oropharyngeal findings in HIV-infected patients with esophageal ulceration. Am J Gastroenterol 90:1938, 1995.
22. Wilcox CM, Diehl DL, Cello JP, et al: Cytomegalovirus esophagitis in patients with AIDS. Ann Intern Med 113:589, 1990.
23. Goodgame RW: Gastrointestinal cytomegalovirus disease. Ann Intern Med 119:924, 1993.
24. Wilcox CM, Schwartz DA: Comparison of two corticosteroid regimens for the treatment of HIV-associated idiopathic esophageal ulcer. Am J Gastroenterol 89:2163, 1994.
25. Paterson DL, Georghiou PR, Allworth AM, Kemp RJ: Thalidomide as treatment of refractory aphthous ulceration related to human immunodeficiency virus infection. Clin Infect Dis 20:250, 1995.
26. Edwards P, Turner J, Gold J, et al: Esophageal ulceration induced by zidovudine. Ann Intern Med 112:65, 1990.
27. Greenspan JS, Greenspan D (eds): Oral Manifestations of HIV Infection: Proceedings of the 2nd International Workshop on the Oral Manifestations of HIV Infection, January 31–February 3, 1993. Carol Stream, IL, Quintessence Publishing, 1995.
28. Wilcox CM: Esophageal disease in acquired immunodeficiency syndrome: Etiology, diagnosis, and management. Am J Med 92:412, 1992.
29. Pape JEW, Liautaud B, Thomas F, et al: The acquired immunodeficiency syndrome in Haiti. Ann Intern Med 103:674, 1985.
30. Malebranche R, Arnoux E, Gerin JM, et al: Acquired immunodeficiency syndrome with severe gastrointestinal manifestations in Haiti. Lancet 2:873, 1985.
31. Clumeck N, Sonnet J, Taelman H, et al: Acquired immune deficiency syndrome in African patients. N Engl J Med 310:492, 1984.
32. Piot P, Quinn TC, Taelman H, et al: Acquired immunodeficiency syndrome in a heterosexual population in Zaire. Lancet 2:65, 1984.
33. Serwadda E, Mugewrwa RD, Sewankambo NK, et al: Slim disease: A new disease in Uganda and its association with HTLV-III infection. Lancet 2:849, 1985.
34. Kotler DP, Orenstein JM: Prevalence of intestinal microsporidiosis in HIV-infected individuals referred for gastroenterological evaluation. Am J Gastroenterol 89:1998, 1994.
35. Ullrich R, Heise W, Bergs C, et al: Gastrointestinal symptoms in patients infected with human immunodeficiency virus: Relevance of infective agents isolated from gastrointestinal tract. Gut 33:1080, 1992.
36. Mayer HB, Wanke CA: Diagnostic strategies in HIV-infected patients with diarrhea. AIDS 8:1639, 1994.
37. Sharpstone D, Gazzard B: Gastrointestinal manifestations of HIV infection. Lancet 348:379, 1996.
38. Bartlett JG, Belitsos PC, Sears CL: AIDS enteropathy. Clin Infect Dis 15:726, 1992.
39. Smith PD, Lane C, Gill VJ, et al: Intestinal infections in patients with the acquired immunodeficiency syndrome (AIDS). Etiology and response to therapy. Ann Intern Med 108:328, 1988.
40. Antony MA, Brandt LJ, Klein RS, Bernstein LH: Infectious diarrhea in patients with AIDS. Dig Dis Sci 33:1141, 1988.
41. Rolston KVI, Rodriguez S, Hernandez M, et al: Diarrhea in patients infected with the human immunodeficiency virus. Am J Med 86:137, 1989.
42. Greenson JK, Belitsos PC, Yardley JH, et al: AIDS enteropathy: Occult enteric infections and duodenal mucosal alterations in chronic diarrhea. Ann Intern Med 114:366, 1991.
43. Choi SW, Choong HP, Silva TMJ, et al: To culture or not to culture: Fecal lactoferrin screening for inflammatory bacterial diarrhea. J Clin Microbiol 34:928, 1996.
44. van Gool T, Snijders F, Reiss P, et al: Diagnosis of intestinal and disseminated microsporidial infections in patients with HIV by a new rapid fluorescence technique. J Clin Pathol 46:694, 1993.
45. Wilcox MC, Schwartz DA, Cotsonis G, Thompson GE: Chronic unexplained diarrhea in human immunodeficiency virus infection: Determination of the best diagnostic approach. Gastroenterology 110:30, 1996.
46. Kotler DP, Giang TT, Thiim M, et al: Chronic bacterial enteropathy in patients with AIDS. J Infect Dis 171:552, 1995.
47. Mathewson JJ, Jiang ZD, Zumla A, et al: HEp-2 cell–adherent *Escherichia coli* in patients with human immunodeficiency virus–associated diarrhea. J Infect Dis 171:1636, 1995.
48. Ullrich R, Zeitz M, Heise W, et al: Small intestinal structure and function in patients infected with human immunodeficiency virus (HIV): Evidence for HIV-induced enteropathy. Ann Intern Med 111:15, 1989.
49. Keating J, Bjarnason I, Somasundaram S, et al: Intestinal absorptive capacity, intestinal permeability and jejunal histology in HIV and their relation to diarrhoea. Gut 37:623, 1995.
50. Fox CH, Kotler D, Tierney A, et al: Detection of HIV-1 RNA in the lamina propria of patients with AIDS and gastrointestinal disease. J Infect Dis 159:467, 1989.
51. Heise C, Dandekar S, Kumar P, et al: Human immunodeficiency virus infection of enterocytes and mononuclear cells in human jejunal mucosa. Gastroenterology 100:1521, 1991.
52. MacDonald TT, Spencer J: Evidence that activated mucosal T cells play a role in the pathogenesis of enteropathy in human small intestine. J Exp Med 167:1341, 1988.
53. Belitsos PC, Greenson JK, Sisler J, et al: Association of chronic wasting diarrhea with gastric hypoacidity and opportunistic enteric infections in patients with acquired immunodeficiency syndrome (AIDS). J Infect Dis 166:277, 1992.
54. Freeman R, Roberts MS, Friedman LS, Broadbridge C: Autonomic function and human immunodeficiency virus infection. Neurology 40:575, 1990.
55. Batman PA, Miller ARO, Sedgwick PM, Griffin G: Autonomic denervation in jejunal mucosa of homosexual men infected with HIV. AIDS 5:1247, 1991.
56. Kaljot KT, Ling JP, Gold JWM, et al: Prevalence of acute enteric viral pathogens in acquired immunodeficiency syndrome patients with diarrhea. Gastroenterology 97:1031, 1989.
57. Schmidt W, Schneider T, Heise W, et al: Stool viruses, coinfections, and diarrhea in HIV-infected patients. J Acquir Immune Defic Syndr 13:33, 1996.
58. Grohmann GS, Glass RI, Pereira HG, et al: Enteric viruses and diarrhea in HIV-infected patients. N Engl J Med 329:14, 1993.
59. Nelson MR, Shanson DC, Hawkins DA, Gazzard BG: *Salmonella*, *Campylobacter* and *Shigella* in HIV-seropositive patients. AIDS 6:1495, 1992.
60. Mundy LM, Sears CL: Small intestinal infections: *Salmonella* and human immunodeficiency virus–associated enteropathy. Curr Opin Gastroenterol 9:77, 1993.
61. Gruenewald R, Blum S, Chan J: Relationship between human immunodeficiency virus infection and salmonellosis in 20- to 59-year-old residents of New York City. Clin Infect Dis 18:358, 1994.
62. Jacobs JL, Gold JWM, Murray HW, Roberts RB: *Salmonella* infections in patients with the acquired immunodeficiency syndrome. Ann Intern Med 102:186, 1985.
63. Smith PD, Macher AM, Bookman MA, et al: *Salmonella typhimurium* enteritis and bacteremia in the acquired immunodeficiency syndrome. Ann Intern Med 102:207, 1985.
64. Salmon D, Detruchis P, Leport C, et al: Efficacy of zidovudine in preventing relapses of *Salmonella* bacteremia in AIDS. J Infect Dis 163:415, 1991.
65. Lu SS, Schwartz JM, Simon DM, Brandt LJ: *Clostridium difficile*–associated diarrhea in patients with HIV positivity and AIDS: A prospective controlled study. Am J Gastroenterol 89:1226, 1994.
66. Bartlett JG: *Clostridium difficile*: History of its role as an enteric pathogen and the current state of knowledge about the organism. Clin Infect Dis 18(Suppl 4):S265, 1994.

67. Shah V, Marino C, Altice FL: Albendazole-induced pseudomembranous colitis. Am J Gastroenterol 91:1453, 1996.
68. Goodgame RW: Understanding intestinal spore-forming protozoa: Cryptosporidia, microsporidia, isospora, and cyclospora. Ann Intern Med 124:429, 1996.
69. Smith PD, Quinn TC, Strober W, et al: Gastrointestinal infections in AIDS. Ann Intern Med 116:63, 1992.
70. Rabeneck L: Diagnostic workup strategies for patients with HIV-related chronic diarrhea. J Clin Gastroenterol 16:245, 1993.
71. Spector SA, McKinley GF, Lalezari JP, et al: Oral ganciclovir for the prevention of cytomegalovirus disease in persons with AIDS. N Engl J Med 334:1491, 1996.
72. Dieterich DT, Kotler DP, Busch DF, et al: Ganciclovir treatment of cytomegalovirus colitis in AIDS: A randomized, double-blind, placebo-controlled multicenter study. J Infect Dis 167:278, 1993.
73. Dieterich DT, Rahmin M: Cytomegalovirus colitis in AIDS: Presentation in 44 patients and a review of the literature. J Acquir Immune Defic Syndr 4(Suppl 1):529, 1991.
74. Rene E, Marche C, Chevalier T, et al: Cytomegalovirus colitis in patients with acquired immunodeficiency syndrome. Dig Dis Sci 33:741, 1988.
75. Rich JD, Crawford JM, Kazanjian SN, Kazanjian PH: Discrete gastrointestinal mass lesions caused by cytomegalovirus in patients with AIDS: Report of three cases and review. Clin Infect Dis 15:609, 1992.
76. Chachoua A, Dieterich D, Krasinski K, et al: 9-(1,3-Dihydroxy-2-propoxymethyl) guanine (ganciclovir) in the treatment of cytomegalovirus gastrointestinal disease with the acquired immunodeficiency syndrome. Ann Intern Med 107:133, 1987.
77. Frager DH, Frager JD, Wolf EL, et al: Cytomegalovirus colitis in acquired immune deficiency syndrome: Radiologic spectrum. Gastrointest Radiol 111:241, 1986.
78. Balthaar EJ, Megibow AJ, Faini E, et al: Cytomegalovirus colitis in AIDS: Radiographic findings in 11 patients. Radiology 155:585, 1985.
79. Bieterich DT, Poles MA, Lew EA, et al: Concurrent use of ganciclovir and foscarnet to treat cytomegalovirus infection in AIDS patients. J Infect Dis 167:1184, 1993.
80. Dieterich DT, Poles MA, Dicker M, et al: Foscarnet treatment of cytomegalovirus gastrointestinal infections in acquired immunodeficiency syndrome patients who have failed ganciclovir induction. Am J Gastroenterol 88:542, 1993.
81. Blanshard C, Benhamou Y, Dohin E, et al: Treatment of AIDS-associated gastrointestinal cytomegalovirus infection with foscarnet and ganciclovir: A randomized comparison. J Infect Dis 172:622, 1995.
82. MacKenzie WR, Hoxie NJ, Proctor ME, et al: A massive outbreak in Milwaukee of *Cryptosporidium* infection transmitted through the public water supply. N Engl J Med 331:161, 1994.
83. Petersen C: Cryptosporidiosis in patients infected with the human immunodeficiency virus. J Infect Dis 15:903, 1993.
84. Flanigan T, Whalen C, Turner J, et al: *Cryptosporidium* infection and CD4 counts. Ann Intern Med 116:840, 1992.
85. Current WL, Garcia LS: Cryptosporidiosis. Clin Microbiol Rev 4:325, 1991.
86. Wuhib T, Silva TM, Newman RD, et al: Cryptosporidial and microsporidial infections in human immunodeficiency virus–infected patients in northeastern Brazil. J Infect Dis 170:490, 1994.
87. DeHovit JA, Pape JW, Boncy M, et al: Clinical manifestations and therapy of *Isospora belli* infection in patients with the acquired immunodeficiency syndrome. N Engl J Med 315:87, 1986.
88. Weber R, Bryan RT, Bishop HS, et al: Threshold of detection of *Cryptosporidium* oocysts in human stool specimens: Evidence for low sensitivity of current diagnostic methods. J Clin Microbiol 29:1323, 1991.
89. Payne P, Lancaster LA, Heinman M, McCutchan JA: Identification of *Cryptosporidium* in patients with acquired immunodeficiency syndrome. N Engl J Med 309:613, 1984.
90. Garcia LS, Brewer TC, Bruckner DA: Fluorescence detection of *Cryptosporidium* oocysts in human fecal specimens by using monoclonal antibodies. J Clin Microbiol 25:119, 1987.
91. Vakil NB, Schwartz SM, Buggy BP, et al: Biliary cryptosporidiosis in HIV-infected people after the waterborne outbreak of cryptosporidiosis in Milwaukee. N Engl J Med 334:19, 1996.
92. Benhamou Y, Caumes E, Gerosa Y, et al: AIDS-related cholangiopathy. Critical analysis of a prospective series of 26 patients. Dig Dis Sci 38:1113, 1993.
93. Cello JP: Acquired immunodeficiency syndrome cholangiopathy: Spectrum of disease. Am J Med 86:539, 1989.
94. Communicable Disease Center: Cryptosporidiosis: Assessment of chemotherapy of males with acquired immune deficiency syndrome (AIDS). MMWR Morbid Mortal Wkly Rep 31:589, 1982.
95. Bissuel F, Cotte L, Rabodonirina M, et al: Paromomycin: An effective treatment for cryptosporidial diarrhea in patients with AIDS. Clin Infect Dis 18:447, 1994.
96. White BC Jr, Chappell CL, Hayat CS, et al: Paromomycin for cryptosporidiosis in AIDS: A prospective, double-blind trial. J Infect Dis 170:419, 1994.
97. French AL, Beaudet LM, Benator DA, et al: Cholecystectomy in patients with AIDS: Clinicopathologic correlations in 107 cases. Clin Infect Dis 21:852, 1995.
98. Soave R, Johnson WD: AIDS commentary: *Cryptosporidium* and *Isospora belli* infections. J Infect Dis 157:225, 1988.
99. Ng E, Markell EK, Fleming RL, Fried M: Demonstration of *Isospora belli* by acid-fast stain in a patient with acquired immune deficiency syndrome. J Clin Microbiol 20:384, 1984.
100. Pape JW, Johnson WD Jr: *Isospora belli* infections. Prog Clin Parasitol 2:119, 1991.
101. Shadduck JA: Human microsporidiosis and AIDS. Rev Infect Dis 11:203, 1989.
102. Orenstein JM, Chiang J, Steinberg W, et al: Intestinal microsporidiosis as a cause of diarrhea in human immunodeficiency virus–infected patients: A report of 20 cases. Hum Pathol 21:475, 1990.
103. Orenstein JM: Microsporidiosis in the acquired immunodeficiency syndrome. J Parasitol 77:843, 1991.
104. Weber R, Bryan RT, Owen RL, et al: Improved light-microscopical detection of microsporidia spores in stool and duodenal aspirates. The Enteric Opportunistic Infections Working Group. N Engl J Med 326:161, 1992.
105. Rabeneck L, Gyorkey F, Genta RM, et al: The role of microsporidia in the pathogenesis of HIV-related chronic diarrhea. Ann Intern Med 119:895, 1993.
106. Weber R, Sauer B, Spycher MA, et al: Detection of *Septata intestinalis* in stool specimens, and coprodiagnostic monitoring of successful treatment with albendazole. Clin Infect Dis 19:242, 1994.
107. Dieterich DT, Lew EA, Kotler DP, et al: Treatment with albendazole for intestinal disease due to *Enterocytozoon bieneusi* in patients with AIDS. J Infect Dis 169:178, 1994.
108. Damsker B: *Mycobacterium avium–Mycobacterium intracellulare* from the intestinal tracts of patients with the acquired immunodeficiency syndrome: Concepts regarding acquisition and pathogenesis. J Infect Dis 151:179, 1985.
109. Roth RI, Owen RL, Keren DF: AIDS with *Mycobacterium avium-intracellulare* lesions resembling those of Whipple's disease. N Engl J Med 309:1324, 1983.
110. Hawkins CC, Gold JWM, Whimbey E, et al: *Mycobacterium avium* complex infections in patients with the acquired immunodeficiency syndrome. Ann Intern Med 105:184, 1986.
111. Stacey AR: Isolation of *Mycobacterium avium-intracellulare-scrofulaceum* complex from faeces of patients with AIDS. Br Med J 293:119A, 1986.
112. Kiehn TE, Edwards FF, Brannon P, et al: Infections caused by *Mycobacterium avium* complex in immunocompromised patients: Diagnosis by blood culture and fecal examination, antimicrobial susceptibility tests, and morphological and seroagglutination characteristics. J Clin Microbiol 21:168, 1985.
113. Baskin DH, Lax JD, Barenberg D: *Shigella* bacteremia in patients with the acquired immune deficiency syndrome. Am J Gastroenterol 82:338, 1987.
114. Blaser MJ, Hale TL, Formal SB: Recurrent shigellosis complicating human immunodeficiency virus infection: Failure of preexisting antibodies to confer protection. Am J Med 86:105, 1989.
115. Dworkin B, Wormser GP, Abdoo RA, et al: Persistence of multiply antibiotic-resistant *Campylobacter jejuni* in a patient with the acquired immune deficiency syndrome. Am J Med 80:965, 1986.
116. Perlman DM, Ampel NM, Schitman RB, et al: Persistent *Campylobacter jejuni* infections in patients infected with human immunodeficiency virus (HIV). Ann Intern Med 108:540, 1988.

117. Evans TG, Riley D: *Campylobacter laridis* colitis in a human immunodeficiency virus–positive patient treated with a quinolone. Clin Infect Dis 15:172, 1992.
118. Esforzado N, Poch E, Almiralli J, et al: Hemolytic uremic syndrome associated with HIV infection (Letter). AIDS 5:1041, 1991.
119. Farina C, Gavazzeni G, Caprioli A, Remuzzi G: Hemolytic uremic syndrome associated with verocytotoxin-producing *Escherichia coli* infection in acquired immunodeficiency syndrome (Letter). Blood 75:2465, 1990.
120. Miller RA, Minshew BH: *Blastocystis hominis*: An organism in search of a disease. Rev Infect Dis 10:930, 1988.
121. Visvesvara GS, Leitch GJ, Wallace S, et al: Adenovirus masquerading as microsporidia. J Parasitol 82:316, 1996.
122. Haggerty CM, Britton MC, Dorman JM, Maroni FA: Gastrointestinal histoplasmosis in suspected acquired immunodeficiency syndrome. West J Med 143:244, 1985.
123. Cappell MS: Extensive gastrointestinal aspergillosis associated with AIDS. Dig Dis Sci 36:1500, 1991.
124. Wheat LJ, Connolly-Stringfield PA, Baker RL, et al: Disseminated histoplasmosis in the acquired immune deficiency syndrome: Clinical findings, diagnosis and treatment, and review of the literature. Medicine (Baltimore) 69:361, 1990.
125. Lemlich G, Schwam L, Lebwohl M: Kaposi's sarcoma and acquired immunodeficiency syndrome. Postmortem findings in twenty-four cases. J Am Acad Dermatol 16:319, 1987.
126. Friedman S, Wright T, Altman D: Kaposi's sarcoma and the gastrointestinal tract: The San Francisco experience. Gastroenterology 84:1160, 1983.
127. Guenter P, Muurahainen N, Simons G, et al: Relationships among nutritional status, disease progression and survival in HIV infection. J Acquir Immune Defic Syndr 6:1130, 1993.
128. Grunfield C, Pang M, Shimizu L, et al: Resting energy expenditure, caloric intake, and short-term weight change in human immunodeficiency virus infection and the acquired immunodeficiency syndrome. Am J Clin Nutr 55:455, 1992.
129. Grunfield C, Kotler DP, Shigenaga JK, et al: Circulating interferon-α levels and hypertriglyceridemia in the acquired immunodeficiency syndrome. Am J Med 90:154, 1991.
130. Macallan DC, McNurlan MA, Milne E, et al: Whole body protein turnover from leucine kinetics and the response to nutrition in human immunodeficiency virus infection. Am J Clin Nutr 61:818, 1995.
131. Macallan DC, Noble C, Baldwin C, et al: Energy expenditure and wasting in human immunodeficiency virus infection. N Engl J Med 333:83, 1995.
132. Macallan DC, Noble C, Baldwin C, et al: Prospective analysis of patterns of weight change in stage IV human immunodeficiency virus infection. Am J Clin Nutr 58:417, 1993.
133. Souba WW: Nutritional support. N Engl J Med 336:41, 1997.
134. Kotter DP, Tierny AR, Ferraro R, et al: Enteral alimentation and repletion of body cell mass in malnourished patients with acquired immunodeficiency syndrome. Am J Clin Nutr 53:149, 1991.

124

Cutaneous Infections in Human Immunodeficiency Virus Disease

Marsha L. Chaffins
Clay J. Cockerell

A wide variety of cutaneous infectious disorders develop in patients infected with the human immunodeficiency virus type 1 (HIV-1). Many of these disorders also occur in immunocompetent patients; however, in HIV-infected hosts, the clinical manifestations are often unusual, severe, or prolonged and may serve as an initial clue to the diagnosis of HIV infection (Table 124–1). Skin or mucosal lesions may reflect the dissemination of an underlying systemic infectious illness or may serve as a prognostic or acquired immunodeficiency syndrome (AIDS)–defining indicator (Tables 124–2 and 124–3). Furthermore, the development of certain cutaneous disorders can be correlated with the $CD4^+$ lymphocyte counts (Table 124–4). Other conditions, however, such as Kaposi's sarcoma (KS), may appear at any time during the course of HIV infection and show little relationship to the level of T-cell depletion. In any event, early recognition and appropriate treatment of cutaneous infections may have a significant impact on lessening morbidity and mortality.

Viral Infections

Acute Exanthem of Human Immunodeficiency Virus Disease

The acute exanthem of HIV infection is an acute reaction that is associated with HIV seroconversion. This phenomenon

TABLE 124–1 ■ Common Cutaneous Infections That Provide Clues to Human Immunodeficiency Virus Infection

CUTANEOUS INFECTION	CLUE
Herpes simplex	Ulcerative lesion(s), lasting >1 mo, especially perianal location
Herpes zoster	Involvement of more than one dermatome; recurrent episodes
Verrucae	Multiple periungual lesions; numerous flat warts on face and beard area
Molluscum contagiosum	Multiple lesions on face, especially periorbital location; giant lesions
Impetigo	Axillary, inguinal, or other intertriginous locations
Staphylococcal folliculitis	Plaquelike folliculitis; progression to botryomycosis
Scabies	Hyperkeratotic crusted lesions (Norwegian scabies)
Oral candidiasis	Refractory or recurrent disease
Onychomycosis	Proximal white subungual involvement
Tinea versicolor	Extensive disease

TABLE 124–2 ■ AIDS-Defining Cutaneous Disorders

Chronic herpes simplex ulceration > 1 mo duration
Kaposi's sarcoma
Cutaneous cytomegalovirus infection, ulceration
Cutaneous cryptococcosis
Cutaneous lesions secondary to disseminated histoplasmosis, coccidioidomycosis, or mycobacterial infections

develops in 10% to 80% of all newly diagnosed cases of HIV infection but is often subclinical.[1–4] It generally occurs after an incubation period of 3 to 6 weeks and is thought to correspond to widespread infection of cells with HIV.[5] This is thought to lead to release of cytokines and inflammatory mediators that result in the expression of this cutaneous manifestation.

CLINICAL MANIFESTATIONS

Patients experience a sensation of malaise and develop fever with a temperature that can be 102°F or higher. Night sweats, pharyngitis, fatigue, lymphadenopathy, and a fine morbilliform eruption involving the trunk, chest, back, and upper arms develop within one to several days[1, 2] (Fig. 124–1). The cutaneous eruption is similar to that seen with other viral illnesses or drug reactions. The entire syndrome lasts for 4 to 14 days and usually resolves without sequelae. Patients are highly infectious during this time and although the $CD4^+$ cell count may remain perfectly normal, it may fall to as low as 200/mm^3.

A severe form of acute HIV infection may develop with persistent HIV p24 antigenemia, recurrent viremia, rapid decline in $CD4^+$ cell numbers, and accelerated disease progression.[6] Systemic manifestations include pneumonitis, esophagitis, meningitis, abdominal pain, and melena. Skin manifestations that may be seen include urticaria, perlèche, palatal and esophageal ulcers, enanthemata, and candidiasis.[6, 7] Herpesvirus infections may also supervene.[6] The prognosis for patients who suffer from prolonged symptomatic primary HIV infection is significantly poorer than for those with asymptomatic or mild primary infection (see Table 124–3).

DIAGNOSIS

The diagnosis of the acute HIV exanthem is based on the presence of a characteristic clinical picture in an individual with risk factors for the development of HIV infection. The histologic features are somewhat nonspecific, consisting of a superficial perivascular dermatitis with occasional necrotic keratinocytes, again similar to those of a drug eruption or other viral exanthem.[8] Immunocytochemistry has revealed that most of the infiltrating cells in skin lesions are $CD4^+$ T cells with an admixture of $CD8^+$ cells.[8]

Because the eruption occurs around the time of HIV seroconversion, the patient may test negatively for HIV antibody; however, HIV p24 antigen may be detected. Elevated erythrocyte sedimentation rate, leukopenia, and cerebrospinal fluid lymphocytic pleocytosis are nonspecific findings that may be observed. In the case of fulminant acute HIV infection, laboratory findings of profound immunosuppression as alluded to earlier may be demonstrated.[5]

TABLE 124–3 ■ Cutaneous Infections That May Predict Progression to AIDS

DISEASE	PERCENTAGE OF PATIENTS PROGRESSING TO AIDS
Severe acute HIV infection	78% within 3 y
Herpes zoster	34% within 3 y
Oral hairy leukoplakia	83% within 3 y

TABLE 124–4 ■ Relationship of Cutaneous Infections to $CD4^+$ Cell Count

CUTANEOUS DISEASE	AVERAGE $CD4^+$ CELL COUNT AT DISEASE PRESENTATION (CELLS/mm^3)
Acute exanthem of HIV	Normal
Bacterial folliculitis, impetigo	>500
Tinea	>500
Seborrheic dermatitis	>500
Intraepithelial neoplasia	<500
Oral hairy leukoplakia	<400
Verrucae	500–250
Herpes zoster	500–250
Herpes simplex	500–250
Scabies	<250
Bacillary angiomatosis	<250
Leishmaniasis	<250
Molluscum contagiosum	<250
Oral candidiasis	<250
Cytomegalovirus infection	<200

TREATMENT

Zidovudine and other antiviral agents have been administered to patients with the acute HIV viral exanthem without repeatable success.[9–11]

Herpesvirus Infections

Infections with human herpesvirus types 1, 2, and 6, varicella-zoster virus, Epstein-Barr virus, and cytomegalovirus (CMV) are commonly encountered with patients infected with HIV. With advanced immunosuppression, the prevalence of infection with these viruses ranges from between 20% and 40% with herpes simplex virus (HSV) to virtually 100% with CMV.[12–14]

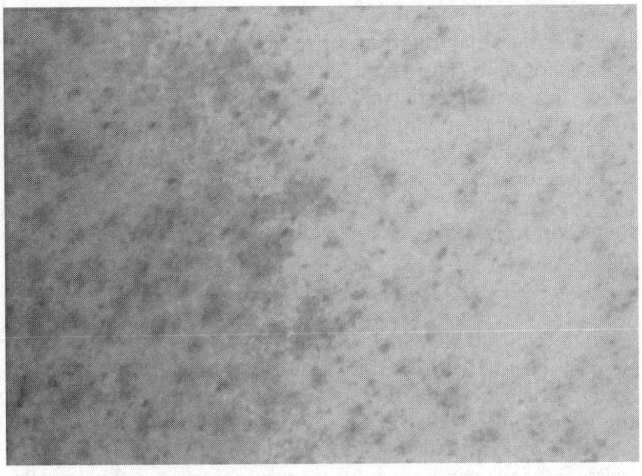

FIGURE 124–1 □ Acute exanthem of HIV infection. A widespread eruption of fine macules and papules distributed over the trunk, extremities, and sometimes the head and neck is characteristic of the viral exanthem of HIV infection. This eruption is seen only rarely and may be confused with other viral exanthems.

HERPES SIMPLEX AND VARICELLA-ZOSTER VIRUS INFECTIONS

HSV and varicella-zoster virus are enveloped double-stranded DNA viruses that may produce both primary and recurrent disease and that have long latency periods. In HIV infection, primary infections tend to be more severe and may be life threatening.[15] Latent virus may be found in the nervous system and reticuloendothelial system as well as in other tissues such as the skin. With the onset of immunosuppression, the herpesvirus may become reactivated and produce recurrent disease.

The presence of a genital herpetic ulcer is a significant risk factor for the acquisition of HIV infection, as the lesions serve as a portal of entry for the virus.[16, 17] In addition, in vitro studies have shown that HSV can potentiate HIV infection.[18]

CLINICAL MANIFESTATIONS

Herpes Simplex

Oral, labial, and genital HSV infections are commonly seen in immunocompetent patients and may be well localized in HIV-infected individuals who are relatively immunocompetent. Characteristically, these are painful grouped vesicles on an erythematous base that rupture, become crusted, and heal within 2 weeks. Once significant immune suppression supervenes, lesions caused by HSV may become progressive and may be manifest as chronic ulcerative mucocutaneous lesions that last for longer than 1 month.[19] Tender, painful ulcerative lesions of the penis, perianal area, lip, perioral area, and digits are quite characteristic. Lesions that are untreated may continue to enlarge dramatically and become deeply situated and extremely painful. Persistent herpetic ulcerations may be recognized by their serpiginous macerated border. Verrucous and hyperplastic changes may also ensue.

Varicella-Zoster

Primary varicella lesions in HIV-infected patients appear like those in non–HIV-infected hosts as clear vesicles on a rose-colored base that heal with crusting and occasionally scars. However, in HIV-infected individuals, varicella is more likely to have a prolonged course and to be associated with systemic complications.[20] In one study, 40% of HIV-positive children who developed primary varicella suffered a complication, and in 5% of these individuals the outcome was fatal.[21] In HIV-infected children, herpes zoster may develop shortly after a course of primary varicella.[22]

Zoster presents as tense vesicles on an erythematous base in a dermatomal distribution and is often associated with significant pain (Fig. 124–2). In the HIV-infected host, lesions involving multiple dermatomes or dissemination of lesions over large areas of the skin may occur.[23, 24] In addition, unusual clinical patterns such as verrucous lesions and crusted, punched-out ulcerations that leave atrophic painful scars have been noted. Postherpetic neuralgia also seems to be more common.

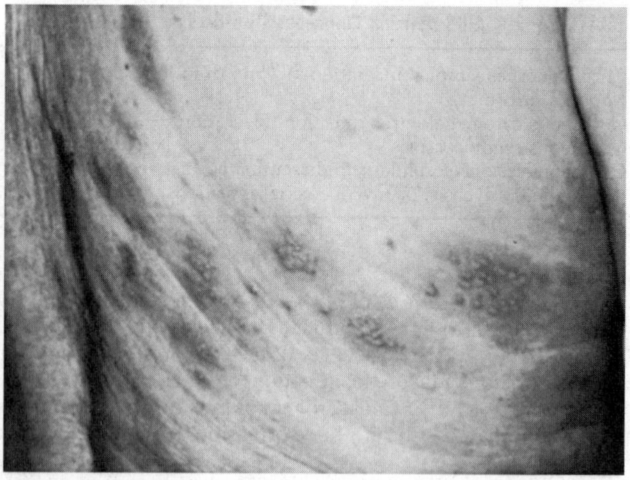

FIGURE 124–2 ☐ Herpes zoster. A linear dermatomal distribution of painful vesicles on erythematous bases is characteristic of herpes zoster. This may be the presenting manifestation of HIV infection and, when present in the proper clinical context, should cause the clinician to perform an HIV test.

DIAGNOSIS

A diagnosis of HSV or varicella-zoster virus infection can usually be made readily by the performance of the Tzanck smear. The specimen to be examined is obtained by scraping the base and/or the roof of a blister, and when it is stained with the Wright-Giemsa stain, ballooned and multinucleated epithelial cells can be visualized microscopically. Histopathologic examination of lesions reveals an intraepidermal acantholytic vesicular dermatitis associated with characteristic cytopathic effects in epithelial cells. Careful inspection of dermal inflammatory infiltrates may demonstrate perineural and intraneural inflammation associated with degeneration of nerves.[25]

TREATMENT

First-line therapy for herpesvirus infections is acyclovir administered orally (Table 124–5). Acyclovir-resistant strains of HSV can develop, however, and require treatment with intravenous foscarnet sodium or vidarabine.[26–28] On occasion, patients with seemingly resistant HSV or varicella-zoster virus infection may be suffering from atrophic gastritis that prevents absorption of acyclovir, so a change to intravenous administration may be necessary. Those suffering from frequent recurrent HSV infections may benefit from prophylactic acyclovir (600 to 800 mg/d).[29]

Herpes zoster should be treated with higher doses of acyclovir, 800 mg orally (PO) every 4 hours while the patient is awake. Nonsteroidal antiinflammatory agents or narcotics may be necessary to help relieve associated pain. Topical therapy with cool compresses or sitz baths and topical anesthetics may also be helpful. Postherpetic neuralgia often responds poorly to treatment. Topical application of capsaicin-containing compounds, eutectic mixture of local anesthetics (EMLA) cream, low-dose tricyclic antidepressants, carbamazepine, fentanyl patches, nerve blocks, biofeedback, and hypnosis have been reported to be effective in some cases. Varicella immune globulin should be given to HIV-seropositive patients at risk for primary varicella if exposure to the virus occurs.[29]

Cytomegalovirus Infections

Despite the high frequency of systemic CMV infections in the HIV-positive population, cutaneous involvement is rarely seen. However, when skin involvement does occur, it usually portends a poor prognosis.

CLINICAL MANIFESTATIONS

Cutaneous lesions of CMV infection that have been reported include localized and diffuse ulcerations, keratotic verrucous lesions, and palpable purpuric papules[30, 31] (Fig. 124–3). CMV-associated perianal ulcerations most often represent contiguous spread from the gastrointestinal tract.[32] Coinfection with

TABLE 124–5 ■ Treatment of Common Cutaneous Infections in Human Immunodeficiency Virus–Infected Patients*

VIRAL INFECTION	TREATMENT OF CHOICE	COMMENT
Herpes simplex	Acyclovir, 200–600 mg PO q 4 h while awake Famciclovir, 500 mg PO tid	Higher doses may be required. Acyclovir-resistant cases require foscarnet, vidarabine, or trifluorthymidine.
Primary varicella ? Vaccine	Acyclovir, 200–800 mg q 4 h while awake	Patients at risk for primary varicella should be given varicella-zoster immune globin within 96 h of known exposure to varicella.
Herpes zoster	Acyclovir, 800–1000 mg q 4 h while awake	In severe cases, IV therapy may be required. Topical anesthetics, nonsteroidal antiinflammatory drugs, and narcotics may be needed for pain control.
Verrucae vulgares	Liquid nitrogen cryotherapy; 16%–40% salicylic acid, liquid or plaster	Interferon alfa may be helpful in recalcitrant cases.
Flat verrucae	Tretinoin 0.05% cream or 0.01% gel applied bid 5% 5-fluorouracil cream applied bid Light liquid nitrogen cryotherapy	Recurrences are common.
Condylomata accuminata	Podofilox 0.5% applied bid 3 d of each week for 7 wk Liquid nitrogen cryotherapy	Multiple treatments usually are necessary.
Molluscum contagiosum	Liquid nitrogen cryotherapy Curettage	Topical tretinoin cream or gel is a useful adjunctive therapy. Recurrence is the rule.
Oral hairy leukoplakia	None Topical podophyllum 20% q d Acyclovir, 200–400 mg q 4 h while awake for 14 d	After discontinuation of therapy, recurrence is usual.
Bacterial folliculitis	Dicloxacillin, erythromycin, or cephalexin, 250–500 mg qid with daily Hibiclens baths	Culture confirmation should be obtained although most cases are due to *Staphylococcus aureus*. Mupirocin bid to the nares or rifampin 300 mg bid for 10–14 d can decrease carriage.
Impetigo	After culture, dicloxacillin, 250–500 mg q 6 h for 7–10 d	
Syphilis	Uncomplicated primary and secondary: benzathine penicillin G, 2.4 million units IM q wk × 3; serology checks at 1, 3, 6, 9, and 12 mo; 4× decrease in titer within 6 mo Primary or secondary with positive lumbar puncture: procaine penicillin G, 2.4 million units IM q d for 10–14 d followed by benzathine penicillin, 2.4 million units IM q wk for 3 wk	Lumbar puncture is advised to rule out neurosyphilis.
Tinea versicolor	Ketoconazole, 200 mg q d for 3–5 d Selenium sulfide 2.5% q d topically, left on 15–20 min	
Dermatophytosis	Topical application of clotrimazole, econazole, cyclopirox, nafitine bid until resolved Griseofulvin, 500 mg bid for 1–2 wk Sporanox, 100 mg bid for 2 wk	Longer courses of therapy may be required. Should not be used in patients with liver disease or porphyria.
Onychomycosis	Itraconazole, 200 mg q d 1 wk/mo for 4 mo	
Oral candidiasis	Miconazole troches four or five times a day Nystatin oral suspension, 100,000 units/mL, gargle and swallow qid Ketoconazole, 200 mg/d Fluconazole, 100 mg/d Itraconazole, 100 mg/d	For all mentioned medications, continued maintenance therapy is often needed. Fluconazole resistance may emerge.
Scabies	5% permethrin cream or gamma benzene hexachloride applied from neck to toes and left on 8–12 h; repeat application in 1 wk Postscabetic pruritus and nodular scabies: crotamiton (Eurax) lotion applied bid Oral antihistamines q 4–6 h with topical triamcinolone 0.025% cream applied bid	Treatment of household contacts is required. Careful laundering of linen and clothing as well as vacuuming is recommended.

*PO, Oral; tid, three times a day; IV, intravenous; bid, twice a day; IM, intramuscular.

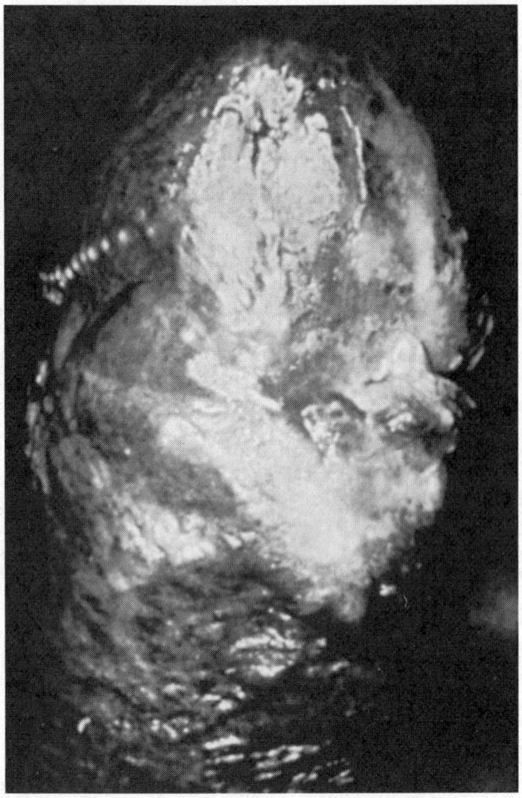

FIGURE 124–3 □ CMV infection. This nondescript penile ulceration was due to cutaneous CMV infection. Biopsy and cultures are necessary to establish this diagnosis.

CMV and HSV occurs not infrequently.[33, 34] CMV has been reported to induce hyperpigmented plaques, diffuse morbilliform eruptions, and vesicular lesions, as well as a bullous toxic epidermal necrolysis–like reaction.[31, 35–37] Adrenal infection may be associated with diffuse hyperpigmentation.

DIAGNOSIS

Skin biopsy is necessary for definitive diagnosis of cutaneous disease. CMV characteristically infects dermal fibroblasts and endothelial cells, resulting in ulceration of the epidermis. CMV-infected cells are enlarged to several times their normal diameter and develop purplish intracytoplasmic and intranuclear inclusions that have a somewhat crystalline shape. Immunoperoxidase antibody stains to CMV may be used to confirm the diagnosis. When a biopsy specimen for CMV is evaluated, it is important to search for other pathogens, as coinfections are not uncommon.[33, 34]

TREATMENT

Ganciclovir at doses of 5 mg/kg per day is needed for the treatment of CMV infection.[38] The combination of ganciclovir and foscarnet may be more effective than either agent alone, and continued prophylactic treatment with ganciclovir may be indicated for severely immunocompromised patients.[29]

Oral Hairy Leukoplakia

Oral hairy leukoplakia (OHL) is caused by infection with the Epstein-Barr virus, and although initially described only in HIV-infected patients, it may be seen in other diseases associated with immunosuppression.[39, 40] The incubation period from primary HIV infection to the detection of OHL varies from 5 to 10 years. Development of this condition is thought to correlate with progression from HIV infection to AIDS[41] (see Table 124–3).

CLINICAL MANIFESTATIONS

OHL presents as one or more whitish corrugated plaques usually on the lateral margins of the tongue. These lesions are generally asymptomatic, although rarely they may become verrucous and lead to dysphagia.

DIAGNOSIS

Characteristically, OHL does not rub off when scraped with a tongue depressor, which is helpful in distinguishing it from candidiasis. Scrapings also yield negative results when examined microscopically after treatment with potassium hydroxide. Histopathologically, OHL is characterized by epithelial hyperplasia with pale-staining, ballooned keratinocytes. The lack of cytologic atypia differentiates it from premalignant leukoplakia, and Epstein-Barr virus particles may be demonstrated with electron microscopy and in situ hybridization techniques.[42, 43]

TREATMENT

No treatment of the condition is usually required; however, lesions may respond temporarily to acyclovir at a dosage of 200 to 400 mg five times a day. Topical application of podophyllum resin, 20% in alcohol, two or three times daily also leads to resolution but recurrence after discontinuation is usual.[44, 45] Local destructive measures may also be beneficial.

Human Papillomavirus Infections

The human papillomavirus (HPV) is a double-stranded DNA virus that characteristically infects epithelial cells, producing hyperplastic changes. HPV infection is one of the most common viral infections of humans and is transmitted by close repeated contact, which may be sexual in nature.[46] After internalization, the virus enters the nucleus, where it either produces productive infection or undergoes latency.

In HIV-infected individuals, HPV infection is quite prevalent. In one study, 48% of HIV-seronegative homosexual men and 54% of homosexual men with AIDS were shown to have evidence of HPV infection.[47] Defective cell-mediated immunity and up-regulation of HPV expression induced by HIV Tat protein may be responsible for the high incidence of HPV-induced lesions in HIV-positive patients.[48–50]

CLINICAL MANIFESTATIONS

Verrucae vulgares are manifest by skin-colored to reddish verrucous hyperkeratotic papules or plaques that may occur on any surface of the skin. The glabrous skin is commonly involved, especially the skin around the fingers and on the extremities, although the face and head and neck area are also common sites of involvement. Individual small blackish bleeding points are often seen that correlate with dilated blood vessels and intraepidermal hemorrhage. Multiple verrucae vulgares, especially in periungual locations, and extensive flat and filiform warts on the bearded area of the face are commonly seen in HIV-infected individuals. Exuberant cauliflower-like plaques of condylomata acuminata involving the perianal region as well as flexural areas such as the axillae and oral commissures are also common findings. Difficulty with defecation and secondary constipation may result from extensive perianal condylomata.

Epidermodysplasia verruciformis (EDV) has been reported

in association with HIV infection.[51] This condition is manifest as a widespread maculopapular eruption of reddish to skin-colored, flat, wartlike lesions involving mostly the sun-exposed areas of the skin. In addition to harboring HPV, individual lesions may be associated with cytologic atypia and may develop into squamous cell carcinoma (see later).

Bowenoid papulosis that is related to HPV types 16 and 18 may also be seen in HIV-infected hosts.[52, 53] This condition classically presents as multiple 2- to 5-mm red-brown papules involving the shaft of the penis. Bowenoid papulosis of the anus has been reported in association with the development of squamous cell carcinoma of the anus in an HIV-positive patient.[53]

DIAGNOSIS

Diagnosis of HPV infection is based on clinical features in the context of characteristic histopathologic findings. Verrucae and condylomata are characterized by marked epithelial hyperplasia, papillomatosis, and koilocytosis. EDV is manifest as koilocytic changes in conjunction with keratinocyte atypia that is suggestive of evolving squamous cell carcinoma in situ. Histopathologically, bowenoid papulosis demonstrates the features of condyloma acuminatum combined with atypical keratinocytic proliferation involving the full thickness of the epithelium. In difficult cases, immunoperoxidase stains for HPV antigens, DNA in situ hybridization, and the polymerase chain reaction can be performed to increase the sensitivity of diagnosis.[52, 54, 55]

TREATMENT

Treatment generally consists of destructive measures such as application of topical agents or surgery. Podophyllum resin (20% to 50%) in tincture of benzoin, 35% trichloroacetic acid, or salicylic acid (6% to 40%) may successfully be used to destroy verruca or condyloma; however, repeated applications are almost always necessary. Podofilox (Condylox) applied twice a day for 3 days a week for 3 to 4 weeks is a regimen that can be used by the patient at home.[56] Verruca plana and filiform verrucae may be treated with tretinoin (Retin-A), 0.05% cream or 0.01% gel, and/or topical 5-fluorouracil cream (Efudex). Cryosurgery with liquid nitrogen, electrodesiccation and curettage, and carbon dioxide laser vaporization are other treatment modalities commonly employed. Intralesional, subcutaneous, and parenteral interferon alfa has been shown to be effective against recalcitrant condyloma and acral verruca; however, the use of this agent usually entails repeated visits to the physician and significant cost.[57, 58] The lesions of EDV and bowenoid papulosis may respond to 5-fluorouracil cream, cryotherapy, electrodesiccation, or other destructive modalities.

Poxvirus Infections

Poxviruses are complex DNA viruses that are transmitted by direct contact. These viruses replicate in the cytoplasm and are especially adapted to epidermal cells. Molluscum contagiosum develops in 10% to 20% of patients with AIDS.[3, 59] Most patients who develop widespread molluscum contagiosum are severely immunocompromised at the time of infection, with $CD4^+$ cell counts less than 200 to 250/mm^3.[59] Vaccinia virus infection occurs only sporadically in patients who have been occupationally exposed or are accidental hosts.[60]

CLINICAL MANIFESTATIONS

Molluscum contagiosum is characterized by dome-shaped umbilicated translucent 2- to 4-mm papules that may occur on any part of the body but localize especially around the eyes. Lesions may number in excess of 100, and individual lesions may become quite large, expanding to more than 1 cm in diameter.[61] In addition, clusters of lesions may coalesce, forming large plaques. In some cases, molluscum contagiosum may induce a localized dermatitis known as molluscum dermatitis.[62] In HIV-infected patients, molluscum tends to erupt during a short time, from 2 to 4 weeks, and then persists for months to years.

Vaccinia lesions are characterized by widespread, uniform, tense umbilicated vesicles and pustules. Patients are often clinically ill with fever and acute toxic symptoms associated with viremia.[60]

DIAGNOSIS

Diagnosis of molluscum is generally established on the basis of clinical appearance. In atypical cases, a biopsy may be necessary to rule out other disorders. Lesions that occur in HIV-positive patients and may appear similar to molluscum include those of cryptococcosis, cutaneous pneumocystosis, pyogenic granulomata, keratoacanthoma, and basal cell carcinoma. Histopathologically, molluscum lesions are characterized by a dome-shaped papule with a central crater that arises as a consequence of coalescence of infected keratinocytes. Viral particles fill the cells, forming the pathognomonic molluscum body, which is a pinkish, hyaline-like, oval structure within the cytoplasm of keratinocytes.

Vaccinia is diagnosed on the basis of the clinical appearance of the eruption in the context of a history of exposure to the causative agent. Virtually all cases develop in patients with occupational exposure or who have recently been vaccinated for smallpox. Histologically, prominent intraepidermal ballooning and reticular degeneration are seen.

TREATMENT

Treatment of molluscum contagiosum is generally accomplished by using destructive measures similar to those used to treat HPV infection. Cryotherapy, electrosurgery, topical keratolytic preparations, cantharidin, and curettage are standard effective therapies. Tretinoin cream, 0.025%, may be applied to decrease recurrence. Vaccinia infection is associated with a high mortality rate, and treatment is generally ineffective. Administrations of semithiocarbazone may sometimes be beneficial.[63]

Other Viral Infections

There are sporadic reports of other viral infections occurring in HIV-positive patients. Parvovirus B19, the cause of erythema infectiosum (fifth disease), has been reported to cause an exanthem in patients with HIV infection as well as leading to persistent and occasionally fatal aplastic anemia.[64] Paramyxovirus (measles), some coxsackieviruses, and enteroviruses may cause an exanthem in HIV-infected individuals. The clinical course of such infections varies greatly and depends on the background immune status of the host.[65, 66]

Bacterial Infections

Pyogenic Infections

Staphylococcus aureus is the most common cutaneous and systemic bacterial pathogen of the HIV-infected adult. Defective neutrophil chemotaxis and decreased oxidative burst in conjunction with other immune alterations may lead to defective eradication of organisms.[67, 68] A nasal carriage rate of approximately 50% has been observed in HIV-infected hosts, which is twice that of HIV-seronegative homosexual and heterosexual men.[69] Multiple breaks in the skin from needlesticks, dermatoses, and immunodeficiency are risk factors for the development of *S. aureus* infection. Up to 83% of patients with AIDS may suffer from some form of *S. aureus* infection at some point during the course of their disease.[70, 71] Infections with gram-negative organisms occur less frequently but still represent a significant proportion of skin infections in HIV disease.[72–74]

CLINICAL MANIFESTATIONS

Gram-Positive Infections

Folliculitis is generally manifest as widely distributed acneiform papules and pustules that may be pruritic and excoriated. Although in most cases infections are confined to the skin, occasionally sepsis may develop. In some cases, the bacterial density may increase significantly, leading to botryomycosis or ecthyma.[75, 76] These disorders appear as nondescript verrucous papules or as necrotic, deeply seated chronic ulcerations, respectively. An atypical form of folliculitis manifested as plaques may develop that presents as large violaceous plaques with superficial pustules and crusts occurring in the groin, axilla, or scalp.[77]

Soft tissue and deeply seated bacterial infections such as cellulitis, pyomyositis, deep soft tissue abscesses, and necrotizing fasciitis may also develop.[78, 70] Extreme toxemia is often associated with deeper infections such as these, so early recognition is essential. A characteristic infection, streptococcal axillary lymphadenitis, presents as a usually bilateral diffuse, painful swelling of lymph nodes in the axillae.[79] Impetigo is manifest as localized or erythematous areas of the skin associated with yellowish surface crusts and, rarely, intact bullae and pustules. In patients with HIV infection, it may be seen in unusual locations such as axillary, inguinal, and other intertriginous locations. In addition, secondary infection of other primary dermatoses with *S. aureus* occurs frequently.

Toxin-producing strains of *Streptococcus pyogenes* and *S. aureus* may produce a toxic shock–like syndrome.[80, 81] Diffuse cutaneous erythema followed by desquamation, fever, and shock is seen.

Gram-Negative Infections

Pseudomonas aeruginosa and *Pseudomonas cepacia* may produce clinical conditions similar to those described earlier, so culture of lesions is essential.[72–74] An unusual form of cellulitis of the head and neck caused by *Haemophilus influenzae* may develop in patients with HIV infection.[82] This infection tends to be aggressive and may become disseminated or involve deeper soft tissues and vital structures. Infections with *Streptomyces, Nocardia,* and *Actinomyces* may produce thickened verrucous plaques and chronic draining sinuses.[83, 84] Deeply seated abscesses caused by *Rhodococcus equi* have been observed on multiple occasions.[85] *Corynebacterium diphtheriae* may cause bullous lesions that ulcerate and become covered with a grayish pseudomembrane.[86]

DIAGNOSIS

Gram stains and cultures are extremely important in evaluating pyogenic infections in HIV-infected individuals, as they often have unusual or mixed infections. A characteristic leukocytosis and "left shift" may not occur in some patients despite significant infections.

Skin biopsy may be helpful in establishing diagnoses. Histopathologic findings generally seen are dense collections of neutrophils in conjunction with bacterial organisms. Bacterial colonies may actually grow in the skin of immunocompromised patients and form grains of botryomycosis that can be seen grossly. Secondary changes such as vasculitis and ulceration can also occur.

TREATMENT

Treatment of each of the aforementioned disorders is based on accurate diagnosis and identification of causative microorganisms and their sensitivities to antibiotics. Pyogenic bacterial infections generally respond to treatment with dicloxacillin, cephalexin, or ciprofloxacin. Chlorhexidine gluconate washes of the skin and application of topical antibiotics such as polymyxin B sulfate, bacitracin, or mupirocin ointment preparations into the nostrils may help to eradicate bacterial colonization. Unfortunately, in immunocompromised hosts, recurrence is the rule.

Bacillary Angiomatosis

Bacillary angiomatosis is a rare condition caused by rickettsia-like organisms of the genus *Bartonella* (formerly *Rochalimaea*) *henselae* and *Bartonella quintana*.[87–89] The pathogenesis is not completely known but it has been postulated that a vasoproliferative factor is produced or is induced as a consequence of bacterial infection. Sound epidemiologic evidence has demonstrated an association between exposure to cats and bacillary angiomatosis.[90, 91] However, one third of patients have no history of prior feline contact, so infection from another source such as the soil may also be important.

CLINICAL MANIFESTATIONS

Small pinpoint reddish to purple papules that resemble angiomata or pyogenic granulomata are the most common lesions. They range in number from one to several thousand and in size from 1 mm to several centimeters. Subcutaneous nodules are seen in approximately 50% of patients with skin lesions.[92] They may be located deep in the subcutis and extend to involve soft tissue and bone.[93] When bone is involved, lesions are generally osteolytic in nature. Nondescript crusted ulcerations, plaques, and cellulitis may also be seen in 5% to 10% of patients.[92]

Visceral involvement may occur as well. The most common sites of involvement are the liver and spleen, in which dilated blood-filled vascular spaces develop as a consequence of infection with *Bartonella*. These conditions are known as bacillary peliosis hepatis and splenis, respectively.[94, 95] In addition, patients with bacillary angiomatosis may develop a bacteremic syndrome of fever, weight loss, and night sweats.[95, 96] Endocarditis has been reported in both immunocompromised and immunocompetent patients.[97–99]

DIAGNOSIS

The diagnosis of bacillary angiomatosis can usually be established on the basis of characteristic histopathologic findings in the context of clinical ones. Lesions show a lobular proliferation of capillaries admixed with neutrophils and granular masses of bacteria. Organisms appear as black tangled strands after staining with the Warthin-Starry stain. *B. henselae* can be isolated from blood if lysis centrifugation blood cultures are used, and *B. quintana* can be isolated from cutaneous lesions by cocultivation with an endothelial cell monolayer.[100, 101] Serum may be sent to the Centers for Disease Control and Prevention for determination of antibody titers to the bacillary angiomatosis organisms.

TREATMENT

Bacillary angiomatosis responds well to treatment with erythromycin ethylsuccinate at doses of 500 mg PO four times a day (qid) for 4 weeks to 6 months depending on the tendency to relapse, which may be substantial.[102] Doxycycline hydrochloride, 100 mg PO twice a day (bid), is also effective.[103] Azithromycin and roxithromycin have also been used with good response.[104, 105]

Mycobacterial Infections

Skin lesions are seen in up to 10% of patients with systemic mycobacterial infections and may be caused by *Mycobacterium tuberculosis, Mycobacterium avium-intracellulare,* and other atypical mycobacteria. A significant percentage of *M. tuberculosis* infections represent reactivation of a preexisting infectious focus. Leprosy has been observed only rarely in patients with HIV infection, the reason for which remains unknown.

CLINICAL MANIFESTATIONS

Mycobacterial skin lesions may assume a number of different appearances. The lesions may present as small papules and pustules that resemble folliculitis, verrucous papules, localized cutaneous abscesses, suppurative lymphadenitis, ulcerations, or sporotrichoid nodules (Fig. 124–4). Tuberculous lymphadenitis, in particular, is a characteristic finding of disseminated tuberculosis in intravenous drug users with AIDS and is manifested as suppurative draining lymph nodes in the neck, axillae, or groin.[106] *Mycobacterium marinum* may cause classic swimming pool granulomata in patients with HIV disease manifested as verrucous nodules classically extending up one extremity in a linear arrangement. *Mycobacterium haemophilum* may cause cutaneous infections in AIDS patients, which usually present as painful erythematous papules and nodules on the distal extremities and ears.[107]

DIAGNOSIS

In cases of suspected mycobacterial infections, cultures and smears for acid-fast organisms should be performed, keeping in mind that these organisms have special growth requirements and are slow growers. Biopsy generally shows a suppurative granulomatous infiltrate. Acid-fast stains may be used to identify organisms; however, these stains may be negative even in an ongoing active infection.

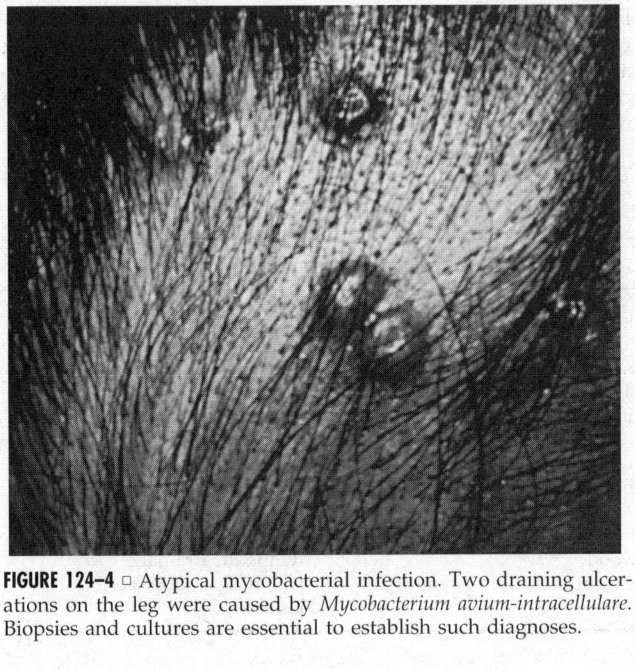

FIGURE 124–4 ▫ Atypical mycobacterial infection. Two draining ulcerations on the leg were caused by *Mycobacterium avium-intracellulare.* Biopsies and cultures are essential to establish such diagnoses.

TREATMENT

Cutaneous mycobacterial infections demonstrate variable responses to antibiotics, so it is important to determine sensitivities. In general, cutaneous tuberculosis responds to antituberculous regimens of isoniazid and ethambutol with or without pyrazinamide. Multidrug-resistant tuberculosis has been described and may not respond to any medication currently available.[108] Clarithromycin, rifabutin (Ansamycin), clofazimine, minocycline, and trimethoprim-sulfamethoxazole all have variable degrees of efficacy in the treatment of atypical mycobacterial infections. *M. haemophilum* is usually sensitive to ciprofloxacin and rifampin, but even in cases in which both antibiotics are used, chronic relapse may be noted.[107]

Syphilis

Syphilis is common in patients with HIV infection, and of all reported cases of syphilis, 25% occur in HIV-infected hosts.[109]

CLINICAL MANIFESTATIONS

Syphilis may occur in a number of forms in patients with HIV infection, ranging from classic papulosquamous forms with involvement of the palms and soles and mucous membranes to unusual forms such as sclerodermiform lesions, rupial verrucous plaques, extensive oral ulcerations, keratoderma, deep cutaneous nodules, rubeoliform eruptions, and widespread gummata.[110] Rapid progression from the primary chancre to gummatous tertiary lues or lues maligna (syphilis with vasculitis) may occur. Central nervous system disease has been noted more frequently and with greater severity.[111]

DIAGNOSIS

Serology is the most important parameter in establishing a diagnosis of syphilis; however, HIV-positive patients with syphilis may have negative serologic tests for syphilis as well as a negative antibody test despite the presence of active infection. Seronegativity may be due to either a prozone phenomenon or true absence of antibody. In these cases a skin biopsy may be helpful. Histopathologic examination usually shows a prominent infiltrate of plasma cells arranged around swollen endothelial cells. It is worth mentioning that in about one fourth of cases, plasma cells are few or absent. Warthin-Starry stains can be used to demonstrate the organisms.

TREATMENT

Syphilis responds to penicillin at higher doses and must be continued for longer courses than in immunocompetent hosts. Recommended treatment regimens are summarized in Table 124–5. Lumbar puncture is recommended to rule out concomitant neurosyphilis. Careful follow-up with repeated serologic testing is recommended. In patients who are allergic to penicillin, tetracycline or erythromycin at doses of 500 mg PO qid for up to 30 days may be substituted.

Other Venereal Diseases

Multiple sexually transmitted diseases are commonly seen in association with HIV infection. This phenomenon may be decreasing somewhat with improved education about safe sex, however. In addition to the more common sexually transmitted diseases, less common ones may be encountered in HIV-positive patients.

Chancroid, caused by the gram-negative coccobacillus *Haemophilus ducreyi,* has been reported in a number of patients with HIV infection, especially in those from Africa. Lesions most often present as a solitary, painful penile or labial ulceration, although widespread ulcerations may develop.[112] Granuloma inguinale caused by *Calymmatobacterium granulomatis* may also occur. This disorder is characterized by vegetating lesions of the penis and vulva associated with pseudobuboes in the inguinal crease. Although uncommon, lymphogranuloma venereum has also been associated with HIV infection and is manifested as generalized lymphadenopathy accompanied by vulvar or penile edema with ulcerations and erosions. Severe gonococcemia with gonococcal arthritis has also been reported.[113]

DIAGNOSIS

Appropriate smears and cultures are important in evaluating these disorders. Granuloma inguinale is characteristically diagnosed by crush preparations of a friable skin lesion followed by histologic examination. Chancroid is diagnosed by microscopic examination of gram-stained smears of lesions that demonstrate clusters of thin gram-negative rods, the characteristic "schools of fish."

TREATMENT

Chancroid is treated with erythromycin, 500 mg PO qid for 7 days; alternatively, a single intramuscular injection of ceftriaxone, 250 mg, may be administered. Lymphogranuloma venereum responds to erythromycin in the same dosage, although doxycycline, 100 mg PO bid for 7 days, and ofloxacin, 300 mg PO bid for 7 days, are also quite effective. Granuloma inguinale responds to treatment with erythromycin or trimethoprim-sulfamethoxazole. Gonorrhea is treated with regimens generally consisting of penicillin, spectinomycin, or ceftriaxone.

Fungal Infections

Deep Fungal Diseases

The systemic fungal infections associated with HIV infection are summarized in Table 124–6. The most common opportunistic fungal infections to involve the skin are histoplasmosis and cryptococcosis. Nearly 20% of HIV-positive patients with disseminated histoplasmosis and up to 10% of those with disseminated cryptococcosis develop mucosal or cutaneous lesions. Mucocutaneous lesions associated with systemic fungal infections may assume a number of different features. The most common lesions are pustules and ulcers, although papules and nodules are also frequently observed. Less often, patches, plaques, and verrucous lesions are seen. It is important to recognize that cutaneous lesions caused by disseminated fungi may mimic the appearance of other diseases.

CLINICAL MANIFESTATIONS

Histoplasmosis

In one review, 17% of HIV-positive patients with disseminated histoplasmosis developed cutaneous lesions.[114] Clinically, the lesions had highly variable clinical appearances. Cutaneous histoplasmosis commonly presents with cutaneous or mucosal ulcerations, although erythematous macules, papules, nodules, and verrucous plaques may also occur. *Histoplasma capsulatum* and KS were found to coexist in a single skin lesion, and coexistent psoriasis and histoplasmosis have also been observed.[115, 116] The possibility of human-to-human transmission of histoplasmosis between two HIV-seropositive individuals via close skin contact has been postulated but not proved.[117]

Cryptococcosis

Cryptococcosis develops not uncommonly in HIV-infected individuals. Up to 10% of patients with disseminated *Cryptococcus* infection develop skin involvement. Mucocutaneous lesions of cryptococcosis are polymorphous and may appear as erythematous papules, nodules, pustules, and/or ulcers as well as cellulitis of the skin and mucosa (Fig. 124–5). The clinical appearance of cutaneous cryptococcosis has been reported to mimic lesions of HSV infection and molluscum contagiosum as well as soft tissue hypertrophic lesions such as rhinophyma and KS.[118, 119]

Sporotrichosis

Clinical forms of sporotrichosis include fixed cutaneous, lymphocutaneous, disseminated cutaneous, and systemic. Fixed cutaneous forms consist of a solitary lesion; lymphocutaneous forms are manifest as multiple lesions developing along the lines of lymphatic drainage. Disseminated cutaneous lesions occur over widespread areas.[120] Systemic disease may present as either localized pulmonary disease or wide-

TABLE 124–6 ■ Summary of Deep Fungal Infections

DISEASE	CAUSATIVE ORGANISM	ENDEMIC AREA	DISTINCTIVE CUTANEOUS LESION(S)
Cryptococcosis	*Cryptococcus neoformans*	Widespread distribution; found in pigeon excrement	Cellulitis, purpura, molluscum contagiosum–like lesions
Histoplasmosis	*Histoplasma capsulatum*	Central river valleys of United States; in droppings of blackbirds	Acneiform lesions, oral ulcerations
Blastomycosis	*Blastomyces dermatitidis*	Southeastern and south-central North America	Raised plaque with heaped-up border; skin and mucosal ulcerations
Coccidioidomycosis	*Coccidioides immitis*	Lower Sonoran life zones	Verrucous plaques, erythema nodosum
Sporotrichosis	*Sporothrix schenckii*	Tropical or subtropical Americas; found in soil and wood	Linear nodules in line of lymphatic drainage
Paracoccidioidomycosis	*Paracoccidioides brasiliensis*	Latin America, from Mexico to Argentina	Mucosal ulceration, periorificial lesions

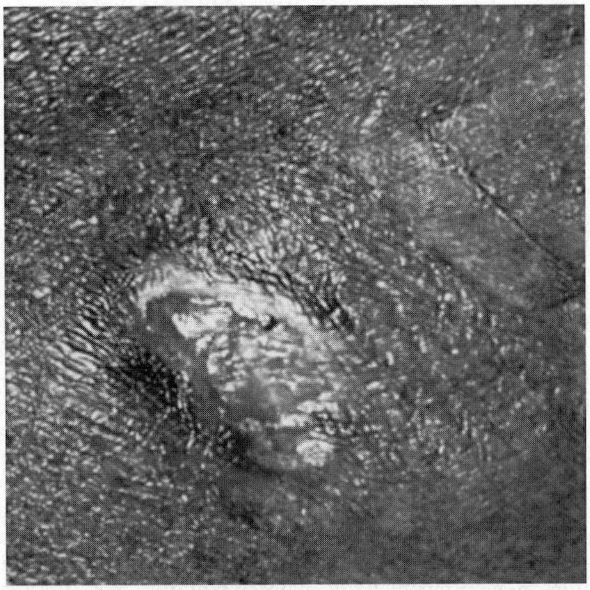

FIGURE 124–5 ◻ Cutaneous cryptococcosis. This somewhat yellowish translucent crusted papule with a nondescript appearance was caused by *Cryptococcus neoformans*. This emphasizes the need to perform biopsies and cultures of virtually any lesion in a patient with HIV infection.

spread involvement of numerous organs. Skin lesions may be ulcers, papules, nodules, plaques, and/or pustules.[121]

Less Common Deep Fungal Infections

Penicillium marneffei, a fungus that is endemic in Asia, causes an infection that has been reported with increasing frequency in patients with AIDS in Thailand.[122] Systemic manifestations include fever, weight loss, anemia, and lymphadenopathy. Seventy-six percent of affected individuals develop skin disease. The most characteristic lesions are umbilicated papules that resemble molluscum contagiosum. Ecthyma-like lesions, folliculitis, subcutaneous nodules, and abscesses may also occur.

Sporadic reports of disseminated coccidioidomycosis, blastomycosis, and paracoccidioidomycosis with cutaneous involvement in HIV-infected hosts have appeared in the literature. Infection with *Coccidioides immitis* has produced leukocytoclastic vasculitis, subcutaneous abscesses, ulcerations, and nodules.[123] Fatal disseminated blastomycosis with cutaneous pustules, nodules, and ulcers has been observed.[124] An HIV-positive patient from Brazil with painful ulcerations of the face and thigh caused by *Paracoccidioides brasiliensis* has been described as well.[125] Disseminated *Scedosporium inflatum*, *Pseudallescheria boydii*, and *Microsporum canis* infections have been observed in these patients, as have infections with zygomycotic organisms.[126–129] The clinical lesions seen most often in these cases were ulcerations.

DIAGNOSIS

When the possibility is considered that a mucocutaneous lesion in an HIV-infected patient is secondary to dissemination of a systemic fungal infection, a tissue biopsy and potassium hydroxide preparation or tissue smear, as well as culture, should be performed. Biopsies and smears can often yield a more rapid diagnosis than is possible with cultures, which may take up to several weeks. Histology characteristically reveals epithelial hyperplasia with suppurative granulomatous inflammation. The number of organisms may vary, so special staining for fungi with either periodic acid–Schiff or Gomori methenamine silver stain is necessary. A diligent search for concurrent infectious organisms is warranted, as HIV-infected individuals often harbor more than one pathogen.

TREATMENT

Intravenous amphotericin B remains the drug of choice for the treatment of most deep fungal infections. Ketoconazole, fluconazole, or itraconazole may be effectively used in the treatment of sporotrichosis. In some cases, the lymphocutaneous form can be treated successfully with potassium iodide, although careful monitoring is necessary to avoid recurrences. Fluconazole and itraconazole are promising less toxic alternatives for the initial and/or maintenance therapy of these systemic fungal infections in HIV-infected patients.

Superficial Fungal Infections

YEAST INFECTIONS

Oral thrush involving the tongue and/or buccal mucosa is the most common manifestation of candidiasis in HIV-seropositive patients and may be the initial sign of HIV infection in many individuals[130, 131] (Fig. 124–6). Candidal infection may also produce chronic paronychia and onychodystrophy, chronic refractory vaginal candidiasis, distal urethritis, and persistent monilial infection of the axilla, glans penis, groin, or inframammary area. Despite the high prevalence of mucocutaneous candidiasis, disseminated candidiasis is quite rare in this population. Broad-spectrum antibiotics, indwelling catheters, and parenteral nutrition are risk factors that predispose one to the development of disseminated disease.

Pityrosporum ovale and *Pityrosporum orbiculare (Malassezia*

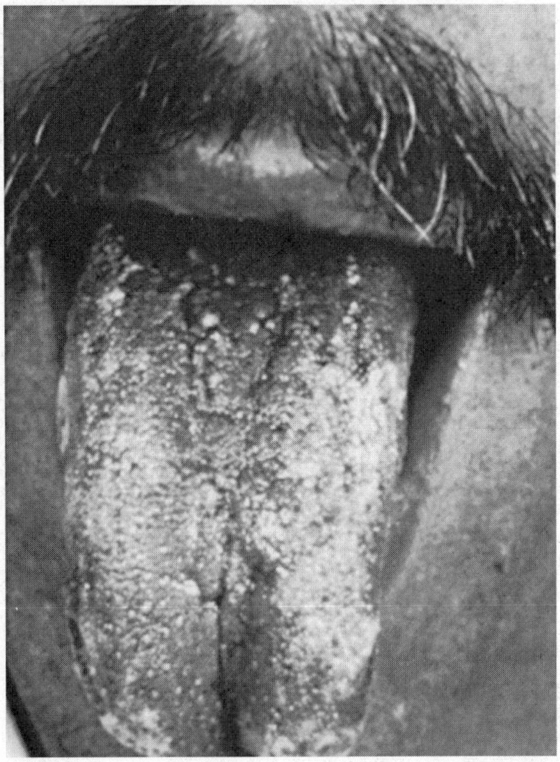

FIGURE 124–6 ◻ Candidiasis. Whitish curdlike exudates present on mucous membranes that are easily scraped off with a tongue depressor are characteristic of candidiasis. This is often associated with candidal esophagitis, which may result in severe dysphagia.

fur fur) are normal residents of the hair follicles of the scalp and have been suggested to cause or exacerbate seborrheic dermatitis in patients with HIV infection. In one study, the density of *P. ovale* on the involved skin was found to correlate with the severity of seborrheic dermatitis.[132] *Pityrosporum* folliculitis characterized by pruritic papules and pustules on the trunk and extremities may also develop in HIV-infected hosts. Extensive tinea versicolor, also caused by *P. ovale*, may occur in patients with HIV infection.

DERMATOPHYTE INFECTIONS

Any cornified epithelial surface may be involved by a dermatophyte. Tinea pedis and onychomycosis are commonly found in HIV-infected individuals.[133] Proximal white subungual onychomycosis of the toenails characteristically occurs in patients with HIV infection, in contrast to the classic form of distal subungual onychomycosis.[134] More than 50% of these infections are caused by *Trichophyton rubrum*.[133] Extensive widespread tinea corporis should raise the possibility of underlying HIV infection.

Trichosporosis caused by infection with *Trichosporon beigelii* generally causes white piedra, a superficial infection of the hair endemic to tropical and subtropical regions of the world and regions of the southeastern United States. Carriage of this organism has been shown to be increased in homosexual men, and several cases of invasive disease with positive blood and urine cultures have been reported.[135]

Dematiaceous fungi can also be a cause of cutaneous fungal infections. *Cladosporium cladosporioides* has been reported to cause pustular nodules in an HIV-infected patient.[136] Surgical excision in this case was curative. Cutaneous alternariosis presenting as an eschar on the leg and *Curvularia* phaeohyphomycosis causing a keratotic lesion on the scrotum have both been observed in HIV-infected individuals.[137, 138]

DIAGNOSIS

Microscopic examination of potassium hydroxide preparations of skin scrapings and cultures should establish the diagnosis in most if not all cases. Cultures from lesions of onychomycosis are often negative despite active clinical infection. In these cases, histopathologic examination of the nail plate may be helpful.

TREATMENT

Appropriate treatment regimens are summarized in Table 124–5. Topical antifungal agents may be effective and are first-line therapy. Many patients require oral medications, and continued prophylactic therapy may be necessary as well.[139–141] Fluconazole-resistant *Candida albicans* is well documented in HIV-positive patients and may necessitate therapy with alternative agents such as itraconazole.[142] Onchyomycosis is best treated with pulse therapy with itraconazole at doses of 200 mg PO bid for 1 week per month for 3 to 4 months or terbinafine at 250 mg PO bid for 1 week per month for 3 to 4 months.

Parasitic Infections and Ectoparasitic Infestations

Scabies

Scabies, caused by the mite *Sarcoptes scabiei* var. *humanus*, is the most common ectoparasitic infection in HIV-infected individuals, occurring in approximately 20% of patients.[143] Severe infestation with scabies often develops as a consequence of impaired cell-mediated immunity and impaired Langerhans cell function.[144] In immunocompetent hosts, the number of infesting mites ranges from 10 to 20, whereas in HIV-infected patients they may number in the millions.

CLINICAL MANIFESTATIONS

Clinical manifestations vary and range from a few scattered pruritic papules to thick hyperkeratotic plaques covering palms, soles, extremities, and trunk. The latter variant is commonly referred to as crusted, or Norwegian, scabies. Characteristically, scabies lesions are localized to intertriginous sites and the genitalia, although typical lesions may not be found in HIV-infected hosts. In addition to the crusted variant, widespread papulosquamous eruptions resembling atopic dermatitis and scalp and facial scaling resembling seborrheic dermatitis have been reported.[143, 145] Associated pruritus is particularly severe at night. Characteristic burrows may be difficult to identify, so that virtually any patient with a scaly persistent pruritic eruption should have skin lesions scraped and examined histologically in search of scabies mites. When scabies has been treated, persistent pruritic nodules may occur, usually in intertriginous sites (nodular scabies). Severe forms of scabies may be associated with secondary infection, bacteremia, and fatal septicemia, especially in severely immunocompromised hosts.[146]

DIAGNOSIS

The diagnosis of scabies depends primarily on the clinical appearance and distribution of the skin eruption as well as demonstration of mites on microscopic examination of skin scrapings. In Norwegian scabies, multiple mites are usually visible in the stratum corneum of the skin biopsy specimen. In nodular scabies, there is a dense infiltrate in the dermis containing numerous eosinophils, but the number of mites is few and they are not often seen.

TREATMENT

Scabies generally responds to treatment with lindane lotion or 5% permethrin cream applied from head to toe, left in place for 8 to 12 hours, then washed off and repeated in 1 week. Patients should be given careful instructions to ensure that sites such as under the fingernails are treated and that linens and clothing are laundered. Household contacts should be treated as well. In HIV-infected individuals, multiple treatments may be required. Postscabetic pruritus is common and must be treated with antihistamines such as doxepin, 10 to 25 mg PO three to four times a day, with topical application of corticosteroid preparations to diminish inflammation. Crotamiton (Eurax) lotion may also be effective in controlling pruritus and in preventing reinfestation.

Less Common Infestations

One hundred fifty cases of leishmaniasis in HIV-infected hosts have been diagnosed in India, Southeast Asia, and the Mediterranean coast.[147] The most common agent reported is *Leishmania donovani*. Papular demodicidosis, which is the result of an excess proliferation of *Demodex folliculorum*, has also been reported sporadically in patients with HIV infection.[148] There are rare reports of cutaneous *Pneumocystis carinii* infection, disseminated strongyloidiasis caused by *Strongyloides stercoralis*, acanthamebiasis caused by *Acanthamoeba castellani*, and disseminated *Toxoplasma gondii*.[149–152]

CLINICAL MANIFESTATIONS

Leishmaniasis usually appears as scaly lichenified plaques with dyspigmentation. Demodicidosis generally consists of a persistent pruritic follicular eruption that may involve the face, trunk, and extremities. *P. carinii* infection of the skin may present as friable reddish papules or nodules seen in the ear canal or the nares. Small translucent molluscum contagiosum–like papules, bluish cellulitic plaque–like lesions, and deeply seated abscesses have also been observed. The one case of toxoplasmosis that has been reported had an appearance of a papular dermatitis, whereas strongyloidiasis gives rise to a rapidly migrating serpiginous urticarial eruption known as larva currens. Acanthamebiasis manifests as painful nodular lesions with ulcerations usually on the trunk or extremities.

DIAGNOSIS

In these unusual conditions, the diagnosis rests on histology with confirmatory cultures when possible. Careful inspection of skin biopsy specimens usually reveals the characteristic organism.

TREATMENT

Leishmaniasis is best treated with stibogluconate sodium at a dosage of 20 mg/kg per day for 3 to 4 weeks. Systemic metronidazole at doses of 250 to 750 mg PO bid should be used to treat amebiasis; however, response to therapy is often quite poor. Demodicosis may be treated with either topical or systemic metronidazole. Strongyloidiasis requires treatment with thiabendazole, 25 mg/kg bid for 4 to 5 days to several weeks. Cutaneous *Pneumocystis* infection responds to usual *Pneumocystis* treatments.

Cutaneous Infections in Human Immunodeficiency Virus–Infected Children

The spectrum of cutaneous infections that occur in HIV-infected children is similar to that of adults; however, the frequency of some disorders differs between the two populations. For example, cutaneous neoplasms are rarely a manifestation of pediatric HIV infection but multiple cutaneous infections are commonly seen.

Viral Infections

Herpetic gingivostomatitis and herpes zoster are common in HIV-infected children and may be severe.[153, 154] Measles without the characteristic rash has been reported with progression to giant cell pneumonia.[66] OHL has rarely been reported in children.[155] The clinical manifestations of molluscum, condyloma, and verrucae are similar to those in the adult population.

Bacterial Infections

As previously mentioned, HIV-infected children frequently suffer from severe recurrent bacterial infections. This is most likely the result of HIV infection occurring before the development of memory cells to bacterial antigens.[153] The most common pathogen is *S. aureus*, the most common clinical manifestations of which are impetigo, cellulitis, and folliculitis. Intravenous immune globulin may have some benefit in the treatment of severe recurrent infections, although one large study has shown that the overall mortality rate after its administration was unchanged.[156–158] For unknown reasons, mycobacterial skin infections and bacillary angiomatosis are rare in HIV-infected children.

Fungal Infections

C. albicans is the most common fungal infection in the pediatric HIV-infected population, and oral thrush or severe diaper dermatitis may be the first manifestation of the disease.[130, 153] In children older than 1 year of age, recalcitrant thrush or diaper dermatitis should raise suspicion of possible HIV infection. Angular cheilitis and onychomycosis secondary to *Candida* may also occur.[153] As in adults, disseminated deep fungal infections with cutaneous involvement are extremely uncommon in children. Treatment regimens are similar for adults and children, with appropriate dosage adjustments.

Virus-Related Neoplasms

A variety of different neoplastic disorders may develop in patients with HIV disease, many of which have been associated with a viral agent. Impaired and altered immunity that results from HIV infection may be important in the genesis of these neoplasms, as may be direct interaction between HIV and other viral agents.

Squamous Cell Carcinoma and Other Epithelial Neoplasms

The frequency of intraepithelial neoplasia of both the uterine cervix in women and the anorectal mucosa in homosexual men is markedly increased in HIV-infected individuals.[159, 160] Women with AIDS have a twofold increased risk for the development of cervical cancer, and cervical cancer is now included as an AIDS-defining illness in women.[161] In American patients with AIDS, there is a 40-fold increased risk for the development of anal cancer, with most of the cases occurring in homosexual men.[160, 162] Nearly 50% of HIV-positive men and women have evidence of HPV infection.[47, 159] Cervical and anal cancers have both been associated with infection with HPV types 16, 18, and 31.[160, 162] In HIV-infected women, cervical cancer may demonstrate rapid progression and a greater tendency to recurrence, and close surveillance and follow-up are particularly important. Less is known concerning the natural history of anal carcinoma, although it might be expected that these lesions would be more aggressive in AIDS patients.

As mentioned previously, epidermodysplasia verruciformis (EDV) has been associated with immunosuppression, including HIV disease.[51, 163, 164] Non–HIV-infected individuals with EDV have been found to have defective cell-mediated immune responses against HPV as well as other antigens, so it is not surprising that EDV has been seen in association with HIV. HPV types 5 and 8 are unique to this disorder and are strongly associated with neoplastic transformation. The combination of oncogenic viral infection, ultraviolet radiation from sun exposure, and altered immune surveillance induces neoplastic epithelial changes.

Because HPV-associated neoplasia also occurs in immunocompetent patients, it is unlikely that there is a direct association between HIV and malignant progression. Rather, decreased cell-mediated immunity and tumor surveillance most likely are permissive for neoplastic transformation. In addition, as previously mentioned, HIV Tat protein up-regulates the expression of HPV in tissue, which may augment the development of HPV-induced neoplasia.[50]

Kaposi's Sarcoma

EPIDEMIOLOGY AND PATHOGENESIS

KS was first described by Moritz Kaposi in 1872, and before the onset of the AIDS pandemic, it was observed only in a small subset of individuals. This vascular neoplastic proliferative disorder is the most frequent neoplastic disorder to develop in patients with AIDS.[165, 166] In the early years of the AIDS epidemic, KS was observed in approximately 50% of the male homosexual AIDS patients in San Francisco.[166] This incidence has dropped significantly, and KS is now reported in only 15% of HIV-seropositive patients, almost all of them homosexual men. The reason for this is not entirely known, but it may be related to the assumption of safer sexual practices in the homosexual community. In the United States, the disorder is far less common among intravenous drug users and is rare in women, hemophiliacs, and their sexual partners. In addition to HIV-positive homosexual men, KS has been reported in a group of homosexual men with no HIV infection but with risk factors for it.[167] In these patients, KS tends to have a more indolent course, similar to that observed in elderly Italian and Jewish men.

These epidemiologic features suggest that KS may be related to a sexually transmitted infectious agent. The association of KS with immunosuppression and its capacity for spontaneous regression also support an infectious etiology. Genomic sequences of type 16 HPV DNA have previously been identified in KS lesions, but these have since been shown to be not significant.[168] A unique herpesvirus, closely related to *Herpesvirus saimiri,* a virus of squirrel monkeys, has been identified in lesions of HIV-associated KS, HIV-negative homosexuals with KS, and classic KS.[169–172] This virus, known as human herpesvirus type 8 or KS-associated herpesvirus, is now believed to be the cause of KS. Altered levels of cytokines such as transforming growth factor-β and oncostatin M, which can occur in HIV-infected individuals, have been shown to promote the growth of KS cells.[173, 174] In addition, HIV Tat protein can stimulate the growth of AIDS-associated KS cells in vitro.[175]

CLINICAL MANIFESTATIONS

Clinically, KS skin lesions may be pink, red, brown, or purple macules, patches, or plaques. Purplish to brown-black nodules and tumors may also develop. Lesions are commonly oriented along the lines of skin tension and may spread locally in areas of trauma. Favored sites include mucous membranes, nose, and trunk. Internal organ involvement, particularly of the gastrointestinal tract and lymphatics, is common, and as a rule one internal lesion is present for every five skin lesions.

DIAGNOSIS

Diagnosis is generally based on the characteristic clinical features of purplish skin lesions in the appropriate clinical setting in conjunction with histopathologic findings. Skin biopsy typically shows a proliferation of spindle-shaped endothelial cells forming irregular jagged vascular slits. There are often associated hemosiderin deposition and an infiltrate of plasma cells. The diagnosis of HIV-related KS should be made with caution in women and children from the United States as the neoplasm occurs only rarely in these populations of patients.

TREATMENT

Treatment of uncomplicated KS is done for cosmesis only. Local destructive measures are generally most effective. Liquid nitrogen cryotherapy can be used for early, flat lesions. Radiotherapy is also quite effective. Intralesional injections of vinblastine, interferon alfa (Intron A), and daunorubicin are promising alternatives, as is infusion of liposome-encapsulated daunorubicin and doxorubicin, which localizes to the skin.[176–178] Systemic chemotherapy is reserved for patients with widespread disease caused by associated immunosuppression.

Leiomyoma and Leiomyosarcoma

Smooth muscle tumors, leiomyomas and leiomyosarcomas, have been described in children with HIV infection and in immunosuppressed children.[179] Reported sites include gastrointestinal tract, lung, and subcutaneous tissue, where multiple subcutaneous nodules have been described.[179–181] Interestingly, Epstein-Barr virus has been demonstrated in leiomyomas and leiomyosarcomas from HIV-infected and immunosuppressed children; however, it has not been found in these tumors occurring in immunocompetent patients.[182–183] These studies suggest that Epstein-Barr virus plays a direct role in the genesis of these neoplasms.

T-Cell Leukemia and Lymphoma

Human T-cell lymphotropic virus type I (HTLV-I) is a retrovirus that is endemic to southern Japan, northern South America, southern North America, and areas of Africa. Less than 1% of carriers develop an aggressive T-cell leukemia that is characterized by multiple skin lesions and lytic bone lesions. Tropical spastic paraparesis may also be a rare complication of infection with this virus. A few patients have been observed who have dual infection with HTLV-I and HIV, and in these patients the HIV appeared to accelerate the appearance of T-cell leukemia and tropical spastic paraparesis.[184–187] In addition, two patients have been reported with dual HTLV-I and HIV infection who developed cutaneous lesions similar to those in mycosis fungoides. Sézary cells were demonstrated in peripheral blood and skin.[188]

Human T-cell lymphotropic virus type II (HTLV-II) is closely related to but distinct from HTLV-I. This virus is found in the Native American and Brazilian Indian populations as well as among intravenous drug users and may rarely be associated with hairy cell leukemia. No cases of hairy cell leukemia have been found in patients with concomitant HTLV-II and HIV infection, although a cutaneous disorder resembling mycosis fungoides has been described.[189] The eruption was characterized by extensive scaling, lichenified plaques, peripheral eosinophilia, and dermatopathic lymphadenopathy. Histologically, a dermal infiltrate of $CD8^+$ lymphocytes and giant cells was seen.

The effects of concurrent retroviral infections are just beginning to be observed and studied; however, combined adverse effects are expected. In vitro, HTLV-I has been shown to promote penetration of HIV into $CD4^+$ cells and to enhance HIV proliferation.[190, 191] In addition, both HTLV and HIV can activate Epstein-Barr virus.[192]

Conclusions

The diagnosis and management of HIV infection have evolved dramatically since its initial recognition. Early diagnosis and prevention of opportunistic infections as well as treatment of HIV disease itself have become significant priorities. A wide variety of cutaneous infections occur in HIV disease and can be the source of significant morbidity. By recognizing these signs and symptoms and by performing appropriate diagnostic testing to establish correct diagnoses, these complications can be minimized significantly.

References

1. Tindall B, Barker S, Donovan B, et al: Characterization of the acute clinical illness associated with human immunodeficiency virus infection. Arch Intern Med 148:945–949, 1988.

2. Sinicco A, Palestro G, Caramello P, et al: Acute HIV-1 infection: Clinical and biologic study of twelve patients. J Acquir Immune Defic Syndr 3:260–265, 1990.
3. Gaines H: Primary HIV infection. Clinical and diagnostic aspects. J Infect Dis 61(Suppl):1–46, 1989.
4. Ho DD, Sarngadharan MG, Reznick, L, et al: Primary human T-lymphocyte virus type III infection. Ann Intern Med 103:880–883, 1985.
5. Isaksson B, Albert J, Chiodi F, et al: AIDS two months after primary human immunodeficiency virus infection. J Infect Dis 158:866–868, 1988.
6. Kinlock S, de Saussure PH, Vanhems PH, et al: Primary HIV infection: A prospective and retrospective study. Poster presented at the VIII International Conference on AIDS; July 19–24, 1992; Amsterdam.
7. Rabeneck L, Popovic M, Gartner S, et al: Acute HIV infection presenting with painful swallowing and esophageal ulcers. JAMA 263:2318–2322, 1990.
8. McMillan A, Bishop PE, Aw D, Peutherer JF: Immunohistology of the skin rash associated with acute HIV infection. AIDS 3:309–312, 1989.
9. Henderson DK, Gerberding JL: Prophylactic zidovudine after occupational exposure to the human immunodeficiency virus: An interim analysis. J Infect Dis 160:321–323, 1989.
10. Looke DFM, Grove DI: Failed prophylactic zidovudine after needle-stick injury (Letter). Lancet 335:1280, 1990.
11. Lange J, Boucher CAB, Hollack CEM, et al: Failure of zidovudine prophylaxis after accidental exposure to HIV-1. N Engl J Med 322:1375–1377, 1990.
12. Safran S, Ashley R, Houlihan C, et al: Clinical and serologic features of herpes simplex virus infection in patients with AIDS. AIDS 5:1107–1110, 1991.
13. Klatt EC, Shibata D: Cytomegalovirus infection in the acquired immunodeficiency syndrome. Arch Pathol Lab Med 112:540–544, 1988.
14. Masur H: Clinical implications of herpesvirus infections in patients with AIDS. Am J Med 92(2A):1S-2S, 1992.
15. Corey YL, Spear PG: Infections with herpes simplex viruses (Part II). N Engl J Med 314:749–756, 1986.
16. Simonson JN, Cameron WD, Gakenya MN, et al: Human immunodeficiency virus infection among men with sexually transmitted diseases: Experience from a center in Africa. N Engl J Med 319:274–278, 1988.
17. Stamm WE, Hansfield HH, Rompalo AM, et al: The association between genital ulcerative disease and acquisition of HIV infection in homosexual men. JAMA 260:1429–1433, 1988.
18. Lawrence J: Perspective. Molecular interactions among herpes viruses and human immunodeficiency viruses. J Infect Dis 162:338–347, 1990.
19. Siegal FP, Lopez C, Hammer GS, et al: Severe acquired immunodeficiency in male homosexuals, manifested by chronic perianal ulcerative herpes simplex lesions. N Engl J Med 305:1439–1444, 1981.
20. Buchbinder SP, Katz MH, Hessal NA, et al: Herpes zoster and human immunodeficiency virus infection. J Infect Dis 166:1153–1156, 1992.
21. Leibovitz E, Cooper D, Giurgiutiu D, et al: Varicella-zoster virus infection in Romanian children infected with the human immunodeficiency virus. Pediatrics 92:838–842, 1993.
22. Jura E, Chadwick EG, Josephs HS, et al: Varicella zoster virus infections in children infected with human immunodeficiency virus. Pediatr Infect Dis J 8:856–590, 1989.
23. Gilson IH, Barnett JH, Conans MA, et al: Disseminated ecthymatous varicella-zoster virus infection in patients with acquired immunodeficiency syndrome. J Am Acad Dermatol 20:637–642, 1989.
24. Cohen PR, Beltranny VP, Grossman ME: Disseminated herpes zoster in patients with immunodeficiency virus infection. Am J Med 84:1076–1080, 1988.
25. Worrell JT, Cockerell CJ: Histopathology of peripheral nerves in cutaneous herpesvirus infection. Am J Dermatopath 19:133–137, 1966.
26. Jacobson MA, Berger TG, Fikrig S, et al: Acyclovir-resistant varicella zoster virus infection after chronic oral acyclovir therapy in patients with the acquired immunodeficiency syndrome (AIDS). Ann Intern Med 112:187–191, 1990.
27. Hardy WD: Foscarnet treatment of acyclovir-resistant herpes simplex virus infection in patients with acquired immunodeficiency syndrome: Preliminary results of a controlled, randomized, regimen-comparative trial. Am J Med 92:30s–35s, 1992.
28. Chatis PA, Miller CH, Schrager LE, et al: Successful treatment with foscarnet of an acyclovir-resistant mucocutaneous infection with herpes simplex virus in a patient with acquired immunodeficiency syndrome. N Engl J Med 1989;320:297–300.
29. Gallant JE, Moore RD, Chaisson RE: Prophylaxis for opportunistic infections in patients with HIV infection. Ann Intern Med 120:932–944, 1994.
30. Lin CS, Pinha PD, Krishnan MN, et al: Cytomegalic inclusion disease of the skin. Arch Dermatol 117:282–284, 1981.
31. Feldman PS, Walker AN, Baker R: Cutaneous lesions heralding disseminated cytomegalovirus infections. J Am Acad Dermatol 7:545–548, 1982.
32. Horn TD, Hood AF: Cytomegalovirus is predictably present in perineal ulcers from immunosuppressed patients. Arch Dermatol 126:642–644, 1990.
33. Lee JY, Peel R: Concurrent cytomegalovirus and herpes simplex virus infections in skin biopsy specimens from two AIDS patients with fatal CMV infection. Am J Dermatopathol 11:136–143, 1989.
34. Smith KJ, Skelton HG, James WD, et al: Concurrent epidermal involvement of cytomegalovirus and herpes simplex virus in two HIV-infected patients. J Am Acad Deramtol 25:500–506, 1991.
35. Muehler-Stamou A, Sen HJ, Emodi G: Epidermolysis in a case of severe cytomegalovirus infection. Br Med J 3:609–611, 1974.
36. Minars N, Silverman JF, Escobar NR, et al: Fatal cytomegalic inclusion disease: Associated skin manifestations in a renal transplant patient. Arch Dermatol 113:1569–1571, 1977.
37. Jacobson MA, Mills J: Serious cytomegalovirus disease in the acquired immunodeficiency syndrome (AIDS). Ann Intern Med 108:585–594, 1988.
38. Treatment of serious cytomegalovirus infections with 9-(1,3-dihydroxy-2-propoxymethyl)guanine in patients with AIDS and other immunodeficiencies. Collaborative DHPG Treatment Study Group. N Engl J Med 314:801–805, 1986.
39. Greenspan JS, Greenspan D, Lenette ET, et al: Replication of Epstein-Barr virus within epithelial cells of oral "hairy" leukoplakia and AIDS associated lesion. N Engl J Med 313:1564–1571, 1985.
40. Itin PH: Oral hairy leukoplakia—10 years on. Dermatology 187:159–163, 1993.
41. Greenspan D, Greenspan JS, Overby G, et al: Risk factors for rapid progression from hairy leukoplakia to AIDS: A nested case-control study. J Acquir Immune Defic Syndr 4:652–658, 1991.
42. Fowler CD, Reed KD, Brannon RB: Intranuclear inclusions correlate with the ultrastructural detection of herpes-type virions in oral hairy leukoplakia. Am J Surg Pathol 13:114–119, 1989.
43. DeSouza YG, Greenspan D, Feltzen JR, et al: Localization of Epstein-Barr virus DNA in the epithelial cells of oral hairy leukoplakia via in situ hybridization of tissue sac (Letter). N Engl J Med 320:1559, 1989.
44. Gaglioti D, De Pietro M, Ficarra G, Alder-Storthz K: Oral hairy leukoplakia: Clinical appearance and treatment results (Abstr). Presented at the V International Conference on AIDS; June 4–9, 1989; Montreal; p 473.
45. Schofer H, Ochsendorf FR, Elm EB, et al: Treatment of oral hairy leukoplakia in AIDS patients with vitamin A acid (topically) or acyclovir (systemically) (Letter). Dermatologica 174:150–151, 1987.
46. Beutner KR, Becker TM, Stone KM: Epidemiology of HPV infections. Dermatol Clin 9:211–218, 1991.
47. Palefsky JM, Gonzales J, Greenblatt RM, et al: Anal intraepithelial neoplasia and anal papillomavirus infection among homosexual males with group IV HIV disease. JAMA 263:2911–2916, 1990.
48. Chardonnet Y, Viac J, Staqnet MJ: Cell mediated immunity to human papillomavirus. Clin Dermatol 3:156–161, 1985.
49. Doherty R, Tanskanen E, Churchill MJ, Deacon NJ: Interactions between human immunodeficiency virus and human papillomavirus. Poster presented at the VIII International Conference on AIDS; July 19–24, 1992; Amsterdam.

50. Tornesello ML, Buonaguro FM, Galloway DA, Beth-Giraldo E: Human immunodeficiency virus type 1 *tat* gene enhances human papillomavirus early gene expression. Intervirology 36(2):57–64, 1993.
51. Berger TG, Sawchuk WS, Leonardi C, et al: Epidermodysplasia verruciformis–associated papillomavirus infection complicating human immunodeficiency virus disease. Br J Dermatol 126:79–83, 1991.
52. Braun L, Farmer ER, Shah KV: Immunoperoxidase localization of papillomavirus antigen and cutaneous warts in bowenoid papulosis. J Med Virol 12:187–193, 1983.
53. Rudlinger R, Buchmann P: HPV 16–positive bowenoid papulosis and squamous-cell carcinoma of the anus in an HIV-positive man. Dis Colon Rectum 32:1042–1045, 1989.
54. Beckmann AM, Myerson D, Daling JR, et al: Detection and localization of human papillomavirus DNA in human genital condylomas by in situ hybridization with biotinylated probes. J Med Virol 16:265–273, 1985.
55. Shibata KK, Arnheim M, Martin WJ: Detection of human papillomavirus in paraffin-embedded tissue using the polymerase chain reaction. J Exp Med 167:225–230, 1988.
56. Beutner KR, Conant M, Friedman-Kien AE, et al: Patient-applied podofilox for treatment of genital warts. Lancet 1:831–838, 1989.
57. Lane HC: Interferons in HIV and related diseases. AIDS 8:19–23, 1994.
58. Friedman-Kien AE, Eron LJ, Conant M, et al: Natural interferon alfa for treatment of condylomata acuminata. JAMA 259:533–538, 1988.
59. Stern RS: Epidemiology of skin disease in HIV infection: A cohort study of health maintenance organization members. J Invest Dermatol 102:34S–37S, 1994.
60. Redfield RR, Wright DC, James WD, et al: Disseminated vaccinia in a military recruit with human immunodeficiency virus (HIV) disease. N Engl J Med 316:673–676, 1987.
61. Fivenson DP, Weltman RE, Gibson SH: Giant molluscum contagiosum presenting as basal cell carcinoma in an AIDS patient (Letter). J Am Acad Dermatol 19:912–914, 1988.
62. Berger TG, Greene I: Bacterial, viral, fungal and parasitic infections in HIV disease and AIDS. Dermatol Clin 3:465–492, 1991.
63. Ross LA, Kim KS, Comport Z: Successful treatment of disseminated measles in a patient with acquired immune deficiency syndrome: Consideration of anti-viral and passive immunotherapy. Am J Med 88:313–314, 1990.
64. Torok TJ: Parvovirus and human disease. Adv Intern Med 37:431–455, 1992.
65. Coldiron BM, Freeman RG, Beaudoing DL: Isolation of adenovirus from a granuloma annulare–like lesion in the acquired immunodeficiency syndrome-related complex. Arch Dermatol 124:654–655, 1988.
66. Markowitz LE, Chandler FW, Roldan EO, et al: Fatal measles and pneumonia without rash in a child with AIDS. J Infect Dis 158:480–483, 1988.
67. Ellis M, Gupta S, Gellant S, et al: Neutrophil function in patients with AIDS or AIDS-related complex: A comprehensive evaluation. J Infect Dis 158:1268–1276, 1988.
68. Pahwa SG, Quilop MT, Lange M, et al: Defective B-lymphocyte function in homosexual men in relation to acquired immune deficiency syndrome. Ann Intern Med 101:757–763, 1984.
69. Ganesh R, Castle D, Gibbon D, et al. Staphylococcal carriage in HIV infection (Letter). Lancet 2:558, 1989.
70. Nichols SL, Balog K, Silverman M: Bacterial infection and AIDS. Clinical pathologic correlations in a series of autopsy cases. Am J Clin Pathol 92:787–790, 1989.
71. Raviglione MC, Battan R, Pablos-Mendez A, et al: Infections associated with Hickman catheters in patients with acquired immune deficiency syndrome. Am J Med 86:780–786, 1989.
72. el Baze P, Thyss A, Vinti H, et al: A study of nineteen immunocompromised patients with extensive skin lesions caused by *Pseudomonas aeruginosa* with and without bacteremia. Acta Derm Venereol (Stockh) 71:411–415, 1991.
73. Kielhofner M, Atmar RL, Hamill RF, Musher DM: Life-threatening *Pseudomonas aeruginosa* infections in patients with human immunodeficiency virus infection. Clin Infec Dis 14:403-411, 1992.
74. Sangeorzan JA, Bradley SF, Kaufman CA: Cutaneous manifestation of *Pseudomonas* infection in the acquired immune deficiency syndrome. Arch Dermatol 126:832–833, 1990.
75. Patterson JW, Kitces EN, Neafie RC: Cutaneous botryomycosis in a patient with acquired immunodeficiency syndrome. J Am Acad Dermatol 16:238–242, 1987.
76. Weitzner JM, Dhawan SS, Rosen LB, et al: Successful treatment of botryomycosis in a patient with acquired immunodeficiency syndrome. J Am Acad Dermatol 21:1312–1314, 1989.
77. Becker BA, Odom RB, Berger TG: Atypical plaque-like staphylococcal folliculitis in human immunodeficiency virus infected persons. J Am Acad Dermatol 21:1024–1026, 1989.
78. Gaut P, Wong PK, Meyer RD: Pyomyositis in a patient with the acquired immunodeficiency syndrome. Arch Intern Med 148:1608–1610, 1988.
79. Janssen F, Zelinsky-Gurung A, Caumes E, Decazed JM: Group A streptococcal cellulitis-adenitis in a patient with the acquired immunodeficiency syndrome. J Am Acad Dermatol 24:363–365, 1991.
80. Kline MW, Dunkle LM: Toxic shock syndrome in the acquired immunodeficiency syndrome. Pediatr Infect Dis J 7:736–738, 1988.
81. Cipriano J, Feranno J, Ferranti E: Acquired immunodeficiency syndrome in non-menstrual toxic shock syndrome (Letter). Ann Intern Med 105:300, 1986.
82. Steinhart R, Reingold AL, Taylor F, et al: Invasive *Haemophilus influenzae* infections in men with HIV infection. JAMA 268:3350–3352, 1992.
83. Javaly K, Horowitz HW, Wormser GP: Nocardiosis in patients with human immunodeficiency virus Infection. Medicine (Baltimore) 71:128–138, 1992.
84. Watkins KV, Richmond AS, Langstein IM: Nonhealing extraction site due to *Actinomyces naeslundii* in patients with AIDS. Oral Surg Oral Med Oral Pathol 71:675–677, 1991.
85. Drancourt M, Bonnet E, Gallais H, et al: *Rhodococcus equi* infection in patients with AIDS. J Infect 24:123–131, 1992.
86. Patey O, Halioua B, Casciani JP, et al: *Corynebacterium diphtheriae* septicemia in an AIDS patient (Abstr). Presented at the VIII International Conference on AIDS; July 19–24, 1992; Amsterdam.
87. Cockerell CJ, Whitlow MA, Webster GF, Friedman-Kien AE: Epithelioid angiomatosis: A distinct vascular disorder in patients with acquired immunodeficiency syndrome or AIDS-related complex. Lancet 329:654–656, 1987.
88. Relman DA, Loutit JS, Schmidt TM, et al: The agent of bacillary angiomatosis: An approach to the identification of uncultured pathogens. N Engl J Med 323:1573–1580, 1990.
89. Relman DA, Lepp PW, Sadler KN, Schmidt TM: Phylogenetic relationships among the agents of bacillary angiomatosis. Mol Microbiol 6:1801–1807, 1992.
90. Tappero JW, Mohle-Boetani JM, Koehler JE, et al: The epidemiology of bacillary angiomatosis and bacillary peliosis. JAMA 269:770–775, 1993.
91. Koehler JE, Claser CA, Tappero JW: *Rochalimaea henselae* infection: A new zoonosis with the domestic cat as reservoir. JAMA 271:531–535, 1994.
92. Webster GF, Cockerell CJ, Friedman-Kien AE: The clinical spectrum of bacillary angiomatosis. Br J Dermatol 126:535–541, 1992.
93. Schinella RA, Alba-Greco M: Bacillary angiomatosis presenting as a soft-tissue tumor without skin involvement. Hum Pathol 21:567–569, 1990.
94. Perkocha LA, Geaghan SM, Yen TS, et al: Clinical and pathological features of bacillary peliosis hepatis in association with human immunodeficiency virus infection. N Engl J Med 323:1581–1586, 1990.
95. Welch DF, Pickett DA, Slater LN, et al: *Rochalimaea henselae* sp. nov., a cause of septicemia, bacillary angiomatosis and parenchymal bacillary peliosis. J Clin Microbiol 30:275–280, 1992.
96. Slater LN, Welch DF, Hensel D, Coody DW: A newly recognized fastidious gram-negative pathogen as a cause of fever and bacteremia. N Engl J Med 323:1587–1593, 1990.
97. Daly JS, Worthington MG, Brenner DJ, et al: *Rochalimaea elizabethae* sp. nov. isolated from a patient with endocarditis. J Clin Microbiol 31:872–881, 1993.
98. Draincort M, Mainardi JL, Brouqui P, et al: *Bartonella (Rochalimaea) quintana* endocarditis in three homeless men. N Engl J Med 332:419–423, 1995.

99. Spach DH, Kanter AS, Doughtery ML, et al: *Bartonella (Rochalimaea) quintana* bacteremia in innter-city patients with chronic alcoholism. N Engl J Med 332:424–428, 1995.
100. Koehler JE, Quinn FD, Berger TG, et al: Isolation of *Rochalimaea* species from cutaneous and osseous lesions of bacillary angiomatosis. N Engl J Med 327:1625–1631, 1992.
101. Regnery RL, Anderson BE, Clarridge JEI, et al: Characterization of a novel *Rochalimaea* species, *R. henselae* sp. nov., isolated from blood of a febrile human immunodeficiency virus–seropositive patient. J Clin Microbiol 30:265–274, 1992.
102. Lucey D, Dolan MJ, Moss CW, et al: Relapsing illness due to *Rochalimaea henselae* in immunocompetent hosts: Implication for therapy and new epidemiological associations. Clin Infect Dis 14:683–688, 1992.
103. Mui BSK, Mulligan ME, George WL: Response of HIV-associated disseminated cat-scratch disease to treatment with doxycycline. Am J Med 89:229–231, 1990.
104. Guierra LG, Neka CJ, Boman D, et al: Rapid response of AIDS-related bacillary angiomatosis to azithromycin. Clin Infect Dis 17:264–266, 1993.
105. Duong M, Dalao S, Chavanet P, et al: Angiomatose bacillair au cours de l'infection à VIH. Mise au point à propos d'un cas traité par la roxithromycine. Ann Intern Med 143:107–112, 1992.
106. Barbaro DJ, Orcutt VL, Colder BM: *Mycobacterium avium-intracellulare* infection limited to the skin and lymph nodes in patients with AIDS. Rev Infect Dis 11:625–6281989.
107. Rogers PL, Walker RE, Wayne HC, et al: Disseminated *Mycobacterium haemophilum* infection in two patients with AIDS. Am J Med 84:640–642, 1988.
108. Geman MD: Treatment of multidrug resistant tuberculosis. N Engl J Med 329:784–791, 1993.
109. Quinn TC, Cannon RO, Glasser D, et al: The association of syphilis with risk of human immunodeficiency virus in patients attending sexually transmitted disease clinics. Arch Intern Med 159:1297–1302, 1990.
110. Gregory N, Sanchez M, Buchness MR: The spectrum of syphilis in patients with human immunodeficiency virus infection. J Am Acad Dermatol 22:1061–1067, 1990.
111. Johns DR, Tierney M, Felsenstein D: Alteration of the natural history of neurosyphilis by concurrent infection with the human immunodeficiency virus. N Engl J Med 316:1569–1572, 1987.
112. Quale J, Tepletts E, Augenbraun F: Atypical presentation of chancroid in a patient infected with the human immunodeficiency virus. Am J Med 88(Suppl 5):43–44, 1990.
113. Strongin IS, Kale SA, Raymond MK, et al: An unusual presentation of gonococcal arthritis in an HIV-positive patient. Ann Rheum Dis 50:572–573, 1991.
114. Cohen PR, Grossman ME, Silvers DN: Disseminated histoplasmosis and human immunodeficiency virus infection. Int J Dermatol 30:614–622, 1991.
115. Cole MC, Cohen PR, Satra KH, Grossman ME: The concurrent presence of systemic disease pathogens and cutaneous Kaposi's sarcoma in the same lesion: *Histoplasma capsulatum* and Kaposi's sarcoma coexisting in a single skin lesion in a patient with AIDS. J Am Acad Dermatol 26:285–287, 1992.
116. Chaker MB, Cocerell CJ: Concommitant psoriasis, seborrheic dermatitis and disseminated cutaneous histoplasmosis in a patient infected with the human immunodeficiency virus. J Am Acad Dermatol 29:311–13, 1993.
117. Cohen PR, Held JL, Grossman ME, et al: Disseminated histoplasmosis presenting as an ulcerated verrucous plaque in a human immunodeficiency virus–infected man: Report of a case possibly involving human-to-human transmission of histoplasmosis. Int J Dermatol 30:104–108, 1991.
118. Rico NJ, Penneys NS: Cutaneous cryptococcosis resembling molluscum contagiosum in a patient with AIDS. Arch Dermatol 121:901–902, 1985.
119. Mares M, Sartori MT, Carretta M, et al: Rhinophyma-like cryptococcal infection as an early manifestation of AIDS in a hemophilia B patient. Acta Haematol 84:101–103, 1990.
120. Bibler MR, Luber HJ, Glueck HI, Estes SA: Disseminated sporotrichosis in a patient with HIV infection after treatment for acquired factor VIII inhibitor. JAMA 256:3125-3126, 1986.
121. Shaw JC, Levinson W, Montanara A: Sporotrichosis in the acquired immunodeficiency syndrome. J Am Acad Dermatol 21:1145–1147, 1989.
122. Borradori L, Schmit J-C, Stetzkowski M, et al: Penicilliosis *marneffei* infection in AIDS. J Am Acad Dermatol 31:843–846, 1994.
123. Fish DG, Ampel NM, Galgiani JN, et al: Coccidioidomycosis during human immunodeficiency virus infection: A review of 77 patients. Medicine (Baltimore) 69:384–391, 1990.
124. Fraser VJ, Keath EJ, Powderly WG: Two cases of blastomycosis from a common source: Use of DNA restriction analysis to identify strains. J Infect Dis 163:1378–1381, 1991.
125. Bakos L, Kronfeld M, Hampe S, et al: Disseminated paracoccidioidomycosis with skin lesions in a patient with acquired immunodeficiency syndrome (Letter). J Am Acad Dermatol 20:854–855, 1989.
126. Wood GM, McCormack JG, Muir DB, et al: Clinical features of human infection with *Scedosporium inflatum*. Clin Infect Dis 14:1027–1033, 1992.
127. Scherr GR, Evans SG, Kiyabu MT, Klatt EC: *Pseudallescheria boydii* in the acquired immunodeficiency syndrome. Arch Pathol Lab Med 116:535–536, 1992.
128. Hevia O, Kligman D, Penneys NS: Non-scalp hair infection caused by *Microsporum canis* in a patient with acquired immunodeficiency syndrome. J Am Acad Dermatol 24:789–790, 1991.
129. Frazer R, Stoole E, et al. Head and neck Zygomycetes/*Aspergillus* infections in patients with AIDS. Poster presented at the IX International Conference on AIDS; June 6–12, 1993; Berlin.
130. British Society for Antimicrobial Chemotherapy Working Group: Antifungal chemotherapy in patients with acquired immunodeficiency syndrome. Lancet 340:648–651, 1992.
131. Klein RS, Harris CA, Small CB, et al: Oral candidiasis in high-risk patients as the initial manifestation of the acquired immunodeficiency syndrome. N Engl J Med 311:354–358, 1984.
132. Hing MCY, Henderson CL, Barker DC, et al: Correlation of *Pityrosporon ovale* density with clinical severity of seborrheic dermatitis as assessed by simplified technique. J Am Acad Dermatol 23:82–86, 1990.
133. Torssander J, Karlsson A, Morfeldt-Manson L, et al: Dermatophytosis and HIV infection. A study in homosexual men. Acta Derm Venereol (Stockh) 68:563–565, 1988.
134. Noppakun N, Head ES: Proximal white subungual onychomycosis in a patient with acquired immunodeficiency syndrome. Int J Dermatol 25:586–587, 1986.
135. Lief HL, Semperkopf MS: Invasive trichosporonosis in a patient with AIDS. J Infect Dis 160:356–357, 1989.
136. Drabick JJ, Gomatos PJ, Solis JB: Cutaneous cladosporiosis as a complication of skin testing in a man positive for HIV. J Am Acad Dermatol 22:135–136, 1990.
137. Lavy-Clotz B, Badillet G, Cavelier-Balloy, et al: Alternariose cutanée au cours d'un SIDA. Arch Derm Venereol 112:739–740, 1985.
138. Duvic M, Lowe L, Rios A, et al: Superficial phaeohyphomycosis of the scrotum in a patient with AIDS (Letter). Arch Dermatol 123:1597–1599, 1987.
139. Pons V, Greenspan D, Debruin M: Therapy for oropharyngeal candidiasis in HIV-infected patients: A randomized, prospective multicenter study of oral fluconazole versus clotrimazole troches. J Acquir Immune Defic Syndr 6:1311–1316, 1993.
140. Odom R: Common superficial fungal infections in immunosuppressed patients. J Am Acad Dermatol 31(Suppl):56–59, 1994.
141. Greenspan D: Treatment of oropharyngeal candidiasis in HIV positive patients. J Am Acad Dermatol 31(Suppl):51–55, 1994.
142. Sanguineti A, Carmichael K, Campbell D: Fluconazole-resistant *Candida albicans* afer long-term suppressive therapy. Arch Intern Med 153:1122–1124, 1993.
143. Sadick N, Kaplan MH, Pahwa SG, et al: Unusual features of scabies complicating human T-lymphotrophic virus type III infection. J Am Acad Dermatol 15:482–486, 1986.
144. Belsito DB, Sanchez MR, Baer RL, et al: Reduced Langerhans' cell Ia antigen and ATPase activity in patients with the acquired immunodeficiency syndrome. N Engl J Med 310:1279–1282, 1984.
145. Jucowics P, Ramon ME, Donn PC, et al: Norwegian scabies in an infant with acquired immunodeficiency syndrome. Arch Dermatol 125:1670–1671, 1989.
146. Skinner SM, DeVillez RL: Sepsis associated with Norwegian scabies in patients with acquired immunodeficiency syndrome. Arch Dermatol 50:213–216, 1992.

147. Montelban C, Martinez-Fernandez R, Calleja JL, et al: Visceral leishmaniasis (kala-azar) as an opportunistic infection in patients with HIV disease in Spain. Rev Infect Dis 11:655–660, 1989.
148. Dominey A, Roen R, Tschen J: Papulonodular demodicidosis associated with acquired immunodeficiency syndrome. J Am Acad Dermatol 20:197–201, 1989.
149. Hennessey NP, Parro EL, Cockerell CJ: Cutaneous *Pneumocystis carinii* infection in patients with acquired immunodeficiency syndrome. Arch Dermatol 127:1699–1701, 1991.
150. Hirschmann JV, Chu AC: Skin lesions with disseminated toxoplasmosis in a patient with the acquired immunodeficiency syndrome. Arch Dermatol 124:1446–1447, 1988.
151. Portnoy BL, Micheletti GA: *Acanthamoeba* infection of skin and sinuses in an AIDS patient: Diagnosis and treatment (Abstr). Presented at the VIII International Conference on AIDS; July 19–24, 1992; Amsterdam.
152. Glezerov V, Masci JR: Disseminated strongyloidiasis and other selected unusual infections in patients with acquired immunodeficiency syndrome. Prog AIDS Pathol 2:137–142, 1990.
153. Nickles SW: The opportunistic and bacterial infections associated with pediatric human immunodeficiency virus disease. Acta Paediatr (Suppl 400):46–50, 1994.
154. Silverman S Jr, Wara D: Oral manifestations of pediatric AIDS. Pediatrician 16:185–187, 1989.
155. Greenspan JS, Masrucci, Legott PF, et al: Hairy leukoplakia in a child (Letter). AIDS 2:143, 1988.
156. Mofenson LM, Moye J Jr: Intravenous immune globulin for the prevention of infections in children with symptomatic human immunodeficiency virus infection. Pediatr Res 33(Suppl):80–89, 1993.
157. Intravenous immune globulin for the prevention of bacterial infection in children with symptomatic human immunodeficiency virus infection. The National Institute of Child Health and Human Developement Immunoglbulin Study Group. N Engl J Med 325:73–80, 1991.
158. Spector SA, Gelber RD, McGrath N, et al: Results of the ACTG 051: A Double Blind Placebo Controlled Trial to Evaluate Intravenous Gammaglobulin (IVIG) in Children with Symptomatic HIV Infection Receiving Zidovudine. Anaheim, CA, Infectious Disease Society of America. N Engl J Med 331:1181–1187, 1994.
159. Feingold AR, Vermund SH, Burk RD, et al: Cervical cytologic abnormalities and papillomavirus in women infected with human immunodeficiency virus. J Acquir Immune Defic Syndr 3:896–903, 1990.
160. Palefsky JM, Holly EA, Gonzales J, et al: Detection of human papilloma DNA in anal intra-epithelial neoplasial and anal cancer. Cancer Res 51:1014–1019, 1991.
161. 1993 revised classification system for HIV infection and expanded surveillance case definition for AIDS among adolescents and adults. MMWR Morbid Mortal Wkly Rep 41(RR-17):1–19, 1992.
162. Beckmann AM, Daling JR, Sherman KJ, et al: Human papillomavirus infection and anal cancer. Int J Cancer 43:1042–1049, 1989.
163. Majewski S, Jablonska S: Epidermodysplasia verruciformis as a model of human papillomavirus-induced genetic cancers: The role of local immunosurveillance. Am J Med Sci 304:174–179, 1992.
164. Lutzner M, Croisant O, Ducasse MF, et al: A potentially oncogenic human papillomavirus (HPV5) found in two renal allograft recipients. J Invest Dermatol 75:353–356, 1980.
165. Haverkos HW: Factors associated with the pathogenesis of AIDS. J Infect Dis 156:251–257, 1987.
166. Rutherford GW, Payne SF, Lemp GF, et al: The epidemiology of AIDS-related Kaposi's sarcoma in San Francisco. J Acquir Immune Defic Syndr 3(Suppl 1):S4–S7, 1990.
167. Friedman-Kien AE, Saltzman BR, Cao YZ, et al: Kaposi's sarcoma in HIV-negative homosexual men. Lancet 335:168–169, 1990.
168. Huang YQ, Li JJ, Rush MG, et al: HPV-16–related DNA sequences in Kaposi's sarcoma. Lancet 339:515–518, 1992.
169. Chang Y, Cesarman E, Pessin MS, et al: Identification of herpes virus–like DNA sequences in AIDS-associated Kaposi's sarcoma. Science 266:1865–1869, 1994.
170. Su I-J, Hsu Y-S, Chang Y-C, Wang I-W: Herpesvirus-like DNA sequences in Kaposi's sarcoma from AIDS and non-AIDS patients in Taiwan (Letter). Lancet 345:722–723, 1995.
171. Huang Y-Q, Li JJ, Kaplan MH, et al: Human herpesvirus-like nucleic acid in various forms of Kaposi's sarcoma. Lancet 345:759–761, 1995.
172. Moore PS, Chang Y: Detection of herpesvirus-like DNA sequences in Kaposi's sarcoma in patients with and those without HIV infection. N Engl J Med 332:1181–1185, 1995.
173. Roth WK: TGF-beta and FGF-like growth factors involved in the pathogenesis of AIDS-associated Kaposi's sarcoma. Res Virol 144:105–109, 1993.
174. Miles SA, Matrinez-Maza O, Rezai A, et al: Oncostatin M as a potent mitogen for AIDS–Kaposi's sarcoma–derived cells. Science 255:1432–1434, 1992.
175. Ensoli B, Barillari S, Salahuddin SZ, et al: Tat protein of HIV-I stimulates growth cells derived from Kaposi's sarcoma lesions of AIDS patients. Nature 345:84–86, 1990.
176. Serfing U, Hood AF: Local therapies for cutaneous Kaposi's sarcoma in patients with AIDS. Arch Dermatol 127:1479–1481, 1991.
177. Sturzl M, Zietz C, Eisenburg B, et al: Liposomal doxorubicin in the treatment of AIDS-associated Kaposi's sarcoma: Clinical histological and cell biological evlauation. Res Virol 145:261–269, 1994.
178. Newman S: Treatment of epidemic Kaposi's sarcoma with intralesional vinblastine injection (Abstr). Proc Am Soc Clin Oncol 7:19, 1988.
179. Chadwick EG, Conner EG, Guerra-Hanson IC, et al: Tumors of smooth-muscle origin in HIV-infected children. JAMA 263:3182–3184, 1990.
180. van Hoeven KH, Factor SM, Kress Y, Woodruff JM: Visceral myogenic tumors: A manifestation of HIV infection in children. Am J Surg Pathol 17:1176–1186, 1993.
181. Orlow SJ, Kamino H, Lawrence RL: Multiple leiomyosarcomas in an adolescent with AIDS. Am J Pediatr Hematol Oncol 14:265–268, 1992.
182. McClain KL, Leach CT, Jenson HB, et al: Association of Epstein-Barr virus with leiomyosarcomas in young people with AIDS. N Engl J Med 332:12–18, 1995.
183. Lee ES, Locker J, Nalesnik M, et al: The association of Epstein-Barr virus with smooth-muscle tumors occurring after organ transplantation. N Engl J Med 332:19–25, 1995.
184. Harper ME, Kaplan MH, Marselle LM, et al: Concomitant infection of HTLV-I and HTLV-III in a patient with T8 lymphoproliferative disease. N Engl J Med 315:1073–1078, 1986.
185. Shibata D, Brynes RK, Rabinowitz A, et al: Human T-cell lymphotropic virus type I (HTLV-I)–associated adult T-cell leukemia-lymphoma in a patient infected with human immunodeficiency virus type 1 (HIV-1). Ann Intern Med 111:871–875, 1989.
186. Getchell JP, Heath JL, Hicks DR, et al: Detection of human T cell leukemia virus type I and human immunodeficiency virus in cultured lymphocytes of a Zairian man with AIDS. J Infect Dis 155:612–616, 1987.
187. vonder Helm K, vonder Helm D, Deinhardt F: Simultaneous infection with the human immunodeficiency virus and HTLV-I in a patient with AIDS (Letter). J Infect Dis 157:205–207, 1988.
188. Zucker-Franklin D, Pancake B, Friedman-Kien AE: Cutaneous disease resembling mycosis fungoides in HIV-infected patients whose skin and blood cells also harbor proviral HTLV type I. AIDS Res Hum Retroviruses 10:1173–1177, 1994.
189. Kaplan MH, Hall WW, Susin M, et al: Syndrome of severe skin disease, eosinophilia and dermatopathic lymphadenopathy in patients with HTLV-II complicating human immunodeficiency virus infection. Am J Med 91:300–309, 1991.
190. Siekevitz M, Josephs SF, Dukovich M, et al: Activation of the HIV-1 LTR by T cell mitogens and the transactivator protein of HTLV-I. Science 238:1557–1559, 1987.
191. Zack JA, Cann AJ, Lugo JP, Chen IS: HIV-I production from infected peripheral blood T cells after HTLV-I mitogenic stimulation. Science 240:1026–1028, 1988.
192. Pagano JS, Kenny S, Markowitz D, Kamine J: Epstein-Barr virus and interaction with human retroviruses. J Virol Methods 21:29–39, 1988.

125

Neurologic Complications of Human Immunodeficiency Virus Infections

Justin C. McArthur

The initial descriptions of the acquired immunodeficiency syndrome (AIDS) appeared in 1981 with the recognition of clusters of a previously unusual form of pneumonia caused by *Pneumocystis carinii*. Described initially among previously healthy young homosexual men, the new syndrome included opportunistic infections, depletion of helper T ($CD4^+$) lymphocytes, and a previously rare skin cancer—Kaposi's sarcoma. Within a few months, the epidemic was also recognized among users of intravenous drugs and their heterosexual contacts, recipients of blood transfusions, hemophiliacs, children, and Haitians.

In the early years of the epidemic, before human immunodeficiency virus type 1 (HIV-1) was identified as the cause of AIDS, a variety of opportunistic infections involving the central nervous system (CNS) were described. The severe disruption of cellular immunity permitted reactivation of latent infections (e.g., toxoplasmosis) or development of truly opportunistic processes (e.g., cryptococcosis).[1] As experience grew with the clinical manifestations of AIDS, it became obvious not only that neurologic disorders were common in patients with HIV infection but also that some of them could not be ascribed to opportunistic processes and appeared to represent novel conditions (Table 125–1). These disorders probably represent the direct or indirect effects of HIV infection on the nervous system. There are important parallels between these human conditions and the animal lentivirus infections, because all lentiviruses cause a degree of neurologic damage.[2, 3] The lentiviruses, or slow viruses, of which HIV-1 is a member, share certain pathogenic similarities, including mechanisms by which they evade host defenses and immune clearance and cause persistent infection. They typically have long incubation periods and are associated with chronic diseases occurring in nature: visna virus, with which HIV-1 shares morphologic and genomic characteristics; caprine arthritis encephalitis virus; equine infectious anemia virus; feline immunodeficiency virus; and bovine visna. Human infection with HIV-2 and simian disease with simian immunodeficiency virus type 1, which produces an AIDS-like syndrome after experimental inoculation in macaques, complete the currently recognized list.

TABLE 125–1 ■ Major Neurologic Complications of Human Immunodeficiency Virus Type 1

HIV-1 RELATED	OPPORTUNISTIC PROCESSES
Acute aseptic meningitis	Cryptococcal meningitis* or other fungal meningitides
Chronic meningitis	Toxoplasmosis*
HIV-1 encephalopathy*	Cytomegalovirus retinitis or encephalitis*
Vacuolar myelopathy	Tuberculous meningitis
Predominantly sensory neuropathy	Neurosyphilis
	Herpes group encephalitis or radiculitis
Inflammatory demyelinating polyneuropathy	Progressive multifocal leukoencephalopathy*
	Primary CNS lymphoma*
Mononeuritis multiple	Systemic lymphoma*
Myopathy	

*AIDS-defining illnesses (see Centers for Disease Control and Prevention: 1993 revised classification system for HIV infection and expanded surveillance case definition for AIDS among adolescents and adults. MMWR Morbid Mortal Wkly Rep 41:1–19, 1993.)

Neuroepidemiology of Human Immunodeficiency Virus Type 1 Infection

As experience with the spectrum of HIV-1 infection has grown, it has become clear that the nervous system is involved frequently, sometimes before the development of opportunistic infections and frank AIDS. Surveillance data from the Centers for Disease Control and Prevention (CDC) indicate that CNS complications (including HIV-1 encephalopathy [HIVE]) made up 6419 (8%) of all AIDS-defining diseases in the 79,674 patients with AIDS in 1994.[4] These data do not capture neurologic diseases developing as secondary AIDS illnesses. A retrospective series from the University of California at San Francisco found that 39% of patients with AIDS or AIDS-related complex had neurologic symptoms and estimated that 10% of all AIDS patients presented with complaints referable to the nervous system.[5] A similar proportion was reported from New York,[6] and other investigators have confirmed the frequency and diversity of neurologic disorders associated with HIV-1 infection. Table 125–1 shows the neurologic disorders that are considered as AIDS indicator diseases.[7]

Sources of Information

Both the prevalence and course of neurologic illness vary with respect to geographic distribution and the risk factor for infection. Some results of prospective neurologic studies designed to measure both prevalence and incidence are available for cohorts of homosexual or bisexual men, intravenous drug users, and children; however, most of the existing neuroepidemiologic data have been derived from three sources:

1. Institutional series. Interpretation may be biased by selective referral patterns to specific institutions or by differences in definitional criteria between centers.[5, 8]
2. National surveillance data from the CDC. These data suffer from inaccuracies and from underreporting, representing only about 75% of all U.S. cases. Secondary diagnoses developing after the initial AIDS illness are seldom reported, and there is also a substantial delay in reporting. Until 1987, HIVE and HIV dementia were not included in the list of AIDS-defining neurologic illnesses.[9]
3. Autopsy series. Numerous autopsy studies[10, 11] have documented pathologic abnormalities in 90% of patients; however, clinical correlations are frequently incomplete or absent. Autopsy series may reflect opportunistic processes, particularly lymphoma, that have been clinically silent.

Diagnosis

Several of the neurologic diagnoses, for example, cryptococcal meningitis, can be accurately diagnosed because reliable and specific diagnostic tests are available. Diagnoses of other disorders, for example, cerebral toxoplasmosis, rely on presumptive evidence, often from a clinical or radiologic re-

TABLE 125–2 ■ Epidemiologic Features of the Neurologic Manifestations of Acquired Immunodeficiency Syndrome

HIV dementia	Bimodal age distribution No predilection for sex or risk group
Opportunistic infections or neoplasms	Injecting drug users (12.5%) > homosexuals (5.3%) Adults (7.5%) > children (1.2%)
Cryptococcal meningitis	Common in Africa Injecting drug users or blacks > homosexuals or whites
Cerebral toxoplasmosis	Florida (4.9%) > United States (1.8%) Hispanics (3.0%) > non-Hispanics (1.5%)
Progressive multifocal leukoencephalopathy or primary lymphoma	Uniform distribution

Adapted from Levy RM, Janssen RS, Bush TJ, Rosenblum ML: Neuroepidemiology of acquired immunodeficiency syndrome. J Acquir Immune Defic Syndr 1:31–40, 1988.

sponse to empirical antimicrobial therapy. HIVE poses particular problems because definitional criteria have not been established and it is possible to attribute neurocognitive symptoms to HIV dementia when, in fact, alternative explanations for the patient's complaints exist. Increasingly in patients with AIDS, pathologic evidence is not available, either because brain biopsy is not needed or autopsy is declined. The autopsy rate has dropped to less than 10% in some centers, in part because of concerns about transmission of HIV infection to pathologists and autopsy room staff.

Epidemiologic Features

Table 125–2 gives some of the specific epidemiologic features of neurologic characteristics of AIDS,[9] and Table 125–3 shows the range of prevalence figures of these neurologic manifestations. The frequency of the different disorders varies with the geographic, racial, and age characteristics of the population. For example, HIVE has a bimodal distribution, occurring more frequently at the extremes of age. There is, however, no obvious predilection for dementia to occur in certain risk groups or geographic regions, nor is there any obvious difference between men and women.[12] It is not yet clear whether there is a true rise in the incidence of HIVE with age or whether this rise reflects confounding conditions such as Alzheimer disease or multiinfarct dementia. By contrast, there are epidemiologic differences for the AIDS-related opportunistic processes. For example, cryptococcal meningitis occurs significantly more frequently in injecting drug users than in other risk groups. Racial factors appear to be important too, as the prevalence of cryptococcal meningitis is highest among black persons and lowest among white, with Hispanic persons being at intermediate risk. These differences may reflect differences in access to and use of antifungal prophylaxis. Toxoplasmosis is much more common in Europe, Africa, the Caribbean, and Latin America than in the United States. Within the United States, toxoplasmosis is three times more common in Florida (4.9%) than the rest of the country (1.8%) and in patients with Hispanic origin, probably because of the increased exposure to *Toxoplasma gondii* organisms in tropical and subtropical areas. Both progressive multifocal leukoencephalopathy (PML) and primary CNS lymphoma have a uniform distribution across the United States but may be underreported because they are difficult to diagnose reliably without a brain biopsy.

TABLE 125–3 ■ Frequency of Neurologic Complications of Human Immunodeficiency Virus Infection

COMPLICATION	FREQUENCY (%)
Sensory neuropathy	20–30
Dementia	15–20
Minor cognitive impairment	20
Myelopathy	5–10
Myopathy	5
Progressive multifocal leukoencephalopathy	5
Toxoplasmosis	5
Primary CNS lymphoma	5
Cryptococcal meningitis	5
Cytomegalovirus encephalitis	5

Spectrum of Human Immunodeficiency Virus Type 1–Related Neurologic Disorders

Nervous system invasion probably occurs in most individuals during the first weeks or months after infection. In some, entry of the virus into the brain is manifest at the time of seroconversion as acute meningitis; in others silent cerebrospinal fluid (CSF) abnormalities are the only evidence of CNS involvement. Many of the neurologic disorders that affect patients with HIV-1 infection appear to be related primarily to CNS infection with HIV-1 itself rather than being opportunistic infections, that is, complications of the immune deficiency. A progressive dementia, probably caused by direct brain infection with HIV-1, is the most frequent neurologic disorder, affecting between 15% and 20% of individuals with AIDS. Spinal cord dysfunction, manifest as spastic paraparesis, and a variety of peripheral neuropathies have also now been described. In large part, the pathogenetic mechanisms of these HIV-1-related neurologic disorders are poorly understood. The complete spectrum of nervous system involvement with HIV-1 infection remains unclear, and characterization of the clinical presentations and correlation with pathologic patterns are incomplete.

Some of these disorders occur at an early stage in HIV-1 infection in the absence of any constitutional symptoms (Fig. 125–1). For example, inflammatory demyelinating neuropathies (IDPs), including Guillain-Barré syndrome and chronic

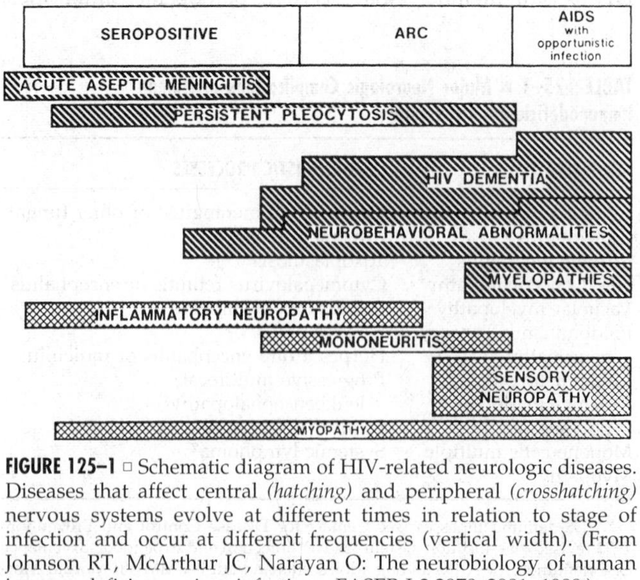

FIGURE 125–1 □ Schematic diagram of HIV-related neurologic diseases. Diseases that affect central *(hatching)* and peripheral *(crosshatching)* nervous systems evolve at different times in relation to stage of infection and occur at different frequencies (vertical width). (From Johnson RT, McArthur JC, Narayan O: The neurobiology of human immunodeficiency virus infections. FASEB J 2:2970–2981, 1988.)

inflammatory demyelinating polyneuropathies (CIDPs), have been described in otherwise asymptomatic individuals. They are often treatable and do not necessarily presage a more aggressive course of HIV-1 infection. Other disorders, for example, HIV-related myelopathy, occur typically in patients with symptomatic HIV disease (AIDS-related complex) or AIDS and usually accompany the progressive dementia. The differences in timing of these specific disorders, in their courses and natural history, and among the pathologic features suggest that different pathogenetic mechanisms underlie these disorders.

There have been preliminary reports of neurologic disease appearing with HIV-2, a distinct type of retrovirus prevalent in western Africa.[13] As yet, however, the spectrum of clinical disease with HIV-2 has not been mapped, but it does not appear to be important in the United States.

Human Immunodeficiency Virus–Related Meningitis

A proportion of individuals undergoing primary HIV-1 infection develop symptoms similar to those of infectious mononucleosis, including fever, myalgias, and rash.[14] This acute and usually self-limited illness coincides with HIV-1 seroconversion, and there may be transient p24 (HIV-1 capsid protein) antigenemia. About 1% to 2% of recently infected individuals develop acute aseptic meningitis with headache, meningismus, cranial neuropathies, and occasionally transient encephalopathy.[14, 15] This disorder appears to represent the initial response of the CNS to viral invasion, but it is uncertain whether the development of symptomatic meningitis portends subsequent progressive neurologic involvement. Typically, the acute symptoms of HIV-1–related meningitis are self-limited, require only symptomatic treatment with analgesics and antipyretics, and resolve within a few weeks. Up to 60% of HIV-1 carriers develop a more indolent variant of HIV-1–related meningitis, with chronic pleocytosis and other CSF abnormalities, that is either clinically silent or associated only with nonspecific headaches.[8, 16] Serologic testing for HIV-1 (and probably human T-lymphotropic virus type I) should be added to the evaluation of patients with aseptic meningitis or chronic pleocytosis.

Human Immunodeficiency Virus Type 1 Encephalopathy

CLINICAL FEATURES

Within the first year or two of clinical experience with HIV-1 infection it became apparent that many patients developed cognitive impairment.[5, 6] At first, the psychomotor slowing and mental dulling were mistakenly attributed to "depression," "delirium," or an "adjustment disorder" or confused with opportunistic infections of the nervous system. It is obvious now, however, that a definable dementia develops in association with infection with HIV-1, known as HIV-1 encephalopathy, or HIVE.[7, 17] This is also variously termed HIV-related dementia, HIV-associated dementia complex, subacute encephalitis, AIDS encephalopathy, and AIDS dementia complex. Clinical manifestations of dementia are evident in 20% of patients with AIDS by the time of death. In adults, HIVE develops only rarely before constitutional symptoms, immune deficiency, and systemic opportunistic processes.[8, 18] More commonly, HIVE develops and progresses in parallel with the later stages of AIDS, usually developing as a secondary AIDS illness and thus being underreported in CDC surveillance figures.

HIV-Associated Minor Cognitive-Motor Disorder

Whereas the incidence and prevalence of frank dementia have been well studied and are clearly delineated now, the frequency and clinical significance of minor neuropsychologic abnormalities detected earlier in HIV infection remain contentious. The introduction of the American Academy of Neurology definition of "HIV-associated minor cognitive/motor disorder"[19] has in some ways hindered rather than helped this field because it lends a concrete terminology to a group of vague symptoms and signs that probably have heterogeneous etiologies. Because of the vague nature of this entity, reliable estimates of its incidence and prevalence are not yet available, nor has its natural history or significance been characterized. Clinical experience suggests that it is even more common than HIV dementia, although the precise relationship of these two disorders is not understood. A number of observations in prospective studies indicate that minor cognitive-motor disorder may remain stable for many months or years, even without antiretroviral therapy. Mayeux and colleagues[20] have found that minor cognitive impairment is a marker for reduced survival, and it is likely that at least for some individuals these neuropsychologic deficits reflect evolving dementia.

Neuropsychologic Studies in HIV Infection

Many groups of investigators (both in the United States and abroad) have used neuropsychologic test batteries for asymptomatic HIV-seropositive individuals to probe for "early" HIV-associated cognitive deficits. Some general statements may be made. First, although some studies have detected a higher frequency of neuropsychologic test abnormalities in asymptomatic HIV-infected subjects than in seronegative control subjects, none has shown that these cognitive "deficits" are progressive or indicative of the later development of clinical dementia. The clinical significance of acquired cognitive symptoms or test impairment in asymptomatic HIV infection is uncertain because the reported neuropsychologic abnormalities do not necessarily progress and may reflect the effects of low education, age, and alcohol and drug use. Second, most of the studies that indicate a higher frequency of abnormalities have used extensive test batteries with relatively small numbers of subjects. By contrast, large studies, in general, have failed to detect differences. Newman and colleagues[21] show a peculiar inverse relationship between the size of the study and the likelihood of detecting a difference in neuropsychologic performance. For example, among several hundred asymptomatic HIV-1–seropositive men without AIDS or constitutional symptoms in the Multicenter AIDS Cohort Study (MACS), the prevalence of HIV dementia was less than 1% (1 in 270 HIV-seropositive men) and overall the frequency of neuropsychologic impairment was not significantly higher in medically healthy HIV-seropositive subjects than in HIV-1–seronegative control subjects.[22] Similar results have been described for injecting drug users.[23] These results stand in contrast to those of other, smaller studies that have demonstrated differences in the frequency of neuropsychologic test abnormalities.[24] The 1988 World Health Organization report on neuropsychiatric aspects of HIV-1 infection concluded that "there is no evidence for an increase of clinically significant neuropsychiatric abnormalities in asymptomatic individuals as compared to HIV-1 seronegative controls."[25] More direct evidence comes from several longitudinal studies with data extending over several years. For example, from longitudinal neuropsychologic evaluation both in the MACS and from a cohort of injecting drug users, no evidence for cognitive decline was detected during the asymptomatic phase of infection.[26, 27] In a prolonged longitudinal study within the MACS,[28] changes in cognitive function were examined before and after development of clinical AIDS or a count of $CD4^+$ cells lower than 200/mm^3. Before AIDS, the dementia group showed a significant decline only on measures of psychomotor speed. For all other measures, there was no evidence of decline in performance before AIDS in the other groups. The group with clinical AIDS showed a significant decline in psychomotor speed after the development of AIDS but no decline on the other cognitive measures. The group with a CD4+ cell count less than 200/mm³ did not show significant decline on any of the cognitive measures after the development of AIDS (defined by a CD4+ cell count less than 200/mm³). Sensory neuropathy was associated with a significant decline in performance on measures of psychomotor speed. Antiretroviral therapy was not associated with any measurable changes in neuropsychologic performance. Overall, these results suggest that there is no significant decline in cognitive function before AIDS, unless overt dementia develops.[26]

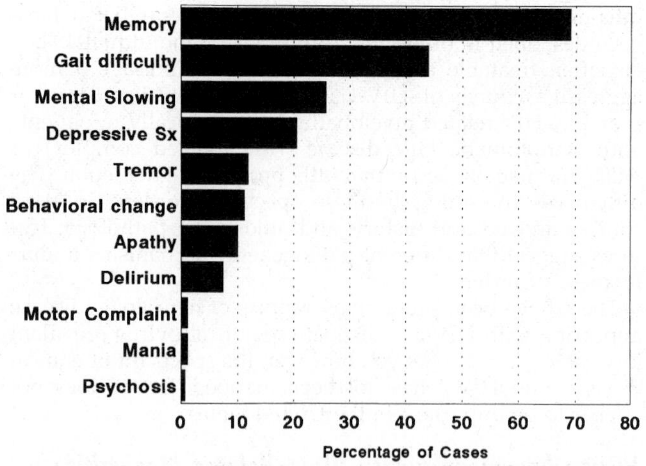

FIGURE 125–3 ▫ Presenting symptoms in HIV dementia (Johns Hopkins University, n = 299). (From McArthur JC, Selnes OA: HIV-associated dementia. *In* Levy RM, Berger JR, Janssen RS [eds]: AIDS and the Nervous System, ed 2. Philadelphia, Lippincott-Raven, 1997, pp 527–567.)

HIV-Associated Dementia

On the basis of epidemiologic studies, the annual incidence of dementia after AIDS is 7%, and approximately 15% to 20% of individuals with AIDS develop this condition. The incidence rates have remained flat in the past few years[29, 30] (Fig. 125–2). The clinical syndrome of HIVE occurs in all groups at risk for HIV-1 infection, including children. In fact, in children, progressive encephalopathy occurs more commonly than do opportunistic infections, in up to 60% of pediatric cases.[31, 32] Clinical features in children include microcephaly, developmental delay leading to loss of milestones, and death occurring within the first few years of life.

Typically, HIVE develops and progresses in parallel with the later stages of AIDS and is associated with marked immune deficiency. The clinical manifestations of HIVE suggest predominantly subcortical involvement in the early stages.[17] A typical presentation includes apathy and inertia, memory loss and cognitive slowing, depressive symptoms, and withdrawal from usual activities. The early symptoms are often subtle and may be overlooked or confused with those of depression or fatigue (Fig. 125–3). Patients complain of slowing of mental processing, gait instability, a reduction in mental flexibility, poor short-term memory, and difficulties with reading comprehension. Family and friends notice behavioral changes such as a loss of initiative or "spark," depressive symptoms, social withdrawal, and a decline in spontaneity. Specific neuropsychologic features include psychomotor slowing, memory disturbance, and visuospatial disturbance. With advancing dementia, new learning and memory deteriorate, there is a further slowing of mental processing, and language impairment becomes more obvious. Seizures occur in about 10% but are usually easily controlled. Nonspecific tremor may also develop. The terminal phases of the syndrome are characterized by a global deterioration of cognitive function with severe psychomotor retardation and mutism. The dementia may progress over a few weeks or months. For example, in one series of 30 patients with HIVE the mean interval from first symptoms to death was 5.6 months[8]; however, there is substantial variability, and a proportion of patients remain relatively stable for months or years.[33] Price and Brew[34] have developed a staging scheme (Table 125–4) that is useful both in clinical practice and in conducting research studies.

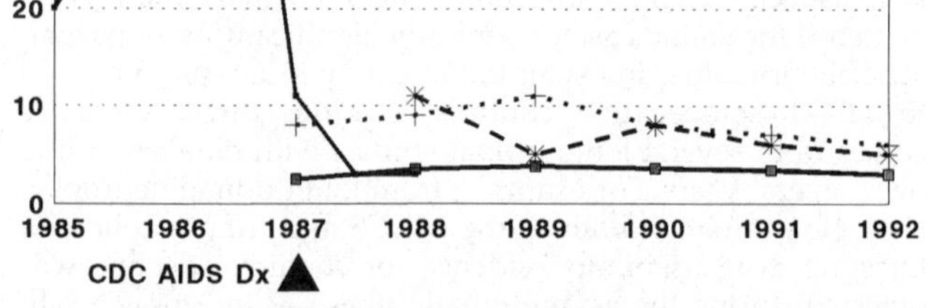

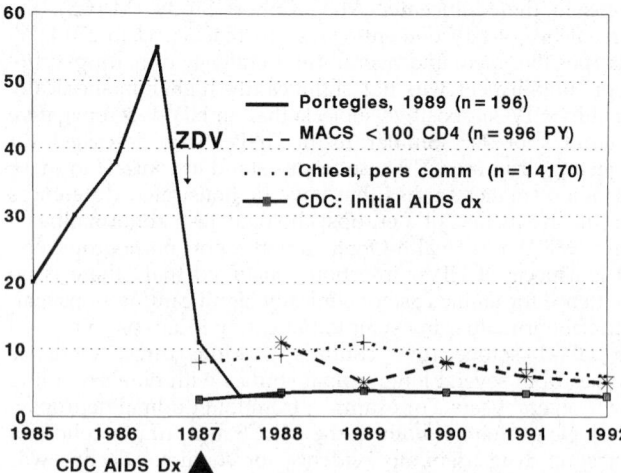

FIGURE 125–2 ▫ Incidence of HIV dementia. Comparison of early data on incidence of dementia (Portegies) compared with later data showing flat incidence rates. (From McArthur JC, Selnes OA: HIV-associated dementia. *In* Levy RM, Berger JR, Janssen RS [eds]: AIDS and the Nervous System, ed 2. Philadelphia, Lippincott-Raven, 1997, pp 527–567.)

Neurologic examination is often normal in the early stages of HIVE, although careful examination frequently demonstrates impairments of rapid eye and limb movements and diffuse hyperreflexia (Fig. 125–4). Abnormalities of eye movements, including impaired smooth tracking, slowing of saccades, and inaccuracy of antisaccades, are common. Retinal changes may be seen, most commonly the presence of cotton-wool spots; however, these are not pathognomonic for HIVE and frequently occur in nondemented individuals.[35] As HIVE progresses, increased tone develops, particularly in the lower extremities, and is usually associated with tremor, clonus, frontal release signs, and hyperactive reflexes. These signs may reflect the effects of an accompanying AIDS-related myelopathy.[36] Sensory neuropathy may also cooccur in patients with advanced immunodeficiency.

In the early stages of HIVE, differential diagnosis is particularly difficult because the initial symptoms can be confused with those of depression, anxiety disorders, or the effects of psychoactive substances (Table 125–5). Often detailed historic information from friends, family, or coworkers is helpful and psychiatric consultation may be indicated. Differentiation from infections such as cerebral toxoplasmosis, neurosyphilis, and cryptococcal or tuberculous (TB) meningitis is critical because specific therapies are available for these conditions. HIVE is not an inevitable consequence of HIV infection and altered mental status in any patient should be evaluated thoroughly and not simply ascribed to the effects of HIVE. A useful screen for the memory disturbance and psychomotor slowing of HIVE is the HIV Dementia Scale, a modification

TABLE 125–4 ■ Clinical Staging of the Acquired Immunodeficiency Syndrome Dementia Complex

STAGE	DEMENTIA	MYELOPATHY
0	Normal mental and motor function. Neurologic signs are within the normal age-appropriate spectrum.	Normal.
0.5	(Equivocal or subclinical): Absent, minimal, or equivocal symptoms without impairment of work or capacity to perform activities of daily living (ADL). Examination may be normal or mildly abnormal; signs may include reflex changes (e.g., generalized increase in deep tendon reflexes with active jaw jerk, snout or glabellar sign) or mildly slowed ocular movements but without clear slowing of extremity movements or loss of their dexterity or strength.	
1	(Mild): Able to perform all but the more demanding aspects of work or ADL but with unequivocal evidence (symptoms or signs including performance on neuropsychologic tests) of intellectual or motor impairment. The abnormal motor signs usually include slow or clumsy movements of extremities.	Tandem gait may be impaired, but the patient can walk without assistance.
2	(Moderate): Able to perform basic activities of self-care at home but cannot work or maintain more demanding aspects of daily life (e.g., maintain finances, read text more complex than a tabloid newspaper).	The patient is ambulatory but may require single prop (e.g., cane).
3	(Severe): Major intellectual incapacity (cannot follow news or personal events, cannot sustain complex conversation, considerable slowing of all output) or motor disability.	The patient cannot walk unassisted, requiring walker or personal support, usually with slowing and clumsiness of arms as well.
4	(End stage): Nearly vegetative. Intellectual and social comprehension and output are at a rudimentary level. Nearly or absolutely mute.	The patient is paraparetic or paraplegic with double incontinence.

Modified from Price RW, Brew BJ: The AIDS dementia complex. J Infect Dis 158:1079–1083, 1988. © by The University of Chicago, publisher.

of the Mini-Mental Status Examination[37] (Fig. 125–5). Neuropsychologic testing is extremely useful as an adjunct to the neurologic examination, and short test batteries focusing on psychomotor speed, memory, and reaction time are particularly valuable for detecting and quantifying early changes.

Definitional criteria have been developed for diagnosing HIVE,[19] and dementia has been included by the CDC as one of the conditions to establish a diagnosis of AIDS.[7] Table 125–6 lists features that may be helpful in establishing this diagnosis in clinical practice.

LABORATORY FINDINGS

CSF abnormalities are frequently found in neurologically normal HIV carriers and also in subjects with minor neuropsychologic abnormalities. Thus, CSF analysis is not specific for the diagnosis of HIVE (Fig. 125–6). CSF analysis is important, however, for excluding opportunistic infections, such as cryptococcosis, TB meningitis, or neurosyphilis, in the patient with suspected HIVE. The most frequent CSF abnormalities in HIVE are an elevated total protein level in about 65% and immunoglobulin G (IgG) fraction in up to 80%.[8] Oligoclonal bands are found in up to 35%, but the myelin basic protein value is usually not elevated. Intrathecal synthesis of anti–HIV-1 IgG is not specific for dementia because intrathecal synthesis can be detected in up to 45% of neurologically normal HIV carriers.[38] The CSF is usually acellular or shows a mild lymphocytic pleocytosis (<15 white cells per mm^3). CSF β_2-microglobulin appears to be a useful marker for the presence of HIVE, elevated levels correlating with the clinical severity of the dementia.[39] At present, no single CSF test or combination of tests can reliably diagnose HIVE; however, a completely normal CSF profile, with no abnormalities of β_2-microglobulin, protein, or IgG, points away from the diagnosis.

Radiologic features include cerebral atrophy and white matter rarefaction. Imaging studies are important in the evaluation of suspected HIVE to exclude mass lesions. Central and cortical atrophy[17, 40] can often be observed to progress in parallel with clinical deterioration (Fig. 125–7*A* and *B*). Computed tomography (CT) and magnetic resonance imaging (MRI) appear to be equally sensitive in demonstrating

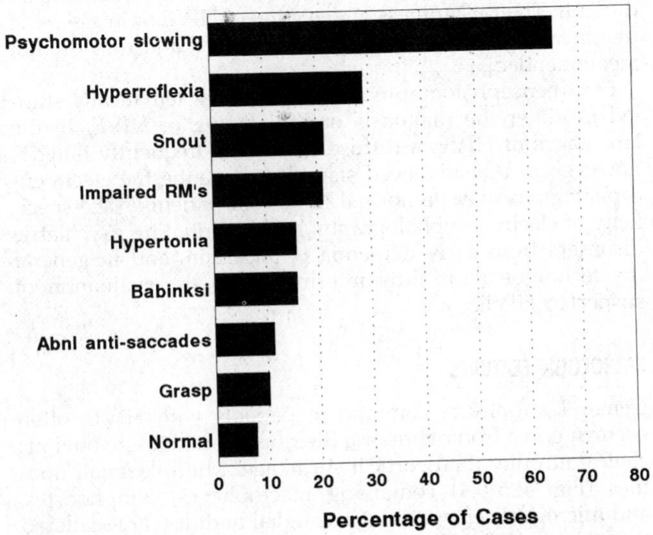

FIGURE 125–4 □ Presenting signs of HIV dementia (Johns Hopkins University, n = 299). (From McArthur JC, Selnes OA: HIV-associated dementia. *In* Levy RM, Berger JR, Janssen RS [eds]: AIDS and the Nervous System, ed 2. Philadelphia, Lippincott-Raven, 1997, pp 527–567.)

TABLE 125–5 ■ Differential Diagnosis of Early Human Immunodeficiency Virus–Associated Dementia Complex

Bereavement
Depression
Anxiety
Alcohol
Recreational drugs
Medication
Metabolic encephalopathy

From Harrison MJG, McArthur JC: AIDS and Neurology. Churchill Livingstone, 1995, p 36.

HIV DEMENTIA SCALE

Max Score	Score	
		MEMORY - REGISTRATION Give four words to recall (dog, hat, green, peach) - 1 second to say each. Then ask the patient all 4 after you have said them.
4	( )	**ATTENTION** Anti-saccadic eye movements: 20 (twenty) commands. ______errors of 20 trials ≤3 errors = 4; 4 errors = 3; 5 errors = 2; 6 errors = 1; >6 errors = 0
6	( )	**PSYCHOMOTOR SPEED** Ask patient to write the alphabet in upper case letters horizontally across the page (use back of this form) and record time: ________ seconds. ≤21 sec = 6; 21.1 - 24 sec = 5; 24.1 - 27 sec = 4; 27.1 - 30 sec = 3; 30.1 - 33 sec = 2; 33.1 - 36 sec = 1; >36 sec = 0
4	( )	**MEMORY - RECALL** Ask for 4 words from Registration above. Give 1 point for each correct. For words not recalled, prompt with a "semantic" clue, as follows: animal (dog); piece of clothing (hat), color (green), fruit (peach). Give 1/2 point for each correct after prompting.
2	( )	**CONSTRUCTION** Copy the cube below; record time: ____ seconds. <25 sec = 2; 25 - 35 sec = 1; >35 sec = 0

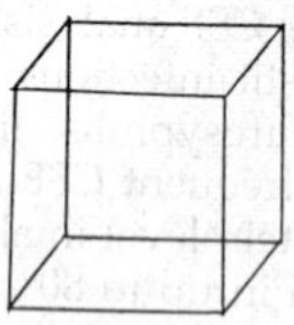

TOTAL SCORE: ____/16

Department of Neurology
Johns Hopkins University

FIGURE 125–5 ▫ The HIV Dementia Scale. (From Power C, Selnes OA, Grim JA, McArthur JC: The HIV Dementia Scale: A rapid screening test. J Acquir Immune Defic Syndr 8:273–278, 1995.)

the atrophy in early HIVE.[8] MRI, however, more readily demonstrates white matter abnormalities in HIVE, which appear as ill-defined areas of increased signal intensity on T2-weighted images.[40, 41] These often evolve from small ill-defined hyperintensities seen in deep white matter in patients with early HIVE (Fig. 125–8*A*) to more diffuse abnormalities in severely demented individuals (Fig. 125–8*B*). MRI abnormalities are rarely identified before the development of cognitive symptoms. In fact, discrete white matter hyperintensities ("unidentified bright objects") are relatively common, even in the age group at most risk for HIV infection, and are probably of no pathologic significance.[42]

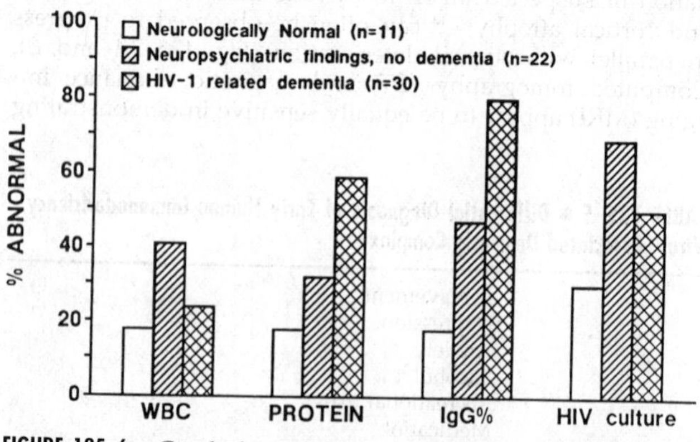

FIGURE 125–6 ▫ Graph depicting the frequency of CSF abnormalities among 11 neurologically normal HIV-1–seropositive men, 22 seropositive with minor neuropsychologic abnormalities, and 30 with HIVE.

TABLE 125–6 ▪ Clinical Features Useful for Diagnosis of Human Immunodeficiency Virus Type 1 Dementia

HIV-1 seropositivity (Western blot confirmation)
History of progressive cognitive or behavioral decline with apathy, memory loss, slowed mental processing
Neurologic examination: diffuse CNS signs including slowed rapid eye or limb movements, hyperreflexia, hypertonia, and release signs
Neuropsychologic assessment: progressive deterioration on serial testing in at least two areas including motor speed, nonverbal memory, and frontal lobe.
CSF analysis: elevated β_2-microglobulin, nonspecific abnormalities of immunoglobulin G and protein, exclusion of cytomegalovirus encephalitis, neurosyphilis, tuberculosis, and cryptococcal meningitis
Imaging studies: diffuse cerebral atrophy with ill-defined white matter hyperintensities at magnetic resonance imaging, exclusion of opportunistic processes
Absence of major psychiatric disorder or intoxication
Absence of metabolic derangement (e.g., hypoxia, sepsis)
Absence of active CNS opportunistic processes

Both single photon emission computed tomography (SPECT) and positron emission tomography (PET) have been studied in small numbers of individuals with HIVE. Using PET, Rottenberg and colleagues[43] demonstrated subcortical hypermetabolism in the early stages of HIVE, with later progression to cortical and subcortical hypometabolism. Normalization of PET abnormalities has also been shown with zidovudine (azidothymidine [AZT], Retrovir) administration.[44] With SPECT, abnormalities in cerebral blood flow have been identified in most individuals with HIVE and in neurologically normal HIV-1–seropositive individuals but also in HIV-seronegative cocaine users, raising concerns about the specificity of these changes.[45] Neither of these techniques is widely available and their interpretation and quantitation are difficult. Their usefulness in detection of HIVE or in assessing treatment effects remains to be determined and they are not recommended.

Electroencephalography has not been systematically studied in either the diagnosis or the staging of HIVE. In the late stages of HIVE, a diffuse slowing is frequently noted[17]; however, in less advanced stages of dementia the electroencephalogram may be normal in 50% of patients.[8] The specificity of electroencephalography in differentiating psychiatric disorders from early dementia is uncertain, and in general the technique adds little information to the evaluation of suspected HIVE.

PATHOLOGIC FEATURES

Cerebral atrophy is common in patients with HIVE, often occurring in a frontotemporal distribution with more obvious central atrophy than cortical shrinkage. Multiple small nodules (Fig. 125–9*A*) containing macrophages, lymphocytes, and microglial cells (termed microglial nodules) are scattered throughout both gray and white matter of the brain, appearing more commonly in white matter and the subcortical gray matter of the thalamus, basal ganglia, and brain stem.[10] Although these inflammatory nodules are frequently identified in HIVE, they are not specific for this disorder and

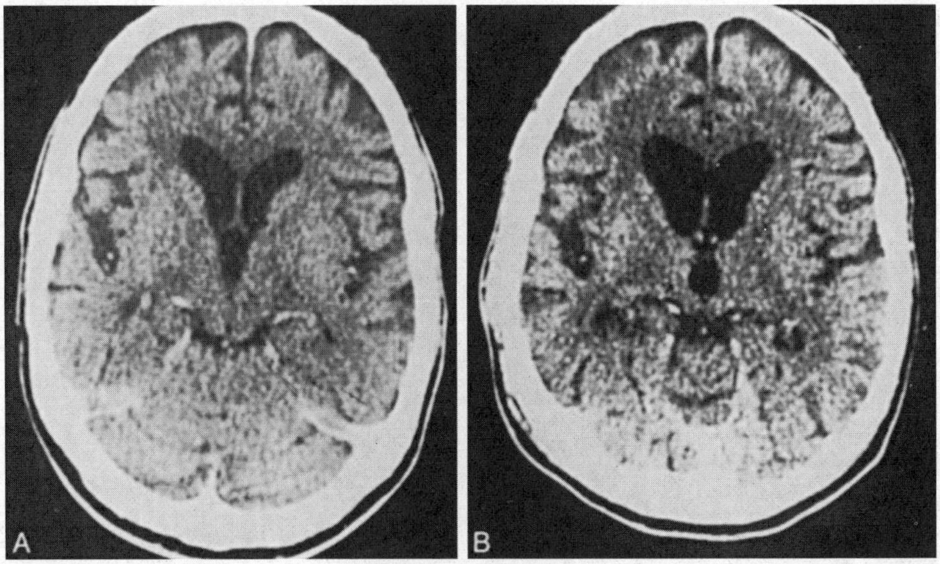

FIGURE 125–7 ▫ HIVE. *A*, CT scan from a 36-year-old intravenous drug user with AIDS-related complex and early HIVE. Mild frontotemporal atrophy and ventricular enlargement are seen. *B*, CT scan from the same patient 3 months later with far advanced HIVE. Severe frontotemporal atrophy and ventriculomegaly are noted with attenuation of the periventricular white matter.

have been described with other CNS infections, including toxoplasmosis and infections not associated with AIDS such as cytomegalovirus (CMV) encephalitis occurring after renal transplantation.[46] The number of nodules does not correlate with the severity of the dementia.[47] Multinucleated giant cells are characteristically seen[48–50] (Fig. 125–9*B*), and the combination of multinucleated giant cells, microglial nodules, and perivenular inflammation has been termed subacute encephalitis.[6, 47, 51, 52] The presence of multinucleated giant cells correlates with both the degree of dementia and the detection of HIV-1 nucleic acid sequences by Southern blot analysis.[53, 54] These giant cells have been posited as markers of HIV-1 replication, because HIV-1 forms giant multinucleated cells in macrophage culture.[55] Perivascular infiltrations of lymphocytes and monocyte/macrophages are also frequently seen.[10, 47, 49, 56] The inflammatory infiltrates, multinucleated giant cells, and endothelial cells have been demonstrated to contain viral nucleic acid sequences,[56] but productive infection of astrocytes appears to be rare. In general, these pathologic changes affect white matter more than gray.

Another striking pathologic feature is the involvement of white matter predominantly and includes relatively discrete areas of focal demyelination[51] or more commonly widespread and diffuse rarefaction or vacuolation of white matter.[47, 57] This leukoencephalopathy is not caused by demyelination but results from a breakdown of the blood-brain barrier[58] and probably gives rise to the abnormal appearance of white matter at MRI. In a prospective series, Glass and coworkers[59] detected either multinucleated giant cells or white matter pallor in only 50% of demented individuals at autopsy. This suggests that indirect mechanisms leading to neuronal dysfunction are important.

A vacuolar (spongiform) myelopathy has been described in association with HIVE[10, 36] and is discovered in about 50% of all autopsies.

EVIDENCE FOR HIV-1 AS THE CAUSATIVE AGENT

Initially CMV was incriminated as the cause of HIVE.[40] Although disseminated systemic CMV infection is frequent in advanced AIDS, in only a minority of cases of HIVE can CMV be identified within the CNS.[47, 51] Using immunocyto-

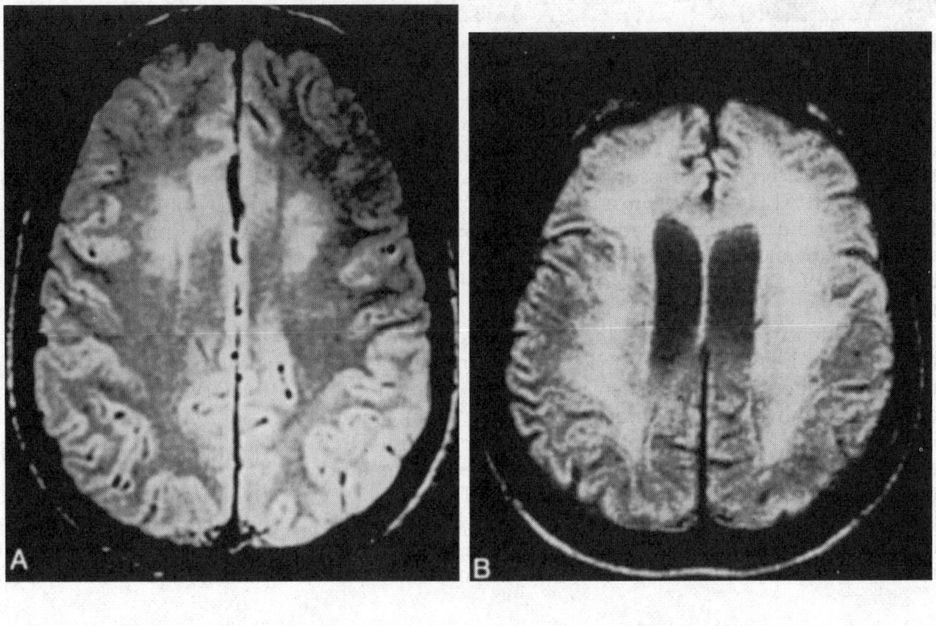

FIGURE 125–8 ▫ HIVE. *A*, MRI scan (T2-weighted image) from a 33-year-old homosexual man, showing large areas of abnormal signal intensity in the white matter. No mass effect is present. *B*, MRI scan (T2-weighted image) from a 38-year-old bisexual man with late HIVE demonstrating enlargement of the ventricles, cerebral atrophy, and diffuse abnormalities throughout the white matter.

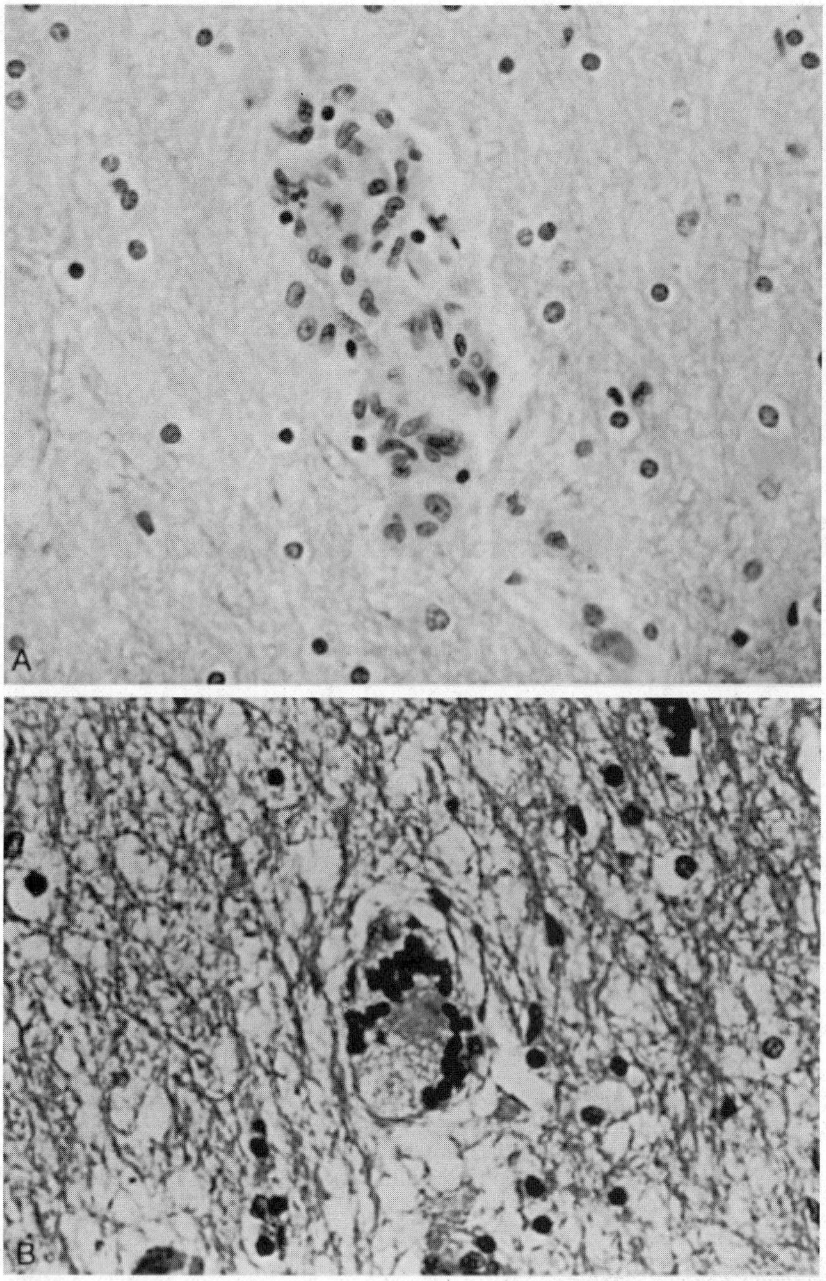

FIGURE 125–9 □ HIVE. *A,* High-power photomicrograph from the centrum semiovale (hematoxylin-eosin) from a patient who died with advanced HIVE demonstrating a microglial nodule. (H&E, × 800.) *B,* High-power photomicrograph from the centrum semiovale of the same patient showing a multinucleated giant cell. (H&E, × 800.)

chemical staining, Wiley and Nelson[60] demonstrated CMV antigens in 31 of 93 (33%) brains at autopsy, with two histopathologic patterns: microscopic infarctions and microglial nodules. HIV-1 is now presumed to be the cause of HIVE,[50, 61–63] but the actual pathogenetic mechanisms remain unexplained[3] and it is possible that an in vivo interaction between HIV-1 and other viruses such as CMV may be important.[60]

The evidence for HIV-1 as the causative agent rests on morphologic identification of the virus,[64, 65] intrathecal synthesis of antibody,[38, 66, 67] virus isolation,[10, 61, 63, 68] immunocytochemical staining for viral antigens,[10, 54, 56, 65, 69–71] and in situ hybridization.[53, 56, 72] In one of the first reports, viral DNA and RNA sequences were detected within the inflammatory nodules in brains from patients with HIVE.[72] The viral DNA, by Southern blot analysis, was present in higher concentrations in the brain than in samples of spleen, lymph node, liver, or lung. Other investigators have demonstrated HIV-1–like particles within multinucleated giant cells and also free in the extracellular space.[64, 65]

A number of virus isolation studies have demonstrated culture of HIV-1 from brain biopsy,[63] CSF, and autopsy specimens.[61] Primary cultures obtained from a brain biopsy specimen of an individual with HIVE revealed that the cells expressing virus in the primary explant cultures are derived from a monocyte/macrophage lineage.[62] HIV-1 can be isolated from a significant proportion of neurologically normal individuals,[73, 74] confirming that the brain is an early target for HIV-1 infection.

LOCALIZATION AND NEUROTROPISM OF HIV-1

By immunocytochemical identification of viral structural proteins and by in situ hybridization, HIV-1 has been localized in macrophages and multinucleated cells in the microglial nodules and areas of perivascular inflammation.[10, 47, 53, 54, 56,

[65, 69–71] Two groups of investigators have reported involvement of capillary endothelial cells.[56, 75] The virus is found with greater frequency in the white matter and subcortical areas than in the cortex,[68] and the predominant target for productive infection is the macrophage or microglial cell. Work using the sensitive technique of in situ polymerase chain reaction has demonstrated HIV DNA and RNA within neurons,[76] but this has not yet been confirmed independently. In summary, the majority of studies have consistently shown that most productive HIV-1 replication occurs in macrophages and multinucleated giant cells and that the deep white matter is more commonly involved than the gray matter. It remains uncertain whether parenchymal cells such as oligodendrocytes or neurons ever contain replicating virus.

HIV-1 probably gains access to the CNS from the blood stream, either by direct infection of capillary endothelial cells[3] or more likely by ingress of infected macrophages, the Trojan horse hypothesis.[77] It is unclear whether certain strains of HIV-1 have a propensity to invade and cause damage in the nervous system. The term neurotropic is often used broadly to describe the biologic properties of HIV-1, implying that the virus has a predilection or tropism for the nervous system. Johnson and McArthur[2] further divided this term into (1) neuroinvasiveness, the ability of a virus to invade the nervous system; (2) neurovirulence, the ability of a virus to cause neurologic disease; and (3) the capacity to replicate in neural cells. Strains isolated from the brain tend to grow more readily in macrophages than in lymphocytes,[55] and specific sequences in the envelope have been detected that may correlate with the development of dementia.[78] These observations need to be confirmed and expanded with in vitro studies, but it is to be hoped that these avenues of research may eventually help explain the differences among patients in susceptibility to HIVE.

PATHOGENETIC MECHANISMS

The pathogenetic mechanisms involved in the production of HIV dementia remain obscure because even in advanced dementia there may be only relatively mild neuropathologic changes[10, 54] and only a small fraction of cells within inflammatory nodules or perivenular infiltrates contain viral antigens.[69] (For reviews, see Epstein and Gendelman[79] and Lipton and Rosenberg.[80]) For example, in one study of 10 demented patients, moderate or severe subacute encephalitis was observed in 8, yet 2 had only mild pathologic abnormalities.[10] By contrast, up to 90% of patients with AIDS have some neuropathologic abnormalities, but not all display manifestations of dementia.[10] In the nervous system, only a small fraction of cells within inflammatory nodules or capillary endothelial cells contain viral antigens, even in individuals with advanced dementia.[69] This discrepancy between the small amounts of replicating HIV-1 and the severity of the dementia suggests that other factors besides direct cellular damage by HIV-1 may be important in pathogenesis.[3] Macrophages and microglial cells in the brain and spinal cord are activated even though productive HIV expression is noted in only a minority of these cells. The most likely possibility is that the release of cytokines locally from infected or activated macrophages might impair cellular functioning or modify neurotransmitter function.[3, 47] Alternatively, these soluble factors might cause the leukoencephalopathy and neuronal loss that are observed both focally and diffusely and probably contribute significantly to the clinical manifestations. Direct neural cell infection with cell damage or killing does not appear to occur, and there is little evidence for productive infection in neurons, although there is a drop in neuronal density and dendritic complexity.[81–84] It has been suggested that intracellular calcium is important, with the description that gp120 (the envelope glycoprotein of HIV-1) increases the amount of free calcium within neurons.[85, 86] This increase in free intracellular calcium might lead to neuronal damage in the same way that calcium is thought to be neurotoxic in other neurologic disorders. Last, the potential for brain dysfunction to result from exposure to toxins has been raised by studies demonstrating greatly elevated levels of quinolinic acid (an excitatory neurotoxic metabolite of tryptophan).[87, 88] Some of these mechanisms may act via the *N*-methyl-D-aspartate (NMDA) receptor,[89] and this could be the final common pathway for several mechanisms of neuronal injury.

The frequent CSF abnormalities in the early stages of infection and the neuropathologic abnormalities in more than 90% of patients who die with AIDS suggest that viral invasion of the nervous system occurs in the majority of HIV-1–infected patients, yet not all develop progressive dementia. Differences in neurotropism and neurovirulence or in rates of replication among strains of HIV-1 may be important in explaining this discrepancy. The clinical, radiologic, and pathologic features of HIV dementia suggest a predominantly subcortical pattern of neurocognitive deficits, with prominent leukoencephalopathy, but radiologic and pathologic studies have demonstrated involvement of the cortex with neuronal loss. Because of the absence of multinucleated giant cells or diffuse myelin pallor in 50% of demented individuals, indirect mechanisms of neuronal damage are probably important, including perhaps local cytokine release from activated macrophages or effects on the NMDA receptors of HIV proteins.

Table 125–7 summarizes the interactions between infected and activated macrophages and microglial cells within the CNS and neural cells. It appears likely that after productive HIV infection within the CNS there is activation of macrophages and microglial cells with release of cytokines into the brain parenchyma. The cytokines may play a number of roles including the amplification of HIV replication, stimulation of astrocytosis, and, via autocrine feedback loops, additional production of cytokines and arachidonic acid metabolites. Activated astrocytes may play a role in modulating and amplifying the release of neurotoxic substances. Stimulation of the NMDA receptor may be the final common pathway for neuronal damage.

In summary, the clinical, radiologic, and pathologic features of HIVE suggest predominantly subcortical involvement with prominent leukoencephalopathy and relative sparing of the cortex. The frequent CSF abnormalities in the early stages of infection and the neuropathologic abnormalities in more than 90% of patients who die with AIDS suggest that viral invasion of the nervous system occurs in the majority of HIV-1–infected patients, yet not all develop progressive dementia. The role of differences in neurovirulence among strains of HIV-1 may be of great importance in explaining this discrepancy. It seems likely that an indirect effect of HIV-1 on neural cells leads to HIVE, mediated through the release of soluble factors or toxic viral proteins.

TREATMENT OF HIVE

Despite the unresolved questions of pathogenesis, antiretroviral agents are currently used in the treatment of HIV dementia. Five antiretroviral agents are currently licensed in the United States—zidovudine, didanosine (ddI, Videx), dideoxycytidine (ddC, Hivid), stavudine (d4T, Zerit), and lamuvidine (3TC, Epivir). All are nucleoside analogs that act by inhibiting reverse transcriptase, an enzyme critical in HIV's life cycle. An important point is that these agents act at a preintegration site in the replicative life cycle of HIV and are less likely to be effective in cells with slow turnover, including macrophages and microglial cells. This has im-

TABLE 125–7 ■ Possible Factors in the Pathogenesis of Human Immunodeficiency Virus–Associated Dementia

FACTORS	CONSEQUENCE
Direct effects of HIV infection of neural cells	
Cytopathic effect	Activation of macrophages or microglial cells with secretion of soluble substances
Noncytopathic effect	Viral proteins—gp120, Nef, Tat—may be neurotoxic or interfere with neuronal function
Cytokines and other macrophage productions	
Toxic effects of monokines	On neurons and oligodendrocytes (tumor necrosis factor-α)
Astrocytic activation and proliferation	Stimulating further cytokine release from macrophages and production of arachidonic acid metabolites
Blood-brain barrier perturbation	Exposure of parenchymal cells to circulating systemic factors and ingress of infected monocytes
Toxic effects of other soluble factors	On neurons, astrocytes, and oligodendrocytes
gp120 release from infected cells	Possible interference with astrocyte-derived neuronal protective factor or other neurotropic factors Possible interference with neurotransmitters (e.g., vasoactive intestinal polypeptide)
Increased HIV load in CNS	
Other infectious agents	CMV, JC virus stimulate transactivation of HIV
Cytokine induced	Tumor necrosis factor-α and other cytokines stimulate transactivation
Autoimmunity	Common immunologic determinants between gp41 and astrocytes

Modified from Johnson RT, McArthur JC, Narayan O: The neurobiology of human immunodeficiency virus infections. FASEB J 2:2970–2981, 1988.

portant implications for infection in the CNS, where these cells are the principal targets. The nucleoside analogs are active only against replicating HIV and not latent provirus. Different toxicities are seen with each: zidovudine, anemia, myopathy; ddI, pancreatitis, neuropathy; ddC, stomatitis, neuropathy; and d4T, neuropathy. The frequency of neuropathy is about 20% with ddC and 10% to 15% with ddI and d4T. The CSF penetrances of zidovudine and d4T are about 25%; of ddI, about 10% to 15%; and of 3TC, about 5%. In vitro resistance can develop to all of them within 6 to 12 months of use, although the clinical significance of this is uncertain.

Neuroprotective Effects of Antiretrovirals

More widespread and earlier use of zidovudine may have reduced the incidence of HIV dementia; a drop in the incidence of HIV dementia from 53% before zidovudine was available to 10% has been reported.[90] Whether this represents a true prophylactic effect or simply an attenuation of the neurologic disease is unclear. Studies have shown stable incidence rates in the past few years and have not shown any definite neuroprotective effects of antiretrovirals.[30] Evidence from the multicenter licensing trial[91] of zidovudine for patients with AIDS or AIDS-related complex suggests that this drug improves neuropsychologic function even without frank dementia.[92] In this study, the zidovudine-treated patients showed significant improvements in cognitive performance, particularly in measures of psychomotor speed, which were sustained for the 16 weeks of the study. Unfortunately, the study was terminated early after only 16 weeks, so the long-term effects of antiretrovirals on cognition are not yet known.

Treatment of Established Dementia

Early open-label studies with zidovudine in demented individuals showed promising improvements in clinical functioning, neuropsychologic performance, and, in one case, normalization of PET scans.[44] The optimal dose of zidovudine for treatment of HIV dementia has not been determined. Most of the studies used doses of 1000 to 1500 mg/d; however, the recommended dose of zidovudine for general use has now been reduced to 600 mg because this dose has equivalent efficacy in preventing systemic infections.[93] Children treated with intravenous zidovudine showed dramatic improvements in neuropsychologic performance and, in some cases, reversal of cerebral atrophy.[94, 95] Improvements in adaptive behavior have also been demonstrated in encephalopathic children.[96]

Data from the only placebo-controlled trial of zidovudine in HIV dementia have suggested that the greatest neurocognitive improvement is seen with high doses of zidovudine, about 2000 mg/d.[97] The effect was modest, however, and no change in clinical severity of dementia was demonstrated. Whether significant improvement can be induced with lower doses remains to be determined, although experience with open-label use of zidovudine suggests that cognitive function is improved with doses of 800 to 1000 mg, particularly in a zidovudine-naive patient. Current practice for treatment of established dementia is to start zidovudine at 1000 mg/d, or if zidovudine is already in use, to increase the dose to 1000 mg. Lamivudine (150 mg twice a day [bid]) and indinavir (Crixivan, 800 mg three times a day [tid]) should also be used in a combination with zidovudine. This combination is suggested on the basis of CSF penetration tolerability and an attempt to minimize the number of capsules and potential interactions. Blood counts should be checked regularly (Fig. 125–10), and anemia or neutropenia can be controlled by dose reduction or the use of a hematopoietic growth factor such as erythropoietin (Procrit) or granulocyte colony-stimulating factor (Neupogen).

In patients with HIV dementia who are zidovudine intolerant, substitution of d4T at 40 mg bid is appropriate, although as yet there is no definite proof of its efficacy. There is little information about the CNS efficacy of the other dideoxynucleosides, and CNS penetrance of ddI and ddC is limited—about 15%, compared with about 25% with zidovudine or d4T. ddI has been shown to improve IQ scores in children in whom the plasma concentration of ddI correlated with both IQ improvement and decline in p24 antigen.[98] For adults, there is limited information about the therapeutic effects of ddI, d4T, or ddC for dementia.[99]

In our own open-label studies and also in studies by Portegies[100] and Tozzi[101] and their colleagues, it has been observed that dementia can be reversed with antiretroviral therapy but that the duration of treatment response varies and, for unexplained reasons, some individuals fail to respond. Whether this is because of irreversible neuronal loss or the

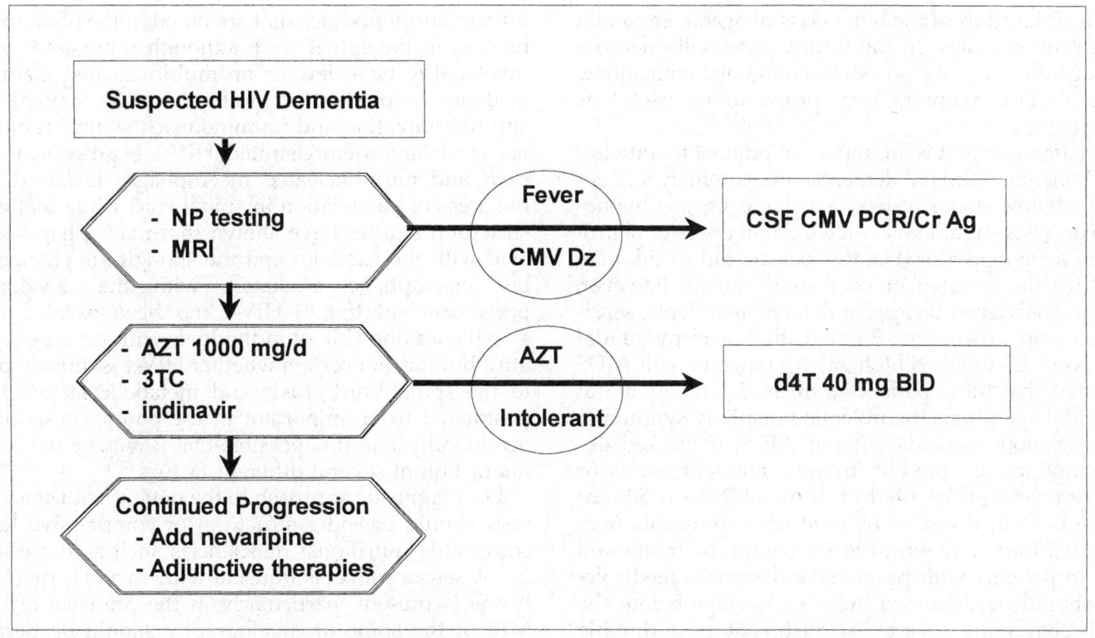

FIGURE 125–10 □ Algorithm for treatment of HIV dementia. ZDV, Zidovudine; NP, neuropsychologic testing; CBC, complete blood count; G-CSF, granulocyte colony-stimulating factor. (From McArthur JC, Selnes OA: HIV-associated dementia. *In* Levy RM, Berger JR, Janssen RS [eds]: AIDS and the Nervous System, ed 2. Philadelphia, Lippincott-Raven, 1997, pp 527–567.)

development of resistance to antiretroviral agents is uncertain. Few studies have examined why some demented patients respond and others fail to, and there has been little study of patterns of response for longer than a few months of treatment. Tartaglione and coworkers[102] noted neurologic improvement in most patients with mild neurologic abnormalities but no relationship between treatment response and CSF zidovudine concentration, cumulative zidovudine dose, or HIV isolation from CSF.

In an open-label study of 30 patients with HIV dementia, Tozzi and colleagues[101] observed improvements in clinical severity in 50% after 1 month of therapy and 83% after 6 months, using doses of 500 to 1000 mg/d. Survival was predicted by clinical severity at entry, and eight patients who had initially responded showed deterioration after 6 to 12 months. Interestingly, MRI white matter hyperintensities improved in 6 of 13 patients and SPECT scans showed reductions in uptake deficits in 9 of 13. This study is one of the most comprehensive to date and shows that, at least for patients with mild to moderate HIV dementia, clinical improvements can be sustained for several months.

Most observations of treatment response have relied on changes in neuropsychologic or neurologic testing. Other outcome measures may be helpful, particularly in the research setting. For example, several studies have shown improvements in markers of immune activation in the CSF.[87, 103] Neurophysiologic measurements may improve with zidovudine treatment,[104] and several studies have shown improvements in MRI white matter hyperintensities (McArthur JC, personal observation),[101] cerebral atrophy,[94] or PET scans.[105] Several autopsy series have suggested a beneficial effect of the use of antiretrovirals by observing reductions in the frequency of multinucleated giant cells with antiretroviral use.[59, 106, 107]

Another large group of adjunctive agents has been developed on the basis of advances in our understanding of the pathophysiologic mechanisms of HIV dementia. It seems likely that in the future, effective and sustained treatment of established dementia will require both antiretroviral agents and agents targeting neuron-damaging mechanisms. Several experimental treatments have been tried in dementia or trials are planned.

For one agent, a synthetic pentapeptide, peptide T,[108] there is suggestive anecdotal evidence of efficacy in treating HIV dementia, purportedly by blocking the actions of tumor necrosis factor-α. This agent was tested in the United States in a large placebo-controlled trial and was found to be ineffective (National Institute of Mental Health press release, 1996). Alternative treatments currently being explored include calcium channel antagonists, such as nimodipine, which may block viral protein–induced neurotoxicity.[86] In the AIDS Clinical Trials Group protocol 162, a phase I double-blind, placebo-controlled trial, patients with AIDS dementia were randomized to receive nimodipine at 60 mg five times daily, or nimodipine at 30 mg tid, or placebo, with antiretrovirals. In this study, nimodipine was well tolerated and there was some improvement in neurocognitive performance. Although efficacy data are not yet available, nimodipine is a licensed drug (but quite expensive) and can be prescribed for the patient with progressive dementia. Other potential agents are listed in Table 125–8 and include cytokine antagonists and

TABLE 125–8 ■ Potential Novel Treatments for Human Immunodeficiency Virus Dementia

Antiretrovirals	Calcium channel blockers
Nucleoside reverse transcriptase inhibitor	Nimodipine
Nonnucleoside reverse transcriptase inhibitor	Glutamate, NMDA antagonists
Protease inhibitors	Memantine
Cytokine blockers	Antioxidants
Pentoxifylline	OPC-14117
Thalidomide	Antiapoptotic agents
Peptide T	Deprenyl
Lexipafant	

From McArthur JC, Selnes OA: HIV-associated dementia. *In* Levy RM, Berger JR, Janssen RS (eds): AIDS and the Nervous System, ed 2. Philadelphia, Lippincott-Raven, 1997, pp 527–567.

antioxidants. Pilot trials of the latter class of agents are under way in the United States. In the future, potentially neuron-protective agents, such as the NMDA antagonist memantine, that block NMDA receptors may prove to be useful as adjunctive therapy.[109]

Symptomatic treatment is an important adjunct to antiviral treatment. Patients with HIV dementia are extremely susceptible to the adverse effects of psychoactive drugs, so hypnotics and anxiolytics should be avoided. Small doses of neuroleptics, such as haloperidol (Haldol), 0.5 mg bid to tid, may be needed for the agitated or combative patient; however, patients with HIV dementia appear to have neuroleptic sensitivity. Hriso and coworkers[110] found that extrapyramidal symptoms were 2.5 times as high among patients with AIDS and suggested that these patients were more susceptible to extrapyramidal symptoms (neuroleptic sensitivity syndrome) than were psychotic patients without AIDS. If marked depressive symptoms are present, tricyclic antidepressants or fluoxetine (Prozac) can be tried at doses of 25% to 50% of the usual dose. Full doses of tricyclic antidepressants may precipitate delirium, and serum levels should be monitored frequently. In patients with progressive dementia, medicolegal issues should be discussed at an early stage before the dementia becomes too severe: establishment of a durable power of attorney, completion of a living will, and arrangement for the dispersal of assets.

Human Immunodeficiency Virus Type 1–Associated Myelopathies

The characterization of the full range of clinical features of the different myelopathies associated with HIV-1 infection is as yet incomplete. The most common of the myelopathies associated with HIV-1 infection is termed vacuolar myelopathy and affects about 10% of patients with AIDS, although it is detected in up to 50% of autopsies. It is manifest clinically with a progressive spastic paraparesis and sensory ataxia, and in about 60%, HIVE develops concurrently. Occasionally, the myelopathy develops before dementia, but usually the two develop and progress in parallel. Often a peripheral neuropathy coexists, so a typical clinical picture can include cognitive deficits as well as myeloneuropathy. The major pathologic finding is vacuolation in the spinal white matter, particularly in the lateral and posterior columns of the thoracic spinal cord (Fig. 125–11). This is distinct from the pathologic picture of HIVE. The multinucleated giant cells and inflammatory nodules that are noted in the brain in HIVE can be seen in the spinal cord, although some cases of vacuolar myelopathy have few or no multinucleated giant cells and evidence of productive viral replication may be scarce. In situ hybridization and immunohistochemical staining of spinal cord have demonstrated HIV-1 expression in mononuclear and multinucleated macrophages localized mainly to the areas of vacuolation in spinal cord white matter.[111] Ultrastructural studies have shown that macrophages are associated with the vacuoles and the spongiform change is probably macrophage mediated, with the development of periaxonal splitting.[112] HIV-1 has been isolated from both spinal cord and CSF of individuals with progressive myelopathy, but it is not certain whether HIV-1 is directly pathogenic to the spinal cord. Toxic and metabolic factors have been postulated to be important in the pathogenesis of vacuolar myelopathy, and it is possible that it may be the result of the interaction of several different factors.

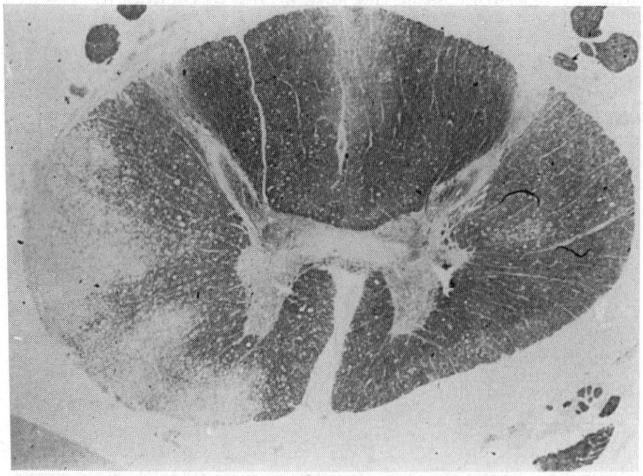

FIGURE 125–11 □ Pathology of vacuolar myelopathy, showing vacuolation in the spinal white matter, particularly in the lateral and posterior columns of the thoracic spinal cord.

The diagnostic approach to the patient with spastic paraparesis should consider structural or compressive lesions and correctable nutritional deficiencies such as those of vitamin B_{12}. A sensory level is unusual with vacuolar myelopathy, so if one is present, particularly in the presence of back pain, MRI of the spine or myelography should be performed to exclude extrinsic cord compression. Nonspecific CSF abnormalities are frequently present but are not diagnostic. Zidovudine is not usually effective in reversing the myelopathy, which usually progresses inexorably. Antispasticity agents such as baclofen (Lioresal) may relieve some of the spasticity.

Peripheral Nerve Disorders Associated with Human Immunodeficiency Virus Type 1

Although the CNS complications of HIV-1 infection constitute the most significant neurologic disorders with respect to morbidity and mortality, the peripheral nervous system can be involved in diverse ways and the incidence of sensory neuropathy is rising rapidly.[30] Not only do novel and distinct clinical syndromes exist, but the frequency and timing of onset vary (see Fig. 125–1), suggesting that diverse pathogenetic mechanisms may produce the different peripheral neuropathies.

PREDOMINANTLY SENSORY NEUROPATHY

Up to 30% of patients with AIDS develop a neuropathy characterized by painful sensory symptoms in the feet.[6, 113, 114] Most individuals develop this neuropathy late in the course of HIV-1 infection, usually in association with systemic opportunistic infections and profound immunodeficiency (see Fig. 125–1). This disorder can be recognized by characteristic complaints of dysesthesias and contact hypersensitivity in the feet with reduced or absent ankle reflexes and elevated sensory thresholds. Electrophysiologic studies are helpful but not essential in diagnosis and usually reveal a neuropathy affecting sensory more than motor fibers, suggestive of a dying-back axonopathy. Nerve biopsies are not usually helpful in the clinical setting and typically show a mixed picture of axonal loss with patchy demyelination. In some patients, a striking selective degeneration of the gracile tract has been observed at autopsy. One hypothesis is that infection of dorsal root ganglion neurons by HIV-1 might lead to central-peripheral axonal degeneration.[115] Consideration should be given to contributing factors, including nutritional and toxic causes of sensory neuropathy, such as alcohol, diabetes, pyridoxine excess, and vitamin B_{12} deficiency. The dideoxynucleosides ddI, ddC, and d4T cause toxic painful neuropathy in 15% to 20% of patients, usually after several weeks of treatment.[99, 116–120]

Patients who develop predominantly sensory neuropathy are often already taking zidovudine because of their advanced immune deficiency. Occasionally, symptoms of peripheral neuropathy improve with zidovudine; however, more often there is no dramatic response. Symptomatic relief with pain-modifying agents, such as amitriptyline (Elavil), mexiletine (Mexitil), or phenytoin (Dilantin), may be useful. Because of their potential for causing delirium in patients with concurrent HIVE, tricyclic antidepressants should be started only at a low dose, for example, amitriptyline at 10 to 25 mg at bedtime and gradually increased to 50 to 100 mg. An algorithm for management is presented in Figure 125–12. In severe neuropathies narcotic analgesics may be required. Transdermal fentanyl or methadone is particularly useful. A new nonnarcotic, centrally acting analgesic, tramadol (Ultram), may be useful because it does not cause tolerance and dependence.

INFLAMMATORY DEMYELINATING POLYNEUROPATHIES

Besides the relatively well characterized opportunistic infections and neoplastic involvement of the nervous system, a number of possible immune-mediated phenomena have been described in association with HIV infection, including IDPs[113, 121–123] and thrombocytopenia.[124, 125] Both disorders often occur at a relatively early stage of HIV infection without profound immunoincompetence and probably result from immunopathic mechanisms. In one autopsy series of 30 patients who died with AIDS, patchy demyelinative peripheral neuropathy was observed in 8 of 16 specimens (50%),[10] suggesting that subclinical IDP may be common in AIDS. Clinically recognized IDP is uncommon, however, and the majority of patients have presented in the early stages of HIV infection without constitutional symptoms.[126] Sometimes the neuropathy is a manifestation of the acute seroconversion illness.[121] This contrasts with the patients with sensory neuropathy, who usually have advanced immune deficiency. The presentations of IDP take two forms, either an acute demyelinating neuropathy (Guillain-Barré syndrome) or a more chronic, sometimes relapsing course with predominantly motor weakness (CIDP). Among the CSF changes that distinguish patients with HIV-1–related IDP from those with IDP unrelated to HIV infection is the presence of a CSF pleocytosis (mean, 23 white cells per mm^3 in one series).[121] This contrasts with the normocellular CSF found in a group of HIV-seronegative patients with IDPs.[121] In HIV-related IDP, CD4/CD8 ratios are reversed in CSF, paralleling the changes in peripheral blood.[127] The CSF total protein is usually markedly elevated (mean, 178 mg/dL) as in IDPs occurring in uninfected individuals. Nerve biopsies disclose mononuclear macrophage infiltration and internodal demyelination, typical of IDP.[121]

The pathogenesis of the demyelinating process is unclear even though circulating anti–peripheral nerve antibodies have been identified in some patients.[122, 128] These probably represent an epiphenomenon rather than being the primary cause of the neuropathy.

The recognition of this association between HIV-1 and IDPs means that a careful search for risk factors for HIV-1 infection and serologic testing should be made for any patient presenting with IDP. At present, plasmapheresis is the treatment of choice because it is less likely than corticosteroids to aggravate existing immunologic dysfunction. The response appears to be just as good as in HIV-seronegative patients. In Guillain-Barré syndrome, a course of five plasma exchanges is given.[121] With CIDP, an induction course is followed by maintenance exchanges as needed. When plasmapheresis is impractical or unavailable, short courses of corticosteroids are generally tolerated well by patients without advanced immunodeficiency without triggering opportunistic infections. For CIDP, a 4-day course of methylprednisolone, 15 mg/kg intravenously in 4 hours, can be used, followed by a tapering schedule of oral prednisone at 60 mg for up to 2 months. This course can be repeated when symptoms recur.

MONONEUROPATHIES

Mononeuritis multiplex is another type of peripheral neuropathy that has been recognized in HIV-1 infection. It is uncommon and typically affects patients with symptomatic HIV-1 disease[121] (see Fig. 125–1). Lipkin and colleagues[129] described 11 patients with AIDS-related complex with mononeuritis

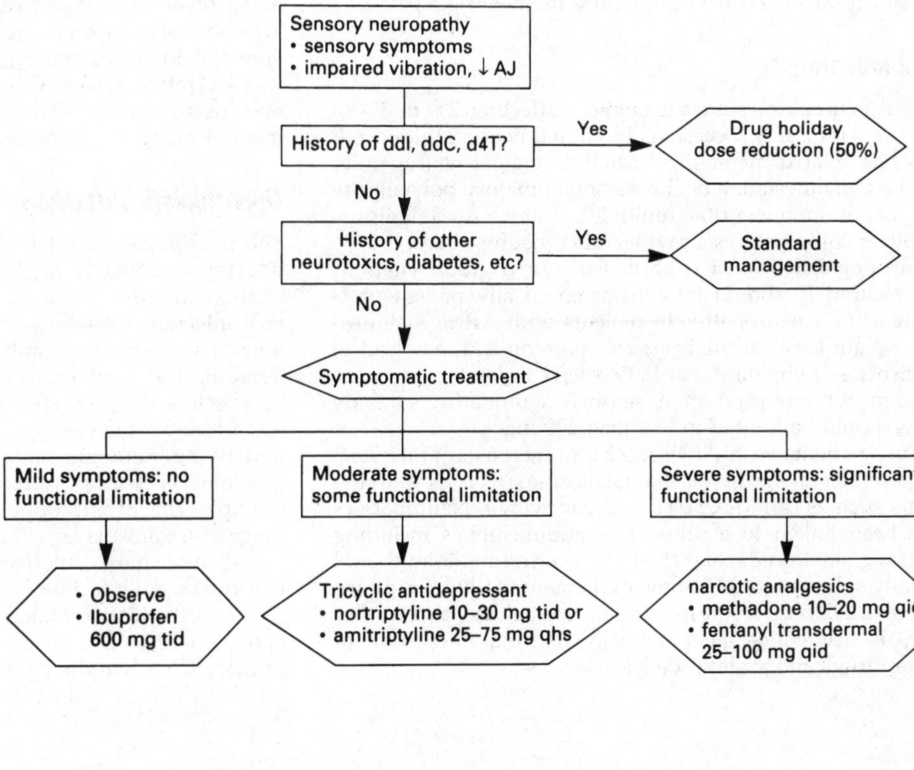

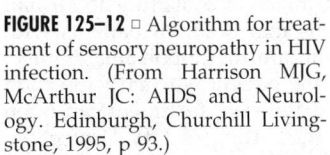

FIGURE 125–12 □ Algorithm for treatment of sensory neuropathy in HIV infection. (From Harrison MJG, McArthur JC: AIDS and Neurology. Edinburgh, Churchill Livingstone, 1995, p 93.)

multiplex who had occasional CNS findings, mixed axonal-demyelinating conduction studies, and nerve biopsies showing a spectrum of pathologic changes ranging from axonal degeneration to mixed axonal degeneration and demyelination. One third of these patients later progressed to AIDS and several appeared to develop a more widespread peripheral neuropathy with features of CIDP. It is unclear, therefore, whether mononeuritis multiplex represents a variant of HIV-related CIDP or is a separate entity. Because some cases have marked vasculitic changes and centrofascicular degeneration, it has been speculated that circulating immune complexes might play a causative role and hepatitis B should be searched for.

HERPES GROUP RADICULITIS

CMV has been identified as causing a progressive radiculopathy involving lumbar and sacral roots.[121, 122, 130] It is the most common cause of subacute leg weakness in advanced HIV infection. Typically occurring in patients with advanced immune deficiency, there is usually flaccid paralysis of the lower extremities with sacral pain and paresthesias and sphincter dysfunction. Disseminated CMV infection with viremia and CMV retinitis are frequent concomitants. Usually there are a polymorphonuclear pleocytosis and hypoglycorrhachia, and CMV can be isolated by culture from the CSF in 50% to 60%. CMV polymerase chain reaction is positive in most cases and is extremely useful for rapid diagnosis. An acyclovir analog, ganciclovir (Cytovene), appears to have some effect, producing stabilization or even improvement, particularly in patients whose course is more indolent.[131, 132]

At least 10% of patients with HIV-1 infection develop herpes zoster radiculitis representing reactivation of latent herpes zoster. The lesions heal more quickly and the frequency of postherpetic neuralgia is reduced if acyclovir (Zovirax) is used. Dermatomal herpes zoster does not require parenteral treatment unless cervical or lumbar dermatomes are involved. In this setting, a severe myeloradiculitis can develop and lead to permanent motor deficits, and intravenous acyclovir (30 mg/kg per day) should be used.[8] The development of postherpetic neuralgia may require the use of pain-modifying agents such as amitriptyline (Elavil) or carbamazepine (Tegretol). After the vesicles have completely healed, topical capsaicin (Zostrix) can reduce the neuralgic pains.

OTHER NEUROPATHIES

Cranial neuropathies are uncommon, affecting 2% to 3% of patients with AIDS. Occasionally, cranial neuropathies occur with HIV-related meningitis.[5] Multiple cranial neuropathies may be a manifestation of chronic inflammatory polyneuropathy or of mononeuritis multiplex. Rarely does lymphomatous meningitis present with cranial neuropathies.

Nutritional deficiencies, particularly of B group vitamins and vitamin E, should be considered in any patient presenting with a neuropathy. In patients with AIDS, malnutrition, weight loss, and diarrhea are common and may lead to deficiencies of vitamin B_{12} or E. Excessive doses of pyridoxine (vitamin B_6) can produce a sensory neuropathy, so daily doses should be limited to less than 200 mg.

Many patients with AIDS receive numerous antimicrobial drugs, either alone or in combination, as well as antiviral agents such as ddI, ddC, d4T, and ganciclovir. Neuropathies have been linked to a number of antimicrobials including isoniazid, metronidazole (Flagyl),[133] nitrofurantoin,[134] and possibly sulfonamides.[135] Some of the neuropathic symptoms seen in AIDS may result from antimicrobial use, and further study is needed of the potentially harmful interaction of certain drugs and vitamin deficiencies.

The patient who has suffered profound weight loss and who is bed bound is susceptible to nerve compression. The most common symptom complexes are (1) ulnar nerve compression at the elbow producing pain and paresthesias in the forearm and fourth and fifth digits, sometimes with weakness in the intrinsic hand muscles, and (2) common peroneal nerve compression at the fibula head resulting in footdrop with numbness over the lateral lower extremity and dorsum of the foot. These are recognizable clinically and can be confirmed with electrophysiologic testing. Treatment consists of appropriate padding, splints, and limb positioning to avoid further trauma.

Myopathies

Two types of myopathy occur in patients with HIV-1 infection. The first, HIV-1–associated myopathy, is uncommon and has been described at all stages of systemic disease[136] (see Fig. 125–1). Like IDP, it appears to be immune mediated. It presents as polymyositis with myalgias, proximal weakness, and elevated serum creatine kinase levels, and there is usually electromyographic evidence of an irritative myopathy. Muscle biopsies show inflammation and necrosis. The second type of myopathy has been associated with the long-term use of zidovudine (cumulative doses >400 g) and was more common in the 1980s when patients received high doses of zidovudine (>1000 mg/d) for months or years. The spectrum of clinical features has been well defined by Simpson and coworkers.[137] Some patients present with marked myopathy, clinically indistinguishable from the HIV-1–associated myopathy. Others simply have mild proximal weakness and myalgias with a moderately elevated creatine kinase values (two to four times normal). Neither electromyographic findings nor biopsy is specific enough to distinguish reliably between the two conditions. In practice, a drug "holiday," stopping zidovudine for 2 to 4 weeks, should result in some clinical improvement and a drop in creatine kinase value if the myopathy is a toxic effect of zidovudine. If there is severe and function-limiting myopathy with biopsy evidence of inflammatory necrosis, immunosuppressive agents such as corticosteroids can be used.[136] In the patient with advanced immune deficiency, the use of steroids may lead to a variety of infectious complications including worsening of oropharyngeal candidiasis and *Listeria* meningitis. Their use should therefore be restricted to patients with severe and life-threatening muscle weakness with greatly elevated creatine kinase values and biopsy documentation of fiber necrosis and inflammation. An algorithm for management of myopathy is presented in Figure 125–13.

Opportunistic Infections

The neurologic disorders discussed earlier that are related directly or indirectly to HIV-1 infection constitute about half of the neurologic complications that occur in patients with HIV infection. Equally common are the opportunistic infections. These are important in the patient with HIV infection because, if they are correctly diagnosed, treatment can often be effective (Fig. 125–14). In the setting of HIV-1 infection, opportunistic infections of the nervous system reflect the underlying immunoincompetence produced by infection and lysis of $CD4^+$ lymphocytes. Individuals with AIDS may have multiple concurrent opportunistic infections with a wide range of organisms (see Table 125–1).

The two most frequent CNS opportunistic infections worldwide are infections with *Cryptococcus neoformans* and *T. gondii*. In the United States, each affects approximately 5% of patients with AIDS, but rising most rapidly in incidence are primary CNS lymphoma and PML. Incidence data from the

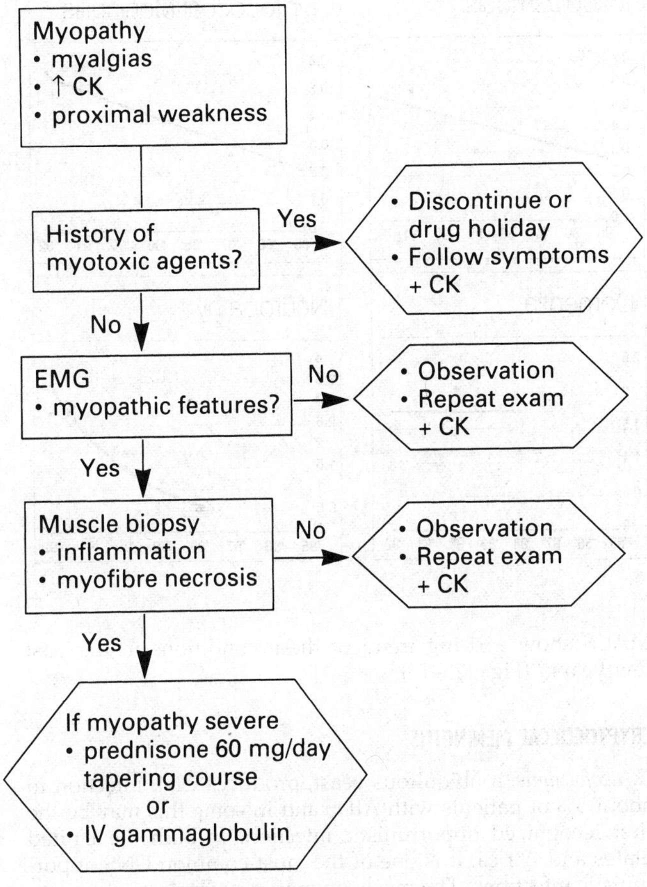

FIGURE 125–13 □ Algorithm for treatment of myopathy in HIV infection. CK, Creatine kinase; EMG, electromyography. (From Harrison MJG, McArthur JC: AIDS and Neurology. Edinburgh, Churchill Livingstone, 1995, p 116.)

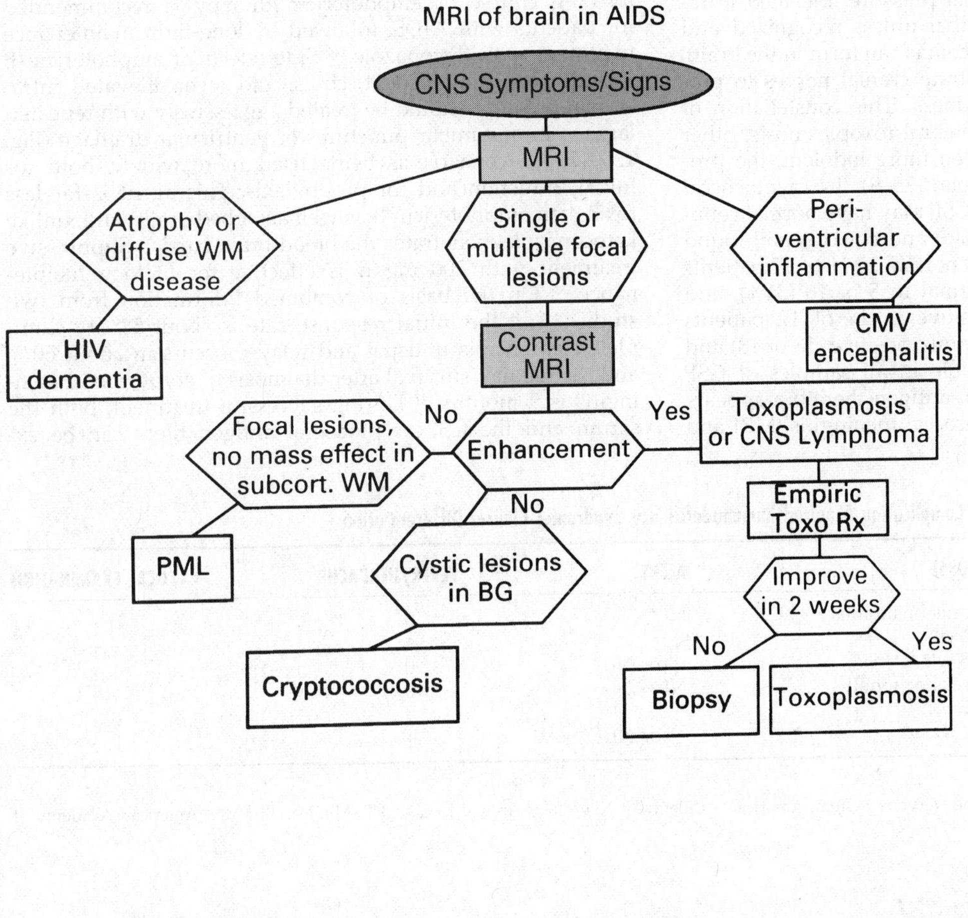

FIGURE 125–14 □ Algorithm for radiologic assessment of neurologic complications in HIV infection. WM, White matter; BG, basal ganglia. (From Harrison MJG, McArthur JC: AIDS and Neurology. Edinburgh, Churchill Livingstone, 1995, p 225.)

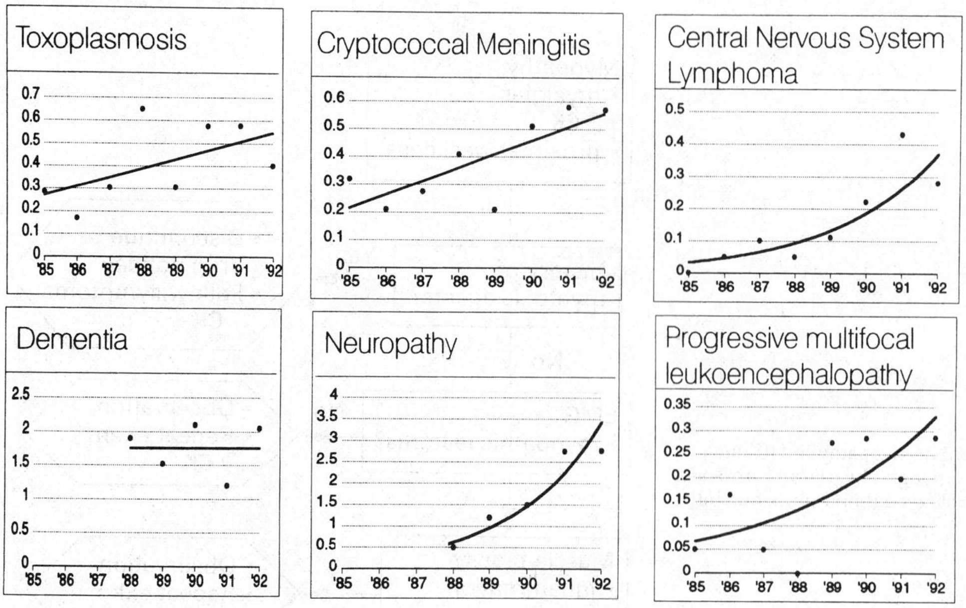

FIGURE 125–15 □ Rising incidence rates of CNS opportunistic processes.

MACS show a rising trend of these conditions in the past few years[30] (Fig. 125–15).

CRYPTOCOCCAL MENINGITIS

C. neoformans, a ubiquitous yeast, produces CNS infection in about 5% of patients with AIDS and in some this may be the first recognized opportunistic infection. In both the United States and Africa, it is one of the most common CNS opportunistic infections. The most common presentation is as meningitis with headache, meningismus, altered mentation, fever, and nausea.[138, 139] About 10% of patients develop papilledema as a result of elevated intracranial pressure. Elevated intracranial pressure is frequently lethal unless recognized and treated aggressively.[140] Cryptococcomas can form in the brain, producing a mass effect, or infiltrate cranial nerves to produce deafness, diplopia, or blindness. This constellation of symptoms can mimic those of cerebral toxoplasmosis, other opportunistic processes, and, when more indolent, the progressive dementia of HIVE (Table 125–9). In cryptococcal meningitis occurring with AIDS, CSF may have normal cellular and protein constituents. Kovacs and coworkers[141] found that the CSF leukocyte count was normal in 11 of 17 patients (65%), CSF protein level was normal in 5 of 16 (31%), and the CSF India ink test was positive in 14 of 17 patients (82%). Fungal cultures were uniformly positive (18 of 18) and cryptococcal antigen was detectable in all samples of CSF and serum. Assay of cryptococcal antigen therefore appears to be highly predictive for cryptococcal meningitis. MRI and CT findings may be normal in cryptococcal meningitis or alternatively may show meningeal enhancement, elevated intracranial pressure, or cryptococcomas typically involving basal ganglia structures[142] (Table 125–10 and Fig. 125–16).

Antifungal therapy is of only moderate efficacy in AIDS-related cryptococcal meningitis and is not well tolerated. Either amphotericin B alone (0.6 to 0.9 mg/kg per day) or, in fulminant cases, a combination of amphotericin B (0.6 to 0.9 mg/kg per day) and flucytosine (Ancobon; 150 mg/kg per day) is used. One study has shown no added benefit from flucytosine, and this drug causes side effects in some, including diarrhea and bone marrow suppression.[143] A total 0.75- to 1.0-g course of amphotericin therapy is recommended for patients with AIDS, followed by long-term maintenance treatment with fluconazole.[144] Side effects of amphotericin B include renal impairment, chills, and fever. Elevated intracranial pressure should be treated aggressively with repeated large-volume lumbar punctures or ventricular drainage (Fig. 125–17). Fluconazole is being used more widely, both for initial induction and for prophylaxis. This agent is far less toxic than amphotericin B, is well absorbed orally, and, unlike ketoconazole, penetrates the blood-brain barrier. Suppressive treatment with 200 mg/d is effective for lifelong maintenance.[145] On the basis of combined information from two studies,[138, 141] the initial response rate is about 58%.[146] Complete clearance is unusual and relapse occurs in about 60%, and the median survival after diagnosis of cryptococcal meningitis is 9 months.[147] During successful treatment, both the serum and the CSF cryptococcal antigen titers can be ex-

TABLE 125–9 ■ Common Brain Diseases Complicating Acquired Immunodeficiency Syndrome: Clinical Differentiation

DISORDER	COURSE	ALERT	FEVER/HEADACHE	FOCAL EXAMINATION
HIV dementia	Weeks or months	NL*	0	0
Toxoplasmosis	<2 wk	↓	+	+ + +
Primary lymphoma	2–8 wk	↓ or NL	0	+
PML	Weeks or months	NL	0	+ +
Cryptococcosis	<2 wk	↓	+ + +	0
CMV encephalitis	<2 wk	↓ or NL	+	0

*NL, Normal.

Modified from Price RW: Infections of the Nervous System, American Academy of Neurology Annual Course 347. Minneapolis, MN, American Academy of Neurology, May 5, 1990.

TABLE 125–10 ■ Radiologic Pattern of Human Immunodeficiency Virus–Related Central Nervous System Disease

DISORDER	NUMBER OF LESIONS	PATTERN	ENHANCEMENT	LOCATION
HIV encephalitis	Diffuse	Ill defined	0	Deep white
Toxoplasmosis	1–many	Ring mass	++	Basal ganglia
Primary lymphoma	1–several	Solid mass	+++	Periventricular
PML	1–several	No mass	0	Subcortical white
Cryptococcosis	1–many	Punctate	0	Basal ganglia
CMV encephalitis	1–several	Confluent	++	Periventricular

Modified from Price RW: Infections of the Nervous System, American Academy of Neurology Annual Course 347. Minneapolis, MN, American Academy of Neurology, May 5, 1990.

pected to fall by at least four dilutions and cultures become negative. The CSF should be reexamined at the end of therapy and if symptoms recur. Retreatment of those who have a relapse is less successful than primary induction and ultimately cryptococcal meningitis is directly fatal in about 30%. In those refractory to intravenous amphotericin, administration of amphotericin B via an intrathecal route or into the ventricles through an indwelling Ommaya reservoir can be considered. These alternative routes of administration are associated with numerous side effects, and their use does not seem justified by any difference in outcome in the small numbers reported to date.[146]

HISTOPLASMOSIS

Histoplasmosis occurs in 2% to 5% of AIDS patients from endemic areas of the central United States, Latin America, and the Caribbean. Cases may occur outside endemic areas. Outdoor workers, such as those in construction and farming, with contact with the soil containing spores, are at particularly high risk. The majority of AIDS-related histoplasmosis occurs with a CD4$^+$ cell count less than 100/mm^3. *Histoplasma capsulatum* is a typical dimorphic yeast present in soil and bird and bat feces in endemic areas, which are usually river valleys, including Ohio, Mississippi, and St. Lawrence. Infection develops after inhalation of airborne spores. Although histoplasmosis remains a common cause of deep-seated fungal infections in North America, CNS abscesses or histoplasmomas are unusual.[148, 149] A more common neurologic manifestation is meningitis, which is seen in up to 8% of all cases and 25% of those with disseminated disease. In 1987, extrapulmonary histoplasmosis was added to the CDC list of AIDS-defining illnesses.[7] Histoplasmosis in AIDS is usually a severe disseminated infection, often resembling septicemia. In the largest review,[150] 72 patients with AIDS and histoplasmosis were reviewed. Fifty-three percent had pulmonary involvement, 13% a septicemia-like syndrome, 26% hepatomegaly, and 18% CNS involvement. These included encephalopathy, meningitis, and focal abscesses. Eight of 13 patients

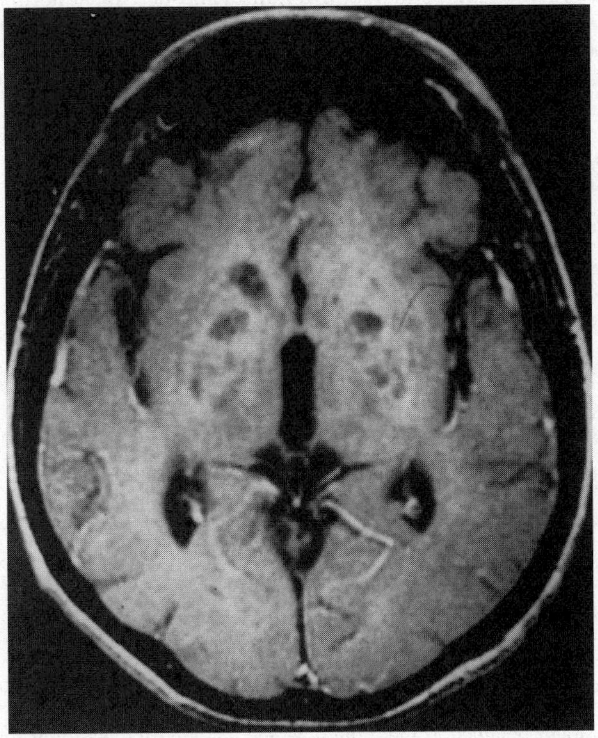

FIGURE 125–16 □ MRI scan in cryptococcal meningitis showing discrete areas of low density in basal ganglia representing cryptococcomas.

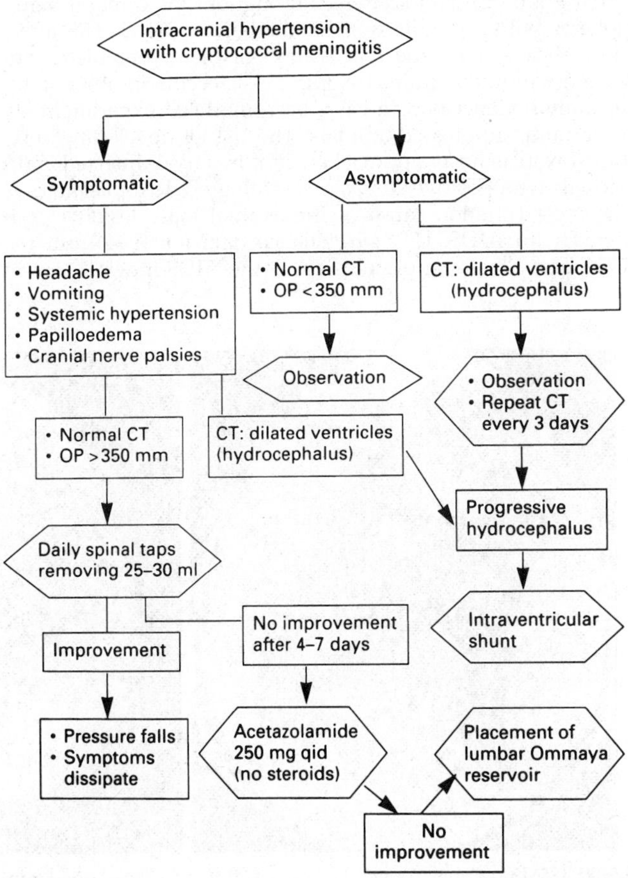

FIGURE 125–17 □ Algorithm for management of elevated intracranial pressure in cryptococcal meningitis. OP, Opening pressure. (From Harrison MJG, McArthur JC: AIDS and Neurology. Edinburgh, Churchill Livingstone, 1995, p 120.)

with CNS histoplasmosis died of the infection. The diagnosis of histoplasmosis was made by positive fungal cultures for *H. capsulatum* in more than 90% of the cases and in the remainder by the detection of *Histoplasma* polysaccharide antigen (HPA) in body fluids (detected in 97%). Regular measurement of HPA in serum and urine is helpful in identifying a relapse of disseminated histoplasmosis in AIDS. An increase in HPA in urine or serum of 2 units or more heralded the majority of relapses in this series. HPA was detected in six of nine cases in this series. Eighty percent of cases improved after induction therapy with amphotericin B, the majority defervescing within 1 week. Ketoconazole was effective in preventing relapse. The organism can be cultured from bone marrow, nodes, or ulcers. However, the most sensitive test is the radioimmunoassay or enzyme immunoassay to detect HPA in urine. Results are expressed as HPA units and values of 1 or more are considered positive. Sensitivity is 90% to 97%.[151] Serologic diagnosis by antibody detection is not reliable because of high false-positive rates in patients from endemic areas and in patients with other fungal or bacterial infections. In patients with AIDS and histoplasmosis, increases in antigenuria or antigenemia herald relapses.[152] Histoplasmoma is treated by a combination of surgical drainage and intravenous amphotericin, 0.6 to 1.0 mg/kg per day, extended until there has been radiologic improvement.

CEREBRAL TOXOPLASMOSIS

CNS infection with *T. gondii,* an obligate intracellular protozoan, causes necrotic and inflammatory abscesses that are often multifocal and scattered throughout the cerebral hemispheres with a predilection for the basal ganglia. The infection is caused by the reactivation of latent organisms encysted within the brain. Toxoplasmosis occurs in other states of immunodeficiency and has been modeled experimentally in immunosuppressed animals. The risk of developing cerebral toxoplasmosis approaches 20% in HIV-1–infected individuals with positive *Toxoplasma* serology.[153] Toxoplasmosis is the most common cause of intracranial mass lesion in patients with AIDS. U.S. surveillance data for 1994 from the CDC show that toxoplasmosis was the AIDS index illness in 2% of patients with AIDS. However, in Europe and Africa, toxoplasmosis is seen much more frequently.

Toxoplasmosis typically presents with the development of fever (about 30% to 40%), altered mentation, seizures, and focal neurologic signs developing in a few days[154] (see Table 125–9). Despite the propensity for toxoplasmosis to develop subacutely and to cause focal neurologic deficits, the clinical features are not specific enough to distinguish it reliably from primary CNS lymphoma.[155] Imaging studies demonstrate multiple contrast-enhanced mass lesions; however, the radiologic appearances are not definitive for toxoplasmosis and can be mimicked by lymphoma or other causes of abscess (see Table 125–10). Areas of edema usually surround *Toxoplasma* lesions, sometimes producing a mass effect and shift of surrounding structures (Fig. 125–18*A*). The abscesses show a predilection for the basal ganglia regions.[155] Other areas affected, in order of frequency, are frontal, parietal, and occipital lobes and occasionally cerebellum. MRI is more sensitive than CT, frequently showing lesions that are not identifiable even with contrast CT[5, 40, 146] (Fig. 125–18*B*). The use of gadolinium, a paramagnetic contrast agent for MRI, has improved our ability to delineate both anatomic detail and the presence of altered blood-brain barrier permeability (Fig. 125–18C). Unfortunately, the number of discrete CT or MRI lesions, their location, or their radiologic characteristics do not allow reliable differentiation of toxoplasmosis from lymphoma. CSF is usually abnormal, with elevated protein and pleocytosis. However, because of the mass effect associated with *Toxoplasma* abscesses, lumbar puncture often has to be deferred to avoid herniation. Prompt initiation of treatment with pyrimethamine (Daraprim) and sulfadiazine leads to clinical improvement in 80% of cases within 1 to 4 weeks.[8, 154] In one series, 86% had responded by day 7 and 91% by day 14.[156] Pyrimethamine is administered orally with a loading dose of 200 mg and continued at 75 mg/d with 5 mg of folinic acid (leucovorin). Sulfadiazine is given orally at a dose of 1.5 g every 6 hours. About 40% of patients develop a reaction to the sulfa component, usually within 7 to 10 days, with development of fever, rash, and hepatic abnormalities. Clindamycin (Cleocin) can be substituted at a dose of 900 mg every 6 hours either orally or intravenously and appears to have equivalent efficacy.[155, 157] After this induction

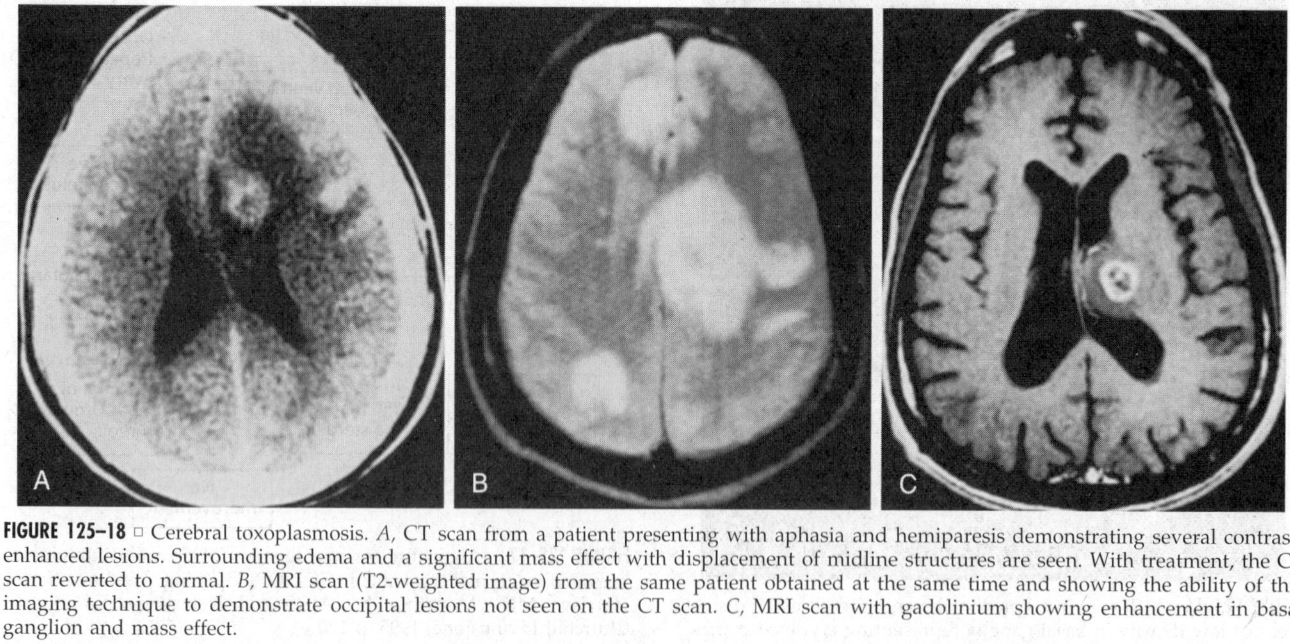

FIGURE 125–18 □ Cerebral toxoplasmosis. *A*, CT scan from a patient presenting with aphasia and hemiparesis demonstrating several contrast-enhanced lesions. Surrounding edema and a significant mass effect with displacement of midline structures are seen. With treatment, the CT scan reverted to normal. *B*, MRI scan (T2-weighted image) from the same patient obtained at the same time and showing the ability of this imaging technique to demonstrate occipital lesions not seen on the CT scan. *C*, MRI scan with gadolinium showing enhancement in basal ganglion and mass effect.

therapy for 6 weeks, maintenance therapy of pyrimethamine, 25 mg/d, with folinic acid and a second agent, either sulfadiazine or clindamycin at 300 mg every 6 hours, needs to be continued lifelong. Alternative agents that are under study include atovaquone, trimetrexate, and spiramycin.[146] Azithromycin does not appear to be effective.[158] Corticosteroids should be avoided for at least two reasons, unless the mass effect is pronounced. First, they add to the existing immunologic dysfunction. Second, any mass lesion may show nonspecific improvement after steroids, which masks any effect of the antimicrobial drugs. In patients with large mass lesions with prominent shift and potential for herniation, dexamethasone (Decadron) can be used at doses of 10 mg every 6 hours.

The role of brain biopsy in the management of patients with AIDS and intracranial mass lesions has changed in the past few years, as experience has accumulated with empirical *Toxoplasma* therapy, and, increasingly, thallium 201 SPECT scans can be used to distinguish between toxoplasmosis and primary CNS lymphoma. Macapinlac and coworkers[159] showed that the radioisotope is taken up by viable neoplastic cells, producing a "hot" spot, whereas infection remains "cold." Stereotactic CT-guided biopsy is, in general, preferable to open biopsy and allows precise biopsy of even deep-seated lesions with minimal morbidity. Unfortunately, in cerebral toxoplasmosis, biopsies can fail to provide a definitive pathologic diagnosis for several reasons. First, the biopsy may miss the lesion or sample only the necrotic core of the abscess. Second, therapy has often been started at the time of biopsy, making it difficult to recognize the tachyzoites histologically. Last, routine hematoxylin-eosin staining is insensitive. In one series, the sensitivity of the brain biopsy in autopsy-proven toxoplasmosis was only 40%.[155] Experience with both stereotactic and open biopsies has led to recommendations to use immunoperoxidase staining routinely.[160, 161] At present, for patients with AIDS presenting with intracranial mass lesions, whether single or multiple, empirical therapy for toxoplasmosis is started. This policy is satisfactory for most patients,[162] and biopsy can be reserved for individuals who (1) are intolerant of or refractory to empirical therapy or (2) have atypical presentations, such as single lesions developing during several months (Table 125–11).

Serologic testing is not diagnostic; however, most patients with toxoplasmosis have detectable antitoxoplasma IgG, and a negative serologic titer (<1:4) should suggest an alternative diagnosis.[155] Measurement of intrathecal synthesis of *Toxoplasma* antibody has been suggested as a useful diagnostic test, but in practice lumbar puncture cannot always be safely performed.

Lifelong suppressive therapy with pyrimethamine, 50 mg/d, and a second agent is necessary—preferably sulfadiazine if tolerated or clindamycin. Relapse occurs in about 10% treated with pyrimethamine plus sulfa and 22% of those receiving pyrimethamine plus clindamycin and is usually linked to noncompliance.[163] In *Toxoplasma*-seropositive patients, trimethoprim-sulfamethoxazole appears to be effective primary prophylaxis for both toxoplasmosis and *P. carinii* pneumonia. Although an effective prophylactic agent, pyrimethamine was actually associated with a higher death rate in one study, possibly because of its hematologic toxicity.[164]

TABLE 125–11 ■ Indications for Brain Biopsy in Acquired Immunodeficiency Syndrome

Failed empirical antitoxoplasma therapy
Accessible lesion, no coagulopathy
Karnovsky function scale >70, that is, independent
No immediate life-threatening systemic disease
Radiation therapy acceptable to patient

From Harrison MJG, McArthur JC: AIDS and Neurology. Edinburgh, Churchill Livingstone, 1995, p 192.

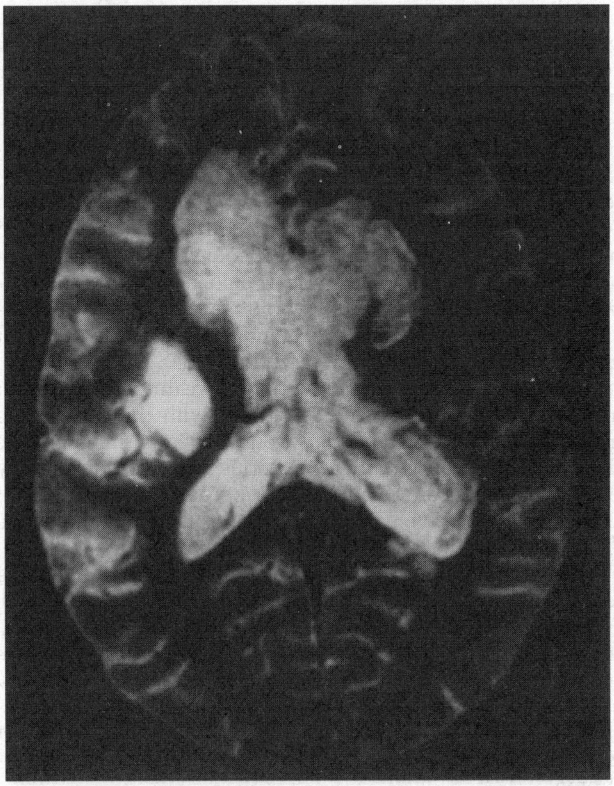

FIGURE 125–19 □ CMV encephalitis. Cranial MRI scan of fulminant CMV encephalitis showing prominent inflammation in ependymal and periventricular area.

CYTOMEGALOVIRUS ENCEPHALITIS AND RETINITIS

CMV also frequently causes CNS opportunistic infection leading to encephalitis.[5, 6, 165–168] The frequency of this complication can only be estimated, because often CMV is not identified ante mortem and CMV infection may exist concurrently with other pathogens.[169–171] The development of CMV encephalitis is more rapid than the slowly progressive dementia of HIVE. The course is often rapidly downhill during 1 to 4 weeks with delirium, memory impairment, and cranial nerve deficits developing with periventriculitis and encephalitis in the setting of disseminated CMV infection (see Table 125–9). Radiologic studies may be normal in the early stages or may show ventricular enlargement, periventricular white matter abnormalities, and contrast-enhanced lesions in subependymal and cortical regions[172] (Fig. 125–19; see Table 125–10). CSF analysis usually provides clues to the presence of encephalitis with a high protein level, pleocytosis, and positive CMV polymerase chain reaction.[173] The virus is rarely isolated from CSF by culture[5] and radiologic findings are absent in 40% to 50%.[174] Neuropathologic findings are variable, in one series[168] ranging from rare isolated CMV inclusions to severe necrotizing ependymitis and meningoencephalitis. The acyclovir analog ganciclovir has been used to suppress active CMV infection and offers one form of specific treatment.[146] In severe cases, combination therapy with ganciclovir and foscarnet can be attempted.

CMV retinitis is the most common ocular infection in patients with AIDS and causes a hemorrhagic retinitis. It has been reported to occur in 4% to 38% of AIDS patients.[175–181]

CMV retinitis is recognized by its characteristic appearance of retinal necrosis admixed with hemorrhage on ophthalmoscopy. In up to 60% it becomes bilateral.[181] Untreated, CMV retinitis is a progressive disease that can lead to blindness. It is important but sometimes difficult to distinguish CMV retinitis from cotton-wool spots. Cotton-wool spots are microinfarcts of the nerve fiber layer of the retina that do not interfere with vision. They occur in 40% to 92% of patients with AIDS,[17, 182] are noninfectious in origin, and may be related to immune complex deposition. Available forms of treatment for CMV retinitis include the antiviral agent ganciclovir, phosphonoformic acid (foscarnet), cidofovir, and intraocular ganciclovir. Several studies have demonstrated the efficacy of ganciclovir in suppressing CMV infection, with a clinical response observed in about 80%.[183–185] Treatment consists of an initial induction phase for 2 weeks with the drug being given intravenously twice daily. Subsequently, maintenance therapy, using a once-daily intravenous infusion 5 days every week, must be continued lifelong because interruption of therapy almost universally results in the reactivation of active CMV retinitis.[181]

The most significant side effect of ganciclovir is reversible leukopenia, which occurs to a mild degree in most patients. Foscarnet can cause nephrotoxicity and electrolyte abnormalities. Cidofovir is a new nucleoside analog with no requirement for thymidine kinase. It has potent anti-CMV activity and is already phosphorylated so does not require triphosphorylation as does ganciclovir. The major limiting side effect is nephrotoxicity; some patients can develop Fanconi syndrome.

PROGRESSIVE MULTIFOCAL LEUKOENCEPHALOPATHY

Reactivation of latent papovavirus (usually the JC strain) under conditions of immune deficiency leads to this progressive demyelinating disorder, PML.[186] Serologic studies have shown that about 70% of all adults have antibodies to JC virus, implying that the infection is common in humans, although the primary infection is usually silent. Before AIDS, the condition had been reported most frequently in patients with lymphoma or leukemia or in those receiving immunosuppressive drugs for the treatment of rheumatoid arthritis or sarcoidosis or after organ transplantation. AIDS is now the most common cause of PML.

About 5% of patients with AIDS develop PML, which typically presents with a progressive accumulation of focal neurologic deficits—aphasia, hemiparesis, or ataxia. A typical presentation is the evolution during 1 to 4 weeks of focal deficits without headache, seizures, or (initially) altered mentation (see Table 125–9). The reactivated papovavirus affects the hemispheric white matter, cerebellum, or brain stem and causes patches of demyelination, which may become confluent. Giant atypical astrocytes and oligodendroglia with markedly enlarged nuclei are seen and inflammatory infiltrates may appear. Electron microscopy may reveal intranuclear papovavirions. The lesions of PML in AIDS are often more destructive than PML not associated with HIV infection.

PML typically presents with focal neurologic deficits that progress inexorably during weeks or a few months to death.[5, 6, 187] The median survival in one series was only 16 weeks[187]; however, spontaneous improvements in patients with AIDS have been documented.[188] Characteristic presentations include aphasia, ataxia, and hemiparesis, and the diagnosis is usually made clinically by recognition of a clinical course with imaging studies demonstrating multiple abnormal areas in the white matter. Generally the lesions cause no mass effect, are confined to the subcortical white matter, and are not enhanced with injection of contrast medium (Fig. 125–20; see Table 125–10). CSF assays and electroencephalography show nonspecific abnormalities or may be normal. CSF polymerase chain reaction has a sensitivity of 30% to 70% but is not widely available outside research settings.[189] Biopsy may be necessary to differentiate PML from cerebral toxoplasmosis, other opportunistic infections, or CNS lymphoma. Immunostaining with antibody to simian virus 40 or electron microscopy is necessary for definitive pathologic diagnosis.

There is no effective treatment, and the neurologic disorder usually progresses inexorably to death in weeks or a few months. A variety of antivirals including amantadine, interferon-α, adenosine arabinoside, and cytarabine have been tried with little success.[190, 191] Clinical trials of high-dose intravenous or intrathecal cytarabine with the AIDS Clinical Trials Group showed no effect on survival (Hall C, personal communication, 1996).

TUBERCULOUS MENINGITIS

Tuberculosis of the meninges results from the rupture of small subependymal foci. The meninges become thickened and opaque, and cranial nerves and roots can be affected as they penetrate the meninges, which contain caseating granulomata. The other mechanism of symptom production is the direct effect of a granuloma in the brain parenchyma or an endarteritis with ischemic foci.

Immunosuppression need not be severe, and in one series[192] counts of $CD4^+$ cells varied from 7 to 251/mm^3. This has been contrasted with the situation in cryptococcal infection, in which $CD4^+$ cell counts tend to be lower. Bishburg and colleagues[193] found 10 patients with CNS involvement among 52 cases of TB from a population of approximately 420 patients with AIDS.

TB meningitis is usually preceded by a period of malaise, fatigue, and headache. A review of 26 HIV-related cases by Shafer and coworkers[194] and of 15 cases by Dube and associates[192] demonstrated that most patients had confusion and/or headache. Less than half had neck stiffness, but 11 from the combined series had focal signs such as a hemiparesis or cranial nerve lesion. By the time meningitis has developed fever is to be expected. The CSF in the two studies showed a pleocytosis in all but five instances with predominantly a lymphocytosis of up to 1000 cells per mm^3. Cases with normal cell counts tended to have miliary infection with positive blood cultures. The protein level was normal or up to 1000 mg/dL. CSF cultures were positive in cases with and without a pleocytosis. CT with use of contrast material had been performed for all but two of Shafer's patients and revealed meningeal enhancement in five. Dube and colleagues reported focal lesions in 9 of their 15 cases on either CT or MRI scans. Several patients had hydrocephalus. At least two had normal scans. Berenguer and coworkers[195] reported mass lesions in 8 of 10 cases, with ring enhancement on CT scans in 5. Interestingly, 52 HIV-infected patients with no evidence of CNS TB had scans and 4 of these had enhancing brain lesions that responded to anti-TB treatment.[194] Clearly, this suggests that HIV-infected patients who develop TB at any site should probably have cranial CT (or MRI). It also means that ring-enhancing lesions may be due to TB if they do not respond to antitoxoplasma treatment or the patient has pulmonary TB.[193]

The clinical presentation does not appear to differ in a major way from that seen in patients without AIDS. Dube and colleagues[192] addressed this issue directly, comparing 15 patients with culture-proven meningitis caused by *Mycobacterium tuberculosis* who were HIV-positive or had AIDS with 16 from the same institution who were not HIV infected. There were no differences in the incidence of the major symptoms of headache, confusion, and fever. Physical signs were equally common in the two groups (papilledema, focal

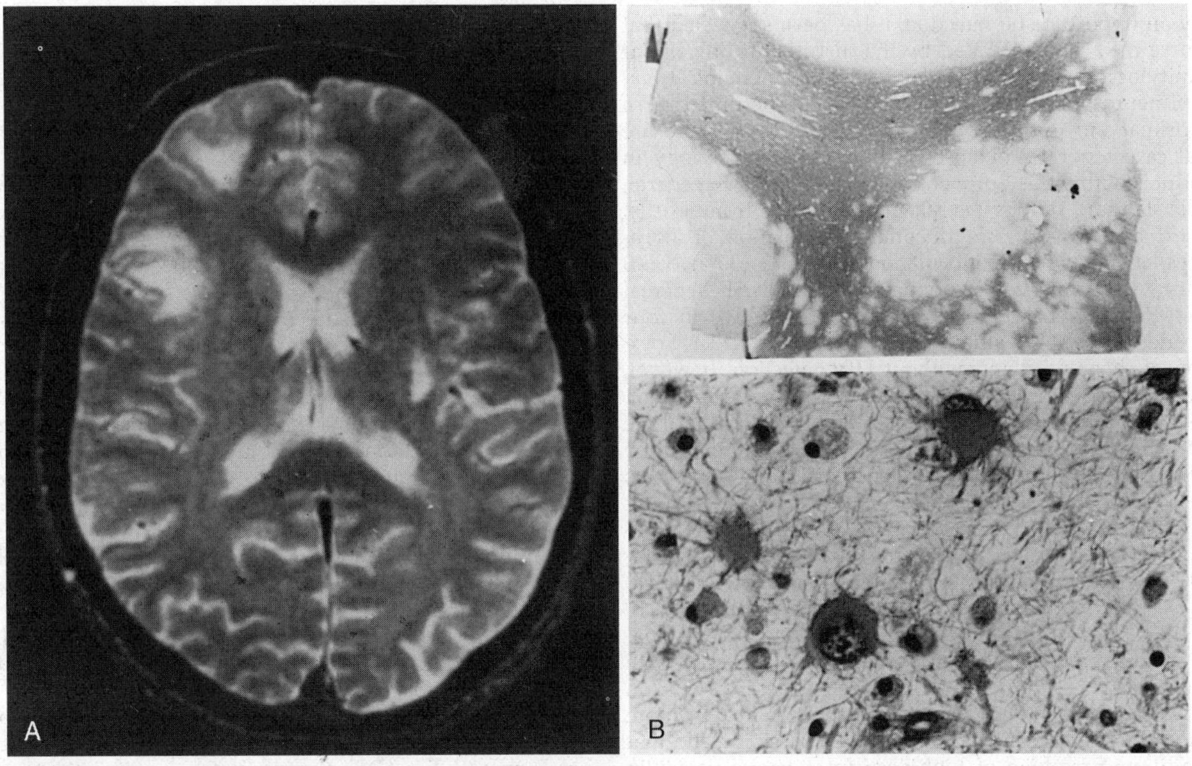

FIGURE 125–20 □ PML. *A*, MRI scan showing multiple areas of hyperintensity confined to the subcortical white matter in the frontoparietal area. No mass effect and no enhancement with contrast medium are seen. *B*, Luxol fast blue stain of brain showing multiple demyelinative foci. High power shows transformed bizarre-looking astrocytes and inclusion-bearing oligodendrocytes.

findings, and depressed consciousness), except for the presence of neck stiffness, which was less common in the HIV-infected patients. However, this difference was barely significant (47% instead of 80%, $P = .06$) and in the context of a large number of comparisons in a small number of cases may well be fortuitous. CSF findings were similar in the two groups, except for the opening pressure, which was lower in the HIV cases (7 to 24 cm H_2O compared with 9 to 55 cm H_2O, $P = .03$). This might reflect a somewhat blunted meningeal response to infection in the immunocompromised patient and support the difference in neck stiffness, but the cellular response did not confirm this, being just as active. In cryptococcal infection with more advanced immunosuppression, there is a tendency for HIV-related cases to show less CSF reaction than non-HIV cases.[139]

Neuroimaging revealed a significant difference in the incidence of mass lesions. Nine of 15 HIV-infected patients but only 2 of 14 non-HIV patients had scans showing such lesions ($P < .01$). Such lesions are sometimes large enough to behave as space-occupying abscesses.[193] Vertebral and spinal cord abscesses have also been described.[196] MRI shows enhanced lesions when the meningitis is accompanied by tuberculomata as in non–HIV-related TB meningitis.

Diagnosis depends on a high index of suspicion, the chest radiograph, and the CSF findings with a reduced glucose level. In the absence of pulmonary tuberculosis, ring-enhancing lesions in the brain in a febrile patient are usually treated as possible *Toxoplasma* infection. When there is no response to *Toxoplasma* treatment, a biopsy is indicated to reveal the caseating TB lesion. In the presence of active pulmonary infection and a negative *Toxoplasma* antibody test, focal neurologic or brain imaging findings would be sufficiently suggestive of CNS tubercle to limit treatment to standard anti-TB therapy.

Treatment with standard quadruple regimes is successful, although the mortality remains higher than in non-AIDS patients. A diagnostic reduction in fever can be expected within a week in 85% of pulmonary cases,[197] and a therapeutic trial may point to the diagnosis before bacteriologic confirmation. Mortality after discharge from the hospital depends primarily on the $CD4^+$ cell count,[198] but rates of drug resistance as high as 30% are reported from some areas.[199] Initial treatment is with isoniazid at 300 mg/d, rifampin up to 600 mg/d, pyrazinamide at 20 to 30 mg/kg per day, and ethambutol at 15 to 25 mg/kg. Monno and colleagues[200] suggested that when in vitro drug resistance is a problem, rifabutin (450 mg/d) may be successful. Pyrazinamide should be given for the first 2 months or longer if resistance or allergy develops to isoniazid or rifampin. Noncompliance is a problem in some AIDS patients, and supervised ambulatory treatment may be necessary. Zidovudine can be continued, but ketoconazole inhibits the absorption of rifampin, and the two should not be prescribed together. Minor changes in liver function tests should not be allowed to cause cessation of use of first-line anti-TB drugs. As noted, treatment is usually successful, but after a course of 9 months or more with culture conversion, isoniazid should probably be continued lifelong, because of the risk of relapse in the immunocompromised individual. Obstruction of CSF pathways related to meningitis may cause hydrocephalus with declining consciousness level. Such a deterioration during drug treatment is therefore an indication for repeated imaging in case a ventricular shunt is needed. This would be likely only in the first days or weeks of TB meningitis. Later deterioration suggests relapse, a second opportunistic infection, or an additional pathologic condition.

NEUROSYPHILIS

Nationwide, the rates of syphilis have increased since 1986, after 5 years of steady decline. Although syphilis is not strictly an opportunistic infection, it has been suggested that its course may be accelerated by the disturbance in cellular immunity accompanying HIV-1 infection.[201] The clinical features of neurosyphilis may be modified and the time course from primary to tertiary syphilis shortened.[202, 203] There are several case reports[204] of false-negative syphilis serology in individuals with biopsy-proven syphilis; however, in general, syphilis standard serology is reliable. In studies from Seattle, Lukehart and coworkers[205] documented isolation of *Treponema pallidum* by rabbit inoculations from 12 (30%) of 40 patients with primary or secondary syphilis. CSF Venereal Disease Research Laboratory (VDRL) was reactive in four (14%) and the protein value was elevated in six (21%). Comparison of those with and without HIV infection, however, showed that isolation of *T. pallidum* was not more frequent. Despite this, there was evidence of treatment failure in three of four HIV-1–seropositive patients treated with benzathine penicillin. In two there was persistence of viable *T. pallidum*; in one, serum and CSF VDRL titers rose.

Gordon and coworkers[206] identified 11 HIV-infected patients with symptomatic neurosyphilis. Five had been previously treated for early syphilis with penicillin G benzathine. Despite treatment with intravenous penicillin G for 10 days, the CSF VDRL titer remained unchanged in two patients and increased in two. One patient had a relapse with meningovascular syphilis 6 months after therapy. Gordon and coworkers concluded that treatment failure may be more common in patients with syphilis and HIV infection and that the traditional regimen of high-dose intravenous penicillin recommended for neurosyphilis is not consistently effective.

In a neurologically normal HIV-1 carrier with a history of treated syphilis who is serofast (rapid plasma reagin ≤ 1:8 consistently), there is probably no indication for additional therapy or lumbar puncture.[207] In fact, the CSF is likely to be abnormal with pleocytosis and protein elevation because of early HIV-1 infection of the CNS.[72] When neurologic symptoms are present, however, even if not typical of neurosyphilis, the CSF should be examined. If CSF VDRL is positive or serum rapid plasma reagin is high or rising (>1:16) and clinical features suggest neurosyphilis, treatment with intravenous penicillin (24 million units for 10 days) should be given. An alternative regimen is 2.4 million units of procaine penicillin with probenecid for 10 days. CSF should be reexamined at 3 to 6 months. Benzathine penicillin should not be used for treatment of neurosyphilis because of poor CSF penetrance.

OTHER INFECTIONS

CNS infection with other opportunistic organisms occurs but is much less frequent than infection with *T. gondii* or *C. neoformans*.[1, 5, 49] Isolates have included *Candida albicans, Coccidioides immitis, T. pallidum, Aspergillus fumigatus,* and *Mycobacterium*.[170] The presentations are not pathognomonic and cannot be differentiated clinically from each other. Experience with the spectrum of pathologic findings in AIDS indicates that multiple intracranial infections are not uncommon.[5, 170] Bacterial infections, either cerebral abscesses or meningitis, are rare in this population.[5, 6] Herpes zoster and herpes simplex can both cause encephalitis and respond to acyclovir.[5]

Opportunistic Neoplasms

PRIMARY CENTRAL NERVOUS SYSTEM LYMPHOMA

Before AIDS, primary CNS lymphoma was a rare tumor developing in immunosuppressed hosts, such as transplant recipients. Up to 5% of patients with AIDS develop primary CNS lymphoma, making AIDS now the most common associated disease. About half of all primary CNS lymphomas are clinically silent and are detected only at autopsy. The typical presentation is with slowly progressive neurologic deterioration leading to death within 3 months. The most common presentation is altered mental status (60%) developing over several weeks, usually without headache, fever, or seizures.[208] Focal neurologic signs can develop in about 40%, but the clinical presentation is not specific enough to differentiate lymphoma from toxoplasmosis[155] (see Table 125–9). The topographic distribution, multicentricity, and pattern of contrast enhancement (Fig. 125–21; see Table 125–10) cannot reliably distinguish lymphoma from toxoplasmosis, so biopsy confirmation is often necessary, particularly if empirical treatment with antimicrobials fails. Thallium SPECT shows some usefulness in distinguishing toxoplasmosis from primary CNS lymphoma (Fig. 125–22). CSF cytology is rarely diagnostic (less than 5%), and lumbar puncture is often contraindicated because of a mass effect and the risk of herniation. The response to whole-brain radiation or chemotherapy is poor, with a median survival of 4 months.[209] The tumors are multicentric and of B-cell origin and are similar in histologic appearance to those observed in immunosuppressed renal allograft recipients.[210] Epstein-Barr virus has been linked with its development, as this agent has been implicated in producing lymphoma in patients without HIV infection.[211] A number of mechanisms for B-cell activation have been postulated, including direct antigenic stimulation by HIV, defective immune surveillance, and direct HIV infection of B cells.[212] The CNS also presents a unique sanctuary for B-cell proliferation because of the absence of an intrinsic immunoregulatory system.

METASTATIC SYSTEMIC LYMPHOMA

Most lymphomas are extranodal diffuse high-grade malignant lymphomas of B-cell origin. CNS involvement occurs in

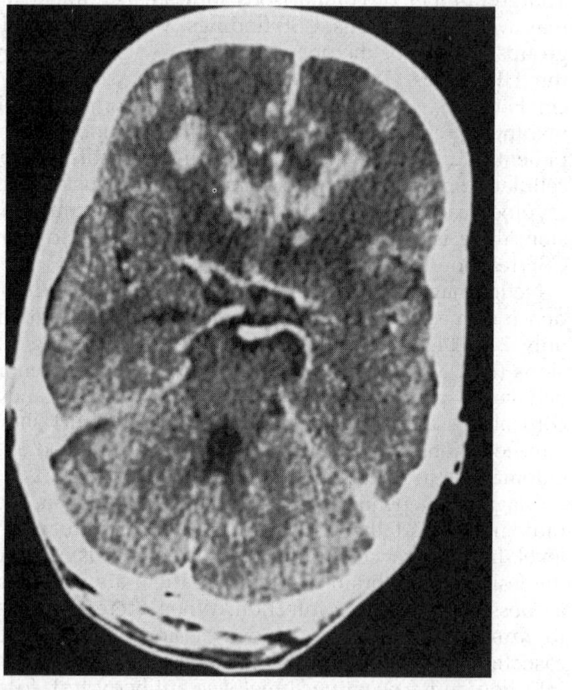

FIGURE 125–21 □ Primary CNS lymphoma. CT scan from a patient with autopsy-proven primary CNS lymphoma. There is a multicentric contrast-enhanced lesion in the frontal lobes with massive surrounding edema and posterior displacement of the middle cerebral arteries.

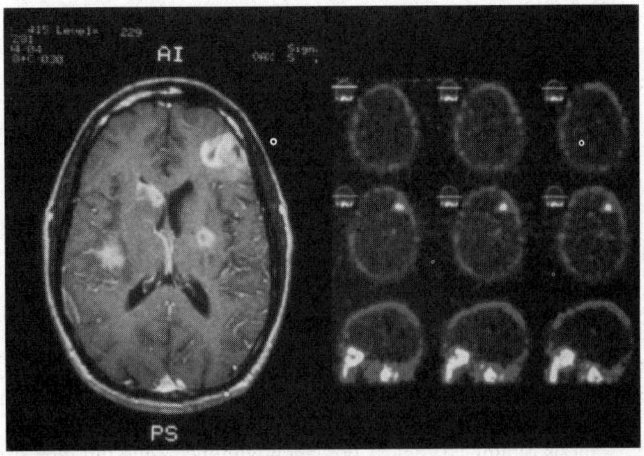

FIGURE 125–22 □ Thallium SPECT scan in primary CNS lymphoma. The area of positive uptake in the frontal lobe corresponds to the focus of lymphoma.

more than 50% of patients with systemic lymphoma. Complications include cranial neuropathies, meningeal involvement, cerebral metastasis, and spinal cord compression.

Metabolic Encephalopathies

These occur frequently in patients with AIDS, particularly when opportunistic infections with *P. carinii* cause hypoxia or when multisystem failure develops.[5, 6] A number of the therapeutic agents, including zidovudine and ganciclovir, have been linked to reversible delirium.[213, 214] Patients with HIVE are particularly predisposed to developing delirium with psychoactive medications, infection, or metabolic derangements.

Cerebrovascular Disease

Cerebrovascular accidents were noted in 9 of 124 (7%) AIDS patients in one series,[5] including examples of both cerebral infarction and hemorrhage. Engstrom and coworkers[215] reviewed the registry of 1600 AIDS patients at the University of California, San Francisco and identified 12 with cerebral infarction. Compared with the annual incidence of stroke of 0.025% in the general population between 35 and 45 years old, this frequency (0.75%) suggests a substantially increased risk of stroke in patients with AIDS. Pathologic series have documented cerebrovascular lesions in one third of patients with AIDS.[216] The thrombocytopenia that sometimes accompanies HIV infection may contribute to an increased incidence of intracranial hemorrhage. Other causes of intraparenchymal or subarachnoid hemorrhage include ruptured mycotic aneurysms or hemorrhage into intracerebral Kaposi's sarcoma. Cerebral infarctions can occur as a result of nonbacterial thrombotic endocarditis[5] or as a consequence of bacterial endocarditis in intravenous drug users. There are scattered case reports of cerebral granulomatous angiitis developing in association with HIV infection.[5, 217] The exact role of HIV in causing this disorder remains uncertain.

Neurologic Projections

The World Health Organization estimates that there are at least 20 million individuals already infected worldwide. Although there is some uncertainty about the ultimate numbers who will develop AIDS, it is clear that large numbers of relatively young individuals are already infected with HIV-1 and are thus at risk for subsequent development of a wide variety of neurologic problems. Extrapolating from the current CDC or World Health Organization estimates and from current prevalence figures for the different neurologic disorders, the following numbers of neurologic cases might be expected in the United States annually:

AIDS cases	140,000
Dementia	20,000
Sensory neuropathy	40,000
Cryptococcosis	7,000
CNS lymphoma	6,000
CNS toxoplasmosis	5,000

Perhaps the most terrifying prospect of all is that, as individuals with advanced AIDS live longer in an era of potent combination therapies, we may face an unprecedented epidemic of progressive dementia, which will place additional burdens on the health care system and caregivers.

Conclusion

We are battling an epidemic of potentially devastating proportions, rivaled perhaps only by the influenza epidemic of 1918 and 1919. The human and social consequences have already touched us all. Worldwide, the problem is enormous, particularly in Africa, where a significant proportion of the population is already infected with HIV-1 and medical resources are inadequate to deal with a health problem of this magnitude. Beyond the biologic and scientific issues there are many unanswered questions related to legal, ethical, and economic aspects of the epidemic.

Acknowledgments

Drs. Jack Griffin, Ola Selnes, Richard Johnson, and Jonathan Glass are acknowledged for helpful discussions. This work is dedicated to the memory of Dr. B. Frank Polk, whose energy, enthusiasm, and compassion continue to inspire. Supported by National Institute of Allergy and Infectious Diseases grant AI-35042, National Institute of Neurological Diseases and Stroke grants 1 PO1 NS 26643 and RR 00722, and a grant from the Charles A. Dana Foundation.

References

1. Pitlik SD, Fainstein V, Bolivar R, et al: Spectrum of central nervous system complications in homosexual men with acquired immune deficiency syndrome (Letter). J Infect Dis 148:771–772, 1983.
2. Johnson RT, McArthur JC: AIDS and the brain. Trends Neurosci 9:1–4, 1986.
3. Johnson RT, McArthur JC, Narayan O: The neurobiology of human immunodeficiency virus infections. FASEB J 2:2970–2981, 1988.
4. Centers for Disease Control and Prevention: HIV/AIDS Surveillance Report 6: Atlanta, Centers for Disease Control and Prevention, 1994, pp 1–39.
5. Levy RM, Bredesen DE, Rosenblum ML: Neurological manifestations of the acquired immunodeficiency syndrome (AIDS): Experience at UCSF and review of the literature. J Neurosurg 62:475–495, 1985.
6. Snider WD, Simpson DM, Nielsen S, et al: Neurological complications of acquired immune deficiency syndrome: Analysis of 50 patients. Ann Neurol 14:403–418, 1983.
7. Centers for Disease Control: Revision of the CDC surveillance case definition for acquired immunodeficiency syndrome. MMWR Morb Mortal Wkly Rep 36(Suppl 1S):3S–15S, 1987.
8. McArthur JC: Neurologic manifestations of AIDS. Medicine (Baltimore) 66:407–437, 1987.

9. Levy RM, Janssen RS, Bush TJ, Rosenblum ML: Neuroepidemiology of acquired immunodeficiency syndrome. J Acquir Immune Defic Syndr 1:31–40, 1988.
10. de la Monte SM, Ho DD, Schooley RT, et al: Subacute encephalomyelitis of AIDS and its relation to HTLV-III infection. Neurology 37:562–569, 1987.
11. Vinters HV, Tomiyasu U, Anders KH: Neuropathologic complications of infection with the human immunodeficiency virus (HIV). Prog AIDS Pathol 1:101–130, 1989.
12. Janssen RS, Nwanyanwu OC, Selik RM, Stehr-Green JK: Epidemiology of human immunodeficiency virus encephalopathy in the United States. Neurology 42:1472–1476, 1992.
13. Brun-Vezinet F, Katlama C, Roulot D, et al: Lymphadenopathy-associated virus type 2 in AIDS and AIDS-related complex. Lancet 1:128–132, 1987.
14. Cooper DA, Gold J, Maclean P, et al: Acute AIDS retrovirus infection: Definition of a clinical illness associated with seroconversion. Lancet 1:537–540, 1985.
15. Ho DD, Sarngadharan MG, Resnick L, et al: Primary human T-lymphotropic virus type III infection. Ann Intern Med 103:880–883, 1985.
16. Hollander H, Stringari S: Human immunodeficiency virus–associated meningitis. Clinical course and correlations. Am J Med 83:813–816, 1987.
17. Navia BA, Jordan BD, Price RW: The AIDS dementia complex: I. Clinical features. Ann Neurol 19:517–524, 1986.
18. Navia BA, Price RW: The acquired immunodeficiency syndrome dementia complex as the presenting or sole manifestation of human immunodeficiency virus infection. Arch Neurol 44:65–69, 1987.
19. Janssen RS, Cornblath DR, Epstein LG, et al: Nomenclature and research case definitions for neurological manifestations of human immunodeficiency virus type-1 (HIV-1) infection. Report of a Working Group of the American Academy of Neurology AIDS Task Force. Neurology 41:778–785, 1991.
20. Mayeux R, Stern Y, Tang MX, et al: Mortality risks in gay men with human immunodeficiency virus infection and cognitive impairment. Neurology 43:176–182, 1993.
21. Newman SP, Lunn S, Harrison MJG: Do asymptomatic HIV-seropositive individuals show cognitive deficit? AIDS 9:1211–1220, 1995.
22. McArthur JC, Cohen BA, Selnes OA, et al: Low prevalence of neurological and neuropsychological abnormalities in otherwise healthy HIV-1–infected individuals: Results from the multicenter AIDS Cohort Study. Ann Neurol 26:601–611, 1989.
23. Royal W, Updike M, Selnes OA, et al: HIV-1 infection and nervous system abnormalities among a cohort of intravenous drug users. Neurology 41:1905–1910, 1991.
24. Grant I, Atkinson JH, Hesselink JR, et al: Evidence for early central nervous system involvement in the acquired immunodeficiency syndrome (AIDS) and other human immunodeficiency virus (HIV) infections. Studies with neuropsychologic testing and magnetic resonance imaging [published erratum in Ann Intern Med 108:496, 1988]. Ann Intern Med 107:828–836, 1987.
25. World Health Organization: Report on the Consultation on the Neuropsychiatric Aspects of HIV Infection. Geneva, World Health Organization, 1988.
26. Selnes OA, Miller E, McArthur JC, et al: HIV-1 infection: No evidence of cognitive decline during the asymptomatic stages. Neurology 40:204–208, 1990.
27. Selnes OA, McArthur JC, Royal W, et al: HIV-1 infection and intravenous drug use: Longitudinal neuropsychological evaluation of asymptomatic subjects. Neurology 42:1924–1930, 1992.
28. Selnes OA, Galai N, Bacellar H, et al: Cognitive performance after progression to AIDS: A longitudinal study from the Multicenter AIDS Cohort Study. Neurology 45:267–275, 1995.
29. McArthur JC, Hoover DR, Bacellar H, et al: Dementia in AIDS patients: Incidence and risk factors. Neurology 43:2245–2252, 1993.
30. Bacellar H, Munoz A, Miller EN, et al: Temporal trends in the incidence of HIV-1 related neurologic diseases: Multicenter AIDS Cohort Study, 1985–1992. Neurology 44:1892–1900, 1994.
31. Belman AL, Ultmann MH, Horoupian D, et al: Neurological complications in infants and children with acquired immune deficiency syndrome. Ann Neurol 18:560–566, 1985.
32. Epstein LG, Sharer LR, Joshi VV, et al: Progressive encephalopathy in children with acquired immune deficiency syndrome. Ann Neurol 17:488–496, 1985.
33. McArthur JC, Harrison MJG: HIV-associated dementia. *In* Appel S (ed): Current Neurology. Chicago, Mosby–Year Book, 1994, p 290.
34. Price RW, Brew BJ: The AIDS dementia complex. J Infect Dis 158:1079–1083, 1988.
35. Pomerantz RJ, Kuritzkes DR, de la Monte SM, et al: Infection of the retina by human immunodeficiency virus type 1. N Engl J Med 317:1643–1647, 1987.
36. Petito CK, Navia BA, Cho ES, et al: Vacuolar myelopathy pathologically resembling subacute combined degeneration in patients with the acquired immunodeficiency syndrome. N Engl J Med 312:874–879, 1985.
37. Power C, Selnes OA, Grim JA, McArthur JC: The HIV Dementia Scale: A rapid screening test. J Acquir Immune Defic Syndr Hum Retrovirol 8:273–278, 1995.
38. Van Wielink G, McArthur JC, Moench T, et al: Intrathecal synthesis of anti–HIV-IgG: Correlation with increasing duration of HIV-1 infection. Neurology 40:816–819, 1990.
39. McArthur JC, Nance-Sproson TE, Griffin DE, et al: The diagnostic utility of elevation in cerebrospinal fluid β_2 microglobulin in HIV-1 dementia. Neurology 42:1707–1712, 1992.
40. Levy RM, Rosenbloom S, Perrett LV: Neuroradiologic findings in AIDS: A review of 200 cases. AJR 147:977–983, 1986.
41. Price RW, Navia BA: Infections in AIDS and in other immunosuppressed patients. *In* Kennedy PGE, Johnson RT (eds): Infections of the Nervous System. London, Butterworth, 1987, p 255.
42. McArthur JC, Kumar AJ, Johnson DW, et al: Incidental white matter hyperintensities on magnetic resonance imaging in HIV-1 infection. Multicenter AIDS Cohort Study. J Acquir Immune Defic Syndr 3:252–259, 1990.
43. Rottenberg DA, Moeller JR, Strother SC, et al: The metabolic pathology of the AIDS dementia complex. Ann Neurol 22:700–706, 1987.
44. Yarchoan R, Berg G, Brouwers P, et al: Response of human-immunodeficiency-virus–associated neurological disease to 3′-azido-3′-deoxythymidine. Lancet 1:132–135, 1987.
45. Holman BL, Barada B, Johnson KA, et al: A comparison of brain perfusion SPECT in cocaine abuse and AIDS dementia complex. J Nucl Med 33:1312–1315, 1992.
46. Dorfman LJ: Cytomegalovirus encephalitis in adults. Neurology 23:136–144, 1973.
47. Navia BA, Cho ES, Petito CK, Price RW: The AIDS dementia complex: II. Neuropathology. Ann Neurol 19:525–535, 1986.
48. Budka H: Multinucleated giant cells in brain: A hallmark of the acquired immune deficiency syndrome (AIDS). Acta Neuropathol (Berl) 69:253–258, 1986.
49. Rhodes RH: Histopathology of the central nervous system in the acquired immunodeficiency syndrome. Hum Pathol 18:636–643, 1987.
50. Sharer LR, Cho ES, Epstein LG: Multinucleated giant cells and HTLV-III in AIDS encephalopathy. Hum Pathol 16:760, 1985.
51. Nielsen SL, Petito CK, Urmacher CD, Posner JB: Subacute encephalitis in acquired immune deficiency syndrome: A postmortem study. Am J Clin Pathol 82:678–682, 1984.
52. Sharer LR, Kapila R: Neuropathologic observations in acquired immunodeficiency syndrome (AIDS). Acta Neuropathol (Berl) 66:188–198, 1985.
53. Koenig S, Gendelman HE, Orenstein JM, et al: Detection of AIDS virus in macrophages in brain tissue from AIDS patients with encephalopathy. Science 233:1089–1093, 1986.
54. Price RW, Sidtis J, Rosenblum M: AIDS dementia complex: Some current questions. Ann Neurol 23(Suppl):S27–S33, 1988.
55. Gartner S, Markovits P, Markovitz DM, et al: The role of mononuclear phagocytes in HTLV-III/LAV infection. Science 233:215–219, 1986.
56. Wiley CA, Schrier RD, Nelson JA, et al: Cellular localization of human immunodeficiency virus infection within the brains of acquired immune deficiency syndrome patients. Proc Natl Acad Sci USA 83:7089–7093, 1986.
57. Kleihues P, Lang W, Burger PC, et al: Progressive diffuse leukoencephalopathy in patients with acquired immune deficiency syndrome (AIDS). Acta Neuropathol (Berl) 68:333–339, 1985.
58. Power C, Kong P-A, Crawford TO, et al: Cerebral white matter changes in HIV dementia: Alterations in the blood-brain barrier. Ann Neurol 34:339–350, 1993.

59. Glass JD, Wesselingh SL, Selnes OA, McArthur JC: Clinical-neuropathologic correlation in HIV-associated dementia. Neurology 43:2230–2237, 1993.
60. Wiley CA, Nelson JA: Role of human immunodeficiency virus and cytomegalovirus in AIDS encephalitis. Am J Pathol 133:73–81, 1988.
61. Ho DD, Rota TR, Schooley RT, et al: Isolation of HTLV-III from cerebrospinal fluid and neural tissues of patients with neurologic syndromes related to the acquired immunodeficiency syndrome. N Engl J Med 313:1493–1497, 1985.
62. Gartner S, Markovits P, Markovitz DM, et al: Virus isolation from and identification of HTLV-III/LAV–producing cells in brain tissue from a patient with AIDS. JAMA 256:2365–2371, 1986.
63. Levy JA, Shimabukuro J, Hollander H, et al: Isolation of AIDS-associated retroviruses from cerebrospinal fluid and brain of patients with neurological symptoms. Lancet 2:586–588, 1985.
64. Epstein LG, Sharer LR, Cho ES, et al: HTLV-III/LAV–like retrovirus particles in the brains of patients with AIDS encephalopathy. AIDS Res 1:447–454, 1984.
65. Gyorkey F, Melnick JL, Gyorkey P: Human immunodeficiency virus in brain biopsies of patients with AIDS and progressive encephalopathy. J Infect Dis 155:870–876, 1987.
66. Resnick L, diMarzo-Veronese F, Schupbach J, et al: Intra–blood-brain-barrier synthesis of HTLV-III–specific IgG in patients with neurologic symptoms associated with AIDS or AIDS-related complex. N Engl J Med 313:1498–1504, 1985.
67. Elovaara I, Iivanainen M, Valle SL, et al: CSF protein and cellular profiles in various stages of HIV infection related to neurological manifestations. J Neurol Sci 78:331–342, 1987.
68. Stoler MH, Eskin TA, Benn S, et al: Human T-cell lymphotropic virus type III infection of the central nervous system. A preliminary in situ analysis. JAMA 256:2360–2364, 1986.
69. Gabuzda DH, Ho DD, de la Monte SM, et al: Immunohistochemical identification of HTLV-III antigen in brains of patients with AIDS. Ann Neurol 20:289–295, 1986.
70. Pumarola-Sune T, Navia BA, Cordon-Cardo C, et al: HIV antigen in the brains of patients with the AIDS dementia complex. Ann Neurol 21:490–496, 1987.
71. Vazeux R, Brousse N, Jarry A, et al: AIDS subacute encephalitis. Identification of HIV-infected cells. Am J Pathol 126:403–410, 1987.
72. Shaw GM, Harper ME, Hahn BH, et al: HTLV-III infection in brains of children and adults with AIDS encephalopathy. Science 227:177–182, 1985.
73. McArthur JC, Cohen BA, Farzedegan H, et al: Cerebrospinal fluid abnormalities in homosexual men with and without neuropsychiatric findings. Ann Neurol 23:S34–S37, 1988.
74. Hollander H, Levy JA: Neurologic abnormalities and recovery of human immunodeficiency virus from cerebrospinal fluid. Ann Intern Med 106:692–695, 1987.
75. Ward JM, O'Leary TJ, Baskin GB, et al: Immunohistochemical localization of human and simian immunodeficiency viral antigens in fixed tissue sections. Am J Pathol 127:199–205, 1987.
76. Nuovo GJ, Gallery F, MacConnell P, Braun A: In situ detection of polymerase chain reaction–amplified HIV-1 nucleic acids and tumor necrosis factor-α RNA in the central nervous system. Am J Pathol 144:659–666, 1994.
77. Haase AT: Pathogenesis of lentivirus infection. Nature 322:130–136, 1986.
78. Power C, McArthur JC, Johnson RT, et al: Demented and non-demented patients with AIDS differ in brain-derived human immunodeficiency virus type 1 envelope sequences. J Virol 68:4643–4649, 1994.
79. Epstein LG, Gendelman HE: Human immunodeficiency virus type 1 infection of the nervous system: Pathogenetic mechanisms. Ann Neurol 33:429–436, 1993.
80. Lipton SA, Rosenberg PA: Excitatory amino acids as a final common pathway for neurologic disorders. N Engl J Med 330:613–622, 1994.
81. Everall IP, Luthert PJ, Lantos PL: Neuronal loss in the frontal cortex in HIV infection. Lancet 337:1119–1121, 1991.
82. Wiley CA, Masliah E, Morey M, et al: Neocortical damage during HIV infection. Ann Neurol 29:651–657, 1991.
83. Ketzler S, Weis S, Haug H, Budka H: Loss of neurons in the frontal cortex in AIDS brains. Acta Neuropathol (Berl) 80:92–94, 1990.
84. Masliah E, Ge N, Morey M, et al: Cortical dendritic pathology in human immunodeficiency virus encephalitis. Lab Invest 66:285–291, 1992.
85. Dreyer EB, Kaiser PK, Offermann JT, Lipton SA: HIV-1 coat protein neurotoxicity prevented by calcium channel antagonists. Science 248:364–367, 1990.
86. Lipton SA: HIV-related neurotoxicity. Brain Pathol 1:193–199, 1991.
87. Heyes MP, Brew BJ, Martin A, et al: Quinolinic acid in cerebrospinal fluid and serum in HIV-1 infection: Relationship to clinical and neurologic status. Ann Neurol 29:202–209, 1991.
88. Heyes MP, Mefford IN, Quearry BJ, et al: Increased ratio of quinolinic acid to kynurenic acid in cerebrospinal fluid of D retrovirus–infected rhesus macaques: Relationship to clinical and viral status. Ann Neurol 27:666–675, 1990.
89. Lipton SA: Models of neuronal injury in AIDS: Another role for the NMDA receptor? Trends Neurosci 15:75–79, 1992.
90. Portegies P, de Gans J, Lange JM, et al: Declining incidence of AIDS dementia complex after introduction of zidovudine treatment [published erratum in BMJ 299:1141, 1989]. BMJ 299:819–821, 1989.
91. Fischl MA, Richman DD, Grieco MH, et al: The efficacy of azidothymidine (AZT) in the treatment of patients with AIDS and AIDS-related complex. N Engl J Med 317:185–191, 1987.
92. Schmitt FA, Bigley JW, McKinnis R, et al: Neuropsychological outcome of zidovudine (AZT) treatment of patients with AIDS and AIDS-related complex. N Engl J Med 319:1573–1578, 1988.
93. Volberding PA, Lagakos SW, Koch MA, et al: Zidovudine in asymptomatic human immunodeficiency virus infection. A controlled trial in persons with fewer than 500 CD4-positive cells per cubic millimeter. N Engl J Med 322:941–949, 1990.
94. Pizzo PA, Eddy J, Falloon J, et al: Effect of continuous intravenous infusion of zidovudine (AZT) in children with symptomatic HIV infection. N Engl J Med 319:889–896, 1988.
95. DeCarli C, Fugate L, Falloon J, et al: Brain growth and cognitive improvement in children with human immunodeficiency virus–induced encephalopathy after 6 months of continuous zidovudine therapy. J Acquir Immune Defic Syndr 4:585–592, 1991.
96. Wolters PL, Brouwers P, Moss HA, Pizzo PA: Adaptive behavior of children with symptomatic HIV infection before and after zidovudine therapy. J Pediatr Psychol 19:47–61, 1994.
97. Sidtis JJ, Gatsonis C, Price RW, et al: Zidovudine treatment of the AIDS dementia complex: Results of a placebo-controlled trial. Ann Neurol 33:343–349, 1993.
98. Butler KM, Husson RN, Balis RM, et al: Dideoxyinosine in children with symptomatic human immunodeficiency virus infection. N Engl J Med 324:137–144, 1991.
99. Yarchoan R, Pluda JM, Thomas RV, et al: Long-term toxicity/activity profile of 2′,3′-dideoxyinosine in AIDS and AIDS-related complex. Lancet 336:526–529, 1990.
100. Portegies P, Enting RH, de Gans J, et al: Presentation and course of AIDS dementia complex: Ten years of follow-up in Amsterdam, The Netherlands. AIDS 7:669–675, 1993.
101. Tozzi V, Narciso P, Galgani S, et al: Effects of zidovudine in 30 patients with mild to end-stage AIDS dementia complex. AIDS 7:683–692, 1993.
102. Tartaglione TA, Collier AC, Coombs RW, et al: Acquired immunodeficiency syndrome: Cerebrospinal fluid findings in patients before and during long-term oral zidovudine therapy. Arch Neurol 48:695–699, 1991.
103. Brew BJ, Bhalla RB, Paul M, et al: Cerebrospinal fluid neopterin in human immunodeficiency virus type-I infection. Ann Neurol 28:556–560, 1990.
104. Arendt G, Hefter H, Hilperath F, et al: Motor analysis predicts progression in HIV-associated brain disease. J Neurol Sci 123:180–185, 1994.
105. Ell PJ, Costa DC, Harrison M: Imaging cerebral damage in HIV infection (Letter). Lancet 2:569–570, 1987.
106. Vago L, Castagna A, Lazzarin A, et al: Reduced frequency of HIV-induced brain lesions in AIDS patients treated with zidovudine. J Acquir Immune Defic Syndr 6:42–45, 1993.
107. Gray F, Belec L, Keohane C, et al: Zidovudine therapy and HIV encephalitis: A 10-year neuropathological survey. AIDS 8:489–493, 1994.
108. Bridge TP, Heseltine PNR, Parker ES, et al: Results of extended peptide T administration in AIDS and ARC patients. Psychopharmacol Bull 27:237–245, 1991.

109. Lipton SA, Gendelman HE: Dementia associated with the acquired immunodeficiency syndrome. N Engl J Med 332:934–940, 1995.
110. Hriso E, Kuhn T, Masdeu JC, Grundman M: Extrapyramidal symptoms due to dopamine-blocking agents in patients with AIDS encephalopathy. Am J Psychiatry 148:1558–1561, 1991.
111. Eilbott DJ, Peress N, Burger H, et al: Human immunodeficiency virus type 1 in spinal cords of acquired immunodeficiency syndrome patients with myelopathy: Expression and replication in macrophages. Proc Natl Acad Sci USA 86:3337–3341, 1989.
112. Becker PS, Griffin JW, McArthur JC, et al: Vacuolar myelopathy in human immunodeficiency virus (HIV) infection: Central remyelination (Abstr). J Neuropathol Exp Neurol 48:383, 1989.
113. Parry GJ: Peripheral neuropathies associated with human immunodeficiency virus infection. Ann Neurol 23:S49–S53, 1988.
114. Cornblath DR, McArthur JC: Predominantly sensory neuropathy in patients with AIDS and AIDS-related complex. Neurology 38:794–796, 1988.
115. Rance NE, McArthur JC, Cornblath DR, et al: Gracile tract degeneration in patients with sensory neuropathy and AIDS. Neurology 38:265–271, 1988.
116. Moyle GJ, Nelson MR, Hawkins D, Gazzard BG: The use and toxicity of didanosine (DDI) in HIV antibody–positive individuals intolerant of zidovudine (AZT). Q J Med 86:155–163, 1993.
117. Berger AR, Arezzo JC, Schaumburg HH, et al: 2′,3′-Dideoxycytidine (ddC) toxic neuropathy: A study of 52 patients. Neurology 43:358–362, 1993.
118. Kieburtz KD, Seidlin M, Lambert JS, et al: Extended follow-up of peripheral neuropathy in patients with AIDS and AIDS-related complex treated with dideoxyinosine. J Acquir Immune Defic Syndr 5:60–64, 1992.
119. Blum AS, Dal Pan GJ, Feinberg J, et al: Low dose zalcitabine (ddC)–related toxic neuropathy: Frequency, natural history, and risk factors. Neurology 46:999–1003, 1996.
120. Skowron G: Biologic effects and safety of stavudine. Overview of phase I and II clinical trials. J Infect Dis 171(Suppl 2):S113–S117, 1995.
121. Cornblath DR, McArthur JC, Kennedy PG, et al: Inflammatory demyelinating peripheral neuropathies associated with human T-cell lymphotropic virus type III infection. Ann Neurol 21:32–40, 1987.
122. Miller RG, Storey J, Greco C: Successful treatment of progressive polyradiculopathy in AIDS patients. Neurology 39(Suppl):271, 1989.
123. Mishra BB, Sommers W, Koski CK, Greenstein JI: Acute inflammatory demyelinating polyneuropathy in the acquired immune deficiency syndrome. Ann Neurol 18:131–132, 1985.
124. Morris L, Distenfeld A, Amorosi E, Karpatkin S: Autoimmune thrombocytopenic purpura in homosexual men. Ann Intern Med 96:714–717, 1982.
125. Walsh C, Krigel R, Lennette E, Karpatkin S: Thrombocytopenia in homosexual patients. Ann Intern Med 103:542–545, 1985.
126. Griffin JW, Cornblath DR, Wesselingh SL, et al: HIV-associated inflammatory demyelinating polyneuropathy. Changes in clinical and pathologic features with advancing immunodeficiency. Ann Neurol (in press).
127. McArthur JC, Sipos E, Cornblath DR, et al: Identification of mononuclear cells in CSF of patients with HIV infection. Neurology 39:66–70, 1989.
128. Kiprov D, Pfaeffl W, Parry G, et al: Antibody-mediated peripheral neuropathies associated with ARC and AIDS: Successful treatment with plasmapheresis. J Clin Apheresis 4:3–7, 1988.
129. Lipkin WI, Parry G, Kiprov D, Abrams D: Inflammatory neuropathy in homosexual men with lymphadenopathy. Neurology 35:1479–1483, 1985.
130. Eidelberg D, Sotrel A, Vogel H, et al: Progressive polyradiculopathy in acquired immune deficiency syndrome. Neurology 36:912–916, 1986.
131. Cohen BA, McArthur JC, Grohman S, et al: Neurologic prognosis in CMV polyradiculomyelopathy in AIDS. Neurology 43:493–499, 1993.
132. So YT, Olney RK: Acute lumbosacral polyradiculopathy in acquired immunodeficiency syndrome: Experience in 23 patients. Ann Neurol 35:53–58, 1994.
133. Coxon A, Pallis CA: Metronidazole neuropathy. J Neurol Neurosurg Psychiatry 39:403–405, 1976.
134. Lhermitte F, Fritel D, Cambier J: Polyneurites au cours de traitements par la nitrofurantoine. Presse Med 71:767–768, 1963.
135. Goldstick L, Mandybur TI, Bode R: Spinal cord degeneration in AIDS. Neurology 35:103–106, 1985.
136. Simpson DM, Bender AN: Human immunodeficiency virus–associated myopathy: Analysis of 11 patients. Ann Neurol 24:79–84, 1988.
137. Simpson DM, Citak KA, Godfrey E, et al: Myopathies associated with human immunodeficiency virus and zidovudine—Can their effects be distinguished? Neurology 43:971–976, 1993.
138. Zuger A, Louie E, Holzman RS, et al: Cryptococcal disease in patients with the acquired immunodeficiency syndrome. Diagnostic features and outcome of treatment. Ann Intern Med 104:234–240, 1986.
139. Dismukes WE: Cryptococcal meningitis in patients with AIDS. J Infect Dis 157:624–628, 1988.
140. Denning DW, Armstrong RW, Lewis BH, Stevens DA: Elevated cerebrospinal fluid pressures in patients with cryptococcal meningitis and acquired immunodeficiency syndrome. Am J Med 91:267–272, 1991.
141. Kovacs JA, Kovacs AA, Polis M, et al: Cryptococcosis in the acquired immunodeficiency syndrome. Ann Intern Med 103:533–538, 1985.
142. Mathews VP, Alo PL, Glass JD, et al: AIDS-related CNS cryptococcosis—Radiologic-pathologic correlation. AJNR 13:1477–1486, 1992.
143. Larsen RA, Bozzette SA, Jones BE, et al: Fluconazole combined with flucytosine for treatment of cryptococcal meningitis in patients with AIDS. Clin Infect Dis 19:741–745, 1994.
144. Dismukes WE, Cloud G, Gallis HA, et al: Treatment of cryptococcal meningitis with combination amphotericin B and flucytosine for four as compared with six weeks. N Engl J Med 317:334–341, 1987.
145. Saag MS, Powderly WG, Cloud GA, et al: Comparison of amphotericin B with fluconazole in the treatment of acute AIDS-associated cryptococcal meningitis. N Engl J Med 326:83–89, 1992.
146. Krol G, Becker R, Zimmerman R, et al: Contribution of MRI to the diagnosis of intracranial complications of acquired immune deficiency syndrome. Neuroradiology 99–104, 1985/1986.
147. Zuger A, Schuster M, Simberkoff MS, et al: Maintenance amphotericin B for cryptococcal meningitis in the acquired immunodeficiency syndrome (AIDS). Ann Intern Med 109:592–593, 1988.
148. Goodwin RA, Shapiro JL, Thurman GH, et al: Disseminated histoplasmosis: Clinical and pathological correlations. Medicine (Baltimore) 59:1–33, 1980.
149. Walpole HT, Gregory DW: Cerebral histoplasmosis. South Med J 80:1575–1577, 1987.
150. Wheat LJ, Connolly-Stringfield PA, Baker RL, et al: Disseminated histoplasmosis in the acquired immune deficiency syndrome: Clinical findings, diagnosis and treatment, and review of the literature. Medicine (Baltimore) 69:361–374, 1990.
151. Wheat LJ, Kohler RB, Tewari RP: Diagnosis of disseminated histoplasmosis by detection of *Histoplasma capsulatum* antigen in serum and urine specimens. N Engl J Med 314:83–88, 1986.
152. Wheat LJ, Connolly-Stringfield P, Blair R, et al: Histoplasmosis relapse in patients with AIDS: Detection using *Histoplasma capsulatum* variety *capsulatum* antigen levels. Ann Intern Med 115:936–941, 1991.
153. Grant IH, Gold JWM, Rosenblum M, et al: *Toxoplasma gondii* serology in HIV-infected patients: The development of central nervous system toxoplasmosis in AIDS. AIDS 4:519–521, 1990.
154. Navia BA, Petito CK, Gold JW, et al: Cerebral toxoplasmosis complicating the acquired immune deficiency syndrome: Clinical and neuropathological findings in 27 patients. Ann Neurol 19:224–238, 1986.
155. Marks WJ Jr, McArthur JC, Royal WR, et al: Intracranial mass lesions in AIDS: Diagnosis and response to therapy (Abstr). Neurology 39(Suppl):380, 1989.
156. Luft BJ, Hafner R, Korzun AH, et al: Toxoplasmic encephalitis in patients with the acquired immunodeficiency syndrome. N Engl J Med 329:995–1000, 1993.
157. Rolston KV, Hoy J: Role of clindamycin in the treatment of central nervous system toxoplasmosis. Am J Med 83:551–554, 1987.

158. Saba J, Moriat P, Raffi F, et al: Pyrimethamine plus azithromycin for treatment of acute toxoplasmic encephalitis in patients with AIDS. Eur J Clin Microbiol Infect Dis 12:853–856, 1993.
159. Macapinlac HA, Scott AM, Caluser CI, et al: Utility of Tl-201 SPECT and F-18 FDG PET as an adjunct to CT and MR imaging in the evaluation of metastatic brain tumors (Abstr). Radiology 185(P):233, 1992.
160. Luft BJ, Brooks RG, Conley FK, et al: Toxoplasmic encephalitis in patients with acquired immune deficiency syndrome. JAMA 252:913–917, 1984.
161. Moskowitz LB, Hensley GT, Chan JC, et al: Brain biopsies in patients with acquired immune deficiency syndrome. Arch Pathol Lab Med 108:368–371, 1984.
162. Cohn JA, McMeeking A, Cohen W, et al: Evaluation of the policy of empiric treatment of suspected *Toxoplasma* encephalitis in patients with the acquired immunodeficiency syndrome. Am J Med 86:521–527, 1989.
163. Porter SB, Sande MA: Toxoplasmosis of the central nervous system in acquired immunodeficiency syndrome. N Engl J Med 327:1643–1648, 1992.
164. Jacobson MA, Besch CL, Child C, et al: Primary prophylaxis with pyrimethamine for toxoplasmic encephalitis in patients with advanced human immunodeficiency virus disease: Results of a randomized trial. J Infect Dis 169:384–394, 1994.
165. Edwards RH, Messing R, McKendall RR: Cytomegalovirus meningoencephalitis in a homosexual man with Kaposi's sarcoma: Isolation of CMV from CSF cells. Neurology 35:560–562, 1985.
166. Hawley DA, Schaefer JF, Schulz DM, Muller J: Cytomegalovirus encephalitis in acquired immunodeficiency syndrome. Am J Clin Pathol 80:874–877, 1983.
167. Moskowitz LB, Gregorios JB, Hensley GT, Berger JR: Cytomegalovirus. Induced demyelination associated with acquired immune deficiency syndrome. Arch Pathol Lab Med 108:873–877, 1984.
168. Vinters HV, Kwok MK, Ho HW, et al: Cytomegalovirus in the nervous system of patients with the acquired immune deficiency syndrome. Brain 112:245–268, 1989.
169. Laskin OL, Stahl-Bayliss CM, Morgello S: Concomitant herpes simplex virus type 1 and cytomegalovirus ventriculoencephalitis in acquired immunodeficiency syndrome. Arch Neurol 44:843–847, 1987.
170. Levy RM, Bredesen DE, Rosenblum ML: Opportunistic central nervous system pathology in patients with AIDS. Ann Neurol 23:S7–S12, 1988.
171. Pepose JS, Hilborne LH, Cancilla PA, Foos RY: Concurrent herpes simplex and cytomegalovirus retinitis and encephalitis in the acquired immune deficiency syndrome (AIDS). Ophthalmology 91:1669–1677, 1984.
172. Post MJ, Hensley GT, Moskowitz LB, Fischl M: Cytomegalic inclusion virus encephalitis in patients with AIDS: CT, clinical, and pathologic correlation. AJR 146:1229–1234, 1986.
173. Clifford DB, Buller RS, Mohammed S, et al: Use of polymerase chain reaction to demonstrate cytomegalovirus DNA in CSF of patients with human immunodeficiency virus infection. Neurology 43:75–79, 1993.
174. Holland NR, Power C, Mathews VP, et al: CMV encephalitis in acquired immunodeficiency syndrome (AIDS). Neurology 44:507–514, 1994.
175. Egbert RP, Pollard RB, Gallagher JG, Merigan TC: Cytomegalovirus retinitis in immunosuppressed hosts. II. Ocular manifestations. Ann Intern Med 93:664–670, 1980.
176. Freeman WR, Lerner CW, Mines JA, et al: A prospective study of the ophthalmologic findings in the acquired immune deficiency syndrome. Am J Ophthalmol 97:133–142, 1984.
177. Holland GN, Pepose JS, Pettit TH, et al: Acquired immune deficiency syndrome: Ocular manifestations. Ophthalmology 90:859–873, 1983.
178. Holland GN, Sakamoto MJ, Hardy D, et al: Treatment of cytomegalovirus retinopathy in patients with acquired immunodeficiency syndrome. Arch Ophthalmol 104:1794–1800, 1986.
179. Khadem M, Kalish SB, Goldsmith J, et al: Ophthalmologic findings in acquired immune deficiency syndrome (AIDS). Arch Ophthalmol 102:201–206, 1984.
180. Rosenberg PR, Uliss AE, Friedland GH, et al: Acquired immunodeficiency syndrome: Ophthalmic manifestations in ambulatory patients. Ophthalmology 90:874–878, 1983.
181. Jabs DA, Enger C, Bartlett JG: Cytomegalovirus retinitis and acquired immunodeficiency syndrome. Arch Ophthalmol 107:75–80, 1989.
182. Newsome DA, Green WR, Miller ED, et al: Microvascular aspects of acquired immune deficiency syndrome retinopathy. Am J Ophthalmol 98:590–601, 1984.
183. Roarty JD, Fisher EJ, Nussbaum JJ: Long-term visual morbidity of cytomegalovirus retinitis in patients with acquired immune deficiency syndrome. Ophthalmology 100:1685–1688, 1993.
184. Spector SA, Weingeist T, Pollard RB, et al: A randomized, controlled study of intravenous ganciclovir therapy for cytomegalovirus peripheral retinitis in patients with AIDS. Aids Clinical Trials Group and Cytomegalovirus Cooperative Study Group. J Infect Dis 168:557–563, 1993.
185. Jabs DA: Mortality in patients with the acquired immunodeficiency syndrome treated with either foscarnet or ganciclovir for cytomegalovirus retinitis. N Engl J Med 326:213–220, 1992.
186. Narayan O, Peeney JB, Johnson RT, et al: Etiology of progressive multifocal leukoencephalopathy. Identification of papovavirus. N Engl J Med 289:1278–1282, 1973.
187. Berger JR, Kaszovitz B, Post MJ, Dickinson G: Progressive multifocal leukoencephalopathy associated with human immunodeficiency virus infection. A review of the literature with a report of sixteen cases. Ann Intern Med 107:78–87, 1987.
188. Berger JR, Mucke L: Prolonged survival and partial recovery in AIDS-associated progressive multifocal leukoencephalopathy. Neurology 38:1060–1065, 1988.
189. Telenti A, Marshall WF, Aksamit AJ, et al: Detection of JC virus by polymerase chain reaction in cerebrospinal fluid from two patients with progressive multifocal leukoencephalopathy. Eur J Clin Microbiol Infect Dis 11:253–254, 1992.
190. Jakobsen J, Diemer NH, Gaub J, et al: Progressive multifocal leukoencephalopathy in a patient without other clinical manifestations of AIDS. Acta Neurol Scand 75:209–213, 1987.
191. Speelman JD, ter Schegget J, Bots GT, et al: Progressive multifocal leukoencephalopathy in a case of acquired immune deficiency syndrome. Clin Neurol Neurosurg 87:27–33, 1985.
192. Dube MP, Holtom PD, Larsen RA: Tuberculous meningitis in patients with and without human immunodeficiency virus infection. Am J Med 93:520–524, 1992.
193. Bishburg E, Sunderam G, Reichman LB, Kapila R: Central nervous system tuberculosis with the acquired immunodeficiency syndrome and its related complex. Ann Intern Med 105:210–213, 1986.
194. Shafer RW, Kim DS, Weiss JP, Quale JM: Extrapulmonary tuberculosis in patients with human immunodeficiency virus infection. Medicine (Baltimore) 70:384–397, 1991.
195. Berenguer J, Moreno S, Laguna F, et al: Tuberculous meningitis in patients infected with the human immunodeficiency virus. N Engl J Med 326:668–672, 1992.
196. Doll DC, Yarbro JW, Phillips K, Klott C: Mycobacterial spinal cord abscess with an ascending polyneuropathy (Letter) [published erratum in Ann Intern Med 106:784, 1987]. Ann Intern Med 106:333–334, 1987.
197. Kramer F, Modilevsky T, Waliany AR, et al: Delayed diagnosis of tuberculosis in patients with human immunodeficiency virus infection. Am J Med 89:451–456, 1990.
198. Stoneburner R, Laroche E, Prevots R, et al: Survival in a cohort of human immunodeficiency virus–infected tuberculosis patients in New York City. Implications for the expansion of the AIDS case definition. Arch Intern Med 152:2033–2037, 1992.
199. Chawla PK, Klapper PJ, Kamholz SL, et al: Drug-resistant tuberculosis in an urban population including patients at risk for human immunodeficiency virus infection. Am Rev Respir Dis 146:280–284, 1992.
200. Monno L, Angarano G, Carbonara S, et al: Emergence of drug-resistant *Mycobacterium tuberculosis* in HIV-infected patients (Letter). Lancet 337:852, 1991.
201. Hook EW: Syphilis and HIV infection. J Infect Dis 160:530–534, 1989.
202. Johns DR, Tierney M, Felsenstein D: Alteration in the natural history of neurosyphilis by concurrent infection with the human immunodeficiency virus. N Engl J Med 316:1569–1572, 1987.
203. Passo MS, Rosenblum JT: Ocular syphilis in patients with human immunodeficiency virus infection. Am J Ophthalmol 106:1–6, 1988.

204. Hicks CB, Benson PM, Lupton GP, Tramont EC: Seronegative secondary syphilis in a patient infected with the human immunodeficiency virus (HIV) Kaposi sarcoma. Ann Intern Med 107:492–495, 1987.
205. Lukehart SA, Hook EW 3d, Baker-Zander SA, et al: Invasion of the central nervous system by *Treponema pallidum*: Implications for diagnosis and treatment. Ann Intern Med 109:855–862, 1988.
206. Gordon SM, Eaton ME, George R, et al: The response of symptomatic neurosyphilis to high-dose intravenous penicillin G in patients with human immunodeficiency virus infection. N Engl J Med 331:1469–1473, 1994.
207. Centers for Disease Control: Leads from the MMWR. Recommendations for diagnosing and treating syphilis in HIV-infected patients. JAMA 260:2488–2489, 1988.
208. Rosenblum ML, Levy RM, Bredesen DE, et al: Primary central nervous system lymphomas in patients with AIDS. Ann Neurol 23:S13–S16, 1988.
209. Baumgartner JE, Rachlin JR, Beckstead JH, et al: Primary central nervous system lymphomas: Natural history and response to radiation therapy in 55 patients with acquired immunodeficiency syndrome. J Neurosurg 73:206–211, 1990.
210. Snider WD, Simpson DM, Aronyk KE, Nielsen SL: Primary lymphoma of the nervous system associated with acquired immune-deficiency syndrome (Letter). N Engl J Med 308:45, 1983.
211. Hochberg FH, Miller G, Schooley RT, et al: Central nervous system lymphoma related to Epstein-Barr virus. N Engl J Med 309:745–748, 1983.
212. Ziegler JL, Beckstead JA, Volberding PA, et al: Non-Hodgkin's lymphoma in 90 homosexual men. Relation to generalized lymphoadenopathy and the acquired immunodeficiency syndrome. N Engl J Med 311:565–570, 1984.
213. Collaborative DHPG Treatment Study Group: Treatment of serious cytomegalovirus with 9-(1,2-dihydroxy-2-propoxymethyl)-guanine in patients with AIDS and other immunodeficiencies. N Engl J Med 314:801–805, 1986.
214. Richman DD, Fischl MA, Grieco MH, et al: The toxicity of azidothymidine (AZT) in the treatment of patients with AIDS and AIDS-related complex. N Engl J Med 317:192–197, 1987.
215. Engstrom JW, Lowenstein DH, Bredesen DE: Cerebral infarctions and transient neurologic deficits associated with acquired immunodeficiency syndrome. Am J Med 86:528–532, 1989.
216. Mizusawa H, Hirano A, Llena JF, Shintaku M: Cerebrovascular lesions in acquired immune deficiency syndrome (AIDS). Acta Neuropathol (Berl) 76:451–457, 1988.
217. Yankner BA, Skolnik PR, Shoukimas GM, et al: Cerebral granulomatous angiitis associated with isolation of human T-lymphotropic virus type III from the central nervous system. Ann Neurol 20:362–364, 1986.

126

Human Immunodeficiency Virus Serology and Viral Burden

John G. Bartlett

Human immunodeficiency virus (HIV) is usually detected with HIV serology, although it is occasionally desirable to use other methods to demonstrate antibody or antigen. There has been interest in and emphasis on measurement of viral concentration in plasma as a measure of viral "burden" to facilitate decisions regarding antiviral therapy.

Human Immunodeficiency Virus Serology

Standard criteria for a positive test are a repeatedly positive enzyme-linked immunosorbent assay (ELISA) followed by a positive Western blot (Table 126–1). Criteria for a positive test are somewhat variable for interpretation of Western blots. The criteria of the Centers for Disease Control and Prevention and the Association of State and Territorial Public Health Laboratory Directors are based on two of the following: p24, gp41, and gp120/160.

The predictive value depends on seroprevalence rates in the population of patients being tested. False-negative results for a high-prevalence population such as injection drug users with a seroprevalence rate of about 30% occur in 0.3%[1] and for a low-prevalence population such as Red Cross blood donors in 0.001%.[2, 3] The usual cause of false-negative test results is the window period between the time of viral transmission and seroconversion, a period that occasionally exceeds 3 months and rarely exceeds 6 months. An occasional cause of false-negative results is related to the subtype of HIV. Subtypes are designated A-H, M, and O on the basis of genetic variation; the distribution varies with geography. The predominant subtypes are B in North America and Europe, B and F in South America, B and F in Asia, and A-H in Africa. The routine serologic test readily detects A-H but does not detect subtype O, found primarily in Cameroon.[4, 5] Rare cases of subtype O have been found in the United States, and there is concern that this or another genetic variant in the future may reduce the sensitivity of routine HIV serology. HIV type 2 (HIV-2) is another genetic variant with a distinctive serologic pattern, reduced virulence, reduced efficiency of transmission, and a source primarily in West Africa.[6, 7] As of June 30, 1995, there were 62 patients in the United States with this strain and most could be traced to a West African contact.[8] About 80% of HIV-2–infected patients have a positive ELISA with routine HIV type 1 (HIV-1) serology and Western blots that are weakly reactive, so most are either negative or have indeterminate results.[6] Serologic tests for HIV-2 and for combined HIV-1 and HIV-2 are available and routinely used in Red Cross screening.[7] Another cause of false-negative results is the presence of agammaglobulinemia.

The frequency of false-positive results in a low-prevalence population is 1 per 135,000 or 0.0007%.[9] A single case of a false-positive test ascribed to autoantibodies has been reported for a patient with lupus erythematosus.[10] The most common cause of false-positive tests is vaccination. A review of 266 volunteers in vaccine studies showed that 68% had a positive ELISA and 0% to 44% had a positive Western blot, depending on the criteria used for interpretation and the immunogen used for vaccination.[11] Occasional patients report factitious positive HIV serology, emphasizing the need to repeat tests for some patients with unverified claims.[12]

Results showing a positive ELISA and a single band on a Western blot are usually reported as indeterminate results. Studies with blood donors show that this occurs in approximately 2 per 10,000; results in the Johns Hopkins Hospital laboratory indicate that about 10% of the specimens that are positive with ELISA screening are indeterminate by the Western blot. Possible causes are the following: seroconversion is occurring, usually with p24 antibody as the first to appear; there is advanced HIV infection with decreased titers of antibodies, primarily anti-p24; there are cross-reacting alloantibodies from blood transfusions, pregnancy, or organ transplantation; there are autoantibodies as seen with some collagen-vascular diseases, malignancy, or autoimmune diseases; there is infection with HIV-2 or there is HIV vaccine exposure. The most important factor in the interpretation of indeterminate results is a careful review of the risk profile.

TABLE 126–1 ■ Tests for Human Immunodeficiency Virus Type 1 and Viral Burden*

ASSAY	$CD4^+$ CELL COUNTS	% POSITIVE (SENSITIVITY)	COMMENTS
Routine serology	>3 mo after viral transmission	99.7%–99.99%	Readily available and inexpensive.
Rapid tests SUDS (Murex) RLAA (Cambridge Biotech)	>3 mo after viral transmission	99.95%	Advantage is that test results are available in ≤10 min. There are two commercial suppliers of FDA-approved reagents. Specificity is 99.6%, so positive tests should be confirmed. Tests are highly sensitive, so negative tests do not usually require confirmation.[18, 19]
p24 antigen	200–500/mm^3	20%	Measures free viral antigen by EIA and indicates a high viral load.[20]
	<200/mm^3	37%–95%	Infrequently used in practice because of relative insensitivity and lack of clear guidelines for using results. Potential advantages are that it is inexpensive and readily available with numerous suppliers of commercial kits. It is most useful for detecting acute retroviral syndrome, staging, evaluating the rate of progression, and therapeutic monitoring in clinical trials. A 50% decrease (×2) indicates a significant response to treatment. Newer techniques (quantitative PCR and bDNA) have largely replaced p24 antigen for therapeutic monitoring.
Immune complex–dissociated p24 (ICD p24)	200–500/mm^3 <200/mm^3	45%–70% 75%–100%	Acid treatment increases detection of p24 antigen because of its release from immune complexes.
Plasma RNA viremia	>500/mm^3 <200/mm^3	Rare 75%–100%	Detection of cell-free virus in plasma indicates active replication; persistence of plasma viremia is a sign of poor prognosis. Rates of recovery are inversely related to $CD4^+$ cell counts. Samples containing >30 pg of p24 antigen by EIA are usually positive.
Peripheral blood mononuclear cell culture	<500/mm^3	95%–100%	Expensive and labor-intensive. The test is nearly always positive at all stages and during treatment. Quantitative yield correlates with stage: mean titer 20 per 10^6 cells in asymptomatic patients and 2200 per 10^6 cells in patients with AIDS.[21, 30] The greatest potential use is for therapeutic monitoring. A 10-fold decrease in titer is significant. Quantitative RNA PCR and bDNA assays are less expensive and generally preferred.
DNA PCR assay	All stages	99%–100%	Qualitative DNA PCR is used to detect cell-associated proviral DNA; primers are commercially available from Roche Laboratories. Sensitivity approaches 100%, but rigorous quality assurance is necessary. Its main use is in viral detection: acute viral syndrome, neonatal HIV infection, and confused or challenged serologic assays.
Quantitative RNA PCR			RNA PCR to detect proviral RNA shows good reproducibility (≤twofold differences between laboratories; three- to fourfold changes or 0.5 log considered significant). Threshold for detection is 200–500 copies per mL.[34] Most laboratories report titers ranging from 10^2 to 10^6 copies per mL.
Quantitative bDNA			Quantitative bDNA shows reproducibility comparable to that of quantitative RNA PCR. Its major use is for therapeutic monitoring and for staging.[21, 26] The detection threshold with first-generation tests is 10,000 copies per mL; for second-generation tests it is about 200 copies per mL; for third-generation tests it is about 25 copies per mL.

*FDA, U.S. Food and Drug Administration; EIA, enzyme immunoassay; PCR, polymerase chain reaction; bDNA, branched chain DNA; AIDS, acquired immunodeficiency syndrome.

Patients in low-risk categories with indeterminate tests are almost never infected with HIV; repeated tests often show persistence of a single band, and the cause of this pattern is usually not determined.[13] The usual recommendation is to repeat tests to detect patients who are in the process of seroconverting at 2 to 3 months, when definitive results are expected.

Alternative Human Immunodeficiency Virus Antibody Detection Methods

The usual justifications for using alternative techniques for detecting HIV antibody are to improve acceptance by patients, to clarify inconsistent or challenged serologic results, and to decrease the lag time for results.

Home test kits have been developed that show good sensitivity and specificity. These are available in drug stores with blood samples submitted on filter strips for enzyme immunoassay and Western blot. The consumer mails the sample to a reference laboratory and obtains results by telephone.[14] Acceptance by the public has been good.[15] The initial experience is that about 1% of samples are positive. One concern is emotional reactions and possible suicides, although there is currently no evidence that this would be problematic.[14] In a population-based survey, 42% of respondents indicated that they would consider use of this test.[15]

Salivary tests and urine tests have been developed for detection of HIV antibody. The goal here is to improve patients' acceptance of testing by offering an alternative to blood sampling. This may be used for a screening ELISA or more definitive tests using the screening ELISA plus Western blotting.[16, 17]

Rapid tests are available that provide preliminary results within 10 minutes with accuracy analogous to that of ELISA screening.[18] Initial results with 6200 samples showed 100% sensitivity and a specificity of 98.9% to 100%.[18] These tests are attractive for use in clinical settings, where immediate results are often important for management decisions. An example is an occupational needlestick exposure involving a source with unknown HIV serologic status; the results of the rapid test would be used to assist counseling and the decision about prophylaxis. The rapid test might also be useful for screening in clinical settings in which compliance with follow-up visits may be difficult to achieve, such as emergency rooms or sexually transmitted disease clinics.[19]

Viral Detection

Alternatives to serology for HIV detection include techniques for detecting HIV antigen, viral isolation, or HIV polymerase chain reaction (PCR) (see Table 126–1). These tests are considered inferior to routine serology in terms of sensitivity, specificity, technical requirements, and/or cost. For this reason, use is usually restricted to the following clinical situations: routine serologic tests provide confusing results or results that are challenged; there is a need to clarify indeterminate serology; the patient has a cause for false-negative tests such as agammaglobulinemia; the patient is seen early in the course of infection before seroconversion; or there is a need for detection of neonatal infection. Viral culture may also be desirable for genetic mapping to determine the source of infection, as in the case of the Florida dentist who became the source of infection for six of his patients. In some therapeutic trials, viral culture is performed to determine phenotype (such as syncytium-inducing strains versus non–syncytium-inducing strains) and it may be used to determine antiviral susceptibilities; these studies are not used routinely for clinical monitoring but may be in the future. None of these alternative tests for HIV detection should be done to circumvent the informed consent process required for HIV serology.

The sensitivity of these tests for HIV detection depends on the test method and the stage of disease. It is usually reported as higher than 99% for DNA PCR and 95% to 100% for viral culture of peripheral blood mononuclear cells, and it is substantially less for plasma cultures or p24 antigen detection.[20–24] The p24 antigen assay is often used to establish the diagnosis of the acute HIV syndrome noted before seroconversion because of sensitivity, ease of performance, and low cost. This test measures free viral antigen by enzyme immunoassay, and a positive assay generally indicates a relatively high viral load. The test is positive for nearly all patients with acute HIV infection when concentrations of HIV in plasma are high; the sensitivity is only about 20% for asymptomatic patients with $CD4^+$ cell counts of 200 to 500/mm^3, and the test is positive for 37% to 95% of patients with a $CD4^+$ cell count less than 200/mm^3. Acid treatment to disrupt antigen-antibody complexes increases the sensitivity at least twofold. Detection of cell-free virus in plasma indicates active replication, so persistence of this observation is thought to be a poor prognostic sign.[25] HIV RNA viremia is rarely found in asymptomatic patients in early-stage disease ($CD4^+$ cell count greater than 500/mm^3), and it is found in 75% to 100% of patients with $CD4^+$ cell counts less than 200/mm^3. Cultures of peripheral blood mononuclear cells are nearly always positive throughout the course of HIV infection, but the test is expensive and labor-intensive. HIV DNA PCR assays are used to detect cell-associated proviral DNA. Sensitivities approach 100%, but there is a need for rigorous quality assurance.

Measurement of Viral Burden

There is rapidly increasing interest in monitoring concentrations of HIV in blood as a reflection of the viral burden. This information is potentially useful for determining the clinical staging of a patient with HIV infection, evaluating the response to experimental drugs, and therapeutic monitoring. There are four major methods for assessing the viral burden in peripheral blood: quantitative culture of HIV in plasma, quantitative culture of HIV in peripheral blood mononuclear cells, quantitation of p24 antigen, and measurement of plasma RNA levels (see Table 126–1).

A p24 antigen assay is often favored for the diagnosis of the acute retroviral syndrome, because the high levels of plasma viremia ensure positive results with a test that is readily available, technically easy, and inexpensive. During the acute infection, the antigen levels are usually in the range of 1200 to 4200 pg/mL; levels become undetectable 7 to 12 days after symptoms resolve.[24]

Cultures of HIV in peripheral blood mononuclear cells may be done with titration to determine the number of infected cells. The mean titer is about 20 per 10^6 cells in asymptomatic patients and 2200 per 10^6 cells in patients with acquired immunodeficiency syndrome.[21] The problem is that the work is labor-intensive and expensive.

Measurement of plasma RNA levels is the most practical way to evaluate viral load for the purposes of therapeutic monitoring and staging HIV infection. The viral load is determined by measuring branched chain DNA or quantitative RNA PCR. Reagents for these assays are now commercially available, although the threshold for detection indicating sensitivity of the assay is variable, depending on the methods and reagents used. With quantitative PCR and second-generation branched chain DNA tests, the threshold for detection is approximately 200 to 500 copies per milliliter. Studies of the natural history of HIV and cross-sectional studies show high viral concentrations of 10^5 to 10^8 copies per milliliter during the acute HIV syndrome, a rapid decrease to 10^2 to 10^5 per milliliter after recovery, and a direct correlation between viral concentration or set point and rate of progression based on time of survival, time to an acquired immunodeficiency syndrome–defining diagnosis and rate of $CD4^+$ cell decline.[25–32] Quality assurance testing shows good reproducibility between laboratories performing these tests and a three- to fourfold change (0.5 log) is considered significant.[33] In terms of interpretation, the goal of therapy is often "no detectable virus" indicating a concentration below the threshold of detection. Therapeutic trials show that the decrease usually achieved with antiviral agents is 0.5 to 0.7 log/mL for nucleoside analogs, 0.8 to 1.5 log/mL for nucleoside analog combinations, and up to 2 to 3 log/mL for protease inhibitors combined with nucleoside analogs. The time to respond to treatment begins within hours and approaches a maximum at 3 to 4 weeks. In general, a 1-log decrease corresponds to an average increase in $CD4^+$ cell count of approximately 50 to 80/mm^3.[28, 30] Sequential samples over time showed relatively stable HIV RNA levels with increases exceeding 10-fold (1 log) in only 6 of 42 subjects followed for 3 to 11 years.[34] This study also showed that the mean level among patients who progressed to the acquired immunodeficiency syndrome in less than 4 years was about 10^4 per mL; it was about 10^3 per mL for those who progressed in 4 to 9 years and about 10^2 per mL for those who did not develop the acquired immunodeficiency syndrome within 6 to 11 years. The four factors associated with substantial increases in viral burden are disease progression, a failing treatment regimen, an intercurrent infection such as tuberculosis or cytomegalovirus disease, and immunizations.

References

1. Farzadegan H, Vlahov D, Solomon L, et al: Detection of human immunodeficiency virus type 1 infection by polymerase chain reaction in a cohort of seronegative intravenous drug users. J Infect Dis 168:327–331, 1993.
2. Van de Perre P, Simonon A, Msellati P, et al: Postnatal transmission of human immunodeficiency virus type 1 from mother to infant. N Engl J Med 325:593–598, 1991.
3. Busch MP, Eble BE, Khayam-Bashi H, et al: Evaluation of screened blood donations for human immunodeficiency virus type 1 infection by culture and DNA amplification of pooled cells. N Engl J Med 325:1–5, 1991.
4. Loussert-Ajaka I, Ly TD, Chaix ML, et al: HIV-1/HIV-2 seronegativity in HIV-1 subtype O infected patients. Lancet 343:1393–1394, 1994.
5. De Cock KM, Adjorlolo G, Ekpini E, et al: Epidemiology and transmission of HIV-2. Why there is no HIV-2 pandemic. JAMA 270:2083–2086, 1993.
6. Markovitz DM: Infection with the human immunodeficiency virus type 2. Ann Intern Med 118:211–218, 1993.
7. George JR, Rayfield MA, Phillips S, et al: Efficacies of U.S. Food and Drug Administration–licensed HIV-1 screening enzyme immunoassays for detecting antibodies to HIV-2. AIDS 4:321–326, 1990.
8. Centers for Disease Control and Prevention: Update: HIV-2 infection among blood and plasma donors—United States, June 1992–June 1995. MMWR Morb Mortal Wkly Rep 44:603–606, 1995.
9. Burke DS, Brundage JF, Redfield RR, et al: Measurement of false positive rate in a screening program for human immunodeficiency virus infection. N Engl J Med 319:961–964, 1988.
10. Jindal R, Solomon M, Burrows L: False positive tests for HIV in a woman with lupus and renal failure. N Engl J Med 328:1281–1282, 1993.
11. Belshe RB, Clements ML, Keefer MC, et al: Interpreting HIV serodiagnostic test results in the 1990s: Social risks of HIV vaccine studies in uninfected volunteers. Ann Intern Med 121:584–589, 1994.
12. Craven DE, Steger KA, La Chappelle R, Allen DM: Factitious HIV infection: The importance of documenting infection. Ann Intern Med 121:763–766, 1994.
13. Jackson JB, MacDonald KL, Cadwell J, et al: Absence of HIV infection in blood donors with indeterminate Western blot tests for antibody to HIV-1. N Engl J Med 322:217–222, 1990.
14. Bayer R, Stryker J, Smith MD: Testing for HIV infection at home. N Engl J Med 332:1296–1299, 1995.
15. Phillips KA, Flatt SJ, Morrison KR, Coates TJ: Potential use of home HIV testing. N Engl J Med 332:1308–1310, 1995.
16. Ishikawa S, Hashida S, Hashinaka K, et al: Diagnosis of HIV-1 infection with whole saliva by detection of antibody IgG to HIV-1 with ultrasensitive enzyme immunoassay using recombinant reverse transcriptase as antigen. J Acquir Immune Defic Syndr Hum Retrovirol 10:41–47, 1995.
17. Emmons WW, Paparello SF, Decker CF, et al: A modified ELISA and Western blot accurately determine anti–human immunodeficiency virus type 1 antibodies in oral fluids obtained with a special collecting device. J Infect Dis 171:1406–1410, 1995.
18. Malone JD, Smith ES, Sheffield J, et al: Comparative evaluation of six rapid serological tests for HIV-1 antibody. J Acquir Immune Defic Syndr 6:115–119, 1993.
19. Kassler WJ, Haley C, Jones WK, et al: Performance of a rapid, on-site human immunodeficiency virus antibody assay in a public health setting. J Clin Microbiol 33:2899–2902, 1995.
20. Hammer S, Crumpacker C, D'Aquila R, et al: Use of virologic assays for detection of human immunodeficiency virus in clinical trials: Recommendation of the AIDS Clinical Trials Group Virology Committee. J Clin Microbiol 31:2557–2564, 1993.
21. Ho DD, Moudgil T, Alam M: Quantitation of human immunodeficiency virus type 1 in the blood of infected persons. N Engl J Med 321:1621–1625, 1989.
22. Burke DS, Fowler AK, Redfield RR, et al: Isolation of HIV-1 from the blood of seropositive adults: Patient stage of illness and sample inoculum size are major determinants of a positive culture. J Acquir Immune Defic Syndr 3:1159–1167, 1990.
23. Aoki-Sei S, Yarchoan R, Kageyama S, et al: Plasma HIV-1 viremia in HIV-1 infected individuals assessed by polymerase chain reaction. AIDS Res Hum Retroviruses 8:1263–1270, 1992.
24. Daar ES, Moudgil T, Meyer RD, Ho DD: Transient high levels of viremia in patients with primary human immunodeficiency virus type 1 infection. N Engl J Med 324:961–964, 1991.
25. Ruffault A, Michelet C, Jacquelinet C, et al: The prognostic value of plasma viremia in HIV-infected patients under AZT treatment: A two-year follow-up study. J Acquir Immune Defic Syndr Hum Retrovirol 9:243–248, 1995.
26. Dewar RL, Highbarger HC, Sarmiento MD, et al: Application of branched DNA signal amplification to monitor human immunodeficiency virus type 1 burden in human plasma. J Infect Dis 170:1172–1179, 1994.
27. Henrard DR, Daar E, Farzadegan H, et al: Virologic and immunologic characterization of symptomatic and asymptomatic primary HIV-1 infection. J Acquir Immune Defic Syndr Hum Retrovirol 9:305–310, 1995.
28. Ho DD, Neumann AU, Perelson AS, et al: Rapid turnover of plasma virions and CD4 lymphocytes in HIV-1 infection. Nature 373:123–126, 1995.
29. Pantaleo G, Graziosi C, Fauci AS: The immunopathogenesis of human immunodeficiency virus infection. N Engl J Med 328:327–335, 1993.
30. Wei X, Ghosh SK, Taylor ME, et al: Viral dynamics in human immunodeficiency virus type 1 infection. Nature 373:117–122, 1995.
31. Mellors JW, Kingsley LA, Rinaldo CR, et al: Quantitation of HIV-1 RNA in plasma predicts outcome after seroconversion. Ann Intern Med 122:573–579, 1995.
32. Lee T-H, Sheppard HW, Reis M, et al. Circulating HIV-1 infected cell burden from seroconversion to AIDS. J Acquir Immune Defic Syndr 7:381–389, 1994.
33. Lin HJ, Myers LE, Yen-Lieberman B, et al: Multicenter evaluation of methods for the quantitation of plasma human immunodeficiency virus type 1 RNA. J Infect Dis 170:194–198, 1994.
34. Henrard DR, Phillips JF, Muenz LR, et al: Natural history of HIV-1 cell-free viremia. JAMA 274:554–558, 1995.

127

Antiretroviral Treatment

John G. Bartlett

Treatment of human immunodeficiency virus (HIV) infection began with zidovudine (azidothymidine, AZT) with the demonstration in 1986 that this drug reduced rates of progression to acquired immunodeficiency syndrome (AIDS) and increased survival.[1] The next 9 years of drug development and therapeutic trials resulted in a lineage of new drugs in the nucleoside analog class including didanosine (ddI), zalcitabine (ddC), stavudine (d4T), and lamivudine (3TC). These drugs provided the foundation for recommendations for antiviral treatment by the expert panel representing guidelines of the U.S. Public Health Service made in June 1993.[2] During the next 3 years, there were dramatic changes that notably altered therapeutic recommendations. These changes are in five major categories:

1. Studies of HIV kinetics showed rapid replication of HIV throughout the course of the disease with an average of approximately 10^{10} new virions daily.[3] Conclusions are that the mean half-life of HIV in plasma is 6 hours and the half-life of the infected CD4$^+$ cell is only 1.6 days. The implication is that 99% of viral production is from recently infected cells. Furthermore, each cycle of HIV replication is associated with the production of genetic variants, so high levels of replication result in enormous genetic diversity, including strains that are drug resistant.

2. The second major development was the use of quantitative methods to determine concentrations of HIV RNA in plasma referred to as viral load or viral burden. Using stored serum samples collected during 10 years in a natural history study of HIV, Mellors and colleagues[4, 5] defined the history of HIV infection in terms of viral burden. This work demonstrated that acute HIV infection is associated with high-level HIV viremia in concentrations that often exceed 10^7 per mL. After immune response, primarily a cytotoxic T-cell response, the patient establishes a "set point" that remains relatively stable for a period of years in the absence of treatment. This set point appears to dictate the rate of disease progression independently of the CD4$^+$ cell count. The average patient, in the absence of treatment, progresses to an AIDS-defining diagnosis during 9 to 10 years after viral transmission and has an average viral burden of 10^3 to 10^4 copies per mL. Higher concentrations are associated with a more rapid progression, and "chronic nonprogressors" (patients with a normal CD4$^+$ cell count for 8 years in the absence of treatment) have mean concentrations lower than 10^2 per mL. Studies of antiviral agents show significant changes in viral burden within days, and this test is consequently favored for therapeutic monitoring.

3. The third development was the introduction of a new series of drugs for HIV, protease inhibitors, that became available in late 1995.[6, 7] The protease inhibitors are much more potent against HIV than are nucleoside analogs, especially with combination treatment. These second-generation drugs were then followed by additional agents including nonnucleoside reverse transcriptase inhibitors, hydroxyurea, and invirase inhibitors. By 1997, there were nine U.S. Food and Drug Administration (FDA)–approved drugs available for HIV infection and a long list of additional drugs in therapeutic trials.

4. Concurrent with the increasing availability of new drugs were several studies demonstrating superiority of combination therapy in terms of viral burden, CD4$^+$ cell slope (the rate of decline of the number of CD4$^+$ cells), and rates of progression.[8–10] By 1996, it became clear that the original guidelines of the U.S. Public Health Service from 1993 were badly antiquated. Their major recommendation was for zidovudine monotherapy until there was clinical failure or toxicity, but several studies showed that this tactic could no longer be recommended.

5. The foregoing sequence of events was also accompanied by a disturbing trend in resistance ascribed to point mutations on specific codons that reduced susceptibility to specific agents with variable frequency and severity.[11–14] Many authorities pointed to analogies with tuberculosis in terms of concerns about resistance in community strains as well as individual patients. With selected agents (protease inhibitors, nonnucleoside reverse transcriptase inhibitors, zidovudine, and lamivudine), there was emphasis on the critical importance of rigid adherence to guidelines using combination treatment with appropriate dosage, uninterrupted treatment, and compliance.

This evolution of events transformed HIV therapeutics from a simplistic strategy with limited options and limited benefits to highly complex, although often controversial, treatments involving multiple combinations of drugs with complicated patterns of toxicity, drug interactions, resistance profiles, and efficacy based on viral burden, CD4$^+$ cell slope, or clinical progression. Although complicated, the new therapeutic regimens appeared to be on the horizon of transforming HIV from an inevitably progressive disease to one in which appropriate therapy offered the probability of clinical stability for sustained periods for most patients. Some even entertained the notion of a cure with aggressive therapy, especially if applied in early-stage disease. A major limitation in formulating generally accepted guidelines based on consensus has been the fact that observations of in vitro activity, studies of natural history and pathogenesis, and trials using viral burden end points evolved far more rapidly than did controlled trials to confirm clinical benefit.

Natural History

The natural history of HIV[15] is summarized in Figure 127–1. This shows the sequence of events from transmission of virus to death for the average patient in the absence of antiviral therapy. After viral acquisition, there is the acute retroviral syndrome accompanied by high-level viremia and variable expression of symptoms[16, 17] (Table 127–1). This syndrome is an acute febrile illness that is often accompanied by pharyngitis, lymphadenopathy, aphthous ulcers, variable neurologic complications, lymphopenia with a low CD4$^+$ cell count, and high-level HIV viremia detected with p24 antigen or quantitative HIV polymerase chain reaction. Standard serologic test results are negative or indeterminate. Symptoms last 1 to 3 weeks and are usually accompanied by weight loss. Occasional patients develop opportunistic infections during the acute illness stage, including thrush or *Pneumocystis carinii* pneumonia. Recovery from the acute illness is largely ascribed to immune response, especially cytotoxic T-cell response, followed by seroconversion and reduced viral load.

The subsequent course of HIV infection is determined by multiple factors that are independent of antiviral therapy. The major correlates with rate of progression are the viral

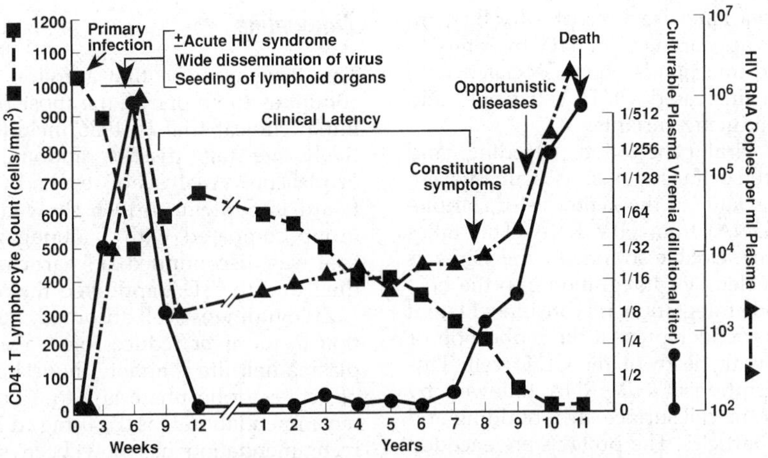

FIGURE 127–1. □ Natural history of HIV infection showing CD4$^+$ cell count *(squares)*, plasma HIV RNA concentrations *(triangles)*, and cultivable plasma viremia *(circles)*. The initial event at 5 to 30 days after virus transmission is the acute retroviral syndrome associated with high concentrations of plasma HIV RNA and a decline in the CD4$^+$ cell count. This is followed by the cytotoxic CD8$^+$ cell response with clinical recovery and a decrease in plasma concentrations of HIV RNA copies. The decline in CD4$^+$ cell count averages 30 to 60/mm^3 per year in the absence of antiretroviral treatment. The rate of progression averages 9.1 years from the time of seroconversion to an AIDS-defining diagnosis, the median survival after the CD4$^+$ cell count reaches 200/mm^3 or less is 2.7 years, and the median survival after an AIDS-defining event is 1.3 years. The viral load reaches a plateau at about 6 months after the acute retroviral syndrome; this concentration, or set point, correlates directly with rates of progression.[4] Individual patients show great variation in viral RNA concentrations and rates of progression presumably related to variations in HIV virulence,[21] immune response,[19] genetic determination of receptor sites,[22] age,[23] and therapy.[25] (Reprinted with permission from Haynes BF, Panteleo G, Fauci AS: Toward an understanding of the correlates of protective immunity to HIV infection. Science 271:324–328, 1996. Copyright 1996 American Association for the Advancement of Science.)

burden or set point[5] established at about 6 months after the acute retroviral syndrome and the CD4$^+$ cell slope.[18] Large population-based studies show the average CD4$^+$ cell count slope is a reduction of 30 to 60 cells per mm^3 per year and the mean viral burden is stable at 10^3 to 10^4 copies per mL. Lymphoid tissue (e.g., lymph nodes, tonsils, spleen) is the primary site of HIV replication. Virus produced in lymphatic tissue is rapidly transmitted to the plasma compartment, so that quantitative plasma HIV RNA reflects the number of infected cells. Patients who have rapid progression of illness usually have a steep CD4$^+$ cell slope accompanied by high viral burden, often 10^5 to 10^6 copies per mL. At the other extreme are chronic nonprogressors, sometimes defined as patients with CD4$^+$ cell counts in the normal range (usually exceeding 500/mm^3) for 8 to 10 years after HIV transmission in the absence of antiviral treatment.[19] Some patients have a relatively stable CD4$^+$ cell count for years and then experience a continuous decline; others have a gradual decline with a change toward a more rapid decline. This change in the CD4$^+$ cell slope is referred to as the inflection point.

TABLE 127–1 ■ Clinical Features of Acute Human Immunodeficiency Virus Syndrome

Symptomatic disease: 50%[17]–89%[16]
Frequency of correct diagnosis with medical consultation: 25%[16]
Incubation period (HIV exposure to onset of symptoms): 2–6 wk[17]
Symptoms and signs[17*]

Fever	96%	Diarrhea	32%
Adenopathy	74%	Nausea or vomiting	27%
Pharyngitis	70%	Hepatosplenomegaly	14%
Rash	70%	Thrush	12%
Myalgias	54%	Meningoencephalitis	6%
Headache	32%	Peripheral neuropathy	6%

Duration of symptoms (mean): 1–2 wk
Laboratory tests: p24 antigenemia (1200–4200 pg/mL), plasma viremia with high titer (peak of 10^5–10^7 copies per mL), high-titer HIV-1 in peripheral blood mononuclear cells (10^2–10^4 tissue culture infective doses per mL), HIV-1 serologic test negative

*Metaanalysis of 209 reported cases.[17]

Longitudinal, cohort studies such as the Multicenter AIDS Cohort Study show that the median time from seroconversion to an AIDS-defining diagnosis in the absence of therapy is 9.1 years; the frequency of a delay of 12 years or more is 32% to 40%, of a delay of 16 years is 19% to 25%, and of a delay of 20 or more years is 10% to 17%. There is no discrete group in this cohort with no eventual CD4$^+$ cell decline, suggesting that the great majority eventually have progressive disease. Others have shown that 10% to 15% of untreated patients are chronic nonprogressors, but after 16 years only 3% to 5% are in this category.[20] Variables that dictate rates of progression are incompletely understood, although it is known that defective viruses explain slow progression in occasional patients[21] and genetic variation in susceptibility of receptor sites may play a role[22]; the most important factor appears to be the host antiviral immune response,[15] which is influenced by age[23] and major histocompatibility complex genes.[24] In general, the CD4$^+$ cell slope and the viral burden are independent predictors of progression, but they also show the anticipated correlation with high HIV counts correlated with rapid declines in CD4$^+$ cell slope and low counts correlated with relatively stable CD4$^+$ cell counts. Nevertheless, there are notable exceptions in both directions, for example, patients with rapid CD4$^+$ cell decline despite relatively low viral burden and those with stable CD4$^+$ cell counts in the presence of a high viral burden.

HIV infection is largely an infection of CD4$^+$ cells, resulting in progressive destruction of this cell population. The events at the cellular level may be divided into the establishment phase and the expressive phase. The initial event is attachment reflecting the affinity between HIV envelope *(env)* glycoprotein and the CD4$^+$ surface receptor molecule.[25] The process of cell fusion that results in syncytium formation requires a specific CD4-HIV *env* interaction as well. This represents a distinct cytopathic effect. HIV variants that induce syncytium use a coreceptor called LESTR (leukocyte-derived seven-transmembrane-domain receptor) or fusin.[26]

Non–syncytium-inducing variants use a receptor for B chemokines; thus, B chemokines appear to inhibit HIV by competitive inhibition. Accelerated infection is often associated with increases in viral burden, increased CD4+ cell slope, and emergence of syncytium-inducing variants.

Fusion is followed by viral penetration, encoding, and reverse transcription. Reverse transcriptase is a unique enzyme of retroviruses that results in the synthesis of complementary DNA (proviral DNA) from HIV RNA. This takes place in the cell cytoplasm. Double-stranded viral DNA is then transported to the nucleus for integration into the host genome. Events that precede integration are considered latent infection, and subsequent events represent the replication or expressive phase of HIV with death of the CD4+ cell. This last stage includes transcription of HIV RNA followed by translation into proteins at the cell surface, then budding and release of immature viral particles. The proteins are encoded as large precursor polyproteins. HIV protease catalyzes cleavage of these polyproteins to mature structural proteins and enzymes that are necessary for the formation of infectious particles.

Nucleoside Analogs (Table 127–2)

Nucleoside analogs inhibit reverse transcriptase by competitive binding to the reverse transcriptase enzyme and/or act as an alternative substrate leading to viral DNA chain termination. Drugs in this class are essentially prodrugs that must be metabolically activated by intracellular enzymes to 5′-triphosphates. Variations in intracellular metabolism including variations in affinity for converting enzymes account for some differences in potency and toxicity. A major limitation with some nucleoside analogs is the development of resistance, which occurs at variable rates of frequency and severity.[11, 12, 14, 27]

Zidovudine

This drug was the first antiviral agent tested for HIV and continues to be one of the most frequently used drugs. The initial clinical trial in 1986 included 282 patients with relatively late-stage disease randomized to receive zidovudine or placebo.[1] Analysis of results by the Data and Monitoring Board in September 1986 showed 19 deaths in the placebo group compared with 1 among zidovudine recipients; the trial was discontinued, all participants were offered zidovudine, and the FDA approved the agent in early 1987.

Zidovudine is well absorbed, but extensive glucuronidization in the liver reduces bioavailability to about 60%.[28] The plasma half-life is about 1 hour, but the intracellular half-life of active triphosphate is 3 to 4 hours.[29] The original dosing recommendation was 1500 mg/d in five divided doses; this recommendation has now been supplanted with 600 mg/d in two divided doses. Zidovudine (and other nucleoside analogs) appears to achieve a threshold for efficacy, meaning that doses above the recommendation of 600 mg/d do not increase potency. Exceptions are HIV-associated dementia, in which higher doses may be required to achieve adequate levels at the target site, and possibly HIV-associated idiopathic thrombocytopenic purpura. The major toxicity of zidovudine is bone marrow suppression with neutropenia or anemia; these are dose dependent and stage related, with a higher frequency in late-stage disease.[30] Both complications respond to reduced dosage, discontinuation of drug, or use of cytokines: erythropoietin for anemia and granulocyte colony-stimulating factor for neutropenia. Other common side effects include gastrointestinal intolerance (nausea, vomiting, diarrhea, anorexia), myalgias, fatigue, and headache. These symptoms tend to be dose related and stage related. The minimal effective dose, when dose reduction is necessary, is 300 mg/d.[29] Occasional patients develop zidovudine-associated myopathy accompanied by elevated levels of creatine

TABLE 127–2 ■ Comparison of Nucleoside Analogs

CHARACTERISTIC	ZIDOVUDINE (AZT, RETROVIR)	DIDANOSINE (ddI, VIDEX)	ZALCITABINE (ddC, HIVID)	STAVUDINE (d4T, ZERIT)	LAMIVUDINE (3TC, EPIVIR)
Usual dose	200 mg three times daily (tid) or 300 twice daily (bid)	Tablets >60 kg: 200 mg bid <60 kg: 125 mg bid	0.75 mg tid	>60 kg: 40 mg bid <60 kg: 30 mg bid	150 mg bid
Minimal effective dose	300 mg/d	200 mg/d (powder)	Not studied	Not studied	Not studied
Oral bioavailability	60%	Tablet: 40% Powder: 30%	85%	86%	86%
Serum half-life	1.1 h	1.6 h	1.2 h	1.0 h	3–6 h
Intracellular half-life	3 h	12 h	3 h	3.5 h	12 h
Central nervous system penetration (% serum levels)	60%	20%	20%	30%–40%	10%
Elimination	Metabolized to zidovudine glucuronide; Renal excretion zidovudine glucuronide	Renal excretion, 50%	Renal excretion, 70%	Renal excretion, 50% unchanged	Renal excretion
Major toxicity	Bone marrow suppression: anemia and/or neutropenia; Subjective complaints: gastrointestinal intolerance, headache, insomnia, asthenia	Pancreatitis; Peripheral neuropathy	Peripheral neuropathy; Stomatitis	Peripheral neuropathy	Minimal toxicity
Mutations conferring resistance (codon)	41,* 67, 70,* 215,* 219	65, 69, 74, 75, 184	65, 69, 74, 75, 184, 215	41, 50, 70, 75	65, 184*

*Mutations considered most clinically significant.

kinase.[31] These patients usually respond with discontinuation of zidovudine unless there is confusion with HIV-associated myopathy. Most studies show that 10% to 20% of patients are not able to tolerate zidovudine.

Zidovudine has established efficacy in properly controlled trials demonstrating the following: decrease in viral burden (mean decrease of approximately 0.5 log), increase in CD4$^+$ cell count (mean increase of 30 to 50/mm^3), delay in progression to an AIDS-defining opportunistic infection, prolonged survival, improvement in HIV-associated dementia, increased platelet count in HIV-associated idiopathic thrombocytopenic purpura, prevention of vertical transmission, safety during the second and third trimesters of pregnancy, and reduction in rates of HIV transmission to health care workers after needlestick exposure to HIV.[1, 29, 32] In many categories, this remains the only agent with demonstrated benefit. Zidovudine is also favored in many or most combination treatment regimens and is the only drug with demonstrated efficacy in combination with 3TC.

The benefit of zidovudine in therapeutic trials appears to be "time limited," that is, at least partly related to the development of resistance.[11, 12, 14, 27] Resistant phenotypes show site-directed mutations with amino acid substitutions at codons 41, 67, 70, 215, and 219.[12] Three that are particularly important in terms of frequency and the severity of accompanying resistance are at codons 41, 70, and 215.[33] The multiplicity of resistance mutations is especially important. The time of emergence of zidovudine resistance is earlier with late-stage disease and with a high viral burden; in general, resistance is initially seen at 6 months and about 50% of patients receiving monotherapy have resistant strains at 2 years. The prevalence of zidovudine resistance in community strains was 5% to 20% in industrialized countries in 1996. Most authorities believe that the true rate of clinically significant resistance in newly infected people is about 5% and that this should not dissuade use of zidovudine as initial treatment. Discontinuation of zidovudine after resistance develops results in predominance of zidovudine-sensitive strains, but resistant strains reemerge rapidly with reintroduction of zidovudine. Resistance does not clearly explain all therapeutic failures. Other factors that may account for reduced efficacy are the relative lack of activity of zidovudine against syncytium-inducing isolates and reduced efficacy with a high viral burden.[34]

Didanosine

This is the second nucleoside analog approved by the FDA and has proved to be an effective agent with modest but sustained antiviral activity. ddI is acid labile, so it must be administered with buffering and an empty stomach. The plasma half-life is about 1.6 hours, but the intracellular half-life is 8 to 24 hours.[35, 37] Major toxicities are gastrointestinal intolerance, peripheral neuropathy, and pancreatitis. The neuropathy is reversible if it is recognized early and the drug is discontinued.[38] Patients should be warned of this side effect and promptly discontinue the drug when pain or paresthesias are noted, most frequently in the distal lower extremities. Pancreatitis occurs in 4% to 5% of patients, and some suggest monitoring of serum amylase levels at monthly intervals during administration of ddI.[37] The frequency of pancreatitis increases with alcohol abuse, a history of prior episodes of pancreatitis, or the concurrent use of other drugs associated with this complication and with late-stage HIV infection. Many patients have difficulty with gastrointestinal intolerance to ddI. All of these complications are dose related. The usual dose for an adult weighing more than 60 kg is two 100-mg tablets twice daily or 250 mg of the sachet twice daily. The minimal effective dose is about one half of this suggested dose. The lack of overlapping toxicity with zidovudine makes this combination attractive.

Resistance to ddI is noted with mutations at codons 65, 69, 74, 75, and 184, but these are relatively infrequent or the reduction in sensitivity is only four- to fivefold, making the significance enigmatic.[12, 14, 39] Strains of HIV resistant to zidovudine retain sensitivity to ddI.[12, 40] Prolonged treatment with ddI may result in emergence of strains resistant to zidovudine.[41] Therapeutic trials suggest that monotherapy with zidovudine has a greater initial antiviral effect in nucleoside analog–naive patients, but ddI has a more prolonged or sustained antiviral effect.[9, 32, 43] AIDS Clinical Trials Group (ACTG) trial 175 showed that monotherapy with ddI was comparable to combination treatment with nucleoside analogs (zidovudine plus ddC or zidovudine plus ddI) and was superior to prolonged treatment with zidovudine in terms of rates of clinical progression.[9] Nevertheless, studies of viral burden showed that the combination regimens were superior to ddI alone and that this combination is synergistic in vitro.[43]

Zalcitabine

This drug is the third nucleoside analog approved by the FDA and has been used primarily in combination with zidovudine or protease inhibitors. The combination with zidovudine has documented superiority compared with zidovudine monotherapy in zidovudine-naive patients.[9] The drug is well absorbed, with a bioavailability of about 80%, but this is substantially reduced when it is taken with food.[37] The plasma half-life is 1 to 2 hours, and the intracellular half-life of the triphosphate is about 2.5 hours. Urinary excretion is the major mechanism of excretion, and this is one of the few nucleoside analogs that has precise recommendations for dose adjustment in patients with renal failure.[44] The major side effect of ddC is peripheral neuropathy that is related to dose and duration of treatment and stage of disease.[37] Less common side effects include pancreatitis and oral or esophageal ulcers. As with ddI, ddC has no significant hematologic toxicity, no overlapping resistance with zidovudine, and in vitro synergy with zidovudine, favoring its use in this combination.[12] Resistance mutations are noted at codons 65, 69, 74, 75, and 184, thus overlapping with ddI. These are generally infrequent or they impart only modest resistance, so their significance is unclear. The clinical results with ddC plus zidovudine have been variable.[9, 45]

Stavudine

This drug is the fourth nucleoside analog approved by the FDA, and it has proved to have modest antiviral activity; it is well tolerated and resistance is relatively uncommon.[7, 46] The drug is well absorbed with a bioavailability of 90%.[46] The plasma half-life is about 1 hour and the intracellular half-life of the triphosphate is about 32 hours. The major side effect is peripheral neuropathy. Use in combination with ddI does not appear to magnify the frequency of peripheral neuropathy despite this overlapping toxicity. Resistance is noted with a mutation at codon 75, but the clinical relevance is unclear.[47] Initial trials with d4T showed sustained benefit in a fashion somewhat suggestive of the performance of ddI as monotherapy in ACTG 175.[48] Attractive features of d4T are the twice-daily dosing schedule, low pill burden, and good acceptance by patients.

Lamivudine

Lamivudine is the fifth nucleoside analog approved by the FDA. Early studies showed rapid development of high-grade resistance ascribed to a rapid selection of strains with a mutation at codon 184, and this was associated with a 10,000-fold decrease in susceptibility.[12, 14] The initial prognosis was poor, but two subsequent observations rejuvenated this drug to an anticipated billion dollar market: First, the codon 184 mutation is accompanied by enhanced susceptibility to zidovudine among strains previously resistant to that agent.[49] Second, this drug is remarkably well tolerated with good oral bioavailability, a relatively long plasma half-life, and a twice-daily dosing recommendation.[50, 51] The codon 184 mutation that confers high-grade resistance to 3TC also imparts modest resistance to ddI and ddC, although the therapeutic implications of this observation are not clear.[12] In general, 3TC is advocated for combination use primarily with zidovudine rather than other nucleoside analogs on the basis of demonstrated efficacy in terms of clinical outcome, impact on viral burden, and $CD4^+$ cell slope, as well as the enhanced susceptibility to zidovudine in vitro.[49, 51]

Nonnucleoside Reverse Transcriptase Inhibitors

This category of drugs also inhibits reverse transcriptase, but by an alternative mechanism compared with nucleoside analogs: the nonnucleoside reverse transcriptase inhibitors inactivate the enzyme by conformational change. They do not require cellular processing to become active, whereas nucleosides require cellular phosphorylation. Activity is highly selective for HIV-1, and these drugs are not active versus HIV-2 or other retroviruses. Initial drugs in this class are nevirapine and delaviridine. Both are associated with relatively high rates of a rash reaction, they are active against HIV strains that are resistant to nucleoside analogs, they are synergistic with nucleosides in vitro, and use is complicated by rapid evolution of resistance when they are given as monotherapy.[52–55]

Nevirapine

This drug has a bioavailability greater than 90%, it is largely metabolized by cytochrome P-450, and metabolic products are eliminated primarily in the urine. Nevirapine autoinduces metabolism by inducing cytochrome P-450 enzymes so that the half-life is reduced from 45 to 25 hours after 2 to 4 weeks of treatment. This drug also decreases the plasma levels of other drugs that utilize this metabolic pathway, including protease inhibitors. The major side effect is a morbilliform rash, which develops in about 18% of patients, and a Stevens-Johnson–like reaction in about 0.5%. The rash is dose related and can be reduced with a graduated dose regimen. The standard dose is 200 mg/d for 2 weeks and then 200 mg twice daily. A major problem is rapid evolution of high-grade resistance when this drug is used as monotherapy. Within 2 weeks, there is reduced in vitro activity ascribed to one or more reverse transcriptase mutations at codons 103, 106, 108, 181, 188, and/or 190. By 8 weeks of monotherapy, there is a greater than 100-fold decrease in susceptibility, and this may occur with a single mutation. There does not appear to be cross-resistance between these strains and nucleoside analogs or protease inhibitors. Thus, nevirapine (as well as others in this class) must be used in combination, usually with nucleoside analogs[56] and preferably with nucleosides that have not been used previously. Superior results with profound decreases in viral burden for sustained periods were seen in nucleoside-naive patients treated with combination regimens.[57] The advantages of these regimens are the twice-daily dosing regimen, a relatively low pill burden, good tolerance, pronounced antiviral activity in combination therapy, good central nervous system penetration, and relatively low cost.

Delaviridine (Rescriptor)

This agent is another potent nonnucleoside reverse transcriptase inhibitor for use in combination with nucleoside analogs.[58, 59] Clinical trials show that delaviridine in combination with zidovudine produced a 0.5 $\log_{10}$ per mL decrease that persisted more than 1 year and better results with triple therapy including zidovudine, ddI, and delaviridine. As with nevirapine, rash is the major side effect (in 12% to 18% of patients) but usually does not require drug discontinuation. In vitro synergy is shown with nucleoside analogs. Bioavailability is good and the plasma half-life is relatively long. The standard dose is 400 mg three times a day. As with nevirapine, resistance develops rapidly and is high level, but there is no cross-resistance with protease inhibitors or with nucleoside analogs. Metabolism is largely by cytochromes P-450IIIA (CYP3A) and P-450IID6 (CYP2D6). Drugs that induce CYP3A reduce delaviridine concentrations and should not be used concurrently. These include rifabutin, rifampin, carbamazepine, phenobarbital, and phenytoin. Inhibitors of CYP3A and CYP2D6 (ritonavir, saquinavir, indinavir, ketoconazole, fluconazole, clarithromycin, and fluoxetine) do not alter delaviridine concentrations. Other drug interactions include those with the following agents, which should not be used concurrently: terfenadine, astemizole, cisapride, triazolam, alprazolam, and midazolam.

Protease Inhibitors (Table 127–3)

Intracellular replication of HIV results in two types of polyproteins: the *gag* gene encodes structural proteins of the viral core, and *gag* and *pol* encode retroviral enzymes including reverse transcriptase, protease, and integrase. These precursor proteins align on the viral envelope and are cleaved by protease to mature structural proteins and enzymes, a critical component of viral maturation. HIV protease is a symmetric homodimer containing 99 amino acids. Protease inhibitors are peptide derivatives that competitively inhibit HIV protease. This enzyme was characterized by crystallography in 1989,[60] but subsequent development of protease inhibitors was hampered by multiple obstacles in drug development: poor oral bioavailability because of poor absorption and/or rapid metabolism by hepatic cytochrome P-450 enzymes, unexpected toxicity, high degree of plasma protein binding, rapid development of resistance, and poor penetration of the central nervous system.[61] Some but not all of these obstacles have subsequently been overcome, and a large number of protease inhibitors are either FDA approved or in some stage of development toward that goal.[7, 62–64]

Saquinavir (Invirase)

This drug was the first protease inhibitor approved by the FDA, in late 1995.[6, 62] Saquinavir has potent anti-HIV activity in vitro but limited activity in vivo that is ascribed to poor bioavailability. Maximal absorption is achieved with concurrent administration of a high-fat meal, but the bioavailability is still only about 4%.[65–67] Tactics that may be used to increase serum levels include use of an alternative preparation with better bioavailability, concurrent use with ketoconazole, grapefruit juice, delaviridine, and/or ritonavir to inhibit cytochrome P-450 hepatic enzymes, or use of extraordinarily high doses.[6, 66] The drug is generally well tolerated, although occasional patients have gastrointestinal intolerance or diarrhea. The major disadvantage of the drug is its poor bioavailability. A potential advantage is concurrent administration with ritonavir to make use of the drug interaction to magnify antiviral activity while possibly reducing the total daily dose of rito-

TABLE 127–3 ■ Comparison of Protease Inhibitors

CHARACTERISTIC	SAQUINAVIR	RITONAVIR	INDINAVIR	NELFINAVIR
Trade name	Invirase	Norvir	Crixivan	Viracept
Supplier	Hoffman-LaRoche	Abbott	Merck	Agouron
Form	200-mg capsules	100-mg capsules	100-, 200-, 400-mg capsules	250-mg capsules
Usual dose	600 mg three times daily (tid)*	600 mg twice daily (bid)*	800 mg q 8 h	750 mg tid
Bioavailability (recommendations)	Hard capsule: 4% Soft capsule: 12% (with high-fat meal)	70%–90% (taken with food)	60%–70% (empty stomach)	60%–80% (with food)
Serum half-life	1–2 h	3–4 h	1.5–2 h	
Central nervous system penetration	Poor	Poor	Moderate (?)	Slight
Elimination	Biliary metabolism Cytochrome P-450IIIA	Biliary metabolism Cytochromes P-450IIIA, P-450IID, P-450IIC	Biliary metabolism Cytochrome P-450IIIA	Biliary metabolism Cytochrome P-450IIIA
Toxicity	Gastrointestinal intolerance (nausea and diarrhea) (5%) Headache	Gastrointestinal intolerance (nausea, vomiting, diarrhea) (30%–50%) Paresthesias—circumoral and extremities (10%) Asthenia (10%–15%) Taste perversion (5%–10%) Laboratory: triglyceride increase >200% (60%), transaminase elevation (10%–15%), elevated creatine kinase and uric acid	Nephrolithiasis (5%–15%) Gastrointestinal intolerance (10%–15%) Laboratory: increased indirect bilirubinemia (inconsequential) Miscellaneous: headache (6%), asthenia, blurred vision, dizziness, rash, metallic taste, thrombocytopenia	Diarrhea (10%–30%)
Drug interactions	Increased levels of saquinavir: ritonavir, ketoconazole, grapefruit juice Reduced saquinavir levels: rifampin, rifabutin, and (?) phenobarbital, phenytoin, dexamethasone, and carbamazepine Forbidden drugs: terfenadine, astemizole, cisapride	Inhibits cytochrome P-450 (potent inhibitor) Increase levels of multiple drugs that are "forbidden" for concurrent use†	Inhibits cytochrome P-450 (less than ritonavir) Increase levels of rifampin, rifabutin, terfenadine, astemizole, cisapride, calcium channel blockers Increase indinavir levels: ketconazole, delaviridine Reduce indinavir levels: rifampin, rifabutin, nevirapine	Inhibits cytochrome P-450 (less than ritonavir) Decrease nelfinavir: rifampin Increase levels of rifabutin, terfanadine, astemizole, calcium channel blockers, cisapride, saquinavir, indinavir Increase levels of nelfinavir: ritonavir, indinavir
Codon mutations associated with resistance; parentheses indicate most significant	10, 36, 46, 48, 63, 71, 84, (90)	20, (36), 46, (54), 63, 71, (82), 84, 90	(10), 20, 24, 36, (46), 54, (63), 66, 71, (82), 84, 90	(30), 35, 36, (71), 77, 84

*Dose escalation for ritonavir: days 1–2: 300 mg bid; days 3–5: 400 mg bid; days 6–13: 500 mg bid; day ≥14: 600 mg bid. Combination treatment regimen with saquinavir (400 mg orally bid) plus ritonavir (400–600 mg orally bid).

†Drugs contraindicated for concurrent use with ritonavir: alprazolam (Xanax), amiodarone (Cordarone), astemizole (Hismanal), bepridil (Vascor), bupropion (Wellbutin), cisapride (Propulsid), clorazepate (Tranxene), clozapine (Clozaril), diazepam (Valium), encainide (Enkaid), estazolam (ProSom), flecainide (Tambocor), flurazepam (Dalmane), meperidine (Demerol), midazolam (Versed), piroxicam (Feldene), propoxyphene (Darvon), propafenone (Rythmol), quinidine, rifabutin (Mycobutin), terfenadine (Seldane), triazolam (Halcion), zolpidem (Ambien). Decreased levels of clarithromycin (Biaxin), ethinyl estradiol (contraceptives), theophylline, sulfamethoxazole, and AZT.

navir, an advantage because of the poor tolerance that is a dose-dependent side effect. Additional potential advantages compared with other protease inhibitors are a limited number of identified codon mutations that impart resistance and the relative lack of demonstrated cross-resistance with other protease inhibitors.[14, 68, 69]

Ritonavir (Norvir)

This protease inhibitor shows potent antiviral activity in vitro and in vivo. Oral bioavailability is approximately 70%, the plasma half-life is approximately 1 to 2 hours, and the major mechanism of excretion is hepatic metabolism via the CYP3A4 isoform.[70–72] Ritonavir is an exceptionally potent inhibitor of cytochrome P-450 and can also serve as an inducer of cytochrome P-450 isoforms.[63, 64] This leads to potent drug interactions when ritonavir is given in combination with agents that are metabolized by cytochrome P-450, accounting for a long list of drugs that need to be avoided among recipients of ritonavir.[70] This type of drug interaction may be exploited by combining ritonavir with saquinavir, because the latter shows poor bioavailability, but the area under the curve increases by a factor of up to 300-fold when saquinavir is given concurrently with ritonavir. The major side effects associated with ritonavir are diarrhea, nausea, headache, and weakness; all are dose related and many patients have improved tolerance with a graduated dosing regimen and continued use.[70] The graduated dose regimen for 2 weeks is justified because hepatic metabolism is increased by autoinduction during treatment; thus, the serum concentrations with 600 mg/d for initial treatment are comparable to those achieved with 1200 mg/d on treatment day 14.

Therapeutic trials with ritonavir showed that when it was used in combination with nucleoside analogs or saquinavir, there was a two- to three-log reduction in quantitative HIV RNA that was sustained for at least 1 year in a large cohort and up to 2 years in a smaller number of patients.[63, 64, 70, 72] The largest clinical trial included patients with relatively late-stage disease (average $CD4^+$ cell count ~20/mm^3) who continued their standard treatment with nucleoside analogs and were randomized to the addition of either ritonavir or placebo; results showed a statistically significant advantage with ritonavir treatment in terms of survival and reduction in AIDS-defining complications.[72] Treatment of recent seroconverters with ritonavir, zidovudine, and 3TC resulted in a reduction in plasma HIV RNA to undetectable levels (<25 copies per mL), negative cultures of peripheral blood mononuclear cells and lymph nodes, and, in some cases, seroreversion[73]; durability of these results is unknown. Advantages of this agent include evidence of statistically significant benefit in terms of clinical end points including survival, a substantial antiviral effect according to quantitative HIV virology, and a good safety profile in terms of objective adverse drug reactions. Disadvantages include a multitude of potentially serious interactions with drugs including several agents that are commonly used by patients with HIV infection and poor gastrointestinal tolerance.

Indinavir (Crixivan)

Indinavir is the third protease inhibitor approved by the FDA and is a potent inhibitor of HIV both in vitro and in vivo when used in combination with nucleoside analogs.[74] Oral bioavailability is about 60%, the half-life is 1.5 to 2 hours, and excretion is primarily by hepatic metabolism. Indinavir inhibits cytochrome P-450, but the inhibition is less profound than that with ritonavir.[74, 75] The major toxicity is nephrolithiasis, noted in 5% to 10% of patients. This is dose related and presumably reduced by use of large volumes of oral fluid. The presumed mechanism is crystallization of indinavir. Acidification of urine is an unrealistic method of prevention. Many patients also have gastrointestinal intolerance with nausea and vomiting, although these reactions are less severe and frequent than with ritonavir. Some patients have an increased indirect bilirubin value that is unexplained and inconsequential.[73] Therapeutic trials showed that indinavir in combination with nucleoside analogs was associated with a decrease in quantitative HIV by up to 10^2 to 10^3 log (2 to 3 $\log_{10}$) copies per mL, up to 86% of patients in some trials had undetectable virus (<200 copies per mL), and this antiviral effect was sustained for up to 1 year in a large cohort and up to 2 years in a smaller sample.[76–78] As with ritonavir, indinavir in combination with zidovudine and 3TC in recent seroconverters has been shown to produce a reduction in plasma HIV RNA to undetectable levels, negative cultures of peripheral blood mononuclear cells, negative lymph node biopsies, and, in some cases, seroreversion.[77] Exposure to indinavir is associated with at least 11 mutations that confer resistance to this agent and possibly to other protease inhibitors as well.[13] Resistance in vivo depends on the multiplicity of mutations, as no single mutation appears to confer clinically significant resistance. A concern is that these mutations overlap with those that impart resistance to other protease inhibitors including ritonavir.[13] As with other protease inhibitors, it is assumed that resistance is obviated by long-term viral suppression.[78] The major advantages of indinavir are the potency of the antiviral effect when it is given in combination regimens and relatively good tolerance. Major disadvantages are nephrolithiasis and multiple mutations conferring resistance that may reduce activity of multiple other protease inhibitors.

Recommendations

The protease inhibitors, unlike nucleoside analogs, show potency that is dose dependent with no apparent threshold for maximal activity. Thus, higher doses yield increased antiviral activity and the limitations to increased doses are cost and toxicity. A major concern with this class is the evolution of drug resistance ascribed to codon mutations on the protease gene, and these occur with variable frequency and induce variable degrees of resistance.[13] Of particular concern is possible cross-resistance, implying that resistance to one agent may alter susceptibility to others in this class. Rules for protease inhibitor administration are stringent and include the following:

1. These drugs should always be given in combination with other antiretroviral agents.
2. Full dosage should be used.
3. Treatment should not be interrupted.
4. Management of a failing regimen should include changes with introduction of at least two new antiretroviral drugs.
5. Patients should be instructed well in the importance of compliance.

Treatment Guidelines

The goal of antiviral treatment is to minimize virus replication and increase the complexity of resistance mutations required for viral escape. This implies a reduction in viral burden to undetectable levels for as long as possible. A second goal is to reconstitute or preserve immune competence.[79] A practical issue is the ability to achieve viral suppression for sustained periods using drugs that may lose activity because of resistance, are poorly tolerated, and require compliance that is difficult to achieve.

Therapeutic Monitoring

The CD4+ cell count has been the standard parameter for evaluating immune competence. Use of the CD4+ cell slope is a way to monitor progression. Care needs to be exercised in drawing conclusions from sequential CD4+ cell counts because of large variations in test results. A recommendation for therapeutic monitoring introduced in 1996 was quantitative HIV RNA as a method for determining prognosis and response to therapy.[4–5] The usual methods for measurement are HIV RNA polymerase chain reaction, branched chain DNA assay, and the nucleic acid sequence–based amplification assay. Correlation between measurements with these techniques is reasonably good, and changes of 0.3 to 0.5 $\log_{10}$ copies per mL are considered significant. The threshold for detection is variable depending on the test used, but 1997 assay systems will detect HIV at a threshold of 25 to 200 copies per mL. Drug susceptibility testing may be done using phenotypic in vitro testing (like bacterial testing) or genetic sequencing, but these are generally reserved for research laboratories, and quantitative HIV RNA assay is preferred. Recommendations for use[80] are summarized in Table 127–4. Factors that increase viral load are the following: disease progression, intercurrent illness (e.g., tuberculosis, pneumonia, cytomegalovirus disease), failure of antiviral treatment, and immunizations. Response to treatment with antiviral agents is prompt, usually within hours[3]; the downward slope levels off after 10 to 14 days and then declines more gradually during a period of months. These two posttreatment slopes are called phases 1 and 2, and the transition period is referred to as the inflection point. The usual standard for quantitative virology measurements is to obtain two baseline measurements and monitor response to a new regimen at 3 to 4 weeks, with subsequent monitoring at 3- to 4-month intervals. The anticipated response with zidovudine monotherapy is a maximal decrease of about 0.5 $\log_{10}$ copies per mL, with nucleoside analog combinations it is a decrease of 1.0 to 2.0 $\log_{10}$ copies per mL, and for protease inhibitor combinations it is a decrease of up to 2 to 3 $\log_{10}$ copies per mL. Treatment failure is defined as an inability to achieve a decrease exceeding 0.5 $\log_{10}$ copies per mL or a return to a value of 0.3 to 0.5 $\log_{10}$ copies per mL below baseline. The goal of treatment is to reduce viral burden to threshold values that are poorly defined, but many authorities conclude that the goal should be less than 200 copies per mL or "undetectable" concentrations. The use of CD4+ cell counts and viral burden measurements for decisions regarding initiation of treatment is arbitrary. Recommendations of the International AIDS Society–U.S.A. are to initiate treatment of any patient with a viral burden exceeding 30,000 to 50,000 copies per mL.[80] For patients with a CD4+ cell count less than 500/mm³ or with clinical symptoms, the recommendation is to initiate treatment when the viral burden exceeds 5000 to 10,000 copies per mL.

TABLE 127–4 ■ Recommendations for Viral Load Monitoring

VARIABLE	VIRAL LOAD MONITORING
Frequency	Baseline × 2 separated by 2–4 wk Routine testing: every 3–4 mo Monitoring response to treatment: 3–4 wk after initiating or changing therapy
Goal of therapy	"Undetectable" using an assay that detects <400 copies per mL
Minimal detectable change	≥0.5 log
Treatment failure	Viral load within 0.3–0.5 log baseline

From Saag MS, Holodniy M, Kuritzkes DR, et al: Viral load markers in clinical practice: Recommendations of the International AIDS Society—USA Expert Panel. Nat Med 2:625–629, 1996.

Initiation of Antiviral Therapy

Guidelines are summarized in Table 127–5. The recommendation to initiate treatment rapidly after the acute retroviral syndrome is based on the assumption that this treatment can reestablish the set point that dictates the subsequent course. Some authorities have concluded that aggressive early therapy may achieve cure.[73] Additional guidelines are based on CD4+ cell count and viral burden as defined earlier. The large study of early treatment with zidovudine monotherapy in patients who were asymptomatic (ACTG 019) showed that this treatment delayed the onset of an AIDS-defining diagnosis but was not associated with prolongation of survival.[81, 82] Since that time, there has been substantial progress in new drug development, far more potent antiviral regimens are now readily available, and more aggressive treatment is more widely accepted despite the lack of evidence of long-term benefit.

Initial Regimen

The standard regimens for treatment are various drugs in combination, usually two nucleoside analogs combined with a nonnucleoside reverse transcriptase inhibitor or a protease inhibitor. Monotherapy with zidovudine is advocated only for pregnant patients to prevent perinatal transmission. Alternative less potent treatment is two nucleoside analogs. Monotherapy with ddI or possibly d4T may be used[9] in selected patients who do not accept more complicated regimens. The choice of combination nucleoside analogs versus a protease inhibitor combination for initial treatment is arbitrary. Most authorities prefer a regimen likely to reduce the viral burden to undetectable levels for a sustained period, and this is most likely with triple therapy. Others favor a more conservative approach with simplified, more easily tolerated regimens, with subsequent decisions based on sequential measurements of viral burden, CD4+ cell slope, and/or evidence of clinical progression. Treatment in late-stage disease as indicated by CD4+ cell counts less than 200/mm³ is often complicated by drug toxicity and extensive prior exposure to antiretroviral drugs used in commonly advocated regimens. Studies of immune response suggest that immune reconstitution is not an achievable goal in late-stage disease even when the viral burden is reduced to undetectable levels. Instead, the rise in CD4+ cells is often limited to an increase of about 100 to 150/mm³, and most of the increase is in memory cells rather than naive cells. These observations indicate a greater challenge with antiviral agents in terms of long-term benefits and drug tolerance.[83, 84]

Changing Therapy

One major reason for altering antiretroviral regimens is toxicity, intolerance, or nonadherence. A second reason is treatment failure as indicated by increases in viral burden, progressive decline in the number of CD4+ cells (CD4+ cell slope), or clinical progression (new AIDS-defining diagnosis). In general, the CD4+ cell count is the mirror image of viral burden, with a decrease of one log in viral burden equal to a CD4+ cell count increase of 50 to 100/mm³.[3, 85] As noted, reduction in viral burden to undetectable levels or to a threshold below 5000 to 10,000 copies per mL is the highest priority.[79, 80] With regard to CD4+ cell response, there appears to be a limit in the reconstitution that is quantitative (usually a limit to increase of 100 to 150/mm³) and possibly qualita-

TABLE 127–5 ■ Recommendations for Antiretroviral Therapy

INDICATIONS TO INITIATE TREATMENT

Symptomatic disease
Asymptomatic with CD4+ cell count <500/mm³
Asymptomatic with CD4+ cell count >500/mm³ plus viral load > 10,000 copies per mL (viral load >5000–10,000 copies per mL—consider)

INITIAL REGIMEN

Preferred: two nucleoside analogs plus a protease inhibitor or two nucleoside analogs plus nevirapine
Alternative: two nucleoside analogs
Substandard: ddI or d4T
Contraindicated: monotherapy with zidovudine, 3TC, ddC, nevirapine or a protease inhibitor

INDICATIONS TO CHANGE THERAPY

Treatment failure: detectable virus
- Viral burden: increase or return to within 0.3–0.5 $\log_{10}$ of pretreatment levels
- CD4+ cell count: return to pretreatment levels or CD4+ cell decline
- Clinical criteria: HIV-associated complications

Toxicity, intolerance, or nonadherence
Current use of a suboptimal regimen

OPTIONS FOR DRUG CHANGES (TREATMENT FAILURE)

Initial Regimen	New Therapy
Two nucleoside analogs plus a protease inhibitor	Two nucleosides (including ≥ one new) plus nevirapine Two protease inhibitors ± a nucleoside analog*
Two nucleoside analogs plus nevirapine	Two nucleosides (including ≥ one new) plus a protease inhibitor
Two nucleoside analogs	Two nucleosides (including ≥ one new) plus a protease inhibitor or nevirapine

*Experience limited but appropriate in some patients with extensive exposure or toxicity with nucleosides.

tive (functional capacity). Some patients have a paradoxical increase in both CD4+ cell count and viral burden or the reverse—both parameters decline. The viral burden is presumed to be the best indicator of antiviral activity, but the CD4+ cell response is considered a secondary factor in assessing response.

What to Change to

A multitude of drugs are now available, so options are extensive. These include multiple agents that are available as investigational new drugs or through therapeutic trials. An obvious concern is anticipated resistance to drugs of prior exposure, although this is highly variable depending on the agent, stage of disease, duration of treatment, and combination used. Rapid and high-grade resistance is the rule with monotherapy using lamivudine, nonnucleoside reverse transcriptase inhibitors, and protease inhibitors. Resistance is relatively modest and delayed with ddI, ddC, d4T, and hydroxyurea. One caveat regarding treatment changes is that when this decision is based on a failing regimen, the patient should receive at least two new drugs that have not been previously used.[79] The overlapping resistance of protease inhibitors is a great concern because exposure to some agents (ritonavir, indinavir) may preclude use of most or all agents in the class. Some patients are unresponsive to standard regimens or have problems with intolerance or toxicity that precludes use of nucleoside analogs. Salvage therapy in these cases often includes combinations of protease inhibitors.

Recommendations to Reduce Perinatal Transmission of Human Immunodeficiency Virus

ACTG 076 was designed to determine the efficacy of zidovudine for reducing vertical transmission of HIV.[86] This was a placebo-controlled trial with the following eligibility criteria: pregnancy of 14 to 34 weeks' gestation, no antiretroviral therapy during the current pregnancy, and CD4+ cell count exceeding 300/mm³. The drug regimen was the following:

Before delivery: zidovudine (100 mg five times a day) initiated at 14 to 34 weeks of gestation and continued to the onset of labor.

During labor: intravenous zidovudine (loading dose of 2 mg/kg for 1 hour followed by continuous infusion of 1 mg/kg per hour until delivery).

Infant: zidovudine for the newborn (zidovudine syrup at 2 mg/kg every 6 hours) for the first 6 weeks of life beginning 8 to 12 hours after birth.

The rate of transmission was 28% in the placebo group compared with 8% among zidovudine recipients. Further observations included the following: (1) zidovudine did not appear to delay the diagnosis of HIV infection in the infant; (2) there was no significant zidovudine toxicity to pregnant women; (3) there was no evidence in this study or in prior reports of congenital malformations that could be ascribed to zidovudine; (4) the only adverse effect observed among infants who received zidovudine was a mild, transient anemia. Although this study was limited to women with CD4+ cell counts above 200/mm³, subsequent analyses have shown that zidovudine is protective across all CD4+ cell counts.[87] The potential impact of these observations is apparent from current estimates that about 6530 HIV-infected women give birth annually in the United States. A vertical transmission rate of 25% yields an estimated 1630 HIV-infected infants a year; at 8%, this estimate is reduced to 522 a year. Subsequent studies have shown that the rate of HIV transmission is only partially correlated with viral burden.[88] Furthermore, analysis of data from ACTG 076 showed that a benefit of zidovudine was independent of a significant effect on viral burden.[89] The role of viral burden monitoring as a method for determining changes in therapy to prevent vertical transmission is consequently controversial. There is also limited experience with drugs other than zidovudine in pregnancy, and their safety has not been established. The U.S. Public Health Service guideline is to utilize zidovudine according to the regimen employed in the study, although many authorities advocate the standard zidovudine regimen of 600 mg/d in two or three divided doses to improve compliance.[89] Effective implementation of this recommendation requires HIV serologic testing of pregnant women as advocated by the U.S. Public Health Service.[90] Cost analysis of these recommendations shows that they are highly cost-effective.[91] Results of following the recommendations in the first year in North Carolina showed that 82% of pregnant women were tested for HIV and the rate of vertical transmission was reduced from 21% to 8%.[92]

Occupational Exposure of Health Care Workers

As of June 1996, 49 health care workers had been reported to the Centers for Disease Control and Prevention with occupationally acquired HIV confirmed by seroconversion in the context of HIV exposure. An additional 120 cases of probable HIV transmission in the workplace were not confirmed by documented seroconversion. The occupations most at risk were nurses and laboratory technicians. All transmissions involved blood or bloody body fluids except for three laboratory workers who were exposed to HIV cultures. Most transmissions followed needlestick injuries, although five documented cases involved mucocutaneous exposures. Numerous studies indicate that the risk of acquiring HIV with needlestick injury from an HIV-infected source is 0.3% and the risk with mucocutaneous exposure is less than 0.1%.[93] Factors associated with increased risk were examined in a retrospective case-control trial of health care workers with occupational percutaneous HIV exposures including 31 with seroconversion and 679 control subjects.[94] Odds ratios for risk are summarized in Table 127–6. This table shows that significant risks were associated with deep injury, visible blood on the device, terminal illness in the source, and needle placement in an artery or vein. These observations are not surprising; they simply verify that the inoculum size of HIV and the depth of challenge correlate with the efficiency of transmission. An additional observation in this study was that zidovudine prophylaxis reduced the risk of transmission by fivefold. On the basis of these observations, the U.S. Public Health Service now recommends the use of prophylaxis with antiviral agents for health care workers who have occupational exposures[94] using a standard regimen of zidovudine (600 mg/d) combined with 3TC (300 mg/d) for 4 weeks. Health care workers who have high-risk exposures based on relative risk as just defined should receive a protease inhibitor as well. The addition of a protease inhibitor should also be considered when the source has received zidovudine and/or 3TC for extended periods, suggesting possible resistance in the transmitted strain.

TABLE 127–6 ■ Risk Factors for Human Immunodeficiency Virus Transmission in Health Care Workers with Needlestick Injuries from an Infected Source*

RISK	ODDS RATIO
Deep injury (not further defined)	16.1
Visible blood on the device	5.2
Needle placement in artery or vein	5.1
Source with late-stage disease (died within 2 mo of HIV-related complications)	8.2
Zidovudine prophylaxis	0.2

*Case-control retrospective analysis of 31 cases showing seroconversion compared with 679 control subjects who did not seroconvert. The source in all cases and control subjects was known to have HIV infection.

Adapted from Centers for Disease Control and Prevention: Update: Provisional recommendations for chemoprophylaxis after occupational exposure to human immunodeficiency virus. MMWR Morbid Mortal Wkly Rep 45:468–472, 1996.

Primary Human Immunodeficiency Virus Infection

Aggressive treatment of HIV in early stages offers what many believe is the optimal opportunity to have a major impact on long-term outcome.[95] This is the setting in which aggressive therapy is theoretically justified by the relative lack of drug-resistant mutants and an opportunity for immune salvage before possibly irreversible depletion of useful $CD4^+$ clones. Some authorities think that extremely aggressive treatment with three or four drugs for 1.5 to 3 years has the potential to achieve cure.[72, 73, 96] The treatment is in two stages, the first directed at productively infected cells, which account for 99% of the total viral burden and are largely depleted within 1 to 2 weeks with arrested replication. The second phase is directed against latently infected cells, such as tissue macrophages, which account for 1% of the viral burden and require a much longer period for depletion by cell death. No long-term studies have documented this outcome, but substantial anecdotal and short-term experience supports the concept that early and aggressive therapy may result in sustained periods in which there is no detectable virus by culture of peripheral blood mononuclear cells, plasma HIV RNA polymerase chain reaction, and culture of lymph node biopsy specimens.[72, 73, 96] Early treatment requires detection of HIV in early stages, which represents a major challenge: many patients do not seek medical consultation at the time of the acute retroviral syndrome either because it is asymptomatic or because the symptoms are mild or nonspecific. When medical care is sought, only about 25% of cases are correctly diagnosed.[16] Symptoms suggesting the acute HIV infection are summarized in Table 127–1. Particularly important observations that distinguish this syndrome from other common viral infections are the relatively long duration of fever, accompanying weight loss, frequent oral or esophageal ulcers, and rash. Sequential serology in the context of a defined exposure is another option for detection. An alternative is frequent serologic testing in patients with high-risk behavior. Additional components of this tactic that require emphasis are the importance of compliance with treatment regimens and aggressive monitoring of viral burden with appropriate changes in therapy as indicated by viral burden and/or toxicity.

Resistance

Resistance appears to be an inevitable consequence of antiviral treatment for HIV, although there is substantial variation in rates of resistance with different drugs, viral burdens, and various combination regimens. The initial infection involves a homogeneous population of HIV, and resistance is determined by selection of naturally occurring variants. The transcription error rate is 3×10^{-5}, which translates to an average of one mutation for every three 10,000 base pair genomes. The implication is that resistant strains are constantly being produced. For drugs such as 3TC (lamivudine) and nevirapine, a single mutation may cause a 100-fold or greater decrease in susceptibility. For drugs such as zidovudine and protease inhibitors, multiple mutations are usually required for high-level resistance. Resistance can be measured by genetic analysis to detect codon mutations associated with resistance (genotypic analysis) or by in vitro analysis to determine minimal inhibitory concentrations (phenotypic analysis).[98–104]

Nucleoside Analogs

Resistance to nucleoside analogs results from amino acid substitutions and structural changes in HIV reverse transcriptase. This enzyme is error prone, with an average of one mutant base pair per genome in converting RNA to DNA. Thus, all patients with prolonged infection have swarms of viral variants, including some defective virions and multidrug-resistant strains that can be selected. With zidovudine, susceptibility is phenotypically defined as follows: sensitive, 0.2 μM or less; partially resistant, 0.21 to 0.99 μM; and resistant, greater than 1.0 μM. Assays for measuring phenotypic resistance generally require 4 to 6 weeks.[99] The alternative and generally preferred technique is determination of genotypic resistance by detection of mutations associated with phenotypic resistance (see Table 127–2). The technology uses amplification of HIV RNA or DNA and then probes or differential polymerase chain reaction to detect specific amino acid substitutions that confer resistance.[102–104] At least five mutations are associated with zidovudine resistance, and the frequency and level of resistance are variable with each mutation. Resistance is cumulative,[107] so multiple mutations confer high-grade resistance. The most common genotypes associated with high-level resistance involve codons 41 plus 215 and the combination of 67, 70, and 215.[108] Approximately 50% of patients receiving zidovudine monotherapy for 2 years have resistant strains. The frequency of zidovudine resistance in community strains indicates that 10% to 20% were resistant by 1995; resistance to zidovudine and to most other drugs is associated with accelerated decreases in the CD4$^+$ cell count, clinical progression, and death.[105, 108, 110, 111] Neither combination nucleoside analog treatment nor sequential (alternating) therapy appears to prevent resistance.[106] Detection of resistance during the course of treatment may predict failure to respond before changes in viral burden or clinical progression.[112] The technology for detecting these changes is currently available, but its role in therapeutic monitoring is not established. With 3TC, the codon 184 mutation confers high-grade resistance with a 1000-fold reduction in susceptibility within weeks of treatment using 3TC monotherapy, but these strains acquire sensitivity to zidovudine, making this combination particularly attractive both in vitro and in vivo.[49–51, 113, 114] With other nucleoside analogs including ddI, ddC, and d4T, resistance has been noted but the level of resistance is modest, with 5- to 10-fold reductions in susceptibility, or the mutations are rare, so the clinical significance is often vague.[115–119] Some authorities believe that this difference compared with zidovudine accounts for the apparent greater durability of ddI compared with zidovudine.[9]

Nonnucleoside Reverse Transcriptase Inhibitors

Resistance to nevirapine and delaviradine develops rapidly and is profound when these drugs are used as monotherapy.[120] There is no cross-resistance with nucleoside analogs, but there may be cross-resistance between agents in this class. The nonnucleoside reverse transcriptase inhibitors should consequently never be used as monotherapy because benefit is only transient, with high-grade resistance developing within weeks. In combination with zidovudine, there is delayed resistance to the nonnucleoside reverse transcriptase inhibitors and to the nucleoside analogs.

Protease Inhibitors

Mutations in the protease enzyme are responsible for resistance, and these have been observed in vitro and in vivo with all agents tested to date. Resistance develops within days after monotherapy, especially with suboptimal doses.[13] The codon mutations on the protease gene associated with resistance to this class include multiple amino acid substitutions that confer graded levels of reduced activity (see Table 127–3). Multiple mutations are usually associated with therapeutic failure[13, 121, 122] (Condra JH, et al, manuscript submitted). There is overlap in resistance between some agents associated with the possibility of class resistance, implying resistance to all protease inhibitors.[13] In general, indinavir is associated with multiple resistance mutations that affect multiple other compounds in the class.[13] In contrast, saquinavir and nelfinavir have relatively modest numbers of resistance mutations and minimal cross-resistance. These patterns of cross-resistance and variations in severity of resistance presumably play an important but poorly understood role in drug sequencing. The acquisition of resistance with mutations at multiple sites is accompanied by rapid dominance of resistant strains and clinical deterioration. With discontinuation of the protease inhibitor, there is rapid loss of resistant strains, suggesting that the mutations conferring resistance are associated with reduced virulence. With reintroduction of the same protease inhibitor, there is rapid evolution of resistant strains. Because of overlapping resistance, there is little rationale for substituting ritonavir in cases of indinavir failure or for changing ritonavir to indinavir on the basis of clinical failure or demonstration of reduced in vitro activity. Factors associated with resistance are suboptimal doses, noncompliance, monotherapy, and incomplete viral suppression. These observations account for current guidelines that emphasize full doses, combination treatment, and uninterrupted therapy with a high priority for halting virus replication to reduce the frequency of mutations.

Alternative Treatments

The first decade of drug development and therapeutic trials for HIV-infected patients was dominated by antiretroviral agents. This approach is likely to be inadequate for many or most patients for several reasons. One is the genetic instability of HIV, resulting in great genomic variation imparting resistance that develops during the course of treatment, cross-resistance that limits utility of multiple agents, and resistance in community strains. Many patients do not tolerate the currently recommended regimens, and others tolerate the drugs but fail to respond. Among those who respond, there appears to be a threshold for immune reconstitution with a peak CD4$^+$ cell response of 100 to 150/mm^3 in most patients. Analysis of functional status shows that most of the reconstituted CD4$^+$ cell population is composed of memory T cells, although their functional capacity is poorly defined. These observations indicate that currently recommended antiviral regimens have limitations in their capacity to inhibit HIV for sustained periods and the reconstituted T-cell repertoire appears limited in quantity and possibly in quality. It is also unclear that the drug costs of $10,000 to $12,000 per year and the reduction in quality of life experienced by asymptomatic patients taking multiple drugs are justified on the basis of long-term benefits. The result is that alternative treatment strategies need to be pursued.

Cytokines

Interleukin-2 is produced by T cells and has potent effects on the growth and maturation of T cells, B cells, and natural killer cells. It is commercially available as Aldesleuken to treat renal cell carcinoma. A placebo-controlled trial in HIV-infected persons with $CD4^+$ cell counts greater than 200/mm^3 showed a brisk response with mean increases in $CD4^+$ cells from 428 to 916/mm^3.[123] This activity does not decrease with continued use for up to 1 year. The regimen used was 8 million IU/d given intravenously for 5 days every 2 months. The most common side effects were fatigue and malaise. Because the target of the therapy is $CD4^+$ cells instead of virus, there should be no problem with resistance. Dose-limiting toxicity was unusual, and HIV RNA levels were stable during interleukin-2 therapy.

Interleukin-12 is another cytokine with limited studies that appear promising. This agent promotes the cellular or Th1 response in place of Th2 or antibody response; it blocks interleukin-4 and interleukin-10 (Th2 cytokines) and blocks apoptosis of $CD4^+$ cells.[124]

Chemokine Antagonists

Chemokine receptors serve as cofactors for HIV entry into $CD4^+$ cells. RANTES (regulated on activation, normal T-cell expressed and secreted) is a CC chemokine that inhibits HIV infection of $CD4^+$ cells by interaction with the CCR5 receptor.[125] The initial experience with RANTES and RANTES analogs with high affinity for chemokine receptors in in vitro studies appears promising.

Gene Therapy

Gene therapy uses transfer of therapeutic genes into target cells to make them resistant to HIV. Attempts are being made to give HIV-resistant genes to pluripotent hematopoietic stem cells to ensure persistence. Another approach is to use RNA decoys that compete with viral RNAs for essential binding sites[125] and ribozymes that cleave HIV RNAs.[127] Transdominant mutant proteins such as Rev M10 are mutant forms of HIV proteins that compete with wild-type protein and suppress virus replication.[128] HIV may also be inhibited by intracellular single-chain antibiotics or intracellular toxins ("suicide" molecules).[129]

Adoptive cell transfer involves selection of T-cell populations with expansion and reinfusion. Cytotoxic T cells may be redirected by introducing genes that encode chimeric receptors.[130] Alternatively, there may be HIV-specific cytotoxic T lymphocyte clones with a marker or suicide gene that imparts sensitivity to ganciclovir to permit elimination through adverse effects.[131] Ex vivo expansion and reinfusion of $CD4^+$ cells is another option.

Nucleic acid–based vaccines utilize HIV genes for delivery into the patient to promote immune response. Both cellular and humoral responses may be elicited by this technique.[132]

Other Antiviral Agents

Few data suggest that hydroxyurea is a promising antiretroviral agent; it acts by blocking cellular ribonucleotide reductase with a consequent reduction in intracellular deoxynucleotides. In vitro activity against HIV in quiescent or activated human lymphocytes has been shown.[133] Preliminary clinical results obtained with hydroxyurea (500 mg twice daily) in combination with ddI showed a significant decrease in viral burden.[134] Many patients do not experience a change in $CD4^+$ cell count, a paradox that is presumably explained by inhibition of $CD4^+$ cell expansion by hydroxyurea. Possible advantages of hydroxyurea are a relatively low toxicity profile, good penetration of the central nervous system, and minimal resistance with sequential transfer in vitro.

Foscarnet possesses anti-HIV activity in vitro, and this may explain the prolonged survival among foscarnet recipients in a comparative trial of foscarnet versus ganciclovir in cytomegalovirus retinitis.[135, 136] The drug is too toxic for use except when indicated by opportunistic infections.

Inhibition of growth regulatory genes, including *tat*, *rev*, and *nef*, is another potential target of antiviral agents.[19, 137] The *tat* gene produces a regulatory protein that accelerates transcription of HIV provirus, resulting in a 1000-fold increase in virus replication. The *rev* gene acts by switching the processing of RNA transcripts to promote production of HIV proteins. The third growth regulatory gene, *nef*, was originally thought to inhibit transcription but has subsequently been shown to be required for progression to AIDS.[21]

Summary

Antiviral therapy for HIV infection is a rapidly changing field that has shown exponential growth in the past few years. The theory and practice have far exceeded the clinical trials to confirm the recommendations. Virtually all authorities recognize great potential value of an aggressive attack on HIV; the major controversies concern the timing and the appropriate combinations. An ideal objective is to have no detectable virus for a sustained period; the rationale is the assumption that there would be no disease progression and no viral escape with the consequence of resistant mutants. The problems with this tactic are that the ability to achieve these goals for sustained periods is not established and the aggressive treatment strategies considered necessary are problematic in terms of toxicity, compliance, resistance, and cost. There is near consensus that patients with advanced disease and those with high viral burdens need treatment with multiple drugs, but there is a large middle zone in which expert opinion is quite diverse.

References

1. Fischl MA, Richman DD, Grieco MH, et al: The efficacy of azidothymidine (zidovudine) in the treatment of patients with AIDS and AIDS-related complex. A double-blind, placebo-controlled trial. N Engl J Med 317:185–191, 1987.
2. Sande MA, Carpetner CCJ, Cobbs CG, et al: Antiretroviral therapy for adult HIV-infected patients. Recommendations from a state-of-the-art conference. National Institute of Allergy and Infectious Diseases State-of-the-Art Panel on Anti-Retroviral Therapy for Adult HIV-Infected Patients. JAMA 270:2583–2589, 1993.
3. Ho DD, Neumann QU, Perelson AS, et al: Rapid turnover of plasma virions and CD4 lymphocytes in HIV-1 infection. Nature 373:123–126, 1995.
4. Mellors JW, Kingsley LA, Rinaldo CR Jr, et al: Quantitation of HIV-1 RNA plasma predicts outcome after seroconversion. Ann Intern Med 122:573–579, 1995.
5. Mellors JW, Rinaldo CR Jr, Gupta P, et al: Prognosis in HIV-1 infection predicted by the quantity of virus in plasma. Science 272:1167–1170, 1996.
6. Bartlett JG: Protease inhibitors for HIV infection. Ann Intern Med 124:1086–1087, 1996.
7. Lipsky JJ: Antiretroviral drugs for AIDS. Lancet 348:800–803, 1996.
8. Wilson CC, Hirsch MS: Combination antiretroviral therapy for the treatment of human immunodeficiency virus type-1 infection. Proc Assoc Am Physicians 107:19–27, 1995.
9. Hammer SM, Datzenstein DA, Hughes MD, et al: A trial com-

paring nucleoside monotherapy with combination therapy in HIV-infected adults with CD4 cell counts from 200 to 500 per cubic millimeter. N Engl J Med 335:1081–1090, 1996.

10. Delta Coordinating Committee: Delta: A randomised double-blind controlled trial comparing combinations of zidovudine plus didanosine or zalcitabine with zidovudine alone in HIV-infected individuals. Lancet 348:283–291, 1996.
11. Shirasaka T, Kavlick MF, Ueno T, et al: Emergence of human immunodeficiency virus type 1 variants with resistance to multiple dideoxynucleosides in patients receiving therapy with dideoxynucleosides. Proc Natl Acad Sci USA 92:2398–2402, 1995.
12. Arts EJ, Wainberg MA: Mechanisms of nucleoside analog antiviral activity and resistance during human immunodeficiency virus reverse transcription. Antimicrob Agents Chemother 40:527–540, 1996.
13. Condra JH, Schleif WA, Blahy OM, et al: In vivo emergence of HIV-1 variants resistant to multiple protease inhibitors. Nature 374:569–571, 1995.
14. Richmond DD: Resistance, drug failure and disease progression. AIDS Res Hum Retroviruses 10:901–905, 1994.
15. Pantaleo G, Graziosi C, Fauci AS: New concepts in the immunopathogenesis of human immunodeficiency virus infection. N Engl J Med 328:327–335, 1993.
16. Schacker T, Collier AC, Hughes J, et al: Clinical and epidemiologic features of primary HIV infection. Ann Intern Med 125:257–264, 1996.
17. Niu MT, Stein D, Schnittman SM: Primary human immunodeficiency virus type 1 infection: Review of pathogenesis and early treatment intervention in humans and animal retrovirus infections. J Infect Dis 168:1490–1501, 1993.
18. Stein DS, Korvick JA, Vermund SH: $CD4^+$ lymphocyte cell enumeration for prediction of clinical course of human immunodeficiency virus disease: A review. J Infect Dis 165:352–363, 1992.
19. Haynes BF, Panteleo G, Fauci AS: Toward an understanding of the correlates of protective immunity to HIV infection. Science 271:324–328, 1996.
20. Buchbinder SP: Long-term non-progression in the San Francisco City Clinical Cohort (Abstr Tu C553). Presented at the 11th International Conference on AIDS; July 7–12, 1996; Vancouver, British Columbia, Canada.
21. Learmont J, Tindall B, Evans L, et al: Long term symptomless HIV-1 infection in recipients of blood products from a single donor. Lancet 340:863–867, 1992.
22. Fauci AS: Resistance to HIV-1 infection: It's in the genes. Nat Med 2:966–967, 1996.
23. Darby SC, Ewart DW, Giangrande PLF, et al: Importance of age at infection with HIV-1 for survival and development of AIDS in UK haemophilia population. UK Haemophilia Centre Directors' Organisation. Lancet 347:1573–1579, 1996.
24. Kaslow RA, Carrington M, Apple R, et al: Influence of combinations of human major histocompatibility complex genes on the course of HIV infection. Nat Med 4:405–411, 1996.
25. Feinberg MB: Changing the natural history of HIV disease. Lancet 348:239–246, 1996.
26. Weiss RA: HIV receptors and the pathogenesis of AIDS. Science 272:1885–1886, 1996.
27. D'Aquila RT, Johnson VA, Welles SL, et al: Zidovudine resistance and HIV-1 disease progression during antiretroviral therapy. Ann Intern Med 122:401–408, 1995.
28. Tadepalli SM, Puckett L, Jeal S, et al: Differential assay of zidovudine and its glucuronide metabolite in serum and urine with a radioimmunoassay kit. Clin Chem 36:897–900, 1990.
29. McLeod GX, Hammer SM: Zidovudine: Five years later. Ann Intern Med 117:487–501, 1992.
30. Fischl MA, Richman DD, Hansen N, et al: The safety and efficacy of zidovudine (zidovudine) in the treatment of subjects with mildly symptomatic human immunodeficiency virus type 1 (HIV) infection: A double-blind, placebo-controlled trial. Ann Intern Med 112:721–723, 1990.
31. Mhiri C, Baudrimont M, Bonne G, et al: Zidovudine myopathy: A distinctive disorder associated with mitochondrial dysfunction. Ann Neurol 29:606–614, 1991.
32. Spooner KM, Lane C, Masur H: Antiretroviral therapy: Reference guide to major clinical trials in patients infected with human immunodeficiency virus. Clin Infect Dis 20:1145–1151, 1995.
33. Edlin BR, St. Clair MH, Pitha PM, et al: In vitro resistance to zidovudine and alpha-interferon in HIV-1 isolates from patients: Correlations with treatment duration and response. Ann Intern Med 117:457–460, 1992.
34. Boucher CAB, Lange JMA, Miedema FF, et al: HIV-1 biological phenotype and the development of zidovudine resistance in relation to disease progression in asymptomatic individuals during treatment. AIDS 6:1259–1264, 1992.
35. Cooley TP, Kunches LM, Saunders CA, et al: Once-daily administration of 2′,3′-dideoxyinosine (ddI) in patients with the acquired immunodeficiency syndrome or AIDS-related complex. Results of a phase I trial. N Engl J Med 322:1340–1345, 1990.
36. Yarchoan R, Mitsuya H, Myers CE, et al: Clinical pharmacology of 3′-azido-2′,3′-dideoxythymidine (zidovudine) and related dideoxynucleosides. N Engl J Med 321:726–738, 1989.
37. Lipsky JJ: Zalcitabine and didanosine. Lancet 341:30–32, 1993.
38. Kieburtz KD, Seidlin M, Lambert JS, et al: Extended follow-up of peripheral neuropathy in patients with AIDS and AIDS-related complex treated with dideoxyinosine. J Acquir Immune Defic Syndr 5:60–64, 1992.
39. Martin JL, Wilson JE, Haynes RL, et al: Mechanism of resistance of human immunodeficiency virus type 1 to 2′,3′-dideoxyinosine. Proc Natl Acad Sci USA 90:6135–6139, 1993.
40. St. Clair MH, Martin JL, Tudor-Williams G, et al: Resistance to ddI and sensitivity to AZT induced by a mutation in HIV-1 reverse transcriptase. Science 253:1557–1559, 1991.
41. Demeter LM, Nawaz T, Morse G, et al: Development of zidovudine resistance mutations in patients receiving prolonged didanosine monotherapy. J Infect Dis 172:1480–1485, 1995.
42. Martin JL, Wilson JE, Haynes RL, Furman PA: Mechanism of resistance of human immunodeficiency virus type 1 to 2′,3′-dideoxyinosine. Proc Natl Acad Sci USA 90:6135–6139, 1993.
43. Johnson V, Merrill D, Videler J, et al: Two-drug combinations of zidovudine, didanosine and recombinant interferon-α A inhibit replication of zidovudine-resistant human immunodeficiency virus type 1 synergistically in vitro. J Infect Dis 164:646–655, 1991.
44. Shelton MH, O'Donnell AM, Morse GD: Zalcitibine. Ann Pharmacother 27:480–489, 1993.
45. Fischl MA, Stanley K, Collier K, et al. Combination and monotherapy with zidovudine and zalcitabine in patients with advanced HIV disease. Ann Intern Med 122:24–32, 1995.
46. Dudley MN, Graham KK, Kaul S, et al: Pharmacokinetics of stavudine in patients with AIDS or AIDS-related complex. J Infect Dis 166:480–485, 1992.
47. Lin P-F, Samanta H, Rose RE, et al: Genotypic and phenotypic analysis of human immunodeficiency virus type 1 isolates from patients on prolonged stavudine therapy. J Infect Dis 170:1157–1164, 1994.
48. Merrill DP, Moonis M, Chou T-C, Hirsch MS: Lamivudine or stavudine in two- and three-drug combinations against human immunodeficiency virus type 1 replication in vitro. J Infect Dis 173:355–364, 1996.
49. Larder BA, Kemp SD, Harrigan PR: Potential mechanism for sustained antiretroviral efficacy of AZT-3TC combination therapy. Science 269:696–699, 1995.
50. Eron JJ, Benoit SL, Jemsek J, et al: Treatment with lamivudine, zidovudine, or both in HIV-positive patients with 200 to 500 $CD4^+$ cells per cubic mullimeter. N Engl J Med 333:1662–1669, 1995.
51. Staszewski S, Loveday C, Picazo JJ, et al: Safety and efficacy of lamivudine-zidovudine combination therapy in zidovudine-experienced patients. JAMA 276:111–117, 1996.
52. Saag MS, Emini EA, Laskin OL, et al: A short term clinical evaluation of L-697,661, a non-nucleoside inhibitor of HIV-1 reverse transcriptase. N Engl J Med 329:1065–1072, 1993.
53. Dueweke TJ, Pushkarskaya T, Poppe SM, et al: A mutation in reverse transcriptase of bis(heteroaryl)piperazine-resistant human immunodeficiency virus type 1 that confers increased sensitivity to other nonnucleoside inhibitors. Proc Natl Acad Sci USA 90:4713–4717, 1993.
54. Richman DD, Rosenthal AS, Skoog M, et al: BI-RG-587 is active against zidovudine-resistant HIV-1 and synergistic with zidovudine. Antimicrob Agents Chemother 35:305–308, 1991.
55. Havilar D, Cheeseman SH, McLaughlin M, et al: High dose nevirapine: Safety, pharmacokinetics and antiviral effect in patients with HIV infection. J Infect Dis 171:537–545, 1995.

56. Spence RA, Kati WM, Anderson KS, Johnson KA: Mechanism of inhibition of HIV-1 reverse transcriptase by nonnucleoside inhibitors. Science 267:988–993, 1995.
57. D'Aquilla RT, Hughes MD, Johnson VA, et al: Nevirapine, zidovudine, and didanosine compared with zidovudine and didanosine in patients with HIV-1 infection: A randomized, double-blind, placebo-controlled trial. Ann Intern Med 124:1019–1030, 1996.
58. Campbell TB, Young RK, Eron JJ, et al: Inhibition of human immunodeficiency virus type 1 replication in vitro by the bis-(heteroaryl)piperazine atevirdine (U-87201E) in combination with zidovudine or didanosine. J Infect Dis 168:318–326, 1993.
59. Romero D, Morge R, Biles C, et al: Discovery, synthesis, and bioactivity of bis(hetero)piperazines: A novel class of non-nucleoside HIV-1 reverse transcriptase inhibitors. J Med Chem 37:999–1014, 1994.
60. Wlodawer A, Miller M, Jaskolski M, et al: Conserved folding in retroviral proteinases: Crystal structure of a synthetic HIV-1 protease. Science 245:616–621, 1989.
61. Wlodawer A: Rational drug design: The proteinase inhibitors. Pharmacotherapy 14:9S–20S, 1994.
62. Kitchen VS, Skinner C, Ariyoshi K, et al: Safety and activity of saquinavir in HIV infection. Lancet 345:952–955, 1995.
63. Markowitz M, Saag M, Powderly WG, et al: A preliminary study of ritonavir, an inhibitor of HIV-1 protease, to treat HIV-1 infection. N Engl J Med 333:1534–1539, 1995.
64. Danner SA, Carr A, Leonard JM, et al: A short-term study of the safety, pharmacokinetics, and efficacy of ritonavir, an inhibitor of HIV-1 protease. N Engl J Med 333:1528–1533, 1995.
65. Jacobsen H, Yasargil K, Winslow D, et al: Characterization of human immunodeficiency virus type-1 mutants with decreased sensitivity to proteinase inhibitor Ro31-8959. Virology 206:527–534, 1995.
66. Schapiro JM, Winters MA, Steward F, et al: The effect of high-dose saquinavir on viral load and $CD4^+$ T-cell counts in HIV-infected patients. Ann Intern Med 124:1039–1050, 1996.
67. Saquinavir (Invirase™) package insert, Nutley, NJ, Roche Laboratories, 1995.
68. Vella S: Clinical experience with saquinavir. AIDS 9:21–25, 1996.
69. McMahon DK, Mellors JW: Resistance to protease inhibitors. HIV: Advances in Research and Therapy, Vol 6. Greenwich, CT, Cliggott Communications, 1996, p 9.
70. Ritonavir (Norvir™) package insert, North Chicago, IL, Abbott Laboratories, 1996.
71. Kumar GN, Rodrigues AD, Buko AM, et al: Cytochrome P450–mediated metabolism of the HIV-1 protease inhibitor ritonavir (ABT 538) in human liver microsomes. J Pharmacol Exp Ther 277:423–431, 1996.
72. Cameron B, Heath-Chiozzi M, Kravcik S, et al: Prolongation of life and prevention of AIDS in advanced HIV immunodeficiency with ritonavir (Abstr MoB 411). Presented at the 11th International Conference on AIDS; July 7–12, 1996; Vancouver, British Columbia, Canada.
73. Markowitz M, et al: Triple therapy with AZT, 3TC and ritonavir in 12 patients newly infected with HIV-1 (Abstr ThB 933). Presented at the 11th International Conference on AIDS; July 7–12, 1996; Vancouver, British Columbia, Canada.
74. Indinavir (Crixivan™) package insert, West Point, PA, Merck, Sharp and Dohm, 1996.
75. Bilello JA, Bilello PA, Prichard M, et al: Reduction of the in vitro activity of A77093, an inhibitor of human immunodeficiency virus protease, by α1-acid glycoprotein. J Infect Dis 171:559–565, 1995.
76. Gulick R, Mellors J, Havlir D, et al: Potent and sustained antiretroviral activity of indinavir (IDV) in combination with zidovudine (ZDV) and lamivudine (3TC) (Abstr LB7). *In* Program and Abstracts of the 3rd Conference on Retroviruses and Opportunistic Infections; January 28–February 1, 1996; Washington, DC.
77. Condra JH, et al: Bidirectional inhibition of HIV-1 drug resistance selection by combination therapy with indinavir and reverse transcriptase inhibitors (Abstr ThB 932). Presented at the 11th International Conference on AIDS; July 7–12, 1996; Vancouver, British Columbia, Canada.
78. Emini EA: Maintenance of long-term virus suppression in patients treated with the protease inhibitor Crixivan (indinavir) (Abstr MoB 170). Presented at the 11th International Conference on AIDS; July 7–12, 1996; Vancouver, British Columbia, Canada.
79. Carpenter CC, Fischl MA, Hammer SM, et al: Antiretroviral therapy for HIV infection in 1996. JAMA 276:146–154, 1996.
80. Saag MS, Holodniy M, Kuritzkes DR, et al: Viral load markers in clinical practice: Recommendations of the International AIDS Society–USA Expert Panel. Nat Med 2:625–629, 1996.
81. Volberding PA, Lagakos SW, Grimes JM, et al: A comparison of immediate with deferred zidovudine therapy for asymptomatic HIV-infected adults with CD4 cell counts of 500 or more per cubic millimeter. N Engl J Med 333:401–407, 1995.
82. Concorde Coordinating Committee: Concorde: MRC/ANRS randomised double-blind controlled trial of immediate and deferred zidovudine in symptom-free HIV infection. Lancet 343:871–881, 1994.
83. Saravolatz LD, Winslow DL, Collins G, et al: Zidovudine alone or in combination with didanosine or zalcitabine in HIV-infected patients with the acquired immunodeficiency syndrome or fewer than 200 CD4 cells per cubic millimeter. N Engl J Med 335:1099–1106, 1996.
84. Corey L, Holmes KK: Therapy for human immunodeficiency virus infection—what have we learned? N Engl J Med 335:1142–1143, 1996.
85. Katzenstein DA, Hammer SM, Hughes MD, et al: The relation of virologic and immunologic markers to clinical outcomes after nucleoside therapy in HIV-infected adults with 200 to 500 CD4 cells per cubic millimeter. N Engl J Med 335:1091–1098, 1996.
86. Connor EM, Sperling RS, Gelber R, et al: Reduction of maternal-infant transmission of human immunodeficiency virus type 1 with zidovudine treatment. N Engl J Med 331:1173–1180, 1994.
87. Wiznia AA, Crane M, Lambert G, et al: Zidovudine use to reduce perinatal HIV type 1 transmission in an urban medical center. JAMA 275:1504–1506, 1996.
88. Dickover RE, Garratty EM, Herman SA, et al: Identification of levels of maternal HIV-1 RNA associated with risk of perinatal transmission: Effect of maternal zidovudine treatment on viral load. JAMA 275:599–605, 1996.
89. Sperling RS, Shapiro DE, Coombs RW, et al: Maternal viral load, zidovudine treatment, and the risk of transmission of human immunodeficiency virus type 1 from mother to infant. N Engl J Med 335:1621–1629, 1996.
90. Centers for Disease Control and Prevention: Recommendations of the U.S. Public Health Service Task Force on the use of zidovudine to reduce perinatal transmission of human immunodeficiency virus. MMWR Morbid Mortal Wkly Rep 43(RR-11):1–19, 1994.
91. Mauskopf JA, Paul JE, Wickman DS, et al: Economic impact of treatment of HIV-positive pregnant women and their newborns with zidovudine. JAMA 276:132–138, 1996.
92. Fiscus SA, Adimora AA, Schoenbach VJ, et al: Perinatal HIV infection and the effect of zidovudine therapy on transmission in rural and urban counties. JAMA 275:1483–1488, 1996.
93. Henderson DK, Fahey BJ, Willy M, et al: Risk for occupational transmission of human immunodeficiency virus type 1 (HIV-1) associated with clinical exposures: A prospective evaluation. Ann Intern Med 113:740–746, 1990.
94. Centers for Disease Control and Prevention: Update: Provisional recommendations for chemoprophylaxis after occupational exposure to human immunodeficiency virus. MMWR Morbid Mortal Wkly Rep 45:468–472, 1996.
95. Ho D: Time to hit HIV, early and hard. N Engl J Med 333:450–451, 1995.
96. Havlir DV, Richman DD: Viral dynamics of HIV: Implications for drug development and therapeutic strategies. Ann Intern Med 124:984–994, 1996.
97. Mansky LM, Temin HM: Lower in vivo mutation rate of human immunodeficiency virus type 1 than predicted from the fidelity of purified reverse transcriptase. J Virol 69:5087–5094, 1995.
98. O'Brien WA, Hartigan PM, Martin D, et al: Changes in plasma HIV-1 RNA and $CD4^+$ lymphocyte counts and the risk of progression to AIDS. N Engl J Med 334:426–431, 1996.
99. Japour AJ, Mayers DL, Johnson VA, et al: A standardized peripheral blood mononuclear cell culture assay for determination of drug susceptibilities of clinical human immunodeficiency virus (HIV-1) isolates. Antimicrob Agents Chemother 37:1095–1101, 1993.
100. Kellam P, Larder BA: Recombinant virus assay: A rapid phenotypic assay for assessment of drug susceptibility of human

immunodeficiency virus type 1 isolates. Antimicrob Agents Chemother 38:23–30, 1994.
101. Gingeras TR, Prodanovich P, Latimer T, et al: Use of self-sustained sequence replication amplification reaction to analyze and detect mutations in zidovudine-resistant human immunodeficiency virus. J Infect Dis 164:1066–1074, 1991.
102. Richman DD, Guatelli JC, Grimes J, et al: Detection of mutations associated with zidovudine resistance in human immunodeficiency virus by use of the polymerase chain reaction. J Infect Dis 164:1075–1081, 1991.
103. Eastman PS, Boyer E, Mole L, et al: Nonisotopic hybridization assay for determination of relative amounts of genotypic human immunodeficiency virus type 1 zidovudine resistance. J Clin Microbiol 33:2777–2780, 1995.
104. Kozal MJ, Shah N, Shen N, et al: Expensive polymorphisms observed in HIV-1 clade B protease gene using high-density oligonucleotide assays. Nat Med 2:753–759, 1996.
105. Larder BA, Darby G, Richman DD: HIV with reduced sensitivity to zidovudine isolated during prolonged therapy. Science 243:1731–1734, 1989.
106. Richman DD: Resistance of clinical isolates of human immunodeficiency virus to antiretroviral agents. Antimicrob Agents Chemother 37:1207–1213, 1993.
107. Kellam P, Boucher CA, Larder BA: Fifth mutation in human immunodeficiency virus type 1 reverse transcriptase contributes to the development of high-level resistance to zidovudine. Proc Natl Acad Sci USA 89:1934–1938, 1992.
108. Boucher CAB, O'Sullivan E, Mulder JW, et al: Ordered appearance of zidovudine-resistant mutations during treatment of 18 human immunodeficiency virus–positive subjects. J Infect Dis 165:105–110, 1992.
109. Erice A, Mayers DL, Strike DG, et al: Brief report: Primary infection caused by zidovudine-resistant human immunodeficiency virus type 1 (HIV-1). N Engl J Med 328:1163–1165, 1993.
110. Montaner JSG, Singer J, Schechter MT, et al: Clinical correlates of in vitro HIV-1 resistance to zidovudine. Results of the multicentre Canadian zidovudine trial. AIDS 7:189–196, 1993.
111. Tudor-Williams G, St. Clair MH, McKinney RE, et al: HIV-1 sensitivity to zidovudine and clinical outcome in children. Lancet 339:15–19, 1992.
112. Kozal MJ, Shafer RS, Winters MA, et al: A mutation in HIV reverse transcriptase and decline in CD4 lymphocyte numbers in long-term zidovudine recipients. J Infect Dis 167:526–532, 1993.
113. Tisdale M, Kemp SD, Parry NR, Larder BA: Rapid in vitro selection of human immunodeficiency virus type 1 resistant to 3′-thiacytidine inhibitors due to a mutation in the YMDD region of reverse transcriptase. Proc Natl Acad Sci USA 90:5653–5656, 1993.
114. Schuurman R, Nijhuis M, van Leeuwen R, et al: Rapid changes in human immunodeficiency virus type 1 RNA load and appearance of drug-resistant populations in persons treated with lamivudine (3TC). J Infect Dis 171:1411–1419, 1995.
115. St. Clair MH, Martin JL, Tudor WG, et al: Resistance to ddI and sensitivity to AZT induced by a mutation in HIV-1 reverse transcriptase. Science 253:1557–1559, 1991.
116. Fitzgibbon JE, Howell RM, Haberzettl CA, et al: Human immunodeficiency virus type 1 *pol* gene mutations which cause decreased susceptibility to 2′,3′-dideoxycytidine. Antimicrob Agents Chemother 36:153–157, 1992.
117. Zhang D, Caliendo AM, Eron JJ, et al: Resistance to 2′,3′-dideoxycytidine conferred by a mutation in codon 65 of the HIV-1 reverse transcriptase. Antimicrob Agents Chemother 38:282–287, 1994.
118. Lacey SF, Larder BA: A novel mutation (V75T) in the HIV-1 reverse transcriptase confers resistance to 2′,3′-didehydro-2′,3′-dideoxythymidine (d4T) in cell culture. Antimicrob Agents Chemother 38:1428–1432, 1994.
119. Lin P-F, Samanta H, Rose RE, et al: Genotypic and phenotypic analysis of human immunodeficiency virus type 1 isolates from patients on prolonged stavudine therapy. J Infect Dis 170:1157–1164, 1994.
120. Larder BA: 3′-Azido-3′-deoxythymidine resistance suppressed by a mutation conferring human immunodeficiency virus type 1 resistance to non-nucleoside reverse transcriptase inhibitors. Antimicrob Agents Chemother 36:2664–2669, 1992.
121. Jacobsen H, Hanggi M, Ott M, et al: In vivo resistance to a human immunodeficiency virus type-1 proteinase inhibitor: Mutations, kinetics, and frequencies. J Infect Dis 173:1379–1387, 1996.
122. Patick AK, Mo H, Markowitz M, et al: Antiviral and resistance studies of AG1343, an orally bioavailable inhibitor of human immunodeficiency virus protease. Antimicrob Agents Chemother 40:292–297, 1996.
123. Kovacs JA, Vogel S, Albert JM, et al: Controlled trial of interleukin-2 infusions in patients infected with the human immunodeficiency virus. N Engl J Med 335:1350–1356, 1996.
124. Normile D: IL-12 at the crossroads. Science 268:1432, 1995.
125. Arenzana-Selsdedos F, Virelizier J-L, Rousset D, et al: HIV blocked by chemokine antagonist (Letter). Nature 383:400, 1996.
126. Bridges SH, Sarver N: Gene therapy and immune restoration for HIV disease. Lancet 345:427–432, 1995.
127. Rossi JJ, Sarver N: Catalytic antisense RNA (ribozymes): Their potential and use as anti-HIV therapeutic agents. Adv Exp Med Biol 312:95–109, 1992.
128. Nabel GJ, Fox BA, Post L, et al: A molecular genetic intervention for AIDS—Effects of a transdominant negative form of Rev. Hum Gene Ther 5:79–92, 1994.
129. Duan L, Bagasra O, Laughlin MA, et al: Potent inhibition of human immunodeficiency virus type 1 replication by an intracellular anti-Rev single-chain antibody. Proc Natl Acad Sci USA 91:5075–5079, 1994.
130. Roberts MR, Qin L, Smith DH, et al: Immunotherapy for HIV: Targeting of HIV-infected cells by $CD8^+$ T lymphocytes armed with universal T cell receptors. Blood 84:2787–2789, 1994.
131. Riddell SR, Greenberg PD, Overell RW, et al: Phase I study of cellular adoptive immunotherapy using genetically modified $CD8^+$ HIV-specific T cells for HIV seropositive patients undergoing allogeneic bone marrow transplant. Hum Gene Ther 3:319–38, 1992.
132. Ulmer JB, Donnelly JJ, Parker SE, et al: Heterologous protection against influenza by injection of DNA encoding a viral protein. Science 259:1745–1749, 1993.
133. Lori F, Malykh A, Cara A, et al: Hydroxyurea as an inhibitor of human immunodeficiency virus-type 1 replication. Science 266:801–805, 1994.
134. Biron F, Lucht F, Peyramond D, et al: Anti-HIV activity of the combination of didanosine and hydroxyurea in HIV-1 infected individuals. J Acquir Immune Defic Syndr Hum Retrovirol 10:36–40, 1995.
135. Mortality in patients with the acquired immunodeficiency syndrome treated with either foscarnet or ganciclovir for cytomegalovirus retinitis. Studies of Ocular Complications of AIDS Research Group, in collaboration with the AIDS Clinical Trials Group [published erratum in N Engl J Med 326:1172, 1992]. N Engl J Med 326:213–220, 1992.
136. Sandstrom EG, Kaplan JC, Byington RE, Hirsch MS: Inhibition of human T-cell lymphotropic virus type III in vitro by phosphonoformate. Lancet 1:1480–1482, 1985.
137. Feinberg M, Greene W: Molecular insights into human immunodeficiency virus type-1 pathogenesis. Curr Opin Immunol 4:466–474, 1992.

128

Prevention of Human Immunodeficiency Virus Transmission

Jonathan M. Zenilman

Efforts to prevent human immunodeficiency virus (HIV) infection are based on altering the known modes of transmission. Because HIV infection is a dynamic epidemic, effective prevention programs depend on continuous surveillance to elucidate the modes of HIV transmission and on understanding of the risk behaviors that promote transmission.

"Primary" prevention is based on eliminating behavioral risk factors. For example, primary prevention would be the goal of sexual abstinence or of preventing intravenous drug use. From a practical perspective, primary prevention is an option only in the long term. Drug use and sexual behaviors are widespread, are conducted within social situations that are supportive of these behaviors, and are pleasurable. Reducing the frequency of these activities is therefore difficult even under optimal circumstances; behavior change, when it occurs, is a gradual process for most individuals. Equally difficult is maintaining and sustaining these changes (intervention "maintenance"). The objective of most intervention efforts is therefore to reduce risk. Risk reduction can be effected through decreasing the frequency of risky behaviors or by intervening to decrease the transmission efficiency during the behavior. Decreasing sexual partner turnover, intercourse frequency, or drug use frequency exemplifies decreased risky behavior—analogous to a simplistic dose-response model. Two examples of settings in which behavior frequency remains the same but transmission efficiency is reduced are condom use, which reduces the efficiency of sexual transmission, and needle exchange programs, which decrease transmission among intravenous drug users.

Vertical transmission prevention and control of sexually transmitted diseases (STDs) are biomedical approaches that have an impact on HIV transmission efficiency. For vertical transmission, treatment with antiretrovirals during pregnancy and the peripartum period decreases HIV transmission to the fetus—a pharmacologic intervention that is directed specifically at HIV. STDs have been recognized as biologic cofactors in facilitating HIV transmission. Community-based STD treatment has the potential to reduce HIV transmission efficiency—an indirect pharmacologic intervention. Development of comprehensive HIV prevention programs requires a complex menu of services, including individual-based interventions; community-wide education; health care services, especially HIV counseling, testing, and treatment services; drug treatment services; and STD diagnostic and treatment services.

Epidemiologic Issues Relevant to Prevention

Effective prevention and risk reduction intervention approaches require a current understanding of HIV epidemiology, in particular the groups at highest risk for infection. Behavioral and risk reduction interventions designed for one ethnic, cultural, or sexual preference group may be inappropriate or ineffective in other groups, which highlights the need for continuous epidemiologic monitoring and program effectiveness evaluation. Evaluation of intervention effectiveness is often difficult because the HIV epidemic is dynamic. For example, in the past 10 years, the proportion of cases in homosexual men has been decreasing, whereas cases in intravenous drug users, heterosexual contacts, and women have increased. At the end of 1995, more than 506,000 cases of surveillance-definition acquired immunodeficiency syndrome (AIDS) were reported to the Centers for Disease Control and Prevention (CDC).[1] Homosexual men accounted for 51% of cases, a marked decrease from 64% in 1981 to 1987,[2] and women, predominantly infected through heterosexual contact, accounted for 19% of cases. When prevalent HIV cases are considered (rather than surveillance-definition AIDS), the estimates of infection are between 650,000 and 900,000,[3] with a higher prevalence in women and minorities.

Early in the epidemic, most HIV intervention programs targeted homosexual men and intravenous drug users. As the epidemic evolves, messages of safer sex for gay men and safer injecting practice for heterosexual intravenous drug users, or vice versa, are often not appropriate. In fact, unless carefully conceived, intervention programs targeting one risk group have the potential to alienate or marginalize other risk group members from the prevention effort. As another example, the initial HIV prevention efforts in gay men resulted in greater than 80% reductions of incident infections and risky behaviors by the late 1980s. However, in 1989 and the early 1990s, rectal gonorrhea and other markers of high-risk behavior in homosexual men[4] began to increase substantially. This was interpreted by some observers as a cohort effect of younger gay men becoming sexually active or, in some situations, as a reaction of younger gay men to the safer sex culture that had developed. HIV prevention programs must therefore be flexible.

Biologic Approaches to Reducing Disease Transmission: A Brief Summary

Blood and Biologic Product Screening

Universal screening of blood and biologic products has essentially eliminated transmission through transfusion. Blood-borne transmission infected more than 50% of hemophiliacs until blood screening tests became available in 1985. Although there continues to be concern about the possibility of false-negative results due to either HIV variants or the seroconversion "window" period, the risk has been substantially reduced by the use of new-generation screening tests and the application of stringent blood donor screening procedures, the heat treatment of clotting concentrate products, and the accelerated development of recombinant nonhuman-derived clotting factor replacements. A CDC study estimated the HIV risk through blood products to be less than 1 per 493,000.[5] Similar procedures have also been instituted to reduce risk through other biologic products, such as from allogeneic organ transplantation and artificial insemination.[6] In developing countries, however, testing of blood products is not universal, even in areas with high HIV seroprevalence rates.

Vaccines[9]

Primary prevention through vaccination is an attractive theoretical option[8] that will not, however, be realized in the near future. Developing HIV vaccines has proved to be an enormous technical challenge. Some of the approaches taken have included whole inactivated virus; subunit vaccines based on *env, pol,* or *gag* components or component combinations; and DNA vaccines. The challenges to development include elucidating the protective immune response, the high antigenic variation of the virus, the role of immune modulators, and the rapid neurotropism of the virus. Even if a vaccine were developed, difficult epidemiologic issues and ethical problems are incurred in the clinical trials that would be necessary.[9] For even in high-risk communities, HIV seroconversion (HIV incidence) is a relatively rare event. Seroincidence rates of 1% to 2% are typical of communities that are considered for vaccine trials. A randomized, placebo-controlled trial of a candidate vaccine would require enormous sample sizes. By definition, only HIV-seronegative individuals could be enrolled in a trial, necessitating pretest and posttest counseling and counseling on risk reduction—which in itself may be a confounding effect.

Preventing Vertical Transmission: Development of a Pharmacologic Prevention Intervention

Nearly all HIV cases in children are acquired through vertical transmission. Vertical transmission has been demonstrated perinatally or postnatally through breast-feeding.[10–12] Without intervention, HIV transmission occurs in 15% to 35%.[13–17] In developing countries, the fraction attributable to breast-feeding is estimated at 22%.[18] Reducing breast-feeding poses profound ethical dilemmas, because sanitary and socioeconomic conditions often preclude the availability of safe formula feeding. Obstetric complications, such as premature rupture of membranes, nearly doubles the transmission risk.[19]

Pharmacologic intervention with zidovudine during pregnancy, perinatally, and postnatally has been found to profoundly reduce the vertical transmission rate. In a placebo-controlled double-blind trial (AIDS Clinical Trials Group Protocol 076),[20] the vertical transmission rate was reduced threefold, from 25% to 8%, providing the first evidence that pharmacologic interventions can be effective in preventing HIV transmission. Nevertheless, substantial barriers prevent use of zidovudine for all HIV-infected pregnant women. In developing countries, the cost of the medications is prohibitive and will limit the implementation. Even when cost is not a factor, this intervention requires that women be enrolled in a prenatal care program; that they be offered and accept HIV counseling and testing; that on the basis of a positive HIV test result, they be offered the zidovudine protocol; and that they be compliant with the medication regimen. Successful implementation of this pharmacologic intervention is dependent on a well-functioning medical care system and access to it. There was initial concern about the acceptability of HIV counseling and testing and zidovudine therapy in pregnant women who are HIV infected, especially the ethics of performing "blinded" serosurveys in pregnant women and neonates. Studies in the Bronx, New York,[21] and in North Carolina[22] found that the majority of pregnant women diagnosed with HIV infection antenatally accepted the zidovudine therapy option. In response, the CDC and other federal agencies have expanded the availability of HIV voluntary counseling and testing available to pregnant women.[23] A major problem, however, appears to be lack of access to and use of prenatal care and HIV testing resources, especially in urban areas. The zidovudine protocol requires frequent visits and monitoring after the 20th week of gestation; therefore, referral to perinatal centers experienced in HIV management is often required.

Behavioral Intervention Approaches[24, 25]

Population-Based Mass Media Campaigns

Initial approaches to HIV control used educational approaches, the intervention hypothesis being that provision of accurate information would induce a rational change in individuals' behavior. Included within this were mass media campaigns and a national mailout of HIV education materials, school-based HIV prevention education, and incorporation of HIV-based themes into the popular media. These efforts increased the knowledge base of the population as measured in national surveys[26] and local studies and may have reduced HIV-related discrimination; there are few data to suggest that these had an impact on high-risk behaviors related to HIV transmission.[27] As the epidemic progressed, it also became clear that more sophisticated approaches were required to develop and evaluate behavioral interventions.

Surveys of Sexual Behavior

Because most HIV transmission is through either homosexual or heterosexual behavior, reducing sexual risk is a logical approach to disease control efforts. Designing interventions to reduce high-risk sexual behavior requires an accurate definition of the "baseline" state, without which program effectiveness evaluation would be impossible. In 1985, the descriptive epidemiology of sexual behavior in the United States was not known, and the only large-scale surveys of sexual behavior were Kinsey's original work conducted in the 1940s and 1950s. Sexual behavior modules were therefore incorporated into large national health surveys.

The General Social Survey, which is a national probability sample of 2896 adults (1988–1990), estimated that 3 to 6 million adults had five or more sex partners in the past year and that alcohol consumption doubled the incidence of high-risk sexual behavior.[27] Similar data were found in the National Survey of Family Growth, which surveyed reproductive health issues in women aged 15 to 44 years. These data indicated that 23% of all women surveyed had more than 5 lifetime sexual partners and that 8% of unmarried women had three or more sexual partners within the past 3 months.[28, 29] An important finding in the National Survey of Family Growth was that the age at first heterosexual intercourse actually decreased by nearly a full year between 1982 and 1988. In the National Survey of Adolescent Males, which is a nationally representative interview study of adolescent men 15 to 19 years old, the average age at first intercourse was 15.6 years.[30] Condom use was higher than in surveys done in previous years. However, as adolescents age, the proportion using condoms during each sexual act decreases. This finding is also associated with an increased level of drug and alcohol use. The largest set of sexual behavior data is from the National AIDS Behavioral Surveys of more than 10,000 respondents collected in 1990 to 1991. Initial reports of the data found that in the heterosexual population, 15% to 31% of heterosexuals nationally and 20% to 41% of those in cities with high AIDS prevalence reported an HIV risk factor. Condom use was low; only 12% of respondents reported consistent condom use.[31] In a longitudinal component of that survey, little change occurred in these proportions from 1990 to 1992.[32] To assess HIV and STD risk behaviors in adolescents, the CDC has conducted behavioral risk factor surveillance in the National Youth Risk Behavior Survey, which is a periodic self-administered survey conducted in schools.[33, 34] In 1993, 53% of high-school students reported being sexually experienced, 18.8% had four or more partners, and 11% had used alcohol and drugs before the last intercourse. These data in 1993 were not different from those of the survey conducted in 1990. However, a small increase in reported condom use was observed; 46% to 53% reported condom use at last intercourse. Similar results were found in a series of longitudinal studies conducted among college students in Rhode Island and Maryland; although the rate of sexual behavior and partner turnover was essentially unchanged over time, marked increases in the use of condoms were noted.[35–37]

In summary, the behavioral surveys are a useful population-based baseline state for the evaluation of HIV prevention interventions directed at sexual behaviors and, to a lesser extent, drug-using behavior. These surveys also demonstrate the high rate of sexual activity among adolescents, underscoring the need for prevention efforts in these groups. Behavioral surveys have evolved as one potential method for evaluating the impact of interventions on large proportions of the population.

Adaptation of Behavioral Deterministic Models to Intervention Efforts

More sophisticated efforts at developing behavioral interventions require a model of human behavior and action. A behavioral model provides

- A rational explanation of the determinants of behavior. This in turn provides insight into how an intervention should be developed.
- A qualitative and quantitative framework for evaluation of intervention effectiveness. In HIV prevention interventions, direct measurement of HIV seroincidence is rarely used as an intervention outcome. HIV seroincidence is a relatively rare event (in a statistical sense) and would require a long follow-up time. Program evaluation measures often focus on changes in either high-risk behaviors or other correlates (such as attitudes and beliefs). For example, if self-efficacy in using condoms was shown to correlate highly with HIV and STD risk, an intervention may focus its efforts and evaluation on improving condom use self-efficacy. This is especially important because HIV incidence is almost never measurable in an intervention to reduce high-risk sexual behaviors. In addition, fully controlled studies of sexual behavior interventions, in which the control condition receives no intervention, are unethical. Therefore, behavioral models offer a series of behavioral variables that can be evaluated in place of the biologic HIV outcome. No one model is accepted as a standard for HIV risk reduction interventions, and often, elements of multiple models are blended in an intervention program.[38]

In adapting behavioral models for HIV interventions, several themes predominate. Successful intervention efforts are developed by multidisciplinary teams including physicians, epidemiologists, behavioral scientists, and often anthropologists and social workers. For example, anthropologists can provide crucial information by elucidating deep-seated cultural attitudes toward sexual behaviors and which behaviors are amenable to intervention. In terms of developing intervention approaches, several themes predominate, all of which are interrelated.

Increasing Knowledge Base. Providing accurate information about sexuality, HIV, STDs, and drug use is important. At-risk individuals often have poor access to accurate information. This includes opportunities to explore local beliefs and myths related to sensitive behaviors in a nonjudgmental environment.

Self-esteem. Investigators have focused on developing self-esteem within sexual relationships and especially how this relates to the decision to have sexual intercourse or use drugs.

Communication Skills. Improving communication and negotiation skills, especially within the context of sensitive behaviors such as sexual behaviors, is important for being able to make one's wishes known to sexual partners. Condom use interventions, for example, have stressed development of negotiating skills (i.e., convincing a partner that a condom should be used) as well as increasing self-esteem (including the ability to refuse sexual intercourse if a condom is not used).

Technical Efficacy. In condom use interventions, the technical aspects of using condoms or other barrier methods are important. A flaw in many traditional public health approaches is that "use condom" messages assume that the intended intervention recipients use them correctly.

Social Norms.[39] Behaviors occur within a social environment, usually one's peer group. Individual-based approaches to behavior change are often ineffective if the operative external environment does not change. For example, smoking behaviors in the United States between 1960 and 1995 underwent a drastic transformation from acceptance or promotion in most social settings to a behavior that is actively discouraged in social group settings and in the environment, such as workplaces, restaurants, and public places. This type of social norm change takes time. The most successful approach to changing social norms for sexual behavior has focused on identifying "peer opinion leaders" to whom the group looks for leadership and guidance.

Examples of Behavioral Models Used to Develop Interventions

Interventions to reduce risky behaviors have been developed by use of four major behavioral models. These behavioral models are derived from a variety of health program interventions since the 1960s. The utility of these models is that the frameworks were developed and understood, thereby reducing the development time needed for use in an epidemic that is rapidly progressing. However, the disadvantage is that these models for the most part were not developed to explain the determinants of sexual and other sensitive behavior, which are the core needs of HIV-related prevention interventions.

The Health Belief Model

The health belief model is a "value expectancy" theory.[40] In other words, an individual's actions are driven by

- The desire to avoid illness or get well
- The belief that a specific health action will provide benefit (e.g., prevent illness)

An individual either consciously or unconsciously makes a value judgment for implementing an intervention behavior on the basis of

- Perceived susceptibility to the illness or condition
- Perceived severity of the illness or condition
- Perceived benefits of taking health action (including physical and psychologic benefits)
- Perceived barriers ("costs") to taking health action (e.g., in condom use, the barriers could be reduced sensation or need for negotiation with the partner)
- "Cues to action" (e.g., social triggers)
- Social variables (e.g., socioeconomic status, education)

- Self-efficacy, which is particularly important for the development of long-term behavioral changes

Behavioral interventions organized along the health belief model will focus on increasing awareness of susceptibility, the severity of HIV infection, and the benefits of intervention. The intervention would also strive to identify barriers (such as reduced sensation with condom use) and attempt to ameliorate them.

Social Cognitive Theory

The principles of social cognitive theory[41] are that self-directed behavioral change requires skills in self-motivation, guidance, and the behavioral means and resources and social supports to maintain behavioral change. The theory's central concepts are those of "modeling and efficacy beliefs." In this model, the three determinants of a behavior are

- Personal determinants, such as cognitive, affective, and biologic factors. This would include the availability of information, self-efficacy, self-esteem, and negotiating skills.
- Environmental influences, such as the social environment.
- The behavior itself operating as a reinforcing feedback loop.

The Stages of Change Model

The stages of change model[42, 43] focuses more on the process of behavioral change than on the determinants. The "stages" paradigm offers a temporal sequence for intervention. For example, condom use in heterosexuals may be modeled in five stages:

1. Precontemplative—condom use is not being considered by the individual.
2. Contemplative—condom use is a consideration, but no action is imminent.
3. Ready for action—the individual has synthesized the intervention components and will use condoms if provided the correct trigger event.
4. Action—the individual has initiated using condoms.
5. Maintenance—the intervention has been maintained over time and is stable.

Under this paradigm, a variety of strategies are proposed to facilitate moving from one stage to the next. Some behavioral intervention studies have begun to use this paradigm to describe the target population. In this paradigm, individuals can be staged for a prevention behavior by use of short standardized interviews. For example, in studies conducted in U.S. STD clinics in 1993, 43% of men with a primary partner were precontemplative about condom use; with other partners, it was 14%.[44] Two interesting considerations follow. First, movement between stages can be in both directions. For example, movement from ready for action to action would be defined as a positive step; if this was in response to an intervention, it would define intervention success. Movement in the reverse direction would be considered relapse. Second, from a public health perspective, it may be cost-effective to focus intervention efforts only on a small segment of the population defined by these methods who are most likely going to have a tangible response (e.g., increasing condom use), such as the ready for action group if only limited resources are available.

Theory of Reasoned Action

The theory of reasoned action[45] assumes a causal chain that links beliefs to behavior, that is, performance of a behavior is a direct expression of an individual's intention to perform that behavior. Under this model, the key to intervention would be to alter intention. Determinants of intention include

- Attitude toward the behavior (positive and negative)
- Belief that behavior leads to disease outcome
- Subjective norms (i.e., social peer group considerations)
- Relative importance of attitudes compared with the social norms

In this model, the behavior is predicted by a series of mathematic models that combine the factors described.

Caveats with Behavioral Models

No single behavioral model has been shown to work in all situations. In part, this is due to the cultural diversity of at-risk populations and the need to specifically tailor intervention approaches, which makes comparisons difficult. There are also problems inherent to the models themselves. The models were derived from research in a variety of health areas, such as treatment of phobias, programs designed to increase compliance with no-smoking campaigns, and immunization programs. In contrast, sexual and drug-related behaviors are much more likely to be drive stimulated. Integrated behavioral models, such as the AIDS risk reduction model, incorporate features of several base models.[38]

The models assume that sexual and drug use behavior are rational consequences of a consistent set of determinants that can be defined. This is not the case.

- Sexual and drug-related behaviors present major problems in measurement. For example, in an STD treatment environment, there is an implicit social desirability to overreport condom use because of the context of the setting. These settings cannot usually be controlled in the clinical environment, where disease prevention messages are provided through a variety of venues. Measurement of these behaviors is nearly always by self-report. However, because the disease incidence rate is low, the interventions require that outcomes be measured by self-report in nearly every situation.[46]
- The models make a contextual assumption that risky behaviors can be addressed independently of other needs, such as drug treatment, HIV treatment, medical care, or income maintenance.
- The HIV epidemic is heterogeneous, as are the populations at risk. Each cultural and ethnic group may have different beliefs and customs regarding sexual behavior that need to be addressed in interventions.
- Behavior occurs within a social context. Nearly all of the behavioral models include social norms within one's peer group as a major factor in changing behavior or in maintaining safe behaviors. This has prompted a substantial body of research on the diffusion of knowledge within social groups. An important area in this context is the study of "social networks."[47–49] Social networks are an individual's immediate personal (including sexual) and family relationships. These form the basis of tangible and emotional support and are the basis in many situations for the social norms of behavior. A type of social network analysis is the tracing of sexual contacts, which is often done as part of HIV and STD transmission investigations. Intravenous drug use social networks, which consist of drug-using and sexual partners, are particularly important because they are often close knit. As a consequence of the social network structure, behavior change in key members of the social networks, or opinion leaders,[39] translates into changing social norms and hence behaviors within the group. This approach has the advantage of "leveraging" scarce intervention resources because the intervention is

focused primarily on changing attitudes, norms, and behaviors of the identified group leaders. This approach has been applied successfully in populations of gay men, drug users, and adolescents, in which peer educators have been used to promote STD and HIV control and contraceptive programs.

- Intervention studies must be longitudinal and hence costly because short-term relapse is common. Most intervention approaches still consider behavior amenable to rapid intervention. Sexual and drug-using behavior patterns, however, often develop over long periods and in response to multiple individual-based and community-based stimuli. Not all of these factors can be changed simultaneously.

Interventions to Reduce the Risk for Sexual Exposure

Promotion of Condom Use

Promoting condom use has been one of the central tenets of the HIV and STD risk reduction strategy both in the United States and abroad. Large programs have been developed to ensure the timely distribution of a large number of condoms, and instructions for condom use have been part of the national STD guidelines since 1989.[50] Condoms are effective when they are used correctly and consistently. Studies of HIV discordant heterosexual couples in California[51] and Italy[52, 53] have conclusively demonstrated that consistent use in controlled settings results in an approximately sevenfold decrease in HIV seroconversions. Condoms are also effective in reducing the risk for STDs,[54] which attains an increasing importance as the relationships of STDs as cofactors continue to be elucidated.

Studies of condom use have focused on understanding the determinants and issues related to their use, especially considering the low consistent use rate indicated by the national surveys. Increased condom use is influenced by the appreciation of a perceived benefit (i.e., STD and HIV prevention), the peer group's social norms, and sex education with specific instruction in condom use.[55–57] Challenges to maintain continued use include the need to continually reinforce the perceived benefit; the result of a successful prevention effort is that no adverse event occurs, in contrast to other interventions or commercial marketing strategies in which self-reinforcement of continued behavior is easier. As with other sex education programs, promoting condom use has not been found to increase sexual activity in adolescents or to result in earlier sexual debut.[58] Effective condom promotion requires integration of public health and social marketing efforts. Probably the most intensive and successful effort has been implemented in Thailand, where the "100% condom" program[59] has been implemented since 1991. This program includes open discussion of HIV prevention and condom promotion; intensive advertising; an infrastructure to purchase and distribute condoms; and linkages in promoting condoms with "stakeholders" including the army, provincial and municipal governments, commercial sex workers, and brothel owners. Large-scale reductions in HIV seroincidence in Thailand have in part been attributed to this program.[60] The Thai program provides a useful model on the development of an effective condom promotion and sexual risk reduction campaign. This effective program's major accomplishment was to change the social norms across a broad spectrum of society to encourage condom use.

Targeted Intervention Efforts

Education is often confused with interventions and counseling. Education refers to the transmittal of knowledge—in this case, knowledge of HIV transmission patterns, risks, and methods to avoid risk. In contrast, risk reduction counseling entails a dialogue between the counselor and the counseled, in either an individual or a group format. Structured behavioral interventions may include a combination of counseling, education, and attempts to alter group norms. Multiple sessions, small groups, and individual counseling are the intervention formats that have most frequently been used and appear to be the most effective. Although clinic-based interventions are the types most frequently reported, interventions have been integrated into other venues, such as school curricula. For example, one school-based intervention consisted of six interactive sessions conducted in a traditional high-school classroom environment.[61] Other approaches have used student peer educators, street outreach workers, and coworkers in places of employment.

The longitudinal (i.e., multisession) aspect of these interventions is critical. Evaluation of single-session interventions has demonstrated equivocal efficacy at best. Probably the best example of an unintended single-session intervention occurred in 1991, when basketball player Magic Johnson announced that he was HIV-positive and was retiring from basketball. At that time, a multisession behavioral intervention study was being conducted in high-risk heterosexuals recruited from an STD clinic in Baltimore.[62] Evaluation of participants 1 month after the announcement found a one-third reduction in high-risk behavior. Follow-up 1 year later found that high-risk behavior had returned to baseline levels and that the effect of Mr. Johnson's announcement had dissipated. This example illuminates the need for continued "maintenance" and reinforcement of behavioral risk reduction in any intervention context.

Multisession, longitudinal client-focused, and culturally sensitive approaches have demonstrated reductions in self-reported HIV sexual behavior risks in homosexual men, heterosexuals, and adolescents. For example, in 318 African-American homosexual men recruited from gay bars and bathhouses, a triple-session intervention reduced the rate of self-reported rectal intercourse from 45% to 20%, with no change reported in the control groups.[63] In heterosexuals, studies that compared multisession educational, counseling, and skills-building sessions (which included self-esteem building and condom negotiation skills) were conducted in San Francisco,[64] Milwaukee,[65] and Philadelphia.[66] For example, in the San Francisco study, inner-city women were recruited through street outreach. The intervention group had consistent increases in reported condom use and greater measures of sexual communication between partners (negotiating skills). These results are encouraging and suggest that behavioral change can be induced and maintained in high-risk populations.

Issues in Behavioral Intervention Studies

Advantages

Focused interventions are usually conducted in small group settings, using interventions that are developed specifically for the target populations. The more innovative efforts have used community group members as facilitators or team leaders, which many believe enhances the effectiveness.

Disadvantages

There are three major disadvantages of these interventions, which makes it difficult to generalize their use.

1. The community-based focus makes these interventions extremely expensive. Sexual and drug-using behavior occurs

within a social context, which must be defined for each target group.

2. Intervention effectiveness can be measured only through self-reported change in sexual behavior. Some authorities believe that this may predispose to reporting bias, that is, within an intervention setting, there is bias to overreport condom use and safer sex practices. For example, within Baltimore STD clinics, self-reported condom use was found not to correlate with incident STD.[67]

3. Intervention efforts require enrollment and participation of the community members in a long-term process. This may be difficult, especially in settings where there is substantive competition for an individual's time, such as employment or child care.

It appears that focused behavioral interventions may be an option for specific, high-risk groups. From a physician's perspective, it may be useful to approach high-risk behavioral reduction from a chronic disease model—gradual, incremental improvement when it occurs, requiring continued maintenance, and subject to relapse.

Challenges and Barriers to Implementation of Prevention Efforts

Community-Level Barriers

As demonstrated by the Thai model, effective community-based prevention interventions require a change in social norms and frank, open discussion of sensitive behavioral issues such as sexuality and drug use. Persons with HIV infection or at risk for HIV infection are often at risk for being marginalized from society because of their behaviors. For example, an effective HIV prevention program must include approaches to homosexual men, intravenous drug users, commercial sex workers, adolescents, and minorities.

Patient-Level Barriers

Implementation of HIV prevention interventions at the personal level requires the perception that one is at risk and the technical efficacy to implement these interventions. These issues are independent of the motivations behind sexual and drug use behavior, which must always be recognized as in part pleasure seeking and drive oriented. For example, successful implementation of condom use intervention requires the following steps to occur in sequence:

- Recognition that sexual activity is going to occur, perceiving the need for a condom (judgment)
- Accessibility to a condom (access and availability)
- Negotiation of condom use with partner
- Technical efficacy: removing condom from the package, putting it on correctly, using it during intercourse, and removing it correctly

Conditions that could impede the successful completion of these tasks, as well as other behaviorally oriented interventions, include mental illness and substance abuse (see later). Condom breakage is occasionally cited as a potential problem, especially among patients attending STD clinics. Breakage rates[68, 69] in high-risk patients (i.e., STD clinics) have been found to be 2% to 7%, with higher rates seen in homosexual men and the lowest in commercial sex workers.[70] Partner selection is another factor that could have an impact on effectiveness of a condom intervention. In practice, many individuals use condoms selectively. Typically, the pattern is to use condoms with casual sexual partners but not with regular partners (unless condoms are also being used as a contraceptive method). HIV risk in these situations would be dependent on the HIV seroprevalence in the partner pool with whom the individual is having unprotected intercourse.

Mental Illness

Psychiatric problems are extraordinarily common in HIV-infected patients.[71, 72] Although these disorders may occur as a response to HIV infection, in many cases they are long-standing and probably contribute to the high-risk behaviors that predispose to HIV infection. Studies in homosexual men with HIV infection found the prevalence of any axis I disorder (major depressive disorder, anxiety disorder, or adjustment disorder) to be 47% to 85%,[73, 74] and similarly high rates were found in patients attending an inner-city HIV clinic.[75] More troubling is the high rate of high-risk behaviors found in the chronically mentally ill. For example, of 60 chronic psychiatric outpatients studied in Wisconsin mental health clinics, 42% of men and 19% of women reported multiple sexual contacts with infrequent condom use.[76] A study of more than 600 adolescents in St. Louis similarly found that those with symptoms of mental health disorders were 2 to 11 times as likely to engage in risky sexual behaviors.[77] The highest risk appeared in those who had symptoms of alcohol use and affective illness disorders. Many of these disorders are treatable, and there is disagreement about whether the psychiatric disorder represents the effects of HIV infection or is a substantive contribution to the increased risk-taking behaviors, which in turn increase HIV risk. Nevertheless, whether an individual is HIV infected and continues to be sexually active or is at risk for being infected because of depression or other mental illness, implementation of behavioral interventions is not likely to occur unless the underlying psychiatric disorder is treated.

Substance Use

Substance abuse can impede intervention efforts by two mechanisms. First, substance use may be associated with increased risk-taking behavior, which may include high-risk sexual behavior. Second, substance abuse, especially of alcohol, may impede the technical efficacy in implementing risk reduction, which includes the technical steps in placing a condom correctly and negotiating with sexual partners.

Alcohol is increasingly recognized as a risk factor for HIV infection and high-risk sexual behaviors. Early studies in homosexual men found that heavy alcohol use was associated with general increases in risky sexual behavior,[78] decreased condom use,[79] and increased risk for relapse into risky sexual behavior after successful behavioral intervention.[80] Contextual substance use (i.e., immediately before sexual activity, or being high or intoxicated during intercourse) appears to have the highest risk. Similar results have been found in heterosexual populations. Studies in adolescents[81] and STD patients[82] in San Francisco demonstrated that alcohol use was associated with twofold to fourfold increased risk of not using condoms at last intercourse. A study in Baltimore STD clinics[83] found that heavy alcohol use was strongly associated with prevalent HIV infection and syphilis, a relationship that was present even after adjustment for heroin and crack cocaine use, which are often comorbid conditions.

HIV INFECTION IN SUBSTANCE ABUSERS: IMPACT ON INTERVENTION

The seroprevalence rate in intravenous drug users varies by community. National estimates of HIV seroprevalence in intravenous drug users range as high as 65%.[84, 85] Risks are greatest for those who share injection equipment, for the practices associated with sharing injecting equipment or sharing drug preparations ("back-loading" and "front-loading"), and for those who inject in "shooting galleries."[86–88] For noninjectors, such as crack cocaine smokers, cross-sectional studies have demonstrated that the seroprevalence rate ranges between 0% and 15%, depending on the locality,[89] with highest rates in the Northeast and the South. In intravenous drug users, the barriers to prevention implementation are not the pharmacologic effect of drugs so much as the social milieu. Nevertheless, there are a number of major problems. In a study conducted early in the HIV epidemic, HIV-infected female intravenous drug users in the Bronx were offered intensive HIV counseling and testing and contraceptive counseling; 24% of the HIV-positive women became pregnant within 2 years, compared with 22% of HIV-negative control women.[90] More than 90% of intravenous drug users are sexually active, and more than half identify a primary sexual partner within the previous 6 months. In one study, 19% of intravenous drug users reported having more than five partners in the past year.[91] However, studies of condom use have ranged between 9% and 34% for self-reported consistent condom use.[92–94] In a multicity study conducted of intravenous drug users, HIV infection was found to be associated with increased self-reported condom use.[95] However, 31% of patients in that study still reported unsafe sexual activity. In a large Baltimore longitudinal study,[88] in which more than 2000 active intravenous drug users were recruited who had an initial seroprevalence rate of 30% for those who used shooting galleries, 23% for those who shared needles, and 16% for those who denied either of these activities, the subsequent seroconversion rate has been 4% per year, of which half is estimated to be due to sexual transmission.

NONINJECTION DRUG USE

Noninjection crack cocaine use is a recognized risk factor for HIV infection and other STDs in a variety of populations, including STD clinic attendees and prenatal populations.[96–98] This association was particularly pronounced during the early 1990s, when there was a major crack cocaine epidemic. HIV transmission in this setting is related to the sexual behavior associated with cocaine use, especially drug-related prostitution activities.

Because of the interrelationships between HIV infection, drug use, and sexual transmission, the term intersecting epidemics has been used to describe this constellation of phenomena.[99] The social interactions make intervention difficult, depending on an understanding of the driving forces for the risk behaviors and the underlying social environment that promotes and supports the risk behaviors.[95] Examples of this intersecting characteristic are evident in studies of sexual behavior among drug users, a group that has the potential to spread HIV through high-risk drug and sexual behaviors. In a 1989 to 1991 study of drug users in Bangkok and New York City, an international group of investigators found that only 12% and 20%, respectively, of sexually active intravenous drug users reported always using condoms, a finding that in itself may be subject to overreporting bias.[95] Traditional HIV intervention approaches (behavioral counseling, HIV counseling and testing) have been found to have minimal impact in populations of intravenous drug users.[100]

Drug Use Interventions: Risk Reduction

Primary prevention of HIV transmission through cessation of drug use or through drug treatment is clearly the most preferable policy option. However, the number of active intravenous drug users currently overwhelms the availability of drug treatment,[101] and the medical model of substance abuse recognizes this disorder as a chronic condition that is prone to relapse and exacerbation in many individuals. Therefore, although politically attractive, HIV prevention through cessation of drug use (Just Say No! and its descendants) has inherent practical problems. Recognizing this, many public health officials and substance abuse experts have recommended harm reduction approaches—acknowledging drug use activity and taking interventions to make injection drug use less likely to promote HIV infection. These interventions were guided by the epidemiologic studies demonstrating that needle sharing and its associated practices were the risk most likely to promote HIV transmission.

Comprehensive Efforts

In 1995, an international group of investigators[102] identified five large cities with large populations of intravenous drug users and where HIV seroprevalence remained below 5% for 5 consecutive years. The three common characteristics were implementation of HIV prevention activities directed at intravenous drug use when seroprevalence was low; implementation of a needle exchange or other mechanism to provide sterile injection equipment; and street-level community outreach efforts. These findings underscore the necessity for a multidisciplinary approach to HIV risk reduction in intravenous drug users, even when comprehensive drug treatment options are not available. Studies in even severely affected areas such as New York[85, 95] and Bangkok demonstrated that substantial behavior change has taken place among intravenous drug users, particularly regarding injection practices and sharing of needles. These changes were more pronounced in individuals who had increased interpersonal communication (i.e., talked about HIV prevention with their friends), had previously been tested for HIV, and had a higher educational level. Use of "underground" needle exchanges also contributed to decreased high-risk practices. What evolved from these studies is the following:

1. Drug users can adapt prevention behaviors related to HIV.
2. Prevention activities appear to be more focused on drug use behaviors, although most are sexually active.
3. Drug treatment has a positive impact on implementation of HIV prevention behaviors.[103–105]
4. HIV prevention behaviors are most effectively implemented in a community context. This argues strongly against the marginalization of drug users.

Bleach Distribution

Promoting bleach disinfectant was the initial approach taken and was based on the general infection control procedures recommended by the CDC and other public health agencies. Initial community-based programs were established to distribute bleach kits to intravenous drug users and their social networks, achieving distribution rates as high as 74%. Bleach distribution is inexpensive. Follow-up process evaluation studies of intravenous drug users found that the majority were aware of the bleach distribution programs. Compliance, however, was variable.[106] Despite the widespread implementation of bleach distribution, effectiveness in preventing HIV transmission has been difficult to demonstrate. In part, this may be due to the multifaceted risks in the target population of intravenous drug users; observational studies cannot control for the myriad social, substance abuse, and sexual risks that may be present. A 1995 review from the Institute of Medicine[101] acknowledged these shortcomings.

Needle Exchange

Needle exchange as a means of risk reduction has gained increasing popularity and has been subject to considerable political controversy. In the late 1980s, underground (i.e., "illegal") needle exchange programs developed in a number of large cities. In some areas, these have become legitimatized and are operated by health departments or community groups. The underlying hypothesis of the needle exchange programs is that access to clean injection equipment is attractive to intravenous drug users and that its provision will result in decreased sharing practices. These arguments were strengthened by findings in diabetic intravenous drug users. In the Baltimore longitudinal study,[107] insulin-dependent diabetes was used as a surrogate for the availability of legal injection equipment. Cross-sectional seroprevalence in diabetic drug users was 9.8%, compared with 24.3% in the nondiabetic subjects, despite a similar profile of injection frequency. Diabetic subjects were less likely to share needles and other injection paraphernalia.

Client acceptance rates for syringe and needle exchange programs have consistently been high. For example, surveys of intravenous drug users in San Francisco found that 41% were regular users of the needle exchange and that 65% had visited it within the past year.[108]

The opposing arguments include the potential to increase initiation of drug use and increased occupational risk to medical and law enforcement personnel.[101] In addition, senior law enforcement officials and many legislators have opposed needle exchange for legal and moral grounds. Nevertheless, a report from the Institute of Medicine[101] reviewing all the evidence believed that syringe exchange provided a beneficial health benefit and that the risks cited before were minimal.

Community-based needle exchange programs, often illicit, have been operating since the late 1980s. In April 1995, a CDC survey identified 68 operating syringe exchange programs,[109] which in the previous year distributed more than 8 million syringes. Pilot studies have demonstrated that the HIV seropositivity in needles contributed to syringe exchanges has decreased over time. For example, initial studies in the New Haven, Connecticut, syringe exchange program found that after the first year of operation, the proportion of HIV-infected syringes decreased from 68% to 49%.[110] Despite the attractiveness of this intervention (at least in the absence of effective drug treatment), measuring the effect of needle exchange programs on HIV seroconversion rates will be difficult.

Counseling and Testing Approaches: Diagnosis or Intervention?

Since 1986, testing and counseling programs have been one of the cornerstones of HIV prevention policies and programs. HIV testing must be accompanied by pretest counseling to ensure that patients understand the nature of the test and the potential implications of the results. HIV pretest and posttest counseling protocols vary by locality but consist of the following elements:

1. Ensuring that the testing is voluntary. Mandatory testing occurs only in specific situations, such as the military.
2. Education regarding current concepts of HIV disease. Counselors emphasize that HIV disease is a continuum, that a diagnosis of AIDS represents the late stage of HIV disease. The asymptomatic latent period of HIV disease is stressed, with particular emphasis on the fact that disease transmission can occur while the individual is asymptomatic.
3. Ensuring that the individual understands the impact of a positive test result, including that HIV is a chronic, lifelong disease; that medical therapy is available, which affects the disease course; and, in confidential testing, that the case may be reported to local health authorities, depending on local statute.
4. Prevention messages, including counseling on safer sexual and drug-using behaviors. Unfortunately, what occurs in most settings is education. Counseling, to be effective, requires more time and more interaction with the client than the circumstances typically allow in an HIV counseling and testing setting.
5. Obtaining informed consent.

HIV counseling and testing are offered in three settings. In anonymous testing, no identifiers of the patient are used to ensure absolute confidentiality. Therefore, patients have to return in person for test results, and no follow-up is possible for those who test positive but who do not return. Confidential testing is performed in settings where the test result becomes part of the medical record, for example, in STD clinics, tuberculosis clinics, and private offices of physicians. Follow-up is possible, and many local health departments will use disease intervention outreach personnel to contact individuals who do not return for test results. Interviewing for sexual partners and HIV partner notification are often part of confidential testing protocols. Home HIV testing[111] became licensed in the United States in early 1996 and will be available in states where it is allowed by local law. In home testing, a blood sample is taken on filter paper and sent to a laboratory; the results are available several days later by telephone using a numeric code to ensure anonymity. Pretest and posttest counseling is provided by telephone.

In theory, HIV testing and counseling programs serve three roles: case identification (diagnosis), partner referral, and risk reduction. Through diagnosis, HIV counseling and testing play an important role in facilitating referral for medical care interventions, such as antiretroviral therapy, opportunistic infection prophylaxis, and prenatal therapy for pregnant women. Confidential partner referral is an integral part of the federal counseling and testing program and has been implemented except in states where local statute prohibits reporting of HIV-infected individuals (as opposed to AIDS cases). Of sexual partners interviewed in partner referral programs, 15% will be new, previously undiagnosed cases of HIV infection.[112, 113] As a preventive intervention, the effectiveness of HIV counseling and testing is more controversial. A large review of 66 studies conducted between 1986 and 1990 found reductions in self-reported risk behaviors among intravenous drug users, homosexual men, and heterosexuals.[114] However, the effects and the sample sizes in many of the studies were small. Two studies conducted in STD clinic settings in Miami[115] and Baltimore[116] found that HIV counseling and testing had little impact on subsequent STD incidence rates, a biologic marker of continued high-risk sexual activity. A more in-depth study conducted in women counseled and tested in Connecticut community health centers also found that HIV counseling and testing have minimal effects on subsequent sexual behaviors.[117]

The apparent limited efficacy of HIV counseling and testing in reducing HIV transmission (as opposed to diagnosing cases) is due to a number of factors:

1. Despite the large investment, only approximately one third of HIV-infected individuals have been diagnosed through counseling and testing programs. For example, of

U.S. adults surveyed in the CDC Behavioral Risk Factor Survey in 1993, only 25% reported ever having had an HIV test.[118] By definition, the large number of undiagnosed individuals, presumably unaware of their seropositive status, are still at risk for infecting others through drug and sexual behaviors.

2. Sexual and drug-related behaviors are complex phenomena, driven by both biologic and social cues. Typically, these behavior patterns have developed for a long time. Therefore, it is unlikely that a single, short counseling session will result in sustained changes of risk-taking behaviors.

3. Because of underuse of counseling and testing among those at high risk, persons diagnosed are often found only late in the course of their disease. For example, in an 11-state study of AIDS patients diagnosed between 1990 and 1992, more than half of patients were diagnosed a year or less before their AIDS diagnosis.[119] Thirteen percent were diagnosed with HIV infection at an HIV counseling and testing site, 6% in STD clinics, 4% in emergency departments, and 28% in physicians' offices. More than one third were diagnosed as a result of a hospital admission. These data suggest that counseling and testing resources are being underused by those at highest risk.

Despite these limitations, a number of investigators have attempted to measure the cost-effectiveness of HIV counseling and testing.[120–122] Studies that have used only small incremental behavior change have been found to be cost-effective. In part, these findings are driven by the high medical cost of HIV treatment in developed countries, estimated to be $117,000 per case in 1992.[123] Nevertheless, these types of analyses require assumptions to be made about behavior change that cannot be tested experimentally. Furthermore, the traditional approach of cost-effective analysis, in which the total costs of an outcome are compared with the total costs of intervention, is subject to bias, especially in situations in which large proportions of patients may have poor prospects of income generation. Alternative methods of formulating these analyses, such as in years of life saved per intervention dollar, have therefore been proposed.[124]

Counseling and Testing in Low-Risk Settings

With the exception of blood supply screening and HIV testing in the military, HIV counseling and testing in low-risk settings have been controversial. In the late 1980s, HIV premarital testing was instituted in Louisiana and Illinois. These efforts proved to be enormously expensive and of low yield. For example, during the first 6 months of the Illinois effort, only 8 of 70,846 applicants for marriage license were seropositive, an estimated $312,000 per case diagnosed.[125] Both states have since disbanded these programs.

Patients admitted to the hospital without HIV infection or HIV-related conditions have been found to have HIV seroprevalence rates of 0.1% to 7.8%,[126] prompting calls for routine HIV counseling and testing for all hospitalized inpatients,[127] especially in areas where seroprevalence is greater than 1%.[128] The cost-effectiveness of hospital-based screening has been controversial,[129] especially regarding the ability to implement behavioral interventions in the acute care hospital setting. One study estimated that hospital-based screening in areas with high prevalence rates (greater than 1%), and with effective behavioral intervention, would cost $47,200 per year of life saved.[122] Even if case detection were the only goal, widespread implementation of hospital screening has not occurred. HIV counseling and testing resources within the hospital require trained counseling staff, and often, this may not be a reimbursable procedure.

In summary, HIV counseling and testing are effective as a means of case diagnosis. In terms of behavioral intervention, the data suggest that if counseling and testing are effective, the impact is only marginal. The behavioral literature suggests that a more intensive and longitudinal approach is required.

Early Intervention: Interaction Between Medical Care and Prevention

Programmatic approaches to HIV management have typically separated treatment and prevention functions. For example, HIV prevention initiatives are usually coordinated by local health departments, whereas medical care is provided by the hospital system and physicians.

High-risk behaviors often continue after a diagnosis of HIV infection is made. For example, in Baltimore, 15% of patients tested and counseled after testing for HIV infection in an STD clinic setting returned within 3 months with a new STD diagnosis.[130] In a Los Angeles HIV continuity clinic, unprotected intercourse was reported by 9% of patients with an HIV-negative sexual partner and by 13% with a sexual partner whose HIV status was unknown.[131] In a Boston intervention study, high-risk behavior was consistently found in HIV-seropositive individuals 1 year after diagnosis, and higher rates were found in those individuals with depression or other diagnosable mental illness.[132] These findings highlight the need to develop appropriate interventions for the HIV-infected person, targeting behavioral intervention and the need to reduce risk to their sexual and drug partners. Traditional medical care programs often neglect behavioral intervention strategies but focus solely on the clinical aspects of medication provision and prophylaxis of opportunistic infection. Nevertheless, many HIV-infected patients, even those with low $CD4^+$ cell counts, continue to be sexually active. From an alternative standpoint, all newly infected individuals contracted the disease from an individual with active infection. Focusing prevention efforts on the already infected may, therefore, be an efficient albeit widely neglected approach.

Reducing transmission through medical treatment has been theoretically attractive.[133] Antiretroviral therapy, by reducing the viral load in blood and secretions, could potentially lower transmission risk by lowering the transmission efficiency. This presumes access to and compliance with antiretroviral therapy regimens. There are obvious ethical and practical problems in studying this prospectively, which necessitates consideration only of empirical data. A small study in European HIV discordant couples, controlled for condom use, found that HIV seroconversion was reduced by 50% (confidence limits, 10% to 90%) when the HIV-infected partner was treated with zidovudine,[134] demonstrating that behavioral counseling was still a necessary adjunct. No data are available on the newer combination therapy regimens or the impact of the protease inhibitors on biologic factors of transmission.

Comprehensive early intervention for HIV infection, integrating medical care, case management services, and social support, was proposed by Francis[135, 136] soon after antiretroviral therapy became available. This paradigm integrated medical care, case management, and treatment for comorbid conditions, such as mental illness and substance abuse. Despite the advantages of increased care coordination, this approach is expensive and has not been widely implemented. A number of small studies have documented the effectiveness of this approach. In community health centers, a study of intensive case management for 61 HIV-infected persons found reductions in self-reported high-risk practices and increased condom use; however, no control group was studied.[137] In Baltimore, implementation of HIV early intervention in inner-city patients diagnosed with HIV infection in an STD clinic setting resulted in a 71% decreased incidence of gonorrhea compared with historical HIV-positive control subjects.[130]

Control of Sexually Transmitted Diseases as a Prevention Intervention

Epidemiologic Relationships[138]

As an STD, HIV infection is transmitted by the same risk behaviors as those associated with the traditional STDs, that is, multiple sexual partners, sex with prostitutes, and drug-using sexual partners. Because of these behavioral confounders, establishing the link between STDs and HIV infection has been methodologically difficult. Cross-sectional and prospective studies in the developed and developing world have firmly established that bacterial and viral STDs are biologic cofactors in facilitating HIV transmission. Multiple factors contribute to this biologic relationship, including the following:

1. Facilitated access to the vascular portal of entry. HIV has been cultured from the base of genital ulcers[139] in persons with coexistent genital ulcer disease and HIV infection. Similarly, mucosal inflammation caused by STDs, or increased cervical friability[140] induced by STDs or hormonal contraceptives, may reduce the barriers to vascular entry.
2. Recruitment of target cells. STDs such as syphilis, chancroid, and chlamydial infection induce a lymphocytic response. Theoretically, recruitment of an increased number of $CD4^+$ target lymphocytes into an area that is exposed to HIV could facilitate infection.
3. Potentiation of HIV replication. Studies have demonstrated that HIV replication is potentiated by the presence of herpes simplex virus (viral transactivation). Human challenge studies of gonorrhea in HIV-infected men demonstrated that gonococcal infection increases HIV shedding by 2 logs (100-fold increase).[141] These studies suggest that the presence of other STDs may increase the inoculum size beyond the threshold required for infectivity.
4. HIV subtype. HIV subtype E preferentially infects Langerhans epithelial cells, which are found on surfaces such as skin. Type E has been found to predominate in areas where heterosexual transmission is common, such as in sub-Saharan Africa. STDs, by disrupting the epithelial barrier, may facilitate contact with the Langerhans target cells.

Genital Ulcer Disease[142]

HIV prevalence studies demonstrated a threefold to fivefold increased odds ratio for HIV positivity in a variety of populations of patients with genital ulcer disease. Initial studies were in gay men[143] and were conducted in the early 1980s; this became less of an issue in this population because of the precipitous decrease in STD incidence that occurred during that decade. In contrast, HIV transmission facilitated by genital ulcers is important, especially in developing countries or in impoverished areas of developed countries. These studies included Baltimore syphilis patients,[144] homosexual men with genital ulcers,[143] and Kenyan STD clinic attendees in whom the majority of genital ulcer infections were due to chancroid.[145, 146] In the Nairobi studies, the cross-sectional HIV seroprevalence in persons with genital ulcers was 27% to 33%. In Baltimore, STD clinic patients had an HIV seroprevalence rate three to four times that of the general STD clinic population.[144, 147] In a large survey of New York City STD clinic patients, HIV seroprevalence was found to be 16%, whereas no epidemiologic relationship was demonstrated for nongenital ulcer disease.[148] For genital herpes, establishing the relationship with HIV seroconversion requires reference-based serologic methods, because the majority of herpes simplex virus infections are asymptomatic. Early studies in blood donor populations[149] and STD clinic clients have established that serologic evidence of genital herpes[150] is associated with a twofold to threefold increased odds ratio for HIV infection. Most prospective studies of genital ulcers and increased risk for HIV infection have been performed in commercial sex workers or STD clinic clients. In Kenya, where the population-based prevalence rate for persons aged 15 to 44 years is between 10% and 30%, the 6-month seroconversion rate for prostitutes with genital ulcers was 12%.[151] In India, the overall population-based incidence of HIV was 2.6 times higher in commercial sex workers. Prospectively, genital ulcer disease was associated with a seven times increased seroconversion risk[152]; similar results were found in a large prospective study of Thai army recruits.[153] In the United States, a prospective study conducted in Bronx STD clinic heterosexual patients, during a chancroid outbreak, found that HIV seroconversion risk was three times higher in men with a genital ulcer than in men without genital ulcer disease.[98]

Gonorrhea and Chlamydial Infection

Studies of gonococcal and chlamydial infection are complicated by the high prevalence and incidence of these infections.[154] The cross-sectional Nairobi prostitute studies suggested a twofold increased HIV risk among patients with chlamydial infection; however, this relationship was not stable in a multivariate analysis.[145, 146] In Baltimore, a case-control study of HIV seroconverters found a threefold increased risk in patients who had a diagnosis of gonorrhea at their last STD clinic visit before seroconversion.[155] Prospective studies in India[152] and Zaire[156] conclusively demonstrated an association between exudative STD and HIV seroconversion. In the Zaire study, prostitutes with chlamydial infection had a 4.6 relative risk for seroconversion; for those with gonorrhea, the relative risk was 3.6. Both relationships were stable after controlling for other confounding variables. From a population perspective, gonorrhea and chlamydial infection may be more important because they may be associated with a higher attributable fraction of HIV seroconversion cases. For example, the Baltimore investigators, whose population included a large number of intravenous drug users, concluded that the adjusted attributable fraction of HIV seroconversions related to coexistent gonococcal infection was 18%.

Control of Sexually Transmitted Diseases as an Intervention

The epidemiologic evidence suggests that control of STDs may reduce HIV seroincidence. Because behavioral change is a long-term and incremental process, this option is increasingly attractive. A large population-based study in Tanzania has demonstrated that this approach may be feasible.[157] In the Tanzanian study, STD clinical facilities were upgraded, and drug treatment regimens were upgraded to be in concordance with World Health Organization guidelines.[158] In control communities, no changes were made. This intervention resulted in a 42% decrease in HIV seroconversions after 2 years, despite no change in sexual behavior patterns or condom use rates. Most of the decrease was due to either decreased STD incidence or duration of STD infections.

STD screening tests have been developed that use DNA

amplification technology and can diagnose gonococcal and chlamydial infection in urine, eliminating the need for invasive procedures and examinations. STD treatment protocols have been developed with a focus on single-dose oral regimens.[159] These developments have simplified STD clinical management in the primary care setting. STD control therefore needs to be incorporated as an integral part of HIV prevention efforts. Effective integrated STD and HIV control efforts require

1. Implementation of an effective HIV and STD screening strategy for populations at high risk
2. HIV counseling and testing offered to individuals evaluated for STD
3. Rapid access to STD diagnosis and treatment
4. Effective integration of STD diagnosis and treatment facilities with other components of the medical care system

Prevention Issues Specific to Women

Women are at higher risk for HIV and STD transmission because of both biologic and behavioral factors. During unprotected intercourse, women are potentially exposed to a higher viral inoculum through the ejaculate than their male partner is. Inflammatory changes in the vaginal and cervical mucosa or hormonally induced changes can increase the tissue's friability and therefore its ability to act as a conduit to the host's vasculature. Inflammation occurs most frequently in the setting of lower reproductive tract infection. Hormonal contraceptives, including oral contraceptives, cause an increased proliferation of columnar epithelium in the cervix (ectropion), which is more friable. Hormonal contraceptives have been epidemiologically associated with increased risk for HIV transmission,[151, 160] which coincidentally causes a major policy dilemma in developing countries where overpopulation and the HIV epidemic coexist.

Nevertheless, women are at significant risk. In many sexual relationships, women may not be able to refuse sexual relations or require their male partner to use a condom because of either economic circumstance or fear of physical or emotional abuse.[161, 162] For example, commercial sex workers may be at an economic disadvantage if the client's preference is for unprotected intercourse. These issues have intensified the need for development of female-controlled disease prevention methods.

TABLE 128–1 ■ Essential Elements of Prevention Programs for Human Immunodeficiency Virus Transmission

Epidemiologic Assessment: Human Immunodeficiency Virus (HIV) Infection
Frequent assessment of risk groups, incidence rates, and changing demographics is important for planning intervention approaches. HIV incidence is the best marker; acquired immunodeficiency syndrome incidence is most frequently used as a surrogate marker.

Epidemiologic Assessment: Behaviors and Risks
Community assessments of prevalence of risk-taking behaviors, such as drug and sexual behaviors.

Screening of Biologic Products (e.g., blood, tissues)

Public Information Campaigns
Periodic information campaigns including school- and media-based approaches.

Prevention Interventions: Primary Prevention
Interventions to reduce sexual behavior (especially risky or undesired sexual behavior) and to prevent intravenous and other drug use. These interventions are typically resource intensive, require multiple sessions, and may require reinforcement for intervention maintenance.

Prevention Interventions: Changing Social Norms
Community-based approaches to encourage risk reduction and prevention-oriented behaviors as the social norms within the community are essential to reinforce individual-based interventions.

Risk Reduction: Sexual Behavior
Interventions to reduce sexual behavior risk, including the reduction in number of partners and the widespread use of condoms.

Risk Reduction: Drug-Using Behaviors
Interventions to reduce the risk for infection in active substance abusers through the provision of injection equipment (needle exchange).

Risk Reduction: Medical Treatment Interventions
Treatment on demand for sexually transmitted diseases (STDs) to reduce transmission efficiency.

Risk Reduction: Treatment of Comorbid Conditions
Treatment availability for common comorbid conditions, especially mental illness and substance abuse.

HIV Counseling and Testing
HIV counseling and testing programs offer HIV education and an accessible means for case identification and diagnosis.

HIV Treatment
Individuals undergoing HIV treatment have lower rates of risky behaviors than do those without access to treatment.

World Health Organization HIV Program Prevention Indicators
(for use in community assessment)
Knowledge of prevention practices
Condom availability
Reported nonregular sexual partners
Reported condom use in relationships of risk
STD case management
STD prevalence (women)
STD incidence (men)
HIV prevalence (women)

From Mertens T, Carael M, Sato P, et al: Prevention indicators for evaluating the progress of national AIDS programmes. AIDS 8:1359–1369, 1994.

Female Condoms

Female condoms are one approach and have been approved in the United States since 1993. The female condom is essentially a double-ring latex pouch, with one ring adjacent to the cervix and the other to the introitus, that is inserted before intercourse.[163] Evaluations of the device have been mixed. Cost is the major barrier to its increased use; the cost per device ranges from $2 to $4 in the United States.

Vaginal Microbicides

These methods should demonstrate physical and chemical stability in the vaginal environment, allowing insertion some time before intercourse; should not interfere with sexual intercourse; and should also be inexpensive.[164] The ideal compound would be bactericidal and virucidal while being nontoxic to the host epithelium. Besides the potential toxic injury to host epithelium, another consideration is the potential effect on the commensal vaginal microflora and the consequent bacterial vaginosis and inflammation. To date, vaginal microbicides have been chemical detergents that are water soluble and can solubilize the lipid membranes of bacteria and spermatozoa. Nonoxynol 9 is the prototype. Initial enthusiasm for the nonoxynol 9 contraceptive sponge has been dampened. Nonoxynol 9 is effective against common bacterial STD pathogens.[165, 166] However, studies in African prostitutes have demonstrated that nonoxynol 9 is associated with more genital ulcer disease and is associated with increased risk for HIV seroconversion, most likely because of chemical irritation of the vaginal mucosa.[167] There has therefore been increased research interest in developing chemically stable, buffered, nonionic compounds that could potentially be used as vaginal microbicides. Current experimental approaches have included organic polymers, dextran congeners, and reverse transcriptase inhibitors incorporated into a biologically inert matrix.[168]

Establishment of Comprehensive Prevention Programs

Role of Physicians

Primary care physicians have the opportunity to counsel patients at risk for HIV infection through a large variety of interactions, and HIV testing and counseling have been recommended for pregnant women and all individuals who are homosexual, drug users, or heterosexual with multiple partners.[169, 170] In the current medical care environment, primary care providers will often need to play a major role in the treatment of HIV-infected patients. Overall, patients feel more comfortable discussing HIV infection and sexual issues with their physicians than with other individuals.[171] Surveys have shown that physicians offer HIV counseling to more than 90% of homosexual men or drug users, but they offer HIV counseling to only two thirds of heterosexuals with multiple partners and to less than half of noninjection drug users or sexually active adolescents.[172] Provider educational interventions using interactive formats have been found to increase both the providers' comfort level in addressing sensitive behavioral issues and the patients' compliance with STD and HIV screening recommendations.[173, 174]

One of the impediments to extensive implementation of effective HIV prevention programs within traditional health care settings is time and reimbursement. Effective HIV intervention requires education, counseling, trust, and intensive behavioral intervention—little of which is reimbursable under current payment schemes. This issue will pose a major challenge to the health care system, especially because the financial expense alone of HIV infections is extraordinarily high.

On a community-wide basis, developing and maintaining a comprehensive HIV prevention program necessitate a multidisciplinary approach—from the policy perspective, identification of target populations, behaviors, and defining outcome indicators. For example, an intervention in a developing country would focus predominantly on heterosexual transmission and STD treatment; in the United States and Western Europe, intervention needs of intravenous drug users and homosexual men must be addressed. Guidance in developing large-scale intervention programs has been provided by the World Health Organization,[175] which can be used to assess program effectiveness while at the same time being flexible enough to be adapted to a large variety of operating environments (Table 128–1). These program effectiveness guidelines encompass aspects of epidemiologic surveillance, risk assessment, STD and drug treatment, risk reduction, and behavioral intervention—the critical components of effective prevention of HIV infection.

References

1. Centers for Disease Control and Prevention: HIV/AIDS Surveillance Report. 7:1–24, 1995.
2. Centers for Disease Control and Prevention: First 500,000 AIDS cases—United States, 1995. MMWR Morbid Mortal Wkly Rep 44:849–853, 1995.
3. Karon JM, Rosenberg PS, McQuillan GM, et al: Prevalence of HIV infection in the United States, 1984 to 1992. JAMA 276:126–131, 1996.
4. Centers for Disease Control: Trends in gonorrhea in homosexually active men—King County, Washington. MMWR Morbid Mortal Wkly Rep 38:762–764, 1989.
5. Schreiber GB, Busch MP, Kleinman SH, Korelitz JJ, Retrovirus Epidemiology Study Group: The risk of transfusion-transmitted viral infections. N Engl J Med 334:1685–1690, 1996.
6. Stewart GJ, Tyler JPP, Cunningham AL, et al: Transmission of human T-cell lymphotropic virus type III (HTLV-III) by artificial insemination by donor. Lancet 2:581–585, 1985.
7. Graham BS, Wright PF: Candidate AIDS vaccines. N Engl J Med 333:1331–1339, 1995.
8. Travers K, Mboup S, Marlink R, et al: Natural protection against HIV-1 infection provided by HIV-2. Science 268:1612–1615, 1995.
9. Koopman JS, Little RJ: Assessing HIV vaccine effects. Am J Epidemiol 142:1113–1120, 1995.
10. Peckham C, Gibb D: Mother-to-child transmission of human immunodeficiency virus. N Engl J Med 333:298–303, 1995.
11. Dunn DT, Newell ML, Ades AE, Peckham CS: Risk of human immunodeficiency virus type 1 transmission through breastfeeding. Lancet 340:585–588, 1992.
12. St. Louis ME, Kamenga M, Brown C, et al: Risk for perinatal HIV-1 transmission according to maternal immunologic, virologic, and placental factors. JAMA 269:2853–2859, 1993.
13. Ryder RW, Nsa W, Hassig SE, et al: Perinatal transmission of the human immunodeficiency virus type 1 to infants of seropositive women in Zaire. N Engl J Med 320:1637–1642, 1989.
14. Blanche S, Rouzioux C, Moscato MG, et al: A prospective study of infants born to women seropositive for human immunodeficiency virus type 1. N Engl J Med 320:1643–1648, 1989.
15. European Collaborative Study: Risk factors for mother-to-child transmission of HIV-1. Lancet 339:1007–1012, 1992.
16. Gabbiano C, Tovo P-A, deMartino M, et al: Mother-to-child transmission of human immunodeficiency virus type 1: Risk and correlates of infection. Pediatrics 90:369–374, 1992.
17. Datta P, Embree JE, Kreiss JK, et al: Mother-to-child transmission of human immunodeficiency virus type 1: Report from the Nairobi study. J Infect Dis 170:1134–1140, 1994.
18. Van de Perre P, Simonon A, Msellati P, et al. Postnatal transmission of human immunodeficiency virus type 1 from mother to infant: A prospective cohort study in Kigali, Rwanda. N Engl J Med 325:593–598, 1991.

19. Landesman SH, Kalish L, Burns DN, et al: Obstetrical factors and the transmission of human immunodeficiency virus type 1 from mother to child. N Engl J Med 334:1617–1623, 1996.
20. Connor EM, Sperling RS, Gelbert R, et al: Reduction of maternal-fetal transmission of human immunodeficiency virus type 1 with zidovudine treatment: Pediatric AIDS Clinical Trials Group Protocol 076 Study Group. N Engl J Med 331:1173–1180, 1994.
21. Wiznia AA, Crane M, Lambert G, et al: Zidovudine use to reduce perinatal HIV type 1 transmission in an urban medical center. JAMA 275:1504–1506, 1996.
22. Fiscus SA, Adimora AA, Schoenbach VJ: Perinatal HIV infection and the effect of zidovudine therapy on transmission in rural and urban counties. JAMA 275:1483–1488, 1996.
23. Centers for Disease Control and Prevention: U.S. Public Health Service recommendations for human immunodeficiency virus counseling and voluntary testing for pregnant women. MMWR 44(RR-7):1–15, 1995.
24. Office of Technology Assessment, US Congress: The Effectiveness of AIDS Prevention Efforts. Washington, DC, US Congress, Office of Technology Assessment, 1995. Publication OTA-BP-H-172.
25. Auerbach JD, Wypijewska C, Brodie HKH (eds): AIDS and Behavior—An Integrated Approach. Washington, DC, National Academy Press, 1994.
26. Schoenborn CA, Marsh SL, Hardy AM: AIDS knowledge and attitudes for 1992: Data from the National Health Interview Survey. Advance Data from Vital and Health Statistics, No. 243. Hyattsville, MD, US Department of Health and Human Services, 1994. USDHHS publication 94-1250.
27. Anderson JE, Dahlberg LL: High-risk sexual behavior in the general population. Sex Transm Dis 19:320–325, 1992.
28. Kost K, Forrest JD: American women's sexual behavior and exposure to risk of sexually transmitted diseases. Fam Plann Perspect 24:244–254, 1992.
29. Seidman SN, Mosher WD, Aral SO: Women with multiple sexual partners: United States, 1988. Am J Public Health 82:1388–1394, 1992.
30. Ku L, Sonenstein FL, Pleck JH: Young men's risk behaviors for HIV infection and other sexually transmitted diseases, 1988 through 1991. Am J Public Health 83:1609–1615, 1993.
31. Catania JA, Coates TJ, Stall R, et al: Prevalence of AIDS-related risk factors and condom use in the United States. Science 258:1101–1106, 1992.
32. Catania JA, Binson D, Dolcini MM, et al: Risk factors for HIV and other sexually transmitted disease and prevention practices among U.S. heterosexual adults: Changes from 1990 to 1992. Am J Public Health 85:1492–1499, 1995.
33. Centers for Disease Control and Prevention: Trends in sexual risk behavior among high school students—United States, 1990, 1991, and 1993. MMWR Morbid Mortal Wkly Rep 44:124–132, 1995.
34. Centers for Disease Control and Prevention: HIV instruction and selected HIV risk behaviors among high school students—United States, 1989–1991. MMWR Morbid Mortal Wkly Rep 41:866–868, 1992.
35. Peipert JF, Domagalski L, Boardman L, et al: College women and condom use, 1975–1995 (Letter). N Engl J Med 335:211, 1996.
36. Kotloff KL, Tacket CO, Wasserman SS, et al: A voluntary serosurvey and behavioral risk assessment for human immunodeficiency virus infection among college students. Sex Transm Dis 18:223–227, 1991.
37. Debuono BA, Zinner SH, Daamen M, McCormack WM: Sexual behavior of college women in 1975, 1986, and 1989. N Engl J Med 322:821–825, 1990.
38. Catania J, Kegeles J, Coates T: Towards an understanding of AIDS risk behavior: An AIDS risk-reduction model. Health Educ Q 17:53–72, 1990.
39. Kelly J, St. Lawrence J, Diaz Y, et al: HIV risk behavior reduction following intervention with key opinion leaders of population: An experimental analysis. Am J Public Health 81:168–171, 1991.
40. Rosenstock IM, Strecher VJ, Becker MH: The health belief model and HIV risk behavior change. *In* DiClemente RJ, Peterson JL (eds): Preventing AIDS—Theories and Methods of Behavioral Interventions. New York, Plenum Publishing, 1994, pp 5–24.
41. Bandura A: Social cognitive theory and exercise of control over HIV infection. *In* DiClemente RJ, Peterson JL (eds): Preventing AIDS—Theories and Methods of Behavioral Interventions. New York, Plenum Publishing, 1994, pp 25–59.
42. Prochaska J, DiClemente C: Stages and processes of self-change in smoking: Toward an integrative model of change. J Consult Clin Psychol 5:390–395, 1983.
43. Prochaska J, DiClemente C: In search of how people change. Am Psychol 47:1102–1114, 1992.
44. Centers for Disease Control and Prevention: Distribution of STD clinic patients along a stages-of-behavioral-change continuum—Selected sites, 1993. MMWR Morbid Mortal Wkly Rep 42:880–883, 1993.
45. Fishbein M, Middlestadt SE, Hitchcock PJ: Using information to change sexually transmitted disease–related behaviors. An analysis based on the theory of reasoned action. *In* Wasserheit JN, Aral SO, Holmes KK, Hitchcock PJ (eds): Research Issues in Human Behavior and Sexually Transmitted Diseases in the AIDS Era. Washington, DC, American Society for Microbiology, 1991, pp 243–266.
46. Catania JA, Gibson DR, Chitwood DD, Coates TJ: Methodological problems in AIDS behavioral research: Influences on measurement error and participation bias in studies of sexual behavior. Psychol Bull 108:339–362, 1990.
47. Laumann E, Gagnon S, Michaels S, et al: Monitoring AIDS and other rare population events: A network approach. J Health Soc Behav 34:7–22, 1993.
48. Neaigus A, Friedman S, Curtis R, et al: The relevance of drug injectors' social and risk networks for understanding and preventing HIV infection. Soc Sci Med 38:67–78, 1994.
49. Klovdahl A, Potterat J, Woodhouse D, et al: Social networks and infectious disease: The Colorado Springs study. Soc Sci Med 38:79–88, 1994.
50. Centers for Disease Control: Sexually transmitted disease treatment guideline. MMWR 38(Suppl 8):1–43, 1989.
51. Padian NS, O'Brien TR, Chang Y, et al: Prevention of heterosexual transmission of human immunodeficiency virus through couple counseling. J Acquir Immune Defic Syndr 6:1043–1048, 1993.
52. Saracco A, Musicco M, Nicolosi A, et al: Man-to-woman sexual transmission of HIV: Longitudinal study of 343 steady partners of infected men. J Acquir Immune Defic Syndr 6:497–502, 1993.
53. deVincenzi I: A longitudinal study of human immunodeficiency virus transmission by heterosexual partners. N Engl J Med 331:341–346, 1994.
54. Weller SC: A meta-analysis of condom effectiveness in reducing sexually transmitted HIV. Soc Sci Med 36:1635–1644, 1993.
55. Orr DP, Langefeld CD: Factors associated with condom use by sexually active male adolescents at risk for sexually transmitted disease. Pediatrics 91:873–879, 1993.
56. Cohen DA, Dent C, MacKinnon D, Hahn G: Condoms for men, not women—results of brief promotion programs. Sex Transm Dis 19:245–250, 1992.
57. Ku LC, Sonenstein FL, Pleck JH: The association of AIDS education and sex education with sexual behavior and condom use among teenage men. Fam Plann Perspect 24:100–106, 1992.
58. Sellers DE, McGraw SA, McKinlay JB: Does the promotion and distribution of condoms increase teen sexual activity? Evidence from an HIV prevention program for Latino youth. Am J Public Health 84:1952–1959, 1994.
59. Rojanapithayakorn W, Hanenberg R: The 100% condom program in Thailand. AIDS 10:1–7, 1996.
60. Nelson KE, Celentano DD, Eiumtrakol S, et al: Changes in sexual behavior and a decline in HIV infection among young men in Thailand. N Engl J Med 335:297–303, 1996.
61. Walter HJ, Vaughan RD: AIDS risk reduction among a multiethnic sample of urban high school students. JAMA 270:725–730, 1993.
62. Centers for Disease Control and Prevention: Sexual risk behaviors of STD clinic patients before and after Earvin "Magic" Johnson's HIV-infection announcement—Maryland, 1991–1992. MMWR Morbid Mortal Wkly Rep 42:45–48, 1993.
63. Peterson JL, Coates TJ, Catania J, et al: Evaluation of an HIV risk reduction intervention among African-American homosexual and bisexual men. AIDS 10:319–325, 1996.
64. DiClemente RJ, Wingood GM: A randomized controlled trial of an HIV sexual risk-reduction intervention for young African-American women. JAMA 274:1271–1276, 1995.

65. Kelly JA, Murphy DA, Washington CD, et al: The effects of HIV/AIDS intervention groups for high risk women in urban clinics. Am J Public Health 84:1918–1922, 1994.
66. Jemmott J, Jemmott L, Fong G: Reductions in HIV risk-associated sexual behaviors among black male adolescents: Effects of an AIDS prevention intervention. Am J Public Health 82:372–377, 1992.
67. Zenilman JM, Smith P, Shepard M, Celentano DA: Alcohol and other substance use in STD clinic patients: Relationships with STDs and prevalent HIV infection. Sex Transm Dis 21:220–225, 1994.
68. Steiner M, Trussell J, Glover L, et al: Standardized protocols for condom slippage and breakage trials: A proposal. Am J Public Health 84:1897–1900, 1994.
69. Richters J, Donovan B, Gerofi J: How often do condoms break or slip off in use? Int J STD AIDS 4:90–94, 1993.
70. Albert AE, Warner DL, Hatcher RA, et al: Condom use among female commercial sex workers in Nevada's legal brothels. Am J Public Health 85:1514–1520, 1995.
71. Lyketsos CG, Treisman GJ: Psychiatric disorders in HIV-infected patients: Epidemiology and issues in drug treatment. CNS Drugs 4:195–206, 1995.
72. Treisman G, Fishman M, Lyketsos CG, et al: Evaluation and treatment of psychiatric disorders associated with HIV infection. *In* Price RW, Perry SW (eds): HIV, AIDS and the Brain. New York, Raven Press, 1994, pp 249–250.
73. Chuang EA, Jason GW, Pajurkova EM, et al: Psychiatric morbidity in patients with HIV infection. Can J Psychiatry 37:109–115, 1992.
74. Perkins DO, Davidson EJ, Leserman J, et al: Personality disorder in patients infected with HIV: A controlled study with implications for clinical care. Am J Psychiatry 150:309–315, 1993.
75. Lyketsos CG, Hanson AL, Fishman M, et al: Screening for psychiatric morbidity in a medical outpatient clinic for HIV infection: The need for a psychiatric presence. Int J Psychiatry Med 24:103–113, 1994.
76. Kelly JA, Murphy DA, Bahr R, et al: AIDS/HIV risk behavior among the chronic mentally ill. Am J Psychiatry 149:886–889, 1992.
77. Stiffman AR, Dore P, Earls F, Cunningham R: The influence of mental health problems on AIDS-related risk behaviors in young adults. J Nerv Ment Dis 180:314–320, 1992.
78. Siegel K, Mesagno FP, Chen JY, Christ G: Factors distinguishing homosexual males practicing risky and safer sex. Soc Sci Med 28:561–569, 1989.
79. Valdiserri RO, Arena VC, Proctor D, Bonati FA: The relationship between women's attitudes about condoms and their use: Implications for condom promotion programs. Am J Public Health 79:499–501, 1989.
80. Ekstrand M, Coates TJ: Maintenance of safer sexual behaviors and predictors of risky sex: The San Francisco men's health study. Am J Public Health 80:973–977, 1990.
81. Shafer M-A, Hilton JF, Ekstrand M, et al: Relationship between drug use and sexual behaviors and the occurrence of sexually transmitted diseases among high-risk male youth. Sex Transm Dis 20:307–313, 1993.
82. Weinstock HS, Lindan C, Bolan G, et al: Factors associated with condom use in a high-risk heterosexual population. Sex Transm Dis 20:14–20, 1993.
83. Zenilman JM, Hook EW III, Shepherd M, et al: Alcohol and other substance use in STD clinic patients: Relationship with STDs and prevalent HIV infection. Sex Transm Dis 21:220–225, 1994.
84. Hahn RA, Onorato IM, Jones TS, Dougherty J: Prevalence of HIV infection among intravenous drug users in the United States. JAMA 261:2677–2684, 1989.
85. Des Jarlais DC, Friedman SR, Sotheran JL, et al: Continuity and change within an HIV epidemic. JAMA 271:121–127, 1994.
86. Chitwood DD, Griffin DK, Comerford M, et al: Risk factors for HIV-1 seroconversion among injection drug users: A case-control study. Am J Public Health 85:1538–1542, 1995.
87. Schoenbaum EE, Hartel D, Selwyn PA, et al: Risk factors for human immunodeficiency virus infection in intravenous drug users. N Engl J Med 321:874–879, 1989.
88. Vlahov D, Munoz A, Anthony JC, et al: Association of drug injection patterns with antibody to human immunodeficiency virus type 1 among intravenous drug users in Baltimore, Maryland. Am J Epidemiol 132:847–856, 1990.
89. Lehman JS, Allen DM, Green TA, Onorato IM, and the Field Services Branch: HIV infection among non-injecting drug users entering drug treatment, United States, 1989–1992. AIDS 8:1465–1469, 1994.
90. Selwyn PA, Schoenbaum EE, Davenny K, et al: Prospective study of human immunodeficiency virus infection and pregnancy outcomes in intravenous drug users. JAMA 261:1289–1294, 1989.
91. Saxon AJ, Caslyn DA, Whittaker S, Freeman G: Sexual behaviors of intravenous drug users in treatment. J Acquir Immune Defic Syndr 4:938–944, 1991.
92. Watkins KE, Metzgre D, Woody G, McLellan AT: Determinants of condom use among intravenous drug users. AIDS 7:719–723, 1993.
93. Centers for Disease Control: Condom use among male injecting-drug users—New York City, 1987–1990. MMWR Morbid Mortal Wkly Rep 41:617–620, 1992.
94. Centers for Disease Control: Drug use and sexual behaviors among sex partners of injecting-drug users—United States 1988–1990. MMWR Morbid Mortal Wkly Rep 40:855–860, 1991.
95. Des Jarlais DC, Friedman SR, Friedmann P, et al: HIV/AIDS-related behavior change among intravenous drug users in different national settings. AIDS 9:611–617, 1995.
96. Minkoff HL, McCalla S, Delke I, et al: The relationship of cocaine use to syphilis and human immunodeficiency virus infections among inner city parturient women. Am J Obstet Gynecol 163:521–526, 1990.
97. Chirgwin K, DeHovitz JA, Dillon S, McCormack WM: HIV infection, genital ulcer disease, and crack cocaine use among patients attending a clinic for sexually transmitted diseases. Am J Public Health 81:1576–1579, 1991.
98. Telzak EE, Chiasson MA, Bevier PJ, et al: HIV-1 seroconversion in patients with and without genital ulcer disease. Ann Intern Med 119:1181–1186, 1993.
99. Edlin BR, Irwin KL, Faruque S, et al: Intersecting epidemics: Crack cocaine use and HIV infection among inner-city young adults. The multicenter crack cocaine and HIV infection study team. N Engl J Med 331:1422–1427, 1994.
100. Calsyn DA, Saxon AJ, Freeman G, Whittaker S: Ineffectiveness of AIDS education and HIV antibody testing in reducing high-risk behaviors among injection drug users. Am J Public Health 82:573–575, 1992.
101. Normand J, Vlahov D, Moses LE (eds): Preventing HIV Transmission: The Role of Sterile Needles and Bleach. Washington, DC, Institute of Medicine, National Academy Press, 1995.
102. Des Jarlais DC, Hagan H, Friedman SR, et al: Maintaining low HIV seroprevalence in populations of injecting drug users. JAMA 274:1226–1231, 1995.
103. Centers for Disease Control: Risk behaviors for HIV transmission among intravenous-drug users not in drug treatment—United States, 1987–1989. MMWR Morbid Mortal Wkly Rep 39:273–275, 1990.
104. Friedman SR, Jose B, Deren S, et al: National AIDS Research Consortium: Risk factors for human immunodeficiency virus seroconversion among out-of-treatment drug injectors in high and low seroprevalence cities. Am J Epidemiol 142:864–874, 1995.
105. National Commission on AIDS: The Twin Epidemics of Substance Use and HIV. Washington, DC, US Government Printing Office, 1991.
106. Centers for Disease Control and Prevention: Knowledge and practices among injection-drug users of bleach use for equipment disinfection—New York City, 1993. MMWR 43:439–446, 1994.
107. Nelson KE, Vlahov D, Cohn S, et al: Human immunodeficiency virus infection in diabetic intravenous drug users. JAMA 266:2259–2261, 1991.
108. Watters JK, Estilo MJ, Clark GL, Lorvick J: Syringe and needle exchange as HIV/AIDS prevention for injection drug users. JAMA 271:115–120, 1994.
109. Centers for Disease Control and Prevention: Syringe exchange programs—United States 1994–1995. MMWR Morbid Mortal Wkly Rep 44:684–691, 1995.
110. Heimer R, Kaplan EH, Cadman EC: Prevalence of HIV-infected

syringes during a syringe-exchange program. N Engl J Med 327:1883–1884, 1992.
111. Bayer R, Stryker J, Smith MD: Testing for HIV infection at home. N Engl J Med 332:1296–1299, 1995.
112. Jones JL, Wykoff RF, Hollis SL, et al: Partner acceptance of health department notification of HIV exposure, South Carolina. JAMA 264:1284–1286, 1990.
113. Wykoff RF, Jones JL, Longshore ST, et al: Notification of the sex and needle-sharing partners of individuals with human immunodeficiency virus in rural South Carolina: 30 months experience. Sex Transm Dis 18:217–222, 1991.
114. Higgins DL, Galavotti C, O'Reilly KR, et al: Evidence for the effects of HIV antibody counseling and testing on risk behaviors. JAMA 266:2419–2429, 1991.
115. Otten MW, Zaidi AA, Wroten JE, et al: Changes in sexually transmitted disease rates after HIV testing and counseling, Miami 1988 to 1989. Am J Public Health 83:529–533, 1993.
116. Zenilman JM, Erickson B, Fox R, et al: Effect of HIV posttest counseling on STD incidence. JAMA 267:843–845, 1992.
117. Ickovics JR, Morrill AC, Beren SE, et al: Limited effects of HIV counseling and testing for women. JAMA 272:443–448, 1994.
118. Centers for Disease Control and Prevention: HIV counseling and testing—United States, 1993. MMWR Morbid Mortal Wkly Rep 44:169–174, 1995.
119. Wortley PM, Chu SY, Diaz T, et al: HIV testing patterns: Where, why, and when were persons with AIDS tested for HIV? AIDS 9:487–492, 1995.
120. Holtgrave DR, Qualls NL, Curran JW, et al: An overview of the effectiveness and efficiency of HIV prevention programs. Public Health Rep 110:134–146, 1995.
121. Holtgrave DR, Valdiserri RO, Gerber AR, Hinman AR: Human immunodeficiency virus counseling, testing, referral, and partner notification services: A cost-benefit analysis. Arch Intern Med 153:1225–1230, 1993.
122. Owens DK, Nease RF, Harris RA: Cost-effectiveness of HIV screening in acute care settings. Arch Intern Med 156:394–404, 1996.
123. Hellinger FJ: The lifetime cost of treating a person with HIV. JAMA 270:474–478, 1993.
124. Holtgrave DR, Qualls NL: Threshold analysis and programs for prevention of HIV infection. Med Decis Making 15:311–317, 1995.
125. Turnock BJ, Kelly CJ: Mandatory premarital testing for human immunodeficiency virus: The Illinois experience. JAMA 261:3415–3418, 1989.
126. St. Louis ME, Rauch KJ, Petersen LR, et al: Seroprevalence rates of human immunodeficiency virus infection at sentinel hospitals in the United States. N Engl J Med 323:213–218, 1990.
127. Centers for Disease Control and Prevention: Recommendations for HIV testing services for inpatients and outpatients in acute-care hospital settings. MMWR Morbid Mortal Wkly Rep 42 (RR-2):1–6, 1993.
128. Janssen RS, St. Louis ME, Satten GA, et al: HIV infection among patients in U.S. acute care hospitals: Strategies for the counseling and testing of hospital patients. N Engl J Med 327:445–452, 1992.
129. Lurie P, Avins AL, Phillips KA, et al: The cost-effectiveness of voluntary counseling and testing of hospital inpatients for HIV infection. JAMA 272:1832–1838, 1994.
130. Golden MR, Rompalo AM, Fantry L, et al: Early intervention for human immunodeficiency virus in Baltimore sexually transmitted disease clinics. Sex Transm Dis 23:370–377, 1996.
131. Wenger NS, Kusseling FS, Beck K, Shapiro MF: Sexual behavior of individuals infected with the human immunodeficiency virus—The need for intervention. Arch Intern Med 154:1849–1854, 1994.
132. Cleary PD, Van Devanter N, Steilen M, et al: A randomized trial of an education and support program for HIV-infected individuals. AIDS 9:1271–1278, 1995.
133. Anderson RM, Gupta S, May RM: Potential of community-wide chemotherapy or immunotherapy to control the spread of HIV-1. Nature 350:356–359, 1991.
134. Musicco M, Lazzarin A, Nicolosi A, et al, Italian Group on HIV Heterosexual Transmission: Antiretroviral treatment of men infected with human immunodeficiency virus type 1 reduces the incidence of heterosexual transmission. Arch Intern Med 154:1971–1976, 1994.
135. Francis DP, Anderson RE, Gorman ME, et al: Targeting AIDS prevention and treatment toward HIV-1 infected persons: The concept of early intervention. JAMA 262:2572–2576, 1989.
136. Francis DP: Every person infected with HIV-1 should be in a lifelong early intervention program. Sex Transm Dis 23:351–352, 1996.
137. Centers for Disease Control and Prevention: HIV prevention through case management for HIV-infected persons—Selected sites. MMWR Morbid Mortal Wkly Rep 42:448–449, 455–456, 1993.
138. Wasserheit JN: Epidemiological synergy. Sex Transm Dis 19:61–77, 1992.
139. Kreiss JK, Coombs R, Plummer F, et al: Isolation of human immunodeficiency virus from genital ulcers in Nairobi prostitutes. J Infect Dis 160:380–384, 1989.
140. Kreiss J, Willerford DM, Hensel M, et al: Association between cervical inflammation and cervical shedding of human immunodeficiency virus DNA. J Infect Dis 170:1597–1601, 1994.
141. Moss GB, Overbaugh J, Welch M, et al: Human immunodeficiency virus DNA in urethral secretions in men: Association with gonococcal urethritis and CD4 cell depletion. J Infect Dis 172:1469–1474, 1995.
142. Dickerson MC, Johnston J, Delea TE, et al: The causal role for genital ulcer disease as a risk factor for transmission of human immunodeficiency virus. Sex Transm Dis 23:429–439, 1996.
143. Stamm WE, Handsfield HH, Rompalo AM, et al: The association between genital ulcer disease and acquisition of HIV infection in homosexual men. JAMA 260:1429–1433, 1988.
144. Quinn TC, Cannon RO, Glasser D, et al: The association of syphilis with risk of human immunodeficiency virus in patients attending sexually transmitted disease clinics. Arch Intern Med 150:1297–1302, 1990.
145. Plourde PJ, Plummer FA, Pepin J: Human immunodeficiency virus type 1 infection in women attending a sexually transmitted disease clinic in Kenya. J Infect Dis 166:86–92, 1992.
146. Plummer FA, Simonsen JN, Cameron DW, et al: Cofactors in male-female sexual transmission of human immunodeficiency virus type 1. J Infect Dis 163:233–239, 1991.
147. Hutchinson CM, Rompalo AM, Reichart CA, Hook EW III: Characteristics of patients with syphilis attending Baltimore STD clinics. Arch Intern Med 151:511–516, 1991.
148. Torian LV, Weisfuse IB, Makki HA, et al: Increasing HIV-1 seroprevalence associated with genital ulcer disease, New York City, 1990–1992. AIDS 9:177–181, 1995.
149. Holmberg SD, Stewart JA, Gerber AR, et al: Prior herpes simplex virus type 2 infection as a risk factor for HIV infection. JAMA 259:1048–1050, 1988.
150. Hook EW, Cannon RO, Nahmias AJ, et al: Herpes simplex infection as a risk factor for human immunodeficiency virus infection in heterosexuals. J Infect Dis 165:251–255, 1992.
151. Plourde PJ, Pepin J, Agoki E, et al: Human immunodeficiency virus type 1 seroconversion in women with genital ulcers. J Infect Dis 170:313–317, 1994.
152. Mehendale SM, Rodrigues JJ, Brookmeyer RS, et al: Incidence and predictors of human immunodeficiency virus type 1 seroconversion in patients attending sexually transmitted disease clinics in India. J Infect Dis 172:1486–1491, 1995.
153. Celentano DD, Nelson KE, Suprasert S, et al: Risk factors for HIV-1 seroconversion among young men in northern Thailand. JAMA 275:122–127, 1996.
154. Weir SS, Feldblum PJ, Roddy RE, Zekeng L: Gonorrhea as a risk factor for HIV acquisition. AIDS 8:1605–1608, 1994.
155. Kassler WK, Zenilman JM, Erickson B, et al: Seroconversion in patients attending sexually transmitted disease clinics. AIDS 8:351–355, 1994.
156. Laga M, Manoka A, Kivuvu M, et al: Non-ulcerative sexually transmitted diseases as risk factors for HIV-1 transmission in women: Results from a cohort study. AIDS 7:95–102, 1993.
157. Grosskurth H, Mosha F, Todd J, et al: Impact of improved sexually transmitted disease treatment on HIV infection in rural Tanzania: Randomised controlled trial. Lancet 346:530–536, 1995.
158. Hayes R, Mosha F, Nicoll A, et al: A community trial of the impact of improved sexually transmitted disease treatment on the HIV epidemic in rural Tanzania: Design. AIDS 9:919–926, 1995.

159. Centers for Disease Control and Prevention: 1993 sexually transmitted diseases treatment guidelines. MMWR Morbid Mortal Wkly Rep 42(RR-14):1–102, 1993.
160. Marx PA, Spira AI, Getie A, et al: Progesterone implants enhance HIV vaginal transmission and early virus load. Nat Med 2:1084–1089, 1996.
161. Rothenberg KH, Paskey SJ: The risk of domestic violence and women with HIV infection: Implications for partner notification, public policy, and the law. Am J Public Health 85:1569–1576, 1995.
162. Padian N: Prostitute women and AIDS: Epidemiology. AIDS 2:413–419, 1988.
163. Leeper M: Preliminary evaluation of REALITY: A condom for women to wear. AIDS Care 2:287–290, 1990.
164. Stein ZA: HIV prevention: The need for methods women can use. Am J Public Health 80:460–462, 1990.
165. Niruthisard S, Roddy RE, Chutivongse S: Use of nonoxynol-9 and reduction in rate of gonococcal and chlamydial cervical infections. Lancet 339:1371–1375, 1992.
166. Louv WC, Austin H, Alexander WJ, et al: A clinical trial of nonoxynol-9 for preventing gonococcal and chlamydial infections. J Infect Dis 158:518–523, 1988.
167. Kreiss J, Ngugu E, Holmes K, et al: Efficacy of nonoxynol-9 contraceptive sponge use in preventing heterosexual acquisition of HIV in Nairobi prostitutes. JAMA 268:477–482, 1991.
168. Paukels R, DeClercq E: Development of vaginal microbicides for the prevention of heterosexual transmission of HIV. J Acquir Immune Defic Syndr 11:211–221, 1996.
169. Sox HC Jr: Preventive health services in adults. N Engl J Med 330:1589–1595, 1994.
170. U.S. Preventive Services Task Force: Guide to Clinical Preventive Services: An Assessment of the Effectiveness of 169 Interventions. Report of the U.S. Preventive Services Task Force. Baltimore, Williams & Wilkins, 1989.
171. Gerbert B, Maguire BT, Coates TJ: Are patients talking to their physicians about AIDS? Am J Public Health 80:467–468, 1990.
172. Centers for Disease Control and Prevention: HIV prevention practices of primary-care physicians—United States, 1992. MMWR Morbid Mortal Wkly Rep 42:988–992, 1994.
173. American College of Physicians, Infectious Diseases Society of America: Human immunodeficiency virus infection (position paper). Ann Intern Med 120:310–319, 1994.
174. Rabin DL, Boekeloo BO, Marx ES, et al: Improving office-based prevention practices for sexually transmitted diseases. Ann Intern Med 121:513–519, 1994.
175. Mertens T, Carael M, Sato P, et al: Prevention indicators for evaluating the progress of national AIDS programmes. AIDS 8:1359–1369, 1994.

129

Pediatric Human Immunodeficiency Virus Infection

Brigitta U. Mueller
Philip A. Pizzo

History

The observation of a cluster of cases of *Pneumocystis carinii* pneumonia (PCP) occurring in young homosexual men in Los Angeles in June 1981 was followed in 1982 by the description of an unusual syndrome of immunodeficiency in children, which shortly thereafter was recognized as part of the same syndrome, the acquired immunodeficiency syndrome (AIDS).[1–4] After the discovery of the human immunodeficiency virus type 1 (HIV-1) as the causative agent and the subsequent development of antibody tests (enzyme-linked immunosorbent assay and Western blot), as well as culture and later polymerase chain reaction (PCR) assays, the diagnosis of HIV infection has become relatively easy, although the tests are still not performed on a routine basis (see later). Pediatric HIV infection and AIDS have been recognized as part of the same disease process observed in adults but also as being different, because the child's organs (both before and after birth) and especially the immune system are not yet mature when the infection occurs. This has opened unique opportunities to study the immunopathogenesis of HIV infection as well as the intricacies of immune defense and repair mechanisms of the body and also has resulted in an accelerated drug approval process for children.[5] The HIV epidemic, although affecting a relatively small proportion of the population, has not only advanced our knowledge far beyond this specific disease and led to the development of new tools but also created a new and productive basis for interactions among physicians, scientists, drug companies, and members of the community. This model is now being applied to other diseases, such as breast cancer and heart disease.

As we learned more about the relationship between clinical symptoms and immune status, the definition of AIDS in children younger than 13 years has undergone several revisions.[6–8] The current definition of the Centers for Disease Control and Prevention (CDC)[8] is shown in Tables 129–1, 129–2, and 129–3.

Epidemiology

Through September 1996, 7472 children younger than 13 years and 2574 adolescents between 13 and 19 years old were diagnosed with AIDS in the United States (Fig. 129–1). In addition, 19,997 young adults between 20 and 24 years old have been registered with AIDS, and given the long clinical development until the development of AIDS, it has to be

TABLE 129–1 ■ Pediatric Human Immunodeficiency Virus Classification for Children Younger Than 13 Years*†

	CLINICAL CATEGORY			
IMMUNE CATEGORY	(N) No Symptoms	(A) Mild Symptoms	(B)‡ Moderate Symptoms	(C)‡ Severe Symptoms
(1) No suppression	N1	A1	B1	C1
(2) Moderate suppression	N2	A2	B2	C2
(3) Severe suppression	N3	A3	B3	C3

*Using this system children are classified according to three parameters: infection status, clinical status, and immunologic status. The categories are mutually exclusive. Once classified in a more severe category, a child is not reclassified in a less severe category even if the clinical or immunologic status improves.

†Children whose HIV infection status is not confirmed are classified by using this grid with a letter E (for vertically exposed) placed before the appropriate classification code (e.g., EN2).

‡Both category C and lymphoid interstitial pneumonitis in category B are reportable to state and local health departments as acquired immunodeficiency syndrome.

From Centers for Disease Control and Prevention: Revised classification system for human immunodeficiency virus infection in children less than 13 years of age. MMWR Morbid Mortal Wkly Rep 43(RR-12):1–12, 1994.

TABLE 129–2 ■ Immunologic Categories Based on Age-Specific CD4+ T-Lymphocyte Counts and Percentage of Total Lymphocytes*

	AGE GROUP		
IMMUNOLOGIC CATEGORY	0–11 Months	1–5 Years	>6 Years
(1) No suppression	>1500 cells per mm³ (>25%)	>1000 cells per mm³ (>25%)	>500 cells per mm³ (>25%)
(2) Moderate suppression	750–1499 cells per mm³ (15%–24%)	500–999 cells per mm³ (15%–24%)	200–499 cells per mm³ (15%–24%)
(3) Severe suppression	<750 cells per mm³ (<15%)	<500 cells per mm³ (<15%)	<200 cells per mm³ (<15%)

*The immunologic category classification is based on age-specific CD4+ T-lymphocyte count or percentage of total lymphocytes and is designed to determine severity of immunosuppression attributable to HIV for age. If either CD4+ cell count or percentage results in classification in a different category, the child should be classified in the more severe category. A value should be confirmed before reclassification of the child into a more severe category. Regardless of subsequent CD4+ cell count determinations, children should not be reclassified into a less severe category.

From Centers for Disease Control and Prevention: Revised classification system for human immunodeficiency virus infection in children less than 13 years of age. MMWR Morbid Mortal Wkly Rep 43(RR-12):1–12, 1994.

assumed that these men and women acquired HIV infection during childhood or adolescence.[9] The World Health Organization assumes that 27.9 million people have been infected with HIV-1, 2.4 million of them children. More than 1.3 million children have already died of HIV infection, 300,000 children younger than 5 years in 1995 alone. It was estimated that more than 3.1 million new infections would occur in 1996, at a rate of 8500 per day, more than 1000 per day in children. More than 1 million children are presumed to be living currently with HIV and AIDS, 65% of them in sub-Saharan Africa. But the epidemic also affects children who are not infected: it was estimated that more than 9 million children have lost their mothers to HIV and/or AIDS (source: Internet Web pages of UNAIDS and World Health Organization).[10]

In the United States, more than 90% of the AIDS cases in children are the result of vertical (i.e., mother-to-infant) transmission.[9] The mothers acquired their infection either through heterosexual contact (34%) or through a nonspecified mode (22%), most of which is likely to include heterosexual activity. Almost 80% of the children diagnosed with AIDS are younger than 5 years, and males and females are equally affected. HIV infection and AIDS disproportionally affect minorities: 84% of the children diagnosed with AIDS in 1995 were of either African-American or Hispanic origin, but these groups account for only 31% of the children in the United States. The World Health Organization estimates that the pediatric prevalence of HIV and AIDS in the developing world is about 35 times higher than that in industrialized countries. HIV-1 infection is currently the seventh leading cause of death in children in the United States, and in some cities, such as Newark and New York, AIDS has become the first or second leading cause of death in black or Hispanic children between 1 and 4 years old.[11, 12] Infant mortality in Africa is projected to be more than 4% higher than it would have been in the absence of AIDS, and it has been predicted that by the mid-1990s the increase in childhood mortality related to AIDS would start to negate the public health progress that has been achieved during the past decades through programs of better nutrition and immunization.[10]

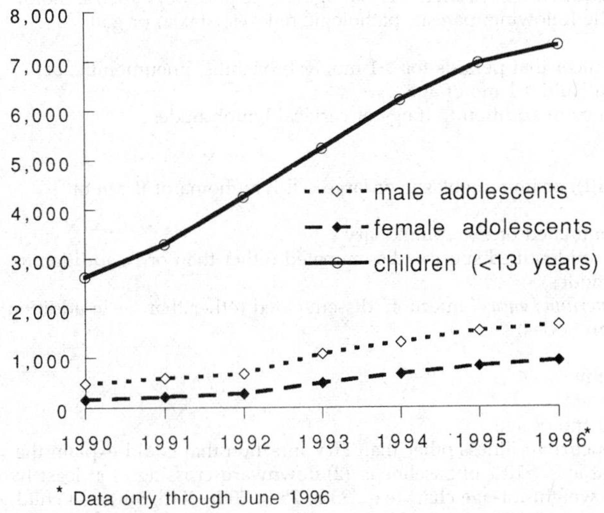

FIGURE 129–1 □ Cumulative AIDS cases in children and adolescents in the United States as reported to the CDC since 1990. (Adapted from data published by the Centers for Disease Control and Prevention in the MMWR year-end reports of AIDS cases occurring in the United States between 1990 and mid-1996.)

Thirty-three percent of the adolescent males (13 to 19 years old) with AIDS report homosexual contacts as their risk factor, and 55% of the females acquire HIV infection through heterosexual contact. The incidence of infection has increased markedly from 0.20 per 100,000 in 1985 to 0.72 per 100,000 diagnosed in 1992.[13] In a study of 79,802 runaway youth, 0.74% were found to be HIV infected, with the highest incidence found among adolescents living in shelters for homeless youth (1.1%).[14] Sexual transmission appears to be the main mode of infection, and national data indicate that the age of first sexual (often unprotected) contact is steadily decreasing, rendering more adolescents at risk for HIV infection. HIV infection and AIDS combined are the sixth leading cause of death in young people between 15 and 24 years old.[13]

Pathogenesis

The pathogenesis of HIV infection in infants and children has some unique features that not only may help us understand HIV disease in this age group but also continue to provide insights into the intricacies of the interactions between immune surveillance and the infectious agent that might be applicable to other diseases as well. The damage that this infection can cause during a vulnerable phase of organ development and maturation is balanced by an astounding potential for compensation and a number of repair mechanisms.

Perinatal Transmission

It is still not clear at what point in time and through which mechanism(s) vertical transmission occurs, and the CDC has

TABLE 129–3 ■ Clinical Categories for Children with Human Immunodeficiency Virus

CATEGORY	DESCRIPTION
N: Not symptomatic	Children who have no signs or symptoms considered to be the result of HIV infection or who have only one of the conditions listed in category A
A: Mildly symptomatic	Children with two or more of the following conditions but none of the conditions listed in categories B and C Lymphadenopathy (>0.5 cm at more than two sites; bilateral = one site) Hepatomegaly Splenomegaly Dermatitis Parotitis Recurrent or persistent respiratory infection, sinusitis, or otitis media
B: Moderately symptomatic	Children who have symptomatic conditions other than those listed for category A or C that are attributed to HIV infection. Examples of conditions in clinical category B include but are not limited to Anemia (<8 g/dL), neutropenia (<1000/mm³), or thrombocytopenia (<100,000/mm³) persisting >30 d Bacterial meningitis, pneumonia, or sepsis (single episode) Candidiasis, oropharyngeal thrush, persisting for >2 mo in children >6 mo of age Cardiomyopathy Cytomegalovirus infection, with onset before 1 mo of age Diarrhea, recurrent or chronic Hepatitis Herpes simplex virus (HSV) stomatitis, recurrent (more than two episodes within 1 y) HSV bronchitis, pneumonitis, or esophagitis with onset before 1 mo of age Herpes zoster (shingles) involving at least two distinct episodes or more than one dermatome Leiomyosarcoma Lymphoid interstitial pneumonia (LIP) or pulmonary lymphoid hyperplasia complex Nephropathy Nocardiosis Persistent fever (lasting >1 mo) Toxoplasmosis, onset before 1 mo of age Varicella, disseminated (complicated chickenpox)
C: Severely symptomatic	Children who have any condition listed in the 1987 surveillance case definition for AIDS, with the exception of LIP Serious bacterial infections, multiple or recurrent (i.e., any combination of at least two culture-confirmed infections within a 2-y period, of the following types: septicemia, pneumonia, meningitis, bone or joint infection, or abscess of an internal body organ or body cavity (excluding otitis media, superficial skin or mucosal abscesses, and indwelling catheter–related infections) Candidiasis, esophageal or pulmonary (bronchi, trachea, lungs) Coccidioidomycosis, disseminated (at site other than or in addition to lungs or cervical or hilar nodes) Cryptococcosis, extrapulmonary Cryptosporidiosis or isosporidiosis with diarrhea persisting >1 mo Cytomegalovirus disease with onset of symptoms at age >1 mo (other than liver, spleen, or lymph nodes) Encephalopathy (at least one of the following progressive findings present for at least 2 mo in the absence of a concurrent illness other than HIV infection that could explain the findings): (1) failure to attain or loss of developmental milestones or loss of intellectual ability, verified by standard developmental scale or neuropsychologic tests; (2) impaired brain growth or acquired microcephaly demonstrated by head circumference measurements or brain atrophy demonstrated by computed tomography or magnetic resonance imaging (serial imaging is required for children <2 y of age; (3) acquired symmetric motor deficit manifested by two or more of the following: paresis, pathologic reflexes, ataxia, or gait disturbance HSV infection causing a mucocutaneous ulcer that persists for >1 mo, or bronchitis, pneumonitis, or esophagitis for any duration affecting a child >1 mo of age Histoplasmosis, disseminated (other than or in addition to lungs or cervical lymph nodes) Kaposi's sarcoma Lymphoma, primary, in brain Lymphoma, small, noncleaved cell (Burkitt), or immunoblastic or large cell lymphoma of B-cell or unknown immunologic phenotype *Mycobacterium tuberculosis* infection, disseminated or extrapulmonary *Mycobacterium* infection, other species or unidentified species, disseminated (other than or in addition to lungs, skin, or cervical or hilar lymph nodes) *Mycobacterium avium* complex or *Mycobacterium kansasii* infection, disseminated (other than or in addition to lungs, skin, or cervical or hilar lymph nodes) *Pneumocystis carinii* pneumonia Progressive multifocal leukoencephalopathy *Salmonella* (nontyphoid) septicemia, recurrent Toxoplasmosis of the brain with onset >1 mo of age Wasting syndrome in the absence of a concurrent illness other than HIV infection that could explain the following findings: (1) persistent weight loss >10% of baseline *or* (2) downward crossing of at least two of the following percentile lines on the weight-for-age chart (e.g., 95th, 75th, 50th, 25th, 5th) in a child >1 y of age *or* (3) <5th percentile on weight-for-height chart on two consecutive measurements >30 d apart *plus* (1) chronic diarrhea (i.e., at least two loose stools per day for >30 d) *or* (2) documented fever (for >30 d, intermittent or constant)

proposed the term perinatal to describe this route of infection, because this includes the prenatal, intrapartum, and postpartum periods. An infant would be considered to have in utero infection if the HIV-1 genome could be detected by PCR or be cultured from blood within 48 hours of birth. In contrast, a child would be considered to have intrapartum infection if results of diagnostic assays such as culture, PCR, and serum p24 antigen assay were negative in blood samples obtained during the first week of life but became positive during the period from day 7 to day 90 and the infant had not been breast-fed.[15]

Without therapeutic intervention, the perinatal transmission rate ranges from 13% in Europe to about 30% in African countries.[16–18] Several studies have suggested that breast-feeding may increase the risk for infection by an additional 15%.[19–21] HIV-1 has been demonstrated by culture or PCR in up to 73% of breast milk specimens from HIV-1–seropositive women.[20, 22] Anecdotal reports have documented the transmission of HIV through breast milk to infants, sometimes correlated with the duration of exposure.[19, 23–25] However, there is a substantial risk associated with the use of contaminated water to prepare powdered infant formulas, which outweighs the risk for HIV infection from breast milk.[26] Ryder and colleagues[27] did not find a statistically significant difference in infection rates between breast-fed and bottle-fed children in Zaire but found a significantly higher morbidity among bottle-fed children. The World Health Organization therefore recommends that women in developing nations whose water supplies are unsafe continue to breast-feed their infants.[28]

Only about a fourth to a third of infants who become vertically infected are thought to acquire HIV during the intragestational period. HIV does not infect the sperm or oocytes directly; however, semen does contain white blood cells, including granulocytes, macrophages, and CD4+ and CD8+ lymphocytes and thus plays a role in the transmission of HIV infection to women.[29] HIV has been cultured from vaginal and cervical fluid, as well as from macrophages and lymphocytes of the cervix, potentially exposing the ovum and the developing embryo shortly after implantation to the proximity of HIV-infected tissue.[30, 31] Virus has been detected in some aborted fetuses of 8 to 20 weeks' gestational age, as well as in amniotic fluid.[32–36] Maternal decidual leukocytes, villous macrophages (Hofbauer cells), and endothelial cells stain positive for gp41 antigen and HIV nucleic acids.[37] The placenta can be infected through the CD4+ trophoblasts or through the occasional occurrence of a chorioamnionitis.[38–41] However, identification of HIV in the placenta does not have a clear predictive value for the infection of the fetus or newborn.[42] There are important technical limitations to studies of fetal or placental tissues that have to be taken into account, particularly the difficulty of excluding contamination of fetal tissue with maternal blood.

Two thirds to three fourths of infants appear to become infected during labor and delivery, as it was observed that in twin pregnancies the first-born infant, whether delivered vaginally or by cesarean section, has a substantially higher risk of becoming infected with HIV than does the second born.[43–45] The risk for an HIV-positive mother to transmit HIV infection is higher if she has p24 antigenemia, a CD4+ cell count less than 400/mm^3, a high HIV replication rate in viral cultures, and an elevated plasma HIV-1 RNA level of more than 50,000 to 100,000 copies per mL.[17, 46–50] This is consistent with the observation that at an advanced clinical stage of disease the transmission rate approached 100% in 10 patients with CDC class IV (symptomatic) disease, versus 13% in 56 patients with CDC class II (asymptomatic) or class III (i.e., lymphadenopathy as the only symptom) disease.[51] Some investigators, albeit not supported by others, have suggested that high antibody titers to certain epitopes of the gp 120 envelope protein, especially the V3 loop, are associated with a lower transmission rate.[52–55] One study has also shown that the risk for transmission nearly doubles in the presence of ruptured membranes for more than 4 hours, regardless of the mode of delivery.[56]

Fortunately, the rate of transmission can be decreased substantially by therapeutic intervention. In a double-blind, placebo-controlled study (AIDS Clinical Trials Group [ACTG] 076) the mothers were treated with oral zidovudine or placebo, starting at 14 to 34 weeks of gestation, and they received intravenous zidovudine (or placebo) during labor and delivery. Their infants received oral zidovudine (or placebo) for the first 6 weeks of life. The perinatal transmission rate was decreased by 67% in the group of mothers and infants who received zidovudine treatment.[57] The CDC has published guidelines, based on these results, to recommend HIV counseling and voluntary testing for all pregnant women.[58] However, this intensive and expensive prophylactic regimen is not easily applicable to the situation in developing countries, and more feasible interventional strategies are currently under study.

Immune System

Flow cytometric analysis of lymphocyte subpopulations in healthy children has revealed age-related changes in the numbers of the different subgroups.[59–63] The percentage of T cells within the lymphocyte population increases with age, and percentages of B cells and natural killer cells are higher in newborns than in adults.[60] Healthy, noninfected infants younger than 1 year have an absolute CD4+ lymphocyte count of 2200/mm^3 (range 1700 to 2800), compared with 1600 cells per mm^3 (range 1000 to 1800) for children between 1 to 6 years old and 800 cells per mm^3 (range 700 to 1100) for children older than 6 years and adults. The percentage of CD4+ cells in children younger than 5 years decreases from a median of 52% (range 33% to 68%) in children younger than 3 months to 42% (range 34% to 52%) in children between 2 and 5 years old.[61] These differences have been taken into account in the latest CDC definition of AIDS in children[8] (see Table 129–2).

Comparison of lymphocyte subsets in HIV-infected versus noninfected children younger than 2 years demonstrates no difference for absolute CD8+ counts but clearly decreased levels of CD4+ cells.[64] In one study, an abnormal CD4+ cell count (less than the 10th percentile for uninfected children) was found in 83% and an abnormally low absolute CD4+ cell count was observed in 67% of the infected children. After 4 years of age, the mean levels of naive (CD45RA) and memory (CD45RO, CD29) markers on CD4+ and CD8+ cells are markedly altered in HIV-infected children.[63] The loss of CD4+ CD45RA+ cells appears to be more marked in children than adults.[65] Lymphoproliferative responses to tetanus toxoid, diphtheria toxoid, and *Candida* often remain relatively normal during the first 2 years of life, but accumulating abnormalities lead to an increased susceptibility to infections.[66, 67] HIV-specific cytotoxic T lymphocyte responses can occur early in infancy; however, they are not as consistently present as they are in adult primary infection.[68] In fact, children with vertically acquired HIV infection appear to have a lesser degree of HIV-1 *gag*-specific cytolysis than do adults, possibly contributing to the more rapid course of disease in children.[69, 70]

Other immune abnormalities include a polyclonal B-cell activation resulting in hypergammaglobulinemia and altered function of monocytes and neutrophils.[67, 71–73] In the European Collaborative Study, hypergammaglobulinemia (immunoglobulin [Ig] G, IgM, and IgA) identified 77% of infected children at the age of 6 months with 97% specificity.[74] In a group of 47 HIV-infected children (17 asymptomatic and 30 symptomatic), Roilides and colleagues[75] found an abnormality of at least one IgG subclass in 83%, including some patients who had IgG2, IgG4, or combined IgG2-IgG4 deficiencies without a clear correlation between the incidence of bacterial infections and specific subclass deficiencies. Children with vertically acquired HIV infection also exhibit decreased production of interferon-γ and interleukin-2 (type 1 cytokines) and increased production of interleukin-4 and interleukin-10 (type 2 cytokines).[76] As with adults, lymph node biopsies of children revealed a progressive loss of an organized structure, especially of the follicular dendritic network, which is correlated with the decrease of CD4+ T cells in the peripheral blood.[77, 78]

Virology

Plasma viral load and its relationship to other surrogate markers, such as CD4+ cells, as well as to disease stage and progression of symptomatic disease and ultimately duration of survival, have become an area of intensive research.[79–83] Because data for HIV-infected adults show that viral load can be used as a prognostic indicator, preliminary guidelines for integrating plasma viral load measurements into clinical decision-making have been developed.[84–88] However, the natural course of viremia is clearly different in perinatally infected children. In adults, a distinct phase of viremia can be seen during the first few weeks of primary HIV infection.[89–91] As an HIV-specific immune response emerges, the viral replication rate is down-regulated and plasma viremia levels off to a relatively low level. Only at later stages, after a major loss of CD4+ cells, does the viral load in the peripheral blood increase again. This is probably partly due to an initial sequestration of virus in lymphoid tissue, leading to a distinct dichotomy between peripheral and central viral burden.[92–97]

In children who acquired HIV infection in the perinatal period (two thirds of them during birth), high levels of plasma RNA, often more than 1 million copies per mL, as well as proviral DNA can be detected for several years and can persist without evidence of an accelerated loss of CD4+ cells.[98, 99] This indicates that, although the principles used in adults might be applicable to children, the viral "set-point" definitions (i.e., the level achieved during chronic infection) might be different. Furthermore, this prolonged viremic phase is possibly detrimental to the developing immune system, and early aggressive intervention with antiretroviral agents is probably warranted. Intriguing results appear to indicate that clearance of HIV infection (as measured by currently available techniques) might be achievable in children with perinatally acquired infection.[100–102]

Prognostic Factors

Advances in supportive care as well as in antiretroviral therapy have improved both the quality and the duration of life of HIV-infected infants and children. In a study from New York City, the survival trends for children reported with AIDS before August 1987 (the time of the first revision of the CDC classification system) were compared with the survival for children diagnosed later.[103] The overall rate of children surviving more than 12 months after birth increased from 32% to 65%. In another study, 56.5% of the children died within the first year after the diagnosis of AIDS, and the median time of survival after the diagnosis of AIDS was 26 months.[104] Mortality is highest when AIDS-related symptoms (e.g., PCP, other opportunistic infections, or encephalopathy) emerge during the first year of life ($P < .001$).[105–109] In contrast, a later onset of symptoms or specific disease manifestations (e.g., lymphocytic interstitial pneumonitis [LIP]) have been reported to be correlated with a better prognosis.[107] In children with vertically acquired HIV infection, the rate of disease progression is correlated with the severity of disease in the mother at the time of delivery.[110] The risk of opportunistic infections or encephalopathy within the first 18 months of life was 50% in the infants whose mother had advanced disease, compared with 14% in children whose mother had mild or moderate disease. Interestingly, there are significant survival differences between children with perinatally acquired HIV disease and children who were infected through a blood transfusion during the neonatal period. The time point at which 25% of children had died of AIDS was 44 months for children with vertically acquired disease compared with 71 months for transfusion-associated infection.[111]

Rapid progression of disease is strongly correlated with an absolute CD4+ cell count below 500/mm³ in untreated infants, and the presence of an extremely low CD4+ cell count (less than 21% of the lower limit of normal for age, which is equivalent to 50/mm³ in adults) is significantly associated with an increased risk of death within 2 years.[108, 112] Seventy-five percent of children who develop a pattern of lymphocyte depletion of the thymus, reminiscent of DiGeorge syndrome, progress to AIDS within 12 months of age, compared with only 14% of children without this pattern.[113] Serum p24 antigen levels are often positive in HIV-infected neonates and children and have been used widely as surrogate markers.[114] However, when CD4+ cell counts and p24 antigen were compared, p24 antigen did not add any predictive value to the CD4+ cell counts.[112] HIV-1 culture or PCR assay positivity at birth probably identifies children with intrauterine infection and is correlated with a higher risk of early, symptomatic HIV infection.[115, 116] Children with advanced disease generally have higher plasma viremia levels, possibly because of a loss of the filter capacity of the follicular dendritic cells in the lymph nodes.[77, 78]

Diagnosis

Because of the high risk for the development of infectious complications (especially PCP) in the undiagnosed infant, as well as the proven reduction in perinatal transmission with the use of zidovudine during pregnancy and the first 6 weeks of life in the infant, testing of all pregnant women is strongly encouraged.[58, 117] A child older than 18 months can be reliably diagnosed with a positive enzyme immunoassay and confirmatory test (e.g., Western blot or indirect fluorescent antibody test).[8] However, the diagnosis of HIV infection in infants is complicated by the fact that maternal antibodies are transmitted through the placenta and are measurable in the child for a median of 13.3 months (range 10.4 to 15.6 months).[118] Virus culture and PCR can identify 30% to 50% of infected infants shortly after birth and nearly 100% by 3 to 6 months of age.[114, 119, 120] The CDC has therefore issued guidelines for the diagnosis of HIV infection in infants[7] (Table 129–4).

Clinical Manifestations

Children show a number of differences in the rate of disease progression and the type of specific symptom complexes[121] (Table 129–5). Recurrent bacterial infections, encephalopathy, and failure to thrive are typical and often early manifestations of HIV disease in children; severe opportunistic infections occur mainly in children with advanced impairment of the immune system.[122]

TABLE 129–4 ■ Diagnosis of Human Immunodeficiency Virus Infection in Children*

INFECTION STATUS	DIAGNOSTIC CRITERIA
HIV infected	1) A child <18 mo of age who is known to be HIV-seropositive or born to an HIV-infected mother **and** • has positive results on two separate determinations (excluding cord blood) from one or more of the following HIV detection tests: —HIV culture —HIV polymerase chain reaction —HIV antigen (p24) • meets criteria for acquired immunodeficiency syndrome (AIDS) diagnosis based on the 1987 AIDS surveillance case definition 2) A child >18 mo of age born to an HIV-infected mother or any child infected by blood products, or other known modes of transmission (e.g., sexual contact) who • is HIV antibody–positive by repeatedly reactive enzyme immunoassay (EIA) and confirmatory test (e.g., Western blot or immunofluorescence assay [IFA]); **or** • meets any of the criteria in 1) above
Vertically exposed (prefix E)	A child who does not meet the criteria above who • is HIV-seropositive by EIA and confirmatory test (Western blot or IFA) and <18 mo old at the time of the test **or** • was born to an HIV-infected mother but has unknown antibody status
Seroreverter (SR)	A child born to an HIV-infected mother who • has been documented to be HIV antibody–negative (two or more negative EIA tests after 6 mo of age) **and** • has no other laboratory evidence of infection (has not had two positive viral detection tests performed) **and** • has had no AIDS-defining condition

*This definition of HIV infection replaces that published in the 1987 AIDS surveillance case definition.
From Centers for Disease Control and Prevention: Revised classification system for human immunodeficiency virus infection in children less than 13 years of age. MMWR Morbid Mortal Wkly Rep 43(RR-12):1–12, 1994.

Onset of Clinical Symptoms

Overall, children have more rapidly progressing HIV disease than do adults. In perinatally infected children, three distinct patterns of disease progression can be observed: most children who become infected intragestationally become symptomatic within the first few months of life and are considered rapid progressors. Approximately 70% of vertically infected children are less rapid progressors, becoming symptomatic within the first several years of life. These children presumably acquired their infection during the intrapartum period. A small but growing percentage of children with vertically acquired infection do not develop evidence of disease progression until after 8 to 10 years of age, following an adult-equivalent course.[105, 107, 108, 111, 123]

Infectious Complications

Many infectious complications are considered AIDS indicator diseases (see Table 129–3). Fortunately, considerable progress has been made in the diagnosis, prevention, and treatment of infections. However, the emergence of resistant organisms may diminish these accomplishments in the near future and poses a threat worldwide.

Bacterial Infections

Recurrent and serious bacterial infections such as sepsis, pneumonia, meningitis, osteomyelitis, and abscesses are often the first indication of symptomatic HIV infection and may be a persistent problem throughout the course of the

TABLE 129–5 ■ Differences in Human Immunodeficiency Virus Disease Between Children and Adults

CHARACTERISTIC	ADULTS	CHILDREN
Transmission	70% sexually, 25% intravenous drug use	90% vertically
Clinical course	Acute retroviral syndrome a few weeks after infection, then many years without symptoms	Rapid progressors (symptomatic within the first few months of life) in 10%–30% Intermediate course (symptomatic within first few years) in 70%–85% Slow progressors (adult equivalent)
Viral profile	Peak a few weeks after infection (primary HIV infection, acute retroviral syndrome), after a few weeks leveling off at relatively low levels (5,000–50,000 copies per mL); increase after years during late stages of disease	Extremely high levels of viremia reached within first few weeks of life (intrapartum infection); high levels (often >1 million copies per mL) maintained for 3–4 y
Main problems	Opportunistic infections, malignancies	Encephalopathy, recurrent bacterial and opportunistic infections, failure to thrive

illness.[124, 125] Common invading organisms include pathogens associated with childhood: *Streptococcus pneumoniae*, *Staphylococcus aureus*, *Neisseria meningitidis*, and *Salmonella* spp. Gram-negative organisms, other than *Salmonella*, assume importance in patients who are hospitalized, have central lines in place, or are neutropenic, and infections with these organisms appear to increase in frequency[125–129] (Table 129–6). Because of the impaired immune surveillance or because of the acquisition of unusual strains, it is possible for HIV-infected children to develop an infection with an organism against which they have previously been vaccinated.[130, 131]

Atypical mycobacterial infections contribute to the morbidity and mortality of children with HIV infection and can result in localized or more often disseminated disease.[132, 133] Infection with the *Mycobacterium avium-intracellulare* complex (MAC) occurs in nearly 20% of HIV-infected children with a $CD4^+$ cell count below $50/mm^3$ and presents with nonspecific symptoms such as night sweats, weight loss, and low-grade fevers.[133, 134] Although most children do not develop MAC infection unless their $CD4^+$ cell count is less than 50 to $75/mm^3$, infection has been reported to occur at higher levels as well. Virtually every organ system can be involved; common clinical manifestations of systemic involvement include fever, anorexia, pneumonia, enteropathy, hepatitis, and bone marrow suppression. Diagnosis and treatment are similar in children and adults, with administration of three or more drugs (e.g., clarithromycin or azithromycin, ethambutol, rifampin and/or amikacin, ciprofloxacin, clofazimine).[135, 136] Although controlled clinical trials with children have not been performed, prophylaxis with rifabutin appears to be safe and efficacious in children and its use for prophylaxis of MAC infection is recommended.[135, 137, 138]

The number of HIV-infected children in the United States who are infected with *Mycobacterium tuberculosis* is still relatively small, but as the number of infected adults grows, more children will be infected.[139–143] In a New York City cohort of HIV-positive adolescents and young adults, 19% had a positive Mantoux skin test and half of them had a history or chest radiographic finding suggestive of active *M. tuberculosis* infection.[144] In a study of 12 children between 2 months and 13 years old with culture-proven *M. tuberculosis* infection, the mean time between the diagnosis of AIDS and the infection was 20 months.[145] The most common presenting symptoms were fever (75%) and tachypnea (33%); extrapulmonary disease was present in 25% of the patients. The diagnosis of *M. tuberculosis* infection is difficult in the HIV-infected child (as in adults) because of the anergy that is frequently associated with AIDS, leading to a negative Mantoux test even in the presence of infection.[146] In the foregoing study, none of the children had a positive skin test with 5 tuberculin units of purified protein derivative.[145] Despite that, it is recommended that HIV-infected children be tested annually with a Mantoux skin test, preferably together with a *Candida* or other control.[147] Gastric lavage appears to be more sensitive than bronchoalveolar lavage for diagnosing mycobacterial disease in children.[148] Treatment of *M. tuberculosis* infection in children is complicated by the lack of suitable pediatric formulations of a number of effective drugs but should include isoniazid, rifampin, and, during the first 2 months, pyrazinamide.[149, 150] If multidrug-resistant *M. tuberculosis* is suspected, initial therapy should include a minimum of four or five drugs.[151]

Viral Infections

Viral infections can cause significant morbidity and mortality in HIV-infected children. In most HIV-infected children, primary varicella-zoster virus infection does not appear to follow a more aggressive course than in HIV-negative children, but with progressive immune deficiency it often manifests as recurrent episodes of shingles or an atypical, folliculitis-like picture with few disseminated and pruritic lesions.[152–155] The virus may become resistant to standard treatment with acyclovir or foscarnet.[156, 157]

Cytomegalovirus (CMV) infection can result in esophagitis, hepatitis, enterocolitis, retinitis, or other complications.[158–161] CMV can become resistant to treatment with ganciclovir, necessitating the use of foscarnet or even combination regimens.[162, 163] HIV-infected children with high levels of CMV DNAemia have been shown to have significantly shorter mean survival times (42.5 versus 60 months; $P < .01$) and a higher mortality rate than CMV-seropositive children without CMV DNAemia.[164]

Other commonly encountered viruses in the HIV-infected infant and child are hepatitis viruses A, B, and C, often associated with a more fulminant or chronic aggressive course than in the non–HIV-infected patient.[165, 166] Both hepatitis B and hepatitis C can be transmitted transplacentally and children can therefore be born infected with both HIV and a hepatitis virus.[167] Measles is associated with a high mortality in HIV-infected children and often presents without the typical rash and may result in a fatal giant cell pneumonia.[168–171] The high morbidity and mortality rates for both hepatitis and measles infections have led to a change in the recommendations for immunization practice in children.[172–175] Infection with respiratory syncytial virus or adenovirus, alone or in combination, can also result in rapid and sometimes fatal respiratory compromise, as well as in chronic or persistent virus shedding or infection.[176–178]

Fungal Infections

Several functional defects of the myeloid phagocytes have been observed in HIV-infected children, including impaired bacterial killing, decreased chemotaxis, and decreased phagocytosis of *Candida albicans* and *Aspergillus fumigatus*.[73, 179–181] Clinically, HIV-infected children are susceptible to mucosal infections with *Candida* spp. and can develop particularly severe and chronic thrush and esophagitis, which can present as failure to thrive and a decreased appetite, without the typical retrosternal burning and dysphagia commonly observed in cancer patients.[182] Recurrence or persistence of infections is more likely in HIV-infected children, and maintenance therapy may be necessary. Fungemia in HIV-infected children is relatively uncommon, but the incidence increases significantly in the presence of an indwelling central venous catheter.[183] Twenty-two cases of fungemia were observed in a study of 347 children with HIV infection, and the presence of an intravenous catheter for more than 90 days was the best predictor ($P > .00001$).[184]

Cryptococcal infections, especially meningitis, often affect adults with AIDS but are uncommon in children.[185–187] However, the diagnosis should be considered in patients with central nervous system symptoms, new pulmonary infiltrates, unexplained fever or respiratory distress, or a mediastinal mass. If they are present, lifelong maintenance therapy with fluconazole with or without flucytosine is necessary.[187] Coccidioidomycosis and infection with *Histoplasma capsulatum* are rare in young children but may be seen in the older child, especially in an endemic area.[186, 188–190] Both can result in localized or disseminated infections and are included in category C of the pediatric HIV classification system[8] (see Table 129–3).

Pulmonary and extrapulmonary *Aspergillus* infections have been observed in AIDS patients but are rare in children.[182, 191, 192] *Aspergillus* spp. can cause an exit site or tunnel infection around an indwelling central line, and we have observed an infant with perinatally acquired HIV infection and associated

TABLE 129–6 ■ Examples of Common Infectious Problems in Human Immunodeficiency Virus–Infected Children*

SYNDROME	SYMPTOM	ORGANISM(S)	TREATMENT
Otitis media	Often chronic or recurrent	Respiratory viruses, *Branhamella (Moraxella) catarrhalis, Streptococcus pneumoniae, Haemophilus influenzae, Staphylococcus epidermidis, Pseudomonas aeruginosa, Escherichia coli, Enterococcus*	Same as in immunocompetent patients In chronic or recurrent cases consider placement of tubes
Sinusitis	Often chronic or recurrent	*S. pneumoniae, H. influenzae, B. catarrhalis, P. aeruginosa,* and MAC *Aspergillus* spp. and *Mucor* possible in patients with prolonged neutropenia	Acute disease: same as in immunocompetent patients; intravenous antibiotics during neutropenia Chronic or recurrent disease: consider surgical intervention for diagnosis and treatment (mandatory for fungal disease); often long-term (i.e., months) treatment with antibiotics necessary
Meningitis	Can be AIDS indicator disease	*S. pneumoniae, H. influenzae, Neisseria meningitidis* *Toxoplasma gondii* (rare in children), *Cryptococcus neoformans* *Mycobacterium tuberculosis* CMV, HSV	Same as in other immunocompromised patients Lifelong maintenance therapy indicated for fungal, parasitic, and some viral infections
Chorioretinitis	Retinitis common in patients with low CD4$^+$ cell counts	CMV, HIV, *T. gondii* (rare in children), VZV, *P. carinii*	Aggressive induction and lifelong maintenance therapy necessary
Pneumonia	Relatively common, may be recurrent PCP can follow indolent or rapidly progressive course Chronic infection or carrier status demonstrated for respiratory viruses	*Common:* Respiratory viruses (RSV, adenovirus, influenza and parainfluenza viruses) Bacteria (*S. pneumoniae, H. influenzae*) *P. carinii* *Less common but still important:* *Staphylococcus aureus, Streptococcus viridans, Klebsiella pneumoniae, P. aeruginosa, Enterococcus, Bordetella pertussis, Legionella* spp., *Aspergillus* spp., mycobacterial infections (especially MAC and *M. tuberculosis*) *Histoplasma capsulatum, C. neoformans, Coccidioides immitis* (in patients from endemic regions) CMV	Viral infections: same as in other immunocompromised patients Bacterial infections: same as in other immunocompromised patients; intravenous antimicrobial therapy at least for the first few days PCP: treatment for 3 wk, possibly combined with steroids Prophylaxis for PCP is indicated according to age and/or CD4$^+$ cell counts (see Table 129–7) Fungal or mycobacterial infections: same as in other immunocompromised patients
Stomatitis, esophagitis	Chronic and often treatment-resistant thrush Oral ulcers	*Candida* spp., HSV, rarely aeorbic and/or anaerobic bacteria CMV	Viral infections: same as in other immunocompromised patients Fungal infections: often continued maintenance therapy with various agents (e.g., azoles) or intermittent courses of amphotericin B necessary
Diarrhea	Often chronic, resulting in severe wasting, sometimes associated with chronic pancreatitis	*Clostridium difficile* *Salmonella* spp., *Shigella* spp., MAC, *Cryptosporidium, Giardia lamblia,* Microsporida, CMV	Same as in other immunocompromised patients
Hepatitis	Common	HIV; CMV; EBV; hepatitis virus A, B, or C; MAC; *P. carinii*	Treatment of underlying cause, if possible
Pancreatitis	Can be common, recurrent or chronic	CMV, HIV, MAC, *Cryptosporidium*	Treatment extremely difficult
Other intraabdominal infections	Diffuse infiltration of mesenteric lymph nodes, resulting in chronic pain Uncommon: abscess formation	Disseminated MAC	Treatment with three or four antimicrobial agents plus analgesic therapy, if necessary with continuous infusion of morphine
Infections of the genitourinary tract	Increased incidence of sexually transmitted diseases in adolescents Pelvic inflammatory disease, condylomata accuminata	*E. coli, Klebsiella* spp., *Enterobacter* spp., *Enterococcus, Candida* spp. In sexually active HIV-infected adolescents: *Treponema pallidum, Neisseria gonorrhoeae, Chlamydia, Trichomonas,* HPV, HSV	Same as in other immunocompromised patients
Skin and soft tissue infections	Quite common and often chronic or recurrent Bacterial infections: folliculitis, exit site infection, cellulitis Viral infections: exanthem, papules (Molluscum, warts), vesicles (chickenpox or shingles) Fungal infections: cheilitis, onychomycosis, tinea capitis or corporis	Bacteria: *S. epidermidis, S. aureus, H. influenzae* (cellulitis), atypical mycobacteria Viruses: VZV, HSV, molluscum contagiosum, HPV, parvovirus, measles virus Fungi: *Candida* spp., *Aspergillus* (rare), dermatophytes Mites (scabies), lice (infestations)	Same as in other immunocompromised patients Chronic suppressive therapy sometimes necessary
Fever	Common in patients with advanced HIV disease	Bacteria, viruses (including HIV), mycobacteria (especially MAC), fungi (*C. neoformans* or *Candida* spp.)	Broad-spectrum antibiotics, aggressive search for origin of fever

*PCP, *Pneumocystis carinii* pneumonia; MAC, *Mycobacterium avium-intracellulare* complex; CMV, cytomegalovirus; VZV, varicella-zoster virus; HPV, human papillomavirus; RSV, respiratory syncytial virus; HSV, herpes simplex virus; EBV, Epstein-Barr virus.

myelodysplastic syndrome who developed fatal pulmonary aspergillosis, as well as another child who developed sphenoid sinusitis caused by *A. fumigatus*.[193]

Parasitic and Protozoal Infections

PCP was the AIDS indicator disease in 27% of the pediatric cases reported to the CDC in 1995, an encouraging downward trend compared with 1990 (36%).[9] Infection with *P. carinii* and subsequent pneumonia are unfortunately still associated with high mortality in young children. Too many children are not diagnosed with HIV infection (and given PCP prophylaxis) until they present with respiratory distress and PCP, making it the major cause of death in HIV-infected children younger than 1 year.[9, 117] Although *P. carinii* can be transmitted transplacentally, infection is rare in the newborn period.[194] The peak incidence of PCP occurs between 3 and 6 months of age, presumably representing primary infection.[194, 195] In infants, PCP has been associated with a mortality rate of 39% to 65%, with a median survival after the diagnosis of PCP as short as 1 month.[107, 196, 197]

The initial presentation of PCP in children can be insidious, with gradually worsening cough, tachypnea, and fever, or acute, with emergence of symptoms in hours.[198, 199] In the assessment of a tachypneic HIV-infected child, PCP must always be considered a possibility. Tachypnea and cough are the key symptoms; fever, although usually present, may be of relatively low grade initially. Cyanosis, usually not apparent at rest, may develop during bouts of coughing or exertion. When present, the radiologic appearance of a diffuse interstitial pneumonitis is helpful in reaching a diagnosis. However, radiologic change may lag behind the clinical presentation, be atypical, or be confounded by the presence of chronic interstitial changes.[199]

Diagnosis rests on the recovery of the organism. This has been greatly facilitated by techniques of sputum induction, whereby the use of nebulized saline results in vigorous coughing and sputum production. In our hands this technique has been diagnostic in children as young as 18 months.[200] Failing this, bronchoalveolar lavage is a highly sensitive method of diagnosing PCP.[200–202] Only rarely is it necessary to resort to open lung biopsy, except perhaps for extremely young patients to whom the former techniques may not be applicable or, as is more commonly the case, when it is necessary to ensure that no concomitant process is contributing to respiratory deterioration despite appropriate *Pneumocystis* therapy.

As in adult patients, there is a marked correlation between $CD4^+$ cell counts and the occurrence of PCP. Guidelines for PCP prophylaxis in children have been developed[117] (Table 129–7). The recommended regimen for prophylaxis is trimethoprim-sulfamethoxazole (TMP-SMX) with TMP at 150 mg/m^2 per day and SMX at 750 mg/m^2 per day given orally in divided doses twice a day for 3 consecutive days per week or on a Monday, Wednesday, Friday schedule.[203] Alternative regimens, if TMP-SMX is not tolerated, include oral dapsone (2 mg/kg per day) or aerosolized pentamidine.[117, 203–205] However, breakthrough infections can occur with every regimen, most commonly with intravenous pentamidine.[206–208] TMP-SMX and parenteral pentamidine are effective therapeutic agents, producing overall survival rates on the order of 75% in adults and children. As in adults, the addition of steroids for moderate to severe cases of PCP has been shown to be highly efficient.[209, 210]

Infectious complications related to *Toxoplasma gondii*, relatively common in adults with HIV infection, are rarely seen in children.[211] Cerebral toxoplasmosis (with or without ocular involvement) is observed either as a congenital infection in the extremely young child or as a newly acquired infection in older adolescents but is exceedingly rare in the other age groups.[211–213] Difficult diagnostic and therapeutic problems, especially for child care settings, can arise from protozoal infections of the gastrointestinal tract, caused by *Cryptosporidium*, *Isospora belli*, Microsporida, or *Giardia*, which are often associated with intractable diarrhea.[214, 215]

Central Nervous System

Encephalopathy is a common manifestation of pediatric HIV infection and is the AIDS-defining diagnosis in 17% of children, a number that probably greatly underestimates the true incidence.[9] Over time, neuroencephalopathy may occur in 40% to 90% of HIV-infected children.[216–221] The risk of developing encephalopathy appears to be especially high for infants born to mothers with far advanced or rapidly progressing disease, probably because of in utero infection occurring during a vulnerable phase of brain development.[110] In the older child, impairment of cognitive, behavioral, and motor functions becomes apparent, manifested by a loss of or failure to attain normal developmental milestones, as well as weakness, intellectual deficits noted as impaired school performance, or even neurologic symptoms such as ataxia and pyramidal tract signs including spasticity or rigidity. However, seizures are usually not part of the HIV-related encephalopathy complex.[217, 220] A marked discrepancy has been found between receptive and expressive language faculties, with expressive language apparently significantly more impaired than receptive language.[222] This difference is observed in both encephalopathic and putatively nonencephalopathic HIV-infected children. Encephalopathy can also af-

TABLE 129–7 ■ Guidelines for *Pneumocystis carinii* Pneumonia Prophylaxis in Children

AGE AND HIV INFECTION STATUS	PROPHYLAXIS
Birth to 4–6 wk, HIV exposed	No prophylaxis, because of low risk of infection with *P. carinii* and possibility of kernicterus with the use of trimethoprim-sulfamethoxazole
4–6 wk to 4 mo, HIV exposed	Prophylaxis for all children born to HIV-infected mothers, regardless of $CD4^+$ cell counts
4–12 mo	
HIV infected or indeterminate status	Prophylaxis
HIV infection reasonably excluded*	No prophylaxis
1–5 y, HIV infected	Prophylaxis, if $CD4^+$ cell count $< 500/mm^3$ ($<15\%$)
>6 y, HIV infected	Prophylaxis, if $CD4^+$ cell count $< 200/mm^3$ ($<15\%$)
Prior episode of PCP	Prophylaxis, regardless of age and $CD4^+$ cell count

*HIV infection reasonably excluded: one or more negative diagnostic HIV tests (i.e., HIV culture or PCR), performed at ≥1 mo of age and one of which was performed at ≥4 mo of age.

From Centers for Disease Control and Prevention: 1995 revised guidelines for prophylaxis against *Pneumocystis carinii* pneumonia for children infected with or perinatally exposed to human immunodeficiency virus. MMWR Morbid Mortal Wkly Rep 44(RR-4):1–11, 1995.

fect the extremely young child and, in fact, be one of the first symptoms of HIV infection. HIV-1 can be detected in fetal brain tissue, and an HIV-associated meningoencephalitis has been described in a newborn child.[223, 224] Encephalopathy in the newborn or young infant includes problems such as delayed head control or delayed acquisition of a social smile and variable degrees of truncal hypotonia.[225] The course can be static (delayed milestones), reach a plateau (no new milestones), or, in the most severe form, be subacute but progressive (loss of previously acquired capabilities).[216, 226]

Radiologic examination often demonstrates cerebral atrophy, calcifications in the basal ganglia, and periventricular frontal white matter.[227] Postmortem examination shows variable degrees of white matter abnormalities, calcific deposits in the wall of blood vessels of the basal ganglia and the frontal white matter, and subacute encephalitis.[228] Children with encephalopathy have significantly lower $CD4^+$ cell counts than do age-matched children without central nervous system involvement, and a detectable serum p24 antigen level, indicating active viral replication, has also been associated with more severe radiologic abnormalities.[229–231] However, there is no "threshold" effect (as described for several opportunistic infections in regard to $CD4^+$ cell counts), nor does an improvement in neuropsychometric testing necessarily correlate with an increase in $CD4^+$ cell counts or decrease in serum p24 antigen level. Quinolinic acid, a relatively unspecific cytokine marker, appears to have a positive correlation with the presence of encephalopathy when measured in the cerebrospinal fluid.[232] It is possible that the direct measurement of viral RNA in plasma (or cerebrospinal fluid) with more sensitive assays (PCR) may reveal a correlation between the course of central nervous system disease and amount of virus burden.[233, 234]

Successful therapy not only can ameliorate the clinical symptoms but also is often accompanied by an improvement of the radiologic manifestations, especially a decrease in atrophy.[235, 236] It is also important to remember that, although HIV infection is the most common reason for the neuropsychologic impairment in an HIV-infected infant, other etiologies must be excluded. We have observed a relatively high incidence of hypothyroidism, an easily treatable disease.[237] Congenital infection with CMV or rubella can present in a way similar to HIV infection. In addition, many children born to HIV-infected mothers were exposed to recreational drugs in utero, and some of them suffer social neglect that can affect their behavior and developmental potential.

It is presumed that HIV infection interferes with the normal myelination of the spinal cord, and in fact spinal and corticospinal tract degeneration can be observed in HIV-infected children affecting the myelin, the axon, or both.[217, 218] Other spinal cord lesions are less common in children than in adults but a vacuolar myelopathy has been described.[238] Peripheral neuropathy in HIV-infected children, presenting as tingling or numbness in hands and feet, is most commonly a side effect of the treatment with antiretroviral agents (e.g., zalcitabine, didanosine, and stavudine).[239, 240]

Respiratory Tract

Respiratory tract involvement is common in HIV infection.[241, 242] Early manifestations of infection are often concentrated in the upper respiratory tract with frequent bouts of otitis and sinusitis. Recurrent episodes of bacterial pneumonias with normal childhood pathogens are a frequent problem; however, the two main pulmonary pathologic processes in HIV-infected children are LIP and PCP (see earlier). LIP, which may affect as many as 50% of the HIV-infected children, is no longer considered to be an indicator for severe clinical disease but is still reportable in children younger than 13 years.[8, 243] The etiology of LIP is poorly understood, but coinfection with HIV and Epstein-Barr virus has been implicated. On biopsy specimens, peribronchiolar lymphoid aggregates or a diffuse lymphoid infiltration of the alveolar septa and peribronchiolar areas can be observed.[244, 245] LIP appears to be part of the group of lymphoproliferative disorders, which range from hypergammaglobulinemia and generalized lymphadenopathy to malignant non-Hodgkin's lymphoma (NHL). LIP can be a major cause of morbidity or can remain relatively asymptomatic and be detectable only by chest radiography. A diffuse, interstitial, often reticulonodular infiltrative process is typically observed, sometimes with hilar or mediastinal lymphadenopathy.[246] Rarely, bronchiectases can develop and be associated with secondary infections, including those with *Pseudomonas* spp.[247] Clinical symptoms can include progressively more debilitating dyspnea, resulting in digital clubbing as a sign of chronic hypoxia. Acute or chronic treatment with steroids may be indicated.

Other lung diseases range from infectious to neoplastic disorders. We have seen several cases of pulmonary mucosa–associated lymphoid tumors in HIV-infected children.[248] Although our ability to diagnose pulmonary disease with noninvasive measures has improved markedly, in certain circumstances it is still necessary to perform either fine-needle aspiration or open lung biopsy.[249]

Cardiovascular System

Wide differences in the incidence of cardiac disease in HIV-infected children have been reported (14% to 93% of children), probably because some estimates were based on the prospective monitoring of children with echocardiograms and ultrasonography, whereas others were based on cardiac evaluations that were performed in the presence of clinical symptoms.[107, 250, 251] Clinically, the most common findings include symptoms of congestive heart failure, such as hepatosplenomegaly, tachypnea, tachycardia, and an S_3 gallop. Signs of left and/or right ventricular dysfunction, as well as T wave abnormalities, can be demonstrated by electrocardiography.[252, 253] With echocardiography and Doppler studies, the most common abnormality found is progressive left ventricular dysfunction, often combined with an increase in ventricular afterload.[254] Treatment of HIV-infected children for cardiomyopathy is the same as that for noninfected children and the patients usually respond well to therapy, but hemodynamic abnormalities and dysrhythmias occur not infrequently and can lead to sudden death.[251, 253]

Although HIV-1 RNA and DNA are present in cardiac tissue of some children, the typical changes of viral myocarditis or endocarditis are rarely observed.[255–257] Zidovudine is known to cause a reversible myopathy of skeletal muscle; however, its contribution to cardiomyopathy is more controversial. Lipshultz and colleagues[254] were not able to define any positive or negative effects of zidovudine on cardiac function in children, but Domanski and coworkers[258] noted a significant increase in the incidence of decreased ejection fraction and cardiomyopathy in children who had ever been treated with zidovudine compared with those receiving didanosine.

Another intriguing finding that has also been described in several HIV-infected children is the occurrence of an arteriopathy affecting various organs, including cardiac and cerebral vessels.[259] This can lead to the formation of giant aneurysms, which, if localized in the brain, can result in neurologic and endocrinologic deficits or even sudden death with hemorrhage.[260]

Gastrointestinal Tract

Some HIV-infected children present with an asymptomatic, unilateral or bilateral enlargement of the parotid glands that may be part of a lymphoproliferative disorder also involving the lungs (manifested as LIP).[261–264]

Diarrhea and malabsorption are frequent problems in children with AIDS, occurring in up to 40% of children and often resulting in either a failure to gain weight or weight loss.[265–269] In 1995, wasting was the AIDS indicator disease in 18% of the children compared with 9% of the adults.[9] A number of organisms have been associated with chronic diarrhea syndromes, including *Cryptosporidium*, Microsporida, *Salmonella, Shigella*, mycobacteria, and a number of viruses (especially rotavirus and adenovirus).[270–273] It is also important to note that the gut is the largest lymphoid reservoir in the body and therefore harbors a large number of HIV-1 particles, possibly contributing to the syndrome of chronic diarrhea.[256] Primary or secondary lactose intolerance is a common finding in HIV-infected children but is not clearly correlated with the presence of chronic diarrhea.[266, 274]

Hepatobiliary abnormalities similar to the presentation in HIV-infected adults have been described in children.[268] A clinical syndrome characterized by cholestasis and hepatitis may be the first manifestation of vertically acquired HIV disease in some children, even before a significant decline in the $CD4^+$ cell count has occurred.[275–277] Chronically elevated transaminase levels have been found in up to 20% of infants perinatally exposed to HIV infection and may be correlated with poor outcome.[278] In a study of 15 pediatric AIDS patients (21 to 48 months old) who presented with hepatomegaly, 56% had a histopathologic diagnosis of reactive hepatitis. Eight-seven percent of the patients had an abnormally elevated alkaline phosphatase level.[277] Although infectious hepatitis can be caused by hepatitis A, B, or C; MAC; or a number of noninfectious agents (e.g., didanosine, rifabutin, dapsone), it is not uncommon that the specific etiology of the transaminitis remains undefined.

The frequency of pancreatitis in HIV-infected children is notable, because this is an uncommon disease in non–HIV-infected children. Pancreatitis can be caused by drugs (e.g., didanosine, zalcitabine, pentamidine) or infections (e.g., CMV, MAC).[279–282] Pancreatitis may become chronic and be associated with persistently elevated amylase levels and intermittent clinical symptoms.

Genitourinary Tract

Renal disease in children with HIV infection presents most often as focal glomerulosclerosis or mesangial hyperplasia.[283] It can be characterized by proteinuria and may result in life-threatening renal failure.[284, 285] In a study of 62 pediatric patients with AIDS, all children with AIDS who exhibited clinical nephropathy died ($n = 16$), with a mean survival time of 55.3 months.[286] In contrast, 70% of the children who did not manifest nephropathy were alive at the end of the study period. Patients with nephropathy were noted to have significantly lower $CD4^+$ lymphocyte counts than those without nephropathy. In another study, 12 of 155 children between the ages of 7 months and 8 years were found to have proteinuria, and 5 of them developed severe renal failure within a year of diagnosis.[287] This nephrotic syndrome is often resistant to the treatment with steroids, but cyclosporine may induce a remission.[285] In addition, HIV can be associated with an IgA nephropathy, manifested by hematuria and proteinuria, possibly induced by an immune complex mechanism involving IgA antibodies against HIV antigens.[288, 289] A syndrome of painful urinary frequency, suprapubic pain, and microscopic or macroscopic hematuria has been described in HIV-positive adult patients, without any histologic evidence for any infections other than HIV, and we have observed an HIV-infected child with ureteritis caused by CMV infection.[290, 291]

Hematopoietic System

Hematologic problems are common in HIV-infected children and adolescents. In a study of 78 bone marrow biopsies and aspirates from 60 HIV-infected children, we found that most patients (84%) had a normal or hypercellular marrow, despite peripheral cytopenias.[291] Dysplastic features of the erythroid, myeloid, and megakaryocytic lineages, including megaloblastosis, a leftward shift, and nuclear and cytoplasmic abnormalities, were common in the bone marrow of our patients.

Anemia, the most common hematologic disorder observed in HIV-infected children, occurs in 16% to 94% of patients, its frequency depending on the severity of HIV disease, the age group, and the use of antiretroviral therapy.[106, 292–295] In some HIV-infected children, pure red cell aplasia secondary to acute or persistent parvovirus B19 infection has been described, and hemolytic anemia, as part of a hemolytic-uremic syndrome, an autoimmune process, or a virus-associated hemophagocytic syndrome, has been observed as well.[294, 296–299] Erythropoietin given as a thrice-weekly injection subcutaneously or intravenously has been used to treat anemia in some HIV-infected children.[300, 301]

Neutropenia, defined as an absolute neutrophil count of less than 1500/mm^3, has been observed in 43% of untreated pediatric patients, and a white cell count of less than 3000/mm^3 was present in 26% to 38%.[240, 302] The cause may be the infection with HIV per se or the involvement of the bone marrow with opportunistic pathogens such as MAC or CMV. Iatrogenic causes, such as agents that have myelosuppressive effects, including zidovudine, must also be ruled out. Treatment with subcutaneous granulocyte colony-stimulating factor at doses between 1 and 20 μg/kg per day has been demonstrated to be effective in many HIV-infected children with neutropenia.[303]

Thrombocytopenia, a symptom included in the CDC classification, is relatively common and has even been described in HIV-infected infants.[304–306] Treatment options include intravenous immune globulin, anti-D immunoglobulin (WinRho), or a short course of steroids. Some children improve with more active antiretroviral therapy alone.[307, 308]

Apart from hemophilia, deficiencies of the vitamin K–dependent factors II, VII, IX, and X are the most common coagulopathies in HIV-infected children, possibly because of malnutrition and malabsorption, as well as liver dysfunction. Acquired protein S and protein C deficiency is increasingly recognized as a complication of pediatric HIV disease.[309] Disseminated intravascular coagulation has been described as a complication of fulminant infectious conditions, but there are no data to indicate that this complication occurs more frequently in HIV-infected individuals. We have observed a case of disseminated intravascular coagulation in conjunction with granulocyte colony-stimulating factor treatment for neutropenia.[310] However, a coagulopathy that is caused by the presence of a lupus-like anticoagulant is more frequent in HIV-infected children.

Endocrine System

Dysregulation of thyroid function appears to be more common than expected in HIV-infected children and can easily be corrected.[311] In a study of 167 children with HIV infection (age, 1 to 19 years; mean, 9.15 years), Hirschfeld and colleagues[237] found that the free thyroxine value was at or below the lower limit of normal in 18% of the children and thyrotropin and thyroid-binding globulin levels were above the normal range in 31% and 30%, respectively. Failure to thrive or grow is commonly observed in children with HIV infection, often with no definable endocrine cause but associated with a worse prognosis.[312–316] In a study of nine children with AIDS and failure to thrive there were one case of primary hypothyroidism, six cases of deficient nocturnal thyroid-stimulating hormone increase, and one child with growth hormone deficiency.[312] Adrenal insufficiency may be caused by CMV infection of the adrenal gland, and we have observed at least one child with severe salt craving who required therapy with fluorocortisol.[317]

Malignancies

Cancer is the AIDS-defining illness in only 2% of children, compared with 14% of the adults.[9, 318] The most common malignancy in HIV-infected children is NHL, presenting either as a systemic disease or as a primary central nervous system tumor; Kaposi's sarcoma is rare in children in industrialized countries.[319–323] However, an increase in the incidence of Kaposi's sarcoma in HIV-infected children has been described in studies from Africa.[324, 325] Leiomyomas and leiomyosarcomas, soft tissue tumors rarely associated with immunodeficiency, have been reported to occur in HIV-infected children, and this tumor is now included in the CDC classification system for children younger than 13 years[8, 322, 326] (see Table 129–3). Interestingly, an apparent correlation with Epstein-Barr virus infection was established not only in HIV-infected children with smooth muscle tumors but also in patients who developed leiomyomatous tumors after an organ transplantation.[327, 328]

Systemic NHL can occur at any stage during the course of HIV infection but a primary NHL of the central nervous system is usually seen only after a severe depletion of $CD4^+$ cells. Clinical manifestations range from a localized lymphadenopathy to disseminated disease with cachexia, night sweats, and pain. The diagnosis is often delayed because HIV or associated infections (especially with MAC) can cause similar symptoms. NHL of the central nervous system can be difficult to distinguish radiologically from toxoplasmosis, and an empirical antibiotic treatment for 10 to 14 days is an appropriate approach.

Although most NHL in HIV-infected children follows an aggressive course, we have observed several children with relatively indolent, low-grade tumors, possibly representing a transition state between a benign lymphoproliferative disorder and malignant NHL. Two children presented with a localized, slowly growing intrapulmonary mass, not associated with any clinical symptoms, a mucosa-associated lymphoid tumor.[248] In another child, we observed multiple cutaneous $CD30^+$ lesions that clinically followed the typical waxing and waning course described for lymphomatoid papulosis, a disease that usually occurs in elderly adults.[329, 330] Furthermore, if rapid growth of the tumor necessitates chemotherapy, these HIV-infected children can tolerate cytotoxic agents fairly well when appropriate supportive care is provided. We therefore initiate chemotherapy with therapeutic intent in children who have an adequate performance status and, to date, our preliminary experience with nine children has been promising.

Lymphoproliferative syndromes occur in HIV-infected children in the form of hypergammaglobulinemia, LIP, localized or generalized lymphadenopathy, or NHL. A new syndrome of cystic tumors arising in the anterior mediastinum of clinically asymptomatic children has been described, histologically consistent with a polyclonal B-cell lymphoproliferative disorder.[331–333] The distinction between a self-limited benign hyperproliferation and the development of a monoclonal lymphoid malignancy is crucial for treatment and prognosis.[245]

Therapy and Prevention

The care of HIV-infected children is complex and includes antiretroviral therapy, prophylaxis for opportunistic infections, and management of acute problems, as well as intervention on the child's behalf with school officials, daycare centers, the legal system, or insurance companies. Although HIV infection in children can be an acute event with high morbidity and mortality, in the past few years it has for many patients become a more chronic condition, and therapy should therefore not only include antiretroviral agents but also be directed at the preservation of normal development and lifestyle. If possible, the HIV-infected child should be allowed to participate in normal childhood activities, such as kindergarten or school, and, if feasible, the care of the infected parent should be coordinated with the child's care. Because the standards of care are still evolving, collaboration between the child's primary health care provider and an HIV treatment center is important.

When to initiate antiretroviral therapy in children has been a topic of discussion and is still not definitively determined. An HIV-infected child with normal age-adjusted $CD4^+$ cell counts who is asymptomatic (CDC stage N0) or has only lymphadenopathy, hepatomegaly, or hypergammaglobulinemia (A1) may not need antiretroviral therapy. Symptomatic children, regardless of their $CD4^+$ cell count, or children with a significantly decreased $CD4^+$ cell count for age should receive treatment. In the infant younger than 12 months with proven infection (i.e., HIV culture or PCR result positive on two occasions), it is currently recommended that therapy be initiated when the $CD4^+$ cell percentage falls below 30% or the absolute $CD4^+$ cell count below 1750/mm^3. In the child between 1 and 6 years old, therapy should be initiated if the $CD4^+$ cell percentage falls below 25% or the absolute CD^+ cell count below 750/mm^3. This is intentionally above the level for the initiation of PCP prophylaxis and should be based on at least two different measurements of $CD4^+$ cell counts within a 2-week interval. Furthermore, new evidence suggests that early and aggressive intervention might be of benefit, and the role of viral load (measured most commonly as plasma HIV RNA levels) must be taken into account in the future; specific guidelines for children are currently being developed.

Monitoring of the HIV-infected child includes many of the same laboratory tests used for adults but also should include careful documentation of growth and developmental parameters. Regular ophthalmologic examinations, especially of the child with extremely low $CD4^+$ cell counts (i.e., for CMV retinitis) or those receiving therapy with didanosine (i.e., retinal depigmentation), should be part of the routine for young children who are unable to call attention to visual impairments.

The life cycle of HIV-1 offers many sites for possible pharmacologic intervention. Active therapy to date employs reverse transcriptase inhibitors, which, although not able to eradicate the infection, provide temporary control of the viral replication process. Their potency can be enhanced when combined with protease inhibitors, which act at a later stage of the viral life cycle. So far, only three drugs have been approved for the use in children: zidovudine, didanosine, and lamivudine in combination with zidovudine. It is hoped that several more drugs will be approved for use in pediatrics in the near future, including stavudine, nevirapine (a nondideoxynucleoside reverse transcriptase inhibitor), and the protease inhibitors ritonavir and indinavir.

Reverse Transcriptase Inhibitors

Six reverse transcriptase inhibitors are currently available for the treatment of HIV-infected adults, but only half of them (zidovudine, didanosine, and lamivudine) have also been approved for the use in children.[334] Stavudine, zalcitabine, and nevirapine are being used in children but do not have official pediatric labeling (Table 129–8).

DIDEOXYNUCLEOSIDES

Zidovudine. In May 1990, zidovudine was approved for use in children with symptomatic HIV infection. Although no longer recommended for single-agent therapy, zidovudine continues to play an important role in the treatment of HIV disease in children because of its significant and reliable penetration of the cerebrospinal fluid, an important feature in children with encephalopathy.[335, 336] Zidovudine does cross the placenta and can be measured in amniotic fluid, cord blood, and fetal organs, and it has been successfully used to decrease the rate of transmission from mother to fetus (ACTG 076).[57, 337, 338] A 67% reduction in perinatal transmission (decreased from 25% to 8.3%, $P = .00006$) was achieved when pregnant mothers received oral zidovudine starting at 14 to 34 weeks of gestation and intravenous zidovudine during labor and delivery, and the children were treated with 6 weeks of oral zidovudine after birth.[57, 339] The elimination of zidovudine and its main metabolite was markedly prolonged during the first 24 to 36 hours of life in newborns whose mothers had been treated with oral zidovudine during pregnancy until delivery (mean serum half-life after maternal ingestion of 14.4 ± 7.5 hours).[337, 340] Zidovudine in a dose range of 2 to 4 mg/kg administered to infants resulted in linear pharmacokinetics in 23 asymptomatic children younger than 3 months, and no side effects were observed.[338, 341] Pharmacokinetic parameters for children older than 12 months are similar to those for adults.[342]

Zidovudine has been evaluated as a continuous infusion, designed to maintain a minimal constant level of 1 μM, the inhibitory concentration in vitro.[302] In all 13 children who had presented with encephalopathy, improvement in neurodevelopmental status was demonstrated after 6 months, and follow-up examination after a year of treatment indicated that these patients had maintained their gains in IQ points and improvements in general cognitive functioning.[302, 343] Furthermore, the degree of cerebral atrophy as measured by computed tomography decreased, accompanied by a decrease in cerebrospinal fluid protein level, a nonspecific marker for HIV-related encephalopathy.[235] Children with mild to moderate impairment of neuropsychometric function showed no difference in outcome when treated with either high doses (180 mg/m^2 every 6 hours) or low doses (90 mg/m^2 every 6 hours) of zidovudine (ACTG 128).[344] However, in a double-blind trial including 831 children with a history of no or minimal prior antiretroviral therapy (ACTG 152) randomly assigned to receive zidovudine (180 mg/m^2 every 6 hours), didanosine (120 mg/m^2 every 12 hours), or the combination of zidovudine (120 mg/m^2 every 6 hours) and didanosine (90 mg/m^2 every 12 hours), significantly more children in the zidovudine monotherapy arm reached a primary end point, defined as death or clinical progression. Didanosine monotherapy was less toxic and had equal efficacy in regard to clinical end points.[345]

Didanosine. In 1991, didanosine was approved simultaneously for use in symptomatic children and adults. Didanosine has a high interpatient variability in bioavailability and a low penetration rate of cerebrospinal fluid.[346] Pharmacokinetic data for neonates or young infants are not yet available. Therapy with didanosine is generally well tolerated; however, a reversible pancreatitis develops in about 7% of children.[280, 347] In a French study of children who had previously been treated with zidovudine and then received didanosine at a daily dose of 120 or 270 mg/m^2, liver function abnormalities developed in 5 of 34 children and 1 died of unexplained hepatocellular failure, suggesting the possibility of liver toxicity.[348] In addition, peripheral retinal depigmentation has been described in children receiving didanosine, especially at doses above 270 mg/m^2 per day.[349] Improvements in clinical and immunologic parameters occurred in both previously treated and untreated patients in a phase I-II study of 43 children with symptomatic HIV infection.[240] Patients with a CD4$^+$ cell count above 200/mm^3 were more likely to show an increase after 24 weeks of treatment than were patients with lower counts; this increase was sustained for several years of therapy in children who started didanosine therapy with more than 100 CD4$^+$ cells per mm^3.[347]

Lamivudine. The combination of zidovudine and lamivudine was approved in 1995 for both children and adults with HIV disease. Lamivudine has been studied both as monotherapy and in combination with zidovudine, didanosine, and stavudine, as well as with protease inhibitors.[350–357] Two daily doses of lamivudine at a total daily dose of 0.5 to 20 mg/kg have been well tolerated by children.[356] During the pediatric phase I-II study we observed hyperactivity (in 2%), an increase in liver function to more than 10 times normal (in 3%), neutropenia (in 3%), and reversible pancreatitis (in 8%). The occurrence of pancreatitis did not seem to be dose related and occurred after a median of 38 weeks of the study. Most children had other risk factors for the development of pancreatitis, such as concurrent medications or a history of prior pancreatitis. Children and parents commonly reported an increase in appetite and energy level, although the change in height and weight parameters did not reach statistical significance. In this monotherapy study, both serum p24 antigen levels and plasma HIV RNA levels decreased significantly and CD4$^+$ cell counts remained relatively stable.[356] However, lamivudine is clearly more active when given in combination with zidovudine or another antiretroviral agent.

Stavudine and Dideoxycytidine. On the basis of the demonstration of an increase in CD4$^+$ cell counts, stavudine was granted accelerated approval by the U.S. Food and Drug Administration for the treatment of adults with advanced HIV infection.[358, 359] Doses of 0.125 to 4 mg/kg per day (in two daily doses) were well tolerated by 37 children entered into a phase I-II study of stavudine, and none of the clinical or laboratory adverse events was thought to be due to study drug.[360] A small study of eight children receiving stavudine (2 mg/kg per day divided in two doses) to which didanosine (180 mg/m^2 per day divided in two doses) was added after 19 to 33 weeks of monotherapy has been published.[361] No pharmacokinetic interactions were observed and the combination was well tolerated, without any occurrence of peripheral neuropathy. Increases in absolute CD4$^+$ cell counts were variable; however, plasma HIV RNA levels showed a median decline of 0.88 $\log_{10}$ (range, -3.41 $\log_{10}$ to 0.31 $\log_{10}$), which is more than seen with dideoxynucleoside monotherapy.

NONNUCLEOSIDE REVERSE TRANSCRIPTASE INHIBITORS

Nevirapine was the first nonnucleoside reverse transcriptase inhibitor to obtain U.S. Food and Drug Administration approval for the treatment of HIV-infected adults. Nevirapine is rapidly absorbed after an oral dose and has a prolonged terminal half-life (>24 hours), making once- or twice-daily administration feasible.[362] The main side effect of nevirapine

TABLE 129–8 ■ Reverse Transcriptase Inhibitors for the Treatment of Human Immunodeficiency Virus–Infected Children

CHARACTERISTIC	ZIDOVUDINE	DIDANOSINE	ZALCITABINE	STAVUDINE	LAMIVUDINE	NEVIRAPINE
Trade name	Retrovir	Videx	HIVID	Zerit	Epivir	Viramune
Bioavailability	68% (±25%)	19% (±17%)	88% (few data for children)	61%–78% (few data for children)	70% (15%–126%)	>90%
CNS penetration	24% (±19%)	Minimal	Minimal	16%–97%	11%	≈9% in children
Toxicities	Neutropenia, anemia, skeletal myopathy (possibly cardiomyopathy)	Pancreatitis (in 7%), peripheral retinal depigmentation, peripheral neuropathy (rare in children)	Peripheral neuropathy, mouth ulcers, rash, pancreatitis	Peripheral neuropathy, hepatotoxicity, anemia	Pancreatitis (8%) hyperactivity	Rash, transaminitis
Main benefits	Improvement of encephalopathy; decrease in p24 antigen; transient increase in CD4$^+$ cell counts; weight gain	Sustained increase in CD4$^+$ cell counts; decrease in p24 antigen; weight gain	Decrease in p24 antigen; increase in CD4$^+$ cell counts	Increase in CD4$^+$ cell counts; decrease in p24 antigen and plasma HIV-1 RNA	Decrease in p24 antigen and plasma RNA; weight gain; subjective increase in energy and appetite	Rapid decrease in plasma RNA; decrease in p24 antigen
Recommended pediatric dose	0–2 wk of age: 2 mg/kg q 6 h 2–4 wk of age: 3 mg/kg q 6 h >4 wk: 360–720 mg/m^2/d (q 6–8 h)	270–360 mg/m^2/d (twice or three times daily)	Few data for children, doses studied between 0.06 and 0.16 mg/kg/d (q 6 h)	Few data for children, between 0.125 and 2 mg/kg/d (twice daily)	4–8 mg/kg/d (twice daily)	Few data for children, doses between 120 and 400 mg/m^2/d (twice daily) commonly used
Comments	Should be used only in combination Lower doses can be used in combination (240 mg/m^2/d)	Increase in antacid may improve absorption in selected children	Approved only in combination with zidovudine and only for adults	Approved only for use in adults Combination with lamivudine or didanosine promising	Approved in combination with zidovudine	Rapid emergence of resistant virus strains Approved for adults Currently being studied in combination with zidovudine and didanosine

is the occurrence of a rash, sometimes even Stevens-Johnson syndrome, but the frequency of this side effect can be greatly decreased by giving half the target dose for the first 2 weeks. Nevirapine leads to a rapid decrease in virus RNA concentration; however, this response does not last long, as resistance emerges within a few weeks of continued monotherapy.[363, 364] This potent albeit short-lived activity makes this compound interesting for further evaluation for the reduction of perinatal transmission or the early and aggressive treatment of infected neonates. Only few data are available so far regarding the use of nevirapine in children. Preliminary results from a randomized, double-blind, placebo-controlled trial in HIV-infected children (ACTG 245) comparing the triple combination of zidovudine, didanosine, and nevirapine with both zidovudine-didanosine and didanosine-nevirapine therapy look promising. A small study of eight children who had nevirapine added to their regimen of zidovudine and didanosine demonstrated a transient decrease in viral load as measured by HIV culture, plasma HIV RNA levels, and serum p24 antigen assays.[78]

Protease Inhibitors

The protease inhibitors are a new class of drugs that exert their potent antiviral activity by interfering with the cleavage of the Gag-Pol polypeptide into its functional parts, which results in decreased production of mature virions. Synergistic activity with reverse transcriptase inhibitors has been demonstrated.[365] The three currently available protease inhibitors, saquinavir, indinavir, and ritonavir, have different toxicity profiles but cross-resistance develops to a certain degree.[366] None of them has been approved for the use in children.

Indinavir sulfate is rapidly absorbed after oral administration with a terminal half-life of approximately 2 hours. The occurrence of an asymptomatic indirect hyperbilirubinemia without any increase in liver transaminase levels and the appearance of kidney stones have been associated with the use of indinavir. The incidence of kidney stones in adults is estimated as 10% at the dose level of 2400 mg/d. Data for adults indicated that at doses of indinavir sulfate between 400 mg every 6 hours and 600 mg every 8 hours there were decreases in p24 antigen and viral RNA ($>1 \log_{10}$), as well as an increase in $CD4^+$ cell counts ($>50/mm^3$).[367]

Only few data are available regarding the use of indinavir for children.[368] Three dose levels (250, 350, and 500 mg/m^2 given orally every 8 hours) are being evaluated in an ongoing phase I-II study. All children receive monotherapy with indinavir for 16 weeks, and then zidovudine and lamivudine are added to their regimen. Preliminary evaluation of the pediatric pharmacokinetics revealed lower bioavailability of the indinavir suspension compared with the capsules, with wide interpatient variability (range 15% to 50% compared with the capsule formulation).[368] Indinavir has so far been well tolerated by most children and hyperbilirubinemia does not appear to be a clinically significant problem. However, hematuria and rarely kidney stones appear to be more common at the highest dose level. In this preliminary evaluation, the $CD4^+$ cell count response appeared more durable than the viral RNA response. Further evaluations of the safety and efficacy of the capsule formulation, as well as the development of a better absorbed liquid formulation suitable for use in children, are ongoing.

Ritonavir is another protease inhibitor with good oral bioavailability and potent antiretroviral activity.[369, 370] The liquid and capsule formulations of ritonavir are often associated with nausea and vomiting and circumoral paresthesias, especially during the first few weeks of therapy. Other side effects include elevation of liver enzyme values, as well as an increase in triglyceride and cholesterol levels. Ritonavir (like all protease inhibitors) is a potent inhibitor of the cytochrome P-450IIIA enzyme system, which can lead to numerous interactions with other drugs that are commonly used to treat HIV-infected patients.

A phase I-II study in HIV-infected children is evaluating the liquid formulation of ritonavir at dosages between 250 and 400 mg/m^2 given orally every 12 hours).[371] In this study, ritonavir is given alone for the first 12 weeks and then in combination with zidovudine and/or didanosine. Overall, ritonavir was well tolerated and the side effects were comparable to those described in adults (nausea and occasional increases in hepatic enzyme values). By day 28, the absolute $CD4^+$ cell count had increased by a median of $38/mm^3$ in the children at the first dose level and $148/mm^3$ at the fourth dose level. Plasma HIV RNA levels decreased rapidly to 0.5 to 2 $\log_{10}$ below baseline and remained below baseline for at least 24 weeks.

Saquinavir was the first protease inhibitor to be approved by the U.S. Food and Drug Administration for the treatment of HIV-infected adults. However, no pediatric trials have been published to date.

Other Agents

In addition to agents that suppress or alter the HIV life cycle, strategies for improving or boosting the immune system are being explored in children. These include, among others, the use of interleukin-2 in combination with reverse transcriptase inhibitors (National Cancer Institute protocol), the evaluation of HIV-1 immunogen, a gp120-depleted inactivated HIV-1 preparation (National Cancer Institute protocol), the use of recombinant interferon-α (ACTG 153) or interferon-γ (ACTG 211), and a study of hyperimmune intravenous immune globulin (ACTG 273). Data are not yet available from any of these studies.

Prevention

One of the most gratifying results in clinical AIDS research was the recognition that a significant amount of HIV transmission can potentially be prevented with the ACTG 076 regimen, the treatment of pregnant women and their children with zidovudine. However, the need for less expensive and cumbersome schedules is evident, especially for the developing countries that are hit hardest by the AIDS pandemic. To be successful we have to understand more about the timing of transmission, the route of acquisition of HIV by the fetus and newborn, and the reasons why only a minority of children are infected. Unfortunately, to develop a preventive vaccine has proved to be much more challenging than initially assumed.[372–375] Coupled with any preventive strategies, a sustained and increased effort at education and behavioral modification is necessary to be able to reduce the high-risk behaviors that perpetuate the pandemic. Nowhere are these efforts more necessary than in the adolescent population.

Summary

HIV infection is usually more accelerated in children, and because many organs, especially the brain, are not yet mature, it can have devastating effects on growth and development. The pathogenesis, course of disease, and response to treatment can differ between children and adults. Studies in adults have reflected only modest gains with dideoxynucleosides, but the progress in children has been more gratifying, with improvements in weight gain and growth velocity, reversal of neurodevelopmental deficits, and sustained improvements in CD4$^+$ cell counts. The nondideoxynucleoside reverse transcriptase inhibitors may have their most important role in the prevention of perinatal transmission. Protease inhibitors, combined with reverse transcriptase inhibitors, may even be able to eradicate HIV infection in some children treated early and aggressively. During the past years, both frustration and progress have characterized the field of HIV infection and AIDS in children. Effective antiretroviral agents have been developed, and many drugs are now being developed simultaneously for children and adults. However, there is still a lack of suitable pediatric formulations not only for antiretroviral agents but also for many drugs used to treat or prevent infectious complications. Children with AIDS are clearly living longer, with an improved quality of life. Nonetheless, to date AIDS remains an inevitably fatal disease and new agents and therapeutic strategies are urgently needed.

References

1. Centers for Disease Control: Unexplained immunodeficiency and opportunistic infections in infants—New York, New Jersey, California. MMWR Morbid Mortal Wkly Rep 31:665–667, 1982.
2. Ammann AJ, Cowan MJ, Wara DW, et al: Acquired immunodeficiency in an infant: Possible transmission by means of blood products. Lancet 1:956–958, 1983.
3. Oleske J, Minnefor A, Cooper R, et al: Immune deficiency syndrome in children. JAMA 249:2345–2349, 1983.
4. Rubinstein A, Sicklick M, Gupta A, et al: Acquired immunodeficiency with reversed T4/T8 ratios in infants born to promiscuous and drug-addicted mothers. JAMA 249:2350–2356, 1983.
5. Ammann AJ: Human immunodeficiency virus infection/AIDS in children: The next decade. Pediatrics 93:930–935, 1994.
6. Centers for Disease Control: Revision of the case definition of acquired immunodeficiency syndrome for national reporting—United States. MMWR Morbid Mortal Wkly Rep 34:373–375, 1985.
7. Centers for Disease Control: Revision of the CDC surveillance case definition for acquired immunodeficiency syndrome. MMWR Morbid Mortal Wkly Rep 36(Suppl 1):1S–15S, 1987.
8. Centers for Disease Control and Prevention: Revised classification system for human immunodeficiency virus infection in children less than 13 years of age. MMWR Morbid Mortal Wkly Rep 43(RR-12):1–12, 1994.
9. Centers for Disease Control and Prevention: US HIV and AIDS cases reported through December 1995. HIV/AIDS Surveillance Report. Year-end Edition. 7:1–38, 1996.
10. Chin J, Remenyi MA, Morrison F, Bulatao R: The global epidemiology of the HIV/AIDS pandemic and its projected demographic impact in Africa. World Health Stat Q 45:220–227, 1992.
11. Gayle JA, Selik RM, Chu SY: Surveillance for AIDS and HIV infection among black and Hispanic children and women of childbearing age, 1981–1989. MMWR CDC Surveill Summ 39:23–30, 1990.
12. Chu SY, Buehler JW, Oxtoby MJ, Kilbourne BW: Impact of the human immunodeficiency virus epidemic on mortality in children, United States. Pediatrics 87:806–810, 1991.
13. Lindegren ML, Hanson C, Miller K, et al: Epidemiology of human immunodeficiency virus infection in adolescents, United States. Pediatr Infect Dis J 13:525–535, 1994.
14. Sweeney P, Lindegren ML, Buehler JW, et al: Teenagers at risk of human immunodeficiency virus type 1 infection. Results from seroprevalence surveys in the United States. Arch Pediatr Adolesc Med 149:521–528, 1995.
15. Bryson YJ, Luzuriaga K, Sullivan JL, Wara DW: Proposed definition for in utero versus intrapartum transmission of HIV-1. N Engl J Med 327:1246–1247, 1992.
16. Blanche S, Rouzioux C, Guihard Moscato M-L, et al: A prospective study of infants born to women seropositive for human immunodeficiency virus type 1. N Engl J Med 320:1643–1648, 1989.
17. Ryder RW, Nsa W, Hassig SE, et al: Perinatal transmission of the human immunodeficiency virus type 1 to infants of seropositive women in Zaire. N Engl J Med 320:1637–1642, 1989.
18. Adjorlolo-Johnson G, De Cock KM, Ekpini E, et al: Prospective comparison of mother-to-child transmission of HIV-1 and HIV-2 in Abidjan, Ivory Coast. JAMA 272:462–466, 1994.
19. de Martino M, Tovo P-A, Tozzi AE, et al: HIV-1 transmission through breast-milk: Appraisal of risk according to duration of feeding. AIDS 6:991–997, 1992.
20. Ruff AJ, Halsey NA, Coberly J, Boulos R: Breast-feeding and maternal-infant transmission of human immunodeficiency virus type 1. J Pediatr 121:325–329, 1992.
21. Nicoll A, Newell M-L, Van Praag E, et al: Infant feeding policy and practice in the presence of HIV-1 infection. AIDS 9:107–119, 1995.
22. Thiry L, Sprecher-Goldberger S, Jonckheer T, et al: Isolation of AIDS virus from cell-free breast milk of three healthy virus carriers. Lancet 2:891–892, 1985.
23. Ziegler JB, Johnson RO, Cooper DA, Gold J: Postnatal transmission of AIDS-associated retrovirus from mother to infant. Lancet 1:896–897, 1985.
24. Hira SK, Mangrola UG, Mwale C, et al: Apparent vertical transmission of human immunodeficiency virus type 1 by breast-feeding in Zambia. J Pediatr 117:421–424, 1990.
25. Datta P, Embree JE, Kreiss JK, et al: Resumption of breast-feeding in later childhood: A risk factor for mother to child human immunodeficiency virus type 1 transmission. Pediatr Infect Dis J 11:974–976, 1992.
26. Van de Perre P, Simonon A, Hitimana D-G, et al: Infective and anti-infective properties of breastmilk from HIV-1 infected women. Lancet 341:914–918, 1993.
27. Ryder RW, Manzila T, Baende E, et al: Evidence from Zaire that breast-feeding by HIV-1–seropositive mothers is not a major route for perinatal HIV-1 transmission but does decrease morbidity. AIDS 5:709–714, 1991.
28. World Health Organization: Global program on AIDS. Consensus statement from the WHO/UNICEF consultation on HIV transmission and breast-feeding. Wkly Epidemiol Rec 67:177–179, 1992.
29. Douglas GC, King BF: Maternal-fetal transmission of human immunodeficiency virus: A review of possible routes and cellular mechanisms of infection. Clin Infect Dis 15:678–691, 1992.
30. Pomerantz RJ, de la Monte SM, Donegan SP, et al: Human immunodeficiency virus infection of the uterine cervix. Ann Intern Med 108:321–327, 1988.
31. Vogt MW, Witt DJ, Craven DE, et al: Isolation patterns of human immunodeficiency virus infection from cervical secretions during the menstrual cycle of women at risk for the acquired immunodeficiency syndrome. Ann Intern Med 106:380–382, 1987.
32. Sprecher S, Soumenkoff G, Puissant F, Degueldre M: Vertical transmission of HIV in 15-week fetus. Lancet 2:288–289, 1986.
33. Jovaisas E, Koch MA, Schäfer A, et al: LAV/HTLV-III in 20-week fetus (Letter). Lancet 2:1129, 1985.
34. Courgnaud V, Laure F, Brossard A, et al: Frequent and early in utero HIV-1 infection. AIDS Res Hum Retroviruses 7:337–341, 1991.
35. Mano H, Chermann J-C: Fetal human immunodeficiency virus type 1 infection of different organs in the second trimester. AIDS Res Hum Retroviruses 7:83–88, 1991.
36. Mundy DC, Schinazi RF, Gerber AR, et al: Human immunodeficiency virus isolated from amniotic fluid. Lancet 2:459–460, 1987.
37. Lewis SH, Reynolds-Kohler C, Fox HE, Nelson JA: HIV-1 in trophoblastic and villous Hofbauer cells, and haematological precursors in eight-week fetuses [published erratum in Lancet 335:1046, 1990]. Lancet 335:565–568, 1990.
38. Amirhessami-Aghili N, Spector SA: Human immunodeficiency virus type 1 infection of human placenta: Potential route for fetal infection. J Virol 65:2231–2236, 1991.
39. Douglas GC, Fry GN, Thirkill T, et al: Cell-mediated infection of human placental trophoblast with HIV in vitro. AIDS Res Hum Retroviruses 7:735–740, 1991.
40. Maury W, Potts BJ, Rabson AB: HIV-1 infection of first trimester and term human placental tissue: A possible mode of maternal-fetal transmission. J Infect Dis 160:583–588, 1989.
41. Chandwani S, Greco MA, Mittal K, et al: Pathology and human immunodeficiency virus expression in placentas of seropositive women. J Infect Dis 163:1134–1138, 1991.

42. Mattern CFT, Murray K, Jensen A, et al: Localization of human immunodeficiency virus core antigen in term human placentas. Pediatrics 89:207–209, 1992.
43. Goedert JJ, Duliege AM, Amos CI, et al: High risk of HIV-1 infection for first-born twins. The International Registry of HIV-exposed Twins. Lancet 338:1471–1475, 1991.
44. Duliege A-M, Amos CI, Felton S, et al: Birth order, delivery route, and concordance in the transmission of human immunodeficiency virus type 1 from mothers to twins. J Pediatr 126:625–632, 1995.
45. Mofenson LM: A critical review of studies evaluating the relationship of mode of delivery to perinatal transmission of human immunodeficiency virus. Pediatr Infect Dis J 14:169–177, 1995.
46. Boue F, Pons J, Keros L, et al: Risk for HIV-1 perinatal transmission varies with the mother's stage of HIV infection. Presented at the Sixth International Conference on AIDS; July 1990; San Francisco.
47. Borkowsky W, Krasinski K, Cao Y, et al: Correlation of perinatal transmission of human immunodeficiency virus type 1 with maternal viremia and lymphocyte phenotypes. J Pediatr 125:345–351, 1994.
48. Thomas PA, Weedon J, Krasinski K, et al: Maternal predictors of perinatal human immunodeficiency virus transmission. Pediatr Infect Dis J 13:489–495, 1994.
49. Fang G, Burger H, Grimson R, et al: Maternal plasma human immunodeficiency virus type 1 RNA level: A determinant and projected threshold for mother-to-child transmission. Proc Natl Acad Sci USA 92:12100–12104, 1995.
50. Dickover RE, Garratty EM, Herman SA, et al: Identification of levels of maternal HIV-1 RNA associated with risk of perinatal transmission. Effect of zidovudine treatment on viral load. JAMA 275:599–605, 1996.
51. D'Arminio Monforte A, Ravizza M, Muggiasca ML, et al: HIV-infected pregnant women: Possible predictors of vertical transmission. Presented at the Seventh International Conference on AIDS; July 1991; Florence, Italy.
52. Rossi P, Moschese V, Broliden PA, et al: Presence of maternal antibodies of human immunodeficiency virus 1 envelope glycoprotein gp 120 epitopes correlates with the uninfected states of children born to seropositive mothers. Proc Natl Acad Sci USA 86:8055–8058, 1989.
53. Halsey NA, Markham R, Wahren B, et al: Lack of association between maternal antibodies to V3 loop peptides and maternal-infant HIV-1 transmission. J Acquir Immune Defic Syndr 5:153–157, 1992.
54. Goedert JJ, Drummond JE, Minkoff HL, et al: Mother-to-infant transmission of human immunodeficiency virus type 1: Association with prematurity or low anti-gp120. Lancet 2:1351–1354, 1989.
55. Devash Y, Calvelli TA, Wood DG, et al: Vertical transmission of human immunodeficiency virus is correlated with the absence of high-affinity/avidity maternal antibodies to the gp120 principal neutralizing domain. Proc Natl Acad Sci USA 87:3445–3449, 1990.
56. Landesman SH, Kalish LA, Burns DN, et al: Obstetrical factors and the transmission of human immunodeficiency virus type 1 from mother to child. N Engl J Med 334:1617–1623, 1996.
57. Connor EM, Sperling RS, Gelber R, et al: Reduction of maternal-infant transmission of immunodeficiency virus type 1 with zidovudine treatment. N Engl J Med 331:1173–1180, 1994.
58. Centers for Disease Control and Prevention: Recommendations of the U.S. Public Health Service Task Force on the use of zidovudine to reduce perinatal transmission of human immunodeficiency virus. MMWR Morbid Mortal Wkly Rep 43(RR-11):1–20, 1994.
59. Yanase Y, Tango T, Okumura K, et al: Lymphocyte subsets identified by monoclonal antibodies in healthy children. Pediatr Res 20:1147–1151, 1986.
60. Erkeller-Yuksel FM, Deneys V, Hannet I, et al: Age-related changes in human blood lymphocyte subpopulations. J Pediatr 120:216–222, 1992.
61. Denny T, Yogev R, Gelman R, et al: Lymphocyte subsets in healthy children during the first 5 years of life. JAMA 267:1484–1488, 1992.
62. The European Collaborative Study: Age-related standards for T lymphocyte subsets based on uninfected children born to human immunodeficiency virus 1–infected mothers. Pediatr Infect Dis J 11:1018–1026, 1992.
63. Aldhous MC, Raab GM, Doherty KV, et al: Age-related ranges of memory, activation, and cytotoxic markers on CD4 and CD8 cells in children. J Clin Immunol 14:289–298, 1994.
64. McKinney RE, Wilfert CM: Lymphocyte subsets in children younger than 2 years old: Normal values in a population at risk for human immunodeficiency virus infection and diagnostic and prognostic application to infected children. Pediatr Infect Dis J 11:639–644, 1992.
65. Ibegbu C, Spira TJ, Nesheim S, et al: Subpopulations of T and B cells in perinatally HIV-infected and noninfected age-matched children compared with those in adults. Clin Immunol Immunopathol 71:27–32, 1994.
66. Borkowsky W, Rigaud M, Krasinski K, et al: Cell-mediated and humoral immune responses in children infected with human immunodeficiency virus during the first four years of life. J Pediatr 120:371–375, 1992.
67. Roilides E, Clerici M, DePalma L, et al: Helper T-cell responses in children infected with human immunodeficiency virus type 1. J Pediatr 118:724–730, 1991.
68. Luzuriaga K, Holmes D, Hereema A, et al: HIV-1–specific cytotoxic T lymphocyte responses in the first year of life. J Immunol 154:433–443, 1995.
69. Luzuriaga K, Koup RA, Pikora CA, et al: Deficient human immunodeficiency virus type 1–specific cytotoxic T cell responses in vertically infected children. J Pediatr 119:230–236, 1991.
70. Buseyne F, Blanche S, Schmitt D, et al: Detection of HIV-specific cell-mediated cytotoxicity in the peripheral blood from infected children. J Immunol 8:3569–3581, 1993.
71. Forte M, Maartens G, Campbell F, et al: T-lymphocyte responses to *Pneumocystis carinii* in healthy and HIV-positive individuals. J Acquir Immune Defic Syndr 5:409–416, 1992.
72. Madhok R, Gracie JA, Forbes CD, Lowe GDO: B cell dysfunction in haemophilia in the absence and presence of HIV-1 infection. Thromb Haemost 65:7–10, 1991.
73. Ellis M, Gupta S, Galant S, et al: Impaired neutrophil function in patients with AIDS or AIDS-related complex: A comprehensive evaluation. J Infect Dis 158:1268–1276, 1988.
74. European Collaborative Study: Children born to women with HIV-1 infection: Natural history and risk of transmission. Lancet 337:253–260, 1991.
75. Roilides E, Black C, Reimer C, et al: Serum immunoglobulin G subclasses in children infected with human immunodeficiency virus type 1. Pediatr Infect Dis J 10:134–139, 1991.
76. Vigano A, Principi N, Villa ML, et al: Immunologic characterization of children vertically infected with human immunodeficiency virus, with slow or rapid disease progression. J Pediatr 126:368–374, 1995.
77. Sei S, Akiyoshi H, Bernard J, et al: Dynamics of virus versus host interaction in children with human immunodeficiency virus type 1 infection. J Infect Dis 173:1485–1490, 1996.
78. Mueller BU, Sei S, Anderson B, et al: Comparison of virus burden in blood and sequential lymph node biopsy specimens from children infected with human immunodeficiency virus. J Pediatr 129:410–418, 1996.
79. Coffin JM: Plasma viral load. CD4+ cell counts, and HIV-1 production by cells. Science 271:670–671, 1996.
80. Coffin JM: HIV population dynamics in vivo: Implications for genetic variation, pathogenesis, and therapy. Science 267:483–489, 1995.
81. Ho DD, Neumann AU, Perelson AS, et al: Rapid turnover of plasma virions and CD4 lymphocytes in HIV-1 infection. Nature 373:123–126, 1995.
82. Ho DD: Viral counts count in HIV infection. Science 271:1124–1125, 1996.
83. Wei X, Ghosh SK, Taylor ME, et al: Viral dynamics in human immunodeficiency virus type 1 infection. Nature 373:117–122, 1995.
84. Cao Y, Qin L, Zhang L, et al: Virologic and immunologic characterization of long-term survivors of human immunodeficiency virus type 1 infection. N Engl J Med 332:201–208, 1995.
85. Pantaleo G, Menzo S, Vaccarezza M, et al: Studies in subjects with long-term nonprogressive human immunodeficiency virus infection. N Engl J Med 332:209–216, 1995.

86. O'Brien TR, Blattner WA, Waters D, et al: Serum HIV-1 RNA levels and time to development of AIDS in the Multicenter Hemophilia Cohort Study. JAMA 276:105–110, 1996.
87. Mellors JW, Rinaldo JCR, Gupta P, et al: Prognosis of HIV-1 infection predicted by the quantity of virus in plasma. Science 272:1167–1170, 1996.
88. Saag MS, Holodniy M, Kuritzkes DR, et al: HIV viral load markers in clinical practice. Nat Med 2:625–629, 1996.
89. Daar ES, Moudgil T, Meyer RD, Ho DD: Transient high levels of viremia in patients with primary human immunodeficiency virus type 1 infection. N Engl J Med 324:961–964, 1991.
90. Clark SJ, Saag MS, Decker WD, et al: High titers of cytopathic virus in plasma of patients with symptomatic primary HIV-1 infection. N Engl J Med 324:954–960, 1991.
91. Graziosi C, Pantaleo G, Butini I, et al: Kinetics of human immunodeficiency virus type 1 (HIV-1) DNA and RNA synthesis during primary HIV-1 infection. Proc Natl Acad Sci USA 90:6405–6409, 1993.
92. Graziosi C, Pantaleo G, Demarest JF, et al: HIV-1 infection in the lymphoid organs. AIDS 7(Suppl 2):S53–S58, 1993.
93. Spiegel H, Herbst H, Niedobitek G, et al: Follicular dendritic cells are a major reservoir for human immunodeficiency virus type 1 in lymphoid tissues facilitating infection of $CD4^+$ T-helper cells. Am J Pathol 140:15–22, 1992.
94. Fox CH, Tenner-Racz K, Racz P, et al: Lymphoid germinal centers are reservoirs of human immunodeficiency virus type 1 RNA. J Infect Dis 164:1051–1057, 1991.
95. Fox CH, Cottler-Fox M: In situ hybridization in HIV research. Microsc Res Tech 25:78–84, 1993.
96. Pantaleo G, Graziosi C, Butini I, et al: Lymphoid organs function as major reservoirs for human immunodeficiency virus. Proc Natl Acad Sci USA 88:9838–9842, 1991.
97. Pantaleo G, Graziosi C, Demarest JF, et al: HIV infection is active and progressive in lymphoid tissue during the clinically latent stage of disease. Nature 362:355–358, 1993.
98. Palumbo PE, Kwok S, Wesley Y, et al: Viral measurement by polymerase chain reaction–based assays in human immunodeficiency virus–infected infants. J Pediatr 126:592–595, 1995.
99. Luzuriaga K, McQuilken P, Alimenti A, et al: Early viremia and immune responses in vertical human immunodeficiency virus type 1 infection. J Infect Dis 167:1008–1013, 1993.
100. Bryson YJ, Pang S, Wei LS, et al: Clearance of HIV infection in a perinatally infected infant. N Engl J Med 332:833–838, 1995.
101. Roques PA, Gras G, Parnet-Mathieu F, et al: Clearance of HIV infection in 12 perinatally infected children: Clinical, virological and immunological data. AIDS 9:F19–F26, 1995.
102. Bakshi SS, Tetali S, Abrams EJ, et al: Repeatedly positive human immunodeficiency virus type 1 DNA polymerase chain reaction in human immunodeficiency virus–exposed seroreverting infants. Pediatr Infect Dis J 14:658–662, 1995.
103. Thomas P, Singh T, Williams R, Blum S: Trends in survival for children reported with maternally transmitted acquired immunodeficiency syndrome in New York City, 1982 to 1989. Pediatr Infect Dis J 11:34–39, 1992.
104. Morris CR, Araba-Owoyele L, Spector SA, Maldonado YA: Disease patterns and survival after acquired immunodeficiency syndrome diagnosis in human immunodeficiency virus–infected children. Pediatr Infect Dis J 15:321–328, 1996.
105. Blanche S, Tardieu M, Duliege A-M, et al: Longitudinal study of 94 symptomatic infants with perinatally acquired human immunodeficiency virus infection. Am J Dis Child 144:1210–1215, 1990.
106. Tovo PA, De Martino M, Gabiano C, et al: Prognostic factors and survival in children with perinatal HIV-1 infection. Lancet 339:1249–1253, 1992.
107. Scott GB, Hutto C, Makuch RW, et al: Survival in children with perinatally acquired human immunodeficiency virus type 1 infection. N Engl J Med 321:1791–1796, 1989.
108. Duliege A-M, Messiah A, Blanche S, et al: Natural history of human immunodeficiency virus type 1 infection in children: Prognostic value of laboratory tests on the bimodal progression of disease. Pediatr Infect Dis J 11:630–635, 1992.
109. Forsyth BW, Andiman WA, O'Connor T: Development of a prognosis-based clinical staging system for infants infected with human immunodeficiency virus. J Pediatr 129:648–655, 1996.
110. Blanche S, Mayaux M-J, Rouzioux C, et al: Relation of the course of HIV infection in children to the severity of the disease in their mothers at delivery. N Engl J Med 330:308–312, 1994.
111. Frederick T, Mascola L, Eller A, et al: Progression of human immunodeficiency virus disease among infants and children infected perinatally with human immunodeficiency virus or through neonatal blood transfusion. Pediatr Infect Dis J 13:1091–1097, 1994.
112. Butler KM, Husson RN, Lewis LL, et al: CD4 status and p24 antigenemia. Are they useful predictors of survival in HIV-infected children receiving antiretroviral therapy? Am J Dis Child 146:932–936, 1992.
113. Kourtis AP, Igegbu C, Nahmias AJ, et al: Early progression of disease in HIV-infected infants with thymus dysfunction. N Engl J Med 335:1431–1436, 1996.
114. Burgard M, Mayaux M-J, Blanche S, et al: The use of viral culture and p24 antigen testing to diagnose human immunodeficiency virus infection in neonates. N Engl J Med 327:1192–1197, 1992.
115. Dickover RE, Dillon M, Gillette SG, et al: Rapid increases in load of human immunodeficiency virus correlate with early disease progression and loss of CD4 cells in vertically infected infants. J Infect Dis 170:1279–1284, 1994.
116. Mayaux M-J, Burgard M, Teglas J-P, et al: Neonatal characteristics in rapidly progressive perinatally acquired HIV-1 disease. JAMA 275:606–610, 1996.
117. Simonds RJ, Lindegren ML, Thomas P, et al: Prophylaxis against *Pneumocystis carinii* pneumonia among children with perinatally acquired human immunodeficiency virus infection in the United States. N Engl J Med 332:786–790, 1995.
118. Palasanthiran P, Robertson P, Ziegler JB, Graham GG: Decay of transplacental human immunodeficiency virus type 1 antibodies in neonates and infants. J Infect Dis 170:1593–1596, 1994.
119. Siena Consensus Workshop II: Strategies for prevention of perinatal transmission of HIV infection. J Acquir Immune Defic Syndr 8:161–175, 1993.
120. McIntosh K, Pitt J, Brambilla D, et al: Blood culture in the first 6 months of life for the diagnosis of vertically transmitted human immunodeficiency virus infection. J Infect Dis 170:996–1000, 1994.
121. Turner BJ, Eppes S, McKee LJ, et al: A population-based comparison of the clinical course of children and adults with AIDS. AIDS 9:65–72, 1995.
122. Englund JA, Baker CJ, Raskino C, et al: Clinical and laboratory characteristics of a large cohort of symptomatic, human immunodeficiency virus–infected infants and children. Pediatr Infect Dis J 15:1025–1036, 1996.
123. The European Collaborative Study: Natural history of vertically acquired human immunodeficiency virus-1 infection. Pediatrics 94:815–819, 1994.
124. Principi N, Marchisio P, Tornaghi R, et al: Occurrence of infections in children infected with human immunodeficiency virus. Pediatr Infect Dis J 10:190–193, 1991.
125. Andiman WA, Mezger J, Shapiro E: Invasive bacterial infections in children born to women infected with human immunodeficiency virus type 1. J Pediatr 124:846–852, 1994.
126. Krasinski K, Borkowsky W. Bonk S. et al: Bacterial infections in human immunodeficiency virus–infected children. Pediatr Infect Dis J 7:323–328, 1988.
127. Roilides E, Marshall D, Venzon D, et al: Bacterial infections in human immunodeficiency virus type 1–infected children: The impact of central venous catheters and antiretroviral agents. Pediatr Infect Dis J 10:813–819, 1991.
128. Janoff EN, Breiman RF, Daley CL, Hopewell PC: Pneumococcal disease during HIV infection. Epidemiology, clinical, and immunologic perspectives. Ann Intern Med 117:314–324, 1992.
129. Farley JJ, King JC, Nair P, et al: Invasive pneumococcal disease among infected and uninfected children of mothers with human immunodeficiency virus infection. J Pediatr 124:853–858, 1994.
130. Adamson PC, Wu TC, Meade BD, et al: Pertussis in a previously immunized child with human immunodeficiency virus infection. J Pediatr 115:598–592, 1989.
131. Hirschfeld S, Schiffman G, Tudor-Williams G, Pizzo PA: Pneumonia and bacteremia by pneumococcal serotype 16 in a human immunodeficiency virus–infected child with normal serum antibody response to 23-valent pneumovax vaccine (Letter). J Infect Dis 171:761–762, 1995.

132. Nadal D, Caduff R, Kraft R, et al: Invasive infection with *Mycobacterium genavense* in three children with the acquired immunodeficiency syndrome. Eur J Clin Microbiol Infect Dis 12:37–43, 1993.
133. Lewis LL, Butler KM, Husson RN, et al: Defining the population of human immunodeficiency virus–infected children at risk for *Mycobacterium avium-intracellulare* infection. J Pediatr 121:677–683, 1992.
134. Rutstein RM, Cobb P, McGowan KL, et al: *Mycobacterium avium intracellulare* complex infection in HIV-infected children. AIDS 7:507–512, 1993.
135. Masur H, The Public Health Service Task Force on Prophylaxis and Therapy for Mycobacterium Avium Complex: Recommendations on prophylaxis and therapy for disseminated *Mycobacterium avium* complex disease in patients infected with the human immunodeficiency virus. N Engl J Med 329:898–904, 1993.
136. Husson RN, Ross LA, Sandelli S, et al: Orally administered clarithromycin for the treatment of systemic *Mycobacterium avium* complex infection in children with acquired immunodeficiency syndrome. J Pediatr 124:807–814, 1994.
137. Lewis L, Jacobsen F, Mueller B, et al: Phase I/II assessment of oral rifabutin suspension for the prophylaxis of *Mycobacterium avium* complex (MAC) bacteremia in HIV-infected children. Presented at the First National Conference on Human Retroviruses and Related Infections; 1993; Washington, DC.
138. Nightingale SD, Cameron W, Gordin FM, et al: Two controlled trials of rifabutin prophylaxis against *Mycobacterium avium* complex infection in AIDS. N Engl J Med 329:828–833, 1993.
139. Braun MM, Cauthen G: Relationship of the human immunodeficiency virus epidemic to pediatric tuberculosis and bacillus Calmette-Guérin immunization. Pediatr Infect Dis J 11:220–227, 1992.
140. Dumois JA: Tuberculosis in children with HIV infection. Pediatr AIDS HIV Infect Fetus Adolesc 3:177–182, 1992.
141. Moss WJ, Dedyo T, Suarez M, et al: Tuberculosis in children infected with human immunodeficiency virus: A report of five cases. Pediatr Infect Dis J 11:114–120, 1992.
142. Khoury YF, Mastrucci MT, Hutto C, et al: *Mycobacterium tuberculosis* in children with human immunodeficiency virus type 1 infection. Pediatr Infect Dis J 11:950–955, 1992.
143. Gutman LT, Moye J, Zimmer B, Tian C: Tuberculosis in human immunodeficiency virus–exposed or –infected United States children. Pediatr Infect Dis J 13:963–968, 1994.
144. Hoffman ND, Kelly C, Futterman D: Tuberculosis infection in human immunodeficiency virus–positive adolescents and young adults: A New York City cohort. Pediatrics 97:198–203, 1996.
145. Chan SP, Birnbaum J, Rao M, Steiner P: Clinical manifestations and outcome of tuberculosis in children with acquired immunodeficiency syndrome. Pediatr Infect Dis J 15:443–447, 1996.
146. Starke JR, Jacobs RF, Jereb J: Resurgence of tuberculosis in children. J Pediatr 120:839–855, 1992.
147. Committee on Infectious Diseases: Update on tuberculosis skin testing of children. Pediatrics 97:282–284, 1996.
148. Abadco DL, Steiner P: Gastric lavage is better than bronchoalveolar lavage for isolation of *Mycobacterium tuberculosis* in childhood pulmonary tuberculosis. Pediatr Infect Dis J 11:735–738, 1992.
149. Starke JR: Multidrug therapy for tuberculosis in children. Pediatr Infect Dis J 9:785–793, 1990.
150. Starke JR, Correa AG: Management of mycobacterial infection and disease in children. Pediatr Infect Dis J 14:455–470, 1995.
151. Centers for Disease Control and Prevention: Initial therapy for tuberculosis in the era of multidrug resistance. Recommendations of the Advisory Council for the Elimination of Tuberculosis [published erratum in MMWR 42(27):536, 1993]. MMWR Morbid Mortal Wkly Rep 42(RR-7):1–7, 1993.
152. Srugo I, Israele V, Wittek AE, et al: Clinical manifestations of varicella-zoster virus infections in human immunodeficiency virus–infected children. Am J Dis Child 147:742–745, 1993.
153. Penney NS: Skin Manifestations of AIDS. Philadelphia, JB Lippincott, 1990.
154. Jura E, Chadwick EG, Josephs SH, et al: Varicella-zoster virus infections in children infected with human immunodeficiency virus. Pediatr Infect Dis J 8:586–590, 1989.
155. Pahwa S, Biron K, Lim W, et al: Continous varicella-zoster infection associated with acyclovir resistance in a child with AIDS. JAMA 260:2879–2882, 1988.
156. Leibovitz E, Kaul A, Rigaud M, et al: Chronic varicella zoster in a child infected with human immunodeficiency virus: Case report and review of the literature. Cutis 49:27–31, 1992.
157. Hirsch MS, Schooley RT: Resistance to antiviral drugs: The end of innocence. N Engl J Med 320:313–314, 1989.
158. Frenkel LD, Gaur S, Tsolia M. et al: Cytomegalovirus infection in children with AIDS. Rev Infect Dis 12:820–826, 1990.
159. Mueller BU, MacKay K, Cheshire LB, et al: Cytomegalovirus ureteritis as a cause of renal failure in a child infected with the human immunodeficiency virus. Clin Infect Dis 20:1040–1043, 1995.
160. Belec L, Tayot J, Tron P, et al: Cytomegalovirus encephalopathy in an infant with congenital acquired immuno-deficiency syndrome. Neuropediatrics 21:124–129, 1990.
161. Kitchen BJ, Engler HD, Gill VJ, et al: Cytomegalovirus infection in children with HIV infection. Pediatr Infect Dis J (in press).
162. Butler KM, De Smet MD, Husson RN, et al: Treatment of aggressive cytomegalovirus retinitis with ganciclovir in combination with foscarnet in a child infected with human immunodeficiency virus. J Pediatr 120:483–486, 1992.
163. Walton RC, Whitcup SM, Mueller BU, et al: Combined intravenous ganciclovir and foscarnet for children with recurrent cytomegalovirus retinitis. Ophthalmology 102:1865–1870, 1995.
164. Nigro G, Krysztofiak A, Castelli Gattinara G, et al: Rapid progression of HIV disease in children with cytomegalovirus DNAemia. AIDS 10:1127–1133, 1996.
165. Martin P, Di Bisceglie AM, Kassianides C, et al: Rapidly progressive non-A, non-B hepatitis in patients with human immunodeficiency virus infection. Gastroenterology 97:1559–1561, 1989.
166. Bodsworth NJ, Cooper DA, Donovan B: The influence of human immunodeficiency virus type 1 infection on the development of the hepatitis B virus carrier state. J Infect Dis 163:1138–1140, 1991.
167. Paccagnini S, Principi N, Massironi E, et al: Perinatal transmission and manifestation of hepatitis C virus infection in a high risk population. Pediatr Infect Dis J 14:195–199, 1995.
168. Kaplan LJ, Daum RS, Smaron M, McCarthy CA: Severe measles in immunocompromised patients. JAMA 267:1237–1241, 1992.
169. Nadel S, McGann K, Hodinka RL, et al: Measles giant cell pneumonia in a child with human immunodeficiency virus infection. Pediatr Infect Dis J 10:542–544, 1991.
170. Markowitz LE, Chandler FW, Roldan EO, et al: Fatal measles pneumonia without rash in a child with AIDS. J Infect Dis 158:480–483, 1988.
171. Krasinski K, Borkowsky W: Measles and measles immunity in children infected with human immunodeficiency virus. JAMA 261:2512–2516, 1989.
172. Centers for Disease Control and Prevention: Recommendations of the Advisory Committee on Immunization Practices (ACIP): Use of vaccines and immune globulins for persons with altered immunocompetence. MMWR Morbid Mortal Wkly Rep 42(RR-4):1–18, 1993.
173. Ambrosino DM, Molrine DC: Critical appraisal of immunization strategies for prevention of infection in the compromised host. Hematol Oncol Clin North Am 7:1027–1050, 1993.
174. Palumbo P, Hoyt L, Demasio K, et al: Population-based study of measles and measles immunization in human immunodeficiency virus–infected children. Pediatr Infect Dis J 11:1008–1014, 1992.
175. Centers for Disease Control: Hepatitis B virus: A comprehensive strategy for eliminating transmission in the United States through universal childhood vaccination. Recommendations of the Immunization Practices Advisory Committee (ACIP). MMWR Morbid Mortal Wkly Rep 40(RR-13):1–25, 1991.
176. Ellaurie M, Schutzbank TE, Rakusan TA, Lipson SM: Spectrum of adenovirus infection in pediatric HIV infection. Pediatr AIDS HIV Infect Fetus Adolesc 4:211–214, 1993.
177. King JC Jr, Burke AR, Clemens JD, et al: Respiratory syncytial virus illnesses in human immunodeficiency virus– and noninfected children. Pediatr Infect Dis J 12:733–739, 1993.
178. Chandwani S, Borkowsky W, Krasinski K, et al: Respiratory syncytial virus infection in human immunodeficiency virus–infected children. J Pediatr 117:251–254, 1990.
179. Roilides E, Mertins S, Eddy J, et al: Impairment of neutrophil

chemotactic and bactericidal function in children infected with human immunodeficiency virus type 1 and partial reversal after in vitro exposure to granulocyte-macrophage colony-stimulating factor. J Pediatr 117:531–540, 1990.
180. Roilides E, Pizzo PA: Modulation of host defense by cytokines: Evolving adjuncts in prevention and treatment of serious infections in immunocompromised hosts. Clin Infect Dis 15:508–524, 1992.
181. Roilides E, Holmes A, Blake C, et al: Impairment of neutrophil antifungal activity against hyphae of *Aspergillus fumigatus* in children infected with human immunodeficiency virus. J Infect Dis 167:905–911, 1993.
182. Walsh TJ: Fungal infections complicating pediatric HIV infection. *In* Pizzo PA, Wilfert CM (eds): Pediatric AIDS. The Challenge of HIV Infection in Infants, Children, and Adolescents. Baltimore, Williams & Wilkins, 1994, pp 321–347.
183. Walsh TJ, Gonzales C, Roilides E, et al: Fungemia in children infected with the human immunodeficiency virus: New epidemiologic patterns, emerging pathogens, and improved outcome with antifungal therapy. Clin Infect Dis 20:900–906, 1995.
184. Gonzales CE, Venson D, Lee S, et al: Risk factors for fungemia in children infected with human immunodeficiency virus: A case control study. Clin Infect Dis 23:515–521, 1996.
185. Clark RA, Greer D, Atkinson W, et al: Spectrum of *Cryptococcus neoformans* infection in 68 patients infected with human immunodeficiency virus. Rev Infect Dis 12:768–777, 1990.
186. Leggiadro RJ, Kline MW, Hughes WT: Extrapulmonary cryptococcosis in children with acquired immunodeficiency syndrome. Pediatr Infect Dis J 10:658–662, 1991.
187. Gonzales GE, Shetty D, Lewis LL, et al: Cryptococcosis in human immunodeficiency virus–infected children. Pediatr Infect Dis J 15:796–800, 1996.
188. Ting SF, Glader BE, Prober CG: *Cryptococcus* infection in a nine-year-old child with hemophilia and the acquired immunodeficiency syndrome. Pediatr Infect Dis J 10:76–77, 1991.
189. Butcher JD, Krober MS: Cryptococcal meningitis in a child with acquired immunodeficiency syndrome. Pediatr AIDS HIV Infect Fetus Adolesc 2:134–136, 1991.
190. Byers M, Feldman S, Edwards J: Disseminated histoplasmosis as the acquired immunodeficiency syndrome–defining illness in an infant. Pediatr Infect Dis J 11:127–128, 1992.
191. Minamoto GY, Barlam TF, Vander Els NJ: Invasive aspergillosis in patients with AIDS. Clin Infect Dis 14:66–74, 1992.
192. Denning DW, Follansbee SE, Scolaro M, et al: Pulmonary aspergillosis in the acquired immunodeficiency syndrome. N Engl J Med 324:654–662, 1991.
193. Ashdown BC, Tien RD, Felsberg GJ: Aspergillosis of the brain and paranasal sinuses in immunocompromised patients: CT and MR imaging findings. AJR 162:155–159, 1994.
194. Mortier E, Pouchot J, Bossi P, Molinié V: Maternal-fetal transmission of *Pneumocystis carinii* in human immunodeficiency virus infection. N Engl J Med 332:825–826, 1995.
195. Leibovitz E, Rigaud M, Pollack H, et al: *Pneumocystis carinii* pneumonia in infants infected with the human immunodeficiency virus with more than 450 CD4 T lymphocytes per cubic millimeter. N Engl J Med 323:531–533, 1990.
196. Bernstein LJ, Bye MR, Rubinstein A: Prognostic factors and life expectancy in children with acquired immunodeficiency syndrome and *Pneumocystis carinii* pneumonia. Am J Dis Child 143:775–778, 1989.
197. Kovacs A, Frederick T, Church J, et al: CD4 T-lymphocyte counts and *Pneumocystis carinii* pneumonia in pediatric HIV infection. JAMA 265:1698–1703, 1991.
198. Bye MR, Bernstein LJ, Glaser J, Kleid D: *Pneumocystis carinii* pneumonia in young children with AIDS. Pediatr Pulmonol 9:251–253, 1990.
199. Connor E, Bagarazzi M, McSherry G, et al: Clinical and laboratory correlates of *Pneumocystis carinii* pneumonia in children infected with HIV. JAMA 265:1693–1697, 1991.
200. Ognibene FP, Gill VJ, Pizzo PA, et al: Induced sputum to diagnose *Pneumocystis carinii* pneumonia in immunosuppressed pediatric patients. J Pediatr 115:430–433, 1989.
201. Gosey LL, Howard RM, Witebsky FG, et al: Advantages of a modified toluidine blue O stain and bronchoalveolar lavage for the diagnosis of *Pneumocystis carinii* pneumonia. J Clin Microbiol 22:803–807, 1985.
202. Amaro-Galvez R, Rao M, Abadco D, et al: Nonbronchoscopic bronchoalveolar lavage in ventilated children with acquired immunodeficiency syndrome: A simple and effective diagnostic method for *Pneumocystis carinii* infection. Pediatr J Infect Dis 10:473–475, 1991.
203. Rigaud M, Pollack H, Leibovitz E, et al: Efficacy of primary chemoprophylaxis against *Pneumocystis carinii* pneumonia during the first year of life in infants infected with human immunodeficiency virus type 1. J Pediatr 125:476–480, 1994.
204. Bozzette SA, Finkelstein DM, Spector SA, et al: A randomized trial of three antipneumocystis agents in patients with advanced human immunodeficiency virus infection. N Engl J Med 332:693–699, 1995.
205. Cruciani M, Concia E, Gatti G, et al: Dapsone prophylaxis against *Pneumocystis carinii* pneumonia in human immunodeficiency virus–infected children. Pediatr Infect Dis J 13:80–81, 1994.
206. Mueller BU, Pizzo PA, Steinberg S: Failure of intravenous pentamidine prophylaxis for *Pneumocystis carinii* pneumonia (Reply to letter). J Pediatr 122:163–164, 1993.
207. Mueller BU, Butler KM, Husson RN, Pizzo PA: *Pneumocystis carinii* pneumonia despite prophylaxis in children with human immunodeficiency virus infection. J Pediatr 119:992–994, 1991.
208. Nachman SA, Mueller BU, Mirochnik M, Pizzo PA: High failure rate of dapsone and pentamidine as *Pneumocystis carinii* pneumonia prophylaxis in human immunodeficiency virus–infected children. Pediatr Infect Dis J 13:1004–1006, 1994.
209. The National Institutes of Health–University of California Expert Panel for Corticosteroids as Adjunctive Therapy for Pneumocystis Pneumonia: Consensus statement on the use of corticosteroids as adjunctive therapy for pneumocystis pneumonia in the acquired immunodeficiency syndrome. N Engl J Med 323:1500–1504, 1990.
210. Sleasman JW, Hemenway C, Klein AS, Barrett DJ: Corticosteroids improve survival of children with AIDS and *Pneumocystis carinii* pneumonia. Am J Dis Child 147:30–34, 1993.
211. Miller MJ, Remington JS: Toxoplasmosis in infants and children with HIV infection or AIDS. *In* Pizzo PA, Wilfert CM (eds): Pediatric AIDS. The Challenge of HIV Infection in Infants, Children, and Adolescents. Baltimore, Williams & Wilkins, 1991, pp 299–307.
212. Bottoni F, Gonnella P, Autelitano A, Orzalesi N: Diffuse necrotizing retinochoroiditis in a child with AIDS and toxoplasmic encephalitis. Graefes Arch Clin Exp Ophthalmol 228:36–39, 1990.
213. Medlock MD, Tilleli JT, Pearl GS: Congenital cardiac toxoplasmosis in a newborn with acquired immunodeficiency syndrome. Pediatr Infect Dis J 9:129–132, 1990.
214. Curry A, Turner AJ, Lucas S: Opportunistic infections in human immunodeficiency virus disease: Review highlighting diagnostic and therapeutic aspects. J Clin Pathol 44:182–193, 1991.
215. Cordell RL, Addiss DG: Cryptosporidiosis in child care settings: A review of the literature and recommendations for prevention and control. Pediatr Infect Dis J 13:310–317, 1994.
216. Belman AL, Diamond G, Dickson D, et al: Pediatric acquired immunodeficiency syndrome. Neurologic symptoms. Am J Dis Child 142:29–35, 1988.
217. Civitello LA. Neurologic complications of HIV infection in children. Pediatr Neurosurg 17:104–112, 1991.
218. Dickson DW, Belman AL, Park YD, et al: Central nervous system pathology in pediatric AIDS: An autopsy study. APMIS Suppl 8:40–57, 1989.
219. Schmitt B, Seeger J, Kreuz W, et al: Central nervous system involvement of children with HIV infection. Dev Med Child Neurol 33:535–540, 1991.
220. The European Collaborative Study: Neurologic signs in young children with human immunodeficiency virus infection. Pediatr Infect Dis J 9:402–406, 1990.
221. DeCarli C, Civitello LA, Brouwers P, Pizzo PA: The prevalence of computed tomographic abnormalities of the cerebrum in 100 consecutive children symptomatic with the human immunodeficiency virus. Ann Neurol 34:198–205, 1993.
222. Wolters PL, Brouwers P, Moss HA, Pizzo PA: Adaptive behavior of children with symptomatic HIV infection before and after zidovudine therapy. J Pediatr Psychol 19:47–61, 1994.
223. Lyman WD, Kress Y, Kure K, et al: Detection of HIV in fetal central nervous system tissue. AIDS 4:917–920, 1990.

224. Srugo I, Wittek AE, Israele V, Brunell PA: Meningoencephalitis in a neonate congenitally infected with human immunodeficiency virus type 1. J Pediatr 120:93–95, 1992.
225. Belman AL: AIDS and pediatric neurology. Neurol Clin 8:571–603, 1990.
226. Epstein LG, Sharer LR, Goudsmit J: Neurological and neuropathological features of human immunodeficiency virus infection in children. Ann Neurol 23(Suppl):S19–S23, 1988.
227. Kauffman WM, Sivit CJ, Fitz CR, et al: CT and MR evaluation of intracranial involvement in pediatric HIV infection: A clinical-imaging correlation. Am J Neuroradiol 13:949–957, 1992.
228. Kure K, Llena JF, Lyman WD, et al: Human immunodeficiency virus-1 infection of the nervous system: An autopsy study of 268 adult, pediatric, and fetal brains. Hum Pathol 22:700–710, 1991.
229. Lobato MN, Caldwell MB, Ng P, Oxtoby MJ: Encephalopathy in children with perinatally acquired human immunodeficiency virus infection. Pediatric Spectrum of Disease Clinical Consortium. J Pediatr 126:710–715, 1995.
230. Brouwers P, Tudor-Williams G, DeCarli C, et al: Relation between stage of disease and neurobehavioral measures in children with symptomatic HIV disease. AIDS 9:713–720, 1995.
231. Gallo P, Laverda AM, De Rossi A, et al: Immunological markers in the cerebrospinal fluid of HIV-1 infected children. Acta Paediatr Scand 80:659–666, 1991.
232. Brouwers P, Heyes MP, Moss HA, et al: Quinolinic acid in the cerebrospinal fluid of children with symptomatic human immunodeficiency virus type 1 disease: Relationships to clinical status and therapeutic response. J Infect Dis 168:1380–1386, 1993.
233. Sei S, Saito K, Stewart SK, et al: Increased human immunodeficiency virus (HIV) type 1 DNA content and quinolinic acid concentration in brain tissues from patients with HIV encephalopathy. J Infect Dis 172:638–647, 1995.
234. Sei S, Stewart SK, Farley M, et al: Evaluation of HIV-1 RNA levels in cerebrospinal fluid and viral resistance to zidovudine in children with HIV encephalopathy. J Infect Dis 174:1200–1206, 1996.
235. DeCarli C, Fugate L, Falloon J, et al: Brain growth and cognitive improvement in children with human immunodeficiency virus–induced encephalopathy after 6 months of continuous infusion zidovudine therapy. J Acquir Immune Defic Syndr 4:585–592, 1991.
236. Brouwers P, DeCarli C, Civitello L, et al: Correlation between computed tomographic brain scan abnormalities and neuropsychological function in children with symptomatic human immunodeficiency virus disease. Arch Neurol 52:39–44, 1995.
237. Hirschfeld S, Laue L, Cutler GB Jr, Pizzo PA: Thyroid abnormalities in children infected with human immunodeficiency virus. J Pediatr 128:70–74, 1996.
238. Sharer LR, Dowling PC, Michaels J, et al: Spinal cord disease in children with HIV-1 infection: A combined molecular biological and neuropathological study. Neuropath Appl Neurobiol 16:317–331, 1990.
239. Pizzo PA, Butler K, Balis F, et al: Dideoxycytidine alone and in an alternating schedule with zidovudine in children with symptomatic human immunodeficiency virus infection. J Pediatr 117:799–808, 1990.
240. Butler KM, Husson RN, Balis FM, et al: Dideoxyinosine in children with symptomatic human immunodeficiency virus infection. N Engl J Med 324:137–144, 1991.
241. Marolda J, Bonforte RJ, Kotin NM, et al: Pulmonary manifestations of HIV infection in children. Pediatr Pulmonol 10:231–235, 1991.
242. Moran CA, Suster S, Pavlova Z, et al: The spectrum of pathological changes in children with the acquired immunodeficiency syndrome: An autopsy study of 36 cases. Hum Pathol 25:877–882, 1994.
243. Pitt J: Lymphocytic interstitial pneumonia. *In* Edelson PJ (ed): Childhood AIDS. Philadelphia, WB Saunders, 1991, pp 89–96.
244. Joshi VV, Oleske JM, Connor EM: Morphologic findings in children with acquired immune deficiency syndrome: Pathogenesis and clinical implications. Pediatr Pathol 10:155–165, 1990.
245. Joshi VV: Systemic lymphoproliferative lesions in children with AIDS. Pediatr AIDS HIV Infect Fetus Adolesc 1:44–48, 1990.
246. Connor EM, Marquis J, Oleske JM: Lymphoid interstitial pneumonitis. *In* Pizzo PA, Wilfert CM (eds): Pediatric AIDS. The Challenge of HIV Infection in Infants, Children, and Adolescents. Baltimore, Williams & Wilkins, 1991, pp 343–354.
247. Amorosa JK, Miller RW, Laraya-Cuasay L, et al: Bronchiectasis in children with lymphocytic interstitial pneumonia and acquired immune deficiency syndromes. Plain film and CT observations. Pediatr Radiol 22:603–607, 1992.
248. Teruya-Feldstein J, Temeck BK, Sloas MM, et al: Pulmonary malignant lymphoma of mucosa-associated lymphoid tissue (MALT) arising in a pediatric HIV-positive patient. Am J Surg Pathol 19:357–363, 1995.
249. Izraeli S, Mueller BU, Ling A, et al: Role of tissue diagnosis in pulmonary involvement in pediatric human immunodeficiency virus infection. Pediatr Infect Dis J 15:112–116, 1996.
250. Lipshultz SE, Chanock S, Sanders SP, et al: Cardiovascular manifestations of human immunodeficiency virus infection in infants and children. Am J Cardiol 63:1489–1497, 1989.
251. Luginbuhl LM, Orav EJ, McIntosh K, Lipshultz SE: Cardiac morbidity and related mortality in children with HIV infection. JAMA 269:2869–2875, 1993.
252. Steinherz LJ, Brochstein JA, Robins J: Cardiac involvement in congenital acquired immunodeficiency syndrome. Am J Dis Child 140:1241–1244, 1986.
253. Stewart JM, Kaul A, Gromisch DS, et al: Symptomatic cardiac dysfunction in children with human immunodeficiency virus infection. Am Heart J 117:140–144, 1989.
254. Lipshultz SE, Orav EJ, Sanders SP, et al: Cardiac structure and function in children with human immunodeficiency virus infection treated with zidovudine. N Engl J Med 327:1260–1265, 1992.
255. Lipshultz SE, Fox CH, Perez-Atayde AR, et al: Identification of human immunodeficiency virus-1 RNA and DNA in the heart of a child with cardiovascular abnormalities and congenital acquired immune deficiency syndrome. Am J Cardiol 66:246–250, 1990.
256. Sei S, Kleiner DE, Kopp JB, et al: Quantitative analysis of viral burden in tissues from adults and children with symptomatic human immunodeficiency virus type I infection assessed by polymerase chain reaction. J Infect Dis 170:325–333, 1994.
257. Joshi VV, Gadol C, Connor E, et al: Dilated cardiomyopathy in children with acquired immunodeficiency syndrome: A pathologic study of five cases. Hum Pathol 19:69–73, 1988.
258. Domanski MJ, Sloas MM, Follmann DA, et al: Effect of zidovudine and didanosine treatment on heart function in children infected with human immunodeficiency virus. J Pediatr 127:137–146, 1995.
259. Joshi VV, Pawel B, Connor E, et al: Arteriopathy in children with acquired immune deficiency syndrome. Pediatr Pathol 7:261–275, 1987.
260. Husson RN, Saini R, Lewis LL, et al: Cerebral artery aneurysms in children infected with human immunodeficiency virus. J Pediatr 121:927–930, 1992.
261. Soberman N, Leonidas JC, Berdon WE, et al: Parotid enlargement in children seropositive for human immunodeficiency virus: Imaging findings. AJR 157:553–556, 1991.
262. Schiødt M: HIV-associated salivary gland disease: A review. Oral Surg Oral Med Oral Pathol 73:164–167, 1992.
263. Sperling NM, Lin P-T: Parotid disease associated with human immunodeficiency virus infection. Ear Nose Throat J 69:475–477, 1990.
264. Sperling NM, Lin P-T, Lucente FE: Cystic parotid masses in HIV infection. Head Neck 12:337–341, 1990.
265. Fischer GD, Rinaldo CR, Gbadero D, et al: Seroprevalence of HIV-1 and HIV-2 infection among children diagnosed with protein-calorie malnutrition in Nigeria. Epidemiol Infect 110:373–378, 1993.
266. Miller TL, Orav EJ, Martin SR, et al: Malnutrition and carbohydrate malabsorption in children with vertically transmitted human immunodeficiency virus 1 infection. Gastroenterology 100:1296–1302, 1991.
267. Kotloff KL, Johnson JP, Nair P, et al: Diarrheal morbidity during the first 2 years of life among HIV-infected infants. JAMA 271:448–452, 1994.
268. Lewis JD, Winter HS. Intestinal and hepatobiliary diseases in HIV-infected children. Gastroenterol Clin North Am 24:119–132, 1995.
269. Miller TL: Nutritional assessment and its clinical application in children infected with the human immunodeficiency virus. J Pediatr 129:633–636, 1996.

270. Nicholas SW: The opportunistic and bacterial infections associated with pediatric human immunodeficiency virus disease. Acta Paediatr Suppl 400:46–50, 1994.
271. Oshitani H, Kasolo FC, Mpabalwani M, et al: Association of rotavirus and human immunodeficiency virus infection in children hospitalized with acute diarrhea, Lusaka, Zambia. J Infect Dis 169:897–900, 1994.
272. Thea DM, St. Louis ME, Atido U, et al: A prospective study of diarrhea and HIV-1 infection among 429 Zairian infants. N Engl J Med 329:1696–702, 1993.
273. Yolken RH, Li S, Perman J, Viscidi R: Persistent diarrhea and fecal shedding of retroviral nucleic acids in children infected with human immunodeficiency virus. J Infect Dis 164:61–66, 1991.
274. Yolken RH, Hart W, Oung I, et al: Gastrointestinal dysfunction and disaccharide intolerance in children infected with human immunodeficiency virus. J Pediatr 118:359–363, 1991.
275. Persaud D, Bangaru B, Greco A, et al: Cholestatic hepatitis in children infected with the human immunodeficiency virus. Pediatr Infect Dis J 12:492–498, 1993.
276. Leggiadro RJ, Lewis D, Whitington GL, et al: Chronic hepatitis associated with perinatal HIV infection. AIDS Reader March/April:57–61, 1992.
277. Della Negra M, Queiroz W, Taveras RCJ, et al: Liver disorders in pediatric AIDS patients. Pediatr AIDS HIV Infect Fetus Adolesc 4:222–226, 1993.
278. de Martino M, Tovo P-A, Zuccotti GV, et al: Transferase values in infants at risk from human immunodeficiency virus type 1 perinatal infection. Pediatr Infect Dis J 12:248–250, 1993.
279. Miller TL, Winter HS, Luginbuhl LM, et al: Pancreatitis in pediatric human immunodeficiency virus infection. J Pediatr 120:223–227, 1992.
280. Butler KM, Venzon D, Henry N, et al: Pancreatitis in human immunodeficiency virus–infected children receiving dideoxyinosine. Pediatrics 91:747–751, 1993.
281. Hart CC: Aerosolized pentamidine and pancreatitis (Letter). Ann Intern Med 111:691, 1989.
282. Kumar S, Schnadig VJ, MacGregor MG: Fatal acute pancreatitis associated with pentamidine therapy. Am J Gastroenterol 451:451–453, 1989.
283. Zilleruelo G, Strauss J: HIV nephropathy in children. Pediatr Clin North Am 42:1469–1485, 1995.
284. Strauss J, Zilleruelo G, Abitbol C, et al: Human immunodeficiency virus nephropathy. Pediatr Nephrol 7:220–225, 1993.
285. Ingulli E, Tejani A, Fikrig S, et al: Nephrotic syndrome associated with acquired immunodeficiency syndrome in children. J Pediatr 119:710–716, 1991.
286. Rajpoot D, Kaupke CJ, Vaziri ND, et al: Childhood AIDS nephropathy: A 10-year experience. J Natl Med Assoc 88:493–498, 1996.
287. Strauss J, Abitol C, Zilleruelo G, et al: Renal disease in children with the acquired immunodeficiency syndrome. N Engl J Med 321:625–630, 1989.
288. Kimmel PL, Phillips TM, Ferreira-Centeno A, et al: Brief report: Idiotypic IgA nephropathy in patients with human immunodeficiency virus infection. N Engl J Med 327:702–706, 1992.
289. Schoeneman MJ, Ghali V, Lieberman K, Reisman L: IgA nephritis in a child with human immunodeficiency virus: A unique form of human immunodeficiency virus–associated nephropathy? Pediatr Nephrol 6:46–49, 1992.
290. Elem B, Patil PS, Lucas SB: Haematuria frequency syndrome in patients with positive HIV serology: Observations in Zambia. Br J Urol 67:146–149, 1991.
291. Mueller BU, Tannenbaum S, Pizzo PA: Bone marrow aspirates and biopsies in children with human immunodeficiency virus infection. J Pediatr Hematol Oncol 18:266–271, 1996.
292. Scott GB, Buck BE, Leterman JG, et al: Acquired immunodeficiency syndrome in infants. N Engl J Med 310:76–81, 1984.
293. McKinney RE, Pizzo PA, Scott GB, et al: Safety and tolerance of intermittent intravenous and oral zidovudine therapy in human immunodeficiency virus–infected pediatric patients. J Pediatr 116:640–647, 1990.
294. Ellaurie M, Burns ER, Rubinstein A: Hematologic manifestations in pediatric HIV infection: Severe anemia as a prognostic factor. Am J Pediatr Hematol Oncol 12:449–453, 1990.
295. Hilgartner M: Hematologic manifestations in HIV-infected children. J Pediatr 119:S47–S49, 1991.
296. Griffin TC, Squires JE, Timmons CF, Buchanan GR: Chronic human parvovirus B19–induced erythroid hypoplasia as the initial manifestation of human immunodeficiency virus infection. J Pediatr 118:899–901, 1991.
297. Parmentier L, Boucary D, Salmon D: Pure red cell aplasia in an HIV-infected patient. AIDS 6:234–235, 1992.
298. Frickhofen N, Abkowitz JL, Safford M, et al: Persistent B19 parvovirus infection in patients infected with human immunodeficiency virus type 1 (HIV-1): A treatable cause of anemia in AIDS. Ann Intern Med 113:926–933, 1990.
299. Dalle JH, Dollfus C, Courpotin C, et al: Human immunodeficiency virus–associated hemophagocytic syndrome in children (Letter). Pediatr Infect Dis J 13:1159, 1994.
300. Mueller BU, Jacobsen F, Jarosinski P, et al: Erythropoietin for zidovudine-associated anemia in children with HIV-infection. Pediatr AIDS HIV Infect Fetus Adolesc 5:169–173, 1994.
301. Zuccotti GV, Plebani A, Biasucci G, et al: Granulocyte-colony stimulating factor and erythropoietin therapy in children with human immunodeficiency virus infection. J Int Med Res 24:115–121, 1996.
302. Pizzo PA, Eddy J, Falloon J, et al: Effect of continuous intravenous infusion of zidovudine (AZT) in children with symptomatic HIV infection. N Engl J Med 319:889–896, 1988.
303. Mueller BU, Jacobsen F, Butler KM, et al: Combination treatment with azidothymidine and granulocyte colony-stimulating factor in children with human immunodeficiency virus infection. J Pediatr 121:797–802, 1992.
304. Mueller BU: Hematological problems and their management in children with HIV infection. *In* Pizzo PA, Wilfert CM (eds): Pediatric AIDS. The Challenge of HIV Infection in Infants, Children, and Adolescents, ed 2. Baltimore, Williams & Wilkins, 1994, pp 591–602.
305. Labrune P, Blanche S, Catherine N, et al: Human immunodeficiency virus–associated thrombocytopenia in infants. Acta Paediatr Scand 78:811–814, 1989.
306. Rigaud M, Leibovitz E, Sin Quee C, et al: Thrombocytopenia in children infected with human immunodeficiency virus: Long term follow-up and therapeutic considerations. J Acquir Immune Defic Syndr 5:450–455, 1992.
307. Bussel JB, Graziano JN, Kimberly RP, et al: Intravenous anti-D treatment of immune thrombocytopenic purpura: Analysis of efficacy, toxicity, and mechanism of effect. Blood 77:1884–1893, 1991.
308. Pollak AN, Janinis J, Green D: Successful intravenous immune globulin therapy for human immunodeficiency virus–associated thrombocytopenia. Arch Intern Med 148:695–697, 1988.
309. Sugerman RW, Church JA, Goldsmith JC, Ens GE: Acquired protein S deficiency in children infected with human immunodeficiency virus. Pediatr Infect Dis J 15:106–111, 1996.
310. Mueller BU, Burt R, Gulick L, et al: Disseminated intravascular coagulation associated with granulocyte colony-stimulating factor therapy in a child with human immunodeficiency virus infection. J Pediatr 126:749–752, 1995.
311. Blethen SL, Nachman S, Chasalow FI: Thyroid function in children with perinatally acquired antibodies to human immunodeficiency virus. J Pediatr Endocrinol 7:1–4, 1994.
312. Laue L, Pizzo PA, Butler K, Cutler GB: Growth and neuroendocrine dysfunction in children with acquired immunodeficiency syndrome. J Pediatr 117:541–545, 1990.
313. Schwartz LJ, St. Louis Y, Wu R, et al: Endocrine function in children with human immunodeficiency virus infection. Am J Dis Child 145:330–333, 1991.
314. Brettler DB, Forsberg A, Bolivar E, et al: Growth failure as a prognostic indicator for progression to acquired immunodeficiency syndrome in children with hemophilia. J Pediatr 117:584–588, 1990.
315. McKinney RE Jr, Robertson JW: Effect of human immunodeficiency virus infection on the growth of young children. Duke Pediatric AIDS Clinical Trials Unit. J Pediatr 123:579–582, 1993.
316. McKinney RE, Wilfert C: Growth as a prognostic indicator in children with human immunodeficiency virus infection treated with zidovudine. AIDS Clinical Trials Group Protocol 043 Study Group. J Pediatr 125:728–733, 1994.
317. Grinspoon SK, Bilezikian JP: HIV disease and the endocrine system. N Engl J Med 327:1360–1365, 1992.
318. Mueller BU, Pizzo PA: Malignancies in pediatric AIDS. Curr Opin Pediatr 8:45–49, 1996.

319. Arico M, Caselli D, D'Argenio P, et al: Malignancies in children with human immunodeficiency virus type 1 infection. Cancer 68:2473–2477, 1991.
320. DiCarlo FJ, Joshi VV, Oleske JM, Connor EM: Neoplastic diseases in children with acquired immunodeficiency syndrome. Prog AIDS Pathol 2:163–185, 1990.
321. Epstein LG, DiCarlo FJ, Joshi VV, et al: Primary lymphoma of the central nervous system in children with acquired immunodeficiency syndrome. Pediatrics 82:355–363, 1988.
322. Connor E, Boccon-Gibod L, Joshi V, et al: Cutaneous acquired immunodeficiency syndrome–associated Kaposi's sarcoma in pediatric patients. Arch Dermatol 126:791–793, 1990.
323. Serraino D, Franceschi S: Kaposi's sarcoma and non-Hodgkin's lymphomas in children and adolescents with AIDS. AIDS 10:643–647, 1996.
324. Athale UH, Patil PS, Chintu C, Elem B: Influence of HIV epidemic on the incidence of Kaposi's sarcoma in Zambian children. J Acquir Immune Defic Syndr Hum Retrovirol 8:96–100, 1995.
325. Ziegler JL, Katongole-Mbidde E: Kaposi's sarcoma in childhood: An analysis of 100 cases from Uganda and relationship to HIV infection. Int J Cancer 65:200–203, 1996.
326. Mueller BU, Butler KM, Feuerstein IM, et al: Smooth muscle tumors in children with human immunodeficiency virus infection. Pediatrics 90:460–463, 1992.
327. McClain KL, Leach CT, Jenson HB, et al: Association of Epstein-Barr virus with leiomyosarcomas in young people with AIDS. N Engl J Med 332:12–18, 1995.
328. Lee ES, Locker J, Nalesnik M, et al: The association of Epstein-Barr virus with smooth muscle tumors occurring after organ transplantation. N Engl J Med 332:19–25, 1995.
329. Cabanillas F, Armitage J, Pugh WC, et al: Lymphomatoid papulosis: A T-cell dyscrasia with a propensity to transform into malignant lymphoma. Ann Intern Med 122:210–217, 1995.
330. Tirelli U, Vaccher E, Zagonel V, et al: CD30 (Ki-1)–positive anaplastic large-cell lymphomas in 13 patients with and 27 patients without human immunodeficiency virus infection: The first comparative clinicopathological study from a single institution that also includes 80 patients with other human immunodeficiency virus-related systemic lymphomas. J Clin Oncol 13:373–380, 1995.
331. Mishalani SH, Lones MA, Said JW: Multilocular thymic cyst. A novel thymic lesion associated with human immunodeficiency virus infection. Arch Pathol Lab Med 119:467–470, 1995.
332. Kontny HU, Sleasman JW, Kingma DW, et al: Multilocular thymic cysts in children with human immunodeficiency virus infection. Clinical and pathological aspects. J Pediatr (in press).
333. Avila NA, Mueller BU, Carrasquillo J, et al: Multilocular thymic cysts: Imaging features in children with human immunodeficiency virus (HIV) infection. Radiology 201:130–134, 1996.
334. Dudley MN: Clinical pharmacokinetics of nucleoside antiretroviral agents. J Infect Dis 171(Suppl 2):S99–S112, 1995.
335. Balis FM, Pizzo PA, Eddy J, et al: Pharmacokinetics of zidovudine administered intravenously and orally in children with human immunodeficiency virus infection. J Pediatr 114:880–884, 1989.
336. Balis FM, Pizzo PA, Murphy RF, et al: The pharmacokinetics of zidovudine administered by continuous infusion in children. Ann Intern Med 110:279–285, 1989.
337. Lyman WD, Tanaka KE, Kress Y, et al: Zidovudine concentrations in human fetal tissue: Implications for perinatal AIDS. Lancet 335:1280–1281, 1990.
338. Chavanet P, Diquet B, Waldner A: Perinatal pharmacokinetics of zidovudine. N Engl J Med 321:1548–1549, 1989.
339. Connor EM, Mofenson LK: Zidovudine for the reduction of perinatal human immunodeficiency virus transmission: Pediatric AIDS Clinical Trials Group protocol 076—Results and treatment recommendations. Pediatr Infect Dis J 14:536–541, 1995.
340. Watts DH, Brown ZA, Tartaglione T, et al: Pharmacokinetic disposition of zidovudine during pregnancy. J Infect Dis 163:226–232, 1991.
341. Boucher FD, Modlin JF, Weller S, et al: Phase I evaluation of zidovudine administered to infants exposed at birth to the human immunodeficiency virus. J Pediatr 122:137–144, 1993.
342. Balis FM, Poplack DG: Drug development and clinical pharmacology. *In* Pizzo PA, Wilfert CA (eds): Pediatric AIDS. Baltimore, Williams & Wilkins, 1991, pp 457–477.
343. Brouwers P, Moss H, Wolters P, et al: Effect of continuous-infusion zidovudine therapy on neuropsychologic functioning in children with symptomatic human immunodeficiency virus infection. J Pediatr 117:980–985, 1990.
344. Brady MT, McGrath N, Brouwers P, et al: Randomized study of the tolerance and efficacy of high versus low-dose zidovudine in human immunodeficiency virus–infected children with mild to moderate symptoms (AIDS Clinical Trial Group 128). J Infect Dis 173:1097–1106, 1996.
345. Englund JA, Baker CJ, McKinney RE Jr, et al: ACTG 152: A randomized comparative trial of zidovudine (ZDV) vs didanosine (DDI) vs combination ZDV + DDI in symptomatic HIV-infected children. Presented at the Third Conference on Retroviruses and Opportunistic Infections; January 1996; Washington, DC.
346. Balis FM, Pizzo PA, Butler KM, et al: Clinical pharmacology of 2′,3′-dideoxyinosine in human immunodeficiency virus–infected children. J Infect Dis 165:99–104, 1992.
347. Mueller BU, Butler KM, Stocker VL, et al: Clinical and pharmacokinetic evaluation of long-term therapy with didanosine in children with HIV infection. Pediatrics 94:724–731, 1994.
348. Blanche S, Calvez T, Rouzioux C, et al: Randomized study of two doses of didanosine in children infected with human immunodeficiency virus. J Pediatr 122:966–973, 1993.
349. Whitcup SM, Butler KM, Caruso R, et al: Retinal toxicity in human immunodeficiency virus–infected children treated with 2′,3′-dideoxyinosine. Am J Ophthalmol 113:1–7, 1992.
350. van Leeuwen R, Lange JMA, Hussey EK, et al: The safety and pharmacokinetics of a reverse transcriptase inhibitor, 3TC, in patients with HIV infection: A phase I study. AIDS 6:1471–1475, 1992.
351. Pluda JM, Cooley TP, Montaner JSG, et al: A phase I/II study of 2′-deoxy-3′-thiacytidine in patients with advanced human immunodeficiency virus infection. J Infect Dis 171:1438–1447, 1995.
352. Lewis L, Mueller B, Schock R, et al: A phase I/II study to evaluate the safety, toxicity and preliminary efficacy of combination of lamivudine (3TC), zidovudine (AZT) and didanosine (ddI) in children with HIV infection. Presented at the Second National Conference on Human Retroviruses and Related Infections; February 1995; Washington, DC.
353. Eron JJ, Benoit SL, Jemsek J, et al: Treatment with lamivudine, zidovudine, or both in HIV-positive patients with 200 to 500 $CD4^+$ cells per cubic millimeter. N Engl J Med 333:1662–1669, 1995.
354. Ingrand D, Weber J, Boucher CAB, et al: Phase I/II study of 3TC (lamivudine) in HIV-positive, asymptomatic or mild AIDS-related complex patients: Sustained reduction in viral markers. AIDS 9:1323–1329, 1995.
355. Bartlett JA, Benoit SL, Johnson VA, et al: Lamivudine plus zidovudine compared with zalcitabine plus zidovudine in patients with HIV infection. A randomized, double-blind, placebo-controlled trial. Ann Intern Med 125:161–172, 1996.
356. Lewis LL, Venzon D, Church J, et al: Lamivudine in children with human immunodeficiency virus infection: A phase I/II study. J Infect Dis 174:16–25, 1996.
357. Merrill DP, Moonis M, Chou T-C, Hirsch MS: Lamivudine or stavudine in two- and three-drug combinations against human immunodeficiency virus type 1 replication in vitro. J Infect Dis 173:355–364, 1996.
358. Browne MJ, Mayer KH, Chafee SBD, et al: 2′,3′-Didehydro-3′-deoxythymidine (d4T) in patients with AIDS or AIDS-related complex: A phase I trial. J Infect Dis 167:21–29, 1993.
359. Petersen EA, Ramirez-Ronda CH, Hardy WD, et al: Dose-related activity of stavudine in patients infected with human immunodeficiency virus. J Infect Dis 171(Suppl 2):S131–S139, 1995.
360. Kline MW, Dunkle LM, Church JA, et al: A phase I/II evaluation of stavudine (d4T) in children with human immunodeficiency virus infection. Pediatrics 96:247–252, 1995.
361. Kline MW, Fletcher CV, Federici ME, et al: Combination therapy with stavudine and didanosine in children with advanced human immunodeficiency virus infection: Pharmacokinetic properties, safety, and immunologic and virologic effects. Pediatrics 97:886–890, 1996.
362. Cheeseman SH, Hattox SE, McLaughlin MM, et al: Pharmacoki-

netics of nevirapine: Initial single-rising-dose study in humans. Antimicrob Agents Chemother 37:178–182, 1993.
363. Richman DD, Havlir D, Corbeil J, et al: Nevirapine resistance mutations of human immunodeficiency virus type 1 selected during therapy. J Virol 68:1660–1666, 1994.
364. Havlir D, Cheeseman SH, McLaughlin M, et al: High-dose nevirapine: Safety, pharmacokinetics, and antiviral effect in patients with human immunodeficiency virus infection. J Infect Dis 171:537–545, 1995.
365. Johnson VA, Merrill DP, Chou TC, Hirsch MS: Human immunodeficiency virus type 1 (HIV-1) inhibitory interactions between protease inhibitor Ro-31-8959 and zidovudine, 2′,3′-dideoxycytidine, or recombinant interferon-alpha A against zidovudine-sensitive or resistant HIV-1 in vitro. J Infect Dis 166:1143–1146, 1992.
366. Condra JH, Schleif WA, Blahy OM, et al: In vivo emergence of HIV-1 variants resistant to multiple protease inhibitors. Nature 374:569–571, 1995.
367. Stein DS, Fish DG, Bilello JA, et al: A 24-week open-label phase I/II evaluation of the HIV protease inhibitor MK-639 (indinavir). AIDS 10:485–492, 1996.
368. Mueller BU, Smith S, Sleasman J, et al: A phase I/II study of the protease inhibitor indinavir (MK-0639) in children with HIV infection. Presented at the 11th International Conference on AIDS; July 7–12, 1996; Vancouver, British Columbia, Canada.
369. Danner SA, Carr A, Leonard JM, et al: A short-term study of the safety, pharmacokinetics, and efficacy of ritonavir, an inhibitor of HIV-1 protease. N Engl J Med 333:1528–1533, 1995.
370. Markowitz M, Saag M, Powderly WG, et al: A preliminary study of ritonavir, an inhibitor of HIV-1 protease, to treat HIV-1 infection. N Engl J Med 333:1534–1539, 1995.
371. Mueller BU, Zuckerman J, Nelson JRP, et al: A phase I/II study of the protease inhibitor ritonavir (ABT-538) in children with HIV infection. Presented at the 11th International Conference on AIDS; July 7–12, 1996; Vancouver, British Columbia, Canada.
372. Koff WC, Fauci AS: Human trials of AIDS vaccines: Current status and future directions. AIDS 3(Suppl 1):S125–S129, 1989.
373. Letvin NL: Vaccines against human immunodeficiency virus—Progress and prospects. N Engl J Med 329:1400–1405, 1993.
374. Weniger BG: Experience from HIV incidence cohorts in Thailand: Implications for HIV vaccine efficacy trials. AIDS 8:1007–1010, 1994.
375. Graham BS, Wright PF: Candidate AIDS vaccines. N Engl J Med 333:1331–1339, 1995.

130

Human T-Cell Lymphotropic Virus Type I and Neurologic Diseases

Richard T. Johnson

In 1985, human T-cell lymphotropic virus type I (HTLV-I) was associated with a chronic inflammatory myelopathy known in tropical areas as tropical spastic paraparesis (TSP) and in Japan and temperate zones as HTLV-I–associated myelopathy (HAM). A variety of tropical myeloneuropathies have been described in different geographic regions of the world during the past century. Some are peripheral neuropathies associated with ataxia that have nutritional and toxic causes such as those affecting Far East prisoners of war during World War II, those associated with dietary insufficiency of tropical malabsorption, and those that appear during famines when cassava consumption leads to cyanide poisoning. The chronic tropical diseases include outbreaks of lathyrism related to the consumption of peas that contain a neurotoxic amino acid and endemic TSP recognized in the Caribbean, Africa, India, and South America.[1]

In 1985, a French research group on Martinique found that nearly 60% of patients with endemic spastic paraparesis had antibodies to HTLV-I virus, whereas only 4% of the general population had these antibodies.[2] Within months a similar association of seroprevalence of antibody to HTLV-I was shown in patients with TSP in Jamaica and Colombia, and high levels of antibody were also found in cerebrospinal fluid.[3] The following year, patients with HAM were reported from Kyushu, the southern island of Japan, where one of the highest antibody prevalences against HTLV-I was known.[4, 5] Similar patients were found among Caribbean immigrants to England and local populations of Africa, North America, South America, Europe, and the Seychelles.[6] The demonstration of abnormal lobulated lymphocytes in the cerebrospinal fluid, the recovery of virus from cerebrospinal fluid, and the demonstration of HTLV-I sequences in affected spinal cord have provided further evidence for the association of HTLV-I with many cases of chronic spastic paraparesis.[5, 7–9]

Etiology

HTLV-I viruses recovered from patients with spastic paraparesis and proviral DNAs found in peripheral blood and cerebrospinal fluid lymphocytes of these patients appear to be the same as those recovered from acute T-cell leukemia.[10] In HTLV-I–induced neoplasms, however, the integration site in an individual patient is the same in all malignant T cells, indicating a monoclonal origin of the leukemia or lymphoma. The pathogenesis of TSP is obviously different with HTLV-I provirus integrated at random sites[11] (Table 130–1). In Japan some common human leukocyte antigen haplotypes are found in the majority of HAM cases,[12] but other studies have lent little support for the role of host genetic determinants. Nevertheless, the difference in disease expression is assumed to be due to host and environmental factors rather than strain differences of the virus. Factors leading to malignancy or TSP are not exclusive; however, one Caribbean patient and several Japanese patients were described in whom acute T-cell leukemia or lymphoma and chronic spastic paraparesis developed in the same patient.[13]

Epidemiology

The modes of transmission of HTLV-I are (1) from mother to child either across the placenta or from breast milk; (2) sexual transmission, with the higher prevalence of antibody in women indicating greater transmissibility from men to women; and (3) from direct inoculation by transfusions or contaminated needles and syringes.

The distribution of HTLV-I virus is worldwide, although it is more common in the southern islands of Japan, the Caribbean, the Seychelles, the Pacific coast of Colombia, and areas of Africa. It is rare in North America and is exceedingly rare in China and Korea. Specific ethnic groups, such as immigrants from Surinam to Holland, Ethiopian Jews in Israel, and a Jewish population from Marhad, Iran, have higher prevalence rates of antibody. Rates worldwide vary between less than 1% and 15%. The distribution of TSP/HAM reflects the distribution of HTLV-I, although studies of this association in Africa and India are incomplete.

TABLE 130–1 ■ Human T-Cell Lymphotropic Virus Type I–Associated Leukemia or Lymphoma and Myelopathy

OBSERVATION	LEUKEMIA OR LYMPHOMA	MYELOPATHY
Demographic		
Male/female ratio	1.4:1	1:1.4
Mean age at onset (y)	40–45	40–45
Place of birth	Southern Japan Seychelles Caribbean basin Equatorial Africa Southeastern United States	Same
Risk factors		
Risk in seropositive persons	2.5%	0.3%
Blood transfusion of HTLV-I$^+$ blood	No observed effect	Increases risk to 20%
Disease	Aggressive: mean survival 10 mo	Indolent: long life expectancy
Virology		
Viral DNA	CD4$^+$ lymphocytes	CD4$^+$ lymphocytes (? astrocytes)
Integration	At same site in malignant cells of individual (clonal origin)	Random site (polyclonal)
Immune responses	Immunosuppression	Enhanced humoral and some cellular response to HTLV-I

Conversely, among patients with all forms of chronic spastic paraparesis the role of HTLV-I varies with geography. For example, none of 29 Canadian patients with chronic myelopathy had antibodies to HTLV-I,[14] 10 of 37 in France had antibodies,[15] 8 of 15 in Peru had antibodies (Johnson RT, personal observation), and in the areas of high HTLV-I antibody prevalence the rates range from 75% to 90%.

Pathology and Pathogenesis

Because death during the early years of the disease is rare, complete pathologic studies have been limited to persons who have had the disease for long periods. The meninges may be thickened and the cord may show gross atrophy. A mild mononuclear cell inflammatory response is found in the meninges and in perivascular spaces within the spinal cord. Inflammation is more intense in the thoracic than in cervical and lumbar areas. Inflammatory changes are more focal and sparse in the brain. There is secondary degeneration and demyelination of the long tracts, particularly the lateral columns. Hyalinization of blood vessels and perivascular gliosis are found in the cord.[16, 17] In one patient who had a spinal cord biopsy during the first year of symptoms, a more intense inflammatory response was found, including the infiltration of many inflammatory cells into thickened vessel walls. This active vasculitis was associated with severe necrosis of the thoracic spinal cord.[18]

Patients with chronic myelopathy show intrathecal synthesis of antibodies to HTLV-I virus. Compared with HTLV-I–seropositive persons without disease, TSP patients have higher levels of serum antibodies to HTLV-I, ratios of CD4$^+$ to CD8$^+$ cells are elevated, and there are many activated T cells in the peripheral blood and cerebrospinal fluid.[19]

These factors and the therapeutic response to steroids and plasmapheresis suggest immunopathogenic mechanisms. Most studies have indicated that HTLV-I infection in the cord is limited to inflammatory cells, supporting this autoimmune hypothesis[8]; however, a study localizing HTLV-I messenger RNA and using cell type–specific counterstains has shown astrocytic infection, indicating that a cytotoxic mechanism remains possible.[9] Regardless of the mechanism of tissue damage, several enigmatic questions remain: Why is disease, when it occurs, delayed until middle age? Why is pathologic change localized largely to the thoracic spinal cord? Why does disease progress relentlessly and then decelerate without dissemination throughout the neuraxis?

Clinical Manifestations

Onset is usually in the third and fourth decades of life, although it has been described in children as young as 6 years of age. TSP/HAM occurs more frequently in women than in men, consistent with the greater female seroprevalence of HTLV-I antibody. The onset is usually subacute and insidious but occasionally is abrupt. Fever or systemic symptoms are not reported. Initial symptoms are heaviness, stiffness, and weakness in the lower extremities and urgency and frequency of urination. Impotence develops in most men. Dysesthesias may be distressing but are usually limited to the lower part of the trunk and legs; occasionally a bandlike sensation involves thoracic dermatomes, similar to the dysesthesias in acute transverse myelitis.

Physical findings are weakness of the legs with spasticity, hyperreflexia, and extensor plantar responses. Strength in the arms is relatively spared, but deep tendon reflexes tend to be brisk in the upper extremities with a brisk jaw jerk. Despite frequent sensory symptoms, sensory findings are usually minor. Some loss of position and vibratory sense in the lower extremities may be evident, but a profound sensory loss or sensory level is rare. A small number of patients also have loss of the ankle deep tendon reflexes, which suggests peripheral nerve involvement. Cranial nerve function is usually normal but rare patients have been reported with retrobulbar neuritis, nerve deafness, seizures, or cerebellar ataxia. The disease may be asymmetric at onset, with one leg more affected than the other. Progression after a few years tends to stabilize, and most patients have functional use of spastic arms and normal cognition after many years.

Peripheral blood studies are normal except for the presence of lobulated nuclei that may be found in some lymphocytes. Early in disease, cerebrospinal fluid may show a pleocytosis and may contain abnormal cells. The cerebrospinal fluid protein level is usually moderately elevated; immunoglobulin G is increased, and oligoclonal bands are present. Levels of antibody to HTLV-I virus in the cerebrospinal fluid are higher than can be accounted for by increased permeability of the blood-brain barrier. Oligoclonal bands of immunoglobulin G have been shown to be directed against polypeptides of HTLV-I.[20]

In the majority of patients, results of magnetic resonance imaging of the brain are normal, but some patients have subcortical bright foci on T2-weighted images. Foci are only rarely in a periventricular distribution typical of multiple sclerosis. The cerebral lesions are more frequent in long-standing disease,[21] which correlates with increasing age, when bright white matter lesions become frequent in the general population. Magnetic resonance imaging of the spinal cord usually fails to show discrete lesions, presumably because of the diffuse nature of inflammation and scarring.

Diagnosis

Diagnosis of HAM depends on the typical clinical findings and the demonstration of antibody to HTLV-I in serum and excessive levels of antibody in cerebrospinal fluid. The demonstration of abnormal lobulated nuclei and lymphocytes in blood and cerebrospinal fluid may assist in this diagnosis, and virus may be cultured from the cerebrospinal fluid or detected by polymerase chain reaction.[22]

Differential diagnosis includes nutritional and toxic myelopathies as well as meningovascular syphilis, which was for many years thought to be a major cause of TSP. In more temperate zones, the major differential diagnosis is multiple sclerosis, and the chronic spinal forms of that disease may be quite similar to TSP/HAM. TSP/HAM associated with retrobulbar neuritis or cerebral lesions at magnetic resonance imaging may mimic progressive multiple sclerosis. The vacuolar myelopathy of human immunodeficiency virus infections produces similar clinical findings, and dual infections are well known. Other infections including spinal cysticercosis, tuberculosis, *Brucella melitensis* infections, and *Borrelia* infections; vascular disease including anterior spinal artery occlusions and arterial venous malformations; and spinocerebellar degenerations and neoplasms may enter in the differential diagnosis.

Treatment

The value of zidovudine in the treatment of TSP/HAM is uncertain.[23] A marked improvement has been documented in some patients with corticosteroids, but this treatment appears effective only in patients who are in the early stages of disease, in which there is rapid progression and the presence of a pleocytosis.[5] Transient improvement has also been shown with plasmapheresis.[24]

Other Neurologic Diseases

Polymyositis. In a serologic survey of other neurologic diseases in Jamaica, 7% to 18% of persons showed antibody to HTLV-I, which is the expected frequency for that geographic area, but seven of seven patients with polymyositis were found to have antibodies.[25] Subsequent Japanese studies have shown a less convincing correlation. In one report, a young man in the United States who had received multiple blood transfusions for trauma 4 years previously developed proximal muscle weakness, muscle tenderness, and elevated creatine kinase levels. He was seropositive for both human immunodeficiency virus and HTLV-I. Muscle biopsies showed an inflammatory myopathy with fiber atrophy and necrosis. Immunocytochemical staining showed antigen of HTLV-I, but not human immunodeficiency virus, in fibers with fiber atrophy and in the areas of inflammation. In situ hybridization confirmed this localization.[26]

Multiple Sclerosis. Antibody to p24 protein of HTLV-I and detection of sequences of HTLV-I by polymerase chain reaction in blood cells have been reported in patients with multiple sclerosis.[27, 28] Most subsequent studies have failed to confirm these findings.[29] In general, these studies do not suggest a role for HTLV-I in multiple sclerosis but do raise the intriguing question of the presence of a related but distinct retrovirus.

References

1. Roman GC, Spencer PS, Schoenberg BS: Tropical myeloneuropathies: The hidden endemias. Neurology 35:1158–1170, 1985.
2. Gessain A, Barin F, Vernant JC, et al: Antibodies to human T-lymphotropic virus type I in patients with tropical spastic paraparesis. Lancet 2:407–409, 1985.
3. Rodgers-Johnson P, Gajdusek DC, Morgan OS, et al: HTLV-I and HTLV-III antibodies and tropical spastic paraparesis (Letter). Lancet 2:1247–1248, 1985.
4. Osame M, Usuku K, Izumo S, et al: HTLV-I–associated myelopathy, a new clinical entity. Lancet 1:1031–1032, 1986.
5. Osame M, Matsumoto M, Usuku K, et al: Chronic progressive myelopathy associated with elevated antibodies to human T-lymphotropic virus type I and adult T-cell leukemialike cells. Ann Neurol 21:117–122, 1987.
6. Montgomery RD: The epidemiology of myelopathy associated with human T-lymphotropic virus 1. Trans R Soc Trop Med Hyg 87:154–159, 1993.
7. Hirose S, Uemura Y, Fujishita M, et al: Isolation of HTLV-I from cerebrospinal fluid of a patient with myelopathy. Lancet 2:397–398, 1986.
8. Hara H, Morita M, Iwaki T, et al: Detection of human T lymphotrophic virus type I (HTLV-I) proviral DNA and analysis of T cell receptor Vβ CDR3 sequences in spinal cord lesions of HTLV-I–associated myelopathy/tropical spastic paraparesis. J Exp Med 180:831–839, 1994.
9. Lehky TJ, Fox CH, Koenig S, et al: Detection of human T-lymphotropic virus type I (HTLV-I) tax RNA in the central nervous system of HTLV-I–associated myelopathy/tropical spastic paraparesis patients by in situ hybridization. Ann Neurol 37:167–175, 1995.
10. Nishimura M, McFarlin DE, Jacobson S: Sequence comparisons of HTLV-I from HAM/TSP patients and their asymptomatic spouses. Neurology 43:2621–2624, 1993.
11. Greenberg SJ, Jacobson S, Waldmann TA, McFarlin DE: Molecular analysis of HTLV-I proviral integration and T cell receptor arrangement indicates that T cells in tropical spastic paraparesis are polyclonal. J Infect Dis 159:741–744, 1989.
12. Usuku K, Sonoda S, Osame M, et al: HLA haplotype–linked high immune responsiveness against HTLV-I in HTLV-I–associated myelopathy: Comparison with adult T-cell leukemia/lymphoma. Ann Neurol 23(Suppl):S143–S150, 1988.
13. Bartholomew C, Cleghorn F, Charles W, et al: HTLV-I and tropical spastic paraparesis. Lancet 1:99–100, 1986.
14. Rice GPA, Armstrong HA, Bulman DE, et al: Absence of antibody to HTLV-I and III in sera of Canadian patients with multiple sclerosis and chronic myelopathy. Ann Neurol 20:533–534, 1986.
15. Gout O, Gessain A, Bolgert F, et al: Chronic myelopathies associated with human T-lymphotropic virus type I. A clinical, serologic, and immunovirologic study of ten patients in France. Ann Neurol 46:255–260, 1989.
16. Akizuki S, Setoguchi M, Nakazato O, et al: An autopsy case of human T-lymphotropic virus type I–associated myelopathy. Hum Pathol 19:988–990, 1988.
17. Rosenblum MK, Brew BJ, Hahn B, et al: Human T-lymphotropic virus type I–associated myelopathy in patients with the acquired immunodeficiency syndrome. Hum Pathol 23:513–519, 1992.
18. Johnson RT, Griffin DE, Arregui A, et al: Spastic paraparesis and HTLV-I in Peru. Ann Neurol 23:S151–S155, 1988.
19. Itoyama Y, Minato S, Kira J, et al: Altered subsets of peripheral blood lymphocytes in patients with HTLV-I associated myelopathy (HAM). Neurology 38:816–818, 1988.
20. Grimaldi LME, Roos RP, Devare SG, et al: HTLV-I–associated myelopathy: Oligoclonal immunoglobulin G bands contain anti–HTLV-I p24 antibody. Ann Neurol 24:727–731, 1988.

21. Kira J, Minato S, Itoyama Y, et al: Leukoencephalopathy in HTLV-I–associated myelopathy: MRI and EEG data. J Neurol Sci 87:221–232, 1988.
22. Bhagavati S, Ehrlich G, Kula RW, et al: Detection of human T-cell lymphoma/leukemia virus type I DNA and antigen in spinal fluid and blood of patients with chronic progressive myelopathy. N Engl J Med 318:1141–1147, 1988.
23. Gout O, Gessain A, Iba-Zizen M, et al: The effect of zidovudine on chronic myelopathy associated with HTLV-I. J Neurol 238:108–109, 1991.
24. Matsuo H, Nakamura T, Tsujihata M, et al: Plasmapheresis in treatment of human T-lymphotropic virus type I associated myelopathy. Lancet 2:1109–1113, 1988.
25. Mora CA, Garruto RM, Brown P: Seroprevalance of antibodies to HTLV-I in patients with chronic neurological disorders other than tropical spastic paraparesis. Ann Neurol 23:S192–S195, 1988.
26. Wiley CA, Nerenberg M, Cros D, Soto-Aguilar MC: HTLV-I polymyositis in a patient also infected with the human immunodeficiency virus. N Engl J Med 320:992–995, 1989.
27. Koprowski H, DeFreitas EC, Harper ME, et al: Multiple sclerosis and human T-lymphotropic retroviruses. Nature 318: 154–160, 1985.
28. Reddy EP, Sandberg-Wollheim M, Mettus RV, et al: Amplification and molecular cloning of HTLV-I sequences from DNA of multiple sclerosis patients. Science 243:529–533, 1989.
29. Ehrlich GD, Glaser JB, Vryz-Gronia B, et al: Multiple sclerosis, retroviruses, and PCR. Neurology 41:335–343, 1991.

131

Women with Acquired Immunodeficiency Syndrome

Deborah Cotton

Acquired immunodeficiency syndrome (AIDS) is now one of the five leading causes of death in U.S. women of childbearing age. In 1994, 18% of all reported AIDS cases in the United States were in women,[1] and this percentage is likely to continue to increase in coming years. Worldwide, the number of women infected with the human immunodeficiency virus (HIV) is roughly equal to that of men. Although questions have been raised about how HIV infection is manifested in women compared with men, data on HIV infection in women have been too limited in the past to permit such analysis.

Women with AIDS are largely young, poor, and living in communities beset by a variety of public health problems, including substance abuse and domestic violence. These conditions have led to major barriers in their access to early diagnosis and treatment and has made prevention efforts difficult. Because HIV infection is vertically transmitted, the epidemic in women has led to a corresponding pediatric epidemic. Reflecting increased interest in these issues, several books on the subject of AIDS in women have now been published.[2–4]

Epidemiology and Transmission

Worldwide, HIV infection is a heterosexually transmitted disease. Whereas illicit drug use has accounted for about half of the cumulative cases of AIDS in women in the United States to date, the proportion of AIDS cases in women due to heterosexual transmission reached 38% in 1994, and heterosexual transmission has surpassed drug use as the most common means of acquisition of HIV infection in women in some areas of the country.[5] In addition, drug-using women often have intercourse with HIV-infected male drug users; thus, cases in women ascribed to drug use may in fact have been sexually acquired. Alcohol consumption and the use of inhaled crack are also significant risk factors for infection because of their disinhibiting effects and the fact that women may exchange sex for drugs and alcohol.[6]

Women are at greater risk for acquiring HIV during vaginal intercourse than are men.[7] HIV infection requires rapid entry of the virus into the blood stream, and the friction of intercourse may produce abrasions in the vagina, thus facilitating such entry through infected semen. Women who are the passive partners in anal intercourse are at greatest risk for acquiring HIV infection because of the fragility of the anal mucosa.[8–10] The role of menstruation in HIV transmission is only partially understood.[11] It appears to increase risk for transmission to men, but it is uncertain whether it increases transmission to women. Genital ulcerations increase risk for infection during vaginal intercourse for both men and women. Rates of woman-to-woman sexual transmission appear low.[12]

HIV infection occurs predominantly in women of childbearing age, as is typical of a sexually transmitted disease.[1] Women of color are at far greater risk for HIV infection than are white women; African-American and Latina women account for nearly three quarters of cases. Thus far, women with AIDS reside predominantly in U.S. cities of the eastern seaboard, where the prevalence of illicit drug use is high. However, there is a growing epidemic among women in the rural southeastern United States due to heterosexual transmission, and every state has reported female cases of the disease.[13]

Natural History

Whereas small early reports concluded that women had shorter survival than did men with AIDS, better designed studies suggest that poorer access to primary care and therapy accounts for this discrepancy, rather than true biologic differences.[14–16] Data compiled to date suggest that women have a pattern of presenting opportunistic infection similar to that of men. However, some manifestations including esophageal candidiasis, wasting syndrome, and recurrent herpes simplex virus infection may be more common among women.[17] Kaposi's sarcoma is distinctly unusual in women.

Proposed gynecologic manifestations of HIV infection in women have included vaginal candidiasis, cervical dysplasia and neoplasia, pelvic inflammatory disease, and menstrual abnormalities. Although vaginal candidiasis may be the first clinical manifestation of HIV infection in women, appearing before oral candidiasis,[18] studies suggest that the risk for vaginal candidiasis increases above that of the general population only when the $CD4^+$ cell count falls below 200/mm^3.[19] Cervical dysplasia and neoplasia, which have been etiologically linked to human papillomavirus, appear more common in HIV-infected women than in women matched for other known risk factors for these conditions.[20, 21] A direct causal role for HIV in producing cervical dysplasia and neoplasia is less certain. However, it is generally believed that the immunosuppression caused by HIV facilitates the expression and progression of cervical dysplasia as has been seen in women who have received transplants accompanied by immunosuppressive drugs or intensive chemotherapy. The majority of experts in the United States believe that Papanicolaou smear screening is sufficiently sensitive to detect cervical intraepithelial neoplasia in women with HIV infection.[22, 23] A minority favor periodic colposcopy.[24] Although most centers caring for women do not report an unexpected prevalence of overt cervical cancer, as women with HIV infection live longer, this may become a more frequently seen manifestation of the disease, especially among women with poor access to preventive services including Papanicolaou smear screening.

At this writing, it is unclear whether pelvic inflammatory disease is more common among HIV-infected women than among demographically matched HIV-negative women, although it is probably more severe in the presence of HIV infection, especially among women with low CD4$^+$ cell counts. Studies support the use of the same criteria for hospitalization, surgery, and duration of antibiotic therapy in pelvic inflammatory disease in HIV-positive women as in HIV-negative women.[25]

A wide array of menstrual abnormalities are reported by women with HIV infection, including amenorrhea, hypermenorrhea, and painful menstrual cramps. More data are needed to ascertain the true prevalence of these conditions in HIV-infected women and to determine if this differs from rates seen among matched HIV-negative women. The Centers for Disease Control and Prevention now includes gynecologic conditions in its revised classification system for HIV infection, although only invasive cervical cancer is considered to be an AIDS-defining condition.[26]

Diagnosis of Human Immunodeficiency Virus Infection in Women

The two major impediments to care for HIV-infected women are failure to suspect the diagnosis and poor access to early intervention. Older women are the most likely to be misdiagnosed.[27] Women who present with a history of sexually transmitted disease, a large number of sexual partners, or illicit drug use should be considered at high risk, even if these risks were in the distant past. In my opinion, women who do not have these risks but who live in communities where HIV infection is prevalent should also be offered testing regardless of known personal risk factors.

In addition, any woman who presents with cervical dysplasia, recurrent pneumonia, tuberculosis, recurrent vaginal candidiasis without known predisposing cause, severe genital herpes, shingles, diffuse adenopathy, or unexplained weight loss should also be considered possibly HIV infected. HIV infection should also be included in the differential diagnosis of fever of unknown origin, interstitial pulmonary infiltrates, and non-Hodgkin's lymphoma. The possibility of acute HIV seroconversion should be considered in work-up of all women presenting with mononucleosis-like illnesses or viral meningitis.

Finally, because zidovudine has been shown to dramatically lessen the risk for perinatal transmission of HIV, the Centers for Disease Control and Prevention now recommends that all pregnant women in the United States be offered HIV antibody testing, the first low-prevalence population to be recommended for mass screening.[28] However, it is imperative that pregnant women with unexpected positive or indeterminate results on HIV antibody tests have further testing performed, especially because multiparous women may have antibodies to human leukocyte antigens that cross-react in some enzyme-linked immunosorbent assays and all Western blot kits.[29]

At present, women who are found to be HIV infected should be managed in a nearly identical fashion to men. A detailed baseline history and physical examination including pelvic examination should be performed, routine immunizations given as appropriate, and tuberculin skin test performed. A baseline CD4$^+$ cell count should be obtained and prophylaxis against opportunistic infections recommended as indicated by results. HIV-infected women are not universally positive for cytomegalovirus (CMV) antibody, as has been reported for gay men; ascertaining CMV serostatus is therefore useful in the event that transfusion is needed, in which case CMV-negative or leukocyte-filtered blood should be given, or for future reference should the patient become pregnant. CMV-negative women with young children or who work in daycare or health care settings should have good hand-washing practices reinforced. *Toxoplasma* serostatus should also be ascertained, and prevention of acquisition of toxoplasmosis stressed in seronegative women, who are usually the family members responsible for preparation of meals and care of pets. Similarly, women need to be counseled about the risks for infection from other sources of food and water, both for themselves and for other HIV-positive family members for whom they are responsible.

Antiretroviral Therapy in Nonpregnant Women

In general, antiretroviral therapy in the woman who is not pregnant and is not contemplating a future pregnancy should be identical to that in men. Currently licensed antivirals appear to be well tolerated in women, although one study has suggested that women may experience more side effects leading to discontinuation of therapy with didanosine.[30] However, a rare complication of zidovudine, hepatic steatosis, may be more frequent in women, especially obese women, and more frequent monitoring of liver function may be indicated in this setting.[31] Few clinical trials of these agents included many women.[32]

Management of Pregnancy in Human Immunodeficiency Virus–Infected Women

Natural History

Women now often learn that they are HIV infected when they are screened during pregnancy, and this "dual diagnosis" poses significant challenges to the practitioner. Women in this circumstance need to be rapidly educated about HIV infection so that they can make informed decisions regarding both the pregnancy itself and their own medical care needs. For women with more than 200 CD4$^+$ cells per mm^3, pregnancy does not appear to increase maternal morbidity or mortality during the pregnancy or after.[33, 34] However, there are anecdotal reports of women with more advanced HIV disease having increased morbidity and mortality when they are pregnant.[35] In addition, adequate nutrition for both mother and fetus may be compromised when pregnancy occurs in the woman with advanced disease; because maternal survival is likely to be short, important issues are raised about who will care for the child.

The best current evidence supports an overall vertical transmission rate of HIV infection between 15% and 30% in the absence of treatment. A more advanced stage of disease in the mother as evidenced by low CD4$^+$ cell numbers may increase the risk for vertical transmission, as may high viral burden in the mother.[36, 37] However, there does not appear to be a "threshold" viral load below which transmission does not occur. Whereas the precise time of transmission is not known, there is increasing evidence that viral transmission often occurs in the peripartum period.[38, 39] One study found that among women with advanced disease, prolonged rupture of membranes and hard drug use were also associated with increased vertical transmission.[40]

Breast-feeding is also a significant means of infection of the infant, and in developed countries where formula can be safely stored and prepared, breast-feeding should be strongly discouraged.[41] However, the situation and thus decision-making are far more complex in areas of the world where there is inadequate access to properly prepared infant feeding alternatives and where breast-feeding many also have the desired effect of reducing fertility.[42]

Antiviral Therapy During Pregnancy

A large well-designed and well-conducted clinical trial has demonstrated that administration of zidovudine to the mother during pregnancy and labor followed by treatment of the infant for 6 weeks after birth resulted in an 8% rate of HIV transmission to infants compared with a rate of 24% among infants in the placebo arm.[43] Of note, the effect of zidovudine was only partially explained by a reduction in maternal viral load.[44] No maternal side effects were noted, and only mild, reversible anemia occurred in the neonates. At 2 years, both infected and uninfected children who received zidovudine did not appear to have had any long-term adverse outcomes related to zidovudine use. Although the clinical trial establishing the benefit of zidovudine during pregnancy enrolled only women with more than 200 CD4$^+$ cells per mm^3, an analysis concluded that this benefit extends to women with CD4$^+$ cell levels of 200/mm^3 or lower. Thus, all pregnant women should be offered zidovudine in this setting, with use of the regimen that was employed in the clinical trial (Table 131–1). To improve compliance, some experts use a dosing schedule of 200 mg orally three times daily rather than the dose of 100 mg five times per day used in the trial. Treatment is generally instituted after the 14th week of gestation or at any time after that when the patient presents for care. Therapy is given intravenously during labor and delivery and continued in the infant for 6 weeks after birth. However, many experts argue that nucleoside analogs should not be used as monotherapy because of development of drug resistance and favor combination therapy during pregnancy.

TABLE 131–1 ■ Use of Zidovudine in Pregnancy: Results of AIDS Clinical Trials Group Protocol 076

STUDY POPULATION

Pregnant women at 14–34 wk of gestation with CD4$^+$ T cell count at study entry of 200/mm^3 or more

STUDY REGIMEN

During Pregnancy

100 mg of zidovudine orally five times daily

During Labor

Loading dose of zidovudine of 2 mg/kg intravenously, followed by continuous intravenous infusion of 1 mg/kg/h until the cord is clamped

For Newborns

Zidovudine oral syrup at 2 mg/kg every 6 h starting 8–12 h after birth and continuing until the infant is 6 wk old

STUDY RESULTS

Placebo Group

Estimated transmission rate: 25.5% (confidence interval, 18.4%–32.5%)

Zidovudine-Treated Group

Estimated transmission rate: 8.3% (confidence interval, 3.9%–12.8%)

Zidovudine Side Effects

No significant difference between treated and untreated mothers
Mild, transient anemia greater in treated infants
No other differences

Data from Connor E, Sperling R, Gelber R, et al: Reduction of maternal-infant transmission of human immunodeficiency virus type 1 with zidovudine treatment. Pediatric AIDS Clinical Trials Group Protocol 076 Study Group. N Engl J Med 331:1173–1180, 1994.

Pregnant women who have had prolonged treatment with zidovudine or were infected by a partner who has been receiving prolonged treatment with zidovudine may harbor a zidovudine-resistant strain. Experts are divided as to the best means of preventing perinatal transmission in this setting, but many favor switching to two nucleoside analogs to which the patient has not yet been exposed. Early studies suggest that the nonnucleoside reverse transcriptase inhibitor nevirapine in combination with nucleoside reverse transcriptase inhibitors is well tolerated in late pregnancy and can result in dramatic decreases in maternal HIV viral load.[45] To date, there are reports of only a few women being treated with protease inhibitors during pregnancy. Saquinavir has poor oral bioavailability in its present formulation, and its use may therefore be limited in this setting. On the other hand, ritonavir is associated with significant gastrointestinal intolerance even in nonpregnant subjects, and indinavir routinely results in hyperbilirubinemia that could have deleterious effects in the perinatal period. It is likely that antiviral therapy for pregnant women will evolve rapidly during the next several years, and thus it is important that clinicians caring for pregnant women with HIV infection continue to stay up-to-date with new studies in this fast-changing area.

CD4$^+$ Cell Counts and Prophylaxis of Opportunistic Infection

Normal pregnancy is accompanied by mild immunosuppression, and a significant decline in CD4$^+$ cell number may occur in the third trimester in HIV-infected women.[46–48] A CD4$^+$ cell count should be obtained during the first trimester or at the first pregnancy visit and repeated during the third trimester. At present, the same CD4$^+$ cell count thresholds as in the nonpregnant state should be used to determine appropriate opportunistic infection prophylaxis. For almost all drugs used for prophylaxis, there are only few data on use in pregnancy, including information on teratogenicity.[49] Because the blood plasma volume is increased in pregnancy, drug concentrations tend to be lower than in the nonpregnant state, and doses of drugs at the high end of recommended ranges should generally be used in prophylactic regimens.

Prophylaxis for *Pneumocystis carinii* pneumonia should be started when the CD4$^+$ cell count is less than 200/mm^3 in an asymptomatic pregnant woman or less than 250/mm^3 in women who have had recurrent oral or vaginal candidiasis, shingles, or other clinical manifestations of HIV infection. Trimethoprim-sulfamethoxazole is preferred throughout pregnancy, even at term, despite theoretical concerns regarding neonatal kernicterus.[50] It has efficacy superior to other agents in preventing *P. carinii* pneumonia and has the added advantage of providing prophylaxis against toxoplasmosis. The higher maintenance dose of one double-strength tablet daily should be used during pregnancy. In pregnant women who are allergic to trimethoprim-sulfamethoxazole or cannot tolerate it, dapsone is thought to be both effective and safe, although data are limited. There are as yet no controlled data on the use of atovaquone in pregnancy. Aerosolized pentamidine is clearly inferior to systemic regimens for prophylaxis of *P. carinii* pneumonia and should be avoided except for patients who cannot tolerate systemic regimens. When used, it does have the advantage of low teratogenic potential because there is no systemic absorption.

The guidelines of the U.S. Public Health Service/Infectious Diseases Society of America suggest that pyrimethamine-containing compounds be avoided for primary toxoplasmosis prophylaxis during pregnancy.[52] No recommendations were made by this group for prophylaxis against *Mycobacterium avium* complex infection in pregnancy. However, in my opinion, in asymptomatic women with less than 50 $CD4^+$ cells per mm^3 or in those women with less than 100 $CD4^+$ cells per mm^3 who have had an AIDS-defining opportunistic infection, the risk for development of *M. avium* complex infection during the subsequent year and the devastating consequences of such an infection for both mother and fetus warrant the use of prophylactic therapy. Clarithromycin and azithromycin are closely related to erythromycin, which is thought to be safe in pregnancy. Rifabutin is similar to rifampin, which has also been used without apparent toxic effects during pregnancy. If it is feasible, initiation of prophylaxis should be delayed until after the first trimester. For pregnant women with a positive tuberculin skin test reaction or at high risk for having acquired tuberculosis, isoniazid should be employed after the first trimester.

Listeriosis may pose a special threat to women who are both pregnant and HIV infected, and women should be specifically educated about how to avoid this infection. For recurrent oral or vaginal candidiasis requiring systemic therapy, the lowest dose and frequency of fluconazole to control disease should be used; for many women, 100 mg/wk orally of fluconazole prevents recurrent vaginal candidiasis. Oral ganciclovir is not currently recommended during pregnancy for prevention of CMV retinitis or other CMV disease because of its bone marrow suppressive effect. Instead, women with advanced HIV infection should have a dilated ophthalmologic examination at least every 3 months during pregnancy.

Treatment of Opportunistic Infection During Pregnancy

For women who develop opportunistic infections during pregnancy, the risk from the infection itself, which is almost always life threatening, usually far outweighs any real or theoretical adverse drug effects for the mother or fetus. The same philosophy holds for most instances in which maintenance therapy is needed to prevent a recurrence of opportunistic infections. The least teratogenic drugs should be chosen of those that are effective.

A special issue is raised by primary or recurrent toxoplasmosis during pregnancy. Pyrimethamine is teratogenic and should not be used during the first trimester. For therapy of primary toxoplasmosis, spiramycin in combination with sulfadiazine has been shown to be efficacious in non–HIV-infected pregnant women and can be obtained from the U.S. Food and Drug Administration or from outside the United States. The management of the more common situation in HIV infection of reactivation of toxoplasmosis (usually manifested as encephalitis) is more difficult.[52] Therapy could be started with spiramycin in the first trimester and then switched, after 12 weeks of gestation, to pyrimethamine-sulfadiazine. However, spiramycin may not effectively treat maternal toxoplasmosis encephalitis.

In the acute management of and maintenance therapy for systemic mycoses, many favor avoiding fluconazole at least during the first trimester because it has been reported to cause fetal osseous abnormalities and loss in rats attributed to inhibition of estrogen synthesis. These effects have not been seen in women treated with fluconazole. In my opinion, after the first trimester, fluconazole (or itraconazole in maintenance therapy for histoplasmosis) should be used because it is less likely than amphotericin B to cause maternal anemia or renal toxic effects, does not require permanent venous access, and has been shown to be superior to amphotericin B in maintenance therapy for cryptococcal meningitis.

Management of Labor and Delivery

Labor and delivery should be managed for the most part without regard to HIV status. However, if possible, fetal scalp electrodes should be avoided. The role of cesarean section is controversial. Two metaanalyses demonstrated a statistically significant benefit compared with vaginal delivery.[53, 54] In women receiving zidovudine in whom the risk for transmission is already low, any additional advantage of cesarean section may be small, and the procedure has obvious maternal morbidity. However, in women who have not received antiviral therapy or who are otherwise at greater risk for transmission because of high maternal viral load or low $CD4^+$ cell count, and in whom rupture of membranes for 4 hours or more is anticipated, cesarean section should be considered. Otherwise, cesarean section should be performed for the usual indications, regardless of HIV status. Breast-feeding should be strongly discouraged among HIV-infected women giving birth in developed countries where there is ready access to safely prepared formula because breast-feeding is a relatively efficient means of HIV transmission.

Prevention of Human Immunodeficiency Virus Infection in Women

Behavioral intervention must at present be the mainstay of prevention of HIV infection for women.[55] However, a reality that must be dealt with is that women often do not determine how or when they have sex. In addition, many women who are HIV infected are in situations in which the risk for domestic violence is high, and demands for safe sex can precipitate such violence.[56] Condoms are highly effective in preventing transmission through vaginal intercourse; however, many women are unable to get their male partners to use them. Because a relatively high percentage of heterosexual couples practice anal sex, the risky nature of this behavior should be emphasized with patients, who should also be cautioned that condoms are more likely to break during anal intercourse. Controversy persists as to whether nonoxynol 9, the most commonly used spermicide in condoms, as well as contraceptive creams, jellies, and foams (which can kill HIV-1 in vitro) may paradoxically increase the risk for transmission of HIV in vivo because of vaginal irritation and inflammation[57]; thus, they should always be used in conjunction with a condom. The female condom, a sheath attached at one end to a diaphragm-like device with a lip at the other end that covers the perineum, is now approved for sale in the United States.[58] However, the efficacy of this device for either interruption of HIV transmission or pregnancy prevention has not been demonstrated, and discontinuation rates may be high. Condoms or dental dams should be used for oral-genital or oral-anal contact.

Conclusion

More attention to the unique needs of women in preventing acquisition of HIV infection, the continued conduct of large natural history studies of women with HIV infection, and the development of systems of care that can ensure the early and appropriate treatment of women with HIV infection including pregnant women could lead to a sharp reduction in the death rates of both women and children caused by AIDS.

References

1. Wortley PM, Chu SY, Berkelman RC: The epidemiology of HIV/AIDS in women and the impact of the expanded 1993 CDC surveillance definition of AIDS. *In* Cotton D, Watts DH (eds): The Medical Management of AIDS in Women. New York, Wiley-Liss, 1997, pp 3–14.
2. Johnson MA, Johnstone FD (eds): HIV Infection in Women. Edinburgh, Churchill Livingstone, 1993.
3. Minkoff H, DeHovitz J, Duerr A: HIV Infection in Women. New York, Raven Press, 1994.
4. Cotton D, Watts DH (eds): The Medical Management of AIDS in Women. New York, Wiley-Liss, 1997.
5. Centers for Disease Control and Prevention: Update: Acquired immune deficiency sydrome. MMWR Morbid Mortal Wkly Rep 42:547–557, 1993.
6. Minkoff HL, McCalla S, Delke I, et al: The relationship of cocaine use to syphilis and human immunodeficiency virus infections among inner city parturient women. Am J Obstet Gynecol 163:521–526, 1990.
7. European Study Group on Heterosexual Transmission of HIV: Comparison of female-to-male and male-to-female transmission of HIV in 563 stable couples. BMJ 304:809–813, 1992.
8. Bolling DR: Prevalence, goals and complications of heterosexual anal intercourse in a gynecologic population. Adv Contracept 6:41–45, 1977.
9. Bolling DR, Voeller B: AIDS and heterosexual anal intercourse (Letter). JAMA 258:474, 1987.
10. Padian N: Heterosexual transmission: Infectivity and risks. *In* Alexander NJ, Gabelnick HL, Spieler JM (eds): Heterosexual Transmission of AIDS. New York, Wiley-Liss, 1990, pp 25–34.
11. Stratton P, Alexander NJ: Heterosexual transmission of HIV infection. *In* Cotton D, Watts DH (eds): The Medical Management of AIDS in Women. New York, Wiley-Liss, 1997, pp 15–43.
12. Chu SY, Hammett TA, Buehler JW: Update: Epidemiology of reported cases of AIDS in women who report sex only with other women, United States, 1980–1991 (Letter). AIDS 6:518–519, 1992.
13. Ellerbrock TV, Lieg S, Harrington PE, et al: Heterosexually transmitted human immunodeficiency virus infection among pregnant women in a rural Florida community. N Engl J Med 327:1704–1709, 1992.
14. Friedland GH, Saltzman B, Vileno J, et al: Survival differences in patients with AIDS. J Acquir Immune Defic Syndr 4:144–153, 1991.
15. Chaisson RE, Keruly JC, Moore RD: Race, sex, drug use, and progresssion of human immunodeficiency virus disease. N Engl J Med 333:751–756, 1995.
16. Rothenberg R, Woelfel M, Stoneburner R, et al: Survival with the acquired immunodeficiency syndrome. N Engl J Med 317:1297–1302, 1987.
17. Fleming PL, Ciesielski CA, Byers RH, et al: Gender differences in reported AIDS-indicative diagnoses. J Infect Dis 168:61–67, 1993.
18. Imam N, Carpenter CC, Mayer KH, et al: Hierarchical patterns of mucosal *Candida* infections in HIV-seropositive women. Am J Med 89:142–146, 1990.
19. Clark RA, Brandon W, Dumestre J, Pindara C: Clinical manifestations of infection with the human immunodeficiency virus in women in Louisiana. Clin Infect Dis 17:173–177, 1993.
20. Safrin S, Dattel BJ, Hauer L, Sweet RL: High frequency of latent and clinical human papillomavirus cervical infections in immunocompromised human immunodeficiency virus–infected women. Obstet Gynecol 79:321–327, 1992.
21. Vermund SH, Kelley KF, Klein RS, et al: High risk of human papillomavirus infection and cervical squamous intraepithelial lesions among women with symptomatic human immunodeficiency virus infection. Am J Obstet Gynecol 165:392–400, 1991.
22. Wright TC Jr, Ellerbrock TV, Chaisson MA, et al: Cervical intraepithelial neoplasia in women infected with human immunodeficiency virus: Prevalence, risk factors, and validity of Papanicolaou smears. New York Cervical Disease Study. Obstet Gynecol 84:591–597, 1994.
23. Korn A, Autry M, De Remer P: Sensitivity of the Papanicolaou smear in human immunodeficiency virus–infected women. Obstet Gynecol 83:401–404, 1994.
24. Maiman M, Tarricone N, Vieira J, et al: Colposcopic evaluation of human immunodeficiency virus–seropositive women. Obstet Gynecol 78:84–88, 1991.
25. Celum C: Diagnosis and treatment of STDs in HIV-infected women. *In* Cotton D, Watts DH (eds): The Medical Management of AIDS in Women. New York, Wiley-Liss, 1997, pp 235–251.
26. Centers for Disease Control and Prevention: 1993 revised classification system for HIV infection and expanded surveillance case definition for AIDS among adolescents and adults. MMWR Morbid Mortal Wkly Rep 41(RR-17):1–19, 1992.
27. Schoenbaum EE, Webber MP: The underrecognition of HIV infection in women in an inner-city emergency room. Am J Public Health 83:363–368, 1990.
28. U.S. Public Health Service recommendations for human immunodeficiency virus counseling and voluntary testing for pregnant women. MMWR Morbid Mortal Wkly Rep 44:1–15, 1995.
29. Pins MR, Teruya J, Stowell C: Human immunodeficiency virus testing and case detection: Pragmatic and technical issues. *In* Cotton D, Watts DH (eds): The Medical Management of AIDS in Women. New York, Wiley-Liss, 1997, pp 163–175.
30. Currier JS, Spino CS, Grimes J, Cotton D: Gender differences in toxicity rates and CD4 responses to nucleoside analogue therapy in ACTG 175 (Abstr 290). Presented at the XI International Conference on AIDS, Vol 1; July 7–12, 1996; Vancouver, British Columbia, Canada; p 224.
31. Freiman SP, Helfert KE, Hamrell MR, Stein J: Hepatomegaly with severe steatosis in HIV-seropositive patients. AIDS 7:379–385, 1993.
32. Cotton DJ, Finkelstein DM, He W, Feinberg J: Determinants of accrual of women to a large, multicenter clinical trials program of human immunodeficiency virus infection. J Acquir Immune Defic Syndr 6:1322–1328, 1993.
33. Berrebi A, Kobuch WE, Ruel J, et al: Influence of pregnancy on human immunodeficiency virus disease. Eur J Obstet Gynecol Reprod Biol 37:211–217, 1990.
34. Johnstone FD, Willox L, Brettle R: Survival time after AIDS in pregnancy. Br J Obstet Gynaecol 99:633–636, 1992.
35. Minkoff H, Willoughby A, Mendez H, et al: Serious infections during pregnancy among women with advanced human immunodeficiency virus infection. Am J Obstet Gynecol 162:30–34, 1990.
36. European Collaborative Study: Risk factors for mother-to-child transmission. Lancet 339:1007–1012, 1992.
37. Hague RA, Mok JY, Johnstone FD, et al: Maternal factors in HIV transmission. Int J STD AIDS 4:142–146, 1993.
38. Ehrnst A, Lindgren S, Dictor M, et al: HIV in pregnant women and their offspring: Evidence for late transmission. Lancet 338:203–207, 1991.
39. Goedert JJ, Duliege AM, Amos CT, et al: High risk of HIV-1 infection for first-born twins. Lancet 338:1471–1475, 1991.
40. Landesman SH, Kalish LA, Burns DN, et al: Obstetrical factors and the transmission of human immunodeficiency virus type I from mother to child. N Engl J Med 334:1617–1623, 1996.
41. Dunn DT, Newell MC, Ades AE, Peckham CS: Risk of human immunodeficiency virus type I transmission through breastfeeding. Lancet 340:585–588, 1992.
42. Heymann SJ: Modeling the impact of breast-feeding by HIV-infected women on child survival. Am J Public Health 80:1305–1309, 1990.
43. Connor E, Sperling R, Gelber R, et al: Reduction of maternal-infant transmission of human immunodeficiency virus type 1 with zidovudine treatment. Pediatric AIDS Clinical Trials Group Protocol 076 Study Group. N Engl J Med 331:1173–1180, 1994.
44. Sperling RS, Shapiro DE, Coombs RW, et al: Maternal viral load, AZT treatment and the risk of transmission of human immunodeficiency virus type I from mother to infant. N Engl J Med 335:1621–1629, 1996.
45. Miroch-Nick M, Sullivan J, Cort S, et al: Safety and pharmokinetics (pK) of nevirapine (NVP) in HIV-1 infected pregnant women and their newborns (Abstr 403). Presented at the 3rd Conference on Retro and Opportunistic Infections. January 28–February 1, 1996; Washington, DC.

46. Brette RP, Raab GM, Ross A, et al: HIV infection in women: Immunological markers and the influence of pregnancy. AIDS 9:1177–1184, 1995.
47. Brunham RC, Martin DH, Hubbard T, et al: Depression of the lymphocyte transformation response to microbial antigens and to phytohemagglutinin during pregnancy. J Clin Invest 72:1629–1638, 1983.
48. Vanderbeeken Y, Vlieghe MP, Delespesse G, et al: Characterization of immunoregulatory T cells during pregnancy by monoclonal antibodies. Clin Exp Immunol 48:118–120, 1982.
49. Biggar RJ, Pahwa S, Minkoff H, et al: Immunosuppression in pregnant women infected with human immunodeficiency virus. Am J Obstet Gynecol 161:1239–1244, 1989.
50. Briggs GG, Freeman RK, Yaffe SJ: Drugs in Pregnancy and Lactation. Baltimore, Williams & Wilkins, 1986, p 364.
51. Kaplan JF, Masur H, Holmes KK, et al: USPHS/IDSA guidelines for the prevention of opportunistic infections in persons infected with human immunodeficiency virus: An overview. Clin Infect Dis 21(Suppl 1):S12–S31, 1995.
52. Mariuz P, Bosler E, Luft B: Toxoplasmosis in HIV-infected women. *In* Cotton D, Watts DH (eds): The Medical Management of AIDS in Women. New York, Wiley-Liss, 1997, pp 321–343.
53. Villari P, Spino C, Chalmers TC, et al: Caesarean section to reduce perinatal transmission of human immunodeficiency virus: A metaanalysis. Online J Curr Clin Trials July 8, 1993. Document 74.
54. Dunn DT, Newell ML, Mayoux MJ, et al: Mode of delivery and vertical transmission of HIV-1: A review of prospective studies. J Acquir Immune Defic Syndr 7:1064–1066, 1994.
55. Guinan ME, Leviton L: Prevention of HIV infection in women: Overcoming barriers. J Am Med Wom Assoc 50:74–77, 1995.
56. Rothenberg KH, Paskey JJ, Reuland MM, et al: Domestic violence and partner notification: Implication for treatment and counseling of women with HIV. J Am Med Wom Assoc 50:87–93, 1995.
57. Rekart ML: The toxicity and local effects of the spermicide nonoxynol 9. J Acquir Immune Defic Syndr 5:425–427, 1992.
58. Gollub EL, Stein ZA: Commentary: The new female condom—Item 1 on a woman's AIDS prevention agenda. Am J Public Health 83:498–500, 1993.

IMMUNOCOMPROMISED HOSTS

132

Approach to the Immunocompromised Patient

Michael H. Grieco

The first step in approaching management of an immunodeficient patient is to recognize what defects are likely to be present in a host. This exercise is useful in forming a basis for the second step: deducing the probability of infectious complications. The third step involves the selection of empirical therapy for patients presumed to be infected.

Classification of Immunodeficiency Disorders

Immunodeficiency disorders include afferent and efferent abnormalities of immunity involved in the development of antigen-specific primary or secondary immune responses and aberrations of inflammatory cells functioning in effector mechanisms. Table 132–1 outlines some of the major defects of phagocytes, complement, antibody formation, and cell-mediated immunity and associated categories of congenital and/or hereditary, acquired, and drug-induced clinical disorders.[1, 2]

Phagocytic Disorders[3, 4]

After the natural barriers of the skin or the mucociliary apparatus have been penetrated, the phagocyte system, including neutrophils and monocytes and macrophages, constitutes the next line of defense. Neutropenia, resulting from inadequate production or excessive destruction, is the most frequent abnormality that leads to complicating infections. Reduction of the number of circulating granulocytes to less than 400/mm^3 is associated with increased rates of infection, but a critical decrease to less than 100/mm^3 is associated with bacteremia. Abnormalities of chemotaxis, adherence, and phagocytosis and bactericidal disorders are common manifestations of several metabolic, inflammatory, and neoplastic diseases listed in Table 132–1 and may also contribute to secondary infections.

Phagocytic deficiency states result in infections that are often recurrent and respond poorly to antibiotic therapy. As can be seen in Table 132–1, a wide variety of disorders are associated with compromise of phagocyte function.

Complement Disorders

Complement activity results from the sequential interaction of approximately 25 plasma and cell membrane–interactive proteins.[5] Two pathways of complement activation are recognized, the classical and the alternative. The classical pathway is activated by antigen-antibody complexes or antibody-coated particles, and the alternative pathway by antibodies or other mechanisms not involving antibodies. Both pathways form C3 convertases, which cleave the C3 component of complement, a key protein common to both pathways. The two pathways then proceed in identical fashion to bind late-acting components to form a membrane attack complex (C5b,6,7,8,9), which results in target cell lysis.

Inherited disorders of complement may result in a propensity for infection. Typically, only deficiencies of C3 and of late-acting components and some nonregulatory components of the alternative pathway are associated with infectious sequelae. Recurrent pyogenic infections are associated with inherited deficiency of C3, properdin, factor D, and factor I, whereas recurrent disseminated meningococcal infections are reported with deficiencies of alternative pathway properdin and late complement components C5, C6, C7, and C8. Patients with late complement component deficiencies have intact complement-enhanced phagocytosis. This may account

TABLE 132–1 ■ Congenital, Acquired, and Drug-Induced Inflammatory and Immunodeficiency Disorders*

PHAGOCYTES (NEUTROPHILS, MONOCYTES)	COMPLEMENT COMPONENTS		ANTIBODY-MEDIATED IMMUNITY	CELL-MEDIATED IMMUNITY
Defense Mechanisms				
Chemotactic responsiveness	Kinin activity, C4		Interfere with adherence, SIgA	Delayed-type hypersensitivity (T lymphocyte, macrophage)
Adherence	Viral neutralization, C1, C4		Neutralization of viruses, SIgA	Direct cytotoxicity (T lymphocyte)
Vacuole formation	Opsonization, C3b		Microbicidal, IgG, IgM	NK cells
Degranulation	Chemotaxis, C3a, C5a		Immune adherence, IgG, IgM	
Microbicidal activity	Anaphylatoxin, C3a, C5a		Antibody-dependent cellular cytotoxicity, IgG (NK cell, macrophage, neutrophil, eosinophil)	
	Neutrophil activation, C5a			
	Cytolysis, C5b,6,7,8,9			
Congenital or Hereditary Disorders				
Neutropenia	C3	AR	Reticular dysgenesis, U	Reticular dysgenesis, AR
Infantile genetic agranulocytosis	C5	AR	SCID (thymid dysplasia), AR, occasionally XLR	SCID (thymic dysplasia), AR, XLR
	C6	AR		
Autoimmune neutropenia	C7	AR	SCID with ADA deficiency, AR	SCID with ADA deficiency, AR
	C8	AR		
Isoimmune neonatal neutropenia	Factor I	AR		DiGeorge syndrome, V
	Properdin	XLR	X-linked agammaglobulinemia, XLR	Nezelof syndrome, U
Kostmann syndrome				
Abnormal chemotaxis	CR3 (LAD)	AR	CVID, U	Chronic mucocutaneous candidiasis, V
Chédiak-Higashi, AR			Congenital hypogammaglobulinemia, AR	
Lazy leukocyte, U			IgA deficiency, V	Wiskott-Aldrich syndrome, XLR
Hyper IgE, U			IgM deficiency, U	Ataxia-telangiectasia, AR
				Cartilage-hair hypoplasia, AR
Abnormal digestion			Hyper-IgM, XLR	CVID, U
Actin-myosin dysfunction, AR				Nucleoside phosphorylase deficiency, U
Abnormal microbicidal				
CGD, XLR				X-linked recessive lymphoproliferative syndrome, Duncan syndrome, XLR
MPD, AR				
G6PD, XLR				
Abnormal adherence				Bare lymphocyte syndrome, AR
LAD, AR				
Acquired Disorders				
Neutropenia	Factor B		Multiple myeloma	Hodgkin's disease
Acute leukemia	Splenectomy		Macroglobulinemia	Sézary syndrome
Chronic leukemia	Sickle cell disease		Heavy chain diseases	Organ transplantation
Alcoholism	Hypocomplementemia		Non-Hodgkin's lymphoma	Bone marrow transplantation
Nutritional deficiency (vitamin B_{12}, folate)	SLE		Chronic lymphatic leukemia	AIDS
Infectious diseases (e.g., HIV-1)	Protein-calorie malnutrition		AIDS	
Bone marrow transplant–related suppression				

Abnormal chemotaxis		
Intrinsic		
Diabetes mellitus		
Rheumatoid arthritis, Felty syndrome, SLE		
Acute infections		
Burn injuries		
Alcoholism (chronic)		
Job syndrome		
Circulating inhibitor to CF		
Renal disease		
Hepatic cirrhosis		
Hodgkin's disease		
Lepromatous leprosy		
Sarcoidosis		
Circulating inhibitor to cells		
Hepatic cirrhosis		
Sarcoma		
Carcinoma		
Anergy		
Abnormal granulocyte adherence		
Alcoholism (acute)		
Abnormal phagocytosis		
Rheumatoid arthritis		
Acute infections		
Hyperosmolar states		
Abnormal microbicidal		
Malakoplakia		
Felty syndrome		
Drug-Induced Disorders		
Neutropenia	Cyclophosphamide (alkylating agent)	Cyclophosphamide (alkylating agent)
Cytoxic drugs (e.g., cyclophosphamide)	Azathioprine (antimetabolite)	Azathioprine (antimetabolite)
Noncytotoxic drugs (chloramphenicol)		
Abnormal phagocytosis		Corticosteroids
Colchicine		Cyclosporine
Tetracycline		Tacrolimus
Cyclophosphamide		
Abnormal granulocyte adherence		
Corticosteroids		
Aspirin		
Abnormal microbicidal		
Phenylbutazone		
Chloramphenicol		

*ADA, Adenosine deaminase; AIDS, acquired immunodeficiency syndrome; AR, autosomal recessive; CFs, chemotactic factors; CGD, chronic granulomatous disease; CVID, common variable immunodeficiency; G6PD, glucose-6-phosphate dehydrogenase deficiency; HIV, human immunodeficiency virus; IgA, IgE, IgG, IgM, immunoglobulins A, E, G, M; LAD, leukocyte adhesion disorder; MPD, myeloperoxidase deficiency; NK, natural killer; SCID, severe combined immunodeficiency disease; SIgA, secretory IgA; SLE, systemic lupus erythematosus; U, unknown; V, variable; XLR, X-linked recessive.

Adapted from Grieco MH: Introduction to the abnormal host and complicating infections. *In* Grieco MH (ed): Infections in the Abnormal Host. New York, Yorke Medical Books, 1980.

for the low case-fatality rate of 2.9% with the latter, which contrasts with the 64% rate associated with infection in properdin-deficient persons.[6] Laboratory tests of total hemolytic complement activity, if results are normal, do not exclude alternative pathway deficiency, evaluation for which requires a specific assay.

Patients with leukocyte adhesion deficiency have a hereditary disorder involving the β_2-leukocyte integrins lymphocyte function antigen-1, CR3/MAC-1, and p150,95, which function as adhesion molecules on neutrophils. This is a rare disorder in which β-chain synthesis is abnormal and interferes with expression of these three heterodimers on neutrophil and monocyte membrane surfaces. Both CR3 and p150,95 contain CR3 moieties, so that binding to iC3b is defective and may contribute to clinical infections. Patients with this disorder have markedly depressed inflammatory responses, recurrent bacterial and fungal infections, retarded healing, and severe gingivitis and periodontal disease.[7] Complement disorders associated with infection are principally hereditary and thus relatively infrequent.

Antibody Disorders

Antibody deficiency reduces the host's resistance to infection through lack of a secretory antibody, which favors mucosal attachment by pathogens and by reduced circulatory antibodies that provide protective neutralizing, microbicidal, phagocytic, and cytotoxic actions. Respiratory and gastrointestinal infections predominate. Agammaglobulinemia and hypogammaglobulinemia result primarily from congenital hereditary disorders and from some hematologic malignancies, such as chronic lymphatic leukemia. Drug-induced hypogammaglobulinemia is rarely of clinical importance.

Cell-Mediated Immunity Disorders

Monocytes, lymphocytes, and natural killer cells play critical roles in the control of intracellular pathogens. This category of protective mechanisms accounts for many infectious sequelae associated with modern immunosuppressive medical therapy and includes bacterial, fungal, viral, and protozoan infections. Both primary pathogenic and opportunistic pathogens are incriminated. The organisms that cause disseminated infection in these circumstances are able to proliferate within cells, including monocytes, and are protected from cytolytic destruction by cytotoxic T cells and natural killer cells as well as from lymphokines that would normally activate monocytes to control intracellular infections that are less susceptible to the effects of serum factors such as antibody and complement.

Infectious Syndromes and Infectious Agents

Categorization of the underlying disorder or disorders is important in assessment because of the associations with various infectious syndromes and agents. In other chapters, inherited immunodeficiency states, acquired malignancy, and organ and bone marrow transplantation and the infectious complications of therapy with corticosteroid and immunosuppressive agents are discussed. Here I attempt to summarize the types of infections seen in association with various immunodeficiencies (Table 132–2).

Phagocytic Disorders

Functional or quantitative defects of neutrophils result in complicating infections with pyogenic bacteria, including *Streptococcus pneumoniae, Staphylococcus aureus, Staphylococcus epidermidis, Klebsiella pneumoniae, Enterobacter cloacae, Pseudomonas aeruginosa*, and *Acinetobacter calcoaceticus* var. *anitratus*. There is some variation among the primary phagocytic disorders, depending on the particular stage of impairment of granulocyte function; however, a wide variety of infections may result. A case in point is chronic granulomatous disease, which consists of a group of rare disorders (incidence of 1 in 1 million persons) of phagocytic cell superoxide production that lead to recurrent infections with catalase-positive organisms and chronic inflammation. Chronic granulomatous disease is transmitted by X-linked inheritance in 66% and by autosomal recessive inheritance in 33%. Neutrophils from most patients with X-linked chronic granulomatous disease lack a membrane-associated cytochrome *b*-558, which is required for production of superoxide. Some variants lack cytosolic components of the NADPH oxidase system.[8] Fourteen patients with the disease who were followed up at the National Institutes of Health had a severe infection approximately once every 10 months: 119 major infectious episodes occurred, and for more than 55% of episodes, no organism was recovered. Most of the identified infectious agents were catalase-positive microorganisms capable of destroying hydrogen peroxide, most commonly, *S. aureus* (16%). Less frequent infectious agents were *Aspergillus* species, *Chromobacterium violaceum, Pseudomonas cepacia, Nocardia* species, *Salmonella typhimurium, Serratia marcescens, Mycobacterium fortuitum, Klebsiella* species, *Escherichia coli, Actinomyces* species, *Legionella bosmanii, Clostridium difficile*, and *S. pneumoniae*.[9]

Patients with neoplastic diseases often develop neutropenia complicated by bacterial and fungal infections. Neutropenic patients usually become infected with their endogenous flora, most often bacteria from the gastrointestinal tract. In a study of septicemia in patients with leukemias and lymphomas reported from Memorial Sloan-Kettering in 1977,[10] Singer and coworkers noted *E. coli* in 24%, *P. aeruginosa* in 15%, *Klebsiella* or *Enterobacter* in 11%, *S. aureus* in 9%, *Candida* species in 5%, *Streptococcus pyogenes* in 3%, other organisms in 15%, and polymicrobial sepsis in 17%; the overall mortality rate was 40.5%. The source of infection is often obscure and may not be detectable in more than 35% of patients. The most common sites identified are the lungs, urinary tract, wounds, perineum, and perirectal areas. The principal change that has occurred since that study is that gram-positive organisms (particularly *S. epidermidis*; groups A, B, C, and D α-hemolytic streptococci; and corynebacteria) have become responsible for an increasing proportion of blood stream infections in cancer patients[11–13] and have led to a great deal of concern about recommendations for empirical therapy.

Complement Disorders

Primary deficiencies of late complement components have been linked to infectious sequelae but rarely acquired defects. C3 is positioned at a critical point for both the classical and alternative complement pathways. A deficiency of C3 is associated with serious recurrent infection with *S. pneumoniae* and *Neisseria meningitidis*.

Deficiencies of the later acting components, C5, C6, C7, and C8, as well as of properdin, are linked to life-threatening infections with *N. meningitidis* and *Neisseria gonorrhoeae*.[14] *E. coli* and *Brucella, Toxoplasma*, and *Staphylococcus* organisms have been isolated less frequently. The neisserial infections are usually in the meninges, associated with bacteremia. Pneumonia, otitis media, pyelonephritis, and endocarditis have been reported infrequently. Homozygotic late component deficiencies are complicated by neisserial infections at some time in more than 40% of subjects (mean of 17 years of age at the time of neisserial infection). Mortality resulting

TABLE 132–2 ■ Frequent Infectious Complications of Inflammatory and Immunodeficiency Disorders

MICROBE	PHAGOCYTES (NEUTROPHILS, MONOCYTES)	COMPLEMENT COMPONENTS	ANTIBODY-MEDIATED IMMUNITY	CELL-MEDIATED IMMUNITY
Bacteria				
Gram-positive cocci	+++	++	+++	
Enterobacteriaceae	+++	+	+	
Pseudomonas aeruginosa	+++	+	+	
Haemophilus influenzae	+	+	+++	
Salmonella species				+++
Listeria monocytogenes				+++
Mycobacterium species				+++
Mycobacterium tuberculosis				+++
Nocardia asteroides				+++
Legionella species				++
Rhodococcus species				++
Fungi				
Candida species				
Sytemic	++			
Chronic mucocutaneous				+++
Aspergillus species	+++			+++
Mucor, Absidia, Rhizopus	+++			
Cryptococcus neoformans				+++
Coccidioides immitis				+++
Histoplasma capsulatum				+++
Viruses				
Herpes simplex virus type 1			+	+++
Herpes simplex virus type 2			+	+++
Varicella-zoster virus				+++
Cytomegalovirus				+++
Vaccinia virus				+++
Rubella virus				+++
Papovaviruses				++
Enteroviruses			++	+
Hepatitis B virus			++	+
Influenza virus			+	+
Adenoviruses			+	+
Rotavirus			+	
Respiratory syncytial virus				+
Parasites				
Pneumocystis carinii			++	+++
Giardia lamblia			++	+
Toxoplasma gondii				+++
Strongyloides stercoralis				+++
Cryptosporidium			+	+
Isospora			+	+
Microsporida *(Enterocytozoan, Septata)*			+	+
Cyclospora				+

Adapted from Grieco MH: Introduction to the abnormal host and complicating infections. *In* Grieco MH (ed): Infections in the Abnormal Host. New York, Yorke Medical Books, 1980.

from meningococcal infection is higher in properdin deficiency than in disorders of the late complement components.[14] Recurrent pyogenic infections with encapsulated bacteria complicate other alternative complement pathway deficiencies, such as diminished C3 in partial lipodystrophy and chronic membranoproliferative nephritis and low titer of factor B in newborns.

Antibody Disorders

Table 132–2 lists bacterial, viral, and parasitic agents associated with antibody deficiencies that produce respiratory, diarrheal, and central nervous system (CNS) syndromes.

Respiratory Syndromes. In patients with X-linked agammaglobulinemia, infections with encapsulated pneumococci and *Haemophilus influenzae,* and to a lesser extent streptococci and staphylococci, result in pneumonia, recurrent otitis media, purulent sinusitis, meningitis, and furunculosis. Subjects with common variable immunodeficiency were also noted to have pneumonia (87%), sinusitis (60%), and bronchiectasis (53%).

Diarrheal Syndromes. Chronic diarrhea, the second most important sequela of antibody deficiency, may result from rotavirus and enterovirus infections, from parasites such as *Cryptosporidium, Isospora, Giardia lamblia, Cyclospora,* and Microsporida,[15, 16] and from gram-negative bacteria such as *Salmonella* and *Campylobacter.*

CNS Syndromes. Viral infections of the CNS are severe infectious sequelae of hypogammaglobulinemia. Patients with X-linked agammaglobulinemia are susceptible to chronic echovirus infection of the CNS and less frequently to infections with other viruses, including herpes simplex virus, coxsackievirus, and adenovirus.[17] In addition, these patients are more likely to develop paralytic poliomyelitis after live poliovirus vaccination. CNS syndromes rarely complicate common variable immunodeficiency.

Other Syndromes. Other infections described in association with severe hypogammaglobulinemia include progressive vaccinia, disseminated adenovirus infection, and *Pneumocystis carinii* pneumonia.

Cell-Mediated Immunity Disorders

A wide variety of infectious agents, bacteria, fungi, viruses, and parasites cause disease in patients with defective cell-mediated immunity (see Table 132–2). Most of these agents are sequestered in intracellular sites, where they are protected from the effects of serum factors such as antibody and complement.

In adults, the acquired immunodeficiency syndrome is complicated by infectious syndromes that are primarily the result of defective cell-mediated immunity, and this syndrome serves as a model that is readily applicable to other conditions of immune suppression such as neoplastic diseases, primary immunodeficiency disorders, and drug- and radiation-induced suppression, as for transplant recipients. Some infectious syndromes and implicated organisms are outlined in Table 132–3.

TABLE 132–3 ■ Infectious Syndromes and Organisms Associated with Defective Cell-Mediated Immunity

SYNDROME	COMMON PATHOGENS	LESS COMMON PATHOGENS
Mucocutaneous infections	Herpes simplex virus *Candida albicans*	Varicella-zoster virus
Esophagitis	*C. albicans*	Herpes simplex virus Cytomegalovirus
Enteritis	*Cryptosporidium parvum*	*Isospora belli* *Giardia lamblia* *Campylobacter* species Microsporida *Salmonella* species *Shigella* species *Strongyloides stercoralis*
Pneumonia	*Pneumocystis carinii* Cytomegalovirus	*Cryptococcus neoformans* *Mycobacterium tuberculosis* *Mycobacterium avium-intracellulare* *Histoplasma capsulatum* *Legionella* species *S. stercoralis* *Coccidioides immitis* *Rhodococcus bronchialis*
Meningitis	*Cryptococcus neoformans*	*Listeria monocytogenes*
Encephalitis	*Toxoplasma gondii*	*Nocardia asteroides* *Aspergillus* species *Mucor, Absidia, Rhizopus* Cytomegalovirus Human immunodeficiency virus types 1 and 2 Papovavirus
Retinitis	Cytomegalovirus	Herpes simplex virus *Treponema pallidum* *T. gondii* Herpes zoster virus
Septicemia	*Mycobacterium avium-intracellulare* *Salmonella* species	*L. monocytogenes*

Empirical Therapy in the Case of Presumed Infection

Neutropenia

Empirical Multiple Antimicrobial Agent Therapy. In immunosuppressed patients with neutropenia, less than 60% of episodes of fever are ever associated with bacterial infection, but rapid institution of antibiotic programs improves these patients' prognosis. More than a decade ago, combination therapy with carbenicillin (5 g every 4 hours), gentamicin, and cephalothin or cephapirin (2 g every 4 hours) was utilized to cover likely gram-negative and gram-positive bacteria. Later, results of large prospective comparative trials suggested that three-drug combination therapy might not be necessary.[18, 19] In fact, cephalosporins appeared to be more nephrotoxic than carbenicillin or ticarcillin combined with an aminoglycoside. A combination of carbenicillin or ticarcillin with an aminoglycoside has appeared to have a good ratio of efficacy to toxicity for initial empirical therapy of infection in granulocytopenic cancer patients. Alternative options, depending on clinical assessment (renal failure, hospital-acquired infection, vascular catheter) include two β-lactam agents (e.g., ceftazidime plus piperacillin), a single broad-spectrum drug (imipenem, cefoperazone, or ceftazidime), or vancomycin combined with an aminoglycoside plus an antipseudomonad penicillin.[20]

A study of 747 febrile granulocytopenic patients with cancer randomized to receive ceftazidime plus amikacin with or without vancomycin as initial therapy did not support the empirical addition of vancomycin to the initial antibiotic therapy in cancer patients with fever and granulocytopenia.[21]

It is reasonable to continue treatment for a total of 5 days after fever subsides if cultures do not grow the organism and for 10 days if an organism is isolated. Antibiotics should not be continued longer than 1 week in a persistently positive febrile patient without positive blood cultures. These recommendations are based on the observation that the risk of superinfection increases after 7 days of therapy if an organism is not isolated.

The choice of a specific aminoglycoside is based on consideration both of relative nephrotoxicity and of effectiveness in the presence of profound neutropenia. Although gentamicin and amikacin demonstrate similar nephrotoxicity, a controlled study in nonneutropenic patients suggested that tobramycin is less nephrotoxic than gentamicin.[22, 23] Amikacin has been advocated for use over gentamicin and tobramycin because resistance to it is less common and there is greater appreciation of the role of multidrug-resistant bacteria in late-breakthrough gram-negative rod bacteremia.[24, 25]

One of the most important developments in the treatment of serious gram-negative infections is the establishment of the relationship of elevated trough levels of aminoglycosides to nephrotoxicity. Aminoglycoside properties of dose-dependent killing and postantibiotic suppression of bacterial growth remain valuable. Several clinical trials using once-daily dosing of aminoglycosides, rather than more frequent conventional dosing, have shown that once-daily aminoglycoside therapy appears to be as effective as standard therapy and is associated with reduced toxicity.[26, 27] Single daily dosing of amikacin and ceftriaxone appeared to be as effective and no more toxic than were multiple daily doses of amikacin and ceftazidine for the empirical therapy of infection in patients with cancer and granulocytopenia.[27]

During the 1980s, the availability of new therapeutic agents, particularly those of the cephalosporin class, has revived the question of whether therapy with a single potent agent might be as effective as combination antimicrobial therapy. Cefotaxime,[28] imipenem-cilastin,[29] and ceftazidime[11, 30–32] have been studied. The reports have not concurred, possibly because of differences between institutions in the patterns of resistant strains of bacteria and in the epidemiologic settings of individual oncology centers. A report by Kramer and coworkers[32] summarized the principal complication of monotherapy: superinfection with gram-positive organisms. They noted that 5 of 21 patients assigned to receive ceftazidime alone contracted bacteremic superinfections with a total of eight organisms, including four *Clostridium* species and three enterococci. All the superinfections in the triple-therapy arm were with either gram-negative bacteria or fungi. A report from the European Organization for Research and Treatment of Cancer (EORTC) disclosed response rates of single-organism gram-negative bacteremia of 81% with ceftazidime and long-course (at least 9 days) amikacin, 48% with ceftazidime and short-course (3 days) amikacin, and 40% with azlocillin and long-course amikacin. Among patients with less than 100 neutrophils per mm^3, the response rate was 6% to ceftazidime and 50% to ceftazidime and long-course amikacin.

At this point the case for monotherapy is not compelling. Continued use of an anti-*Pseudomonas* β-lactamase–resistant antibiotic and an aminoglycoside should be instituted empirically, the specific choice of drugs depending on local institutional resistance patterns. Once-daily dosing of the aminoglycoside agent should be considered as an alternative.

Because of a shift toward gram-positive bacteremia in patients with neutropenia, there has been controversy as to whether vancomycin should be included as a component of initial empirical antibiotic therapy. Again, the use of vancomycin varies with the prevalence of gram-positive bacteremias at various institutions. Rubin and coworkers[33] found evidence to support adding vancomycin to ceftazidime on the basis of clinical or microbiologic findings. Shenep and colleagues[34] reported unsatisfactory responses in 15% of febrile, neutropenic children treated initially with vancomycin, ticarcillin, and amikacin, compared with 38% in the group who received ticarcillin-clavulanate and amikacin. Nine of 10 breakthrough bacteremias with *S. epidermidis* and α-hemolytic streptococci occurred in the ticarcillin-clavulanate arm, even though most of the isolates were susceptible in vitro. However, the EORTC study reported in 1991 failed to confirm a benefit related to the use of vancomycin as a component of combination empirical therapy.[21]

Empirical amphotericin B therapy trials have been summarized by Holleran and associates.[35] Blood cultures for fungi give positive results in only 12% to 34% of cases of acute leukemia with documented fungal infection, usually *Candida* or *Aspergillus*. Although criteria for initiating empirical therapy with amphotericin B have varied, it would appear reasonable to add this drug for patients who remain febrile with neutropenia (cell count less than 500/mm^3) and after receiving 7 days of multidrug combination therapy.

Treatment of Complement Disorders

Primary deficiencies of complement components are relatively rare. Patients with known disorders of properdin, factor B, C3b, and the later acting components should be treated for presumed pyogenic infections, including *N. meningitidis* and *N. gonorrhoeae*, before culture identification is complete, especially for life-threatening infections such as meningitis. Ampicillin should be instituted immediately if there is a history of severe recurrent infection.

Treatment of Antibody Disorders

Conventional antibiotic therapy directed against probable encapsulated pneumococci and *H. influenzae* is usually indicated soon after the onset of clinical signs of respiratory infection. Replacement γ-globulin therapy, as well as prophylactic antibiotics, usually decreases the severity and frequency of these infections. Therapy of diarrheal syndromes usually depends on the initial identification of an agent.

Devastating CNS echovirus infections are usually not responsive to γ-globulin replacement, because the blood-brain barrier prevents accumulation of high concentrations of antibody in the CSF. Control of CNS infection has been reported with intraventricular administration of immune serum globulin via a permanent Ommaya reservoir.[36]

Treatment of Cell-Mediated Immunity Disorders

In general, therapy is dependent on identification of a specific agent by culture, stain, or serologic or histopathologic examination.[37, 38] There are at least three situations in which empirical therapy is indicated before there is a definitive diagnosis. Therapy should be initiated presumptively whenever it is likely that a patient may have pneumonitis due to *P. carinii*, encephalitis due to *Toxoplasma gondii*, or retinitis due to cytomegalovirus. Early treatment of these infections has been associated with improved clinical outcome in immunodeficient patients, including those who have acquired immunodeficiency syndrome.[39–42]

References

1. Grieco MH (ed): Infections in the Abnormal Host. New York, Yorke Medical Books, 1980.
2. Grieco MH: Introduction to the abnormal host and complicating infections. *In* Grieco MH (ed): Infections in the Abnormal Host. New York, Yorke Medical Books, 1980, pp 2–3.
3. Malech HL, Gallin JI: Neutrophils in human diseases. N Engl J Med 317:687, 1987.
4. Cohen MS: Molecular events in the activation of human neutrophils for microbial killing. Clin Infect Dis 18(Suppl 2): S 170, 1994.
5. Frank MM: Complement in the pathophysiology of human disease. N Engl J Med 316:1525, 1987.
6. Densen P, Weiler JM, McLeod Griffiss J, Hoffman LG: Familial properdin deficiency and fatal meningococcemia. Correction of the bactericidal defect vaccination. N Engl J Med 316:922, 1987.
7. Gallin JI: Leukocyte adherence–related glycoproteins LFA-1 MO1, and p150,95: A new group of monoclonal antibodies, a new disease, and a possible opportunity to understand the molecular basis of leukocyte adherence. J Infect Dis 152:661, 1985.
8. Clark RA, Malech HL, Gallin JJ, et al: Genetic variants of chronic granulomatous disease: Prevalence of deficiencies of two cytosolic components of the NADPH oxidase system. N Engl J Med 321:647, 1989.
9. Gallin JI, Buescher, ES, Seligman BE, et al: Recent advances in chronic granulomatous disease. Ann Intern Med 99:657, 1983.
10. Singer C, Kaplan MH, Armstrong D: Bacteremia and fungemia complicating neoplastic disease: A study of 364 cases. Am J Med 62:731, 1977.
11. Pizzo PA, Hathorn JW, Hiemenz J, et al: A randomized trial comparing ceftazidime alone with combination antibiotic therapy in cancer patients with fever and neutropenia. N Engl J Med 315:552, 1986.
12. Klastersky J, Glauser MP, Schimpff SC, et al: Prospective randomized comparison of three antibiotic regimens for empirical therapy of suspected bacteremic infection in febrile granulocytopenic patients. Antimicrob Agents Chemother 29:263, 1986.
13. Langley J, Gold R: Sepsis in febrile neutropenia children with cancer. Pediatr Infect Dis 7:34, 1988.
14. Ross SC, Densen P: Complement deficiency states and infection: Epidemiology, pathogenesis, and consequences of neisserial and other infections in an immune deficiency. Medicine (Baltimore) 63:243, 1984.
15. Weber R, Bryan RT, Schwartz DA, Owen RL: Human microsporidial infections. Clin Microbiol Rev 7:426, 1994.
16. Shadduck JA: Human microsporidiosis and AIDS. Rev Infect Dis 11:203, 1989.

17. Stiehm ER, Chin TW, Haas A, Peerless AG: Infectious complications of the primary immunodeficiencies. Clin Immunol Immunopathol 40:69, 1986.
18. European Organization for Research on Treatment of Cancer: Three antibiotic regimens in the treatment of infection in febrile granulocytopenic patients with cancer. J Infect Dis 137:14, 1987.
19. Wade JC, Petty BF, Conrad G, et al: Cephalothin plus an aminoglycoside is more nephrotoxic than methicillin plus aminoglycoside. Lancet 2:604, 1978.
20. Hughes WT, Armstrong D, Bodey G, et al: Guidelines for the use of antimicrobial agents in neutropenic patients with unexplained fever. J Infect Dis 161:381, 1990.
21. EORTC and National Cancer Institute of Canada: Vancomycin added to empirical combination therapy for fever in granulocytopenic cancer patients. J Infect Dis 163:951, 1991.
22. Smith CR, Maxwell RR, Edwards CO, et al: Nephrotoxicity induced by gentamicin and amikacin. Johns Hopkins Med J 142:85, 1978.
23. Smith CR, Lipsky JJ, Laskin OL, et al: Double-blind comparison of the nephrotoxicity and auditory toxicity of gentamicin and tobramycin. N Engl J Med 302:1105, 1980.
24. Anderson ET, Young LS, Hewitt WL: Simultaneous antibiotic levels in "breakthrough" gram-negative rod bacteremia. Am J Med 61:493, 1976.
25. Meyer RD, Lewis RP, Carmalt ED, et al: Amikacin therapy for serious gram-negative bacillary infections. Ann Intern Med 83:790, 1975.
26. Prins JM, Bueller HR, Kuijper EJ, et al: Once versus thrice daily gentamicin in patients with serious infections. Lancet 341:335, 1993.
27. International Antimicrobial Therapy Cooperative Group of the European Organization for Research and Treatment of Cancer: Efficacy and toxicity of single daily doses of amikacin and ceftriazone versus multiple daily doses of amikacin and ceftazidine for infection in patients with cancer and granulocytopenia. Ann Intern Med 119:584, 1993.
28. Smith CR, Ambinder R, Lipsky JJ, et al: Cefotaxine compared with nafcillin plus tobromycin for serious bacterial infections: A randomized, double-blind trial. Ann Intern Med 101:469, 1984.
29. Bodey GP, Alvarez ME, Jones PG, et al: Imipenem-celastin as initial therapy for febrile cancer patients. Antimicrob Agents Chemother 30:211, 1986.
30. de Jongl CA, Joshi JH, Newman KA, et al: Antibiotic synergism and response in gram-negative bacteremia in granulocytopenic patients with fever and neutropenia. N Engl J Med 315:552, 1986.
31. The EORTC International Antimicrobial Therapy Cooperative Group: Ceftazidime combined with a short or long course of amikacin for empirical therapy of gram-negative bacteremia in cancer patients with granulocytopenia. N Engl J Med 317:1692, 1987.
32. Kramer BS, Ramphal R, Rand K: Antibiotic therapy in cancer patients with fever and neutropenia (Letter). N Engl J Med 316:410, 1987.
33. Rubin M, Hathorn JW, Marshall D, et al: Gram-positive infections and the use of vancomycin in 550 episodes of fever and neutropenia. Ann Intern Med 108:30, 1988.
34. Shenep JL, Hughes WT, Roberson PK, et al: Vancomycin, ticarcillin, and amikacin compared with ticarcillin-clavulanate and amikacin in the empirical treatment of febrile, neutropenic children with cancer. N Engl J Med 319:1053, 1988.
35. Holleran WM, Wilbur JR, DeGregorio WM: Empiric amphotericin B therapy in patients with acute leukemia. Rev Infect Dis 7:619, 1989.
36. Erlendsson K, Swartz T, Dwyer JM: Successful reversal of echovirus encephalitis in X-linked hypergammaglobulinemia by intraventricular administration of immunoglobulin. N Engl J Med 312:351, 1985.
37. Glatt AE, Chirgwin K, Landesman SH: Treatment of infections associated with human immunodeficiency virus. N Engl J Med 318:1439, 1988.
38. Young LS: Treatable aspects of infections due to human immunodeficiency virus. Lancet 2:1503, 1987.
39. Sattler FR, Cowan R, Nielsen DM, Ruskin J: Trimethoprim-sulfamethoxazole compared with pentamidine for treatment of *Pneumocystis carinii* pneumonia in AIDS. Ann Intern Med 109:280, 1988.
40. Luft BJ, Brooks RG, Conley FK, et al: Toxoplasmic encephalitis in patients with AIDS. JAMA 252:913, 1984.
41. Drew WL: Cytomegalovirus infection in patients with AIDS. J Infect Dis 158:449, 1988.
42. Reed EC, Bowden RA, Dandliker PS, et al: Treatment of CMV pneumonia with ganciclovir and intravenous CMV immunoglobulin in patients with bone marrow transplants. Ann Intern Med 109:783, 1988.

133

Infections Associated with Malignancy

Shahe Vartivarian
Gerald P. Bodey

Infection is the most common complication of cancer patients and especially among those receiving antitumor chemotherapy. The fatality rate from infectious complications has been reduced substantially during the past three decades, mainly due to the recognition of the need for the prompt administration of empirical antibiotic therapy and the introduction of a variety of potent broad-spectrum antimicrobial agents. Nevertheless, infection remains a frequent and serious complication in cancer patients because of advances in the management of malignant diseases, such as the administration of intensive chemotherapeutic regimens, the extended use of bone marrow transplantation, and the routine insertion of intravascular catheters. Antimicrobial prophylaxis has reduced the frequency of gram-negative bacterial infections but has been associated with an increase in the number of gram-positive and fungal infections. Growth factors such as granulocyte colony-stimulating factor and granulocyte-macrophage colony-stimulating factor have become available that stimulate earlier recovery from chemotherapy-induced neutropenia. The use of these agents may reduce the frequency of infection in some populations of patients.

Factors Associated with Infection in Cancer Patients

A variety of factors have been associated with certain malignancies or their therapies that predispose to infectious complications. Table 133–1 lists some of the most common of these factors and the malignancies with which they occur. Most infections occur in patients undergoing chemotherapy for cancer, because most of these agents cause myelosuppression, immunosuppression, and mucosal damage.[1, 2]

A temperature of 38.5°C or higher is usually the earliest manifestation of infection in the cancer patient, although some therapeutic agents such as adrenal corticosteroids may suppress the febrile reaction. Fever may be due to other causes, such as the administration of blood products, biologic agents, or an allergic reaction. Fever secondary to a malignancy has been observed most frequently in Hodgkin's disease, malignant lymphoma, and chronic myelogenous leukemia. Possible mechanisms for malignancy-induced fever include tumor emboli, tumor necrosis, or a circulating meta-

TABLE 133–1 ■ Factors Predisposing to Infection in Cancer Patients

FACTOR	MALIGNANCY OR THERAPY
Neutropenia	Acute leukemia, chemotherapy
Deficient neutrophil function	Radiation
Monocytopenia	Hairy cell leukemia
Impaired cellular immunity	Lymphoma, Hodgkin's disease
Increased suppressor T-lymphocyte activity	Bone marrow transplantation
Splenectomy	Hodgkin's disease, myelodysplastic syndrome
Impaired macrophage function	Adrenal corticosteroid therapy
Hypogammaglobulinemia	Multiple myeloma, chronic lymphocytic leukemia
Mucositis	Chemotherapy
Tumor necrosis	Various malignancies
Bronchial obstruction	Bronchogenic carcinoma
Gastrointestinal ulceration	Acute leukemia, chemotherapy

bolic product. Only 5% of febrile episodes occurring in cancer patients are caused by the malignancy.[3]

The type of neoplasm (and its therapy) determines the frequency of fever and infections (Table 133–2). Patients with acute leukemia spend about half of their hospital stay with fever, whereas those with lymphoma and solid tumors have fever for 25% and 10% of their hospital days, respectively. Autopsy studies show that infection is responsible for the death of 75% of patients with leukemia, 50% of patients with lymphoma, and 50% of patients with solid tumors.[4–6] One review of failures of initial induction of remission in acute myelogenous leukemia documented death from infection in approximately 70% of the patients.[7]

Neutropenia

Neutropenia is the most common predisposing factor for infection in the cancer patient. Occasionally, it is a consequence of the disease process itself, which occurs in acute leukemia or when a malignant neoplasm invades the bone marrow. More often, neutropenia is associated with cancer chemotherapy. As demonstrated in patients with acute leukemia, the risk of infection is related to the degree and duration of neutropenia. In the leukemic patient, the risk begins to increase when the neutrophil count falls below 1000/mm^3 and increases precipitously when the neutrophil count falls below 500/mm^3.[8] However, in patients with solid tumors or in patients who are in remission of leukemia, although this relationship remains, the risk at any level of neutrophil count is less than that in patients with active leukemia. Furthermore, it is not the amount of the decline in the neutrophil count after chemotherapy but rather the nadir that determines the risk of infection.

Another important consideration in neutropenic patients is the fact that the response to appropriate antimicrobial therapy depends on whether or not the neutrophil count recovers during therapy.[9] This is especially true if the patient's neutrophil count is less than 100/mm^3 at the onset of infection. The importance of neutrophil recovery on outcome has been demonstrated for both bacterial and fungal infections. Although the impact of neutrophil recovery has been observed with all antibacterial agents, it is especially true for aminoglycosides. Only about 25% of infections caused by susceptible organisms respond to aminoglycoside therapy if the patient's neutrophil count remains less than 100/mm^3. For these reasons, patients with acute leukemia have a poorer prognosis when they become infected than do most other cancer patients, because they are likely to experience prolonged periods of neutropenia.

Deficiencies in neutrophil function have been described in some cancer patients, although their role in predisposing to infection is less important than the role of neutropenia. For example, some patients with acute leukemia produce nearly adequate numbers of circulating neutrophils but still develop frequent infections. Children who are administered radiotherapy to prevent central nervous system leukemia may develop abnormalities in neutrophil function. Chemotherapeutic agents may also interfere with neutrophil function when administered at doses that do not cause neutropenia.

Because neutropenic patients are unable to mount an adequate inflammatory reaction, the characteristic signs and symptoms associated with infection may be absent in these patients. For example, among patients with urinary tract infections, pyuria was observed in 97% of patients whose neutrophil count exceeded 1000/mm^3 but was observed in only 11% of patients whose neutrophil counts were less than 100/mm^3.[10] Among patients with pneumonia, 84% of the former group produced purulent sputum compared with only 8% of the latter group. In a study of cancer patients with gram-negative pneumonia, almost 40% of patients whose neutrophil count was less than 1000/mm^3 had a normal chest radiograph at the onset of infection.[11] In a study of febrile neutropenic patients, the physician failed to detect the presence of infection in 28% of those patients who proved ultimately to be infected.[12]

Because antibiotic therapy is instituted promptly when fever occurs in neutropenic patients, the presence of infection as the cause of fever often cannot be documented. In most series, infection is documented in only 40% to 50% of febrile episodes. The organism responsible for infection can be determined in only about 50% of documented infections. In most cases, the organism is cultured from blood specimens. Cultures from other sites, such as sputum, are seldom useful, and the ability to obtain biopsy specimens is often limited

TABLE 133–2 ■ Relation of Neoplasm to Fever and Infection

	ACUTE LEUKEMIA	CHRONIC LYMPHOCYTIC LEUKEMIA	LYMPHOMA	SOLID TUMOR
Febrile episodes*	5	1	2	1
Febrile days*	48	14	23	11
Death from infection (%)	75	80	50	50
Agent of fatal infections (%)				
Bacteria	66		86	94
Fungi	33		13	6
Viruses	0.2		0.3	0
Protozoa	0.1		0.6	0.4

*Per 100 hospital days.

From Bodey GP: Infections in patients with cancer. *In* Holland JF, Frei E III (eds): Cancer Medicine, ed 2. Philadelphia, Lea & Febiger, 1982.

because of concurrent thrombocytopenia. Consequently, the majority of cases of pneumonia, cellulitis, and some other infections are only clinically documented. It is not surprising that therapy is often ineffective when it has been selected without knowledge of the infecting pathogen. For example, less than 50% of pneumonias in neutropenic patients respond to initial antibiotic therapy.

MICROBIOLOGY

Neutropenic patients are susceptible to infection caused by a wide variety of organisms (Table 133–3). Before the availability of antibiotic therapy, many neutropenic patients died of pneumococcal and streptococcal infections. After the introduction of penicillin G, *Staphylococcus aureus* emerged as the most common cause of fatal infection. The introduction of the antistaphylococcal penicillins resulted in a dramatic decline in these infections and the emergence of gram-negative bacilli, and especially *Pseudomonas aeruginosa*, as the predominant pathogens.[5] With the availability of regimens producing broad-spectrum activity and the widespread use of intravascular catheters, gram-positive organisms have reemerged as important pathogens, accounting for about 60% to 70% of microbiologically documented infections.[13] Some of these infections are caused by organisms generally considered to be nonvirulent, such as *Bacillus cereus, Corynebacterium jeikeium*, and *Streptococcus viridans*. In addition, organisms that are resistant to the antibiotic regimens routinely utilized have emerged as significant pathogens in some institutions, such as *Stenotrophomonas* (formerly *Xanthomonas*) *maltophilia, Pseudomonas* species, and *Acinetobacter* species.

Several types of infection represent special problems for neutropenic patients. Pneumonia causes at least 25% of documented infections and is associated with a high mortality rate. Because neutropenic patients are unable to produce purulent sputum and invasive procedures often fail to identify the causative organism, selection of an appropriate therapy is often problematic, especially because a diversity of bacterial, viral, and fungal organisms can cause this infection.

Typhlitis, or necrotizing enterocolitis, is a life-threatening infection in neutropenic patients.[14] This infection presents with fever, watery or bloody diarrhea, and abdominal pain. The abdomen is distended; bowel sounds are diminished or absent; and there is tenderness often localized to the right lower quadrant. The infection is often associated with septicemia caused by *P. aeruginosa, Escherichia coli, Klebsiella* species, or *Clostridium septicum*. The infection typically involves the cecum but may be much more extensive. Some patients have responded to conservative therapy; surgery should be considered only in patients with localized infection.

Neutropenic patients are susceptible to perianal infections, which are especially common in patients with acute monocytic leukemia.[15] The patient presents with hectic or septic fever, rectal pain, and pain on defecation. The lesions are erythematous, indurated, or ulcerated; however, abscess formation occurs infrequently. These lesions are often associated with a fissure or a hemorrhoid. Tissue necrosis and septicemia, usually caused by aerobic gram-negative bacilli, are common. In addition to symptomatic therapy and broad-spectrum antibiotics, a surgical incision may be beneficial.

Several bacterial organisms pose special threats to the neutropenic patient. These patients are especially susceptible to infections caused by *P. aeruginosa*, although the frequency of these infections has declined. If not treated promptly, these infections can be fulminant.[16] Patients with *Pseudomonas* septicemia may develop characteristic skin lesions known as ecthyma gangrenosa, which usually arise in the groin, axilla, or perianal area. The lesion begins as a red macule, becomes pustular, and eventually evolves into a central bluish black necrotic area surrounded by an erythematous halo. Fulminant septicemia caused by *Clostridium* species, especially *Clostridium perfringens* and *C. septicum*, occur in neutropenic patients, often originating from an abdominal source.[17] These infections may be associated with acute hemolysis, gas gangrene, or spreading cellulitis and, when these complications occur, the outcome is almost always fatal despite appropriate therapy. Fulminant infections caused by several species of α-hemolytic streptococci have been recognized in patients with leukemia and also in bone marrow transplant recipients.[18] Although most cases of α-hemolytic streptococcus bacteremia respond promptly to appropriate therapy, patients occasionally develop rapidly fatal infections or infections associated with acute respiratory distress syndrome or renal failure. Some patients develop an erythematous rash that desquamates. Some of the infecting organisms are susceptible to penicillin G, but others are tolerant or resistant and require therapy with vancomycin.

Fungal organisms have emerged as significant pathogens in neutropenic patients during the past three decades. These infections occur most often in patients with prolonged severe neutropenia; hence, they are diagnosed most often in patients with acute leukemia or in bone marrow transplant recipients. It has become apparent that these latter patients remain susceptible to fungal infections for several months after their marrow has successfully engrafted and their neutropenia has resolved. For many years the majority of fungal infections were caused by *Candida albicans*. *Candida tropicalis* is now as common as *C. albicans* in many cancer centers, and other species such as *Candida parapsilosis, Candida krusei*i, and *Torulopsis glabrata* are not uncommon at some institutions. *Aspergillus* species, once a rare cause of infection, are now a common cause of respiratory infections in neutropenic patients. Other important fungal pathogens include *Fusarium* species and *Trichosporon* species. Less commonly, other molds such as Mucorales, *Bipolaris* species, and *Alternaria* species may cause serious infections.[19]

Oropharyngeal candidiasis and esophageal candidiasis are relatively common in neutropenic patients and usually respond promptly to antifungal therapy. Disseminated candidiasis is a serious and often fatal infection. The infection is difficult to diagnose, because most patients present with persistent fever unresponsive to antibacterial antibiotics and deteriorating organ function without any characteristic clinical findings. The organism is cultured from blood specimens in less than 50% of infected patients. Antifungal therapy is seldom effective unless the patient's neutropenia resolves.[20] A chronic form of disseminated candidiasis, usually involv-

TABLE 133–3 ■ Organisms Causing Infection in Neutropenic Patients

FREQUENT	LESS COMMON
	Bacteria
Staphylococcus aureus	*Corynebacterium jeikeium*
Staphylococcus epidermidis	*Bacillus* spp.
Streptococcus viridans	*Enterococcus* spp.
Pseudomonas aeruginosa	*Clostridium* spp.
Enterobacteriaceae	*Capnocytophaga* spp.
	Stenotrophomonas (formerly *Xanthomonas*) *maltophilia*
	Pseudomonas spp.
	Aeromonas spp.
	Fungi
Candida spp.	*Trichosporon* spp.
Aspergillus spp.	*Fusarium* spp.
	Mucorales

ing the liver and spleen, has been recognized in neutropenic patients.[21] Characteristically, these patients have a persistent fever that originates while they are neutropenic and continues after their neutrophil counts recover. At this time they may develop hepatosplenomegaly, and most will have a highly elevated serum alkaline phosphatase value. Multiple lesions are found in the liver and spleen at abdominal imaging. The disease is often chronic, and although it responds to amphotericin B therapy, fluconazole appears to be more effective.

Aspergillus species are respiratory pathogens; hence, most infections involve the lung.[22] Because the organisms invade blood vessels and cause thrombosis and infarction, some patients present with symptoms suggestive of acute pulmonary embolism. The earliest manifestation of aspergillosis on chest x-ray examination is the appearance of single or multiple nodular lesions. Approximately 30% of patients develop infections of the sinus and orbit. These infections may destroy the eye or erode into the brain, causing cerebral infarction. Primary cutaneous aspergillosis has been associated with intravascular catheters. Disseminated aspergillosis occurs in about 30% of infected patients. Fusariosis resembles aspergillosis, but dissemination occurs in approximately 75% of cases and is often associated with skin lesions.[23] These mold infections rarely respond to therapy unless neutropenia resolves.

TREATMENT

Initial empirical antibacterial therapy for the febrile neutropenic patient must provide broad-spectrum activity against the most likely bacterial pathogens. For many years, the combination of a broad-spectrum penicillin or cephalosporin with antipseudomonal activity plus an aminoglycoside was the standard regimen.[24] Studies indicate that some antibiotics (e.g., imipenem and ceftazidime) may be used without an aminoglycoside. Almost all infected patients have intravascular catheters in place; therefore, coverage against methicillin-resistant gram-positive organisms is often necessary. Vancomycin is usually included as part of the initial regimen, but this drug should be discontinued promptly if not needed to avoid problems with vancomycin resistance.[25] Patients who fail to respond after 3 to 4 days of broad-spectrum antibacterial therapy should be considered candidates for empirical antifungal therapy; however, a careful evaluation of these patients is necessary, because some patients may be infected by antibiotic-resistant bacterial or viral pathogens.[26]

Impairments in Cell-Mediated Immunity

Other cellular elements, in addition to the neutrophil, play an important role in host defenses against infection. These elements include the T lymphocyte, monocyte, and macrophage. Deficiencies in cell number or function may result from the malignant disease or its therapy. Diseases that are characteristically associated with deficiencies in cellular immunity include lymphomas, Hodgkin's disease, chronic lymphocytic leukemia, and hairy cell leukemia. Adrenal corticosteroids interfere with several aspects of cell-mediated immunity, including causing lympholysis and interfering with macrophage function. Antitumor agents also affect various aspects of cellular immunity, different agents having different effects.[1] Although some of these effects can be detected at doses of drugs that do not cause myelosuppression, immunosuppression often occurs concomitantly with myelosuppression.

CLINICAL FEATURES AND MICROBIOLOGY

Patients with impaired cell-mediated immunity are susceptible to a different group of pathogens than are neutropenic patients (Table 133–4). Most of these organisms are intracellular pathogens. Brucellosis used to be a relatively common infection in patients with Hodgkin's disease but occurs rarely in the United States at present. *Listeria monocytogenes* most frequently causes meningitis or septicemia.[27] It is important to recognize patients who are at risk of this infection, because the therapies of choice (ampicillin, trimethoprim-sulfamethoxazole) are often not included in antibiotic regimens commonly used as empirical therapy in cancer patients, and these infections can be rapidly fatal. Although *Nocardia* infections have been associated historically with patients with lymphoma, these infections are also found in patients with solid tumors. The organisms can cause infections of the lung or central nervous system. *Salmonella* infections have been associated with malignant lymphoma. *Salmonella typhimurium* is a common cause of serious infection in these patients, whereas it usually causes only gastroenteritis in normal individuals. *Salmonella* species may cause septicemia, pneumonia, urinary tract infection, osteomyelitis, or meningitis.

Patients with impaired cellular immunity are at increased risk of contracting tuberculosis. Most of these are pulmonary infections but some patients develop disseminated infection. At some cancer institutions, atypical mycobacterial infections are almost as common as tuberculosis. For example, disseminated *Mycobacterium kansasii* and *Mycobacterium avium-intracellulare* infections have been described in patients with hairy cell leukemia, a disease characterized by monocytopenia.

Cryptococcosis is the most common fungal infection in these patients. It is a respiratory pathogen, so infection begins in the lung.[28] Some patients develop a rapidly progressive pneumonia that can terminate fatally despite appropriate therapy. More often, patients present with disseminated infection, which is usually manifested as meningitis. Other organs involved in disseminated infection include lymph nodes, liver, kidneys, bone, and skin. Histoplasmosis and coccidioidomycosis may cause serious problems in patients with impaired cellular immunity. Patients may have latent

TABLE 133–4 ■ Organisms Causing Infection in Patients with Impaired Cellular Immunity

BACTERIA	FUNGI	VIRUSES	PARASITES
Listeria monocytogenes	*Cryptococcus neoformans*	Cytomegalovirus	*Pneumocystis carinii*
Mycobacterium tuberculosis	*Histoplasma capsulatum*	Herpes simplex virus	*Toxoplasma gondii*
Legionella spp.	*Coccidioides immitis*	Herpes zoster virus	*Strongyloides stercoralis*
Nocardia spp.	*Candida* spp. (superficial infection)	Respiratory syncytial virus	
Brucella spp.	*Aspergillus* spp.	Influenza virus	
Mycobacterium spp.		Parainfluenza virus	
		JC virus*	

*Cause of progressive multifocal leukoencephalopathy.

foci from infection acquired while they were immunocompetent that reactivate when they become immunocompromised, resulting in disseminated disease. Patients who acquire their infection when immunocompromised may develop fulminant pneumonia or acute disseminated infection.

Viral infections are prevalent in many cancer patients but are a special problem in patients with hematologic malignancies and in bone marrow transplant recipients. Although many of these infections occur in severely neutropenic patients, deficiencies in host defenses other than neutropenia are most likely responsible for the patient's susceptibility to these infections. The most common viral infections are those caused by herpesviruses. Varicella epidemics have occurred in pediatric cancer services. Patients occasionally develop rapidly progressive infection with circulatory collapse and death shortly after the vesicles appear. Disseminated infection may result in widespread pneumonia or focal necrosis of the liver, pancreas, or adrenal glands. The vesicular skin lesions may become necrotic and hemorrhagic, especially in thrombocytopenic patients. Herpes zoster may arise at sites where the tumor is close to a nerve trunk or at sites of recent radiotherapy. Localized herpes zoster often causes no special problems, but slow healing, necrosis, and scarring may result. Postherpetic neuralgia appears to be more common, and some patients develop disseminated cutaneous infection. Dissemination to internal organs is uncommon.

Lesions caused by herpes simplex virus most often involve the lips or oral mucosa and occasionally the genitalia. The lesions may become quite large and painful. Multiple lesions may coalesce and become superinfected with bacteria, especially *S. aureus*. Oral ulcerations due to cancer chemotherapy may be more severe in patients with a history of herpes simplex. Patients sometimes develop herpetic esophagitis. Pneumonia and disseminated infection occur rarely. Acyclovir and famcyclovir are useful for therapy for all of these herpesvirus infections.

Cytomegalovirus infection is a special problem among bone marrow recipients, although it occurs occasionally in patients with hematologic malignancies.[29] The risk of this infection in transplant recipients has been reduced by screening of donors, recipients, and blood products and by the use of prophylaxis. A variety of syndromes have been due to cytomegalovirus. Some patients develop a relatively benign viremia that is associated with fever and occasionally an elevation of liver function test results. Other patients may develop a mononucleosis syndrome or delayed marrow recovery. The most serious infections that are likely to occur in cancer patients are pneumonitis and colitis; rarely, these patients develop hepatitis, myocarditis, retinitis, or encephalitis.

It has become apparent that community respiratory viruses can cause serious pulmonary infections in immunocompromised hosts.[30] Although the majority of these infections have been recognized in neutropenic patients, especially in bone marrow recipients and patients with acute leukemia, it is likely that deficiencies other than neutropenia are responsible for these infections. Respiratory syncytial virus infection is the most prevalent of these infections, and epidemics have been detected on transplant and leukemia services during the respiratory syncytial virus season. The patient may acquire infection from members of the community, from other patients, or from hospital personnel. Some patients may suffer only upper respiratory tract infection, but once the disease progresses to the tracheobronchial tree and the lung, the fatality rate is high if the disease is not treated promptly with aerosolized ribavirin. High-titer immunoglobulin may also play an important role in successful therapy. Strict infection control measures during the season of infection with this virus can greatly reduce the extent of this problem. Influenza virus and parainfluenza virus can also cause serious infection in these patients.

Pneumocystis carinii causes pneumonia in some cancer patients with impaired cellular immunity. In some institutions, until prophylactic programs were introduced, this infection was common among children with acute leukemia who had achieved remission of their disease but were receiving intensive consolidation therapy. In most patients the pneumonitis represents reactivation of latent infection, but in some cases it is newly acquired. The infection may be insidious or rapidly progressive and often presents initially as fever and nonproductive cough with progression to tachypnea, dyspnea, and cyanosis with the slightest exertion. Characteristically, the chest radiograph reveals more extensive pneumonitis than is suspected by the physical examination. The diagnosis is usually confirmed by bronchoalveolar lavage, and therapy with trimethoprim-sulfamethoxazole is generally effective.

Toxoplasmosis in cancer patients may represent reactivation or newly acquired infection. The infection disseminates to many organs, but approximately 60% of patients present with central nervous system infection—some with signs of encephalitis and others with focal neurologic defects.[31] Some patients develop pneumonia, myocarditis, or hepatitis. The diagnosis is established by identification of the organisms in clinical specimens or by serologic tests. Therapy with pyrimethamine and sulfadiazine is effective in about half of infected cancer patients, and the prognosis is especially poor in the case of central nervous system infection.

Because of the wide diversity of organisms causing infection in patients with impaired cell-mediated immunity, it is not possible to devise an empirical regimen that will provide adequate coverage for these patients. Consequently, the focus in these patients must be on the institution of appropriate diagnostic procedures. It is critically important, however, that these procedures are performed expeditiously, because even apparently inconsequential infections can progress rapidly and cause death.

Hypogammaglobulinemia and Splenectomy

Deficiencies in the production of normal immunoglobulins are characteristic of multiple myeloma and Waldenström macroglobulinemia but can also occur in chronic lymphocytic leukemia and in some lymphomas. The frequency of infectious complications has been related to the patient's ability to produce an antibody to antigenic stimuli. The pathogens that classically cause infection in patients with impaired humoral immunity are the encapsulated organisms, *Streptococcus pneumoniae, Haemophilus influenzae*, and *Neisseria meningitidis*. These organisms can cause fulminant septicemia, resulting in a fatal outcome despite appropriate therapy. Intravenous γ-globulin prophylaxis is effective in these patients. The use of more intensive chemotherapeutic regimens has altered the types of infections prevalent in these populations.

Some patients with hematologic malignancies require splenectomy as management of their disease. This results in deficiencies of tuftsin, a phagocytosis-stimulating peptide. Their antibody response to new antigens is also deficient. These patients are also susceptible to fulminant infections caused by encapsulated organisms, especially during the first 6 months after splenectomy. Babesiosis can also be a severe infection in these patients.

Other Predisposing Factors to Infection

Numerous other factors predispose to infection in the cancer patient (Table 133–5). Many of these factors are not unique to the cancer population, but a few are a consequence of the

TABLE 133–5 ■ Organisms Causing Infection Related to Therapeutic Interventions

CHEMOTHERAPY
Interleukin-2: Gram-positive cocci
Fludarabine: *Listeria monocytogenes, Pneumocystis carinii*
Adrenal corticosteroids: *Aspergillus* spp., *L. monocytogenes, P. carinii*
MUCOSITIS
Streptococcus viridans
Capnocytophaga spp.
Candida spp.
Herpes simplex virus
Stomatococcus spp.
INTRAVASCULAR CATHETERS
Staphylococcus epidermidis
Staphylococcus aureus
Corynebacterium jeikeium
Bacillus spp.
Pseudomonas aeruginosa
Acinetobacter spp.
Stenotrophomonas (formerly *Xanthomonas*) *maltophilia*
Candida spp.

malignancy or its therapy. Among the unique factors are some that are directly related to the tumor. Bronchogenic carcinomas may cause obstruction to bronchi, resulting in postobstructive pneumonia that is often difficult to treat successfully unless the obstruction can be eliminated. Obstruction to the urinary tract may be caused by tumors of these organs or by tumor-bearing lymph nodes. Ulceration or necrosis of tumor masses frequently leads to superinfection. Long-term successful management of such infections depends on the ability to remove the tumor mass. Shunts, stints, ileal bladders, hepatobiliary drains, and other devices may lead to infectious complications that are difficult to manage. These types of infection can often be treated successfully initially; however, antibiotic-susceptible organisms are eventually replaced by resistant organisms that fail to respond to therapy.

Chemotherapy-induced mucositis is a frequent cause of infection. Although attention is focused on the oropharynx where mucositis is easily visualized and frequently symptomatic, often the entire gastrointestinal mucosa is involved. A physical examination of the oropharynx cannot always discriminate between tissue damage and infection. Septicemia related to mucositis has been associated with *S. viridans, Capnocytophaga* species, and *Stomatococcus mucilaginosus*. Herpes simplex virus and *Candida* species contribute to the severity of local symptoms and tissue damage.

Factors that are common to other hospitalized patients also have an impact on infection in cancer patients. Patients are exposed to nosocomial pathogens on admission to the hospital and especially to the intensive care unit. The administration of broad-spectrum antibiotic regimens facilitates colonization by resistant organisms. The widespread use of intravascular catheters has had a major impact on the types of organisms causing bacteremia. Organisms associated with catheter-related infections include *Staphylococcus epidermidis, S. aureus, S. maltophilia, Enterococcus* species, *P. aeruginosa*, and *Candida* species. The use of specially trained personnel, meticulous catheter care, implantable devices, and more extensive outpatient management have helped to reduce these problems.

Prophylaxis of Infection

Various measures have been introduced to prevent infections in cancer patients (Table 133–6). The decision to use such

TABLE 133–6 ■ Approaches to Infection Prophylaxis

Antibacterial agents (fluoroquinolones, trimethoprim-sulfamethoxazole)
Antifungal agents (fluconazole, nystatin, clotrimazole)
Antiviral agents (acyclovir, ganciclovir)
γ-Globulin
Air filtration (high-efficiency particulate air units, laminar airflow)
Isolation units (protected environments)
Specially prepared food
Dental care (topical antimicrobials)
Immunization
Growth factors (granulocyte colony-stimulating factor; granulocyte-macrophage colony-stimulating factor)

measures should take into consideration the frequency of the infection, the usual outcome of therapy, the potential adverse effects, and the cost of prophylaxis. For example, antifungal prophylaxis is indicated in many leukemia services because the frequency of major *Candida* infections exceeds 20%, and the mortality rate exceeds 80% among persistently neutropenic patients. Some investigators have espoused the concept of selective decontamination whereby antibacterial agents are administered that suppress the aerobic gram-negative flora but preserve the anaerobic flora. This theory proposes that the anaerobic flora prevents acquisition of resistant organisms, an attractive concept that has not been adequately demonstrated in patients. The use of growth factors in association with intensive antitumor or marrow transplant regimens can shorten the duration of neutropenia and, in some cases, reduce the frequency of infectious complications.[32] Simple measures such as meticulous hand washing, appropriate infection control measures, and proper air filtration can have a substantial impact on infection prophylaxis and are sometimes neglected by hospital personnel.

References

1. Bodey GP, Hersh EM, Valdivieso M, et al: Effects of cytotoxic drugs and immunosuppressive agents on the immune system. Postgrad Med 58:67, 1975.
2. Pickering LK, Ericsson CD, Hohl S: Effect of chemotherapeutic agents on metabolic and bactericidal activity of polymorphonuclear leukocytes. Cancer 42:1741, 1978.
3. Browder AA, Huff JW, Petersdorf RD: The significance of fever in neoplastic disease. Ann Intern Med 55:932, 1961.
4. Casazza AT, Duvall CP, Carbone PP: Infection in lymphoma—histology, treatment and duration in relation to incidence and survival. JAMA 197:710, 1966.
5. Hersh EM, Bodey GP, Nies BA, et al: Causes of death in acute leukemia: A ten year study of 414 patients from 1954–1963. JAMA 198:105, 1965.
6. Feld R, Bodey GP, Rodriguez V, et al: Causes of death in patients with malignant lymphoma. Am J Med Sci 268:97, 1974.
7. Estey EH, Keating MJ, McCredie KB, et al: Causes of initial remission induction failure in acute myelogenous leukemia. Blood 60:309, 1982.
8. Bodey GP, Buckley M, Sathe YS, et al: Quantitative relationships between circulating leukocytes and infection in patients with acute leukemia. Ann Intern Med 64:328, 1966.
9. Bodey GP: Antibiotics in patients with neutropenia. Arch Intern Med 144:1845, 1984.
10. Sickles EA, Greene WH, Wiernik PH, et al: Clinical presentation of infection in granulocytopenic patients. Arch Intern Med 135:715, 1975.
11. Valdivieso M, Gil-Extremera B, Zornoza J, et al: Gram-negative bacillary pneumonia in the compromised host. Medicine (Baltimore) 56:241, 1977.
12. Lawson RD, Gentry LO, Bodey GP, et al: Randomized study of tobramycin plus ticarcillin, tobramycin plus cephalothin and

ticarcillin, or tobramycin plus mezlocillin in the treatment of infection in neutropenic patients with malignancies. Am J Med Sci 287:16, 1984.
13. Viscoli C, Van der Auwera P, Meunier F: Gram-positive infections in granulocytopenic patients: An important issue? J Antimicrob Chemother 21(Suppl C):149, 1988.
14. Dosik GM, Luna M, Valdivieso M, et al: Necrotizing colitis in patients with cancer. Am J Med 67:646, 1979.
15. VanHeuverzwyn R, Delannoy A, Michaux JL, Dive C: Anal lesions in hematologic diseases. Dis Colon Rectum 23:310, 1980.
16. Bodey GP, Jadega L, Elting L: *Pseudomonas* bacteremia: Retrospective analysis of 410 episodes. Arch Intern Med 145:1621, 1985.
17. Bodey GP, Rodriguez S, Fainstein V, Elting LS: Clostridial bacteremia in cancer patients. A 12 year experience. Cancer 67:1928, 1991.
18. Bochud PY, Calandra T, Francioli P: Bacteremia due to viridans streptococci in neutropenic patients: A review. Am J Med 97:256, 1994.
19. Anaissie E, Bodey GP, Kantarjian H, et al: New spectrum of fungal infections in patients with cancer. Rev Infect Dis 11(Suppl 7):369, 1989.
20. Bodey GP: Hematogenous and major organ candidiasis. *In* Bodey GP (ed): Candidiasis: Pathogenesis, Diagnosis, and Treatment. New York, Raven Press, 1992, pp 279–329.
21. Haron E, Feld R, Tuffnell P, et al: Hepatic candidiasis: An increasing problem in immunocompromised hosts. Am J Med 83:17, 1987.
22. Bodey GP, Vartivarian S: Aspergillosis. Eur J Clin Microbiol Infect Dis 8:413, 1989.
23. Rabodonirina M, Piens MA, Monier MF, et al: Fusarium infections in immunocompromised patients: Case reports and literature review. Eur J Clin Microbiol Infect Dis 13:152, 1994.
24. Hughes WT, Armstrong D, Bodey GP, et al: Guidelines for the use of antimicrobial agents in neutropenic patients with unexplained fever. J Infect Dis 161:381, 1990.
25. EORTC. Vancomycin added to empirical combination antibiotic therapy for fever in granulocytopenic cancer patients. J Infect Dis 163:951, 1991.
26. EORTC International Antimicrobial Therapy Cooperative Group: Empiric antifungal therapy in febrile granulocytopenic patients. Am J Med 86:668, 1989.
27. Louria DB, Henselee T, Armstrong D, et al: Listeriosis complicating malignant disease. Ann Intern Med 67:261, 1967.
28. Zimmerman LE, Rappoport H: Occurrence of cryptococcosis in patients with malignant disease of the reticuloendothelial system. Am J Clin Pathol 24:1050, 1954.
29. Zaia JA, Churchill MA: Human cytomegalovirus infection after bone marrow transplantation. *In* Lode H, Huhn D, Molzahn M (eds): Infections in Transplant Patients. International Symposium, Berlin. Stuttgart, Georg Thieme Verlag, 1987, pp 116–126.
30. Whimbey E, Bodey GP: Viral pneumonia in the immunocompromised adult with neoplastic disease: The role of common community respiratory viruses. Semin Respir Infect 7:122, 1992.
31. Vietzke WM, Gelderman AH, Grimley PM, Valsamis MD: Toxoplasmosis complicating malignancy: Experience at the National Cancer Institute. Cancer 21:816, 1968.
32. Maher DW, Lieschke GJ, Green M, et al: Filgrastin in patients with chemotherapy-induced febrile neutropenia. Ann Intern Med 121:492, 1994.

134

Infections in Organ Transplant Recipients

Nina E. Tolkoff-Rubin
Robert H. Rubin

One of the major triumphs of 20th century biomedical science is the successful rehabilitation of patients with end-stage renal, hepatic, and cardiac disease after organ transplantation. At transplant centers around the world, 1-year allograft survival rates are better than 80% for each of these organs (in the case of kidney allograft recipients, for whom life-sustaining dialysis is available when the allograft fails, the 1-year survival rate exceeds 90%), and the drop-off in survival of allografts and patients thereafter is small. This remarkable achievement can be attributed to advances in both the technical and the "immunologic" aspects of organ transplantation, because impeccable management of both is essential if the two major barriers to successful transplantation, allograft rejection and infection, are to be overcome. It is important to emphasize that in transplant recipients infection and rejection are closely linked by the requirement for lifelong immunosuppressive therapy to combat rejection. Because of this requirement, infection remains the leading cause of death at all times after transplantation, and more than two thirds of transplant recipients endure at least one significant infection.[1]

The risk of infection in organ transplant recipients is determined principally by the interaction of two major factors: the epidemiologic exposures that the patient encounters and the net state of immunosuppression. Epidemiologic exposures can be divided into three general categories (Table 134–1). (1) Remote infections are ones that were acquired months to years earlier, have incited a protective host immunologic response, and are dormant at the time of transplantation.

TABLE 134–1 ■ Epidemiologic Exposures of Importance to Transplant Recipients

Exposure before transplantation
Mycobacterium tuberculosis
Histoplasma capsulatum
Coccidioides immitis
Blastomyces dermatitidis
Stronglyloides stercoralis
Hepatitis B and C viruses
Human immunodeficiency virus
Community-acquired exposure after transplantation
Influenza virus (and other respiratory viruses)
Varicella-zoster virus (primary infection)
Nontyphoidal *Salmonella*
M. tuberculosis (and the fungal infections listed above)
Legionella species
Nocardia asteroides
Cryptococcus neoformans
Nosocomial epidemiologic exposure
Aspergillus species
Legionella species
Pseudomonas aeruginosa and other gram-negative bacilli

The initiation of immunosuppressive therapy results in an attenuation of the host response and the potential for reactivation and systemic dissemination as well as superinfection if another exposure should occur. Tuberculosis, the geographically restricted systemic mycoses, and strongyloidiasis are prime examples of this phenomenon. (2) Community-acquired infections circulate in the general population, but their impact is much greater on the transplant recipient, with disseminated or complicated infection (e.g., bacterial superinfection of viral respiratory processes) being more common than in the general population. In addition, exposure to tuberculosis and the systemic mycoses after transplantation can result in both progressive primary infection and systemic dissemination at a rate and to an extent that are not observed in the general population. (3) Nosocomial infections are acquired when immunosuppressed transplant recipients are exposed to air or potable water that is contaminated with infectious agents such as *Aspergillus* species, *Legionella* species, and gram-negative organisms such as *Pseudomonas aeruginosa*.[1–4] Such outbreaks are of two types: domiciliary, in which patients are exposed to contaminated air on the wards where they reside in the hospital, and nondomiciliary, in which the patients are exposed to the contaminated air at central locations in the hospital, such as radiology or surgical suites, where they are taken for essential procedures. Domiciliary epidemics are relatively easy to detect because of clustering of cases in time and space and can be effectively prevented by the provision of high-efficiency particle air filtration to patients' rooms, but nondomiciliary outbreaks are much more difficult to detect and to prevent. They are also probably more common. Immunosuppressed patients such as transplant recipients have been likened to sentinels, who signal any excessive exposure to microorganisms in the hospital environment by developing life-threatening infection.[5, 6]

The net state of immunosuppression is a complex function that is determined by a variety of factors: the type, dose, and temporal sequence of immunosuppressive therapy being administered; the presence or absence of such factors as granulocytopenia, injury to the primary mucocutaneous barriers to infection, and indwelling foreign bodies such as vascular, urinary, and biliary catheters; and metabolic factors such as malnutrition, and possibly uremia and hyperglycemia. In addition, it is now apparent that certain immunomodulating viruses contribute significantly to the net state of immunosuppression—cytomegalovirus (CMV), Epstein-Barr virus (EBV), the hepatitis viruses, and the human immunodeficiency virus (HIV), among them. The important contribution of these agents to the net state of immunosuppression is underlined by the following observation: the only transplant recipients with invasive, opportunistic infection identified over a period of several years who did not have preexisting viral infection were those who were exposed to an unusually intense nosocomial hazard. Indeed, this can be an important clue to the presence of a nosocomial epidemic.[1, 2]

Expected Timetable of Infection in Organ Transplant Recipients

As the approach to immunosuppressive therapy and to surgical management of organ transplant recipients has become standardized, a stereotyped timetable describing when in the posttransplant course a given infection is likely to occur has emerged (Fig. 134–1). This timetable can be utilized in two ways: to establish the possible cause of an infectious disease syndrome in an individual patient (e.g., the causes of pneumonia in the first month after transplantation are quite different from those in the third month), and as the basis of a system for monitoring excessive environmental hazards (exceptions to the timetable are almost invariably due to unusual and unexpected epidemiologic exposures, usually within the hospital environment). It is useful, in terms of etiologic considerations, to divide the posttransplantation course into three different periods.[1, 2]

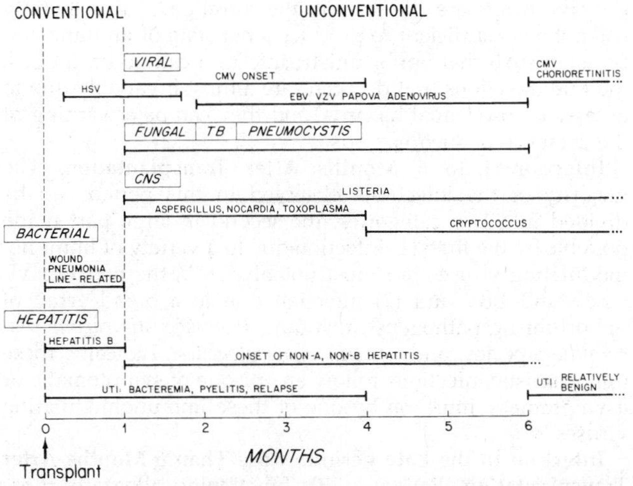

FIGURE 134–1 ▫ Timetable for the occurrence of infection in the organ transplant recipient. Exceptions to this timetable should prompt a search for an unusual hazard. CMV, Cytomegalovirus; HSV, herpes simplex virus; EBV, Epstein-Barr virus; VZV, varicella-zoster virus; CNS, central nervous system; UTI, urinary tract infection. (From Rubin RH, Wolfson JS, Cosimi AB, Tolkoff-Rubin NE: Infection in the renal transplant recipient. Am J Med 70:405–411, 1981.)

Infection in the First Month After Transplantation. Three categories of infection should be considered in transplant recipients who present with clinical syndromes of possible infectious origin. (1) Infection that was present in the transplant recipient before the transplant operation and that is exacerbated by the operation, anesthesia, or the institution of immunosuppressive therapy. This is a particular problem with liver and cardiac transplant candidates, who may require life support systems, with all of the infectious disease problems inherent with such intensive care, before transplantation. Thus, pneumonia, intravenous access–related infection, and smouldering infections such as tuberculosis and strongyloidiasis are of concern. (2) Infection can be transmitted with a contaminated allograft (usually due to an undetected blood stream infection in the donor). Whether blood stream infection is occurring in the donor or recipient at the time of transplantation, the vascular anastamoses are at risk for microbial seeding. When such seeding occurs, mycotic aneurysms with the risk of catastrophic rupture will result. (3) More than 95% of the infections that occur in this time period are the same bacterial or candidal infections of the surgical wound, lungs, urine, vascular access, or drainage catheters observed in nonimmunosuppressed patients undergoing comparable forms of surgery, although the consequences in transplant recipients can be much greater. Although appropriate antimicrobial prophylaxis offers some protection against these infections, the major determinant is the technical skill with which the surgery is performed and the various invasive lines and catheters are managed. Because of the particular technical demands associated with liver and lung transplantation, these transplant recipients are at greatest risk for this form of infectious complication.[1, 2]

Noteworthy by their absence in this period are opportunistic infections. Even though the daily doses of immunosuppressive drugs are the largest, the duration of this therapy has not been sufficient to produce a net state of immunosuppression such that opportunistic infection can occur. Indeed, the rare infections that do occur are almost invariably due to excessive nosocomial hazards, and they can be a warning of the presence of such hazards.

Infection 1 to 6 Months After Transplantation. The majority of the infections observed in this period can be divided into two categories, the second in large part made possible by the first: (1) infection due to a variety of immunomodulating viruses but most notably CMV, the hepatitis viruses, and EBV and (2) infection due to a broad array of opportunistic pathogens, including *Pneumocystis carinii*, *Aspergillus* species, and *Listeria monocytogenes*. Typically, these opportunistic infections follow an episode of symptomatic or asymptomatic infection by one of these immunomodulating viruses.[1, 2, 7]

Infection in the Late Period, More Than 6 Months After Transplantation. Patients with functioning allografts more than 6 months after transplantation can be divided into three major categories in terms of infectious disease risk. (1) The patients who have good allograft function, are receiving only maintenance immunosuppressive therapy, and are free of chronic viral infection (70% to 80% of this population) are at risk primarily for the same infections that affect the general community (e.g., influenza, pneumococcal pneumonia, urinary tract infection). (2) The patients with chronic viral infection (5% to 15% of this population) are at risk for progressive destruction of the target organ (e.g., the liver from hepatitis B virus [HBV] or hepatitis C virus [HCV]; the retina from CMV), malignancy (e.g., hepatocellular carcinoma due to HBV or HCV infection), or overt acquired immunodeficiency syndrome (AIDS) (from HIV infection). (3) The patients whom we have called "chronic n'er do wells," with less than ideal allograft function, a history of excessive immunosuppressive therapy, and a high incidence of chronic viral infection (5% to 10% of this population), are at the highest risk of any organ transplant group for opportunistic infection with such pathogens as *P. carinii*, *L. monocytogenes*, and *Nocardia asteroides*.[1, 2, 7]

TABLE 134–2 ■ Categories of Infection in Organ Transplant Recipients

Infections related to technical complications*
Transplantation of a contaminated allograft
Anastomotic leaks or stenosis
Inappropriate management of endotracheal tube
Wound hematoma
Contamination of intravenous or intraarterial line
Contamination of urinary, biliary, or drainage catheter
Iatrogenic damage to the skin
Infections related to excessive nosocomial hazard
Aspergillus spp.
Legionella spp.
Pseudomonas aeruginosa and other gram-negative bacilli
Nocardia asteroides
Infections related to particular exposure in the community
Systemic mycotic infections in certain geographic areas
Histoplasma capsulatum
Coccidioides immitis
Blastomyces dermatitidis
Community-acquired opportunistic infection due to ubiquitous saprophytes in the environment†
Cryptococcus neoformans
Aspergillus spp.
N. asteroides
Pneumocystis carinii
Typical and atypical mycobacterial infections
Strongyloides stercoralis
Respiratory infections circulating in the community
Influenza virus
Streptococcus pneumoniae
Infections acquired by ingestion of contaminated food or water
Salmonella spp.
Listeria monocytogenes
Viral infections of particular importance to transplant patients
Herpes simplex viruses
Hepatitis viruses
HIV
Papovaviruses

*All lead to infection with gram-negative bacilli, *Staphylococcus*, or *Candida* species.

†The incidence and severity of these infections (and, to a lesser extent, the other infections listed) are directly related to the net state of immunosuppression in the particular patient.

Modified from Rubin RH: Infection in organ transplant recipients. *In* Rubin RH, Young LS (eds): Clinical Approach to Infection in the Compromised Host, ed 3. New York, Plenum Publishing, 1994, pp 629–705.

Infections of Special Importance in Organ Transplant Recipients

From the preceding comments it is clear that infections of transplant recipients can be divided into four major categories: those related to technical complications, those related to particular epidemiologic exposures, those due to certain viruses, and opportunistic infections due to organisms that are essentially nonpathogenic for normal hosts (Table 134–2). Although viruses are the single most important group of microbial pathogens for transplant recipients, bacterial, fungal, and parasitic infections must be considered as well, because their occurrence is much influenced by technical and epidemiologic factors as well as the immunomodulating effects of certain viruses.

Viral Infections

The most important form of infection affecting organ transplant recipients is that caused by viruses. The potential clinical impact of viral infections for these patients is much broader than for immunocompetent hosts.[2] Viral infections can directly cause syndromes such as fever, pneumonia, and hepatitis. They can produce a global state of immunosuppression that makes possible superinfection by opportunistic pathogens such as *P. carinii*, *L. monocytogenes*, and various fungal organisms. They can initiate a series of pathogenic events that damage the allograft by mechanisms other than those of classic allograft rejection. Finally, in persons whose immune function is permanently suppressed, a virus can contribute to the development of malignancies. Of the viruses that occur in transplant recipients, the herpesviruses, the hepatitis viruses, the papovaviruses, and HIV have had the greatest clinical impact.

Herpesviruses. The human herpesviruses share several characteristics that make them particularly well adapted to cause significant disease in transplant recipients, as follows.

Latency. Once infected with a herpesvirus, an individual forever harbors nonreplicating virus that is capable of being reactivated by factors such as certain forms of immunosuppression and certain cytokines released during allograft rejection, systemic sepsis, and other processes. (Serologic positivity in the absence of replicating virus is the laboratory marker of latent infection.)

Cell Association. The virus spreads from cell to cell by direct contact, rendering neutralizing antibody relatively inefficient and cell-mediated immunity, particularly virus-specific cytotoxic T cells, of critical importance in the control of such infections.

Oncogenicity. All herpesviruses should be considered potentially oncogenic, the clearest evidence of this phenomenon being the association of EBV with B-cell lymphoproliferative disease.

Cytomegalovirus. CMV is the single most important infectious agent affecting organ transplant recipients: at least two thirds of them manifest at least laboratory evidence of CMV infection. The direct clinical effects of CMV are outlined in Table 134–3 and are similar in all forms of organ transplantation, with one possible exception: a transplanted organ may be more affected than an endogenous organ. Thus, CMV hepatitis is an important problem in liver transplantation, but a relatively minor one in transplantation of other organs. Similarly, CMV myocarditis in heart transplant patients and CMV pancreatitis in pancreas transplant recipients can be significant problems, whereas they are rarely problems in recipients of other organs. It should be emphasized that CMV is the predominant cause of infectious disease syndromes in the second through the sixth month after transplantation.[1, 7–9]

It has become apparent that the indirect effects of CMV are probably even more important than the direct effects.[10] Infection with CMV clearly predisposes to potentially lethal superinfection by agents such as *P. carinii, L. monocytogenes,* and a variety of fungi.[1, 10–12] In addition, there is increasing evidence that CMV may play a role in the pathogenesis of allograft injury. Thus, a particular form of glomerulopathy in kidney allograft recipients,[13] both a distinct histologic picture associated with acute liver allograft dysfunction[14] and the disappearing bile duct syndrome of chronic dysfunction,[15] both acute allograft dysfunction and accelerated coronary artery atherosclerosis in heart allograft recipients, and bronchiolitis obliterans in lung allograft recipients[16–20] have been associated with CMV infection.[12] The role and the mechanism by which CMV exerts its effects on these processes are currently unclear, with two major but not necessarily mutually exclusive theories being proposed.[1, 12] One theory is that CMV infection results in direct immune injury of the allograft by a process of molecular mimicry. Sequence homology and immune cross-reactivity between an immediate early antigen of human CMV and the human leukocyte antigen DR β-chain have been demonstrated. In addition, CMV-infected cells produce a glycoprotein homologous to major histocompatibility complex class I antigens. The hypothesis, then, would be that an immune response to the virus would also affect allograft cells that bear either the appropriate human leukocyte DR antigen or the particular class I antigen. Another theory is that CMV infection has a more indirect effect on the pathogenesis of these processes. Studies have demonstrated that CMV infection of both vascular smooth muscle and endothelium is a regular occurrence during CMV infection, thus providing a mechanism for vascular injury, which is an important aspect of chronic allograft rejection.[21–23] Infected cells manifest a down-regulation of major histocompatibility complex class I antigens, but surrounding cells, because of the local elaboration of cytokines, manifest an up-regulation of these antigens as well as adhesion molecules such as intercellular adhesion molecule-1 and leukocyte function–associated antigen-3.[24] Together, these events may facilitate an immune-mediated attack on the infected allograft. One advantage of this cytokine hypothesis is that it would provide a plausible explanation for the occurrence of similar forms of allograft injury in patients with or without CMV infection. The key step is the local elaboration of cytokines; CMV infection is just one process, although a common and an important one, in which cytokine elaboration occurs.[1, 12]

TABLE 134–3 ■ Clinical Effects of Cytomegalovirus Infection in Organ Transplant Recipients

Early manifestations (1–6 mo after transplantation)
Fever
Pneumonia
Hepatitis
Gastrointestinal ulceration, with bleeding or perforation or both
Leukopenia and thrombocytopenia
Encephalitis*
Transverse myelitis*
Cutaneous vasculitis*
Late manifestations (more than 6 mo after transplantation)
Progressive chorioretinitis

*Rare.

Three patterns of CMV transmission are noted. (1) In primary infection, a seronegative transplant recipient receives cells latently infected with the virus from a seropositive donor (more than 90% of the time these cells are within the allograft; in the remainder of cases, viable leukocytes administered with blood products are the source of latent virus). (2) In reactivated infection, a seropositive recipient's endogenous virus is reactivated after the transplant operation. (3) In superinfection, a seropositive recipient is superinfected with virus of donor origin. The incidence of clinical disease is different in these three forms of CMV infection: approximately 60% for patients at risk for primary disease (seropositive donor and seronegative recipient), 20% to 50% for those at risk for superinfection (seropositive donor and recipient), and less than 20% for those at risk for reactivation (seronegative or seropositive donor and seropositive recipient).[1, 7]

The key steps in the pathogenesis of CMV infection in transplant recipients are as follows: reactivation of the virus from latency, systemic dissemination of replicating virus, and development of a host response, both humoral, and, more important, cellular—particularly virus-specific, major histocompatibility complex–restricted cytotoxic T cells.[1] Evidence suggests that tumor necrosis factor is a key mediator in the reactivation process, which explains the association of viral reactivation with a diverse array of clinical events: allograft rejection, antilymphocyte antibody therapy of rejection (fever, chills, and a measurable cytokine response being regular features of such therapy), and systemic sepsis. Each of these results in tumor necrosis factor release and the potential for CMV reactivation.[25–27] This analysis also explains the different effects of the various immunosuppressive agents on the course of CMV infection. Whereas cyclosporine, FK-506 (tacrolimus), and corticosteroids have no ability to reactivate latent virus, they are quite potent in amplifying the level of virus and its extent due to the profound inhibitory effect on the key cytotoxic T-cell response. In contrast, antilymphocyte antibody therapy is potent at reactivating virus but has only minor effects on systemic dissemination and the host response to the virus. Thus, one would predict that the treatment of rejection with antilymphocyte antibody therapy followed by cyclosporine-based immunosuppression would be the scenario that would be most likely to lead to CMV disease. Indeed, this has been confirmed: CMV-seropositive transplant recipients who were treated only with cyclosporine, prednisone, and azathioprine have an incidence of clinical CMV disease of approximately 10%; if antilymphocyte antibody therapy of rejection is needed as well, the incidence of symptomatic disease rises to 65%.[28]

Intravenous ganciclovir remains the treatment of choice for symptomatic CMV disease, with some groups advocating the addition of hyperimmune anti-CMV globulin therapy in patients with primary infection and in those with life-threatening CMV disease. To date, ganciclovir-resistant CMV infection has not been documented in the transplant recipient (unlike the situation in the patient with AIDS), and alternative anti–CMV drugs such as foscarnet have not received much attention in this population of patients. Not surprisingly, efforts to prevent CMV disease have received a great deal of attention, with hyperimmune globulin, high-dose oral acyclovir, combination therapy with these, and sequential therapy, often with 1 to 4 weeks of intravenous ganciclovir followed by oral therapy, being advocated by different groups. The optimal regimen is still being defined. What is clear, however, is that in different periods of intense immunosuppression, such as during the antilymphocyte antibody treatment of rejection, intravenous ganciclovir should be added to whatever prophylactic program is being used. For example, in the seropositive patient, this practice eliminated the excessive occurrence of CMV disease that was previously cited. The therapeutic principle here is that the intensity of the antiviral program should be linked to the intensity of the immunosuppressive program.[1, 28, 29]

Epstein-Barr Virus. In both normal and immunosuppressed persons, EBV infection produces clinical effects quite similar to those of CMV, and it is likely that in transplant recipients EBV contributes to the net state of immunosuppression and to the causation of mononucleosis-like syndromes. Whether it can play a role in the pathogenesis of allograft injury and its quantitative importance (evidence of active EBV replication can be found in at least 50% of organ transplant recipients) have been difficult to discern because of the ubiquity of CMV infection.[1, 30] One aspect of EBV infection in organ transplant recipients is uniquely important: it can cause the B-cell lymphoproliferative syndrome. This entity, which has the histologic appearance of a polymorphic B-cell lymphoma, commonly presents with invasion of the central nervous system, nasopharynx, liver, small bowel, heart, or allograft in addition to lymphoid tissue. It appears that EBV-associated lymphoproliferative disease represents a continuum of clinical disease ranging from benign EBV-dependent polyclonal B-cell hyperplasia to malignant EBV-independent monoclonal B-cell lymphoma.[31–36]

B-cell lymphoproliferative disease is more common with primary than with reactivated EBV infection, and it is directly related to the type and intensity of immunosuppressive therapy. The current concept of pathogenesis is as follows. In healthy immunocompetent persons who have latent EBV infection (and are therefore antibody-positive), circulating cytotoxic T lymphocytes specific for EBV antigens on the surface of infected B lymphocytes prevent the outgrowth of virally induced, transformed cells that are believed to initiate the oncogenic process that culminates in lymphoproliferative disease. In immunosuppressed patients, especially those with primary infection, this defense system is defective. Thus, drugs such as cyclosporine and FK-506 will inhibit the recipient's ability to eliminate the outgrowth of EBV-transformed B lymphocytes. In contrast, antilymphocyte antibodies exert their primary effect on the pathogenesis of this process by increasing the amount of virus that has been reactivated and is actively replicating, thus increasing the level of transformed B lymphocytes. Accordingly, the occurrence of EBV-related B-cell lymphoproliferative disease should be regarded as a consequence, rather than one single component, of the net state of immunosuppression. Indeed, there is evidence that preceding symptomatic CMV disease is an important risk factor for the subsequent development of lymphoproliferative disease (presumably related to the elaboration of cytokines in the course of CMV infection and the immunomodulating effects of this virus).[1, 31–37]

The optimal treatment of EBV-associated lymphoproliferative disease remains to be defined. All patients should have a major reduction of immunosuppressive therapy; most centers prescribe high-dose acyclovir or ganciclovir as well, although it is unclear what role such therapy plays because antivirals have no effect on the episomal form of the virus present in the infected B cells. Approximately 25% of patients respond to these maneuvers. In patients with localized disease, particularly of the gastrointestinal tract, surgery and local radiotherapy have had significant success. In patients with more generalized disease, a variety of regimens including antilymphoma chemotherapy, the infusion of clones of anti-EBV T cells, anti–B-cell monoclonal antibodies, and interferon alfa are all being evaluated, with no clear-cut best strategy emerging as of the present.[1, 37–42]

Varicella-Zoster Virus. Reactivation varicella-zoster virus (VZV) infection, in the form of dermatomal zoster, affects at least 10% of organ transplant recipients. Visceral dissemination of VZV is uncommon in organ transplant recipients with reactivated infection (these patients are, by definition, seropositive for VZV before reactivation). Therapy with high-dose acyclovir or famciclovir shortens the duration of this entity, leading to more rapid healing, although it is unclear that any therapy will influence the duration of zoster-induced neuralgic pain.[1]

Primary VZV infection is a rapidly lethal visceral infection characterized by pneumonia, pancreatitis, hepatitis, encephalitis, and disseminated intravascular coagulation. Large doses of intravenous acyclovir can be lifesaving in the treatment of primary VZV infection of organ transplant recipients, *provided that it is initiated early in the clinical course.* The VZV serologic status of all transplant candidates should be determined before transplantation, and the newly licensed varicella vaccine should be offered to all seronegative individuals. Proof of seroconversion should be obtained after immunization. For seronegative transplant recipients, immunization is also recommended with a close follow-up, because it is not yet clear whether acyclovir will be needed to treat any clinical effects of this live, attenuated vaccine. Again, proof of seroconversion is recommended. For seronegative individuals who are exposed to VZV, immediate zoster immune prophylaxis is essential, with close clinical follow-up to detect failures of such prophylaxis, to ensure early antiviral intervention.[1, 43, 44]

Herpes Simplex Virus. Reactivated herpes simplex virus (HSV) type 1 or 2 infection is quite common after organ transplantation, especially with intensive antirejection therapy. Localized mucocutaneous infection of either the oral or the anogenital area is the usual result, although the lesions, especially in the anogenital area, often have an atypical appearance, ulcers being more common than vesicles. Rare instances of disseminated primary infection, probably transmitted by the allograft, have been described, which produce a clinical syndrome similar to that described earlier for primary VZV infection. Other uncommon manifestations of HSV infection in transplant recipients that have been described include (1) tracheal (and even bronchopulmonary) and esophageal infection, which almost invariably is due to the combination of a nasogastric or endotracheal tube traumatizing these sites in the face of active oral HSV infection in any transplant recipient but with particular impact on the lung transplant recipients and their bronchial anastomosis; (2) eczema herpeticum (also called Kaposi's varicelliform eruption), a disseminated skin infection without visceral involvement in patients with such underlying dermatologic conditions as eczema; (3) meningoencephalitis due to HSV type 2 in patients with anogenital infection; and (4) a zosteriform dermatomal rash akin to that of VZV.[1]

HSV is quite sensitive to both acyclovir and ganciclovir, so either drug may be used both prophylactically or therapeutically, depending on the clinical situation. As with CMV, antiviral-resistant HSV infection has not been a problem in the organ transplant recipient. Because of the particular impact of both CMV and HSV on the lung transplant recipient, most groups use prophylactic intravenous ganciclovir in the first 2 to 6 weeks after transplantation. Anti–HSV prophylaxis can easily be accomplished with oral acyclovir or oral ganciclovir for the other organ transplant groups, although many centers prefer to treat symptomatic HSV disease as it occurs (with oral acyclovir for 5 to 10 days) rather than specifically design a prophylaxis program just for HSV. In the future, it is likely that prophylactic programs will be designed to prevent all forms of herpes group viral infections, not just CMV, EBV, or HSV.[1, 29]

Hepatitis Viruses. The prevalence of chronic liver disease in organ transplant recipients is approximately 10%, with virtually all of it caused by HBV and HCV. The impact of these viruses on the transplant recipient is threefold: (1) both HBV and HCV are immunomodulating viruses that contribute significantly to transplant patients' net state of immunosuppression; (2) the combination of infection with these agents and chronic immunosuppressive therapy leads to chronic infection and progressive liver damage; and (3) chronic infection with both of these agents is associated with the development of hepatocellular carcinoma.[1, 45]

The efficiency of transmission of HBV with organ transplantation from an infected donor approaches 100%, with a relatively high rate of acute, fulminant hepatitis associated with the acquisition of HBV in the peritransplant period. Accordingly, every effort should be made to screen both organ and blood donors to prevent this event. In addition to donors who have hepatitis B surface antigen, it is important to recognize that donors negative for this antigen but positive for hepatitis B core antibody can occasionally transmit the virus. We restrict the use of organs from such donors to individuals at imminent risk of death without a transplant.[1, 45, 46]

Patients who come to transplantation with chronic HBV infection will exhibit an increase in the level of HBV replication because of the exogenous immunosuppressive therapy, and, in some individuals, an acceleration of the course of hepatitis. Thus, in one important study, it was noted that 8 to 10 years after kidney transplantation, 42% of patients positive for hepatitis B surface antigen had cirrhosis and 54% had died of either chronic liver disease or hepatocellular carcinoma (in contrast, for HCV, approximately 20% of patients will have serious consequences after this time).[47] In the special case of liver transplantation in the treatment of patients with HBV infection, reinfection of the new liver is universal if no anti–HBV therapy is administered, with significant consequences to the transplant recipient (decreased survival of both patient and allograft). It has been shown that the long-term administration of hepatitis B hyperimmune globulin offers significant protection against the consequences of reinfection in these patients.[48, 49]

Hepatitis C is responsible for more than 80% of the chronic liver disease that occurs in transplant recipients. The clinical effects have been noted earlier. The biggest issue regarding HCV in transplantation involves the approach to possible organ donors who are anti–HCV positive (1% to 5% of the donor pool). The risk of transmitting the virus with transplantation of an organ from an anti–HCV positive donor is approximately 50%. If the PCR assay for HCV RNA in the serum of the donor is positive, the rate of transmission with transplantation approaches 100%. Given the relatively slow course of HCV in the transplant recipient, as well as the failure of the anti–HCV assay to predict transmissibility in 50% of individuals, there has been considerable argument over the appropriate approach to such donors. Our own policy is to reserve organs from anti–HCV positive donors for critically ill recipients or for older individuals, with the belief that the several years necessary for HCV to become clinically apparent after transplantation offers a tradeoff that is acceptable for these two population groups.[1, 47, 50, 51]

Papovaviruses. More than 25% of transplant recipients show evidence of infection with one or both of the two major human papovaviruses, BK and JC virus. In general, it has not been clear exactly what their clinical effects might be; they seem to have some association in transplant recipients with ureteral stenosis, both endocrine and exocrine pancreatic dysfunction, and accelerated atherosclerosis. JC virus is known to be the agent of the uncommon but lethal neurologic disease progressive multifocal leukoencephalopathy. In addition, these viruses (which are quite similar to simian virus 40 should be regarded as potentially oncogenic.[1] Indeed, the closely related wart viruses (papillomaviruses) not only produce severe warts in many transplant recipients but also have been implicated in the pathogenesis of squamous cell carcinoma of the skin in these patients. In the latter case, it is believed that the virus, in association with chronic immunosuppression and the effects of ultraviolet irradiation, are responsible for the development of this serious form of malignancy in transplant recipients.[1]

Human Immunodeficiency Virus. Organ transplant recipients have not been spared the impact of the worldwide epidemic of HIV infection. Primary acquisition of HIV infection at the time of transplantation has been documented. The efficiency of transmission from an infected donor approaches 100%. After primary infection, all manifestations of HIV infection in persons who are not receiving immunosuppressive therapy have been observed in transplant recipients: asymptomatic seroconversion; an acute mononucleosis-like syndrome 1 to 3 months after infection; prolonged, unexplained fevers (the so-called AIDS-related complex); conjugal transmission of the virus to the spouse; and full-blown AIDS. Immunosuppressive therapy may cause a false-negative result when transplant recipients with HIV infection undergo routine antibody tests. Clearly, this form of infection must be prevented by careful screening of donors, and great care must be taken to ensure that the donor blood specimen tested is a representative sample. On several occasions, HIV has been transmitted because a potential donor was screened only after receiving at least 50 units of blood, which rendered the HIV test result invalid.[1]

Although careful screening of donors (and blood products) should essentially eliminate the risk of primary HIV infection for transplant recipients, an increasing problem is the management of patients with end-stage kidney, liver, or heart disease who have asymptomatic HIV infection. Currently available data, although incomplete, suggest that about 25% of such persons will die within 6 months of receiving an organ; 50% do well for 3 to 5 years and then develop full-blown AIDS; and 25% are still doing well more than 5 years after transplantation. How prophylactic anti-HIV and anti–*P. carinii* therapies will influence these statistics is not known, and there remains considerable controversy over whether such patients should receive a transplant.[1]

Bacterial Infections

Bacterial infections in organ transplant recipients can be divided into four general categories: infection of the transplanted organ, due in large part to catheters placed to protect the surgical anastomoses; infection secondary to technical complications related to the transplant operation and postoperative management; infection of the gastrointestinal tract; and opportunistic infection by *L. monocytogenes, N. asteroides,* and *Mycobacterium* species (both typical and atypical).

The prime example of bacterial infection of a transplanted organ is urinary tract infection in kidney transplant recipients. The prevalence of such infections in the first 4 months after transplantation is approximately 35%, with a relatively high rate of transplant pyelonephritis, bacteremia, and relapse after a 10-day course of antibiotic therapy. Careful study has revealed that prophylaxis with such drugs as trimethoprim-sulfamethoxazole, trimethoprim, or ciprofloxacin can effectively prevent such infections. In addition, at least in the case of trimethoprim-sulfamethoxazole, there appears to be the added benefit of preventing *P. carinii, L. monocytogenes,* and *N. asteroides* infection at the same time. The optimal duration of prophylaxis is not clear, as the risk of all infections is significantly less after 6 months, although some groups continue prophylaxis for significantly longer periods.[1]

Cholangitis after liver transplantation is uncommon in the absence of technical complications, despite the presence of a catheter in the biliary tract for many weeks after transplantation, but colonization of the biliary tract by staphylococcal species, enterococci, and gram-negative bacilli is to be expected. This becomes clinically important if the liver transplant is "injured," as by formation of a hematoma after biopsy, or if the biliary tree is manipulated, as by cholangiography. Because of the risk of liver abscesses in the first instance and cholangitis in the second, antibiotic prophylaxis aimed at the biliary flora (e.g., single doses of vancomycin and aztreonam) is usually given in association with such procedures.[1]

Technical complications of organ transplantation are invariably associated with secondary infection with bacteria or *Candida* species. Such technical complications include urine and biliary leaks or obstruction, tissue infarction due to clotting of vascular anastamoses (particularly important in liver transplantation), lymphoceles, wound hematomas, and mismanagement of endotracheal tubes or vascular or drainage catheters. There is no less forgiving form of surgery than organ transplantation, as a technical problem guarantees potentially life-threatening infection. Management of such problems requires early diagnosis, prompt drainage and correction of the problem, and aggressive, prolonged specific antimicrobial therapy.[1]

The principal type of gastrointestinal bacterial infection observed in transplant recipients is the result of acute diverticulitis. Corticosteroid-treated patients with underlying diverticulosis are at risk of developing diverticulitis, which is associated with a high incidence of perforation. The initial clinical presentation can be quite insidious in these patients, owing to suppression of the inflammatory response by immunosuppressive therapy. Pain but no signs of frank peritonitis, unexplained change in bowel habits, and fever are common initial findings. Prompt surgical therapy with broad-spectrum antibiotic coverage is mandatory to save these patients. In addition, the gastrointestinal tract of transplant recipients is particularly susceptible to invasion by nontyphoidal salmonellae and *L. monocytogenes.* Both infections can present as acute diarrheal syndromes that progress to bacteremia alone, or, in the case of *Listeria,* bacteremia with central nervous system infection.[1]

N. asteroides infection usually presents as a subacute pulmonary process. Cough, fever, purulent sputum production, and pleurisy are common presenting features. Once pulmonary infection develops, metastatic infection to the brain, skin, and other sites is common, and on occasion such metastatic infection is the cause of the presenting clinical complaint (e.g., seizures or subcutaneous nodules). Early diagnosis and therapy with large doses of sulfasoxazole or trimethoprim-sulfamethoxazole for a minimal period of 4 to 6 months are quite effective.[1]

Mycobacterial infection remains a significant problem in organ transplant recipients for several reasons. It is much more frequent in these patients than in the general population. Antituberculosis therapy with isoniazid or rifampin is often difficult because of hepatic dysfunction and the effects on metabolism of the immunosuppressive drugs (see later). Finally, even disseminated disease can be clinically silent. A variety of forms of tuberculosis have been observed in these patients, from cavitary pulmonary disease to miliary disease and from bowel disease to skin disease. An unusually high rate of bone and joint involvement has been reported in this group of patients.[43] Clearly, active disease must be treated aggressively, but which patients should be placed on isoniazid prophylaxis in the face of inactive infection is the subject of controversy. Our approach is not to use such prophylaxis for patients whose only evidence of mycobacterial infection is a long-standing positive skin test result and who can be followed closely clinically. Prophylaxis is prescribed for patients who have other risk factors such as non-Caucasion racial status, another immunosuppressive illness, malnutrition, a clearly abnormal chest radiograph, or a history of active tuberculosis.[1]

Atypical mycobacterial infection has also been observed in transplant recipients—pulmonary, skin, skeletal, and disseminated infection due to *Mycobacterium kansasii*; or isolated skin infection (usually after injury to the skin, often due to water immersion) by any of a variety of relatively less virulent mycobacterial species, including *Mycobacterium marinum, Mycobacterium haemophilum,* and *Mycobacterium chelonae.* Management of such infections often requires a combination approach: decreasing the dose of immunosuppressive drugs, surgical débridement or ablation, and appropriate chemotherapy.[1]

Fungal Infections

Two principal types of fungal infections affect transplant recipients: disseminated primary or reactivated infection with one of the geographically restricted systemic mycoses (histoplasmosis, blastomycosis, coccidioidomycosis) and invasive infection by the opportunistic pathogens *Candida* species, *Aspergillus* species, *Cryptococcus neoformans,* and the Mucoraceae. Clinical syndromes that suggest the first category (in persons with a history of recent or remote epidemiologic exposure) include subacute respiratory illness, with focal, disseminated, or miliary infiltrates on chest radiographs; a nonspecific systemic febrile illness; unexplained pancytopenia; and an illness in which metastatic aspects of the infection predominate (e.g., mucocutaneous manifestations in histoplasmosis and blastomycosis or central nervous system manifestations in coccidioidomycosis or histoplasmosis).[1, 3]

Much more common is infection with one of the opportunistic fungi. Three types of opportunistic fungal infection are observed in transplant recipients: (1) *P. carinii* pneumonia, which often complicates the course of CMV infection, is the most common form of life-threatening fungal infection occurring in transplant recipients, with an frequency of at least 10% unless prophylaxis is administered to patients at high risk for this infection. High-risk groups include the following: all transplant recipients in the 1 to 6 months after transplantation, especially those with active viral infection; and the chronic n'er do wells more than 6 months after transplantation. In both of these groups, low-dose trimethoprim-sulfamethoxazole prophylaxis essentially eliminates not only this infection but also nocardiosis and listeriosis. When *Pneumocystis* pneumonia does develop, it is a subacute disease characterized by fever, nonproductive cough, and progressive dyspnea over several days in conjunction with an interstitial infiltrate on chest radiographs—an identical presentation to that of CMV, both clinically and radiographically (Fig. 134–2). (2) Primary infection, usually of the lungs but occasionally of the nasal sinuses, caused most commonly by *C. neoformans* or *Aspergillus* species, with the most common clinical manifestation of such infections often being metastatic disease to sites such as the central nervous system or

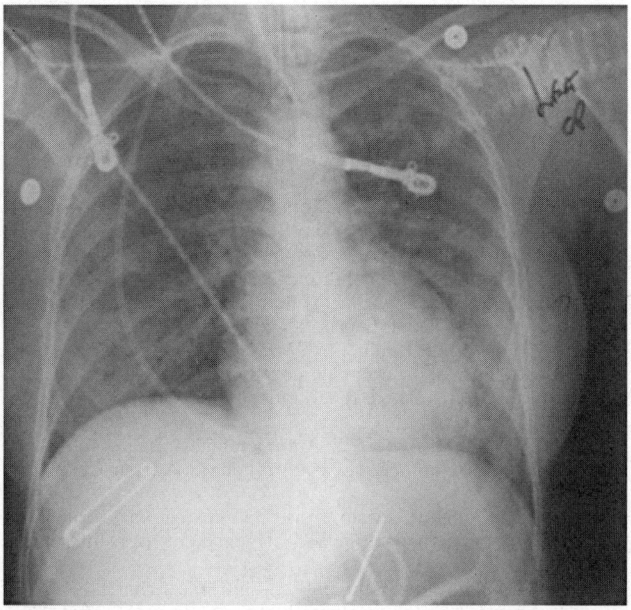

FIGURE 134–2 □ Chest x-ray film of a liver transplant recipient with pneumonia 6 weeks after transplantation, shown on biopsy to be caused by simultaneous infection with cytomegalovirus and *Pneumocystis carinii.* The patient responded to therapy with ganciclovir and trimethoprim-sulfamethoxazole.

skin. (3) Sequential and concurrent secondary infections of technically compromised wounds, the lungs, or infected intravenous lines by *Candida* or *Aspergillus* species or *Torulopsis glabrata.*[1, 3]

The traditional cornerstone of antifungal therapy for the last two categories of fungal infection has been amphotericin B, the toxicities of which are well recognized. Unfortunately, in the presence of cyclosporine, the incidence and severity of nephrotoxicity are greatly increased, and increased attention has been paid to alternative therapies. Fluconazole has proved to be extremely useful in the management of cryptococcal and candidal disease in the transplant recipient, with its form of interaction with cyclosporine being to decrease the metabolism, necessitating a decrease in the dose of cyclosporine. Unfortunately, an alternative to amphotericin as a primary therapy for invasive aspergillosis in transplant recipients has not yet emerged, with itraconazole being reserved for "wrap-up" therapy.[1, 52]

Parasitic Infections

Two types of parasitic infection are particularly important for transplant recipients: disseminated toxoplasmosis and strongyloidiasis. Although disseminated toxoplasmosis has been reported in recipients of kidney and liver transplants, it is a particular problem with heart transplantation. Transplantation of a heart from a donor who is seropositive for toxoplasmosis (connoting latent infection with this organism, particularly in the heart) into a seronegative recipient is associated with a high rate of disseminated toxoplasmosis in recipients. Such a syndrome has a particular clinical impact on the heart (myocarditis, which has been mistakenly diagnosed and treated as rejection, with disastrous consequences) and the brain (focal abscesses or diffuse encephalitis). It is now accepted practice to screen heart donors and recipients serologically for toxoplasmosis and to administer prophylactic pyrimethamine and sulfasoxazole for 3 to 6 months to recipients at risk for primary toxoplasmosis.[1, 3]

Strongyloids stercoralis is an intestinal nematode that is endemic in many areas of the world. Because of its ability to be maintained in the gastrointestinal tract for decades, owing to an autoinfection part of its life cycle, silent infection may be sustained long after the host has taken up residence outside endemic areas. Tissue invasion is normally prevented by an intact cell-mediated immune system. After transplantation and the initiation of immunosuppressive therapy, a disastrous hyperinfection syndrome or disseminated strongyloidiasis, or both, can develop. The hyperinfection syndrome, an exaggeration of the normal life cycle of the parasite, has major impact on the gastrointestinal tract (necrotizing, hemorrhagic enterocolitis) and lungs (hemorrhagic pneumonia). Disseminated strongyloidiasis consists of extension of the infection outside its normal habitat: the larvae invade all portions of the body. Both entities are associated with recurrent gram-negative bacteremia, meningitis, or both. Although, this severe disease can theoretically be treated with large doses of thiabendazole and anti–gram-negative antibacterial agents, emphasis should be placed on prevention. It is strongly recommended that residents or former residents of areas where *S. stercoralis* is endemic be screened before transplantation by examination of Papanicolaou smears of sputum and duodenal aspirates and of purged stool specimens. Preventive therapy is then a simple 3-day course of thiabendazole.[1, 53, 54]

Special Considerations of Antimicrobial Therapy for Transplant Recipients

The guiding principle for the infectious disease clinician in approaching a transplant recipient is that prevention is much better than treatment. An important reason is that many of the antimicrobial agents commonly used to treat the infections interact adversely with cyclosporine, the mainstay of current immunosuppressive regimens. Three types of cyclosporine interactions can be observed with antimicrobial agents. First, and most important, is synergistic nephrotoxicity, which is most often associated with amphotericin B, aminoglycosides, high-dose trimethoprim-sulfamethoxazole therapy (as used to treat *Pneumocystis* pneumonia), and perhaps other drugs such as vancomycin. Second, increased blood levels of cyclosporine increase the potential for profound immunosuppression and nephrotoxicity (caused by inhibition of the hepatic cytochrome P-450 system responsible for cyclosporine metabolism), most notably by erythromycin, ketoconazole, and, to a lesser extent, fluconazole. Finally, certain drugs, most notably rifampin, up-regulate the hepatic enzymes, resulting in increased cyclosporine metabolism, decreased blood levels of cyclosporine, and an increased risk of allograft rejection. As a result, for treating bacterial infections in these patients there is an increased reliance on β-lactam–based therapies (including drugs such as ceftazadime, ampicillin-sulbactam, aztreonam, and imipenem), despite their costliness.[1, 29]

As a corollary to the principle that prevention is much better than treatment, when allograft recipients regularly manifest infectious disease problems, every effort is made to develop an effective prophylactic strategy. Examples of success in this area include prophylaxis against urinary tract infections after kidney transplantation, against primary CMV infection, against primary toxoplasmosis after heart transplantation, and against *Pneumocystis* in all transplant recipients.[1, 29]

Finally, when infection does develop the key to effective therapy is early diagnosis and initiation of effective treatment. This objective can be a challenging one, as the signs of infection in these patients are frequently blunted by an impaired inflammatory response. The responsible clinician must take seriously the most innocuous-looking skin lesion, pulmonary nodule, or other sign. A policy of aggressive observation will translate into increased survival of patients and increased success of organ transplantation, results that are worth the effort.[1, 29]

References

1. Rubin RH: Infection in the organ transplant recipient. *In* Rubin RH, Young LS (eds): Clinical Approach to Infection in the Compromised Host, ed 3. New York, Plenum Publishing, 1994, p 629.
2. Rubin RH, Wolfson JS, Cosimi AB, Tolkoff-Rubin NE: Infection in the renal transplant recipient. Am J Med 70:405, 1981.
3. Rubin RH, Tolkoff-Rubin NE: Opportunistic infections in renal allograft recipients. Transplant Proc 20:12, 1988.
4. Rubin RH, Tolkoff-Rubin NE: Infection: The new problems. Transplant Proc 21:1440, 1989.
5. Hopkins CC, Weber DJ, Rubin RH: Invasive aspergillus infection: Possible non-ward common-source within the hospital environment. J Hosp Infect 27:211, 1989.
6. Rubin RH: The compromised host as sentinel chicken (editorial). N Engl J Med 317:1151, 1987.
7. Rubin RH: Infectious disease complications of renal transplantation. Kidney Int 44:221, 1993.
8. Peterson PK, Balfour HH Jr, Marker SC, et al: Cytomegalovirus disease in renal allograft recipients: A prospective study of the clinical features, risk factors, and impact on renal transplantation. Medicine (Baltimore) 59:283, 1980.
9. Marker SC, Howard RJ, Simmons RL, et al: Cytomegalovirus infection: A quantitative prospective study of 320 consecutive renal transplants. Surgery 89:660, 1981.
10. Rubin RH: The indirect effects of cytomegalovirus infection on the outcome of organ transplantation. JAMA 261:3607, 1989.
11. Rand KH, Pollard RB, Merigan TC: Increased pulmonary superinfection in cardiac transplant patients undergoing primary cytomegalovirus infection. N Engl J Med 298:951, 1978.
12. Grattan MT, Moreno-Cabral CE, Stames VA, et al: Cytomegalovirus infection is associated with cardiac allograft rejection and atherosclerosis. JAMA 261:3561, 1989.
13. Richardson WP, Colvin RB, Cheeseman SH, et al: Glomerulopathy associated with cytomegalovirus viremia in renal allografts. N Engl J Med 305:57, 1981.
14. Paya CV, Hermans PE, Wiesner RH, et al: Cytomegalovirus hepatitis in liver transplantation: Prospective analysis of 93 consecutive orthotopic liver transplantations. J Infect Dis 160:752, 1989.
15. O'Grady JG, Alexander GJM, Sutherland S, et al: Cytomegalovirus infection and donor/recipient HLA antigens: Interdependent co-factors in pathogenesis of vanishing bile duct syndrome after liver transplantation. Lancet 2:302, 1988.
16. Milne DS, Gascoigne A, Wilkes J, et al: The immunohistopathology of obliterative bronchiolitis following lung transplantation. Transplantation 54:748, 1992.
17. Reinsmoen NL, Bolman RM, Savik K, et al: Are multiple immunopathogenetic events occurring during the development of obliterative bronchiolitis and acute rejection? Transplantation 55:1040, 1993.
18. Nakhleh RE, Bolman RM 3rd, Henke CA, et al: Lung transplant pathology. A comparative study of pulmonary acute rejection and cytomegaloviral infection. Am J Surg Pathol 15:1197, 1991.
19. Scott JP, Higenbottam TW, Sharples L, et al: Risk factors for obliterative bronchiolitis in heart-lung transplant recipients. Transplantation 51:813, 1991.
20. Keenan RJ, Lega ME, Dummer JS, et al: Cytomegalovirus serologic status and postoperative infection correlated with risk of developing chronic rejection after pulmonary transplantation. Transplantation 51:433, 1991.
21. Melnick JL, Dreesman G, McCollum CH, et al: Cytomegalovirus antigen within human arterial smooth muscle cells. Lancet 2:644, 1983.
22. Tumilowicz JJ, Gawlick MF, Powell BB, et al: Replication of cytomegalovirus in human arterial smooth muscle cells. J Virol 56:839, 1985.
23. Smiley ML, Mar EC, Huang ES: Cytomegalovirus infection and viral-induced transformation of human endothelial cells. J Med Virol 25:213, 1988.
24. Hosenpud JD, Chou S, Wagner CR: Cytomegalovirus-induced regulation of major histocompatibility complex class I antigen expression in human aortic smooth muscle cells. Transplantation 52:896, 1991.
25. Stein J, Volk H, Liebenthal C, et al: Tumor necrosis factor alpha stimulates the activity of the human cytomegalovirus major and immediate early enhancer/promoter in immature monocytic cells. J Gen Virol 74:2333, 1993.
26. Fietze E, Prosch S, Reinke P: Cytomegalovirus infection in transplant recipients. Transplantation 58:675, 1994.
27. Docke W, Prosch S, Fietze E: Cytomegalovirus reactivation and tumour necrosis factor. Lancet 343:268, 1994.
28. Hibberd P, Tolkoff-Rubin N, Conti D, et al: Preemptive ganciclovir therapy to prevent cytomegalovirus disease in cytomegalovirus antibody-positive renal transplant recipients. Ann Intern Med 123:18, 1995.
29. Rubin RH, Tolkoff-Rubin NE: Antimicrobial strategies in the care of organ transplant recipients. Antimicrob Agents Chemother 37:619, 1993.
30. Strauss SE, Cohen JI, Tosato G, Meier J: Epstein-Barr virus infections: Biology, pathogenesis, and management. Ann Intern Med 118:45, 1993.
31. Morrison V, Dunn D, Manivel C, et al: Clinical characteristics of post-transplant lymphoproliferative disorders. Am J Med 97:14, 1994.
32. Walker R, Marshall W, Strickler J, et al: Pretransplantation assessment of the risk of lymphoproliferative disorder. Clin Infect Dis 20:1346, 1995.
33. Sullivan JL, Medveczky P, Forman SJ, et al: Epstein-Barr virus induced lymphoproliferation. Implications for antiviral chemotherapy. N Engl J Med 311:1163, 1984.
34. Randhawa P, Yousem S: Epstein-Barr virus–associated lymphoproliferative disease in a heart-lung allograft. Transplantation 49:126, 1990.
35. Ho M, Miller G, Atchison W, et al: Epstein-Barr virus infections and DNA hybridization studies in posttransplantation lymphoma and lymphoproliferative lesions: The role of primary infection. J Infect Dis 152:876, 1985.
36. Nalesnik M, Jaffe R, Starzl T, et al: The pathology of posttransplant lymphoproliferative disorders occurring in the setting of cyclosporine A–prednisone immunosuppression. Am J Pathol 133:173, 1988.
37. Preiskaitis JK, Diaz-Mitoma F, Mirzayans F, et al: Quantitative oropharyngeal Epstein-Barr virus shedding in renal and cardiac transplant recipients: Relationship to immunosuppressive therapy, serologic responses, and the risk of posttransplant lymphoproliferative disorder. J Infect Dis 166:986, 1992.
38. Kuo P, Dafoe D, Alfrey E, et al: Posttransplant lymphoproliferative disorders and Epstein-Barr virus prophylaxis. Transplantation 59:135, 1995.
39. Pirsch J, Stratta R, Sollinger H, et al: Treatment of severe Epstein-Barr virus–induced lymphoproliferative syndrome with ganciclovir: Two cases after solid organ transplantation. Am J Med 86:241, 1989.
40. Hanto D, Frizzera G, Gajl-Peczalska K, et al: Acyclovir therapy of Epstein-Barr virus–induced posttransplant lymphoproliferative diseases. Transplant Proc 27:89, 1985.
41. Starzl T, Porter K, Iwatsuki S: Reversibility of lymphomas and lymphoproliferative lesions developing under cyclosporin-steroid therapy. Lancet 1:583, 1984.
42. Papadoulos E, Ladanyi M, Emanuel D, et al: Infusions of donor leukocytes to treat Epstein-Barr virus–associated lymphoproliferative disorders after allogeneic bone marrow transplantation. N Engl J Med 330:1185, 1994.
43. Lynfield R, Herrin JT, Rubin RH: Varicella in pediatric renal transplant recipients. Pediatrics 90:216, 1992.
44. Kitai I, King S, Gafni A: An economic evaluation of varicella vaccine for pediatric liver and kidney transplant recipients. Clin Infect Dis 17:441, 1993.
45. Katkov W, Rubin R: Liver disease in the organ transplant recipient: Etiology, clinical impact, and management. Transplant Rev 5:200, 1991.
46. Wachs M, Amend W, Ascher N, et al: The risk of transmission of hepatitis B from $HBsAg^-$, $HBcAb^+$, $HBIgM^-$ organ donors. Transplantation 59:230, 1995.

47. Rao K, Kasiske B, Anderson W: Variability in the morphological spectrum and clinical outcome of chronic liver disease in hepatitis B–positive and B–negative renal transplant recipients. Transplantation 51:391, 1991.
48. Samuel D, Bismuth A, Mathieu D, et al: Passive immunoprophylaxis after liver transplantation in HBsAg-positive patients. Lancet 1:813, 1991.
49. Lauchait W, Müller R, Pichlmayr R: Long-term immunoprophylaxis of hepatitis B virus (HBV) reinfection in recipients of human liver allografts. Transplant Proc 19:4051, 1987.
50. Periera B, Milford E, Kirkman R, et al: Prevalence of hepatitis C virus RNA in organ donors positive for hepatitis C antibody and in the recipients of their organs. N Engl J Med 327:910, 1992.
51. Chan T, Lok A, Cheng I, Chan R: A prospective study of hepatitis C virus infection among renal transplant recipients. Gastroenterology 104:862, 1993.
52. Conti DJ, Tolkoff-Rubin NE, Baker GP Jr, et al: Successful treatment of invasive fungal infections with fluconazole in organ transplant patients. Transplantation 47:692, 1989.
53. Morgan JS, Schaffner W, Stone WJ: Overwhelming strongyloidiasis in renal transplant recipients. Transplantation 42:518, 1986.
54. De Vauly GA Jr, King JW, Rorh MS, et al: Opportunistic infections with *Strongyloides stercoralis* in renal transplantation. Rev Infect Dis 12:653, 1990.

135

Infections Associated with Bone Marrow Transplantation

Richard T. Ellison, III

Bone marrow transplantation with intravenous infusion of bone marrow stem cells was first attempted in humans in 1939 and was performed successfully in the 1960s.[1] As knowledge developed regarding the supportive and immunosuppressive approaches necessary for success, bone marrow transplantation became an established clinical therapy in the 1970s. There are now approximately 15,000 transplantations performed annually.[2]

Three basic forms of bone marrow transplantation are performed. *Syngeneic* transplantation involves the infrequent circumstance of transplantation of bone marrow from a genetically identical twin and is a preferred option when feasible. *Autologous* transplantation involves the transplantation of the recipient's own bone marrow that has been harvested before bone marrow ablative treatment. This therapeutic approach is now used to allow the administration of otherwise lethal doses of chemotherapy and radiation therapy for the treatment of different forms of neoplasia, predominantly lymphoma and solid tumors, but occasionally leukemia and multiple myeloma. In addition, this approach may be used in the future for gene replacement therapy involving hematopoietic stem cells. *Allogeneic* transplantation involves the transplantation of bone marrow from a human leukocyte antigen (HLA)–matched nonidentical donor. The principal indications for allogeneic transplantation are severe aplastic anemia, acute leukemia, chronic myelogenous leukemia, lymphoma, multiple myeloma, immunodeficiency syndromes, thalassemia, and genetic-metabolic disorders. Whenever possible, allogeneic transplantation is performed with an HLA-matched sibling donor to decrease the risk of graft-versus-host disease (GVHD). Less desirable options are transplantation from an unrelated closely HLA–matched donor or from a relative with a partial HLA match.

There are significant differences in the relative risks of autologous and allogeneic transplantation. Because there is no risk of GVHD, the degree of immunosuppression is less with autologous transplantation. This allows the technique to be performed routinely in individuals up to the age of 60 to 70 years. In contrast, because of the increasing incidence of GVHD with advancing age, the upper age limit for allogeneic transplantation is 40 to 55 years. The major concern with autologous transplantation is the relapse of the original malignancy, and numerous methods are used and are under development to purge the autologous graft of tumor cells. The most serious complication arising from allogeneic transplantation is the development of GVHD. This disease primarily presents with skin disease, gastrointestinal disease, and hepatitis (Table 135–1). However, GVHD is also accompanied by profound immunosuppression and increases the risk of infectious complications. It can be characterized as two different clinical entities—acute GVHD, arising in the first 30 to 60 days after transplantation, and chronic GVHD, developing more than 60 days after transplantation. Most patients who receive allogeneic transplantation have some degree of acute GVHD, even though standard treatment now includes prophylactic therapy against this complication with cyclosporine with or without methotrexate, prednisone, and the removal of T cells from the graft.[1, 3] Therapy for severe acute GVHD includes a high dose of corticosteroids, antithymocyte globulin, and monoclonal antibody therapy.[3] Chronic GVHD arises most commonly in older patients and shares clinical features with scleroderma. However, it is also associated with immunosuppression, thrombocytopenia, and liver disease, all of which portend a poor prognosis.

The risk of infection for the transplant recipient follows directly from the loss and reconstitution of various components of host defenses.[1, 4] The sequence of immune injury and gradual recovery gives a temporal pattern to the infectious and noninfectious complications of transplantation (Table 135–2).

Infection During the Immediate Transplantation Period

Host Defense Defects

Patients undergoing transplantation are typically at some risk of systemic or localized infection based on their underlying disease. Once the transplant procedure is initiated, all bone marrow transplant recipients are at significantly increased risk of infection during a period of profound leukopenia with both absolute neutropenia and lymphocytopenia. The duration of leukopenia depends on the conditioning regimen used, the use of ex vivo marrow treatments to prevent GVHD, and whether colony-stimulating factors (CSF) are used.[5, 6] Although the period of profound leukopenia typically lasts approximately 3 to 4 weeks, it can be shortened by approximately 1 week by treatment with CSF.[5] The major risk of infection begins to resolve as the neutrophil count increases. Still, in vitro studies have shown that qualitative defects in neutrophil and macrophage function persist even though there is a quantitative recovery in circulating cells.[4, 7, 8] In addition, B-cell and $CD4^+$ T lymphocyte number and function appear to remain dysfunctional for up to 1 year after transplantation.[4, 9]

TABLE 135–1 ■ Clinical Classification of Acute Graft-Versus-Host Disease

	ORGAN INJURY		
LEVEL OF INJURY	Skin	Liver (Bilirubin Level)	Gastrointestinal Tract
1	Maculopapular rash on <25% of body surface	2–3 mg/dL	500–1000 mL of liquid stool per day
2	Maculopapular rash on 25%–50% of body surface	>3–6 mg/dL	>1000 and <1500 mL of liquid stool per day
3	Generalized erythroderma	>6–15 mg/dL	>1500 mL of liquid stool per day
4	Generalized erythroderma with formation of bullae and desquamation	>15 mg/dL	Severe abdominal pain with or without ileus
	LEVEL OF INJURY		
CLINICAL GRADE*	Skin	Liver	Gastrointestinal Tract
I	1 or 2	0	0
II	1–3	1	1
III	2 or 3	2 or 3	2 or 3
IV	2–4	2–4	2–4

*A grade of II or higher requires skin injury plus liver or intestinal injury, or both. A grade of IV requires an extreme decrease in performance status.
Adapted from Armitage JO: Bone marrow transplantation. N Engl J Med 330:827–838, 1994. Reprinted by permission of The New England Journal of Medicine. Copyright 1994, Massachusetts Medical Society.

Other major predisposing factors for infection in this period include the presence of indwelling intravenous catheters and damage to the oropharyngeal and gastrointestinal mucosal surfaces arising as a complication of conditioning radiation and chemotherapy. Xerostomia, increased mucus production, and reactivated herpes simplex virus (HSV) infections also contribute to oral mucosal injury that occurs in approximately 70% of allogeneic transplant recipients and a small percentage of autologous and syngeneic transplant recipients.[2]

Bacterial Infections

During this period of severe immunodeficiency, the major infectious complications are bacteremia, fungal infections with *Candida* and *Aspergillus*, and recurrent herpes. Bacterial infections are the most common identified illnesses, and the spectrum of pathogens is comparable to that in other neutropenic hosts. They consist predominantly of Enterobacteriaceae and *Pseudomonas aeruginosa* from the gastrointestinal tract, and gram-positive organisms (*Staphylococcus aureus*, coagulase-negative staphylococci, and viridans streptococci) from the skin, indwelling catheters, and oropharynx. The exact spectrum of organisms as well as their patterns of antimicrobial susceptibility varies significantly from one institution to another, and selection of empirical antimicrobial therapy should be based on the epidemiology of the individual transplant center. Infection caused by anaerobic organisms is infrequent, as is bacterial pneumonias in the absence of bacteremia.[10] Infectious gastroenteritis may be due to ade-

TABLE 135–2 ■ Temporal Pattern of Infectious and Noninfectious Complications of Bone Marrow Transplantation

	PREENGRAFTMENT (0–30 DAYS)	EARLY POSTENGRAFTMENT (31–100 DAYS)	LATE POSTENGRAFTMENT (100+ DAYS)
Host defense defect	Neutropenia Mucositis Indwelling venous catheters	Acute GVHD Indwelling venous catheters	Chronic GVHD
Bacterial infections	*Staphylococcus aureus* *Pseudomonas aeruginosa* Viridans streptococci	Coagulase-negative staphylococci	Encapsulated bacteria (*Streptococcus pneumoniae, Haemophilus influenzae)*
Fungal infections	*Candida* species *Aspergillus* species *Torulopsis glabrata** *Mucorales* species* *Fusarium* species* *Pityrosporum* species*	*Candida* species *Aspergillus* species *Cryptococcus neoformans** *Histoplasma capsulatum** *Coccidioides immitis**	*Candida* species
Viral infections	Herpes simplex virus Adenovirus* Rotavirus* Coxsackievirus*	Cytomegalovirus Herpes simplex virus* Adenovirus* BK virus* Respiratory syncytial virus* Parainfluenza virus*	Varicella-zoster virus
Other infections		*Pneumocystis carinii* toxoplasmosis Nocardiosis	
Other noninfectious complications	Venoocclusive disease of the liver	Interstitial pneumonitis	

*Uncommon pathogens that may occur in these time periods.

novirus, rotavirus, coxsackievirus, and *Clostridium difficile*.[11] The course of these gastroenteric infections can be quite prolonged, and the infections are associated with an increased mortality rate.

The general approach to management of bacterial infections and indwelling catheters is comparable to that used with other neutropenic patients, with empirical antibiotic therapy directed against the predominant pathogens initiated after the collection of appropriate samples for microbiologic cultures. During the past several years there has been both a decrease in the incidence of bacteremia and a shift from a predominance of infections with *S. aureus* and gram-negative bacilli to disease due to coagulase-negative staphylococci and viridans streptococci.[2, 12] These shifts appear to be related to improved supportive care, the general use of prophylactic antibiotic therapy, and the greater reliance on indwelling catheters. A number of potential empirical antibiotic regimens can be utilized when patients have fever and there are no localizing signs or symptoms. Appropriate regimens that have been found to be effective include (1) an aminoglycoside and an antipseudomonal β-lactam antibiotic (e.g., mezlocillin, azlocillin, piperacillin, ceftazidime); (2) monotherapy with ceftazidime or imipenem-cilastatin; (3) vancomycin plus an aminoglycoside and an antipseudomonal penicillin (or third-generation cephalosporin); and (4) an antipseudomonal ureidopenicillin and an antipseudomonal third-generation cephalosporin.[13] The choice of any specific regimen should be based on knowledge of a center's own microbiologic epidemiology. If a patient continues to be febrile for 3 days, the patient should be reevaluated, and modification of antibiotic therapy should be considered. If unexplained fever persists for 7 days, amphotericin B therapy should be initiated to treat for occult fungal disease.[13]

Fungal Infections

Fungal infection, predominantly with *Candida* species, also occurs frequently in this immediate posttransplant period before engraftment. Without prophylaxis, invasive candidal infection occurred in 11% of transplant recipients with a median time of onset of 2 weeks and a mortality rate of 75%.[10] Hepatosplenic candidiasis is an increasingly recognized complication arising from seeding of the portal circulation with *Candida* after gastrointestinal mucosal injury. This syndrome presents with fever, hepatosplenomegaly, and an elevated alkaline phosphatase level as the neutrophil count begins to normalize.[14] Multiple round defects are demonstrable in the liver and spleen by hepatic ultrasound of computed tomographic evaluation. Fluconazole has been shown to be an alternative agent for treatment of candidemia in the nonimmunocompromised patient, but its therapeutic efficacy for this infection remains undefined in the transplant recipient.[15] *Aspergillus* is the second principal fungus causing infection during periods of profound neutropenia; less commonly, infections occur with Mucorales, *Fusarium*, *Trichosporon*, *Pityrosporum*, and other soil saphrophytic fungi.[16–19] The incidence of invasive *Aspergillus* infection increases greatly in patients with neutropenia that persists longer than 21 days; infection usually involves the sinuses, lungs, or central nervous system, and blood cultures are rarely positive.[2, 20] In general, amphotericin B remains the drug of choice for treatment of invasive fungal disease even though the use of cyclosporine and other nephrotoxic drugs complicates treatment in allogeneic transplant recipients. Oral itraconazole has been shown to have efficacy in the treatment of invasive aspergillosis in immunocompromised hosts; however, its efficacy has not been compared with that of amphotericin B in controlled trials, and the mortality rate associated with this infection remains high.[20, 21]

Viral Infections

Before the use of acyclovir prophylaxis there was a 75% incidence of HSV reactivation in seropositive marrow transplant recipients during the early posttransplant period correlating with suppression in HSV specific immunity.[2, 22] Reactivation characteristically occurred with oral or genital lesions, although the appearance is often atypical. HSV reactivation could be complicated by HSV esophagitis, HSV pneumonitis, or bacterial superinfection; the incidence of these complications is decreased by routine acyclovir prophylaxis.[23]

Hepatic Venoocclusive Disease

A major noninfectious complication of the early preengraftment period that may simulate an infectious illness is hepatic venoocclusive disease (VOD). This presents as sudden weight gain, hepatomegaly or right upper quadrant pain, and hyperbilirubinemia. It appears to arise from damage to hepatocytes and the endothelium of hepatic venules from conditioning chemotherapy. Postsinusoidal venous occlusion occurs, and the condition can progress to hepatic failure. Other diagnostic considerations include viral hepatitis, acute GVHD, toxic effects of drugs, and bacterial or fungal infection. The incidence of VOD has increased during the past decade, and up to 50% of marrow transplant patients have some evidence of VOD.[24] Risk factors for VOD are pretransplant elevation of serum transaminase levels, high-dose conditioning chemotherapy, and persistent fever during the chemotherapy period. Unfortunately, only supportive therapy is currently available for the condition, and the mortality rate before day 100 for patients with VOD is approximately 40%.[24]

Antimicrobial Prophylaxis

Several modalities have been used among marrow transplant recipients to prevent infection in this time period with varying results.[6] Although the use of protective isolation procedures including laminar airflow rooms reduces the risk of infection, this approach has not substantially altered the outcome among patients undergoing transplantation for leukemia. A protective environment does decrease the incidence of acute GVHD among patients who undergo transplantation for aplastic anemia, although this effect has not been noted among leukemia patients.[6, 8, 10] Prophylactic oral and systemic antibiotics are used commonly; oral quinolone therapy appears to be comparable in efficacy to oral treatment with neomycin–polymyxin–nalidixic acid with better acceptance by patients.[25] Both low-dose intravenous amphotericin B (0.1 to 0.25 mg/kg per day) and oral fluconazole (400 mg/d) have been shown to be effective in preventing both superficial and invasive fungal disease.[16, 26–28] In a multicenter randomized, double-blind, placebo-controlled trial, fluconazole prophylaxis was further found to decrease day 110 mortality.[28] In contrast to fluconazole, amphotericin B can provide effective prophylaxis against aspergillosis, but it is associated with a greater risk of toxicity and has not been shown to clearly decrease mortality. In selected institutions where fluconazole prophylaxis has been used routinely, there has been the emergence of infections due to fluconazole-resistant organisms including *Candida krusei* and *Candida albicans*. Prophylactic therapy with high-dose intravenous immunoglobulin is also used in some transplant centers,[29] although one randomized trial found that weekly therapy did not reduce the incidence of bacterial or fungal infections or in-hospital mortality.[30]

Colony-Stimulating Factors

The use of the granulocyte and granulocyte-macrophage CSFs, in marrow transplant recipients has now been studied relatively extensively, and guidelines for the use of these agents in the management of marrow transplant recipients have been published by both the American Society for Clinical Oncology and the Eastern Cooperative Oncology Group.[29, 31] Both of these CSFs appear to enhance neutrophil number and function without increasing the rate of relapse of underlying disease or the risk of GVHD. There is strong evidence that use of these hematopoietic growth factors is safe and effective in shortening the period of neutropenia in patients undergoing autologous transplantation. The agents are also likely to be safe and effective in this role for allogeneic transplant recipients, although the evidence for this is not conclusive at this time. They appear to be safe and effective in treating both autologous and allogeneic transplant recipients who do not show engraftment by 21 to 28 days. There remains a concern that these CSFs could stimulate residual leukemia in patients with acute myeloid leukemia, and CSFs should therefore be used with caution in this disease.

Infection Early After Transplant Engraftment (Days 30 to 100)

Host Defense Defects

Once marrow engraftment occurs, the risk of infection associated with leukopenia decreases significantly, as does the incidence of serious HSV mucosal infection. However, there are still profound abnormalities in host defense, and the kinetics of immune reconstitution follow normal immune ontogeny.[4, 10] The more general early immune mechanisms such as cytotoxic and phagocytic cells recover first, followed by the more specialized humoral and cell-mediated immune systems. Multiple defects exist in the function of effector and accessory cells as well as in cytokine regulation. There are prolonged delays in the development of antibody production to specific antigens as well as in the development of antigen-specific T-cell responses. The response to some antigens appears to require reexposure in the form of active infection for reconstitution of immunity.[22] Another major factor that influences the rate of full immunologic recovery is the occurrence of acute GVHD, which directly prolongs the period of immunosuppression. Moreover, all of the therapeutic interventions used to treat GVHD (e.g., corticosteroids, cyclosporine, methotrexate, antithymocyte globulin, or anti–T-cell monoclonal antibodies) suppress the cell-mediated immune response.[3, 17] The damage that acute GVHD does to the integrity of the skin and gastrointestinal mucosa further predisposes to bacterial and fungal infection. In addition, acute GVHD appears to alter neutrophil function.[7]

Bacterial, Fungal, and Parasitic Infections

Bacterial, fungal, and protozoal infections will all occur during this period after transplantation. Bacterial disease typically occurs either as a complication of indwelling central venous catheters or as a complication of GVHD-mediated skin or gastrointestinal damage. The same spectrum of nosocomial bacterial pathogens that cause illness during the neutropenic period can produce illness early in this period, although overwhelming infection is unusual except in patients with severe GVHD, graft rejection, or graft failure.[10] Fungal infections continue to be common, with the predominant pathogens remaining *Candida* and *Aspergillus* species. Systemic aspergillosis usually arises slightly later in the course than candidal disease. The median onset is at 6 to 8 weeks after transplantation.[10] Aspergillosis occurs more commonly with allogeneic than autologous transplants, related to the greater degree of immunosuppression. Infections with *Cryptococcus neoformans* and the focally endemic fungi *Histoplasma capsulatum* and *Coccidioides immitis* also occur occasionally. *Pneumocystis carinii* pneumonia can occur in this period, but its incidence has fallen dramatically with the standard use of prophylaxis with trimethoprim-sulfamethoxazole.[32] Cerebral toxoplasmosis can also be seen infrequently in patients with severe acute GVHD; it typically presents as an intracranial lesion with headache, focal neurologic findings, and a ring-enhancing lesion on a computed tomographic scan of the head or a magnetic resonance image.

Viral Infections

Infections with DNA viruses also become a significant concern in this period. The most frequent problems arise from cytomegalovirus (CMV) disease; however, infections with herpes zoster virus, Epstein-Barr virus, human herpesvirus type 6, BK polyoma virus (hemorrhagic cystitis), and adenoviruses also occur.[33–37] Varicella-zoster occurs in approximately 30% of seropositive transplant recipients who do not receive any antiviral prophylaxis. The majority of these infections are cutaneous, although disseminated disease can be seen with severe GVHD. Treatment of herpes zoster is with acyclovir. Reactivation of Epstein-Barr virus is usually noted through asymptomatic shedding or seroconversion. Human herpesvirus type 6 infection is an occasional cause of acute febrile illness with rash and continued bone marrow suppression; the value of antiviral treatment for this complication is unknown.[34, 38] BK virus and adenovirus have both been associated with the development of hemorrhagic cystitis. Adenovirus has also been associated with pneumonia, renal insufficiency, gastroenteritis, and hepatitis. No definitive therapy for these last two viral pathogens is currently available.

CMV is the most frequent cause of severe viral disease in the transplant recipient.[39] The incidence of CMV disease depends on the serologic status of the marrow recipient and donor before transplantation, the use of unscreened blood products, the degree of immunosuppression of the recipient, and the presence of GVHD. More frequent and more serious disease is seen in patients receiving allogeneic transplants and in those with significant GVHD.[40–42] In marrow recipients who are seronegative at the time of transplantation, the incidence of CMV disease is approximately 28% when unscreened or non–leukocyte-depleted blood products are used. The incidence of disease is approximately 50% in seronegative recipients who receive a transplant from a seropositive donor and approximately 70% in seropositive marrow recipients.

The clinical manifestations of CMV infection are quite diverse in the transplant recipient. Seroconversion with asymptomatic virus shedding was historically noted in 30% to 90% of these patients. Clinical syndromes that arise include persistent unexplained fever, leukopenia, thrombocytopenia, esophagitis, gastroenteritis, retinitis, hepatitis, polyarthritis, central nervous system disease, and pneumonia. Of these syndromes, the most serious is CMV pneumonia. Despite advances in therapy, the mortality rate of this illness remains approximately 50%. It develops in 15% to 25% of seropositive allogenic transplant recipients and in 1% to 2% of autologous transplant recipients and appears to be more frequent in seropositive patients receiving antithymocyte globulin.[40, 42] The high frequency of CMV pneumonia in transplant recipients with GVHD in comparison to its rarity in patients with the acquired immunodeficiency syndrome has suggested that the pulmonary disease is mediated by an aberrant immunopathogenic response and not by direct viral injury.[43] In support of this premise, treatment of CMV pneumonia with ganciclovir therapy alone has little effect, whereas combined therapy with both ganciclovir and intravenous CMV immune globulin reduced mortality from 85% to 50%.[44] Foscarnet is a second antiviral agent that is effective for treatment of CMV disease, but its relative utility in the management of transplant recipients remains undefined except for the treatment of ganciclovir-resistant CMV infection.

CMV is the most common cause of severe gastroenteritis after marrow transplantation, usually presenting with protracted nausea, vomiting, or diarrhea; esophageal involvement is characterized by dysphagia and retrosternal pain. However, the incidence of CMV colitis, retinitis, and central nervous system infection is lower than that in patients with acquired immunodeficiency syndrome.

CMV disease can be prevented on a primary basis in seronegative patients either by screening all blood products for CMV or by removing leukocytes from blood products by filtration.[45] In addition, prophylactic ganciclovir therapy reduces the rate of symptomatic CMV disease in seropositive allogeneic marrow transplant recipients, although the treatment is complicated by neutropenia.[46–48] The beneficial effect of ganciclovir prophylaxis may be enhanced by the concurrent administration of granulocyte or granulocyte-macrophage CSF or by targeting ganciclovir prophylaxis to patients who have a positive culture or who are CMV antigen-positive.[46, 47] Intravenous anti-CMV immunoglobulin and acyclovir have also been used to prevent CMV, but their efficacy remains controversial.[10, 39]

Interstitial Pneumonitis

In addition to these defined infectious processes, diffuse interstitial pneumonitis is a frequent complication of allogeneic marrow transplantation and occurs in 15% to 40% of patients approximately 6 to 7 weeks after transplantation.[49] It is defined as the presence of tachypnea, hypoxemia, and interstitial pulmonary infiltrates in the absence of obvious bacterial or fungal infection, pulmonary edema, or pulmonary hemorrhage. Approximately half of these pneumonias are due to CMV, with the majority of the remainder being classified as idiopathic. Risk factors for this complication include methotrexate therapy, older age, severe GVHD, a prolonged period after diagnosis before transplantation, and a poor performance status before the transplant procedure.[49] Unfortunately, this complication continues to have a high mortality rate.

Infection Late After Transplant Engraftment (After Day 100)

Chronic Graft-Versus-Host Disease

After 100 days following engraftment, there has usually been resolution of both the leukopenic period and the immunosuppression of acute GVHD. The major risks of infection relate to the development of chronic GVHD as well as to delays in the development of antigen-specific humoral and T-cell–mediated immunity. The majority of syngeneic, autologous, and allogeneic transplant recipients without chronic GVHD will experience only one or two late infections other than recurrent herpes zoster.[50] Chronic GVHD arises in approximately 30% to 60% of allogeneic transplants as either a continuation of acute GVHD or de novo. It resembles a mixed autoimmune disease with multiorgan involvement, predominantly of the immune system, skin, mucous membranes, liver, and bone marrow. Immunologic abnormalities include impaired proliferation of B cells and decreased antibody production to specific antigens, as well as a decrease in the number and function of $CD4^+$ T cells.[3] Skin and mucous membrane changes can be limited to mild dermatitis or evolve into a scleroderma-like pattern with severe destruction of dermal appendages and a sicca syndrome. A cholestatic hepatitis can develop and progress to cirrhosis. Hematopoietic involvement is characteristically manifested as thrombocytopenia. Further, most patients with chronic GVHD appear to be functionally asplenic.

Viral, Bacterial, and Fungal Infections

Infections that arise in patients during this late phase reflect breaches in anatomic host defenses and the defects in humoral and cell-mediated immunity. The most frequent infection seen in this period is recurrent varicella-zoster due to reactivation of latent virus. The median time to onset is 5 months after transplantation, and 80% of episodes occur within 9 months.[33] The majority of episodes appear as zoster, but 15% of the episodes are varicella and 35% of the episodes of zoster are associated with dissemination. Acyclovir treatment has demonstrated efficacy in treating zoster in this population; newer antiviral agents (ganciclovir, famciclovir, and foscarnet) are also likely to be effective, but their use in treating varicella-zoster virus has not been well studied in transplant recipients. Bacterial infections that occur are predominantly sinusitis and pneumonia due to encapsulated organisms (*Streptococcus pneumoniae* and *Haemophilus influenzae*) related to abnormalities associated with chronic GVHD and immunoglobulin A deficiency. Systemic pneumococcal infection can occur and is associated with an inability to produce opsonizing antibody, even after systemic infection.[51] Patients with significant skin and mucous membrane damage from chronic GVHD also suffer cutaneous infection with *S. aureus* and group A streptococci. Severe fungal disease is quite rare at this stage, but impaired cell-mediated immunity contributes to continued problems with oropharyngeal or vaginal candidiasis.

Prevention of Infection

Prophylactic measures can lower the incidence of late infectious complications. Oral acyclovir will prevent recurrent HSV and varicella-zoster virus disease as long as patients receive therapy.[22, 52] The use of oral trimethoprim-sulfamethoxazole chemoprophylaxis has lowered the incidence of bacterial infections due to *S. pneumoniae* and *H. influenzae*, while also providing prophylaxis against late cases of *P. carinii* pneumonia.[53] Unfortunately, immunization with the pneumococcal vaccine does not appear to be beneficial.

References

1. Armitage JO: Bone marrow transplantation. N Engl J Med 330:827, 1994.
2. Sable CA, Donowitz GR: Infections in bone marrow transplant recipients. Clin Infect Dis 18:273, 1994.
3. Ferrara JLM, Deeg HJ: Graft-versus-host disease. N Engl J Med 324:667, 1991.
4. Lum LG: The kinetics of immune reconstitution after human marrow transplantation. Blood 69:369, 1987.
5. Nemunaitis J, Rabinowe SN, Singer JW, et al: Recombinant granulocyte-macrophage colony-stimulating factor after autologous bone marrow transplantation for lymphoid cancer. N Engl J Med 324:1773, 1991.
6. Petersen F, Thornquist M, Buckner C, et al: The effects of infection prevention regimens on early infectious complications in marrow transplant patients: A four armed randomized study. Infection 16:199, 1988.
7. Clark RA, Johnson FL, Klebanoff SJ, Thomas ED: Defective neutrophil chemotaxis in bone marrow transplant recipients. J Clin Invest 58:22, 1976.
8. Storb R, Prentice RL, Buckner CD, et al: Graft-versus-host disease

and survival in patients with aplastic anemia treated by marrow grafts from HLA-identical siblings. Beneficial effect of a protective environment. N Engl J Med 308:302, 1983.
9. Mackall CL, Fleisher TA, Brown MR, et al: Age, thymopoiesis, and CD4+ T-lymphocyte regeneration after intensive chemotherapy. N Engl J Med 332:143, 1995.
10. Meyers JD: Infections associated with bone marrow transplantation. *In* Gorbach SL, Bartlett JG, Blacklow NR (eds): Infectious Diseases. Philadelphia, WB Saunders, 1992, pp 1047–1050.
11. Yolken RH, Bishop CA, Townsend TR, et al: Infectious gastroenteritis in bone-marrow transplant patients. N Engl J Med 306:1009, 1982.
12. Bochud P-Y, Eggiman P, Calandra T, et al: Bacteremia due to viridans streptococcus in neutropenic patients with cancer: Clinical spectrum and risk factors. Clin Infect Dis 18:25, 1994.
13. Hughes WT, Armstrong D, Bodey GP, et al: Guidelines for the use of antimicrobial agents in neutropenic patients with unexplained fever. J Infect Dis 161:381, 1990.
14. Thaler M, Pastakia B, Shawker TH, et al: Hepatic candidiasis in cancer patients: The evolving picture of the syndrome. Ann Intern Med 108:88, 1988.
15. Rex JH, Bennett JE, Sugar AM, et al: A randomized trial comparing fluconazole with amphotericin B for the treatment of candidemia in patients without neutropenia. N Engl J Med 331:1325, 1994.
16. Goodman JL, Winston DJ, Greenfield RA, et al: A controlled trial of fluconazole to prevent fungal infections in patients undergoing bone marrow transplantation. N Engl J Med 326:845, 1992.
17. Pirsch JD, Maki DG: Infectious complications in adults with bone marrow transplantation and T-cell depletion of donor marrow. Increased susceptibility to fungal infections. Ann Intern Med 104:619, 1986.
18. Blazar BR, Hurd DD, Snover DC, et al: Invasive *Fusarium* infections in bone marrow transplant recipients. Am J Med 77:645, 1984.
19. Bufill JA, Lum LG, Caya JG, et al: *Pityrosporum* folliculitis after bone marrow transplantation. Ann Intern Med 108:560, 1988.
20. Wingard JR, Beals SU, Santos GW, et al: *Aspergillus* infections in bone marrow transplant recipients. Bone Marrow Transplant 2:175, 1987.
21. Denning DW, Lee JY, Hostetler JS, et al: NIAID mycoses study group multicenter trial of oral itraconazole therapy for invasive aspergillosis. Am J Med 97:135, 1994.
22. Meyers JD, Flournoy N, Thomas ED: Infection with herpes simplex virus and cell-mediated immunity after marrow transplant. J Infect Dis 142:338, 1980.
23. Ringden O, Heimdahl A, Lonnqvist B, et al: Decreased incidence of viridans streptococcal septicaemia in allogenic bone marrow transplant recipients after the introduction of acyclovir. Lancet 1:744, 1984.
24. McDonald GB, Hinds MS, Fisher LD, et al: Veno-occlusive disease of the liver and multiorgan failure after bone marrow transplantation: A cohort study of 355 patients. Ann Intern Med 118:255, 1993.
25. Jansen J, Cromer M, Akard L, et al: Infection prevention in severely myelosuppressed patients: A comparison between ciprofloxacin and a regimen of selective antibiotic modulation of the intestinal flora. Am J Med 96:335, 1994.
26. Rousey SR, Russler S, Gottlieb M, Ash RC: Low-dose amphotericin B prophylaxis against invasive *Aspergillus* infections in allogeneic marrow transplantation. Am J Med 91:484, 1991.
27. Riley DK, Pavia AT, Beatty PG, et al: The prophylactic use of low-dose amphotericin B in bone marrow transplant patients. Am J Med 97:509, 1994.
28. Slavin MA, Osborne B, Adams R, et al: Efficacy and safety of fluconazole prophylaxis for fungal infections after marrow transplantation—a prospective, randomized, double-blind study. J Infect Dis 171:1545, 1995.
29. Rowe JM, Ciobanu N, Ascensao J, et al: Recommended guidelines for the management of autologous and allogenic bone marrow transplantation. A report from the Eastern Cooperative Oncology Group (ECOG). Ann Intern Med 120:143, 1994.
30. Wolff SN, Fay JW, Herzig RH, et al: High-dose weekly intravenous immunoglobulin to prevent infections in patients undergoing autologous bone marrow transplantation or severe myelosuppressive therapy. A study of the American Bone Marrow Transplant Group. Ann Intern Med 118:937, 1993.
31. American Society for Clinical Oncology: American Society for Clinical Oncology recommendations for the use of hematopoietic colony-stimulating factors: Evidence-based, clinical practice guidelines. J Clin Oncol 12:2471, 1994.
32. Tuan IZ, Dennison D, Weisdorf DJ: *Pneumocystis carinii* pneumonitis following bone marrow transplantation. Bone Marrow Transplant 10:267, 1992.
33. Locksley RM, Flournoy N, Sullivan KM, Meyers JD: Varicella zoster virus infection after marrow transplantation. J Infect Dis 152:1172, 1985.
34. Yoshikawa T, Suga S, Asano Y, et al: Human herpesvirus-6 infection in bone marrow transplantation. Blood 78:1381, 1991.
35. Russell SJ, Vowels MR, Vale T: Hemorrhagic cystitis in pediatric bone marrow transplant patients: An association with infective agents, GVHD and prior cyclophosphamide. Bone Marrow Transplant 13:533, 1994.
36. Arthur RR, Shah KV, Baust SJ, et al: Association of BK viruria with hemorrhagic cystitis in recipients of bone marrow transplants. N Engl J Med 315:230, 1986.
37. Shields AF, Hackman RC, Fife KH, et al: Adenovirus infections in patients undergoing bone marrow transplantation. N Engl J Med 312:529, 1985.
38. Drobyski WR, Dunne WM, Burd EM, et al: Human herpesvirus-6 (HHV-6) infection in allogenic bone marrow transplant recipients: Evidence of a marrow-suppressive role for HHV-6 in vivo. J Infect Dis 167:735, 1993.
39. Meyers JD: Prevention of cytomegalovirus infection after marrow transplantation. Rev Infect Dis 11(Suppl 7):S1691, 1989.
40. Meyers JD, Flournoy N, Thomas ED: Risk factors for cytomegalovirus infection after human marrow transplantation. J Infect Dis 153:478, 1986.
41. Miller W, Flynn P, McCullough J, et al: Cytomegalovirus infection after bone marrow transplantation: An association with acute graft-v-host disease. Blood 67:1162, 1986.
42. Wingard JR, Chen D, Burns WH, et al: Cytomegalovirus infection after autologous bone marrow transplantation with comparison to infection after allogeneic bone marrow transplantation. Blood 71:1432, 1988.
43. Grundy JE, Shanley JD, Griffiths PD: Is cytomegalovirus interstitial pneumonitis in transplant recipients an immunopathological condition? Lancet 2:996, 1987.
44. Reed EC, Bowden RA, Dandliker PS, et al: Treatment of cytomegalovirus pneumonia in marrow transplant patients with ganciclovir and intravenous cytomegalovirus immunoglobulin. Ann Intern Med 109:783, 1988.
45. Sayers MH, Anderson KC, Goodnough LT, et al: Reducing the risk for transfusion-transmitted cytomegalovirus infection. Ann Intern Med 116:55, 1992.
46. Goodrich JM, Bowden RA, Fisher L, et al: Ganciclovir prophylaxis to prevent cytomegalovirus disease after allogenic marrow transplant. Ann Intern Med 118:173, 1993.
47. Winston DJ, Ho WG, Bartoni K, et al: Ganciclovir prophylaxis of cytomegalovirus infection and disease in allogeneic bone marrow transplant recipients. Results of a placebo-controlled, double-blind trial. Ann Intern Med 118:179, 1993.
48. Schmidt GM, Horak DA, Niland JC, et al: A randomized, controlled trial of prophylactic ganciclovir for cytomegalovirus pulmonary infection in recipients of allogeneic bone marrow transplants. N Engl J Med 324:1005, 1991.
49. Weiner RS, Bortin MM, Gale RP, et al: Interstitial pneumonitis after bone marrow transplantation. Ann Intern Med 104:168, 1986.
50. Atkinson K, Farewell V, Storb R, et al: Analysis of late infections after human bone marrow transplantation: Role of genotypic nonidentity between marrow donor and recipient and of nonspecific suppression cells in patients with chronic graft-versus-host disease. Blood 60:714, 1982.
51. Winston DJ, Schiffman G, Wang DC, et al: Pneumococcal infections after human bone-marrow transplantation. Ann Intern Med 91:835, 1979.
52. Ljungman P, Wilczek H, Gahrton G, et al: Long-term acyclovir prophylaxis in bone marrow transplant recipients and lymphocyte proliferation responses to herpes virus antigens in vitro. Bone Marrow Transplant 1:185, 1986.
53. Wingard JR, Santos GW, Saral R: Late-onset interstitial pneumonia following allogeneic bone marrow transplantation. Transplantation 39:21, 1985.

136

Infections Associated with Corticosteroids and Immunosuppressive Therapy

Neil L. Barg
Robert Fekety

In this chapter we focus on infections in immunocompromised hosts that result not from factors inherent in their underlying disease but instead from the immunosuppressive effects of treatment of those diseases. The chapter concerns iatrogenic infectious diseases or so-called diseases of medical progress, which result from violations, albeit well intentioned, of a fundamental tenet of therapy: "Above all, do no harm." These diseases illustrate all too well that many therapeutic measures are undertaken despite their striking an uncertain compromise between risks and benefits. As the costs of keeping such immunosuppressed persons alive escalate, medical scientists and society as a whole will have to make difficult choices about who will live and who will die; these decisions will unfortunately be based on financial considerations as often as on humanitarian principles.

Infections in immunosuppressed hosts have many features that overlap with infections in compromised hosts, but the latter may suffer from even broader and more diverse derangements in host defenses. Infections in immunosuppressed hosts most often result from treatment-induced reductions in granulocyte numbers or function or both or from impairment of cellular immunity related to effects upon lymphocytes, monocytes, or macrophages. In addition, immunocompromised patients may have deficiencies in immunoglobulins, the complement system, and other key defensive mechanisms. Significantly, these patients are also subject to infections related to the presence of catheters, prostheses, other foreign bodies, tissue damage, obstruction, and bleeding from the underlying disease. Whereas in clinical practice problems associated with granulocytopenia and impaired cellular immunity are even more complex than the terms imply, it is useful to consider them here as isolated problems. More details concerning the diagnosis and management of the specific infections seen in these patients are provided in other chapters of this book.

Infections in Patients Receiving Glucocorticosteroid Therapy

Short- or long-term administration of adrenal glucocorticosteroids results in a wide range of dose-related negative effects on inflammatory and immune defenses against infections. The most important mechanism by which steroids suppress inflammation and enhance susceptibility to infection is by impairing the mobilization and function of neutrophils and mononuclear cells at sites of primary lodgment of microorganisms in tissues. Thus, even though corticosteroids may cause leukocytosis, these patients actually have a risk of infection similar to that of neutropenic patients but with three important additional features. First, these deficiencies in neutrophil mobilization may persist for long periods if steroid therapy is continued; second, neutrophil deficiencies are often accompanied by lymphopenia, monocytopenia, or deficiencies in monocyte, macrophage, and lymphocyte function, with resultant impairment of important cellular immune mechanisms that are normally effective in preventing infections with certain pathogens (Table 136–1); and third, these patients often have all the infection-related risks of the anatomic abnormalities of the underlying disease and also those resulting from treatment with immunosuppressive or cytostatic agents, radiation, implantation of foreign bodies, and surgical procedures. Consequently, multiple sequential infections or polymicrobial infections frequently afflict these patients, especially those undergoing organ transplantation.[1]

Fever and Infection in Neutropenic Patients

With the increasing use of myelosuppressive and immunosuppressive agents or radiation for the treatment of neoplastic diseases and in transplantation, infections in granulocytopenic patients have become more common. Experience has shown that appropriate empirical therapy must be started early during the course of infections in neutropenic patients if a fatal outcome is to be prevented.[2] Antibiotics should not be withheld because the infection and its pathogens have not been documented precisely. Unfortunately, the usual manifestations of infection typically are absent during the early stages in patients with marked neutropenia, for whom a temperature higher than 101.5°F, erythema, local pain, and tenderness are often the only signs of infection.[3]

The frequency of infections during neutropenia is inversely proportional to the absolute neutrophil count (Fig. 136–1). They begin to increase when the neutrophil count falls below 500/mm^3, and both the frequency and severity of infection

TABLE 136–1 ■ Pathogens That Often Cause Infections in Patients with Deficiencies of Cell-Mediated Immunity

Bacteria
Legionella pneumophila
Listeria monocytogenes
Mycobacterium tuberculosis
Mycobacterium avium-intracellulare
Nocardia asteroides
Pseudomonas species
Salmonella species
Viruses
Cytomegalovirus
Herpes simplex virus
Varicella-zoster virus
Epstein-Barr virus
Fungi
Aspergillus
Blastomyces dermatitidis
Candida species
Coccidioides immitis
Cryptococcus neoformans
Histoplasma capsulatum
Zygomycetes *(Mucor)*
Protozoa
Toxoplasma gondii
Giardia lamblia
Entamoeba histolytica
Helminths
Strongyloides stercoralis

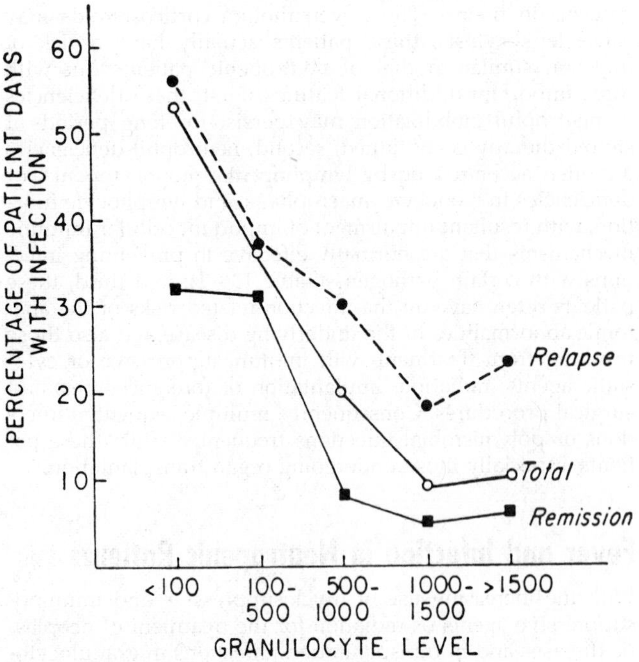

FIGURE 136–1 □ Quantitative relationship between various degrees of neutropenia and infection. (From Bodey GP, Buckely M, Sathe YS, Freireich EJ: Quantitative relationships between circulating leukocytes and infection in patients with acute leukemia. Ann Intern Med 64:328–340, 1966.)

increase steadily as the granulocyte count approaches zero. Severe infections with bacteremia tend to occur when the granulocyte count is below 100 to 200/mm^3. Because corticosteroid therapy impairs granulocyte mobilization and function,[4] the risk of infection at a given level of granulocytopenia is further increased when these patients are also treated with corticosteroids. The frequency of infectious complications of steroid therapy rises with doses of prednisone equivalents of more than 20 mg/d, or a total of more than 700 mg, and with treatment for longer than 30 days. Susceptibility may be reduced by using alternate-day dosing and by keeping the dose as small as possible.[4–6] The duration of the neutropenic state also is directly related to the infection rate; neutropenia is usually sustained longer and infections are more frequent after treatment of leukemia or after bone marrow transplantation (about 2 to 4 weeks) than after treatment of most carcinomas and solid tumors, in which profound neutropenia usually lasts only 7 to 10 days on the average.

Pathogens

Although many different kinds of organisms have been isolated from the blood and infected sites of neutropenic patients, certain organisms are more common than others (Table 136–2). Most of these organisms normally colonize areas adjacent to the site of infection. Although they may be considered part of the normal flora, they have often been acquired nosocomially and are also resistant to antibiotics, especially if the patient received broad-spectrum antibiotic therapy before the onset of the infection.[7] In addition, a shift of the normal oropharyngeal flora toward more resistant gram-negative organisms has correlated with increasing severity of the underlying diseases, use of nasogastric tubes, and use of antacid medications, even in the absence of antibiotic exposure. Suppression of the "colonization resistance" provided normally by intestinal anaerobes also favors a shift in the intestinal flora toward pathogenic, antibiotic-resistant aerobes; this is usually the result of treatment with antibiotics that have good activity against colonic anaerobes. Fungal infections typically occur as complications or as superinfections that follow successful treatment of bacterial infections in these patients.

Increasingly, unusual organisms, recognized now primarily because of their isolation from patients with acquired immunodeficiency syndrome, cause infections in neutropenic patients and patients treated for prolonged periods with corticosteroids. For example, atypical mycobacteria,[8] the fungus *Fusarium solani*,[9, 10] *Prototheca*,[11] and *Bartonella henselae* (the agent of bacillary angiomatosis and cat-scratch disease),[12] and *Rhodococcus equi*[13] have been isolated from blood, catheters, or wounds in these patients.

Sites of Infection

In most studies of infection in febrile neutropenic patients, about 20% of patients are found to have bacteremia, often from perirectal infection, an intravascular line, or an inapparent source in the gastrointestinal tract; 20% have microbiologically defined infections at a site such as the lungs, skin, oral cavity, or urinary tract; 20% have a recognizable probable site of infection but a specific bacterial pathogen cannot be determined; 20% have fever caused by factors unrelated to infection; and the remaining 20% have fever of unknown cause. Many of the last are probably caused by common viruses. Infections of the oral cavity, sinuses, skin, or perirectal area are often minor in appearance and are thus overlooked, but they are important nonetheless in neutropenic patients.[14] Oral mucositis in association with cytarabine therapy seems uniquely associated with a high frequency of viridans streptococcal bacteremia and especially with *Streptococcus mitis*, *Streptococcus sanguis*, and *Streptococcus oralis*. Fortunately, these organisms are usually susceptible to the antimicrobials in the usual regimens started empirically for neutropenic fever.[15]

Diagnosis

Cultures should be propagated with blood, material from intravenous access sites, and exudate from sites of infection as soon as possible after infection is suspected; aspirates or biopsy specimens from cutaneous lesions should also be cultured. Chest radiography should be performed even if there are no pulmonary symptoms, because minimal infiltrates may be an early clue to pneumonitis. Routine surveillance cultures from asymptomatic body sites do not appear

TABLE 136–2 ■ Pathogens That Most Often Infect Granulocytopenic Patients

Bacteria
Gram-negative bacilli
Common: *Escherichia coli, Pseudomonas aeruginosa, Klebsiella pneumoniae, Enterobacter cloacae, Enterobacter aerogenes, Proteus* species
Less common: *Serratia marcescens, Aeromonas, Bacteroides, Capnocytophaga* species
Gram-positive cocci and bacilli
Common: *Staphylococcus aureus, Staphylococcus epidermidis, Enterococcus faecalis*
Less common: corynebacteria JK, *Bacillus* species, *Clostridium* species
Polymicrobial infections of yeasts and molds
Common: *Candida, Aspergillus*, zygomycetes (*Mucor, Rhizopus*) species
Less common: *Fusarium, Trichosporon* species, *Pseudallescheria boydii*

to be worthwhile as a guide to empirical therapy, because it is common for many organisms to be isolated, which makes selecting the probable opportunistic pathogen difficult, and because of the expense and inherent delay in obtaining results of these cultures[16].

More rapid and sensitive tools have become available with use of polymerase chain reaction–based techniques for diagnosis of toxoplasmosis[17] and for infections with viruses such as cytomegalovirus (CMV),[18] parvovirus,[19] and hepatitis C virus.[20]

Therapy

EMPIRICAL THERAPY

Because bacteremia is relatively common in neutropenic patients, empirical therapy should be instituted promptly after blood cultures have been obtained, especially if the granulocyte count is lower than 200/mm^3 or if the patient appears to be in a toxic state. If there is a suspected site of infection, therapy should be based on knowledge of the normal flora at contiguous areas and on the results of Gram staining or other stain examination when exudate is available. Previous antibiotic therapy and hospitalization favoring selection of resistant organisms should be taken into consideration.

Because both gram-positive and gram-negative organisms are common causes of these infections, empirical therapy should be broad and designed to cover both kinds of organisms. Usually two antimicrobials are given simultaneously, one primarily for gram-positive organisms and another for gram-negative. Many different regimens have been studied and recommended, and in general none is clearly superior. In individual patients and in specific places, some regimens may be clearly better than others.[21] Unless intravascular lines are the probable source of the infection or Gram stain examination suggests staphylococci, many experts prefer to direct empirical therapy primarily toward gram-negative aerobic or facultative anaerobic pathogens because of their greater occurrence. Infections with strict anaerobes do occur, but they are both rare and rarely associated with signs of severe sepsis in neutropenic patients unless there are localizing findings that suggest intraabdominal or necrotizing infection. Therefore, current empirical therapy often ignores the possibility of obligate anaerobes as the etiologic agents. Some prefer, in fact, to use drugs with poor activity against anaerobic organisms (such as aztreonam or ceftazidime), because they may preserve colonization resistance in the intestines, thus reducing the likelihood of sepsis caused by gram-negative enteropathogens. Therapy should be bactericidal if possible, because granulocytes present in small numbers cannot be relied on to kill bacteria. This means that large doses of parenteral antibiotics designed to achieve bactericidal serum levels may be needed. Combination antibiotic therapy employing an antipseudomonal β-lactam agent plus an aminoglycoside is favored by most experts because it may result in synergistic or at least additive effects.[22] Neutropenic patients who exhibit bacteremia or are in shock as a result of infection (which is relatively uncommon in neutropenic patients) have better response rates when treated with a synergistic combination of antimicrobials.[23, 24] Other experts prefer to use an antipseudomonal β-lactam or carbapenem alone initially for febrile neutropenic patients who do not appear to be in a toxic condition or severely ill; aminoglycosides, vancomycin, or antifungal therapy is added later as needed, on the basis of culture results, clinical findings, and the course of the illness. Vancomycin should be added to the regimen when methicillin-resistant coagulase-positive or -negative staphylococci are either definitely implicated or strongly suspected. Serum levels of aminoglycosides and vancomycin, as well as renal function, may need to be monitored to minimize toxicity and maximize therapeutic responses. After the infecting organisms and their susceptibility patterns have been determined and the patient's condition begins to improve, it may be possible and in fact desirable to discontinue aminoglycosides or other unnecessary antibiotics or to reduce the dosage so as to minimize toxicity. The antimicrobials used most often for these infections are listed in Table 136–3.

Some studies of empirical therapy for neutropenic fever indicate that results with single agents (usually a β-lactam such as ceftazidime) are as good as those with a combination of drugs. Most of these studies can be criticized on the grounds that they have included too few cases of either documented gram-negative bacteremia or sustained neutropenia (because such patients are at greatest risk of a bad outcome) or because they included too many patients with minor infections or no proven infection or patients with only brief episodes of neutropenia, as this last group has done relatively well even when given no antibiotic therapy. In one well-controlled study by the European Organization for Research and Treatment of Cancer that compared empirical combination therapy of febrile neutropenic patients with amikacin given for either 3 or 9 days in addition to ceftazidime given to both groups for 9 days, the overall response rate was 64% in 266 patients given amikacin for 3 days and 68% in 368 patients given amikacin for 9 days, an insignificant difference.[25] However, in the 80 patients with documented gram-negative bacteremia, the response rate was only 48% in those given amikacin for 3 days but 81% in those given amikacin for 9 days. The difference favoring the longer course of amikacin in patients with bacteremia was seen with each of the most frequent specific organisms (*Escherichia coli*, *Klebsiella pneumoniae*, and *Pseudomonas aeruginosa*). Although a comparison of short-course versus long-course therapy with an aminoglycoside is not entirely relevant to the issue of combination therapy versus monotherapy, these results do demonstrate the importance of analyzing data according to specific pathogens and sites instead of looking only at overall

TABLE 136–3 ■ Antibiotics Most Often Used in Combination for Empirical Therapy of Suspected Infection in Granulocytopenic Patients

Antibacterials (usually initial therapy is with an antipseudomonal β-lactam plus an aminoglycoside)	
Penicillins	Cephalosporins
Ticarcillin	Ceftazidime
Timentin	Cefotaxime
Piperacillin	Cefoperazone
Azlocillin	Ceftizoxime
Mezlocillin	Monobactams
Carbapenems	Aztreonam
Imipenem-cilastatin	
Aminoglycosides	
Gentamicin	
Tobramycin	
Amikacin	
Netilmicin	
Agents usually added in special circumstances	
Vancomycin (methicillin-resistant *Staphylococcus aureus*, *Staphylococcus epidermidis*, enterococci, corynebacteria JK)	
Erythromycin (*Legionella*)	
Ciprofloxacin, ofloxacin (*Pseudomonas*)	
Metronidazole (anaerobes)	
Ampicillin-sulbactam (anaerobes)	
Trimethoprim-sulfamethoxazole (*Pneumocystis carinii*)	
Antifungals	
Amphotericin B	Itraconazole
Flucytosine	Fluconazole
Ketoconazole	Miconazole

results. Conversely, in another study that is often cited to support monotherapy with ceftazidime for neutropenia and fever, a large proportion of patients eventually required modification of monotherapy to achieve a good response (for example, vancomycin may have been added because a gram-positive infection was documented). Patients who required such a modification of therapy were not considered treatment failures by the investigators, as they survived despite delayed initiation of appropriate therapy.[26] Unfortunately, only a relatively small number of patients in this study had documented bacteremia, and the number was too small to permit valid statistical tests to determine significant differences in outcome. Because imipenem-cilastatin (Primaxin) has a broad spectrum of activity and is resistant to inducible β-lactamases, it has been considered attractive for monotherapy.[16] In one study, imipenem-cilastatin yielded as good results as the double β-lactam combinations studied for comparison, but it produced seizures when given in a dose of 1.0 g intravenously every 6 hours.[27] Finally, resistant organisms are reported to emerge more rapidly with monotherapy,[28] and combination therapy may be better in that regard.[2, 29–31]

Currently, for initial therapy of febrile neutropenic patients, most experts recommend either an aminoglycoside or fluoroquinolone plus an antipseudomonal β-lactam or carbapenem antimicrobial. No single combination of antibiotics seems clearly superior to other popular ones when response rates, toxicity, and cost are taken into consideration.[30, 31] When neutropenic patients are given appropriate antibiotics for a documented infection, it usually takes at least 3 or 4 days for a good response to become evident; therefore, unless new diagnoses are made, antibiotic regimens should probably not be altered more often than that when fever persists. When modifications are indicated during the course of empirical therapy, anaerobic coverage should be added when necrotizing gingivitis or perirectal cellulitis is present. Vancomycin or teicoplanin should be added when methicillin-resistant *Staphylococcus aureus* or *Staphylococcus epidermidis* infection is identified. Likely pathogens and local susceptibility patterns should be taken into consideration. The use of fluoroquinolone prophylaxis in patients with neutropenic fever has been reported to reduce the duration and amount of antibiotic therapy required but is likely to select for quinolone-resistant organisms, particularly α-hemolytic streptococci such as *S. mitis*, *S. oralis*, and *S. sanguis*.[15] Fluconazole may be useful in treatment of fungal infections and reduce the need for treatment with amphotericin B, but both therapy and prophylaxis with fluconazole have been followed by the emergence of fluconazole-resistant *Candida* species; consequently, most authorities discourage the use of fluconazole prophylaxis during neutropenic fever. Detailed discussions of the advantages and disadvantages of various popular regimens have been published.[30, 31]

Another still controversial area in the management of neutropenic fever concerns the use of so-called double β-lactam therapy, that is, two β-lactam drugs given simultaneously, such as ceftazidime plus piperacillin or aztreonam plus cefoperazone. Double β-lactam combinations are used most often in the hope of achieving better coverage against *Pseudomonas* and other resistant gram-negative pathogens without incurring the toxicity risks of aminoglycosides. Reasons for *not* using double β-lactam therapy include possible antagonism, undesirable alterations in fecal anaerobic flora,[32] the possibility of promoting resistance (because two β-lactamase inducers are present or because more penicillin binding sites are blocked), the possibly greater frequency of coagulation defects, more frequent side effects such as rash, and increased expense.[29, 33, 34] In favor of the practice of using double β-lactam therapy are a few encouraging but not conclusive studies. Results of controlled studies that are now under way may provide better guidelines.

Some experts have begun cautiously to treat low-risk patients with neutropenic fever as outpatients, using agents such as oral quinolones, clindamycin, aztreonam, ceftriaxone, or once-daily aminoglycosides.[35] Most of these patients do not have serious, documentable bacterial infections. Although some patients did not respond to such therapy and later required admission to the hospital for more aggressive antiinfective therapy, the overall results were surprisingly good and mortality rates were low (2%). Advantages included lower costs, lower exposure to nosocomial organisms, fewer superinfections, and improved quality of life. A variant of this that is becoming popular is the early discharge from the hospital of patients with neutropenic fever who are doing well, whose cultures and other diagnostic studies do not reveal anything alarming, and who are reliable and able to take antibiotics orally or parenterally at home.

Granulocyte colony-stimulating factor and granulocyte-macrophage colony-stimulating factor are being used with increasing frequency to produce early return of granulocytes in the peripheral blood of patients with neutropenic fever. This is an expensive innovation and one that has not yet been clearly shown to reduce mortality rates, even though the duration of neutropenia, fever, and hospitalization is shortened during their use.[36, 37] Additional studies are indicated to determine their role.

MODE OF ADMINISTRATION OF ANTIBIOTICS

Although some experts prefer to give aminoglycosides by continuous infusion, evidence supports the notion that the efficacy of aminoglycosides in immunocompromised patients is related more to peak concentrations than to sustained concentrations and that the reverse is true for β-lactams, possibly because they have a brief postantibiotic effect. Thus, it has been recommended that β-lactams be given to neutropenic patients by continuous infusion and that aminoglycosides be given intravenously, either once or more times per day or continuously.[38]

DURATION OF THERAPY

Whatever empirical regimen is used, it is clear that persistent profound granulocytopenia is associated with substantially lower favorable response rates than those seen in patients with rising granulocyte counts. In a study that compared three β-lactam plus aminoglycoside combinations, only 27% of patients with persistent granulocytopenia had good responses, whereas 73% of those whose granulocyte counts rose during therapy responded well.[39] Patients who respond and become afebrile and whose neutropenia resolves need not be treated longer than 10 days in most cases. The proper duration of therapy for persistently neutropenic patients whose disease has responded to antimicrobials is still controversial. Most authorities recommend therapy for 10 to 14 days or for 1 week after the fever subsides. In contrast, others advocate continuing therapy until neutropenia resolves, as determined by the granulocyte count rising to 500 to 1000/mm^3, despite the attendant risks of possibly increased toxicity, antibiotic resistance, and expense. Still others believe that therapy should be discontinued despite persistent neutropenia after 7 to 10 afebrile days if the patient has no other significant complaints or problems and that diagnostic studies and therapy should be reinstituted if fever returns or the patient's clinical status deteriorates.[40–42]

Prophylaxis with oral quinolones or trimethoprim-sulfamethoxazole, with or without antifungal prophylaxis with ketoconazole or fluconazole, is frequently given instead of continued treatment to afebrile but persistently neutropenic patients, particularly those who have leukemia, who tend to have more profound and prolonged neutropenia than that induced by drugs in patients with solid tumors.[23, 43, 44] A regimen of oral ciprofloxacin or ofloxacin and amphotericin may provide better results than other prophylactic regimens, with less risk of emergence of resistant strains.[43] Intensive gut decontamination regimens employing oral drugs such as vancomycin, erythromycin, neomycin, colistin, framycetin, nystatin, or amphotericin B with or without a parenteral third-generation cephalosporin can also be effective in preventing infection during persistent neutropenia,[24] but they are no longer used at most centers unless patients are also in a total protective environment designed to limit exposure to resistant organisms. In addition, such regimens are likely to favor the emergence and spread of antibiotic-resistant organisms.

Persistent Fever and Neutropenia Despite Broad Antibacterial Therapy

When fever persists more than 4 to 7 days in neutropenic patients despite treatment and despite failure to diagnose a specific infection, most physicians recommend adding antifungal therapy with amphotericin B or fluconazole, even though this practice may not increase survival rates.[45] Empirical antibacterial therapy is also continued in most cases, but superinfections are common in this setting. Table 136–4 is a modification of a published algorithm for managing persistent neutropenia and fever in the presence of empirical therapy.[46] Granulocyte transfusions are no longer employed often in these cases, although they may given when patients with documented gram-negative bacteremia fail to respond to intensive and appropriate antibiotic therapy.

Fungal Infections

The diagnosis of invasive fungal infection in an immunosuppressed host is often difficult, and dissemination may occur while therapy is being withheld for fear of the toxicity of amphotericin B or while awaiting a definitive diagnosis.[7] *Candida* ophthalmitis is a definite indication for therapy with parenteral amphotericin or parenteral fluconazole, and these agents are often used for *Candida* pyelonephritis or fungemia with cutaneous lesions. As is the case with bacterial infections, the outcome of treatment of fungal infections in neutropenic patients is improved with early therapy. Earlier antifungal therapy may become more popular as confidence increases in the efficacy of oral antifungals, especially fluconazole. Once begun, amphotericin B therapy should be continued for a total dose of 500 mg or more or for 10 to 14 days unless there is toxicity or the granulocytopenia resolves. Patients with documented invasive or disseminated fungal infection should be treated according to the usual guidelines, generally with 1 to 2 g of amphotericin B. In patients without neutropenia or major immunodeficiency, parenteral fluconazole, given as 400 mg/d for at least 14 days after the last positive culture, has also been reported to be effective.[47]

FOCAL HEPATIC AND SPLENIC CANDIDIASIS

Focal hepatic and splenic *Candida* infection has been recognized with increasing frequency in neutropenic patients.[48, 49] Patients usually present with persistent fever of unknown origin that is not responsive to antibiotic therapy. The syndrome usually does not occur until the neutrophil count has returned to normal. It most often affects patients with leukemia but has also been associated with neutropenia and solid tumors or aplastic anemia. There is usually a history of *Candida* infection during the neutropenic period, but there is little or no evidence of an active *Candida* infection when the syndrome is recognized. Abdominal pain and enlargement of the liver and spleen may occur, along with leukocytosis and an elevated serum alkaline phosphatase level. Characteristic lesions are seen in the liver at ultrasonography (bull's-eye, or target, lesions) or computed tomography (Fig. 136–2). Liver biopsy examination shows yeasts or pseudohyphae in the center of granulomatous lesions; surprisingly, cultures of the biopsy specimen and blood are usually sterile, especially if the patient was previously treated with antifungal therapy. *Candida albicans* is most often implicated. Treatment is frequently unsuccessful unless it is aggressive: more than 2 g of amphotericin B (with or without flucytosine) is given to most patients. Multiple biopsy examinations and scans and multiple courses of therapy are frequently required because of treatment failure or relapse. Liposomal amphotericin B may prove superior to ordinary amphotericin because of enhanced delivery of liposomes to the sites of infection in the liver and spleen as well as reduced toxicity. Some patients who failed to respond to amphotericin or suffered toxicity were treated successfully with fluconazole, 200 to 400 mg/d for 6 to 12 months.[50] Both the increasing efficacy of therapy of leukemia or solid tumors and the availability of ultrasonography and computed tomography have probably combined to increase the apparent frequency of this syndrome.

TABLE 136–4 ■ Modifications of Therapy That May Be Required in Cases of Persistent Fever and Neutropenia

CLINICAL PROBLEM	SUGGESTED MODIFICATION
Persistent unexplained fever and neutropenia	After 4–7 d, add antifungal therapy and continue antibiotics.
Breakthrough bacteremia	Add vancomycin if isolate is gram-positive. Switch to new, more intensive regimen if isolate is gram-negative.
Intravenous catheter-related infection	Add vancomycin or gram-negative coverage if not already being given. Add amphotericin B or fluconazole if there is evidence of *Candida* retinitis, pyelonephritis, fungemia, or skin infection.
Severe oral mucositis or gingivitis	Add coverage specific for anaerobes if not already being given.
Perianal tenderness or infection	Add specific anaerobe coverage if not already being given.
Esophagitis	Add oral clotrimazole, amphotericin, or fluconazole.
Pneumonitis	
New infiltration	Watch and wait if granulocyte count is rising and patient is otherwise doing well. If granulocyte count is not rising, obtain sputum or biopsy sample and add amphotericin or fluconazole while awaiting results.
Diffuse or interstitial infiltrates	Add trimethoprim-sulfamethoxazole and erythromycin.

Adapted from Pizzo PA: After empiric therapy: What to do until the granulocyte comes back. Rev Infect Dis 9:214–219, 1987.

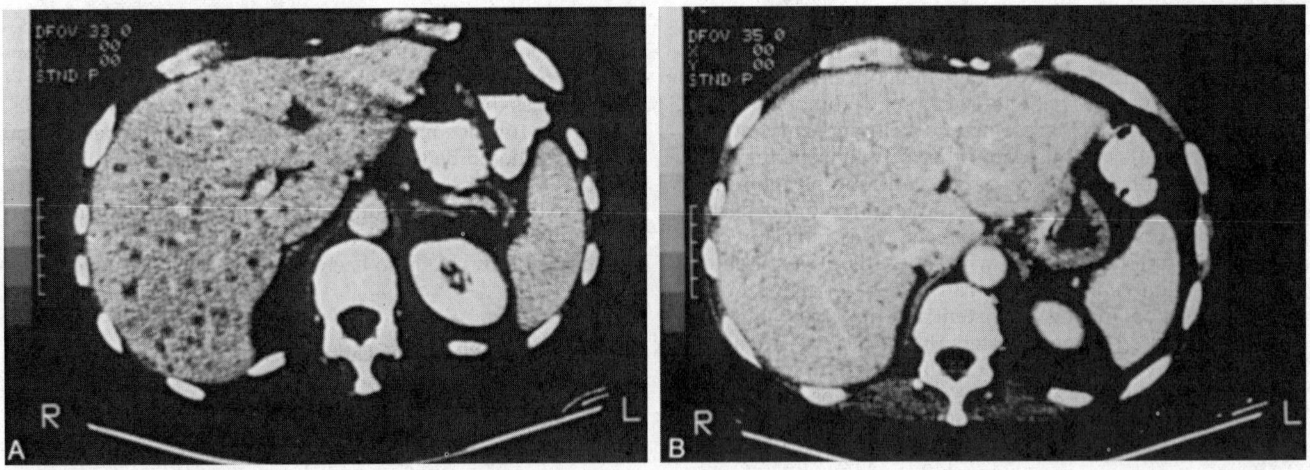

FIGURE 136–2 □ Computed tomographic scan of the liver of a patient with hepatic candidiasis after recovery from neutropenia. *A*, At time of diagnosis. *B*, One month later, after treatment with intravenous amphotericin B.

Infections and Renal Transplantation

A retrospective review of infections in 162 renal allograft recipients studied before 1976 at the University of Michigan showed that 83% of patients developed an infection during the first year after transplantation (during which the mean daily dose of prednisone was 50 mg), and infection was an important contributory cause in 73% of deaths.[5] Urinary tract, pulmonary, surgical wound, blood stream, meningeal, and shunt infections were most common. *S. aureus*, enteric bacteria, *Pseudomonas*, and *Candida* species were most frequently implicated, but a wide variety of conventional and opportunistic pathogens were detected. *Cryptococcus neoformans* was the most common cause of meningitis, which often presented as a chronic or subacute illness characterized by headache and low-grade fever.

The frequency of fatal infections after renal transplantation has declined markedly because lower maintenance doses (less than 20 mg of prednisone per day) of steroids are now used, because of less frequent production of neutropenia by cytotoxic immunosuppressive agents, and because of less frequent use of vigorous immunosuppressive therapy designed to save the kidney from being rejected at all costs. Newer pathogens, such as *Rhodococcus equi*, first recognized in patients with acquired immunodeficiency syndrome, are being reported in patients with renal transplants. This gram-positive coccus is resistant to most antibiotics except vancomycin and rifampin, and infections with it are usually associated with cavitary pulmonary lesions.[51] Tuberculosis, usually reactivation, is also seen in renal transplant patients, particularly after a period of intensive immunosuppression. Twenty-five percent of infections were disseminated on presentation in one report.[52]

It is noteworthy that the acquired immunodeficiency syndrome is a recognized complication of renal transplantation. Human immunodeficiency virus has usually been transmitted along with the transplanted kidney, which has generally shown remarkably little evidence of rejection. Acquired immunodeficiency syndrome usually pursues a rapid course in these patients.[53] This complication has become uncommon after routine testing for human immunodeficiency virus of all organ donors and of blood for transfusion.

CMV infections are important in renal transplant recipients, partly because primary CMV infection in a transplant recipient is associated with doubling of the rate of rejection, although causality has not been proved. Several studies have shown that CMV infection is more likely to occur after therapy for rejection with antilymphocyte preparations such as OKT3 or antilymphoblast globulin.[54] Preemptive therapy with ganciclovir may prevent severe CMV infection in this setting.[55] Primary CMV infection tends to be more serious than reactivation of a latent infection in these patients. Its major manifestations, in addition to rejection, are fever of unknown origin and leukopenia.[56] Administration of prophylactic anti-CMV immunoglobulin has been shown to prevent severe CMV-related disease in seronegative recipients of grafts from seropositive donors, even when they are being treated for rejection.[57] Ganciclovir may also be useful in treatment of these infections when they are documented early during rejection.

Other viral infections that are more common in renal transplant patients include hepatitis B and C and parvovirus infections. Since the advent of screening for hepatitis B, most cases are associated with progressive worsening of preexisting infections in the recipient after immunosuppression.[58] After CMV, hepatitis C virus is the next most common cause of hepatitis in transplant patients. Approximately 25% of patients have positive tests for hepatitis C by 1 year after transplantation.[59] Their illness is often mild and may not cause elevated transaminase values. However, its progression may be insidious and patients with elevated transaminase levels are at increased risk of complications.[60] Parvovirus can cause red blood cell aplasia and unresponsive anemia in immunosuppressed transplant patients, especially if they are children or young adults.[61, 62] There is an absence of reticulocytes during infection. Unless treated with intravenous immuneglobulin, parvovirus infection may be fatal.

Infections and Liver Transplantation

Although mortality rates associated with serious infections in patients with liver transplants have declined, such infections are still common. Their frequency is related directly to operative time and difficulties with this surgical procedure involving clean-contaminated sites. The most serious infections are polymicrobial peritonitis, cholangitis, and hepatic or other intraabdominal abscesses and are associated with anastomotic leakage of bacteria from the intestinal tract, leakage of bile, or fungal superinfections. Cholangitis as a result of stricture or instrumentation of the bilary tract may resemble rejection clinically.

Gram-positive bacteremias (especially with *S. aureus* and *Enterococcus*) are notably more common in patients with liver transplants than in patients with other solid organ transplants.[63] Bacterial infections within the first posttransplantation month are often mixed, along with fungal infection.[64] Unusual bacteria may be isolated because of the nature of the surgery. Roux-en-Y anastomoses may permit easy bacterial access to the biliary tree, and concomitant treatment with vancomycin may select for vancomycin-resistant organisms such as lactobacilli.[65] Use of granulocyte colony-stimulating factor for 7 to 10 days postoperatively to keep the total leukocyte count between 10,000 and 20,000/mm^3 has been reported to reduce significantly the incidence of sepsis and sepsis-related deaths as well as the rate of rejection, even though these patients were never neutropenic.[66] *Candida* and *Aspergillus* infections are particularly frequent after liver transplantation and may cause fungemia, infection of the central nervous system, or severe wound infections.[67] Prolonged treatment with ciprofloxacin appears to be a risk factor for developing candidal infections.[63] *Aspergillus* infections have been reported despite the prophylactic postoperative administration of amphotericin B (0.5 mg/kg).[68] Mycotic aneurysms caused by either *Aspergillus* or *Candida* are a cause of intracerebral hemorrhage in these patients. Concomitant diabetes is an associated risk factor.[69] Cryptococcosis has also been reported to cause severe cellulitis indistinguishable from bacterial skin and soft tissue infections in these patients.[70] The incidence of postoperative fungal infections may be reduced by the administration of liposomal amphotericin B to patients with liver transplants.[71] *Pneumocystis carinii* pneumonia, a late infection after liver transplantation, has been effectively prevented by the prophylactic administration of trimethoprim-sulfamethoxazole.[72]

Acute severe viral hepatitis is frequent after a patient with chronic active hepatitis B receives a liver transplant, even when hyperimmune globulin is also given. Hepatitis C is also seen in liver transplant patients and is surpassed in frequency only by CMV infection. Almost all of these represent relapses of infection acquired before the transplantation.[73] Pretransplantation screening for hepatitis C can identify the patients at risk for this complication. As in renal transplant patients, the infection may be indolent, and severe liver damage may result.[60] An association has been noted between CMV hepatitis, rejection, and the need for retransplantation; treatment of severely ill patients with ganciclovir or foscarnet can successfully control the CMV infection but is often associated with severe side effects. The risk of CMV infection is also associated with the use of OKT3.[74] Prophylaxis of patients at high risk of reactivation of CMV infection with 2 weeks of intravenous ganciclovir followed by high-dose oral acyclovir may be effective in patients not at risk for primary CMV infection.[75]

Infections and Heart and Heart-Lung Transplantation

Infections are a major cause of morbidity and mortality after heart transplantation, and in some centers more than half of early deaths resulted from infection. Infecting organisms may be transmitted via the graft, transfused blood, direct contact, or environmental reservoirs or may come from the endogenous flora or prior infections. Most of the nosocomial bacterial infections are encountered principally in the first 30 to 60 days after transplantation, and their frequency appears to be reduced by perioperative antibiotic prophylaxis; no single regimen is widely applicable, but one popular regimen consists of trimethoprim-sulfamethoxazole or a fluoroquinolone plus penicillin V plus nystatin or clotrimazole orally. Opportunistic infections with relatively weak pathogens usually do not occur during this early period unless the patient has been treated for acute rejection. The frequency of infection after the first month or two is directly related to the intensity of the immunosuppressive therapy required to prevent rejection. The use of antilymphocyte preparations for the treatment of rejection is also associated with increased severity of infections in the first 3 months postoperatively.[76] Protective isolation has not been shown to have a favorable effect on morbidity or mortality resulting from infection of these patients. Heart transplant recipients who require mechanical support with an intraaortic balloon pump, a left ventricular assist device, or a total artificial heart are at high risk for severe infection and death. Protocols utilizing cyclosporines to prevent rejection have been associated with a lowering of rates of severe infection. A multicenter report of patients who underwent transplantation in the cyclosporine era indicated that 58% of 384 patients developed infection, but there were only 20 infection-related deaths (5%).[76] All classes of organisms were involved, but the most frequent pathogens were *Staphylococcus*, gram-negative enterics, *Nocardia*, *Aspergillus*, *Cryptococcus*, CMV, other herpesviruses, *P. carinii*, and *Toxoplasma gondii*. Pulmonary infections are more common and more serious after heart or heart-lung transplantation than with other organ allografts. *Nocardia*, *Aspergillus*, and *P. carinii* pneumonia and *Pseudomonas* bronchitis are frequent. CMV pneumonia, enteritis, and retinitis are also common and can be treated with ganciclovir or foscarnet, but it is not certain that these infections adversely affect survival. A syndrome of unexplained fever, hepatitis, interstitial pneumonitis, leukopenia, and atypical lymphocytosis is common in heart transplant patients with primary CMV infection. CMV may also be associated with gastrointestinal bleeding in heart transplant patients; this may present with abdominal pain and refractory nausea. This infection does respond to treatment with gancylovir.[77] Accelerated coronary atherosclerosis has been linked to CMV infection in a group of young transplant patients, especially if infection occurs within the first year.[78, 79] It is likely that immune globulin prophylaxis of CMV infections in patients undergoing cardiac or bone marrow transplantation will result in decreased morbidity and mortality, but further documentation is needed. Pulmonary infections in heart transplant recipients frequently disseminate and are associated with a high rate of intracranial infection with opportunistic pathogens (Table 136–5). *Nocardia* and *Aspergillus* infections have been noted to cause intracranial abscesses with poorly developed capsules and extensive tissue necrosis in heart transplant recipients; the cerebrospinal fluid is usually normal in these patients. Infections of the nervous system tend to occur within the first 3 months after transplantation and in association with treatment of episodes of rejection. The routine use of prophylaxis with trimethoprim-sulfamethoxazole postoperatively has markedly reduced the incidence of *Pneumocystis* pneumonia; similarly, the prophylactic administration of pyrimethamine has reduced the incidence and severity of *Toxoplasma* infection.[80, 81]

TABLE 136–5 ■ Causes of Central Nervous System Infection in Transplant Patients

Cryptococcus neoformans
Listeria monocytogenes
Toxoplasma gondii
Nocardia asteroides
Zygomycetes *(Mucor)*
Aspergillus fumigatus
Candida species
Varicella-zoster virus
Progressive multifocal leukoencephalopathy

Infections and Bone Marrow Transplantation

See Chapter 135.

References

1. Korvick J, Yu VL: Simultaneous infection with *Cryptococcus neoformans* and *Legionella pneumophila*. In vivo expression of common defects in cell-mediated immunity. Respiration 53:132, 1988.
2. Schimpff SC: Overview of empiric therapy for the febrile neutropenic patient. Rev Infect Dis 7(Suppl 4):S734, 1985.
3. Sickles EA, Greene WH, Wiernik PH: Clinical presentation of infection in granulocytopenic patients. Arch Intern Med 135:715, 1975.
4. Fauci AS, Dale DC, Balow JE: Glucocorticosteroid therapy: Mechanisms of action and clinical considerations. Ann Intern Med 84:304, 1976.
5. Murphy JF, McDonald FD, Dawson M, et al: Factors affecting the frequency of infection in renal transplantation recipients. Arch Intern Med 136:670, 1976.
6. Stuck AE, Minder CE, Frey FJ: Risk of infectious complications in patients taking glucocorticosteroids. Rev Infect Dis 11:954, 1989.
7. Whimbey E, Kiehn TE, Brannon P, et al: Bacteremia and fungemia in patients with neoplastic disease. Am J Med 82:723, 1987.
8. Ingram CW, Tanner DC, Durack DT, et al: Disseminated infection with rapidly growing mycobacteria. Clin Infect Dis 16:463, 1993.
9. Bushelman SJ, Callen JP, Roth DN, et al: Disseminated *Fusarium solani* infection. J Am Acad Dermatol 32:346, 1995.
10. Ammari LK, Puck JM, McGowan KL et al: Catheter-related *Fusarium solani* fungemia and pulmonary infection in a patient with leukemia in remission. Clin Infect Dis 16:148, 1993.
11. Tsuji K, Hirohara J, Fukui Y, et al: Protothecosis in a patient with systemic lupus erythematosus. Intern Med 32:540, 1993.
12. Koehler JE, Glaser CA, Tappero JW: *Rochalimaea henselae* infection. A new zoonosis with the domestic cat as reservoir. JAMA 271:531, 1994.
13. Novak RM, Polisky EL, Janda WM, et al: Osteomyelitis caused by *Rhodococcus equi* in a renal transplant recipient. Infection 16:186, 1988.
14. Glenn J, Cotton D, Wesley R, Pizzo P: Anorectal infections in patients with malignant diseases. Rev Infect Dis 10:42, 1988.
15. Richard P, Amador Del Valle G, Moreau P, et al: Viridans streptococcal bacteraemia in patients with neutropenia. Lancet 345:1607, 1995.
16. Daw MA, Munnely P, McCann SR, et al: Value of surveillance cultures in the management of neutropenic patients. Eur J Clin Microbiol Infect Dis 7:742, 1998.
17. Holliman J, Johnson D, Savva D, et al: Diagnosis of toxoplasma infection in cardiac transplant recipients using the polymerase chain reaction. J Clin Pathol 45:9331, 1992.
18. Drouet I, Michelson S, Denoyel G, Colimon R: Polymerase chain reaction detection of human cytomegalovirus in over 2000 blood specimens correlated with virus isolation and related to urinary virus excretion. J Virol Methods 45:259, 1993.
19. Heegaard ED, Hornsleth A: *Parvovirus*: The expanding spectrum of disease. Acta Paediatr 84:109, 1995.
20. Wright TL, Donegan E, Hsu HH, et al: Recurrent and acquired hepatitis C viral infection in liver transplant recipients. Gastroenterology 103:317, 1992.
21. Bodey GP: Infection in cancer patients. A continuing association. Am J Med 81:11, 1986.
22. Gaya H: Combination therapy and monotherapy in the treatment of severe infection in the immunocompromised host. Am J Med 80(Suppl 6B):149, 1986.
23. Young LS: Antimicrobial prophylaxis in the neutropenic host: Lessons of the past and perspectives for the future. Eur J Microbiol Infect Dis 7:93, 1988.
24. Gava H: Rational basis for the choice of regimens for empirical therapy of sepsis in granulocyctopenia patients. Clin Hematol 13:573, 1984.
25. Ceftazidime combined with a short or long course of amikacin for empirical therapy of gram-negative bacteremia in cancer patients with granulocytopenia. The EORTC International Antimicrobial Therapy Cooperative Group. N Engl J Med 317:1692, 1987.
26. Pizzo PA, Hathorn JW, Hiemenz J, et al: A randomized trial comparing ceftazidime alone with combination antibiotic therapy in cancer patients with fever and neutropenia. N Engl J Med 315:552, 1986.
27. Mortimer J, Millar S, Black D, et al: Comparison of cefoperazone and mezlocillin with imipenem as empiric therapy in febrile neutropenic cancer patients. Am J Med 85:17, 1988.
28. Gribble MJ, Chow AW, Naiman SC, et al: Prospective randomized trial of piperacillin monotherapy versus carboxypenicillin/aminoglycoside combination regimens in the empirical treatment of serious bacterial infections. Antimicrob Agents Chemother 24:388, 1983.
29. Brown AE: Management of the febrile, neutropenic patient with cancer: Therapeutic considerations. J Pediatr 106:1035, 1985.
30. Wade JS: Antibiotic therapy for the febrile granulocytopenic patient: Combination therapy vs monotherapy. Rev Infect Dis 11(Suppl 7):S1572, 1989.
31. Young LS: Neutropenia: Antibiotic combinations for empiric therapy. Eur J Clin Microbiol Infect Dis 8:118, 1989.
32. Meijer-Severs GJ, Joshi JH: The effect of new broad-spectrum antibiotics on faecal flora of cancer patients. J Antimicrob Chemother 24:605, 1989.
33. Anaissie EJ, Fainstein V, Bodey GP, et al: Randomized trial of β-lactam regimens in febrile neutropenic cancer patients. Am J Med 84:581, 1988.
34. Jones P, Bodey GP, Rolston K, et al: Cefoperazone plus mezlocillin for empiric therapy of febrile cancer patients. Am J Med 85:3, 1988.
35. Malik IA, Khan WA, Karim M, et al: Feasibility of outpatient management of fever in cancer patients with low-risk neutropenia: Results of a prospective randomized trial. Am J Med 98:224, 1995.
36. Mayordomo JI, Rivera F, Diaz-Puente MT, et al: Improving treatment of chemotherapy-induced neutropenic fever by administration of colony-stimulating factors. J Natl Cancer Inst 87:803, 1995.
37. Riikonen P, Saarinen UM, Makipernaa A, et al: rhGM-CSF in the treatment of fever and neutropenia: A double-blind placebo controlled study in children with malignancy. Proc Annu Meet Am Soc Clin Oncol 12:A1532, 1993.
38. Bakker-Woudenberg IAJM, Roossendaal R: Impact of dosage regimens on the efficacy of antibiotics in the immunocompromised host. J Antimicrob Chemother 21:145, 1988.
39. Klastersky J, Glauser MP, Schimpff SC, et al: Prospective randomized comparison of three antibiotic regimens for empirical therapy of suspected bacteremic infection in febrile granulocytopenic patients. Antimicrob Agents Chemother 29:263, 1986.
40. DiNubile MJ: Stopping antibiotic therapy in neutropenic patients. Ann Intern Med 108:289, 1988.
41. Talbot GH, Provencher M, Cassileth PA: Persistent fever after recovery from granulocytopenia in acute leukemia. Arch Intern Med 148:129, 1988.
42. Talcott JA, Finberg R, Mayer RL, Goldman L: The medical course of cancer patients with fever and neutropenia. Arch Intern Med 148:2561, 1988.
43. Dekker AW, Rosenberg-Arska M, Verhoef J: Infection prophylaxis in acute leukemia: A comparison of ciprofloxacin with trimethoprim-sulfamethoxazole and colistin. Ann Intern Med 106:7, 1987.
44. Karp JE, Merz WG, Hendricksen C, et al: Oral norfloxacin for prevention of gram-negative bacterial infections in patients with acute leukemia and granulocytopenia. Ann Intern Med 106:1, 1987.
45. EORTC Cooperative Group: Empiric antifungal therapy in febrile granulocytopenic patients. Am J Med 86:668, 1989.
46. Pizzo PA: After empiric therapy: What to do until the granulocyte comes back. Rev Infect Dis 9:214, 1987.
47. Rex JH, Bennett JE, Pappas PG, et al: A randomized trial comparing fluconazole with amphotericin B for the treatment of candidemia in patients without neutropenia. N Engl J Med 331:1325, 1994.
48. Tashjian LS, Abramson JS, Peacock JE: Focal hepatic candidiasis. A distinct clinical variant of candidiasis in immunocompromised patients. Rev Infect Dis 6:689, 1984.
49. Thaler M, Pastakian B, Shawku TH, et al: Hepatic candidiasis in cancer patients. The evolving picture of the syndrome. Ann Intern Med 108:88, 1988.

50. Kauffman CA, Bradley SF, Ross SS, Weber DR: Hepatosplenic candidiasis: Successful treatment with fluconazole. Am J Med 91:137, 1991.
51. Lezama JA, Garcia-Arenzana JM, Viedma PI, Aznar MS: Pulmonary infection caused by *Rhodococcus equi* in a renal transplant recipient. Med Clin (Barc) 99:143, 1992.
52. Hall CM, Willcox PA, Swanepoel CR, et al: Mycobacterial infection in renal transplant recipients. Chest 106:435, 1994.
53. Briner V, Zimmerli W, Cathomas G, et al: HIV infection caused by kidney transplant: Case report and review of 18 published cases. Schweiz Med Wochenschr 119:1046, 1989.
54. Bailey TC, Powderly WG, Storch GA, et al: Symptomatic cytomegalovirus infection in renal transplant recipients given either Minnesota antilymphoblast globulin (MALG) or OKT3 for rejection prophylaxis. Am J Kidney Dis 21:196, 1993.
55. Hibberd PL, Rubin RH: Renal transplantation and related infections. Semin Respir Infect 8:216, 1993.
56. Bosch FH, Hoctsma AJ, Janssen HP, et al: Cytomegalovirus infection and diseases in renal transplant patients treated with cyclosporine. A prospective study. Transplant Int 2:92, 1989.
57. Metselaar HJ, Rothbart PH, Browwer RM, et al: Prevention of cytomegalovirus-related death by passive immunization. A double-blind placebo-controlled study in kidney transplant recipients treated for rejection. Transplantation 48:264, 1989.
58. Hamada T, Kumashiro MR, Koga Y, et al: Fatal acute hepatitis B virus infection while receiving immunosuppressants after renal transplantation. Intern Med 32:547, 1993.
59. Brunson ME, Lau JY, Davis GL, et al: Non-A, non-B hepatitis and elevated serum aminotransferases in renal transplant patients. Correlation with hepatitis C infection. Transplantation 56:1364, 1993
60. Chan TM, Wu PC, Lau JY, et al: Clinicopathologic features of hepatitis C virus infection in renal allograft recipients. Transplantation 58:996, 1994.
61. Rao SP, Miller ST, Cohen BJ: B19 parvovirus infection in children with malignant solid tumors receiving chemotherapy. Med Pediatr Oncol 22:255, 1994.
62. Uemura N, Ozawa K, Tani K, et al: Pure red cell aplasia caused by parvovirus B19 infection in a renal transplant recipient. Eur J Haematol 54:68, 1995.
63. Wade JJ, Rolando N, Hayllar K, et al: Bacterial and fungal infections after liver transplantation: An analysis of 284 patients. Hepatology 21:1328, 1995.
64. Barkholt L, Ericzon BG, Tollemar J, et al: Infections in human liver recipients: Different patterns early and late after transplantation. Transplant Int 6:77, 1993.
65. Patel R, Cockerill FR, Porayko MK, et al: Lactobacillemia in liver transplant patients. Clin Infect Dis 18:207, 1994.
66. Foster PF, Mital D, Sankary HN, et al: The use of granulocyte colony-stimulating factor after liver transplantation. Transplantation 59:1557, 1995.
67. Pla MP, Berenguer J, Arzuaga JA, et al: Surgical wound infection by *Aspergillus fumigatus* in liver transplant recipients. Diagn Microbiol Infect Dis 15:703, 1992.
68. Singh N, Mieles L, Yu VL, Gayowski T: Invasive aspergillosis in liver transplant recipients: Association with candidemia and consumption coagulopathy and failure of prophylaxis with low-dose amphotericin B. Clin Infect Dis 17:906, 1993.
69. Wijdicks EF, de Groen CF, Wiesner RH, Krom RA: Intracerebral hemorrhage in liver transplant recipients. Mayo Clin Proc 70:443, 1995.
70. Singh N, Rihs JD, Gayowski T, Yu VL: Cutaneous cryptococcosis mimicking bacterial cellulitis in a liver transplant recipient: Case report and review in solid organ transplant recipients. Clin Transplant 8:365, 1994.
71. Tollemar J, Hockerstedt K, Ericzon BG, et al: Liposomal amphotericin B prevents invasive fungal infections in liver transplant recipients. A randomized, placebo-controlled study. Transplantation 59:45, 1995.
72. Hayes MJ, Torzillo PJ, Sheil AG, McCaughan GW: *Pneumocystis carinii* pneumonia after liver transplantation in adults. Clin Transplant 8:499, 1994.
73. Weinstein JS, Poterucha JJ, Zein N, et al: Epidemiology and natural history of hepatitis C infections in liver transplant recipients. J Hepatol 22:154, 1995.
74. Stratta RJ, Shaeffer MS, Markin RS, et al. Cytomegalovirus infection and disease after liver transplantation. An overview. Dig Dis Sci 37:673, 1992.
75. Martin M, Manez R, Linden P, et al: A prospective randomized trial comparing sequential ganciclovir–high dose acyclovir to high dose acyclovir for prevention of cytomegalovirus disease in adult liver transplant recipients. Transplantation 58:779, 1994.
76. Grossi P, De Maria R, Caroli A, et al: Infections in heart transplant recipients: The experience of the Italian heart transplantation program. Italian Study Group on Infections in Heart Transplantation. J Heart Lung Transplant 11:847, 1992.
77. Arabia FA, Rosado LJ, Huston CL, et al: Incidence and recurrence of gastrointestinal cytomegalovirus infection in heart transplantation. Ann Thorac Surg 55:8, 1993.
78. Dummer S, Lee A, Breinig MK, et al: Investigation of cytomegalovirus infection as a risk factor for coronary atherosclerosis in the explanted hearts of patients undergoing heart transplantation. J Med Virol 44:305, 1994.
79. Koskinen PK, Nieminen MS, Krogerus LA, et al: Cytomegalovirus infection accelerates cardiac allograft vasculopathy: Correlation between angiographic and endomyocardial biopsy findings in heart transplant patients. Transplant Int 6:341, 1993.
80. Wreghitt TG, Gray GG, Pavel P, et al: Efficacy of pyrimethamine for the prevention of donor-acquired *Toxoplasma gondii* infection in heart and heart-lung transplant patients. Transplant Int 5:197, 1992.
81. Keating MR, Wilhelm MP, Walker RC: Strategies for prevention of infection after cardiac transplantation. Mayo Clin Proc 67:676, 1992.

Bibliography

- Bodey GP, Buckely M, Sathe YS, Freireich EH: Quantitative relationships between circulating leukocytes and infection in patients with acute leukemia. Ann Intern Med 64:328, 1966.
- Goering P, Berlinger NT, Weisdorf DJ: Aggressive combined modality treatment of progressive sinonasal fungal infections in immunocompromised patients. Am J Med 85:619, 1988.
- Hertz MI, Englund JA, Snover D, et al: Respiratory syncytial virus–induced acute lung injury in adult patients with bone marrow transplants: A clinical approach and review of the literature. Medicine (Baltimore) 68:269, 1989.
- Linder J: Infection as a complication of heart transplantation. J Heart Transplant 7:390, 1988.
- Melewski DJ, Higby DJ, Reese PA: Infectious complications in neutropenic patients. Clinical-laboratory correlations. J Med 19:1, 1988.
- Meyers JD, Leszcynski J, Zaia JA, et al: Prevention of cytomegalovirus infection by cytomegalovirus immune globulin after marrow transplantation. Ann Intern Med 98:442, 1983.
- van der Meer JWM, Guiot HFL, van den Broek PJ, van Furth R: Infections in bone marrow recipients. Semin Hematol 21:123, 1984.
- Watson JG: Problems of infection after bone marrow transplantation. J Clin Pathol 36:683, 1983.
- Winston DJ, Ho WG, Lin CH, et al: Intravenous immune globulin for prevention of cytomegalovirus infection and interstitial pneumonia after bone marrow transplantation. Ann Intern Med 106:12, 1987.

137

Treatment and Prevention of Infections in Immunocompromised Hosts

Stephen H. Zinner

The acquired immunodeficiency syndrome (AIDS) epidemic has highlighted the critical role of the intact immune system in the prevention of infection. This chapter focuses on a general approach to the treatment of infection in patients with immune defects (other than AIDS) and reviews the several methods reported to prevent infection in such patients.

Specific Defects Predict Infecting Organisms

The approach to the treatment of infections in the immunocompromised patient depends on an understanding of the specific immune defect. The nature of the immune defect roughly predicts the most likely infecting organisms (Table 137–1).

The white blood cell is critically important in maintaining an infection-free state. A variety of conditions may impair white blood cell number and function. Neutropenia is among the most common defects in host response. It may be found in patients with leukemia, AIDS, carcinoma metastatic to the bone marrow, and tuberculosis or other infections involving the marrow-forming elements. Neutropenia may also occur in patients receiving cytotoxic chemotherapy or radiation therapy. Many drugs may cause granulocytopenia, including penicillins, cephalosporins, rifampin, chloramphenicol, nonsteroidal antiinflammatory drugs, some antihypertensive drugs, and others; however, these effects are usually reversible on discontinuation of the agent.[1]

The risk of infection increases as the granulocyte count falls below 1000 cells per mm^3, but the most severe risk occurs at counts below $100/mm^3$, especially if prolonged for several days or weeks.[2, 3] Patients with prolonged neutropenia are subject to bacterial infections; *Escherichia coli, Klebsiella pneumoniae, Pseudomonas aeruginosa, Staphylococcus aureus*, and *Staphylococcus epidermidis* used to be isolated most frequently.[4–6] Gram-positive cocci have become more frequent than gram-negative rods, and viridans streptococci, coagulase-negative staphylococci, *Streptococcus* sp., and *Enterococcus* sp. play a major role.[7–10] Factors responsible for this shift include mucositis produced by intensive chemotherapy regimens (especially those containing cytosine arabinoside), long-term indwelling vascular cannulas, fluoroquinolone and other antibiotic prophylaxis, and perhaps the use of histamine type 2 blockers.[10] Shock and the acute respiratory distress syndrome have been associated with bacteremia caused by viridans streptococci.[10] Bacteremia caused by gram-negative rods continues to occur, and organisms such as *Stenotrophomonas* (formerly *Xanthomonas*) *maltophilia* may be particularly difficult to eradicate. Some organisms described in neutropenic patients include *Legionella* sp., *Leptotrichia buccalis, Capnocytophaga* sp., *Corynebacterium jeikeium, Stomatococcus mucilaginosus, Leuconostoc* sp., *Rhodococcus equi*, and *Bartonella henselae*. Neutropenic patients are also subject to infections with fungi such as *Candida* and *Aspergillus* spp., often after antibiotic therapy. Unusual fungal infections with *Drechslera, Trichosporon, Fusarium*, and *Geotrichum* spp., among others, may occur in patients with malignancies.[11]

Defects in the ability of granulocytes to move to sites of infection may also be associated with various bacterial infections.[12] Defective chemotactic activity is described in patients with diabetes mellitus,[13] alcoholism,[14] chronic renal failure,[15] systemic lupus erythematosus, Hodgkin's disease, C3A or C5A deficiency, Job syndrome, and corticosteroid therapy, as well as in a variety of congenital immunodeficiencies including congenital ichthyosis, lazy leukocyte syndrome, and hyperimmunoglobulinemia E or A.[12] Defective chemotaxis is associated with infections of the skin and respiratory system, usually caused by staphylococci, streptococci, and yeasts.[12]

In the presence of normal numbers of neutrophils, defects in the ability of the neutrophil to kill ingested bacteria are well described in chronic granulomatous disease,[16] myeloper-

TABLE 137–1 ■ Specific Defects in Host Response and the Likely Infecting Organisms

DEFECTS	CONDITIONS	ASSOCIATED INFECTING ORGANISMS
Neutropenia	Leukemia, cytotoxic chemotherapy, AIDS, systemic lupus erythematosus, Felty syndrome, drugs	*Escherichia coli, Klebsiella pneumoniae, Pseudomonas aeruginosa, Staphylococcus aureus, Staphylococcus epidermidis*, streptococci, yeasts, *Aspergillus* spp. and other fungi
Defective chemotaxis	Diabetes, alcoholism, renal failure, systemic lupus erythematosus, Hodgkin's disease, trauma, lazy leukocyte syndrome	Staphylococci, streptococci, yeasts
Defective neutrophil killing	Chronic granulomatous disease, Down syndrome, myeloperoxidase deficiency	Catalase-positive bacteria (e.g., *S. aureus, E. coli, Candida* spp.)
B-lymphocyte defects	Congenital and acquired agammaglobulinemia, burns, enteropathies, myeloma, lymphocytic leukemia	Encapsulated organisms, e.g., *Streptococcus pneumoniae, Haemophilus influenzae, Neisseria* spp.; also *Salmonella* and *Campylobacter* spp.
T-lymphocyte defects	Congenital immunodeficiencies, AIDS, lymphoma, sarcoidosis, Epstein-Barr virus infection, systemic lupus erythematosus, cytomegalovirus infections	Intracellular infections with bacteria, mycobacteria, viruses, parasites, fungi
Complement components	Congenital absence	Miscellaneous bacterial infections

oxidase deficiency,[17] and sometimes Down syndrome.[18] Neutrophils from patients with chronic granulomatous disease are unable to produce toxic oxygen radicals with their resultant microbicidal activity. This may be due to the absence of cytochrome *b*, which is responsible for early activation of the intracellular respiratory burst.[19] These patients have subcutaneous, lung, and bone infections with organisms that produce catalase or are unable to generate hydrogen peroxide, such as *S. aureus, E. coli*, other gram-negative rods, and *Candida albicans*.[16] Patients with a defect in the lysosomal enzyme myeloperoxidase, including patients with Chédiak-Higashi syndrome, are frequently infected with *Candida* spp. and staphylococci.[17]

Several conditions affect the number and function of B lymphocytes responsible for the production of specific immunoglobulin antibodies. These disorders include congenital agammaglobulinemias; primary immunodeficiencies of the major immunoglobulins G, A, and M (IgG, IgA, and IgM); multiple myeloma; some forms of lymphocytic leukemia; nephrotic syndrome; severe burns; and protein-losing enteropathies. Humoral immunity may also be deficient after splenectomy. Patients with B-cell deficiency states and hypogammaglobulinemia are subject to pyogenic infections, especially those caused by *Streptococcus pneumoniae, Haemophilus influenzae*, and *Neisseria meningitidis*,[20] although infections with *Neisseria gonorrhoeae* and *Salmonella* and *Campylobacter* spp. may occur.[21, 22] IgM deficiency is associated with infections caused by encapsulated bacteria. *Giardia* spp. infections may be particularly difficult for patients with selective IgA deficiency. Deficiencies in IgG subclasses may result in recurrent infections with *S. pneumoniae* and *H. influenzae* (especially if also associated with IgA deficiency).[12]

Defective T-lymphocyte–mediated immunity may occur in several congenital immunodeficiency states, including congenital thymic aplasia, combined immunodeficiency, Swiss-type agammaglobulinemia, adenosine deaminase deficiency, nucleoside phosphorylase deficiency, ataxia-telangiectasia, and DiGeorge syndrome.[21] Some of these conditions also cause humoral immune defects. Acquired defects in T-cell numbers or function include AIDS; sarcoidosis; Hodgkin's disease; systemic lupus erythematosus; non-Hodgkin's lymphoma; cytomegalovirus (CMV) and Epstein-Barr virus infections; pregnancy; and immunosuppressive therapy with corticosteroids, cyclophosphamide, cyclosporine, azathioprine, and antilymphocyte globulin.

Patients with defective T-cell–mediated immunity are subject to a broad spectrum of infection with intracellular pathogens, including such bacteria as *Mycobacterium tuberculosis* and other mycobacteria, *Salmonella* spp., *Listeria monocytogenes*, and *Bacillus* and *Nocardia* spp. These patients are infected with herpesviruses, including herpes simplex virus, varicella-zoster virus, and CMV. Patients with T-cell defects are also subject to fungal infections, including cryptococcal meningitis, candidal esophagitis, and disseminated candidiasis. *Pneumocystis carinii, Toxoplasma gondii, Isospora belli*, and *Cryptosporidium* spp. cause serious infections in these patients.

The complement system is critically important in mediating humoral defense mechanisms.[23] The complement system may be activated via the alternative pathway by bacterial products in the absence of specific immune responses. Specific defects of many complement components have been described that predispose patients to bacterial infections. Deficiencies in the terminal complement components C5 through C8 are associated with *Neisseria* infection.[24] Defects in the early components are associated with serious pneumococcal infections. Some enteric pathogens and C3 deficiencies commonly lead to recurrent respiratory and skin infections with pneumococci, streptococci, some enteric bacteria, and *H. influenzae*.[25]

As mentioned in Chapter 135, the patient undergoing bone marrow transplantation for the treatment of leukemia or other malignant diseases has several infectious risks. These risks vary with time since transplantation.

Approach to the Treatment of Infections in the Immunocompromised Patient

According to the cause and extent of immunosuppression, an immunocompromised patient may have infection in any of several sites. The skin may be the focus of recurrent pyogenic infections such as furuncles caused by staphylococci, cellulitis associated with streptococci, or zoster caused by reactivation of varicella-zoster virus in a dermatomal distribution. Disseminated herpesvirus infection may occur in severely immunocompromised patients and extensive or confluent warts caused by human papillomavirus are not uncommon in these patients, especially after renal transplantation.[26] Patients may develop mucocutaneous candidiasis or necrotizing superficial erosive infections with *Mucor* spp. or other fungi. Solitary or multiple cryptococcal lesions may occur on the skin,[26] and these may antedate systemic infection.[27] Conditions such as these should be diagnosed by aspiration, biopsy, and/or direct culture from the lesion.

Respiratory infections are common in the immunocompromised patient, including otitis media, pharyngitis, bronchitis, and pneumonia. Interstitial infiltrates may be due to *P. carinii*, CMV, or less commonly *T. gondii*. Bronchopneumonia and lobar pneumonia may be due to pyogenic bacteria, including *S. pneumoniae, S. aureus, P. aeruginosa, Legionella pneumophila*, and *M. tuberculosis*. Extensive multilobar bronchopneumonia and necrotizing pneumonitis may occur with *C. albicans, Aspergillus* spp., or other fungi. *Nocardia asteroides* may produce lobar or segmental infiltrates with nodular densities and ultimately may form thick-walled abscess cavities. Solitary nodules may be seen with *Cryptococcus neoformans, Nocardia* spp., and so forth.

When possible, coughed or induced sputum should be examined for the usual bacterial pathogens; however, fiberoptic bronchoscopy with washings and biopsies may be necessary to establish a diagnosis. Transthoracic needle aspiration or biopsy is quite useful for peripheral lung lesions and is relatively safe if at least 75,000 platelets per mm^3 are present.[28] Open-lung biopsy remains controversial, but Rubin and Green[28] effectively argued that this and other aggressive or invasive procedures are most likely to be successful and useful in patients whose underlying disease prognosis is good (e.g., renal transplantation, Hodgkin's disease, collagen-vascular diseases) but not in patients with advanced leukemia or AIDS.[29, 30]

The gastrointestinal tract may be involved with a variety of pathogenic organisms including *Salmonella* and *Shigella* spp. and *Strongyloides stercoralis*. Disseminated infection may occur with any of these organisms. *I. belli* and *Cryptosporidium* spp. are not infrequent causes of infection in severely immunocompromised patients. Infections of the upper gastrointestinal tract occur, including esophagitis caused by herpes simplex virus, CMV, or *Candida* spp. and other fungi. Hepatitis may be due to CMV or the hepatitis viruses. Fungal and mycobacterial infections may disseminate and involve the liver. Biopsy may be necessary to establish the diagnosis.

Central nervous system infections include meningitis caused by *L. monocytogenes, C. neoformans*, and other more usual causes of meningitis. Meningoencephalitis may be caused by herpes simplex virus; varicella-zoster virus; *T.*

gondii; tuberculous and nontuberculous mycobacteria; human polyomavirus (progressive multifocal leukoencephalopathy); and disseminated infections with *Candida*, *Aspergillus*, or other fungal species. Lumbar puncture may establish a diagnosis in some of these conditions, but brain scans, computed tomography with use of contrast medium, magnetic resonance imaging, and brain biopsy may be required.

Fever in the Neutropenic Patient

Neutropenic patients spend approximately 50% of their hospital days with fever.[31] Fever may be the only manifestation of infection in a granulocytopenic patient.[32]

Fever in the neutropenic patient (Table 137–2) is associated with a microbiologically documented infection in approximately 40% of patients; bacteremia accounts for about half of these.[5, 6] Clinically documented infections such as pneumonia without definitive microbiologic identification account for another 20% of fevers, and possible infections for another 20%. Only 20% of fevers in neutropenic patients are presumed to be due to the underlying disease or to other noninfectious causes, although the specific cause of the febrile episode is not always identified.

The diagnosis of infection in a severely granulocytopenic patient may be difficult because of the lack of typical physical findings. Classic signs of fluctuance, calor, rubor, and lymphadenopathy are found less frequently in neutropenic than in nonneutropenic patients, although pain may be a presenting symptom.[33] Neutropenic patients with pneumonia may not show an initial infiltrate on a chest radiograph. Frequent radiographs may be needed to localize infection to the lung. Exudates may be less common in pharyngeal infections, and patients with urinary infections may not have pyuria. Even in some meningitides, the meningeal reaction may be limited by the inability to mobilize granulocytes to the site of infection.

In evaluating a febrile granulocytopenic patient, frequent physical examinations should emphasize examination of mucosal sites, including the perianal area. The examination should also include the liberal use of blood, urine, and sputum cultures, if available, as well as cerebrospinal fluid cultures when symptoms point to the nervous system. Routine lumbar punctures are not recommended, especially in the presence of thrombocytopenia.

The organisms usually responsible for bacterial infections in the febrile, neutropenic patient include *E. coli*, *K. pneumoniae*, *P. aeruginosa*, and *S. aureus*. However, most centers have noted a dramatic increase in the relative frequency of gram-positive coccal bacteremia,[7–10, 34] including infections with viridans streptococci, pneumococci, *S. pyogenes*, *Enterococcus* spp., and staphylococci. The mortality in gram-negative bacteremia is greater than that in gram-positive coccal bacteremia, although the latter may be more difficult to eradicate.[8, 9]

TABLE 137–2 ■ Causes of Fever in Neutropenic Patients

CONDITION	APPROXIMATE RATE (%)
Bacteremia	15–29
Microbiologically documented infections	6–20
Clinically documented infections	20–26
Possible infection	20–39
Infection doubted	15–25

Based on several therapeutic trials by the European Organization for Research and Treatment of Cancer's International Antimicrobial Therapy Cooperative Group (see references 5, 6, 8, 9, 44, and 45).

TABLE 137–3 ■ Current Antibiotics Used as Empirical Therapy for Fever in Granulocytopenic Patients

COMBINATIONS*		SINGLE-DRUG THERAPY
Azlocillin	plus aminoglycoside†	Ceftazidime
Carbenicillin	plus aminoglycoside†	Imipenem
Mezlocillin	plus aminoglycoside†	Meropenem
Piperacillin	plus aminoglycoside†	Cefepime
Ticarcillin‡	plus aminoglycoside†	
Ceftazidime§	plus aminoglycoside†	
Cefoperazone‡	plus aminoglycoside†	
Piperacillin-tazobactam	plus aminoglycoside†	
Meropenem	plus aminoglycoside†	
Ceftazidime plus piperacillin		
Azlocillin plus ceftazidime		

*Some authors have also used a cephalosporin plus a penicillin plus an aminoglycoside. Vancomycin is often added.
†Amikacin, gentamicin, netilmicin, tobramycin.
‡With or without clavulanate or sulbactam.
§Other cephalosporins such as ceftriaxone, cefotaxime, ceftizoxime, and the cefamycin moxalactam have been used, but they have no activity against *P. aeruginosa*.

Considerable controversy exists about the optimal treatment of febrile neutropenic patients.[35–38] There is clearly no single drug or drug combination of choice. Most investigators agree with early empirical institution of antibiotics after obtaining specimens for cultures.[32] Formerly, most authorities instituted treatment with a combination of an aminoglycoside plus a β-lactam compound, such as an antipseudomonal penicillin or cephalosporin.[32, 38] Several drugs have been used for this purpose (Table 137–3). Double β-lactam combinations, such as a penicillin and a cephalosporin (e.g., piperacillin plus ceftazidime, cephalothin plus carbenicillin),[5, 39–41] may be used; however, these combinations may not have optimal activity against *S. aureus* and *P. aeruginosa*, and they have the potential to induce β-lactamase production in gram-negative rods.

Aminoglycosides provide rapid bactericidal activity against most gram-negative rods, and patients with persistent profound granulocytopenia and gram-negative rod bacteremia respond better to two antimicrobial agents that are active or synergistically active against the infecting organism[42, 43]; therefore, aminoglycoside-containing combinations are still useful. In a trial of ceftazidime plus amikacin, neutropenic patients with gram-negative rod bacteremia did better with a full course of both antibiotics than when the aminoglycoside was discontinued after 3 days.[44] This finding was most prominent in patients with profound and prolonged granulocytopenia.[44] Susceptibility to the β-lactam is an important determinant of outcome in gram-negative rod bacteremia treated with an aminoglycoside-containing regimen.[45] Depending on local susceptibility patterns, reasonable initial drug combinations include ceftazidime or piperacillin-tazobactam plus an aminoglycoside. If gram-negative rod bacteremia is not documented, the aminoglycoside can be discontinued.[44]

Several studies of single-drug empirical therapy have been performed using ceftazidime or imipenem alone.[34, 46, 47] These broad-spectrum active drugs might be as effective as aminoglycoside–β-lactam combinations, but some patients require additional specific therapy (e.g., vancomycin) if staphylococci or other gram-positive cocci are isolated from blood. Aminoglycosides may be required for bacteremia with *P. aeruginosa* and other gram-negative rods, especially in profoundly neutropenic patients.[44] In a study comparing ceftazidime with imipenem as monotherapy, both drugs were effective with similar modifications of initial therapy in both groups.[47] Meropenem also has been used to treat febrile neutropenic patients and in one study compared favorably to ceftazidime plus amikacin.[47a] Centers with large numbers of *S. aureus* infections might consider starting with a vancomycin-containing regimen,[48] but several studies support the later addition of this drug if nonresponse to empirical antibiotics is due to gram-positive coccal infection.[49, 50]

One study reported the clinical equivalence of single daily doses of ceftriaxone plus amikacin and multiple daily dosing of ceftazidime plus amikacin.[51] The single daily dose of amikacin was given as an intravenous infusion of 20 mg/kg during 1 hour. The regimens had similar associated nephrotoxicity (2% to 3%), but nephrotoxicity was associated with additional nephrotoxic agents and occurred later in patients receiving single daily doses. In another trial, piperacillin-tazobactam plus single daily doses of amikacin was more effective than ceftazidime plus amikacin.[8]

The duration of empirical therapy for fever in the granulocytopenic patient is also controversial.[39, 52, 53, 54] If the patient responds, therapy can continue until the granulocyte count has increased above 500 cells per mm^3.[53, 54] Some authors treat documented gram-negative rod bacteremia for 10 to 14 days, regardless of the granulocyte count.[38] Pizzo and colleagues[53, 54] showed that patients who remain granulocytopenic and febrile who had antibiotics discontinued after 7 days developed rebound infection and/or shock. However, Pennington[52] had suggested that antibiotics could be discontinued after 7 days if no infection had been documented. Young[38] has suggested that antibiotics could be stopped in febrile patients with no bacterial diagnosis after 7 days if the granulocyte count exceeds 500/mm^3 for 2 days. However, if further chemotherapy or profound granulocytopenia is expected, antibiotic use should continue. Surveillance cultures of *P. aeruginosa, K. pneumoniae, Aeromonas* sp., or *Enterobacter* sp. would mitigate toward continued empirical antibiotics.[38] Concern must be given to the potential for invasive fungal infections during prolonged antibiotic treatment.

Patients with documented bacteremia generally respond to appropriate antimicrobial agents within 4 to 5 days. However, failure to respond should prompt a search for loculated infections such as perirectal, intraabdominal, or subcutaneous abscesses. Antimicrobial activity can be adjusted to increase serum bactericidal activity, and granulocyte transfusions can be considered. Patients without documented bacterial sepsis who remain febrile after 4 to 7 days of empirical antibiotics should be considered for empirical antifungal therapy with amphotericin B.[54, 55] Fluconazole is useful in the treatment of candidal infections in the immunocompromised host. Some species, notably *Candida krusei* and *Candida glabrata*, may be resistant. Leukemic patients with hepatosplenic candidiasis have been successfully treated with fluconazole,[56] and a comparative trial of empirical fluconazole versus amphotericin B in febrile neutropenic patients is in progress. Itraconazole may be effective for patients with aspergillosis, and new preparations of amphotericin B are undergoing evaluation.

Although enthusiasm had been raised for adjunctive treatments with antiendotoxin antibodies, antibodies to tumor necrosis factor, and interleukin-1 receptor antagonist, results of clinical trials have been disappointing.[57–59] Further investigation of the molecular biology of endotoxin should reveal potentially useful interventions for sepsis in neutropenic and other patients. Several authors have reviewed their general approach to the treatment of febrile neutropenic patients.[60–62]

Risk factor analyses have been used to identify patients at highest risk for bacteremia (and therefore needing aggressive intravenous treatment with potent antibiotics) and those who probably would be neutropenic for a short time and have a lower risk of serious infection. In the patients at high risk, duration of granulocytopenia before fever, low platelet counts, high fever, shock, and clinical evidence of localized infection are some of the predictive factors that have been identified.[63] Similarly, patients at low risk for bacteremia (excluding those with resistant bacterial infections, abnormal hepatic function, shock, hypercalcemia, altered mental state, tachypnea and hyponatremia) have been safely treated at home with intravenous or oral therapy, often with a fluoroquinolone.[64–66] This approach is interesting and needs further study. A report on patients who received selective antibiotic decontamination advocated the use of specific antibiotic therapy only for demonstrated or proven infection.[67] This approach needs further documentation.

Prevention of Infection in the Immunocompromised Patient

Prevention of infection in immunosuppressed patients depends in part on the specific host defect and the likely source of infection. For example, neutropenic patients are primarily infected with organisms that colonize body sites, including the oropharynx, gastrointestinal tract, and skin.[4, 68, 69] Most of the approaches to infection prevention have been developed for granulocytopenic patients, and some also apply to other immunosuppressed patients (Table 137–4).

All attempts should be made to improve or eliminate the defect in host defenses. Patients who are hypogammaglobulinemic can be treated effectively with maintenance doses of intravenous immunoglobulins.[70, 71] Patients with leukemia can be treated to achieve remission, rendering them nonneutropenic and lowering their risk of infection.

Methods for improving nutritional status are worthwhile. Careful attention should be paid to adequate protein, vitamin, and calorie intake. Peripheral hyperalimentation may be necessary in some circumstances, but this carries its own risk of infection.[72] Although vaccinations are effective to prevent a variety of infectious diseases in immunocompetent patients, many immunocompromised patients are less able to respond appropriately.[73] Pneumococcal vaccination and *H. influenzae* type b vaccination might be useful to patients

TABLE 137–4 ■ General Considerations for Infection Prevention in Immunocompromised Patients

I. Improve host defenses
   A. Treat underlying disease
   B. Improve nutrition, protein, vitamin, and calorie intake
   C. Vaccines: influenza, pneumococcal, hepatitis B, varicella-zoster virus, varicella-zoster immune globulin on exposure
   D. Immunomodulators: lithium, intravenous immune globulin, GM-CSF, G-CSF
II. Minimize invasive procedures and maximize care for indwelling intravenous and bladder catheters
III. Reduce acquisition of new pathogens
   A. Hand washing and cleansing of patient's skin
   B. Low-bacterial foods and fluids
   C. Housekeeping
   D. Laminar airflow
IV. Reduce colonizing bacterial load
   A. Nonabsorbable oral antibiotics, antifungal agents, antiseptics
   B. Absorbable antibiotics
   C. Selective gastrointestinal bacterial suppression
   D. Systemic antibacterial prophylaxis
   E. Local or systemic antifungal prophylaxis
   F. Acyclovir prevention of dissemination of herpesvirus infections

before splenectomy. Influenza vaccine may minimize risk of this disease, and hepatitis B vaccine also may have a role.[12, 74, 75] CMV pneumonia has been prevented with anti-CMV–IgG and seronegative blood products in some but not all bone marrow transplant recipients.[76, 77] Currently, ganciclovir is used in conjunction with anti-CMV–IgG to treat CMV pneumonia in transplant recipients.[12]

Many attempts at modifying the immune defect are under study. Lithium has been used to stimulate the bone marrow[78] and recombinant granulocyte-macrophage colony-stimulating factor (GM-CSF) and granulocyte colony-stimulating factor (G-CSF) have been widely used to minimize the period of neutropenia after cancer chemotherapy and to reduce granulocytopenia-associated infection.[79, 80] These cytokines are frequently used to elevate peripheral granulocyte counts after treatment for lymphomas and solid tumors. These drugs reduce the incidence of febrile neutropenia by a factor of 2 in adults, with a 40% incidence occurring in patients not treated with CSFs.[81] Reports of the use of G-CSF as an adjunct to chemotherapy for acute lymphoblastic leukemia in adults suggested that the degree of neutropenia was reduced and more therapy could be given.[81] Although these hematopoietic cytokines decrease the duration of neutropenia after induction therapy, beneficial effects on the incidence of severe infection and long-term results of antileukemia treatment have not been definitively determined; therefore, CSFs are not routinely recommended for the treatment of patients with acute myelocytic leukemia. However, one study suggested that low-dose, continuous infusion of G-CSF did reduce the duration of neutropenia.[82] Further studies are needed to establish appropriate doses and indications for these cytokines in acute myeloid leukemia.

The guidelines of the American Society of Clinical Oncology recommend the routine use of CSFs for patients expected to develop prolonged and profound neutropenia with an anticipated fever incidence of 40% or greater.[81] They do not support the use of CSFs for all patients with cancer who receive chemotherapy. Special risk might exist for patients with extensive prior chemotherapy, recurrent febrile neutropenia, existing wounds, active infections, and other risk-enhancing situations.[81] More clinical study is needed to determine the use of CSFs as adjuncts to antibiotics in the treatment of fever or established infection in neutropenic patients.[80] GM-CSF also raises peripheral blood leukocyte counts in neutropenic patients with AIDS.[83] Intravenous IgG has been used successfully to protect chronic lymphocytic leukemia patients from bacterial infection.[84]

It is important to minimize invasive procedures and maximize care of indwelling intravenous and urinary catheters. Use of Hickman, Broviac, and Port-A-Cath long-term indwelling devices for patients with hematologic and other malignancies is increasing, and these devices have a real potential for infection.

Several measures are useful for reducing the acquisition of new pathogenic bacteria. Obviously, careful hand washing is required. Skin cleansing with soap and antiseptic solutions is recommended for the patient. An often-overlooked area of infection prevention is the provision of low-bacterial food and fluids. Foods such as natural cheeses, uncooked vegetables, raw meats or salads, cold soups, and uncooked herbs and spices are notoriously high in bacteria. These are well tolerated by immunocompetent hosts but are potential sources of infection for neutropenic patients.[85]

Laminar airflow units are clearly effective in providing a low-particle-count atmosphere for patients.[86, 87] These rooms are essential for patients undergoing bone marrow transplantation. Patients are usually also treated with nonabsorbable or other antibiotics (discussed later).[88]

A major effort to prevent infection in granulocytopenic patients involves reduction of bacterial colonization of the gastrointestinal tract.[79] Several methods are available, including use of nonabsorbable or absorbable antibiotics, selective microbial suppression, or partial antimicrobial decontamination.[88–97] Compliance of patients is critical for success of these regimens.[97] The efficacy of prophylactic regimens can be measured in terms of reduction of infection, with its associated morbidity and mortality, and the degree to which additional cancer chemotherapy can be administered.[98] Although no preventive approach is perfect, well-tolerated regimens such as those using trimethoprim-sulfamethoxazole (TMP-SMX) or an oral fluoroquinolone are preferred.

Nonabsorbable oral antibiotics include combinations of gentamicin, vancomycin plus nystatin, and framycetin or neomycin plus colistin and nystatin.[90, 93] These antibiotics are given every 4 or 6 hours. Treatment may include the application of antimicrobial ointments to the vagina or rectum, nares, auditory canals, and gums. Povidone-iodine and chlorhexidine are used as douches, swabs, or mouthwashes. Although some studies have shown dramatic reductions in infection rates with oral nonabsorbable antibiotics, side effects of nausea, vomiting, and abdominal cramps limit compliance and patients' acceptance. Rebound overgrowth and infection have been reported after discontinuation of these regimens, and the gastrointestinal tract may be colonized with resistant bacteria.[93, 99] These agents are not inexpensive. With appropriate support from nursing and medical staffs, the benefits may outweigh the unpleasant side effects and high costs.[93, 94] Most of these preparations have been studied in conjunction with protective environment units and are not recommended for sporadic use.

Several studies have compared TMP-SMX with placebo or with other regimens.[97, 99–106] Hughes and colleagues[103] observed that TMP-SMX reduced bacterial infections in patients with acute leukemia during prophylaxis against *P. carinii* pneumonia. In a large number of granulocytopenic patients with solid tumors, leukemia, and lymphomas, Pizzo and coworkers[97] showed a reduction in febrile episodes and infection in totally compliant recipients of TMP-SMX plus erythromycin. The European Organization for Research and Treatment of Cancer study of 342 patients who were granulocytopenic for at least 6 days showed a reduction of infection with TMP-SMX compared with placebo from 39% to 26% (P = .016).[100] However, reduction in bacteremia by TMP-SMX was seen only in patients who did not have acute nonlymphocytic leukemia. (Bacteremia occurred in 17 of 101 placebo-treated patients and in 4 of 102 TMP-SMX–treated patients, $P < .001$.[100])

Although widely used for the prevention of infection in granulocytopenic patients, TMP-SMX is not without dermatologic side effects. It has been reported to prolong granulocytopenia, delay marrow engraftment, and result in the emergence of resistant organisms.[99–107] A randomized, double-blind comparative trial of bone marrow transplant patients showed similar prophylactic efficacy of TMP-SMX and ciprofloxacin, but TMP-SMX recipients had more *Clostridium difficile* colitis, slightly more gram-negative rod infections, and a trend for prolonged granulocytopenia.[108]

Another approach has been to individualize antibiotic prophylaxis and eliminate susceptible enteric flora while preserving the anaerobic flora, with its property of colonization resistance. Antibiotics such as TMP-SMX, colistin, neomycin, and nalidixic acid have been used.[95, 96, 104, 109]

Several studies of prophylaxis with fluoroquinolone drugs have been reported. Bow and colleagues[110] randomized 63 neutropenic patients to receive norfloxacin or TMP-SMX. Gram-negative rod infections were not observed in the 31 norfloxacin-treated patients compared with 4 of 32 TMP-SMX recipients. However, gram-positive coccal bacteremias were found more frequently with quinolone therapy. Karp and coworkers[111] treated 35 neutropenic leukemic patients with norfloxacin and 33 with placebo. This study also showed a decrease in gram-negative rod bacteremia in the quinolone group. Dekker and colleagues[112] treated 28 patients with ciprofloxacin and 28 with TMP-SMX plus colistin and noted no gram-negative rod bacteremias with the quinolone. However, they did report gram-positive coccal bacteremias. Too few placebo-controlled studies with fluoroquinolones exist to recommend these antibiotics definitively for prophylaxis in neutropenic patients. In addition, quinolones may increase and certainly do not decrease the incidence of gram-positive coccal bacteremias.[10, 110, 112] However, the addition of penicillin V to a fluoroquinolone significantly reduced streptococcal bacteremias in one trial.[113] Two studies reported similar results when a macrolide was added to a quinolone for prophylaxis.[114, 115] Also, the use of prophylactic acyclovir was shown to reduce bacteremia during acute leukemia induction therapy, possibly through the prevention of ulcerative herpes simplex lesions.[116]

Prevention of Fungal Infections

Invasive fungal infections are major problems in immunocompromised patients. Despite advances in antifungal chemotherapy, the overall prognosis remains poor for profoundly neutropenic patients infected with fungi. Several approaches directed at preventing these infections in immunocompromised patients have met with minimal success.

The polyenes nystatin and amphotericin B have been evaluated as oral antifungal prophylactic agents. These drugs are not substantially absorbed from the gastrointestinal tract, and colonization and invasive candidiasis have been reported despite varying doses.[117] The imidazoles clotrimazole, miconazole, and ketoconazole reduce yeast colonization of the skin and nasopharynx. One study demonstrated a reduction in disseminated candidiasis in 61 patients who received 600 mg of ketoconazole daily, but *C. glabrata* colonization was not infrequent.[117] Oral polyenes and ketoconazole do not reduce *Aspergillus* infection; only high-efficiency particulate air filters do. However, preliminary data suggest that amphotericin B nasal spray might decrease *Aspergillus* colonization.[118]

Administration of clotrimazole troches every 4 hours while the patient is awake minimizes oropharyngeal candidiasis. However, it must be recognized that this does not prevent disseminated fungal infection. Fluconazole, an oral triazole antifungal agent, reduced superficial fungal infections in bone marrow transplant recipients from 33% to 8.4% ($P <$ .001) and systemic fungal infections from 15.8% to 2.8% ($P <$ .001) when administered at 400 mg/d compared with placebo.[119] In a similar trial in patients with acute leukemia, fluconazole reduced fungal colonization and superficial infection with *Candida* sp. but not invasive infection, use of amphotericin B, or death.[120] In some centers, fluconazole prophylaxis has been associated with increased infection with *C. krusei, C. glabrata*, and other resistant yeasts.[121, 122]

Antiviral Prophylaxis

With the introduction of acyclovir, effective antiviral prophylactic therapy is available. Acyclovir is used intravenously (250 mg/m^2 every 8 hours) and orally (200 mg four times daily) to prevent herpes simplex virus infections in patients undergoing bone marrow or kidney transplantation or high-dose cancer chemotherapy.[123] Varicella-zoster virus infection in immunocompromised patients can be minimized within 72 hours of exposure with varicella-zoster immune globulin, 1 vial (1.25 mL)/10 kg up to a maximum of 5 vials (6.25 mL), intramuscularly.[124] A live varicella-zoster virus vaccine resulted in seroconversion in children with acute leukemia who were in remission. This vaccine may modify disease[125] and is now licensed for use. Both vidarabine and acyclovir prevent dissemination of zoster in compromised patients.[126, 127] Intravenous acyclovir (10 to 12 mg/kg intravenously three times a day for 7 days) is used to treat chickenpox in these patients.[128, 129] Oral therapy is also used. Oral acyclovir is effective in preventing CMV infections in bone marrow and kidney transplant recipients, although it is largely ineffective as therapy for CMV infections.[130] Although intravenous immunoglobulin reduced non-CMV viral infections, it did not add prophylactic activity for CMV infection to that obtained with the use of CMV-seronegative blood products alone.[131] Ganciclovir at 2.5 mg/kg every 8 hours for the week before transplantation followed by 6 mg/kg per day for 5 days per week after transplantation reduces the incidence and severity of CMV infection in bone marrow transplant recipients.[132]

Summary

In summary, each center must develop an organized approach to the prevention of infection in immunocompromised patients. General measures include awareness of infection control techniques, proper hand washing, vaccines where applicable, use of appropriate food, and reduction of bacterial colonization. Because specific antimicrobial agents are developed against the usual causes of infection in immunocompromised hosts, careful studies to evaluate their prophylactic role are necessary.

References

1. Vincent PC: Drug-induced aplastic anaemia and agranulocytosis: Incidence and mechanisms. Drugs 31:32, 1986.
2. Bodey GP, Buckley M, Sathe YS, et al: Quantitative relationships between circulating leukocytes and infection in patients with acute leukemia. Ann Intern Med 64:328, 1966.
3. Schimpff SC, Hahn DM, Brouillet MD, et al: Infection prevention in acute leukemia: Comparison of basic infection prevention techniques with standard room reverse isolation or with reverse isolation plus added air filtration. Leuk Res 2:231, 1978.
4. Schimpff SC, Young VM, Greene WH, et al: Origin of infection in acute nonlymphocytic leukemia: Significance of hospital acquisition of potential pathogens. Ann Intern Med 77:707, 1972.
5. The EORTC International Antimicrobial Therapy Project Group: Three antibiotic regimens in the treatment of infection in febrile granulocytopenic patients with cancer. J Infect Dis 137:14, 1978.
6. The International Antimicrobial Therapy Project Group of the European Organization for Research and Treatment of Cancer: Combination of amikacin and carbenicillin with or without cefazolin as empirical treatment of febrile neutropenic patients. J Clin Oncol 1:597, 1983.
7. Gibson J, Johnson L, Snowdon L, et al: Trends in bacterial infection in febrile neutropenic patients: 1986–1992. Aust N Z J Med 24:374, 1994.
8. Cometta A, Zinner S, deBock R, et al: Piperacillin-tazobactam versus ceftazidime plus amikacin as empiric therapy for fever in granulocytopenic patients with cancer. Antimicrob Agents Chemother 39:445, 1995.
9. EORTC International Antimicrobial Therapy Cooperative Group and the National Cancer Institute of Canada-Clinical Trials Group: Vancomycin added to empirical combination antibiotic therapy for fever in granulocytopenic cancer patients. J Infect Dis 137:14, 1991.
10. Elting LS, Bodey GP, Keefe BH: Septicemia and shock syndrome due to viridans streptococci: A case-control study of predisposing factors. Clin Infect Dis 14:1201, 1992.
11. Anaissie E, Bodey GP, Kantarjian H, et al: New spectrum of fungal infections in patients with cancer. Rev Infect Dis 11:369, 1989.
12. Van der Meer JWM: Defects in host-defense mechanisms. *In*

Rubin RH, Young LS (eds): Clinical Approach to Infections in the Compromised Host, ed 3. New York, Plenum Publishing, 1994, pp 33–66.
13. Mowat AG, Baum J: Chemotaxis of polymorphonuclear leukocytes from patients with diabetes mellitus. N Engl J Med 284:621, 1971.
14. Brayton RG, Stokes PE, Schwartz MS, et al: Effect of alcohol and various diseases on leukocyte mobilization, phagocytosis and intracellular bacterial killing. N Engl J Med 282:123, 1970.
15. Salant DF, Glover AM, Anderson R, et al: Depressed neutrophil chemotaxis in patients with chronic renal failure and after renal transplantation. J Lab Clin Med 88:536, 1976.
16. Johnston RB Jr, Baehner RL: Chronic granulomatous disease: Correlation between pathogenesis and clinical findings. J Pediatr 75:300, 1969.
17. Salmon SE, Cline MJ, Schultz J, et al: Myeloperoxidase deficiency. N Engl J Med 282:250, 1970.
18. Rosner F, Kozinn PJ, Jervis GA: Leukocyte function and serum immunoglobulins in Down's syndrome. N Y State J Med 73:672, 1973.
19. Segal AW, Cross AR, Garcia RC, et al: Absence of cytochrome *b*-245 in chronic granulomatous disease. N Engl J Med 308:245, 1983.
20. Ochs HD, Wedgwood RJ: Disorders of the B-cell system. *In* Stiehm ER (ed): Immunologic Disorders in Infants and Children. Philadelphia, WB Saunders, 1989, pp 226–256.
21. Christenson JC, Hill HR: Infections complicating congenital immunodeficiency syndromes. *In* Rubin RH, Young LS (eds): Clinical Approach to Infection in the Compromised Host, ed 3. New York, Plenum Publishing, 1994, pp 521–549.
22. Rosen FS, Cooper MD, Wedgewood RJP: The primary immunodeficiencies. N Engl J Med 311:235, 1984.
23. Joiner KA, Brown EJ, Frank MM: Complement and bacteria: Chemistry and biology in host defense. Annu Rev Immunol 2:46, 1984.
24. Petersen BH, Lee JJ, Snyderman RJ, et al: *Neisseria meningitidis* and *Neisseria gonorrhoeae* bacteremia associated with C6, C7 or C8 deficiency. Ann Intern Med 90:917, 1979.
25. Alper CA, Colten HA, Gear JSS, et al: Homozygous human C3 deficiency. J Clin Invest 57:222, 1976.
26. Kaye ET, Johnson RA, Wolfson JS, Sober AJ: Dermatologic manifestations of infection in the compromised host. *In* Rubin RH, Young LS (eds): Clinical Approach to Infection in the Compromised Host, ed 3. New York, Plenum Publishing, 1994, pp 105–119.
27. Kerkering TM, Duma RJ, Shadomy S: The evolution of pulmonary cryptococcosis. Ann Intern Med 94:611, 1981.
28. Rubin RH, Green R: Clinical approach to the compromised host with fever and pulmonary infiltrates. *In* Rubin RH, Young LS (eds): Clinical Approach to Infection in the Compromised Host, ed 3. New York, Plenum Publishing, 1994, pp 121–161.
29. Cockerill FR III, Wilson WR, Carpenter HA, et al: Open lung biopsy in immunocompromised patients. Arch Intern Med 145:1398, 1985.
30. Cheson BD, Samlowski WE, Tang TT, et al: Value of open lung biopsy in 87 immunocompromised patients with pulmonary infiltrates. Cancer 55:453, 1985.
31. Gurwith MJ, Brunton JL, Lank BA, et al: Granulocytopenia in hospitalized patients. 1. Prognostic factors and etiology of fever. Am J Med 64:121, 1978.
32. Schimpff S, Satterlee W, Young VM, et al: Empiric therapy with carbenicillin and gentamicin for febrile patients with cancer and granulocytopenia. N Engl J Med 284:1061, 1971.
33. Sickles EA, Greene WH, Wiernik PH: Clinical presentation of infection in granulocytopenic patients. Arch Intern Med 135:715, 1975.
34. Pizzo A, Hathorn JW, Hiemenz J, et al: A randomized trial comparing ceftazidime alone with combination antibiotic therapy in cancer patients with fever and neutropenia. N Engl J Med 315:552, 1986.
35. Bodey GP: Antibiotics in patients with neutropenia. Arch Intern Med 144:1845, 1984.
36. Anaissie E, Rolston K, Bodey GP: Treatment of gram-negative bacteremia in patients with neutropenia and cancer (Letter). N Engl J Med 318:1964, 1988.
37. Hughes WT, Armstrong D, Bodey GP, et al: Guidelines for the use of antimicrobial agents in neutropenic patients with unexplained fever. J Infect Dis 161:381, 1990.
38. Young LS: Fever and septicemia. *In* Rubin RH, Young LS (eds): Clinical Approach to Infections in the Compromised Host, ed 3. New York, Plenum Publishing, 1994, pp 67–104.
39. Bodey GP, Valdivieso M, Feld R, et al: Carbenicillin plus cephalothin or cefazolin as therapy for infections in neutropenic patients. Am J Med Sci 273:309, 1977.
40. Young LS: Double beta-lactam therapy in the immunocompromised host. J Antimicrob Chemother 16:4, 1985.
41. DeJongh CA, Joshi JH, Newman KA, et al: Antibiotic synergism and response in gram-negative bacteremia in granulocytopenic cancer patients. Am J Med 80(Suppl 5C):96, 1986.
42. Joshi JH, Newman KA, Brown BW, et al: Double beta-lactam regimen compared to an aminoglycoside/beta-lactam regimen as empiric antibiotic therapy for febrile granulocytopenic cancer patients. Support Care Cancer 1:186, 1993.
43. Klastersky J, Zinner SH: Synergistic combinations of antibiotics in gram-negative bacillary infections. Rev Infect Dis 4:294, 1982.
44. The EORTC International Antimicrobial Therapy Cooperative Group: Ceftazidime combined with a short or long course of amikacin for empirical therapy of gram-negative bacteremia in cancer patients with granulocytopenia. N Engl J Med 317:1692, 1987.
45. Klastersky J, Glauser MP, Schimpff SC, et al: European Organization for Research on Treatment of Cancer Antimicrobial Therapy Project Group: Prospective randomized comparison of three antibiotic regimens for empirical therapy of suspected bacteremic infection in febrile granulocytopenic patients. Antimicrob Agents Chemother 29:263, 1986.
46. Bodey GP, Alvarez ME, Jones PG, et al: Imipenem-cilastatin as initial therapy for febrile cancer patients. Antimicrob Agents Chemother 30:211, 1986.
47. Freifeld AG, Walsh T, Marshall D, et al: Monotherapy for fever and neutropenia in cancer patients: A randomized comparison of ceftazidime versus imipenem. J Clin Oncol 13:165, 1995.
47a. Cometta A, Calandra T, et al: Monotherapy with meropenem versus combination therapy with ceftazidime plus amikacin as empiric therapy for fever in granulocytopenic patients with cancer. Antimicrob Agents Chemother 50:1108, 1996.
48. Shenep JL, Hughes WT, Roberson PK, et al: Vancomycin, ticarcillin, and amikacin compared with ticarcillin-clavulanate and amikacin in the empirical treatment of febrile, neutropenic children with cancer. N Engl J Med 319:1053, 1988.
49. Rubin M, Hathorn JW, Marshall D, et al: Gram-positive infections and the use of vancomycin in 550 episodes of fever and neutropenia. Ann Intern Med 108:30, 1988.
50. Ramphal R, Bolger M, Oblon DJ, et al: Vancomycin is not an essential component of the initial empiric treatment regimen for febrile neutropenic patients receiving ceftazidime: A randomized prospective study. Antimicrob Agents Chemother 36:1062, 1992.
51. International Antimicrobial Therapy Cooperative Group of the EORTC: Efficacy and toxicity of single daily dose of amikacin and ceftriaxone versus multiple daily doses of amikacin and ceftazidime for infection in patients with cancer and granulocytopenia. Ann Intern Med 119:584, 1983.
52. Pennington JE: Fever, neutropenia, and malignancy: A clinical syndrome in evolution. Cancer 39:1345, 1977.
53. Pizzo PA, Robichaud KJ, Gill FA, et al: Duration of empiric antibiotic therapy. Am J Med 67:194, 1979.
54. Pizzo PA, Robichaud KJ, Gill FA, et al: Empiric antibiotic and antifungal therapy for cancer patients with prolonged fever and granulocytopenia. Am J Med 72:101, 1982.
55. EORTC International Antimicrobial Therapy Cooperative Group: Empiric antifungal therapy in febrile granulocytopenic patients. Am J Med 86:668, 1989.
56. Flannery MT, Simmons DB, Saba H, et al: Fluconazole in the treatment of hepatosplenic candidiasis. Arch Intern Med 152:406, 1992.
57. Calandra T, Glauser MP, Schellekens J, et al: Treatment of gram negative septic shock with human IgG antibody to *Escherichia coli* J5: A prospective, double-blind randomized trial. J Infect Dis 158:312, 1988.
58. Ziegler EJ, Fisher CJ Jr, Sprung CL, et al: Treatment of gram-negative bacteremia and septic shock with HA-1A human

monoclonal antibody against endotoxin—A randomized, double-blind, placebo-controlled trial. N Engl J Med 324:429, 1991.
59. Greenman RI, Schein RMH, Martin MA, et al: A controlled clinical trial of E5 murine monoclonal IgM antibody to endotoxin in the treatment of gram-negative sepsis. JAMA 266:1097, 1991.
60. Klastersky J: Empirical therapy for bacterial infections in neutropenic patients. Support Care Cancer 2:347, 1994.
61. Lee JW, Pizzo PA: Management of the cancer patient with fever and prolonged neutropenia. Hematol Oncol Clin North Am 7:937, 1993.
62. Bodey GP: Empirical antibiotic therapy for fever in neutropenic patients. Clin Infect Dis 17(Suppl 2):S378, 1993.
63. Viscoli C, Bruzzi P, Castagnola E, et al: Factors associated with bacteraemia in febrile, granulocytopenic cancer patients. The International Antimicrobial Therapy Cooperative Group (IATCG) of the European Organization for Research and Treatment of Cancer (EORTC). Eur J Cancer 30A:430, 1994.
64. Talcott JA, Siegel RD, Finberg R, Goldman L: Risk-assessment in cancer patients with fever and neutropenia: A prospective, two-center validation of a prediction rule. J Clin Oncol 10:316, 1992.
65. Rubenstein EB, Rolston K, Benjamin RS, et al: Outpatient treatment of febrile episodes in low-risk neutropenic patients with cancer. Cancer 71:3640, 1993.
66. Malik IA, Khan WA, Karim M, et al: Feasibility of outpatient management of fever in cancer patients with low-risk neutropenia: Results of a prospective randomized trial. Am J Med 98:224, 1995.
67. de Marie S, van den Broek PJ, Willemze R, van Furth R: Strategy for antibiotic therapy in febrile neutropenic patients on selective antibiotic decontamination. Eur J Clin Microbiol Infect Dis 12:897, 1993.
68. Newman KA, Schimpff SC, Young VM, et al: Lessons learned from surveillance cultures from patients with acute nonlymphocytic leukemia: Usefulness for epidemiologic prevention and therapeutic research. Am J Med 70:423, 1982.
69. Cohen ML, Murphy MT, Counts GW, et al: Prediction by surveillance cultures of bacteremia among neutropenic patients treated in a protective environment. J Infect Dis 147:489, 1984.
70. Eibl MM, Cairns L, Rosen FS: Safety and efficacy of a monomeric, functionally intact intravenous IgG preparation in patients with primary immunodeficiency syndromes. Clin Immunol Immunopathol 31:151, 1984.
71. Bjorkander J, Wadsworth C, Hanson LA: 1040 prophylactic infusions with an unmodified intravenous immunoglobulin product causing few side-effects in patients with antibody deficiency syndromes. Infection 13:102, 1985.
72. Shamberger RC, Pizzo PA, Goodgame JT, et al: The effect of total parenteral nutrition on chemotherapy induced myelosuppression: A randomized study. Am J Med 74:40, 1983.
73. Siber GR, Weitzman SA, Aisenberg AC, et al: Impaired antibody response to pneumococcal vaccine after treatment for Hodgkin's disease. N Engl J Med 299:442, 1978.
74. Ortbals DW, Liebhaber H, Presant CA, et al: Influenza immunization of adult patients with malignant diseases. Ann Intern Med 87:552, 1977.
75. Dienstag JL, Katkov WN: Viral hepatitis in the compromised host. *In* Rubin RH, Young LS (eds): Clinical Approach to Infection in the Compromised Host, ed 3. New York, Plenum Publishing, 1994, pp 355–377.
76. Meyers JD, Leszczynski J, Zaia JA, et al: Prevention of cytomegalovirus infection by cytomegalovirus immune globulin after marrow transplantation. Ann Intern Med 98:442, 1983.
77. Bowden RA, Sayers M, Fluornoy N, et al: Cytomegalovirus immune globulin and seronegative blood products to prevent primary cytomegalovirus infection after marrow transplantation. N Engl J Med 314:1006, 1986.
78. Stein RS, Beamon C, Ali MY, et al: Lithium carbonate attenuation of chemotherapy-induced neutropenia. N Engl J Med 297:427, 1977.
79. Dale DC: Potential role of colony-stimulating factors in the prevention and treatment of infectious diseases. Clin Infect Dis 18(Suppl 2):180, 1994.
80. Roilides E, Pizzo PA: Perspectives on the use of cytokines in the management of infectious complications of cancer. Clin Infect Dis 17(Suppl 2):85, 1993.
81. American Society of Clinical Oncology: Recommendations for the use of hematopoietic colony-stimulating factors: Evidence-based, clinical practice guidelines. J Clin Oncol 12:2471, 1994.
82. Ikeda K, Tasaka T, Sasaki K, et al: Low-dose continuous subcutaneous infusion of granulocyte colony-stimulating factor for chemotherapy-induced neutropenia in acute myelogenous leukemia and its pharmacokinetics. Leukemia 8:1838, 1994.
83. Groopman JE, Mitsuyasu RT, DeLeo MJ, et al: Effect of recombinant human granulocyte-macrophage colony-stimulating factor on myelopoiesis in the acquired immunodeficiency syndrome. N Engl J Med 317:593, 1987.
84. Cooperative Group for the Study of Immunoglobulin in Chronic Lymphocytic Leukemia: Intravenous immunoglobulin for the prevention of infection in chronic lymphocytic leukemia: A randomized, controlled clinical trial. N Engl J Med 319:902, 1988.
85. Remington JS, Schimpff SC: Please don't eat the salads. N Engl J Med 304:433, 1981.
86. Bodey GP, Johnson D: Microbiological evaluation of protected environment during patient occupancy. Appl Microbiol 22:828, 1971.
87. Yates JW, Holland JF: A controlled study of isolation and endogenous microbial suppression in acute myelocytic leukemia patients. Cancer 32:1490, 1973.
88. Levine AS, Siegel SE, Schreiber AD, et al: Protected environments and prophylactic antibiotics: A prospective controlled study of their utility in the therapy of acute leukemia. N Engl J Med 288:477, 1973.
89. Pizzo PA: Antimicrobial prophylaxis in the immunosuppressed cancer patient. Curr Clin Top Infect Dis 4:153, 1983.
90. Storring RA, Jameson B, McElwain TJ, et al: Oral non-absorbable antibiotics prevent infection in acute non-lymphoblastic leukaemia. Lancet 2:837, 1977.
91. Cohen MH, Creaven PJ, Fosseick BE Jr, et al: Effect of oral prophylactic broad spectrum nonabsorbable antibiotics on the gastrointestinal absorption of nutrients and methotrexate in small cell bronchogenic carcinoma patients. Cancer 38:1556, 1976.
92. Klastersky J, Debusscher L, Weerts D, et al: Use of oral antibiotics in protected units environment: Clinical effectiveness and role in the emergence of antibiotic-resistant strains. Pathol Biol (Paris) 22:5, 1973.
93. Schimpff SC, Greene WH, Young VM, et al: Infection prevention in acute nonlymphocytic leukemia: Laminar air flow room reverse isolation with oral, nonabsorbable antibiotic prophylaxis. Ann Intern Med 82:351, 1975.
94. Schimpff SC: Infection prevention during profound granulocytopenia: New approaches to alimentary canal microbial suppression. Ann Intern Med 93:358, 1980.
95. Hargadon MT, Young VM, Schimpff SC, et al: Selective suppression of alimentary tract microbial flora as prophylaxis during granulocytopenia. Antimicrob Agents Chemother 20:620, 1981.
96. Sleijfer DTH, Mulder NH, de Vries-Hospers HG, et al: Infection prevention in granulocytopenic patients by selective decontamination of the digestive tract. Eur J Cancer 16:859, 1980.
97. Pizzo PA, Robichaud KJ, Edwards BK, et al: Oral antibiotic prophylaxis in patients with cancer: A double-blind randomized placebo-controlled trial. J Pediatr 102:125, 1983.
98. Pizzo PA, Schimpff SC: Strategies for the prevention of infection in the myelosuppressed or immunosuppressed cancer patient. Cancer Treat Rep 67:223, 1983.
99. Wade JC, Schimpff SC, Hargadon MT, et al: A comparison of trimethoprim-sulfamethoxazole plus nystatin with gentamicin plus nystatin in the prevention of infection in acute leukemia. N Engl J Med 304:1057, 1981.
100. EORTC International Antimicrobial Therapy Project Group: Trimethoprim-sulfamethoxazole in the acute nonlymphocytic leukemia: A double-blind, placebo-controlled study. J Infect Dis 150:372, 1984.
101. Estey E, Maksymiuk A, Smith T, et al: Infection prophylaxis in acute leukemia: Comparative effectiveness of sulfamethoxazole and trimethoprim, ketoconazole, and a combination of the two. Arch Intern Med 144:1562, 1984.
102. Gurwith MJ, Brunton JL, Lank BA, et al: A prospective controlled investigation of prophylactic trimethoprim/sulfamethoxazole in hospitalized granulocytopenic patients. Am J Med 66:248, 1979.

103. Hughes WT, Kuhn S, Chaudhary S, et al: Successful prophylaxis for *Pneumocystis carinii* pneumonitis. N Engl J Med 297:1419, 1977.
104. Wade JC, de Jongh CA, Newman KA, et al: Selective antimicrobial modulation as prophylaxis against infection during granulocytopenia: Trimethoprim-sulfamethoxazole vs. nalidixic acid. J Infect Dis 147:624, 1983.
105. Gualtieri RJ, Donowitz GR, Kaiser DL, et al: Double blind randomized study of prophylactic trimethoprim/sulfamethoxazole in granulocytopenic patients with hematologic malignancies. Am J Med 74:934, 1983.
106. Watson JG, Jameson B, Powles RL, et al: Co-trimoxazole versus non-absorbable antibiotics in acute leukaemia. Lancet 1:6, 1982.
107. Wilson JM, Guiney DG: Future of oral trimethoprim-sulfamethoxazole prophylaxis in acute leukemia: Isolation of resistant plasmids from strains of Enterobacteriaceae causing bacteremia. N Engl J Med 306:16, 1982.
108. Lew MA, Kehoe K, Ritz J, et al: Ciprofloxacin versus trimethoprim/sulfamethoxazole for prophylaxis of bacterial infections in bone marrow transplant recipients: A randomized controlled trial. J Clin Oncol 13:239, 1995.
109. Bow EJ, Rayner E, Scott BA, et al: Selective gut decontamination with nalidixic acid or trimethoprim-sulfamethoxazole for infection prophylaxis in neutropenic cancer patients: Relationship of efficacy to antimicrobial spectrum and timing of administration. Antimicrob Agents Chemother 31:551, 1987.
110. Bow EJ, Rayner E, Louie TJ: Comparison of norfloxacin with cotrimoxazole for infection prophylaxis in acute leukemia. Am J Med 84:847, 1988.
111. Karp JE, Merz WG, Hendricksen C, et al: Oral norfloxacin for prevention of gram-negative bacterial infections in patients with acute leukemia and granulocytopenia: A randomized, double-blind, placebo-controlled trial. Ann Intern Med 106:1, 1987.
112. Dekker AW, Rozenberg-Arska M, Verhoef J: Infection prophylaxis in acute leukemia: A comparison of ciprofloxacin with trimethoprim-sulfamethoxazole and colistin. Ann Intern Med 106:7, 1987.
113. International Antimicrobial Therapy Cooperative Group of the European Organization for Research and Treatment of Cancer: Reduction of fever and streptococcal bacteremia in granulocytopenic patients with cancer: A trial of oral penicillin V or placebo combined with pefloxacin. JAMA 272:1183, 1994.
114. Rozenberg-Arska M, Dekker A, Verdonck L, Verhoef J: Prevention of bacteremia caused by alpha-hemolytic streptococci by roxithromycin (RU28 965) in granulocytopenic patients receiving ciprofloxacin. Infection 17:240, 1989.
115. Kern WV, Hay B, Kern P, et al: A randomized trial of roxithromycin in patients with acute leukemia and bone marrow transplant recipients receiving fluoroquinolone prophylaxis. Antimicrob Agents Chemother 38:465, 1994.
116. Lonnqvist B, Palmblad J, Ljungman P, et al: Oral acyclovir as prophylaxis for bacterial infections during induction therapy for acute leukaemia in adults. The Leukemia Group of Middle Sweden. Support Care Cancer 1:139, 1993.
117. Meunier F: Prevention of mycoses in immunocompromised patients. Rev Infect Dis 9:408, 1987.
118. Meunier-Carpentier F, Snoeck R, Gerain J, et al: Amphotericin B nasal spray as prophylaxis against aspergillosis in patients with neutropenia (Letter). N Engl J Med 311:1006, 1984.
119. Goodman JL, Winston DH, Greenfield RA, et al: A controlled trial of fluconazole to prevent fungal infections in patients undergoing bone marrow transplantation. N Engl J Med 326:845, 1992.
120. Winston DJ, Chandrasekar PH, Lazarus HM, et al: Fluconazole prophylaxis of fungal infections in patients with acute leukemia. Results of a randomized placebo-controlled, double-blind, multicenter trial. Ann Intern Med 118:495, 1993.
121. Wingard JR, Merz WG, Rinaldi MG, et al: Increase in *Candida krusei* infection among patients with bone marrow transplantation and neutropenia treated prophylactically with fluconazole. N Engl J Med 325:1274, 1991.
122. Wingard JR, Merz WG, Rinaldi MG, et al: Association of *Torulopsis glabrata* infections with fluconazole prophylaxis in neutropenic bone marrow transplant patients. Antimicrob Agents Chemother 37:1847, 1993.
123. Gold D, Corey L: Acyclovir prophylaxis for herpes simplex virus infection. Antimicrob Agents Chemother 31:361, 1987.
124. Varicella-zoster immune globulin: United States. MMWR Morbid Mortal Wkly Rep 30:15, 1981.
125. Sawyer MH: Treatment and prevention of varicella-zoster virus infections. Ann Intern Med 108:221, 1988.
126. Whitley RJ, Soong SJ, Dolin R, et al: Early vidarabine therapy to control the complications of herpes zoster in immunosuppressed patients. N Engl J Med 307:971, 1982.
127. Balfour HH Jr, Bean B, Laskin OL, et al: Acyclovir halts progression of herpes zoster in immunocompromised patients. N Engl J Med 308:1448, 1983.
128. Shepp DH, Dandliker PS, Meyers JD: Treatment of varicella-zoster virus infection in severely immunocompromised patients: A randomized comparison of acyclovir and vidarabine. N Engl J Med 314:208, 1986.
129. Balfour HH Jr: Varicella zoster virus infections in immunocompromised hosts: A review of the natural history and management. Am J Med 85(Suppl 2A):68, 1988.
130. Balfour HH Jr, Chace BA, Stapleton JT, et al: A randomized placebo-controlled trial of oral acyclovir for the prevention of cytomegalovirus disease in recipients of renal allografts. N Engl J Med 320:1381, 1989.
131. Winston DJ, Ho WG, Bartoni K, Champlin RE: Intravenous immunoglobulin and CMV-seronegative blood products for prevention of CMV infection and disease in bone marrow transplant recipients. Bone Marrow Transplant 12:283, 1993.
132. Winston DJ, Ho WG, Bartoni K, et al: Ganciclovir prophylaxis of cytomegalovirus infection and disease in allogeneic bone marrow transplant recipients. Results of a placebo-controlled, double-blind trial. Ann Intern Med 118:179, 1993.

SKIN AND SOFT TISSUE

138

Approach to the Patient with Skin or Soft Tissue Infection

David S. Feingold
Jan V. Hirschmann

Because the skin is the major interface between humans and their environment, it is not surprising that bacterial, fungal, and viral infections of the skin and the underlying soft tissues are the most common human infections. A knowledge of the anatomy of the skin and soft tissues is central to understanding their vulnerability to infection and their defenses against it (Fig. 138–1).

The skin is composed of the epidermis, the dermis, and subcutaneous fat. The epidermis is an avascular, proliferating layer that generates on its surface a constantly renewing tough barrier of protein and lipid, the stratum corneum. The stratum corneum, a protective sheath all over the body, is both an important permeability barrier and a wall that excludes most environmental pathogens. The epidermis is, on average, the thickness of a piece of paper.

The dermis, deep to the epidermis, contains blood vessels and lymphatics as well as fibroblasts, which synthesize the collagen and elastic tissue that impart strength and resilience to the skin. The skin "appendages," that is, eccrine sweat glands, sebaceous glands, and hair follicles, originate in the dermis. The skin appendages may contain organisms of the normal skin microbial flora but also are susceptible to invasion by pathogens because they create gaps in the protective stratum corneum. The subcutaneous fat is of variable thickness over the body. It is both an effective cushion and an energy storage reserve; for better or worse, its distribution sculpts our appearance. Beneath the subcutaneous fat, the superficial fascia, which must be penetrated by all the important vessels and nerves, separates the skin from underlying muscle. All these layers may become infected, often by predictable microorganisms, causing distinct syndromes.

Specific infections may involve one or more layers of soft tissue. For example, impetigo is restricted to the epidermis; folliculitis involves hair follicles; erysipelas is a superficial cellulitis of the dermis that spreads along the dermal lymphatics; acute cellulitis affects the subcutaneous fat and the dermis; necrotizing fasciitis centers in the superficial fascia; and myositis involves muscle. Pyoderma is a general term referring to bacterial infections of the skin caused by pyogenic organisms.

Table 138–1 lists factors to consider when bacterial infection of the soft tissues is suspected clinically. Primary cutaneous infections of the skin originate in grossly healthy skin. They usually have a characteristic morphologic appearance and are caused by a single organism. The portal of entry for the pathogen is often not obvious, although minor trauma is suspected. Secondary infections develop in preexisting lesions, which serve as portals of entry for the organisms.

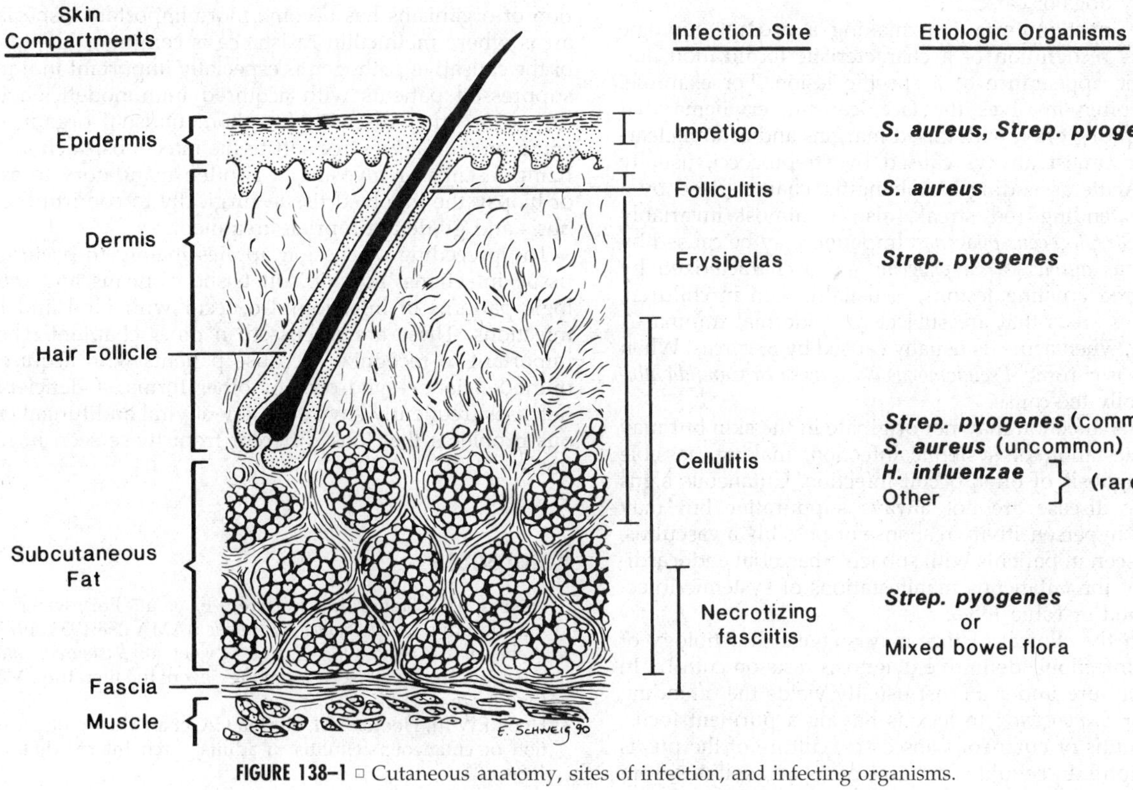

FIGURE 138–1 □ Cutaneous anatomy, sites of infection, and infecting organisms.

TABLE 138–1 ■ Some Considerations in Managing Bacterial Skin and Soft Tissue Infections

Primary versus secondary
Infection, portal of entry
Impaired host defenses against infection
Associated signs and symptoms
Localization and morphology of lesion
Recent environmental exposure

TABLE 138–2 ■ Some Cutaneous Signs in Systemic Infection

NONINFECTIOUS
Erythema nodosum
Erythema multiforme
Necrotizing vasculitis
Osler nodes
Janeway lesions
Disseminated intravascular coagulation
INFECTIOUS
Purulent petechiae in meningococcemia
Cutaneous abscesses in staphylococcal sepsis
Ecthyma gangrenosum in *Pseudomonas* sepsis
Cellulitis in *Vibrio vulnificus* septicemia
Erythema migrans in Lyme disease *(Borrelia burgdorferi)*

Atopic dermatitis and other eczematous lesions are the most common cutaneous lesions that become secondarily infected. Various lesions that interrupt the integrity of the stratum corneum, for example, surgical or traumatic wounds, burns, insect bites, and ulcers, are prone to secondary infection. Secondary infections are frequently polymicrobial and more likely to be caused by organisms less pathogenic for the normal soft tissues.

When a patient has impaired phagocytic or immune defenses, secondary infections are much more likely to develop and to progress rapidly. Thus, in leukopenic or immunosuppressed patients or in poorly controlled diabetic persons, scrupulous skin care to minimize portals for pathogen entry and aggressive treatment of early infections are indicated.

Most cutaneous infections in the normal host are self-limited. Early treatment is indicated when the tempo of extension is rapid or when associated fever or chills suggest a failure to contain the infection. It is always important to try to establish a specific etiology of the infection but even more so in this instance; blood cultures as well as local cultures and Gram stains are indicated before initiating antibiotic therapy.

Knowledge of recent environmental exposure may be critical to making a correct etiologic diagnosis. There are many examples of zoonoses or environmental contamination with pathogens. For example, one must consider *Aeromonas hydrophila* when severe cellulitis follows traumatic exposure to fresh water[1] and *Pasteurella multocida* infection after bites or scratches by dogs or cats.[2]

Probably most important in making a prompt etiologic diagnosis is recognition of a characteristic localization and morphologic appearance of a specific lesion. For example, erysipelas often involves the face, causing erythema that expands rapidly, often with raised margins and central clearing; this is almost always caused by streptococci, usually group A. Acute ascending lymphangitis, characterized by a centrally extending red streak, also is almost invariably caused by *Streptococcus pyogenes*. Impetigo may be caused by *Staphylococcus aureus* or *S. pyogenes*. It is characterized by honey-colored crusting lesions, is usually seen in children, and involves areas that are subject to epidermal trauma. A paronychia, when acute, is usually caused by *S. aureus*. When paronychia is chronic, *Pseudomonas aeruginosa* or *Candida albicans* is usually the cause.

Cutaneous infection may not originate in the skin but may be a manifestation of systemic infection, making possible prompt diagnosis of often occult infection. Cutaneous signs in systemic disease are not always suppurative but may represent a hypersensitivity response or possibly a vasculitis, as may be seen in patients with subacute bacterial endocarditis. Some of the cutaneous manifestations of systemic infection are listed in Table 138–2.

Although the clinical picture may suggest the etiology of soft tissue infections, definitive diagnosis rests on culture. In impetigo, culture under a crust usually yields the offending *S. aureus* or *S. pyogenes*. In lesions having a purulent focus, as in folliculitis or cutaneous abscesses, culture of the pus is usually helpful. In cellulitis, cultures of tissue aspirates from the lesion have been productive in a minority of the cases, unless a primary focus was present, when the culture usually yielded a pathogen and agreed with a positive aspirate, if obtained.[3, 4] In a prospective study of erysipelas and cellulitis of the leg reported from France in 1989, direct immunofluorescence assays were positive for group streptococcal antigen in 29 of the 42 cases. In combination with culture, direct immunofluorescence studies identified a causative agent in 37 of the cases.[5] Search for bacterial antigen in tissue is an experimental procedure but some day may become a clinically useful diagnostic test.

Specific DNA can now be amplified in vitro and identified by using the polymerase chain reaction. Although the polymerase chain reaction is still primarily a research tool at the time of this writing, it is likely that it will be used routinely to diagnose many infectious diseases in the near future, when procedures to ensure specificity of diagnosis are standardized.[6]

In summary, when there is an open or a purulent cutaneous lesion, culture is usually productive. Aspiration of inflammatory lesions has a low yield. Because of the increasing problem of methicillin-resistant *S. aureus* in pyodermas, isolation of organisms has become more important, especially in areas where methicillin resistance is common. Identification of the causative pathogen is especially important in immunosuppressed patients with acquired immunodeficiency syndrome or other diseases, in whom unusual organisms are common. For aggressive soft tissue infections, such as necrotizing fasciitis or myositis, it is often mandatory to aspirate or biopsy the involved tissue surgically to confirm the diagnosis and guide appropriate treatment.

The preceding discussion applies mainly to bacterial soft tissue infections. Specific soft tissue tropisms and morphologic patterns of infection also occur with viral and fungal infections. These are discussed in other chapters. They are important to recognize, because patients with acquired immunodeficiency syndrome or other forms of deficient host defenses frequently have a variety of viral and fungal cutaneous problems that look different from those seen in normal hosts.

References

1. Hanson PG, Standridge J, Jarrett F, et al: Freshwater wound infection due to *Aeromonas hydrophila*. JAMA 238:1053, 1977.
2. Weber DJ, Wolfson JS, Swartz MN, et al: *Pasteurella multocida* infections, report of 34 cases and review of the literature. Medicine (Baltimore) 63:133, 1984.
3. Hook EW III, Hooton TM, Horton CA, et al: Microbiologic evaluation of cutaneous cellulitis in adults. Arch Intern Med 146:295, 1986.

4. Duvanel T, Auckenthaler R, Rohrer P, et al: Quantitative cultures of biopsy specimens from cutaneous cellulitis. Arch Intern Med 149:293, 1989.
5. Bernard P, Bedane C, Mounier M, et al: Streptococcal cause of erysipelas and cellulitis in adults: A microbiologic study using direct immunofluorescence technique. Arch Dermatol 125:779, 1989.
6. Ehrlich GD, Greenberg ST: PCR-Based Diagnosis in Infectious Diseases. Boston, Blackwell Scientific Publications, 1994.

139

Normal Cutaneous Flora and Infections They Cause

Jan V. Hirschmann
David S. Feingold

The normal cutaneous flora[1–3] is a teeming population of microorganisms belonging to relatively few species. Aerobes vary in density from 10^2 per cm^2 on dry skin to 10^7 per cm^2 in moist areas such as the axilla and toe web spaces. Anaerobes, infrequent in other sites, reach concentrations of 10^4 to 10^6 per cm^2 in areas rich in sebaceous glands. The sweat glands and ducts are ordinarily sterile, but anaerobes populate the deeper parts of the hair follicles and sebaceous glands. Table 139–1 lists the resident cutaneous flora and the skin diseases associated with each.

The reason that the permanent cutaneous flora persists is partly related to the organisms' ability to attach to skin cells. "Transients," organisms that are found temporarily on the skin, usually originate from the environment or from adjacent, noncutaneous surfaces such as mucous membranes. However, these organisms do not adhere well to cutaneous cells and cannot thrive or reproduce on the skin for sustained periods. A third subpopulation of cutaneous organisms is temporary residents or nomads. These organisms, often because of changes in the environment or the population of the permanent residents, attach to the cells and multiply only for brief durations.

Several factors other than epithelial cell adherence limit the normal flora to only a few species and prevent colonization and invasion by pathogens. The most important is probably an intact stratum corneum. Its overlapping cells form a barricade to impede entry of microorganisms into the epidermis below, and its dryness discourages growth of many microbes, such as gram-negative bacilli and *Candida* species, that require moisture to thrive. The cell remnants in the stratum corneum constantly shed, making it difficult for most organisms to establish permanent residence. Another factor is the low pH of normal skin (about 5.5), which results from the resident cutaneous flora's ability to produce acids from the lipids of sebum. The host's immune system also seems important, because defects in cell-mediated immunity, granulocyte function, or secretion of antibodies (ordinarily present in sweat as immunoglobulins A and G) may predispose to recurrent, severe cutaneous infection. In addition, the resident flora itself may inhibit colonization with other microorganisms by occupying binding sites, exhausting nutrients, or elaborating antimicrobial substances.

TABLE 139–1 ■ Resident Cutaneous Flora and Associated Skin Disorders

ORGANISMS	ASSOCIATED CUTANEOUS DISORDER
Gram-Positive Cocci	
Staphylococcus aureus	Impetigo, ecthyma, blistering distal dactylitis, pustules, folliculitis, cutaneous abscesses
Coagulase-negative staphylococci	—
Micrococcus species	—
M. sedentarius	Pitted keratolysis
Gram-Positive Bacilli	
Corynebacterium species	Trichomycosis axillaris,
C. minutissimum	dermatophytosis complex, axillary odor, erythrasma, pitted keratolysis
Brevibacterium species	Cheesy foot odor
Propionibacterium species	—
P. acnes	Acne
Gram-Negative Bacilli	
Acinetobacter species	—
Fungi	
Pityrosporum orbiculare (ovale)	Tinea (pityriasis) versicolor Seborrheic dermatitis *Pityrosporum* folliculitis

Identity of the Normal Flora

Gram-Positive Cocci

Staphylococcus aureus usually does not colonize the skin, but up to 20% of normal people harbor it in the intertriginous areas, especially the perineum, and 20% to 40% carry it in the nares. In contrast, coagulase-negative staphylococci are the most numerous organisms of the skin flora. Prominent among these is *Staphylococcus epidermidis*, which tends to colonize the upper body and represents more than half of the resident staphylococci. Other *Staphylococcus* species include *S. hominis, S. haemolyticus, S. capitis, S. warneri, S. cohnii, S. simulans,* and *S. saphrophyticus*, which is often a resident of the perineum and a common cause of urinary tract infections in females.

The related gram-positive cocci, *Micrococcus* species, primarily *M. luteus* and *M. varians*, are also commonly present on the skin. The anaerobic staphylococcus *Peptococcus saccharolyticus* is part of the normal flora in 20% of the population, especially on the forehead and in the antecubital fossa.

Streptococci are not members of the normal skin flora, although oral streptococci may occur transiently on the perioral skin. The cutaneous pathogen *Streptococcus pyogenes* (group A streptococcus) usually dies quickly on normal, intact skin; disruption of the stratum corneum is necessary for infection to occur. In some normal hosts, however, it can survive for a few days, but most develop impetigo shortly afterward.[4]

Gram-Positive Bacilli

The coryneforms are gram-positive pleomorphic bacilli that include primarily *Corynebacterium* and *Brevibacterium* species. *Corynebacterium* species are lipophilic—they thrive in areas of high lipid content—and are a major component of the normal flora. This is so particularly in moist areas, including the interdigital toe spaces. Group JK coryneforms appear to be antibiotic-resistant *Corynebacterium* species that colonize intertriginous areas and are especially prevalent among immunocompromised hosts. *Brevibacterium* species inhabit the skin of many normal people, particularly in moist areas. They are frequently isolated from the toe webs, especially in patients with tinea pedis, and probably cause the cheesy odor of sweaty feet.

Propionibacterium species, which are normal inhabitants of hair follicles and sebaceous glands, are the most common anaerobes of the permanent cutaneous flora. *Propionibacterium acnes,* which is present in almost all adults, is most numerous on the scalp, forehead, and back; its density correlates directly with the quantity of sebum present. Other *Propionibacterium* species are *P. granulosum,* present in small numbers at all skin sites, and *P. avidum,* usually found in moist areas, especially the anterior nares, axilla, and perineum.

Gram-Negative Bacilli

In part because they flourish best only in moist areas, gram-negative bacilli are unusual in the normal flora, although they occasionally become residents in intertriginous sites. The most common of these is *Acinetobacter* species, found in up to 25% of the population. They are especially common in summer, probably because increased sweating provides a moist milieu for their growth.

Fungi

Pityrosporum orbiculare and *Pityrosporum ovale,* probably the same organism, are lipophilic yeasts that are densest on the back and chest, areas of greatest sebum excretion. *Candida* species, although common in the oral cavity and elsewhere in the alimentary tract, rarely reside on the normal skin.

Resident Flora as Cutaneous Pathogens

Coryneforms

Erythrasma is a common and usually asymptomatic superficial cutaneous infection that is apparently caused by *Corynebacterium minutissimum.*[5] Erythrasma especially affects intertriginous areas such as the groin, axillae, and toe webs. In tropical climates, extensive disease can occur anywhere on the body. In the most common form of erythrasma, scaling, fissuring, and maceration occur in the toe webs, especially the fourth interspace. In other areas the lesions are scaly, slightly brown or red patches that are irregular in shape but have well-delineated borders. In all locations, the involved skin fluoresces red to pink with ultraviolet light from a Wood lamp because the organisms produce porphyrins. This procedure is the major diagnostic test. Treatment consists of vigorous washing with soap; topical imidazoles, such as miconazole,[6] which have antibacterial (gram-positive) as well as antifungal properties; oral erythromycin; topical erythromycin or clindamycin, or Whitfield ointment.[7]

Trichomycosis axillaris is the presence of yellow, red, or black nodules on the axillary hair. This condition is caused by large colonies of *Corynebacterium* species of several biochemical types on the outside of the hair shaft.[7] Because the bacteria can invade the cuticle, the hair may become brittle. The same process may affect the pubic or facial hair.[8] Increased sweating, poor hygiene, and failure to use an axillary deodorant are predisposing factors. Shaving the hair eliminates the disease, although topical clindamycin or erythromycin may also be effective.[8]

Pitted keratolysis consists of multiple pitted erosions of the soles that measure 1 to 7 mm in diameter or, occasionally, collarettes on the palms. The lesions become more prominent if soaked in water for 10 to 15 minutes.[9] Usually asymptomatic, pitted keratolysis seems to occur in settings of increased moisture resulting from excessive sweating, occlusive footwear, or frequent contact with water. An intense malodor of the feet is common, and some victims develop reddened plaques, scaling, pruritus, and tenderness of the soles. Some studies have implicated coryneform bacteria as the cause; organisms are recovered from the erosion or pit rather than the adjacent normal skin. The bacteria may produce enzymes that digest keratin and create excavations of the stratum corneum.[9] One study found both *C. minutissimum* and *Micrococcus sedentarius* in all cases of pitted keratolysis. The authors reproduced the disease experimentally in a volunteer by using *M. sedentarius* in pure culture under occlusion over the surface of the heel.[10] Coryneform bacteria and *M. sedentarius* may be synergistic, or each organism may be able to produce the disorder. Several treatments are effective, including topical imidazoles such as miconazole and clotrimazole, topical erythromycin and clindamycin, antiseptics such as glutaraldehyde and formaldehyde, and systemic erythromycin.[9]

The term dermatophytosis complex applies to dermatophyte infection combined with bacterial overgrowth in the moist, partially occluded interdigital toe spaces.[11] Scaling produced by the fungal infection, combined with occlusion, maceration, and wetness, promotes the growth of coryneforms, especially *Brevibacterium* species. The result is white maceration, soggy scaling, pruritus, and malodor in the interdigital space. Redness, tenderness, edema, and fissuring may occur in severe cases. The dermatophytes, forced lower in the stratum corneum, become more difficult to isolate from superficial scrapings. However, dermatophytes are detectable on biopsy of the deepest portion of the stratum corneum. Effective antimicrobial therapy requires agents active against both the fungi and the bacteria, such as the imidazoles (e.g., clotrimazole or miconazole). Drying of the area by removing the shoe, separating the interspaces with soft pads, and applying astringents such as aluminum chloride are also useful measures.

Propionibacterium *Species*

The presence of *P. acnes* in the sebaceous follicle is a critical element in the development of acne vulgaris. This organism produces certain extracellular factors that may initiate the inflammatory phase of acne. Papules and pustules result from rupture of the follicular wall and inflammation of the surrounding dermis. Therapies for acne involve decreasing one or more of the three basic pathogenetic elements: sebum production, hyperkeratosis of the follicular duct, and *P. acnes* population. Diminishing the number of *P. acnes* organisms can be accomplished with oral antibiotics such as tetracycline or topical antibiotics such as erythromycin or clindamycin, which are therapeutically equivalent to the oral agents.[12] Other topical antibacterial substances such as benzoyl peroxide are also effective.[12]

Pityrosporum *Species*

Certain factors cause *P. orbiculare (P. ovale* or *Malessezia furfur)* to transform from a saprophyte into a pathogen. The transformation is often, but not always, accompanied by a morphologic change from yeasts to hyphal forms. These conditions include high temperature and humidity, increased sweating, occlusive clothing, greasy skin, and certain systemic conditions such as depressed cellular immunity and excessive exogenous or endogenous corticosteroids.[13] When the mycelial form of *P. orbiculare* involves the stratum corneum, tinea (or pityriasis) versicolor results. This condition is usually asymptomatic, but pruritus sometimes occurs. Mildly scaly macules or large patches of hypopigmented or hyperpigmented skin develop, predominantly on the trunk but also on the neck, and upper arms. Occasionally the perineum, genitalia, axillae, and thighs may be involved. The lesions may be white, red, or yellowish tan to brown. On white skin they tend to be hyperpigmented, but on tanned or dark skin the lesions are paler than the surrounding skin. With ultraviolet light from the Wood lamp, the lesions usually show pale yellow-green fluorescence. The diagnosis is established by finding mycelia and yeast ("spaghetti and meatballs") on potassium hydroxide preparations. Treatment is topical application of selenium sulfide left overnight and washed off in the morning. Propylene glycol, 50% in water twice daily, is effective, as are the topical imidazoles; however, the imidazoles are more expensive. Oral ketoconazole, 200 to 400 mg in a single dose or for a few days, is another approach. Ketoconazole may be repeated for relapses or used for monthly prophylaxis.

P. orbiculare can also cause an itchy folliculitis, usually on the upper back, chest, and upper arms and usually in adults 30 years of age or older.[14] The lesions are small, dome-shaped follicular papules or pustules. Lesions are occasionally present on the forearms, hands, legs, and face. Direct microscopy of material examined with potassium hydroxide, methylene blue, or Gram stain shows budding yeasts, which are also visible by skin biopsy. Topical therapy is effective, consisting of selenium sulfide for 30 minutes daily for 3 days then once weekly; propylene glycol, 50% in water twice daily for 3 weeks; or a topical imidazole daily for 1 week, followed by treatment once a week for several months.[13] Oral ketoconazole also clears the infection.

P. orbiculare probably causes seborrheic dermatitis, a scaly erythematous disorder that involves the scalp, face, sternal and interscapular regions of the chest, and intertriginous areas. The scale tends to have a greasy appearance and may form crusts. The scalp lesions usually respond to treatment with selenium sulfide, although a potent corticosteroid such as fluocinolone may be necessary. Lesions on the face, ears, and groin are controlled by hydrocortisone; those on the trunk may require more potent corticosteroids. The evidence that *Pityrosporum* species cause the seborrheic dermatitis consists not only of the consistent isolation of the organism from lesions but also of the successful treatment of this disorder with topical miconazole and oral or topical ketoconazole.[15–17] Corticosteroids are superior to topical ketoconazole, however, in controlling the disease,[18] which tends to be chronic and relapsing.

References

1. Noble WC: Microbiology of Human Skin, ed 2. London, Lloyd-Luke, 1981.
2. Leyden JJ, McKinley KJ, Nordstrom KM, et al: Skin microflora. J Invest Dermatol 88:65s, 1987.
3. Roth RR, James WD: Microbiology of the skin: Resident flora, ecology, infection. J Am Acad Dermatol 20:367, 1989.
4. Ferrieri P, Dajani AS, Wannamaker LW, et al: Natural history of impetigo. I. Site sequence of acquisition and familial patterns of spread of cutaneous streptococci. J Clin Invest 51:2851, 1972.
5. Sarkany I, Taplin D, Blank H: The etiology and treatment of erythrasma. J Invest Dermatol 37:283, 1961.
6. Pitcher DG, Noble WC, Seville RH: Treatment of erythrasma with miconazole. Clin Exp Dermatol 4:453, 1979.
7. Freeman RG, McBride ME, Know JM: Pathogenesis of trichomycosis axillaris. Arch Dermatol 100:95, 1969.
8. White SW, Smith J: Trichomycosis pubis. Arch Dermatol 115:444, 1979.
9. Zaias N: Pitted and ringed keratolysis: A review and update. J Am Acad Dermatol 7:787, 1982.
10. Nordstrom KM, McGinley KJ, Capiello L, et al: Pitted keratolysis: The role of *Micrococcus sedentarius*. Arch Dermatol 123:1320, 1987.
11. Leyden JJ, Kligman AM: Interdigital athlete's foot. Arch Dermatol 114:1691, 1988.
12. Hirschmann JV: Topical antibiotics in dermatology. Arch Dermatol 14:1466, 1989.
13. Faergemann J: Lipophilic yeasts in skin disease. Semin Dermatol 4:173, 1985.
14. Back O, Faergemann J, Hornqvist R: Pityrosporum folliculitis: A common disease of the young and middle-aged. J Am Acad Dermatol 12:56, 1985.
15. Ford GP, Farr PM, Ive FA, et al: The response of seborrheic dermatitis to ketoconazole. Br J Dermatol 111:603, 1984.
16. Faergemann J: Seborrheic dermatitis and *Pityrosporum orbiculare*: Treatment of seborrhoeic dermatitis of the scalp with miconazole-hydrocortisone (Daktacort), miconazole and hydrocortisone. Br J Dermatol 114:695, 1986.
17. Skinner RB, Noah PW, Taylor RM, et al: Double-blind treatment of seborrheic dermatitis with 2% ketoconazole cream. J Am Acad Dermatol 12:852, 1985.
18. Stratigos JD, Antoniou C, Katsambas A, et al: Ketoconazole 2% cream versus hydrocortisone 1% cream in the treatment of seborrheic dermatitis: A double-blind comparative trial. J Am Acad Dermatol 19:850, 1988.

140

Staphylococcal and Streptococcal Skin or Soft Tissue Infections

Jan V. Hirschmann
David S. Feingold

Cutaneous pyogenic infections usually occur where the skin's protective stratum corneum has been disrupted by inflammation, trauma, maceration from excessive moisture, or other factors. Although the normal resident flora can sometimes cause the ensuing infectious complications, especially cutaneous abscesses, organisms acquired from elsewhere are usually responsible, particularly *Staphylococcus aureus* and *Streptococcus pyogenes* (group A streptococcus).

S. aureus is present in the anterior nares of 20% to 40% of the normal population.[1] From this reservoir it can cause persistent skin colonization in some people and, occasionally, a predisposition to recurrent staphylococcal skin infections. The rate of colonization of the anterior nares and skin may be increased in intravenous drug abusers, diabetics requiring insulin, hospital workers, patients receiving allergy injections, and those undergoing hemodialysis.[2] The bacterium frequently resides on areas damaged by dermatitis. The degree of colonization directly correlates with the severity of exudation. *S. aureus* is present on the skin of most patients with atopic dermatitis, nummular eczema, and lichen simplex chronicus. It is present in about 20% of those with seborrheic dermatitis and, in low numbers, in about 50% of patients with psoriasis.[3] *S. aureus* can spread from person to person, but in previously uncolonized people it typically appears first in the nose and only later on normal skin. It usually colonizes the skin before causing cutaneous infection.

S. pyogenes, by contrast, rarely persists for long on mucocutaneous surfaces. It is usually acquired from others whose skin or pharynx is infected or briefly colonized with the organism. In those who develop cutaneous infection, it typically appears on the skin first and only later spreads to the respiratory tract, which is opposite to the order of spread in *S. aureus* infection.[4]

Impetigo

S. pyogenes and *S. aureus,* separately or together, cause several types of skin infections. Their clinical appearance depends on the depth and anatomic location of the inflammation. The most superficial of these is impetigo, which involves the formation beneath the stratum corneum of vesicles and pustules containing numerous neutrophils and occasional gram-positive cocci. In the bullous variety the fluid collection is also below the stratum corneum, but it contains few or no neutrophils. Other histologic features of impetigo are neutrophilic and lymphocytic inflammation of the upper dermis and epidermal edema (spongiosis).

In nonbullous impetigo, thin-walled vesicles and pustules form on an erythematous base. They rupture and release their liquid contents, which dry to create yellow-brown ("honey-colored") scabs. Most common on the face and extremities, the lesions usually occur on skin that is damaged by minor trauma, such as cuts, abrasions, and insect bites. The crusts later separate from the underlying skin, which does not scar because the infection is so superficial. Impetigo may be pruritic and regional lymphadenitis may occur, but systemic manifestations such as fever are rare.

In bullous impetigo superficial flaccid bullae form. When they rupture, the released liquid dries to become a thin, brown covering like lacquer. Lesions several centimeters wide may occur through coalescence of many smaller areas.

Impetigo may complicate underlying dermatitis, particularly atopic eczema. The clinical distinction between an exudative dermatitis and superimposed impetigo may be difficult, because a weeping, crusted skin surface may be present in both. Yellow-brown scales should suggest the possibility of superinfection. However, that diagnosis is most convincing when pustules, surrounding cellulitis, contiguous lymphangitis, or regional lymphadenitis is present, in addition to positive skin cultures for *S. aureus* or *S. pyogenes.*

Poor personal hygiene, crowded living conditions, and hot, humid climates predispose to impetigo, which can occur in outbreaks among family members or populations in closed institutions. Carriers of *S. pyogenes* or *S. aureus* and those with infected skin may transmit the organism to others, in whom the bacteria reside briefly on normal skin. Minor trauma such as insect bites, often complicated by scratching, disrupts the cutaneous surface, allowing the bacteria to enter the skin. In nonbullous impetigo, either *S. pyogenes* or *S. aureus* can be the initial pathogen, but combined infection with both organisms is frequent. Bullous impetigo, however, is a primary infection with certain strains of *S. aureus,* usually group II phage type 71. These strains produce a toxin, exfoliatin, that causes cleavage beneath the stratum corneum. The same toxin is responsible for the staphylococcal scalded skin syndrome. Impetigo complicating eczema and other skin disorders is typically staphylococcal, but *S. pyogenes* is sometimes present.

The definitive diagnosis of the various forms of impetigo requires isolation of *S. pyogenes* or *S. aureus* from cultures of the involved skin. However, microbiologic studies are frequently unnecessary in clinically obvious cases.

Although impetigo may resolve spontaneously, treatment is indicated to relieve symptoms more rapidly, halt the formation of new lesions, and prevent potentially serious infectious complications, such as cellulitis. Whether antimicrobial therapy decreases the risk of poststreptococcal glomerulonephritis, a rare immunologic reaction provoked by certain "nephritogenic" strains of *S. pyogenes,* is uncertain. Often, the renal disorder is already evident when the patient comes to medical attention.[5]

Nonbullous impetigo of limited extent may respond well to topical antibiotics.[6] Bacitracin or neomycin-bacitracin formulations may be useful, but mupirocin is the best topical agent. When applied to the lesions three times a day for 7 to 8 days, mupirocin is as effective as oral erythromycin.[7] Unlike systemic antimicrobials, however, topical agents are inconvenient to use with widespread disease or when several family members are simultaneously infected, and they are not very effective in bullous impetigo. Furthermore, they do not eradicate streptococci in the respiratory tract, an important reservoir for spread of infection to others, especially in epidemic situations or when nephritogenic strains are involved. In these circumstances, systemic antibiotics are indicated to minimize contagion.

When systemic antimicrobials are warranted (Table 140–1), oral or intramuscular penicillin usually cures nonbullous impetigo, even when resistant *S. aureus* is present with *S. pyogenes.* Intramuscular benzathine penicillin has the advantage of affording successful treatment with a single injection, eliminating the necessity of further therapy. Penicillin-resistant *S. aureus* is now frequently the *sole* pathogen isolated in nonbullous impetigo, however, a change from previous experience. Accordingly, many clinicians treat all forms of impetigo, including bullous impetigo and impetigo complicating underlying dermatologic diseases, with an agent effective against penicillin-resistant *S. aureus* rather than with penicillin. Two studies demonstrated the superiority of such an approach.[8, 9] Dicloxacillin is a good choice. In patients allergic to penicillin, clindamycin is an acceptable alternative, or, if the allergy is not life threatening, an oral cephalosporin is reasonable. Erythromycin is usually successful, but in some locales *S. aureus* is commonly resistant to it. For disease caused by methicillin-resistant staphylococci, trimethoprim-sulfamethoxazole should be effective. The duration of oral therapy for impetigo with any of these agents should be about 1 week. When the risk of impetigo is high, such as for young children living in a hot, humid climate, the frequency of impetigo can be reduced by prophylactically applying topical neomycin-bacitracin to areas of minor trauma, such as insect bites and abrasions.[10]

Ecthyma

Ecthyma, the Greek word for pustule, is a streptococcal or staphylococcal infection causing dermal ulceration. Ecthyma

TABLE 140–1 ■ Systemic Antibiotic Therapy for Streptococcal and Staphylococcal Pyoderma

AGENT	USUAL ADULT DOSE*
Benzathine penicillin	1.2 million units IM as single dose
Penicillin V	250 mg PO qid
Cloxacillin, dicloxacillin	250 mg PO qid
Cephradine, cephalexin	250 mg PO qid
Clindamycin	150 mg PO qid
Trimethoprim-sulfamethoxazole	160 mg trimethoprim, 800 mg sulfamethoxazole PO bid
Erythromycin	500 mg PO qid

*IM, Intramuscularly; PO, orally; qid, four times a day; bid, twice a day.

often occurs in patients with preceding trauma, malnutrition, or poor hygiene. In alcoholics, the lesions have sometimes been labeled "wine sores." Like impetigo, it begins with vesicles that form crusts, but the infection causes ulceration beneath the adherent scabs. Ecthyma usually occurs on the lower extremities, appearing as single or multiple erythematous ulcerations with overlying crusts. Because of the deeper level of infection, ecthyma, unlike impetigo, causes scarring. Appropriate therapy should be an antibiotic that is effective against both *S. aureus* and *S. pyogenes*, such as dicloxacillin.[11]

Blistering Distal Dactylitis

Blistering distal dactylitis, an infection with *S. pyogenes*, or less commonly *S. aureus*, usually occurs in children.[12] A superficial, tender or nontender bulla with an erythematous base appears over the anterior fat pad of the distal phalanx of a finger, thumb, or toe and may extend to the nailfolds. Gram staining of the blister fluid demonstrates gram-positive cocci in chains or clusters. Clusters yield *S. pyogenes* or *S. aureus*. Incision and drainage are appropriate for painful lesions. When *S. pyogenes* is responsible, penicillin is the drug of choice; for *S. aureus* an antistaphylococcal agent such as dicloxacillin is indicated.

Folliculitis

Folliculitis is an inflammation of the ostium of a hair follicle. The pathogenesis apparently involves a combination of ostial occlusion and superficial follicular inflammation, which may be caused by bacteria, fungi, chemicals, or other agents. Among the many causes of folliculitis is *S. aureus*, most commonly in children but rarely in adults, in whom other causes of folliculitis predominate. Erythematous papules or pustules develop around individual hairs, often in crops and usually on the scalp or extremities. They tend to subside rapidly with systemic antistaphylococcal antibiotics.

Furuncles and Carbuncles

S. aureus can cause infections of the hair follicle. Inflammation extends deeper than in folliculitis to involve the dermis. There is an inflammatory nodule surmounted by a pustule through which the hair emerges. Discrete lesions, whether single or multiple, are called furuncles. They are called carbuncles when the infection affects several adjacent follicles, producing a coalescent inflammatory mass with pus draining from multiple follicular orifices. Furuncles can occur anywhere on hairy skin. Carbuncles tend to develop on the back of the neck. For small furuncles, moist heat, which seems to promote drainage, is satisfactory. Larger furuncles and carbuncles require incision and drainage. Systemic antistaphylococcal antibiotics are usually unnecessary unless extensive surrounding cellulitis or fever occurs.

Recurrent Staphylococcal Skin Infections

Some patients have recurrent episodes of furunculosis or other staphylococcal skin infections. Diabetes mellitus, chronic hemodialysis, and intravenous drug abuse are predisposing factors. Occasionally, a disorder of immune or granulocytic function is present, but it is important to recognize that most victims are apparently healthy. These patients are usually chronic nasal carriers of *S. aureus*, and they probably repetitively inoculate the organism onto the skin from this nasal reservoir.

Many topical antibiotics applied to the anterior nares eliminate *S. aureus* during use; however, once the drug is discontinued, the organism quickly returns. Mupirocin is the most effective topical agent and can eradicate nasal carriage for a protracted period. However, resistant *S. aureus* has emerged during mupirocin use.[5] Oral therapy with penicillinase-resistant penicillins such as cloxacillin is not effective alone. Rifampin by itself or combined with an antistaphylococcal penicillin is successful, and eradication can persist for many weeks after drug discontinuation. With rifampin alone, however, development of resistance is common. The quinolones, such as ciprofloxacin or ofloxacin, may be effective, but resistance is again a concern.[13] Clindamycin appears to be the most useful oral antimicrobial. In a controlled trial of 150 mg daily for 3 months, clindamycin eliminated recurrent staphylococcal skin infections in 82% of patients with a previous history of them, whereas 64% of those receiving placebo continued to have infections.[14] Furthermore, most of those receiving clindamycin had no recurrent infections for at least 9 months after discontinuation of the drug. This suggests long-term eradication of nasal carriage, although nasal cultures were not performed.

References

1. Roth RR, James WD: Microbiology of the skin: Resident flora, ecology, infection. J Am Acad Dermatol 20:367, 1989.
2. Sheagren JN: *Staphylococcus aureus:* The persistent pathogen. N Engl J Med 310:1368, 1984.
3. Leyden JJ, McGinley KJ, Nordstrom KM, et al: Skin microflora. J Invest Dermatol 88:65s, 1987.
4. Ferrieri P, Dajani AS, Wannamaker LW, et al: Natural history of impetigo. I. Site sequence of acquisition and familial patterns of spread of cutaneous streptococci. J Clin Invest 51:2851, 1972.
5. Hirschmann JV: Topical antibiotics in dermatology. Arch Dermatol 124:1691, 1988.
6. Dillon HC: The treatment of streptococcal skin infections. J Pediatr 76:676, 1970.
7. Barton LL, Friedman AD, Sharkey AM, et al: Impetigo contagiosa. III. Comparative efficacy of oral erythromycin and topical mupirocin. Pediatr Dermatol 6:134, 1989.
8. Barton LL, Friedman AD: Impetigo: A reassessment of etiology and therapy. Pediatr Dermatol 4:185, 1987.
9. Dagan R, Bar-David Y: Comparison of amoxicillin and clavulinic acid (Augmentin) for the nonbullous impetigo. Am J Dis Child 143:916, 1989.
10. Maddox JS, Ware JC, Dillon HC: The natural history of streptococcal skin infection: Prevention with topical antibiotics. J Am Acad Dermatol 13:207, 1985.
11. Musher DM, McKenzie SO: Infections due to *Staphylococcus aureus.* Medicine (Baltimore) 56:383, 1977.
12. Norcross ML Jr, Mitchell DF: Blistering distal dactylitis caused by *Staphylococcus aureus.* Cutis 51:353, 1993.
13. Chow JW, Yu VL: *Staphylococcus aureus* nasal carriage in hemodialysis patients: Its role in infection and approaches to prophylaxis. Arch Intern Med 149:1258, 1989.
14. Klempner MS, Styrt B: Prevention of recurrent staphylococcal skin infections with low-dose oral clindamycin therapy. JAMA 260:2682, 1988.

141

Gram-Negative Bacillary Skin or Soft Tissue Infections

David S. Feingold
Jan V. Hirschmann

Pseudomonas aeruginosa causes several characteristic cutaneous infections. The organism is common in moist environmental niches and colonizes moist areas of the body. Typical *Pseudomonas* infections include external otitis or swimmer's ear, paronychia and erosive interdigital infections in patients whose hands are frequently in water, and folliculitis associated with hot tub use. Drying the skin and eliminating the exposure are often adequate to cure these infections.

Malignant (sometimes called invasive) external otitis is a serious, locally invasive *Pseudomonas* infection that typically occurs in elderly diabetic patients.[1, 2] Reported predisposing factors in addition to diabetes include chronic external otitis and ear trauma, as may be seen in hearing aid users or with irrigation for cerumen impaction. Severe otalgia is the regular presenting complaint of malignant external otitis. Purulent drainage and granulation tissue in the external auditory canal are usually found on examination. Local cellulitis and bone destruction are best documented by radiographic imaging techniques. Extension to the central nervous system may cause neurologic deficit and even death.

In the past, successful treatment of malignant external otitis required prolonged hospitalization of at least 6 weeks for débridement and parenteral antipseudomonas therapy. The availability of the fluoroquinolone antibiotics with excellent antipseudomonas activity and tissue penetration after oral administration has obviated the need for prolonged hospitalization and parenteral therapy with the associated complications. A series of 23 consecutive patients with malignant external otitis treated with oral ciprofloxacin (usually 750 mg twice daily) and local surgical débridement was reported from Israel.[3] Twenty-one patients were cured. Ciprofloxacin therapy was continued for at least 6 weeks, but hospitalization averaged only 17 days.

P. aeruginosa may colonize the soles of used, not new, shoes; nail puncture wounds may cause inoculation of the organism into the foot, with resultant cellulitis and osteomyelitis.[4] Surgical débridement and antibiotics are required.

During *Pseudomonas* sepsis, usually in impaired hosts, skin lesions that yield the organism on culture occasionally occur. Four types have been described: vesicles and bullae, gangrenous cellulitis, macular or papular lesions, and ecthyma gangrenosum (a black eschar with surrounding erythema).[5] These lesions may be important clues for the diagnosis of *Pseudomonas* sepsis. Of the gram-negative bacilli, *Pseudomonas* spp. show a tropism for the skin during sepsis that is rarely seen with other gram-negative organisms. In typhoid fever, rose-colored spots may occur on the skin. In systemic *Vibrio vulnificus* infection, metastatic areas of cutaneous cellulitis are common.[6] Also in the differential diagnosis of metastatic cutaneous lesions in sepsis are *Escherichia coli* (rare), *Neisseria meningitidis*, *Neisseria gonorrhoeae*, and fungi of the *Aspergillus* and *Rhizopus* groups.

V. vulnificus and *Aeromonas hydrophila* are water-borne organisms that cause cutaneous infection. *V. vulnificus* is commonly found in seawater and fish, especially in the southern United States but as far north as New England in the summer.[7] Two types of *V. vulnificus* cutaneous involvement occur.[6] Wounds incurred in seawater may become contaminated and culminate in aggressive *V. vulnificus* cellulitis. Areas of cutaneous cellulitis may also develop as part of a life-threatening sepsis that occurs when susceptible patients, particularly those with liver disease, ingest *Vibrio*-contaminated seafood. Aggressive therapy with tetracyclines or other appropriate antibiotics based on sensitivities is mandatory. *A. hydrophila* grows in fresh or brackish water. It may contaminate preexisting wounds or traumatic wounds incurred in water. The severe cellulitis that may occur requires antibiotic treatment; gentamicin and chloramphenicol are good choices.

Pasteurella multocida is a normal inhabitant of the oral flora of dogs and cats. Many cases of localized soft tissue or bone infection have occurred after dog or cat bites or scratches.[8] Generalized sepsis is rare. Penicillin is the treatment of choice.

Haemophilus influenzae type b is a common cause of infection in young children.[9] One characteristic form of this infection is a facial cellulitis, presumably because the respiratory tract is the source of the organism. The lesions may be violaceous, but in most patients, *H. influenzae* cellulitis is difficult to distinguish from that due to streptococci or other causes. Because bacteriologic testing often yields no pathogen, it is wise to treat facial cellulitis in children with an antibiotic regimen that is effective against *H. influenzae*.

Gram-negative folliculitis is seen mostly by dermatologists as a complication of antibiotic therapy for acne. When acne patients receiving antimicrobials (usually tetracyclines) develop worsening "acne" with pustular lesions, superinfection of the follicles with gram-negative bacilli, including *E. coli* or *Klebsiella* and *Pseudomonas* spp., may have occurred. The diagnosis depends on history, Gram stain, and culture. At times, discontinuing the antibiotic may allow spontaneous clearing of the infection, but more often, appropriate antimicrobial agents, based on sensitivity tests, are indicated. Oral therapy is preferred, and trimethoprim-sulfamethoxazole, ciprofloxacin, or oral cephalosporins may be helpful.

References

1. Chandler JR: Malignant external otitis. Laryngoscope 78:1257, 1968.
2. Doroghaji RM, Nadol JB, Hyslop NE Jr, et al: Invasive external otitis. Am J Med 71:603, 1981.
3. Lang R, Goshan S, Kitzes-Cohen R, et al: Successful treatment of malignant external otitis with oral ciprofloxacin: Report of experience with 23 patients. J Infect Dis 161:537, 1990.
4. Fisher MC, Goldsmith JF, Gilligan PH: Sneakers as a source of *Pseudomonas aeruginosa* in children with osteomyelitis following puncture wounds. J Pediatr 106:607, 1985.
5. Weinberg AN, Swartz MN: Gram-negative coccal and bacillary infections. *In* Fitzpatrick TB, et al (eds): Dermatology in General Medicine, ed 3. New York, McGraw-Hill, 1987, p 2127.
6. Hill MK, Sanders CV: Localized and systemic infection due to *Vibrio* species. Infect Dis Clin 1:687, 1987.
7. Oliver JD, Warner RA, Deland DR: Distribution of *Vibrio vulnificans* and other lactose fermenting vibrios in the marine environment. Appl Environ Microbiol 45:985, 1983.
8. Weber DJ, Wolfson JJ, Swartz MN, Hooper DC: *Pasteurella multocida* infections: Report of 34 cases and review of the literature. Medicine (Baltimore) 63:133, 1984.
9. Dajani AS, Asmar BI, Thirumoorthi MC: Systemic *Hemophilus influenzae* disease: An overview. J Pediatr 94:355, 1979.

142

Cutaneous Abscesses and Ulcers

Jan V. Hirschmann
David S. Feingold

Abscesses

Staphylococcus aureus can cause cutaneous abscesses; however, it is isolated, usually in pure culture, in only about 25% of all cases.[1] The location of the abscess is the most important determinant of the infecting flora. *S. aureus* is present in half or more of axillary abscesses,[1–3] finger paronychia,[4] and breast abscesses in puerperal women.[5] It is isolated in about 20% to 40% of toe paronychia[4] and breast abscesses in nonpuerperal women.[5] It is present in about the same percentage of abscesses of the trunk, extremities, hands, buttocks, and inguinal regions. This organism is even less frequent in abscesses of the head and neck, vulvovaginal, scrotal, and perianal areas.[1, 2, 6, 7]

When *S. aureus* is not the cause, the usual infecting bacteria are anaerobes alone or a mixture of aerobic and anaerobic organisms. These organisms may constitute the normal regional skin flora or include transients from adjacent mucous membranes. Abscesses on the head, neck, and trunk, for example, commonly contain *Staphylococcus epidermidis* and *Propionibacterium* and *Peptococcus* spp., all part of the resident skin bacteria of those areas.[1] Perineal abscesses involving the vulvovaginal, inguinal, scrotal, perianal, and buttocks regions, by contrast, typically yield cultures containing fecal flora, such as *Bacteroides* spp., anaerobic gram-positive cocci, and α-hemolytic or nonhemolytic streptococci.[1, 2, 6, 7] *S. aureus* and β-hemolytic streptococci (isolated commonly only in hand abscesses) are clearly capable of causing disease by themselves. The other aerobic and anaerobic organisms grown from most cutaneous abscesses possess little virulence individually. When several of these species are combined and inoculated into the dermis or subcutaneous tissue by trauma or other mechanisms, however, they can produce inflammation and purulence.

Cutaneous abscesses are usually painful, tender, fluctuant, erythematous nodules, often with a pustule on top. In some cases, extensive surrounding cellulitis, lymphangitis, lymphadenitis, and fever may be present. Evacuation of the pus by incision and drainage ordinarily provides effective therapy.[1] Some clinicians leave the incision open, others pack the cavity with gauze for a few days, and still others suture the incision immediately after drainage. In any event, Gram stain and culture of the pus are usually unnecessary. Systemic antibiotics are also unnecessary,[1, 8] unless extensive surrounding cellulitis, cutaneous gangrene, seriously impaired host defenses, or systemic manifestations of infection are present.

Ulcers

Some organisms, such as mycobacteria, can cause primary cutaneous ulcers; more commonly, however, bacteria colonize or infect ulcers of noninfectious causes. Most frequent in clinical practice are those due to pressure (decubitus ulcers or bedsores), neuropathic changes (e.g., diabetic ulcers), or vascular insufficiency from venous or arterial disease. In all these types of ulcers, bacteria, often of several different species, flourish.

In ulcers due to venous insufficiency, *S. aureus* and various gram-negative bacilli alone or in combination are the usual isolates.[9, 10] The flora of an individual ulcer generally remains constant, regardless of local therapy or systemic antibiotics, until healing occurs. The species and concentration of the bacteria do not correlate well with either the degree of purulence or the rate of healing.[9] In a randomized trial, oral antibiotic treatment of the organisms isolated from the ulcers did not accelerate resolution of the ulcers or alter their bacteriologic findings in comparison to a control group receiving no antimicrobial therapy.[10] These findings indicate that routine cultures of venous ulcers are unrewarding and that purulent exudation in the wound by itself does not warrant antibiotics. Antibiotics should be reserved for ulcers complicated by extensive surrounding cellulitis, lymphangitis, or systemic signs of infection.

Diabetic foot ulcers tend to have a complex flora of both aerobic and anaerobic bacteria. The number of isolates tends to be lower in chronic stable ulcers than in those with extensive surrounding cellulitis.[11] Among the aerobic microbes are *S. aureus*, *S. epidermidis*, streptococci, *Corynebacterium* spp., and gram-negative bacilli. The predominant anaerobes are *Peptococcus* and *Bacteroides* spp. With more severe infection, such as gangrene, clostridia may become more common. The number and identity of the organisms isolated depend on the site and sampling technique of the cultures. When complications of soft tissue or bone infection occur, the bacteriologic findings of swabs obtained from the ulcer correlate poorly with those of aspirates of bullae or abscesses or with deep tissue specimens from biopsy or curettage during surgery. The latter methods more often yield a single species from specimens, especially *S. aureus* and *S. epidermidis*. *S. epidermidis* by itself is evidently a pathogen in this setting.[12]

In general, chronic, stable diabetic ulcers do not require routine cultures or systemic antibiotic therapy. These measures should be reserved for substantial inflammation of adjacent soft tissues, osteomyelitis, or signs of systemic infection. When these are present, abscesses or bullous lesions should be aspirated for culture. With mild cellulitis, an agent effective against staphylococci and streptococci may be adequate. With more extensive disease, surgical therapy in addition to antibiotics is often necessary. The antimicrobial regimen empirically chosen in this setting should be active against staphylococci, streptococci, anaerobes, and aerobic gram-negative bacilli until culture results are available to help determine the optimal choice.[13] A reasonable selection, among many, is an aminoglycoside such as gentamicin plus clindamycin or monotherapy with cefoxitin or cefotetan.

The bacteriologic findings of decubitus ulcers are similar to those of diabetic foot ulcers, that is, a mixture of aerobic and anaerobic bacteria. Blood cultures from patients who are bacteremic from decubitus ulcers reflect this complex flora, often yielding more than one organism. The most common anaerobes are *Bacteroides fragilis* and *Peptococcus* and *Peptostreptococcus* spp. The most common aerobes are *S. aureus*, streptococci, *Proteus mirabilis*, and other gram-negative bacilli.[14] The principles of diagnosis and management of decubitus ulcers are the same as those of diabetic foot ulcers, discussed previously.

References

1. Meislin HW, Lerner SA, Graves MH, et al: Cutaneous abscesses: Anaerobic and aerobic bacteriology and outpatient management. Ann Intern Med 87:145, 1977.

2. Ghoneim ATM, McGoldrick J, Blick PWH, et al: Aerobic and anaerobic bacteriology of subcutaneous abscesses. Br J Surg 68:498, 1981.
3. Leach RD, Eykyn SJ, Phillips I, et al: Anaerobic axillary abscess. Br Med J 2:5, 1979.
4. Whitehead SM, Eykyn SJ, Phillips I: Anaerobic paronychia. Br J Surg 68:420, 1981.
5. Leach RD, Eykyn SJ, Phillips I, et al: Anaerobic subareolar breast abscess. Lancet 1:35, 1979.
6. Whitehead SM, Leach RD, Eykyn SJ, et al: The aetiology of perirectal sepsis. Br J Surg 69:166, 1982.
7. Whitehead SM, Leach RD, Eykyn SJ, et al: The aetiology of scrotal sepsis. Br J Surg 69:729, 1982.
8. Macfie J, Harvey J: The treatment of acute superficial abscesses: A prospective clinical trial. Br J Surg 64:264, 1977.
9. Erickson G, Eklund AE, Kallinger LO: The clinical significance of bacterial growth in venous leg ulcers. Scand J Infect Dis 16:175, 1984.
10. Alinovi A, Bassissi P, Pini M: Systemic administration of antibiotics in the management of venous ulcers: A randomized clinical trial. J Am Acad Dermatol 15:186, 1986.
11. Louie TJ, Bartlett JG, Tally FP, et al: Aerobic and anaerobic bacteria in diabetic foot ulcers. Ann Intern Med 85:461, 1976.
12. Sapico FL, Canawati HN, Witte JL, et al: Quantitative aerobic and anaerobic bacteriology of infected diabetic feet. J Clin Microbiol 12:413, 1980.
13. Fierer J, Daniel D, David C: The fetid foot: Lower-extremity infections in patients with diabetes mellitus. Rev Infect Dis 1:210, 1979.
14. Galpin JE, Chow AW, Bayer AS, et al: Sepsis associated with decubitus ulcers. Am J Med 61:356, 1976.

143

Foot Infections in the Diabetic Patient and Infections Associated with Pressure Sores

Francisco L. Sapico
Alice N. Bessman

Foot Infections in the Diabetic Patient

The economic, social, and personal costs of foot infections in diabetic patients are considerable. In the United States alone, at least 20% of hospital admissions among diabetic patients are for foot problems. Fifty percent to 70% of all nontraumatic amputations are performed on patients with diabetes.[1–3] This increased susceptibility to foot infection has been attributed to several factors: immune dysfunction, neuropathy, and vascular insufficiency. The same factors also play important roles in the poor healing often observed in this population of patients.

Microbiology

Minor foot trauma and improperly fitting footwear contribute to the initiation and perpetuation of early lesions. Early lesions are characterized by local cellulitis, non–foul-smelling drainage, and poorly healing tissue defects without tissue necrosis and gangrene. These infections are usually monomicrobial in origin (i.e., *Staphylococcus aureus*, coagulase-negative staphylococci, enterococci, and aerobic streptococci).[4, 5] Moderate to severe infections (especially when tissue necrosis or gangrene is present) are usually characterized by a polymicrobial picture. Table 143–1 shows the dominant microorganisms isolated from uncontaminated deep tissue specimens in these types of infections.[6, 7] They are characteristically polymicrobial (average of about five different species per lesion, approximately equal numbers of aerobes and anaerobes) and with a heavy density of growth (approximately 7.0 $\log_{10}$ per g of tissue). The most common organisms isolated from blood cultures in diabetic patients with foot infections have been *Bacteroides fragilis* and *S. aureus*.[8]

Collection of specimens for culture necessitates removal of superficial necrotic tissue overlying the base of the ulcer (usually by sharp débridement). Bits of tissue can be obtained from the underlying tissue by using a sharp instrument such as a dermal curette or a scalpel.[9] Aerobic and anaerobic cultures should be performed and aerobic transport media used. Pus obtained by needle aspiration is an excellent material for culture, but results obtained after injection of nonbacteriostatic normal saline and subsequent reaspiration have been disappointing.[7]

Certain variants of necrotizing soft tissue infections have been shown to be more prevalent in diabetic patients. Necrotizing fasciitis (usually polymicrobial), nonclostridial anaerobic myonecrosis, spontaneous (hematogenous) clostridial my-

TABLE 143–1 ■ The Most Common Deep Tissue Isolates from 32 Diabetic Patients with Moderate to Severe Foot Infections

MICROORGANISMS ISOLATED	PERCENTAGE OF PATIENTS STUDIED
Aerobes	
Gram-negative bacilli	
Proteus mirabilis	28
Escherichia coli	16
Pseudomonas aeruginosa	16
Enterobacter aerogenes	12
Enterobacter cloacae	6
Citrobacter freundii	6
Gram-positive cocci	
Enterococcus spp.	41
Staphylococcus aureus	25
Group B streptococci	16
Other streptococci	12
Group E nonenterococci	12
Coagulase-negative staphylococci	10
Anaerobes	
Gram-negative bacilli	
Bacteroides fragilis	19
Bacteroides ovatus	9
Bacteroides ureolyticus	9
Prevotella melaninogenica (formerly *Bacteroides melaninogenicus*)	7
Bacteroides capillosus	7
Gram-positive cocci	
Peptostreptococcus magnus	28
Peptostreptococcus anaerobius	19
Peptostreptococcus asaccharolyticus	9
Gram-positive bacilli	
Clostridium bifermentans	9

Data from Sapico FL, Witte JL, Canawati HN, et al: The infected foot of the diabetic patient: Quantitative microbiology and analysis of clinical features. Rev Infect Dis 6(Suppl 1):171–176, 1984.

onecrosis (usually caused by *Clostridium septicum*), and the less virulent crepitant anaerobic cellulitis have been observed to occur with increased frequency in the diabetic host.[10]

Diagnostic Evaluation

The status of the neurologic and vascular systems should be evaluated thoroughly in diabetic patients with foot infections. Noninvasive tests, such as Doppler ultrasonography with waveform analysis, as well as transcutaneous oximetry can help assess the patients' vascular status. Plain radiographs, computed tomographic scans, technetium bone and gallium scans, and white blood cell scans have had problems with lack of sensitivity and/or specificity for the diagnosis of osteomyelitis. Enthusiasm for magnetic resonance imaging has been generated by some studies.[11, 12]

Management

Antimicrobial therapy should be directed at the most likely organisms involved. Milder cases of localized cellulitis or infected ulcers (without gangrene, tissue necrosis, or foul smell) generally necessitate therapy directed primarily at gram-positive aerobic cocci (i.e., *S. aureus*). A first-generation cephalosporin such as cefazolin may be used if there are no contraindications. Moderate to more severe infections that are not immediately limb threatening or life threatening may necessitate wider spectrum coverage such as parenteral ampicillin-sulbactam,[13] ticarcillin-clavulanate, or pipericillin-tazobactam.[14] Severe limb-threatening and life-threatening infections may require even broader coverage such as the combination of either ampicillin-sulbactam or ticarcillin-clavulanate with ceftazidime, aztreonam, or ciprofloxacin given parenterally. High doses of imipenem-cilastatin or piperacillin-tazobactam are also viable alternatives. The antimicrobial regimen may be changed later on the basis of the culture results. It should be remembered, however, that the reliability of anaerobic cultures depends on the techniques of culture collection and may vary from one laboratory to another and that the presence of gangrene, tissue necrosis, and/or foul-smelling discharge strongly suggests the presence of anaerobes regardless of culture results. The length of therapy can vary depending on the severity of infection, from 7 to 10 days for mild cellulitis to several weeks for more severe infections. The presence of osteomyelitis dictates longer therapy if complete ablation of infected bone is not performed. A minimum of 4 weeks of parenteral therapy or a combination of parenteral and oral therapy totaling 10 weeks has been suggested for osteomyelitis.[15]

Surgical removal of necrotic and devitalized tissue and drainage of pus are essential. Opinions vary as to how surgically aggressive one has to be in removing infected bone. Limited ablative surgery removing as much infected bone as possible (e.g., toe amputation, metatarsal ray resection) may shorten the course of antibiotic therapy, shorten hospital stay, and result in the patient's earlier return to normal living.[16] The level of necessary surgical amputation is dictated by the extent of soft tissue and bone involvement, as well as the vascular status of the extremity. Vascular reconstruction may be necessary in the presence of vascular insufficiency, and healing of some persistent ulcers may be accelerated by this surgical procedure.

There appears to be no clear-cut superiority of any form of local therapy. Normal saline wet-to-dry dressings accompanied by meticulous surgical débridement and removal of offending external pressures plus avoidance of dependent position generally help accelerate wound healing.

Infected Pressure Sores

It has been estimated that more than 1 million patients in hospitals and nursing homes in the United States suffer from pressure sores and that at least 3% of patients in acute care hospitals are similarly afflicted.[17, 18]

The pathophysiology of pressure sore formation involves an interplay of several factors, including pressure, shearing forces, friction, excess moisture, local spasticity, and local blood supply deficiency.[17–19] Because more than 90% of pressure sores are located on the lower part of the body (the most common location being sacral, trochanteric, and ischial), and especially because these patients are often fecally incontinent, these sores are colonized by a variety of microorganisms. Continued worsening of tissue necrosis may then lead to soft tissue infection, osteomyelitis of adjacent bone, and septic complications of the infection.

Microbiology

Moderate to severely infected pressure sores show polymicrobial flora similar to that seen in infected feet in diabetic patients.[20–22] The dominant microorganisms are microorganisms that constitute fecal flora. *Escherichia coli* and *Proteus mirabilis* are the most common gram-negative aerobic enteric bacilli seen, with *Pseudomonas aeruginosa, Klebsiella, Enterobacter,* and other enterics seen less often. Among the gram-positive aerobic cocci, *S. aureus, Enterococcus* spp., and coagulase-negative staphylococci are the most common organisms isolated. Anaerobes are clearly dominant organisms in this disease entity, especially when the sores are close to the perianal area.[22] *B. fragilis*, other *Bacteroides* spp., and *Peptostreptococcus* spp. are the most common isolates. Bacteremic sepsis associated with infected pressure sores is most often associated with *B. fragilis, P. mirabilis, Peptostreptococcus* spp., and *S. aureus*.[20, 23] As the pressure sore heals and necrotic and gangrenous tissue is eliminated, anaerobic microorganisms gradually disappear, but gram-negative bacilli and gram-positive cocci continue to be isolated. When the sore is almost healed and a smaller lesion with healthy granulation tissue remains, fewer microorganisms may be seen, primarily *P. aeruginosa* and *Enterococcus* spp.[21]

Proper culture collection includes submission of material such as aspirated pus or deep tissue or bone obtained after overlying superficial necrotic tissue is removed. Anaerobic transport media should be utilized at all times.

Diagnostic Evaluation

Pressure sores may be classified into four stages. Stage I represents nonblanchable erythema of intact skin, stage II involves partial-thickness skin loss involving epidermis and/or dermis, stage III involves full-thickness skin loss with damage or necrosis of subcutaneous tissue down to but not through underlying fascia, and stage IV represents extensive destruction with damage to muscle, bone, or supporting structures.[24]

As with the evaluation for osteomyelitis in foot infections, plain radiographs may be limited in sensitivity and specificity. Lack of specificity has also hampered the use of radionuclide scans, and there has been little experience with the use of magnetic resonance imaging in this disease entity. Bone biopsy for histologic examination is still considered to be the "gold standard" in the establishment of the diagnosis of osteomyelitis in this disease entity.[25–27] Quantitative microbiology of bone was disappointing in one study.[27]

Management

Surgical removal of dead, necrotic tissue is of paramount importance in the management of infected pressure sores.

These surgical procedures may have to be performed repeatedly to keep up with continuing advance of tissue necrosis. Liquid purulent material should be drained as completely as possible. Infected bone should be removed or scraped off until healthy bone is encountered.

Empirical antimicrobial coverage before knowing the culture results should address the potential presence of polymicrobial flora. The choice of antimicrobial agents for moderate to severe infections would be similar to the choice in the case of moderate to severe foot infections in diabetic patients. Initial coverage should include *S. aureus*, *B. fragilis*, gram-negative enterics such as *E. coli* and *P. mirabilis*, and *Enterococcus* spp. and *P. aeruginosa*. The antimicrobial regimen can be changed later depending on the culture results. Again, the presence of tissue gangrene, necrosis, and foul smell should strongly suggest the presence of anaerobic microorganisms. There is no consensus on the length of antimicrobial therapy. One study found no necessity to treat longer than 3 weeks as long as there is thorough surgical removal of infected bone.[26] Another study recommended 6 weeks of antimicrobial therapy.[27]

There is also no clear consensus on the most efficacious type of local therapy.[28] As with diabetic foot ulcers, normal saline wet-to-dry dressings are often used. The use of silver sulfadiazine has achieved some popularity.[29] Frequent turning, proper positioning, pressure dispersion, and the use of specialized beds and mattresses are of paramount importance in the prevention and therapy of pressure sores. Control of muscle spasticity and surgical release of flexion contractures are likewise important measures in preventing, as well as alleviating, pressure sores.

Besides removal of necrotic tissue, infected bone, and bony prominences, surgical management includes the use of a variety of musculocutaneous flaps once the wound has been cleaned up and shows healthy granulation tissue.[30, 31]

References

1. Sapico FL: Foot infections in patients with diabetes mellitus. J Am Podiatr Med Assoc 79:482–485, 1989.
2. Levin ME, O'Neal LW (eds): Preface. *In* The Diabetic Foot, ed 2. St. Louis, CV Mosby, 1988, pp ix–x.
3. Gibbons GW, Eliopoulos GM: Infections of the diabetic foot. *In* Kozak GP, Hoar CS, Rawbottom JL, et al (eds): Management of Diabetic Foot Problems. Philadelphia, WB Saunders, 1984, p 97.
4. Leslie CA, Sapico FL, Ginunas VJ, et al: Randomized, controlled trial of topical hyperbaric oxygen for the treatment of diabetic foot ulcers. Diabetes Care 11:111–115, 1988.
5. Lipsky BA, Pecoraro RE, Larson SA, et al: Outpatient management of uncomplicated lower-extremity infections in diabetic patients. Arch Intern Med 150:790–797, 1990.
6. Sapico FL, Canawati HN, Witte JL, et al: Quantitative aerobic and anaerobic bacteriology of infected diabetic feet. J Clin Microbiol 12:413–420, 1980.
7. Sapico FL, Witte JL, Canawati HN, et al: The infected foot of the diabetic patient: Quantitative microbiology and analysis of clinical features. Rev Infect Dis 6(Suppl 1):171–176, 1984.
8. Sapico FL, Bessman AN, Canawati HN: Bacteremia in diabetic patients with infected lower extremities. Diabetes Care 5:101–104, 1982.
9. Louie TJ, Bartlett JG, Tally FP, et al: Aerobic and anaerobic bacteria in diabetic foot ulcers. Ann Intern Med 85:461–463, 1976.
10. Leslie CA, Sapico FL, Bessman AN: Infections in the diabetic host. Compr Ther 15(7):23–32, 1989.
11. Yuh WTC, Corson JD, Baraniewski HM, et al: Osteomyelitis of the foot in diabetic patients: Evaluation with plain film, ^{99m}Tc-MDP bone scintigraphy, and MR imaging. AJR 152:795–800, 1989.
12. Wang A, Weinstein D, Greenfield L, et al: MRI and diabetic foot infections. Magn Reson Imaging 8:805–809, 1990.
13. Grayson ML, Gibbons GW, Habershaw GM, et al: Use of ampicillin/sulbactam versus imipenem/cilastatin in the treatment of limb-threatening foot infections in diabetic patients. Clin Infect Dis 18:683–693, 1994.
14. Tan JS, Wishnow RM, Talan DA, et al: Treatment of hospitalized patients with complicated skin and skin structure infections: Double-blind randomized, multicenter study of piperacillin-tazobactam versus ticarcillin-clavulanate. Antimicrob Agents Chemother 37:1580–1586, 1993.
15. Bamberger DM, Dans GP, Gerding DN: Osteomyelitis in the feet of diabetic patients: Long-term results, prognostic factors, and the role of antimicrobial and surgical therapy. Am J Med 83:653–660, 1987.
16. Tan JS, Miller C, File TM, et al: Can aggressive therapeutic intervention of diabetic foot infection reduce the length of hospitalization (Abstr)? Clin Infect Dis 19:620, 1994.
17. Reuler JB, Cooney TG: The pressure sore: Pathophysiology and principles of management. Ann Intern Med 94:661–666, 1981.
18. Allman RM, Laprade CA, Noel LB, et al: Pressure sores among hospitalized patients. Ann Intern Med 105:337–342, 1986.
19. Cooney TG, Reuler JB: Pressure sores. West J Med 940:622–624, 1984.
20. Galpin JE, Chow AW, Bayer AS, et al: Sepsis associated with decubitus ulcers. Am J Med 61:345–350, 1975.
21. Sapico FL, Ginunas VJ, Thornhill-Joynes M, et al: Quantitative microbiology of pressure sores in different stages of healing. Diagn Microbiol Infect Dis 5:31–38, 1986.
22. Brook I: Microbiological studies of decubitus ulcers in children. J Pediatr Surg 26:207–209, 1991.
23. Bryan CS, Dew CE, Reynolds KL: Bacteremia associated with decubitus ulcers. Arch Intern Med 143:2093–2095, 1983.
24. Pressure ulcer prevalence, cost and risk assessment: Consensus development conference statement—The National Pressure Ulcer Advisory Panel. Decubitus 2:24–28, 1989.
25. Sugarman B, Hawes S, Musher DM, et al: Osteomyelitis beneath pressure sores. Arch Intern Med 143:683–688, 1983.
26. Thornhill-Joynes M, Gonzales F, Stewart CA, et al: Osteomyelitis associated with pressure sores. Arch Phys Med Rehab 67:314–318, 1986.
27. Darouiche RO, Landon GF, Klima M, et al: Osteomyelitis associated with pressure sores. Arch Intern Med 154:753–758, 1994.
28. DeLisa JA, Mikulic MH: Pressure ulcers: What to do if preventive management fails. Postgrad Med 77:209–220, 1985.
29. Kucan JO, Robson MC, Heggers JP, et al: Comparison of silver sulfadiazine, povidone-iodine and physiologic saline in the treatment of chronic pressure ulcers. J Am Geriatr Soc 29:232–235, 1981.
30. Mathes SJ, Nahai F: Clinical Applications for Muscle and Musculocutaneous Flaps. St. Louis, CV Mosby, 1982.
31. Rubayi S, Cousins S, Valentine WA: Myocutaneous flaps. AORN J 52:40–55, 1990.

144

Infections of Muscle

Dave Hollander
Theodore L. Munsat

Skeletal muscle displays a variable susceptibility to different infectious agents. It is quite resistant to bacterial infection, but it is a major site of parasitic infection and encystation. Viruses can produce a clinical picture ranging from benign myositis to life-threatening rhabdomyolysis. Fungi rarely infect muscle, usually in immunocompromised hosts. In this chapter, we discuss the different infectious myositides. These are to be differentiated from idiopathic polymyositis, which is an idiopathic inflammatory myopathy of uncertain cause.

Bacterial Myositis

Bacterial infections of muscle are uncommon in the United States and other temperate regions of the world. By contrast, in tropical regions such infections are common and have been called tropical pyomyositis by some.

Pyomyositis most frequently involves the quadriceps muscle, although others may also be affected. Most infections are solitary abscesses, but in 40% of cases multiple abscesses are found.[1] All ages are affected, with males below the age of 40 years forming the largest group. Muscle pain precedes fever and swelling by several days to weeks. The muscle is initially indurated and "woody," without frank pus. Later, a fluctuant mass develops. The infections are typically deep in location. As a consequence, classic signs of inflammation are not seen early and muscle pain is ill-defined. These factors may obscure the diagnosis initially, especially in North America, where most physicians are not familiar with this infection. Limb pyomyositis may be confused with hematomas, thrombophlebitis, and soft tissue sarcomas. Truncal abscesses may be mistakenly diagnosed as intraabdominal processes or pneumonia.

Laboratory findings include an elevated white cell count and increased erythrocyte sedimentation rate. Eosinophilia is frequently seen in tropical cases and probably reflects concurrent parasitic infection. Lymphadenopathy may not be present. The serum creatine kinase value is usually normal despite muscle necrosis. Blood cultures are usually negative. Ultrasonography, computed tomography, and magnetic resonance imaging are extremely useful for visualizing abscesses and ruling out other pathologic conditions, as well as guiding needle aspiration.

The majority of cases are due to *Staphylococcus aureus*, the remainder to *Streptococcus* and other organisms. The pathogenesis of pyomyositis is poorly understood. Most patients are healthy, without underlying predisposing conditions. Antecedent trauma has been identified in 25%,[2] providing a possible portal of entry for an organism, but most cases remain unexplained. The occurrence of multiple abscesses suggests bacteremia with muscle seeding. As blood cultures are positive in less than 5% of cases,[1] bacteremia must occur early and not persistently. Pyomyositis may develop in patients infected with the human immunodeficiency virus (HIV). It has been suggested that the frequency of colonization with *S. aureus* and the impaired activity of neutrophils against *S. aureus* in patients infected with HIV may contribute to the development of pyomyositis in these cases.[3]

The propensity for pyomyositis to occur in tropical climates is also not understood. Some have proposed that the high rate of coincidental parasitic infections in tropical regions decreases resistance to *S. aureus*, possibly by generating a strong local immunoglobulin E response that secondarily impairs the neutrophil response.[4] Others have invoked poor nutrition as a predisposing factor.[2]

Treatment consists of drainage of the abscess and antibiotic therapy, usually with a β-lactamase–resistant penicillin. Cases diagnosed before fluctuance develops may be successfully treated with antibiotics alone. Untreated patients may develop metastatic abscesses to other organs.

Fungal Myositis

Fungal infections of muscle are rare. They are usually seen in immunosuppressed patients as part of a disseminated fungal disease. Muscle involvement in these cases is often an incidental postmortem finding. Occasional patients develop prominent muscle symptoms. In some, this may be the sole clinical manifestation of their disseminated disease. Microscopic examination of muscle reveals fungal infiltration, inflammation, and necrosis.

Viral Infections

Myositis is an uncommon complication of viral infections, occurring most commonly in children as benign acute childhood myositis (BACM). The mean age of patients is 9 years. The illness usually begins with an upper respiratory tract viral prodrome that lasts several days. This prodrome almost completely resolves by the time muscle pain develops. The calves are most commonly affected, followed by the thighs. Pain is progressive and may become severe, to the point that the child refuses to walk. The muscles are tender to palpation, but swelling is uncommon. Weakness in BACM, if present, is mild and may result from pain. The creatine kinase level is significantly elevated, but myoglobinuria does not occur.

Electromyographic studies have been reported for few patients. The results have been normal or have shown patchy myopathic changes. Serologic and virus isolation studies have most often linked BACM to influenza A virus and especially influenza B virus, usually during an epidemic. Other viruses, such as parainfluenza virus and adenovirus, have occasionally been implicated. Acute-phase antibody titers are lacking in these cases, suggesting that myositis follows only first-time infection of a particular virus strain. In many cases, the responsible agent is not identified. Muscle biopsies have been done rarely. These have been normal or have shown nonspecific muscle fiber necrosis or interstitial inflammation. Virus-like particles have not been seen, and virus has only rarely been cultured from muscle. This syndrome has a benign course, with complete recovery within a week. Treatment is supportive: bed rest, fluids, and analgesia.

In adults, viral myositis is less common but more severe and usually leads to rhabdomyolysis and myoglobinuria. In most patients, muscle symptoms coincide with an influenza-like illness. This is in contrast to BACM, in which they occur during the convalescent phase. Muscle involvement is more widespread than in BACM and weakness more severe, but pain is less prominent. Myoglobinuria occurs in most cases and can result in acute tubular necrosis. The creatine kinase level is elevated. Recovery may be prolonged and incomplete, and death may result from cardiopulmonary complications. Similar cases have been described, less frequently, in children. Most cases have been associated with influenza, particularly influenza A virus, or with coxsackievirus infection. Cases associated with Epstein-Barr virus, herpes simplex virus type 2, parainfluenza virus types 2 and 3, adenovirus type 21, echovirus 9, HIV, and cytomegalovirus have also been reported. Virus has occasionally been isolated from muscle, but specific identification usually rests on serology or isolation from nasopharyngeal secretions. Muscle biopsies have demonstrated necrosis without prominent inflammation. Treatment is supportive; dialysis may be necessary for renal failure. Antiviral agents have not been assessed, but amantadine has been suggested for adults with acute influenza A myositis.[5]

A number of reports in the past have attempted to link the chronic inflammatory myopathies with viral infections. Mumps virus in inclusion body myositis and coxsackievirus in polymyositis or dermatomyositis were particularly implicated. However, sensitive polymerase chain reaction studies have failed to confirm these findings.[6]

Retroviruses

HIV and human T-cell lymphotropic virus type I (HTLV-I) are pathogenic retroviruses of humans. A myopathic picture resembling that of idiopathic polymyositis is a well-described complication of HIV infection. This may occur in patients with full acquired immunodeficiency syndrome or with acquired immunodeficiency syndrome–related complex, or it may be the first and only expression of disease in HIV-seropositive patients. Painless, progressive proximal weakness may rarely be accompanied by a rash simulating dermatomyositis. Muscle enzyme levels are elevated, and electromyography shows myopathic changes and fibrillation potentials, as in polymyositis. Two patterns of abnormalities have been described in muscle biopsies.[7] Most commonly, muscle fiber necrosis with inflammatory infiltrates is seen (Fig. 144–1). In the second pattern, nemaline rod bodies and necrosis are found, with or without inflammation. HIV has been found in lymphoid cells and macrophages within muscle, but most studies have failed to detect direct muscle invasion by HIV. However, a study using the polymerase chain reaction has reported the presence of amplified HIV-1 nucleic acids in some myocyte nuclei,[8] suggesting that active infection of muscle by HIV may occur. Treatment with corticosteroids has been advocated,[7] but controlled trials are lacking.

HTLV-I infection has been associated with inflammatory myopathy in Jamaica, an area in which the virus is endemic.[9] A single report has documented direct viral infection of muscle fibers in a patient with HTLV-I–associated polymyositis, coinfected with HIV.[10]

Parasitic Infections

In certain geographic areas, parasites are an important cause of infectious myositis. The muscle involvement may be isolated or part of a systemic illness. The spectrum of disease ranges from asymptomatic infection to frank polymyositis. Parasitic infections may be grouped into three categories: protozoan, cestode, and nematode infections (Table 144–1). Toxoplasmosis, cysticercosis, and trichinosis account for the majority of such cases.

Protozoan Infections

Toxoplasmosis is the most important of the protozoan myositides. The causative agent is *Toxoplasma gondii*, an obligate intracellular parasite with a worldwide distribution. Infection with *T. gondii* cysts or oocysts is followed by dissemination and encystation. Brain, heart, and skeletal muscle are the most common sites of cyst formation. Chronic asymptomatic infection is common; up to 50% of the U.S. population is estimated to be affected.[11] Cysts may persist in a viable state in human muscle for years, without provoking an inflammatory response. Acute symptomatic infection is much less common, occurring in only 10% to 20% of *Toxoplasma* infections in adults.[12] This is usually a benign, self-limited illness, most commonly manifesting as cervical lymphadenopathy.

Toxoplasmic polymyositis may occur in association with or may be part of a systemic illness that includes meningoencephalitis, pneumonitis, pericarditis, or myocarditis. In such cases, muscle biopsy may show inflammatory infiltrates with foci of necrosis. *T. gondii*, as either free tachyzoites or cysts, may be found (Fig. 144–2), but identification is often difficult and may require special staining. Frequently, no organism is seen, and the diagnosis is made on serologic grounds alone. A number of reports have documented an association between toxoplasmosis and idiopathic polymyositis. A causal relationship between acute infection and polymyositis is lacking in these cases, however. Instead, it has been proposed that the altered immune state associated with polymyositis,

TABLE 144–1 ■ Parasitic Infections Affecting Muscle

DISEASE	ORGANISM
Protozoan Infections	
Toxoplasmosis	*Toxoplasma gondii*
African trypanosomiasis	*Trypanosoma brucei rhodesiense*
	Trypanosoma brucei gambiense
American trypanosomiasis	*Trypanosoma cruzi*
Sarcosporidiosis	*Sarcocystis lindemanni*
Cestode Infections	
Cysticercosis	*Taenia solium*
Hydatidosis	*Echinococcus granulosus*
	Echinococcus multilocularis
Sparganosis	*Spirometra mansonoides*
Coenurosis	*Multiceps brauni*
Nematode Infections	
Trichinosis	*Trichinella spiralis*
Toxocariasis	*Toxocara canis*
	Toxocara cati

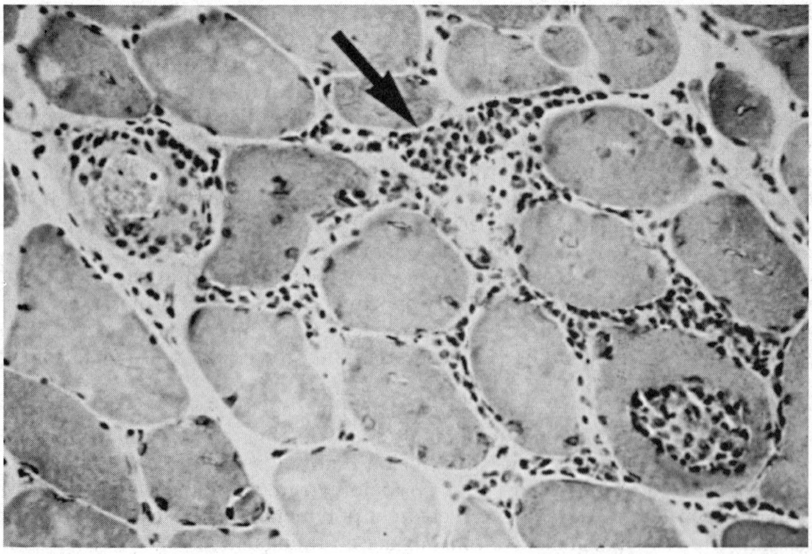

FIGURE 144–1 □ HIV-associated myopathy. Interstitial, perivascular, and intrafibrillar inflammatory infiltrates are seen. One muscle fiber has been completely replaced by inflammatory cells *(arrow)*. (Courtesy of Dr. M. Dalakas, National Institutes of Health, Bethesda, MD.)

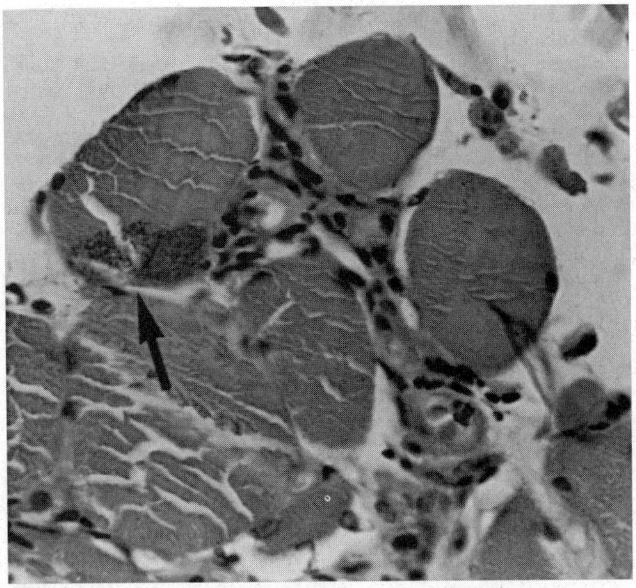

FIGURE 144–2 □ Toxoplasmosis. Within a muscle fiber, there is a *Toxoplasma* cyst containing numerous organisms *(arrow)*. There is an adjacent perivascular lymphocytic infiltrate. (Courtesy of Dr. L. Adelman, New England Medical Center, Boston, MA.)

or its treatment, may predispose to acute *Toxoplasma* infection or to reactivation of latent infection.[13] The latter mechanism may be particularly important in immunocompromised patients.

Treatment should be reserved for patients with severe and persistent symptoms and for all immunocompromised patients. Mild symptoms in immunologically normal patients do not require treatment. Pyrimethamine, with sulfadiazine or trisulfapyrimidine, is the treatment of choice.

African and American trypanosomiasis can cause polymyositis. Sarcosporidiosis, a rare infection in humans, occasionally causes painful muscle masses.

Cestode Infections

Cysticercosis, the most important of the cestode infections in humans, is due to infection with the tapeworm *Taenia solium*. It is common in South America, Central America, Asia, Africa, and Eastern Europe but rare in the United States. Cysticercosis develops when humans, who normally serve as the definitive host of the tapeworm, ingest ova and become intermediate hosts. Embryos released from the eggs are transported via the blood stream and lymphatic system to various tissues, where they encyst as cysticerci within 2 to 3 months. Skeletal muscle and the central nervous system (CNS) are the most common sites of infection. CNS symptoms include seizures, meningoencephalitis, and hydrocephalus. Muscle involvement may be seen in isolation or with CNS disease. There may be weakness, pain, and palpable nodules. Plain radiographs of muscle often reveal calcified cysticerci. Pseudohypertrophy is seen rarely. Patients may develop massive hypertrophy of pelvic and shoulder girdle muscles and the gastrocnemius muscles in a symmetric, bilateral fashion. Weakness is often present, but pain is usually absent. Eosinophilia is commonly seen in cysticercosis, and serologic testing is often positive. Biopsy of the involved muscle demonstrates cysticerci and an associated inflammatory response. Treatment of CNS cysticercosis with praziquantel is effective. Its role in muscle disease has not yet been defined.

Human hydatid disease occurs after ingestion of ova of *Echinococcus granulosus* and *Echinococcus multilocularis*. It is seen most frequently in sheep-rearing areas. Muscle is exceeded only by liver and lung as the most frequent site of hydatid cyst formation. The most common muscle sites are the paravertebral gutters and limb girdle muscles, especially in the thighs. Distal muscle involvement is rare. As the cysts grow, they cause painless, localized swellings. Exercise may produce dull muscle aches, but weakness is not characteristic. Secondary infection may lead to abscess formation. Pathologically, the hydatid cyst provokes a granulomatous inflammatory reaction. Unilocular cysts are surrounded by a limiting membrane that prevents outward growth. Multilocular cysts are not bound by their membrane; they expand aggressively in muscle, behaving like tumors. Diagnosis is aided by serologic testing, which is positive in most patients with hydatid disease. Cysts may be demonstrated by routine radiographs. Ultrasonography and computed tomography may identify specific hydatid features in them. Eosinophilia is seen in a minority of cases. Treatment is surgical excision of the cyst.

Sparganosis refers to infection by the plerocercoid larva (sparganum) of the pseudophyllidean tapeworm *Spirometra mansonoides*. Human infection may occur as a result of drinking contaminated water, such as unboiled well or river water containing infected copepods. Infection may also follow ingestion of the flesh of infected intermediate hosts such as the pig or frog or application of poultices of infected animal meat to open wounds. This is a result of the migratory capability of the encysted larvae, which reencyst in their new host. Most sparganosis infections are seen in the Far East. Only a few cases have been reported in North America. They usually cause subcutaneous or muscle masses that grow slowly in size and may actually move within a muscle. Ocular sparganosis may also occur. Treatment is surgical removal of the lesion or alcohol injection of the nodule, which kills the resident parasite.

Coenurosis is a rare disease in humans that follows ingestion of ova of the dog tapeworm *Multiceps multiceps* or *Multiceps brauni*. Whereas *M. multiceps* usually causes CNS disease, infection with *M. brauni* causes a solitary, slowly growing mass in muscle and subcutaneous tissue, usually over the trunk. Treatment is surgical excision of the lesion.

Nematode Infections

The most important of the nematode infections is trichinosis, which is due to *Trichinella spiralis*. This worm is found worldwide except for Australia. Most human infection follows ingestion of undercooked pork containing the *Trichinella* cysts. In the stomach, *Trichinella* larvae are released and migrate to the intestine, where they develop into male and female forms. After copulation, the female burrows into the intestinal tract and releases her larvae. These enter the systemic circulation and become distributed among the tissues, chiefly skeletal muscle. In muscle, the larvae penetrate single muscle fibers and grow within them. A cellular inflammatory reaction develops, walling off the worm and leading to cyst formation (Fig. 144–3). Cysts begin to calcify after 6 to 9 months, but larvae may remain viable within them for years.

Infection may be heralded by a prodrome of abdominal pain and diarrhea. Fever and myalgias follow. Periorbital edema is a frequent early feature; rashes, conjunctivitis, and petechial hemorrhages may also be seen. The most striking features are muscle pain and weakness, which may be severe. Muscle swelling may occur. The muscles most commonly affected are the diaphragm and extraocular, masseter, tongue, laryngeal, intercostal, neck, back, and deltoid muscles. Dyspnea may result from diaphragmatic lesions. Masseter muscle involvement causes pain on jaw opening or chewing. Dysphagia may follow tongue and pharyngeal muscle involvement. Muscle symptoms may last several weeks, al-

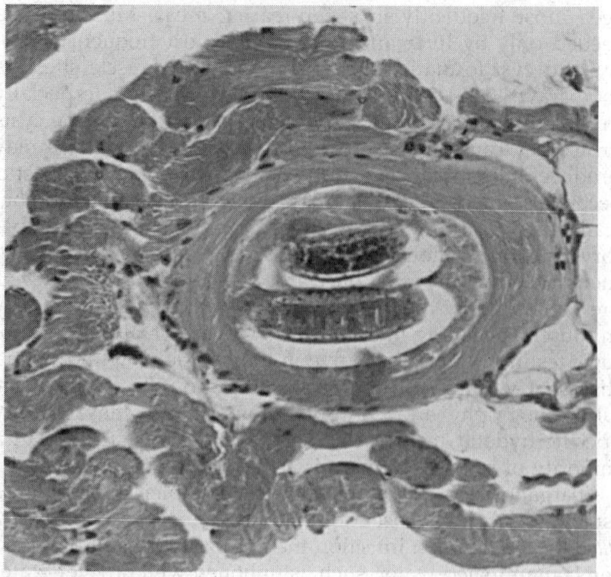

FIGURE 144–3 □ Trichinosis. The larva is coiled within a well-developed fibrous capsule and cut across twice. A few chronic mononuclear cells surround the cyst. (Courtesy of Dr. L. Adelman, New England Medical Center, Boston, MA.)

though most *Trichinella* infections are asymptomatic. Uncommonly, in severe cases with massive infestation, there may be CNS involvement, resulting in headache, seizures, encephalopathy, and focal deficits. Myocarditis, with tachyarrhythmias and congestive failure, may occur.

Laboratory abnormalities include a significant eosinophilia (4% to 60% of total white cell count) and an elevated creatine kinase level. Antibody titers rise fourfold or more in acute infections. Electromyography shows myopathic changes and fibrillations, consistent with an inflammatory myopathy. Muscle biopsy demonstrates the larvae within muscle fibers, muscle fiber necrosis, and inflammation. Polymorphonuclear cells and eosinophils are seen early. Older lesions are associated with mononuclear infiltrates and may be calcified.

The preferred treatment is thiabendazole. Because of the Herxheimer-like reaction that may follow larval disintegration, steroids should be given concurrently.

Toxocariasis may result from ingestion of the ova of *Toxocara canis* and, less frequently, *Toxocara cati*. Embryos are widely distributed to many tissues, including skeletal muscle. Manifestions range from asymptomatic eosinophilia to a severe systemic illness with fever, organomegaly, pneumonitis, and seizures. Myalgias reflect muscle involvement. Pathologically, one finds myofiber necrosis with a surrounding granulomatous reaction that may include eosinophils.

References

1. Levin MJ, Gardner P, Waldvogel FA: "Tropical" pyomyositis: An unusual infection due to *Staphylococcus aureus*. N Engl J Med 284:196, 1971.
2. Chiedozi LC: Pyomyositis: Review of 205 cases in 112 patients. Am J Surg 137:255, 1979.
3. Schwartzman WA, Kennedy CA, Goetz MB: Staphylococcal pyomyositis in patients infected by the human immunodeficiency virus. Am J Med 90:595, 1991.
4. Sheagren JN: *Staphylococcus aureus*: The persistent pathogen. N Engl J Med 310:1368, 1984.
5. Hays AP, Gamboa ET: Acute viral myositis. *In* Engel AG, Franzini-Armstrong C (eds): Myology, ed 2. New York, McGraw-Hill, 1994, pp 1399–1418.
6. Dalakis MC: Immunopathogenesis of inflammatory myopathies. Ann Neurol 37(S1):S74, 1995.
7. Simpson DM, Bender AN: Human immunodeficiency virus–associated myopathy: Analysis of 11 patients. Ann Neurol 24:79, 1988.
8. Seidman R, Peress NS, Nuovo GJ: In situ detection of polymerase chain reaction–amplified HIV-1 nucleic acids in skeletal muscle in patients with myopathy. Mod Pathol 7:369, 1994.
9. Morgan OS, Rodgers-Johnson P, Mora C, Char G: HTLV-1 and polymyositis in Jamaica. Lancet 2:1184, 1989.
10. Wiley CA, Nerenberg M, Cros D, et al: HTLV-I polymyositis in a patient also infected with the human immunodeficiency virus. N Engl J Med 320:992, 1989.
11. Krick JA, Remington JS: Toxoplasmosis in the adult—An overview. N Engl J Med 298:550, 1978.
12. McCabe RE, Remington JS: Toxoplasmosis. *In* Warren KS, Mahmoud AAF (eds): Tropical and Geographical Medicine. New York, McGraw-Hill, 1984, pp 281–292.
13. Behan WMH, Behan PO, Draper IT, et al: Does *Toxoplasma* cause polymyositis? Report of a case of polymyositis associated with toxoplasmosis and a critical review of the literature. Acta Neuropathol (Berl) 61:246, 1983.

145

Fungal Infections of the Skin

Jill R. Rosenthal

Cutaneous fungal infections are common in all age groups worldwide; the superficial mycoses include infections caused by dermatophytes, *Candida* species, *Pityrosporum* yeasts, several nondermatophyte molds, and the agents of black and white piedra. Other conditions include infections caused by dematiaceous fungi, which cause chromoblastomycosis, phaeohyphomycosis, and mycetoma (see Chapter 282). Candidiasis and deep infections caused by other agents, including cryptococcosis, aspergillosis, histoplasmosis, coccidioidomycosis, sporotrichosis, blastomycosis, paracoccidioidomycosis, and the phycomycoses, are covered elsewhere.

Dermatophytoses

Dermatophytes are extremely common causes of infection in humans. They are aerobic fungi that produce proteases that digest keratin, allowing colonization, invasion, and infection of the stratum corneum of the skin, the hair shaft, and the nail.[1] Many can infect multiple cutaneous structures, causing a variety of clinical syndromes; similarly, a given skin structure or site may be infected by more than one species. For example, hair infections can be caused by *Microsporum* and *Trichophyton* species, nail infections by *Trichophyton* and *Epidermophyton* species, and skin infections by fungi of all three genera. In addition, different species predominate as causes

Some of the material in this chapter has previously been published by the author in *Current Opinion in Pediatrics* (Rosenthal JR: Pediatric fungal infections from head to toe: What's new? Curr Opin Pediatr 6:435–441, 1994).

of each clinical type of infection in different parts of the world; even in a given geographic location, species predominance may change in time.[1–8] For these reasons, dermatophytoses are classified by anatomic site rather than by species.

Dermatophytes are preferentially distributed in certain habitats and, depending on the species (Table 145-1), may be found in the soil (geophilic), on animals (zoophilic), or on humans (anthropophilic). Anthropophilic species are transmitted from person to person and often cause chronic infections, but geophilic and zoophilic dermatophytes are more frequently acquired as sporadic, incidental infections and often tend to produce more inflammatory host responses than their anthropophilic counterparts.[9] This difference in host response appears to be due in part to differences in protease production by zoophilic dermatophytes, depending on the keratin source on which the fungus is growing.[10] There are approximately 40 dermatophyte species.[10] However, most infections are caused by 11 species, and within the continental United States, most infections are caused by 6 species.[11] The spread of anthropophilic species is more common in the presence of close contact, such as the transmission of tinea capitis due to *Trichophyton tonsurans* within the family unit or in conditions of social crowding; this is paralleled in the animal kingdom, where dermatophyte infections are more commonly seen in social animals that live together than in species that tend to be solitary.[11]

Diagnosis of dermatophyte infections is made by microscopic examination of scrapings from the involved site, placed in potassium hydroxide (KOH) solution, which allows visualization of fungal hyphae and spores. In culture, structures such as macroconidia, microconidia, and specialized vegetative structures such as pectinate or spiral hyphae are seen, which along with nutritional requirements and morphologic features in culture allow species identification. However, these specialized structures are not present in keratinized tissues, and thus precise identification of dermatophyte species cannot be based on KOH microscopy alone.[12(p1136)]

Dermatophyte Infections of the Hair

TINEA CAPITIS

Tinea capitis (ringworm of the scalp), caused by *Microsporum* and *Trichophyton* species, is by far the most common pediatric dermatophyte infection worldwide, accounting for up to 92.5% of dermatophytoses in children younger than 10 years; the disease is rare in adults.[2, 6, 13, 14] In the United States, tinea capitis is most common in school-age black males and is usually caused by *T. tonsurans*, although all races and age groups can be affected.[4] The age predilection is thought to be due to the presence of *Pityrosporum orbiculare* (also known as *Pityrosporum ovale*), part of the normal flora, and the fungistatic properties of short and medium chain saturated fatty acids in postpubertal sebum.[5, 15–17] Fatty acids present in hair oils commonly applied in India are thought to contribute to the low frequency of tinea capitis there.[18] Some authors postulate that tinea capitis is more common in boys with short hair than in girls because the stratum corneum is relatively more accessible for the initial colonization.[11]

During the second half of this century, *T. tonsurans* has replaced *Microsporum audouinii* and *Microsporum canis* as the most common cause of tinea capitis in the United States; it now causes more than 90% of cases of tinea capitis.[4] However, in other parts of the world, other species still predominate, including zoophilic species such as *M. canis*, usually because of acquisition by direct contact with infected animals, in particular with stray cats, which in some areas are the source for 70% of infections.[2, 6, 16, 19] In other areas, *Trichophyton violaceum, Trichophyton rubrum, Trichophyton schoenleinii*, and *M. audouinii* are more common, varying by country.[2] In Africa, *Trichophyton soudanense, Trichophyton yaoundei*, and *Trichophyton gourvilii* predominate.[20]

The clinical presentation may vary from a mildly scaly noninflammatory dermatosis with patchy or diffuse seborrheic dermatitis–like scaling with variable alopecia, to black-dot tinea capitis (in which the infected hairs fracture, leaving the infected dark stubs visible in the follicular orifices), to a more inflammatory pattern with pustules and oozing, to the highly inflammatory boggy mass known as a kerion (Fig. 145–1 [see Color Plate 1]). Cervical lymphadenopathy is common. The host's response is thought to determine the degree of inflammation, in part influenced by the infecting species, but the possible role of secondary bacterial infection has been postulated by some authors.[21, 22] Permanent scarring alopecia may result, particularly with more inflammatory presentations such as kerion.

Inflammatory pustules and kerions have in general been presumed to be the result of the host's immune response to the fungus. Although bacteria may sometimes be cultured, it is not clear whether they represent contamination, colonization, or secondary infection or whether they are actually pathogenic.[14] Cultures from 44 patients with kerions grew *Staphylococcus aureus* in 50% of cases and gram-negative rods in 27%.[21] However, addition of oral antibiotics and oral steroids to griseofulvin in the treatment of kerions does not hasten flattening of kerions, although it may help to decrease scaling and pruritus.[22] Because griseofulvin monotherapy

TABLE 145–1 ■ Classification of Dermatophytes

ANTHROPOPHILIC	ZOOPHILIC	GEOPHILIC
Microsporum audouinii	*Trichophyton verrucosum*	*Microsporum vanbreuseghemii*
Epidermophyton floccosum	*Microsporum persicolor*	*Microsporum fulvum*
Trichophyton megninii	*Trichophyton mentagrophytes* var. *mentagrophytes*	*Microsporum gypseum*
Trichophyton gourvilii	*Trichophyton mentagrophytes* var. *erinacei*	*Microsporum racemosum*
Trichophyton soudanense	*Trichophyton mentagrophytes* var. *quinckeanum*	*Trichophyton ajelloi*
Trichophyton yaoundei	*Microsporum canis*	*Microsporum nanum*
Trichophyton violaceum	*Microsporum distortum*	*Trichophyton terrestre*
Trichophyton concentricum	*Microsporum (?Trichophyton) gallinae*	*Microsporum cookei*
Microsporum ferrugineum	*Trichophyton equinum*	
Trichophyton mentagrophytes var. *interdigitale*	*Trichophyton verrucosum*	
Trichophyton rubrum	*Trichophyton simii*	
Trichophyton schoenleinii		
Trichophyton tonsurans		

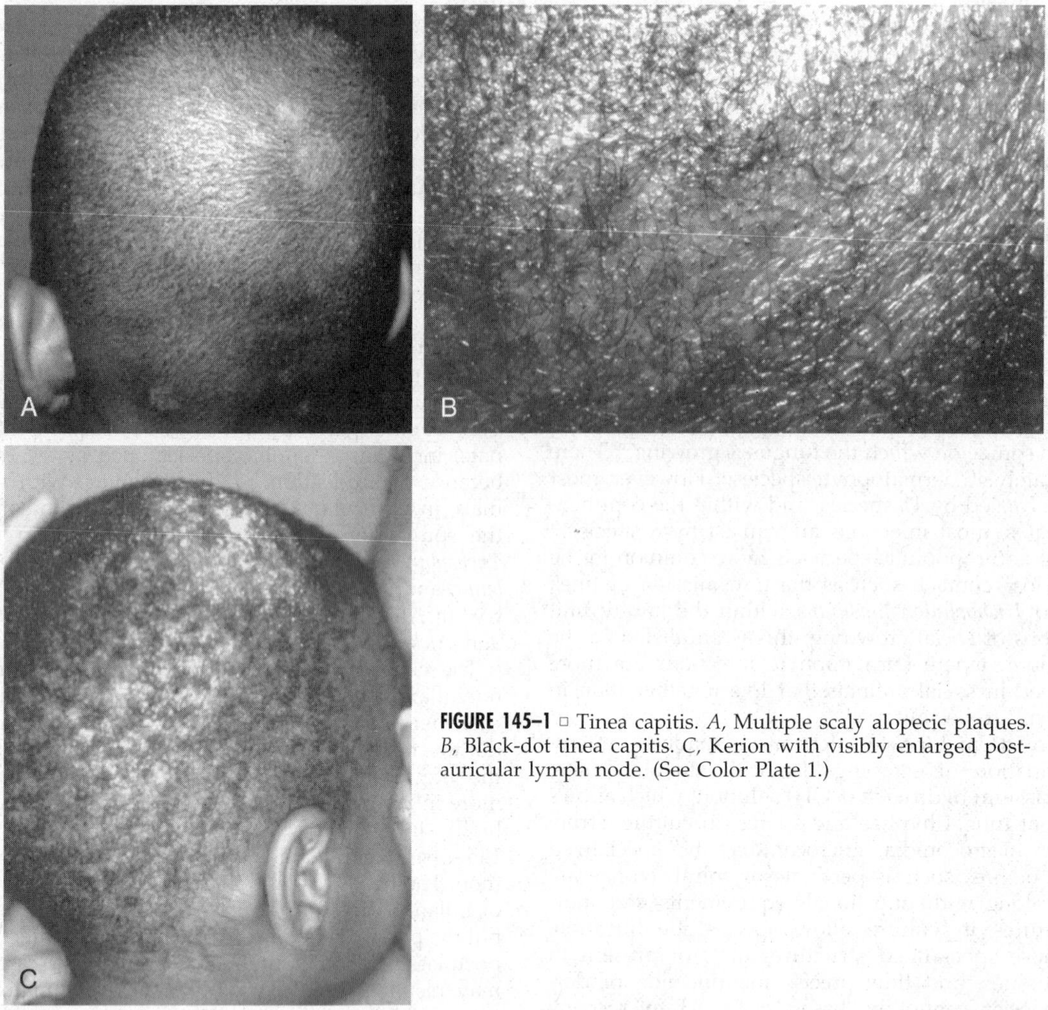

FIGURE 145–1 □ Tinea capitis. *A*, Multiple scaly alopecic plaques. *B*, Black-dot tinea capitis. *C*, Kerion with visibly enlarged post-auricular lymph node. (See Color Plate 1.)

cures almost all cases of tinea capitis, and the addition of oral antibiotics does not hasten this, it remains to be seen whether *S. aureus* or gram-negative organisms, when present, play a pathogenic role.[14] Similarly, whether steroids decrease the extent or frequency of permanent scarring alopecia in patients with kerion remains to be proved, but given the relative safety of a 1- or 2-week course of oral steroids in an otherwise healthy young person, it is appropriate to consider oral steroid therapy in this setting.[14, 23]

Tinea capitis has also been reported in other age groups. Both tinea capitis and tinea faciei due to *M. canis* have occurred in infants as young as 16 days old, acquired from mothers and siblings; dermatophyte infections have also been reported in even younger infants.[24–28] A nosocomial outbreak of *M. canis* tinea capitis and tinea corporis in six premature infants in a level II intermediate care nursery was traced to a nurse; what is most striking about this report is that the infections were acquired from an asymptomatic human carrier of this zoophilic fungus, which is usually acquired by direct contact with infected animals.[29] A more typical nosocomial outbreak is exemplified by one involving the anthropophilic dermatophyte *T. tonsurans* in nine hospital staff and one family member who cared for a child with tinea capitis and tinea corporis before a diagnosis of dermatophyte infection was made.[30]

Although tinea capitis in adults is more common in women than in men, possibly owing to increased exposure to infected children and hormonal factors, a healthy 52-year-old black man acquired tinea capitis caused by *T. tonsurans* from contaminated haircutting instruments.[5] *T. rubrum* tinea capitis was reported in a 67-year-old black woman with systemic lupus erythematosus after treatment with topical and intralesional corticosteroids; *T. rubrum* rarely causes scalp infections in the United States but is the most commonly isolated cause of tinea capitis in Benghazi, Libya, and in Bangkok, Thailand.[15] Several children with Langerhans cell histiocytosis were noted to have secondary infections with tinea capitis, and it should be kept in mind that the clinical appearance may be similar, potentially delaying the diagnosis of either condition.[31]

Endothrix infections, in which arthrospores are present within the hair shaft, involve hairs in both anagen and telogen phases, contributing to the chronicity of these infections. *T. tonsurans*, the most common cause of tinea capitis in the United States, belongs to this group, along with *T. violaceum* and other *Trichophyton* species. Endothrix infection begins in the surface stratum corneum, followed by follicular invasion and colonization of the hair cortex. As the hair grows out, the hyphae break up into arthrospores; the cortex is replaced by spores and swells, and the hair weakens and fractures as it emerges from the scalp. The swollen cortex forms a coiled plug in the infundibulum, producing the clinically visible black dot.[3] Hair invasion in ectothrix infections produces arthrospores both within the hair shaft and on its surface. Wood light fluorescence occurs in the ectothrix infections caused by *M. audouinii, M. canis, Microsporum distortum*, and *Microsporum ferrugineum* as well as in favus caused by *T. schoenleinii*.

Historically, when tinea capitis was more commonly caused by *M. audouinii and M. canis,* Wood lamp examination could be used to rapidly screen large numbers of children in schools for infection, but this is no longer useful now that *T. tonsurans*, a nonfluorescing endothrix infection, is responsible for most tinea capitis in the United States. Rapid diagnosis of tinea capitis is made by KOH examination of infected hairs (visible as black dots) and surrounding scale—a sensitive and specific examination in the hands of an experienced practitioner—or by culture on Sabouraud agar, which takes several weeks. Samples for KOH examination or culture may be obtained with a sterile toothbrush, a moistened cotton swab or gauze pad, or a No. 15 blade.[14, 32] Because oral therapy for at least 8 weeks is required, it is important to document the presence of fungal infection.

The differential diagnosis of tinea capitis includes other scalp dermatoses characterized by scaling, alopecia, or pustule formation. Depending on the clinical presentation, these may include seborrheic dermatitis, atopic dermatitis, psoriasis, alopecia areata, bacterial folliculitis, trichotillomania, lichen planopilaris, discoid lupus erythematosus, secondary syphilis, and Langerhans cell histiocytosis. However, most of these can often be ruled out on clinical grounds, and definitive diagnosis of tinea can usually be documented with KOH examination or culture.

Treatment of dermatophyte infections of the hair and nails requires systemic therapy. Griseofulvin remains the treatment of choice, given for 8 to 12 weeks, although longer courses are occasionally necessary. The usual adult dosage is 500 mg microcrystalline orally twice a day or 250 mg ultramicrosized orally twice a day. Children should be treated with 15 to 20 mg/kg per day microcrystalline or 7.5 to 10 mg/kg per day ultramicrosized, usually given as a single daily dose with a fatty meal to increase enteric absorption and decrease the risk of gastrointestinal side effects. Higher doses are occasionally necessary.[33] Other adverse effects may include headache in 10% to 15% of patients (usually only for the first few days of therapy), photosensitivity, and exacerbation of systemic lupus erythematosus and porphyrias.

Shampooing twice weekly with a sporicidal shampoo containing selenium sulfide 2.5%, zinc pyrithione, or ketoconazole may help to decrease contagion by lowering spore counts. However, topical therapy alone is inadequate to treat tinea capitis, and oral ketoconazole is less effective than is griseofulvin in the treatment of tinea capitis. A few reports suggest that the triazoles fluconazole and itraconazole may be useful in some patients with tinea capitis who cannot tolerate or fail to respond to griseofulvin.[20, 34–36] Oral terbinafine also appears promising as a potential therapy, although additional studies with larger numbers of patients are necessary to document safety in children and efficacy against *T. tonsurans* tinea capitis.[37–41] Itraconazole at 5 mg/kg per day for 6 weeks also appears effective in the treatment of tinea capitis in children.[42] If kerion is present, oral or intralesional steroid use should be considered; when secondary bacterial infection is present, appropriate cultures should be performed, and antibiotic therapy may be added to the antifungal regimen.[23]

Even when the presentation is inflammatory, *T. tonsurans* frequently causes chronic infections that do not necessarily resolve after puberty, as *M. audouinii* infections may; adults may thus be infected or colonized and may serve as carriers.[4, 43] The carriage rate in family members of all ages can be high; 48% of 31 children with *T. tonsurans* tinea capitis had at least one additional family member from whom *T. tonsurans* could be cultured.[4] Positive cultures were found in 20 (63%) of 32 siblings and 5 (14%) of 35 adult family members. Twenty-five percent of the culture-positive siblings and 80% of the culture-positive adults were asymptomatic—important because asymptomatic carriers of *T. tonsurans* may transmit this anthropophilic fungus to other persons. Family members of affected children should be examined if at all possible, and consideration should be given to possible culture and treatment of these individuals; whether asymptomatic carriers should be treated with oral griseofulvin or with ketoconazole shampoo requires further study.[4, 16] Sharing of combs, brushes, hats, and other fomites should be avoided until the infection has cleared.

FAVUS

Favus is a severe, chronic scalp ringworm caused by *T. schoenleinii*, characterized by yellow cup-shaped crusts called scutula that surround the hair follicles. Rarely, it may be caused by *T. violaceum* or *Microsporum gypseum*. The name comes from the Latin word for honeycomb. Infection begins with a small yellow-red papule that develops surrounding erythema and scaling, spreading to give a patchy distribution. Scarring alopecia may result. Favus is seen mostly in Africa, the Mediterranean, and the Middle East, with rare cases in North and South America, usually in descendants of immigrants from endemic areas. It is generally acquired early in life and tends to cluster in families. Diagnosis is made by the clinical appearance, mousy odor, dull fluorescence on Wood light examination, KOH preparation, and culture. Treatment consists of long-term griseofulvin.

TINEA BARBAE

Tinea barbae refers to infections of the beard and mustache hair in adult men. It is most commonly caused by *Trichophyton verrucosum* or *Trichophyton mentagrophytes*, which produce a large-spore ectothrix infection similar to that seen in tinea capitis caused by the same organisms. *T. verrucosum* infection is especially common in dairy farmers and cattle ranchers, who may acquire an intensely inflammatory zoophilic infection from infected cows, but the infection can also be acquired from horses or dogs.

Tinea barbae presents clinically as an inflammatory pustular folliculitis in the beard or mustache area, often with exudate and crusting and sometimes with draining sinuses. It may be accompanied by systemic symptoms such as fever, malaise, and regional lymphadenopathy. Occasionally, the lesions are less inflammatory, consisting of scaling red plaques with broken-off hairs (Fig. 145–2). Tinea barbae may heal with scarring.

The differential diagnosis includes sycosis barbae (caused by *S. aureus*), bacterial folliculitis, acne, rosacea, pseudofolliculitis barbae, actinomycosis, and herpes simplex. A history of animal contact should raise the index of suspicion for tinea barbae. As with tinea capitis, diagnosis is made by the demonstration of arthroconidia in involved hairs and pus with a KOH preparation or culture. Treatment consists of oral griseofulvin, in regimens similar to those used for tinea capitis, and epidemiologic control of infection in the animal population. As with tinea capitis, itraconazole, fluconazole, or terbinafine may be considered alternative therapies.[23]

Dermatophyte Infections of the Skin

TINEA CORPORIS

Tinea corporis (ringworm) refers to dermatophyte infections of the glabrous skin other than specialized sites such as the scalp, groin, palms, and soles. It may be caused by any species of *Trichophyton*, *Microsporum*, or *Epidermophyton*, but the most common agents are *T. rubrum*, *T. mentagrophytes*, *Epidermophyton floccosum*, and *M. canis*. Infections are com-

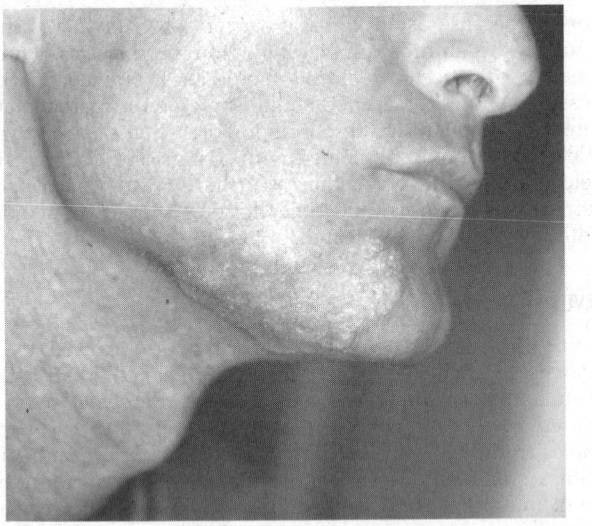

FIGURE 145–2 □ Tinea barbae. Pink scaly plaque with raised red border in the beard area.

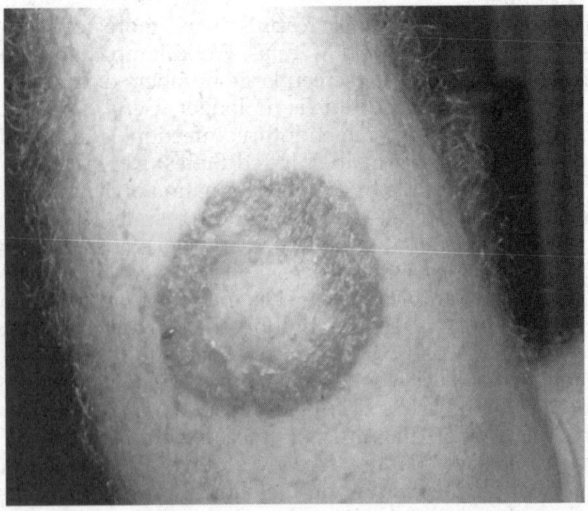

FIGURE 145–4 □ Tinea corporis. Inflammatory annular plaque with vesicular border on the forearm.

mon worldwide but may be more common in hot, humid areas and may be acquired by humans from other people, animals, fomites, or soil. The species most frequently acquired from animals are *M. canis* and *T. mentagrophytes*. Inflammatory infections with *T. verrucosum* or *Trichophyton equinum* may result from exposure to infected cattle or horses.[44, 45]

In tinea corporis, infection is limited to the top layer of the epidermis, the stratum corneum, but involvement of follicles may lead to persistent or recurrent infection. Infection begins with inoculation of fungal spores or hyphae from an infected person, animal, fomite, or soil or from lesions elsewhere on the body. Lesions begin as pruritic erythematous papules that spread outward to form sharply marginated annular plaques, usually with central clearing and red, raised scaly borders (Fig. 145–3 [see Color Plate 1]). Central postinflammatory hyperpigmentation or hypopigmentation is common. Vesicles or pustules are sometimes seen at the border in more inflammatory lesions (Fig. 145–4). Frankly bullous lesions of tinea corporis from which *M. canis* was cultured were reported in a 63-year-old woman who also had classic annular lesions.[46] Thicker psoriasiform or granulomatous lesions may occasionally be seen, and verrucous lesions may occur in immunocompromised hosts; a deeper form, tinea profunda, which is analogous to kerion formation on the scalp, also exists.[11] Lesions may coalesce to form larger lesions with serpiginous borders. More inflammatory lesions may be seen with zoophilic or geophilic species, although the infected animal may have disease that is inconspicuous or even subclinical.[47]

A granulomatous perifollicular form of tinea corporis known as Majocchi granuloma may be seen on the lower legs in women as the result of shaving. This appears as multiple inflammatory follicular papules coalescing into irregular plaques. It may also be seen if lesions of tinea corporis are occluded or treated with topical corticosteroids. A suppurative folliculitis with rupture of the follicles results in release of fungal elements into the dermis, causing a granulomatous inflammatory response[48] (Fig. 145–5). Majocchi granuloma is usually caused by *T. violaceum*, *T. rubrum*, *E. floccosum*, or *T. mentagrophytes*.[48] A deep form may be seen in patients treated with systemic steroids or other immunosuppressive medications and in patients with acquired immunodeficiency syndrome (AIDS).[49]

The differential diagnosis depends on the body site and morphologic features of the lesions but may include contact dermatitis, nummular dermatitis, the herald patch of pityriasis rosea, seborrheic dermatitis, *Candida* infection, psoriasis, and other skin diseases. The diagnosis of tinea corporis is

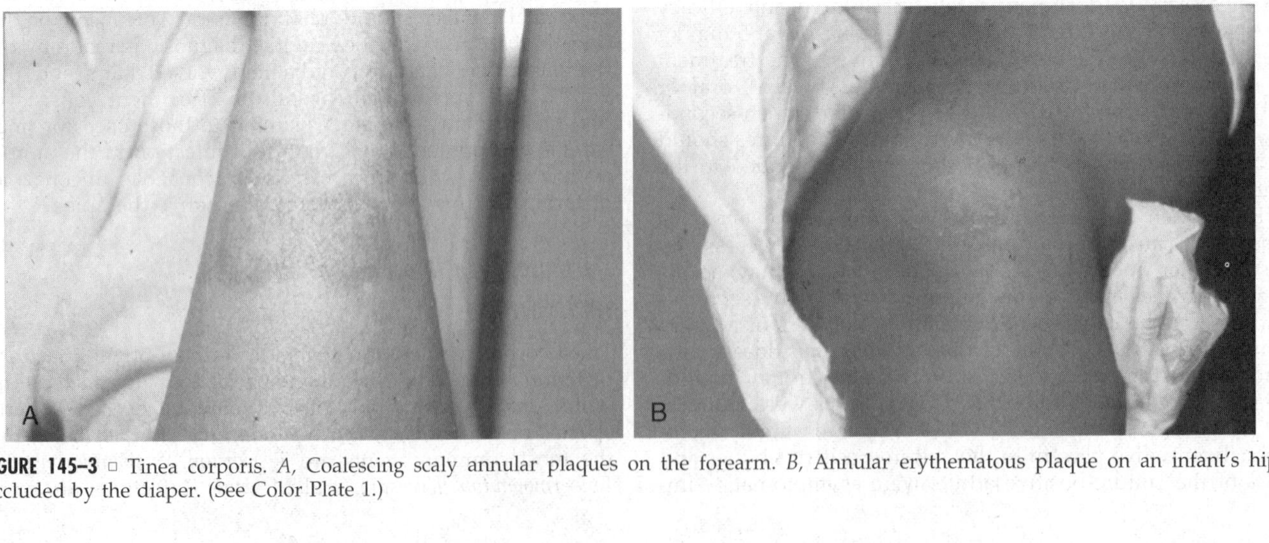

FIGURE 145–3 □ Tinea corporis. *A*, Coalescing scaly annular plaques on the forearm. *B*, Annular erythematous plaque on an infant's hip, occluded by the diaper. (See Color Plate 1.)

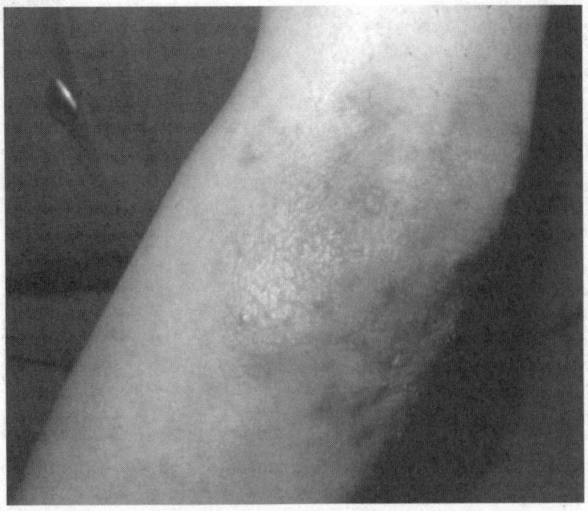

FIGURE 145–5 □ Majocchi granuloma. Coalescing plaques with follicular papules on the elbow.

established by KOH examination of infected scale scraped with a No. 15 blade from the active border of the lesion (Fig. 145–6). Culture of infected material may also be performed on Sabouraud agar with antibiotics to suppress bacterial overgrowth.

Tinea corporis may be treated with a variety of topical antifungal agents; oral therapy should be considered for patients with extensive disease or infections that are resistant to therapy.[50] If the infection was acquired from a zoonotic source, the infected animal should also be treated. Therapy is discussed in more detail later.

TINEA CORPORIS GLADIATORUM

Epidemics of tinea corporis and tinea capitis in wrestlers, caused by *T. tonsurans* or *T. verrucosum*, have been termed tinea corporis gladiatorum.[51–55] Lesions are typically seen on the shoulders, face, neck, and scalp—areas that are frequently abraded and may be inoculated by direct contact with opponents' skin; contact with wrestling mats or sharing of headgear may also contribute to the spread of infection but this mode of transmission is less likely.[51, 52, 55] Control of tinea corporis gladiatorum requires regular screening of wrestlers and participants in other contact sports for signs of dermatophyte infection and exclusion of infected athletes from practice and competition, analogous to precautions taken for herpes simplex gladiatorum. As for all dermatophyte infections, therapy is determined by the site and extent of infection; most patients can be treated topically, although scalp infections must obviously be treated with oral griseofulvin.

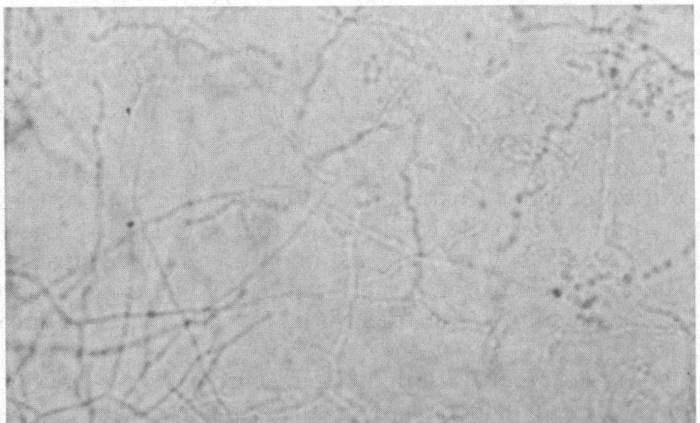

FIGURE 145–6 □ KOH preparation. Dermatophyte hyphae visualized on microscopic examination in KOH. (Courtesy of Victor Newcomer, MD, Santa Monica, CA.)

TINEA IMBRICATA

Tinea imbricata (tokelau ringworm) is a distinctive infection caused by the anthropophilic dermatophyte *Trichophyton concentricum* seen only in the Pacific Islands, Southeast Asia, and Central and South America. Multiple concentric brownish scaly rings are seen, resembling the rings of a tree. There appears to be a genetic predisposition, probably inherited as an autosomal recessive trait. Relapses after treatment are common and may be characterized by the intense pruritus and inflammation normally seen only in the early stages of infection. Systemic terbinafine seems slightly superior to itraconazole in the treatment of tinea imbricata.[56]

TINEA FACIEI

Tinea corporis of the face, excluding the beard and mustache area of adult men, is known as tinea faciei. The usual causative agents are *T. mentagrophytes* and *T. rubrum*; infections with *M. canis* acquired from kittens are not uncommon. Tinea faciei tends to be erythematous but much less scaly than other forms of tinea corporis, leading to frequent misdiagnosis (Fig. 145–7). In addition to seborrheic dermatitis, tinea faciei has been mistaken for lupus erythematosus, polymorphous light eruption, rosacea, and perioral dermatitis. A history of animal contact, particularly with kittens, should raise the clinical suspicion for tinea and prompt a careful search for fungal elements on a KOH scraping. Successful treatment is usually accomplished with topical antifungal agents.

TINEA CRURIS

Tinea cruris (jock itch, dhobie itch) refers to dermatophyte infection of the groin, perineum, or perianal area; infection also commonly spreads to the buttocks. Infection is seen almost exclusively in adolescent and adult men. *E. floccosum*, *T. rubrum*, and *T. mentagrophytes* are the most commonly isolated agents, presumably because they are also the usual causes of tinea pedis, which is often the source of infection. Tinea cruris presents with pruritic, well-demarcated scaly erythematous and hyperpigmented plaques with central clearing and scalloped borders and tends to involve the inner thighs and inguinal creases but spares the scrotum and penis, unlike *Candida* infections. Diagnosis and treatment are the same as for tinea corporis.

In infants, diaper dermatitis due to dermatophyte infection is rare. However, cases due to *T. rubrum* and *E. floccosum*, which commonly cause tinea cruris in adults, and also *T. verrucosum*, in an infant whose father was a cattle farmer,[57] have been reported.

TINEA MANUUM

Tinea manuum refers to dermatophyte infection of the palmar surfaces, although infection may also occur on the dorsal hands. It is most commonly seen in association with tinea pedis, and therefore the most common pathogen is *T. rubrum*, followed by *E. floccosum* and *T. mentagrophytes* var. *interdigitale*. It frequently presents in a two-feet–one-hand distribution, for unknown reasons. Lesions most commonly consist of dry, powdery, hyperkeratotic scale accentuated in the creases; there is usually little to no erythema, although inflammatory and vesicular forms occasionally occur (Fig. 145–

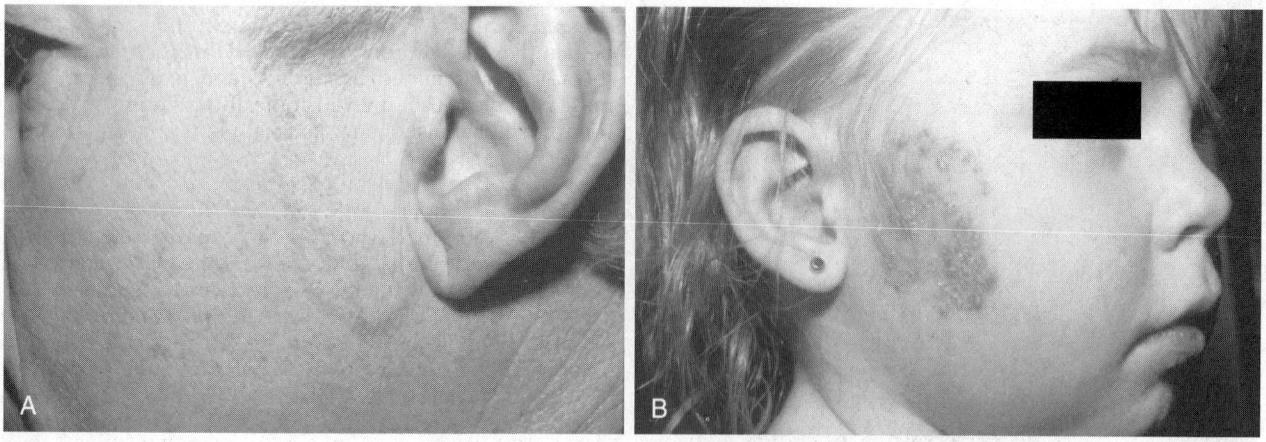

FIGURE 145–7 ▫ Tinea faciei. *A*, Erythematous annular plaque in the left preauricular area. Note the relative absence of scale. *B*, Inflammatory, erythematous, slightly scaly plaques and papules on the face of a 2-year-old girl.

8). One or more fingernails may be involved as well. The differential diagnosis includes xerosis, irritant contact dermatitis, other forms of hand dermatitis, and palmar keratodermas. The presence of a unilateral hand dermatitis should prompt a search for tinea, especially if the feet are also involved. Diagnosis and treatment are the same as for tinea pedis, consisting of KOH examination, culture, and topical antifungal agents; oral therapy is occasionally required.

TINEA PEDIS

Tinea pedis (athlete's foot) is the most common fungal infection in adults. The most common etiologic agents are *T. rubrum*, *T. mentagrophytes* var. *interdigitale*, and *E. floccosum*. Tinea pedis is primarily a dermatosis of shoe-wearing populations, illustrating the importance of local factors such as maceration, heat, moisture, and occlusion. Acquisition of tinea pedis commonly occurs at communal athletic and bathing facilities, locker rooms, and swimming pools, where infected individuals walk barefoot and floors are frequently wet.[58, 59]

Fungal infections of the feet and nails occur less frequently in children than in adults, the incidence rising with age. However, foot and nail infections are not uncommonly observed in children and seem to occur with some frequency in children with trisomy 21, as do other chronic dermatophytoses.[14, 60–62] Clearly, tinea must be considered in the differential diagnosis of children with foot dermatitis. Twenty-five

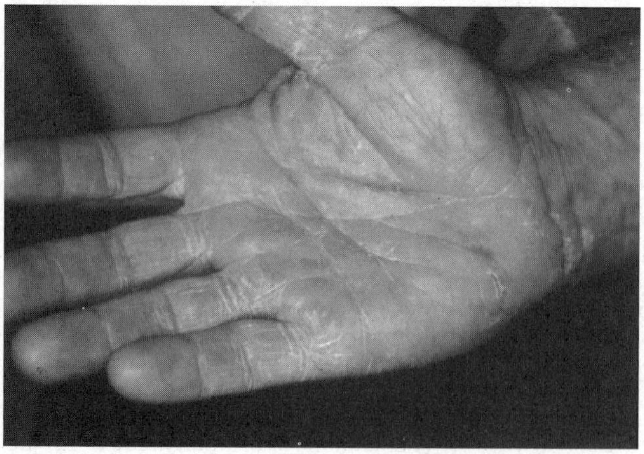

FIGURE 145–8 ▫ Tinea manuum. (Courtesy of Nellie Konnikov, MD, New England Medical Center Hospital, Boston, MA.)

percent of cases of childhood tinea pedis are associated with a positive family history, usually in a parent, suggesting genetic as well as environmental factors.[63]

There are three main clinical types of tinea pedis. The most common is an infection limited to the interdigital web spaces, most commonly involving only the fourth web space, between the fourth and fifth toes (Fig. 145–9). This area is thought to be predisposed because it lacks sebaceous glands that produce fungistatic lipids, which help to prevent infection in other areas. Tinea pedis presents clinically with peeling, maceration, erythema, and fissuring and is often pruritic. The differential diagnosis of interdigital tinea pedis includes candidiasis, bacterial infections, and erythrasma. Normally a mild infection, this type, known as dermatophytosis simplex, may, in the setting of occlusion and secondary bacterial growth, develop into dermatophytosis complex, a mixed infection characterized by maceration, pruritus, and malodor produced by various bacterial products[14, 64] (Fig. 145–10). Bacterial superinfection due to *S. aureus*, *Micrococcus sedentarius*, *Brevibacterium epidermidis*, *Corynebacterium minutissimum*, *Pseudomonas*, and *Proteus* may occur, which may mask the underlying fungal infection both clinically and when cultures are performed because of production of antifungal sulfur compounds, which may allow the gradual conversion from fungal to bacterial infection.[64] Similarly, the bacteria are frequently antibiotic resistant owing to prior exposure to antibiotic substances produced by the fungi.[64, 65] In addition to antifungal and antibacterial therapy, treatment requires agents that dry the web space, such as aluminum chloride, gentian violet, or Castellani paint.[14] Ciclopirox olamine and terbinafine are two antifungal agents that also have antibacterial properties in vitro and in vivo against gram-positive and gram-negative organisms, making them useful in the treatment of mixed fungal and bacterial infections such as interdigital dermatophytosis complex.[66]

The second type of tinea pedis is the acute vesicular type, a pruritic eruption characterized by erythema and vesicles commonly seen on the instep of the foot (Fig. 145–11). Diagnosis is established by demonstration of fungal hyphae on the undersurface of the blister roof on a KOH examination or by fungal culture. Treatment is as for other types of tinea pedis.

The third type of tinea pedis is the chronic hyperkeratotic form, often called moccasin-type tinea pedis because of its distribution. Dry hyperkeratotic scale and variable erythema are present on the soles and along the sides of the feet and toes (Fig. 145–12). This infection is usually caused by *T. rubrum*. Recurrences are common and are the rule when nail involvement is present, as it frequently is. Interestingly, al-

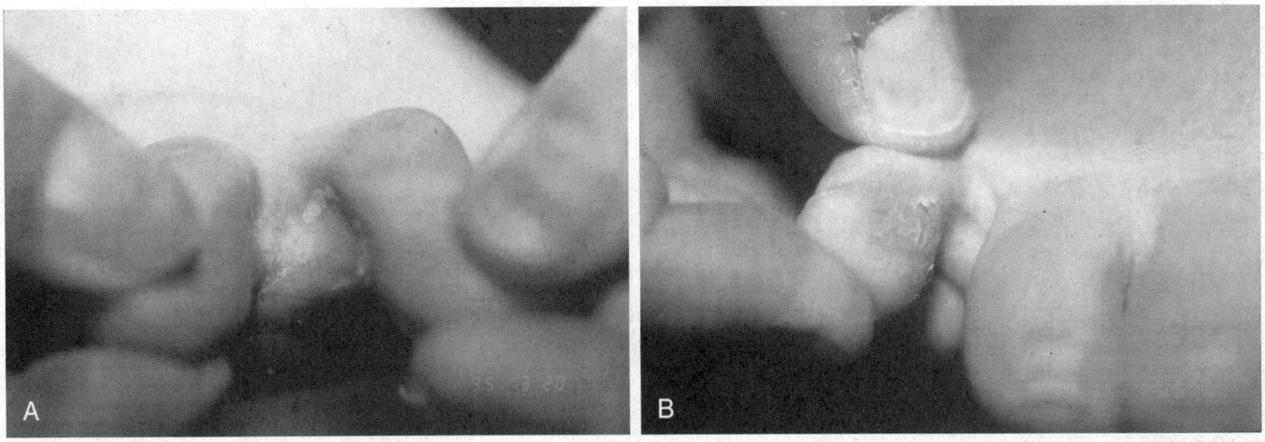

FIGURE 145–9 □ Tinea pedis. *A,* Interdigital maceration and scaling. (Courtesy of Nellie Konnikov, MD, New England Medical Center Hospital, Boston, MA.) *B,* Interdigital maceration and scaling.

most all chronic dermatophyte infections involving the skin and nails are due to *T. rubrum*. Several reasons are postulated that may help to explain this phenomenon. First, *T. rubrum* cell wall mannan inhibits the immune response; second, in some people, *T. rubrum* does not elicit a cell-mediated response adequate to clear the infection but rather preferentially activates specific suppressor T cells; third, the fungus is nonaggressive and remains in the stratum corneum, rather than attempting to invade the dermis where it might encounter complement, neutrophils, and other immune defenses; and finally, it is stable in the environment in a spore form for long periods.[67]

TINEA INCOGNITO

Tinea that has been treated with topical corticosteroids is known as tinea incognito because of the suppression of the usual inflammatory response, resulting in an altered morphologic appearance. In addition to making the diagnosis more difficult clinically, the steroid use, by blunting the immune response, potentiates the underlying infection. The patient is frequently led to believe that the steroid is treating the condition because inflammation and pruritus appear to subside, but when treatment is discontinued, the rash recurs. Corticosteroid-treated lesions tend to be less raised and less scaly; scaling is one of the host defenses by which the infectious organisms are normally shed (Fig. 145–13). The appearance may be further modified by the development of steroid side effects, such as atrophy and telangiectasia, or by the development of perioral dermatitis on the face. Diagnosis is made by KOH examination, which may be easier to perform a few days after the steroid is discontinued, when scaling resumes.[12(p1160)]

Treatment consists of discontinuing steroid use and implementing appropriate topical antifungal therapy. If infection has invaded the follicles under the influence of the steroid, leading to the development of Majocchi granuloma, oral therapy may be required to eradicate infection. Combination agents containing both antifungal and corticosteroid medications should be avoided; permanent scars may result from the exacerbation of tinea corporis due to such agents.[68] The potential risks of using potent topical steroids, and the potential decreased efficacy of the antifungal agent in the presence of steroid-impaired host defenses, make it difficult to justify use of these combination agents in the treatment of dermatophyte infections. In cases in which it is unclear whether a lesion is fungal or inflammatory, it is preferable to document fungal infection with a KOH examination and employ specific antifungal treatment once an accurate diagnosis has been made.[69]

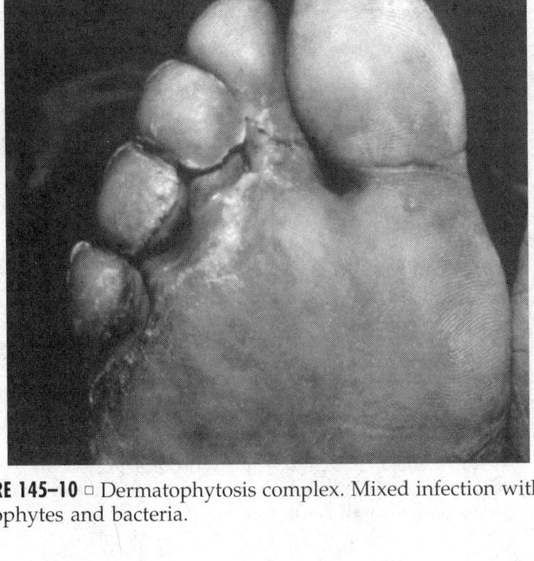

FIGURE 145–10 □ Dermatophytosis complex. Mixed infection with dermatophytes and bacteria.

DERMATOPHYTID REACTIONS

Dermatophytids, also known as id reactions, are uncommon cutaneous allergic responses to dermatophyte infections, usually occurring in the setting of inflammatory tinea. The id reaction occurs at a site distant from the infection, and cultures of the lesions are negative. The classically described id reaction consists of a pompholyx-like vesicular hand dermatitis in response to tinea pedis; the id reaction resolves when the underlying infection is treated. Many children with tinea capitis will develop a pruritic eruption of pinpoint lichenoid papules over the face and upper body when therapy for the tinea is initiated (Fig. 145–14 [see Color Plate 2]). This reaction is self-limited and appears to be an immune response to fungal antigens; it is important to continue treatment and not to misdiagnose it as a drug eruption due to griseofulvin. True allergy to griseofulvin is rare.[33]

Dermatophyte Infections of the Nails

Onychomycosis refers to any fungal infection of the nails; tinea unguium refers specifically to those nail infections caused by dermatophytes. Fungal nail infections are chronic

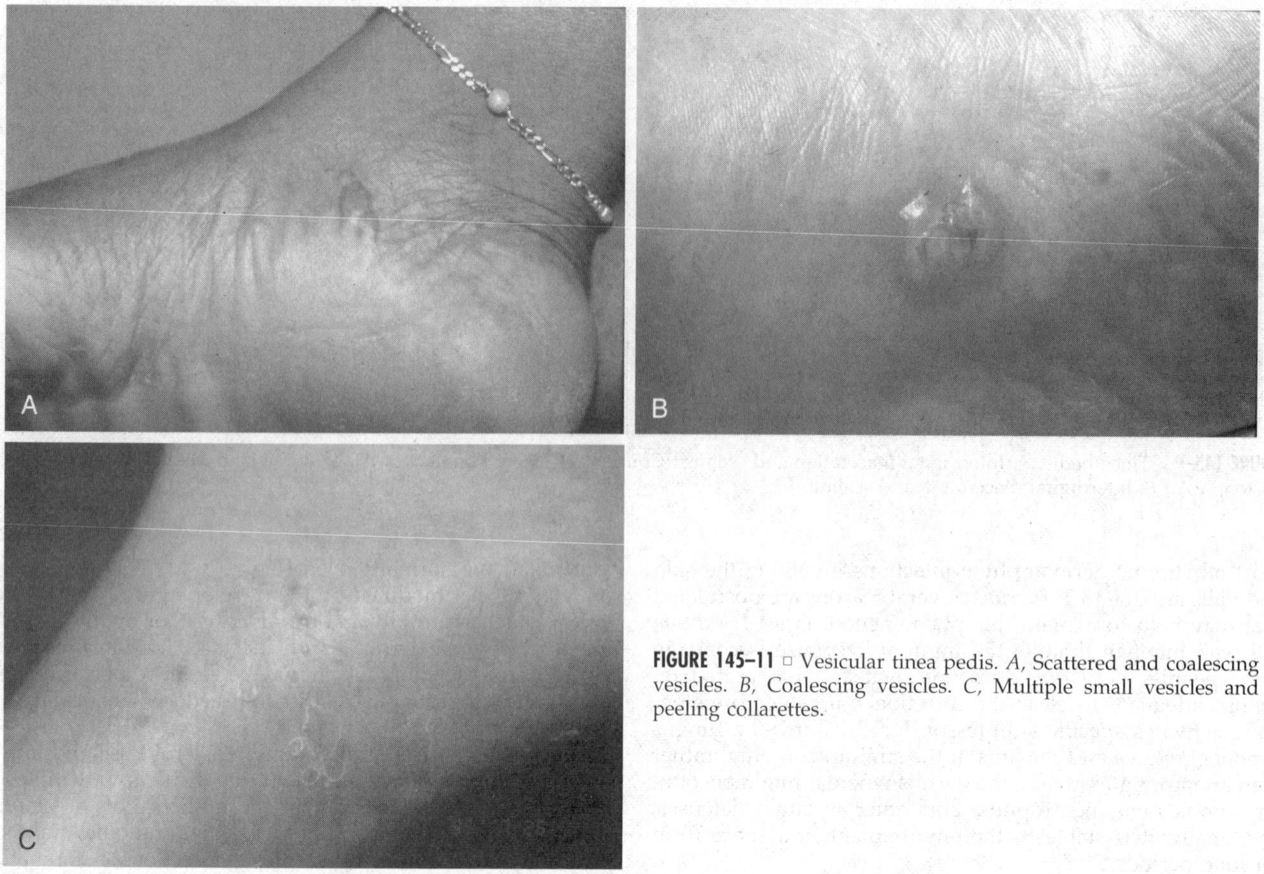

FIGURE 145–11 ▫ Vesicular tinea pedis. *A*, Scattered and coalescing vesicles. *B*, Coalescing vesicles. *C*, Multiple small vesicles and peeling collarettes.

and respond poorly to therapy, although newer agents that persist in the nail plate, some of which are fungicidal, are proving useful. Onychomycosis may cause a great deal of morbidity in terms of discomfort, functional impairment, and psychologic distress.[59] Nail infection is relatively uncommon in children in general but appears common in children with trisomy 21 (Fig. 145–15).

Tinea unguium is usually seen in association with tinea pedis or tinea manuum and is most commonly caused by *T. rubrum* or *T. mentagrophytes* var. *interdigitale*, with some cases caused by *E. floccosum*. *Microsporum* species do not invade the nail. Infection usually starts in one nail and may spread to involve others over a period of years. Although many saprophytic nondermatophyte molds can also cause nail infections, and *Candida* can produce onychomycosis in patients with chronic mucocutaneous candidiasis, there are three clinical types of true dermatophyte nail infection.

DISTAL SUBUNGUAL ONYCHOMYCOSIS

Distal subungual onychomycosis is the most common type of tinea unguium and is characterized by distal subungual hyperkeratosis, onycholysis, and thickening of the nails (Fig. 145–16). Infection begins in the keratin of the hyponychium

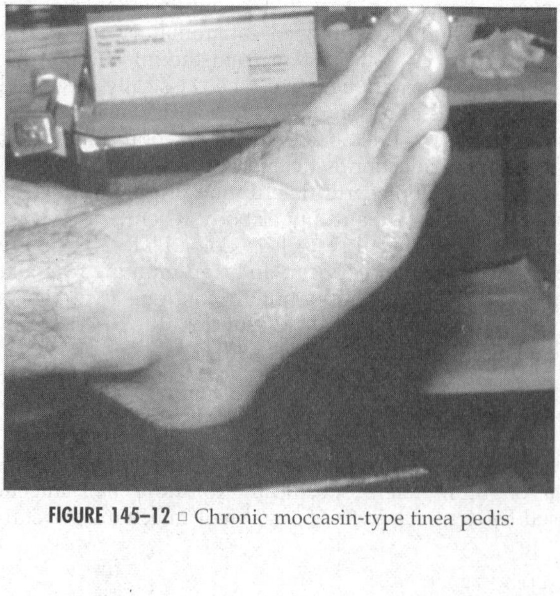

FIGURE 145–12 ▫ Chronic moccasin-type tinea pedis.

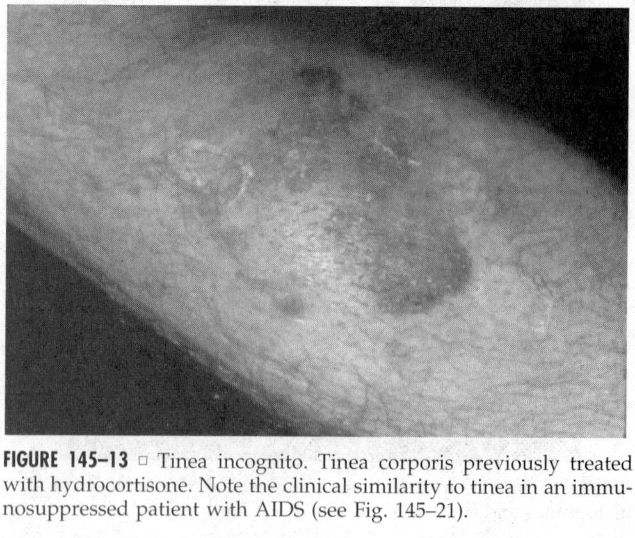

FIGURE 145–13 ▫ Tinea incognito. Tinea corporis previously treated with hydrocortisone. Note the clinical similarity to tinea in an immunosuppressed patient with AIDS (see Fig. 145–21).

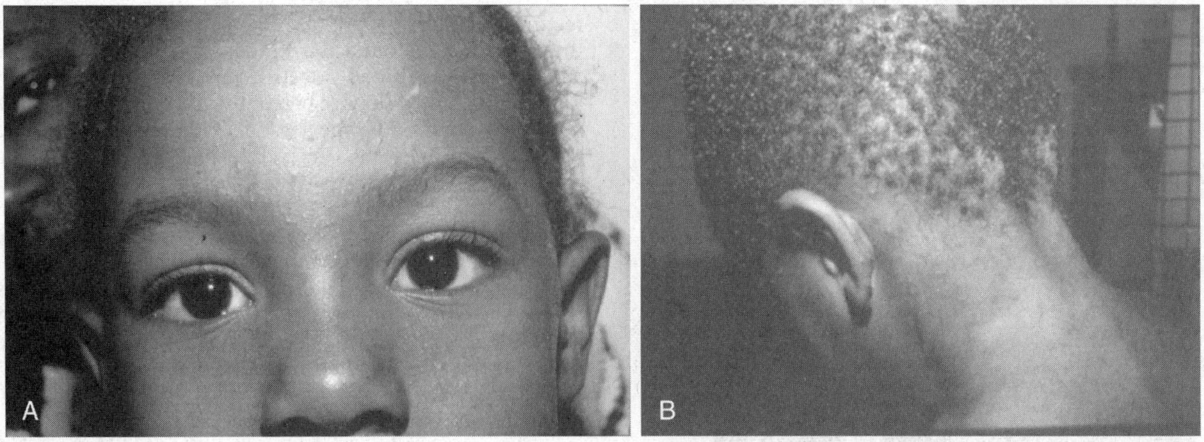

FIGURE 145–14 □ Id reaction. *A,* Fine papular eruption on the face in a 3-year-old girl with tinea capitis. *B,* Tinea capitis with fine papular id reaction on the neck. (See Color Plate 2.)

and spreads proximally to the nail bed and nail plate. Subungual hyperkeratosis, the nail equivalent to scaling as an attempt to rid the body of infection, ultimately results in the lifting up of the nail plate from the nail bed (onycholysis). The nail may become thickened and crumbly; secondary infection with bacteria or nondermatophytic fungi may also occur. The dystrophic nail that results may be painful when shoes are worn.

PROXIMAL SUBUNGUAL ONYCHOMYCOSIS

Proximal subungual onychomycosis is the rarest type of tinea unguium. The organism invades under the cuticle, and infection involves the ventral surface of the nail, creating irregular white spots under the nail that begin proximally and spread distally with the nail (Fig. 145–17). This type of tinea unguium appears to occur more commonly in human immunodeficiency virus–positive patients.[70] It may occur without involvement of the skin and is usually caused by *T. rubrum,* although *T. schoenleinii, Trichophyton megninii,* and *E. floccosum* have also been reported.[71]

SUPERFICIAL WHITE ONYCHOMYCOSIS

Superficial white onychomycosis occurs in toenails and is usually caused by *T. mentagrophytes,* which directly infects the nail plate. Other etiologic agents may include nondermatophyte molds such as *Acremonium* spp., *Fusarium oxysporum,* and *Aspergillus terreus.*[72, 73] Involved nails develop dull opaque superficial white patches, which may be focal or may involve the entire nail (Fig. 145–18). In human immunodeficiency virus–positive patients, *T. rubrum* may cause superficial white onychomycosis.[70]

ONYCHOMYCOSIS CAUSED BY NONDERMATOPHYTE MOLDS

Nondermatophyte molds that commonly cause onychomycosis include *Acremonium, Aspergillus,* and *Fusarium* species and *Onycochola canadensis, Scopulariopsis brevicaulis, Hendersonula toruloidea (Scytalidium dimidiatum),* and *Scytalidium hyalinum.*[73, 74] *Scytalidium* is an especially important pathogen in tropical and subtropical countries.[74] It is important to distinguish these agents by culture because they do not respond to the agents usually used to treat dermatophyte infections of the skin and nails. Clues to the diagnosis of nail infections with nondermatophyte molds may include the involvement of only one nail, frequently after trauma because these agents tend to invade only previously damaged nails, or the presence of brown or black pigmentation of the nail.[59] Some of these agents may respond to long-term oral terbinafine.[75] Onychomycosis caused by *Aspergillus flavus* has been successfully treated with itraconazole.[76]

DIAGNOSIS

The differential diagnosis of tinea unguium includes psoriasis, traumatic nail dystrophy, fungal infections other than those caused by dermatophytes, congenital deformities such

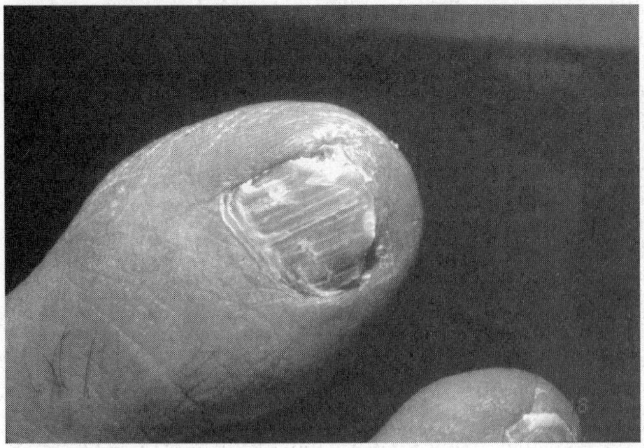

FIGURE 145–15 □ Onychomycosis in a patient with trisomy 21.

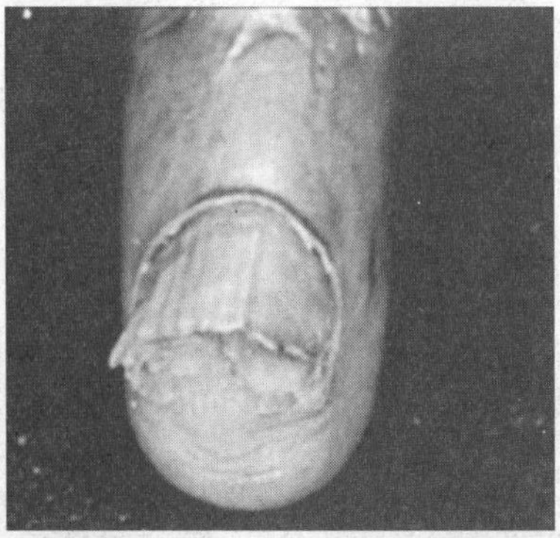

FIGURE 145–16 □ Distal subungual onychomycosis. Note the distal subungual hyperkeratosis.

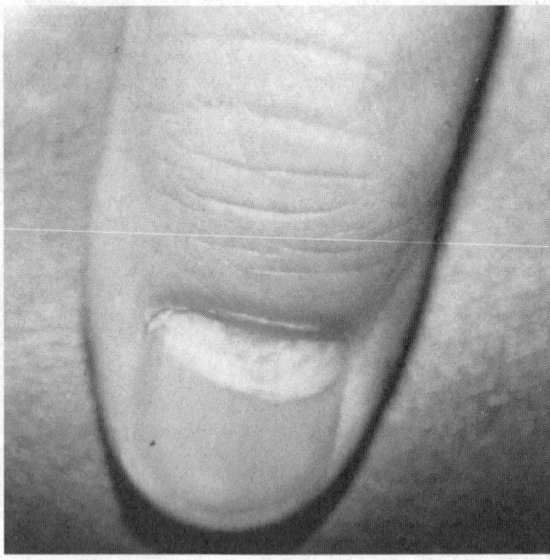

FIGURE 145–17 ▫ Proximal subungual onychomycosis. This type of onychomycosis occurs more commonly in AIDS. (Courtesy of Nellie Konnikov, MD, New England Medical Center Hospital, Boston, MA.)

as pachyonychia congenita, and nail changes due to systemic diseases. KOH examination, culture, or both are required to confirm a diagnosis of tinea unguium. An alternative diagnostic method involves clipping a piece of the involved nail and sending it for histologic mounting and periodic acid–Schiff or silver staining to identify fungal elements. If necessary, nail biopsy may be performed.

TREATMENT

Tinea unguium cannot be cured with topical agents currently available, although amorolfine and tioconazole are under investigation and may prove useful in the treatment of mild to moderate infections in which the lunula and matrix remain uninvolved.[77–79] Although they are not curative, ciclopirox olamine and naftifine appear to have some nail penetration and may be helpful in some patients.[80] Surgical avulsion or chemical avulsion may be a useful adjunctive therapy in some patients in combination with topical or oral therapy.[81]

Oral agents that can be used include griseofulvin, ketoconazole, fluconazole, and itraconazole.[72] Griseofulvin must be given for 6 to 12 months for fingernail infections and for 12 to 18 months for toenail involvement, because the agent is fungistatic and nails grow so slowly. Griseofulvin is also limited by its effectiveness only against dermatophytes, because other fungi may also infect nails, either alone or coinfecting with dermatophytes.[82] Ketoconazole use is limited by the risk for hepatotoxicity. Itraconazole and fluconazole are active against a broad spectrum of fungi and can be used to treat nail infections caused by dermatophytes, *Candida*, *Aspergillus*, and other species.[80, 83] Both, particularly itraconazole, may be prescribed in pulsed-dose regimens, as well as continuous ones, because they persist in the nail plate.[84] Adverse effects of itraconazole and fluconazole include gastrointestinal symptoms, headache, rashes, and hepatotoxic reactions, although the last appear to be less common with the triazoles than with ketoconazole; drug interactions are common with all three agents because they work by interfering with the cytochrome P-450 system, which many other drugs depend on for their metabolism.[42, 85, 86]

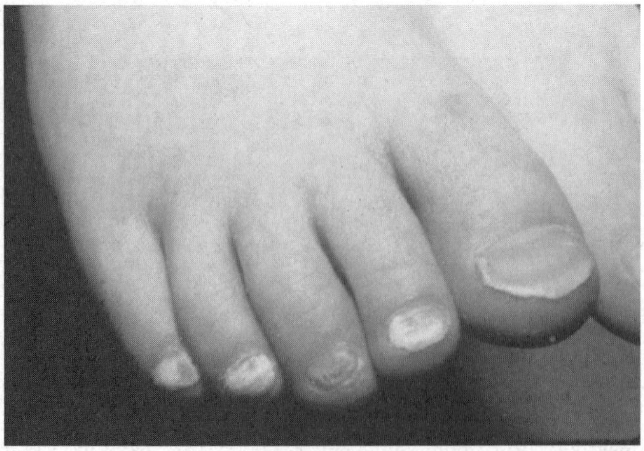

FIGURE 145–18 ▫ Superficial white onychomycosis.

The most promising breakthrough will probably be oral terbinafine, because it is fungicidal and persists for long periods in the nail (see later).[14, 84] Either terbinafine, 250 mg daily, or itraconazole, 200 mg daily, achieves rapid penetration and prolonged persistence in nails, enabling treatment periods to be shortened to as little as 6 weeks for fingernails and 12 weeks for toenails; the fungicidal nature of terbinafine also enables shortened treatment schedules.[83] Mycologic cure rates of about 80% and low relapse rates of about 10% at 12 months after short courses of these two drugs appear to be much better than those for previously available therapies for the treatment of tinea unguium and chronic moccasin-type tinea pedis.[83, 87] Intermittent, pulsed-dose regimens can also be used. Some patients require a second course of treatment.[88] It is anticipated that terbinafine will be extremely useful in the treatment of fungal infections of the hair and nails.[89] Studies in several countries indicate that oral terbinafine is the most cost-effective therapy for dermatophyte infections of both toenails and fingernails.[90, 91]

Superficial Mycoses Caused by Nondermatophytes

Piedra

Piedra refers to a rare infection of hair characterized by the presence of localized nodules consisting of fungal spores or hyphae attached to the hair shaft. There are two forms, each produced by different organisms, neither of which is a dermatophyte.

White piedra is caused by *Trichosporon beigelii*, a fungus that may be isolated from soil, air, and skin in endemic areas. It is usually seen in South America, central and eastern Europe, and Japan but has rarely been reported in the United States. Infection may involve the scalp but more commonly affects beard, mustache, axillary, or pubic hairs and produces white to tan, red, brown, or greenish nodules up to 1 mm in diameter that are easily detached from the hairs. Eyebrow and eyelash hairs may also be involved. Because the fungus grows inside and outside the hair shaft, the hair is weakened and may fracture. Diagnosis is made by KOH examination, which will distinguish white piedra from trichomycosis axillaris or pubis caused by several *Corynebacterium* species. Pruritus and the distinctive shape and adherence of nits should help to distinguish pediculosis from white piedra. Microscopic examination also rules out trichorrhexis nodosa.

In the last decade, the role of *T. beigelii* as a sole pathogen in white piedra has come into question. There appears to be an increased rate of carriage of bacteria, in particular of coryneform bacteria distinct from those causing trichomycosis axillaris, in hairs infected with *T. beigelii*; it has been proposed that white piedra results from a synergistic infection of *T. beigelii* and a specific type III coryneform bacterium, a newly characterized species of *Brevibacterium* called *Brevibacterium mcbrellneri*.[92–95]

T. beigelii has also been reported to cause onychomycosis in healthy adults and systemic opportunistic infection in immunocompromised hosts.[93, 96–99] Culture media without cycloheximide are necessary for the isolation of this organism.[96]

Black piedra is characterized by adherent, hard, gritty black nodular concretions on the hair shaft; these concretions may vary in size from microscopic to more than 1 mm in diameter. Invasion of the shaft may result in hair breakage. Black piedra usually involves the scalp but may involve other sites, such as the mustache, beard, and pubic area. It is caused by *Piedraia hortae*, another soil fungus, and is rare in the United States, occurring mainly in tropical areas of South America and Southeast Asia, the Pacific Islands, and Africa.

Treatment of piedra consists primarily of shaving or cutting the affected hair. Terbinafine has been reported as a successful treatment for black piedra, with demonstration of in vitro susceptibility of the isolate corresponding to the clinical and mycologic cure.[92, 100] Treatment of white piedra is difficult. In addition to shaving the affected hairs, reported treatments have included topical and oral imidazoles, ciclopirox olamine, selenium sulfide, bichloride of mercury, benzoic acid, salicylic acid, 3% to 6% precipitated sulfur ointment, chlorhexidine, Castellani paint, zinc pyrithione, amphotericin B lotion, 2% to 10% glutaraldehyde, and 2% formalin.[92, 101(p165)] In view of the location of infection within and on the hair, and the likely involvement of both *T. beigelii* and *B. mcbrellneri*, consideration should be given to a combination of shaving, oral and topical antifungal therapy, and topical antibacterial soaps or topical antibiotics effective against coryneform bacteria.

Tinea Nigra

Although it is not a dermatophyte infection, tinea nigra is included in this discussion because it is another superficial fungal infection involving only the stratum corneum. The disease is caused by *Exophiala werneckii* and occurs sporadically throughout the world but most commonly in tropical and subtropical areas. It presents as a well-demarcated but irregularly shaped superficial nonscaly brown or black macule, usually on the palm but occasionally on the sole and rarely on other body sites. The differential diagnosis includes melanoma, junctional nevus, lentigo, postinflammatory hyperpigmentation, and chemical staining. Diagnosis is easily made when the KOH preparation reveals pigmented septate hyphae or budding forms, and culture on Sabouraud glucose agar can be done to confirm the diagnosis. Treatment consists of scraping of the lesion, followed by application of a topical imidazole or a keratolytic agent such as benzoic acid or salicylic acid.

Nondermatophyte Molds

H. toruloidea (S. dimidiatum) and *S. hyalinum* are nondermatophyte molds that may cause infections clinically identical to tinea pedis, tinea manuum, and tinea unguium. A patient with a tinea capitis–like infection due to *H. toruloidea* has also been described.[102] These infections are technically referred to as dermatomycoses. *H. toruloidea* has been found in the southeastern United States and the western states; outside the United States, it has been found in Canada, South America, the Caribbean, Africa, India, and the Far East, and most infections have been reported in these areas.[103] Clinical presentations of tinea pedis due to these agents include interdigital and moccasin types. Mixed infections with true dermatophytes are common. Microscopic examination with KOH reveals narrow, septate, branching hyphae that are similar to those of the dermatophytes. Because these infections fail to respond to conventional antifungal agents, they must be distinguished from true tinea. Growth of these agents is inhibited by cycloheximide, so it is important to perform cultures on cycloheximide-free media in addition to the traditional dermatophyte media that contain cycloheximide to eliminate overgrowth of contaminants.[103] A positive finding on the KOH examination, coupled with a negative culture on cycloheximide-containing agar (e.g., dermatophyte test medium, Mycosel, Mycobiotic) should raise the clinical suspicion for one of these agents, especially with a history of treatment failure or living in or visiting an endemic area.[74, 103] Terbinafine, amorolfine, tioconazole, econazole, or benzoic acid (Whitfield ointment) may be effective topical therapies, but to date there is no one reliable agent for treating these dermatomycoses.[12(pp1170–1171), 59, 104–106]

Pityrosporum *Infections*

Pityrosporum ovale (P. orbiculare, Malassezia furfur) is a lipophilic yeast present as normal postpubertal skin flora in the hair follicles in sites rich in sebaceous glands, such as the face, scalp, and upper trunk. The amount of *P. ovale* present in different age groups seems to correlate with variations in sebum production that are age dependent.[107] Under certain host conditions, however, it causes diseases such as tinea versicolor (pityriasis versicolor) and *Pityrosporum* folliculitis and appears to be involved in the pathogenesis of seborrheic dermatitis.[16] It has also been postulated to play a role in some patients with atopic dermatitis and in confluent and reticulated papillomatosis of Gougerot and Carteaud, although the latter association has come into question.[107, 108] Finally, *Pityrosporum* is rarely the cause of disseminated infection.[16, 101(p157), 109, 110]

TINEA VERSICOLOR

Tinea versicolor is a common scaling dermatosis that occurs when *Pityrosporum* overgrowth extends from the follicles to adjacent skin, resulting in hyperpigmented or hypopigmented, thin, finely scaly 0.5- to 1-cm papules that may coalesce to form larger plaques, usually on the upper trunk and proximal upper extremities (Fig. 145–19*A*). Lesions on tanned skin tend to be hypopigmented, and both hyperpigmented and hypopigmented lesions may be seen in the same patient in different locations (Fig. 145–19*B*). In children, involvement occasionally extends onto the face and scalp, especially in tropical climates (Fig. 145–19*C*). In early cases, the lesions may be seen to be perifollicular in origin. It is occasionally pruritic but is often asymptomatic.

Hot, humid environments favor the development of tinea versicolor, and the disease is more common in tropical and subtropical climates than in temperate ones, where it may appear only during the summer and may be quiescent during the winter months. Heredity, glucocorticosteroid medications, hyperhidrosis, greasy skin, and exogenously applied oils can also be predisposing factors.[107, 111, 112] Tinea versicolor occurs most commonly in adolescents and young adults, in whom sebum production is higher than that in other age groups, and seems to correlate with increased colonization by *Pityrosporum* with increasing age (5% to 15% in 0- to 10-year-old children compared with 56% to 90% for 11- to 20-year-old individuals).[108] Because tinea versicolor is a disease produced by normal flora, it is not contagious.

The diagnosis of tinea versicolor is usually straightforward, but in some cases the differential diagnosis may include pityriasis alba, seborrheic dermatitis, tinea corporis, vitiligo, or postinflammatory hyperpigmentation or hypopig-

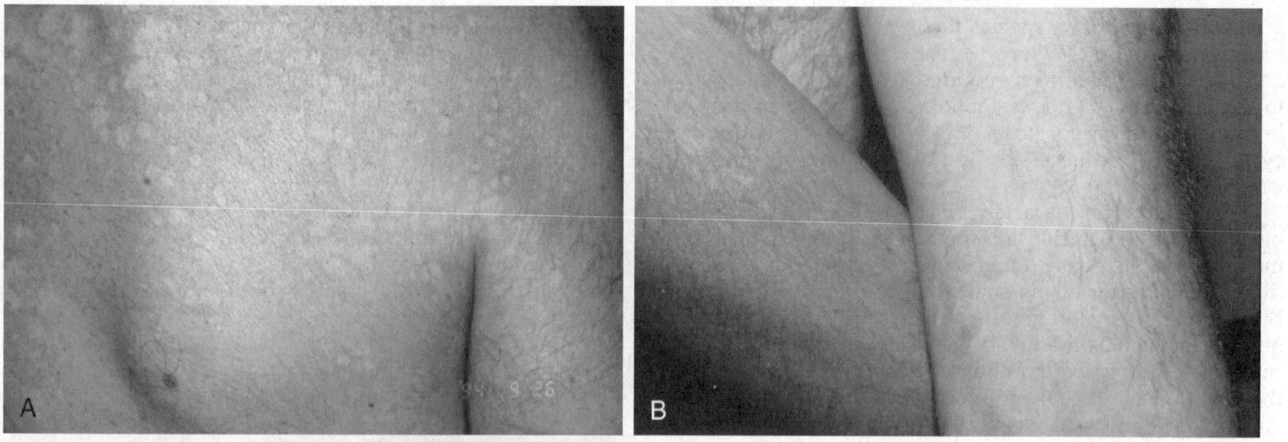

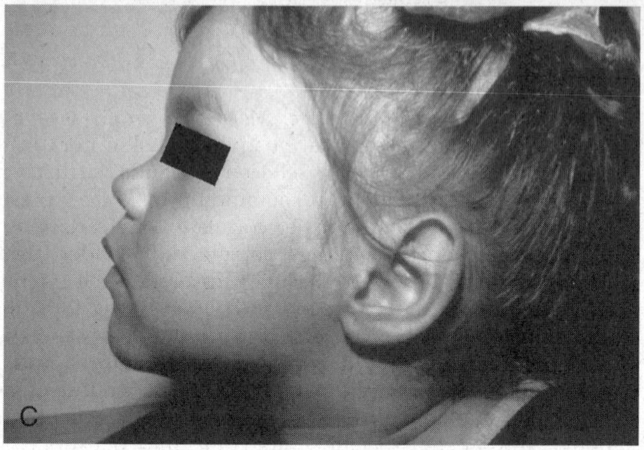

FIGURE 145–19 □ Tinea versicolor. *A,* Innumerable finely scaly hypopigmented thin papules on the trunk and proximal extremities. *B,* Hypopigmented and hyperpigmented lesions in the same patient. The lesions on the sun-exposed dorsal forearms were hypopigmented, whereas those on the relatively sun-protected volar forearms were hyperpigmented compared with normal skin. *C,* Hypopigmented finely scaly papules extending onto the face of a 3-year-old child.

mentation. Diagnosis is confirmed by the classic "spaghetti and meatballs" appearance of abundant short stubby hyphae and spores seen on KOH microscopic examination of scrapings. Culture is not routinely performed because special oil-containing medium is required.

Treatment consists of topical agents such as selenium sulfide lotion applied for 10 to 20 minutes nightly to the trunk and proximal extremities for 1 to 2 weeks. Other topical therapies include the imidazoles, ciclopirox olamine, zinc pyrithione, sulfur or salicylic acid preparations, propylene glycol, benzoyl peroxide, sodium hyposulfite, and the allylamines naftifine and terbinafine, which work topically but not orally to treat tinea versicolor.[87, 111, 112] Extensive cases, or those in which lesions extend into the hairline, may be treated with brief courses of oral ketoconazole, itraconazole, or fluconazole.[111, 112] One or two weekly oral doses of ketoconazole 400 mg, or itraconazole 200 mg daily for 5 days, is an effective regimen in the treatment of tinea versicolor.[42, 113] Ketoconazole should be taken with breakfast, including an acidic juice, and the patient should avoid bathing for at least 12 hours because the drug is delivered to the skin primarily in the sweat. Griseofulvin is effective only for treatment of dermatophyte infections and cannot be used to treat tinea versicolor. Because the disease is caused by endogenous flora, recurrence is common but may be prevented or delayed with once-monthly prophylactic topical treatment.

Pigment alteration may take months to resolve after treatment, especially for patients with hypopigmented forms. Hypopigmentation is thought to result from the organism's production of azelaic acid, which interferes with melanin synthesis; the cause of hyperpigmentation is unknown but does not appear to involve the production of melanin.[112, 114]

PITYROSPORUM FOLLICULITIS

P. ovale may cause a folliculitis characterized by pruritic follicular erythematous papules and pustules on the trunk, especially on the back (Fig. 145–20). Like tinea versicolor, it occurs more frequently in hot, humid environments.[107] It appears to be more common in diabetic patients, in immunocompromised hosts, in circumstances where skin is occluded, and after systemic steroid or antibiotic therapy.[107] The differential diagnosis includes bacterial folliculitis due to *S. aureus* or gram-negative organisms such as in hot tub folliculitis due to *Pseudomonas*, eosinophilic folliculitis, and acne vulgaris. It

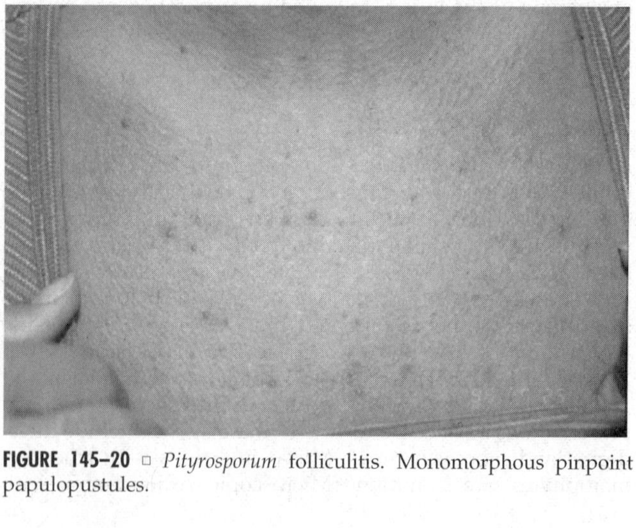

FIGURE 145–20 □ *Pityrosporum* folliculitis. Monomorphous pinpoint papulopustules.

is possible that steroid acne is a variant of *Pityrosporum* folliculitis. Diagnosis is usually made by skin biopsy with use of special stains to demonstrate the presence of budding yeast forms in the follicle, but the organism can occasionally be identified by a KOH examination of the contents of a pustule. Treatment is as for tinea versicolor, but oral therapy, at least initially, may be required. Topical amphotericin B can also be used.

SEBORRHEIC DERMATITIS

P. ovale has been implicated in both infantile and adult seborrheic dermatitis.[16] Characterized by orange-red to dull red plaques with greasy scale, seborrheic dermatitis typically involves the scalp and hairline, ears and retroauricular folds, forehead, glabella, eyebrows, nasolabial folds, and beard and mustache areas. Blepharitis may be seen, and fissuring below the earlobe is common when this site is involved. The central chest and back and the axillae and groin may also be involved. Cultures have repeatedly demonstrated increased carriage of *Pityrosporum* in patients with seborrheic dermatitis compared with unaffected patients, and topical agents such as ketoconazole are efficacious in treating the disease.[73] The condition is also seen with increased frequency and severity in patients with AIDS. It is believed that abnormal host immune response to *Pityrosporum* causes the aberrant inflammatory reaction and dermatitis, possibly through the alternative pathway of complement activation.[71, 101(p157), 107]

The differential diagnosis of seborrheic dermatitis includes psoriasis, tinea corporis, tinea capitis, and occasionally lupus erythematosus. Effective treatments include antifungal preparations such as ketoconazole cream and shampoo, selenium sulfide, and zinc pyrithione; keratolytics such as salicylic acid and sulfur; and tars and mild topical steroids, which suppress inflammation.

ATOPIC DERMATITIS

Evidence that *Pityrosporum* may be an important allergen in some patients with atopic dermatitis is mounting. In both children and young adults with atopic dermatitis, there appears in general to be increased sensitization to *P. ovale;* in particular, sensitization to *P. ovale* appears to correlate with atopic dermatitis involving the face, scalp, neck, and upper back of adults. Whether hypersensitivity to *P. ovale* is pathogenic or is merely an epiphenomenon due to altered skin barrier function leading to increased sensitization has not yet been determined.[108] Reports of clearance of dermatitis with ketoconazole treatment suggest that *P. ovale* may be pathogenic.[107] In addition, although colonization is not increased in patients with atopic dermatitis, specific immunoglobulin E antibodies to *P. ovale* are found only in atopic individuals and occur more frequently in children with atopic dermatitis than in patients with other forms of atopy.[14, 108] Positive skin prick test responses to *P. ovale* are also seen only in patients with atopic dermatitis, primarily in adolescents and adults.[107, 108]

CONFLUENT AND RETICULATED PAPILLOMATOSIS

Confluent and reticulated papillomatosis of Gougerot and Carteaud is characterized by the presence of hyperpigmented thin scaly or hyperkeratotic papules that become confluent centrally, with a reticulated pattern peripherally, primarily over the chest and central back. It is usually seen in adolescents and young adults. The clinical appearance, coupled with reports of patients with this condition in whom *M. furfur* was demonstrated on biopsy and who responded to ketoconazole or other treatments for tinea versicolor, has led to speculation by some authors that this condition may be caused by *P. ovale* or by an abnormal host response to this normal inhabitant of the skin.[107, 115] However, in most patients, the presence of *Pityrosporum* cannot be demonstrated and treatment directed against this agent is unsuccessful. On the basis of histologic and electron microscopic data as well as response to retinoids and other agents that work by altering keratinization, numerous reports have suggested that this disease is instead a disorder of abnormal keratinization.[116–121] Possibly, abnormal keratinization predisposes patients with this condition to infection with *Pityrosporum*, leading to the early hypothesis that it was causative.

DISSEMINATED INFECTIONS

Pityrosporum, presumably because of its lipophilic nature, has been reported as a cause of sepsis in premature neonates and adults with underlying gastrointestinal disease, associated with intravenous intralipid feeding.* It presents with fever, leukocytosis, and thrombocytopenia, sometimes with pulmonary infiltrates; lipid-rich culture media are necessary for the isolation of the organism from blood cultures.[101(p157), 109, 110, 122] Yeast may sometimes be visualized on Gram stain of the buffy coat from central venous blood specimens.[110] When blood specimens are drawn from patients receiving parenteral lipids, consideration should be given to the possibility of sepsis with a lipophilic fungus such as *M. furfur*, and special lipid-supplemented media should be employed to assist in the isolation of such organisms; Sabouraud medium covered with a thin layer of sterile olive oil may suffice.[109, 110] Treatment consists of removal of the infected catheter, withdrawal of intralipid therapy, and chemotherapy with azoles or amphotericin B.[109, 110]

Host Immune Response and Pathophysiology

Various factors contribute to the host's resistance to dermatophyte infection. The local environment may be made less hospitable by medium chain free fatty acids on the skin surface, which potentiate the growth of *Pityrosporum* and inhibit that of dermatophytes; these free fatty acids may also interfere with fungal adhesion to keratinocytes.[16] However, it is primarily the host's cell-mediated immunity that clears the skin of dermatophyte infections, in part by producing keratinocyte proliferation, epidermal thickening, and scaling, leading to desquamation of infected skin, perhaps mediated by lymphocyte or monocyte cytokines.[9, 14, 16, 124] Immunophenotyping of dermal cellular infiltrates in two studies of biopsy specimens of tinea revealed helper T lymphocytes, with some Langerhans cells and macrophages, but essentially no B cells.[125, 126]

Nonspecific host immune defenses also play a role. Unsaturated transferrin (serum inhibitory factor) in sweat and serum produces inhibition of fungal growth by binding iron and making it unavailable to the fungus.[16, 124, 127] Growth is also inhibited by complement activation through the alternative pathway by products in fungal cell walls.[127] Neutrophil adhesion to opsonized and unopsonized hyphae also results in fungal growth inhibition but does not necessarily cause fungal killing.[127] Polymorphonuclear leukocyte activation and inhibition of fungal growth may occur even in the absence of cell-mediated immunity and appears to involve the myeloperoxidase–hydrogen peroxide–halide system.[127] Similarly, although dermatophytes will invade viable epidermis in tissue culture, they do not do so in vivo, even in the absence of

*References 16, 101(p157), 109, 110, 122, 123.

cell-mediated immunity, possibly because of this complement activation and neutrophil attack.[124]

Fungal substances such as cell wall mannans appear to suppress the host's immune response, preventing eradication of infection or predisposing to reinfection. Mannans inhibit turnover of the stratum corneum and in vitro suppress the immune response in several ways, possibly inhibiting lymphoproliferation by interfering with antigen presentation.[124, 128] Interestingly, *T. rubrum* mannans produce greater in vitro suppression of cell-mediated immune responses than do mannans from zoophilic dermatophytes.[124] This correlates clinically with the observation that zoophilic dermatophytes tend to produce inflammatory responses, whereas *T. rubrum*, an anthropophilic fungus, tends to produce chronic, noninflammatory infections such as moccasin-type tinea pedis. *T. rubrum* mannans may enable infections with other dermatophytes, because inoculation of the usually highly inflammatory *T. mentagrophytes* into patients chronically infected with *T. rubrum* produces only slight inflammation.[129] However, this could be due either to suppression by *T. rubrum* mannan or to an inherent host unresponsiveness that allowed chronic infection in the first place.[14]

An example of the give and take between dermatophyte and host is illustrated by tinea pedis due to *T. mentagrophytes*, which may consist of chronic low-grade scaling punctuated by acute episodes of vesicular tinea pedis. When local environmental factors tip the balance in favor of the fungus and proliferation and penetration into the stratum corneum lead to contact of the epidermis with fungal antigens, T-cell–mediated immune response is triggered, resulting in a vesicular dermatitis analogous to allergic contact dermatitis; the blistering and scaling serve to shed the fungus from the skin.[64]

Studies of such inflammatory infections show that clearing of experimental *T. mentagrophytes* infections in previously uninfected individuals is associated with the development of cell-mediated immunity, acute inflammatory reaction, and conversion to a positive response to the trichophytin intradermal test; subsequent reinfection requires a much larger inoculum and clears spontaneously.[124, 129] In contrast, chronic infections are associated with immunodeficiency, atopy, or predisposing local cutaneous environmental factors.[124] Poor cell-mediated immunity, the presence of an immunoglobulin E response, and negative trichophytin test result tend to be associated with chronic infections, requiring treatment, both in humans and in athymic rats.[129]

Specific immunoglobulin E antibodies to dermatophytes may block interactions between T cells and antigen-presenting cells, thus interfering with the development of delayed hypersensitivity.[129] Th1 cells produce interferon-γ, which promotes the development of delayed hypersensitivity and cell-mediated immunity; Th2 cells produce interleukin-4, which promotes immunoglobulin E production; preferential sensitization or response of either cell type may determine whether dermatophyte infections will be quickly cleared or will result in an immunoglobulin E host response and chronic infection.[14, 129] Interferon-γ, interleukin-2, and granulocyte-macrophage colony-stimulating factor were detected in the culture supernatant after incubation of trichophytin with peripheral blood mononuclear cells obtained from a patient with a dermatophyte infection; the authors postulated that these cytokines may play a role in the development of delayed-type hypersensitivity to trichophytin.[130]

Immunocompromised Hosts

Extensive, severe, recalcitrant dermatophyte infections may be seen in the setting of abnormal T-cell function, such as in patients with AIDS or other T-cell immune deficiencies.[16, 131] The sites and organisms are the same as those involved in normal patients, but infections are often more extensive and more chronic, and the appearance may be atypical; superficial fungal infections occur early in the clinical course of human immunodeficiency virus infection and affect almost all patients with advanced disease[71, 73, 132] (Fig. 145–21). Even dermatophytes as nonaggressive and noninvasive as *T. rubrum* may cause atypical, aggressive infections such as deep folliculitis, granuloma formation, and even abscesses in neutropenic or otherwise immunocompromised patients; other dermatophytes reported to cause local invasion in immunocompromised patients include *M. audouinii, T. schoenleinii, T. violaceum*, and *E. floccosum*.[70, 133] Dermatophyte infections in human immunodeficiency virus–positive patients, especially infections of a deep type, may require systemic oral therapy as well as topical treatment.[70] Patients treated with immunosuppressive agents for organ transplantation or hematologic malignant neoplasms, or those receiving systemic corticosteroids, may be at risk for extensive dermatophyte infections (Fig. 145–22). These may culminate in dermal invasion, usually presenting with erythematous papules or nodules within an area of chronic *T. rubrum* infection but sometimes appearing as firm or fluctuant dusky or hemorrhagic nodules.[134] Long-term topical steroid therapy or radiation therapy can also predispose to locally invasive disease.[135] The dematiaceous fungi can also cause abscesses in such hosts.[133] Invasive

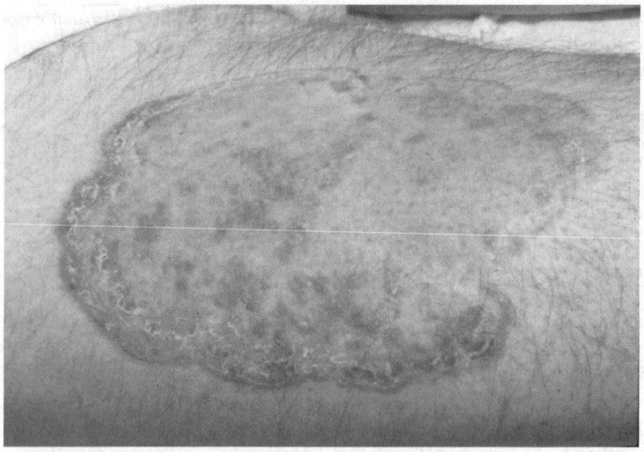

FIGURE 145–21 □ Tinea corporis on the thigh of a patient with AIDS. Large scaling erythematous plaque with numerous papules within it.

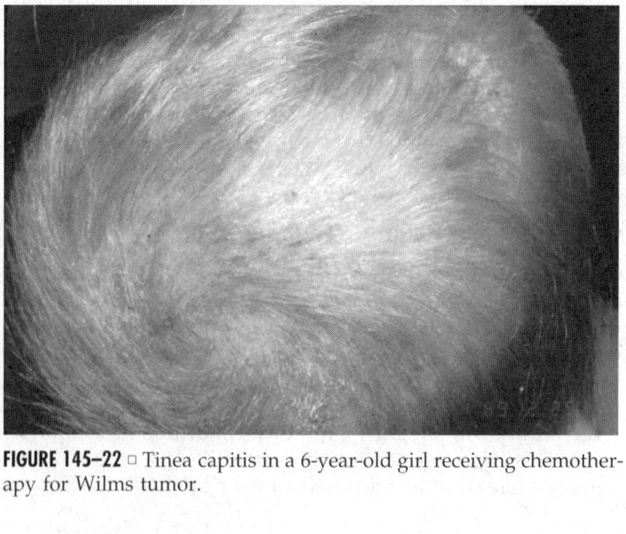

FIGURE 145–22 □ Tinea capitis in a 6-year-old girl receiving chemotherapy for Wilms tumor.

dermatophyte infections may occur while patients are receiving systemic therapy with amphotericin B, which, although it has in vitro activity against dermatophytes, is not effective in vivo against dermatophytes because it is not secreted in sweat or sebum and minimal tissue levels are obtained in the stratum corneum by passive diffusion. Consideration should be given to combined therapy with fluconazole and topical agents in such infections.[133] Candidal infections of various types are also common.

Organisms such as *P. ovale* and *T. beigelii*, which ordinarily cause benign superficial infections (tinea versicolor and white piedra, respectively), have been reported to cause systemic opportunistic infections in immunocompromised patients as well as in a neutropenic murine model.[16, 97–99, 136] Opportunistic infections with *T. beigelii* occur most commonly in neutropenic patients with underlying neoplasms but have also been reported in patients with AIDS and in those with a history of intravenous drug use, organ transplantation, and chronic active hepatitis.[97, 137] Infection often involves the lungs, kidneys, liver, spleen, and heart as well as the skin in approximately 30% of patients.[137] *T. beigelii* septic arthritis has been reported in a patient with acute leukemia.[138] The prognosis for disseminated trichosporosis is poor.[97] Several authors have found an increased frequency of rectal carriage of *T. beigelii* in homosexual men, as high as 15.5% compared with 3.1% for other hospitalized patients, raising the possibility of sexual transmission of this organism; not surprisingly, white piedra has also been reported to be sexually transmitted in heterosexuals.[97, 136, 139–141] *T. beigelii* has been found to colonize normal perigenital skin in about 12% of patients, more commonly in men than in women.[142]

Hosts who otherwise have normal immune systems but who have abnormal skin may also be predisposed to dermatophyte infections, which may be more dificult to diagnose because of the underlying skin disease. These include patients with various types of ichthyosis.[143–146] The apparent increased occurrence in patients with trisomy 21 may in part be due to the retention hyperkeratosis commonly seen in these patients, which provides a thickened stratum corneum that the fungus may invade. Increased occurrence has also been noted in hereditary palmoplantar keratodermas, in which the amount of keratin was considered the most important factor for dermatophyte affinity for the palms and soles.[147]

Nondermatophyte infections of many types are also common in immunocompromised patients, including candidiasis, which may involve multiple mucocutaneous sites, and disseminated fungal infections, including histoplasmosis, cryptococcosis, coccidioidomycosis, sporotrichosis, aspergillosis, and other infections that are covered elsewhere. As a general rule, however, fungal infections in patients with AIDS and other immunocompromised patients may present with atypical findings; therefore, the index of suspicion must be high and the threshold for biopsy and culture low.

Antifungal Agents and Therapy for Dermatophytoses

The choice of therapeutic agents in the treatment of dermatophyte infections is influenced by site affected, pathogen, severity, extent of infection, drug spectrum and efficacy, drug safety profile, potential drug interactions, dosage schedule and drug pharmacokinetics, patient's compliance, and cost. Required duration of therapy may also be a factor and varies with the agent, its antifungal mechanism, and the site of infection. For example, therapy with fungistatic drugs must be continued until the infected tissue has been shed, resulting in longer treatment courses for infections of the hair and nails than are required for infections involving only the skin. This can cause problems with the patient's compliance even in treating skin infections, because patients frequently discontinue therapy once symptoms have improved but before the infection has been adequately treated, increasing the risk for recurrence.[148, 149] For similar reasons, negative cultures generally precede negative results of the KOH examination by several weeks because of the delay in stratum corneum turnover.[150]

Routine fungal sensitivity testing is generally not available but may be of potential clinical use in the treatment of selected patients. Methods of assessing in vitro susceptibility of dermatophytes to antifungal agents include a simple disk diffusion method that measures growth inhibition zones and the more complicated dilution method for measuring minimal inhibitory concentrations.[151, 152] Staining with neutral red can also be used as an in vitro method of assessing the viability of fungal cells after exposure to antifungal agents.[153] In areas where routine testing is not available, awareness of patterns of drug susceptibility may help to guide therapy.

Many classes of antifungal agents are active against dermatophytes, and most are fungistatic and appear to work by interfering in fungal cell wall synthesis. The azoles include both the older imidazoles, such as clotrimazole, miconazole, and ketoconazole, and the newer triazoles itraconazole, terconazole, and fluconazole. These drugs inhibit cytochrome P-450 14-α-demethylase, blocking demethylation of lanosterol in membrane ergosterol biosynthesis.[42] The triazoles are slightly more specific for inhibition of fungal sterols compared with human sterols than are the original azole compounds.[105] Other types of compounds include the thiocarbamate tolnaftate, which inhibits squalene epoxidase and is active only against growing dermatophytes; ciclopirox olamine, which blocks membrane protein synthesis; and griseofulvin, which inhibits microtubule polymerization.[42] Griseofulvin is normally administered orally and delivered to the stratum corneum by sweat, but a few studies of this agent against experimentally induced *T. mentagrophytes* and various dermatophytes in tinea pedis and tinea corporis suggested that topical use may also be possible.[154, 155] Nystatin and amphotericin B are polyene antibiotics, which bind to ergosterol and disrupt fungal cell membrane transport and are generally active only against yeasts.[80] Newer classes of drugs that are fungicidal include the dimethylmorpholines (amorolfine) and the allylamines (naftifine, terbinafine). Dimethylmorpholines inhibit ergosterol synthesis at two steps, 14-reduction and 7-8–isomerization, causing accumulation of ignosterol and depletion of ergosterol in the fungal cell membrane.[42] Allylamines are broad-spectrum fungicidal agents; without inhibiting the host's cytochrome P-450, they inhibit squalene epoxidase, the enzyme that catalyzes the conversion of squalene to squalene-2,3-epoxide in the ergosterol synthetic pathway.[148] Interference with cell wall structure, and presumably function, by naftifine and terbinafine has been demonstrated by scanning electron microscopy, which revealed structural abnormalities of *E. floccosum* cell walls after treatment with these drugs.[156] In addition, some naturally occurring products, such as azelaic acid, have been shown to have in vitro activity against dermatophytes and several other fungi and may deserve further investigation.[14, 157]

Topical therapies currently available in the United States include the imidazoles, ciclopirox olamine, the allylamines, and tolnaftate, which is somewhat less effective. Most infections of the skin can be treated with these agents. In part because it is fungicidal, topical terbinafine produces high clinical and mycologic cure rates in brief treatment courses for interdigital tinea pedis, tinea cruris, tinea corporis, and chronic moccasin-type tinea pedis, with more rapid attainment of a higher cure rate and a lower relapse rate than traditional longer courses with clotrimazole.[149, 150, 158–162] One study suggested that terbinafine cream may be effective after a single application in the therapy of tinea pedis.[163] With moccasin-type tinea pedis, higher cure rates and lower relapse rates are obtained in patients without onychomycosis, because reinfection tends to occur owing to seeding from infected nails.[150] The other allylamine, naftifine, is also usually fungicidal and is frequently superior to other agents; however, a report of naftifine failure in two children with tinea corporis due to *T. tonsurans* suggested the need for additional in vivo studies in children with *T. tonsurans* infections.[164, 165] Another promising topical agent is amorolfine, not yet available in the United States, which is active against molds and *Candida* as well as dermatophytes; it produces excellent results in all types of tinea pedis, including infections with yeasts, mixed infections, and dermatophyte infections, including chronic *T. rubrum* moccasin-type tinea pedis.[166]

Oral therapy for dermatophyte infections is necessary for treatment of infections that involve the hair, nails, extensive areas of the skin, or multiple inoculation sites and often in recalcitrant infections such as chronic moccasin-type tinea pedis, although topical allylamines may suffice in the latter.[148] Griseofulvin is currently the treatment of choice for tinea capitis, although itraconazole, fluconazole, and oral terbinafine may become useful. Griseofulvin can also be used for extensive cutaneous infections, although it has a lower rate of clinical and mycologic cure and a higher relapse rate than oral terbinafine or itraconazole after a 2-week course.[167–169] Once-weekly doses of fluconazole for 1 to 4 weeks are also effective as therapy for tinea corporis and tinea cruris and slightly less so for tinea pedis.[170–172] The possible utility of oral ketoconazole for cutaneous dermatophyte infections is usually outweighed by the potential risk for hepatotoxic effects, even more so when the long treatment course necessary for nail infections is considered, but once-weekly dosing of 400 mg for 3 to 8 weeks can be used for dermatophyte infections of the skin.[42, 82, 173] Itraconazole in a dosage regimen of 100 mg daily for 2 weeks, or 200 mg daily for 1 week, is extremely effective in the treatment of tinea corporis and tinea cruris; tinea pedis can be treated with 200 mg twice daily for 1 week.[174–177]

Terbinafine, the newest allylamine, is lipophilic and keratinophilic and achieves excellent and persistent penetration into sebum and keratin, including nails; it is also rapidly fungicidal and highly active.[37] The drug persists in stratum corneum, nails, hair, and sebum for months after discontinuation of a 4-week oral course of 250 mg daily.[178] It is fungicidal against dermatophytes, molds, dimorphic fungi, and some yeasts but not against *Candida albicans*, and it is highly effective in the treatment of dermatophyte infections of the hair and nails.[38, 89] These characteristics allow brief treatment schedules that may enhance the patient's compliance. Although oral therapy would obviously be unnecessary for most patients with skin infections, terbinafine is also highly effective in 1- to 2-week courses for the treatment of tinea corporis, tinea cruris, and tinea pedis, and some patients may prefer the convenience of a brief course of oral medication to the use of a topical agent.[42, 179] Terbinafine may be slightly more effective than itraconazole in the treatment of tinea pedis and has a much lower relapse rate than griseofulvin in this condition.[180, 181] Adverse effects occur in about 10% of patients treated with oral terbinafine but tend to be mild; these effects include abdominal pain, nausea, rash, pruritus, headache, dizziness, fatigue, and anorexia.[38, 87]

Oral steroids may help to reduce the risk for and extent of permanent alopecia in the treatment of kerion, but the use of topical corticosteroids should be avoided in the treatment of dermatophyte infections. Combination products containing both a topical antifungal medication and a potent topical steroid have been advocated by some for treatment of inflammatory tinea to provide more rapid symptomatic relief. However, there is ample evidence that the steroid agents frequently impair the host's natural cell-mediated immunity to the point that the ability of the antifungal agent to eradicate the infection is overwhelmed.[68, 182] This may be even more of a problem with organisms that are less sensitive to the antifungal agent, as in the case of *M. canis* and clotrimazole.[182] In these cases, substitution of the identical antifungal ingredient without the steroid is often adequate to clear the infection, although when the infection has progressed to Majocchi granuloma, oral therapy may be required.

References

1. Macura AB: Dermatophyte infections. Int J Dermatol 32:313, 1993.
2. Al-Fouzan AS, Nanda A: Dermatophytosis of children in Kuwait. Pediatr Dermatol 9:27, 1992.
3. Lee JYY, Hsu ML: Pathogenesis of hair infection and black dots in tinea capitis caused by *Trichophyton violaceum*: A histopathological study. J Cutan Pathol 19:54, 1992.
4. Vargo K, Cohen BA: Prevalence of undetected tinea capitis in household members of children with disease. Pediatrics 92:155, 1993.
5. Hayes AG, Buntin DM, Wible LO: Black dot tinea capitis in a man. Int J Dermatol 32:740, 1993.
6. Venugopal PV, Venugopal TV: Tinea capitis in Saudi Arabia. Int J Dermatol 32:39, 1993.
7. Rippon JW: Forty-four years of dermatophytes in a Chicago clinic (1944–1988). Mycopathologia 119:25, 1992.
8. Rogers M, Muir D, Pritchard R: Increasing importance of *Trichophyton tonsurans* in childhood tinea in New South Wales. The pattern of childhood tinea in New South Wales, Australia, 1979–1988: The emergence of *Trichophyton tonsurans* as an important pathogen in tinea capitis in white children. Australas J Dermatol 34:5, 1993.
9. Odom R: Pathophysiology of dermatophyte infections. J Am Acad Dermatol 28:S2, 1993.
10. Aly R: Ecology and epidemiology of dermatophyte infections. J Am Acad Dermatol 31:S21, 1994.
11. Rippon JW: Dermatophytosis and dermatomycosis. *In* Rippon JW (ed): Medical Mycology: The Pathogenic Fungi and the Pathogenic Actinomycetes, ed 3. Philadelphia, WB Saunders, 1988, pp 175–177.
12. Hay RJ, Roberts SOB, MacKenzie DWR: Mycology. *In* Champion RH, Burton JL, Ebling FJG (eds): Textbook of Dermatology, ed 5. Boston, Blackwell Scientific Publications, 1992, pp 1127–1216.
13. Venugopal PV, Venugopal TV: Superficial mycoses in Saudi Arabia. Australas J Dermatol 33:45, 1992.
14. Rosenthal JR: Pediatric fungal infections from head to toe: What's new? Curr Opin Pediatr 6:435, 1994.
15. Stiller MJ, Rosenthal SA, Weinstein AS: Tinea capitis caused by *Trichophyton rubrum* in a 67 year old woman with systemic lupus erythematosus. J Am Acad Dermatol 29:257, 1993.
16. Hay RJ: Fungal skin infections. Arch Dis Child 67:1065, 1992.
17. Garg AP, Muller J: Fungitoxicity of fatty acids against dermatophytes. Mycoses 36:51, 1993.
18. Garg AP, Muller J: Inhibition of growth of dermatophytes by Indian hair oils. Mycoses 35:363, 1992.
19. Lunder M, Lunder M: Is *Microsporum canis* infection about to become a serious dermatological problem? Dermatology 184:87, 1992.
20. López-Gómez S, Del Palacio A, Van Cutsem J, et al: Itraconazole versus griseofulvin in the treatment of tinea capitis: A double-blind randomized study in children. Int J Dermatol 33:743, 1994.
21. Honig PJ, Caputo GL, Leyden JJ, et al: Microbiology of kerions. J Pediatr 123:422, 1993.
22. Honig PJ, Caputo GL, Leyden JJ, et al: Treatment of kerions. Pediatr Dermatol 11:69, 1994.
23. American Academy of Dermatology: Guidelines of care for

superficial mycotic infections of the skin: Tinea capitis and tinea barbae. *In* Dermatology World/Guidelines (Supplement). Schaumburg, IL, American Academy of Dermatoloy, 1995, pp 39–43.
24. Gondim-Goncalves HM, Mapurunga ACP, Melo-Monteiro C, et al: Tinea capitis caused by *Microsporum canis* in a newborn. Int J Dermatol 31:367, 1992.
25. Virgili A, Corazza M, Zampino MR: Atypical features of tinea in newborns. Pediatr Dermatol 10:92, 1993.
26. Cabon N, Moulinier C, Taieb A, et al: Tinea capitis and faciei caused by *Microsporon langeronii* in two neonates. Pediatr Dermatol 11:281, 1994.
27. Hiruma M, Kukita A: Tinea faciei caused by *Microsporum canis* in a newborn. Dermatologica 176:130, 1988.
28. Johnson ML, Anderson LL: Papulosquamous plaques in a mother and newborn son. Pediatr Dermatol 12:281, 1995.
29. Snider R, Landers S, Levy ML: The ringworm riddle: An outbreak of *Microsporum canis* in the nursery. Pediatr Infect Dis J 12:145, 1998.
30. Arnow PM, Houchins SG, Pugliese G: An outbreak of tinea corporis in hospital personnel caused by a patient with *Trichophyton tonsurans* infection. Pediatr Infect Dis J 10:355, 1991.
31. Pakula AS, Paller AS: Langerhans cell histiocytosis and dermatophytosis. J Am Acad Dermatol 29:340, 1993.
32. Hubbard TW, de Triquet JM: Brush-culture method for diagnosing tinea capitis. Pediatrics 90:416, 1992.
33. Frieden IJ, Howard R: Tinea capitis: Epidemiology, diagnosis, treatment, and control. J Am Acad Dermatol 31:S42, 1994.
34. Gatti S, Marinaro C, Bianchi L, et al: Treatment of kerion with fluconazole. Lancet 338:1156, 1991.
35. Elewski B: Tinea capitis: Itraconazole in *Trichophyton tonsurans* infection. J Am Acad Dermatol 31:65, 1994.
36. Legendre R, Escola-Macre J: Itraconazole in the treatment of tinea capitis. J Am Acad Dermatol 23:559, 1990.
37. Haroon TS, Hussain I, Mahmood A, et al: An open clinical pilot study of the efficacy and safety of oral terbinafine in dry noninflammatory tinea capitis. Br J Dermatol 126(Suppl 39):47, 1992.
38. Terbinafine for dermatophytes in skin and nail. Drug Ther Bull 30:47, 1992.
39. Derrick EK, Voyce ME, Price ML: *Trichophyton tonsurans* kerion in an elderly woman. Br J Dermatol 130:683, 1994.
40. Gordon PM, Stankler: Rapid clearing of kerion ringworm with terbinafine. Br J Dermatol 129:503, 1993.
41. Goulden V, Goodfield MJD: Treatment of childhood dermatophyte infections with oral terbinafine. Pediatr Dermatol 12:53, 1995.
42. Degreef HJ, De Doncker PRG: Current therapy of dermatophytosis. J Am Acad Dermatol 31:S25, 1994.
43. DeHart DJ: Tinea capitis. N Engl J Med 329:849, 1993.
44. Halasz CLG: Successful treatment with fluconazole of tinea corporis caused by *Trichophyton verrucosum* (barn itch). Cutis 54:207, 1994.
45. Shwayder T, Andreae M, Babel D: *Trichophyton equinum* from riding bareback: First reported U.S. case. J Am Acad Dermatol 30:785, 1994.
46. Terragni L, Marelli MA, Oriani A, et al: Tinea corporis bullosa. Mycoses 36:135, 1993.
47. Katoh T, Maruyama R, Nishioka K, et al: Tinea corporis due to *Microsporum canis* from an asymptomatic dog. J Dermatol 18:356, 1991.
48. Janniger CK: Majocchi's granuloma. Cutis 50:267, 1992.
49. Radentz WH, Yanase DJ: Papular lesions in an immunocompromised patient. Arch Dermatol 129:1189, 1993.
50. American Academy of Dermatology: Guidelines of care for superficial mycotic infections of the skin: Tinea corporis, tinea cruris, tinea faciei, tinea manuum, and tinea pedis. *In* Dermatology World/Guidelines (Supplement). Schaumburg, IL, American Academy of Dermatology, 1995, pp 22–26.
51. Stiller MJ, Klein WP, Dorman RI, et al: Tinea corporis gladiatorum: An epidemic of *Trichophyton tonsurans* in student wrestlers. J Am Acad Dermatol 27:632, 1992.
52. Cohen BA, Schmidt C: Tinea gladiatorum. N Engl J Med 327:820, 1992.
53. Werninghaus K: Tinea corporis in wrestlers (Letter). J Am Acad Dermatol 28:1022, 1993.
54. Cohen D, Foa H, Sangueza OP: Trichophytosis gladiatorum (Letter). J Am Acad Dermatol 28:1022, 1993.
55. Beller M, Gessner BD: An outbreak of tinea corporis gladiatorum on a high school wrestling team. J Am Acad Dermatol 31:197, 1994.
56. Budimulja U, Kuswadji K, Bramono S, et al: A double-blind, randomized, stratified controlled study of the treatment of tinea imbricata with oral terbinafine or itraconazole. Br J Dermatol 130(Suppl 43):29, 1994.
57. Baudraz-Rosselet F, Ruffieux P, Mancarella A, et al: Diaper dermatitis due to *Trichophyton verrucosum*. Pediatr Dermatol 10:368, 1993.
58. Education called best means of controlling tinea pedis. Mycology Observer 13:4, 1995.
59. Elewski B, Hay RJ: International Summit on Cutaneous Antifungal Therapy. Boston, Massachusetts, Nov. 11–13, 1994. J Am Acad Dermatol 33:816, 1995.
60. Roberts DT: Prevalence of dermatophyte onychomycosis in the United Kingdom: Results of an omnibus survey. Br J Dermatol 126(Suppl 39):23, 1992.
61. Williams HC: The epidemiology of onychomycosis in Britain. Br J Dermatol 129:101, 1993.
62. Kearse HL, Miller OF: Tinea pedis in prepubertal children: Does it occur? J Am Acad Dermatol 19:619, 1988.
63. McBride A, Cohen BA: Tinea pedis in children. Am J Dis Child 146:844, 1992.
64. Leyden JL: Tinea pedis pathophysiology and treatment. J Am Acad Dermatol 31:S31, 1994.
65. Leyden JJ: Progression of interdigital infections from simplex to complex. J Am Acad Dermtol 28:S7, 1993.
66. Nolting S, Bräutigam M: Clinical relevance of the antibacterial activity of terbinafine: A contralateral comparison between 1% terbinafine cream and 0.1% gentamicin sulphate cream in pyoderma. Br J Dermatol 126(Suppl 39):56, 1992.
67. Dahl MV, Grando SA: Chronic dermatophytosis: What is special about *Trichophyton rubrum*? Adv Dermatol 9:97–99, discussion 110, 1994.
68. Reynolds RD, Boiko S, Lucky AW: Exacerbation of tinea corporis during treatment with 1% clotrimazole/0.05% betamethasone dipropionate (Lotrisone). Am J Dis Child 145:1224, 1991.
69. Amantea MA, Drutz DJ, Rosenthal JR: Antifungals: A primary care primer. Patient Care 24:58, 1990.
70. Elmets CA: Management of common superficial fungal infections in patients with AIDS. J Am Acad Dermatol 31:S60, 1994.
71. Odom RB: Common superficial fungal infections in immunosuppressed patients. J Am Acad Dermatol 31:S56, 1994.
72. American Academy of Dermatology: Guidelines of care for superficial mycotic infections of the skin: Onychomycosis. *In* Dermatology World/Guidelines (Supplement). Schaumburg, IL, American Academy of Dermatology, pp 27–32.
73. Diagnosis and management of cutaneous fungal infections: *Pityrosporum* infections, onychomycosis, common superficial fungal infections in patients with HIV infections. *In* Clinical Mycology Update. Fairlawn, OH, Research Center, 1995, pp 1–7.
74. Midgley G, Moore MK, Cook JC, et al: Mycology of nail disorders. J Am Acad Dermatol 31:S68, 1994.
75. Nolting S, Bräutigam M, Weidinger G: Terbinafine in onychomycosis with involvement by non-dermatophytic fungi. Br J Dermatol 130(Suppl 43):16, 1994.
76. Scher RK, Barnett JM: Successful treatment of *Aspergillus flavus* onychomycosis with oral itraconazole. J Am Acad Dermatol 23:749, 1990.
77. Lauharanta J: Comparative efficacy and safety of amorolfine nail lacquer 2% versus 5% once weekly. Clin Exp Dermatol 17(Suppl 1):41, 1992.
78. Reinel D: Topical treatment of onychomycosis with amorolfine 5% nail lacquer: Comparative efficacy and tolerability of once and twice weekly use. Dermatology 184(Suppl 1):21, 1992.
79. Haria M, Bryson HM: Amorolfine. A review of its pharmacological properties and therapeutic potential in the treatment of onychomycosis and other superficial fungal infections. Drugs 49:103, 1995.
80. Goldgeier MH: Fungal infections of the skin, hair, and nails. Pediatr Ann 22:253, 1993.
81. Cohen PR, Scher RK: Topical and surgical treatment of onychomycosis. J Am Acad Dermatol 31:S74, 1994.
82. Piérard GE, Arrese-Estrada J, Piérard-Franchimont C: Treatment of onychomycosis: Traditional approaches. J Am Acad Dermatol 29:S41, 1993.

83. Roseeuw D, De Doncker P: New approaches to the treatment of onychomycosis. J Am Acad Dermatol 29:S45, 1993.
84. Roberts DT: Oral therapeutic agents in fungal nail disease. J Am Acad Dermatol 31:S78, 1994.
85. Systemic antifungal drugs. Med Lett Drugs Ther 36:16, 1994.
86. Bickers DR: Antifungal therapy: Potential interactions with other classes of drugs. J Am Acad Dermatol 31:S87, 1994.
87. Villars VV, Jones TC: Special features of the clinical use of oral terbinafine in the treatment of fungal diseases. Br J Dermatol 126(Suppl 39):61, 1992.
88. Watson A, Marley J, Ellis D, et al: Terbinafine in onychomycosis of the toenail: A novel treatment protocol. J Am Acad Dermatol 33:775, 1995.
89. Tüzün Y, Kotogyan A, Oguz O: Terbinafine: Efficacy and safety in the treatment of dermatophytosis. Int J Dermatol 31:720, 1992.
90. Arikian SR, Einarson TR, Kobelt-Nguyen G, et al: A multinational pharmacoeconomic analysis of oral therapies for onychomycosis. The onychomycosis study group. Br J Dermatol 130 (Suppl 43):35, 1994.
91. Einarson TR, Arikian SR, Shear NH: Cost-effectiveness analysis for onychomycosis therapy in Canada from a government perspective. Br J Dermatol 130(Suppl 43):32, 1994.
92. American Academy of Dermatology: Guidelines of care for superficial mycotic infections of the skin: Piedra. *In* Dermatology World/Guidelines (Supplement). Schaumburg, IL, American Academy of Dermatology, 1995, pp 33–35.
93. Kalter DC, Tschen JA, Cernoch PL, et al: Genital white piedra: Epidemiology, microbiology, and therapy. J Am Acad Dermatol 14:982, 1986.
94. Ellner KM, McBride ME, Kalter DC, et al: White piedra: Evidence for a synergistic infection. Br J Dermatol 123:355, 1990.
95. McBride ME, Ellner KM, Black HS, et al: A new *Brevibacterium* sp. isolated from infected genital hair of patients with white piedra. J Med Microbiol 39:255, 1993.
96. Fusaro RM, Miller NG: Onychomycosis caused by *Trichosporon beigelii* in the United States. J Am Acad Dermatol 11:747, 1984.
97. Nahass GT, Rosenberg SP, Leonardi CL, et al: Disseminated infection with *Trichosporon beigelii*. Arch Dermatol 129:1020, 1993.
98. Hospenthal D, Belay T, Lappin P, et al: Disseminated trichosporonosis in a neutropenic murine model. Mycopathologia 122:115, 1993.
99. El-Ani AS, Castillo NB: Disseminated infection with *Trichosporon beigelii*. N Y State J Med 84:457, 1984.
100. Gip L: Black piedra: The first case treated with terbinafine (Lamisil®). Br J Dermatol 130(Suppl 43):26, 1994.
101. Rippon JW: Superficial infections. *In* Rippon JW (ed): Medical Mycology: The Pathogenic Fungi and the Pathogenic Actinomycetes, ed 3. Philadelphia, WB Saunders, 1988, pp 154–168.
102. Frankel DH, Rippon JW: *Hendersonula toruloidea* infection in man. Index cases in the non-endemic North American host, and a review of the literature. Mycopathologia 105:175, 1989.
103. Elewski BE, Greer DL: *Hendersonula toruloidea* and *Scytalidium hyalinum*: Review and update. Arch Dermatol 127:1041, 1991.
104. Gupta AK, Sauder DN, Shear NH: Antifungal agents: An overview. Part II. J Am Acad Dermatol 30:911, 1994.
105. Hay RJ: Antifungal drugs on the horizon. J Am Acad Dermatol 31:S82, 1994.
106. Clayton YM: Relevance of broad-spectrum and fungicidal activity of antifungals in the treatment of dermatomycoses. Br J Dermatol 130(Suppl 43):7, 1994.
107. Faergemann J: *Pityrosporum* infections. J Am Acad Dermatol 31:S18, 1994.
108. Broberg A, Faergemann J, Johansson S, et al: *Pityrosporum ovale* and atopic dermatitis in children and young adults. Acta Derm Venereol (Stockh) 72:187, 1992.
109. Garcia CR, Johnston BL, Corvi G, et al: Intravenous catheter–associated *Malassezia furfur* fungemia. Am J Med 83:790, 1987.
110. Long JG, Keyserling HL: Catheter-related infection in infants due to an unusual lipophilic yeast—*Malassezia furfur*. Pediatrics 76:896, 1985.
111. American Academy of Dermatology: Guidelines of care for superficial mycotic infections of the skin: Pityriasis (tinea) versicolor. *In* Dermatology World/Guidelines (Supplement). Schaumburg, IL, American Academy of Dermatology, 1995, pp 36–38.
112. Fungal infections. *In* Arndt KA, Bowers KE, Chuttani AR: Manual of Dermatologic Therapeutics, ed 5. Boston, Little, Brown, 1995, pp 75–89.
113. Delescluse J: Itraconazole in tinea versicolor: A review. J Am Acad Dermatol 23:551, 1990.
114. Galadari I, El Komy M, Mousa A, et al: Tinea versicolor: Histologic and ultrastructural investigation of pigmentary changes. Int J Dermatol 31:253, 1992.
115. Griffiths WAD, Leigh IM, Marks R: Disorders of keratinization. *In* Champion RH, Burton JL, Ebling FJG (eds): Textbook of Dermatology, ed 5. Boston, Blackwell Scientific Publications, 1992, p 1390.
116. Lee MP, Stiller MJ, McClain SA, et al: Confluent and reticulated papillomatosis: Response to high-dose oral isotretinoin therapy and reassessment of epidemiologic data. J Am Acad Dermatol 31:327, 1994.
117. Hodge JA, Ray MC: Confluent and reticulated papillomatosis: Response to isotretinoin. J Am Acad Dermatol 24:654, 1991.
118. Barnette DJ Jr, Yeager JK: A progressive asymptomatic hyperpigmented papular eruption. Confluent and reticulated papillomatosis (CRP) of Gougerot and Carteaud. Arch Dermatol 129:1608, 1993.
119. Baalbaki SA, Malak JA, Al-Khars MAA: Confluent and reticulated papillomatosis. Treatment with etretinate. Arch Dermatol 129:961, 1993.
120. Jimbow M, Talpash O, Jimbow K: Confluent and reticulated papillomatosis: Clinical light and electron microscopic studies. Int J Dermatol 31:480, 1992.
121. Lee SH, Choi EH, Lee WS, et al: Confluent and reticulated papillomatosis: A clinical, histopathological, and electron microscopic study. J Dermatol 18:725, 1991.
122. Redline RW, Redline SS, Boxerbaum B, et al: Systemic *Malassezia furfur* infections in patients receiving intralipid therapy. Hum Pathol 16:815, 1985.
123. Powell DA, Aungst J, Snedden S, et al: Broviac catheter–related *Malassezia furfur* sepsis in five infants receiving intravenous fat emulsions. J Pediatr 105:987, 1984.
124. Dahl MV: Suppression of immunity and inflammation by products produced by dermatophytes. J Am Acad Dermatol 28:S19, 1993.
125. Brasch JB, Sterry W: Immunophenotypical characterization of inflammatory cellular infiltrates in tinea. Acta Derm Venereol (Stockh) 72:345, 1992.
126. Szepes E, Magyarlaki M, Battyani Z, et al: Immunohistochemical characterization of the cellular infiltrate in dermatophytosis. Mycoses 36:203, 1993.
127. Dahl MV: Dermatophytosis and the immune response. J Am Acad Dermatol 31:S34, 1994.
128. Blake JS, Dahl MV, Herron MJ, et al: An immunoinhibitory cell wall glycoprotein (mannan) from *Trichophyton rubrum*. J Invest Dermatol 96:657, 1991.
129. Jones HE: Immune response and host resistance of humans to dermatophyte infection. J Am Acad Dermatol 28:S12, 1993.
130. Koga T, Ishizaki H, Matsumoto T, et al: Cytokine production of peripheral blood mononuclear cells in a dermatophytosis patient in response to stimulation with trichophytin. J Dermatol 20:441, 1993.
131. Ohashi DK, Crane JS, Spira TJ, et al: Idiopathic $CD4^+$ T-cell lymphocytopenia with verrucae, basal cell carcinomas, and chronic tinea corporis infection. J Am Acad Dermatol 31:889, 1994.
132. Smith KJ, Skelton HG, Yeager J, et al: Cutaneous findings in HIV-1–positive patients: A 42-month prospective study. J Am Acad Dermatol 31:746, 1994.
133. Elewski BE, Sullivan J: Dermatophytes as opportunistic pathogens. J Am Acad Dermatol 30:1021, 1994.
134. Grossman ME, Pappert AS, Garzon MC, et al: Invasive *Trichophyton rubrum* infection in the immunocompromised host: Report of three cases. J Am Acad Dermatol 33:315, 1995.
135. Cohen PR, Maor MH: Tinea corporis confined to irradiated skin: Radiation port dermatophytosis. Cancer 70:1634, 1992.
136. Walzman M, Leeming JG: White piedra and *Trichosporon beigelii*: The incidence in patients attending a clinic in genitourinary medicine. Genitourin Med 65:331, 1989.
137. Walsh TJ: Trichosporonosis. Infect Dis Clin North Am 3:43, 1989.
138. McWhinney PH, Madgwick JC, Hoffbrand AV, et al: Successful

surgical management of septic arthritis due to *Trichosporon beigelii* in a patient with acute myeloid leukemia. Scand J Infect Dis 24:245, 1992.
139. Grainger CR: White piedra: A case with evidence of spread by contact. Trans R Soc Trop Med Hyg 80:87, 1986.
140. Torssander J, Carlsson B, Von Krogh G: *Trichosporon beigelii*: Increased occurrence in homosexual men. Mykosen 28:355, 1985.
141. Stenderup A, Schønheyder H, Ebbesen P, et al: White piedra and *Trichosporon beigelii* carriage in homosexual men. J Med Vet Mycol 24:401, 1986.
142. Ellner K, McBride ME, Rosen T, et al: Prevalence of *Trichosporon beigelii*. Colonization of normal perigenital skin. J Med Vet Mycol 29:99, 1991.
143. Moreno-Giménez JC: Infections by *Trichophyton rubrum* (Letter). J Am Acad Dermatol 24:323, 1991.
144. Sheetz K, Lynch PJ: Ichthyosis and dermatophyte fungal infection (Letter). J Am Acad Dermatol 24:321, 1991.
145. Shelley ED, Shelley WB, Schafer RL: Generalized *Trichophyton rubrum* infection in congenital ichthyosiform erythroderma. J Am Acad Dermatol 20:1133, 1989.
146. Agostini G, Geti V, Difonzo EM, et al: Dermatophyte infection in ichthyosis vulgaris. Mycoses 35:197, 1992.
147. Nielsen PG: Hereditary palmoplantar keratoderma and dermatophytosis in the northernmost county of Sweden (Norrbotten). Acta Derm Venereol Suppl (Stockh) 188:1, 1994.
148. Smith EB: Topical antifungal drugs in the treatment of tinea pedis, tinea cruris, and tinea corporis. J Am Acad Dermatol 28:S24, 1993.
149. Berman B, Ellis C, Leyden J, et al: Efficacy of a 1-week, twice-daily regimen of terbinafine 1% cream in the treatment of interdigital tinea pedis. J Am Acad Dermatol 26:956, 1992.
150. Savin R, Atton AV, Bergstresser PR, et al: Efficacy of terbinafine 1% cream in the treatment of moccasin-type tinea pedis: Results of placebo-controlled multicenter trials. J Am Acad Dermatol 30:663, 1994.
151. Macura AB: In vitro susceptibility of dermatophytes to antifungal drugs: A comparison of two methods. Int J Dermatol 32:533, 1993.
152. Venugopal PV, Venugopal TV: Disk diffusion susceptibility testing of dermatophytes with allylamines. Int J Dermatol 33:730, 1994.
153. Nishikawa T, Naka W: Evaluation of antifungal effects of terbinafine and itraconazole using neutral red staining. Br J Dermatol 130(Suppl 43):4, 1994.
154. Aly R, Bayles CI, Oakes RA, et al: Topical griseofulvin in the treatment of dermatophytoses. Clin Exp Dermatol 19:43, 1994.
155. Macasaet EN, Pert P: Topical (1%) solution of griseofulvin in the treatment of tinea corporis (Letter). Br J Dermatol 124:110, 1991.
156. Butty P, Mallie M, Bastide JM: Antifungal activity of allylamines on *Epidermophyton floccosum*: Scanning electron microscopy study. Mycopathologia 120:147, 1992.
157. Brasch J, Christophers E: Azelaic acid has antimycotic properties in vitro. Dermatology 186:55, 1993.
158. Zaias N, Berman B, Cordero CN, et al: Efficacy of a 1-week, once-daily regimen of terbinafine 1% cream in the treatment of tinea cruris and tinea corporis. J Am Acad Dermatol 29:646, 1993.
159. Evans EGV, Dodman B, Williamson DM, et al: Comparison of terbinafine and clotrimazole in treating tinea pedis. Br Med J 307:645, 1993.
160. Bergstresser PR, Elewski B, Hanifin J, et al: Topical terbinafine and clotrimazole in interdigital tinea pedis: A multicenter comparison of cure and relapse rates with 1- and 4-week treatment regimens. J Am Acad Dermatol 28:648, 1993.
161. Elewski BE, Bergstresser PR, Hanifin J, et al: Long-term outcome of patients with interdigital tinea pedis treated with terbinafine or clotrimazole. J Am Acad Dermatol 32:290, 1995.
162. Evans EG: A comparison of terbinafine (Lamisil) 1% cream given for one week with clotrimazole (Canesten) 1% cream given for four weeks, in the treatment of tinea pedis. Br J Dermatol 130(Suppl 43):12, 1994.
163. Evans EGV, Seaman RAJ, James IGV: Short-duration therapy with terbinafine 1% cream in dermatophyte skin infections. Br J Dermatol 130:38, 1994.
164. Rabinowitz L, Esterly NB: Naftifine (Naftin) in pediatrics. Pediatrics 90:652, 1992.
165. Turkish Multicenter Dermatophytosis Study Group: Naftifine treatment for dermatophytosis: Multicenter clinical investigations in Turkey. Int J Dermatol 31:247, 1992.
166. Nolting S, Reinel D, Semig G, et al: Amorolfine spray in the treatment of foot mycoses (a dose-finding study). Br J Dermatol 129:170, 1993.
167. Voravutinon V: Oral treatment of tinea corporis and tinea cruris with terbinafine and griseofulvin: A randomized double blind comparative study. J Med Assoc Thai 76:388, 1993.
168. Lachapelle JM, De Doncker P, Tennstedt D, et al: Itraconazole compared with griseofulvin in the treatment of tinea corporis/cruris and tinea pedis/manus: An interpretation of the clinical results of all completed double-blind studies with respect to the pharmacokinetic profile. Dermatology 184:45, 1992.
169. Katsambas A, Antoniou C, Frangouli E, et al: Itraconazole in the treatment of tinea corporis and tinea cruris. Clin Exp Dermatol 18:322, 1993.
170. Suchil P, Gei FM, Robles M, et al: Once-weekly oral doses of fluconazole 150 mg in the treatment of tinea corporis/cruris and cutaneous candidiasis. Clin Exp Dermatol 17:397, 1992.
171. Montero-Gei F, Perera A: Therapy with fluconazole for tinea corporis, tinea cruris, and tinea pedis. Clin Infect Dis 14(Suppl 1):S77, 1992.
172. Stengel F, Robles-Soto M, Galimberti R, et al: Fluconazole versus ketoconazole in the treatment of dermatophytoses and cutaneous candidiasis. Int J Dermatol 33:733, 1994.
173. Segal R, Trattner A, Alteras I, et al: Once-weekly treatment with oral ketoconazole for superficial fungal infections. J Am Acad Dermatol 28:126, 1993.
174. Decroix J: Tinea pedis (moccasin-type) treated with itraconazole. Int J Dermatol 34:122, 1995.
175. Pariser DM, Pariser RJ, Ruoff G, et al: Double-blind comparison of itraconazole and placebo in the treatment of tinea corporis and tinea cruris. J Am Acad Dermatol 31:232, 1994.
176. Ketele A, Moens M, Stoops K, et al: International Registration File R 51211/86. Titusville, NJ, Janssen Pharmaceutica, 1987.
177. Parent D, Decroix J, Heenen M: Clinical experience with short schedules of itraconazole in the treatment of tinea corporis and/or tinea cruris. Dermatology 189:378, 1994.
178. Faergemann J, Zehender H, Denouël J, et al: Levels of terbinafine in plasma, stratum corneum, dermis-epidermis (without stratum corneum), sebum, hair and nails during and after 250 mg terbinafine orally once per day for four weeks. Acta Derm Venereol (Stockh) 73:305, 1993.
179. Farag A, Taha M, Halim S: One-week therapy with oral terbinafine in cases of tinea cruris/corporis. Br J Dermatol 131:684, 1994.
180. De Keyser P, De Backer M, Massart DL, et al: Two-week oral treatment of tinea pedis, comparing terbinafine (250 mg/day) with itraconazole (100 mg/day): A double-blind, multicentre study. Br J Dermatol 130(Suppl 43):22, 1994.
181. Hay RJ, Logan RA, Moore MK, et al: A comparative study of terbinafine versus griseofulvin in 'dry-type' dermatophyte infections. J Am Acad Dermatol 24:243, 1991.
182. Rosen T, Elewski B: Failure of clotrimazole–betamethasone dipropionate cream in treatment of *Microsporum canis* infections. J Am Acad Dermatol 32:1050, 1995.

VIRAL EXANTHEMS AND LOCALIZED VIRAL SKIN INFECTIONS

146

Measles

David I. Bernstein
Gilbert M. Schiff

Measles (rubeola) is a highly contagious disease that produces a distinct clinical syndrome. Measles has been recognized since the 7th century, although it was first described as a distinct disease by Rhazes in the 10th century. Measles virus is a singular entity belonging to the family Paramyxoviridae, genus *Morbillivirus.* It is an enveloped single-stranded RNA virus similar to other animal viruses, such as canine distemper virus and bovine rinderpest virus (see discussions of RNA viruses and Chapter 253 for details of the history and physical and biologic properties).

The epidemiologic picture of measles in developed countries has been altered dramatically by the introduction of effective vaccines.[1] Instead of being one of the most common childhood exanthems, it is now associated with outbreaks among adolescents and young adults or unvaccinated children younger than school age who remain susceptible because they lack either proper childhood immunizations or natural exposure. In developing nations, measles is usually acquired before the age of 5 years and remains a leading cause of death[2] (see discussions of RNA viruses and Chapter 253 for details of the epidemiology and pathogenesis).

Clinical Manifestations

The incubation period for measles is 10 to 14 days and may be somewhat longer in adults than in children (Fig. 146–1). This period is usually asymptomatic, although some patients develop mild transient respiratory symptoms, fever, or a morbilliform rash shortly after infection.[3] The prodromal phase, probably coinciding with the secondary viremia,[4] follows and persists for 2 to 4 days. Initial manifestations include malaise and fever accompanied within 24 hours by coryza, conjunctivitis, and cough. These symptoms gradually increase in severity and peak with the onset or height of the exanthem on the fourth to sixth day. A typical case of measles lasts 7 to 10 days.

Fever usually increases in a stepwise fashion. Maximal temperature coincides with the peak of the rash, followed by a rapid decline to normal. Occasionally the temperature is elevated for the first day or two, followed by an afebrile period of a day and then a rapid rise up to 40.5°C at the peak of the rash. In some patients, the temperature may peak by the end of the first day and remain elevated at 39.5°C to 40.5°C for the next 5 to 6 days. Defervescence usually occurs by lysis over 24 hours. Fever that persists after the third or fourth day of the rash should raise suspicion of a complication.

Respiratory symptoms are similar to those produced during a severe common cold. Coryza begins with frequent sneezing followed by nasal congestion and a copious mucopurulent discharge, which becomes most prominent at the peak of the exanthem. Continued nasal discharge after defervescence suggests a secondary bacterial infection. The cough has a brassy quality, suggesting laryngeal and tracheal involvement, and is caused by the inflammatory reaction in the respiratory tract. Although there is usually marked improvement when the fever subsides, a mild cough may persist for a week or two.

The degree of conjunctivitis can be quite variable. A transverse marginal line of conjunctival injection can be seen during the early prodromal period[5] but is obscured later by the marked injection of the conjunctiva and caruncle. Conjunctivitis is associated with edema of the lids and increased lacrimation. Photophobia is common and may be severe in older patients.

Koplik spots, the pathognomonic lesions of measles, were originally described by Koplik in 1896.[6] They are faint, white 1- to 2-mm elevated lesions on an erythematous background that occur on the buccal mucosa. They first appear 2 days before the onset of rash opposite the lower molars. Within 24 hours they increase dramatically in number to involve most of the buccal and lower labial mucosa. The erythematous background is bright red and granular in appearance. The erythematous areas coalesce to form a diffuse bright red background, so that the Koplik spots resemble grains of salt on a red background. They fade rapidly and are difficult to see after 3 days. By the end of the third day of rash the mucous membranes appear normal, although the posterior pharyngeal wall may be injected and symptoms of a sore throat may appear by the end of the prodromal period.

The rash of measles appears about the 14th day after exposure, 3 to 4 days after the onset of illness. The erythematous maculopapular eruption begins behind the ears and involves the forehead at the hairline and upper part of the neck. It then spreads centrifugally, and by the third day the face, neck, trunk, upper extremities, buttocks, and lower extremities are involved. The soles of the feet and the palms of the hands are not involved. The initial lesions are light pink and discrete, but they become confluent at the earliest involved sites. Those on the extremities remain fairly discrete.

The exanthem begins to fade by 3 days, following the same sequence as its appearance. Thus, the face and upper trunk may be clear by the fourth day, although lesions are still present on the lower extremities. The initial color of the rash is red, and lesions blanch with pressure. After 3 to 4 days as the rash begins to fade it assumes a brownish coppery appearance. The brownish discoloration (staining) does not clear with pressure and is probably the result of capillary hemorrhages. The exanthem typically lasts 6 to 7 days; its end is marked by a fine desquamation most frequently involving the confluent areas. In contrast to scarlet fever, the skin of the hands and feet does not desquamate.

Malaise and anorexia are also common during the febrile period. Young children may occasionally have diarrhea, vomiting, and abdominal pain. Pharyngitis is common during the exanthem period and may be accompanied by enlargement of the cervical and posterior-auricular nodes. Generalized lymphadenopathy and splenomegaly may occur in severe cases.

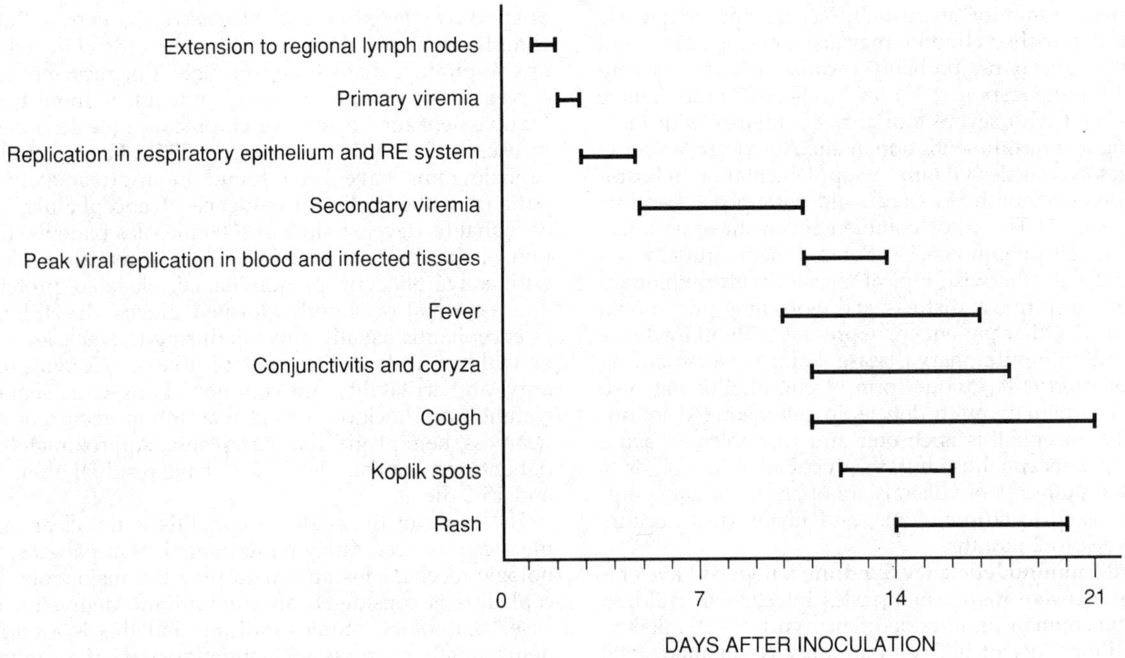

FIGURE 146–1 □ After inoculation of the epithelial surface of the nasopharynx, this sequence of events takes place during uncomplicated measles. RE, Reticuloendothelial.

At the height of the illness, usually the second day of the rash, the patient appears to be quite miserable. He or she has a diffuse rash, high temperature, malaise, copious nasal discharge, cough, and conjunctivitis. These symptoms are followed by a relatively uneventful short convalescence unless complications occur. Persistence of fever beyond the third day of rash should arouse suspicion of a complication. Although nutritional status and age are commonly thought of as the major risk factors for severe infections, other researchers have suggested that overcrowding and intensive exposure may be more important.[7, 8]

Atypical Measles

In 1965, Rauh and Schmidt[9] reported a severe atypical form of measles occurring in children who had received inactivated measles vaccine 2 to 4 years previously. These findings were later confirmed by others.[10, 11] In 1968, killed measles vaccine was discontinued in the United States. Although most commonly associated with the previous administration of killed measles vaccine, a similar atypical syndrome occurred in some children who received live measles vaccine.[12, 13]

The incubation period of atypical measles is similar to that of typical measles. The prodromal period is marked by the acute onset of high fever and headache. The rash appears after a prodrome of 1 to 3 days. Unlike that in typical measles, the rash begins peripherally and progresses in a cephalad direction. The rash is usually maculopapular but can be urticarial, petechial, or purpuric. In some cases this rash becomes vesicular, which may lead to confusion with varicella. The rash is most prominent on the ankles and wrists and may involve the palms and soles, similar to the exanthem of Rocky Mountain spotted fever. Koplik spots are a rare manifestation.

Respiratory distress is common, although coryza and conjunctivitis are less prominent. Radiographic evaluation reveals pulmonary involvement in virtually all cases. Lobar or segmental lesions are often nodular in appearance. Pleural effusions are common. Patients are frequently severely ill, with high fever and edema of the extremities accompanying the respiratory problems. Illness may last 2 weeks or more.

Measles virus has not been isolated from these patients but measles antibody patterns are characteristic. Before infection, antibody levels are low or undetectable. Antibody levels then increase rapidly and become quite high, especially levels of antibody to the H protein, which exceed those seen after recovery from typical measles. In contrast, little if any antibody to the F and P proteins is seen.[14, 15] A preferential induction of Th1 cells by the inactivated vaccine, as opposed to the Th2-like response seen with natural infection, could also potentiate a response like that of delayed-type hypersensitivity and be responsible for the symptoms observed.[14, 15]

Modified Measles

Modified measles is a mild form that occurs in partially immune individuals. Partial immunity can result from the presence of maternally derived transplacental antibody (infants younger than 9 months old), administration of serum immune globulin (IG) to exposed susceptible children, or varying immunity in those previously immunized with live viral vaccines.[16–18] Modified measles may also rarely occur as a reinfection in those with documented previous measles and secondary immunologic responses.[19, 20]

The symptoms of modified measles are similar to but milder than those of measles. The incubation period may be longer (14 to 21 days) and the prodromal period slightly shorter. Cough, coryza, conjunctivitis, and fever are minimal and Koplik spots are few in number or absent. Similarly, the exanthem follows the same progression as that in measles but is milder and confluence of lesions does not occur.

Measles in Immunocompromised Patients and in Patients with Acquired Immunodeficiency Syndrome

Measles infections in patients who are immunocompromised by chemotherapy or by inherited or acquired disorders of cell-mediated immunity are usually severe and frequently fatal.[21, 22] Malnourished children may also develop severe and fatal measles infections, probably because of deficient cell-mediated immune responses.[23] Low levels of vitamin A have been associated with severe mortality in children with measles, leading to a recommendation by the American Academy of Pediatrics to consider vitamin A supplementation in hospitalized patients 6 months to 2 years old with measles and its complications.[24, 25] The most common severe measles infection is giant cell pneumonia.[22, 23] Some patients initially develop severe but otherwise typical measles with pulmonary involvement, respiratory distress, and worsening pneumonia during 1 week. Other patients may present without evidence of a rash and with pulmonary disease that gets worse during 1 month or more.[26] A unique form of encephalitis has also been noted in patients with deficits in cell-mediated immunity.[27, 28] The encephalitis is chronic and resembles subacute sclerosing panencephalitis, but the incubation period is 5 weeks to 6 months.[27] Convulsions are often the initial symptom. Progression to stupor, coma, and finally death occurs within 1 week to 2 months.

Acquired Immunodeficiency Syndrome. Reports have emphasized the severe nature of measles infection in children infected with human immunodeficiency virus.[28, 29] Similar to other conditions in which T-cell immunity is impaired, fatal measles infection can develop in the absence of a rash.[30] Because there have been no reports of complications resulting from measles vaccination in infants with human immunodeficiency virus infection, present recommendations are to immunize these children.[31] However, a case of severe measles pneumonitis[31a] in a revaccinated 20-year-old man has prompted a reevaluation of this policy (see the later section on active immunization). Because documented immunization and low antibody level do not guarantee protection after exposure, infants with human immunodeficiency virus infection should be given IG prophylaxis after measles exposure.[32]

Measles in Pregnant Women

Unlike rubella, measles infection during pregnancy does not appear to cause congenital malformation. Measles infection of a pregnant woman can, however, lead to spontaneous abortion prematurely[33] and stillbirth.[4]

Complications

Complications of measles may be due to the direct consequences of viral infection, secondary bacterial infection, or both. Sudden appearance of leukocytosis and prolonged fever should alert the physician to the possibility of complications.

Otitis media is the most common complication of measles and the most likely cause of a persistent fever. It is more common in infants, those with previous episodes of otitis, and those with severe disease. The usual pathogens responsible for otitis media are involved. Laryngitis and laryngotracheitis are also common, but mastoiditis has declined dramatically with the use of antibiotics.

Some pulmonary involvement occurs in the majority of cases of measles and accounts for more than 90% of measles deaths.[34] Pulmonary involvement is seen as bronchiolitis in infants or as bronchopneumonia or lobar pneumonia. Pneumonia caused by direct viral invasion is characterized by bilateral hyperinflation with diffuse, fluffy infiltrates. Bacterial superinfection of the respiratory tract is difficult to distinguish from the primary viral infection and is caused by the common respiratory pathogens *Haemophilus influenzae*, *Streptococcus pyogenes*, and *Staphylococcus aureus*. Pulmonary complications should be considered in the child who develops respiratory distress and persistent or recurrent fevers.

Neurologic complications are not uncommon in measles. Involvement can be acute or chronic (see the section on RNA viruses in Part VIII and Chapter 253). Abnormal electroencephalograms have been found in approximately 50% of patients without clinical evidence of encephalitis.[35] Clinical encephalitis develops in 1 in 1000 measles patients. Examination of the cerebrospinal fluid usually reveals a pleocytosis with a lymphocytic predominance, elevated protein level, and a normal or slightly elevated glucose level. Symptoms of encephalitis usually develop during the measles exanthem or within 8 days of the onset of illness.[36] Convulsions, lethargy, and irritability are common. Long-term sequelae are common and include mental retardation, recurrent seizures, deafness, hemiplegia, and paraplegia. Approximately 60% of patients recover completely, 25% have residual brain damage, and 15% die.

The cause of the acute encephalitis is not clear. Although measles virus can rarely be recovered from patients,[37] immunologic mechanisms appear to play the major role. This encephalitis is considered an autoimmune demyelinating disease.[38] Pathologic studies indicate that this is a perivenular demyelinating disease with the induction of an immune response to myelin basic protein.

Less frequent complications include myocarditis, pericarditis,[39] and transient hepatitis.[40]

Diagnosis

The diagnosis of typical measles in an epidemic setting is straightforward and based on history and physical findings. Sporadic cases in a highly immunized population may be difficult to diagnose. Laboratory tests may be of value in this situation.

The differential diagnosis of measles should include all illnesses associated with an erythematous maculopapular rash. The brown discoloration and intensity of the measles rash—in the presence of a history of typical febrile prodrome (3 to 4 days) with cough, coryza, conjunctivitis, and caudal progression of the rash—make differentiation from rubella, erythema infectiosum, roseola infantum, and enteroviral infection relatively simple. A history of possible exposure should always be sought. The exanthems produced by Epstein-Barr virus and *Mycoplasma pneumoniae* infections, Rocky Mountain spotted fever, and drug eruption may be the most difficult to differentiate from measles. The presence of Koplik spots is considered pathognomonic.

Laboratory confirmation can be of value in suspected cases. Virus isolation or rapid detection of measles antigens in nasopharyngeal secretions can be attempted, but these techniques are difficult and not readily available.[41, 42] Therefore, laboratory confirmation of measles is usually accomplished by serologic tests that document a significant rise in antibody titer.[41] The hemagglutination inhibition assay has been the most commonly used test but is now being replaced by the enzyme-linked immunosorbent assay.[43] Serum antibodies usually appear 1 to 3 days after onset of the rash and peak 3 to 4 weeks later. Paired serum samples obtained early in the course of illness and 7 to 14 days later usually show a significant rise in antibody, confirming the diagnosis, although a single specimen can be used to detect the presence of immunoglobulin M antibody.[43]

Treatment

No specific antiviral drugs or agents have been shown to be effective for the treatment of typical and atypical measles or the viral complications of measles. Therapy with intravenous ribavirin has, however, been associated with reversal of respiratory compromise in adults with severe measles pneumonitis.[44] High doses of vitamin A also appear to reduce the morbidity and mortality of young children hospitalized with measles in developing countries.[45, 46] The World Health Organization has therefore recommended vitamin A for children with acute measles in areas with high measles mortality.[24, 25] Antibiotics are indicated when secondary bacterial infection occurs.

Prevention

Effective methods (passive and active prophylaxis) are available for the prevention of measles.

Passive Immunization

It is desirable to prevent or modify measles infection after exposure of children younger than 1 year old; chronically ill patients; immunosuppressed patients, including symptomatic human immunodeficiency virus–infected patients; and pregnant women. Human IG administered intramuscularly within 6 days after exposure has been shown to be effective.[47] A single dose of 0.25 mL/kg is recommended. For immunocompromised patients, in whom the consequences of measles infection are serious, the dose should be 0.5 mL/kg. If active disease is prevented by the administration of IG, follow-up active immunization is necessary unless contraindicated. The vaccine should be administered at least 3 months later in these patients provided they are 15 months of age or older.

Active Immunization

Highly effective, safe vaccines have been available to prevent measles since 1963. Initially, both inactivated and attenuated live measles vaccines were developed.[48] The inactivated vaccines required a series of inoculations, and the early live attenuated vaccines were administered simultaneously with IG to avoid a high rate of side effects. In 1965, further attenuated live measles vaccines were developed. When used properly, these vaccines are 90% to 95% effective. Factors that must be considered at the time of vaccination include age, interval since use of other blood products (e.g., IG), concurrent illness, and storage conditions.

Although a goal of eliminating measles from the United States by 1982[49] has not been realized, its incidence has been dramatically lowered.[14] Continued outbreaks of measles with an increase in annual cases have been the result of failure to immunize preschool and inner city children sufficiently, the residual effect of immunization of children at less than 12 months of age, use of killed IG in the 1960s, and poor stability and storage of vaccine lots in the past.[48] The increased number of outbreaks during the winter and spring of 1989 prompted new recommendations by the American Academy of Pediatrics and the Advisory Committee on Immunization Practices.[24, 50]

The new recommendations include two doses of vaccine for all children. The policy initially recommended that the first dose be given as a combined measles, mumps, and rubella vaccination at 15 months of age. In 1993, the recommendation for the first dose of measles vaccine was extended to allow vaccination at 12 to 15 months of age. This is at least partially due to the fact that infants now receive less maternal antibody, probably because it is largely vaccine-induced rather than infection-induced antibody and higher rates of seroconversion at 12 months have been detected in infants born to mothers with vaccine-induced immunity.[51] The recommendations by the two groups differ with regard to the age for the second immunization. The Advisory Committee on Immunization Practices recommends the second dose at school entry (4 to 6 years of age), whereas the American Academy of Pediatrics recommends the second dose at entry into middle school or junior high school (11 to 12 years of age). The recommendation of the Advisory Committee on Immunization Practices is based on use and feasibility, whereas the American Academy of Pediatrics recommendations are designed to decrease the number of outbreaks occurring in junior high and high schools. Children vaccinated before their first birthday should have another vaccination at 15 months of age, using measles, mumps, and rubella vaccine and a third dose as described earlier.

Recipients of killed vaccine, those who received live vaccine before their first birthday, those who were born after 1957 who have no history of measles or vaccination, those who received an unknown type of measles vaccine from 1963 to 1967 or received an unknown type of vaccine and simultaneous IG, those who were immunized before 1979, and all known susceptible individuals within 72 hours of exposure to measles should receive vaccine. Contraindications include anaphylaxis to egg ingestion and allergy to neomycin, recipients of IG within 3 months, altered immunity, and pregnancy. The last is on theoretical grounds alone.

The available data suggest that human immunodeficiency virus–infected children can be vaccinated safely.[47, 52–54] One case of severe measles pneumonitis after the second dose of measles-mumps-rubella vaccine prompted the following change in recommendations from the American Advisory Committee on Immunization Practices.[31a] The committee suggested that it may be prudent to withhold measles-mumps-rubella or measles vaccine from human immunodeficiency virus–infected persons with evidence of severe immunosuppression based on $CD4^+$ cell counts. Measles-mumps-rubella vaccine is still recommended for human immunodeficiency virus–infected persons who are not severely immunocompromised. Because measles is a severe disease in human immunodeficiency virus–infected patients, measles vaccine is recommended for children infected with the virus.[24] These patients may, however, respond poorly to vaccination[53–55] and should be given IG if exposed.[24] Measles vaccination is not recommended for other patients with significant immunodeficiency.

In underdeveloped countries, where measles is a major cause of death in young children, vaccine recommendations are different. Thus, efforts are largely directed to immunization of younger children using methods that are designed to overcome the protection provided by maternally derived antibody. These efforts have included multiple doses of vaccine, use of aerolization, or the Edmonston-Zagreb strain of measles.[14, 56, 57] Use of high-titer vaccine in children at 6 months initially appeared to be promising but later was associated with higher than usual mortality, not from measles but from other concurrent infections.[58, 59] This increased mortality was especially evident in girls.[59, 60] The use of high-titer vaccine has now been discouraged by the World Health Organization.[61] The World Health Organization's expanded program on immunization currently recommends standard-titer live attenuated measles vaccine at 9 months of age in developing countries.[62]

References

1. Markowitz LE, Preblud SR, Orenstein WA, et al: Patterns of transmission in measles outbreaks in the United States 1985–1986. N Engl J Med 320:75, 1989.
2. World Health Organization: Expanded Programme on Immuni-

zations. Global Advisory Group. Revised Plan of Action for Global Measles Control. Geneva, World Health Organization, 1993. Working paper 10.
3. Partington MW, Quinton JFP: The preeruptive illness of measles. Arch Dis Child 34:149, 1959.
4. Kempe CH, Fulginiti VA: The pathogenesis of measles virus infection. Arch Virusforsch 16:103, 1965.
5. Stimson PM: The earlier diagnosis of measles. JAMA 90:660, 1928.
6. Koplik H: The diagnosis of the invasion of measles from a study of the exanthema as it appears on the buccal mucous membrane. Arch Pediatr 13:918, 1896.
7. Aaby P: Malnutrition and overcrowding/intensive exposure in severe measles infection: Review of community studies. Rev Infect Dis 10:478, 1988.
8. Lamb WH: Epidemic measles in a highly immunized rural West African (Gambian) village. Rev Infect Dis 10:457, 1988.
9. Rauh LW, Schmidt R: Measles immunization with killed virus vaccine: Serum antibody titers and experience with exposure to measles epidemic. Am J Dis Child 109:232, 1965.
10. Nader PR, Horwitz MS, Rousseau J: Atypical exanthem following exposure to natural measles: Eleven cases in children previously inoculated with killed vaccine. J Pediatr 72:22, 1968.
11. Fulginiti VA, Eller JJ, Downie AW, et al: Altered reactivity to measles virus: Atypical measles in children previously immunized with inactivated measles virus vaccines. JAMA 202:1075, 1967.
12. Cherry JD, Feigin RD, Lobes LA Jr, et al: Atypical measles in children previously immunized with attenuated measles virus vaccines. Pediatrics 50:712, 1972.
13. Linneman CC Jr, Rotte TC, Schiff GM, et al: A seroepidemiologic study of a measles epidemic in a highly immunized population. Am J Epidemiol 95:238, 1972.
14. Gellin BG, Katz SI: Measles: State of the art and future directions. J Infect Dis 170(Suppl 1):S3, 1994.
15. Griffin DE, Ward BJ, Esolen LM: Pathogenesis of measles virus infection: An hypothesis for altered immune responses. J Infect Dis 170(Suppl 1):S24, 1994.
16. Cherry JD, Feigin RD, Shackelford PG: A clinical and serologic study of 103 children with measles vaccine failure. J Pediatr 82:802, 1973.
17. Barsegar B, Hofmann H, Zweymuller E: The diagnosis of measles in the newborn and infant age groups. Z Kinderheilkd 113:175, 1972.
18. Janeway CA: Use of concentrated human serum gamma globulin in the prevention and attenuation of measles. Bull N Y Acad Med 21:202, 1945.
19. Cherry JD, Feigin RD, Lobes LA Jr, et al: Urban measles in the vaccine era: A clinical, epidemiologic, and serologic study. J Pediatr 81:217, 1972.
20. Schaffner W, Schluederberg AES, Byrne EB: Clinical epidemiology of sporadic measles in a highly immunized population. N Engl J Med 279:783, 1968.
21. Siegel MM, Walter TK, Ablin AR: Measles pneumonia in childhood leukemia. Pediatrics 60:38, 1977.
22. Meadow SR, Weller RO, Archibald RWR: Fatal systemic measles in a child receiving cyclophosphamide for nephrotic syndrome. Lancet 2:876, 1969.
23. Katz M, Stiehm ER: Host defense in malnutrition. Pediatrics 59:490, 1977.
24. Peter G (ed): Report of the Committee on Infectious Diseases (The Red Book). *In* Measles, ed 23. Elk Grove Village, IL, American Academy of Pediatrics, 1994, pp 1014–1015.
25. Committee on Infectious Diseases, American Academy of Pediatrics: Vitamin A treatment of measles. Pediatrics 91:1014, 1993.
26. Enders JF, McCarthy K, Mitus A: Isolation of measles virus at autopsy in cases of giant cell pneumonia without rash. N Engl J Med 261:875, 1959.
27. Aicardi J, Goutieres F, Arsenio-Nunes ML, et al: Acute measles encephalitis in children with immunosuppression. Pediatrics 59:232, 1977.
28. Krasinski K, Borkowsky W: Measles and measles immunity in children infected with human immunodeficiency virus. JAMA 261:2512, 1989.
29. Centers for Disease Control: Epidemiologic notes and reports: Measles in HIV-infected children, United States. MMWR Morbid Mortal Wkly Rep 37:183, 1988.
30. Markowitz LE, Chandler FW, Roldan EO, et al: Fatal measles pneumonia without rash in a child with AIDS. J Infect Dis 158:480, 1988.
31. McLaughlin M, Thomas P, Onorato I, et al: Live virus vaccines in human immunodeficiency virus–infected children: A retrospective survey. Pediatrics 82:229, 1988.
31a. Centers for Disease Control and Prevention: Measles pneumonitis following measles-mumps-rubella vaccination of a patient with HIV infection. MMWR Morbid Mortal Wkly Rep 45:603, 1996.
32. Centers for Disease Control: Immunization of children infected with human immunodeficiency virus: Supplementary ACIP statement. MMWR Morbid Mortal Wkly Rep 37:181, 1988.
33. Atmar RL, Englund JA, Hammill H: Complications of measles in pregnancy. Clin Infect Dis 14:217, 1992..
34. Murphy JV, Unis EJ: Encephalopathy following measles infection in children with chronic illness. J Pediatr 88:937, 1976.
35. Gibbs FA, Gibbs EL, Carpenter PR, et al: Electroencephalographic abnormality in "uncomplicated" childhood diseases. JAMA 171:1050, 1959.
36. LaBoccetta AC, Tornay AS: Measles encephalitis: Report of 61 cases. Am J Dis Child 107:247, 1964.
37. Meulen VT, Kackell Y, Muller D, et al: Isolation of infectious measles virus in measles encephalitis. Lancet 2:1172, 1972.
38. Johnson RT, Griffin DE, Hirsch RL, et al: Measles encephalomyelitis: Clinical and immunologic studies. N Engl J Med 310:137, 1984.
39. Finkel HE: Measles myocarditis. Am Heart J 67:679, 1964.
40. McLellan RK, Gleiner JA: Acute hepatitis in an adult with rubeola. JAMA 247:2000, 1982.
41. Fucillo DA, Sever JL: Measles virus. *In* Schmidt NJ, Emmons RW (eds): Diagnostic Procedures for Viral Rickettsial and Chlamydial Infections, ed 6. Washington, DC, American Public Health Association, 1989, pp 713–730.
42. Forthal DN, Blanding J, Aarnaes S, et al: Comparison of different methods and cell lines for isolating measles virus. J Clin Microbiol 31:695, 1993.
43. Rossier E, Miller H, McCulloch B, et al: Comparison of immunofluorescence and enzyme immunoassay for detection of measles-specific immunoglobulin M antibody. J Clin Microbiol 9:1069, 1991.
44. Forni AL, Schluger NW, Roberts B: Severe measles pneumonitis in adults. Evaluation of clinical characteristics and therapy with intravenous ribavirin. Clin Infect Dis 19:454, 1994.
45. Hussey GD, Klein M: A randomized, controlled trial of vitamin A in children with severe measles. N Engl J Med 323:160, 1990.
46. Barclay AJG, Foster A, Sommer A: Vitamin A supplements and mortality related to measles: A randomized clinical trial. Br Med J (Clin Res Ed) 294:294, 1987.
47. Centers for Disease Control: Recommendations of the Immunization Practices Advisory Committee: Measles prevention. MMWR Morbid Mortal Wkly Rep 36:409, 423, 1987.
48. Markowitz LE, Katz SL: Measles vaccine. *In* Plotkin SA, Mortimer EA Jr (eds): Vaccines. Philadelphia, WB Saunders, 1994, pp 229–276.
49. Hinman AR, Brandling-Bennett AD, Nieburg PI: The opportunity and obligation to eliminate measles from the United States. JAMA 242:1157, 1979.
50. Centers for Disease Control: Measles prevention: Recommendation of the Immunization Practices Advisory Committee (ACIP). MMWR 38(S-9):1, 1989.
51. Markowitz AE, Albrecht P, Demonteverde R, et al: Declining measles antibody titers in mothers and infants, United States (Abstr). Presented at the 32nd Interscience Conference on Antimicrobial Agents and Chemotherapy; October 11–14, 1992; Anaheim, CA.
52. Krasinski K, Borkowsky W: Measles and measles immunity in children infected with human immunodeficiency virus. JAMA 261:2512, 1989.
53. McLaughlin M, Thomas P, Onorato I, et al: Live viral vaccines in human immunodeficiency virus–infected children: A retrospective survey. Pediatrics 82:229, 1988.
54. Onorato IM, Markowitz LE, Oxtoby MJ: Childhood immunization, vaccine-preventable diseases and infection with human immunodeficiency virus. Pediatr Infect Dis J 7:588, 1988.
55. Palumbo P, Hoyt L, Demasio K, et al: Population-based study of

measles and measles immunization in human immunodeficiency virus–infected children. Pediatr Infect Dis J 11:1008, 1992.
56. Osterhaus A, deVries P, van Binnendyk N: Measles vaccines: Novel generations and new strategies. J Infect Dis 170(Suppl): S42, 1994.
57. Cutts FT, Markowitz LE: Successes and failures in measles control. J Infect Dis 170(Suppl):S32, 1994.
58. Garenne M, Leroy O, Beau JP, Sene I: Child mortality after high-titre measles vaccines: Prospective study in Senegal. Lancet 338:903, 1991.
59. Aaby P, Knudsen K, Whittle H, et al: Long-term survival after Edmonston-Zagreb measles vaccination in Guinea-Bissau: Increased female mortality rate. J Pediatr 122:904, 1993.
60. Holt EA, Moulton LH, Siberry GK, Halsey NA: Differential mortality by measles vaccine titer and sex. J Infect Dis 168:1087, 1993.
61. World Health Organization Expanded Programme on Immunization. Measles control in the 1990: Plan of action for global measles control. Geneva, World Health Organization, 1992. Publication WHO/EPI/Gen/92.3.
62. World Health Organization: Expanded programme on immunization. Global Advisory Group—Part II. Wkly Epidemiol Rec 66:9, 1991.

147

Rubella (German Measles)

Alexander Rakowsky
John L. Sever

Background

Rubella is usually a mild illness known more for its sequelae than for the actual acute infection. The major interest in rubella, and in the development of vaccines against it, may have not arisen if not for the devastating consequences of congenital rubella infection.

Epidemiology

Distribution

Since the introduction of the first rubella vaccine in the United States in 1969, the rates of both rubella and its associated congenital rubella syndrome (CRS) have decreased dramatically.[1] However, it is still an illness with a worldwide distribution,[2] and in countries where the vaccine is distributed it still occurs in certain high-risk populations such as religious communities whose members, because of their beliefs, are not routinely vaccinated.[1]

Before the vaccine, in the Northern Hemisphere, peak attack rates were seen from March through May. Worldwide, notable epidemics can be seen every 6 to 9 years and pandemics occur every 10 to 30 years. The last such worldwide pandemic lasted from 1962 to 1964, and there were 12.5 million cases of acquired rubella and more than 30,000 affected infants in the United States during that time.[3] Since the introduction of the rubella vaccine, the rates in the United States have been less than 1% of those in the prevaccine age.[1, 4]

Transmission

Humans appear to be the only natural host for the rubella virus, although certain animals can be infected in the laboratory setting. The mode of transmission for acquired cases is respiratory. Prolonged exposure to an infected person is required, with a single, brief exposure to an infected person appearing to be relatively inefficient in transmitting disease.[5] In closed populations of susceptible people, such as military recruits and prisoners, the infection rate has been as high as 90% to 100%.[6] In people with a history of either past infection or appropriate vaccination, reinfection can occur, but rarely, after prolonged or repeated exposures.

Congenitally infected infants can serve as a potential reservoir because they cannot fully neutralize the virus for prolonged periods. Up to half of infants shed virus until the sixth month of life, and a percentage of such infants are found to be actively shedding virus up to 1 year of age.[7] However, the overall contribution of these infants to the spread of infection is considered minimal compared with the higher prevalence of asymptomatic infections: 50% of serologically detected infections in children result in inapparent illness.

Prevalence

Before mass immunization was practiced, rubella was typically a childhood disease seen predominantly in the 5- to 14-year age group.[8] It was and still is rarely seen in infants younger than 1 year. With efficacious mass immunization programs, the demographics of rubella infections have changed. The overall number of cases is down dramatically, and the infection is seen more commonly in the young adult and teenage years.[1] This is believed to be due to missed immunizations combined with a much lower background prevalence of the illness in communities.[9]

As noted before, the overall rate of both acquired and congenital rubella has declined dramatically since the advent of the rubella vaccine in 1969. As seen in Figure 147–1, the rates for both are less than 1% of the total seen in prevaccine years. However, occasional outbreaks have led to elevated total numbers of cases in the past few years. In 1990 and 1991, there were outbreaks of rubella in Amish communities in Ohio and Pennsylvania,[1, 10] which contributed to a total increase in congenital rubella cases in those 2 years to 25 and 31, respectively, compared with only 1 case in 1989.[1] In fact, according to the Centers for Disease Control and Prevention,[1] the vast majority of acquired and congenital rubella cases seen in the United States in the past few years were confined to either a small, unimmunized population (such as the Amish in the previously noted cases) or recent immigrants or visitors from countries where rubella vaccination is not widely distributed.

A concerning statistic is the continued susceptibility to rubella infection of women of childbearing age. Serologic surveys have shown that 10% to 20% of such women in the United States are susceptible, percentages virtually unchanged from those seen in similar surveys done in the years before mass vaccination.[11] Similar results are seen in countries that have used different vaccination strategies. In 1969, when the first rubella vaccine became available, the United States adopted a policy of mass vaccination of young children and infants in the hope of lessening the circulation of wild rubella virus in the community and thus preventing children from transmitting rubella infection to their susceptible mothers and other pregnant women. The United Kingdom adopted a

The information contained in this manuscript reflects the views of the authors only and not necessarily those of the Food and Drug Administration.

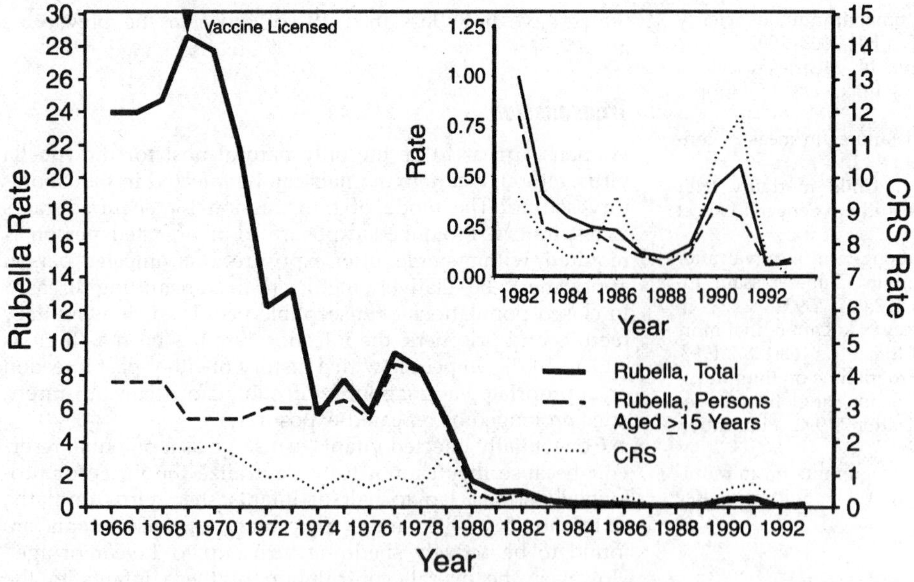

*Cases reported to the National Notifiable Disease Surveillance System per 100,000 population.
†Cases reported to the National CRS Registry per 100,000 live births.

FIGURE 147–1 □ Incidence rates of rubella* and CRS†—United States, 1966 to 1993. (From Rubella and congenital rubella syndrome—United States, January 1, 1991–May 7, 1994. MMWR Morbid Mortal Wkly Rep 43:391, 397–401, 1994.)

different approach, aiming to vaccinate all 12-year-old schoolgirls to ensure that they were immune before reaching childbearing age. In addition, vaccines were offered to nonpregnant adult women found to be rubella-seronegative. In both countries, the number of both acquired and congenital rubella cases dropped significantly, with the United States showing a larger decrease in acquired cases.[12, 13] However, because of the persistence of rubella susceptibility in a significant number of women of childbearing age, the official policy in both countries now is to vaccinate young children and infants and to find seronegative young women so as to vaccinate them as well[11] (more details are given in the later section on management).

With regard to newborns, estimates of the risk of developing a congenital rubella infection after maternal infection vary considerably among different studies. Complicating this matter is the definition of congenital rubella infection. In one approach, serologic studies have been done to determine whether the timing of the maternal infection affects the rate of developing congenital infection, with "congenital infection" being based on serologic changes. Using another approach, other studies have determined the risk of an infant's being born with stigmata of a congenital infection in relation to the timing of the maternal infection. Still other studies have investigated the long-term sequelae of congenital rubella infections. However, it is clear that the risk of developing congenital rubella infection depends on the month of pregnancy in which the maternal infection occurred, and the following overall statements can be made[11, 13–21] (Table 147–1):

1. The highest rate of serologically proven congenital infection is associated with maternal infection in the 4th through 6th (and probably as high as the 10th) weeks of gestation.
2. The rates of serologic conversion consistent with a congenital infection after a maternal infection drop significantly toward the latter part of the first trimester and throughout the second trimester, reaching a low at the end of the second trimester.[14]
3. During the third trimester, the risk of developing congenital infection (determined by serology) after a maternal infection starts to rise again, reaching approximately 60% for the 31st through 36th weeks of gestation and close to 100% at term.[14]
4. The highest risk of developing both stigmata of the CRS noticeable at birth and long-term complications of congenital infection exists during the first trimester. The risk rates drop considerably during the second trimester and stay low in the third trimester, despite the increasing seroprevalence rates. In fact, in a study by Miller and colleagues,[15] no defects were seen in 63 children infected after the 16th week of gestation, and in a study by Cradock-Watson and associates[22] there appeared to be little, if any, risk of congenital anomalies in infants infected beyond weeks 16 to 20 of gestation.

In a review by Ghidini and Lynch,[14] estimated fetal infection rates after confirmed maternal rubella infections were presented, with data from studies by Miller,[15] Enders,[16] Munro,[17] Grillner,[18] and their colleagues being used. The au-

TABLE 147–1 ■ Fetal Infection Rates After Confirmed Maternal Rubella Infection

GESTATIONAL AGE (WK)	FETAL INFECTION, NO. INFECTED/NO. EXPOSED (%)	RUBELLA-ASSOCIATED DEFECTS/SEROPOSITIVE INFANTS, NO./NO. (%)	OVERALL RISK*
2–3	4/13 (31)	NA†	NA
4–6	10/10 (100)	11/11 (100)	100
7–10	9/9 (100)	24/29 (83)	83
11–12	8/13 (62)	20/25 (80)	55
13–14	16/25 (64)	16/31 (52)	33
15–16	24/46 (52)	17/38 (45)	23
17–20	13/33 (39)	2/33 (6)	2
21–23	6/35 (17)	0/16 (0)	0
24–30	19/63 (30)	(0)	0
31–36	15/25 (60)	(0)	0
>36	8/8 (100)	(0)	0

*The overall risk was calculated as follows: % seropositive fetuses with defects × % infants infected.
†NA, Not available.
Reprinted by permission of The Western Journal of Medicine (Ghidini A, Lynch L, Prenatal diagnosis and significance of fetal infections, 1993, September, volume 159, p 370).

thors divided the risk rates into three categories: risk of developing rubella infection as shown by serologic changes; risk of developing defects (seen either at birth or later in life) consistent with a congenital rubella infection; and an "overall risk," which was defined as the percentage of seropositive infected infants times the percentage of these infants with defects (for example, if 90% of infants born to mothers with acquired rubella infection during a certain gestational age show serologic infection but only 50% of these congenitally infected infants have defects consistent with congenital infection, the overall risk is 45%).

Pathogenesis

Acquired Infection

The portal of entry for the virus appears to be the upper respiratory tract. From there, via the lymphatic system and/or by transient viremia, the virus spreads to lymph nodes, where replication occurs.[23, 24] Approximately 7 to 9 days after exposure, the virus disseminates hematogenously and may infect multiple tissues, including the placenta. The peak of viremia occurs between 10 and 17 days after exposure, and this is followed by the onset of rash on days 16 to 18.[23, 25] The virus is cleared from the serum in a few days, as antibody levels rise, but may persist in peripheral blood lymphocytes and monocytes for 1 to 4 weeks.[26] Virus excretion occurs from the nasopharynx, kidneys, cervix, and gastrointestinal tract starting on postexposure days 9 to 11. Nasopharyngeal virus shedding, usually copious, typically persists for 2 weeks, with the highest rate of nasopharyngeal excretion being from 5 days before to 6 days after the appearance of rash.

The etiology of the rash is unclear. Some investigators speculate that the rash may result from circulating immune complexes. However, rubella virus has been isolated from both involved and uninvolved skin, and circulating immune complexes containing rubella virus antigen are detectable in only 16% of patients.[27]

Immune mechanisms may also play a role in the development of arthralgias and arthritis, but the incidence of arthritis and arthralgias varies considerably among different studies. Tingle and coworkers[28] noted the development of acute polyarticular arthritis in 30% of a mixed adult population with acquired rubella infection. The rates of both arthralgias and arthritis after natural infection are higher in females, suggesting a hormonal influence on their development. Other studies have shown the presence of virus in joint fluid, leading to the possibility that an active infection is the actual cause of the arthritis or arthralgias.[29–34] Finally, an immune mechanism may play a major role.

Immune mechanisms are also thought to play a major role in the development of acute rubella encephalitis and in the late complication of diabetes mellitus after natural rubella infection.[20]

The pathogenesis of rubella has been studied in animal models, particularly primates and small animals.[35] Of the small laboratory animals, the ferret appears to be the most useful animal model in rubella studies, although no one animal model completely mimics either the acquired or congenital disease seen in humans.[36]

Congenital Infection

Rubella virus is transmitted in utero to the fetus via the placenta during primary maternal infection.[37] There are rare reports of maternal reinfection leading to fetal infection, but the rate of risk in such cases is considered to be exceptionally low.[38, 39] With regard to the primary maternal infection, it does not matter whether the infection is asymptomatic or symptomatic; fetal infection rates are the same for both groups.

Congenital infection may give rise to multiple outcomes[39, 40]: no fetal evidence of infection, resorption of the embryo if infection occurs early, spontaneous abortion, stillbirth, isolated placental infection without involvement of the fetus, and involvement of both fetus and placenta. Outcomes of infected infants may also range from severe multiple-organ involvement to apparent absence of disease. A variable outcome is further demonstrated by viral infection of one monozygotic twin that leaves the other twin unaffected.

It has long been recognized that the younger the gestational age at the time of infection, the higher the risk of congenital anomalies.[15] These defects are more severe and more likely to involve multiple organs if acquired during the first 8 weeks of gestation. This is related to the mechanism of damage. There are two ways in which the rubella virus can lead to cellular damage in the fetus. The first involves infection of fetal cells by actual cytolysis, generalized vasculitis, or genetic disruptions.[41] It appears that only a small, variable number of fetal cells are infected (from 1 in 1000 to 1 in 250,000, of which cytolysis is fairly rare)[41] and inflammation secondary to cellular destruction is minimal. In contrast, generalized vasculitis leading to small blood vessel thrombosis is common, and vascular insufficiency is a more important cause of congenital defects. Congenital defects may also be attributed to chromosome breaks and the mitotic arrest of certain cell types by the increased production of protein inhibitor.[42]

The second method of damage is by continued viral presence leading to inflammatory responses and damage via immune mechanisms.[14] Rubella virus is known to persist in congenitally infected infants, and the virus can be found throughout gestation[43] and for many months postnatally. By 1 year of age, up to 10% of infants still shed virus,[25] and virus shedding may continue beyond 2 years of age. Virus can be recovered from the nasopharynx (most prominent, at 85%), urine, conjunctival fluid, stool, cerebrospinal fluid, bone marrow, and peripheral leukocytes.[44]

Because of these two mechanisms of damage, clinical manifestations can be divided into transient, permanent, and late emerging (delayed)[20, 45] (Table 147–2). Transient features, including low birth weight, thrombocytopenia, hepatitis, and some instances of meningoencephalitis, and permanent features, including cardiac defects (such as atrial septal defects and pulmonary pulmonic stenosis), eye lesions, and sensorineural deafness, appear to be caused by either the first mechanism of damage or a combination of the two. Late-emerging features, such as sensorineural deafness, endocrine abnormalities, and progressive panencephalitis, appear to be secondary to persistence of virus (second method of damage). In fact, more than half of all newborn infants with congenital rubella syndrome appear normal at birth and may still develop late-emerging deficits years later.[20]

Pathology of Acquired Infection

Because of the frequently benign course of acquired rubella, little pathologic experience exists. Lymphoreticular tissues demonstrate mild edema, nonspecific follicular hyperplasia, and some loss of follicular morphology. Examination of brain tissue of patients with encephalitis reveals diffuse swelling, nonspecific degeneration, and little meningeal or perivascular infiltration.[46]

Pathology of Congenital Infection

Much more is known of the histopathologic appearance of congenital infection than of acquired infection. Predominant

TABLE 147–2 ■ Congenital Rubella: Transient (T), Permanent (P), and Developmental (D) Manifestations

COMMON		UNCOMMON OR RARE	
Low birth weight	T	Jaundice	T
Thrombocytopenic purpura	T	Dermatoglyphic "abnormality"	P
Hepatosplenomegaly	T		
Bony "lesions"	T	Glaucoma	P
Large anterior fontanelle	T	Cloudy cornea	T
Meningoencephalitis	T	Severe myopia	P, D
Hearing loss	P, D	Myocardial abnormalities	P
Cataract (and microphthalmia)	P	Hepatitis	T
		Generalized lymphadenopathy	T
Retinopathy	P		
Patent ductus arteriosus	P	Hemolytic anemia	T
Pulmonic stenosis	P, D	Rubella pneumonitis	T
Mental retardation	P, D	Diabetes mellitus	P, D
Behavior disorders	P, D	Thyroid disorders	D, P
Central language disorders	P, D	Seizure disorders	D
Cryptorchidism	P	Precocious puberty	D
Inguinal hernia	P	Degenerative brain disease	D
Splastic diplegia	P		
Microcephaly	P		

From Cooper LZ: Congenital rubella in the United States. *In* Krugman S, Gershon A (eds): Infections of the Fetus and the Newborn Infant. New York, Alan R. Liss, 1975. Copyright © 1975 Wiley-Liss. Reprinted by permission of Wiley-Liss, Inc., a subsidiary of John Wiley & Sons, Inc.

normal tissue cells are interspersed with small foci of infected cells,[47] and cellular necrosis and secondary inflammation are minimal. However, a generalized vasculitis is present. Virtually every organ is involved to some degree, and hypoplasia is a characteristic finding.[48] Owing to the nature of a chronic, persistent infection, the pathologic process is progressive. Both healing and new lesions can be found in the same specimen. Perivascular calcifications in the brain, giant cell hepatitis, and micronecrosis in autopsy specimens have been reported.

The placenta typically shows hypoplasia, inflammatory foci, granulomatous changes, mild edema, focal hyalinization and necrosis, and an extensive necrotizing angiopathy in the chorion.[49] Placental infections appear to be more extensive when infection occurs in the last trimester of pregnancy.

Clinical Manifestations

Acquired Infection

Rubella is typically a mild disease with few complications, and the symptoms are typically more pronounced in adults than in children. Studies have estimated that the ratio of subclinical to clinical infection ranges from 1:9 (civilian or open population) to 7:1 (military recruits or closed population).[50, 51]

The incubation period for the virus is usually 16 to 18 days but it can last 14 to 21 days.[48] For children, the first symptom is typically the rash. In adults, the rash is preceded by 1 to 5 days of prodromal symptoms, such as low-grade fever, headache, malaise, anorexia, mild conjunctivitis, coryza, pharyngitis, cough, and lymphadenopathy (suboccipital, postauricular, and/or cervical nodes).[48] Once the rash becomes apparent, and it is usually pruritic in adults, the prodromal symptoms subside. An enanthema (Forschheimer spots) consisting of small, red macules on the soft palate occasionally precedes or accompanies the rash. The rash itself can last 1 to 5 days or longer but frequently may not be present. The rash is morbilliform, but with more coalescence than is seen with rubeola, and typically begins on the face and behind the ears, spreading downward during the next 1 or 2 days. Peeling of affected skin usually does not occur. The tip of the spleen is often palpable, and a transient hepatitis can occur. This hepatitis peaks 3 to 10 days after the onset of rash and in one study was noted in 7.5% of 241 children with acute rubella infection.[52]

There are numerous possible complications of acquired rubella infection, with arthralgias and arthritis being the most common. Complications are more common in adults, particularly in women and even more so younger women (young adult age). The joint manifestations can appear at any time from when the rash subsides up to several weeks later. The arthritis or arthralgias last from 5 to 10 days in the majority of affected subjects but may persist, resembling rheumatoid arthritis. This has raised interest in the possible role of rubella virus in chronic rheumatic disease in children,[53] but no definitive ties have been described.

With regard to the development of arthritis or arthralgias after vaccination, the evidence indicates a causal relation between the currently used rubella vaccine strain (RA 27/3) and acute arthritis.[54] Incidence rates are estimated to average 13% to 15% among adult women, with much lower rates among children, adolescents, and adult men.[54] With regard to chronic arthritis, the Institute of Medicine's official stance is that "the evidence is consistent with a causal relation between the currently used rubella vaccine strain (RA 27/3) and chronic arthritis in adult women, although the evidence is limited in scope and confined to reports from one institution."[54] The "one institution" refers to Tingle's group[28, 55, 56] in Vancouver, which has published several articles on the possible association between the currently used rubella vaccine and the development of chronic arthritis.

Other, rarer complications of acquired rubella infection include thrombocytopenia (less than 1 in 3000 cases; may persist up to 6 months), myocarditis, Guillain-Barré syndrome, relapsing encephalitis, optic neuritis, and bone marrow aplasia.[20] Acute postrubella encephalitis, occurring in 1 of every 5000 to 6000 cases, is clinically similar to but less common than postmeasles encephalitis.[20] Unlike the findings in postmeasles encephalitis, demyelination of nerves is not seen.

Congenital Infection

In 1941, Gregg,[57] an Australian ophthalmologist, reported congenital defects, which included eye cataracts, cardiac defects, and low birth weight, in infants born to mothers who had had clinically apparent rubella in the early months of pregnancy. This report was met with initial skepticism, but by 1947 the medical literature included 28 reports, describing more than 500 children with severe CRS.[20] Subsequently, CRS was described as a collection of defects, including cardiac, eye, and hearing abnormalities, with or without mental retardation and microcephaly. With the isolation of the virus in 1962 and the advent of more sophisticated virus isolation techniques and diagnostic antibody studies, the spectrum of the CRS was further expanded and the reality of chronic persistent infection was acknowledged.

Multiple defects are associated with congenital rubella infection. The most common manifestations, with their frequencies, are as follows[20, 58]:

Auditory nerve deafness	80%–90%
Intrauterine growth retardation	50%–85%
Eye cataracts	35%
Retinopathy	35%
Patent ductus arteriosus	30%
In utero death	10%–30%
Pulmonary arterial hypoplasia	25%

Mental retardation	10%–20%
Meningoencephalitis	10%–20%
Behavior disorders	10%–20%
Hepatosplenomegaly	10%–20%
Bone radiolucencies	10%–20%

However, the time at which these various defects manifest themselves varies. In fact, silent infections, which may become clinically apparent later, are more common than early symptomatic cases. Of congenitally infected neonates who appeared normal, 71% developed manifestations of infection during the first 5 years of life.[59] In addition, existing defects may progress or become manifest at any time throughout life because of continued active infection (for example, a normal hearing test in a child with CRS does not preclude subsequent development of deafness).

The best way to grasp the myriad of defects associated with CRS is to divide them into three groups: transient manifestations, permanent manifestations, and developmental or delayed manifestations. In Table 147–3, the most common defects are divided into these three groups.[45]

Transient manifestations are seen in neonates and infants and in some circumstances may represent circulating immune complexes in the presence of active infection.[40] These findings usually resolve within days to weeks, and most have little prognostic significance. However, in the presence of extreme prematurity, several of these manifestations can be life threatening.[60] Included in this group are gross cardiac defects or myocarditis with congestive heart failure, progressive hepatitis, extensive meningoencephalitis, and interstitial pneumonitis.[40] In general, transient manifestations of CRS can include hepatitis, hepatosplenomegaly, jaundice, thrombocytopenia with petechiae, "blueberry muffin" lesions (violaceous lesions of dermal erythropoiesis), chronic rubelliform rash, hemolytic anemia, hypogammaglobulinemia, lymphadenopathy, meningoencephalitis, large anterior fontanelle, interstitial pneumonitis, myositis, myocarditis, chronic diarrhea, cloudy cornea, and osteopathy.[40] Intrauterine growth retardation is present in more than half of all cases.[20]

Permanent manifestations may be present at birth or develop during the first year of life and represent defects in organogenesis (except for the case of deafness); thus, they are uncommon if infection occurred after the eighth week of gestation. Included in this group, in decreasing order of frequency, are hearing problems, central nervous system disorders, ocular defects, and cardiovascular system defects.[20, 21, 40, 61]

Deafness is the most common manifestation of CRS[40] (occurring in 80% to 90% of subjects), and it is usually bilateral.[62] Deafness can occur alone, with no other stigmata of congenital rubella infection, and can develop at any point in an affected subject's life. Thus, the true incidence of deafness related to congenital rubella infection was not appreciated in the past. The deafness is due to either central or peripheral neurologic damage, with the organ of Corti being specifically affected. The hearing loss is usually across all frequencies, and asymptomatic vestibular dysfunction can accompany it.

Central nervous system abnormalities are also common, and approximately three fourths of children with confirmed CRS attend special schools.[17] These abnormalities can manifest themselves at any time during life, but the vast majority are noted in the first year after birth. Included among central nervous system abnormalities are microcephaly, psychomotor retardation, behavioral and psychiatric disorders, spastic diplegia, meningoencephalitis, and chronic encephalitis.[63] Psychomotor retardation is common, and there is a strong correlation between the magnitude of cognitive defects and the degree of growth failure.[64] It appears that the most profoundly affected children are those infected early in the first trimester, suggesting an organogenesis defect, but active and persistent rubella infection can also play a major role, as seen in the manifestations of both meningoencephalitis and chronic encephalitis.[20, 61]

The most common ocular findings are cataracts and retinopathy, both of which are usually present at birth, although the cataracts may not appear until several months of age in some cases.[20] The retinopathy has a characteristic pigmentary "salt-and-pepper" appearance[46, 65, 66] and is not an active process (retinitis). In fact, in a study of patients with confirmed retinopathy and CRS initially seen by either Swan or Gregg in Australia, there were no cases in which the retinopathy had progressed when the patients were reexamined 50 years later.[65] The retinopathy usually involves only one eye, except when cataracts are also present, in which case the retinopathy tends to be bilateral. Cataracts are bilateral half of the time and are often associated with microophthalmos. Glaucoma does not appear to affect a cataractous eye and is an uncommon manifestation of CRS.[65]

Cardiovascular defects are frequently associated with other major organ defects, and this is related to the time of infection. Cardiac defects are rare in infants infected after the first trimester but are present more than 50% of the time in children infected in the first 8 weeks of gestation, the time of major organogenesis.[20] The most common cardiovascular defects are patent ductus arteriosus and pulmonary arterial hypoplasia, including supravalvular stenosis, valvular stenosis, and peripheral branch stenosis. Other "permanent" cardiovascular defects are rare, with atrial septal defects, ventricular septal defects, aortic stenosis, and tetralogy of Fallot each occurring 2% to 5% of the time.[20] A more common "transient" cardiovascular defect is myocarditis, which can be present in up to 10% of newborns with CRS and is more indicative of an active rubella infection.[67]

Developmental or delayed manifestations of congenital rubella infection usually appear later in childhood and are progressive in nature.[68] The etiology of these defects appears to be continued subacute active rubella infection leading to direct viral damage, vascular insufficiency, and triggering of autoimmune mechanisms. This group of manifestations includes endocrinopathies, deafness, ocular damage, and central nervous system disease progression. Of these, endocrinopathies are the most common.

Various endocrinopathies, including growth hormone deficiency, hypoadrenalism, and precocious puberty, can occur, but only insulin-dependent diabetes mellitus and thyroid dysfunction are common. Insulin-dependent diabetes mellitus has been reported to occur in as many as 20% of CRS patients by age 35 years.[61, 69] The risk of developing it is approximately 100 to 200 times that observed for the general population. The exact etiology of insulin-dependent diabetes mellitus development is not clear, but it can occur in all congenitally infected patients, regardless of the timing of infection. Approximately 5% of CRS patients develop thyroid dysfunction, which can be manifest as hyperthyroidism, hypothyroidism, or thyroiditis, and this is believed to be secondary to autoantibody production.[70]

With regard to deafness, hearing deficits can increase over time and acute-onset sensorineural deafness can occur years after birth. Late-onset ocular defects include myopia, glaucoma, keratic precipitates, keratoconus, corneal hydrops, spontaneous lens absorption, and delayed visual defects caused by subretinal neovascularization.[65] However, as seen in the study that followed up the patients with CRS and ocular defects initially described by Gregg or Swan, these delayed ocular manifestations are uncommon.[65]

Rubella virus can be reactivated in the central nervous system and lead to a progressive rubella panencephalitis, which clinically resembles the subacute sclerosing panencephalitis seen with measles.[68] The number of patients who have developed this devastating and fatal delayed manifestation is less than 20.[71] In these cases, ataxia and loss of intellectual function were the first manifestations, usually occurring in the second decade of life, progressing to a vegetative state and eventually death.[71]

Diagnosis

Suspicion

Because acquired rubella infection often presents subclinically and is no longer a common illness in the United States, a high index of suspicion is needed. In older children and young adults, a clinical picture consisting of prodromal symptoms followed by postauricular or occipital lymphadenopathy and/or a rash (usually pruritic) should lead one to suspect rubella, especially in high-risk populations such as recent immigrants or visitors from countries where mass immunization against rubella is not practiced. In children, the prodromal symptoms are not seen as often, and the postauricular or occipital lymphadenopathy and coalescing, morbilliform rash originating on the head may be the only clinical clues to an active rubella infection.

A high index of suspicion is also necessary for diagnosis of congenital rubella infections. A classic CRS picture in a severely affected neonate leads to an easy diagnosis, but, unfortunately, the delayed manifestations of rubella may occur without any prior stigmata of congenital infection. Thus, in children who present with sensorineural deafness, especially if bilateral, or with ocular signs such as cataracts, congenital rubella infection should be considered as a possible etiology.

In general, the most important information needed in case of a suspected rubella infection, be it acquired or congenital, is the immunization status of either the subject (for acquired) or the mother (for congenital).

Differential Diagnosis

It was believed that postauricular or occipital lymphadenopathy occurring together with a rash is pathognomonic for acquired rubella infection. However, enteroviruses, adenoviruses, and human parvovirus B19 (of the more clinically common viral agents) can cause a similar clinical picture.[20, 21] In addition, mild cases of measles, scarlet fever, and allergic reactions can present with a rash similar to that seen in patients with acquired rubella infection. In smaller children, Kawasaki disease (mucocutaneous lymphadenopathy syndrome) must also be considered when the patient has occipital or postauricular lymphadenopathy and a rash.

CRS is quite similar to the clinical picture seen with any one of many agents known to cause congenital or perinatal infections. Included in this list are syphilis, toxoplasmosis, herpes simplex, and cytomegalovirus infection, all of which can lead to intrauterine growth retardation, deafness, mental retardation, and thrombocytopenic purpura. In addition, several of the enteroviruses can cause an acute hepatitis and thrombocytopenia in the affected neonate.

Specific Diagnosis

ACQUIRED INFECTION

Because the presentation of infection may be either subclinical or nonspecific, laboratory diagnosis is essential to the diagnosis of acquired rubella infection. Routine laboratory tests are of little value, as a low to normal leukocyte count is the norm. Plasma cells and atypical lymphocytes are frequently noted, but these are nonspecific findings. Thus, more specific laboratory techniques are required to diagnose acquired rubella infection. The three methods employed are

1. Virus isolation
2. Observation of a significant change (usually at least a fourfold increase) in the value of immunoglobulin G (IgG) antibody in two sequential serum samples[48]
3. Demonstration of specific rubella immunoglobulin M (IgM) antibody in a single serum sample[48]

Virus isolation is the least used method for diagnosis of acquired rubella infection because of the frequency with which rubella presents in a subclinical fashion. When it is utilized, specimens are obtained from the throat or nasopharynx and plated out in African green monkey kidney tissue culture or a similar sensitive tissue culture system. Virus shedding usually stops several days after the attenuation of the rash, so cultures must be obtained during the acute illness to be of good sensitivity.[20]

The majority of rubella infections are now diagnosed serologically. Initially developed were the hemagglutination inhibition (HI) and neutralization tests.[72, 73] The neutralization test determines the capacity of rubella virus antibody to prevent rubella virus infectivity. It is a sensitive test but expensive, time-consuming, and not available in most clinical laboratories. Thus, the HI test became the "gold standard" initially.[72, 73] This assay is based on the ability of rubella virus to hemagglutinate erythrocytes from specific animal sources. If specific rubella virus antibodies are present, hemagglutination does not occur in the test specimen. Like the neutralization test, it is sensitive but also time-consuming and difficult to perform and to standardize. Thus, other serologic methods were developed with which to determine antibody against rubella virus; among these are complement fixation tests, passive agglutination, and enzyme immunoassay (EIA) or enzyme-linked immunosorbent assay (ELISA). Complement fixation tests are not used frequently because they are less sensitive than the other accepted methods and because complement fixation antibodies appear later in the course of the disease than do antibodies measured by other assays.[72–74] Passive agglutination tests are fast and convenient and are useful for detecting evidence of immunity. However, they are difficult to quantitate and thus not of much service in diagnosing recent rubella infection. The present standard technique for serologically determining rubella infection is thus the ELISA.[75]

Rubella IgM antibody can be detected by EIA from early after the onset of illness through the peak at 7 to 10 days and for up to 4 weeks after the appearance of rash. Thus, a single serum specimen obtained within this period, if positive, can be viewed as serologic confirmation of a clinically suspected rubella infection. However, the IgM determination may yield false-positive results, especially if there is concomitant exposure to cytomegalovirus or parvovirus B19.[20, 72–75] Also, in some laboratories, a false-positive result can be obtained if the ELISA technique used does not avoid nonspecific reactions caused by complexes with rheumatoid antibody.[76]

The other way to confirm a suspected rubella infection serologically is to measure acute- and convalescent-phase IgG levels using the ELISA technique. A single measurement is not helpful, because up to 15% of the normal population may have a high baseline IgG level by this method.[11] The acute-phase serum should be collected within 7 days of appearance of the rash, and the convalescent-phase serum should be obtained 10 to 14 days later. The serum samples should be tested in tandem.[48]

There are several new developments in serologic testing for rubella virus. A major problem with currently available

EIAs (or ELISAs) is the difficulty of obtaining rubella virus antigens of reliable quality. Rubella virus is both difficult to grow and difficult to purify of cellular debris. Thus, false-positive reactions of immunoglobulins with nonviral contaminants are reported.[72–75] Several studies have compared the use of a synthetic peptide–based EIA with that of the traditional rubella virus lysate–based EIA in detecting rubella antibodies, and the results have been promising. Also, tests that use oral fluid samples or saliva to determine the presence of rubella antibody by using either antibody capture radioimmunoassay or enzyme-linked immunoassay methods have been developed and show good reliability.[77, 78] More work is being done to see if these tests can be used to quantitate the antibody levels and thus be of use in confirming clinically suspected rubella infections.

CONGENITAL INFECTION

A diagnosis of CRS should be entertained for any infant born with stigmata compatible with intrauterine rubella infection. The Centers for Disease Control and Prevention has formulated case definitions for either confirmed or compatible cases of CRS,[47] and these are shown in Table 147–3.

In contrast to the situation in acquired rubella infection, virus is frequently isolated from congenitally infected infants and may persist in the majority of such patients for up to 1 year. The virus may be isolated from the nasopharynx and less reliably from conjunctival secretions, cerebrospinal fluid, or urine. However, in patients with eye involvement, conjunctival cultures alone may be sufficient, and virus has been detected in cataractous lens at age 3 to 4 years.

In addition, polymerase chain reaction techniques have been studied for the diagnosis of congenital rubella infection in utero. By using this method, viral RNA has been detected in specimens of chorionic villus specimens from infected infants as early as 15 weeks of gestation.[79]

As with acquired rubella infection, the majority of congenital infections are determined by serologic studies. Serologic diagnosis may be made by determining the rubella-specific IgM titer in cord serum.[11, 79] However, there is a risk of false-positive results. If the maternal infection occurred late in the pregnancy, there may not have been sufficient time for the neonate to mount an immune response. Also, IgM is not present in neonates until approximately the fifth month in utero, so the determination of IgM levels before this time leads to a negative result.[79] Still, the determination of anti–rubella virus IgM by EIA is currently the accepted and best available way of diagnosing congenital rubella infection in the newborn.[79]

An alternative method is to follow sequential IgG levels. Because levels of maternally transferred IgG drop as the infant becomes older, the persistence or rise of specific anti–rubella virus IgG would be consistent with a congenital infection.[11]

The biggest challenge, however, lies in diagnosing congenital rubella infection in patients who present with delayed manifestations, such as sensorineural deafness. Positive IgG levels are not diagnostic because of the routine immunization of young children. Occasionally, rubella virus can be cultured from persistently infected sites, such as cerebrospinal fluid and cataractous lenses, for up to 3 to 4 years after birth. However, in cases in which a delayed manifestation such as bilateral hearing loss develops in the preschool age or later, an epidemiologic history is still the only way to "confirm" rubella as the cause.

TABLE 147–3 ■ Summary of Centers for Disease Control and Prevention Criteria for the Classification of Congenital Rubella Syndrome Cases

CRS confirmed
- Presence of defects and at least one of the following:
  - A. Isolation of rubella virus
  - B. Detection of rubella-specific IgM antibodies
  - C. Rubella-specific HI titer in the infant persisting beyond the period expected from that of passively transferred maternal antibodies

CRS compatible
- Insufficient laboratory data for confirmation of diagnosis and any two complications from A or one from A and one from B:
  - A. Cataracts or congenital glaucoma, congenital heart disease, hearing loss, pigmentary retinopathy
  - B. Purpura, splenomegaly, jaundice, radiolucent bone disease, meningoencephalitis, microcephaly, mental retardation

CRS possible
- Presence of some compatible clinical findings but insufficient criteria for either the confirmed or compatible categories

Congenital rubella infection only
- No defects are present, but laboratory evidence of infection is found

Stillbirths
- Stillbirths believed to be a consequence of maternal rubella infection

Not CRS
- At least one of the following inconsistent laboratory findings in an immunocompetent child:
  - A. Absence of rubella-specific HI titer in a child younger than 2 y of age
  - B. Absence of rubella-specific HI titer in the mother
  - C. Decline in rubella-specific HI titer in an infant in a manner consistent with what is expected from passively transferred maternal antibodies (a twofold dilution drop per month)

From Freij BJ, South MA, Sever JL: Maternal rubella and the congenital rubella syndrome. Clin Perinatol 15:247–257, 1988.

Prevention and Management

General Comments

Acquired rubella infection is essentially a fairly benign illness, and management usually involves time to allow the virus to run its course. The greatest damage done by the rubella virus is in developing fetuses; thus, the vital aspect of rubella infection management is to prevent acquired rubella infection in women of childbearing age. Because acquired rubella infection often presents subclinically, the only adequate way to prevent the devastating effects of congenital rubella infections is by immunization. The importance of this cannot be overemphasized.

Immunization

GENERAL COMMENTS

Rubella virus was isolated in 1962 and attenuated in 1966.[20] In 1969, three live attenuated rubella vaccines were licensed for use in the United States: the HPV-77 (DE-5 and DK-12) vaccines and the Cendehill vaccine.[20] In 1979, the RA 27/3 vaccine was licensed, and it is currently the only available vaccine.[80] It was found to be more immunogenic than the three previous vaccines and elicits an immune response more closely resembling the response seen after natural infection. All four vaccines have been shown to produce a good immune response, with RA 27/3–induced antibody levels present in at least 95% of vaccinees. Likewise, all four vaccines produce persisting immunity, with 92% of vaccinees who had originally seroconverted after a dose of the RA 27/3 vaccine showing serologic evidence of immunity up to 18 years after receipt of the vaccine.[20] It appears that one dose of vaccine is adequate to produce this high level of long-lasting immunity. However, two doses of rubella vaccine are now recommended.[75] Although primary rubella vaccine failures have not been a major problem, the potential consequences of rubella vaccine failure are substantial (i.e., congenital rubella), and thus an additional dose of rubella vaccine should provide an added safeguard against such failures.[11, 75]

WHOM TO VACCINATE

It is currently recommended that rubella vaccine be administered in combination with measles and mumps vaccine when a child is 12 months of age or older, with a second dose (again, as part of the measles-mumps-rubella vaccine) being given in the early school-age years.[75] Special emphasis must continue to be placed on the immunization of postpubertal males and females, especially those living in closed settings, such as in the military or in a college. In general, for this age group immunization should be performed unless documented evidence of rubella immunization or serologic evidence of naturally acquired immunity is provided.[11] A history of acquired rubella infection is not adequate, as studies have shown a poor correlation between recollection of a rubella infection and confirmation via serologic tests.[11]

For the postpubertal population, the Red Book Committee of the American Academy of Pediatrics published the following specific recommendations[75]:

1. Postpubertal females who are not known to be immunized to rubella should be immunized. They should not receive vaccine if they are known to be pregnant and should be warned not to become pregnant for 3 months after vaccine receipt (more details of the theoretical risks of the vaccine when given during pregnancy are discussed in the next section).
2. Premarital serologic screening for rubella immunity enhances efforts to identify and vaccinate susceptible women before pregnancy.
3. Prenatal or antepartum serologic screening for rubella immunity should be routinely undertaken, and rubella vaccine should be administered to susceptible women in the immediate postpartum period before discharge. Receipt of $Rh_0(D)$ immune globulin is not a contraindication to vaccination, nor should breast-feeding be a deterrent.
4. A special effort should be made to be certain that all individuals are protected who plan to attend or work in educational institutions, child care centers, health care facilities, or other places where they are likely to be exposed to or spread rubella.

CONTRAINDICATIONS

Pregnancy. Rubella vaccine should not be given to pregnant women, because of a theoretical risk of the occurrence of congenital rubella, especially if the vaccine is given in the first trimester.[75] However, as of 1993 the Centers for Disease Control and Prevention had received reports of 226 susceptible women who received the RA 27/3 vaccine during the first trimester and none of whose infants had congenital defects. Of these infants, 2% had asymptomatic infection (as shown by serologic determinations), which led the Centers for Disease Control and Prevention to estimate a maximal theoretical risk of 1.6% for the occurrence of congenital rubella after administration of the presently used vaccine during the first trimester.[11, 75]

Recent Receipt of Immune Globulin. Because of the potential for antibodies to neutralize the vaccine virus, it is recommended that rubella vaccine not be given in the 2 weeks before or the 3 months after the administration of immune globulin or blood transfusion.[75]

Altered Immunity. Patients with immunodeficiency diseases (except human immunodeficiency virus infection) or who are receiving immunosuppressive therapy or large, systemic doses of corticosteroids, alkylating agents, antimetabolites, or radiation should not be recipients of the rubella vaccine.[75] It is recommended that patients with human immunodeficiency virus infection receive rubella vaccine, and several studies have shown that these patients have the highest rate of serologic conversion to the rubella component of the measles-mumps-rubella vaccine.[81–83] For patients who are receiving immunosuppressive therapy (such as for leukemia or lymphoma), the interval between cessation of such therapy and rubella vaccine receipt should be approximately 3 months to allow the immune system to be properly restored.[75]

In general, fever per se is not a contraindication to rubella vaccine administration. If the fever is a manifestation of a more serious condition, the vaccine should be withheld until resolution of the problem. However, mild childhood illnesses (such as upper respiratory infections) should not be perceived as contraindications to measles-mumps-rubella vaccine administration.[75]

ADVERSE EVENTS

By day 5 to 7 after vaccination, virus may be detected in peripheral blood lymphocytes, and thus the main complications of a naturally acquired rubella infection can occur.[63] All complications secondary to rubella vaccine are more common in adults than in children and most common in women older than 25 years. Overall, the vaccine is safe and complications after vaccination are but a percentage of those seen after natural infection.

Fever, rash, and/or lymphadenopathy can develop in 5% to 15% of children who receive the vaccine, and the rate is higher in adults.[75] Joint pain, usually affecting small peripheral joints in children, is seen in 0.5% of child vaccine recipients.[75] However, in women, this complication is much more common, with approximately 25% developing arthralgias and/or arthritis.[54–56, 75] This complication usually develops 1 to 3 weeks after vaccine receipt, and in the vast majority of cases the arthritis and arthralgias are mild to moderate in severity and resolve in several days to 1 week.[54–56, 75] There are reports in the literature of chronic arthritis developing in women,[55, 56] but the official stance of the Institute of Medicine is that "the evidence is consistent with a causal relation between the currently used rubella vaccine strain (RA 27/3) and chronic arthritis in adult women, although the evidence is limited in scope and confined to reports from one institution."[54, 75]

Other rare complications include transient peripheral neuritic complaints, central nervous system manifestations, and thrombocytopenia, although a causal relationship to vaccine receipt has not been firmly established for the last two.[75]

In an effort to reduce the adverse effects seen with the presently used rubella vaccine, several investigators are studying the efficacy of a vaccine based on rubella virus structural proteins instead of the presently used attenuated live whole virus particle. Ou and colleagues[84] mapped T-cell epitopes of the three major rubella structural proteins, E1, E2, and C, and found that more T-cell epitopes were present in E1 and C than in E2. With more work, the identification of such T-cell sites may provide the basis for selecting candidate T-cell epitopes for the development of an effective synthetic vaccine against rubella.[84] Hobman and colleagues[85] developed a Chinese hamster ovary cell line from which rubella virus proteins C, E1, and E2 are secreted in the form of rubella virus–like particles, which form by budding into the cisterna of the Golgi complex. According to their results, these particles may serve as a convenient source of rubella virus antigen, which may become an alternative to live attenuated vaccine strains.[85]

Chemotherapy

Chemotherapy is rarely needed in acquired infection, considering the typical uncomplicated clinical course seen with rubella infection. For patients with chronic arthritis secondary to natural infection, there has been some success with systemic steroid therapy, but this course of therapy is not routinely recommended.[20, 55, 56]

For patients with CRS, the experience with chemotherapeutic agents is also limited. Trials with amantadine or interferon therapy did not show an improvement in clinical outcome,[86, 87] and at present the number of children affected by CRS is so small that future clinical trials may be difficult to conduct.

Immunoglobulin was advocated at one point for the prevention or modification of rubella in susceptible pregnant women who were exposed to the infection. However, it was discovered that although immune globulin may suppress symptoms, it does not necessarily prevent viremia. Also, most commercially available immunoglobulins have varying concentrations of antibody to rubella, and thus the use of immune globulin is not recommended.[11, 75]

Isolation

Patients with acquired rubella infection continue to shed virus for 5 to 7 days after the onset of rash and thus should be isolated from susceptible subjects, especially women of childbearing age. In addition, hospitalized exposed patients should be placed under contact isolation until the 21st day after exposure. Only health care workers with serologically proven immunity should work with patients infected or potentially infected with rubella.

Infants with CRS can shed virus for the first year of life[7] and occasionally even longer. Thus, these infants should be considered potentially infectious until results of repeated nasopharyngeal and urine viral cultures are negative. Until that time, appropriate isolation measures should be used.

Congenitally Infected Infants

Owing to the chronic, persistent nature of congenital rubella infection, patients must be viewed as having a continually evolving disease. A multidisciplinary approach is often needed because of the broad range of potential problems, and defects must be looked for aggressively and often in infants known to be infected in utero.[20] Children in whom congenital rubella infection was not suspected but who develop a delayed manifestation should also be examined thoroughly for other potential defects.

Hearing disability is the most common abnormality seen after congenital rubella infection, with more than 80% of infants having some degree of hearing disability. Proper hearing is paramount to language and communication development, and thus hearing should be tested definitively as soon as possible in the infant suspected to have had congenital rubella infection.[20] Unfortunately, many physicians believe that hearing cannot be adequately tested in infants. However, in proper centers specific audiometric testing of infants can be performed, and infants found to be severely affected should be enrolled in specially designed programs of education. Also, children should be fitted with a proper auditory amplification device.

Even though congenital rubella infection can lead to a decrease in intelligence, at times an infant's lack of or delayed development is secondary to hearing or vision defects, and thus a full ophthalmologic examination is also indicated.

Summary

Rubella, in its acquired form, is a rather benign infection. However, congenital infection can lead to devastating consequences and thus it is imperative to eliminate it through continued mandatory immunization of infants and aggressive immunization of postpubertal people who have no documentation of rubella immunity. Since 1969, when the first rubella vaccines were introduced, there has been a remarkable decrease in the number of both acquired and congenital rubella infections, but epidemics in closed communities should remind us that this illness is still a potential problem in this country. Work is being done on the development of better EIA tests for rubella detection and better vaccines against rubella by using synthetic peptide chains, and these future advances should help the effort to eliminate rubella totally.

References

1. Centers for Disease Control and Prevention: Rubella and congenital rubella syndrome—United States, January 1, 1991–May 7, 1994. MMWR Morbid Mortal Wkly Rep 43:391, 1994.
2. Assad R, Ljungars-Esteves K: Rubella—World impact. Rev Infect Dis 7(Suppl 1):S29, 1985.
3. Bart KJ, Ortenstein NA, Preblud SR, et al: Universal immunization to interrupt rubella. Rev Infect Dis 7(Suppl 1):S177, 1985.
4. Centers for Disease Control: Update: Changes in notifiable disease surveillance data—United States, 1992–1993. MMWR Morbid Mortal Wkly Rep 42:824, 1993.
5. Marcy SM, Jordan MC: Rubella. *In* Hoeprich PD, Jordan MC (eds): Infectious Diseases: A Modern Treatise of Infectious Processes, ed 4. Philadelphia, JB Lippincott, 1989, p 866.
6. Pollard RB, Edwards EA: Epidemic survey of rubella in a military recruit population. Am J Epidemiol 101:435, 1975.
7. Garner JS, Simmons BP: CDC guidelines for isolation precautions in hospitals. Infect Control 4:245, 1983.
8. Witte JJ, Karchmer AW, Case G, et al: Epidemiology of rubella. Am J Dis Child 118:107, 1969.
9. Preblud SR, Serdual MK, Frank JA Jr, et al: Rubella vaccination in the United States: A ten-year review. Epidemiol Rev 2:171, 1980.
10. Jackson B, Payton T, Horst G, et al: An epidemiologic investigation of a rubella outbreak among the Amish of northeastern Ohio. Public Health Rep 108:436, 1993.
11. The American College of Obstetricians and Gynecologists (ACOG): Rubella and pregnancy: ACOG technical bulletin number 171—August 1992. Int J Gynecol Obstet 42:60, 1993.
12. Condon RJ, Bower C: Rubella vaccination and congenital rubella syndrome in Western Australia. Med J Aust 158:379, 1993.
13. Ostlere LS, Stevens HP, Dillon MJ, et al: Chronic rash associated with congenital rubella. J R Soc Med 87:242, 1994.
14. Ghidini A, Lynch L: Prenatal diagnosis and significance of fetal infections. West J Med 159:366, 1993.
15. Miller E, Cradock-Watson JE, Pollock TM: Consequences of confirmed maternal rubella at successive stages of pregnancy. Lancet 2:781, 1982.
16. Enders G, Nickerl-Pacher U, Miller E, Cradock-Watson JE: Outcome of confirmed periconceptional maternal rubella. Lancet 1:1445, 1988.
17. Munro ND, Sheppard S, Smithells RW, et al: Temporal relations between maternal rubella and congenital defects. Lancet 2:201, 1987.
18. Grillner L, Forsgren M, Barr B, et al: Outcome of rubella during pregnancy with special reference to the 17th–24th weeks of gestation. Scand J Infect Dis 15:321, 1983.
19. Grangeot-Keros L: Rubella and pregnancy. Pathol Biol (Paris) 40:706, 1992.
20. Cherry J: Rubella. *In* Feigin R, Cherry J (eds): Textbook of Pediat-

ric Infectious Diseases, ed 3. Philadelphia, WB Saunders, 1992, pp 1792–1817.
21. Gershon A: Rubella virus (German measles). *In* Mandell G, Bennett J, Dolin R (eds): Principles and Practice of Infectious Disease, ed 4. New York, Churchill Livingstone, 1995, pp 1242–1247.
22. Cradock-Watson JE, Ridehalgh MKS, Anderson MJ, et al: Fetal infection resulting from maternal rubella after the first trimester of pregnancy. J Hyg (Lond) 83:381, 1980.
23. Green RH, Balsame MR, Giles JP, et al: Studies of the natural history and prevention of rubella. Am J Dis Child 110:348, 1965.
24. Halstead SB, Diwan AR, Oda AI: Susceptibility to rubella among adolescents and adults in Hawaii. JAMA 210:1881, 1969.
25. Sever JL, Monif G: Limited persistence of virus in congenital rubella. Am J Dis Child 110:452, 1965.
26. O'Shea S, Mutton D, Best JM: In vivo expression of rubella antigens on human leukocytes: Detection by flow cytometry. J Med Virol 25:297, 1988.
27. Ziola B, Lund G, Meurman O, et al: Circulating immune complexes in patients with acute measles and rubella virus. Infect Immun 41:578, 1983.
28. Tingle AJ, Allen M, Petty RE, et al: Rubella associated arthritis. Comparative study of joint manifestations associated with natural rubella infection and RA 27/3 rubella immunization. Ann Rheum Dis 45:110, 1986.
29. Graham R, Armstrong R, Simmons NA, et al: Isolation of rubella virus from synovial fluid in five cases of seronegative arthritis. Lancet 2:649, 1981.
30. Phillips CA, Behbehani AM, Johnson LW, et al: Isolation of rubella virus: An epidemic characterized by rash and arthritis. JAMA 191:615, 1965.
31. Ogra PL, Herd JK: Arthritis associated with induced rubella infection. J Immunol 107:810, 1971.
32. Smith CA, Petty RE, Tingle AJ: Rubella virus and arthritis. Rheum Dis Clin North Am 13:265, 1987.
33. Graham R, Armstrong R, Simmons NA, et al: Chronic arthritis associated with the presence of intrasynovial rubella virus. Ann Rheum Dis 42:2, 1983.
34. Chantler JK, Ford DK, Tingle AJ: Persistent rubella infection and rubella-associated arthritis. Lancet 1:1323, 1982.
35. Parkman PD, Phillips PE, Kirchstein RL, et al: Experimental rubella virus infection in the rhesus monkey. J Immunol 95:743, 1965.
36. Fabiyi A, Gitnick GL, Sever JL: Chronic rubella infection in the ferret *(Mustela putorius fero)* puppy. Proc Soc Exp Biol Med 125:766, 1967.
37. Rawls WE, Desmyter J, Melnick JL: Serologic diagnosis and fetal involvement in maternal rubella. JAMA 203:627, 1968.
38. Grangeot-Keros L, Nicolas JC, Bricout F, et al: Rubella reinfection and the fetus. N Engl J Med 313:1547, 1985.
39. Weber B, Enders G, Schlosser R, et al: Congenital rubella syndrome after maternal reinfection. Infection 21:118, 1993.
40. Hanshaw JB, Dudgeon JA: Rubella. *In* Hanshaw JB, Dudgeon JA, Marshall WC (eds): Viral Diseases of the Fetus and Newborn, ed 2. Philadelphia, WB Saunders, 1985, p 13.
41. Thompson KM, Tobin J: Isolation of rubella virus from abortion material. Br Med J 2:264, 1970.
42. Nusbacher J, Hirschhorn K, Cooper LZ: Chromosomal studies on congenital rubella. N Engl J Med 276:1409, 1967.
43. Krugman S: Rubella symposium. Am J Dis Child 110:345, 1965.
44. Schiff GM, Dine MS: Transmission of rubella from newborns. A controlled study among young adult women and report of an unusual case. Am J Dis Child 110:447, 1965.
45. Cooper LZ: Congenital rubella in the United States. *In* Krugman S, Gershon A (eds): Infections of the Fetus and the Newborn Infant. New York, Alan R Liss, 1975, pp 1–22.
46. Cherry JD: Rubella. *In* Feigin RD, Cherry JD (eds): Textbook of Pediatric Infectious Diseases, ed 2. Philadelphia, WB Saunders, 1987, p 1810.
47. Freij BJ, South MA, Sever JL: Maternal rubella and the congenital rubella syndrome. Clin Perinatol 15:247, 1988.
48. Preblud SR, Alford CA Jr: Rubella. *In* Remington JS, Klein JO (eds): Infectious Diseases of the Fetus and Newborn, ed 3. Philadelphia, WB Saunders, 1990, p 196.
49. Garcia AGP, Marques RLS, Lobato YY, et al: Placental pathology in congenital rubella. Placenta 6:281, 1985.
50. Horstmann DM, Leibhaber H, LeBouvier GL, et al: Rubella. Reinfection of vaccinated and naturally immune persons exposed in an epidemic. N Engl J Med 283:771, 1970.
51. Brody JA: The infectiousness of rubella and the possibility of reinfection. Am J Public Health 56:1082, 1966.
52. Sugaya N, Nirasawa M, Mitamura K, et al: Hepatitis in acquired rubella infection in children (Letter). Am J Dis Child 142:817, 1988.
53. Chantler JK, Tingle AJ, Petty RE: Persistent rubella virus infection associated with chronic arthritis in children. N Engl J Med 313:1117, 1985.
54. Howson CP, Howe CJ, Fineberg HV (eds): Adverse Effects of Pertussis and Rubella Vaccine. Washington DC, Institute of Medicine, National Academy Press, 1991, pp 195–197.
55. Tingle AJ, Chantler JK, Pot KH: Postpartum rubella immunization: Association with development of prolonged arthritis, neurological sequelae, and chronic rubella viremia. J Infect Dis 152:606, 1985.
56. Mitchell LA, Tingle AJ, Shukin R, et al: Chronic rubella vaccine–associated arthropathy. Arch Intern Med 153:2268, 1993.
57. Gregg NM: Congenital cataracts following German measles in the mother. Trans Ophthalmol Soc Aust 3:35, 1941.
58. South MA, Sever JL: Teratogen update: The congenital rubella syndrome. Teratology 31:297, 1985.
59. Schiff GM, Sutherland J, Light I: Congenital rubella. *In* Thalhamer O (ed): Prenatal Infections. International Symposium of Vienna, September 2–3, 1970. Stuttgart, Georg Thieme, 1971, p 31.
60. Cooper LZ: The history and medical consequences of rubella. Rev Infect Dis 7(Suppl 1):S1, 1985.
61. Williams LL, Shannon BT, Leguire LE, et al: Persistently altered T cell immunity in high school students with the congenital rubella syndrome and profound hearing loss. Pediatr Infect Dis J 12:831, 1993.
62. Kobayashi H, Suzuki A, Nomura Y: Unilateral hearing loss following rubella infection in an adult. Acta Otolaryngol Suppl (Stockh) 514:49, 1994.
63. Cooper LZ, Buimovici-Klein E: Rubella. *In* Fields BN, Knipe DM (eds): Virology. New York, Raven Press, 1985, p 1005.
64. Chiriboga-Klein S, Oberfield SE, Casullo AM, et al: Growth in congenital rubella syndrome and correlation with clinical manifestations. J Pediatr 115:251, 1989.
65. Arnold JJ, McIntosh EDG, Martin FJ, et al: A fifty-year follow-up of ocular defects in congenital rubella: Late ocular manifestations. Aust N Z J Ophthalmol 22:1, 1994.
66. Yoser SL, Forster DJ, Rao NA: Systemic viral infections and their retinal and choroidal manifestations. Surv Ophthalmol 37:339, 1993.
67. Baley JE, Goldfarb J: The immune system, viral infections. *In* Fanaroff AA, Martin RJ (eds): Neonatal-Perinatal Medicine, Diseases of the Fetus and Infant, ed 5. St. Louis, Mosby–Year Book, 1992, pp 113–117.
68. Sever JL, South MA, Shaver KA: Delayed manifestations of congenital rubella. Rev Infect Dis 7(Suppl 1):S164, 1985.
69. Menser MA, Forrest JM, Bransby RD, et al: Long-term observation of diabetes and the congenital rubella syndrome in Australia. *In* Mimura G, Baba S, Goto Y, et al (eds): Clinicogenetic Genesis of Diabetes Mellitus. Amsterdam, Excerpta Medica, 1982, p 221.
70. Rubenstein P, Walker ME, Fedun B, et al: The HLA system in congenital rubella patients with and without diabetes. Diabetes 31:1088, 1982.
71. Waxham MN, Wolinsky JS: Rubella virus and its effect on the nervous system. Neurol Clin 2:367, 1984.
72. Zrein M, Joncas JH, Pedneault L, et al: Comparison of a whole-virus enzyme immunoassay (EIA) with a peptide-based EIA for detecting rubella virus immunoglobulin G antibodies following rubella vaccination. J Clin Microbiol 31:1521, 1993.
73. Pedneault L, Zrein M, Robillard L, et al: Comparison of novel synthetic peptide–based DETECT-RUBELLA enzyme immunoassays with Enzygnost and IMx for detection of rubella-specific immunoglobulin G. J Clin Microbiol 32:1085, 1994.
74. Condorelli F, Ziegler T: Dot immunobinding assay for simultaneous detection of specific immunoglobulin G antibodies to measles virus, mumps virus, and rubella virus. J Clin Microbiol 31:717, 1993.
75. Committee on Infectious Diseases of the American Academy of Pediatrics: Report of the Committee on Infectious Diseases (The Red Book), ed 23. Elk Grove Village, IL, American Academy of Pediatrics, 1994, pp 406–412.

76. Meurman OH, Ziola BR: IgM-class rheumatoid factor interference in the solid-phase immunoassay of rubella-specific IgM antibodies. J Clin Pathol 31:483, 1978.
77. Thieme T, Piacentini S, Davidson S, et al: Determination of measles, mumps, and rubella immunization status using oral fluid samples. JAMA 272:219, 1994.
78. Perry KR, Brown DWG, Parry JV, et al: Detection of measles, mumps, and rubella antibodies in saliva using antibody capture radioimmunoassay. J Med Virol 40:235, 1993.
79. Valente P, Sever JL: In utero diagnosis of congenital infections by direct fetal sampling. Isr J Med Sci 30:416, 1994.
80. Wharton M, Cochl SL, Williams WW: Measles, mumps, and rubella vaccines. Infect Dis Clin North Am 4:47, 1990.
81. Frenkel LM, Nielsen K, Garakian A, et al: A search for persistent measles, mumps, and rubella vaccine virus in children with human immunodeficiency virus type I infection. Arch Pediatr Adolesc Med 148:57, 1994.
82. Sprauer MA, Markowitz LE, Nicholson JKA, et al: Response of human immunodeficiency virus–infected adults to measles-rubella vaccination. J Acquir Immune Defic Syndr 6:1013, 1993.
83. Brena AE, Cooper ER, Cabral HJ, et al: Antibody response to measles and rubella vaccine by children with HIV infection. J Acquir Immune Defic Syndr 6:1125, 1993.
84. Ou D, Chong P, Tingle AJ: Mapping T-cell epitopes of rubella virus structural proteins E1, E2, and C recognized by T-cell lines and clones derived from infected and immunized populations. J Med Virol 40:175, 1993.
85. Hobman TC, Lundstrom ML, Mauracher CA, et al: Assembly of rubella virus structural proteins into virus-like particles in transfected cells. Virology 202:574, 1994.
86. Arvin AM, Schmidt NJ, Cantell K, et al: Alpha interferon administration to infants with congenital rubella. Antimicrob Agents Chemother 21:259, 1982.
87. Plotkin SA, Klaus RM, Whitely JA: Hypogammaglobulinemia in an infant with congenital rubella syndrome: Failure of 1-adamantanamine to stop virus excretion. J Pediatr 69:1085, 1966.

148

Varicella and Herpes Zoster

John A. Zaia
Charles Grose

In memory of Stephen R. Preblud, MD, who was an expert among workers in this field.

Historical Background

Varicella is the vesicular exanthem caused by primary infection with varicella-zoster virus (VZV), commonly termed chickenpox. Herpes zoster is the clinical syndrome of segmental vesicular exanthem and pain associated with reactivation of latent VZV infection in a nerve ganglion, commonly termed shingles.

The history and epidemiology of varicella have been reviewed in detail.[1, 2] The documented record of varicella dates from the ninth century AD, when the Persian physician Rhazes noted the mild pustular skin eruption that was not protective against smallpox.[3] It was formally differentiated in the medical literature from scarlet fever in the 16th century but was not distinguished from smallpox until the late 17th century.[2, 3] The vernacular term chickenpox seems to derive from the Old English *gican*, meaning "to itch" or "to scratch,"[4] although other derivations from folklore have been suggested.[5] The itching rash of chickenpox was termed varicella in the mid-18th century, formally distinguishing it from the severe morbidity of variola.[2] More than a century later, varicella became epidemiologically linked to herpes zoster.

Herpes zoster has been recognized from antiquity as the creeping eruption that girdles the body; from this characteristic feature, the common name shingles is derived (Latin *cingulum*, a "girdle").[1] It was not until 1892, however, that the observation was made by von Bokay that varicella can develop after exposure to shingles.[6] Subsequently, varicella was observed to occur after inoculation of susceptible children with zoster vesicle fluid.[7] In addition, the histopathology of these two entities was noted to be virtually identical.[8] It was later suggested by Garland[9] that this relationship reflected the reactivation of a latent virus. Not until Weller[10] and coworkers demonstrated the method for isolation and serial propagation of VZV were these two clinical syndromes conclusively shown to be due to the same viral agent. Viral isolates obtained from varicella and from zoster were demonstrated to be identical on the basis of cytopathic effect,[11] antigen reactivity,[12] viral morphology,[13, 14] identity of DNA molecular weight,[15] and restriction fragment length polymorphism.[16–18]

Epidemiology

Transmission and Communicability

The spread of infectious VZV is by air droplets from nasopharyngeal secretions; this usually requires face-to-face exposure but can also occur without direct contact through air currents to susceptible individuals.[19] The period of infectivity is generally considered to be between 48 hours before and 4 days after appearance of the exanthem; this is derived from published observations of varicella in cohorts of children quarantined for other infections. In this setting, it was rare to observe spread of varicella from a child who exposed other wardmates more than 2 days before the onset of rash.[20, 21] Although there is a single report that infectivity could occur 4 days before exanthem,[22] this case is suspect and would be the exception to the common experience, which suggests that exposure more than 1 day before exanthem is unlikely to be infectious.[20, 21] The recommendation of the Centers for Disease Control and Prevention is to consider the period of infectivity 48 hours before rash until the skin lesions are crusted.[23]

Herpes zoster is spread by direct contact or by exposure to airborne infectious material.[24, 25] The incubation period for chickenpox after exposure to zoster[24] is the same as that after exposure to varicella[21] (median time, 15 days; range, 10 to 21 days). The clinical varicella attack rate after household zoster, however, is only 15% among history-negative children,[24] compared with an attack rate of 87% after exposure to household chickenpox.[26] This difference is thought to be due to a shorter infectious period (approximately 2 days) in herpes zoster.

Incidence and Morbidity Data

There are approximately 3.5 million cases of varicella and 300,000 cases of herpes zoster in the United States per year.[27] The age-specific epidemiologic analysis is shown in Table 148–1. More than 90% of all cases of varicella occur in per-

TABLE 148–1 ■ Epidemiologic Data for Varicella and Herpes Zoster in the United States

VARICELLA*						HERPES ZOSTER¶		
Age (y)	Susceptibility† (%)	Incidence‡	Total Cases (%)	Hospitalization Rate§	Mortality‖	Age (y)	General Incidence‡	Incidence After Varicella**
<1	100	3377	3.3	10	7.2			
1–4	97	8214	32.3	9	1.4	<5	20	110
5–9	64	9027	49.9	8	1.4	5–9	30	51
10–14	18	1753	11.1	12	1.4	10–14	59	69
15–19	10	291	1.9	42	1.3	15–19	63	70
>20	8	33	1.5	127	30.9	20–50	42	68

*Modified from population-based data in Guess HA, Broughton DD, Melton LJ III, Kurland LT: Population-based studies of varicella complications. Pediatrics 78(Suppl):723–727, 1986; and Guess HA, Broughton DD, Melton LJ 3d, Kurland LT: Chickenpox hospitalizations among residents of Olmsted County, Minnesota, 1962 through 1981. A population-based study. Am J Dis Child 138:1055–1057, 1984.
†Based on serologic surveys and comparison to incidence rates.
‡Incidence = cases per 100,000 persons per year.
§Hospitalization per 10,000 varicella cases.
‖Mortality = deaths per 100,000 varicella cases. From Preblud SR: Varicella: Complications and costs. Pediatrics 78(Suppl):728–735, 1986; ages 1 to 4 combined.
¶Based on published data from Ragozzino MW, Melton LJ 3d, Kurland LT, et al: Population-based study of herpes zoster and its sequelae. Medicine (Baltimore) 61:310–316, 1982; and Guess HA, Broughton DD, Melton LJ III, Kurland LT: Epidemiology of herpes zoster in children and adolescents: A population-based study. Pediatrics 76:512–517, 1985.
**Incidence = cases per 100,000 persons per year with prior varicella.

sons younger than 15 years, and nearly half of all cases in children occur between the ages of 5 and 9 years. On the basis of public records, the incidence of herpes zoster is constant for each age group through middle adulthood. Thereafter, the incidence of zoster increases with age, such that persons in their 80s have a 1 in 100 chance per year of developing zoster.[28] When it is adjusted for prior occurrence of varicella, the incidence of zoster in younger children it is also higher, a known association in children who have acquired varicella before their first year of life.[29]

Data from population-based studies of hospital discharges show a relatively constant rate of serious varicella-related complications for each age group up to 14 years, but the rate increases by more than 10-fold for persons older than 20 years. The types of complications that lead to hospitalization in VZV infection have been reviewed[2, 27, 30–32] and are summarized in Table 148–2. Bacterial skin infections and bacterial pneumonias occur in the youngest groups, and before the antibiotic era, severe bacterial infections, including osteomyelitis, were not uncommonly associated with varicella. With

TABLE 148–2 ■ Age-Specific Complication Rate of Varicella in the United States

AGE (y)	COMPLICATION	RATE
<5	Bacterial skin infections	1:3,800*
	Pneumonia	1:7,700
5–9	Encephalitis	1:11,100
	Reye's syndrome	1:16,700†
10–14	Encephalitis	1:11,100
	Reye's syndrome	1:6,700†
15–19	Encephalitis	1:3,400
	Varicella pneumonia	1:4,100
>20	Encephalitis	1:3,000
	Varicella pneumonia	1:375

*Hospitalization rate per number of varicella cases.
†Rates calculated before 1982 and exceed currently reported rates (see text).
Modified from Preblud SR: Varicella: Complications and costs. Pediatrics 78(Suppl):728–735, 1986; and Guess HA, Broughton DD, Melton LJ III, Kurland LT: Population-based studies of varicella complications. Pediatrics 78(Suppl):723–727, 1986.

the development of antibiotics, however, the major complications of VZV infection in childhood have been encephalitis and Reye's syndrome. Encephalitis occurs in approximately 1 in 11,000 cases in the group aged 5 to 14 years and is described later. Reye's syndrome was associated with the use of aspirin during varicella and had been observed to occur at a rate as high as 1 in 6600 cases in certain regions of the United States.[30] The occurrence of Reye's syndrome is waning since the recommendation that aspirin be avoided in children with varicella.[27, 33]

In older teenagers and adults, the primary complications are encephalitis and varicella pneumonia.[30] Encephalitis occurs in approximately 1 in 3000 cases of varicella in persons older than 15 years. Varicella pneumonia occurs at a constant rate in those aged 15 to 19 years, but thereafter the pneumonia rate is much higher. Clinically significant disease is seen in 1 in 375 cases of varicella, and asymptomatic disease with radiographic changes is common, occurring in as many as 16% of adults.[34]

Mortality and Estimated Cost

The case reports to public health agencies of deaths due to varicella have indicated a range slightly below 100 fatalities per year in the United States. It is possible that this rate is falling with the increased ability to treat the infection.[27] The mortality rate for all cases of chickenpox in normal children 1 to 14 years of age is estimated to be 0.0014% (1.4 per 100,000 cases), and the estimated rate is 31 per 100,000 in normal adults.[27] Pregnant women are at increased risk for complications during varicella.[35, 36] The two highest risk groups for lethal complications of varicella are susceptible immunosuppressed persons and neonates born within 5 days of onset of maternal varicella; these groups are discussed in detail later.

The cost of hospitalization for VZV infections is estimated to be $17 million per year.[27] However, the more significant cost of this infection in an industrialized society is lost wages by parents for home care of their sick children. In the United States, this totals approximately $380 million per year.[27] The major cost of VZV infection, therefore, is not related to the severity of disease but to lost income in affected families; these losses support the effort to develop a vaccine for prevention of this disease.

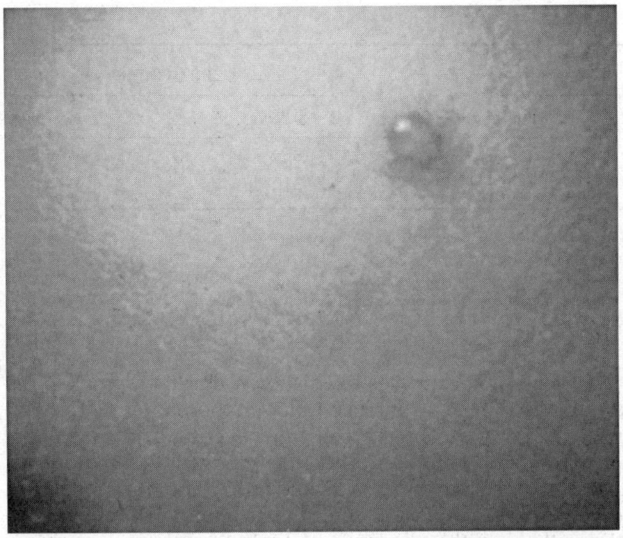

FIGURE 148–1 ▫ Initial vesicular lesion of varicella, appearing as a dewdrop on a rose petal.

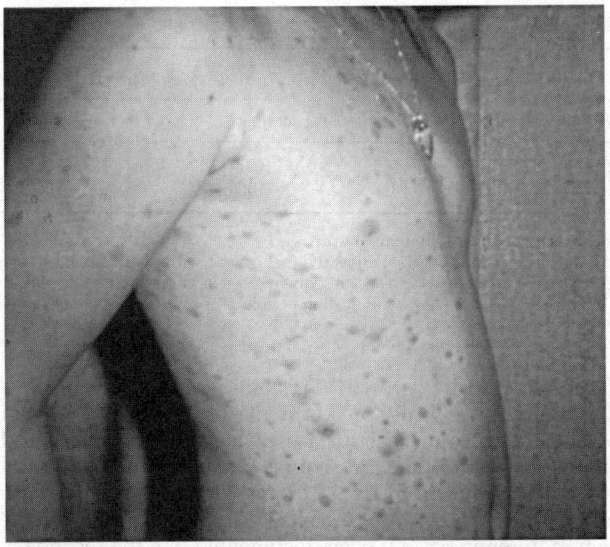

FIGURE 148–3 ▫ Varicella, day 2; note truncal distribution and lesions in multiple stages of development.

Pathophysiology

Primary Infection: Varicella

Clinical Features. In most healthy children, the clinical features of VZV infection appear at a median time of 15 days after exposure[21, 24, 26] and present as a mild exanthem often associated with prodromal malaise, pharyngitis, and rhinitis. The rash is characterized as a vesicular eruption that emerges in successive crops during the first 3 to 4 days of illness, usually with concomitant enanthema. Each skin vesicle appears on an erythematous base—hence the simile "a dewdrop on a rose petal" to describe this lesion (Fig. 148–1). However, it is difficult to see this stage of infection because of the rapid progression of the skin changes. Within 12 hours, this lesion becomes an umbilicated papule (Fig. 148–2); the involved area then undergoes leukocytic infiltration and develops into a pustule, which evolves into a hardened, crusted papule. This rapid progression from stage to stage characterizes the clinical syndrome of varicella and enables it to be distinguished from certain other vesicular eruptions. The exanthem usually begins on the head and quickly progresses to the trunk and arms, finally appearing on the legs (Figs. 148–3 and 148–4). Because of the rapid progression of individual lesions, it is common to see all stages of the exanthem, including macules, vesicles, papules, and crusts, in the same region of the skin. The most definitive clinical description of varicella was made by Ross,[26] and a summary of the fever and rash of chickenpox is shown in Table 148–3. Fever can be expected to be elevated for the first 4 days of the exanthem. Much of the morbidity is associated with the extent of the cutaneous exanthem. The average number of pox per child is variable, apparently depending on the child's age and on whether the infection occurred as a secondary case within a family.[26]

Pathogenesis. The events leading to the clinical syndrome of varicella are thought to be similar to those that were first proposed by Fenner[37] to explain an animal model of viral exanthem. In this schema, virus enters the host from an exogenous source, spreads locally to a site of initial augmentation, and then, by a primary viremia, spreads to a location

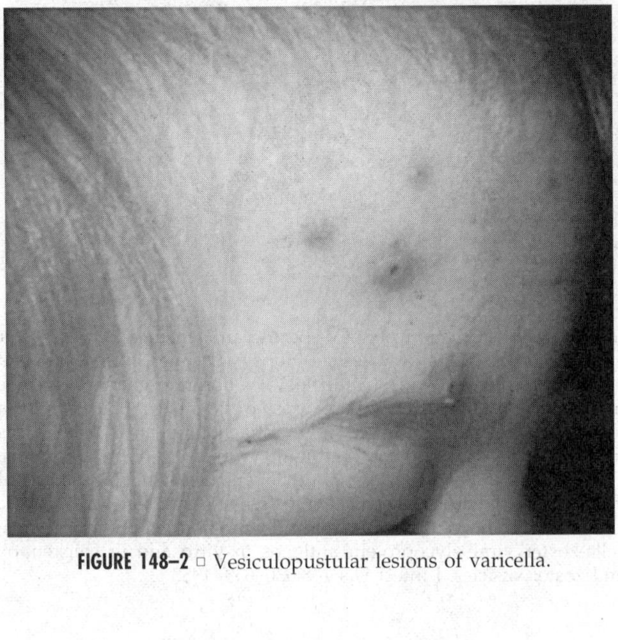

FIGURE 148–2 ▫ Vesiculopustular lesions of varicella.

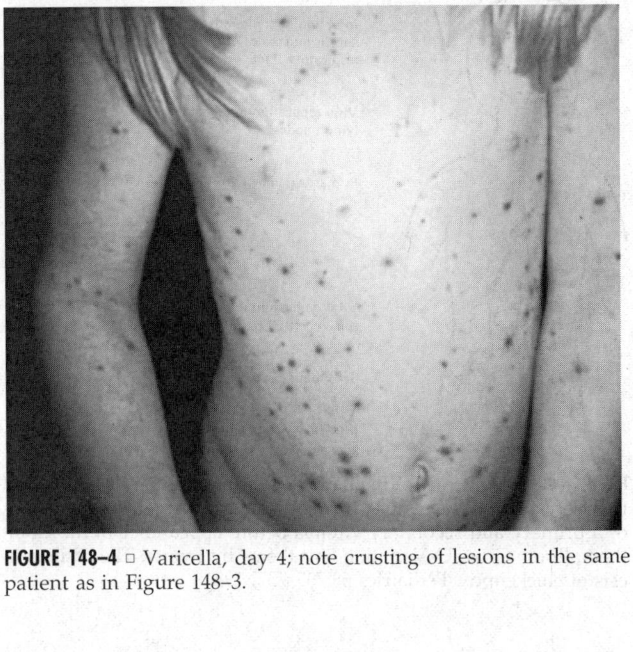

FIGURE 148–4 ▫ Varicella, day 4; note crusting of lesions in the same patient as in Figure 148–3.

TABLE 148–3 ■ Clinical Course of Varicella in Children

GROUP	T_{max} (°F)* Day 2	Day 4	Day 6	POX COUNT <5 Years	>5 Years
Primary infection†	101.0	100.2	99.3	207	258
Secondary infections‡	100.8	100.5	99.4	310	510

*Average maximal daily temperature.
†Primary infection was defined as the first case of varicella in a child having clinically well siblings.
‡Secondary infections were all subsequent cases of varicella in siblings of the primary case.
Modified from Ross AH: Modification of chicken pox in family contacts by administration of gamma globulin. N Engl J Med 267:369–376, 1962.

of subsequent viral growth (Fig. 148–5). After several days of replication, the virus spreads by means of a second viremia to the skin and mucosal surfaces, where the exanthem and enanthema occur.[37] The time course for such virus replication and spread varies from 10 to 21 days, the range observed for the incubation period of varicella.[21, 24, 26] The existence of the primary viremia has not been documented, but the secondary viremia is well described.[38] Virus spreads to endothelial cells of the skin and then infects the basal and deep malpighian layers of the epidermis. Here "ballooning degeneration" of these cells occurs, and local collection of extracellular edema results in unilocular and multilocular vesicles[1, 8] (Fig. 148–6). In addition to swelling of infected cells, multinucleation occurs, forming the basis for the Tzanck assay, and condensation of viral proteins within the nuclei results in intranuclear inclusions.

Reactivation Infection: Herpes Zoster

Clinical Features. The initial symptom of herpes zoster is pain, which is usually localized to a single spinal nerve dermatome. In 1900, Head and Campbell[39] described the anatomic pathology of this syndrome and its precise localization to single dermatomes, which permitted a mapping of the cutaneous distribution of the spinal nerves. The clinical morbidity of herpes zoster is determined largely by the involved dermatome, cranial nerve syndromes being particularly severe. The distribution mimics that of varicella, with thoracolumbar dermatomes being most frequently involved, followed by cranial dermatomes, and then by cervical and lumbar dermatomes.[39–41]

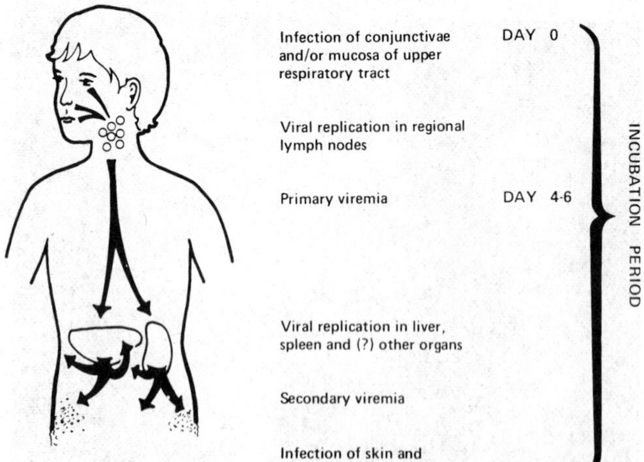

FIGURE 148–5 □ Schema for the pathogenesis of varicella. It is assumed to involve a biphasic course during the incubation period consisting of a primary and secondary viremia before appearance of the exanthem. (From Grose C: Variation on a theme by Fenner: The pathogenesis of chickenpox. Pediatrics 68:735–737, 1981.)

Histopathologic studies have shown that the dorsal spinal ganglion is the site of intense inflammation, often with hemorrhagic necrosis of nerve cells and eventual destruction of portions of the ganglion. There is intense inflammatory response to the site of VZV reactivation, and this results in nerve damage manifested clinically as meningitis or encephalitis, with or without paresis of limbs, face, gut, or urinary bladder.[42–49] In addition, there can be considerable inflammation and scarring of the involved epidermis (Figs. 148–7 and 148–8), resulting in loss of epidermal appendages, corneal clouding, and vascularization of ophthalmic structures.[46] In addition to severe inflammation, it is associated with postherpetic neuralgia, which occurs with increasing frequency in older persons and can be a significant problem lasting for many months.[28, 41, 49] VZV-associated central nervous system (CNS) complications observed with varicella and herpes zoster are compared in Table 148–4. Varicella complications present equally as cerebral or cerebellar abnormalities, the latter being a more benign disease.[45, 50, 51] Rarer CNS disorders, such as granulomatous angiitis, have been observed after herpes zoster, but these are poorly understood syndromes that have not been etiologically related to reactivation of VZV infection.[52] In immunodeficient persons, CNS disease is an important problem in herpes zoster, as with varicella, and progressive CNS disease occurs in persons with human immunodeficiency virus type 1 infection.[53, 54]

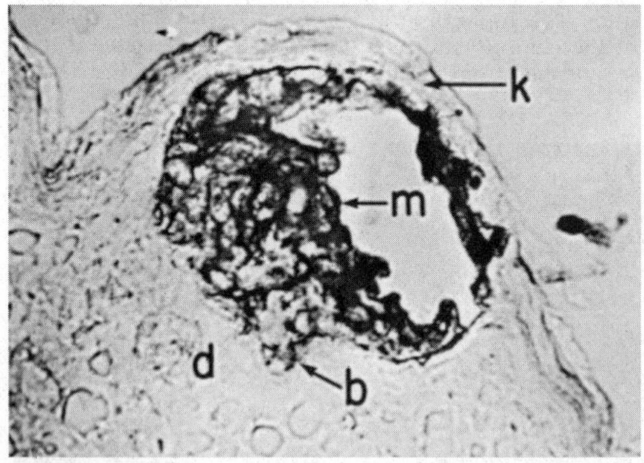

FIGURE 148–6 □ Location of VZV-specific antigen in a herpes zoster vesicle. Thin sections of a vesicle biopsy specimen were examined by indirect staining with a murine VZV immune globulin–specific monoclonal antibody and a peroxidase-conjugated rabbit antiserum to mouse immunoglobulin G. VZV antigens appear as black areas throughout the basal (b) and malpighian (m) layers of the epidermis. The outer granular and keratin (k) layers overlying the emergent vesicle and the inner dermis (d) were negative for VZV-specific antigens. (From Weigle KA, Grose C: Common expression of varicella-zoster viral glycoprotein antigens in vitro and in chickenpox and zoster vesicles. J Infect Dis 148:630–638, 1983.)

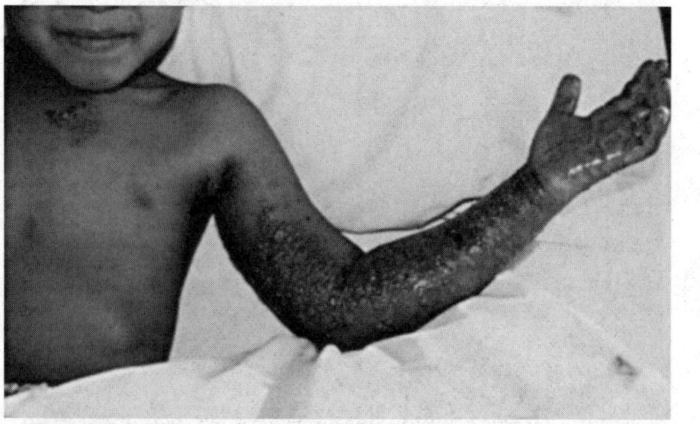

FIGURE 148–7 □ Herpes zoster in an otherwise healthy child. Note the dermatomal distribution of this unusually severe form, which required skin grafts to restore full range of motion.

TABLE 148–4 ■ Clinical Features of Varicella-Zoster Virus–Associated Neurologic Complications

FEATURE	VARICELLA (%)* (N = 52)	HERPES ZOSTER (%)† (N = 39)
Mild confusion	7	18
Altered sensorium or hallucinations	15	46
Stupor, semicoma	30	15
Meningismus	26	10
Headache	32	13
Ataxia	48	10
Seizure	17	10
Cranial nerve palsies	5	10
Extracranial nerve palsies	0	21
Cerebrospinal fluid findings		
Glucose	Normal	Normal
Protein	5.2–76 mg/dL	48–123 mg/dL
Cells	0–260	20–800

*Modified from Johnson R, Milbourn PE: Central nervous system manifestations of chickenpox. Can Med Assoc J 102:831–834, 1970.

†Modified from Jemsek J, Greenberg SB, Taber L, et al: Herpes zoster–associated encephalitis: Clinicopathologic report of 12 cases and review of the literature. Medicine (Baltimore) 62:81–97, 1983.

As with varicella, zoster-related neurologic disease can occur either before or after the acute infection[55, 56] and can occur with VZV reactivation in the absence of skin eruption, an entitity called zoster sine herpete.[57] Several CNS syndromes, including aseptic meningitis, polyneuropathy, myelitis, and encephalitis, have been observed in normal persons in association with otherwise occult VZV infection.[58]

Pathogenesis. Two factors important in the pathogenesis of herpes zoster are recognized: VZV becomes latent in dorsal spinal ganglia after primary VZV infection,[14, 59, 60] and clinical zoster presents after reactivation of this latent infection.[43, 61] But the additional factors involved in controlling this reactivation are not understood. The virus is thought to reactivate in either the ganglion cell or the perineuronal cells.[62] The disease process involves demyelination as well as active replication of virus.[63] When reactivation occurs, the virus spreads within the ganglion and within the distribution of that spinal nerve.

Because of its tropism for nervous tissue, in persons with profound immunodeficiency, VZV can spread transsynaptically within specific neuronal systems, producing necrosis of brain.[64] In general, however, the immune system generates intense inflammation at the initial site of virus reactivation, and the tissue reaction leads to nerve damage with pain syndrome and to damage in the epidermal structures with functional abnormalities. A generalized vesicular rash appears during the first week of herpes zoster in approximately 10% of normal adults,[40, 41, 65, 66] suggesting that failure to control the virus at the initial site of reactivation permits spread in a manner similar to that of varicella. This rash consists of a single crop of vesicles, which lack the polymorphism of varicella unless continued dissemination occurs.[66] Furthermore, in recipients of bone marrow transplantation, disseminated vesicular exanthem without primary dermatomal skin eruption can follow reactivation.[67] This and the observation of frequent subclinical VZV viremia in marrow transplant recipients[68] suggest that VZV latency might occur in sites other than dorsal spinal ganglia and that reactivation at extraneuronal sites could lead to viremia and generalized spread.

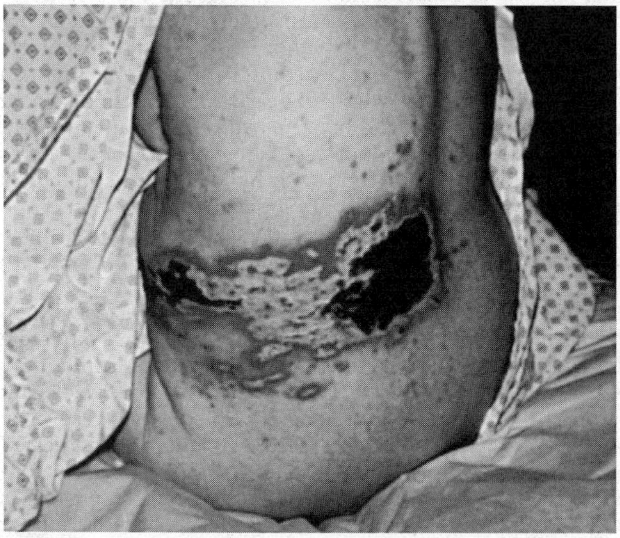

FIGURE 148–8 □ Herpes zoster in same patient as in Figures 148–10 and 148–11, day 18. Note necrosis and scarring of skin of this person, who developed postherpetic neuralgia.

Varicella-Zoster Virus Infection in the Immunocompromised Host

Clinical Features of Progressive VZV Infection. With the initiation of anticancer therapy and the use of immunosuppressive agents, progressive VZV infection has been observed.[69] Here, severe skin eruption occurs with or without hemorrhage (Fig. 148–9). There is high fever with dissemination of infection to visceral organs, producing hepatitis, pneumonitis, pancreatitis, small bowel obstruction, and encephalitis.[70, 71] A major manifestation of visceral dissemination in addition to fever is severe abdominal or back pain.[72] In the pre-antiviral era, visceral dissemination occurred in 30% of children with chickenpox while they were receiving active cancer therapy.[70] Pneumonitis occurred between 3 and 7 days after onset of varicella in 25% of such patients. Without antiviral therapy, the overall mortality in such cases is approximately 7%. In placebo-controlled trials of antiviral agents in similar patients, a fatal outcome occurred in 17% and visceral dissemination in 52% of the placebo groups.[73–75] In addition to virus dissemination, bacterial superinfection was a problem, and bacteremia accounted for significant morbidity during VZV dissemination.[70]

The severity of herpes zoster is less predictable in patients receiving immunosuppressive agents (Fig. 148–10). Persons

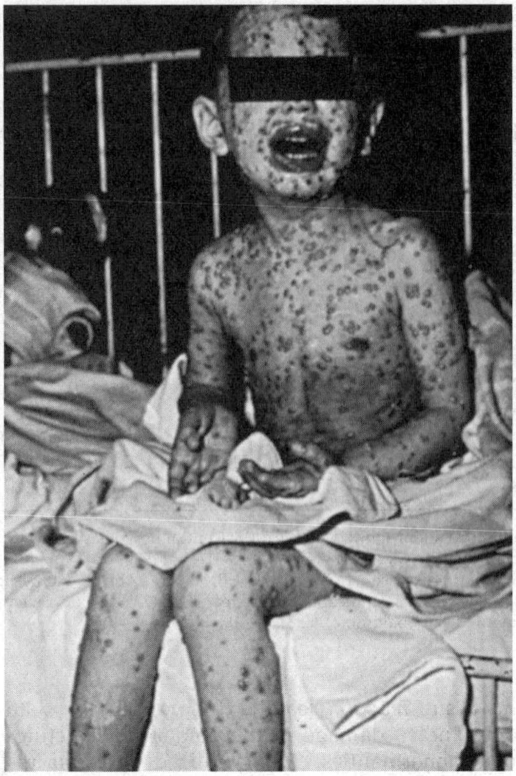

FIGURE 148–9 ▫ Disseminated varicella in child with leukemia receiving chemotherapy in 1950s. (Courtesy of Dr. Thomas Weller, Harvard University School of Public Health, Boston.)

undergoing treatment for cancer are at higher risk for developing herpes zoster than are others. Certain of these patients, such as those with Hodgkin's disease and those undergoing bone marrow transplantation, will reactivate VZV in 35% to 50% of cases during the first year of treatment.[67, 76–79] In the pre-antiviral era, the significant feature of herpes zoster was interruption of cancer therapy and further hospitalization. In general, mortality was low compared with disseminated VZV infection occurring during varicella; yet in the immunosuppressed person, herpes zoster can be associated with prolonged infection, delayed healing, and chronic postherpetic

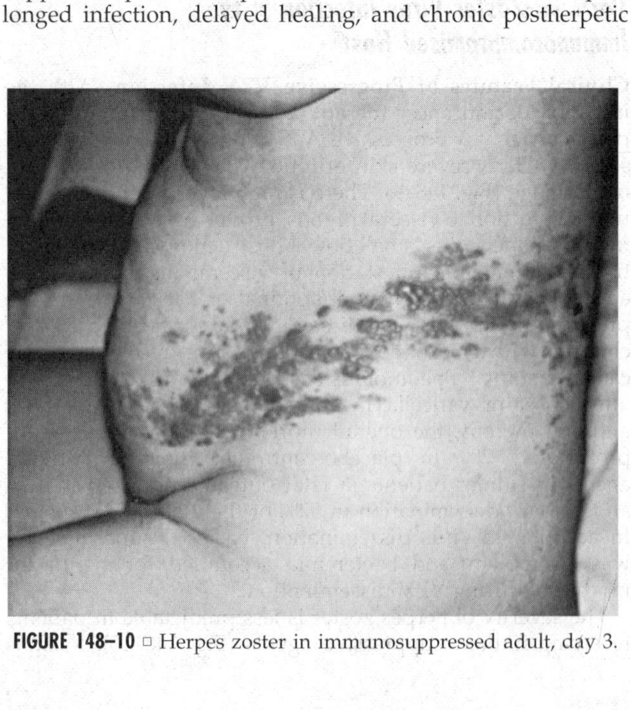

FIGURE 148–10 ▫ Herpes zoster in immunosuppressed adult, day 3.

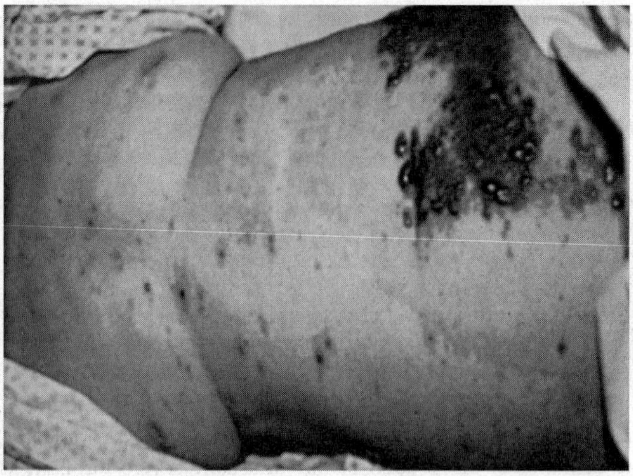

FIGURE 148–11 ▫ Herpes zoster in same patient as in Figure 148–10, day 8; note cutaneous dissemination of vesicular rash and hemorrhage into dermatomal lesion.

neuralgia. General cutaneous dissemination of virus will occur in 30% to 50% of these patients (Fig. 148–11), and although most can be expected to have a relatively benign illness, in certain groups, up to 10% will have significant visceral involvement with hepatitis, pneumonitis, and occasionally encephalitis.[76, 78, 79] In addition, in the neutropenic patient, bacterial superinfection and staphylococcal sepsis can be a particular threat.[77] The mortality rate for immunosuppressed patients with disseminated herpes zoster was 3% to 5% in the pre-antiviral era.[76, 77] Antiviral therapy significantly reduces this morbidity and, when it is used early in reactivation, can usually eliminate mortality.[74, 80, 81]

Pathogenesis of VZV Dissemination. The relationship between immunosuppression and VZV reactivation supports the view that the host's immune function controls both reactivation and dissemination of VZV infections. The explanation for this control is poorly understood. It has been observed that herpes zoster occurs in children when primary VZV infection has occurred in the first year of life[29] and in the elderly[28, 49] at times when immune regulation may not be completely functional.[82] The reactivation associated with bone marrow transplantation occurs between 3 and 9 months after the initial radiochemotherapy for bone marrow transplantation; this interval suggests that immune factors involved in control of reactivation are lost after marrow engraftment.[67, 68] It is recognized that humoral factors can influence blood-borne virus dissemination,[83] but declining humoral immunity in the bone marrow transplant recipient probably does not account for the reactivation of herpes zoster. Furthermore, children with hypogammaglobulinemia usually have no difficulty controlling primary VZV infection and have no recognized increased incidence of herpes zoster.[84] Progressive VZV dissemination is observed in children with primary cell-mediated immune deficiency[85] and in children and adults with acquired immunodeficiency syndrome.[53, 54, 86, 87] It appears that VZV antibody can moderate the extent or duration of viremia and that cellular immunity is required to prevent VZV replication.[83–89] In the elegant studies of Arvin and coworkers,[89] it was shown that severity of disease is a function of T-cell activation, as indicated by proliferative responses in vitro. In addition, interferon-α production can play a role in limiting virus spread[73, 90]; immunosuppressed children with severe varicella have been shown to have diminished production of interferon-α and significantly reduced lymphocyte proliferative response to VZV antigen.[89]

Management

Diagnosis

The diagnosis of VZV infection is discussed in Chapter 243. The primary reason for documenting this diagnosis is to confirm the need for antiviral therapy or for control of nosocomial infection. Basically, the diagnosis of VZV infection rests on three pieces of information: (1) the history of exposure and the clinical appearance of exanthem; (2) the presence of virus, viral antigens, or virus-associated cytopathic effect within the lesion; and (3) the subsequent documentation of antibody production to VZV. From a practical standpoint, the diagnosis can often be made on clinical grounds, and this is especially true for secondary cases of varicella and for herpes zoster. However, because other vesicular exanthems, such as streptococcal impetigo, poison ivy, and coxsackievirus infections, can mimic VZV infection, it is sometimes necessary to document the diagnosis of infection more exactly (Fig. 148–12).

Antiviral Therapy

General Approach. The initial assessment of the patient with VZV infection should include (1) determination of diagnosis by history, physical examination, and laboratory tests; (2) determination of whether the individual is at higher than normal risk for severe infection; and (3) characterization of current status of the infection (see Fig. 148–12). Once a tentative diagnosis is established, the critical information on which antiviral therapy hinges is whether there is risk for complications of infection and whether there is existing evidence of virus dissemination. Persons at risk for complications* are those receiving immunosuppressive medication or those who are immunodeficient from prior medication or radiotherapy; those with congenital or acquired immunodeficiency, including acquired immunodeficiency syndrome; adults with varicella; and premature infants with varicella or neonates with varicella acquired from a maternal source (Table 148–5). Because the increased risk is not easy to assess in many persons, especially in normal adults with varicella or with cutaneous dissemination of zoster, it is necessary to base the clinical decision to treat with an antiviral agent on the course of infection. In doing this, it is necessary to determine the progression of the illness using parameters such as fever, continued development of new vesicles on skin, change in hepatic enzyme levels, pulmonary examination and chest radiographic findings, and physical and laboratory evidence of specific organ involvement. Fever several days into the course of infection, especially in association with abdominolumbar pain, can be an indication of visceral dissemination.[72] Hepatic enzyme levels will be mildly elevated in most cases of varicella, even in nonimmunodeficient persons,[91] but can be useful to observe disease progression. Certain organ involvement, such as eye, lung, or brain, should always be treated with antiviral medication.

Recommended Use of Antiviral Agents. Although five

*References 23, 27, 30, 67, 69, 70, 76, 78, 83, 86, 87.

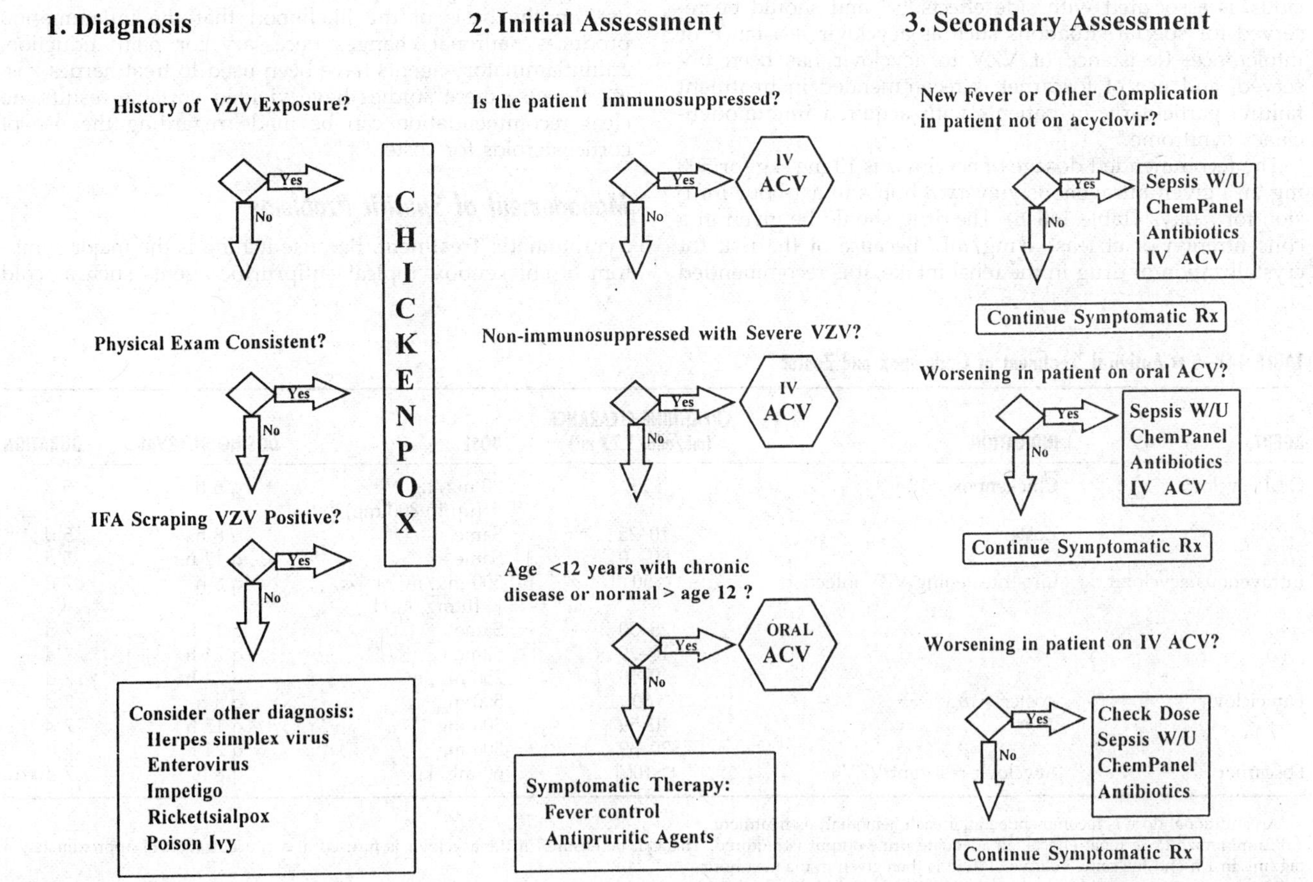

FIGURE 148–12 □ Flow chart for guiding the management of chickenpox. The three steps include establishing the diagnosis, making the initial assessment of the patient, and then making secondary assessments, as described in text. IFA, Indirect fluorescent antibody assay; IV ACV, intravenous acyclovir; W/U, work-up. (From Zaia JA: Varicella-zoster virus. *In* Schlossberg D [ed]: Current Therapy of Infectious Disease. Philadelphia, Mosby–Year Book, 1995, p 501.)

TABLE 148–5 ■ Groups at Risk for Complications of Varicella-Zoster Virus Infection*

Susceptible persons receiving immunosuppressive therapy†
Persons with congenital cellular immunodeficiency
Persons with an acquired immunodeficiency, including acquired immunodeficiency syndrome
Persons older than 20 y
Newborn infants exposed to onset of maternal varicella <5 d before or shortly after birth
Premature infants‡

*Susceptible (antibody-negative) persons exposed to VZV by indoor face-to-face contact with an infected person less than 2 d before or anytime during vesiculopustular stage of varicella rash are at highest risk.

†In general, all types of cytoreductive therapy and radiotherapy are considered immunosuppressive. The dose of prednisone that is immunosuppressive can vary in individual cases but is in the range of 1 mg/kg/d.

‡The risk for complications of VZV infection in this group is poorly defined and is based on the likelihood of protective maternal antibody versus gestational age at birth.

commercially available antiviral drugs—acyclovir, vidarabine, interferon alfa, foscarnet, and famciclovir—are active against VZV, acyclovir is the only agent licensed in the United States for the treatment of chickenpox or of disseminated VZV infection in immunosuppressed persons.[73–75, 80, 81, 92–95] For the treatment of zoster, both acyclovir and famciclovir are licensed agents.[96–99] It has been shown in comparative studies of vidarabine and acyclovir for the treatment of herpes zoster in immunosuppressed patients that acyclovir produces a more complete clinical and antiviral response.[81] Treatment with vidarabine or interferon alfa is less efficacious, is associated with side effects,[81, 95] and should be reserved for special situations such as acyclovir resistance or intolerance. Resistance of VZV to acyclovir has been observed, and use of foscarnet is recommended in treatment failure, particularly in patients with acquired immunodeficiency syndrome.[92]

The recommended dosage of acyclovir is 10 mg/kg (or 500 mg/m^2) given intravenously every 8 hours in a 1-hour infusion for 7 days (Table 148–6). The drug should be given in a concentration of at least 4 mg/mL. Because of the risk for crystallization of drug in the renal intake, it is recommended that serum creatinine levels be obtained every 3 days, and dosage modification is necessary for renal failure (see Table 148–6). To minimize the occurrence of renal complications during therapy, it is useful to give a volume of intravenous fluid equal to the volume of acyclovir, if tolerated, to initiate a diuresis before the infusion of acyclovir.

Acyclovir (800 mg five times daily) and famciclovir (500 mg three times daily) have been licensed in the United States by oral route of administration for the treatment of herpes zoster in otherwise healthy adults.[96–99]

Oral acyclovir can lessen the fever and the number and duration of skin lesions and is licensed for the treatment of chickenpox.[100] However, the American Academy of Pediatrics does not recommend that it be used for this indication in otherwise healthy children younger than 12 years. It recommends, instead, that oral acyclovir be used to treat chickenpox in those with chronic cutaneous or pulmonary disorders, in those receiving chronic salicylate therapy, in those receiving short or intermittent courses of corticosteroids or aerosolized corticosteroids, and in otherwise healthy persons older than 12 years.[101] The use of oral acyclovir for chickenpox in immunodeficient persons is not generally recommended because of inadequate experience with the oral formulation in this situation. However, as noted by the American Academy of Pediatrics, with case-by-case evaluation of risk versus benefit and with assurance of follow-up, oral acyclovir is used by some experts for treatment of chickenpox in selected immunosuppressed persons.[101]

For herpes zoster, postherpetic neuralgia is probably not prevented by the use of antiviral agents, although some studies suggest an effect with acyclovir therapy.[98, 99] The pathogenesis of postherpetic neuralgia is not understood[102]; yet, on the basis of the likelihood that the inflammation produces neuronal changes necessary for pain induction, antiinflammatory agents have been used to treat herpes zoster. Because these studies have yielded variable results, no clear recommendation can be made regarding the use of corticosteroids for zoster.[103–105]

Management of Specific Problems

Symptomatic Treatment. Because itching is the major symptom of chickenpox, topical antipruritic agents such as cold

TABLE 148–6 ■ Antiviral Treatment of Chickenpox and Zoster

AGENT	INDICATION	CREATININE CLEARANCE (mL/min/1.73 m^2)	DOSE	DOSING INTERVAL	DURATION
Oral acyclovir	Chickenpox >12 y	>25	20 mg/kg (up to 800 mg)	q 6 h	5 d
	Zoster	10–25	Same	q 8 h	5 d
		0–10*	Same	q 12 h	5 d
Intravenous acyclovir	Life-threatening VZV infection	>50	500 mg/m^2 or 10 mg/kg†‡	q 8 h	7 d
		25–50	Same	q 12 h	7 d
		10–25	Same	q 24 h	7 d
		0–10*	250 mg/m^2	q 24 h	7 d
Famciclovir	Zoster >18 y	>60	500 mg	q 8 h	7 d
		40–59	500 mg	q 12 h	7 d
		20–39	500 mg	q 24 h	7 d
Foscarnet	Acyclovir-resistant VZV§	>100‖	60 mg/kg	q 8 h	7–10 d

*An additional dose is recommended after each hemodialysis treatment.

†To minimize toxic renal effects, an adequate urine output is required. This can be ensured if the acyclovir is infused at a concentration of approximately 4 mg/mL in 1 h and the same volume of fluid is then given in the next hour.

‡ In obese persons, use ideal body weight for calculating dose.

§ Foscarnet is recommended by experts for treatment of life-threatening acyclovir-resistant VZV infection, but this is not an indication approved by the U.S. Food and Drug Administration for foscarnet use. Appropriate informed consent should be obtained before such use.

‖Foscarnet is nephrotoxic, and dosage should be determined on the basis of creatinine clearance. Guidelines for dosage adjustment are listed in the package information.

calamine lotion with diphenhydramine (Benadryl) are often helpful. Warm baths containing baking soda (⅓ cup per tub of water) can temporarily relieve pruritus and should be combined with use of oral antihistamines. Antipyretics should be given to reduce fever, but aspirin must be avoided because of the association with Reye's syndrome.[105, 106] In herpes zoster and disseminated VZV infection, pain is a major symptom and must be treated with vigorous and effective analgesia; however, narcotic analgesics must be used at reduced dosage in the presence of hepatitis.

Bacterial Infection. Pyoderma is the most frequently observed bacterial complication of varicella[2, 31] and causes the poxlike scars associated with varicella. This problem can be minimized by attention to good hygiene, including daily bathing with bacteriostatic soap, trimming of children's fingernails to minimize excoriation of itchy skin, and early recognition and treatment of superinfection. Bacterial infection should be treated with appropriate oral antibiotics, usually either erythromycin or a β-lactamase–resistant semisynthetic penicillin. Because of the persistence of infection beneath crusted lesions, débridement with salt solution soaks can be helpful.

Respiratory Tract Infection. Laryngitis and laryngotracheobronchitis can occur during varicella and may require treatment with analgesics and humidification of air. Bacterial superinfection can also involve the lower respiratory tract, producing pneumonia and bronchitis, and pneumonia in the otherwise healthy child with varicella is usually due to the respiratory pathogens, including *Streptococcus pneumoniae, Haemophilus influenzae,* and *Staphylococcus aureus.*[31]

Mucositis. Varicella is a generalized infection involving all epithelial areas, including mucosal surfaces of respiratory, alimentary, and genitourinary systems. Involvement of the bladder and urethra can result in severe dysuria with functional bladder obstruction. Urinary analgesics and, occasionally, bladder drainage may be required.

Gastrointestinal Complications and Reye's Syndrome. Some of the most serious complications of VZV infection occur in the gastrointestinal system. Vomiting is not usually part of the clinical course, and this symptom should alert the physician to abdominal or CNS complications. As with other viral infections, surgical emergencies such as appendicitis and intussusception can occur during varicella. Mild hepatic involvement is seen in a majority of children with varicella and is usually manifested by asymptomatic elevation of hepatic enzyme values, for which no treatment is necessary.[91] As noted earlier, Reye's syndrome has been described in association with varicella, often with concomitant use of aspirin in the child older than 5 years.[105, 106] Reye's syndrome and other metabolic diseases must be excluded in any child with varicella in whom there is vomiting and changes in mental status.[107] Since 1980, when the use of aspirin during respiratory infections was actively discouraged, the incidence of postvaricella Reye's syndrome has decreased so significantly that its presence should suggest an inborn error of metabolism as the primary diagnosis.[107]

Encephalitis or Myelitis. VZV infection involving the CNS is of two types: cerebellar or cerebral complications during varicella, and cranial or peripheral nerve complications during herpes zoster (see Table 148–4). Cerebellar ataxia is the most common syndrome associated with varicella encephalitis. It is generally a benign entity that is thought to be due to postinfectious demyelination.[50, 51, 63] Cerebral involvement is more serious, although it, too, has a favorable outcome in the normal child. However, in the immunosuppressed patient, cerebral involvement with seizures and altered mental status occurs and has a grave prognosis. Antiviral therapy is indicated in patients with CNS syndromes in which there is reason to suspect continued replication of virus, such as in any immunosuppressed person, any person with congenital or acquired immunodeficiency, and anyone in whom there is clinical evidence of continued new cutaneous vesicular lesions. From a practical standpoint, any major disorder of cerebral function occurring in association with acute VZV infection should be treated with acyclovir until diagnostic evaluation indicates that there is another explanation for the disease.

Thrombocytopenia and Bleeding Disorders. Bleeding disorders can occur during varicella and are due to disseminated intravascular coagulation, vasculitis, or idiopathic thrombocytopenia. The syndrome of purpura fulminans must be treated with supportive and antibiotic therapy until sepsis is ruled out. Anaphylactoid purpura can follow an otherwise uncomplicated case of varicella and must be managed with appropriate attention to the status of renal function and the possibility of occult intraabdominal hemorrhage. Idiopathic thrombocytopenic purpura can occur during active infection or during convalescence. Mild hemorrhage into vesicles during active infection does not require specific treatment, but excessive hemorrhage and profound thrombocytopenia should be treated with platelet infusions, intravenous immune globulin, and antiviral therapy.

Maternal, Congenital, and Perinatal VZV Infection. The most significant danger of VZV infection during pregnancy is to the health of the mother, who has nearly a 10% risk for severe pneumonia.[36] Therefore, antiviral therapy should be instituted immediately if the pregnant woman develops any signs of respiratory distress. Early induction of labor, if appropriate, should be a consideration in the management of this infection. In addition, there is a risk of VZV infection to the unborn infant; this can be in the form of either congenital teratogenic infection[36, 108–110] or perinatal infection.[36, 111] If maternal varicella occurs less than 5 days before or shortly after delivery, there is an increased mortality associated with subsequent VZV infection in the infant.[111] The risk of severe VZV infection appears to be a function of the level of transplacental maternal antibody to VZV in the infant.[111, 112] It is recommended that such high-risk neonates exposed to maternal varicella, as well as premature infants likely to lack such maternal antibody, be given passive immunization with varicella-zoster immune globulin (VZIG).[23] Maternal herpes zoster presents no significant risk to mother or infant.[36]

A pregnant woman with significant exposure to VZV infection should be evaluated for susceptibility to VZV with appropriate antibody assay (see Chapter 243) if she has a negative or unknown history of having had varicella as a child. Seronegative women should receive passive immunization with VZIG.[23]

Intrauterine VZV infection can occur after maternal varicella in all trimesters of gestation, but teratogenic or developmental damage results from infection before the third trimester.[36, 110] The rate of transplacental infection is 24%, but clinically apparent disease is approximately 3% for maternal varicella in early pregnancy.[36] The stigmata of early fetal infection include defects of the extremities, skin, and eyes as well as microcephaly, hydrocephalus, and brain calcifications.[108, 109] The abnormalities of the extremities derive from hypoplasia during development and appear as limb shortening and deformity. The characteristic cutaneous manifestations are deep cicatricial scarring, often in association with the limb abnormalities. The eye defects include microphthalmos, cataracts, and chorioretinitis. Virtually all the defects can be attributed to an interruption in the developing neurologic system of the fetus; the period of greatest risk for severe disease is the first trimester, when the fetal limb muscles are formed and innervated by nerves from the developing spinal cord. This represents a process in which the known neurotropism of the virus manifests itself in its most virulent form.[110]

Approach to the Immunocompromised Host

General Management. In the pre-antiviral era, the management of the immunocompromised child focused on the prevention of exposure to VZV infection. This strategy relied on awareness by parents, friends, and school personnel of the importance of early notification of possible varicella contagion. This system aimed at passive immunization of high-risk groups, but because it depended on timely reaction to exposure, it was less than optimal and resulted in prolonged absences from school. With the introduction of antiviral therapy and active immunization, we are closer to the elimination of VZV as a cause of morbidity and mortality in immunosuppressed children, and there is less emphasis on the importance of varicella awareness. The VZV vaccine is not indicated for routine use in immunosuppressed persons, but children with acute lymphoblastic leukemia can and should receive this form of protection by use of an investigational protocol available from the manufacturer. Parents and school personnel must continue to be aware of exposure to VZV and of the importance of actual VZV rash in unvaccinated high-risk children so that VZIG or early antiviral treatment can be given in the most timely fashion.

Use of Varicella-Zoster Immune Globulin. It has been recognized for decades that convalescent serum from persons with VZV infection could protect from severe clinical disease.[21] Ross[26] demonstrated that immune serum globulin would modify infection in otherwise healthy children. Subsequently, it was shown that the effective administration of passive antibody to immunosuppressed persons failed unless convalescent antibody was used.[113] With the development of efficient screening procedures for selection of high-titer outdated donor blood units,[114] VZIG became commercially available. VZIG has been demonstrated to be effective for the prevention of severe varicella in the immunosuppressed person.[83] Any susceptible person at risk for complications of varicella (see Table 148–5) should receive passive immunization if exposure to VZV was adequate and occurred within approximately 4 days. VZIG should not be used in the person with prior history of varicella; sensitive serologic testing for VZV antibody, using an enzyme immunoassay, a fluorescent antibody assay, or a rapid slide agglutination test, is available to make this distinction.

Antiviral Therapy. The specific use of acyclovir was described earlier, but management of individual patients may be less straightforward. Not all immunosuppressed persons with VZV infection need to be treated with acyclovir, and case-by-case evaluation of risk versus benefit is necessary. For certain groups, the risk of disseminated infection is so high or so unpredictable that treatment is recommended in all cases, for example, varicella in children receiving treatment for leukemia, varicella in profound immunodeficiency states, and herpes zoster in the first 6 months after bone marrow transplantation.[67, 101, 115] The use of oral instead of intravenous acyclovir is never recommended in the immunocompromised individual with life-threatening infection, because the intravenous formulation. is the only clearly efficacious treatment in this setting.[74, 80, 101] Famciclovir has not been licensed for use in immunosuppressed persons.

Management of Nosocomial Infections

Nosocomial VZV infection is a well-recognized problem, particularly in tertiary care centers for immunosuppressed patients.[116, 117] Clusters of varicella can be difficult to eradicate from chronic care facilities for children and frequently affect paramedical staff from foreign countries where the rate of susceptibility among adults is higher than in the United States.[118] Interestingly, herpes zoster cases have been described after exposure to VZV infection; there is no explanation for these occurrences.[24, 119]

Control of nosocomial infections involves three actions: (1) surveillance of susceptibility and use of VZV vaccine in susceptible or history-negative hospital staff, (2) adequate isolation of contagious VZV infections, and (3) rapid evaluation and response to reported VZV exposure. Hospitals that care for immunodeficient patients should screen staff at the time of employment for susceptibility. This can be done efficiently by performing antibody tests on those who have a negative or unknown history of prior varicella. Susceptible employees should be excluded from care of patients with VZV infection. Recommended isolation procedures for varicella are respiratory precautions, including double-door isolation, with gown, gloves, and mask for persons in the patient's room.[120, 121] Recommended isolation procedures for herpes zoster vary on the basis of a report that airborne spread of VZV can be associated with reactivated virus infection. However, for practical reasons in cancer centers, contact precautions are sufficient unless there is a threat of viral dissemination due to the presence of VZV pneumonia.[116, 117]

Varicella Vaccine

A live attenuated VZV vaccine was developed by Takahashi[122] and coworkers in 1974; since that time, there has been extensive experience with live virus vaccination for prevention of VZV infection. This vaccine was prepared by attenuation of a VZV isolate (Oka strain) in human embryonic lung cells, in guinea pig embryonic cells, and then in human diploid fibroblasts.[123] The vaccine virus is biologically different from wild VZV in its growth characteristics and DNA restriction enzyme profile.

This vaccine has been used extensively in Japan in healthy children and has been demonstrated to be effective for the prevention of varicella after exposure and for curtailment of outbreaks of VZV infection.[124–126] A live attenuated VZV vaccine (Varivax) was approved in the United States in 1995.[127–130] A single dose of vaccine results in seroconversion in 97% of susceptible children 1 to 12 years old, in 79% of children 13 to 17 years old, and in 82% of adults. Two doses of vaccine result in seroconversion in 94% of adults. Antibody is known to persist for at least 6 years. The rate of zoster has not been shown to be influenced by vaccination. VZV vaccine is recommended for all healthy children 12 months to 12 years of age in chickenpox history–negative persons, especially health care and daycare workers, college students, prisoners, military recruits, nonpregnant women of childbearing age, and international travelers. The vaccine is not recommended for infants younger than 1 year; for immunosuppressed persons; for those receiving salicylate therapy; for pregnant women; or for persons allergic to components of the vaccine, including neomycin, gelatin, and monosodium glutamate.

In children with leukemia studied in the United States, Gershon and Steinberg[131] have given either one or two doses of vaccine to those in remission. At 5-year follow-up, seropositivity was lost in 30%, but after household exposure to VZV, the attack rate for varicella was only 14% and disease was usually mild.[131, 132]

Acknowledgments

The authors express their gratitude to Ms. Diane Schulz for her assistance in the preparation of the manuscript.

References

1. Taylor-Robinson D, Caunt AE: Varicella Virus. Vienna, Springer-Verlag, 1972.

2. Gordon JE, Ingalls TH: Chickenpox: An epidemiologic review. Am J Med Sci 244:362, 1962.
3. Bett WR: A Short History of Some Common Diseases. London, Oxford University Press, 1934.
4. Scott-Wilson JH: Why 'chicken' pox? (Letter). Lancet 1:1152, 1978.
5. Lerman SJ: Why is chickenpox called chickenpox? Clin Pediatr 20:1111, 1981.
6. von Bokay J: Das Auftreten von Varizellen unter Eigentumlichen. Magy Orvosi Arch, November 3, 1892. As cited in Blatt ML, Zeldes M, Stein AF: Chickenpox following contact with herpes zoster. J Lab Clin Med 25:951, 1940.
7. Lipschutz B, Kundratit K: Über die Aetiologie des Zoster und uber seine Beziehungen zu Varizellen. Wien Klin Wochenschr 38:499, 1925.
8. Tyzzer EE: The histology of the skin lesions in varicella. J Med Res 14:361, 1906.
9. Garland J: Varicella following exposure to herpes zoster. N Engl J Med 1228:336, 1943.
10. Weller TH: Serial propagation in vitro of agents producing inclusion bodies derived from varicella and herpes zoster. Proc Soc Exp Biol 83:340, 1953.
11. Weller TH, Witton HM, Bell EJ: The etiologic agents of varicella and herpes zoster: Isolation, propagation, and cultural characteristics in vitro. J Exp Med 108:843, 1958.
12. Weller TH, Coons AH: Fluorescent antibody studies with agents of varicella and herpes zoster propagated in vitro. Proc Soc Exp Biol Med 86:789, 1954.
13. Kimura A, Tosaka K, Nakao T: An electron microscopic study of varicella skin lesions. Arch Gesamte Virusforsch 36:1, 1972.
14. Esiri MM, Tomlinson AH: Herpes zoster—Demonstration of virus in trigeminal nerve and ganglion by immunofluorescence and electron microscopy. J Neurol Sci 15:35, 1972.
15. Iltis JP, Oakes JE, Hyman RW, Rapp F: Comparison of the DNAs of varicella-zoster viruses isolated from clinical cases of varicella and herpes zoster. Virology 82:345, 1977.
16. Richards JC, Hyman RW, Rapp F: Analysis of the DNAs from seven varicella-zoster virus isolates. J Virol 32:812, 1979.
17. Pichini B, Ecker JR, Grose C, Hyman RW: DNA mapping of paired varicella-zoster virus isolates from patients with shingles. Lancet 2:1223, 1983.
18. Straus SE, Reinhold W, Smith HA, et al: Endonuclease analysis of viral DNA from varicella and subsequent zoster infections in the same patient. N Engl J Med 311:1362, 1984.
19. Leclair JM, Zaia JA, Levin MJ, et al: Airborne transmission of chickenpox in a hospital. N Engl J Med 302:450, 1980.
20. Thomson FH, Aberd CM: The aerial conveyance of infection. Lancet 1:341, 1916.
21. Gordon JE, Meader FM: The period of infectivity and serum prevention of chickenpox. JAMA 93:2013, 1929.
22. Evans P, Mane MB: An epidemic of chickenpox. Lancet 2:339, 1940.
23. Prevention of varicella: Recommendations of the Advisory Committee on Immunization Practices (ACIP). Centers for Disease Control and Prevention. MMWR Morbid Mortal Wkly Rep 45:1, 1996.
24. Seiler HE: A study of herpes zoster particularly in its relationship to chickenpox. J Hyg 47:253, 1949.
25. Josephson A, Gombert ME: Airborne transmission of nosocomial varicella from localized zoster. J Infect Dis 158:238, 1988.
26. Ross AH: Modification of chickenpox in family contacts by administration of gamma globulin. N Engl J Med 267:369, 1962.
27. Preblud SR: Varicella: Complications and costs. Pediatrics 78(Suppl):728, 1986.
28. Hope-Simpson RE: Herpes zoster in the elderly. Geriatrics 22:151, 1967.
29. Brunell PA, Kotchmar GS: Zoster in infancy: Failure to maintain virus latency following intrauterine infection. J Pediatr 98:71, 1981.
30. Guess HA, Broughton DD, Melton LJ III, Kurland LT: Population-based studies of varicella complications. Pediatrics 78(Suppl):723, 1986.
31. Bullowa JGM, Wishik SM: Complications of varicella: I. Their occurrence among 2,534 patients. Am J Dis Child 49:923, 1935.
32. Preblud SR: Age-specific risks of varicella complications. Pediatrics 68:14, 1981.
33. Barret MJ, Hurwitz ES, Schonberger LB, Rogers MR: Changing epidemiology of Reye syndrome in the United States. Pediatrics 77:598, 1986.
34. Weber DM, Pellechia JA: Varicella pneumonia: Study of prevalence in adult men. JAMA 192:572, 1965.
35. Pearson HE: Parturition varicella-zoster. Obstet Gynecol 23:21, 1964.
36. Paryani SG, Arvin AM: Intrauterine infection with varicella-zoster virus after maternal varicella. N Engl J Med 314:1542, 1986.
37. Grose C: Variation on a theme by Fenner: The pathogenesis of chickenpox. Pediatrics 68:735, 1981.
38. Ozaki T, Ichikawa T, Matsui Y, et al: Viremic phase in non-immunocompromised children with varicella. J Pediatr 104:85, 1984.
39. Head H, Campbell AW: The pathology of herpes zoster and its bearing on sensory localization. Brain 23:353, 1900.
40. Hope-Simpson RE: The nature of herpes zoster: A long-term study and a new hypothesis. Proc R Soc Med 58:9, 1965.
41. Burgoon DF Jr, Burgoon JS, Baldridge GD: The natural history of herpes zoster. JAMA 164:265, 1957.
42. Denny-Brown D, Adams RD, Fitzgerald PJ: Pathologic features of herpes zoster—A note on "geniculate herpes." Arch Neurol Psychol 51:216, 1944.
43. Gold E: Serologic and virus-isolation studies of patients with varicella or herpes-zoster infection. N Engl J Med 274:181, 1966.
44. Jellinek EH, Tulloch WS: Herpes zoster with dysfunction of bladder and anus. Lancet 2:1219, 1976.
45. Jemsek J, Greenberg SB, Taber L, et al: Herpes zoster–associated encephalitis: Clinicopathologic report of 12 cases and review of the literature. Medicine (Baltimore) 62:81, 1983.
46. Womack LW, Liesegang TJ: Complications of herpes zoster ophthalmicus. Arch Ophthalmol 101:42, 1983.
47. Winkelmann RK, Perry HO: Herpes zoster in children. JAMA 171:376, 1959.
48. Guess HA, Broughton DD, Melton LJ III, Kurland LT: Epidemiology of herpes zoster in children and adolescents: A population-based study. Pediatrics 76:512, 1985.
49. Ragozzino ME, Melton LJ III, Kurland LT, et al: Population-based study of herpes zoster and its sequelae. Medicine (Baltimore) 61:310, 1982.
50. Johnson R, Milbourn PE: Central nervous system manifestations of chickenpox. Can Med Assoc J 102:831, 1970.
51. Underwood EA: The neurological complications of varicella—A clinical and epidemiologic study. Br J Child Dis 32:83, 177, 241, 1935.
52. Blue MC, Rosenblum WI: Granulomatous angiitis of the brain with herpes zoster and varicella encephalitis. Arch Pathol Lab Med 107:126, 1983.
53. Cole EL, Meisler DM, Calabrese LH, et al: Herpes zoster ophthalmicus and acquired immune deficiency syndrome. Arch Ophthalmol 102:1027, 1984.
54. Gilden DH, Murray RS, Wellish M, et al: Chronic progressive varicella-zoster virus encephalitis in an AIDS patient. Neurology 38:1150, 1988.
55. Goldston AS, Millichap JG, Miller RH: Cerebellar ataxia with preeruptive varicella. Am J Dis Child 106:111, 1963.
56. McCarthy JT, Amer J: Postvaricella acute transverse myelitis: A case presentation and review of the literature. Pediatrics 62:202, 1978.
57. Lewis GW: Zoster sine herpete. Br Med J 2:418, 1958.
58. Mayo DR, Booss J: Varicella zoster–associated neurologic disease without skin lesions. Arch Neurol 46:313, 1989.
59. Hyman RW, Ecker JR, Tenser RB: Varicella-zoster virus RNA in human trigeminal ganglia. Lancet 2:814, 1983.
60. Gilden DH, Rozenman Y, Murray R, et al: Detection of varicella-zoster virus nucleic acid in neurons of normal human thoracic ganglia. Ann Neurol 22:377, 1987.
61. Pichini B, Ecker JR, Grose C, Hyman RW: DNA mapping of paired varicella-zoster virus isolates from patients with shingles. Lancet 2:1223, 1983.
62. Croen KD, Ostrove JM, Dragovic LJ, Straus SE: Patterns of gene expression and sites of latency in human nerve ganglia are different for varicella-zoster and herpes simplex viruses. Proc Natl Acad Sci USA 85:9773, 1988.
63. McCormick WF, Rodnitzky RL, Schochet SS, McKee AP: Varicella-zoster encephalomyelitis. Arch Neurol 26:559, 1969.

64. Rostad SW, Olson K, McDougall J, et al: Transsynaptic spread of varicella zoster virus through the visual system: A mechanism of viral dissemination in the central nervous system. Hum Pathol 20:174, 1989.
65. Oberg G, Svedmyr A: Varicelliform eruption in herpes zoster—Some chemical and serological observations found. Scand J Infect Dis 1:47, 1969.
66. Hutton PW: Bilateral zoster and zoster varicellosus. Lancet 2:302, 1935.
67. Locksley RM, Flournoy N, Sullivan KM, Meyers JD: Infection with varicella-zoster virus after marrow transplantation. J Infect Dis 152:1172, 1985.
68. Wilson A, Sharp M, Koropchak CM, et al: Subclinical varicella-zoster viremia, herpes zoster, and T lymphocyte immunity to varicella-zoster viral antigens after bone marrow transplantation. J Infect Dis 165:119, 1992.
69. Cheatham WJ, Weller TH, Dolan TF Jr, et al: Varicella: Report of 2 fatal cases with necroscopy, virus isolation, and serologic studies. Am J Pathol 32:1015, 1956.
70. Feldman S, Hughes WT, Daniel CB: Varicella in children with cancer: Seventy-seven cases. Pediatrics 56:388, 1975.
71. Chang AE, Young NA, Reddick RL, et al: Small bowel obstruction as a complication of disseminated varicella-zoster infection. Surgery 83:371, 1978.
72. Simmons RL, Balfour HH Jr: Complication of disseminated varicella-zoster infection. Surgery 83:486, 1978.
73. Arvin AM, Kusher JH, Feldman S, et al: Human leukocyte interferon for treatment of varicella in children with cancer. N Engl J Med 306:761, 1982.
74. Prober DG, Kirk LE, Keeney RE: Acyclovir therapy of chickenpox in immunosuppressed children—A collaborative study. J Pediatr 101:622, 1982.
75. Whitley RJ, Hilty M, Haynes R, et al: Vidarabine therapy of varicella in immunosuppressed patients. J Pediatr 1:125, 1982.
76. Feldman S, Hughes WT, Kim HY: Herpes zoster in children with cancer. Am J Dis Child 126:178, 1973.
77. Schimpff SC, Fortner WH, Greene WH, Wiernik P: Cytosine arabinoside for localized herpes zoster in patients with cancer: Failure in a controlled trial. J Infect Dis 130:673, 1974.
78. Schimpff S, Serpick A, Stoler B, et al: Varicella-zoster infection in patients with cancer. Ann Intern Med 76:241, 1972.
79. Sokol JE, Firat D: Varicella-zoster infection in Hodgkin's disease. Am J Med 39:452, 1965.
80. Balfour HH Jr, Bean B, Laskin OL, et al: Acyclovir halts progression of herpes zoster in immunocompromised patients. N Engl J Med 308:1448, 1983.
81. Shepp DH, Dandliker PS, Meyers JD: Treatment of varicella-zoster virus infection in severely immunocompromised patients—A randomized comparison of acyclovir and vidarabine. N Engl J Med 314:208, 1986.
82. Hayward AR, Herberger M: Lymphocyte reponses to varicella zoster virus in the elderly. J Clin Immunol 7:174, 1987.
83. Zaia JA, Levin MJ, Preblud SR, et al: Evaluation of varicella-zoster immune globulin—Protection of immunosuppressed children after household exposure to varicella. J Infect Dis 147:737, 1983.
84. Good RA, Zak SJ: Disturbances in gamma globulin synthesis as "experiments of nature." Pediatrics 18:109, 1956.
85. Lux SE, Johnston RB, August CS, et al: Chronic neutropenia and abnormal cellular immunity in cartilage-hair hypoplasia. N Engl J Med 282:231, 1970.
86. Cohen PR, Beltrani VP, Grossman ME: Disseminated herpes zoster in patients with human immunodeficiency virus infection. Am J Med 14:1076, 1988.
87. Jura E, Chadwick EG, Josephs SH, et al: Varicella-zoster virus infections in children infected with human immunodeficiency virus. Pediatr Infect Dis J 8:586, 1989.
88. Giller RH, Bowden RA, Levin MJ, et al: Reduced cellular immunity to varicella zoster virus during treatment for acute lymphoblastic leukemia of childhood: In vitro studies of possible mechanisms. J Clin Immunol 6:472, 1986.
89. Arvin AM, Koropchak CM, Williams BRG, et al: Early immune response in healthy and immunocompromised subjects with primary varicella-zoster virus infection. J Infect Dis 154:422, 1986.
90. Patel PA, Yoonessi S, O'Malley J, et al: Cell-mediated immunity to varicella-zoster virus infection in subjects with lymphoma or leukemia. J Pediatr 94:223, 1979.
91. Pitel PA, McCormick KL, Fitzgerald E, Orson JM: Subclinical hepatic changes in varicella infection. Pediatrics 65:631, 1980.
92. Pahwa S, Biron K, Lim W, et al: Continuous varicella-zoster infection associated with acyclovir resistance in a child with AIDS. JAMA 260:2879, 1988.
93. Crumpacker CS, Schnipper LE, Zaia JA, Levin MJ: Growth inhibition by acycloguanosine of herpesviruses isolated from human infections. Antimicrob Agents Chemother 15:642, 1979.
94. Merigan TC, Rand KH, Pollard RB, et al: Human leukocyte interferon for the treatment of herpes zoster in patients with cancer. N Engl J Med 298:981, 1978.
95. Winston DJ, Eron LJ, Ho M, et al: Recombinant interferon alpha-2a for treatment of herpes zoster in immunosuppressed patients with cancer. Am J Med 85:147, 1988.
96. McKendrick MW, McGill JI, White JE, Wood MJ: Oral acyclovir in acute herpes zoster. Br Med J 293:1529, 1986.
97. Cobo LM, Foulks GN, Liesegang T, et al: Oral acyclovir in the treatment of acute herpes zoster ophthalmicus. Ophthalmology 93:763, 1986.
98. Huff JC, Bean B, Balfour HH, et al: Therapy of herpes zoster with oral acyclovir. Am J Med 85(Suppl 2A):84, 1988.
99. Tyring S, Barbarash RA, Nahlik JE, et al: Famciclovir for the treatment of acute herpes zoster: Effects on acute disease and postherpetic neuralgia, a randomized, double-blind, placebo-controlled trial. Ann Intern Med 123:89, 1995.
100. Balfour HH, Kelly JM, Suarez CS, et al: Acyclovir treatment of varicella in otherwise healthy children. J Pediatr 116:633, 1990.
101. American Academy of Pediatrics: Varicella zoster infections. *In* Peter G (ed): 1994 Red Book: Report of the Committee on Infectious Diseases, ed 23. Elk Grove Village, IL, American Academy of Pediatrics, 1994, pp 512–513.
102. Schon F, Mayer ML, Kelly JS: Pathogenesis of post-herpetic neuralgia. Lancet 2:366, 1987.
103. Eaglstein WH, Katz R, Brown JA: The effects of early corticosteroid therapy on the skin eruption and pain of herpes zoster. JAMA 211:1681, 1970.
104. Esmann V, Kroon S, Peterslund NA, et al: Prednisolone does not prevent postherpetic neuralgia. Lancet 2:126, 1987.
105. McGowan JE Jr, Chesney PJ, Crossley KB, LaForce FM: Guidelines for the use of systemic glucocorticoids in the management of selected infections. J Infect Dis 165:1, 1992.
106. Hurwitz ES, Barrett MJ, Bregman D, et al: Public Health Service study of Reye syndrome and medications: Report of the main study. JAMA 257:1905, 1987.
107. Rowe PC, Valle D, Bruislowo SW: Inborn errors of metabolism in children referred with Reye's syndrome: A changing pattern. JAMA 260:3168, 1988.
108. Laforet EG, Lynch CL: Multiple congenital defects following maternal varicella. N Engl J Med 236:534, 1947.
109. Williamson AP: The varicella-zoster virus in the etiology of severe congenital defects. Clin Pediatr 14:553, 1975.
110. Grose C, Itani O: Pathogenesis of congenital infection with three diverse viruses: Varicella-zoster virus, human parvovirus, and human immunodeficiency virus. Semin Perinatol 13:278, 1989.
111. Meyers JD: Congenital varicella in term infants: Risk reconsidered. J Infect Dis 129:215, 1974.
112. Gershon AA, Raker R, Steinberg S, et al: Antibody to varicella-zoster virus in parturient women and their offspring during the first year of life. Pediatrics 58:692, 1976.
113. Gershon AA, Steinberg S, Brunell PA: Zoster immunoglobulin: A further assessment. N Engl J Med 290:243, 1974.
114. Zaia JA, Levin MJ, Wright GG, Grady GF: A practical method for the preparation of varicella-zoster immune globulin. J Infect Dis 137:601, 1978.
115. Balfour HH Jr: Intravenous acyclovir therapy for varicella in immunocompromised children. J Pediatr 104:134, 1984.
116. Preblud SR: Nosocomial varicella: Worth preventing, but how? Am J Public Health 78:13, 1988.
117. Myers MG, Rasley DA, Hierholzer WJ: Hospital infection control for varicella zoster virus infection. Pediatrics 70:199, 1982.
118. Sinha DP: Chickenpox—A disease predominantly affecting adults in rural West Bengal, India. Int J Epidemiol 5:367, 1976.
119. Berlin BS, Campbell T: Hospital-acquired herpes zoster following exposure to chickenpox. JAMA 211:1831, 1970.

120. Garner JS, Simmons BP: Guideline for isolation precautions in hospitals. Infect Control 4(Suppl 4):245, 1983.
121. Williams WW: Guideline for infection control in hospital personnel. Infect Control 4(Suppl 4):326, 1983.
122. Takahashi M: Clinical overview of varicella vaccine: Development and early studies. Pediatrics 78(Suppl):736, 1986.
123. Takahashi M, Okuno Y, Otsuka T, et al: Development of a live attenuated varicella vaccine. Biken J 18:25, 1975.
124. Takahashi M, Otuska T, Okuna Y, et al: Live vaccine used to prevent the spread of varicella in children in hospital. Lancet 2:1288, 1974.
125. Asano Y, Yazaki T, Miyata T, et al: Application of a live attenuated varicella vaccine to hospitalized children and its protective effect on spread of varicella infection. Biken J 18:35, 1975.
126. Asano Y, Nagai T, Miyata T, et al: Long-term protective immunity of recipients of the OKA strain of varicella vaccine. Pediatrics 75:667, 1985.
127. Varicella vaccine. Med Lett Drugs Ther 37:55, 1995.
128. Arbeter AM, Starr SE, Plotkin SA: Varicella vaccine studies in healthy children and adults. Pediatrics 78(Suppl):748, 1988.
129. Gershon AA, Steinberg SP, Gelb L, and the National Institute of Allergy and Infectious Diseases Varicella Vaccine Collaborative Study Group: Live attenuated varicella vaccine use in immunocompromised children and adults. Pediatrics 78(Suppl):757, 1986.
130. Brunell PA, Novelli VM, Lipton SV, et al: Combined vaccine against measles, mumps, rubella, and varicella. Pediatrics 81:779, 1988.
131. Gershon AA, Steinberg SP: Persistence of immunity to varicella in children with leukemia immunized with live attenuated varicella vaccine. N Engl J Med 320:892, 1989.
132. Lawrence R, Gershon AA, Holzman R, Steinberg SP, and the NIAID Varicella Vaccine Collaborative Study Group: The risk of zoster after varicella vaccination in children with leukemia. N Engl J Med 318:543, 1988.

149

Smallpox

John Noble
Joseph J. Esposito

Smallpox was one of the most dreaded diseases of humans. It raged in epidemic and endemic forms for more than 3000 years. Smallpox "exerted a singular influence on human history through the ages before its extinction in 1977—suddenly removing or temporarily indisposing leaders of nations, destroying armies, disrupting cities, and laying waste to ordinary citizens, devastating virgin populations and influencing fateful decisions . . . ."[1]

The high mortality of smallpox caused an average of 10% of all deaths each year in towns and cities where the disease was endemic. Mortalities up to 100% were recorded in the devasting epidemics of smallpox that swept through Native American populations of North, Central, and South America. The disease continued into the 20th century; there were 65 cases with 20 deaths in Seattle in 1945, 12 cases with 2 deaths in New York City in 1947, and 8 cases with 1 death in Texas in 1949. These were the last reported cases of smallpox in the United States.

An Intensified Smallpox Eradication Program was established by the World Health Organization (WHO) in 1966, with the goal of attaining global eradication of smallpox in 10 years. At that time, smallpox was reported in 41 countries, extending from Afghanistan to Malaysia and Indonesia; throughout most of Africa south of the Sahara; and in Brazil, Argentina, and other dispersed locations. National eradication campaigns were conducted in more than 80 countries between 1966 and 1977. Using standardized potent vaccine in well-organized vaccination campaigns, intensive surveillance for smallpox outbreaks, and extensive public education, this program eradicated smallpox. The last case of naturally occurring smallpox was reported in Somalia in October 1977. This remarkable accomplishment, the first disease to be eradicated by humans, was comprehensively chronicled by Fenner and colleagues.[2]

Smallpox was produced by the variola virus, a member of the genus *Orthopoxvirus*. It was a human virus with no known nonhuman reservoir of disease. A narrow range of laboratory animals were susceptible to experimental infection. There were at least three distinct subspecies, variola major, intermedius, and minor (alastrim), which produced illness of varying severity and mortality. The DNA and neutralizing antibodies of these viruses revealed many similarities between variola virus and the other orthopoxviruses, including ectromelia, cowpox, monkeypox, taterapox, camelpox, and vaccinia viruses. However, variola produced distinctive lesions when inoculated on the chorioallantoic membrane of an embryonated egg. This test served for many years as the confirmatory laboratory test for smallpox.

The clinical illness variola major varied in prognosis, differential diagnosis, and transmissibility (Table 149–1). In ordinary smallpox, infection was transmitted by the aerosol route through droplet nuclei, dust, and fomites.

The virus was shed in large quantities in nasal and oropharyngeal secretions at the end of the 12- to 14-day incubation period. Infectious virus was present in the vesicular fluid and scabs of cutaneous lesions and could be readily cultured from bed linen and clothing. The capacity for this virus to spread through convection currents of air within buildings and by contaminated articles, clothing, and so forth was the basis for the repeated widespread epidemics that occurred throughout human history until 1977.

The site of initial infection was usually the oropharynx, nasopharynx, or lower respiratory tract. Proliferation of virus in macrophages led to lymph node infection and viremia, with diffuse involvement of the reticuloendothelial system.

Patients became febrile and often developed severe consti-

TABLE 149–1 ■ A Classification of Clinical Types of Variola Major

Ordinary types	Raised pustular skin lesions; three subtypes: Confluent—confluent rash on face and forearms Semiconfluent—confluent rash on face, discrete elsewhere Discrete—areas of normal skin between pustules, even on face
Modified types	Like ordinary type but with an accelerated course
Variola sine eruptione	Fever without rash caused by variola virus; serologic confirmation required
Flat type	Pustules remained flat; usually confluent or semiconfluent
Hemorrhagic type	Widespread hemorrhages in skin and mucous membrane; two subtypes: Early, with purpuric rash; always fatal Late, with hemorrhages into base of pustules; usually fatal

From Fenner R, Henderson DA, Arita I, et al: Smallpox and Its Eradication. Geneva, World Health Organization, 1988.

tutional symptoms at the end of the incubation period. Splitting headache, backache, and malaise were common. Vomiting and colicky abdominal pain, occasionally suggestive of appendicitis, often occurred, and a few patients developed seizures. A diffuse erythematous "allergic" rash was noted in some fair-skinned patients in the preeruptive phase. The true maculopapular rash of smallpox began 2 to 3 days after the onset of the prodrome, at a time when the patient was defervescing. Lesions on mucous membranes in the oropharynx and the upper and lower airway appeared first. Skin lesions appeared predominantly on the head, torso, and extremities in a centrifugal distribution. The reason for this pattern of involvement and for the dermatotropism of the variola virus is not known.

The rash of smallpox became apparent during 2 to 4 days. Although lesions on the face were often more advanced than those on the legs, all of the lesions in an area of the body evolved as a single crop (Fig. 149–1). Most patients had lesions on the palms and soles. Papules evolved into vesicles by day 3 or 4 and into pustules by day 5 or 6 of the rash. The lesions were firm to the touch, domed, or umbilicated. When extensive, they often coalesced and became confluent. Pustules reached their maximal size on or about the ninth day of the rash. Fever often returned during the pustular stage and persisted until the lesions had become inspissated, scabbed over, and sloughed off. By the 20th day, all of the scabs had usually separated except for those embedded in the thick corneum stratum of the palms and soles. Depigmentation persisted at the base of skin lesions for 3 to 6 months after illness. Smallpox left permanent scars depressed 1 to 2 mm below the surface of the skin. These pockmarks resulted from fibrosis in the dermis and sebaceous glands. Scarring was usually most extensive on the face.

Smallpox, especially variola major, produced a rapidly fatal toxemic illness in some patients. Diagnosis was difficult when death occurred from hemorrhagic complications before the appearance of the rash. Pneumonia, dehydration, and septicemia secondary to denuded, sloughed skin were other serious complications (Fig. 149–2). Conjunctivitis, corneal ulceration, and blepharitis occurred, producing corneal opacity in between 1.0% and 4.4% of cases. Osteomyelitis variolosa was a rare complication that produced deformities in children, afflicting the elbows more often than other joints.

In reviewing this illness and virus, it is important to consider those factors that made eradication possible:

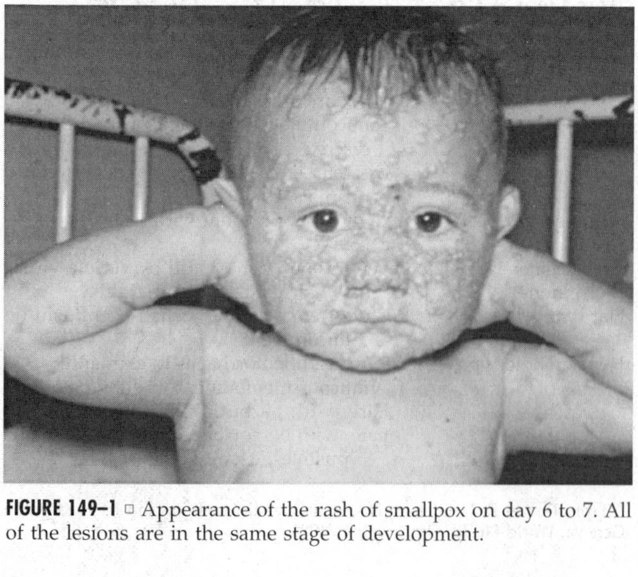

FIGURE 149–1 ▫ Appearance of the rash of smallpox on day 6 to 7. All of the lesions are in the same stage of development.

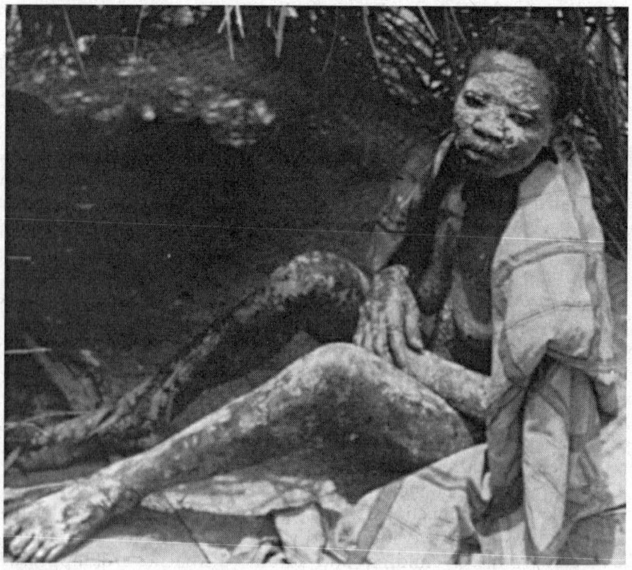

FIGURE 149–2 ▫ Denuded areas of skin produced by the sloughing of confluent smallpox lesions.

1. It produced a distinctive, easily recognizable acute illness.
2. It had no chronic or carrier stage.
3. There was no nonhuman reservoir of endemic disease.
4. A stable, inexpensive vaccine was produced that conveyed long-term immunity.
5. Large-scale vaccination campaigns and intensive case reporting and surveillance were conducted in more than 80 countries.
6. Public education was actively promoted in all of these countries to overcome the hiding of cases and to break the cycle of smallpox transmission.

Current Status of the Destruction of the Known Samples of Smallpox Virus

The eradication of smallpox from the world was announced by the WHO in 1979 and certified by a Global Commission with sanction by the World Health Assembly in 1980. By 1982, after efforts of nearly 100 WHO authentication teams, all known samples of variola virus were either destroyed or sent to repositories at the WHO Collaborating Centers for Smallpox and Other Poxvirus Infections at the Centers for Disease Control and Prevention (CDC) in Atlanta or the Research Institute for Viral Preparations in Moscow. The CDC retains about 400 samples, including samples collected by the CDC, the U.S. Army, the United Kingdom, the Netherlands, Japan, and the American Type Culture Collection; the Research Institute for Viral Preparations retains about 100 diagnostic samples.

After the breakup of the Soviet Union, situations in Moscow raised fears that the collection of the Research Institute for Viral Preparations could come into jeopardy. Thus, in 1994, a decision was made by the Russian government to move the stocks to the Russian State Research Center for Virology and Biotechnology at NPO Vector, Koltsovo, Novosibirsk Region, Russia. The WHO was then informed, and after a WHO biosafety team was dispatched in the summer of 1995 to evaluate the facility, the new repository location was approved.

As part of the posteradication strategy, the WHO Committee on Orthopoxvirus Infections recommended destruction of the stocks at least three times: in 1986, coincident with recommending production of a set of reference bacterial plasmids containing variola DNA fragments representing the entire genome; in 1990, destruction by December 31, 1993, was proposed after an announcement by the U.S. Secretary of Health and Human Services at the World Health Assembly that the stocks at the CDC would be destroyed after determination of a complete genome DNA sequence of variola virus[3]; and in 1994, after the determination of more than 650,000 base pairs of genome DNA sequences of one alastrim and two major strains plus parts of other strains from research collaborations mainly involving the CDC, the National Institutes of Health, and the Russian State Research Center for Virology and Biotechnology.[4, 5]

In 1994, 8 of 10 scientists who composed the committee recommended destruction on June 30, 1995, because they believed that the risks associated with smallpox return by inadvertent escape or an unforseen malevolent act involving repository samples far outweighed any benefits of further research with live virus. Two members recommended destruction in 5 years, after considering publicly professed opinions of several scientists who urged that the virus be used to gain valuable scientific knowledge. For example, resolving the molecular basis of virulence and strict human host range of variola virus in light of the sequences would be enormously beneficial to the public health; they predicted enhanced development of new therapies for various diseases based on knowledge of variola immune evasion and pathobiologic components.

Nonetheless, the recommendation for destruction in 1995 was sent for sanction by the WHO executive board. However, at the board meeting in January 1995, endorsement was postponed because the British and U.S. military raised serious concerns about the potential for smallpox terrorism or biologic warfare should a diabolical source of virus emerge. The issue did not come up for a vote at the 1995 World Health Assembly despite prodestruction efforts led by the Australian contingent. To address the concerns, the U.S. Departments of Defense and Health and Human Services are now conducting the following research toward diminishing the odds of malevolent use of variola virus from unknown or uncompromised known sources of infectious material: (1) testing of potential orthopoxvirus antiviral compounds using drugs already in human clinical trials for other reasons; (2) development of rapid, highly sensitive diagnostics that could be used at stages before appearance of rash when an antiviral could be effective, and potentially for detecting traces of virus; and (3) determination of the efficacy of a new cell culture–based vaccine and lot of vaccinia immunoglobulin produced by the U.S. Department of Defense. The 1996 World Health Assembly recommended "that the remaining stocks . . . should be destroyed on 30 June 1999 after a decision has been taken by the Health Assembly, that being a moratorium of five-and-a-half years from the deadline of 31 December 1993 proposed by the ad hoc committee on orthopoxvirus infections, with a view of taking action to achieve broader consensus. . . ."

References

1. Hopkins DR: Princes and Peasants: Smallpox in History. Chicago, University of Chicago Press, 1983.
2. Fenner F, Henderson DA, Arita I, et al: Smallpox and Its Eradication. Geneva, World Health Organization, 1988.
3. Mahy BWJ, Esposito JJ, Venter JC: Sequencing the smallpox virus genome: Prelude to destruction of a virus species. Am Soc Microbiol News 57:577–580, 1991.
4. Massung RF, Esposito JJ, Liu L, et al: Potential virulence determinants in terminal regions of variola smallpox virus genome. Nature 366:748–751, 1993.
5. Massung RF, Loparev VN, Knight JC, et al: Terminal region sequence variations in variola virus DNA. Virology 221:291–300, 1996.

150

Mumps

Adriano Arguedas
Hillel K. Janai
Melvin I. Marks

Mumps is an acute, contagious, generalized viral disease that usually causes painful enlargement of the salivary glands, most commonly the parotids.

History

Mumps was first described as a clinical entity by Hippocrates in 500 BC. The viral origin was firmly established in 1934 when Johnson and Goodpasture[1] successfully reproduced the disease in monkeys. In 1945, the virus was grown in hen eggs, and the viral property of hemagglutination was described. Subsequently, the virus was successfully attenuated in 1960, and the live mumps virus vaccine was prepared in chick embryo tissue culture by Hilleman and Buynack[2] in 1966.

Microbiology

Mumps is caused by a member of the paramyxovirus group. The virus particle contains a single-stranded RNA enclosed in an envelope of protein and lipid. The viral envelope contains three proteins: (1) HN protein, which has both hemagglutinin and neuraminidase activity; (2) F protein, which has hemolytic and cell fusion activity; and (3) M protein, which forms the inner layer of the viral envelope. There is only one known serotype. For more information, refer to Chapter 252.

Epidemiology

Mumps is endemic in heavily populated areas but may occur in epidemic areas when susceptible individuals are crowded together. The virus is spread from its human reservoir by direct contact through infected saliva and urine. Incidence peaks occur in late winter and early spring.

The disease has a worldwide distribution and affects both sexes equally. Infection is uncommon during the early months of life owing to infrequent exposure and to protection conferred by transplacental passage of maternal antibodies. Although the majority of cases occur in children younger than 15 years (85%), there are rare reports of neonatal cases,[3] and an increase in the number of cases in adolescents between 15 and 19 years of age was noticed during the 1986 to 1987 period. This phenomenon was attributed to a failure in the vaccination programs between the 1968 and 1977 period.[4] The source of infection is not always found because 25% to 30% of cases are clinically inapparent.[5, 6]

It is not known how long a patient may be infectious. However, transmission does not seem to occur longer than 24 hours before the appearance of the swelling or later than 3 days after it has subsided. Virus has been isolated from saliva as long as 7 days before and 8 days after the appearance of salivary swelling. Urine cultures have shown the presence of the virus from 1 to 14 days after the onset of the salivary gland swelling.[7]

Lifelong immunity is usually achieved after a clinical or subclinical infection.

Pathogenesis

Humans are the only reservoir for mumps virus, and person-to-person contact is essential for spreading to occur. The mumps virus initially attaches to the epithelial cells of the respiratory tract, producing, in both immune and nonimmune individuals, upper (e.g., common cold and pharyngitis) and lower (e.g., bronchopneumonia, croup, and bronchiolitis) respiratory symptoms. This virus–epithelial cell interaction induces local immunologic responses characterized by secretion of secretory immunoglobulin A, edema, lymphocyte infiltration, and increased vascular permeability.[8] After the initial multiplication in the respiratory tract, the virus is blood-borne to many tissues and glands (e.g., salivary glands).

Infection with mumps virus stimulates humoral and cell-mediated immune responses. Levels of immunoglobulins G and M as well as interferon and local immunoglobulin A are increased in patients after mumps infection.[9] Lymphocyte proliferation to mumps antigen has been documented in response to cutaneous hypersensitivity.[10]

Parotid swelling is produced by interstitial edema. The main changes occur in the salivary ducts, ranging from mild epithelial swelling with sparse polymorphonuclear cell infiltration to complete desquamation of the epithelium resulting in dilated lumens choked with debris.

Changes in the brain may occur in acute viral meningoencephalitis. These include neuronal destruction and inflammation with lymphocyte infiltration, perivascular edema, and vasculitis. After the acute process, perivascular demyelination and glial reaction follow recovery. Occasionally, mumps meningoencephalitis may cause hydrocephalus due to aqueductal stenosis secondary to scarring at the sites of necrotic ependymal cells.[11]

In orchitis, there are massive interstitial edema and perivascular lymphocyte exudate. The histologic changes are characterized by a patch destruction of the epithelium of some seminiferous tubules; the Leydig cells are usually both histologically normal and functional. These changes are usually focal and unilateral (80% to 90%), accompanied by epididymitis in 85% of cases.[12]

Rarely, acute self-limited inflammation of the pancreas (less than 10%), thyroid, joints (0.4%), or labyrinth may develop.[13] On histologic examination, there is an acute inflammatory response in the interstitium consisting of mononuclear cells with edema and swelling.

Intrauterine infection with mumps virus has been associated with multiple anomalies, including endocardial fibroelastosis; imperforate anus; spina bifida; auditory, optic, and urogenital deformities; and abortions.[14] Animal studies have suggested the possible association between mumps infection during pregnancy and congenital hydrocephalus, probably secondary to obstructive lesions in the spinal canal.[15]

Clinical Manifestations of Parotitis

The incubation period of mumps ranges from 14 to 24 days, most commonly 17 to 18 days. In children, prodromal symptoms and signs are rare and may be manifested by 2 to 3 days of malaise, anorexia, headache, muscle pain, and fever. Orchitis or meningitis may precede parotitis or may be the sole manifestation of mumps. Approximately 20% to 30% of all mumps infections are subclinical. This group of patients represents a significant risk for spread of the disease.

The onset of illness is usually characterized by pain and swelling in one or both parotid glands (Fig. 150–1). The parotid swelling begins by filling the space between the posterior border of the mandible and the mastoid and then extends downward and forward, being limited above by the zygoma. Local heat and erythema are absent. The swollen tissues push the earlobe upward and outward as the angle of the mandible is no longer visible. Swelling is usually maximal during a 2- to 3-day period and disappears by 7 to 10 days. Redness and swelling are commonly noted around the opening of the Stensen or Wharton duct. Because salivary gland ducts may be partially occluded by inflammation, pain can be experienced on exposure to acid drinks and other stimulants of salivary secretion.

Swelling of the sublingual and submaxillary glands is frequently associated with mumps. In 10% to 15% of patients, only the submandibular gland is swollen. The inflammation is usually an ovoid enlargement extending forward and downward from the angle of the mandible. Submandibular infection is usually not as painful as when the parotid is involved, but the swelling subsides more slowly. Less commonly, only the sublingual glands may be infected. The infection is usually bilateral and noted in the submental region and on the floor of the mouth.

Complications

Complications of mumps virus infection can occur during the acute, convalescent, or postconvalescent phase. Viremia,

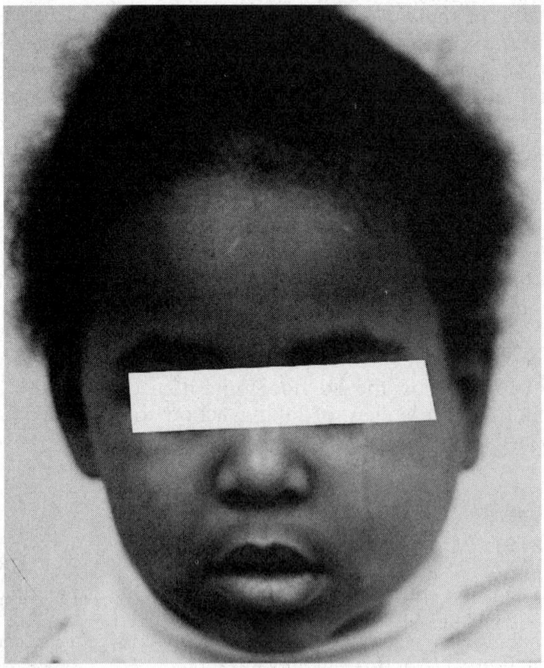

FIGURE 150–1 □ Female patient with swelling of left parotid gland due to parotitis. Note the difference with the right parotid gland. (Courtesy of Dr. A. Deveikis, Memorial Miller Children's Hospital and Health System, Long Beach, CA.)

early in the infection, is the route of infection in organs other than the salivary glands (Table 150–1). The frequency of mumps-related complications is higher in the postpubertal population than in the prepubertal group. It is also higher in males than in females.[16]

Acute meningoencephalitis is the most frequent complication in childhood. The true frequency is difficult to estimate, but clinical central nervous system involvement during the infection occurs in 15% of cases reported to the Centers for Disease Control and Prevention in the United States.[17] The mortality rate is about 2%, and males are affected three to five times more frequently than females are.[16] A case of chronic mumps encephalitis with mental deterioration and recurrent seizures that may have responded to antiviral therapy was reported.[18]

In most cases, central nervous system signs become evident 1 to 6 days after the onset of parotitis and are characterized by fever (94%), vomiting (84%), nuchal rigidity (71%), lethargy (69%), parotid swelling (47%), headache (47%), convulsions (18%), and delirium (6%).[19] The cerebrospinal fluid usually contains less than 500 cells per mm^3, almost exclusively lymphocytes; the protein concentration is slightly elevated, and the glucose concentration is usually normal. However, hypoglycorrhachia has been reported in some patients with mumps meningitis.[20] Mumps virus can be isolated from the cerebrospinal fluid in the illness. The prognosis is favorable in most cases, although permanent sequelae, such as unilateral (rarely bilateral) nerve deafness or facial paralysis, may result.[21, 22] The incidence of deafness after mumps is approximately 1 in 20,000, but findings suggest that because of diagnostic problems it may be higher.[13] The pathogenesis is not completely understood but appears to be secondary to hematogenous viral invasion of the labyrinth.[23, 24] Other unusual central nervous system manifestations include acute cerebellar ataxia, transverse myelitis, and polyneuritis.[25, 26] Ependymitis appears to be a common finding in patients with central nervous system involvement. Ependymal cells and cytoplasmic inclusions of viral nucleocapsid-like material are usually found in the cerebrospinal fluid of these patients and have been implicated in the pathogenesis of hydrocephalus.[11]

TABLE 150–1 ■ Complications of Mumps

NEUROLOGIC	**HEMATOLOGIC**
Meningoencephalitis	Thrombocytopenia
Guillain-Barré syndrome	Hemolysis
Myelitis	Leukemoid reaction
Neuropathies	Paroxysmal cold hemoglobinuria
Deafness	Splenomegaly
Labyrinthitis	
Hydrocephalus	**OTHER**
Diabetes insipidus	Pancreatitis
	Thyroiditis
OCULAR	Mastitis
Conjunctivitis	Hepatitis
Scleritis	Polyarthritis
Keratitis	Myocarditis
Optic neuritis	Laryngitis
Iritis	Psychosis
Iridocyclitis	Teratogenicity (microcephaly,
Dacryoadenitis	hydrocephalus, endocardial
	fibroelastosis, abortion)
GENITOURINARY	
Orchitis	
Epididymitis	
Oophoritis	
Nephritis	
Priapism	
Bartholinitis	
Prostatitis	

Adapted from Marks MI: Mumps. *In* Braude AI, Davis CE, Fierer J (eds): Infectious Diseases and Medical Microbiology, ed 2. Philadelphia, WB Saunders, 1986, pp 776–782.

Orchitis is a complication that is most commonly observed during adolescence and young adulthood. About 20% of postpubertal male patients develop orchitis.[5] It is usually unilateral, and therefore sterility is rare.[12] Bilateral involvement has been reported to occur in 17% to 38% of cases.[27, 28] Orchitis may occur before or in the absence of parotitis, but the majority of cases become clinically apparent 3 to 7 days after the parotid swelling has subsided.[29] The onset is usually abrupt with a rise in temperature, chills, headache, nausea, vomiting, and lower abdominal pain. Within 12 to 24 hours, the affected gonad displays an inflammatory reaction characterized by marked swelling, warmth, and pain. The average duration of illness is 4 days. The risk for testicular neoplasia has been found to be higher for men with history of mumps orchitis.[30] Despite the rare complications of sterility and neoplasia, the course of mumps orchitis is generally self-limited. Appropriate therapy includes use of analgesics and adequate support of the testes. Steroids are not effective and may potentiate the parotitis or increase the rate of secondary infection.[29] Nerve blocks should be reserved for patients with intractable pain.

Oophoritis may be a complication of mumps infection and is noted in about 7% of postpubertal female patients. The clinical manifestations are less dramatic than in orchitis, and the main complaints are usually pelvic pain and tenderness in the lower abdominal quadrants. There is no evidence of impairment of fertility after infection.

Mumps-induced pancreatitis has been reported in less than 10% of patients and is usually a late effect of the infection, developing days or weeks after the parotid swelling. Approximately one third of the cases have occurred in the absence of parotitis.[29] It is more common in young adults. Nausea, vomiting, fever, chills, and epigastric pain are usually the main complaints. These symptoms disappear in 1 week, and most of the patients recover completely. Serum amylase determination is not a helpful diagnostic tool in the early-onset cases because it is normally elevated with parotitis in the absence of pancreatic inflammation. Serum lipase determination may be more helpful. Epidemiologic and serologic correlations between mumps and type I diabetes mellitus have been suggested; however, controlled studies have failed to confirm this association.[31–34]

Thyroid inflammation has been reported to occur about 1 week after the onset of parotitis. Although it is uncommon in children, the appearance of a diffuse, tender, swollen thyroid is suggestive of this complication.

Arthritis has been observed in 0.4% of patients with mumps.[35] Arthritic complaints are more common in men during the third decade of life, usually starting 10 to 14 days after parotid swelling and persisting an average of 12 days.[36] The large joints (e.g., knees, ankles, and shoulders) are most frequently involved, but any joint can be affected. The arthritic pain is migratory and self-limited, resolving after a few days without any residual joint damage or recurrence.[37]

Mumps myocarditis is a rare complication. However, fatal cases have been reported in the literature.[38]

Viruria has frequently been noted. The frequency of renal involvement in children is unknown, but the virus is isolated from the urine of 72% of patients during the first 5 days of mumps parotitis.[39, 40] Cases of symptomatic nephritis after mumps are unusual, but fatal cases have been reported.[41]

Rare complications of mumps virus include mastitis, prostatitis, dacryoadenitis, transient abnormalities in liver function tests, and thrombocytopenic purpura.

Diagnosis

Diagnosis of clinical cases during an epidemic is simple, based on the epidemiologic condition, the history, and the physical examination. When clinical manifestations are limited to one of the less common sites of infection, or when the case is sporadic, the diagnosis is more difficult to establish.

Swelling of the parotid or other salivary glands due to mumps virus must be distinguished from other causes of parotid swelling. Infectious, noninfectious, and nonparotid causes of swelling should always be excluded (Table 150–2).

Routine laboratory tests are usually nonspecific. The white cell count is usually within the normal range, although leukopenia with lymphocytosis may occur. A polymorphonuclear leukocytosis is more commonly present with extraparotid involvement.

The serum amylase value is above normal in mumps and usually parallels the parotid swelling, reaching its peak in 1 week and returning to normal in the course of the next 2 weeks. Serum and urine amylase values can be used to differentiate between parotid and nonparotid swelling. Both values are increased when parotid involvement is present and are normal when the swelling is due to extraparotid disease.

TABLE 150–2 ▪ Differential Diagnosis of Parotid Swelling

INFECTIOUS
Mumps
Parainfluenza
Influenza
Cytomegalovirus infection
Coxsackievirus infection
Lymphocytic choriomeningitis
Echovirus infection
Suppuration (bacterial)
Actinomyces infection
Mycobacterial infection
Cat-scratch disease
NONINFECTIOUS
Drug hypersensitivity (thiouracil, phenothiazines, thiocyanate, iodides, copper, isoprenaline, lead, mercury, phenylbutazone)
Sarcoidosis
Tumors, mixed
Hemangioma, lymphangioma
Sialectasis
Sjögren syndrome
Mikulicz syndrome (scleroderma, mixed connective tissue disease, systemic lupus erythematosus)
Recurrent idiopathic parotitis
Pneumoparotitis
Trauma
Sialolithiasis
Foreign body
Cystic fibrosis
Malnutrition (marasmus, alcohol cirrhosis)
Dehydration
Diabetes mellitus
Waldenström macroglobulinemia
Reiter syndrome
Amyloidosis
NONPAROTID SWELLING
Hypertrophy of masseter muscle
Lymphadenopathy
Rheumatoid mandibular joint swelling
Tumors of jaw
Infantile cortical hyperostosis

Adapted from Marks MI: Mumps. *In* Braude AI, Davis CE, Fierer J (eds): Infectious Diseases and Medical Microbiology, ed 2. Philadelphia, WB Saunders, 1986, pp 776–782.

The definitive diagnosis of mumps is established by a positive viral culture or by serologic methods. Publications[42] have suggested that the salivary detection of mumps-specific immunoglobulin M may be a noninvasive, sensitive, and specific method to diagnose mumps under specific circumstances. For details, refer to Chapter 252.

Treatment and Prevention

Treatment of parotitis and the majority of its complications is entirely symptomatic. Bed rest may help reduce discomfort, and diet should be adjusted according to the ability of the patient to chew. As mentioned before, patients may have difficulty with acid foods; therefore, diet should be light, with generous offering of fluids to preserve good hydration.

Analgesics, such as acetaminophen, may be used for headache and general malaise. Potent analgesics, such as morphine, are sometimes useful for orchitis or pancreatitis. Patients with orchitis require bed rest. Measures to minimize testicular tension, such as supporting the scrotum in a sling on an adhesive tape bridge between the thighs, and applying ice packs often help relieve pain. Pancreatic inflammation is treated with bed rest, withholding of oral feeding for 48 to 72 hours, and intravenous administration of dextrose and saline solutions. Electrolyte imbalance and metabolic alkalosis should be suspected when vomiting is severe. Headaches associated with meningoencephalitis may be relieved by oral analgesics; in intractable cases, lumbar puncture may be considered.

The patient should remain in isolation until glandular swelling subsides. Usually, patients can be considered noncontagious 9 days after the onset of parotid swelling. Susceptible contacts should be observed closely from 14 to 28 days after exposure. Mumps immune globulin and immune serum globulin are not helpful in preventing the disease.

Live mumps virus vaccine (5000 $TCID_{50}$ [median tissue culture infective dose]/dose) is the agent of choice for active immunization. The commercially available vaccine is grown in chick embryo cell cultures and contains no penicillin. The commercially available mumps vaccine is administered in a single subcutaneous injection of 0.5 mL, either alone or in combination with measles and rubella vaccines. The vaccine is immunogenic in 93% to 98% of subjects and has a protective efficacy of about 95%.[6] Mumps vaccine should be routinely given after the first birthday. Simultaneous administration of mumps with measles and rubella at 13 to 15 months of life is safe and has been shown, if properly used, to reduce the number of mumps cases and related diseases.[43, 44]

Serologic and epidemiologic evidence suggests that vaccine-induced immunity is long lasting and may be lifelong. Vaccine-induced antibody may develop slowly (14 to 28 days) and, therefore, may not prevent infection during the first few weeks after vaccination.

Adverse reactions attributed to live mumps vaccine are extremely rare. The vaccine may produce a noncommunicable, subclinical infection and may induce reactions in patients allergic to the egg protein or neomycin (vaccine contains 25 μg of neomycin). In view of the possible teratogenic effect of all live virus vaccines, mumps vaccines are contraindicated in pregnancy.

The vaccine should not be given within 3 months after administration of immune globulin or blood transfusion because of the possible neutralization of the vaccine; it should also not be given to immunosuppressed patients. It is recommended, however, for patients with symptomatic human immunodeficiency virus infection. Rare complications after administration of mumps vaccine include nerve deafness, encephalitis, purpura, and orchitis.[6, 7]

References

1. Johnson CD, Goodpasture EW: An investigation of the etiology of mumps. J Exp Med 59:1–20, 1934.
2. Hilleman MR, Buynack EB, Weibel RE, et al: Live attenuated mumps-virus vaccine. N Engl J Med 278:227–233, 1968.
3. Lacour M, Maherzi M, Vienny H, et al: Thrombocytopenia in a case of neonatal mumps infection: Evidence of further clinical presentations. Eur J Pediatr 152:739–741, 1993.
4. Cochi SL, Preblud SR, Orenstein WA: Perspectives on the relative resurgence of mumps in the United States. Am J Dis Child 142:499–507, 1988.
5. Brunell PA: Mumps. *In* Feigin RD, Cherry JD (eds): Textbook of Pediatric Infectious Diseases. Philadelphia, WB Saunders, 1987, pp 1628–1632.
6. Marks MI: Mumps. *In* Braude AI, Davis CE, Fierer J (eds): Infectious Diseases and Medical Microbiology, ed 2. Philadelphia, WB Saunders, 1986, pp 776–782.
7. Tolipn MD, Schauf V: Mumps virus. *In* Belshe RB (ed): Textbook of Human Virology. Littleton, MA, PSG Publishing, 1985, pp 311–331.
8. Friedman MG: Salivary IgA antibodies to mumps virus during and after mumps. J Infect Dis 143:617, 1981.
9. Glikmann G, Mordhorst CH: Serological diagnosis of mumps and parainfluenza type-1 virus infections by enzyme immunoassay, with a comparison of two different approaches for detection of mumps IgG antibodies. Acta Pathol Microbiol Immunol Scand 94:157–166, 1986.
10. Chiba Y, Dzierba JL, Morag A, et al: Cell-mediated immune response to mumps virus infection in man. J Immunol 116:12–15, 1976.
11. Herndon RM, Johnson RT, Davis LE, et al: Ependymitis in mumps virus meningitis. Arch Neurol 30:475–479, 1974.
12. Tsvetkov D: Spermatological disorders in patients with post mumps orchitis. Akush Ginekol (Sofiia) 29:46–49, 1990.
13. Yamamoto M, Watanabe Y, Mizukoshi K: Neurotological findings in patients with acute mumps deafness. Acta Otolaryngol Suppl (Stockh) 504:94–97, 1993.
14. Garcia AGP, Pereira JMS, Vidigal N, et al: Intrauterine infection with mumps virus. Obstet Gynecol 156:756–759, 1980.
15. London WT, Ken SG, Palmer AE, et al: Induction of congenital hydrocephalus with mumps virus in rhesus monkeys. J Infect Dis 139:324–328, 1979.
16. Donald PR, Burger PJ, Becker WB: Mumps meningoencephalitis. S Afr Med J 71:283–285, 1987.
17. Centers for Disease Control: Mumps vaccine. MMWR Morbid Mortal Wkly Rep 26:393–394, 1977.
18. Ito M, Go T, Okuno T, et al: Chronic mumps virus encephalitis. Pediatr Neurol 7:467–470, 1991.
19. Azimi PH, Cramblett HG, Haynes RE: Mumps meningoencephalitis in children. JAMA 207:509–512, 1969.
20. Wilfert CM: Mumps meningoencephalitis with low cerebrospinal-fluid glucose, prolonged pleocytosis and elevation of protein. N Engl J Med 280:855–859, 1969.
21. Kirk M: Sensorineural hearing loss and mumps. Br J Audiol 21:227–228, 1987.
22. Yanagita N, Nakashima T, Ohno Y, et al: Estimated annual number of patients treated for sensorineural hearing loss in Japan. Results of a nationwide epidemiological survey in 1987. Acta Otolaryngol Suppl (Stockh) 514:9–13, 1994.
23. Izushima N, Murakami Y: Deafness following mumps: The possible pathogenesis and incidence of deafness. Auris Nasus Larynx 1:S55–S57, 1986.
24. Fukuda S: Experimental viral labyrinthitis—An immunohistochemical investigation of the cochlear lesion. Hokkaido Igaku Zasshi 61:58–71, 1986.
25. Nussinovitch M, Brand N, Frydman M, et al: Transverse myelitis following mumps in children. Acta Paediatr 81:183–184, 1992.
26. Cohen HA, Ashkenazi A, Nussinovitch M, et al: Mumps-associated acute cerebellar ataxia. Am J Dis Child 146:930–931, 1992.
27. Beard CM, Benson RC, Kelalis PP, et al: The incidence and outcome of mumps orchitis in Rochester, Minnesota, 1935 to 1974. Mayo Clin Proc 52:3–7, 1977.
28. Philip RN, Reinhard KR, Lackman DB: Observations on a mumps epidemic in a "virgin" population. Am J Hyg 69:91–111, 1959.
29. Lerner AM: Guide to immunization against mumps. J Infect Dis 122:116–121, 1970.
30. Swerdlow AJ, Huttly SR, Smith PG: Testicular cancer and antecedent diseases. Br J Cancer 55:97–103, 1987.
31. Levy NL, Notkins AL: Viral infections and diseases of the endocrine system. J Infect Dis 124:94–103, 1971.
32. Schulz B, Michaelis D, Hildmann W, et al: Islet cell surface antibodies (ICSA) in subjects with a previous mumps infection—A prospective study over a 4 year period. Exp Clin Endocrinol 90:62–70, 1987.
33. Ratzman KP, Jahr H, Richter KV: Complement-mediated cytotoxic effects of islet cell surface antibodies in non-diabetic subjects with antecedent mumps infection and diabetic risk. Exp Clin Endocrinol 91:176–182, 1988.
34. Toniolo A, Conaldi PG, Garzelli C, et al: Role of antecedent mumps and reovirus infections on the development of type 1 (insulin-dependent) diabetes. Eur J Epidemiol 1:172–179, 1985.
35. Gold HE, Boxerbeum B, Leslie HJ: Mumps arthritis. Am J Dis Child 116:547–548, 1968.
36. Caranasos GJ, Felker JR: Mumps arthritis. Arch Intern Med 119:394–398, 1967.
37. Hyer FH, Gottlied NL: Rheumatic disorders associated with viral infection. Semin Arthritis Rheum 8:17–31, 1978.
38. Brown NJ, Richmond SJ: Fatal mumps myocarditis in an 8-month old child. Br Med J 281:356–357, 1980.
39. Eknoyan G, Dillman RO: Renal complications of infectious disease. Med Clin North Am 52:979–1002, 1978.
40. Lin CY, Chen WP, Chiang H: Mumps associated with nephritis. Child Nephrol Urol 10:68–71, 1990.
41. Hughes WT, Steigman AJ, Delong HF: Some implications of fatal nephritis associated with mumps. Am J Dis Child 111:297–301, 1966.
42. Perry KR, Brown DN, Parry JV, et al: Detection of measles, mumps and rubella antibodies in saliva using antibody capture radioimmunoassay. J Med Virol 40:235–240, 1993.
43. Kanesaki T, Baba K, Tsuda N, et al: Protection of mumps in children with various underlying diseases: Application of a live attenuated mumps and trivalent measles-rubella-mumps vaccines in these children. Biken J 29:63–71, 1986.
44. Peltola H, Heinonen OP, Valle M, et al: The elimination of indigenous measles, mumps, and rubella from Finland by a 12-year, two-dose vaccination program. N Engl J Med 331:1397–1402, 1994.

151

Warts

Karen F. Rothman
Jeffrey D. Bernhard

History

Warts were first described by the ancient Greeks and Romans. *Verruca* is the Latin word for a "warty excrescence." Wart derives from the Anglo-Saxon *wearte*, a "callosity." The Romans believed that genital warts were sexually transmitted, but it was not until the late 1800s that the contagious nature of all warts was appreciated. In 1907, Cuiffo produced warts by injecting himself with a wart extract from which bacteria and fungi had been eliminated, implying that warts had a viral origin. In 1950, Strauss and coworkers saw viral wart particles by electron microscopy. In the last few years, advances in DNA sequencing and viral culturing have increased our understanding of differences in the clinical manifestations, anatomic distribution, and oncogenic potential of certain strains of verrucae.[1] The complete DNA sequencing of several wart viruses is known.[2]

Characteristics of the Pathogen

Papillomavirus is a genus comprising more than 60 DNA viruses in the Papovaviridae family. The viruses are 50 to 55 nm in diameter and contain double-stranded DNA folded tightly into 72 capsomeres.[3] They are named according to their natural host (e.g., human papillomavirus [HPV] indicates that the virus infects humans). They are further classified according to their extent of DNA sequence homology. If there is less than 50% cross-hybridization between two types, they are assigned different numbers. Viruses that have less than 30% DNA sequence homology show clear-cut biologic differences; however, some viral types with even less DNA similarity seem to be identical in pathogenicity.

The virulence of a wart depends on specific characteristics of the HPV type as well as host factors. Plantar warts may contain more viral DNA than other types and may proliferate rapidly. Warts present for less than a year contain more viral particles than older warts do. Children's lesions regress more quickly. Patients whose immune system is compromised are particularly prone to develop multiple, rapidly progressive warts that are difficult to eradicate.

Specific HPV types may be divided into two general categories on the basis of whether they usually infect the skin or mucosal surfaces. Occasionally, however, mucosal HPV types affect the skin and vice versa. Although certain mucosal HPV types are commonly found in premalignant and malignant lesions, nonmucosal HPV types are rarely associated with malignant neoplasia in the normal host. This chapter focuses on HPV types affecting the skin only.

HPV may be studied in vitro by use of xenograft cultures,[4] cell line grafting,[5] or raft cultures. The last system allows investigators to manipulate the entire HPV life cycle and may also be used to test new therapies in vitro.[6]

Epidemiology

To develop warts, one must either have direct contact with an infected person or touch contaminated material. A lesion develops at the site of inoculation. Warts may then be spread by touching. The virus can survive for many months and at extremely low temperatures without a host but is inactivated at temperatures above 55°C.[1] A barefoot person with plantar warts may infect many others through shed scales.

Approximately 7% to 10% of the population have warts. Their frequency varies widely with the population studied. They are less common in black than in white persons.[7] Teenagers are most commonly afflicted. Adults in certain occupations, such as meat, poultry, and fish handlers, have infection rates up to 50%.[8, 9] Patients with hereditary or acquired forms of cell-mediated immunodeficiency get more warts and have more difficulty eradicating the virus. Patients receiving immunosuppressive drugs, particularly organ transplant recipients, are especially susceptible.

Pathogenesis

HPV penetrates the skin through small fissures and travels down to the granular cell layer of the epidermis, where virus replication occurs. Infected cells continue their normal migration to the stratum corneum. When corneocytes are shed, infectious virus is released into the environment.

Lesions appear 1 to 20 months after exposure. HPV DNA can survive in the host's cells without replicating or producing viral antigens on the host's cell surfaces. The virus can thus escape the host's immune response. This may explain why warts can reappear years after they clinically regress.[10, 11]

Immune Response

Wart regression involves both humoral and cell-mediated immunity, although the latter is more important. Patients with regressing warts often have immunoglobulin M and G antibodies to HPV.[1] These are not usually found in persons with proliferating or persistent warts. Approximately 15% of people with no history of wart infection have specific immunoglobulin G anti-HPV antibodies.[12] Patients who have demonstrable antibody to HPV can develop new verrucae.[13]

Patients with defective cell-mediated immunity frequently cannot resolve wart infections.[1, 14, 15] Patients with active atopic dermatitis have a lower frequency of warts than that in the normal population.[16, 17] Immunologically competent patients with multiple warts have demonstrable defects in cell-mediated immunity, which normalize when the warts regress.[18] As warts regress, lymphocytes in the dermis migrate to the epidermis and cause keratinocytes bearing the virus to degenerate.[19] Langerhans cells carry antigens and help to target immune reactions. Their numbers are markedly decreased within warts, suggesting that perhaps a decrease in the host's immune surveillance allows warts to develop or spread.[19, 20]

Clinical Manifestations

More than 60 wart types have been recognized. The clinical appearance of the lesion depends on its location on the body rather than on the specific viral type.[21] Warts usually have a rough, somewhat irregular, "verrucous" surface. Warts disrupt normal skin lines. When they are pared with a blade, thrombosed capillaries may be seen as pinpoint, red to black dots. Further paring often leads to pinpoint bleeding. Warts are usually asymptomatic, except when they occur in an area of pressure, such as on the foot or periungual area. Scratching may produce a linear array of new lesions by autoinoculation. This phenomenon is described as an isomorphic response. Histologic findings vary somewhat with the HPV type[22]; however, all warts have hyperkeratosis and papillomatosis with areas of parakeratosis in the stratum corneum. Vacuolated cells and clumped keratohyaline granules are seen within the stratum granulosum.

Myrmeciae are deep plantar warts caused by HPV-1. They occur most commonly in teenagers and are usually solitary lesions. They may become black and painful just before spontaneous regression.

The agent of verruca vulgaris, the common wart, is usually HPV-2 but may also be HPV-4. Exophytic papules may coalesce into small plaques. Hand lesions are most common. Periungual lesions may cause nail dystrophy (Fig. 151–1). When located on the face, neck, or groin, they may be filiform (Fig. 151–2). When large plaques develop, they are known as mosaic warts.

Verrucae in butchers, fish handlers, and poulterers are associated with HPV types 2, 4, or 7. Infection with HPV-7 is nearly unique to this population and may cause large, cauliflower-like plaques.[23, 24] HPV-7 is also epidemiologically linked to an increased frequency of lung cancer in butchers.[25]

Verrucae planae, flat warts, are caused by HPV types 3 and 10. They are flat, 1- to 3-mm papules with little overlying scale. They are virtually always multiple and may be grouped. They occur most commonly on the dorsum of the

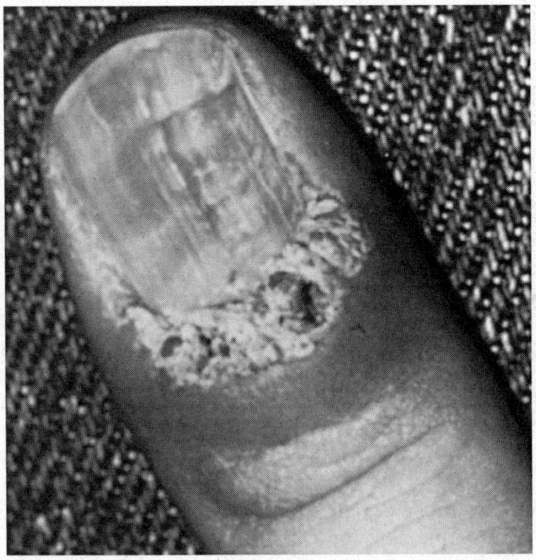

FIGURE 151–1 □ Periungual warts result in nail dystrophy.

hands and on the face. Verrucae planae eventually undergo spontaneous regression after a number of years, signaled by the development of erythema or pruritus around each wart and the disappearance of all the warts within 2 or 3 weeks.[1]

Epidermodysplasia verruciformis is a noncontagious autosomal recessive condition characterized by innumerable small papules that develop in early childhood and are clinically and histologically identical to flat warts.[26] Slightly elevated scaling plaques resembling tinea versicolor may also be seen. Lesions are usually caused by HPV types 3, 5, and 8. About 35% of these patients develop cutaneous squamous cell carcinomas at the sites of previous warts. These can occur as early as the second decade of life. Patients with epidermodysplasia verruciformis infected with HPV-5 are at greatest risk for developing skin cancer. Ultraviolet light seems to act as a cofactor for malignant transformation, because the cancers occur in sun-exposed areas. These patients have depressed cell-mediated immunity. Epidermodysplasia verruciformis–like lesions have been described in patients with human immunodeficiency virus disease.

Although patients with epidermodysplasia verruciformis and those patients with anogenital or laryngeal papillomas may develop malignant neoplasms, most HPV infections are not premalignant. Forty percent of renal transplant patients, however, develop squamous cell carcinomas in preexisting warts 10 years after transplantation.[27, 28] Sun exposure markedly increases a patient's risk for cutaneous malignant disease. HPV was found in 62% of benign proliferations in renal transplant patients.[29] HPV types normally seen in only mucosal verrucae may be detected in some benign, premalignant, and malignant growths in organ transplant patients.[30, 31] This is not caused by *HRAS* gene mutations.[32] HPV has occasionally been found in patients with a normal immune system in squamous cell carcinomas,[33] keratoacanthomas,[34] verrucous carcinomas,[35] and actinic keratoses,[36] but this is probably an unusual event.

Diagnosis

Warts rarely pose a diagnostic dilemma for the clinician. They may be confused with skin tags, seborrheic keratoses, molluscum contagiosum, and corns. A skin biopsy can be performed if the diagnosis is uncertain. To identify the specific HPV type, Southern blot, in situ hybridization, or polymerase chain reaction techniques may be used with the electron microscope. Paraffin-embedded sections are preferred, but even formalin-embedded sections may be used.[37]

Treatment

Most cutaneous warts regress on their own in the immunologically normal host,[38] and except in immunodeficient patients in whom oncogenic potential exists, they pose no threat to physical well-being. They can, however, be painful and disfiguring. Treatments can be painful, time-consuming, and expensive and do not confer lifelong immunity to HPV infections. However, the longer warts persist, the harder they are to eradicate and the more they are likely to spread. Patients must be told that regardless of the method chosen, multiple treatments are usually required and recurrences are common. Treatments that cause scarring or prolonged discomfort are probably not justifiable. All of the treatments discussed have a 65% to 85% cure rate if they are used for 12 weeks. Clinicians vary in their preferences for treatment modality, with no single modality being clearly superior. Gloves should always be worn by the physician in examining or treating warts. Practitioners unfamiliar with a technique discussed should watch a clinician perform it or consult a more detailed text[39, 40] before treating patients. Particular care should be exercised in treating patients with diabetes, Raynaud phenomenon, or peripheral vascular disease. Although the majority of warts may be taken care of by primary care physicians and physician extenders, patients who fail to respond to treatment in the expected manner should be referred to a dermatologist.

Treatments used may be conveniently divided into topical treatments applied by the patient (under the supervision of a practitioner), treatments applied by the practitioner, surgical options, and systemic therapies.

Topical Treatments Applied by the Patient

Topical preparations applied by the patient are usually repeated daily. Efficacy is increased if the lesions are soaked and pared with pumice before medication application. Occlusion by tape increases the efficacy of treatment but increases the potential for irritation. Individual response and degree of

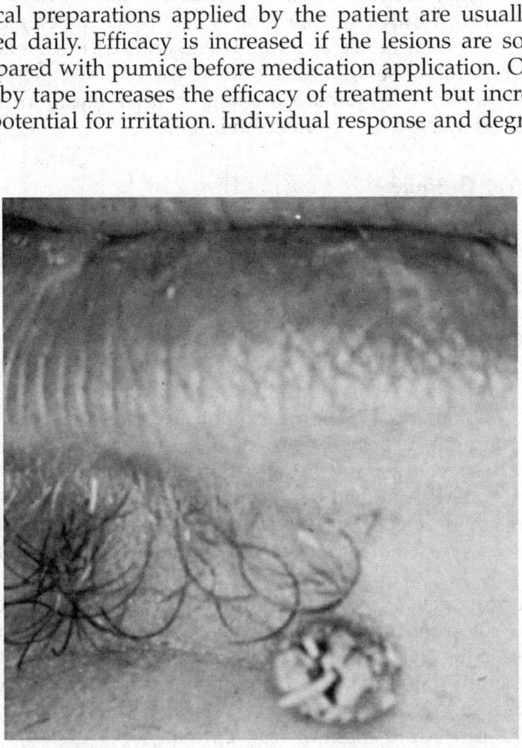

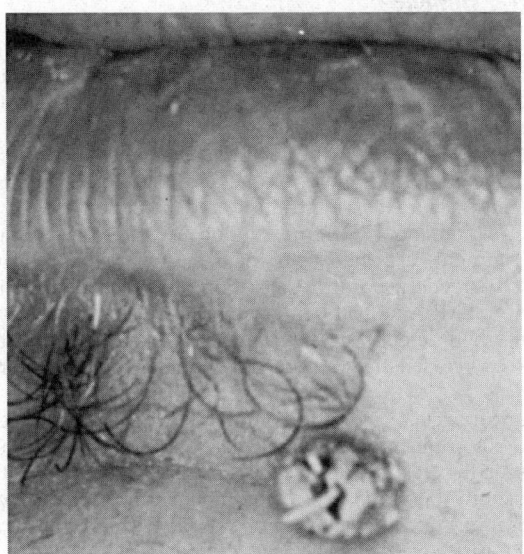

FIGURE 151–2 □ Filiform warts on the chin.

irritation are extremely variable. Patients' progress should be monitored every 4 to 6 weeks by the prescribing practitioner.

Salicylic acid preparations in collodion or impregnated tape are available in the United States without a prescription. Lactic acid is added to some salicylic acid preparations and may increase their efficacy. Formalin,[1] glutaraldehyde,[41] squaric acid,[42] diphenylcyclopropenone,[43] and dinitrochlorobenzene[44] are useful in some patients but may cause pruritus secondary to the contact dermatitis they cause. The practitioner must inform the patient that future exposure to these chemicals will induce the same contact dermatitis. Dinitrochlorobenzene use is controversial, because it is mutagenic in vitro. Topical retinoids may be effective, particularly for flat warts. Topical retinoids may also decrease papillomas and premalignant lesions in renal transplant patients.[45]

Treatments Applied by the Practitioner

Treatments applied by the practitioner should be repeated at 1- to 3-week intervals, depending on the patient's tolerance. Cantharidin[1] is extremely useful for some periungual warts, particularly in children, but is no longer available in the United States. Painful blisters and circles of warts around the original treated lesion may develop. Monochloroacetic, dichloroacetic, and trichloroacetic acid preparations are useful but may be irritating in high concentrations. Silver nitrate sticks also have their proponents.[46] Podophyllum resin, commonly used to treat genital warts, is extremely irritating to the skin and may cause vomiting, lethargy, neuropathy, and even death if excessive amounts are used. It is antimitotic and should not be used in infants and pregnant women.[1] Localized controlled heat therapy may also be used.[47]

Intralesional bleomycin has gained popularity as a treatment for warts. A multiple puncture technique is particularly useful.[48] Small doses are used, and a systemic toxic effect has not been reported; however, permanent nail dystrophy and Raynaud phenomenon may occur rarely.[49] Because significant absorption of bleomycin occurs after intralesional injection,[50] the medication should not be used in pregnancy.

Both interferon alfa-2a and interferon alfa-2b have been used systemically, intralesionally, and as a cream for warts.[51, 52] Treatments are expensive and tedious, because injections must be repeated one to three times per week. Influenza-like symptoms are common after injections; liver and bone marrow toxic effects are rare.

Surgical Options

Cryosurgery with liquid nitrogen is probably the most commonly used office technique for treating warts. It is painful on application and may cause blistering. Four or five treatments, repeated at 1- to 3-week intervals, cure about 45% of patients.[53] Although the technique is simple, appropriate training is required. Hypopigmented and hyperpigmented scars may occur. It is contraindicated in patients with Raynaud phenomenon. Extreme caution must be used to avoid overtreatment, especially on the feet, where complications such as infection, painful ulceration, and scarring are more common. EMLA, eutectic mixture of local anesthetics, a topical anesthetic cream, applied an hour or more before treatment may lessen the discomfort of the treatment considerably.

Surgical excision is not recommended because recurrences (up to 30%) are more frequent than with other techniques,[54] and scarring results. However, curettage with or without cauterization alone is useful, particularly for solitary warts. Injection of lidocaine is superior to EMLA cream for controlling the procedural pain of wart curettage.[55]

The carbon dioxide laser may be used to vaporize intractable warts,[56] particularly on the soles. It causes prolonged morbidity and is expensive. The recurrence rate is about 35%.[57] Furthermore, aerosolized virus in the carbon dioxide laser plume may pose a risk to the treating physician.[58] This treatment is recommended only in unusually recalcitrant warts. More recently, the pulsed dye laser has been used for recalcitrant warts with preliminary encouraging results.[59] However, larger studies are needed before the role of this laser in wart therapy can be adequately evaluated.

Systemic Therapies

Systemic therapies may be used as an adjunct to topical wart therapy or reserved for those patients in whom other treatment modalities have failed. With the exception of cimetidine, they are used primarily in immunocompromised patients in whom the risk for malignant transformation warrants aggressive wart therapy. Oral cimetidine is well tolerated by most patients and is reported to be effective in about three quarters of patients after 3 months of use,[60] although the authors have found it somewhat less effective. Cimetidine is particularly useful in children with multiple lesions. Interferon therapy is discussed earlier. Oral retinoids, particularly etretinate,[61] and interleukin-2[62] help temporarily, but warts usually recur after treatment is stopped.

Hypnosis may be tried in some patients when other modalities have failed or are contraindicated. Hypnosis may decrease blood flow to the warts or may alter the immune response.[63, 64] Treatment is painless but special training is required, and patients may not be willing to try the technique.

Prevention

Because HPV is so ubiquitous, it is difficult to prevent contact, either directly or indirectly, through infected people or contaminated objects. Patients with warts should use their own towels and should not walk barefoot around pools or in showers. Patients with warts in hairy areas should be discouraged from shaving, because this may cause warts to disseminate. No vaccine is available for warts, but because they are not debilitating for most patients and are premalignant in only unusual circumstances, vaccination is probably unnecessary.

References

1. Bunney MH, Benton C, Cubie HA: Viral Warts: Biology and Treatment, ed 2. New York, Oxford University Press, 1992.
2. Devillers EM: Heterogeneity of the human papillomavirus group. J Virol 63:4898, 1989.
3. Lutzner MA: The human papillomaviruses: A review. Arch Dermatol 119:631, 1983.
4. Krieder JW, Patricks D, Cladel NM, Welsh PA: Experimental infection with human papillomavirus type I of human hand and foot skin. Virology 177:415, 1990.
5. Sterling J, Stanley M, Gatward ZG, Minson T: Production of human papillomavirus type 16 virions in a keratinocyte cell line. J Virol 64:6305, 1990.
6. Laimins LA: The biology of human papillomaviruses: From warts to cancer. Infect Agents Dis 2:74, 1993.
7. Mallory SB, Baugh LS, Parker RK: Warts in blacks versus whites. Pediatr Dermatol 8:91, 1991.
8. Jablonska S, Obalek S, Golebiowska A, et al: Epidemiology of butcher's warts. Arch Dermatol Res 280:S24, 1988.
9. Keefe M, al-Glamdi A, Coggon D, et al: Cutaneous warts in butchers. Br J Dermatol 130:9, 1994.
10. Bender M: Concepts of wart regression. Arch Dermatol 122:644, 1986.

11. Amella CA, Lofgren LA, Ronn AM, et al: Latent infection induced with cottontail rabbit papillomavirus. A model for human papillomavirus latency. Am J Pathol 144:1167, 1994.
12. Haftek M, Jablonska S, Orth G: Specific cell-mediated immunity in patients with epidermodysplasia verruciformis and plane warts. Dermatologica 170:213, 1985.
13. Cubie HA: Serological studies in a student population prone to infection with human papillomavirus. J Hyg 70:677, 1972.
14. Williams L, Webster G: Warts and molluscum contagiosum. Clin Dermatol 9:87, 1991.
15. Yell JA, Burge SM: Warts and lupus erythematosus. Lupus 2:21, 1993.
16. Williams H, Pottier A, Strachan D: Are viral warts seen more commonly in children with eczema? Arch Dermatol 129:717, 1993.
17. Beltrani VS: Warts and the atopic. Arch Dermatol 130:388, 1994.
18. Rogozinski TT, Jablonska SS, Jarabek-Chorzelska M: Role of cell-mediated immunity in spontaneous regression of plane warts. Int J Dermatol 27:322, 1988.
19. Iwatsuki K, Tagami H, Takigawa M, et al: Plane warts under spontaneous regression. Arch Dermatol 122:655, 1986.
20. Bergfelt L: Langerhans cells, immunomodulation and skin lesions. A quantitative, morphologic and clinical study. Acta Derm Veneriol (Stockh) 180:1, 1993.
21. Egawa K, Inaba Y, Yoshimura K, Ono T: Varied clinical morphology of HPV-1–induced warts, depending on anatomical factors. Br J Dermatol 128:271, 1993.
22. Egawa K: New types of human papillomaviruses and intracytoplasmic inclusion bodies: A classification of inclusion warts according to clinical features, histology, and associated HPV types. Br J Dermatol 130:158, 1994.
23. Melchers W, de Mare S, Kuitert E, et al: Human papillomavirus and cutaneous warts in meat handlers. J Clin Microbiol 31:2547, 1993.
24. Stehr-Green PA, Hewer P, Meeking F, Judd LE: The aetiology and risk factors for warts among poultry processing workers. Int J Epidemiol 22:294, 1993.
25. Benton EC: Warts in butchers—A cause for concern? Lancet 343:1114, 1994.
26. Lynch P: Warts and cancer. Am J Dermatopathol 4:55, 1982.
27. Barr BB, McLaren K, Smith IW, et al: Human papillomavirus infection and skin cancer in renal allograft patients. Lancet 1:124, 1989.
28. Leigh IM, Glover MP: Cutaneous warts and tumors in immunosuppressed patients. J R Soc Med 88:61, 1995.
29. Shamanin V, Glover M, Proby C, et al: Specific types of human papillomavirus found in benign proliferations and carcinomas of the skin in immunosuppressed patients. Cancer Res 54:4610, 1994.
30. Saler C, Chardonnet Y, Allibert P, et al: Detection of mucosal human papillomavirus types 6/11 in cutaneous lesions from transplant recipients. J Invest Dermatol 100:286, 1993.
31. Viac J, Chardonnet Y, Chignot MC, Schmitt D: Papilloma viruses, warts, carcinoma and Langerhans cells. In Vivo 7:207, 1993.
32. Pelisson I, Chardonnet Y, Euvrard S, Schmitt D: Low incidence of c-Ha-*ras* gene mutations in benign and malignant cutaneous lesions from transplant recipients. Int J Cancer 55:915, 1993.
33. Moy RL, Eliezri YD, Nuovo GJ, et al: Human papillomavirus type 16 DNA in periungual squamous cell carcinoma. JAMA 261:2669, 1989.
34. Gassenmaier A, Pfister H, Hornstein OP: Human papillomavirus 25–related DNA in solitary keratoacanthoma. Arch Dermatol Res 279:73, 1986.
35. Noel JC, Penny MO, Detremmerie O, et al: Demonstration of human papillomavirus type 2 in a verrucous carcinoma of the foot. Dermatology 187:58, 1993.
36. Kawashima M, Favre M, Jablonska S, et al: Characterization of a new type of papillomavirus (HPV) related to HPV 5 from a case of actinic keratosis. Virology 154:389, 1986.
37. Hagari Y, Shibata M, Mihara M, et al: Detection of human papillomavirus type 2a DNA in verrucae vulgaris by electron microscopic in situ hybridization. Arch Dermatol Res 285:255, 1993.
38. Massing AM, Epstein WL: Natural history of warts. Arch Dermatol 87:74, 1963.
39. Goldfarb MT, Gupta AK, Gupta MA, Sawchuk WS: Office therapy for human papillomavirus infection in nongenital sites. Dermatol Clin 9:287, 1991.
40. Bolton RA: Nongenital warts: Classification and treatment options. Am Fam Physician 43:2049, 1991.
41. Hirose R, Hori M, Shukuwa T, et al: Topical treatment of resistant warts with glutaraldehyde. J Dermatol 21:248, 1994.
42. Iijima S, Otsuka F: Contact immunotherapy with squaric acid dibutyl ester for warts. Dermatology 187:115, 1993.
43. van der Steen P, van de Kerkhof P, der Kinderen D, et al: Clinical and immunohistochemical responses of plantar warts to topical immunotherapy with diphenylcyclopropenone. J Dermatol 18:330, 1991.
44. Campbell BJ: The treatment of warts. Prim Care 13:465, 1986.
45. Euvrard S, Verschoore M, Touraine JL, et al: Topical retinoids for warts and keratoses in transplant recipients (Letter). Lancet 340:48, 1992.
46. Yazar S, Basaran E: Efficacy of silver nitrate pencils in the treatment of common warts. J Dermatol 21:329, 1994.
47. Halasz CL: Treatment of common warts using the infrared coagulator. J Dermatol Surg Oncol 20:252, 1994.
48. Shelley WB, Shelley ED: Intralesional bleomycin sulfate therapy for warts. Arch Dermatol 127:234, 1991.
49. Hayes ME, O'Keefe EJ: Reduced dose of bleomycin in the treatment of recalcitrant warts. J Am Acad Dermatol 15:1002, 1986.
50. James MP, Collier PM, Aherne W, et al: Histologic, pharmacologic, and immunochemical effects of injection of bleomycin into viral warts. J Am Acad Dermatol 28:933, 1993.
51. Landow RK: The interferons; a clinician's view. Dermatol Clin 6:569, 1988.
52. Finter NB, Chapman S, Dowd P, et al: The use of interferon-alpha in virus infections. Drugs 42:749, 1991.
53. Bourke JF, Berthe-Jones J, Hutchinson PE: Cryotherapy of common warts at intervals of 1, 2, and 3 weeks. Br J Dermatol 132:433, 1995.
54. Vickers CFH: Treatment of plantar warts in children. Br Med J 2:743, 1961.
55. Vesterager L, Petersen KP, Nielsen R, et al: EMLA-induced analgesia inferior to lignocaine infiltration in curettage of common warts—A randomized study. Dermatology 188:32, 1994.
56. Lim JT, Goh CL: Carbon dioxide laser treatment of periungual and subungual viral warts. Australas J Dermatol 33:87, 1992.
57. Street ML, Roenigk RK: Recalcitrant periungual verrucae: The role of carbon dioxide laser vaporization. J Am Acad Dermatol 23:115, 1990.
58. Garden JM, O'Banion K, Shelnitz LS, et al: Papillomavirus in the vapor of carbon dioxide laser–treated verrucae. JAMA 259:1199, 1988.
59. Tan OT, Hurwitz RM, Stafford TJ: Pulsed dye laser treatment of recalcitrant verrucae: A preliminary report. Lasers Surg Med 13:127, 1993.
60. Orlow SJ, Paller A: Cimetidine therapy for multiple viral warts in children. J Am Acad Dermatol 28:794, 1993.
61. Gelmetti C, Cerri D, Schiuma AA, et al: Treatment of extensive warts with etretinate: A clinical trial in 20 children. Pediatr Dermatol 4:254, 1987.
62. Ades EW, Gillespie T: Resolution of warts during interleukin-2 immunotherapy. Pathobiology 58:88, 1990.
63. Morris BA: Hypnotherapy of warts using the Simonton visualization technique: A case report. Am J Clin Hypn 27:237, 1985.
64. Ewin DM: Hypnotherapy for warts (verruca vulgaris): 41 consecutive cases with 33 cures. Am J Clin Hypn 35:1, 1992.

152

Erythema Infectiosum, Roseola, and Enteroviral Exanthems

Walter W. Tunnessen, Jr.

Erythema Infectiosum

Fifth disease (erythema infectiosum) is the only exanthem that retains the numerical eponym assigned to it during the late 1800s and early 1900s. This distinctive exanthem was first described by Tschamer in 1886, and the label erythema infectiosum was applied by Stricker in 1899.[1] The first report in the American literature appeared in 1905, but the cases described were actually seen in Vienna.[2] Herrick's careful description of 74 cases provided the first record of a large outbreak in the United States.

The cause of erythema infectiosum defied discovery until 1984, when the sera of 36 children involved in an outbreak of this exanthem were tested for the presence of specific immunoglobin M (IgM) antibody to human parvovirus (HPV) and all showed significant titers.[3] A number of reports confirmed this association.[4–6]

HPV-B19 was discovered in 1975 in blood obtained from adult donors who were asymptomatic or had mild symptoms during an evaluation of hepatitis B detection tests.[7] HPV-B19 has since then been incriminated as the cause of aplastic crises in persons with hemolytic anemias; it has been found to be a cause of acute arthritis in some adults; it has been associated with spontaneous abortions, stillbirths, and hydrops fetalis; and it may lead to chronic marrow hypoplasia from persistent red blood cell precursor lysis in immunocompromised patients who develop persistent infections.[8]

Epidemiology

The mode of spread of HPV is presumed to be person to person through the respiratory tract. Erythema infectiosum has a worldwide distribution. It tends to occur in epidemics, most commonly in the late winter and early spring. The exanthem seems to be fairly well confined to school-age children. Herrick[1] found all but 4 of his 74 cases in the 6- to 15-year age bracket. Ager and coworkers[9] similarly observed the peak attack rate between 5 and 14 years, with 80% of 364 patients younger than 15 years. School attack rates during epidemics have varied between 13% and 43.9%.[3, 10, 11] Antibody to HPV increases with age. Almost 20% of children 10 to 14 years of age, 35% of adults 30 to 39 years of age, and 50% of persons older than 50 years will demonstrate antibody.[4] This suggests that adults may acquire the infection but frequently do not manifest the exanthem.

Pathogenesis

Healthy adult volunteers inoculated intranasally with HPV obtained from an asymptomatic blood donor demonstrated a two-phase illness. A week after inoculation, during intense viremia, the volunteers had a mild illness with fever, malaise, myalgia, and itching. At 17 to 18 days, the second phase occurred when three of four volunteers developed a fine maculopapular rash and arthralgias that lasted 3 to 4 days.[12] During the latter phase, viral secretion was absent, suggesting that infected persons are not contagious when the rash appears. The appearance of the rash coincided with high titers of IgM antibodies to HPV, suggesting an immune-mediated rash.

Clinical Manifestations

The most characteristic feature of erythema infectiosum is the striking erythematous eruption on the face, which creates a "slapped cheek" appearance. The borders of the erythema are sharp, and the eruption is often raised. The malar areas and chin are usually involved, and the bright red color fades to a violet hue in a few days. The second stage occurs about 1 day later, when an erythematous, maculopapular rash erupts on the trunk, buttocks, and extremities. This rash is less characteristic and has been described as morbilliform, confluent, circinate, or anular.[9] The individual lesions measure 2 mm to as much as 30 mm in diameter, and they are not confluent. This stage lasts for a few days to 1 week.

The third stage of the rash is perhaps the most pathognomonic. The eruption on the trunk fades, but it persists on the extremities, particularly the thighs and forearms (Fig. 152–1). Areas of clearing develop in the macular confluence, creating a reticular or lacy appearance. An unusual feature of this stage is the rash's tendency to fade and reappear. Whereas the rash disappears in the majority of cases in less than 10 days, it persists or recurs in 15% for more than 20 days and in 1% for longer than 80 days. The longest reported case lasted 95 days.[9] The evanescent character of the rash is ob-

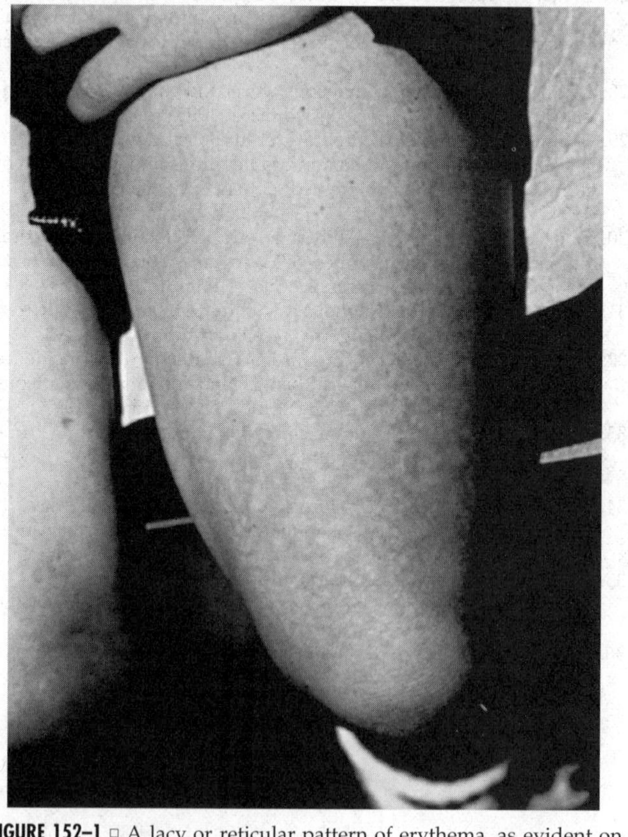

FIGURE 152–1 □ A lacy or reticular pattern of erythema, as evident on the thigh, is characteristic of erythema infectiosum.

served in about one third of cases. The reappearance is often precipitated by chilling, sunlight, bathing, exercise, or emotional stress. An enanthema consisting of macular areas of erythema is occasionally described. Papular, vesicular, and purpuric variants of the rash have also been described.[13, 14]

Erythema infectiosum is most often a mild illness. A prodrome consisting of malaise, low-grade fever, sore throat, and nasal stuffiness may herald the appearance of the rash. Table 152–1 summarizes the signs and symptoms associated with erythema infectiosum. The frequency of many symptoms, particularly arthralgia and arthritis, varies with the age of the infected person. Whereas Ager and colleagues[9] found that 77.2% of adults 20 years and older complained of joint pain and 59.6% had joint swelling, only 5.1% of children 9 years or younger complained of joint pain and 2.8% had joint swelling. Similarly, in the 10- to 19-year age group, 11.5% and 5.3%, respectively, had these complaints.

Complications of erythema infectiosum are uncommon. Two children have been reported who developed an encephalopathy with erythema infectiosum, one with persistent neurologic sequelae.[14, 15] Children with chronic hemolytic anemias who develop erythema infectiosum rarely develop aplastic crises.[16]

Two different cutaneous eruptions attributed to HPV-B19 are worth noting. One is a purpuric, petechial, and pseudopustular rash involving the buttocks and wrists, followed by the development of a morbilliform rash and Koplik spots in the mouth. The other is a petechial glove and sock rash with the hallmarks of fever, pruritic edema followed by pain, and petechial rash of the hands and feet with sharp demarcation at the wrist and ankle and an enanthema consisting of petechiae and oral erosions.[17, 18]

Diagnosis

Serologic testing for HPV IgG and IgM antibodies by use of indirect immunofluorescence is more readily available than are nucleic acid hybridization probes to detect B19 DNA. HPV-B19 IgM antibody can be detected by the third day of symptoms of erythema infectiosum or transient aplastic crisis and can persist for 2 to 3 months after infection. IgG antibody is usually present by the seventh day of illness and persists for years. Routine laboratory tests provide no specific clues to the diagnosis. The differential diagnosis of erythema infectiosum includes rubella, which should easily be separated on the basis of its short duration, and scarlet fever, which shares the slapped cheek appearance.

TABLE 152–1 ■ Signs and Symptoms of Erythema Infectiosum

SIGN OR SYMPTOM	REPORTED FREQUENCY (%)
Rash	
Face	52–87
Arms	78–87
Legs	74–77
Chest	48–71
Pruritus	46–71
Fever	20–44
Headache	23–51
Sore throat	8–44
Nasal stuffiness	3–44
Cough	8–32
Anorexia	13–24
Arthralgia	5–77
Joint swelling	3–60

Compiled from references 3, 9, 10, 11.

Treatment and Prevention

No antiviral therapy for or immunization against erythema infectiosum is available. Because the disease is benign, often lasts for weeks, and is probably not communicable a few days after the rash appears, there is no reason to exclude infected persons from school or work.

Roseola

Zahorsky[19] is credited with separating roseola from other exanthems with which it previously had been included. The benign nature of this disease and its frequent occurrence were soon recognized. In 1921, Veeder and Hempelmann[20] suggested the name exanthem subitum (sudden) to separate roseola from rubella. Although this distinctive exanthematous disorder has received many appellations, including sixth disease, roseola is the name most often used. The discovery of a viral cause for roseola in 1988 has finally completed the etiologic identification of the numbered exanthems.

Microbiology

The agent responsible for roseola has eluded investigators for years. The exanthem was thought to be a hypersensitivity response to a number of different viruses, because roseola-like rashes were identified with several echoviruses and coxsackieviruses. In 1988, Yamanishi and coworkers[21] isolated a virus from cultured lymphocytes from four infants with roseola. The virus was cultured in cord blood lymphocytes and shown to be antigenically related to human herpesvirus 6 (HHV-6). The morphologic features of the virus on thin-section electron microscopy resembled those of the herpesvirus group, and convalescent serum samples demonstrated seroconversion against HHV-6. In a subsequent report, 11 of 12 infants observed serologically developed antibody titers to HHV-6, 7 of whom had documented roseola within 9 months of birth.[22] An infant who had typical roseola at 6 months had a second roseola-like illness at age 13 months. Seroconversion to HHV-7 was found.[23] HHV-7 will probably be found to be the cause of more roseola-like illnesses.

HHV-6 is a new human B lymphotropic virus isolated in 1986.[24] It is interesting that both Breese[25] and Kempe[26] considered herpes simplex virus the possible agent of roseola.

Epidemiology

It was suspected early in the history of roseola that the agent responsible was ubiquitous, because adults and older children rarely developed the disease and most children affected were younger than 3 years but older than 4 months. It was also noted that cases were almost always sporadic with rare outbreaks in hospitals or foundling homes, which suggested carriage of the infectious agent by healthy adults or older children.[27] Serum from an 18-month-old infant with roseola injected intravenously into a 6-month-old infant produced the typical disease course 9 days later.[26] Three of 14 infants injected intramuscularly with blood from persons with typical cases of roseola developed a similar illness 6 to 9 days later.[28]

Roseola is thought to be the most common infectious exanthem affecting children in the first 2 years of life. Breese[25] observed 70 newborn infants in his practice for 1 year and found that 16% developed roseola. He concluded that approximately 30% of children eventually contract clinical roseola. Of 1653 children presenting to an emergency department with an acute febrile illness 10% of those up to 2 years of age and 21% of those 6 to 12 months of age had documented HHV-6 infections. Only 17% of these HHV-6–infected children developed a rash.[29] One third of children younger than 2 years who suffered febrile seizures were HHV-6–positive. The majority of infants affected are between 6 months and 2 years of age, with 80% younger than 2 years and 90% younger than 3 years. The reduced frequency in infants younger than 6 months suggests protection from transmitted maternal antibodies. Rare cases have been reported in older children.[20, 30]

The illness may occur at any time of year, although late winter–early spring and fall seem to produce more cases. The incubation period appears to average 10 days, ranging from 5 to 15 days.[27]

Clinical Manifestations

The typical clinical picture is the abrupt onset of fever in a young child; the temperature remains elevated for 3 to 5 days, then rapidly falls to normal and is followed by the appearance of the rash. Children with roseola usually have little or no prodrome. They may have mild malaise. The fever starts suddenly, and temperature generally ranges from 38.8°C to above 40°C. It tends to be constant rather than intermittent. Despite the fever, affected infants do not act ill. They may be more listless or irritable during peak fever, but appetite is not severely affected. Infants may occasionally have some vomiting, diarrhea, or mild cough and coryza.

Early in the illness, the physical examination is not of much diagnostic help. Palpebral edema has been reported in some infants early in the illness, but rarely later than day 3.[31] An occasional child may have a bulging fontanel.[32] Mild inflammation of the pharynx and tonsils and erythematous macules on the soft palate are sometimes seen. The tympanic membranes may be mildly injected. Some observers have noted posterior occipital, auricular, and cervical adenopathy in infants with roseola.[19, 30, 33]

The frequency of signs and symptoms in infants with virologically confirmed exanthem subitum is shown in Table 152–2.[34]

The fever falls to normal rapidly (crisis) in about half the cases and more gradually (lysis) in the other half.[27] The rash, which consists of discrete 1- to 5-mm pink macules, may appear just before the fever breaks or within 12 hours after it disappears. The rash is frequently sparse and is first noted on the neck and back. It rapidly spreads to the chest and extremities, the face and feet almost always being spared (Fig. 152–2). The lesions are occasionally papular and frequently have a whitish halo. The duration of the rash may be as short as a few hours or as long as 2 days.

TABLE 152–2 ■ Frequency of Signs and Symptoms in Infants with Virologically Confirmed Exanthem Subitum

SIGN OR SYMPTOM	FREQUENCY (%)
Fever	98
Rash	98
Diarrhea, mild	68
Erythematous pharyngeal papules	65
Cough	50
Edematous eyelids	30
Mild cervical lymphadenopathy	31
Bulging fontanelle	26
Seizures	8

Adapted from Asano Y, Yoshikawa T, Suga S, et al: Clinical features of infants with primary human herpesvirus 6 infection (exanthem subitum, roseola infantum). Reproduced by permission of Pediatrics, Vol 93, Page 104. Copyright 1994.

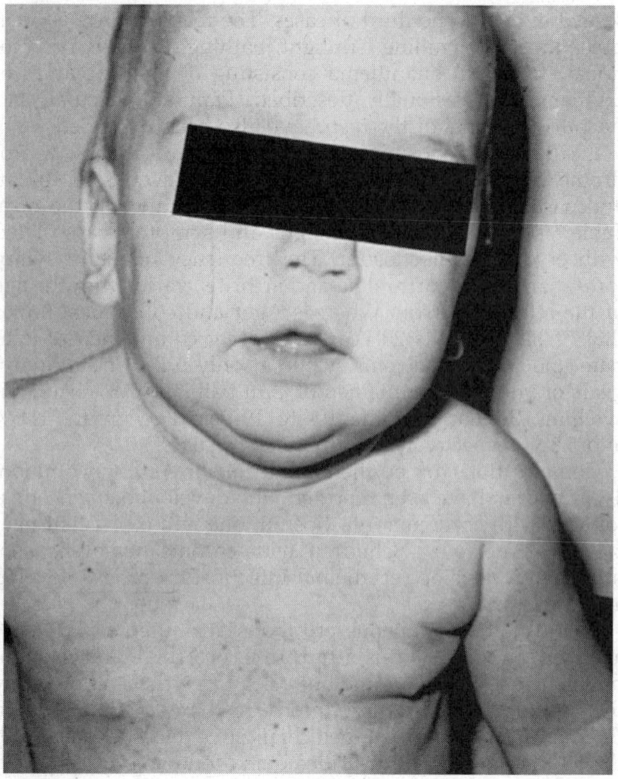

FIGURE 152–2 ▫ The scattered maculopapular rash of roseola is most evident on the trunk, the face being relatively spared.

Diagnosis

The diagnosis of roseola is a clinical one. There are no helpful laboratory tests. The white cell count is usually elevated (in the range of 12,000 to 15,000/mm^3) in the first 24 to 36 hours of illness; by the third day, there is definite leukopenia and relative lymphocytosis.[35] Rarely, cerebrospinal fluid may show a mild lymphocytic pleocytosis. IgG antibody to HHV-6 may be determined by indirect immunofluorescent antibody assay. Polymerase chain reaction techniques may also be used for identification of this virus.

Complications of roseola are uncommon. Febrile convulsions are the most common adverse association, but their frequency varies with practice or hospital-based reports. Hemiplegia, sometimes persistent, has been reported.[36, 37]

The caveat in the diagnosis of roseola is possible confusion with a drug eruption. The fever and mild tympanic injection in young infants often prompt prescription of antibiotics. The appearance of the rash may be mistaken for a drug eruption. Rubella is unlikely to be associated with such a high fever, and the rash is more diffuse and longer lasting. Rubeola is readily differentiated by its prodrome and course.

Treatment and Prevention

There is no specific therapy for roseola. Antipyretics such as acetaminophen may help make the infant more comfortable during the high fever. No active or passive immunizations are currently available. Lifelong immunity seems to result from active disease.

Enteroviral Exanthems

The enteroviruses of which more than 30 have been associated with rashes, are common causes of exanthematous disease in childhood. Unlike measles, rubella, erythema infectiosum, and other classic exanthems, enteroviral rashes, with the exception of hand-foot-and-mouth disease and herpangina, are not distinctive or specific enough to allow differentiation on clinical grounds, and one virus type may produce various rashes.

Epidemiology

The enteroviruses gain entrance to their human host through the oropharynx, replicate in the epithelial and lymphoid cells of the intestinal tract, and spread to other organ sites through the blood stream. They are shed from the oropharynx and urine for 1 week but in the feces for as long as 1 month.[38] Although they can be disseminated from the respiratory tract, the intestinal route by manual transmission is most common. The incubation period for these viruses appears to be short, 4 to 7 days.

The diseases associated with enteroviruses tend to occur in epidemics, and most appear in the summer months or early fall in temperate climates. There is no seasonal pattern in tropical climates. Crowded conditions and poor hygiene encourage their spread.

Pathogenesis

Direct invasion of the skin or mucous membranes through the blood stream is the most likely mechanism for the production of the vesicular or ulcerative lesions seen in hand-foot-and-mouth disease and herpangina. The more prevalent maculopapular exanthems are probably the result of the skin's reacting with circulating or cell-mediated immune factors. Unfortunately, accurate histologic definition of the viral exanthems is sparse.

Clinical Manifestations

Hand-foot-and-mouth disease, anatomically describing the most common sites of the vesicles and ulcers associated with this illness, is the most readily recognized and distinctive enteroviral exanthem. The first recognized outbreak of this disease occurred in Toronto in 1957.[39] The appellation hand-foot-and-mouth disease was given after an epidemic in Birmingham, England, in 1959.[40] Since then, the disease has occurred worldwide, most often in the summer and early fall.

Coxsackievirus A16 is responsible for the majority of cases of hand-foot-and-mouth disease, but this exanthem has also been described with coxsackievirus types A5, A7, A9, A10, B2, and B5. The virus is highly contagious. Whereas up to 100% of infected preschool-age children develop a rash, only 38% of school-age children and 11% of infected adults have cutaneous manifestations.[41]

The most common presentation is the complaint of a sore throat or mouth, usually without prodrome. The enanthema is vesicular but rapidly ulcerates. Usually, 5 to 10 oral lesions are present; as opposed to herpangina, they may occur anywhere in the mouth.[42] The exanthem, primarily consisting of hand and foot lesions, follows shortly after the oral lesions. The vesicles generally measure 3 to 7 mm and are set on an erythematous base (Fig. 152–3). Frequently, the vesicles take on linear or arcuate forms. The vesicular fluid contains the virus and provides a mode of spread through contact. The vesicles can be found in other body areas, but sparingly. The buttocks are most frequently involved besides the typical sites.

Hand-foot-and-mouth disease usually runs a benign course lasting about 1 week. Rarely, a more severe chronic or relapsing course is seen.[43] The differential diagnosis of hand-foot-and-mouth disease is limited because of the characteristic rash. When oral ulcerations are found, the hands and feet should be inspected for vesicles before a diagnosis of herpes simplex, aphthous stomatitis, or herpangina is assigned.

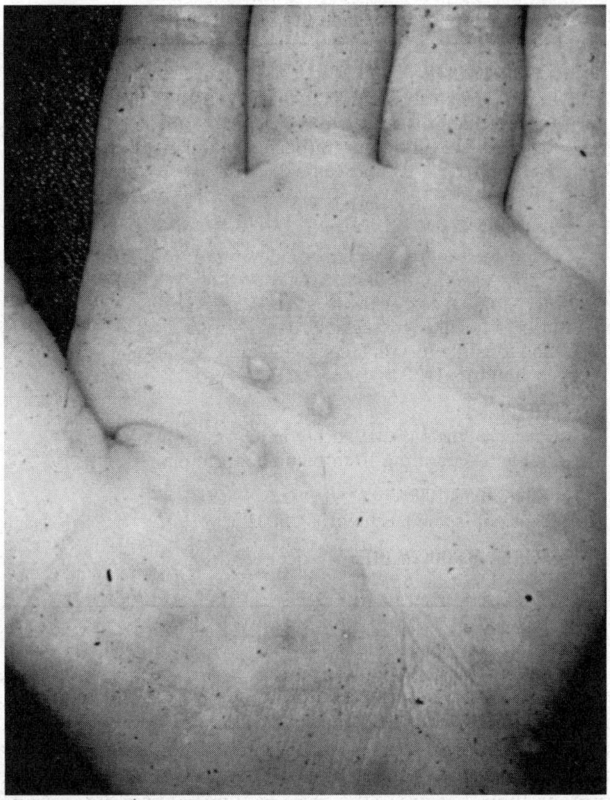

FIGURE 152–3 ▫ Multiple vesicles of hand-foot-and-mouth disease are present on the palm.

Herpangina is caused by several enteroviruses, including coxsackieviruses A1 through A10, A16, and A22, and less commonly by coxsackieviruses B and echoviruses. The characteristic feature of this infection is the presence of small (2- to 4-mm) vesicles or ulcers on the tonsillar pillars, soft palate, or uvula. The lesions are usually few in number (two to six), but they are associated with a sore throat and pain on swallowing. The illness may be heralded by the abrupt onset of fever, vomiting, headache, and myalgia.

Echovirus 16 is best known as the cause of the Boston exanthem, named for the site of the first recorded epidemic in 1951.[44] A subsequent epidemic occurred in Pittsburgh in 1954.[45] The illness is often described as resembling roseola. In children, a temperature of 102°F (39°C) for 24 to 36 hours is common, and associated symptoms are mild. Sore throat is occasionally present, and punched-out ulcers of the soft palate may occur. The exanthem, which consists of pink or salmon-colored, discrete, 0.5- to 1.5-cm macules and maculopapules, appears as the fever declines.[38] The rash almost always involves the face (roseola does not) and lasts 1 to 5 days.

Children are much more likely to develop an exanthem with this illness than are adults; adults are generally sicker than children, with higher fever, prostration, muscle aches, and crampy abdominal pain. A small outbreak was described in the summer of 1974 in 10 children, 5 of whom were neonates.[46] Aseptic meningitis was associated in 6 of the 10.

Echovirus 9 has been described as causing a rubelliform eruption in children and adults and is particularly troublesome when it occurs in pregnant women.[47] Fever, headache, and nuchal rigidity are common in affected persons. The

TABLE 152–3 ■ Enteroviral Exanthems

MACULOPAPULAR
Rubelliform: echovirus 9, also 2, 4, 11, 19, 25 and coxsackievirus A9; size: 1–3 mm
Roseola-like: echovirus 16 (Boston exanthem); also echovirus 11, 25 and coxsackievirus B1, B5; size: 5–15 mm
VESICULAR
Hand-foot-and-mouth: coxsackievirus A16, also A5, A7, A9, A10, B2, B5
Herpangina: coxsackievirus A22, also A1–10, A16
Insect bite–like: coxsackievirus A4, crops, last 1–2 wk[48]
Non–pustule forming: coxsackievirus A9; also echovirus 11, 30[49]
PETECHIAL
Coxsackievirus B5, A9; echovirus 9
Problem separating from meningococcemia
HEMANGIOMA-LIKE
Transient, sparse: echovirus 25, 32[50, 51]
PAPULAR ACRODERMATITIS
Coxsackievirus A16

rash consists of discrete maculopapules 1 to 5 mm in diameter, which appear first on the face and neck shortly after the onset of fever. The exanthem lasts 3 to 5 days and is much more prominent in children, occurring in 57% of those younger than 4 years, 41% of 5- to 9-year-old children, and only 8% of adults. The rash may take on a petechial component, resembling meningococcemia.

Table 152–3 summarizes the most common of the types of rashes associated with coxsackievirus and echovirus infections. Note the diversity of lesions and the different types of rashes caused by the same virus. Exanthems occurring in children during the summer and fall are most likely caused by these viruses.

References

Erythema Infectiosum

1. Herrick TP: Erythema infectiosum. Am J Dis Child 31:486, 1926.
2. Shaw HLK: Erythema infectiosum. Am J Med Sci 129:16, 1905.
3. Anderson MJ, Lewis E, Kidd IM, et al: An outbreak of erythema infectiosum associated with human parvovirus infection. J Hyg (Camb) 93:85, 1984.
4. Nunoue T, Okochi K, Mortimer PP, et al: Human parvovirus (B19) and erythema infectiosum. J Pediatr 107:38, 1985.
5. Okabe N, Koboyashi S, Tatsuzawa O, et al: Detection of antibodies to human parvovirus in erythema infectiosum (fifth disease). Arch Dis Child 59:1016, 1984.
6. Plummer FA, Hammond GW, Forward K, et al: An erythema infectiosum–like illness caused by human parvovirus infection. N Engl J Med 313:74, 1985.
7. Cossart YE, Cant B, Field AM, et al: Parvovirus-like particles in human sera. Lancet 1:72, 1975.
8. Anderson LJ: Role of parvovirus B19 in human disease. Pediatr Infect Dis J 6:711, 1987.
9. Ager EA, Chin TDY, Poland JD: Epidemic erythema infectiosum. N Engl J Med 275:1326, 1966.
10. Brass C, Elliott LM, Stevens DA: Academy rash. JAMA 248:568, 1982.
11. Lauer BA, MacCormack JN, Wilfert C: Erythema infectiosum. An elementary school outbreak. Am J Dis Child 130:252, 1976.
12. Anderson MJ, Higgins PG, Davis LR, et al: Experimental parvoviral infection in humans. J Infect Dis 152:257, 1985.
13. Condon FJ: Erythema infectiosum: Report of an area-wide outbreak. Am J Public Health 49:528, 1959.
14. Balfour HH Jr, Schiff GM, Bloom JE: Encephalitis associated with erythema infectiosum. J Pediatr 77:133, 1970.
15. Hall CB, Horner FA: Encephalopathy with erythema infectiosum. Am J Dis Child 131:65, 1977.
16. Nunoue T, Koike T, Koike R, et al: Infection with human parvovirus (B19), aplasia of the bone marrow, and a rash in hereditary spherocytosis. J Infect 14:67, 1987.
17. Evans LM, Grossman ME, Gregory W: Koplik spots and a purpuric eruption associated with parvovirus B19 infection. J Am Acad Dermatol 27:466, 1992.
18. Halasz CLG, Cormier D, Den M: Petechial glove and sock syndrome caused by parvovirus B19. J Am Acad Dermatol 27:835, 1992.

Roseola

19. Zahorsky J: Roseola infantum. JAMA 16:1446, 1913.
20. Veeder BS, Hempelmann TC: A febrile exanthem occurring in childhood (exanthem subitum). JAMA 77:1787, 1921.
21. Yamanishi K, Okuno T, Shiraki K, et al: Identification of human herpesvirus 6 as a causal agent for exanthem subitum. Lancet 1:1065, 1988.
22. Takahashi K, Sonoda S, Kawakami K, et al: Human herpesvirus 6 and exanthem subitum. Lancet 1:1463, 1988.
23. Asano Y, Suga S, Yoshikawa T, et al: Clinical features and viral excretion in an infant with primary human herpesvirus 7 infection. Pediatrics 95:187, 1995.
24. Salahuddin SZ, Ablashi DV, Markham PD, et al: Isolation of a new virus, HBLV in patients with lymphoproliferative disorders. Science 234:596, 1986.
25. Breese BB Jr: Roseola infantum (exanthem subitum). N Y State J Med 41:1854, 1941.
26. Kempe CH, Shaw EB, Jackson JR, et al: Studies on the etiology of exanthem subitum. J Pediatr 37:561, 1950.
27. Barenberg LH, Greenspan L: Exanthem subitum (roseola infantum). Am J Dis Child 58:983, 1939.
28. Hellstrom B, Vahlquist B: Experimental inoculation of roseola infantum. Acta Paediatr 40:189, 1951.
29. Hall CB, Long CE, Schnabel KC, et al: Human herpesvirus-6 infection in children. N Engl J Med 331:432, 1994.
30. Letchner A: Roseola infantum: A review of fifty cases. Lancet 1:1163, 1955.
31. Berliner BC: A physical sign useful in diagnosis of roseola infantum before the rash. Pediatrics 25:1034, 1960.
32. Oski FA: Roseola infantum. Another cause of bulging fontanel. Am J Dis Child 101:376, 1961.
33. McEnery JT: Postoccipital lymphadenopathy as a diagnostic sign in roseola infantum (roseola subitum). Clin Pediatr 9:512, 1970.
34. Asano Y, Yoshikawa T, Suga S, et al: Clinical features of infants with primary human herpesvirus 6 infection (exanthem subitum, roseola infantum). Pediatrics 93:104, 1994.
35. Berenberg W, Wright S, Janeway CA: Roseola infantum (exanthem subitum). N Engl J Med 241:253, 1949.
36. Burnstine RC, Paine RS: Residual encephalopathy following roseola infantum. Am J Dis Child 98:144, 1959.
37. Holliday PB Jr: Preeruptive neurological complications of the common contagious diseases—Rubella, rubeola, and varicella. J Pediatr 36:185, 1950.

Enteroviral Exanthems

38. Lerner AM, Klein JO, Cherry JD, et al: New viral exanthems. N Engl J Med 269:678, 1963.
39. Robinson CR, Doane FW, Rhodes AJ: Report of an outbreak of febrile illness with pharyngeal lesions and exanthem: Toronto, summer 1957—isolation of group A coxsackievirus. Can Med Assoc J 79:615, 1958.
40. Alsop J, Flewett TH, Foster JR: "Hand-foot-and-mouth disease" in Birmingham in 1959. Br Med J 2:1708, 1960.
41. Cherry JD: Viral exanthems. Curr Probl Pediatr 13:1, 1983.
42. Tindall JP, Callaway JL: Hand-foot-and-mouth disease. It's more common than you think. Am J Dis Child 124:372, 1972.
43. Evans AD, Waddington E: Hand, foot and mouth disease in South Wales, 1964. Br J Dermatol 79:307, 1967.
44. Neva FA, Enders JF: Cytopathogenic agents isolated from patients during unusual epidemic exanthem. J Immunol 72:307, 1954.

45. Neva FA, Feemster RF, Gorback IJ: Clinical and epidemiologic features of unusual epidemic exanthem. JAMA 155:544, 1954.
46. Hall CB, Cherry JD, Hatch MH, et al: The return of the Boston exanthem. Am J Dis Child 131:323, 1977.
47. Bell EJ, Ross CAC, Grist NR: Echo 9 infection in pregnant women with suspected rubella. J Clin Pathol 28:267, 1975.
48. Rouchouse B, Bonnefoy M, Pallot B, et al: Acute generalized exanthematous pustular dermatitis and viral infection. Dermatologica 173:180, 1986.
49. DeChamps C, Peigue-Lafeville HH, Laveran H, et al: Four cases of vesicular lesions in adults caused by enterovirus infections. J Clin Microbiol 26:2182, 1988.
50. Guidotti MB: An outbreak of skin rash by echovirus 25 in an infant home. J Infect 6:67, 1983.
51. Cherry JD, Bobinski JE, Horvath FL, et al: Acute hemangioma-like lesions associated with ECHO viral infection. Pediatrics 44:498, 1969.

BONES AND JOINTS

153

Osteomyelitis

Francis A. Waldvogel

Definitions

Osteomyelitis is an infectious process involving the various components of bone, namely, periosteum, medullary cavity, and cortical bone. The disease is characterized by progressive inflammatory destruction of bone, necrosis, and new bone apposition.

Acute osteomyelitis evolves during several weeks; the term acute is used in opposition to chronic osteomyelitis, a disease characterized by long-standing infection that evolves during months or even years and by the persistence of microorganisms, low-grade inflammation, the presence of dead bone (sequestra) and foreign material, and fistulous tracks. The terms acute and chronic do not have a sharp demarcation and are often used somewhat loosely. Nevertheless, they are useful clinical concepts in infectious disease, because they describe two different patterns of the same disease due to the same microorganisms but with different clinical presentations and pathogenic factors, different evolutions,[1] and different responses to therapy.

Osteomyelitis secondary to bacteremia has to be distinguished from septic arthritis, a condition in which the inflammatory reaction resides in the joint synovium with little bone participation, for instance, as in *Neisseria gonorrhoeae* bacteremia. Occasionally, as in neonates, both the joint and the adjacent bone are involved in the septic process, a condition for which the term osteoarthritis has been coined.

Pathophysiology and Pathology

For many years, most of our information about osteomyelitis was obtained from pathologic observations obtained during surgery or at autopsy. Microscopic examination in the area of acute osteomyelitis has demonstrated an acute suppurative inflammation in which bacteria are embedded. A variety of phlogistic factors, and possibly leukocytes themselves, contribute to the tissue necrosis, the destruction of bone trabeculae, and the removal of bone matrix. Vascular channels are obliterated by the inflammatory process, further contributing to bone necrosis.[2] Segments of bone devoid of blood supply can become separated to form the well-known sequestra. Meanwhile, bone apposition occurs, sometimes exuberantly, causing periosteal apposition and new bone formation in a mosaic pattern similar to that of Paget disease.

Experimental Models

New experimental models of bone infection have established with accuracy the time course of these events and the necessity of producing profound bone trauma (i.e., with morrhuate sodium or other sclerosing agents) to initiate the disease.[3] Intravenous injection of bacteria has consistently produced osteomyelitis in chickens without trauma[4]; abscesses were most commonly observed in the metaphyseal area of long bones within 24 hours of bacterial inoculation, bordering on the epiphyseal growth plate. Sequestra could be observed within 8 days after inoculation.[1] It has been shown, further, that in this area of bone growth, the vascular endothelium is discontinuous, allowing bacteria to escape into adjacent tissue—a valid explanation why bacteremic osteomyelitis so frequently occurs before puberty.

Favoring Factors and Role of Foreign Body

Most cases of osteomyelitis are of bacterial origin. Favoring factors are numerous and include the presence of foreign material such as implants and orthopedic devices.[5] Major contributors to the development of infection in this setting include a striking phagocytic defect of resident polymorphonuclear leukocytes in the vicinity of a foreign body[6] and strong adhesion of bacteria, mostly *Staphylococcus aureus* and coagulase-negative staphylococci, on the foreign body surface through a ligand interaction of the bacterial surface with host proteins such as fibrinogen, fibronectin, and others coating the foreign body.[7] Within a few days, bacteria accumulate on their cell surface a thick layer of extracellular molecules called either slime or glycocalyx, which probably interferes with many host immune functions.[8] Many additional local factors are probably operational in favoring the development and the persistence of infections under these conditions.[9]

Other general contributing conditions to the development of osteomyelitis deserve further study. Patients with sickle cell disease develop, besides intraosseous sickling crises, osteomyelitis due to *Salmonella* species.[10] Patients with diabetes often suffer from microvascular disease and are at risk for developing osteomyelitis of the lower extremities, mostly due to *S. aureus* or to anaerobic organisms. Finally, patients with congenital defects of phagocyte function are frequently observed to develop *S. aureus* osteomyelitis. Thus, the presence of a competent phagocytic axis, good vascular supply to bone, and absence of foreign and necrotic material are important determinants in the clearing of small bacterial inocula within bone structures.

Clinical Manifestations and Characteristics of the Pathogen

From a practical point of view, it is useful to distinguish three types of osteomyelitis, which are described separately. Hematogenous osteomyelitis follows bacteremic spread, is seen mostly in prepubertal children and in elderly patients, and is characterized by local multiplication of bacteria within bone during septicemia. In most cases, infection is located in the metaphyseal area of long bones or in the spine. Osteomyelitis secondary to a contiguous focus of infection follows trauma or an orthopedic procedure. It implies a first infection, which by continuity gains access to bone. By definition, it can occur at any age and can involve any bone. Osteomyelitis secondary to vascular insufficiency is one of the consequences of poor blood supply, usually to the lower extremities. Often associated with diabetes, this disease entity is difficult to analyze as to its most important contributing factors; diabetes and its metabolic consequences, bone ischemia, neuropathy, and infection probably all contribute to bone destruction.

Hematogenous Osteomyelitis

Historically, hematogenous osteomyelitis has been described in children. It involves mostly the metaphysis of long bones (particularly tibia and femur), usually as a single focus. Although rare in adults, it most frequently involves the vertebral bodies.[1]

Bacteria responsible for hematogenous osteomyelitis reflect essentially their bacteremic incidence as a function of age, so the organisms most frequently encountered in neonates include *S. aureus* and group B streptococci; in infants, the majority of infections are due to *S. aureus*, coagulase-negative staphylococci, various streptococci, and *Haemophilus influenzae* (Fig. 153–1). Later in life, *S. aureus* predominates; in elderly persons, who are frequently subject to gram-negative bacteremias, most cases of vertebral osteomyelitis are due to gram-negative rods and only rarely to *S. aureus*.

The clinical features of hematogenous osteomyelitis in long bones are typical: chills, fever, and malaise reflect the bacteremic spread of microorganisms; pain and local swelling are the hallmarks of the local infectious process. Toxic shock, with its characteristic rash, may occasionally occur if *S. aureus* produces the corresponding toxin. Pneumonia, empyema, endocarditis, or subcutaneous abscesses may reflect widespread staphylococcal disease. Microorganisms responsible for acute hematogenous osteomyelitis are summarized in Table 153–1. Their respective frequency depends on the age of the patient. *S. aureus* and *Staphylococcus epidermidis* still account for the majority of these infections (more than 50%) and can be isolated from the blood stream in a large percentage of cases. Not specifically mentioned in Table 153–1 is fungal osteomyelitis, a complication of intravenous device infections or of profound immunodeficiency; *Pseudomonas aeruginosa* hematogenous osteomyelitis is often seen in drug addicts and has a predilection for the spine. Viral osteomyelitis is currently almost nonexistent.

Osteomyelitis Secondary to a Contiguous Infection

The situation and the clinical picture are more complex in cases of osteomyelitis associated with a contiguous focus of infection, for example, as a complication of the insertion of a total hip prosthesis. After a few days' pain that follows surgery, the situation improves and the patient is progressively mobilized. During that period, pain reappears, mostly on weight bearing. The patient is mildly febrile, and the wound is slightly erythematous with a pink discharge. No other clinical signs point toward the diagnosis of osteomyelitis, and no radiographic examination is fully diagnostic. Under such conditions, careful probing of the wound and Gram stains and cultures are the only diagnostic procedures of immediate help.

Similar clinical reasoning has to be used to diagnose osteomyelitis secondary to a contiguous infection such as a comminuted fracture, which can become contaminated by the contiguous wound infection. Any other prosthetic material can become contaminated during surgery and produce signs of infection during the ensuing weeks. Exceptionally, prosthetic material may become seeded by the bacteremic spread from a distant infectious focus. Acute purulent frontal sinusitis can lead to bone involvement, with a characteristic edema of the forehead (Pott puffy tumor). Dental root infection can lead to local bone destruction. Finally, deep-seated decubitus ulcers can lead to local bone destruction, usually of the sacrum.[11] Under all these conditions, the inflammatory reaction may be mild, and the bone destruction difficult to assess, unless the wound is probed and aspirated and the material adequately stained and cultured.

What organisms are responsible for this type of osteomyelitis? In the past, *S. aureus* and coagulase-negative staphylococci were most frequently the culprits. In more recent years, other microorganisms have been isolated: various types of streptococci; *Propionibacterium acnes;* Enterobacteriaceae; and even *P. aeruginosa*, mostly in the setting of chronic osteomyelitis, comminuted fractures, and puncture wounds to the heel. Finally, osteomyelitis of the mandible, secondary to decubitus ulcers, and due to bites, frequently contains anaerobic flora.

Osteomyelitis Secondary to Vascular Insufficiency

Osteomyelitis secondary to vascular insufficiency is a special entity observed in patients with diabetes or vascular impairment and is located almost exclusively on the lower extremities. The disease starts insidiously in a patient who has complained of intermittent claudication in an area of previously traumatized skin. Cellulitis may be kept at a minimum, and infection progressively burrows its way to the underlying bone (e.g., toe, metatarsal head, tarsal bone). Physical examination elicits either no pain (in case of advanced neuropathy) or excruciating pain if bone destruction has been acute; an area of cellulitis may or may not be present; crepitus can be felt occasionally, which points toward the presence of either anaerobes or Enterobacteriaceae. Physical examination includes a careful assessment of the vascular

TABLE 153–1 ■ Microorganisms Responsible for Acute Hematogenous Osteomyelitis of Long Bones

ORGANISMS	COMMENTS
Staphylococcus aureus, *Staphylococcus epidermidis*	Most frequent isolates
Haemophilus influenzae	Mostly in infants
Group B streptococci	Mostly in neonates
Candida species	Mostly associated with intravenous devices
Gram-negative bacilli	Rare, in elderly patients

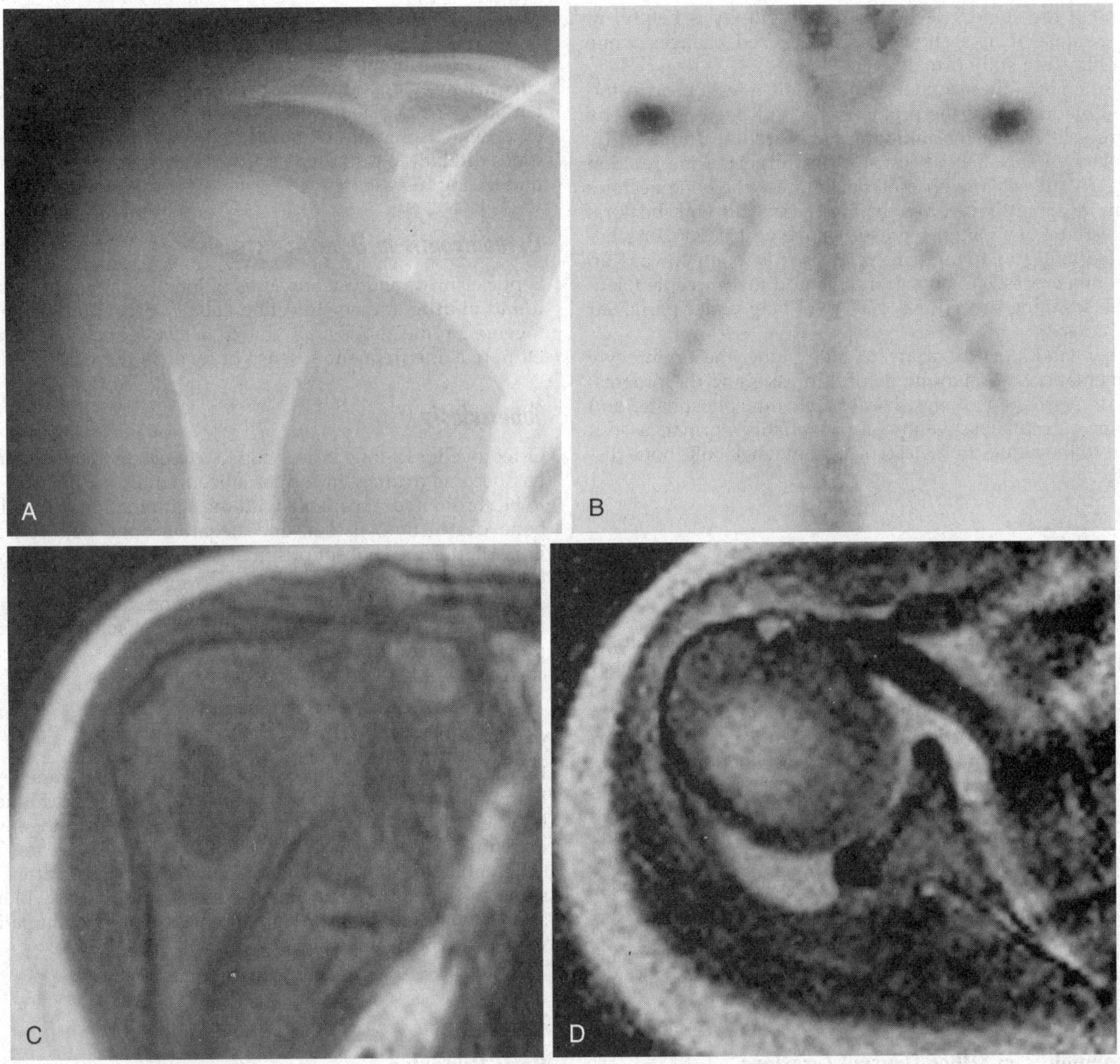

FIGURE 153–1 □ Acute hematogenous osteomyelitis in a 20-month-old child presenting with mild fever and impotence of the right shoulder. *A,* The conventional radiographs on admission do not show major bone modifications. *B,* Technetium scan on the same day demonstrates symmetric uptake of the two shoulder areas. *C,* Nuclear magnetic resonance imaging performed 4 days later is more explicit, showing in a clear metaphyseal ovoid hypointense area on a T1-weighted image. *D,* The transverse section on a T2-weighted image of the same area shows hyperintensity similar to subcutaneous fat tissue. There is also an effusion in the same joint.

supply to the affected limb and the evaluation of a concomitant neuropathy. Here again, the whole gamut of human pathogenic bacteria can be isolated, often in multiple combinations. *S. aureus* still predominates, but any other gram-positive or gram-negative, aerobic or anaerobic bacteria deserve close consideration and treatment, because infection is often the only reversible process in this multifactorial disease.

Diagnostic Procedures

In osteomyelitis of any kind, it is of paramount importance to isolate the offending organisms; this can be done by blood cultures (40% hematogenous cases of disease yield a positive result) or by isolation by direct biopsy from the involved bone. This procedure sometimes has to be performed under regional or general anesthesia, but its importance cannot be overstated.[12] Isolation of microorganisms from material taken from an open sinus track by swab will give conflicting results.[13]

Second in importance are radiographic procedures. The sequence of events observed in hematogenous osteomyelitis is well described and includes irregular bone destruction followed by new bone apposition and end-stage sclerosis. These events extend for a period of many weeks and months, in asynchrony with the clinical evolution; the x-ray appearance is often normal during the acute phase of the disease, whereas "apparent bone destruction" is sometimes observed during the treatment phase. Computed tomography is of little additional help, except for identifying complications such as an intramedullary abscess, a sequestrum, or an early subcutaneous abscess.[14] Intramedullary complications and early edema—a nonspecific but sometimes useful sign—are best seen by magnetic resonance imaging, as are infectious lesions of the spine.[15] Technetium scintigraphy is helpful as well because it also shows early, localized changes while plain films are still normal.[1, 12]

In osteomyelitis secondary to adjacent infection or to impaired blood supply, the problem is complicated not only by the insensitivity of the radiographic procedures but also by their lack of specificity, because prior surgery, bone reaction in the vicinity of foreign material, and aseptic bone necrosis can mimic infection. X-ray changes consistent with bilateral involvement of a joint, progressive bone destruction, or bilateral loosening of foreign material usually point toward an infectious process.[16] Although not yet routinely accepted, leukocyte scanning procedures may be of help under particular conditions.

Other laboratory tests are of little value; the erythrocyte sedimentation rate may be helpful in assessing the progression or regression of the disease; calcium, phosphate, and alkaline phosphatase values are invariably normal, as opposed to the values in metastatic or some metabolic bone diseases.

Specific Clinical Conditions

Vertebral Osteomyelitis

Vertebral osteomyelitis is most frequently of the hematogenous type and usually involves the lower dorsal and lumbar spine; occasional involvement of the cervical spine has been described. The disease usually presents in an adult as a febrile lumbago or torticollis.[12] Radiographs are usually normal on admission, and abnormality in technetium scintigraphy may be the only clue to the diagnosis; later, narrowing of the disk space, mottled destruction of adjacent vertebral plateaus, and anterior bridging may occur. Owing to the many organisms potentially responsible for this type of disease, needle biopsy under computed tomographic guidance has become the diagnostic procedure of choice. Complications, including paraspinal abscess, cord compression, and soft tissue extension, have to be carefully sought and emergency decompression may be dictated by the clinical and radiographic findings.[12, 16]

Osteomyelitis in Other Unusual Locations

Involvement of the sternoclavicular joint area has been described in intravenous drug abusers and in patients with indwelling intravenous devices. Sacral involvement has to be carefully sought in patients with decubitus ulcers of the overlying area. Osteomyelitis of the calcaneus, often due to *P. aeruginosa,* follows apparently innocent puncture wounds. Osteomyelitis of the sternum may follow cardiac surgery; frequently due to coagulase-negative staphylococci, it is difficult to differentiate from delayed healing after sternotomy. Another interesting clinical presentation consists in the development of multiple, well-delineated areas of bone destruction. As documented radiographically, in association with skin disorders such as acne conglobata or palmoplantar pustulosis, acute multifocal osteomyelitis is characterized by negative bone cultures and by spontaneous healing in a period of several months.[17]

Anaerobic Osteomyelitis

Osteomyelitis due to anaerobic organisms has been described in a variety of clinical situations.[18] It may be due to deep inoculation during a human bite, it may follow deep tooth socket infection or radiation therapy to the mandible, and finally it can be observed in diabetic foot infection.

Osteomyelitis in Sickle Cell Anemia

Patients with homozygous sickle cell disease, who under all circumstances are subject to severe *Salmonella* infections, often suffer from osteomyelitis due to this organism. The disease, which presents either acutely or subacutely, is sometimes difficult to differentiate from bone infarction due to the underlying disease.[10]

Osteomyelitis in Drug Addicts

Septic arthritis and osteomyelitis of long bones are frequently found in drug addicts. Infection usually occurs by the hematogenous route and is often due to *S. aureus* and *P. aeruginosa.* Of note is the frequent absence of fever in these cases.[19]

Tuberculosis

Osteomyelitis of long bones due to *Mycobacterium tuberculosis* has become a rarity in industrialized countries but still has to be considered in patients with the combination of localized bone destruction, fistula, and negative bone cultures. Still important is the concept of spinal involvement by *M. tuberculosis;* this entity is characterized by low fever, a subacute course, slow bone destruction, and absence of periosteal reaction. Abscess formation can sometimes be visualized by computed tomography and spine compression is a surgically correctible but feared complication.[20]

Brodie Abscess

Brodie abscess is characterized by bone pain, low-grade fever, if any, and an x-ray picture of central destruction surrounded by sclerosis. Seventy-five percent of cases occur in the lower extremities, usually in patients younger than 20 years. The differential diagnosis encompasses many inflammatory lesions and bone tumors; diagnosis is best resolved by biopsy and isolation of *S. aureus*[1] or another organism compatible with this type of infection.

Treatment

Basic Principles

The many pathogenic factors, modes of contamination, and clinical presentations of osteomyelitis have precluded a scientific approach to therapy, with well-controlled, statistically valid studies. However, experimental models have helped us to understand some basic principles of antibiotic therapy. Thus, except for the fluoroquinolones, which penetrate well into bone, bone antibiotic levels 3 to 4 hours after administration usually do not exceed 20% to 30% of the peak serum levels.[21] Second, antibiotic treatment has to be given for several weeks to achieve an acceptable cure rate. Third, early antibiotic treatment, given before extensive bone destruction has occurred, produces the best results.[22] Finally, a combined antimicrobial and surgical approach should at least be discussed in all cases; whereas at one end of the spectrum (e.g., hematogenous osteomyelitis) surgery is usually unnecessary, at the other end (a consolidated infected fracture) cure may be achieved with minimal antibiotic treatment provided that the foreign material is removed.

Antimicrobial Therapy

Single-agent chemotherapy is usually adequate for the treatment of osteomyelitis of any type. A conventional choice of antimicrobial agents for the most commonly encountered

TABLE 153–2 ■ Parenteral Antibiotic Treatment of Hematogenous Osteomyelitis in Adults

MICROORGANISMS ISOLATED	TREATMENT OF CHOICE	ALTERNATIVES
Staphylococcus aureus		
Penicillin sensitive	Penicillin G (4 million units, q 4 h)	A cephalosporin II* or clindamycin (600 mg, q 6 h)
Penicillin resistant	Nafcillin (2 g, q 4–6 h)	A cephalosporin II or clindamycin (600 mg, q 6 h)†
Methicillin resistant	Vancomycin (1 g, q 12 h)	
Various streptococci (group A or B β-hemolytic; *Streptococcus pneumoniae*)	Penicillin G (3 million units, q 4–6 h)	Erythromycin (500 mg, q 6 h), or clindamycin (600 mg, q 6 h), or newer macrolides
Haemophilus influenzae	Amoxicillin† (2 g, q 6 h)	Cefuroxime (2 g, q 6 h) or ceftriaxone (2 g, q 24 h)
Enteric gram-negative rods *Pseudomonas aeruginosa*	A cephalosporin III† or a quinolone	Piperacillin† (2–4 g, q 4 h) and gentamicin (1.5 mg/kg/d)
Gram-negative anaerobes	Clindamycin (600 mg, q 6 h)	Amoxicillin–clavulanic acid (2.0 and 0.2 g, respectively, q 8 h)

*II indicates second generation; III, third generation.
†Depends on sensitivities.

microorganisms is given in Table 153–2. As a general principle, these antibiotics should be given for 4 to 6 weeks if possible by the intravenous route. Results of serum bactericidal tests, which are notoriously difficult to standardize, have been proposed to monitor therapy efficacy, and trough levels at a dilution higher than 1:2 are associated with a higher cure rate.[23] If signs of infection do not abate after 1 week, possible complications should be sought; such as the presence of a subcutaneous, subperiosteal, or intramedullary abscess; the formation of sequestra; or the presence of foreign material. Most of the time, a surgical intervention solves this problem more radically than the switch to other antibiotics, provided that adequate microbiologic results have led to appropriate chemotherapy.

New approaches to antimicrobial therapy have been developed experimentally and validated clinically. Thus, in hematogenous osteomyelitis of childhood, short parenteral administration of antibiotics may be followed with an equal success rate by oral therapy for several weeks, provided that the organism is known, the clinical signs abate rapidly, the patient's compliance is good, and the serum antibiotic levels can be monitored.[24, 25] This approach has now also been validated in adults.[25, 26] Another approach that has gained acceptance because of its reduced cost is parenteral administration of antibiotics, first in the hospital, then on an outpatient basis; effective as it is for hematogenous osteomyelitis, the question remains open whether this mode can be used for postsurgical osteomyelitis. Long-term oral therapy extending for years is aimed at palliation of acute flare-ups of chronic, refractory osteomyelitis. Local administration of antibiotics, either by instillation or by gentamicin-laden beads, has its advocates both in the United States and in Europe, but it has not been submitted to a critical, controlled study; antibiotic diffusion is limited in time and space but may be of some additional benefit in osteomyelitis secondary to a contiguous focus of infection. Finally, the 8-fluoroquinolones have been shown to be efficient in experimental infections and in selected cases in adults. Whereas their efficacy in the treatment of gram-negative osteomyelitis seems undisputed, their advantage over conventional therapy in osteomyelitis due to gram-positive organisms remains to be demonstrated except for their ease of administration.[27, 28]

Surgical Approaches

It is beyond the scope of this chapter to describe and discuss the many orthopedic procedures used in the treatment of osteomyelitis, and only some general principles are discussed.[12] In hematogenous osteomyelitis, the help of the surgeon is required mainly for the treatment of complications such as abscesses and sequestra. In osteomyelitis secondary to a contiguous focus of infection, the help of the surgeon is almost always required. In acute infection after total hip arthroplasty, for instance, the surgeon delineates the depth of the septic process and evaluates the indication for removal of the prosthesis.[29] Under other conditions, when infection occurs without consolidation of a fracture, removal of the foreign material is mandatory; if consolidation is already present, full mechanical recovery can be achieved in spite of sepsis, and the fixation material may be removed later, complemented by a short course of antibiotics. Finally, under conditions in which foreign material has to remain in place, at least for a certain time, combination therapy with rifampin and quinolones shows promising results.[30, 31]

Prevention

Under many circumstances in which implantation of prosthetic material is necessary, infection should be avoided by all possible means. This is particularly the case in clean orthopedic procedures, such as the implantation of artificial joints. Besides laminar airflow, cleansing techniques, and other general procedures to avoid nosocomial infections, the empirical use during the operating time and on the following day of an antibiotic directed against gram-positive organisms (a semisynthetic penicillin or a cephalosporin) has been associated with a reduced risk of infection. Although criticized and not considered to be applicable to all patients, such a short course of antibiotics is justified in a high-risk population, such as patients with diabetes, rheumatoid arthritis, previous orthopedic surgery, or another favoring factor.

References

1. Waldvogel FA, Medoff G, Swartz MN: Osteomyelitis: A review of clinical features, therapeutic considerations, and unusual aspects. N Engl J Med 282:198, 260, 316, 1970.

2. Trueta J: The three types of acute hematogenous osteomyelitis: A clinical and vascular study. J Bone Joint Surg Br 41:671, 1959.
3. Norden CW: Experimental osteomyelitis. II. Therapeutic trials and measurement of antibiotic levels in bone. J Infect Dis 124:565, 1971.
4. Emslie KR, Nade S: Pathogenesis and treatment of acute hematogenous osteomyelitis: Evaluation of current views with reference to an animal model. Rev Infect Dis 8:841, 1986.
5. Elek SD, Conen PE: The virulence of *Staphylococcus pyogenes* for man: A study of the problems of wound infection. Br J Exp Pathol 38:573, 1957.
6. Zimmerli W, Lew PD, Waldvogel FA: Pathogenesis of foreign body infection. Evidence for a local granulocyte defect. J Clin Invest 73:1191, 1984.
7. Vaudaux P, Waldvogel FA, Morgenthaler JJ, et al: Adsorption of fibronectin onto polymethylmethacrylate and promotion of *Staphylococcus aureus* adherence. Infect Immun 45:768, 1984.
8. Mayberry-Carson KJ, Tober-Meyer B, Smith JK, et al: Bacterial adherence and glycocalyx formation in osteomyelitis experimentally induced with *Staphylococcus aureus*. Infect Immun 43:825, 1984.
9. Bisno AL, Waldvogel FA (eds): Infections Associated with Indwelling Medical Devices. Washington, DC, American Society for Microbiology, 1989.
10. Barrett-Conner E: Bacterial infection and sickle cell anemia: An analysis of 150 infections in 166 patients and a review of the literature. Medicine (Baltimore) 50:97, 1971.
11. Sugarman B, Hawes S, Musher DM, et al: Osteomyelitis beneath pressure sores. Arch Intern Med 143:683, 1983.
12. Waldvogel FA, Vasey H: Osteomyelitis: The past decade. N Engl J Med 303:360, 1980.
13. Mackowiak PA, Jones SR, Smith JW: Diagnostic value of sinus-tract cultures in chronic osteomyelitis. JAMA 239:2772, 1978.
14. Kuhn JP, Berger PE: Computed tomographic diagnosis of osteomyelitis. Radiology 130:503, 1979.
15. Smith FW, Runge V, Permezel M, et al: Nuclear magnetic resonance (NMR) imaging in the diagnosis of spinal osteomyelitis. Magn Reson Imaging 2:53, 1984.
16. Eftekhar NS: The infected total hip. *In* AAOS Instructional Course Lectures, Vol 26. St. Louis, CV Mosby, 1977, pp 66–74.
17. Meller Y, Yagupsky P, Elitsur Y, et al: Chronic multifocal symmetrical osteomyelitis. Am J Dis Child 138:349, 1984.
18. Raff MJ, Melo JC: Anaerobic osteomyelitis. Medicine (Baltimore) 57:83, 1978.
19. Chandrasekar PH, Narula AP: Bone and joint infections in intravenous drug abusers. Rev Infect Dis 8:904, 1986.
20. Hodgson AR, Yau A, Kwon JS, et al: A clinical study of 100 consecutive cases of Pott's paraplegia. Clin Orthop 36:128, 1964.
21. Auckenthaler R, Waldvogel FA: Bone and synovial fluid. *In* Ristuccia AM, Cunha BA (eds): Antimicrobial Therapy. New York, Raven Press, 1984, pp 505–512.
22. Emslie KR, Nade S: Acute hematogenous staphylococcal osteomyelitis: Evaluation of cloxacillin therapy in an animal model. Pathology 16:441, 1984.
23. Weinstein MP, Stratton CW, Hawley HB, et al: Multicenter collaborative evaluation of a standardized serum bactericidal test as a predictor of therapeutic efficacy in acute and chronic osteomyelitis. Am J Med 83:218, 1987.
24. Tetzlaff TR, McCracken GH, Nelson JD: Oral antibiotic therapy for skeletal infections of children. II. Therapy of osteomyelitis and suppurative arthritis. J Pediatr 92:485, 1978.
25. Gentry LO: Oral antimicrobial therapy for osteomyelitis (Editorial) [see comments]. Ann Intern Med 114:986, 1991.
26. Black J, Hunt TL, Godley PJ, et al: Oral antimicrobial therapy for adults with osteomyelitis or septic arthritis. J Infect Dis 155:968, 1987.
27. Waldvogel FA: Use of quinolones for the treatment of osteomyelitis and septic arthritis. Rev Infect Dis 11(Suppl 5):S1259, 1989.
28. Lew DP, Waldvogel FA: Use of quinolones for treatment of osteomyelitis and septic arthritis. *In* Hooper DC, Wolfson JS (eds): Quinolone Antimicrobial Agents. Washington, DC, American Society for Microbiology, 1993, pp 371–379.
29. Fitzgerald RH Jr, Nolan DR, Ilstrup DM, et al: Deep wound sepsis following total hip arthroplasty. J Bone Joint Surg Am 59:693, 1977.
30. Drancourt M, Stein A, Argenson JN, et al: Oral rifampin plus ofloxacin for treatment of *Staphylococcus*-infected orthopedic implants. Antimicrob Agents Chemother 37:1214, 1993.
31. Widmer AF, Gaechter A, Ochsner PE, Zimmerli W: Antimicrobial treatment of orthopedic implant-related infections with rifampin combinations. Clin Infect Dis 14:1251, 1992.

154

Septic Arthritis

Nancy Y. Liu
David F. Giansiracusa

Bacteria are the most common and important cause of joint infections. Acute bacterial arthritis is a medical emergency because of the potential for joint destruction[1] and even mortality if diagnosis and treatment are delayed, particularly in elderly individuals and in patients with preexisting arthritis.[2–8] Early recognition and prompt treatment of septic arthritis reduce the extent of joint damage.[9] In the majority of cases, bacteria gain access to the joints by hematogenous spread.[2, 9–11] Skin flora is the most common source of microorganisms, but the respiratory, gastrointestinal, and genitourinary systems may also be sources. Less frequently, joint sepsis results from penetrating injury; diagnostic and therapeutic procedures, including arthroscopy[12–14]; or extension from contiguous osteomyelitis, cellulitis, soft tissue abscesses, tenosynovitis, or septic bursitis.[11] Factors that increase vulnerability to the development of joint infection include underlying joint disease and seeding of a joint by trauma or intraarticular injection. Predisposing factors affect the types and numbers of joints involved, the nature of the infecting organisms, and the clinical outcomes.[11] Table 154–1 lists the microbiology of bacterial arthritis in relationship to the patient's age.[15]

Nongonococcal Bacterial Arthritis

Nongonococcal bacterial infections are generally the most serious type of septic arthritis because of the potential for cartilage damage within 1 to 2 days.[1, 16] Gram-positive aerobic bacteria compose about 80% of infecting microorganisms. In adults, *Staphylococcus aureus* is the most common cause of primary septic arthritis and of septic arthritis associated with intraarticular injection, trauma or debilitating illness such as diabetes mellitus, rheumatoid arthritis, or systemic lupus erythematosus.[17] Nearly all strains of *S. aureus* are resistant to penicillin, and some strains are resistant to methicillin.[17, 18] Approximately 15% of infecting gram-positive bacteria are group A β-hemolytic streptococci, and 3% are *Streptococcus pneumoniae*.[2] Group B streptococcus is the predominant cause of joint infection in diabetic adults.[9] Fifteen percent to 20% of bacterial infections are caused by gram-negative and anaerobic organisms. These bacteria are an increasing cause of joint infection in debilitated patients, parenteral drug abusers, elderly persons, young children, and immunocompromised hosts.[2, 10] Anaerobic joint infections occur in patients with postoperative wound infections, especially joint replacements and extremity wounds, and in the setting of gastrointestinal malignant neoplasms.[19]

TABLE 154–1 ■ Microbiology of Bacterial Septic Arthritis Related to Age of Patient*

ORGANISM	CHILDREN (6 mo–5 y)	YOUNG ADULT	ADULT	ELDERLY
Staphylococcus aureus	10%–20%	15%–20%	60%–70%	45%–65%
Streptococci	5%–10%	1%–5%	15%–20%	10%–15%
Gram-negative bacteria	1%–5%	Rare	10%–15%	15%–35%
Haemophilus influenzae	30%–50%	1%–5%	1%–5%	Rare
Neisseria gonorrhoeae	1%–5%	60%–80%	1%–5%	Rare

*Percentages were compiled from several studies.
From Zimmermann B, Lally EV, Liu NY: Infectious agents and the musculoskeletal system. *In* Noble J, Greene H, Levinson W, et al (eds): Primary Care and General Medicine, ed 2. St. Louis, Mosby–Year Book, 1996, p 1187.

Pathophysiology

Within hours of entry into a joint, bacteria cause changes in the articular cartilage and synovium.[20, 21] Hematologic seeding of the highly vascular synovial membrane results in bacterial trapping and multiplication in the subsynovium and phagocytosis by polymorphonuclear leukocytes (PMNs) and synovial lining cells. Neovascularization, synovial proliferation, and growth of granulation tissue develop. Proteolytic enzymes released from synovial lining cells and PMNs (particularly when the synovial fluid white cell counts exceed 50,000/mm^3) and increased intracavitary pressure from accumulation of purulent synovial fluid cause necrosis of synovium and cartilage. Vascular plugging of granulation tissue by inflammatory cells and bacteria may also cause necrosis of bone.[20] Proinflammatory cytokines such as interleukin-1 and tumor necrosis factor-α also contribute to joint injury. The degree of synovial, cartilage, and bone destruction is a function not only of the size of the inoculum but also of the virulence of the infecting microorganisms, the host response to the infection, and the rapidity of diagnosis and treatment.[22–24]

Clinical Presentation

Eighty percent to 90% of bacterial arthritis affects one joint; the knees, hips, and shoulders (in decreasing frequency) are the most commonly involved sites. Less frequently involved joints are the elbows, wrists, ankles, and small joints of hands and feet, although any joint may be affected.[2, 10, 22, 24–27] Repeated trauma to the knee may be the explanation for the frequency of involvement.[28] The hip is particularly vulnerable to osteonecrosis of the femoral head secondary to increases in intracavity pressure that may impair blood flow.[2, 11] Infection may also spread to the diaphysis of the bone, especially in children younger than 7 years.[11]

Most patients with septic arthritis present with chills, fever, malaise, and the acute onset of monarticular and less frequently polyarticular arthritis.[22, 29] Localized signs of inflammation and severe, even incapacitating, pain are usually present.[11] However, in elderly, severely ill, bedridden, or immunocompromised patients, symptoms and findings may be subtle.[16, 30]

In cases of polyarticular septic arthritis, the causative bacterium is also *S. aureus* in approximately 80% of cases and streptococcal species in 4%.[3] In one study, approximately a quarter of the patients with polyarticular septic arthritis were not febrile on presentation, and nearly half (10 of 25 patients) had a peripheral white cell count of less than 10,000/mm.[3] Concurrent rheumatic disease, generally advanced, long-standing rheumatoid arthritis, was present in 52% of the patients. (In patient with rheumatoid arthritis, superficial infection of rheumatoid nodules or of ulcerated calluses on feet was the major source of bacteria; joint prostheses were a major site of joint sepsis.[3]) Other studies have also indicated that affected patients with rheumatoid arthritis tend to have long-standing, erosive, destructive joint disease, often in the setting of receiving chronic corticosteroid or cytotoxic drug therapy or intraarticular steroid injections.[11, 22, 31, 32] Mortality secondary to the infection or its consequences was 32% in the 25 patients with polyarticular septic arthritis and as high as 49% in those with rheumatoid arthritis compared with a mortality rate of 4% for 95 cases of monarticular septic arthritis.[3] In another study of polyarticular septic arthritis, the mortality rate among patients with rheumatoid arthritis was as high as 56%.[33]

Other than underlying inflammatory joint disease, host risk factors for developing polyarticular septic arthritis include intravenous drug abuse, cirrhosis, diabetes mellitus, other chronic diseases, and immunosuppression.[3] Because delay in diagnosis and treatment is the major cause for an unfavorable outcome in septic arthritis,[4, 34] prompt arthrocentesis for bacterial cultures and examination of synovial fluid should be performed on all inflamed joints.

Age may also affect clinical presentation. Bacterial arthritis is infrequent in neonates and infants.[35–37] Infections may be community or hospital acquired. Although joints may rapidly become swollen, warm, and erythematous,[38] such signs may not be present, and the child may simply cry and refrain from moving the affected extremity. Systemic features of high fevers rather than local symptoms and signs may predominate, possibly resulting in a delay of diagnosis.[36] Severely ill neonates and infants may develop polyarticular joint sepsis and infection of soft tissues and bone.[39, 40] *S. aureus* and other gram-positive organisms, particularly group B streptococcal species, are the pathogens in the majority of cases (approximately 80%); gram-negative organisms including *Pseudomonas aeruginosa* and other coliform microorganisms constitute a smaller proportion. The severely ill infant may develop polymicrobial joint infections.[38]

In children aged 6 months to 2 years, *Haemophilus influenzae* is the most common isolate causing joint sepsis.[38, 41, 42] The *H. influenzae* vaccine may significantly reduce the frequency of *H. influenzae* septic arthritis. Urinary tract infection rather than meningitis is the common source of *H. influenzae* in about half of the children.[28, 38]

In children 2 years of age and older, the organisms causing septic arthritis and the joints affected are similar to those in adults.[25, 28, 38] As in adults, knees and hips are the most frequently affected joints.[25, 28, 38] Osteomyelitis and adjacent soft tissue infection may accompany septic arthritis, particularly in children younger than 10 years.

Predisposing Factors

PROSTHETIC JOINTS

Prosthetic joint infection is a rare but devastating complication of total joint arthroplasties and contributes to loosening and failure of the prosthetic joint. Infections occurring within 3 to 6 months of surgery are categorized as early and those greater than 6 months postoperatively as late. The incidence of early infections has decreased to less than 2% with the advent of improved surgical techniques and prosthetic hardware, identification of high-risk patients, and use of perioperative antibiotics. Late infections occur at an annual rate of 0.18% to 0.60%.[43] The mechanism of early infection is usually wound contamination or seeding from another infected site, such as the urinary tract, lungs, or dental caries. Late infections are presumed to be secondary to hematogenous seeding from a distant source, usually identifiable if it is sought. Gram-positive organisms (*S. aureus, Staphylococcus epidermidis,* and *Streptococcus*) remain the most common bacteria identified in both early and late infections, with gram-negative and anaerobic organisms constituting the remainder.[44] Fungal infections compose less than 1% of the cases. Treatment with appropriate intravenous antibiotics is similar to that of native septic joints except that surgical intervention with exploration and débridement of the prosthetic joint is usually necessary, followed by an excision arthroplasty or revision arthroplasty.

INTRAVENOUS DRUG ABUSE

S. aureus is the most frequent cause of septic arthritis in intravenous drug abusers, but gram-negative infections also occur, particularly due to *P. aeruginosa.* In addition to the commonly infected joints, the sternoclavicular, sacroiliac, and manubriosternal joints and the symphysis pubis may be infected.[11, 22, 42, 45, 46] Sternoclavicular septic arthritis may present with pain on shoulder motion and a paucity of swelling, warmth, or erythema. Infection at this site may spread to the thoracic wall or into the anterior mediastinum and may require aggressive medical and surgical treatment.[47, 48] Sacroiliac involvement produces poorly localized pain in the buttocks, abdomen, or hip and may cause sciatic pain. Although motion of the ipsilateral hip may be full, the FABER maneuver (hip flexion, abduction, external rotation) often elicits or aggravates pain in the region of the sacroiliac joint, as may direct palpation of the joint or pelvic compression of the lateral iliac wings. Purulent drainage from the sacroiliac joints may extend into the retroperitoneal space and into the psoas muscle.[49]

IMMUNOCOMPROMISED STATES

Immunocompromised hosts, including young or old individuals with multiorgan system disease, patients with human immunodeficiency virus (HIV) infection,[50] transplant recipients, and patients treated with immunosuppressant therapy for malignant and nonmalignant (including collagen-vascular or autoimmune) disease,[51] present an increasing population of individuals susceptible to polyarticular, polymicrobial bacterial arthritis. Patients with HIV infection may have numerous rheumatic manifestations, but septic arthritis is generally caused by the same bacteria that infect joints of immunocompetent hosts.[52–55]

Diagnosis

Arthrocentesis for synovial fluid cultures, smears, and analysis is the single most important diagnostic procedure in the evaluation of possible septic arthritis. The affected joints should be aspirated through noncellulitic skin. In cases of polyarticular involvement, all inflamed joints should be aspirated. Synovial fluid should be sent for Gram stain, culture, white cell count, and differential. In *S. aureus* arthritis, bacteria may be identified on Gram stain in 50% to 75% and on culture in more than 90% of cases.[27] Gram stains are less frequently positive in identifying gram-negative organisms.[10] If synovial fluid is not grossly purulent, Gram stain of the centrifuged synovial fluid pellet may increase the yield of positive findings.[2, 25, 42, 56] Synovial fluid samples should be cultured for aerobic and anaerobic organisms in appropriate media. Bacterial antigen determinations by counterimmunoelectrophoresis may be performed in cases of partially treated bacterial arthritis, but these studies are not routinely done.[2, 25] Cultures of blood and of all suspected extraarticular sites of infection should also be performed. The positive growth of blood cultures in patients with nongonococcal bacterial arthritis occurs in about 50% of cases.[2, 38] Synovial fluid white cell counts generally exceed 50,000/mm^3 with more than 90% PMNs.[2, 22, 24, 25, 29, 38] However, such high cell counts and predominance of PMNs may also occur in rheumatoid arthritis, crystal-induced arthritis, Reiter syndrome (reactive arthritis), and psoriatic arthritis.[27, 57, 58] Synovial fluid glucose and protein levels have not proved helpful in distinguishing septic from noninfectious causes of inflammatory joint disease.[59]

Imaging studies include conventional radiographs, which are rarely diagnostic but provide a baseline status of the joint and adjacent bone and may identify a focus of osteomyelitis. Rarefaction and erosion of subchondral bone may not be present for several (2 to 4) weeks after the onset of joint symptoms.[60] Scintigraphy (radionuclide scans) with technetium diphosphonate reflects the presence of inflammation but does not define a specific cause. Such studies may be particularly helpful in evaluating for inflammation of sacroiliac, sternoclavicular, and facet joints.[61] Indium- or technetium diphosphonate–labeled leukocyte scans may help localize sites of bone and joint infections, but these are much more expensive and of no greater usefulness than radioiodinated monoclonal antigranulocyte antibody studies when such are available.[11] Computed tomography is useful to evaluate sacroiliac and sternoclavicular joints for erosive bone changes and to localize retroperitoneal, intrapsoas, and mediastinal abscesses.[47, 62, 63] Fluoroscopic or computed tomographic guidance is helpful for aspiration of the sacroiliac joints.[49] Magnetic resonance imaging is the method of choice for evaluating deep-seated bone and joint disease because it can demonstrate synovitis, joint effusions, osteonecrosis (avascular-ischemic necrosis of bone), and marrow space edema.[11, 64]

Differential Diagnosis

The differential diagnosis of septic arthritis depends on the presence of monarticular versus polyarticular joint involvement and the age of the patient. Monarticular arthritis in children or adults may be due to juvenile rheumatoid arthritis (in children), Lyme disease, or a spondyloarthropathy. Polyarticular arthritis in children and adults may be caused by rheumatoid arthritis, systemic lupus erythematosus, a spondyloarthropathy, acute rheumatic fever, Kawasaki syndrome, and viral illnesses (particularly parvovirus infection, rubella, and hepatitis B). In older adults, crystal-induced arthritis, "pseudoseptic" rheumatoid arthritis,[58, 65] reactive arthritis,[9] neuropathic arthropathy,[57] and infectious arthritis caused by other microorganisms including mycobacteria and fungi are in the differential diagnosis of septic (bacterial) arthritis.[11]

Treatment

Treatment of bacterial arthritis consists of adequate joint drainage, joint rest and mobilization, and antibiotics.[2, 22, 24, 25, 38, 42, 56] Drainage of the affected joints should be performed daily until synovial fluid is sterile and minimal effusion is evident. Rapid reaccumulation of synovial effusions may

TABLE 154–2 ■ Initial Antibiotic Therapy for Presumed Bacterial Arthritis in an Adult (Pathogen Unknown)

GRAM STAIN	PRESUMED ORGANISM	ANTIBIOTIC
Positive		
Gram-positive cocci	*Staphylococcus aureus*	Oxacillin or nafcillin (alternative: cefazolin or vancomycin)
Gram-positive cocci (prosthetic joint)	*Staphylococcus epidermidis*	Vancomycin
Gram-negative cocci	*Neisseria gonorrhoeae*	Ceftriaxone or cefotaxime
Gram-negative bacilli	*Escherichia coli, Serratia marcescens,* other Enterobacteriaceae	Third-generation cephalosporin, or imipenem, or aztreonam, or ciprofloxacin* (and in cases of bacteremia or severe infection, the addition of an aminoglycoside)
Gram-negative bacilli (thin)	*Pseudomonas aeruginosa*	Ceftazidime (or piperacillin, or imipenem, or aztreonam) plus tobramycin or ciprofloxacin
Negative		
Noncompromised host	*Staphylococcus aureus,* Enterobacteriaceae†	Nafcillin plus gentamicin, or alternatively a third-generation cephalosporin (ceftriaxone or cefotaxime) plus vancomycin
Compromised host	*Staphylococcus aureus,* Enterobacteriaceae, and *Pseudomonas aeruginosa*†	Nafcillin plus gentamicin, or alternatively (ceftazidime or aztreonam) plus vancomycin, or alternatively imipenem plus (tobramycin or ciprofloxacin)

*Ciprofloxacin is available for parenteral use (400 mg intravenously every 12 h).
†Treatment for both gram-positive and gram-negative pathogens must be continued until cultures return.
Modified from Upchurch KS, Giansiracusa DF: Rheumatic diseases in the intensive care unit. *In* Rippe JM, Irwin RS, Fink MP, Cerra FB (eds): Intensive Care Medicine, ed 3. Boston, Little, Brown, 1996, p 2397.

indicate resistance to antibiotics, the presence of more than one microorganism, or loculation of synovial fluid in the joint cavity.[11] Methods of joint drainage include percutaneous needle aspiration, arthroscopic surgical drainage, and open surgical drainage. Percutaneous needle drainage is the procedure of choice for accessible joints in the absence of underlying joint disease such as rheumatoid arthritis. Indications for surgical drainage include all cases of septic arthritis of the hip,[22, 36–38, 66] failure of percutaneous aspiration (generally after 5 to 7 days)[2, 67] and appropriate antibiotics, suspected synovial fluid loculations, and joints anatomically altered by underlying joint diseases. Arthroscopic surgery offers the opportunity to débride and lavage the joint with less extensive surgery than an open procedure. The choice of arthroscopic versus open surgical drainage is generally best made cooperatively by the rheumatologist and orthopedic surgeon.[68–71]

Antibiotic therapy is initially determined by results of the synovial fluid Gram stain and by the clinical setting, for example, the presence of an extraarticular focus such as gram-negative urinary tract infection. If the Gram stain is unrevealing, judicious antibiotics to cover the most likely organisms should be started as soon as appropriate cultures have been obtained. Table 154–2 lists general initial antibiotic recommendations in the setting of the pathogens not being known. Table 154–3 lists antibiotic choices and alternatives in the cases of known bacterial pathogens.[72, 73]

Treatment of bacterial arthritis of hand joints as a result of human or animal bites should include antibiotics effective against oral flora, such as ampicillin or ampicillin-sulbactam. Ceftriaxone and doxycycline are alternatives for the penicillin-allergic patient.[9]

Parenteral antibiotics should be continued for at least 4 weeks at adequate bactericidal blood levels to ensure eradication of the bacteria.[11] Other authorities recommend 2 weeks

TABLE 154–3 ■ Antibiotic Therapy for Acute Bacterial Arthritis in the Critically Ill Adult (Known Pathogen)

ORGANISM	ANTIBIOTIC CHOICE	ALTERNATIVES
Staphylococcus aureus	Nafcillin, 9–12 g/d (q 4 h), or oxacillin, 9–12 g/d (q 4 h)	Cefazolin, 4.5–6 g/d (q 8 h), or vancomycin, 2 g/d (q 12 h)
Staphylococcus aureus, methicillin resistant	Vancomycin, 2 g/d	None
Streptococcus pyogenes, Streptococcus pneumoniae	Penicillin G, 12–18 million units/d (q 4 h)	Cefazolin or vancomycin
Neisseria gonorrhoeae	Ceftriaxone, 1–2 g/d (q 12 h), or cefotaxime, 3–6 g/d (q 8 h)	Tetracycline, aztreonam, or ciprofloxacin or penicillin G if sensitive
Pseudomonas aeruginosa	Piperacillin, 12 g/d (q 4 h), plus tobramycin, 4–5 mg/kg/d (q 4 h)	Ceftazidime, 6 g/d (q 8 h), or imipenem-cilastatin, 2–3 g/d, or ciprofloxacin* plus tobramycin or gentamicin
Enterobacteriaceae	Third-generation cephalosporin, plus gentamicin, 4–5 mg/kg/d (q 8 h)	Aztreonam, 3 g/d (q 8 h), or ciprofloxacin* plus gentamicin or amikacin

*Ciprofloxacin is available for parenteral use (400 mg intravenously every 12 hours).
From Upchurch KS, Giansiracusa DF: Rheumatic diseases in the intensive care unit. *In* Rippe JM, Irwin RS, Fink MP, Cerra FB (eds): Intensive Care Medicine, ed 3. Boston, Little, Brown, 1996, p 2397.

of parenteral antibiotics for septic arthritis due to *H. influenzae,* streptococci, or gram-negative cocci and 3 weeks for staphylococcal or gram-negative bacillary septic arthritis.[9] Sterilization of synovial fluid within 5 days of antibiotic therapy generally indicates a good response to treatment.[9] Home intravenous therapy may be an alternative to long-term hospitalization, particularly in the patient with involvement of a non–weight-bearing joint and a good initial response to antibiotics and drainage. Long-term oral antibiotic therapy may be necessary for protracted bone and prosthetic joint infections.[74]

For years, the practice of choice had been prolonged immobilization of the infected joint until the joint effusion resolved followed by gradual mobilization. However, experimental studies of septic arthritis in animals have indicated that prolonged immobilization is detrimental. As such, immobilization is now recommended only for incapacitatingly painful joints and joints treated with surgical drainage. Passive joint mobilization and functional splinting for the severely ill patient and passive and active range of motion for the less ill patient are recommended to prevent joint contractures and to preserve joint function.[11]

The prognosis of septic arthritis is affected by a number of variables. In general, the sooner the diagnosis is established and appropriate therapy instituted, the better the outcome.[22, 24, 36, 38, 42, 56] Factors indicating poor prognosis include (1) age older than 60 years; (2) comorbid conditions, such as preexisting rheumatoid arthritis; and (3) hip, shoulder, or polyarticular involvement.[9] The infecting organism (specifically *S. aureus* and gram-negative bacteria),[15] persistence of positive synovial fluid cultures after 7 days of appropriate antibiotics, and host-microbial interactions may also adversely influence the outcome.

Major changes in the past decade in nongonococcal bacterial arthritis have been (1) the longer life expectancy, thus increasing the number of elderly patients and those with comorbid conditions; (2) the increased frequency of methicillin-resistant *S. aureus* joint infections; (3) the increased use of arthroscopy, which poses a risk for postprocedure infection as well as being a surgical option for draining septic joints; (4) the increased number of patients with prosthetic joints; and (5) the increasing frequency of septic arthritis in patients infected with HIV.[11]

Gonococcal Arthritis

Gonococcal arthritis is the most common form of septic arthritis among sexually active young adults,[2] constituting up to 66% of the cases of septic arthritis and tenosynovitis in this population.[75] Disseminated gonococcal infection (DGI) may also occur in children and in the elderly,[76, 77] in patients with systemic rheumatic diseases, and in patients with HIV infection.[78, 79] The prevalence of DGI varies from 0.5% to 3%.[80] DGI occurs four times as frequently in women as in men. The risk for dissemination increases during menstruation and pregnancy and in the immediate postpartum period. Approximately one half of women who develop DGI do so in association with one of these risk factors.[81–83] In men, risk factors for dissemination include homosexual activity with asymptomatic rectal or pharyngeal involvement.[84] Less common risk factors for DGI include inherited terminal complement component deficiencies (C5 through C8, especially C8)[85] and more rarely deficiencies of the third and fourth components of complement.[75] Humans are the only known source of the organism, *Neisseria gonorrhoeae.* Disseminated disease occurs only after mucous membrane infection of the endocervix, urethra, pharynx, or rectum. Most cases of DGI result from asymptomatic primary gonococcal infection of the genitourinary tract that has been sexually transmitted days to months previously. Symptomatic genitourinary infection including urethral or vaginal discharge, urethritis, urinary frequency, and dysuria is rarely present.[75]

Pathogenesis

The strains of *N. gonorrhoeae* isolated from patients with DGI and their sexual partners tend to be more invasive, more resistant to natural bactericidal activity of serum, and less associated with salpingitis than other strains are. They can cause asymptomatic urethritis in men.[75] Invasiveness is enhanced by pili, which facilitate bacterial attachment to mucosal surfaces, and by protein 1A in the outer bacterial membrane, which induces epithelial cell endocytosis.[75] That the gonococcus grows well in an iron-rich milieu and that the organism produces a protease that inactivates secretory immunoglobulin A may contribute to increased invasiveness during menses and increased virulence, respectively.[86, 87] The lipooligosaccharide in the gonococcal outer membrane contributes to serum resistance and may induce chronic synovitis when it is injected intraarticularly into rabbits.[86] Formation of immune complexes in the synovium may also contribute to the arthrogenic properties of the bacteria.[75]

Clinical Features

DGI is characterized by the acute onset of oligoarthralgias or polyarthralgias, which may have a diffuse, migratory, or additive pattern generally building to a maximum during several days.[75] Constitutional symptoms with chills and fever, which may be low to moderate, are common. Two thirds of patients develop tenosynovitis, most frequently involving the wrists, fingers, ankles, and toes, with or without the presence of an arthritis. Less than half of patients with DGI develop a true arthritis that is generally monarticular but can be oligoarticular or polyarticular. The most commonly affected joints are the knees, wrists, hands, and ankles,[88–90] although any joint may be involved, including the hip.[91]

Skin involvement occurs in approximately two thirds of patients with DGI. Most lesions are painless and may go unnoticed by the patient. The most common lesions are macules, papules, or pustules on an erythematous base. Lesions may progress to central necrosis. Vesicular lesions and lesions resembling bullae, erythema nodosum, and erythema multiforme have also been described. Lesions are few in number, occurring mostly on the extremities, sometimes on the trunk, and rarely on face, palms, and soles.[80, 90] Skin lesions develop simultaneously with tenosynovitis and arthritis, continue to evolve for 48 hours, and then resolve, even if untreated.[92]

DGI may present in one of two forms, a bacteremic form and a suppurative form. The bacteremic form, which is more common, presents as tenosynovitis, dermatitis, chills, fever, and a true arthritis with joint effusions that are typically culture-negative. In the suppurative form, arthritis is the major clinical manifestation. Joint effusions tend to be large and purulent. Some patients present with both clinical forms.[82]

Differential Diagnosis

The differential diagnosis of DGI includes those conditions manifested by arthritis and dermatitis. These include Reiter syndrome (reactive arthritis), nongonococcal bacterial arthritis, bacterial endocarditis, meningococcal arthritis, chronic meningococcal septicemia, hepatitis B, rheumatic fever, Lyme disease, systemic lupus erythematosus, rheumatoid arthritis, and Still disease.[75] Of these, acute and subacute bacterial endocarditis can be particularly difficult to distinguish from

DGI because patients with endocarditis and DGI may present with arthralgias accompanied by tenosynovitis followed by arthritis. The synovitis in both may be sterile unless hematogenous spread of organisms to the synovium has occurred. Skin lesions, particularly pustules and pustulonecrotic lesions, may occur in both.[75] Splinter hemorrhages, Osler nodes, Janeway lesions, rheumatoid factor, and positive blood cultures help to establish the diagnosis of endocarditis, as does the finding of valvular vegetations. Acute and chronic meningococcemia may also have clinical features resembling DGI. Helpful features in distinguishing meningococcemia are the presence of a greater number of skin lesions and a positive throat culture for the organism. Definitive diagnosis of meningococcemia is established by identification of the organisms in blood or synovial fluid.[75]

Diagnosis

The diagnosis of DGI and gonococcal arthritis is based on an appropriate clinical presentation and positive cultures. A definite diagnosis of DGI is established by positive cultures of *N. gonorrhoeae* or identification of the organism by Gram stain in samples of synovial fluid, blood, or skin lesions. The majority of patients presenting with DGI will have elevated peripheral white cell counts and elevated erythrocyte sedimentation rates. Synovial fluid from joints affected with gonococcal arthritis will frequently contain 30,000 to 100,000 white cells per mm^3, with a PMN predominance, but counts may be much lower.[81, 88] The majority of Gram stain examinations of synovial fluid specimens fail to reveal organisms. Yield may be increased by Gram staining the pellet of centrifuged synovial fluid. Cultures of synovial fluid fail to yield growth in more than 50% of cases, even when they are carefully performed.[93] Fluid from patients with the suppurative form is more likely to yield growth (almost 50% of cases) than is fluid from patients with the bacteremic form.[80, 82] Gram stain and cultures of skin lesions rarely yield positive results.[88] Blood culture positivity occurs in less than 30% of patients, with positive yield being more likely in patients with dermatitis and tenosynovitis.[75, 80, 90, 94]

The highest yields of culture positivity for gonococci are from genitourinary tract samples.[93] In women, cultures of cervical swabs yield growth in 80% to 90% of cases. In men, Gram stain and culture of urethral discharge, or of urethral swab in the absence of a discharge, yield positive results in 50% to 70% of cases.[81, 88] To maximize yield of positive cultures, all potentially infected mucosal sites, including pharynx and rectum, should be sampled. In some situations, all cultures of the presenting patient will be negative, but cultures of the sexual partner may yield growth of the organism.[75] To maximize culture yields, samples from the urethra, endocervix, rectum, and pharynx should be cultured on chocolate agar containing antibiotics (modified Thayer-Martin media); samples of joint fluid, blood, and skin lesions are cultured on plain chocolate agar.[75]

In most patients, a diagnosis of DGI or gonococcal arthritis is made indirectly by the presence of positive urethral, endocervical, rectal, or pharyngeal cultures in patients with appropriate clinical features. A presumptive diagnosis may be made by the typical presentation and rapid response to appropriate antibiotics.[75]

Treatment of Disseminated Gonococcal Infection and Gonococcal Arthritis

Patients should be educated regarding the sexual mode of gonococcal transmission, identification of sexual partners, and risk for other sexually transmitted diseases. Serologic testing for syphilis should be done and testing for HIV infection encouraged.

Initial hospitalization is recommended for management of DGI, particularly if (1) the diagnosis is in question, (2) compliance is uncertain, (3) purulent effusions are present (requiring repeated joint aspirations), and (4) complications of endocarditis, meningitis, or myopericarditis are suspected.[75]

With regard to antibiotic therapy, because a significant number of the infecting strains are penicillin (β-lactamase) resistant,[93, 95–97] initial treatment in the penicillin-tolerant (nonallergic) patient should consist of a third-generation β-lactamase–resistant cephalosporin. Antibiotic therapy for the patient tolerant of penicillins is listed in Table 154–4. Antibiotic therapy for the penicillin-allergic patient is listed in Table 154–5.

Unless *Chlamydia* diagnostic testing is available and yields negative results for coinfection, patients, in addition to being treated for gonococcal infection, should be treated with a 7-

TABLE 154–4 ■ Antibiotic Treatment of Disseminated Gonococcal Infection in Penicillin-Tolerant (Nonallergic) Patients

PARENTERAL THERAPY
Ceftriaxone, 1 g intramuscularly (IM) or intravenously (IV) q 24 h
or
Cefotaxime, 1 g IV q 8 h

Continue parenteral therapy until signs and symptoms of infection resolve or clinical improvement is evident (usually 2–4 d)

ORAL THERAPY (to complete total of 7 d of antibiotics)
Amoxicillin, 500 mg, plus clavulanate, 125 mg, three times daily
or
Cefuroxime axetil, 500 mg twice daily
or
Ciprofloxacin, 500 mg twice daily (in the nonpregnant patient)

Concurrent Treatment of *Chlamydia trachomatis*
Doxycycline, 100 mg orally twice daily for 7 d
or
Erythromycin base, 500 mg 4 times daily for 7 d
or
Azithromycin, 1 g (one dose)

From Centers for Disease Control and Prevention: 1993 sexually transmitted diseases treatment guidelines. MMWR Morbid Mortal Wkly Rep 42(RR-14):1–102, 1993.

TABLE 154–5 ■ Antibiotic Treatment of Disseminated Gonococcal Infection in Penicillin-Allergic Patients

PARENTERAL THERAPY (until clinical improvement)
Spectinomycin, 2 g intramuscularly q 12 h

ORAL THERAPY (to complete a 7-d course of antibiotics)
In the nonpregnant patient
Ciprofloxacin, 500 mg twice daily
In the pregnant patient
Erythromycin base, 500 mg 4 times a day for 7 d

Concurrent Therapy for *Chlamydia trachomatis*
In the nonpregnant patient
Doxycycline, 100 mg twice daily for 7 d
In the pregnant patient
Erythromycin base, 500 mg 4 times a day for 7 d

From Centers for Disease Control and Prevention: 1993 sexually transmitted diseases treatment guidelines. MMWR Morbid Mortal Wkly Rep 42(RR-14):1–102, 1993.

day course of doxycycline, 100 mg twice daily (or the pregnant woman is treated with erythromycin base, 500 mg four times daily).

With appropriate antibiotics, signs and symptoms of DGI generally improve within 48 hours, and dermatitis and arthralgias resolve within 5 days, but joint pain may persist for several weeks. Mean duration of hospitalization in one study was 5.8 days.[93] Management for large, purulent synovial effusions with regard to drainage and immobilization or exercise is similar to that for nongonococcal bacterial arthritis, although the response is generally more rapid in the case of gonococcal arthritis and the eventual outcome is generally excellent.[93] Although the clinical features of gonococcal arthritis have changed little in the past decades, patients presenting with gonococcal arthritis may more commonly have an underlying condition such as intravenous drug abuse or systemic lupus erythematosus and be infected with a penicillin-resistant gonococcal organism.[93]

After completion of antibiotics, patients should be reevaluated, including undergoing repeated sampling of sites that previously yielded positive cultures. Serologic testing for syphilis should be repeated 4 to 6 weeks after completion of antibiotic therapy.

Septic Bursitis

Infections of the subcutaneous bursae (olecranon, prepatellar, and infrapatellar) are common owing to their superficial location and susceptibility to trauma resulting in the percutaneous inoculation of bacteria. The infection may remain contained within the bursal cavity, lined by a thin layer of synovial cells, or may rupture into surrounding soft tissues and clinically resemble cellulitis. Deep bursal infection including the subacromial, trochanteric, and iliopsoas is rare and usually results from hematogenous seeding or underlying joint infection.

Gram-positive bacteria including *S. aureus* (80%) and various streptococcal species (5% to 30%) are the primary causative organisms.[98, 99] However, gram-negative and polymicrobial bacterial infections may occur, especially in immunocompromised or chronically debilitated patients. Fungi and mycobacteria have also been reported.

Clinical presentations may vary from minimal erythema and bursal swelling to systemic symptoms of malaise, fevers, and severe pain in the involved area. On physical examination, discrete swelling over the olecranon or prepatellar areas is often present, but extensive peribursal cellulitis extending beyond the borders of the bursa occurs in other cases.

The diagnosis of septic bursitis is based on aspiration and analysis of bursal fluid for total white cell count, culture, and crystals. In contrast to septic joint fluid, the bursal white cell counts may be low, often less than 10,000/mm^3 with a range from 920 to 300,000/mm^3, but PMNs will predominate.[99] Confirmation of infection is based on positive bursal fluid cultures. Because crystalline bursitis may occur simultaneously with a septic process, infection is not excluded until final cultures are negative.

Treatment of septic bursitis requires appropriate antibiotics, serial closed needle drainage, and immobilization of the joint. In otherwise healthy patients, septic olecranon and sometimes prepatellar bursitis are treated in the outpatient setting with oral antibiotics. The usual length of treatment is 5 days beyond the first sterile bursal fluid (a typical course is 10 to 14 days).[100] Hospital admission and 4 to 7 days of intravenous antibiotics followed by an additional 7 to 14 days of oral antibiotics are required in patients who are immunocompromised, are chronically debilitated, or fail to improve with oral therapy. Cases of septic prepatellar bursitis fail to respond to outpatient therapy more frequently and may require inpatient management. Other risk factors for poor outcome include delay in treatment, prior bursal infection, underlying disease of the bursa, extension of infection beyond the bursal sac, and bacteremia.[99] Rarely, surgical debridement of the bursa is required if (1) serial cultures remain positive despite appropriate antibiotics, (2) loculations or abscesses develop that are inaccessible to closed needle drainage, or (3) foreign material is present. Immobilization of the knee is an important adjunct of treatment for prepatellar bursitis accompanied by isometric strengthening exercises within a few days of immobilization.

Fungal Arthritis

Fungal arthritis is relatively rare and was previously described in patients with endemic mycoses: histoplasmosis, blastomycosis, or coccidioidomycosis. With emergence of a larger number of immunocompromised patients including patients with acquired immunodeficiency syndrome and those treated with immunosuppressive drugs for malignant and nonmalignant disorders, mycotic joint infections including unusual organisms have become more frequent. Maintenance on home total parenteral nutrition or intravenous administration of antibiotics also poses a risk for development of fungal infection.

The most common musculoskeletal fungal infections in immunocompetent hosts include those due to *Coccidioides immitis, Blastomyces dermatitidis, Histoplasma capsulatum, Sporothrix schenckii,* and *Cryptococcus neoformans.*[101] A hypersensitivity reaction with associated polyarthralgias, polyarthritis, and erythema nodosum accompanies primary infections of *H. capsulatum* (0% to 34%) and *C. immitis* (30%).[101] The symptoms are often migratory, self-limited, and without sequelae. Disseminated (or secondary) fungal infections commonly affect the skeletal system with *C. immitis* (10% to 50%), *B. dermatitidis* (25% to 60%), and *C. neoformans* (5%).[101] Septic arthritis typically results from extension of contiguous osteomyelitis.[102] Hematogenous seeding rarely occurs. Whereas *C. immitis* and *C. neoformans* arthritis appears more chronic and indolent with physical findings of monarthritis, *B. dermatitidis* arthritis is often associated with systemic symptoms and may be polyarticular. The knee is the most commonly involved joint followed by ankle, elbow, and wrist. Synovial fluid is moderately inflammatory with a predominance of mononuclear cells, but in *B. dermatitidis* infection, purulent fluid with an elevated number of PMNs is typical. *S. schenckii* infection, in contrast, develops secondary to direct inoculation from trauma. Chronic monarticular or polyarticular arthritis in the hands, wrist, knee, or feet and tenosynovitis are the usual musculoskeletal manifestations.

In immunocompromised or chronically ill patients, *Candida, Aspergillus* (particularly *Aspergillus fumigatus*), *Cryptococcus,* and *Histoplasma* are the most common fungi associated with skeletal infections. The pathogenesis and manifestations of bone and joint disease are similar to those of patients who are immunocompetent.

Candida arthritis develops by direct inoculation or hematogenous seeding, each of which is equally common. Direct inoculation occurs when *Candida* is introduced into osteoarthritic or rheumatoid joints by repeated aspirations or corticosteroid injections. The corticosteroids may alter host defense in an already abnormal joint. Direct inoculation may also occur during prosthetic joint replacement or other surgical procedures. In all these situations, patients are typically healthy but have a pathologic process in the knee, hip, or shoulder. Some patients may be immunocompromised from their rheumatoid arthritis, concomitant corticosteroid therapy, or other immunosuppressive therapy. The arthritis develops insidiously, often without associated systemic symptoms. The course is indolent, and the diagnosis is often delayed. Synovial fluid analysis reveals a variable degree of inflammatory fluid with predominantly PMNs and an associated low glucose level. Blood cultures are usually negative. The diagnosis is established by positive fluid or synovial tissue culture for the fungus. The most common species include *Candida parapsilosis* and *Candida albicans; Candida tropicalis* and *Candida guilliermondii* are rare.[103] Radiographs may reveal changes of the underlying joint disease and, in the case of a prosthetic joint, loosening, sometimes accompanied by osteomyelitis.

Disseminated candidiasis with associated septic arthritis is primarily reported in the pediatric population younger than 6 months. These infants are usually hospitalized and have underlying illnesses. Joint infection is usually associated with osteomyelitis. In adults, septic arthritis secondary to disseminated candidiasis is associated with immunocompromised states, prolonged systemic antibiotics, indwelling catheters, and intravenous drug abuse. In contrast to direct inoculation, the majority of patients (66%) with hematogenously seeded joints are acutely ill; 33% of patients may have an insidious onset.[104] Monarthritis of the knee is most common, although polyarticular infection can occur and is frequent in infants. Other joints involved include the hip, ankle, shoulder, or elbow. *C. albicans* is identified in 70% of the cases; *C. tropicalis, C. parapsilosis,* and *C. guilliermondii* (in order of decreasing frequency) are less common.[104] In intravenous drug abusers, the infection has a predilection for the fibrocartilaginous joints (sacroiliac, costochondral, sternoclavicular, and intervertebral disks).

Diagnosis of fungal arthritis is often delayed but is established by examination of synovial fluid or, more commonly, synovial tissue and bone biopsy specimens for identification of various fungal morphologic phases by culture, histopathology, or cytology. Aside from synovial fluid, candida may be cultured from multiple sites (blood, cerebrospinal fluid, urine, pharynx, stool, catheter tips, bone marrow) in patients with hematogenous dissemination. *C. immitis* and *B. dermatitidis* may have cutaneous lesions such as ulcerations or draining sinus tracks from which fungus may be cultured. Serodiagnosis provides additional confirmation of infection, but discussion of the various methods and their sensitivity and specificity is beyond the scope of this section (refer to Part XI of this book).

Amphotericin B alone or in combination with flucytosine has been the primary treatment of fungal arthritis. Refer to Chapter 33 for details of therapy. With the development of oral azole drugs, new drug regimens have been evaluated for the various mycoses. In disseminated candidiasis, fluconazole and amphotericin B may be equally effective.[105] Fluconazole alone successfully treated two cases of *Candida* arthritis.[106, 107] Itraconazole has in vitro effects against candida, but its potential clinical efficacy remains undefined. However, itraconazole may be an alternative to amphotericin B in the primary treatment of histoplasmosis, blastomycosis, coccidioidomycosis, and sporotrichosis.[108–110] In cryptococcal infections, fluconazole has been effective for meningitis and subsequent prophylaxis, but specific studies on musculoskeletal infections are not available. Itraconazole may potentially also be effective, and further studies are needed.[111] At this time, amphotericin B with or without flucytosine is the recommended regimen.[112]

As an adjunct to antifungal therapies, surgical drainage, débridement, or synovectomy may be necessary in cases of prosthetic joint infection, loculated joint effusions, or failure to respond to medical therapy. Removal of the prosthesis is necessary in the majority of patients with prosthetic *Candida* arthritis.[104]

Viral Arthritis

Various viral infections have been associated with acute arthritis or persistent arthropathy. The pathogenesis includes direct synovial infection, immune complex–mediated inflammation, and mechanisms as yet to be defined. Although most of the viral arthritides are self-limited and present in the prodromal state, rubella and parvovirus may cause chronic arthritis.

Rubella, by natural infection or immunization with attenuated virus, is the most common form of viral arthritis. The pathogenesis of the arthritis is direct infection and viral replication within the joint. A frequency has been reported of 52% in female patients compared with 8.7% in male patients who developed polyarthritis after natural rubella infection; nearly 50% of adult women developed joint disease after immunizations.[113] Polyarthritis of small joints, knees, wrist, ankles, and elbows occurs within 1 week of the rash in natural infections and within 2 to 3 weeks of immunization. The arthritis is typically self-limited, but persistent symptoms beyond 1 year have been described in up to 30% of adult women.[114, 115]

Human parvovirus B19 (HPV-B19) infection, also known as erythema infectiosum, is a common childhood disease that was rarely associated with joint symptoms. However, in a group of 104 pediatric patients with recent onset of arthritis and associated constitutional symptoms with or without exposure to viral illness, 22 children (19%) had serologic evidence of recent HPV-B19 infection.[116] Both polyarticular and pauciarticular joint involvement was described. Although a majority of the children had brief episodes of arthritis with complete resolution, eight children had prolonged (greater than 2 months) symptoms.

In adults, 77% of patients with HPV-B19 infections have associated arthralgias, and 60% of patients develop a brief period of arthritis.[117] Persistent polyarticular arthritis (defined as greater than 2 months) occurred in 17 of 19 patients who had recent serologic evidence of HPV-B19 infection.[118] Joint involvement clinically resembles rheumatoid arthritis with symmetric polyarthritis. However, despite the chronicity and persistent symptoms, neither do erosive changes develop nor is rheumatoid factor present. Arthroscopic findings reveal normal synovium without cartilage damage. Findings on synovial histologic examination are essentially normal.[119] The presence of B19-specific DNA sequences has been demonstrated in bone marrow aspirates of patients with chronic HPV-B19 arthropathy.[120] Initial results of synovial biopsies from the same investigators suggested the presence of HPV-B19 DNA as well. They postulated that chronic arthropathy is associated with persistence of either B19 virus or select B19 DNA sequence. The pathogenetic mechanism may not be immune mediated; rather, it may be direct viral injury of joint tissues.[119]

Hepatitis B–associated arthritis due to antigen-antibody complexes develops during the prodromal phase. The patients typically have polyarthralgias with or without frank polyarthritis. The arthritis usually resolves with the onset of jaundice. Chronic arthritis and other rheumatic syndromes (essential mixed cryoglobulinemia, polyarteritis nodosa, and glomerulonephritis) may develop in the setting of chronic active hepatitis.

With the identification of hepatitis C virus by recombinant antigens and the polymerase chain reaction, essential mixed cryoglobulinemia has been recognized as an extrahepatic manifestation of the disease. Polyarthritis, however, has rarely been reported. Two patients have been described with polyarthritis during acute and chronic hepatitis C.[121] In one patient, hepatitis C virus RNA was demonstrated in both serum and synovial fluid. The significance of anti–hepatitis C antibodies in patients with rheumatoid arthritis remains unclear.

Other viruses that may infrequently produce acute joint inflammation include Epstein-Barr virus,[122] varicella virus,[123] mumps virus,[124] coxsackievirus B,[125] human T-cell leukemia virus type I,[126] herpes simplex virus type 1, and cytomegalovirus.[127] The six arthropod-borne alphaviruses (chikungunya, o'nyong-nyong, Sindbis, Mayaro, Barmah Forest, and Ross River) produce distinct febrile polyarthritis syndromes in endemic regions.

Mycobacterial Infections

The increased frequency of *Mycobacterium tuberculosis* and some of the other atypical mycobacterial infections has been closely associated with the rise in prevalence of HIV infections. Similar to fungal infections, mycobacterial involvement of bone and joints is typically insidious, evolves slowly, and is often not associated with systemic symptoms.

Bone and joint involvement occurs in approximately 2% of all cases of tuberculosis.[128] Osteoarticular involvement typically develops secondary to hematogenous and lymphatic dissemination of tuberculosis, but local extension from an infected site may occur. Initial osteoarticular infection is often silent and remains dormant for a variable time before active symptoms develop. Tuberculosis has a predilection for the axial skeleton and weight-bearing joints, but case reports of numerous other joints, bursae, or tendons exist. The vertebral disk space and the anterior vertebral body (Pott disease) in the thoracic and lumbar regions are the most common osteoarticular sites of infection. Progressive infection results in disk space narrowing and anterior vertebral body collapse producing kyphosis. Paravertebral abscesses may also occur.

Peripheral arthritis is usually monarticular and involves, in order of decreasing frequency, knee, hip, and ankle.[129] The monarthritis is clinically indistinguishable from other forms of chronic infection or chronic inflammatory arthropathies such as the seronegative spondyloarthropathies or rheumatoid arthritis. Synovial fluid analysis is variably inflammatory; synovial fluid white cell counts average 10,000 to 20,000/mm^3.[130] Rice bodies, or fibrin-cellular debris formed into compact masses, may be present in synovial fluid but are not unique to tuberculous arthritis. The yield of synovial fluid acid-fast stains is 20%, positive synovial fluid cultures 80%, and positive synovial tissue biopsy smears and cultures 94%.[130] Biopsies often reveal caseating or noncaseating granulomatous synovitis, but nonspecific inflammatory changes are reported as well. Radiographs of late-stage peripheral joint infection may reveal subchondral erosions before articular cartilage narrowing develops. Computed tomographic scans are the most accurate imaging technique for visualizing the posterior vertebral elements; magnetic resonance imaging is most useful for delineating soft tissue or extradural involvement.[131] A rare form of tuberculous polyarticular arthritis, Poncet disease, previously described as a form of reactive arthritis has been challenged by the findings of granulomata in synovial tissue.[132]

Chemotherapy is the primary form of treatment for osteoarticular tuberculosis (refer to Chapter 34). Controversy exists about the length of therapy. Results from the Medical Research Council Working Party on Tuberculosis from Korea indicate that isoniazid plus rifampin for 6 or 9 months was as effective as 18 months of isoniazid plus *p*-aminosalicylate or ethambutol in the treatment of vertebral tuberculosis.[133] At this time, no reports of skeletal multidrug-resistant *M. tuberculosis* exist. Surgical débridement is a necessary adjunct to chemotherapy if neurologic compromise, spinal instability, large abscesses, proliferative pannus, or loose bodies in peripheral joints develop.

Atypical mycobacterial skeletal infections are rare and primarily involve tendon sheaths and bursae; less commonly, they cause monarthritis of wrist, finger, and knee joints. The pathogenesis is usually through percutaneous inoculation of atypical mycobacteria, which are ubiquitous in soil, water, or animals. Hematogenous seeding is rare and usually occurs in the immunocompromised host. The most common organisms include *Mycobacterium marinum, Mycobacterium avium-intracellulare,* and *Mycobacterium kansasii. M. marinum* typically involves the metacarpophalangeal, proximal interphalangeal, and wrist joints or tendon sheaths of healthy individuals with vocational or avocational contact with fish or water activities. *M. avium-intracellulare* similarly involves the tenosynovia or bursae and rarely involves bones and joints. *M. kansasii* typically infects joints with preexisting abnormalities or immunocompromised hosts.[134] Case reports of other mycobacterial infections have included *Mycobacterium haemophilum, Mycobacterium fortuitum, Mycobacterium chelonae,* and *Mycobacterium terrae.*[135, 136]

Diagnosis of atypical mycobacterial infection is based on isolation of the organism from synovial fluid or tissue samples. Histologic appearance is similar to that of *M. tuberculosis* infection. The sensitivity of granulomata on pathologic examination was 60%, whereas that of acid-fast staining was only 30%.[137] Treatment is primarily with combined chemotherapeutic agents (refer to Chapter 34). Surgical débridement or excision is often necessary.

References

1. Riegels-Nielson P, Frimodt-Moller N, Jensen JS: Rabbit model of septic arthritis. Acta Orthop Scand 58:14, 1987.
2. Goldenberg DL, Reed JI: Bacterial arthritis. N Engl J Med 312:764, 1985.
3. Dubost JJ, Fis I, Denis P, et al: Polyarticular septic arthritis. Medicine (Baltimore) 72:296, 1993.
4. Gardner GC, Weisman MH: Pyarthrosis in patients with rheumatoid arthritis: A report of 13 cases and a review of the literature from the past 40 years. Am J Med 88:503, 1990.
5. Cooper C, Cawley MI: Bacterial arthritis in an English health district: A 10 year review. Ann Rheum Dis 45:458, 1986.
6. Cooper C, Cawley MI: Bacterial arthritis in the elderly. Gerontology 32:222, 1986.
7. Newman ED, Davis DE, Harrington TM: Septic arthritis due to gram-negative bacilli: Older patients with good outcome. J Rheumatol 15:659, 1988.
8. Mateo Soria L, Nolla Sole JM, Rozadilla Sacanell A, et al: Infectious arthritis in patients with rheumatoid arthritis. Ann Rheum Dis 51:402, 1992.
9. Smith JW, Piercy EA: Infectious arthritis. Clin Infect Dis 20:225, 1995.
10. Baker DG, Schumacher HR: Acute monoarthritis. N Engl J Med 329:1013, 1993.
11. Mikhail IS, Alarcon GS: Nongonococcal bacterial arthritis. Rheum Dis Clin North Am 19:311, 1993.
12. Ajemian E, Andrews L, Hryb K, et al: Hospital acquired infections after arthroscopic knee surgery. A probable environmental source. Am J Infect Control 15:159, 1987.
13. D'Angelo GL, Ogilvie-Harris DJ: Septic arthritis following arthroscopy with cost/benefit analysis of antibiotic prophylaxis. Arthroscopy 4:10, 1988.
14. Toye B, Thomson J, Karsh J: *Staphylococcus epidermis* septic arthritis post arthroscopy. Clin Exp Rheumatol 5:165, 1987.
15. Zimmermann B, Lally EV, Liu NY: Infectious agents and the musculoskeletal system. *In* Noble J, Greene H, Levinson W, et al (eds): Primary Care and General Medicine, ed 2. St. Louis, Mosby–Year Book, 1996, pp 1186–1199.

16. Sharp JT, Lidsky MD, Duffy J, Duncan W: Infectious arthritis. Arch Intern Med 139:1125, 1979.
17. Espersen F, Frimodt-Moller, Rosdahl VT, et al: Changing pattern of bone and joint infections due to *Staphylococcus aureus:* Study of cases of bacteremia in Denmark, 1959–1988. Rev Infect Dis 13:347, 1991.
18. Ang-Fonte GZ, Rozboril MB, Thompson GR: Changes in nongonococcal septic arthritis: Drug abuse and methicillin-resistant *Staphylococcus aureus.* Arthritis Rheum 28:210, 1985.
19. Hale BB, Rosenblatt JE, Fitzgerald RH Jr: Anaerobic septic arthritis and osteomyelitis. Orthop Clin North Am 15:505, 1984.
20. Mahowald ML: Animal models of infectious arthritis. Clin Rheum Dis 12:403, 1986.
21. Mahowald ML, Peterson J, Raskind DA, et al: Antigen-induced experimental septic arthritis in rabbits after intraarticular injection of *Staphylococcus aureus.* J Infect Dis 54:273, 1986.
22. Esterhai JL Jr, Gelb I: Adult septic arthritis. Orthop Clin North Am 22:503, 1991.
23. Riegels-Nielson P, Frimodt-Moller N, Sorensen M, Jensen JS: Antibiotic treatment insufficient for established septic arthritis. *Staphylococcus aureus* experiments in rabbits. Acta Orthop Scand 60:113, 1989.
24. Schmid FH: New developments in bacterial arthritis. Bull Rheum Dis 41:1, 1992.
25. Goldenberg DL: The evaluation of patients with nongonococcal bacterial arthritis. *In* Espinoza L, Goldenberg DL, Arnett FC, et al (eds): Infections in the Rheumatic Diseases: A Comprehensive Review of Microbial Relations to Rheumatic Diseases. Orlando, FL, Grune & Stratton, 1988, p 9.
26. Ho G Jr: Bacterial arthritis. Curr Opin Rheumatol 4:509, 1992.
27. Pinals RS: Polyarthritis and fever. N Engl J Med 330:769, 1994.
28. Sequeira W, Swedler WI, Skosey JL: Septic arthritis in childhood. Ann Emerg Med 14:1185, 1985.
29. Goldenberg DL: Pathophysiology—Nongonococcal bacterial arthritis. *In* Espinoza L, Goldenberg DL, Arnett FC, et al (eds): Infections in the Rheumatic Diseases: A Comprehensive Review of Microbial Relations to Rheumatic Diseases. Orlando, FL, Grune & Stratton, 1988, p 3.
30. Yoshikawa TT: Geriatric infectious diseases: An emerging problem. J Am Geriatr Soc 31:34, 1983.
31. Von Essen R, Savolainen HA: Bacterial infection following intraarticular injection. A brief review. Scand J Rheumatol 18:7, 1989.
32. Goldenberg DL: Infectious arthritis complicating rheumatoid arthritis and other chronic rheumatic disorders. Arthritis Rheum 32:496, 1989.
33. Epstein JH, Zimmermann B III, Ho G Jr: Polyarticular septic arthritis. J Rheumatol 13:1105, 1986.
34. Ho G Jr: Bacterial arthritis. *In* McCarty DJ, Koopman WJ (eds): Arthritis and Allied Conditions: A Textbook of Rheumatology, ed 12, Vol 2. Philadelphia, Lea & Febiger, 1993, pp 2003–2023.
35. Peltola H, Vahvanen V: Acute purulent arthritis in children. Scand J Infect Dis 15:75, 1983.
36. Wang CH, Huang FY: Septic arthritis in early infancy. Acta Paediatr Sin 31:69, 1990.
37. Welkon CH, Long SS, Fisher MC, et al: Pyogenic arthritis in infants and children: A review of 95 cases. Pediatr Infect Dis 5:669, 1986.
38. Fink CW, Nelson JD: Septic arthritis and osteomyelitis in children. Clin Rheum Dis 12:423, 1986.
39. Deshpande PG, Wagle SU, Mehta SD, et al: Neonatal osteomyelitis and septic arthritis. Indian Pediatr 27:453, 1990.
40. Morrissy RT: Bone and joint infection in the neonate. Pediatr Ann 18:33, 1989.
41. Spesier JC, Moore TL, Osborn TG, et al: Changing trends in pediatric septic arthritis. Semin Arthritis Rheum 15:132, 1985.
42. Blackburn WD Jr: Gram-negative septic arthritis. *In* Espinoza L, Goldenberg DL, Arnett FC, et al (eds): Infections in the Rheumatic Diseases: A Comprehensive Review of Microbial Relations to Rheumatic Diseases. Orlando, FL, Grune & Stratton, 1988, p 21.
43. Blackburn WD, Alarcon GS: Prosthetic joint infections: A role for prophylaxis. A review. Arthritis Rheum 34:110, 1991.
44. Inman RD, Gallegos KV, Brause BD, et al: Clinical and microbial features of prosthetic joint infection. Am J Med 77:47, 1984.
45. Brancos MA, Peris P, Miro JM, et al: Septic arthritis in heroin addicts. Semin Arthritis Rheum 21:81, 1991.
46. Chandrasekas PH, Narula AP: Bone and joint infections in intravenous drug abusers. Rev Infect Dis 8:904, 1986.
47. Pollack MS: Staphylococcal mediastinitis due to sternoclavicular pyarthrosis. CT appearance. J Comput Assist Tomogr 14:924, 1990.
48. Wohlgethan JR, Newberg AH, Reed JI: The risk of abscess from sternoclavicular septic arthritis. J Rheumatol 15:1302, 1988.
49. Hodgson BF: Pyogenic sacroiliac joint infection. Clin Orthop 246:146, 1989.
50. Bleasel JF, York JR, Rickard KA: Septic arthritis in human immunodeficiency virus infected haemophiliacs. Br J Rheumatol 29:494, 1990.
51. Steinberg AD Jr: Principles in the use of immunosuppressive agents. *In* Schumacher HR (ed): Primer on the Rheumatic Diseases, ed 9. Atlanta, Arthritis Foundation, 1988, p 288.
52. Zimmermann B III, Erickson AD, Mikolich DJ: Septic acromioclavicular arthritis and osteomyelitis in a patient with acquired immunodeficiency syndrome. Arthritis Rheum 32:1175, 1989.
53. Berman A, Espinoza LR, Diaz JD, et al: Rheumatic manifestations of human immunodeficiency virus infection. Am J Med 85:59, 1988.
54. Calabrese LH: The rheumatic manifestations of infection with human immunodeficiency virus. Semin Arthritis Rheum 18:225, 1989.
55. Fernandez SM, Cardenal A, Balsa A, et al: Rheumatic manifestations in 556 patients with human immunodeficiency virus infection. Semin Arthritis Rheum 21:30, 1991.
56. Goldenberg DL: Gram-positive, anaerobic, and mixed bacterial arthritis. *In* Espinoza L, Goldenberg DL, Arnett FC, et al (eds): Infections in the Rheumatic Diseases: A Comprehensive Review of Microbial Relations to Rheumatic Diseases. Orlando, FL, Grune & Stratton, 1988, p 17.
57. Louthrenoo W, Ostrov BE, Park YS, et al: Pseudoseptic arthritis: An unusual presentation of neuropathic arthropathy. Ann Rheum Dis 50:717, 1991.
58. Singleton JD, West SG, Nordstrom DM: "Pseudoseptic" arthritis complicating rheumatoid arthritis. A report of six cases. J Rheumatol 18:1319, 1991.
59. Shmerling RH, Delbanco TL, Tosteson AN, et al: Synovial fluid tests. What should be ordered? JAMA 264:1009, 1990.
60. Mitchell M, Howard B, Haller J, et al: Septic arthritis. Radiol Clin North Am 26:1295, 1988.
61. Kim EE, Haynie TP, Podoloff DA, et al: Radionuclide imaging in the evaluation of osteomyelitis and septic arthritis. Crit Rev Diagn Imaging 29:257, 1989.
62. Hatfield MK, Gross BH, Glazer GM, et al: Computed tomography of the sternum and its articulations. Skeletal Radiol 11:197, 1984.
63. Morgan GJ, Schlegelmilch JG, Spiegel PK: Early diagnosis of septic arthritis of the sacroiliac joint by use of computerized tomography. J Rheumatol 18:979, 1981.
64. Stoller DW, Genant HK, Helms CA, Goumas CG (eds): Magnetic Resonance Imaging in Orthopaedics and Rheumatology. Philadelphia, JB Lippincott, 1989, pp 220–222, 223–229, 239–243, 259–262.
65. Fuchs HA: Polyarticular pseudosepsis in rheumatoid arthritis. South Med J 85:381, 1992.
66. Broy SB, Schmid FR: A comparison of medical drainage (needle aspiration) and surgical drainage (arthrotomy or arthroscopy) in the initial treatment of infected joints. Clin Rheum Dis 12:501, 1986.
67. Rosenthal J, Bole GG, Robinson WD: Acute non-gonococcal infectious arthritis. Evaluation of risk factors, therapy, and outcome. Arthritis Rheum 23:889, 1980.
68. Broy SB, Stulberg SD, Schmid FR: The role of arthroscopy in the diagnosis and management of the septic joint. Clin Rheum Dis 12:489, 1986.
69. Ohl MD, Kean JR, Steensen RN: Arthroscopic treatment of septic arthritic knees in children and adolescents. Orthop Rev 20:894, 1991.
70. Parisien JS, Shaffer B: Arthroscopic management of pyarthrosis. Clin Orthop 275:243, 1992.
71. Theiry JA: Arthroscopic drainage in septic arthritides of the knee: A multicenter study. Arthroscopy 5:65, 1989.
72. Sanford JP: Guide to Antimicrobial Therapy 1992. Dallas, Antimicrobial Therapy, 1992.

73. Symonds J, Geddes AM: Cephalosporins in gram-positive infections. Drugs 34(Suppl 2):121, 1987.
74. Dickie AS: Current concepts in the management of infection in bones and joints. Drugs 32:458, 1986.
75. Scopelitis E, Martinez-Osuna P: Gonococcal arthritis. Rheum Dis Clin North Am 19:363, 1993.
76. Fink CW: Gonococcal arthritis in children. JAMA 194:123, 1965.
77. Shapira O, Bar-On E, Sagiv S, et al: Disseminated gonococcal infection. J Am Geriatr Soc 38:678, 1990.
78. Rowe IF, Forster SM, Seifert MH, et al: Rheumatologic lesions in individuals with human immunodeficiency virus infection. Q J Med 272:1167, 1989.
79. Strogin IS, Kale SA, Raymond MK, et al: Unusual presentation of gonococcal arthritis in an HIV positive patient. Ann Rheum Dis 50:572, 1991.
80. Holmes KK, Counts GW, Beaty HN: Disseminated gonococcal infection. Ann Intern Med 74:979, 1971.
81. Masi AT, Eisenstein BI: Disseminated gonococcal infection and gonococcal arthritis (GCA): II. Clinical manifestations, diagnosis, complications, treatment, and prevention. Semin Arthritis Rheum 10:173, 1981.
82. Keiser H, Ruben FL, Wolinsky E, et al: Clinical forms of gonococcal arthritis. N Engl J Med 279:234, 1968.
83. Zbella EA, Deppe G, Elrad H: Gonococcal arthritis in pregnancy. Obstet Gynecol Surg 39:8, 1984.
84. Wilson J, Zaman AG, Simmon AV: Gonococcal arthritis complicated by acute pericarditis and pericardial effusion. Br Heart J 63:134, 1990.
85. Peterson BH, Lee TJ, Snyderman R, et al: *Neisseria meningitides* and *Neisseria gonorrhoeae* bacteremia associated with C_6, C_7, or C_8 deficiency. Ann Intern Med 90:917, 1979.
86. Mulks MH, Plaut AG: IgA protease production as a characteristic distinguishing pathogenic from harmless Neisseriaceae. N Engl J Med 299:973, 1978.
87. Goldenberg DL, Reed JI, Rice PA: Arthritis in rabbits induced by killed *Neisseria gonorrhoeae* and gonococcal lipopolysaccharide. J Rheumatol 11:3, 1984.
88. O'Brien JP, Goldenberg DL, Rice PA: Disseminated gonococcal infection: A prospective analysis of 49 patients and a review of the pathophysiology and immune mechanisms. Medicine (Baltimore) 62:395, 1983.
89. Grippo GN, Genovese MN, Piccora R: Monarthric gonococcal arthritis involving the calcaneocuboid joint. J Am Podiatr Med Assoc 80:91, 1990.
90. Brogadir SP, Schimmer BM, Myers AR: Spectrum of the gonococcal arthritis-dermatitis syndrome. Semin Arthritis Rheum 8:177, 1979.
91. Lee AH, Chin AE, Ramanujam T, et al: Gonococcal septic arthritis of the hip. J Rheumatol 18:1932, 1991.
92. Koss PG: Disseminated gonococcal infection. The tenosynovitis-dermatitis and suppurative arthritis syndromes. Cleve Clin Q 52:161, 1985.
93. Wise CM, Morris CR, Wasilauskas BL, Salzer WL: Gonococcal arthritis in an era of increasing penicillin resistance. Arch Intern Med 154:2690, 1994.
94. Gelfand SC, Masi AT, Gardia-Kutzbach A: Spectrum of gonococcal arthritis. Evidence for sequential stages and clinical subgroups. J Rheumatol 2:83, 1975.
95. Jaffe HW, Biddle JW, Johnson SR, Wiesner PJ: Infections due to penicillinase producing *Neisseria gonorrhoeae* in the United States 1976–1980. J Infect Dis 144:191, 1981.
96. Centers for Disease Control and Prevention: Sentinel surveillance for antimicrobial resistance in *Neisseria gonorrhoeae*—United States 1988–1991. MMWR CDC Surveill Summ 43(NSS-3):29, 1993.
97. Faruki H, Kohmescher RN, McKinney WP, Sparling PF: A community-based outbreak of infection with penicillin-resistant *Neisseria gonorrhoeae* not producing penicillinase (chromosomally mediated resistance). N Engl J Med 313:607, 1985.
98. Canoso JJ, Barza M: Soft tissue infections. Rheum Dis Clin North Am 19:293, 1993.
99. Zimmermann B 3d, Mikolich DJ, Ho G Jr: Septic bursitis. Semin Arthritis Rheum 24:391, 1995.
100. Ho G, Su EY: Antibiotic therapy of septic bursitis. Arthritis Rheum 24:905, 1981.
101. Cuellar ML, Silveira LH, Citera G, et al: Other fungal arthritides. Rheum Dis Clin North Am 19:439, 1993.
102. MacDonald PB, Black GB, MacKenzie R: Orthopedic manifestations of blastomycosis. J Bone Joint Surg Am 72:860, 1990.
103. Cuende E, Barbadillo C, E-Mazzucchelli R, et al: *Candida* arthritis in adult patients who are not intravenous drug addicts: Report of three cases and review of the literature. Semin Arthritis Rheum 22:224, 1993.
104. Silveira LH, Cuellar ML, Citera G, et al: *Candida* arthritis. Rheum Dis Clin North Am 19:427, 1993.
105. Rex JH, Bennett JE, Sugar AM, et al: Fluconazole vs. amphotericin B for treatment of candidemia: Results of a randomized multicenter trial. *In* Program and abstracts of the 33rd Interscience Conference on Antimicrobial Agents and Chemotherapy; October 17–20, 1993; New Orleans. Washington, DC, American Society for Microbiology, 1993, p 43.
106. Eady JL, Agnew DK: *Candida* infection of a total knee arthroplasty treated with fluconazole. Contemp Orthop 25:483, 1992.
107. O'Meeghan T, Varcoe R, Thomas M, et al: Fluconazole concentration in joint fluid during successful treatment of *Candida albicans* septic arthritis. J Antimicrob Chemother 26:601, 1990.
108. Graybill JR, Stevens DA, Galgiani JN, et al: Itraconzaole treatment of coccidiomycosis. NAIAD Mycoses Study Group. Am J Med 89:282, 1990.
109. Dismukes WE, Bradsher RW Jr, Cloud GC, et al: Itraconazole therapy for blastomycosis and histoplasmosis. NIAID Mycoses Study Group. Am J Med 93:489, 1992.
110. Sharkey-Mathis PK, Kauffman CA, Graybill JR, et al: Treatment of sporotrichosis with intraconazole. NIAID Mycoses Study Group. Am J Med 95:279, 1993.
111. Como JA, Dismukes WE: Oral azole drugs as systemic antifungal therapy. N Engl J Med 330:263, 1994.
112. Behrman RE, Masci JR, Nicholas P: Cryptococcal skeletal infections: Case report and review. Rev Infect Dis 12:181, 1990.
113. Tingle AJ, Allen M, Petty RE, et al: Rubella associated arthritis. I. Comparative study of joint manifestations associated with natural rubella infection RA27/3 rubella immunization. Ann Rheum Dis 45:110, 1986.
114. Howson CP, Katz M, Johnston RB, Fineberg HV: Chronic arthritis after rubella vaccination. Clin Infect Dis 15:307, 1992.
115. Mitchell LA, Tingle AJ, Shukin R, et al: Chronic rubella vaccine-associated arthropathy. Arch Intern Med 153:2268, 1993.
116. Nocton JJ, Miller LC, Tucker LB, Schaller JG: Human parvovirus B19–associated arthritis in children. J Pediatr 122:186, 1993.
117. Ager EA, Chin TDY, Poland JD: Epidemic erythema infectiosum. N Engl J Med 275:1326, 1966.
118. White DG, Woolf AD, Mortimer PP, et al: Human parvovirus arthropathy. Lancet 1:419, 1985.
119. Naides SJ: Parvovirus B19 infection. Rheum Dis Clin North Am 19:457, 1993.
120. Foto F, Saag KG, Scharosch LL, et al: Parvovirus B19–specific DNA in bone marrow from B19 arthropathy patients: Evidence for B19 virus persistence. J Infect Dis 167:744, 1993.
121. Ueno Y, Kinoshita R, Kishimoto I, et al: Polyarthritis associated with hepatitis C virus infection. Br J Rheum 33:289, 1994.
122. Ray GC, Gall EP, Minnich LL, et al: Acute polyarthritis associated with active Epstein-Barr virus infection. JAMA 248:2990, 1982.
123. DiLiberti JH, Bartel SJ, Humphrey TR, et al: Acute monoarticular arthritis in association with varicella: A case report. Clin Pediatr 16:663, 1977.
124. Gordon SC, Lauter CB: Mumps arthritis: A review of the literature. Rev Infect Dis 6:338, 1984.
125. David JJ, Dietz FR, Jones MM: Coxsackie-B monarthritis with hepatitis. J Bone Joint Surg Am 75:1685, 1993.
126. Nishioka K, Nakajima T, Hasunuma T, et al: Rheumatic manifestation of human leukemia virus infection. Rheum Dis Clin North Am 19:489, 1993.
127. Friedman HM, Pincus T, Gibilisco P, et al: Acute monoarticular arthritis caused by herpes simplex virus and cytomegalovirus. Am J Med 69:241, 1980.
128. Meier JL: Mycobacterial and fungal infections of bone and joints. Curr Opin Rheum 6:408, 1994.
129. Evanchick CC, Davis DE, Harrington TM: Tuberculosis of pe-

ripheral joints: An often missed diagnosis. J Rheumatol 13:187, 1986.
130. Wallace R, Cohen AS: Tuberculous arthritis: A report of two cases with a review of biopsy and synovial fluid findings. Am J Med 61:277, 1976.
131. Hoffman EB, Crosier JH, Cremin BJ: Imaging in children with spinal tuberculosis: A comparison of radiography, computed tomography, and magnetic resonance imaging. J Bone Joint Surg Br 75:233, 1993.
132. Hameed K, Karim M, Islam N, Gibson T: The diagnosis of Poncet's disease. Br J Rheumatol 32:824, 1993.
133. Medical Research Council Working Party on Tuberculosis of the Spine: Twelfth report: Controlled trial of short-course regimens of chemotherapy in the ambulatory treatment of spinal tuberculosis: Result of three years of study. J Bone Joint Surg Br 75:240, 1993.
134. Glickstein SL, Nashel DJ: *Mycobacterium kansasii* septic arthritis complicating rheumatic disease: Case report and review of the literature. Semin Arthritis Rheum 16:231, 1987.
135. Wallace RJ, O'Brien R, Glassroth J, et al: Diagnosis and treatment of disease caused by nontuberculous mycobacteria. Am Rev Respir Dis 142:940, 1990.
136. Strauss WL, Ostroff SM, Jernigan DB, et al: Clinical and epidemiologic characteristics of *Mycobacterium haemophilum,* an emerging pathogen in immunocompromised patients. Ann Intern Med 120:118, 1994.
137. Kozin S, Bishop A: Atypical mycobacterial infections of the upper extremity. J Hand Surg 19:480, 1994.

EYE AND PARANASAL SINUSES

155

Infections of the Eye

Jules Baum
Michael Barza

INFECTIONS OF THE ANTERIOR EYE AND ADNEXAE

Most ocular infections involve tissues that are visible to the naked eye, and many have a characteristic appearance that suggests the diagnosis. Additional information may be gained by viewing the external ocular structure with magnification. Whereas the ophthalmologist routinely uses a slit lamp for this purpose, other physicians may use a penlight and hand magnifier or loupe to see, for example, the molluscum nodule partially concealed by the eyelash, follicles on the palpebral conjunctiva suggestive of viral or chlamydial conjunctivitis, or the characteristic dendrite of herpes simplex epithelial keratitis. This chapter provides an overview of a variety of infections of the eyelid, conjunctiva, cornea, and lacrimal apparatus and also of the deeper structures (endophthalmitis). For a more detailed treatment, the reader may consult other publications.[1-4] Figure 155–1 provides a schematic diagram of the structure of the eye for purposes of orientation.

Eyelid Infections

Bacterial Infections

Staphylococcal blepharitis (Fig. 155–2) is among the most common bacterial infections of the eyelids. Because coagulase-negative staphylococci may be grown in cultures from the lids and conjunctiva of as many as 70% of normal persons and *Staphylococcus aureus* may be cultured from these sites in up to 40% of normal persons,[5] it has been difficult to establish the role of these species in the disease. The diagnosis is made on clinical grounds. The disease rarely may be acute, but characteristically it is chronic and bilateral, lasting months to years if not effectively treated. It is often seen in association with rosacea, seborrheic blepharitis, or keratoconjunctivitis

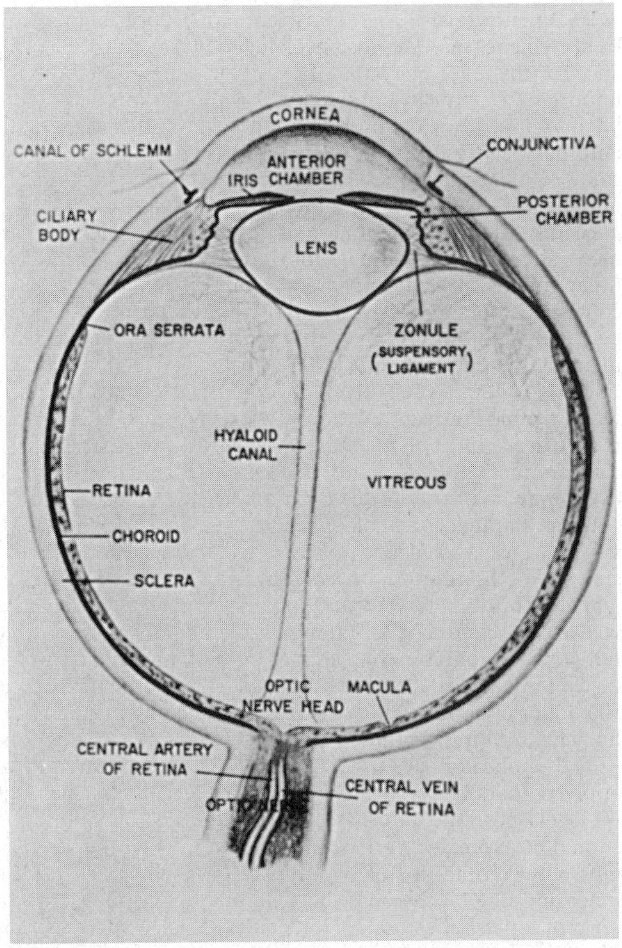

FIGURE 155–1 □ Schematic diagram of the eye. (From Barza M, Baum J: Treatment of bacterial infections of the eye. Curr Clin Top Infect Dis 158:159, 1980.)

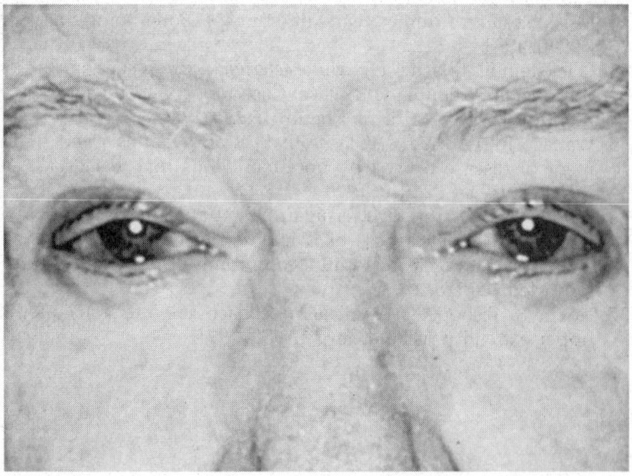

FIGURE 155–2 □ Staphylococcal blepharitis. Note erythema of lid margins.

sicca. The patient usually has only mild discomfort. The eyelid margins of patients with chronic symptoms are diffusely injected, and flakes of keratinized epithelium cling to the lashes. Fibrin exudate is commonly seen at the base of the lashes, often forming a characteristic "collarette." Eyelid margins may be thickened and irregular with telangiectasia, misdirected lashes, and sparse and whitened (poliosis) lashes.

Treatment consists of topical antibiotic applications and local hygiene, in some instances for many months. Compliance for this long period is often difficult to obtain, but it is important. Bacitracin ophthalmic ointment is applied to the lid margin with a cotton-tipped applicator after dried exudate has been wiped off. Depending on the severity of the condition, bacitracin may be applied two to four times a day initially for 1 to 2 weeks; the frequency may then be reduced gradually to once a night at bedtime for 4 to 8 weeks. Treatment should be continued for 1 month after all signs of inflammation have disappeared.[6] If antibiotic therapy is discontinued too soon after a supposed cure, the process may be reactivated. Erythromycin or gentamicin ophthalmic ointment may be used if clinical resistance or a reaction to bacitracin develops. Vancomycin eyedrops, 1%, may be used when methicillin-resistant staphylococci are encountered, but the eyedrops must be formulated as there is no such commercial product. Topical ciprofloxacin or ofloxacin eyedrops, 0.3%, may be of use in this circumstance.

When staphylococcal blepharitis is seen in association with rosacea, oral tetracycline is suggested, because the tetracyclines are thought to be concentrated in the meibomian glands. An initial dose of 250 mg four times daily for 1 to 2 weeks can be reduced to 250 mg once daily for some months, until it is found by trial and error that treatment can be discontinued without reactivating the disease. Doxycycline, 100 mg orally (PO) once or twice daily, is another option. Lid hygiene is an important component of therapy. Moist cotton-tipped applicators are used to keep the eyelids clean and to apply a mild baby shampoo twice a week to the base of the eyelashes. The contents of congested meibomian glands should be expressed periodically by compressing the lid margins between the tips of two applicators, one placed on the inner and one on the outer lid margin, after application of a drop of topical anesthesia. Hordeolum (stye), acute meibomitis, and chalazion, which are, on occasion, associated with staphylococcal blepharitis but also occur independently, are described in the following sections.

Hordeolum and Chalazion

Hordeola (styes) are of two types. An external hordeolum, the more common variety, is a staphylococcal microabscess of one of the glands of Zeis, a series of superficial sebaceous glands at the base of the eyelashes. An acute infection produces localized pain, redness, and swelling. Within a day or two, the 1- to 2-mm milk-white microabscess points at the lid margin. Almost invariably, it ruptures and drains spontaneously, but resolution and relief of pain are hastened if the lesion is pierced with a sterile needle. No antibiotic therapy is required.

An internal hordeolum, a staphylococcal cellulitis-like infection of a meibomian gland, appears clinically as a painful focal area of swelling and induration of the eyelid. The signs and symptoms are more severe than those of a chalazion (see later). Meibomian glands are a series of sebaceous glands whose orifices are visible along the length of the lid margin. We believe, as do others, that acute meibomitis is a better term than internal hordeolum for this minor infection. Because the meibomian glands lie buried in the tarsus, a cartilaginous support of the lid, the abscess of acute meibomitis cannot drain easily, as a stye can. An oral preparation of an antistaphylococcal antibiotic is often used to eradicate the infection.

A chalazion (Fig. 155–3) is a granulomatous nodule that develops in a meibomian gland, often in association with staphylococcal blepharitis. It is not clear why the granuloma forms, but it may be as a response to lipid retained in the gland. Initial mild pain for 24 to 72 hours is followed by the development of a painless lump within the lid. Untreated, 80% of chalazia resolve within a month.[7] For those that persist, the commercial preparation of triamcinolone acetonide, 10 mg/mL, is diluted to 5 mg/mL and 0.1 mL of the dilute solution is injected into the lesion.[8] A second injection may be necessary 3 to 7 days later. This treatment eradicates or greatly reduces the size of the nodule in more than half of cases. Surgical excision may be necessary for lesions that do not respond to corticosteroid injection. Antibiotic treatment is ineffective. Multiple chalazia that develop at different locations in the same lid within a period of several months generally should be treated as if they were staphylococcal blepharitis.

Angular blepharitis is a minor infection of the skin at the lateral canthus. The infection may persist indefinitely without treatment, but it responds rapidly to topical antibiotic therapy. *Moraxella lacunata,* a gram-negative bacillus, had been the major cause, especially among derelicts.[9] For reasons that are not clear, *Moraxella* infections are now less common and *S. aureus* is the major cause. Rarely, angular blepharitis is caused by anaerobic bacteria, mycobacteria, or other agents.

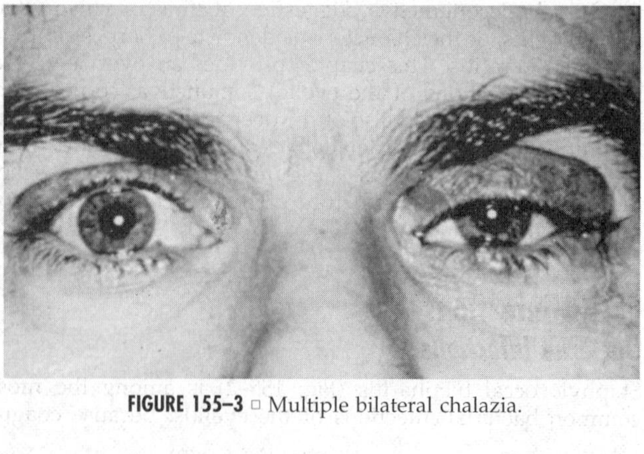

FIGURE 155–3 □ Multiple bilateral chalazia.

TABLE 155–1 ■ Features That Distinguish Bacterial from Viral and Chlamydial Conjunctivitis

FEATURE	BACTERIAL CONJUNCTIVITIS	VIRAL CONJUNCTIVITIS	CHLAMYDIAL CONJUNCTIVITIS
Conjunctival injection	Moderately severe	Minimal	Absent or minimal
Exudate	Moderate to profuse (polymorphonuclear)	Minimal (usually mononuclear)	Minimal in adults, copious in newborns
Sticking of lids on awakening	Yes	No	Absent in adults, present in newborns
Papillae (palpebral conjunctiva)	Present	Usually absent	May be present
Follicles (palpebral conjunctiva)	Usually absent	Present	Present in adults, absent in newborns
Preauricular lymphadenopathy	Absent	Present	Present in adults, absent in newborns
Response to antibiotic therapy	Yes	No	Yes
Duration of untreated disease	Up to several weeks	Several weeks	Persistent

Modified from Barza M, Baum J: Ocular infections. Med Clin North Am 67:131–152, 1983.

Viral Blepharitis

Herpes simplex virus, usually type 1, produces a primary ocular infection in children. Typically, a cluster of umbilicated vesicles forms on the eyelid together with acute follicular conjunctivitis. The cornea is rarely involved in a primary infection, whereas it is invariably affected in recurrent disease in adults. The blepharitis usually heals without treatment in 1 to 2 weeks. In severe cases, ulcerative blepharitis and dendritic keratitis may develop. In such instances, oral acyclovir at 200 to 400 mg or acyclovir ophthalmic ointment (not commercially available in the United States) may be administered four or five times daily. Alternatively, famciclovir at 500 mg PO may be administered three times a day.

Varicella-zoster virus may infect the upper or lower eyelid when, respectively, the ophthalmic or maxillary branch of the trigeminal nerve is involved. For treatment, see the later section on varicella-zoster keratitis.

Molluscum contagiosum, a poxvirus disease, produces white, often umbilicated nodules 2 to 3 mm in diameter on the skin of an eyelid. Small lesions may be obscured by the eyelashes. Characteristic eosinophilic bodies are seen in biopsy specimens. Curettage or incision of the nodule sufficient to produce bleeding cures the infection.

Papillomavirus may produce single or multiple warts on the eyelid. Virus or undetermined products of the infection may cause conjunctival injection or corneal epithelial disease. Vaccinia virus, another poxvirus, may infect the eyelid; this infection usually occurs by inoculation from another site.

Parasitic Infections

Phthirus pubis, the crab louse, may affect the eye, usually after pubic infestation. The major symptom is itching. The transparent adult lice, which are attached to the lashes, are difficult to see, even with magnification, but the nits (eggs) are more readily visible. A bland ophthalmic ointment such as sterile petrolatum may be applied to smother the lice, and the nits can be removed mechanically. In refractory cases, lindane cream, 1%, may be used cautiously on the eyelid margins as a single application, avoiding contact with the eyes. Family members and sexual contacts should also be examined and, if necessary, treated.

Fungal Infections

In warm climates as many as 22% of healthy persons harbor fungi along their eyelid margins,[10] yet fungal infections of the eyelids are unusual. Dermatophytes (ringworm) may produce superficial infection of the eyelids. Fungi that produce systemic infection, such as *Candida albicans* and *Blastomyces dermatitidis,* may cause ulcers and granulomata of the lids.

Infections of the Conjunctiva

Clinical features that help to distinguish bacterial, viral, and chlamydial conjunctivitis are presented in Table 155–1, and features that distinguish conjunctivitis from keratitis and iritis, in Table 155–2. Conjunctival infections are almost always bilateral. In otherwise healthy patients they are also usually self-limited, except for chlamydial and staphylococcal conjunctivitis.

In developed countries most conjunctival infections are caused by viruses. The most common viral agent of conjunctivitis is adenovirus. The infection usually abates spontaneously within several weeks. Follicles (foci of lymphoid hyperplasia that appear as translucent grains of sand on the palpebral conjunctiva) and preauricular lymphadenopathy are the hallmarks of viral conjunctivitis. If follicular conjunctivitis persists longer than 1 month in adults, and especially if the follicles appear relatively large, chlamydial infection should be suspected. Infants with chlamydial conjunctivitis do not exhibit follicles because their lymphoid system is underdeveloped. Conversely, older children with fever of various origins may develop conjunctival follicles as part of a generalized lymphatic response even in the absence of ocular infection.

Bacterial conjunctivitis produces a papillary rather than a follicular conjunctival response. Papillae appear as opaque grains of sand on the palpebral conjunctiva. With magnification, a central blood vessel is seen in each papilla, whereas blood vessels surround a follicle but none are seen centrally.

Infectious conjunctivitis is usually a bilateral disease and is usually transferred to the second eye via fingers, towels, or other objects. Patients should be cautioned about infecting the other eye and other persons. Adenoviral conjunctivitis is especially contagious.

TABLE 155–2 ■ Features That Distinguish Conjunctivitis from Keratitis or Iritis

FEATURE	CONJUNCTIVITIS	KERATITIS OR IRITIS
Vision	Normal	May be reduced
Pain	Gritty irritation	True pain
Conjunctiva	Diffuse injection	Ciliary flush
Exudate	Minimal to profuse	Usually none
Mattering of lids (dried exudate)	May be present	Absent
Photophobia	Absent	Present
Lacrimation	Usually absent	Present
Pupillary diameter	Normal	Usually small

Modified from Barza M, Baum J: Ocular infections. Med Clin North Am 67:131–152, 1983.

Bacterial Conjunctivitis

Bacterial conjunctivitis may be classified by the duration of the illness as acute or chronic and by the nature of the exudate as purulent or mucopurulent. Historically, the names hyperpurulent and purulent conjunctivitis have been used interchangeably, as have the terms acute catarrhal and mucopurulent conjunctivitis.

In this chapter, we use the shorter terms, purulent and mucopurulent. A purulent or mucopurulent discharge and the presence of papillae on the palpebral conjunctiva are the diagnostic signs of bacterial conjunctivitis. The tendency for the eyelids to be stuck together on awakening, which depends on the degree of purulence of the exudate, is usually associated with bacterial, not viral, conjunctivitis. Although the grossly visible inflammatory reaction is not a precise indicator from which the cause of conjunctivitis may be inferred, purulent reactions suggest infection by *Neisseria gonorrhoeae* or *Neisseria meningitidis* or chlamydiae in neonates, whereas most other bacterial conjunctivitides are mucopurulent. Chronic conjunctivitis is most often caused by staphylococci or gram-negative bacilli. Chronic conjunctivitis with blepharitis suggests infection by staphylococci or by *M. lacunata.*

ACUTE CONJUNCTIVITIS

Most cases of acute bacterial conjunctivitis are caused by gram-positive cocci, but when the conjunctiva is abnormal as a result of exposure (e.g., thyroid exophthalmos, coma) or keratinization (e.g., after irradiation), gram-negative bacilli may cause infection.

Different pathogens characteristically produce different degrees of purulence in the secretions. Purulent conjunctivitis with copious exudate is most frequently caused by *N. gonorrhoeae* and less commonly by *N. meningitidis.* Gonococcal infection most often appears in newborns, being acquired during passage through the birth canal. The infection becomes clinically apparent 2 to 5 days after birth. The exudate may become trapped beneath swollen eyelids, causing pressure necrosis of the corneal epithelium. Devitalization of the epithelium renders the cornea more prone to infection. Adults acquire purulent gonococcal conjunctivitis through sexual contact.

Mucopurulent conjunctivitis, known to the laity as pinkeye, is usually caused by *S. aureus, Streptococcus pyogenes, Streptococcus pneumoniae* (in colder climates), or *Haemophilus influenzae* (in warmer climates).

True membranous conjunctivitis is caused by *Corynebacterium diphtheriae* infection but is seen rarely, if ever, today. Pseudomembranes derived from inflammatory debris and fixed loosely to the palpebral conjunctiva occur in β-hemolytic streptococcal and adenoviral conjunctivitis. Conjunctival petechiae may be seen in conjunctivitis caused by streptococci and *H. influenzae. Haemophilus aegyptius,* a close relative of *H. influenzae,* has been implicated as the cause of Brazilian hemorrhagic fever; the conjunctivitis antedates the generalized illness by 3 to 15 days.[11] Other species of gram-negative bacteria, including *Pseudomonas* and *Escherichia coli,* may produce conjunctivitis, especially when the conjunctiva is abnormal. Such gram-negative infections are sometimes difficult to eradicate.

CHRONIC CONJUNCTIVITIS

Chronic bacterial conjunctivitis is most often caused by coagulase-positive staphylococci. It is frequently associated with staphylococcal blepharitis and at times is accompanied by a noninfectious keratitis. As stated earlier, chronic gram-negative bacillary conjunctivitis is seen in patients with devitalized conjunctiva. *M. lacunata* organisms produce both chronic blepharitis and conjunctivitis, most frequently in derelicts; these infections are rare today. Whereas most organisms that cause conjunctivitis do not affect the skin simultaneously, *Moraxella* and staphylococcal organisms can both be involved in chronic conjunctivitis and may simultaneously affect the skin, the lid margin, and the conjunctiva.

TREATMENT OF BACTERIAL CONJUNCTIVITIS

Some general principles for treatment of conjunctivitis should be kept in mind. Although most cases of bacterial conjunctivitis resolve spontaneously within a week or two, appropriate antibiotic therapy shortens the course of the infection. (Exceptions are *Staphylococcus* and *Moraxella* infections, which may become chronic if not adequately treated.) As a rule, conjunctival cultures are not performed, and acute bacterial conjunctivitis is treated empirically. Eyedrops generally are preferred over ointments for adults because ointments blur vision. By contrast, ointments are preferred for infants and children because eyedrops are squeezed out and diluted during crying. Ointments are acceptable for adults at bedtime and are useful because they are eliminated slowly, so their action persists during sleep. Eyedrops containing ciprofloxacin; ofloxacin; gentamicin; tobramycin; a combination of neomycin, gramicidin, and polymyxin B; or a combination of trimethoprim-polymyxin B, applied every 1 to 4 hours, are commonly used, as are ointments containing gentamicin, tobramycin, or bacitracin–polymyxin B. Physicians treating acute bacterial conjunctivitis empirically should remember that aminoglycosides are not effective against streptococci. Vancomycin eyedrops at 5 mg/mL (not available commercially) may be used for methicillin-resistant staphylococcal infections. Although adverse effects of topically applied medications are rare, neomycin may induce a dose-related epithelial keratitis, and chloramphenicol applied topically has caused fatal bone marrow aplasia.[12]

Gonococcal conjunctivitis in neonates is treated primarily by the parenteral route because the swelling of the eyes often makes it difficult to instill drops. Almost all other forms of bacterial conjunctivitis are treated exclusively by the topical route. Although topical antibiotics were often part of the standard treatment of gonococcal conjunctivitis in the past, they are probably unnecessary if the patient is receiving treatment by the parenteral route. A suggested regimen for the treatment of gonococcal conjunctivitis in adults is a single dose of ceftriaxone 1 g intramuscularly. The infected eye should be lavaged with saline once. For neonates, ceftriaxone should be given in a single dose of 25 to 50 mg/kg intravenously (IV) or intramuscularly, not to exceed 125 mg.[13] The mother and her sexual partner should also be evaluated and, if necessary, treated. A neonate born to a mother with proven gonococcal infection should be given the same dosage of ceftriaxone for prophylaxis as for treatment of proven neonatal gonococcal conjunctivitis. Saline irrigation of the eyes is also suggested.[13] Other regimens for the treatment of genital and disseminated gonococcal infections are described in Chapter 110. Their efficacy in gonococcal conjunctivitis has not been well established. Patients with gonococcal eye infection, like patients with other gonococcal infections, should be evaluated for coinfection with *Chlamydia trachomatis* and treated appropriately.[13] The issue of routine topical prophylaxis for neonates is discussed in the section on inclusion conjunctivitis.

Chlamydial Conjunctivitis

Inclusion conjunctivitis and trachoma are caused by various serotypes of chlamydiae, which are grouped under the acronym TRIC (trachoma inclusion conjunctivitis) agent. Trachoma, caused mainly by serotypes A, B, and C, is the leading cause of blindness in the world, whereas inclusion conjunctivitis, caused mainly by serotypes D through K, is almost invariably a benign, self-limited condition.

TRACHOMA

The prevalence of trachoma throughout the world has decreased as a result of improved personal hygiene and sanitation, but millions of people, largely in developing countries, are still afflicted. The disease is spread by person-to-person contact, by fomites, and by flies that carry the chlamydiae from human excrement to the eye and then from eye to eye. Young children in endemic areas are at high risk.

The incubation period is 5 to 14 days. Discomfort is minimal. Follicles develop on the palpebral conjunctiva and may also appear at the limbus. Healed limbal follicles leave the diagnostic scars called Herbert pits. Papillae as well as follicles develop on the palpebral conjunctiva. In short order the cornea is affected with punctate epithelial and subepithelial keratitis. With persistence of the low-grade inflammation for months to years, conjunctival cicatrization develops, along with in-turned eyelashes (trichiasis) and eyelid margins (entropion), obliteration of lacrimal gland ducts, and destruction of conjunctival goblet cells. These abnormalities combine to produce a dry eye, which, along with an abrasive effect from the scarred palpebral conjunctiva, create corneal scarring and vascularization (pannus). These changes eventually lead to blindness. Secondary bacterial keratitis further increases the risk of blindness. Laboratory diagnosis of the infection is made most often by fluorescent antibody examination of conjunctival cells obtained by a scraping.

Treatment of Acute Trachoma

Adults. Doxycycline or minocycline, 100 mg PO twice daily for 3 to 4 weeks, *or* tetracycline, 1.5 to 2.0 g PO in four doses for 3 to 4 weeks. Azithromycin has also been shown to be effective in a single dose of 20 mg/kg PO.[14]

Pregnant Women. Tetracycline or erythromycin ointment, two or three times daily for 2 months, *or* erythromycin, 500 mg PO every 8 hours for 3 to 4 weeks, or a combination of these.

Children Younger Than 8 Years. Tetracycline or erythromycin ophthalmic ointment twice daily for 2 months, *or* erythromycin, 40 mg/kg per day PO for 3 weeks.

The treatment of chronic trachoma is complicated and is best left to those with wide experience. The eradication of trachoma from endemic areas depends less on antibiotic treatment than on improvements in hygiene, including the availability of fresh running tap water.

INCLUSION CONJUNCTIVITIS

Inclusion conjunctivitis in adults is the most common sexually transmitted ocular disease in the United States. Clinically, the disease in adults and neonates is quite different. Adults have bilateral, low-grade, chronic follicular conjunctivitis that produces only mild discomfort and little or no exudate. Follicles larger than those of viral conjunctivitis are characteristically seen on the inferior palpebral conjunctiva (Fig. 155–4). The follicles persist for months without therapy, whereas follicles associated with viral infection resolve in a few weeks. Disease in neonates usually appears 7 to 10 days (range 5 to 13) after birth. A copious purulent exudate is typically seen, but no follicles form because the newborn has yet to develop a lymphoid system. If the disease smolders untreated for some months, epithelial keratitis may ensue and pannus may form. Ten percent to 20% of infected infants develop chlamydial pneumonitis, typically 3 to 6 weeks after birth, as the result of spread of the TRIC agent to the respiratory tract through the lacrimal outflow system. Otitis media is less common.

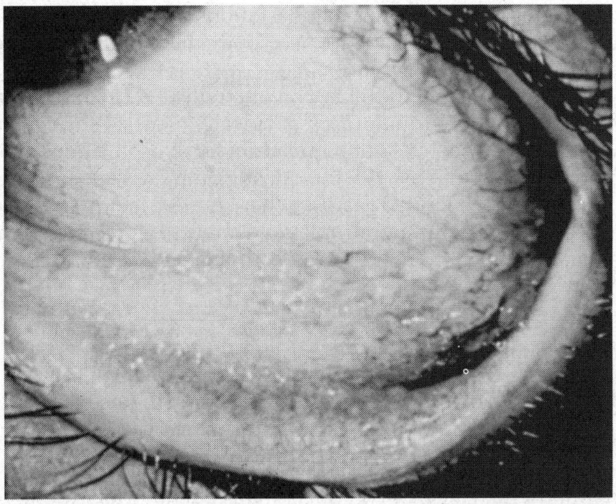

FIGURE 155–4 □ Large follicles on the inferior palpebral conjunctiva, typically seen in adult chlamydial (inclusion) conjunctivitis.

The differential diagnosis of conjunctivitis in the newborn (ophthalmia neonatorum) includes a number of infections that may be distinguished by the interval until onset of signs or symptoms: gonococcal conjunctivitis (2 to 5 days), chlamydial conjunctivitis (7 to 10 days), infection produced by other bacteria and herpes simplex virus (any time), chemical conjunctivitis (day 1) secondary to prophylactic instillation of silver nitrate.

Treatment

Neonates. Erythromycin at 50 mg/kg per day PO in four doses for 2 weeks.

Adults. Doxycycline at 100 mg PO twice daily for 7 days or azithromycin at 1 g PO once.

Pregnant Women. Erythromycin base at 500 mg four times daily for 7 days.

Prophylaxis of Ophthalmia Neonatorum

All infants should receive routine topical prophylaxis, in a single application, to prevent ophthalmia neonatorum.

Silver nitrate 1% drops (Credé method) are the traditional prophylactic for neonatal conjunctivitis. After instillation of the drops, the eyes should not be irrigated. Silver nitrate is active against gonococci but not against the TRIC agent. Because chlamydial conjunctivitis is more common in the United States than is gonococcal infection, some authorities have advocated the use of tetracycline or erythromycin ointment instilled within 1 hour of birth for prophylaxis; however, these two antibiotics are only partially effective in preventing neonates' conjunctivitis either chlamydial or gonococcal. Povidone-iodine 2.5% eyedrops were shown to be more effective than either silver nitrate or erythromycin for prophylaxis against *C. trachomatis* and as effective as the other two agents against *N. gonorrhoeae*.[15] Povidone-iodine was also less toxic and is less expensive than the other two agents.

Other Conjunctival Infections

Lymphogranuloma venereum, another sexually transmitted chlamydial infection, may cause Parinaud oculoglandular conjunctivitis. The ocular manifestations are usually unilateral. If the disease is not treated, both the conjunctiva and cornea may become scarred.

Parinaud oculoglandular conjunctivitis is a unilateral chronic granulomatous process; typically there is severe enlargement of the ipsilateral preauricular lymph node. Cat-scratch disease is by far the most common cause of the syndrome in the United States. Other causes include tuberculosis, syphilis, lymphogranuloma venereum, chancroid, tularemia, infectious mononucleosis, mumps, and various fungal infections.

Viral Conjunctivitis

ADENOVIRAL CONJUNCTIVITIS

In the United States, viral conjunctivitis is more common than either bacterial or chlamydial conjunctivitis. The most common viral cause of conjunctivitis is adenovirus. Adenoviral infection usually presents clinically as epidemic keratoconjunctivitis (EKC) or pharyngoconjunctival fever.

EKC, usually caused by adenovirus serotype 8 or 19, is an acute, usually bilateral infection that often affects persons aged 20 to 40 years. It is highly infectious and typically is seen in epidemics. Patients, their contacts, and school personnel should be educated about the substantial risk from contact with infected persons, contaminated objects, and swimming pools. The virus survives on dry surfaces for long periods. Infections are contagious for about 2 weeks.

The clinical hallmarks are a moderately severe follicular conjunctivitis with preauricular lymphadenopathy. Subconjunctival hemorrhages may also appear. Many patients develop keratitis 1 week after the onset of the conjunctivitis. The keratitis causes pain, photophobia, and increased lacrimation. Characteristic focal subepithelial corneal infiltrates are seen on slit-lamp examination (Fig. 155–5).

These infiltrates usually resolve without scarring after some weeks, but occasionally they persist, either symptomatically or asymptomatically. The conjunctivitis usually abates spontaneously after 2 to 3 weeks. Its course may be prolonged, however, by the development of a pseudomembrane on the palpebral conjunctiva.

Pharyngoconjunctival fever is principally a disease of children younger than 10 years. It is caused epidemically by adenovirus serotypes 3 and 7 and endemically by serotype 4. Typically the conjunctivitis is accompanied by malaise, sore throat, and fever. The ocular findings are similar to those of EKC, but the cornea is involved much less often. The issues of communicability are similar to those for EKC (see earlier). There is no specific therapy.

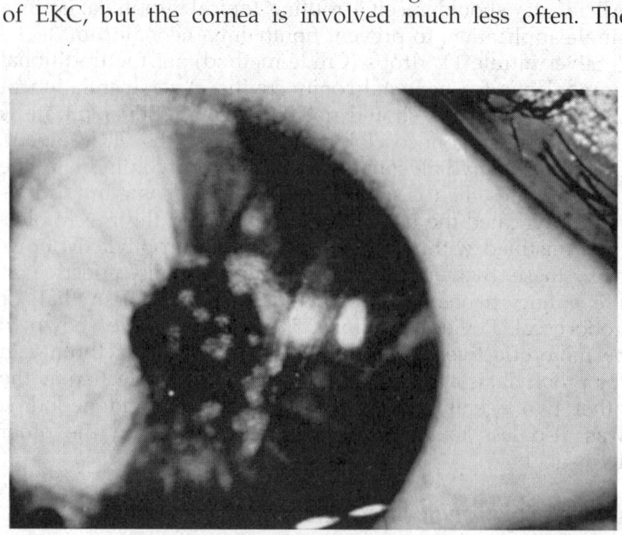

FIGURE 155–5 □ Subepithelial corneal infiltrates in a patient with epidemic keratoconjunctivitis (adenovirus).

OTHER VIRAL CONJUNCTIVITIDES

Acute hemorrhagic conjunctivitis was pandemic in the 1970s but is uncommon at present, for reasons unknown. The first outbreaks were caused by an enterovirus of serotype 70, but subsequent outbreaks were caused by coxsackievirus A24 and adenovirus 11. Typically there is fulminating bilateral conjunctivitis with severe eyelid edema, chemosis, extensive subconjunctival hemorrhage, and copious mucoid exudate. A follicular reaction and preauricular lymphadenopathy occur. Some patients develop punctate keratitis with photophobia, and there may be features suggestive of systemic involvement, including sore throat, malaise, headache, and myalgia. Rarely, Bell palsy and paralysis of the legs may develop. Ocular signs and symptoms generally resolve spontaneously within 2 weeks. There is no specific treatment.

Viruses, including herpes simplex virus, varicella-zoster virus, the agent of molluscum contagiosum, papillomavirus, and vaccinia virus, that produce blepharitis may also produce conjunctivitis. Other viruses that cause conjunctivitis include Epstein-Barr virus, cytomegalovirus, and the agents of measles, mumps, influenza, rubella, smallpox, and Newcastle disease (paramyxovirus). Measles keratitis, a punctate keratitis, resolves spontaneously but may be followed by secondary *H. influenzae* conjunctivitis; this is especially common in developing countries.

Corneal Infections

Corneal infections pose a serious risk of permanent loss of vision and perforation of the globe. Inflammation of the cornea (keratitis) often causes corneal scarring and opacification, and enzymes from microorganisms (e.g., collagenases and proteoglycanases) and neutrophils act to thin the corneal matrix. In developed countries the most common cause of infectious keratitis is herpes simplex virus; in developing countries bacteria and fungi are the usual agents. These latter types of infections are often secondary to trauma and trachoma. Keratitis caused by bacteria is usually more fulminant than infection caused by other agents and requires prompt diagnosis and treatment to reduce the threat to vision and the risk of perforation.

Bacterial Keratitis

The cornea is resistant to bacterial infection, in large part owing to the protective effect of the epithelium. Susceptibility of the cornea to infection is increased by corneal epithelial drying, trauma, or hypoxia. Drying may occur from increased evaporation, as in lagophthalmos or exophthalmos, or from decreased tearing, as in keratoconjunctivitis sicca. Hypoxia of the corneal epithelium may occur in patients who wear soft contact lenses for prolonged periods or during sleep. Diabetes and the use of corticosteroids and immunosuppressive drugs are other risk factors for corneal infection.

The most common bacterial agents of corneal ulcers are *S. aureus* and *Staphylococcus epidermidis.* Other frequently encountered pathogens are *S. pneumoniae,* α- and β-hemolytic streptococci, *Pseudomonas aeruginosa,* and *Bacillus cereus.* An association has been observed between the wearing of extended-wear soft contact lenses and the development of corneal ulcers caused by *P. aeruginosa;* indeed, more than 50% of corneal ulcers in wearers of extended-wear soft contact lenses are caused by *P. aeruginosa.*

P. aeruginosa keratitis must be dealt with promptly, as the organisms produce a proteoglycanase that can cause corneal perforation within a few days.[15, 15a] *B. cereus* keratitis is perhaps the most fulminant of corneal infections; it typically occurs in rural areas after trauma.[16] Less common pathogens include *Serratia marcescens*, other gram-negative bacilli, *Neisseria* species, *M. lacunata* (in derelict populations), *Mycobacterium fortuitum* and *Mycobacterium chelonae*, and anaerobic species of bacteria.

In a typical case of bacterial corneal ulcer, the patient experiences ocular pain, lacrimation, and photophobia. The eye is red and there is a milk-white corneal infiltrate. The surrounding cornea is hazy (edematous; Fig. 155–6), the eyelids are swollen, and the pupil is miotic. A hypopyon may be present.

APPROACH TO THE MANAGEMENT OF CORNEAL ULCER

Identification of the Specific Agent. Before treatment is begun the infiltrate should be scraped with a platinum spatula or a calcium alginate swab to obtain material for Gram stain, Grocott methenamine silver stain to detect fungi,[17] and culture.

Empirical Treatment (Table 155–3). We recommend empirical treatment initially with a broad-spectrum antibiotic regimen. We usually use two antibiotics that are active against the most likely pathogens. This broad-spectrum approach is advocated because of the need to institute therapy before the results of culture are available and because of the relatively poor correlation between the results of Gram stain and culture.[18]

Topical fluoroquinolones are likely to be highly effective against the more commonly encountered gram-positive and gram-negative corneal pathogens, except that streptococcal infections occasionally fail to respond. Third-generation cephalosporins are quite active against gram-negative bacteria, but their efficacy in the treatment of bacterial keratitis has not been proved clinically. Cefazolin plus either gentamicin or tobramycin has been commonly employed.[19] If *P. aeruginosa* infection is suspected initially (e.g., because of extended-wear soft contact lenses), tobramycin plus piperacillin, ticarcillin, or ceftazidime[19, 19a] is suggested.[6] Tobramycin is preferred over gentamicin in this instance because of its greater anti-*Pseudomonas* activity.

Topical Treatment by Frequent Administration of Fortified Antibiotic Eyedrops. Except for the fluoroquinolones, antibiotic eyedrops that are available commercially are not likely to be as effective as the more concentrated solutions that hospital pharmacists can prepare.[6] For initial treatment, eyedrops are usually instilled every 15 to 30 minutes around the clock for the first 2 or 3 days. Another method, perhaps less fatiguing to the patient, hospital staff, and family, is to administer one antibiotic, one drop every minute for five doses, to wait for 5 minutes, and then to instill the second antibiotic in a similar manner. After a period of 45 minutes the process is repeated. It should be remembered that an eye can hold only one drop and that a 5-minute interval should be allowed between the administration of different preparations of eyedrops to avoid a washout effect. Animal studies have verified that when concentrated antibiotic eyedrops are instilled frequently, bactericidal corneal drug levels are achieved and bacterial counts are sharply and promptly reduced.[20, 21] Experimental and clinical studies suggest that dehydrated bovine or porcine collagen corneal shields, when rehydrated in an antibiotic solution and applied as a contact

TABLE 155–3 ■ Treatment of Bacterial Corneal Ulcers

A. *Initial empirical therapy for suspected bacterial corneal ulcers (see text)*
  1. Low suspicion of *Pseudomonas aeruginosa*
     Topical:
       Ciprofloxacin (or ofloxacin), 3 mg/mL* alone
       or
       Ciprofloxacin (or ofloxacin), 3 mg/mL,* *plus* cefazolin drops, 50 mg/mL
       or
       Gentamicin or tobramycin, 10–20 mg/mL, *plus* cefazolin, 50 mg/mL
     In patients allergic to β-lactam drugs, vancomycin (25–50 mg/mL) or bacitracin (10,000 units/mL) can be substituted for cefazolin.
     Subconjunctival (see text for indications): cefazolin, 100 mg, or vancomycin, 25 mg, in 0.5 mL; gentamicin or tobramycin, 40 mg in 0.5 mL
  2. High suspicion of *P. aeruginosa*†
     Topical:
       Tobramycin, 10–20 mg/mL, *plus* ticarcillin or piperacillin, 6–20 mg/mL, or ceftazidime, 50 mg/mL
     In patients allergic to β-lactam drugs, aztreonam, 10–50 mg/mL, might be substituted for ticarcillin, piperacillin, or ceftazidime, but there is no published experience in this regard.
     Subconjunctival (see text for indications): piperacillin or ceftazidime, 100 mg in 0.5 mL; tobramycin, 40 mg in 0.5 mL
  3. Continue treatment or until culture report and clinical conditions suggest change
  4. Cycloplegia
  5. Consider use of anticollagenase treatment and cyanoacrylate glue

B. *Antibiotic choices for defined pathogen*
  Change treatment only if pathogen is resistant in vitro to the antibiotics being administered and there is failure of clinical response.
  1. Staphylococcus (penicillin resistant, oxacillin susceptible)
     Topical: vancomycin, 33 mg/mL, or bacitracin, 10,000 units/mL
     Subconjunctival (see text for indications): cefazolin, 100 mg, oxacillin, 100 mg, or vancomycin, 25 mg
  2. Staphylococcus (penicillin-susceptible) or streptococcus
     Similar to treatment for penicillin-resistant staphylococcus; for subconjunctival injection, penicillin G, 1 million units, may be used instead of the agents listed above
  3. Gram-negative
     Topical: gentamicin or tobramycin, 10–20 mg/mL, or quinolone (ciprofloxacin or ofloxacin), 3 mg/mL*
     Subconjunctival (see text for indications): gentamicin or tobramycin, 40 mg (0.5 mL), *possibly with* ticarcillin or piperacillin or ceftazidime, 100 mg (0.5 mL)

*Commercially available.
†For example, in wearers of extended-wear soft contact lenses.
Modified from Glaser DB, Baum J: Bacterial keratitis. *In* Stenson SM (ed): Surgical Management of External Eye Disease. New York: Igaku-Shoin, 1995, p 127.

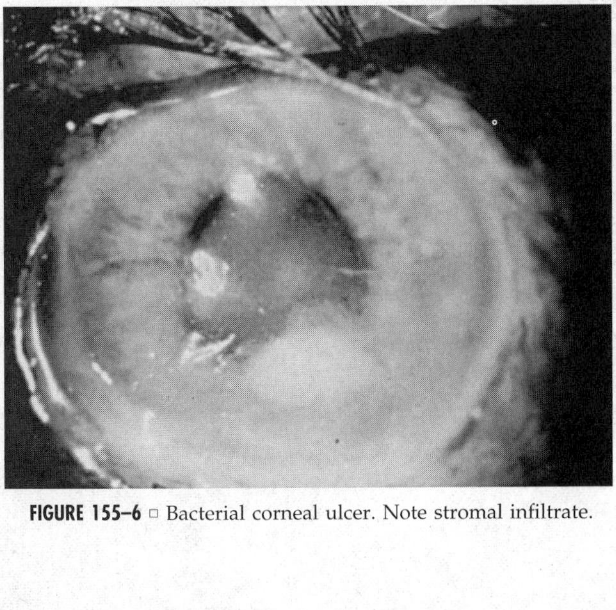

FIGURE 155–6 □ Bacterial corneal ulcer. Note stromal infiltrate.

lens, may be as good as or better than eyedrops as a delivery system.

In studies in animals, subconjunctival injections, which in the past were frequently used for the treatment of corneal ulcers, have been found to be no more effective than frequently administered concentrated antibiotic eyedrops.[20, 21] These injections are now used principally when compliance is in doubt or to treat infections in infants and small children, who frequently squeeze out the eyedrops and dilute them as they cry. Orally or parenterally administered antibiotics produce only modest corneal concentrations and probably offer little or no benefit to patients who are being treated with intensive topical applications of concentrated eyedrops. In special circumstances, however, as in gonococcal keratitis, or when the cornea has perforated, or the infection has spread to involve the sclera, parenteral as well as topical therapy is suggested.

Fungal Keratitis

The incidence of fungal keratitis is lower than that of either bacterial or viral keratitis. Fungal keratitis is more common in warmer climates and in rural areas. It often follows trauma to the cornea, especially by vegetable matter or objects contaminated by soil. Topical application of corticosteroids may predispose to fungal keratitis.[22] Unlike most nonocular fungal infections, many fungal corneal infections are due to filamentous species, particularly the nonpigmented *Fusarium solani.* This species often causes infection after minor trauma to the cornea. In northern climates and in immunosuppressed patients whose corneal epithelium has been compromised by decreased sensation, exposure, or drying, *Candida albicans* infection is not uncommon. Less frequent causes of infection include *Aspergillus fumigatus* and *Alternaria, Curvularia,* and *Acremonium* species.

A corneal fungal infiltrate typically enlarges slowly during a period of weeks and has characteristic fine feathery margins, heaped-up edges, and adjacent satellite lesions (Fig. 155–7). The clinical diagnosis is confirmed by scraping material from the lesion and observing fungal elements with methenamine silver stain[17] and by culture of material in Sabouraud medium without cyclohexamide, an inhibitor to growth of filamentous species. Sometimes the scraping fails to demonstrate the pathogen, which may reside in the posterior corneal stroma, in which case examination of a corneal biopsy specimen may be necessary to prove the diagnosis.

The outcome of treatment of fungal keratitis has often been poor. The laboratory may be slow to identify the pathogen, which delays treatment; in some instances cultures fail to yield the organism, so specific treatment is not given. A corneal biopsy must often be obtained when a scraping for cultural identification is negative. In the past, it was usual to administer amphotericin B in eyedrops in a concentration of 1% to 5%.[23] The high concentration of the desoxycholate solubilizer makes such solutions irritating, and they may damage the cornea. Noncompliance may also have contributed to the unsatisfactory results with these eyedrops. Studies suggest that treatment with eyedrops containing much lower concentrations of amphotericin B (0.05% to 0.15%) produces a good clinical response in keratitis caused by a variety of species of fungi and is tolerated well.[24] Amphotericin B eyedrops usually are given at the rate of one drop each hour while the patient is awake. Treatment should be continued for 3 to 6 weeks if there is improvement, after which time the frequency of administration is gradually reduced. Oral flucytosine has been used on occasion to supplement therapy with amphotericin B in the treatment of *Candida* keratitis. Natamycin eyedrops, in the form of a 5% suspension, are effective in the treatment of superficial *Fusarium* keratitis but less effective for deeper corneal infections because the drug penetrates the corneal stroma poorly. The imidazoles are variably effective against a wide range of pathogens. Ketoconazole, 200 to 400 mg/d PO for adults or as a 2% eyedrop suspension every 30 to 60 minutes for 3 to 6 weeks, has in large part replaced or supplemented miconazole. Fluconazole may be an even better choice. Despite the availability of a number of agents, at present we prefer dilute preparations of amphotericin B eyedrops for the treatment of fungal keratitis.

Viral Keratitis

Of all forms of infectious keratitis in developed countries, herpes simplex keratitis is unquestionably the most prevalent and carries the highest rate of morbidity.[3] This section addresses herpes simplex and herpes zoster keratitis. Other viral diseases that sometimes affect the cornea but primarily affect the conjunctiva are discussed earlier in the section on viral conjunctivitis.

HERPES SIMPLEX KERATITIS

The pathogenesis of herpes simplex keratitis is complex and continues to be the subject of extensive basic investigation.

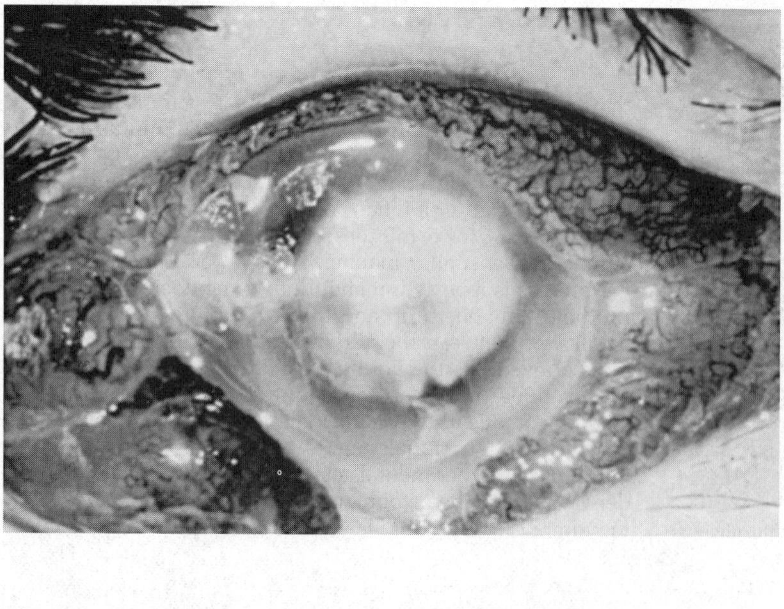

FIGURE 155–7 □ Fungal ulcer of the cornea. Note satellite lesions.

Most clinically significant episodes of herpes keratitis occur in adults, but they are thought to be sequelae of subclinical primary infections that occur quite early in life, perhaps in infancy.[25] Humans are the only natural host for the virus. After the primary infection, the virus becomes dormant in nervous tissue (e.g., trigeminal or ciliary ganglion) for years. Various stimuli—sunlight, fever, trauma, other infection, various forms of stress, and corticosteroid therapy—can trigger the dormant virus to produce infectious particles, which travel from ganglia through nerves to the cornea to produce recurrent corneal infection. Investigations have raised the additional possibility that latent virus resides in corneal stromal cells and that recurrent corneal disease follows reactivation from this source.[26] This hypothesis perhaps better explains recurrent corneal infection but not the recurrent infections in other ocular tissues that are innervated by branches of the trigeminal nerve. There is some evidence to suggest that certain strains of herpes simplex virus are more likely than others to lead to recurrent infection and that infection with a strain with a low potential for recurrence may be protective against infection by a strain with a high potential for recurrence.[25] Evidence also suggests that properties of the individual strain determine the number and shape of the dendritic epithelial lesions and that both the virus and the host response determine the stromal manifestations.[25]

Herpes simplex virus type 1 accounts for the majority of infections seen in children and for the vast majority of those in adults. By contrast, type 2 strains are responsible for most illness in neonates, who are infected during passage through the birth canal. Type 2 strains seem to produce more severe disease than type 1 strains in both adults and neonates.

In children and neonates, clinically evident primary herpes simplex virus infection of the eye characteristically involves the eyelid and conjunctiva but only rarely the cornea. The process is usually benign and self-limited, is most often unilateral, and generally lasts 1 to 2 weeks. The corneal epithelium, when involved in primary infection, displays punctate lesions or typical dendrites with fluorescein staining. Stromal involvement is rare, possibly because it is immunologically mediated and the immune response to the virus is not well developed at the time of primary infection. By contrast, recurrent herpes simplex infection in adults may affect all corneal layers and the uveal tract and almost always is monocular. Typically, the initial attack of keratitis in the adult produces dendritic figures (Fig. 155–8). When the cornea is examined at an early stage of infection after being stained with fluorescein, the dendritic figures are thin and seem to terminate in bulbs. The epithelium is hypoesthetic. With effective antiviral therapy, the dendrites resolve within 1 to 2 weeks but sometimes leave a "ghost" imprint, which fades during a period of weeks. Especially in adults, the stroma may be involved, most often displaying a ground-glass appearance related to edema. Less commonly, cellular infiltration predominates and the infiltrate appears more densely white. Stromal involvement is more serious than epithelial involvement, being more intractable, and scarring of the stroma may result in permanent loss of vision.

The major component of herpetic stromal disease is thought to be a manifestation of delayed hypersensitivity. Viral antigens, arising either from a reservoir in the epithelial cells or by retrograde spread from ganglia via peripheral nerves to the cornea, have been found in the stromal matrix and in stromal keratocytes.[27] Stromal edema (disciform keratitis) develops when sensitized lymphocytes are activated by viral antigen.

Viral subunits have been identified in human stromal tissue at times of reactivation.[26] In addition to stimulating delayed hypersensitivity, particles may trigger complement-mediated damage in the form of corneal infiltrates and "immune

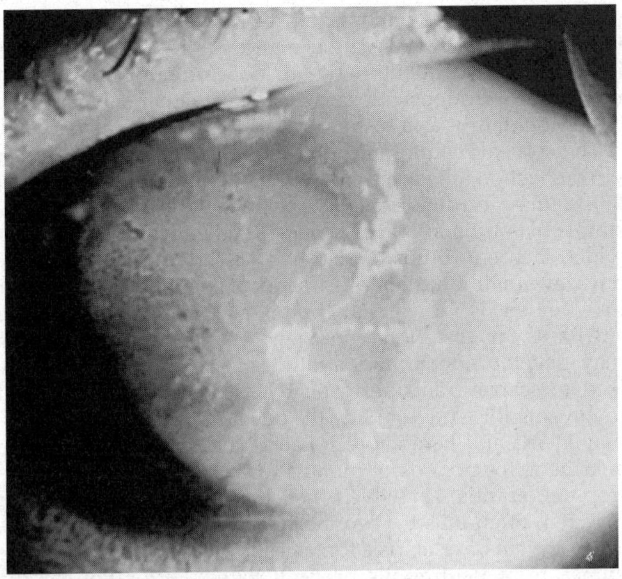

FIGURE 155–8 □ Dendritic figures (stained with fluorescein) characteristic of herpes simplex dendritic (epithelial) keratitis.

rings."[26] Even with optimal treatment, there is a 25% to 50% incidence of stromal reactivation within 2 years of an attack, and often the stromal recurrence may last weeks to months. The development of keratic precipitates on the endothelium, flare and cells in the aqueous humor, and elevated intraocular pressure are manifestations of corneal endothelial and uveal tract involvement.

The treatment of herpes simplex keratitis may be divided into two components, a regimen for epithelial disease, which is relatively easy to treat, and stromal involvement, for which treatment is difficult and multifactorial. Epithelial dendritic keratitis without stromal involvement typically responds well to topical antiviral therapy. Trifluoridine, which is available as an eyedrop, initially is given at a frequency of one drop an hour for 9 hours. It appears to be slightly more effective than vidarabine, which is available topically only as an ointment and is usually given five times a day. The large majority of patients show a good response to treatment as manifested by relief of symptoms and the beginning of resolution of the dendrites within 48 hours. Topical acyclovir, not yet commercially available in the United States, has proved to be at least as effective as trifluorthymidine[3] in the treatment of herpes simplex keratitis and is the least toxic of all the antiviral agents. An oral preparation has therapeutic value in treating severe herpes simplex keratouveitis.[28] In patients whose response is poor, epithelial débridement is usually undertaken to reduce the viral load. Stromal keratitis, a refractory infection with a tendency to recur, is usually treated with topical corticosteroids and a topical antiviral agent. The addition of oral acyclovir to this regimen appears to offer no benefit.[29]

VARICELLA-ZOSTER KERATITIS

Recurrent (recrudescent) varicella-zoster virus infection of the eye occurs 20 times more frequently along the distribution of the ophthalmic division of the trigeminal nerve than in either the maxillary or mandibular branches. Approximately 60% of patients with involvement of the skin in the distribution of the ophthalmic division of the trigeminal nerve develop varicella-zoster virus keratitis. Severe ocular pain may precede signs of ocular and cutaneous infection. Ocular manifestations involve principally the cornea. In immunocompromised patients, most often those afflicted with lymphoma, other ocular tissues and cranial nerves may be involved. Even patients who are not immunocompromised may develop iridocyclitis and glaucoma, either subsequently or concomitantly, as a result of varicella-zoster virus keratitis.

The corneal manifestations of recrudescent varicella-zoster virus infection are varied. The epithelium may develop punctate staining or dendrites (which differ from those of herpes simplex keratitis in that the processes are fewer, shorter, and wider, lack end bulbs, and usually disappear within a few days, even without therapy). The most common site of ocular involvement is the corneal stroma, and involvement of this site has the most serious consequences for vision. The stroma may develop edema and infiltrates, which may eventually lead to scarring and permanent loss of vision. Endothelial involvement is suggested by the development of diffuse stromal edema and keratic precipitates. The cornea may become anesthetic for periods of months to well over a year (neurotrophic keratitis), in which case the corneal epithelium, if abraded, often fails to reepithelialize or does so only slowly. Such patients are at risk for digestion of the cornea by enzymes from neutrophils or keratocytes. Perforation of the cornea may occur unless the process is recognized and arrested.

Acyclovir is effective in treating both ocular and cutaneous components of the infection. A dose of 600 mg PO, five times a day for 10 days, reduces virus shedding and pain, provided that treatment is started within 3 days of the appearance of the skin lesion. Famciclovir, 500 mg PO three times a day for 10 days, appears to be as effective as acyclovir. Oral cimetidine may help reduce pain if started within 2 to 3 days after onset of the infection.

Acanthamoeba *Keratitis*

It has been almost 25 years since the first reports were published of *Acanthamoeba* keratitis.[30, 31] In the past, the disease was often misdiagnosed as herpes simplex keratitis. Fewer than 200 cases have been reported, but many authorities suspect that the disease is more common than the number of reports would suggest.

Acanthamoeba organisms are free-living protozoa commonly found in soil, air, and water. They are hardy and survive extremes of temperature (−20°C to 42°C). Under adverse conditions, the trophozoites revert to an inactive cyst form, both in the cornea and in the environment. *Acanthamoeba polyphaga* and *Acanthamoeba castellani* are the most common isolates from corneal infections.

The risk factors for *Acanthamoeba* keratitis are trauma to the corneal epithelium, which may result from wearing soft contact lenses, and exposure to the parasite, which may occur through swimming or the use of hot tubs or contaminated contact lens solutions. Clinically, the earliest sign of corneal infection is an atypical "abrasion," in which the epithelium appears shaggy and does not heal quickly (Wright P, personal communication, 1990). It is at this stage that the prompt institution of appropriate therapy, after laboratory identification of amoebae, leads to the greatest likelihood of a nonsurgical cure. Without specific therapy, the process waxes and wanes but gradually worsens. A foreign body sensation gives way to intense pain, which is out of proportion to the signs. The epithelium cyclically heals and breaks down and the corneal stroma becomes hazy. Typically, an arclike or anular stromal infiltrate develops (Fig. 155–9) many weeks after the onset of the disease, and there is severe iritis with or without hypopyon.

The diagnosis is confirmed by placing the scraped fragments of infected tissue on a microscope slide, staining the material with calcofluor white, and visualizing the characteristic cysts under a fluorescence microscope.[32, 33] Confocal microscopy is a useful in vivo technique for the visualization of intrastromal cysts. Material may be cultured on nonnutrient agar (e.g., agar seeded with a gram-negative bacterium such as *E. coli*).

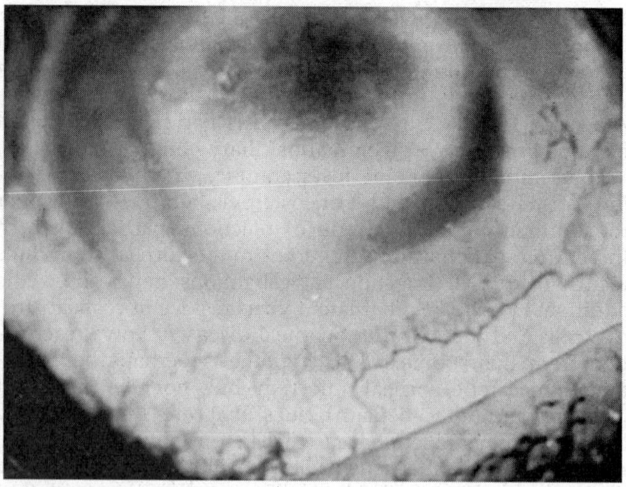

FIGURE 155–9 □ *Acanthamoeba* keratitis. Note typical anular appearance with less dense central area.

The earlier treatment is begun, the greater is the potential for cure by drug therapy. If treatment is delayed, the results of all therapies are usually disappointing but a combination of surgical treatment and chemotherapy appears to be the most effective approach.[34] Although dozens of drugs are active against the protozoa in vitro, most produce a poor response in patients.

Standard therapy consists of 0.1% propamidine isethionate eyedrops, and 5% neomycin eyedrops (or the commercially available combination of neomycin–gramicidin–polymyxin B eyedrops).[35] The drugs are alternated every 15 to 60 minutes for 5 to 7 days, after which the frequency of instillation is decreased gradually during a period of weeks as the clinical condition stabilizes and then improves. It is suggested that treatment be given for 5 to 9 months in an attempt to sterilize the infection.[36, 37] Two new agents, polyhexamethylene biguanide[38] 0.02% and chlorhexidine[39] 0.02%, have been shown to be possibly more effective than other therapies. The former agent is sold in the United States as Bacquicil (ICI Americas, Wilmington, Delaware), a swimming pool disinfectant. Only anecdotal information exists for the efficacy of these new agents in combinations with other drugs. If medical therapy fails, a penetrating keratoplasty followed by additional drug therapy has proved effective.[34] The value of topical corticosteroid therapy is still undetermined. Eyedrops of 1% clotrimazole have also been shown to be effective clinically.[40] The efficacy of topical miconazole or paramomycin and of oral ketoconazole has yet to be clearly defined.

Infection of the Lacrimal Apparatus

Dacryoadenitis

The anatomy of the lacrimal system is shown in Figure 155–10. Infection of the lacrimal gland, dacryoadenitis, is usually caused by bacteria, but occasionally by viruses, fungi, or parasites. Fungal and parasitic infections are rare in developed countries. The most common bacterial cause is *S. aureus*. Less common agents are streptococci, gonococci, *Mycobacterium tuberculosis*, and *Treponema pallidum*. The most common

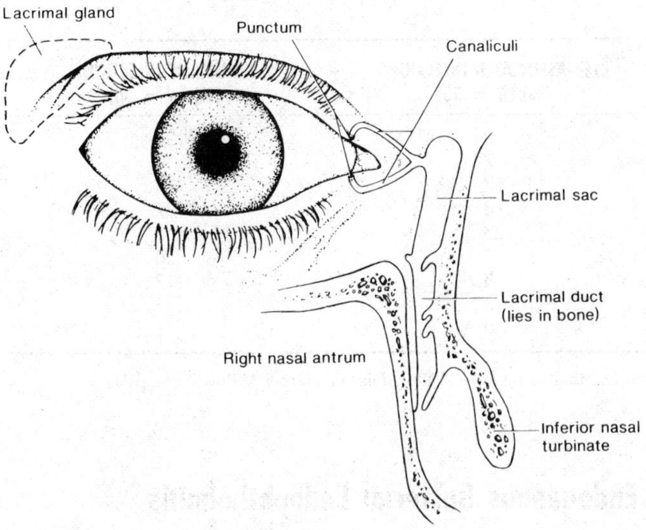

FIGURE 155–10 □ Schematic diagram of the lacrimal apparatus. (From Barza M, Baum J: Ocular infections. Med Clin North Am 67:131–152, 1983.)

viral causes of dacryoadenitis are mumps virus and Epstein-Barr virus.

Acute dacryoadenitis caused by staphylococci and streptococci produces swelling, pain, and tenderness over the lateral portion of the upper lid. Fever and malaise are often present. The other species characteristically produce subacute or chronic disease, with swelling of the gland but few other symptoms. Treatment is usually empirical, because the pathogen is often sequestered in deeper tissue and not evident in conjunctival cultures; however, material for Gram stain examination and culture may be obtained by inserting a fine needle into the gland and aspirating fluid. Treatment should be started immediately after the clinical diagnosis has been made. Acute bacterial infections should be treated for 4 to 7 days with parenteral antibiotics that are active against *S. aureus* and streptococci. If there is an abscess, hot packs should be used and surgical incision may be required.

Canaliculitis

Infection of the small ducts that carry tears from the eye to the lacrimal sac is termed canaliculitis. The most common cause is *Actinomyces israelii.* Fungi (*Candida, Aspergillus*), bacteria (streptococci), viruses (herpes simplex virus, varicella-zoster virus), and TRIC are occasional causes of canaliculitis. Stasis within the outflow tract, which may occur in infants because of congenital pouches, increases the risk of infection.

Pain, swelling, and erythema at the inner third of the upper or lower eyelid accompanied by tearing are present in varying degrees. In some instances, mucopurulent exudate can be expressed through an abnormally dilated lacrimal punctum by finger pressure against the skin overlying the lacrimal sac. When *A. israelii* is the pathogen, cheesy white concretions can often be expressed. The ophthalmologist treats *A. israelii* infection by irrigating the outflow tract with 10% sulfacetamide eyedrops introduced through the punctum using a cannula attached to a syringe. Penicillin G at 100,000 units/mL and clindamycin at 10 mg/mL are alternative antibiotics.

Dacryocystitis

Infection of the lacrimal sac, or dacryocystitis, is the most common infection of the lacrimal system. The most common agents are gram-positive bacteria, especially *S. pneumoniae* and *S. aureus.* Other pathogens include *H. influenzae, P. aeruginosa,* and *Proteus mirabilis.* Fungi such as *C. albicans* and *Aspergillus* species are less frequent causes. As with canaliculitis, stasis within the lacrimal outflow tract increases the risk of infection.

Infection of the lacrimal sac may be either acute or chronic. With acute infection, the patient experiences localized pain and tearing. The lacrimal sac and overlying tissues are erythematous, swollen, and tender. With chronic infection, as is usually the case in newborns, symptoms are typically absent except for tearing. The lacrimal sac area usually looks normal but may be swollen. Clues to chronic infection include a dilated lacrimal punctum and regurgitation of exudate from the punctum after finger pressure applied to the skin overlying the lacrimal sac. When the disease is acute, the organisms are located in the wall of the sac and the infection is best treated by parenteral or oral administration of antibiotics. When the disease is chronic, the organisms reside in the lumen of the sac and are most effectively eradicated by irrigation of antibiotics through the punctum.

ENDOPHTHALMITIS

Endophthalmitis means inflammation *within* the eye. In common usage, the term denotes an intraocular infection involving the vitreous humor. In this chapter, both exogenous and endogenous (metastatic) bacterial and fungal endophthalmitis are discussed. Infections that primarily affect the retina and choroid but not the vitreous humor, such as cytomegalovirus infection and toxoplasmosis, are not addressed. For a more comprehensive review of bacterial endophthalmitis, the reader is referred elsewhere.[41–47]

Most cases of bacterial endophthalmitis arise after cataract surgery and accidental trauma. A smaller number follow infection of a conjunctival bleb constructed surgically to alleviate glaucoma or by hematogenous spread from an infection elsewhere. Endophthalmitis almost never occurs as a complication of periorbital infection and only rarely is the result of bacterial conjunctivitis, mainly meningococcal conjunctivitis. Endophthalmitis is among the most injurious of ocular infections and, except for cytomegalovirus retinitis in a patient with human immunodeficiency virus infection, is the one with the poorest prognosis for vision.

Most studies suggest that the incidence of postcataract bacterial endophthalmitis is approximately 0.1% to 0.5%,[48–50] but these estimates may be too low because of underreporting or too high because some cases are not confirmed by culture and could represent instances of sterile postoperative inflammation (iridocyclitis). The incidence of exogenous bacterial and fungal endophthalmitis after other types of injury is not clear; however, two studies reported a 2% to 3% incidence of bacterial endophthalmitis after traumatic penetration of the globe.[51, 52]

Exogenous Bacterial Endophthalmitis

Table 155–4 shows a comparison of the bacterial species isolated from patients with exogenous endophthalmitis after various forms of surgical and nonsurgical trauma. In endophthalmitis after cataract extraction, *S. epidermidis* is the most common bacterial isolate, followed by *S. aureus,* streptococcal species, and a variety of gram-negative organisms, including

TABLE 155–4 ■ Microbiology of Endophthalmitis

ORGANISM	POSTOPERATIVE INFECTIONS (%) (N = 63)	BLEB-ASSOCIATED INFECTIONS (%) (N = 30)	TRAUMATIC INFECTIONS (%) (N = 30)
Staphylococcus epidermidis	38	0	20
Staphylococcus aureus	21	7	0
Streptococcus spp.	11	57	13
Bacillus spp.	0	0	27
Haemophilus influenzae	3	23	0
Other gram-negative species	13	7	20
Fungi	8	3	17
Other	6	3	3
Mixed flora	2	0	11

Modified from Forster RK: Endophthalmitis. *In* Duane TD, JaegerAE (eds): Clinical Ophthalmology, Vol 4. Philadelphia, Harper & Row, 1994, p 11.

Pseudomonas and *Proteus* species and *H. influenzae, S. marcescens,* and *E. coli.*[53] Data from the Endophthalmitis Vitrectomy Study,[54, 54a] to be discussed in the section on treatment of endophthalmitis, show a similar distribution of pathogens after cataract extraction. Among the approximately 70% of patients in that study with "confirmed" growth from the eye, the major infecting species were coagulase-negative staphylococci (70%), *S. aureus* (10%), and streptococcal species (11.5%); gram-negative species were found in about 6%.[54a] Patients with filtering blebs after surgery for glaucoma are at special risk for streptococcal and *H. influenzae* endophthalmitis, in part because the thin wall of the bleb facilitates penetration of the globe by the pathogen[55] and in part because of the common postoperative prophylactic use of topical aminoglycosides, which have limited activity against streptococci. The most common pathogen in endophthalmitis associated with accidental trauma is *B. cereus,* followed by other *Bacillus* species; staphylococci, especially *S. epidermidis; Streptococcus* species; various gram-negative species; and anaerobes.[52, 56] Endophthalmitis caused by obligately anaerobic bacteria is rare. In a series of 18 cases of endophthalmitis caused by anaerobes, *Propionibacterium acnes* was isolated in 14 cases and, in 10, was the only pathogen isolated.[57] In the remaining cases, it was part of a polymicrobial infection. Polymicrobial infection is uncommon.[58] Of special note are reports of a low-grade *P. acnes* endophthalmitis, appearing as long as 10 months after extracapsular cataract extraction.[59, 60] The bacteria seem to be sequestered in residual lens cortex. The onset of the clinical infection may, at times, be triggered by subtle events such as laser therapy.

TABLE 155–5 ■ Site of Primary Infection in Patients Developing Metastatic Bacterial Endophthalmitis

	108 PATIENTS 1935–1975		72 PATIENTS 1976–1985	
PRIMARY INFECTION	N	%	N	%
Meningitis	59	55	19	26
Endocarditis	1–2	—	10	14
Urinary tract	7	6	10	14
Gastrointestinal tract or abdomen	—	—	8	11
Skin	12	11	5	7
Lungs	9	8	4	6
Puerperium	6	6	—	—
Other	15*	14	16	22

*Including endocarditis.
Data from references 46 and 47.

Endogenous Bacterial Endophthalmitis

Endogenous (metastatic) bacterial endophthalmitis is now much rarer than in the preantibiotic era. Furthermore, the clinical characteristics of patients with this form of endophthalmitis are different from those before the advent of antibiotics.[46, 47] Two risk factors, immunosuppression and IV drug abuse, which were rare 50 years ago, are contributing factors today. The infection is presumed to arise by hematogenous spread although, in some patients, bacteremia cannot be demonstrated. Tables 155–5 and 155–6 compare the sites of primary infection and the pathogens for the years 1935 to 1975 and 1976 to 1985. In the preantibiotic era, meningitis was the most common primary infection associated with endogenous endophthalmitis, and *N. meningitidis* was the most common infecting organism. The pattern has changed and a wide variety of sources and infecting organisms have been reported.[47, 61] A striking association is a fulminant endophthalmitis caused by *B. cereus* in injection drug users. In one series, not shown in the tables, diabetes mellitus was the most common underlying medical disorder, streptococcal species were the most common infecting group of organisms (although *S. aureus* was the most common single species), and endocarditis and the gastrointestinal tract were the most

TABLE 155–6 ■ Pathogens in Metastatic Bacterial Endophthalmitis in Two Time Periods

	1935–1975		1976–1985	
ORGANISM	N	%	N	%
Streptococcus pneumoniae	14	13	2	3
Streptococcus spp.	9	8	10	14
Staphylococcus aureus	11	10	7	10
Bacillus cereus	1		11	15
Listeria monocytogenes	1		3	4
Clostridium perfringens	1		—	
Neisseria meningitidis	56	52	8	11
Haemophilus influenzae	—		7	
Actinobacillus spp.	—		2	
Escherichia coli	4	3.7	5	7
Klebsiella pneumoniae	1		5	
Serratia spp.	—		3	4
Salmonella spp.	—		3	
Pseudomonas aeruginosa	2		2	
Proteus spp.	2		—	
Nocardia asteroides	6	5.5	3	
Unidentified	—		1	

Data from references 46 and 47.

common sources of infection.[61] Vitreous cultures and blood cultures are each positive in about three fourths of patients.[47, 61] Because the ocular symptoms (decreased vision, floaters, redness, discharge, eye pain, headache) and systemic symptoms are usually vague, at least initially, in most patients, the diagnosis of endogenous endophthalmitis is often made relatively late.[61] About 75% to 85% of infections are unilateral, and the right eye is almost twice as likely to be infected as the left,[47, 61] probably because of the shorter, more direct arterial route from the carotid artery to the right eye. The overall visual prognosis for endogenous endophthalmitis is poor. There is some suggestion that early treatment with intravitreal injection of antibiotics and vitrectomy may be of some benefit.[61] Treatment of the primary infection, usually with IV antibiotics, is also indicated.

Fungal Endophthalmitis

There are many fewer cases of fungal than of bacterial endophthalmitis. In contrast to bacterial endophthalmitis, fungal endophthalmitis is more often endogenous than exogenous. The most common pathogen is *C. albicans. Aspergillus* species are the second most common isolates, *A. fumigatus* being more commonly found than *Aspergillus flavus.*[61a] A variety of other fungi occasionally are seen.

The incidence of endogenous fungal endophthalmitis has increased in the past few decades, in large part owing to increased use of parenteral hyperalimentation, hemodialysis, urinary and intravenous catheters, and immunosuppressive agents and a rise in the incidence of immunosuppressive diseases, such as acquired immunodeficiency syndrome, all of which are risk factors for fungal infection. The increased frequency of injection drug use, with the potential for injection of contaminated material, is another important risk factor. In a review of the world's literature on endogenous *Candida* endophthalmitis, blood cultures were positive in 41 of 100 patients.[62]

Exogenous fungal endophthalmitis is most frequently seen after cataract surgery. The pathogens include *Candida, Aspergillus, Cephalosporium, Penicillium,* and *Curvularia* species, among others. Contaminated lots of solutions containing commercial intraocular lenses have been responsible for the two largest series of cases. Thirteen cases of *Paecilomyces lilacinus*[63] and 15 cases of *Candida parapsilosis*[64] infection followed use of contaminated solutions to store intraocular lenses or to adjust the pH of lenses immediately before implantation.

Clinical Manifestations

Bacterial endophthalmitis is most often seen after cataract surgery. Although the clinical presentation is influenced by a variety of factors, the onset of symptoms typically occurs 2 to 5 days after surgery, at which time the patient may experience decreased vision, increased ocular pain, and headache. There are no systemic symptoms except in cases involving *B. cereus,* when fever and malaise may be present. Ocular signs include lid edema, increasing conjunctival injection, corneal haze, increasing flare and cells in the anterior chamber with or without hypopyon, and, most important, increasing haziness of the vitreous humor with a decreased or absent red reflex because of infiltration by polymorphonuclear leukocytes. Organisms of low virulence, such as *S. epidermidis, Achromobacter,* and *P. acnes,*[60] have been associated with a delayed onset of initial signs and symptoms. In one series, the mean interval between cataract surgery and the onset of initial signs and symptoms of *S. epidermidis* endophthalmitis was 7 days.[66] By contrast, a short interval between trauma and onset of clinical infection, averaging 1.5 days, was reported in seven patients with *B. cereus* endophthalmitis.[52]

The usual presentation of fungal endophthalmitis is an insidious, slowly progressive loss of visual acuity with little or no pain beginning a week to several months after surgery or a penetrating injury to the eye. Early in the course of endogenous infection, a number of small whitish lesions are seen around the retinal vessels. During some days to weeks they increase in number and size, becoming more fluffy and finally extending into the vitreous humor. As the disease progresses, the number of vitreal fluffballs increases. The vitreal material is sometimes seen by patients as floaters.

Laboratory Diagnosis

Because the damage caused by endophthalmitis and the difficulty of eradicating the infection increase sharply the longer treatment is delayed, early diagnosis and treatment are crucial. Both experimental[67] and clinical[53] studies confirm that the most fruitful source of material for culture is the vitreous humor. This is true even when the infecting agent is introduced into the anterior chamber and whether or not the lens is present (the lens serving as a barrier to the pathogen), suggesting that vitreous humor is a better culture medium than aqueous humor. Because on rare occasions the aqueous humor may yield organisms when the vitreal sample does not,[41] both aqueous humor and vitreous humor should be harvested for culture. Except in endophthalmitis secondary to an infected bleb, culturing the lids or conjunctiva is unrewarding and has the potential for growth of organisms other than the agent responsible for the infection. Individual drops of each specimen are placed on culture media, which include chocolate agar and liquid thioglycolate. If a more intensive search for anaerobes is desired, solid media that allow growth and recovery of individual colonies are suggested.[57] When a vitreal sample is obtained with an automated vitrectomy apparatus, the inoculum is necessarily diluted by an irrigating solution. In such instances, the diluted specimen can be passed through a membrane filter. With sterile technique, cut portions of the filter paper can be plated for culture. If there is enough material for this purpose, samples of vitreous humor should be subjected to Gram and Giemsa stain examination. If a fungal infection is suspected, culture material is also plated on Sabouraud agar and some of the sample is stained with Grocott methenamine silver.[68] There is a greater chance of obtaining fungi for culture if a vitrectomy unit is used or if the needle point is placed into a vitreal fluffball under direct observation. Vitreal material aspirated between fluffballs is less likely to harbor organisms. When endogenous endophthalmitis is suspected, blood cultures should be obtained.

Treatment

Pharmacologic Principles

Major barriers impede delivery of antibiotic to the vitreous humor, the principal site of infection in endophthalmitis[50, 69] (Fig. 155–11). The corneal epithelial barrier, the lens-iris apparatus, and the diluting effect of the aqueous humor flow combine to prevent topically applied drug from accumulating in therapeutic concentrations in the vitreous. Studies in animals and some data in humans have also established that, for the majority of antimicrobial agents, which are not lipid soluble, therapeutic intravitreal antibiotic concentration cannot be achieved after subconjunctival or parenteral administration.[69]

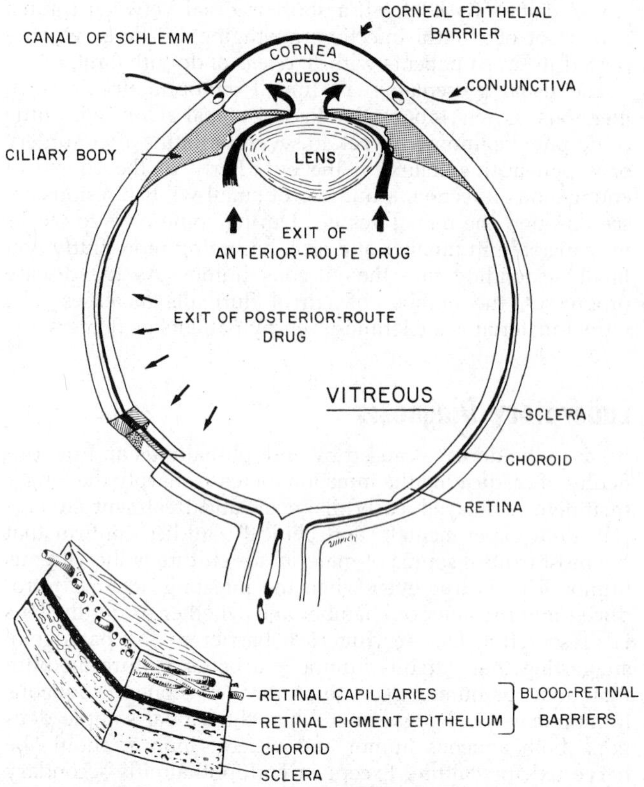

FIGURE 155–11 □ The major pharmacokinetic features of the eye. There are three barriers to ocular penetration: the corneal epithelium, the blood-aqueous barrier (in the ciliary body), and the blood-retinal barriers. The outer blood-retinal barrier is in the retinal pigment epithelium; the inner one lies in the tight junctions of the retinal capillaries. Each contains an active transport pump for organic anions. Anterior-route drugs (aminoglycosides) leave the vitreous by way of the aqueous humor and canal of Schlemm. Posterior-route drugs (penicillins, cephalosporins) leave by active transport across the retina. (From Barza M: Pharmacokinetics of antibiotics. *In* Sabath LD [ed]: Action of Antibiotics in Patients. Bern, Switzerland, Hans Huber, 1982, pp 11–39.)

Drugs injected subconjunctivally pass fairly readily through the sclera but do not traverse the barrier of the retinal pigment epithelium and are probably largely absorbed into the systemic circulation by the uveal, retinal, and orbital vessels. The new third-generation cephalosporins were thought possibly to achieve higher vitreous concentrations than older drugs after subconjunctival injection, especially because their vitreous half-life is longer, but this did not prove to be the case in studies in rabbits.[70, 71] Moreover, in a study of ceftriaxone and ceftazidime in humans with uninfected eyes, vitreous concentrations of ceftriaxone and ceftazidime after a single subconjunctival injection were generally undetectable.[72] Vancomycin was also undetectable in that study.[72]

Most drugs injected systemically do not traverse the tight junctions of the nonfenestrated retinal capillaries and do not reach high vitreal concentrations. Therapeutic intravitreal levels of antibiotics can probably be achieved after subconjunctival or parenteral administration of drugs that are quite lipid soluble such as rifampin, metronidazole, chloramphenicol, minocycline, trimethoprim, and sulfamethoxazole. However, these are not drugs of first choice for most species that cause endophthalmitis and except for few data for trimethoprim-sulfamethoxazole (Barza M, Doft B, manuscript submitted) and chloramphenicol, documentation of their vitreous penetration is lacking.

There are two principal routes of egress of antimicrobial agents from the vitreous humor (see Fig. 155–11). The aminoglycosides and vancomycin are eliminated by diffusion through the vitreous humor into the aqueous humor and through the canal of Schlemm; this is called the anterior route. Because the route is long and relatively confined, the vitreal half-life of anterior-route drugs is comparatively long, about 24 hours in the normal rabbit eye (Table 115–7). Because of the larger volume of the human eye, the half-life of anterior-route drugs is about twice as long in humans as in rabbits.[74] In inflamed eyes the half-life is reduced by about 50%, presumably because the eyes are more "leaky." The half-life is also shortened by extraction of the lens, perhaps because the lens-iris barrier is violated.

The second major route of elimination from the vitreous humor is the so-called posterior, or retinal, route (see Fig. 155–11). This is the route taken by most penicillins and cephalosporins, and probably clindamycin. The retinal route consists of an active transport system[75] that removes weak organic acids from the vitreous humor and transports them into the circulation. Because of the short diffusion distances and the active transport system, drugs eliminated by the retinal route have a relatively short vitreal half-life (see Table 155–7). The active transport pump is probably located in the retinal pigment epithelium, the retinal capillaries, or both sites.[73, 76] Probenecid, even when given systemically, inhibits the pump and prolongs the half-life of β-lactam drugs in the vitreous humor.[77] Inflammation has at least two contradictory effects on transport from the vitreous humor: it impairs the function of the transport pump, which reduces drug elimination, but it makes the eye leaky, which enhances drug elimination from the vitreous humor. The net effect is little change in the vitreal half-life of retinal-route drugs as a result of inflammation.

The effect of protein binding on the ocular pharmacokinetics of antibiotics has not been studied well.[78] On theoretical grounds, one would predict that a high degree of serum protein binding would restrict the passage of drug from the systemic circulation into the ocular tissues and fluids.

Prognosis for Vision

Before the early 1970s, when most treatment was systemic, the visual outcome for patients with bacterial endophthalmitis was dismal. In approximately 75% of patients, the final visual acuity in the affected eye was no better than "light perception."[49] Intravitreal injections of drug and vitrectomy[79] have improved somewhat the prognosis for the restoration of vision. In one series, factors associated with a poor visual result (worse than 20/400) included infection by virulent organisms, poor visual acuity at outset of treatment, and infection secondary to accidental trauma.[80] In many instances, poor initial visual acuity is related to a long interval between onset of infection and initiation of therapy; presumably, the delay allows bacteria to multiply in the vitreous humor, resulting in large inocula and in considerable retinal damage because of bacterial and leukocyte enzymes and toxins. A long interval before onset of treatment has also been shown experimentally to be associated with a poor bactericidal effect of various classes of antimicrobial agents.[82]

Among the common infections, *S. epidermidis* infection has the best prognosis for recovery of vision.[41, 82, 83] This probably results from the relatively low virulence of this species. In one review of postcataract infection, 78% of patients had a final visual acuity of 20/400 or better and 33%, 20/40 or better.[83] Infection caused by other species or in settings other than cataract surgery has a poorer prognosis. In posttraumatic bacterial endophthalmitis caused by *Bacillus* species,[52]

TABLE 155–7 ■ Regimens for Intravitreal Injection in Humans (Pharmacokinetic Data Estimated from Data in Rabbits)

DRUG	DOSE (μg)	PEAK VITREAL CONCENTRATION (μg/mL)	ESTIMATED HALF-LIFE (HOURS) IN VITREOUS HUMOR OF HUMANS*: Uninflamed Eye	ESTIMATED HALF-LIFE (HOURS) IN VITREOUS HUMOR OF HUMANS*: Inflamed Eye	DAYS FOR CONCENTRATION TO FALL BY EIGHTFOLD OR THREE HALF-LIVES*: Uninflamed Eye	DAYS FOR CONCENTRATION TO FALL BY EIGHTFOLD OR THREE HALF-LIVES*: Inflamed Eye
Anterior Route						
Gentamicin	200–400	40–80	40–60	20–40 (less with aphakia)	6	3
Tobramycin	200–400	40–80	Presumably, as for gentamicin		Presumably, as for gentamicin	
Amikacin	400	40	Presumably, as for gentamicin		Presumably, as for gentamicin	
Vancomycin	1000–2000	200–400	40–60	48	6	6
Retinal Route						
Penicillin G	600 units	120	8	—	1	—
Carbenicillin	2000	400	6–8	10	1	1
Cefazolin	2000	400	10–12	18	1.5	2
Ceftizoxime	Not known		10	15	1.5	4.5
Ceftriaxone	3000	600	15	22	2	3
Ceftazidime	2000	400	30	38	4	5
Clindamycin	1000	200	6	—	1	—

*Calculated by multiplying the half-life in rabbits by 2.0 for anterior-route drugs and by 1.7 for retinal-route drugs.
Data from references 69 and 75.

anaerobic infections caused by species other than *P. acnes* (which has a favorable prognosis),[57] and endophthalmitis associated with filtering blebs in which streptococci and *H. influenzae* are often the cause,[55] the final visual acuity for the majority of infected eyes is less than 20/200 and, so, qualifies as legal blindness.

With endogenous bacterial endophthalmitis the chance of having useful vision is even worse than with the exogenous variety because the pathogen is often more virulent, there is a high incidence of immune compromise, and retinal ischemia sometimes occurs as a result of septic embolic occlusion of the central retinal artery.[47] Data on fungal endophthalmitis are meager. The outcome of postoperative fungal infection is better than with the endogenous type, presumably because the latter usually occurs in a setting of poor host defense mechanisms; however, the prognosis for vision recovery in fungal endophthalmitis is guarded because recognition and treatment are often delayed, owing to the insidious nature of the infection and to the problem of delivering high concentrations of effective antifungal agents to the infection site without causing toxicity to the retina.

Treatment of Bacterial Endophthalmitis

As soon as the clinical diagnosis of bacterial endophthalmitis is made, the patient should be brought to the operating room for a diagnostic tap of the vitreous and aqueous humor, intravitreal administration of antibiotics, and possibly vitrectomy. Speed is essential in diagnosis and therapy, because delayed treatment is associated with poorer visual acuity. Experimental[84] and clinical[85] studies attest to the value of corticosteroids in the treatment of this infection, although debate continues on the timing and routes of administration of the drug.[45, 85a]

A plan for initial empirical therapy of postoperative bacterial endophthalmitis when no specific pathogen is implicated is outlined in Table 155–8. Even if the Gram stain examination suggests certain pathogens, we recommend beginning treatment with a regimen that is active against the most common gram-positive and gram-negative pathogens, to reduce the likelihood of inadequate treatment resulting from misinterpretation of the Gram stain. The most popular regimens currently involve a combination of vancomycin and either amikacin or ceftazidime. The vancomycin is directed at strains of staphylococci (coagulase-negative and -positive)[86] and streptococci[55] (including *Enterococcus faecalis*) resistant to β-lactam drugs and, in posttraumatic infections, *B.*

TABLE 155–8 ■ Empirical Initial Therapy for Postoperative Bacterial Endophthalmitis

A. Immediately after diagnosis and aspiration of vitreous and aqueous humor for diagnostic purposes, begin therapy as follows:
   Intravitreal injection: Amikacin, 0.4 mg (400 μg), *or* ceftazidime, 2.25 mg, in 0.1 mL, and vancomycin, 1.0 mg (1000 μg) in 0.1 mL. After aspiration of fluid from the vitreous humor for diagnostic purposes, a 22-gauge needle remains in the midvitreous while two new tuberculin syringes, each containing antibiotic, are exchanged consecutively and the material is slowly injected into the midvitreous. Ensure that the drug is delivered into the vitreous humor and does not remain in the bore of the needle. In phakic eyes, both the diagnostic and therapeutic vitreal aspiration and injections are performed behind the lens, through a track made in the sclera 3.5 mm behind the corneal limbus.
   Periocular injection: Vancomycin, 25 mg in 0.5 mL, and ceftazidime, 100 mg in 0.5 mL. Injections are made with a disposable tuberculin syringe, 25-gauge, ⅝-inch needle.
   Systemic administration: Generally not necessary. If it is desired to give antibiotics systemically, ceftazidime, amikacin, or ciprofloxacin may be given in standard dosages.
B. Twelve hours after the therapy just detailed, repeat the periocular injections and give the following drugs:
   Periocular injection: Dexamethasone phosphate, 4 mg (1 mL), *or* prednisolone succinate, 25 mg (1 mL)
   Systemic administration: Prednisone, 60 mg PO

The periocular injections are given daily for 4–7 d, each drug administered from a separate syringe. Systemic corticosteroid therapy is continued for 10–14 d. Antibiotic therapy is modified if necessary based on the clinical condition and the results of culture and sensitivity studies.

Modified from Baum J: Antibiotic use in ophthalmology. *In* Tasman W, Jaeger AE (eds): Clinical Ophthalmology, Vol 4. Philadelphia, Harper & Row, 1990.

TABLE 155–9 ■ Intravitreal Antibiotic Injection

ANTIBIOTIC	INTRAVITREAL DOSE (mg)	DURATION OF THERAPEUTIC LEVEL IN VITREOUS (h)
Aminoglycosides		
Gentamicin	0.4	48–72
Tobramycin	0.4	48–72
Amikacin	0.4	48–72
Penicillins and cephalosporins		
Oxacillin	0.5	24
Ampicillin	5.0	24
Carbenicillin	2.0	16–24
Cefazolin	2.0	24
Ceftazidime	2.0	36–48
Miscellaneous		
Clindamycin	1.0	16–24
Vancomycin	1.0	72
Antifungal antibiotic		
Amphotericin B	5–15 μg	120–168

Modified from Baum J: Antibiotic use in ophthalmology. *In* Tasman W, Jaeger AE (eds): Clinical Ophthalmology, Vol 4. Philadelphia, Harper & Row, 1990, p 9.

cereus.[52] The drug is well tolerated[87] and its intravitreal half-life is long. Amikacin is preferred over gentamicin or tobramycin because, in experimental animals, it is less toxic to the retina.[88, 89] Because of concerns about rare instances of macular infarction possibly attributable to the intravitreal or subconjunctival injection of aminoglycosides,[90] some ophthalmologists prefer ceftazidime over amikacin, but experience with ceftazidime is limited and the Endophthalmitis Vitrectomy Study (see later) elected to use amikacin for postoperative endophthalmitis.[91]

Initial therapy can be modified in response to an evaluation of the clinical condition and the results of the culture and sensitivity reports. Tables 155–9 and 155–10 list the intravitreal doses of antibiotic when it is given as a single initial injection or delivered as part of a vitrectomy infusion. Any antibiotic solution for intraocular administration is best prepared by the hospital pharmacist. If an anaerobic infection is suspected or documented, penicillin or clindamycin is the drug of choice.[57] Metronidazole would probably be highly effective for infection by strict anaerobes. There are no data for its use by intravitreal injection but, because it is so lipid soluble, it would probably penetrate well by systemic routes. Vancomycin is recommended in infection by *P. acnes*.[60]

TABLE 155–10 ■ Maximal Nontoxic Dose of Antibiotic and Antifungal Agents for Vitrectomy Infusion Fluid for Endophthalmitis

AGENT	MAXIMAL NONTOXIC DOSE (μg/mL)
Chloramphenicol	10
Clindamycin	9
Amikacin	10
Tobramycin	10
Gentamicin	8
Ceftazidime	100
Netilmicin	4
Methicillin	20
Oxacillin	10
Penicillin	80
Amphotericin B methyl ester	75*

*Recommended dose is 10 μg/mL.

Modified from Peyman GA, Schulman JA: Intravitreal Surgery: Principles and Practice, ed 2. Norwalk, CT, Appleton-Century-Crofts, 1994, p 905 © by Appleton & Lange; and Peyman GA, personal communication, regarding ceftazidime.

The role of vitrectomy in the initial treatment of endophthalmitis has been controversial. The procedure has the theoretical advantage of decreasing the infective inoculum and of removing destructive toxins and enzymes, thereby reducing the morbidity of the disease. In addition, by reducing the vitreal opacification, vitrectomy enhances visualization of the retina. Some reports suggest that the procedure improves the final visual acuity,[92] whereas others conclude that the effect is harmful. However, the studies were retrospective and subject to marked allocation bias. Likewise, IV antibiotics may be unnecessary in patients receiving antibiotics by intravitreal and periocular injection for endophthalmitis occurring after cataract extraction.[93] Because of these uncertainties, the Endophthalmitis Vitrectomy Study was undertaken.[54] This was a large, multicenter, randomized trial of both immediate vitrectomy and IV antibiotics in the treatment of endophthalmitis after cataract extraction or secondary lens implantation. All patients received intravitreal injections of vancomycin and amikacin, as well as subconjunctival and topical antibiotics and corticosteroids. Preliminary analysis of the results of the study suggests that immediate vitrectomy (as opposed to delayed vitrectomy done only in eyes in which the response to initial treatment was poor) and IV antibiotics (as opposed to no IV antibiotics) offered no overall benefit. Subgroup analysis post hoc suggests that eyes with light perception only on initial presentation might benefit from immediate vitrectomy. Despite these negative findings, there may be utility to immediate vitrectomy in certain cases, for example, when there has been a long interval between the onset of symptoms and treatment.[92]

Clinical[80] and experimental[81, 92] studies have documented the difficulty of sterilizing the vitreous humor with a single injection, except in infections caused by less virulent organisms such as *S. epidermidis* and *P. acnes*. This underlines the need for repeated injections and vitrectomies in unresponsive cases. In one study, patients who received a series of intraocular injections of antibiotic and multiple vitrectomies had a higher cure rate than those who received a single intravitreal injection of antibiotics and no vitrectomy.[79] The suggested interval of 48 hours between successive injections of gentamicin is based on finding little or no drug in the vitreous humor of humans 48 hours after an injection[94] and by extrapolation (see Table 155–7) from the behavior of various antimicrobial agents in rabbit eyes. The doses recommended for intravitreal injection in humans are generally intended to produce a peak vitreal concentration of 10% of the weakest concentration that produces retinal toxicity in the rabbit eyes.[74] Transscleral iontophoresis, a noninvasive method for driving drug into the vitreous, is under investigation.[95]

Treatment of Fungal Endophthalmitis

At present, amphotericin B is the most reliable drug for the treatment of fungal endophthalmitis. An intravitreal dose of 5 to 10 μg in 0.1 mL is suggested,[41] although the toxic retinal dose is different in various experimental studies: 1 μg[96] and 10 μg in rabbit models[97] and 20 μg in a primate model.[98] The value of parenterally administered amphotericin B to supplement the intravitreal dose is not clear, but the drug has been shown to cure clinical *Candida* endophthalmitis when administered only parenterally.[63] Small incipient intraretinal foci of infection may be treated with IV drug; however, if there is clinical evidence of vitreal infection, in most instances antifungal agents probably should be administered intravitreally.

Other antifungal drugs have been used primarily to supplement amphotericin B.[99] These include miconazole, given by intravitreal or subconjunctival injection,[41] and ketoconazole, given orally.[100] However, more potent azole derivatives such as fluconazole, which penetrates the vitreous well after systemic administration, have considerable promise, especially for *Candida* endophthalmitis. A report and literature review indicates that 15 of 16 (94%) eyes with *Candida* endophthalmitis were cured by treatment with fluconazole alone, in a dosage of 100 to 200 mg daily for about 2 months.[101] This treatment can be combined with pars plana vitrectomy for eyes with moderate to severe vitritis.

References

1. Tabbara KF, Hyndiuk RA: Infections of the Eye, ed 2. Boston, Little, Brown, 1996.
2. Duane TD, Jaeger EA (eds): Clinical Ophthalmology, Vol 4. Philadelphia, Harper & Row, 1988.
3. Easty DL: Virus Disease of the Eye. Chicago, Year Book Medical Publishers, 1985.
4. Pepose JS, Holland GN, Wilhelmus KR: Ocular Infection and Immunity. St. Louis, CV Mosby, 1996.
5. Barza M, Baum J: Ocular infections. Med Clin North Am 67:131, 1983.
6. Baum J: Antibiotic use in ophthalmology. *In* Tassman W, Jaeger EA (eds): Clinical Ophthalmology, Vol 4. Philadelphia, Harper & Row, 1990.
7. Perry HD, Serniuk RA: Conservative treatment of chalazia. Ophthalmology 87:218, 1980.
8. Pizzarello LD, Jakobiec FA, Hoseldt AJ, et al: Intralesional corticosteroid therapy of chalazia. Am J Ophthalmol 85:818, 1978.
9. Baum JL, Fedukowicz HB, Jordan A: A survey of *Moraxella* corneal ulcers in a derelict population. Am J Ophthalmol 90:476, 1980.
10. Wilson LA, Ahearn DG, Jones DE, Sexton RR: The fungi from the normal outer eye. Am J Ophthalmol 67:52, 1969.
11. Brazilian Purpuric Fever Study Group: Brazilian purpuric fever: Epidemic purpura fulminans associated with antecedent purulent conjunctivitis. Lancet 2:757, 1987.
12. Fraunfelder FT, Bagby GC, Kelly DJ: Fatal aplastic anemia following topical administration of ophthalmic chloramphenicol. Am J Ophthalmol 93:356, 1982.
13. Centers for Disease Control and Prevention: 1993 Sexually transmitted diseases treatment guidelines. MMWR Morbid Mortal Wkly Rep 42(RR-14):56, 1993.
14. Bailey R, Arullendran P, Whittle H, Mabey D: Randomised controlled trial of single dose azithromycin in treatment of trachoma. Lancet 342:453, 1993.
15. Isenberg SJ, Apt L, Wood M: A controlled trial of povidone-iodine as prophylaxis against ophthalmia neonatorum. N Engl J Med 332:562, 1995.

15a. Kreger AS, Griffin OK: Physiochemical fractionation of extracellular cornea-damaging proteases of *Pseudomonas aeruginosa.* Infect Immun 9:828, 1974.

16. O'Day DM, Smith RS, Gregg CR, et al: The problem of bacillus species infection with special emphasis on the virulence of *Bacillus cereus*. Ophthalmology 88:833, 1931.
17. Forster RK, Wirta MG, Solis M, et al: Methenamine silver–stained corneal scrapings in keratomycosis. Am J Ophthalmol 82:261, 1976.
18. Jones DB: A plan for antimicrobial therapy in bacterial keratitis. Trans Am Acad Ophthalmol Otolaryngol 79:95, 1973.
19. Baum JL: Initial therapy of suspected microbial corneal ulcers. I. Broad antibiotic therapy based on prevalence of organisms. Surv Ophthalmol 24:97, 1979.

19a. Kremer I, Robinson A, Braffman M, et al: The effect of topical ceftazidime on pseudomonas keratitis in rabbits. Cornea 13:360, 1994.

20. Baum J, Barza M: Topical vs subconjunctival treatment of bacterial corneal ulcers. Ophthalmology 90:162, 1983.
21. Leibowitz HM, Ryan WJ, Kupferman A: Route of antibiotic in bacterial keratitis. Arch Ophthalmol 99:1420, 1981.
22. Koenig SB: Fungal keratitis. *In* Tabbara KF, Hyndiuk RA: Infections of the Eye. Boston, Little, Brown, 1986, p 331.
23. Jones BR: Principles in management of oculomycosis. Trans Am Acad Ophthalmol Otolaryngol 79:15, 1975.
24. Wood TO, Tuberville AW: Keratomycosis and amphotericin B. Trans Am Ophthalmol Soc 83:397, 1985.
25. Rayfield MA, Kaufman HE: Pathogenicity and strain specificity of herpes simplex virus. *In* Duane TD, Jaeger AE (eds): Foundations of Clinical Ophthalmology. Philadelphia, JB Lippincott, 1988.
26. Sabbaga EMH, Pavan-Langston D, Bean KM, Dunkel EC: Detection of HSV nucleic acid sequences in the cornea during acute and latent ocular disease. Exp Eye Res 47:545, 1988.
27. Meyers-Elliot RH, Pettit PH, Maxwell A: Viral antigens in the immune ring of herpes simplex stromal keratitis. Arch Ophthalmol 98:897, 1980.
28. Schwab IR: Oral acyclovir in the management of herpes simplex ocular infections. Ophthalmology 95:423, 1988.
29. Barron BA, Gee L, Hauck WW, et al: Herpetic eye disease study. A controlled trial of oral acyclovir for herpes simplex stromal keratitis. Ophthalmology 101:1871, 1994.
30. Jones DB, Visvesvara GS, Robinson NM: *Acanthamoeba polyphaga* keratitis and *Acanthamoeba* uveitis associated with fatal meningoencephalitis. Trans Ophthalmol Soc UK 95:221, 1975.
31. Nagington J, Watson PG, Playfair TJ, et al: Amoebic infection of the eye. Lancet 2:1537, 1974.
32. Epstein RJ, Wilson LA, Visvesvara GS, et al: Rapid diagnosis of *Acanthamoeba* keratitis from corneal scrapings using indirect fluorescent antibody staining. Arch Ophthalmol 104:1318, 1986.
33. Silvany RE, Luckenbach MW, Moore B: The rapid detection of *Acanthamoeba* in paraffin-embedded sections of corneal tissue with calcofluor white. Arch Ophthalmol 105:1366, 1987.

33a. Pfister DR, Cameron JD, Krachmer JH, Holland EJ: Confocal microscopy findings of *Acanthamoeba* keratitis. Am J Ophthalmol 121:119, 1996.

34. Auran JD, Starr MB, Jakobiec FA: *Acanthamoeba* keratitis. A review of the literature. Cornea 6:2, 1987.
35. Wright P, Warhurst D, Jones BR: *Acanthamoeba* keratitis successfully treated medically. Br J Ophthalmol 69:778, 1985.
36. Cohen EJ, Parlato CJ, Arentsen JJ, et al: Medical and surgical treatment of *Acanthamoeba* keratitis. Am J Ophthalmol 103:615, 1987.
37. Moore MB: *Acanthamoeba* keratitis. Arch Ophthalmol 106:1181, 1988.
38. Larkin DFP, Kilvington S, Dart JKG: Treatment of *Acanthamoeba* keratitis with polyhexamethylene biguanide. Ophthalmology 99:185, 1992.
39. Seal D, Hay J, Kirkness C, et al: Successful medical therapy of acanthamoeba keratitis with topical chlorhexidine and propamidine. Eye 10:413, 1996.
40. Driebe WT Jr, Stern GA, Epstein RJ, et al: *Acanthamoeba* keratitis. Potential role for topical clotrimazole in combination chemotherapy. Arch Ophthalmol 106:1196, 1988.
41. Forster RK: Endophthalmitis. *In* Duane TD, Jaeger AE: Clinical Ophthalmology, Vol 4. Philadelphia, Harper & Row, 1994.

42. Parke DW II, Brinton GS: Endophthalmitis. *In* Tabbara KF, Hyndiuk RA (eds): Infections of the Eye. Boston, Little, Brown, 1986, pp 563–585.
43. Tabbara KF: Endogenous ocular candidosis. *In* Tabbara KF, Hyndiuk RA (eds): Infections of the Eye. Boston, Little, Brown, 1986, pp 511–516.
44. Barza M, Baum J: Ocular pharmacology of antibiotics. *In* Duane TD, Jaeger AE: Foundations of Clinical Ophthalmology, Vol 2. Philadelphia, JB Lippincott, 1988, pp 1–14.
45. Baum J, Peyman GA, Barza M: Intravitreal administration of antibiotic in the treatment of bacterial endophthalmitis. III. Consensus. Surv Ophthalmol 26:204, 1982.
46. Shammas HF: Endogenous *E. coli* endophthalmitis. Surv Ophthalmol 21:429, 1977.
47. Greenwald MJ, Wohl LG, Sell CH: Metastatic bacterial endophthalmitis. A contemporary reappraisal. Surv Ophthalmol 31:81, 1986.
48. Christy NE, Lall P: Postoperative endophthalmitis following cataract surgery. Arch Ophthalmol 90:361, 1973.
49. Allen HF, Mangiaracine AB: Bacterial endophthalmitis after cataract extraction: II. Incidence in thirty-six thousand consecutive operations with special reference to preoperative topical antibiotics. Arch Ophthalmol 91:3, 1974.
50. Fahmay JA: Endophthalmitis following cataract extraction: A study of 24 cases in 4,498 operations. Acta Ophthalmol 53:522, 1975.
51. Barr CC: Prognostic factors in corneoscleral lacerations. Arch Ophthalmol 101:919, 1983.
52. Affeldt JC, Flynn HW Jr, Forster RK, et al: Microbial endophthalmitis resulting from ocular trauma. Ophthalmology 94:407, 1987.
53. Forster RK: Symposium: Postoperative endophthalmitis: Etiology and diagnosis of bacterial postoperative endophthalmitis. Ophthalmology 85:320, 1978.
54. Endophthalmitis Vitrectomy Study Group: Results of the Endophthalmitis Vitrectomy Study. A randomized trial of immediate vitrectomy and of intravenous antibiotics for the treatment of postoperative bacterial endophthalmitis. Arch Ophthalmol 113:1479, 1995.
54a. Han DP, Wisniewski SR, Wilson LA, et al: Spectrum and susceptibilities of microbiologic isolates in the Endophthalmitis Vitrectomy Study. Am J Ophthalmol 122:1, 1996.
55. Mandelbaum S, Forster RK, Gelender H, Culbertson W: Late-onset endophthalmitis associated with filtering blebs. Ophthalmology 92:964, 1985.
56. Brinton GS, Topping TM, Hyndiuk RA, et al: Posttraumatic endophthalmitis. Arch Ophthalmol 102:547, 1984.
57. Ormerod LD, Paton BG, Haaf J, et al: Anaerobic bacterial endophthalmitis. Ophthalmology 94:799, 1987.
58. Jones DB: Polymicrobial keratitis. Trans Am Ophthalmol Soc 79:153, 1981.
59. Meisler DM, Mandelbaum S: *Propionibacterium*-associated endophthalmitis after extracapsular cataract extraction. Review of reported cases. Ophthalmology 96:54, 1989.
60. Winward KE, Pflugfelder SC, Flynn JR HW, et al: Postoperative *Propionibacterium* endophthalmitis. Ophthalmology 100:447, 1993.
61. Okada AA, Johnson RP, Liles WC, et al: Endogenous bacterial endophthalmitis. Report of a ten-year retrospective study. Ophthalmology 101:832, 1994.
61a. Doft BH, Clarkson JG, Rebell T, Forster RD: Endogenous *Aspergillus* endophthalmitis in drug abusers. Arch Ophthalmol 98:859, 1980.
62. Brod RD, Clarkson JG, Flynn H Jr, Green WR: Endogenous fungal endophthalmitis. *In* Duane TD, Jaeger AE: Clinical Ophthalmology, Vol 3. Philadelphia, Harper & Row, 1990.
63. Pettit TH, Olson RJ, Foos RY, Martin WJ: Fungal endophthalmitis following intraocular lens implantation: A surgical epidemic. Arch Ophthalmol 98:1025, 1980.
64. Stern WH, Tamura E, Jacobs RA, et al: Epidemic surgical candida parapsilosis endophthalmitis. Clinical findings and management of 15 consecutive cases. Ophthalmology 92:1701, 1985.
65. Ficker L, Meredith TA, Wilson LA, et al: Chronic bacterial endophthalmitis. Am J Ophthalmol 103:745, 1987.
66. Bode DD Jr, Gelender H, Forster RK: A retrospective review of endophthalmitis due to coagulase-negative staphylococci. Br J Ophthalmol 69:915, 1985.
67. Mayleth FR, Leopold JH: Study of experimental intraocular infection. Am J Ophthalmol 40:86, 1985.
68. Forster RK, Wirta MG, Solis M, et al: Methenamine silver–stained corneal scrapings in keratomycosis. Am J Ophthalmol 82:261, 1976.
69. Barza M: Antibacterial agents in the treatment of ocular infections. Infect Dis Clin North Am 3:533, 1989.
70. Barza M, Lynch E, Baum JL: Pharmacokinetics of newer cephalosporins after subconjunctival and intravitreal injection in rabbits. Arch Ophthalmol 111:121, 1993.
71. Meredith TA: Antimicrobial pharmacokinetics in endophthalmitis treatment: Studies of ceftazidime. Trans Am Ophthalmol Soc 91:653, 1993.
72. Barza M, Doft B, Lynch E: Ocular penetration of ceftriaxone, ceftazidime, and vancomycin after subconjunctival injection in humans. Arch Ophthalmol 111:492, 1993.
73. Ficker L, Meredith TA, Gardner S, Wilson LA: Cefazolin levels after intravitreal injection. Invest Ophthalmol Vis Sci 31:502, 1990.
74. Maurice DM: Injection of drugs into the vitreous body. *In* Leopold IH, Burns RP (eds): Symposium on Ocular Therapy, Vol 9. New York, John Wiley & Sons, 1976, pp 59–72.
75. Forbes M, Becker B: The transport of organic anions by the rabbit eye: II. In vivo transport of iodopyracet (Diodrast). Am J Ophthalmol 50:867, 1960.
76. Cunha-Vaz J: The blood-ocular barriers. Surv Ophthalmol 23:279, 1979.
77. Barza M, Kane A, Baum J: Pharmacokinetics of intravitreal carbenicillin, cefazolin and gentamicin in rhesus monkeys. Invest Ophthalmol Vis Sci 12:1602, 1983.
78. Barza M, Baum J: Penetration of ocular compartments by penicillins. Surv Ophthalmol 18:71, 1973.
79. Stern GA, Engel HM, Driebe WT Jr: The treatment of postoperative endophthalmitis. Ophthalmology 96:62, 1989.
80. Bohigian GM, Olk RJ: Factors associated with a poor visual result in endophthalmitis. Am J Ophthalmol 101:332, 1986.
81. Davey PG, Barza M, Stuart M: Dose response of experimental *Pseudomonas* endophthalmitis to ciprofloxacin, gentamicin and imipenem: Evidence for resistance to "late" treatment of infections. J Infect Dis 155:518, 1987.
82. Rowsey JJ, Newsom DL, Sexton DJ, Harms WK: Endophthalmitis: Current approaches. Ophthalmology 89:1055, 1982.
83. Driebe WT Jr, Mandelbaum S, Forster RK, et al: Pseudophakic endophthalmitis: Diagnosis and management. Ophthalmology 93:442, 1986.
84. Baum JL, Barza M, Lugar J, et al: The effect of corticosteroids in the treatment of experimental bacterial endophthalmitis. Am J Ophthalmol 80:513, 1975.
85. Baum JL, Rao GN: Treatment of postcataract bacterial endophthalmitis with periocular and systemic antibiotics and corticosteroids. Trans Am Acad Ophthalmol Otol 81:151, 1976.
85a. Meredith TA, Aguilar HE, Drews C, et al: Intraocular dexamethasone produces a harmful effect on treatment of experimental *Staphylococcus aureus* endophthalmitis. Trans Am Ophthalmol Soc 94:241, 1996.
86. Davis JC, Koidou-Tsiligianni A, Pflugfelder SC, et al: Coagulase-negative staphylococcal endophthalmitis. Increase in antimicrobial resistance. Ophthalmology 95:1404, 1988.
87. Pflugfelder SC, Hernandez E, Fliesler SJ, et al: Intravitreal vancomycin. Retinal toxicity, clearance and interaction with gentamicin. Arch Ophthalmol 105:831, 1987.
88. D'Amico DJ, Caspers-Velu L, Libert J, et al: Comparative toxicity of intravitreal aminoglycoside antibiotics. Am J Ophthalmol 100:264, 1985.
89. Talamo JH, D'Amico DJ, Kenyon KR: Intravitreal amikacin in the treatment of bacterial endophthalmitis. Arch Ophthalmol 104:1483, 1986.
90. Campochiaro PA, Lim JI: The aminoglycoside toxicity study group. Aminoglycoside toxicity in the treatment of endophthalmitis. Arch Ophthalmol 112:48, 1994.
91. Doft BH, Barza M, for the Endophthalmitis Vitrectomy Study Group. Ceftazidime or amikacin: Choice of intravitreal antimicrobials in the treatment of postoperative endophthalmitis. Arch Ophthalmol 112:17, 1994.
92. Cottingham AJ Jr, Forster RK: Vitrectomy in endophthalmitis: Results of a study using vitrectomy, intraocular antibiotics, or a combination of both. Arch Ophthalmol 94:2078, 1976.

93. Pavan PR, Oteiza EE, Hughes BA, Avni A: Exogenous endophthalmitis initially treated without systemic antibiotics. Ophthalmology 101:1289, 1994.
94. Cobo LM, Forster RK: The clearance of intravitreal gentamicin. Am J Ophthalmol 92:59, 1981.
95. Barza M, Peckman C, Baum J: Transscleral iontophoresis of cefazolin, ticarcillin and gentamicin in the rabbit. Ophthalmology 93:133, 1986.
96. Souri EN, Green WR: Intravitreal amphotericin B toxicity. Am J Ophthalmol 78:77, 1974.
97. Axelrod AJ, Peyman GA, Apple DJ: Toxicity of intravitreal injection of amphotericin B. Am J Ophthalmol 76:578, 1973.
98. Barza M, Baum J, Tremblay C, et al: Ocular toxicity of intravitreally injected liposomal amphotericin B in rhesus monkeys. Am J Ophthalmol 100:259, 1985.
99. Blumenkranz MS, Stevens DA: Therapy of endogenous fungal endophthalmitis. Arch Ophthalmol 98:1216, 1980.
100. Jones DB: Chemotherapy of fungal infections. *In* Srinevasan BD (ed): Ocular Therapeutics. New York, Masson, 1980, pp 35–50.
101. Akler ME, Vellend H, McNeely DM, et al: Use of fluconazole in the treatment of candidal endophthalmitis. Clin Infect Dis 20:657, 1995.

156

Orbital Infections

Christopher T. Westfall
John W. Shore
*Ann Sullivan Baker**

Orbital infections are potentially life-threatening processes historically associated with a 20% incidence of blindness and a 17% mortality rate.[1] Antibiotics and aggressive surgical management have significantly reduced morbidity and mortality.

Anatomy

The orbit is the bony cavity that encompasses the globe and its adnexal structures. The anatomy of this region is central to any discussion of orbital infection, as the anatomy specifically determines how infection reaches the orbit, how it is clinically manifested, and how it may extend to involve the central nervous system (Fig. 156–1).

Seven bones make up the orbit: frontal, zygoma, maxilla, ethmoid, lacrimal, sphenoid, and palatine. Three sides of the orbit are, in fact, represented by sinuses. The roof of the orbit houses the frontal sinus; the medial wall, the ethmoids and sphenoid; and the floor, the maxillary sinus. The ethmoid sinuses are separated from the orbit only by the wafer-thin lamina papyracea. From an anatomic perspective it is little wonder that the majority of orbital infections originate in the sinuses, predominantly in the ethmoids.[2–5]

Anteriorly, the orbit is bounded by the orbital septum, which is contiguous with the periorbita at the orbital rim (arcus marginalis). The septum terminates in the levator aponeurosis of the upper lid and the capsulopalpebral fascia of the lower lid. The orbital septum and periorbita serve as barriers to the extension of orbital infection.

Sinus infection may gain access to the orbit through defects in the orbital bones. Further spread of infection may be halted by the periorbita, giving rise to a subperiosteal abscess. This entity has a tendency for rapid spread in the subperiosteal space and compression of the optic nerve at the apex of the orbit.[6]

The orbital septum defines the orbital space anatomically and clinically. Infections anterior to the septum are termed periorbital or preseptal, whereas those posterior to this barrier are called orbital or postseptal. This anatomic differentiation often determines prognosis and treatment. Clinically, orbital (postseptal) infections may be characterized by a sharp line of demarcation representing the arcus marginalis.

Within the rigid confines of the orbit are the eye and a multiplicity of neurovascular adnexal structures. There is little space to accommodate the additional volume resulting from the inflammation and abscess formation associated with orbital infection. Functional deficit relates directly to anatomic structure in the tightly packed orbital apex.

At the apex of the orbit is the optic canal, which transmits the ophthalmic artery and vein as well as the optic nerve itself. Here at the apex, the four rectus muscles originate at the annulus of Zinn. The superior orbital fissure is temporal to the optic canal. Oculomotor (III), trochlear (IV), trigeminal (V-1), and abducens (VI) nerves, as well as the superior ophthalmic vein, enter the orbit from the middle cranial fossa by way of this fissure. The inferior orbital fissure communicates with the infratemporal fossa but not the cranial vault. It transmits the trigeminal nerve (V-2) as well as the inferior ophthalmic vein.

The valveless nature of the midfacial veins potentiates extension of infection by way of the facial veins and pterygoid plexus. Superior and inferior ophthalmic veins provide a direct conduit to the orbit and to the cavernous sinus beyond.[1–3, 7] This anatomic consideration explains the incidence of cavernous sinus thrombosis associated with orbital infection.[8]

Pathophysiology

Infection reaches the orbit by one of three routes: direct inoculation, extension from a contiguous structure, or hematogenous dissemination.[3] The most common route is by extension from adjacent infection, usually sinusitis. Most series report a 50% to 70% incidence of sinusitis or other upper respiratory tract infection in association with orbital infection.[2, 4, 7, 9] Other sites of contiguous spread include dental abscess,[10, 11] pharyngeal infection,[12] and otitis media.[4] Direct inoculation usually follows penetrating trauma to the eye or skin. This route accounts for about 25% of orbital infections and includes surgical trauma, such as rhinoplasty[13] and blepharoplasty[14, 15] or strabismus surgery.[15–17] Hematogenous dissemination may originate from many sites, including bacterial endocarditis.[18]

Although it is convenient to think of orbital infection as a progression—inflammatory edema, orbital cellulitis, subperiosteal abscess, orbital abscess, and cavernous sinus thrombosis[3, 7, 19] (Fig. 156–2)—this pathophysiologic continuum is not always seen in clinical practice. Orbital apex and sphenoid fissure syndrome[20] is a particularly interesting entity occasionally seen in association with sphenoid sinusitis.[21] These patients evidence oculomotor (III), trochlear (IV), trigeminal (V), and abducens (VI) nerve involvement due to inflammation within the superior orbital fissure, as well as visual loss

The views expressed in this chapter are those of the authors and do not reflect the official policy or position of the U.S. Department of Defense or the U.S. government.

*Deceased.

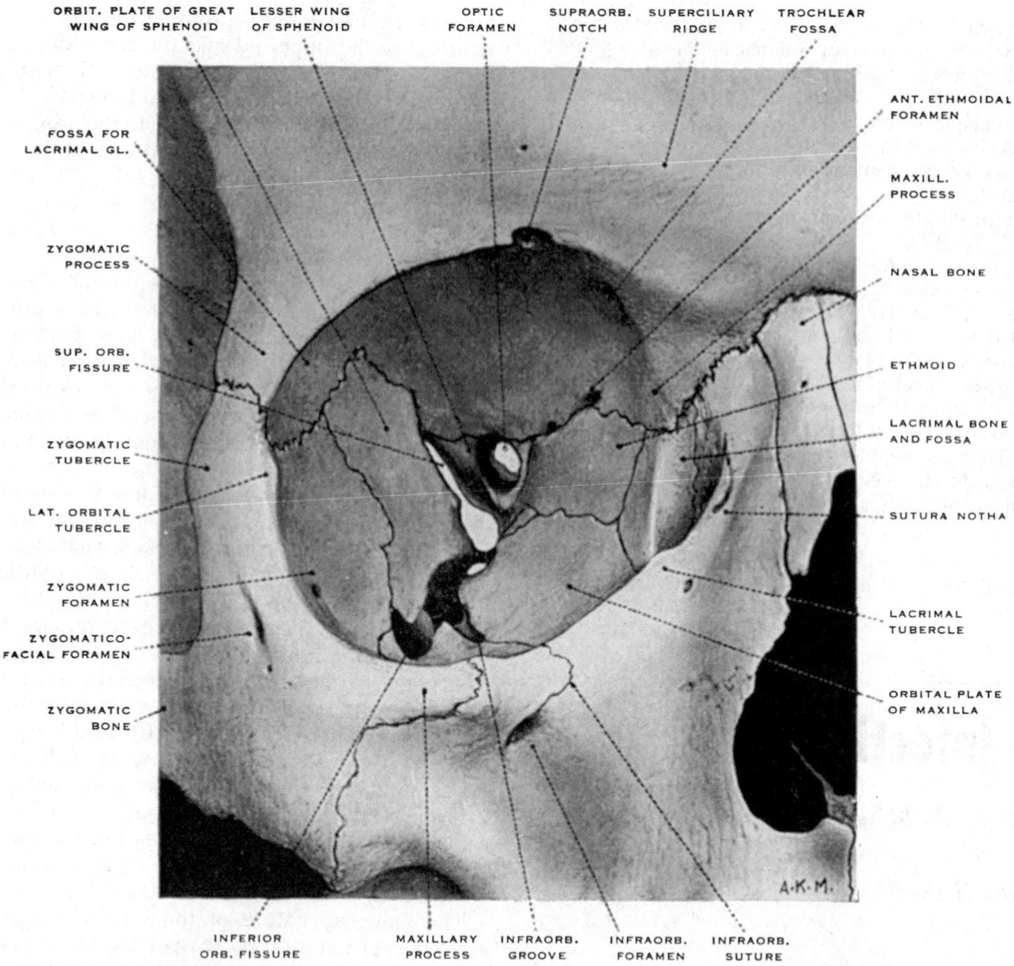

FIGURE 156–1 □ Anatomy of the orbit. (From Last RJ: Eugene Wolff's Anatomy of the Eye and Orbit, ed 6. Philadelphia, WB Saunders, 1968.)

secondary to compression of the optic nerve in its canal. This entity must be differentiated from cavernous sinus thrombosis, which may be associated with an anterior finding such as conjunctival chemosis.

Infectious Agents

The orbit may be infected by bacteria, fungi, or parasites; bacterial infections are by far those most commonly encountered. In diabetic, leukemic, and other immunocompromised hosts, fungal infection must be considered. Parasitic infection is rarely seen in the United States but is not uncommon in other parts of the world.

Isolates from adult and pediatric bacterial orbital infections relate to the site of origin. Organisms isolated after a traumatic break in the skin are inherently different from those associated with ethmoid sinusitis or dental abscess.

A wide variety of aerobic and anaerobic bacteria have been reported to cause orbital cellulitis, but the most commonly encountered bacteria in adult orbital infections are *Staphylococcus aureus, Streptococcus* species, and anaerobic bacteria. *S. aureus* is associated with trauma, whereas streptococci and anaerobic bacteria are most often associated with sinus infection. In children, *Haemophilus influenzae* is a frequent organism in cases involving sinusitis.[22] *Eikenella corrodens* often resists broad-spectrum antibiotic therapy and has been reported to cause orbital cellulitis.[23] Streptococci, especially when associated with staphylococci, may cause a necrotizing infection of the eyelids.[24, 25] Other organisms producing necrosis include *Pseudomonas aeruginosa* and *Peptostreptococcus*.[24, 26]

An unusual infectious process that has been known to occur in periorbital tissues is pseudomycosis or botryomycosis. This infection, postulated to be the result of an encapsulated form of *Staphylococcus,* is particularly resistant to antibiotic and surgical treatment.[27]

Mycobacteria may be responsible for orbital infection.[28–32] Skin testing and cultures are important in an orbital infection that is resistant to treatment or one in which there is bony destruction or fistula formation.

The most commonly encountered mycotic orbital infections are those caused by Phycomycetes, *Mucor* and *Rhizopus* genera; and Ascomycetes, *Aspergillus* and *Bipolaris* genera.[33] Both groups consist of saprophytic fungi that are usually not pathogenic to humans. Infection generally occurs in debilitated individuals after normal phagocytic processes fail to eliminate inhaled spores.[34]

Among the parasites known to infect the orbit are *Echinococcus* and *Taenia solium.* Myiasis may also involve orbital tissues. The clinical features of these infections are inherently different from those of bacterial infections and are beyond the scope of this chapter.

Clinical Presentation

Bacterial infections of the periorbital tissues usually have an acute onset with unilateral periorbital pain, redness, swelling,

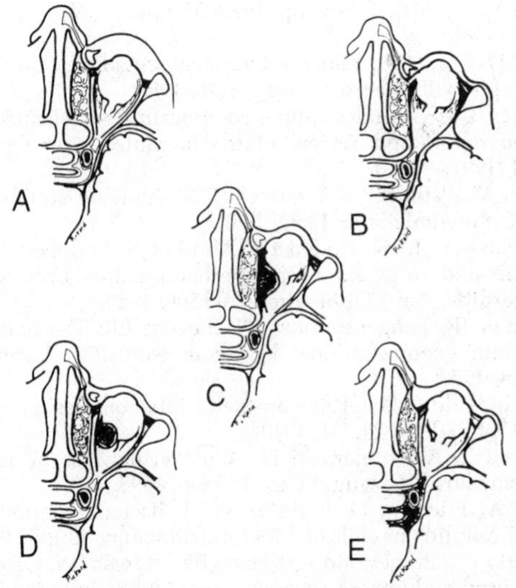

FIGURE 156–2 ▫ Pathologic changes and differences in inflammatory edema *(A)*; orbital cellulitis *(B)*; subperiosteal abscess *(C)*; orbital abscesses *(D)*; and cavernous sinus thrombosis *(E)*. (From Chandler JR, Langenbrunner DJ, Stevens ER: The pathogenesis of orbital complications in acute sinusitis. Laryngoscope 80:1414–1428, 1970.)

heat, and tenderness. Fever and leukocytosis are commonly present. As previously discussed, it is important to determine the presence of postseptal or orbital involvement. Characteristics of orbital infection include proptosis of the globe, ptosis of the eyelid, chemosis, and limitation of ocular motility (Fig. 156–3). Afferent pupillary defect, color vision deficit, visual field defect, and decreased visual acuity may indicate subperiosteal abscess, orbital abscess, sphenoid sinusitis, or cavernous sinus thrombosis. A demarcation line corresponding to the arcus marginalis suggests orbital infection. The absence of any of these findings does not, however, exclude deep orbital infection.

Phycomycetal infection may present with rapid rhinoorbital-cerebral progression,[29, 35, 36] usually in the diabetic or immunocompromised host. Nasal infection leads to involvement of the sinuses, orbit, and finally the central nervous system. Vascular thrombosis and subsequent necrosis of involved tissues underlie the physical findings of a seropurulent nasal discharge and a black eschar overlying nasal mucous membranes. Extension to the orbit leads to the typical findings of orbital inflammation.

In contrast to the rapidly aggressive nature of phycomycetal infection, aspergillosis may present as a more indolent process. *Aspergillus* has a predilection for cancer patients, especially those with lymphoma or leukemia.[37] Gradual visual loss with mild orbital inflammatory changes is a common presentation. Slowly progressive though they may be, these infections are potentially fatal, and a high index of suspicion is necessary to diagnose them early enough to effect a cure.

Diagnosis

The patient's history should provide specific information concerning antecedent infection (upper respiratory tract infection, sinusitis, otitis media, pharyngitis), antecedent trauma or surgery, and predisposing conditions such as diabetes or leukemia. Physical examination should determine whether the infection is pre- or postseptal.

Appropriate laboratory studies include white cell count with differential, serum glucose level, and cultures of blood, infected sinus drainage, and any purulent material. Aspirates from periorbital soft tissues are of little benefit. Purulent material should be Gram stained. Lumbar puncture is reserved for those patients with meningeal signs.[38, 39] Tuberculin skin testing is appropriate in selected cases.

Early biopsy should be performed for patients suspected of harboring fungal infection. Gomori methenamine silver, hematoxylin-eosin, and calcofluor white[40] stains are appropriate in combination with culture on Sabouraud agar without inhibitors such as cycloheximide.

Computed tomography with axial and coronal views, thin (2.5 mm) cuts, with and without use of contrast material, is the imaging study of choice. Plain films, orbital ultrasonography, and magnetic resonance imaging should be used to provide specific additional information. Although the sensitivity and specificity of computed tomography are excellent, the information provided by this modality must be interpreted in the context of the clinical situation.[41–44] Computed tomography should be considered in any patient with a postseptal infection or in one whose condition warrants hospitalization.

Therapy

Treatment of orbital infection is dictated by the site of origin. Sinusitis should be treated with appropriate antibiotics and possibly surgical drainage of the sinus. Dental abscesses should be drained. Consultation with the appropriate surgical specialist is appropriate.

Adults with mild preseptal cellulitis may be treated as outpatients if close clinical follow-up can be ensured. A semisynthetic penicillin is the drug of choice for situations in which *Staphylococcus* or *Streptococcus* is the suspected organism.

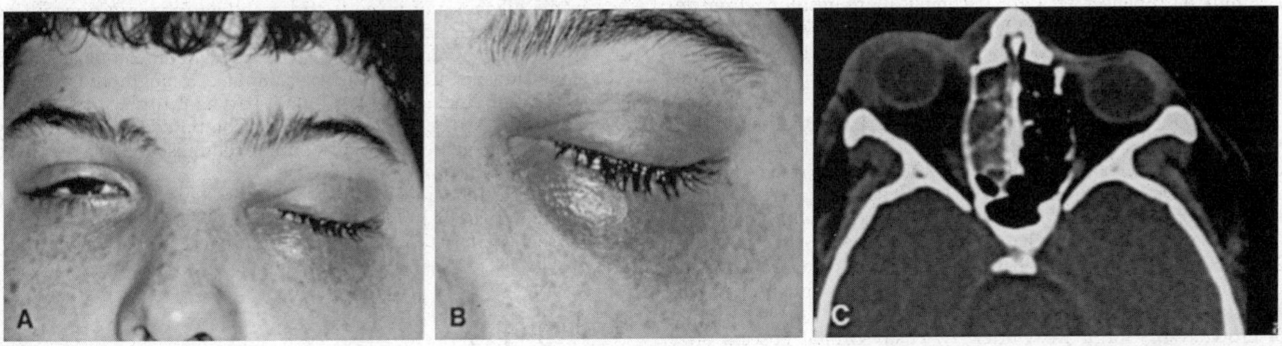

FIGURE 156–3 ▫ *A* and *B*, Orbital cellulitis: patient with left lid swelling, ptosis, and erythema. *C*, CT scan of same patient with left ethmoid sinusitis.

Children with preseptal or postseptal infection should probably be hospitalized for intravenous antibiotic therapy and close clinical observation. If the orbital infection follows trauma or a dermatologic condition, a semisynthetic penicillin such as nafcillin for coverage for staphylococci and streptococci is appropriate. Pediatric sinusitis demands coverage for the three most prevalent organisms seen in children—*Staphylococcus, Streptococcus,* and *Haemophilus* species. Selection must take into account the presence of meningeal signs or drug allergy.[44] Ampicillin and methicillin are no longer drugs of choice because of β-lactamase–producing strains of *Haemophilus* and the emergence of methicillin-resistant strains of *S. aureus.* Subperiosteal and orbital abscesses should, in general, be drained, although successful medical management of orbital abscess has been reported. This may be an acceptable alternative in selected cases, but it demands close follow-up and sound clinical judgment.

Adults with orbital cellulitis resulting from trauma should be hospitalized and treatment should be initiated if there is a strong suspicion of staphylococcal or streptococcal infection. Sinusitis is frequently associated with streptococci, staphylococci, anaerobes, and *Haemophilus* species. Subperiosteal or orbital abscess in an adult should be drained. Clearly, if there is Gram stain or other evidence to suggest a specific bacterium, antibiotic coverage should be tailored to the specific situation.

Fungal infections demand prompt, aggressive surgical debridement in combination with intravenous and topical antifungal therapy.

Management Considerations

Orbital infections can be devastating. The anatomy and function of the eye and orbit are complex. Commonly, management of the patient with orbital infection demands a team approach involving an otorhinolaryngologist, ophthalmologist, and infectious disease consultant.

References

1. Gutierrez Diaz A, del Palacio Hernanz A, Larregla S, Sanz Lopez A: Orbital phycomycosis. Ophthalmologica 182:165, 1981.
2. Clary R, Weber AL, Eavey R, Oot RF: Orbital cellulitis with abscess formation caused by sinusitis. Ann Otol Rhinol Laryngol 97:211, 1988.
3. Hornblass A, Herschorn BJ, Stern K, Grimes C: Orbital abscess. Surv Ophthalmol 29:169, 1984.
4. Jackson K, Baker SR: Periorbital cellulitis. Head Neck Surg 9:227, 1987.
5. Weizman Z, Mussaffi H: Ethmoiditis-associated periorbital cellulitis. Int J Pediatr Otorhinolaryngol 11:147, 1986.
6. Harris GJ: Subperiosteal inflammation of the orbit, a bacteriological analysis of 17 cases. Arch Ophthalmol 106:947, 1988.
7. Smith AT, Spencer JT: Orbital complications resulting from lesions of the sinuses. Ann Otol Rhinol Laryngol 57:5, 1948.
8. Southwick F, Richardson EP, Joseph M, Swartz MN: Septic thrombosis of the dural venous sinuses. Medicine (Baltimore) 65:82, 1986.
9. Bergin DJ, Wright J: Orbital cellulitis. Br J Ophthalmol 70:174, 1986.
10. Allan BP, Egbert MA, Myall RWT: Orbital abscess of odontogenic origin. J Oral Maxillofac Surg 20:268, 1991.
11. Bullock JD, Fleishman JA: Orbital cellulitis following dental extraction. Trans Am Ophthalmol Soc 87:111, 1984.
12. Harbour RC, Trobe JD, Ballinger WE: Septic cavernous sinus thrombosis associated with gingivitis and parapharyngeal abscess. Arch Ophthalmol 102:94, 1984.
13. Erdogan B, Gorgu M, Gurlek A, et al: Orbital abscess after rhinoplasty. Plast Reconstructr Surg 9:528, 1994.
14. Allen MV, Cohen KL, Grimson BS: Periorbital cellulitis secondary to dacryocystitis following blepharoplasty. Ann Ophthalmol 17:498, 1985.
15. Rees TD, Craig SM, Fisher Y: Orbital abscess following blepharoplasty. Plast Reconstruct Surg 73:126, 1983.
16. Weakley DR: Orbital cellulitis complicating strabismus surgery: A case report and review of the literature. Ann Ophthalmol 23:454, 1991.
17. Wilson M, Paul TO: Orbital cellulitis following strabismus surgery. Ophthalmic Surg 18:92, 1987.
18. Hornblass A, To K, Coden DJ, Ahn-Lee S: Endogenous orbital cellulitis and endogenous endophthalmitis in subacute bacterial endocarditis. Am J Ophthalmol 108:196, 1989.
19. Chandler JR, Langenbrunner DJ, Stevens ER: The pathogenesis of orbital complications in acute sinusitis. Laryngoscope 80:1414, 1970.
20. Holt H, de Rotth A: Orbital apex and sphenoid fissure syndrome. Arch Ophthalmol 24:731, 1940.
21. El-Sayed Y, Al-Muhaimeid H: Acute visual loss in association with sinusitis. J Laryngol Otol 107:840, 1993.
22. Weiss A, Friendly D, Eglin K, et al: Bacterial periorbital and orbital cellulitis in childhood. Ophthalmology 90:195, 1983.
23. Hemady R, Zimmerman A, Katzen BW, Karesh JW: Orbital cellulitis caused by *Eikenella corrodens.* Am J Ophthalmol 114:584, 1992.
24. Prendiville KJ, Bath PE: Lateral cantholysis and eyelid necrosis secondary to *Pseudomonas aeruginosa.* Ann Ophthalmol 20:193, 1988.
25. Ross J, Kohlhepp PA: Gangrene of the eyelids. Ann Ophthalmol 5:84, 1983.
26. Jones DB, Steinkuller PG: Strategies for the initial management of acute preseptal and orbital cellulitis. Trans Am Ophthalmol Soc 86:94, 1988.
27. Kallet HA, McKenzie KS, Johnson FD: Bacterial pseudomycosis of the orbit. Am J Ophthalmol 68:504, 1969.
28. Khali M, Lindley S, Matouk E: Tuberculosis of the orbit. Ophthalmology 92:1624, 1985.
29. Kohn R, Hepler R: Management of limited rhino-orbital mucormycosis without exenteration. Ophthalmology 92:1440, 1985.
30. Oakhill A, Shah KJ, Thompson AG, et al: Orbital tuberculosis in childhood. Br J Ophthalmol 66:396, 1982.
31. Sen DK: Tuberculosis of the orbita and lacrimal gland: A clinical study of 14 cases. J Pediatr Ophthalmol Strabismus 17:232, 1980.
32. Spoor TC, Harding SA: Orbital tuberculosis. Am J Ophthalmol 91:644, 1981.
33. Jacobson M, Galetta SL, Atlas SW, et al: Bipolaris-induced orbital cellulitis. J Clin Neuro Ophthalmol 12:250, 1992.
34. Ferry AP, Abedi S: Diagnosis and management of rhinoorbitocerebral mucormycosis (phycomycosis). Ophthalmology 90:1096, 1983.
35. Bray WH, Giangiacomo J, Ide CH: Orbital apex syndrome. Surv Ophthalmol 32:136, 1987.
36. Schwartze GM, Kilgo GR, Ford CS: Internal ophthalmoplegia resulting from acute orbital phycomycosis. J Clin Neuro Ophthalmol 4:105, 1984.
37. Harris G, Will B: Orbital aspergillosis, conservative debridement and local amphotericin irrigation. Ophthal Plast Reconstruct Surg 5:207, 1989.
38. Antoine GA, Grundfast KM: Periorbital cellulitis. Int J Pediatr Otorhinolaryngol 13:273, 1987.
39. Ciarallo LR, Rowe PC: Lumbar puncture in children with periorbital and orbital cellulitis. J Pediatr 3:355, 1993.
40. Marines HM, Osato MS, Font RL: The value of calcofluor white in the diagnosis of mycotic and acanthamoeba infections of the eye and ocular adnexa. Ophthalmology 94:23, 1987.
41. Clary RA, Cunningham MJ, Eavey RD: Orbital complications of acute sinusitis: Comparison of computed tomography scan and surgical findings. Ann Otol Rhinol Laryngol 101:598, 1992.
42. Gold SC, Arrigg PG, Hedges TR: Computerized tomography in the management of acute orbital cellulitis. Ophthalmic Surg 18:753, 1987.
43. Hodges E, Tabbara KF: Orbital cellulitis: Review of 23 cases from Saudi Arabia. Br J Ophthalmol 73:205, 1989.
44. Lessner A, Stern GA: Preseptal and orbital cellulitis. Ocular Infect 6:933, 1992.

Bibliography

□ Ahrens-Palumbo MJ, Ballen PH: Primary dacryocystitis causing orbital cellulitis. Ann Ophthalmol 14:600, 1982.

- Biedner BZ, Marmur U, Yassur Y: *Streptococcus faecalis* orbital cellulitis. Ann Ophthalmol 18:194, 1986.
- Case 38-1982: Case Records of the Massachusetts General Hospital. A 66 year old diabetic woman with sinusitis and cranial nerve abnormalities. N Engl J Med 307:806, 1982.
- Crock GW, Heriot WJ, Janakiraman P, Weiner JM: Gas gangrene infection of the eyes and orbits. Br J Ophthalmol 69:143, 1985.
- Dortzbach R, Segrest DR: Orbital aspergillosis. Ophthalmic Surg 14:240, 1983.
- Gatot A, Tovi F, Moshiashvili A: Periorbital cellulitis: Presenting feature of undiagnosed old maxillary fracture. Int J Pediatr Otorhinolaryngol 11:129, 1986.
- Geggel HS, Isenberg SJ: Cavernous sinus thrombosis as a cause of unilateral blindness. Ann Ophthalmol 14:569, 1982.
- Goodwin WJ Jr: Orbital complications of ethmoiditis. Otolaryngol Clin North Am 1:18, 1985.
- Green WR, Font RL, Zimmerman LE: Aspergillosis of the orbit. Arch Ophthalmol 82:302, 1969.
- Hamed HH: Orbital affection with *Cysticercus cellulosae.* Bull Ophthalmol Soc Egypt 61:253, 1968.
- Harris GJ: Subperiosteal abscess of the orbit. Arch Ophthalmol 101:751, 1983.
- Jakobiec FA, Jones IS: Orbital inflammations. *In* Duane TD (ed): Clinical Ophthalmology. Philadelphia, JB Lippincott, 1988.
- Kars Z, Kansu T, Ozcan OE, Erbengi A: Orbital echinococcosis, report of two cases studied by computerized tomography. J Clin Neuro Ophthalmol 2:197, 1982.
- Kaufman SJ: Orbital mucopyoceles. Two cases and a review. Surv Ophthalmol 25:253, 1981.
- Lazzaro EC, Sloan B: Mucormycosis: Case presentation and discussion. Ann Ophthalmol 14:660, 1982.
- Levine RA: Infection of the orbit by an atypical mycobacterium. Arch Ophthalmol 82:608, 1969.
- Maskin SL, Fetchick RJ, Leone CR Jr, et al: *Bipolaris hawaiiensis*–caused phaeohyphomycotic orbitopathy. Ophthalmology 96:175–179, 1989.
- McNamara MP, Richie M, Kirmani N: Ocular infections secondary to *Pasteurella multocida.* Am J Ophthalmol 106:361, 1988.
- Miller RD, Steinkuller PG, Naegele D: Nonfatal maxillocerebral mucormycosis. Ann Ophthalmol 12:1065, 1980.
- Morales AG, et al: Hydatid cysts of the orbit, a review of 35 cases. Ophthalmology 95:1027, 1988.
- Munford RS: Orbital infections. Curr Clin Top Infect Dis 4:1, 1983.
- Nielsen EW, Weisman RA, Savino PJ, Schatz NJ: Aspergillosis of the sphenoid sinus presenting as orbital pseudotumor. Otolaryngol Head Neck Surg 91:699, 1983.
- O'Keefe M, Haining WM, Young JDH, Guthrie W: Orbital mucormycosis with survival. Br J Ophthalmol 70:634, 1986.
- Partamian LG, Jay WM, Fritz KJ: Anaerobic orbital cellulitis. Ann Ophthalmol 15:123, 1983.
- Rubin SE, Rubin LG, Zito J, et al: Medical management of orbital subperiosteal abscess in children. J Pediatr Ophthalmol Strabismus 26:21, 1989.
- Rubin SE, Slavin ML, Rubin LG: Eyelid swelling and erythema as the only signs of subperiosteal abscess. Br J Ophthalmol 73:576, 1989.
- Scott PM, Bloome MA: Lid necrosis secondary to streptococcal periorbital cellulitis. Ann Ophthalmol 13:461, 1981.
- Slavin ML, Glaser JS: Acute severe irreversible visual loss with sphenoethmoiditis–'posterior' orbital cellulitis. Arch Ophthalmol 105:345, 1987.
- Spoor TC, Hartel WC, Harding S, Kocher G: Aspergillosis presenting as a corticosteroid-responsive optic neuropathy. J Clin Neuro Ophthalmol 2:103, 1982.
- Stankiewicz JA: Sphenoid sinus mucocele. Arch Otolaryngol Head Neck Surg 115:735, 1989.
- Streeten BW, Rabuzzi DD, Jones DB: Sporotrichosis of the orbital margin. Am J Ophthalmol 77:750, 1974.
- Thomas D, Older J, Kandawalla NM, Torczynski E: The *Dirofilaria* parasite in the orbit. Am J Ophthalmol 82:931, 1976.
- Ullman S, Pflugfelder SC, Hughes RS, Forster RK: *Bacillus cereus* panophthalmitis manifesting as an orbital cellulitis. Am J Ophthalmol 103:105, 1987.
- Vida L, Moel SA: Systemic North American blastomycosis with orbital involvement. Am J Ophthalmol 77:240, 1974.
- Wever AL, Mikulis DK: Inflammatory disorders of the paraorbital sinuses and their complications. Radiol Clin North Am 25:615, 1987.
- Wolff E (revised by RJ Last): Eugene Wolff's Anatomy of the Eye and Orbit. Philadelphia, WB Saunders, 1968.
- Yumoto E, Kitani S, Okamura H, Yanagihara N: Sino-orbital aspergillosis associated with total ophthalmoplegia. Laryngoscope 95:190, 1985.
- Zak SM, Katz B: Successfully treated spheno-orbital mucormycosis in an otherwise healthy adult. Ann Ophthalmol 17:344, 1985.

NERVOUS SYSTEM

157

Approach to the Patient with Infection of the Central Nervous System

Diane E. Griffin

Central nervous system (CNS) infections are relatively infrequent, accounting for approximately 1% of hospital admissions and another 2% of nosocomially acquired infections. When encountered, CNS infections often require prompt diagnosis and initiation of treatment. The potential for rapid progression and permanent neurologic damage lends greater urgency to the evaluation and presumptive treatment of a CNS disease than to many other infectious diseases.

CNS infections take a great variety of forms, ranging from acute but benign forms of viral meningitis to rapidly fatal bacterial meningitis, to the slowly progressive mental deterioration from fungal, mycobacterial, or persistent viral infection (Table 157–1). The most common diseases are viral and bacterial meningitis, with the cumulative risk for CNS infection through age 80 years being 2.3% for men and 1.5% for women.[1] Prompt treatment is effective for many of the more severe diseases, and the outcome is often determined by the speed and appropriateness of the therapy.[2–4] Most deaths due to bacterial infection occur within the first 48 hours of hospitalization.[5] For these reasons, CNS infection must be recognized early and the probable infecting agent determined as rapidly as possible, by either laboratory examination or clinical acumen. Proper initial assessment of the patient requires a careful history with attention to the tempo of the disease, exposures to infectious agents, and host factors that may result in increased susceptibility to certain infections. The physical examination is directed at localizing the neurologic disease anatomically and identifying evidence of

TABLE 157–1 ■ Incidence and Mortality Rate for Central Nervous System Infections from 1950 to 1981, in Olmsted County, Minnesota

INFECTION	INCIDENCE (PER 100,000 PERSON-YEARS)	MORTALITY (%)
Aseptic meningitis	10.9	0
Bacterial meningitis	8.6	10
Viral encephalitis	7.4	3.8
Brain abscess	1.1	37
Chronic meningitis	0.4	43

From Nicolosi A, Hauser WA, Beghi E, Kurland LT: Epidemiology of central nervous system infections in Olmsted County, Minnesota, 1950–1981. J Infect Dis 154:399–408, 1986. © by The University of Chicago.

systemic infection. These assessments are supplemented by examination of the cerebrospinal fluid (CSF) and, when indicated, imaging studies.

Anatomic Considerations

The CNS is relatively protected from infection. The scalp, skull, and meninges help to prevent infection from external sources, and the blood-brain barrier helps to prevent infection from blood-borne sources; however, when infection does occur much of the initial evaluation should be directed at determining the anatomic site of infection, because this is important in narrowing the differential diagnosis, determining the type of therapy necessary, and predicting the likely outcome of infection. Although some infections may spread to involve more than one site, initially each is characteristically localized to a particular anatomic area.

Dura

The dura is adjacent to the skull and relatively adherent to it in many places, and epidural abscesses typically spread laterally and are relatively thin. Between the dura and the arachnoid is a potential space with few restraining structures, and subdural abscesses may be relatively large, space-occupying lesions. Infections in both of these parameningeal locations are usually associated with direct invasion by microorganisms secondary to trauma, neurosurgical procedures, or infections of adjacent orifices. Occasionally, blood-borne organisms may localize in a closed sterile area that was previously traumatized.[3, 6, 7]

Leptomeninges

The pia and arachnoid are usually involved together in infectious processes on the surface of the brain and spinal cord. Viruses, mycoplasmas, bacteria, mycobacteria, fungi, and parasites are all capable of causing leptomeningitis. Organisms usually arrive at the meninges from the initial site of replication through the blood,[8] causing a disease that may be acute, subacute, or chronic, depending on the infecting agent and the immune status of the host.

Parenchyma

Infection of the brain parenchyma may be the result of local spread of organisms from a contiguous source of infection (usually resulting in a single lesion) or by hematogenous spread (often resulting in multiple lesions).[9] Bacterial infection in the brain parenchyma from either source begins as a localized cerebritis with focal softening, necrosis, inflammation, and edema. As the process continues, fibroblasts begin to proliferate at the periphery to encapsulate the infected area.[10] Symptoms may be due to local destruction of tissue, but most often they are due to pressure and surrounding edema caused by mass effect from the expanding lesion. Viral infection of the brain parenchyma causes encephalitis, which may be focal or diffuse. Most viruses that cause encephalitis reach the brain from the blood and may infect neurons or glial cells directly, leading to seizures, paralysis, or changes in mental status.[11]

Epidemiologic Considerations

Many viral, rickettsial, and bacterial infections have distinct seasonal and regional variations, which are often helpful in narrowing the differential diagnosis (Fig. 157–1). Arthropod-borne infections are limited to locations where their arthropod vectors are present and to the times of the year when the vectors are active. Tick-borne infections, such as Rocky Mountain spotted fever, tick-borne encephalitis, and Lyme disease, are most common in spring and early summer.[12, 13] Mosquito-borne diseases such as eastern equine, western equine, California, and St. Louis encephalitides occur during the summer and early fall.[14] In addition, enteroviral infections, the most common cause of viral meningitis and encephalitis, have their highest incidence during the late summer and fall months.[15–17] Bacterial meningitis peaks in the winter months[5, 18] and may also occur in outbreaks.[19, 20]

Host Considerations

The host is an important determinant of susceptibility to certain CNS infections. A recent history of open trauma, surgery, or severe burn suggests the possibility of infection with candidal, staphylococcal, or gram-negative organisms from the environment and skin.[4, 7, 21, 22] A history of closed head trauma that resulted in a recognized or unrecognized CSF leak is strongly associated with pneumococcal meningitis.[23] The majority of persons with spinal epidural abscesses

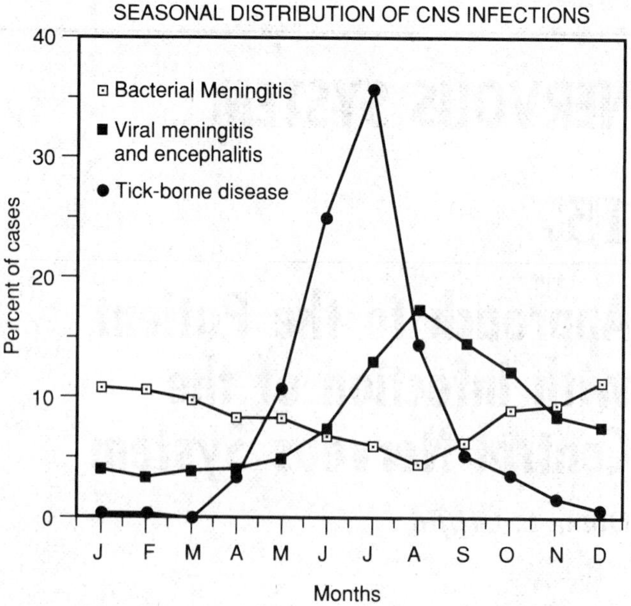

FIGURE 157–1 □ Percentages of the cases of bacterial meningitis, tick-borne disease (Lyme disease and Rocky Mountain spotted fever), and viral meningitis and encephalitis that occur during each month of the year. (Data from references 5, 12, 13, 63 to 65.)

have underlying degenerative joint disease.[3] Brain abscess occurs more frequently in persons with chronic sinusitis or otitis, congenital heart disease, and previous esophageal procedures.[9] CSF shunts and reservoirs are most often associated with staphylococcal infections.[24]

Defenses against invasion of organisms from the blood stream are compromised by abnormalities of cellular immunity, antibody formation, complement production, and phagocytosis, because prevention of CNS infection depends on prompt clearing of the infectious agent from blood and tissue. Different types of immune compromise are preferentially associated with certain types of CNS infections. Genetic and acquired deficiencies in splenic phagocytosis (e.g., sickle cell disease, traumatic or surgical asplenia), in γ-globulin synthesis, or in circulating levels of complement result in inadequate clearance of blood-borne organisms and predispose primarily to CNS infections with encapsulated bacteria.[25, 26] Hypogammaglobulinemia also predisposes to chronic enteroviral infections.[27] Genetic and acquired deficiencies of cellular immunity, which result in inadequate clearance of organisms from tissue and inadequate control of latent or persistent organisms, predispose principally to CNS infection by fungi or intracellular pathogens such as viruses, *Listeria*, mycobacteria, and parasites[28–35] (Table 157–2).

Age is an important host factor in considering the cause of CNS infections[16, 36] (Fig. 157–2 and Table 157–3). Bacterial and viral meningitis and encephalitis are most common in childhood. Infants, possibly because of their immature immune status, are uniquely susceptible to CNS infection with *Listeria*, gram-negative bacilli, group B streptococci, enteroviruses, and herpesviruses.[16, 20, 37–39] As maternal antibody wanes and production de novo of antibody to bacterial polysaccharides lags, susceptibility to other bacterial pathogens, such as *Haemophilus*, pneumococcus, and *Meningococcus*, emerges.[4] With advancing age and increasing prevalence of hepatic disease, susceptibility to gram-negative organisms increases,[40] accounting for 25% of all CNS infections in persons older than 65 years.[41] Spinal epidural abscess is most common in the fifth and sixth decades.[3]

Clinical Assessment

Headache or backache and fever are common, but not universal, indications of CNS infection. Fever generally accompanies acute CNS infection but may be absent in chronic infection. The initial physical evaluation should include evaluation for cranial trauma, level of consciousness, cranial nerve palsy, focal deficits, meningismus, and increased intracranial pressure.

Infection in the subdural or epidural space that has spread

TABLE 157–2 ■ Organisms That Most Often Cause Central Nervous System Infection in Immunocompromised Hosts

Deficiencies in complement and antibody production
Streptococcus penumoniae
Neisseria meningitidis
Haemophilus influenzae
Enterovirus
Deficiencies in cellular immunity
Cryptococcus
Toxoplasma
Nocardia
Listeria
JC virus (progressive multifocal leukoencephalopathy)
Human immunodeficiency virus
Cytomegalovirus

Age-specific Incidence of CNS Infections

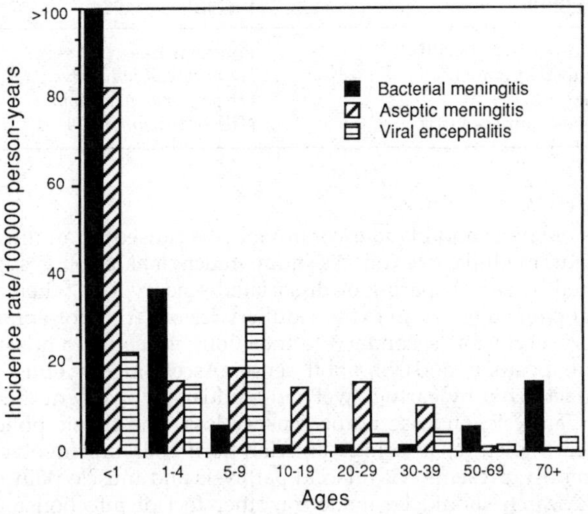

FIGURE 157–2 □ Age-specific incidence of CNS infections based on a population-based study in Olmsted County, Minnesota. (Data from Nicolosi A, Hauser WA, Beghi E, Kurland LT: Epidemiology of central nervous system infections in Olmsted County, Minnesota, 1950–1981. J Infect Dis 154:399, 1986.)

from contiguous areas of infection or previous injury is likely to present as localized pain in the head or spine. Epidural abscesses located near the spine typically progress, at a variable pace, from back pain to root pain, weakness, and paralysis.[3]

Infections limited to the leptomeninges usually present with signs and symptoms of meningeal irritation and altered mental status. Inflammation of the meninges causes reflex paraspinous muscle spasm, which is reflected in an opisthotonic posture (particularly in children), nuchal rigidity, inability to straighten a raised leg, and flexion of the leg when the neck is flexed.[42] Most patients with acute bacterial meningitis after the neonatal period have signs of meningeal irritation at the time of presentation.[4] Those without such signs are more likely to be elderly and to have gram-negative meningitis.[41] Neonates usually exhibit listlessness but no clear CNS signs.[43] Seizures are common. Chronic meningeal inflammation may involve the cranial nerves, resulting in cranial nerve palsies, or produce hydrocephalus (headache, nausea and vomiting, mental deterioration, or spastic paraparesis) or localized infarction secondary to vasculitis.

Disease within the brain parenchyma may result in seizures, altered states of consciousness, acute changes in personality or behavior, or focal neurologic deficits. Patients with viral encephalitis typically progress from lethargy to confusion, stupor, and coma. Signs of meningeal inflammation may or may not be present. Focal neurologic signs usually develop, and seizures are common. The hypothalamic-pituitary axis may be involved, causing severe hyper- or hypothermia and diabetes insipidus.[11] In herpes simplex encephalitis, signs often include bizarre behavior, hallucinations, and aphasia, suggesting the temporal lobe localization typical of that infection.[44] Brain abscess usually presents with headache of increasing severity followed by nausea and vomiting. Fever is often absent, particularly in older patients and those with temporal lobe abscesses.[9] Increased intracranial pressure can cause papilledema and third and sixth cranial nerve palsies.

Myelitis can occur with or without encephalitis. Transverse myelitis resulting in lower limb weakness, sensory loss, and

TABLE 157–3 ■ Organisms That Most Often Cause Central Nervous System Infection in Immunologically Normal Hosts at Different Ages

<1 MONTH	1 MONTH–5 YEARS	6–59 YEARS	>60 YEARS
Gram-negative bacilli	Enteroviruses	Enteroviruses	*S. pneumoniae*
Group B streptococci	*Haemophilus influenzae*	*N. meningitidis*	Gram-negative bacilli
Listeria	*Streptococcus pneumoniae*	*S. pneumoniae*	*Listeria*
Herpes simplex virus	*Neisseria meningitidis*	Herpes simplex virus	

loss of bowel and bladder control may be caused by an intra- or extramedullary lesion. An intraparenchymal lesion is suggested by sacral sparing or dissociated sensory loss, whereas local pain suggests an extramedullary lesion. Anterior spinal artery occlusion secondary to infectious vasculitis tends to spare position and vibration sense. Ascending myelitis is characterized by early bowel and bladder involvement, flaccid paralysis, and ascending sensory loss. The classic poliomyelitis picture, in which anterior horn cells are involved primarily, presents with flaccid paralysis and muscle pain.

A search should be made for other foci of infection and for physical signs that suggest a specific microbial cause. The presence of petechiae may suggest meningococcal infection or Rocky Mountain spotted fever.[45] Exanthems are also found with varicella, herpes zoster, and typhus, and occasionally with *Haemophilus influenzae, Streptococcus pneumoniae, Mycoplasma*, coxsackievirus, and echovirus infections, Lyme disease, and syphilis. Meningitis with pneumonia suggests pneumococcal infection.[5]

The evidences of CNS infection may be masked by other disease processes, especially in elderly persons.[46] Fever may be attributed to a recognized infection elsewhere, such as pneumonia, cellulitis, endocarditis, otitis, or sinusitis, and altered CNS function may be blamed on alcoholism, head trauma, stroke, brain tumor, subarachnoid hemorrhage, or metabolic abnormalities.[40] Treatable CNS infection, particularly bacterial meningitis, must be ruled out in such patients. This is usually done by careful neurologic examination, including lumbar puncture.

Laboratory Studies

Examination of CSF is a mainstay of the diagnostic approach to CNS infection. Careful consideration should be given to the types of information desired and to what supplemental information (such as peripheral glucose values) may be necessary to interpret the results. Normally, CSF is crystal clear; contains less than five mononuclear cells per cubic millimeter; has a protein content less than 4.5 g/L, of which 14% or less is γ-globulin; has a glucose concentration about two thirds that of the blood (except in diabetes patients and those who are receiving glucose intravenously or have recently); and is under pressure of less than 180 mm H_2O.

CNS infection usually produces changes in the CSF (Table 157–4). These may include an increased number of cells, increased protein concentration, and decreased glucose concentration. Total and differential cell counts should be performed. Mononuclear cells usually predominate in mycobacterial, fungal, rickettsial, and viral infections, whereas a predominance of polymorphonuclear cells is typical of bacterial and amebic infections. One polymorphonuclear leukocyte or more than five mononuclear cells in uncentrifuged CSF are abnormal. Early in any of these diseases there may be no increase in cells. Polymorphonuclear cells may be present in large numbers early in viral infections. Repeated examination of the CSF in 8 to 24 hours often is useful.[47] Severely immunocompromised persons may also fail to mount an inflammatory response.[33] A pleocytosis may be found in subacute bacterial endocarditis, after severe seizures, during systemic viral infection such as measles, or after treatment with anti-CD3 antibody for graft rejection. Significant numbers of erythrocytes may be found in herpesvirus infection[48] and in postinfectious and amebic encephalitis.

The fluid should be stained and cultured for the infecting agent. Because CNS infection is frequently a complication of systemic disease, other relevant body fluids (e.g., blood, stool, throat scrapings, sputum, urine) should also be cultured. Short-term antibiotic treatment before admission does not significantly alter the total or differential cell count, or protein or glucose values, but it does reduce the frequency of "positive cultures" and diagnostic Gram strain.[5, 49] Certain microbial antigens (e.g., *Cryptococcus, Haemophilus*, pneumococcus, and *Meningococcus*) may be detected by immunodiagnostic techniques rapidly providing a clue to diagnosis and a potential mechanism for identifying the infecting organism in previously treated persons.[49–51] Polymerase chain reaction is increasingly useful for diagnosis of CNS viral infections.[35, 38, 52]

The CSF protein level increases with most infections, and in chronic infections an increased proportion of this protein may be locally synthesized immunoglobulin. The increase in protein concentration may be slight with viral infections, but it is usually greater with bacterial, fungal, or tuberculous infections. An increased protein value may be the only CSF abnormality in brain abscess and parameningeal infections. The immunoglobulin present is often against the infecting agent and may be a means of diagnosing acute (immunoglobulin M) and chronic (immunoglobulin G) viral[11] and spirochetal[53] infections.

The CSF glucose value is usually low in untreated bacterial meningitis, and frequently in fungal, amebic, and tuberculous meningitis. In many persons, the CSF glucose value can be interpreted only if a plasma glucose level is also available from a sample taken at approximately the same time. The CSF glucose value, usually normal during viral or rickettsial infections of the CNS,[45] may be depressed in some viral encephalitides (particularly those caused by mumps and lymphocytic choriomeningitis viruses), CNS sarcoid, tumors, and subarachnoid hemorrhage.

The major risk in performing a lumbar puncture occurs when there is evidence of increased intracranial pressure due to a mass lesion in the cranial vault. With removal of CSF the intracranial pressure dynamics may be altered and the brain may shift downward through the tentorial notch or foramen magnum. This is particularly likely to happen when there is a large, asymmetric, supratentorial mass or a mass in the posterior fossa.[7, 9, 54, 55] In contrast, herniation is seldom seen with diffuse increases in intracranial volume, as occurs with generalized infection or meningitis. If a mass lesion is suspected based on the history or physical examination or if increased intracranial pressure is evident on funduscopic examination, then an imaging technique such as computed tomography or magnetic resonance imaging should be performed before the lumbar puncture. In other situations the lumbar puncture should not be delayed, because the informa-

TABLE 157–4 ■ Typical Cerebrospinal Fluid Findings in Various Types of Central Nervous System Infections

INFECTION	CELLS/MM³	CELL TYPES*	PROTEIN LEVEL	GLUCOSE LEVEL	CULTURE
Meningitis					
Bacterial	500–10,000	PMNs	High–very high	Low–very low	Positive
Viral	50–1,000	Monocytes	Slightly elevated	Normal	Positive
Tuberculous	50–1,000	Monocytes	High	Low	Positive
Parenchymal					
Brain abscess	5–100	PMNs, monocytes	High–very high	Normal	Negative
Viral encephalitis	5–100	Monocytes	Normal–high	Normal	Negative
Parameningeal					
Epidural	5–100	PMNs, monocytes	High–very high	Normal	Negative
Subdural	5–100	PMNs, monocytes	High	Normal	Negative

* PMNs, Polymorphonuclear leukocytes.

tion gained from examining CSF is crucial for the differential diagnosis and early institution of treatment. The practice of performing computed tomography routinely before lumbar puncture imposes a significant and unnecessary delay in treatment of bacterial meningitis.[56]

Imaging Studies

Plain radiographs of the skull or spine usually are not necessary, but they may help in cases in which trauma or vertebral disease is a predisposing factor to infection. Computed tomography with use of contrast material may or may not confirm meningeal infection, particularly in chronic meningitis,[57] but it is useful in the diagnosis of epidural, subdural, or parenchymal brain abscess[9, 10] and takes less time than magnetic resonance imaging. Magnetic resonance imaging is more sensitive for recognition of many types of parenchymal infection—progressive multifocal leukoencephalopathy, herpes simplex virus encephalitis, human immunodeficiency virus–associated dementia white matter lesions, bacterial cerebritis before the development of the capsule, and spinal cord lesions.[52, 58–60] Myelography is quite sensitive in the diagnosis of spinal epidural abscess.[3]

Initial Management

The first steps in management of suspected CNS infection are dictated by the type and location of the infectious process. For viral infections the most important steps are aimed at diagnosis (collection of "acute-phase serum" and cultures from appropriate sites), supportive therapy (control of seizures, fluid and electrolyte balance, respiratory assistance) if needed, and initiation of acyclovir therapy[52] if herpes simplex virus encephalitis is suspected (temporal lobe localization). It should be noted that herpes simplex virus causes less than 10% of cases of viral encephalitis.

For focal parenchymal bacterial infections the most important initial step is surgical drainage if there is threat of abscess rupture or evidence of mass effect compromising neurologic function. Prompt drainage is also important for subdural empyema and spinal epidural abscesses. Appropriate antibiotic therapy (e.g., metronidazole, penicillin with or without ceftriaxone) alone is often sufficient for treatment of intraparenchymal bacterial abscesses if drainage is not necessary to relieve pressure.[61]

For suspected bacterial meningitis, bactericidal antibiotics that penetrate the CNS (e.g., penicillin or ampicillin, ceftriaxone or cefotaxime) should be initiated as soon as blood and CSF cultures have been obtained.[8] If there is an unavoidable delay in obtaining CSF for culture, antibiotic therapy should be initiated.[49] The antibiotic regimen selected should include coverage for organisms suspected on the basis of CSF Gram stain and antigen detection tests but should also cover other likely possibilities until a definitive diagnosis has been made. In children, routine adjunctive therapy with dexamethasone is controversial[62] now that *H. influenzae* infection is infrequent. If clinical presentation or epidemiologic considerations suggest rickettsial disease, chloramphenicol or tetracycline should be included in the therapeutic regimen.

References

1. Nicolosi A, Hauser WA, Beghi E, Kurland LT: Epidemiology of central nervous system infections in Olmsted County, Minnesota, 1950–1981. J Infect Dis 154:399, 1986.
2. Mauser HW, Van Houwelingen HC, Tullekin CAF: Factors affecting the outcome in subdural empyema. J Neurol Neurosurg Psychiatry 50:1136, 1987.
3. Darouiche RO, Hamill RJ, Greenberg SB, et al: Bacterial spinal epidural abscess: Review of 43 cases and literature survey. Medicine (Baltimore) 71:369, 1992.
4. Swartz MN, Dodge PR: Bacterial meningitis—a review of selected aspects. N Engl J Med 272:725; 779; 842; 954, 1965.
5. Geiseler PJ, Nelson KE, Levin S, et al: Community-acquired purulent meningitis: A review of 1316 cases during the antibiotic era, 1954–1976. Rev Infect Dis 2:725, 1980.
6. Kaufman DM, Mitler MH, Steigbigel NH: Subdural empyema: Analysis of 17 recent cases and review of the literature. Medicine (Baltimore) 54:485, 1975.
7. Dill SR, Cobbs CG, McDonald CK: Subdural empyema: Analysis of 32 cases and review. Clin Infect Dis 20:372, 1995.
8. Tunkel AR, Wispelwey B, Scheld WM: Bacterial meningitis: Recent advances in pathophysiology and treatment. Ann Intern Med 112:610, 1990.
9. Chun CH, Johnson JD, Hofstetter M, Raff MJ: Brain abscess: A study of 45 consecutive cases. Medicine (Baltimore) 65:415, 1986.
10. Britt RH, Enzmann DR: Clinical stages of human brain abscesses on serial CT scans after contrast infusion: Computerized tomographic, neuropathological, and clinical correlations. J Neurosurg 59:972, 1983.
11. Griffin DE: Viral infections of the central nervous system. *In* Galasso GJ, Whitley RJ, Merigan TC (eds): Antiviral Agents and Viral Diseases of Man, ed 3. New York, Raven Press, 1990, pp 461–495.
12. Wilfert CM, MacCormack JN, Kleeman K, et al: Epidemiology of Rocky Mountain spotted fever as determined by active surveillance. J Infect Dis 150:469, 1984.
13. Schmid GP, Horsley R, Steere AC, et al: Surveillance of Lyme disease in the United States, 1982. J Infect Dis 151:1144, 1985.
14. Arboviral infections of the central nervous system—United States, 1989. MMWR Morbid Mortal Wkly Rep 39:407, 1990.
15. Deibel R, Barron A, Millian S, Smith V: Central nervous system infections in New York State. N Y State J Med 74:1929, 1974.
16. Berlin LE, Rorabaugh ML, Heldrich F, et al: Aseptic meningitis

in infants <2 years of age: Diagnosis and etiology. J Infect Dis 168:888, 1993.
17. Koskiniemi M, Rautonen J, Lehtokoski-Lehtiniemi E, Vaheri A: Epidemiology of encephalitis in children: A 20-year study. Ann Neurol 29:492, 1991.
18. Schlech WF, Ward JI, Band JD, et al: Bacterial meningitis in the United States, 1978 through 1981: The national bacterial meningitis surveillance study. JAMA 253:1749, 1985.
19. Greenwood BM: Selective primary health care: Strategies for control of disease in the developing world. XIII. Acute bacterial meningitis. Rev Infect Dis 6:374, 1984.
20. Linnan MJ, Mascola L, Lou XD, et al: Epidemic listeriosis associated with Mexican-style cheese. N Engl J Med 319:823, 1988.
21. Durand ML, Calderwood SB, Weber DJ, et al: Acute bacterial meningitis in adults: A review of 493 episodes. N Engl J Med 328:21, 1993.
22. Winkelman MD, Galloway PG: Central nervous system complications of thermal burns: A postmortem study of 139 patients. Medicine (Baltimore) 71:271, 1992.
23. Pappas DG Jr, Hammerschlag PE, Hammerschlag M: Cerebrospinal fluid rhinorrhea and recurrent meningitis. Clin Infect Dis 17:364, 1993.
24. Morissette I, Gourdeau M, Francoeur J: CSF shunt infections: A fifteen-year experience with emphasis on management and outcome. Can J Neurol Sci 20:118, 1993.
25. Cullingford GL, Watkins DN, Watts AD, Mallon DF: Severe late postsplenectomy infection. Br J Surg 78:716, 1991.
26. Platonov AE, Beloborodov VB, Vershinina IV: Meningococcal disease in patients with late complement component deficiency. Studies in the U.S.S.R. Medicine (Baltimore) 72:374, 1993.
27. McKinney RE Jr, Katz SL, Wilfert CM: Chronic enteroviral meningoencephalitis in agammaglobulinemic patients. Rev Infect Dis 9:334, 1987.
28. Salaki JS, Louria DB, Chmel H: Fungal and yeast infections of the central nervous system: A clinical review. Medicine (Baltimore) 63:108, 1984.
29. Luft BJ, Remington JS: Toxoplasmic encephalitis in AIDS. Clin Infect Dis 15:211, 1992.
30. Peterson PK: Host defense abnormalities predisposing the patient to infection. Am J Med 76:2, 1984.
31. Wong B: Parasitic diseases in immunocompromised hosts. Am J Med 76:479, 1984.
32. Stamm AM, Dismukes WE, Simmons BP, et al: Listeriosis in renal transplant recipients: Report of an outbreak and review of 102 cases. Rev Infect Dis 4:665, 1982.
33. Powderly WG: Cryptococcal meningitis and AIDS. Clin Infect Dis 17:837, 1993.
34. Mischel PS, Vinters HV: Coccidioidomycosis of the central nervous system: Neuropathological and vasculopathic manifestations and clinical correlates. J Infect Dis 20:400, 1995.
35. McCutchan JA: Cytomegalovirus infections of the nervous system in patients with AIDS. Clin Infect Dis 20:747, 1995.
36. Wenger JD, Hightower AW, Facklam RR, et al: Bacterial meningitis in the United States, 1986: Report of a multistate surveillance study. J Infect Dis 162:1316, 1990.
37. Dillon HC Jr, Khare S, Gray BM: Group B streptococcal carriage and disease: A 6 year prospective study. J Pediatr 110:31, 1987.
38. Rotbart HA: Enteroviral infections of the central nervous system. Clin Infect Dis 20:971, 1995.
39. Whitley RJ, Hutto C: Neonatal herpes simplex virus infections. Pediatr Rev 7:119, 1985.
40. Crane LR, Lerner AM: Nontraumatic gram-negative bacillary meningitis in the Detroit Medical Center, 1964–1974 (with special mention of cases due to *Escherichia coli*). Medicine (Baltimore) 57:197, 1978.
41. Behrman RE, Meyers BR, Mendelson MH, et al: Central nervous system infections in the elderly. Arch Intern Med 149:1596, 1989.
42. Verghese A, Gallemore G: Kernig's and Brudzinski's signs revisited. Rev Infect Dis 9:1187, 1987.
43. Rorabaugh ML, Berlin LE, Heldrich F, et al: Aseptic meningitis in infants younger than 2 years of age. Acute illness and neurologic complications. Pediatrics 92:206, 1993.
44. Whitley RJ, Soong S-J, Linneman C Jr, et al: Herpes simplex: Clinical assessment. JAMA 247:317, 1982.
45. Kirk JL, Fine DP, Sexton DJ, Muchmore HG: Rocky Mountain spotted fever: A clinical review based on 48 confirmed cases, 1943–1986. Medicine (Baltimore) 69:35, 1990.
46. Quaade F: Meningitis in the aged. Geriatrics 18:860, 1963.
47. Feigin RD, Shackelford PG: Value of repeat lumbar puncture in the differential diagnosis of meningitis. N Engl J Med 289:571, 1973.
48. Koskiniemi M, Vaheri A, Taskinen E: Cerebrospinal fluid alterations in herpes simplex virus encephalitis. Rev Infect Dis 6:608, 1984.
49. Talan DA, Hoffman JR, Yoshikawa TT, Overturf GD: Role of empiric antibiotics prior to lumbar puncture in suspected bacterial meningitis: State of the art. Rev Infect Dis 10:365, 1988.
50. Granoff DM, Murphy TV, Ingram DL, Cates KL: Use of rapidly generated results in patient management. Diagn Microbiol Infect Dis 4:157S, 1986.
51. Wilson CB, Smith AL: Rapid tests for the diagnosis of bacterial meningitis. Curr Clin Top Infect Dis 7:134, 1986.
52. Whitley RJ, Lakeman F: Herpes simplex virus infections of the central nervous system: Therapeutic and diagnostic considerations. Clin Infect Dis 20:414, 1995.
53. Hansenk, Lebech A-M: Lyme neuroborreliosis: A new sensitive diagnostic assay for intrathecal synthesis of *Borrelia burgdorferi*–specific immunoglobulin G, A, and M. Ann Neurol 30:197, 1991.
54. Garfield J: Management of supratentorial intracranial abscess: A review of 200 cases. Br Med J 2:7, 1969.
55. Duffy GP: Lumbar puncture in the presence of raised intracranial pressure. Br Med J 1:407, 1969.
56. Bryan CS, Reynolds KL, Crout L: Promptness of antibiotic therapy in acute bacterial meningitis. Ann Emerg Med 15:544, 1986.
57. Ogawa SK, Smith MA, Brennessel DJ, Lowy FD: Tuberculous meningitis in an urban medical center. Medicine (Baltimore) 66:317, 1987.
58. Berger JR, Kaszovitz B, Post JD, Dickson G: Progressive multifocal leukoencephalopathy associated with human immunodeficiency virus infection: A review of the literature with a report of sixteen cases. Ann Intern Med 107:78, 1987.
59. McArthur JH: Neurologic manifestations of human immunodeficiency virus infection. Medicine (Baltimore) 66:407, 1987.
60. Buff BL Jr, Mathews VP, Elster AD: Bacterial and viral parenchymal infections of the brain. Top Magn Reson Imaging 6:11, 1994.
61. Rousseaux M, Lesoin F, Destee A, et al: Developments in the treatment and prognosis of multiple cerebral abscesses. Neurosurgery 16:304, 1985.
62. Schaad UB, Kaplan SL, McCracken GH Jr: Steroid therapy for bacterial meningitis. Clin Infect Dis 20:685, 1995.
63. Summary of notifiable diseases, United States, 1987. MMWR Morbid Mortal Wkly Rep 36:1, 1988.
64. Summary of notifiable diseases, United States, 1988. MMWR Morbid Mortal Wkly Rep 37:1, 1989.
65. Summary of notifiable diseases, United States, 1989. MMWR Morbid Mortal Wkly Rep 38:1, 1990.

158

Acute Bacterial Meningitis

Morton Swartz

Bacterial meningitis is a rapidly evolving inflammatory process, affecting the arachnoid, the pia mater, and the intervening cerebrospinal fluid (CSF), that results from invasion by pyogenic bacteria. Onset is usually acute and most often the infection is associated with a predominantly polymorphonuclear pleocytosis. Uncommonly, bacterial meningitis is caused by nonpyogenic bacteria, such as *Mycobacterium tuberculosis*, *Brucella* species, *Borrelia burgdorferi*, *Treponema pallidum*, and *Leptospira interrogans*, or unusual meningeal patho-

TABLE 158–1 ■ Pathogens of Bacterial Meningitis in the United States, 1978 Through 1981

ORGANISM	CASES N	CASES %	CASE-FATALITY RATE (%)
Haemophilus influenzae	6,756	48.3	6
Neisseria meningitidis	2,742	19.6	10.3
Streptococcus pneumoniae	1,865	13.3	26.3
Group B streptococci	476	3.4	22.5
Listeria monocytogenes	265	1.9	28.5
Other	1,043	7.5	33.7
Escherichia coli	115	0.8	
Staphylococcus aureus	84	0.6	
Klebsiella-Enterobacter-Serratia	61	0.4	
Streptococci, unspecified	43	0.3	
Staphylococcus spp.	35	0.3	
Staphylococcus epidermidis	27	0.2	
Streptococcus, group A	25	0.2	
Pseudomonas spp.	25	0.2	
Haemophilus spp.	24	0.2	
Viridans streptococci	20	0.2	
Salmonella and *Arizona* spp.	18	0.1	
Miscellaneous species	76	0.5	
Unidentified species	470	3.3	
Unknown	827	5.9	16.4
Total	13,974	99.9	

Modified from Schlech WF III, Ward JI, Band JD, et al: Bacterial meningitis in the United States, 1978 through 1981. JAMA 253:1749–1754, 1985.

gens such as *Nocardia asteroides* and *Actinomyces* species. In these processes the clinical picture is usually subacute or chronic and the pleocytosis is (in the first five instances) lymphocytic.

The incidence of bacterial meningitis in the United States in the 1970s and 1980s has been estimated to be from 20,000 to 30,000 cases annually.[1] The overall attack rate for bacterial meningitis during the period 1978 to 1981 in the United States was 3.0 per 100,000 population per year, but this figure likely represents underreporting by 60% to 70%.[2] In many cases of bacterial meningitis, initial examination of CSF does not provide identification of the infecting microorganism. Since 1990 in the United States the annual attack rate for bacterial meningitis has declined as a result of a sharp decrease in the incidence of invasive infections with *Haemophilus influenzae* (see later). Classification of bacterial meningitis into categories is helpful, as the relative frequency of individual bacterial species varies among the categories, which are related to age (neonatal, childhood, adult) or setting (community acquired, nosocomial).

Bacteriology

The three most frequent bacterial pathogens of community-acquired meningitis *(H. influenzae, Neisseria meningitidis, Streptococcus pneumoniae)* have been responsible for about 80% of reported cases in the United States (Table 158–1). Until the 1990s *H. influenzae* had been the leading cause of bacterial meningitis, accounting for almost 50% of cases. When age-specific attack rates have been examined, the highest rate, 76.7 per 100,000 population per year, has been among children younger than 1 year of age.[2] The dominant position of *H. influenzae* as the leading cause of bacterial meningitis in infants and young children (and as the most frequent cause of bacterial meningitis when all ages are combined) has been altered dramatically by the widespread use since the late 1980s of *H. influenzae* type b (Hib) conjugate vaccines. In children younger than 5 years of age in the United States in the mid-1980s, the rate of Hib meningitis had been about 40 per 100,000, but by 1993 it had dropped to about 2 per 100,000.[3] As a result, the relative frequencies of *S. pneumoniae* and *N. meningitidis* have increased among children. For example, at one urban children's hospital the number of cases of bacterial meningitis seen annually had decreased by 66% between the periods 1985 to 1987 and 1991 to 1992, primarily as a result of a decline in Hib meningitis. During the same two time periods, the percentage of cases of community-acquired childhood bacterial meningitis caused by *S. pneumoniae* and *N. meningitidis* in the aggregate increased from a mean of 31% to 73%.[4]

The other common bacterial causes are group B streptococci, *Listeria monocytogenes,* and enteric gram-negative bacilli. Whereas formerly *Escherichia coli* and other gram-negative bacilli were the principal agents of meningitis in infants during the first months of life, they have been superseded by group B streptococci.[2] *L. monocytogenes* has assumed an increasing role in bacterial meningitis, owing to the increasing numbers of immunocompromised and otherwise vulnerable persons at risk (e.g., transplant recipients, patients receiving hemodialysis, patients with liver disease)—and, possibly, to changes in dairy food production methods. In New York City, cases of *Listeria* meningitis increased from 0.9% to 3.4% of all reported cases between 1972 and 1979.[5] At Massachusetts General Hospital, *L. monocytogenes* increased about ninefold (0.5% to 4.5%) in relative frequency among bacterial causes of meningitis between the 1950s and the 1980s. Similarly, gram-negative bacillary meningitis (excluding cases caused by *H. influenzae*) increased in New York City from 5.6% to 7.0% of reported cases between 1972 and 1979.[5] At Massachusetts General Hospital, gram-negative bacilli accounted for about 4.5% of cases of bacterial meningitis in the 1950s, whereas more recently they accounted for close to 10%. In any large series of cases of bacterial meningitis, 6% to 10% of cases in which the clinical manifestations are consistent with bacterial meningitis are of unknown cause.[2, 6–8]

The frequencies of the various bacterial species in meningitis are strikingly age related (Table 158–2). In neonatal menin-

TABLE 158–2 ■ Relationship of Bacterial Meningitis Pathogens

PATHOGEN	AGE < 2 MONTHS*	AGE 2 MONTHS THROUGH 15 YEARS† (%)	AGE > 16 YEARS‡
Haemophilus influenzae	2	59	4
Neisseria meningitidis	0.5	24	29
Streptococcus pneumoniae	2	13	46
Escherichia coli	38	0.5	4§ (E. coli and other gram-negative bacilli)
Other gram-negative bacilli	11.5	<0.2	
Group B streptococci	22	1‖ (group B and other streptococci)	4‖ (group B and other streptococci)
Other streptococci	6		
Listeria monocytogenes	6	—	0.5
Staphylococcus aureus and *Staphylococcus epidermidis*	3.5	—	2.5
Miscellaneous	8	2.5	10
	99.5	100	100

*Compilation of 483 cases from six series covering the period 1963–1986.[9–12]

†Compilation of 1657 cases from five series covering the period 1956–1982.[6, 13–17]

‡Compilation of 658 cases from five series covering the period 1950–1987.[6, 7, 14, 18, 19]

§This number is the sum of *E. coli* and other gram-negative bacilli.

‖These numbers are the sums of group B steptococci and other streptococci.

gitis, *E. coli* (and other enteric gram-negative bacilli) and group B streptococci predominate, but other streptococci and *L. monocytogenes* have significant roles as well. During childhood, after age 2 months, Hib has been preeminent, the majority of cases occurring in the first 3 years of life. As noted earlier, the predominant position of Hib as a cause of meningitis in the first few years of life has declined dramatically since 1990 in the United States as a result of widespread immunization, with Hib-protein conjugate vaccines, of children at age 2 to 6 months. *N. meningitidis* is the second most frequent cause of childhood bacterial meningitis. Currently in the United States, serogroups B and C each are responsible for about 45% of cases, and serogroup A (the cause of periodic major epidemics of meningococcal disease in sub-Saharan Africa) is rarely involved in the United States.[20] Serogroups B and C cause primarily sporadic cases, although they are sometimes involved in outbreaks. Since 1986, serogroup C outbreaks in diverse areas of the United States have presented an increasingly important problem. For adult meningitis, *S. pneumoniae* is the principal bacterial agent in about 40% of cases.

The majority of cases of bacterial meningitis occur during childhood, are community acquired, and are caused by the three common pathogens *(N. meningitidis, S. pneumoniae,* and *H. influenzae).* In adults with bacterial meningitis treated in large urban tertiary care institutions, cases of nosocomial as well as community origin are not infrequently seen, and the species of infecting organisms may be more varied as a result.[21] Among community-acquired cases, *S. pneumoniae, N. meningitidis,* and *L. monocytogenes* are the leading causes, accounting for about 40%, 15%, and 10% of cases, respectively (Table 158–3). In contrast, among nosocomial cases, gram-negative bacilli, various streptococcal species, *S. aureus,* and coagulase-negative staphylococci are the principal infecting microorganisms, accounting for about 40%, 10%, 10%, and 10% of cases, respectively. Gram-negative bacillary meningitis is commonly a *postneurosurgical* (nosocomial) complication but may be *spontaneous* (in hospitalized patients or in the community setting). The incidence of both categories is increasing: the former as a result of more frequent and extensive neurosurgical procedures, the latter as a result of a larger, more vulnerable population at risk for gram-negative bacillary bacteremia. *E. coli* and *Klebsiella* infections account for more than half the cases of gram-negative bacillary meningitis in adults (Table 158–4).

TABLE 158–3 ■ Causative Organisms in Episodes (Nonrecurrent) of Bacterial Meningitis in Adults at a Tertiary Care Hospital,* 1962 to 1989

ORGANISM	COMMUNITY ACQUIRED (%) (*N* = 253)	NOSOCOMIAL (%) (*N* = 151)
Streptococcus pneumoniae	38	5
Gram-negative bacilli	4	38
Neisseria meningitidis	14	1
Streptococci†	7	9
Listeria monocytogenes	11	3
Staphylococcus aureus	5	9
Coagulase-negative staphylococci	0	9
Mixed bacterial species	2	7
Haemophilus influenzae	4	4
Enterococci	0	3
Other‡	2	3
Culture-negative	13	11

*Massachusetts General Hospital.
†Including groupable and nongroupable streptococci.
‡Including micrococci, anaerobes, *Neisseria* spp., and diphtheroids.
Modified with permission from Durand ML, Calderwood SB, Weber DJ, et al: Acute bacterial meningitis in adults. A review of 493 episodes. N Engl J Med 328:21–28, 1993. Copyright 1993 Massachusetts Medical Society. All rights reserved.

TABLE 158–4 ■ Agents of Gram-Negative Bacillary Meningitis in Adults*

ORGANISM	CASES *N*	CASES %
Escherichia coli	84	30
Klebsiella spp.	73	26
Pseudomonas spp.	35	12
Enterobacter spp.	26	9
Serratia spp.	19	7
Acinetobacter spp.	15	5
Salmonella spp.	8	3
Proteus spp.	9	3
Pasteurella multocida	3	1
Citrobacter spp.	4	1
Aeromonas spp., *Flavobacterium* spp.	2	1
Mixed	6	2
Total	284	100

*Compilation of 221 cases from seven reported series spanning the period 1961–1984.[5, 21, 22–26] *Haemophilus influenzae* and gram-negative anaerobic bacilli are not included.

S. aureus is the pathogen in 1% to 9% of cases of bacterial meningitis overall.[2, 27] Cases occur in several categories, based on predisposing circumstances: central nervous system (CNS) disorders (usually involving prior neurosurgery) in about 50%, endocarditis in about 20%, and bacteremia from other sites of infection (often in the setting of diabetes, cancer, or alcoholism) in about 25%.

Obligate anaerobic bacteria rarely cause meningitis.[28] Such infections usually occur in the setting of leakage of a brain abscess into the ventricular system, recent neurosurgery or trauma, chronic otitis media,[29] or bacteremia from abdominal infections. The principal organisms involved are anaerobic streptococci, *Fusobacterium necrophorum, Prevotella melaninogenica* (formerly *Bacteroides melaninogenicus*), and *Bacteroides fragilis. Clostridium perfringens* meningitis has been reported in 16 patients, usually in association with penetrating head injury, recent neurosurgery, or bacteremia after gastrointestinal or genitourinary operations.[30]

About 1% of cases of bacterial meningitis are polymicrobial infections.[31] Before the antibiotic era, most cases of mixed bacterial meningitis were associated with otitis media or pharyngeal infection and were caused by respiratory tract pathogens. Subsequently, the common predisposing factors for mixed bacterial meningitis have become CSF fistulae, neoplasms in proximity to the CNS, such as carcinoma of the rectosigmoid eroding through the sacrum to the subarachnoid space, and contiguous sites of infection. Mixtures of Enterobacteriaceae, obligate anaerobes *(B. fragilis, Clostridium* species, *Peptostreptococci), S. aureus, Pseudomonas* species, and *H. influenzae* have been involved most often.[31]

Very rarely, unusual bacterial species of zoonotic importance may produce meningitis in humans, and epidemiologic considerations may provide the clues to the diagnosis. Ingestion of imported (unpasteurized) cheese, travel to Mexico or the Mediterranean littoral, work in an abattoir or as a veterinarian, or work in a bacteriology laboratory might raise suspicion of *Brucella* meningitis.[32] Rarely, meningitis due to *Francisella tularensis* follows exposure to an infected rabbit, squirrel, or cat, although such meningitis usually follows an episode of one of the more typical forms of tularemia (ulceroglandular, oropharyngeal, typhoidal, pneumonic) and is characterized by a predominantly mononuclear pleocytosis.[33] Group R *Streptococcus (Streptococcus suis)* is carried by healthy swine and is the cause of meningitis in young pigs. About 60 cases of *S. suis* meningitis have occurred, principally in pig breeders and abattoir workers.[34]

Epidemiology

Meningococcal meningitis is the major form of meningococcal infection—and the one form of bacterial meningitis capable of producing epidemic disease. Meningococcal infection also occurs as the asymptomatic carrier state, the frequency of which varies with age (0.5% to 1.0% for children of ages 3 to 48 months, 5% for ages 14 to 17 years, 20% to 40% for young adults), endemic disease (sporadic cases), or hyperendemic disease (cyclic waves of increased incidence). The annual attack rate for meningococcal meningitis in the United States is 0.5 cases per 100,000 population (as high as 13 per 100,000 in the first year of life, declining to 2 per 100,000 at 5 years of age, and ultimately reaching the level of 0.2 to 0.6 per 100,000 for adults).[2] Group B and C meningococci are usually associated with endemic or hyperendemic disease. Epidemic meningococcal disease occurs on all continents, is commonly due to type A strains, and tends to recur at 20- to 30-year intervals. Major epidemics in the past 25 years have occurred in Finland (1973), Brazil (1974), northern Nigeria (1977), and Nepal (1983). Annual attack rates may be extremely high: in São Paulo, Brazil, in 1974, the rate was 370 per 100,000. A unique combination of endemic, hyperendemic, and epidemic meningococcal disease is present in the "meningitis belt" of sub-Saharan Africa, where major outbreaks occur in approximately 10-year cycles.

Concentration of large numbers of persons from different geographic origins in proximity, as occurs in training of military recruits, may result in heightened rates of meningococcal transmission via aerosol dispersion and eventuate in outbreaks of meningitis. Under similar conditions of crowding in an elementary school classroom with reduced seat-to-seat distances, an outbreak of five cases of group C meningococcal disease occurred in a 6-day period.[35] In the United States, such outbreaks in the military during World War II were due to group A strains and during the mid-1960s to group B and C strains (commonly sulfonamide resistant). At present this does not appear to be a problem in the military, since introduction of the meningococcal vaccine (groups A, C, Y, W-135) and the demonstrated prophylactic efficacy of newer antimicrobials in eradicating the meningococcal carrier state.

Nasopharyngeal carriage of *N. meningitidis,* the usual means of acquiring immunity, produces an increase in bactericidal antibody within 5 to 12 days after acquisition of the organism. Complement is also an important component of serum bactericidal activity. Isolated congenital late complement component (C5, C6, C7, or C8) deficiency, a rare occurrence, has been associated with repeated *Neisseria (gonorrhoeae)* infections and with chronic meningococcemia.[36, 37] Recurrent episodes of meningococcal meningitis have occurred in patients with such complement deficiencies. Congenital (late component) complement deficiencies, acquired complement (C1, C3, C4) deficiencies, and properdin deficiencies appear to be risk factors for the development of initial episodes of endemic meningococcal meningitis and meningococcemia.[38, 39]

In the endemic setting, household contacts of index cases of meningococcal infection in the United States are at greater risk (up to 1000-fold) of contracting the disease than the general population.[40, 41]

Before the introduction of Hib conjugate vaccines, more than 85% of all invasive *H. influenzae* disease occurred in children younger than 5 years of age, and 95% of disease in this age group was caused by Hib.[42] In fact, most Hib meningitis occurred before 18 months of age. Considerably higher rates of Hib disease are evident in selected populations of children, such as Native Americans in Alaska and Navajos (approximately five times the overall United States incidence). Host factors that may contribute to bacteremic Hib disease and meningitis include sickle cell disease, immunoglobulin deficiencies, history of splenectomy, and CSF fistula.

Unimmunized household contacts younger than 4 years of age of an index case of *H. influenzae* meningitis are at risk for invasive *H. influenzae* disease.[43] The risk is age dependent: 6% before age 1 year, 1.5% from 1 to 4 years, and 0.1% after 4 years. Thus, in the 30 days after onset of Hib meningitis in an index case, the age-adjusted risk is 585 times greater for household contacts than for the general population. The aforementioned data applied to household contacts in the United States in the 1970s and 1980s (before widespread use of Hib conjugate vaccines in children younger than 6 months of age) and are applicable currently to populations elsewhere where such immunization is not yet employed.

The risk of subsequent transmission of Hib disease among unimmunized children younger than 2 years who are daycare contacts of an index case is not clear. Studies from two states (Minnesota and Texas) suggest the risk of disease in the succeeding 60 days is quite low,[44, 45] whereas data from a third study (Oklahoma) suggest that the rate of secondary transmission can be appreciable (5 of 292, or 1.7%).[46] These differences may reflect geographic variation, intensity (duration) of exposure, and type of setting (home care versus large daycare centers).

H. influenzae is an infrequent cause (1% to 4%) of meningitis in adults. The leading predisposing factor in 119 cases was head trauma (20% of cases).[47] Other important predisposing factors were sinusitis (15%), otitis (13%), pneumonia, diabetes, alcoholism, immunodeficiency, and asplenia.

Pathogenesis

General Features

The usual sequence of events in the development of meningitis due to the three common bacterial species *(H. influenzae, N. meningitidis, S. pneumoniae),* all encapsulated organisms, consists of initial mucosal colonization, followed by blood stream invasion, penetration of the blood-brain barrier, and multiplication within the CSF.

Fimbriae, or pili, are involved in the binding of *N. meningitidis* to nonciliated mucosal epithelial cells, the initial step in colonization or invasive infection, but for *H. influenzae* the expression of pili does not appear to be required for such attachment.[48] All three major pathogens *(S. pneumoniae, N. meningitidis,* and *H. influenzae)* in community-acquired bacterial meningitis produce immunoglobulin A proteases, cleaving immunoglobulin A antibody in the hinge region and inactivating this early mucosal defense. The invasion routes taken by these pathogens on their ingress from the mucosal surface differ.[49] For example, meningococci enter nonciliated epithelial cells via endocytosis and are carried in membrane-bound vacuoles to the abluminal side[50]; *H. influenzae,* on the other hand, invades intercellularly by creating gaps in the apical tight junctions between the columnar epithelial cells. In the absence of specific antibody, the factors that determine whether initial exposure to these encapsulated species eventuates in benign nasopharyngeal carrier state or bacteremic invasion are unclear. Undefined strain-specific virulence factors may play a role. In addition, respiratory viruses such as influenza A virus and respiratory syncytial virus can foster acquisition and colonization by Hib.

The incubation period from nasopharyngeal to invasive

infection with *N. meningitidis* is less than 10 days and often only 1 to 4 days. Among prospectively studied military recruits, only about 20% of those whose secretions were cultured within 7 days preceding hospitalization for meningococcal disease were carriers of the implicated strain.

A polysaccharide capsule is a feature of each of the principal meningeal pathogens: *H. influenzae, N. meningitidis, S. pneumoniae, E. coli* K1 (the predominant *E. coli* serotype in neonatal meningitis), and *Streptococcus agalactiae* (group B streptococcus). Such encapsulation inhibits phagocytosis by neutrophils and antibody-independent complement-mediated bactericidal activity in different ways.[48] The capsular sialic acid of *N. meningitidis* appears to facilitate binding of complement factor H to C3b and this interferes with factor B binding and alternative pathway activation. In the case of *S. pneumoniae,* factor B binds poorly to C3b on its capsular surface, and the polyribosyl phosphate capsule of Hib is not able to serve as an acceptor for covalent C3 deposition.

In monkeys younger than 2 months of age, meningitis after intranasal inoculation of Hib develops within hours of bacteremia, reaching a level of 10^6 colony-forming units per milliliter.[51] The initial site of Hib entry into the CNS is the vascular choroid plexus, which shows the earliest histopathologic evidence of inflammation. After egress from the inflamed plexus capillaries, the organisms enter the lateral ventricles and the subarachnoid space. Once infection is introduced into the CSF, bacteria multiply rapidly because of inadequate local defenses: lack of complement-mediated lysis,[52] opsonizing antibody, and neutrophil phagocytosis.

Specific Predisposing Factors

The most common route of entry of bacteria into the CSF is hematogenous, but bacterial meningitis may also result from spread of infection from a contiguous structure or via a CSF fistula. The principal barriers to hematogenous spread to the meninges are circulating antibody and complement-mediated bactericidal activity. Immunoglobulin deficiencies predispose to invasive infection, particularly by encapsulated organisms such as *S. pneumoniae, H. influenzae,* and *N. meningitidis.* Complement deficiencies predispose to systemic infections with *N. meningitidis.* Complement deficiency may also predispose to meningitis caused by nongroupable (unencapsulated) *N. meningitidis* and by *Neisseria*-related bacteria such as *Moraxella* species and *Acinetobacter* species.[53] In patients with decreased spleen function, increased susceptibility to systemic infections with encapsulated organisms occurs, attributed to reduced clearance of intravascular organisms because of lower levels of complement components and tuftsin and decreased antibody formation.

Infection of a parameningeal structure may lead to bacterial penetration into the subarachnoid space. The organisms involved are representative of the species involved in the primary parameningeal infection (e.g., anaerobic bacteria and microaerophilic streptococci in the setting of chronic sinusitis or leakage of a brain abscess into the ventricular system; *S. pneumoniae, H. influenzae,* or *S. aureus* in the setting of acute frontal sinusitis; *S. aureus* or gram-negative bacilli in the setting of vertebral body or cranial osteomyelitis; *S. epidermidis* or *S. aureus* in infections involving CSF shunts).

Meningitis complicating CSF fistulae (congenital, traumatic or postsurgical, spontaneous) is associated with bacterial species that vary with the site of the abnormal communication (e.g., pneumococci with leaks about the cribriform plate and air sinuses, *S. aureus* and facultative gram-negative bacilli with congenital dermal sinuses or meningomyeloceles along the spine, and members of the Enterobacteriaceae and anaerobic intestinal flora with erosion of colonic neoplasms into the lumbosacral subarachnoid space).

Predisposing factors for pneumococcal meningitis are varied (Table 158–5). Antecedent acute otitis media is the most common predisposing factor. In this instance, meningitis follows bacteremia rather than direct invasion through the mastoid. It is important to note that in occasional cases of chronic otitis media in which cultures of drainage material have consistently grown *P. aeruginosa* or *Proteus* species, acute meningitis caused by *S. pneumoniae* has developed. CSF rhinorrhea has been noted in 4% of cases of pneumococcal meningitis (see Table 158–5); however, this is probably an underestimate, because in this compilation a quarter of the cases with head injury had skull fractures (and were likely to have had CSF leaks as well). Also, CSF rhinorrhea is likely to be a more frequent predisposing factor (12%) for pneumococcal meningitis in adults.[6]

At least 18 cases of mixed bacterial-viral meningitis have been reported.[8, 55] Most cases have involved children; the bacterial pathogens have been principally Hib, *N. meningitidis,* and *Salmonella* organisms; and the most frequent viruses have been echovirus, coxsackievirus, and herpes simplex virus. It is impossible to know whether viral aseptic meningitis preceded and predisposed to subsequent bacterial invasion.

Pathophysiology

A multitude of pathophysiologic changes develop as a consequence of bacterial meningitis and involve the brain, its linings, cranial nerves, meningeal and other intracranial blood vessels, and the spinal cord. In experimental animal models, specific bacterial subcapsular components (for *S. pneumoniae,* peptidoglycan or lipoteichoic acid; for Hib, lipopolysaccharide) are the major inducers of the meningeal inflammation that follows bacterial entry and multiplication in the CSF.[48] Ampicillin-induced lysis of pneumococci in the CSF results in a transient increase in polymorphonuclear pleocytosis, consistent with the release of cell wall debris.[56] This inflammatory response is caused by the release into the subarachnoid space of various proinflammatory cytokines such as interleukin-1 and tumor necrosis factor from meningeal cells. These cytokines elicit increased adherence and transendothelial movement of neutrophils by induction of several families of adhesion molecules on endothelium that interact with corresponding leukocytic receptors. These include (1) the selectin family, for example, endothelial-leukocyte adhesion molecule and CD62, and (2) the immunoglobulin superfamily, for example, intercellular adhesion molecules (ICAM-1, ICAM-2). The integrin (CD18) subfamily of adhesion molecules, also known as leukocyte integrins, is expressed only

TABLE 158–5 ■ Predisposing Factors in Pneumococcal Meningitis*

PREDISPOSING FACTOR	FREQUENCY (%)
Otitis media or mastoiditis†	30
Sinusitis‡	3
Previous head trauma†	10
CSF rhinorrhea§	4
Pneumonia†	20
Neoplastic disease, collagen-vascular disease, or immunosuppression‖	5
Alcoholism‖	9
Diabetes mellitus‖	2

*Compilation from four series of cases occurring between 1956 and 1976.[6–8, 54]
†Based on data from a total of 459 cases.
‡Based on data from a total of 119 cases.
§Based on data from a total of 281 cases.
‖Based on data from a total of 234 cases.

on leukocytes and their expression can be increased rapidly by chemoattractants. Another leukocyte adhesion molecule (LAM-1), belonging to the selectin family, mediates adhesion to endothelium even under conditions of flow; its binding affinity for its endothelial receptor is increased by exposure to cytokines (tumor necrosis factor, granulocyte-macrophage colony-stimulating factor), thus furthering neutrophil trafficking into the subarachnoid space.

Once within the subarachnoid space, activated neutrophils release prostaglandins and toxic oxygen metabolites that produce increased vascular permeability and may cause direct neurotoxicity. Early in the course of meningitis, as observed in animal models, changes take place in meningeal and cerebral capillaries. These vessels, which by virtue of their tight intercellular endothelial junctions and their meager rate of pinocytosis constitute the blood-brain barrier, undergo morphologic changes (opening of tight junctions, enhanced pinocytosis) and become permeable to proteins.[56] In experimental Hib meningitis, the increase in permeability in the blood-brain barrier appears to correlate principally with the bacterial titer in the CSF but is augmented by increasing pleocytosis.[57]

A variety of mediators of the inflammatory response, such as interleukin-1, tumor necrosis factor, complement components, and arachidonate metabolites, probably contribute to the breakdown of the blood-brain barrier and the cerebral manifestations of bacterial meningitis.[59, 60] The major physiologic consequence of altered vascular permeability is (vasogenic) cerebral edema.

The brain edema may also have cytotoxic (from inflammatory mediators in the meningeal exudate and from hypoxia) and interstitial (impaired CSF absorption due to arachnoid villus dysfunction from blockage by fibrin and leukocytes) components.[61] Increased intracranial pressure (ICP) due to cerebral edema and reduced CSF resorption produce vomiting and obtundation. In extreme instances cerebral edema may produce temporal lobe or cerebellar herniation with brain stem compression and respiratory arrest.

Cerebral blood flow appears to be enhanced in the early stages of bacterial meningitis but it declines subsequently, reflecting the severity of the inflammatory process. Focal areas of marked hypoperfusion (attributable to local vasculitis or thrombosis) can occur in patients with overall normal blood flow. In some patients, impaired autoregulation of cerebral blood flow may contribute to development of cerebral edema or ischemia by altering cerebral perfusion pressure.

With spread of the meningeal inflammation over the cerebral hemispheres and into the basal cisterns, superficial pial arteries and veins may be subject to thrombosis. Decreased cerebral blood flow due to cerebral edema or vascular thrombosis, plus any element of hypoxia due to pneumonia or respiratory insufficiency, results in enhanced glucose metabolism via the anaerobic glycolytic pathway, with ensuing lactate accumulation in the brain and CSF. This central lactic acidosis may contribute considerably to the obtundation and coma of patients with severe meningitis.[62]

Cranial nerve palsies may be the consequence of accumulation of basilar exudate about these nerves in their course through the subarachnoid space. Seizures may result from a variety of pathophysiologic changes in meningitis: fever in infants and young children, hyponatremia secondary to increased release of antidiuretic hormone,[63] and cerebral infarction due to arteritis or cortical venous thrombophlebitis. Hydrocephalus probably results from choroid plexus necrosis and aqueductal occlusion (obstructive hydrocephalus) or from impaired CSF resorption due to obstruction by exudate of the arachnoid villi. Focal signs of cerebral dysfunction such as hemiparesis, dysphasia, and visual field defects are probably a consequence of arterial vasculitis or venous infarction from cortical thrombophlebitis.

Brain abscess is a rare complication of meningitis; more often bacterial meningitis is a complication of a brain abscess leaking into the ventricular system. When meningitis is complicated by brain abscess it occurs in the neonate and almost invariably is caused by *Citrobacter diversus*.[64] Brain abscess has developed in 41 of 53 (77%) of cases of *C. diversus* neonatal meningitis. The propensity for producing ventriculitis and brain abscess appears to reside in a specific outer membrane protein of the organism.[65]

Clinical Manifestations

History

In community-acquired bacterial meningitis, antecedent upper respiratory tract infection is common (40%); another 10% to 15% of patients have an ill-defined prior illness (often diagnosed as otitis media).[8] Between 25% and 75% of patients have a rapid onset (within 24 hours) of headache, lethargy, and confusion ("meningeal symptoms").[7, 15] Other patients have more prolonged (1 to 7 days) respiratory tract or ear symptoms, and meningeal symptoms develop and progress more slowly. In patients with *L. monocytogenes* meningitis, the prodromal symptomatic period tends to be longer than in patients with other types of pyogenic meningitis; indeed, in about 15% of patients the premonitory symptoms may be present for 7 or more days before hospitalization. Rarely, patients have had meningeal symptoms that predate hospitalization by several weeks. In such instances, parental neglect and, in one case, complement deficiency[66] have been factors.

Fever, vomiting, irritability, lethargy, and headache are features in most patients. Neck stiffness is a symptom in less than half of patients, but nuchal rigidity of some degree is noted as a sign in more than 80%. Myalgias (especially in meningococcal disease) and backache occur less frequently. Photophobia is more often associated with viral meningitis.

In young infants, manifestations of meningitis may be difficult to recognize and interpret. Fever and vomiting, features common to many types of both systemic and local infections, may be the only abnormalities noted by the parents. Nuchal rigidity may be absent on examination of the infant. Bulging of the fontanelle and diastasis of the sutures may suggest the diagnosis but may be absent early in meningitis or if the infant is markedly dehydrated. Occasionally, lumbar puncture performed in the absence of overt signs has revealed a clear CSF without even minor pleocytosis, and the infant has been treated with antipyretic measures and sent home only to return some hours later because of parental concern or a seizure. Another CSF examination may then show pleocytosis, and in the next 24 hours bacteria, usually Hib, are isolated from the initial CSF culture.

General Physical Findings

Drowsiness, reduced cognitive function, stiff neck, and Kernig and Brudzinski signs—all manifestations of meningeal inflammation—are usually present along with fever. These findings may be overlooked or misinterpreted in patients who are obtunded because of other illness or in elders, particularly those with pneumonia or marked congestive failure.

A petechial or purpuric rash, predominantly on the extremities, in a patient with meningeal signs almost always indicates a meningococcal cause and requires immediate treatment because of the rapidity with which this type of infection can advance. About 50% of patients with meningococcal meningitis have such skin lesions. Occasionally a maculopapular rash is seen in patients with meningococcal meningitis. In more severe infections, large purpuric areas with gunmetal gray necrotic or vesicular centers (suggillations) develop, usually accompanying hypotension or shock and evidence of disseminated intravascular coagulation. Although such lesions may provide an initial clue to bacteriologic diagnosis, rarely they occur in meningitis caused by *S. pneumoniae* or *H. influenzae.* Quite rarely, petechial and purpuric skin lesions occur in patients with acute *S. aureus* endocarditis who have meningeal signs and pleocytosis (due to either staphylococcal meningitis or cerebral embolic infarction). In this setting, one or two of the purpuric lesions often contain a purulent center, and aspirated material reveals staphylococci on Gram stain examination. Macular and petechial skin lesions accompanied by meningeal signs may occur with enteroviral aseptic meningitis in summer outbreaks. The presence of an initial pleocytosis of up to several hundred cells, with neutrophils predominating at first, enhances the mimicry of meningococcal disease. Tache cérébrale, an erythematous raised response evoked by stroking the skin with a blunt implement, is a nonspecific sign sometimes observed in children with meningitis.

Neurologic Findings and Complications

Confusion, stupor, or delirium is quite common in bacterial meningitis, but about 20% to 40% of patients are noted on admission to the hospital to have normal consciousness.[6, 21, 54]

CRANIAL NERVE DYSFUNCTION

Ten percent to 20% of patients with bacterial meningitis have cranial nerve dysfunction. Cranial nerves III, VI, and VIII are most often involved. Prospective studies utilizing brain stem evoked potentials indicate that neurosensory deafness affects about 10% of infants and young children with bacterial meningitis.[67] The highest frequency is associated with *S. pneumoniae* meningitis. About 20% of those children who become deaf during Hib meningitis recover their hearing by the time of hospital discharge.[68, 69] Unfortunately, for the remaining children deafness is permanent. Vasculitis-induced infarction of the cranial nerve VIII and necrosis of cells in the organ of Corti may be responsible for such permanent deafness. In studies of an animal model of pneumococcal meningitis, hearing loss could be detected as early as 12 hours after infection; it progressed rapidly, and the severity of meningogenic hearing loss correlated with the degree of inflammation observed on cochlear histopathologic study and the inflammatory changes in CSF cytochemistry.[70, 71] Involvement of the inner ear is not a result of direct extension of infection from the middle ear to the inner ear, even when otitis media precedes meningitis.[72] Rather, contiguous infection is represented by extension of the process from the subarachnoid space to the inner ear via the cochlear aqueduct. This view is supported by studies in infant rats with Hib meningitis produced by intraperitoneal or intranasal inoculation. Labyrinthitis occurs as a result of spread of inflammation from the subarachnoid space with sparing of the middle ear.[73]

SEIZURES

Early seizures occur in 15% to 30% of cases of bacterial meningitis.[6, 7, 21, 74] Seizures may be focal or generalized. In adults with meningitis, *S. pneumoniae* was the cause in a greater percentage of patients who had seizures than of patients who did not, but alcoholism was a confounder.[21] Seizures that occur early in hospitalization do not herald the onset of a permanent seizure disorder, but those that persist beyond the first few days or that develop later during hospitalization may.

FOCAL CEREBRAL SIGNS

Focal cerebral signs (hemiparesis, quadriparesis, visual field defects, disorders of conjugate gaze, dysphasia) occur in 10% to 20% of patients with meningitis, more frequently with pneumococcal than with other types of community-acquired meningitis[6, 7, 16, 21] (Table 158–6). They may appear early in the course of meningitis, or, less frequently, later in the course of the disease due to cortical arteritis or phlebitis. Postictal findings of a hemiparesis (Todd paralysis) must be distinguished from persisting focal cerebral signs. The postictal changes, however, may last several hours.

In the adult the most frequent neurologic complications of bacterial meningitis are cerebrovascular ones, occurring in about 37% of patients with intracranial complications, followed in frequency by brain swelling detected by computed tomography (CT) (34%) and hydrocephalus (29%).[75] These figures are derived from a study of 86 adults with bacterial meningitis in whom cerebral arteriography was performed on those who had focal deficits either clinically or at cranial CT (or both) and in those with persistent coma without apparent cause after 3 days of antimicrobial therapy. The spectrum of cerebrovascular changes includes (1) narrowing and spasm of major arteries at the base of the brain, such as the supraclinoid portion of the internal carotid artery; (2) irregularities or focal aneurysmal dilatations of medium-sized arteries; (3) occlusions of distal branches of the middle cerebral artery with or without retrograde flow; (4) focal abnormal parenchymal blush; (5) marked prolongation of circulation time; and (6) thrombosis of cortical veins or the superior sagittal sinus, or both.

BRAIN SWELLING

Cerebral edema can occur in acute bacterial meningitis. Manifestations include obtundation and coma, third nerve palsies (including dilated, poorly reactive, or nonreactive pupils), abnormal reflexes, hypertension, decerebrate posturing, abnormal respiratory pattern, and bradycardia. Brain edema causes increased ICP, which in older infants has been shown to result in reduced cerebral blood flow velocity.[76] Such decreased cerebral perfusion is another potential cause of brain injury. Papilledema is rare because of the relatively brief duration of the meningeal process and increased CSF pressure. In one study of 279 episodes of community-acquired meningitis in adults, only 1% of patients had findings of "blurred optic disc margins" and "early papilledema" along with extremely high CSF pressures of 440 mm H_2O or higher.[21] Its presence should suggest the possibility of another related or independent suppurative intracranial process, such as brain abscess or subdural empyema. Rarely, rhombencephalitis due to *L. monocytogenes* may accompany listerial meningitis, represent a complication thereof, or occur in the absence of overt meningitis.[77, 78] Its histologic characteristics are those of a suppurative encephalitis with vasculitis and hemorrhages in the pons and medulla.

Markedly increased ICP due to meningitis may lead to impending herniation. Signs of herniation include (1) bradycardia and abnormal respiratory patterns; (2) midposition, nonreactive pupils; (3) unequal or dilated, nonreactive pupils; (4) skew deviation or dysconjugate eye movements; and (5) decorticate or decerebrate posturing.

Marked hyperpnea sometimes occurs in patients with severe bacterial meningitis: CSF acidosis, due mainly to increased lactic acid levels, provides much of the respiratory drive. Persistent or late-developing obtundation without fo-

TABLE 158–6 ■ Focal Cerebral Signs and Seizures in Community-Acquired Bacterial Meningitis in Adults

	EPISODES OF MENINGITIS (%)					
TIME OF ONSET OF FINDINGS	Hemiparesis	Aphasia	Visual Field Defect	Gaze Preference	Seizures	Other*
Early (≤24 h)	9	6	3	10	15	5
Late (>24 h)	2	1	0.3	0	8	1
Total†	11	7	2.3	10	23	6

*These findings included ataxia, dysmetria, nystagmus, monoparesis, hemianesthesia, and central seventh nerve palsy.
†Percentage of 279 episodes in which individual finding occurred.
Modified with permission from Durand ML, Calderwood SB, Weber DJ, et al: Acute bacterial meningitis in adults. A review of 493 episodes. N Engl J Med 328:21–28, 1993.

cal findings might suggest any of several anatomically distinct processes: cerebral swelling (with or without herniation), subdural effusion (particularly in young infants, where it may cause enlargement of the head and abnormal transillumination findings), hydrocephalus, loculated ventriculitis or ventricular empyema, or rarely, subdural empyema or superior sagittal sinus thrombosis. Minor or extensive arteritis or cortical vein thrombophlebitis may be responsible for obtundation, focal cerebral deficits,[79, 80] and seizures as a result of cortical infarction. Rarely, arteritis complicating meningitis involves a spinal or radicular artery and causes paraplegia with a sensory level.[81] The pathologic basis of the neurologic complications (including cerebral vasculitis) in meningitis is provided in the classic study of Adams and coworkers[82] of fatal cases of *H. influenzae* meningitis.

LATE NEUROLOGIC SEQUELAE

The long-term prognosis for neurologic complications has been evaluated mainly in childhood meningitis. In a prospective study of 185 infants and children with acute bacterial meningitis between 1973 and 1977 (mean follow-up of 8.9 years), the percentage of patients with significant neurologic abnormalities decreased from 37% 1 month after the meningitis to 14% with permanent deficits.[83] Only 10% of the study group had permanent sensorineural hearing loss, and other major permanent neurologic deficits such as hemiparesis, quadriparesis, mental retardation, or blindness were present in another 5%. Seizures were noted in 31% of patients during acute bacterial meningitis. Late-onset epilepsy occurred principally in patients with clinical evidence of permanent cerebral dysfunction. Normal results of neurologic examination shortly after meningitis indicate an excellent prognosis for full neurologic recovery, including escaping late-onset epilepsy.[83]

Children who had recovered from *H. influenzae* meningitis 6 to 8 years earlier were found to perform as well as their comparably aged siblings in spelling, reading, and arithmetic, despite having slightly lower IQ scores and mild deficits in neuropsychologic testing.[84] They were able to maintain academic achievement and behavioral performance comparable to their siblings, although they probably needed more family and school support.

Persons who have meningitis as neonates or young infants more frequently have long-term sequelae. Among survivors in a study of group B streptococcal meningitis, only half were judged to be functioning normally when evaluated for long-term sequelae at mean age of 6.0 years.[85]

Recurrent Meningitis

About 8% of adults seen in a large urban general hospital with bacterial meningitis had recurrent episodes, and about 16% of episodes of meningitis in this setting were recurrent.[21] The interval between recurrences is usually months to years. Predisposing circumstances for the development of recurrent bacterial meningitis are generally either anatomic defects, which allow direct ingress of bacteria into the subarachnoid space while circumventing the usual immune defenses of circulating immunoglobulins, or immunodeficiencies (Table 158–7). The principal predisposing factor, CSF leak, is identifiable in about 75% of patients with recurrent meningitis.

The bacteriologic findings in recurrent meningitis differ for community-acquired and nosocomial varieties. *S. pneumoniae* is the agent of about 33% of episodes of the former but less than 5% of the latter.[21] Overall, about two thirds of episodes of community-acquired recurrent meningitis are due to bacterial species that can normally be found in the upper respiratory tract *(S. pneumoniae,* other streptococcal species, meningococci, *H. influenzae).* In adults, *H. influenzae* is the agent of only 4% of cases of bacterial meningitis, yet about two thirds of such patients have CSF leaks. In recurrent episodes of nosocomial meningitis, gram-negative bacilli (other than *H. influenzae*) are the cause in about 45% of cases and staphylococci (coagulase-positive and -negative), another 20% to 25%.

Clinical Course of Infection

Untreated acute bacterial meningitis rapidly progresses to a fatal outcome. With early diagnosis and with appropriate antimicrobial and supportive therapy the case-fatality rate for *H. influenzae* meningitis is 6%; for *N. meningitidis* meningitis, 10%; and for *S. pneumoniae* meningitis, 26%.[2] In adults, the overall meningitis-related case-fatality rate is 19%; for gram-negative bacillary meningitis, 20% to 25%.[21] There appears to have been a decrease in the case-fatality rate for gram-negative bacillary meningitis in the past decade and a half, compared with the two prior decades, but the case-

TABLE 158–7 ■ Predisposing Factors to Recurrent Bacterial Meningitis

Anatomic defects
- CSF fistulae (leak at cribriform plate, leak into nasal air sinus or middle ear, empty sella syndrome)
- Head injury (with CSF otorrhea or rhinorrhea)
- Mastoid erosion by osteomyelitis or cholesteatoma
- Neurosurgical complication (with dural tear)

Immunoglobulin deficiency
Asplenia
Complement deficiencies (congenital deficiencies of late-acting components or acquired deficiencies of early-acting components, predisposing to recurrent *Neisseria* infections and rarely to recurrent meningococcal meningitis)
Failure (rare) to mount specific immune response to *Haemophilus influenzae* type b after *H. influenzae* type b meningitis in an infant

fatality rate for pneumococcal meningitis has not changed. The overall case-fatality rate for recurrent community-acquired meningitis is about one fifth that of nonrecurrent community-acquired meningitis.

Nonneurologic Complications

SHOCK

Shock may develop early in the course of acute bacterial meningitis, usually as a consequence of intense bacteremia, as can occur in meningococcemia-meningitis or in pneumococcal bacteremia in asplenic patients. In these instances the major acute impact of the illness stems from the high-grade bacteremia.

COAGULOPATHIES

In patients with meningitis, coagulation disorders may complicate bacteremias and hypotension. The coagulopathy may be mild and consist only of thrombocytopenia, but in patients with more profound bacteremia the clinical features and laboratory findings may be typically those of disseminated intravascular coagulation.

SEPTIC COMPLICATIONS

Early treatment of pneumococcal meningitis or its initiating infection and bacteremia has made acute bacterial endocarditis an uncommon complication of this form of meningitis. In the rare instance in which endocarditis develops, it usually involves the aortic valve. It may not become evident (recrudescence of fever, a new aortic diastolic murmur) until a few days after conclusion of a course of antibiotic therapy for meningitis. Pyogenic arthritis due to the common agents of community-acquired meningitis may complicate the bacteremia occurring early in the course of CNS infection.

IMMUNE-MEDIATED MANIFESTATIONS

In about 10% of patients with meningococcal meningitis a serum sickness–like syndrome develops 4 to 10 days after initiation of antimicrobial therapy, when the meningitis is clearly responding to treatment. Fever, arthritis, and pericarditis are the principal features, but occasionally pleuritis and new papulobullous skin lesions may appear. The synovial and pericardial fluids are serosanguineous and sterile, unlike the purulent infected effusions that sometimes occur at these sites during the first 2 or 3 days of meningococcal meningitis. Usually, such late-onset pericardial effusions are not hemodynamically significant, but nonetheless they warrant careful monitoring of cardiovascular status. Symptomatic relief is afforded by salicylates and nonsteroidal antiinflammatory agents. A likely role for immune complex formation in the pathogenesis of these sterile processes has been suggested.

PROLONGED FEVER

Most patients with the common types of community-acquired bacterial meningitis become afebrile within 2 to 5 days of initiation of appropriate antimicrobial therapy. Occasionally, fever persists for 8 to 10 days or longer or recurs after initial defervescence. Such a febrile course accompanied by persisting headache, stiff neck, depressed sensorium, and focal cerebral signs suggests that antimicrobial therapy has been inadequate or that a neurologic complication—cortical vein thrombophlebitis and arteritis, ventriculitis, ventricular empyema, subdural effusion or empyema, sagittal sinus thrombosis—has supervened. Reevaluation of CSF findings, particularly Gram-stained smears and cultures, is of paramount importance; appearance of new focal cerebral signs would be an indication for cranial CT.

Drug fever or a serum sickness–like syndrome (see later) should be considered in a patient with persistent fever whose clinical course and CSF findings show continued improvement.

Laboratory Findings

CEREBROSPINAL FLUID EXAMINATION

CSF values characteristic of acute pyogenic meningitis include pleocytosis of 100 to 5000 cells per mm^3 (predominantly neutrophils), elevated opening pressure, elevated protein level, and Gram-stained smear of centrifuged CSF that shows the infecting agent in 60% to 90% of cases (Table 158–8). The frequency of a positive CSF Gram stain in untreated bacterial meningitis is somewhat dependent on the infecting microorganism: *S. pneumonia,* 70% to 90%; *H. influenzae,* about 80%; *N. meningitidis,* 50% to 80%; and group B streptococcus, 60% to 85%.[86] However, in community-acquired meningitis in adults, in which 13% of cases are "culture-negative," the overall frequency of positive Gram stains on initial CSF examination is 60%.[21] More common misinterpretations of Gram-stained smears include mistaking pneumococci for *H. influenzae,* because of bipolar gram-positive staining of the organism due to inadequate decolorizing, or mistaking *Listeria* for pneumococci. *Enterococcus* species in the CSF may occasionally appear primarily as gram-positive diplococci and be mistaken for *S. pneumoniae.* The pleomorphic appearance of *Acinetobacter baumannii* (formerly *Acinetobacter anitratus*) or of *Pasteurella multocida* in the CSF may sometimes suggest on Gram stain the appearance of meningitis due to a mixture of *H. influenzae* and *N. meningitidis.* The acridine orange stain may be slightly more sensitive than the Gram stain for detecting bacteria in CSF specimens.[86]

Initial CSF opening pressures may be markedly elevated (450 to 500 mm H_2O or more) in about 5% of patients (see Table 158–8). Clear CSF with less than 40 to 50 cells per mm^3 may occasionally be seen in early bacterial meningitis, particularly in young infants, or in neutropenic patients. Among 261 cases of meningitis in infants, 2.7% had less than

TABLE 158–8 ■ Cerebrospinal Fluid Findings in Bacterial Meningitis*

PLEOCYTOSIS (831 episodes between 1963 and 1984)

Cell Count	Prevalence (%)
0–100	15
101–1,000	27
1,001–5,000	33
5,001–10,000	14
10,001–50,000	9
>50,000	1

GLUCOSE (681 evaluable episodes)
<40 mg/dL or <40% of level of simultaneous blood glucose in 52% of episodes

OPENING PRESSURE (354 evaluable episodes)

mm H_2O	Prevalence (%)
≤200	36
>200–300	32
>300–450	20
>450–500	6
>500	6

*Episodes of meningitis at Massachusetts General Hospital.

10 leukocytes per mm^3 of CSF, but *H. influenzae, S. pneumoniae, N. meningitidis* and group B streptococci were isolated on initial culture.[87] Rarely, the CSF of a patient who is not neutropenic will be grossly cloudy but contain only a few neutrophils. In this instance the turbidity is due to myriad pneumococci, and this is usually a sign of poor prognosis. Although most patients with pyogenic meningitis have brisk pleocytosis, the cell count in 75% of patients with *L. monocytogenes* meningitis is $1000/mm^3$ or less. Although two thirds of patients with *Listeria* meningitis have neutrophilic pleocytosis of more than 70%, about 10% (usually neonates, neutropenic children or adults, or rarely a nonneutropenic adult) have mononuclear pleocytosis of about 80%. Rarely, lymphocytic pleocytosis is observed in a nonneutropenic child with meningitis due to one of the common bacteria, such as *H. influenzae*.[88]

The CSF protein level is elevated in 95% of patients with bacterial meningitis—in 50%, 200 mg/dL or higher. Latex particle agglutination and other rapid tests to detect bacterial antigens can be used as an adjunct to Gram stain examination and culture to evaluate the cause of a case of presumed bacterial meningitis, particularly in the patient who received prior parenteral antibiotic therapy. However, in view of the sensitivity of the CSF Gram stain and culture in patients who have not received prior parenteral antibiotics, it has been suggested that CSF antigen testing be deferred (with the initial CSF sample stored at 2°C to 8°C) for 48 hours until CSF and blood cultures are determined to be negative.[89] The sensitivity of latex particle agglutination in detecting antigen of the common species of bacteria implicated in community-acquired meningitis varies among organisms. *H. influenzae* antigen can be detected in 95% of cases, including some with negative Gram stain findings[86]; *N. meningitidis,* in 64% to 78% of cases; *S. pneumoniae,* in 67% of cases. The sensitivity of the latex particle agglutination assay depends to a large measure on the potency of the specific antisera employed and the concentration of bacteria in the CSF.[90]

A variety of chemical and enzymatic changes have been noted in the CSF of patients with acute bacterial meningitis. Determination of these values has been suggested as a means of distinguishing acute bacterial from aseptic meningitis. The tests include levels of C-reactive protein,[91, 92] lactate,[86, 91] lactate dehydrogenase,[93] special profiles of fatty acids and carbohydrate metabolites as detected by gas-liquid chromatography,[91] and endotoxin.[86, 93] C-reactive protein levels higher than 100 ng/mL of CSF or a qualitative latex slide agglutination test had a sensitivity of about 95% in patients with pleocytosis greater than 10 leukocytes per mm^3 but a somewhat lower specificity of 86%.[92, 94] The value of the test is limited by the fact that some patients fail to mount a prompt response and that it provides no information on the nature of the infecting bacteria. Levels of CSF lactate above 3.9 mmol/L are usually observed in bacterial meningitis, and levels are generally lower in patients with aseptic meningitis. Occasional patients with bacterial meningitis have normal values, and the level can be elevated independently in the presence of cerebral ischemia, cerebral edema, or brain tumor. An elevated CSF lactate level corresponds with a low CSF glucose level and correlates with numbers of neutrophils greater than $350/mm^3$.[95] Detection of specific metabolites in CSF by gas-liquid chromatography might provide helpful diagnostic information. Increased quantities of succinic acid have been detected in the CSF of patients with *H. influenzae* meningitis but not in the CSF of patients with pneumococcal, meningococcal, tuberculous, or other types of meningitis.[96]

The *Limulus* amoebocyte lysate test for detection of endotoxin of gram-negative bacteria in CSF can provide additional bacteriologic information. It has an overall sensitivity of 99% (100% for *H. influenzae* and *N. meningitidis* meningitis but only 67% for other types of gram-negative bacillary meningitis).[97] The value of this test lies only in its capacity to identify a meningeal pathogen as a gram-negative bacterium.

Although the various tests have their proponents, cell counts and chemistries, the proper interpretation of Gram-stained smears, and culture of CSF provide the needed information for diagnosis and initial treatment in most cases of bacterial meningitis.

OTHER LABORATORY STUDIES

Blood cultures from patients with community-acquired meningitis often reveal the pathogen: 90% of *H. influenzae,* 80% of *S. pneumoniae,* and 90% of *N. meningitidis.*[98] Culture of the nasopharynx cannot be used to identify the specific agent in a given patient with pyogenic meningitis.

Bacteremic skin lesions associated with highly invasive organisms may reveal the agent on Gram-stained smear. Thus, aspiration of the whitish center of the purulent purpura associated with *S. aureus* bacteremia may reveal the pathogen. The purely petechial lesions of the skin in bacterial meningitis, however, are unlikely to be revealing on Gram stain examination.

Gram stain examination and culture of fluid aspirated from a middle-ear effusion may provide a clue to bacteriologic diagnosis when the findings of CSF smear examination are equivocal. The peripheral leukocyte count is commonly elevated in patients with bacterial meningitis, 14,000 to 24,000 cells per mm^3 and generally higher in pneumococcal and meningococcal than in *H. influenzae* disease.[99]

Hyponatremia in the course of bacterial (or tuberculous or fungal) meningitis is commonly due either to the complicating syndrome of inappropriate antidiuretic hormone secretion (SIADH) or to inappropriate fluid administration.

RADIOGRAPHIC FINDINGS

Chest radiography should be performed to discover any predisposing pulmonary portal of infection. Films of the air sinuses and mastoids should be taken at an appropriate time after commencing antimicrobial therapy if history or findings suggest infection of these structures.

When the history, clinical setting, or physical signs (papilledema, focal cerebral findings) suggest a suppurative intracranial collection, cranial CT should be carried out without delay—and *before lumbar puncture (but after blood for cultures has been taken and therapy with appropriate antimicrobials for meningitis of unknown bacterial cause has been instituted).*

A variety of abnormalities detectable by head CT may occur during the course of bacterial meningitis[75, 100–103]: contrast enhancement of the leptomeninges and ventricular lining, cerebral edema, widening of the subarachnoid space, patchy areas of diminished density in the cerebrum from cerebritis or necrosis, multifocal enhancing lesions consistent with cerebral infarcts (arterial or venous), subdural effusion, subdural empyema, ventriculomegaly or hydrocephalus, ventricular empyema, enhancement about the basal cisterns. The rare complication of sagittal sinus thrombophlebitis can be detected by magnetic resonance imaging or cerebral angiography.

Patients with bacterial meningitis rarely have clinically significant CT findings without concomitant focal neurologic abnormalities.[21, 101] In a prospective study of head CT in 43 children with acute bacterial meningitis, abnormalities were noted in 30% of the patients. In the two patients who died within 72 hours of admission, CT showed generalized cerebral edema. Focal infarction was seen in five of the eight patients who developed hemiparesis. CT during the second week of meningitis is most sensitive for cerebral infarction.[102, 103] In the course of community-acquired meningitis in children, CT is most valuable when persistent focal neurologic findings occur, when CSF cultures remain positive, or when meningitis is recurrent.[104]

In about 30% of adults with community-acquired meningitis, CT shows abnormalities related to meningitis or its complications.[21] Cerebral edema and dural enhancement are abnormalities seen on early scans within 72 hours of admission, whereas cerebral infarcts are seen on later scans. Although subdural effusions are often found in infants with meningitis, they are uncommon in adults (in only 2 of 87 adults with meningitis undergoing CT).[21] Ventriculomegaly is the most common CT abnormality in adult meningitis: 15% of all cases, 15% of which require a shunting procedure. In this study of adult meningitis,[21] of the 39 patients who exhibited focal neurologic deficits or seizures, 19 (49%) had CT abnormalities related to meningitis. In contrast, of the 48 patients with nonfocal findings, only 8 (17%) had CT abnormalities. Thus, CT in meningitis should not be routine but should be employed as indicated by the clinical setting, neurologic findings, and clinical course.

Differential Diagnosis

The clinical manifestations of meningeal inflammation (headache, fever, stiff neck, obtundation) are common to various other types of meningitis (viral, fungal, mycobacterial, treponemal, borrelial, parasitic, hypersensitivity) as well as to acute pyogenic bacterial meningitis and to parameningeal infections. Analysis of CSF findings is central to the development of the differential diagnosis (see Chapter 159).

Enteroviral aseptic meningitis usually can be distinguished from bacterial meningitis by its seasonal incidence, somewhat more gradual onset, occasional occurrence in outbreaks, occasional accompanying maculopetechial rash, and a lymphocytic pleocytosis without hypoglycorrhachia. Echovirus 9 aseptic meningitis may produce an initial pleocytosis of up to 500 to 1000 cells per mm^3, with up to 60% to 80% neutrophils, shifting in the next 12 to 36 hours to predominance of lymphocytes. The CSF glucose level is usually higher than 40 mg/dL but may be slightly reduced in occasional patients if the pathogen is the virus of lymphocytic choriomeningitis, mumps, or herpes simplex. Aseptic meningitis may be associated with the acute human immunodeficiency virus mononucleosis-like syndrome, but it is readily distinguished from acute bacterial meningitis by associated risk factors, lymphadenopathy, truncal maculopapular rash, and lymphocytic pleocytosis.[105] Acute herpes simplex virus type 2 aseptic meningitis occurs in sexually active persons and may be distinguished from bacterial meningitis by the presence of clustered vesicular lesions in the genital area or in the L1, L2, S3-5 dermatomes, and by its lymphocytic pleocytosis.

To provide greater accuracy in discriminating between acute bacterial and acute viral meningitis, a retrospective analysis of the predictive value of initial clinical and laboratory observations has been performed in 422 patients with meningitis seen at one hospital between 1969 and 1980.[106] Five CSF values were found to be individual predictors of bacterial infection with 99% or greater certainty: (1) CSF glucose level less than 1.9 mmol/L (34 mg/dL), (2) CSF/blood glucose ratio less than 0.23, (3) CSF protein level greater than 2.2 g/L, (4) greater than 2000/mm^3 CSF leukocytes, or (5) greater than 1180/mm^3 CSF neutrophils. Although any one of the foregoing tests could rule in bacterial meningitis with a high likelihood, none could exclude it. However, a logistic multiple regression model (converted to a nomogram for estimating probability of bacterial versus viral meningitis), utilizing the four parameters of (1) patient's age, (2) month of onset, (3) total neutrophil count in CSF, and (4) CSF/blood glucose ratio could be used to exclude acute bacterial meningitis with a greater than 95% confidence in patients whose CSF Gram stains were negative.[106]

Diagnosis of acute syphilitic meningitis would be suggested by a history of a recent chancre, maculopapular rash or generalized lymphadenopathy, lymphocytic pleocytosis (with or without mildly depressed CSF glucose level), and positive Venereal Disease Research Laboratory (VDRL) tests of serum and CSF. The aseptic meningitis picture of neuroborreliosis can be distinguished from acute pyogenic meningitis by its more subacute onset, exposure to an area endemic for Lyme disease, history of erythema chronicum migrans, lymphocytic pleocytosis, and positive serologic test result for Lyme disease. Leptospiral meningitis might be suggested by a biphasic illness, conjunctivitis, and lymphocytic pleocytosis occurring in a person exposed to rodents, dogs, or cows. Diagnosis is usually made by serologic tests. Tuberculous meningitis occurs in a setting of either past tuberculous infection (breakdown of an old meningeal tuberculoma) or recently acquired infection with miliary dissemination to the meninges in an immunocompetent or immunocompromised (e.g., human immunodeficiency virus–infected) patient. The onset of tuberculous meningitis tends to be less abrupt than that of acute pyogenic meningitis. The characteristic CSF changes are lymphocytic pleocytosis, hypoglycorrhachia, and elevated protein level. Bilateral palsies of cranial nerve VI suggest a basilar meningitis and with the aforementioned CSF formula strongly suggest tuberculous meningitis.

Fungal meningitides are almost always more subacute in onset than bacterial meningitis, produce a lymphocytic pleocytosis with hypoglycorrhachia, and are suggested by epidemiologic clues (immunosuppressed host at risk for cryptococcal meningitis; exposure in areas endemic for coccidioidomycosis, histoplasmosis, or blastomycosis). Fungal meningitides most commonly present the clinical picture of chronic meningitis and are diagnosed by culture and antigen detection *(Cryptococcus neoformans)* in the CSF or by CSF and serum antibody determination. Rarely, chronic meningitis may be characterized by a predominantly neutrophilic CSF formula, and several bacterial and mycotic agents are responsible.[107]

Parameningeal infections (particularly brain abscess, subdural empyema, and cranial and spinal epidural abscess) should be considered in the differential diagnosis of acute bacterial meningitis. These processes might be suspected in a patient with features of meningeal inflammation who also has a chronic ear, sinus, or lung infection. Focal cerebral signs and neurologic symptoms antedating the onset of the acute meningitis suggest a space-occupying intracranial infection, such as a brain abscess. In a patient with presumed bacterial meningitis whose CSF formula shows an atypical neutrophilic pleocytosis, a normal glucose level, and no demonstrable organisms on a Gram-stained smear, parameningeal infections in the differential diagnosis warrant particular attention. Isolation of anaerobic bacteria from CSF, especially in mixed culture, suggests parameningeal infection.

Rarely, a fulminant, acute, and usually fatal purulent meningitis is caused by *Naegleria fowleri*, a species of free-living amoeba. This diagnosis would be considered when the patient had recently swum in warm freshwater. Early symptoms may include an altered sense of smell and taste. In addition to a neutrophilic pleocytosis with a low to normal glucose level, the CSF often contains numerous red blood cells. Diagnosis is made by finding motile amoebic trophozoites on fresh preparations of unspun CSF.

The clinical picture of acute meningitis may develop in bacterial endocarditis. It may represent true bacterial meningitis due to pyogenic organisms (e.g., *S. pneumoniae, Staphylo-*

coccus aureus,) or it may result from cerebral embolic infarctions in endocarditis produced by nonpyogenic organisms such as viridans streptococci. Heart murmurs or peripheral signs of endocarditis suggest this pathogenesis for the meningeal process. CSF findings of cerebral infarction in this setting include pleocytosis of several hundred cells, with varying numbers of neutrophils, a normal glucose level, and absence of bacteria. In occasional patients with meningeal symptoms due to small cerebral embolic infarctions in acute *S. aureus* endocarditis, the diagnosis may sometimes be made by examination of Gram-stained smears of cutaneous lesions of purulent purpura.

Chemical meningitis occasionally results from leakage into the subarachnoid space of debris from an intracranial tumor, commonly a craniopharyngioma or an epidermoid tumor of the posterior fossa. This may produce the picture of recurrent meningitis. CSF findings include an initial neutrophilic (or lymphocytic) pleocytosis, with or without hypoglycorrhachia. Birefringent material (keratinized debris) from an epidermoid tumor or a craniopharyngioma may be observed under polarized light microscopy.

Occasionally, meningitis may be the principal manifestation of hypersensitivity to drugs such as sulfonamides and nonsteroidal antiinflammatory agents. The pleocytosis may be predominantly neutrophilic or lymphocytic, and some eosinophils may be present, but the glucose level in CSF is normal. Another rare, noninfectious cause of meningitis is systemic lupus erythematosus. The CSF formula is usually a lymphocytic pleocytosis with normal glucose, but, rarely, numerous neutrophils and hypoglycorrhachia are features. Antinuclear antibodies are present in high titers. Rarely, unusual acute, recurrent episodes of nonbacterial meningitis of unknown cause occur in the course of Behçet syndrome, Mollaret meningitis, or familial Mediterranean fever. Hypopyon, orogenital lesions, and pathergic skin changes would be indicative of Behçet syndrome. Mollaret meningitis, characterized by self-limited episodes of fever, meningeal findings, mononuclear pleocytosis (sometimes neutrophilic at inception), and the presence in the CSF of unusual cells variously described as "epithelial" or "endothelial," has been associated in some instances with underlying herpes simplex virus type 1 infections[108, 109] or with CNS epidermoid cysts.[110, 111]

Treatment

Essential for prompt treatment of meningitis is early recognition in the ambulatory setting of the development of meningeal signs, particularly the transition from a predisposing illness, such as otitis media, which until now may have been responsible for fever and headache. In the hospital emergency department there is similar need for timely triage of patients with symptoms possibly compatible with a diagnosis of meningitis, rapid contact with a physician, early performance of a lumbar puncture in the absence of clinical suspicion of an intracranial mass lesion, and prompt delivery of appropriate antimicrobial(s). In a study at two busy urban children's hospitals, the median time from triage in an emergency department until administration of parenteral antibiotics was 2.0 hours (interquartile time range, 1.25 to 3.33 hours); only 16% of the children with bacterial meningitis received antibiotics within 1 hour and only 1%, within 30 minutes or less after presentation.[112]

Therapy of acute bacterial meningitis involves (1) rapid identification of the pathogen, (2) *prompt* institution of an appropriate antimicrobial against the etiologic agent, when it can be defined on initial CSF examination, or institution of treatment directed at meningitis of unknown cause (utilizing clues provided by the age of the patient and clinical setting) pending definitive culture information, (3) management of neurologic and systemic complications, and local predisposing conditions (e.g., mastoiditis), and (4) study of predisposing factors, such as CSF fistulae, in the patient with recurrent bacterial meningitis.

General Aspects of Antimicrobial Treatment

The efficacy of antimicrobial therapy in bacterial meningitis depends on a variety of factors: antimicrobial susceptibility of the organism, bactericidal activity of the antimicrobial, capacity of the drug to penetrate the blood-brain barrier, and effectiveness of various modes of antibiotic administration in achieving desired concentrations of the drug in CSF. In view of the lack of intrinsic opsonic and bactericidal activity in CSF early in bacterial meningitis, bactericidal rather than bacteriostatic agents are needed for treatment.[52] CSF concentrations of β-lactam antibiotics or aminoglycosides must be 10 to 20 times higher than the minimal bactericidal concentration for the infecting organism to achieve optimal bactericidal effects.[113] The low pH and abundance of nucleic acids in purulent CSF inhibit rapid bacterial killing by aminoglycosides.

Antagonism by a bacteriostatic drug, chloramphenicol, of the early bactericidal effect of penicillin in experimental canine pneumococcal meningitis and of the bactericidal activity of gentamicin in experimental *Proteus mirabilis* meningitis in rabbits has been demonstrated.[114] Little clinical information on humans bearing on this point is available. There is evidence of antagonism between chlortetracycline and penicillin in the treatment of pneumococcal meningitis.[115] Similarly, in a retrospective study of patients with meningitis due to Enterobacteriaceae, the case-fatality rate was highest when treatment included chloramphenicol, usually in combination with an aminoglycoside.[5]

Most antibiotics employed in treatment of bacterial meningitis, with the exception of chloramphenicol, do not readily penetrate the normal blood-brain barrier. β-Lactam antibiotics penetrate to only 0.5% to 2.0% of peak serum concentrations,[114] but higher levels are achieved when the meninges are inflamed. Clindamycin, erythromycin, and first- and second-generation cephalosporins should not be used to treat bacterial meningitis because effective bactericidal levels cannot be obtained. For antimicrobial drugs such as β-lactams, aminoglycosides, and vancomycin, which poorly penetrate even inflamed meninges, intermittent bolus parenteral administration is preferable to continuous administration because higher peak levels are achieved.

Specific Antimicrobial Therapy

Acute bacterial meningitis requires prompt antimicrobial treatment based on examination of a Gram-stained smear of the spun sediment of CSF (Table 158–9). When clinical evaluation suggests a parameningeal suppurative mass lesion and head CT is needed before performance of a lumbar puncture, antibiotic therapy should be instituted, directed toward meningitis of unknown cause (Table 158–10), after blood cultures have been obtained. If in this situation CT has excluded a mass lesion and the subsequent CSF examination shows bacterial types not treated by the initial empirical program, antimicrobial therapy can be altered. Such initial therapy is unlikely to prevent identification of the pathogen if CSF is sampled within 2 or 3 hours.

COMMUNITY-ACQUIRED MENINGITIS

Streptococcus pneumoniae

Penicillin G and ampicillin have been the drugs of choice for meningitis due to penicillin-susceptible *S. pneumoniae.*

TABLE 158–9 ■ Antimicrobial Therapy of Community-Acquired Bacterial Meningitis*

ORGANISM	PREFERRED THERAPY			ALTERNATIVE THERAPY		
	Antimicrobial	**Adults, 24-Hour Dose**	**Children, 24-Hour Dose**	**Antimicrobial**	**Adults, 24-Hour Dose**	**Children, 24-Hour Dose**
Streptococcus pneumoniae						
Penicillin MIC < 0.1 μg/mL	Penicillin G	24 million units IV, q 4 h aliquots	300,000 units/kg IV, q 4 h aliquots	Cefotaxime	12 g IV, q 4 h aliquots	200 mg/kg IV, q 4–6 h aliquots
	or			*or*		
	Ampicillin	12 g IV, q 4 h aliquots	200–400 mg/kg IV, q 4 h aliquots	Ceftriaxone†	4 g IV, q 12 h aliquots	80–100 mg/kg IV, q 12 h aliquots
				or		
				Vancomycin	2 g IV, q 8–12 h aliquots‡	50–60 mg/kg IV, q 6 h aliquots
				or		
				Chloramphenicol	4–6 g IV, q 6 h aliquots	75–100 mg/kg IV, q 6 h aliquots
Penicillin MIC 0.1–1.0 μg/mL	Ceftriaxone†	4 g IV, q 12 h aliquots	80–100 mg/kg IV, q 12 h aliquots†	Vancomycin‡	2 g IV, q 8–12 h aliquots	50–60 mg/kg IV, q 6 h aliquots
	or			*or*		
	Cefotaxime	12 g IV, q 4 h aliquots	200 mg/kg IV, q 4–6 h aliquots	Imipenem§	2–3 g IV, q 6 h aliquots	—
Penicillin MIC > 1.0 μg/mL	Vancomycin‡‖	2 g IV, q 8–12 h aliquots‡	50–60 mg/kg IV, q 6 h aliquots	Imipenem§	2–3 g IV, q 6 h aliquots	—
Neisseria meningitidis	Penicillin G	24 million units IV, q 4 h aliquots	300,000 units/kg IV, q 4 h aliquots	Ceftriaxone†		80–100 mg/kg IV, q 12 h aliquots
	or			*or*		
	Ampicillin	12 g IV, q 4 h aliquots	200–400 mg/kg IV, q 4 h aliquots	Cefotaxime	Dose as above	200 mg/kg IV, q 4–6 h aliquots
				or		
				Chloramphenicol	4–6 g IV, q 6 h aliquots	75–100 mg/kg IV, q 6 h aliquots
Haemophilus influenzae						
β-Lactamase-negative	Ampicillin	12 g IV, q 4 h aliquots	200–400 mg/kg IV, q 4 h aliquots	Third-generation cephalosporin¶ or chloramphenicol	Dose as above	Dose as above
β-Lactamase-positive	Ceftriaxone†	4 g IV, q 12 h aliquots	80–100 mg/kg IV, q 12 h aliquots	Chloramphenicol	Dose as above	75–100 mg/kg IV, q 6 h aliquots
	or					
	Cefotaxime	12 g IV, q 4 h aliquots	200 mg/kg IV, q 4–6 h aliquots			
Listeria monocytogenes	Ampicillin**	12 g IV, q 4 h aliquots	200–400 mg/kg IV, q 4 h aliquots	TMP-SMX††	10–20 mg/kg IV,‡‡ q 6–8 h aliquots	10–20 mg/kg IV,‡‡ q 6 h aliquots
	or					
	Penicillin G**	24 million units IV, q 4 h aliquots	300,000 units/kg IV, q 4 h aliquots			

*Dosages are those for patients with normal renal and hepatic function. IV, Intravenous.
†Maximal daily dose is 4 g.
‡Monitoring of peak and trough serum levels is advisable; CSF levels may need to be monitored if the patient is not responding well and, if low, the daily dose may need to be increased temporarily by 0.5–1.0 g in adults or adjuvant intrathecal vancomycin added as in treatment of methicillin-resistant *S. aureus* meningitis (see text).
§Use is associated with an increased incidence of seizures.
‖Addition of rifampin should be considered.
¶Ceftriaxone or cefotaxime.
**Addition of IV gentamicin might be considered.
††Trimethoprim-sulfamethoxazole.
‡‡Dosage is based on the trimethoprim component of the combination.

TABLE 158–10 ■ Initial Therapy for Community-Acquired Purulent Meningitis of Unknown Cause

AGE OR CONDITION	LIKELY PATHOGENS	PREFERRED DRUGS	ALTERNATIVE DRUGS
0–4 wk	Group B streptococci, *Escherichia coli, Listeria monocytogenes*	Ampicillin + cefotaxime	Ampicillin + aminoglycoside*
4–12 wk	Group B streptococci, *E. coli, L. monocytogenes, Haemophilus influenzae, Streptococcus pneumoniae*	Ampicillin + either cefotaxime or ceftriaxone	
3 mo through 17 y	*S. pneumoniae,*† *Neisseria meningitidis, H. influenzae*	Cefotaxime or ceftriaxone	Ampicillin + chloramphenicol
18–50 y	*S. pneumoniae,*† *N. meningitidis*	Cefotaxime or ceftriaxone ± ampicillin	Vancomycin + chloramphenicol
>50 y	*S. pneumoniae,*† *N. meningitidis, L. monocytogenes*	Cefotaxime or ceftriaxone + ampicillin	Cefotaxime or ?vancomycin + trimethoprim-sulfamethoxazole
Basilar skull fracture or CSF leak	*S. pneumoniae,*† various streptococci, *H. influenzae, N. meningitidis*	Cefotaxime or ceftazidime	Vancomycin + chloramphenicol
CSF mechanical shunt	*Staphylococcus aureus*, coagulase-negative staphylococci, *Pseudomonas aeruginosa*, Enterobacteriaceae	Vancomycin + ceftazidime	

*Gentamicin or tobramycin (or amikacin in hospitals where gentamicin-resistant enteric organisms are common).
†In communities where highly penicillin resistant or cephalosporin resistant *S. pneumoniae* has occurred (or is likely), vancomycin should be added.

Formerly, *S. pneumoniae* was universally susceptible to penicillin in vitro (MIC [minimal inhibitory concentration] ≤ 0.06 μg/mL), but in the past decade and a half, relatively resistant (MIC 0.1 to 1.0 μg/mL) and very resistant (MIC 1.0 to 2.0 μg/mL or more) strains have been isolated from patients.[114] Such resistance in these strains is chromosomal in origin (alterations in penicillin binding proteins). In other parts of the world (South Africa, Hungary, parts of South America, and Spain), as many as 40% to 50% of strains show moderate or high degrees of resistance.[116–119] Although reports of isolation of penicillin-resistant pneumococci, sometimes resistant as well to other drugs (tetracycline, erythromycin, chloramphenicol, clindamycin), from abroad appeared as early as the 1970s,[120] only 0.02% of isolates of *S. pneumoniae* in a nationwide surveillance program between 1979 and 1987 in the United States showed high-level resistance to penicillin.[121] By 1992 the proportion of such resistant isolates increased to 1.3%; subsequent studies of both children and adults in a variety of regions indicate that the percentage of penicillin-resistant isolates among invasive *S. pneumoniae* ranged from 2% to 17%. Most disturbing is the finding, in a 1994 survey of *S. pneumoniae* isolates from more than 400 patients with invasive infection in the Atlanta area, of resistance to penicillin in 25% (7% high level).[122] Multiple antimicrobial resistance was common among the penicillin-resistant isolates: 75% resistant to trimethoprim-sulfamethoxazole; 41%, to erythromycin; 34%, to cefotaxime; 24%, to tetracycline; 23%, to imipenem; 12%, to chloramphenicol. Among all the 431 isolates analyzed, 9% were resistant to cefotaxime, a proportion identical to that in Barcelona, Spain, in the period 1989 to 1993.[123] Molecular fingerprinting has indicated that a multidrug-resistant clone of *S. pneumoniae* serotype 23F, related to multidrug-resistant isolates from Spain and South Africa, has spread to the United States and become widely disseminated.[124, 125] Other multidrug-resistant strains are particularly prevalent among serotypes 6, 14, 15, and 19 (often found among children).

The increasing prevalence of penicillin resistance (and multidrug resistance) among strains of *S. pneumoniae* mandates susceptibility testing of any isolate from blood or normally sterile body sites. The increase in prevalence of penicillin resistance in *S. pneumoniae* precludes reliance, as in years past, on penicillin for treatment of pneumococcal infections. Although current evidence suggests that penicillin can be used successfully in adults in the treatment of pneumococcal pneumonia due to penicillin-resistant strains (no increased mortality compared with penicillin-susceptible strains), the penicillin must be administered intravenously in high doses (150,000 to 200,000 units/kg daily) and the penicillin MIC should be 2 μg/mL or less.[123] In contrast, penicillin should not be employed as the drug of choice in the empirical treatment of pyogenic meningitis when *S. pneumoniae* is a likely pathogen because even with "meningeal dosages" of penicillin it is difficult to achieve during the first and subsequent days CSF concentrations greater than approximately 1 μg/mL. In view of the widespread and increasing prevalence of relatively penicillin resistant strains in the United States, Europe, and South Africa, third-generation cephalosporins such as cefotaxime or ceftriaxone in high dosage should be used in such regions as initial treatment when *S. pneumoniae* is a suspected cause.[113, 126–128]

During the past 4 years, the occurrence of meningitis caused by strains of *S. pneumoniae* with decreased susceptibility to third-generation cephalosporins (MIC values ≥ 2.0 μg/mL) has presented a new therapeutic problem, and, disturbingly, scattered reports of patients with such infecting strains who have been unsuccessfully treated with such cephalosporins have appeared.[129–131] This has led to the recommendation that *S. pneumoniae* isolates from meningitis with MIC values of 0.5 to 1.0 μg/mL to third-generation cephalosporins be considered as intermediately resistant and those with MIC values of 2.0 μg/mL or greater as fully resistant. This has been debated on the basis of comparable clinical courses and outcomes of *S. pneumoniae* meningitis in five children with relatively or highly penicillin resistant strains that had cefotaxime (or ceftriaxone) MIC values of 0.5 to 2.0 μg/mL and in five children with similar penicillin-resistant strains that were susceptible to cefotaxime concentrations of 0.25 μg/mL or less.[131] Vancomycin has been used successfully, alone or in combination with other drugs such as rifampin, in the treatment of a small number of patients with meningitis who were unsuccessfully treated initially with cefotaxime or ceftriaxone and whose infecting strains of *S. pneumoniae* had MIC values for these third-generation cephalosporins of 2 to 8 μg/mL.[131]

In areas of the United States where cases of pneumococcal meningitis due to strains highly resistant to penicillin and resistant to third-generation cephalosporins are known to have occurred (e.g., Arkansas, California, Indiana, Michigan, Tennessee, Texas), initial treatment before ascertainment of the antimicrobial susceptibility results might include vancomycin along with a third-generation cephalosporin. Indeed, the recommendation has been made to include vancomycin in initial treatment of all cases of pneumococcal meningitis along with a β-lactam before determination of susceptibilities in areas in which intermediately or highly penicillin resistant *S. pneumoniae* have been identified.[132] Experience with vancomycin is still limited in treatment of pneumococcal meningitis caused by penicillin-resistant strains. In one series of 11 patients treated with vancomycin, 10 were eventually cured, but 4 required a shift to other drugs because of failure of vancomycin.[133] Possible causes of therapeutic failure, because vancomycin resistance has not been observed among pneumococci, include inadequate serum levels of vancomycin and poor penetration of the drug into the CSF, possibly abetted by the antiinflammatory effect of adjunctive dexamethasone therapy. At present, vancomycin together with rifampin is the most reasonable therapy for meningitis due to highly penicillin resistant *S. pneumoniae*, but clinical experience is meager. Intrathecal or intraventricular vancomycin may be added in management if the response to intravenous (IV) vancomycin is unsatisfactory. In this situation, measurement of CSF levels may be helpful.

For several decades, chloramphenicol has been the alternative treatment for pneumococcal meningitis in the highly β-lactam allergic patient. Although only 3% of 431 isolates of *S. pneumoniae* from Atlanta in 1994 showed resistance to chloramphenicol (MIC $\geq$ 8 μg/mL), 12% of penicillin-resistant isolates were also resistant to chloramphenicol.[122] In a South African study of pneumococcal meningitis due to strains that were both penicillin resistant and chloramphenicol susceptible, 80% of children who were treated initially with chloramphenicol had an unsatisfactory outcome (death, neurologic deficit, poor clinical response).[134] In contrast, adverse outcomes occurred in only 33% of children with meningitis due to penicillin-susceptible strains who were treated with penicillin. Although all the strains (penicillin susceptible and penicillin resistant) were chloramphenicol susceptible by antibiotic disk testing, the penicillin-resistant strains were more likely to have a higher chloramphenicol minimal bactericidal concentration (4 μg/mL or more), suggesting that the poor clinical results might be attributable to inadequate bactericidal activity of chloramphenicol against penicillin-resistant strains. In view of the increasing frequency of penicillin-resistant strains in *S. pneumoniae* meningitis, initial treatment of the highly β-lactam allergic patient with suspected pneumococcal meningitis might consist of vancomycin along with rifampin or chloramphenicol, but not chloramphenicol alone as in the past. Vancomycin (with or without the addition of rifampin) is the drug of choice for treatment of meningitis caused by highly penicillin resistant pneumococci.

Neisseria meningitidis

Penicillin or ampicillin remains the antimicrobial of choice for treatment of meningitis caused by *N. meningitidis*. Strains with relative resistance to penicillin (MIC 0.1 to 1.0 μg/mL) due to reduced affinity for penicillin binding protein 2 (sometimes designated penicillin binding protein 3) have been reported, particularly from Spain.[135] As with relative penicillin resistance in *S. pneumoniae*, in Spain the prevalence of relative penicillin resistance has increased in the past decade from 0.4% in 1985 to 5.0% in 1986, 20% in 1989, and 46% in 1990.[136, 137] Increased resistance to penicillin has been reported in sporadic cases from elsewhere in Europe (United Kingdom, Belgium, Greece), South Africa, and Canada.[137] Most of these relatively resistant strains have belonged to serogroup B or C, and the DNA fingerprints containing the penicillin binding protein 2 gene of these strains have shown considerable diversity when compared with penicillin-susceptible strains.[138] Although relatively penicillin resistant isolates of *N. meningitidis* have occasionally been noted in surveillance reports in the United States, it is only within the past 5 years that such strains have sporadically been reported responsible for invasive disease (five cases).[137, 139] In treating such infections, cefotaxime or ceftriaxone would be the drugs of choice.[140] A rare β-lactamase–producing strain of *N. meningitidis* has been isolated from the genitourinary tract of one patient[141]; such a highly penicillin resistant strain has been isolated from two bacteremic and meningeal infections in South Africa.[142] The laboratory demonstration of transfer of β-lactamase plasmids from *N. gonorrhoeae* to *N. meningitidis* and commensal *Neisseria* species indicates the potential for development of high-level penicillin resistance among meningococci and the need for active surveillance of such strains.[143]

Haemophilus influenzae

Although ampicillin was the drug of choice in the treatment of Hib meningitis from the late 1960s to the mid-1970s, the emergence and increasing prevalence of β-lactamase–producing strains (approximately 30% of isolates in the United States currently)[144] have required a change in therapy. The approach utilized in the late 1970s was the combination initially of ampicillin with chloramphenicol, with omission of chloramphenicol if the isolate was demonstrated to lack β-lactamase activity. Currently, chloramphenicol resistance occurs in less than 1% of strains of *H. influenzae* in the United States,[145, 146] but it has been observed in more than 50% of isolates in parts of Spain.[147] Therapy of childhood meningitis, caused primarily by *H. influenzae* until widespread immunization with Hib conjugate vaccines, with ceftriaxone or cefotaxime has yielded results superior to those obtained with chloramphenicol, even among patients infected by chloramphenicol-susceptible isolates.[148] Thus, these two third-generation cephalosporins have become the drugs of choice for treatment of Hib meningitis. In a survey of 69 pediatric centers in the United States and Canada in 1992, 93% treated presumed bacterial meningitis in children 5 months of age with either ceftriaxone or cefotaxime, whereas only 2% employed the combination of ampicillin plus chloramphenicol.[149] Another factor contributing to the aforenoted preference for third-generation cephalosporins is the hematotoxicity, albeit rare, and interactions of chloramphenicol with other drugs (phenytoin, phenobarbital, acetaminophen, rifampin), which may contribute to toxicity.[150]

Resistance of *H. influenzae* to ceftriaxone or cefotaxime has not yet been reported as a problem. Cefuroxime, a second-generation cephalosporin, was used in the mid-1980s in the initial treatment of childhood meningitis about as frequently as either cefotaxime or ceftriaxone[149] on the basis of early studies indicating efficacy comparable to that of the combination of ampicillin and chloramphenicol. However, subsequent trials comparing cefuroxime and ceftriaxone in the treatment of childhood bacterial meningitis, although showing no difference in mortality (no deaths in either group), did demonstrate a delay in sterilization of the CSF at 18 to 36 hours with cefuroxime and an increased incidence of sensorineural hearing loss (17% versus 4%).[151, 152] Thus, cefuroxime should not be considered as an initial choice for treatment of childhood meningitis or known Hib meningitis.

ACUTE BACTERIAL MENINGITIS OF UNDEFINED CAUSE

Initial antimicrobial treatment of acute bacterial meningitis of unknown cause is based on coverage of the likely pathogens, as suggested by the age of the patient and the clinical setting (community or nosocomial origin, compromised host; see Table 158–10). In adults, *S. pneumoniae, N. meningitidis,* various streptococci, and *L. monocytogenes* are responsible for most cases of community-acquired meningitis[21]; the combination of a third-generation cephalosporin (ceftriaxone or cefotaxime) with ampicillin is mandated as initial therapy[153] (pending culture results) because of the prevalence of penicillin resistance among *S. pneumoniae,*[121–123] the prominent role of *Listeria* in CNS infections in adults,[21, 154] and the relative insusceptibility of *Listeria* to third-generation cephalosporins. The role of *H. influenzae* and Enterobacteriaceae in 5% to 10% of episodes of community-acquired meningitis in adults further supports the use of ceftriaxone or cefotaxime in an initial combination with ampicillin. The likelihood of *L. monocytogenes* as the cause of meningitis in an adult, and thus the need for addition of ampicillin to a third-generation cephalosporin, is increased in patients older than 50 years, in the presence of immunosuppression or pregnancy, and in the setting of liver disease. In the penicillin-allergic patient, an alternative antimicrobial for treatment of *L. monocytogenes* meningitis is trimethoprim-sulfamethoxazole (TMP-SMX), which is bactericidal in vitro against this organism.[155] In an epidemic of 57 cases of listeriosis in adults (almost 80% with meningitis or meningoencephalitis), seven patients with CNS infection were treated with TMP-SMX and survived.[156] The addition of gentamicin to penicillin or ampicillin might be considered, in view of synergism in vitro and enhanced killing in animal models, in culture-proven cases of severe infection caused by *L. monocytogenes* or if such infections failed to respond to treatment.[154]

NOSOCOMIAL MENINGITIS

The principal agents of nosocomial bacterial meningitis are gram-negative bacilli, *S. aureus,* and *S. epidermidis* (Tables 158–11 to 158–13). A third-generation cephalosporin is the treatment of choice for meningitis caused by Enterobacteriaceae; for *P. aeruginosa* meningitis, IV ceftazidime in combination with an aminoglycoside such as tobramycin is the treatment of choice. Among 24 patients with *Pseudomonas* meningitis treated with ceftazidime alone or in combination with an aminoglycoside, 19 (79%) were cured.[157] Owing to the ready penetration of ceftazidime and other third-generation cephalosporins into CSF in the presence of meningeal inflammation, intrathecal or intraventricular aminoglycoside is infrequently needed to treat meningitis caused by Enterobacteriaceae or *P. aeruginosa.* It may be considered, however, when patients are not responding to parenteral therapy, particularly when ready access to intraventricular administration is available from prior neurosurgery. Limited experience indicates that other drugs may be available as alternatives should a third-generation cephalosporin prove ineffective in gram-negative bacillary meningitis. These include aztreonam, which readily penetrates the blood-brain barrier and has been effective in treatment of meningitis caused by susceptible aerobic gram-negative bacilli,[158] and imipenem, whose usefulness has been limited because of its tendency to induce seizures. Although some fluoroquinolones readily penetrate the CSF in the presence of meningitis (10% to 90% of simultaneous serum levels), there are as yet only few data on their use in bacterial meningitis. Fluoroquinolones have been used successfully in the treatment of some patients with gram-negative bacillary meningitis.[159] Their place in the therapy of meningitis is limited at present to the treatment of infections caused by multidrug-resistant gram-negative bacilli that are susceptible to ciprofloxacin. *Stenotrophomonas* (formerly *Xanthomonas) maltophilia* is increasingly important as a nosocomial pathogen and is often resistant to third-generation cephalosporins and imipenem but susceptible to TMP-SMX. On the basis of in vitro susceptibilities and experience in treatment of several cases of *S. maltophilia* meningitis after neuro-

TABLE 158–11 ■ Antimicrobial Therapy of Nosocomial Bacterial Meningitis

	PREFERRED THERAPY		ALTERNATIVE THERAPY
ORGANISM	**Antimicrobial**	**Adjunctive Intrathecal Therapy**	**Antimicrobial**
Staphylococcus aureus			
Methicillin susceptible	Nafcillin or oxacillin ± rifampin	—	Vancomycin
Methicillin resistant	Vancomycin ± rifampin	Vancomycin, if needed, 5–20 mg/d*	Trimethoprim-sulfamethoxazole + either ciprofloxacin or rifampin
Coagulase-negative *Staphylococcus*	Vancomycin ± rifampin	Vancomycin, if needed, 5–20 mg/d*	—
Enterobacteriaceae	Cefotaxime or ceftriaxone	—	Piperacillin + gentamicin; aztreonam; ciprofloxacin; trimethoprim-sulfamethoxazole
Pseudomonas aeruginosa	Ceftazidime + tobramycin or gentamicin	Gentamicin, if needed, 2–4 mg/d†	Piperacillin + tobramycin or gentamicin; aztreonam; ciprofloxacin; ?imipenem
Streptococcus agalactiae (group B streptococcus)	Ampicillin or penicillin G	—	Cefotaxime or ceftriaxone; vancomycin
Enterococcus spp.	Ampicillin (or penicillin G) + gentamicin	Gentamicin, if needed, 2–4 mg/d†	Vancomycin + gentamicin
Empirical Therapy for Specific Settings (Nosocomial)			
After neurosurgery or head trauma	Vancomycin + ceftazidime	—	—
Immunocompromised host	Vancomycin + ceftazidime + ampicillin	—	—

*Intrathecal vancomycin has been employed as adjunctive therapy when response to IV vancomycin was unsatisfactory. For intrathecal use it should be free of preservative.
†Without preservative, in 5–10 mL of CSF or in a volume of sterile saline (without preservative, comparable to the 5–10 mL of CSF removed from an adult for analysis). Injection should be administered slowly for 10 min.

TABLE 158–12 ■ Dosages for Antimicrobial Agents in Treatment of Nosocomial Meningitis in Adults*

ANTIMICROBIAL AGENT	TOTAL DAILY DOSE†	FREQUENCY OF DOSES
Third-generation cephalosporins		
Cefotaxime	12 g	q 4 h
Ceftriaxone	4 g	q 12 h
Ceftazidime	6 g	q 6–8 h
Penicillins		
Penicillin G	24 million units	q 4 h
Ampicillin	12 g	q 4 h
Nafcillin	9–12 g	q 4 h
Oxacillin	9–12 g	q 4 h
Piperacillin	24 g	q 4 h
Aminoglycosides‡		
Gentamicin	3–5 mg/kg	q 8–12 h
Tobramycin	3–5 mg/kg	q 8–12 h
Amikacin	15 mg/kg	q 8–12 h
Vancomycin§	2 g	q 8–12 h
Chloramphenicol‖	4–6 g	q 6 h
Rifampin	600 mg	q 24 h
Aztreonam	6–8 g	q 6–8 h
Ciprofloxacin	800 mg	q 12 h
Trimethoprim-sulfamethoxazole¶	20 mg/kg	q 6–12 h
Imipenem**	2–4 g	q 6 h

*All dosages are for IV administration.
†Dosages are for adults with normal renal and hepatic function.
‡Aminoglycoside peak and trough serum levels should be monitored for dosage regulation.
§Vancomycin peak and trough serum levels should be monitored for dosage regulation.
‖Chloramphenicol serum levels may need to be monitored for dosage regulation.
¶Dosage refers to trimethoprim component.
**Higher dose (4 g) may induce seizure activity.

surgery, TMP-SMX appears to be the treatment of choice.[160] The value of adjunctive intrathecal therapy with an aminoglycoside is unclear.

Treatment of nosocomial meningitis due to *Enterobacter* species with third-generation cephalosporins may be complicated by the development of resistance to the third-generation cephalosporin during the course of therapy, and by clinical failure. In a study of 12 patients with *Enterobacter* meningitis at one hospital, resistance to the third-generation cephalosporin employed developed in 4 of 10 patients who received initial therapy with the cephalosporin.[161] TMP-SMX appears to be a useful drug when such resistance develops or when *Enterobacter* is isolated from CSF even when the initial CSF isolate is susceptible to third-generation cephalosporins. *A. baumannii* has been involved increasingly in the past decade with outbreaks of nosocomial infections, including meningitis after invasive neurosurgical procedures.[162] Treatment with a combination of an extended-spectrum ureidopenicillin (mezlocillin, piperacillin) and an aminoglycoside (amikacin, tobramycin) has been successful. Because of variable antimicrobial susceptibilities, other drugs may be required. Most clinical isolates have shown susceptibility to

TABLE 158–13 ■ Dosages of Antimicrobial Agents for Neonatal Meningitis*

ANTIMICROBIAL AGENT	NEONATES, 0–1 WEEK†		NEONATES, 1–4 WEEKS†	
	Total Daily Dose	Frequency of Doses	Total Daily Dose	Frequency of Doses
Penicillins				
Penicillin G	100,000–150,000 units/kg	q 8–12 h	150,000–250,000 units/kg	q 6–8 h
Ampicillin	100–150 mg/kg	q 8–12 h	200 mg/kg	q 6 h
Nafcillin	100–150 mg/kg	q 8–12 h	200 mg/kg	q 6 h
Cephalosporins				
Cefotaxime	100 mg/kg	q 12 h	150–200 mg/kg	q 6–8 h
Ceftazidime	60 mg/kg	q 12 h	100–150 mg/kg	q 8 h
Aminoglycosides				
Gentamicin‡	5 mg/kg	q 12 h	5.0–7.5 mg/kg	q 8 h
Tobramycin‡	4 mg/kg	q 12 h	6 mg/kg	q 8 h
Amikacin‡	15–20 mg/kg	q 8–12 h	20–30 mg/kg	q 8 h
Vancomycin§‖	20 mg/kg	q 12 h	30–40 mg/kg	q 8 h
Chloramphenicol¶	25 mg/kg	q 24 h	50 mg/kg	q 12 h

*All drugs are administered IV.
†Smaller doses and less frequent administration are advisable for neonates of <2000 g.
‡Peak and trough serum levels should be monitored.
§Peak and trough serum levels should be monitored, particularly in preterm infants.
‖Should be infused over 1 h.
¶Monitoring serum levels is necessary because of wide variations.

imipenem, ciprofloxacin, ceftazidime, and minocycline.[162] As in treatment of other resistant gram-negative bacillary meningitides, use of intrathecal as well as parenteral aminoglycosides may be indicated.

Treatment of *S. aureus* meningitis involves the use of intravenous nafcillin or oxacillin. For meningitis caused by methicillin-resistant *S. aureus*, or when such methicillin-resistant organisms are likely, or for patients who are allergic to penicillin, vancomycin is the alternative of choice.[27] The addition of rifampin to either nafcillin or vancomycin should be considered when the therapeutic response has been inadequate, or, from the beginning, when the infection is severe. Because coagulase-negative staphylococci are the most frequent causes of CSF shunt infections (and complicating meningitis), and because more than one third of such nosocomial strains are methicillin resistant, vancomycin is the initial drug of choice, although its penetration is limited in the absence of marked meningeal inflammation. If the response to treatment is unsatisfactory, rifampin (which readily penetrates the CSF) might be added.[163]

Meningitis in the presence of an infected CSF shunt requires initial therapy directed by findings on Gram stain of CSF. In the absence of the finding of a likely pathogen on an initial Gram-stained smear, initial antimicrobial treatment should be directed at the most likely pathogens (*S. aureus*, coagulase-negative staphylococci, and aerobic gram-negative bacilli such as Enterobacteriaceae and *P. aeruginosa*) until culture results become available to guide definitive therapy. All components of the infected shunt should be removed at the onset of antimicrobial therapy. External ventriculostomy is recommended at the same time to reduce ventriculitis and for observation of CSF changes.[164] Ventricular irrigation with an antibiotic solution has been used in treatment of severe or difficult to eradicate infections, with amikacin (30 μg/mL) or gentamicin (15 μg/mL) solutions (without preservative) in a continuous flow through a functioning ventriculostomy.[164] Intraventricular antibiotic administration may be used for distribution through the ventricular system and CSF in the absence of external ventriculostomy, to overcome the problem of poor CSF penetration after IV administration of drugs such as gentamicin and vancomycin (see later). When an aminoglycoside is used intraventricularly for treatment of an aerobic gram-negative bacillary infection, it should be combined with a parenteral drug (e.g., a third-generation cephalosporin or an extended-spectrum ureidopenicillin) as well as with a parenteral aminoglycoside.

ADJUNCTIVE INTRATHECAL THERAPY

Intrathecal therapy is unnecessary in the treatment of the common types of community-acquired meningitis. Introduction of third-generation cephalosporins, which achieve CSF levels that are bactericidal for many of the gram-negative bacilli involved in nosocomial meningitis, has eliminated the need for intrathecal aminoglycosides in most situations. Occasionally, with refractory meningitis caused by gram-negative bacilli, adjunctive use of intrathecal (or when appropriate, intraventricular) aminoglycosides might be considered.

The adjunctive use of intrathecal gentamicin occasionally might be indicated in the treatment of enterococcal meningitis when the response to initial treatment with IV penicillin (or ampicillin) and gentamicin has not been satisfactory.

Adjuvant intrathecal vancomycin is occasionally employed in the treatment of meningitis (or CSF shunt infections) caused by methicillin-resistant *S. aureus* or coagulase-negative staphylococci that do not respond satisfactorily to IV vancomycin. Intrathecal, preservative-free vancomycin, in doses up to 20 mg daily for adults (or approximately 0.5 mg/kg for children), is administered slowly or by barbotage after dilution in CSF or preservative-free physiologic diluent.[165]

Adjunctive intraventricular gentamicin has been administered in a daily dosage of 4 to 8 mg in adults (1 to 2 mg in infants).[164, 166, 167] Adjunctive intraventricular vancomycin has been given in doses of 4 to 10 mg daily.[164, 168, 169]

DURATION OF ANTIMICROBIAL THERAPY

Treatment of meningococcal meningitis for 7 days (for 5 days after the patient becomes afebrile) is adequate. Treatment of *H. influenzae* meningitis should continue for 10 days (for 7 days after the patient becomes afebrile). However, studies have shown that 7 days' treatment of childhood meningitis is generally effective and the results are comparable to results from 10 days' treatment.[170] Antimicrobial treatment of pneumococcal meningitis should be continued somewhat longer, for 10 to 14 days, because of the not infrequent presence of a predisposing otitis media and mastoiditis and because of possible metastatic foci of infection. More prolonged therapy is needed in the presence of an accompanying parameningeal infection.

Repeated CSF examination at the conclusion of a course of antimicrobial therapy for *H. influenzae* and *N. meningitidis* meningitis is unnecessary in most instances when there has been a prompt and satisfactory clinical recovery.[171] Follow-up examination should be done for pneumococcal meningitis at the completion of therapy, because of occasional relapse from an associated parameningeal site of infection and because of therapeutic problems with *S. pneumoniae* strains that are relatively or highly resistant to penicillin. In the patient who has not shown satisfactory improvement in the first 24 to 48 hours of treatment, CSF examination should be repeated to determine whether viable bacteria persist. This would apply particularly when the antibiotic employed (e.g., vancomycin) enters the CSF in limited concentrations and when simultaneous use of corticosteroids may reduce its penetrance by attenuating meningeal inflammation.

Treatment of nosocomial meningitis, usually associated with neurosurgical procedures, is more prolonged than that of community-acquired meningitis, because of the associated anatomic changes (subgaleal collections, CSF fistulae) and the antimicrobial resistance patterns of the causative organisms. Gram-negative bacillary meningitis requires treatment for 3 weeks or more because of the frequent association of an infected subgaleal collection communicating with the subarachnoid space.

Management of Acute Brain Swelling and Markedly Heightened Cerebrospinal Fluid Pressure

Markedly elevated CSF pressures (at least 500 mm H_2O) are observed in about 5% of cases of acute bacterial meningitis in the absence of any complicating mass lesion. Such elevated pressure is usually the result of acute cerebral edema; complicating cerebral herniation has been reported in bacterial meningitis in children[172] and adults.[21] Of 27 adults with community-acquired bacterial meningitis who died within the first week of illness, 30% had evidence of temporal lobe herniation with prominent cerebral edema.[21] In the majority, clinical deterioration occurred within several hours of performance of a lumbar puncture that had shown markedly elevated CSF pressure. Herniation has occurred in occasional cases of bacterial meningitis in the absence of a proximate lumbar puncture. Although the relationship is unproved by controlled study, it would seem reasonable to exercise the following precautions in the patient whose CSF pressure is 450 to 500 mm H_2O or higher: (1) removal of only the amount of

CSF in the manometer (sufficient for Gram stain, cell count, culture); (2) IV infusion of 20% mannitol solution (0.25 to 0.5 g/kg; higher doses with evidence of herniation) during 20 to 30 minutes; and (3) continued control of increased ICP, if needed, with subsequent infusions of dexamethasone (10 mg IV, followed by 4 mg every 6 hours) or mannitol. Direct measurement of CSF pressure by an ICP monitoring device may be helpful in management of patients with bacterial meningitis who have clinical (stupor, coma) or neuroimaging signs of markedly increased ICP.[173–175] ICP greater than 20 mm Hg is abnormal and should be treated to forestall herniation and brain stem injury. Treatment of ICP levels even of greater than 15 mm Hg may be warranted to avoid greater elevations or "plateau waves," sustained elevations of ICP that may develop spontaneously or as a consequence of small increments in cerebral blood volume produced by fever, hypoxia, or intratracheal suctioning.[173, 176, 177] The increase in ICP associated with intubation may be blocked by preceding IV lidocaine (1.5 mg/kg), but neuroanesthesiologists now favor use of Pentothal succinylcholine for this purpose. Subsequent transient increases associated with hyperactive airway reflexes can be lessened by intratracheal instillation of lidocaine before vigorous suctioning.[176–179]

If signs suggesting marked increase in ICP or impending herniation develop, a variety of measures may be used to reduce ICP such as (1) elevation of the head of the bed 30 degrees to assist venous drainage; (2) intubation and hyperventilation to maintain the partial pressure of arterial carbon dioxide between 25 and 32 mm Hg to induce vasoconstriction and reduce cerebral blood volume; (3) mannitol infusion IV of 1.0 g/kg during 10 to 15 minutes in an adult (0.5 to 2.0 g/kg during 30 minutes in a child).[177] Reduction of the partial pressure of arterial carbon dioxide to 20 mm Hg or below should be avoided to prevent resultant cerebral ischemia. Hyperventilation becomes less effective with duration of use and may have little effect after 48 hours of use. High-dose pentobarbital therapy has been used in some patients whose elevated ICP has not been controlled by hyperventilation and hyperosmolar agents.[177] Because clinical evaluation of such barbiturate-treated patients is greatly restricted by the depressive effects of the drug, this form of therapy requires an intracranial monitoring device or electroencephalography to monitor cortical activity.

Initial fluid management of the patient with bacterial meningitis involves careful evaluation of the state of hydration. Hypovolemia or shock requires fluid replacement to maintain systemic blood pressure and sustain cerebral perfusion. In children with meningitis, hyponatremia has been observed and attributed to SIADH (low serum sodium level, urine concentrated inappropriately for the degree of hyponatremia or serum hypotonicity, absence of dehydration, normal renal and adrenal function).[180] Studies in the past have shown elevated plasma levels of arginine vasopressin in children with bacterial meningitis.[181] The SIADH might then be expected to be associated with excessive free water retention and contribute to the development of cerebral edema. The frequency of SIADH reported in bacterial meningitis varies widely, from 4% to 88%.[182, 183] This led to conservative fluid administration early in treatment of meningitis in patients who were neither hypotensive nor hypovolemic. It has been suggested that the hyponatremia sometimes observed in patients with meningitis may be the result of a negative sodium balance (fever, vomiting, increased sodium excretion during the early stages of infection) rather than representing dilutional hyponatremia due to water retention as occurs in SIADH. A randomized study of children with meningitis comparing the effect on plasma arginine vasopressin concentrations of giving maintenance fluid requirements plus replacement of any deficit with restricting fluids to two thirds of maintenance for 24 hours supports this hypothesis. Plasma arginine vasopressin concentrations were significantly lower at the end of 24 hours in the children who received maintenance plus replacement fluids than after fluid restriction.[184] Further support for this concept is provided by a prospective study in India examining the effect of fluid restriction on body water and the outcome of children with acute meningitis.[185] The authors concluded that routine fluid restriction did not improve the outcome and that, in fact, a decreased volume of extracellular water at 48 hours increased the possibility of an adverse outcome. Thus, rather than routine fluid restriction (e.g., 800 to 1000 mL/m^2 per day) in a patient with meningitis without obvious shock or dehydration, maintenance plus replacement fluids can be administered in the initial 24 to 48 hours, but with subsequent monitoring for SIADH.

Other Aspects of Treatment

Patients with acute bacterial meningitis require constant nursing attention in an intensive care unit to prevent aspiration and hypoxia and to allow prompt recognition and treatment of seizures. Diazepam (Valium; 5 to 10 mg for adults; 0.3 mg/kg for children to a maximum of 10 mg) should be administered slowly over several minutes for acute control of a seizure. Maintenance anticonvulsant therapy is continued subsequently with IV phenytoin until the medication can be given by mouth. Routine use of sedation should be avoided.

Surgical drainage of an associated pyogenic focus such as mastoiditis should be deferred until full recovery from meningitis. In the rare instance when a mastoid infection is hyperacute (e.g., Bezold abscess), early drainage may be necessary after 48 to 72 hours' antibiotic treatment, when the acute meningeal process will have abated somewhat.

When shock develops early in the course of bacterial meningitis it is usually a consequence of the accompanying bacteremia (meningococcemia) rather than the meningitis itself. Management involves the standard measures employed to treat septic shock (see Chapter 67).

Coagulopathies may occur in patients with meningitis, particularly with the meningococcemia-meningitis syndrome. Clinical and laboratory features of disseminated intravascular coagulation may develop in more severely ill patients. These abnormalities alone do not warrant heparin therapy unless active bleeding supervenes, because they usually subside with control of infection.

Role of Corticosteroids

Corticosteroids reduce the intense leukocyte responses, CSF outflow resistance, and development of brain edema in experimental models of pneumococcal meningitis.[114] In experimental *H. influenzae* meningitis, the combination of dexamethasone with ceftriaxone is more effective than ceftriaxone alone in decreasing brain water content, CSF pressure, and lactate concentration, but the differences do not reach statistical significance.[186] In another study of Hib meningitis in a rabbit model, adjunctive dexamethasone with ceftriaxone caused a lowering of CSF tumor necrosis factor concentrations (over the reduction with ceftriaxone alone), a significant decrease in neutrophilic pleocytosis, and a trend toward earlier improvement in CSF levels of glucose, protein, and lactate, but without any evident decrease in in vivo bacterial killing within the CSF.[187]

Controlled clinical trials of adrenocorticosteroids as adjunctive therapy for acute bacterial meningitis, principally in children in the 1950s and 1960s, failed to show any significant beneficial effect.[188, 189] In 1988, a double-blind placebo-controlled study evaluated 4 days' adjunctive dexamethasone therapy (with either cefuroxime or ceftriaxone) in 200 infants and children with bacterial meningitis.[190] Only one death occurred among the 200, and that was in the placebo group. Those receiving dexamethasone became afebrile more rapidly than those receiving placebo, and they had a more rapid increase in CSF glucose and decrease in CSF lactate and protein levels after 24 hours' treatment. Those treated with dexamethasone developed moderate to severe bilateral sensorineural hearing loss less frequently (3.3% versus 15.5%). The benefit of reduced sensorineural hearing loss was significant only in patients receiving cefuroxime and not ceftriaxone, but the former is now known to be inferior to ceftriaxone in treatment of childhood bacterial meningitis.[152] Gastrointestinal bleeding requiring blood transfusions occurred in two patients receiving adjunctive dexamethasone.

In a subsequent randomized, placebo-controlled, double-blind trial, infants and children in Costa Rica received cefotaxime with either placebo or dexamethasone administered 15 to 20 minutes before the antibiotic.[191] Those receiving adjunctive dexamethasone had a decreased incidence of neurologic sequelae, principally ataxia, but only a trend toward reduction of sensorineural hearing loss. There were no differences in mortality between those receiving cefotaxime with and without dexamethasone.

In two other more recent multicenter controlled trials of ceftriaxone with and without adjunctive dexamethasone, statistically significant differences in the occurrence of sequelae were not demonstrable.[192, 193] However, the relatively small number of neurologic and audiologic sequelae observed and the relatively small numbers of subjects in these studies would have made it difficult to detect any significant differences. A metaanalysis of the results of these two studies and another ceftriaxone trial in Dallas (involving a total of 352 patients, half receiving dexamethasone and half placebo) showed a relative risk for neurologic or audiologic sequelae of 2.29 for those not treated with dexamethasone.[194]

Another trial involving more than 400 children and adults with bacterial meningitis was performed in Egypt, with randomization into groups receiving antibiotics (intramuscular chloramphenicol and ampicillin) with or without adjunctive dexamethasone therapy.[195] No differences in mortality were noted in the subgroups with Hib or meningococcal meningitis, but in the subgroup with pneumococcal meningitis receiving adjunctive dexamethasone there was a significant reduction in mortality rate and neurologic sequelae. However, evaluation of the results of this study is limited by the lack of inclusion of data on possible adverse effects and the high percentage of patients with pneumococcal meningitis who presented in coma.

Adjunctive dexamethasone therapy has usually been administered for a 4-day period. In a study of 118 children in Greece with mainly Hib and meningococcal meningitis, in which conventional initial antimicrobial therapy consisted of ampicillin (or penicillin G) plus chloramphenicol, 2-day and 4-day regimens of adjunctive dexamethasone were compared.[196] On long-term follow-up, neurologic sequelae or hearing impairment was found in 1.8% and 3.8% of patients treated with dexamethasone for 2 and 4 days, respectively, and the 2-day regimen was judged appropriate for treatment of Hib and meningococcal meningitis. Complicating gross gastrointestinal bleeding appeared to be less frequent in patients treated for 2 days (one patient versus three patients).

In most of the studies demonstrating a reduction in sensorineural hearing loss or neurologic sequelae with adjunctive dexamethasone therapy, the majority of cases of childhood meningitis were due to *H. influenzae.* Several studies have attempted to evaluate the possible benefit of adjunctive dexamethasone use in childhood meningitis caused by *S. pneumoniae.* In a retrospective review of 97 infants and children with pneumococcal meningitis (1984 to 1990; Dallas), those who had received adjunctive dexamethasone, who had clinical characteristics similar to those who had not, had a significant reduction in neurologic sequelae and hearing impairment compared with those who had been treated with antibiotics alone.[197] Information on the specific antimicrobials used was not included, and it is now known that sensorineural hearing loss may be more frequent with certain antibiotics (e.g., cefuroxime) than with others (e.g., ceftriaxone).[152] A prospective, double-blind, placebo-controlled trial with limited statistical power involving a total of only 56 children older than 2 years with pneumococcal meningitis was carried out in Turkey.[198] The antimicrobial therapy for all patients was ampicillin-sulbactam, and half the patients received adjunctive dexamethasone for 4 days and the other half received placebo. There were no differences between the two groups in mortality (two deaths in the dexamethasone group and one in the placebo group), duration of fever, or number with seizures, and no patient had clinically evident gastrointestinal bleeding. At 6 weeks after discharge, overall neurologic sequelae (including hearing loss) were not significantly different between the dexamethasone group and the placebo group (18.5% versus 30.7%); at 1 year, there was also no statistical difference between the two treatment groups in adverse neurologic outcomes (7.4% versus 26.9%).

A prospective trial of the effect of several adjunctive therapies along with ceftriaxone in the treatment of childhood bacterial meningitis (primarily due to *H. influenzae* and *N. meningitidis)* in 122 infants and children has been reported from Finland.[199] The children were assigned to one of four groups for adjunctive therapy: (1) dexamethasone IV; (2) glycerol orally or via nasogastric tube; (3) dexamethasone plus glycerol; (4) neither of these drugs. Only two deaths occurred, both in the dexamethasone plus glycerol group, and both patients were in shock before initiation of therapy. Although hearing impairment was most common among patients given neither dexamethasone nor glycerol, the differences among the four groups were not statistically significant. When all those who received adjunctive dexamethasone were compared with those who did not receive dexamethasone, the incidence of neither neurologic nor audiologic sequelae at 3 or 6 months was statistically different. When a similar comparison was made between all those who received glycerol and those who did not receive glycerol, the incidence of any neurologic or audiologic sequelae was statistically greater at 3 or 6 months in those not receiving glycerol (19%) than in those receiving glycerol (7%), and the relative risk was 2.94. Thus, adjunctive dexamethasone was not shown to reduce neurologic or audiologic sequelae in this study, whereas adjunctive glycerol reduced neurologic abnormalities and severe bilateral hearing loss.

On the basis of earlier studies cited before and a metaanalysis of such trials,[200] the use of adjunctive dexamethasone became widespread among pediatricians in the treatment of acute bacterial meningitis by 1992. When the directors of pediatric infectious disease programs were polled in 1992, half stated that they always used adjunctive dexamethasone and the remainder indicated that they used it sometimes.[149] The use of adjunctive dexamethasone (0.15 mg/kg every 6 hours IV) to reduce the frequency of neurologic and audiologic complications in infants and children with Hib meningitis, particularly those patients with elevated ICP, coma, and high concentrations of bacteria in the CSF (per Gram stain), appears warranted. On the basis of animal models and clinical trials, dexamethasone is best administered either 15 minutes before or simultaneously with antimicrobial therapy to lessen the inflammatory response in the CSF to bacterial lysis and release of cell wall components and lipopolysaccharide. Evidence indicates that a 2-day course is comparable in efficacy to one of 4 days and may reduce the possibility of complicating gastrointestinal bleeding.[196] Several caveats should be borne in mind in considering the use of adjuvant corticosteroids in treatment of bacterial meningitis: (1) Clinical data as yet do not support the routine use of adjuvant dexamethasone in treatment of community-acquired bacterial meningitis in adults, although it can be helpful in management of cerebral edema and high CSF pressure. (2) Benefit from adjunctive dexamethasone, although shown for treatment of Hib meningitis in infants and children, has not been demonstrated as yet in treatment of meningitis due to *S. pneumoniae.* (3) Immunization of infants with Hib polysaccharide-protein conjugate vaccines has dramatically reduced the incidence of meningitis caused by *H. influenzae* in this age group and has given *S. pneumoniae* an ascendant position as the cause. (4) Initial favorable clinical response to ceftriaxone and adjuvant dexamethasone in meningitis caused by *S. pneumoniae* with decreased susceptibility to the third-generation cephalosporins may be misleading in that the apparent response may be due to the antiinflammatory effects of dexamethasone rather than to the expected antibiotic effect.[201] This masking effect of the corticosteroid may delay performance of another lumbar puncture (revealing continuing bacterial presence) that would have been mandated earlier by virtue of an unsatisfactory clinical response. (5) Adjunctive dexamethasone may not be beneficial, indeed may be detrimental, in treatment of meningitis caused by highly penicillin resistant *S. pneumoniae* by decreasing meningeal inflammation, reducing vancomycin levels in CSF, and thus delaying bacterial killing.[202] (6) There have been no clinical studies performed demonstrating benefits to the use of adjuvant dexamethasone in the treatment of meningitis caused by gram-negative bacilli (other than *H. influenzae)* or to other microorganisms often involved in nosocomial meningitis or meningitis in immunocompromised hosts.

Use of dexamethasone after initial infusions of mannitol to control brain swelling in patients with bacterial meningitis (caused by highly antibiotic susceptible organisms) and markedly heightened CSF pressure is appropriate on the basis of experimental animal studies and extrapolation from its use in cerebral edema of other causes.

Management of Bacterial Meningitis Associated with a Cerebrospinal Fluid Fistula

Congenital defects along the cerebrospinal axis, particularly persistent dermal sinuses or meningoceles, may predispose to meningitis, especially in neonates or young children. In older children and adults, fistulae occur about the cribriform plate, paranasal sinuses, and temporal bone, resulting from accidental or surgical trauma or from erosion by tumor, sequestrum, or cholesteatoma.[203, 204]

Such a fistula should be suspected in any patient who has recurrent bacterial meningitis, a history of skull fracture or clear rhinorrhea, or a midline dermal sinus. CSF rhinorrhea commonly originates from a defect in the cribriform plate or a paranasal sinus, but it may result from a defect in the temporal bone that allows fluid to pass into the middle ear and down the eustachian tube into the nasopharynx (paradoxic rhinorrhea). CSF otorrhea occurs with a leak into the middle ear. The most common cause of CSF rhinorrhea is trauma, and rhinorrhea complicates 1% to 2% of blunt head injuries.[203] The incidence of CSF rhinorrhea is highest (approximately 25%) when blunt trauma has produced fractures involving the paranasal sinuses.

With the onset of acute bacterial meningitis, CSF rhinorrhea may cease as a result of the increased viscosity of the purulent CSF. Thus, it is important to check all patients with pyogenic meningitis (particularly pneumococcal, especially if recurrent) for CSF rhinorrhea by history and physical examination at the onset of illness and again after recovery. A history of a salty taste and frequent swallowing (due to extra fluid entering the pharynx from above) suggests CSF rhinorrhea. Anosmia might suggest cribriform plate leakage. On examination with the head in the brow-down position, fluid from CSF rhinorrhea may flow from one or both nostrils and, unlike nasal mucus, does not stiffen a handkerchief on drying. Collection of several drops in a test tube for determination of glucose and chloride levels is the preferred method for determining whether a clear nasal secretion is CSF. CSF normally has a glucose content of 50 to 75 mg/dL and a chloride level of about 120 mEq/L. Identification by electrophoresis and immunofixation of a specific isoform of transferrin, present only in CSF, in clear nasal fluid can help define a CSF leak.[205]

Rhinorrhea of an otic or sphenoid origin may be noted with the patient in the lateral decubitus or prone position, respectively. If the tympanic membrane is intact, fluid and air bubbles may be seen behind the eardrum.

Visual fields should be evaluated, as they are frequently abnormal when the cause of CSF rhinorrhea is a pituitary cyst or tumor. Visual fields are normal in the atrophic type of empty sella syndrome, which also can be associated with CSF leakage.

Studies to define an anatomic defect are indicated in patients with CSF rhinorrhea and bacterial meningitis, or in patients with repeated episodes of bacterial meningitis. Skull, sinus, and mastoid films may show a skull fracture, opacification or air-fluid levels in an air sinus or in mastoid air cells, or pneumencephalus. Head CT should be performed for most accurate anatomic definition of the site of leakage, particularly in the case of a nontraumatic leak, when an intracranial mass lesion may be responsible. Contrast cisternography (with iopamidol or iohexal preferred to metrizamide as a contrast agent) may be confirmatory but requires an active CSF leak at the time of testing.[203]

Direct confirmation of the leak exit site is essential for surgical correction. Radiolabeled (iodine 131 or technetium 99m) albumins are used to determine sites of CSF leakage; Cottonoid strips are placed into the sphenoid-ethmoid recess, in the region of the middle meatus, into the anterior superior nasal cavity, and into the ear canal to detect leakage after lumbar injection of the radionuclide. Fluorescein (0.5 mL of 10% fluorescein solution in 10 mL of physiologic diluent injected slowly during 3 to 5 minutes into the lumbar sac) is preferred by some physicians[204] because it can be visualized directly and promptly. Also, fluorescein stains the tympanic membrane in CSF otorrhea, and it can be used intraoperatively to allow direct visualization of the origin of the leak.

Recurrent meningitis is most commonly associated with a CSF leak.[21] The organisms responsible for recurrent meningitis vary depending on whether the episodes are community acquired or nosocomial (Table 158–14). Thus, the setting provides some direction for selection of initial antimicrobial therapy.

Posttraumatic rhinorrhea or otorrhea usually subsides within several weeks of the trauma. Such acute CSF rhinorrhea is treated expectantly with head elevation at 45 degrees and, if required, a spinal drain; this usually eliminates the rhinorrhea within 5 to 7 days.[203] Indications for surgical correction include prior leak and one or more episodes of bacterial meningitis; profuse leakage that does not abate in the 2 weeks after the trauma; and persistent leakage for longer than 6 weeks after the trauma.[204] Prospective study of the value of prophylactic antibiotics (e.g., penicillin) in preventing bacterial meningitis in patients with a CSF leak has not been performed. In a retrospective study of 1192 patients with basilar skull fractures reported in eight nonrandomized

TABLE 158–14 ■ Causative Organisms in Recurrent Meningitis in Adults at Massachusetts General Hospital, 1962 to 1988

ORGANISM	COMMUNITY ACQUIRED (%) (38 EPISODES)	NOSOCOMIAL (%) (41 EPISODES)
Streptococcus pneumoniae	34	2
Gram-negative bacilli*	0	46
Neisseria meningitidis	8	0
Streptococci†	11	2
Staphylococcus aureus	3	15
Haemophilus influenzae	11	0
Mixed bacterial species	0	5
Coagulase-negative	0	7
staphylococci	5	2
Other	29	20
Culture-negative		

*Exclusive of *H. influenzae*.
†Mainly α-hemolytic, nongroupable strains.
Modified with permission from Durand ML, Calderwood SB, Weber DJ, et al: Acute bacterial meningitis in adults. A review of 493 episodes. N Engl J Med 328:21–28, 1993.

series between 1970 and 1988, 8% of 803 patients receiving prophylactic antibiotics and 3% of 389 patients not receiving antibiotic prophylaxis developed meningitis (difference not statistically significant).[206] In the subset of 117 patients with basilar skull fractures who developed obvious CSF otorrhea or rhinorrhea, prophylactic antibiotics did not protect against development of meningitis. In another retrospective study of CSF fistulae (mainly traumatic) from a neurosurgical unit in England, which compared the incidence of meningitis among 106 patients treated with prophylactic antibiotics with 109 patients who were untreated, antibiotic prophylaxis did not reduce the risk of meningitis significantly.[207] Prolonged use of prophylactic antibiotics increases the likelihood of involvement of a resistant organism if meningitis does develop. For example, posttraumatic meningitis caused by *S. aureus* and gram-negative bacilli has developed in patients receiving penicillin prophylaxis. At present, routine prophylactic antibiotic use is not recommended for patients with a traumatic CSF leak. However, this is a considerable problem and merits a multiinstitutional prospective, randomized trial.

The type of surgical repair employed for CSF fistulae depends on the nature of the fistula. Nontraumatic high-pressure fistulae are usually secondary to obstructive hydrocephalus resulting from posterior fossa tumors or basilar arachnoiditis. After treatment of any complicating meningitis, initial neurosurgical management involves CSF shunting or removal of obstruction to CSF flow. For nontraumatic normal-pressure leaks, large CSF leaks, or posttraumatic leaks that persist for 4 to 6 weeks, surgical repair by obliteration of the leak site is indicated. Transsinus approaches have been employed successfully by skilled otolaryngologists to repair leaks through the cribriform plate and sphenoid and frontal sinuses.[203, 204]

Prevention

Meningococcal Disease

The risk of meningococcal disease for household contacts of an initial case is 500 to 800 times greater than the endemic rate for meningococcal disease in the general population. Chemoprophylaxis is indicated for close contacts (e.g., household or daycare center; medical personnel in close direct contact before institution of respiratory precautions) of a patient with meningococcal disease. Rifampin, 80% to 90% effective in eliminating asymptomatic nasopharyngeal carriage, is the recommended drug for chemoprophylaxis, in a dose of 600 mg orally every 12 hours for 2 days for adults (10 mg/kg every 12 hours for children older than 1 month, and 5 mg/kg every 12 hours for children younger than 1 month). Because the carrier state may recur shortly after discontinuation of treatment with high doses of penicillin, rifampin should also be administered to patients with meningococcal disease before discharge from hospital.

Minocycline has been almost as effective as rifampin in eliminating *N. meningitidis* from nasopharyngeal carriers, but it is not commonly used because of reports of vestibular side effects. Although prophylaxis with sulfonamides was effective in the past, it was abandoned because of the emergence of widespread resistance (more than 60% of strains) in the 1960s and 1970s. Although sulfonamide resistance had decreased by 1980 to only 12% of isolates, its use as chemoprophylaxis would be considered only in outbreaks caused by strains known to be susceptible. Given orally, ciprofloxacin achieves concentrations in nasal secretions above the MIC for *N. meningitidis*.[208] Single-dose oral ciprofloxacin, 500 or 750 mg in the adult, is about 90% effective in eradicating pharyngeal carriage.[209, 210] Ciprofloxacin is the alternative of choice for rifampin for prophylaxis in adults and may replace it as the drug of choice if rifampin resistance should become widespread among meningococci. Owing to potential side effects on growing cartilage it would not be recommended for children or pregnant women. Ceftriaxone (250 mg intramuscularly in adults and 125 mg in children) eliminated the carriage of serogroup A meningococci in more than 90% of patients for up to 2 weeks.[211] In pregnant patients and young infants, ceftriaxone is probably the safest alternative to rifampin for prophylaxis.

In the United States, immunoprophylaxis of meningococcal disease currently involves use of a quadrivalent (A/C/Y/W-135) polysaccharide vaccine only in the military, in travelers to countries with hyperendemic or epidemic disease, in aborting outbreaks due to serogroups in the vaccine, and for persons at high risk such as asplenic patients or those who have terminal complement component deficiencies. Routine vaccination with meningococcal vaccine is not warranted because the risk of infection is low in the United States, because a vaccine against serogroup B (responsible for more than 50% of meningococcal disease in this country) is not yet available, and because the meningococcal vaccine is poorly immunogenic for children younger than 2 years. Because the antibody response to group B polysaccharide is almost entirely immunoglobulin M, and because these antibodies are not bactericidal, alternative approaches are necessary for inducing protective immunity to group B *N. meningitidis*. Serotypes 2b and 15 (together responsible for most outbreaks of group B disease) outer membrane protein vaccines induce bactericidal antibodies to these serotypes and may provide protection against some serogroup B disease.[212]

Meningococcal vaccines have been important in quelling epidemics in developing countries (e.g., sub-Saharan Africa) and as a complement to prophylactic chemotherapy in neighborhood or school outbreaks.

Haemophilus influenzae *Disease*

The risk of secondary spread of invasive Hib infection to nonimmunized household contacts younger than 4 years is 2% to 6% during the 30-day period after exposure. The highest rate occurs in contacts younger than 1 year. The majority of secondary cases occur within a week of onset of disease in the index case.

Rifampin is effective in eliminating nasopharyngeal carriage of Hib. If another child (whether previously given Hib vaccine or not) younger than 4 years resides in the household, rifampin prophylaxis is recommended for all household contacts, including adults (except pregnant women), of an index case: 20 mg/kg orally once daily for 4 days (maximal daily dose 600 mg).[213] If the youngest child in the household is 4 years or older, or if more than 2 weeks has elapsed since the onset of the index household illness, rifampin prophylaxis is probably not necessary. Because nasopharyngeal carriage may reappear after discontinuation of antimicrobial therapy for systemic infection, the index patient should receive rifampin before hospital discharge.

Whether contacts of patients in daycare centers outside the home are at greater risk of secondary spread of infection is debatable. Risk may vary from region to region and depends on the age of the exposed children. Children younger than 2 years are at higher risk than those older than 2 years. If two or more cases occur within 60 days in a daycare center, rifampin prophylaxis should be given to all contacts, including adults (except pregnant women). Whether such prophylaxis is indicated after a single case is controversial, but it does seem warranted if any of the exposed classroom contacts is younger than 2 years.

Hib polysaccharide vaccine in Finland had 90% efficacy among children vaccinated between 18 and 71 months of age[214]; it was licensed in the United States in 1985 for children 24 months of age and older. Subsequent studies indicated variability in efficacy of this vaccine in this country and led to a search for more immunogenic polysaccharide-protein conjugate vaccines that would be effective in infants, the age group most susceptible to invasive Hib disease. One such vaccine, an Hib polysaccharide–diphtheria toxoid (PRP-D) conjugate vaccine was licensed and recommended in the United States for routine use in children 18 months of age or older. A large-scale field trial in Finland of this same vaccine in infancy (administered at 3, 4, 6, and 14 months of age) indicated a protective efficacy of 94%.[215] Current recommendations of the American Academy of Pediatrics Committee on Infectious Diseases call for vaccination of all infants beginning at 2 months of age with one of the three licensed Hib PRP (or PRP oligomer)–protein conjugate vaccines[216]: (1) HbOC (HibTITER), diphtheria CRM 197 protein conjugate; (2) PRP-OMP (PedvaxHIB), *N. meningitidis* serogroup B outer membrane protein complex conjugate; (3) PRP-T (ActHIB, OmniHIB), tetanus toxoid protein complex. A primary series of HbOC or PRP-T consists of three doses given at 2, 4, and 6 months of age, whereas for PRP-OMP, only two doses given at 2 and 4 months are recommended. An additional booster dose of a conjugate vaccine should be given at 12 to 15 months of age. A fourth vaccine, PRP-D (ProHIBIT), a dipththeria toxoid–protein conjugate vaccine, is recommended only for use in children 12 months of age and older and can be substituted at that time for one of the other vaccines as the booster dose.

References

1. Centers for Disease Control: Bacterial meningitis and meningococcemia—United States, 1978. MMWR 28:277, 1979.
2. Schlech WF III, Ward JI, Band JD, et al: Bacterial meningitis in the United States, 1978 through 1981. JAMA 253:1749, 1985.
3. Adams WG, Deaver KA, Cochi SL, et al: Decline of childhood *Haemophilus influenzae* type b (Hib) disease in the Hib vaccine era. JAMA 269:221, 1993.
4. Buchanan GA, Darville T: Impact of immunization against *Haemophilus influenzae* type b (HIB) on the incidence of HIB meningitis treated at Arkansas Children's Hospital. South Med J 87:38, 1994.
5. Cherubin CE, Marr JS, Sierra MF, et al: Listeria and gram-negative bacillary meningitis in New York City, 1972–1979. Am J Med 71:199, 1981.
6. Swartz MN, Dodge PR: Bacterial meningitis—A review of selected aspects. N Engl J Med 272:725, 1965.
7. Carpenter RR, Petersdorf RG: The clinical spectrum of bacterial meningitis. Am J Med 33:262, 1962.
8. Geiseler PJ, Nelson KE, Levin S, et al: Community-acquired purulent meningitis: A review of 1,316 cases during the antibiotic era, 1954–1976. Rev Infect Dis 2:726, 1980.
9. Klein JO, Marcy SM: Bacterial sepsis and meningitis. *In* Remington JS, Klein JO (eds): Infectious Diseases of the Fetus and Newborn Infant. Philadelphia, WB Saunders, 1983, pp 680–735.
10. Bell AH, Brown D, Halliday HL, et al: Meningitis in the newborn—A 14 year review. Arch Dis Child 64:873, 1989.
11. Baumgartner ET, Augustine RA, Steele RW: Bacterial meningitis in older neonates. Am J Dis Child 37:1052, 1983.
12. Bortolussi R, Krishnan C, Armstrong D, et al: Prognosis for survival in neonatal meningitis: Clinical and pathologic review of 52 cases. Can Med Assoc J 118:165, 1978.
13. Friedman A, Fleisher G: Meningitis. Update of recommendations for the neonate. Clin Pediatr 19:395, 1980.
14. Underman AE, Overturf GD, Leedom JM: Bacterial meningitis. Dis Mon 24:1, 1978.
15. Salwen KM, Vikerfors T, Olcén P: Increased incidence of childhood bacterial meningitis. Scand J Infect Dis 19:1, 1987.
16. Feigin RD: Bacterial meningitis beyond the neonatal period. *In* Feigin RD, Cherry J (eds): Textbook of Pediatric Infectious Diseases. Philadelphia, WB Saunders, 1981, pp 293–308.
17. Valmari P, Peltola H, Ruuskanen O, et al: Childhood bacterial meningitis: Initial symptoms and signs related to age, and reasons for consulting a physician. Eur J Pediatr 146:515, 1987.
18. Karandanis D, Shulman JA: Recent survey of infectious meningitis in adults: Review of laboratory findings in bacterial, tuberculous and aseptic meningitis. South Med J 69:449, 1976.
19. Harris LF: Bacterial meningitis in adults—A community perspective. Ala Med 58:20, 1988.
20. Jackson LA, Schuchat A, Reeves MW, Wenger JD: Serogroup C meningococcal outbreaks in the United States: An emerging threat. JAMA 273:383, 1995.
21. Durand MI, Calderwood SB, Weber DJ, et al: Acute bacterial meningitis in adults: A review of 493 episodes. N Engl J Med 328:21, 1993.
22. Crane LR, Lerner AM: Nontraumatic gram-negative bacillary meningitis in the Detroit Medical Center, 1964–1974. Medicine (Baltimore) 57:197, 1978.
23. Buckwold FJ, Hand R, Hansebout RR: Hospital-acquired bacterial meningitis in neurosurgical patients. J Neurosurg 46:494, 1977.
24. Mancebo J, Domingo P, Blanch L, et al: Postneurosurgical and spontaneous gram-negative bacillary meningitis in adults. Scand J Infect Dis 18:533, 1986.
25. Gower DJ, Barrows AA III, Kelly DL Jr, et al: Gram-negative bacillary meningitis in the adult: Review of 39 cases. South Med J 79:1499, 1986.
26. Berk SL, McCabe WR: Meningitis caused by gram-negative bacilli. Ann Intern Med 93:253, 1980.
27. Schlesinger LS, Ross SC, Schaberg DR: *Staphylococcus aureus* meningitis: A broad-based epidemiologic study. Medicine (Baltimore) 66:148, 1987.
28. Swartz MN: Central nervous system infections. *In* Finegold SM, George WL (eds): Anaerobic Infections in Humans. San Diego, CA, Academic Press, 1989, pp 155–212.
29. Tärnvik A: Anaerobic meningitis in children. Eur J Clin Microbiol 5:271, 1986.
30. Long JG, Preblud SR, Keyserling HL: *Clostridium perfringens* meningitis in an infant: Case report and literature review. Pediatr Infect Dis J 6:752, 1987.
31. Downs NJ, Hodges GR, Taylor SA: Mixed bacterial meningitis. Rev Infect Dis 9:693, 1987.
32. Bouza E, Garcia de la Torre M, Parras F, et al: *Brucella* meningitis. Rev Infect Dis 9:810, 1987.
33. Lovell VM, Cho CT, Lindsey NJ, et al: *Franciscella tularensis* meningitis: A rare clinical entity. J Infect Dis 154:916, 1986.
34. Arends JP, Zanen HC: Meningitis caused by *Streptococcus suis* in humans. Rev Infect Dis 10:131, 1988.
35. Feigin RD, Baker CJ, Herwaldt LA, et al: Epidemic meningococ-

cal disease in an elementary school classroom. N Engl J Med 307:1255, 1982.
36. Merino J, Rodriques-Valverde V, Lamelas JA, et al: Prevalence of deficits of complement components in patients with recurrent meningococcal infections. J Infect Dis 148:331, 1983.
37. Clough JD, Clough ML, Weinstein A, et al: Familial late complement component (C_6,C_7) deficiency with chronic meningococcemia. Arch Intern Med 140:929, 1980.
38. Ellison RT, Kohler PH, Curd JG, et al: Prevalence of congenital or acquired complement deficiency in patients with sporadic meningococcal disease. N Engl J Med 308:913, 1983.
39. Griffis JM, Brandt BL: Nonepidemic (endemic) meningococcal disease: pathogenic factors and clinical features. Curr Clin Top Infect Dis 7:27, 1986.
40. Meningitis Disease Surveillance Group: Household chemoprophylaxis for meningococcal disease: Observations on the meningococcal secondary attack rate and the practice of chemoprophylaxis in the United States. JAMA 235:261, 1976.
41. DeWSals P, Hertoghe L, Borlée-Grimée, et al: Meningococcal disease in Belgium. Secondary attack rate among household, day-care nursery and preelementary school contacts. J Infect 3(Suppl 1):53, 1981.
42. Wenger JD, Ward JI, Broome CV: Prevention of *Haemophilus influenzae* type b disease: Vaccines and passive prophylaxis. Curr Clin Top Infect Dis 10:306, 1989.
43. Ward JI, Fraser DW, Baraff LJ, et al: *Haemophilus influenzae* meningitis. A national study of secondary spread in household contacts. N Engl J Med 301:122, 1979.
44. Osterholm MT, Pierson LM, White KE, et al: The risk of subsequent transmission of *Haemophilus influenzae* type B disease among children in day care. N Engl J Med 316:1, 1987.
45. Murphy TV, Clements JF, Breedlove JA, et al: Risk of subsequent disease among day-care contacts of patients with systemic *Hemophilus influenzae* type B disease. N Engl J Med 316:5, 1987.
46. Makintubee S, Istre GR, Ward JI: Transmission of invasive *Haemophilus influenzae* type b disease in day-care settings. J Pediatr 111:180, 1987.
47. Spagnuolo PJ, Ellner JJ, Lerner PI, et al: *Haemophilus influenzae* meningitis: The spectrum of disease in adults. Medicine (Baltimore) 61:74, 1982.
48. Quagliarello V, Scheld WM: Bacterial meningitis: Pathogenesis, pathophysiology and progress. N Engl J Med 327:864, 1992.
49. Stephens DS, Farley MM: Pathogenic events during infection of the human nasopharynx with *Neisseria meningitidis* and *Haemophilus influenzae.* Rev Infect Dis 13:22, 1991.
50. McGee AZ, Stephens DS, Hoffman LH, et al: Mechanisms of mucosal invasion by pathogenic *Neisseria.* Rev Infect Dis 5:S708, 1983.
51. Smith AL, Daum RS, Scheifele D, et al: Pathogenesis of *Haemophilus influenzae* meningitis. *In* Sell SH, Wright PF (eds): *Haemophilus influenzae*: Epidemiology, Immunology and Prevention of Disease. New York, Elsevier, 1982, pp 89–109.
52. Simberkoff M, Moldover H, Rahal J Jr: Absence of detectable bactericidal and opsonic activities in normal and infected cerebrospinal fluids: A regional host defense deficiency. J Lab Clin Med 95:362, 1980.
53. Fijen CAP, Kuijper EJ, Tjia et al: Complement deficiency predisposes for meningitis due to nongroupable meningococci and *Neisseria*-related bacteria. Clin Infect Dis 18:780, 1994.
54. Bohr V, Hansen B, Jessen O, et al: Eight hundred and seventy-five cases of bacterial meningitis. Part I of a three-part series: Clinical data, prognosis, and the role of specialized hospital departments. J Infect 7:21, 1983.
55. Sferra TJ, Pacini DL: Simultaneous recovery of bacterial and viral pathogens from cerebrospinal fluid. Pediatr Infect Dis J 7:552, 1988.
56. Tuomanen E, Hengstler B, Rich R, et al: Nonsteroidal antiinflammatory agents in the therapy for experimental pneumococcal meningitis. J Infect Dis 155:985, 1987.
57. Quagliarello VJ, Long WJ, Scheld M: Morphologic alterations of the blood-brain barrier with experimental meningitis in the rat. J Clin Invest 77:1084, 1986.
58. Lesse AJ, Moxon ER, Zwahlen A, et al: Role of cerebrospinal fluid pleocytosis and *Haemophilus influenzae* type b capsule on blood brain barrier permeability during experimental meningitis in the rat. J Clin Invest 82:102, 1988.
59. Leist TP, Frei K, Kam-Hansen S, et al: Tumor necrosis factor α in cerebrospinal fluid during bacterial, but not viral, meningitis. J Exp Med 167:1743, 1988.
60. Tuomanen E: Partner drugs: A new outlook for bacterial meningitis. Ann Intern Med 109:690, 1988.
61. Scheld WM, Dacey R, Winn R, et al: Cerebrospinal fluid outflow resistance in rabbits with experimental meningitis. Alterations with penicillin and methyl-prednisolone. J Clin Invest 66:243, 1980.
62. Posner JB, Plum F: Spinal fluid pH and neurologic symptoms in systemic acidosis. N Engl J Med 277:605, 1967.
63. Kaplan SL, Feigin RD: The syndrome of inappropriate secretion of anti-diuretic hormone in children with bacterial meningitis. J Pediatr 92:758, 1978.
64. Kline MW: *Citrobacter* meningitis and brain abscess in infancy: Epidemiology, pathogenesis, and treatment. J Pediatr 113:430, 1988.
65. Kline MW, Kaplan SL, Hawkins EP, et al: Pathogenesis of brain abscess formation in an infant rat model of *Citrobacter diversus* bacteremia and meningitis. J Infect Dis 157:106, 1988.
66. Rosen MS, Lorber B, Myers AR: Chronic meningococcal meningitis. An association with C5 deficiency. Arch Intern Med 148:1441, 1988.
67. Dodge PR, Davis H, Feigin RD, et al: Prospective evaluation of hearing impairment as a sequela of acute bacterial meningitis. N Engl J Med 311:869, 1984.
68. Vienny H, Despland PA, Lütschz J, et al: Early diagnosis and evolution of deafness in childhood bacterial meningitis: A study using brainstem auditory evoked potentials. Pediatrics 73:579, 1984.
69. Özdamar Ö, Kraus N, Stein L: Auditory brainstem responses in infants recovering from bacterial meningitis: Audiologic evaluation. Arch Otolaryngol 109:13, 1983.
70. Bhatt SM, Halpin C, Hsu W, et al: Hearing loss and pneumococcal meningitis: An animal model. Laryngoscope 101:1285, 1991.
71. Bhatt SM, Lauretano A, Cabellos C, et al: Progression of hearing loss in experimental pneumococcic meningitis: Correlation with cerebrospinal fluid cytochemistry. J Infect Dis 167:675, 1993.
72. Eavey RD, Gao YZ, Schuknecht HF, et al: Otologic features of bacterial meningitis of childhood. J Pediatr 106:402, 1985.
73. Wiedermann BL, Hawkins EP, Johnson GS, et al: Pathogenesis of labyrinthitis associated *Haemophilus influenzae* type b meningitis in infant rats. J Infect Dis 153:27, 1986.
74. Bohr VA, Rasmussen N: Neurologic sequelae and fatality as prognostic measures in 875 cases of bacterial meningitis. Dan Med Bull 35:92, 1988.
75. Pfister H-W, Borasio GD, Dirnagl U, et al: Cerebrovascular complications of bacterial meningitis in adults. Neurology 42:1497, 1992.
76. McMenamin JB, Volpe JJ: Bacterial meningitis in infancy: Effects on intracranial pressure and cerebral blood flow velocity. Neurology 34:500, 1984.
77. Weinstein AJ, Schiavone WA, Furlan AJ: *Listeria* rhombencephalitis: Report of a case. Arch Neurol 39:514, 1982.
78. Bach MC, Davis KM: *Listeria* rhombencephalitis mimicking tuberculous meningitis. Rev Infect Dis 9:130, 1987.
79. Dunn DW, Daum RS, Weisberg L, et al: Ischemic cerebrovascular complications of *Haemophilus influenzae* meningitis. The value of computed tomography. Arch Neurol 39:650, 1982.
80. DiNubile MJ, Boom WH, Southwick FS: Septic cortical thrombophlebitis. J Infect Dis 161:1216, 1990.
81. Glista GG, Sullivan TD, Brumlik J: Spinal cord involvement in acute bacterial meningitis. JAMA 243:1362, 1980.
82. Adams RD, Kubik CS, Bonner FJ: The clinical and pathological aspects of influenzae meningitis. Arch Pediatr 65:354, 408, 1984.
83. Pomeroy SL, Holmes SJ, Dodge PR, Feigin RD: Seizures and other neurological sequeleae of bacterial meningitis in children. N Engl J Med 323:1651, 1990.
84. Feldman HM, Michaels RH: Academic achievement in children 10 to 12 years after *Haemophilus influenzae* meningitis. Pediatrics 81:339, 1988.
85. Edwards MS, Reuch MA, Haffar AAM, et al: Long-term sequelae of group B streptococcal meningitis in infants. J Pediatr 106:717, 1985.
86. Wilson CW, Smith AL: Rapid tests for the diagnosis of bacterial meningitis. Curr Clin Top Infect Dis 7:134, 1986.

87. Polk BP, Steele RW: Bacterial meningitis presenting with normal cerebrospinal fluid. Pediatr Infect Dis J 6:1040, 1987.
88. Ronadio WA: Acute bacterial meningitis: Cerebrospinal fluid differential count. Clin Pediatr 27:445, 1988.
89. Maxson S, Lewno MJ, Schutze GE: Clinical usefulness of cerebrospinal fluid bacterial antigen studies. J Pediatr 125:235, 1994.
90. Ferraro MJ: Rapid immunologic diagnosis of meningitis—Is there a future? *In* Balows A, Tilton RC, Turano A (eds): Rapid Methods and Automation in Microbiology and Immunology. Brescia, Italy, Brixia Academic Press, 1988, pp 481–487.
91. Komorowski RA, Farmer SG, Knox KK: Comparison of cerebrospinal fluid C-reactive protein and lactate for diagnosis of meningitis. J Clin Microbiol 24:982, 1986.
92. Gray BG, Simmons DR, Mason H, et al: Quantitative levels of C-reactive protein in cerebrospinal fluid in patients with bacterial meningitis and other conditions. J Pediatr 108:665, 1986.
93. Martin WJ: Rapid and reliable techniques for the laboratory detection of bacterial meningitis. Am J Med 75:119, 1983.
94. Abramson JS, Hampton KD, Babu S: The use of C-reactive protein from cerebrospinal fluid for differentiating meningitis from other central nervous system diseases. J Infect Dis 151:854, 1985.
95. Kölmel HW, von Maravic M: Correlation of lactic acid level, cell count and cytology in cerebrospinal fluid of patients with bacterial and non-bacterial meningitis. Acta Neurol Scand 78:6, 1988.
96. Thadepalli H, Gangopadhysy PK, Ansari A, et al: Diagnosis of bacterial meningitides by direct gas-liquid chromatography. J Clin Invest 69:979, 1982.
97. Saubolle MA, Jorgenson JH: Use of the *Limulus* amebocyte lysate test as a cost-effective screen for gram-negative agents of meningitis. Diagn Microbiol Infect Dis 7:177, 1987.
98. Bohr V, Rasmussen N, Hansen B, et al: Eight hundred seventy-five cases of bacterial meningitis: Diagnostic procedures and the impact of preadmission antibiotic therapy. J Infect 7:193, 1983.
99. Valmari P: White blood count, erythrocyte sedimentation rate and serum C-reactive protein in meningitis: Magnitude of the response related to bacterial species. Infection 12:328, 1984.
100. Stovring J, Snyder RD: Computed tomography in childhood bacterial meningitis. J Pediatr 96:820, 1980.
101. Cabral DA, Flodmark O, Farrell K, Speert DP: Prospective study of computed tomography in acute bacterial meningitis. J Pediatr 111:201, 1987.
102. Bodino J, Lylyk P, Del Volle M, et al: Computed tomography in purulent meningitis. Am J Dis Child 136:495, 1982.
103. Packer RJ, Bilaniuk LT, Zimmerman RA: CT parenchymal abnormalities in bacterial meningitis: Clinical significance. J Comput Assist Tomogr 6:1064, 1982.
104. Kline MK, Kaplan SL: Computed tomography in bacterial meningitis of childhood. Pediatr Infect Dis J 7:855, 1988.
105. Ho DD, Sarngadharan MG, Resnick L, et al: Primary human T-lymphotropic virus type III infection. Ann Intern Med 103:880, 1985.
106. Spanos A, Harrell FE, Durack DT: Differential diagnosis of acute meningitis. An analysis of the predictive value of initial observations. JAMA 262:2700, 1989.
107. Peacock JE Jr, McGinnis MR, Cohen MS: Persistent neutrophilic meningitis: report of four cases and review of the literature. Medicine (Baltimore) 63:379, 1984.
108. Steel JG, Dix RD, Baringer JR: Isolation of herpes simplex virus type 1 in recurrent (Mollaret) meningitis. Ann Neurol 11:17, 1982.
109. Yamamoto LY, Tedder DG, Ashley R, Levin MJ: Herpes simplex virus type 1 DNA in cerebrospinal fluid of a patient with Mollaret's meningitis. N Engl J Med 325:1082, 1991.
110. Crossly GH, Dismukes WE: Central nervous system epidermoid cyst: A probable etiology of Mollaret's meningitis. Am J Med 89:805, 1990.
111. Archard J-M, Lallement P-Y, Veyssier P: Recurrent aseptic meningitis secondary to intracranial epidermoid cyst and Mollaret's meningitis: Two distinct entities or a single disease? A case report and a nosologic discussion. Am J Med 89:807, 1990.
112. Meadow WL, Lantos J, Tanz RR, et al: Ought 'standard care' be the 'standard of care'? A study of the time to administration of antibiotics in children with meningitis. Am J Dis Child 147:40, 1993.
113. Scheld WM, Sande MA: Bactericidal versus bacteriostatic antibiotic therapy of experimental pneumococcal meningitis in rabbits. J Clin Invest 71:411, 1983.
114. Tunkel AR, Wispelwey B, Scheld WM: Bacterial meningitis: Recent advances in pathophysiology and treatment. Ann Intern Med 112:610, 1990.
115. Lepper MH, Dowling HF: Treatment of pneumococcic meningitis with penicillin compared with penicillin plus aureomycin. Arch Intern Med 88:489, 1951.
116. Latorre C, Juncosa T, Sanfeliu I: Antibiotic resistance and serotypes of 100 *Streptococcus pneumoniae* strains isolated in a children's hospital in Barcelona, Spain. Antimicrob Agents Chemother 28:357, 1985.
117. Friedland IR, McCracken GH Jr: Management of infections caused by antibiotic-resistant *Streptococcus pneumoniae.* N Engl J Med 331:337, 1994.
118. Tomasz A: Multiple-antibiotic resistant pathogenic bacteria—A report on the Rockefeller University workshop. N Engl J Med 330:1247, 1994.
119. Appelbaum PC: Antimicrobial resistance in *Streptococcus pneumoniae*: An overview. Clin Infect Dis 15:77, 1992.
120. Jacobs MR, Koornhof HJ, Robins-Browne RM, et al: Emergence of multiply resistant pneumococci. N Engl J Med 299:735, 1978.
121. Spika JS, Facklam RR, Plikaytis BD, Oxtoby MJ: Antimicrobial resistance of *Streptococcus pneumoniae* in the United States, 1979–1987. J Infect Dis 163:1273, 1991.
122. Hofman J, Cetron MS, Farley MM, et al: The prevalence of drug-resistant *Streptococcus pneumoniae* in Atlanta. N Engl J Med 333:481, 1995.
123. Pallares R, Liñares J, Vadillo M, et al: Resistance to penicillin and cephalosporin and mortality from severe pneumococcal pneumonia in Barcelona, Spain. N Engl J Med 333:474, 1995.
124. McDougal LK, Facklam R, Reeves M, et al: Analysis of multiply antimicrobial-resistant isolates of *Streptococcus pneumoniae* from the United States. Antimicrob Agents Chemother 36:2176, 1992.
125. Tomasz A: The pneumococcus at the gates. N Engl J Med 333:514, 1995.
126. Viladrich PF, Gudiol F, Liñares J, et al: Characteristics and antibiotic therapy of adult meningitis due to penicillin-resistant pneumococci. Am J Med 84:839, 1988.
127. Friedland IR, Istre GR: Management of penicillin-resistant pneumococcal infections. Pediatr Infect Dis J 11:433, 1992.
128. Tan TQ, Mason EO Jr, Kaplan SL: Systemic infections due to *Streptococcus pneumoniae* relatively resistant to penicillin in a children's hospital: Clinical management and outcome. Pediatrics 90:928, 1992.
129. Friedland IR, Shelton S, Paris M, et al: Dilemmas in diagnosis and management of cephalosporin-resistant *Streptococcus pneumoniae* meningitis. Pediatr Infect Dis J 72:196, 1993.
130. Kleiman MB, Weinberg GA, Reynolds JK, et al: Meningitis with beta-lactam resistant *Streptococcus pneumoniae*: The need for early repeat lumbar puncture. Pediatr Infect Dis J 12:782, 1993.
131. Tan TQ, Schutze GE, Mason EO Jr, Kaplan SL: Antibiotic therapy and acute outcome of meningitis due to *Streptococcus pneumoniae* considered intermediately susceptible to broad-spectrum cephalosporins. Antimicrob Agents Chemother 38:918, 1994.
132. Austrian R: Confronting drug-resistant pneumococci (Letter). Ann Intern Med 121:807, 1994.
133. Viladrich PF, Gudiol F, Liñares J, et al: Evaluation of vancomycin for therapy of adult pneumococcal meningitis. Antimicrob Agents Chemother 35:2467, 1991.
134. Friedland IR, Klugman KP: Failure of chloramphenicol therapy in penicillin-resistant pneumococcal meningitis. Lancet 339: 405, 1992.
135. Mendelman PM, Campos DO, Chaffin DA, et al: Relative penicillin G resistance in *Neisseria meningitidis* and reduced affinity of penicillin-binding protein 3. Antimicrob Agents Chemother 32:706, 1988.
136. Siez-Nieto JA, Lujan R, Berron S, et al: Epidemiology and molecular basis of penicillin-resistant *Neisseria meningitidis* in Spain: A 5-year history (1985–1989). Clin Infect Dis 14:394, 1992.
137. Woods CR, Smith AL, Wasilauskas BL, et al: Invasive disease caused by *Neisseria meningitidis* relatively resistant to penicillin in North Carolina. J Infect Dis 170:453, 1994.
138. Zhang Q-Y, Jones DM, Saez Nieto JA, et al: Genetic diversity of penicillin-binding protein 2 genes of penicillin-resistant strains

of *Neisseria meningitidis* revealed by fingerprinting of amplified DNA. Antimicrob Agents Chemother 34:1523, 1990.
139. Jackson LA, Tenover FC, Baker C, et al: Prevalence of *Neisseria meningitidis* relatively resistant to penicillin in the United States. J Infect Dis 169:438, 1994.
140. Trallero EP, Arenzana JMG, Ayestaran I, Baroja IM: Comparative activity in vitro of 16 antimicrobial agents against penicillin-susceptible meningococci and meningococci with diminished susceptibility to penicillin. Antimicrob Agents Chemother 33:1622, 1989.
141. Dillon JR, Pauze M, Yeung KH: Spread of penicillinase-producing and transfer plasmids from the gonococcus to *Neisseria meningitidis*. Lancet 1:779, 1983.
142. Botha P: Penicillin-resistant *Neisseria meningitidis* in Southern Africa. Lancet 1:54, 1988.
143. Roberts MC, Knapp JS: Transfer of β-lactamase plasmids from *Neisseria gonorrheae* to *Neisseria meningitidis* and commensal *Neisseria* species by the 25.2 megadalton conjugative plasmid. Antimicrob Agents Chemother 32:1430, 1988.
144. Jorgensen JH: Update on mechanisms and prevalence of antimicrobial resistance in *Haemophilus influenzae*. Clin Infect Dis 14:1119, 1992.
145. Givner LB, Abramson JS, Wasilauskas B: Meningitis due to *Haemophilus influenzae* type b resistant to ampicillin and chloramphenicol. Rev Infect Dis 11:329, 1989.
146. Jacoby GA: Prevalence and resistance mechanisms of common respiratory pathogens. Clin Infect Dis 18:951, 1994.
147. Campos J, Garcia-Tornel S, Gairi JM, Fabregues I: Multiply resistant *Haemophilus influenzae* type b causing meningitis: Comparative clinical and laboratory study. J Pediatr 108:897, 1986.
148. Peltola H, Anttila M, Renkonen OV: Randomised comparison of chloramphenicol, ampicillin, cefotaxime, and ceftriaxone for childhood bacterial meningitis. Lancet 1:1281, 1989.
149. Klass PE, Klein JO: Therapy of bacterial sepsis, meningitis and otitis media in infants and children: 1992 poll of directors of programs in pediatric infectious diseases. Pediatr Infect Dis J 11:702, 1992.
150. McCracken GH Jr: Current management of bacterial meningitis in infants and children. Pediatr Infect Dis J 11:169, 1992.
151. Lebel MH, Hoyt MJ, McCracken GH Jr: Comparative efficacy of ceftriaxone and cefuroxime for treatment of bacterial meningitis: J Pediatr 114:1049, 1989.
152. Schaad UB, Suter S, Gianella-Borradori A, et al. A comparison of ceftriaxone and cefuroxime for the treatment of bacterial meningitis in children. N Engl J Med 322:141, 1990.
153. The Medical Letter: Choice of antibacterial drugs. *In* Handbook of Microbiology Therapy, rev ed. 1994, p 28.
154. Trautmann M, Wagner J, Chahin M, Weinke T: *Listeria* meningitis: Report of ten recent cases and review of current therapeutic recommendations. J Infect 10:107, 1985.
155. Levitz RE, Quintiliani R: Trimethoprim-sulfamethoxazole for bacterial meningitis. Ann Intern Med 100:881, 1984.
156. Bula CJ, Bille J, Glauser MP: An epidemic of food-borne listeriosis in western Switzerland: Description of 57 cases involving adults. Clin Infect Dis 20:66, 1995.
157. Fong IW, Tomkins KB: Review of *Pseudomonas aeruginosa* meningitis with special emphasis on treatment with ceftazidime. Rev Infect Dis 7:604, 1985.
158. Kilpatrick M, Girgis N, Farid Z, et al: Aztreonam for treating meningitis caused by gram-negative rods. Scand J Infect Dis 23:125, 1991.
159. Tunkel AR, Scheld WM: Treatment of bacterial meningitis. *In* Wolfson JS, Hooper DC (eds): Quinolone Antimicrobial Agents. Washington, DC, American Society for Microbiology, 1993, pp 481–495.
160. Nguyen MH, Muder RR: Meningitis due to *Xanthomonas maltophilia*: Case report and review. Clin Infect Dis 19:325, 1994.
161. Wolff MA, Young CL, Ramphal R: Antibiotic therapy for *Enterobacter* meningitis: A retrospective review of 13 episodes and review of the literature. Clin Infect Dis 16:772, 1993.
162. Siegman-Igra Y, Bar-Yosef S, Avram J: Nosocomial *Acinetobacter* meningitis secondary to invasive procedures: Report of 25 cases and review. Clin Infect Dis 17:843, 1993.
163. Gardner P, Leipzig T, Sadigh M: Infections of mechanical cerebrospinal fluid shunts. Curr Clin Top Infect Dis 9:185, 1988.
164. Kaufman BA, McLone DG: Infections of cerebrospinal fluid shunts. *In* Scheld WM, Whitley RJ, Durack DT (eds): Infections of the Central Nervous System. New York, Raven Press, 1991, pp 561–585.
165. Gump DW: Vancomycin for treatment of bacterial meningitis. Rev Infect Dis 3(Suppl):S289, 1981.
166. McLaurin RL: Infected cerebrospinal fluid shunts. Surg Neurol 1:191, 1973.
167. Wald SL, McLaurin RL: Cerebrospinal fluid antibiotic levels during treatment of shunt infections. J Neurosurg 52:41, 1980.
168. Paul AK, Smego RA, Fisher MA: Intraventricular vancomycin: Observations of tolerance and pharmacokinetics in two infants with ventricular shunt infections. Pediatr Infect Dis J 5:93, 1986.
169. Reesor C, Chow AW, Kureishi A, Jewesson PJ: Kinetics of intraventricular vancomycin in infections of cerebrospinal fluid shunts. J Infect Dis 158:1142, 1988.
170. Lin TY, Chrane DF, Nelson JD, McCracken GH Jr: Seven days of ceftriaxone therapy is as effective as ten days' treatment for bacterial meningitis. JAMA 253:3559, 1985.
171. Durack DT, Spanos A: End-of-treatment spinal tap in bacterial meningitis. Is it worthwhile? JAMA 248:75, 1982.
172. Horwitz SJ, Boxerbaum B, O'Bell J: Cerebral herniation in bacterial meningitis in childhood. Ann Neurol 7:524, 1980.
173. Dacey RG: Monitoring and treating increased intracranial pressure. Pediatr Infect Dis J 6:1161, 1987.
174. Lyons MK, Meyer FB: Cerebrospinal fluid physiology and the management of increased intracranial pressure. Mayo Clin Proc 65:684, 1990.
175. Ashwal S, Perkin RM, Thompson JR, et al: Bacterial meningitis in children: Current concepts of neurologic management. Curr Problems Pediatr 24:267, 1994.
176. Roos KL, Scheld WM: The management of fulminant meningitis in the intensive care unit. Crit Care Clin 4:375, 1988.
177. Roos L, Tunkel AR, Scheld WM: Acute bacterial meningitis in children and adults. *In* Scheld WM, Whitley RJ, Durack DT (eds): Infections of the Central Nervous System. New York, Raven Press, 1991, pp 335–409.
178. Ropper AH: Raised intracranial pressure in neurologic disease. Semin Neurol 4:397, 1984.
179. Marshall LF, Marshall SB: Medical management of intracranial pressure. *In* Cooper PR (ed): Head Injury, ed 2. Baltimore, Williams & Wilkins, 1987, pp 177–196.
180. Brown LB, Feigin RD: Bacterial meningitis: Fluid balance and therapy. Pediatr Ann 23:93, 1994.
181. Kaplan SL, Feigin RD: The syndrome of inappropriate secretion of antidiuretic hormone in children with bacterial meningitis. J Pediatr 92:758, 1978.
182. Feigin RD, Kaplan SL: Inappropriate secretion of antidiuretic hormone in children with bacterial meningitis. Am J Clin Nutr 30:1482, 1977.
183. Prince AS, Neu HC: Fluid management of *Haemophilus influenzae* meningitis: Infection 8:5, 1980.
184. Powell KR, Sugarman LI, Eskenazi AE, et al: Normalization of plasma arginine vasopressin concentrations when children with meningitis are given maintenance plus replacement fluid therapy. J Pediatr 117:515, 1990.
185. Singhi SC, Singhi PD, Srinivas B, et al: Fluid restriction does not improve the outcome of acute meningitis. Pediatr Infect Dis J 14:495, 1995.
186. Syrogiannopoulos GA, Olsen KD, Reisch JS, McCracken GH Jr: Dexamethasone in the treatment of experimental *Haemophilus influenzae* type b meningitis. J Infect Dis 155:213, 1987.
187. Mustafa MM, Ramilo O, Mertsola J, et al: Modulation of inflammation and cachectin activity in relation to treatment of experimental *Haemophilus influenzae* type b meningitis. J Infect Dis 160:818, 1989.
188. de Lemos RA, Haggerty RJ: Corticosteroids as an adjunct to treatment in bacterial meningitis. A controlled clinical trial. Pediatrics 44:30, 1969.
189. Harbin GL, Hodges GR: Corticosteroids adjunctive therapy for acute bacterial meningitis. South Med J 72:977, 1969.
190. Lebel MH, Frey BJ, Syrogiannopoulos GA, et al: Dexamethasone therapy for bacterial meningitis. Results of two double-blind, placebo-controlled trials. N Engl J Med 319:964, 1988.
191. Odio CM, Faingezicht I, Paris M, et al: The beneficial effects of early dexamethesone administration in infants and children with bacterial meningitis. N Engl J Med 324:1525, 1991.

192. Wald E, US Meningitis Study Group: Dexamethasone for children with meningitis. Presented at the 32nd Interscience Conference on Antimicrobial Agents and Chemotherapy; October 11–14, 1992; Anaheim, CA.
193. Schaad UB, Lyss U, Gnehm HE, et al: Dexamethasone therapy for bacterial meningitis in children. Lancet 342:457, 1993.
194. Jafari HS, McCracken GH Jr: Dexamethasone therapy in bacterial meningitis. Pediatr Ann 23:82, 1994.
195. Girgis NI, Farid Z, Mikhail IA, et al: Dexamethasone treatment for meningitis in children and adults. Pediatr Infect Dis J 8:848, 1989.
196. Syrogiannopoulos GA, Lourida AN, Theodoridou MC, et al: Dexamethasone therapy for bacterial meningitis in children: 2- versus 4-day regimen. J Infect Dis 169:853, 1994.
197. Kennedy WA, Hoyt MJ, McCracken GH Jr: The role of corticosteroid therapy in children with pneumococcal meningitis. Am J Dis Child 145:1374, 1991.
198. Kanra GY, Ozen H, Secmeer G, et al: Beneficial effects of dexamethasone in children with pneumococcal meningitis. Pediatr Infect Dis J 14:490, 1995.
199. Kilpi T, Peltola H, Jauhiainen T, et al: Oral glycerol and intravenous dexamethasone in preventing neurologic and audiologic sequelae of childhood bacterial meningitis. Pediatr Infect Dis J 14:270, 1995.
200. Geiman BJ, Smith AL: Dexamethasone and bacterial meningitis. A meta-analysis of randomized control trials. West J Med 157:27, 1992.
201. Paris MM, Hickey SM, Uscher MI, et al: Effect of dexamethasone on therapy of experimental penicillin- and cephalosporin-resistant pneumococcal meningitis. Antimicrob Agents Chemother 38:1320, 1994.
202. Bradley JS: Dexamethasone therapy in meningitis: Potentially misleading anti-inflammatory effects in central nervous system infections. Pediatr Infect Dis J 13:823, 1994.
203. Pappas DG, Hammerschlag PE, Hammerschlag M: Cerebrospinal fluid rhinorrhea and recurrent meningitis. Clin Infect Dis 17:364, 1993.
204. Hyslop NE Jr, Montgomery WM: Diagnosis and management of meningitis associated with cerebrospinal fluid leaks. Curr Clin Top Infect Dis 3:254, 1982.
205. Rouah E, Rogers BB, Buffone GJ: Transferrin analysis by immunofixation as an aid in the diagnosis of cerebrospinal fluid otorrhea. Arch Pathol Lab Med 111:756, 1987.
206. Rathore MH: Do prophylactic antibiotics prevent meningitis after basilar skull fracture? Pediatr Infect Dis J 10:87, 1991.
207. Eljamel MS: Antibiotic prophylaxis in unrepaired CSF fistulae. Br J Neurosurg 7:501, 1993.
208. Darouiche R, Perkins B, Musher D, et al: Levels of rifampin and ciprofloxacin in nasal secretions: Correlation with MIC_{90} and eradication of nasopharyngeal carriage of bacteria. J Infect Dis 1162:1124, 1990.
209. Dworzak DL, Sanders CC, Horowitz EA, et al: Evaluation of single-dose ciprofloxacin in the eradication of *Neisseria meningitidis* from nasopharyngeal carriers. Antimicrob Agents Chemother 32:1740, 1988.
210. Gaunt PN, Lambert BE: Single-dose ciprofloxacin for the eradication of pharyngeal carriage of *Neisseria meningitidis*. J Antimicrob Chemother 21:489, 1988.
211. Schwartz B, Al-Tobaiqi A, Al-Ruwais A, et al: Comparative efficacy of ceftriaxone and rifampicin in eradicating pharyngeal carriage of group A *Neisseria meningitidis*. Lancet 1:1239, 1988.
212. Frasch CE, Zahradnik JM, Wang LY, et al: Antibody response of adults to an aluminum hydroxide–adsorbed *Neisseria meningitidis* serotype 2b protein–group B polysaccharide vaccine. J Infect Dis 158:710, 1988.
213. Lieberman JM, Greenberg DP, Ward JI: Prevention of bacterial meningitis. Vaccines and chemoprophylaxis. Infect Dis Clin North Am 4:703, 1990.
214. Peltola H, Käyhty H, Virtanen M, Makela PH: Prevention of *Haemophilus influenzae* type b bacteremic infections with the capsular polysaccharide vaccine. N Engl J Med 310:1561, 1984.
215. Eskola J, Käyhty H, Takala AK, et al: A randomized, prospective field trial of a conjugate vaccine in the protection of infants and young children against invasive *Haemophilus influenzae* type b disease. N Engl J Med 323:1381, 1990.
216. Committee on Infectious Diseases of American Academy of Pediatrics: Immunization against *Haemophilus influenzae* infections. *In* Red Book Report of Committee of Infectious Diseases, ed 23. Elk Grove Village, IL, American Academy of Pediatrics, 1994, pp 207–216.

159

Acute Viral Meningitis and Encephalitis

Stephen G. Baum

Acute viral meningitis is a subset of the group of central nervous system (CNS) infections known as aseptic meningitis. This latter term antedates the science of virology and signifies syndromes that involve infection of the subarachnoid space and meninges in which no etiologic bacterial pathogen can be isolated or otherwise identified.

If a specific virus can be isolated or identified by molecular biologic techniques from the cerebrospinal fluid (CSF) of a patient with aseptic meningitis syndrome, the physician is entirely justified in diagnosing viral meningitis. Unfortunately, owing to the pathophysiology of many viral infections, the relative inaccessibility and expense of viral isolation procedures, and a lack of interest in pursuing etiologic diagnoses in non–life-threatening illnesses, diagnosis often rests primarily on clinical grounds, substantiated, in retrospect, by serologic responses.

The term encephalitis defines a condition in which there is inflammation in brain tissue, as opposed to meningitis, which involves only the covering of the brain. The sine qua non for the diagnosis of encephalitis is an altered state of consciousness. Although there are noninfectious causes of encephalitis that include allergic reactions and toxins, by far the most common cause is viral infection. A large number of viruses are capable of infecting the brain as part of a multiorgan disease such as measles and mumps. These viruses often cause meningoencephalitis, and grouping for discussion under either site of CNS infection versus the other is artificial. Other viruses, primarily the arboviruses, selectively target the brain and neural tissue during infection. This probably is due to receptor specificity, because initial infection may be at some distance from the CNS. Appropriate chapters of this book should be consulted for complete descriptions of each virus and the diseases it causes.

Owing to advances in molecular biologic techniques such as the polymerase chain reaction (PCR), and the use of monoclonal antibodies and the enzyme-linked immunosorbent assay, we are about to enter an exciting era in the rapid and accurate diagnosis of viral infections of the CNS.

Meningitis

Epidemiology

Many viruses can cause acute meningitis, and the epidemiology of specific syndromes differs with the etiologic agent (Table 159–1). The principal viruses identified with acute meningitis include the enteroviruses (coxsackievirus, echovi-

TABLE 159–1 ■ Epidemiology of Acute Viral Meningitis

EPIDEMIOLOGIC FACTORS*				
Season	**Patient's Age (y)**	**Patient's Sex**	**Risk Factor**	**SUGGESTED VIRAL AGENT**
Summer–fall	Infant	—	Infected mother	Coxsackievirus B
	1–15	—	Swimming pools, closed communities	Enteroviruses
			Geographic area: California, southeastern United States	California serogroup virus
Winter	1–15	—	School exposure	Varicella virus, measles virus
		Male/female 3:1		Mumps virus
	16–21	—	College exposure	Measles virus
		Male/female 3:1		Mumps virus
		—		Epstein-Barr virus (mononucleosis)
	Any	—	Mice, rats, hamsters	Lymphocytic choriomeningitis virus
	Adults	—	Varicella-zoster	Varicella-zoster virus
Any	Any	—	Immunocompromise	Adenovirus
		—	Acquired immunodeficiency syndrome	Human immunodeficiency virus

*Epidemiologic factors are suggestive but should not be used to exclude diagnoses in individual cases.

rus, and poliovirus), the herpesviruses (herpes simplex virus types 1 and 2 [HSV-1 and HSV-2] and varicella-zoster virus), the flaviviruses (which cause St. Louis encephalitis), paramyxoviruses (which cause mumps), bunyaviruses (California group, La Crosse), morbillivirus (which causes measles), arenaviruses (which cause lymphocytic choriomeningitis), and adenoviruses. Less common causative viruses include other herpesviruses (e.g., Epstein-Barr virus and cytomegalovirus) and hepatitis B virus.

Enteroviruses, of which there are more than 70 serotypes,[1, 2] cause more than one half of the cases of acute meningitis in which a specific viral agent is identified,[3] and probably an even greater proportion of unproven cases. As would be expected from the viruses involved, which most often cause infectious diseases in childhood, the majority of cases of acute viral meningitis occur in infants, young children, and adolescents; however, no age group is spared. In infants, eight of the serotypes (five echoviruses and three type B coxsackieviruses) cause about 80% of the cases.[4] In neonates older than 7 days, the enteroviruses would appear to be the most common cause of meningitis, accounting for one third of cases.[5] The mode of spread depends on the agent involved. Enteroviruses are transmitted both by fecal-oral and respiratory routes from person to person; lymphocytic choriomeningitis is transmitted to humans through direct contact with rodents; adenovirus can be spread by the respiratory route or can cause meningitis in immunocompromised persons by reactivation of latent infection. The enteroviruses cause infection during the summer and fall in temperate climates, whereas mumps, measles, and varicella-zoster meningitides peak in the winter and spring months.

Pathogenesis

Involvement of the meninges in the course of viral infection, whether caused by enteroviruses or by one of the other virus groups, is probably secondary to hematogenous dissemination from the primary focus of infection. This has been demonstrated in the case of poliovirus[6] and is suggested by the fact that genital HSV-2 infection is more often associated with meningitis than is oronasal HSV-1 infection.[7] Viremic spread remains hypothetic in other diseases because of a lack of totally applicable animal models and the fact that in humans the viruses that cause meningitis are rarely isolated from the blood stream. The factors that predispose to meningitis as a complication of common viral infections are unclear. In poliomyelitis, involvement of particular segments of the spinal cord appears to relate to limbs that were exercised during the viremic phase of the illness.[8] An analysis of meningitis cases in seven outbreaks of enteroviral illness among high-school students showed a statistically relevant increased attack rate of meningitis among football players.[9] These findings suggest that increased blood flow or minor trauma might predispose to meningitis. Because most viral meningitides have low mortality rates when not complicated by encephalitis, the pathologic changes and the nature of the inflammatory response can be surmised only from the cell content of the CSF. Here, lymphocytes predominate after a 24- to 48-hour polymorphonuclear response. The CSF lymphocytes have been identified as T cells,[10] and one study has shown that suppressor T cells bearing the OKT8 marker predominate.[11] This study found that cell-free CSF from patients with aseptic meningitis could inhibit B-cell generation in vitro.

Lymphocytes of the B-cell line are probably also involved in the CNS immune response, because virus-specific antibody has been detected in the CSF of patients with viral meningitis in excess of the concentration seen in serum.[12, 13] There is controversy surrounding this point, there being some indication that in acute viral meningitis all virus-specific antibody in the CSF derives from loss of the integrity of the blood-brain barrier and leakage of serum.[14] In fatal cases of enteroviral meningitis in infants or in cases in which encephalitis does supervene, the leptomeninges show inflammation, with involvement of the pons, cerebrum, and cerebellum manifested by increased number of microglial cells and perivascular cuffing.[15] Both white matter and gray matter show marked cellular destruction. In these cases of encephalitis compounding meningitis, it is the former involvement that most probably leads to death. In fatal cases, myocarditis often is found, as is inflammation of the liver and lungs.[15] The mortality rate of acute viral meningitis in the absence of brain and other systemic involvement is probably 1% or less.

Diagnosis

Etiologic diagnosis usually rests on clinical and epidemiologic criteria. Features common to cases of acute viral meningitis include headache, fever (usually temperature lower than 102°F), photophobia, mild to moderate meningismus, and irritability. These may be accompanied by findings that are more specific for a given disease, such as parotitis in mumps, a zosteriform eruption in zoster, a typical multiphasic vesiculopustular eruption in varicella, asymmetric paralysis in poliomyelitis and enterovirus 71 infection, gastrointestinal disturbance and rash in other enteroviral illness, and pharyngitis with diffuse adenopathy and psychosis[16] in mononucleosis (Table 159–2). In most cases, however, these helpful concomitant findings are absent.

Signs and symptoms of meningitis should prompt the clinician to perform lumbar puncture. The most important elements of CSF analysis are a search for bacteria or fungal elements and enumeration and differential count of any leukocytes present. The absence of bacteria should be assessed by examination of a Gram-stained preparation of the CSF sediment obtained by centrifuging 1 to 10 mL of CSF in a laboratory centrifuge for 5 minutes. A drop of CSF sediment should be allowed to air-dry on a slide, after which it is heat fixed and stained. The presence or absence of fungi (primarily *Cryptococcus neoformans*) is assessed initially by adding another drop of CSF sediment to a drop of India ink and examining the wet preparation under the microscope. The cryptococci are seen as budding yeast forms in about 50% of proven cases. Cryptococcal antigen assay should be ordered, and results are usually available in 4 to 12 hours. This test has a sensitivity of more than 90%.

The cell count in viral meningitis is variable but usually does not exceed 1000 white cells per mm^3. In most cases the count is less than 200 white cells per mm^3. Although the classic finding in viral meningitis is a predominance of small lymphocytes, polymorphonuclear leukocytes may predominate for the first 24 to 48 hours. The protein content of the CSF is usually normal but may be elevated to about 200 mg/dL. The glucose concentration also is usually normal (at least 50 mg/dL or at least 50% of the value in a simultaneously drawn sample of blood), but hypoglycorrachia has been reported in cases of meningitis due to mumps[17] and lymphocytic choriomeningitis[18] infection. Of the many viruses that cause meningitis, only some of the enteroviruses can be cultured readily from the CSF. Isolation of some type A coxsackieviruses requires inoculation of newborn mice. These isolations are rarely attempted, however, except as part of a virus surveillance study. Most often, if confirmation of the clinical diagnosis is sought, it is through finding a fourfold rise in antibodies to the suspected virus. In the case of enteroviruses, which may be ubiquitous in the oropharynx and stool of children, a diagnostic rise in antibody to the virus isolated from these sites must be demonstrated to ensure a causal relationship. Other specific diagnostic measures are discussed below, and clinical and laboratory findings suggestive of a specific cause are given in Table 159–2. A number of authors have indicated that levels of lactate dehydrogenase,[19] lactate,[20] and other nonspecific acute-phase reactants can be used to differentiate viral from bacterial meningitis. It appears that concentrations of these substances vary directly with the number of leukocytes present and so contribute little additional helpful information. A most promising addition to the diagnostic armamentarium is the application of PCR technology to this problem. Using PCR, several laboratories have demonstrated high degrees of sensitivity and specificity in finding nucleic acid sequences of enteroviruses in CSF with a single pair of oligonucleotide primers that detect the highly conserved 5′ end of the enterovirus sequence.[21–24] This technology not only should improve the epidemiologic accuracy of detecting enteroviral disease but will do so quickly enough to have a major impact on treatment by allowing withdrawal of antimicrobials and discharge from the hospital.

Differential Diagnosis

The most significant decision one can make in evaluating meningitis is whether or not the infection will respond to specific antimicrobial therapy. Once pyogenic bacterial and fungal meningitides are excluded, there remain several causes of the aseptic meningitis syndrome that require specific treatment—tuberculosis, syphilis, leptospirosis, Lyme disease, and far less commonly, protozoal meningitis. In addition, and perhaps more common than any of these, is pyogenic bacterial meningitis in a patient who received some antibiotic treatment before the lumbar puncture. In these cases, bacteria may not be evident on Gram stain, and the initial polymorphonuclear response may have shifted to a mononuclear lymphocytic one. Although assays for bacterial antigens in the CSF, including counterimmunoelectrophoresis and latex agglutination, were developed to assist in just such cases, it has been my experience, substantiated by numerous personal communications, that these assays are no more sen-

TABLE 159–2 ■ Clinical and Laboratory Findings in Viral Meningitis*

CLINICAL PRESENTATION	SUGGESTIVE LABORATORY FINDINGS: CSF	SUGGESTIVE LABORATORY FINDINGS: Other	SUGGESTED VIRAL AGENT
Parotitis, orchitis	Glucose ↓	Amylase ↑	Mumps virus
Diffuse rash, gastroenteritis, upper respiratory tract infection	—	—	Enteroviruses
Herpangina (soft palate enanthem)	—	—	Coxsackievirus A
Hand-foot-mouth rash	—	—	Coxsackievirus A
Pleurisy, orchitis, carditis	—	—	Coxsackievirus B
Orchitis, influenza-like syndrome	>2000 lymphocytes per mm^3, glucose ↓	Leukopenia, thrombocytopenia	Lymphocytic choriomeningitis virus
Zosteriform rash	—	—	Varicella-zoster virus
Encephalitis with focal neurologic signs	Erythrocytes	—	Herpes simplex virus
Pneumonia, immunocompromise	—	—	Adenovirus
Lymphadenopathy, splenomegaly, pharyngitis, psychosis	—	Atypical lymphocytes, monospot	Epstein-Barr virus

*These findings may be present in only a minority of cases but are nevertheless helpful.

sitive than is Gram stain. In other words, it is highly unlikely that results of bacterial antigen tests will be positive if there is a negative Gram stain. One must take careful and sometimes repeated histories to exclude casual prior antibiotic use at the onset of symptoms.

Specific Meningitis Syndromes

Although viral meningitis syndromes are often nonspecific, sometimes a specific viral cause is suggested by the accompanying signs, symptoms, and laboratory findings.

ENTEROVIRUSES

The enteroviruses cause a multiplicity of syndromes in children and young adults. The most common clinical presentation is a febrile illness associated with mild respiratory or gastrointestinal symptoms. Exanthems or enanthemas may be associated with particular virus groups. Herpangina, painful vesicular and ulcerative lesions on the soft palate and tonsillar fauces, is associated with coxsackievirus A, as is the hand-foot-and-mouth syndrome consisting of isolated vesicles on an erythematous base in the aforementioned locations. Type B coxsackieviruses can be associated with pleuritis (pleurodynia, devil's grip), pericarditis, myocarditis, and orchitis. Echovirus, as well as other coxsackievirus, infections can be associated with a generalized macular or vesicular exanthem. Coxsackievirus B infection may be fatal to infants.[15] Enterovirus 71 can cause a paralytic syndrome in young children that is indistinguishable from that caused by poliovirus. This virus has also been associated with Guillain-Barré syndrome, aseptic meningitis, and encephalitis.[25]

MUMPS VIRUS

In the prevaccine era, mumps virus was the most common cause of meningoencephalitis in the United States and accounted for up to 10% of cases of this syndrome. Parotitis, the cardinal sign of mumps, was absent in up to one half of cases, and affected males outnumbered females by 3 to 1.[26] With the advent of live mumps vaccine in 1967, the incidence of mumps and its associated syndromes diminished dramatically; however, a significant number of children born in the late 1960s and early 1970s were not vaccinated. Because of herd immunity, these children had little chance of contracting natural infection. We are, therefore, witnessing a marked upsurge in the incidence of mumps among young adults and may see a reappearance of mumps-related CNS syndromes, which are more common in older age groups. This infection should be suspected in males who develop aseptic meningitis in winter or spring. Evidence of parotitis and epididymoorchitis should be sought, and an elevated serum amylase level may be found even in the absence of overt parotitis.[26]

HERPESVIRUS

Although HSV-1 and HSV-2 can cause CNS infection, data from several studies indicate that HSV-2 is more likely than HSV-1 to cause aseptic meningitis.[7] HSV involvement of the CNS can be the result of either primary or recurrent herpesvirus infection, although it appears to be more common as a complication of primary infection. One study showed that 36% of women and 13% of men with primary genital HSV-2 infection had stiff neck, photophobia, and headache.[7] The absence of herpetic lesions does not exclude the possibility of HSV involvement of the CNS. Herpetic meningitis has a much better prognosis than encephalitis and is almost invariably self-limited and without sequelae. There have been several intriguing reports implicating HSV-2 as a cause of the benign recurrent lymphocytic meningitis syndrome (Mollaret). This association, made possible by the use of PCR, would be entirely consistent with the recurring nature of HSV infections.[27, 28] Varicella-zoster virus, another member of the herpesvirus family, can cause meningitis. This can occur during the course of childhood or adult chickenpox, as a rare complication, or in adult patients with zoster of any dermatome.[29, 30] CSF pleocytosis without meningeal signs or symptoms is probably quite common in zoster.[30] Occasionally, the CNS involvement antecedes the rash in either condition. If there is no encephalitic component, the illness is usually mild and self-limited.[29]

LYMPHOCYTIC CHORIOMENINGITIS VIRUS

Lymphocytic choriomeningitis virus causes sporadic meningitis. Mice and other rodents are colonized with this organism and excrete it in their urine and feces. The peak incidence may occur any time except summer months, and disease occurs in localized areas of the United States and Europe.

The only clue to the diagnosis of this infection is a history of exposure to rodents. Thirty years ago, pet Syrian hamsters were shown to be a source of epidemic human infection, and both a nonmeningitic influenza-like syndrome, accompanied in some cases by orchitis, and meningitic illness have been reported.[18, 31] Exposure to chronically infected nude mice, or mouse tissues, has been shown to transmit the disease to laboratory workers.[32] CSF findings are nonspecific, but elevated protein concentration and lymphocytosis of up to 2000 cells per mm^3 are common. Hypoglycorrachia occurs in about 30% of cases.

ADENOVIRUS

In patients who are immunocompromised as a result of kidney or bone marrow transplantation, adenovirus has been found to be a relatively common cause of CNS infection. Typically, this takes the form of meningoencephalitis and is often associated with acute adenovirus pneumonia. Types 7, 12, and 32 have been implicated (see Chapter 239).

Therapy

There is no effective antiviral therapy for viral meningitis. Adenine arabinoside and acyclovir, which have proved somewhat useful in treating herpes simplex and varicella-zoster encephalitis, are probably not necessary in cases of uncomplicated meningitis.

Prevention

Vaccines are available for the prevention of measles, mumps, varicella, and poliomyelitis. There are no commercially available vaccines for any of the other viruses discussed in this chapter. Spread of the enteroviruses is so ubiquitous during the summer and fall that infection control measures are of little use. One study group has recommended that women in the third trimester of pregnancy avoid swimming in pools to prevent enteroviral vaginal colonization.[33]

Encephalitis

Epidemiology

There are two distinct epidemiologic patterns in viral encephalitis. One is identical to that previously described for the meningitides and involves respiratory or oral person-to-person transmission as exemplified by measlesvirus, mumpsvirus, enteroviruses, and herpesviruses, including varicella-zoster virus. The other, typical of the arboviral diseases, requires inoculation of the virus into the human blood stream through the bite of an infected insect, usually a mosquito (Flaviviridae, Togaviridae, and Bunyaviridae) or tick (tick-borne encephalitis virus). In the case of rabies virus and monkey herpesvirus B, direct inoculation into neural tissue by the bite of an infected animal is the mode of transmission. Table 159–3 gives the taxonomic grouping and vectors of some of the viruses that most commonly cause encephalitis.

The epidemiology of arboviral encephalitis is extremely complex and represents highly specialized adaptation of the virus to replication in a given species of mosquito or tick vector, as well as availability of that insect's preferred blood meal source. These intermediate animal hosts are usually birds or horses. Humans are often incidental and "dead-end" hosts of infection. For these reasons, there is specific geographic localization of the arboviral syndromes based on the presence of insect vector and animal reservoir. On the other hand, the viruses transmitted from person to person, and the diseases they cause, are found worldwide. Table 159–4 summarizes some of the epidemiologic and diagnostic factors useful in assessing the cause of encephalitis in a given patient.

The incidence of viral encephalitis varies greatly with the specific virus, season, geographic location, and climatic conditions (see Table 159–4). Epidemiologic reporting is both deficient and inaccurate, so many cases probably go unreported. In the United States, the most common cause is herpesvirus type 1, of which there are about a thousand cases reported annually. The second most common agents are the arboviruses, especially St. Louis encephalitis virus or California virus, although in any given year other arboviruses such as eastern equine encephalitis virus may predominate.[34–36] The total number of arbovirus cases per year in the United States usually does not exceed 1 to 200; however, there were 3000 cases of St. Louis encephalitis in 1933,[34] and Japanese encephalitis virus is responsible for tens of thousands of cases in Southeast Asia annually.[37, 38] Postinfectious encephalitis has been seen after influenza, but never to the extent seen after the 1918 epidemic attributed to infection with swine influenza virus (von Economo encephalitis).

TABLE 159–3 ■ Grouping and Mode of Transmission of Encephalitis Viruses

FAMILY	MEMBER VIRUS	TRANSMISSION (VECTOR)
Flaviviridae	Japanese encephalitis St. Louis encephalitis Murray Valley encephalitis West Nile encephalitis	*Culex* mosquitos
	Powassan Tick-borne encephalitis	*Ixodes* ticks
Togaviridae (alphaviruses)	Eastern equine encephalitis Western equine encephalitis Venezuelan equine encephalitis	*Culex* mosquitos
Bunyaviridae	California group La Crosse Jamestown Canyon	*Aedes* mosquitos
Herpesviridae	HSV-1 > HSV-2	Person to person
	Cytomegalovirus	Person to person
	Varicella-zoster	Person to person
	Monkey B	Monkey bite
Retroviridae	Human immunodeficiency virus type 1	Person to person

The number of complications associated with the acquired immunodeficiency syndrome (AIDS) is ever growing. Included in these are a multiplicity of CNS syndromes caused by various opportunistic agents such as *Toxoplasma gondii, Mycobacterium tuberculosis,* cytomegalovirus, and *Treponema pallidum.* It is now clear that the human immunodeficiency virus, which is the cause of AIDS, can itself infect neural tissue to produce meningoencephalitis.[39] Diagnosis of this condition rests on excluding the other potential causes of CNS infection. In fact, involvement of the CNS is perhaps the only *direct* result of human immunodeficiency virus infection, the other elements of AIDS being indirect results of damaged immunity. This involvement, with the attendant requirement that anti-AIDS drugs penetrate brain tissue, represents one of the major stumbling blocks to effective treatment of AIDS.

Pathogenesis

In herpesvirus B infection and rabies, the virus travels along peripheral nerves to the CNS. In the arboviral encephalitides and in mumps and measles, viremia is the source of infection of the CNS.[40–42] Encephalitis viruses are neurotropic and apparently replicate in neurons, thereby lysing them. In addition, later in infection, there may be an immune inflammatory component to neuronal damage.[43, 44] Histologically, there is perivascular infiltration by both mononuclear and polymorphonuclear cells. Neuronal cells degenerate and are phagocytosed.

Disease Manifestations

Incubation periods in cases other than those caused by animal bite are difficult to calculate precisely. In cases of arboviral encephalitis, the incubation period may vary from several days to 2 weeks.[34, 37] The vast majority (greater than 90%) of arboviral infections result in mild disease resembling an influenza-like illness. If encephalitis occurs, the syndrome generally consists of fever, headache, malaise, and abnormal mental state progressing during several days to stupor and coma. This syndrome may be accompanied by nuchal rigidity and seizures. After the first week, either flaccid or spastic paralysis may occur. Many patients exhibit electrolyte imbalance caused by the syndrome of inappropriate secretion of antidiuretic hormone. Once signs and symptoms are present, they progress for 1 to 2 weeks, at which time the patient either dies or begins to show signs of recovery. Because of the damage to neurons, which are incapable of regeneration, there are often severe sequelae of infection. Patients may be left with cognitive and cranial nerve deficits, including dysarthria, as well as paralysis and aphasia. Parkinsonian tremors have been noted after recovery from Japanese and postinfluenzal encephalitis.

There are differences in the propensity to develop clinical disease and in the severity of disease after arboviral infection that vary with the virus and with the age and underlying condition of the host. St. Louis encephalitis tends to cause most severe disease in the elderly, especially in black persons and people with hypertension, whereas Japanese B encephalitis and California virus encephalitis are most common in children. The case-fatality rate in Japanese encephalitis and eastern equine encephalitis is in excess of 30%, whereas St. Louis encephalitis has a 7% mortality in young adults and a 20% mortality in the elderly. Most other arboviral encephalitides carry a mortality rate of less than 1%.[34, 37, 45] Herpesvirus B infection and untreated rabies are almost universally fatal; herpes simplex encephalitis has an inherent mortality of 70% to 80%, which has been reduced to less than 30% with the early use of acyclovir.[46]

TABLE 159–4 ■ Epidemiologic Characteristics and Laboratory Diagnosis of Viral Encephalitis*

VIRUS	RECENT TRAVEL	RISKY HABITAT	MONTH OF EXPOSURE†	PATIENT'S AGE	DIAGNOSTIC TEST	RESEARCH LABORATORY
St. Louis encephalitis	United States	Unscreened home	JJA	Older	IgM ELISA	CDC
Japanese encephalitis	Asia	Rice fields	MJJAS	Any	IgM ELISA	WRAIR
Western equine encephalitis	Western North America, South America	Agroecosystems in western United States	JJAS	Any	IgM ELISA	CDC
Eastern equine encephalitis	Eastern United States	Coastal marshland	JJA	<10, >55 y	IgM ELISA	CDC
Venezuelan equine encephalitis	South America to Texas	Rural	Rainy months	Adult men	IgM ELISA CSF	CDC
Tick-borne encephalitis	Central Europe and Asia	Woodlands	JJA	Any	IgM ELISA CSF	U. Vienna
Herpes simplex	Anywhere	None	Any	Any	Brain biopsy	
California encephalitis	Western United States	Rural areas	JJASO	Children	IgM ELISA	CDC
Murray Valley encephalitis	Southern Australia	River valley area	JFMAM	Any	IgM ELISA	CDC
West Nile encephalitis	North Africa, eastern and southern Asia	Rice areas	JJAS	Any	ELISA Virus isolation	WRAIR
Powassan	North Central United States, southern Canada	Rural areas	JJAS	<20 or >50 y	HAI, CF	CDC
La Crosse	U.S. Midwestern	Woodlands	JJAS	Boys <19 y	ELISA	CDC
Rocio	São Paulo, Brazil	Poor rural areas	FMAMJJ	Young men	HAI, ELISA	CDC
Jamestown Canyon	New York and westward	Rural areas	JJAS	Children	CF, NT	
Human immunodeficiency virus type 1	Worldwide	All	Any	Undefined	ELISA Immunoblot	Most
B virus		Monkey colony	Any	Adult	Virus isolation	SFBR

*ELISA, Enzyme-linked immunosorbent assay; HAI, hemagglutination inhibition; CF, complement fixation; NT, neutralization test; IgM, immunoglobulin M; CDC, Fort Collins, CO (303-221-6407); WRAIR, Department of Virus Diseases, Walter Reed Army Institute of Research, Washington, DC (202-576-2054); U. Vienna, University of Vienna, Vienna, Austria; SFBR, Southwest Foundation for Biomedical Research, San Antonio, TX.

†Initial of months in most cases; the first J refers to June in all entries, the first M to March.

Diagnosis

The encephalitis syndrome itself gives little clue in any given case as to the cause. Although localization of neurologic signs to the temporal lobe is probably most common in HSV encephalitis, the absence of this localization does not rule out an HSV cause, and other encephalitides may affect the temporal lobe. The most important factor in establishing a probable cause of encephalitis is the taking of a careful history, including habitation or travel in an area endemic for a particular disease (arboviruses); exposure to animals such as rodents (lymphocytic choriomeningitis), dogs, raccoons, skunks (rabies), and monkeys (herpesvirus B); and the presence of concomitant illness (measles, mumps, varicella, or zoster).

Routine laboratory investigation is not usually helpful. The peripheral white cell count is elevated in most cases, with a relative lymphocytosis present. Examination of the CSF reveals a mild to moderate pleocytosis (25 to 250 white cells per mm^3). Although polymorphonuclear cells may predominate early in infection, by the second or third day of symptoms the majority of cells in the CSF are mononuclear. Protein levels may be slightly elevated and the glucose concentration is usually normal (see the earlier section on meningitis for exceptions). The presence of 100 to 200 erythrocytes per mm^3 in the CSF is more common in HSV encephalitis than in other encephalomeningitides. These are essentially the CSF findings in aseptic meningitis, and attempts should be made to exclude treatable causes of this syndrome before assuming that one is dealing with viral encephalitis. Such treatable causes would include tuberculosis, cryptococcal meningitis, toxoplasmosis in the patient with AIDS, and partially treated bacterial meningitis.

CSF also can be cultured for the presence of specific arboviruses, which grow quite well on a variety of monkey cell cultures, but attempts to culture CSF for HSV have been unsuccessful. One can also assay CSF for the presence of immunoglobulin M antibodies to specific etiologic agents. Although the specificity of these assays is high, antibodies may not be present at the outset of disease, thereby yielding a false-negative result. Because of the importance of arboviral outbreaks, attempts should be made to arrive at specific diagnoses of suspected arboviral encephalitis even if such results would not help the care of the patient at hand. In appropriate geographic locations, state health agencies should be able to provide diagnostic help. Further information can be obtained from the Centers for Disease Control and Prevention, Vector-Borne Diseases Laboratory, Fort Collins, Colorado.

The greatest hope for rapid and accurate etiologic diagnoses in cases of viral encephalitis lies in the commercially available application of the PCR. This test can reveal infinitesimal amounts of nucleic acid with great specificity in CSF and other body fluids. PCR has already been successfully applied experimentally to the diagnosis of HSV, enteroviral, and arboviral CNS diseases.[22, 24, 37, 47]

Ancillary tests may help to confirm a diagnosis of encephalitis, but they do not establish the cause. Electroencephalography is probably the most sensitive early in infection and may show focal slow waves over the affected area of the brain and diffuse delta activity indicating thalamic involvement. Computed tomography is insensitive early, but magnetic resonance imaging has been used successfully to reveal early brain involvement.[47, 48]

Treatment

The only form of viral encephalitis for which effective treatment exists is that caused by the herpesviruses. HSV encephalitis responds well to early (before coma) institution of therapy with acyclovir. The drug is given intravenously at a dose of 30 mg/kg per day in three divided doses for at least 10 days. Before the advent of acyclovir, it was recommended that brain biopsy be performed to obtain tissue for HSV testing by immunofluorescence and electron microscopy. The relative nontoxicity of acyclovir makes this procedure unnecessary in my opinion, unless there is no response to therapy, and one is searching for the presence of another causative agent. It is probably worthwhile to initiate therapy with acyclovir in cases of herpesvirus B encephalitis.[49] Although no controlled studies have been done, patients with zoster encephalitis appear to benefit from treatment with acyclovir. Cytomegalovirus more often causes meningitis than encephalitis in patients with AIDS. However, these patients often have an encephalopathy of undetermined cause. Human immunodeficiency virus encephalopathy may also improve after therapy with zidovudine.

Prevention

Because there is no effective therapy for most causes of viral encephalitis, vaccines would be desirable in protecting against infection. Vaccines have been developed against Japanese B, Venezuelan, and tick-borne encephalitides, but only the first of these (JE-VAX, Connaught Laboratories) is commercially available in the United States. Visitors to endemic areas of Asia should consider obtaining the Japanese B vaccine. However, in Australia, where the vaccine is available, there have been several reports of vaccine-associated severe allergic reactions.[44] Perhaps the best advice would be to take all measures available to prevent exposure to the mosquito or tick vectors.

Mumps and measles vaccinations have decreased markedly the incidence of encephalitis due to these two diseases. The newer rabies vaccine is effective in preventing disease even after the bite of an infected animal.

Acknowledgment

This chapter is affectionately dedicated to the memory of Bernard N. Fields, MD—friend, colleague, and virologist.

References

1. Schmidt NJ, Lennette EH, Ho HH: An apparently new enterovirus isolated from patients with disease of the central nervous system. J Infect Dis 129:304, 1974.
2. Matthews REF: Fourth report of the International Committee on Taxonomy of Viruses. Intervirology 17:1, 1982.
3. Centers for Disease Control: Enterovirus surveillance—United States, 1983. MMWR Morbid Mortal Wkly Rep 32:535, 1983.
4. Berlin LE, Rorabaugh ML, Heldrick F, et al: Asceptic meningitis in infants <2 years of age: Diagnosis and etiology. J Infect Dis 168:888, 1993.
5. Shattuck KE, Chonmaitree T: The changing spectrum of neonatal meningitis over a fifteen-year period. Clin Pediatr 31:130, 1992.
6. Bodian D: Emerging concepts of poliomyelitis infection. Science 122:105, 1955.
7. Corey L, Adams HG, Brown ZA, Holmes KK: Genital herpes simplex virus infections: Clinical manifestations, course and complications. Ann Intern Med 98:958, 1983.
8. Horstmann DM: Acute poliomyelitis. Relation of physical activity at the time of onset to the course of the disease. JAMA 142:236, 1950.
9. Moore M, Baron RC, Filstein MR, et al.: Aseptic meningitis and high school football players. JAMA 249:2039, 1983.
10. Naess A, Solberg CO, Tønder O: Granulocyte and lymphocyte membrane receptors in aseptic meningitis, infectious mononucleosis and other viral infections. Acta Pathol Microbiol Immunol Scand 93:37, 1985.
11. Bertotto A, Stagni G, Fabietti GM: Plasma cell generation inhibition in lymphocyte cultures containing cerebrospinal fluid from children with central nervous system viral infections. Microbiologica 8:11, 1985.
12. Forsberg P, Frydén A, Link H, Örvell C: Viral IgM and IgG antibody synthesis within the central nervous system in mumps meningitis. Acta Neurol Scand 73:372, 1986.
13. Ichimura H, Shimase K, Tamura I, et al.: Neutralizing antibody and interferon-α in cerebrospinal fluids and sera of acute aseptic meningitis. J Med Virol 15:231, 1985.
14. Siemes H, Siegert M: Immune response in the CSF in viral infections. Prog Brain Res 59:133, 1983.
15. Kaplan MH, Klein SW, McPhee J, Harper RG: Group B coxsackie infections in infants younger than three months of age: A serious childhood illness. Rev Infect Dis 5:1019, 1983.
16. Grose CF: Neurologic complications of infectious mononucleosis. *In* Schlossberg D (ed): Infectious Mononucleosis. New York, Springer-Verlag, 1989, pp 49–68.
17. Wilfert CM: Mumps meningoencephalitis with low cerebrospinal fluid glucose, prolonged pleocytosis and elevation of protein. N Engl J Med 280:855, 1969.
18. Biggar RJ, Woodall JP, Walter PD, et al.: Lymphocytic choriomeningitis outbreak associated with pet hamsters: Fifty-seven cases from New York State. JAMA 232:494, 1975.
19. Martin WJ: Rapid and reliable techniques for the laboratory detection of bacterial meningitis. Am J Med 75:119, 1983.
20. Jordan GW, Statland B, Halsted C: CSF lactate in disease of the CNS. Arch Intern Med 143:85, 1983.
21. Rotbart HA: Diagnosis of enteroviral meningitis with the polymerase chain reaction. J Pediatr 117:85, 1990.
22. Sawyer MH, Holland D, Aintablian N, et al: Diagnosis of enteroviral central nervous system infection by polymerase chain reaction during a large community outbreak. Pediatr Infect Dis 13:177, 1994.
23. Schlesinger Y, Sawyer MH, Storch GA: Enteroviral meningitis in infancy: Potential role for polymerase chain reaction in patient management. Pediatrics 94:157, 1994.
24. Rotbart HA, Sawyer MH, Fast S, et al: Diagnosis of enteroviral meningitis by using PCR with a colorimetric microwell detection assay. J Clin Microbiol 32:2590, 1994.
25. Alexander JP, Baden L, Pallansch MA, et al: Enterovirus 71 infections and neurologic disease—United States, 1977–1991. J Infect Dis 169:905, 1994.
26. Baum SG, Litman N: Mumps virus. *In* Mandell GL, Douglas RG Jr, Bennett JE (eds): Principles and Practice of Infectious Diseases, ed 4. New York, John Wiley & Sons, 1995, pp 1496–1501.
27. Tedder DG, Ashley R, Tyler K, et al: Herpes simplex infection as a cause of benign recurrent lymphocytic meningitis. Ann Intern Med 121:334, 1994.
28. Picard FJ, Dekaban GA, Silva J, et al: Mollaret's meningitis associated with herpes simplex type 2 infection. Neurology 43:1722, 1993.
29. Johnson R, Milbourne PE: Central nervous system manifestations of chickenpox. Can Med Assoc J 102:831, 1970.
30. Barnes DW, Whitley RJ: CNS disease associated with varicella zoster virus and herpes simplex infection. Neurol Clin 4:265, 1986.
31. Baum SG, Lewis AM Jr, Rowe WP, et al.: Epidemic nonmeningitic lymphocytic choriomeningitis virus infection. N Engl J Med 274:934, 1966.
32. Dykewicz CA, Dato VM, Fisher-Hock SP: Lymphocytic choriomeningitis outbreak associated with nude mice in a research institute. JAMA 267:1349, 1992.
33. Reyes MP, Zalenski D, Smith F, et al.: Coxsackievirus-positive cervices in women with febrile illnesses during the third trimester in pregnancy. Am J Obstet Gynecol 155:159, 1986.
34. Tsai TF: Arboviral infections in the United States. Infect Dis Clin North Am 1:73, 1991.
35. Centers for Disease Control: Arboviral disease—United States, 1991. MMWR Morbid Mortal Wkly Rep 41:545, 1992.
36. Centers for Disease Control and Prevention: Arboviral Diseases—United States, 1992. MMWR Morbid Mortal Wkly Rep 42:467, 1993.
37. Vaughn DW, Hoke CH: The epidemiology of Japanese encephalitis: Prospects for prevention. Epidemiol Rev 14:197, 1992.
38. Thisyakorn U, Thisyakorn C: Diseases caused by arbovi-

ruses—Dengue hemorrhagic fever and Japanese B encephalitis. Med J Aust 160:22, 1994.
39. Gabuzda DH, Hirsch MS: Neurologic manifestations of infection with human immunodeficiency virus. Ann Intern Med 107:383, 1987.
40. Tsiang H: Pathophysiology of rabies virus infection of the nervous system. Adv Virus Res 42:375, 1993.
41. Dupont JR, Earle KM: Human rabies encephalitis: A study of forty-nine fatal cases with a review of the literature. Neurology 15:1023, 1965.
42. Weigler BJ: Biology of B virus in macaque and human hosts: A review. Clin Infect Dis 14:555, 1992.
43. de la Monte S, Castro F, Bonilla NJ: The systemic pathology of Venezuelan equine encephalitis virus infection in humans. Am J Trop Med Hyg 34:194, 1985.
44. Johnson RT: The pathogenesis of acute viral encephalitis and post infectious encephalomyelitis. J Infect Dis 155:359, 1987.
45. Ohtaki E, Murakami Y, Komori H, et al: Acute disseminated encephalomyelitis after Japanese B encephalitis vaccination. Pediatr Neurol 8:137, 1992.
46. Whitley RJ, Alford CA, Hirsch MS, et al: Vidarabine versus acyclovir therapy in herpes simplex encephalitis. N Engl J Med 314:144, 1986.
47. Schlesinger Y, Buller RS, Brunstrom JE, et al: Expanded spectrum of herpes simplex encephalitis in childhood. J Pediatr 126:234, 1995.
48. Misra UK, Kalita J, Jain SK, et al: Radiological and neurophysiological changes in Japanese encephalitis. J Neurol Neurosurg Psychiatry 57:1484, 1994.
49. Centers for Disease Control: B-virus infection in humans—Pensacola, Florida. MMWR Morbid Mortal Wkly Rep 36:289, 1987.

160

Chronic Meningitis

John C. Pottage, Jr.
Alan A. Harris

Chronic meningitis is generally defined as a constellation of signs and symptoms of meningeal irritation for greater than 4 weeks with an associated cerebrospinal fluid (CSF) pleocytosis.[1] Included in this syndrome is meningitis with an acute onset in which the signs, symptoms, and CSF pleocytosis fail to resolve in the presence of appropriate antibacterial therapy and negative bacterial cultures. Characteristically, the patient remains symptomatic and progressively deteriorates over days to weeks until specific treatment is given. In contrast, relapsing meningitis has asymptomatic periods with normal CSF, even without therapy. Chronic meningitis is less common than acute pyogenic or viral meningitis. There is an extensive literature on specific causes, but the syndrome as a whole had not been considered in the past,[1] reflecting the difficulty in diagnosis and the vast number of possible causes.

History and physical examination are the major tools for focusing the diagnosis. Symptoms of global dysfunction such as headache or alteration in consciousness help in pointing to encephalitis, whereas clues such as cranial nerve deficits or seizures suggest localized cortical, meningeal, or vascular involvement. Evidence of systemic illness such as neoplasm, collagen-vascular disease, oral or genital ulceration, sarcoid, exposure to tuberculosis, or the use of immunosuppressive drugs should be sought. Multiple sexual contacts or a history of other venereal diseases suggests human immunodeficiency virus (HIV) infection, syphilis, or recurrent herpes simplex infection. Travel to areas endemic for illnesses such as Lyme disease, histoplasmosis, blastomycosis, coccidioidomycosis, and parasitic infection suggests important tests that may otherwise be omitted. Symptoms at extraneural sites, such as ears, mouth, and chest, should be elicited. Medications should be documented, including over-the-counter drugs such as ibuprofen, as should surgical procedures or trauma involving the spine or head.

The physical examination should evaluate any focal neurologic findings, particularly cranial neuropathy. Radiculopathy or mononeuritis may suggest spirochetal disease, systemic lupus erythematosus, or sarcoidosis. The ears and nose should be examined for masses or obstruction, the teeth for abscess or cavities, and the sinuses for tenderness or decreased transillumination. Careful examination of the lumbar area and less commonly the occiput may reveal congenital dermal sinuses or fistulae communicating to the subarachnoid space. A detailed ophthalmologic examination should be done to assess for papilledema, granulomatous uveitis, choroidal tubercles, cytoid bodies, and Roth spots. Evaluation of the lymphoreticular, skin, and musculoskeletal systems is necessary, as abnormalities of lymph nodes, skin, and muscle readily lend themselves to biopsy and specific diagnosis. Skin examination may reveal erythema nodosum, vasculitis, septic embolization, or a specific infectious lesion.

Laboratory confirmation of the suspected diagnosis is frequently difficult. Optimally, CSF cultures will be positive or serologic studies will suggest local antibody production. Because these results may be delayed and are frequently not diagnostic, extensive evaluation for extraneural disease should be quickly initiated and the results should help guide early presumptive therapy. A laboratory evaluation is suggested in Table 160–1.[2] The CSF formula comprising cell count and differential, glucose, and protein is rarely diagnostic but prioritizes the differential diagnosis and assists in guiding early empirical therapy. The predominant CSF cell type is the basis for categorization of the specific clinical entities discussed here and in Table 160–2.[3]

Lymphocytic or Mononuclear Cell Predominance

Tuberculosis

Mycobacterium tuberculosis meningitis remains the most common cause of chronic meningitis.[4] CSF inflammation occurs due to breakdown of a meningeal focus that developed at the time of primary dissemination. This breakdown may occur soon after primary spread in children. In 50% of adults, reactivation is associated with an immunocompromising condition such as chemotherapy, alcoholism, diabetes mellitus, gastrectomy, malnutrition, or pregnancy.[5] Only half of all cases have a documented exposure to tuberculosis.[6] Other conditions that depress T-cell immunity such as sarcoidosis, Hodgkin's disease, measles, organ transplantation, and HIV infection predispose to dissemination and therefore meningitis. All patients with a new diagnosis of tuberculosis, regardless of which organ systems are involved, should have a serologic test for HIV. "Atypical" mycobacteria have been documented to cause meningitis[7] but are extremely rare in non–HIV-infected patients. In HIV-infected patients, the most common organism is *Mycobacterium avium* complex. Although *M. avium* complex infection is common in patients with advanced HIV infection, spread to the CNS is uncommon. In addition, most patients have evidence of *M. avium* complex infection elsewhere in the body.[8]

TABLE 160–1 ■ Diagnostic Evaluation of Patients with Chronic Meningitis*

Suggested for all patients
Complete blood count
Chemistry panel, with attention to diabetes insipidus
Cultures of blood, urine, and sputum if possible
Chest radiograph
CT of head with infusion
ANA, rheumatoid factor, erythrocyte sedimentation rate
Serum serology for histoplasmosis, coccidioidomycosis, syphilis, and Lyme disease
Skin test with 5 TU of PPD (second-strength PPD and anergy profile if intermediate test is negative)
CSF for glucose, protein, cell count, India ink; culture for bacteria, fungus, and AFB; cryptococcal antigen and antibody; CSF VDRL; cytology
Additional studies if indicated
CSF serology for histoplasmosis, coccidioidomycosis, *Borrelia,* aspergillosis, sporotrichosis, brucellosis
CSF, blood, and urine for *Histoplasma* antigen
CSF for tuberculous antigens or antibodies, immunoglobulin G/albumin ratio
Cultures of serum or CSF for *Brucella*
MRI of head and spine to evaluate for parameningeal and parenchymal lesions
Electroencephalography
Lymph node biopsy of enlarged node
Bone marrow and liver biopsy for pathologic study and culture
Skin and muscle biopsy for vasculitis or sarcoid
Cerebral angiography

*CT, Computed tomography; ANA, antinuclear antibodies; PPD, purified protein derivative; AFB, acid-fast bacillus; CSF VDRL, cerebrospinal fluid Venereal Disease Research Laboratory; TU, tuberculin units; MRI, magnetic resonance imaging.

Modified from Wilhelm C, Ellner JJ: Chronic meningitis. Neurol Clin 4:115–141, 1986.

Clinical manifestations are not specific. The presentation can be acute, but classically it is subacute, usually spanning weeks. The duration of symptoms is usually less than a month before a physician is contacted. Fever of varying degree is almost always present.[9] Headache, nausea, and vomiting occur in 70% of cases. In a minority of cases, palsies of cranial nerves II, III, IV, VI, and VII are present, suggesting involvement of the basilar meninges. Diabetes insipidus is nonspecifically associated with tuberculous meningitis. Choroidal tubercles are rare but aid significantly in early diagnosis and should be aggressively sought. Manifestations of hydrocephalus and focal neurologic findings from infarction increase with disease progression.

A definitive diagnosis is made by culturing *M. tuberculosis* from CSF. Smears for acid-fast bacilli are positive in only 10% to 40% of patients.[10] Yield may be improved by extensive examination of an auramine-rhodamine fluorochrome stain for 20 to 60 minutes, by obtaining multiple specimens, or by centrifuging the CSF. Up to 80% of CSF samples will be positive by culture,[11] but results may require 2 to 8 weeks. Automated systems with lysis centrifugation can indicate growth within 1 to 2 weeks. DNA probes can be used to identify *M. tuberculosis* once the organism is growing in culture.[12] Polymerase chain reaction techniques are currently investigational but once available may prove to be extremely sensitive. Currently, in the absence of a positive smear, other findings must be used to make an early diagnosis. CSF hypoglycorrhachia is present in 70% to 85% of cases on admission[11, 13] and will be present in 98% of patients some time during hospitalization.[11] Fungal meningitis is also associated with a low CSF glucose level, but this finding does exclude most viral processes. With CSF lymphocytosis and an appropriate syndrome, patients with hypoglycorrhachia warrant empirical antituberculous therapy as the work-up continues. Daily fluctuations in the CSF formula may be a clue to tuberculous meningitis. This same variability limits the value of sequential analysis of CSF in monitoring the early response to therapy.

Several attempts have been made to develop rapid, specific, and sensitive tests of CSF.[14] Indirect tests include adenosine deaminase[15] and bromide partition,[16] with specificity and sensitivity of about 90%. Direct tests using radioimmunoassay[17] and gas chromatography and mass spectrometry[18] to assay tuberculous antigens seem promising. None of these are routinely available. Tests for extraneural disease are important. Chest radiographs reveal evidence of past or present tuberculosis in at least 50% of patients.[9] Sputum analysis is warranted, as 10% to 20% of patients have active pulmonary disease. Skin testing with an intermediate-strength purified protein derivative will be negative in many patients. Tests with second-strength purified protein derivative (250 tuberculin units) will be positive in 80% of patients,[19] but a lack of specificity at this concentration limits its usefulness. A negative second-strength test in the absence of anergy does not exclude tuberculous meningitis.

Outcome is strongly associated with the severity of neurologic symptoms at presentation and any delay in initiation of therapy.[5, 20] When the organism is susceptible, initial treatment consists of isoniazid, rifampin, and a third or fourth antituberculous drug such as ethambutol, pyrazinamide, or ethionamide. In such situations, standard 6- and 9-month regimens for pulmonary and extrapulmonary disease have been deemed acceptable, but data are limited. When isoniazid resistance in an area exceeds 4%, four drugs should be used initially. When a patient has tuberculosis resistant to isoniazid and rifampin, the best therapy is unknown, but three drugs to which the organism is susceptible should be used. Six- and 9-month regimens cannot currently be recommended in the presence of isoniazid or rifampin resistance. In a "trial of therapy," rifampin should be used cautiously because its broad spectrum against bacteria, fungi, and spirochetes may partially treat other infections. A response to treatment may take 2 to 4 weeks. Daily fluctuations in neurologic status and CSF abnormalities do not require alteration in treatment. In the absence of an alternative diagnosis, once initiated, antituberculous therapy should be continued for at least 12 months.

The mortality for tuberculous meningitis is 10% to 30%, and 40% of patients have persisting neurologic deficits. Mental retardation, paralysis and paresis, sphincter incontinence, and seizure disorders may be lasting residua. Severe disease has been associated with cerebral infarctions caused by an arteritis at the circle of Willis.[21] Corticosteroids have been advocated for children with infarction and also for hydrocephalus. With corticosteroids, CSF abnormalities may resolve more quickly and the risk of herniation may be decreased.[22] However, evidence of decreased morbidity and mortality is lacking and we do not support their general use. When the patient is receiving therapy and computed tomography (CT) demonstrates stable or progressive obstructive hydrocephalus and increased intracranial pressure, steroids may be tried. If there is no response, shunting has resulted in decreased mortality compared with historical controls.[23]

Fungal Meningitis

CRYPTOCOCCOSIS

Meningitis caused by *Cryptococcus neoformans* is difficult to distinguish from tuberculous meningitis, but subtle clues are

TABLE 160–2 ■ Differential Diagnoses of Chronic Meningitis by Predominant Cerebrospinal Fluid Inflammatory Cell Type

ETIOLOGY	LYMPHOCYTIC	NEUTROPHILIC	EOSINOPHILIC
Viral	Lymphocytic choriomeningitis; mumps; herpes simplex; herpes zoster; arbovirus, flavivirus, and echovirus infections	Herpes simplex, cytomegalovirus infection	
Bacterial	Tuberculosis, brucellosis, tularemia, syphilis, Lyme disease, leptospirosis, recurrent fever, nocardiosis, actinomycosis, listeriosis, subacute bacterial endocarditis	Tuberculosis, nocardiosis, actinomycosis, brucellosis, meningococcal infection in complement deficiency	Tuberculosis, syphilis
Fungal	Cryptococcosis; coccidiomycosis; histoplasmosis; blastomycosis; *Candida*, *Aspergillus*, *Zygomycetes*, and *Pseudallescheria boydii* infections	*Candida* infection; coccidioidomycosis; histoplasmosis; blastomycosis; *Aspergillus*, dematiaceous fungi, Zygomycetes, *P. boydii* infections	Coccidioidomycosis
Parasitic	Cysticercosis, paragonimiasis, schistosomiasis, *Fasciola hepatica* infection, echinococcosis, trichinosis, visceral larva migrans		*Angiostrongylus cantonensis* infection, cysticercosis, *Gnathostoma spinigerum* infection, paragonimiasis, schistosomiasis, echinococcosis, trichinosis, *Fasciola hepatica* infection, visceral larva migrans
Noninfectious	Solid neoplasm, lymphoma, leukemia, sarcoidosis, vasculitis, collagen-vascular disease, Behçet's disease, Vogt-Koyanagi-Harada syndrome	Foreign body in the central nervous system, sarcoidosis, drug induced, chemical induced, solid neoplasm	Foreign body in the central nervous system, sarcoidosis, lymphoma
Other	Parameningeal focus, benign chronic lymphocytic meningitis	Parameningeal focus	

available.[24] The onset is more gradual, taking up to 20 years from onset to diagnosis. Headache is the most common presenting symptom. Mental status changes and nuchal rigidity occur only half as often as in tuberculous meningitis. Abnormal hosts account for 50% to 80% of patients with *C. neoformans*, and this is the most common cause of subacute and chronic meningitis in this population. Most patients are immunosuppressed as a result of corticosteroids, cytotoxic drugs, hematologic malignancies, or transplants. HIV infection is the major risk factor in many centers. Today, HIV testing is warranted for all patients despite a known alternative immunocompromising condition. Physical findings, especially cranial nerve abnormalities, are less common than in tuberculous meningitis, except for optic nerve invasion with subsequent papilledema and vision loss.[2] Disease outside the CSF is frequently present but may not be clinically apparent. The chest radiograph is helpful, although less commonly than with tuberculosis. Cultures are positive from extrapulmonary sites such as skin, bone marrow, lymph nodes, and prostate in greater than one third of patients.[24]

Early diagnosis is facilitated by positive CSF India ink smear. The sensitivity of the test is unfortunately less than 50%, and false-positive results are common in less experienced laboratories. Cryptococcal antigen in the CSF is present in 85% of patients, and more than 90% of patients have the presence of either CSF or serum cryptococcal antigen. CSF cryptococcal antigen assay is at least 80% specific and is more sensitive than culture. A patient with a CSF cryptococcal antigen titer greater than 1:8 should be treated despite negative cultures.[25] Neither hypoglycorrhachia nor other routine CSF tests help in making an etiologic diagnosis.[26] No skin testing is available. CSF white cell counts greater than 20/mm³ in patients with altered mental status has been a favorable prognostic sign.[27] Hypoglycorrhachia, a positive India ink smear, and high CSF cryptococcal antigen titers portend a poor outcome. Elevated CSF pressure may also be associated with a poor outcome.

The standard treatment for cryptococcal meningitis in non–HIV-infected patients is intravenous amphotericin B (0.3 to 0.5 mg/kg per day). In the absence of preexisting bone marrow suppression, oral flucytosine (150 mg/kg per day) is usually given in combination with amphotericin B. Duration of therapy is 4 to 6 weeks, with a cumulative amphotericin B dose of 1 to 2 g.[27] If therapy is continued until the CSF cryptococcal antigen titer is less than 1:8, the relapse rate is 10%. When cryptococcal antigen titer persists in CSF, the relapse rate is 17% even with prolonged treatment.[27] Immunocompromised patients have even higher relapse rates. Although intraventricular amphotericin B given via an Ommaya reservoir is usually unnecessary, it results in earlier clearing of infection[28] and possibly reduced relapse.[24] The use of fluconazole in the treatment of non–HIV-infected patients with cryptococcal meningitis is not well studied.

Initial therapy for cryptococcal meningitis in HIV-infected patients consists of amphotericin B with or without flucytosine.[29, 30] After successful initial therapy, maintenance therapy with fluconazole is begun and continued for the remainder of the patient's life.[31] Clinical studies evaluating the efficacy of 2 weeks of amphotericin B with or without flucytosine followed by either fluconazole or itraconazole are under way. The combination of fluconazole and flucytosine and the use of the various lipid formulations of amphotericin B are investigational.[32]

COCCIDIOIDOMYCOSIS

Coccidioides immitis is a common cause of pulmonary disease in the southwestern United States, Mexico, and Central America. High skin test positivity rates in local residents indicate self-limited or subclinical infection in most persons. Meningitis may follow a prolonged latent period. Therefore, the diagnosis must be considered in a patient with a prior history of travel to an endemic area. Two thirds of patients have no risk factors for dissemination. One third of patients with meningitis are already known to have disease in other organs, but in two thirds the symptoms of meningitis are the presenting complaints.[33]

Headache, lethargy, disorientation, confusion, and coma are common and may reflect the propensity of this organism to cause hydrocephalus. Constitutional manifestations are usually present. Nodular, ulcerative, and subcutaneous skin lesions should be sought. The chest radiograph is usually abnormal, but sputum and blood cultures are rarely positive. CSF cultures are positive in only one third of patients and smears are rarely positive. Diagnosis rests on finding elevated titers of coccidioidal complement-fixing antibodies in serum or CSF.[33] Skin testing may falsely elevate the titers and should not be used diagnostically. Hypoglycorrhachia is usually present, but the CSF profile is not distinguishable from that of other fungal or mycobacterial causes of chronic meningitis.

The standard therapy for *Coccidioides* meningitis is amphotericin B. Early institution of combined systemic and local therapy is recommended, because the response is poor, especially in compromised hosts. Amphotericin B can be given intrathecally via repeated lumbar, cisternal, or lateral cervical puncture. Placement of an Ommaya reservoir is preferable to minimize arachnoiditis. However, complications such as obstruction occur in up to 85% of reservoirs.[33] Intrathecal amphotericin B is given at doses of 1.0 to 1.5 mg three times weekly for a total of at least 20 mg and preferably more than 40 mg.[34] Intravenous amphotericin B should be given for a total of 3 to 4 g. Local therapy may need to be continued after completion of systemic dosing. Drug-induced arachnoiditis may limit treatment and also makes pleocytosis uninterpretable as a reliable indicator of therapeutic response. Therapeutic response can be assessed clinically and by the disappearance of CSF antibody.

When amphotericin B has failed or is not tolerated, systemic and intrathecal miconazole has been effective.[35] Systemic itraconazole and fluconazole have also been used in the treatment of *Coccidioides* meningitis.[36, 37] Their use is increasing due to the reduced toxicity of the azoles compared with that of amphotericin B. Relapses have occurred once therapy is discontinued. Comparative studies are under way in an effort to define the optimal use of azoles in the treatment of *Coccidioides* meningitis.

INFREQUENT FUNGAL CAUSES

Less common fungal meningitides caused by *Candida* species, *Blastomyces dermatitidis, Histoplasma capsulatum,* and *Sporothrix schenckii* are associated with a predominantly lymphocytic meningitis. The clinical presentation is indistinguishable from that of the previously discussed infections. Although dissemination with these organisms is rare, meningitis is common in disseminated disease. *Candida* is an exception because it disseminates often but is an unusual cause of meningitis. *Candida* meningitis can have an acute presentation and is found in debilitated hospitalized patients with central venous catheters receiving hyperalimentation or corticosteroids. Intravenous drug addicts and premature infants are also at risk.[38] Most patients have received prior antibacterial therapy. CSF cultures are usually positive, with *Candida albicans* being the most frequent isolate. When cultures are negative, the diagnosis is rarely made ante mortem. The role of serology has yet to be defined.

B. dermatitidis has been noted in the CNS in as many as 33% of patients with disseminated disease.[39, 40] A few patients with blastomycosis have concurrent disease due to *M. tuberculosis* or malignancy. The diagnosis is made by demonstrating the organism in skin, sputum, prostatic secretions, or joints. CSF cultures are rarely positive and serology is unreliable.[39, 40] *Blastomyces* is an unusual organism in HIV-infected patients. However, disseminated blastomycosis in the setting of advanced HIV infection is frequently associated with CNS disease.[41]

Histoplasma meningitis occurs in a similar population of patients as blastomycosis. Like cryptococcal meningitis, it may be present for years before detection. The diagnosis is made by culturing the organism from bone marrow, blood, liver, lymph nodes, sputum, or urine.[42, 43] One half of patients have positive CSF cultures. Detection of *H. capsulatum* polysaccharide antigen is also useful. Tests for antigen should be performed on CSF, blood, and urine.[43] CSF antibodies are diagnostically useful with a sensitivity of almost 90%[44]; however, there is cross-reactivity with other fungi.

CNS sporotrichosis is also rare. The organism is difficult to culture, but local CSF antibody production can be used to make the diagnosis.[45] In all CNS fungal infections except for *Candida* infections, the diagnostic yield of cultures is thought to be augmented by sampling large volumes of CSF or by obtaining CSF from the ventricles. A mainstay of antemortem diagnosis is documentation of extraneural infection. Standard therapy is systemic amphotericin B, and the prognosis is related to the patient's status at the time of therapeutic intervention. Local therapy is usually unnecessary. If blastomycotic meningitis is as frequent as has been suggested, lumbar puncture will be necessary in all patients with blastomycosis, as azoles may not predictably treat asymptomatic subclinical meningitis. We currently do not recommend routine lumbar puncture in all patients with blastomycosis.

Patients with HIV infection usually use lifelong maintenance therapy to prevent relapse of disease caused by susceptible fungi. Itraconazole is effective therapy to prevent relapse in histoplasmosis.[46] The preferred agent to prevent relapse in patients with blastomycosis or coccidioidomycosis remains to be determined. In patients with advanced HIV infection ($\leq$50 $CD4^+$ cells per mm^3) who live in endemic areas, primary prophylaxis with azoles may be warranted.[47]

Chronic Bacterial Meningitis

Chronic bacterial infections can mimic tuberculous and fungal meningitis. Meningitis with these infections may be more common than appreciated, because antibiotic therapy given for systemic manifestations in the absence of CSF examination may treat subclinical meningitis. If initial treatment is suboptimal for CNS infection, localized chronic infection can develop.

The classic manifestations of systemic brucellosis are night sweats, fever, adenopathy, and hepatosplenomegaly. Neural involvement occurs in less than 5% of patients. However, one third of patients with neurobrucellosis present with an isolated meningitis syndrome.[48] Cranial nerve abnormalities, seizures, hydrocephalus, radiculopathy, and peripheral neuropathy are frequently present. The key to diagnosis is obtaining a history of exposure to unpasteurized dairy products, travel to an endemic area such as the Mediterranean or South America, or previous infection.[48] The CSF formula is abnormal but nonspecific. Hypoglycorrhachia and increased protein level are present in more than 90% of patients but do not narrow the differential diagnosis. Cultures of blood and CSF require special media and incubation of 2 to 4 weeks and are usually negative. The diagnosis can be established by use of blood or CSF agglutination titers. Although brucellosis is rarely lethal, cure is difficult and usually requires two drugs for at least 6 weeks. Tetracycline or doxycycline with rifampin or streptomycin has been effective. Trimethoprim-sulfamethoxazole may also be effective.

Meningitis caused by *Francisella tularensis* is clinically similar to brucellosis meningitis but is rare. In the setting of chronic meningitis and an appropriate zoonotic exposure, the diagnosis should be attempted by culture or serology.[49] The usual treatment is chloramphenicol. *Listeria monocytogenes* and *Neisseria meningitidis* cause acute meningitis in normal hosts. Rarely, they cause a chronic meningitis, possibly with lymphocytic preponderance, in the immunocompromised host. Isolation of one of these pathogens in association with a benign or prolonged disease course warrants an evaluation for occult immunodeficiency, for example, HIV infection with *Listeria* infection[50] or terminal complement deficiency with *N. meningitidis*.[51] Bacterial encephalitis due to Whipple's disease or cat-scratch disease may cause chronic progressive neurologic deficits with minimal meningeal involvement. Because these disorders are treatable, diagnostic brain biopsy should be performed in patients with a compatible syndrome.

A prolonged clinical course may occur when meningeal irritation is due to the gradual expansion of a parameningeal focus. Patients manifest meningismus and a sterile CSF with pleocytosis. Purulent meningitis occurs if a parameningeal abscess ruptures into the subarachnoid space. The entire neuraxis needs to be evaluated with CT or magnetic resonance imaging (MRI) because spinal epidural[52] or subdural abscess can also cause CSF pleocytosis. Thorough evaluation includes investigation for dental,[53] otic,[54] and sinus disease.

Spirochetal Meningitis

All spirochetes have a neurotropism resulting in many clinical manifestations (Table 160–3). After inoculation, these organisms disseminate hematogenously with meningeal seeding. As host defenses have not yet developed, CSF cultures may be positive at a time when patients have no CSF pleocytosis, have other CSF abnormalities, or have only systemic manifestations. This occurs in 30% of patients with syphilis.[55] Classic manifestations of secondary disease occur when an active host response develops. Relapses of secondary manifestations occur in syphilis and relapsing fever because *Treponema pallidum* and *Borrelia recurensis* alter cell surface antigens, resulting in periodic development of an immune response to new antigens.

SYPHILIS

Meningitis may occur in all spirochetal infections. Syphilitic meningitis usually appears within 2 years of infection. The rash of secondary syphilis is present only 10% of the time.[56] Fever may not be present. Abnormalities of cranial nerves VI, VII, and VIII are common. Patients may present with hydrocephalus in association with papilledema unrelated to optic neuritis.[57] Syphilitic meningitis may be self-limited or present as an acute medical emergency. A CSF pleocytosis with high protein and hypoglycorrhachia occurs, but the fluid characteristics may also mimic a viral process. The diagnosis is suggested by a positive serum treponemal test (e.g., fluorescent treponemal antibody absorption) and a positive CSF Venereal Disease Research Laboratory (VDRL) test. Although the serum VDRL result is almost always positive in patients with active syphilitic meningitis, it may be negative in tertiary disease. Appropriate therapy is high-dose penicillin (10 to 20 million units/d IV) or tetracycline (2 g/d). With suboptimal therapy, symptoms may resolve while CNS infection persists. Third-generation cephalosporins may be effective, but comparative studies with first-line therapy have not been published. Third-generation cephalosporins have failed in patients with concomitant HIV infection.[58] The development of tertiary complications, tabes dorsalis, general paresis, or gummata in a 10- to 30-year period can be considered sequelae of a long-term chronic meningitis.[59] Therefore, we may need to be more aggressive in treating early syphilis.[60]

LYME DISEASE

Lyme disease, caused by *Borrelia burgdorferi*, is an etiologic factor in chronic meningitis. In Europe, Bannwarth syndrome, or lymphocytic meningoradiculitis, is probably the same disease. About 15% of patients who contract Lyme disease develop symptomatic meningitis.[61] This occurs in the second stage of the disease, several months after tick exposure and initial infection; hence, there is a preponderance in late summer and early fall. Patients usually present with headache. Two thirds have symptoms of radiculopathy, usually in a distribution associated with the antecedent tick bite. Cranial and peripheral nerve abnormalities are common, Bell palsy being the most frequent.[62]

Lyme disease should be considered in the differential diagnosis of any aseptic meningitis. Many patients cannot give a history of tick bite or the characteristic rash, erythema chronicum migrans. Therefore, history of exposure in an endemic area needs to be sought. The CSF formula varies widely. Most patients have CSF pleocytosis and elevated protein level; 15% have hypoglycorrhachia.[62] A false-positive CSF VDRL test can occur but false-positive treponemal tests do not. Local CSF antibody production occurs, but serologic studies lack sensitivity. Twelve percent of patients are negative on tests from both serum and CSF.[62] Early treatment may confound serodiagnosis without eradicating infection. Patients respond well to treatment with high-dose intravenous penicillin or ceftriaxone. A 4-week duration of therapy may be preferable to the usually recommended 2 weeks. If the longer duration is used, therapy for at least 14 days should be parenteral. Oral doxycycline or amoxicillin can be used to complete therapy. Later in the infection, patients may have other neurologic manifestations such as chronic fatigue or psychiatric symptoms[51] (see Table 160–3). The pathogenesis of these symptoms is not well understood, but when present, meningeal symptoms or CSF pleocytosis is rare.

TABLE 160–3 ■ Spirochetal Infections Commonly Associated with Neurologic Manifestations

DISEASE	EXPOSURE	PRIMARY LESION	SECONDARY NEUROLOGIC MANIFESTATION	TERTIARY NEUROLOGIC MANIFESTATION
Syphilis	Sexual	Chancre	Meningitis	Meningovascular infarcts Tabes dorsalis General paresis
Lyme disease	*Ixodes* ticks (deer, mice, birds)	Erythema chronicum migrans	Meningitis	Multiple sclerosis–like syndrome Psychiatric changes Chronic fatigue syndrome
Leptospirosis	Rodents, dogs	"Leptospiremia"	Meningitis	None
Relapsing fever	Ticks, lice		Meningitis	None

OTHER SPIROCHETES

Other spirochetal infections also present as acute or subacute meningitis. In 24% of patients hospitalized with Weil disease, clinical meningitis occurs concomitantly with other systemic manifestations of leptospirosis.[64] Dog, animal, or natural water exposures are the epidemiologic clues. Relapsing fever caused by *Borrelia recurensis* is associated with CNS manifestations in 8% of tick-borne and 30% of louse-borne disease.[65] Cranial nerve abnormalities are common. The CSF formula in both these conditions is similar to that observed in other spirochetal diseases. There are no chronic sequelae and the illnesses are ultimately self-limiting. Both respond to appropriate treatment, but evidence that therapy alters long-term neurologic outcome is limited. Any spirochetal illness may be associated with a Jarisch-Herxheimer reaction. Patients should be closely observed for several hours after initiation of therapy.

Viral Central Nervous System Infection

Viral CNS infection usually presents as encephalitis or meningoencephalitis with altered levels of consciousness. CSF pleocytosis may be present. Although the CSF glucose level is usually normal, hypoglycorhachia has been observed with mumps, lymphocytic choriomeningitis, and herpesvirus infection.[66] Chronic viral infection is classically associated with the slow viruses that cause kuru, Creutzfeldt-Jakob disease, or the measles-like virus of subacute sclerosing panencephalitis. Human T-cell lymphotropic virus type I[67] and HIV[68] have become significant causes of encephalitis manifested by a chronic CSF pleocytosis without meningeal symptoms. Immune defects can predispose to chronic infection. Malignancy, organ transplantation, and acquired immunodeficiency syndrome have been associated with progressive multifocal leukoencephalopathy.[69] Agammaglobulinemia predisposes to chronic echovirus or coxsackievirus meningoencephalitis spanning months to years.[70] Some of the abovementioned diagnoses can be made serologically, but often brain biopsy is necessary. Biopsy is generally diagnostic if directed toward regions of abnormality as seen by electroencephalography or MRI. Blind biopsy has a low yield.

Carcinomatous Meningitis

Chronic meningitis occurs without infection. Metastatic malignancy presenting as meningitis before detection of the primary tumor occurs with carcinoma of the breast and lung, lymphoma, and melanoma. Clinical suspicion is increased by noncontiguous focal deficits suggestive of multiple areas of involvement, and by a greater severity of signs and symptoms.[71] Headache, change in mental status, and back or radicular pain are frequent. Fever is rare. On presentation, 52% of patients have mental status changes and 60% have absent reflexes in an extremity.[71] Cranial nerve abnormalities and pareses are common. The CSF formula is nondiagnostic. Pleocytosis may be absent but the profile is rarely normal. Elevation of CSF lactate dehydrogenase is suggestive of malignancy.[72] Cytology is positive in half of initial lumbar punctures, and examining multiple specimens increases the yield to 80%. Imaging studies demonstrate lesions corresponding to cranial or spinal nerve deficits. CT, MRI, and metrizamide myelography are the procedures of choice. Long-term prognosis is poor, but neurologic function can be improved with treatment.[73]

Idiopathic Disorders Causing Meningitis

SARCOIDOSIS

Sarcoidosis has neurologic manifestations in 5% of cases, and in half of these they are the presenting manifestations.[74] Bell palsy or other cranial nerve deficits are typical. Decreased visual acuity, hydrocephalus, diabetes insipidus, and seizures may occur. Single or multiple brain masses can involve any area of the neuraxis. When granulomatous involvement of the basal meninges predominates, the disease is indistinguishable from tuberculous meningitis.[75] There is chest or eye involvement in 88% and 55% of patients, respectively.[74] The CSF findings are normal in half of the patients with neurologic signs or symptoms. Only 9% have hypoglycorrhachia, but results of head CT are abnormal in greater than one third.

Diagnosis is by exclusion of infectious and neoplastic diseases and demonstration of noncaseating granulomata on biopsy. Extraneural tissues such as lung, lymph nodes, conjuctiva, or liver are usually available for biopsy. With isolated CNS disease, the diagnosis may require biopsy of abnormal areas detected by head CT or MRI. Peripheral or spinal nerve biopsies may be positive. Elevation of serum angiotensin-converting enzyme is characteristic but not pathognomonic. Steroids are recommended in neurosarcoidosis but controlled studies of their use are unavailable. Because of the similarity of sarcoidosis, tuberculosis, and fungal meningitis, steroids should not be given until these other diagnoses have been excluded.[76]

SYSTEMIC VASCULITIS

Systemic vasculitides, with the exception of giant cell arteritis, have caused meningeal inflammation with abnormal CSF. Symptoms and signs are usually due to focal ischemia or infarction, but diffuse meningoencephalitis also occurs.[77] Polyarteritis nodosa is characterized by peripheral neuropathies. Hepatitis B surface antigen is present in at least 15% of patients. Muscle biopsy, sural nerve biopsy, or renal angiography may establish the diagnosis.[78] In contrast, Wegener granulomatosis, lymphomatoid granulomatosis, and isolated CNS angiitis have cranial nerve or focal findings. However, clinical overlap is great. In suspected Wegener and lymphomatoid granulomatosis, head CT frequently reveals hypodense lesions consistent with infarction.[77] A thorough search must be made for the expected sites of extraneural disease: lungs, sinuses, and kidneys. If no extraneural disease is present, cerebral angiography will be necessary. A beaded pattern is characteristic.[79] Caution is necessary because many infectious diseases previously discussed can cause a similar arteriographic pattern. If the evaluation is not diagnostic, brain biopsy will be necessary before making a decision to initiate steroids or cytotoxic therapy.[77] During treatment, patients must be monitored for the emergence of disseminated tuberculosis or fungal infection.

Collagen-vascular disease can present with CNS vasculitis associated with CSF pleocytosis.[80] Complement levels, circulating immune complexes, and serologic evaluation for systemic lupus erythematosus, Sjögren syndrome, and rheumatoid arthritis should be performed. CNS vasculitis has also been present in cat-scratch disease, herpes encephalitis, and Hodgkin's disease. Atrial myxoma and subacute bacterial endocarditis may be associated with immune complex disease and vasculitis. Blood cultures, electrocardiography, and cardiac ultrasonography are warranted to evaluate these processes.

BEHÇET'S DISEASE

Behçet's disease usually manifests the triad of oral and genital ulcers, skin lesions, and uveitis. Twenty-five percent of patients develop meningoencephalitis. Neurologic symptoms are nonspecific but are almost always associated with a flare of oral or genital ulcers.[81] These lesions are frequently asymptomatic, necessitating a thorough examination. Ophthalmologic findings occur later in the disease. The CSF usually shows a pleocytosis and increased protein level, even in patients without neurologic symptoms. The CSF glucose value is normal. The clinical course is notable for episodes of deterioration, sometimes acute, alternating with periods of stability but not spontaneous resolution.[81] Most manifestations improve with corticosteroid or cytotoxic therapy.

VOGT-KOYANAGI-HARADA SYNDROME

Vogt-Koyanagi-Harada syndrome is a rare disease of unknown cause characterized by meningoencephalitis, skin lesions, and uveitis. People with darker pigmentation appear more susceptible. Photophobia, headache, ocular pain, bilateral visual impairment, and intracranial hypertension are common.[82] The ophthalmic and neurologic symptoms usually present within days of each other and persist for several weeks. Sensorineural deafness, diabetes insipidus, or other focal findings usually follow meningitis.[83] Alopecia, poliosis (whitened eyebrows and lashes), and vitiligo occur in one third of patients and also typically follow the meningitis.[82] The severity of sequelae does not correlate with the severity of the initial symptoms. On presentation, 81% of patients have a CSF pleocytosis. The diagnosis is primarily clinical but is supported by the ophthalmologic findings of granular inflammation of the iris, ciliary body, and retina. Treatment is with corticosteroids or cytotoxic drugs.

Neutrophilic Predominance

Chronic neutrophilic meningitis is a syndrome with persistent CSF neutrophils for greater than 1 week, negative bacterial cultures, and no response to routine antibacterial therapy.[84] Prolonged CSF neutrophilic pleocytosis is occasionally seen in patients with more typical lymphocytic meningeal processes including candidiasis, brucellosis, tuberculosis, blastomycosis, histoplasmosis, and coccidioidomycosis (see Table 160–2). This usually occurs early in the illness but can be perpetuated by treatment.[85] However, several chronic meningitides are associated with a preponderance of CSF neutrophils throughout the course of the illness.

Bacterial Meningitis

Actinomyces and *Nocardia* species are bacterial causes of this syndrome. Actinomycosis usually occurs in a normal host with a portal of entry.[86] The source is typically the mouth where the organism is normal flora. There may be an otic focus. A primary pulmonary process may result from aspiration in alcoholics. CNS involvement occurs by direct invasion or hematogenous seeding. Although typically associated with abscess formation, 13% of neural actinomycosis was found to be meningitis or meningoencephalitis.[86]

In the absence of trauma, nervous system nocardiosis is associated with disseminated disease in normal patients or those with depressed cell-mediated immunity, typically after transplantation or steroid therapy. Persons with pulmonary alveolar proteinosis, Cushing's disease, and systemic lupus erythematosus are at specific risk. As with actinomycosis, intracerebral abscess formation is a classic finding and should be prospectively sought. Isolated meningitis does occur and the diagnosis can be made by CSF culture.[87]

Fungal Meningitis

Fungal causes of neutrophilic pleocytosis typically present in an indolent fashion. Although most patients with *Candida* meningitis have a lymphocytic predominance, a significant proportion may present with a neutrophilic process.[38] The important fungal diseases that typically present with a neutrophilic predominance include *Aspergillus* infections, zygomycosis, and *Pseudallescheria boydii* infections. CNS infection caused by *Aspergillus* species is usually associated with disseminated disease in a neutropenic patient. Zygomycosis (mucormycosis) is associated with oral, nasal, or facial disease in a diabetic or acidotic host. Altered mental status, stroke syndromes, or space-occupying lesions are more typical presentations. These may present with meningitis without mass effect, particularly if they follow surgery of the neural axis.[84] *P. boydii* and dematiaceous fungi can also cause meningitis without a demonstrable brain mass.[88] These are common soil fungi inoculated after penetrating injuries to the cranial vault or orbit. Disseminated disease occurs in immunosuppressed persons, typically renal or bone marrow transplant recipients. *P. boydii* is important to consider as patients respond to miconazole more predictably than to amphotericin B.[89] Difficulty in establishing disease caused by these fungi is related to the low yield of CSF culture and a lack of sensitive or specific serologic tests.[84] Diagnoses can be made by isolating the organism from an extraneural site such as sinuses, ears, lungs, or wounds. Skin lesions should be sought and biopsies performed. A search for mass lesions along the neuraxis should be done with CT and MRI. If a lesion is seen, surgery may be required for diagnosis and therapy.

Viral Meningitis

A cytomegalovirus-induced polyradiculopathy in patients with advanced HIV infection presents with weakness and sensory loss coupled with a neutrophilic predominant CSF.[90, 91] The diagnosis can be confirmed with viral cultures. Polymerase chain reaction techniques are useful in establishing the diagnosis quickly. Early treatment with ganciclovir may be beneficial.[92]

Drug-Induced Meningitis

Meningitis associated with systemic medications is usually neutrophilic and acute in onset. Common causes include isoniazid, sulfonamides, γ-globulin, and OKT3 monoclonal antibody. Patients with underlying collagen-vascular disease, especially mixed connective tissue disease, appear predisposed to this syndrome associated with nonsteroidal antiinflammatory agents. Occasionally, the disease course is subacute or chronic. Chronic neutrophilic meningitis is more typical when due to contrast myelography or methylprednisolone injections.[75] Other substances used in intrathecal injection, such as antibiotics, methotrexate, or contaminating disinfectants, have also caused neutrophilic meningitis.

Eosinophilic Predominance

Eosinophilic meningitis is rare[93] (see Table 160–2). Peripheral and CSF eosinophilia is well described in coccidioidomycosis but is less common with other nonparasitic causes of chronic meningitis. Helminthic infections predominate. Worldwide, the most frequent cause is *Angiostrongylus cantonensis*, the rat lung worm. This is acquired by ingesting raw fish, mollusks, and snails in the Far East and Pacific Islands, including Hawaii.[94] Patients present subacutely with symptoms of meningitis and fever without other findings. The diagnosis is primarily clinical, based on CSF eosinophilia with an appropriate exposure history. Serologic tests are being developed.[94] In Southeast Asia, *Gnathostoma spinigerum* also presents as an eosinophilic meningitis but in association with painful radiculopathy, subarachnoid hemorrhage, and symptoms of visceral and cutaneous larva migrans.[95]

Cysticercosis is the other parasitic infection that usually presents with isolated CNS findings. Seizures or symptoms associated with increased intracranial pressure and space-occupying lesions are classic, but meningitis occurs.[96] Eosinophilia is present in half of early inflammatory cases and is helpful in suggesting the diagnosis if there has been exposure in an endemic region. The characteristic lesions are usually present at CT or MRI. Diagnosis is assisted by serology.[97] Even with space-occupying lesions, the prognosis is good if hydrocephalus is not present. Praziquantel is currently the therapy of choice. Albendazole may be more efficacious and has been released in the United States.[98]

Other parasitic infections associated with eosinophilic meningitis usually have manifestations outside the CNS and the diagnosis is based on extraneural identification. Fresh stool for ova and parasite examination should be obtained on at least three occasions when a patient has unexplained CSF eosinophilia. Despite an absence of eosinophilia, parasites such as *Schistosoma, Paragonimus westermani,* and *Echinococcus* warrant consideration if patients with unexplained chronic meningitis have traveled to endemic regions. In immunocompromised patients, disseminated strongyloidiasis and strongyloides meningitis occur without eosinophilia.[99] Strongyloidiasis should be considered as a source of persistent or relapsing gram-negative bacteremia or gram-negative bacterial meningitis.

Approach to the Patient

Despite a thorough evaluation for CNS or extraneural diseases, a pathogen will not be identified in 30% to 50% of patients with subacute or chronic meningitis.[4] Many patients respond to empirical antituberculous treatment, particularly children and patients from endemic areas.[4] Undiagnosed patients with CSF pleocytosis and without spontaneous resolution of symptoms should receive empirical treatment with three antituberculous drugs, even in the absence of hypoglycorrhachia. This should be continued for at least 4 weeks before concluding a lack of response. Initiation of empirical therapy should not delay additional diagnostic evaluation. This includes CT or MRI of the entire neural axis, cerebral angiography if vasculitis is suspected, and when feasible, brain biopsy of any lesions seen on these studies. Blind biopsy has a much lower yield and is not generally recommended.[2, 4] If the patient progresses on antituberculous therapy, empirical intravenous amphotericin B should be initiated if there has been a previous exposure to an area endemic for histoplasmosis, blastomycosis, or coccidioidomycosis. Negative serologic evaluation does not preclude a trial of amphotericin B. Again, several weeks are needed to assess a response. Such combinations of empirical therapy can become confusing when a beneficial response occurs. In general, empirical antibiotics should be continued for a full course unless a definitive alternative diagnosis is made.

Trials of steroids may be warranted in the progressively declining patient, but we rarely recommend their empirical use, and then only when the patient is simultaneously receiving antituberculous treatment and amphotericin B. Patients with undiagnosed tuberculosis and fungal infections may progress despite a transient clinical response or improved CSF pleocytosis associated with steroids. Patients with diseases requiring steroid therapy may need indefinite treatment to prevent relapse. More likely they will subsequently tolerate steroid tapering and withdrawal.[4] Many of these patients may have chronic benign lymphocytic meningitis. This entity consists of minimal localizing symptoms, normal CSF glucose value, and a lymphocytic pleocytosis that gradually decreases and resolves without therapy.[100] The cause is presumed to be similar to other aseptic meningitides, but with a prolonged resolution. This diagnosis of exclusion can be made only after the patient has recovered without receiving antimicrobial therapy. If a patient has already received antibiotics, a full course will be necessary as a therapeutic response is indistinguishable from this benign self-limited condition.

Recurrent Meningitis

Recurrent meningitis is a distinctly different syndrome in which episodes are separated by asymptomatic periods with normal CSF. Recurrent infection with *N. meningiditis* suggests a terminal complement deficiency. Although skin flora such as *Staphylococcus epidermidis* or *Propionibacterium acnes* suggests an epidermal fistula, recurrent *Streptococcus pneumoniae*[101] or *Haemophilus influenzae*[102] meningitis suggests a CSF communication to the ears or nasopharynx. Localization of CSF leaks may require an arduous search by metrizamide cisternography, radioiodinated albumin studies, gadolinium MRI, or any combination of these. Other infectious causes of recurrent meningitis include *Brucella, M. tuberculosis, Cryptococcus,* viruses, and hydatid cysts. Noninfectious diseases include migraine, systemic lupus erythematosus, sarcoidosis, Behçet's disease, and Vogt-Koyanagi-Harada syndrome.[103] The intermittent rupture of a dermoid cyst or intracranial tumor can cause an episodic sterile reactive meningitis diagnosed only by thorough physical examination, CT, or MRI.

Mollaret meningitis is a condition frequently considered a chronic meningitis but one that actually has a recurrent presentation. The onset is abrupt and includes transient focal neurologic findings such as seizures, delirium, cranial nerve dysfunction, and abnormal reflexes.[103] The CSF is characterized by pleocytosis, including cells termed "endothelial" by Mollaret but that are actually large monocytes. Both the symptoms and the CSF abnormalities resolve in several days with or without treatment. The cause is unknown, but patients have been reported with polymerase chain reaction evidence of herpes simplex virus type 1 and, more commonly, type 2.[104, 105] Indeed, herpes simplex virus is likely a common cause of relapsing lymphocytic meningitis. Acyclovir may be helpful in acute treatment and possibly in prophylaxis. Further study is needed.[105]

References

1. Ellner JJ, Bennett JE: Chronic meningitis. Medicine (Baltimore) 55:341–369, 1976.
2. Wilhelm C, Ellner JJ: Chronic meningitis. Neurol Clin 4:115–141, 1986.
3. Swartz MN: "Chronic meningitis"—Many causes to consider. N Engl J Med 317:957–959, 1987.
4. Anderson NE, Willoughby EW: Chronic meningitis without predisposing illness—A review of 83 cases. Q J Med 63:283–295, 1987.
5. Klein NC, Damsker B, Hirschman SZ: Mycobacterial meningitis: Retrospective analysis from 1970 to 1983. Am J Med 79:29–34, 1985.
6. Kennedy DH, Fallon RJ: Tuberculous meningitis. JAMA 241:264–268, 1979.
7. Lincoln EM, Gilbert LA: Diseases in children due to mycobacteria other than *Mycobacterium tuberculosis.* Am Rev Respir Dis 105:683–714, 1972.
8. Benson CA: Disease due to the *Mycobacterium avium* complex in patients with AIDS: Epidemiology and clinical syndrome. Clin Infect Dis 18(Suppl 3):S218–S222, 1994.
9. Ogawa SK, Smith MA, Brenuessel DJ, Lowy FD: Tuberculous

meningitis in an urban medical center. Medicine (Baltimore) 66:317–326, 1987.
10. Root TE, Harris AA, Levin S: Diagnosis and treatment of tuberculous and fungal meningitis. *In* Klawans HL (ed): Clinical Neuropharmacology, Vol. 2. New York, Raven Press, 1977, pp 151–177.
11. Lepper MH, Spies HW: The present status of the treatment of tuberculosis of the central nervous system. Ann N Y Acad Sci 106:106–123, 1963.
12. Peterson EM, Lu R, Floyd C, et al: Direct identification of *Mycobacterium tuberculosis, Mycobacterium avium,* and *Mycobacterium intracellulare* from amplified primary cultures in BACTEC media using DNA probes. J Clin Microbiol 27:1542–1547, 1989.
13. Hinman AR: Tuberculous meningitis at Cleveland Metropolitan General Hospital, 1959 to 1963. Am Rev Respir Dis 95:670–673, 1967.
14. Daniel TM: New approaches to the rapid diagnosis of tuberculous meningitis. J Infect Dis 155:599–602, 1987.
15. Rivera E, Martinez-Vazquez JM, Ocana I, et al: Activity of adenosine deaminase in cerebrospinal fluid for the diagnosis and follow-up of tuberculous meningitis in adults. J Infect Dis 155:603–607, 1987.
16. Coovadia YM, Dawood A, Ellis ME, et al: Evaluation of adenosine deaminase activity and antibody to *Mycobacterium tuberculosis* antigen 5 in cerebrospinal fluid and the radioactive bromide partition test for the early diagnosis of tuberculosis meningitis. Arch Dis Child 61:428–435, 1986.
17. Kadival GV, Samuel AM, Mazarelo TBMS, Chaparas SD: Radioimmunoassay for detecting *Mycobacterium tuberculosis* antigen in cerebrospinal fluids of patients with tuberculosis meningitis. J Infect Dis 155:608–611, 1987.
18. French GL, Chan CY, Cheung SW, et al: Diagnosis of tuberculous meningitis by detection of tuberculosteric acid in cerebrospinal fluid. Lancet 2:117–119, 1987.
19. Steiner P, Portugaleza C: Tuberculous meningitis in children. Am Rev Respir Dis 107:22–29, 1973.
20. Freiman I, Geefhuysen J: Evaluation of intrathecal therapy with streptomycin and hydrocortisone in tuberculous meningitis. J Pediatr 76:895–901, 1970.
21. Leiguarda R, Berthier M, Starkstein S, et al: Ischemic infarction in 25 children with tuberculous meningitis. Stroke 19:200–204, 1988.
22. O'Toole RD, Thornton GF, et al: Dexamethasone in tuberculous meningitis. Ann Intern Med 70:39–47, 1969.
23. Bulloch MR, Van Dellen JR: The role of cerebrospinal fluid shunting in tuberculous meningitis. Surg Neurol 18:274–277, 1982.
24. Stockstill MT, Kauffman CA: Comparison of cryptococcal and tuberculous meningitis. Arch Neurol 40:81–85, 1983.
25. Snow RM, Dismukes WE: Cryptococcal meningitis: Diagnostic value of cryptococcal antigen in cerebrospinal fluid. Arch Intern Med 134:1155–1157, 1975.
26. Butler WT, Alling DW, Spickard A, Utz JP: Diagnostic and prognostic value of clinical and laboratory findings in cryptococcal meningitis. N Engl J Med 270:59–67, 1964.
27. Dismukes WE, Cloud G, Gallis HA, et al: Treatment of cryptococcal meningitis with combination amphotericin B and flucytosine for four as compared with six weeks. N Engl J Med 317:334–341, 1987.
28. Polsky B, Depman MR, Gold JWM, et al: Intraventricular therapy of cryptococcal meningitis via a subcutaneous reservoir. Am J Med 81:24–28, 1986.
29. Larsen RA, Leal MAE, Chan LS: Fluconazole compared with amphotericin B plus flucytosine for cryptococcal meningitis in AIDS: A randomized trial. Ann Intern Med 113:183–187, 1990.
30. Saag MS, Powderly WG, Cloud GC, et al: Comparison of amphotericin B with fluconazole in the treatment of acute AIDS-associated cryptococcal meningitis. N Engl J Med 326:83–89, 1992.
31. Powderly WG, Saag MS, Cloud GA, et al: A controlled trial of fluconazole or amphotericin B to prevent relapse of cryptococcal meningitis in patients with the acquired immunodeficiency syndrome. N Engl J Med 326:793–798, 1992.
32. Larsen RA, Bozzette SA, Jones BE, et al: Fluconazole combined with flucytosine for treatment of cryptococcal meningitis in patients with AIDS. Clin Infect Dis 19:741–745, 1994.
33. Bouza E, Dreyer JS, Hewitt WL, Meyer RD: Coccidioidal meningitis: An analysis of thirty-one cases and review of the literature. Medicine (Baltimore) 60:139–172, 1981.
34. Labadie EL, Hamilton RH: Survival improvement in coccidioidal meningitis by high-dose intrathecal amphotericin B. Arch Intern Med 146:2013–2018, 1986.
35. Stevens DA: Miconazole in the treatment of coccidioidomycosis. Drugs 26:347–354, 1983.
36. Tucker RA, Denning DW, DuPont B, et al: Itraconazole therapy of chronic coccidioidal meningitis. Ann Intern Med 112:108–112, 1990.
37. Galgiani JN, Catanzaro A, Cloud GA, et al: Fluconazole therapy for coccidioidal meningitis. Ann Intern Med 119:28–35, 1993.
38. Bayer AS, Edwards JE, Seidrl JS, Guze LB: *Candida* meningitis: Report of seven cases and review of the English literature. Medicine (Baltimore) 55:477–486, 1976.
39. Kravitz GR, Davies SF, Eckman MR, Sarosi GA: Chronic blastomycotic meningitis. Am J Med 71:501–505, 1981.
40. Gonyea EF: The spectrum of primary blastomycotic meningitis: A review of central nervous system blastomycosis. Ann Neurol 3:26–39, 1978.
41. Pappas PG, Pottage JC Jr, Powderly WG, et al: Blastomycosis in patients with the acquired immunodeficiency syndrome. Ann Intern Med 116:847–853, 1992.
42. Karalakulasingam R, Arora KK, Adams G, et al: Meningoencephalitis caused by *Histoplasma capsulatum.* Arch Intern Med 136:217–220, 1976.
43. Wheat LJ, Batteiger BE, Sathapatayovongs B: *Histoplasma capsulatum* infections of the central nervous system: A clinical review. Medicine (Baltimore) 69:244–260, 1990.
44. Wheat J, French M, Batteiger B, Kohler R: Cerebrospinal fluid histoplasma antibodies in central nervous system histoplasmosis. Arch Intern Med 145:1237–1240, 1985.
45. Scott NE, Kaufman L, Brown AC, Muchmore HG: Serologic studies in the diagnosis and management of meningitis due to *Sporothrix schenckii.* N Engl J Med 317:935–940, 1987.
46. Wheat LJ, Hafner R, Wulfsohn M, et al: Prevention of relapse of histoplasmosis with itraconazole in patients with the acquired immunodeficiency syndrome. Ann Intern Med 118:610–616, 1993.
47. USPHS/IDSA, Prevention of Opportunistic Infections Working Group: USPHS/IDSA guidelines for the prevention of opportunistic infections in persons infected with the human immunodeficiency virus: Disease specific recommendations. Clin Infect Dis 21(Suppl 1):32–43, 1995.
48. Bouza E, de la Torre MG, Parras F, et al: Brucellar meningitis. Rev Infect Dis 9:810–822, 1987.
49. Lovell VM, Cho CT, Lindsey NJ, Nelson PL: *Francisella tularesis* meningitis: A rare clinical entity. J Infect Dis 154:916–918, 1986.
50. Harvey RL, Chandrasekar PH: Chronic meningitis caused by *Listeria* in a patient infected with human immunodeficiency virus. J Infect Dis 157:1091–1092, 1988.
51. Rosen MS, Lorber B, Myer AR: Chronic meningococcal meningitis: An association with C5 deficiency. Arch Intern Med 148:1441–1442, 1988.
52. Danner RL, Hartman BJ: Update of spinal epidural abscess: 35 cases and review of the literature. Rev Infect Dis 9:265–274, 1987.
53. Hedstrom SA, Nord CE, Ursing B: Chronic meningitis in patients with dental infections. Scand J Infect Dis 12:117–121, 1980.
54. Habib RG, Girgis NI, Abu El Ella AH, et al: The treatment and outcome of intracranial infection of otogenic origin. J Trop Med Hyg 91:83–86, 1988.
55. Lukehart SA, Hook EW: Invasion of the central nervous system by *Treponema pallidum*: Implications for diagnosis and treatment. Ann Intern Med 109:855–862, 1988.
56. Simon RP: Neurosyphilis. Arch Neurol 42:606–613, 1985.
57. Trenholme GM, Harris AA: Syphilitic meningitis with papilledema. South Med J 70:1013–1014, 1977.
58. Dowell ME, Ross PG, Musher DM, et al: Response of latent syphilis or neurosyphilis to ceftriaxone therapy in persons infected with HIV. Am J Med 93:481–488, 1992.
59. Hotson JR: Modern neurosyphilis: A partially treated chronic meningitis. West J Med 135:191–200, 1981.
60. Musher DM: How much penicillin cures early syphilis? Ann Intern Med 109:849–851, 1988.

61. Pachner AR: Spirochetal diseases of the CNS. Neurol Clin 4:207–222, 1986.
62. Stierstedt G, Gustafsson R: Clinical manifestations and diagnosis of neuroborreliosis. Ann N Y Acad Sci 539:46–55, 1988.
63. Finkel MF: Lyme disease and its neurologic complications. Arch Neurol 45:99–104, 1988.
64. Lecour H, Miranda M: Human leptospirosis—A review of 50 cases. Infection 17:8–12, 1989.
65. Southern PM, Sanford JP: Relapsing fever: A clinical and microbiologic review. Medicine (Baltimore) 48:129–149, 1969.
66. Fishman RA: Cerebrospinal Fluid in Diseases of the Nervous System. Philadelphia, WB Saunders, 1980, pp 269–272.
67. Yokota T, Yamada M, Furukawa T, Tsukagoshi H: HTLV-I associated meningitis. J Neurol 235:129–130, 1988.
68. McArthur JC, Cohen BA, Farzedegan H, et al: Cerebrospinal fluid abnormalities in homosexual men with and without neuropsychiatric findings. Ann Neurol 23(Suppl):S34–S37, 1988.
69. Richardson EP: Progressive multifocal leukoencephalopathy 30 years later. N Engl J Med 315–317, 1988.
70. McKinney RE, Katz SL, Wilfert CM: Chronic enteroviral meningoencephalitis in agammaglobulinemic patients. Rev Infect Dis 9:334–356, 1987.
71. Olson ME, Chernik NL, Posner JB: Infiltration of the leptomeninges by systemic cancer. Arch Neurol 30:122–137, 1974.
72. Twijnstra A, Zanten AP Van, Hart AAM, Ongerboer de Visser BW: Serial lumbar and ventricle cerebrospinal fluid lactate dehydrogenase activities in patients with leptomeningeal metastases from solid and haematological tumours. J Neurol Neurosurg Psychiatry 50:313–320, 1987.
73. Wasserstrom WR, Glass JP, Posner JB: Diagnosis and treatment of leptomeningeal metastases from solid tumors: Experience with 90 patients. Cancer 49:759–772, 1982.
74. Stern BJ, Krumholz A, Johns C, et al: Sarcoidosis and its neurological manifestations. Arch Neurol 42:909–917, 1985.
75. Reik L: Disorders that mimic CNS infections. Neurol Clin 4:223–248, 1986.
76. Cahill DW, Salcman M: Neurosarcoidosis: A review of the rarer manifestations. Surg Neurol 15:204–211, 1981.
77. Moore PM, Cupps TR: Neurological complications of vasculitis. Ann Neurol 14:155–167, 1983.
78. Smith C, Rae SA, Berry H: Polyarteritis nodosa presenting as meningoencephalitis. J R Soc Med 80:704–705, 1987.
79. Calabrese LH, Malleh JA: Primary angiitis of the central nervous system: Report of 8 new cases, review of the literature, and proposal for diagnostic criteria. Medicine (Baltimore) 67:20–39, 1988.
80. Sigal LH: The neurologic presentation of vasculitic and rheumatologic syndromes: A review. Medicine (Baltimore) 66:157–180, 1987.
81. Alema G: Behçet's disease. *In* Vinken RJ, Bruyn GW, Klawans HL (eds): Handbook of Clinical Neurology, Vol 34. Amsterdam, Elsevier, 1978, pp 475–512.
82. Manor RS: Vogt-Koyanagi-Harada syndrome and related diseases. *In* Vinken PJ, Bruyn GW, Klawans HL (eds): Handbook of Clinical Neurology, Vol 34. Amsterdam, Elsevier, 1978, pp 513–544.
83. Pattison EM: Uveomeningoencephalitis syndrome (Vogt-Koyanagi-Harada). Arch Neurol 12:197–205, 1965.
84. Peacock JE, McGinnis MR, Cohen MS: Persistent neutrophilic meningitis: Report of four cases and review of the literature. Medicine (Baltimore) 63:379–395, 1984.
85. Teoh R, O'Mahony G, Yeung VTF: Polymorphonuclear pleocytosis in the cerebrospinal fluid during chemotherapy for tuberculous meningitis. J Neurol 233:237–241, 1986.
86. Smego RA: Actinomycosis of the central nervous system. Rev Infect Dis 9:855–865, 1987.
87. Buggy BP: *Nocardia asteroides* meningitis without brain abscess. Rev Infect Dis 9:228–231, 1987.
88. Kershaw P, Freeman R, Templeton D, et al: *Pseudallescheria boydii* infection of the central nervous system. Arch Neurol 47:468–472, 1990.
89. Lutwick LI, Rytel MW, Yanez JP, et al: Deep infections from *Petriellidium boydii* treated with miconazole. JAMA 241:272–273, 1979.
90. Behar R, Wiley C, McCutchan JA: Cytomegalovirus polyradiculopathy in acquired immunodeficiency syndrome. Neurology 37:557–561, 1987.
91. Said G, LaCroix C, Chemouilli P, et al: Cytomegalovirus neuropathy in acquired immunodeficiency syndrome: A clinical and pathological study. Ann Neurol 29:139–146, 1989.
92. Miller RG, Storey J, Greco C: Ganciclovir treatment of lumbosacral polyradiculopathy in AIDS. Lancet 334:48–49, 1990.
93. Kuberski T: Eosinophils in the cerebrospinal fluid. Ann Intern Med 91:70–75, 1979.
94. Koo J, Pien F, Kliks MM: *Angiostrongylus (Parastrongylus)* eosinophilic meningitis. Rev Infect Dis 10:1155–1161, 1988.
95. Schmutzhard E, Boongird P, Vejjajiva A: Eosinophilic meningitis and radiculomyelitis in Thailand, caused by CNS invasion of *Gnathostoma spinigerum* and *Angiostrongylus catonensis.* J Neurol Neurosurg Psychiatry 51:80–87, 1988.
96. Sotelo J, Guerrero V, Rubio F: Neurocysticercosis: A new classification based on active and inactive forms: A study of 753 cases. Arch Intern Med 145:442–445, 1985.
97. Scharf D: Neurocysticercosis: Two hundred thirty-eight cases from a California hospital. Arch Neurol 45:777–780, 1988.
98. Takayangni OM, Jardim E: Therapy for neurocysticercosis: Comparison between albendazole and praziquantel. Arch Neurol 49:290–294, 1992.
99. Belani A, Leptrone D, Shands JW: *Strongyloides* meningitis. South Med J 80:916–918, 1987.
100. Hopkins AP, Harvey PKP: Benign chronic lymphocytic meningitis. J Neurol Sci 18:443–453, 1973.
101. Levin S, Nelson KE, Spies HW, Lepper MH: Pneumococcal meningitis: The problem of the unseen cerebrospinal fluid leak. Am J Med Sci 264:319–327, 1972.
102. Bol P, Spanjaard L, van Alphen L, Zanen HC: Epidemiology of *Haemophilus influenzae* in patients more than six years of age. J Infect Dis 15:81–94, 1987.
103. Hermans PE, Goldstein NP, Wellman WE: Mollaret's meningitis and differential diagnosis of recurrent meningitis: Report of case with review of the literature. Am J Med 52:128–140, 1972.
104. Yamamoto LJ, Tedder D, Ashley R, Levin MJ: Herpes simplex virus type 1 DNA in cerebrospinal fluid of a patient with Mollaret's meningitis. N Engl J Med 325:1082–1085, 1991.
105. Picard FJ, Dekaban GA, Silva J, Rice GPA: Mollaret's meningitis associated with herpes simplex type 2 infection. Neurology 43:1722–1727, 1993.

161

Central Nervous System Shunt Infections

Majid Sadigh
Pierce Gardner
Thomas J. Leipzig

Hydrocephalus (from the Greek *hydro,* "water," and *kephalē,* "head") is classified as either communicating (no obstruction between the ventricles and the subarachnoid space) or noncommunicating (obstruction between the ventricles and the subarachnoid space).[1] The early Greeks described hydrocephalus and recognized its poor prognosis.[2] Although more than 20 causes of hydrocephalus have been described, the physiologic end result is an abnormal accumulation of cerebrospinal fluid (CSF) in the cerebral ventricles. Attempts to reduce CSF production (normally about 500 mL/d regardless of age)[3] by drugs such as acetazolamide offer only short-term benefits,[4] and surgical decompression is the definitive treatment of hydrocephalus.[1, 5] Many anatomic variations for surgical diversion of CSF from the ventricular system to other compartments have been tried, but currently more than 95% of CSF shunts drain into either the peritoneal cavity (ventriculoperitoneal [VP] shunts) or right atrium (ventriculoatrial [VA] shunts).[4, 6] The standard shunt system consists of a proximal ventricular catheter, a one-way valve, a reservoir, and a distal peritoneal or right atrial catheter (Fig. 161–1). Barium-impregnated Silastic is the usual catheter material.[7, 8]

Shunting has dramatically extended the life span of infants and children with hydrocephalus; survival rates now range from 70% to 85%.[1, 9] Approximately 30% to 40% of patients maintain normal intelligence, and an equal number show no physical abnormalities, but only 20% suffer no mental or physical handicap.[1, 9]

Epidemiology

Incidence

An estimated 10,000 new shunts and 6000 revisions are performed annually in the United States.[10] The frequency of shunt infection varies from 1.5% to 39% (average, 10% to 15%).[9, 11–14] In series measuring an individual patient's lifelong risk for infection, the rates are high compared with series reporting infection rates per procedure with short periods of follow-up.[11, 15, 16] Improved shunt materials, shorter operating time, fewer invasive preoperative tests, and other factors may have contributed to the lower infection rates (generally 3% to 10%) in later reports.[4, 11, 13–15, 17–20]

Host Factors

Infection rates do not appear to vary by the type or severity of hydrocephalus, the underlying cause, or the patient's sex or race.[11, 13, 14] Age, however, is a significant risk factor; infection rates exceed 50% in low-birth-weight infants who require shunts before age 3 months.[11, 13, 14] The increased infection rates observed in neonates may be due to a greater density of colonization with coagulase-negative staphylococci, which have high bacterial adherence properties.[21] Higher infection rates are also reported in elderly patients.[22, 23]

Skin conditions that favor bacterial proliferation are associated with shunt infections by skin microflora. Likewise, the risk for shunt infection is increased by intercurrent infection at other sites or by a history of a previous shunt infection.[13, 14]

Patients with CSF shunts appear to have an increased risk for bacterial meningitis caused by traditional meningitis pathogens (*Haemophilus influenzae, Streptococcus pneumoniae,* and *Neisseria meningitidis*).[11, 24] This suggests that the presence of a shunt may facilitate the entry of organisms into the CSF during bacteremia; this is analogous to the increased risk for meningitis after lumbar puncture in the presence of bacteremia.[25] The meninges, rather than the shunt, appear to be the focus of infection in this situation as evidenced by the high rate of success with antibiotic therapy without shunt revision.[24, 26]

Technical Factors

Rates of infection do not appear to vary with the type of valve used,[11] although favorable experience has been reported with one-piece shunts.[27] Surgical technique and the experience of the neurosurgeon are important determinants of infection rates.[28, 29]

Microbiology

Although a great variety of microorganisms have infected CSF shunts[30–35] (Table 161–1), the majority of VP and VA shunt infections are caused by *Staphylococcus epidermidis* (36% to 80%). *Staphylococcus aureus* accounts for approximately 25% of shunt infections, and gram-negative enteric bacteria cause 5% to 10%. Anaerobic skin flora (mainly *Propionibacterium* species) alone or in mixed culture have been isolated from 2% to 35% of shunt infections.[11, 13, 17, 18, 22, 36]

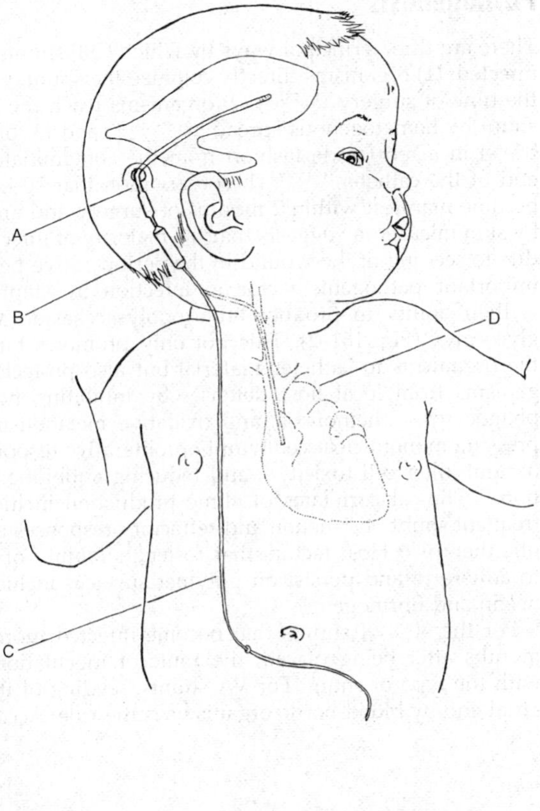

FIGURE 161–1 □ Schematic diagram of a typical CSF shunt system. The shunt is composed of three components: a ventricular catheter (A), a unidirectional flow valve (B), and a distal catheter directed into the peritoneum (C) or the atrium (D). A reservoir may be located in-line as demonstrated in this diagram. (From Gardner P, Leipzig T, Phillips P: Infections of central nervous system shunts. Med Clin North Am 69:297–314, 1985.)

TABLE 161–1 ■ Pathogens Associated with Cerebrospinal Fluid Shunt Infections

GRAM-POSITIVE ORGANISMS	GRAM-NEGATIVE ORGANISMS
Bacillus subtilis	*Achromobacter* species
Corynebacterium jeikeium	*Acinetobacter* species
Enterococci	*Alcaligenes* species
Listeria monocytogenes	*Bacteroides fragilis*
Micrococcus luteus	*Brucella melitensis*
Oerskovia xanthineolytica	*Enterobacter* species
Peptococci	*Escherichia coli*
Propionibacterium	*Flavobacterium*
(anaerobic diphtheroids)	*Haemophilus influenzae* group b
Propionibacterium acnes	and nontypeable groups
*Staphylococcus aureus**	*Hafnia* species
Coagulase-negative	*Klebsiella pneumoniae*
staphylococci†	*Neisseria gonorrhoeae*
Staphylococcus citreus	*Neisseria meningitidis* group C
Staphylococcus epidermidis	*Neisseria mucosa*
Streptococci	*Pasteurella multocida*
α-Hemolytic	*Proteus* species
β-Hemolytic	*Pseudomonas aeruginosa*
Group A	*Salmonella* species
Streptococcus pyogenes	*Serratia marcescens*
Group B	**MYCOBACTERIA**
Viridans streptococci	*Mycobacterium aquae*
Streptococcus pneumoniae	*Mycobacterium fortuitum*
	Mycobacterium tuberculosis
	FUNGI
	Candida albicans
	Candida stellatoides
	Coccidioides immitis
	Histoplasma capsulatum
	Paecilomyces variotii
	Trichosporon beigelii
	POLYMICROBIAL (INCLUDING ANAEROBES)

*Accounts for about 25% of shunt infections.
†Accounts for 36%–80% of shunt infections.

Pathogenesis

There are three principal ways by which CSF shunts become infected: (1) organisms directly colonize the shunt, usually at the time of surgery[6, 11, 28, 37]; (2) organisms reach the CSF and shunt by hematogenous spread[11, 24, 26, 38, 39]; and (3) organisms travel in a retrograde fashion from the contaminated distal end of the catheter.[11, 40–42] The observation that 70% of cases become manifest within 2 months of surgery and are caused by skin microflora suggests that the majority of infections are due to seeding of the wound in the perioperative period. An important pathogenic factor in infection by staphylococci is their ability to produce an exopolysaccharide slime, or glycocalyx (Fig. 161–2). This not only promotes binding of the organisms to catheter material but also protects the organisms from local host defenses by inhibiting neutrophil phagocytosis, chemotaxis, and oxidative metabolism[43]; suppressing mononuclear cell lymphoproliferative responses and natural killer cell toxicity[44]; and reducing antibiotic penetration.[45] Clinical correlates of slime production include more frequent shunt obstruction and refractory responses to antibiotic therapy.[46] Host factors that foster the ability of bacteria to adhere to and persist on polymer surfaces include fibronectin and fibrinogen.[47]

For the 30% of shunts that become infected more than 2 months after being placed, the route of inoculation differs with the type of shunt. For VA shunts, seeding of the distal atrial end by blood-borne organisms is the rule. Accordingly, blood cultures offer greater diagnostic yield than do cultures of CSF obtained by lumbar puncture. In late-onset VP shunt infections, enteric bacteria and enterococci, presumably of intestinal origin, constitute a greater proportion of the infecting organism.[11, 40, 41]

Clinical Manifestations

The clinical presentations of CSF shunt infection are varied and are often subtle and nonspecific. Only a minority of patients present with signs and symptoms that are clearly indicative of meningeal inflammation (severe headache, lethargy, meningismus, photophobia).[11] Almost all patients have a temperature greater than 100°F, and a majority of patients are febrile to 102°F or more.[11, 29, 36] Shunt infection commonly presents as shunt malfunction, so it is recommended that any catheter material removed during revision or replacement be cultured.

In the early postoperative period, infected shunts often show signs of inflammation along the course of the catheter.[48] Frequently, the infection is established first in the distal part of the shunt, and therefore the infectious complications associated with each type of shunt differ. Approximately one third of patients with VP shunts present primarily with abdominal symptoms.[40, 49, 50] Predictably, but infrequently, VP shunts are associated with a number of serious intraabdominal complications, including peritonitis, bowel obstruction or perforation, and peritoneal cysts.[51] Patients with infections of VA shunts may manifest signs of chronic bacteremia with immune complex nephritis,[52–56] hypocomplementemia,[57] and septic pulmonary emboli.[58] Nephritis has also been reported in patients with VP shunts.[54] Surprisingly, the frequency of right-sided endocarditis does not appear to be increased in patients with VA shunts. Fortunately, the clinical manifestations of shunt infection are usually reversible with successful treatment.[52, 59]

Diagnosis

The diagnosis of shunt infection requires a high index of suspicion and a willingness to aggressively collect appropriate specimens for evaluation and culture.[48] Common presentations of shunt infections are listed in Table 161–2, together with suggestions for the appropriate diagnostic steps. Because infection is best established in the distal (nonventricular) catheter, culture of lumbar CSF has a lower yield than does culture of blood in VA shunt infections[11, 60] or needle aspirate of inflamed areas along the distal catheter path in VP shunt infections.[11] However, for any type of shunt infection, culture of CSF obtained by needle aspiration of the shunt reservoir yields a microbial diagnosis in more than 90% of cases.[11, 12, 41, 60] The high diagnostic yield, the ease of the procedure, and the low rate of complications make aspiration of the reservoir the single most useful diagnostic test in the evaluation of possible shunt infection.

The CSF cellular reaction to shunt infection is usually modest, averaging 79 and 156 cells per mm^3 in two large series.[14, 16] The proportion of segmented neutrophils, and in some series eosinophils, is characteristically elevated.[61, 62] Gram-stained smears are usually positive in patients with an active CSF inflammatory response.[41, 60, 63] Positive cultures may be obtained in the absence of CSF pleocytosis,[11, 12, 63] but in general, the more inflammatory cells in CSF, the higher the yield of culture. The presence of more than 100 white cells per mm^3 of CSF correlates with a 90% yield of pathogens by culture.[60, 63] When the white cell count is less than 20/mm^3, fewer than half of CSF cultures grow pathogens.[60, 63]

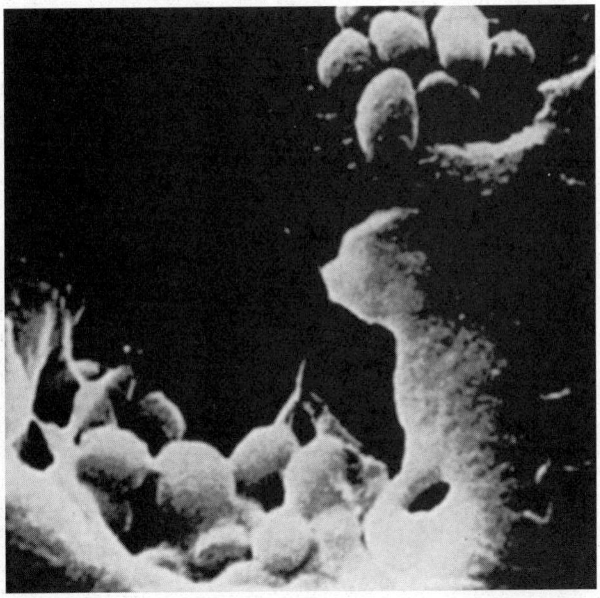

FIGURE 161–2 □ Scanning electron micrograph of *Staphylococcus aureus* cells attached to a CSF shunt. (From Guevara JA, Zuccaro G, Trevisan A, Denoya CD: Bacterial adhesion to cerebrospinal fluid shunts. J Neurosurg 67:438–445, 1987.)

Immunologic tests of CSF for antigen detection of common shunt pathogens have not achieved clinical importance owing to low sensitivity and specificity. CSF protein level is usually high, but hypoglycorrhachia is not a consistent feature and is often mild when present.[12]

In patients with shunt infections, the peripheral white cell count is characteristically elevated, but it is below 10,000/mm^3 in 25% of cases.[11] Elevated levels of serum lactate dehydrogenase and C-reactive protein are common but rarely have significant diagnostic value.[64]

A variety of radiographic studies are useful for evaluating the size of the ventricular system and the location, configuration, and functional status of the shunt[12] or for assessing potential intraabdominal complications of a VP shunt.[65]

Treatment

Variables that influence therapeutic choices for shunt infections include the patency of the shunt system, the necessity for uninterrupted ventricular drainage, the presence of ventriculitis, the infecting pathogen and its antimicrobial susceptibility pattern, and the presence of clinical complications such as bowel obstruction or perforation.[66]

Complete replacement of the shunt system with intensive antibiotic therapy delivered in a dosage and route that will produce effective CSF drug levels consistently yields excellent results and is the therapeutic "gold standard."[6, 9, 11, 19, 29, 40, 67–69] The antibiotics most commonly used are vancomycin by the intraventricular (as well as systemic) route and β-

TABLE 161–2 ■ Clinical Presentation of Shunt Infection and Suggested Diagnostic Steps

CLINICAL PRESENTATION	MAJOR DIAGNOSTIC STEPS
Shunt malfunction	Assessment of shunt malfunction by pumping reservoir Needle aspiration of reservoir (shunt tap) Computed tomography of brain and abdomen, if indicated Contrast radiographic studies of shunt
Wound or shunt track inflammation	Culture of aspirate of inflamed area, shunt tap, lumbar puncture (if no mass present)
Infection of proximal site: meningitis, ventriculitis, brain abscess	Computed tomography of brain, shunt tap Lumbar puncture (if no mass present)
Infection of distal site	
Ventriculoatrial shunt	
Bacteremia (acute or chronic)	Blood cultures, shunt tap, evaluation for right-sided endocarditis
Septic thrombophlebitis	Blood culture, shunt tap
Septic pulmonary embolism	Blood culture, chest radiograph, sputum Gram stain and culture
Circulating immune complex–related diseases: nephritis and arthritis	Blood culture, shunt tap, serum complement, circulating immune complexes, urine sediment examination
Ventriculoperitoneal shunt	
Acute abdomen, peritonitis, obstruction or perforation of bowel, intraabdominal abscess, liver abscess, peritoneal cyst	Shunt tap, aspiration of inflammation along distal ventriculoperitoneal catheter Evaluation for surgical abdomen clinically and radiographically

Adapted from Gardner P, Leipzig TJ, Sadigh M: Infections of mechanical cerebrospinal fluid shunts. Clin Top Infect Dis 9:198–214, 1988.

TABLE 161–3 ■ Antimicrobial Treatment of Common Cerebrospinal Fluid Shunt Pathogens

ORGANISM	ANTIBIOTICS	ROUTE*	INTRAVENTRICULAR OR INTRASHUNT ANTIBIOTICS	REMARKS
Staphylococci (β-lactam resistant)	[Vancomycin, 2 g/d Children: 40 mg/kg/d ± Rifampin, 10–20 mg/kg/d]	IV PO	Vancomycin, 10–20 mg/d Children: 0.5 mg/kg/d	Keep the serum vancomycin level at 10–20 μg/mL Keep the cerebrospinal fluid vancomycin level at 10–20 μg/mL
	or			
	[Trimethoprim, 10–20 mg/kg/d and Sulfamethoxazole, 50–100 mg/kg/d + Rifampin, 10–20 mg/kg/d]	PO		Keep the serum sulfamethoxazole level at 75–150 μg/mL
Staphylococci (β-lactam susceptible)	Nafcillin, 12 g/d Children: 300 mg/kg/d *or*	IV	Methicillin, 1–2 mg/kg/d *or* Nafcillin 1–4 mg/kg/d, both not to exceed 50 mg/d	
	[Trimethoprim 10–20 mg/kg/d and Sulfamethoxazole, 50–100 mg/kg/d + Rifampin, 10–20 mg/kg/d]	PO PO		Keep the serum sulfamethoxazole level at 75–150 μg/mL
Streptococcus pneumoniae *Neisseria meningitidis* *Propionibacterium* species	Penicillin G, 24 million units/d Children: 250,000 units/kg/d	IV		
Haemophilus influenzae Gram-negative enteric bacilli	A third-generation cephalosporin, e.g., ceftriaxone, 2 g q 12 h Children: 50–100 mg/kg/d	IV		
Pseudomonas aeruginosa	An anti-*Pseudomonas* β-lactam agent, e.g., ceftazidime, 2 g q 8 h Children: 150 mg/kg/d +	IV		
	An aminoglycoside, e.g., gentamicin, 2 mg/kg loading dose then 1.5 mg/kg q 8 h	IV	Gentamicin, 4–8 mg/d Children: 1–2 mg/d	Keep the serum gentamicin level at 4–8 μg/mL

*IV, Intravenously; PO, orally.

TABLE 161–4 ■ Standard Treatment of Central Nervous System Shunt Infection

STEP	PROCEDURE
I*	Removal of the entire infected shunt
II	Placement of external ventricular drainage
III	Administration of effective systemic antibiotics (refer to Table 161–3)
IV†	Administration of effective intraventricular antibiotics through external ventricular drainage once or twice daily (refer to Table 161–3)
V	Removal of external ventricular drainage and discontinuation of intraventricular antibiotics, after 3–5 d when ventricular infection is clinically improved
VI	Placement of a new shunt preferably in a site different from the previously removed infected shunt
VII	Continuation of systemic antibiotics for 7–10 d after removal of the infected shunt

*Alternatively, the distal part of the infected shunt can be externalized, followed by steps III to VII.
†Clamp the drain for 30 min after dosage administration.

lactam agents (Table 161–3). When ventriculitis is present, ventricular drainage and intraventricular antibiotic administration are indicated. Although immediate replacement of the entire infected shunt has good cure rates and avoids the risks associated with external ventricular drainage, it can be technically difficult and carries a slightly higher risk for subsequent shunt infection. Therefore, it is preferable either to place a temporary external ventricular catheter or to externalize the distal portion of the infected shunt system to drain the ventricle and to provide easy access for administration of antibiotics. Antibiotics can be given in a retrograde fashion once or twice daily, with the drain clamped for 30 minutes after dosage administration. To prevent superinfection, the external drainage system (ventricular catheter or old infected shunt) should be removed within 3 to 5 days after the infection has been controlled, and a new shunt should be placed at a different site[6, 41, 68, 70–73] (Table 161–4). For patients with functioning shunts infected by non–slime-producing organisms susceptible to bactericidal antibiotics and who have neither active ventricular infection nor other complications requiring surgery (e.g., bowel perforation), it is often possible to cure the infection without completely removing the shunt. The most successful regimen consists of externalization of the distal catheter followed by intraventricular and systemic antimicrobial therapy for 2 to 3 weeks with subsequent replacement of the distal shunt[59] (Table 161–5). Meningitis due to organisms that reach the CSF through the blood stream (e.g., *H. influenzae, S. pneumoniae, N. meningitidis*) can usually be treated without shunt revision or removal.[24, 26, 72] In the future, agents that reduce the formation of the bacterial slime layer and other factors related to pathogenesis may play a role in improving the nonoperative treatment of shunt infections.

Prognosis

Retrospective studies indicate that shunt infections cause deterioration of IQ scores and are associated with increases in both short-term and long-term mortality.[9, 11, 22, 49]

Prevention

Efforts to prevent shunt infections have focused on technical improvements in shunt materials, insertion techniques, and antibiotic prophylaxis during the perioperative period.[74] Studies of systemic and topical antibiotic prophylaxis in the perioperative period have yielded conflicting results.[20, 60–66, 74–83] A metaanalysis of 12 trials with 1359 randomized patients demonstrated that perioperative use of systemic antibiotics significantly reduces the risk for subsequent infection.[83] Therefore, prophylaxis with a β-lactam antibiotic with or without rifampin, vancomycin, or trimethoprim-sulfamethoxazole has become the norm[11, 81] (Table 161–6). Antibiotic prophylaxis is recommended for patients with VA shunts who must undergo dental or other procedures that may cause bacteremia.[10, 84, 85] The value of prophylaxis for patients with VP shunts undergoing similar procedures is not clear. However, when peritoneal infection (e.g., ruptured appendix or diverticulum) is suspected in patients with VP shunts, antibiotic prophylaxis should be given. It would also make good sense to avoid placing VP shunts in women who have a history of recurrent pelvic inflammatory disease or have an intrauterine contraceptive device in place.

TABLE 161–5 ■ Alternative Treatment of Uncomplicated Functioning Shunt Infections Caused by Non–Slime-Producing Organisms

STEP	PROCEDURE
I	Externalization of the distal part of infected shunt
II	Administration of effective systemic antibiotics (refer to Table 161–3)
III*	Administration of effective intraventricular antibiotics once or twice daily (refer to Table 161–3) retrograde through the reservoir
IV	Continuation of systemic and intrashunt antibiotic regimen for 2–3 wk
V	Revision and replacement of the distal shunt

*Clamp the drain for 30 min after dosage administration.

TABLE 161–6 ■ Suggested Prophylactic Antibiotic Regimens for Prevention of Central Nervous System Shunt Infection

Start antibiotics 1 h before operation and continue for 24–48 h

1. Antistaphylococcal β-lactam agents
   Nafcillin: 2 g intravenously (IV) q 6 h (children: 25 mg/kg IV q 6 h)
   or
   Oxacillin: 3 g IV q 6 h (children: 50 mg/kg IV q 6 h)
   ±
   Rifampin: 5–10 mg/kg q 12 h orally (PO)

*2. Vancomycin: 1 g IV q 12 h (children: 20 mg/kg q 12 h IV)

*†3. Trimethoprim: 5–10 mg/kg q 12 h IV or PO and sulfamethoxazole: 25–50 mg/kg q 12 h PO or IV

*Dosage adjustment according to renal function is necessary.
†It is not recommended for newborns.

References

1. Jennett B (ed): An Introduction to Neurosurgery. London, William Heinemann, 1977.
2. Ransohoff J, Shulman K, Fishman R: Hydrocephalus: A review of etiology and treatment. J Pediatr 56:399, 1960.
3. McComb JG: Recent research into the nature of cerebrospinal fluid formation and absorption. J Neurosurg 59:369, 1983.
4. O'Brien MS: Hydrocephalus in children. *In* Youmans JR (ed): Neurological Surgery, ed 2, Vol 3. Philadelphia, WB Saunders, 1982, pp 1381–1422.
5. Matson DD: Hydrocephalus. N Engl J Med 271:1360, 1964.
6. Keucher TR, Mealey J: Long-term results after ventriculoatrial and ventriculoperitoneal shunting for infantile hydrocephalus. J Neurosurg 50:179, 1979.
7. Post EM: Currently available shunt systems: A review. Neurosurgery 16:257, 1985.
8. Shurtleff DB: Characteristics of the various CSF shunt systems. Clin Pediatr 17:154, 1978.
9. Overton MC, Snodglass SR: Ventriculovenous shunts for infantile hydrocephalus: A review of five years' experience with this method. J Neurosurg 23:517, 1965.
10. Croll TP, Greiner DG, Schut L: Antibiotic prophylaxis for the hydrocephalic dental patient with a shunt. Pediatr Dent 1:81, 1979.
11. Schoenbaum SC, Gardner P, Schillito J: Infections of cerebrospinal fluid shunts: Epidemiology, clinical manifestations and therapy. J Infect Dis 131:543, 1975.
12. Noetzel MJ, Baker RP: Shunt fluid examination: Risks and benefits in the evaluation of shunt malfunction and infection. J Neurosurg 61:328, 1984.
13. Renier D, Lacombe J, Pierre-Kahn A, et al: Factors causing acute shunt infection; computer analysis of 1174 operations. J Neurosurg 61:1072, 1984.
14. Spanu G, Karussos G, Achinolfi D, et al: An analysis of cerebro-

spinal fluid shunt infections in adults. A clinical experience of twelve years. Acta Neurochir (Wien) 80:79, 1986.
15. Younger JJ, Simmons JCH, Barrett FF: Operative related infection rates for ventriculoperitoneal shunt procedures in a children's hospital. Infect Control 8:67, 1987.
16. Shurtleff DB, Christie D, Foltz EL: Ventriculoauriculostomy: Associated infection: A 12 year study. J Neurosurg 35:686, 1971.
17. Cotton MF, Hartzenberg B, Donald PR, et al: Ventriculoperitoneal shunt infections in children: A 6-year study. S Afr Med J 79:139, 1991.
18. Kontny U, Hofling B, Gutjahr P, et al: CSF shunt infections in children. Infection 21:89, 1993.
19. Morissette I, Gourdeau M, Francoeur J: CSF shunt infections: A fifteen-year experience with emphasis on management and outcome. Can J Neurol Sci 20:118, 1993.
20. Choux M, Genitori L, Lang D, et al: Shunt implantation: Reducing the incidence of shunt infection. J Neurosurg 77:875, 1992.
21. Pople IK, Bayston R, Hayward RD: Infection of cerebrospinal fluid shunts in infants: A study of etiological factors. J Neurosurg 77:29, 1992.
22. George R, Leibrock L, Epstein M: Long-term analysis of cerebrospinal fluid shunt infections: A 25 year experience. J Neurosurg 51:804, 1979.
23. Salmon JH: Adult hydrocephalus: Evaluation of shunt therapy in 80 patients. J Neurosurg 37:423, 1972.
24. Lerman SJ: *Haemophilus influenzae* infections of cerebrospinal fluid shunts. J Neurosurg 54:261, 1981.
25. Teele DW, Dashefsky B, Rakusa T, et al: Meningitis after lumbar puncture in children with bacteremia. N Engl J Med 305:1079, 1981.
26. Rennels MB, Wald ER: Treatment of *Hemophilus influenzae* type B meningitis in children with cerebrospinal fluid shunts. J Pediatr 97:424, 1980.
27. Haase J, Bang F, Tange M: Danish experience with the one-piece shunt. A long-term follow-up. Childs Nerv Syst 3:93, 1987.
28. Bayston R, Lari J: A study of the sources of infection in colonised shunts. Dev Med Child Neurol 16(Suppl 32):16, 1974.
29. Yogev R, Davis AT: Neurosurgical shunt infections: A review. Childs Brain 6:74, 1980.
30. Ashpole RD, Jacobson K, King AT, et al: Cysto-peritoneal shunt infection with *Trichosporon beigelii*. Br J Neurosurg 5:515, 1991.
31. Chan KH, Mann KS, Seto WH: Infection of a shunt by *Mycobacterium fortuitum*: Case report. Neurosurgery 29:472, 1991.
32. Chowdhary UM, Twum Danso K: *Brucella* meningoencephalitis associated with cerebrospinal fluid shunt in a child: Case report. Surg Neurol 35:468, 1991.
33. Feder HM Jr: *Bacteroides fragilis* meningitis. Rev Infect Dis 9:783, 1987.
34. Lee T, Kerr RS, Adams CB: *Pasteurella multocida*: A rare case of shunt infection. Br J Neurosurg 4:237, 1990.
35. Stotka JL, Rupp ME, Meier FA, et al: Meningitis due to *Neisseria mucosa*: Case report and review. Rev Infect Dis 13:837, 1991.
36. Everett ED, Eickhoff TC, Simon RH: Cerebrospinal fluid shunt infections with anaerobic diphtheroids (*Propionibacterium* species). J Neurosurg 44:580, 1976.
37. Shapiro S, Boaz J, Kleinmann M, et al: Origin of organisms infecting ventricular shunts. Neurosurgery 22:868, 1988.
38. Petrak RM, Pottage JC, Harris AA, et al: *Haemophilus influenzae* meningitis in the presence of a cerebrospinal fluid shunt. Neurosurgery 18:79, 1986.
39. Leggiardo RJ, Atluru VL, Katz SP: Meningococcal meningitis associated with cerebrospinal fluid shunts. Pediatr Infect Dis 3:489, 1984.
40. Brook I, Johnson N, Overturf GD, Wilkins J: Mixed bacterial meningitis: A complication of ventriculo- and lumboperitoneal shunts. J Neurosurg 47:961, 1977.
41. Hubschmann OR, Countee RW: Acute abdomen in children with infected ventriculoperitoneal shunts. Arch Surg 115:305, 1980.
42. Demmler GJ, Wells D, Heitkamp JW, et al: *Neisseria gonorrhoeae* ventriculoperitoneal shunt infection in a child. Pediatr Infect Dis 4:419, 1985.
43. Johnson GM, Lee DA, Regelman WE, et al: Interference with granulocyte function by *Staphylococcus epidermidis* slime. Infect Immun 50:179, 1979.
44. Gray ED, Peters G, Verstegen M, et al: Effect of extracellular slime substance from *Staphylococcus epidermidis* on the human cellular immune response. Lancet 1:365, 1984.
45. Davenport DS, Massanari RM, Pfaller MA, et al: Usefulness of a test for slime production as a marker for clinically significant infections with coagulase-negative staphylococci. J Infect Dis 153:332, 1986.
46. Diaz Mitoma F, Hardking G, Hoban DJ, et al: Clinical significance of a test for slime production in ventriculoperitoneal shunt infections caused by coagulase-negative staphylococci. J Infect Dis 156:555, 1987.
47. Hermann M, Vaudaux PE, Pittet D, et al: Fibronectin, fibrinogen, and laminin act as mediators of adherence of clinical staphylococcal isolates to foreign material. J Infect Dis 158:693, 1988.
48. Haines SJ, Taylor F: Prophylactic methicillin for shunt operations: Effects on incidence of shunt malfunction and infection. Childs Brain 9:10, 1982.
49. Forrest DM, Cooper DGW: Complications of ventriculoatrial shunts: A review of 455 cases. J Neurosurg 29:506, 1968.
50. Reynolds M, Sherman JO, McLane DG: Ventriculoperitoneal shunt as an acute surgical abdomen. J Pediatr Surg 18:951, 1983.
51. Grosfeld JL, Cooney DR, Smith J, et al: Intraabdominal complications following ventriculoperitoneal shunt procedures. Pediatrics 54:791, 1974.
52. Wakabayashi Y, Kobayashi Y, Shigematsu H: Shunt nephritis: Histological dynamics following removal of the shunt. Nephron 40:111, 1985.
53. Noiri E, Kuwata S, Nosaka K, et al: Shunt nephritis: Efficacy of an antibiotic trial for clinical diagnosis. Intern Med 32:291, 1993.
54. Rifkinson Mann S, Rifkinson N, Leong T: Shunt nephritis. Case report. J Neurosurg 74:656, 1991.
55. Samtleben W, Bauriedel G, Bosch T, et al: Renal complications of ventriculoatrial shunts. Artif Organs 17:695, 1993.
56. Ter Borg EJ, Van Rijswijk MH, Kallenberg CG: Transient arthritis with positive tests for rheumatoid factor as presenting sign of shunt nephritis. Ann Rheum Dis 50:182, 1991.
57. Strife CF, McDonald BM, Ruley EJ, et al: Shunt nephritis: The nature of the serum cryoglobulins and their relation to the complement profile. J Pediatr 88:403, 1976.
58. Gibney RTN, Donovan F, Fitzgerald MX: Recurrent symptomatic pulmonary embolism caused by an infected Pudenz cerebrospinal fluid shunt device. Thorax 33:662, 1978.
59. McLaurine RL, Frame PT: Treatment of infections of cerebrospinal fluid shunts. Rev Infect Dis 9:595, 1987.
60. Odio C, McCracken GH, Nelson JD: CSF shunt infections in pediatrics: A seven-year experience. Am J Dis Child 138:1103, 1984.
61. Tung H, Raffel C, McComb JG: Ventricular cerebrospinal fluid eosinophilia in children with ventriculoperitoneal shunts. J Neurosurg 75:541, 1991.
62. Vinchon M, Vallee L, Prin L, et al: Cerebro-spinal fluid eosinophilia in shunt infections. Neuropediatrics 23:235, 1992.
63. Forward KR, Fewer HD, Stiver HG: Cerebrospinal fluid shunt infections: A review of 35 infections in 32 patients. J Neurosurg 59:725, 1983.
64. Bayston R: Serum C-reactive protein test in diagnosis of septic complications of cerebrospinal fluid for hydrocephalus. Arch Dis Child 54:545, 1979.
65. Agha FP, Amendola MA, Shirazi KK, et al: Abdominal complications of ventriculoperitoneal shunts with emphasis on the role of imaging methods. Surg Gynecol Obstet 156:473, 1983.
66. Walters BC: Cerebrospinal fluid shunt infection. Neurosurg Clin North Am 3:387, 1992.
67. Garvey G: Current concepts of bacterial infections of the central nervous system: Bacterial meningitis and bacterial brain abscess. J Neurosurg 59:725, 1983.
68. James HE, Walsh JW, Wilson HD, et al: The management of cerebrospinal fluid shunt infections: A clinical experience. Acta Neurochir (Wien) 59:157, 1981.
69. James HE, Walsh JW, Wilson HD: Prospective randomized study of therapy in cerebrospinal fluid shunt infections. Neurosurgery 7:459, 1980.
70. Mori K, Raimondi AJ: An analysis of external ventricular drainage as a treatment for infected shunts. Childs Brain 1:243, 1975.
71. James HE, Wilson HD, Connor JD, et al: Intraventricular cerebrospinal fluid antibiotic concentrations in patients with intraventricular infections. Neurosurgery 10:50, 1982.

72. Stern S, Bayston R, Hayward RJ: *Haemophilus influenzae* meningitis in the presence of cerebrospinal fluid shunts. Childs Nerv Syst 4:164, 1988.
73. Jacobs F, Delecluse F, Raftopoulos C, et al: Intraventricular vancomycin in CSF shunt infections. Neurosurgery 21:112, 1987.
74. Venes JL: Control of shunt infection: Report of 150 consecutive cases. J Neurosurg 45:311, 1976.
75. Bullock R, van Dellen JR, Ketelbey W, et al: A double-blind placebo-controlled trial of perioperative prophylactic antibiotics for elective neurosurgery. J Neurosurg 69:687, 1988.
76. Lambert M, Mackinnon AE, Vaishanav A: Comparison of two methods of prophylaxis against CSF shunt infection. Z Kinderchir 11(Suppl):109, 1984.
77. Dempsey R, Rapp RP, Young B, et al: Prophylactic parenteral antibiotics in clean neurosurgical procedures: A review. J Neurosurg 60:52, 1988.
78. Slight PH, Gundling K, Plotkin SA, et al: A trial of vancomycin for prophylaxis of infection after neurosurgical shunts. N Engl J Med 312:921, 1985.
79. Wang EEL, Prober CG, Hendrick BE, et al: Prophylactic sulfamethoxazole and trimethoprim in ventriculoperitoneal shunt surgery. JAMA 215:1174, 1984.
80. Schmidt K, Flemming G, Jerris OO, et al: Antibiotic prophylaxis in cerebrospinal fluid shunting. A prospective randomized trial in 1952 hydrocephalic patients. Neurosurgery 17:1, 1985.
81. Goran C, Blomstedt MD: Results of trimethoprim-sulfamethoxazole prophylaxis in ventriculostomy and shunting procedures. A double-blind randomized trial. J Neurosurg 62:694, 1985.
82. Yogev R, Shinco F, McLone D: Prophylaxis for ventriculoperitoneal shunt surgery with nafcillin alone or in combination with rifampin (Abstr 664). Presented at the 23rd Interscience Conference on the Antimicrobial Agents and Chemotherapy; October 1983; Las Vegas, NV.
83. Langley JM, LeBlanc JC, Drake J, et al: Efficacy of antimicrobial prophylaxis in placement of cerebrospinal fluid shunts: Meta-analysis. Clin Infect Dis 17:98, 1993.
84. Monfared AH, Kee SK, Apuzzo MLJ, et al: Obstetric management of pregnant women with extracranial shunts. Can Med Assoc J 120:562, 1979.
85. Redleaf PD, Fodell EJ: Bacteremia during parturition: Prevention of subacute bacterial endocarditis. JAMA 169:1284, 1959.

162

Brain Abscess

Staci A. Fischer
Alan A. Harris

Brain abscess is an important but uncommon disease with an estimated annual incidence in the United States of 1 in 10,000 hospital admissions. Much of the available information is from retrospective studies and reviews.[1–18] Although brain abscess is in the differential diagnosis of all intracranial space-occupying lesions, presenting signs and symptoms frequently provide no clues as to the presence of infection. Advances in computed tomography (CT), magnetic resonance imaging (MRI), and ultrasonography have made important contributions to diagnosis and management and have obviated the need for certain invasive studies such as pneumoencephalography, arteriography, and myelography. CT and MRI may detect small or multiple central nervous system (CNS) lesions and may identify the underlying cause of abscess formation (e.g., chronic otic and sinus abnormalities). As a result of such improvements, the prevalence of cryptogenic abscesses has decreased from 35% to between 15% and 20%.[15] The benefit of earlier detection may explain some of the improved therapeutic results with antimicrobial therapy alone; yet the place of antibiotics, alone or in combination with excisional surgery, needle aspiration, or both, is still evolving.[19–22] Our therapeutic armamentarium has expanded with bactericidal agents whose pharmacokinetic properties allow penetration into abscess cavities and surrounding tissue and that possess a spectrum of activity against the usual agents of brain abscess. The rate of associated mortality has declined in the last two decades, but significant morbidity and mortality persist. Prognosis relates directly to the age of the patient, neurologic function and mental status at the time of diagnosis, and underlying immune compromise.

Pathogenesis

The recognized association of brain abscess with cyanotic heart disease[15, 23–25] and pulmonary arteriovenous malformations[24, 26, 27] provided early pathophysiologic clues that areas of ischemia or infarction were more vulnerable to the development of brain abscess. The presence of polycythemia, local tissue hypoxia, and areas of microinfarction predisposes to bacteremic seeding, often with organisms bypassing the pulmonary filtering process via right-to-left shunting. With hematogenous spread of infection, the junction of gray and white matter, an area with poor collateral circulation, is where most abscesses develop. In the setting of head trauma, otic or sinus infection, or other predisposing factors, an alternative locus minoris resistentiae is present. Abscesses subsequent to open head trauma in humans and to direct inoculation of bacteria in some animal models demonstrate that otherwise normal brain is vulnerable to abscess formation. However, inoculation of α-hemolytic streptococci into the cerebral parenchyma of dogs in one study was followed by eventual resolution of enhancing lesions seen by CT and histopathologic sterile granulomata indicative of spontaneous resolution.[28]

Clearly, organisms vary in their capability to induce brain abscess. In a rat model, inoculation of *Escherichia coli* was more infective than *Pseudomonas* species, *Staphylococcus aureus*, or *Streptococcus pyogenes*. *E. coli* strains with K1 capsules were more infective than unencapsulated forms.[29] *Citrobacter diversus*, a major cause of postmeningitis brain abscess in neonates, demonstrated strain variation in its ability to cause abscess by either hematogenous spread or inoculation.[30] In experimental *S. aureus* brain abscesses, formation of a collagen capsule may serve less of a containment function than was previously thought and the predilection for white matter over gray matter has been apparent.[31] *Streptococcus milleri*, in many series the most commonly isolated bacterial cause of brain abscess, characteristically produces purulence at any site of infection.

Host factors are also important considerations. The immunocompromised host is at risk for infection with opportunistic pathogens and may demonstrate altered clinical and radiographic presentations of brain abscess. In dog studies, the effect of immunosuppression with azathioprine or prednisone on CT monitoring of abscess formation has been evaluated. Immunosuppression retarded abscess formation and decreased maximal abscess size. Initially there was less mass effect, although eventually the abscess was larger than in the immunocompetent animals.[32] Corticosteroids clearly retard the inflammatory response to infection and delay encapsulation, important components in the evolution and therapeutic implications of brain abscess.

Predisposing Factors

Brain abscess occurs most often in males in the second through fourth decades of life.[13, 15, 16, 33] The overall incidence of infection is 0.18% to 1.3% in autopsy studies, with a number of predisposing factors identified. Despite advances in diagnostic technology, cryptogenic abscesses still occur in approximately 15% to 20% of cases.[15]

Ischemia, infarction, and contusion likely provide a fertile soil for inoculation or bacteremic seeding of organisms and resultant brain abscess in humans. They also help explain the rarity of brain abscess after bacteremia due to nonembolic conditions such as pyelonephritis, pneumonitis, cellulitis, and vascular catheter sepsis. Untreated bacterial endocarditis with continuous bacteremia is associated with multiple neurologic complications, although brain abscess is rare.[15, 34] Abscess formation in these patients is usually accompanied by microemboli or cerebrovascular disease resulting in locally decreased oxygenation or perfusion.[35] In watershed areas with little collateral flow, sludging or vascular stasis associated with conditions such as hyperviscosity, cryoglobulinemia, or altered red blood cell rheology may also create an environment conducive to bacterial seeding.

Systemic or localized vascular disorders have been associated with brain abscess. Hereditary hemorrhagic telangiectasia (Osler-Weber-Rendu disease) may involve the CNS or the lung.[36] When the lung is involved, right-to-left shunting occurs with polycythemia and hypoxemia, at times with septic embolization to the brain.[23, 24] It is estimated that 1% of patients with this disorder develop brain abscesses, a risk approximately 1000 times that of the general population.[26, 37] As a brain abscess may be the presenting sign of pulmonary arteriovenous malformations, this condition should be suspected whenever a person has more than one apparently cryptogenic brain abscess during his or her lifetime.[38] Carotid endarterectomy and preeclampsia have been complicated by intracranial hematoma with subsequent hematogenous seeding and development of staphylococcal brain abscess.[39, 40] In addition, it would seem that any CNS hemorrhage may provide a nidus for abscess secondary to bacteremia from another focus.

Suppurative otitis media, paranasal sinusitis, and mastoiditis are the best described localized head and neck infections associated with brain abscess.[13, 14, 16, 17, 41–48] Contiguous spread of infection to brain parenchyma may occur via associated cranial osteitis or osteomyelitis; retrograde spread may occur via thrombophlebitic emissary or diploic veins or via preformed pathways (e.g., dural rents related to prior trauma or the internal auditory canal). Brain abscess complicates chronic otitis media or mastoiditis four to eight times more frequently than their acute counterparts.[15] Cholesteatomas are an additional risk factor, particularly in adults, in whom they have been associated with up to 50% of otogenic brain abscesses.[49, 50] Otogenic infections most commonly produce temporal lobe or cerebellar abscesses and frequently involve multiple pathogens, including anaerobes and gram-negative bacilli. Paranasal sinus infections are an additional predisposing factor, often producing abscesses in predictable locations: with ethmoidal and frontal sinusitis, the frontal lobes, and with sphenoid sinusitis, the pituitary and sella turcica area. As hematogenous spread may occur with otic or sinus infections, the presence of multiple abscesses or lesions in noncontiguous sites does not rule out these underlying processes.[18, 51] In approximately 30% of cryptogenic brain abscesses, the responsible organisms are anaerobic flora usually associated with chronic otic or sinus infections.[52] When extensive evaluation does not reveal disease in these anatomic areas, other upper and lower respiratory tract locations should be considered. Poor dental hygiene with subsequent dental infection, particularly of the molar teeth, may be associated with up to 10% of cases of brain abscess, often affecting the frontal or temporal lobes.[15, 18, 53, 54] With hematogenous spread, multiple lesions may be seen.

Although intracranial neurosurgical procedures may be complicated by wound infections, bone flap osteomyelitis, subdural empyema, or meningitis, brain abscess is rare, occurring in less than 0.2% of clean procedures.[18] Localized intraparenchymal abscesses may develop secondary to deep wound infection or extension of a superficial infection through a dural rent, particularly in the patient with preceding trauma. Surgical procedures such as submucous resection of the nasal septum,[55] ventriculostomy with intracranial pressure monitor placement,[1] or placement of cranial traction with Crutchfield tongs or halo orthoses[56–59] have been complicated by intracranial abscesses.[60] Postoperative brain abscess of uncertain cause should raise concern for an unsuspected source of bacteremia or a microscopic communication between the ears or sinuses and the cranial vault.

Posttraumatic brain abscess may follow penetrating cranial injuries produced by numerous objects, including missiles (e.g., gunshot wounds), lawn darts, and pencil tips.[61–63] Staphylococcal species are most frequently isolated, although with soil contamination, enteric gram-negative bacteria, anaerobes, and fungi may be involved as well. Sharp instruments penetrating the orbital roof can lead to brain abscess, sometimes caused by unusual bacteria and fungi. The presence of a foreign body (most commonly bone fragments) within the brain parenchyma may predispose to abscess formation presenting years after trauma[64]; brain abscess caused by *Clostridium bifermentans* has been reported to be associated with a mortar shell in place for 15 years.[65] Cerebellar abscesses have complicated congenital occipital dermal sinuses and epidermoid cysts.[66, 67]

Multiple series attest to the rarity of brain abscess as a sequela of community-onset meningitis caused by *Streptococcus pneumoniae, Haemophilus influenzae*, and *Neisseria meningitidis* in adults. One important exception to this observation is that of *C. diversus*, a prominent cause of bacterial meningitis in the neonatal period. This organism is associated with necrotizing vasculitis and abscess formation in more than 70% of affected infants and is associated with a significant mortality rate.[15, 68, 69] *Listeria monocytogenes* is the agent most often associated with brain abscess complicating community-onset bacterial meningitis in adults.[70] Brain abscess subsequent to *H. influenzae* type b meningitis in a 7-month-old infant[71] suggests the importance of age as a predisposing factor to brain abscess after bacterial meningitis. Other *Haemophilus* species, specifically *Haemophilus aphrophilus* and *Haemophilus paraphrophilus*,[72–75] have resulted in brain abscess secondary to meningitis or bacteremia. As a cause of bacterial endocarditis, these species have been recognized to cause large vegetations with a predisposition for embolic phenomena. Their association with brain abscess may reflect species virulence. Meningitis caused by group B streptococci, the most common cause of neonatal meningitis, is rarely followed by brain abscess. Certain opportunistic fungi such as *Cryptococcus neoformans* and *Coccidioides immitis* may be associated with meningitis and subsequent abscess formation, along with several other pathogens discussed later.

Hematogenous spread of extraneural infection to the CNS may occur in patients presenting with skin and soft tissue infection, osteomyelitis, intraabdominal infection, pleuropulmonary infection, or pelvic infection.[15, 33] Multiple abscesses may be seen, frequently at the gray matter–white matter junction in the distribution of the middle cerebral artery. Dilatation of esophageal strictures and sclerosis of esophageal varices have been complicated by bacteremia and subsequent development of brain abscess, frequently involving a multitude of oropharyngeal flora.[76–79]

Microbiology

Organisms are usually isolated from brain abscess, even when antibiotic therapy is instituted shortly before the specimen is obtained.[80, 81] Pathogens isolated in brain abscesses are listed in Table 162–1, with pathogens typical of certain underlying causes given in Table 162–2. Improved techniques have demonstrated the role of anaerobic organisms in abscesses at all anatomic sites and markedly decreased the rate of culture negativity of obtained specimens. Polymicrobial flora is to be expected when the abscess is formed by contiguous spread, especially from otic or sinus infections; in some series, 30% to 60% of brain abscesses are polymicrobial.[13]

Streptococci—aerobic, anaerobic, and microaerophilic—are isolated in up to 70% of brain abscesses, with *S. milleri* the most commonly identified aerobic organism.[1–10, 13, 15, 17, 33, 82] *Prevotella* and *Bacteroides* species, including *Prevotella melaninogenica* (formerly *Bacteroides melaninogenicus*), *Prevotella oralis* (formerly *Bacteroides oralis*), and *Bacteroides fragilis*, are found in up to 40% of cases.[13] *Fusobacterium* species are anaerobic oral flora and may be associated with extensive tissue necrosis; *Actinomyces, Eikenella, Veillonella*, and *Clostridium* species may be involved in brain abscesses as well, frequently as part of mixed infections.[13, 24, 33, 47, 83] Infection with *Actinomyces* results from spread from pulmonary or cervicofacial foci, either by direct extension or by hematogenous dissemination; it is often the sole pathogen isolated in these patients.[83] Abscesses complicating bacteremia, or rarely bacterial meningitis, are usually caused by a single agent. Posttraumatic or postneurosurgical abscesses may be associated with either single or multiple organisms. *S. aureus*, once a major cause of brain abscess, has diminished in frequency over the years. It is usually secondary to bacteremia, including acute endocarditis, or complicates local cranial wound infection or neurosurgical procedures. Its diminished frequency likely reflects the use of early broad-spectrum antimicrobial therapy and improved microbiologic techniques to detect other pathogens, including anaerobes.

TABLE 162–1 ■ Bacterial Pathogens Isolated from Brain Abscess

CLASS	ORGANISM
Aerobes	*Streptococcus* spp.
	S. milleri–S. intermedius group
	Other viridans streptococci
	Group C streptococci
	S. pneumoniae
	Staphylococcus aureus
	Coagulase-negative *Staphylococcus*
	Proteus mirabilis
	Klebsiella pneumoniae
	Klebsiella ozaenae
	Escherichia coli
	Citrobacter diversus
	Enterobacter spp.
	Haemophilus spp.
	Salmonella spp.
	Listeria monocytogenes
	Streptobacillus moniliformis
	Nocardia asteroides
	Brucella melitensis
Anaerobes	*Bacteroides fragilis*
	Prevotella melaninogenica
	Prevotella (formerly *Bacteroides*) *oralis*
	Peptostreptococcus spp.
	Clostridium spp.
	Actinomyces israelii
	Fusobacterium spp.
	Eikenella spp.
	Veillonella spp.
	Prevotella spp.

TABLE 162–2 ■ Predominant Pathogens Associated with Specific Conditions That Are Occasionally Followed by Brain Abscess*

PREDISPOSING CONDITIONS	PATHOGENS
Otitis, mastoiditis, invaded paranasal sinus, lung abscess, empyema	Usually polymicrobial—anaerobic and microaerophilic streptococci, *Bacteroides, Prevotella, Fusobacterium, Pseudomonas, Proteus* spp., other Enterobacteriaceae†
Noninvaded paranasal sinus, dental	Usually polymicrobial—anaerobic and microaerophilic streptococci, *Bacteroides, Prevotella, Fusobacterium* spp.
Trauma or neurosurgery	Monomicrobial or polymicrobial—*Staphylococcus aureus*, Enterobacteriaceae, *Pseudomonas* spp.
Meningitis (not surgical or traumatic)	*Listeria monocytogenes, Citrobacter diversus*
Bacteremia	
Without apparent source	*Salmonella* spp., *S. aureus, Listeria monocytogenes*
Genitourinary or gastrointestinal source	Enterobacteriaceae
Wound source	*S. aureus*, Enterobacteriaceae
Endocarditis	Viridans streptococci, enterococci, *S. aureus, Haemophilus aphrophilus, Candida, Aspergillus* spp.

*The extent of the microbiologic evaluation should be dictated by epidemiologic concerns about the potential pathogen. In addition to routine Gram stain, and aerobic and anaerobic cultures, prolonged incubation, special media, and evaluation by smear and culture for mycobacteria, fungi, and *Nocardia* organisms may be appropriate for specific patients.

†*Escherichia, Proteus, Klebsiella, Enterobacter, Serratia, Salmonella, Shigella, Arizona, Citrobacter, Edwardsiella, Hafnia, Morganella, Providencia, Yersinia*, and *Erwinia* spp.

Enterobacteriaceae and Pseudomonadaceae may be isolated in up to 30% to 40% of cases, depending on the underlying cause. When bacteremic in origin, infections are usually monomicrobial and involve *E. coli* or *Proteus* species, the most frequent causes of gram-negative sepsis. After trauma or neurosurgery, single or multiple Enterobacteriaceae or *Pseudomonas* species may be responsible. Chronic otic conditions are usually associated with *Pseudomonas* or *Proteus* species in conjunction with anaerobic flora.[84] *Klebsiella* and *Enterobacter* are observed less frequently in these settings. *C. diversus* and *Proteus mirabilis* are important considerations in the neonate with brain abscess and meningitis.

Salmonella species, an important cause of community-onset bacteremia, exhibit tropism for endothelial surfaces. Systemic disease most frequently involves bones, joints, atherosclerotic aneurysms, and heart valves, but meningitis and brain abscess may occur.[85] *Salmonella* species, including *Salmonella typhi*, have been reported to cause brain abscess during, years after, or without gastrointestinal disease.[86] Lesions are most commonly located in the temporal or parietal lobes. In addition, brain abscess secondary to *Salmonella enteritidis* has occurred within a glioblastoma multiforme.[87] *Klebsiella ozaenae*, a cause of atrophic rhinitis or ozena and a nasal colonizer, has also caused brain abscess, probably through contiguous spread.[88] Infection with *Legionella pneumophila* is commonly associated with encephalopathy, and rarely with brain abscess.[89]

The acquired immunodeficiency syndrome (see Chapter 125) has provided seemingly unending examples of the capability of unusual infectious agents to cause cerebral mass lesions, although given the appropriate predisposing immunosuppressive or anatomic conditions, brain abscess caused by unusual fungal or bacterial agents unrelated to human immunodeficiency virus infections is well known. *Actinomyces* and *Mucorales* species colonize the upper respiratory tract and may cause brain abscess secondary to local invasion.[83, 90] Brain abscess caused by *Pseudoallescheria boydii* complicating infection of an intravenous catheter and penetrating cranial vault injury has also been described.[91] *Nocardia asteroides* causes a lung-brain syndrome, with nodular and/or cavitary pulmonary infiltrates and mass lesions in the brain. A diagnosis of systemic nocardiosis warrants investigation for intracerebral lesions, even if overt clinical signs or symptoms are absent. Cerebral mass lesions caused by *Mycobacterium tuberculosis* or *C. neoformans* typically accompany systemic disease; however, atypical mycobacteria may cause cerebral involvement secondary to trauma, disseminated disease, and, theoretically, wound infection. Table 162–3 lists the additional infectious and noninfectious causes of CNS mass lesions in the immunocompromised host, which are discussed in greater detail in Chapter 137.

The anatomic location should suggest predisposing sources and associated etiologic agents and so may help direct early diagnostic procedures and antibiotic therapy. Cultures of superficial wound material do not always correlate with the organism responsible for deep wound infection. The underlying source of bacteremia resulting in brain abscess may be cryptic or only historically apparent at the time the abscess becomes clinically evident. Our ability to predict the pathogen of brain abscess is poorest when there is no obvious association with otic or paranasal sinus disease or source of bacteremia.

TABLE 162–3 ■ Causes of Mass Lesions of the Brain in the Immunocompromised Host

INFECTIOUS CAUSES		
Type of Organism	**Organism**	**NONINFECTIOUS CAUSES**
Bacteria	*Streptococcus* spp. and other typical pathogens (see Table 162–1)	Neoplasm
		Primary
		Metastatic
	Pseudomonas aeruginosa	Infarction
	Listeria monocytogenes	Aneurysm
	Enterobacteriaceae	Vascular malformation
	Nocardia asteroides	Radiation necrosis
	Stenotrophomonas (formerly *Xanthomonas*) *maltophilia*	
	Gordona terrae	
	Salmonella typhi	
	Rhodococcus equi	
Fungi	*Aspergillus* spp.	
	Mucorales	
	Candida spp.	
	Cryptococcus neoformans	
	Coccidiodes immitis	
	Fusarium oxysporum	
	Pseudoallescheria boydii	
	Fonsecaea pedrosoi	
	Cladosporium trichoides	
	Absidia spp.	
	Scopulariopsis spp.	
	Bipolaris spp.	
	Curvularia spp.	
Mycobacteria	*Mycobacterium tuberculosis*	
	Mycobacterium kansasii	
	Mycobacterium avium complex	
Protozoa	*Toxoplasma gondii*	
	Strongyloides stercoralis	
	Acanthamoeba spp.	
Viruses	Progressive multifocal leukoencephalopathy (JC virus)	
	Cytomegalovirus	

Clinical Manifestations

Signs and symptoms depend on the stage of the abscess, its anatomic location, and the patient's ability to communicate. The classic triad of fever, headache, and focal neurologic deficits is present in less than half of all affected patients, with fever present in only 40% to 50%.[13, 15, 92] Consequently, the clinical findings in the patient with brain abscess are not specific for infection, with most patients presenting with signs of rapidly or slowly expanding mass lesion. Most patients present with a less than 2-week history of symptoms, with headache present in approximately 75% of cases; nausea, vomiting, altered level of consciousness, and seizures are variably present.[1, 15, 93] If present, fever is frequently of low grade. Localizing signs or symptoms may be noted, with ataxia and nystagmus in the patient with cerebellar abscess, hemiparesis in the patient with basal ganglia or thalamic involvement, and altered personality in the patient with a frontal lobe lesion.[33, 94] In neonates, a rapid increase in head circumference has been noted.[95] Systemic cardinal signs and symptoms of inflammation are usually lacking. As a deep infectious problem, localized redness, swelling, and tenderness are uncommon unless the lesion is posttraumatic with overlying soft tissue infection or cranial vault osteomyelitis. Should the abscess be juxtaposed to meningeal surfaces, there may be commensurate meningeal irritation with nuchal rigidity and/or meningismus. If the clinical picture initially suggests a focal lesion but rapid deterioration occurs with fever, headache, and stiff neck, rupture of an abscess into the subarachnoid or intraventricular space should be seriously considered. The vagueness of neurologic signs and symptoms demands consideration of brain abscess in the differential diagnosis of malignancy, aneurysm, infarction, embolism, and a multitude of meningoencephalitides including herpes simplex encephalitis.[1–10, 13]

Peripheral leukocytosis is uncommonly noted, but if present it is generally mild (total white cell count less than 15,000/mm^3) and does not differentiate infection from neoplastic, immune-mediated, or nonneurologic infectious aspects of the differential diagnosis.[33] Absence of fever or leukocytosis should not eliminate brain abscess from diagnostic consideration. Elevation of the serum C-reactive protein has been a "soft" clue for brain abscess in the differential diagnosis of slowly progressive intracranial mass lesions.[96] Erythrocyte sedimentation rates are usually elevated, but this finding is nonspecific. Blood cultures are likely to be negative unless the brain abscess is associated with septic embolization from an intravascular endothelial infection such as endocarditis or aneurysm. Hyponatremia may be seen, concomitant with the syndrome of inappropriate secretion of antidiuretic hormone.

Diagnosis

Despite its essential role in diagnosing other CNS infections, lumbar puncture should not be the initial neurologic diagnostic test when a brain abscess or other intracranial mass lesion is suspected. Signs of increased intracranial pressure or focal neurologic findings have traditionally been contraindications to lumbar puncture. When MRI or CT fails to demonstrate excessive cerebral edema, midline shift, compression of the ventricles, or obstruction of the ventricular system, lumbar puncture is likely to be safe. Herniation, a dread complication with a mortality rate in excess of 25% to 30%, is heralded by bradypnea, bradycardia, and hypertension and is often irreversible; the frequency of this complication in the setting of brain abscess is estimated to be 20%.[13] Children with cyanotic congenital heart disease and brain abscess have suffered herniation after lumbar puncture even in the absence of obvious space-occupying lesions. If performed, lumbar puncture rarely reveals specific information.[13, 15] Hypoglycorrhachia is seen in 10% to 20% of patients. The cerebrospinal fluid (CSF) protein level is mildly elevated in 60% to 80% of cases; marked elevations of protein level should suggest an obstruction. A protein level in excess of 1 g (Froin syndrome) is seen in the presence of low pressure and an essentially complete obstruction. CSF demonstrates a pleocytosis of less than 500 cells per mm^3 in 60% to 70% of cases; lymphocytes usually predominate, although polymorphonuclear cells may be seen.[15] A CSF leukocyte count in excess of $1000/mm^3$ with a predominance of polymorphonuclear forms, if related to brain abscess, suggests meningitis secondary to rupture of the abscess into the ventricular or subarachnoid space. This occurrence is associated with rapid clinical deterioration and the appearance of signs and symptoms of bacterial meningitis. In this setting, Gram stain, culture, counterimmunoelectrophoresis, and limulus testing are important to rapidly establish an etiologic diagnosis (i.e., the meningitis provides a way of sampling the flora of the abscess); as anaerobes are not rapidly or easily identified, the physician must also recall the likely predisposing condition and provide coverage for the expected flora. Gas-liquid chromatography has been valuable in the rapid identification of anaerobes.[97] Importantly, the yield of CSF cultures, even with ventricular rupture of an abscess, is not greater than 20%.[15] In general, lumbar puncture yields little diagnostic information and carries a significant risk of morbidity and mortality in the patient with brain abscess and should be avoided.[98]

Advances in radiologic techniques have aided the diagnosis and management of CNS infections.[99] More invasive techniques such as myelography and pneumoencephalography are rarely necessary or indicated. Arteriography may still be required to help distinguish tumor, abscess, and ruptured aneurysm. Plain skull radiographs occasionally demonstrate air,[100] but they produce such a low yield that they should not be ordered routinely. Importantly, gas noted on skull films or CT scans may result from infection with gas-producing organisms or indicate extracranial communications predisposing to infection and requiring surgical repair.[47] Electroencephalography and ultrasonography are rarely of value in adult patients.[101–103] Indium 111 leukocyte scans have been evaluated as an adjunct to other diagnostic modalities.[104–108] These scans are 50% to 90% sensitive for the presence of infection, although false-positive scans due to infarcts, tumors, and hematomas have been described.[25, 33, 109, 110]

CT was a major advance that obviated the need for many invasive diagnostic techniques. In both animals and humans, CT abnormalities were found to change as the abscess evolved from a stage of cerebritis to a well-formed encapsulated lesion.[111–116] Bone window settings at the time of brain CT allow detection of suspected and occult sinusitis or mastoiditis as a predisposing condition to brain abscess.[117]

Inoculation of brain parenchyma with mixed aerobic and anaerobic flora has been followed by histopathologic correlation with CT findings in a number of animal studies.[114, 115, 118] Histopathologic examination at surgery and autopsy indicates that humans go through a similar staging process.[116] In general, abscesses undergo phases of early and late cerebritis (days 1 to 3, and 4 to 9, respectively), followed by early and late capsule formation between days 10 and 13, and day 14 and later.[119] The early cerebritis stage is marked radiographically by poorly delineated areas of low attenuation at CT, with little to no contrast enhancement. As the capsule begins to form (in the late cerebritis stage), peripheral enhancement may be noted, with a characteristic diffusion of contrast media into the center of the lesion on delayed (e.g., 60-minute) scanning. As the lesion becomes more encapsulated, this centripetal enhancement is lost, signaling the development of a necrotic center with limited vascular supply (a concept with important clinical implications, as noted later). Typically, there is thick smooth ring enhancement when contrast material is used in conjunction with CT, but enhancement may be irregular, especially with smaller lesions, making it difficult to exclude a neoplastic process. Capsules tend to form more readily and to be thicker on the side adjacent to gray matter, which is better vascularized than the white matter.[33] Concurrent antibiotic therapy, steroids, radiation, immunosuppression, or neutropenia may alter the expected staging progression. Steroid therapy may reduce the thickness of the capsule and the degree of ring enhancement present; importantly, capsule size may increase after the discontinuation of steroids, often without clinical deterioration or evidence of abscess expansion. In following the progression of disease and effect of therapy, the size of the enhancing capsule is recommended as a guide.[116]

None of the CT findings are pathognomonic for brain abscess, especially in the early cerebritis stage. Other CNS processes such as primary or metastatic tumor, infarction, resolving hematoma, and radiation necrosis may produce ring-enhancing lesions, further complicating definitive diagnosis.[13, 33, 120, 121] Patients with brain abscess have been empirically treated with irradiation, usually when an extracranial primary neoplasm is diagnosed first and the intracranial lesion is assumed to be metastatic. Conversely, patients with malignancy have received 6 weeks of empirical parenteral antibiotic therapy. Of course, brain abscess and neoplastic processes can coexist.

MRI is a rapidly expanding technology, but CT is the "gold standard" against which future technologies must be compared.[122, 123] The use of contrast enhancement with gadolinium–pentetic acid extends the usefulness of MRI by allowing evaluation of tissue perfusion and disruption of the blood-brain barrier[124] (Figs. 162–1 and 162–2). Studies of humans have corroborated the findings of animal studies of enhanced and earlier sensitivity, leading some authorities to suggest that MRI is now the diagnostic procedure of choice in brain abscess.[125–128] Additional advantages include the ability to better evaluate edema, atrophy, and hemorrhage as intraparenchymal complications of infection. Bone detail and calcification, however, are more difficult to evaluate by MRI than by CT.[125, 129] Cerebritis appears as an area of high signal intensity on T2-weighted images; the subsequent capsule appears as a ringlike area of low signal intensity.[128] As with CT, infection progression and resolution may be followed by using the size of the enhancing rim as a guide. As further studies using MRI to stage abscesses become available, its utility in diagnosing, staging, and following up patients with brain abscesses will become more apparent.

Definitive diagnosis of brain abscess and identification of

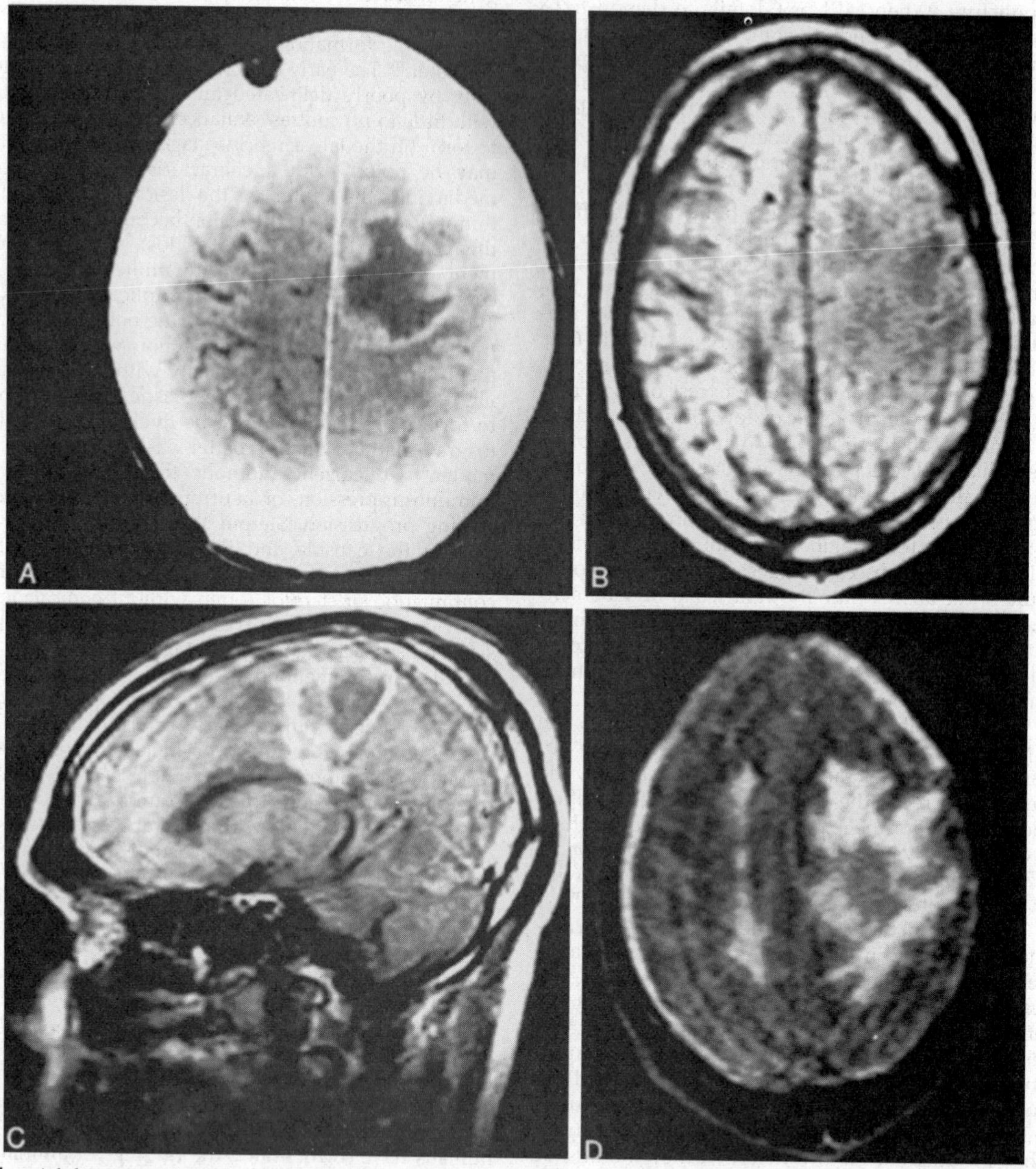

FIGURE 162–1 ▫ Adult man with brain abscess caused by *Listeria monocytogenes*. *A*, Postinfusion CT demonstrates mass lesion with ring enhancement. The serpiginous border is consistent with neoplasia. No lesion was seen on a scan made 1 month previously. Note bony defect from the burr hole for shunt placement. *B*, T1-weighted MRI study with low T1 signal in the region of the abscess as well as surrounding edema. *C*, T1-weighted MRI scan after gadolinium–pentetic acid with high signal intensity in the abscess wall and surrounding edema due to breakdown in the blood-brain barrier. *D*, T2-weighted MRI demonstrates the abscess as an area of low signal intensity and the surrounding edema as an area of high signal intensity. Note the high signal intensity of CSF. Gadolinium–pentetic acid does not affect the T2-weighted images.

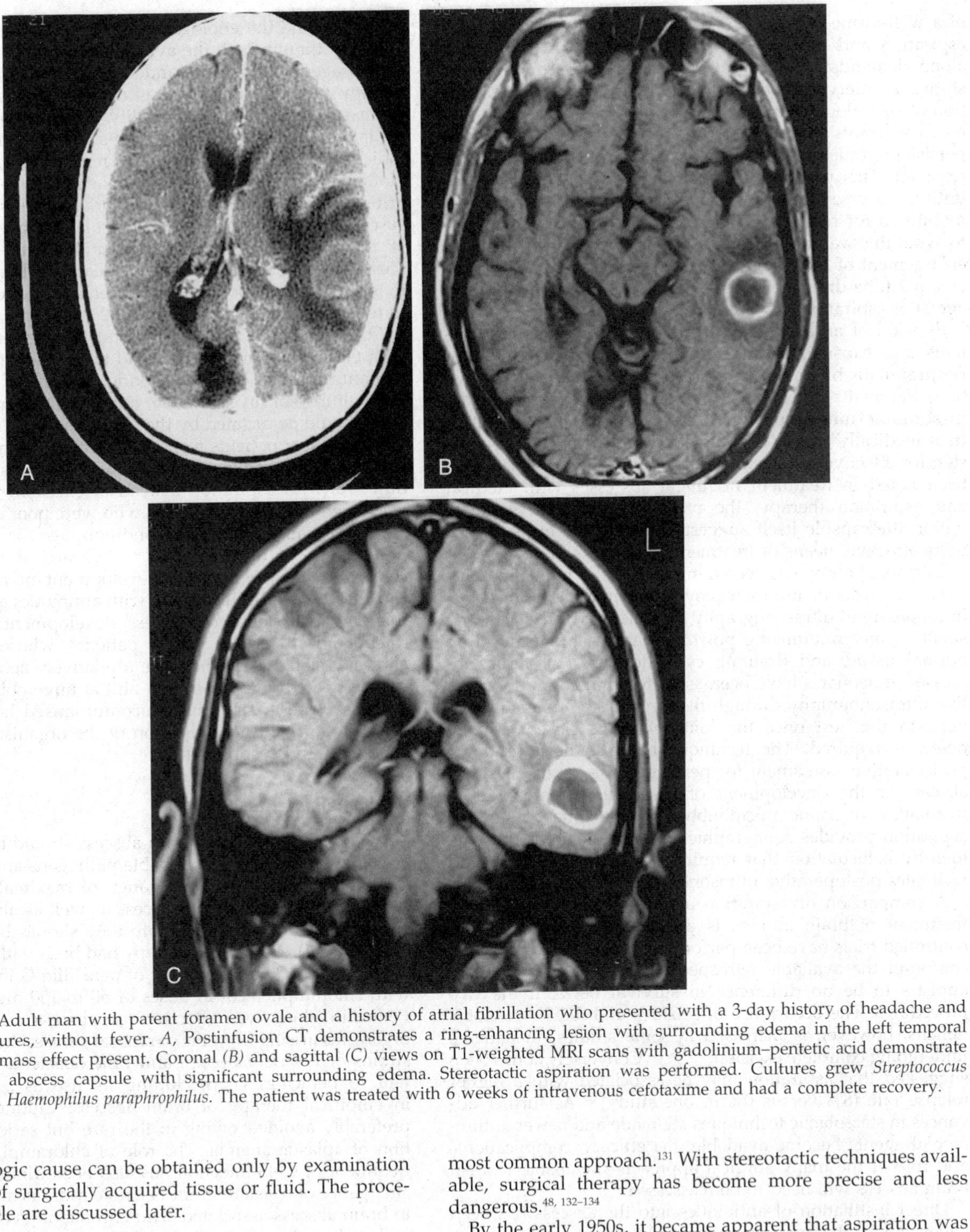

FIGURE 162–2 ▫ Adult man with patent foramen ovale and a history of atrial fibrillation who presented with a 3-day history of headache and new-onset seizures, without fever. *A*, Postinfusion CT demonstrates a ring-enhancing lesion with surrounding edema in the left temporal lobe. Note the mass effect present. Coronal *(B)* and sagittal *(C)* views on T1-weighted MRI scans with gadolinium–pentetic acid demonstrate an asymmetric abscess capsule with significant surrounding edema. Stereotactic aspiration was performed. Cultures grew *Streptococcus intermedius* and *Haemophilus paraphrophilus*. The patient was treated with 6 weeks of intravenous cefotaxime and had a complete recovery.

its microbiologic cause can be obtained only by examination and culture of surgically acquired tissue or fluid. The procedures available are discussed later.

Treatment

Surgical Therapy

Before the advent of antibiotics, surgery was the only therapy available. Potential procedures included aspiration, excision, marsupialization, tube drainage, and tapping.[130] Surgery reduced the nearly 100% mortality to a range of 25% to 60%. With the addition of antibiotics, mortality remained approximately 40%, although with CT and more effective antimicrobial agents, the overall mortality rate has declined to 5% to 10%.[33] Surgery is still the mainstay of therapy, with aspiration or excision combined with prolonged antibiotic courses the most common approach.[131] With stereotactic techniques available, surgical therapy has become more precise and less dangerous.[48, 132–134]

By the early 1950s, it became apparent that aspiration was often as effective as excision and that early antibiotic therapy might diminish a lesion and obviate the need for surgical intervention. Aspiration of a lesion is often necessary for diagnostic purposes and is helpful therapeutically, especially in patients with deep-seated lesions (e.g., in the cerebellum, brain stem, or thalamus).[48, 135–137] Aspiration is often performed in poor surgical candidates, as local anesthesia may be utilized.[48] Removal of purulent material provides a more favorable local environment for antimicrobial activity, in addition to allowing definitive identification of the etiologic organism(s) involved. The most common complication of this procedure is intracranial hemorrhage, which may occur during the cerebritis stage or from the vascularized capsule of a well-formed abscess.[13, 25, 138] A decision to proceed with aspiration and antibiotics, or occasionally with antibiotics alone, demands close clinical observation and sequential CT studies at intervals dictated by the clinical course. Deterioration of neurologic status or enlargement of the abscess seen by CT warrants a more extensive procedure.[139] CT may reveal persistence of a lesion when clinical signs or symptoms have resolved. This poses a dilemma that may not be resolved until the course of antibiotics is completed and the patient is monitored for relapse. A stereotactic procedure can be used to avoid this wait-and-see approach or as soon as there is any enlargement of the lesion after therapy concludes. Although external tube drainage is rarely used, the duration of drainage after aspiration has averaged 14.5 days.[132]

Excision of an abscess (with removal of the abscess contents and capsule) is often required for the treatment of posttraumatic brain abscess, to débride the area and remove bone fragments that may predispose to subsequent infection. In addition, multiloculated abscesses, which are difficult to treat medically and to aspirate effectively, may require excision for effective treatment. Clinical failures or relapses have been noted in treatment of fungal abscesses with medical and aspiration therapy; the presence of fungal elements within the capsule itself suggests that surgical excision is a more effective means of treatment.

Ultrasonography has been minimally useful in the preoperative diagnosis of intraparenchymal neurologic lesions, but intraoperative ultrasonography has assisted in localizing small lesions, minimizing potential damage to surrounding normal tissue, and draining cystic lesions.[140, 141] Brain abscesses in neonates have been aspirated utilizing intraoperative ultrasonography through the fontanels.[142] To adequately perform this test once the fontanels have closed, a bone defect is required. The technique has also been used for postoperative assessment for persistence or expansion of an abscess or the development of ventricular enlargement.[143] Instillation of saline microbubbles at the time of surgical aspiration provides sonographic contrast. At times this will identify a loculation that requires additional drainage and facilitates postoperative ultrasonographic follow-up.[144]

A comparison of aspiration and surgical excision in the treatment of brain abscess is difficult, as no randomized, controlled trials have been performed and selection bias may confound the available retrospective studies. Overall, there appears to be no difference in survival between the two procedures. The occurrence of seizures and focal neurologic deficits, however, is increased in some studies, in patients undergoing complete excision. [25, 145, 146] Conversely, it has been suggested that aspiration may be associated with a higher relapse rate (8% versus 0% in one study).[64] As further advances in stereotactic techniques are made and newer antimicrobial agents become available, the efficacy, complications, and role of the many surgical approaches available to treat brain abscess will need to be reassessed.

Direct instillation of antibiotics into the abscess has been suggested for therapy of pathogens that are particularly virulent or difficult to treat such as *Pseudomonas*.[15] This approach has been limited by the epileptogenic properties of certain instilled agents (e.g., high doses of penicillin or other β-lactam compounds) and, when performed during the early cerebritis stage, potential spread of infection.[25, 92, 147] Of note, there is no evidence that local instillation of antibiotics improves outcome.

A surgical procedure should be considered part of the definitive diagnostic and therapeutic approach to any patient with brain abscess.[148, 149] Improved surgical technique, early diagnosis, and antibiotic therapy have diminished acute surgical mortality from approximately 15% to a rare event.[150–152] Surgery will reduce mass effect, establish a diagnosis, and usually define the etiologic agent and its susceptibility pattern.[153] Although both the available antimicrobial agents and the dosage used have expanded over time, use of antibiotic therapy for brain abscess was not initially associated with decreased morbidity or mortality. As ring enhancement at CT is associated with late cerebritis and does not necessarily indicate capsule formation,[21, 154, 155] reported responses to antibiotic therapy alone may be due partially to therapy of cerebritis rather than to well-defined brain abscess.[20] At surgery, susceptible organisms have been isolated from brain abscess in the presence of therapeutic antimicrobial levels.[147] Abscesses smaller than 3 to 4 cm in diameter have been found to respond to antibiotics alone, whereas larger ones are likely to require excision or drainage.[64, 145, 156]

At a minimum, we recommend a diagnostic aspiration with Gram stain and aerobic and anaerobic culture to facilitate antimicrobial decision-making. The use of special stains and cultures for mycobacteria, fungi, or other unusual pathogens should be dictated by the clinical setting. Yet an increasing number of patients respond to antimicrobial therapy and do not need a diagnostic or therapeutic neurosurgical procedure. As with aspiration instead of excision, this approach was taken initially for patients who were poor candidates for surgery because of general condition, age, or number, location, or size of the lesions.[12, 157–159] Clearly, during the early cerebritis stage, before the development of a well-formed capsule, the possibility of cure with antibiotics alone is higher than in later stages of abscess development. The current dilemma is to decide which patients, whose condition is clinically stable and who have a relatively accessible lesion, can be treated with aspiration and antimicrobials or antimicrobials alone. In the immunocompromised host, the value of aspiration with identification of the organism(s) involved cannot be underestimated.[25]

Antimicrobial Therapy

Antibiotics used to treat brain abscess should be agents that are effective against the probable pathogens and available in parenteral form. Within the range of maximal daily doses, they should penetrate the abscess as well as any underlying site of infection, and preferably they should be bactericidal (Table 162–4). Traditional therapy had been with adult equivalent doses of 20 million units of penicillin G in combination with chloramphenicol in doses of 50 to 100 mg/kg per day. Penicillin alone was effective for abscess associated with organisms arising from the paranasal sinuses; however, many strains of *P. melaninogenica* and Enterobacteriaceae are resistant to penicillin G, precluding its use as a single agent in empirical therapy of brain abscess. Chloramphenicol is preferably avoided owing to the rare but serious complication of aplastic anemia. The role of chloramphenicol in the treatment of CNS infection has also been diminished by the emergence of resistant gram-negative rods, as might be found in brain abscess associated with chronic otitis or mastoiditis, and perhaps because it is usually bacteriostatic. An effective alternative is available. Metronidazole penetrates abscess cavities at levels that are frequently higher than the concurrent serum concentration. It is bactericidal and effective at acid pH in the presence of pus or neutropenia, but it provides no aerobic coverage, and its activity against *Peptococcus* and *Peptostreptococcus* may be marginal.[160–162] Therefore, depending on the likely mixed flora, metronidazole must be accompanied by a second agent, such as penicillin or a third-generation cephalosporin. Doses of 7.5 mg/kg given intravenously every 6 hours are recommended.[33]

New therapeutic agents have become available in the 1990s. Although controlled studies are lacking, the spectrum of activity, pharmacokinetic data, and clinical experience in-

TABLE 162–4 ■ Antibiotic Selection Based on Condition Predisposing to Brain Abscess*

FOCUS	ANTIBIOTIC
Otic Mastoid Paranasal sinus (operated on or irrigated) Empyema Lung abscess	Third-generation cephalosporin† and metronidazole
Dental Paranasal sinus (not operated on or irrigated)	Penicillin‡ and metronidazole
Bacteremia	
Gastrointestinal origin	Third-generation cephalosporin and metronidazole
Urinary tract origin	
Acute	Cefuroxime§ or trimethoprim-sulfamethoxazole
Chronic	Third-generation cephalosporin
Endocarditis	As for the pathogen causing endocarditis
Wounds	
Use Gram stain for early decision	
Pure gram-negative or mixed flora	Third-generation cephalosporin and metronidazole
Gram-positive cocci	Penicillinase-resistant antistaphylococcal penicillin‡‖

*Use maximal daily doses with adjustments as dictated by renal and hepatic function. Therapy should eventually be tailored to results of culture and susceptibility tests. Remember that anaerobes may take weeks to grow.

†Ceftriaxone, ceftazidime, cefotaxime, ceftizoxime, moxalactam; we avoid moxalactam based on the possibility of associated increased clinical bleeding.

‡Vancomycin should be used for penicillin-allergic patients or when methicillin-resistant *Staphylococcus aureus* is a concern. Vancomycin should be the drug of choice when the gram-positive cocci are from a surgical wound.

§Cefuroxime is the only first- or second-generation cephalosporin indicated for bacterial meningitis and the only first- or second-generation cephalosporin we would recommend using in the treatment of brain abscess.

‖Oxacillin, nafcillin, methicillin.

dicate efficacy. Many third-generation cephalosporins and a single second-generation agent, cefuroxime, have become drugs of choice for therapy of pediatric bacterial meningitis. Ceftriaxone, cefotaxime, ceftizoxime, and ceftazidime have been used in many patients with brain abscess; they penetrate the CNS well and cover many methicillin-susceptible *S. aureus*, streptococci, Enterobacteriaceae, and *Pseudomonas* species.[13, 15, 163] In combination with intravenous metronidazole, these agents provide broad-spectrum empirical coverage in many patients with bacterial brain abscess.[164] Ceftriaxone has enjoyed wide use because of its once- or twice-daily administration. It is important to remember that none of these agents has good activity against *L. monocytogenes*, a cause of both meningitis and brain abscess. Imipenem levels in serum, CSF, and brain abscess exceeded the minimal inhibitory concentrations for the infecting organisms in a patient with multiple cerebral abscesses.[165] However, CNS toxicity, manifested by seizures or obtundation, limits the usefulness of imipenem as a drug of choice for brain abscess. Quinolones, DNA gyrase inhibitors, are active against a broad spectrum of gram-negative aerobes and staphylococci and may be useful in some patients; their CNS toxicity profile may be prohibitive in some cases, however.

Expanded-spectrum penicillins, including nafcillin and oxacillin, have also proved efficacious, when given in high doses (e.g., 12 to 18 g/d of nafcillin).[33] For nearly two decades, the aminoglycosides—gentamicin, tobramycin, and amikacin—have been the gold standard of therapy for infections caused by Enterobacteriaceae and *Pseudomonas aeruginosa*. Aminoglycoside penetration of brain abscess is more predictable than penetration of CSF; however, decreased activity at acidic pH as might be encountered within the abscess, the potential renal toxicity and ototoxicity, and the availability of newer agents that do not require as intense monitoring will likely continue to decrease the use of aminoglycosides for empirical gram-negative aerobic coverage. Aminoglycosides may be needed for the therapy of unusual gram-negative organisms or common organisms resistant to broad-spectrum β-lactam agents. Aztreonam is a monocyclic β-lactam with a spectrum of activity against gram-negative aerobic rods similar to that of aminoglycosides. Its role in brain abscess has not been determined. The tetracyclines penetrate CSF poorly and are generally ineffective in brain abscess.

Selection of antibiotics encompasses several possible scenarios. Secretions or drainage from any underlying focus should be obtained for Gram stain and culture if at all possible. Gram stains are helpful in initial decision-making, while culture results are pending. Cultures and antimicrobial susceptibility testing allow tailoring of the antimicrobial regimen to obtain the widest therapeutic/toxic ratio. Rarely, the organism will have already been isolated from abscess, blood, sinus, empyema, or wound, and initial antimicrobial therapy can be based on known susceptibility. More typically, the likely flora is suggested by the anatomic location of the brain abscess and a known underlying cause.

When the origin is related to the ears and mastoids, metronidazole and a third-generation cephalosporin are appropriate. Empyema and lung abscess would be treated as are otic, paranasal sinus, or mastoid foci, with coverage of Enterobacteriaceae, *P. aeruginosa*, aerobic streptococci, and anaerobes. An abscess of dental origin dictates penicillin and metronidazole for streptococci and *Eikenella* and *Bacteroides* species potentially present. An obvious source of bacteremia also indicates coverage of the likely agent (e.g., gram-negative organisms from the abdomen or urinary tract; staphylococcal or streptococcal species from wounds).

The therapy of infections caused by methicillin-susceptible *S. aureus* is best accomplished with a narrow-spectrum β-lactamase–stable penicillin, such as oxacillin or nafcillin. These are preferable to broader spectrum antistaphylococcal β-lactam antibiotics and are more active on a weight basis. Any antistaphylococcal β-lactamase–stable penicillin should be given in intravenous doses of 12 g/d or more.[166] Vancomycin has traditionally been reserved for the therapy of methicillin-resistant *S. aureus*, clinically significant *Staphylococcus epidermidis*, and other gram-positive coccal infections in penicillin-allergic patients. Should clinically significant *S. epidermidis* infections in immunocompetent hosts or the frequency of methicillin-resistant *S. aureus* infections of community onset continue to increase, vancomycin will become a drug of choice when any staphylococcal infection is suspected. Importantly, vancomycin concentrates in brain abscesses with levels 60% to 80% of concomitant serum levels.[167] In addition, as vancomycin-resistant enterococci are an increasing cause of nosocomial bacteremia, these organisms are anticipated to cause brain abscess in the future. Cephalosporins, imipenem, and β-lactams in combination with β-lactamase inhibitors are all active against methicillin-susceptible *S. aureus* strains, but despite reports of laboratory susceptibility, clinical failures may occur. These agents should not be used for treating CNS infections caused by methicillin-resistant *S. aureus*.

Ancillary therapy of brain abscess has included mannitol, hyperventilation, and steroids, which have been used to reduce intracranial swelling and cerebral edema. The osmotic effect of mannitol has been associated with an increase in gentamicin concentrations in the abscess and surrounding tissue, although its role in abscess resolution is unclear. Steroid effects on radiographic appearance and therapy of brain abscess have been discussed. In a rodent model of *E. coli* brain abscess, steroids were associated with an increase in the evident number of bacteria while there was decreased collagen formation and macrophage and glial response, as well as overall diminished survival. The delivery of gentamicin was inconsistent and not obviously affected by steroid therapy, although it has been suggested by a number of authors[33, 168–170] that steroids decrease antibiotic penetration into abscesses. In patients with bacterial meningitis, the use of steroids has been associated with decreased levels of antibiotics in CSF. When *P. melaninogenica* was inoculated stereotactically to produce abscess, concomitant use of corticosteroids significantly reduced the local concentrations of benzyl penicillin, but not of metronidazole.[171] Methylprednisolone has been found to decrease collagen deposition 8 days after inoculation of organisms, but no effect on capsule thickness was apparent by 18 days after inoculation.[172] In one patient, steroid therapy decreased ring enhancement and was associated with clinical improvement in the absence of concomitant antimicrobial therapy.[173] After discontinuation of the steroid therapy, enhancement increased and the patient's clinical condition deteriorated. In addition, no studies have demonstrated a benefit regarding survival, neurologic sequelae, or length of hospital stay in patients treated with steroids.[1, 169] When steroids are indicated to decrease cerebral edema and increased intracranial pressure, they should be used for as brief a time as possible. If brain abscess is suspected, these agents should not be given without concurrent effective antimicrobial therapy.

Duration of antibiotic therapy should be 4 to 6 weeks for most pathogens. In the immunocompromised host, more prolonged antibiotic courses may be necessary, based on the organisms involved and the particular immunosuppressed state of the host. If the abscess is excised completely, a shorter course is more likely appropriate, yet in the absence of specific data, we recommend at least 4 weeks of therapy after complete excision. Oral therapy has been suggested,[174] although we currently avoid it unless 4 weeks of parenteral therapy has been completed. If this is accomplished, no further therapy may be necessary. If an oral agent is prescribed, documentation of high therapeutic serum levels is recommended. Most agents used as initial parenteral therapy are either not available in oral form or cannot be given in oral doses approximating those administered parenterally. CT should be used in addition to clinical follow-up, with most authors recommending CT every 2 weeks while the patient receives therapy or as clinically indicated.[64, 175] Ring-enhancing lesions may persist as long as 3 to 4 months and are not by themselves an indication for prolonging therapy.[25] Radiographic techniques and multiple scans potentially expose the patient to doses of radiation (200 cGy) that are theoretically capable of initiating cataract formation,[176] an important consideration in follow-up evaluations. Surgical intervention is indicated if, either during or after completion of therapy, symptoms recur or progress, or the lesion enlarges.

Prognosis

Recurrences occur in 5% to 10% of patients, usually within 6 weeks of completion of antibiotic therapy.[14, 25] Occasional cases of recurrent infection have been noted years after presumed adequate therapy. Relapses may be related to inadequate antimicrobial therapy (e.g., ineffective agents, poor abscess penetration at doses prescribed, development of resistance), failure to aspirate a lesion or treat the underlying cause, or the presence of a foreign body or persistent extracranial communication. The evaluation and treatment of the patient with recurrent abscess should include an extensive search for and eradication of the underlying cause of failure.

Morbidity related to brain abscess may be substantial, with epilepsy noted in as many as 72% of patients after effective therapy.[25, 146] Since the advent of CT, patients are more alert and have fewer lesions and a better-defined surgical site at the time of diagnosis. Postoperative complications such as recurrence, hemorrhage, and cerebral edema are more specifically and easily identified by CT or MRI.[177] Focal neurologic sequelae are usually minor and infrequent but have occurred in up to 24% of patients. The prevalence of mental retardation has averaged about 16% and is correlated with disease in childhood and underlying cyanotic congenital heart disease.[146, 178] Seizures have been reported in 10% to 72% of patients, with mean onset in the third year after abscess treatment.[25, 179] Studies documenting long-term follow-up of patients indicate that seizures may develop years after therapy and are most frequent in those with temporal or frontal lesions.[146] Severity of disability related to epilepsy varies; 3 to 7 years after diagnosis and therapy, two thirds of affected patients were able to work without restriction. Electroencephalographic abnormalities have not correlated directly with overall prognosis. Electroencephalographic abnormalities have persisted in up to 50% of patients who initially had abnormalities.[180] Rarely, gliosarcoma has followed brain abscess associated with injection of Thorotrast into the lesion and surgical decompression.[181, 182] Meningioma after abscess treatment has also been described.[183]

Mortality is currently 5% to 10% overall.[16, 33, 150–152, 184] The operative mortality rate has usually been the same or less than the nonoperative mortality. Misdiagnosis accounts for a significant percentage of cases diagnosed at autopsy. Multiple lesions, deep-seated lesions, abscess rupture, and age older than 40 years portend higher risk of death, although in many studies the only factor predictive of mortality or sequelae is level of consciousness at presentation.[93, 172, 185–187] The prognosis is poorer with diminishing state of consciousness at presentation—from lethargy to obtundation, stupor, and coma. Patients who present in coma usually have no antecedent focal signs or symptoms, no history of seizures, and no symptoms suggestive of meningitis and have a significantly worse prognosis overall. The treatment route chosen does not appear, in most studies,[145, 188] to affect overall mortality rates.

Brain abscess remains a disease of low frequency but significant morbidity and mortality. Further advances in surgical and neuroradiologic techniques are anticipated, as are additional antibiotic agents with favorable antimicrobial spectra and pharmacokinetic properties. Only time will tell whether the outcome for patients will continue to improve.

References

1. Chun CH, Johnson JD, Hofstetter M, et al: Brain abscess: A study of 45 consecutive cases. Medicine (Baltimore) 65:415, 1986.
2. Harris LF, Maccubbin DA, Triplett JN, et al: Brain abscess: Recent experience at a community hospital. South Med J 78:704, 1985.
3. Garvey G: Current concepts of bacterial infections of the central nervous system. Bacterial meningitis and bacterial brain abscess. J Neurosurg 59:735, 1983.
4. Renier D, Flandin C, Hirsch E, et al: Brain abscesses in neonates: A study of 30 cases. J Neurosurg 69:877, 1988.
5. Sutton DL, Ouvrier RA: Cerebral abscess in the under 6 month age group. Arch Dis Child 58:901, 1983.
6. Theophilo F, Markakis E, Theophilo L, et al: Brain abscess in childhood. Childs Nerv Syst 1:324, 1985.
7. Hegde AS, Venkataramana NK, Das BS: Brain abscess in children. Childs Nerv Syst 2:90, 1986.

8. Tavora L, Antunes JL: Brain abscesses and ischemic necrotic lesions during early childhood. Neurosurgery 21:923, 1987.
9. Small M, Dale BA: Intracranial suppuration 1968–1982—A 15 year review. Clin Otolaryngol 9:315, 1984.
10. Molavi AA, Dinubile MJ: Brain Abscess. *In* Harris AA (ed): Handbook of Clinical Neurology. Amsterdam, Elsevier, 1988, pp 143–166.
11. Samson DS, Clark K: A current review of brain abscesses. Am J Med 54:201, 1973.
12. Donald FE, Firth JL, Holland IM, et al: Brain abscess in the 1980's. Br J Neurosurg 4:265, 1990.
13. Wispelwey B, Scheld WM: Brain abscess. Semin Neurol 12:273, 1992.
14. Beller AJ, Sahar A, Praiss I: Brain abscess: Review of 89 cases over a period of 30 years. J Neurol Neurosurg Psychiatry 36:757, 1973.
15. Wispelwey B, Scheld WM: Brain abscess. Clin Neuropharmacol 10:483, 1987.
16. Lakshmi V, Rao RR, Dinakar I: Bacteriology of brain abscess—Observations on 50 cases. J Med Microbiol 38:187, 1993.
17. Richards J, Sisson PR, Hickman JE, et al: Microbiology, chemotherapy and mortality of brain abscess in Newcastle-upon-Tyne between 1979 and 1988. Scand J Infect Dis 22:511, 1990.
18. Kangsanarak J, Fooanant S, Ruckphaopunt K, et al: Extracranial and intracranial complications of suppurative otitis media. Report of 102 cases. J Laryngol Otol 107:999, 1993.
19. Hervas JA, Ciria L, Henales V, et al: Nonsurgical management of neonatal multiple brain abscesses due to *Proteus mirabilis*. Helv Paediatr Acta 42:451, 1987.
20. Neuwelt EA, Lawrence MS, Blank NK: Effect of gentamicin and dexamethasone on the natural history of the rat *Escherichia coli* brain abscess model with histopathological correlation. Neurosurgery 15:475, 1984.
21. Mathisen GE, Meyer RD, George WL, et al: Brain abscess and cerebritis. Rev Infect Dis 6:S101, 1984.
22. Boom WH, Tuazon CU: Successful treatment of multiple brain abscesses with antibiotics alone. Rev Infect Dis 7:189, 1985.
23. Kagawa M, Takeshita M, Yato S, et al: Brain abscess in congenital cyanotic heart disease. J Neurosurg 58:913, 1983.
24. Coroli M, Arienta C, Rampini PM, et al: Recurrence of brain abscess associated with asymptomatic arteriovenous malformation of the lung. Neurochirurgia 35:167, 1992.
25. Osenbach RK, Loftus CM: Diagnosis and management of brain abscess. Neurosurg Clin North Am 3:403, 1992.
26. Hall WA: Hereditary hemorrhagic telangiectasia (Rendu-Osler-Weber disease) presenting with polymicrobial brain abscess: Case report. J Neurosurg 81:294, 1994.
27. Román G, Fisher M, Perl DP, et al: Neurological manifestations of hereditary hemorrhagic telangiectasia (Rendu-Osler-Weber disease): Report of two cases and review of the literature. Ann Neurol 4:130, 1978.
28. Kurzydlowski H, Wollenschlager C, Venezio FR, et al: Reevaluation of an experimental streptococcal canine brain abscess model. J Neurosurg 67:717, 1987.
29. Costello GT, Heppe R, Winn HR, et al: Susceptibility of brain to aerobic, anaerobic, and fungal organisms. Infect Immun 41:535, 1983.
30. Kline MW, Kaplan SL, Hawkins EP, et al: Pathogenesis of brain abscess formation in an infant rat model of *Citrobacter diversus* bacteremia and meningitis. J Infect Dis 157:106, 1988.
31. Enzmann DR, Britt RR, Obana WB, et al: Experimental *Staphylococcus aureus* brain abscess. AJNR 7:395, 1986.
32. Obana WB, Britt RH, Placone RC, et al: Experimental brain abscess development in the chronically immunosuppressed host. J Neurosurg 65:382, 1986.
33. Kaplan K: Brain abscess. Med Clin North Am 69:345, 1985.
34. Kanter MC, Hart RG: Neurologic complications of infective endocarditis. Neurology 41:1015, 1991.
35. Lerner PI: Neurologic complications of infective endocarditis. Med Clin North Am 69:385, 1985.
36. Gelfand MS, Stephens DS, Howell EI, et al: Brain abscess: Association with pulmonary arteriovenous fistula and hereditary hemorrhagic telangiectasia: Report of three cases. Am J Med 85:719, 1988.
37. Press OW, Ramsey PG: Central nervous system infections associated with hereditary hemorrhagic telangiectasia. Am J Med 77:86, 1984.
38. Gibbons JR, McIlrath TE, Bailey IC: Pulmonary arteriovenous fistula in association with recurrent cerebral abscess. Thorac Cardiovasc Surg 33:319, 1984.
39. Biller J, Baker WH, Quinn JP, et al: Intracranial hematoma with subsequent brain abscess after carotid endarterectomy. Surg Neurol 23:605, 1984.
40. Biller J, Adams HP Jr, Godersky JC, et al: Preeclampsia complicated by cerebral hemorrhage and brain abscess. J Neurol 232:378, 1985.
41. Gower D, McGuirt WF: Intracranial complications of acute and chronic infectious ear disease: A problem still with us. Laryngoscope 93:1028, 1983.
42. Gower DJ, McGuirt WF, Kelley DL Jr: Intracranial complications of ear disease in a pediatric population with special emphasis on subdural effusion and empyema. South Med J 78:429, 1984.
43. Bradley PJ, Manning KP, Shaw MD: Brain abscess secondary to otitis media. J Laryngol Otol 98:1185, 1984.
44. Samuel J, Fernandes CM, Steinberg JL: Intracranial otogenic complications: A persisting problem. Laryngoscope 96:272, 1986.
45. Venezio FR, Naidich TP, Shulman ST: Complications of mastoiditis with special emphasis on venous sinus thrombosis. J Pediatr 101:509, 1982.
46. Nunez DA, Browning GG: Risks of developing an otogenic intracranial abscess. J Laryngol Otol 104:468, 1990.
47. Jurado R, Garcia-Herola A, Garcia-Lazaro M, et al: Brain abscess with intracranial gas formation: Case report. Clin Infect Dis 19:219, 1994.
48. Kondziolka D, Duma CM, Lunsford LD: Factors that enhance the likelihood of successful stereotactic treatment of brain abscesses. Acta Neurochir 127:85, 1994.
49. Mathews TJ: Acute and acute-on-chronic mastoiditis (a five year experience at Groote Schuur Hospital). J Laryngol Otol 102:115, 1988.
50. Nalbone VP, Kuruvilla A, Gacek RR: Otogenic brain abscess: The Syracuse experience. Ear Nose Throat J 71:238, 1992.
51. Kratimenos G, Crockard HA: Multiple brain abscess: A review of fourteen cases. Br J Neurosurg 5:153, 1991.
52. Yogev R: Suppurative intracranial complications of upper respiratory tract infections. Pediatr Infect Dis J 6:324, 1987.
53. Aldous JA, Powell GL, Stensaas SS: Brain abscess of odontogenic origin: Report of case. J Am Dent Assoc 115:861, 1987.
54. Ingham, HR, Kalbag RM, Tharagonnet D, et al: Abscesses of the frontal lobe of the brain secondary to covert dental sepsis. Lancet 2:497, 1978.
55. Haddad FS, Hubballa J, Zaytoun G, et al: Intracranial complications of submucous resection of the nasal septum. Am J Otolaryngol 6:443, 1985.
56. Celli P, Palatinsky E: Brain abscess as a complication of cranial traction. Surg Neurol 23:594, 1985.
57. Martinez-Lage JF, Perez-Espejo MA, Masegosa J, et al: Bilateral brain abscesses complicating the use of Crutchfield tongs. Childs Nerv Syst 2:208, 1986.
58. Goodman ML, Nelson PB: Brain abscess complicating the use of a halo orthosis. Neurosurgery 20:27, 1987.
59. Williams FH, Nelms DK, McGaharan KM: Brain abscess: A rare complication of halo usage. Arch Phys Med Rehabil 73:490, 1992.
60. Blomstedt GC: Infections in neurosurgery: A retrospective study of 1143 patients and 1517 operations. Acta Neurochir 78:81, 1985.
61. Tay JS, Garland JS: Serious head injuries from lawn darts. Pediatrics 79:261, 1987.
62. Foy P, Sharr M: Cerebral abscesses in children after pencil-tip injuries. Lancet 2:662, 1980.
63. Bank DE, Carolan PL: Cerebral abscess formation following ocular trauma: A hazard associated with common wooden toys. Pediatr Emerg Care 9:285, 1993.
64. Rosenblum ML, Mampalam TJ, Pons VG: Controversies in the management of brain abscesses. Clin Neurosurg 33:603, 1986.
65. Pancek TL, Burchiel KJ: Delayed brain abscess related to a retained foreign body with culture of *Clostridium bifermentans*. Case report. J Neurosurg 64:813, 1986.
66. Schijman E, Monges J, Cragnaz R: Congenital dermal sinuses, dermoid and epidermoid cysts of the posterior fossa. Childs Nerv Syst 2:83, 1986.

67. Martens F, Ectors P, Noel P, et al: Unusual cause of cerebellar abscess. Occipital dermal sinus and dermoid cyst. Neuropediatrics 18:107, 1987.
68. Morgan MG, Stuart C, Leanord AT, et al: *Citrobacter diversus* brain abscess: Case reports and molecular epidemiology. J Med Microbiol 36:273, 1992.
69. Curless RG: Neonatal intracranial abscess: Two cases caused by *Citrobacter* and a literature review. Ann Neurol 8:269, 1980.
70. Dee RR, Lorber B: Brain abscess due to *Listeria monocytogenes*: Case report and literature review. Rev Infect Dis 8:968, 1986.
71. Feldman WE, Schwartz J: *Haemophilus influenzae* type b brain abscess complicating meningitis: Case report. Pediatrics 72:473, 1983.
72. Abla AA, Maroon JC, Slifkin M: Brain abscess due to *Haemophilus aphrophilus*: Possible canine transmission. Neurosurgery 19:123, 1986.
73. Jensen KT, Hojbjerg T: Meningitis and brain abscess due to *Haemophilus paraphrophilus*. Eur J Clin Microbiol 4:419, 1985.
74. Habib M, Fosse T, Pellissier JF, et al: Metastatic cerebral abscesses due to *Haemophilus paraphrophilus*. Arch Neurol 41: 1290, 1984.
75. Pajeau AK, Yu PK, Ebersold MJ: *Haemophilus paraphrophilus* frontal lobe abscess: Case report. Neurosurgery 23:643, 1988.
76. Schlitt M, Mitchem L, Zorn G, et al: Brain abscess after esophageal dilation for caustic stricture: Report of three cases. Neurosurgery 17:947, 1985.
77. Cohen FL, Koerner RS, Taub SJ: Solitary brain abscess following endoscopic injection sclerosis of esophageal varices. Gastrointest Endosc 31:331, 1985.
78. Algoed L, Boon P, De Vos M, et al: Brain abscess after esophageal dilatation for stenosis. Clin Neurol Neurosurg 94:169, 1992.
79. Robert JY, Raoul JL, Bretagne JF, et al: Unusual presentation of a case of brain abscess after endoscopic injection sclerotherapy of esophageal varices. Endoscopy 23:237, 1991.
80. De Louvois J, Gortvai P, Hurley R: Bacteriology of abscesses of the central nervous system: A multicentre prospective study. Br Med J 2:981, 1977.
81. Szuwart U, Bennefeld H: Bacteriologic analysis of pyogenic infections of the brain. Neurosurg Rev 13:113, 1990.
82. Ariza J, Casanova A, Fernandez Viladrich P, et al: Etiological agent and primary source of infection in 42 cases of focal intracranial suppuration. J Clin Microbiol 24:899, 1986.
83. Smego RA: Actinomycosis of the central nervous system. Rev Infect Dis 9:855, 1987.
84. Gupta SK, Mohanty S, Tandon SC, et al: Brain abscess: With special reference to infection by *Pseudomonas*. Br J Neurosurg 4:279, 1990.
85. Rodriguez RE, Valero V, Watanakunakorn C: *Salmonella* focal intracranial infections: Review of the world literature (1884–1984) and report of an unusual case. Rev Infect Dis 8:31, 1986.
86. Iplikcioglu AC, Kokes F, Bayar MA, et al: Brain abscess caused by *Salmonella typhimurium*: Case report and review of the literature. J Neurosurg Sci 35:165, 1991.
87. Noguerado A, Cabanyes J, Vivancos J, et al: Abscess caused by *Salmonella enteritidis* with a glioblastoma multiforme. J Infect 15:61, 1987.
88. Strampfer MJ, Schoch PE, Cunha BA: Cerebral abscess caused by *Klebsiella ozaenae*. J Clin Microbiol 25:1553, 1987.
89. Andersen BB, Sogaard I: Legionnaire's disease and brain abscess. Neurology 37:333, 1987.
90. Couch L, Theilen F, Mader JT: Rhinocerebral mucormycosis with cerebral extension successfully treated with adjunctive hyperbaric oxygen therapy. Arch Otolaryngol Head Neck Surg 14:791, 1988.
91. Perez RE, Smith M, McClendon J, et al: *Pseudallescheria boydii* brain abscess. Complication of an intravenous catheter. Am J Med 84:359, 1988.
92. Yang SY: Brain abscess: A review of 400 cases. J Neurosurg 55:794, 1981.
93. Bidzinski J, Koszewski W: The value of different methods of treatment of brain abscess in the CT era. Acta Neurochir 105:117, 1990.
94. Brydon HL, Hardwidge C: The management of cerebellar abscess since the introduction of CT scanning. Br J Neurosurg 8:447, 1994.
95. Lahat E, Livneh M, Schiffer J, et al: Rapidly growing head circumference as an isolated presenting symptom of brain abscesses in an infant. Clin Neurol Neurosurg 89:269, 1987.
96. Hirschberg H, Bosnes V: C-reactive protein levels in the differential diagnosis of brain abscesses. J Neurosurg 67:358, 1987.
97. Gupta U, Murugesan K, Bhatia R, et al: Gas liquid chromatography in rapid diagnosis of anaerobic brain abscess. Indian J Med Res 84:502, 1986.
98. Nielsen H: Cerebral abscess in children. Neuropediatrics 14:76, 1983.
99. Sarwar M, Falkoff G, Naseem M: Radiologic techniques in the diagnosis of CNS infections. Neurol Clin 4:41, 1986.
100. Young RF, Frazee J: Gas within intracranial abscess cavities: An indication for surgical excision. Ann Neurol 16:35, 1984.
101. Kawamura H, Umezawa Y, Amano K, et al: EEG topographic changes of brain abscesses in children. No Shinkei Geka 15:381, 1987.
102. Frank JL: Sonography of intracranial infection in infants and children. Neuroradiology 28:440, 1986.
103. Gray PH, O'Reilly C: Neonatal *Proteus mirabilis* meningitis and cerebral abscess: Diagnosis by real-time ultrasound. J Clin Ultrasound 12:441, 1984.
104. Rehncrona S, Brismar J, Holtas S: Diagnosis of brain abscesses with indium-111–labeled leukocytes. Neurosurgery 16:23, 1985.
105. Bellotti C, Aragno MG, Medina M, et al: Differential diagnosis of CT-hypodense cranial lesions with indium-111-oxine–labeled leukocytes. J Neurosurg 64:750, 1986.
106. Dudiak CM, Ali A, Dickerson M, et al: Acute tentorial subdural hematoma as a false-positive in indium-111 leukocyte scintigraphy. Clin Nucl Med 10:513, 1985.
107. Balachandran S, Husain MM, Adametz JR, et al: Uptake of indium-111–labeled leukocytes by brain metastasis. Neurosurgery 20:606, 1987.
108. Shih WJ, DeLand FH: Equivocal findings on cranial CT but apparent cerebral lesion(s) on conventional radionuclide imaging. Clin Nucl Med 12:219, 1987.
109. Palestro CJ, Swyer AJ, Kim CK, et al: Role of In-111 labeled leukocyte scintigraphy in the diagnosis of intracerebral lesions. Clin Nucl Med 16:305, 1991.
110. Whelan MA, Hilal SK: Computed tomography as a guide in the diagnosis and follow-up of brain abscesses. Radiology 135:663, 1980.
111. Enzmann DR, Placone RC, Britt RH: Dynamic computed tomographic scans in experimental brain abscess. Neuroradiology 26:309, 1984.
112. Enzmann DR, Britt RH, Placone R: Staging of human brain abscess by computed tomography. Radiology 146:703, 1983.
113. Weisberg LA: The role of CT in the evaluation of patients with intracranial CNS infectious-inflammatory disorder. Comput Radiol 8:29, 1984.
114. Britt RH, Enzmann DR, Yeager AS: Neuropathological and computerized tomographic findings in experimental brain abscess. J Neurosurg 55:590, 1981.
115. Enzmann DR, Britt RH, Yeager AS: Experimental brain abscess evolution: Computed tomographic and neuropathologic correlation. Radiology 133:113, 1979.
116. Enzmann DR. Britt RH, Placone R: Staging of human brain abscess by computed tomography. Radiology 146:703, 1983.
117. Carter BL, Bankoff MS, Fisk JD: Computed tomographic detection of sinusitis responsible for intracranial and extracranial infections. Radiology 147:739, 1983.
118. Britt RH, Enzmann DR, Placone RC Jr, et al: Experimental anaerobic brain abscess: Computerized tomographic and neuropathological correlations. J Neurosurg 60:1148, 1984.
119. Britt RH, Enzmann DR: Clinical stages of human brain abscesses on serial CT scans after contrast infusion. Computerized tomographic, neuropathological, and clinical correlations. J Neurosurg 59:972, 1983.
120. Piszczor M, Thornton G, Bia FJ: The evaluation of contrast-enhancing brain lesions: Pitfalls in current practice. Yale J Biol Med 58:19, 1985.
121. Berry AD III, Reintjes SL, Kepes JJ: Intracranial malignant fibrous histiocytoma with abscess-like tumor necrosis. Case report. J Neurosurg 69:780, 1988.
122. Bydder GM: Magnetic resonance imaging of the brain. Radiol Clin North Am 22:779, 1984.
123. Sze G, Zimmerman RD: The magnetic resonance imaging of

infections and inflammatory diseases. Radiol Clin North Am 26:839, 1988.
124. Runge VM, Clanton JA, Price AC, et al: The use of Gd DTPA as a perfusion agent and marker of blood-brain barrier disruption. Magn Reson Imaging 31:43, 1985.
125. Davidson HD, Steiner RE: Magnetic resonance imaging in infections of the central nervous system. AJNR 6:499, 1985.
126. Schroth G, Kretzschmar K, Gawehn J, et al: Advantage of magnetic resonance imaging in the diagnosis of cerebral infections. Neuroradiology 29:120, 1987.
127. Bertorini TE, Laster RE, Thompson BF, et al: Magnetic resonance imaging of the brain in bacterial endocarditis. Arch Intern Med 149:815, 1989.
128. Enzmann DR: Magnetic resonance imaging update on brain abscess and central nervous system aspergillosis. Curr Clin Top Infect Dis 13:269, 1993.
129. Gooding CA, Brasch RC, Lallemand DP, et al: Nuclear magnetic resonance imaging of the brain in children. J Pediatr 104:509, 1984.
130. Stephanoy S: Surgical treatment of brain abscess. Neurosurgery 22:724, 1988.
131. Garfield J: Management of supratentorial intracranial abscess: A review of 200 cases. Br Med J 2:7, 1969.
132. Itakura T, Yokote H, Ozaki F, et al: Stereotactic operation for brain abscess. Surg Neurol 28:196, 1987.
133. Stephanov S: Surgical treatment of brain abscess. Neurosurgery 22:724, 1988.
134. Whittle IR, Denholm SW, Elshunnar K: CT-guided stereotactic neurosurgery using the Brown-Roberts-Wells system: Experience with 125 procedures. Aust N Z J Surg 61:919, 1991.
135. Coin CG, Hucks-Folliss AG, Mahegan CC: Computed-tomographically guided percutaneous transmastoid drainage of a cerebellar abscess. Surg Neurol 20:387, 1983.
136. Hollander D, Villemure JG, Leblanc R: Thalamic abscess: A stereotactically treatable lesion. Appl Neurophysiol 50:168, 1987.
137. Nauta HJ, Briner RP, Eisenberg HM: Computed tomogram-guided stereotactic brain biopsy in the pediatric patient. Pediatr Neurosci 12:63, 1985–86.
138. Stroobandt G, Zech F, Thauvoy C, et al: Treatment by aspiration of brain abscesses. Acta Neurochir 85:138, 1987.
139. Johnson DL, Markle BM, Wiedermann BL, et al: Treatment of intracranial abscesses associated with sinusitis in children and adolescents. J Pediatr 113:15, 1988.
140. Knake JE, Bowerman RA, Silver TM, et al: Neurosurgical applications of intraoperative ultrasound. Radiol Clin North Am 23:73, 1985.
141. Pery M, Borovich B, Kaftori JK, et al: Intraoperative ultrasonography in cystic brain lesions. Isr J Med Sci 24:405, 1988.
142. Theophilo F, Burnett A, Juca Filho G, et al: Ultrasound-guided brain abscess aspiration in neonates. Childs Nerv Syst 3:371, 1987.
143. Portafaix M, Motuo-Fosto MJ: Postoperative echographic surveillance. Neurochirurgie 32:568, 1986.
144. Scatamacchia SA, Raptopoulos V, Davidson RI: Saline microbubbles monitoring sonography-assisted abscess drainage. Invest Radiol 22:868, 1987.
145. Leys D, Christiaens JL, Derambure P, et al: Management of focal intracranial infections: Is medical treatment better than surgery? J Neurol Neurosurg Psychiatry 53:472, 1990.
146. Nielsen H, Harmsen A, Gyldensted C: Cerebral abscess: A long-term follow-up. Acta Neurol Scand 67:330, 1983.
147. Black P, Graybill JR, Charache P: Penetration of brain abscess by systemically administered antibiotics. J Neurosurg 38:705, 1973.
148. De Louvois J: The bacteriology and chemotherapy of brain abscess. J Antimicrob Chemother 4:395, 1978.
149. Choudhury AR, Taylor JC, Whitaker R: Primary excision of brain abscess. Br Med J 2:1119, 1977.
150. Mampalam TJ, Rosenblum ML: Trends in the management of bacterial brain abscesses: A review of 102 cases over 17 years. Neurosurgery 23:451, 1988.
151. Freeman J: Changing concepts in the management of otitic intracranial infection: Use of computerized axial tomography in early detection and monitoring of cerebritis. Laryngoscope 94:907, 1984.
152. Patrick CC, Kaplan SL: Current concepts in the pathogenesis and management of brain abscesses in children. Pediatr Clin North Am 35:625, 1988.
153. Villar LA, Massanari RM, Koontz FP: Brain abscess due to penicillin- and clindamycin-resistant *Bacteroides melaninogenicus*. Surg Neurol 20:453, 1983.
154. Rennels MB, Woodward CL, Robinson WL, et al: Medical cure of apparent brain abscesses. Pediatrics 72:220, 1983.
155. Dobkin JF, Healton EB, Dickinson PC, et al: Nonspecificity of ring enhancement in "medically cured" brain abscess. Neurology 34:139, 1984.
156. Petit H, Rousseaux M, Lesoin F, et al: Primacy of medical treatment of cerebral abscesses (19 cases). Rev Neurol (Paris) 139:575, 1983.
157. De Louvois J, Gortvai P, Hurley R: Antibiotic treatment of abscesses of the central nervous system. Br Med J 2:985, 1977.
158. Yoshikawa TT, Goodman SJ: Brain Abscess—Teaching Conference. University of California, Los Angeles, and Harbor General Hospital, Torrance (Specialty Conference). West J Med 121:207, 1974.
159. Daniels SR, Price JK, Towbin RB, et al: Nonsurgical cure of brain abscess in a neonate. Childs Nerv Syst 1:346, 1985.
160. Barling RWA, Selkon JB: The penetration of antibiotics into cerebrospinal fluid and brain tissue. J Antimicrob Chemother 4:203, 1978.
161. Warner JF, Perkins RL, Cordero L: Metronidazole therapy of anaerobic bacteremia, meningitis, and brain abscess. Arch Intern Med 139:167, 1979.
162. Ingham HR, Selkon JB, Roxby CM: Bacteriological study of otogenic cerebral abscesses: Chemotherapeutic role of metronidazole. Br Med J 2:991, 1977.
163. Sjolin J, Eriksson N, Arneborn P, et al: Penetration of cefotaxime and desacetylcefotaxime into brain abscesses in humans. Antimicrob Agents Chemother 35:2606, 1991.
164. Sjolin J, Lilja A, Eriksson N, et al: Treatment of brain abscess with cefotaxime and metronidazole: Prospective study on 15 consecutive patients. Clin Infect Dis 17:857, 1993.
165. Carton JA, Perez F, Maradona JA, et al: Successful treatment of recurrent cerebral empyema and brain abscesses with imipenem. Eur J Clin Microbiol 6:578, 1987.
166. Fong IW: Staphylococcal central nervous system infections treated with cloxacillin. J Antimicrob Chemother 12:607, 1983.
167. Levy RM, Gutin PH, Baskin DS, et al: Vancomycin penetration of a brain abscess: Case report and review of the literature. Neurosurgery 18:632, 1986.
168. Neuwelt EA, Baker DE, Pagel MA, et al: Cerebrovascular permeability and delivery of gentamicin to normal brain and experimental brain abscess in rats. J Neurosurg 61:430, 1984.
169. McGowan JE, Chesney PJ, Crossley KB, et al: Guidelines for the use of systemic glucocorticosteroids in the management of selected infections. J Infect Dis 165:1, 1992.
170. Seydoux C, Francioli P: Bacterial brain abscesses: Factors influencing mortality and sequelae. Clin Infect Dis 15:394, 1992.
171. Kourtopoulos H, Holm SE, Norrby SR: The influence of steroids on the penetration of antibiotics into brain tissue and brain abscesses. An experimental study in rats. J Antimicrob Chemother 11:245, 1983.
172. Schroeder KA, McKeever PE, Schaberg DR, et al: Effect of dexamethasone on experimental brain abscess. J Neurosurg 66:264, 1987.
173. Black KL, Farhat SM: Cerebral abscess: Loss of computed tomographic enhancement with steroids. Case report. Neurosurgery 14:215, 1984.
174. Smith AL: Oral antibiotic therapy for serious infections. Annu Rev Med 39:171, 1988.
175. Rousseaux M, Lesoin F, Destee A, et al: Developments in the treatment and prognosis of multiple cerebral abscesses. Neurosurgery 16:304, 1985.
176. Moseley IF, Zilkha E: Considerations of radiation dose in the management of intracranial abscesses by computed tomography. Br J Radiol 57:303, 1984.
177. Rosenblum ML, Hoff JT, Norman D, et al: Decreased mortality from brain abscesses since advent of computerized tomography. J Neurosurg 49:658, 1978.
178. Hirsch JF, Roux FX, Sainte-Rose C, et al: Brain abscess in childhood. A study of 34 cases treated by puncture and antibiotics. Childs Brain 10:251, 1983.
179. Legg NJ, Gupta PC, Scott DF: Epilepsy following cerebral abscess: A clinical and EEG study of 70 patients. Brain 96:259, 1973.

180. Mises J, Daviet F, Moussalli-Salefranque F, et al: Brain abscess in the newborn infant (27 cases: initial electroclinical study, course). Rev Electroencephalogr Neurophysiol Clin 17:301, 1987.
181. Reid PM, Barber PC: Gliosarcoma developing in close relationship to an abscess cavity injected with Thorotrast. Surg Neurol 29:67, 1988.
182. Prager J, Zaret BS, Davidson R, et al: Gliosarcoma at the site of a surgically treated *Actinomyces* cerebral abscess. Neurosurgery 15:868, 1984.
183. Reichenthal E, Rubenstein AB, Shevach I, et al: Meningioma presenting at a site of previously aspirated brain abscess. Acta Neurochir 109:142, 1991.
184. Jefferson AA, Keogh AJ: Intracranial abscesses: A review of treated patients over 20 years. J Med 183:389, 1977.
185. Dohrmann PJ, Elrick WL: Observations on brain abscess. Review of 28 cases. Med J Aust 2:81, 1982.
186. Karandanis D, Shulman JA: Factors associated with mortality in brain abscess. Arch Intern Med 135:1145, 1975.
187. Witzmann A, Beran H, Bohm-Jurkovic H, et al: Brain abscess. Prognostic factors. Dtsch Med Wochenschr 20:114, 1989.
188. Mampalam TJ, Rosenblum ML: Trends in the management of bacterial brain abscesses: A review of 102 cases over 17 years. Neurosurgery 23:451, 1988.

163

Slow Viral Infections of the Central Nervous System

David M. Asher

Several neurologic diseases once considered to be degenerative are caused by infections with asymptomatic incubation periods of months or years and durations of overt clinical illness that may also be quite long. Although the infectious agents may be latent in other organs of the body, pathologic changes are found only in the nervous system. Sigurdsson[1, 1a, 1b] studied such diseases of sheep and coined the term slow infection to describe them. Some slow infections—the spongiform encephalopathies (Chapter 272)—are caused by unique infectious agents of unknown structure,[2] variously called prions[3] or infectious amyloids.[4] Other slow infections of the human nervous system are caused by viruses with conventional physical properties—viruses that more often cause acute, self-limited illnesses. This chapter reviews five such slow viral infections of humans (Table 163–1): progressive multifocal leukoencephalopathy (PML), subacute sclerosing panencephalitis (SSPE), rubella panencephalitis (RPE), tropical spastic paraparesis (TSP; also called human T-cell leukemia virus–associated myelopathy), and chronic tick-borne encephalitis (TBE). Other viral infections causing human neurologic diseases after prolonged latent periods—with human immunodeficiency virus (HIV), cytomegalovirus, herpes simplex virus, varicella-zoster virus, and rabies virus—are considered elsewhere in this book (Chapters 125, 130, 148, 170, 186, 240, 243, 264, 270).

History

Progressive Multifocal Leukoencephalopathy

PML[5] is a progressive demyelinating disease of the nervous system caused by activation of a latent infection with the JC papovavirus[6, 7] in immunosuppressed subjects, for whom it is invariably fatal. PML was first recognized complicating leukemia and Hodgkin's disease.[5] It is now most often recognized as an opportunistic infection with acquired immunodeficiency syndrome (AIDS) in adults and, rarely, children.[8] In 1969, structures resembling virions of papovaviruses (Fig. 163–1) were detected by electron microscopy in oligodendrocytes of patients with PML.[7] Two years later the causative agent, the JC virus (JCV), was isolated in cultures of fetal spongioblasts (glial precursor cells).[6]

Subacute Sclerosing Panencephalitis

SSPE is caused by a persistent measles virus infection. It was first clearly described by Dawson,[9] who postulated its viral etiology. Bouteille and colleagues[10] observed that brain cells of patients with SSPE contained tubular structures (Fig. 163–2) similar to those seen in cells infected with measles virus, and Connolly and coworkers[11] showed that patients with SSPE had high levels of antibodies to measles virus in serum and cerebrospinal fluid (CSF) and measles viral antigens in brain cells. Measles virus was isolated from brains of patients with SSPE in 1969.[12–15]

Rubella Panencephalitis

RPE was first described in 1974 by Lebon and Lyon[16] affecting a boy with typical congenital rubella syndrome, an association that suggested that rubella virus might be the causative agent. Rubella virus was isolated from the brain of a patient with RPE by Cremer and coworkers in 1975.[17]

Tropical Spastic Paraparesis

TSP was long known as a chronic neurologic disease affecting the spinal cord in adolescents and adults living in several tropical regions. A serologic study on the island of Martinique led Gessain and coworkers[18] to recognize that most subjects with TSP had antibodies to the oncogenic retrovirus human T-cell leukemia (or lymphotropic) virus type I (HTLV-I), whereas normal subjects and those with other neurologic diseases rarely did. That finding was confirmed for patients with TSP in other tropical populations as well as in patients with a similar condition in Japan, where the condition was designated HTLV-I–associated myelopathy (HAM). Soon afterward, Hirose and coworkers[19] isolated HTLV-I (Fig. 163–3) from the CSF of a patient with HAM.

Chronic Tick-Borne Encephalitis

Chronic progressive neurologic diseases have been described in patients who recovered from acute TBE in Europe and Asia, and limited evidence suggests that the syndromes may be associated with persistence of virus in the central nervous system.[20, 21]

Microbiology

Properties of the viruses are summarized in Table 163–1. JCV is a member of the family Papovaviridae in the genus *Polyomavirus*—a small double-stranded circular DNA with unenveloped icosahedral nucleocapsid sharing some anti-

TABLE 163–1 ■ Slow Infections of the Human Nervous System Caused by Five Conventional Viruses

DISEASE	CAUSATIVE VIRUS	VIRUS GENUS AND FAMILY	VIRUS SIZE AND MORPHOLOGY	VIRAL NUCLEIC ACID*
Progressive multifocal leukoencephalopathy (PML)	JC	*Polyomavirus*, Papovaviridae	45 nm, spherical, nonenveloped	dsDNA, circular, 5 kbp
Subacute sclerosing panencephalitis (SSPE)	Measles	*Morbillivirus*, Paramyxoviridae	150–300 nm, spherical or filamentous (pleomorphic), enveloped	ssRNA, negative sense, 16 kb
Rubella panencephalitis (RPE)	Rubella	*Rubivirus*, Togaviridae	60–70 nm, spherical, enveloped	ssRNA, positive sense, 10 kb
Tropical spastic paraparesis (TSP)/HTLV-I–associated myelopathy (HAM)	Human T-cell lymphotropic virus type I (HTLV-I)	[Undecided], Retroviridae	80–100 nm, spherical, enveloped	ssRNA, positive sense, homodimer, 9 kb
Kozhevnikov epilepsy and other chronic forms of tick-borne encephalitis (TBE)	Tick-borne encephalitis (Russian spring–summer encephalitis)	*Flavivirus*, Flaviviridae	45–60 nm, spherical, enveloped	ssRNA, positive sense, 10.7 kb

*ss, Single stranded; ds, double stranded; kb, kilobase; kbp, kilobase pair.

gens with other members of that genus.[22] JCV strains causing PML are heterogeneous and presumably generated from ordinary archetypal strains during asymptomatic persistence[23] rather than from especially neurovirulent progenitors. JCV isolates from brain shared certain similarities in DNA sequences and differed from strains found in kidney,[24, 25] especially in the noncoding region of the genome, prompting the hypothesis that mutations in regulatory genes play an important role in establishing viral latency and reactivation in the nervous system.[26] A synergy was demonstrated between a host protein that activates promoters of JCV, expressed on oligodendrocytes, and the JCV large-tumor antigen[27] suggesting another potential mechanism by which lytic infection of those cells might be established.

Measles virus is a morbillivirus of the family Paramyxoviridae, a negative-sense enveloped RNA virus that forms pleomorphic spherical and filamentous particles.[28] The genomes of strains of measles virus isolated from patients with SSPE contain multiple mutations.[29] No consistent genomic abnormalities have been identified in strains of measles virus iso-

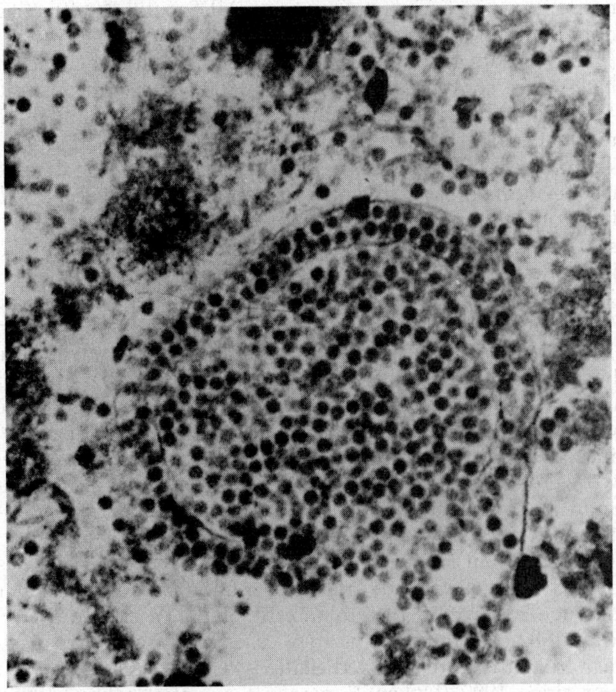

FIGURE 163–1 ▫ PML. Crystalloid array of JC virus particles in the nucleus of an oligodendrocyte. (Courtesy of Dr. E. O. Major, National Institutes of Health, Bethesda, MD. From Major EO, Amemiya K, Tornatore CS, et al: Pathogenesis and molecular biology of progressive multifocal leukoencephalopathy, the JC virus–induced demyelinating disease of the human brain. Clin Microbiol Rev 5:49–73, 1992.)

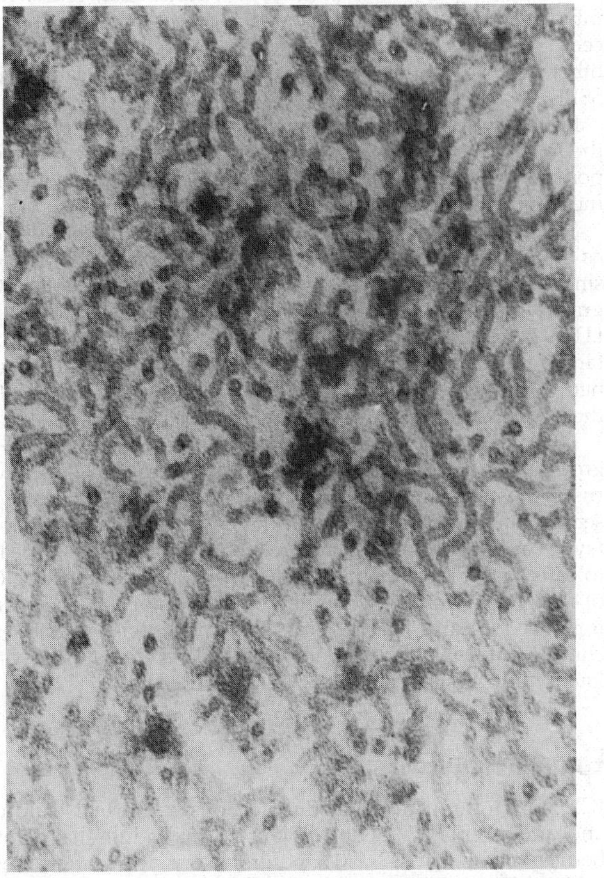

FIGURE 163–2 ▫ SSPE. Measles nucleocapsids in the nucleus of a cell from the brain of a patient with SSPE. (Courtesy of Dr. Jerzy Kulczycki, Institute of Psychiatry and Neurology, Warsaw, Poland.)

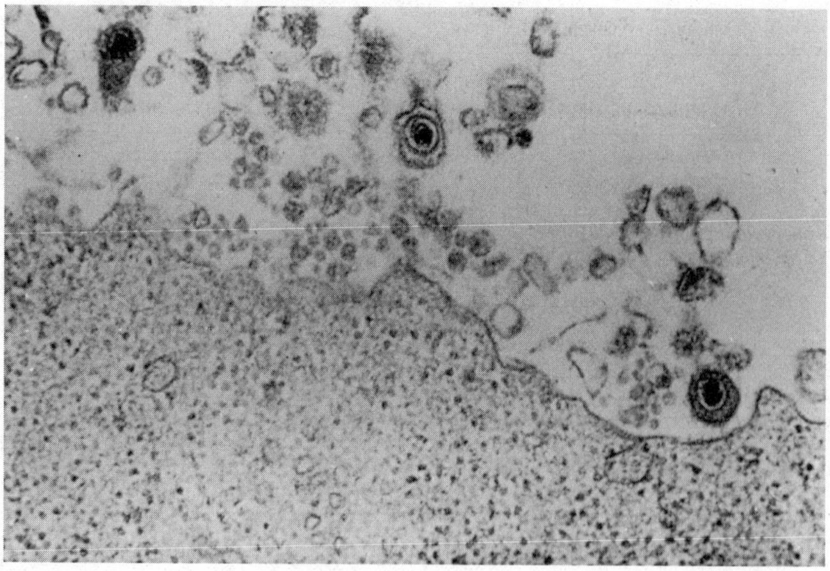

FIGURE 163–3 □ TSP/HAM. Extracellular particles of HTLV-I from the spinal cord of a patient with TSP/HAM, cultured in normal human peripheral blood cells. (Courtesy of Dr. C. J. Gibbs, Jr., National Institutes of Health, Bethesda, MD.)

lated from brains of SSPE patients. (One cluster of SSPE cases suggestive of a point-source outbreak caused by a strain of special virulence has been described.[30, 31]) Complete measles virus particles are not found in the brains of patients with SSPE, and the matrix (M) protein required for the final assembly and budding of virus from the host cells is reduced or missing, not only from brain tissues of patients but also from cells cultured from their brains; however, the full complement of genetic material needed to code for all proteins, including M protein, is present and functional, and when infected brain cells are cultivated together with permissive cells, complete measles virus often emerges. Mutations in other genes of measles virus have also been associated with SSPE.[28]

Rubella virus is the sole member of the genus *Rubivirus* in the family Togaviridae, a group of small spherical enveloped positive-sense RNA viruses. Nothing is known about the mechanism by which rubella virus causes RPE.[32]

HTLV-I, the first human retrovirus to be identified, occurs as spherical enveloped particles containing homodimers of single-stranded RNA[33] as well as in DNA transcripts integrated into host genomic DNA. No molecular changes in HTLV-I associated with neurotropism are known. The distantly related virus HTLV-II has not been associated with neurologic disease. Leukemias and other diseases caused by these viruses are described elsewhere (Chapter 264).

TBE virus is a flavivirus of the family Flaviviridae—a group of antigenically related small spherical enveloped viruses, mostly arthropod-borne, with single-stranded positive-sense genomes. A mutation in the envelope gene of yellow fever vaccine virus—distantly related to TBE virus—appears to cause acute encephalitis in humans,[34] and the same region of the genome may encode neurovirulence of the TBE virus for mice.[35] Strains of TBE virus that cause delayed onset of chronic movement disorders in monkeys have been isolated,[21] but the molecular basis is unknown.

Epidemiology

JCV most often causes silent infections in normal children and adolescents[36, 37]; about 75% of normal adults have antibodies to the virus.[22] PML occurs many years after those initial infections, affecting primarily adults with immune systems compromised for a variety of reasons—congenital or acquired immunodeficiency syndromes, leukemias and lymphomas, immunosuppressive therapy for tumors or transplantation, miliary tuberculosis, sarcoidosis, and others. A few patients have PML without any other diagnosis.[26, 38] Possibly because of the lower prevalence of latent infections with JCV in the early years of life, only a few cases of PML have been recognized in children with congenital immunodeficiencies[38] and AIDS,[8, 38, 39] in whom it may represent a primary infection.[22] The epidemiology of PML reflects that of its underlying conditions; the spread of AIDS resulted in a dramatic increase in cases of PML recognized as well as a reduction in mean age of patients (from the sixth to the fifth decade of life) and relative increase in proportion of males affected.[40] Although PML remains rare overall, it is a common opportunistic infection among AIDS patients, affecting more than 4% in some series.[41]

SSPE occurs throughout the world. Data for the United States were compiled for more than 600 cases with onset in 1956 or later by the U.S. National SSPE Registry[42] (maintained by Dr. Paul R. Dyken, Institute for Research in Childhood Neurodegenerative Diseases, Mobile, Alabama). The disease has been diagnosed in patients younger than 1 year[43] to those older than 30 years,[44] but it affects primarily children and young adolescents. More than 85% of cases in the National Registry had onset between 5 and 15 years of age.[42] The average age at onset of SSPE in cases reported before 1980 was about 10 years; between 1980 and 1984 it rose to almost 14 years. The risk of SSPE for boys is more than twice that for girls and the risk is higher for rural children than for urban children. Cases have become more frequent in the western United States, especially among Hispanic children[42]; since 1990 all cases reported to the National Registry except two were among immigrant children. Acquisition of measles before the age of 18 months increased the risk of SSPE substantially.[43]

Mean annual incidence rates of SSPE in the United States fell markedly from 0.61 case per million persons younger than age 20 years in 1960 to an estimated 0.06 case in 1980.[45] After 1982, fewer than five new cases were registered each year from the entire United States—only two or three each year since 1990 (Dyken P, personal communication, 1995). This drop presumably resulted from the decline in measles cases after the introduction of live attenuated measles vaccine in 1963. The risk of SSPE was estimated as 8.5 SSPE cases per million cases of measles for a 6-year period during which the estimated risk after measles vaccination was only 0.7 case per million doses of vaccine. Of the patients with SSPE reported to the National Registry since 1969, only 14% had a history of measles vaccination without also having clinically apparent measles, and a roughly equal number had no history of either acute measles illness or receiving vaccine.[45] SSPE has never been demonstrated to result from persistent infection with measles vaccine virus; more likely, SSPE in vaccinated subjects resulted from undiagnosed wild-type measles infection either preceding vaccination or after unsuccessful immunization. Lack of measles vaccination itself constituted a highly significant risk factor in one study of SSPE.[46] In a survey of England and Wales, the overall risk of SSPE after measles was 29 compared with that after measles vaccination, and the relative risk for children who had measles before the age of 1 year was more than 100.[47, 48]

RPE[32, 49] is exceedingly rare; since its first description in 1974[16] fewer than 20 cases have been reported. All patients were males 8 to 21 years old; most had typical stigmata of the congenital rubella syndrome, including cataracts, deafness, and mental retardation, but several had recovered completely from childhood rubella.[16, 50–52] Cases of RPE may be expected where rubella still occurs.[53]

TSP/HAM has been recognized most frequently in the West Indies, Colombia, and other countries of Central and South America, West Africa, the Seychelles, and southern Japan as well as in migrants from those areas[54]; the asymptomatic carriage rate of HTLV-I is quite high in affected populations. The overall prevalence of HTLV-I antibodies among healthy blood donors in the United States was estimated to be 0.025%. The estimated lifetime risk of myelopathy among those infected is less than 1%—substantially lower than the risk of leukemia. Mechanisms of transmission of HTLV-I are similar to those for HIV: from mother to child in breast milk, sexually, by transfusion, and by use of shared needles. Unlike HIV, HTLV-I appears to be transmitted only by infected cells. Transfusion-acquired cases of TSP/HAM had relatively short incubation periods, probably because of the large infecting dose of virus. Women are more frequently affected by TSP/HAM than men and adults more often than children. The distantly related virus HTLV-II, with similar epidemiology, has not been recognized to cause myelopathy.

Most cases of chronic progressive TBE have been reported from Russia,[55] affecting mainly young adults from rural villages, especially in Siberia.[21, 56] Two typical patients were described in Japan.[57] In most areas the chronic illness is an uncommon late complication of acute TBE, although in some clinical series as many as 20% of patients recovering from acute encephalitis were reported to develop new signs of neurologic disease months or years later.[20, 21] TBE virus is spread by tick bites or, less frequently, by ingesting milk from infected animals.[58]

Pathology and Pathogenesis

The histopathologic picture of PML[59] is characterized by diffusely scattered demyelinated lesions, variable in size and distribution—generally most numerous in the cerebral hemispheres (Fig. 163–4), less in brain stem and cerebellum, and tending to spare the spinal cord. Myelin sheaths within the lesions are degenerated and replaced by lipid-bearing phagocytes, leaving neuronal axis cylinders. Oligodendroglial cells at the margins of lesions are abnormal, with enlarged degenerated nuclei and intranuclear eosinophilic inclusions. Astrocytes are enlarged with abnormal or multiple nuclei. Perivascular lymphocytic cuffing occurs. In electron micrographs from AIDS patients with PML, virions of papovavirus are observed not only in oligodendrocytes and astroglial cells but also in macrophages and neurons.[60, 61] The histopathologic findings of PML complicating AIDS are the same as with other predisposing conditions.[62] JCV has been found in kidneys and circulating B lymphocytes of asymptomatically infected subjects.[63] One hypothesis holds that latently infected B lymphocytes are activated during immune suppression and carry JCV from the blood into the brain to infect oligodendrocytes and astrocytes, causing loss of myelin and functional impairments of neurons.[26] Lymphocytes, primarily T cells, found in the brains of patients with PML in areas of inflammation are reported to contain JCV consistently, but only rarely are they infected with HIV, opportunistic viruses other than JCV, or *Toxoplasma*.[64] Phagocytosis of papovaviral particles by macrophages has been observed.[61] The role of those cells and of JCV-infected neurons[60] in the pathogenesis of PML remains uncertain.

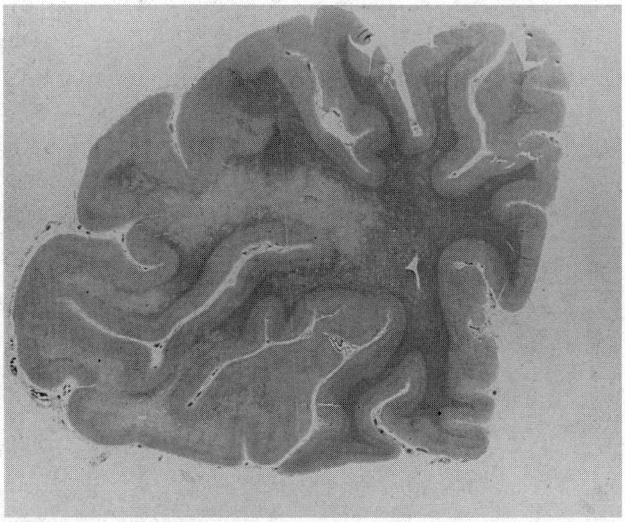

FIGURE 163–4 □ PML. Patchy demyelination in the cerebrum of a patient with PML. (Courtesy of Dr. C. J. Gibbs, Jr., National Institutes of Health, Bethesda, MD.)

The histopathologic characteristics of SSPE consist of inflammation, necrosis, and repair.[42, 65, 66] Brain biopsy performed in the early stages of SSPE shows mild inflammation of meninges and a panencephalitis involving cortical and subcortical gray matter as well as white matter, with cuffs of plasma cells and lymphocytes around blood vessels (Fig. 163–5) and increased numbers of glial cells throughout. Neuronal loss may not be marked until later in the course of illness. Loss of myelin secondary to neuronal degeneration may be apparent. Intranuclear Cowdry type A inclusion bodies surrounded by clear halos (Fig. 163–6), noted by Dawson[9] in his original description, may be seen in hematoxylin-eosin–stained sections within the nuclei of neurons, astrocytes, and oligodendrocytes, but they are sometimes difficult to find. By electron microscopy, the inclusions are found to contain tubular structures[10] (see Fig. 163–2) typical of paramyxoviral nucleocapsids. Measles viral antigens can be demonstrated by labeled antibody techniques within the inclusions as well as in cells without inclusions. Lesions may be unevenly distributed throughout the brain, so biopsy is not always diagnostic, particularly when small samples of tissue are obtained. The same findings of inclusion body panencephalitis are generally present in the brain at autopsy; however, late in disease it may be difficult to find typical areas of inflammation, and the main histopathologic changes are necrosis and gliosis. SSPE is believed to begin in the cortical gray matter, subsequently progressing to white matter and subcortical gray matter and, finally, to lower structures.[65] (Myoclonus probably results from extrapyramidal involvement.) Although persistent infection of lymphoid tis-

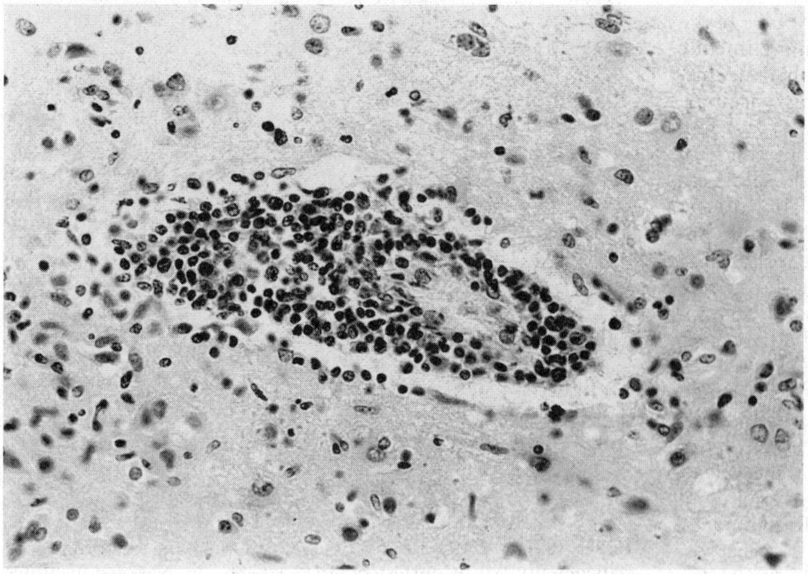

FIGURE 163–5 □ SSPE. A cuff of inflammatory cells surrounding a blood vessel in the cerebral cortex of a child with SSPE. (Courtesy of Dr. P. Swoveland, University of Maryland, Baltimore, MD. From Asher DM: Slow viral infections. *In* Scheld WM, Whitley RJ, Durack DT [eds]: Infections of the Nervous System, ed 2. New York, Raven Press, 1997, pp 199–221.)

sues with measles virus has been claimed,[67–69] those tissues show no pathologic changes. Cerebral vascular endothelial cells may be infected without showing structural abnormalities[70–72] (Fig. 163–7) and might constitute a portal of entry into the central nervous system for measles virus. The increased risk in children who had measles as infants implies that either their immunologic immaturity or low levels of residual maternal antibodies predispose them to SSPE. The frequent finding in the nucleic acid sequences of measles virus isolated from SSPE of mutations in the M gene, with reduced expression of M protein, or of other mutations interfering with viral assembly and budding suggests that the progressive encephalitis may result from intracellular accumulation of incomplete measles virus not cleared by antibodies or cell-mediated immunity.

Histopathologic changes in brains of patients with RPE[73, 74] are similar to those in SSPE, with cuffs of lymphocytes and plasma cells around blood vessels, glial nodules in the cortex, some loss of neurons, and an increase in numbers of astrocytes throughout gray matter and white matter. The histopathologic picture of RPE differs from that of SSPE in two important respects: no inclusion bodies have been recognized in RPE, and deposits of amorphous material stained by the periodic acid–Schiff reaction are found around vessels in subcortical white matter.

The histopathologic changes in spinal cords (and, to a lesser extent, brains) of patients with TSP/HAM from Jamaica and from Japan are similar: chronic inflammation (Fig. 163–8), perivascular cuffing with mononuclear cells, loss of neurons, and proliferation of astrocytes and microglial cells.[75] Inflammatory changes in spinal cords of TSP patients who survived for many years were minimal, but there was a vacuolar myelopathy resembling that seen in AIDS.[76]

Although patients with TSP/HAM generally have no other evidence of leukemia, atypical T cells resembling those in adult T-cell leukemia have been observed in their blood and CSF.[54] One study suggested that 1 or 2 in 10,000 peripheral blood lymphocytes from patients with TSP/HAM contained viral transcripts[77]—somewhat less than previously thought. These cells may be the progeny of a few infected founder cells.[78] Infected lymphocytes are predominantly CD4^{+}, although CD4 is not a receptor for HTLV-I.[54] Virus-infected lymphocytes from patients with TSP/HAM express activation markers on their surfaces and proliferate spontaneously

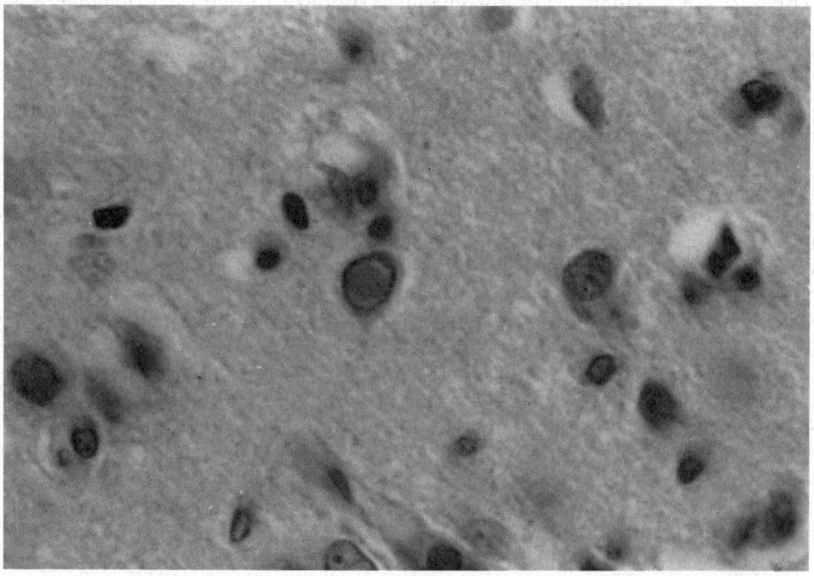

FIGURE 163–6 □ SSPE. An intranuclear inclusion in the cerebral cortex of a child with SSPE. (Courtesy of Dr. P. Swoveland, University of Maryland, Baltimore, MD. From Asher DM: Slow viral infections. *In* Scheld WM, Whitley RJ, Durack DT [eds]: Infections of the Nervous System, ed 2. New York, Raven Press, 1997, pp 199–221.)

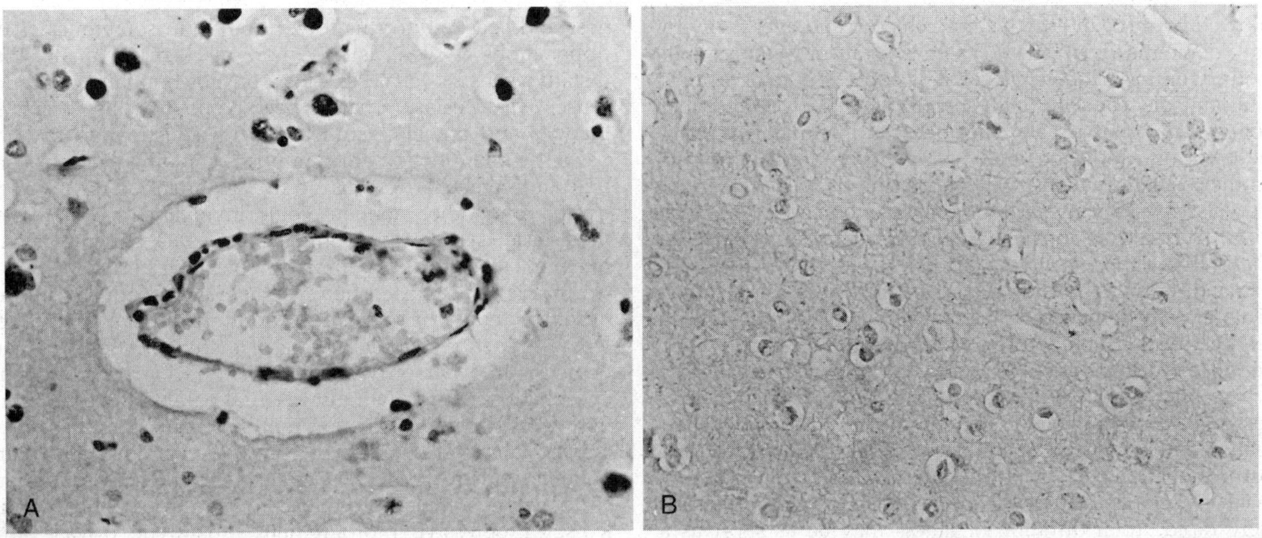

FIGURE 163–7 □ SSPE. In situ reverse transcriptase–PCR and labeled-probe hybridization followed by immunostaining[72] from formalin-fixed, paraffin-embedded sections of brain. *A*, Measles virus–infected neurons, oligodendrocytes, astrocytes, and vascular endothelial cells in SSPE are stained. *B*, A section from a control patient shows no staining.

in culture. The role of infected lymphocytes in the pathogenesis of TSP/HAM is not yet understood; they have been postulated to provoke an autoimmune demyelinating process. Uninfected CD8$^+$ lymphocytes, common in the CSF of patients with TSP/HAM, are cytotoxic to HTLV-I–infected cells and might cause demyelination by killing of infected glial cells, although it remains unclear if neurons and glial cells are actually infected.[54]

Brain tissues from biopsies of patients with Kozhevnikov epilepsy[79] and progressive bulbar paralysis[57] after TBE contained perivascular cuffs and parenchymal infiltrates of inflammatory cells, with loss of neurons and sclerosis; no inclusion bodies were described.

Clinical Manifestations

PML causes a variety of clinical abnormalities, reflecting the multifocal distribution of lesions; findings include pareses, sensory deficits, seizures, dementia, dysarthria and other bulbar signs, and cerebellar signs. Progression is relatively rapid. Average survival in one series of AIDS patients was less than 3 months after onset of PML.[41] Although most patients with PML live less than a year, an occasional patient with PML has survived longer.[80]

Most children with SSPE recovered from typical measles several years before the onset of neurologic disease. Measles may not have been especially severe. Some patients with SSPE had measles pneumonia, but none had a history of typical measles encephalitis. The mean interval between measles and onset of SSPE in the United States was formerly about 7 years,[45] later increasing to 12 years.[42] The National SSPE Registry divided the clinical course of typical SSPE into four stages marked by the onset and disappearance of myoclonic jerks and the degree of disability, with several patterns of progression depending on degree of chronicity and occurrence of remissions. Most cases were classified as acute, subacute, or chronic progressive, and only a few were remitting. The onset of SSPE is usually insidious, marked by subtle changes in behavior and deterioration of schoolwork,

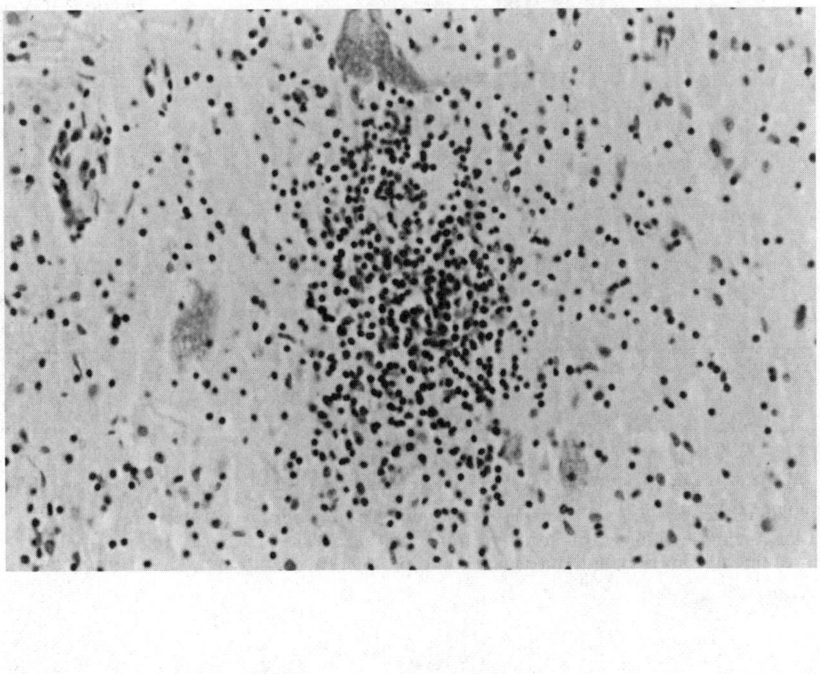

FIGURE 163–8 □ TSP/HAM. An infiltrate of inflammatory cells in the spinal cord. (Courtesy of Dr. C. J. Gibbs, Jr., National Institutes of Health, Bethesda, MD.)

followed by more overtly bizarre behavior and eventually by frank dementia (Fig. 163–9). There is no fever, photophobia, or other finding of acute encephalitis except for an occasional complaint of headache. Diffuse neurologic disease becomes progressively more severe. The appearance of massive repetitive myoclonic jerks, generally symmetric, especially involving the axial musculature and occurring at 5- to 10-second intervals, marks the onset of the second clinical stage of SSPE. True convulsions may also appear at any stage of illness. In addition to myoclonic jerks, which tend to disappear as disease progresses, a variety of other abnormal movements and dystonias have been observed. Cerebellar ataxia may be noted as well.[42, 65] Retinopathy and optic atrophy may occur at any time, sometimes preceding behavioral changes[81]; cortical blindness has also been described.[82] Dementia progresses to stupor and coma, sometimes with autonomic insufficiency. Patients may be rigid or spastic with decorticate postures or may be flaccid. The rate of progression is highly variable; but most often the course is inexorable and relatively rapid. Total duration of illness may be as short as a few months, but most patients live more than a year after diagnosis, with a mean survival of about 18 months.[42] Occasional patients show some spontaneous improvement and have lived for more than 10 years. In the mid-1980s, the few patients diagnosed with SSPE in the United States had a relatively long survival, perhaps because of improvements in chronic care. Patients with SSPE have the usual secondary complications associated with incapacitating neurologic diseases, including pneumonia and decubitus ulcers.

The onset of RPE resembles that of SSPE,[83–85] with insidious changes in behavior and deterioration of intellectual performance. Those are followed by dementia and other signs of multifocal brain disease, including seizures, cerebellar ataxia, and spastic weakness. Myoclonus and other abnormal movements may occur,[84, 86] but those are not as common as in SSPE. Retinopathy (similar to that of acute rubella) and optic atrophy may be found.[51, 84, 85] The course of RPE is similar to that of SSPE, with progression to coma, spasticity, brain stem involvement, and death in 2 to 5 years.

TSP/HAM also begins insidiously with progressive weakness and spasticity of the lower limbs and sometimes of the upper limbs as well, usually more marked proximally than distally; sensory changes—loss of position and vibration sense, dysesthesias, radiating back pain—may also occur.[54, 75] Bladder and bowel dysfunction with constipation and impaired sexual function are common complaints. Various cerebral and cerebellar lesions occur less often, as do myositis, uveitis, and other nonneurologic involvement. Progression of disease is typically indolent, and some patients remain relatively stable or even improve over long periods.[87]

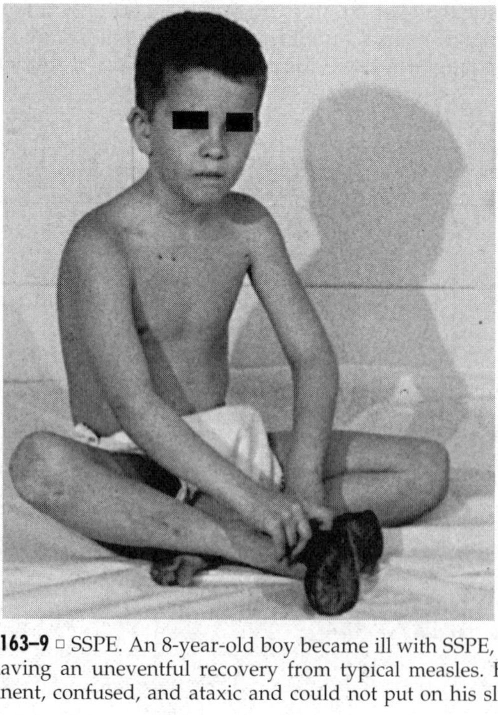

FIGURE 163–9 □ SSPE. An 8-year-old boy became ill with SSPE, 7 years after having an uneventful recovery from typical measles. He was incontinent, confused, and ataxic and could not put on his slipper.

Chronic TBE most often begins with relatively sudden onset of epilepsia partialis continua (Kozhevnikov epilepsy)—repetitive clonic jerking of the extremities or of face or neck—in a person who previously recovered from acute encephalitis, with or without residual paralysis; the condition may also begin with major motor seizures, or those may appear later. The course of illness is variable, and some patients with Kozhevnikov epilepsy after TBE have apparently made sufficient recovery to lead reasonably normal lives.[56] Progressive ("progredient") paralytic disease after TBE more often begins insidiously and runs a long but inexorable course; in one typical case, progressive deafness and tinnitus appeared 13 years after recovery from acute TBE, followed soon after by hallucinations and other mental changes and later by diplopia, optic atrophy, ataxia and intention tremor, scanning speech, and a variety of other signs of cerebral, cerebellar, and bulbar involvement that progressed during a 10-year period.[57]

Diagnosis

The diagnosis of PML is suggested by signs of multifocal neurologic disease in an immunodeficient patient. Cranial imaging typically reveals the presence in various areas of the brain of multiple noncompressing lesions[88] that enlarge as disease progresses.[38] Measurement of serum antibodies to JCV in AIDS patients was of no value in diagnosing PML.[89] JCV genomic sequences were successfully amplified by polymerase chain reaction (PCR) from specimens of CSF of patients with PML,[90–93] although that did not always provide a sensitive diagnostic test. One study demonstrated papovavirus particles in CSF of patients by electron microscopy.[94] Isolation of virus from the brain, requiring human fetal brain cultures, is rarely available. Negative-stain electron microscopy augmented by incubation with immune serum was useful for detecting JCV particles in suspensions of brain tissue.[95] JCV is now most easily detected by amplification of viral DNA using PCR.[26, 96–98]

The diagnosis of SSPE should be suspected in young patients with progressive encephalopathy and a history of measles or residence in measles endemic areas. The electroencephalogram is useful in supporting the diagnosis of SSPE (Fig. 163–10), although early in disease it may be normal or show only moderate nonspecific slowing.[99] In the myoclonic stage, most patients with SSPE have episodes of "suppression burst"—high-amplitude slow and sharp waves recurring at intervals of 3 to 5 seconds on a slow background; however, that pattern is not unique to SSPE.[100] Later in the illness the electroencephalogram becomes increasingly disorganized, with high-amplitude random dysrhythmic slowing; in terminal disease the amplitude may fall.[42, 65] Computed tomograms or magnetic resonance images of patients with SSPE may show variable cortical atrophy and ventricular enlargement, and there may be focal or multifocal low-density lesions in white matter. Those studies may also be normal, especially early in the disease.[101]

The blood of patients with SSPE has elevated titers of antibodies to measles virus; antibodies are of the immuno-

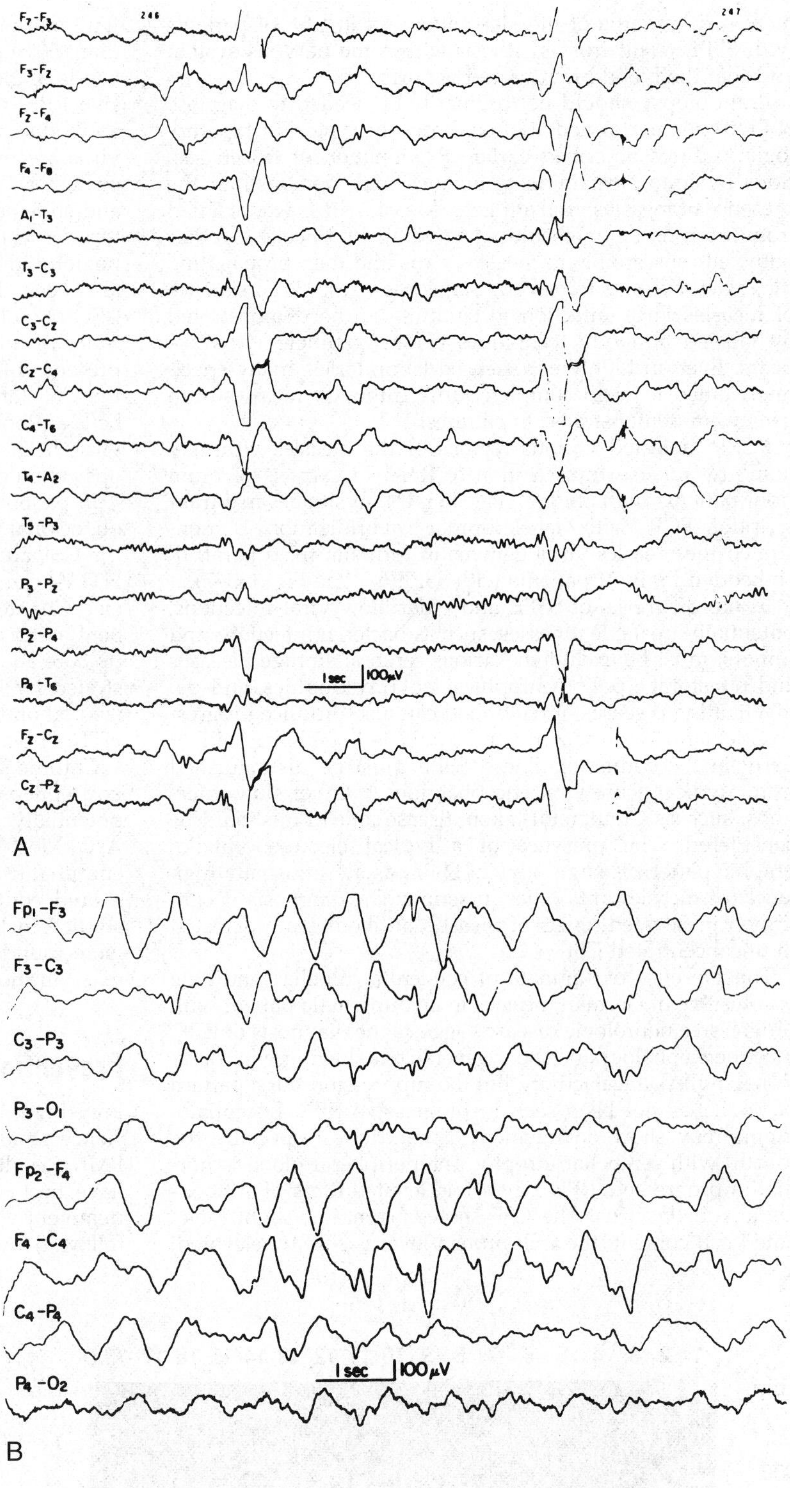

FIGURE 163–10 □ SSPE. Electroencephalograms from several patients with SSPE. (Courtesy of Drs. E. Niedermeyer and E. Vining, Johns Hopkins University School of Medicine, Baltimore, MD. From Asher DM: Slow viral infections. *In* Scheld WM, Whitley RJ, Durack DT [eds]: Infections of the Nervous System, ed 2. New York, Raven Press, 1997, pp 199–221.)

globulin G and immunoglobulin M classes and are directed against all the component proteins of measles virus except the M protein. Examination of the CSF has been most useful for establishing the diagnosis of SSPE. Cell content of the CSF is generally normal, although stained sediments were reported to show plasma cells. Total protein content of the CSF is generally normal or only slightly elevated; however, the γ-globulin fraction is greatly elevated (usually constituting at least 20% of total protein in CSF), resulting in a paretic type of colloidal gold curve. When the CSF is examined by electrophoresis or isoelectric focusing, "oligoclonal" bands of immunoglobin are usually observed. Immunoglobulin G and immunoglobulin M antibodies to measles virus, not normally found in unconcentrated CSF, make up most of the immunoglobulin, and these may often be detected in dilutions of 1:8 or higher. Complement fixation, hemagglutination inhibition, immunofluorescence, and other serologic tests, including enzyme-linked immunosorbent assay, demonstrate increased levels of measles antibodies in the CSF. The normal ratio of titer in serum to titer in CSF is reduced (below 200) for measles antibodies, whereas serum/CSF ratios are normal for other viral antibodies and for albumin, indicating that the increased amounts of measles antibodies in CSF of patients with SSPE result from synthesis within the nervous system and that the blood-brain barrier is normal.[102]

Brain biopsy should not ordinarily be needed to diagnose SSPE. When performed, it often shows the typical histopathologic findings described earlier. Examination of frozen sections by immunostaining techniques may demonstrate the presence of measles viral antigens. Measles virus was isolated from brain tissue by cocultivating viable brain cells together with cells susceptible to measles virus and then propagating the mixed cultures for several serial passages.[12–15] Persistence of measles virus infection in cultures can be demonstrated by labeled antibody techniques before complete virus appears. Even in highly experienced laboratories, many specimens failed to yield complete virus, although measles antigens were demonstrated in cultures.[103]

PCR[104] detected various regions of the measles virus genome by reverse transcription of RNA in extracts of brain from patients with SSPE[105] (Fig. 163–11); in situ reverse transcription–PCR with labeled-probe hybridization demonstrated the measles virus genome in formalin-fixed paraffin-embedded brain of patients with SSPE[71, 72] (see Fig. 163–7).

In the diagnosis of SSPE and other slow viral infections, potentially treatable illnesses, such as bacterial infections and tumors, must be excluded. Various cerebral storage diseases and nonstorage poliodystrophies, leukodystrophies, and demyelinating diseases of childhood can also produce progressive dementia with seizures and paralysis resembling SSPE.[101] Early in the course of illness, SSPE must be distinguished from atypical acute viral encephalitides.[106] Other slow infections, such as Creutzfeldt-Jakob disease and RPE, should be considered. The presence of a typical electroencephalographic pattern is suggestive of SSPE, as are unusually high levels of measles antibodies in serum. The diagnosis is confirmed if elevated levels of measles antibodies are detected in unconcentrated CSF.

The presence of stigmata of congenital rubella syndrome or a history of German measles in a young male patient with progressive neurologic disease suggests the diagnosis of RPE. Electroencephalograms show generalized slowing with occasional high-voltage activity, but the suppression-burst pattern of SSPE has not been seen in progressive RPE. Encephalograms may show enlargement of ventricles (especially the fourth) with cerebellar atrophy. The peripheral blood is normal in progressive RPE except for elevated titers of antibodies to rubella virus. The CSF shows normal or slightly elevated cell content; the CSF protein level is slightly elevated, with marked increase in globulin, which may make up more than 50% of total protein.[52, 83] Oligoclonal electrophoretic bands of globulin are found in CSF of patients with progressive RPE; the bands resemble those in SSPE but consist of antibodies to rubella virus antigens.[85] Antibodies to rubella virus are readily detectable in CSF, often at dilutions of 1:8 or higher. Complement fixation, hemagglutination inhibition, and enzyme-linked immunosorbent assay should be satisfactory for testing CSF. Most of the rubella antibodies are immunoglobulin G, although immunoglobulin M antibodies have also been detected early in the course of RPE; the serum/CSF ratio of antibody titers to rubella virus is reduced[85] while ratios of titers to measles and other viruses are normal. The presence of elevated levels of antibodies to rubella virus in the CSF (and reduction of normal serum/CSF ratio for rubella antibodies) establishes the diagnosis. Isolation of rubella virus from blood lymphocytes may be attempted. Brain biopsy should not be required.

In patients with clinical illnesses suggestive of TSP/HAM, oligoclonal immunoglobulin bands and antibodies to HTLV-I in CSF are highly suggestive of TSP/HAM.[54] Infection with HTLV-I can be confirmed by the presence of serum antibodies (see Chapter 264), detected by enzyme-linked immunosorbent assay or gel agglutination test; specificity of antibodies (to core and envelope antigens of HTLV-I) should be demonstrated by immunoblotting or a comparable assay. Specialized laboratories can isolate HTLV-I and distinguish it from HTLV-II by PCR amplification.

Chronic TBE may be suspected in patients with Kozhevnikov epilepsy or progessive paralytic syndrome who were potentially exposed to infected ticks or milk in Europe or Asia. Most patients have a history of recovering from acute encephalitis with onset in the spring or summer. The serum should contain antibodies to TBE virus. In one case, well studied in Japan, elevated levels of antibodies to TBE virus were found in the CSF.[57] Chronic TBE has not been recognized in the United States.

Prevention, Treatment, and Precautions

Prevention of the underlying predisposing immunodeficiency state is the most promising approach to control of PML. Results of therapy for PML, even after early diagnosis, have been discouraging,[41] although reports suggested that treatment with interferon-α, with or without cytarabine, was followed by clinical improvement.[107, 108] No special precau-

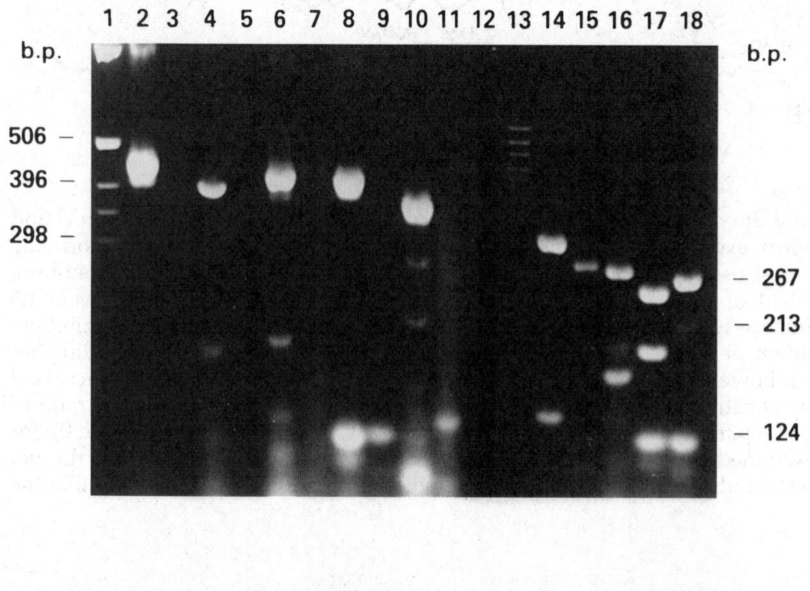

FIGURE 163–11 □ SSPE. Electrophoresis in agarose gel, stained with ethidium bromide and visualized under ultraviolet light, showing products amplified by PCR with complementary DNA transcribed from RNA extract of brain from a patient with SSPE (lanes 2, 4, 6, 8, 10). RNA from the brain of a control patient (lanes 3, 5, 9, 11) was included in the same study. Lanes 1 and 13 contain nucleic acid size markers (b.p., number of base pairs). Pairs of oligonucleotide primers amplifying five regions of measles viral genes were selected. Digestion of the complementary DNA products displayed in lanes 2, 4, 6, 8, 10 with restriction enzyme *Alu*I or *Ava*II yielded smaller fragments of sizes predicted for measles viral genome (lanes 14–18), confirming identity as measles. Lane 12 is blank. (From Godec MS, Asher DM, Masters CL, et al: Detection of measles virus genomic sequences in SSPE brain tissue. J Med Virol 30:237–244, 1990. Copyright © 1990 Wiley-Liss. Reprinted by permission of Wiley-Liss, Inc., a subsidiary of John Wiley & Sons, Inc.)

tions are indicated for PML, although they may be for the underlying conditions.

As noted earlier, not only does successful immunization prevent measles, it also protects children from SSPE.[42] It has been reported that treatment of SSPE with inosiplex increased the number of patients with prolonged survival and some clinical improvement in degree of disability.[42, 109] Several groups claimed to have slowed progression of SSPE after intrathecal or intraventricular injections of interferon-α.[110–114] However, in other trials no improvement in CSF abnormalities in SSPE followed treatment with inosiplex alone[30] or with inosiplex plus interferon.[115] One report claimed to have stabilized the rate of clinical deterioration in SSPE by immunomodulation with cimetidine.[116] A single attempt to treat SSPE by immune reconstitution using transfused cells from an unaffected sibling failed.[117] The use of anticonvulsants, maintenance of nutritional status, prompt treatment of secondary bacterial infections, physical therapy, and other supportive care may prolong survival and improve the quality of life. Information on current therapeutic trials may be sought through the National SSPE Registry.

The persistent measles infection in SSPE produces no complete virus particles. Patients with SSPE should pose no hazard of infecting others, and no special precautions need ordinarily be taken. Claims that measles virus was present in blood of SSPE patients were not confirmed.[118] In any case, universal blood and body fluid precautions should be observed for all patients[119] including those with SSPE.

Immunization with currently recommended measles-mumps-rubella vaccine probably protects children against RPE as well as SSPE. No successful therapy has been reported. Patients with RPE should pose no substantial risk of infection to others, although isolation of rubella virus from separated blood lymphocytes of a patient with RPE has been claimed.[52] Rubella virus has not been detected in urine of patients with panencephalitis, and their secretions have apparently never been studied.

TSP/HAM may be prevented by interfering with transmission of HTLV-I—screening and discarding potentially infected blood and blood products, discouraging infected mothers from breast-feeding (where social conditions allow that to be done), and promoting the same methods used to reduce sexual and drug-related spread of HIV. Although there is no specific therapy for TSP/HAM, some patients may benefit from corticosteroid treatment[54]; other therapies have also been attempted.[87] Blood precautions should be observed.

Infection with TBE virus can be prevented by immunization with inactivated vaccines[58] as well as by preventing exposure to infected ticks and milk. There is no documented effective therapy for the acute or chronic encephalitis. Patients with chronic TBE syndromes should not pose any risk of infecting others.

Other Possible Slow Infections of the Human Central Nervous System: Rasmussen Encephalitis

Patients with chronic encephalitis not associated with known viral infection have been recognized throughout the world. In North America, a syndrome of seizures (especially epilepsia partialis continua), spastic paralysis, and mental retardation associated with chronic encephalitis was described by Rasmussen and colleagues[120–126] in children, adolescents, and young adults. Patients had no history of preceding acute encephalitis. Computed tomograms of patients with Rasmussen encephalitis show cerebral cortical atrophy and ventricular dilatation, and, when brain tissue was resected, a panencephalitis without inclusion bodies or without virus-like particles was found. Later reports implicated the Epstein-Barr virus in two cases of Rasmussen encephalitis[127, 128] and cytomegalovirus in several other cases of the disease[129, 130]; those findings remain unconfirmed.[131, 132] Efforts to isolate viruses from brains of patients with Rasmussen encephalitis were unsuccessful.[21] A report that chronic encephalitis with seizures was produced in experimental animals immunized with a glutamate receptor and that patients with Rasmussen syndrome had antibodies to glutamate receptor in their serum suggests that the disease may be autoimmune and not caused by a persistent infection.[133]

A variety of other chronic neurologic diseases—multiple sclerosis best known among them—have been postulated to be caused by slow infections, but, in spite of a variety of intriguing but unconfirmed preliminary reports,[134] their etiology remains unknown.[33, 135]

References

1. Sigurdsson B: Observations on three slow infections of sheep. 1. Maedi, a slow progressive pneumonia of sheep: An epizootological and a pathological study. Br Vet J 110:255, 1954.
1a. Sigurdsson B: Observations on three slow infections of sheep. 2. Paratuberculosis (Johne's disease) of sheep in Iceland. Immunological studies and observations on its mode of spread. Br Vet J 110:307, 1954.
1b. Sigurdsson B: Observations on three slow infections of sheep. 3. Rida, a chronic encephalitis of sheep, with general remarks on infections which develop slowly and some of their special characteristics. Br Vet J 110:341, 1954.
2. Kimberlin RH: Scrapie: How much do we really understand? Neuropathol Appl Neurobiol 12:131, 1986.
3. Prusiner SB: Novel proteinaceous infectious particles cause scrapie. Science 216:136, 1982.
4. Gajdusek DC: Infectious amyloids. Subacute spongiform encephalopathies as transmissible cerebral amyloidoses. *In* Fields BN, Knipe DM, Howley PM (eds): Fields Virology, ed 3, Vol 2. Philadelphia, Lippincott-Raven, 1996, pp 2851–2900.
5. Aström K, Mancall EL, Richardson EP: Progressive multifocal leukoencephalopathy. A hitherto unrecognized complication of chronic lymphatic leukemia and Hodgkin's disease. Brain 81:93, 1958.
6. Padgett BL, Zu Rhein GM, Walker DL, et al: Cultivation of papova-like virus from human brain with progressive multifocal leukoencephalopathy. Lancet 1:1257, 1971.
7. Zu Rhein GM: Association of papova-virions with a human demyelinating disease (progressive multifocal leucoencephalopathy). Prog Med Virol 11:185, 1969.
8. Vandersteenhoven JJ, Dbaibo G, Boyko OB, et al: Progressive multifocal leukoencephalopathy in pediatric acquired immunodeficiency syndrome. Pediatr Infect Dis J 11:232, 1992.
9. Dawson JR: Cellular inclusions in cerebral lesions of lethargic encephalitis. Am J Pathol 9:7, 1933.
10. Bouteille M, Fontaine C, Verenne C, et al: Sur un cas d'encephalite subaigue à inclusions. Étude anatamoclinique et ultrastructurale. Rev Neurol (Paris) 118:454, 1965.
11. Connolly JH, Allen IV, Hurwitz LJ: Measles-virus antibody and antigen in subacute sclerosing panencephalitis. Lancet 1:542, 1967.
12. Chen TT, Watanabe I, Zeman W, et al: Subacute sclerosing panencephalitis: Propagation of measles virus from brain biopsy in tissue culture. Science 163:1193, 1969.
13. Horta-Barbosa L, Fuccillo DA, Sever JL, et al: Subacute sclerosing panencephalitis: Isolation of measles virus from a brain biopsy. Nature 221:974, 1969.
14. Horta-Barbosa L, Fuccillo DA, London WT, et al: Isolation of measles virus from brain cell cultures of two patients with subacute sclerosing panencephalitis. Proc Soc Exp Biol Med 132:272, 1969.
15. Payne FE, Baublis JV, Itabashi HH: Isolation of measles virus

from cell cultures of brain from a patient with subacute sclerosing panencephalitis. N Engl J Med 281:585, 1969.
16. Lebon P, Lyon G: Non-congenital rubella encephalitis. Lancet 2:468, 1974.
17. Cremer NE, Oshiro LS, Weil ML, et al: Isolation of rubella virus from brain in chronic progressive panencephalitis. J Gen Virol 29:143, 1975.
18. Gessain A, Barin F, Vernant JC, et al: Antibodies to human T-lymphotropic virus type-I in patients with tropical spastic paraparesis. Lancet 2:407, 1985.
19. Hirose S, Uemura Y, Fujishita M, et al: Isolation of HTLV-I from cerebrospinal fluid of a patient with myelopathy. Lancet 2:397, 1986.
20. Asher DM: Chronic encephalitis. *In* Boese A (ed): Search for the Cause of Multiple Sclerosis and Other Chronic Diseases of the Central Nervous System (Proceedings of the First International Symposium of the Hertie Foundation). Weinheim, Verlag Chemie, 1980, pp 272–279.
21. Asher DM, Gajdusek DC: Virologic studies in chronic encephalitis. *In* Andermann F (ed): Chronic Encephalitis and Epilepsy: Rasmussen's Syndrome. Boston, Butterworth-Heinemann, 1991, pp 147–158.
22. Shah KV: Polyomaviruses. *In* Fields BN, Knipe DM, Howley PM (eds): Fields Virology, ed 3, Vol 2. Philadelphia, Lippincott-Raven, 1996, pp 2027–2043.
23. Iida T, Kitamura T, Guo J, et al: Origin of JC polyomavirus variants associated with progressive multifocal leukoencephalopathy. Proc Natl Acad Sci USA 90:5062, 1993.
24. Ault GS, Stoner GL: Two major types of JC virus defined in progressive multifocal leukoencephalopathy brain by early and late coding region DNA sequences. J Gen Virol 73:2669, 1992.
25. Ault GS, Stoner GL: Human polyomavirus JC promoter/enhancer rearrangement patterns from progressive multifocal leukoencephalopathy brain are unique derivatives of a single archetypal structure. J Gen Virol 74:1499, 1993.
26. Major EO, Amemiya K, Tornatore CS, et al: Pathogenesis and molecular biology of progressive multifocal leukoencephalopathy, the JC virus–induced demyelinating disease of the human brain. Clin Microbiol Rev 5:49, 1992.
27. Renner K, Leger H, Wegner M: The POU domain protein Tst-1 and papovaviral large tumor antigen function synergistically to stimulate glia-specific gene expression of JC virus. Proc Natl Acad Sci USA 91:6433, 1994.
28. Griffin DE, Bellini WJ: Measles virus. *In* Fields BN, Knipe DM, Howley PM (eds): Fields Virology, ed 3, Vol 1. Philadelphia, Lippincott-Raven, 1996, pp 1267–1312.
29. Cattaneo R, Schmid A, Billeter MA, et al: Multiple viral mutations rather than host factors cause defective measles virus gene expression in a subacute sclerosing panencephalitis cell line. J Virol 62:1388, 1988.
30. Beersma MF, Galama JM, Van Druten HA, et al: Subacute sclerosing panencephalitis in The Netherlands—1976–1990. Int J Epidemiol 21:583, 1992.
31. Sie TH, Weber W, Freling G, et al: Rapidly fatal subacute sclerosing panencephalitis in a 19-year-old man. Eur Neurol 31:94, 1991.
32. Wolinsky JS: Rubella. *In* Fields BN, Knipe DM, Howley PM (eds): Fields Virology, ed 3, Vol 1. Philadelphia, Lippincott-Raven, 1996, pp 899–929.
33. Cann AJ, Chen ISY: Human T-cell leukemia virus types I and II. *In* Fields BN, Knipe DM, Howley PM (eds): Fields Virology, 3rd ed., Vol 2. Philadelphia, Lippincott-Raven, 1996, pp 1849–1880.
34. Jennings AD, Gibson CA, Miller BR, et al: Analysis of a yellow fever virus isolated from a fatal case of vaccine-associated human encephalitis. J Infect Dis 169:512, 1994.
35. Pletnev AG, Bray M, Lai CJ: Chimeric tick-borne encephalitis and dengue type 4 viruses: Effects of mutations on neurovirulence in mice. J Virol 67:4956, 1993.
36. Taguchi F, Kajioka J, Miyamura T: Prevalence rate and age of acquisition of antibodies against JC virus and BK virus in human sera. Microbiol Immunol 26:1057, 1982.
37. Padgett BL, Walker DL: Prevalence of antibodies in human sera against JC virus, an isolate from a case of progressive multifocal leukoencephalopathy. J Infect Dis 127:467, 1973.
38. Katz DA, Berger JR, Hamilton B, et al: Progressive multifocal leukoencephalopathy complicating Wiskott-Aldrich syndrome. Report of a case and review of the literature of progressive multifocal leukoencephalopathy with other inherited immunodeficiency states. Arch Neurol 51:422, 1994.
39. Berger JR, Scott G, Albrecht J, et al: Progressive multifocal leukoencephalopathy in HIV-1–infected children. AIDS 6:837, 1992.
40. Stoner GL, Walker DL, Webster HD: Age distribution of progressive multifocal leukoencephalopathy. Acta Neurol Scand 78:307, 1988.
41. Karahalios D, Breit R, Dal Canto MC, et al: Progressive multifocal leukoencephalopathy in patients with HIV infection: Lack of impact of early diagnosis by stereotactic brain biopsy. J Acquir Immune Defic Syndr 5:1030, 1992.
42. Dyken PR, Cunningham SC, Ward LC: Changing character of subacute sclerosing panencephalitis in the United States. Pediatr Neurol 5:339, 1989.
43. Modlin JF, Halsey NA, Eddins DL, et al: Epidemiology of subacute sclerosing panencephalitis. J Pediatr 94:231, 1979.
44. Cape CA, Martinez AJ, Roberston JT, et al: Adult onset of subacute sclerosing panencephalitis. Arch Neurol 28:124, 1973.
45. Centers for Disease Control: Subacute sclerosing panencephalitis—United States. MMWR Morbid Mortal Wkly Rep 31:585, 1982.
46. Halsey NA, Modlin JF: Subacute sclerosing panencephalitis. Pediatr Neurol 7:151, 1991.
47. Miller C, Farrington CP, Harbert K: The epidemiology of subacute sclerosing panencephalitis in England and Wales 1970–1989. Int J Epidemiol 21:998, 1992.
48. Farrington CP: Subacute sclerosing panencephalitis in England and Wales: Transient effects and risk estimates. Stat Med 10:1733, 1991.
49. Wolinsky JS: Subacute sclerosing panencephalitis, progressive rubella panencephalitis, and multifocal leukoencephalopathy. Res Publ Assoc Res Nerv Ment Dis 68:259, 1990.
50. Dayras JC, Lyon G, Ponsot G, Allemon MC: Progressive chronic rubella encephalitis. Report of a personal case. Sem Hop 56:1703, 1980.
51. Wolinsky JS, Bedrg BO, Maitland CJ: Progressive rubella panencephalitis. Arch Neurol 33:722, 1976.
52. Wolinsky JS, Dau PC, Buimovici-Klein E, et al: Progressive rubella panencephalitis: Immunovirological studies and results of isoprinosine therapy. Clin Exp Immunol 35:397, 1979.
53. Guizzaro A, Volpe E, Lus G, et al: Progressive rubella panencephalitis. Follow-up EEG study of a case. Acta Neurol (Napoli) 14:485, 1992.
54. Höllsberg P, Hafler DA: Pathogenesis of diseases induced by human lymphotropic virus type I infection. N Engl J Med 368:1173, 1993.
55. Brody JA, Hadlow WJ, Hotchin J, et al: Soviet search for viruses that cause chronic neurologic diseases. Science 147:1114, 1965.
56. Asher DM: Persistent tick-borne encephalitis infection in man and monkeys: Relation to chronic neurologic disease. *In* Kurstak E (ed): Arctic and Tropical Arboviruses. New York, Academic Press, 1979, pp 179–195.
57. Ogawa M, Okubo H, Tsuji Y, et al: Chronic progressive encephalitis occurring 13 years after Russian spring-summer encephalitis. J Neurol Sci 19:363, 1973.
58. Monath TP, Heinz FX: Flaviviruses. *In* Fields BN, Knipe DM, Howley PM (eds): Fields Virology, ed 3, Vol 1. Philadelphia, Lippincott-Raven, 1996, pp 961–1034.
59. Richardson EP: Progressive multifocal leukoencephalopathy. N Engl J Med 265:815, 1961.
60. Boldorini R, Cristina S, Vago L, et al: Ultrastructural studies in the lytic phase of progressive multifocal leukoencephalopathy in AIDS patients. Ultrastruct Pathol 17:599, 1993.
61. Mesquita R, Parravicini C, Bjorkholm M, et al: Macrophage association of polyomavirus in progressive multifocal leukoencephalopathy: An immunohistochemical and ultrastructural study. Case report. APMIS 100:993, 1992.
62. Kuchelmeister K, Gullotta F, Bergmann M, et al: Progressive multifocal leukoencephalopathy (PML) in the acquired immunodeficiency syndrome (AIDS). A neuropathological autopsy study of 21 cases. Pathol Res Pract 89:163, 1993.
63. Tornatore C, Berger JR, Houff SA, et al: Detection of JC virus DNA in peripheral lymphocytes from patients with and without

progressive multifocal leukoencephalopathy. Ann Neurol 31:454, 1992.
64. Hair LS, Nuovo G, Powers JM, et al: Progressive multifocal leukoencephalopathy in patients with human immunodeficiency virus. Hum Pathol 23:663, 1992.
65. Dyken PR: Subacute sclerosing panencephalitis. Current status. Neurol Clin 3:179, 1985.
66. Sever JL: Persistent measles infection of the CNS: Subacute sclerosing panencephalitis. Rev Infect Dis 5:467, 1983.
67. Brown HR, Goller NL, Rudelli RD, et al: Postmortem detection of measles virus in non-neural tissues in subacute sclerosing panencephalitis. Ann Neurol 26:263, 1989.
68. Fournier JG, Tardieu M, Lebon P, et al: Detection of measles virus RNA in lymphocytes from peripheral-blood and brain perivascular infiltrates of patients with subacute sclerosing panencephalitis. N Engl J Med 313:910, 1985.
69. Fournier JG, Gerfaux J, Joret AM, et al: Subacute sclerosing panencephalitis: Detection of measles virus sequences in RNA extracted from circulating lymphocytes. Br Med J (Clin Res Ed) 296:684, 1988.
70. Kirk J, Zhou AL, McQuaid S, et al: Cerebral endothelial cell infection by measles virus in subacute sclerosing panencephalitis: Ultrastructural and in situ hybridization evidence. Neuropathol Appl Neurobiol 17:289, 1991.
71. Isaacson SH, Asher DM, Gajdusek DC, et al: Detection of RNA viruses in archival brain tissue by in situ RT-PCR amplification and labeled-probe hybridization. CellVision 1:25, 1994.
72. Isaacson SH, Asher DM, Godec MS, et al: Widespread, restricted low-level measles virus infection of brain in a case of subacute sclerosing panencephalitis. Acta Neuropathol (Berl) 91:135, 1996.
73. Townsend JJ, Stroop WG, Baringer JR, et al: Neuropathology of progressive rubella panencephalitis after childhood rubella. Neurology 32:185, 1982.
74. Townsend JJ, Wolinsky JS, Baringer JR: The neuropathology of progressive rubella panencephalitis of late onset. Brain 99:81, 1976.
75. Rodgers-Johnson PEB, Ono SG, Asher DM, et al: Tropical spastic paraparesis and HTLV-I myelopathy: Clinical features and pathogenesis. *In* Waksman BH (ed): Immunologic Mechanisms in Neurologic and Psychiatric Disease. New York, Raven Press, 1990, pp 117–130.
76. Petito CK, Navia BA, Cho ES, et al: Vacuolar myelopathy pathologically resembling subacute combined degeneration in patients with the acquired immunodeficiency syndrome. N Engl J Med 312:874, 1985.
77. Levin MC, Fox RJ, Lehky T, et al: PCR–in situ hybridization detection of human T-cell lymphotropic virus type 1 (HTLV-1) tax proviral DNA in peripheral blood lymphocytes of patients with HTLV-1–associated neurologic disease. J Virol 70:924, 1996.
78. Utz U, Banks D, Jacobson S, et al: Analysis of the T-cell receptor repertoire of human T-cell leukemia virus type 1 (HTLV-1) Tax-specific $CD8^+$ cytotoxic T lymphocytes from patients with HTLV-1–associated disease: Evidence for oligoclonal expansion. J Virol 70:843, 1996.
79. Omorokov LI: Kozhevnikov's epilepsy in Siberia. Originally published in Zh Nevropatol Psikhiatr 20:13, 1927. *In* Andermann F (ed): Chronic Encephalitis: Rasmussen's Syndrome. Boston, Butterworth-Heinemann, 1991, pp 263–269.
80. Hedley-White ET, Smith BP, Tyler HR, et al: Multifocal leukoencephalopathy with remission and five year survival. J Neuropathol Exp Neurol 25:107, 1966.
81. Johnston HM, Wise GA, Henry JG: Visual deterioration as presentation of subacute sclerosing panencephalitis. Arch Dis Child 55:899, 1980.
82. Kabra SK, Bagga A, Shankar V: Subacute sclerosing panencephalitis presenting as cortical blindness. Trop Doct 22:94, 1992.
83. Townsend JJ, Baringer JR, Wolinski JS, et al: Progressive rubella panencephalitis: Late onset after congenital rubella. N Engl J Med 292:990, 1975.
84. Weil ML, Itabashi HH, Cremer NE, et al: Chronic progressive panencephalitis due to rubella virus simulating subacute sclerosing panencephalitis. N Engl J Med 292:994, 1975.
85. Wolinsky JS: Progressive rubella panencephalitis. *In* Vinken PJ, Bruyn GW (ed): Handbook of Clinical Neurology, Vol 34. Amsterdam, Elsevier North Holland, 1978, pp 331–341.
86. Abe T, Nukada T, Hatanaka H, et al: Myoclonus in a case of suspected rubella panencephalitis. Arch Neurol 40:98, 1983.
87. Kuroda Y, Yukitake M, Kurohara K, et al: A follow-up study on spastic paraparesis in Japanese HAM/TSP. J Neurol Sci 132:174, 1995.
88. Whiteman ML, Post MJ, Berger JR, et al: Progressive multifocal leukoencephalopathy in 47 HIV-seropositive patients: Neuroimaging with clinical and pathologic correlation. Radiology 187:233, 1993.
89. Gillespie SM, Chang Y, Lemp G, et al: Progressive multifocal leukoencephalopathy in persons infected with human immunodeficiency virus, San Francisco, 1981–1989. Ann Neurol 30:597, 1991.
90. Gibson PE, Knowles WA, Hand JF, et al: Detection of JC virus DNA in the cerebrospinal fluid of patients with progressive multifocal leukoencephalopathy. J Med Virol 39:278, 1993.
91. Henson J, Rosenblum M, Armstrong D, et al: Amplification of JC virus DNA from brain and cerebrospinal fluid of patients with progressive multifocal leukoencephalopathy. Neurology 41:1967, 1991.
92. Moret H, Guichard M, Matheron S, et al: Virological diagnosis of progressive multifocal leukoencephalopathy: Detection of JC virus DNA in cerebrospinal fluid and brain tissue of AIDS patients. J Clin Microbiol 31:3310, 1993.
93. Telenti A, Marshall WF, Aksamit AJ, et al: Detection of JC virus by polymerase chain reaction in cerebrospinal fluid from two patients with progressive multifocal leukoencephalopathy. Eur J Clin Microbiol Infect Dis 11:253, 1992.
94. Orefice G, Campanella G, Cicciarello S, et al: Presence of papova-like viral particles in cerebrospinal fluid of AIDS patients with progressive multifocal leukoencephalopathy. An additional test for in vivo diagnosis. Acta Neurol (Napoli) 15:328, 1993.
95. Weiner LP, Narayan O, Penney JB Jr, et al: Papovavirus of JC type in progressive multifocal leukoencephalopathy. Rapid identification and subsequent isolation. Arch Neurol 29:1, 1973.
96. Aksamit AJ Jr: Nonradioactive in situ hybridization in progressive multifocal leukoencephalopathy. Mayo Clin Proc 68:899, 1993.
97. Buckle GJ, Godec MS, Rubi JU, et al: Lack of JC viral genomic sequences in multiple sclerosis brain tissue by polymerase chain reaction. Ann Neurol 32:829, 1992.
98. von Einsiedel RW, Fife TD, Aksamit AJ, et al: Progressive multifocal leukoencephalopathy in AIDS: A clinicopathologic study and review of the literature. J Neurol 240:391, 1993.
99. Gimenez-Roldan S, Martin M, Mateo D, et al: Preclinical EEG abnormalities in subacute sclerosing panencephalitis. Neurology 31:763, 1981.
100. Gloor P, Kalabay O, Giard N: The electroencephalogram in diffuse encephalopathies: Electroencephalographic correlates of grey and white matter lesions. Brain 91:779, 1968.
101. Duda E, Huttenlocher P, Patronas N: CT of subacute sclerosing panencephalitis. AJNR 1:35, 1980.
102. Tourtellotte WW, Ma BI, Brandes DB, et al: Quantification of de novo central nervous system IgG measles antibody synthesis in SSPE. Ann Neurol 9:551, 1981.
103. Katz M, Koprowski H: The significance of failure to isolate infectious viruses in cases of subacute sclerosing panencephalitis. Arch Ges Virusforsch 41:390, 1973.
104. Saiki RK, Gelfand DH, Stoffel S, et al: Primer-directed enzymatic amplification of DNA with a thermostable DNA polymerase. Science 239:487, 1988.
105. Godec MS, Asher DM, Masters CL, et al: Detection of measles virus genomic sequences in SSPE brain tissue. J Med Virol 30:237, 1990.
106. Whitley RJ: Viral encephalitis. N Engl J Med 323:242, 1990.
107. Colosimo C, Lebon P, Martelli M, et al: Alpha-interferon therapy in a case of probable progressive multifocal leukoencephalopathy. Acta Neurol Belg 92:24, 1992.
108. Steiger MJ, Tarnesby G, Gabe S, et al: Successful outcome of progressive multifocal leukoencephalopathy with cytarabine and interferon. Ann Neurol 33:407, 1993.
109. Dyken PR, Swift A, Durant RH: Long-term follow-up of patients with subacute sclerosing panencephalitis treated with inosiplex. Ann Neurol 11:359, 1982.
110. Anlar B, Yalaz K, Imir T, et al: The effect of inosiplex in subacute

sclerosing panencephalitis: A clinical and laboratory study. Eur Neurol 34:44, 1994.
111. Gascon GG, Yamani S, Cafege A, et al: Treatment of subacute sclerosing panencephalitis with alpha interferon. Ann Neurol 30:227, 1991.
112. Miyazaki M, Hashimoto T, Fujino K, et al: Apparent response of subacute sclerosing panencephalitis to intrathecal interferon alpha. Ann Neurol 29:97, 1991.
113. Steiner I, Wirguin I, Morag A, et al: Intraventricular interferon treatment for subacute sclerosing panencephalitis. J Child Neurol 4:20, 1989.
114. Wirguin I, Steiner I, Brenner T, et al: Intraventricular interferon treatment for subacute sclerosing panencephalitis. Ann Neurol 30:227, 1991.
115. Mehta PD, Kulczycki J, Patrick BA, et al: Effect of treatment on oligoclonal IgG bands and intrathecal IgG synthesis in sequential cerebrospinal fluid and serum from patients with subacute sclerosing panencephalitis. J Neurol Sci 109:64, 1992.
116. Anlar B, Gucuyener K, Imir T, et al: Cimetidine as an immunomodulator in subacute sclerosing panencephalitis: A double blind, placebo-controlled study. Pediatr Infect Dis J 12:578, 1993.
117. Bakheit AM, Behan PO: Unsuccessful treatment of subacute sclerosing panencephalitis treated with transfusion of peripheral blood lymphocytes from an identical twin. J Neurol Neurosurg Psychiatry 54:377, 1991.
118. Schneider-Schaulies S, Kreth HW, Hofmann G, et al: Expression of measles virus RNA in peripheral blood mononuclear cells of patients with measles, SSPE, and autoimmune diseases. Virology 182:703, 1991.
119. Occupational, Safety and Health Administration (United States Department of Labor): Occupational exposure to bloodborne pathogens; final rule (29 CFR Part 1910.1030). Fed Regist 56:64175, 1991.
120. Aguilar MJ, Rasmussen T: Role of encephalitis in pathogenesis of epilepsy. Arch Neurol 2:663, 1960.
121. Andermann F: Epilepsia partialis continua and other seizures arising from the precentral gyrus: High incidence in patients with Rasmussen syndrome and neuronal migration disorders. Brain Dev 14:338, 1992.
122. Rasmussen T, Olszewski J, Lloyd-Smith D: Focal seizures due to chronic localized encephalitis. Neurology 8:435, 1958.
123. Rasmussen T, McCann W: Clinical studies of patients with focal epilepsy due to "chronic encephalitis." Trans Am Neurol Assoc 93:89, 1968.
124. Rasmussen T: Further observations on the syndrome of chronic encephalitis and epilepsy. Appl Neurophysiol 41:1, 1978.
125. Rasmussen T: Hemispherectomy for seizures revisited. Can J Neurol Sci 10:89, 1983.
126. Rasmussen TB: Chronic encephalitis and seizures: Historical introduction. *In* Andermann F (ed): Chronic Encephalitis and Epilepsy: Rasmussen's Syndrome. Boston, Butterworth-Heinemann, 1991, pp 1–4.
127. Walter GF, Renella RR, Hori A, et al: Detection of Epstein-Barr viruses in Rasmussen's encephalitis. Report of 2 cases. Nervenarzt 60:168, 1989.
128. Walter GF, Renella RR: Epstein-Barr virus in brain and Rasmussen's encephalitis. Lancet 1:279, 1989.
129. Power C, Poland SD, Blume WT, et al: Cytomegalovirus and Rasmussen's encephalitis. Lancet 336:1282, 1990.
130. McLachlan RS, Girvin JP, Blume WT, et al: Rasmussen's chronic encephalitis in adults. Arch Neurol 50:269, 1993.
131. Cytomegalovirus and Rasmussen's encephalitis (Letter). Lancet 337:239, 1991.
132. Farrell MA, Cheng L, Cornford ME, et al: Cytomegalovirus and Rasmussen's encephalitis. Lancet 337:1551, 1991.
133. Rogers SW, Andrews PI, Gahring LC, et al: Autoantibodies to glutamate receptor GluR3 in Rasmussen's encephalitis. Science 265:648, 1994.
134. Haas AT: Slow virus infections of the central nervous system. *In* Gorbach SL, Bartlett JG, Blacklow NR (eds): Infectious Diseases. Philadelphia, WB Saunders, 1992, pp 1206–1216.
135. Taller AM, Asher DM, Pomeroy KL, et al: Search for viral nucleic acid sequences in brain tissues of patients with schizophrenia using nested polymerase chain reaction. Arch Gen Psychiatry 53:32, 1996.

164

Infectious Diseases of the Spinal Cord and Peripheral Nervous System

Newton E. Hyslop, Jr.
Timothy S. Leach

In this chapter, we review the common infectious diseases associated with neurologic findings arising from damage to the spinal cord or its radicles, plexuses, and peripheral nerves.

Infectious disorders affecting the cord include spinal epidural abscess, spinal subdural empyema, several patterns of myelitis, and intramedullary abscess. Infectious diseases affecting peripheral nerves include direct infection, disorders caused by toxins produced by organisms, and "postinfection" syndromes.[1]

The clinical patterns of these diseases are a combination of the location of the process within the nervous system itself and the other manifestations of the specific infectious agent. Familiarity with the neuropathic syndromes shown in Tables 164–1 to 164–7 allows the clinician to categorize the possible infectious causes. A suggested approach to the patient with bilateral neurologic deficits that could be compatible with spinal cord or peripheral nerve disorders concludes this discussion. A neurology text should be consulted to encompass complete differential diagnosis, because patterns seen with infectious causes may also be produced by nutritional deficiencies, toxic metals and drugs, diabetes mellitus, malignant neoplasms, metabolic diseases, trauma, reaction to vaccines, and other causes. Furthermore, details of special studies that may pinpoint the anatomic site of the disease process, such as nerve conduction velocity and electromyography, are not discussed; they are the province of experts in these technologies.[1(pp1124–1133)]

PERIPHERAL NERVOUS SYSTEM INFECTIONS: MONONEUROPATHIES AND POLYNEUROPATHIES

Diseases of the peripheral nervous system (PNS) are clinically complex because a wide range of genetic and acquired disorders acting at several potential target sites produce a limited spectrum of clinical findings. Hence, the expression of clinical disorders is limited to isolated nerve palsies (mononeuropathies), unilateral plexus lesions, combinations of cranial palsies, and asymmetric and symmetric polyneuropathies. For simplicity, we consider diseases affecting the cranial nerves as a subdivision of those affecting peripheral nerves originating from the spinal cord.

Infectious agents are known or suspected causes within each clinical pattern and operate by several mechanisms.[1(pp1124–1133)] They may act by local compression or destruction of a nerve itself; through toxic effects on Schwann cells; by immune complex damage of the vasa nervorum; by inflammatory injury to sensory ganglia and nerve roots, accompanied by cells in the cerebrospinal fluid (CSF); by perivenous lymphocytic demyelination of ventral and dorsal columns of the cord, causing interruption of neuronal transmission along exiting and entering nerve fibers; or finally, by irreversible cytopathic damage to nerve cells located in anterior or lateral horns of cord, dorsal root ganglia, or sympathetic ganglia.

Anatomy

The nervous system is separated anatomically into central, peripheral, and autonomic categories. The central nervous system (CNS) consists of the brain and spinal cord and is covered by the pia-arachnoid membrane. The PNS consists of all nervous structures lying outside the pia-arachnoid with the exception of the optic nerves and olfactory bulbs, which are considered extensions of the brain. Hence, the PNS comprises cranial nerves III to XII; the brachial, crural, and lumbosacral plexuses; and all other spinal nerves, including their sensory and motor roots and their ganglia.

The peripheral nerves arise as pairs of roots from brain stem and cord (Fig. 164–1). The dorsal (sensory) roots carry axonal processes of ganglion cells located in the cranial and spinal ganglia. Sensory ganglion cell axons project peripherally (to sensory organs) and centrally (through sensory tracts in cord and brain stem) to the brain. The ventral (motor) roots consist of axon processes emerging from brain stem and from the anterior and lateral horn cells of the cord.

After traversing the subarachnoid space, bathed in CSF and covered only by a thin layer of arachnoid, each pair of roots is joined by unmedullated fibers from autonomic ganglia. At the exit point, fibers that are to be myelinated are now enveloped by Schwann cells, which produce and maintain the myelin, and the neural bundle is then wrapped in a thick supportive sheath of well-vascularized perineurium and epineurium as it passes to the periphery.

The autonomic nervous system is anatomically distinct from the PNS. However, the autonomic nervous system receives and sends impulses to the CNS by the PNS through the white and gray communicating rami, which intersect the anterior roots and spinal nerves, respectively.

Pathogenesis

Infectious causes of peripheral nerve injury fall into five main categories:

1. Focal external compression or invasion of a nerve by infection in adjacent structures, usually after producing a unique constellation of findings (e.g., Gradenigo cranial nerve syndrome, tuberculoid leprosy mononeuropathy)
2. Interruption of nutrient blood supply by vasculitis involving the vasa nervorum (e.g., polyarteritis nodosa, granulomatous arteritis)
3. Demyelination by lymphocytic invasion (e.g., polyneuritis) or toxic injury to Schwann cells (e.g., diphtheria)
4. Direct invasion and proliferation within nerve sheaths (e.g., lepromatous leprosy)
5. Inflammatory injury to ganglion and associated sensory and motor roots in response to viral replication in a cranial or spinal ganglion (e.g., herpes zoster)

Certain drugs commonly used in treating infectious diseases are also capable of producing symptoms and signs of peripheral neuropathy. Some interfere with normal metabolic

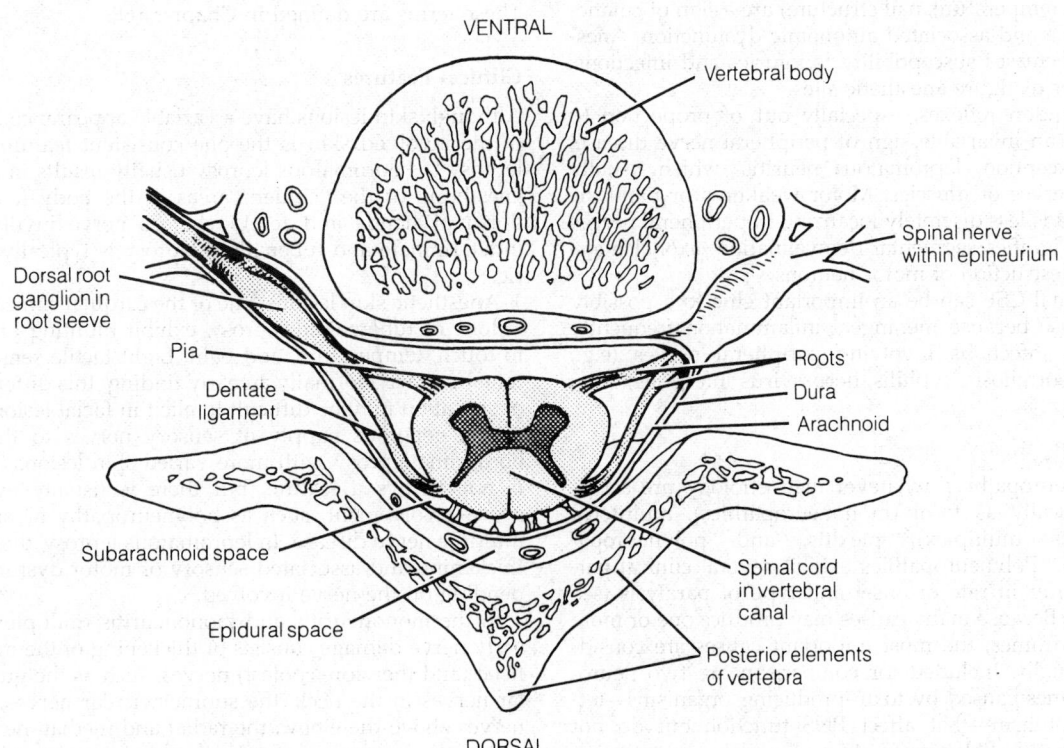

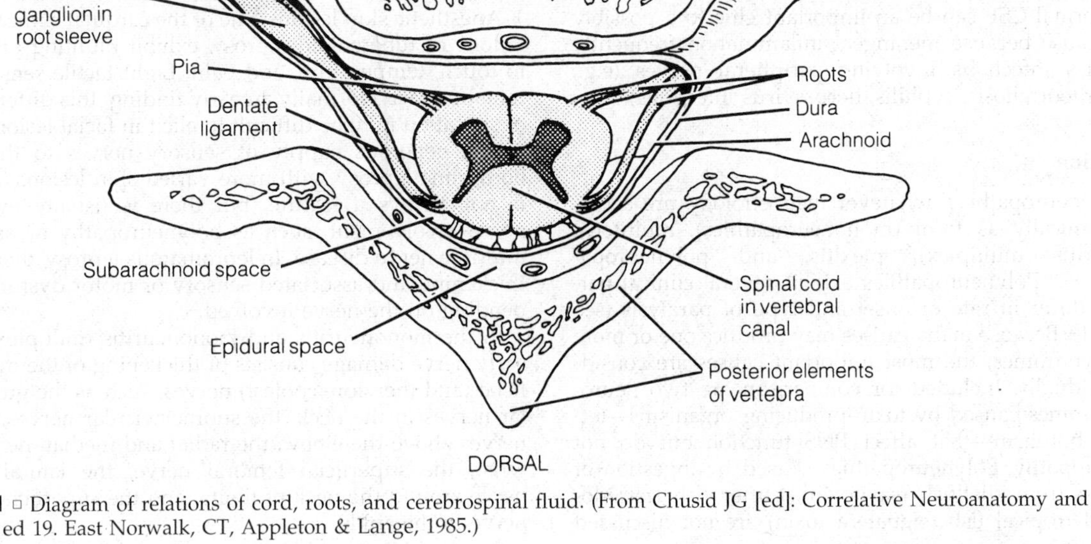

FIGURE 164–1 □ Diagram of relations of cord, roots, and cerebrospinal fluid. (From Chusid JG [ed]: Correlative Neuroanatomy and Functional Neurology, ed 19. East Norwalk, CT, Appleton & Lange, 1985.)

processes required to maintain myelin (e.g., isoniazid), whereas others may produce their effect by interference with axonal transport (e.g., the antivirals dideoxycytidine and dideoxyinosine); in both instances, symptoms arise first in areas served by the longest nerves and thus initially cause stocking-glove patterns of sensory and motor dysfunction. Antibiotics that produce concentration-dependent neuromuscular blockade (e.g., aminoglycosides, polymyxins) may closely mimic the polyneuropathy syndromes (Table 164–1).

Clinical Features

Whereas motor dysfunction or paralysis ultimately dominates the signs of most peripheral nerve disorders, sensory disturbances usually herald the onset. Characteristic symptoms are paresthesia (tingling, electric, numb feelings or, alternatively, aching, cutting, crushing pains) and dysesthesia (e.g., burning, tingling provoked by light touch). Spontaneous unprovoked pain and perversion of sensation are particularly characteristic of tabes dorsalis and postzoster neuralgia, both of which are associated with inflammatory changes predominantly in the dorsal root. Inflammation always extends into the dorsal column in tabes and may also be a factor in the pathogenesis of postzoster neuralgia.

Seemingly paradoxical dissociations of sensory losses may be helpful in evaluating the site of lesion. When the disease process mainly targets myelin, pain and temperature sensation are spared, but deep tendon reflexes and proprioceptive functions (pressure-touch, vibration, joint pressure sensations, and two-point discrimination) are abnormal. Conversely, when nerve itself is invaded and if invasion is limited by the organism's requirement for localizing in superficial nerves (e.g., lepromatous leprosy), proprioceptive functions and tendon reflexes remain intact in the presence of widespread cutaneous anesthesia. Sensory ataxia (brusque, flinging, slapping movements, especially of legs) results when motor function is relatively spared, which is characteristic of tabes dorsalis. Trophic skin changes (alteration of color, turgor, temperature, nail structure) are a sign of cutaneous anesthesia and associated autonomic dysfunction. Anesthesia also increases susceptibility to injuries and infections, which further disfigure anesthetic sites.

Loss of tendon reflexes, especially out of proportion to weakness, is an invariable sign of peripheral nerve disease, with one exception: lepromatous neuritis, which usually spares the nerves of muscles. Motor weakness or paralysis with areflexia is less discretely localizing to peripheral nerves but always signifies segmental demyelination, axonal interruption, or destruction of motor neurons.

An abnormal CSF can be an important clue to a possibly treatable cause because meningeal inflammation frequently accompanies infections involving peripheral nerves (e.g., Lyme neuroborreliosis, syphilis, herpesvirus infections).

Classification

Peripheral neuropathies, whatever their etiology, are classified anatomically as focal (mononeuropathies), multifocal (mononeuritis multiplex), plexitis, and polyneuropathies.[1(pp1124–1133)] Polyneuropathies exhibit several clinical patterns that differ in rate of onset and type of paralysis (see Table 164–1). Because many causes may produce one or more of these syndromes, the most important causes are considered individually. Included for comparison are two neurologic syndromes caused by toxin-producing organisms—tetanus and botulism—that affect PNS function but do not cause neuropathy. Polyneuropathies caused by ingestion of neurotoxins from shellfish (saxitoxin), puffer fish (tetrodotoxin), and tropical fish (ciguatera toxin) are not discussed but must be considered in the differential diagnosis of acute polyneuropathy.

Specific Diseases

Direct Invasion

LEPROSY

Cause

Leprosy (or Hansen disease) is a chronic mycobacterial infection in which *Mycobacterium leprae* primarily affects the PNS and secondarily involves skin and other tissues.[2] The three characteristics of leprosy are anesthetic skin lesions, palpably enlarged peripheral nerves, and acid-fast bacilli on slit skin smear.

Epidemiology

M. leprae is shed from skin and mucous membranes and transmitted from person to person by prolonged physical contact. The World Health Organization (WHO) estimates the current prevalence of leprosy at 10 to 12 million cases.[3, 3a] Worldwide, leprosy remains one of the most common diseases of the PNS. Although it is a rare endemic disease in the United States, new cases are still diagnosed regularly, particularly among immigrants from Southeast Asia.[3, 4]

Pathogenesis

Ranging from tuberculoid through lepromatous disease, leprosy represents a spectrum of illness resulting from a complex interaction between the organism and the host's immune response. The pathogenesis of neurologic lesions (see Table 164–1) depends on the stage of leprosy that is present: lepromatous, tuberculoid, or indeterminate (borderline). Lepromatous patients are anergic, whereas tuberculous patients are intensely immune. Borderline states fall in between. These terms are defined in Chapter 168.

Clinical Features

Although skin lesions have a variable appearance, anesthesia of the involved skin is the one consistent feature in typical leprosy.[5, 6] Lepromatous leprosy usually results in symmetric anesthesia of the "colder" areas of the body (e.g., pinnae, dorsa of hands and feet), whereas nerve involvement in indeterminate and tuberculoid leprosy is typically asymmetric.

Anesthetic skin lesions, one of the cardinal clinical manifestations of tuberculoid leprosy, exhibit blunting of sensation to touch, temperature, and pain. Light tactile sensation may remain intact. Normally an early finding, this differential loss of sensation may be difficult to elicit in facial lesions because of the generous supply of sensory nerves to the face. In borderline leprosy with more varied skin lesions, anesthesia is not always a feature, but there is usually evidence of nerve involvement, such as polyneuropathy or asymmetric multiple nerve disease. In lepromatous leprosy, there is nerve thickening and associated sensory or motor dysfunction, depending on the nerve involved.[2]

In the mononeuritis and mononeuritis multiplex patterns, early nerve damage consists of thickening of the most superficial (and therefore coolest) nerves, such as the great auricular nerves in the neck, the supraclavicular nerves, the ulnar nerves above the elbow, the radial and median nerves at the wrist, the superficial femoral nerve, the lateral popliteal nerve around the neck of fibula, and the superficial peroneal nerve in the ankle.

TABLE 164–1 ■ Polyneuropathy Syndromes of Infectious Etiology or Complicating Antimicrobial Therapy

	SYMPTOMS	SIGNS	DIAGNOSIS*
ACUTE ASCENDING MOTOR PARALYSIS WITH VARIABLE SENSORY DYSFUNCTION			
Acute Inflammatory Demyelinating Polyneuritis: Guillain-Barré Syndrome			
Idiopathic	*Progressive ascending symmetric weakness* involving distal then proximal limbs, truncal and cranial muscles in 10–14 d *Paresthesias* common *Autonomic dysfunction* variable—cardiovascular, gastrointestinal *Variants* Descending paralysis Complete ophthalmoplegia, ataxia, and areflexia without progression (Miller-Fisher syndrome)	*Hypotonia* without atrophy (initially) *Facial diplegia* (50%) No sphincteric paralysis *Areflexia* *Sensory loss:* minimal to variable	*CSF* Cells: 0–5/mm³ lymphocytes (90%), 10–50 (10%) Protein: elevated, peak at 4–6 wk Antibody studies: negative *Nerve conduction:* slowed *CT and MRI* Absence of myelitis, intramedullary or extramedullary mass Enhancement with gadolinium on MRI Spinal and cranial nerve roots Spinocerebellar tract in Miller-Fisher variant Correlates with location of symptoms
Infection Associated			
Viral Infectious mononucleosis Viral hepatitis HIV Other Brucellosis *Campylobacter* Lyme borreliosis Psittacosis	*Symptoms and signs of primary illness* precede onset of neurologic symptoms *Progressive ascending symmetric weakness* in 10–14 d Distal → proximal limbs Truncal → cranial muscles *Paresthesias* common	*Acute ascending sensorimotor paralysis:* identical to idiopathic Guillain-Barré	*CSF* Cells 0-200/mm³ lymphocytes B cells (primarily) IgM-positive early in disease Protein: elevated Oligoclonal banding on electrophoresis IgM, IgG increased Specific antibody ELISA positive in many infections IgM early, then IgG Immunoblot: positive if antibody in high titer Identification of organism PCR: for specific antigen (where available) Culture: insensitive *Blood serology:* diagnostic of primary infection *CT and MRI:* same as for idiopathic form
Diphtheritic Polyneuropathy			
Prodromal infection	*Pharyngitis*—usual *Wound infection*—rare	*Diphtheritic membrane*	*Culture: Corynebacterium diphtheriae* (toxin producing)
Early *local* findings	*Incubation period* after onset of primary infection 1–2 wk Nasal voice Nasal regurgitation Dysphagia Numb lips 2–3 wk Blurred vision	*"Bulbar" symptoms* (if pharynx is site of infection) Laryngeal, pharyngeal, and palatal paralysis *Ciliary paralysis* Loss of accommodation	*CSF* Cells: 0–5/mm³ Protein: 50–200/mm³ *Blood serology:* absent antitoxin titer in early disease *Culture: C. diphtheriae:* primary infection site remains positive for weeks
Later *systemic* findings	*Acute or subacute progression* 5–8 wk Ascending, symmetric progressive weakness (descending pattern also occurs) Paresthesias in extremities Weakness, dyspnea	*Motor weakness* Extremities and trunk Paralysis variable if site of primary infection not in throat *Proprioceptive loss:* distal Vibration and position sense *Carditis* Resting tachycardia Congestive heart failure	*EMG:* mixed pattern *Nerve conduction:* abnormal *ECG:* abnormal conduction *ECHO:* cardiomyopathy (20%)

Table continued on following page

TABLE 164–1 ■ Polyneuropathy Syndromes of Infectious Etiology or Complicating Antimicrobial Therapy *Continued*

	SYMPTOMS	SIGNS	DIAGNOSIS*
ACUTE DESCENDING MOTOR PARALYSIS WITH PRESERVED SENSORY FUNCTION			
Botulism	*Prodrome* Gastroenteritis: in food-borne source only, 12–36 h before onset of paralysis *Neurologic phase* *Early* Blurred vision, diplopia Dry mouth, painful tongue Nasal voice Hoarseness, dysphagia Dysarthria *Later* Rapid progression (2–4 d) of symmetric weakness, including muscles of respiration No paresthesias or numbness	*Autonomic dysfunction* Dry mouth: no saliva Beefy red, tender tongue Constipation Dilated pupils Ptosis *Early bulbar signs* Extraocular muscles weak Bulbar paralysis *Motor weakness:* progressive Myasthenia-like fatigability Respiratory insufficiency Absent tendon reflexes *Intact sensation*	*CSF:* normal *EMG:* characteristic *Nerve conduction:* normal *Microbiology* Toxin identification in food source, serum, or stool *Clostridium botulinum* culture: in wound or stool *Vital capacity:* reduced in severe cases
Neuromuscular Blockade by Antibiotics			
Concentration dependent Reversible Aminoglycosides Polymyxins	*Myasthenia-like weakness* *Circumoral paresthesias*	*Progressive motor fatigue* On repetitive movement Progressing to paralysis at high blood levels of drug *Intact sensation*	*CSF:* normal *EMG:* characteristic *Nerve conduction:* normal *Blood level of drug:* toxic
SUBACUTE SENSORIMOTOR PARALYSIS			
Neurotoxic Antiinfectives			
Chloramphenicol Isoniazid Dideoxycytidine Dideoxyinosine Nitrofurantoin Metronidazole	*Symmetric,* distal pattern Distal paresthesia: tingling, aching, burning of toes and feet Hyperesthesia Footdrop, weakness of hands and wrist follow sensory symptoms	*Minimal objective loss* in early stages Loss of ankle jerk Distal weakness Appears first in lower then upper extremities	*CSF:* normal *EMG:* normal *Nerve conduction:* abnormal
Vasculitis			
Infections associated with circulating immune complexes HIV-associated vasculitis Polyarteritis nodosa Wegener granulomatosis	*Asymmetric,* mononeuritis multiplex pattern Distribution Two or more nerves, cranial or peripheral Tempo Abrupt onset Sequential attacks Symptoms Pain or numbness Weakness	*Matched motor and sensory deficits* Distribution of specific peripheral nerves	*CSF:* normal *Serology:* immune complexes may be present *EMG:* abnormal in distribution of specific peripheral nerves *Nerve conduction:* abnormal in distribution of specific peripheral nerves *Biopsy* Muscle is normal Vaculitis of vasa vasorum rarely seen
CHRONIC SENSORIMOTOR POLYNEUROPATHY			
Leprosy			
Lepromatous polyneuritis	*Symmetric,* proximal and distal pattern Cutaneous anesthesia: initially in limited areas but eventually symmetric Trophic dyshidrotic changes in skin Relative sparing of motor functions *Unrecognized cutaneous injury* Burns, abrasions, and infections	*Objective anesthesia to pain and temperature in "colder" areas* Pinnae of ears Dorsum of hands Forearms Anterolateral legs and feet *Loss of sweating in affected areas* *Motor loss restricted to muscles innervated by nerves close to skin* (e.g., ulnar nerve) *Tendon reflexes intact* (unique feature of leprosy)	*CSF:* normal *Nerve biopsy:* abnormal *Skin biopsy* or *slit skin technique* High-yield areas: anesthetic sites, macules AFB stain: positive Culture for mycobacteria: negative

TABLE 164–1 ■ Polyneuropathy Syndromes of Infectious Etiology or Complicating Antimicrobial Therapy *Continued*

	SYMPTOMS	SIGNS	DIAGNOSIS*
Indeterminate Leprosy Neuritis	*Asymmetric* pattern Anesthetic hypopigmented macules or papules	*Selective sensory loss* Loss of pain and temperature sensation	
Tuberculoid Leprosy Neuritis	*Asymmetric* pattern Anesthetic lesions as above Weakness of muscles innervated by ulnar, median, peroneal, or facial nerves	*Palpable subcutaneous sensory nerves* (e.g., greater auricular) *Limited sensory and motor loss* Only in distribution of involved nerves	*EMG:* abnormal *Nerve biopsy:* abnormal

*AFB, Acid-fast bacilli; CSF, cerebrospinal fluid; CT, computed tomography; ECG, electrocardiography; ECHO, echocardiography; ELISA, enzyme-linked immunosorbent assay; EMG, electromyography; HIV, human immunodeficiency virus; IgG, immunoglobulin G; IgM, immunoglobulin M; MRI, magnetic resonance imaging; PCR, polymerase chain reaction.

Two other patterns may occur: sensory polyneuropathy, more common in lepromatous leprosy, and neuralgia.[4] Three types of neuralgia are recognized: one type is associated with nerve swelling, especially in nerve reactions; a second type is dull pain in the extremities and trigeminal territory in disease-arrested patients; and the third type is phantom pain neuralgia at the site of artificial limbs, which is not unique to leprosy.[2]

Involvement of the autonomic nervous system supplying the skin results in anhidrosis with impaired sweat response. Eye involvement causes denervation of the iris and reduced intraocular pressure.[6a]

Diagnosis

The peripheral nerves most commonly involved are the facial, ulnar, median, common peroneal, and posterior tibial nerves. Superficial nerves, such as the ulnar and posterior auricular nerves, are readily accessible to palpation and are often enlarged and tender.

Sensory impairment should be evaluated for loss of light touch, pain, and temperature. The ability to distinguish between hot and cold is usually the first modality to be lost. Vibration and position senses can be conserved until a later stage. Damage to motor nerves is manifested by weakness and paralysis (facial palsy, clawhand, ape hand, dropped foot). Retention of deep tendon reflexes is a unique feature and relates to the differential susceptibility of deep and superficial nerves to invasion by *M. leprae*.[1(pp1124–1133)]

Neurophysiologic studies are helpful in preliminary diagnosis, but nerve biopsy is often necessary for precise diagnosis, especially in the absence of skin lesions.[4]

In areas of the world where the disease is rare, such as the United States, skin biopsy should be performed.[4–6] Slit skin smears are usually positive in lepromatous and borderline lepromatous leprosy but are typically negative in tuberculoid and borderline tuberculoid disease. Slit skin smears are performed by making small incisions into the dermis at multiple sites. The fluid is then stained for acid-fast bacilli. The organism cannot be cultured in vitro. Skin testing with lepromin is not useful in diagnosis.

Treatment

Treatment regimens for leprosy are based on the burden of infecting organisms and on host immune status.[5–7, 7a] Because neuropathic mutilation of the hands and feet is a significant cause of disability, a complete motor and sensory examination of the hands and feet should be performed before therapy is begun and appropriate preventive measures taken to prevent injury to anesthetic extremities.

Treatment is discussed in detail in Chapter 168.

Neuritis as a Complication of Treatment

After the initiation of specific chemotherapy, patients must be monitored closely for development of two immunologic disturbances, reversal reaction and erythema nodosum leprosum.[4, 7b] Neuritis is one of the most serious complications of these reactions. If it is unrecognized or untreated, permanent neurologic sequelae may result. Neuritis presents as pain and tenderness in the peripheral nerves commonly affected in tuberculoid leprosy. Reversal reaction neuritis usually occurs within the first year of treatment, but neuritis may be delayed up to several years in erythema nodosum leprosum. Patients at high risk for reversal reaction and neuritis are those with three or more palpable nerves and borderline patients with more than 10 skin lesions. These patients may benefit from corticosteroid prophylaxis during the first 6 months of antileprosy chemotherapy.[7c] Although nerve damage occurs much more slowly in erythema nodosum leprosum, the sequelae are no less severe if left untreated. Erythema nodosum leprosum, unlike reversal reactions, responds to thalidomide, which is considered the drug of choice if it is not contraindicated because of its teratogenicity.[7, 7d]

Severe immunologic reactions, including neuritis, require the immediate administration of prednisone at 40 to 60 mg/d. Steroids should be gradually tapered in the ensuing 2 to 3 months.[7]

Neuropathies Due to Bacterial Toxins

Diphtheria, tetanus, and botulism are neurologic disorders caused by bacterial toxins elaborated by metabolically active bacteria. Diphtheria toxin causes direct damage to Schwann cells, affecting conduction; botulinal and tetanus toxins act on nerve-nerve and neuromuscular junctions to interrupt normal function.

Tetanus and botulinum neurotoxins are produced by *Clostridium* and share certain molecular characteristics despite their disparate clinical features. Both bind to nerve cells, penetrate the cytosol, and release zinc proteases, which cleave key components in the protein complex controlling the docking of synaptic vesicles with the cell membrane, processes critical to exocytosis of neurotransmitters. Both neurotoxins consist of two polypeptide chains: one contains the metalloendopeptidase activity specific to the toxin and its subtype; the other determines the tropism for specific neural cells, such that tetanus neurotoxin acts mainly at CNS synapses, whereas the several botulinum neurotoxin subtypes act peripherally.[7e]

BOTULISM

Cause and Pathogenesis

Clostridium botulinum is a spore-forming, anaerobic gram-positive rod that lives in soil. It produces a potent toxin capable of blocking acetylcholine release at the neuromuscular junction. Eight subtypes of toxin are known: A, B, C1, C2, D, E, F, and G.[7e] Human disease usually results from ingestion of toxin-containing contaminated food and rarely from contamination of a wound.[8] Types A, B, and E are the most frequently implicated in human disease.[9, 10] Toxin production has also been identified in other *Clostridium* species *(Clostridium baratii)* associated with toxicoinfectious botulism.[11, 12] Purified botulinum neurotoxin has been mass produced for aerosol use in biologic warfare and for treatment of dystonias and repetitive muscular spasms through selective injection of toxin.[12a, 12b]

Epidemiology

Infant botulism occurs in infants between 1 and 6 months of age after contamination of the gut by spores of *C. botulinum*. Honey has been implicated as the source of spores in some cases. Gastrointestinal colonization of adults with *C. botulinum* also occurs. In these rare cases, there is an initial gastroenteritis prodrome, after which progression of symptoms follows the usual adult pattern of food-borne botulism.[13]

Food-borne botulism, by far the most common form, is rare because of stringent regulations governing commercial food processing and as a result of public education about food storage and home canning processes. First recognized in 1897 by E. van Ermengem in a group of musicians who ate improperly cured ham at a wake,[13a] food-borne botulism, as in this classic outbreak, in most instances involves several persons who share the same food and then develop disease. Traditional salted foods, such as uneviscerated fish[14] and home-cured ham,[15] continue to be important sources of botulism. Antimicrobial growth inhibitors or acidifying agents are commonly added to commercial processed food products capable of providing an anaerobic environment supportive of germination of ubiquitous *C. botulinum* spores, because contamination may occur before and after products are in use.[15a, 15b]

Wound botulism has the same clinical pattern as food botulism but arises from the proliferation of *C. botulinum* in a contaminated wound.[8] The wound is frequently not inflamed and therefore not overtly suggestive of being infected. Posttraumatic wounds and subcutaneous injection ("skin popping") sites in drug users are the most common sources, but paranasal sinuses have been the site of infection in cocaine snorters.[16, 17]

Clinical Features

Neuromuscular symptoms of botulism vary with the age of the patient; whether the exposure results from ingestion of preformed prototoxin or from active toxin production after colonization of gut or wound; and toxin type.[9] Infants first develop constipation, then hypotonia (floppy baby syndrome) and ophthalmoplegia.[18] In the adult form, most patients present a "descending" symmetric form of paralysis, because the eye and facial muscles are relatively more sensitive than skeletal muscles to any form of neuromuscular blockade. Sensory examination is always normal. Wound botulism has the same clinical pattern as food botulism.

If the source is food, there is a predictable interval from exposure to onset of disease. Sixteen to 60 hours after ingestion, signs of autonomic dysfunction (abdominal cramps, dry mouth, blurred vision, inability to accommodate, abnormal pupillary reflexes, urinary difficulty, diarrhea or constipation) are followed by descending muscle weakness, first in the ocular and bulbar musculature, then in the whole body. In severe disease, paralysis involves the diaphragm and other muscles of respiration[10] (see Table 164–1). Because neurologic effects are dose dependent, members of groups with a common-source exposure will exhibit different degrees of neurologic findings depending on the amount of prototoxin ingested. Toxin type also affects the rate and extent of progression of symptoms.[9] Type E has the shortest incubation period, but type A produces more severe illness and requires intubation more frequently (67%).

Diagnosis

CSF is normal. The edrophonium chloride (Tensilon) test result for myasthenia gravis is negative. Electrophysiologic testing is helpful in distinguishing this disorder from other causes of motor weakness with preserved sensation.[19] Diagnosis can be confirmed by measuring toxin in stool and blood and in the food source, if it is available.[20] Stool cultures may contain the organism in food-borne disease as well as in infant botulism.[13] Any suspicious wounds should be cultured.

Treatment

Public health authorities should always be notified immediately of any suspected case.[17] Specific treatment of adult botulism includes administration of polyvalent antitoxin, released on request by the Centers for Disease Control and Prevention (CDC). Wounds suspected of contamination should be widely débrided and irrigated, but ideally after administration of antitoxin. Penicillin, 10 to 20 million units per day, is considered the antibiotic of choice. Transitory neurologic deterioration may occur despite early administration of antitoxin.[21] Vital capacity should be closely monitored and intubation performed if necessary. Intubation is preferred to tracheostomy because of lower complication rates and relatively short duration of need (mean interval, 8.6 days).[21]

DIPHTHERIA

Cause and Pathogenesis

Neurologic and cardiac complications of diphtheria are due to the elaboration by the microorganism of an extremely potent protein toxin that acts on the elongation factor, a critical protein needed for mammalian protein synthesis.[22] The two major fragments (A and B) of the toxin secreted by *Corynebacterium diphtheriae* are excluded by the blood-brain barrier, which explains the preferential involvement of peripheral and cranial nerves. The organism remains localized, in either the throat (faucial diphtheria) or the wound, releasing its toxin for local and systemic effects. The toxin causes a noninflammatory demyelinization of the cranial and peripheral nerves through its toxic effect on Schwann cells.

Epidemiology

Diphtheria is rarely seen in the United States and occurs primarily in unimmunized children or in adults with waning immunity.[23] However, omission of routine immunization of children with diphtheria toxoid has been associated with diphtheria outbreaks in many developed and developing countries.[23–25] Diphtheria is of increasing concern to developed countries owing to outbreaks in Eastern Europe, where the reported incidence rate of diphtheria increased 2-fold to 10-fold between 1989 and 1994.[25] In the Newly Independent States of the former Soviet Union, the number of cases grew from 839 in 1989 to 47,802 in 1994, and case-fatality rates ranged from 2.8% to 23.0%. Approximately 70% of reported cases were among persons older than 15 years, presumably because of the large number of nonimmune susceptible adults. Highest age-specific incidences occurred among those 4 to 10 years, 15 to 17 years, and 40 to 49 years of age.[25] International governmental and private volunteer agencies provided needed materials (vaccine, syringes, needles, antitoxin, and antibiotics) to assist the Newly Independent States in implementing control measures, which by 1996 began to show evidence of slowing the epidemic.[25a]

Prevention

In 1995, the WHO declared the rapidly expanding diphtheria epidemic an international public health emergency, because serologic studies in the Newly Independent States, Western Europe, and the United States indicated that 20% to 60% of adults older than 20 years were susceptible to diphtheria.[25] The potential for importing diphtheria underscored the importance of maintaining high levels of diphtheria immunity among the total populations of countries currently not experiencing outbreaks of diphtheria. To minimize the risk in the United States, the CDC advised that all U.S. residents be up-to-date for diphtheria vaccination, regardless of whether they plan international travel.[26] All children younger than 7 years should receive a routine series of five doses of diphtheria-pertussis-tetanus vaccine (DPT) or diphtheria and tetanus toxoids for pediatric use (DT) if pertussis vaccine is contraindicated. All unimmunized persons older than 7 years should receive a series of three doses of tetanus and diphtheria toxoids, adult type (Td), and boosters of the vaccine are recommended every 10 years for all newly and previously immunized persons. Further, travelers to areas with outbreaks, or endemic diphtheria, should have either completed a primary immunization series or received a booster dose within the last 10 years and should be advised to report promptly if they develop a sore throat during travel or within 2 weeks afterward. Empirical antibiotic treatment is recommended for close contacts of persons with diphtheria, regardless of immunity status.[25a]

Clinical Features

In the absence of treatment, the frequency of neurologic complications is about 20%.[22] In faucial diphtheria, the most common form, local production of toxin in the pharynx causes early paralysis of the pharyngeal and laryngeal muscles, and the earliest neurologic manifestation is palatal weakness. The patient speaks with a nasal voice and complains of dysphagia and nasal regurgitation. Within days, the trigeminal, facial, vagal, and hypoglossal nerves are affected (bulbar phase). By the third week, ciliary paralysis with loss of accommodation and blurring of vision are evident. On occasion, paralysis of the extraocular muscles occurs.[22]

The onset of sensorimotor polyneuropathy of the trunk and extremities (systemic paralysis) is delayed and usually appears 2 to 3 months after the primary infection (see Table 164–1). The polyneuropathy may occur simultaneously in all extremities, or it may descend. Sensory findings include paresthesias; loss of superficial touch, joint, and position senses; and impaired or lost tendon reflexes. Severity of motor weakness varies from a mild deficit with maximal distal involvement to a rapidly ascending paralysis. Respiratory paralysis occasionally develops.[1, 27] In diphtheritic myocarditis, electrocardiographic changes precede abnormal contractile activity detectable by echocardiography by 3 weeks.[27a]

Diagnosis

The diagnosis is established by recovering the organism from the source: from throat culture in pharyngitis or from the wound in the case of cutaneous diphtheria. Isolation of *C. diphtheriae* from blood cultures indicates possible endocarditis.[27b, 27c] Assays for circulating antitoxin antibody support the diagnosis when the level is nonprotective (less than 0.01 IU/mL).[27] Analysis of the CSF is normal except for an elevated protein level.

Treatment

Early recognition and treatment of local infection with antibiotics and antitoxin may avoid neurologic and cardiac complications. Antitoxin therapy is not effective once polyneuropathy begins in late disease, but booster vaccination with age-appropriate diphtheria toxoid–containing vaccine is recommended during convalescence.[23] Although antitoxin is of no value in late disease, antibiotics are still indicated to prevent further elaboration of toxin and to prevent transmission of the infection. Immunity against the toxin protects only against disease; it does not protect against local infection and secondary transmission to nonimmune persons.

TETANUS

Cause

Tetanus is caused solely by the toxic action on the nervous system of tetanospasmin produced by the anaerobic spore-forming rod *Clostridium tetani*, which is widely distributed in nature.[28] *C. tetani* is usually introduced into an area of injury as an anaerobic spore. Disease develops only if anaerobic conditions obtain, which permits growth of the toxin-producing vegetative form.

Pathogenesis

The incubation period in humans is usually 3 to 21 days but may be as short as 1 day or as long as several months.[28] Toxin reaches the CNS by retrograde, intraaxonal transport. It is taken up distally by motor, sensory, and autonomic nerve terminals and is carried to the spinal cord and brain stem before transsynaptic transfer to presynaptic terminals in the neuropil of the ventral horn. The mode of toxin transport to the CNS explains the variable onset of symptoms: the shorter the axon, the earlier the involvement.[29] A significant amount of toxin remains bound to nerve terminals at the neuromuscular junction in the infected site, which interferes with acetylcholine release by means indistinguishable from botulinal toxin. Tetanus toxin is the next most potent toxin after botulinal toxin.

The tetanic syndrome is believed to originate from the toxin's disinhibitory action.[28] Its effects on the spinal cord are similar to those of strychnine and lead to dysfunction of polysynaptic reflexes that involve inhibition of antagonists. Tetanic muscle spasms arise from the accumulation of toxin in presynaptic terminals of the spinal inhibitory interneurons, blocking release of inhibitory neurotransmitters. Disturbance of the sympathetic nervous system may occur, including labile hypertension, cardiac tachyarrhythmias, peripheral vasoconstriction and profuse sweating. Neuronal cell death may occur from unopposed excitation.[30] The toxin also has direct effects on the neuromuscular junction.

The brain is minimally affected, except in cephalic tetanus, in which instead of spasm, there is initially paralysis of muscles closest to the site of injury but spasm affecting adjacent muscles. Paralysis, which gives way to spasm during the recovery phase, is considered to be due to higher concentrations of toxin in the brain stem, which cause paralysis instead of abolishing inhibition. Correspondingly, the paralytic phase is associated with electrophysiologic findings of lower motor neuron injury, such as denervation potentials, hyperirritability, loss of motor units, and marginally increased latencies.

Epidemiology

Worldwide, about 500,000 deaths annually are attributable to tetanus; most are of neonates born to unimmunized mothers.[31, 31a, 31b] Neonatal tetanus results when a neonate without passively transferred maternal anti–tetanus toxin antibody sustains a *C. tetani* infection in the umbilical cord stump, most commonly as a result of unclean childbirth conditions or of unsanitary cord care practices, such as application of dung or grease to the wound.[31a] Of all vaccine-preventable diseases, neonatal tetanus is second only to measles as a cause of childhood mortality worldwide.[31b] Although deep, penetrating necrotizing wounds are especially supportive of growth of *C. tetani*, a minor wound is the most common portal of entry in cases of childhood and adult tetanus. Tetanus, like botulism, also occurs in nonimmune drug users who contaminate an injection site.

In the United States during the years 1965 to 1974, tetanus cases averaged 176 per year and occurred mainly among unimmunized and partially immunized populations in the Gulf South.[32] Since 1975, reported cases of tetanus have been less than 100 per year and falling.[33] However, in 1995, it was estimated that more than 10% of the U.S. population was not properly immunized and that any significant reduction in preventive medical services would be likely to return nationwide tetanus rates to the levels seen in the 1950s of approximately 500 cases per year.[33, 34]

Despite the availability of effective and inexpensive tetanus toxoid vaccines, cases of tetanus continue to occur in the United States and are fatal in nearly 25%.[34a] Risk for tetanus increases with age, corresponding to a low prevalence of protective antibody titers among elderly populations.[34b, 34c] Other potentially vulnerable groups include recipients of autologous and heterologous bone marrow transplants.[34d, 34e]

During 1991 to 1994, 54% of 188 patients were age 60 years and older and 5% were 20 years old and younger, and the risk for tetanus among persons 80 years old and older was more than 10 times greater than for persons aged 20 to 29 years.[34a] Tetanus followed an acute injury in 77% of cases, and less than half received tetanus toxoid as part of their wound prophylaxis.

Prevention

Primary prevention of tetanus is accomplished by active immunization with vaccines. Combined vaccines containing tetanus toxoid, diphtheria, and pertussis (DPT) are used in children 7 years and older; the Td vaccine is given to persons 7 years and older and is recommended for tetanus boosters to maintain protective immunity to both diphtheria and tetanus.[34f] Primary immunization of those 7 years and older consists of two doses of Td 1 to 2 months apart, followed by a third dose after 6 to 12 months. Booster doses should be administered every 10 years.[34f]

Secondary prevention refers to postwound tetanus prophylaxis and varies with vaccine history and type of wound. Persons with unclean or major wounds and who have unknown or uncertain vaccination histories should be considered unvaccinated and be given passive immune protection with human tetanus immune globulin (HTIG, 250 to 500 IU, given intramuscularly). Simultaneous primary active immunization should be initiated by injection of Td at a separate intramuscular site and arrangements made for completion of the primary series. Passive immunity in addition to tetanus booster should also be provided to persons vaccinated more than 5 years previously if the type of wound sustained is considered tetanus prone, such as wounds contaminated with dirt, saliva, or feces; puncture wounds, including unsterile injections; missile injuries; burns; frostbite; avulsions; and crush injuries.[34g]

Clinical Features

There are three alternative presentations: (1) local tetanus with muscle contraction at the site of injury, which may persist or progress to the generalized form; (2) cephalic tetanus affecting cranial nerves, mostly the seventh pair; and (3) generalized tetanus with lockjaw, reflex spasms easily provoked by external stimuli, opisthotonos, and risus sardonicus.[1(pp1124–1133)]

In localized tetanus, a mild form of the disease, unyielding rigidity of muscle groups close to the injury site may persist for weeks or months, finally disappearing without residua.[28] Localized disease may occur in a partially immune individual or when a nonimmune individual sustaining a wound at high risk for growth of *C. tetani* receives hyperimmune serum at protective rather than therapeutic dosage. Localized tetanus sometimes precedes the generalized form.

In generalized tetanus, the most common form of the disease, trismus is the presenting complaint in more than 50% of cases. Associated or alternative initial complaints are restlessness, irritability, neck stiffness, abdominal rigidity, dysphagia, or preexisting localized tetanus. Tonic contractions of muscles of jaw, face, neck, abdomen, and back are common, and abdominal and lumbar muscles may become rigid. Opisthotonos results from viselike persistent constriction of chest and back muscles. The typical tetanic seizure is characterized by a sudden burst of tonic contraction of muscle groups causing opisthotonos, flexion and adduction of the arms, clenching of the fists on the thorax, and extension of the lower extremities. The patient is completely conscious during such episodes and experiences intense pain. Glottal or laryngeal spasm and urinary retention may occur. If intensive care is not available, death occurs from spasm in respiratory muscles. Autonomic involvement results in generalized sympathetic overactivity with hypertension, tachycardia, and arrhythmias.[28, 35] Convulsions are uncommon.

Case-fatality rates in generalized tetanus can be more than 50% when sophisticated intensive care is not available.[31] The most important prognostic factor for generalized tetanus is not the incubation period, but the rate of progression from onset of symptoms to full development of disease, called the invasion period or period of onset.[32] The shorter this interval, the higher the mortality.

Cephalic tetanus, an unusual form of the disease characterized by local muscle paralysis after injuries of the head or otitis media, commonly has an incubation period of only 1 or 2 days. Muscle paralysis is maximal close to the site of injury, whereas spasm is evident at more distal sites. As paralysis recedes with time, it is succeeded by spasm before the muscle returns to normal. Lockjaw is the usual presenting symptom, associated with hemifacial spasm, weakness, paresis, or paralysis. Whereas cranial nerve VII is the one most commonly affected, depending on the site of the infected wound, nerves IX, X, and XII may be affected singly or in combination. Extraocular movements are generally unaffected.[36] Cephalic tetanus generally has a good prognosis if treatment is begun early.

Diagnosis

Diagnosis is confirmed by the characteristic neurophysiologic findings and the absence of serum antitetanus antibody. The CSF is normal. Gram stain and anaerobic cultures of the wound may or may not reveal the organism.[32]

Treatment

Treatment has four components: (1) appropriate care of the local wound with débridement and systemic antibiotics; (2) systemic administration of human antitoxin; (3) control of spasms, with associated intensive care support until the effects of bound toxin are no longer detectable, using sedation with benzodiazepines and adding neuromuscular blockade to the level of paralysis when necessary; and (4) α- and β-adrenergic blockade to prevent secondary autonomic hyperactivity.[34g] Prevention of future risk requires a primary vaccination series for active immunization.

When infected wounds are the source of intoxication, débridement of necrotic tissue removes the site of continued toxin production, and antibiotics directed against mixed organisms characteristic of synergistic infections prevent progression of infection at the excision margins.

Although retrograde axonal transport is the primary means by which tetanus neurotoxin reaches its CNS targets, antitoxin is given systemically to bind any toxin absorbed into the circulation from the primary site. Human antitoxin is given intramuscularly at 500 to 3000 IU, depending on the severity of the primary wound. Commercial preparations of hyperimmune antitetanus immune globulin should not be given intravenously. Intravenous preparations of normal immune globulins do contain antitetanus antibody and may be substituted when necessary, although commercial lots do not contain specified titers.[34g]

The theoretical possibility that some circulating toxin may reach the CSF before binding to the CNS led at one time to the regular administration of antitoxin intrathecally as well as systemically. However, intrathecal injection of tetanus antitoxin has been shown to be of no benefit in established severe tetanus (hourly generalized spasms, plus trismus, dysphagia, and generalized rigidity), whereas passive immunization systemically with human antitoxin ($\geq$500 IU HTIG) may shorten its course.[36a] Higher doses of systemic antitoxin do not appear to provide any further benefit.[34g]

Mild tetanus at entry (trismus, dysphagia, and localized rigidity without spasms) is more responsive to systemic antitoxin therapy. Intrathecal antitoxin is not recommended in mild tetanus, although in one alternating case trial among 97 adolescents and adults well matched for age, mode of infection, and incubation period, parenteral antitoxin was significantly less effective than intrathecal antitoxin in preventing progression to moderate (generalized rigidity, occasional spasms) or severe tetanus or death.[36a] Of those given intrathecal HTIG (250 IU) alone, only 2% died and 6% progressed, compared with 21% deaths and 31% progression among those receiving intramuscular HTIG antitoxin (1000 IU) alone.

Human Immunodeficiency Virus Type 1–Associated Neuropathies

Neuropathy is one of the most common disorders associated with human immunodeficiency virus (HIV) disease.[37–39] On occasion, neuropathy occurs before overt immunosuppression and represents the initial manifestation of HIV infection itself, such as Bell palsy[40] or Guillain-Barré syndrome.[41] Late-onset neuropathy, which is probably nearly universal at the time of death,[42] is frequently overshadowed by the more striking CNS complications of HIV infection, such as vacuolar myelopathy and acquired immunodeficiency syndrome (AIDS) dementia complex, or by opportunistic infections such as toxoplasmic encephalitis or cytomegalovirus (CMV) infection of the nervous system.

The HIV-associated neuropathies consist of several distinctive clinical patterns, each of which may be caused by any one of several infectious agents (Table 164–2), some of them eminently treatable. Some of these agents also produce overlap syndromes, because they may also attack brain, cord, and ganglia. In evaluating individual HIV-infected patients, it is well to remember also that two or more simultaneous infections may be the cause of the particular clinical syndrome presented by the patient.[37]

PREDOMINANTLY SENSORY NEUROPATHY

Cause and Pathogenesis

Predominantly sensory neuropathy is one of the most common and most debilitating aspects of advanced HIV infection.[42, 43] Its exact etiology is unclear, although immune complex vasculitis has been suggested by pathologic studies.[39, 42, 44] Late in HIV infection, neuropathic findings are more common, but multiple factors, including vitamin deficiency and drug toxicity, may contribute to the process.

Clinical Findings

Patients usually complain of painful paresthesias and burning of the distal extremities, primarily of the soles of the feet.[42] On examination, only patients with advanced HIV neuropathy will have demonstrable generalized decrease in sensation in the affected areas or atrophy of the intrinsic muscles of the feet. Deep tendon reflexes of the ankles are eventually lost, but patellar reflexes may be exaggerated because of coexisting myelopathy.

Diagnosis

When ankle reflexes are affected, nerve conduction studies are consistent with distal axonal degeneration of any cause.[42]

TABLE 164–2 ■ Etiology of Neuropathic Syndromes in Human Immunodeficiency Virus Infection

Immune-mediated response to human immunodeficiency virus
Bell palsy
Acute inflammatory demyelinating neuropathy (Guillain-Barré syndrome)
Chronic inflammatory demyelinating neuropathy
Vasculitis
Bell palsy
Ataxic dorsal radiculopathy
Mononeuritis multiplex: hepatitis B virus–associated cryoglobulinemia
Opportunistic invasive herpesvirus infections
Cytomegalovirus
Polyradiculopathy
Multiple mononeuropathy
Herpes simplex virus
Polyradiculopathy
Varicella-zoster virus
Herpes zoster
Polyradiculopathy
Meningitis
Cryptococcal
Neurosyphilitic
Tuberculous
Malignant neoplasm
Lymphoma
Nutritional
Multiple vitamin deficiencies: folate, pyridoxine
Vitamin B_{12} deficiency
Drug toxicity from concurrent antiinfectives
Antiretroviral nucleoside analogs
Dideoxycytidine
Dideoxyinosine
Stavudine
Niacin analogs: isoniazid
Idiopathic
Predominantly sensory neuropathy of acquired immunodeficiency syndrome

Therefore, reversible causes of neuropathy should be excluded before the diagnosis of HIV neuropathy is made.

Treatment

Treatment of HIV predominantly sensory neuropathy is generally unsatisfactory.[39, 42, 43] The nonneurotoxic antiretrovirals, such as zidovudine and lamivudine, are of no therapeutic benefit, nor are they preventive.[42, 43] Because subclinical disease is probably universal in advanced HIV infection,[42] long-term therapy with those antiretroviral agents that have dose-dependent neurotoxicity, such as didanosine, zalcitabine, and stavudine, should include regular monitoring for development of clinical neuropathy.[42, 43] Symptomatic medical therapy with antidepressants and carbamazepine may be employed, but significant improvement is unusual. Placebo-controlled trials comparing palliative effects of amitriptyline with mexiletine are currently under way, as are therapeutic protocols using human nerve growth factor.

ISOLATED CRANIAL NEUROPATHIES

Causes

Cranial neuropathies, particularly involving the facial nerve, may also occur at any stage of HIV infection.[43] Bell palsy usually occurs early in HIV infection and is often associated with a lymphocytic meningitis.[43] In advanced HIV infection, the differential diagnosis of cranial neuropathies includes CNS opportunistic infections such as neurosyphilis, cryptococcosis, acute herpes zoster, and meningeal lymphomatosis[43] as well as disorders seen in normal hosts, such as neuroborreliosis.

POLYRADICULOPATHY

Causes and Pathogenesis

Polyradiculopathy, the most dramatic of syndromes caused by herpesvirus invasion in advanced HIV disease, is caused by CMV more often than by other herpesviruses.[45, 46] Essentially unknown before AIDS, CMV invasion of the CNS and PNS in advanced HIV disease is the consequence of systemic infection and is often associated with evidence of active infection in other systems, particularly retinitis.[47] The capacity of CMV to invade both endothelial and Schwann cells accounts for its varied clinical manifestations,[42] which range from mononeuritis multiplex to acute inflammatory polyradiculitis and ascending myelitis.

Clinical Findings

Like the Guillain-Barré syndrome, polyradiculitis is characterized by a subacute onset of ascending motor weakness, areflexia, incontinence or urinary retention, paresthesias, and variable sensory dysfunction.[47] Patients often complain of pain in the back and legs.[42] Neurologic findings are usually more asymmetric than in Guillain-Barré syndrome.

Diagnosis

The CSF mirrors the intense neutrophilic inflammation of the lumbar nerve roots and dorsal root ganglia and later the spinal cord and yields characteristic CSF findings mimicking bacterial meningitis: polymorphonuclear predominance (up to 90%), hypoglycorrhachia, and elevated protein levels.[42, 47] CSF white cell counts can vary from less than $50/mm^3$ to greater than $3000/mm^3$.

Magnetic resonance imaging (MRI) contrast enhancement of the lumbosacral plexus and cauda equina has been noted in multiple cases of polyradiculopathy due to CMV and other herpesviruses as well as to a wide range of other causes of polyneuritis, and it has shown improvement after specific therapy.[48, 49]

CMV inclusions have been seen in cytologic examination of CSF and in biopsy specimens.[42] Specific herpesviruses have been successfully identified in CSF by polymerase chain reaction (PCR), but viral cultures are generally negative.[50]

Treatment

If diagnosed and treated early, some cases of CMV polyradiculopathy have responded partially to early treatment with ganciclovir at dosages of 5 mg/kg intravenously twice daily for 2 weeks, followed by a maintenance dose of 5 mg/kg daily.[47] If ganciclovir resistance is suspected because of prior use of ganciclovir or persistent CSF abnormalities with ganciclovir therapy, foscarnet is the only alternative at present.[46, 48] Pharmacokinetic studies have demonstrated that CSF concentrations, relative to plasma, vary between 24% and 70% for ganciclovir and 13% and 68% for foscarnet.[51] Common dose-dependent side effects of ganciclovir are leukopenia and thrombocytopenia, which require frequent monitoring. Leukopenia can be treated with granulocyte colony-stimulating factor (filgrastim) at doses appropriate to maintain the absolute granulocyte count at 1000 cells/mm^3 or greater. With use of standard dosing for CMV retinitis, foscarnet's primary toxic effect is renal failure.

Differential Diagnosis

Other causes of subacute polyradiculopathy in HIV infection include *Treponema pallidum* and two other herpesviruses, herpes simplex virus type 2 (HSV-2) and varicella-zoster virus (VZV).[42] HSV and VZV cause an acute inflammatory radiculomyelitis in AIDS patients that may be confused with CMV polyradiculopathy, whereas neurosyphilis has a lymphocytic profile. These agents are discussed in more detail elsewhere in this chapter (see sections on Guillain-Barré syndrome, primary ascending myelitis, and polymorphic infections).

MONONEURITIS MULTIPLEX

Causes

Mononeuritis multiplex is characterized by patchy and asymmetric motor and sensory nerve dysfunction, possibly the result of ischemic injury from viral infection of the endothelium of the vasa nervorum.[42] Mononeuritis multiplex may be seen early in HIV infection even before immunosuppression has occurred. Some cases are associated with cryoglobulinemia in persons dually infected with hepatitis B virus, in which the course is often benign and generally does not require specific therapy.[43, 52] In patients with advanced HIV infection and CD4$^+$ cell counts less than 50/mm^3, CMV is the most likely cause.

Clinical Findings

Mononeuritis multiplex is defined as a simultaneous or sequential neuropathy of noncontiguous nerve trunks evolving during days to years.[1(pp1124–1133)]

Diagnosis

Definitive diagnosis requires biopsy, although the characteristic histologic lesions may be missed because of their patchy distribution.[42, 43] CSF abnormalities, if present, probably reflect a coexisting pathologic process.[43] Nerve conduction studies show asymmetric axonal loss rather than demyelination, although considerable overlap does occur.[42, 45, 47, 53]

Treatment

Treatment depends on identifying a specific cause. In 47 patients with advanced HIV disease in which mononeuritis multiplex was suspected of being caused by CMV, intravenous ganciclovir was used successfully, but the prognosis, in general, is poor.[42]

Inflammatory Demyelinating Polyneuropathies: Polyneuritis

Two syndromes of inflammatory polyneuritis are recognized on the basis of differences in tempo and persistence of paralysis: acute inflammatory demyelinating polyneuropathy, or Guillain-Barré syndrome, and chronic inflammatory demyelinating polyneuropathy (CIDP). Both syndromes are characterized by an ascending or descending generalized sensorimotor demyelinating polyneuropathy, with elevated protein level and variable lymphocytosis in the CSF[54] (see Table 164–1). Most cases are classified as idiopathic and are treated empirically, primarily with plasmapheresis. However, there are well-known associations with certain infectious agents that also require specific therapy.

ACUTE INFLAMMATORY DEMYELINATING POLYNEUROPATHY (GUILLAIN-BARRÉ SYNDROME)

Causes and Epidemiology

Guillain-Barré syndrome is the most frequent cause of acute paralytic illness in young adults.[55] In the United States, the frequency is 9.5 cases per million. It occurs worldwide with a slightly greater prevalence in males and has no seasonal preference.[56] Frequency peaks between ages 16 and 25 years with a second smaller peak at ages 45 to 60 years.

Guillain-Barré syndrome has a well-known association with a variety of infectious agents, such as the herpesviruses Epstein-Barr virus and CMV, and with HIV, hepatitis C virus,[57] *Mycoplasma pneumoniae, Chlamydia psittaci* (psittacosis), *Borrelia burgdorferi* (Lyme disease), and particularly *Campylobacter jejuni*.[58–60]

It is unclear whether the occurrence of Guillain-Barré syndrome during HIV infection represents a causal or merely a chance relationship.[39] Guillain-Barré syndrome in HIV disease typically develops before the onset of advanced immunosuppression.[39] The course of the illness is similar to that found in HIV-negative patients, except for the finding of up to 50 white cells per mm^3 in the CSF and a higher frequency of coexisting CNS dysfunction.[42] However, the illness responds to standard therapy, and prognosis is generally favorable.[43]

More frequently, the acute polyneuritis is idiopathic, although in many instances it appears after a precipitating factor. The precipitating factors, or antecedent events, of this acute idiopathic inflammatory demyelinating polyneuropathy are numerous—infections with agents other than those noted before, vaccinations, malignant neoplasm, surgery, and other stressful events. Patients having an antecedent event frequently mention a virus-like illness: respiratory (58%), gastrointestinal (22%), or both (10%).[61] *C. jejuni* has been noted in several persons with a gastrointestinal prodrome.[60] According to the U.S. national Guillain-Barré syndrome surveillance, the "event," always diagnosed in retrospect, usually occurs within 1 to 2 months preceding the syndrome and is present in approximately 80% of patients.[61]

Pathogenesis

Two types of lesions have been observed. By far the most common is infiltration by lymphocytic and monocytic inflammatory cells within roots and nerves of the PNS, followed by widespread segmental demyelination, with sparing of axons and of the CNS.[62] Remyelination then slowly takes place by Schwann cell proliferation. Nerve biopsies show subperineural edema, macrophage infiltration, and complete demyelination of axon with intratubal macrophages, which is characteristic of primary demyelination rather than axonal degeneration.[63] The intensity of the inflammatory infiltrate varies according to duration of disease, with more leukocytes and T cells in the endoneurium in the first month than later.[64] The second type of lesion, dominated by macrophages and early marked inflammation and suggestive of antibody-mediated immune destruction, may be the hallmark of the uncommon form of Guillain-Barré syndrome that has both demyelination and severe axonal degeneration and results in severe residual disability.[65] Both types of lesions are seen in the experimental allergic neuritis animal model. A third mechanism is suggested by occasional patients who have extensive axonal degeneration, indicating either "innocent bystander" injury by inflammation or a direct attack on axons. A search for viral genomes in the myelin sheaths of affected nerves and in infiltrating cells in biopsy specimens from typical Guillain-Barré syndrome cases has failed to reveal CMV or any other suspects.[66]

Clinical Features

Guillain-Barré syndrome is a rapidly progressive and slowly reversible motor neuropathy and usually follows an ascending pattern, although descending patterns occur (see Table 164–1). The common ascending pattern starts with progressive and often symmetric weakness in the distal lower limbs, ascends over the entire body within days or may progress for up to a month, and often results in respiratory failure. Facial weakness is often present. Tendon reflexes are usually absent. Approximately 90% of untreated patients reach maximal impairment within 4 weeks; the remainder fluctuate for up to 8 weeks. The progressive paralytic phase is followed by a plateau phase and then a variable period of recovery.

Sensory symptoms are mild and do not usually progress, although transient paresthesias and pain in the back and legs are common complaints. Objective sensory loss is variable and, when present, tends to affect deep sensibility more than superficial. Autonomic involvement (e.g., hypotension or hypertension, cardiac arrhythmias, abnormalities of sweating, gastric atony) is not uncommon. Constitutional symptoms are usually absent.

It is stated that two thirds of the patients recover within a year and that the other third usually have mild residual disability.[67] The relapse rate is approximately 3%. Overall mortality even with excellent supportive care is approximately 5%.[58, 59]

There are three distinctive variant forms of acute idiopathic inflammatory demyelinating polyneuropathy: the Miller-Fisher syndrome (acute ophthalmoplegia, ataxia, and generalized areflexia)[68]; cranial polyneuritis (polyneuritis cranialis), in which only cranial nerves are involved; and CIDP, in which patients continue to deteriorate after 4 weeks (see later). In a retrospective analysis of 266 cases of inflammatory polyneuropathy covering 33 years, 84% had typical Guillain-Barré syndrome, 13% CIDP, 1.5% cranial polyneuritis, and 0.8% each of Miller-Fisher syndrome and predominantly sensory neuropathy.[69] Some of these cases undoubtedly represented undiagnosed neuroborreliosis, which is a relatively recently recognized infectious cause of a Guillain-Barré syndrome–like polyneuritis pattern.

Diagnosis

The laboratory hallmark of Guillain-Barré syndrome is called in French *dissociation albumino-cytologique*: a rise in CSF protein level (which can be normal during the first days of illness) with minimal concomitant rise of CSF white cells, although lymphocytosis is not uncommon in the earliest phase of disease.[59] CSF protein values peak at 3 to 4 weeks. The protein consists of elevated concentrations of albumin and immunoglobulins G, A, and M without unique κ/λ ratios, suggesting that the elevated immunoglobulin concentrations may not be due to intrathecal synthesis.[70] The absence of significant lymphocytosis in the CSF is a major distinction between idiopathic Guillain-Barré syndrome and the infectious causes of polyneuritis (see Table 164–1). Serum immunoglobulin concentrations are elevated and increasing numbers of immunoblasts circulate in the blood in the acute phase; reductions in immunoblasts seem to correlate with recovery. Antimyelin antibodies are present in the serum of many acute cases, which might explain some of the good results obtained with plasmapheresis. Findings include circulating immune complexes.[71]

MRI has found increasing application in diagnosis of acute and chronic inflammatory demyelinating polyneuropathies. T1-weighted spinal MRI shows characteristic enhancement of the pial lining of involved nerve roots, cauda equina, and conus medullaris. Enhancement is able to demonstrate greater involvement than is apparent from symptoms or electrodiagnostic studies,[72, 73] correlates well with stage and presentation of disease,[74] and changes with its progression and remission.[75] In the Miller-Fisher variant, nerve enhancement is confined to the cranial nerves but may also involve the spinocerebellar tracts in the lower medulla and demonstrate other findings compatible with brain stem encephalitis.[76, 77] Enhancement of nerve roots and cord structures is not unique to idiopathic Guillain-Barré syndrome, however, and has been documented in AIDS-related polyradiculopathy associated with CMV, as described before,[49] and with neuroborreliosis (see later).

Differential Diagnosis

Idiopathic Guillain-Barré syndrome must be distinguished from the known causes of acute polyneuritis, from other neurologic illnesses (such as myasthenia gravis), and from uncommon infectious diseases that mimic polyneuropathy: botulism, diphtheria, poliomyelitis, and the polyradiculitis and myelitis of advanced HIV infection due to herpesviruses and neurosyphilis. In botulism, the pupillary reflexes are lost early in the illness and are accompanied progressively by other significant autonomic dysfunctions (e.g., bradycardia, dry mouth, abdominal cramps, urinary difficulty).[1(pp1124–1133)] Poliomyelitis presents with meningeal symptoms, fever, and an asymmetric paralysis. Diphtheria should be considered when bulbar paralysis precedes descending paralysis.

Concomitant HIV infection extends the range of possible causes. Herpesvirus radiculitis and myelitis are typically subacute, ascending, and asymmetric; occur only in advanced immunosuppression ($CD4^+$ cell count less than $50/mm^3$); and have CSF changes of acute inflammation mimicking bacterial infection. Neurosyphilis in HIV infection has a neurologic pattern similar to the subacute onset of herpesvirus infection,[47] but the CSF contains lymphocytes instead of neutrophils, and blood and CSF usually test positive for reaginic antibodies (automated reagin test, Venereal Disease Research Laboratory [VDRL] test). When the CSF VDRL test response is negative, but *Treponema*-specific blood serology points to prior syphilis, the patient should be treated empirically for neurosyphilis, because HIV infection regardless of $CD4^+$ cell count may contribute to an unacceptably high number of treatment failures of primary and secondary syphilis with conventional therapy.[78]

Other disorders to consider in patients initially presenting only with symptoms of weakness are hypokalemia; tick paralysis; porphyria and toxic neuropathies, including antibiotic toxicity; and food source toxins from shellfish, puffer fish, and tropical fish. In tick paralysis, symptoms begin 2 to 4 days after the bite, and recovery begins within 24 hours of tick removal.[79] Chronic or chronic relapsing inflammatory neuropathy may initially be indistinguishable from Guillain-Barré syndrome but declares itself in its relenting or relapsing fashion.[80]

Treatment

Therapy for idiopathic Guillain-Barré syndrome consists of respiratory monitoring, with support as necessary, and early plasmapheresis.[58, 59] About 80% of patients have a complete recovery, but the fatality rate remains 5% even when specialized care is available.[55] Because the patient's condition can deteriorate rapidly, management normally requires immediate hospitalization and surveillance of respiratory function (vital capacity, arterial blood gases, cough reflex, swallowing). Intubation, fluid management, parenteral feeding, prevention of deep venous thrombosis, and physical therapy are usually required. Nosocomial pneumonia, urinary tract infection, and pulmonary emboli are significant complications of the illness.

Plasmapheresis has shown significant benefit in 70% of patients in a controlled, collaborative trial, provided that it was applied early in the course. Several studies suggest that intravenous immune globulin (IVIG) at 0.4 g/kg per day for 5 days is as effective as plasmapheresis[81–83]; however, plasmapheresis remains the current recommended treatment of choice.[53, 58, 59, 84, 85] A multicenter randomized trial determined that plasma exchange alone, IVIG alone, and plasma exchange followed by IVIG were equally effective treatments.[55, 85a]

According to several well-controlled trials, glucocorticosteroids alone are not beneficial in Guillain-Barré syndrome[22, 86]; their role in combination therapy with IVIG is under investigation.[55]

CHRONIC INFLAMMATORY DEMYELINATING POLYNEUROPATHY

Causes and Epidemiology

CIDP occurs spontaneously and is also seen in patients infected with HIV.[42] CIDP occurs in the early stages of HIV infection, although with the development of immunosuppression, the disease tends to improve.

Clinical Features

Like Guillain-Barré syndrome, CIDP presents primarily as weakness with varying degrees of sensory loss. Physical examination reveals proximal muscle weakness of both the upper and lower extremities. Weakness of the neck flexors is particularly suggestive.[87]

Diagnosis

As in Guillain-Barré syndrome, CSF analysis is remarkable for an elevated protein level and the absence of cells; the presence of cells should raise the suspicion of concurrent HIV infection. CD4 levels in CSF may be a sensitive indicator.[88] MRI enhancement of lumbosacral roots, similar to findings in Guillain-Barré syndrome, is characteristically present.[89] Electrodiagnostic studies may show relapsing cycles of demyelination and remyelination. Complete diagnostic criteria are discussed in the review by Mendell.[87]

Treatment

Plasmapheresis, IVIG, and steroids have been used therapeutically,[42] but plasmapheresis is the current treatment of choice.[42, 83] Some investigators cite a potential risk for renal failure if IVIG is administered to AIDS patients, particularly if underlying renal disease is present, because AIDS patients often already have high levels of serum immunoglobulins.[42] Steroids are best avoided, if possible, in these patients.

Postinfectious Peripheral Neuropathy

The term postinfectious indicates that neurologic findings usually follow the appearance of the characteristic nonneurologic clinical features of the disease and may also occur in only a small proportion of infected patients. Further, although the pathogenesis of these lesions usually involves inflammation in the nervous system, the causative agent is not always identifiable in the lesions. Guillain-Barré syndrome is the principal postinfectious peripheral neuropathy syndrome recognized and is discussed earlier.

Parameningeal Infections: Cranial Nerve Syndromes

(Table 164–3)

Bacterial and fungal infections of the skull produce characteristic groupings of cranial nerve involvement, usually unilateral because of their origin in air sinuses or middle ear. The cause of nerve dysfunction is a combination of inflammatory damage to vasa vasorum and nerve and also invasion by organisms. Bacterial and fungal infections are the most common causes and frequently occur in persons with diabetes or immunosuppression as part of the syndrome of rhinocerebral infections.

Causes and Pathogenesis

Bacterial and fungal infections of the ethmoid-sphenoid complex of air sinuses that extend into the adjacent cavernous venous sinuses cause two characteristic unilateral cranial nerve syndromes, depending on the extent of invasion: the Tolosa-Hunt and the Foix-Jefferson.

Bacterial infections of the middle ear or postoperative infections of the temporal (petrous) bone also have two patterns of cranial nerve involvement. Gradenigo syndrome (cranial nerves V and VI) results when the apex of the temporal bone is the site of inflammation. A peripheral seventh nerve palsy results when inflammation in the attic of the middle ear invades cranial nerve VII as it passes through the thin bony roof of the middle ear—the tegmen tympani.

Infections involving the base of the skull produce two unique patterns of cranial nerve palsies. When malignant otitis externa or mastoiditis extends subperiosteally (Bezold abscess) and into the soft tissues beneath the temporal bone, extension to the jugular foramen affects cranial nerves IX, X, and XI (Vernet syndrome). If the location of the infection is in the retropharyngeal tissues (retropharyngeal abscess or retroparotid lymphadenitis), cranial nerve XII and the cervical sympathetic nerve outflow as well as cranial nerves IX, X, and XI are affected (Villaret syndrome).

Table 164–4 presents the more common unilateral cranial nerve syndromes that may be caused by localized infections.

Diagnosis and Treatment

Diagnosis and treatment are discussed in Chapter 157.

SPINAL CORD INFECTIONS: PRIMARY AND SECONDARY MYELITIS

Infections involving the spinal cord may be subdivided into those that directly attack cord structures (primary myelitis) and those that begin as adjacent infections but progress to alter cord function and may ultimately produce irreversible damage (secondary myelitis).[1(pp1124–1133)]

TABLE 164–3 ■ Cranial Nerve Syndromes

NERVE	FUNCTIONS	DISTRIBUTION	NEURONAL LOCATION	PERIPHERAL NERVES OR DIVISIONS	SIGNS OF PERIPHERAL NERVE DYSFUNCTION	COMMON INFECTIOUS CAUSES OF FINDINGS
III Oculomotor	Somatic motor	Superior, inferior, and medial rectus muscles Inferior oblique muscle Levator of lid	Brain stem	Oculomotor	*Abducted eye at rest* *Inability to rotate eye up, down, or medially* *Ptosis*	*Herpes zoster* (gasserian) *Meningitis* *Mononeuritis* *Cavernous sinus syndrome*
	Visceral motor	Sphincter pupillae Ciliary body			*Dilated nonreactive pupil* *Paralysis of accommodation*	
IV Trochlear	Motor	Superior oblique muscle	Brain stem	Trochlear	*Extortion of eye* *Weak downward gaze*	*Herpes zoster* (gasserian) *Meningitis* *Cavernous sinus syndrome*
V Trigeminal	Sensory	Skin: face, scalp (anterior two thirds) Mucosa: nose, mouth, cornea, conjunctiva	Gasserian ganglion	Ophthalmic n. Maxillary n. Mandibular n.	*Pain*	*Herpes zoster* *Petrositis* *Cavernous sinus syndrome*
	Motor	Masseter muscles Pterygoid muscles	Midpons	Mandibular n.	*Trismus*	*Central:* tetanus *Local:* adjacent inflammation
VI Abducens	Motor	External rectus muscles	Brain stem	Abducens	*Paralysis of abduction* *Partially abducted eye at rest*	*Herpes zoster* (gasserian) *Meningitis* *Mononeuritis* *Cavernous sinus syndrome* *Petrositis*
VII Facial	Sensory	Tongue (anterior two thirds): taste	Geniculate ganglion	Nervus intermedius and branches	*Loss of taste on hemitongue*	*Herpes zoster* (Ramsay Hunt syndrome)
		Ear (anterior wall, external auditory canal): all sensations		Lingual n. Mandibular n.		
	Secretomotor	Lacrimal gland Sublingual glands Submaxillary glands	Brain stem	Chorda tympani n.	*Reduced lacrimation* *Reduced salivary mucus*	*Herpes zoster* (Ramsay Hunt syndrome)
	Motor	Facial muscles Stylomastoid muscle Posterior belly, digastric muscle Stapedius muscle	Brain stem (adjacent to VI n. nuclei)	Facial n. and branches	*Facial palsy or paralysis* *Eyelids will not close, eye rolls up* *Creaseless brows* *Recovery: weeks to months* *Late complications* *Hemifacial spasm* *Crocodile tears*	*Otitis media,* mastoiditis Bell palsy pattern (no vesicles) *of mononeuritis or bilateral neuritis* Brucellosis Cat scratch disease Human immunodeficiency virus infection Lyme borreliosis Relapsing fever
VIII Cochleovestibular	Sensory	Spiral organ of Corti	Spiral ganglion (in cochlea)	Cochlear n.	*Deafness*	*Otitis media* *Meningitis*
		Semicircular canal			*Vertigo* *Nystagmus*	*Mastoiditis*
		Saccule Utricle	Scarpa vestibular ganglion (internal auditory meatus)	Vestibular n.	*Absent response to caloric stimulation*	*Mastoiditis* *Meningitis*
IX Glossopharyngeal	Sensory	Tonsils, soft palate, posterior pharynx	Petrosal ganglion Superior ganglion	Glossopharyngeal n.	*Anesthetic posterior pharynx*	*Herpes zoster (rare)*
	Secretory	Pharyngeal mucosa	Medulla		*Palatal paralysis (deviation)* *Hoarseness* *Dysphagia*	*Herpes zoster (rare)* *Meningitis*
	Motor	Pharyngeal striated muscle	Medulla		*Weakness upper trapezoid and sternomastoid*	*Skull base infections*

TABLE 164–3 ■ Cranial Nerve Syndromes *Continued*

NERVE	FUNCTIONS	DISTRIBUTION	NEURONAL LOCATION	PERIPHERAL NERVES OR DIVISIONS	SIGNS OF PERIPHERAL NERVE DYSFUNCTION	COMMON INFECTIOUS CAUSES OF FINDINGS
X Vagus	Sensory	Ear (posterior wall of canal, concha and pinna)	Jugular ganglion	Posterior auricular n.	*Decreased sensation in auditory canal and back of pinna*	*Herpes zoster (infrequent)*
		Pharynx, larynx, trachea, esophagus	Nodose ganglion	Pharyngeal branch of vagus n.	*Loss of gag reflex (affected side)*	
	Somatic motor	Thoracic and abdominal viscera	Medulla	Thoracoabdominal branch of vagus n.	*Palatal paralysis: complete*	*Herpes zoster (infrequent)*
					Loss of curtain movement of lateral pharyngeal walls	*Skull base infections*
		Larynx, pharynx, and palate (striated muscle)		Pharyngeal branch of vagus n.	*Nasal regurgitation* *Voice nasal, hoarse* *Abducted vocal cord*	
	Visceral motor	Heart, other thoracic organs Abdominal viscera	Medulla	Thoracoabdominal branch of vagus n.		
XI Accessory	Motor	Sternocleidomastoid muscle Trapezius muscle	High cervical cord (C1–5)	Accessory n.	*Partial paralysis: trapezius and sternocleidomastoid muscles* *Wing scapula*	*Skull base infections*
XII Hypoglossal	Motor	Tongue muscles Genioglossus Styloglossus Hypoglossus	Medulla	Hypoglossal n.	*Hemiparalysis of tongue (deviation to affected side)*	*Basilar meningitis*
					Progression to wrinkling, atrophy, fibrillary twitches	*Skull base infections*

Anatomy

The anatomic relationship between the spinal cord and its coverings explains the classification of spinal cord infections (see Fig. 164–1). The spinal cord lies in the vertebral canal and is protected by three layers of membranous meninges. The outermost layer is the dura mater. The epidural or extradural space is the potential space between the fibrous dura and the bony vertebral column. The subdural space is also a potential space and is located between the dura and the thin arachnoid membrane. The arachnoid is separated from the pia mater, the innermost layer, by the subarachnoid space, which contains the CSF. The pia closely surrounds the spinal cord and extends into Virchow spaces together with the vessels nourishing the cord. The pia mater also covers the ventral and dorsal roots branching from the cord until they are covered by the perineurium and epineurium of the peripheral nerves.

Pathology

Primary myelitis refers to either infectious or noninfectious inflammation of the spinal cord. Inflammation is referred to as poliomyelitis if it involves only the gray matter and as leukomyelitis if it is confined to the white matter. Transverse myelitis is defined as inflammation of an entire cross-section of the spinal cord, although it is not necessarily limited to one spinal segment.[1(pp1124–1133)] Inflammatory diseases of the spinal cord that also involve adjacent nerve roots and meninges are referred to as radiculomyelitis and meningomyelitis, respectively.[1(pp1124–1133), 90] The spinal cord pathologic change in primary myelitis depends on the cause and ranges from isolated injury to motor neurons, with or without cytolysis, to predominating demyelination associated with focal inflammatory infiltrates, and to more severe, diffuse destruction, as shown in Figure 164–2.

Classification

Three relatively discrete clinical patterns of primary myelitis are based on the type and location of cord lesions: the syndromes of (1) anterior poliomyelitis, (2) leukomyelitis, and (3) transverse myelitis.[1] Whereas anterior poliomyelitis is almost invariably due to acute infection with poliovirus, the cause of the other syndromes varies and in many cases may remain unknown.

Secondary myelitis arises from focal infections located either inside or outside the subarachnoid space. Two infections located within the subarachnoid space commonly have some degree of inflammatory involvement of adjacent cord: infection of the dorsal root ganglion in herpes zoster syndrome, caused by VZV, and infection of posterior roots in the tabes dorsalis syndrome, caused by *T. pallidum*. Although neurologists call these disorders more properly infections of the PNS, inflammatory responses to these infections do directly affect the cord. Spinal intramedullary abscesses are focal inflammatory responses to hematogenous or posttraumatic infection of the cord or infection in a congenital dermal sinus.

Infections arising outside the subarachnoid space that secondarily affect the cord are (1) spinal subdural empyema, (2) spinal epidural abscess or granulations, and (3) vertebral osteomyelitis. Extraarachnoid infections affect cord function by a combination of mass effect and interference with venous and arterial circulation, causing edema and tissue hypoxia. These focal infections are usually caused by bacteria and less commonly by *Mycobacterium tuberculosis*, but opportunistic fungi are important causes in immunocompromised patients. If therapy is delayed or unsuccessful, the ultimate sequela is

TABLE 164–4 ■ Unilateral Cranial Nerve Syndromes Caused by Cranial and Extracranial Focal Infections

SITE OF LESION	EPONYM	CRANIAL NERVE INVOLVED	CLINICAL SIGNS AND SYMPTOMS	INFECTIOUS CAUSE
Cavernous Sinus				
Lateral wall	Tolosa-Hunt	III, IV, VI Ophthalmic V	*Orbital pain* *Sensory loss over upper face* *Ophthalmoparesis* Then *ophthalmoplegia* and *exophthalmos* develop	*Sinusitis* (ethmoid-sphenoid) *Rhinocerebral mycosis*
Cavernous sinus invasion	Foix-Jefferson	III, IV, VI Ophthalmic V Maxillary V ± Mandibular V	*Same complex* *plus* *More extensive area of sensory loss*	*Sinusitis* (ethmoid-sphenoid) *Rhinocerebral mycosis*
Petrous Bone				
Apex	Gradenigo	V, VI	*Facial neuralgia* *Double vision* *Abducens palsy*	*Petrositis* complicating otitis
Middle ear	—	VII	*Facial paresis, palsy* *Ear pain ± drainage* *Deafness*	*Otitis media*
Jugular Foramen				
Base of skull	Vernet	IX, X, XI	*Dysphagia* *Paralysis curtain motion* of lateral pharyngeal wall *Oropharyngeal sensory loss* Posterior tongue Soft palate Pharynx Larynx *Hoarseness* *Weak sternocleidomastoid* and trapezius	*Bezold subperiosteal abscess* Complication of otitis externa or mastoiditis
Posterior Retroparotid Space (Retropharyngeal Syndrome)				
Base of skull	Villaret	IX, X, XI, XII, and cervical sympathetic nerves	*Jugular foramen syndrome* *plus* *Loss of normal tongue mobility* *and* *Horner syndrome* (ipsilateral ptosis, miosis, and enophthalmos)	*Retroparotid lymphadenitis* *or* *Retropharyngeal abscess*

permanent cord injury. Spinal subdural empyemas affect cord function mainly by secondary vasospasm and thrombosis of the cord's venous and arterial circulation, including anterior spinal artery thrombosis, but may extend into the cord to create an intramedullary abscess. Epidural abscess or granulations compress the cord and interfere with venous and arterial circulation. Vertebral osteomyelitis can be complicated by pathologic vertebral fracture and traumatization of the cord by dislocation of bone fragments into the spinal canal.

Clinical Patterns

The several patterns of clinical findings associated with primary and secondary cord injury caused by infections are described in Tables 164–5 and 164–6. Some authors group leukomyelitis and transverse myelitis together,[1(pp1124–1133), 91] whereas others believe it useful to make the distinction because of the difference in pace and type of onset and possible difference in pathogenesis and prognosis.[1] Not included in this discussion is multiple sclerosis,[92] which may ultimately prove to be infectious in etiology.[93] Newer imaging techniques, especially contrast-enhanced MRI, allow precise determination of extent of involvement.[94, 95]

Primary Myelitis

The enteroviruses are well known causes of infectious myelitis, of which poliovirus is most common worldwide.[96, 97] In developed nations, poliomyelitis is now unusual, but sporadic cases of myelitis due to other enteroviruses still occur (e.g., coxsackieviruses A and B, echoviruses, and other enteroviruses).[97] Myelitis due to the nonpoliovirus enteroviruses is generally less severe than that due to poliovirus and presents with weakness rather than paralysis.

Myelitis in severely immunosuppressed persons has been temporally related to other viral infections, particularly aggressive invasive infections caused by CMV, HSV, and VZV.

In some cases of primary myelitis, it may be difficult to distinguish between postinfectious, immune-mediated cord injury and direct viral invasion. Primary myelitis may be caused by several classes of infectious agents besides viruses. Of particular note are chlamydiae (psittacosis), mycoplasmas, spirochetes (Lyme neuroborreliosis, relapsing fever, neurosyphilis), and parasites embolizing to cord (ova of schistosomes and *Taenia* species).[91, 92] Some agents affect peripheral and cranial nerves in addition to the cord and therefore are discussed later in the section on polymorphic infections.

Etiologic diagnosis of primary myelitis is possible for sev-

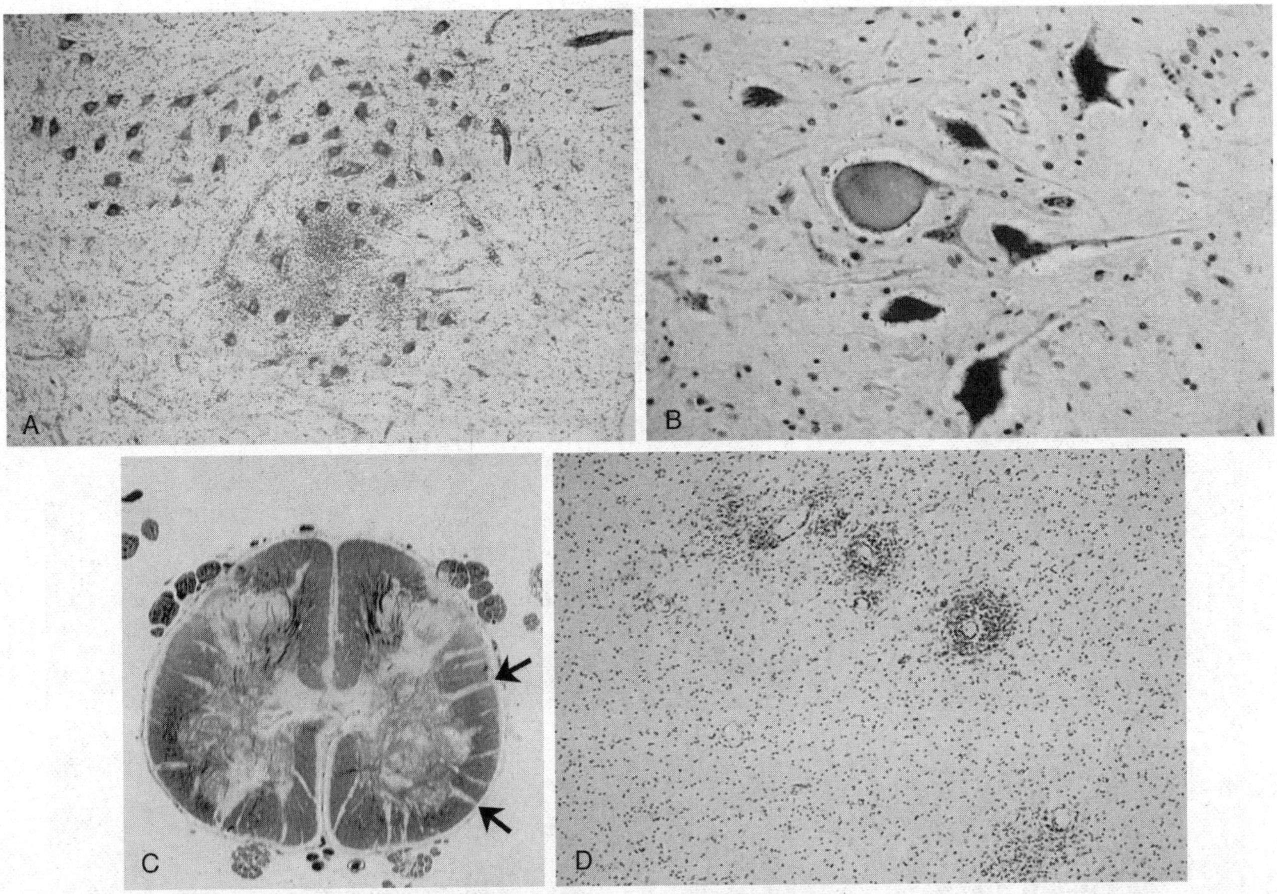

FIGURE 164–2 ◻ Pathology of infectious and postinfectious myelitis. *Poliomyelitis:* Direct irreversible injury of cells infected by poliovirus and reversible demyelination from perivascular lymphocytic infiltration. *A,* Anterior horn: neuronophagia and lymphocytic perivascular cuffing in postcapillary venules (×40). *B,* Motor neurons: central chromatolysis of acutely infected cells (×100). *Acute disseminated encephalomyelitis, postinfectious (measles):* Demyelination follows a pattern of perivascular invasion by lymphocytes and macrophages. *C,* Myelin stain of cord: arrows mark pale linear streaks that follow radiating postcapillary venules in white matter (×10). *D,* Dense clusters of perivenular lymphocytes and macrophages (×40).

Illustration continued on following page

eral agents. Enteroviruses can be recovered in the CSF as well as in blood, pharynx, and stool, and acute infection can be established by comparison of specific antibody titers in acute and convalescent sera. The presence of virus in the CSF is supportive of direct viral invasion. The detection of organisms by PCR and the measurement in CSF of specific antibodies by enzyme-linked immunosorbent assay and immunoblot assay have significantly improved the ability to assign specific causes to cases of primary myelitis.

Enteroviral Myelitis

ACUTE POLIOMYELITIS

Cause

Poliomyelitis is a clinicopathologic syndrome caused by enteroviruses (Table 164–5). Within a few days of the onset of an acute febrile illness, it presents with varying degrees of flaccid paralysis, usually asymmetric, of various striated muscles. Although this syndrome can be caused by the three types of poliovirus (type 1, Brunhilde; type 2, Lansing; and type 3, Leon) and by coxsackieviruses A and B, echoviruses, and enterovirus types 70 and 71 (the so-called new enteroviruses), about 85% of the persistent paralytic cases and most of the epidemics through the years have been caused by poliovirus type 1.[98, 98a]

Pathogenesis

The portal of entry of the virus is the alimentary tract. The virus multiplies in the lymphoid tissue of the pharynx and gut during the incubation period (usually 7 to 14 days, with a range of 2 to 35 days) before viremia occurs. Viremia may be followed by involvement of several target organs in the nervous system—the spinal cord, brain, and meninges—but this happens in only a small proportion of the infected. The motor neurons of the anterior horn cells of the spinal cord, especially in its lumbosacral and cervical enlargements, are most often affected. Cells in the intermediate, intermediolateral, and posterior horns can also be affected, and lesions may even extend into the dorsal root ganglia. In the brain, the hypothalamus, precentral motor cortex, and rarely the cerebellar roof nuclei and cerebellar vermis may be involved. The disease can also affect several brain stem motor nuclei (ambiguous, facial, hypoglossal, more rarely trigeminal). Involvement of the reticular formation in the medulla, pons, and midbrain can cause ventilatory failure and central cardiorespiratory dysfunction.[1(pp1124–1133)]

Immunity

In nonimmunized immunocompetent individuals who are naturally infected, postinfection immunity to the poliovirus

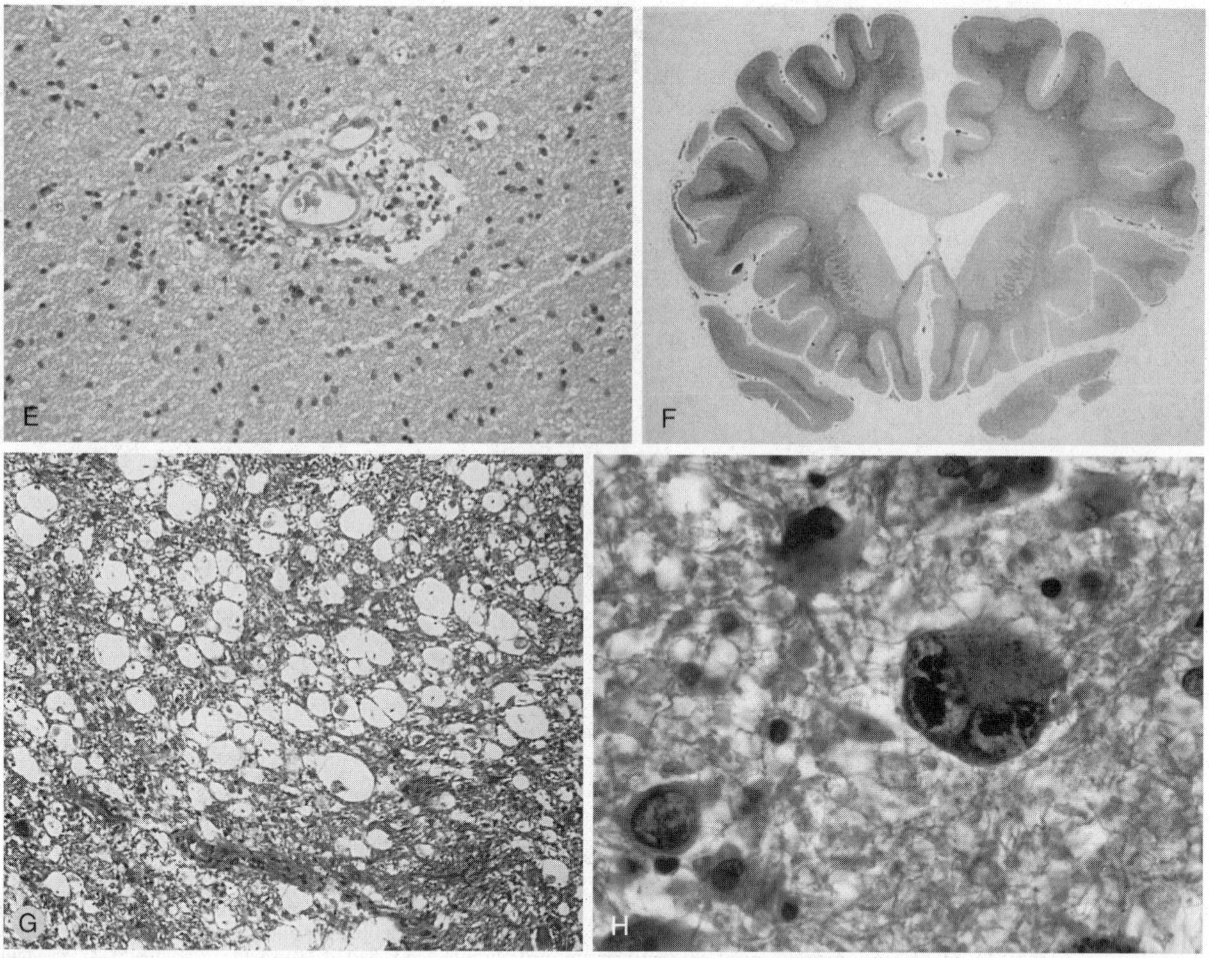

FIGURE 164–2 □ *Continued. E,* Detail of perivascular infiltrate in postcapillary venule (×100). *HIV-associated encephalomyelopathy:* Demyelination is symmetric and in the spinal cord is associated with vacuolar degeneration of myelin with a paucity of inflammation. *F,* Myelin stain of whole brain: extensive loss of normal staining pattern (×1). *G,* Myelin stain of cord: vacuolization of white matter (×40). *CMV myelitis and radiculitis:* Viral replication within several cell types produces direct cytopathic effects and stimulates acute inflammation. *H,* Single and multinucleated cells with intranuclear inclusions (×100). (*A* to *E* courtesy of Dr. E. P. Richardson, Department of Neuropathology, Harvard Medical School and Massachusetts General Hospital. *F* to *H* courtesy of Drs. F. Aydin and S. Mitruka, Department of Pathology, Tulane University School of Medicine, New Orleans, LA.)

type causing the infection is permanent. After primary infection, viral neutralizing antibodies are detectable in serum within a few days after exposure, often before the onset of illness. Natural infection and oral immunization with live attenuated poliovirus vaccine both induce mucosal immunity and local antibody production, which protects against intestinal reinfection. Passive immunity is transferred from mother to offspring transplacentally and by breast milk. However, maternal antibodies gradually disappear during the first 6 months of life, and the infant is no longer protected.

Epidemiology

Acute paralytic poliomyelitis is not an extinct disease. It remains a major health problem in tropical and less developed areas,[99] and cases have been encountered annually even in the United States and Europe until more recent years. Until 1985, vaccine programs were not always available or effective in the developing world, and underreporting was common, as it still is in some areas.[100] The WHO estimated that the report of 39,361 cases worldwide for 1985 represented less than 5% of the actual cases.[98] Case rates decreased 84% to 6241 in 1994 after the initiation of the WHO global poliomyelitis eradication program in 1985,[100] which raised routine vaccination coverage worldwide from 47% to 80% to 81% through national immunization days and promoted special vaccination campaigns in areas where wild poliovirus transmission persisted at low levels. To detect all cases meeting the WHO case definition of poliomyelitis, the WHO eradication program introduced surveillance in 94 cooperating countries for all cases of acute flaccid paralysis. The WHO also created the Global Polio Laboratory Network of certified reference laboratories to perform viral isolations on specimens from cases of acute flaccid paralysis and to confirm and type isolates. The WHO's goal is global eradication of poliomyelitis by the year 2000.[101] Three years after the last case of paralytic poliomyelitis caused by wild poliovirus occurred in 1991 in Peru, the Western Hemisphere was certified free of wild poliovirus by an international commission in 1994.[100]

Despite extensive use of poliovirus vaccines in developed countries, poliomyelitis has not been completely eradicated. Imported wild poliovirus from poliomyelitis endemic countries, the source of many outbreaks and sporadic cases of poliomyelitis since 1988 in previously poliomyelitis-free countries of Europe, the Middle East, and North America,

TABLE 164–5 ■ Primary Myelitis Syndromes*

ACUTE ANTERIOR POLIOMYELITIS

Etiology: Enteroviruses
Usual cause: polioviruses 1, 2, 3
Milder disease: coxsackieviruses A, B; echovirus; enterovirus types 70, 71

Pathogenesis: Combination of irreversible cytolytic destruction of lower motor neurons and reversible inflammatory damage to anterior and intermediate horns; also involves hypothalamus, thalamus, motor nuclei of brain stem and reticular formation, vestibular nuclei, and roof nuclei of cerebellum

Clinical pattern: *Biphasic disease*

	Symptoms	*Neurologic Findings*	*Laboratory*
Viremia phase: "minor illness" (lasts 3–4 d)	*Influenza-like syndrome* Listlessness Fever (38°C–40°C) Sore throat Anorexia, nausea, vomiting Generalized headache Muscle stiffness, aching	Normal	*Virus* detectable in blood, throat washings, stool
CNS phase: "major illness" (evolves in 5–7 d) *Nonparalytic stage:* Aseptic meningitis	*Recrudescence of headache and fever* if asymptomatic period (3–5 d) is followed by minor illness; otherwise, headache intensifies *Pain in back and neck* *Muscles tender, painful*	*Encephalopathic* signs Irritable Restless Emotionally labile *Meningeal* signs Kernig and Brudzinski signs present *Muscle spasm* (e.g., tight hamstring)	*CSF* Cells: pleocytosis—PMNs initially, then lymphocytes Glucose: normal Protein: elevated *Serology:* neutralizing and CF antibody present *Virus:* detectable in blood, throat washings, stool, and CSF (except polioviruses rarely isolated from CSF)
Paralytic stage: Meningomyeloencephalitis	*Weakness* Rapid, progressive onset of weakness that continues until afebrile for 48 h *Extent of weakness:* dependent on age of patient *Infants:* trunk and extremities *Children* <5 y: often one leg only *Older children:* arm + both legs *Adolescents and adults:* asymmetric weakness of all four extremities	*"Spinal paralysis"* pattern *Muscles* Coarse fasciculations initially (transient —days) Atrophy—detectable within 3 wk (permanent) *Reflex losses* Abdominal musculature: cremasteric and abdominal reflexes Limbs—DTRs *Subjective paresthesias* Objectively normal *"Bulbar paralysis"* pattern Hiccup Dysphagia, dysphonia, aspiration Respiratory insufficiency; irregular respiration Dysregulation of blood pressure (hypertension, hypotension)	*CSF* Cells: lymphocytosis Glucose: normal Protein: elevated; normalizes in 4–5 wk

LEUKOMYELITIS

Etiology

Acute invasive infections: Mycoplasma pneumoniae; monkey B virus; CMV, HSV, EBV in advanced immunosupression from HIV; postinfectious or postvaccinial
Subacute with variable chronic meningitis: HIV vacuolar myelopathy, HTLV-I, Lyme borreliosis, relapsing fever, neurosyphilis

Associations

Postinfectious: rubeola, varicella, variola, rubella, influenza, mumps, WEE, HTLV-I, brucellosis, psittacosis, cat-scratch disease
Postvaccinial: Japanese B encephalitis vaccine, vaccinia virus, Pasteur rabbit cord rabies vaccine

Pathogenesis: Lesions in cord involve demyelination or necrosis of white matter tracts. Only demyelination is potentially reversible. Herpesviruses ascend neurons, replicate in myelin, cause necrosis of white matter with acute cellular infiltration; HIV is found in phagocytic mononuclear cells associated with myelin destruction. Perivascular demyelination with lymphocytic cuffing is characteristic of postinfectious and postvaccinial disease.

Table continued on following page

TABLE 164–5 ■ Primary Myelitis Syndromes* *Continued*

Symptoms	***Neurologic Findings***	***Diagnosis***
Prodromal event or *risk factors* (potential associations include host factors) Travel or residence in endemic area Tick bite or louse bite Macaque monkey exposure (bite or contamination with tissues) Unpasteurized dairy products STD risk Exanthem, e.g., erythema chronicum migrans Advanced immunosuppression (HIV, transplant) Vaccine (neurotropic) administration recently (e.g., 10–20th day of serial Pasteur vaccinations)	*Ascending paralysis* until it reaches *spinal sensory and motor level* All function below abolished Progressive sensory and motor weakness Beginning in sacral level Progressing to lumbar then thoracic level Bladder paralysis Spinal shock (flaccid areflexia) may occur initially *Differential features* Encephalopathic findings common Absence of spinal ache and root pain Recovery to "minimal reflex" activity after spinal shock	*CT-myelography or MRI* No block or external mass Variable swelling of cord Enhancement of cord at MRI (gadolinium) *CSF* *Acute invasive form* Cells Lymphocytes and PMNs B cells: IgM dominantly Glucose: low or normal Protein Normal or elevated Oligoclonal banding (on electrophoresis) Immunoglobulins: IgM then IgG Cultures: negative
Onset over days Weakness in legs, feet Numbness in legs, feet (bilateral); may extend to trunk Difficulty voiding *Monophasic course* if postinfectious or postvaccinial Single attack Several weeks' duration Variable recovery No relapse		*Subacute form* Cells Lymphocytosis B cells: IgG Glucose: normal Protein Normal or slightly elevated Oligoclonal banding on electrophoresis Immunoglobulins: IgG Cultures: negative *Blood serology:* diagnostic for neuroborreliosis

TRANSVERSE MYELITIS

Etiology: Varicella-zoster virus (rarely), postmeningococcal meningitis, spirochetal infection, schistosomiasis, delayed treatment of epidural abscess

Pathology: Inflammatory injury to white and gray matter in spinal cord at segmental level; in some instances due to infarct after arteriospasm or thrombosis of anterior spinal artery, in which case posterior columns are relatively spared. Irreversible changes.

Symptoms	***Neurologic Findings***	***Diagnosis***
Prodromal event (potential associations related to primary illness) Lyme borreliosis: prior erythema chronicum migrans Leptospirosis: hepatitis Meningococcal meningitis: early phase Relapsing fever: pattern of periodic fevers Schistosomiasis: acute illness weeks to months after infected Zoster: single or multiple dermatome skin eruption	*Flaccid motor paralysis* of extremities related to level *C4–5:* complete *C5–6:* arms, abduct, flex *C6–7:* arms intact, except hands *Below C-7, above conus:* legs only *Conus medullaris syndrome* Weak muscles in lower legs Sphincteric paralysis only (bladder, bowel) Lax anal sphincter Sacral dermatome sensory loss Absent sphincteric sensory reflexes	*CSF:* dependent on infectious cause *CT-myelography or MRI* No block or external mass Variable swelling of cord Enhancement of cord at affected levels at MRI (gadolinium) *Serology:* dependent on infectious cause
Rapid onset of sensorimotor level Loss of voluntary movement Loss of sensation No recovery	*Sensory level:* parallels motor level *"Spinal shock"* *Initial loss* (related to level) of reflexes Visceral, genital, cutaneous, and DTRs Vasomotor tone *Return of reflex activity in 1–6 wk* ("minimal reflex activity") *Later progression to hyperreflexia below level* Babinski flexion reflexes Tendon reflexes Reflex urination, defecation, sweating Mass reflex responses	

*CF, Complement-fixing; CMV, cytomegalovirus; CNS, central nervous system; CSF, cerebrospinal fluid; CT, computed tomography; DTRs, deep tendon reflexes; EBV, Epstein-Barr virus; HIV, human immunodeficiency virus; HSV, herpes simplex virus; HTLV-I, human T-cell lymphotropic virus type I; IgG, immunoglobulin G; IgM, immunoglobulin M; MRI, magnetic resonance imaging; PMNs, polymorphonuclear leukocytes; STD, sexually transmitted disease; WEE, western equine encephalomyelitis.

TABLE 164–6 ■ Myelitis Secondary to Adjacent Intrathecal Infection*

DORSAL ROOT GANGLION INFECTION: *HERPES ZOSTER SYNDROME*

Etiology: VZV

Pathogenesis: Inflammatory injury to (1) isolated cranial or spinal sensory ganglion that is site of recrudescent VZV replication; (2) related spinal cord segment, especially posterior gray matter and dorsal roots; (3) leptomeninges of involved cord segment and roots; and (4) spinal roots and peripheral nerve contiguous to involved ganglia

	Symptoms and Signs	*Neurologic Findings*	*Diagnosis*
General features	*Constitutional symptoms* Fever, malaise *Prodromal segmental dysesthesias* Itching, tingling, burning *Radicular pain* Onset 72–96 h before eruption Persists 1–4 wk in 70%–80% Chronic pain, hypersensitivity in remainder *Skin lesions* Segmental unilateral distribution Vesicles on erythematous base Progress to pustules then crusts Extensive dermal swelling, tenderness, inflammatory changes at site *Mucous membrane lesions* Aphthous-like clusters of unroofed vesicles Unilateral distribution Only occur with ganglia supplying mucosa *Gasserian (V):* conjunctival, corneal, buccal *Geniculate (VII):* tongue, anterior palate *IX and X:* soft palate, pharynx *Sacral:* bladder	*Segmental, ipsilateral* distribution of *Vesicles* (variable numbers) *Superficial sensory loss* (common) *Motor weakness* (~5%) *Patterns* *Thoracic zoster*—65% Single dermatome when immunocompetent Between T-5 and T-10 most common *Craniocervical*—20% One or more adjacent dermatomes Motor involvement frequent Adjacent cranial nerves without ganglia affected by inflammation (e.g., III, IV, VI) *Limb* One or more adjacent dermatomes *Sacral* Bladder paralysis, with hematuria *Disseminated* Two or more dermatomes heavily involved *or* Generalized varicella-like eruption	*Vesicle:* scrape base or biopsy Tzanck prep: multinucleated giant cells DFA: positive with anti-VZV EM: positive Viral culture: often negative *Blood serology:* ELISA—anamnestic response noted if patient is immunocompetent (requires paired sera 10 d apart) *CSF* Cells: lymphocytosis in 40% Glucose: normal Protein: elevated Culture: negative for virus Antibody: ELISA and immunoblot positive for VZV antibody
Cranial syndromes			
Ophthalmic zoster (zoster ophthalmicus) Gasserian (V) ganglion	*Frequency:* 10%–15% of all zoster *Skin lesions* Anterior scalp Forehead Periorbital skin Nose tip (nasociliary branch) *Mucous membrane lesions:* conjunctiva	*Pain* in scalp, forehead *Corneal lesions* and *iridocyclitis* if nasociliary branch involved *Ipsilateral cranial neuritis:* commonly associated ipsilateral cranial nerve palsies when III, IV, and VI motor roots or brain stem involved *Extraocular paresis* *Ptosis* *Mydriasis*	*Eye:* slit-lamp examination Corneal and ciliary evaluation
Geniculate zoster (Ramsay Hunt syndrome) Geniculate (VIIth) ganglion	*Skin lesions* External auditory canal Pinna and adjacent scalp (variable) *Mucous membrane lesions* Hemitongue—ipsilateral *Neurologic symptoms*—variable Tinnitus, vertigo, deafness	*Pain:* in ear canal, pinna, and adjacent scalp *Ipsilateral cranial neuritis:* variable *VII:* facial nerve palsy (common) *VIII:* auditory-vestibular involvement: tinnitus, vertigo, deafness *IX, X:* dysphagia	*ENT examination* External auditory canal examination Audiogram
Vagal and glossopharyngeal zoster IX and X ganglia	*Mucous membrane lesions only* Ipsilateral Soft palate Posterior pharynx	*Pain in throat* *Dysphagia*	*ENT examination:* evaluate for mucosal lesions
Upper cervical zoster (herpes occipitocollaris) C-1, C-2 ganglia	*Skin lesions* Retroauricular and occipital	*Pain in occiput*	*Vesicles:* evaluate as above

Table continued on following page

TABLE 164–6 ■ Myelitis Secondary to Adjacent Intrathecal Infection* *Continued*

POSTERIOR ROOT INFECTION: TABES DORSALIS SYNDROME

Etiology: *Treponema pallidum*

Pathology: Form of neurosyphilis—thinning of posterior roots of lumbosacral cord, with dominant secondary destruction of proprioceptive fibers in radicular nerves with associated degeneration of posterior columns in cord

	Symptoms and Signs	Neurologic Findings	Diagnosis
Cardinal features	*Lightning (lancinating) pains* Legs especially Repetitive for hours to days *Ataxia* Broad-based gait Flinging movements of legs *Urinary incontinence*	*Sensory ataxia* Impaired vibration and position sense in feet and legs Positive Romberg test response *Intact muscle power and mass* *Absent knee* and *ankle reflexes*	*CSF* Lymphocytosis common Abnormal protein Normal glucose VDRL: result usually positive if previously untreated *Blood serology* Reaginic test (ART) result variable, but usually positive Specific antibody tests (TPHA and FTA-ABS) positive
Other common findings	*Visceral crises* Epigastric pain Nausea Vomiting *Constipation*	*Neuroophthalmologic* abnormalities Abnormal pupils in 90%, including Argyll Robertson Ophthalmoplegia—variable Optic atrophy Ptosis *Insensitive hypotonic bladder* Overflow incontinence *Megacolon* *Secondary trophic ulcers* *Advanced osteoarthritis* Charcot joints: 1%–10% Hips, knees, and ankles	

*ART, Automated reagin test; CSF, cerebrospinal fluid; DFA, direct fluorescent antibody assay; ELISA, enzyme-linked immunosorbent assay; EM, electron microscopy; ENT, ear, nose, and throat; FTA-ABS, fluorescent treponemal antibody absorption; TPHA, *Treponema pallidum* hemagglutination; VDRL, Venereal Disease Research Laboratory test; VZV, varicella-zoster virus.

has frequently originated from Southeast Asia, which in 1994 accounted for 73% of the global reported cases.[100] These outbreaks occurred mainly in nonimmunized persons who belonged predominantly to groups that oppose vaccination.

The other source of cases in developed countries is immunodeficient individuals who directly receive, or secondarily acquire, oral poliovirus vaccine strains and then develop acute paralytic poliomyelitis. In the period 1973 through 1984, 76% of 138 cases of paralytic poliomyelitis in the United States were vaccine associated.[91] However, oral poliovirus vaccine–associated paralytic poliomyelitis is rare (one case per 2.6 million doses distributed).[102]

Demographic Patterns

There are three demographic patterns of poliomyelitis:

1. The endemic pattern is seen in areas with limited sanitation and without vaccine programs. This is the true infantile paralysis syndrome that is seen sporadically. In these countries, virtually all children older than 4 years are naturally immune. Because passive immunity is transferred from mother to offspring, many infants experience poliovirus infection while still partially protected by maternal antibodies. Consequently, the ratio of inapparent to apparent infection is highest in infants and young children, and paralytic disease is relatively rare despite common exposure to wild-type virus.

2. The second or epidemic pattern was seen during the first half of the 20th century in many areas of temperate zones with good standards of community and household hygiene before vaccine became available. A generally accepted explanation is that improved sanitation and hygiene reduced opportunities for infection among the young. Thus, increasing numbers of persons encountered poliovirus for the first time in later childhood or adult life, when infection is more likely to take the paralytic form. This pattern has been seen in developing countries with rising levels of sanitation, where vaccine programs are incompletely effective.

3. The third pattern is the postvaccination pattern in which outbreaks of poliomyelitis occur in a vaccinated population, the result either of unique host defense defects (vaccine-related virus) or of noncompliance with vaccine programs (wild-type virus), as described before.

Clinical Features

Approximately 90% to 95% of patients have an inapparent infection.[1(pp1124–1133)] Only 4% to 8% of patients have what has been called minor illness, non-CNS symptoms and signs such as sore throat, headache, nausea, vomiting, anorexia, and abdominal pain, which generally last 1 to 4 days. Only 1% to 2% of these patients develop the so-called major illness consisting of aseptic meningitis. It presents with fever, meningeal signs, paresthesias, and neck and back pains and has an associated CSF pleocytosis with normal or slightly elevated CSF protein and normal CSF glucose levels (see Table 164–5).

The paralytic disease is occasionally preceded by the minor illness and usually by the major illness. In most cases, the meningitic phase lasts for a day or two before the first signs of paralysis are seen. Severe muscle pain and spasms precede or accompany onset of paralysis in the extremities. Fasciculations and hyperactive deep tendon reflexes are transient and are followed by loss of reflexes and flaccid paralysis, progressing usually from 1 to 4 days. In the spinal form, there is asymmetric weakness or paralysis of muscle groups of the extremities or trunk. Transient urinary retention also occurs in about 30% of patients. In the bulbar form, there is weakness or paralysis of the soft palate, pharynx, and vocal cords. Peripheral facial paralysis and transient oculomotor palsies (rarely) may be seen. There can be disturbances of breathing and circulation due to neuronal damage in the respiratory and vasomotor centers of the medulla.

Paralysis remains fixed for a period of days or weeks, after which improvement slowly follows; 60% of eventual recovery is achieved by 3 months and 80% by 6 months.[1(pp1124–1133)] Minimal further improvement continues for 18 months to 2 years, probably mostly due to learning more effective use of weakened muscles. The so-called post-polio syndrome of return of weakness or paralysis in later life after childhood or adolescent poliomyelitis and in the same distribution as the original attack is due not to relapse or reacquisition of poliovirus infection but rather to gradual loss of the compensatory neuronal and muscle activities that mark the muscle retraining and recovery process.[91, 102a, 102b]

During acute poliomyelitis, there are also rare cases of encephalitis and a variable degree of autonomic disturbance with regional hyperhidrosis or hypohidrosis, transient urinary retention, constipation, labile hypertension, and gastric atony.[1(pp1124–1133)]

Diagnosis

In early poliomyelitis, the CSF contains an excess of cells (neutrophils in the first 72 hours, then lymphocytes) and slightly more protein than normal. Virus can usually be grown in tissue culture from pharyngeal swabs or throat washings in the first week of the acute stage of the illness. It can be recovered from the feces for at least 3 weeks and often longer. It has only rarely been grown from the CSF. Diagnosis can also be made retrospectively by demonstrating a fourfold or greater rise in specific antibodies in the convalescent serum. In certifying acute flaccid paralysis cases as poliomyelitis, the standard WHO case definition permits any of four criteria to confirm the diagnosis, including isolation of poliovirus from a stool specimen.[100]

Treatment

The treatment of the paralytic form is entirely supportive.

Prevention

Two types of vaccine have been developed to prevent poliomyelitis.[99, 103, 104] The killed inactivated poliovirus (IPV, Salk) vaccine, the first to be available, reduced the number of annual cases in the United States from an average of approximately 31,000 cases per year between 1945 and 1955 to 2545 by 1960. It induced good humoral immunity and could be used in immunosuppressed patients. However, repeated boosters were required to maintain detectable antibody levels. The enhanced inactivated poliovirus vaccine (E-IPV), made by a different process and introduced in 1988, proved to be more potent and more consistently immunogenic, produced higher titers of neutralizing antibody after fewer doses, and is now the standard inactivated poliovirus vaccine. However, inactivated vaccines do not induce mucosal immunity in vaccinees, who remain susceptible at least once to subsequent local infection with wild-type polioviruses, during which they are transiently capable of transmitting them to nonimmune persons.[104a]

The attenuated live oral poliovirus vaccine (OPV, Sabin), licensed in the United States in the early 1960s, rapidly brought the number of annual cases to approximately 12 a year. Easy to administer, it induces humoral, cellular, and intestinal mucosal immunity (which may be lifelong) but cannot be administered to immunosuppressed patients. Whereas oral poliovirus vaccine has the potential to mutate and revert to sufficient neurovirulence to cause paralytic poliomyelitis in recipients or their contacts, this has not been observed in mass vaccination programs.

Enhanced inactivated poliovirus vaccine is recommended for boosters for a variety of previously immunized persons. It should always be used for primary immunization of households with immunodeficient individuals, because live oral poliovirus vaccine, which is excreted in the stool by healthy vaccinees, can infect immunoincompetent persons and may result in paralytic disease.

In 1997, the CDC Advisory Committee for Immunization Practices recommended changes in poliovirus vaccine policy that place increased reliance on inactivated poliovirus vaccine for routine immunization in the United States, because of the relative increased risk of vaccine-associated poliomyelitis in the face of elimination of wild-type virus–associated poliomyelitis from the Western Hemisphere and the reduced threat of its importation into the United States.[104b] Revised recommendations include three options for poliovirus vaccination: sequential vaccination with inactivated poliovirus vaccine followed by oral poliovirus vaccine, oral poliovirus vaccine alone, or inactivated poliovirus vaccine alone. For overall public benefit, this CDC committee recommended two doses of inactivated poliovirus vaccine followed by two doses of oral poliovirus vaccine for routine childhood vaccinations. Exceptions are oral poliovirus vaccine for children beginning a vaccination schedule after 6 months of age, and inactivated poliovirus vaccine for children who are immunosuppressed and unvaccinated adults. Adults vaccinated in childhood who are at increased risk for exposure to poliovirus may receive another dose of oral or inactivated vaccine.[104c]

Herpesvirus Myelitis

MACAQUE MONKEY B VIRUS *(HERPESVIRUS SIMIAE)* MYELITIS

Cause

Cercopithecine herpesvirus 1 (B virus), *H. simiae*, was first isolated in 1933 from the brain and spinal cord of a researcher who died of rapidly progressive meningoencephalitis after being bitten by a macaque.[105] B virus occurs naturally among primates of the genus *Macaca*. It is the biologic counterpart of herpes simplex virus in humans and usually causes minimal or undetectable morbidity in its natural host.[106] No other Old World and no New World monkeys are known to harbor B virus. Indeed, infections in several non-*Macaca* species cause fatal disease, as in humans. In well-documented human cases, the incubation period between exposure and onset of clinical disease has ranged from 5 to 30 days.[105] More than 25 proven cases have been described in persons who handled monkeys or their tissues. Infection in untreated persons has a fatality rate of approximately 70%.[105]

Epidemiology

The prevalence of infection is low among immature macaques but reaches more than 80% as animals reach sexual maturity. Latently infected monkeys shed virus only intermittently in conjunctiva, buccal mucosa, and genital areas and primarily during the breeding season or when ill, stressed (e.g., after transport, anesthesia, or invasive procedures), or immunocompromised. Macaques are native to Asia and northern Africa, but thousands are housed in research facilities and zoos and are kept as pets in private homes throughout the world.[105] Persons at risk are those experiencing macaque-related injuries and laboratory workers exposed to B virus–contaminated primary rhesus monkey cell cultures.

Seroprevalence studies among primate handlers indicate that asymptomatic infection does not occur.[105] Monkey-related injuries at U.S. research facilities have been monitored closely since 1987. During the interval between 1987 and 1994, while several hundred persons were treated empirically for B virus infection after high-risk injuries, only eight infections were confirmed. Infection with B virus must be considered an uncommon result of macaque-related human injuries, because disease is rare despite the annual occurrence of several thousand monkey-inflicted bites, scratches, and other exposures.[105]

Pathogenesis

Studies in mice on the pathogenesis of B virus infection of the nervous system indicate that route of inoculation controls mode of spread to CNS. Virus introduced intramuscularly in the leg ascends the ipsilateral dorsal column, the bilateral spinothalamic and spinoreticular systems, and central autonomic pathways. Subcutaneous inoculation spares the dorsal column, but virus otherwise follows the same routes. However, virus introduced intraperitoneally spreads in the cord bilaterally, mainly along the spinothalamic and central autonomic pathways.

Ascent to the brain in mice is mainly orthograde along ascending systems, regardless of method of inoculation. In brain, virus first accumulates in thalamus, hypothalamus, and motor cortex and then spreads retrograde along the pyramidal tract and central autonomic systems.[107] MRI findings suggest a similar pattern of spread in human cases.[105]

Clinical Features

Humans infected with B virus have a prodromal illness of early and then intermediate manifestations before progression to aseptic meningitis and rapidly ascending encephalomyelitis. Early manifestations, when present, are vesicular eruptions or ulcerations at or near the exposure site, often accompanied by severe pain or itching and regional lymphadenopathy. Intermediate manifestations include local development of numbness, paresthesia, or other neuresthesias, which progress proximally with associated muscle weakness, plus findings compatible with viremia (fever, conjunctivitis) and early brain stem involvement (persistent hiccup). Late manifestations, which are avoidable if therapy begins early, include sinusitis and central neurologic involvement. Meningitis (headache, stiff neck) progresses to encephalitis, manifested initially as brain stem and cerebellar findings before evidence of cortical involvement (altered mentation, seizures, hemiparesis, hemiplegia, coma, respiratory failure, and urinary retention).[105]

Diagnosis

Human B virus infections are diagnosed by viral culture and serology. These studies must be performed in certified laboratories because of the dangers of viral cultivation, which requires biosafety level 4 facilities, and the potential for incorrect interpretation of serologic results due to the cross-reaction of human antibodies to HSV with B virus. Serology is performed on paired acute and convalescent sera, separated by 2 to 3 weeks. False-positive results are reduced by using the monoclonal competitive radioimmunoassay, or by enzyme-linked immunosorbent assay combined with Western blot.[105]

Viral isolation is required for definitive diagnosis. Serial cultures of high-risk asymptomatic and symptomatic exposed persons are recommended. If the initial postinjury wound cultures from an asymptomatic person turn positive for B virus, or if shedding was documented in the source monkey exposure of a symptomatic person, regardless of results of initial wound cultures, additional swab specimens should be collected for viral cultures from the individual's wound, oropharynx, and conjunctiva and from the bases of any papular, vesicular, or ulcerative herpes-like lesions. If the first set of cultures is still negative for B virus after 5 days, at least two additional sets of cultures should be obtained. Detailed instructions for collecting and sending specimens for viral culture are described in published guidelines.[105]

CSF in patients with neurologic symptoms contains rising titers of specific antibody, which precedes appearance of detectable serum antibody. Antibody in CSF may inhibit virus recovery. PCR assay for B virus is under development.[105]

MRI has proved helpful in diagnosing involvement of meninges and cord and early brain stem encephalitis. The ascending nature of B virus infections, characterized by preferential early involvement of cerebellum, hypothalamus, thalamus, brain stem, medulla, and pons, may be detected as enhancing lesions by MRI. By contrast, HSV encephalitis localizes early in the temporal lobe.[105]

Differential Diagnosis

When B virus is not isolated from either a monkey or a high-risk exposed person, neurologic symptoms may still reflect undetected B virus infection. However, other diseases must be considered, such as reactivated HSV infection, herpes zoster, or, in severely immunocompromised persons, CMV infection. When serial specimens fail to yield B virus from monkey or patient, definitive diagnosis of encephalitis requires brain biopsy for proper treatment, especially when there is temporal lobe involvement, because an alternative diagnosis may be found in up to 20% of suspected cases of B virus infection.[105]

Treatment

The CDC recommends that asymptomatic persons with an initially positive wound site culture for B virus be treated with oral acyclovir (800 mg five times daily) and that aggressive efforts be made to confirm evidence of active infection, because an initial positive culture could indicate viral contamination of the site. Absence of continued virus shedding or of clear-cut seroconversion permits omission of therapy after 14 days. However, the individual should remain under medical supervision to detect recurrence of virus shedding, late seroconversion, or onset of clinical disease.[105]

All symptomatic individuals should be hospitalized for medical evaluation and for isolation with barrier precautions. Treatment of symptomatic patients should begin empirically while awaiting culture and serology results. Recommended dosages, routes, and duration are related to the risk for encephalitis on admission. Low-risk individuals are those with herpetiform lesions limited to the trunk or extremities and only peripheral neurologic symptoms and signs. High-risk persons are those with herpetiform lesions on the head or neck or who have signs or symptoms of CNS involvement.

The dosage of acyclovir, the current drug of choice, should be adjusted for renal function, and the intravenous route should always be used in initial treatment of symptomatic persons. Recommended for those at low risk is a moderate dose of intravenous acyclovir (at least 10 mg/kg every 8 hours, if renal function is normal). High-risk cases should receive maximal dosing intravenously (15 mg/kg every 8 hours). Intravenous treatment should continue until symptoms resolve and until serial viral cultures for virus shedding are consistently negative for 14 days. Thereafter, oral acyclovir (800 mg five times daily) may be used, with serial monitoring for B virus shedding after the change in route and dose. When viral cultures are negative, the patient can be discharged. Long-term suppressive therapy and continued intermittent monitoring for virus shedding are recommended.[105] Acyclovir-resistant strains of B virus have not yet been described.

Prevention

Fortunately, human infections with B virus remain an uncommon result of macaque-related injuries, and thus optimal diagnostic and therapeutic approaches are unclear.[106] Experimental evidence suggests that early therapy with acyclovir or postexposure chemoprophylaxis should decrease morbidity and mortality. Clinical experience with acyclovir postexposure chemoprophylaxis and treatment of early disease has been encouraging.[108]

Guidelines established by the CDC for prevention and treatment of B virus infections in exposed persons include standard operating procedures and quality-control interventions for institutions handling macaques, and instructions for physicians evaluating and treating persons with potential B virus exposure.[105] Updated information and any changes in the guidelines are available from the Division of Viral and Rickettsial Diseases at the National Center for Infectious Diseases, CDC, Atlanta.[106]

See Chapter 240 for further details of management of asymptomatic exposed persons.

HUMAN HERPESVIRUS MYELITIS

Cause and Epidemiology

Acute transverse myelitis caused by human herpesviruses, once a rare manifestation, is of increasing etiologic importance in the era of AIDS.[109] HSV-1 and HSV-2,[110–115] VZV,[116–119] CMV,[120–123] and Epstein-Barr virus[124] have all been associated with myelitis, usually in immunocompromised patients.[125] Mixed herpesvirus infections have also been observed.[126]

Clinical Features

The myelitis is often nonspecific, although severe ascending necrosis of the cord appears to be most typical.[127] Skin lesions characteristic of HSV-1 and HSV-2 and VZV may be of help in suggesting these causes, but absence of rash cannot reliably exclude them.[128–131] Patients may present with fever and rapidly progressive neurologic deficits.

Diagnosis

In acute myelitis due to herpesviruses, the CSF usually shows a lymphocytic pleocytosis, elevated protein level, and normal glucose value, in contrast to the polymorphonuclear predominance when CMV and HSV cause plexitis or polyneuritis. Recovery of the virus in CSF culture is insensitive but helpful if it is positive. Epstein-Barr virus cannot be routinely cultured. PCR may enable rapid, definitive diagnosis when it becomes routinely available in the near future. Information is lacking on detectability of specific antibody in the CSF when herpesvirus causes invasive myelitis in persons with advanced HIV immunosuppression.

MRI findings are similar to those described for B virus.[132]

Treatment

In immunocompromised patients presenting with acute transverse myelitis of unknown etiology, early empirical therapy with intravenous acyclovir, ganciclovir, or foscarnet may preserve cord function pending definitive diagnosis.

Human Retroviral Myelitis

Causes

Two human lymphotropic retroviruses have been clearly associated with myelitis. HIV-1 has been reported to cause acute myelopathy[133] and acute peripheral neuropathy in primary infection, as discussed before. Chronic vacuolar myelopathy with spastic paralysis commonly precedes or accompanies the AIDS dementia syndrome.[134] Human T-cell lymphotropic virus type I (HTLV-I) is associated with a syndrome characterized by slowly progressive paralysis called either tropical spastic paraparesis or, in Japan, HTLV-I–associated myelopathy.[135] The tropical spastic paraparesis/HTLV-I–associated myelopathy neurologic syndrome usually begins in middle age after a prolonged incubation period; it has a female predominance and previously had a restricted geographic distribution, mainly in the Caribbean, South America, Africa, India, and Japan. However, increasing numbers of cases of HTLV-I–associated myelopathy in the presence of HIV-1 coinfection have been described in the United States.[136]

Laboratory Diagnosis

HIV-1 may be isolated from the CSF of some asymptomatic individuals, whereas HTLV-I is primarily cell associated. Specific diagnosis of retroviral myelitis requires demonstration of virus-specific oligoclonal immunoglobulins in CSF or detection of retrovirus in tissue by nucleic acid probes.[137] Whereas risk for a retroviral cause in cases of myelitis may be assessed by detecting serum antibodies with standard serologic tests, caution must be observed in using serology alone to diagnose myelitis in populations with high seroprevalence for HIV-1 or HTLV-I infection. HTLV has a low frequency of myelitis among HTLV-I–infected persons, and HIV-1–infected persons are at risk for several other causes of myelitis.[40]

HIV-1 VACUOLAR MYELOPATHY

Pathology

Vacuolar myelopathy is associated with advanced HIV infection and has been found in up to 50% of AIDS patients undergoing autopsy.[138] On pathologic examination, the white matter of the cord is vacuolated, primarily in the thoracic segments, with a cellular infiltrate of myelin-containing macrophages (see Fig. 164–2*G*).

Clinical Features

In severe cases, patients develop spastic paraparesis of the lower extremities with or without involvement of the arms. The weakness may be asymmetric and evolves during a period of weeks. Coexisting neuropathy is often present. A discrete sensory level is unusual, and sphincter dysfunction occurs later in the course of the disease. It is also frequently associated with HIV dementia.[139]

Diagnosis

Vacuolar myelopathy remains a histopathologic diagnosis and, at present, is a clinical diagnosis of exclusion. CSF findings are nonspecific, and the CSF examination is often normal. MRI does not show the enhancement characteristic of acute ascending myelitis. Treatable causes of spinal cord diseases should be excluded, including myelitis due to herpesviruses or syphilis, epidural abscess, tumor, and vitamin B_{12} deficiency.[90–92]

Treatment

There is no known effective treatment, and long-term prognosis is poor.

TROPICAL SPASTIC PARAPARESIS/HTLV-I–ASSOCIATED MYELOPATHY

Epidemiology

HTLV-I is a retrovirus associated with adult T-cell leukemia and tropical spastic paraparesis/HTLV-I–associated myelopathy.[140] Asymptomatic infection is endemic in the Caribbean basin and southern Japan. In the southeastern United States, seroprevalence may be as high as 2.1%. Intravenous drug users appear to have the highest prevalence of infection. Neurologic disease occurs in less than 1% of those infected with HTLV and without concomitant HIV infection. The mean age at onset of neurologic disease is 40 to 50 years; women are more commonly affected than men are (by approximately 2.5:1).

Pathology

HTLV-I causes a chronic meningomyelitis with focal destruction of the gray matter and demyelination, located primarily in the spinal cord and especially in the thoracic portion. Capillary proliferation and perivascular cuffing of lymphocytes with demyelination and axonal loss may be seen. The posterior columns and corticospinal tracts are primarily affected. Demyelination of long presynaptic motor neurons leads to spastic paraparesis particularly in the lower limbs. Widespread inflammatory changes involve the meninges, brain stem, and white matter of the cerebrum and cerebellum. Thickening of media and adventitia of blood vessels in the subarachnoid space, cord, and brain suggests vasculitis.[141]

Clinical Features

Patients typically complain of bilateral weakness and stiffness of the lower extremities but may also complain of difficulty ambulating and pain in the back. Later in the disease, neurogenic bladder may develop. Physical examination shows spastic paraparesis, hyperreflexia, and extensor plantar reflexes. Vibratory sensation and proprioception are reduced. Typically, the disease is slowly progressive, although the upper extremities are usually not affected. Autonomic neuropathy, manifested by impotence and incontinence, is sometimes also present.

Diagnosis

The CSF may demonstrate a lymphocytic pleocytosis, elevated immunoglobulin G, and oligoclonal banding. Anti–HTLV-I antibodies are also demonstrable in the CSF. Diagnosis is established clinically in the presence of HTLV-I seropositivity in conjunction with CSF findings. Limited numbers of studies with long TR/long TE MRI of brain have identified discrete punctate and nodular foci of hyperintensity in periventricular and subcortical white matter without mass effect that are of uncertain correlation with HTLV-induced lesions. No data are available regarding visible changes in MRI of the cord.

The differential diagnosis includes multiple sclerosis, syphilitic meningomyelitis, and adhesive arachnoiditis. Because the virus is also associated with polymyositis, weakness secondary to myopathy must also be excluded. Because risk factors for HTLV-I infection overlap with HIV, patients should also be tested for coexisting HIV infection.

Treatment

High-dose steroids (prednisone at 60 mg/d for 4 weeks, then tapered for 2 weeks) may have significant benefit in some patients, especially those with concomitant myositis.[142] At present, therapeutic trials using antiviral agents have not been performed.

Postinfectious and Postvaccinial Myelitis

Myelitis has been reported after rubeola, varicella, influenza, and mumps (postinfectious) and after certain vaccines no longer in general use (postvaccinial: vaccinia virus, Pasteur-type rabbit cord rabies vaccine). These usually take the form of leukomyelitis or transverse myelitis (see Table 164–5), depending on the severity and extent of inflammatory response.[90–92]

Secondary Myelitis

Infections of Dorsal Root Ganglion and Posterior Spinal Root

The syndromes of herpes zoster and tabes dorsalis commonly involve the spinal cord and therefore represent mixed root and cord disorders (Table 164–6). Because of the multiple target sites of *T. pallidum* in the central nervous system, tabes dorsalis is discussed later under polymorphic infections.

HERPES ZOSTER (VARICELLA-ZOSTER VIRUS)

VZV causes disease of sensory nerves though its attack on the dorsal ganglia. It can also affect motor functions of cranial and peripheral nerves and is a cause of polyneuritis. In HIV-infected asymptomatic persons, zoster is usually the first opportunistic infection; in those with far-advanced disease, it can cause myelitis and encephalitis.[117–119]

Pathogenesis

After childhood varicella, VZV is thought to be sequestered and dormant in the dorsal root ganglia,[143] kept in check by cell-mediated immunity.[119, 143] Depression of cell-mediated immunity, particularly due to HIV infection or lymphoma, allows the virus to become reactivated in the dorsal ganglion, which causes the clinical syndrome of zoster or shingles, a sensory neuropathy with skin manifestations[144] (see Table 164–6).

The pathologic findings include virus replication in the dorsal ganglion and axonal transport of virus to the skin area served by the ganglion. A lymphocytic inflammatory response is common in the ganglion and CSF.[131] Frequently, inflammation extends to the adjacent spinal cord segment as well as to sensory and motor roots and their peripheral nerve, which explains the various combinations of motor and sensory findings in the zoster syndrome. In myelitis, focal demyelination and vasculitis of the cord are most severe in the dorsal root entry zone and in the posterior horn of the spinal cord segment corresponding to the dermatome of the zosteriform skin eruption. VZV is visible in oligodendrocytes and vascular lesions as Cowdry type A bodies and by immunostaining.[131]

Clinical Features

The first sign of sensory radiculitis is pain in the affected dermatome with focal cutaneous inflammation and maculopapular rash preceding the typical vesicles. The lesions are characteristically, but not exclusively, unilateral and normally limited to a single dermatome. Among 116 patients in one series,[145] the most common location of zoster was in the thoracic area (53%) followed by cervical (22%), lumbar (18%), facial (15%), and sacral (8%) locations, which closely parallel data from Adams and Victor[1(pp1124–1133)] shown in Table 164–6. Zoster involving sacral plexus outflow may produce vesicles in bladder wall mucosa and symptomatic cystitis with hematuria.

Motor deficits, when present, usually involve only the motor root from the same segment as the sensory ganglion, except in cranial neuritis in which ipsilateral nerves without sensory ganglia may be affected. Motor symptoms may be delayed and not develop until 2 weeks after onset of the rash.

Zoster may directly involve sensory ganglia of cranial nerves V, VII, VIII, IX, and X, producing the cranial syndromes shown in Tables 164–3 and 164–6. Cranial neuritis caused by VZV most commonly involves the gasserian ganglion of cranial nerve V; if the ophthalmic branch of the first division (V1) is affected, the eye is susceptible to the complications of corneal ulcer, necrotizing angiitis, and uveitis. Involvement of cranial nerve VIII produces deafness or vestibular symptoms. Multiple ipsilateral cranial nerves may be affected in geniculate ganglion zoster (Ramsay Hunt syndrome), especially cranial nerves VII, VIII, and IX (zoster oticus).

Myelitis is a rare complication that can occur in normal patients but seems to be more common in immunosuppressed patients, especially those with AIDS. In the rare instances in which brain stem or cord is extensively involved in the inflammatory response to recrudescent VZV, rapidly developing segmental paralysis may occur together with diaphragmatic paralysis, neurogenic bladder, or hypotonia, depending on the extent of cord involvement.[129–131] Presenting neurologic complaints of motor dysfunction, spinothalamic dysfunction, and posterior column dysfunction are ipsilateral to the skin eruption, which precedes onset of myelitis by 12 days, after which it progresses another 10 days to maximal deficit.[131]

Diagnosis

In most patients, the combination of dermatomal sensory disturbances followed by vesicular eruption is the primary clue to diagnosis of herpes zoster. Laboratory confirmation is usually based on immunodiagnosis of VZV in scrapings from the base of the lesions and lack of growth of HSV in cultures. Cases of VZV myelitis preceding cutaneous eruption have been described. The CSF normally contains lymphocytes with elevated protein and normal glucose levels. Virus usually cannot be recovered but is detectable with PCR. MRI demonstrates enhancement of involved nerve roots. In myelitis, focal swelling of involved spinal cord may be visible.

Treatment

Treatment is recommended for persons with facial zoster and for immunosuppressed persons. Although it is not always necessary in otherwise healthy individuals, it can be extremely helpful in reducing morbidity, provided that therapy can be started within 72 hours after the beginning of the eruption or if crops of lesions are continuing to appear. Acyclovir is the drug of choice; valacyclovir should be used only in immunocompetent persons with normal renal function.

Postherpetic neuralgia is a frequent and disabling complication. Antiviral treatment has no effect on its frequency. Controlled trials with short-course steroid therapy early during the eruption have failed to show that steroids prevent this sometimes long-term consequence of zoster.

Intraspinal Abscess and Infections of Subdural and Epidural Spaces

INTRASPINAL (INTRAMEDULLARY) ABSCESS

Causes and Pathogenesis

Intramedullary abscess is a rare condition and was usually a discovery by necropsy until the advent of MRI and computed tomography (CT) imaging technology.[146, 147] These abscesses occur most often in the thoracic segment of the cord and usually involve two or three spinal segments. Half are believed to be of hematogenous origin, the primary source being most often the respiratory tract.[146] Subacute endocarditis and vertebral osteomyelitis are frequently concomitant complications. Pathogens reported include *Staphylococcus aureus*, various streptococci, *Listeria monocytogenes*, and hematogenous larval forms of parasites (schistosomiasis and cysticercosis).[148] Intramedullary abscess may also complicate congenital dermal sinuses, which are also causes of recurrent bacterial meningitis.[149, 149a]

Clinical Features

The symptoms are indistinguishable from those of epidural abscess.[150] Because intramedullary abscess is often complicated by cerebral meningitis, bouts of meningitis with sudden onset of transverse myelitis should raise the twin possibilities of congenital dermal sinus with intramedullary abscess.

Diagnosis and Treatment

Diagnosis is usually by myelography. CT and MRI are of value, although the disease process is so rare that there is relatively little accumulated experience.[150] Treatment of suppurative abscess consists of surgical débridement and prolonged antibiotic therapy.[150a] Schistosomiasis is treated with a combination of corticosteroids and praziquantel.

SPINAL EPIDURAL ABSCESS

Cause

Although epidural abscess is a rarely diagnosed condition (0.2 to 1.2 cases per 10,000 admissions in a large tertiary care hospital), the high morbidity and mortality from this infection necessitate familiarity with its presentation, because it warrants prompt diagnosis and immediate medical and surgical attention.[151, 152, 152a] *S. aureus* has been implicated in half of the cases.[153] Other pathogens include *Escherichia coli; Pseudomonas* species; streptococci, including microaerophilic *Streptococcus milleri*[154] and anaerobic species[155]; *Salmonella typhi*[156]; coagulase-negative staphylococci[157]; *Nocardia asteroides*[158]; *Actinomyces israelii;* and *Fusobacterium necrophorum.*[155] *M. tuberculosis*[159] and fungi, especially *Aspergillus* species,[159a] remain important pathogens in immunocompromised patients.[160] Echinococcal cysts may mimic the symptoms and findings of chronic epidural abscess.[161]

Epidemiology

Until the epidemic of intravenous and injection drug use with its secondary bacteremias,[162] the most frequent primary sources of acute epidural abscess were bacteremias from skin and soft tissue infections, followed by osteomyelitis, recent spinal surgery, and respiratory tract infections.[163–166] Injection drug use has become a major risk factor for spinal epidural abscess, subdural empyema, and vertebral osteomyelitis. Nosocomial intravenous catheter–related sepsis in immunocompromised persons and infected arteriovenous shunts for chronic hemodialysis have also become important sources of these infections.[166a–166d]

Pathogenesis

Epidural abscesses are located predominantly anterior or posterior to the cord, depending on pathogenesis. Abscesses in the anterior location are commonly complications of vertebral osteomyelitis or of intervertebral disk space infections and have varying degrees of purulence and associated granulation tissue, depending on the causative organisms and host responsiveness. Posterior epidural abscesses do not normally involve bone, unless they are postsurgical. They are usually hematogenous in origin and often associated with prior trauma and possible hematoma formation or with intravenous drug use.

Clinical Features

Signs and symptoms of epidural abscess relate to the location of the abscess (cervical, thoracic, lumbar, sacral) and to the underlying cause, which influences the tempo of the process. Table 164–7 describes the findings of radicular cord and cauda equina syndromes that accompany symptomatic spinal epidural abscess.

Classically, acute disease progresses in four stages: (1) spinal ache; (2) pain; (3) weakness, bowel and bladder dysfunction; and (4) paralysis, unless the cause is recognized and treated surgically and medically.[167] Patients with acute epidural abscess may develop complete paralysis in less than 2 hours.[168] Subacute and chronic forms may follow the same sequence but during a period of weeks to months, and the pathologic findings may be dominated by granulation tissue rather than frank abscess.[169]

Diagnosis

Leukocytosis and other signs of acute infection are common in acute epidural abscess but are frequently absent in chronic cases.[163] The erythrocyte sedimentation rate is almost always uniformly elevated. CSF examination usually shows evidence of a parameningeal irritation; an elevated protein level and pleocytosis are common. CSF glucose determination, Gram stain, and culture should be normal unless the abscess is entered inadvertently.

CT with myelography will identify an extradural mass and demonstrate a block when they are present.[169] Air may be visualized in the abscess if organisms are gas forming.[170] MRI permits detection of smaller abscesses not seen by CT.[171, 172, 172a] MRI also has the advantage of avoiding one of the possible dangers of lumbar puncture preceding myelography: contamination of the subarachnoid space by inadvertent entry into abscess.[173, 174] However, if meningitis is already present, MRI may not be able to demonstrate epidural collections, whereas CT can. Further, because preexisting vertebral osteomyelitis is the source of epidural abscess in a large proportion of cases, CT is also helpful in identifying bone changes not visualized on routine spinal films. The combination of CT with MRI gives complementary information.

Treatment and Prognosis

Acute epidural abscess normally mandates simultaneous intravenous antibiotic therapy and immediate surgical decompression by bilateral laminectomy. Before cultures become available, initial therapy should include an antistaphylococcal agent (e.g., penicillinase-resistant penicillin or cephalosporin; or vancomycin if methicillin-resistant *S. aureus* or *Staphylococcus epidermidis* is a risk) and coverage for gram-negative rods (e.g., third-generation cephalosporin plus aminoglycoside) and anaerobes (e.g., metronidazole), unless tuberculous or fungal etiology is more likely. Antibiotic treatment is then adjusted on the basis of results of pretreatment blood cultures and cultures taken at operation. Therapy should continue for a minimum of 3 to 4 weeks and up to 8 weeks if there is associated osteomyelitis.

Outcome in acute epidural abscess strongly correlates with severity of neurologic involvement at the initiation of treatment, hence the importance of early diagnosis. In a review of 35 patients,[163] all those with normal neurologic function at the time of diagnosis and treatment recovered. Of 12 patients with radicular pain only, 10 recovered completely and 2 died. Of 12 patients with weakness, 6 recovered completely, 4 had residual weakness, and 2 died. Of eight patients who had paralysis, none recovered completely: four improved partially, three remained paralyzed, and one died. Functional improvement was closely related to duration of deficit; only 2 of 11 patients with weakness or paralysis lasting more than 1.5 days improved.[163] These data emphasize the crucial necessity of rapid diagnosis and surgical intervention in epidural abscess, although consideration may be given in selected instances to antibiotic treatment alone.[175, 175a, 175b]

Chronic epidural abscess and mass effect from granulation tissue are more characteristic of brucellosis and fungal and tuberculous infections, in which once the etiology is clarified, surgical intervention can be guided by the rate of progression of symptoms and signs. Unexpected reversal of long-standing myelopathic signs by judicious surgical removal of granulation tissues has been reported in tuberculous epidural masses that were unresponsive to antituberculous therapy.[176]

SPINAL SUBDURAL EMPYEMA

Causes and Pathogenesis

Spinal subdural empyema is an uncommon condition with many similarities to spinal epidural abscess in pathogenesis, microbiology, and clinical findings.[177–179] It is often a complication of retropharyngeal abscess, vertebral osteomyelitis, intravenous drug use, or surgery.[173, 180] *S. aureus, Streptococcus pneumoniae*, and *Streptococcus viridans* have been reported pathogens, although anaerobes and microaerophilic organisms should also be suspected from respiratory sources.

Diagnosis and Therapy

Diagnosis and therapy are similar to those for epidural abscess. Unlike epidural abscesses, which remain relatively localized, subdural infection tends to extend longitudinally, producing the appearance of multiple defects at myelography, a diagnostic finding highly suggestive of subdural empyema.[181–183] MRI is the most sensitive technique for diagnosis. Prognosis depends on duration and extent of neurologic impairment before initiation of combined medical and surgical therapy. Nonoperative therapy may be appropriate for certain cases.[184–186]

TABLE 164–7 ■ Secondary Myelitis Syndromes

SPINAL EPIDURAL ABSCESS OR GRANULATIONS

Syndromes of *Radicular–Spinal Cord* and *Cauda Equina* Compression

Etiology: Determined by risk factors for (1) associated original hematogenous osteomyelitis, (2) contaminated lumbar puncture needles, (3) contamination of operative field in back surgery, (4) intravenous drug use

Pathogenesis: Bacterial, fungal, mycobacterial, or parasitic infection accessing epidural space from (1) adjacent vertebral disk space or osteomyelitic vertebrae and extending secondarily into epidural space (*anterior* epidural abscess) or (2) hematogenous seeding of epidural blood clot (most commonly in *posterior* location), then encroaching on root and cord by mass effect and interference with venous return, with potential involvement of anterior spinal artery producing focal infarction

Site of Cord Compression	*Symptoms*	*Neurologic Findings*	*Diagnosis**
Radicular–spinal cord syndrome with irritative root *Between C-1 and L-1 vertebrae*	*Constitutional symptoms* Weight loss—variable Fever—variable Chills—variable *Segmental (root) symptoms initially* *Pain*—knifelike, dull ache Intensified by cough, sneeze, movement Radiates away from spine distally *Paresthesias*—same distribution *"Spinal ache"*—at site *Onset of cord signs below lesion* *Difficulty walking* *Muscle weakness* below level of lesion *Sphincteric weakness* (especially bladder)	*Local findings* in involved area of vertebral spine Limited range of motion Paravertebral muscle spasm Spine tender to palpation or percussion *Progressive segmental abnormalities* Limited to root distribution, rarely bilateral *Deep tendon reflexes:* reduced/lost *Muscle groups:* decreased tone and strength; fasciculation, then atrophy *Sensory* Pinprick, touch impaired Posterior column dysfunction: position, vibration sense Romberg sign Sensory level (pain, temperature) on trunk *Paraparesis: asymmetric spastic weakness* Arms and legs = cervical lesions Legs only = thoracolumbar lesion *Progression to paralysis*	*CSF* Protein: elevated Glucose: normal Cells: lymphocytes or PMNs, depending on cause *Culture:* negative *Pressure:* dynamic block (Queckenstedt sign) may be present *CT and MRI* Anterior lesion: epidural mass ± dislocated vertebral bone fragment Posterior lesion: epidural mass enhances with gadolinium *CT-myelography:* spinal stenosis ± block *Microbiology* Blood cultures: detect acute bacterial causes only Tissues: from operation (decompression or laminectomy) or Craig needle biopsy should be cultured for bacteria (aerobic and anaerobic), fungi, mycobacteria
Cauda equina syndrome *Between T-10 and L-1* (with mixed cord signs) *or* *Below L-1* (cord terminus)	*Legs and buttocks* *Muscle fatigue:* tiredness, weakness *Paresthesias:* on standing, walking, heavy exertion; relieved by laying down *Sphincteric dysfunction* *Pain*	*Asymmetric findings below waist* Radicular sensory loss Progressive motor loss Atrophy Areflexia Paralysis (late)	*Radiologic findings:* as above *Lumbar puncture:* may yield pus if posterior epidural abscess is as low as L3–5 level *Microbiology:* tissues from aspiration or operation (decompression or laminectomy) should be cultured for bacteria (aerobic and anaerobic), fungi, mycobacteria

*CSF, Cerebrospinal fluid; CT, computed tomography; MRI, magnetic resonance imaging; PMNs, polymorphonuclear leukocytes.

POLYMORPHIC INFECTIONS THAT AFFECT CORD, PERIPHERAL NERVES, AND CRANIAL NERVES

Causes

Several infectious agents affect two or more parts of the nervous system, producing findings in any given individual in which disorders of the PNS, cord, or brain may dominate or in which all three are sequentially or simultaneously involved to different degrees. Normal hosts infected by either of two spirochetes, *B. burgdorferi* and *T. pallidum*, frequently have polymorphic involvement of the nervous system, whereas symptomatic invasion of the nervous system by *Brucella* species and *M. pneumoniae* is rare. Other organisms of note not discussed here, but which in normal hosts infrequently involve the PNS, cord, or brain, are *Chlamydia* (psittacosis)[187] and the agents of louse-borne[188, 189] and tick-borne relapsing fever[190, 191] and murine typhus.[192] Both normal and immunosuppressed persons are susceptible to polymorphic infections by VZV. In severely immunosuppressed hosts, polymorphism is particularly characteristic of opportunistic infections by several herpesviruses, as discussed before.

This section focuses on patterns of polymorphic infections seen in normal hosts.

NEUROBORRELIOSIS (LYME BORRELIOSIS)

Cause

Lyme disease, caused by the spirochete *B. burgdorferi*, was initially recognized after an outbreak in Old Lyme, Connecticut. It was subsequently recognized that *B. burgdorferi* infection can result in acute and chronic peripheral neuropathies as well as in other neurologic patterns, leading to its designation as the great imitator.[193–203]

Epidemiology

B. burgdorferi is distributed worldwide and is transmitted from rodent to humans by tick bite. Neuroborreliosis has increased to become the most frequent arthropod-borne infection in North America and Europe. The tick vectors and genotypes of *B. burgdorferi* vary geographically. Genotypic variants may have different phenotypic expressions in infected humans. The hard tick *Ixodes ricinus*, the vector for *B. burgdorferi* in Sweden, is most abundant in the southern and central parts of Sweden, where there are an estimated 2000 cases of Lyme borreliosis annually. Seroprevalence surveys in Sweden indicate that many persons have asymptomatic infections, because although risk for positive serologic responses in the endemic areas increased with age and ranged from 7% to 29%, only 1% to 21% reported having had symptoms consistent with clinical disease. By contrast, symptomatic disease was 2.5 times more frequent than asymptomatic infection in an endemic area of southeastern Connecticut, where a prospective study of 410 teenagers found the incidence of asymptomatic infection and clinical Lyme disease to be, respectively, 3.8 and 10.1 cases per 1000 person-years.

In 1994, 13,083 cases of Lyme disease were reported to CDC by 44 state health departments, with highest incidences ranging from 15 to 62 per 100,000 population in Delaware, New Jersey, New York, Rhode Island, and Connecticut.[203a] However, the risk for exposure can be highly focused, as illustrated by the location of the county with the highest incidence (1197.6): Nantucket, Massachusetts. Because human infection with *B. burgdorferi* results from exposure to nymphal and adult forms of *Ixodes* species, risk in the United States correlates with the prevalence of black-legged tick vectors, *Ixodes scapularis* in the northeastern and upper north-central states and *Ixodes pacificus* in the Pacific coastal states. Prevalence of tick infection with *B. burgdorferi* can reach 15% in endemic areas for Lyme disease.[203a]

Prevention

The risk for infection in areas endemic for Lyme disease can be reduced by avoidance of known tick habitats and by proper protection when in areas of risk, such as wearing long-sleeved shirts and long pants, tucking pants into socks, applying tick repellants to clothing and exposed skin, checking regularly and thoroughly for ticks, and promptly removing any attached ticks.[203a] A vaccine is in clinical trials.

The efficacy of chemoprophylaxis given shortly after a presumed tick bite and using limited doses of long-acting drugs, such as doxycycline, has not yet been determined, but observational studies to date show that erythema migrans does not develop frequently enough to warrant routine chemoprophylaxis.[203b]

Treatment of early Lyme disease presenting as erythema migrans is effective in preventing progression to neurologic disease. Erythema migrans may precede symptomatic neuroborreliosis and is frequently accompanied by nonspecific viral-like symptoms, particularly fatigue (54%), myalgia (44%), arthralgia (44%), headache (42%), and fever and/or chills (39%). In the 50% of patients without specific antibodies at presentation, treatment must be presumptive; most of these will progress to seropositivity within the first month.[203b] Erythema migrans must be distinguished from streptococcal and staphylococcal cellulitis, hypersensitivity to arthropod bites, plant dermatitis, tinea, and granuloma annulare. History of a tick bite should lead to consideration of other tick-borne diseases in endemic areas, such as Rocky Mountain spotted fever, babesiosis, ehrlichiosis, and in Europe tick-borne encephalitis.[203b]

Oral therapy for 14 days[203b] to 28 days[204] is recommended for uncomplicated erythema migrans. Doxycycline at 100 mg twice daily or amoxacillin at 500 mg three times daily is preferred, but penicillin VK at 500 mg four times daily and tetracycline at 500 mg four times daily are less expensive and apparently equally effective alternatives.[203b] Evidence of extracutaneous disease, characterized by advanced heart block, arthritis refractory to oral antibiotics, or neurologic disease other than cranial nerve VII palsy, is presumed to require intravenous treatment for 2 to 3 weeks, as indicated later. For this reason, some authorities recommend CSF examination in all patients with isolated cranial nerve VII palsy.[204]

Pathogenesis

Neuroborreliosis has been well studied in the adult rhesus macaque, which provides a highly predictable model for neuroborreliosis after cutaneous inoculation of a highly infective strain of *B. burgdorferi*.[204] Erythema migrans first appears at the inoculation site at 1 to 2 weeks, followed at weeks 3 to 4 by appearance of detectable serum antibody and spirochetemia. CNS invasion occurs predictably within 1 month and consists of CSF pleocytosis, elevated protein level, and intrathecally produced specific antibody to *B. burgdorferi*.

C3H/HeNCrIBR mice reproducibly develop persistent infection and have been used to study the efficacy of different antibiotics in eradicating the spirochetes.[205]

Clinical Features

The primary disease is characterized by an early skin lesion called erythema chronicum migrans, which develops at the site of a tick bite in days to 1 month (median, 7 to 10 days). Multiple skin lesions occur in 20%.[206] Several weeks to months thereafter, the second stage of neurologic and cardiac manifestations occurs.[201] The later third stage is marked by arthritis. Instances of neurologic disease without initial skin lesions have been recorded.[202] The spirochete invades the eye early but remains dormant until later onset of keratitis and neuroretinitis.[203]

Acute disseminated disease is usually characterized by peripheral and cranial neuropathies, with or without meningoencephalitis, and normally occurs within 4 to 12 weeks after tick bite.[197] Acute infection may also present as myelitis.[198–200] Unilateral or bilateral facial palsies, the result of chronic basilar meningitis, are the most frequent neurologic manifestations and may be seen in 50% of patients.[51, 204] The most common findings in one series were aseptic meningitis (89%), encephalitis (29%), unilateral facial palsy (32%), bilateral facial palsy (18%), abducens nerve palsy (3%), and peripheral neuropathy (32%). Peripheral nerve involvement is typically asymmetric and usually presents as a motor, sensory, or mixed radiculoneuropathy expressed in patterns of mononeuropathy multiplex and radiculitis. Brachial radiculitis and crural radiculitis, also called plexitis, cause paralysis of muscles in arms and legs, respectively. In contrast to Guillain-Barré syndrome, paralysis due to plexitis of neuroborreliosis is usually accompanied by sensory loss.

Months to years after infection, chronic Lyme borreliosis can cause intermittent distal paresthesias and radicular pain. Physical examination findings may be normal, but nerve conduction studies demonstrate axonal neuropathy.

Differential Diagnosis

Other infectious causes of the neurologic syndromes associated with neuroborreliosis include the known causes of Guillain-Barré syndrome (see earlier), Bell palsy (see Table 164–3), and HIV-associated disorders (see Table 164–2).

Diagnosis

The CSF formula is that of an aseptic meningitis, with lymphocytosis, increased protein level, and normal glucose value. Proof of diagnosis and determination of stage of disease have been evaluated by several groups. Acute disease is characterized by elevated CSF cell count with predominance of T lymphocytes, large numbers of plasma cells and immunoglobulin M–positive B lymphocytes, *B. burgdorferi*–specific immunoglobulin M antibody by enzyme-linked immunosorbent assay, and a high specific antibody index (ratio of CSF titers to blood, corrected for albumin content).[207, 208] The CSF of untreated past disease, by contrast, contains immunoglobulin G–bearing B cells and immunoglobulin G–specific antibody.

Presumptive diagnosis of active neuroborreliosis may be based on clinical and epidemiologic criteria, following recommendations from the American Academy of Neurology.[208a] Specific diagnosis of early or late-stage prior infection is made most reliably by serology, as culture and current molecular identification methods are relatively insensitive.[208b] Positive CSF antibody is almost universal in patients with Lyme meningitis.[204] A completely normal CSF is strong evidence against the diagnosis of Lyme meningitis or encephalomyelitis.[204, 208c]

Serologic diagnosis requires initial testing with a sensitive screening assay, either an enzyme immunoassay or immunofluorescent assay, followed by standardized Western blot testing for recognition of *B. burgdorferi* antigens by immunoglobulins M and G. Patients with suspected disease in the early stages (first 4 weeks of symptoms) but negative serology should be retested, and acute and convalescent sera run in parallel. Sera from persons with disseminated disease or late-stage disease almost always have a strong immunoglobulin G–specific immune response.[208d] Those with high antibody titers at the time of diagnosis will remain seropositive for years, even after a clinical response to treatment.[204]

Patients with disseminated disease may have anicteric hepatitis, splenomegaly, and an associated myositis visible by gallium Ga 67 nuclear imaging and located near an involved joint or localized neuropathy.[209]

Treatment

Neurologic disease should probably be treated with intravenous antibiotics, except that oral antibiotics have generally been used for facial palsy with a normal CSF. In endemic areas, Bell facial palsy with a history of tick bite is sufficient to warrant empirical therapy, even in the absence of meningitis.[52, 210]

Current recommendations for optimal treatment of neuroborreliosis vary according to duration of infection (acute versus chronic disease); differences among antibiotics in their dosage, route of administration, penetration of CSF and brain, and efficacy in eradicating infection; duration of treatment; and length and type of follow-up. On the basis of experience with neurosyphilis, intravenous antibiotic therapy for 2 to 3 weeks is recommended for treatment of Lyme meningitis, meningoradiculitis, and other neurologic complications.[204, 208a] The optimal intravenous regimen has not been defined, but currently recommended agents are cephalosporins (ceftriaxone, 1 g every 12 hours or cefotaxime, 6 g/d in divided doses) or penicillin G (4 million units every 4 hours). Oral doxycycline (100 mg twice daily) for 2 weeks has also been reported to be successful.[204, 208c, 211] One randomized controlled study of 54 neuroborreliosis patients in Sweden showed 14 days of treatment with oral doxycycline or intravenous penicillin G to be equivalent and without treatment failures.[211]

Symptomatic response to therapy is slow and may take weeks, even after completion of antibiotic treatment. The most common cause of treatment failure is incorrect diagnosis, particularly in seronegative patients. In general, 86% of patients with facial palsy achieve complete recovery. Prognosis can be predicted with nerve conduction studies[51] and correlates with whether the nerve lesion is demyelinative or axonopathic, with demyelination conferring a favorable outcome.[210] Steroids do not appear to hasten resolution of facial palsy.

NEUROBRUCELLOSIS

Cause

Brucella melitensis, Brucella abortus, and *Brucella suis* are all capable of producing neurologic disease in humans.[212–214] *Brucella* organisms can also cause spondylitis,[215] which may progress to epidural abscess.[216]

Epidemiology

Brucellosis exists worldwide and is especially prevalent in countries of the Mediterranean basin, Arabian Gulf, Indian subcontinent, and parts of Mexico and Central and South America. Occupational risk for human brucellosis is primarily related to the livestock industry (ranchers, dairy farmers, veterinarians, abattoir workers).[217] Food-borne transmission results from consumption of unpasteurized infected dairy products from areas of enzootic *B. melitensis*, especially camel's milk and milk cheeses from goat and sheep. The incubation period after exposure is 2 to 3 weeks. Hence, travelers and immigrants may develop symptoms only after returning from endemic areas.[218]

Pathology

A systemic infection, brucellosis can involve any organ of the body.[214] *Brucella* species replicate intracellularly in macrophages and monocytes; are widely distributed in the reticuloendothelial system; and may be associated with inflammatory lesions in liver, spleen, lymph nodes, bone marrow, joints, and epididymis. The type of inflammatory response evoked varies from granulomata to abscess formation, depending on the infecting species. *B. abortus* characteristically elicits a sarcoid-like noncaseating, epithelioid granuloma and *B. melitensis* a more heterologous response, including a loose granuloma. *B. suis* is associated with abscess formation, which commonly occurs in liver and spleen. Leukoclastic vasculitis, thrombocytopenia, and splenomegaly are common findings in children with brucellosis.

In neurobrucellosis, the intrathecal roots of cranial nerves and spinal roots may be invaded by granulomatous reactions, producing radiculopathy and polyneuritis that commonly involve the lumbosacral roots.[219] Direct involvement of the CNS results in encephalitis or myelitis. Myelopathy typically involves the corticospinal tracts and produces a pure upper motor neuron syndrome without sensory findings. Vasculitis may result in infarction and formation of mycotic aneurysms.

Clinical Features

Approximately 2% to 5% of patients with brucellosis develop a wide array of neurologic complications, often with considerable clinical overlap.[220] Neurologic involvement is often subacute or chronic and encompasses encephalitis, myelitis, meningitis, and radiculitis. Meningitis is the most common neurologic presentation and may result in cranial nerve palsies and vasculitis. Intracerebral mycotic aneurysms may be complicated by stroke and intracerebral hemorrhage.

Diagnosis

The CSF usually reveals a lymphocytic pleocytosis, elevated protein level, and hypoglycorrhachia, comparable to findings in fungal and mycobacterial meningitis.[214] Specific antibodies are detectable in CSF with the serum agglutination test. When CSF is cultured without special provision for isolation of fastidious organisms, CSF cultures are positive in less than 50% of cases.

Presumptive diagnosis of systemic brucellosis is based on rising titers of specific antibody in the serum, generally assessed with the serum agglutination test, together with fractionation of any specific antibody into immunoglobulin M and immunoglobulin G components. False-negative results due to the prozone phenomenon can occur in infection by *B. melitensis*, *B. abortus*, and *B. suis* if the serum agglutination test is performed on inadequately diluted, high-titered serum (above 1:160). A falsely negative serum agglutination test result will also occur on the rare occasion when the infecting agent is *Brucella canis*, which cannot be detected by the serum agglutination test.

Proof of diagnosis requires isolation of *Brucella* species from blood, bone marrow, liver, or other tissue. Cultures of blood and tissue fluids may become positive in 2 to 4 days with modern automated liquid culture systems, particularly when specimens are first processed to release intracellular organisms.[221] Otherwise, incubation may be prolonged (14 to 21 days) with nonradiometric liquid culture detection systems[222, 223] and more than 4 weeks with enriched solid media (*Brucella* agar). The laboratory receiving specimens for culture should be alerted to the provisional diagnosis to avoid misidentification of isolates as *Branhamella (Moraxella)* or *Haemophilus* species and because *Brucella* species constitute an important biohazard for laboratory-acquired infections.[224]

Treatment

Treatment is with antibiotics alone, unless there is a symptomatic epidural abscess, in which case surgical exploration and decompression may be advisable. Prolonged antibiotic treatment is necessary to avoid relapse.

Antibiotic treatment of brucellosis currently consists of multidrug therapy. Established therapies incorporate a tetracycline (tetracycline HCl, 500 mg four times daily or doxycycline, 100 mg twice daily) with a second drug, which is either an aminoglycoside (streptomycin, 1 g/d intramuscularly, or gentamicin, 1.5 mg/kg every 8 hours intravenously, for 2 to 3 weeks) or rifampin (600 to 900 mg/d throughout). Standard treatment for uncomplicated brucellosis is 6 weeks of antibiotics. Doxycycline-streptomycin may be superior to doxycycline-rifampin in the treatment of spondylitis.[224a] For meningitis or other CNS involvement, there is no uniform treatment due to the lack of controlled studies. Common practice is three-drug therapy with a tetracycline, aminoglycoside, and rifampin, with or without trimethoprim-sulfamethoxazole, with duration of treatment 2 to 4 months.[220] Ceftriaxone has been recommended as alternative therapy during pregnancy.[220] Adjunctive use of steroids early in meningitis may reduce complications resulting from immune vasculitis.[220]

NEUROSYPHILIS

Pathogenesis

Spirochetemia and dissemination occur in every instance of *T. pallidum* infection.[224b] Hence, any organ can become infected. In at least 40% of secondary syphilis cases, the CNS is invaded. Because of inadequate drug concentrations, viable spirochetes may not be eradicated by low-dose antibiotic treatment in those with infections of the CNS or the eye.[224b] Unlike immunocompetent individuals whose immune systems may successfully eradicate residual infection, immunologically dysfunctional persons may permit more aggressive or chronic infection and thus are more likely to develop disease in these organs even after treatment for early syphilis.[224b]

Obliterative endarteritis, a consequence of the tropism of *T. pallidum* for arterioles, accounts for the progressive microscopic tissue destruction, with associated lesions of the aorta, cerebral vessels, and micro- and macroscopic infarctions of neural tissues.[224b]

Pathology

Four types of spinal cord involvement are associated with *T. pallidum* infections: (1) tabes dorsalis, a form of chronic meningoradiculitis that affects the posterior root predominantly; (2) syphilitic meningomyelitis (often called Erb spastic paraplegia), a chronic fibrosing meningitis in which myelinated fibers are lost owing to bilateral involvement of the corticospinal tract; (3) anterior spinal artery syndrome caused by meningovascular syphilis; and (4) gummata of the spinal meninges and cord.[225, 226] Because of its varied pathogenesis, syphilis should be considered in the differential diagnosis of nearly all diseases of the spinal cord.[227, 228]

Clinical Features

There are three clinical patterns of CNS involvement: (1) asymptomatic neurosyphilis (abnormal CSF only), (2) acute syphilitic meningitis, and (3) symptomatic neurosyphilis. Findings in symptomatic neurosyphilis are classified as (1) meningovascular manifestations (seizures and/or focal neurologic signs due to multiple microscopic infarcts in the cortex and cord, (2) behavioral abnormalities (dementia, general paresis, and temporal lobe or amygdala dysfunction, resulting from infarcts and/or parenchymatous disease), (3) abnormalities of spinal cord function due to tabes dorsalis and myelopathy, (4) hearing loss (often unilateral, due to cranial nerve VIII damage and/or labyrinthitis[228a, 228b]), and (5) ophthalmologic manifestations. Involvement of the eye is common among patients whose CNS has been invaded by *T. pallidum*, especially those concomitantly infected by HIV or receiving corticosteroids. Anterior uveitis is most common, followed by posterior uveitis, chorioretinitis, and optic atrophy. Blurred vision is the most common symptom.[224b]

The clinical features of tabes dorsalis include lightning (lancinating) pains, especially in the legs and repetitive for hours to days; broad-based gait with flinging movements of legs (sensory ataxia); visceral crises (e.g., epigastric pain, nausea and vomiting); and urinary incontinence. Neurologic findings include absent knee and ankle reflexes; impaired vibration and position sense in feet and legs; a positive Romberg test response; intact muscle power and mass; abnormal pupils in 90% (e.g., Argyll Robertson), ptosis, variable ophthalmoplegia, optic atrophy; insensitive hypotonic bladder with overflow incontinence; megacolon; secondary trophic ulcers; and advanced osteoarthritis in hips, knees, and ankles (Charcot joints, 1% to 10%).

Diagnosis

Diagnosis is by evidence of active infection in the CNS (pleocytosis in CSF, usually with positive VDRL test result), together with serologic evidence of prior syphilis (positive results of *T. pallidum* hemagglutination or treponemal fluorescent antibody tests). The CSF usually shows a lymphocytic pleocytosis, elevated protein level, and normal glucose value. The CSF VDRL test is specific but generally insensitive. More recently, testing CSF for local production of antitreponema antibody has been advocated.[228c] PCR and immunoglobulin M immunoblotting are both sensitive and specific but are not widely available.[228d] The intrathecal *T. pallidum* antibody index is a ratio comparing CSF and serum immunoglobulin G levels and is more widely used.[228e, 228f]

Neuroradiologic studies with MRI, although relatively insensitive in recognizing meningovascular syphilis involving the cord, may demonstrate cerebral infarcts, nonspecific white matter lesions, and meningeal enhancement. Magnetic resonance angiography or conventional angiography can detect arteritis in large vessels but does not disclose the small vessel obliterative endarteritis characteristic of syphilitic leptomeningitis.[228c]

Treatment

Neurosyphilis and syphilitic eye disease in HIV-infected patients generally appear to respond as well to standard intravenous penicillin regimens (12 to 24 million units/d for 10 to 14 days) as disease in HIV-negative patients. Both HIV-positive and -negative groups may relapse after standard treatments.[228g] Recommended alternative nonintravenous penicillin-related regimens include: (1) procaine penicillin G (2 to 4 million units/d intramuscularly) plus probenecid (500 mg orally four times daily) for 10 to 14 days; (2) benzathine penicillin G (4.8 million units/wk) for 3 weeks; and (3) amoxacillin (3 g/d orally twice daily) and probenecid (500 mg orally twice daily) for 15 days. Penicillin-allergic patients without history of anaphylaxis may receive ceftriaxone (1 g/d intravenously) for 14 days,[224b, 228g] or oral therapy with doxycycline (100 mg orally twice daily) for 21 days. There are limited data on the efficacy of oral regimens in HIV-positive patients with neurosyphilis.

The response to treatment is judged by peripheral blood serology and CSF abnormalities and, except for syphilitic meningitis, not by reversal of clinical findings, which may be permanent due to the common vascular nature of the injuries. Most HIV-negative patients with neurosyphilis resolve all CSF and serum abnormalities by 30 weeks.[228h] High, persistent nontreponemal titers and slower peripheral blood serologic responses to treatment of early and late syphilis distinguish HIV-infected patients from uninfected patients.[224b, 228g, 228i] HIV-infected patients may also have higher relapse rates after standard therapy, although it can be difficult to distinguish relapse from reinfection.[228g, 228j] CSF abnormalities are slower to reverse.[228h] Follow-up of CSF for at least 2 years after normalization is recommended.[228h]

Close posttreatment follow-up of syphilis reaginic antibodies in serum and CSF is warranted, because HIV infection regardless of $CD4^+$ cell count may contribute to an unacceptably high number of treatment failures.[229]

NEUROLOGIC SYNDROMES ASSOCIATED WITH *MYCOPLASMA* INFECTION

Cause

CNS complications of *M. pneumoniae* infection are probably the most frequent extrapulmonary manifestation of this disease but are rare.[230] Although encephalitis is the most common neurologic complication, meningitis, polyradiculitis, and myelitis have also been reported.[231, 232]

Pathogenesis

The exact pathogenesis of CNS disease is unknown but may be secondary to direct invasion, elaboration of neurotoxins, autoimmune complexes, or vasculitis.

Diagnosis

A history of recent or concurrent respiratory tract infection, especially in a child or young adult, should suggest the diagnosis.[233] Serologic diagnosis requires a fourfold increase in antibody titer in paired sera or a single titer greater than 1:64. Acute titers may in fact be greater than convalescent levels, because neurologic disease may present several weeks after respiratory symptoms have resolved. Standard complement fixation assays for *M. pneumoniae* are nonspecific and can cross-react with a variety of other antigens. More specific tests for *Mycoplasma* are not yet widely available.

Treatment

If active infection is present, antibiotic therapy may be effective. Tetracycline penetrates the CNS more effectively than erythromycin does but is contraindicated in young children. Steroids and plasmapheresis have also been advocated but remain controversial. About 15% of patients have a poor outcome with little or no improvement in neurologic deficits.

WHIPPLE'S DISEASE

Cause

Whipple's disease is a systemic illness characterized by fever, systemic lymphadenopathy, malabsorption, and variable neurologic manifestations.[234] Considered infectious in nature and usually responsive to antibiotic therapy, the causative agent has not yet been cultivated in vitro, although with electron microscopy it can be seen intracellularly in macrophages within the diagnostic periodic acid–Schiff–positive material. Molecular techniques have been used to identify and speciate a proposed agent, *Tropheryma whippelii*, which by ribosomal RNA sequence and phylogenetic analysis is consistent with a gram-positive actinomycete.[235] The pathogenesis of associated focal cranial and peripheral neuropathies is not clear, because periodic acid–Schiff–positive material has been found only in the CNS[236] and not in peripheral nerve biopsy specimens.

Clinical Features

Several neuropathic syndromes may accompany Whipple's disease, including instances of peripheral neuropathy preceding other signs of the disease.[237] Other neurologic manifestations include progressive dementia, myoclonus of face and arms, ophthalmoplegia, nystagmus, and ataxia. The associated polyneuropathy is possibly related to vitamin deficiencies secondary to malabsorption.

Diagnosis and Treatment

Diagnosis is suggested by diarrhea, weight loss, and lymphadenopathy and, until recently, proved by finding periodic acid–Schiff–positive macrophages in jejunal biopsy material. Molecular probes have been used to detect Whipple's agent in blood and other fluids as well as in tissues.[238, 239] In a biopsy proven case of Whipple's disease with dementia, multiple lesions in white matter and in the gray-white matter junction were seen with gadolinium-enhanced MRI.[240]

Diagnosis and treatment of Whipple's disease are discussed in Chapter 84.

APPROACH TO THE PATIENT

The cardinal features that distinguish disorders affecting peripheral nerve, plexus, root, and cord from symptoms and signs resulting from cerebral lesions are

1. Distribution and nature of abnormal sensations, when present
2. Hyporeflexia or areflexia in the presence of weakness, or flaccid paralysis, which is characteristic of all plexus, nerve, and root lesions but occurs only in the initial stages of cord injury ("spinal shock")
3. Distribution and nature of abnormal tendon reflexes

Distribution of Motor Function Abnormalities

Examination of motor function should answer the following questions.

Symmetry. Is the weakness or paralysis symmetric or asymmetric? If it is asymmetric, is there evidence of bilateral lesions (crossover)?

Distribution. Is the weakness or paralysis distal or generalized ("systemic")? If it is generalized, did its onset begin in the lower extremities (ascending) or initially with bulbar signs (descending)? If it is ascending, is there evidence of involvement of the trunk, the neck, and the muscles of respiration?

Anatomic Correlations. If distal, does weakness or paralysis follow anatomic patterns compatible with a spinal segment (or adjacent segments) or root, a plexus (brachial or crural), the cauda equina, or a peripheral or cranial nerve or its branches?

Reflex and Autonomic Function. What are the activity levels (absent, depressed, normal, hyperactive) of deep tendon reflexes and other reflex responses (Babinski response to noxious stimuli; anogenital and abdominal responses to cutaneous stimuli)? Is there sphincter dysfunction or paralysis of bladder or bowel?

Spasticity or Flaccidity. Is there evidence of denervation (e.g., fasciculation, atrophy, or fatigue on repetitive effort)?

Distribution and Type of Sensory Abnormalities

Somatic sensory symptoms (pain versus numbness and anesthesia; dysesthesias, such as tingling, numbness, burning) may be the only abnormality reported by the patient in the early phase of several disorders and may precede objectively demonstrable sensory loss. In such cases, diminished or absent deep tendon reflexes in the same distribution as sensory symptoms may be the only objective neurologic finding despite disabling symptoms.

Examination should separately evaluate responses to light touch (cotton wisp), pain (pinprick), temperature (cold or hot), and proprioception (vibration, joint position, Romberg) and answer the following questions.

Presence or Absence of Sensory Involvement. Is sensation normal by history and examination?

Distribution of Objective Findings. If the patient is symptomatic, are objective abnormalities present? If so, are all modalities affected or only selective defects? Do they match the distribution of symptoms? Do they match the distribution of any motor weakness or paralysis?

Symmetry. Are the symptoms and signs symmetric or asymmetric? Are they distal or generalized? If they are generalized, are they ascending or descending? If they are symmetric, is there a sensory level on the trunk?

Pain Evaluation. Is pain one of the sensory symptoms? Are there predictable aggravating factors (certain movements; percussion or palpation tenderness over focal areas of the spine), or is the pain constant or unpredictably intermittent?

Anatomic Correlation. Does the distribution of pain or sensory defect follow anatomic patterns compatible with a cranial or spinal segment or root, a plexus, the cauda equina, the conus medullaris, or a peripheral or cranial nerve or its branches?

Associated Skin and Mucous Membrane Findings. Are there skin lesions in the area of abnormal sensation (macules,[5] vesicles; trophic changes; ulcers)? If complaints are of a painful unilateral cranial neuropathy, do those areas served by the nerve contain ipsilateral cutaneous vesicles (scalp, face, external auditory canal) or mucosal ulcerations (conjunctiva, tongue, palate, pharynx) that do not cross the midline?

Figure 164–3 uses the answers to these questions in the evaluation of a patient as an example of application of the neurologic data to determine possible infection-related causes of the syndrome.

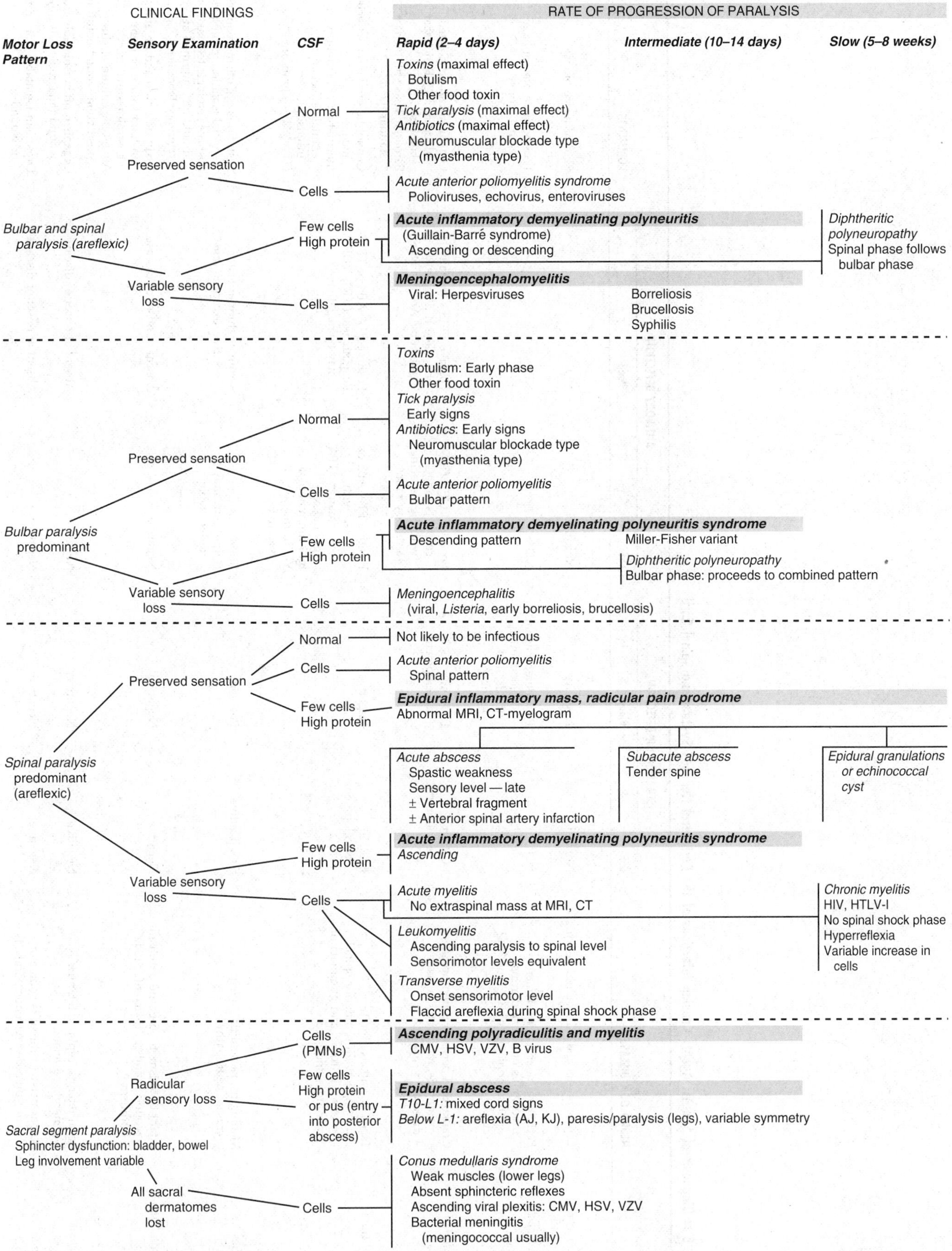

FIGURE 164–3 □ Evaluation of patient with bilateral symmetric weakness or paralysis for possible infection-related cause. CSF, Cerebrospinal fluid; MRI, magnetic resonance imaging; CT, computed tomography; HIV, human immunodeficiency virus; HTLV-I, human T-cell lymphotropic virus type I; PMNs, polymorphonuclear leukocytes; CMV, cytomegalovirus; HSV, herpes simplex virus; VZV, varicella-zoster virus; AJ, ankle jerk; KJ, knee jerk.

TABLE 164–8 ■ Diagnosis of Specific Agents Causing Infections of the Peripheral Nervous System and Spinal Cord

ORGANISM	NEUROLOGIC DISEASE	ISOLATION OR DETECTION		ANTIBODY DETECTION		COMMENTS
		CSF	Blood	CSF	Blood	
Mycobacteria						
Mycobacterium leprae	Lepromatous and tuberculoid neuritis	Normal	Negative	Negative	ND	Skin or nerve biopsy
Actinomycetes						
Tropheryma whippelii	Peripheral neuropathy, dementia, myoclonus of face and arms, ophthalmoplegia, nystagmus, and ataxia	PCR: in development	PCR detects agent in blood, other fluids, and tissues	ND	ND	PAS-positive macrophages in jejunal biopsy
Spirochetes						
Borrelia burgdorferi	Cranial and peripheral neuropathies, meningitis, radiculitis in acute disease	PCR: in development	PCR: in development	Positive ELISA (IgM converts to IgG) with high specific antibody ratio	Positive ELISA (usually IgG) by stage II disease) Confirm by Western blot	Organism can be isolated from blood and CSF in research laboratories Serologic tests still being standardized
Treponema pallidum	Tabes dorsalis, syphilitic meningomyelitis, anterior spinal artery syndrome, and gummata of meninges and cord	PCR: in development	Negative	Positive FTA-ABS or TPHA, with confirmatory ITPA IgG index IgM immunoblot VDRL may be negative	Positive FTA-ABS or TPHA Reaginic test (ART, VDRL) may be negative	Cannot be grown on artificial media Inoculation of laboratory animals effective but insensitive ITPA ≥3 is significant[224b]
Bacteria						
Brucella species	Meningitis, radiculitis, myelitis, cranial neuropathy	50% positive	Positive	ELISA positive Agglutinins may be undetectable	Serum agglutinin test is positive, except *B. canis*	Fastidious organism: requires special isolation techniques Positive serologic test results should be confirmed at reference laboratory
Clostridium botulinum	Infant botulism, food-borne botulism, wound botulism, toxicoinfectious botulism	Negative	Negative	Negative	Absent at onset of disease	Toxin detection and organism in food source or from gastrointestinal tract Anaerobic culture of site positive in wound botulism
Clostridium tetani	Local tetanus, cephalic tetanus, generalized tetanus	Negative	Negative	Negative	Absent at onset of disease	Organism often isolatable from wound (anaerobic culture)
Corynebacterium diphtheriae	Bulbar palsy (if throat is source of toxin) precedes systemic paralysis	Negative	Negative	Negative	Absent at onset of disease	Organism isolatable from throat or wound

Mycoplasma						
Mycoplasma pneumoniae	Encephalitis, meningitis, polyradiculitis, and myelitis	ND	ND	ND	Fourfold increase in antibody titer in paired sera or a single titer greater than 1:64	Complement fixation assays for *M. pneumoniae* are nonspecific and can cross-react with a variety of other antigens Acute titers may be greater than convalescent levels, because neurologic disease occurs weeks after respiratory symptoms
Enteroviruses						
Poliovirus	Aseptic meningitis, bulbar or spinal paralysis (poliomyelitis)	Low yield	Negative	Positive	Positive rise in type-specific neutralization titer	Virus is isolatable from stool and throat washings
Herpesviruses						
B virus	Aseptic meningitis, ascending encephalomyelitis	Low yield PCR under development	Negative	Positive before serum	ELISA with Western blot or RIA	Virus isolation is dangerous! Isolatable from wound site or mucous membranes and pustules
CMV	Radiculitis, ascending myelitis, acute transverse myelitis, encephalitis	Low yield PCR under development	Viral antigen detectable by FAB PCR under development	ND	Positive rise unless severely immunosuppressed	Virus isolatable from buffy coat of peripheral blood cells in chronic disseminated CMV CSF cytology positive in some cases
EBV	Radiculitis, ascending myelitis, acute transverse myelitis	Low yield PCR under development	ND	ND	Positive rise unless severely immunosuppressed	EBV expressed in AIDS-associated B-cell lymphomas of central nervous system
HSV-1 and HSV-2	Radiculitis, ascending myelitis, acute transverse myelitis, encephalitis	Low yield PCR under development	ND	ND	Positive rise unless severely immunosuppressed	Virus isolatable from skin lesions Skin scraping/biopsy positive for immunodiagnosis
VZV	Radiculitis, ascending myelitis, acute transverse myelitis, cranial neuritis, encephalitis	Low yield PCR under development	ND	ND	Positive rise unless severely immunosuppressed	Skin scraping/biopsy positive for immunodiagnosis
Retroviruses						
HIV-1	*Early:* aseptic meningitis, cranial neuropathies, Guillain-Barré syndrome *Late:* sensory neuropathy, mononeuropathy multiplex, vacuolar myelopathy	Early: p24 antigen and vRNA Late: variable	Positive cultures from PBMs Plasma vRNA	Early: rising ELISA titer Late: low-level titers	Positive ELISA and confirmatory test	HIV-1 isolatable from CSF of some asymptomatic persons $CD4^+$ cell count correlates with stage of disease
HTLV-I	Chronic meningitis, spastic paraparesis	PCR under development	Positive cultures from PBMs	Oligoclonal banding ELISA and Western blot positive	ELISA and Western blot positive	

*AIDS, Acquired immunodeficiency syndrome; ART, automated reagin test; CSF, cerebrospinal fluid; EBV, Epstein-Barr virus; ELISA, enzyme-linked immunosorbent assay; FAB, fluorescent antibody; FTA-ABS, fluorescent treponemal antibody absorption; HIV, human immunodeficiency virus; HSV, herpes simplex virus; HTLV-I, human T-cell lymphotropic virus; IgG, immunoglobulin G; IgM, immunoglobulin M; ITPA, intrathecal *T. pallidum* antibody index; ND, not detectable; PAS, periodic acid–Schiff; PBMs, peripheral blood mononuclear cells; PCR, polymerase chain reaction; RIA, radioimmunoassay; TPHA, *T. pallidum* hemagglutination; VDRL, Venereal Disease Research Laboratory test; VZV, varicella-zester virus.

Clues to Neuropathy

Neuropathy refers to injury to one or more nerves at any level along their pathways and is termed cranial or peripheral on the basis of the nerve involved. When the level of nerve injury is proximal, the pathogenic process usually involves nerve roots and sensory ganglia. It may also extend to involve adjacent CNS structures, producing overlap syndromes in which peripheral neuropathy accompanies myelitis or meningitis.

Causes of neuropathy—both infectious and noninfectious—often prefer one of four anatomic patterns, as described in Table 164–1, and are further classified on the basis of the type of functional nerve involvement: purely motor, sensory, or autonomic or mixed with one functional type predominating. Whereas motor dysfunction is the most obvious sign of peripheral nerve disease, sensory disturbances often herald its onset. When the level of nerve injury is proximal, involving nerve roots, dorsal ganglia, or the course of the nerve within the subarachnoid space, the composition of the CSF will usually reflect the method of injury.

In classifying the neuropathy, the physical examination should attempt to answer the following questions: Does the involvement include more than one functional nerve type? Is involvement symmetric or asymmetric, distal or generalized, ascending or descending? Is there a sensory level on the trunk? Do motor and sensory deficits overlap and do they match subjective complaints? What are the activity levels of the deep tendon reflexes and other reflexes (e.g., Babinski, genitoanal, and abdominal responses)? Is sphincter function normal? Is there evidence of denervation (e.g., fasciculation, atrophy, fatigability)? Are any nerves palpable? Are there skin lesions associated with the nerve deficits (e.g., anesthetic macules)?

The underlying cause determines the characteristic time course and associated clinical findings. To identify the pattern of disease, the history should focus on the rate of progression of neuropathic symptoms and their relation to antecedent or comorbid illnesses.[241] An acute onset is highly suggestive of an infectious cause; the majority of neuropathies due to infectious diseases will present acutely or subacutely. Chronic neuropathies of infectious cause are less common but do occur, as exemplified by leprosy and Lyme borreliosis.

Diagnostic clues of an infectious cause in PNS disorders may be suggested by finding risks from inadequate immunizations (diphtheria, tetanus, poliomyelitis); a recent or current systemic illness, such as pharyngitis in diphtheritic neuropathy, *Campylobacter* gastroenteritis (Guillain-Barré syndrome), or lymphadenopathy with malabsorption (Whipple's disease); epidemiologic exposures, such as tick bites (Lyme disease) or consumption of unpasteurized dairy products (brucellosis) or of home-canned or salted foods (botulism); and risks for sexually transmitted diseases (syphilis, HIV or HTLV infection) or for autoinfection from injection drug use (wound botulism, tetanus). The travel and residence history is of great diagnostic importance in suggesting geographically focused causes (Lyme borreliosis, brucellosis).

In general, an acute onset suggests a more favorable prognosis and should prompt a timely search for the underlying cause to prevent permanent neurologic sequelae. By establishing the rate of onset and anatomic pattern of illness, the neuropathic syndrome can be identified and appropriate studies obtained to diagnose the cause.

Clues to Myelitis

The five cardinal manifestations of spinal cord disease are pain, motor deficits, sensory deficits, abnormalities of reflexes or muscle tone, and bladder dysfunction. The distribution of neurologic deficits depends on the spinal segments affected. Local pain occurs at the site of the lesion and can assume a radicular quality if the nerve roots are involved. Paresthesias also occur and have greater localizing value than does radicular pain. Weakness is present in virtually all disorders of the spinal cord and, in myelitis, may progress for a period of hours, days, or weeks. Paraplegia and spinal shock can develop and are characterized by areflexia, atony, and absent plantar reflexes. More slowly progressive lesions are associated with hyperreflexia and hypertonia. Bladder dysfunction is usually not an early sign of spinal cord disease, although if spinal shock develops, flaccid bladder paralysis ensues with urinary retention and overflow incontinence. Chronic myelopathies cause a small spastic bladder and result in urgency, frequency, and incontinence.

The history should explore risks for immunosuppression (low $CD4^+$ cell count in HIV infection, chronic suppression for transplantation), hematogenous infections (injection drug use), recent exposure to macaque monkeys (B virus), travel to areas endemic for Lyme disease, schistosomiasis, or cysticercosis. A history of distant and recent vaccinations should be obtained to assess the risk for poliovirus infection and possible postvaccinial myelitis or encephalitis, now uncommon since discontinuation of the older rabies and cowpox vaccines. The history or other clinical findings may suggest infectious agents known to cause or to be associated with acute or chronic primary myelitis, such as skin lesions (human or simian herpesviruses, syphilis, Lyme borreliosis). An immediately preceding illness may suggest *Mycoplasma* myelitis or postinfectious transverse myelitis, an uncommon complication of rubeola, varicella, rubella, influenza, and mumps that is more common in younger patients.

Secondary myelitis due to inflammatory and compressive infections, such as epidural abscess, spinal subdural empyema, and intraspinal abscess, must be distinguished from primary myelitis of an infectious cause. MRI with or without myelography should be performed early to exclude an operable compressive lesion.[242]

Differential Diagnosis

Because weakness or paralysis may also arise from disorders affecting the neuromuscular junction (e.g., myasthenia gravis, neurotoxins, and drugs) or from disease of muscle itself, measurement of nerve conduction velocity and electromyography are required to assess whether symptoms and signs are due to demyelination or result from degeneration, neuromuscular blockade, or primary muscle disease. Noninfectious myelopathies include tumor and other causes of myelitis such as multiple sclerosis and systemic lupus erythematosus.

The differential diagnosis of neurologic symptoms and signs requires consultation with a neurologist. However, the precise location of peripheral lesions and possible infectious causes can be surmised by careful examination of the patient, analysis of CSF, and use of relevant imaging techniques, as indicated in Table 164–8 and Figure 164–3.

Acknowledgment

We gratefully acknowledge assistance in the 1992 version by Pierre DeJace, MD; the computer assistance of Marcia E. H. Rezza, MA; and the many years of stimulation and encouragement by Morton N. Swartz, MD, Raymond D. Adams, MD, and other colleagues at the Massachusetts General Hospital.

References

1. Adams RD, Victor M: Principles of Neurology, ed 5. New York, McGraw-Hill, 1993.
2. Jopling WH, McDougall AC: Handbook of Leprosy. Oxford, Heinemann, 1988.
3. World Health Organization: Expert Committee on Leprosy. 6th Report, Technical Report Series 768, 1988.

3a. World Health Organization: Chemotherapy of leprosy. Report of a WHO Study Group. WHO Tech Rep Ser 847:1, 1994.

4. Yoder LJ: Leprosy (Hansen's disease). *In* Rakel RE (ed): Conn's Current Therapy, ed 45. Philadelphia, WB Saunders, 1993, pp 94–99.
5. Pattyn SR: Future trends in the treatment of leprosy. Trop Geogr Med 46:85, 1994.
6. Grosset J-H: Progress in the chemotherapy of leprosy. Int J Lepr 62:269, 1994.

6a. Katoch K: Autonomic nerve affection in leprosy. Indian J Lepr 68:49, 1996.

7. Kaplan G: Recent advances in cytokine therapy in leprosy. J Infect Dis 167(Suppl 1):S18, 1993.

7a. Gelber RH: Chemotherapy of lepromatous leprosy: Recent developments and prospects for the future. Eur J Clin Micro Infect Dis 13:942, 1994.

7b. Duncan ME: Pregnancy and leprosy neuropathy. Indian J Lepr 68:23, 1996.

7c. Job CK: Nerve in reversal reaction. Indian J Lepr 68:43, 1996.

7d. Crawford CL: Use of thalidomide in leprosy. Adverse Drug React Toxicol Rev 13:177, 1994.

7e. Montecucco C, Schiavo G: Structure and function of tetanus and botulinum neurotoxins. Q Rev Biophys 28:423, 1995.

8. Thorne FL, Kropp RJ: Wound botulism: A life-threatening complication of hand injuries. Plast Reconstr Surg 71:548, 1983.
9. Woodruff BA, Griffin PM, McCroskey LM, et al: Clinical and laboratory comparison of botulism from toxin types A, B, and E in the United States, 1975–1988. J Infect Dis 166:1281, 1992.
10. Hughes JM, Blumenthal JR, Merson JM, et al: Clinical features of type a and b botulism. Ann Intern Med 95:442, 1981.
11. Gimenez JA, Gimenez MA, DasGupta BR: Characterization of the neurotoxin isolated from a *Clostridium baratii* strain implicated in infant botulism. Infect Immun 60:518, 1992.
12. McCroskey LM, Hatheway CL, Woodruff BA, et al: Type F botulism due to neurotoxigenic *Clostridium baratii* from an unknown source in an adult. J Clin Microbiol 29:2618, 1991.

12a. Wiener SL: Strategies for the prevention of a successful biological warfare aerosol attack. Mil Med 161:251, 1996.

12b. Cardoso F, Jankovic J: Clinical use of botulinum neurotoxins. Curr Top Microbiol Immunol 195:123, 1995.

13. Chia JK, Clark JB, Ruan CA, Pollack M: Botulism in an adult associated with food-borne intestinal infection with *Clostridium botulinum*. N Engl J Med 315:239, 1986.

13a. Van Ermengem E: Classics in infectious diseases. A new anaerobic bacillus and its relation to botulism. Rev Infect Dis 1:701, 1970. Originally published as Ueber einen neuen anaeroben Bacillus und seine Beziehungen zum Botulismus. Z Hyg Infektionskr 26:1, 1897.

14. Weber JT, Hibbs RG Jr, Darwish A, et al: A massive outbreak of type E botulism associated with traditional salted fish in Cairo. J Infect Dis 167:451, 1993.
15. Roblot P, Roblot F, Fauchere JL, et al: Retrospective study of 108 cases of botulism in Poitiers, France. J Med Microbiol 40:379, 1994.

15a. Centers for Disease Control and Prevention: Type B botulism associated with roasted eggplant in oil—Italy, 1993. MMWR Morbid Mortal Wkly Rep 44:33, 1995.

15b. Townes JM, Cieslak PR, Hatheway CL, et al: An outbreak of type A botulism associated with a commercial cheese sauce. Ann Intern Med 125:558, 1996.

16. Mechem CC, Walter FG: Wound botulism. Vet Hum Toxicol 36:233, 1994.
17. Centers for Disease Control and Prevention: Wound botulism—California, 1995. MMWR Morbid Mortal Wkly Rep 44:889, 1995.
18. Arnon SS: Infant botulism. Annu Rev Med 31:541, 1980.
19. Cherington M: Electrophysiologic methods as an aid in diagnosis of botulism: A review. Muscle Nerve 5:528, 1982.
20. Hatheway CL: Laboratory procedures for cases of suspected infant botulism. Rev Infect Dis 1:647, 1979.
21. Barrett DH: Endemic food-borne botulism: Clinical experience, 1973–1986 at Alaska Native Medical Center. Alaska Med 33:101, 1991.
22. Salazar-Grueso EF, Arnason BGW: Peripheral nerve disease caused by infection, toxins and post infectious syndromes. *In* Schlossberg D (ed): Clinical Topics in Infectious Diseases: Infections of the Nervous System. New York, Springer-Verlag, 1990, pp 192–206.
23. Dixon JMS: Diphtheria. *In* Topley WWC, Parker MY, Collier L, Wilson G (eds): Topley and Wilson's Principles of Bacteriology, Virology, and Immunity. Philadelphia, BC Decker, 1990, pp 56–75.
24. Harnisch JP, Tronca E, Nolan CM, et al: Diphtheria among alcoholic urban adults; a decade of experience in Seattle. Ann Intern Med 111:71, 1989.

24a. Galazka AM, Robertson SE, Oblapenko GP: Resurgence of diphtheria. Eur J Epidemiol 11:95, 1995.

25. Centers for Disease Control and Prevention: Diphtheria epidemic—New Independent States of the former Soviet Union, 1990–1994. MMWR Morbid Mortal Wkly Rep 44:177, 1995.

25a. Centers for Disease Control and Prevention: Update: Diphtheria epidemic—New Independent States of the Former Soviet Union, January 1995–March 1996. MMWR Morbid Mortal Wkly Rep 45:693, 1996.

26. Centers for Disease Control and Prevention: Diphtheria acquired by U.S. citizens in the Russian Federation and Ukraine—1994. MMWR Morbid Mortal Wkly Rep 44:237, 1995.
27. Farizo KM, Strebel PM, Chen RT, et al: Fatal respiratory disease due to *Corynebacterium diphtheriae*: Case report and review of guidelines for management, investigation and control. Clin Infect Dis 16:59, 1993.

27a. Groundstroem KW, Molnar G, Lumio J: Echocardiographic follow-up of diphtheritic myocarditis. Cardiology 87:79, 1996.

27b. Booth LV, Ellis C, Wale MC, et al: An atypical case of *Corynebacterium diphtheriae* endocarditis and subsequent outbreak control measures. J Infect 31:63, 1995.

27c. Pennie RA, Malik AS, Wilcox L: Misidentification of toxigenic *Corynebacterium diphtheriae* as a *Corynebacterium* species with low virulence in a child with endocarditis. J Clin Microbiol 34:1275, 1996.

28. Weinstein L: Current concepts: Tetanus. N Engl J Med 289:1293, 1973.
29. Fernandez JM, Ferrandiz M, Larrea L, et al: Cephalic tetanus studied with single fibre EMG. J Neurol Neurosurg Psychiatry 46:862, 1983.
30. Bagetta G, Nistico G: Tetanus toxin as a neurobiological tool to study mechanisms of neuronal cell death in the mammalian brain. Pharmacol Ther 62:29, 1994.
31. Schofield F: Selective primary health care strategies for control of disease in the developing world XXII: Tetanus a preventable problem. Rev Infect Dis 8:144, 1986.

31a. Centers for Disease Control and Prevention: Progress towards global elimination of neonatal tetanus, 1989–1993. MMWR Morbid Mortal Wkly Rep 43:885, 1994.

31b. Centers for Disease Control and Prevention: Progress towards elimination of neonatal tetanus—Egypt, 1988–1994. MMWR Morbid Mortal Wkly Rep 45:89, 1996.

32. Faust RA, Vickers OR, Cohn I Jr: Tetanus: 2,449 cases in 68 years at Charity Hospital. J Trauma 16:704, 1976.
33. Centers for Disease Control and Prevention: Summary of notifiable diseases, United States 1994. MMWR Morbid Mortal Wkly Rep 43:1, 1994.
34. Gergen PJ, McQuillan GM, Kiely M, et al: A population-based survey of immunity to tetanus in the United States. N Engl J Med 332:761, 1995.

34a. Centers for Disease Control and Prevention: Tetanus surveillance—United States, 1991–1994. MMWR CDC Surveill Summ 46(SS-2):15, 1997.

34b. Middlebrook JL, Brown JE: Immunodiagnosis and immunotherapy of tetanus and botulinum neurotoxins. Curr Top Microbiol Immunol 195:89, 1995.

34c. Alagappan K, Rennie W, Kwiatkowski T, et al: Seroprevalence of tetanus antibodies among adults older than 65 years. Ann Emerg Med 28:18, 1996.

34d. Ljungman P, Cordonnier C, de Bock R, et al: Immunisations after bone marrow transplantation: Results of a European sur-

vey and recommendations from the infectious diseases working party of the European Group for Blood and Marrow Transplantation. Bone Marrow Transplant 15:455, 1995.
34e. Somani J, Larson RA: Reimmunization after allogeneic bone marrow transplantation. Am J Med 98:389, 1995.
34f. Centers for Disease Control and Prevention: Diphtheria, tetanus and pertussis: Recommendations for vaccine use and other preventive measures. Recommendations of the Advisory Committee on Immunization Practices (ACIP). MMWR Morbid Mortal Wkly Rep 40:1, 1991.
34g. Bleck TP: *Clostridium tetani. In* Mandell GL, Bennett JE, Dolin R (eds): Principles and Practice of Infectious Diseases. Churchill Livingstone, ed 4, 1995, pp 2173–2182.
35. Wesley AG, Hariparsad D, Dather M, Rocke DA: Labetalol in tetanus: The treatment of sympathetic nervous system overactivation. Anesthesia 38:243, 1983.
36. Dastur FD, Shahan MT, Dastoor DH, et al: Cephalic tetanus: Demonstration of a dual lesion. J Neurol Neurosurg Psychiatry 40:782, 1977.
36a. Gupta PS, Kapoor R, Goyal S, et al: Intrathecal human tetanus immunoglobulin in early tetanus. Lancet 2:439, 1980.
37. Miller RG, Kiprov DD, Barry G, Bredesen DE: Peripheral nervous system dysfunction in acquired immunodeficiency syndrome. *In* Rosenblum ML, Levey RM, Bredesen DE (eds): AIDS and the Nervous System. New York, Raven Press, 1988, pp 65–78.
38. Dalakas MC, Pezeshkpour GH: Neuromuscular diseases associated with human immunodeficiency virus infection. Ann Neurol 23(Suppl):S38, 1988.
39. Parry GJ: Peripheral neuropathies associated with human immunodeficiency virus infection. Ann Neurol 23(Suppl):S49, 1988.
40. Brew BJ, Sidtis JJ, Petito CK, Price RW: The neurologic complications of AIDS and human immunodeficiency virus. *In* Plum F (ed): Advances in Contemporary Neurology. Philadelphia, FA Davis, 1988, pp 1–49.
41. McArthur JC: Neurologic manifestations of AIDS. Medicine (Baltimore) 66:407, 1987.
42. Griffin JW, Wesselingh SL, Griffin DE, et al: Peripheral nerve disorders in HIV infection. Similarities and contrasts with CNS disorders. *In* Price RW, Perry SW (eds): HIV, AIDS and the Brain. New York, Raven Press, 1994, pp 159–182.
43. Lange DJ: AAEM Minimonograph 41: Neuromuscular diseases associated with HIV-1 infection. Muscle Nerve 17:16, 1994.
44. Lipkin WI, Parry G, Kiprov D, Abrams D: Inflammatory neuropathy in homosexual men with lymphadenopathy. Neurology 35:1479, 1985.
45. Morgello S, Simpson DM: Multifocal cytomegalovirus demyelinative polyneuropathy associated with AIDS. Muscle Nerve 17:176, 1994.
46. Said G, Lacroix C, Chemouilli P, et al: Cytomegalovirus neuropathy in acquired immunodeficiency syndrome: A clinical and pathological study. Ann Neurol 29:139, 1991.
47. Cohen BA, McArthur JC, Grohman S, et al: Neurologic prognosis of cytomegalovirus polyradiculopathy in AIDS. Neurology 43:493, 1993.
48. Karmochkine M, Molina J-M, Scieux C, et al: Combined therapy with ganciclovir and foscarnet for cytomegalovirus polyradiculomyelitis in patients with AIDS. Am J Med 97:196, 1994.
49. Talpos D, Tien RD, Hesselink JR: Magnetic resonance imaging of AIDS-related polyradiculopathy. Neurology 41:1995, 1991.
50. Gozlan J, Salord J-M, Roullet E, et al: Rapid detection of cytomegalovirus DNA in cerebrospinal fluid of AIDS patients with neurologic disorders. J Infect Dis 166:1416, 1992.
51. Hayden FG: Antiviral agents. *In* Mandell GL, Bennett JE, Dolin R (eds): Principles and Practice of Infectious Diseases, ed 4. New York, Churchill Livingstone, 1995, pp 411–450.
52. Simpson DM, Olney RK: Peripheral neuropathies associated with human immunodeficiency virus infection. Neurol Clin 10:685, 1992.
53. Gilchrist JM: AAEM Case Report 26: Seventh cranial neuropathy. Muscle Nerve 16:447, 1993.
54. Asbury AK: Diagnostic considerations in Guillain-Barré syndrome. Ann Neurol 9(Suppl):1, 1981.
55. Rees J: Guillain-Barré syndrome. Clinical manifestations and directions for treatment. Drugs 49:912, 1995.
56. Schoenberger LB, Hurwitz ES, Katona P, et al: Guillain-Barré syndrome: Its epidemiology and associations with influenza vaccines. Ann Neurol 9(Suppl):31, 1981.
57. De Klippel N, Hautekeete ML, De Keyser J, Ebinger G: Guillain-Barré syndrome as the presenting manifestation of hepatitis C infection. Neurology 43:2143, 1993.
58. Feasby TE: Inflammatory-demyelinating polyneuropathies. Neurol Clin 10:651, 1992.
59. Ropper AH: Current concepts: The Guillain-Barré syndrome. N Engl J Med 326:1130, 1992.
60. Ropper AH: *Campylobacter* diarrhea and Guillain-Barré syndrome. Arch Neurol 45:655, 1988.
61. Hurwitz ES, Holman RC, Nelson DB, Berger LB: National surveillance for Guillain-Barré syndrome. Neurology 33:150, 1983.
62. Prineas JB: Pathology of the Guillain-Barré syndrome. Ann Neurol 9(Suppl):6, 1981.
63. Hall SM, Hughes RA, Atkinson PF, et al: Motor nerve biopsy in severe Guillain-Barré syndrome. Ann Neurol 31:441, 1992.
64. Honavar M, Tharakan JK, Hughes RA, et al: A clinicopathologic study of the Guillain-Barré syndrome. Nine cases and literature review. Brain 114:1245, 1991.
65. Feasby TE, Hahn AF, Brown WF, et al: Severe axonal degeneration in acute Guillain-Barré syndrome: Evidence of two different mechanisms? J Neurol Sci 116:185, 1993.
66. Hughes R, Atkinson P, Coates P, et al: Sural nerve biopsies in Guillain-Barré syndrome: Axonal degeneration and macrophage-associated demyelination and absence of CMV genome. Muscle Nerve 15:568, 1992.
67. Dowling PC, Blumberg GM, Cook SD: Guillain-Barré syndrome. *In* Vinken PJ, Bruyn GW: Handbook of Clinical Neurology, Vol 7. Amsterdam, Elsevier North Holland, 1987, p 239.
68. Sauron B, Bouche P, Cathala HP, et al: Miller-Fisher syndrome: Clinical and electrophysiological evidence of peripheral origin in 10 cases. Neurology 34:953, 1984.
69. Gibbels E, Giebisch U: Natural course of acute and chronic monophasic inflammatory demyelinating polyneuropathies (IDP). A retrospective analysis of 266 cases. Acta Neurol Scand 85:282, 1992.
70. Araga S, Kagimoto H, Adachi A, et al: Kappa/lambda ratios of IgG, IgA and IgM in the cerebrospinal fluid of patients with Guillain-Barré syndrome. Jpn J Med 30:118, 1991.
71. Cook SD, Dowling PC: The role of autoantibodies and immune complexes in the pathogenesis of Guillain-Barré syndrome. Ann Neurol 9:70, 1981.
72. Fulbright RK, Erdum E, Sze G, Byrne T: Cranial nerve enhancement in the Guillain-Barré syndrome. AJNR 16(Suppl 4):923, 1995.
73. Georgy BA, Chong B, Chamberlain M, et al: MR of the spine in Guillain-Barré syndrome. AJNR 15:300, 1994.
74. Patel H, Garg BP, Edwards MK: MRI of Guillain-Barré syndrome. J Comput Assist Tomogr 17:651, 1993.
75. Crino PB, Zimmerman R, Laskowitz D, et al: Magnetic resonance imaging of the cauda equina in Guillain-Barré syndrome. Neurology 44:1334, 1994.
76. Petty RK, Duncan R, Jamal GA, et al: Brainstem encephalitis and the Miller-Fisher syndrome. J Neurol Neurosurg Psychiatry 56:201, 1993.
77. Urushitani M, Udaka F, Kameyama M: Miller-Fisher–Guillain-Barré overlap syndrome with enhancing lesions in the spinocerebellar tracts. J Neurol Neurosurg Psychiatry 58:241, 1995.
78. Gordon SM, Eaton ME, George R, et al: The response of symptomatic neurosyphilis to high-dose intravenous penicillin G in patients with human immunodeficiency virus infection. N Engl J Med 331:1469, 1994.
79. Kincaid JC: Tick bite paralysis. Semin Neurol 10:32, 1990.
80. Schaumburg HH, Spencer PS, Thomas PK: Disorders of peripheral nerves. Contemp Neurol Ser 24, 1983.
81. Van der Meche FGA, Schmitz PIM, and the Dutch Guillain-Barré Study Group: A randomized trial comparing intravenous immune globulin and plasma exchange in Guillain-Barré syndrome. N Engl J Med 326:1123, 1992.
82. Van der Meche FGA, Schmitz PIM, Kleyweg RP for the Dutch Guillain-Barré Study Group: Intravenous immune globulin versus plasma exchange in Guillain-Barré syndrome (Letter). N Engl J Med 327:817, 1992.
83. van Doorn PA, Brand A, Strengers PFW, et al: High-dose intra-

venous immunoglobulin treatment in chronic inflammatory demyelinating polyneuropathy: A double blind, placebo-controlled, cross-over study. Neurology 40:209, 1992.
84. Raphael J-C, Chastang C, Chevret S, Gajdos P: Intravenous immune globulin versus plasma exchange in Guillain-Barré syndrome (Letter). N Engl J Med 327:816, 1992.
85. Ellie E, Combe C, Ferrer X: High dose intravenous immunoglobulin and acute renal failure (Letter). N Engl J Med 327:1032, 1992.
85a. Plasma Exchange/Sandoglobulin Guillain-Barré Syndrome Trial Group: Randomized trial of plasma exchange, intravenous immunoglobulin, and combined treatments in Guillain-Barré syndrome. Lancet 349:225, 1997.
86. Guillain-Barré Syndrome Steroid Trial Group: Double-blind trial of intravenous methylprednisolone in Guillain-Barré syndrome. Lancet 341:586, 1993.
87. Mendell JR: Chronic inflammatory demyelinating polyradiculopathy. Annu Rev Med 44:211, 1993.
88. Koguchi Y, Yamada T, Kuwabara S, et al: Increased CD4 in demyelinating neuropathy indicates radicular involvement. Acta Neurol Scand 91:58, 1995.
89. Bertorini T, Halford H, Lawrence J, et al: Contrast-enhanced magnetic resonance imaging of the lumbosacral roots in the dysimmune inflammatory polyneuropathies. J Neuroimaging 5:9, 1995.
90. Woolsey RM, Young RR: The clinical diagnosis of disorders of the spinal cord. Neurol Clin 9:573, 1991.
91. Nordli DR, Bello JA, DeVivo DC: Myelitis. *In* Schlossberg D (ed): Clinical Topics in Infectious Diseases: Infections of the Nervous System. New York, Springer-Verlag, 1990, pp 179–191.
92. Jeffrey DR, Mandler RN, Davis LE: Transverse myelitis. Retrospective analysis of 33 cases, with differentiation of cases associated with multiple sclerosis and parainfectious events. Arch Neurol 50:532, 1993.
93. Stoner GL: Implications of progressive multifocal leukoencephalopathy and JC virus for the etiology of MS. Acta Neurol Scand 83:20, 1991.
94. Cumming WJ: Myelitis and toxic, inflammatory and infectious disorders. Curr Opin Neurol Neurosurg 5:549, 1992.
95. Corboy JR, Price RW: Myelitis and toxic, inflammatory and infectious disorders. Curr Opin Neurol Neurosurg 6:564, 1993.
96. Graber D, Fossoud C, Grouteau E, et al: Acute transverse myelitis and coxsackie A9 virus infection. Pediatr Infect Dis 13:77, 1990.
97. Modlin JF: Coxsackie viruses, echoviruses and newer enteroviruses. *In* Mandell GL, Bennett JE, Dolin R (eds): Principles and Practice of Infectious Diseases, ed 4. New York, Churchill Livingstone, 1995, pp 1620–1636.
98. World Health Organization: Poliomyelitis. Wkly Epidemiol Rec 64:273, 1989.
98a. Melnick JL: Current status of poliovirus infections. Clin Microbiol Rev 9:293, 1996.
99. Assaad F, Ljungars-Esteves K: World overview of poliomyelitis: Regional patterns and trends. Rev Infect Dis 6(Suppl):S302, 1984.
100. Centers for Disease Control and Prevention: Progress toward global poliomyelitis eradication, 1985–1994. MMWR Morbid Mortal Wkly Rep 44:273, 1995.
101. Centers for Disease Control and Prevention: Mass vaccination with oral poliovirus vaccine—Asia and Europe, 1995. MMWR Morbid Mortal Wkly Rep 44:234, 1995.
102. Strebel PM, Sutter RW, Cochi SL, et al: Epidemiology of poliomyelitis in the United States: One decade after the last reported case of indigenous wild virus–associated disease. Clin Infect Dis 14:568, 1992.
102a. Windebank AJ, Litchy WJ, Daube JR, Iverson RA: Lack of progression of neurologic deficit in survivors of paralytic polio: A 5-year prospective population-based study. Neurology 46:80, 1996.
102b. Kidd D, Williams AJ, Howard RS: Poliomyelitis. Postgrad Med J 72:641, 1996.
103. Hatch MH, Marchetti GE, Nottay BK, et al: Strain characterization studies of poliovirus type I isolates from poliomyelitis cases in the United States in 1979. Dev Biol Stand 47:307, 1981.
104. Jacob J: Poliomyelitis in India; prospects and problems of control. Rev Infect Dis 6(Suppl 2):438, 1984.
104a. Centers for Disease Control and Prevention: Paralytic poliomyelitis—United States, 1980–1994. MMWR 46:79, 1997.
104b. Centers for Disease Control and Prevention: Poliomyelitis prevention in the United States: Introduction of a sequential vaccination schedule of inactivated poliovirus vaccine followed by oral poliovirus vaccine. Recommendations of the Advisory Committee on Immunization Practices (ACIP). MMWR Morbid Mortal Wkly Rep 46:1, 1997.
104c. Conyn-van Spaendonck MA, Oostvogel PM, van Loon AM, et al: Circulation of poliovirus during the poliomyelitis outbreak in the Netherlands in 1992–1993. Am J Epidemiol 143:929, 1996.
105. Holmes GP, Chapman LE, Stewart JA, et al and the B Virus Working Group: Guidelines for the prevention and treatment of B-virus infections in exposed persons. Clin Infect Dis 20:421, 1995.
106. Centers for Disease Control and Prevention: Publication of guidelines for the prevention and treatment of B virus infections in exposed persons. MMWR Morbid Mortal Wkly Rep 45:96, 1995.
107. Gosztonyi G, Falke D, Ludwig H: Axonal and transsynaptic (transneuronal) spread of *Herpesvirus simiae* (B virus) in experimentally infected mice. Histol Histopathol 7:63, 1992.
108. Artenstein AW, Hicks CB, Goodwin BS Jr, Hilliard JK: Human infection with B virus following a needle stick injury. Rev Infect Dis 13:288, 1991.
109. Berman M, Feldman S, Alter M, et al: Acute transverse myelitis: Incidence and etiologic considerations. Neurology 31:966, 1981.
110. Folpe A, Lapham LW, Smith HC: Herpes simplex myelitis as a cause of acute necrotizing myelitis syndrome. Neurology 44:1955, 1994.
111. Farkkila M, Koskiniemi M, Vaheri A: Clinical spectrum of neurologic herpes simplex infection. Acta Neurol Scand 87:325, 1993.
112. Ellie E, Rozenberg F, Dousset V, Beylot-Barry M: Herpes simplex type 2 ascending myeloradiculitis: MRI findings and rapid diagnosis by the polymerase chain method. J Neurol Neurosurg Psychiatry 57:869, 1994.
113. Iwamasa T, Yoshitake H, Sakuda H, et al: Case report. Acute ascending necrotizing myelitis in Okinawa caused by herpes simplex virus type 2. Virchows Archiv A Pathol Anat 418:71, 1991.
114. Shyu W-C, Lin J-C, Chang B-C, et al: Recurrent ascending myelitis: An unusual presentation of herpes simplex virus type 1 infection. Ann Neurol 34:625, 1993.
115. Ahmed I: Survival after herpes simplex type 2 myelitis. Neurology 38:1500, 1988.
116. Barnes DW, Whitley RJ: CNS diseases associated with varicella zoster virus and herpes simplex infection. Pathogenesis and current therapy. Neurol Clin 4:265, 1986.
117. Gray F, Belec L, Lescs MC, et al: Varicella-zoster virus infection of the central nervous system in the acquired immune deficiency syndrome. Brain 117:987, 1994.
118. Rosenfeld J, Taylor CL, Atlas SW: Myelitis following chickenpox: A case report. Neurology 43:1834, 1993.
119. Gilden DH, Beinlich BR, Rubinstein EM, et al: Varicella-zoster virus myelitis: An expanding spectrum. Neurology 44:1818, 1994.
120. Miles C, Hoffman W, Lai C-W, Freeman JW: Cytomegalovirus-associated transverse myelitis. Neurology 43:2143, 1993.
121. Holland NR, Power C, Mathews VP, et al: Cytomegalovirus encephalitis in acquired immunodeficiency syndrome (AIDS). Neurology 44:507, 1994.
122. Barohn RJ, Bazan C, Jackson CE: Cytomegalovirus radiculomyelitis (Letter). Neurology 43:2421, 1993.
123. Tyler KL, Gross RA, Cascino GD: Unusual viral causes of transverse myelitis: Hepatitis A and cytomegalovirus. Neurology 36:855, 1986.
124. Caldas C, Bernicker E, Dal Nogare A, Luby JP: Case report: Transverse myelitis associated with Epstein-Barr virus infection. Am J Med Sci 307:45, 1994.
125. Rubin RH, Young LS: Clinical Approach to Infection in the Compromised Host, ed 2. New York, Plenum Publishing, 1988.
126. Tucker T, Dix RD, Katzen C, et al: Cytomegalovirus and herpes simplex ascending myelitis in a patient with AIDS. Ann Neurol 18:74, 1985.
127. Dawson DM, Potts F: Acute nontraumatic myelopathies. Neurol Clin 9:585, 1991.

128. Wiley CA, VanPatten PD, Carpenter PM, et al: Acute ascending necrotizing myelopathy caused by herpes simplex virus type 2. Neurology 37:1791, 1987.
129. Heller HM, Carnevale NT, Steigbigel RT: Varicella zoster virus transverse myelitis without cutaneous rash. Am J Med 88:550, 1990.
130. Gomez-Tortosa E, Gadea I, Gegundez MI, et al: Development of myelopathy before herpes zoster rash in a patient with AIDS. Clin Infect Dis 18:810, 1994.
131. Devinsky O, Cho E-S, Petito CK, Price RW: Herpes zoster myelitis. Brain 114:1181, 1991.
132. Whiteman ML, Dandapani BK, Shebert RT, Post MJ: MRI of AIDS-related polyradiculomyelitis. J Comput Assist Tomogr 18:7, 1994.
133. Denning DA, Anderson J, Rudge P, Smith H: Acute myelopathy associated with primary infection with human immunodeficiency virus. Br Med J 294:143, 1987.
134. Petito CK, Naviax BA, Cho ES, et al: Vacuolar myelopathy pathologically resembling subacute combined degeneration in patients with AIDS. N Engl J Med 312:874, 1985.
135. Blattner WA: Human T-lymphotrophic viruses and diseases of long latency. Ann Intern Med 111:4, 1989.
136. Beilke MA, Greenspan D, Thompson J, et al: Laboratory study of HIV-1 and HTLV-I/II coinfection. J Med Virol 44:131, 1994.
137. Rogers-Johnson PEB, Ono S, Gibbs CJ Jr, Gajdusek DG: Tropical spastic paraparesis and HTLV-I–associated myelopathy: Clinical and laboratory diagnosis. *In* Blattner WA (ed): Human Retrovirology. New York, Raven Press, 1990, pp 205–212.
138. Dal Pan GJ, Glass JD, McArthur JC: Clinicopathologic correlations of HIV-1–associated vacuolar myelopathy: An autopsy-based case control study. Neurology 44:2159, 1994.
139. Berger JR, Levy RM: The neurologic complications of human immunodeficiency virus infection. Med Clin North Am 77:1, 1993.
140. Stoeckle MY: Introduction—Type C oncoviruses including human T-cell lymphotropic viruses types I and II. *In* Mandell GL, Bennett JE, Dolin R (eds): Principles and Practice of Infectious Diseases, ed 4. New York, Churchill Livingstone, 1995, pp 1579–1584.
141. Bowen BC, Post MJD: Diagnostic imaging of CNS infection and inflammation. *In* Schlossberg D (ed): Infections of the Nervous System. New York, Springer-Verlag, 1990, pp 315–389.
142. McArthur JC, Griffin JW, Cornblath DR, et al: Steroid-responsive myeloneuropathy in a man dually infected with HIV-1 and HTLV-I. Neurology 40:938, 1990.
143. Gilden DH, Vafai A, Shram Y, et al: Varicella zoster virus in human sensory ganglia. Nature 306:478, 1983.
144. Weller TH: Varicella and herpes zoster, part I and part II. N Engl J Med 309:1302, 1434, 1983.
145. Brunell PA: Varicella zoster virus. *In* Mandell GL, Gordon Douglas R, Bennett J (eds): Principles and Practice of Infectious Diseases, ed 2. New York, John Wiley & Sons, 1985, pp 952–959.
146. Menezes AH, Graf CJU, Perret GE: Spinal cord abscess: A review. Surg Neurol 8:461, 1977.
147. Heindel CC, Fergerson JP, Kumarasamy T: Spinal subdural empyema complicating pregnancy. Case report. J Neurosurg 40:654, 1974.
148. Cohen J, Capildeo R, Rose FC, Pallis C: Schistosomal myelopathy. Br Med J 1:1258, 1977.
149. Maurice-Williams RS, Pamphilon D, Coakham HB: Intramedullary abscess: A rare complication of spinal dysraphism. J Neurol Neurosurg Psychiatry 43:1045, 1980.
149a. Gurbani SG, Cho CT, Lee KR: *Staphylococcus epidermidis* meningitis and an intraspinal abscess associated with a midthoracic dermal sinus tract. Clin Infect Dis 19:1138, 1994.
150. DiTullio MV Jr: Intramedullary spinal abscess: A case report with review of 53 previously described cases. Surg Neurol 7:351, 1977.
150a. Martin RJ, Yuan HA. Neurosurgical care of spinal epidural, subdural, and intramedullary abscesses and arachnoiditis. Orthop Clin North Am 27:125, 1996.
151. Darouiche RO, Hamill RJ, Greenberg SB, et al: Bacterial spinal epidural abscess. Review of 43 cases and literature survey. Medicine (Baltimore) 71:369, 1992.
152. Nussbaum ES, Rigamonti D, Standiford H, et al: Spinal epidural abscess: A report of 40 cases and review. Surg Neurol 38:225, 1992.
152a. Tacconi L, Johnston FG, Symon L: Spinal epidural abscess—Review of 10 cases. Acta Neurochir (Wien) 138:520, 1996.
153. Bleck TP, D'Angelo CM, Whistler WW: Bacterial infections of the spinal cord and its coverings. *In* Vinken PJ, Bruyn GW: Handbook of Clinical Neurology, Vol 8. Amsterdam, Elsevier North Holland, 1988, p 185.
154. Gelfand MS, Bakhtian BJ, Simmons BP: Spinal sepsis due to *Streptococcus milleri*: Two cases and review. Rev Infect Dis 13:559, 1991.
155. Guerrero IC, Slap GB, MacGregor RR, et al: Anaerobic spinal epidural abscess. J Neurosurg 48:465, 1978.
156. Herbert DA, Ruskin I: *Salmonella typhi* and staphylococcal epidural abscess occurring 47 years after typhoid fever. J Neurosurg 57:719, 1982.
157. Brian JE, Westerman GR, Chadduck WM: Septic complications of chemonucleolysis. Neurosurgery 15:730, 1989.
158. Saio P, McCabe P, Yagnik P: Nocardial spinal epidural abscess. Neurology 39:996, 1989.
159. Kaufman DM, Kaplan JG, Littman N: Infectious agents in spinal epidural abscess. Neurology 30:844, 1980.
159a. Witzig RS, Greer DL, Hyslop NE Jr: *Aspergillus flavus* mycetoma and epidural abscess successfully treated with itraconazole. J Med Vet Mycol 34:133, 1996.
160. Hershkowitz S, Link R, Lipons K: Spinal empyema in Crohn's disease. J Clin Gastroenterol 12:67, 1990.
161. Rayport M, Wisoff HS, Zaiman H: Vertebral echinococcosis: Report of case of surgical and biological therapy with review of the literature. J Neurosurg 21:647, 1969.
162. Koppel BS, Tuchman AJ, Mangiardi JR, et al: Epidural spinal infection in intravenous drug abscess. Arch Neurol 45:1331, 1988.
163. Danner RL, Hartman BJ: Update of spinal epidural abscess: 35 cases and review of the literature. Rev Infect Dis 9:265, 1987.
164. Fischer EG, Greene CS, Winston KR: Spinal epidural abscess in children. Neurosurgery 9:257, 1981.
165. Laster BR, Harter DH: Cervical epidural abscess. Neurology 37:1747, 1987.
166. Feldenzer JA, McKeever PE, Schaberg DR, et al: The pathogenesis of spinal epidural abscess: Microangiographic studies in an experimental model. J Neurosurg 69:110, 1988.
166a. Kovalik EC, Raymond JR, Albers FJ, et al: A clustering of epidural abscesses in chronic hemodialysis patients: Risks of salvaging access catheters in cases of infection. J Am Soc Nephrol 7:2264, 1996.
166b. Obrador GT, Levenson DJ: Spinal epidural abscess in hemodialysis patients: Report of three cases and review of the literature. Am J Kidney Dis 27:75, 1996.
166c. Ozuna RM, Delamarter RB: Pyogenic vertebral osteomyelitis and postsurgical disc space infections. Orthop Clin North Am 27:87, 1996.
166d. Broner FA, Garland DE, Zigler JE: Spinal infections in the immunocompromised host. Orthop Clin North Am 27:37, 1996.
167. Schmutzhard E, Aichner F, Dierckx RA, et al: New perspectives in acute spinal epidural abscess. Acta Neurochir (Wien) 80:105, 1986.
168. Baker AS, Ojemann RG, Swartz MN, Richardson EP: Spinal epidural abscess. N Engl J Med 293:463, 1975.
169. DiNubile MJ: Spinal epidural abscess. *In* Schlossberg D (ed): Clinical Topics in Infectious Diseases: Infections of the Nervous System. New York, Springer-Verlag, 1990, pp 171–178.
170. Kirzner H, Oh YK, Lee H: Intraspinal air: A CT finding of epidural abscess. AJR 151:1217, 1988.
171. Masaryk TJ, Nodic MT, Geisinger MA, et al: Cervical myelopathy: A comparison of magnetic resonance and myelopathy. J Comput Assist Tomogr 10:184, 1986.
172. Erntell M, Haltas S, Norlink, et al: MRI in the diagnosis of spinal epidural abscess. Scand J Infect Dis 20:323, 1988.
172a. Villoria MF, Fortea F, Moreno S, et al: MR imaging and CT of central nervous system tuberculosis in the patient with AIDS. Radiol Clin North Am 33:805, 1995.
173. Post EM, Modesti LM: Subacute postoperative subdural empyema. J Neurosurg 55:761, 1981.
174. Post MJD, Quencer RM, Montalvo BM, et al: Spinal infection: Evaluation with MR imaging and intraoperative ultrasound. Radiology 169:765, 1988.

175. Lees D, Lesoin F, Viaud C, et al: Decreased morbidity from acute bacterial spinal epidural abscesses using computed tomography and nonsurgical treatment in selected patients. Ann Neurol 17:350, 1985.
175a. Sapico FL: Microbiology and antimicrobial therapy of spinal infections. Orthop Clin North Am 27:9, 1996.
175b. Lang IM, Hughes DG, Jenkins JP, et al: MR imaging appearances of cervical epidural abscess. Clin Radiol 50:466, 1995.
176. Janssens JP, de Haller R: Spinal tuberculosis in a developed country. A review of 26 cases with special emphasis on abscesses and neurologic complications. Clin Orthop 257:67, 1990.
177. Harrier-Jones R, Hernandez-Bronchud M, Anslow P, Davies CJ: Meningitis and spinal subdural empyema as a complication of sinusitis. J Neurol Neurosurg Psychiatry 58:441, 1990.
178. Dill SR, Cobbs CG, McDonald CK: Subdural empyema: Analysis of 32 cases and review. Clin Infect Dis 20:372, 1995.
179. Levy ML, Wieder BH, Schneider J, et al: Subdural empyema of the cervical spine: Clinicopathological correlates and magnetic resonance imaging. Report of three cases. J Neurosurg 79:929, 1993.
180. Lownie SP, Fergerson GG: Spinal subdural empyema complicating cervical discography. Spine 14:1415, 1989.
181. Knudsen LL, Volby B, Stagaard M: Computed tomographic myelography in spinal subdural empyema. Neuroradiology 29:99, 1987.
182. Patronas NJ, Marx WJ, Duda EE: Radiographic presentation of spinal abscess in the subdural space. AJR 132:138, 1979.
183. Theodotou B, Woosley RE, Whaley RA: Spinal subdural empyema: Diagnosis by spinal computed tomography. Surg Neurol 21:610, 1984.
184. Obana WG, Rosenblum ML: Nonoperative treatment of neurosurgical infections. Neurosurg Clin North Am 3:359, 1992.
185. Sathi S, Schwartz M, Cortez S, Rossitch E Jr: Spinal subdural abscess: Successful treatment with limited drainage and antibiotics in a patient with AIDS. Surg Neurol 42:425, 1994.
186. Bartels RH, de Jong TR, Grotenhuis JA: Spinal subdural abscess. Case report. J Neurosurg 76:307, 1992.
187. Williams W, Sunderland R: As sick as a pigeon: Psittacosis myelitis. Arch Dis Child 64:1626, 1989.
188. Seboxa T, Rahlenbeck SI: Treatment of louse-borne relapsing fever with low dose penicillin or tetracycline: A clinical trial. Scand J Infect Dis 27:29, 1995.
189. Borgnolo G, Hailu B, Ciancarelli A, et al: Louse-borne relapsing fever. A clinical and epidemiological study of 389 patients in Asella Hospital, Ethiopia. Trop Geogr Med 45:66, 1993.
190. Southern PM, Sanford JP: Relapsing fever: A clinical and microbiological review. Medicine (Baltimore) 48:129, 1969.
191. Rawlings JA: An overview of tick-borne relapsing fever with emphasis on outbreaks in Texas. Tex Med 91:56, 1995.
192. Samara Y, Saked Y, Maier MK: Delayed neurologic display in murine typhus. Report of two cases. Arch Intern Med 149:949, 1989.
193. Reik L, Steere AC, Bartenhagen NH, et al: Neurologic abnormalities of Lyme disease. Medicine (Baltimore) 58:281, 1979.
194. Pachner AR, Steere AC: The triad of neurologic manifestations of Lyme disease: Meningitis, cranial neuritis and radiculoneuritis. Neurology 35:47, 1985.
195. Halperin JJ: Neurologic manifestations of Lyme disease. *In* Schlossberg D (ed): Clinical Topics in Infectious Diseases: Infections of the Nervous System. New York, Springer-Verlag, 1990, pp 304–314.
196. Belman AL, Iyer M, Coyle PK, Dattwyler R: Neurologic manifestations in children with North American Lyme disease. Neurology 43:2609, 1993.
197. Pfister H-W, Wilske B, Weber K: Lyme borreliosis: Basic science and clinical aspects. Lancet 343:1013, 1994.
198. Steere AC: Medical progress. Lyme disease. N Engl J Med 321:586, 1989.
198a. Nocton JJ, Steere AC: Lyme disease. Adv Intern Med 40:69, 1995.
199. Vallat JM, Hugon J, Lubeau M, et al: Tick-bite meningoradiculitis: Clinical, electrophysiologic and histologic findings in 10 cases. Neurology 7:749, 1987.
200. Garcia-Monco JC, Beldarrain MG, Estrade L: Painful lumbosacral plexitis with increased ESR and *Borrelia burgdorferi* infection. Neurology 43:1269, 1993.
201. Pachner AR: Neurologic manifestations of Lyme disease, the new "great imitator." Rev Infect Dis 11:S1482, 1989.
202. Reik L, Burgdorfer W, Donaldson JD: Neurologic abnormalities of Lyme disease without erythema chronicum migrans. Am J Med 81:73, 1986.
203. Lesser RL: Ocular manifestations of Lyme disease. Am J Med 98:60S, 1995.
203a. Centers for Disease Control and Prevention: Lyme disease—United States, 1994. MMWR Morbid Mortal Wkly Rep 44:459, 1995.
203b. Nadelman RB, Wormser GP: Erythema migrans and early Lyme disease. Am J Med 98(Suppl 4A):15S, 1995.
204. Pachner AR: Early disseminated Lyme disease: Lyme meningitis. Am J Med 98:30S, 1995.
205. Moody KD, Adams RL, Barthold SW: Effectiveness of antimicrobial treatment against *Borrelia burgdorferi* infection in mice. Antimicrob Agents Chemother 38:1567, 1994.
206. Nadelman RB, Wormser GP: Erythema migrans and early Lyme disease. Am J Med 98:15S, 1995.
207. Tumani H, Nolker G, Reiber H: Relevance of cerebrospinal fluid variables for early diagnosis of neuroborreliosis. Neurology 45:1663, 1995.
208. Sindern E, Malin JP: Phenotypic analysis of cerebrospinal fluid cells over the course of Lyme meningoradiculitis. Acta Cytol 39:73, 1995.
208a. Halperin JJ, Logigian EL, Finkel MF, Pearl RA: Practice parameters for the diagnosis of patients with nervous system Lyme borreliosis (Lyme disease). Quality Standards Subcommittee of the American Academy of Neurology. Neurology 46:619, 1996.
208b. Magnarelli LA: Current status of laboratory diagnosis for Lyme disease. Am J Med 98:10S, 1995.
208c. Halperin JJ: Neuroborreliosis. Am J Med 98(Suppl 4A):52S, 1995.
208d. Centers for Disease Control and Prevention: Recommendations for test performance and interpretation from the Second National Conference on Serologic Diagnosis of Lyme Disease. MMWR Morbid Mortal Wkly Rep 44:590, 1995.
209. Ilowite NT: Muscle, reticuloendothelial, and late manifestations of Lyme disease. Am J Med 98:638, 1995.
210. Weber K, Pfister H-W: Clinical management of Lyme borreliosis. Lancet 343:1017, 1994.
211. Karlsson M, Hammers-Berggren S, Lindquist L, et al: Comparison of intravenous penicillin G and oral doxycycline for treatment of Lyme neuroborreliosis. Neurology 44:1203, 1994.
212. Shakir RA, Al-Din AS, Araj GF, et al: Clinical categories of neurobrucellosis. Brain 110:213, 1987.
213. Pascual J, Combarros O, Polo JM, et al: Localized CNS brucellosis: Report of 7 cases. Acta Neurol Scand 78:282, 1988.
214. Young EJ: *Brucella* species. *In* Mandell GL, Bennett JE, Dolin R (eds): Principles and Practice of Infectious Diseases, ed 4. New York, Churchill Livingstone, 1995, pp 2053–2060.
215. Ariza J, Pujol M, Valverde J, et al: Brucellar sacroiliitis: Findings in 63 episodes and current relevance. Clin Infect Dis 16:761, 1993.
216. Nelson-Jones SA: Neurological complication of undulant fever: The clinical picture. Lancet 1:495, 1951.
217. Robson JM, Harrison MW, Wood RN, et al: Brucellosis: Re-emergence and changing epidemiology in Queensland. Med J Aust 159:153, 1993.
218. Chomel BB, DeBess EE, Mangiamele DM, et al: Changing trends in the epidemiology of human brucellosis in California from 1973 to 1992: A shift toward foodborne transmission. J Infect Dis 170:1216, 1994.
219. Larbrisseau A, Maraui E, Aguilhera F, Martinez-Lage JM: The neurological complications of brucellosis. Can J Neurol Sci 5:369, 1978.
220. McLean DR, Russell N, Khan MY: Neurobrucellosis: Clinical and therapeutic features. Clin Infect Dis 15:582, 1992.
221. Navas E, Guerrero A, Cobo J, Loza E: Faster isolation of *Brucella* spp. from blood by isolator compared with BACTEC NR. Diagn Microbiol Infect Dis 16:79, 1993.
222. Yagupsky P: Detection of *Brucella melitensis* by BACTEC NR660 blood culture system. J Clin Microbiol 31:1899, 1994.
223. Gamazo C, Vitas AI, Lopez-Goni I, et al: Factors affecting detection of *Brucella melitensis* by BACTEC. NR730, a nonradiometric system for hemocultures. J Clin Microbiol 31:3200, 1993.

224. Stszkiewicz J, Lewis CM, Colville J, et al: Outbreak of *Brucella melitensis* among microbiology laboratory workers in a community hospital. J Clin Microbiol 29:287, 1991.
224a. Young EJ: An overview of human neurobrucellosis. Clin Infect Dis 21:283, 1995.
224b. Tramont EC: Syphilis in adults: From Christopher Columbus to Sir Alexander Fleming to AIDS. Clin Infect Dis 21:1361, 1995.
225. Goodman LJ, Karakosis PU: Neurosyphilis. *In* Handbook of Clinical Neurology, Vol 8. Amsterdam, Elsevier North Holland, 1988, p 273.
226. Tramont EC: *Treponema pallidum* (syphilis). *In* Mandell GL, Bennett JE, Dolin R (eds): Principles and Practice of Infectious Diseases, ed 4. New York, Churchill Livingstone, 1995, pp 2117–2133.
227. Strom T, Schneck SA: Syphilitic meningomyelitis. Neurology 41:325, 1991.
228. Harrigan EP, McLaughlin TJ, Feldman RG: Transverse myelitis due to meningovascular syphilis. Arch Neurol 41:337, 1984.
228a. Chan YM, Adams DA, Kerr AG: Syphilitic labyrinthitis—An update. J Laryngol Otol 109:719, 1995.
228b. Little JP, Gardner G, Acker JD, Land MA: Otosyphilis in a patient with human immunodeficiency virus: Internal auditory canal gumma. Otolaryngol Head Neck Surg 112:488, 1995.
228c. Brightbill TC, Ihmeidan IH, Post MJ, et al: Neurosyphilis in HIV-positive and HIV-negative patients: Neuroimaging findings. Am J Neuroradiol 16:703, 1995.
228d. Marra CM, Critchlow CW, Hook EC 3rd, et al: Cerebrospinal fluid treponemal antibodies in untreated early syphilis. Arch Neurol 52:68, 1995.
228e. Marra CM, Gary DW, Kuypers J, Jacobsen MA: Diagnosis of neurosyphilis in patients infected with human immunodeficiency virus type 1. J Infect Dis 174:219, 1996.
228f. Larsen SA, Steiner BM, Rudolph AH: Laboratory diagnosis and interpretation of tests for syphilis. Clin Microbiol Rev 8:1, 1995.
228g. Rolfs RT: Treatment of syphilis, 1993. Clin Infect Dis 20(Suppl 1):S23, 1995.
228h. Marra CM, Longstreth WT Jr, Maxwell CL, Lukehart SA: Resolution of serum and cerebrospinal fluid abnormalities after treatment of neurosyphilis. Influence of concomitant human immunodeficiency virus infection. Sex Transm Dis 23:184, 1996.
228i. Yinnon AM, Coury-Doniger P, Polito R, Reichman RC: Serologic response to treatment of syphilis in patients with HIV infection. Arch Intern Med 156:321, 1996.
228j. Malone JL, Wallace MR, Hendrick BB, et al: Syphilis and neurosyphilis in a human immunodeficiency virus type-1 seropositive population: Evidence for frequent serologic relapse after therapy. Am J Med 99:55, 1995.
229. Gordon SM, Eaton ME, George R, et al: The response of symptomatic neurosyphilis to high-dose intravenous penicillin G in patients with human immunodeficiency virus infection. N Engl J Med 331:1469, 1994.
230. Koskiniemi M: CNS manifestations associated with *Mycoplasma pneumoniae* infections: Summary of cases at the University of Helsinki and review. Clin Infect Dis 17(Suppl 1):S52, 1993.
231. Mills RW, Schoolfield L: Acute transverse myelitis associated with *Mycoplasma pneumoniae* infection: A case report and review of the literature. Pediatr Infect Dis 11:228, 1992.
232. Heller L, Keren O, Mendelson L, Davidoff G: Transverse myelitis associated with *Mycoplasma pneumoniae*: Case report. Paraplegia 28:522, 1990.
233. Case records of the Massachusetts General Hospital. Weekly clinicopathological exercises. Case 42-1994. A 19-year-old man with rapidly progressive lower-extremity weakness and dysesthesias after a respiratory tract infection. N Engl J Med 331:1437, 1994.
234. Knox DL, Bayless TM, Pittman FE: Neurologic disease in patients with treated Whipple's disease. Medicine (Baltimore) 55:467, 1976.
235. Relman DA, Schmidt TM, MacDermott RP, Falkow S: Identification of the uncultured bacillus of Whipple's diseases. N Engl J Med 327:293, 1992.
236. Knox DL, Green WR, Troncoso JC, et al: Cerebral-ocular Whipple's disease: A 62-year odyssey from death to diagnosis. Neurology 45:617, 1995.
237. Halperin JJ, Dennis DMD, Kleinman GM: Whipple's disease of the nervous system. Neurology 32:612, 1982.
238. Lowsky R, Archer GL, Fyles G, et al: Brief report: Diagnosis of Whipple's disease by molecular analysis of peripheral blood. N Engl J Med 331:1343, 1994.
239. Dobbins WO 3rd: The diagnosis of Whipple's disease. N Engl J Med 332:390, 1995.
240. Erdem E, Carlier R, Delvalle A, et al: Gadolinium-enhanced MRI in cerebral Whipple's disease. Neuroradiology 35:581, 1993.
241. Hyslop NE Jr, DeJace P: Infectious diseases of the spinal cord and peripheral nervous system. *In* Gorbach SL, Bartlett JG, Blacklow N (eds): Infectious Diseases. Philadelphia, WB Saunders, 1992, pp 1216–1235.
242. Smith AS, Blaser SI: MR of infectious and inflammatory diseases of the spine. Crit Rev Diagn Imaging 32:165, 1991.

165

Reye's Syndrome

Bruce G. Gellin
John R. La Montagne

First described in 1929,[1] the syndrome originally known as encephalopathy with fatty degeneration of the viscera— actually a triad of postinfectious encephalopathy, microvesicular fat infiltration of hepatic parenchyma, and elevated serum transaminase values—was thought to be a rare event until the reports by Reye and coworkers in 1963[2] and later by Johnson and associates.[3] Reye's group reported a series of cases of fatal encephalopathy with associated fatty degeneration of the liver that occurred in 21 Australian children. This report focused on the pathologic manifestations of this clinical presentation and gave rise to the term Reye's syndrome. (Although the preferred term is Reye's syndrome, it has also been called Reye syndrome and Reye-Johnson syndrome.) The report by Johnson and coworkers in 1970 analyzed a cluster of 16 cases of this syndrome that occurred during an outbreak of influenza B in a community in North Carolina and focused attention on the potential role of epidemic viral infections as important triggering factors in the etiology of Reye's syndrome. In the days after an uncomplicated viral infection, these cases developed an acute onset of persistent, intractable vomiting and dehydration and the development of neurologic signs and symptoms, including encephalopathy and coma. One of the important early observations was that the disease almost always occurred in children who were otherwise healthy and were in the recovery period after an influenza virus infection, although only a small proportion of influenza virus–infected children (1 in 20,000) developed this complication.[4]

Epidemiology

After the description of this syndrome by Reye and colleagues in 1963, there was a dramatic increase in reporting of Reye's syndrome cases to the Centers for Disease Control (now the Centers for Disease Control and Prevention [CDC]) during the 1970s,[5–11] particularly during influenza B epidemics.[12, 13] In 1974, before the establishment of CDC's Reye's Syndrome Surveillance in December 1976, 83% of the 379 cases reported that year occurred over a 2-month period during an epidemic of influenza B (Hong Kong/5/72). An increase in Reye's syndrome reports also occurred in 1977 and 1980, 454 and 555 cases, respectively, both coincident with significant influenza B epidemics.[7] Although influenza A had been identified as a risk factor for Reye's syndrome in 1967,[14] this association was further strengthened by the appearance of a cluster of 85 cases linked to influenza virus A(H1N1) activity during the winter of 1978 to 1979.[6] Subsequent reports also confirmed the association of Reye's syndrome with influenza A virus, with varicella-zoster virus, and with dengue virus.[15–18]

Because of its association with both influenza and varicella, Reye's syndrome exhibits a distinct seasonal pattern and most cases occur during the winter and spring months. Reye's syndrome principally affects children 18 years old and younger, although it has been reported in adults.[19–23]

In 1981, the U.S. Public Health Service Task Force on Reye's Syndrome initiated and reviewed a series of retrospective case-control studies and demonstrated that, of the medications commonly used to treat influenza or chickenpox, aspirin was significantly associated with the development of Reye's syndrome.[24, 25] Since the publication of the results of the U.S. Public Health Service study and the development and dissemination of recommendations against the use of aspirin in children in the setting of a presumed viral infection,[26] the incidence of Reye's syndrome has decreased dramatically in the United States, despite the significant influenza B epidemics in 1987 and 1988. In 1987 and 1988, only 36 and 25 cases, respectively, were reported to CDC.[8–10] Since then, reports to CDC have dropped off substantially, with an average of fewer than 20 reports a year, although clusters continue to occur[9, 11] (Table 165–1).

In the United Kingdom, nationwide Reye's syndrome surveillance was initiated in 1981. During the 1980s the annual incidence ranged between 0.16 and 0.61 per 10^5 children younger than 16 years.[27] A similar pattern in the reduction of reported Reye's syndrome cases was noted in the United Kingdom after both a public education campaign highlighting the risk of aspirin in children after viral illnesses and the withdrawal of children's aspirin formulations. In the United Kingdom and the United States, males and females are equally affected; however, in the United Kingdom the age distribution of cases is younger (33 to 54 months of age) than that observed in the United States (6 to 8 years of age), a feature that has been attributed in part to differences in the investigation and reporting of inborn errors of metabolism as Reye's syndrome.

Since the initial reports of Reye's syndrome, improved diagnosis of inborn errors of metabolism with the increased availability of gas chromatography and mass spectrometry may have facilitated a more accurate accounting of Reye's syndrome cases.[28, 29] Since 1985, 25% of cases initially meeting the case definition of Reye's syndrome were subsequently reclassified as having an inborn error of metabolism.[30] Although the reduction in the number of cases of Reye's syndrome has been largely attributed to the significant reduction in the use of aspirin for treatment of fever during influenza and varicella-zoster, not all groups have been able to demonstrate this association.[31, 32]

Etiology

The temporal association of Reye's syndrome with influenza and varicella prompted speculation that viral factors are important, but none have been identified. Studies aimed at identifying influenza or varicella virus variants that exhibit hepatotropic properties were fruitless.[33] The use of common medications, particularly aspirin, was suggested by many workers.[34–37] Through epidemiologic studies, the U.S. Public Health Service Task Force demonstrated a statistically significant association between Reye's syndrome and the use of aspirin or salicylate medications. Several reports that examined the possible role of environmental toxins in Reye's syndrome, especially in areas of the world where contamination of foods with toxins such as aflatoxin B1[38] and pesticides[39] is more common, were unable to demonstrate consistently that they were risk factors for this syndrome.[33] However, several toxins have been noted to produce similar pathologic changes in the liver, including hypoglycin A poisoning (Jamaican vomiting sickness after the ingestion of akee apples) and salicylate intoxication.[23, 40]

TABLE 165–1 ■ Reye's Syndrome in the United States: 1974 to 1993

YEAR	INFLUENZA STRAIN	TOTAL	VARICELLA*	INCIDENCE†	CASE-FATALITY RATE (%)
1974	B	379	NA‡	0.6	41
1977	B	454	73	0.7	42
1978	A(H3N2)	236	69	0.4	29
1979	A(H1N1)	389	113	0.6	32
1980	B	555	103	0.9	23
1981	A(H3N2)	293	73	0.5	28
1982	B	211	45	0.3	33
1983	A(H3N2)	199	28	0.3	29
1984	A(H1N1)/B	203	26	0.3	24
1985	A(H3N2)	95	15	0.2	29
1986	B	100	5	0.2	25
1987	A(H1N1)	36	7	0.1	31
1988	A(H3N2)	25	4	<0.1	40
1989	A(H1N1)/B	25	3	<0.1	40
1990	A(H3N2)	19	3	<0.1	53
1991	B	15	3	<0.1	40
1992	A(H3N2)/A(H1N1)	13	1	<0.1	46
1993	B/A(H3N2)	19	1	<0.1	56

*Number of Reye's syndrome cases associated with varicella, by year.
†Incidence per 100,000 persons younger than 18 years.
‡Not available.
Courtesy of Dr. J. Bresee, Centers for Disease Control and Prevention, Atlanta, GA, 1995.

Pathology and Pathogenesis

Given the severity of the clinical syndrome, the absence of inflammatory changes in the liver is the most striking feature of this disorder.[41] There is a panlobular, microvesicular infiltration of the hepatocytes and hepatic mitochondria are swollen with a diffuse matrix, an absence of dense bodies, and few cristae on ultrastructural examination. The nature of this injury and its cause have been the subject of many reports.[42–49] These changes are not limited to hepatocytes, as mitochondria from the pancreas and muscle have also been shown to exhibit similar structural abnormalities.[50] Correlating with these ultrastructural abnormalities, mitochondrial function is also affected with reduced activity of inner membrane and internal mitochondrial enzymes while outer membrane and cytosolic enzyme activities are preserved.[50] Elevated levels of aspartate and alanine aminotransferases are characteristic in Reye's syndrome patients, and levels of mitochondrial isozymes are specifically elevated.[51] In addition, liver mitochondria are depleted of adenosine triphosphate relative to hepatocyte cytosol, suggesting that the level of endogenous biochemical activity in the mitochondria is low. This is also supported by the increase in serum levels of known mitochondrial substrates, such as lactate, pyruvate, alanine, and free fatty acids. The mitochondrial injury appears to be completely reversible. In general, the severity with which mitochondria are affected is directly related to the clinical manifestations of Reye's syndrome; the hepatic mitochondrial changes in patients in coma are substantially greater than among patients with less severe clinical manifestations.

Neuropathologic examination is most consistent with secondary effects from the metabolic derangements and features cerebral edema and anoxic neuronal degeneration without evidence of inflammatory changes, although these changes may be related to a generalized mitochondrial insult.[52]

The pathogenesis of Reye's syndrome is complex and is incompletely understood. The lack of inflammatory changes and the profound metabolic changes (Table 165–2) that result in hepatic encephalopathy appear to be more consistent with a toxin than the direct result of an infection. However, the consistent association of Reye's syndrome with antecedent viral infections and concomitant treatment with salicylate-containing medications has led to the hypothesis that the infection acts in some way to predispose to this syndrome, possibly by uncoupling of oxidative phosphorylation and a blockade of β-oxidation leading to a buildup of short and medium chain acyl coenzyme A esters that trap free coenzyme A within the mitochondria and interrupt mitochondrial metabolic pathways and respiration.[20, 30, 53, 54]

The possible role of mitochondrial toxins in the pathogenesis of Reye's syndrome was first suggested by Aprille,[42] who used a bioassay of rat liver mitochondria to search for substances in the serum of patients with Reye's syndrome that affected mitochondrial respiration. It was noted that serum from patients with Reye's syndrome stimulated stage IV mitochondrial respiration in their isolated rat liver mitochondria. Segalman and Lee[46] later showed that this stimulation was only transitory and was followed by inhibition of respiration. Subsequent studies suggested that the injury to the mitochondria in Reye's syndrome may be due to the presence of allantoin.[47–49] They also showed that calcium ions were important in this process, as the toxic effect of allantoin on mitochondrial respiration could be specifically inhibited by adding inhibitors of calcium transport across the mitochondrial membrane or chelating agents with high affinity for calcium such as ethylene glycol-bis(β-aminoethyl ether)-*N,N'*-tetraacetic acid (egtazic acid, EGTA). Allantoin is an intermediate of purine degradation that is highly toxic and not normally present in human serum, because uric acid is the final product of purine metabolism. Other species of mammals produce allantoin from uric acid by the action of uricase. The source of allantoin in the serum of Reye's syndrome patients is not known, but Segalman and Lee[46] showed that allantoin could be generated by the direct oxidation of urate by cytochrome c_3 in their mitochondrial assay system in vitro.

TABLE 165–2 ■ Metabolic and Pathologic Findings in Reye's Syndrome

Morphologically abnormal mitochondria in liver, muscle, and pancreas
Panlobar microvesicular infiltration of hepatocytes
Hepatomegaly
Ammonemia
Hypoglycemia (especially in young infants)
Elevated levels of aspartate and alanine aminotransferase, usually three times the limit of normal
Elevated serum levels of lactate, pyruvate, alanine, and free fatty acids

Clinical Manifestations

Usually Reye's syndrome develops in the days after a child's recovery from an uncomplicated viral infection, in most instances influenza or varicella. The child is usually afebrile and not jaundiced, although hepatomegaly is common. Initial manifestations of the disorder include nausea and 1 to 2 days of intractable vomiting, which may lead to dehydration and contribute to hypoglycemia, particularly in children younger than 4 years. Although featured in the initial description of patients with Reye's syndrome, profound hypoglycemia is uncommon and more likely to be attributed to the underlying metabolic stress, as normal glucose levels are easily maintained by use of glucose-containing intravenous fluids.[4] Increased lethargy, confusion, combativeness, drowsiness, and sleepiness usually follow. The child may become increasingly difficult to arouse and may eventually lapse into coma. The staging system (Table 165–3) developed for Reye's syndrome is a prognostic indicator.[52, 55] In general, the more profound the coma, the worse the prognosis, with a mortality rate from 10% to 60%.[12, 16, 19, 28, 56, 57] Although complete neurologic recovery can be expected, neurologic sequelae can be severe, especially in those who develop seizures or decerebrate posturing during hospitalization, although all other organ systems appear to recover fully among survivors.[58, 59]

Differential Diagnosis

Many inborn errors of metabolism, especially those associated with elevated serum ammonia levels and/or neurologic manifestations (e.g., ornithine transcarbamylase deficiency, carnitine deficiency, glutaric aciduria) can complicate the diagnosis.[4, 60, 61] These should be considered, especially in situations in which Reye's syndrome appears to be recurrent or has been seen previously in a sibling. Therefore, initial diagnostic investigations should include tests that can establish the diagnosis of an inborn error of metabolism as well as Reye's syndrome, including a urine specimen for organic acid analysis, plasma for acylcarnitine analysis, and skin biopsy specimens for fibroblast culture and enzyme analysis.[28, 30] The most common mimics of Reye's syndrome are listed in Table 165–4.[62–67]

TABLE 165–3 ■ Staging of Reye's Syndrome

SIGN	STAGE I	STAGE II	STAGE III	STAGE IV	STAGE V
Level of consciousness	Lethargy; but follows verbal commands	Combative or stuporous; verbalizes inappropriately	Coma	Coma	Coma
Posture	Normal	Normal	Decorticate	Decerebrate	Flaccid
Response to pain	Purposeful	Purposeful or nonpurposeful	Decorticate	Decerebrate	None
Pupillary reaction	Brisk	Sluggish	Sluggish	Sluggish	None
Oculocephalic (doll's eye reflex)	Normal	Conjugate deviation	Conjugate deviation	Inconsistent or absent	None

Diagnosis

The CDC's case definition of Reye's syndrome (Table 165–5) was developed as an epidemiologic tool for surveillance and reporting.[10] The clinical diagnosis of Reye's syndrome is based on the clinical manifestations and medication history of the child, liver biopsy, cerebrospinal fluid examination, and biochemical markers. Reye's syndrome should be actively considered when an afebrile child presents in a state of altered consciousness after a period of intractable vomiting in the setting of a recent febrile illness treated with aspirin or salicylate-containing products. A clinical diagnosis is more difficult in children younger than 1 year, because respiratory disturbances such as hyperventilation or apneic episodes and seizures occur more frequently. Elevations of serum transaminase (aspartate and alanine aminotransferases) and ammonia levels occur, and the bilirubin value may be only mildly elevated but is often normal. Other laboratory abnormalities, which may include elevations of creatine kinase and lactate dehydrogenase values as well as decreased prothrombin activity, are supportive of the diagnosis but not definitive. Hypoglycemia may occur in infants, but glucose levels are usually normal in children older than 4 years. The cerebrospinal fluid usually supports the clinical impression of encephalopathy rather than encephalitis or meningoencephalitis, and protein and glucose concentrations are normal, except in cases with concurrent hypoglycemia. Serum should also be analyzed for levels of salicylate and acetaminophen. Liver biopsy is usually not necessary and should be considered only for infants and children with recurrent or familial Reye's syndrome for a more definitive diagnosis of the underlying hepatic pathologic condition.

TABLE 165–4 ■ Metabolic Disorders That May Mimic Reye's Syndrome

- Disorders of ureagenesis
  - Ornithine transcarbamylase deficiency
  - Carbamoylphosphate synthetase deficiency
  - Argininosuccinic acid synthetase deficiency
  - Lysineuric protein intolerance
- Disorders of branched chain amino acid catabolism
  - Propionyl-CoA* carboxylase deficiency
  - Methylmalonyl-CoA mutase deficiency
  - Methylmalonyl-CoA racemase deficiency
  - Isovaleryl-CoA dehydrogenase deficiency
- Disorders of ketogenesis
  - Various acyl-CoA dehydrogenase deficiencies
  - 3-Hydroxy-3-methyglutaryl-CoA lyase deficiency
  - Systemic carnitine palmitoyltransferase deficiency
- Disorders of carbohydrate metabolism
  - Fructose-1,6-diphosphatase deficiency
- Intoxications
  - Salicylate or amiodarone intoxication
  - Jamaican vomiting sickness
  - Dipropyl acetate intoxication

*CoA, Coenzyme A.

Treatment

Therapy for Reye's syndrome is primarily supportive and closely tied to the stage of coma (see Table 165–3). As with all patients with severe metabolic derangements and altered consciousness, hemodynamic monitoring, including careful monitoring of fluid and electrolyte balance, is crucial, as are ventilatory support and protection of the airway, when appropriate. Although continuous monitoring of blood gas values has been recommended,[52] anecdotally reported attempts to reverse the metabolic derangements typical of Reye's syndrome by heroic interventions such as hypothermic total-body washout, exchange transfusions, dialysis, barbiturate coma, bowel sterilization, charcoal hemoperfusion plasmapheresis, amino acid and phosphate infusions, and insulin administration have not been demonstrated to be efficacious.[4, 51, 68, 69] However, a report of the experimental effect of interferon alfa in prevention of mitochondrial swelling induced by acetylsalicylates suggests that this may offer a specific therapy in the treatment of Reye's syndrome.[70] With progressive neurologic deterioration, administration of intravenous fluids should be adjusted to minimize episodes of hypotension and to sustain organ function while not exacerbating the potential of increased intracranial pressure that results from cerebral edema. Intracranial pressure should be carefully monitored because it is the principal contributor to the mortality of Reye's syndrome, and aggressive efforts must be made to control it with mannitol or glycerol or controlled hyperventilation.[71]

TABLE 165–5 ■ Reye's Syndrome: Case Definition

According to the CDC's case definition, the following conditions must be met for consideration as a Reye's syndrome case:

1. Acute noninflammatory encephalopathy documented by
   a. Alteration in the level of consciousness and, if available, a record of cerebrospinal fluid containing ≤8 leukocytes per mm^3 *or*
   b. Histologic specimen demonstrating cerebral edema without perivascular or meningeal inflammation
2. Hepatopathy documented either by a liver biopsy or autopsy considered to be diagnostic of Reye's syndrome or by a threefold or greater rise in the levels of serum aspartate aminotransferase, serum alanine aminotransferase, or serum ammonia *and*
3. No more reasonable explanation for the cerebral and hepatic abnormalities

From Reye syndrome—United States, 1985. MMWR Morbid Mortal Wkly Rep 35:66, 1986.

Prevention

The results of the U.S. Public Health Service study clearly demonstrated that aspirin use was significantly related to development of Reye's syndrome. The wide publicity that this study received has resulted in a dramatic reduction in the use of aspirin in children and in a parallel drop in cases of Reye's syndrome[72, 73] (see Table 165–1). It is clear from this experience that Reye's syndrome can be effectively prevented by avoiding aspirin and acetylsalicylate-containing medications in the treatment of symptoms during a typical viral infection. Nevertheless, children who receive aspirin routinely for treatment of various connective tissue diseases appear to be at an increased risk for Reye's syndrome.[74, 75] This includes children with juvenile rheumatoid arthritis. A CDC analysis demonstrated that since 1990, 39% of Reye's syndrome cases were linked to antecedent aspirin use, with the majority of cases in children without chronic underlying conditions that would necessitate the use of aspirin, further demonstrating that Reye's syndrome continues to be a preventable disease, by restricting the use of aspirin during periods when influenza and varicella are epidemic, by substituting non–aspirin-containing medications, or by immunizing these children against influenza or varicella.[9] Although the number of varicella-associated cases has been insignificant during the past decade, increasing use of the varicella vaccine should continue to minimize the risk that this may contribute to overall Reye's syndrome morbidity and mortality.

References

1. Brain WR, Hunter D, Turnbull HM: Acute meningoencephalomyelitis of childhood. Lancet 1:221, 1929.
2. Reye RDK, Morgan G, Baral J: Encephalopathy and fatty degeneration of the viscera: A disease entity in childhood. Lancet 2:749, 1963.
3. Johnson GM, Scurleyis TD, Carroll NB: A study of 16 fatal cases of encephalitis-like disease in North Carolina children. N C Med J 24:464, 1970.
4. Keating JP: Reye syndrome. *In* Feigin RD, Cherry JD (eds): Textbook of Pediatric Infectious Diseases, ed 3. Philadelphia, WB Saunders, 1992, pp 705–708.
5. Barrett MJ, Hurwitz ES, Schonberger LB, Rogers MF: Changing epidemiology of Reye's syndrome in the United States. Pediatrics 77:598, 1986.
6. Centers for Disease Control: Reye syndrome—United States. MMWR Morbid Mortal Wkly Rep 28:97, 1979.
7. Reye syndrome surveillance—United States, 1989. MMWR Morbid Mortal Wkly Rep 40:88, 1991.
8. Reye syndrome surveillance—United States, 1986. MMWR Morbid Mortal Wkly Rep 36:689, 1986.
9. Bresee JS, Khan AS, Strine T, et al: Reye syndrome surveillance—United States. Sixty-third Annual Meeting of the Society for Pediatric Research; May 1994; Seattle, WA; p 110A.
10. Reye syndrome—United States, 1985. MMWR Morbid Mortal Wkly Rep 35:66, 1986.
11. Poss WB, Vernon DD, Dean JM: A reemergence of Reye's syndrome. Arch Pediatr Adolesc Med 148:879, 1994.
12. Corey L, Rubin RJ, Hattwick MAE, et al: A nationwide outbreak of Reye's syndrome: Its relationship with influenza B. Am J Med 61:615, 1976.
13. Corey L, Rubin RJ, Bregman D, et al: Diagnostic criteria for influenza B–associated Reye's syndrome: Clinical vs. pathologic criteria. Pediatrics 60:602, 1977.
14. Hall BD, Hughes WT, Kmetz D: Reye's syndrome: An association with influenza A infection. J Ky Med Assoc 4:269, 1967.
15. Linnemann CC, Shea L, Partin JC, et al: Reye's syndrome: Epidemiological and viral studies, 1963–1974. Am J Epidemiol 101: 517, 1975.
16. Lichetenstein PK. Heubi JE, Caughety CC, et al: Grade I Reye's syndrome: A frequent cause of vomiting and liver dysfunction after varicella and upper respiratory-tract infections. N Engl J Med 309:133, 1983.
17. Iyngkaran N, Yadav M, Harun F, et al: Augmented tumour necrosis factor in Reye's syndrome associated with dengue virus. Lancet 340:1466, 1992.
18. Hukin J, Junker AK, Thomas EE, et al: Reye syndrome associate with subclinical varicella zoster virus and influenza A infection. Pediatr Neurol 9:134, 1993.
19. Varma RR, Riedel DR, Komorowski RA, et al: Reye's syndrome in nonpediatric age groups. JAMA 242:1373, 1979.
20. Peters LJ, Wiener GJ, Gilliam J, et al: Reye's syndrome in adults, a case report and review of literature. Arch Intern Med 146:2401, 1986.
21. Atkins JN, Haponik EF: Reye's syndrome in the adult patient. Am J Med 67:672, 1979.
22. Al-Tikriti SA, Rowe PA, Munro AJ: Adult Reye's syndrome. J R Soc Med 77:694, 1984.
23. Chan D: Reye's syndrome in a young adult. Mil Med 158:65, 1993.
24. Hurwitz ES, Barrett MJ, Bergman D, et al: Public Health Service study on Reye's syndrome and medications: Report of the pilot phase. N Engl J Med 313:849, 1985.
25. Hurwitz ES, Barrett MJ, Bregman D, et al: Public Health Service study of Reye's syndrome and medications. JAMA 257:1905, 1987.
26. Surgeon General's advisory on the use of salicylates and Reye syndrome. MMWR Morbid Mortal Wkly Rep 31:289, 1982.
27. Porter JDH, Robinson PH, Glasgow JFT, et al: Trends in the incidence of Reye's syndrome and the use of aspirin. Arch Dis Child 65:826, 1990.
28. Glasgow JFT, Moore R: Current concepts in Reye's syndrome. Br J Hosp Med 50:599, 1993.
29. Green A, Hall SM: Investigation of metabolic disorders resembling Reye's syndrome. Arch Dis Child 67:1313, 1992.
30. Glasgow JFT, Moore R: Reye's syndrome 30 years on. BMJ 307:950, 1993.
31. Center for Disease Control: Reye syndrome surveillance—United States, 1987 and 1988. MMWR Morbid Mortal Wkly Rep 38:325, 1989.
32. Orlowski JP, Campbell P, Goldstein S: Reye's syndrome: A case control study of medication used and associated viruses in Australia. Cleve Clin J Med 57:323, 1990.
33. La Montagne JR: Summary of a workshop on disease mechanisms and prospects for prevention of Reye's syndrome. J Infect Dis 148:943, 1983.
34. Mortimer EA Jr, Lepow ML: Varicella with hypoglycemia possibly due to salicylate use. Am J Dis Child 103:583, 1962.
35. Starko KM, Ray CG, Dominguez LB, et al: Reye's syndrome and salicylate use. Pediatrics 66:859, 1980.
36. Waldman RJ, Hall WN, McGee N, et al: Aspirin as a risk factor in Reye's syndrome. JAMA 247:3089, 1982.
37. Halpin TJ, Holtzhauer FJ, Campbell RJ, et al: Reye's syndrome and medication use. JAMA 248:687, 1982.
38. Bourgeois CH: Encephalopathy and fatty viscera: A possible response to acute aflatoxin poisoning. *In* Pollack JD (ed): Reye's Syndrome. New York, Grune & Stratton, 1975, pp 131–134.
39. Rozee KR, Laltoo M, Lee SHS, et al: Emulsifiers as enhancement factors in virus virulence. *In* Crocker JFS (ed): Reye's Syndrome II. New York, Grune & Stratton, 1979, pp 443–457.
40. Makela AL, Lang H, Koppella P: Toxic encephalopathy with hyperammonemia during high-dose salicylate therapy. Acta Neurol Scand 61:146, 1980.
41. Chaves-Carballo E, Gomez MR, Sharbrough FW: Encephalopathy and fatty infiltration of the viscera (Reye-Johnson syndrome): A 17-year experience. Mayo Clin Proc 50:209, 1975.
42. Aprille JR: Reye's syndrome: Patient serum alters mitochondrial function and morphology in vitro. Science 197:908, 1977.
43. Aprille JR, Austin J, Costello C, et al: Identification of the Reye's syndrome "serum factor." Biochem Biophys Res Commun 94: 381, 1980.
44. Aprille JR: Salicylate has several effects on mitochondrial function. J Natl Reye's Syndr Found 2:56, 1981.
45. Asimakis GK, Aprille JR: Reye's syndrome: The effect of patient serum on mitochondrial respiration in vitro. Biochem Biophys Res Commun 79:1222, 1977.
46. Segalman TY, Lee CP: Reye's syndrome: Plasma-induced alter-

ation in mitochondrial structure and function. Arch Biochem Biophys 214:522, 1982.
47. Martens ME, Lee CP: Reye's syndrome: Salicylates and mitochondrial functions. Biochem Pharmacol 33:2869, 1984.
48. Martens ME, Chang CH, Lee CP: Reye's syndrome: Mitochondrial swelling and Ca^{2+} release induced by Reye's plasma, allantoin, and salicylate. Arch Biochem Biophys 244:773, 1986.
49. Martens ME, Storey BT, Lee CP: Generation of allantoin from the oxidation of urate by cytochrome *c* and its possible role in the Reye's syndrome. Arch Biochem Biophys 252:91, 1987.
50. Partin JC, Schubert WK, Partin JS: Mitochondrial ultrastructure in Reye's syndrome. N Engl J Med 285:1339, 1971.
51. Thaler MM: Clinical and enzymatic indices of hepatic dysfunction in Reye's syndrome. *In* Crocker JFS (ed): Reye's Syndrome II. New York, Grune & Stratton, 1979, pp 443–457.
52. The diagnosis and treatment of Reye's syndrome. Natl Inst Health Consensus Dev Conf Summ 4(1):7, 1981.
53. Deshmukh DR, Maassab HF, Mason M: Interactions of aspirin and other potential etiologic factors in an animal model of Reye's syndrome. Proc Natl Acad Sci USA 79:755, 1982.
54. Corkey BE, Hale DE, Glennon MC, et al: Relationship between unusual hepatic acyl coenzyme A profiles and the pathogenesis of Reye syndrome. J Clin Invest 88:782, 1988.
55. Corey L, Rubin RJ, Hatwick MAW: Reye's syndrome: Clinical progression and evaluation of therapy. Pediatrics 60:708, 1977.
56. Smith AL: Ammonia disposal in Reye's syndrome. N Engl J Med 294:855, 1976.
57. Consensus Development Conference: Diagnosis and treatment of Reye's syndrome. JAMA 247:3089, 1982.
58. Benjamin PY, Levinsohn M, Drotar D, et al: Intellectual and emotional sequelae of Reye's syndrome. Crit Care Med 10:583, 1982.
59. Brunner RL, O'Grady DJ, Partin JC, et al: Neuropsychologic consequences of Reye syndrome. J Pediatr 95:706, 1979.
60. Chapoy PR, Amgelini C, Brown WJ, et al: Systemic carnitine deficiency: A treatable inherited lipid-storage disease presenting as Reye's syndrome. N Engl J Med 303:1389, 1990.
61. Rowe PC, Valle D, Brusilow SW: Inborn errors of metabolism in children with Reye's syndrome: Differential diagnosis. J Pediatr 113:156, 1988.
62. Greene CL, Blitzer MG, Shapira E: Inborn errors of metabolism and Reye syndrome: Differential diagnosis. J Pediatr 113:156, 1988.
63. Rowe PC, Valle D, Brusilow SW: Inborn errors of metabolism in children referred with Reye's syndrome: A changing pattern. JAMA 260:3167, 1988.
64. Jones DB, Mullick FG, Hoofnagle JH, et al: Reye's syndrome–like illness in a patient receiving amiodarone. Am J Gastroenterol 83:967, 1988.
65. Noda S, Umezaki H, Yamamoto K, et al: Reye-like syndrome following treatment with the pantothenic acid antagonist, calcium hopantenate. J Neurol Neurosurg Psychiatry 51:582, 1988.
66. Shahar E, Brand N, Shapira Y, et al: Familial carnitine deficiency: Further evidence for autosomal recessive transmission with variable expression. J Neurol Neurosurg Psychiatry 51:298, 1988.
67. Treem WR, Witzleben CA, Picolli DA, et al: Medium chain and long chain acyl CoA dehydrogenase deficiency: Clinical, pathologic and ultrastructural differentiation from Reye's syndrome. Hepatology 6:1270, 1986.
68. Hottenlocher RP: Reye's syndrome: Relation of outcome to therapy. J Pediatr 80:845, 1970.
69. Trey C, Burns DG, Saunder SJ: Treatment of hepatic coma by exchange blood transfusion. N Engl J Med 294:473, 1966.
70. Tomoda T, Takeda K, Kurashige T, et al: Experimental study on Reye's syndrome: Inhibitory effect of interferon alfa on acetylsalicylate-induced injury to rat liver mitochondria. Metabolism 41:887, 1992.
71. Kindt GW, Waldman J, Kohl S, et al: Intracranial pressure in Reye's syndrome: Monitoring and control. JAMA 231:822, 1975.
72. Pinsky PF, Hurwitz ES, Schonberger LB, et al: Reye's syndrome and aspirin: Evidence for a dose-response effect. JAMA 260:657, 1988.
73. Khan AS, Kent J, Schonberger LB: Aspirin and Reye's syndrome. Lancet 341:968, 1993.
74. Sullivan KM, Remington PL, Hurwitz ES, et al: Reye's syndrome among patients with juvenile rheumatoid arthritis. JAMA 260:3434, 1988.
75. Rennebohm RM, Heubi JE, Daugherty CC: Reye syndrome in children receiving salicylate therapy for connective tissue disease. J Pediatr 107:877, 1985.

TUBERCULOSIS AND LEPROSY

166

Tuberculosis

Zahra Toossi
Jerrold J. Ellner

Tuberculosis is the oldest documented infectious disease, and it remains an important global health problem. An estimated 1 billion people worldwide are infected with *Mycobacterium tuberculosis;* 8 to 10 million new cases of tuberculosis occur each year, and the number of new cases is estimated to increase to 12 million in the year 2005.[1] Inadequacy of diagnosis and prevention and inefficient treatment programs account for uncontrolled infection in developing countries. In the United States, the incidence of tuberculosis had been in decline. However, between 1985 and 1993, a 14% increase was documented.[2] Several factors including the epidemic of human immunodeficiency virus (HIV) infection, occurrence of disease in foreign-born residents, and transmission of tuberculosis in congregate settings such as prisons and shelters for the homeless account for the increase in incidence. The unusual presentation of disease among special groups (e.g., elderly individuals, immunocompromised persons) and disease due to multidrug-resistant strains of *M. tuberculosis* compound the problem of eradicating tuberculosis in the United States. These challenges have been addressed with intensified control efforts; the result is a 6.4% decrease in reported cases in the United States from 24,361 in 1994 (9.4 per 100,000 population) to 22,812 new cases in 1995 (8.7 per 100,000). See Chapter 273 for discussions of bacteriology, epidemiology, environmental control, and prevention.

Pulmonary Tuberculosis

The predominant portal of entry for *M. tuberculosis* is the respiratory route. The lungs are also the main site of expression of clinical tuberculosis: 82% of patients manifest pulmonary disease. The spectrum of the interactions of the host immune factors with tubercle bacilli is reflected in the distinct clinical forms of pulmonary disease.

Once virulent tubercle bacilli gain access to the alveoli, they are subjected to phagocytosis by tissue macrophages. In nonimmune persons, bacilli evade destruction within macrophages, replicate, and eventually destroy the cells. Circulating phagocytes, initially polymorphonuclear but then chiefly mononuclear, are attracted to this area of primary infection. With the enlargement of the inflammatory focus, central necrosis occurs, which may become caseous. Although pulmonary infection remains restricted anatomically, organisms spread to the draining hilar lymph nodes and then through the thoracic duct to the blood stream. Within 4 to 6 weeks, cellular immunity develops. Protective immunity, mediated by subsets of T lymphocytes producing macrophage-activating polypeptide factors (cytokines), in particular interferon-γ, enables the phagocytes to destroy intracellular bacilli. Thus, regression and healing of both primary and disseminated foci are seen. Bacilli are not totally eradicated, however, and the lifelong potential for reactivation is maintained. The long-term survival of *Mycobacterium* organisms is favored at sites of high tissue oxygen tension, such as subapical regions of the lungs, cortices of the kidneys, and vertebral bodies. Both in progressive primary disease and in reactivated tuberculosis, the existing cellular immunity of the *M. tuberculosis*–infected person is inadequate to inhibit bacillary growth. In addition, exaggerated aspects of delayed-type hypersensitivity contribute to disease. Macrophage production of cytokines, such as tumor necrosis factor, proteases, and lipases, enhances liquefaction of caseous foci, favoring extracellular bacillary growth and cavity formation. Other cytokines, such as transforming growth factor, may favor local bacillary growth, suppress T-cell responses, and promote fibrosis.[3] On pathologic examination, inflammation, caseation necrosis, cavity formation, and fibrosis occur sequentially; however, they may be simultaneous to different degrees. Cavities are kept open by their fibrous capsules and elasticity of the pulmonary tissue. Spread within the lungs is by bronchial channels (bronchogenic spread) or directly to neighboring alveoli. Progression from minimal disease to advanced disease may occur within months.

Primary infection with tubercle bacilli is most often silent clinically and is identified only by development of skin test reactivity to tuberculin purified protein derivative. Occasionally, more commonly in children, fever, a nonproductive cough, and shortness of breath develop. Physical examination may reveal posttussive rales or signs of consolidation. Chest radiographs are normal in most patients with primary tuberculosis, perhaps because films are obtained after the pulmonary process has resolved. Infiltration without cavitation, in the anterior segment of the upper lobes or in the middle or lower lobes, with unilateral hilar or paratracheal adenopathy may be seen (Fig. 166–1*A*). In 15% of patients with radiographic abnormalities, mediastinal adenopathy that is often bilateral is seen. Massive hilar adenopathy can lead to atelectasis, commonly involving the anterior segment of the right upper lobe or the medial segment of the right middle lobe. Bronchiectasis may follow. More commonly, calcification of both the lymph node lesion and the parenchymal lesion, known as the Ghon complex, occurs. Primary tuberculosis is paucibacillary. Bacteriologic confirmation by culture of sputum or bronchial washings can be achieved in 25% to 30% of cases. At times, allergic nonpulmonary manifestations are the only evidence of a primary infection. Erythema nodosum, phlyctenular conjunctivitis, and a sterile polyarthritis known as Poncet disease[4] are various syndromes resulting from systemic tuberculin hypersensitivity. Tuberculous pleuritis occurs months after primary infection, and its clinical manifestations are mainly a reflection of a cell-mediated immune response to mycobacterial antigens in the pleural space (see later).

Progressive primary tuberculosis results from the failure of the timely development of a sufficient immune response to limit bacillary growth. In young or elderly persons and those with immunodeficiency, such as HIV-infected individuals, massive lymphohematogenous dissemination can occur, resulting in miliary and meningeal disease. Approximately 10% of young adults with symptomatic primary infection progress to the chronic destructive phase of tuberculosis within a relatively short time. Presentation is similar to that of patients with reactivation tuberculosis. Chest radiographs show upper lobe apical and posterior segment disease, often cavitary, and at times concomitant evidence of primary disease, such as hilar adenopathy. Lower lobe tuberculosis, usually a manifestation of progressive primary disease, constitutes 10% of all pulmonary tuberculosis.[5] It is more common in elderly persons and in patients with diabetes mellitus. There are frequently associated endobronchial lesions.[6] Chest radiographs sometimes show a single cavity, which may have an air-fluid level (Fig. 166–1*B*). Diagnosis may be particularly difficult in such cases, because sputum may contain only few bacilli or none.

Reactivation tuberculosis develops at foci of hematogenous dissemination after a period of dormancy. In the apices of the lungs, small tubercles or fibrotic areas (Simon foci), occasionally seen on chest radiographs, are the sites of development of disease. Factors associated with attenuation of the host cellular immune response favor reactivation of tuberculosis in latent foci. The symptoms of pulmonary tuberculosis are insidious in onset, generally occurring only after the disease has progressed to some extent. Fever (44%), night sweats or chills (60%), fatigue (60%), anorexia, and weight loss are reported. Twenty percent, however, lack such symptoms. Cough, chest pain, and sputum production are common. Hemoptysis, usually moderate, is reported in 25% of cases; it occurs with advanced disease and may indicate endobronchial involvement. On initial examination, only 15% of patients are febrile, whereas 40% manifest fever during hospitalization. Rales over the upper lung fields (at times heard only after coughing), amphoric breathing sounds, and dullness to percussion may be present. On chest radiographs, there is typically a patchy or confluent consolidation with increased linear densities extending to the ipsilateral hilum, and thick-walled cavities without air-fluid levels are common (Fig. 166–1*C*). The apical or posterior segments of the upper lobes or the superior segments of the lower lobes are commonly involved. With bronchogenic spread, multiple alveolar densities can be seen. Lymph node enlargement is rare. Fibrosis with loss of volume and calcification can be seen in chronic disease. Laboratory abnormalities include a normochromic, normocytic anemia; normal to minimally elevated white cell count; and, in 20% of patients, monocytosis. Hypercalcemia, hyponatremia, and elevated serum globulin values can be detected. The tuberculin skin test (5 tuberculin units) result is positive in the majority of patients but may be negative in up to 25%. Diagnosis of tuberculosis is usually achieved by demonstration of acid-fast bacilli (AFB) in expectorated sputum and is confirmed by growing the organisms in culture. For microscopy, fluorescent staining is preferable because it is more sensitive and less time-consuming. Early growth detection using the BACTEC system coupled with the highly specific and sensitive DNA probe (GenProbe) identification of *M. tuberculosis* aids in the rapid diagnosis of tuberculosis. If the patient cannot produce a sputum specimen, induction of sputum should be attempted by having the patient inhale saline aerosol for 10 minutes. Morning

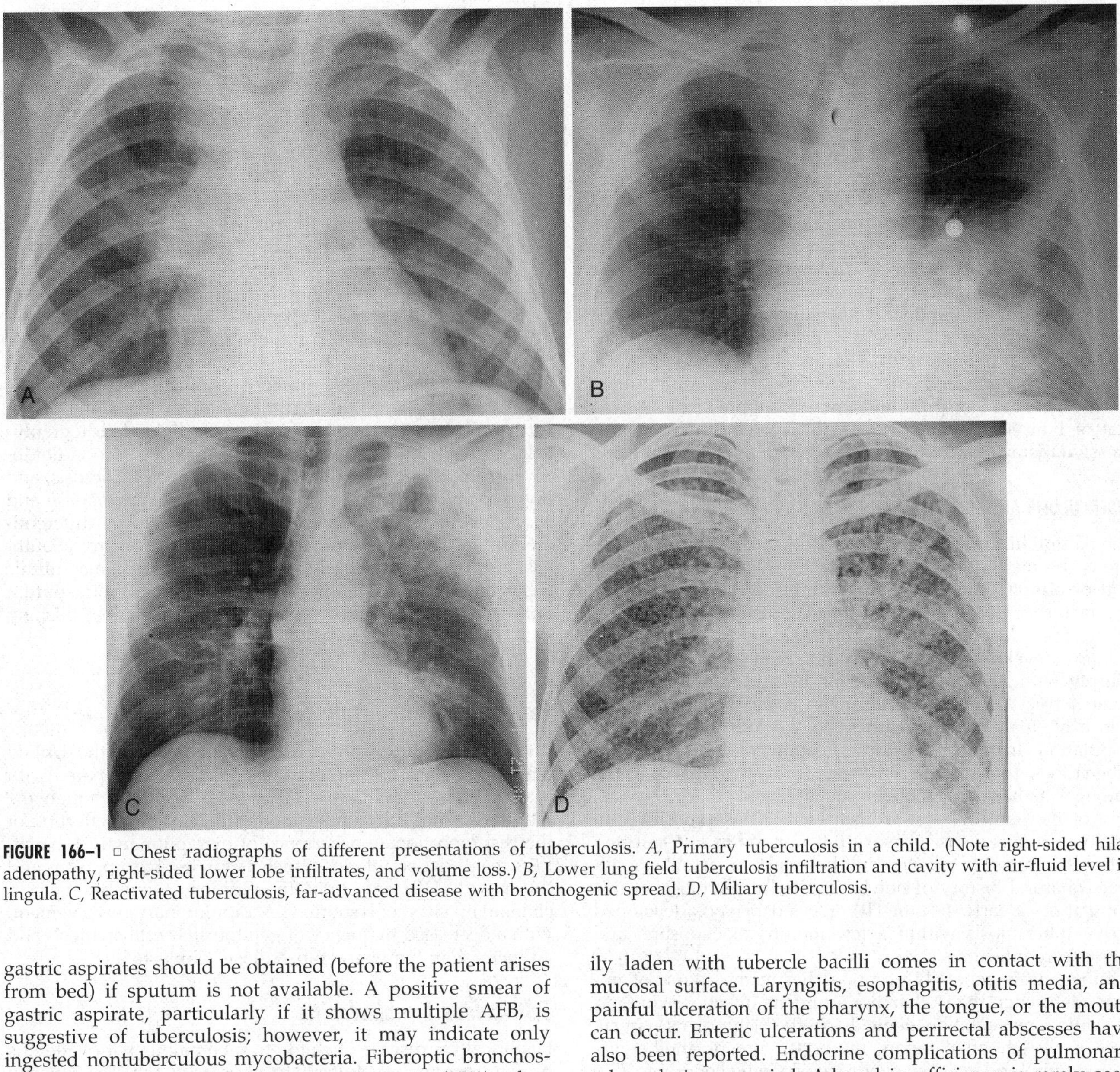

FIGURE 166–1 □ Chest radiographs of different presentations of tuberculosis. *A,* Primary tuberculosis in a child. (Note right-sided hilar adenopathy, right-sided lower lobe infiltrates, and volume loss.) *B,* Lower lung field tuberculosis infiltration and cavity with air-fluid level in lingula. *C,* Reactivated tuberculosis, far-advanced disease with bronchogenic spread. *D,* Miliary tuberculosis.

gastric aspirates should be obtained (before the patient arises from bed) if sputum is not available. A positive smear of gastric aspirate, particularly if it shows multiple AFB, is suggestive of tuberculosis; however, it may indicate only ingested nontuberculous mycobacteria. Fiberoptic bronchoscopy is efficient in establishing the diagnosis (95%) when sputum is unavailable or when smears are negative on repeated examination.[7] Culture of bronchoalveolar lavage material is particularly helpful. Postbronchoscopy sputum was the only source of positive material in 13% of patients in one study.[8] Granulomata can be identified in 20% of transbronchial biopsy specimens. The diagnostic value of fiberoptic bronchoscopy and biopsy is mainly in miliary tuberculosis, or lower lobe disease, in which the number of AFB is small.

Complications

Empyema can complicate extensive parenchymal cavitary tuberculosis, either by contiguous extension or as a result of a bronchopleural fistula. Pneumothorax is uncommon. Pleural fibrosis may lead to trapping and restriction of lung expansion. Massive hemoptysis secondary to the erosion of a pulmonary artery by a cavity (Rasmussen aneurysm) is rare. Hemoptysis, moderate to severe, may occur secondary to an aspergilloma in a healed tuberculous cavity. Mild hemoptysis may be associated with bronchiectasis, a complication of healed tuberculosis. Involvement of the upper respiratory tract or gastrointestinal tract may result when sputum heavily laden with tubercle bacilli comes in contact with the mucosal surface. Laryngitis, esophagitis, otitis media, and painful ulceration of the pharynx, the tongue, or the mouth can occur. Enteric ulcerations and perirectal abscesses have also been reported. Endocrine complications of pulmonary tuberculosis are varied. Adrenal insufficiency is rarely seen in patients with pulmonary tuberculosis. In a retrospective analysis, none of 86 cases of Addison disease was attributable to tuberculosis.[9] In disseminated disease, however, adrenal gland involvement is not uncommon. Hyponatremia secondary to the syndrome of inappropriate antidiuretic hormone secretion is seen occasionally but is rarely symptomatic. Hypercalcemia is present in up to 25% of patients with active pulmonary tuberculosis and disappears with treatment of the infection. Similar to the situation with other granulomatous diseases, hypercalcemia in tuberculosis is associated with high serum calcitriol (1,25-dihydroxycholecalciferol) levels.[10, 11]

EXOGENOUS REINFECTION

In geographic areas of low tuberculosis transmission, tuberculin reactors with a history of prior clinical tuberculosis are in general resistant to reinfection; however, rare instances of reinfection tuberculosis, established by phage typing and drug resistance pattern of the isolate, have been described,[12] and they may be more common in malnourished or immunosuppressed persons. In geographic areas of high transmission, reinfection may be more common. Presentation is similar to that of far-advanced tuberculosis.

TUBERCULOSIS AND CANCER

Patients with pulmonary tuberculosis have a 20-fold greater risk for lung cancer. Tuberculous patients older than 55 years, especially those who are heavy smokers, should have cytologic examination of their sputum. Isolated involvement of the anterior segment of the upper lobes, lower lobe involvement, presence of a mass larger than 3 cm in diameter, or presence of cavities with irregular boundaries should trigger evaluation for complicating cancer despite the presence of AFB on sputum. Pulmonary tuberculosis may also complicate other neoplasia, especially Hodgkin's disease, non-Hodgkin's lymphoma, and head and neck malignant neoplasms. Disseminated disease or extensive pulmonary disease is typical of profound immunosuppression, such as that of lymphoma patients who are receiving immunosuppressive therapy, and it is associated with a poor prognosis.

TUBERCULOSIS AND HUMAN IMMUNODEFICIENCY VIRUS INFECTION

The natural history of *M. tuberculosis* infection is dramatically altered by the presence of HIV infection.[13] In fact, the reduction of cellular immunity by HIV infection is the strongest risk factor for progression of a tuberculous infection to frank tuberculosis. In HIV-infected individuals, a 4% to 8% yearly risk for development of reactivation tuberculosis contrasts sharply with a 5% to 10% lifetime risk in immunologically intact subjects. The risk for tuberculosis varies with the prevalence of dual infection with *M. tuberculosis* and HIV in a population. In many developing countries, 40% to 70% of tuberculous patients are HIV-seropositive. In this country, among U.S.-born tuberculous patients aged 30 to 39 years, 35% of men and 20% of women were HIV-seropositive. In addition, outbreaks of primary tuberculosis in HIV-infected subjects in housing facilities and hospitals indicate the accelerated natural history of newly acquired tuberculosis in this population. Nearly 40% of HIV-infected persons developed active tuberculosis within a few months of exposure, and many were infectious cases.

Tuberculosis generally occurs earlier in the course of immunodeficiency than other opportunistic infections do, and its clinical presentation depends on the stage of HIV infection. Early on, often before the occurrence of another acquired immunodeficiency syndrome–defining condition, 75% to 100% of tuberculosis manifests as pulmonary disease, whereas 25% to 70% of patients who develop tuberculosis late in the course of HIV infection have extrapulmonary involvement.[14] Unusual radiographic features, such as lower lung field involvement, diffuse infiltration, noncavitary disease, intrathoracic adenopathy, and pleural effusions, are often seen.[15] Symptoms may be indistinguishable from those of other opportunistic infections. Tuberculous lymphadenitis and meningitis are not infrequent, and brain abscesses and vertebral, pericardial, peritoneal, and gastric involvement have been reported. In HIV-infected patients with extrapulmonary tuberculosis, active pulmonary tuberculosis is also likely. The yield of positive sputum smears varies but is typically lower in HIV-infected tuberculous patients, particularly if nonfluorescent stains are used.[16] Bronchoscopy with biopsy may be necessary for diagnosis in some cases. High-yield sources for establishing the diagnosis of disseminated tuberculosis include lymph node, blood, bone marrow, and urine samples. Results of tuberculin skin tests may be negative in up to 60% of patients. Treatment directed against *M. tuberculosis* should be initiated promptly once AFB have been identified in any specimen, despite that *Mycobacterium avium-intracellulare* complex infection may still be a consideration. The response to therapy is in general good; however, instances of progression of infection or relapse have been reported. Whether maintenance therapy to prevent recurrence of *M. tuberculosis* infection is necessary after completion of successful treatment is not known.

Differential Diagnosis

The major entity to be distinguished from pulmonary tuberculosis is carcinoma of the lung. The two may be present concurrently, and in such cases, delayed radiographic evidence of healing despite antituberculous therapy necessitates further diagnostic work-up. Bacterial lung abscesses can usually be differentiated from tuberculous infection by their lower lobe distribution and the presence of air-fluid levels in cavities and the frequent presence of putrid odor indicating anaerobic infection. Other granulomatous infections of the lung can be similar to tuberculosis clinically and radiographically. Fungal processes, such as histoplasmosis, coccidioidomycosis, blastomycosis, and occasionally cryptococcosis, and atypical mycobacterioses, such as *Mycobacterium kansasii* and *M. avium-intracellulare* infections, also have to be differentiated from tuberculosis. In veterans or in refugees from Southeast Asia, infection with *Pseudomonas pseudomallei* may mimic tuberculosis. Culture of the causative organism from sputum and occasionally serologic studies are helpful in establishing these other diagnoses.

Extrapulmonary Tuberculosis

The decline of extrapulmonary tuberculosis in the United States in the last two decades has been slow compared with that of pulmonary disease (1% versus 5%).[17] Although the reasons are not fully understood, this may be a reflection of the disproportionate occurrence of extrapulmonary tuberculosis in special populations, such as foreign-born persons and those with HIV infection. In addition, there has been a change in sites of reported extrapulmonary involvement, with a decreased frequency of genitourinary tuberculosis and an increase in lymphatic tuberculosis (Table 166–1).

Tuberculous Lymphadenitis

Historically a disease of children, tuberculous lymphadenitis presently occurs in adults 20 to 40 years of age. The majority of patients are Asian or African-American, and there is a 2:1 female-to-male predilection. In clinical presentation, more than 90% of tuberculous adenitis involves the lymph nodes of the head and neck, a reflection of recrudescence of tubercu-

TABLE 166–1 ■ Percent Distribution of Tuberculosis Cases by Site of Disease, United States

SITE OF TUBERCULOSIS	%
Pulmonary	82.5
Lymphatic	5.2
Pleural	4.0
Genitourinary	2.0
Bone and joint	1.7
Miliary	1.3
Meningeal	0.8
Peritoneal	0.6
Other	1.7

Data from Rieder HL, Snider DE Jr, Cauthen GM: Extrapulmonary tuberculosis in the United States. Am Rev Respir Dis 141:347–351, 1990.

losis in areas infected during generalized lymphatic spread of a primary pulmonary infection. Anterior and posterior cervical, supraclavicular, or submandibular nodes and occasionally submental and preauricular lymph nodes are involved. Although mediastinal nodes are the primary regional draining sites for pulmonary infection, only 5% of lymphatic tuberculosis is accounted for by such involvement. Multiple nodes within a group are involved, and bilateral involvement is common (25%). Generalized lymphadenopathy and hepatosplenomegaly occur in less than 5% of cases. When the focus of infection is on an extremity, such as in primary cutaneous inoculation, axillary or inguinal lymph nodes may be involved. Patients present with painless swelling of nodes, and only 20% have constitutional symptoms. Chronic draining ulcers are rare. Airway compromise secondary to enlarging and eroding parabronchial or paratracheal nodes in young children may lead to paroxysmal cough, wheezing, dyspnea, and finally respiratory distress. In adults, however, mediastinal involvement is commonly asymptomatic. Uncommon presentations include progressive jaundice due to biliary obstruction,[18] dysphagia due to cervical adenitis,[19] and chyluria due to obstruction of the thoracic duct.[20] Physical examination reveals discrete, rubbery, nontender lymph nodes. The result of tuberculin testing is positive in more than 90% of cases, and chest radiographs are abnormal in 30% of adults and the majority of children younger than 6 years. Biopsy and culture of the involved node are necessary to differentiate adenitis due to *M. tuberculosis* from that due to atypical *Mycobacterium* species, a more common problem in children.[21]

The clinical presentation is dramatically different in HIV-infected patients; two thirds have constitutional symptoms, and almost all have abnormalities on chest radiographs. The adenopathy may be painful. In one study, mean $CD4^+$ cell counts were less than 50/mm^3, and all patients were anergic.[22] In HIV-infected patients, fine-needle aspiration of the involved node is often diagnostic.

Management of adenitis caused by *M. tuberculosis* requires antituberculous chemotherapy, even when it is complicated by chronic drainage and sinus tracks. Excisional surgery should be reserved for cases that do not respond to chemotherapy.

Tuberculous Pleuritis

Involvement of the pleural space in tuberculosis most commonly results from rupture of a subpleural caseous focus, usually several months after a primary infection; however, it may occur any time in the course of tuberculosis. Host hypersensitivity to mycobacterial antigens initiates a brisk local cell-mediated immune response, resulting in an exudative pleural effusion and systemic stigmata of acute inflammation. Overall, pleuritis occurs in 10% of untreated tuberculin skin test "converters." In areas of the world where exposure to *M. tuberculosis* is common, tuberculous pleuritis affects a younger population; in the United States, it is seen in middle-aged and older persons. Tuberculosis may also involve the pleura, as a consequence of progressive primary disease or as a manifestation of disseminated disease; in these instances, the host generally has ineffective cellular immune responses, as do patients with HIV disease and other conditions associated with immunosuppression.

Two thirds of patients with tuberculous pleurisy present clinically with symptoms of less than 1 month's duration, at times mimicking acute bacterial pneumonia. Fever, pleuritic chest pain, and a nonproductive cough are present. In one series, 14% of the patients had no fever.[23] Weight loss, malaise, and night sweats are usually seen in patients who present with a more chronic illness. Up to 30% of tuberculin skin test results are negative or less than 5 mm early in disease; however, by 2 months, virtually all patients have positive reactions. Effusions are moderate in volume, are unilateral in 90% of cases, and for unknown reasons occur most often in the right hemithorax. Parenchymal disease may be evident in 30%, especially in older patients. The pleural fluid is an exudate with an abundance of lymphocytes; however, polymorphonuclear leukocytes may predominate initially. A small number of mesothelial cells (less than 5%) is consistent with the diagnosis of tuberculosis; fluid examination must be performed by an expert cytologist, however. The pleural fluid glucose value is depressed (below 50 mg/dL) in 20% of cases. A pleural fluid pH value below 7.3 favors the diagnosis of tuberculosis over malignant effusion. AFB are rarely identified in pleural fluid; mycobacterial cultures, however, are positive in 20% to 50% of cases, especially when larger volumes are cultured. Pleural biopsy is most helpful in establishing the diagnosis. Granulomatous pleuritis is seen in more than 60% of biopsy specimens, and AFB are seen in the material in 5% to 18%. Tissue cultures grow the organism in 55% of cases but less commonly in biopsy specimens that reveal nonspecific inflammation. Cumulatively, the diagnosis can be made on the initial pleural biopsy in 69% of cases—and in more than 95% if two or more specimens are procured.[24] Sputum and gastric aspirates demonstrate the organism in up to one third of patients, mostly those with clinically apparent pulmonary disease. Tuberculous pleuritis commonly resolves spontaneously within 2 to 4 months; however, there is a major risk for reactivation or miliary tuberculosis during the first 5 years of follow-up (65%).[23]

Genitourinary Tuberculosis

Involvement of the kidneys occurs as a sequela of blood-borne dissemination from a distant primary tuberculous focus. Tubercles are initially formed in the renal cortices and may undergo healing or progressive, gradual destruction with further spread to the medulla, renal pelvis, ureter, and bladder. Although tuberculosis usually involves both kidneys, progression of disease is asymmetric. Inflammation and fibrosis lead to urethral obstruction and ultimately hydronephrosis and a thick-walled, nondistensible bladder. Active renal parenchymal disease is usually silent; two thirds of cases present 5 years after the primary infection with *M. tuberculosis*.[25] Dysuria, gross hematuria, and occasionally flank pain are reported. Fever and systemic symptoms are infrequent, and 20% of patients are asymptomatic at the time of diagnosis. Chest radiographs show evidence of old tuberculosis in 50% of cases. The urinary sediment shows pyuria (46%), hematuria (12%), or both (34%), and AFB can be identified in 80%. Culture of early morning urine specimens (at least three samples) grows *M. tuberculosis* in 90% of cases. Patients' tuberculin skin test results are usually positive. Intravenous pyelography may suggest tuberculosis, showing renal calcification, cavitation, urethral stricture with beading, or a rigid, short, pipe-stem ureter.[26]

Tuberculous involvement of the female genital tract usually occurs secondary to hematogenous dissemination, although it may result from local spread of peritoneal, intestinal, or renal tuberculosis. Presenting symptoms may be abnormal menstrual bleeding, pelvic pain, or infertility. The fallopian tubes are most commonly involved (85%), followed by the endometrium (70%), the ovaries (35%), and the vagina or vulva in rare instances. Male genital tuberculosis is usually a consequence of descending infection from renal tuberculosis.[27] In about 10%, however, there is no evidence of renal disease, suggesting possible hematogenous origin. A palpable scrotal mass, painful in 40%, is the most common presentation. Epididymitis, orchitis, and prostatitis are frequent. Urethral and penile involvement have been reported. Oligospermia and infertility are common. When prostatitis is present, sexual transmission of mycobacteria can occur.

Miliary Tuberculosis

Miliary tuberculosis results from the hematogenous dissemination of large numbers of tubercle bacilli within a brief period, leading to heavy seeding of tissues and the emergence of innumerable small lesions widespread throughout the body. This may occur at the time of primary infection or at some time remote from that period. In one autopsy study, a nonpulmonary source was identified in three fourths of cases of disseminated tuberculosis.[28] The frequency of organ involvement in miliary disease parallels blood flow, the most common sites being (in order) the spleen, liver, lungs, bone marrow, kidney, adrenals, and eyes. Miliary tuberculosis has occurred with increased frequency in patients with leukemia and lymphoma, in those undergoing cancer chemotherapy or renal dialysis, in transplant recipients, and in HIV-infected persons. In the past, the highest prevalence was among children, and this is still the case in developing countries; currently in the United States, cases occur at all ages, 30% after age 65 years.

The presentation of miliary tuberculosis is often indolent, with a low-grade intermittent or continuous fever, anorexia, weight loss, fatigue, and weakness. Cough is present in up to 60%, whereas dyspnea and hemoptysis are less common. Headache occurs in 15% and signifies meningeal involvement in more than 90% of patients. Hepatomegaly occurs in 30%. Lymphadenopathy and splenomegaly are common in children. Choroidal tubercles are multiple, grayish white lesions around the optic disk, usually bilateral, and occur in 50% of cases. Their occurrence, however, is not specific for miliary disease. Anemia, leukocytosis with monocytosis, and less frequently leukopenia are seen in miliary tuberculosis. Coagulopathies, including disseminated intravascular coagulation, and leukemoid reactions, pancytopenia, and aplastic anemia have been reported. Liver function abnormalities and hyponatremia are common. Results of purified protein derivative skin tests are positive in 55% of patients, and some develop a positive reaction while receiving therapy. The classic chest film pattern—diffuse, bilateral, pinpoint 2- to 3-mm densities (Fig. 166–1*D*)—may be absent at presentation (30%), and the diagnosis may become evident only after repeated examinations.[29] Chest radiographs, in fact, may remain normal. Focal parenchymal lesions of pulmonary tuberculosis, including cavities, and pleural effusions may be present. Bilateral pleural effusions in a patient with tuberculosis indicate miliary dissemination. Sputum examination shows AFB in up to 30% of patients, mostly those with concomitant pulmonary disease. Cultures from urine and gastric aspirates are positive for *M. tuberculosis* in 10% to 20% of cases. Cerebrospinal fluid should be examined in patients with headaches. Histologic examination of the bone marrow is positive in 35% of cases of miliary tuberculosis, and the yield is higher with biopsy material than with aspirate, especially in patients with hematologic abnormalities.[30] Histologic examination of liver biopsy material reveals granulomata, most often noncaseating, in 50% to 90% of cases. In 20% of liver biopsy specimens, AFB are detected, and sometimes cultures are positive when no granuloma is demonstrable.[31] Fiberoptic bronchoscopy and transbronchial biopsy are highly diagnostic.[32]

Mortality in miliary tuberculosis remains high (25%). Meningitis, extremes of age, severe underlying disease, rapid development of symptoms, and delay in diagnosis are associated with poor outcome.

Tuberculosis of Bones and Joints

Skeletal tuberculosis tends to involve weight-bearing joints; vertebral column (50%), hip (15%), and knee (15%) joints are affected most often. Infection in unusual sites such as ribs (5%) has been reported, as has multiple skeletal involvement. On pathologic examination, the disease is a combination of osteomyelitis and arthritis. Tuberculosis involves the anterior part of the vertebral body subchondrally and subsequently progresses to the intervertebral disk and adjacent vertebral body. The lower thoracic and lumbar vertebrae are often involved. Patients complain of back pain and at times fever and weight loss of several weeks to months in duration. In the thoracic spine, destruction can lead to kyphosis with characteristic gibbous deformity. Paraplegia and paraparesis may occur in 4% to 38% of cases.[33] Paravertebral abscesses (cold abscesses) occur in 50% of patients and may cause sinus track formation; the presenting sign may be empyema or a retropharyngeal mass. Tuberculin skin test results of patients with skeletal tuberculosis are usually positive, and there is evidence of old or active tuberculosis on chest radiographs in 50% of cases. Diagnosis requires biopsy and culture of the bone.

Tuberculous arthritis presents as an indolent monarticular arthritis with swelling, pain, and limitation of motion. One fourth of patients report history of antecedent trauma. Synovial fluid has 25,000 to 100,000 white cells per mm^3, only about 30% mononuclear cells, and a low glucose value. Fibrin precipitates (rice bodies) may be seen. Culture of synovial fluid grows the organism in up to 80% of cases, whereas AFB can be seen in less than 20%. Histologic examination and culture of synovial biopsy material establish the diagnosis in 95% of cases.

Central Nervous System Tuberculosis

Tuberculous involvement of the brain occurs during the hematogenous spread of mycobacteria from a primary pulmonary infection or, less frequently, during the course of chronic tuberculosis. Meningitis follows the rupture or leakage of the contents of such subependymal lesions (Rich foci) into the subarachnoid space.[34] This may occur soon after the lesions are formed or after a latent period of months to years. Infrequently, infection spreads to the meninges from tuberculous otitis or spondylitis. Tuberculous meningitis is characterized by a basilar, exudative inflammation, entrapping the cranial nerves, and a severe arteriolitis, with subsequent thrombosis, most commonly of the branches of the middle and anterior cerebral arteries.

A 2-week history of vague symptoms and feeling ill but no neurologic complaints is common. Signs of meningeal irritation and minor cranial nerve deficits then develop. Patients may have slight clouding of consciousness; without treatment, stupor, coma, cranial nerve palsies, and convulsions may occur. Acute onset of symptoms has been reported in 50% of cases in children, whereas the disease is more often indolent in adults. Fever is present in 95% of children and 90% of adults. Cranial nerve deficits, commonly of the sixth, third, and fourth nerves and occasionally of the seventh (facial) nerve, occur in 30% of cases. Defective resorption of cerebrospinal fluid leads to hydrocephalus with diplopia, visual blurring, and papilledema. Hemiplegia, and less commonly paraplegia, due to ischemia or infarction secondary to vasculitis can occur. Abnormal movements (choreiform or hemiballistic), myoclonic jerks, and ataxia may occur in the late phases of illness and are more common in children. Inflammation of the spinal meninges, a rare entity, can lead to spinal block, radiculomyelopathy, or acute transverse myelitis. In children, tuberculous encephalopathy has been reported, with generalized seizures, stupor, and coma but no signs of meningitis. The cerebrospinal fluid may initially show predominance of granulocytes; however, on serial examinations, a shift to mononuclear cells and a drop in the glucose level occur. Smears of cerebrospinal fluid reveal *M. tuberculosis* in 10% to 20% of cases. Repeated examinations may increase the yield to more than 80%. The neuroradiologic techniques of computed tomography and magnetic resonance imaging are helpful in the diagnosis of neurotuberculosis. Computed tomography detects meningeal enhancement in 60% to 86% of cases and tuberculomas in less than half of patients. Both meningeal enhancement and tuberculomas (especially less than 1 cm) are, however, more frequently seen by magnetic resonance imaging.[35] Hydrocephalus occurs in 40% to 100% of cases; it appears to increase with duration of illness and portends a poor prognosis. Mortality in tuberculous meningitis is adversely affected by a delay in instituting therapy, extremes of age, and the degree of mental status aberration at presentation.

Intracranial tuberculomas can manifest with headache, focal and generalized seizures, proptosis, papilledema, and transient neurologic deficits and occasionally mimic pyogenic brain abscesses. In 30% of patients, tuberculomas remain asymptomatic during life. On skull radiographs, up to 5% of tuberculomas are calcified. Computed tomography usually shows multiple, avascular, masslike lesions. Antituberculous therapy, as opposed to surgical resection, is the treatment of choice. Corticosteroids may be helpful if brain edema is present. Intramedullary tuberculomas are a rare cause of spinal cord compression.[36]

Gastrointestinal Tuberculosis

Tuberculous enteritis appears to occur concurrently with pulmonary tuberculosis in endemic areas; its frequency correlates with the severity of lung disease: 1% with minimal disease and 25% with extensive pulmonary disease.[37] Primary tuberculous enteritis represents only about 20% of all cases of gastrointestinal tuberculosis. The resistance of mycobacterial lipid-laden cell wall to digestion allows organisms to reach and invade bowel mucosa. The most common site of disease is the ileum; the cecum, jejunum, colon, rectum, and anus are infected less often. Anorexia, weight loss, abdominal pain, nausea, vomiting, night sweats, and diarrhea or constipation are reported; however, 15% of patients with gastrointestinal involvement remain asymptomatic and their disease is discovered at autopsy or during surgery for other reasons.

The onset of illness may be acute, with bowel perforation or obstruction, but more often it is indolent. Physical examination is not usually helpful in diagnosis. Tuberculous enteritis may be complicated by formation of fistulae to adjacent organs and by gastrointestinal hemorrhage. Differential diagnosis includes inflammatory and neoplastic diseases of the bowel. Chest radiographs are normal in 50%, and results of tuberculin skin tests are positive in 75% of patients. Iron deficiency anemia commonly develops because of occult gastrointestinal bleeding. Barium radiographic studies of the gastrointestinal tract commonly reveal a nodular or ulcerated mucosa, bowel wall edema, and abnormal motility, but such findings are nonspecific. Colonoscopy is of limited usefulness in establishing the diagnosis, because tuberculous granulomata are commonly submucosal, as opposed to the mucosal location of granulomata in Crohn disease. Caseating granulomata are found in a minority of patients, and growth of mycobacteria from bowel specimens is infrequent. The response to antituberculous therapy also supports the diagnosis of enteric tuberculosis. Abdominal tuberculosis in HIV-infected patients is almost invariably a manifestation of disseminated disease and is associated with significant mortality.[38]

Tuberculous Peritonitis

Peritonitis is a rare manifestation of tuberculosis. Peritoneal involvement is believed to result from extension of a caseous mesenteric node infected during primary hematogenous dissemination. Involvement of the peritoneum secondary to an intestinal or fallopian tube lesion is uncommon. One third of patients have concomitant pulmonary disease, and another third have residual evidence of an earlier pulmonary infection. Concurrence of tuberculous peritonitis with alcoholism and Laënnec cirrhosis has been well established.[39] Two forms of disease have been identified clinically: the wet or ascitic type and the dry form with scant or localized effusion. Fever and abdominal pain occur frequently. Only 60% of patients' tuberculin skin test results are positive. Peritoneal fluid is exudative, with 200 to 2000 white cells per mm^3, and lymphocytes predominate. The peritoneal fluid may, however, have some transudative characteristics when tuberculous peritonitis occurs in patients with cirrhosis and preexisting ascites. AFB are rarely identified in the ascites fluid, and the yield of mycobacterial culture depends on the amount of sample submitted; more than 80% of cultures are positive if 1 L of peritoneal fluid is cultured. Computed tomography of the abdomen may reveal nodular peritoneal densities not easily distinguished from malignant neoplasm. Differential diagnosis of tuberculous peritonitis also includes sarcoidosis and foreign body (starch) peritonitis. Histologic demonstration of granulomata in specimens can be achieved by percutaneous needle biopsy or during laparoscopy; however, the former involves the risk of fatal hemorrhage.

Pericardial Tuberculosis

Involvement of the pericardium is rare; however, it is associated with mortality of 30% to 40%, despite chemotherapy. Rupture of a tuberculous mediastinal or paratracheal lymph node into the pericardial sac initiates the disease. The patient presents with cough, dyspnea, orthopnea, chest pain, and weight loss. Fever, tachycardia, hepatomegaly (60%), peripheral edema (50%), distant heart sounds, and jugular venous distention are present on examination. Pericardial rub is heard in 35% of patients, and pulsus paradoxus is found in 23% of cases. Chest radiographs reveal cardiomegaly and often a left-sided pleural effusion. Electrocardiographs are abnormal (nonspecific ST-T wave changes); however, ST segment elevation is seen in only 10% of patients. Pericardial biopsy establishes the diagnosis in the majority of patients, and cultures of pericardial fluid can be positive in 50% of cases.[40] In some series, however, diagnosis has been made at autopsy, after examination of the entire pericardium, with a yield of only 10% on percutaneous pericardial biopsy.[41] Hemodynamic compromise is present in half of patients, and recurrent tamponade is common after pericardiocentesis. To remove purulent effusion, and for recurrent tamponade, drainage procedures (pericardial window) are indicated. In addition to antituberculous therapy, adjunctive corticosteroids are necessary to curtail signs of inflammation and control associated arrhythmias.

Treatment of Tuberculosis

The approach to treatment of tuberculosis is based on several principles that have evolved during the last four decades. First, spontaneous, random, chromosomal mutations that confer resistance to each antituberculous drug prohibit the use of a single agent for treatment. Such mutations occur at different frequencies for each agent: isoniazid (INH), 1 of 10^6 organisms; rifampin, 1 of 10^8; ethambutol, 1 of 10^6; streptomycin, 1 of 10^5. However, because mutation sites are not linked, spontaneous evolution of multidrug-resistant strains is unlikely. Therefore, for drug-susceptible tuberculosis, use of two agents effectively prevents the emergence of resistant strains and is successful. Drug-resistant tuberculosis is usually a result of the patient's noncompliance (i.e., taking one rather than two agents prescribed) coupled with inappropriate use of chemotherapy by physicians (i.e., adding one new agent, rather than two at a time, to a failing regimen). Single drug–resistant and multidrug-resistant strains thus emerge. The molecular basis of drug resistance has been elucidated.[42] Loss or dysfunction of the *katG* gene, which encodes catalase positivity, is seen in 10% to 25% of INH-resistant strains. A second gene, *inhA*, confers resistance to INH and ethionamide. The gene product of *inhA* is involved in mycolic acid synthesis, which may well be the target of INH. Resistance to rifampin is due to mutations in a 250 base pair region of the *rpo* gene. A remarkable number of multidrug-resistant cases and several outbreaks in hospitals and prisons have been reported.[43] Outbreaks of multidrug-resistant tuberculosis are characterized by a high association with HIV infection, rapid progression, and high case-fatality rates. Spread of resistant strains occurs among contacts, accounting for high prevalences of drug-resistant disease among recent immigrants, HIV-infected patients, and indigent and minority populations. Variability in frequency of drug resistance depends on a number of factors, for example, concentration of individuals dually infected with HIV and tuberculosis, and the effectiveness of the tuberculosis control program of the area. The treatment of drug-resistant tuberculosis should include two agents to which the organism is susceptible. In case of resistance to both INH and rifampin, surgery may be necessary for control of tuberculosis.

The second principle is that for treatment of smear-positive tuberculosis to succeed (the acceptable relapse rate is less than 5%), the regimen must be continued well beyond the point at which organisms are no longer present in sputum. Thus, three- or four-drug regimens for less than 6 months' duration have been associated with high rates of both failure and relapse of disease.[44, 45] Because relapse usually occurs within the first 12 months after completion of a chemotherapeutic regimen, bacteriologic monitoring is in order throughout this period. Third, whereas presently available data on pretreatment susceptibility testing in initial treatment of tuberculosis indicate a marginal impact on the outcome of therapy, such testing should be employed where it is available. The public health benefits clearly outweigh the inconvenience and economic burden of testing. Susceptibility testing is mandatory for patients suspected of having drug-resistant tuberculosis, those who suffer relapse, those whose sputum smears are still positive 2 months after treatment, and those whose results of acid-fast sputum stains revert to positive while they are receiving treatment.

The first-line agents in the treatment of tuberculosis (INH, rifampin, pyrazinamide, ethambutol, and streptomycin) are potent drugs, associated with little toxicity, and highly effective in combination in the majority of cases. Second-line agents (*p*-aminosalicylic acid, ethionamide, cycloserine, capreomycin, kanamycin, and thiacetazone) should be employed when resistance or toxic response to first-line agents occurs. Currently, the regimen of choice for drug-susceptible tuberculosis includes INH plus rifampin plus pyrazinamide for 2 months, then INH plus rifampin for 4 months.[46] A second regimen includes INH and rifampin for 9 months. Studies that directly compare these two regimens indicate that they are equivalent, with no failures and relapse rates of 1.5%. The first regimen is less expensive and may be slightly less toxic to the liver. Addition of another first-line agent, ethambutol or streptomycin, to either regimen is warranted until susceptibility results are available, particularly if there is a possibility of drug resistance, more than 4% primary INH resistance in the community, prior treatment of tuberculosis, exposure to a drug-resistant case of tuberculosis, and country of origin with high prevalence of drug resistance. In the United States, inclusion of ethambutol is recommended. When the combination of INH and rifampin cannot be used, the duration of therapy should be extended to 12 to 18 months, because adequate experience with other regimens for shorter periods is not available. Success of any regimen depends on compliance, so close follow-up is advisable, and directly observed therapy should be administered when possible. Hepatotoxicity, which may be associated with three of the four first-line agents and two of the second-line agents, is the main concern of antituberculous therapy. Patients must be advised of symptoms of hepatotoxicity (nausea, vomiting, anorexia, malaise, jaundice, dark urine) and instructed to promptly discontinue treatment and inform their physician when they occur. Deaths due to INH hepatotoxicity are associated with continuation of taking the drug despite symptoms. In general, adverse drug effects are best detected clinically by health care providers at monthly visits rather than by routine monitoring of laboratory values in the absence of symptoms. Treatment of tuberculosis caused by resistant strains is best dictated by the results of drug susceptibility testing and should be administered for 18 to 24 months. Tuberculin-reactive patients with chest radiographic patterns consistent with tuberculosis (pleural residues, pulmonary infiltrates, hilar adenopathy) who have smear- and culture-negative sputum on multiple examinations can be treated with INH alone for 6 to 12 months or INH and rifampin for 4 to 6 months if drug resistance is unlikely.[47] Successful treatment of extrapulmonary tuberculosis involving the meninges, lymph nodes, and genitourinary system with 9 to 12 months of INH and rifampin has been well documented[48]; however, bone and joint involvement requires longer therapy.[49] The regimen currently recommended for the treatment of tuberculosis in HIV-infected and uninfected patients is similar. However, in the presence of HIV infection, assessment of bacteriologic and clinical responses is critical and the duration of treatment is based on the rapidity of optimal response.

Corticosteroids may be beneficial in the initial management of pulmonary tuberculosis in some patients with hypoxemia, hypoalbuminemia, persistent fever, and weight loss.[50] Daily doses of 20 to 60 mg of prednisone have not been complicated by opportunistic infection, other than in drug-resistant tuberculosis; however, corticosteroids must be used for only a limited time (2 weeks). The use of corticosteroids in tuberculous constrictive pericarditis has been associated with better survival, normalization of rhythm, and fewer requirements for pericardiectomy.[51] In tuberculous meningitis and tuberculomas, corticosteroids may promote reduction of cerebral edema, vasculitis, and cranial nerve entrapment.

References

1. Dolin PJ, Raviglione MC, Kochi A: Global tuberculosis incidence and mortality during 1990–2000. Bull World Health Organ 172:213, 1994.
2. Centers for Disease Control and Prevention: Expanded tuberculosis surveillance and tuberculosis mortality—United States, 1993. MMWR Morbid Mortal Wkly Rep 43:361, 1994.
3. Toossi Z: Cytokine circuits in tuberculosis. Infect Agents Dis 5:98, 1996.

4. Dall L, Long L, Stanford J: Poncet's disease: Tuberculous rheumatism. Rev Infect Dis 11:105, 1989.
5. Stead WW, Kerby GR, Schlueter DP, Jordahl CW: The clinical spectrum of primary tuberculosis in adults. Ann Intern Med 68:731, 1968.
6. Chang S, Lee P, Pemg R: Lower lung field tuberculosis. Chest 91:230, 1987.
7. Danek SJ, Bower JS: Diagnosis of pulmonary tuberculosis by flexible fiberoptic bronchoscopy. Am Rev Respir Dis 119:677, 1979.
8. Wallace JM, Deutsch AL, Harrell JH, Moser KM: Bronchoscopy and transbronchial biopsy in evaluation of patients with suspected active tuberculosis. Am J Med 70:1189, 1981.
9. Kong MF, Coate JW: Eighty six cases of Addison's disease. Clin Endocrinol (Oxf) 41:757, 1994.
10. Abassi A, Chanplavil JK, Farah S: Hypercalcemia in active pulmonary tuberculosis. Ann Intern Med 90:324, 1979.
11. Gkonos PJ, London R, Mendler ED: Hypercalcemia and elevated 1,25 dihydroxy vitamin D levels in a patient with end stage renal disease and active tuberculosis. N Engl J Med 311:1683, 1984.
12. Nardell E, McInnis B, Thomas B, Weidhaas J: Exogenous reinfection with tuberculosis in a shelter for the homeless. N Engl J Med 315:1570, 1986.
13. Shafer RW, Edlin BR: Tuberculosis in patients infected with human immunodeficiency virus: Perspective on the past decade. Clin Infect Dis 22:683, 1996.
14. Barnes PF, Bloch AB, Davidson PT, Snider DE: Tuberculosis in patients with human immunodeficiency virus. N Engl J Med 324:1664, 1991.
15. Hopewell P: Tuberculosis and human immunodeficiency virus infection. Semin Respir Infect 4:111, 1989.
16. Long R, Scalcini M, Manfreda J, et al: The impact of HIV on the usefulness of sputum smears for the diagnosis of tuberculosis. Am J Public Health 81:1326, 1991.
17. Rieder HL, Snider DE Jr, Cauthen GM: Extrapulmonary tuberculosis in the United States. Am Rev Respir Dis 141:347, 1990.
18. Kohn MD, Altman KA: Jaundice due to rare causes: Tuberculous lymphadenitis. Am J Gastroenterol 59:48, 1973.
19. Case records of the Massachusetts General Hospital weekly clinicopathological exercise: Case 7-1977. N Engl J Med 296:384, 1977.
20. Wilson RS, White RI: Lymph node tuberculosis presenting as chyluria. Thorax 31:617, 1976.
21. Appling D, Miller RH: Mycobacterial cervical lymphadenopathy. Laryngoscope 91:1259, 1981.
22. Artenstein AW, Kim JH, Williams WJ, Chung RC: Isolated peripheral tuberculous lymphadenitis in adults: Current clinical and diagnostic issues. Clin Infect Dis 20:876, 1995.
23. Berger HW, Mejia E: Tuberculous pleurisy. Chest 63:88, 1973.
24. Levine H, Metzger W, Lacera W, Kav L: Diagnosis of tuberculous pleurisy by culture of pleural biopsy specimen. Arch Intern Med 126:269, 1970.
25. Horne NW: Renal tuberculosis. Br J Hosp Med 14:158, 1975.
26. Tonkin AK, Witten DM: Genitourinary tuberculosis. Semin Roentgenol 14:305, 1979.
27. Gorse GI, Belshe RB: Male genital tuberculosis: A review of literature with instructive case reports. Rev Infect Dis 7:511, 1985.
28. Slavin RE, Walsh TJ, Pollack AD: Late generalized tuberculosis. Medicine (Baltimore) 59:352, 1980.
29. Munt PW: Miliary tuberculosis in the chemotherapy era. Medicine (Baltimore) 51:139, 1972.
30. Berger HW, Samartin HW: Miliary tuberculosis. Chest 58:586, 1976.
31. Cucin Coleman M, Eckardt JJ: The diagnosis of miliary tuberculosis. Utility of peripheral blood abnormalities, bone marrow and liver biopsy. J Chronic Dis 26:355, 1973.
32. Wilcox PA, Potgieter PD, Bateman ED: Rapid diagnosis of sputum negative miliary tuberculosis using the flexible fiberoptic bronchoscope. Thorax 41:681, 1986.
33. Gorse GJ, Pais MJ, Kusske JA: Tuberculous spondylitis. Medicine (Baltimore) 62:178, 1983.
34. Verdon R, Chevret S, Laissy JP, Wolff M: Tuberculous meningitis in adults; review of 48 cases. Clin Infect Dis 22:882, 1996.
35. Gupta RK, Gupta S, Singh D, et al: Imaging in tuberculous meningitis. Neuroradiology 36:87, 1994.
36. MacDonell AH, Baird RW, Bronze M: Intramedullary tuberculomas of the spinal cord: Case report and review. Rev Infect Dis 12:432, 1990.
37. Theoni RF, Margulis AR: Gastrointestinal tuberculosis. Semin Roentgenol 14:283, 1979.
38. Singh M, Bhargave AN, Jain KP: Tuberculous peritonitis. N Engl J Med 231:1091, 1969.
39. Fee MJ, Oo MM, Gabayan AE, et al: Abdominal tuberculosis in patients infected with human immunodeficiency virus. Clin Infect Dis 20:938, 1995.
40. Rooney JJ, Crocco JA: Tuberculous pericarditis. Ann Intern Med 72:73, 1970.
41. Fredriksen RT, Cohen LS, Mullins CB: Pericardial windows or pericardiocentesis for pericardial effusions. Am Heart J 82:158, 1970.
42. Ellner JJ: Multidrug-resistant tuberculosis. Adv Intern Med 40:155, 1995.
43. Pearson ML, Jereb JA, Frieden TR, et al: Nosocomial transmission of multidrug-resistant *Mycobacterium tuberculosis.* A risk to patients and health care workers. Ann Intern Med 117:191, 1992.
44. Tripathy SP: Controlled clinical trial of a 3 month and two 5 month regimens in pulmonary tuberculosis. Bull Int Union Tuberc 38:97, 1983.
45. Controlled clinical trial of five short-course (4-month) chemotherapy regimens in pulmonary tuberculosis. East African/British Medical Research Councils Study. Am Rev Respir Dis 123:165, 1981.
46. Ad Hoc Committee of the Scientific Assembly on Microbiology, Tuberculosis and Pulmonary Infections: Treatment of tuberculosis and tuberculosis infection in adults and children. Clin Infect Dis 21:9, 1995.
47. Dutt AK, Moers D, Stead WW: Smear- and culture-negative pulmonary tuberculosis: Four-month short course chemotherapy. Am Rev Respir Dis 139:867, 1989.
48. Dutt AK, Moers D, Stead WW: Short-course chemotherapy for extrapulmonary tuberculosis. Nine years' experience. Ann Intern Med 104:7, 1986.
49. Dutt AK, Moers D, Stead WW: Results of therapy in tuberculosis of bones and joints. Am Rev Respir Dis 137:24A, 1988.
50. Johnson JR, Taylor BC, Morissey JF: Corticosteroids in pulmonary tuberculosis. Am Rev Respir Dis 92:376, 1965.
51. Strang JI, Kakaza HH, Gibson DG, et al: Controlled trial of prednisolone as adjuvant in treatment of tuberculous constrictive pericarditis in Transkei. Lancet 2:1418, 1987.

167

Nontuberculous Mycobacterial Infections

Michael D. Iseman

Mycobacteria are slender, raylike bacilli that are obligate aerobes; they are tinctorially characterized by retention of dyes despite exposure to the potent decolorizing agent acid alcohol, an attribute that gives rise to the informal designation acid-fast bacilli. The most widely recognized human pathogens among the genus *Mycobacterium* are *Mycobacterium tuberculosis,* the bacillus that causes the classic pulmonary and extrapulmonary diseases referred to collectively as tuberculosis, and *Mycobacterium leprae* or Hansen bacillus, the microbe that causes the cutaneous and neural disorder known as leprosy. In this chapter, I deal with the other mycobacterial species that are associated with human disease, both pulmonary and extrapulmonary. Controversy exists over the aggregate designation of these organisms. In the past, they have variously been referred to as anonymous, environmental, unclassified, or atypical. More recently, there have been movements in favor of using the term nontuberculous mycobacteria or mycobacteria other than tuberculosis (MOTT). As an adjective, nontuberculous is fundamentally inaccurate, because these organisms typically do elicit gross and histologic "tubercles" in infected tissues. The designation mycobacteria other than *M. tuberculosis* is substantially correct and inclusive; hence, MOTT, including *Mycobacterium bovis,* is used in this chapter. The term tuberculosis is reserved for disease due to *M. tuberculosis*; mycobacterial infection due to MOTT, including *Mycobacterium bovis,* is referred to as mycobacteriosis.

Unlike *M. tuberculosis* and *M. leprae,* MOTT are generally found free in the natural environment. Falkinham[1] has published an extraordinarily thorough and informative review of the environmental sources, biology, and clinical epidemiology of these organisms. It is reasonably assumed that they are contracted from these environmental sources and not from other infected humans, as in the case of tuberculosis or leprosy. There are often demonstrable abnormalities in local host defenses or deficits of immunity associated with the development of MOTT disease; however, it is also apparent that some MOTT disease occurs among persons who have no discernible alterations in structural defenses or immune capacity.

Epidemiology

Whereas each species should be considered separately, some observations on the prevalence and distribution of MOTT disease in the aggregate may be made. Because reporting of MOTT infections is not mandatory, we do not have data with accuracy comparable to those for *M. tuberculosis,* but national surveys from the United States[2] and Japan[3] showed remarkably similar profiles of MOTT disease (Table 167–1).

Given the ambiguities of the data, it is difficult to offer a precise assessment of the extent of the MOTT, but it seems probable that there has been an increase in both the absolute and the relative (to tuberculosis) incidence of disease due to *Mycobacterium avium* complex (MAC) and the rapidly growing mycobacteria (RGM). Note that these increases are *not* due to the impact of human immunodeficiency virus (HIV) infection; they occurred before the appearance of acquired immunodeficiency syndrome (AIDS). An overall upward trend for *Mycobacterium kansasii* disease is not apparent, although in some communities it has become the dominant mycobacterial pathogen.[4] Sporadic cases or focal outbreaks of the other mycobacterioses are the rule.

Disease Forms

For the purposes of this chapter, pulmonary disease, localized extrapulmonary infection, and disseminated or multifocal extrapulmonary disease are discussed separately.

TABLE 167–1 ■ National MOTT Disease Incidence Surveys

ORGANISM	UNITED STATES, 1981 TO 1983 (CASES/100,000)	JAPAN, 1981 TO 1984 (CASES/100,000)
MOTT aggregate	1.78	1.73 ± 0.25
M. avium complex	1.28	1.29 ± 0.24
M. kansasii	0.33	0.34 ± 0.11
M. fortuitum-chelonae	0.19	Not calculated

Data from O'Brien and colleagues[2] and Tsukamura and colleagues.[3]

Pulmonary MOTT Disease

Lung infections due to MOTT range in severity from rapidly progressive, destructive pneumonic disease to indolent disorders with minimal physical manifestations elicitable in the short term. Predisposing conditions or discrete precipitating events may be identified in many cases. Therapy is generally far less predictable than with disease caused by *M. tuberculosis* owing to substantially greater levels of drug resistance as well as underlying lung disorders.

MYCOBACTERIUM AVIUM COMPLEX

Episodic cases of human disease due to *M. avium* were described in Europe and North America in the middle part of this century. A series of patients with pulmonary disease was reported from the Battey Hospital in Georgia in 1957[5]; the organism responsible in this group was subsequently named *Mycobacterium intracellulare* or, informally, the Battey bacillus. Bacteriologists found these organisms, *M. avium* and *M. intracellulare,* to be almost indistinguishable by routine laboratory criteria (colonial morphology, biochemical testing, drug resistance patterns). Distinguishing various strains by their animal virulence and thermal adaptability, Schaefer developed a carbohydrate antigen rabbit antiserum typing system that for years was the primary arbiter of species.[6] In the original Schaefer schema, serotypes 1, 2, and 3 were regarded as *M. avium,* whereas 4 and above were deemed *M. intracellulare.* Molecular biologic genetic analyses have allowed rapid and clear distinction of species; such testing has revealed that serotypes 1 through 6, 8, 10, and 11 are *M. avium* strains.[7] Both species are clearly capable of producing severe illness in both normal and impaired hosts. However, for unclear reasons, people with AIDS who develop disseminated mycobacterial disease are much more likely to be infected with *M. avium,* whereas HIV-negative persons with pulmonary disease are slightly more likely to harbor *M. intracellulare.*[8] At this time, the principal importance of species and serotype distinctions lies with tracing sources and routes of transmission.

A reported series of patients from Philadelphia with pulmonary disease due to MAC highlighted several important aspects of these infections.[7] Of particular note, in contrast to prior reports that had emphasized underlying lung disorders, this study observed that the disease occurred among patients without identifiable predisposing conditions. These "normal" patients have, in fact, been present among MAC series for years; however, they were not explicitly noted.[10] Historically, such cases have been said often to reflect preexisting but cryptic bronchiectasis that rendered the lungs vulnerable to MAC, but other possibilities of pathogenesis must be considered. At the National Jewish Center, we have observed an excess of thoracic skeletal anomalies, including pectus excavatum and scoliosis, among MAC patients (particularly female patients); our preliminary survey also suggests an excess of mitral valve prolapse among these pulmonary MAC patients.[11] We have hypothesized that these thoracic anomalies mark persons who, through mechanisms yet unknown, are vulnerable to environmental mycobacteria such as MAC. Reich and Johns[12] have suggested that some of these female patients become ill from MAC because of their reluctance to cough—the so-called Lady Windermere syndrome. However, we view this explanation with considerable skepticism.[13, 14]

The majority of patients with pulmonary MAC disease do have underlying lung disease or other predisposing factors. Prominent are cigarette-induced chronic bronchitis and emphysema, history of tuberculosis with resultant scarring and bronchiectasis, inorganic dust exposure, and fibrotic disorders including idiopathic fibrosing alveolitis and those associated with rheumatoid arthritis or ankylosing spondylitis. We have also seen pulmonary MAC after radiation therapy treatments to the chest wall and mediastinal ports for breast cancer and other malignancies. In addition, preliminary observations by our group have raised the possibility of vulnerability to MAC or bronchiectasis mediated through subtle heritable lung disorders including heterozygous cystic fibrosis state and heterozygous α_1-antiprotease deficiency.

Furthermore, we have noted a potential association between prior infection with *Histoplasma capsulatum* and vulnerability to MAC lung disease.[15] In a limited number of pulmonary MAC patients, we have observed large, calcified peribronchial lymph nodes surrounding or impinging on airways, including those that subserve lung regions involved with MAC (Fig. 167–1). We believe that these calcified nodes reflect prior histoplasmosis, which facilitates MAC by causing parenchymal scarring with bronchiectasis or impaired drainage owing to bronchial compromise. Although we do not have direct evidence that these calcified nodes are due to histoplasmosis, we infer that this is so because pulmonary MAC is not seen in association with such calcifications except for in patients who have resided for considerable periods in regions indigenous for *H. capsulatum* infections.

Presumed but unproven is the concept that those disorders predispose to MAC primarily by disrupting mucociliary clearance. Because MAC are widely distributed in the environment, presumably everyone inhales these microbes into their lungs. In patients with excessive mucus production (chronic bronchitis), abnormally thick or tenacious secretions (cystic fibrosis), or anatomic distortions that retard mucus clearance (bronchiectasis), stagnation allows the slowly replicating, low-virulence mycobacteria to proliferate, adhere, and invade. In the case of silicosis, and perhaps other diseases, there may also be an element of macrophage dysfunction that potentiates invasive disease.

Active or invasive disease due to MAC (or any of the MOTT) is more difficult to diagnose than tuberculosis, because recovery of the *M. tuberculosis* organism from respiratory secretions or tissue is tantamount to the diagnosis of disease. Given the wide distribution of MAC in nature, it is vital that clinicians realize that MAC recovered from any nonsterile space may reflect colonization. Considerable effort must be made to distinguish a saprophytic state from invasive disease. Failure to appreciate active disease and withholding therapy put a patient at risk for progressive lung destruction and even death; on the other hand, an erroneous assumption of disease commits a patient to extended use of medication, which entails predictable side effects, significant risk for toxic effects, and a considerable financial burden. Because MAC pulmonary disease generally advances slowly, there is a tendency for clinicians who see patients during a short span, even up to 3 to 6 months, to fail to appreciate that there is progressive damage. Alternatively, the disease does not advance in a linear manner but stepwise, with periods of indolence followed by a spate of activity. What should be appreciated is the clear fact that there is considerable morbidity and even mortality from untreated or inadequately treated pulmonary MAC disease.

Criteria for the diagnosis of active disease usually include clinical signs and symptoms, sputum bacteriology, and chest radiography. The spectrum of symptoms includes the classic finding of malaise, fever, chills, night sweats, cough, sputum production, hemoptysis, pleuritic and nonpleuritic chest pain; dyspnea, weight loss, and fever are common as the disease progresses. Early in the course of MAC disease, however, there may be minimal manifestations, such as a chronic nonproductive cough and mild malaise (described as just not feeling well or lack of energy). A possible source of confusion is the predisposing diseases associated with MAC vulnerability. Chronic bronchitis or emphysema, chronic bronchiectasis, pneumoconiosis, and a variety of other diseases may mimic these manifestations, so the clinician must seek recent quantitative changes in symptoms to discern the contribution of MAC.

Sputum studies are obviously central to the issue of active disease. Authorities have sought multiple isolations of MAC, spread out in time and substantial in terms of the numbers of mycobacteria recovered.[16] This is certainly a reasonable system to employ; however, it poses risks for both false-negative and false-positive results. Early in the course of the infection, it may be more difficult to recover the microbes. In some cases of noncavitary disease, the patient may not pro-

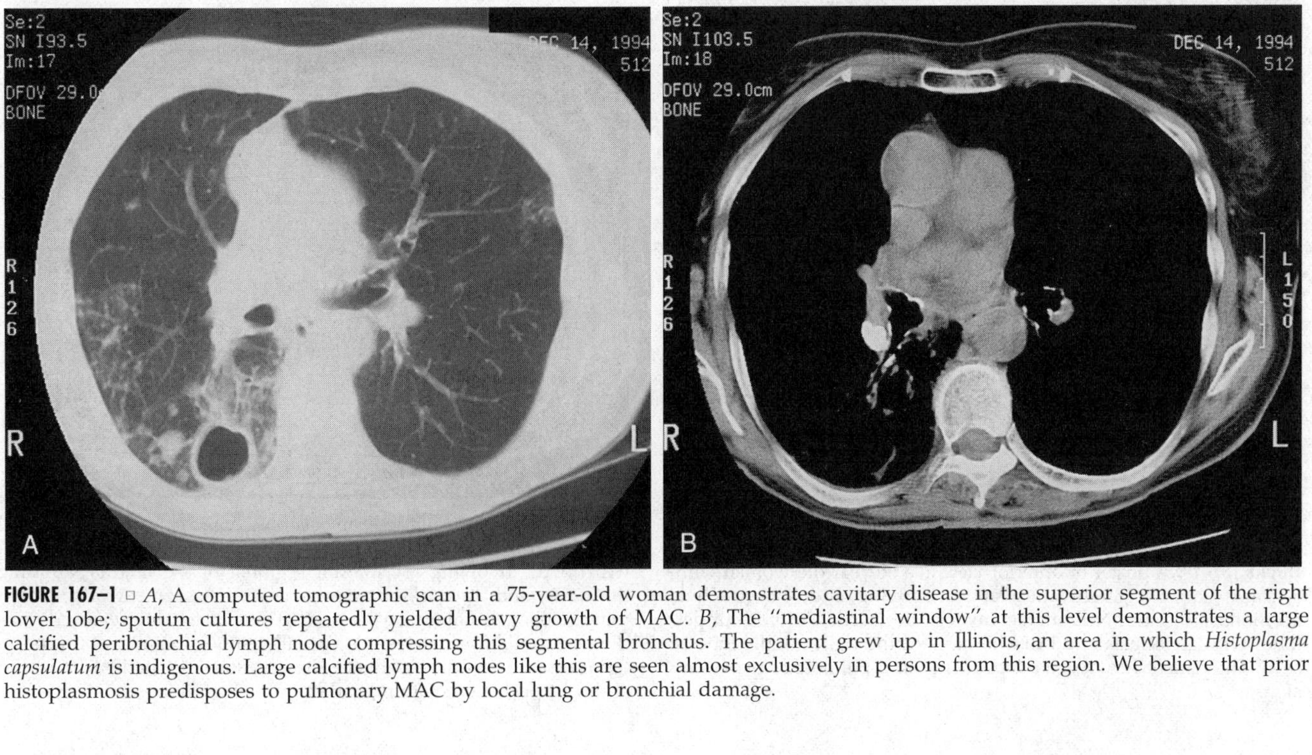

FIGURE 167–1 □ *A*, A computed tomographic scan in a 75-year-old woman demonstrates cavitary disease in the superior segment of the right lower lobe; sputum cultures repeatedly yielded heavy growth of MAC. *B*, The "mediastinal window" at this level demonstrates a large calcified peribronchial lymph node compressing this segmental bronchus. The patient grew up in Illinois, an area in which *Histoplasma capsulatum* is indigenous. Large calcified lymph nodes like this are seen almost exclusively in persons from this region. We believe that prior histoplasmosis predisposes to pulmonary MAC by local lung or bronchial damage.

duce sputum; bronchoscopy is typically done in this situation. Recovery of MAC in this situation is a problem. Although bronchoscopic retrieval of mycobacteria potentially enhances the sensitivity of diagnosis, it can also diminish the specificity by resulting in a positive culture with few organisms. Biopsy of the lung region in question may be extremely useful, because demonstration of granulomatous inflammation, with or without caseation or acid-fast bacilli, strongly supports the diagnosis. However, among patients with scattered, smaller areas of disease, the risk of sampling error makes bronchoscopic biopsy a somewhat insensitive tool. For particularly problematic cases, thoracoscopic biopsy may be required to establish or refute the diagnosis.

Pulmonary MAC disease produces a wide spectrum of radiographic abnormalities. In 1995, Lynch and colleagues[17] published an excellent review of these findings. A substantial proportion of pulmonary MAC patients' chest films are suggestive of classic tuberculosis: unilateral or bilateral upper lobe, apical posterior, fibronodular, partially consolidated, cavitary shadowing (Fig. 167–2). A subset of MAC patients have a distinct radiographic pattern, mainly lower zone, nodular subpleural shadowing, typically bilateral (Fig. 167–3); this seems more common among women. In addition to a number of patients with this pattern, we have encountered women who presented with the predominant abnormality of coarse, saccular bronchiectasis of both the lingula and right middle lobe (Fig. 167–4). Although patchy abnormalities were typically scattered elsewhere, the most dramatic findings were restricted to these regions. By history, it was not possible to determine absolutely whether the bronchiectasis antedated or was caused by the MAC; but in the absence of a clear history of remote, recurrent infections in several of these patients, it seems that MAC may play a major role in the pathogenesis of such bronchiectasis.

Regardless of a primary or secondary role, once established, MAC definitely is part of the ongoing clinical illness with which these patients present. Of interest, in our experience, these bronchiectatic subjects were all women. Their symptom complex usually consisted of low-grade fever, malaise, and relentless productive cough with purulent phlegm, and, rarely, hemoptysis. Associated conditions in our patients variably included pectus excavatum, scoliosis, and mitral valve prolapse. A few of these patients have gastroesophageal reflux; the potential role of recurrent aspiration in the

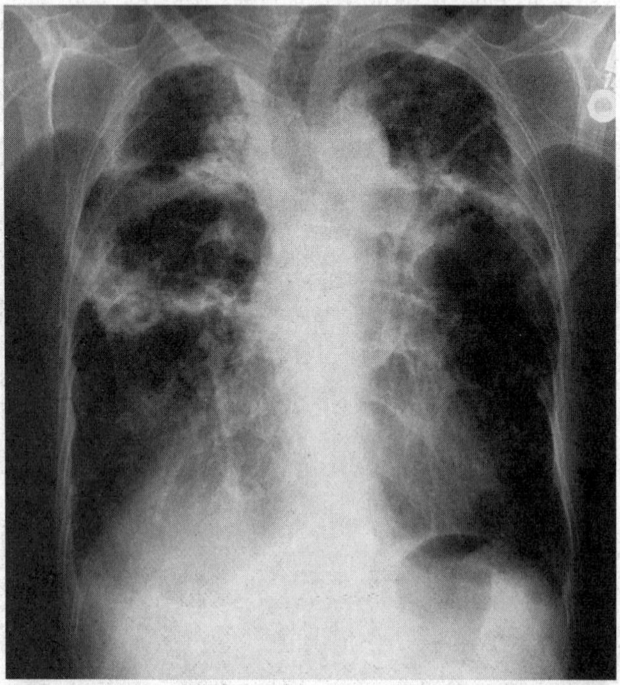

FIGURE 167–2 □ A posterior-anterior view in a 60-year-old woman with 50 pack-years of cigarette abuse and underlying chronic obstructive pulmonary disease. Necrotizing cavitary destruction of both upper lobes with atelectasis and bronchiectasis of the right middle lobe is seen. The patient has oxygen dependency and pulmonary hypertension.

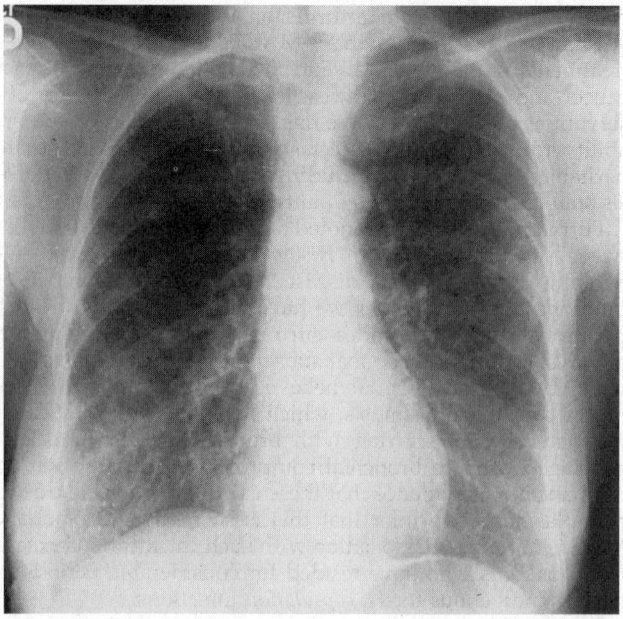

FIGURE 167–3 □ A posterior-anterior view in a 47-year-old woman, a nonsmoker, with bilateral lower zone patchy infiltrates. Early cavitary formation is seen in the right lower lobe and left upper lobe. A computed tomographic scan confirmed extensive bronchiectasis in the right middle lobe with scattered nodular shadowing. This less distinctive pattern is being seen with increasing frequency among patients, especially females, referred to our institution.

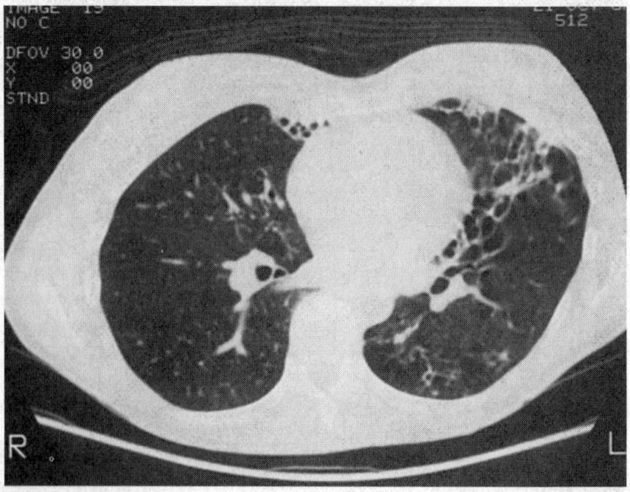

FIGURE 167–4 □ A computed tomographic lung scan of a 43-year-old woman, a nonsmoker, with cystic-sacular bronchiectasis associated with MAC involving the inferior segment of the lingula, abutting the heart, and, to a lesser extent, the medial segment of the right middle lobe, also abutting the heart. This pattern, lingular and middle lobe focal bronchiectasis, is virtually pathognomonic of mycobacterial disease in our experience. In addition, this patient had mild scoliosis, pectus excavatum, and mitral valve prolapse.

pathogenesis of such bronchiectasis has not been proved but should be considered. One further novel clinical-radiographic presentation of pulmonary MAC should be discussed. We and others[18, 19] have seen patients with an illness marked by relentless dry cough, severe dyspnea, hyperinflation on chest radiography and pulmonary function testing, hypoxemia, and computed tomographic findings most mindful of bronchiolitis with or without organizing pneumonia. In several cases, open lung biopsies have revealed features of bronchiolitis obliterans with organizing pneumonia and scattered granulomata. We believe, based on multiple isolations of MAC and responses to antimycobacterial therapy, that these cases represent exhuberant inflammation of the small airways—possibly triggered by the mycobacteria. Theoretically, we believe that such cases most closely fit the model of hypersensitivity pneumonitis and suspect that they may develop from inhalation of environmental aerosols contaminated by the mycobacteria; in one series, the lung disorder improved without chemotherapy, simply on termination of exposure to the aerosol.[19]

Therapy for pulmonary MAC disease is difficult and controversial. Because of the extraordinary number of variables involved, no randomized controlled clinical trials have been conducted to determine whether therapy is better than no therapy, whether any drug or drug regimen is superior to another, or whether resection surgery is a useful adjunct. On the basis of a flawed amalgam of data, I believe that the answer in all three cases is yes.

The natural history of pulmonary MAC disease has not been carefully studied, but one may conclude from several series of patients that a significant proportion of pulmonary MAC cases progress to death that the clinician attributes substantially to the effects of MAC: 14% of 100 patients in Milwaukee,[20] 17% of 86 patients in Alabama,[21] and 19% of 21 patients in Philadelphia[9] died within 10 years. In none of these series were patients left untreated; however, in retrospective analyses, it appeared that the patients who received minimal or ineffective therapy were more likely to die of the MAC disease.

The role of drug susceptibility testing in selecting a regimen for a MAC patient is a problem. Unlike the situation with tuberculosis, for which a wealth of experience has shown a correlation between susceptibility testing results in vitro and response to treatment, only one study has shown such an association with pulmonary MAC disease. In this series of 76 patients from the National Jewish Center, there was a statistically significant association between the initial bacteriologic response and the administration of drugs to which the patients' MAC strains were sensitive in vitro.[22] Similarly, Tsukamura[23] in Japan studied 26 patients with pulmonary MAC. Seven patients were considered treatment failures, and six of these had highly resistant strains of MAC. Nine patients were rendered culture-negative, and all had been treated with regimens that included drugs to which their MAC strain was relatively susceptible. This study also revealed that during treatment minimal inhibitory concentrations to the drugs employed drifted upward, indicating killing of vulnerable populations.

A group from California has reported that in vitro susceptibility testing did not predict response to chemotherapy with rifampin, ethambutol, and clofazimine for patients with AIDS and disseminated MAC.[24] Indeed, the only surrogate marker that did correspond with treatment of disease outcomes was ex vivo macrophage. Although the observations of these authors may be accurate among persons with AIDS and disseminated MAC, our clinical experience and analogy to other pulmonary mycobacterioses indicate that in vitro testing is an appropriate element of treatment for pulmonary MAC.

American Thoracic Society guidelines[25] have suggested an empirical initial regimen, but given the probability that the patient will experience either initial treatment failure, intolerance to the initial regimen, or relapse with such drug therapy, obtaining a comprehensive panel of drug susceptibility studies to plan possible retreatment seems prudent.

The choice of drugs for MAC disease is controversial. Because of a strong natural resistance to most of the antimycobacterial drugs, multidrug regimens employing five to seven agents were used empirically at the National Jewish Hospital for many years.[22, 26] Despite extended hospital stays to cope with the considerable morbidity attendant to this polypharmacy, success rates were only modestly better than those in other programs that employed fewer drugs (Table 167–2).

Unfortunately, owing to three major variables—the extreme heterogeneity in resistance patterns for various MAC strains, the high probability of intolerance to or toxicity of one or more drugs, and a wide range of extent or type of disease—it seems unlikely that a well-controlled clinical trial could be conducted to clearly identify the best regimen or regimens. As noted, only two retrospective studies have shown a statistically significant relationship between susceptibility in vitro and response to therapy. Animal model studies offer some potential utility in refining chemotherapy, but interspecies variation in drug activity limits their applicability. Thus, we are left with a combination of empiricism and clinical data for guidance in choosing a drug regimen. On the basis of a mixture of demonstrated efficacy and predictable tolerance, a 1985 consensus panel advocated initial therapy with isoniazid, rifampin, and ethambutol, including an initial 2- to 4-month phase of streptomycin for the usual case of newly diagnosed pulmonary MAC disease.[27] The 1990 American Thoracic Society recommendations also include these four drugs.[25] We believe that there are sufficient in vitro data showing absent or limited activity of isoniazid against MAC isolates to avoid including it in a treatment plan for MAC.[28, 29]

Multiple studies have shown that the new macrolide, clarithromycin, is quite active in vitro against MAC isolates.[30, 31] See Table 167–3 for in vitro susceptibility testing results for large numbers of MAC strains isolated from patients mainly with pulmonary disease. A 1994 clinical study demonstrated

TABLE 167–2 ■ Results of Chemotherapy for Pulmonary MAC Disease

STUDY	INITIAL RESPONSE (%)	SUBSEQUENT RELAPSE (%)	OVERALL SUCCESS (%)	COMMENTS
Arkansas,[116] 1979	68/85 (80)	16/68 (24)	39/85 (46)	Four or five drugs, no rifampin
Milwaukee,[20] 1979	46/82 (56)	9/46 (20)	37/82 (45)	Two to five drugs, rare rifampin
Wales,[117] 1981	22/40 (55)	3/22 (14)	19/40 (48)	Better response with more drugs
Alabama,[21] 1984	52/86 (60)	10/52 (20)	42/86 (49)	Better response with more drugs
National Jewish Center,[26] 1981	63/81 (78)	10/63 (16)	53/81 (65)	Five or six drugs on average
National Jewish Center,[22] 1987	52/76 (68)	6/52 (12)	46/76 (61)	Five or six drugs; response correlated with susceptibility in vitro

TABLE 167–3 ■ Broth-Determined Minimal Inhibitory Concentrations of Some Antituberculosis Drugs for MAC Isolates in Comparison with Those for *Mycobacterium tuberculosis* Isolates

	MIC RANGE (μg/mL)		DISTRIBUTION (%) OF MAC ISOLATES BY MICs			
DRUG	*M. tuberculosis*	MAC	Low*	Intermediate	High†	REFERENCE
Isoniazid	0.025–0.05	0.6–>10.0	0	32	68	39, 118
Pyrazinamide	<100.00	>100.00	0	0	100	29
Rifampin	0.06–0.25	0.12–16.0	14	74	12	118–120
Ethambutol	0.94–3.8	0.94–15.0	67	24	9	35, 118, 120
Ethionamide	0.3–1.2	0.3–≥10.0	32	16	52	39, 120
Streptomycin	0.5–2.0	1.0–8.0	36	61	13	39, 118, 120, 121
Amikacin	0.5–2.0	1.0–16.0	3	65	32	39, 121
Capreomycin	1.25–2.5	5.0–40.0	0	29	71	39
Ofloxacin	0.25–2.0	4.0–>32.0	0	11	89	122
Ciprofloxacin	0.25–2.0	0.5–16.0	28	33	39	122
Clofazimine	0.06–0.25	0.06–0.25	15.6	59.4	25.0	123, 124
Clarithromycin‡	—§	0.12–8.0	99	1	0	30, 125
Azithromycin‡	—	4.0–16.0	96	4	0	125

*Low, within the range for wild *M. tuberculosis* strains except for clarithromycin and azithromycin.
†High, at or greater than the C_{max}.
‡Shown for pretreatment isolates only.
§—, Not tested in comparison with MAC isolates.
Modified from Heifets L: Susceptibility testing of *Mycobacterium avium* complex isolates. Antimicrob Agents Chemother 40:1759–1767, 1996.

substantial efficacy of clarithromycin in monotherapy in patients with pulmonary MAC.[32] Azithromycin is somewhat less active on in vitro testing.[33] However, its greater concentration and dwell time in macrophages, as well as generally better tolerance by patients, may justify its use. As in the study of clarithromycin cited here, a 1996 report documented clear-cut efficacy of azithromycin monotherapy in a group of patients with pulmonary MAC.[34] Ethambutol is moderately active in vitro against roughly 40% to 50% of MAC isolates.[35] However, it plays an amplified role in treatment because of its complementary relationship to macrolides or azolides, with which it is predictably additive (Heifets L, personal communication) or the rifamycins, with which it is commonly additive and often synergistic.[36] Ethambutol was shown to retard the evolution of resistance to clarithromycin when used in combination in persons with AIDS.

Clofazimine, used for decades as an antileprosy agent, was found to have in vitro activity against a majority of clinical MAC isolates at low concentrations.[37] We have employed it for more than 10 years at the National Jewish Hospital, with generally good tolerance and apparent utility. However, studies of the chemotherapy of disseminated MAC in persons with AIDS have raised the issue of an unexplained negative or adverse impact of clofazimine in this setting.[38] We cannot reconcile the apparent differences in the utility of this agent but continue to use it in selected cases. The quinolones, particularly ciprofloxacin, may also show in vitro activity against MAC.[39] On the basis of various reported series, in vitro activity, and our clinical experience, we have developed the regimen choices seen in Tables 167–4 and 167–5.

One must always be aware of drug-drug interactions when using multiple antibiotics as well as other medications. Data from Wallace and colleagues[40] reveal that, through its induction of the cytochrome P-450 system, rifampin, when administered concomitantly with clarithromycin, actually decreases serum levels of clarithromycin. While this group of pulmonary MAC patients from Texas was given monotherapy, their mean serum level of clarithromycin was 5.4 μg/mL. However, after rifampin was added, the mean clarithromycin concentration fell to 0.7 μg/mL; similarly, if rifabutin (a less potent inducer of the cytochrome system) was added, the clarithromycin level fell to 2.2 μg/mL. Therefore, one might consider eliminating rifamycin antibiotics from a MAC regimen that contains clarithromycin. Alternatively, one might choose to use azithromycin with a rifamycin, because it may be influenced less by this drug interaction.[41]

An additional drug-drug interaction between these two groups of antimicrobials merits attention. Clarithromycin, by slowing the cytochrome P-450 system, delays the catabolism of the rifamycins, resulting in higher drug concentrations; this has resulted in various side effects or toxicities, including uveitis, prominent skin pigmentation, and lupus-like reactions.[42–44]

For persons with AIDS who are receiving polypharmacy for various reasons, both the rifamycins and the macrolides may result in clinically significant drug interactions. (See the later discussion of mycobacterioses and HIV and AIDS for more details.)

For patients with more extensive disease or for those for whom initial therapy has failed, a more aggressive regimen should be employed, including routine use of aminoglycosides. Some would simply add drugs empirically, but we believe that susceptibility testing, including drug combination studies, should be performed to aid with the selections.

Patients must be monitored closely for systemic toxicities associated with antimycobacterial treatment. Hepatitis, bone marrow suppression, ototoxicity, and optic neuritis are among the more common complications associated with antimycobacterial agents. It is prudent, therefore, to monitor complete blood counts, liver function tests, visual acuity testing, and audiograms on a regular basis (see Table 167–4).

Surgery in Pulmonary MAC Disease. Refractoriness to drug therapy necessitated surgical resection at the Battey Hospital in Georgia, where the first large group of pulmonary MAC cases was reported.[45] In this series, the operative mortality rate was 7% and major morbidity rate was 24%, including prolonged air leakage requiring thoracoplasty. This series commenced in the 1950s, when surgical approaches were evolving, anesthesia techniques were less safe, and postoperative intensive care was far less sophisticated. As these elements improved, both morbidity and mortality diminished during the later years of the series. A later series of patients who underwent resectional surgery was reported from Duke University; of 175 pulmonary MAC patients, 37

TABLE 167–4 ■ Drug Options for Pulmonary MAC Disease*

DRUG	DOSE AND SCHEDULE	COMMENTS
Clarithromycin (CLR)	500 mg PO bid or 750 to 1000 mg PO qd	Predictable dysgeusia. Intolerance may evolve after early therapy (? tissue accumulation), requiring reduced dosage. Absorbed well with food; this may reduce side effects.
Azithromycin (AZI)	250 mg PO qd	Extremely long serum and tissue half-life. May accumulate with prolonged use. Generally is better tolerated than CLR. Is absorbed well with food.
Ethambutol (EMB)	25 mg/kg of body weight for initial 2 mo; then reduce dose to 15–20 mg/kg to reduce risk of ocular toxicity (reduce dose with renal impairment)	Predictable additive effect with CLR or AZI. Must test or interrogate carefully for signs of optic neuritis on a *monthly* basis. Is absorbed in the presence of food.
Rifampin (RIF) Rifabutin (RBT)	RIF 600 mg qd, 450 mg if <50 kg of body weight RBT 450 mg qd, 300 mg if <50 kg	May result in clinically significant interactions with CLR; therefore, their use in this setting is disputed (see text). Is poorly absorbed in presence of food. May be synergistic with EMB.
Clofazimine (CFZ)	100–200 mg PO qd for 2–3 mo, then reduce to 50 mg PO qd to prevent excessive pigment and/or gastrointestinal intolerance	Predictably causes reversible skin bronzing; wear ultraviolet light sun block to lessen effect. May cause progressive gastrointestinal intolerance or pain over months.
Amikacin (AK) Streptomycin (SM)	AK or SM, 12–15 mg/kg IV or IM daily; 15–22 mg/kg IV or IM three or two times weekly; usually give for initial 2–6 mo	Tend to use for patients with more extensive or symptomatic disease. Must monitor for hearing impairment, vestibular dysfunction, and renal impairment.
Ciprofloxacin (CIP)	500 mg PO bid or 750 mg qd	Is less likely to be active in vitro than above-listed agents. Is poorly absorbed with food. May alter rifamycin metabolism.

*PO, Orally; bid, twice daily; qd, daily; IV, intravenously; IM, intramuscularly.

were selected to undergo surgery.[46] Elements in selection included localized disease, freedom from major complicating diseases, and younger age. Among these patients, 33 were available for long-term follow-up; two who had relapse responded to retreatment. There were no operative deaths or serious morbidity in this series. We have employed resection for pulmonary MAC disease at the National Jewish Hospital.[47] Basically, we have used surgery in two groups—patients with localized, lobar disease and those with total destruction of one lung. Among those patients with destroyed lungs, the decision to resect was based principally on the extreme morbidity of this condition and only secondarily on the desire to eradicate the MAC. Such patients' lungs are totally devitalized, which not only makes it more difficult to control the mycobacteria but makes the lung vulnerable to chronic polymicrobial superinfection. Unfortunately, our preliminary efforts at resecting the destroyed lung have met with considerable morbidity and even mortality. It has been

TABLE 167–5 ■ Suggested Regimens for Pulmonary MAC Disease

REGIMEN	COMMENTS
Clarithromycin (or azithromycin) Ethambutol Clofazimine	Clarithromycin is more active in vitro but azithromycin may be preferred in some cases because of favorable gastrointestinal tolerance and favorable pharmacokinetics.
Amikacin (or streptomycin)	Initial use of amikacin (or streptomycin) may substantially enhance the response to therapy. Intermittent use (less than daily) delays or obviates toxicity. Amikacin typically affects high-frequency hearing; streptomycin tends to disturb vestibular function initially. Because hearing is more easily and quantitatively monitored than is vestibular function, amikacin may be used more safely.

our experience that right-sided resections, particularly right pneumonectomies, have been associated with a much higher incidence of morbidity and mortality than left pneumonectomies. Despite aggressive measures, including grafting muscle pedicles to the bronchial stump, our complication rate was nearly 50%. We have modified our surgical approach, utilizing a two-stage procedure for many of our pneumonectomies, which includes an initial pneumonectomy with an omental wrap around the bronchial stump. An Eloesser flap is created, and the hemithorax is then packed with gauze soaked with Dakins solution. The hemithorax is left open for 4 to 6 weeks. The second stage involves closure of the Eloesser opening. We have experienced a lower incidence of bronchial stump breakdown since we started using this procedure. Although these results are encouraging, right-sided pneumonectomies still represent a potentially hazardous procedure to be approached with caution.

Although there are no randomized, controlled studies to document the advantage of surgical resection, our clinical experience and analysis of the literature suggest that resection of localized disease coupled with chemotherapy affords a patient the best chance for long-standing control of such disease. When such a patient is encountered, we initially seek to make the chemotherapy regimen optimal while entering into discussions about the possible utility of surgery. If the patient is willing to contemplate this option, we perform careful pulmonary function testing, arterial blood gas analysis, and radionuclide ventilation-perfusion lung scans. The timing of surgery is somewhat arbitrary. In general, we prefer to reduce the number of mycobacteria in the sputum to the minimum: ideally, culture negativity. However, sterilization of the sputum may not be achieved predictably, so surgery is usually performed while sputum cultures still yield mycobacteria and occasionally when the large burden of mycobacteria is large enough to be detectable on examination of smears.

MYCOBACTERIUM KANSASII

The second most common cause of MOTT pulmonary disease is *M. kansasii,* a photochromogenic organism of Runyon's group I. In the survey of MOTT disease by the Centers for Disease Control (CDC), the incidence was 0.33 case per 100,000 during the years 1981 to 1983.[2] *M. kansasii* is recovered most often from water[1] and is therefore believed to be transmitted by this route. In a survey in Texas, substantially different patterns of distribution of *M. kansasii* and MAC pulmonary cases were observed, *M. kansasii* being clustered in larger cities. This raises the question of whether there is a unique urban source[48] or possibly some human-to-human transmission.[49] In a Nebraska Veterans Affairs hospital, *M. kansasii* was the leading cause of pulmonary mycobacterial disease, outnumbering *M. tuberculosis* and MAC during the period of 1976 to 1990 by 118 to 67 and 15, respectively.[4] Predisposing factors, including chronic obstructive pulmonary disease, smoking-induced chronic bronchitis, and chronic inorganic dust exposure, are associated with 50% or more cases in several reports.[50–52] There was a strong male preponderance in all of these series.

The clinical presentation of *M. kansasii* patients ranges from asymptomatic (detected on routine chest radiography) to various combinations of sparsely productive chronic cough, low-grade fever, malaise, and nonpleuritic chest pain. The chest film typically shows upper zone disease with less fibronodular and confluent shadowing than is typical of *M. tuberculosis* or MAC disease. In addition, the cavities seen in *M. kansasii* disease may have thin walls.[53] Pleural effusions are uncommon.

Because of the relative paucity of *M. kansasii* in the environment in the United States, recovery of this organism from a patient's respiratory secretions is more likely to indicate invasive disease than is the recovery of MAC.[52] On staining, *M. kansasii* organisms tend to be longer and slimmer (almost filamentous) as well as more beaded than *M. tuberculosis* or MAC; however, whereas this finding is suggestive, it is not possible to establish the species from the organism's morphologic features. Tuberculin skin testing with purified protein derivative (the antigen derived from *M. tuberculosis*) may produce a reaction in a substantial portion of *M. kansasii* patients because of cross-reactivity.

Chemotherapy. The typical native strain of *M. kansasii* shows partial resistance to low concentrations of isoniazid and streptomycin; high-level resistance to pyrazinamide and *p*-aminosalicylic acid is the rule. Nonetheless, a standard daily regimen of isoniazid, rifampin, and ethambutol for 18 months cures roughly 95% of pulmonary *M. kansasii* cases[52]; the doses of these drugs were not specified in this series. Because of low-level resistance to isoniazid, higher doses (450 to 600 mg) are sometimes used. The efficacy of this tactic is unknown; modestly higher drug toxicity should be anticipated. The addition of streptomycin, 1 g intramuscularly thrice weekly for 3 months, allowed reduction of the duration of therapy to 12 months, and 40 of 41 patients in one series enjoyed a cure.[54] The British Thoracic Society published a study in 1994 of a regimen that featured 9 months of therapy with rifampin and ethambutol. Of note, most of these patients received additional unspecified medications for the initial few months before the mycobacterial species was identified.[55] Of the initial 173, 154 patients completed 9 months of chemotherapy, with 87 patients completing 5 years of follow-up. At the completion of the 5-year follow-up, 15 patients (9.7%) were noted to have relapsed with positive cultures.

On the basis of these studies, we would suggest a hybrid regimen that incorporates various features of previously reported experience. In many cases, the patient is treated on the presumption or possibility of having *M. tuberculosis* disease, probably with a four-drug regimen including isoniazid, rifampin, pyrazinamide, and either ethambutol or streptomycin. If the patient is responding well to this regimen (with diminishing symptoms, diminishing bacillary load, and improving chest radiographs), we would discontinue the isoniazid (and pyrazinamide). If the fourth drug is streptomycin and not ethambutol, we would add ethambutol while continuing the streptomycin through 3 months. Depending on the extent of disease and rate of improvement, we would employ rifampin and ethambutol through 12 months or longer.

Thus chemotherapy of the usual case of *M. kansasii* pulmonary disease is relatively straightforward. However, drug toxicity or acquired drug resistance can substantially complicate management. Loss of rifampin is the biggest hurdle because this agent is the keystone in *M. kansasii* treatment. Toxic reactions may preclude the use of rifampin in a number of patients, or inadequate therapy may lead to the acquisition of resistance to rifampin. If, for instance, patients are started with isoniazid and rifampin on the assumption that they have tuberculosis, resistance to rifampin may evolve.[56] In the situation of toxicity from or resistance to rifampin, careful selection of a regimen is critical, lest further drug resistance evolve. For example, some patients in an early series from Texas were shown to respond to sulfonamide-containing regimens.[57] A more recent report from Texas described an aggressive regimen for the management of rifampin-resistant disease: isoniazid, 900 mg daily, ethambutol, 25 mg/kg daily, sulfamethoxasole, 1000 mg three times a day, and an initial course of amikacin or streptomycin. Although this regimen was apparently successful in this small series, I have misgivings about the prolonged use of these agents in such high doses. Ciprofloxacin and clarithromycin also have excellent activity against most strains of *M. kansasii;* these drugs are generally well tolerated and are thus attractive alternative agents.[56] Other agents with activity against the usual strain of *M. kansasii* include ethionamide and cycloserine.[58]

In cases of extensive drug resistance or toxic effect, it may be appropriate to consider resectional surgery for localized disease. Although experience with surgery for *M. kansasii* is limited, I believe that these broad principles should be observed: remove cavities and grossly devitalized tissue, do lobectomies or pneumonectomies—avoid wedge or segmental resectionism, and only perform the surgery under optimal antimicrobial coverage.[47]

PULMONARY DISEASE CAUSED BY RAPIDLY GROWING *MYCOBACTERIA*

These RGM, particularly *Mycobacterium abscessus, Mycobacterium chelonae,* and *Mycobacterium fortuitum,* are being reported more frequently in association with invasive lung disease in the United States. In the CDC's 1981 to 1983 survey, there were 441 cases, an incidence of 0.19 per 100,000 population.[2] Unpublished data from the CDC's Public Health Laboratory Information System for 1992 revealed that of the more than 13,000 mycobacterial isolates identified, 5% were *M. fortuitum.* Although the number is small, this is a vexing disease that is difficult to treat and associated with considerable morbidity.

M. chelonae and *M. fortuitum* organisms are recovered from water and soil in environmental surveys.[1] Experience with contaminated wounds indicates that soil may well be a source of these infections. The mode of transmission of human disease is unclear; however, some patients with pulmonary disease due to these microbes have underlying esophageal disease, typically achalasia, marked by dilation and high risk for aspiration.[59] This association suggests colonization of the upper alimentary canal with introduction by aspiration of esophagogastric contents. To some extent, women with the high-risk phenotype for MAC described previously appear to be vulnerable to RGM disease as well. We have seen a dual-infection pattern in which MAC and RGM present simultaneously or metachronously in the same patient as pathogens. RGM organisms also seem to have a propensity for contaminating various medical devices and supplies and have been associated with an array of nosocomial infections (see the section on extrapulmonary disease).

A variety of radiographic presentations are noted with lung disease caused by RGM. Most common is the diffuse, irregular, patchy nodular shadowing without frank cavitation. In addition, we have noted upper zone cavitary lesions, bilateral butterfly airspace–consolidating shadows (probably representing acute aspiration pneumonia), and rarely, minimal airspace infiltration with diffuse bronchial or peribronchial thickening as noted with lung computed tomography.

The patients usually manifest symptoms of persistent, hacking cough productive of modest amounts of mucopurulent secretions; low-grade fever, chills, sweats, and malaise are variably present.[60] Chest pain, except that associated with violent coughing, is uncommon. Rarely do patients appear acutely ill or toxic. Examination of sputum smears may demonstrate the organisms but, owing to the rarity of cavitation, less frequently than with other mycobacterial lung diseases. Whereas the organisms grow rapidly once recovered, initial isolation from sputum or tissue may take several weeks for substantial growth.

The majority of patients with pulmonary disease due to RGM are infected with *M. abscessus.*[61] This is unfortunate, because both *M. abscessus* and *M. chelonae* organisms are considerably more resistant to drugs than are *M. fortuitum* organisms.[62] Agents that are potentially active against the RGM include parenterally administered compounds as well as a variety of other drugs (Table 167–6). Of note, the standard antimycobacterial agents have virtually no activity against *M. abscessus* or *M. chelonae* and limited impact on *M. fortuitum.*

M. abscessus organisms are extremely drug resistant, usually being variably susceptible in vitro to only cefoxitin and amikacin. Owing to the toxicity-limited period during which these agents may be used, treatment typically results in a gratifying clinical and bacteriologic response only to be followed by a relapse, usually within weeks to months. Furthermore, these relapses are often marked by evolution of resistance to the drugs employed, so therapy is highly problematic and the decision to initiate treatment should be analyzed carefully. For those whom we have elected to treat, two elements have played major roles. Disabling symptoms, most commonly a relentless racking cough that has seriously interfered with or precluded usual activities including sleep, are the most common indication to treat. In such cases, we explain to the patient the high probability of relapse and the potential for emerging drug resistance and try to clarify whether the symptoms are disruptive enough to justify the risk. In other instances, progressive necrotizing lung disease results in severe constitutional symptoms or threatens to produce respiratory insufficiency. In such cases, the decision to treat is straightforward.

For treatment, our practice has been to hospitalize the patient to place an indwelling, multiport central line and to

TABLE 167–6 ■ Usual Patterns of Activity of Chemotherapeutic Agents Against Rapidly Growing Mycobacteria*

AGENT	*MYCOBACTERIUM CHELONAE*	*MYCOBACTERIUM ABSCESSUS*	*MYCOBACTERIUM FORTUITUM*	*MYCOBACTERIUM SMEGMATIS*
Cefoxitin	+ + +	+ + +	+ +	±
Amikacin	+ +	+ + +	+ + +	+ +
Tobramycin	+ + +	±	X	+ +
Imipenem	+	+ +	+ + +	+ + +
Sulfonamides	0	0	+ + +	+ + +
Azithromycin or clarithromycin	+ + +	+	+ +	0
Doxycycline	+	0	+ +	+ + +
Minocycline	+	0	+ +	X
Ciprofloxacin	+	±	+ + +	+ + +
Rifampin	0	0	±	0
Rifabutin	0	0	+	0
Ethionamide	+	±	+	X
Ethambutol	0	0	±	+ +

*+ + +, Active against the clear majority of strains; + +, active against most strains; +, active against some strains; ±, rarely active; 0, not active; X, unknown.

initiate intravenous therapy with cefoxitin, 2 g every 8 hours, and amikacin, 12 to 15 mg/kg every 24 hours (dosage adjusted for age and renal function and monitored by serum levels). If possible, the patient is instructed in self-administration of the drug, or arrangements are made for in-home health professional assistance. Careful monitoring for drug toxicity is vital lest suppressive treatment result in enduring morbidity. The major problems to be avoided are *Clostridium difficile* colitis associated with cefoxitin and eighth nerve damage secondary to amikacin. The duration of therapy is usually delimited by the appearance of toxic effects, although among younger patients, we have been able to extend medication to some 12 to 16 weeks. Although we believe that protracted treatment may delay recurrence, the mycobacterial infection has always reappeared except when there was an oral antimicrobial regimen to continue or in the rare case in which disease was so localized that resection could be performed.[61] If the strain is susceptible to clarithromycin, we follow the parenteral phase with long-term oral suppressive therapy with the agent; however, the utility of this practice is not established. In addition to drug therapy for RGM, careful attention should be paid to possible coinfection, most notably *Pseudomonas aeruginosa* bronchitis. Also, bronchial hygiene, including flutter valve and β-agonist aerosols to promote sputum clearance, is a beneficial element of management.

Owing to the availability of effective parenteral and oral antibiotics, it is feasible to attempt curative chemotherapy for the occasional patient with pulmonary *M. fortuitum* disease. Depending on the severity of symptoms, the extent of disease, and drug susceptibility data in vitro, therapy might commence with either a parenteral regimen or a multidrug oral regimen including such agents as ciprofloxacin, 500 to 750 mg twice daily, doxycycline, 50 to 100 mg twice daily, or clarithromycin, 500 to 750 mg twice a day. If parenteral therapy is initiated, transition to the oral regimen should commence within 2 weeks, with introduction of an oral regimen dictated by susceptibility in vitro. The duration of treatment has not been established, but by extrapolation from other pulmonary mycobacterioses, it would be desirable to continue antibiotics for 3 to 6 months after sputum cultures have become negative.

UNCOMMON MYCOBACTERIA

Although the majority of MOTT pulmonary disease is caused by MAC, *M. kansasii,* or *M. abscessus,* sporadic cases and occasional clusters of disease are due to other MOTT organisms.

Mycobacterium xenopi, a niacin-negative nonchromogenic organism, was noted to cause an outbreak of pulmonary disease among a group of patients at the Veterans Administration Hospital in West Haven, Connecticut.[63] Many of these patients had underlying chronic bronchitis and emphysema, had been hospitalized previously, and were believed to have acquired the disease from shower water at the institution—water that was subsequently proved to be contaminated with *M. xenopi.* Another cluster of disease due to *M. xenopi* was reported from Canada, in the province of Ontario, where in the period 1981 to 1985, 38% of 89 cases of pulmonary MOTT disease were caused by these organisms[64]; like the West Haven patients, most had underlying chronic obstructive pulmonary disease. Treatment of *M. xenopi* has not been systematically evaluated. The organisms show variable resistance in vitro, typically with partial resistance to isoniazid, resistance to pyrazinamide, and susceptibility to other standard agents. *M. xenopi* pulmonary disease appears to respond poorly to chemotherapy, less predictably than would be anticipated from the pattern of resistance in vitro. Initial therapy might include rifampin, ethambutol, ciprofloxacin, and an introductory 2- to 4-month phase of streptomycin. If the disease is particularly extensive or rapidly progressive, other agents can be added on the basis of susceptibility in vitro. Agents likely to be active include ethionamide, cycloserine, and clarithromycin or azithromycin. Among patients with persistent, localized disease, resectional surgery should be considered. One additional aspect of *M. xenopi* should be mentioned: certain strains do not grow at 37°C, the standard mycobacterial culture incubation temperature. Rather, they grow between 42°C and 45°C. Thus, in cases of acid-fast smear-positive disease when growth cannot be elicited, the laboratory should incubate at the higher temperature as well.

Mycobacterium malmoense is similar to MAC and to *Mycobacterium terrae. M. malmoense* pulmonary disease has been reported infrequently in North America but has been seen with increasing frequency in northern Europe.[65–67] These organisms grow timidly on standard media, typically forming small colonies after a long period of incubation. Also, they may be more vulnerable to killing during decontamination of sputum. Data on resistance patterns and response to the therapy among patients infected with *M. malmoense* are limited. In general, the organisms are somewhat more susceptible in vitro than are MAC strains, and responses to multidrug chemotherapy regimens containing rifampin, ethambutol, and isoniazid have been observed. On the basis of their similarity to MAC and available in vitro susceptibility data, clarithromycin or azithromycin should be considered as first-line therapy. In one series, outcome appeared better when therapy was extended to 18 months; surgery was used to treat patients refractory to drugs.[66]

Mycobacterium simiae and *Mycobacterium africanum* are infrequently associated with human pulmonary disease. Both organisms share with *M. tuberculosis* the property of elaborating niacin during growth, giving a positive niacin test result. *M. africanum,* a nonpigmented organism, is by DNA homology a member of *M. tuberculosis* complex. Like *M. tuberculosis,* most strains of *M. africanum* are susceptible to the standard antituberculosis drugs; however, limited clinical experience suggests that pulmonary disease caused by these microbes is less responsive than would be anticipated by susceptibility in vitro alone. *M. africanum,* as might be surmised, is seen principally among persons who have resided in Africa. *M. simiae,* by contrast, is highly resistant in vitro and is refractory to chemotherapy. Most active agents in vitro include the newer macrolides, fluoroquinolones, and aminoglycosides. It has been reported in geographic clusters, most recently in the southwestern United States.[68, 69] In one center in San Antonio, Texas, positive cultures for *M. simiae* were obtained from clinical specimens of 75 patients.[69] However, clinicians believed that only 15 of 62 (24%) evaluable patients had definite or probable disease. Most people with pulmonary disease had preexisting respiratory disorders.

Mycobacterium szulgai and *Mycobacterium scrofulaceum* are scotochromogenic mycobacteria, group II, that are occasionally associated with pulmonary disease. Both pulmonary disease and extrapulmonary disease due to *M. szulgai* have been well reviewed[70]; the organisms are variably susceptible to standard agents, and therapy based on susceptibility in vitro appears to be effective. Disease due to *M. scrofulaceum* appears to be diminishing in frequency in the United States. Pulmonary disease is uncommon, which is fortunate because the microbes are extremely drug resistant.

M. bovis, although niacin-negative, is also part of *M. tuberculosis* complex. Although no distinguishable differences exist between *M. bovis* and *M. tuberculosis* by DNA homology, consistent phenotypic differences exist that merit continued distinction as separate species. Since the advent of tuberculin testing for dairy herds, *M. bovis* is far less common as a human pathogen in the United States and Canada. In fact, most patients seen in these countries with *M. bovis* disease have immigrated from areas where such testing is not done. *M. bovis* is believed to be transmitted in most cases by ingestion, possibly of unpasteurized milk, cheese, or otherwise contaminated fluids or foodstuff. This presumably results in bacteremic dissemination, with seeding of the lungs and various extrapulmonary sites. However, reports have documented human *M. bovis* disease after animal exposure, including exposure to a variety of ruminants[71] and seals.[72] Aerogenic spread may be responsible for some of these cases, with animal-to-human transmission occurring. The issue of human-to-human transmission has not been resolved. Among adults, types of extrapulmonary disease are diverse and include mesenteric adenitis, osseous disease, and pleural disease; miliary or central nervous system disease is rare. In children, *M. bovis* more commonly presents with cervical lymphadenitis or mesenteric lymph node involvement. Disseminated infection is reported in small numbers of persons with AIDS. Treatment of *M. bovis* disease should take into account uniform resistance to pyrazinamide, a considerable likelihood of resistance to *p*-aminosalicylic acid, and a small risk of primary resistance to isoniazid. *M. bovis* disease has been comprehensively reviewed in a superb article by Dankner and colleagues.[73]

Extrapulmonary MOTT Disease

Other than cervical lymphadenitis, extrapulmonary disease has historically constituted a relatively smaller percentage of all MOTT disease; however, with the appearance of AIDS and the extraordinary prevalence of disseminated MAC disease in these patients, a substantial portion of MOTT disease now is primarily extrapulmonary. For the sake of clarity, this section is broken into two parts: localized single-site extrapulmonary infection, and multifocal or disseminated disease.

LOCALIZED NONPULMONARY MOTT DISEASE

In large measure, this type of infection reflects direct inoculation, soft tissue or skeletal infection, or cervical lymphadenitis, presumably due to spread from contamination of the oropharynx.

Soft Tissue and Skeletal Infection

Environmental mycobacteria may cause localized infection when introduced directly into skin, soft tissues, bone, or joints. This may occur through accidental trauma or iatrogenically through either contamination of medical devices or disruption of defense barrier by invasive procedures. RGM, including *M. chelonae, M. fortuitum,* and *M. abscessus,* have a striking propensity for iatrogenic infections; they have been associated with corneal abrasions and ulcerations after ophthalmic procedures,[74] hypodermic injection site abscesses, monarticular arthritis after intraarticular steroid injections, mastitis after silicone implant mammaplasty,[75] otitis media after placement of tympanotomy tubes,[76] skin infection after cosmetic surgery in which the gentian violet used to outline the incisions was contaminated,[77] and injection of contaminated preparations of adrenocortical extract prescribed by alternative healers.[78] Also, there have been a variety of infections after open heart surgery (including sternal osteomyelitis, mediastinitis, and endocarditis).[79] *Mycobacterium smegmatis,* an organism similar to *M. fortuitum,* has been reported in association with a variety of soft tissue, bone, and other infections[80]; in several instances, it appeared to be iatrogenic in origin.

M. kansasii can produce both nodular (sporotrichoid) and diffuse (cellulitis) cutaneous disease.[81] Most of these cases appear in persons who have impaired immunity, because of either an immunosuppressive disease or medications. Diagnosis may be delayed by failure of the hosts to form destructive granulomata. Treatment entails antibiotics, reduction of immunosuppressive therapy, and local heat.

Mycobacterium marinum infections—swimming pool granulomata, fish-handler's nodules, surfer's nodules—are acquired principally in natural settings. These cases are primarily reported in coastal areas of North America or among individuals who, through hobby or employment, are exposed to fish tanks or fishing paraphernalia. A report from a coastal county abutting the Chesapeake Bay offered useful insights into this infection[82]; there was a strong preponderance of males, and the primary involvement was cutaneous, although joints and tendons were included in some cases. A previous report in which *M. marinum* infections were acquired from a mineral springs pool documented a high percentage of patients with substantial reactions to purified protein derivative tuberculin skin testing.[83]

A similar problem, originally reported from Africa as Buruli ulcers, is a nodular cutaneous scarring process resulting from direct inoculation of *Mycobacterium ulcerans,* typically via grass cuts. Cases of *M. ulcerans* disease have also been reported from Australia.[84] A report has noted disseminated osteomyelitis due to *M. ulcerans* in an African child after an alleged snake bite.[85] The organisms are closely related to *M. marinum,* but *M. ulcerans* produces a much more virulent, necrotizing, invasive infection. Although some response to antimicrobials may be seen, surgical débridement is the central element of therapy. Both of these cutaneous pathogens have strong growth preferences for lower temperatures, presumably associated with their predilection for superficial infections. If incubated at the standard 37°C, they may not grow. The clinician who suspects a cutaneous mycobacteriosis should request that the specimen also be cultivated between 27°C and 33°C.

Monarticular arthritis and localized tenosynovitis have also been reported with MAC, *M. terrae,*[86] *M. marinum,*[87] and, as noted, RGM.[62] In some instances, it seems probable that the process began as a noninfectious condition and was complicated by the iatrogenic introduction of the mycobacteria, often during steroid injections. Because of the immense potential for iatrogenic morbidity, this issue is worth amplification. During the past decade at the National Jewish Hospital, we have seen an increasing number of cases in which it appears probable that MAC organisms have been introduced into wrists, hands, or bursae during steroid injections. In other cases, the infection may have been initiated with a puncture wound resulting in local spread to the joint or tendinous structure. In other instances, no discrete inciting event can be identified, raising the question of transient mycobacteremia with seeding of a single site.[86]

Because, in general, patients with single-site extrapulmonary MOTT disease *do not* have deficits of immunity, initial screening including serologic tests for HIV is not indicated unless the patient comes from a high-risk group. Management usually consists of chemotherapy and surgical extirpation or débridement. If the species and susceptibility pattern are known, drugs may be selected as noted in the section on pulmonary disease. If the species is not yet known or susceptibility has not been determined, one may be forced to begin empirical therapy. Broadly speaking, much empirical therapy might best consist of a macrolide or rifampin, ethambutol, and ciprofloxacin; amikacin should be included in cases in which major joints or vital sites are involved. Such a regimen should be reasonably active against such a diverse group of mycobacteria. Although there is no clear evidence associating response to therapy among MOTT infections with susceptibility in vitro, experience in the treatment of tuberculosis, few clinical data, and common sense dictate that careful, quantitative susceptibility testing be performed to aid in the management of these tenacious infections.

Cervical Lymphadenitis

MOTT infection of lymph nodes is primarily a disease of children aged 1 to 5 years; rarely is it seen in adults.[88] MAC is by far the most common pathogen, in contrast to earlier reports with higher percentages of *M. kansasii* or *M. scrofulaceum*.[88, 89] Typically, it presents as unilateral, anterior cervical, preauricular, or submandibular erythematous swelling in an asymptomatic child with a normal chest radiograph.[90] In contrast, lymphadenitis caused by *M. tuberculosis* more commonly involves supraclavicular or posterior cervical sites. Occasionally, the nodes drain spontaneously or ulcerate. Biopsy typically demonstrates granulomata with or without caseation; in some early lesions, a dimorphic response (mixed granulomatous and pyogenic) is seen. Acid-fast bacilli stains are positive in only about half the cases. Skin testing is a problem. In the past, most children have reacted to MOTT antigens; however, these are no longer available. Owing to cross-reactivity, a portion of MOTT patients react to purified protein derivative, the antigen of *M. tuberculosis.* Indeed, in Wolinsky's series,[90] 35% of children showed induration of 10 mm or more to this antigen; conversely, 29% showed reactivity of 0 to 5 mm. Thus, neither a positive nor a negative reaction to purified protein derivative has much sensitivity or specificity in the etiologic diagnosis of cervical adenitis. Perhaps the most meaningful result of tuberculin skin testing is an intense reaction (20 mm or more of induration), which points toward tuberculosis rather than MOTT infection. Culture of lymph node biopsy material is vital, because the management of cervical adenitis due to MOTT is vastly different from that of disease due to *M. tuberculosis.* Unlike *M. tuberculosis* infection of children or adults, which definitely should receive chemotherapy, the local MOTT infection may require only careful observation, or it may be sufficiently controlled with excisional surgery. Although chemotherapy has been administered to many children with MOTT adenitis, it is not clear that it was beneficial.[89] If a biopsy is performed and demonstrates histopathologic features consistent with mycobacterial lymphadenitis, it is appropriate to initiate chemotherapy until cultures distinguish between MOTT and tuberculosis. This is especially true for persons with a high-risk epidemiologic profile, such as Hispanic, black, or Asian children. If the culture is positive for MOTT, therapy may be terminated, or if a distinctly favorable clinical response is seen, chemotherapy may be continued. If it grows nothing and there are insufficient grounds to rule out tuberculosis, therapy might be continued for 9 months. Until tuberculosis has been excluded, empirical agents of choice are isoniazid and rifampin; ethambutol is an excellent MOTT agent in general, but it is difficult to monitor children who cannot comply with standard tests for visual impairment. However, some experience suggests that, when clearly indicated, ethambutol can be given to children with reasonable expectations for safety.[91] If MAC is identified, clarithromycin or azithromycin—because of the likelihood of in vitro activity and a generally benign profile of toxicity—might be employed. Because of the paucibacillary disease and negligible risk of disseminated infection, monotherapy is justified in our opinion. Neither the ideal duration nor proof of efficacy of this approach has been established.

It is important to distinguish these relatively benign, localized cases of lymphadenitis from the disseminated forms of MAC or *M. tuberculosis* lymphohematogenous disease seen in AIDS patients (see later).

DISSEMINATED OR MULTIFOCAL EXTRAPULMONARY MOTT DISEASE

In the majority of instances, patients with disseminated or multifocal extrapulmonary disease due to MOTT either are immunodeficient or suffer iatrogenic disease. The distinction between disseminated and multifocal disease is a subtle but significant one. Persons with disease involving many different organs (bone marrow, liver, spleen) generally have a more profound deficit of immunity and a worse prognosis than those who have, for instance, multifocal osteomyelitis without other organ involvement. Generally recognized syndromes due to the various MOTT are grouped here by organism.

Disseminated Disease Due to MAC

Before the advent of AIDS, cases of disseminated MAC disease were reported sporadically.[92] Among the younger population, there have been a number of cases that presented with multifocal osteomyelitis without other organ involvement or apparent increased vulnerability to other infections. Studies of their immune system have demonstrated a variety of abnormalities of cellular immunity, including failure of macrophages to limit intracellular replication and absence of serum factors that facilitate macrophage function.

Disseminated MAC disease is the most common systemic bacterial infection in patients with AIDS in the United States and has been reported in as many as 20% to 30% of patients living with AIDS.[93] At highest risk are those individuals with $CD4^+$ T cell counts of less than 50 to 75/mm^3.[94] In the absence of chemoprophylaxis, the yearly rate of development of MAC bacteremia is 20%, after an initial AIDS-defining opportunistic infection and a decline in the $CD4^+$ T cell count to less than 100/mm^3.[95] MAC organisms are known to be ubiquitous in the environment and can be readily isolated from the soil and potable water.[96] Many MAC serotypes have been isolated and characterized, and it is probable that most individuals are frequently exposed to both pathogenic and nonpathogenic strains. Several investigators have studied how an individual becomes infected with MAC. Chin and colleagues[97] reported that the risk of MAC bacteremia was around 60% within 1 year for patients with MAC in either the respiratory or gastrointestinal tract, although the gastrointestinal tract is the likely portal of entry. Once MAC organisms are in the gastrointestinal tract, an intestinal inflammatory process occurs in the lymph nodes. This process appears to be the first phase of localized disease before dissemination through intestinal lymphatics and, ultimately, the blood stream. When dissemination occurs, virtually every organ in the body may become involved. Clinical findings associated with MAC in AIDS patients include constitutional symptoms (fever, sweats, inanition), diffuse peripheral lymphadenitis, massive retroperitoneal and mesenteric lymphadenitis, mediastinal or hilar lymphadenitis, infiltrative hepatosplenomegaly, anemia or cytopenia secondary to massive infiltration of the bone marrow, and refractory diarrhea due to massive infiltration of intestinal and colonic mucosa by mycobacteria-laden macrophages. Although diarrhea is common in disseminated MAC disease, it is by no means specific. Other pathogens such as *Cryptosporidium, Isospora,* or cytomegalovirus may coexist with MAC. Laboratory findings routinely found in disseminated MAC disease include anemia, neutropenia, and an elevated serum alkaline phosphatase level.

In contrast to the non–HIV-infected elderly patient with chronic pulmonary MAC infection, HIV-infected individuals rarely have clinically significant pulmonary disease secondary to MAC. One report found pulmonary MAC disease in only 2.5% of 200 patients with disseminated MAC disease.[98] When MAC does cause clinically significant pulmonary disease, parenchymal infiltrates or nodules are typically seen. Cavitary lesions are uncommon. Airway compromise secondary to endobronchial MAC lesions has been reported. Isolation of the organism from blood is the most reliable method for the diagnosis of disseminated MAC disease in patients with AIDS. Isolation of MAC organisms from bone marrow or other normally sterile sites (lymph node, liver, spleen, cerebrospinal fluid) may precede recovery from the blood; recovery from such sites should be interpreted as indicative of disseminated disease. Cultures of either respiratory secretions or stool specimens that yield MAC organisms are not diagnostic of disseminated disease.

During the early years of the HIV epidemic, management of disseminated MAC disease was hampered by relatively ineffective diagnostic methods, uncertainty regarding its clinical significance, and lack of effective chemotherapeutic agents. Now it is clear that untreated disseminated MAC disease is associated with reduced survival in AIDS patients, and new combination antimicrobial therapy provides clinical and microbiologic responses and improved survival in the majority of patients. Monotherapy was initially thought to be effective in providing clinical stabilization in patients with disseminated MAC disease. Kemper and coworkers[99] evaluated the efficacy of individual drugs in which patients with disseminated MAC disease were given ethambutol, 15 mg/kg per day, clofazimine, 200 mg/d, or rifabutin, 600 mg/d. Of the three drugs, only ethambutol was associated with a microbiologic and clinical response. The most significant advance in MAC therapy has been the introduction of clarithromycin and azithromycin. Both drugs are similar in that they are able to be concentrated within the macrophage and therefore are quite effective against MAC because it is an intracellular pathogen.[100, 101] Dautzenberg and associates[101] conducted a crossover study in which for the first 6 weeks, clarithromycin therapy was compared with placebo. Blood sterilization occurred in six of eight clarithromycin-treated patients, whereas the placebo-treated group experienced increasing levels of bacteremia. Chaisson and others[102] conducted a dose-ranging study with clarithromycin used as monotherapy. Important findings from this study were that patients given 500 mg twice daily had a reduction in adverse effects and mortality. Perhaps just as important was the development of high-level clarithromycin resistance (minimal inhibitory concentration, > 32 μg/mL) in 46% of patients in the study. This finding indicated the need for combination therapy for disseminated MAC disease, with clarithromycin or the newer macrolide azithromycin as the backbone of the regimen. Rifabutin has also shown promise as an effective agent in the treatment of MAC; however, studies have now demonstrated significant drug-drug interactions between clarithromycin and rifabutin, which may limit their coadministration.[40] Rifabutin, by its interaction with the cytochrome P-450 system, induces the metabolism of clarithromycin, thereby decreasing effective serum levels. Clarithromycin inhibits the cytochrome P-450 system and, by virtue of this when coadministered with rifabutin, has been shown to cause a twofold increase in serum rifabutin concentrations.[42] Havlir and colleagues[103] were the first to report the development of uveitis secondary to increased rifabutin levels when rifabutin and clarithromycin were administered together. Chaisson and coworkers[38] reported that the addition of clofazimine to a clarithromycin and ethambutol regimen did not improve bacteriologic outcomes and was associated with a significantly shorter survival. Current recommendations for the treatment of disseminated MAC disease are that at least two drugs should be used in any treatment regimen.[104] The preferred first and second drugs are clarithromycin, 500 mg twice daily, plus ethambutol, 15 mg/kg per day. The recommended alternative regimen is azithromycin, 500 mg/d plus ethambutol. The addition of a third drug (rifabutin, 300 mg/d, ciprofloxacin, or amikacin) should be considered. Because of continued immunosuppression, treatment of disseminated MAC infection in AIDS patients should be lifelong.

Because morbidity and mortality from disseminated MAC disease are so high, prophylaxis is now routinely recommended with a $CD4^+$ count of 75 cells per mm^3 or less in patients with an AIDS-defining illness and at 50 cells per mm^3 or less in those without.[105] Nightingale and colleagues[106] demonstrated a 50% decrease in the development of MAC bacteremia in people with AIDS when rifabutin (300 mg/d) was used. Rifabutin is associated with substantial alterations in the antiretroviral protease inhibitors ritonavir and indinavir and perhaps less so with saquinavir. Rifabutin is therefore not currently used as a first-line agent for disseminated MAC disease prophylaxis. Clarithromycin (500 mg twice daily) has a much less dramatic interaction with the protease inhibitors and is therefore the agent of choice.[105] Studies are currently being evaluated to assess whether azithromycin once weekly versus daily is as effective as the current clarithromycin regimen.

Disseminated Disease Due to MOTT Other Than MAC

Before the AIDS era, disseminated MOTT infections were associated with immunodeficiency states such as lymphatic and hematopoietic malignancies, cytotoxic and corticosteroid therapy, renal failure, and organ transplantation. *M. kansasii* remains the most common mycobacterial species in this setting as well as in the setting of HIV. It has been reported to account for 2.9% of the MOTT species that cause disseminated infection in patients with AIDS.[101] Unlike MAC, *M. kansasii* is a cause of serious pulmonary disease in people with advanced HIV disease.[108] Pulmonary disease appears to be more common than disseminated infection. Radiographic features include cavities and diffuse nodular, interstitial, or parenchymal infiltrates. *M. kansasii* has shown susceptibility in vitro to clarithromycin, ethambutol, rifampin, ciprofloxacin, and amikacin. *M. xenopi* pulmonary disease often mimics tuberculosis in the early stages of HIV infection and may disseminate in patients with advanced disease.[109] Effective antimicrobials are similar to those used against *M. kansasii*. *Mycobacterium haemophilum* most commonly presents with raised, violaceous, fluctuant cutaneous lesions but has also been reported to cause destructive bone and joint disease in advanced HIV disease.[110] The incidence of *M. haemophilum* infection has likely been underreported because of the organism's fastidious growth requirements. To facilitate isolation in the laboratory, media must be iron supplemented (such as chocolate agar) and must also be incubated at a lower temperature. Drugs that have been shown to have susceptibility in vitro include clarithromycin, azithromycin, ciprofloxacin, rifabutin, cycloserine, and amikacin. Despite adequate treatment, however, infection may flare once antibiotics are discontinued.[111] *Mycobacterium genavense* was first reported to cause infection in an AIDS patient in 1990.[112] Symptoms are similar to those seen in disseminated MAC infection and include fever, inanition, weight loss, abdominal pain, splenomegaly, and diarrhea. This organism grows only in liquid media, which makes it difficult to isolate in many laboratories that use only solid agar isolation systems.[113] Susceptibility data are similar to those for MAC. *Mycobacterium gordonae* has more often been regarded as a nonpathogenic mycobacterial species that may act as a laboratory contaminant. Many reports have appeared in the literature describing pulmonary, soft tissue, and disseminated infections in patients with AIDS.[114] *Mycobacterium celatum* is a newly described species. It is easily misidentified as *M. xenopi* when identification is based on biochemical testing alone. Genomic analysis or high-performance liquid chromatography is necessary to distinguish the two species. Zurawski and colleagues[115] have described two AIDS patients with significant pulmonary and disseminated disease. A review of the literature reveals case reports of mycobacterial infections with *M. szulgai, M. scrofulaceum, M. simiae,* and *M. fortuitum.*[40, 106, 107, 113] Given the extraordinary vitiation of cellular immunity in AIDS, it is likely that in the future we will encounter disseminated infection with virtually all known mycobacterial species as well as with exotic species yet to be identified.

References

1. Falkinham J: Epidemiology of infection by nontuberculous mycobacteria. Clin Microbiol Rev 9:177, 1996.
2. O'Brien RJ, Geiter LJ, Snider DE: The epidemiology of nontuberculous mycobacterial diseases in the United States: Results from a national survey. Am Rev Respir Dis 135:1007, 1987.
3. Tsukamura M, Kita N, Shimoide H, et al: Studies on the epidemiology of nontuberculous mycobacteriosis in Japan. Am Rev Respir Dis 137:1280, 1988.
4. Bittner M, Horowitz E, Safranek T, Preheim L: Emergence of *Mycobacterium kansasii* as the leading mycobacterial pathogen isolated over a 20-year period at a midwestern Veterans Affairs hospital. Clin Infect Dis 22:1109, 1996.
5. Crowe HE, King CT, Smith E, et al: A limited clinical, pathologic, and epidemiologic study of patients with pulmonary lesions associated with atypical acid-fast bacilli in the sputum. Am Rev Tuberc 75:199, 1957.
6. Schaefer W: Type-specificity of atypical mycobacteria in agglutination and antibody absorption test. Am Rev Respir Dis 96: 1165, 1967.
7. Baess I: Deoxyribonucleic acid relationships between different serotypes of *Mycobacterium avium, Mycobacterium intracellulare,* and *Mycobacterium scrofulaceum.* Acta Pathol Microbiol Immunol Scand B 91:210, 1983.
8. Guthertz L, Damsker B, Bottone E, et al: *Mycobacterium avium* and *Mycobacterium intracellulare* infections in patients with and without AIDS. J Infect Dis 160:1037, 1989.
9. Prince DS, Peterson DD, Steiner RM, et al: Infection with *Mycobacterium avium* complex in patients without predisposing conditions. N Engl J Med 321:863, 1989.
10. Iseman M: *Mycobacterium avium* complex and the normal host. The other side of the coin (Editorial). N Engl J Med 321:896, 1989.
11. Iseman M, Buschman D, Ackerson L: Pectus excavatum and scoliosis: Thoracic anomalies associated with pulmonary disease due to *M. avium* complex. Am Rev Respir Dis 144:914, 1991.
12. Reich J, Johns N: *Mycobacterium avium* complex pulmonary disease presenting as isolated lingular or middle lobe pattern: The Lady Windermere syndrome. Chest 101:1605, 1992.
13. Iseman M: That's no lady (Letter). Chest 109:1411, 1996.
14. Iseman M: That's no lady, revisited (Letter). Chest 111:255, 1997.
15. Chan E, Iseman M: Hypothesis: Prior infection with *Histoplasma capsulatum* predisposes to pulmonary *Mycobacterium avium* complex infection? Am J Respir Crit Care Med 153:A329, 1996.
16. Ahn CH, McLarty JW, Ahn SS, et al: Diagnostic criteria for pulmonary disease caused by *Mycobacterium kansasii* and *Mycobacterium intracellulare.* Am Rev Respir Dis 125:388, 1982.
17. Lynch D, Simone P, Fox M, et al: CT features of pulmonary *Mycobacterium avium* complex infection. J Comput Assist Tomogr 19:353, 1995.
18. Scully R, Mark E, McNeely W, Ebeling S: Case records of the Massachusetts General Hospital: Weekly clinicopathological exercises. N Engl J Med 334:521, 1996.
19. Embil J, Warren P, Yakrus M, et al: Pulmonary illness associated with exposure to *Mycobacterium avium* complex in hot tub water. Hypersensitivity pneumonitis or infection? Chest 111:813, 1997.
20. Rosenzweig DY: Pulmonary mycobacterial infections due to *Mycobacterium intracellulare-avium* complex. Clinical features and course in 100 consecutive cases. Chest 75:115, 1979.
21. Barnard M, Hawkins E, Bass JB: *Mycobacterium avium-intracellulare* in Alabama, 1970–1980 (Abstr). Am Rev Respir Dis 129:187, 1984.
22. Horsburgh CR Jr, Mason UG, Heifets LB, et al: Response to therapy of pulmonary *Mycobacterium avium intracellulare* infection correlates with results of in vitro susceptibility testing. Am Rev Respir Dis 135:418, 1987.
23. Tsukamura M: Evidence that antituberculosis drugs are really effective in the treatment of pulmonary infection caused by *Mycobacterium avium* complex. Am Rev Respir Dis 137:144, 1988.
24. Sison J, Yao Y, Kemper C, et al: Treatment of *Mycobacterium avium* complex infection: Do the results of in vitro susceptibility tests predict therapeutic outcome in humans? J Infect Dis 173:677, 1996.
25. American Thoracic Society: Diagnosis and treatment of disease caused by nontuberculous mycobacteria. Am Rev Respir Dis 142:940, 1990.
26. Davidson PT, Kanijo V, Goble M, Moulding TS: Treatment of disease due to *Mycobacterium intracellulare.* Rev Infect Dis 3:1052, 1981.
27. American College of Chest Physicians, Consensus Conference: Disease due to *Mycobacterium avium intracellulare.* Chest (Suppl 87):139S, 1985.
28. Heifets L, Lindholm-Levy P, Flory M: Comparison of bacteriostatic and bactericidal activity of isoniazid and ethionamide against *Mycobacterium avium* and *Mycobacterium tuberculosis.* Am Rev Respir Dis 143:268, 1991.
29. Heifets L, Iseman M: Choice of antimicrobial agents for *M. avium* disease based on quantitative tests of drug susceptibility. N Engl J Med 323:419, 1990.
30. Heifets L, Lindholm-Levy P, Comstock R: Clarithromycin minimal inhibitory and bactericidal concentrations against *Mycobacterium avium.* Am Rev Respir Dis 145:856, 1992.
31. Heifets L: Clarithromycin against *Mycobacterium avium* complex infections. Tuber Lung Dis 77:19, 1996.
32. Wallace R Jr, Brown B, Griffith D, et al: Initial clarithromycin monotherapy for *Mycobacterium avium-intracellulare* complex lung disease. Am J Respir Crit Care Med 149:1335, 1994.
33. Heifets L: Susceptibility testing of *Mycobacterium avium* complex isolates. Antimicrob Agents Chemother 40:1759, 1996.
34. Griffith D, Brown B, Girard W, et al: Azithromycin activity against *Mycobacterium avium* complex lung disease in patients who were not infected with human immunodeficiency virus. Clin Infect Dis 23:983, 1996.
35. Heifets L, Iseman M, Lindholm-Levy P: Ethambutol MICs and MBCs for *Mycobacterium avium* complex and *Mycobacterium tuberculosis.* Antimicrob Agents Chemother 30:927, 1986.
36. Heifets L, Iseman M, Lindholm-Levy P: Combinations of rifampin or rifabutin plus ethambutol against *Mycobacterium avium* complex: Bactericidal synergistic, and bacteriostatic additive or synergistic effects. Am Rev Respir Dis 137:711, 1988.
37. Lindholm-Levy P, Heifets L: Clofazimine and other riminocompounds: Minimal inhibitory and minimal bactericidal concentrations at different pHs for *Mycobacterium avium* complex. Tubercle 69:179, 1988.
38. Chaisson R, Kaiser P, Pierce M, et al: Controlled trial of clarithromycin/ethambutol with or without clofazimine for *Mycobacterium avium* complex bacteremia in AIDS. *In* Third National Conference on Human Retroviruses and Related Infections; January 28–February 1, 1996; Washington, DC.
39. Heifets L: MIC as a quantitative measurement of the susceptibility of *Mycobacterium avium* strains to seven antituberculosis drugs. Antimicrob Agents Chemother 32:1131, 1988.
40. Wallace R Jr, Brown B, Griffith D, et al: Reduced serum levels of clarithromycin in patients treated with multidrug regimens including rifampin or rifabutin for *Mycobacterium avium–Mycobacterium intracellulare* infection. J Infect Dis 171:747, 1995.
41. Periti P, Mazzei T, Mini E, Novelli A: Pharmacokinetic drug interactions of macrolides. Clin Pharmacokinet 23:106, 1992.
42. Fuller J, Stanfield L, Craven D: Rifabutin prophylaxis and uveitis (Letter). N Engl J Med 330:1315, 1994.
43. Shafran S, Deschenes J, Miller M, et al: Uveitis and pseudojaundice during a regimen of clarithromycin, rifabutin, and ethambutol. N Engl J Med 330:438, 1994.
44. Berning S, Iseman M: Rifamycin-induced lupus syndrome. Lancet (in press).

45. Corpe RF: Surgical management of pulmonary disease due to *Mycobacterium avium intracellulare.* Rev Infect Dis 3:1064, 1981.
46. Moran JF, Alexander LG, Staub EW, et al: Long-term results of pulmonary resection for atypical mycobacterial disease. Ann Thorac Surg 35:597, 1983.
47. Pomerantz M, Madsen L, Goble M, Iseman M: Surgical management of resistant mycobacterial tuberculosis and other mycobacterial pulmonary infections. Ann Thorac Surg 52:1108, 1991.
48. Ahn CH, Lowell JR, Onstad GD, et al: A demographic study of disease due to *Mycobacterium kansasii* or *M. intracellulare-avium* in Texas. Chest 75:120, 1979.
49. Onstad G: Familial aggregations of group I atypical mycobacterial disease. Am Rev Respir Dis 99:426, 1969.
50. Johanson WB Jr, Nicholson D: Pulmonary disease due to *Mycobacterium kansasii.* An analysis of some factors affecting prognosis. Am Rev Respir Dis 99:73, 1969.
51. Pezzia W, Raleigh J, Bailey M, et al: Treatment of pulmonary disease due to *Mycobacterium kansasii:* Recent experience with rifampin. Rev Infect Dis 3:1035, 1981.
52. Banks J, Hunter A, Campbell I, et al: Pulmonary infection with *Mycobacterium kansasii* in Wales, 1970–9: Review of treatment and response. Thorax 38:271, 1983.
53. Zvetina JR, Demos TC, Maliwan N, et al: Pulmonary cavitations in *Mycobacterium kansasii:* Distinctions from *M. tuberculosis.* AJR 143:127, 1984.
54. Ahn CH, Lowell JR, Ahn SS, et al: Short-course chemotherapy for pulmonary disease caused by *Mycobacterium kansasii.* Am Rev Respir Dis 128:1048, 1983.
55. British Thoracic Society: *Mycobacterium kansasii* pulmonary infection: A prospective study of the results of nine months of treatment with rifampicin ethambutol. Thorax 49:442, 1994.
56. Wallace RJ Jr, Dunbar D, Brown B, et al: Rifampin-resistant *Mycobacterium kansasii.* Clin Infect Dis 18:736, 1994.
57. Ahn CH, Wallace RJ Jr, Steele LC, Murphy DT: Sulfonamide-containing regimens for disease caused by rifampin-resistant *Mycobacterium kansasii.* Am Rev Respir Dis 135:10, 1987.
58. Ahn CH, Lowell JR, Ahn SA, et al: Chemotherapy for pulmonary disease due to *Mycobacterium kansasii*: Efficacies of some individual drugs. Rev Infect Dis 3:1028, 1981.
59. Varghese G, Shepherd R, Watt P, Bruce J: Fatal infection with *Mycobacterium fortuitum* associated with oesophageal achalasia. Thorax 43:151, 1988.
60. Wallace RJ Jr: The clinical presentation, diagnosis, and therapy of cutaneous and pulmonary infections due to the rapidly growing mycobacteria, *M. fortuitum* and *M. chelonae.* Clin Chest Med 10:419, 1989.
61. Griffith D, Girard W, Wallace RJ Jr: Clinical features of pulmonary disease caused by rapidly growing mycobacteria. An analysis of 154 patients. Am Rev Respir Dis 147:1271, 1993.
62. Wallace RJ Jr: Treatment of infections caused by rapidly growing mycobacteria in the era of newer macrolides. Res Microbiol 147:30, 1996.
63. Costrini AM, Mahler DA, Gross WM, et al: Clinical and roentgenographic features of nosocomial pulmonary disease due to *Mycobacterium xenopi.* Am Rev Respir Dis 123:104, 1981.
64. Contreras MA, Cheung OT, Sanders DE, Goldstein RS: Pulmonary infection with the nontuberculous mycobacteria. Am Rev Respir Dis 137:149, 1988.
65. Jenkins PA: *Mycobacterium malmoense.* Tubercle 66:193, 1985.
66. Banks J, Jenkins PA, Smith AP: Pulmonary infection with *Mycobacterium malmoense*—A review of treatment and response. Tubercle 66:197, 1985.
67. Katila M, Brander E, Viljanen T: Difficulty with *Mycobacterium malmoense.* Lancet 2:510, 1989.
68. Bell RC, Higuchi JH, Donovan WN, et al: *Mycobacterium simiae:* Clinical features and follow-up of twenty-five patients. Am Rev Respir Dis 127:35, 1983.
69. Valero G, Peters J, Jorgensen JH, Graybill JR: Clinical isolates of *Mycobacterium simiae* in San Antonio, Texas. An 11-yr review. Am J Respir Crit Care Med 152:1555, 1995.
70. Maloney JM, Gregg CR, Stephens DS, et al: Infections caused by *Mycobacterium szulgai* in humans. Rev Infect Dis 9:1120, 1987.
71. O'Reilly L, Daborn C: The epidemiology of *Mycobacterium bovis* infection in animals and man: A review. Tubercle Lung Dis 76(Suppl 1):1, 1995.
72. Thompson P, Cousins D, Gow B, et al: Seals, seal trainers, and mycobacterial infection. Am Rev Respir Dis 147:164, 1993.
73. Dankner W, Waecker N, Essey M, et al: *Mycobacterium bovis* infections in San Diego: A clinicoepidemiologic study of 73 patients and a historical review of a forgotten pathogen. Medicine (Baltimore) 72:11, 1993.
74. LaFlamme MY, Poisson M, Chehade N: *Mycobacterium chelonei* keratitis following penetrating keratoplasty. Can J Ophthalmol 22:178, 1987.
75. Clegg HW, Foster MT, Sanders WE Jr, Baine WB: Infection due to organisms of the *Mycobacterium fortuitum* complex after augmentation mammaplasty: Clinical and epidemiologic features. J Infect Dis 147:427, 1983.
76. Lowry PW, Jarvis WR, Oberle AD, et al: *Mycobacterium chelonae* causing otitis media in an ear-nose-and-throat practice. N Engl J Med 319:978, 1988.
77. Safraneck TJ, Jarvis WR, Carson LA, et al: *Mycobacterium chelonae* wound infections after plastic surgery employing contaminated gentian violet skin-marking solution. N Engl J Med 317:197, 1987.
78. Centers for Disease Control and Prevention: Infection with *Mycobacterium abscessus* associated with intramuscular injection of adrenal cortex extract—Colorado and Wyoming, 1995–1996. MMWR Morbid Mortal Wkly Rep 45:713, 1996.
79. Robicsek F, Hoffman PC, Masters TN, et al: Rapidly growing nontuberculous mycobacteria: A new enemy of the cardiac surgeon. Ann Thorac Surg 46:703, 1988.
80. Wallace RJ Jr, Nash DR, Tsukamura M, et al: Human disease due to *Mycobacterium smegmatis.* J Infect Dis 158:52, 1988.
81. Breathnach A, Levell N, Munro C, et al: Cutaneous *Mycobacterium kansasii* infection: Case report and review. Clin Infect Dis 20:812, 1995.
82. Jõe L, Hall R: *Mycobacterium marinum* disease in Anne Arundel County: 1995 update. Md Med J 24:1043, 1995.
83. Judson F, Feldman R: Mycobacterial skin tests in humans 12 years after infection with *M. marinum.* Am Rev Respir Dis 109:544, 1974.
84. Goutzamanis G: *Mycobacterium ulcerans* infection in Australian children: Report of eight cases and review. Clin Infect Dis 21:1186, 1995.
85. Hofer M, Hirschel B, Kirschner P, et al: Brief report: Disseminated osteomyelitis from *Mycobacterium ulcrans* after a snakebite. N Engl J Med 328:1007, 1993.
86. Petrini B, Svartengren G, Hoffner SE, et al: Tenosynovitis of the hand caused by *Mycobacterium terrae.* Eur J Clin Microbiol Infect Dis 8:722, 1989.
87. Jones MW, Wahid IA, Matthews JP: Septic arthritis of the hand due to *Mycobacterium marinum.* J Hand Surg 13:333, 1988.
88. Lai KK, Stottmeier KD, Sherman IH, McCabe WR: Mycobacterial cervical lymphadenopathy. JAMA 251:1286, 1984.
89. Schaad UB, Votteler TP, McCracken GH, Nelson JD: Management of atypical mycobacterial lymphadenitis in childhood: A review based on 380 cases. J Pediatr 95:356, 1979.
90. Wolinsky E: Mycobacterial lymphadenitis in children: A prospective study of 105 nontuberculous cases with long-term follow-up. Clin Infect Dis 20:954, 1995.
91. Trébucq A: Should ethambutol be recommended for routine treatment of tuberculosis in children? A review of the literature. Int J Tuberc Lung Dis 1:12, 1997.
92. Horsburgh CR Jr, Mason UG, Farhi DC, Iseman MD: Disseminated infection with *Mycobacterium avium intracellulare.* Medicine (Baltimore) 64:36, 1985.
93. Horsburgh C Jr, Hanson D, Jones J, Thompson S: Protection from *Mycobacterium avium* complex disease in human immunodeficiency virus–infected persons with a history of tuberculosis. Clin Infect Dis 174:1212, 1996.
94. Ostroff S, Ra S, Feinberg J, et al: Preventing disseminated *Mycobacterium avium* complex disease in patients infected with human immunodeficiency virus. Clin Infect Dis 21(Suppl 1):572, 1995.
95. Nightingale S, Byrd L, Southern P, et al: Incidence of *Mycobacterium avium-intracellulare* complex bacteremia in human immunodeficiency virus–positive patients. J Infect Dis 165:1082, 1992.
96. von Reyn CF, Maslow JN, Barber TW, et al: Persistent colonisation of potable water as a source of *Mycobacterium avium* infection in AIDS. Lancet 343:1137, 1994.
97. Chin D, Hopewell P, Yajko D, et al: *Mycobacterium avium* complex in the respiratory or gastrointestinal tract and the risk of

M. avium complex bacteremia in patients with human immunodeficiency virus infection. J Infect Dis 169:289, 1994.
98. Kalayjian R, Toossi Z, Tomachefski J, et al: Pulmonary disease due to infection by *Mycobacterium avium* complex in patients with AIDS. Clin Infect Dis 20:1186, 1995.
99. Kemper C, Havlir D, Haghighat D, et al: The individual microbiologic effect of three antimycobacterial agents, clofazimine, ethambutol, and rifampin on *Mycobacterium avium* complex bacteremia in patients with AIDS. J Infect Dis 170:157, 1994.
100. Dautzenberg B, Truffot C, Legis S, et al: Activity of clarithromycin against *Mycobacterium avium* infection in patients with the acquired immunodeficiency syndrome. Am Rev Respir Dis 144:564, 1991.
101. Young LS, Wiviott L, Wu M, et al: Azithromycin for treatment of *Mycobacterium avium-intracellulare* complex infection in patients with AIDS. Lancet 338:1107, 1991.
102. Chaisson R, Benson C, Duke M, et al: Clarithromycin therapy for bacteremic *Mycobacterium avium* complex disease. A randomized, double-blind, dose-ranging study in patients with AIDS. Ann Intern Med 121:905, 1994.
103. Havlir D, Torriani F, Dube M: Uveitis associated with rifabutin prophylaxis. Ann Intern Med 121:510, 1994.
104. Masur H: Public Health Service Task Force on prophylaxis and therapy for *Mycobacterium avium* complex. Recommendations on prophylaxis and therapy for disseminated *Mycobacterium avium* complex disease in patients infected with the human immunodeficiency virus. N Engl J Med 329:898, 1993.
105. Pierce M, Crampton S, Henry D, et al: A randomized trial of clarithromycin as prophylaxis against disseminated *Mycobacterium avium* complex infection in patients with advanced acquired immunodeficiency syndrome. N Engl J Med 335:384, 1996.
106. Nightingale S, Cameron D, Gordin F, et al: Two controlled trials of rifabutin prophylaxis against *Mycobacterium avium* complex infection in AIDS. N Engl J Med 329:828, 1993.
107. Horsburgh CR Jr, Selik RM: The epidemiology of disseminated nontuberculous mycobacterial infection in the acquired immunodeficiency syndrome (AIDS). Am Rev Respir Dis 139:4, 1989.
108. Witzig R, Fazal B, Mera R, et al: Clinical manifestations and implications of coinfection with *Mycobacterium kansasii* and human immunodeficiency virus type 1. Clin Infect Dis 21:77, 1995.
109. Jiva T, Jacoby H, Weymouth L, et al: *Mycobacterium xenoi:* Innocent bystander or emerging pathogen? Clin Infect Dis 24:226, 1997.
110. Straus W, Ostroff S, Jernigan D, et al: Clinical and epidemiologic characteristics of *Mycobacterium haemophilum,* an emerging pathogen in immunocompromised patients. Ann Intern Med 120:118, 1994.
111. Dever L, Martin J, Seaworth B, Jorgensen J: Varied presentations and responses to treatment of infections caused by *Mycobacterium haemophilum* in patients with AIDS. Clin Infect Dis 14: 1195, 1992.
112. Pechere M, Opravil M, Wald A, et al: Clinical and epidemiological features of infection with *Mycobacterium genavense.* Arch Intern Med 155:400, 1995.
113. Bottger E, Teske A, Kirschner P, et al: Disseminated *M. genavense* infection in patients with AIDS. Lancet 340:76, 1992.
114. Weinberger M, Berg S, Feurstein I, et al: *Mycobacterium gordonae:* Report of a case and critical review of the literature. Clin Infect Dis 14:1229, 1992.
115. Zurawski C, Cage G, Rimland D, Blumberg H: Pneumonia and bacteremia due to *Mycobacterium celatum* masquerading as *Mycobacterium xenopi* in patients with AIDS: An underdiagnosed problem? Clin Infect Dis 24:140, 1997.
116. Dutt AK, Stead WW: Long-term results of medical treatment in *Mycobacterium intracellulare* infection. Am J Med 67:449, 1979.
117. Hunter AM, Campbell IA, Jenkins PA, Smith AP: Treatment of pulmonary infections caused by mycobacteria of the *Mycobacterium avium-intracellulare* complex. Thorax 36:326, 1981.
118. Heifets LB: Qualitative and quantitative drug susceptibility tests in mycobacteriology. Am Rev Respir Dis 37:1217, 1988.
119. Heifets LB, Lindholm-Levy PJ, Flory MA: Bactericidal activity in vitro of various rifamycins agains *M. avium* and *M. tuberculosis.* Am Rev Respir Dis 141:626, 1990.
120. Lee CN, Heifets LB: Determination of minimal inhibitory concentrations of antituberculosis drugs. Am Rev Respir Dis 136: 349, 1987.
121. Heifets L, Lindholm-Levy P: Comparison of bactericidal activities of streptomycin, amikacin, kanamycin, and capreomycin against *M. avium* and *M. tuberculosis.* Antimicrob Agents Chemother 33:1298, 1989.
122. Heifets LB, Lindholm-Levy PJ: Bacteriostatic and bactericidal activities of ciprofloxacin and ofloxacin against *Mycobacterium tuberculosis* and *Mycobacterium avium* complex. Tubercle 68:267, 1987.
123. Heifets LB: Antituberculosis drugs: Antimicrobial activity in vitro. *In* Heifets LB (ed): Drug Susceptibility in the Chemotherapy of Mycobacterial Infections. Boca Raton, FL, CRC Press, 1991, pp 89–122.
124. Heifets LB: Dilemmas and realities in drug susceptibility testing of *M. avium–M. intracellulare* and other slowly growing nontuberculous mycobacteria. *In* Heifets LB (ed): Drug Susceptibility in the Chemotherapy of Mycobacterial Infections. Boca Raton, FL, CRC Press, 1991, pp 123–146.
125. Heifets L, Mor N, Vanderkolk J: *Mycobacterium avium* strains resistant to clarithromycin and azithromycin. Antimicrob Agents Chemother 37:2364, 1993.

168

Leprosy

Diana N. J. Lockwood
Keith P. W. J. McAdam

Leprosy is a chronic granulomatous disease caused by *Mycobacterium leprae.* The principal manifestations of disease are anesthetic skin lesions and peripheral neuropathy with peripheral nerve thickening. The clinical form of the disease in any individual depends on the degree of cell-mediated immunity expressed by that individual toward *M. leprae.* High levels of cell-mediated immunity with elimination of leprosy bacilli produce the tuberculoid form of disease, whereas absent cell-mediated immunity results in lepromatous leprosy. The medical complications of leprosy are due to nerve damage, immunologic reactions, and bacillary infiltration. Nerve damage accompanying leprosy is a particularly serious complication because this remains with the patient for the rest of life and causes considerable morbidity. Currently available drug treatments are highly effective in clearing viable bacilli but do not prevent nerve damage. Leprosy has a long history as a deforming disease, and leprosy patients the world over are frequently stigmatized and ostracized. Words such as "leper" should be avoided, and naming the disease Hansen disease may reduce stigmatization.

Epidemiology

The introduction of the World Health Organization (WHO) multidrug regimen for treatment of leprosy has had a major impact on the global picture of leprosy, with the estimated number of patients worldwide falling from 10 to 12 million in 1988 to 2.7 million in 1994.[1] The burden of leprosy patients is unevenly distributed through the tropics and subtropics; 72% of patients live in Asia and Oceania, 18% in Africa, and 7% in the Americas[2]; 80% of all leprosy patients reside in just six countries (Bangladesh, Brazil, India, Indonesia, Myanmar, and Nigeria).[3] Leprosy has not always been a tropical disease;

it was widespread in medieval Europe and was endemic in Norway until the early 20th century. In North America, small foci of infection are still found in Texas and Louisiana. Virtually all new cases of infection now seen in North America and Europe have been acquired abroad.

Leprosy is a chronic disease with a long incubation period, relatively chronic progress, and slow spread through human communities. The rarity of leprosy in children younger than 5 years reflects the long incubation time. U.S. military personnel who developed leprosy after serving in the tropics presented up to 20 years after their presumed exposure.[4] An average incubation time has been calculated of 2 to 5 years for tuberculoid cases and 8 to 12 years for lepromatous cases.

Although leprosy is rarely a primary cause of death, patients have a standardized death rate at least twice that of the general population as a result of the indirect secondary effects of the disease.[5] It is estimated that 1 million disability-adjusted life-years are lost globally each year because of leprosy; 6.3 years of healthy life are lost per patient.[3]

Age, sex, household contact, and bacille Calmette-Guérin vaccination are important determinants of leprosy risk; leprosy incidence reaches a peak at the ages of 10 to 14 years, then dips only to rise again for 30- to 60-year-old persons.[6] An excess of male cases has been demonstrated in many studies, although it remains unclear whether this is a true finding or a cultural artifact due to the reluctance of women to present with skin lesions.[7] Clustering of cases is well recognized, particularly in low endemic areas such as Louisiana, and may be due to either locally increased exposure to *M. leprae* or shared genetic predisposition to leprosy.[8] Although poor nutritional status was thought to predispose to leprosy, no good evidence substantiates this.[6] There is consistent evidence that improved socioeconomic conditions contribute to a reduction of leprosy in the community, regardless of leprosy control operations involved,[2] and a study from Malawi showed that extended schooling and good housing conditions are associated with reduced risk for leprosy.[9] It was feared that human immunodeficiency virus infection might be a risk factor for leprosy, with human immunodeficiency virus–induced immune paresis causing increased numbers of lepromatous cases. Although studies from Malawi,[10] Uganda,[11] and South India[12] have not shown human immunodeficiency virus infection to be a risk factor for the development of leprosy, human immunodeficiency virus infection may be a risk factor for the development of neuritis.

There is no reliable test for determining whether a person has encountered *M. leprae* without developing disease. Several pieces of evidence suggest that infection occurs more readily than was previously thought. In contacts of leprosy patients, there is frequently evidence of specific sensitization to *M. leprae* with use of markers of infection such as serum antibody levels,[12] in vitro lymphocyte transformation test results,[13] and skin test responses to soluble *M. leprae* antigen. An immunologic study of contacts of an untreated elderly man with borderline lepromatous leprosy in a British residential home showed that 23 of 30 and 25 of 30 contacts had positive Mitsuda skin test and positive lymphocyte transformation test responses to *M. leprae* sonicate, respectively, but only two contacts had positive antibody (immunoglobulin M phenolic glycolipid [PGL]) responses.[14] It has also been shown that self-healing often occurs in early monomacular tuberculoid cases.[15] By use of polymerase chain reaction detection methods, *M. leprae* products have been found in nasal swabs from 19% of occupational contacts of leprosy patients.[16] Leprosy is probably analogous to tuberculosis, in which only 10% of infections manifest as clinical disease.[17]

Transmission

Leprosy is an almost exclusively human disease; human cases are the only important source and reservoir of infection. Leprosy occurs naturally in nine-banded armadillos in the southern United States, and transmission to armadillo handlers has been reported rarely.[18, 19] An untreated lepromatous leprosy patient may discharge up to 6.8×10^{10} acid-fast bacilli (AFB) in a single nose blow.[17] The importance of the nasal discharge in excreting AFB into the environment was recognized in 1898 by Schäffer,[20] who demonstrated that leprosy patients shed large numbers of AFB while coughing, sneezing, and even speaking normally. Despite this evidence, the importance of the nose in the transmission of leprosy was overlooked for much of this century, interest focusing instead on possible excretion of bacilli from the skin, despite bacilli rarely being found in or on the epidermis. In 1960, Shepard[21] showed that AFB in nasal washings from lepromatous patients were viable in mouse footpad inoculation and that the growth pattern resembled that of *M. leprae*.[21] Lepromatous granulomata and abundant macrophages containing AFB have been demonstrated in the larynx.[22]

Infection probably also occurs through the nose. The cool, moist environment of the turbinates favors growth of *M. leprae*. The turbinates are encountered early by inhaled organisms and are consistently involved in early lepromatous disease.[23] Experimental transmission through the nasal mucosa in nude mice is particularly successful if the mucosa is lightly abraded.[24] The nasal mucosa is probably diseased or damaged more often than is generally appreciated; up to 15% of the population are affected by the common cold at any one time, and perhaps even picking of the nose can enable *M. leprae* to breach the nasal mucosa.

Although entry of bacilli through the skin was traditionally considered important, the only evidence to support this view consists of occasional case reports of direct inoculation. Leprosy has been transmitted to nude mice through pricks from infected cactus thorns,[25] and this raises the possibility that transmission may be reduced by increased wearing of shoes. Biting arthropods could theoretically transmit leprosy, but there is no evidence to support this route of transmission. Attempted experimental transmission through the lungs and gastrointestinal tract in experimental animals has not been successful. It is surprising that in contrast to tuberculosis, there are few documented cases of leprosy occurring in both medical and nonmedical attendants of leprosy patients.

Pathology

The pathologic process of infection with *M. leprae* is profoundly influenced by three unusual factors. First, *M. leprae* is not toxic to its host cells, and the pathologic process reflects the immune response of the patient to the organism. Second, the bacillus is able to establish itself in protected sites, notably peripheral nerves. Third, it has a long generation time, and this together with the immune response determines the distribution and chronicity of the disease.

Peripheral nerves and skin are the organs principally affected by leprosy. The most common sites of early infection with *M. leprae* are Schwann cells, subepidermal cells, and superficial perivascular skin macrophages. A mild lymphocytic infiltrate frequently accompanies these early lesions, which may resolve spontaneously when bacilli die. If bacilli persist and multiply, an inflammatory reaction occurs with granuloma formation, and leprosy develops. Once an infection is established, the host immune response determines not only the histologic picture but also the clinical features of disease and the prognosis. The concept of a spectrum of responses to *M. leprae* was developed by Ridley and Jopling[26] in 1966. The two poles of the spectrum are tuberculoid (paucibacillary) and lepromatous (multibacillary) leprosy. At the tuberculoid pole, well-expressed cell-mediated immunity and

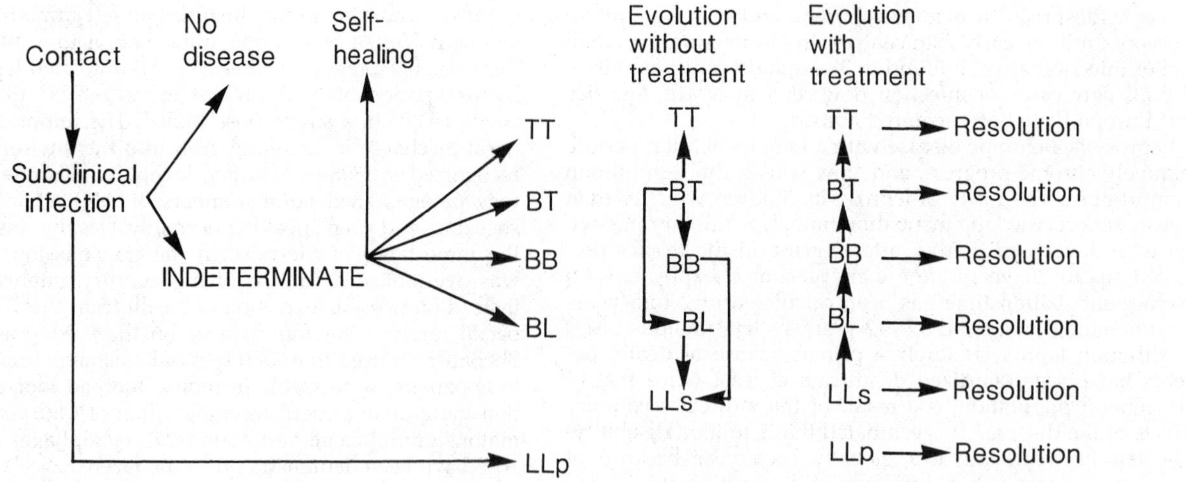

FIGURE 168–1 □ The evolution of leprosy infection in untreated patients and after treatment. TT, Tuberculoid leprosy; BT, borderline tuberculoid leprosy; BB, borderline leprosy; BL, borderline lepromatous leprosy; LLp, lepromatous leprosy (polar); LLs, lepromatous leprosy (subpolar). (From Ridley DS [ed]: Pathogenesis of Leprosy and Related Diseases. London, Wright, 1988, p 100.)

delayed hypersensitivity effectively control bacillary multiplication with the formation of organized epithelioid cell granulomata; by contrast, in the lepromatous form, there is cellular anergy toward *M. leprae* with resultant abundant bacillary multiplication and unactivated macrophages. Between these two poles is a continuum, varying from the patient with moderate cell-mediated immunity (borderline tuberculoid leprosy), through true borderline leprosy, to the patient with little T-lymphocyte response (borderline lepromatous leprosy). Figure 168–1 shows the possible routes in the evolution of infection in an untreated person. The polar groups (tuberculoid, lepromatous) are stable, but within the central groups (borderline tuberculoid, borderline, borderline lepromatous), downgrading toward the lepromatous pole will occur without treatment, and upgrading (reversal reactions) toward the tuberculoid pole may occur during or after treatment. Table 168–1 lists the histologic and immunologic features seen in biopsy specimens across the spectrum. Figures 168–2 to 168–5 show typical skin biopsy specimens from patients at various points on the spectrum.

The systemic nature of infection with *M. leprae* with hematogenous spread of bacilli is not always well appreciated. In patients who have tuberculoid leprosy, granulomata may also be found in lymph nodes and liver.[22, 27] In those who have lepromatous disease, bacilli-laden macrophages are found in lymph nodes, liver, spleen, bone marrow, muscle, testes, kidneys, adrenals, and eyes.[28]

Neuropathology

Neural involvement in leprosy is not a single entity; different types of nerve fibers are involved, the pathologic change seen varies with the chronicity of disease, and the histopathologic features are different at the tuberculoid and lepromatous ends of the spectrum. Nerve damage occurs in two settings, skin lesions and peripheral nerve trunks. In skin lesions, the small dermal sensory and autonomic nerve fibers supplying dermal and subcutaneous structures are damaged, causing local sensory loss and loss of sweating within the area of the skin lesion.[29] Peripheral nerve trunks are vulnerable at sites where they are superficially placed or are in fibroosseous tunnels. At these points, a small increase in nerve diameter leads to raised intraneural pressure with consequent neural compression and ischemia. Damage to peripheral nerve trunks produces characteristic lesions with regional sensory loss and dysfunction of muscles supplied by that peripheral nerve. Physiologic evidence of central and peripheral autonomic nerve involvement has also been reported.[30, 31]

Studies of patients with early leprosy of both tubercu-

TABLE 168–1 ■ Major Histologic and Immunologic Features of the Disease Spectrum in Leprosy*

CHARACTERISTICS	TT	BT	BB	BL	LL
Histologic and Microbial					
Epithelioid cells, mature	++	±	–	–	–
Epithelioid cells, immature	+	++	++	±/–	–
Langhans giant cells, large	++	±/–	–	–	–
Macrophages	–	–	±	++	++
Lymphocytes	+/±	++/±	±	++	±
Bacterial index	0	0–2	3–4	4–5	5–6+
Bacilli in nasal smears	–	–	–	±	++
Immunologic					
Lepromin, Fernandez reaction	++/–	++/–	+/–	–	–
Lepromin, Mitsuda reaction	++/±	++/+	–	–	–
LTT, percent lymphocyte transformation	10	5.7	2.0	0.4	0.2
Antibody, anti–*M. leprae*	–/+	–/++	++	+++	+++

*TT, Tuberculoid leprosy; BT, borderline tuberculoid leprosy; BB, borderline leprosy; BL, borderline lepromatous leprosy; LL, lepromatous leprosy; LTT, lymphocyte transformation test; +++, strongly positive; +, positive; ±, indeterminate; –, negative.

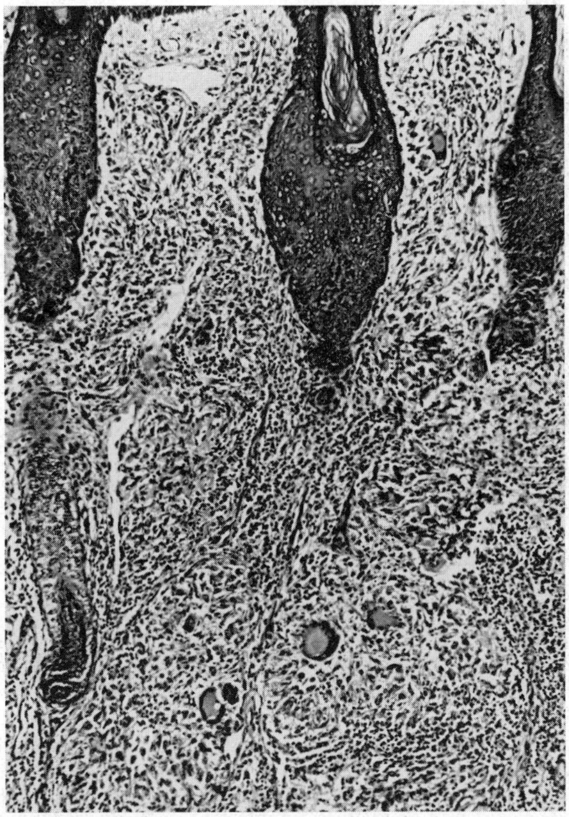

FIGURE 168–2 □ Skin biopsy specimen, tuberculoid leprosy. There is a heavy dermal infiltrate with numerous granulomata in the deep dermis. No bacilli are visible. (Hematoxylin and eosin [H&E], × 100.) (Courtesy of Professor Sebastian Lucas, Department of Pathology, United Medical and Dental School, London.)

loid[32, 33] and lepromatous types show abnormalities in nerve conduction and a histologic picture of small fiber loss with segmental demyelination and remyelination.[34] In established tuberculoid disease, there is gross destruction with a heavy lymphocytic infiltrate producing a fibrosed epineurium and replacement of the endoneurium with epithelioid granulomata.[35] In lepromatous neuropathy, there is quiet asymptomatic bacillation of Schwann cells leading to foamy degeneration of these cells. Demyelination, damage, and destruction of the axis cylinder are prominent features, and later wallerian degeneration occurs.[36] Despite the large numbers of organisms in the nerve, there is only a small inflammatory response; ultimately, the nerve fibroses and is hyalinized.[37] Both these mechanisms of nerve destruction are present in patients with borderline disease. The formation of small granulomata is characteristic of borderline leprosy, and granulomatous regions may abut strands of normal-looking but heavily bacillated Schwann cells.[38] Nerve damage in borderline leprosy results from a combination of lepromatous bacillation and a tuberculoid tissue-damaging response producing widespread and crippling nerve damage. Acute neuritis damage occurs particularly during reversal reactions; edema of the epithelioid cell granuloma compresses the remaining Schwann cells, causing rapid functional loss in an already compromised nerve. The damage may be compounded by new granuloma formation. In erythema nodosum leprosum (ENL), nerve damage occurs more slowly and is probably due to inflammation associated with ENL nodule formation in nerve trunks.

Immunology

The host immune response to *M. leprae* is preeminent in determining not only whether disease will develop but also which type of leprosy will result. Both T cells and macrophages play important roles in the processing, recognition, and response to *M. leprae* antigens.

Lepromin skin testing assesses in vivo responses to a heat-killed suspension of *M. leprae*. This test can be read at 48 to 72 hours (Fernandez reaction) and again at 21 to 28 days (Mitsuda reaction). Both tests reflect the patient's cellular response to *M. leprae*; the Fernandez response is a delayed hypersensitivity reaction to the soluble components of lepromin, and the Mitsuda reaction is a granulomatous response to particulate antigenic material. Results of both tests are positive in tuberculoid patients and negative in lepromatous patients. Neither test is diagnostic because results of both may be positive in people with no evidence of leprosy. However, the close contacts of a multibacillary patient who

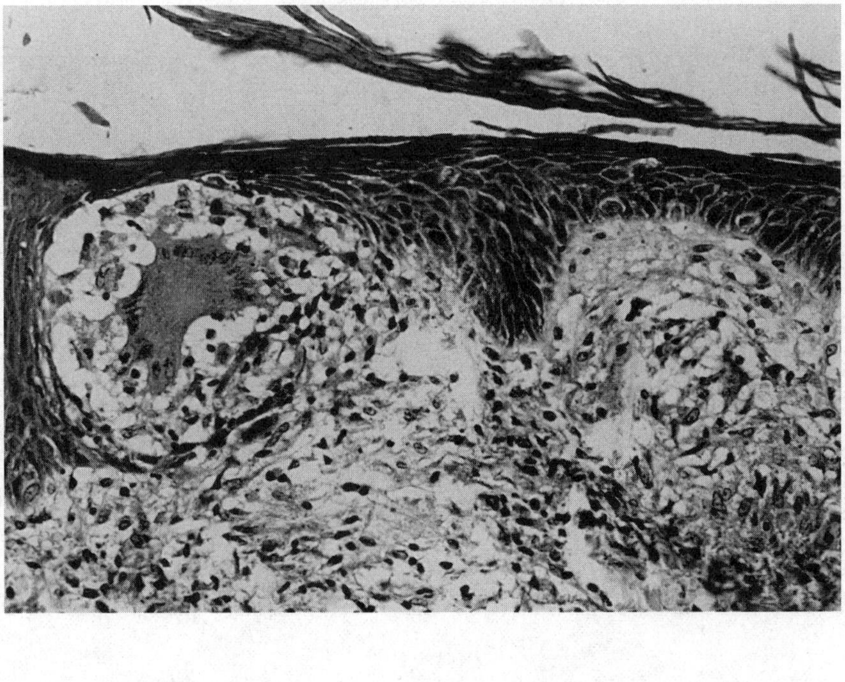

FIGURE 168–3 □ Skin biopsy specimen, borderline tuberculoid leprosy in reversal reaction. New active, edematous granulomata are visible and are eroding the epidermal and subepidermal zones. (H&E, × 400.) (Courtesy of Professor Sebastian Lucas, Department of Pathology, United Medical and Dental School, London.)

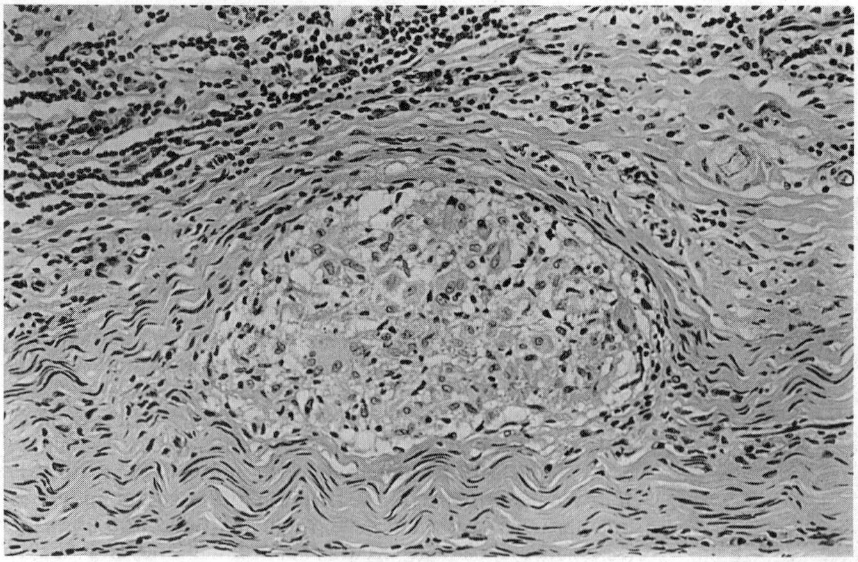

FIGURE 168–4 □ Nerve biopsy specimen, borderline tuberculoid leprosy. This large granuloma in a peripheral nerve is distorting the normal neural architecture; a perineurial lymphocytic infiltrate is also present. (H&E, × 600.) (Courtesy of Professor Sebastian Lucas, Department of Pathology, United Medical and Dental School, London.)

have negative lepromin test results are at high risk for development of disease.

Why one individual develops tuberculoid leprosy and another lepromatous disease is at best only partially understood. Human leukocyte antigen (HLA)–linked genes do not confer susceptibility to leprosy but do at least partially control the type of disease that develops. HLA-DR2 and HLA-DR3 occur at a relatively high frequency in tuberculoid leprosy patients with a corresponding deficit in lepromatous and borderline lepromatous patients in at least two populations,[39] whereas HLA-DQ1 is associated with susceptibility to borderline lepromatous and lepromatous leprosy in three different countries.[40]

The T-cell response to mycobacteria is initiated with the presentation of processed *M. leprae* antigens in association with HLA class II molecules on the macrophage cell surface to the cellular immune system. The HLA–*M. leprae* antigen complex is then recognized by $CD4^+$ lymphocytes bearing the $\alpha\beta$ T-cell receptor. Binding of the antigen-specific T-cell receptor to the *M. leprae* peptide–HLA class II complex leads to activation and proliferation of $\alpha\beta$ T cells with release of interleukin-2 (IL-2). This cytokine amplifies the local response producing recruitment and activation of T cells. In addition, IL-2 stimulates the expansion of $\alpha\beta$ $CD8^+$ T cells and antigen-nonspecific natural killer cells in the lesion. All three types of cell can produce interferon-γ, the major cytokine responsible for activating bactericidal mechanisms within the parasitized macrophage.[41]

This model of the interaction of *M. leprae* and T cells has as its end point establishment of protective immunity to *M. leprae* with the elimination of *M. leprae* and the establishment of immunologic memory at a T-cell level. In those who develop clinical leprosy, this series of immunologic events is in some way impaired. In tuberculoid leprosy, there is good evidence of a strong cell-mediated immune response. Tests of T-cell function such as lymphocyte proliferation assays show that tuberculoid leprosy patients recognize and respond to *M. leprae* antigens, both whole *M. leprae* and separated *M. leprae* antigens[42] and cloned antigens such as the 18-kDa[43] and the 65-kDa antigens.[44] Skin test results with lepromin, a soluble *M. leprae* sonicate preparation, are strongly positive in these patients. Staining of skin biopsy specimens from tuberculoid lesions with T-cell markers shows highly organized granulomata composed predomi-

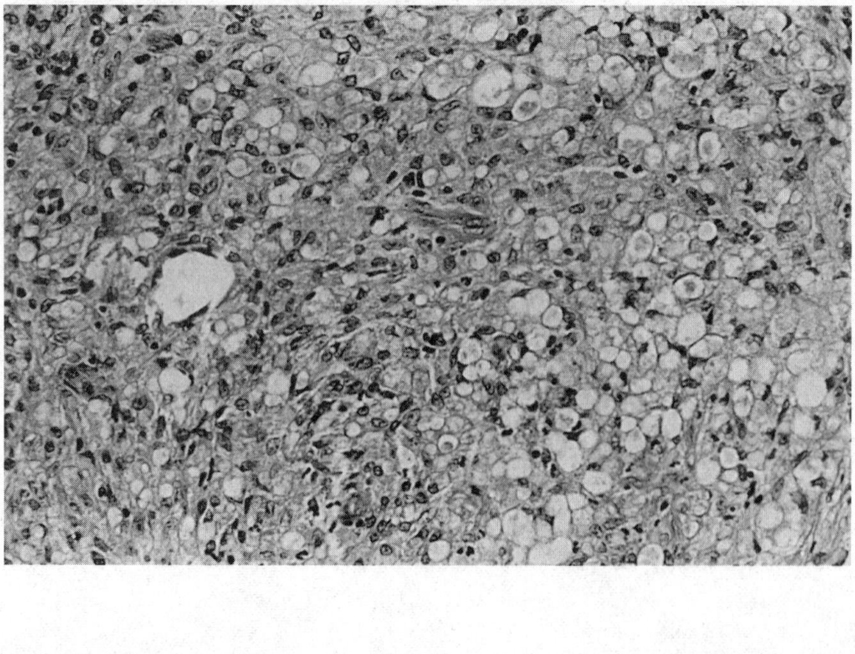

FIGURE 168–5 □ Skin biopsy specimen, lepromatous leprosy. Numerous rounded foamy macrophages with few lymphocytes and no granulomata. (H&E, × 400.) (Courtesy of Professor Sebastian Lucas, Department of Pathology, United Medical and Dental School, London.)

nantly of CD4+ cells and macrophages with a peripheral mantle of suppressor-cytotoxic CD8+ cells.[45] However, this strong cell-mediated immune response has clearly been misdirected at some stage; perhaps the lesion in tuberculoid leprosy is a failure of T cells to respond at a critical moment, or alternatively the failure might be to respond to one or several particular antigens. Whatever the cause for the failure, the end result is that the late strong cell-mediated response, while clearing antigen, does so at the expense of local tissue destruction.

Lepromatous leprosy patients are unable to mount a cell-mediated immune response to *M. leprae* with a failure of the T-cell response, and lymphocytes from lepromatous leprosy patients respond poorly if at all in lymphocyte proliferation assays to whole *M. leprae* and cloned antigens. Similarly, lepromatous leprosy patients are unable to mount a skin test response to intradermal challenge with lepromin. This anergy of the lepromatous patient is striking because it is specific for the leprosy mycobacterium; lepromatous leprosy patients can respond to other mycobacterial antigens such as *Mycobacterium tuberculosis*, in both in vitro lymphocyte studies and skin tests using other mycobacterial antigens.[46] Identification of cell types in lepromatous leprosy granulomata shows them to be disorganized with a random admixture of macrophages and T cells, of which CD8+ cells predominate.[47]

Dysfunction of both T cells and macrophages occurs in lepromatous patients. Britton[41] has reviewed the possible mechanisms underlying the T-cell unresponsiveness in lepromatous leprosy and considered three possible mechanisms: functional inactivation or clonal anergy of reactive T cells; active suppression of reactive T cells, perhaps by lipoarabinomannan or PGL-1; and failure of development (clonal deletion) of *M. leprae*–reactive T cells. Because lepromatous patients may convert from being lepromin skin test–negative to lepromin-positive after prolonged antileprosy drug therapy,[48] it seems likely that either clonal anergy or active suppression is the prime T-cell defect in lepromatous leprosy. Possible mechanisms for the induction of immunologic anergy include oral presentation of mycobacterial antigens, presentation of mycobacterial antigens by nonprofessional cells that lack the second signal required to activate T cells, and blocking of the second signal by molecules that stick to these activation proteins (intercellular adhesion molecules).

Defects in cytokine production have been demonstrated in lepromatous patients; addition of IL-2 to T-cell culture media restored the proliferative response to *M. leprae*,[49] and giving lepromatous patients intralesional injections of recombinant IL-2 led to a reconstitution of the local immune response with elimination of *M. leprae* from macrophages.[50]

Several macrophage defects have been described in lepromatous disease, including defective antigen presentation and recognition, defective IL-1 production, failure of macrophages to kill *M. leprae*, and macrophage suppression of the T-cell response.[51] It seems likely that several immunologic defects may lead to lepromatous disease rather than one defect accounting for this clinical entity.

Studies of circulating cytokines in leprosy patients and cytokine production in skin lesions show that tuberculoid patients have a Th1-type response to *M. leprae* with predominant IL-2 and interferon-γ production; lepromatous patients have a response characterized by Th2-type cytokines.

Serology

Antibody responses are intact and correlate with the number of bacilli present; thus, the highest antibody levels are found in lepromatous patients and the lowest in tuberculoid patients.[52] All leprosy patients mount appropriate antibody responses to bacterial vaccines such as typhoid. Lepromatous patients produce a range of predominantly immunoglobulin M autoantibodies, both organ specific (directed against thyroid, nerve, testis, and gastric mucosa) and nonspecific, such as rheumatoid factors, anti-DNA, cryoglobulins, and cardiolipin. None of these antibodies plays a role in the elimination of *M. leprae*, quite the converse because they are implicated in pathologic processes such as ENL and amyloidosis, which occur only in lepromatous patients.

Specific anti–*M. leprae* antibodies are produced against lipoarabinomannan, PGL, and the protein antigens of *M. leprae*. During the 1980s, many studies were done measuring the serologic responses to separate *M. leprae* antigens. The initial hope had been that there would be one or more antigens that on infection with *M. leprae* would induce a specific antibody response. Identifying such an antibody response would have enabled development of specific serologic tests that could be used to confirm disease and detect early subclinical infection. Unfortunately, none of the serologic tests has proved adequate to meet these needs. For all three types of antigen, lepromatous patients produce antibodies most prolifically; tuberculoid patients have a variable and often undetectable response. The findings from the evaluation of PGL serology in extensive field studies are typical; in most studies, more than 90% of untreated lepromatous patients have positive serologic responses, but 40% to 50% of tuberculoid patients do not have elevated antibody levels, and the proportion of healthy individuals with PGL antibodies is about 5% to 10%.[53] The problems are illustrated well by data from a prospective study of contacts of patients in Venezuela. In a cohort of 9545 contacts, 20 cases of leprosy occurred; of these 20 cases, 15 did not have elevated antibody levels, and only 2 cases of multibacillary disease developed in the 10 contacts with the highest levels of PGL antibodies.[54]

Reactions

Patients in the nonpolar borderline groups are immunologically unstable and are at risk for developing immune-mediated reactions. Reversal reactions or type 1 reactions occur when patients move toward the tuberculoid pole and are an expression of increased delayed hypersensitivity toward *M. leprae* antigens in skin and nerve sites. This is mediated through T-cell activity, with enhanced T-cell proliferation toward *M. leprae* antigens, increased numbers of CD4+ and IL-2–producing cells in granulomata, and local production of cytokines such as interferon-γ and tumor necrosis factor-α. Reversal reactions are probably associated with a switch from production of Th2-type to Th1-type cytokines. Although the end result is an elimination of mycobacteria, this is achieved only at the expense of severe local tissue damage, particularly in nerves.

ENL reactions occur in borderline leprosy and lepromatous leprosy patients who have depressed cellular immunity and a large antigen load. ENL has classically been regarded as an immune complex disorder. This is supported by the presence of immunoglobulin and complement in the lesions and circulating immune complexes.[55] There is now accumulating evidence of enhanced T-cell activity during ENL episodes, although the role of the T cell in the immunopathologic process of ENL remains unclear.[56, 57] Despite the evidence of increased immune activity during ENL episodes, lepromatous patients revert to a state of immunologic unresponsiveness after an episode.

Clinical Features

The cardinal signs of leprosy are hypopigmented, anesthetic skin lesions and thickened peripheral nerves.

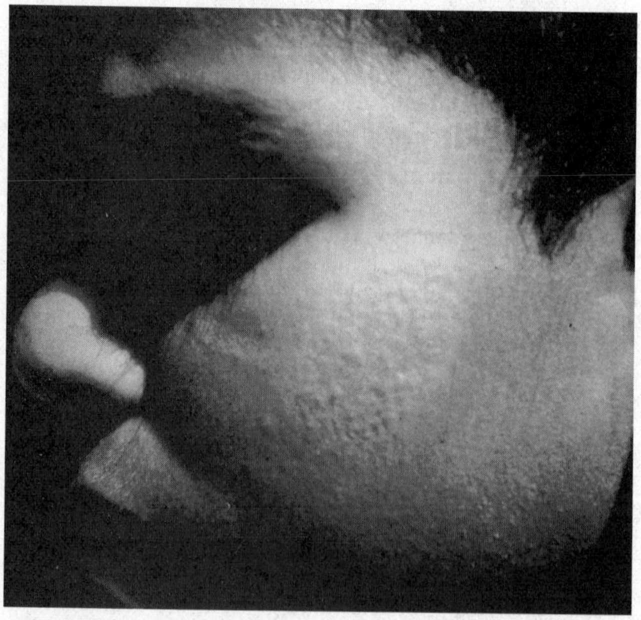

FIGURE 168–6 □ Tuberculoid skin lesion. This young boy has a single, well-defined anesthetic hypopigmented patch on his cheek.

Skin Lesions

The most common skin lesions are macules or plaques; more rarely, papules and nodules are seen. In lepromatous leprosy, a diffuse infiltration of the skin often occurs. Lesions may be found anywhere, although rarely in the axillae, perineum, or hairy scalp. The number of lesions indicates the ability of the cell-mediated immunity to limit the spread of bacilli. Tuberculoid patients have few, hypopigmented lesions; lepromatous patients have numerous, sometimes confluent lesions. The few tuberculoid lesions are usually asymmetric; more numerous lesions are likely to be distributed symmetrically.

Anesthesia

Anesthesia may occur in skin lesions when dermal nerves are involved or in the distribution of a large peripheral nerve.

Peripheral Nerve Involvement

The sites of predilection for peripheral nerve involvement are ulnar (at the elbow), median (at the wrist), radial, radial cutaneous (at the wrist), common peroneal (at the knee), posterior tibial and sural (at the ankle), facial (over the zygomatic arch), supraorbital (on the eyebrow ridge), and great auricular (in the posterior triangle of the neck). All these nerves should be examined for enlargement and tenderness.

Classification of Disease

Classifying patients according to the Ridley-Jopling scale is clinically useful. Lepromatous patients require longer treatment with more drugs than do tuberculoid patients. Tuberculoid leprosy is associated with rapid, severe nerve damage. Lepromatous disease is associated with chronicity and long-term complications. Borderline disease is unstable and may be complicated by reactions.

Tuberculoid Leprosy

Infection is localized and asymmetric. The skin lesions are few and hypopigmented, and they have sharp borders (Fig. 168–6). Anesthesia is usually present in the lesion and is often accompanied by loss of sebaceous gland secretion and sweat, indicating local autonomic nerve damage. The cutaneous nerve on the proximal side of the lesion is frequently thickened; if peripheral nerve trunk involvement is present, usually only one nerve trunk is enlarged. No *M. leprae* organisms are found in the skin, and the lepromin test result is strongly positive. True tuberculoid leprosy has a good prognosis; many infections resolve without treatment, and peripheral nerve trunk damage is limited.[58]

Borderline Tuberculoid Leprosy

The skin lesions are similar to tuberculoid leprosy but are larger and more numerous. The margins are less well defined, and there may be satellite lesions (Fig. 168–7). Damage to peripheral nerves is widespread and severe, usually with several thickened nerve trunks (see Fig. 168–12). It is important to recognize borderline tuberculoid leprosy because these patients are prone to reversal reactions leading to rapid deterioration in nerve function with consequent disability.

Borderline Leprosy

Borderline disease is the most unstable part of the spectrum, and patients usually downgrade toward lepromatous leprosy if they are not treated or upgrade toward tuberculoid leprosy as part of a reversal reaction. There are numerous skin lesions, which may be macules, papules, or plaques, and they vary in size, shape, and distribution. The edges of the lesions may have streaming, irregular borders. Anular lesions with a broad, irregular edge and a sharply defined punched out center are characteristic of borderline disease (Fig. 168–8). Nerve damage is variable with either asymmetric nerve enlargement in a downgrading patient or symmetric neuritis in patient upgrading from the lepromatous end of the spectrum.

Borderline Lepromatous Leprosy

Borderline lepromatous leprosy is characterized by widespread, small but variable macules all over the body; with

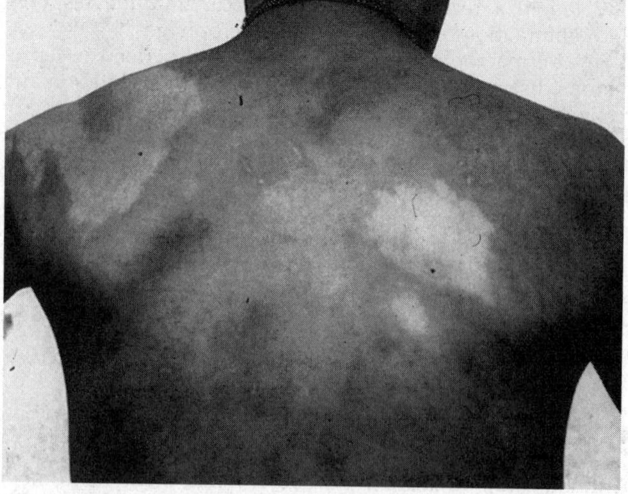

FIGURE 168–7 □ Borderline tuberculoid skin lesion. This patient has several large, hypopigmented anesthetic skin lesions; satellite lesions are also visible.

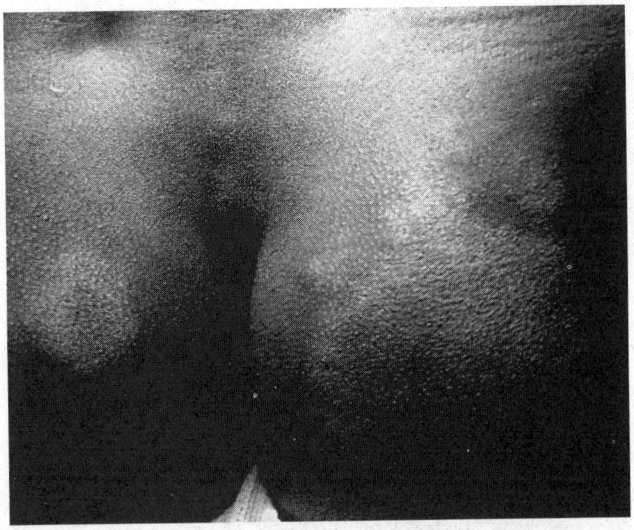

FIGURE 168–8 ▫ Borderline leprosy lesion. Numerous skin lesions of all sizes are seen, some with healing centers on this patient's back and buttocks.

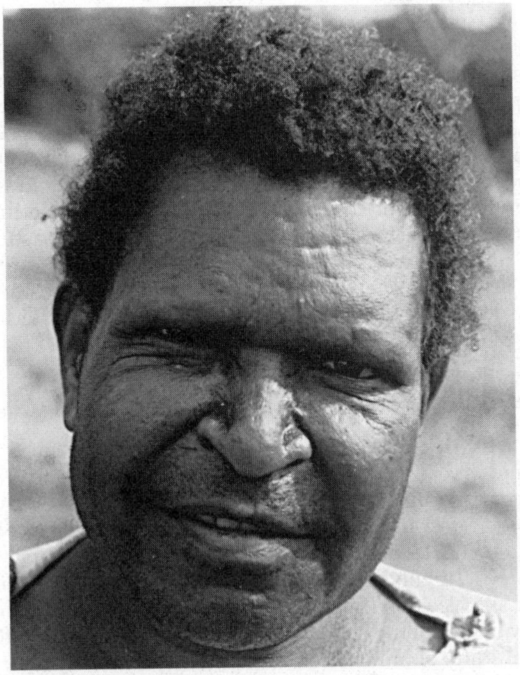

FIGURE 168–10 ▫ Moderately advanced lepromatous leprosy. There is symmetric infiltration of the face with particular involvement of the eyebrows, nose, and cheek creases. Eyebrow loss (madarosis) is also present.

disease progression, the macules become infiltrated (Fig. 168–9). Peripheral nerve involvement is widespread but not as symmetric as in lepromatous disease. Whereas patients with borderline lepromatous leprosy do not suffer the extreme consequences of bacillary multiplication that are seen in lepromatous disease, they may experience both reversal and ENL reactions.

Lepromatous Leprosy

The patient with polar lepromatous leprosy may be carrying 10^{11} leprosy bacilli, and the dissemination of these organisms throughout the body produces the characteristic symptoms and signs of the condition. The onset of disease is frequently insidious, the earliest lesions being ill-defined, hypopigmented papules or macules often first seen on the ears. The skin gradually becomes infiltrated and thickened; facial skin thickening causes the characteristic leonine facies (Figs. 168–10 and 168–11). Hair is lost, especially the lateral third of the eyebrows (madarosis). Dermal nerves are destroyed, and sensory loss (light touch, pain, and temperature) that begins at the hands and feet gradually extends to the whole body except for the axillae, groin, and scalp. Sweating is lost; this can cause profound discomfort in a tropical climate because massive compensatory sweating occurs in the remaining intact areas. Nerve damage to large peripheral nerves does not occur until late in the disease.

Nasal symptoms (stuffy nose, nosebleeds, loss of sense of smell) can often be elicited early in the disease, and 80% of newly diagnosed lepromatous patients have invasion of the nasal mucosa.[23] Septal perforation may occur. The pathognomic collapse of the bridge of the nose is secondary to

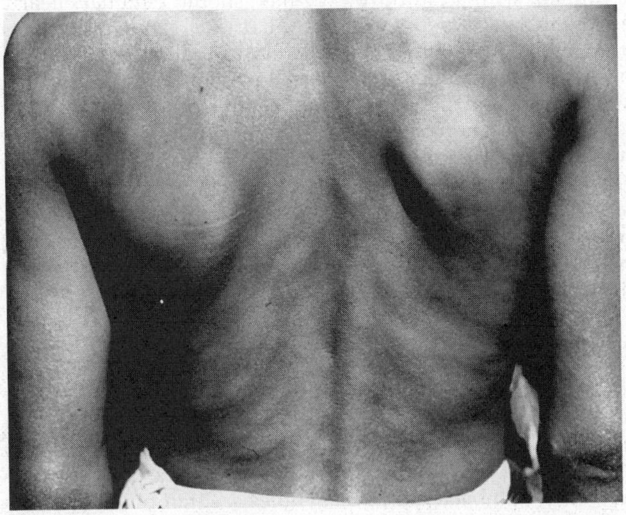

FIGURE 168–9 ▫ Multiple ill-defined lesions typical of borderline lepromatous leprosy are present on this patient's back.

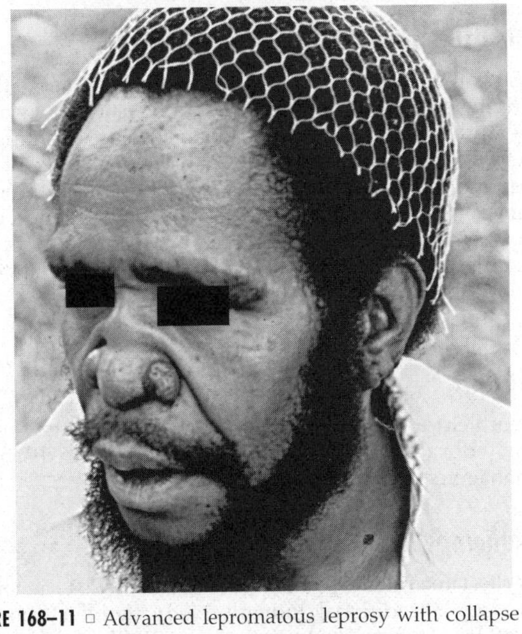

FIGURE 168–11 ▫ Advanced lepromatous leprosy with collapse of the nasal septum.

bacillary destruction of the bony nasal spine. Bone involvement is common, with osteoporosis and fractures. Renal disease is common in lepromatous patients; all types of glomerulonephritis have been reported.[59] Testicular atrophy results from diffuse infiltration and the acute orchitis that occurs with ENL reactions. The consequent loss of testosterone leads to azoospermia and gynecomastia. Secondary amyloidosis of the amyloid A protein variety (AA) is a frequent finding in lepromatous patients who suffer repeated ENL reactions.[60] Acute-phase proteins, including serum amyloid A, are elevated during ENL episodes, with subsequent deposition of the insoluble amyloid derivative, protein AA, in kidneys, liver, spleen, adrenals, and thyroid.

Other Forms of Leprosy

There are three variant forms of leprosy, histoid, pure neuritic, and Lucio leprosy. Histoid lesions are distinctive nodules occurring in lepromatous cases that have relapsed owing to dapsone resistance or noncompliance with chemotherapy. Pure neuritic leprosy is recognized mainly in India, with asymmetric involvement of peripheral nerve trunks and no visible skin lesions. Lucio leprosy is a form of lepromatous leprosy found only in Latin Americans, with a uniform, diffuse, shiny skin infiltration.[61]

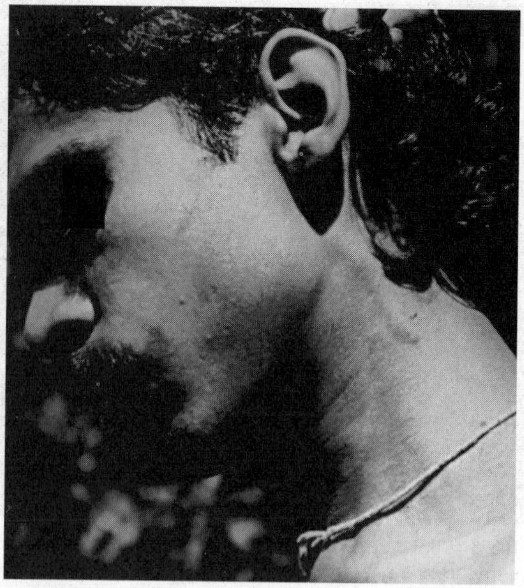

FIGURE 168–12 □ Visible thickening of the great auricular nerve.

Diagnosis

Leprosy should be considered a possible diagnosis in anyone with peripheral nerve or skin lesions who has lived in a leprosy endemic area. The diagnosis is essentially a clinical one based on finding one or more of the cardinal signs of leprosy (see earlier) and supported by the finding of AFB on slit skin smears. It is important to inspect the whole body in a good light because otherwise one may easily miss lesions, particularly on the buttocks in borderline disease. Skin lesions should be tested for anesthesia to light touch, pinprick, and temperature. Loss of sweating may be elicited easily after exercise in a hot climate. The peripheral nerves should be palpated systematically. If the diagnosis remains in doubt, skin biopsy and lepromin testing may provide further evidence of infection.

Differential Diagnosis

Leprosy is the most common cause of peripheral nerve thickening (Fig. 168–12). Other rare conditions, such as Charcot-Marie-Tooth disease and Dejerine-Sottas disease, are differentiated from leprosy by the family history, the absence of skin lesions, and the absence of AFB. The anesthesia of tuberculoid and borderline tuberculoid lesions differentiates them from other conditions with an appearance similar to leprosy (e.g., vitiligo, mycotic skin infections, psoriasis, and systemic lupus erythematosus).

Treatment

The treatment of leprosy has four main components: chemotherapy, education of the patient, prevention of disability, and management of complications.

Chemotherapy

The earliest recorded specific treatment of leprosy is chaulmoogra oil, a traditional Indian remedy derived from the seeds of the *Hydnocarpus* tree, used topically and orally.[62] This was unpleasant to take, and relapse was common. Old leprosaria records suggest that it was partially effective,[63] and an anti–*M. leprae* effect has been demonstrated.[64] Interest in the sulfonamides in the 1930s led to the development of sulfone drugs for use in leprosy. In 1947, dapsone was first used, and its effectiveness and cheapness led to global use of dapsone monotherapy in the 1950s. In 1964, patients relapsing with dapsone-resistant leprosy were first reported[65]; at that time, such cases were rare (1 in 1000). However, during the next 10 years, relapses with dapsone resistance became more common, and primary dapsone resistance was reported in Ethiopia in 1977. WHO surveys in 1981 found that dapsone resistance was present wherever it was sought, with high-grade resistant organisms in relapsing patients and low-grade resistant organisms in cases of primary resistance.[66]

In response to the failure of dapsone monotherapy, the WHO proposed a multidrug regimen for the treatment of leprosy (Table 168–2). It is postulated that in a multibacillary patient, there are three distinguishable types of bacilli: fully drug-sensitive bacteria; drug-resistant mutants; and a small population of "persisters," dormant nonmultiplying bacilli. Treatment with a multidrug regimen should eliminate nearly all organisms. For the purpose of drug treatment, patients are classified as either paucibacillary or multibacillary. The multibacillary category includes all patients with positive slit skin smears and slit skin smear–negative borderline tuberculoid patients with more than 15 skin lesions or widespread nerve damage because nerve biopsy in such patients often shows multibacillary pathologic characteristics. Paucibacillary patients receive a two-drug combination for 6 months, whereas multibacillary patients are treated with a triple-drug combination for at least 24 months. The first-line antileprotic drugs are rifampin, dapsone, and clofazimine.

RIFAMPIN

Rifampin is a potent bactericidal agent for *M. leprae*. Four days after a single 600-mg dose, bacilli from a previously untreated multibacillary patient are no longer viable.[67] It acts by inhibiting DNA-dependent RNA polymerase, thereby interfering with bacterial RNA synthesis. Rifampin is well absorbed orally and is excreted principally in the bile after deacetylation in the liver. Hepatotoxicity is the most common

TABLE 168–2 ■ World Health Organization Multidrug Therapy Regimen

TYPE OF LEPROSY	DRUG TREATMENT		DURATION OF TREATMENT (mo)	DURATION OF FOLLOW-UP (y)
	Monthly Supervised	Daily Self-Administered		
Paucibacillary	Rifampin, 600 mg	Dapsone, 100 mg	6	2
Multibacillary	Rifampin, 600 mg Clofazimine, 300 mg	Clofazimine, 50 mg Dapsone, 100 mg	24	5

side effect; a mild transient elevation of hepatic transaminase values frequently occurs and is not an indication for stopping treatment. Because rifampin induces liver enzymes, the metabolism of other drugs may be affected, so dosages should be reviewed and increased if necessary. Because *M. leprae* resistance to rifampin can develop as a one-step process, rifampin should always be given in combination with other antileprotics.[68] The fever and influenza symptom syndrome seen with intermittent rifampin used in other clinical situations does not seem to be a problem in leprosy patients.

DAPSONE

Dapsone (4,4′-diaminodiphenyl sulfone) acts by blocking folic acid synthesis. It is only weakly bactericidal. Oral absorption is good, and it has a long half-life, averaging 28 hours. It is conjugated in the bile and after enterohepatic circulation is excreted in the urine. Patients' compliance may be monitored by measuring urinary dapsone levels. Hemolytic anemia is the most common side effect of dapsone treatment, and patients with glucose-6-phosphate dehydrogenase deficiency are particularly at risk. The "dapsone syndrome," which is occasionally seen in leprosy, starts 6 weeks after commencing dapsone and manifests as exfoliative dermatitis associated with lymphadenopathy, hepatosplenomegaly, fever, and hepatitis.[69] Agranulocytosis, hepatitis, and cholestatic jaundice occur rarely with dapsone therapy.

CLOFAZIMINE

Clofazimine has a weakly bactericidal action, the mechanism of which is not known. It has an inherently antiinflammatory effect that makes it useful in the management of ENL reactions. The most noticeable side effect is of skin discoloration, ranging from red to purple-black; the degree of discoloration depends on the dose and the amount of leprous infiltration. The pigmentation usually clears up within 6 to 12 months of stopping clofazimine, although traces of discoloration may remain for up to 4 years. Clofazimine also produces a characteristic icthyosis on the shins and forearms. Gastrointestinal side effects, ranging from mild cramps to diarrhea and weight loss, may occur as a result of clofazimine crystal deposition in the wall of the small bowel.

WORLD HEALTH ORGANIZATION MULTIDRUG THERAPY

Since the introduction of multidrug therapy, about 4.2 million patients have been treated successfully. Clinical improvement has been rapid and toxicity rare. Although initial reports suggested that relapse after multidrug therapy is rare, with the WHO reporting cumulative rates of 1% relapse in 9 years of follow-up,[70] one should interpret these figures with caution because such a slowly growing organism will cause relapse only after several years. Patients with high initial bacillary loads may be at a much greater risk for relapse and may warrant longer antibiotic treatment.[71] Susceptibility testing of *M. leprae* strains from relapsed multibacillary patients has shown them to remain drug sensitive.

There have been a number of attempts to develop short-course chemotherapy for paucibacillary leprosy with either rifampin in weekly doses or single-dose chemotherapy in a combination of currently used drugs. So far, all of these regimens have had higher relapse rates than the current WHO paucibacillary regimen.[72] Several new drugs bactericidal for *M. leprae* have been identified: fluoroquinolones, minocycline, and clarithromycin. The fluoroquinolones pefloxacin and ofloxacin have a remarkable degree of bactericidal activity, with 22 daily doses killing 99.99% of viable *M. leprae* organisms present in multibacillary cases at the start of treatment.[73] Multicenter trials of daily rifampin-ofloxacin are being conducted by the WHO and afford the possibility of considerably shortening the duration of multidrug therapy. Daily minocycline treatment of multibacillary patients for 3 months resulted in killing of all viable *M. leprae* organisms.[74] Clarithromycin, given in daily doses of 500 mg to multibacillary patients, has a similar bactericidal effect. Antagonism between these new drugs has not been demonstrated. Ofloxacin, minocycline, and clarithromycin are natural candidates for replacing dapsone and clofazimine, and various options for modifying the current WHO regimen are being developed.

Education of the Patient

Educating leprosy patients about their disease is the key to successful management. Patients need to be reassured that within a few days of chemotherapy, they will not be infectious and can lead a normal social life. A clear explanation of the disease and refutation of myths about leprosy will help patients come to terms with the diagnosis and may well improve compliance. It is important to emphasize that gross deformities are not the inevitable end point of disease and that care and awareness of their limbs is as important as chemotherapy. Appropriate physiotherapy can prevent contractures, muscle atrophy, and overstretching of paralyzed muscles.

Prevention of Disability

Nerve damage produces anesthesia, dryness, and muscle weakness. These three factors lead to misuse of the affected limb, with resultant ulceration, infection, and ultimately severe deformity. Figure 168–13 illustrates the interaction of factors combining to produce deformity. Dryness, particularly of the feet in agricultural workers, predisposes to cracking of the skin and secondary infection. This risk can be reduced by encouraging patients to soak their feet in a warm water-oil mixture and to put petroleum jelly on their hands and feet. Disabilities and deformities are prevented by educating patients to avoid misusing their anesthetic limbs, to recognize infection early, and to protect their hands and feet. Simple advice such as always using gloves for handling hot pans when cooking, checking feet for early signs of damage from foreign bodies and ill-fitting shoes, wearing soft shoes or slippers whenever possible, and wearing in new shoes carefully is worth reiterating regularly.[75]

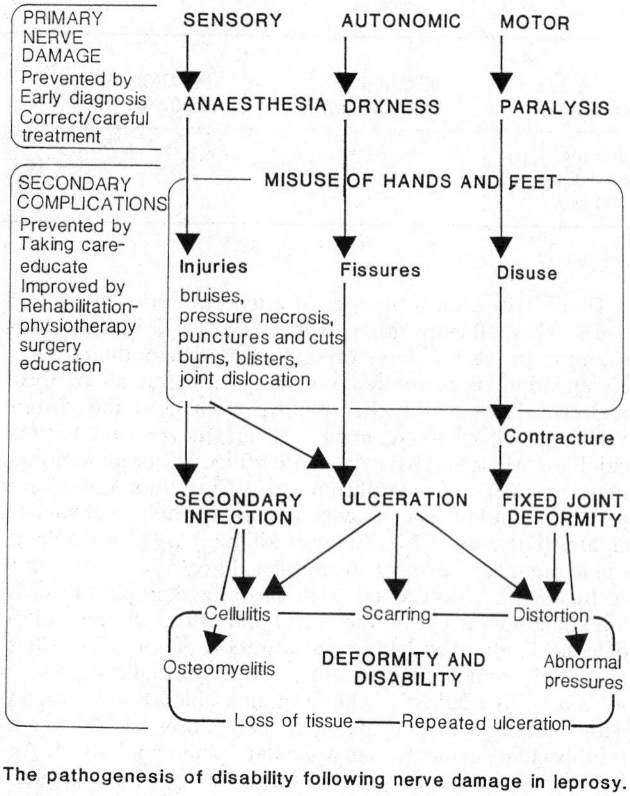

FIGURE 168–13 □ The interaction of factors producing deformities in leprosy. (From Bryceson A, Pfaltzgraff RE [eds]: Leprosy. Edinburgh, Churchill Livingstone, 1979, p 138.)

Foot ulcers arise quickly in anesthetic, deformed feet; hospital admission may be required to ensure adequate rest, soaking, and physiotherapy of the affected limb. Plaster casts are useful for protecting injured limbs and altering weight-bearing stresses during healing. Unfortunately, amputation is sometimes the only feasible treatment for a damaged, infected limb if any function in that limb is to be preserved.

Management of Complications

REACTIONS

Reversal reactions occur in patients with borderline leprosy (borderline tuberculoid, borderline, and borderline lepromatous) and manifest clinically with erythema, swelling, and tenderness of skin lesions (Fig. 168–14) and swelling, pain, and tenderness of peripheral nerves. Loss of nerve function can be dramatic, with footdrop occurring overnight secondary to lateral popliteal nerve involvement.[76] Nerve pain and tenderness are prominent and distressing symptoms, most commonly affecting the ulnar nerve[77] (Fig. 168–15). Severe reactions may be accompanied by fever, malaise, and anorexia. Awareness of the early symptoms by both patient and physician is important because if the reversal reaction is left untreated, severe nerve damage may occur. Patients frequently seek medical advice for their leprosy lesions only when a reversal reaction develops in a previously quiescent skin lesion. The peak time for reversal reactions is in the first 6 months of treatment,[78] so it is important to warn patients about reactions early because the sudden development of reactional lesions soon after starting treatment is distressing and undermines the patient's confidence. Reactions occurring after completion of treatment are not uncommon, and differentiation of reaction from relapse can be difficult and often only resolved by histologic examination of a lesional skin biopsy.

ENL reactions occur only in multibacillary patients, with a frequency of 50% in lepromatous leprosy and 25% in borderline lepromatous leprosy patients.[79] Skin lesions are the most common manifestation (Fig. 168–16), but ENL nodules may occur in any organ in which *M. leprae* organisms are found. Crops of small pink nodules appear on the skin of the face and the extensor surfaces of the limbs. New crops appear as old lesions subside, and a chronic painful panniculitis may develop. Neuritis may occur but is less dramatic than that seen in reversal reactions. Iritis and episcleritis are common and should be treated promptly. The patient is usually unwell with malaise and fever. Other accompanying signs are acute lymphadenitis, orchitis, bone pain, dactylitis, arthritis, and proteinuria. ENL usually starts during the second year of chemotherapy and despite treatment may continue on a relapsing and remitting course for several years.

The Lucio phenomenon is a variant of ENL. It is regarded as a distinct entity because it occurs only in patients with Lucio leprosy and presents with small pink lesions that become hemorrhagic bullae. Microscopic examination shows epidermal necrosis and necrotizing vasculitis with large numbers of AFB in endothelial cells.[80]

The treatment of reactions is guided by the need to control the acute inflammation and neuritis, ease the pain, halt eye damage, and prevent extension of the disease. Standard antileprotic chemotherapy should be continued. Simple antiinflammatory measures, rest, analgesics, and antiinflammatory drugs should be instituted. Clinical evidence of ongoing neuritis (nerve pain and tenderness, loss of function) should be carefully sought, and if it is present, corticosteroid treatment should be started. Reversal reactions respond to treatment with oral prednisolone at an initial daily dose of 30 to 40 mg, reduced by 5 mg/mo.[81] Affected limbs should be splinted and appropriate physiotherapy started. The treatment of ENL should start with simple measures: bed rest and analgesia.

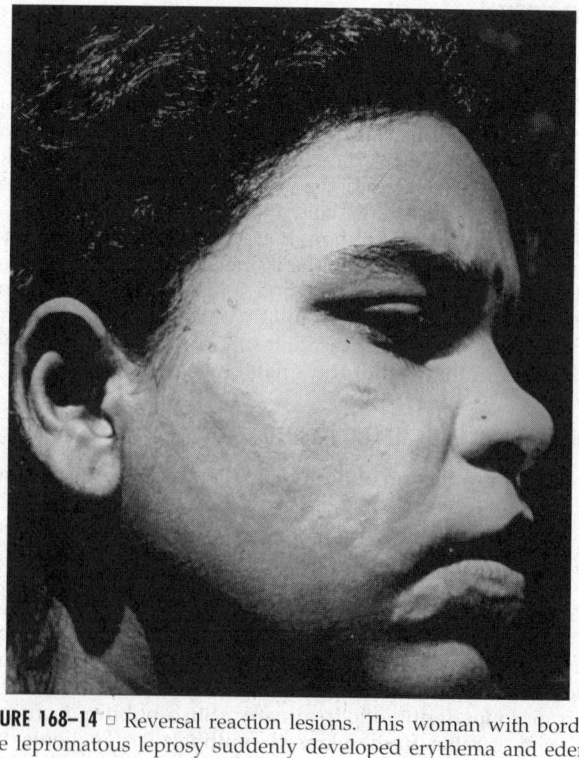

FIGURE 168–14 □ Reversal reaction lesions. This woman with borderline lepromatous leprosy suddenly developed erythema and edema of her previously quiescent facial lesions 6 weeks after delivery.

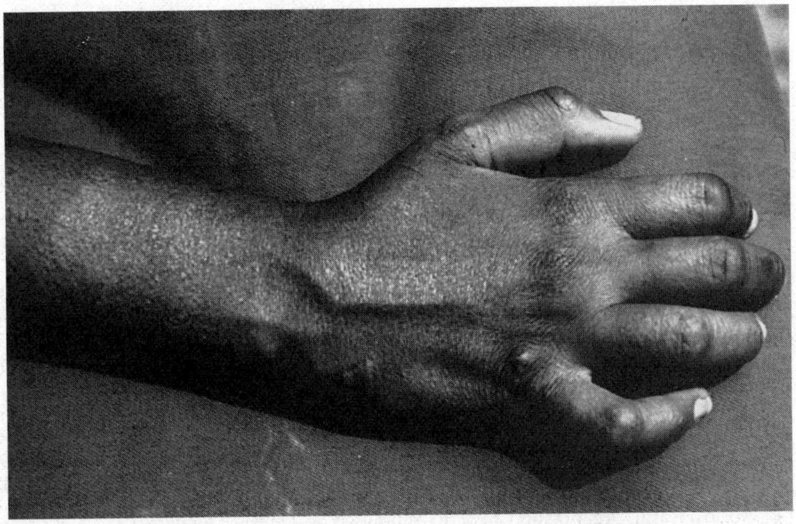

FIGURE 168–15 ▫ Reversal reaction acute neuritis. The hand is swollen with clawing of the fingers, indicating involvement of both the ulnar and median nerves.

In moderate and severe ENL, corticosteroids are useful and may be necessary in initial high doses (60 mg daily), tapered down rapidly in a month. Oral chloroquine, 150 mg of base twice daily, may also reduce symptoms of inflammation. Because ENL tends to recur, there is a serious risk for development of steroid dependency in these patients. Clofazimine has a useful antiinflammatory effect in ENL and can be used at 300 mg/d for several months. Thalidomide (100 mg every 8 hours) has a dramatic effect in controlling ENL and may be useful in preventing recurrent ENL, but its teratogenic side effects in early pregnancy preclude its use in women of childbearing age; it is unavailable in several countries despite its undoubted value in the management of ENL.[82] Cyclosporine has been shown to have a steroid-sparing effect in the treatment of steroid-dependent ENL reactions, but this requires further evaluation.[83]

THE EYE IN LEPROSY

Blindness due to leprosy, which occurs in at least 2.5% of patients,[84] is a devastating complication for a patient who probably already has sensory loss due to anesthesia of the hands and feet. Eye damage results from both nerve damage and bacillary invasion.

Lagophthalmos results from paresis of the orbicular muscle of the eye due to involvement of the zygomatic and temporal branches of the facial (seventh) nerve. These superficial branches are frequently involved in borderline tuberculoid cases, particularly if there are facial skin lesions. In lepromatous disease, lagophthalmos occurs later and is usually bilateral. Damage to the ophthalmic branch of the trigeminal (fifth) nerve causes anesthesia of the cornea and conjunctiva, which results in drying of the cornea and a reduction in blinking; this leaves the cornea at risk for minor trauma and ulceration. Autonomic nerve involvement leads to altered pupillary reflexes. Lepromatous infiltration may occur: in corneal nerves, producing visible beading; and on the conjunctiva, producing avascular punctate keratitis, corneal lepromas, and lepromatous pannus. Invasion of the iris and ciliary body makes them extremely susceptible to reactions.

Iridocyclitis is a common manifestation of an ENL reaction. Edema and hyperemia produce a painful "red eye." The sphincter and ciliary muscles go into reflex spasm, producing blurred vision. Inflammatory cells are deposited on the corneal epithelium as keratitic precipitates. The iritis may result in synechiae, either posterior to the lens or anterior to the cornea, with subsequent iridal atrophy and glaucoma. The effects of lagophthalmos can be mitigated by massage and active forced closure of the lids. Corneal protection can be achieved by wearing spectacles and using tear substitutes. Specific treatment of the ocular complications of ENL reactions consists of 1% atropine eyedrops to dilate the pupil and relax the ciliary muscle and 1% cortisone drops every 4 hours to suppress the inflammation. Chronic iridocyclitis and scleritis also respond to this regimen.

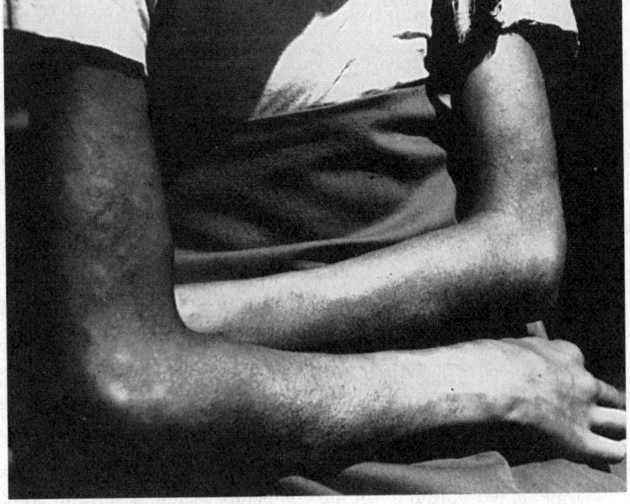

FIGURE 168–16 ▫ Typical cutaneous lesions of ENL.

RECONSTRUCTIVE SURGERY

Reconstructive surgery has a role in improving both function and appearance. Lagophthalmos can be ameliorated by either tarsorrhaphy or temporal muscle transfer. Appropriate tendon transfers can reduce the effects of ulnar and median nerve paralysis and improve footdrop and claw toes. Cosmetic surgery, in particular eyebrow replacement, nasal reconstruction, and reduction of gynecomastia, is important in the rehabilitation of severely affected patients.

Leprosy Control Programs

The current strategy of vertical control programs dedicated to leprosy with case detection, treatment with the WHO drug regimen, and contact examination has been successful.

Efficient treatment is not merely restricted to chemotherapy; it also involves good case management with effective monitoring and supervision. An important secondary role of leprosy control programs is the prevention of disabilities and education of the population about leprosy.

The WHO has declared that "the elimination of leprosy as a public health problem" (defined as 1 case per 100,000 population) should be achieved by the year 2000. Although this will not be possible for all areas, major progress has been made toward this goal. Important future challenges are ensuring that those patients disabled by leprosy have good care and maintaining prompt diagnosis and treatment of patients in areas of low endemicity where they will in future not be seen by specialist leprosy health workers.

References

1. World Health Organization Expert Committee on Leprosy: Chemotherapy of leprosy. World Health Organ Tech Rep Ser 847, 1994.
2. Noordeen SK: Epidemiology and control of leprosy—A review of progress over the last 30 years. Trans R Soc Trop Med Hyg 87:515, 1993.
3. Noordeen SK: Elimination of leprosy as a public health problem. Int J Lepr 62:279, 1994.
4. Brubaker ML, Binford CH, Trautman JR: Occurrences of leprosy in US veterans after service in endemic areas abroad. Public Health Rep 84:1057, 1969.
5. Noordeen SK: Mortality in leprosy. Indian J Med Res 60:439, 1972.
6. Fine PEM: The epidemiology of a slow bacterium. Epidemiol Rev 4:161, 1982.
7. Noordeen SK: The epidemiology of leprosy. *In* Hastings RC (ed): Leprosy. Edinburgh, Churchill Livingstone, 1994, pp 29–48.
8. Feldman RA, Sturdivant M: Leprosy in Louisiana 1855–1970. An epidemiologic study of long term trends. Am J Epidemiol 102:303, 1975.
9. Ponnighaus JM, Fine PEM, Sterne JAC, et al: Extended schooling and good housing conditions are associated with reduced risk of leprosy in rural Malawi. Int J Lepr 62:345, 1994.
10. Ponnighaus JM, Mwanjasi JL, Fine PEM, et al: Is HIV infection a risk factor for leprosy? Int J Lepr 59:221, 1991.
11. Kawuma HJS, Bwire R, Adatu-Engwau F: Leprosy and infection with the human immunodeficiency virus in Uganda; a case-control study. Int J Lepr 62:521, 1994.
12. Sekar B, Jayasheela M, Chattopadhya D, et al: Prevalence of HIV infection and high-risk characteristics among leprosy patients of south India; a case control study. Int J Lepr 62:527, 1994.
13. Godal T: Immunological detection of subclinical infection in leprosy. Lepr Rev 45:22, 1974.
14. Dockrell HM, Eastcott H, Young SK, et al: Possible transmission of *Mycobacterium leprae* in a group of UK leprosy contacts. Lancet 338:739, 1991.
15. Scott GC, Russell DA, Boughton CR, Vincin DR: Untreated leprosy: Probability for shifts in Ridley-Jopling classification. Development of "flares" or disappearance of clinically apparent disease. Int J Lepr 44:110, 1976.
16. De Wit MYL, Douglas JT, McFadden J, Klatser PR: Polymerase chain reaction for detection of *Mycobacterium leprae* in nasal swab specimens. J Gen Microbiol 31:502, 1993.
17. Rees RJW, Meade T: Comparison of the modes of spread and transmission of leprosy and TB. Lancet 7:47, 1974.
18. Lumpkin LRI, Cox GF, Wolf JE: Leprosy in five armadillo handlers. Am J Epidemiol 9:899, 1983.
19. Truman RW, Shannon EJ, Hagstad HV, et al: Evaluation of the origin of *Mycobacterium leprae* in the wild armadillo, *Dasypus novemcinctus*. Am J Trop Med Hyg 35:588, 1986.
20. Schäffer X: On the spread of leprosy bacilli from the upper parts of the respiratory tract. Arch Dermat Syph 44:159, 1898.
21. Shepard CC: Acid-fast bacilli in nasal excretions in leprosy and results of inoculation of mice. Am J Hyg 71:147, 1960.
22. Desikan KV, Job CK: A review of postmortem findings in 37 cases of leprosy. Int J Lepr 36:32, 1968.
23. Barton RPE: A clinical study of the nose in lepromatous leprosy. Lepr Rev 45:135, 1974.
24. McDermott-Lancaster RD, McDougall AC: Mode of transmission and histology of *M. leprae* infection in nude mice. Int J Exp Pathol 71:689, 1990.
25. Job CK, Chehl SK, Hastings RC: Transmission of leprosy in nude mice through thorn pricks. Int J Lepr 62:395, 1994.
26. Ridley DS, Jopling WH: Classification of leprosy according to immunity. Int J Lepr 34:255, 1966.
27. Karat ABA, Job CK, Rao PSS: Liver in leprosy: Histological and biochemical findings. Br Med J 307:307, 1971.
28. Ridley DS: Pathogenesis of Leprosy and Related Diseases. London, Wright, 1988.
29. Dastur DK: Cutaneous nerves in leprosy: The relationship between histopathology and cutaneous sensibility. Brain 78:615, 1955.
30. Shah PKD, Malhotra YK, Lakhotia M., et al: Cardiovascular dysautonomia in patients with lepromatous leprosy. Indian J Lepr 62:91, 1990.
31. Abbot NC, Beck JS, Samson PD, et al: Impairment of fingertip vasomotor reflexes in leprosy patients and apparently healthy contacts. Int J Lepr 59:537, 1991.
32. Antia NH, Mehta LN, Shetty VP, Irani PF: Clinical, electrophysiological, quantitative, histologic and ultrastructural studies of the index branch of the radial cutaneous nerve in leprosy. 1. Preliminary report. Int J Lepr 43:106, 1975.
33. Mehta LN, Shetty VP, Antia NH, Irani PF: Quantitative, histologic and ultrastructural studies of the index branch of the radial cutaneous nerve in leprosy and its correlation with electrophysiologic study. Int J Lepr 43:256, 1975.
34. Shetty VP, Mehta LN, Irani PF, Antia NH: Study of the evolution of nerve damage in leprosy. Part 1—Lesions of the index branch of the radial cutaneous nerve in early leprosy. Indian J Lepr 52:5, 1980.
35. Pearson JMH, Weddell AGM: Perineurial changes in untreated leprosy. Lepr Rev 46:51, 1975.
36. Job CK, Desikan KV: Pathologic changes and their distribution in peripheral nerves in lepromatous leprosy. Int J Lepr 36:257, 1968.
37. Job CK: Pathology of peripheral nerve lesions in lepromatous leprosy—A light and electron microscopic study. Int J Lepr 39:251, 1971.
38. Job CK: Mechanism of destruction in tuberculoid-borderline leprosy. An electron-microscopic study. J Neurosci 20:25, 1973.
39. Ottenhoff THM, Converse PJ, Bjune G, De Vries RRP: HLA antigens and neural reversal reactions in Ethiopian borderline tuberculoid leprosy patients. Int J Lepr 55:261, 1987.
40. de Vries RR: Genetic control of immunopathology induced by *Mycobacterium leprae*. Am J Trop Med Hyg 44:12, 1991.
41. Britton WJ: Immunology of leprosy. Trans R Soc Trop Med Hyg 87:508, 1993.
42. Lee SP, Stoker NG, Grant KA, et al: Cellular immune responses of leprosy contacts to fractionated *Mycobacterium leprae* antigens. Infect Immun 57:2475, 1989.
43. Dockrell HM, Stoker NG, Lee SP, et al: T-cell recognition of the 18-kilodalton antigen of *Mycobacterium leprae*. Infect Immun 57:1979, 1989.
44. Ilangumaran S, Shanker-Narayan NP, Ramu G, Muthukkaruppan VR: Cellular and humoral responses to recombinant 65-kD antigen of *Mycobacterium leprae* in leprosy patients and healthy controls. Clin Exp Immunol 96:79, 1994.
45. Modlin RL, Hofman FM, Horwitz DA, et al: In situ identification of cells in human leprosy granulomas with monoclonal antibodies to interleukin 2 and its receptors. J Immunol 132:3085, 1984.
46. Paul RC, Stanford JL, Carswell JW: Multiple skin testing in leprosy. J Hyg (Camb) 75:57, 1975.
47. Modlin RL, Rea TH: Immunopathology of leprosy granulomas. Springer Semin Immunopathol 10:359, 1988.
48. Waters MFR, Ridley DS, Lucas SB: Positive Mitsuda lepromin reactions in long term treated lepromatous leprosy. Lepr Rev 61:347, 1990.
49. Haregewoin A, Godal T, Mustafa AS, et al: T-cell conditioned media reverse T-cell unresponsiveness in lepromatous leprosy. Nature 303:342, 1983.
50. Kaplan G, Kiessling R, Teklemariam S, et al: The reconstitution of cell-mediated immunity in the cutaneous lesions of lepromatous leprosy by recombinant interleukin 2. J Exp Med 169:893, 1989.

51. Birdi TJ, Antia NH: The macrophage in leprosy: A review on the current status. Int J Lepr 57:511, 1989.
52. Yoder L, Naafs B, Harboe M, Bjune G: Antibody activity against *Mycobacterium leprae* antigen 7 in leprosy: Studies on variation in antibody content throughout the spectrum and on the effect of DDS treatment and relapse in BT leprosy. Lepr Rev 50:113, 1979.
53. Smith PG: The serodiagnosis of leprosy. Lepr Rev 63:97, 1992.
54. Ulrich M, Smith PG, Zuniga M, et al: IgM antibodies to native phenolic glycolipid 1 in contacts of leprosy patients in Venezuela: Epidemiological observations and a prospective study of the risk of leprosy. Int J Lepr 59:405, 1991.
55. Wemambu SNC, Turk JL, Waters MFR: Erythema nodosum leprosum: A clinical manifestation of the Arthus phenomenon. Lancet 2:933, 1969.
56. Dharma Rao T, Ramchander Rao P: Enhanced cell-mediated immune responses in erythema nodosum leprosum reactions of leprosy. Int J Lepr 55:36, 1987.
57. Filley E, Andreolli A, Steele J, Rook GAW: A transient rise in agalactosyl IgG correlating with free interleukin-2 receptors during episodes of erythema nodosum. Clin Exp Immunol 76:343, 1989.
58. Mehra V, Modlin RL: T lymphocytes in leprosy lesions. Curr Top Microbiol Immunol 155:97, 1990.
59. Date A, Harihar H, Jeyavarthini SE: Renal lesions and other major findings in necropsies of 133 patients with leprosy. Int J Lepr 53:455, 1985.
60. McAdam KPWJ, Anders RF, Smith SR: Association of amyloidosis with erythema nodosum leprosum reactions and recurrent neutrophil leucocytosis in leprosy. Lancet 2:572, 1975.
61. Latapi L, Chevez Zamora A: The 'spotted' leprosy of Lucio (la lepra 'manchada' de Lucio). An introduction to its clinical and histological study. Int J Lepr 16:421, 1948.
62. Mouat FJ: Notes on native remedies. No 1. The chaulmoogra. Indian Ann Med Sci 1:646, 1854.
63. Schujman S: Therapeutic value of chaulmoogra in the treatment of leprosy. Int J Lepr 15:135, 1947.
64. Levy L: The activity of chaulmoogra acids against *Mycobacterium leprae*. Am Rev Respir Dis 111:703, 1975.
65. Petit JH, Rees RJW: Sulphone resistance in leprosy. An experimental and clinical study. Lancet 2:673, 1964.
66. Ji Bahong JBH: Drug resistance in leprosy—A review. Lepr Rev 56:265, 1985.
67. Levy L, Shepard CC, Fasal P: The bactericidal effect of rifampicin on *M. leprae* in man: (a) Single doses of 600, 900, and 1200 mg; (b) daily doses of 300 mg. Int J Lepr 44:183, 1976.
68. Jacobson RR, Hastings RC: Rifampicin-resistant leprosy. Lancet 2:1304, 1976.
69. Frey HM, Gershon AA, Borkowsky W, Bullock WE: Fatal reaction to dapsone during treatment of leprosy. Ann Intern Med 94:777, 1981.
70. Grosset JH: Progress in the chemotherapy of leprosy. Int J Lepr 62:268, 1994.
71. Jamet P, Ji B, Marchoux Chemotherapy Study Group: Relapse after long-term follow-up of multibacillary patients treated by WHO multidrug regimen. Int J Lepr 63:195, 1995.
72. Pattyn SR, Ghys P, Janssens L, et al: A randomised clinical trial of two single-dose treatments for paucibacillary leprosy. Lepr Rev 65:45, 1994.
73. N'Deli LN, Guelpa-Lauras CC, Perani EG, Grosset JH: Effectiveness of pefloxacin in the treatment of lepromatous leprosy. Int J Lepr 58:12, 1990.
74. Gelber RH, Fukuda K, Byrd S, et al: A clinical trial of minocycline in lepromatous leprosy. BMJ 304:91, 1992.
75. Srinivasan H: Prevention of Disabilities in Patients with Leprosy: A Practical Guide. Geneva, World Health Organization, 1993.
76. Rose P, Waters MFR: Reversal reactions in leprosy and their management. Lepr Rev 62:113, 1991.
77. Lockwood DNJ, Vinayakumar S, Stanley JNA, et al: Clinical features and outcome of reversal (type 1) reactions in Hyderabad, India. Int J Lepr 60:8, 1993.
78. Lienhardt C, Fine PEM: Type 1 reaction, neuritis and disability in leprosy. What is the current epidemiological situation? Lepr Rev 65:9, 1994.
79. Bryceson A, Pfaltzgraff RE: Leprosy. Edinburgh, Churchill Livingstone, 1990.
80. Rea TH, Ridley DS: Lucio's phenomenon: A comparative histological study. Int J Lepr 47:161, 1979.
81. Kiran KU, Stanley JNA, Pearson JMH: The outpatient treatment of nerve damage in patients with borderline leprosy using a semi-standardised steroid regime. Lepr Rev 56:127, 1985.
82. Jakeman P, Smith WCS: Thalidomide in leprosy reaction. Lancet 343:432, 1994.
83. Miller RA, Shen J, Rea TH, Harnisch JP: Treatment of chronic erythema nodosum leprosum with cyclosporine A produces clinical and immunohistologic remission. Int J Lepr 55:441, 1987.
84. Ocular complications of leprosy. Lancet 340:642, 1992.

ZOONOSES

169

Approach to the Patient with Zoonotic Infection

David R. Stone
Leonard C. Marcus

Our susceptibility to disease from a wide range of zoonotic organisms soberly reminds us that we are members of the animal kingdom. Epidemics due to the emergence of new pathogens as well as the recrudescence of more established pathogens have drastic effects on society. Exploration, deforestation, and manipulation of our wetlands brings us in contact with organisms rarely seen before. War, lack of sanitation, overcrowding, and ease of travel play a major role in the dissemination of these new diseases. Our increasing contact with exotic animals for pets and research and our need to herd ever-increasing populations of farm animals facilitate the transmission of zoonoses to humans.

We are not totally to blame. Mutation, recombination, and reassortment of genetic material, as well as environmental factors, have led some organisms to infect species never affected previously. Changes in the arthropod vector populations also play an important role in the dissemination of these diseases.[1]

Zoonotic diseases have been described since antiquity; more than 200 have been documented.[2] They include viral, bacterial, mycotic, protozoan, and helminthic infections and arthropod infestations. They are transmitted to humans either directly through skin contact, bite or scratch, inhalation, and ingestion, or indirectly through an arthropod intermediate host. Humans usually serve as an accidental host for infection. Occasionally humans serve along with animals as a reservoir for disease (e.g., yellow fever virus, pneumonic plague). To understand and prevent these illnesses, we often need the expertise of molecular biologists, ecologists, entomologists, epidemiologists, and veterinarians.

In this chapter, we highlight some of the unique clinical aspects that need to be considered when zoonotic infections are evaluated. We categorize some of the more common zoonoses by their modes of transmission and discuss preventive measures that can be used to avoid infection. Finally, we consider the special risks that patients with immunodeficiency have for developing zoonotic illnesses from pets and from travel abroad.

Questions about zoonoses are usually presented to the clinician in one of three contexts. In the first instance, an animal was known to have been ill, and the question arises whether humans can become ill because of contact with that animal. This is clearly a question that should be addressed by a veterinarian. Animals may develop many diseases that are not transmitted to humans.

In the second situation, an ill person has a history of contact with animals or insects (bites) and the question arises whether the illness could be related to that contact. In this instance, we should first consider the patient's age. Children are often intimate and careless in their contact with pets. Their failure to wash hands before eating puts them at risk for developing zoonotic infections transmitted by the fecal-oral route, for example, with *Toxocara canis* and *Toxocara cati* (visceral larva migrans), *Ancylostoma caninum* (dog hookworm), *Salmonella*, and *Campylobacter*.[3–6] Their behavior and small size also puts them at increased risk for bite-transmitted diseases such as rabies.

In adults, occupational hazards must be considered. Examples include anthrax in wool sorters, leptospirosis in dairy farmers and sewer workers, tularemia in trappers and hunters, and erysipeloid in fishers.

The species of the contact animal is important. Some zoonoses are highly host specific (e.g., *Taenia solium* in swine), whereas others have a broad range of hosts (e.g., salmonellosis in reptiles, birds, and mammals). Some monkey species (e.g., *Macaca*) in the wild are assumed to be infected with herpes B virus and are excluded from general research unless proper precautions can be taken.[7]

Whenever possible, a description or identification of an arthropod that bit someone should be obtained for help in anticipating or diagnosing zoonotic illness. A febrile illness after an *Ixodes dammini* tick bite in the northeastern United States would make one consider the possibility of Lyme disease or babesiosis. If the tick were *Dermacentor variablis* (dog tick), one would be concerned about Rocky Mountain spotted fever or tularemia.

Zoonotic infections are often limited to certain geographic areas, so a travel history is pertinent. For example, *Taenia saginata*, the beef tapeworm, is commonly transmitted in East Africa but is rare in cattle in the United States. *Trypanosoma cruzi*, the etiologic agent of Chagas disease, is found in South and Central America. It is rarely found in the United States. Glanders, a disease caused by *Pseudomonas mallei*, was once common throughout the world but is now found only in a few countries in Asia and Africa.

It is necessary to inquire where the animal came from and whether it was quarantined. Pet stores, zoos, laboratories, and livestock dealers import animals from foreign countries. Import regulations do not guarantee that the animals are free of exotic zoonoses. Outbreaks of Marburg and Ebola virus infections, transmitted from imported nonhuman primates, have been documented.[8, 9] Wild and domestic canids from regions enzootic for hydatid disease may carry adult *Echinococcus* tapeworms in their gut and become an imported source of human disease.[10]

It should be determined whether the animal has been vaccinated or tested for specific diseases. Dogs and cats should be vaccinated for rabies. Cattle are routinely tested for tuberculosis and brucellosis.

It is pertinent to inquire about the health of the contact animal before, during, and after human exposure. Signs of illness may be similar in human and animal (e.g., skin lesions in ringworm, neurologic signs in rabies). In such situations, demonstration of similar lesions or clinical history in the animal and person may help establish the diagnosis. It is also important to inquire as to whether the animal has given birth recently and whether there was a stillbirth, illness in the newborn, or evidence of an infected placenta (e.g., Q fever, *Leptospirosis* and *Brucella* infections).

For some diseases, the signs of illness may be totally different in humans and animals. For example, a cow transmitting bovine tuberculosis through her milk might have mastitis, whereas the infected person might have tuberculous spondylitis. Many animals with the potential to transmit zoonoses to humans may not appear ill at all. For example, in cats, *Bartonella henselae* bacteremia or *Toxoplasma gondii* infections are usually subclinical.[11]

The third zoonotic context occurs when a patient or a population is documented to have a zoonotic illness and it is necessary to trace the origin of the disease and to institute control and preventive measures. This often requires the cooperation of officials in agriculture or public health at the municipal, state, or federal level. An outbreak of cryptosporidiosis in Milwaukee affecting more than 400,000 people was caused by contamination of the water supply and the failure of authorities to monitor the turbidity of water in one of the city's water treatment plants.[12] In the southwestern United States, an outbreak of respiratory failure with a high mortality rate was traced within months to a new strain of *Hantavirus*.[13] Using polymerase chain reaction technology, molecular biologists were able to determine that the virus was transmitted by aerosolized excreta from local field mice.[14]

Transmission of Zoonoses

Discussion of zoonoses according to their route of transmission is useful in establishing occupational preventive medicine programs, for example, in zoos, veterinary hospitals, stockyards, and laboratories. It is also important in establishing public health guidelines in matters such as the care of animals and the inspection and preparation of food. Tables 169–1 through 169–7 are organized by means of transmission, with some examples and appropriate preventive measures.

Zoonotic Diseases in Immunocompromised Patients

Is your patient with human immunodeficiency virus infection or any other immunodeficiency at risk by owning a pet?

TABLE 169–1 ■ Zoonoses Transmitted by Bite or Scratch

BACTERIA	VIRUSES	FUNGI
Pasteurella multocida *Bartonella henselae* *Spirillum minus* *Streptobacillus moniliformis* *Francisella tularensis* *Yersinia pestis*	Rabies virus Lymphocytic choriomeningitis virus	*Sporothrix schenckii*

Prevention:
1. Reduce risk with proper animal-handling techniques.
2. Wash all bites and scratches as soon as possible.
3. Animal workers or travelers at risk need rabies preexposure prophylaxis and checks of serum immunity every other year.

TABLE 169–2 ■ Zoonoses Transmitted by Direct Contact or Contact with Products of Conception, Urine, Blood, Saliva, and Feces

BACTERIA	VIRUSES	FUNGI	HELMINTHS	OTHER
Bacillus anthracis *Brucella* spp. *Francisella tularensis* *Coxiella burnetii* *Pasteurella multocida* *Leptospira* spp. *Mycobacterium marinum* *Yersinia pestis*	Herpes B virus Vesicular stomatitis virus Orthopoxvirus (monkeypox) Parapoxvirus (orf) Marburg and Ebola viruses	*Microsporum canis* *Trichophyton mentagrophytes*	*Ancylostoma* spp.	*Sarcoptes scabei* var. *canis*

Prevention:
1. Reduce risk by prompt diagnosis, isolation, and treatment of infected animals.
2. With animal contact, use good hand washing, gloves, aprons, and protective clothing. Preferably, wash clothes at work.
3. Clean and disinfect fomites.
4. Use special care when assisting with animal deliveries, surgery, necropsy, and slaughterhouse work.

There have been many reviews of this issue.[15–17] A number of diseases transmitted by pets are particularly serious in immunocompromised patients. The risks can be lowered as long as the pet owners use good hygiene after touching their pets, avoid handling the feces, and take the animal promptly to the veterinarian if it gets sick.

T. gondii oocysts can be shed in the feces of cats (usually kittens) and spread to those in contact with the cat litter or infected soil. Most human infections, however, are due to consumption of cysts in undercooked lamb or pork. Most infections in immunocompromised patients in the United States are a reactivation of a latent infection. It is prudent for patients at risk (including pregnant women) to know their *Toxoplasma* titer and, if susceptible, use extreme caution when cleaning the litter box. The owner should attempt to limit the possibility of infection in the cat by keeping it inside and feeding it well-cooked food, or dry or canned food.[18]

Bacillary angiomatosis is caused by *B. henselae* and *Bartonella quintana*.[11] It is a rare disease even among immunocompromised patients. It can be transmitted by a cat scratch or possibly a bite from an infected flea. Cat owners should make sure that their cats are protected from fleas. Any scratches should be cleaned promptly with soap and water. Risks of *Bartonella* infection are diminished in cats older than 1 year of age. Immunocompromised cat owners must be aware that any unusual skin lesions should be examined promptly by a physician.

A number of zoonotic diarrheal illnesses are associated with significant morbidity in immunocompromised persons. The risks of transmission can be minimized by avoiding contact with animal feces.

Cryptosporidiosis is known to be transmitted from infected farm animals and from contamination of drinking water. Dogs and cats have been shown to shed the organism occasionally, but there is no evidence that having these pets at home increases the likelihood of developing this illness. The younger the pet, the greater the potential for infection. Animals with diarrhea should be removed from the house. A pet owner purchasing a puppy or kitten may wish to have the animal's stool screened for *Cryptosporidium*.[18] Giardiasis may also be present in household pets, but it is unlikely the pet owner is at a significantly increased risk for infection.

Campylobacter and *Salmonella* species are present in many animal species, any of which could potentially spread disease to immunocompromised patients. The most common route of infection is from contaminated and poorly cooked food.

TABLE 169–3 ■ Fecal-Oral Transmission of Zoonoses

BACTERIA	HELMINTHS	PROTOZOA
Salmonella spp. *Shigella* spp. *Escherichia coli* O157:H7 *Campylobacter* spp. *Yersinia pseudotuberculosis* *Yersinia enterocolitica*	*Toxocara canis, Toxocara cati* *Echinococcus* spp.	*Giardia lamblia* *Cryptosporidium* spp. *Toxoplasma gondii* *Baylisascaris procyonis* *Trichostrongylus*

Prevention:
1. Reduce risk as for direct contact (see Table 169–2).
2. Use face mask when hosing cages.
3. Avoid eating, drinking, or smoking in potentially contaminated areas.
4. Culture or examine stools of potentially infectious animals, especially if they have diarrhea.

TABLE 169–4 ■ Zoonoses Transmitted by Consumption of Infected Meat, Poultry, Fish, and Dairy Products

BACTERIA	HELMINTHS	PROTOZOA
Salmonella spp. *Yersinia* spp. *Campylobacter* spp. *Shigella* spp. *Escherichia coli* O157:H7 *Brucella* spp. *Bacillus anthracis* *Vibrio parahaemolyticus* *Francisella tularensis* *Listeria monocytogenes* *Streptobacillus moniliformis*	*Taenia solium* *Trichinella spiralis* *Taenia saginata* *Diphyllobothrium latum* *Anisakis* *Clonorchis sinensis* *Angiostrongylus cantonensis* *Opisthorchis* spp. *Paragonimus* spp. *Capillaria philippinensis*	*Toxoplasma gondii*

Prevention:
1. Use sanitary milking procedures, dairy inspection, mastitis control, brucellosis and tuberculosis testing of dairy animals, and pasteurization of milk.
2. Institute rodent control on farms (to reduce *Salmonella* and *Trichinella* in livestock), sanitary human sewage disposal (to reduce cysticercosis in cattle and swine), meat inspection, proper refrigeration and freezing of meat.
3. Prevent salmonellosis by washing eggs and disposing of cracked eggs.
4. Instruct the public about the need for adequate cooking of all animal products.

TABLE 169–5 ■ Respiratory Transmission of Zoonoses

BACTERIA	VIRUSES
Mycobacterium tuberculosis	Rabies virus
Bacillus anthracis	Influenza virus (swine, humans)
Coxiella burnetii	Lymphocytic choriomeningitis virus
Yersinia pestis	*Hantavirus*
Rhodococcus equi	
Pseudomonas mallei	
Chlamydia psittaci	
Francisella tularensis	
Pasteurella multocida	
Brucella spp.	

Prevention:
1. Reduce risk with use of face masks and proper air circulation and filtration (e.g., in laboratories).
2. Test primates and cattle for tuberculosis. Tuberculin-positive animals are usually killed; rarely is any attempt made to treat them.

TABLE 169–7 ■ Zoonotic Risks for Patients with Immunodeficiency

BACTERIA	PROTOZOA	FUNGI
Salmonella (dog, cat, bird)	*Toxoplasma* (cat)	*Cryptococcus*
Campylobacter (dog, cat)	*Cryptosporidium* (dog, cat)	
Bartonella (cat)		
Rhodococcus (horse)*		
Mycobacterium avium (bird)*		
Mycobacterium marinum (fish)		

*More often from soil or other environmental sources.

Campylobacter infection in humans has also been associated with contact with infected dogs and cats, and *Salmonella* infection in humans has been associated with infected pet birds, turtles, lizards, dogs, and cats. Animals with diarrhea should be taken to the veterinarian. Puppies and kittens may be at higher risk of carrying these infections than older animals.

Inhalation has been considered the primary route of infection by *Cryptococcus* and *Rhodococcus. Mycobacterium avium* complex infections are thought to enter via the gastrointestinal tract or the lungs. *Cryptococcus neoformans* is present in areas polluted with pigeon and other wild bird excrement. Patients who are immunocompromised should refrain from exposure to areas that may be contaminated with bird feces. *M. avium* complex infections occur in pet birds, but birds are rarely the source of infection in immunocompromised patients. *Rhodococcus equi* infection is rare, even in immunocompromised patients. The organism is probably transmitted from the soil more frequently than it is transmitted directly from farm animals.

Home aquariums have been documented as the source of infections by *Mycobacterium marinum.*[19] In immunocompromised patients at risk for disseminated disease, use of gloves is recommended.

Is your patient with an immunodeficiency at risk of developing a zoonotic illness while traveling? There is a risk associated with traveling, especially to developing countries, in patients who are immunodeficient. Patients should be fully immunized before travel; however, the response to immunization may be inadequate.

Extra care should be taken to avoid food-borne infections such as salmonellosis, especially because of the high incidence of bacteremia that occurs in human immunodeficiency virus–positive patients. This population also should be warned about the increased incidence of drug reactions to sulfa-containing medications, which may be prescribed for some of these gastrointestinal infections. Cryptosporidiosis is a concern in countries where water treatment does not exist. Use of a portable water filtration system would make good sense for the immunodeficient traveler. It is not guaranteed that bottled water is safer than tap water in many instances.

TABLE 169–6 ■ Arthropod-Borne Zoonoses

BACTERIA	VIRUSES	PROTOZOA	HELMINTHS
Tick-Borne			
Borrelia burgdorferi	Orbivirus (Colorado tick fever)	*Babesia microti*	
Borrelia spp.		*Babesia divergens*	
Ehrlichia chaffeensis			
Francisella tularensis			
Coxiella burnetii			
Rickettsia ricketsii			
Rickettsia spp.			
Mosquito-Borne			
	Flavivirus (yellow fever, St. Louis encephalitis)		*Brugia* spp.
	Bunyavirus (California and La Crosse encephalitis, Rift Valley fever)		*Dirofilaria immitis*
	Alphavirus (eastern and Venezuelan equine encephalitis)		
Other Insect or Mite			
Rickettsia akari (mite)		*Trypanosoma rhodesiense* (tsetse fly)	
Yersinia pestis (flea)		*Trypanosoma cruzi* (reduviid bug)	
		Leishmania spp. (sandfly)	

Prevention:
1. The risk of transmission can be reduced by wearing protective clothing, using insect repellants, and using environmental insecticides in an appropriate way.
2. Mosquito bed netting should be used in some areas.
3. Ticks should be removed as soon as possible.
4. Pets should be protected from flea and tick infestations.

Arthropod-borne infections pose a risk to patients with immunodeficiency. Inadequate antibody response to yellow fever vaccination puts travelers at risk for the development of disease in South America and Africa. Overwhelming parasitemia caused by *Babesia* species has been seen in asplenic patients and patients with human immunodeficiency virus infection. Immunodeficient patients traveling to areas where arthropod vectors of disease are present should take every precaution to limit the number of insect bites. Protective clothing, repellant with diethyltoluamide (DEET), and bed netting are recommended.

Research Areas and Conclusion

The need for, and benefit of, basic research is exemplified by work on the *Hantavirus* isolated in the southwestern United States in 1993.[14] Within months of its clinical appearance, this new virus was discovered along with an identification of its environmental reservoir and its mode of transmission.

Vaccines are available for yellow fever, Japanese encephalitis, anthrax, and Lyme disease (research stage). Recombinant rabies vaccines have been developed using vaccinia vectors carrying rabies glycoprotein.[20] After ingestion, the vaccine is protective in wild animals. Influenza researchers using yearlong worldwide surveillance can predict upcoming strains of virus for vaccine production.[21] Research is needed to develop vaccines to prevent or control other zoonoses.

We also need to provide adequate water purification, rubbish removal, and rodent and mosquito control. Public health inspections of the food industry are important to keep standards high. Animals from other countries need to be examined and possibly quarantined. The best protection from zoonoses is to ensure good hand washing after handling animals, to clean and cook all food well, and to use insect repellant and protective clothing in mosquito- and tick-infested areas. Education, especially for pet owners who have children or who are immunocompromised, is of great importance.

References

1. Morse SS: Examining the origins of emerging viruses. *In* Morse SS (ed): Emerging Viruses. New York, Oxford University Press, 1993, p 10.
2. McNeill WH: Patterns of disease emergence in history. *In* Morse SS (ed): Emerging Viruses. New York, Oxford University Press, 1993, pp 29–36.
3. Glickman LT, Schantz PM: Epidemiology and pathogenesis of zoonotic toxocariasis. Epidemiol Rev 3:230–250, 1981.
4. Croese J, Loukas A, Opdebeeck J, et al: Human enteric infection with canine hookworms. Ann Intern Med 120:369–374, 1994.
5. Alterkruse SF, Hunt JM, Tollefson LK, et al: Food and animal sources of human *Campylobacter jejuni* infection. J Am Vet Med Assoc 204:57–61, 1994.
6. Saeed AM, Harris NV, DiGiacomo RF: The role of exposure to animals in the etiology of *Campylobacter jejuni/coli* enteritis. Am J Epidemiol 137:108–114, 1993.
7. The B Virus Working Group: Guidelines for prevention of *Herpesvirus simiae* (B virus) infection in monkey handlers. J Med Primatol 17:77–83, 1988.
8. Peters CJ, Johnson ED, Jahrling PB: Filoviruses. *In* Morse SS (ed): Emerging Viruses. New York, Oxford University Press, 1993, pp 159–175.
9. Centers for Disease Control: Update: Filovirus infection in animal handlers. MMWR Morbid Mortal Wkly Rep 39:221, 1990.
10. Gamble WG, Segal M, Schantz PM, Rausch RL: Alveolar hydatid disease in Minnesota. First human case acquired in the contiguous United States. JAMA 241:904–907, 1979.
11. Koehler JE, Glaser CA, Tappero JW: *Rochalimaea henselae* infection: A new zoonosis with the domestic cat as reservoir. JAMA 271:531–535, 1994.
12. Mackenzie WR, Hoxie NJ, Proctor ME, et al: A massive outbreak in Milwaukee of *Cryptosporidium* infection transmitted through the public water supply. N Engl J Med 331:161–167, 1994.
13. Centers for Disease Control and Prevention: Update: Hantavirus pulmonary syndrome—United States, 1993. MMWR Morbid Mortal Wkly Rep 42:816–820, 1993.
14. Nichol ST, Spiropoulou CF, Morzunov S, et al: Genetic identification of a hantavirus associated with an outbreak of acute respiratory illness. Science 262:914–917, 1993.
15. Glaser CA, Angulo FJ, Rooney JA: Animal-associated opportunistic infections among persons infected with the human immunodeficiency virus. Clin Infect Dis 18:14–24, 1994.
16. Mayr B: Pets as permanent excretors of zoonoses pathogens. Zentralbl Hyg Umweltmed 194:214–222, 1993.
17. Parenti DM, Snydman DR: *Capnocytophaga* species: Infections in nonimmunocompromised and immunocompromised hosts. J Infect Dis 151:140–147, 1985.
18. USPHS/IDSA guidelines for the prevention of opportunistic infections in persons with human immunodeficiency virus: Disease-specific recommendations. Clin Infect Dis 21(Suppl 1):S32–S43, 1995.
19. Ries KM, White GL Jr, Murdock RT: Atypical mycobacterial infection caused by *Mycobacterium marinum* (Letter). N Engl J Med 322:633, 1990.
20. Ruppert CE, Wiktor TJ, Johnston DH, et al: Oral immunization and protection of raccoons *(Procyon lotor)* with a vaccinia-rabies glycoprotein recombinant virus vaccine. Proc Natl Acad Sci USA 83:7947–7950, 1986.
21. Kilbourne ED: Epidemiology of influenza. *In* Kilbourne ED (ed): Influenza Viruses and Influenza. New York, Academic Press, 1975, pp 483–538.

170

Rabies

James E. Childs
Donald Z. Noah
Charles E. Rupprecht

Rabies holds a special position in the universe of infectious diseases. The frightening circumstances leading to virus transmission, most often the bite from a "mad" dog, the fear of ensuing madness, and the nearly inevitable death that follows once clinical disease is apparent all contribute to the unique horror with which we regard rabies. It is a disease with one of the oldest pedigrees, recognizable as a malady of humans and animals from European, Middle Eastern, and Eastern texts dating from many centuries BC. Historical descriptions of the disease process have influenced the lexicon of modern microbiology; the Latin word *virus* means "poison" or "slimy liquid"[1] and was used to describe the saliva of rabid dogs, which was identified as an infectious material centuries ago.

Rabies has been eliminated as a significant cause of human death in developed areas of the world. It is the only disease for which a vaccine is usually employed after the exposure, although preexposure prophylaxis is recommended for certain high-risk groups. Treatment with modern tissue culture vaccines, coupled with the appropriate use of immune globulin, is regarded as essentially 100% effective. Yet rabies remains a constant threat and the cause of more than 35,000 potentially preventable deaths per year in the developing and underdeveloped world.[2] Where human rabies has been eliminated or greatly reduced from historical levels, the economic costs of maintaining the programs that control and prevent the chain of events leading to human disease are formidable and beyond the grasp of many nations struggling with a host of other epidemic diseases. Thus, human rabies is essentially a disease of poverty. The frustrations and conflict generated by the gap between scientific knowledge and product development and their practical public health applications are nowhere more evident than with rabies. It is a preventable disease that has not been, and may not be, prevented for the foreseeable future over much of the globe. Rabies is an ancient disease that continues to challenge the way public health is practiced.

History

The earliest known reference to rabies comes from the Eshnunna Code of Babylon from the 23rd century BC, which details the responsibility of a dog owner whose pet is involved in biting and causing the death of another human by rabies.[3] The Greeks Democritus and Aristotle, writing before 400 BC, provided detailed descriptions of dog rabies.[4] Rabies was called *lytta* or *lyssa* by the Greeks, meaning "madness," and the genus to which the rabies virus now belongs, *Lyssavirus*, derives its name from this ancient description. European and Middle Eastern authors were not alone in recognizing the clinical disease rabies and its association with dogs. In seventh century China, a record in the "Zuo Zhuan" Xiang Gong indicated that rabies prevention was effected by hunting rabid dogs.[5] Ge Hong (AD 281 to 341) observed the prolonged incubation period of rabies after a bite from a rabid dog and noted, "If no sickness occurs after a hundred days the patient can be considered safe from the illness."[5] Although much longer incubation periods are now recognized, these observations demonstrate that considerable knowledge of rabies was available in many cultures dating back thousands of years.

The history of rabies as a major cause of human disease is closely linked to the domestication of the dog. Although other carnivores, such as wolves, mongooses, and foxes, have played a role and continue to cause human exposures,[6] no animal other than the dog has assumed this central role in maintaining and transmitting rabies virus to humans. In the Americas, the earliest report of rabies came in 1703 from Mexico,[7] although fox rabies in Arctic regions may have been introduced across the Bering strait at earlier times.[8] By the mid-1700s, rabies was common from Massachusetts to Virginia, involving primarily dogs.[9] During the 18th century, rabies was a frequent occurrence among dogs in British and French colonies of the Caribbean, including Barbados, Jamaica, and Guadeloupe.[9] In South America, reports suggesting vampire bat–transmitted rabies date from the 1500s,[10] and dog rabies appeared in Peru in 1803[4] and in sporting dogs belonging to English officers in La Plata, Argentina, in 1806.[11] It is now apparent that most of the dog rabies encountered by colonialists in the New World was initially imported from Europe with the transportation of domestic dogs incubating the infection. Comparisons of enzootic variants of dog rabies viruses collected from Asia, Africa, Europe, and the Americas by sequence analysis of the nucleocapsid (N) gene revealed that over broad geographic regions (including Europe, Africa, and the Americas), the limited variation of rabies virus strongly suggested a common European origin.[12] Dogs have been imported into the New World since the 16th century[13]; most of the world is still suffering the repercussions of this early transportation of animals.

The development of effective rabies vaccines for humans and domestic animals is one of the major success stories in infectious disease control and prevention. Louis Pasteur and his colleagues developed a "fixed" virus of high virulence and short incubation period by serial intracerebral passages of wild-type or street virus in rabbits.[14] Through progressive attenuation of this virus in air-dried spinal cords of inoculated rabbits, Pasteur produced by a series of inoculations a refractory state in dogs to subsequent intracerebral challenge with fully virulent rabies virus. Of additional major significance, Pasteur also demonstrated that his vaccine, consisting of progressively less attenuated preparations, was effective when used on dogs previously inoculated with rabies, demonstrating efficacy of the vaccine in postexposure treatment. This vaccine was first used on a human, Joseph Meister, on July 6, 1885.[15] Meister survived, and similar treatments were used on thousands of exposed humans.[16] Fermi and Semple introduced two improvements on the nervous tissue vaccines of Pasteur that allowed greater standardization of production; phenol was used as an attenuating agent and tissues used for vaccine were harvested at the same attenuation level and used for all injections in the series. The Fermi and Semple vaccines, made from sheep and goat brain, respectively, as well as the later Fuenzalida suckling mouse brain vaccine, have been used extensively in the past 80 years and still represent the most widely used rabies vaccines in Asia, Africa, and Latin America (approximately 90% of vaccine made and reported to the World Health Organization [WHO]). However, the high probability of adverse reactions associated with nervous tissue–derived vaccines, including neurologic complications such as meningitis and meningoencephalitis,[17] gave added impetus to the development of highly immunogenic avian embryo– and cell culture–derived vaccines. Highly potent vaccines of tissue culture origin are now used to the exclusion of other rabies vaccines in developed nations, although the cost of these vaccines and the technology required to produce them have limited their availability in countries that require them most. The recommendation that immune globulin against rabies of human or equine origin should be given in conjunction with vaccine[18] to ensure efficacy approaching 100% was a milestone in the evolution of effective treatment, although the use of immune globulin was considered as early as the 19th century.

To date, the pathophysiology of rabies infection remains incompletely understood, although aspects of the molecular biology of viral replication and subsequent spread have been elucidated in detail. Some of the first observations of rabies at the cellular level were made in 1903 when Negri[19] published his observations on pathology and described the cytoplasmic inclusion bodies that bear his name. Experiments involving amputations or neurectomies indicated that virus remained at local wound sites for prolonged periods[20] and spread as an ascending infection via retrograde axoplasmic flow[21] to the central nervous system, followed by centrifugal peripheral (anterograde) neural spread.[22, 23] The absolute neurotropism of rabies virus has been questioned, because the initial site of replication may include myocytes in addition to neural tissue,[22] although direct entry into nervous tissue with only secondary replication in myocytes has been observed in a mouse model.[24] The long-term retention of virus within myocytes represents an attractive hypothesis to explain the long incubation periods that occur with rabies,[25] as has sequestering of virus in macrophages.[26] A putative rabies virus receptor has been identified in the nicotinic acetylcholine receptor,[27, 28] although this binding site may not be unique, as virus binds to cells lacking acetylcholine receptors.[29]

In the past two decades, a major leap in our understanding of the epidemiology of rabies has resulted from advances in the fields of immunology and molecular biology. In the late 1970s, monoclonal antibodies were used to demonstrate that antigenically unique variants of rabies virus circulate in different geographic areas and are usually associated with a primary reservoir species of carnivore or bat.[30–32] In the 1990s, genetic analyses utilizing the reverse transcription–polymerase chain reaction (RT-PCR) and nucleic acid sequencing have permitted greater elucidation of the variability and specificity of rabies virus–host coevolution and show promise in the area of disease diagnosis.[12, 33, 34] These analyses have fundamentally changed the understanding of how different rabies viral variants are maintained and transmitted in distinct geographic regions (see later). Finally, only within the past few decades have methods been developed and adapted to the industrial scale, permitting public health officials to consider eliminating rabies within some terrestrial wildlife reservoirs. The rabies virus glycoprotein was one of the first genes to be incorporated into the vaccinia virus genome.[35, 36] These genetic constructs are now delivered in oral baits to wildlife in Europe[37, 38] and the United States,[39, 40] an application of historic dimensions as the first use of a recombinant vaccine in the field. Research into rabies remains a dynamic field centuries after the disease was first described.

Epidemiology

Rabies is a zoonosis and is passed from human to human only under extraordinary circumstances. The epidemiology of human rabies is intimately linked to the cycles of virus maintenance in animals, and to understand the natural history of rabies that leads to human disease requires insight into wildlife ecology and animal behavior.[41] Domestic carnivores (dogs and cats) and wild carnivores (e.g., foxes, skunks, raccoons) are the major reservoirs of terrestrial variants of the rabies virus (Table 170–1). Rabies in humans or animals is almost always the result of a bite containing rabies virus in the saliva. Perhaps this tight linkage between animal rabies and human disease is best illustrated by the dramatic declines in human rabies that followed the initiation of effective animal control programs and the development of canine vaccines and vaccination campaigns.[2, 42] In the United States, the annual number of human rabies cases dropped from 100 per year during the early 1900s to 20 in 1951; during the past two decades, an average of less than one indigenously acquired case has been reported annually. The cases of indigenously acquired rabies in the United States since 1980 have been caused primarily by virus variants maintained by insectivorous bats and only rarely by variants associated with dogs. In some cases of human rabies determined to be of canine origin, laboratory and epidemiologic data indicate that the exposures were received outside the United States.[43, 44] This decrease in the occurrence of human and domestic dog rabies has been accomplished at a time when wildlife rabies is at historically high levels, with 8889 cases reported in 1993.[45] Thus, a central theme in the epidemiology of rabies has been established and used to guide our prevention strategies: effective control of dog-to-dog transmission prevents human disease. An immune barrier in dogs also blocks the chain of events that could result in indirect transmission of wildlife variants of rabies virus to humans. The cost of this barrier is not trivial; estimates exceed $300 million annually.[46]

In most areas of the world, accurate estimates of human rabies deaths or cases in animals are difficult to obtain because surveillance systems and regional laboratories are inadequate or nonexistent. Annual reports of 2000 human deaths in Bangladesh, 1014 in China, and 30,000 in India in the 1990s convey a sense of the magnitude of the problem.[2] In addition to deaths, 6.4 million persons received treatment for rabies exposure in the 60 of 92 rabies endemic countries reporting to the WHO in 1992.[17] Most of these individuals received vaccines of nervous tissue origin, which translates into thousands of potentially serious adverse reactions. The incidence of rabies is highest among males and among individuals younger than 20 years old.[47–50] Exposure to rabies has a seasonal and in some areas a cyclic component; cases of dog rabies occur most commonly in the spring or early summer[51, 52] and epizootics have a period of 5 years in Chile.[52] Bites to humans from dogs are also seasonal[53] and, like rabies,

TABLE 170–1 ■ Worldwide Distribution of Animal Rabies

GEOGRAPHIC REGION	PREDOMINANT ANIMAL CYCLE	MAJOR ANIMAL AFFECTED	COMMENTS
North America	Wildlife	Raccoons, foxes, skunks, bats	Of 8230 reported rabid animals in 1994, >92% wildlife in United States*
Central America (including Mexico and the Caribbean islands)	Domestic	Dogs; cats and farm animals secondarily; vampire bat and mongoose rabies locally	Dog bite accounted for approximately 95% of reported human rabies
South America	Domestic	Dogs; cats and farm animals secondarily; vampire bat rabies locally	Dog bite accounted for approximately 85% of reported human rabies
Africa	Domestic	Dogs; cats and farm animals secondarily	Dog bite accounted for approximately 96% of reported human rabies
Asia	Domestic	Dogs; cats and farm animals secondarily	Dog bite accounted for approximately 97% of reported human rabies
Europe (Western)	Wildlife	Foxes, badgers, stone martens, bats	Human cases split between domestic animal (50% of 14) and wildlife exposures
Europe (Eastern including Russian Federation)	Domestic	Dogs, cats, and farm animals	
Oceania	Domestic	Dogs; cats and farm animals secondarily	Dog bite accounted for approximately 100% of reported human rabies

*Krebs JW, et al, unpublished data.
Except where noted, based on 1992 data from World Health Organization: World Survey of Rabies 28 for Year 1992. Geneva, World Health Organization, 1994, p 24.

usually involve children.[54] The risk of developing disease depends on the anatomic site and severity of the bite, the species inflicting the wound, and the virus variant (see later). However, in the United States a clear history of animal bite has not been obtained in 19 of 25 cases occurring between 1980 and 1995. The indication that unnoticed or trivial contact with bats may result in rabies transmission to humans has resulted in the additional recommendation to treat individuals when bat bite cannot be ruled out[55] (Fig. 170–1).

Although the animal bite remains the most important route of rabies virus transmission, cases of human rabies have been described after a variety of exposures. The best documented reports of human-to-human transmission involved eight recipients of transplanted corneas in France,[56] the United States,[57] Thailand,[58] India,[59] and Iran.[60] Although human transplacental transmission of rabies virus has been reported in a single case,[61] infants have survived delivery from mothers infected with rabies, when the child received postexposure treatment.[62] Rabies infection presumably acquired by aerosol has been described in two persons visiting Frio cave in Texas, where millions of Mexican free-tailed bats congregate and rabies virus is present in the bat population.[63, 64] Experimental studies with animals support the possibility of aerosol transmission under these exceptional circumstances.[65]

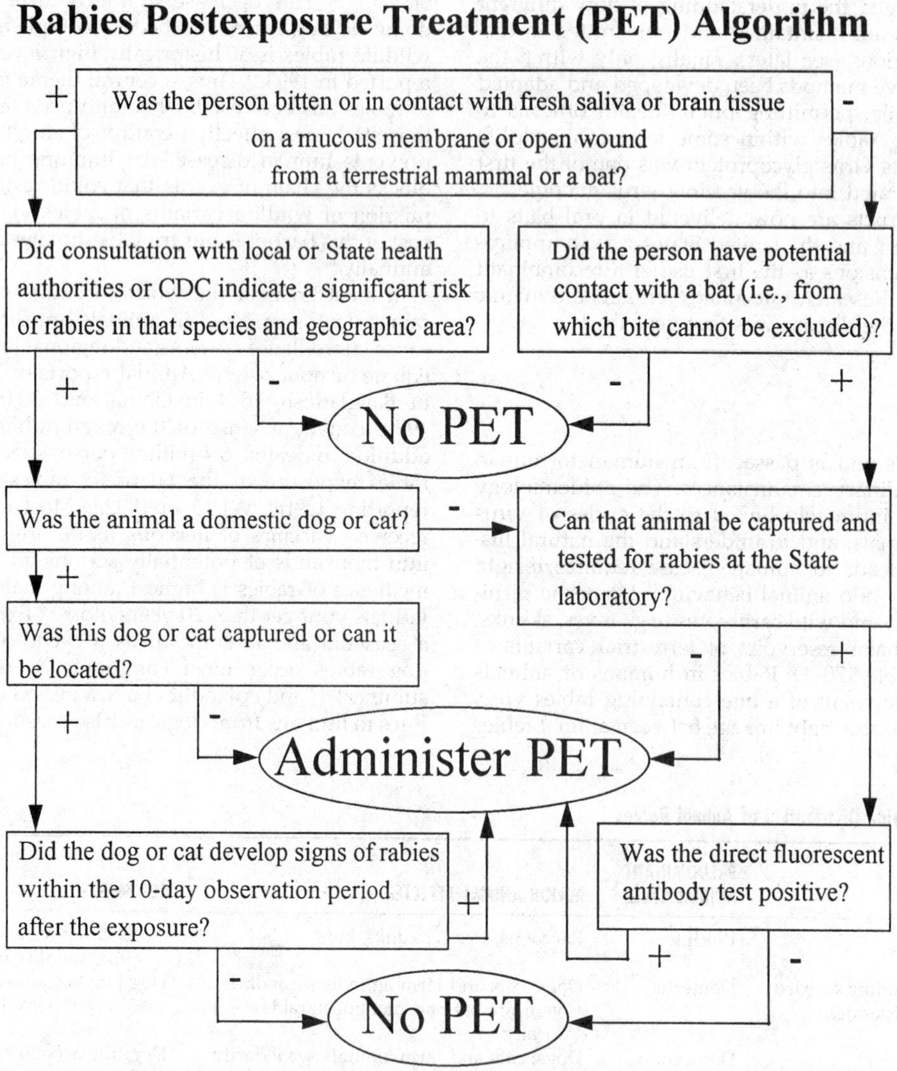

NOTES:

1. Unless person previously received rabies immunoprophylaxis, PET consists of 5 doses (IM in the deltoid region) of HDCV or RVA on days 0,3,7,14, and 28 and 1 dose of HRIG (divided between IM in the gluteal region and at the bite site) on day 0.
2. This algorithm only addresses rabies prevention. Obviously, other treatments such as wound care and antibiotics may be indicated.
3. In the event that the biting animal is captured and tests negative for rabies after PET has begun, PET may be discontinued.

FIGURE 170–1 □ An algorithm for the administration of rabies postexposure prophylaxis. PET, Postexposure treatment; CDC, Centers for Disease Control and Prevention; RVA, rabies vaccine absorbed; HDCV, human diploid cell vaccine; IM, intramuscularly; HRIG, human rabies immune globulin. (Adapted with permission from Fishbein DB: Rabies in humans. *In* Baer GM [ed]: The Natural History of Rabies, ed 2. Boca Raton, FL, CRC Press, 1991, pp 519–549. Copyright © 1991 CRC Press, Boca Raton, Florida.)

Laboratory exposure to aerosols has also resulted in infection.[66] There is little documentation for natural rabies transmission by simple contact with virus-laden saliva or tissue,[67] although isolated reports suggest infection after butchering of infected carcasses.[68, 69] Scratches from a rabid animal could potentially be contaminated with virus shed in saliva and in the United States are treated as an exposure, but documented cases of this injury leading to rabies are rare.[68, 70, 71]

In developing areas of the world, domestic dog rabies remains the most serious problem and results in tens of thousands of deaths and millions of postexposure treatments.[48, 68] Preliminary data suggest that the prevalence of rabies in free-ranging dogs can reach 10% in cities such as Bangkok[72]; in countries with enzootic canine rabies, past recommendations that advocated withholding postexposure treatment until a dog developed clinical rabies during a 10- to 14-day quarantine period are being abandoned in favor of treatment because of the high probability of rabies in dogs and the shorter incubation after bites.[72, 73] Control of dog rabies in developing countries has been difficult to achieve for economic[74] as well as cultural[41] reasons. For example, in the Philippines and China[68] dogs may be raised for food; in the Philippines some dog owners even refused free vaccine because they believed it might adversely affect the flavor of the meat (Robinson L, unpublished data, 1994). However, when large-scale canine vaccine campaigns are mounted in developing countries, they have the same dramatic effect on terminating epidemics of human and canine rabies.[75, 76] Vaccines designed for oral uptake and delivered in baits show promise for immunizing free-ranging dogs in developing countries.[77–79]

Although dogs may in certain circumstances survive rabies infection and carry virus asymptomatically in their tonsils,[80] this finding has not been shown to be epidemiologically important. Dogs can be naturally infected with two other lyssaviruses, Mokola[81] and Lagos bat,[82] but a significant role as reservoirs or vectors has not been suggested.

Wildlife species involved in rabies cycles vary with region, but virus variants associated with terrestrial mammals are maintained primarily by carnivores. In North America, raccoons, skunks, foxes, and bats (several species) are the major wildlife reservoirs of rabies. Less is known about terrestrial wildlife reservoirs in Latin America, although vampire bat–transmitted rabies, which affects cattle and occasionally humans, is of special concern in some regions from northern Mexico to northern Argentina.[83, 84] Mongooses on some islands in the Caribbean (e.g., Puerto Rico), introduced to control rats and snakes in sugarcane fields, have provided a wildlife reservoirs for rabies.[85] Globally, rabies and other *Lyssavirus* infections of bats are widespread and, although transmission cycles are distinct from those of terrestrial rabies, can spill over to terrestrial mammals.

Rabies in animals is a density-dependent disease. Population dynamics of reservoir hosts are regarded as critical to understanding the temporal and spatial patterns of wildlife rabies.[86, 87] Rabies epizootics in European red foxes spread across the landscape in an apparent wavelike fashion, with the area experiencing the current epizootic as the crest and the locale with depleted reservoir host populations the trough.[88] Environmental factors, including habitat heterogeneity, play a major role in the rate of spread and persistence of the disease.[89, 90] Furthermore, multispecies interactions complicate the understanding of the ecology and epidemiology of rabies.[91] Spillover of infection from the dominant reservoir of a region to other species is well documented,[45] but the processes by which new epizootics and variants of rabies virus emerge in different reservoir species are unknown. After epizootic rabies has abated, terrestrial reservoir populations are decreased. Reports of animal rabies in a given locale can decline precipitously; rabies may disappear from regions for some time before reappearing. Some countries have eliminated or remain free of rabies for extended periods[17] (Table 170–2).

Rabies viruses isolates from different geographic areas can be antigenically and genetically variable; five antigenic variants from terrestrial carnivores are currently defined by monoclonal antibody analysis from 10 distinct, although occasionally geographically overlapping, areas of enzootic rabies in the United States[45, 92] (Fig. 170–2). European isolates of rabies from terrestrial mammals are predominantly the red fox rabies virus variant.[30]

Rabies virus variants circulating in bats are antigenically and genetically distinct from those associated with terrestrial carnivores and indicate largely independent transmission cycles of rabies.[93, 94] Rabies has been reported in more than 30 species of bats in the United States since the 1950s and occurs in each of the contiguous 48 states.[95] Variants of rabies virus associated with bats have been responsible for 12 of 25 cases of human rabies reported from the United States since 1980. The rabies variant most commonly associated with human cases is recovered primarily from silver-haired bats,[94] a species rarely encountered or tested.[96] Two cases of human infection with rabies-related viruses have been reported from Europe.[97] The viruses in European bats have been shown to be genetically unique, and perhaps most similar to Duvenhage virus,[97] and may constitute two unique genotypes of *Lyssavirus*.[98] There have been scattered reports of "rabid" bats from Asia, and bats infected with other lyssaviruses are found in Africa, but no isolates of rabies virus, serotype 1, have been collected from bats from either continent.[99]

Clinical Presentation

The clinical presentation of rabies is commonly reported as falling into one of two categories—"furious" and "paralytic" or "dumb."[100–104] The description given here of rabies deemphasizes that dichotomy, as the distinction between these two forms is often unclear. Persons with rabies commonly present with a combination of symptoms, and attempts to distinguish between furious and paralytic forms may not serve to aid the diagnosis. Human disease resulting from exposures to the same animal species, and even the same

TABLE 170–2 ■ Countries Not Reporting Animal or Human Rabies in 1992*

GEOGRAPHIC REGION	COUNTRIES
Americas	Bahamas, Barbados, British Virgin Islands, Cook Islands, French Polynesia, St. Vincent and Grenada, Uruguay, Vanuatu
Africa	Djibouti, Lesotho, Libyan Arab Jamah, Mauritius, Seychelles
Asia	Bahrain, Indonesia, Kuwait, Maldives, Taiwan
Europe	Cyprus, Denmark, Finland, Gibraltar, Greece, Iceland, Ireland, Malta, Norway (except Svalbard Island group), Portugal, Spain (except Ceuta/Melilla), Sweden, United Kingdom
Oceania	Australia, Fiji, Hong Kong, Japan, Malaysia (island), New Caledonia, New Zealand, Niue island, Papua New Guinea, Republic of Korea, Singapore, Solomon Islands, Tonga

*Surveillance for rabies varies by country. Inclusion in this table does not necessarily indicate rabies-free status.

Based on 1992 data from World Health Organization: World Survey of Rabies 28 for Year 1992. Geneva, World Health Organization, 1994, p 24.

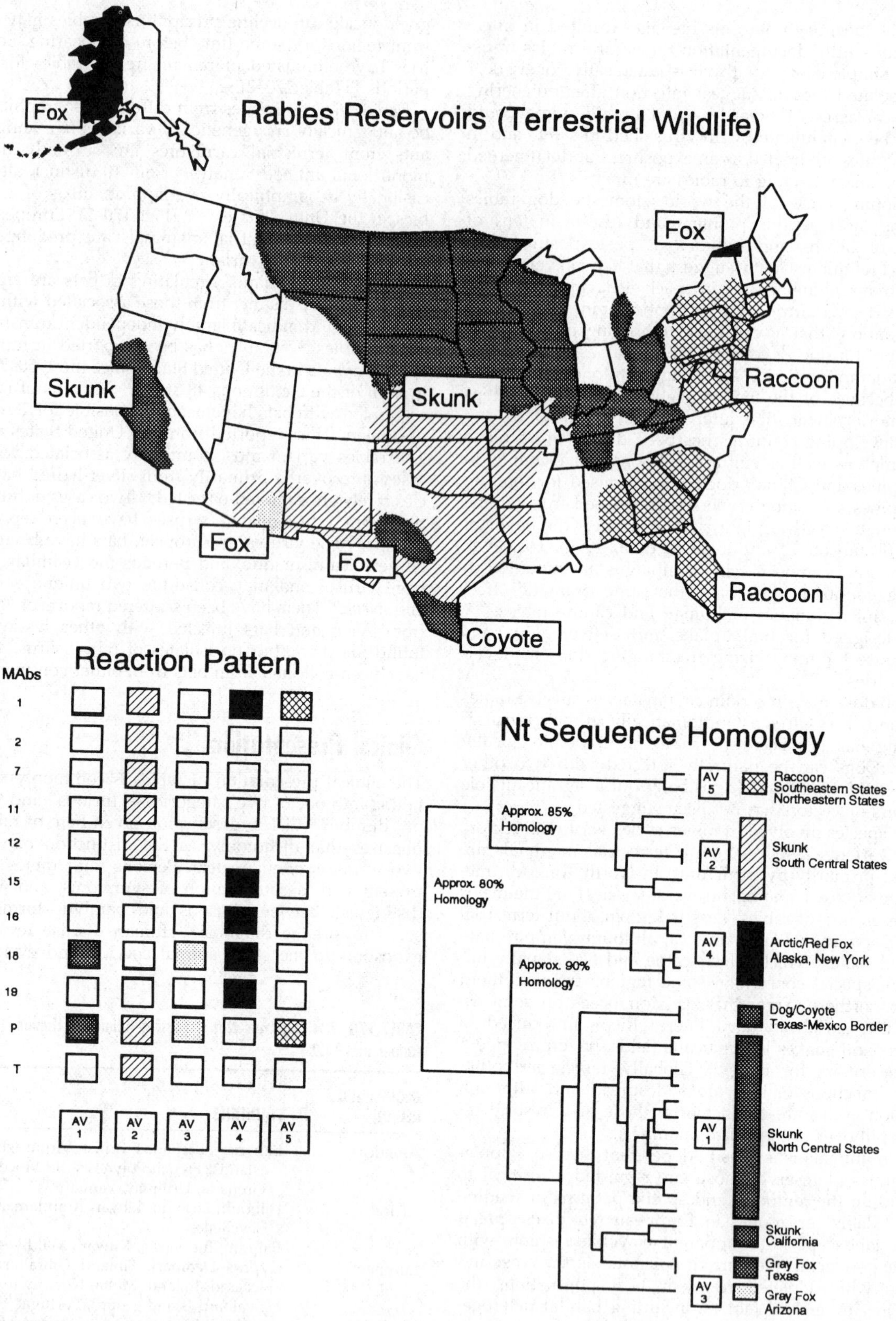

FIGURE 170–2 □ Distribution of five antigenically distinct rabies virus variants and the predominant terrestrial carnivores affected in the United States. Filled boxes to the left indicate negative reactions of monoclonal antibodies (MAbs) used for typing. The genetic variability of these antigenic variants is demonstrated in the tree to the right. AV, Antigenic variant; Nt, nucleotide.

animal, has resulted in cases with both clinical presentations, further clouding the distinction.[104] Therefore, the true determinant of human clinical presentation may be more dependent on inherent host factors than on animal species source or virus virulence.[102, 105]

The course of human rabies infection generally progresses through five clinical phases[106]: incubation, prodrome, neurologic phase, coma, and either death or recovery. The temporal lines separating phases are indistinct; however, each phase is marked by differentiating clinical presentations (Table 170–3).

Incubation

Although the usual period of incubation of rabies is 30 to 90 days, this phase is highly variable.[48, 100, 104, 106] In the extremes, incubation periods from 5 days to more than 19 years have been reported, but the chance of unknown or unreported exposures must be considered in these cases.[25]

The period of incubation seems dependent on several factors. First, the site of virus inoculation is important. Victims of head and neck attacks from rabid animals tend to experience shorter incubations than those experiencing more peripheral attacks.[48, 103, 106] Second, the quantity of virus introduced into a wound (generally paralleling the severity of the attack) is inversely proportional to the incubation period. Third is the relative innervation of the inoculation site. Victims sustaining attacks in highly innervated areas, such as the face, hands, or genitalia, commonly exhibit shorter incubation times.[100, 103] Fourth, the age of the victim is directly proportional to the incubation time as illustrated by the fact that children generally progress more quickly through the clinical stages.[100, 103, 106] Finally, virus virulence and host immune status undoubtedly play important, although as yet undetermined, roles in disease progression. The administration of a full or partial course of postexposure treatment did not appear to alter the incubation period among those who subsequently developed rabies.[48, 105, 107]

Prodrome

After the subclinical incubation period, the prodrome is the phase of initial (but nonspecific) symptoms. Manifested by a combination of local and systemic symptoms lasting from several hours to several days, they are not pathognomonic for rabies and usually serve to direct the clinician's initial diagnostic efforts away from rabies. A common symptom is pain, numbness, or tingling at or near the inoculation site.[100, 101, 103, 105, 106] Additional manifestations may include vomiting, abdominal pain, muscle pain, weakness, and general malaise (fever, chills, headache).[100, 101, 103, 104, 106] Both local and systemic signs are probably due to the virus' initial appearance, and subsequent replication, in dorsal root ganglia and the central nervous system.[106] The nonspecific nature of the initial presentation of the disease coupled with the relative rarity of rabies in developed countries helps to explain why many rabies diagnoses are made only post mortem.[44, 108]

Neurologic Phase

The neurologic phase begins when central nervous system dysfunction dominates the clinical picture and generally lasts from 2 to 7 days. Hyperactivity and restlessness are common early manifestations, which progress to marked agitation and nervousness. Extreme nervousness is perhaps the salient sign that initially resulted in the description as furious.

Hydrophobia presents in variable degrees and may not be initially obvious. Rather than a true fear of water, the response more probably represents a respiratory tract reflex resulting from central nervous system dysfunction. In addition to the mere proximity to water or liquid, reflex gagging and muscle fasciculations may be triggered by an attendant's touch or even the threat of being touched, especially on the head or neck. Mental status continues to deteriorate until sudden death or coma results.

Ascending paralysis similar to that in Guillain-Barré syndrome is a less common manifestation of rabies,[100, 102, 105, 106, 109] in which mental status is preserved until much later in the clinical course and, although average survival times are longer than in the more common hyperactive form, the disease runs an invariably fatal course.[101, 103, 105] This clinical presentation occurs only rarely in the United States, and no clear molecular or epidemiologic explanation for this difference in presentation has been described. Finally, cardiac involvement with or without accompanying cardiovascular signs[110–113] and sexual manifestations such as penile hyperexcitability and priapism have been reported.[114–116]

Tetanus, delirium tremens, poliomyelitis, Guillain-Barré syndrome, herpesvirus encephalitis, and arbovirus encephalitis should be differentiated from rabies early in the clinical course to focus treatment efforts and to minimize exposures among attending medical personnel.

Coma

Heralded by apneustic breathing patterns, this phase is reached when the central nervous system dysfunction results in generalized paralysis.

TABLE 170–3 ■ Hypothetic Human Rabies Clinical Time Line

	EXPOSURE Incubation*	FIRST SYMPTOM Prodrome*	FIRST NEUROLOGIC SIGN Neurologic Phase*	COMA ONSET Coma*	DEATH OCCURS OR RECOVERY BEGINS Recovery*
Usual duration	30–80 d (variable)	Hours to days	2–7 d	0–14 d	Months
Main clinical signs	None	Fever Anorexia, nausea, vomiting Headache Malaise, lethargy Pain or paresthesia at site Anxiety, agitation Depression	Hyperventilation Hypoxia Aphasia Incoordination Paresis, paralysis Pharyngeal spasms Hydrophobia Marked hyperactivity Confusion, delirium Hallucinations	Pituitary dysfunction Hypoventilation Apnea Hypotension Cardiac arrhythmias Cardiac arrest Coma Pneumothorax Intravascular thrombosis Secondary infections	

*Clinical phases.
Modified from Hattwick MAW: Human rabies. Public Health Rev 3:229–274, 1994.

Death or Recovery

Death related to cerebral or cardiovascular dysfunction follows coma within hours or a few days unless intensive medical assistance is available. In 25 human cases in the United States since 1980, the average time from onset of clinical signs to death was 15.7 days (range 6 to 32 days).

There have been only four recorded instances of recovery from clinical rabies. The first involved a 6-year-old boy who developed clinical rabies 20 days after being bitten on the thumb by a bat and 2 days after completing a 14-day course of duck embryo vaccine prophylaxis.[117] After a partial coma of 7 days' duration, he experienced a progressive improvement to full neurologic capacity.

The second was a 45-year-old woman who developed rabies 21 days after being severely bitten by a dog.[118] She also had received 12 daily doses of suckling mouse brain rabies vaccine. She recovered during a 13-month period.

The third case was a 32-year-old male laboratory technician who developed rabies approximately 45 days after exposure to modified live rabies vaccine and work with a laboratory strain of rabies virus.[119] Residual neurologic impairment remained after recovery.

The final case was a 9-year-old boy who was severely bitten by an infected dog 17 days before the development of symptoms.[120] The boy was treated with Vero rabies vaccine and a final dose of human diploid cell vaccine (HDCV), but no immune globulin was administered. Although saliva, corneal impressions, and nuchal biopsy specimens were negative for rabies virus isolation or antigen testing, cerebrospinal fluid (CSF) antibody indicated a diagnosis of rabies. Severe neurologic sequelae persist.

Treatment of Clinical Rabies

Intensive therapy for rabies patients is costly and nearly always futile, and some physicians have questioned its rationale.[121] Nevertheless, such therapeutic efforts can delay the disease progression, and care providers continue to gain experience in preventing and controlling the many presenting complications.

Early consideration of rabies as a differential diagnosis is essential in anticipating these complications and instituting isolation procedures for the protection of attending medical personnel.[104, 122, 123] These isolation precautions should be aimed at preventing contact with potentially infectious body fluids including saliva, CSF, tears, and centrifuged urine.[106, 122, 124] Blood and feces are not considered infectious.[122, 124]

Once the neurologic phase is reached, intensive care and isolation become necessary.[123] Because of the altered mentation and involuntary muscle activity associated with rabies, sedation and analgesia are important, but they do not alter the clinical course. Respiratory, cardiovascular, and neurologic complications require the most therapeutic attention (Table 170–4). A common neurologic complication is increased intracranial pressure. Potential causes include cerebral edema resulting from viral inflammation; cerebral edema caused by hypoxia; and viral inflammation of the brain stem resulting in localized swelling, occlusion of the cerebral aqueduct, and internal hydrocephalus.[106] When hypoxia is successfully managed, cerebral edema does not seem to be a problem.[106]

Death most commonly results from the complications of hypoxemia, cardiac arrhythmias, cerebral edema, fluid imbalance, and hypotension.[121] The concurrent presentation of multiple complications further frustrates therapy. Iatrogenic and nosocomial complications may appear at any time, although they are most common during the coma phase.[106] These include thrombosis of the superior vena cava secondary to indwelling cardiac catheters, bilateral tension pneumothorax secondary to cardiac resuscitation, and opportunistic bacterial infections during prolonged disease progression.[106]

Intravenous and intrathecal ribavirin therapy has not proved successful against human rabies infections.[104, 125] Similarly, vaccine and immune globulin administration, initiated after the onset of clinical signs, has not shown any positive effect and may quicken the disease progression.[121, 122, 126] Finally, although high-dose interferon alfa has not altered the eventual outcome,[125] its use may delay the clinical progression, thus allowing more intensive and specific therapies.[121, 122]

Laboratory Diagnosis

In most countries of the world the majority of human and animal rabies cases reported to the WHO are diagnosed solely on the basis of clinical presentation.[17] This section deals with laboratory methods used to confirm a clinical diagnosis.

The diagnosis of human rabies depends on the isolation of virus or the demonstration of viral antigen or nucleic acid in saliva, corneal impressions, or tissue biopsy material or the finding of specific antibody in serum (of previously unvaccinated persons) or in CSF.[127] Fluorescent antibody methods for antigen detection are the best available tests for the rapid diagnosis of rabies, and since the 1980s the use of monoclonal antibodies has allowed further epidemiologic typing of rabies viruses by their antigenic profiles.[30, 31, 128, 129] Virus isolation remains an important complement to direct fluorescent antibody (DFA) testing and provides material to further characterize the isolate. Nucleic acid–based detection systems using RT-PCR amplification are theoretically more sensitive than is antigen-based detection and are being used by many laboratories as investigational new diagnostic tests,[33, 108, 130] but their cost, analysis time, and potential for contamination are drawbacks.

Virus isolation from infected tissues, saliva, throat swabs, and swabs of the nasal mucosa or eyes can be achieved by using a variety of cell lines or by direct intercerebral inoculation of laboratory rodents.[131] The preferred cell line in the United States is mouse neuroblastoma,[132] although BHK-21, CER, and WI-38 lines are also employed. Virus isolated in culture is usually further identified in infected cells by the DFA test, but genetic assays may be employed. Infected tissues may also be examined with hematoxylin-eosin or the Mann stain for the presence of pink-, lilac-, or red-staining cytoplasmic inclusions (Negri bodies).[19] Negri bodies are pathognomonic for rabies; however, they are not present or are difficult to locate in some cases and may be confused with other viral inclusions in some species (e.g., the Lentz bodies of canine distemper[131]). Intracerebral mouse inoculation using the specimens previously mentioned is a reliable method for isolating rabies virus and was the "gold standard" for rabies diagnosis to which DFA and cell culture isolation were compared. Weanling mice are preferred and should be checked daily until day 28 for paralysis, which typically occurs between days 5 and 12.[131, 133] Confirmation of rabies in mice is usually performed with the DFA test on brain tissue.

The most widely used diagnostic test is the DFA test for detection of rabies antigen contained in intracytoplasmic inclusions, but cellular morphology may not be preserved by all preparations.[134] The test requires a microscope with an ultraviolet source and therefore the cost may be prohibitive for some laboratories, but the sensitivity (compared with intracerebral inoculation of mice) and specificity approach 100% when guidelines for its use are followed.[134, 135] When it is applied ante mortem, the materials most commonly tested

TABLE 170–4 ■ Complications and Interventions in Human Rabies

COMPLICATION	INTERVENTION
Neurologic	
Hyperactivity	Thorazine, diazepam
Hydrophobia	Nothing by mouth
Focal seizures	Phenytoin (Dilantin), diazepam
Localized neurologic signs	None
Cerebral edema	Diuretics, intraventricular catheterization
Aerophobia	Avoid stimulation
Extreme excitation	Avoid stimulation, protect from injury
Pituitary	
Increased antidiuretic hormone	Fluid restriction
Diabetes insipidus	Fluid balance, vasopressin (Pitressin) or furosemide
Pulmonary	
Hyperventilation	None
Hypoxemia	Airway maintenance (tube, tracheostomy with suction), oxygen, ventilation, positive end-expiratory pressure, blood gas monitoring
Atelectasis	Mechanical ventilation
Apnea	Mechanical ventilation
Pneumonia	Respiratory therapy, antibiotics, turn q 2 h
Pneumothorax	Reexpansion
Cardiovascular	
Arrhythmias	Oxygen therapy, drugs as indicated
Hypotension	Fluid balance, drugs as indicated
Congestive heart failure	Fluid restriction, drugs as indicated
Arterial or venous thrombosis	Heparin
Superior vena cava obstruction	Prevention
Cardiac arrest	Resuscitation
Other	
Anemia	Transfusion
Gastrointestinal bleeding	Transfusion
Hyperthermia	Cooling mattress
Hypothermia	Heating blankets
Hypo- or hypervolemia	Fluid balance
Paralytic ileus	Parenteral fluids
Urinary bladder paralysis	Catheterization
Acute renal failure	Hemodialysis
Abnormal biting or chewing	Protect tongue (airway or padded tongue blade)

Data from Fishbein,[121] Hattwick,[106] and Bernard.[122]

are skin biopsy specimens (frequently obtained from the neck or scalp where the density of hair follicles is high[136, 137]) and corneal impressions.[138, 139] A positive test result with these specimens is adequate to confirm a diagnosis of rabies, but a negative finding does not exclude the diagnosis. In a series of 40 rabies patients studied in India, positive corneal impressions were obtained from only 13 cases (32.5%); patients with longer incubation times were more likely to have a positive result.[140] The sensitivity of all assays varies with the laboratory, the timing of specimen collection with regard to disease onset and viral dissemination, and the condition of the specimens when tested.[141] For optimal postmortem diagnosis of rabies, samples of the hippocampus, cerebellum, and brain stem or spinal cord from both sides of the cerebrum should be tested.[134] Monoclonal antibodies applied to fresh-frozen tissues can be used to characterize the antigenic variant responsible for infection and provide inferences about the animal species responsible for the exposure. Other labeled antibodies, such as with horseradish peroxidase, have been applied to the diagnosis of rabies with good results[142–144]; these methods have the advantage of employing conventional microscopy.

Serologic tests that measure antibody binding (e.g., indirect fluorescent antibody or enzyme immunoassay tests) or function (e.g., complement fixation or neutralization) can be useful in the diagnosis of human or animal rabies. Assays exist that readily distinguish between immunoglobulin G and immunoglobulin M.[145] The finding of antibody in CSF can be an indication of intrathecal production and interpreted as indicating central nervous system infection. The finding of CSF antibody with oligoclonal bands has been used to support a documented human survival from rabies.[120] Care must be taken in interpreting CSF results because of the risk of introducing serum antibody into the sample during the procedure and leakage across the blood-brain barrier.[137] Binding assays, such as the indirect fluorescent antibody test or enzyme immunoassay, may be more sensitive than neutralizing assays in detecting early antibody,[146] which in three patients appeared 6 to 7 days before neutralizing antibody was detected.[145] Serologic methods are also employed in documenting the immune response after rabies vaccination and in monitoring the immunologic status of individuals in high-risk professions to determine the necessity for boosters.[55] In the United States, the test of choice is the rapid fluorescent focus inhibition test,[147] a modified standard neutralization assay that replaced the in vivo mouse neutralization test; antibody titers can be converted to international units. Successful immunization is measured by the presence of a titer of 1:5 or greater (complete neutralization) with this fluorescent inhibition test, or approximately 0.5 IU, in sera collected 2 to 4 weeks after preexposure or postexposure prophylaxis.[55]

Nucleic acid detection (based on RT-PCR) potentially offers considerable advantages in sensitivity over other assay systems and may be the test of choice for slightly decomposed tissue.[130] Single-step and nested RT-PCR methods have been developed.[130, 148] The added advantage of obtaining DNA fragments that can be sequenced and analyzed with existing databases of rabies virus variants is also appealing, as this method discriminates between virus variants that are identical by monoclonal antibody techniques.[12, 34] RT-PCR has already taken a place in many diagnostic laboratories as a complementary, but not a replacement, diagnostic and epidemiologic tool. The specialized equipment, expense of reagents, and potential for contamination of samples limit the widespread use of these methods in many laboratories without strong research missions.

Prevention

Prevention of rabies is best achieved by eliminating human exposure to rabid animal vectors through both effective vaccination programs for domestic species and education concerning the hazards of contact with certain wildlife. Mention has already been made of the effectiveness of rabies control efforts aimed at canine populations in both developed and developing nations. This section concentrates on pre- and postexposure prophylaxis of individuals potentially exposed to the rabies virus and emerging methods for control of rabies in wildlife reservoirs.

Human-to-human transmission of rabies through the transplantation of corneas has been well documented, and recommendations for prevention exist.[149] Transmission through bites, saliva, or other contact with humans is poorly documented and best prevented by the early consideration of rabies in any patient with clinical encephalitis and initiation of contact isolation to exclude exposure to the patient's infectious tissues or fluids.[124] Laboratory transmission of rabies is preventable through preexposure prophylaxis and appropriate biosafety recommendations.[150] The overwhelming majority of individuals who receive immunotherapy for prevention of rabies are vaccinated after the exposing event. Because the most important route of rabies transmission is through animal bite, essential prevention therapy begins with the careful cleansing of the wound with a 20% solution of soap and water (or the cationic detergent benzalkonium chloride).[55, 151, 152] The first problem facing the care provider is to assess the need for treatment (Table 170–5; see Fig. 170–1) and whether treatment should be initiated immediately (e.g., is the biting animal a healthy dog or cat available for 10-day quarantine or a wild animal unavailable for testing?). If treatment is required, human rabies immune globulin (HRIG) and the first of five vaccine doses are administered simultaneously.[55] Equine immune globulin is less expensive than HRIG and is used in many parts of the world. The new purified equine immune globulin is considered a safe and effective product, although adverse reactions such as serum sickness are reported in 1% to 6% of recipients, depending on the product manufacturer.[153, 154] HRIG is administered at 20 IU/kg and equine immune globulin at 40 IU/kg, with up to one half the dose infiltrated around the wound sites. HRIG should never be administered in the same syringe or at the same anatomic site as vaccine. If HRIG administration is delayed, it can be used up through day 7 after the initial vaccine dose[55] but is not indicated after that because of potential interference with normal immune responses.[155] Two vaccines, HDCV and rabies vaccine absorbed, are licensed for pre- and postexposure treatment in the United States and either can be used in the postexposure regimens described in Table 170–5.[55] It is important for physicians in the United States to recognize that the recommendations of the Advisory Committee on Immunization Practices for rabies postexpo-

TABLE 170–5 ■ Postexposure Treatment (PET) Guide for the United States (ACIP) and Other Countries (WHO)*

	EXPERT COMMITTEES	
GUIDELINE	**ACIP**	**WHO**
Categories for assessing need for PET	Two categories considered, bite and nonbite. PET warranted if potential exposure to rabies virus by either route. Bite includes any penetration of skin. Nonbite exposures include scratches, abrasions, open wounds, or mucous membrane contaminated with saliva or other potentially infectious material (such as brain) from a rabid animal.	Three categories of exposure (I–III). Category I (touching or feeding of rabid animal or licks on intact skin) does not warrant PET. Category II includes nibbling of uncovered skin, minor scratches or abrasions without bleeding, or licks on broken skin. Category III includes single or multiple transdermal bites or scratches or contamination of mucous membrane with saliva.
Recommended use of rabies immune globulin	Always given as part of PET, except when appropriate or proven effective preexposure prophylaxis has been previously given (see Table 170–6). Only products of human origin (HRIG; 20 IU/kg body weight) used in the United States.	Only given immediately with category III exposures. Both equine (40 IU/kg body weight) and human (20 IU/kg) products are recommended.
Use of rabies vaccine	Always part of PET and given intramuscularly. Can be halted if subsequent information indicates that animal is not rabid.†	Administered immediately with category II and III exposures. Can be given intradermally with rabies immune globulin. Can be halted if subsequent information indicates that animal is not rabid.†
Vaccine regimens	If previously vaccinated, then HRIG is not administered and vaccine (HDVC or RVA) is given at 1.0 mL on d 0 and 3 (see Table 170–6). If not previously vaccinated, HRIG is administered and vaccine is given at 1.0 mL on d 0, 3, 7, 14, and 28. Vaccine is never given intradermally.	Various tissue culture or purified duck or chick embryo vaccines are considered appropriate. A schedule similar to that of ACIP and an abbreviated schedule are recognized for 1.0-mL intramuscular applications. An intradermal schedule using 0.1 mL of vaccine is also appropriate. For nervous tissue–derived vaccines, national authorities must be consulted.

*ACIP, Advisory Committee on Immunization Practices; WHO, World Health Organization; HRIG, human rabies immune globulin; HDCV, human diploid cell vaccine; RVA, rabies vaccine adsorbed.

†If a previously healthy dog or cat is involved in the biting incident, treatment can be delayed in some situations and in some countries during a 10-d observation period. If the dog or cat remains healthy during the 10-d incubation period, treatment can be stopped. If the animal is killed, tested for rabies, and found to be negative, treatment can be stopped.

Data from Centers for Disease Control[55] and World Health Organization.[156]

sure treatment differ from those promulgated by the WHO.[156] HRIG is used whenever vaccine is warranted according to Advisory Committee on Immunization Practices guidelines but restricted to category III exposures by the WHO.

Preexposure prophylaxis (Table 170–6) is offered only to individuals in high-risk occupational groups (veterinarians, animal handlers, and certain laboratory workers) and persons spending more than 1 month in countries where canine rabies is endemic.[55] Preexposure vaccination does not eliminate the need for wound treatment and vaccination after exposure; however, the requirement for HRIG is obviated and the postexposure series is reduced to two 1.0-mL doses (see Table 170–5). Booster doses of vaccine are recommended for some individuals who have received the preexposure series if their serum antibody titer falls to less than 1:5[55] (see Table 170–5). There is no requirement to test serum directly after the preexposure series, as numerous studies have indicated nearly 100% immunologic response[55, 157]; immunity is long term, perhaps lifelong in many recipients, and repeated boosters offer an additional measure of security.[158]

Although not necessarily cost-effective,[159] the preexposure prophylaxis of travelers is a luxury that many individuals choose; in a survey of foreign travelers to Thailand, dog bite and dog lick were experienced by 1.3% and 8.9%, respectively, of more than 1800 persons traveling a mean of 17 days in country.[160] An important complication for preexposure vaccination that is most relevant to foreign travelers is the effect of antimalarial drugs (e.g., chloroquine phosphate) on the development of the immune response.[161, 162] The 1.0-mL intramuscular route of vaccination should be employed, with individuals receiving concurrent chloroquine, or the intradermal 0.1-mL schedule should be completed before antimalarial prophylaxis begins.[55]

Postexposure protection achieved by proper wound treatment and use of modern tissue culture–derived vaccines with immune globulin is considered near 100%.[157] However, postexposure vaccine failures have been reported when immune globulin has not been given[18] or when inadequate wound care, delay of immunoprophylaxis, or improper administration of immune globulin has occurred.[163] Surgery under ketamine anesthesia, possibly resulting in depression of the immune response, may also contribute to postexposure treatment failure.[164] Strict adherence to recognized protocols for rabies management is critical.[46, 165] Elderly, obese, or immunocompromised individuals may not respond optimally to rabies preexposure (or postexposure) immunization, and a sixth dose of vaccine has been suggested for individuals older than 50 years.[166] Young age[55] and pregnancy[167] are not reasons to withhold treatment.

Both local and systemic adverse reactions are reported in pre- and postexposure vaccinations. Local reactions among recipients of HDCV and HRIG include pain, redness, swelling, and itching; systemic reactions include fever, nausea, vomiting, lethargy, anorexia, general malaise, headache, immune complex–like disease, and rarely Guillain-Barré syndrome.[168–172] Local reactions have been reported among 19% to 74% of recipients, whereas systemic reactions have been reported among 5% to 40% of recipients.[55, 169–171, 173] Local reactions are usually manifested within a day or two, but the usual period between immunization and onset of systemic reactions is within 21 days, although periods of 45 days and 5 months have been reported.[168, 174, 175]

Common local adverse reactions are treated symptomatically, if at all, and only rarely justify discontinuation of preventive immunotherapy.[176]

Systemic reactions seem to occur without relation to age, route, or timing of primary or booster vaccination, history of allergies, or history of immunization with products other than HDCV.[177] As with local reactions, systemic reactions rarely preclude the necessity of continuing with a postexposure treatment regimen.

The ultimate prevention strategy for rabies is to eliminate the infection in animal reservoirs. Although control programs aimed at domestic animal populations dramatically reduce human deaths, they are expensive and must be maintained indefinitely in countries like the United States, where wildlife rabies is a constant threat. The successful use of modified live rabies vaccines designed for oral immunization and distributed in baits to immunize red foxes in Europe has demonstrated the potential to control terrestrial cycles of rabies.[178, 179] Efforts to control fox and skunk rabies in Ontario, Canada, are promising and illustrate the difficulties in designing control programs when multiple species are involved.[180] Recombinant rabies vaccines are now being used against red foxes in several countries in Europe,[37, 38, 181] raccoons in several states in the eastern United States,[182] and coyotes in Texas.[183]

The Future

It has been more than 20 years since the advent of the HDCV, which revolutionized rabies postexposure treatment, but the

TABLE 170–6 ■ Preexposure Prophylaxis Requirements and Schedules*

REQUIREMENT FOR PREEXPOSURE IMMUNIZATION	ROUTE	SCHEDULE
Preexposure vaccination should be given if exposure is continuous (e.g., rabies research laboratory workers, rabies biologics production workers), frequent (rabies diagnostic laboratory workers, mammalogists, spelunkers, veterinarians and staff; animal control and wildlife workers in rabies epizootic areas; travelers visiting foreign areas of enzootic rabies for more than 30 d), or in some cases infrequent (veterinarians and animal control and wildlife workers in areas of low endemicity or veterinary students).	IM	HDCV or RVA, 1.0 mL in deltoid region on d 0, 7, and 21 or 28
	ID	HDCV, 0.1 mL on d 0, 7, and 21 or 28
Routine boosters after primary series†	IM	HDCV or RVA, 1.0 mL in deltoid area on d 0
	ID	HDCV, 0.1 mL on d 0
Postexposure treatment for previously vaccinated persons	IM	HDCV or RVA, 1.0 mL in deltoid area on d 0 and 3; HRIG or other immune globulins not administered

*ID, Intradermal; IM, intramuscular; RVA, rabies vaccine adsorbed.

†For continuous exposures, booster is recommended if the antibody titer falls below 1:5 by rapid fluorescent focus inhibition testing done at 6-mo intervals. For frequent exposures, serologic testing and boosting, if necessary, are done at 2-y intervals.

Data from Centers for Disease Control: Rabies prevention—United States, 1991. Recommendations of the Immunization Practices Advisory Committee (ACIP). MMWR Morbid Mortal Wkly Rep 40(RR-3):1, 1991.

majority of the world continues to use multiple inoculations of neural tissue–based biologics.[184] Although the HDCV and its modern progenitors from Vero cells and avian embryo–derived sources were important advances,[185] issues of cost and availability are matters of major concern. Potent, safe, and inexpensive human rabies vaccines are still needed throughout the world. Less expensive but equally efficacious replacements for immune globulins of human or animal origin are also necessary, perhaps via murine, humanized, or human monoclonal antibodies.[186] This development depends on identifying conserved *Lyssavirus* epitopes of immunologic relevance, to limit the number of hybridomas contained within any treatment "cocktail," without sacrificing efficacy or cost. The current Advisory Committee on Immunization Practices 5-dose cell culture vaccine treatment protocol is a major improvement over the required 14 to 28 doses of neural vaccines of the past century, but in the near future it may be feasible to reconsider a further reduction in schedules and the potential elimination of immune globulin; if efficacious cytokine inducers or related immune mediators[187] are identified as the critical elements of human immunoprotection against rabies, a single inoculation with protection of lifetime duration may be within reach.

Concomitant with a heightened focus on prevention of rabies among humans should be increased concentration on disease control in the animal reservoirs. Currently, wildlife rabies constitutes the ultimate source of most human and domestic exposures in the United States, Canada, and much of Europe. Research has progressed rapidly on the development of attenuated and genetically engineered vaccines for rabies in the past three decades. These products show great promise of being safe and effective oral vaccines for foxes, raccoons, and related wild carnivores, with more than 70 million doses delivered over 5 million km^2 to date.[188] However, little attention has been paid to the feral dog in the same capacity, despite the paramount role of canine rabies in human mortality. In contrast to the more than half-dozen different vaccine types used in the field for wildlife, only two biologics have demonstrated preliminary oral efficacy in the dog under laboratory conditions.[189] Given the close relationship between humans and domestic animals, additional safety considerations are inherent in the environmental release of organisms intended for canine use. Once this challenge is met, oral vaccination of the free-ranging dog may become a critical adjunct to traditional parenteral induction of herd immunity in the pariah animal.

References

1. Webster's Ninth New Collegiate Dictionary. Springfield, MA, Merriam-Webster, 1989.
2. World Health Organization: Report of the Symposium on Rabies Control in Asian Countries. Geneva, World Health Organization, 1993, p 42.
3. Tierkel ES: Rabies. Adv Vet Sci 5:183, 1959.
4. Steele JH, Fernandez PJ.: History of rabies and global aspects. *In* Baer GM (ed): The Natural History of Rabies, ed 2. Boca Raton, FL, CRC Press, 1991, p 24.
5. Yu WZ: Notes on Chinese medical history. J Tradit Chin Med 5:232, 1985.
6. Fleming G: Animal Plagues. London, Bailliere, 1882.
7. Malága-Alba A: Factores epidemiologicos que rigen el control de la rabia. Bull Pan Am Health Organ 53:105, 1962.
8. Blancou J, Aubert MFA, Artois M.: Fox rabies. *In* Baer GM (ed): The Natural History of Rabies, ed 2. Boca Raton, FL, CRC Press, 1991, p 290.
9. Fleming G: Rabies and Hydrophobia. London, Chapman & Hall, 1872.
10. Baer GM.: Vampire bat and bovine paralytic rabies. *In* Baer GM (ed): The Natural History of Rabies, ed 2. Boca Raton, FL, CRC Press, 1991, p 403.
11. Malága-Alba A: Rabies in wildlife in middle America. J Am Vet Med Assoc 130:386, 1957.
12. Smith JS, Orciari LA, Yager PA, et al: Epidemiologic and historical relationships among 87 rabies virus isolates as determined by limited sequence analysis. J Infect Dis 166:296, 1992.
13. Varner JG, Varner JJ: Dogs of Conquest. Norman, OK, University of Oklahoma Press, 1983, p 238.
14. Pasteur L: Nouvelle communication sur la rage. C R Acad Sci 98:457, 1884.
15. Pasteur L: Méthode pour prévenir la rage après morsure. C R Acad Sci 101:765, 1885.
16. Perrin P, Lafon M, Sureau P: Rabies vaccines from Pasteur's time up to experimental subunit vaccines today. Adv Biotechnol Processes 14:325, 1990.
17. World Health Organization: World Survey of Rabies 28 for Year 1992. Geneva, World Health Organization, 1994, p 24.
18. Devriendt J, Staroukine M, Costy F, et al: Fatal encephalitis apparently due to rabies. JAMA 248:2304, 1982.
19. Negri A: Beitrag zum Studium der Aetiologie der Tollwurth. Z Hyg Infektionskr 43:507, 1903.
20. Baer GM, Cleary WF: A model in mice for the pathogenesis and treatment of rabies. J Infect Dis 125:520, 1972.
21. Tsiang H: Evidence for an intraaxonal transport of fixed and street rabies virus. J Neuropathol Exp Neurol 38:286, 1979.
22. Murphy FA, Bauer SP, Harrison AK, et al: Comparative pathogenesis of rabies: Viral infection and transit from inoculation site to the central nervous system. Lab Invest 28:361, 1973.
23. Tsiang H, Lycke E, Ceccaldi PE, et al: The anterograde transport of rabies virus in rat sensory dorsal root ganglia neurons. J Gen Virol 70:2075, 1989.
24. Shankar V, Dietzschold B, Koprowski H: Direct entry of rabies virus into the central nervous system without prior local replication. J Virol 65:2736, 1991.
25. Charlton KM: The pathogenesis of rabies and other lyssaviral infections: Recent studies. Curr Top Microbiol Immunol 187:95, 1994.
26. Ray NB, Ewalt LC, Lodmell DL: Rabies virus replication in primary murine bone marrow macrophages and in human and murine macrophage-like cell lines: Implications for viral persistence. J Virol 69:764, 1995.
27. Burrage TG, Lentz TL, Moreno K, et al: Binding of rabies virus to sites of high acetylcholine receptor density on cultured chick myotubes. J Cell Biol 91:86A, 1981.
28. Lentz TL, Burrage TG, Smith AL, et al: The acetylcholine receptor as a cellular receptor for rabies virus. Yale J Biol Med 56:315, 1983.
29. Reagan KJ, Wunner WH: Rabies virus interaction with various cell lines is independent of the acetylcholine receptor. Arch Virol 84:277, 1985.
30. Sureau P, Rollin P, Wiktor TJ: Epidemiologic analysis of antigenic variations of street rabies virus: Detection by monoclonal antibodies. Am J Epidemiol 117:605, 1983.
31. Rupprecht CE, Glickman LT, Spencer PA, et al: Epidemiology of rabies virus variants. Differentiation using monoclonal antibodies and discriminant analysis. Am J Epidemiol 126:298, 1987.
32. Smith JS, Reid Sanden FL, Roumillat LF, et al: Demonstration of antigenic variation among rabies virus isolates by using monoclonal antibodies to nucleocapsid proteins. J Clin Microbiol 24:573, 1986.
33. Sacramento D, Bourhy H, Tordo N: PCR technique as an alternative method for diagnosis and molecular epidemiology of rabies virus. Mol Cell Probes 5:229, 1991.
34. Nadin-Davis SA, Casey GA, Wandeler AI: A molecular epidemiological study of rabies virus in central Ontario and western Quebec. J Gen Virol 75:2575, 1994.
35. Wiktor TJ, Macfarlan RI, Reagan KJ, et al: Protection from rabies by a vaccinia virus recombinant containing the rabies virus glycoprotein gene. Proc Natl Acad Sci USA 81:7194, 1984.
36. Kieny MP, Lathe R, Drillien R, et al: Expression of rabies virus glycoprotein from a recombinant vaccinia virus. Nature 312:163, 1984.
37. Pastoret PP, Brochier B, Languet B, et al: First field trial of fox vaccination against rabies using a vaccinia-rabies recombinant virus. Vet Rec 123:481, 1988.

38. Brochier B, Kieny MP, Costy F, et al: Large-scale eradication of rabies using recombinant vaccinia rabies vaccine. Nature 354:520, 1991.
39. Rupprecht CE, Wiktor TJ, Johnston DH, et al: Oral immunization and protection of raccoons *(Procyon lotor)* with a vaccinia-rabies glycoprotein recombinant virus vaccine. Proc Natl Acad Sci USA 83:7947, 1986.
40. Rupprecht CE, Hanlon CA, Hamir AN, et al: Oral wildlife rabies vaccination: Development of a recombinant rabies vaccine. Trans North Am Wildl Natl Res Conf 57:439, 1992.
41. Wandeler AI, Budde A, Capt S, et al: Dog ecology and dog rabies control. Rev Infect Dis 10(Suppl 4):S684, 1988.
42. Beran GW, Frith M: Domestic animal rabies control: An overview. Rev Infect Dis 10(Suppl 4):S672, 1988.
43. Smith JS, Fishbein DB, Rupprecht CE, et al: Unexplained rabies in three immigrants in the United States. A virologic investigation. N Engl J Med 324:205, 1991.
44. Centers for Disease Control and Prevention: Human rabies—Miami, 1994. MMWR Morbid Mortal Wkly Rep 43:773, 1994.
45. Krebs JW, Strine TW, Smith JS, et al: Rabies surveillance in the United States during 1993. J Am Vet Med Assoc 205:1695, 1994.
46. Fishbein DB, Arcangeli S: Rabies prevention in primary care. A four-step approach. Postgrad Med 82:83, 1987.
47. Bhatia R, Bhardwaj M, Sehgal S: Canine rabies in and around Delhi—A 16 years study. J Commun Dis 20:104, 1988.
48. Lakhanpal U, Sharma RC: An epidemiological study of 177 cases of human rabies. Int J Epidemiol 14:614, 1985.
49. Eng TR, Fishbein DB, Talamante HE, et al: Urban epizootic of rabies in Mexico: Epidemiology and impact of animal bite injuries. Bull World Health Organ 71:615, 1993.
50. Swaddiwudhipong W, Tiyacharoensri C, Singhachai C, et al: Epidemiology of human rabies post-exposure prophylaxis in Bangkok, 1984–1986. Southeast Asian J Trop Med Public Health 19:563, 1988.
51. Kappus KD: Canine rabies in the United States, 1971–1973: Study of reported cases with reference to vaccination history. Am J Epidemiol 103:242, 1976.
52. Ernst SN, Fabrega F: A time series analysis of the rabies control programme in Chile. Epidemiol Infect 103:651, 1989.
53. Beck AM, Loring H, Lockwood R: The ecology of dog bite injury in St. Louis, Missouri. Public Health Rep 90:262, 1975.
54. Bhanganada K, Wilde H, Sakolsataydorn P, et al: Dog-bite injuries at a Bangkok teaching hospital. Acta Trop (Basel) 55:249, 1993.
55. Centers for Disease Control: Rabies prevention—United States, 1991. Recommendations of the Immunization Practices Advisory Committee (ACIP). MMWR Morbid Mortal Wkly Rep 40(RR-3):1, 1991.
56. Centers for Disease Control: Human-to-human transmission of rabies via a corneal transplant—France. MMWR Morbid Mortal Wkly Rep 29:25, 1980.
57. Houff SA, Burton RC, Wilson RW, et al: Human-to-human transmission of rabies virus by corneal transplant. N Engl J Med 300:603, 1979.
58. Centers for Disease Control: Human-to-human transmission of rabies via corneal transplant—Thailand. MMWR Morbid Mortal Wkly Rep 30:473, 1981.
59. Gode GR, Bhide NK: Two rabies deaths after corneal grafts from one donor. Lancet 2:791, 1988.
60. WHO: Two rabies cases following corneal transplantation. Wkly Epidemiol Rec 44:330, 1994.
61. Sipahioglu U, Alpaut S: Transplacental rabies in humans (in Turkish). Mikrobiyol Bul 19:95, 1985.
62. Lumbiganon P, Wasi C: Survival after rabies immunisation in newborn infant of affected mother (Letter). Lancet 336:319, 1990.
63. Irons JV, Eads RB, Grimes JE, et al: The public health importance of bats. Tex Rep Biol Med 15:292, 1957.
64. Humphrey GL, Kemp GE, Wood EG: A fatal case of rabies in a woman bitten by an insectivorous bat. Public Health Rep 75:317, 1960.
65. Constantine DG: Rabies transmission by nonbite route. Public Health Rep 77:287, 1962.
66. Winkler WG, Fashinell TR, Leffingwell L, et al: Airborne rabies transmission in a laboratory worker. JAMA 226:1219, 1973.
67. Leach CN, Johnson HN: Human rabies with special reference to virus distribution and titer. Am Soc Trop Med Hyg 20:335, 1940.
68. Kureishi A, Xu LZ, Wu H, et al: Rabies in China—Recommendations for control. Bull World Health Organ 70:443, 1992.
69. Tariq WU, Shafi MS, Jamal S, Ahmad M: Rabies in man handling infected calf (Letter). Lancet 337:1224, 1991.
70. Tuncman ZM: A rare case of rabies without a bite. Trop Dis Bull 46:139, 1949.
71. Babes V: Traité de la Rage. Paris, Bailliere, 1921, p 119.
72. Wilde H, Chutivongse S, Hemachudha T: Rabies and its prevention. Med J Aust 160:83, 1994.
73. Wilde H, Choomkasien P, Hemachudha T, et al: Failure of rabies postexposure treatment in Thailand. Vaccine 7:49, 1989.
74. Bogel K, Meslin FX: Economics of human and canine rabies elimination: Guidelines for programme orientation. Bull World Health Organ 68:281, 1990.
75. Chomel B, Chappuis G, Bullon F, et al: Mass vaccination campaign against rabies: Are dogs correctly protected? The Peruvian experience. Rev Infect Dis 10(Suppl 4):S697, 1988.
76. Belotto AJ: Organization of mass vaccination for dog rabies in Brazil. Rev Infect Dis 10(Suppl 4):S693, 1988.
77. Perry BD, Johnston DH, Jenkins SR, et al: Studies on the delivery of oral rabies vaccines to wildlife and dog populations. Acta Vet Scand Suppl 84:303, 1988.
78. Haddad N, Ben Khelifa R, Matter H, et al: Assay of oral vaccination of dogs against rabies in Tunisia with the vaccinal strain SADBern. Vaccine 12:307, 1994.
79. Frontini MG, Fishbein DB, Garza Ramos J, et al: A field evaluation in Mexico of four baits for oral rabies vaccination of dogs. Am J Trop Med Hyg 47:310, 1992.
80. Fekadu M, Shaddock JH, Chandler FW, et al: Rabies virus in the tonsils of a carrier dog. Arch Virol 78:37, 1983.
81. Foggin CM: Mokola virus infection in cats and a dog in Zimbabwe. Vet Rec 113:115, 1983.
82. Mebatsion T, Cox JH, Frost JW: Isolation and characterization of 115 street rabies isolates from Ethiopia by using monoclonal antibodies. J Infect Dis 166:972, 1992.
83. Pawan JL: The transmission of paralytic rabies in Trinidad by the vampire bat (*Desmodus rotundus murinus* Wagner, 1840). Ann Trop Med Parasitol 30:101, 1936.
84. Lopez A, Miranda P, Tejada E, et al: Outbreak of human rabies in the Peruvian jungle. Lancet 339:408, 1992.
85. Everard CO, Everard JD: Mongoose rabies. Rev Infect Dis 10(Suppl 4):S610, 1988.
86. Bacon PJ: Population Dynamics of Rabies in Wildlife. New York, Academic Press, 1985, p 358.
87. Clark WR, Fritzell EK.: A review of population dynamics of furbearers. *In* McCollough DR, Barett RH (eds): Wildlife 2001: Populations. London, Elsevier, 1992, p 910.
88. Bogel K, Moegle F, Knorpp F, et al: Characteristics of the spread of a wildlife rabies epidemic in Europe. Bull World Health Organ 54:433, 1976.
89. Carey AB, Giles RH Jr, McLean RG: The landscape epidemiology of rabies in Virginia. Am J Trop Med Hyg 27:573, 1978.
90. Wandeler AI, Capt S, Gerber H, et al: Rabies epidemiology, natural barriers and fox vaccination. Parassitologia 30:53, 1988.
91. Carey AB, McLean RG: The ecology of rabies: Evidence of co-adaptation. J Appl Ecol 20:777, 1983.
92. Smith JS: Rabies virus epitopic variation: Use in ecologic studies. Adv Virus Res 36:215, 1989.
93. Smith JS: Monoclonal antibody studies of rabies in insectivorous bats of the United States. Rev Infect Dis 10(Suppl 4):S637, 1988.
94. Baer GM, Smith JS: Rabies in nonhematophagous bats. *In* Baer GM (ed): The Natural History of Rabies, ed 2. Boca Raton, FL, CRC Press, 1991, p 366.
95. Constantine DG: An updated list of rabies-infected bats in North America. J Wildl Dis 15:347, 1979.
96. Childs JE, Trimarchi CV, Krebs JW: The epidemiology of bat rabies in New York State, 1988–1992. Epidemiol Infect 113:501, 1994.
97. Schneider LG, Cox JH: Bat lyssaviruses in Europe. Curr Top Microbiol Immunol 187:207, 1994.
98. Bourhy H, Kissi B, Tordo N: Molecular diversity of the *Lyssavirus* genus. Virology 194:70, 1993.
99. Pal SR, Arora B, Chuttani PN, et al: Rabies virus infection of a flying fox bat, *Pteropus poliocephalus* in Chandigarh, northern India. Trop Geogr Med 32:265, 1980.
100. Toltzis P: Viral encephalitis. Adv Pediatr Infect Dis 6:111, 1991.

101. Hatchett RP: Rabies: The disease and the value of intensive care treatment. Intensive Care Nurs 7:53, 1991.
102. Tirawatnpong S, Hemachudha T, Manutsathit S, et al: Regional distribution of rabies viral antigen in central nervous system of human encephalitic and paralytic rabies. J Neurol Sci 92:91, 1989.
103. Warrell DA: The clinical picture of rabies in man. Trans R Soc Trop Med Hyg 70:188, 1976.
104. Hemachudha T: Human rabies: Clinical aspects, pathogenesis, and potential therapy. Curr Top Microbiol Immunol 187:121, 1994.
105. Chopra JS, Banerjee AK, Murthy JMK, et al: Paralytic rabies—A clinico-pathological study. Brain 103:789, 1980.
106. Hattwick MAW: Human rabies. Public Health Rev 3:229, 1974.
107. Held JR, Tierkel ES, Steele JH: Rabies in man and animals in the United States, 1946–1965. Public Health Rep 82:1009, 1967.
108. Centers for Disease Control and Prevention: Human rabies—New York, 1993. MMWR Morbid Mortal Wkly Rep 42:799, 1993.
109. Verma AK, Maheswari MC, Chawdhary C, et al: Acute ascending motor paralysis due to rabies: A clinicopathological report. Eur Neurol 24:160, 1985.
110. Morais CF, Assis RVC: Cardiac involvement in human rabies—Case report. Rev Inst Med Trop Sao Paulo 27:145, 1985.
111. Araujo MF, Brito T, Machado CG: Myocarditis in human rabies. Rev Inst Med Trop Sao Paulo 13:99, 1971.
112. Cheetham HD, Hart J, Coghill NF, et al: Rabies with myocarditis. Two cases in England. Lancet 1:921, 1970.
113. Raman GV, Prosser A, Spreadbury PL, et al: Rabies presenting with myocarditis and encephalitis. J Infect 17:155, 1988.
114. Madhusudana SN: Rabies presenting with sexual manifestations. J Indian Med Assoc 86:43, 1988.
115. Bhandari M, Kumar S: Penile hyperexcitability as the presenting symptom of rabies. Br J Urol 58:224, 1986.
116. Udwadia ZF, Udwadia FE, Rao PP, et al: Penile hyperexcitability with recurrent ejaculations as the presenting manifestation of a case of rabies. Postgrad Med J 64:85, 1988.
117. Hattwick MAW, Weiss TT, Stechsulte CJ, et al: Recovery from rabies: A case report. Ann Intern Med 76:931, 1972.
118. Porras C, Barboza JJ, Fuenzalida E, et al: Recovery from rabies in man. Ann Intern Med 85:44, 1976.
119. Centers for Disease Control: Rabies in a laboratory worker—New York. MMWR Morbid Mortal Wkly Rep 76:183, 1977.
120. Alvarez L, Fajardo R, Lopez E, et al: Partial recovery from rabies in a nine-year-old boy. Pediatr Infect Dis J 13:1154, 1994.
121. Fishbein DB: Rabies in humans. *In* Baer GM (ed): The Natural History of Rabies, ed 2. Boca Raton, FL, CRC Press, 1991, p 549.
122. Bernard KW: Clinical rabies in humans. *In* Fishbein DB, Sawyer LA, Winkler WG (eds): Rabies Concepts for Medical Professionals, ed 2. Miami, Mérieux Institute, 1986, p 48.
123. Ferguson CF: Human rabies. Am J Nurs 81:1175, 1981.
124. Helmick CG, Tauxe RV, Vernon AA: Is there a risk to contacts of patients with rabies? Rev Infect Dis 9:511, 1987.
125. Warrell MJ, White NJ, Looareesuwan S, et al: Failure of interferon alfa and tribavirin in rabies encephalitis. BMJ 299:830, 1989.
126. Dutta JK, Dutta TK: Treatment of clinical rabies in man: Drug therapy and other measures. Int J Clin Pharmacol Ther 32:594, 1994.
127. Baer GM (ed): The Natural History of Rabies, ed 2. Boca Raton, FL, CRC Press, 1991.
128. Smith JS, Sumner JW, Roumillat LF, et al: Antigenic characteristics of isolates associated with a new epizootic of raccoon rabies in the United States. J Infect Dis 149:769, 1984.
129. Rollin PE, Sureau P: Monoclonal antibodies as a tool for rabies epidemiological studies. Dev Biol Stand 57:193, 1984.
130. Kamolvarin N, Tirawatnpong T, Rattanasiwanmoke R, et al: Diagnosis of rabies by polymerase chain reaction with nested primers. J Infect Dis 167:207, 1993.
131. Sureau P, Ravisse P, Rollin PE: Rabies diagnosis by animal inoculation, identification of Negri bodies, or ELISA. *In* Baer GM (ed): Natural History of Rabies, ed 2. Boca Raton, FL, CRC Press, 1991, p 217.
132. Rudd RJ, Trimarchi CV: Development and evaluation of an in vitro virus isolation procedure as a replacement for the mouse inoculation test in rabies diagnosis. J Clin Microbiol 27:2522, 1989.
133. Johnson HN, Emmons RW: Rabies virus. *In* Lennette EH (ed): Laboratory Diagnosis of Viral Infections, ed 2. New York, Marcel Dekker, 1992, p 684.
134. Trimarchi CV, Debbie JG: The fluorescent antibody in rabies. *In* Baer GM (ed): The Natural History of Rabies, ed 2. Boca Raton, FL, CRC Press, 1991, p 233.
135. McQueen JL, Lewis AL, Schneider NJ: Rabies diagnosis by fluorescent antibody. Its evaluation in a public health laboratory. Am J Public Health 50:1743, 1960.
136. Blenden DC, Bell JF, Tsao AT, et al: Immunofluorescent examination of the skin of rabies-infected animals as a means of early detection of rabies virus antigen. J Clin Microbiol 18:631, 1983.
137. Warrell MJ, Looareesuwan S, Manatsathit S, et al: Rapid diagnosis of rabies and post-vaccinal encephalitides. Clin Exp Immunol 71:229, 1988.
138. Schneider LG: The cornea test; a new method for the intravitam diagnosis of rabies. Zentralbl Veterinarmed [B] 16:24, 1969.
139. Larghi OP, Gonzalez E, Held JR: Evaluation of the corneal test as a laboratory method for rabies diagnosis. Appl Microbiol 25:187, 1973.
140. Mathuranayagam D, Rao PV: Antemortem diagnosis of human rabies by corneal impression smears using immunofluorescent technique. Indian J Med Res 79:463, 1984.
141. Lewis VJ, Thacker WL: Limitations of deteriorated tissue for rabies diagnosis. Health Lab Sci 11:8, 1974.
142. Hamir AN, Moser G: Immunoperoxidase test for rabies: Utility as a diagnostic test. J Vet Diagn Invest 6:148, 1994.
143. Zimmer K, Wiegand D, Manz D, et al: Evaluation of five different methods for routine diagnosis of rabies. Zentralbl Veterinarmed [B] 37:392, 1990.
144. Fekadu M, Greer PW, Chandler FW, et al: Use of the avidin-biotin peroxidase system to detect rabies antigen in formalin-fixed paraffin-embedded tissues. J Virol Methods 19:91, 1988.
145. Savy V, Atanasiu P: Rapid immunoenzymatic technique for titration of rabies antibodies IgG and IgM. Dev Biol Stand 40:247, 1978.
146. Smith JS: Rabies serology. *In* Baer GM (ed): The Natural History of Rabies, ed 2. Boca Raton, FL, CRC Press, 1991, p 252.
147. Smith JS, Yager PA, Baer GM: A rapid reproducible test for determining rabies neutralizing antibody. Bull World Health Organ 48:535, 1973.
148. Ermine A, Larzul D, Ceccaldi PE, et al: Polymerase chain reaction amplification of rabies virus nucleic acids from total mouse brain RNA. Mol Cell Probes 4:189, 1990.
149. Gottesdiener KM: Transplanted infections: Donor-to-host transmission with the allograft. Ann Intern Med 110:1001, 1989.
150. Richardson JH, Barkeley WEE: Biosafety in Microbiological and Biomedical Laboratories, ed 2. Washington, DC, US Government Printing Office, 1988, p 100. Department of Health and Human Services Publication (CDC) 88-8395.
151. Dean DJ, Baer GM, Thompson WR: Studies on local treatment of rabies infected wounds. Bull World Health Organ 28:477, 1963.
152. Wiktor T, Koprowski H: Action locale de certains médicaments sur l'infection rabique de la souris. Bull World Health Organ 28:487, 1963.
153. Wilde H, Chomchey P, Prakongsri S, et al: Adverse effects of equine rabies immune gobulin. Vaccine 7:10, 1989.
154. Wilde H, Chutivongse S: Equine rabies immune globulin: A product with an undeserved poor reputation. Am J Trop Med Hyg 42:175, 1990.
155. Glhck R, Wegmann A, Keller H, et al: Human rabies immunoglobulin assayed by the rapid fluorescent focus inhibition test suppresses active rabies immunization. J Biol Stand 15:177, 1987.
156. World Health Organization: Expert Committee on Rabies. Eighth report. Geneva, World Health Organization, 1992, p 84.
157. Thraenhart O, Marcus I, Kreuzfelder E: Current and future immunoprophylaxis against human rabies: Reduction of treatment failures and errors. Curr Top Microbiol Immunol 187:173, 1994.
158. Thraenhart O, Kreuzfelder E, Hillebrandt M, et al: Long-term humoral and cellular immunity after vaccination with cell culture rabies vaccines in man. Clin Immunol Immunopathol 71:287, 1994.

159. Bernard KW, Fishbein DB: Pre-exposure rabies prophylaxis for travellers—Are the benefits worth the cost? Vaccine 9:833, 1991.
160. Phanuphak P, Ubolyam S, Sirivichayakul S: Should travellers in rabies endemic areas receive pre-exposure rabies immunization? Ann Med Interne (Paris) 145:409, 1995.
161. Bernard KW, Fishbein DB, Miller KD, et al: Pre-exposure rabies immunization with human diploid cell vaccine: Decreased antibody responses in persons immunized in developing countries. Am J Trop Med Hyg 34:633, 1985.
162. Pappaioanou M, Fishbein DB, Dreesen DW, et al: Antibody response to preexposure human diploid-cell rabies vaccine given concurrently with chloroquine. N Engl J Med 314:280, 1986.
163. Wright J: The threat of rabies. Prof Nurse 4:536, 1989.
164. Fescharek R, Franke V, Samuel MR: Do anaesthetics and surgical stress increase the risk of post-exposure rabies treatment failure? Vaccine 12:12, 1994.
165. Baer GM, Fishbein DB: Rabies post-exposure prophylaxis. N Engl J Med 316:1270, 1987.
166. Mastroeni I, Vescia N, Pompa MG, et al: Immune response of the elderly to rabies vaccines. Vaccine 12:518, 1994.
167. Chutivongse S, Wilde H, Benjavongkulchai M, et al: Postexposure rabies vaccination during pregnancy: Effect on 202 women and their infants. J Infect Dis 20:818, 1995.
168. Dreesen DW, Bernard KW, Parker RA, et al: Immune complex–like disease in 23 persons following a booster dose of rabies human diploid cell vaccine. Vaccine 4:45, 1986.
169. Anderson LJ, Winkler WG: The Center for Disease Control's experience with a human diploid cell rabies vaccine. Curr Chemother Infect Dis 1357, 1980.
170. Anderson LJ, Winkler WG, Hafkin B, et al: Clinical experience with a human diploid cell rabies vaccine. JAMA 244:781, 1980.
171. Fishbein DB, Dreesen DW, Holmes DF, et al: Human diploid cell rabies vaccine purified by zonal centrifugation: A controlled study of antibody response and side effects following primary and booster pre-exposure immunizations. Vaccine 7:437, 1989.
172. Bernard KW, Mallonee J, Wright JC, et al: Preexposure immunization with intradermal human diploid cell rabies vaccine. Risks and benefits of primary and booster vaccination. JAMA 257:1059, 1987.
173. Anderson LJ, Sikes RK, Langkop CW, et al: Postexposure trial of a human diploid cell strain rabies vaccine. J Infect Dis 142:133, 1980.
174. Gamboa ET, Cowen D, Eggers A, et al: Delayed onset of post–rabies vaccination encephalitis. Ann Neurol 13:676, 1983.
175. Appelbaum E, Greenberg M, Nelson J: Neurological complications following antirabies vaccination. JAMA 151:188, 1953.
176. Nicholson KG, Turner GS, Aoki FY: Immunization with a human diploid cell strain of rabies virus vaccine: Two year results. J Infect Dis 137:783, 1978.
177. Nicholson KG: Rabies. Lancet 335:1201, 1990.
178. Brochier B, Thomas I, Iokem A, et al: A field trial in Belgium to control fox rabies by oral immunisation. Vet Rec 123:618, 1988.
179. Aubert MF, Masson E, Artois M, et al: Oral wildlife rabies vaccination field trials in Europe, with recent emphasis on France. Curr Top Microbiol Immunol 187:219, 1994.
180. Campbell JB: Oral rabies immunization of wildlife and dogs: Challenges to the Americas. Curr Top Microbiol Immunol 187:245, 1994.
181. Brochier B, Boulanger D, Costy F, et al: Towards rabies elimination in Belgium by fox vaccination using a vaccinia–rabies glycoprotein recombinant virus. Vaccine 12:1368, 1994.
182. Rupprecht CE, Smith JS: Raccoon rabies: The re-emergence of an epizootic in a densely populated area. Semin Virol 5:155, 1994.
183. Clark KA, Neill SU, Smith JS, et al: Epizootic canine rabies transmitted by coyotes in south Texas. J Am Vet Med Assoc 204:536, 1994.
184. World Health Organization: World Survey of Rabies. Geneva, World Health Organization, 1993, p 37.
185. Celis E, Rupprecht CE, Plotkin S: New and improved vaccines against rabies. *In* Woodrow GC, Levine MM (eds): New Generation Vaccines. New York, Marcel Dekker, 1990, p 438.
186. Rupprecht CE, Shankar V, Hanlon CA, et al: Beyond Pasteur to 2001: Future trends in lyssavirus research? Curr Top Microbiol Immunol 187:325, 1994.
187. Baer GM: Animal models in the pathogenesis and treatment of rabies. Rev Infect Dis 10(Suppl 4):S739, 1988.
188. World Health Organization: Oral immunization of foxes in Europe in 1994. Wkly Epidemiol Rec 70:89, 1995.
189. World Health Organization: Report of the 5th Consultation on Oral Immunization of Dogs Against Rabies. Geneva, World Health Organization, 1994, p 24.

171

Animal Bites

Kenneth W. Kizer

America's pet population numbers well above 100 million cats and dogs and many more millions of rodents, reptiles, birds, horses, tropical fish, and other animals. The ecologic, socioeconomic, legal, and health consequences of this sometimes poorly controlled pet population are many and oftentimes a problem for clinicians, public health agencies, and elected officials.[1–10] Animal bites are a particularly notable problem because of their frequency, preventability, and potential severity. Indeed, animal bites have been characterized as an "unrecognized epidemic."[11, 12]

Epidemiology

Incidence and Prevalence

Of the approximately 4400 species of mammals in the world, fewer than 10 account for the overwhelming majority of animal bites encountered in North America. Although the number of species that inflict bites is small, the magnitude of the problem is not.

Detailed national data on the occurrence of animal bites are not available in the United States or elsewhere, although more than a million bite injuries are known to be treated in the United States each year, at an estimated cost of well above $100 million.[1, 9, 13–17] The actual number of such injuries is believed to be much greater, because less than half of bite injuries are actually reported. In fact, one study documented a 36-fold occurrence of underreporting.[18]

In U.S. communities where it has been specifically studied, the animal bite attack rate ranges from about 300 to 1200 cases per 100,000 population.[1, 11, 13, 19–23] Rates as high as 2059 per 100,000 have been reported.[14]

Predisposing Factors

Mail delivery and animal control personnel, veterinarians, laboratory technicians, police officers, and some other types of workers are at risk for occupationally related animal bites, but these are not the persons who incur the greatest number of bites. Most animal bite victims are children and adolescents, and small children are at especially high risk for serious injury. Dogs most often bite males, and cats most often bite females, at a ratio of about 3:1 in each case. Bites of other animals are apportioned about evenly between the sexes.

Offending Animals

Dogs are identified as the offending animal in 80% to 85% of bite incidents in the United States. Cats account for about

10%. Rodents, rabbits, raccoons, skunks, horses, monkeys, and bats are responsible for the majority of the remaining cases.

Mongrels, German shepherds, and Doberman pinschers have been especially frequently identified as types of dogs that bite; pit bulls have been disproportionately involved in severe and fatal maulings.[1, 24] Unfortunately, detailed statistics on breed of biting dog and the circumstances attendant to the incident are inadequate to reliably apportion bite risk according to breed.

Clinical Considerations

Animal bites were recognized as a public health and clinical management problem at least as far back as ancient Egypt, with numerous prescriptions for treating them being expressed throughout recorded medical history. Despite the long history of this problem and its frequency and magnitude, the medical literature on treatment of animal bites is surprisingly anecdotal. Few controlled studies of the treatment of animal bites were undertaken until the 1980s, and even with the interest demonstrated in more recent years, there remains much controversy about the proper management of this common clinical problem.

Fortunately, most animal bites cause relatively minor injury. Only a small portion produce severe trauma or lead to serious local or systemic infections. Bite incidents leading to permanent disability or death, however, are markedly disproportionate among small children. Overall, in the United States, about 1% of emergency department visits are for animal bites, and 1% to 2% of those patients require hospitalization.[1, 16, 19, 25]

Infectious Complications

Animal bites have a substantial potential for infectious complications, although this has been investigated in detail only for dog bites. The infectious complication most often seen is local wound cellulitis, with or without lymphangitis and regional adenitis. Infection is due to numerous organisms, and at least one fourth of infected wounds grow out multiple species. *Pasteurella multocida, Staphylococcus aureus,* and *Pseudomonas* and *Streptococcus* species are identified relatively often from infected wounds. Anaerobic species are also commonly present, but they are mixed with aerobic species, so their precise pathogenic role is usually indeterminate.

The typical dog's mouth harbors more than 60 species of bacteria.[16, 26–30] Of particular concern are *S. aureus, Streptococcus pyogenes, Pseudomonas* species, *Aeromonas hydrophilia, Capnocytophaga canimorsus, Eikenella corrodens, Proteus mirabilis, Enterobacter* and *Klebsiella* species, *Clostridium tetani* and *Clostridium perfringens, Bacteroides* species, and *P. multocida.* Table 171–1 lists microorganisms recovered from domestic animal bites. The pathogenic behavior of some of these bacteria is relatively poorly understood.

The flora in animals' mouths is also known to change in the course of the year and to vary according to geographic location and the animal's health and diet. Thus, predicting what organism is likely to cause a wound infection in any given case is difficult.

Illustrative of the variable presence of known pathogens is *P. multocida. P. multocida* in animals is similar to the pneumococcus in humans in that it is a common commensal and pathogen of the respiratory tract. It has been isolated from many animal species, but the frequency of its presence varies widely.[30–32] For example, it has been cultured from the upper respiratory tract of about 20% of dogs and 50% to 70% of healthy domestic cats, but the isolation rate from sick cats may be as high as 100%. *P. multocida* is of particular concern as a bite wound pathogen because of its frequent isolation from infected bites, its potential to cause rapid cellulitis and disseminated infection, and its opportunistic nature.[1, 30–32] This microbe has been identified as the pathogen in 10% to 20% of infected dog bites and 30% to 50% of infected cat bites.

TABLE 171–1 ■ Illustrative Microorganisms Recovered from Domestic Animal Bites

Acinetobacter spp.	*Micrococcus* spp.
Actinobacillus spp.	*Moraxella* spp.
Aeromonas hydrophila and other spp.	*Mucor* spp.
Alcaligenes spp.	*Mycobacterium* spp.
Bacillus spp.	*Neisseria* spp.
Bacteroides spp.	*Nocardia* spp.
Bartonella henselae	*Pasteurella multocida* and other spp.
Blastomyces dermatitidis	*Peptococcus* spp.
Bordetella spp.	*Peptostreptococcus* spp.
Brucella canis	*Porphyromonas* spp.
Campylobacter spp.	*Prevotella* spp.
Capnocytophaga canimorsus	*Propionibacterium* spp.
Chromobacterium spp.	*Proteus mirabilis* and other spp.
Clostridium perfringens, Clostridium tetani, and other spp.	*Pseudomonas aeruginosa* and other spp.
Corynebacterium spp.	*Salmonella* spp.
Eikenella corrodens	*Serratia* spp.
Enterobacter cloacae and other spp.	*Sporothrix schenckii*
Enterococcus spp.	*Staphylococcus aureus, Staphylococcus epidermidis, Staphylococcus intermedius,* and other spp.
Escherichia coli	*Streptobacillus moniliformis*
Flavobacterium spp.	*Streptococcus* spp. (α-hemolytic, group A β-hemolytic, nonhemolytic, non–group A)
Fusobacterium spp.	*Veillonella parvula* and other spp.
Francisella tularensis	*Weeksella zoohelcum*
Haemophilus influenzae and other spp.	*Yersinia pestis* and other spp.
Klebsiella spp.	
Leptospira spp.	
Leptotrichia buccalis	
Listeria monocytogenes	

In addition to local wound cellulitis, the infectious complications of animal bites include osteomyelitis and septic arthritis; meningitis, brain abscess, and subdural empyema; endocarditis; pyelonephritis; peritonitis; appendicular abscess; pneumonia and lung abscess; mycotic aneurysm; infection of vascular grafts and prosthetic heart valves; and bacteremia and sepsis. Various species have been identified in these situations. Fatal shock and disseminated intravascular coagulation have been reported after bacteremia with both *Capnocytophaga* and *Bacteroides.*

Animal bites may also transmit a number of zoonotic diseases, including leptospirosis, listeriosis, salmonellosis, cat-scratch fever, campylobacteriosis, brucellosis, tuberculosis, bubonic plague, tularemia, erysipelothrix, rat-bite fever, rabies, cryptosporidiosis, sporotrichosis, and blastomycosis, to name some that have been reported.

The Animal Bite Medical History

Distinguishing innocuous from high-risk bite wounds is an essential component of the initial management of these injuries. Several factors guide such a determination, including the characteristics of the bite incident, the age and health status of the victim, and the nature of the wound. Specific details about these things should be recorded in the patient's medical record. The medical history of any animal bite injury should include, at a minimum, the information listed in Table

171–2. Recording such information is important not only for the management of the patient but also because these cases usually prompt some type of public health investigation and often lead to civil action or litigation in which the medical record is important.

The Nature of Bite Wounds

The wounds caused by animal bites are of four main types: lacerations (often of a tearing or avulsing nature), crush injuries, punctures, and abrasions. Depending on the offending animal, the wound typically involves a combination of two or more of these types of trauma; some degree of crush injury is present in most bite wounds inflicted by dogs or larger animals. Dogs typically exert a bite force of between 200 and 450 pounds per square inch, which is sufficient to cause significant crush injury in addition to other tissue damage. Bites from cows, horses, and other ungulates typically do not break the skin, but they do cause severe crush injuries. Fatal fat embolism has resulted from donkey bites. In contrast, bites from rodents and domestic cats usually produce puncture wounds, which may be deep and susceptible to infection.

The extremities are most often bitten in adolescents and adults, principally the hands and arms. In contrast, facial and cranial bites are especially common in small children, accounting for more than 60% of bites in children younger than 10 years. Because of the greater potential need to administer postexposure rabies prophylaxis in cases of facial bites and their greater potential for cosmetic sequelae and intracranial injury, their high frequency in children is of special concern.

Clinical Management of Animal Bites

As with any trauma patient, management of bite wounds begins with an assessment of the airway, breathing, and circulation.[16, 33] Most bite wounds do not immediately threaten life or limb, but serious injury occurs often enough that attention should be directed initially to determining whether there has been, or is likely to be, significant blood loss, airway compromise, or severe occult injuries. For example, bites to the face or head of infants or small children may penetrate or disrupt the skull, with resultant intracranial injury and severe infectious complications.[34–37] Patients with neck wounds may have underlying damage to vital neurovascular structures. Similarly, pneumothorax may occur in patients with bites to the chest; fractures, tendon injuries, or nerve damage may result from bites to the distal extremities or joints. Depending on the location, nature, and extent of the wound, occult injuries need to be specifically sought with appropriate radiographic and other studies.

After ensuring that the patient's condition is stable and determining the extent, if any, of injury to underlying structures, the physician should focus attention on the wound itself, with the understanding that the major clinical significance of animal bites relates to their potential for local or systemic infectious complications.

TABLE 171–2 ■ The Animal Bite Medical History

Type of offending animal, including breed when known
Relationship of the animal to the victim
Specific circumstances antecedent to the bite
Time of the incident
Exact location of the incident
Health status of the animal (as best as can be determined), including the status of its rabies vaccination, if known
Current location of the animal
First aid given, if any
Patient's tetanus immunization status
Patient's medical history, especially with regard to asplenia, chronic debilitating disease, or other cause of impaired immunocompetence

Risk Factors

The first step in managing the bite wound is identifying the relative risk for infection. The major variables in this regard are the type and anatomic location of the bite, the victim's age and preexisting health status, and the type of offending animal.[38] As noted before, bites to the head or face of small children should be considered high risk because of their potential for causing injury to deep structures and because of the likelihood that pathogens have been deposited deep in vital structures. Likewise, bites of the hands and wrists, of the feet and ankles, or over major joints are considered high-risk wounds because of the frequency with which deep structures—bones, joint spaces, tendons, and neurovascular bundles—are injured or become infected. Tendon sheaths, bursae, and joint spaces are not well vascularized and are easily inoculated with bacteria as a result of the movement of anatomic planes over the affected part.

Because of the difficulty of cleansing them, bites that produce puncture wounds—independent of species—are considered at high risk for infection regardless of location (infection rate, about 25%). Similarly, any bite for which initial treatment is delayed 8 to 10 hours or longer should be considered at increased risk for infection.

Persons who are immunocompromised because of chronic illness, corticosteroid therapy, or other immunosuppressive treatment should be considered at high risk for infection from any bite. Prominent among the preexisting conditions of concern are asplenia (from any cause), cirrhosis or other chronic liver disease, alcoholism, diabetes mellitus, human immunodeficiency virus disease, peripheral vascular insufficiency, and valvular heart disease. Persons older than 55 years and those who have prosthetic joints or heart valves should also be considered at higher risk for infectious complications.

About 5% of dog bites and approximately 30% of cat bites become infected.[1, 16, 30, 38, 39] Consequently, cat bites, including those from species of large felines, should be considered high-risk wounds. Limited experience with pig and monkey bites suggests that they are also associated with a relatively high rate of infection, and alligator bites have a propensity to develop infections with gram-negative organisms.

Additional Treatment Issues

After distinguishing high-risk from low-risk bites, the physician should direct further evaluation to six key issues:

1. Is tetanus prophylaxis needed?
2. Is rabies prophylaxis needed?
3. Does material from the wound need to be cultured?
4. How should the wound be cleaned and débrided?
5. Are prophylactic antibiotics indicated?
6. If necessary, can the wound be safely sutured?

Tetanus Prophylaxis. Because dogs and other animals ingest dirt and, occasionally, feces, and because bite wounds are often contaminated with soil and other materials, the possibility of infection with *C. tetani* must be considered in all animal bites. Consequently, tetanus prophylaxis is an essential aspect of managing any bite wound. The patient must be specifically queried about the status of tetanus immunization, and immunoprophylaxis must be administered according to standard guidelines, as discussed elsewhere in this text (see Chapter 220).

Rabies Prophylaxis. Rabies must be considered in all unprovoked animal bites and in all cases of bites by bats, skunks, foxes, raccoons, ferrets, coyotes, and bobcats. Domestic and farm animals, rodents, and rabbits and other lagomorphs are considered low risk for rabies.

Many persons are administered postexposure rabies prophylaxis unnecessarily, although this is to some degree understandable. A detailed discussion of rabies and its prevention and management is presented in Chapter 170.

Wound Culture. Because all penetrating bite wounds are contaminated by bacteria from the offending animal's mouth, the victim's skin or clothing, and ambient environmental materials, cultures of fresh wounds typically yield multiple bacterial species; such cultures have been found to be unreliable predictors of infection, reflecting only what organisms were present at the time the culture was taken. So, they are not recommended.[16, 30, 39–42] Similarly, Gram stain examinations of fresh wounds are not considered useful predictors of infection.[42]

In contrast, wound cultures are indicated for all infected bites in high-risk patients and when initial antibiotic therapy fails in low-risk patients. Likewise, both aerobic and anaerobic cultures should be obtained of the wound discharge or abscess drainage and of blood from any patient who is thought to have septic complications of bite wounds.

Wound Toilet. Whenever the skin is broken, there is a risk for local wound infection or the transmission of systemic disease from any of the numerous pathogens contaminating the wound. Prompt and thorough cleansing of the wound substantially reduces the risk for infection.[43]

Although it is a routine practice, soaking wounds in antiseptic solution has not been proved to be effective and may even increase microbial contamination. Gently scrubbing with a sponge and dilute povidone-iodine solution is effective in decontaminating the skin around the wound, but the wound itself should not be scrubbed, because this may cause further tissue injury.

Irrigation is the most effective means of decontaminating bite wounds, and the most effective method of irrigating them is with a 19-gauge needle on a 12- or 20-mL syringe using moderate hand pressure. This delivers the irrigant at a pressure of about 15 to 20 pounds per square inch, sufficient to dislodge contaminants but not so great as to force the irrigant into surrounding tissues. For most bite wounds, a volume of 150 to 200 mL of irrigant is adequate to accomplish decontamination.

Although the matter is still somewhat controversial, the preferred irrigant is a solution of povidone-iodine diluted to 1% to 5%. This provides a good balance between bactericidal capacity and tissue toxicity. Normal saline is an effective irrigant that is not tissue toxic, but it is less desirable because it has no bactericidal properties.

Débridement of visibly devitalized tissue further reduces the risk for infection and creates a sharper and typically straighter wound margin that is easier to suture and that tends to heal with less scarring. All blunt, ragged, and crushing wounds should be sharply débrided unless skin tension or the presence of subjacent vital structures makes this impossible or inappropriate.

Irrigation combined with sharp débridement of crushed and devitalized tissue is the most important and effective intervention for preventing wound infection. This combination reduces the infection rate of animal bite wounds to that typically found in other types of lacerations.[16, 30, 39, 44]

Prophylactic Antibiotics. For some procedures, antibiotics given before surgery seem to reduce the rate of infection. However, studies have not demonstrated the efficacy of prophylactic antibiotics in animal bites, except in high-risk wounds.[16, 30, 39, 45–48]

Primary Wound Repair. Although it is still somewhat controversial, the consensus today is that low-risk bite wounds can be safely sutured if they are first cleansed well and débrided.[16, 30, 39] Good wound toilet is essential to success in this regard. Because of the impossibility of thoroughly irrigating puncture wounds, they should not be sutured. Similarly, wounds that are more than 8 to 10 hours old when they first come to medical attention should probably not be sutured.

Data on the desirability of primarily closing hand wounds remain inconclusive. Bite wounds of the hands have a high rate of infection (about 30%), but it is not clear whether the risk is actually increased by primary closure. At this time, nontrivial bite wounds of the hand should be treated aggressively with irrigation and débridement (if indicated and possible to do), complete immobilization of the hand, elevation, and prophylactic antibiotics. Unless it is critical to achieving a satisfactory result, primary closure should be avoided.

Choice of Antibiotic

The antibiotic of choice for the initial treatment of local bite wound infections, or for prophylaxis in cases when indicated, has not been established by controlled comparative studies. Because of the wide spectrum of potential pathogens present in bite wounds, no single antibiotic will be effective in all cases.

As many as half of local bite wound infections are likely to result from *P. multocida,* which is sensitive to penicillin, and the overwhelming majority of others will be caused by organisms susceptible to plain penicillin. Only about 3% to 5% of infections are likely to be caused by penicillin-resistant organisms, so penicillin or one of its analogs is the initial agent of choice for treating these infections. Dicloxacillin, 500 mg orally four times a day for adults, 50 to 100 mg/kg per day in four divided doses for children, is the generally preferred agent because of its effectiveness against most staphylococci. Likewise, cephalexin, 500 mg orally four times a day for adults, 50 to 100 mg/kg per day in four divided doses for children, is a good choice, but it may be more expensive than dicloxacillin. Erythromycin, 500 mg orally four times a day for adults, 30 to 50 mg/kg per day in four doses for children, is a reasonable substitute in cases of penicillin allergy, although this agent may not be effective against *P. multocida.*[49] Tetracycline may be used if the pathogen has been proved to be *P. multocida* and there are no contraindications to the use of this drug. Although they are effective, second- and third-generation cephalosporins and the quinolones should be reserved for special situations because of their cost and the desirability of reserving them for second-line use.

Patients with seriously infected bites or septicemia need to be hospitalized for parenteral antibiotic treatment. In such cases, a cephalosporin (e.g., cefazolin, 25 to 50 mg/kg per day intravenously in three or four doses) combined with gentamicin, 3.0 to 5.0 mg/kg per day intravenously in three doses, is the initial regimen of choice. Diabetic patients with hand infections are often found to have gram-negative infection and should start receiving a parenteral aminoglycoside early on, along with a cephalosporin or penicillin analog, especially if *Pseudomonas* infection is suspected. Clindamycin, 20 to 40 mg/kg per day intravenously in three or four doses, or chloramphenicol, 50 to 100 mg/kg per day intravenously in four doses, is indicated if *Bacteroides* infection is suspected.

Because penicillin and antistaphylococcal drugs will effectively treat nearly all local wound infections, cultures are not routinely indicated. They are, of course, indicated for refractory infections and should be used to guide specific antibiotic therapy in cases of sepsis or other serious infection.

Prevention

The majority of dog and other animal bites could be prevented if greater care were taken in interacting with animals. This is especially so for infants and small children.

Young children are at higher risk for animal bites because of their curiosity; their tendency to engage in active and aggressive play, which often excites animals; their inexperience in handling animals, which may result in abusive or threatening behavior; and their small size and relative inability to defend themselves. Children are particularly likely to be bitten when they disturb animals that are eating or sleeping; when they try to separate fighting animals; when they try to catch, tease, kiss, or pet animals; and when they play recklessly around them. Most of these circumstances and the resulting untoward events could be prevented by instructing children in appropriate ways to interact with animals and by proper adult supervision of children when they are around animals, particularly when the animals and children are unfamiliar with each other.

Similarly, keeping only such pets as are appropriate to the child's age and living situation could prevent many untoward child-pet encounters. Keeping wild or exotic pets in households with small children or keeping animals such as ferrets that have a long history of unprovoked, vicious attacks on infants should be emphatically discouraged.[31, 50, 51]

References

1. Kizer KW: Epidemiologic and clinical aspects of animal bite injuries. JACEP 8:134, 1979.
2. Klein D: Friendly dog syndrome. N Y State J Med 66:2306, 1966.
3. Cohen D: Community health and animal populations. Arch Environ Health 17:1, 1968.
4. Beck AM: The public health implications of urban dogs. Am J Public Health 65:1315, 1975.
5. Feldman BM, Carding TH: Free-roaming urban pets. Health Serv Rep 88:956, 1973.
6. Robinson D: Canis familiaris. N Engl J Med 290:1378, 1974.
7. Carithers HA: Pets in the home: Incidence and significance. Pediatrics 21:840, 1958.
8. Sheridan JP: Dogs, cats and other pets. Practitioner 215:172, 1975.
9. Bennett JS: Man's best friend? Can Med Assoc J 116:126, 1977.
10. Seah SKK, Hucal G, Law C: Dogs and intestinal parasites: A public health problem. Can Med Assoc J 112:1191, 1975.
11. Harris D, Imperato PJ, Oken B: Dog bites: An unrecognized epidemic. Bull N Y Acad Med 50:981, 1974.
12. Lauer EA, White WC, Lauer BA: Dog bite: A neglected problem in accident prevention. Am J Dis Child 136:202, 1982.
13. Beck AM, Loring H, Lockwood R: The ecology of dog bite injury in St. Louis, Missouri. Public Health Rep 90:262, 1975.
14. Newman EC: Animal bites as a public health disease. Tex Med 73:49, 1977.
15. Arena JM: Bites, zoonoses and rabies. Clin Pediatr 6:259, 1967.
16. Callaham ML: Emergency medical management: Dog bite wounds. JAMA 244:2327, 1980.
17. Pinckney LE, Kennedy LA: Traumatic deaths from dog attacks in the United States. Pediatrics 69:193, 1982.
18. Beck AM, Jones BA: Unreported dog bites in children. Public Health Rep 100:315, 1985.
19. Berzon DR, Farber RE, Gordon J, et al: Animal bites in a large city: A report of Baltimore, Maryland. Am J Public Health 62:422, 1972.
20. Morton C: Dog bites in Norfolk, Va. Health Serv Rep 88:59, 1973.
21. Mayers SP, Beachley RG: A survey of dog bites in Arlington. Va Med 82:317, 1955.
22. Olsen CD: Epidemiology of animal exposures. Nebr Med J 46:143, 1961.
23. Parrish HM, Clark FB, Brobst D, et al: Epidemiology of dog bites. Public Health Rep 74:891, 1959.
24. Sacks JJ, Sattin RW, Bonzo SE: Dog bite–related fatalities from 1979 through 1988. JAMA 262:1489, 1989.
25. Aghababian RV, Conte JE: Mammalian bite wounds. Ann Emerg Med 9:79, 1980.
26. Clapper WE, Meade GH: Normal flora of the nose, throat, and lower intestine of dogs. J Bacteriol 85:643, 1963.
27. Bailie WE, Stowe EC, Schmitt AM: Aerobic-bacterial flora of oral and nasal fluids of canines with reference to bacteria associated with bites. J Clin Microbiol 7:223, 1978.
28. Saphir DA, Carter GR: Gingival flora of the dog with special reference to bacteria associated with bites. J Clin Microbiol 3:344, 1976.
29. Goldstein EJC, Citran DM, Wield B, et al: Bacteriology of human and animal bite wounds. J Clin Microbiol 8:667, 1978.
30. Callaham ML: Wild and domestic animal attacks. *In* Auerbach PS, Geehr EC (eds): Management of Wilderness and Environmental Emergencies, ed 2. St. Louis, CV Mosby, 1989, pp 683–726.
31. Kizer KW: *Pasteurella multocida* infection from a cougar bite: A review of cougar attacks. West J Med 150:87, 1989.
32. Weber DJ, Wolfson JS, Swartz MN, et al: *Pasteurella multocida* infections: Report of 34 cases and review of the literature. Medicine (Baltimore) 63:133, 1984.
33. Kizer KW, Callaham ML: A new look at managing mammalian bites. Emerg Med Rep 5:53, 1984.
34. Chait LA, Spitz L: Dog bite injuries in children. S Afr Med J 49:718, 1975.
35. Klein DM, Cohen ME: *Pasteurella multocida* brain abscess following perforating cranial dog bite. J Pediatr 92:588, 1978.
36. Wilberger JE, Pang D: Craniocerebral injuries from dog bites. JAMA 249:2685, 1983.
37. Watson DW: Severe head injury from dog bites. Ann Emerg Med 9:28, 1980.
38. Callaham ML: Treatment of common dog bites: Infection risk factors. JACEP 7:83, 1978.
39. Callaham ML: Prophylactic antibiotics in common dog bite wounds: A controlled study. Ann Emerg Med 9:410, 1980.
40. Ordog GJ: The bacteriology of dog bite wounds. Ann Emerg Med 15:1324, 1986.
41. Callaham M: Controversies in antibiotic choices for bite wounds. Ann Emerg Med 17:1321, 1988.
42. Feder HM, Shanley JD, Baerberg JA: Review of 59 patients hospitalized with animal bites. Pediatr Infect Dis J 6:24, 1987.
43. Dire DJ, Hogan DE, Riggs MW: A prospective evaluation of risk factors for infections from dog-bite wounds. Acad Emerg Med 1:258, 1994.
44. Zook EG, Miller M, Van Beek AL, et al: Successful treatment protocol for canine fang injuries. J Trauma 20:243, 1980.
45. Rosen RA: The use of antibiotics in the initial management of recent dog-bite wounds. Am J Emerg Med 3:19, 1985.
46. Boenning DA, Fleisher GR, Campos JM: Dog bites in children: Epidemiology, microbiology, and penicillin prophylactic therapy. Am J Emerg Med 1:17, 1983.
47. Elenbaas RM, McNabney WK, Robinson WA: Evaluation of prophylactic oxacillin in cat bite wounds. Ann Emerg Med 13:155, 1984.
48. Elenbaas RM, McNabney WK, Robinson WA: Prophylactic oxacillin in dog bite wounds. Ann Emerg Med 11:248, 1982.
49. Levin JM, Talan DA: Erythromycin failure with subsequent *Pasteurella multocida* meningitis and septic arthritis in a cat-bite victim. Ann Emerg Med 19:1458, 1990.
50. Constantine DG, Kizer KW: Pet European Ferrets: A Hazard to Public Health, Small Livestock and Wildlife. Sacramento, CA, California Department of Health Services, 1988.
51. Paisley JW, Lauer BA: Severe facial injuries to infants due to unprovoked attacks by pet ferrets. JAMA 259:2005, 1988.

172

Tularemia

*Jay P. Sanford**

Tularemia is an acute infectious disease caused by the aerobic gram-negative bacillus *Francisella tularensis.* It is a typical zoonosis, a disease of animals transmissible to humans.

History

In 1837, Homma Soken, a Japanese physician, described an unusual illness:

> *Those who eat hare meat have often been found to suffer from poisoning. . . . The symptoms appear on the day following, or even dozens of days after, eating the meat. At first the patient is attacked with chills and fever. . . . Then several glandular tumors will form on the neck, throat, arms, and armpits, resembling scrofula. For many days the tumors will not disappear nor suppurate. . . . Once the tumor suppurates and discharges, the symptoms will disappear and the tumors will cure.*[1]

In 1907, Dr. Martin of Phoenix, Territory of Arizona, wrote to Dr. F. G. Novy at the University of Michigan:

> *There have been during the summer several individuals . . . who have suffered from an infection as a result of skinning and dressing wild rabbits. Three of these persons have had their primary lesions in or about the eye, the preauricular gland being involved. In one instance infection took place in the foot, and others in the hands, the adjacent lymphatics of course being involved.*[2]

In 1911, McCoy and Chapin,[3] who were investigating potential outbreaks of bubonic plague after the 1906 San Francisco earthquake, discovered the causative bacterium of the "plaguelike disease of rodents" prevalent among ground squirrels from Tulare, California. They named the organism *Bacterium tularense.* Working with infected rodents, Chapin had a febrile episode and subsequently found his serum to have antibodies to *B. tularense.* Thus, from the beginning, the laboratory hazard of *F. tularensis* was apparent. In Utah in 1911, Pearse[4] described six cases of an illness that occurred in August caused by the bites of a fly. After an incubation period of 2 to 5 days, the lymph glands that drained the bitten area became markedly swollen and went on to suppuration in three patients. The site of the fly bite progressed from a red infiltration to a punched-out, circular ulcer. Most patients had severe chills during the incubation period. Temperatures varied from 37°C to 40°C. Intrigued by the disease called deer fly fever, the U.S. Public Health Service Surgeon Dr. Edward Francis went to Utah in 1919 to find the cause. In 1921, he published "The Occurrence of Tularemia in Nature as a Disease of Man."[5] He named the disease for the organism, *B. tularense,* and for its occurrence in blood, "-emia." (The name Tulare derives from the Aztec name for the tule reed, which grew in extensive marshes about Tulare Lake, California.[6]) In 1925, a Japanese physician, Ohara,[7] described three patients who developed an illness after they had skinned, cooked, and eaten a dead hare. Ohara named the disease *yato byo* (wild hare disease). In collaboration with Ohara, Francis confirmed that *yato byo* was tularemia. In 1924, Parker and colleagues[8] discovered the role of ticks in transmission. Francis' landmark paper of 1925 describes most of the known aspects, except those relating to treatment.[2]

*Deceased.

Etiology

F. tularensis is a small (1 to 2 μm), pleomorphic, gram-negative coccobacillus, an intracellular pathogen. It is a strict aerobe, grows optimally at 37°C, and requires cysteine for growth. It grows poorly or not at all on most ordinary media. The usual medium used for growth is glucose-cysteine blood agar. It will grow in thioglycolate broth or other sulfhydryl media. Selective media containing cycloheximide and penicillin facilitate isolation from contaminated specimens such as sputum or ulcers. Isolations are reported on charcoal–yeast extract inoculated with specimens from patients with suspected legionellosis. A few cases have been diagnosed by use of radiometric blood culture systems.[9]

All isolates are serologically homogeneous; however, two subtypes (biotypes) are recognized. Biotype *tularensis* (Jellison type A), isolated in nature only in North America, ferments glycerol to produce acid and contains the enzyme citralline ureidase. *F. tularensis* biotype *palaearctica* (Jellison type B) is found in North America, Europe, and Asia. Type B strains do not ferment glycerol and lack citralline ureidase. Type A strains cause more severe disease than type B strains do. A majority of strains of *F. tularensis* produce β-lactamase.

The organism has multiple antigenic components, including multiple outer membrane antigens and lipopolysaccharide (endotoxin). Patients with tularemia show individual variations in humoral antibody responses to the various antigens, suggesting that the use of less refined antigens is advantageous in serologic diagnostic tests.[10] There is cross-reactivity between antigens of *F. tularensis, Brucella abortus,* and *Yersinia enterocolitica.* The cross-reactive antibodies are susceptible to reduction by dithiothreitol.[11]

F. tularensis is readily killed by heat but is not destroyed by freezing. Organisms may remain viable in frozen animal carcasses as long as 3 weeks. Exposure to 56°C for 10 minutes is sufficient for killing, so adequate cooking renders the meat of animals and game birds safe.

Epidemiology

Tularemia occurs in the Northern Hemisphere between 30 and 71 degrees north latitude, worldwide except in the United Kingdom. It has been reported in the United States, Canada, Mexico, the Far East (Japan, the former Soviet Union), and Europe, especially in Scandinavia and Finland, but not from South America or Africa. In the United States, tularemia has been reported from all states except Hawaii. Between a third and half of all reported cases are from Missouri and Arkansas, followed by Tennessee, Oklahoma, Kansas, and Utah.[12]

F. tularensis has been isolated from more than 100 species of wild mammals (rabbits, hares, squirrels, moles, muskrats, beavers), at least 9 species of domestic animals (sheep, cattle, dogs, cats), 25 species of birds (mallards, owls, crows, hawks), amphibians, fish, and more than 50 species of arthropods (ticks, deer flies, mosquitos), as well as from mud and water.

The most common sources of infection in the United States are bites by ticks or deer flies and contact with infected animals or their carcasses. In Scandinavia and Finland, mosquitos are the most important arthropod vector.[13] In the United States, the seasonal occurrence shows a bimodal distribution, with peaks in July and December. The summer peak reflects tick-associated disease, whereas the winter peak is associated with animal contact, especially rabbits.[14] Less often, people acquire infection from the bite of an infected animal or one whose mouth has become contaminated through ingestion of a diseased animal; this mechanism accounts for most instances of cat-bite tularemia. Numerous outbreaks associated with exposure to water contaminated by beavers or muskrats have been reported.[15] Infection may also occur through aerosolization of organisms. Aerosol transmission was postulated for an outbreak of pneumonic tularemia on Martha's Vineyard, Massachusetts, in 1978 and outbreaks in Sweden and Finland associated with handling stored hay or cutting fresh hay.[16–18] Aerosol transmission is also responsible for most laboratory-acquired cases.[19] Human-to-human transmission has been reported only rarely and has no epidemiologic importance.

In the United States, most cases of tularemia associated with rabbits are associated with contact with cottontail rabbits (*Sylvilagus* species). The organism is transmitted between animals by the rabbit tick (*Haemaphysalis leporis-palustris*), which only rarely bites humans. Cottontail rabbits are extremely susceptible to infection and regularly die. Jackrabbits (*Lepus* species) are also a source, whose importance was stressed in the early studies. Snowshoe hares (*Lepus americanus bairdi*) are relatively resistant to infection. Domestic rabbits have not been implicated in natural disease, although they are responsible for some laboratory-associated cases.[20]

In the United States, the incidence and apparent epidemiology of tularemia are changing. During 1930 to 1940, 85% to 90% of cases were associated with rabbits.[21] Tick exposure has now become most common, being responsible for 71% of cases in one report.[22] The reported incidence of tularemia has steadily declined in the United States since 1950. In the 1940s, between 1000 and 2000 cases were reported annually; now between 150 and 300 are reported. A number of factors may be responsible for this decline. There may be less rabbit illness. In 1920, Francis found that 3% of 556 jackrabbits were infected. In contrast, only 0.3% of 5168 animals from the same areas surveyed from 1951 to 1964 were infected.[23] The increased use of antimicrobial agents other than β-lactam antibiotics may also have led to early cure, nonrecognition, and lack of reporting.

In the United States, at least 13 species of ticks have been found to be naturally infected. The important species in transmission to humans are the wood tick (*Dermacentor andersoni*), the dog tick (*Dermacentor variabilis*), and the Lone Star tick (*Amblyomma americanum*). Tick transmission may be associated with injection of saliva during feeding or contamination with tick feces. Transovarial transmission occurs, and because ticks can live as long as 21 years, the potential for transmission is great.

Pathogenesis and Pathology

As with other infectious agents, disease reflects the balance among virulence, number of infecting organisms, and immune status of the host. Jellison type B strains (biotype *palaearctica*) are less virulent in rabbits, and disease in humans is less severe. Disease due to Jellison type A strains, which have been predominant in the United States, is more severe. As few as 10 organisms inoculated intracutaneously may produce systemic disease in humans.[24] The aerosol inoculum required to produce disease is 15 to 50 organisms.[25] By mouth, 10^8 organisms are required to produce disease. Granulomata in wild animals contain up to 10^9 organisms per gram. Portals of entry include the skin, mucous membranes, and respiratory tract. *F. tularensis* is reported to be able to penetrate intact skin but more likely enters through inapparent breaks. Organisms spread through blood or lymphatics. The incubation period between inoculation and onset of disease is usually 3 to 5 days (range, 1 to 14 days). After introduction, the organisms spread through blood or lymphatics. Bacteremia has been detected as early as 3 days and as late as 12 days after onset of illness. After inoculation, organisms evoke a response by neutrophilic leukocytes, macrophages, and T lymphocytes. Neutrophils cannot phagocytose *F. tularensis* in the absence of antibody. Macrophages ingest the organisms, which multiply intracellularly and may kill the host cell. After about 2 weeks, T lymphocytes are activated. This response correlates with the development of reactivity to the tularemia skin test and blast transformation by T lymphocytes on exposure in vitro to tularemia antigens. Cell-mediated immunity persists for at least 25 years after natural infection, with reexposure; agglutinating antibody titers decline or become negative.[26] Humoral antibodies appear between the 11th day and as late as the third week. In most cases, immunoglobulin G, M, and A antibodies appear simultaneously.[10] Early lesions reveal areas of focal necrosis surrounded by neutrophilic leukocytes and a few macrophages. Later, the necrotic areas become surrounded by lymphocytes and epithelioid cells. Caseating granulomata, with or without multinucleated giant cells, occur in some lesions. Viable *F. tularensis* organisms may persist in tissues for long periods. Growth on cultures of biopsy specimens has been obtained as long as 22 months after clinical onset.[27]

Clinical Manifestations

Tularemia has been classified into six clinical constellations: ulceroglandular, glandular, oculoglandular, typhoidal, oropharyngeal (anginose), and pneumonic. The classification is a matter of convenience and does not indicate any fundamental difference in source of infection or even course of illness or prognosis. In fact, the preconception that tularemia is an ulceroglandular disease may result in failure to recognize it in its other presentations, which represent a quarter to half of all cases.

Regardless of portal of entry, the mode of onset and general features of tularemia remain the same. The usual incubation period is 3 to 5 days (range, 1 to 21 days).[21] Onset of symptoms is abrupt. Symptoms consist of fever (85%), with the temperature usually higher than 38.3°C (101°F); chills (52%); headache (45%); cough (38%); pharyngitis (35%); generalized myalgia (31%); and vomiting (17%).[1, 28] The high temperature and symptoms usually subside after 24 to 96 hours. After a remission of 1 to 3 days, the fever and symptoms recur. Illness then typically continues for 2 to 3 weeks longer. During this interval, weakness, sweating, chilliness, and weight loss are common.

Ulceroglandular Disease

Forty-five percent to 85% of patients have the ulceroglandular form of tularemia.[21, 22, 27] Twenty-four to 48 hours after the onset of fever, the area of the lymph nodes draining the site of inoculation becomes painful. The nodes are enlarged, firm, and tender; the overlying skin is usually inflamed. The inflamed nodes are usually axillary or inguinal, although with tick or mosquito bites on the head, cervical lymphadenopathy occurs. Concurrently or within a day, a local lesion or lesions (about 10% are multiple) are noted. They begin as painful, small, red papules, which progress to a pustule, then to an ulcer with sharp undermined borders and a flat base. Local lesions may occasionally consist of cracked dry skin resembling chapped skin but associated with regional nodes. In the course of 1 or 2 weeks, the ulcers become covered with a dark-colored crust; eventually they heal with a residual scar. Lymphangitis with tularemia is rare. "Sporotrichoid" nodules along lymphatics may occasionally develop. If the site of ulceration is an unusual one, such as the shaft of the penis, it is usually misdiagnosed as chancroid or primary syphilis.

Common concurrent findings include pharyngitis (one third of patients) and respiratory problems (one half of patients).[1] Sore throat occurs in the absence of a clear reason (e.g., having eaten potentially infected rabbit). Patients may complain of pharyngitis but have no physical signs on examination, but half have erythema and some have an exudate. Findings on chest radiographs are abnormal in half of patients, including those who have no symptoms or physical findings. Radiographic findings consist of parenchymal infiltrates, usually in one lower lobe (two thirds of cases).[1] About a third of patients also have pleural effusions. Hilar adenopathy occurs with variable frequency (3% to 30%).[1, 18] Uncommon associated findings include pericarditis, erythema nodosum, and erythema multiforme.

The nodes may persist for long periods, the mean being 3 months. Half become fluctuant regardless of treatment and may develop fistulae. The method of incision and drainage has on occasion been associated with bacteremia and sepsis.[25] Without treatment, enlarged nodes have persisted as long as 3 years.[29]

Glandular Disease

The glandular form (8% to 25% of patients) is virtually identical to the ulceroglandular disease in symptoms and signs, except that an ulcerative lesion is not found.

Oculoglandular Disease

Oculoglandular tularemia is uncommon—less than 5% of reported cases. The portal of entry is the conjunctival sac. Symptoms include inflamed, edematous eyelids and conjunctivitis. Small, yellowish nodules and ulcers may be seen on the palpebral conjunctiva. Affected regional nodes include the preauricular, submandibular, and cervical.

Typhoidal Disease

Typhoidal tularemia represents less than 5% of reported cases. It presents clinically as sepsis without localizing features or as a less acute fever of unknown origin. It is not associated with lymphadenopathy.[30] Patients frequently have underlying medical disorders. The diagnosis is often made fortuitously by blood culture. Features in such patients include sterile pyuria (one third of patients), hyponatremia, and elevated serum levels of creatine kinase (with or without rhabdomyolysis).[30] Pulmonary infiltrates occur in half to three fourths of these patients. Typhoidal tularemia is easily mistaken for severe legionellosis. Thorough questioning for a history of exposure to rabbits or tick bites is essential.

Oropharyngeal (Anginose) Disease

Less than 5% of tularemia is oropharyngeal. It usually represents ulceroglandular disease, the oropharynx being the portal of entry for organisms growing in inadequately cooked meat or rarely in contaminated fruit or vegetables (strawberries, in one report). The usual features are pharyngitis and tonsillitis with cervical lymphadenopathy. Occasional patients present with stomatitis and lymphadenopathy.[31]

Pneumonic Disease

Pneumonic tularemia is a blanket term that encompasses both pulmonary involvement with other clinical types and airborne transmission, either induced in the laboratory or acquired naturally. Depending on the pathogenesis, the prognosis differs. As with the ulceroglandular and typhoidal types, pulmonary involvement is common—single, or multiple-lobe infiltrates, often associated with pleural effusion at radiography.[32] The observation of pneumonic tularemia in sheep shearers suggests inhalation associated with shearing.[27] Two epidemics, one in Sweden and one in Finland, have affected farmers exposed to airborne organisms in stored hay contaminated with dead voles and hay fields with many vole mounds.[17, 18] In these outbreaks, symptoms included fever, headache, myalgias, and arthralgias. Half the patients experienced dry cough, retrosternal discomfort, pleural pain, or dyspnea. A fourth had sore throat. The most common radiographic findings were hilar adenopathy (36%) and pulmonary infiltrates (14%). Almost all patients were treated with tetracycline or streptomycin. There were no fatalities. Radiographic changes cleared within 3 months. The relatively benign course probably reflects infection with the biotype *palaearctica* as well as appropriate treatment. In the laboratory-acquired cases reported by Overholt and colleagues,[19] 15 of 17 patients with pneumonia had oval, 2- to 8-cm infiltrates (12 single, 3 multiple). Similar lesions have been reported by others, but not in more recent series.[33]

Laboratory Features

Laboratory findings are not helpful in a positive sense. Hematologic test values are usually normal. Leukocyte counts vary from 5000 to 20,000/mm^3 (median, 10,000/mm^3).[1] Urinalysis reveals sterile pyuria in 20% to 30% of patients.[1, 30] The basis and significance of this finding are unclear, but recognition of its occurrence may help avoid unnecessary diagnostic studies. Serum enzyme determinations—alanine aminotransferase, aspartate aminotransferase, lactate dehydrogenase, and alkaline phosphatase—are often abnormal (5% to 15% of patients) but do not correlate with clinical abdominal findings.[1] Increases in creatine kinase have been noted, especially with typhoidal tularemia.[30, 34]

Diagnosis

The diagnosis of tularemia is usually based on serologic test results rather than other culture. *F. tularensis* requires a medium containing cysteine for growth, and successful cultivation poses a laboratory hazard. Diagnosis is based on bacterial agglutination tests. A fourfold increase in titer is required to confirm the diagnosis. An acute-phase titer of 1:160 or greater is presumptive, but such levels seldom develop before the 11th day of illness and sometimes not until the third week. Positive agglutination titers of 1:10 to 1:80 occur in about 1% of the general U.S. population.[1] Detection of cellular immune responses by skin testing is both sensitive and specific, but skin test antigens are not available commercially.[15]

Treatment and Prognosis

Before streptomycin was introduced in 1947, the course of tularemia was described as 31 days of fever, 31 days in bed, and a total duration of disability of about 3.5 months.[1] *F. tularensis* strains are susceptible in vitro to a number of antimicrobial agents. They are resistant to natural penicillins and first-generation cephalosporins. Agents for which minimal inhibitory concentrations for 90% of strains can be achieved in blood include the aminoglycosides (streptomycin, gentamicin, amikacin, tobramycin, netilmicin), tetracyclines (tetracycline, doxycycline), chloramphenicol, third-generation cephalosporins (cefotaxime, ceftriaxone), rifampin, and erythromycin.[35] Minimal bactericidal concentrations for ciprofloxacin, norfloxacin, pefloxacin, and ofloxacin are within achievable blood levels.[36] Streptomycin has remained the drug of choice, and various regimens have been used: 30 mg/kg per 24 hours, in two doses intramuscularly at 12-hour intervals for 3 days, followed by 15 mg/kg per 24 hours in two doses for another 3 days; others have used 15 mg/kg per day at 12-hour intervals for 10 to 14 days. The response is prompt; 80% of patients' fever drops within 48 hours. Gentamicin, 3 to 5 mg/kg per day intravenously, has been used successfully to treat a smaller number of patients.[35] There are no data that address once-daily dosing of gentamicin. Tetracycline is effective but requires a longer course of treatment, and relapses are common after 1.0 g/d for 15 days or 2.0 g/d for 10 days. If tetracycline is used, the dosage should be 2 g/d for 15 days. In a small number of patients, oral fluoroquinolones (ciprofloxacin, 750 mg orally twice daily) have been effective.[36, 37] Erythromycin (intravenous) has been reported effective in several instances when it was prescribed for suspected legionellosis. Although effective in vitro, ceftriaxone (50 to 75 mg/kg daily for 4 to 7 days) was not clinically effective; eight of eight patients had clinical deterioration. Data on ceftazidime are not known.[39]

The overall mortality rate for untreated tularemia (type A, presumably) was 8%. For typhoidal tularemia, it was two to three times greater. Today, with early diagnosis and appropriate treatment, the mortality is less than 1%, but there remains a group of patients with underlying medical disorders whose treatment is often delayed and among whom the mortality rate remains 6%.[30]

Prevention

To minimize the risk of tularemia, persons should wear gloves to skin or eviscerate wild rabbits. Avoiding tick-infested areas and using tick repellents such as permethrin reduce the risk. It is widely accepted that one attack of tularemia confers permanent immunity. Although there are documented cases of reinfection, efforts to develop an effective tularemia vaccine began early. An investigational live attenuated vaccine provides partial protection and reduces the severity of disease. Its use is limited to persons at high risk, such as laboratory workers handling *F. tularensis* and persons whose occupations bring them into repeated contact with wild mammals or vectors. The vaccine is available from the Centers for Disease Control and Prevention in Atlanta.

References

1. Evans ME, Gregory DW, Schaffner W, McGee ZA: Tularemia: A 30 year experience with 88 cases. Medicine (Baltimore) 64:251, 1985.
2. Francis E: Tularemia. JAMA 84:1243, 1925.
3. McCoy GW, Chapin CW: Further observations on a plague-like disease of rodents with a preliminary note on the causative agent *Bacterium tularense.* J Infect Dis 10:61, 1912.
4. Pearse RA: Insect bites. Northwest Med 3:81, 1911. Cited by Francis E: Medicine (Baltimore) 7:411, 1928.
5. Francis E: The occurrence of tularemia in nature as a disease of man. Public Health Rep 36:1731, 1921.
6. Rockwood SW: Tularemia: What's in a name? ASM News 49:63, 1983.
7. Ohara S: Studies on yato-byo (Ohara's disease) tularemia in Japan, report I. Jpn J Exp Med 24:69, 1954.
8. Parker RR, Spencer RR, Francis E: Tularemia XI. Tularemia infection in ticks of the species *Dermacentor andersoni Stiles* in the Bitter Root Valley, Montana. Public Health Rep 39:1057, 1924.
9. Provenza JM, Klotz SA, Penn RL: Isolation of *Francisella tularensis* from blood. J Clin Microbiol 24:453, 1986.
10. Bevanger L, MacLand JA, Naess AI: Agglutinins and antibodies to *Francisella tularensis* outer membrane antigens in early diagnosis of disease during an outbreak of tularemia. J Clin Microbiol 26:433, 1988.
11. Behan KA, Klein GC: Reduction of *Brucella* species and *Francisella tularensis* cross-reacting agglutinins by dithiothreitol. J Clin Microbiol 16:756, 1982.
12. Taylor JP, Istre GR, McChesney TC, et al: Epidemiologic characteristics of human tularemia in the Southwest-Central States, 1981–1987. Am J Epidemiol 133:1032, 1991.
13. Uhari M, Syrjala H, Salminen A: Tularemia in children caused by *Francisella tularensis* biovar *palaearctica.* Pediatr J Infect Dis 9:80, 1990.
14. Guerrant RL, Humphries MK Jr, Butler JE, Jackson RS: Tick-borne oculoglandular tularemia. Arch Intern Med 136:811, 1976.
15. Young LS, Bickness DS, Archer BG, et al: Tularemia epidemic Vermont, 1968. N Engl J Med 280:1253, 1969.
16. Teutsch SM, Martona WJ, Brink EW, et al: Pneumonic tularemia on Martha's Vineyard. N Engl J Med 301:826, 1979.
17. Dahlstrand S, Ringertz O, Zetterberg B: Airborne tularemia in Sweden. Scand J Infect Dis 3:7, 1971.
18. Syrjala H, Kujala P, Myllyla V, Salminen A: Airborne transmission of tularemia in farmers. Scand J Infect Dis 17:371, 1985.
19. Overholt EL, Tigertt WD, Kadull PJ, et al: An analysis of forty-two cases of laboratory-acquired tularemia. Am J Med 30:785, 1961.
20. Jellison WL: Tularemia in North America 1930–1974. Missoula, MT, University of Montana, 1974.
21. Sanders CV, Hahn R: Analysis of 106 cases of tularemia. J La State Med Soc 120:381, 1969.
22. Jacobs RF, Condrey YM, Yamauchi T: Tularemia in adults and children: A changing presentation. Pediatrics 76:818, 1985.
23. Thorpe BD, Sidwell RW, Johnson DE, et al: Tularemia in the wildlife and livestock of the great Salt Lake desert region, 1951 through 1964. Am J Trop Med Hyg 14:622, 1965.
24. Saslaw S, Eigelsbach HT, Wilson HE, et al: Tularemia vaccine study. I. Intracutaneous challenge. Arch Intern Med 107:689, 1961.
25. Saslaw S, Eigelsbach HT, Prior JA, et al: Tularemia vaccine study. II. Respiratory challenge. Arch Intern Med 107:702, 1961.
26. Ericsson M, Sandstrom G, Sjostedt A, Tarnvik A: Persistence of cell-mediated immunity and decline of humoral immunity to the intracellular bacterium *Francisella tularensis* 25 years after natural infection. J Infect Dis 170:110, 1994.
27. Larsen CL: Tularemia. *In* Tices Practice of Medicine, Vol 3. New York, Harper & Row, 1973, pp 663–676.
28. Jacobs RF, Narain JP: Tularemia in children. Pediatr Infect Dis J 2:487, 1983.
29. Foshay L: Tularemia: A summary of certain aspects of the disease including methods for early diagnosis and the results of serum treatment in 600 patients. Medicine (Baltimore) 19:1, 1940.
30. Penn RL, Kinasewitz GT: Factors associated with a poor outcome in tularemia. Arch Intern Med 147:265, 1987.
31. Luotonen J, Syrjala H, Jokinen K, et al: Tularemia in otolaryngologic practice. Arch Otolaryngol Head Neck Surg 112:77, 1986.
32. Stuart BM, Pullen RL: Tularemic pneumonia. Am J Med Sci 210:223, 1945.
33. Dennis TM, Boudreau RP: Pleuropulmonary tularemia: Its roentgen manifestations. Radiology 68:25, 1957.
34. Kaiser AB, Rieves D, Price AH, et al: Tularemia and rhabdomyolysis. JAMA 253:241, 1985.
35. Enderlin G, Morales L, Jacobs RF, Cross JT: Streptomycin and alternative agents for the treatment of tularemia: Review of the literature. Clin Infect Dis 19:42, 1994.
36. Syrjala H, Schildt R, Raisainen S: In vitro susceptibility of *Francisella tularensis* to fluoroquinolones and treatment of tularemia with norfoxacin and ciprofloxacin. Eur J Clin Microbiol Infect Dis 10:68, 1991.
37. Risi GF, Pombo DJ: Relapse of tularemia after aminoglycoside therapy: Case report and discussion of therapeutic options. Clin Infect Dis 20:174, 1995.
38. Harrell RE Jr, Simmons HF: Pleuropulmonary tularemia: Successful treatment with erythromycin. South Med J 83:1363, 1990.
39. Cross JT, Jacobs RF: Tularemia: Treatment failures with outpatient use of ceftriaxone. Clin Infect Dis 17:976, 1993.

173

Plague

Darwin Palmer

Plague is an infection caused by *Yersinia pestis*, a gram-negative coccobacillary organism of the family Enterobacteriaceae. This zoonosis is endemic in a wide array of rodents and is spread both among them and to humans by fleas. The rat-borne plague epidemics of Europe, with enormous population die-offs in the Middle Ages, made the disease synonymous (as the Black Death) with pestilential horror and biologic calamity. The organism was ineradicably established in enzootic rodent foci on every continent during the three pandemics of the Christian era. Sporadic spread to humans as rodent epidemics wax and wane and as humankind increasingly encroaches on rural habitats is a current problem in much of the world as well as in the western United States. However, early diagnosis and modern treatment have reduced the untreated 40% to 90% mortality of bubonic and pneumonic plague to approximately 5% to 10%.

History

Although biblical writings document a pestilence with high mortality among the Philistines in 1320 BC, the description is so incomplete that one can only suspect plague as the cause. The first pandemic undoubtedly caused by plague occurred during the reign of Justinian starting in AD 542.[1, 2] In this as in subsequent pandemics, plague was imported from Asia Minor during periods of social disruption and war; it was also later spread by travelers and merchant ships. This first pandemic lasted for about 100 years and devastated the populations of the Middle East and the Mediterranean. Not again recorded in the ensuing centuries in Europe, it probably was reimported with the black rat from Asia by the returning crusaders in the 13th century. The black rat, inhabiting the walls and roofs of human habitations, spread throughout Europe. In 1347, plague was imported by traders from the Crimea to Italy, where it rapidly invaded the cities of Genoa, Rome, Naples, and Venice (Fig. 173–1). In the ensuing 3 years, the pandemic reached the rest of Europe, causing an estimated 25 million deaths, a reduction of one quarter of the total population. Known as the Black Death, because of either popular dread or possibly a hemorrhagic diathesis in some victims, the disease became well established in urban rat populations. For the next three centuries, periodic rat die-offs accompanied human outbreaks. Gradual decline in disease then occurred, often preceded regionally by a major epidemic. Thus, the Great Plague of London in 1665 was followed by a virtual absence of English cases until 1909. During the 17th century, the brown sewer rat *(Rattus norvegicus)* replaced the black house rat *(Rattus rattus)* in Europe. Because the brown rat does not frequent house roofs and walls, and its fleas prefer it to humans, this change in rat ecology may have been instrumental in halting this second pandemic.[3]

The third pandemic had its origins, like the others, in the Far East, where plague apparently smoldered until the late 19th century when it erupted in refugees from war in the Yunnan province of China. With spread of the disease first to Canton and then Hong Kong in 1894, its dissemination to the rest of the world was immensely enhanced by international shipping. Initially infecting waterfront areas of major world cities, *Y. pestis* was then spread inland by rats and other rodents. In Hong Kong, the hospital death rate was 95% for plague patients, and the disease was rampant in the slums of neighboring Canton, where 60,000 people had died in 1 year. Alexander Yersin, a French ship's doctor who had worked previously on diphtheria toxin and trained with Pasteur, isolated, cultured, and demonstrated animal pathogenicity in a gram-negative bacillus that he grew from bubo pulp from patients dead of plague in Hong Kong. He published his data on his return to Paris in 1894, naming the organism *Pasteurella pestis* in honor of his mentor. Returning to Vietnam, Yersin spent the rest of his life attempting to develop a plague vaccine. The genus *Yersinia* was renamed in the 1960s to give more authenticity to its origin.

Rapidly spreading throughout the world, the plague bacillus reached India, where it was causing more than a million deaths annually by 1903. Many nations, including the United States, sent plague commissions to India to study the disease. The U.S. Surgeon General mailed a pamphlet alerting his medical officers and commenting on its first appearance in the New World in Santos, Brazil, in 1899; it was also found in islands of the Pacific, including the Philippines and Hawaii.[4]

In 1900, bubonic plague was detected in San Francisco, having been identified from the bubo of a dead Chinese worker discovered in the basement of the house in which he worked.[1] The case was astutely recognized and bacteriologically confirmed as plague by the chief quarantine officer, Joseph Kinyoun, who recommended antipest serum, fumigation, and quarantine of Chinatown. In the next 5 days, two more plague deaths were detected and confirmed in Chinese workers. However, the governor of California, concerned about the effect of adverse publicity on tourism, conducted an investigation sponsored by big business, the chamber of

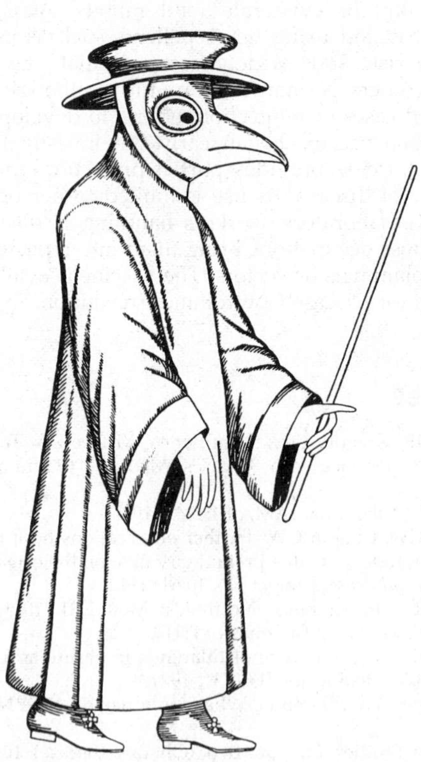

FIGURE 173–1 ▫ Antiplague costume of 16th century. The nasal piece contained herbs to prevent inhaled contagion.

commerce, and the railroad industry and concluded that plague "did not and never had existed." The control measures were halted by his mandate, and the warning concerning plague was officially scoffed at in the newspapers. By 1904, however, after 118 deaths due to plague, the new governor of California officially recognized the presence of the disease in San Francisco and the state of California. Ratproofing of buildings and cleanup then commenced aggressively in the slums of San Francisco. By 1905, the local medical authorities had started rat eradication, and medical ecobiologists first recognized fleas as the vector between infected rats and humans. Despite the waning rat plague epidemic in the city, however, the lack of early disease containment may have assisted in transmitting plague to a focus of ground squirrels in the hills to the east of San Francisco. Detection of wild rodents as carriers (and transmitters) of plague bacillus led to the first understanding of sylvatic (rural) as opposed to urban rat propagation of plague.

This sylvatic focus was the source of the last known epidemic of pneumonic plague in the Western Hemisphere. In August 1919, a man contracted bubonic plague while hunting squirrels in the Berkeley hills. Developing secondary plague pneumonia, he subsequently transmitted primary plague pneumonia to 13 others (including two physicians), of whom 12 died. The epidemic was controlled only by hospitalization and isolation of the patients.

From this wild rodent population, it is suspected that the plague bacillus spread among other wild rodents including ground squirrels, voles, chipmunks, and prairie dogs in California and in neighboring states.[5, 6] Causing only sporadic human cases (5 to 10 per year), it gradually spread to the Pacific Northwest and inland to Nevada, Utah, Arizona, Colorado, and New Mexico. By 1960, plague was present in rodent populations as far east as North Dakota, Kansas, Oklahoma, and Texas and had caused 523 human cases with 340 deaths from 1900 to 1951. The reason for the limitation of spread at the 100th meridian is unclear; possibly the density of susceptible rodents (e.g., ground squirrels, prairie dogs) is sparse beyond this geographic boundary.

Transiently infesting the waterfront areas of New York City, New Orleans, and Galveston, plague did not cause major human outbreaks. The disease in the coastal cities was contained by rat-proofing buildings, and by not spreading to sylvatic rodents, plague eventually disappeared. Similar efforts to rat-proof ships halted new spread to other cities in the United States, and the disease in this country is now confined to the western United States, most particularly the Southwest.

Epidemiology

The plague bacillus exists on all continents of the world except for Australia and Antarctica. It is permanently established in more than 200 sylvatic rodent species in Eurasia, Africa, and North and South America. Whereas human cases must be reported to the World Health Organization, its presence among rodents often goes unrecognized because it circulates unobtrusively in discontinuous and enzootic foci. The periodic increase and plague-associated die-off of rodent populations in the wild are the occasion for greater or lesser contact with rural-dwelling humans.[7] Once established, sylvatic plague rarely completely disappears; an apparent exception may exist in Hawaii.[4] There, 410 human plague cases with a mortality of 90% were recorded between 1899 and 1949. However, since 1957, continuous surveys of rats, other rodents, and carnivores (the mongoose) have failed to detect either plague bacillus or any serologic evidence of infection. Reports from other regions of the world, as in Greater Russia or India, have shown reappearance of human plague after an absence of 30 years, possibly due to inattention to sylvatic sources.

Three separate biogroups of *Y. pestis*—*antiqua, medievalis,* and *orientalis*—have distinctive DNA homology, world localization, and sylvatic hosts, lending credence to the spread and establishment of plague bacilli in three pandemic waves.[8] In Russia, tarbagans, marmots, and gerbils are infected; in Africa, spiny mice, giant grass rats, and insectivorous rodents are plague reservoirs. In the United States, prairie dogs, ground squirrels, and rock squirrels are the most commonly involved species, whereas voles, chipmunks, deer mice, and rabbits are less frequent hosts.[5, 7] Rodents and their fleas vary in sensitivity to *Y. pestis;* thus, peridomestic rats, *R. rattus* and *R. norvegicus,* are readily killed, and their flea, *Xenopsylla cheopis,* carries and transmits plague bacillus well, both between rats and to humans. The bandicoot rat of India is relatively more resistant to lethal infection with *Y. pestis* and may serve as a permanent resident focus for infection. More susceptible species, such as ground squirrels of the western United States, may amplify the organism as the population of rodents increases. The prairie dog, if infected during fall, may overwinter the organism in a dormant phase during hibernation only to develop clinical disease and die with massive replication of *Y. pestis* during the spring. Rodent burrows are also able to maintain viable *Y. pestis* in cool, moist soil for many months.

Rodent fleas are partially specific for rodent species and have relative specificity for carriage of *Y. pestis.* Carriage of *Y. pestis* may persist for many weeks without death of the flea, and flea vector efficiency is variably dependent on environmental temperature and relative humidity.[9] In addition, adverse conditions such as cold may enhance *Y. pestis* dormancy and maintenance in the flea. Fleas suck directly from venules, with the ingested blood going through the proventriculus to the stomach. Replication of *Y. pestis* in the proventriculus closes off this entranceway to the stomach. The flea, now unable to ingest a blood meal, will repeatedly attempt to feed and, because of the blocked proventriculus, will regurgitate infected material directly into the wound. Whereas *X. cheopis* is a good vector, other flea species, such as *Pulex irritans,* the human flea, carry and transmit *Y. pestis* less well.

Human plague has two epidemiologic forms (Fig. 173–2), the sporadic, acquired from endemic rural foci, and the epidemic, acquired from urban rat infestation. Sporadic human disease is probably underreported, especially in Africa, Asia, and Latin America. However, where epidemiologic tracking is precise, as in the southwestern United States, disease in humans closely follows that in wild rodent vectors.[6, 7] Thus, as rodent populations increase because of climatologic variation in foodstuffs, human disease will show resurgence. This has resulted in irregular periodicity in the southwestern United States, with cases in humans varying from 1 or 2 to 40 or 50 per year. The periodicity of such outbreaks in both rodents and humans is not regular but varies according to unpredictable ecologic factors.

Epidemic disease in city-dwelling humans usually erupts after the infestation of large numbers of peridomestic urban rats. An often observed "rat fall," in which rats inhabiting the walls and ceilings of slum homes become infected, die, and drop to the ground, may precede the development of an urban epidemic in humans. This was noted before the 1994 epidemic of pneumonic plague in south-central India.[10] Human plague occurs in settings of war and social disruption in cities; it almost always occurs among conditions of intense poverty, poor sanitation, and absence of control of rats and other vermin. Disease manifestations are identical in sylvatic plague and urban plague, that is, mostly bubonic disease with occasional secondary pneumonic illness.[5, 11] On occasion,

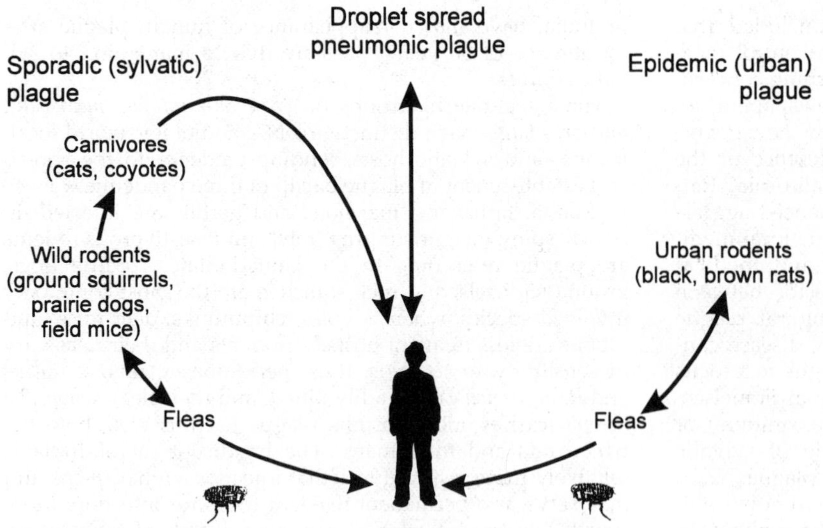

FIGURE 173–2 ▫ Human plague interaction with animal sources of fleas. Sylvatic plague is ecologically distinct from urban plague.

urban population density may foster human-to-human spread of primary pneumonic plague from cough-generated aerosols of *Y. pestis,* with devastating consequences. Bubonic plague is essentially nontransmissible from person to person, whereas primary pneumonic plague is among the most contagious of all illnesses. With an accompanying mortality of almost 100% if untreated, pneumonic plague has been the apparent reason for extremely widespread die-off of human populations in past pandemics.

Plague occurs in zoonotic locations around the world; most cases are reported from the developing countries of Asia and Africa. In the decade of 1980 through 1989, 8554 cases of human plague were reported from 17 countries to the World Health Organization, with an 11% mortality.[2] Sizable outbreaks, often after years of absence, have been reported from Angola, Tanzania, and Brazil. During this same decade, Tanzania, Vietnam, Zaire, Brazil, Madagascar, Peru, Uganda, Burma, Bolivia, and the United States each reported more than 100 cases of plague.

During the 25-year period from 1970 to 1994 (Fig. 173–3), cases in the United States ranged from a low of 1 case in 1972 and 1990 to a maximum of 40 cases in 1983, for a total of 333 cases or a mean of 13 cases per year.[7] In the United States, rural homes and their surroundings accounted for

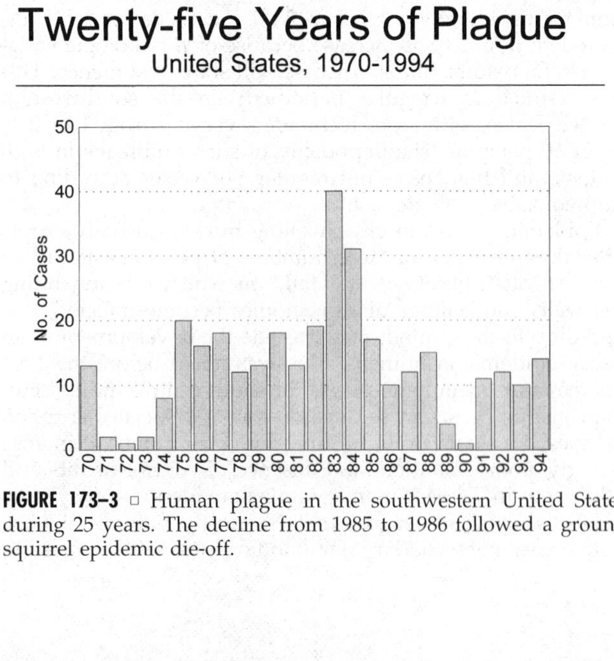

FIGURE 173–3 ▫ Human plague in the southwestern United States during 25 years. The decline from 1985 to 1986 followed a ground squirrel epidemic die-off.

75% of the exposures. Indigenous cases were reported from 12 western states, with New Mexico having more than 50% of the total and Arizona, Colorado, and California with less than 15% each. Mortality was 14.5%; greater mortality occurred in patients in whom there was a delay in diagnosis, often occasioned by an atypical presentation or travel away from the endemic location during incubation of the illness. Approximately 60% of cases were found in males and in those younger than 20 years,[7, 12] possibly reflecting greater outdoor activity. Ground squirrels were the most frequently implicated source of infection, although the absence of a known rodent source or an insect bite was extremely common.[13] Domestic cats have been recognized as increasingly important sources of infection.[14] Cats catch wild rodents and eat them or carry them back to the household, transmitting *Y. pestis* either by rodent fleas or, after developing illness, by a direct contact. A cat with secondary plague pneumonia was the source in three cases of human acquisition of pulmonary plague. Plague has also been acquired from rabbits during the winter months and from carnivores (coyotes and bobcat).[7, 13] Native Americans have had an especially high attack rate (30% of all U.S. cases) because of their close contact with wild animals in a rural setting.[15] In addition, the Navajo have used prairie dogs as a food source. Finally, as humans move from cities to more rural environments, they acquire sporadic cases of plague where either their direct contact or that occasioned by their domestic pets has increased the risk for exposure.

The bulk of the cases in the United States have occurred between the months of May and October, when both human activity in the open and rodent activity are highest.[7] Whereas the cat species usually become ill with plague, with a mortality of 70%, the dog species are more resistant to clinical illness.[14] As a consequence, both feral dogs and coyotes have been used as serologic sentinels to detect resurgent plague in the surrounding rodent populations in both Oregon and New Mexico.[16]

The continued residential expansion into high-risk areas of the rural environment has led to specific recommendations for control of human plague. These include increased surveillance of the rodent populations near human habitation; advice concerning decrease in rodent harborage and food sources surrounding households; control of wild rodents and their fleas by the use of appropriate insecticides; and information to rural dwellers about the significance of sick and dying rodents or the signs and symptoms of human plague.

Etiologic Agent

Y. pestis is a pleomorphic, gram-negative coccobacillus that is facultatively anaerobic and grows readily on most culture media.[5] It is closely related to the pathogens *Yersinia enterocolitica* and *Yersinia pseudotuberculosis* but distinct from them in pathology, specific antigens, and certain culture characteristics.[17] With Wayson or Giemsa stain, it shows characteristic bipolar staining, which gives it a characteristic "safety pin" appearance (Fig. 173–4).

Y. pestis tends to grow aerobically but slowly on blood agar and MacConkey agar, does not ferment lactose, and forms small colonies after 48 hours of incubation. Optimal temperature for growth is 28°C. Hence, prolonged incubation at temperatures below 37°C produces small, semitranslucent colonies that are gray and somewhat mucoid in appearance. The organism is nonmotile and urease-negative and does not use citrate or indole. Automated laboratory diagnostic equipment may fail to properly identify *Yersinia* species or differentiate one *Yersinia* member from the other members of the genus. For definitive identification, the cultures should be forwarded to a reference laboratory, and a public health official should be notified about the possibility of a *Y. pestis* isolate.

The plague bacillus produces several virulence factors that correlate well with its antigenic, immunologic, and invasive characteristics. The organism has a temperature-dependent outer membrane capsule that contains an envelope antigen known as fraction one (F1). This is a protein-polysaccharide complex that is expressed at 37°C and appears to increase resistance to phagocytosis. V and W antigens are mediated by a 45-MDa plasmid and encode for dependence on calcium for growth of the bacterium at 37°C but not at lower temperatures. These V and W antigens confer virulence by enabling the organism to survive and grow intracellularly. Other virulence factors include a lipopolysaccharide endotoxin, the ability to absorb iron in the form of hemin from its surroundings, and the temperature-dependent enzymes coagulase and fibrinolysin. The last two characteristics are also plasmid mediated. Laboratory identification can be achieved by culture and by demonstration of a serologic response by using passive hemagglutination and enzyme-linked immunosorbent assay, both directed toward the F1 antigen of *Y. pestis*. A fourfold rise in titer from acute- to convalescent-phase serum, or a presumptive titer of 1:16, is diagnostic of infection.[5] For definitive identification, cultures can be sent to either one's state laboratory or the Centers for Disease Control and Prevention, Plague Branch. Drug resistance has been detected only once with this organism; however, antibiotic sensitivity testing may reveal misleading sensitivities to the penicillins.

Pathogenesis

Infection with *Y. pestis* is initiated when an infected flea attempts to feed on a human. Organisms are introduced into the blood stream of the recipient host when the flea regurgitates *Y. pestis* organisms from the blocked proventriculus. If the proventriculus is unblocked, the flea may contaminate the bite site after feeding by deposited fecal material, which is then scratched into the wound. On entering the vasculature of the infected host, the organisms migrate to the nearest regional lymph node. Containing only small amounts of the F1 antigen because of their growth in the flea at temperatures of 30°C to 35°C, the organisms are readily phagocytosed by polymorphonuclear or mononuclear cells. Because of contained V and W antigens, however, the *Y. pestis* organisms are able to grow and resist intracellular killing, with eventual destruction and lysis of the cell. At this point, at the end of a 3- to 6-day incubation period, organisms are released into surrounding tissue. With large amounts of F1 antigen now present because of growth in the mammalian host at 37°C, the organisms resist phagocytosis. With continued rapid growth in a lymph node, the node becomes enlarged, inflamed, necrotic, and hemorrhagic. Vast numbers of these phagocytosis-resistant organisms are now released into the circulation, producing bacteremia in almost all infected humans. Clinical manifestations are those due to the typical gram-negative endotoxemia. These include fever, tachycardia, hypotension, leukocytosis, and laboratory evidence of disseminated intravascular coagulation. In the skin, purpura may be seen secondary to hemorrhage after disseminated intravascular coagulation. Splenic tissue may be engorged, inflamed, and hemorrhagic; the liver may show inflammation; and the kidneys often have glomerular fibrin thrombi as a manifestation of disseminated intravascular co-

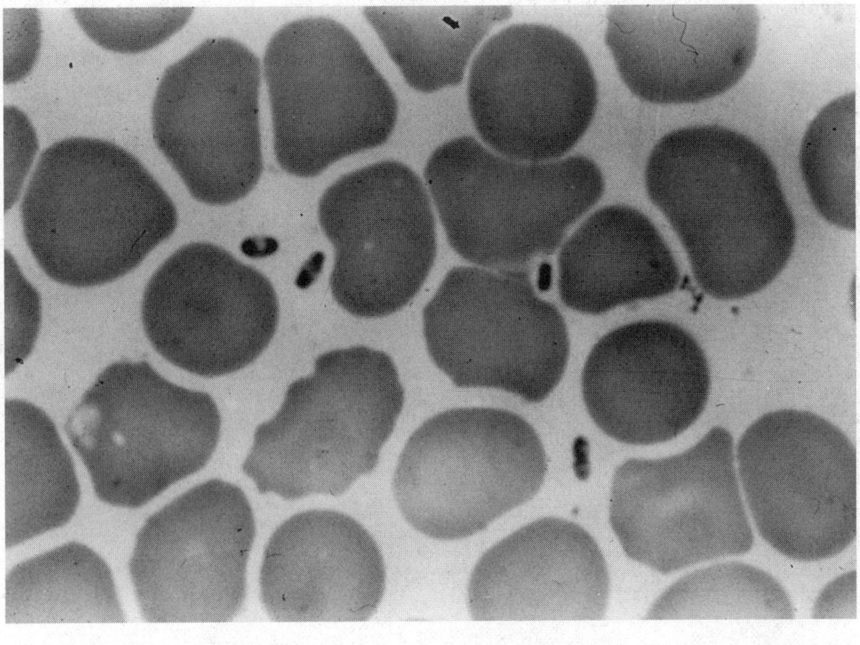

FIGURE 173–4 □ Peripheral blood smear in bacteremic *Y. pestis* infection shows characteristic bipolar (safety pin) staining.

agulation. If the host does not recover, organisms are found in most tissues but in highest concentrations in blood, lymph nodes, and splenic tissue.

Clinical Features

Plague in humans generally presents as bubonic disease, in at least 75% of most sporadic presentations. The so-called septicemic form of plague is most probably a variation of bubonic plague with buboes located intraabdominally or a more fulminant course.[18] Pneumonic plague, developing in about 20% of humans, is secondary to plague bacteremia with dissemination to the lung.[19] However, once established as secondary pneumonia, plague can be transmitted from person to person by cough-generated aerosols of *Y. pestis* to cause primary plague pneumonia. Meningeal plague, like the secondary pneumonia, is due to localization during bacteremia.[20] Pharyngeal plague may be due to direct contact with infected tissues.

Bubonic plague occurs after an incubation period of 2 to 8 days after exposure, presenting with an abrupt onset of fever, chills, weakness, and headache. Although there is generally a history of possible animal exposure, more than 50% of patients do not remember or have physical evidence of an insect bite. Twelve to 24 hours after onset of fever, the patient will note painful adenopathy, the bubo. Found in a single anatomic region, the painful node is so tender that the patient typically avoids any movement that will provoke pain. Buboes are most commonly found in the groin (60%) (Fig. 173–5) but can be seen in the axilla (30%) or cervical area (10%).[5, 11, 13] The distribution of buboes is presumably due to the site of flea inoculation, and buboes at more than one anatomic site are unusual. When intraabdominal nodes are involved, which may either accompany or occur independently of an inguinal bubo, the patient may have severe abdominal pain, nausea, vomiting, and diarrhea that may be so intense as to mimic an acute abdomen.[21] Buboes are swellings that vary from 1 to 10 cm in size and elevate the overlying skin, which is often red and stretched intensely. The surrounding tissue may be edematous, and there may be irregular smaller nodes surrounding the main nodular involvement. At presentation, the bubo is generally not fluctuant.

Depending on how early the patient has sought medical attention, the accompanying clinical manifestations may be severe and include modest hypotension with apprehension, tachycardia, high fever, and shaking chills. As noted, more than 70% of patients with plague may have gastrointestinal complaints.[21] Sometimes overriding the other symptoms, neurologic complaints including insomnia, mental confusion, stupor, weakness, staggering gait, and speech disorders are found. The majority of patients with bubonic plague do not have skin lesions, but approximately 25% of the patients in Vietnam presented with dermatologic findings, including pustules, vesicles, eschars, or papules, presumably the site of the flea bite.[11] These occasionally progress to cellulitis or abscesses. Less commonly, as a consequence of their systemic illness, patients develop purpuric skin lesions that involve the extremities and can become necrotic, resulting in gangrene of the toes, hands, nose, or penis. On abdominal examination, patients with bubonic plague frequently show hepatic and splenic enlargement. Aside from tachycardia, the findings on cardiac examination are usually normal.

Accompanying these physical manifestations, laboratory findings are nondescript. A leukocytosis with a count of between 10,000 and 20,000 white cells per mm^3 is present, although occasionally patients may have a leukemoid reaction with counts as high as $100,000/mm^3$. The peripheral smear will often reveal toxic granulations and Döhle bodies. Platelet counts may be normal or low, depending on the presence of disseminated intravascular coagulation. Disseminated intravascular coagulation may also be manifested by fibrin degradation products, sometimes even with normal platelet counts. Abnormal liver enzyme activities, elevated bilirubin concentration, and hypoglycemia may be seen; with fever and dehydration, there may be a concentrated urine, elevation of the blood urea nitrogen value, and some degree of proteinuria.

Although sometimes described as a separate syndrome, septicemic plague most probably represents a fulminant course with the sepsis and bacteremia often found in bubonic plague. Bacteremia is seen in at least 30% of all patients, and bacteremia without buboes is seen in approximately 10% of all patients. Bacteremia with sepsis is, like other gram-negative sepsis, manifested by hypotension, increased cardiac output, and depressed systemic vascular resistance. Multiorgan system failure results in an overall mortality rate in excess of 50% despite therapy.

Pneumonic plague is one of the most feared complications of this disease and occurs in approximately 20% of all patients with *Y. pestis* infection.[19] Plague pneumonia is generally

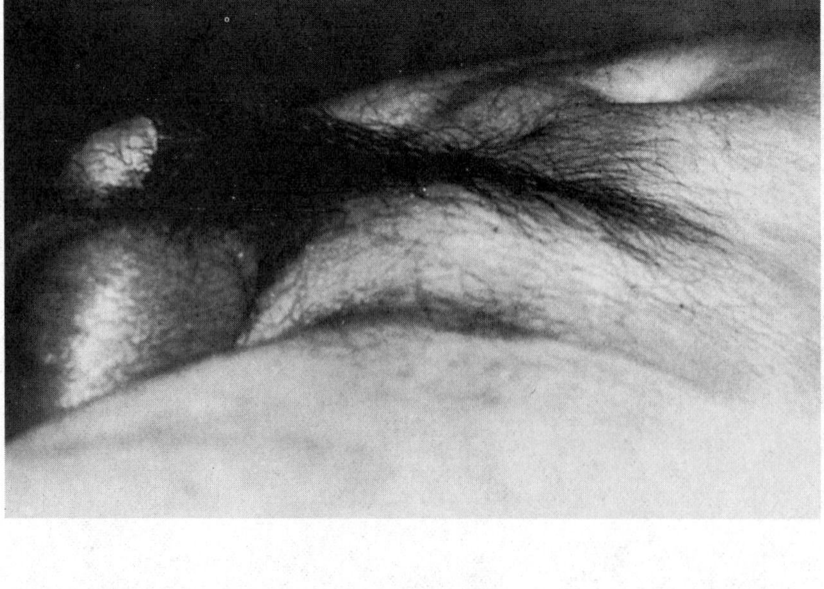

FIGURE 173–5 □ Inguinal bubo in a young man with bacteremic plague.

a complication of bacteremia with secondary involvement of the lung. Some studies have demonstrated that fully 20% of all patients with classic bubonic plague, presumably accompanied or preceded by bacteremia, will develop pulmonary involvement. In half of these, or 10% of all, there is no evidence of an infection, and the pathologic process resembles that of classic endotoxin-associated adult respiratory distress syndrome. In both secondary plague pneumonia and adult respiratory distress syndrome, however, the clinical manifestations may initially be similar (i.e., the patient presents with cough; thin, watery, blood-tinged sputum; and shortness of breath). The radiographic picture is that of a generalized, multilobed, patchy pneumonitis with consolidation in the case of secondary pneumonia and a generalized "whiteout" of the lung in adult respiratory distress syndrome. In plague pneumonia, the consolidation may occasionally progress to cavitation with air-fluid levels and involvement of the adjacent pleura with an exudative plural effusion (Fig. 173–6). In adult respiratory distress syndrome, frank respiratory failure needing ventilatory support may supervene. The difference between the two is manifested by the presence of purulent sputum with white blood cells and *Y. pestis* in the case of secondary plague pneumonia. This condition is contagious because of the generation of *Y. pestis*–containing cough-generated aerosols. Person-to-person transmission with the development of primary plague pneumonia may result in a major, rapidly spreading epidemic disease with a mortality in excess of 90%. Cases of primary plague pneumonia in the United States have been acquired from cats with secondary pneumonia or submandibular abscesses. Many of these cat-acquired cases were fatal owing to lack of early recognition and delay in initiating therapy. Feline plague has been detected in large numbers of cats in the hyperendemic region of New Mexico (60 cases of cat plague) and presents a high risk to both pet owners and veterinarians to whom the sick cats are taken.[5, 14, 16]

Plague meningitis is an uncommon complication of bubonic plague, classically following an axillary bubo.[20] It usually starts 1 week or more after the onset of plague, after antibiotic therapy has been given. Presumably, the plague bacillus, reaching the meninges during the early septicemia phase, is inadequately treated owing to the poor nervous system penetration of antibiotic, which is ordinarily effective for other forms of plague. It may also appear without local adenitis, and it may occur more commonly in those individuals who have handled infected animals than in those who have been bitten by a flea. Patients typically have fever, headache, and a stiff neck.

On rare occasions, mild plague is seen that presents as minor episodes of fever with local lymph node enlargement and minimal systemic disease. In addition, occasional cases present as pharyngeal plague; the patient has sore throat and enlarged tonsils, and *Y. pestis* is cultivated from the throat.

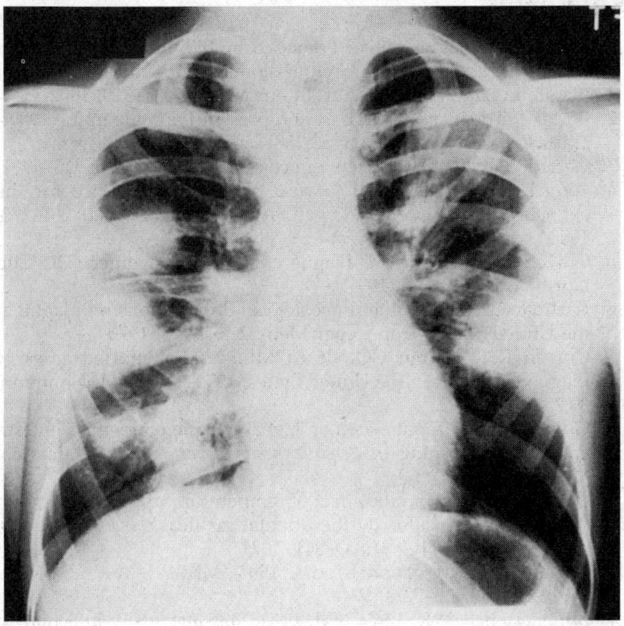

FIGURE 173–6 □ Chest radiograph of patient with secondary plague pneumonia demonstrates cavitary changes.

Diagnosis

The diagnosis of plague is critically dependent on obtaining a careful history to document the possibility of exposure to animals or their fleas in a plague endemic area. In a classic presentation with a bubo, fever, and appropriate travel or residence, the clinical diagnosis can be readily made and bacteriologically confirmed. However, not infrequently, patients have traveled to a nonplague location during the incubation period, an exposure history is not taken, and the connection with bubonic plague is not made. Such patients have had a 50% death rate, most commonly as a result of misdiagnosis and inappropriate therapy. Physical examination is usually dramatic and revealing in a patient presenting with an exquisitely painful, erythematous bubo, although the differential diagnosis can include an incarcerated inguinal hernia, lymphogranuloma venereum, or localized lymphadenopathy due to regional infection. Finally, in the patient with prominent gastrointestinal symptoms and no bubo, the exposure history may be vital.

When a bubo is present, diagnostic confirmation is made by needle aspiration, using a 20-gauge needle while wearing gloves and taking reasonable precautions not to create an infectious aerosol. Because the bubo does not contain liquid material, aspiration of diagnostic material is enhanced by injecting 1 mL of nonbacteriostatic saline and applying suction multiple times until a blood-tinged specimen is obtained. Aspirated material should be plated on blood and MacConkey agar and into an infusion broth. Slides should be prepared, and microscopic examination should be carried out. Gram stain shows white blood cells and characteristic gram-negative bacteria. Wayson (or Giemsa)–stained aspirate shows coccobacillary organisms with bipolar bodies characteristic of *Y. pestis*. Direct fluorescent antibody staining is confirmatory. Direct fluorescent antibody staining, directed at F1 capsular antigen, should be available through state health laboratories in endemic areas; if it is not locally available, the diagnostic material should be sent to the Plague Branch of the Centers for Disease Control and Prevention. Blood cultures and, when indicated, sputum cultures should also be obtained. Blood, sputum, bubo aspirate, or other cultures should be cultivated at 28°C. Because the definitive culture identification of *Y. pestis* may be confused with that of *Y. pseudotuberculosis*, specific identification by bacteriophage and direct fluorescent antibody test of suspicious colonies is necessary. This may be conducted in special laboratories in states having endemic plague or by the Plague Branch of the Centers for Disease Control and Prevention. If pneumonic plague is suspected, sputum should similarly be examined by Gram and Wayson stains and by fluorescent antibody staining. Routine laboratory findings are nonspecific, with a moderate leukocytosis present and evidence of organ system impairment and acidosis if sepsis has occurred. The visually examined peripheral blood smear may show bacteria in as many as 10% of patients. A serologic diagnosis is made by the passive hemagglutination test using the F1 antigen of *Y. pestis*, which demonstrates an antibody rise in 2 weeks. A fourfold or greater increase in the titer of antibody is considered positive, as is a single titer of 1:16 or greater. When meningitic plague is suspected, lumbar puncture should be done and cerebrospinal fluid examined for cell count, glucose, protein, and Gram stain and culture characteristics. Cerebrospinal fluid should show moderate pleocytosis with polymorphonuclear cells, low glucose level, and modest elevation of protein.

Treatment

Untreated plague has a mortality rate of greater than 50%; when there is a high degree of clinical suspicion for this illness, treatment of patients should be started as soon as cultures have been obtained. With appropriate early antibiotic therapy, bubonic plague mortality may be reduced to approximately 5% to 10%. Most plague deaths in the United States are due to inappropriate delays in diagnosis or incorrect choice of antibiotic therapy. A delay in diagnosis is incurred because it is not recognized that plague may be indirectly transmitted to humans by their pets; that plague can present without development of a bubo (septicemic plague); that plague can present with pulmonary symptoms; and that plague may present with severe gastrointestinal symptoms. Streptomycin is the drug of choice for plague and should be administered intramuscularly in two divided doses totaling 30 mg/kg of body weight per day for 10 days. The patient should become afebrile in 3 to 4 days after starting treatment; the full 10-day course is necessary to prevent relapses because plague bacilli may remain viable in buboes during therapy for several days. If streptomycin is not available, gentamicin appears to be effective, although experience with use of other aminoglycosides has been limited to date. In patients with renal functional impairment or preexisting ototoxic effects, the dose may be appropriately reduced, but alternatives should not be used unless patients have had a known, severe allergic reaction to streptomycin. In the case of known ototoxic response, the patient may be switched to tetracycline for the remainder of the 10-day course after 3 to 4 days or after becoming afebrile. For patients in whom an oral drug is strongly preferred, tetracycline can be given orally in a dose of 2 to 4 g/d. Tetracycline is contraindicated in children younger than 7 years because of tooth staining and bone growth retardation, in pregnant women, and in patients with renal failure. However, a single course of tetracycline is probably safe. Neither the penicillins nor the cephalosporins have been proved to be effective therapy for plague and should not be used. Tetracycline may also be administered as prophylactic therapy for individuals who have had face-to-face contact with a patient with pneumonic plague. In this case, it should be administered for 3 to 5 days, with the same concern for toxic effects in children and pregnant women. Alternative drugs for preventive treatment of case contacts may be trimethoprim-sulfamethoxazole or sulfonamides, although neither of these has had extensive use. Contacts of bubonic plague patients without pneumonic involvement should be instructed to return in 1 week and given preventive treatment only if they develop a fever. Because as many as 20% of patients with bubonic plague may develop pulmonary complications, it is probably wise to place all plague patients in respiratory isolation for observation for the first 48 hours of their hospitalization.

Buboes generally resolve during the course of therapy. However, they may occasionally become secondarily infected, most commonly with *Staphylococcus aureus*. If a fluctuant bubo is noted during treatment, surgical incision and drainage may be necessary.

For patients with plague meningitis, neither streptomycin nor tetracycline will penetrate the cerebrospinal fluid adequately, and chloramphenicol is the antibiotic of choice. This can be administered intravenously with a loading dose of 25 mg/kg of body weight followed by 60 mg/kg per day in four divided doses. A similar intravenous regimen may be used in patients with hypotension, in whom intramuscular uptake of streptomycin may be a problem. After clinical improvement, chloramphenicol can be given orally to complete a 10-day course. Whereas reversible bone marrow suppression may be seen at this dosage, it is infrequent, and irreversible bone marrow suppression is extremely rare. Antibiotic resistance in human isolates of *Y. pestis* has been seen only once (in Vietnam), and this has not been documented in other clinical settings during the course of therapy. There is no indication for dual-drug treatment of this disease.

Prevention

Other than respiratory isolation precautions in patients with pneumonic plague and the use of tetracycline or trimethoprim-sulfamethoxazole for case contacts of a pneumonic plague patient, no prophylaxis is necessary. Patients with bubonic plague are not contagious to health care workers or others around them. A formalin-killed vaccine is available for laboratory workers who deal continuously with *Y. pestis* and for wildlife biologists working in plague endemic regions.[22] The vaccine must be administered in two divided doses as a primary series with a 1-month interval between them. Booster injections must be given at 6-month intervals thereafter to maintain immunity. Because the risk is low, travelers or tourists to plague endemic areas are generally not advised to use this vaccine. Individuals living in rural, plague endemic locations should reduce rodent harborage near their homes, keep pet foods stored in rodent-proof containers, and ensure that housing is rat-proof. Use of flea-directed insecticides (but not rodent poisons) may be warranted around houses and on pets.

References

1. Lipson LG: Plague in San Francisco in 1900. The United States Marine Hospital Service Commission to study the existence of plague in San Francisco. Ann Intern Med 77:303–310, 1972.
2. Butler T: The black death past and present I. Plague in the 1980s. Trans R Soc Trop Med Hyg 83:458–460, 1989.
3. Christie AB: Plague: Review of ecology. Ecol Dis 1:111–115, 1982.
4. Tomich PQ, Barnes AM, Devick WS, et al: Evidence for the extinction of plague in Hawaii. Am J Epidemiol 119:261–273, 1984.
5. Craven RB, Barnes AM: Plague and tularemia. Infect Dis Clin North Am 5:165–175, 1991.
6. Kartman L: Historical and oecological observations on plague in the United States. Trop Geogr Med 22:257–275, 1970.
7. Craven RB, Maupin GO, Beard ML, et al: Reported cases of plague infections in the United States, 1970–1991. J Med Entomol 30:758–761, 1993.
8. Guiyoule A, Grimont F, Iteman I, et al: Plague pandemics investigated by ribotyping of *Yersinia pestis* strains. J Clin Microbiol 32:634–641, 1994.
9. Cavanaugh DC: Specific effect of temperature upon transmission of the plague bacillus by the oriental rat flea *Xenopsylla cheopis*. Am J Trop Med Hyg 31:839–841, 1971.
10. Update: Human plague—India, 1994. MMWR Morbid Mortal Wkly Rep 43:722–723, 1994.
11. Butler T, Bell WR, Link NM, et al: *Yersinia pestis* infection in Vietnam. I. Clinical and hematologic aspects. J Infect Dis 129:s78–s83, 1974.

12. Mann JM, Shandler L, Cushing AH: Pediatric plague. Pediatrics 69:762–767, 1982.
13. Palmer DL, Kisch AL, Williams RL Jr, Reed WP: Clinical features of plague in the United States: The 1969–70 epidemic. J Infect Dis 124:367–371, 1971.
14. Eidson M, Tierney LA, Rollag OJ, et al: Feline plague in New Mexico: Risk factors and transmission to humans. Am J Public Health 78:1333–1335, 1988.
15. Crook LD, Tempest B: Plague. A clinical review of 27 cases. Arch Intern Med 152:1253–1256, 1992.
16. Hopkins DD, Gresbrink RA: Surveillance of sylvatic plague in Oregon by serotesting carnivores. Am J Public Health 72:1295–1297, 1982.
17. Ferber DM, Brubaker RR: Plasmids in *Yersinia pestis*. Infect Immun 31:839–841, 1981.
18. Hull HF, Montes JM, Mann JM: Septicemic plague in New Mexico. J Infect Dis 155:113–118, 1987.
19. Alsofrom DJ, Mettler FA, Mann JM: Radiographic manifestations of plague in New Mexico, 1975–1980. Radiology 139:561–565, 1981.
20. Becker TM, Poland JD, Quan TJ, et al: Plague meningitis—A retrospective analysis of cases reported in the United States, 1970–1979. Clin Med 147:554–557, 1987.
21. Hull HF, Montes JM, Mann JM: Plague masquerading as gastrointestinal illness. West J Med 145:485–487, 1986.
22. Plague. Guide for Adult Immunizations, ed 2. Philadelphia, American College of Physicians, 1989, pp 89–91.

174

Anthrax

Christopher C. Penn
Stephen A. Klotz

A disease of great antiquity, anthrax occupies an important place in the history of infectious diseases because it was the first human disease to be attributed to a specific pathogen. The causative organism is *Bacillus anthracis*, an aerobic, gram-positive rod measuring 3 to 8 μm by 1 to 1.5 μm that forms a large polypeptide capsule detectable in clinical specimens. Although the frequency of anthrax in industrialized nations has been reduced sharply in the 20th century, it retains a certain fascination and notoriety, partly because of the potential for use of the bacillus spores in biologic warfare. Anthrax remains an important disease of livestock in many arid and semiarid countries. It is especially prevalent in areas where poverty and nomadic grazing of unvaccinated livestock are the rule. Shipment of contaminated hides, hair, and wool throughout the world gives rise to industry-related anthrax, often in industrialized, nonagrarian countries.

Epidemiology

It has been proposed, but not proved, that *B. anthracis* undergoes an independent propagation cycle in wet alkaline soils in North America, and it is believed to undergo sporulation with the onset of dry weather.[1] However, it has been well shown that anthrax spores can survive for years in ecologically sparse xeric soils and even in workplaces. Some authorities attribute the persistence of anthrax in a geographic region to an environmental cycle that involves contaminated soil and susceptible wild animals and livestock (Fig. 174–1).

Such a cycle, coupled with civil war, led to an epidemic in Zimbabwe from 1978 to 1982 with more than 10,000 human cases of anthrax. In southern Africa, spore counts in the soil can reach prodigious numbers. Disease is spread to animals and humans in these areas not only by contact with contaminated soil or infected carcasses but also by the bites of tabanid flies (deer flies and horseflies). After feeding on infected carcasses, tabanid flies deposit feces and vomitus containing spores on leaves that are subsequently ingested by browsing herbivores. Furthermore, vultures may spread disease from one location to another after feeding on infected carcasses.[2] When spores are ingested by susceptible herbivores, these animals may die in epizootic proportions. Such has occurred in Africa with kudu and hippopotamuses and in west Texas with white-tailed deer. Cases of livestock anthrax occur regularly, if not yearly, on the Edwards plateau in west Texas and in South Dakota, indicating that the microorganism persists in these geographic regions. Contact with carcasses of infected livestock leads to disease in animal husbandry workers and butchers. However, human cases in the United States, even among unvaccinated animal husbandry workers and veterinarians, are exceedingly uncommon, which may be a reflection of greater care surrounding dead livestock, the relative resistance of humans to anthrax, and diminishing contact with anthrax spores as urbanization continues.

The industrial use of contaminated animal products such as hides, hair, and bone meal introduces a risk for persons who are far removed from the agrarian setting. Textile industries and tanneries are historically the principal sources of outbreaks in industrialized areas; therefore, the increasing use of synthetic fibers in the textile industry has undoubtedly contributed to the decline in the number of human cases of industrial anthrax. The report of anthrax in a craftsman working at home (in the United States) with contaminated animal products may signal a change in the type of activities that place individuals at risk for this disease. In recent decades, disease has affected humans in Asia Minor, particularly Iran and Turkey; in southern Europe, principally Greece; and in southern Africa as previously mentioned. Owing to inadequate reporting, the true worldwide frequency of disease in humans is unknown. In this century, the majority of anthrax cases in the United States have been industry related. The frequency has been declining in part as a result of preventive health measures such as dust control in workplaces, import restrictions where they are deemed appropriate, and decontamination of raw materials.

Anthrax can also be spread by biologic weapons. This form of warfare was a perceived threat in the Persian Gulf War that was not realized. However, the accidental expulsion of spores from a biologic weapons plant in Sverdlovsk, now Ekaterinburg, in central Russia resulted in significant mortality in livestock and humans.[3]

Pathogenesis

Inoculation of spores into the skin or contamination of preexisting abrasions leads to germination and vegetative reproduction. The capsule is antiphagocytic. The resulting skin lesion is known as a malignant pustule, even though pus is not a hallmark of cutaneous anthrax unless there is secondary infection. Biopsy of cutaneous lesions reveals extensive tissue destruction with marked subepidermal edema, thrombosis of vessels, and hemorrhagic interstitium.[4] Nonpitting edema around the lesion and a more generalized edema are thought to be due to toxin production. The draining lymph nodes of

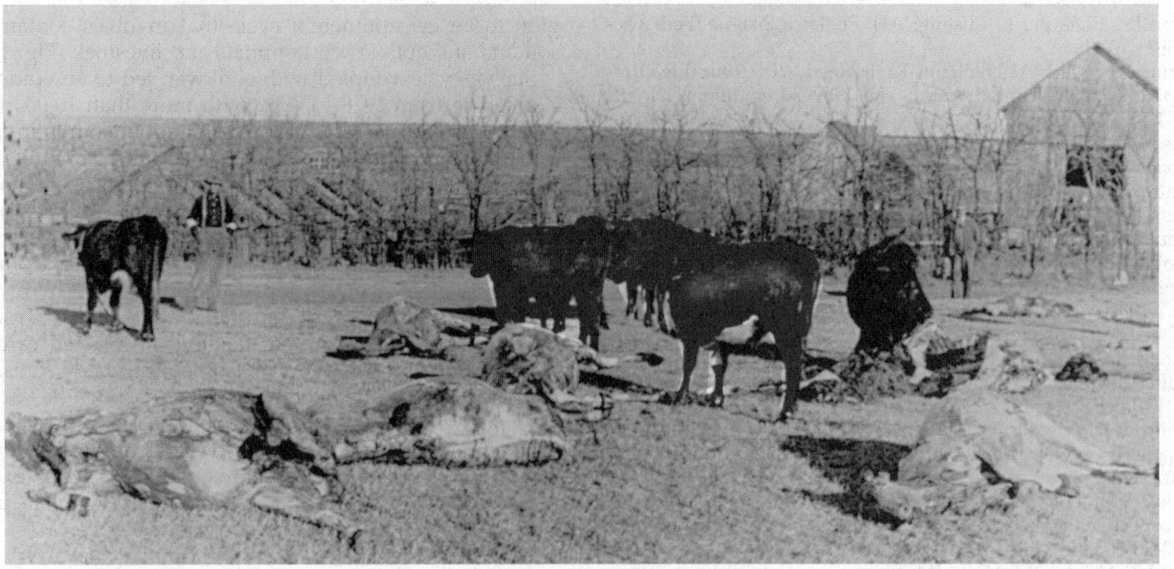

FIGURE 174–1 □ The headquarters of a Smith Center, Kansas, ranch in 1911 showing cattle dead from anthrax. Characteristic of this illness is the inability of the blood to clot, as demonstrated by blood draining from natural orifices and the skinned carcasses. The hides will naturally be contaminated. The same ranch experienced another outbreak of anthrax in cattle in 1990, probably due to persisting spores. (Courtesy of M. W. Vorhies, DVM, Kansas State University, Manhattan, KS.)

cutaneous lesions are avid scavengers of *B. anthracis*, but spread beyond this barrier may give rise to bacteremia.

Inhalation of large numbers of spores leads to their phagocytosis by alveolar macrophages and transport to mediastinal lymph nodes, where the spores germinate. Mediastinal widening then ensues, usually followed by bacteremia. Bacteria are not found in sputum even though autopsy of inhalational anthrax victims in Sverdlovsk demonstrated primary pneumonia.[5]

Gastrointestinal anthrax results from the ingestion of contaminated meat containing large numbers of bacilli or spores. Points of entry into the submucosa appear, particularly in the oropharynx and the ileocecal region. Ulceration develops at the point of inoculation, and hemorrhage occurs in the draining lymph nodes along with local edema. Disease in bowel segments can be accompanied by hemorrhagic ascites. Bacteremia is common in this form of the disease.

Meningitis, when it occurs, is hemorrhagic and secondary to bacteremia, which may arise in any form of the disease.

Immunity may develop from subclinical infection. Disease is thought to confer lasting protection, although reinfection with *B. anthracis* has been reported. Antibodies to toxin and capsule are measurable after infection. A skin test for delayed-type hypersensitivity, Anthraxin, developed in the former Soviet Union, has been reported to be useful in surveys of vaccinated humans and livestock alike.

Clinical Manifestations

Anthrax in humans occurs in three principal forms: cutaneous, inhalational, and gastrointestinal. The majority of cases, 95% or more, are cutaneous disease. Inhalational anthrax comprises the remainder of cases in North America. Gastrointestinal or oropharyngeal anthrax is extremely rare and has not been reported from North America, although an outbreak of gastrointestinal anthrax occurred in northern Thailand in 1982[6] and in India in 1989. Anthrax meningitis, when it occurs, is always secondary to one of the three forms and is hemorrhagic.

Cutaneous Anthrax

Cutaneous anthrax begins as a painless, pruritic papule that appears at the site of inoculation within 3 to 10 days. Lesions usually occur on the upper extremities, neck, and face. Several days later, a vesicle or ring of vesicles develops, along with enlargement of the original lesion to 4 to 6 cm (Fig. 174–2*A*). The base of the vesicle bleeds and may spontaneously discharge clear fluid, which on Gram stain demonstrates numerous microorganisms. The lesion ulcerates, and a central eschar is formed, which may remain in situ for up to 3 weeks (Fig. 174–2*B*). Healing usually results in scar formation, and reconstructive surgery may be required for lesions involving the face, particularly the eyelids. Painful regional adenopathy may persist long after successful treatment. Perilesional edema may be extensive, especially if the lesion is located on the face, neck, or upper chest. On occasion, edema may be so extensive as to embarrass respiratory function. Only about 50% of patients have fever, malaise, or leukocytosis. Untreated, cutaneous anthrax may have a mortality rate as high as 20%, probably related to the development of bacteremia. Rarely, multiple skin lesions occur. The evolution of the cutaneous lesion to an eschar is not interrupted by the use of antibiotics, although bacteremia is probably prevented. The appearance of the skin lesion of cutaneous anthrax may vary, and this, combined with its rarity, may make diagnosis difficult in nonagricultural settings[7] (Table 174–1).

Inhalational Anthrax

Inhalational anthrax is usually peculiar to the textile industry[8] and is frequently biphasic in nature. After inhalation of large numbers of spores, patients often complain of upper respiratory symptoms within 3 to 5 days. This viral illness–like prodrome is followed, often within hours, by dyspnea, diaphoresis, cyanosis, shock, and death (Fig. 174–3). Chest radiographs may show characteristic widening of the mediastinum, pneumonitis, and pleural effusion. Bacteremia and occasionally splenomegaly accompany this form of the dis-

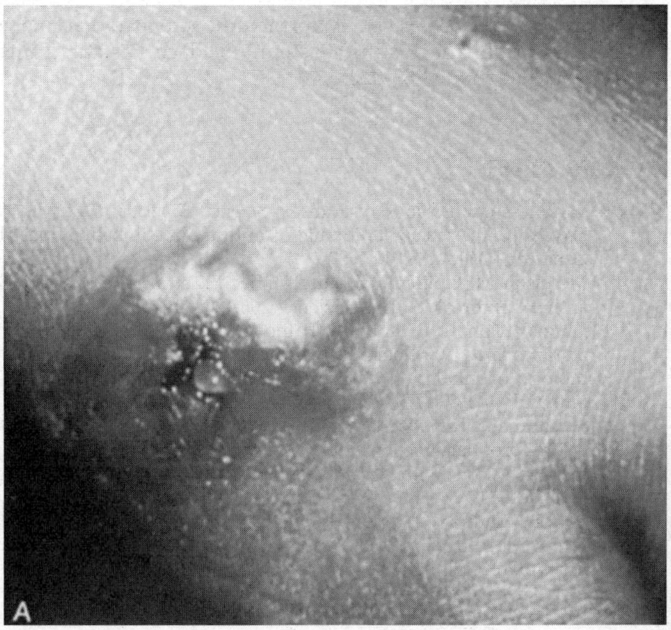

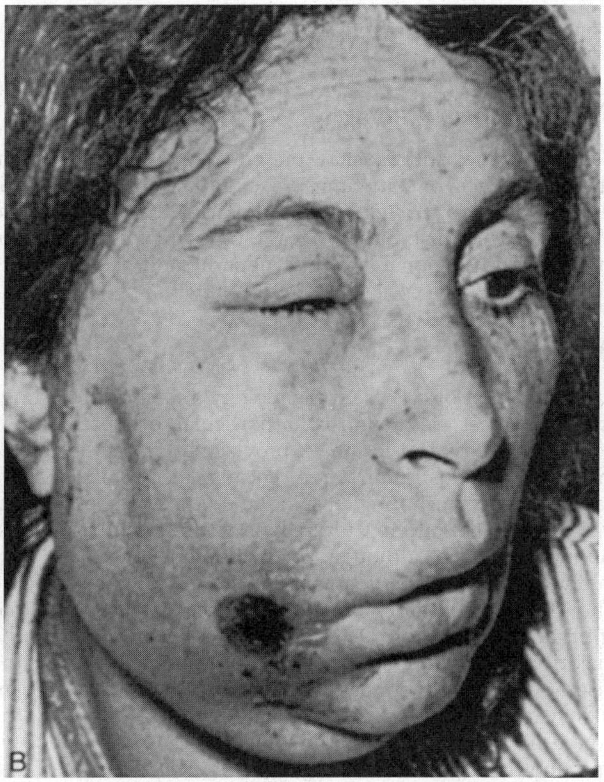

FIGURE 174–2 □ *A*, Early cutaneous lesion on thumb of 6-year-old boy from Zimbabwe. (Courtesy of Wilhelm Kobuch, Toulouse, France.) *B*, Eschar on the face with surrounding edema. (From Dutz W, Kohout E: Anthrax. Pathol Annu 6:209–248, 1971.)

TABLE 174–1 ■ Evolution of Skin Lesions of Anthrax

FEATURES	PAPULE	PAPULE WITH VESICLES	ESCHAR
Size (cm)	1	4–6	4–6
Characteristics	Pruritic, painless	Base of lesion becomes hemorrhagic	On occasion may be quite large
Duration of lesion (d)	2–3	3–5	7–21
Recovery of bacteria	?	Gram stain and culture of vesicular fluid, positive	Gram stain may show bacteria and culture may be positive if material is obtained from base of eschar
Can be confused with	Orf	Staphylococcal skin lesions, bullous impetigo	Tularemia, plague, burn, cutaneous diphtheria

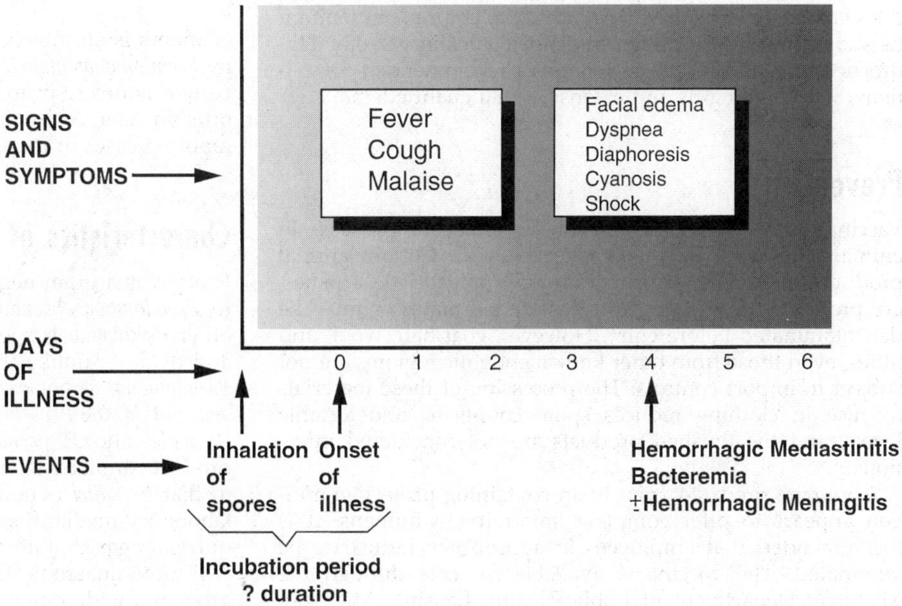

FIGURE 174–3 □ Chronology of clinical signs and symptoms of inhalational anthrax. (From Penn CC, Klotz SA: Anthrax pneumonia. Semin Respir Infect 12:1–5, 1997.)

ease. Diagnosis is often made only at postmortem examination.

Gastrointestinal Anthrax

Gastrointestinal anthrax may present as an acute abdomen, bloody diarrhea, or sometimes a cholera-like syndrome. Ascites may develop. Bacteremia usually accompanies this form of the disease. The oropharyngeal form manifests as a mucosal ulcer, with regional lymphadenopathy and neck edema.[6]

Diagnosis

A combination of clinical epidemiology and clinical findings should suggest the diagnosis, in particular, occupational exposure and a typical lesion. A provisional diagnosis can be made by demonstrating large, encapsulated gram-positive bacilli, usually in short chains, in the fluid of vesicles or from the base of the ulcer. Culture will yield growth on most laboratory media, although prior antibiotic treatment may inhibit growth of the organism and make isolation difficult. The clinical laboratory should be alerted to the fact that anthrax is suspected. Detectable bacteremia occurs in the majority of inhalational and gastrointestinal forms of the disease but in only about 10% of the cutaneous cases. Gram stain examination of cerebrospinal fluid demonstrates the organism in patients with meningitis. The electrophoretic immunotransblot test demonstrates serologic evidence of disease and is available through the Bacteriology Division of the Centers for Disease Control and Prevention in Atlanta.

Treatment

Penicillin is the drug of choice even though mean inhibitory concentrations can be as high as 1.0 μg/mL.[9] Mild forms of cutaneous anthrax can be treated with potassium penicillin V, 2 g/d orally for 5 to 7 days. Intravenous or intramuscular routes may be needed for more severe cases, 6 to 8 million units of penicillin G per day. Tetracycline and erythromycin, 2 g/d, are effective alternatives for penicillin-allergic patients. In vitro, ciprofloxacin demonstrates mean inhibitory concentrations similar to those of tetracycline and therefore may be a suitable alternative drug.[10] The skin lesion should be covered with a sterile bandage. Human-to-human transmission does not occur. Patients with inhalational anthrax or meningitis should receive 20 million units of penicillin per day. Hydrocortisone, 100 to 200 mg, is often recommended for patients with meningitis and extensive, malignant edema.

Prevention

Vaccination of livestock is effective in eradicating disease in animals but must be repeated every year. Certain animal products, such as goat skin from Haiti and bristle brushes, are prohibited from entry into the United States or must be decontaminated before entry. However, goat hair, wool, and hides, even those from other known endemic regions, are not subject to import controls. The processing of these materials for use in clothing reduces spore counts to undetectable levels, and the finished products are not considered infectious.

A vaccine prepared from toxin containing protective antigen appears to offer complete immunity to humans. It is recommended that employees in appropriate industries be vaccinated. The vaccine is available for cost through the Michigan Department of Public Health, Lansing, Michigan (telephone 517-335-8119). A formalin-inactivated vaccine is available from the Institut Pasteur, 13 Place Pasteur, Tunis, Tunisia (telephone 283-022).

References

1. Van Ness GB: Ecology of anthrax. Science 172:1303, 1971.
2. Davies JCA: A major epidemic of anthrax in Zimbabwe, part I. Cent Afr J Med 28:291, 1982.
3. Meselson M, Guillemin J, Hugh-Jones M, et al: The Sverdlovsk anthrax outbreak of 1979. Science 266:1202, 1994.
4. Dutz W, Kohout E: Anthrax. Pathol Annu 6:209, 1971.
5. Abramova FA, Grinberg LM, Yampolskaya OV, Walker DH: Pathology of inhalation anthrax in 42 cases from the Sverdlovsk outbreak of 1979. Proc Natl Acad Sci USA 90:2291, 1993.
6. Sirisanthana T, Navachareen N, Tharavichitkul P, et al: Outbreak of oral-oropharyngeal anthrax: An unusual manifestation of human infection with *Bacillus anthracis*. Am J Trop Med Hyg 33:144, 1984.
7. Gold H: Anthrax. A report of one hundred-seventeen cases. Arch Intern Med 96:387, 1955.
8. Brachman PS: Inhalation anthrax. N Y Acad Sci 353:83, 1980.
9. Gold H: Treatment of anthrax. Fed Proc 26:1563, 1967.
10. Doganay M, Aydin N: Antimicrobial susceptibility of *Bacillus anthracis*. Scand J Infect Dis 23:333, 1991.

Bibliography

- LaForce FM: Anthrax. Clin Infect Dis 19:1009, 1994.
- Whitford HW: A Guide to the Diagnosis, Treatment, and Prevention of Anthrax. WHO/ZOON./87.163, 1987.

175

Glanders

John G. Bartlett

Glanders is an infection with varied clinical features caused by *Pseudomonas mallei*. The organism is usually acquired from equine sources, primarily horses. Glanders is found most often in Asia, Africa, and South America; there have been no reported cases in the United States since 1939.

Characteristics of the Pathogen

P. mallei is a gram-negative aerobic bacterium that is related to *Pseudomonas pseudomallei*, the agent of melioidosis. Like other *Pseudomonas* species, both organisms produce catalase and oxidase; unlike the fluorescent pseudomonads, such as *Pseudomonas aeruginosa*, *Pseudomonas fluorescens*, and *Pseudomonas putida*, the *P. pseudomallei* group do not produce pigment. *P. mallei* and *P. pseudomallei* are antigenically related and produce similar lesions in experimental animals; they differ in that *P. mallei* is nonmotile and grows poorly on ordinary laboratory media. Both organisms grow better on blood and nutrient agar containing glycerol; both are strict aerobes that will grow anaerobically in the presence of nitrate; and both grow at a wide range of temperatures but optimally at 41°C.

History

P. mallei was originally isolated by Loeffler and Schutz in 1882 from a horse that died with glanders.[1] The name *Bacillus mallei* was applied by Zopf in 1885. A related organism was isolated from a man with a disease resembling glanders by Whitmore and Krishnaswami in 1912; that organism was designated *Bacillus pseudomallei* by Whitmore in 1913; Stanton and Fletcher subsequently applied the name melioidosis to the disease and *whitmori* to the agent. Both organisms were initially thought to be animal parasites, but it was subsequently found that *P. pseudomallei* was a natural inhabitant of soil in tropical areas. The close relationship of these two organisms was initially based on the fact that they were similar microbiologically and caused similar diseases, but there was considerable uncertainty about their taxonomic position, and consequently they were placed in numerous genera. By the early 1930s, it was recognized that both organisms had metabolic activity and biochemical features similar to those of other pseudomonads. *P. mallei* and *P. pseudomallei* are closely related biochemically and have a guanine plus cytosine content of 68% to 69%. *P. mallei* infection differs in that it has always been a rare disease in humans; it remains primarily a disease of horses, and infrequently it is found in soil and other environmental sources.

At one time, glanders was a severe and often lethal disease in horses throughout the world. It has been largely eliminated from the developed world through infection control measures as well as replacement of horse-drawn vehicles. Control of glanders in horses was achieved in England through the British Glanders or Farcy Order of 1907, which mandated that every animal with clinical evidence of these conditions was to be slaughtered and the carcass destroyed or buried. Mallein, a product of *P. mallei* grown in glycerol broth, was often used as an intradermal or conjunctival test for case detection in animals, and all positive reactors were also killed. Glanders was never a common disease of humans. Robins succeeded in finding 156 reported cases in 1906. By contrast, *P. pseudomallei* does not appear to have a natural animal reservoir but is readily recovered from environmental sources including soil and water in tropical areas. The disease is relatively common in Southeast Asia and other tropical and subtropical areas.

Epidemiology

Glanders is a serious infection of equine animals, principally horses but also mules and donkeys. The disease may occasionally affect goats, sheeps, dogs, and cats.

The major diseases in horses are glanders and farcy. Glanders may be acute or chronic with primary involvement of the lung. Lung involvement may consist of an acute pneumonic infiltrate; more commonly, there are nodular granulomata in the lungs. There may also be nodular or ulcerative lesions of the nasal or tracheal mucosa. Many animals show subcutaneous abscesses, and there may be widespread dissemination with involvement of the spleen, liver, and other organs. With farcy, the typical lesions are found in the skin or subcutaneous tissue, primarily on the extremities and flanks, which appear as nodules that subsequently ulcerate. Involvement of lymphatic channels results in firm cords, sometimes referred to as farcy pipes, and large lymph nodes referred to as farcy buds.

Glanders has largely been eliminated from the industrialized world. The major sources of infection in humans and animals at present are in Asia, Africa, and South America.

The disease is transmitted to humans by contact with infected animals, primarily horses. The disease may also be transmitted from person to person. This emphasizes the importance of isolation of the patient. The animal source may have clinically silent infection. Infectious material includes nasal and pulmonary discharges and infected urine or stool from animals with glanders. Farcy is transmitted by subcutaneous inoculation. The most frequent source is by contamination of a wound. It is unclear whether the pulmonary form of the disease is acquired by inhalation or by migration from intestinal or cutaneous contamination. The organism also represents a laboratory hazard; several cases have been reported in laboratory workers.[2]

Clinical Features

Symptoms are varied and may be classified in four categories. (1) Localized infection reflects a cutaneous or mucosal site of inoculation that results in a nodule with lymphangitis. The usual incubation period is 1 to 5 days. The typical lesion is a nodule with cordlike induration of lymphatic channels, similar to farcy in animals. The nodules frequently break down and ulcerate. (2) Inoculation of the mucous membranes may cause localized infection of the eye, nose, or oral cavity, resulting in a similar type of ulcerating, granulomatous reaction, with or without a systemic response, including fever. (3) The septicemic form of the disease may result in a generalized papular rash that progresses to a pustular rash. This may be accompanied by widespread involvement of internal organs. (4) The pulmonary form shows an incubation period of 10 to 14 days, followed by fever, malaise, headache, and pleurisy. As noted in animals, it is often uncertain whether the lung is involved through inhalation of the organism or by secondary invasion from other sites of involvement. There are often lymphadenopathy and splenomegaly. The chest radiograph may show lobar pneumonia, bronchopneumonia, or nodular densities. With all forms of glanders, the leukocyte count may show slight leukocytosis, there may be leukopenia, there may be a relative lymphocytosis, or the peripheral leukocyte counts and differential may be entirely normal. The course of the disease is variable. Acute glanders with septicemia is usually fatal within 7 to 10 days. With chronic disease, there may be subcutaneous and muscle abscesses with lymphadenopathy and ulcerating lesions of mucosal surfaces. Abscesses should undergo surgical drainage. The disease may remain active for months or years. There may be apparent spontaneous recovery with subsequent relapse, and there may be latent periods for up to 10 years.

Diagnosis

Gram stain examination of exudates may show typical small, gram-negative, slender bacilli, but the organisms are often present in small numbers and may be difficult to detect with direct stains. *P. mallei* and *P. pseudomallei* cannot be distinguished by Gram stain. *P. mallei* will grow slowly on most nutrient agar; growth is improved with media containing glycerol. Blood cultures usually fail to propagate the organism. Serologic tests include agglutination assays that demonstrate increased titers to 1:640 and greater in the second week of infection. The complement fixation test is more specific but less sensitive. The mallein intradermal test has been applied mostly to detecting the disease in animals.

Treatment

The only antimicrobial agent with established merit is sulfadiazine, which has proved useful in experimentally infected hamsters and in a limited experience in patients with glanders.[3] The organism is resistant to penicillin; it can be grown selectively in media containing penicillin. It is sensitive in vitro to chloramphenicol, streptomycin, and tetracycline. The use of these drugs in experimental animals has given variable results. There is minimal information on the utility of newer drugs.

References

1. Wilson GS, Miles A: Diseases due to pseudomonads, including melioidosis and glanders. *In* Wilson GS (ed): Topley and Wilson's Principles of Bacteriology, Virology and Immunology, Vol 2. Baltimore, Williams & Wilkins, 1975, pp 18–43.
2. Howe C, Miller WR: Human glanders: Report of six cases. Ann Intern Med 26:93, 1947.
3. Miller WR, Pannell L, Ingalls MS: Experimental chemotherapy in glanders and melioidosis. Am J Hyg 47:205, 1948.

176

Leptospirosis

Patrick W. Kelley

Leptospirosis is a spirochetal infection that is acquired by animals and humans, primarily through direct or indirect contact of skin or mucous membranes with the contaminated urine of infected wild and domestic mammals. It can develop clinically as an asymptomatic or influenza-like infection, or it may present with severe hemorrhagic manifestations and associated meningism, jaundice, and renal failure. The more severe presentation, which Adolph Weil described in 1886, became known as Weil disease. As clinical understanding of leptospirosis has grown in the last 100 years, it has become clear that the majority of human leptospiral infections represent the milder, self-limited end of the clinical spectrum. Today, more than 200 serovars, or serologically distinct strains, of the pathogenic *Leptospira* have been described in humans and in more than 180 species of animals throughout the tropical and temperate world. Transmission has been well documented in urban, suburban, and rural settings. Antibiotic therapy is efficacious in at least some situations. Efforts at prevention may include immunization of domestic animals, rodent control, antibiotic prophylaxis, surface decontamination, use of protective clothing, and education to reduce needless exposures.

History

Currently, leptospirosis is considered one of the most geographically widespread of the contemporary zoonoses, yet its recognition as a clinical entity dates only to the 1800s.[1, 2] In 1886, Weil lent his name to the most intense presentation of leptospirosis when he described four febrile men with a distinct syndrome characterized by "particularities of an acute infectious illness with spleen tumor, jaundice, and nephritis."[2] In addition, each patient had "severe nervous symptoms" and hepatomegaly. After relatively short periods of illness, the patients recovered. Three of the four men had a biphasic course, with fever recurring after an afebrile period of 1 to 7 days.[3]

Landouzy may actually have been the first to describe leptospirosis. Three years before Weil, he published a report on two sewer workers who had a syndrome that affected the liver, lungs, and kidneys.[3] Before Weil and Landouzy, various other 19th century observers described clinically compatible cases involving military troops; in contrast to Weil's, however, these reports do not afford a clear differentiation from other causes of jaundice.[2] During the period 1914 to 1916, Inada and Ino concluded that the cause of leptospirosis was a spirochete; they found the organisms in the blood of jaundiced Japanese miners and in the livers of guinea pigs inoculated with blood from infected patients but not in the livers of guinea pigs inoculated with blood from control subjects.[2] In 1916, Ido and coworkers reported that 40% of 86 house and ditch rats carried these spirochetes and thus implicated rats in the transmission cycle of leptospirosis.[3]

In 1917 and 1918, Ido, Ito, and Wani concluded that a similar spirochete was associated with an anicteric illness called the 7-day fever.[2] This spirochete (then termed *Leptospira hebdomadis*) was serologically differentiated from the organism associated with Weil syndrome (then termed *Leptospira icterohaemorrhagiae*); the field mouse *(Microtus montebelli)* was viewed as its animal host. The first U.S. case of leptospirosis was recognized in 1922. Numerous leptospiral serovars were later identified around the world and were associated with a variety of clinical presentations and animal carriers. Up to the late 1940s, most reported U.S. cases were icteric, whereas in Europe, most leptospiral illnesses were known to be anicteric.[1] Although not always recognized, anicteric cases were occurring in the United States. This was documented in the 1950s by retrospective studies that proved that during the early 1940s at Fort Bragg, North Carolina, several summer outbreaks of a self-limited, anicteric, febrile illness accompanied by a pretibial rash were due to the *autumnalis* serovar.[4] Numerous sporadic cases and other outbreaks have resulted in many colorful appellations, such as sugarcane illness, swineherd's meningitis, rice-field fever, swamp fever, fish-handler disease, Japanese autumnal fever, and mouse fever.[5] As knowledge of leptospirosis has evolved, the exclusive association of specific leptospiral serotypes with a distinct clinical presentation and animal host is no longer appropriate.

Characteristics of the Pathogen

Taxonomy and Morphology

Pathogenic manifestations of leptospirosis can result from infection with any of more than 200 antigenically distinct serovars classified traditionally under the species *Leptospira interrogans*.[6, 7] At least 99 serovars have been isolated from humans, and at least 27 have been found in the United States.[5] The genus also contains *Leptospira biflexa*, a free-living nonpathogenic species found in natural water and wet soil. These traditional taxonomic divisions are undergoing revision on the basis of genetic relatedness studies with the result that many new species classifications are being described that do not relate to the traditional serologic groupings. Pathogenic and saprophytic leptospires are morphologically indistinguishable.

Leptospires are obligate aerobes and appear as motile, flexible, tightly coiled, helicoid rods 0.1 to 0.2 μm in diameter and 6 to 20 μm in length. One or both ends of the cells are usually hooked. Virulence does not necessarily correlate with serovar. For example, a nonvirulent *hebdomadis* serovar in one part of the world would be classified as identical to a virulent *hebdomadis* serovar from another region. Also, "identical" serovars from different regions may in one case be pathogenic for humans and not cattle and in the other case be pathogenic for cattle and not humans.[5]

Laboratory Isolation

Media such as Fletcher semisolid or Tween 80–albumin (EMJH) allow leptospiral organisms to be isolated from blood and cerebrospinal fluid during the first 7 to 10 days of illness and from urine after the first week of illness.[6, 8] Kidney or liver tissue can also be cultured. Minimal inocula (1 mL of blood or urine in 10 mL of medium and diluted serially to produce three concentrations of 1:10, 1:100, and 1:1000) of blood, urine, or tissue are recommended to dilute out inhibitory substances. Multiple specimens should be taken for culture over time. In one study in which blood and urine cultures were obtained within 3 days of fever onset, more than 94% of the patients' cultures were positive.[9] Because leptospires are relatively slow growing, cultures should be incubated for at least 5 or 6 weeks in the dark at 28°C to 30°C. If an appropriate medium is not readily available, blood may be collected before antibiotic therapy in a tube containing heparin or sodium oxalate as an anticoagulant. Viable leptospires may be recoverable from such specimens for more than a week after collection. Leptospires can also be isolated from contaminated specimens by passage through weanling hamsters or guinea pigs.[7]

Epidemiology

Transmission

The occurrence of human cases of leptospirosis reflects the phenomenon that animals that survive the acute infection can harbor the spirochete in their renal tubules for months and even years without suffering any significant adverse consequences. Chronic urinary shedding of leptospires can lead to further human or animal infections either through direct urinary contact or by contamination of soil and surface waters. Dogs immunized with canine bacterins to prevent clinical disease can still develop renal infections and leptospiruria.[10] In fact, one study showed no difference in leptospiruria rates between vaccinated and unvaccinated dogs after challenge with the serovar *canicola*.[11] At least one outbreak of leptospirosis has been attributed to contact with the urine of immunized pet dogs.[10] Mammals appear to be the only epidemiologically significant transmitters of leptospirosis, although the spirochetes have been isolated from birds, reptiles, amphibians, arthropods, mollusks, and helminths. In an analysis by Heath and coworkers[12] of 483 U.S. human cases of leptospirosis reported from 1949 to 1961, rats and dogs were implicated most often and about equally as the source of infection. Cattle, swine, raccoons, goats, and mice followed in importance. Carnivores, marsupials, insectivores, rabbits, and deer are also potential carriers.[6] In the United States from 1965 to 1974, dogs were implicated in transmission to humans about twice as often as rodents were. Cattle displaced rodents to third place in importance.[11] The epidemiologic importance of any specific animal source at a given time is probably a function of the local ecology, the nature of human activities in that environment, and the dynamic shifts in the prevalence and virulence of different *Leptospira* serovars. Although a particular host may harbor one or more serovars and a given serovar may occur in a variety of hosts, certain animals tend to serve as principal hosts for particular serovars.

Distribution

Leptospirosis has been reported in humans and animals in almost every country.[5] Maintenance of leptospires in a particular area is a function of the presence of an appropriate animal host and local environmental conditions. In most countries, there are a few regions with many cases and many areas with few cases. In the United States, cases of leptospirosis have been reported from virtually all states, although the majority are recorded in Hawaii and in the less arid states in the southern half of the country.[11] Various biologic factors have a bearing on the efficiency of transmission between animals and to humans. A wet, alkaline environment favors survival. Because the optimal temperature for survival in the environment is 28°C to 32°C, tropical, unpolluted, nonsaline waters with a slightly alkaline pH provide a highly favorable situation. Pathogenic leptospires can survive a few hours in acid urine, but they survive much longer when the urine is diluted and less acid. Flooding after heavy tropical rains is particularly favorable to the survival of leptospires in that it allows saturation of the environment by subsurface leptospires, enhances the flushing of leptospires into surface waters, and draws rodents and other animals to swampy areas.[6]

In the United States, leptospirosis cases occur year-round, but approximately half occur from July to October.[11] Seasonality may be a function of agricultural cycles and increased levels of outdoor recreation in the warmer months; in some tropical countries, however, temporal increases in frequency coincide with the rainy season. Given the right association of animals and humans, even arid regions of the world can sustain significant levels of transmission.[13] A drought may also create local conditions that can facilitate transmission.[14]

Leptospirosis has traditionally been associated with occupations that bring people into direct or indirect contact with contaminated animal urine or infectious tissues. Leptospires enter through breaks in the skin or mucous membranes. Skin changes resulting from prolonged immersion in water may enhance the entrance of leptospires through otherwise intact skin. Occupational groups at particular risk for leptospirosis include persons employed in agriculture and aquaculture, sewer workers, construction workers, livestock handlers, abattoir workers, laboratory personnel, veterinarians, miners, and soldiers. In the last 20 years, avocational pursuits have been as epidemiologically important as occupational exposures and include the care of household pets, hunting, trapping, fishing, swimming in ponds or bodies of freshwater, rafting, and sports that result in contact with muddy fields.[11, 15, 16] Contaminated well water, spring water, and food preparation surfaces have also been implicated in transmission to humans, as have animal bites and stagnant pools of water.[1, 3, 6, 17] Although young men still account for the majority of leptospirosis cases, the shift in occurrence away from occupational groups and toward avocational settings has been reflected in a trend toward more cases in females and in teenagers.[11, 16] Human-to-human transmission has been attributed to urine, breast milk, and sexual intercourse, but transmission by these routes is extremely rare.[6, 18]

Occurrence

During the mid-1980s, the number of cases of leptospirosis reported annually in the United States was in the range of 35 to 60.[19] Because the customary presentation of leptospirosis is fairly nonspecific and the index of suspicion is often low, this incidence should be regarded as a gross underestimate. In 1988, for example, when much attention was drawn to leptospirosis in Hawaii, 58 cases were reported from that state (Centers for Disease Control and Prevention, unpublished data). Throughout the world, leptospirosis occurs both sporadically and in common-source outbreaks associated with immersion in or drinking of water.[9, 11, 17] Incidence rate estimates for various occupations can be high: 11,000 per 100,000 person-years for New Zealand dairy farmers; 3700 per 100,000 person-years for Glasgow sewer workers; and 2200 per 100,000 person-years for Hawaiian taro farmers.[20] Between 1977 and 1982, surveillance of seven U.S. Army units undergoing a 3-week jungle warfare course in Panama during the fall rainy season yielded 91 confirmed and probable cases, for an annualized incidence estimate of 41,000 per 100,000 person-years (Takafuji E, unpublished data). This most likely underestimated the true risk, because potential exposures did not occur every day.

Pathogenesis

The primary pathogenic manifestations of acute leptospirosis result from damage to the endothelial lining of capillaries coupled with renal tubular dysfunction and subcellular hepatic dysfunction.[1] In many ways, it resembles other systemic infectious vasculitides. Many authors have suggested that a toxin elaborated by leptospires may mediate some of the pathophysiologic effects, but putative toxins have been difficult to characterize and have not been found to occur with all serovars that can cause severe disease. In general, there is a marked disparity between the severity of leptospirosis patients' symptoms and the histologic appearance of their tissues. Among patients who die with severe leptospirosis, widespread hemorrhagic signs are evident and may include petechiae of skin, mucosal, and serosal surfaces. In some cases, gross visceral hemorrhage is also noted. One autopsy series found the cut surfaces of the lungs to be hemorrhagic in 60% of the cases.[21] Cardiac, adrenal, and skeletal muscle hemorrhages also occur. These hemorrhagic findings appear to reflect primarily endothelial damage rather than problems with blood clotting. In addition to hemorrhage, the endothelial changes in leptospirosis may facilitate fluid shifts from intravascular to extracellular spaces and thus contribute to hypovolemia.[1] Cardiovascular abnormalities in addition to hemorrhage can include myocarditis, coronary arteritis, aortitis, pericarditis, and arrhythmias.[22]

Historically, renal failure has been the cause of most leptospirosis-associated deaths, but hemodialysis and peritoneal dialysis have to some extent reduced the importance of this factor in causing death. The central pathogenic mechanism of renal failure in leptospirosis is probably ischemia, with consequent tissue hypoxia and renal tubule damage.[1] Interstitial nephritis may follow this hypoxic effect and becomes most evident during the second week of illness. Histologic examination of autopsy specimens within the first week of illness shows cloudy swelling or isolated epithelial cell necrosis, mainly involving the distal convoluted tubule and the ascending loop of Henle. Congestion and hemorrhagic foci may be evident. Later in the clinical course, fatal cases show numerous foci of tubular epithelial necrosis, with distention of the lumen by casts of amorphous material and degenerating cells. Basement membrane damage is evident, and the interstitium is edematous and infiltrated with mononuclear cells.[21] Proteinuria, pyuria, hematuria, hyaline and granular casts, oliguria, and subsequent uremic manifestations clinically complement this pathologic picture.

Jaundice is extremely common in fatal leptospirosis, although the overall architecture of the liver is fairly well preserved. When jaundice does occur, it appears related to hepatic cell dysfunction more than to hemolysis. Increased absorption of blood from tissue hemorrhage may contribute to the jaundice. Even in fatal leptospirosis, the extent of the liver abnormalities is variable. The histologic changes seen in mild and severe cases include disorganization of the liver cell plates, marked variation in the size and shape of parenchymal cells, mitotic figures, bizarre multinucleated cells, Kupffer cell hypertrophy, and evidence of cholestasis.[21] Liver cell necrosis is uncommon, and liver transaminase values are increased only slightly. Leptospires are rarely visualized in liver tissue. Deficiencies in serum prothrombin activity may be detected and can be corrected with vitamin K. Survivors of severe leptospirosis generally enjoy complete return of hepatic and renal function.

Myalgias may be prominent early in the clinical course of leptospirosis. Pathologic findings seen in muscle include hemorrhages and partial or complete necrosis of myofibrils.[21] Meningeal irritation is another hallmark of leptospirosis, although pathologic findings tend to be minimal.[1] During the first week, when spirochetes can be cultured from the cerebrospinal fluid, the fluid is often normal otherwise. Meningismus tends to occur during the second week coincident with the development of serum antibody and the disappearance of leptospires from the cerebrospinal fluid. Similarly, leptospires may penetrate the anterior chamber of the eye and cause inflammation of the anterior uveal tract during the second week of the illness or as late as 1 year into the infection.[6]

Antigen-antibody complexes or autoimmune responses may play a role in some of the effects observed in the eyes, nervous system, and kidney after the first week of illness.[1] Immunity in leptospirosis is largely humoral, with circulating antibodies leading to opsonization of leptospires. The use of antibiotics may blunt the production of antibodies.[1] Subsequent to the initial infection, second attacks due to the same serovar do not seem to occur, but cross-immunity against other serovars is limited.[3, 23] Intrauterine infections can result in fetal death and abortion, stillbirth, premature labor, and signs of congenital leptospirosis within a few weeks of delivery.[24] Lactating mothers may secrete leptospires in their milk during the septicemic phase.

Clinical Manifestations (Table 176–1)

The incubation period of leptospirosis is 7 to 12 days (range, 2 to 26 days). Short incubation has been associated with laboratory and animal bite exposures.[3] The variability in symptoms associated with infection is considerable, although few cases are thought to be entirely asymptomatic, as supported by the observation that in one prospective serosurvey only 1 of 24 infected persons denied any symptoms.[9] About 90% of cases present as a self-limited febrile illness that often escapes specific diagnosis because of a low index of suspicion or because the patient does not seek medical care. The other 10% of cases meet the description of Weil disease and are often marked by fever, jaundice, hemorrhage, renal failure, and neurologic findings.

Patients with mild, anicteric leptospirosis often describe sudden onset of fever, mild to severe headache, profound myalgia, chills, back pain, joint pain, neck stiffness, and prostration. The fever may peak with temperature in the 38°C to 40°C (100°F to 105°F) range. The myalgias are often intense and most prominent in the lumbosacral spine, thighs, and calves. Merely lightly touching the skin over a muscle may cause pain. Conjunctival findings have been rarely noted in some series, yet other authors report them in virtually all cases.[11, 13, 25] The most characteristic ocular finding during the first 3 days of the illness is conjunctival suffusion, a dilatation of the conjunctival vessels without associated signs of inflammation. Generalized abdominal pain is not unusual and has led clinicians to suspect an acute abdomen or enteric fever. The pain may in fact be muscular, although gastrointestinal tract disease has been documented.[1] Acalculous cholecystitis may be a particular problem in children with leptospirosis.[26] Nausea and vomiting are commonly noted and may be accompanied by diarrhea or constipation. A nonpro-

TABLE 176–1 ■ Clinical and Laboratory Manifestations of Leptospirosis in Six Published Series

	PREVALENCE OF FINDINGS (%) BY INVESTIGATORS*					
FINDINGS	Berman et al[28] *150, Vietnam*	Heath et al[12] *483, United States*	Kaufmann[11] *368, United States*	Alexander et al[25] *106 (Anicteric), Puerto Rico*	Alexander et al[25] *102 (Icteric), Puerto Rico*	Alston and Broom[3] *600 (Weil), United Kingdom*
Abrupt onset	—	78	—	—	—	62
Fever	97	100	62	100	99	—
Chills	78	66	16	84	90	—
Headache	98	77	50	82	95	87
Meningismus, stiff neck	12	37	40	12	5	34
Myalgias	79	68	29	97	97	—
Muscle tenderness	42	—	—	70	79	69
Nausea, vomiting	41/33	60	28	71/65	81/75	—
Diarrhea	29	15	5	25	30	—
Jaundice	2	43	33	0	100	74
Hepatomegaly	15	18	—	60	80	—
Splenomegaly	22	5	—	2	5	—
Abdominal tenderness	27	30	5	—	—	—
Conjunctival injection	42	33	8	100	98	72
Rash	7	9	9	—	—	—
Petechiae, ecchymoses	—	3	—	4	29	—
Anuria, oliguria	—	10	15	20	30	—
Azotemia	26	26	26	42	71	—
Albuminuria	≥67	19	21	64	79	75
Hematuria	5	27	22	9	13	—
Relapse (second pyrexia)	48	—	—	4	23	32
Case-fatality rate	0	7	8	0	13	—

*Number of subjects and location of the study are provided after the reference. Some reported percentages are based on a larger or smaller sample than that used to assess most manifestations.

ductive cough may also be reported. Skin manifestations associated with mild leptospirosis can include a transient macular, maculopapular, erythematous, purpuric, or urticarial rash, the distribution of which is mainly truncal but can also include other areas of the body. Hepatomegaly may be noted in more than 50% of cases.[25] Epistaxis and slightly bloody sputum may occur, but frank hemoptysis is rare. Central nervous system effects may be reflected in meningeal irritation, photophobia, or mild to severe physiologic dysfunction. A case of male hypogonadism after severe leptospirosis has been reported.[27] Variation in the clinical presentations reported by different authors may reflect differences in the prevalent serovars or in approaches to case identification.[3, 11, 13, 25, 28]

Leptospirosis is classically described as a biphasic illness with an initial leptospiremic phase, a brief and fairly asymptomatic period, and then a secondary leptospiruric or "immune" phase[1–3] (Fig. 176–1). This classic course has been

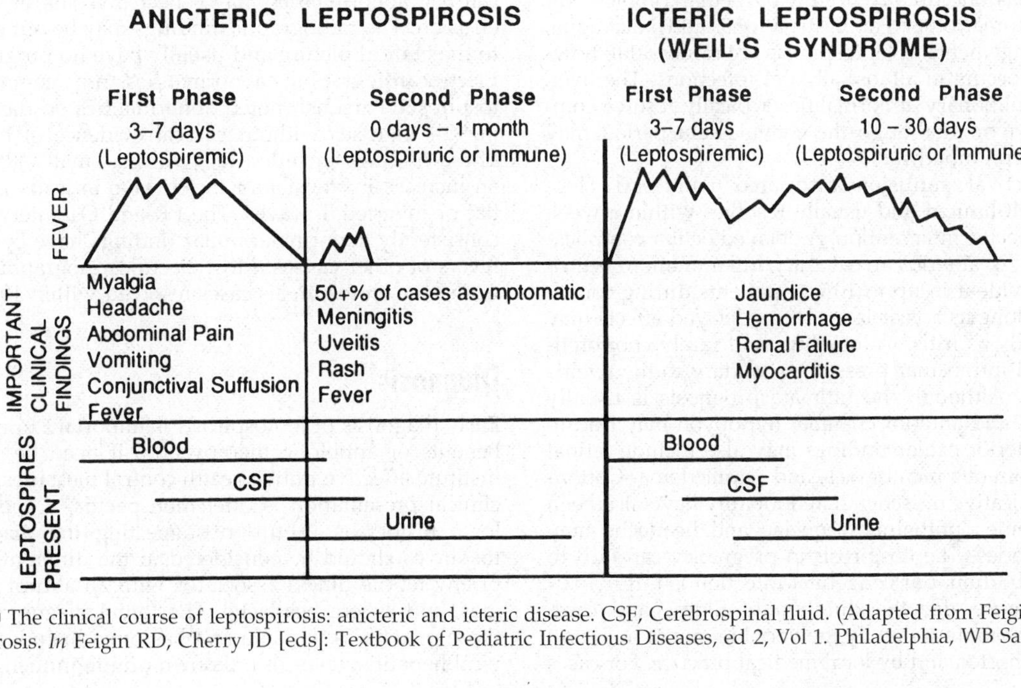

FIGURE 176–1 □ The clinical course of leptospirosis: anicteric and icteric disease. CSF, Cerebrospinal fluid. (Adapted from Feigin RD, Anderson DC: Leptospirosis. *In* Feigin RD, Cherry JD [eds]: Textbook of Pediatric Infectious Diseases, ed 2, Vol 1. Philadelphia, WB Saunders, 1987, pp 1190–1205.)

infrequently appreciated by some authors.[25, 29] In a review of 150 cases among U.S. soldiers in Vietnam by Berman and colleagues,[28] only 48% of cases were marked by recurrence of fever, and that usually lasted only 1 day. The initial phase of leptospirosis is notable for the presence of leptospires in the blood and cerebrospinal fluid and typically lasts 4 to 7 days. The intervening asymptomatic period may last 1 to 5 days. Resolution of fever at the end of the initial phase has been noted to coincide with the appearance of agglutinating antibodies independent of the duration of the illness.[28] The appearance of antibody also correlates with the disappearance of leptospiremia. The leptospiruric phase typically begins with recurrence of fever and otherwise may be highly variable clinically. Headache and other signs of aseptic meningitis are frequent and prominent in the second phase. Meningeal symptoms can actually appear to be the initial manifestation of leptospirosis. The severity of the meningitis is variable and does not correlate with the severity of the other disease manifestations. The leptospiruric phase may last 4 to 30 days or longer.

In the minority of patients whose disease is at the most severe end of the clinical spectrum (those with Weil disease), the initial fever and generalized abnormalities can progress after several days to a life-threatening illness characterized by jaundice, azotemia, hemorrhage, anemia, shock, and severe mental status changes. The disease progresses during the second week, often without any significant interphase clinical improvement. Hemorrhagic signs may include petechiae, purpura, conjunctival hemorrhages, and bloody sputum. Clinical abnormalities peak in the second week, which is when fatally afflicted patients tend to expire.[3] Renal failure may be accompanied by normal or reduced urine output or none. Low urine output may reflect volume depletion, hypotension, or acute tubular necrosis. In survivors, oliguria and anuria usually resolve during the second and third weeks, sometimes in association with notable diuresis. The leading cause of death has historically been renal failure. The availability of dialysis has reduced the magnitude of this factor. Other potentially fatal complications include adult respiratory distress syndrome, congestive heart failure, and arrhythmias.[30–32] Rarely, adrenal hemorrhage may result in sudden death. A severe hemorrhagic pneumonitis occurs occasionally, usually during the second week. Hemorrhagic pneumonitis has anecdotally been a particular problem for strains from Korea, other Far East nations, and Nicaragua. The liver derangements in leptospirosis are rarely fatal; however, jaundice occurs in almost all fatal infections. The liver, cardiac, and pulmonary abnormalities typically resolve completely in survivors, although the convalescent period may extend for several months.

The conjunctival suffusion associated with early leptospirosis is self-limited and usually resolves within a week without any specific intervention. A delayed ocular complication, however, is anterior uveal tract inflammation, which may become evident in up to 10% of patients during convalescence or as long as a year later. These delayed effects may present clinically as iritis, iridocyclitis, and rarely chorioretinitis. Increased intraocular pressure secondary to the uveitis may be noted. Although the ultimate prognosis is usually good, cataracts and anterior chamber hypopyon may lead to blindness. Posterior ocular findings may also include retinal hemorrhage, vitreous membranes, and papilledema. Cotton-wool spots indicative of ischemic retinopathy have also been described.[33] Some ophthalmic sequelae and headache may persist for decades.[34] Leptospirosis in pregnancy can lead to spontaneous abortion, but congenital infection is rare.[35]

Published figures for the duration of illness and case-fatality rates are confounded by the variable mix of mild and severe cases reported and by local medical practice. For cases reported in the United States in 1978, the median hospital stay was 6 days and the median duration of illness was 13 days (range, 1 to 34 days).[36] The case-fatality rate for U.S. cases reported in 1977 through 1983 ranged from 2.4% to 11.3%.[37] In aggressive surveillance efforts in which the proportion of mild cases reported is likely to be increased, the case-fatality rate is less than 1.0%. Reports from several tropical countries have noted case-fatality rates for severe leptospirosis of up to 18.8%.[38] Historically, mortality rates have been reported to be as high as 40%.[3, 6]

Key laboratory abnormalities in leptospirosis include mild proteinuria, which is present in the majority of patients at some time during the clinical course.[6, 28] Pyuria, granular casts, and microscopic hematuria may be seen. Blood urea nitrogen levels vary with the severity of illness but are below 100 mg/100 mL in most cases.[39] In assessing the cause of the azotemia, it is important to discriminate between volume depletion and tubular dysfunction.[1] Results of liver function tests are usually normal in anicteric illness. In jaundiced patients, transaminase and alkaline phosphatase levels may be increased twofold to threefold. The bilirubin level in icteric cases remains below 20 mg/dL in at least two thirds of cases and is predominantly conjugated.[39] Although prothrombin levels are usually normal, vitamin K can correct the prothrombin deficiency that is sometimes seen. Creatine kinase and amylase levels are commonly elevated.[40, 41] A complete blood count typically indicates a white cell count of 5000 to 15,000/mm^3, although it may be increased to above 49,000/mm^3 in severe disease. Neutrophilia is common. Anemia may be present, especially with more severe illness. The erythrocyte sedimentation rate is elevated in half of cases. Thrombocytopenia is common, although the platelet count is usually above 50,000/mm^3; rarely, the thrombocytopenia is severe.[42, 43] Examination of the cerebrospinal fluid during the immune phase commonly shows pleocytosis, with generally less than 500 cells per mm^3. Early in the course of the immune phase, the pleocytosis is mainly polymorphonuclear, but mononuclear cells subsequently predominate. The cerebrospinal fluid glucose value is usually normal, and protein is not infrequently elevated.[39]

Chest x-ray abnormalities have been noted in 23% to 67% of patients.[44, 45] Pulmonary abnormalities include nonsegmental opacities, basal linear opacities, and pleural effusions. Cardiac abnormalities may reflect myositis or a pericardial effusion. The radiographic findings may be out of proportion to the clinical picture and usually have no prognostic value.[1] Electrocardiographic abnormalities are common in leptospirosis. Parsons[46] noted abnormalities on the first records in 90% of cases without clinical evidence of heart disease. These findings included tachycardia, small QRS complexes, an increase in the size of the S wave in leads I and V_7, and flat or inverted T waves. The PR and QT intervals were not consistently abnormal. Similar findings have been seen with fevers of other causes. Most electrocardiographic abnormalities in the leptospirosis cases resolved within 10 days.[46]

Diagnosis

Early diagnosis of leptospirosis is important to maximize the benefits of antibiotic therapy and, if need be, to promptly institute effective public health control measures. Because the clinical presentation is often nonspecific, a good epidemiologic history is useful in suggesting the diagnosis. Leptospirosis should be considered in the differential diagnosis of any febrile illness associated with an abrupt onset, myalgias, and severe headache. The initial diagnosis in most of these patients is variable and has often included meningitis, viral hepatitis, fever of unknown origin, influenza, nephritis, encephalitis, and viral illness.[36, 39] Other illnesses in the differential diagnosis can include heat injury, rickettsioses, typhoid fever, brucellosis, relapsing fever, toxoplasmosis, malaria, yellow fever, septicemia, Kawasaki syndrome, toxic shock syndrome, Hantaan virus infection, and Legionnaires' disease. Atypical pneumonia is a rare presentation.[47] Leptospirosis can be differentiated from purulent bacterial meningitis by examination of the cerebrospinal fluid and by the presence of severe myalgias, conjunctival suffusion, a suggestive epidemiologic history, and results of serologic tests. In contrast to viral hepatitis patients, those with leptospirosis are more likely to have prolonged fever, conjunctival suffusion, proteinuria, elevated creatine kinase levels, and only modest transaminase elevations.

A specific diagnosis is usually based on demonstrating a fourfold rise in antibody titer. Many laboratories screen with a commercially prepared slide macroagglutination test that employs pooled antigens from selected serovars of *Leptospira*. Although this test is easy to use, it lacks the sensitivity and specificity of the microagglutination test, the current reference standard. The microagglutination test is generally limited to reference institutions because it can require the maintenance in live culture of more than 15 different serovars representing the serogroups prevalent in the particular geographic region that generates patients for the laboratory.[6] The importance of having local serovars in the microagglutination test battery is emphasized by Gray's report, discussed by Thiermann,[48] that 70% of U.S. soldiers' leptospirosis acquired in Panama could be diagnosed serologically only when Panamanian isolates were used as antigen for the microagglutination test. A presumptive diagnosis can be made if the patient has compatible clinical findings and either a positive result on the slide test or a microagglutination test titer of at least 1 in 100. The microagglutination test often lacks sensitivity in early disease. A sensitive and specific immunoglobulin M enzyme-linked immunosorbent assay is also available.[49] A variety of other assays including a dot enzyme-linked immunosorbent assay, an immunohemagglutination assay, an immunofluorescent assay, a microcapsule agglutination assay, and a gold immunoblot technique have been described.[50–54] Polymerase chain reaction methods under development hold promise for early diagnosis.[55] As noted before, cultures on specific media of blood and cerebrospinal fluid during the first week of illness and urine cultures thereafter can be useful to confirm the diagnosis; however, it may take 6 to 8 weeks for leptospires to grow out. Serologic studies of routine acute and convalescent specimens may fail to detect infection in up to 10% of patients whose cultures are positive.

Therapy (Table 176–2)

Recommendations concerning the antibiotic therapy for leptospirosis have historically been controversial owing to conflicting results of numerous clinical studies. On the basis of several published controlled trials, most consultants agree that antibiotic treatment of leptospirosis within the first 4 days of illness is beneficial.[56–59] McClain and colleagues,[56] for example, studied the effect of 100 mg doxycycline, orally twice a day for 7 days, in 29 U.S. soldiers with anicteric leptospirosis acquired in Panama. On average, therapy was initiated 45 hours after onset of illness. In comparison with the placebo group, the treated group received statistically significant benefits that included an overall 2.1-day reduction in illness, a 1.7-day reduction of fever, approximately 1 day less of headache and myalgia, and prevention of leptospiruria. No adverse effects of treatment were noted. Penicillin has also been used with success to treat leptospirosis within the first week of illness.[57] Erythromycin, some of the newer penicillins, and cephalosporins may also have a role in specific treatment.[60]

Unfortunately, in clinical practice, the diagnosis of leptospirosis is often not made within the first 4 days of illness. To evaluate the benefits of therapy in severe and late leptospirosis, Watt and coworkers[61] in a double-blind study in the Philippines randomized 42 patients (76% with severe

TABLE 176–2 ■ Duration of Fever in Seven Controlled Antibiotic Treatment Trials for Leptospirosis

INVESTIGATOR	DRUG AND DOSAGE REGIMEN*	TREATED PATIENTS/ CONTROL SUBJECTS	LOCATION	DAY OF ILLNESS WHEN TREATED (MEAN)	TOTAL MEAN DURATION OF FEVER IN DAYS† (ANTIBIOTIC VS. CONTROL)	COMMENTS
Kocen[57]	Penicillin, 600,000 units q 4 h × 1 d, then q 6 h × 4 d	15/23	Malaya	≤4	3.7 vs 8.1	Nonrandom
Kocen[57]	Penicillin, 600,000 units q 4 h × 1 d, then q 6 h × 4 d	13/10	Malaya	>4	6.4 vs 8.6	Nonrandom
Edwards et al[62]	Penicillin, 2 million units q 6 h × 5 d	38/41	Barbados	6.4	12.9 vs. 13.3	Randomized
Watt et al[61]	Penicillin, 1.5 million units q 6 h × 7 d	23/19	Philippines	9	13.7 vs. 20.6	Randomized, blinded
McClain et al[56]	Doxycycline, 100 mg PO bid × 7 d	14/15	Panama	1.9	3.7 vs. 5.4	Randomized, blinded
Russell[58]	Oxytetracycline, 1.5 mg PO, then 0.5 g q 6 h × 5+ d or until afebrile × 48 h (or similar IV regimen prn)	27/25	Malaya	3.5	6.4 vs. 9.4	No effect on jaundice and renal failure
Hall et al[59]	Penicillin, total of 1.5–16.9 million units in 5–20 d	5/12	Puerto Rico	4.2	7.9 vs. 8.6	Nonrandom, no placebo, control subjects' infections milder

*IV, Intravenously; PO, orally; bid, twice daily; prn, as required.
†For references 61 and 62, fever durations are approximate, because either the overlap between the last day before treatment and the first day of treatment could not be determined or the mean pretreatment interval was not separately reported for antibiotic-treated and untreated groups.

disease) to receive a 7-day course of either intravenous penicillin (1.5 million units every 6 hours) or placebo. On average, the patients had been ill for 9 days before enrollment, and about half had received antibiotics. Treatment reduced the duration of fever from 11.6 to 4.7 days ($P < .005$). Creatinine elevations persisted more than three times longer in the placebo group (8.3 versus 2.7 days, $P < .01$), and penicillin markedly reduced the frequency of leptospiruria. By contrast, Edwards and colleagues[62] enrolled 79 icteric patients in Barbados in a randomized controlled trial of penicillin (2 million units every 6 hours for 5 days) or no antibiotic treatment. The mean duration of illness in both groups was 6 to 7 days. With the exception of eliminating leptospiruria, penicillin afforded these patients no measurable clinical benefit. Factors to explain the contrasting conclusions from different studies may include geographic differences in serovar virulence, differences in clinical status or prior antibiotic therapy at enrollment, dosage considerations, and random events. In a few reports, Jarisch-Herxheimer–type reactions (a sharp temperature rise, a marked drop in blood pressure, and precipitation or aggregation of symptoms and signs) have been reported to occur after antibiotic therapy for leptospirosis.[62–64] This unusual phenomenon does not justify withholding antibiotics.[65] Nonspecific therapy for leptospirosis is supportive and may include measures to manage pain, fever, vomiting, mental status changes, fluid and electrolyte imbalances, renal failure, hyperbilirubinemia, hypotension, and hemorrhage. A short course of steroids may be useful for bleeding associated with severe thrombocytopenia.[42, 43]

Prevention

Effective prevention requires tailoring control measures to the epidemiology of leptospirosis in a particular situation. Efforts to control infection in domestic animal hosts can include isolation, chemotherapy, and selective slaughter of infected animals in addition to annual immunization.[6] Immunization of animals, which can prevent disease but not necessarily chronic leptospiruria, requires use of biologicals that protect against the serovars endemic in the animal's locale. Physical barriers and various methods of habitat alteration or poisoning may be necessary to limit human exposure to free-living animal carriers such as rodents. Recognition of the hazards associated with certain swamps or bodies of water may necessitate putting those areas off-limits. Protective clothing (provided that it does not hold contaminated water near the skin or lead to skin conditions that would enhance penetration of leptospires), appropriate use of surface disinfectants, and other hygienic practices are useful in some occupational settings. Chemoprophylaxis with 200 mg of doxycycline once a week has been effective in preventing leptospirosis among U.S. troops training in Panama during the rainy season; use of such a regimen should, however, be limited to prevention in the setting of short, high-risk exposures.[9, 16] Human vaccines have been used for some overseas populations, but no licensed preparation is available for use in the United States.[1, 23] Public and professional education is another important component of prevention.

Acknowledgment

The manuscript review as well as other advice concerning this chapter provided by Drs. George Watt and Bruce McLain is gratefully acknowledged.

References

1. Feigin RD, Anderson DC: Human leptospirosis. Crit Rev Clin Lab Sci 5:413, 1975.
2. Gsell O: The history of leptospirosis: 100 years. Zentralbl Bakteriol Mikrobiol Hyg A 257:473, 1984.
3. Alston JM, Broom JC: Leptospirosis in man and animals. Edinburgh, E & S Livingstone, 1958.
4. Gochenour WS Jr, Smadel JE, Jackson EB, et al: Leptospiral etiology of Fort Bragg fever. Public Health Rep 67:811, 1952.
5. Torten M: Leptospirosis. *In* Steele JH (ed): Handbook Series in Zoonoses, Vol I. Boca Raton, FL, CRC Press, 1979, pp 363–421.
6. Faine S (ed): Guidelines for the Control of Leptospirosis. Geneva, World Health Organization, 1982.
7. Johnson RC, Faine S: Family II. Leptospiraceae Hovind-Hougen. *In* Krieg NR, Holt JG (eds): Bergey's Manual of Systematic Bacteriology, Vol 1. Baltimore, Williams & Wilkins, 1984, pp 62–67.
8. Ellinghausen HC, McCullough WG: Nutrition of *Leptospira pomona* and growth of 13 other serotypes: Fractionation of oleic albumin complex and a medium of bovine albumin and polysorbate 80. Am J Vet Res 26:45, 1965.
9. Takafuji ET, Kirkpatrick JW, Miller RN, et al: An efficacy trial of doxycycline chemoprophylaxis against leptospirosis. N Engl J Med 310:497, 1984.
10. Feigin RD, Lobes LA, Anderson D, Pickering L: Human leptospirosis from immunized dogs. Ann Intern Med 79:777, 1973.
11. Kaufmann AF: Epidemiologic trends of leptospirosis in the United States, 1965–1974. *In* Johnson RC (ed): The Biology of Parasitic Spirochetes. New York, Academic Press, 1976, pp 177–190.
12. Heath CW, Alexander AD, Galton MM: Leptospirosis in the United States: Analysis of 483 cases in man, 1949–1961. N Engl J Med 273:857, 1965.
13. Cacciapuoti B, Nuti M, Pinto A, Sabrie AM: Human leptospirosis in Somalia: A serological survey. Trans R Soc Trop Med Hyg 76:178, 1982.
14. Jackson LA, Kaufmann AF, Adams WG, et al: Outbreak of leptospirosis associated with swimming. Pediatr Infect Dis 12:48, 1993.
15. Wilkins E, Cope A, Waitkins S: Rapids, rafts, and rats. Lancet 2:283, 1988.
16. Sanford JP: Leptospirosis—Time for a booster. N Engl J Med 310:524, 1984.
17. Cacciapuoti B, Ciceroni L, Maffei C, et al: A waterborne outbreak of leptospirosis. Am J Epidemiol 126:535, 1987.
18. Bolin CA, Koellner P: Human-to-human transmission of *Leptospira interrogans* by milk. J Infect Dis 158:246, 1988.
19. Centers for Disease Control: Summary of notifiable diseases, United States, 1987. MMWR Morbid Mortal Wkly Rep 36:1, 1987.
20. Gill ON, Coghlan JD, Calder IM: The risk of leptospirosis in United Kingdom fish farm workers. J Hyg (Camb) 94:81, 1985.
21. Arean VM: The pathogenic anatomy and pathogenesis of fatal human leptospirosis (Weil's disease). Am J Pathol 40:393, 1962.
22. DeBrito T, Morais CF, Yasuda PH, et al: Cardiovascular involvement in human and experimental leptospirosis: Pathologic findings and immunohistochemical detection of leptospiral antigen. Ann Trop Med Parasitol 81:207, 1987.
23. Alexander AD: Immunity in leptospirosis. *In* Johnson RC (ed): The Biology of Parasitic Spirochetes. New York, Academic Press, 1976, pp 339–349.
24. Faine S, Adler B, Christopher W, Valentine R: Fatal congenital human leptospirosis. Zentralbl Bakteriol Mikrobiol Hyg 257:548, 1984.
25. Alexander A, Benenson A, Byrne R, et al: Leptospirosis in Puerto Rico. Zoonoses Res 2:153, 1963.
26. Wong ML, Kaplan S, Dunkle LM, et al: Leptospirosis: A childhood disease. J Pediatr 90:532, 1977.
27. Panidis D, Vavilis D, Rousso D, et al: Hypothalamic-pituitary deficiency after Weil's syndrome: A case report. Fertil Steril 62:1077, 1994.
28. Berman SJ, Tsai C, Holmes K, et al: Sporadic anicteric leptospirosis in Viet Nam: A study in 150 patients. Ann Intern Med 79:167, 1973.
29. Nelson KE, Ager EA, Galton MM, et al: An outbreak of leptospirosis in Washington State. Am J Epidemiol 98:336, 1973.
30. Ramachandran S, Perera M: Cardiac and pulmonary involvement in leptospirosis. Trans R Soc Trop Med Hyg 71:56, 1977.
31. Chee H, Ossenkoppele G, Bronsveld W, Thijs L: Adult respiratory distress syndrome in *Leptospira icterohaemorrhagiae* infection. Intensive Care Med 11:254, 1985.

32. O'Neil KM, Rickman LS, Lazarus AA: Pulmonary manifestations of leptospirosis. Rev Infect Dis 13:705, 1991.
33. Gutman I, Walsh JB, Knapp AB: Cotton-wool spots as a sign in leptospirosis (Weil's disease). Ophthalmologica 187:133, 1983.
34. Shpilberg O, Shaked Y, Maier MK, et al: Long-term follow-up after leptospirosis. South Med J 83:405, 1990.
35. Shaked Y, Shpilberg O, Samra D, Samra Y: Leptospirosis in pregnancy and its effect on the fetus: Case report and review. Clin Infect Dis 17:241, 1993.
36. Centers for Disease Control: Leptospirosis surveillance: Annual Summary 1978 (issued August 1979). Washington, DC, Public Health Service, US Department of Health, Education, and Welfare, 1979.
37. Centers for Disease Control: Annual summary 1984. Reported morbidity and mortality in the United States. MMWR Morbid Mortal Wkly Rep 33:1, 1986.
38. Everard COR, Edwards CN, Webb GB, et al: The prevalence of severe leptospirosis among humans on Barbados. Trans R Soc Trop Med Hyg 78:596, 1984.
39. Heath CW, Alexander AD, Galton MM: Leptospirosis in the United States (concluded): Analysis of 483 cases in man, 1949–1961. N Engl J Med 273:915, 1965.
40. Johnson WD, Coelho I, Rocha H: Serum creatinine phosphokinase in leptospirosis. JAMA 233:981, 1975.
41. Kuriakose M, Eapen CK, Punnoose E, Koshi G: Leptospirosis—Clinical spectrum and correlation with seven simple laboratory tests for early diagnosis in the Third World. Trans R Soc Trop Med Hyg 84:419, 1990.
42. Edwards CN, Nicholson GD, Hassell TA, et al: Thrombocytopenia in leptospirosis: The absence of evidence for disseminated intravascular coagulation. Am J Trop Med Hyg 35:352, 1986.
43. Kahn JB: A case of Weil's disease requiring steroid therapy for thrombocytopenia and bleeding. Am J Trop Med Hyg 31:1213, 1982.
44. Lee R, Terry S, Walter T, Urquhart A: The chest radiograph in leptospirosis in Jamaica. Br J Radiol 54:939, 1981.
45. Wang C, Ch C, Lu F: Studies on anicteric leptospirosis. III. Radiographic observation of pulmonary changes. Chin Med J (Engl) 84:298, 1965.
46. Parsons M: Electrocardiographic changes in leptospirosis. Br Med J 2:201, 1965.
47. Alani FS, Mahoney MP, Ormerod LP, et al: Leptospirosis presenting as atypical pneumonia, respiratory failure and pyogenic meningitis. J Infect 27:281, 1993.
48. Thiermann AB: Leptospirosis: Current developments and trends. J Am Vet Med Assoc 184:722, 1984.
49. Terpstra W, Ligthart G, Schoone G: ELISA for the detection of specific IgM and IgG in human leptospirosis. J Gen Microbiol 131:377, 1985.
50. Pappas MG, Ballou WR, Gray MR, et al: Rapid serodiagnosis of leptospirosis using the IgM-specific dot ELISA: Comparison with the microscopic agglutination test. Am J Trop Med Hyg 34:346, 1985.
51. Petchclai B, Hiranras S, Kunakorn M, et al: Enzyme-linked immunosorbent assay for leptospirosis immunoglobulin M specific antibody using surface antigen from a pathogenic *Leptospira*: A comparison with indirect hemagglutination and microagglutination tests. J Med Assoc Thai 75:203, 1992.
52. Appassakij H, Silpapojakul K, Wansit R, Woodtayakorn J: Evaluation of the immunofluorescent antibody test for the diagnosis of human leptospirosis. Am J Trop Med Hyg 52:340, 1995.
53. Arimitsu Y, Kmety E, Ananyina Y, et al: Evaluation of the one-point microcapsule agglutination test for diagnosis of leptospirosis. Bull World Health Organ 72:395, 1994.
54. Petchclai B, Hiranras S, Potha U: Gold immunoblot analysis of IgM-specific antibody in the diagnosis of human leptospirosis. Am J Trop Med Hyg 45:672, 1991.
55. Merien F, Amouriaux P, Perolat P, et al: Polymerase chain reaction for detection of *Leptospira* spp. in clinical samples. J Clin Microbiol 30:2219, 1992.
56. McClain JB, Ballou WR, Harrison SM, Steinweg DL: Doxycycline therapy for leptospirosis. Ann Intern Med 100:696, 1984.
57. Kocen RS: Leptospirosis: A comparison of symptomatic and penicillin therapy. Br Med J 1:1181, 1962.
58. Russell RW: Treatment of leptospires with oxytetracycline. Lancet 2:1143, 1958.
59. Hall H, Hightower J, Diaz-Rivera R, et al: Evaluation of antibiotic therapy in human leptospirosis. Ann Intern Med 35:981, 1951.
60. Alexander AD, Rule PL: Penicillins, cephalosporins, and tetracyclines in treatment of hamsters with fatal leptospirosis. Antimicrob Agents Chemother 30:835, 1986.
61. Watt G, Padre LP, Tuazon ML, et al: Placebo-controlled trial of intravenous penicillin for severe and late leptospirosis. Lancet 1:433, 1988.
62. Edwards CN, Nicholson GD, Hassell TA, et al: Penicillin therapy in icteric leptospirosis. Am J Trop Med Hyg 39:388, 1988.
63. Mackay-Dick J, Robinson JF: Penicillin in the treatment of 84 cases of leptospirosis in Malaya. J R Army Med Corps 103:186, 1957.
64. Friedland JS, Warrell DA: The Jarisch-Herxheimer reaction in leptospirosis: Possible pathogenesis and review. Rev Infect Dis 13:207, 1991.
65. Watt G, Padre LP, Tuazon M, Calubaquib C: Limulus lysate positivity and Herxheimer-like reactions in leptospirosis: A placebo-controlled study. J Infect Dis 1662: 564, 1990.

177

Relapsing Fever

Thomas Butler

History

The agent of relapsing fever was first established in Berlin in 1873 by Obermeier, who used a microscope to observe spirochetes in the blood of patients. Between 1910 and 1945, epidemics of louse-borne relapsing fever occurred in North Africa, Sudan, Ethiopia, West Africa, central Africa, eastern Europe, and Russia. In these epidemics, there were an estimated 15 million cases, more than 5 million deaths, and case-fatality rates as high as 73%.[1]

Characteristics of the Pathogen

Borrelia spirochetes are spiral bacteria that measure 5 to 40 μm long and about 0.5 μm in diameter. They are too thin to be seen reliably by light microscopy of wet preparations, but they are easily visible when viewed by darkfield or phase-contrast microscopy. They are visible with aniline dyes, such as Wright or Giemsa stains, and stain well in tissue with silver stains, such as the Dieterle or Warthin-Starry stain.

Borrelia recurrentis is the cause of louse-borne relapsing fever. The species names of the tick-borne *Borrelia* are derived from the species names of *Ornithodorus* tick vectors that carry them, rather than from biochemical or antigenic characteristics. The more common ones are *Borrelia turicatae, Borrelia hermsii*, and *Borrelia parkeri* in North America and *Borrelia duttonii* in Africa. Each of the 25 serotypes of *B. hermsii* expresses different variable major proteins that are encoded by genes located on linear plasmids in the spirochete.[2]

Epidemiology

Louse-borne and tick-borne relapsing fevers differ so much in their epidemiology that they must be considered separately. Epidemic relapsing fever refers to the louse-borne kind, and endemic or sporadic relapsing fever to the tick-borne variety.

The geographic distribution of the relapsing fevers remains widespread, occurring in most areas of the world. Louse-borne relapsing fever has disappeared from the United States but still occurs in parts of Latin America, such as the Guatemalan and Andean highlands. During 1960 to 1979, louse-borne relapsing fever was documented in Ethiopia and Sudan.[1] Although accurate statistics on the incidence of this disease are not available, Ethiopia appears to be the country with the highest incidence, estimated at approximately 10,000 or more cases per year.

Tick-borne relapsing fever occurs in endemic foci in southern British Columbia, the western United States, the plateau regions of Mexico, and Central and South America. This disease is present in all areas of Africa except for the Sahara desert and the rain forest belt. It also occurs in Spain and Portugal. In Asia, tick-borne relapsing fever has been reported in Cyprus, Israel, Syria, Turkey, Iraq, Iran, southern Russia, China, Afghanistan, and India. Accurate statistics on tick-borne relapsing fever are not available, but the small numbers of established diagnoses suggest that this form of relapsing fever occurs less frequently in humans than does louse-borne relapsing fever.

The persons at greatest risk for acquiring louse-borne relapsing fever are those living under crowded, unhygienic conditions that favor infestation with body lice. Migrant workers and soldiers in war are particularly susceptible to this infection. Males are at much greater risk than are females, presumably because their lives more often expose them to infected lice. A strain-specific and short-lived acquired immunity develops after infection. This immunity helps to explain why migrant workers coming into an endemic area are more susceptible to infection than are the permanent inhabitants. In some endemic areas, such as Addis Ababa, Ethiopia, there is an increase in frequency during the cool winter season, when people wear heavier clothing that becomes louse infested.

Persons at greatest risk for tick-borne infection are those who come into contact with infected ticks from wild rodents. In the United States, the largest outbreak of tick-borne relapsing fever occurred in 62 campers and employees in the national park at the northern rim of the Grand Canyon, Arizona, in 1973. Another outbreak in Washington State affected 42 boy scouts who also camped out in a log cabin. In tropical countries, people who live in dwellings that are not rodent-proof are susceptible to infection.

Pathogenesis

After exposure to an infected louse or tick, spirochetes enter the skin and gain access to the blood and lymphatic circulations. The incubation period lasts 4 to 18 days after exposure, during which time the spirochetes divide in the blood plasma. After concentration has built up to 10^6 to 10^8 spirochetes per mL of blood, the illness begins. *Borrelia* spirochetes do not possess any known endotoxins or exotoxins. In general, *Borrelia* spirochetes do not produce abscesses and are confined predominantly to the plasma space of their mammalian hosts. Symptoms are caused by elevated concentrations of tumor necrosis factor, interleukin-1, interleukin-6, and interleukin-8.[3]

Clinical Manifestations

The typical patient suffers abrupt onset of shaking chills, fever, headache, and fatigue. Most patients have these symptoms almost continuously throughout the day, whereas some report the intermittent appearance of these symptoms several times a day. Patients complain frequently of myalgia, arthralgia, anorexia, dry cough, and abdominal pains. These symptoms are usually mild on the first day of illness and increase in intensity for a few days, leading to prostration. The nonspecific nature of these symptoms leads patients or their physicians to believe they have an influenza-like illness. In the differential diagnosis of relapsing fever in tropical regions, the most common diseases are malaria and typhoid fever.

The temperature is elevated in the range of 38.5°C to 40°C, and the pulse rate increases to about 115 beats per minute. The blood pressure drops to about 105/70 mm Hg. Patients appear lethargic or may be delirious. Physical signs that are common but not necessarily present include conjunctival injection, petechial rash that is usually truncal in distribution, and hepatosplenomegaly with occasional jaundice.[4–7] Disseminated intravascular coagulation also contributes to a decrease in platelets as well as producing prolonged prothrombin and partial thromboplastin times and elevated titers of fibrinogen-fibrin degradation products.[8]

Untreated patients experience relapses after recovery. The first attack of louse-borne relapsing fever lasts about 6 days and is followed by an afebrile period of about 9 days. There is usually only one relapse, which characteristically lasts only 2 days. The first attack of tick-borne relapsing fever lasts about 3 days and is followed by an interval of about 7 days, after which an average of three relapses occur, each lasting about 2 days. Relapses are usually milder than the first attacks.[9]

Autopsies performed in fatal cases of louse-borne relapsing fever show that the immediate cause of death varies. The spleen is enlarged to as much as 900 g, and the cut surface shows white microabscesses that consist of necrosis and hemorrhage in the white pulp. The liver is also enlarged, and the midzonal regions show scattered necrosis and hemorrhage. The heart is normal sized but frequently shows myocarditis consisting of interstitial edema and a cellular infiltrate of lymphocytes and plasma cells. The brain usually shows cerebral edema, and in some cases there is hemorrhage into the subarachnoid space or cerebrum.[10]

Diagnosis

The diagnosis of relapsing fever depends on the demonstration of spirochetemia (Fig. 177–1). In most patients, this is readily accomplished by obtaining peripheral blood by either finger stick or venipuncture and preparing a thin film on a microscope slide. A routine blood smear stained with Wright or Giemsa stain is adequate, but blood smears prepared for examination for malaria parasites are also satisfactory. Smears from patients who are in the interval between relapses will not demonstrate the organism, and the examination should be repeated when the fever reappears.

Spirochetemia may be detected, alternatively, by darkfield or phase-contrast microscopy. A drop of fresh blood is diluted with a drop of 0.9% sodium chloride solution and overlaid with a coverslip. Spirochetes are readily identified by their characteristic rotational motility.

Borrelia can be cultivated in Kelly broth medium or inoculated intraperitoneally into laboratory mice or rats, whose blood is examined daily for 14 days for spirochetes. Tick-borne *Borrelia* organisms are more readily cultivated and recovered from laboratory animals than is the louse-borne *B. recurrentis*. Louse-borne and tick-borne relapsing fevers are usually differentiated on epidemiologic grounds. If vectors can be collected from the patient or his or her household,

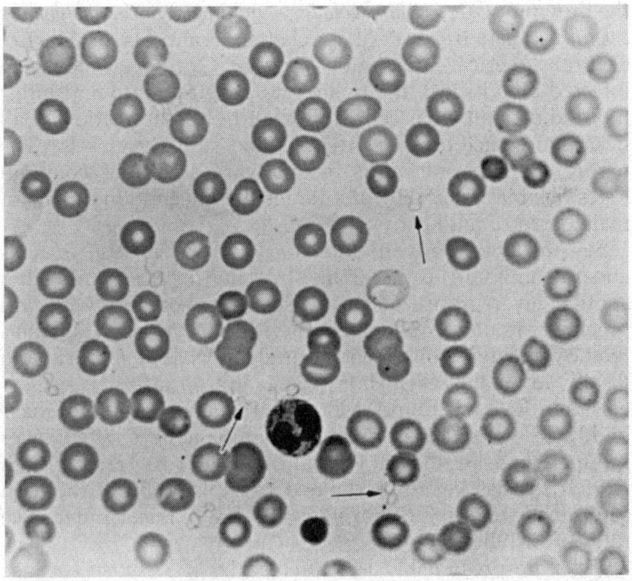

FIGURE 177–1 □ Blood smear from a patient with louse-borne relapsing fever shows spirochetes *(arrows)*. (Wright stain, × 600.)

they can be dissected and the hemolymph or coxal fluid examined microscopically for the presence of spirochetes.

Serologic testing by agglutination, complement fixation, and immobilization of living spirochetes has been employed in endemic areas for purposes of seroepidemiology and examining convalescent patients. None of these tests, however, is standardized or available for general use.

Treatment

The relapsing fevers respond to tetracycline and erythromycin. Tetracycline is the treatment of choice except for children younger than 7 years and pregnant women. A single oral dose of tetracycline, 500 mg, is as effective in clearing spirochetemia and preventing relapse as are longer courses. Erythromycin, 500 mg, given orally as a single dose is a satisfactory alternative to tetracycline.[11] For patients who are unable to take oral medication, intravenous injection of 250 mg of tetracycline or erythromycin is curative. For children smaller than 30 kg, the dose of tetracycline or erythromycin should be reduced to approximately 10 mg/kg. Penicillin G therapy results in slow clearance of spirochetes and frequent relapses.[12]

In most patients with louse-borne relapsing fever and in some with tick-borne relapsing fever,[13] antibiotic treatment provokes a distressing Jarisch-Herxheimer reaction. Rigor occurs 2 to 3 hours after treatment. Subsequently, the temperature rises sharply and the blood pressure drops while spirochetes are cleared from the blood. Patients may require intravenous infusions of 0.9% sodium chloride solution to maintain adequate blood pressure. During several hours, the temperature declines and the patient feels better.

Attempts to ameliorate the severity of the reaction by giving antipyretic or antiinflammatory drugs have not been successful. The best approach is to anticipate the reaction and to provide intensive nursing care and intravenous fluid support during the first day of treatment.

Complete recovery occurs in at least 95% of adequately treated cases of relapsing fever. The prognosis for untreated disease is variable, particularly for louse-borne relapsing fever, during epidemics of which mortality rates of 40% have been reported. The illness is usually fatal in neonates.

Prevention

Available approaches for control of the relapsing fevers include the detection and treatment of human cases, vector control, rodent control, and public health education. Vaccines are not available.

For louse-borne relapsing fever, the detection and treatment of cases have the effect of reducing the reservoir of infection and, consequently, reducing transmission. More important is the control of louse infestation. Instructing people to bathe and wash their clothes is the rational approach, but compliance is likely to be poor. Clothing and bodies can be deloused with insecticides or with insect repellents. In known epidemic situations, prophylactic antibiotics are a temporary measure to contain spread of infection to persons at high risk. The eventual control of this disease requires improvements in personal hygiene and housing conditions.

For tick-borne relapsing fever, the treatment of human cases has no impact on the animal reservoirs. Campers and hikers going into endemic areas should be advised to avoid staying in cabins that are inhabited by rodents and their ticks and to apply topical tick repellents to their skin. In endemic areas of Africa, people need to be assisted in building rodent-proof houses.

References

1. Ahmed MAM, Abdel Wahab SM, Abdel Malik MD, et al: Louse-borne relapsing fever in the Sudan. A historical review and a clinicopathological study. Trop Geogr Med 32:106, 1980.
2. Barbour AG, Hayes SF: Biology of *Borrelia* species. Microbiol Rev 50:381, 1986.
3. Negussie Y, Remick DG, DeForge LE, et al: Detection of plasma tumor necrosis factor, interleukins 6, and 8 during the Jarisch-Herxheimer reaction of relapsing fever. J Exp Med 175:1207, 1992.
4. Butler T, Hazen P, Wallace CK, et al: *Borrelia recurrentis* infection: Pathogenesis of fever and petechiae. J Infect Dis 140:665, 1979.
5. Mekasha A: Louse-borne relapsing fever in children. J Trop Med Hyg 95:206, 1992.
6. Barclay AJG, Coulter JBS: Tick-borne relapsing fever in central Tanzania. Trans R Soc Trop Med Hyg 84:852, 1990.
7. Lovett MA, Goldstein EJC, Fleischmann J: Fever in a couple vacationing in the mountains of southern California. Clin Infect Dis 14:1254, 1992.
8. Galloway RE, Levin J, Butler T, et al: Activation of protein mediators of inflammation and evidence for endotoxemia in *Borrelia recurrentis* infection. Am J Med 63:933, 1977.
9. Southern PM, Sanford JP: Relapsing fever: A clinical and microbiological review. Medicine (Baltimore) 48:129, 1969.
10. Judge DM, Samuel I, Perine PL, et al: Louse-borne relapsing fever in man. Arch Pathol 97:136, 1974.
11. Butler T, Jones PK, Wallace CK: *Borrelia recurrentis* infection: Single-dose antibiotic regimens and management of Jarisch-Herxheimer reaction. J Infect Dis 137:573, 1978.
12. Warrell DA, Perine PL, Krause DW, et al: Pathophysiology and immunology of the Jarisch-Herxheimer–like reaction in louse-borne relapsing fever: Comparison of tetracycline and slow-release penicillin. J Infect Dis 147:898, 1983.
13. Horton JM, Blaser MJ: The spectrum of relapsing fever in the Rocky Mountains. Arch Intern Med 145:871, 1985.

178

Rocky Mountain Spotted Fever

J. Stephen Dumler

Rocky Mountain spotted fever (RMSF) is a potentially severe, tick-borne, febrile illness caused by infection with *Rickettsia rickettsii*. Despite wide general awareness of the local prevalence, the manifestations, and the availability of highly effective therapeutic antimicrobial agents for RMSF, the disease is still frequently fatal.[1, 2] Why this situation exists is not completely understood, but it can be partly explained by generally unrecognized differences between the classic presentation described in medical textbooks and the actual situation in which the clinical diagnostic clues, such as rash, are often not present at the time of initial presentation.[3, 4] Regardless, RMSF can be severe and rapidly fatal if it is not recognized and treated early. It is the often undifferentiated presentation that can cause significant problems; thus, a complete understanding of the clinical manifestations, the appropriate historical and epidemiologic circumstances, the appropriate use and interpretation of laboratory results, and the pathophysiologic process of the infection provides the real key to early recognition and cure.

Ecology and Transmission of *Rickettsia rickettsii*

RMSF is caused by *R. rickettsii*, a small, obligate intracellular bacterium that usually occupies part of its life cycle in tick tissues or in small rodents and other small wild animals.[5] The rickettsiae are in fact well adapted to this propagation cycle and pass into subsequent life stages of the ticks after molting; infection of subsequent tick generations is predominantly maintained by dissemination of the rickettsiae into the tick's ovarian tissues and transmission into the next generation of larval ticks (transovarian or vertical transmission). A smaller percentage of infected tick cohorts survive than do uninfected ticks, and consequently, propagation of the rickettsiae and the resulting rickettsemia in small rodents and other small animals allow uninfected ticks to acquire the agent (horizontal transmission) and the establishment of newly infected tick generations. Such small animals as voles (*Microtus pennsylvanicus, Pitymys pinetorum*), white-footed mice (*Peromyscus leucopus*), cotton rats (*Sigmodon hispidus*), rabbits and hares (*Sylvilagus floridanus, Lepus americanus*), opossums (*Didelphis marsupialis virginiana*), chipmunks (*Eutamias amoenus*), and squirrels (*Spermophilus lateralis tescorum*) may be important, if transient, natural reservoirs that maintain an interval of rickettsemia. Humans, when infected, represent a simple dead-end host and offer no survival advantage for *R. rickettsii*.

Important tick species that are involved in the transmission of RMSF vary over geographic regions, including the American dog tick (*Dermacentor variabilis*) in much of the eastern and midwestern parts of the United States and the wood tick (*Dermacentor andersoni*) in the Rocky Mountain regions.[5] Both the brown dog tick (*Rhipicephalus sanguineus*) and *Amblyomma cajennense* can transmit the rickettsiae in parts of Mexico, Central America, and South America. Once acquired in an infected blood meal, the rickettsiae penetrate into and infect the midgut epithelial cells, followed by dissemination to all tick tissues including the ovaries and salivary glands.[6] The regurgitation of infectious tick salivary secretions contaminates tick bite wounds and initiates the infection in the mammalian or human host.

Several factors govern infection with *R. rickettsii* in ticks and transmission to mammals. Infection of ticks with other spotted fever group rickettsiae seems to compete with and preclude simultaneous infection with *R. rickettsii*.[7] This interference phenomenon is poorly understood but may explain locally low rates of RMSF where appropriate tick vectors exist and RMSF is found. Moreover, the contribution of these highly prevalent, presumably nonpathogenic spotted fever group rickettsiae that induce antibodies cross-reactive with *R. rickettsii* has yet to be defined in explanation of the high seroprevalence of RMSF versus the low clinical prevalence rates of RMSF.

Ticks are presumably less affected by *R. rickettsii* because virulence of this agent is minimal at the relatively low ambient temperatures at which ticks live. After exposure to more elevated temperatures or exposure to blood, *R. rickettsii* becomes activated to a more virulent state, a process that may take hours to occur.[8] As for other tick-transmitted agents, there is an interval ranging up to 48 hours or longer during which exchange of potentially infectious tick saliva is minimal and rickettsiae are not reactivated. Thus, attached ticks removed within this interval, particularly if they are still flat, are less likely to have transmitted *R. rickettsii* to the host.

Mammalian host factors also influence transmission in that previously infected, immune animals will not support rickettsemia or horizontal amplification of *R. rickettsii*.[5, 9] Thus, risk for transmission in any given area is determined by multiple factors, including (1) the local prevalence of appropriate tick species that contain *R. rickettsii*[10]; (2) the local prevalence of ticks that contain nonpathogenic "interfering" spotted fever group rickettsiae[7]; (3) the number of, density of, and immune status of appropriate susceptible small mammals that support local amplification of *R. rickettsii*[5]; (4) the presence of appropriate larger animals that support propagation of adult-stage ticks[5]; and (5) the likelihood that humans accidentally interrupt this natural ecologic cycle.[11]

Distribution and Prevalence

RMSF is the second most frequently diagnosed tick-borne disease next to Lyme disease in the United States, with 590 cases diagnosed in 1995.[1] The national rate of infection in 1995 was 0.23 case per 100,000 population reported to the Centers for Disease Control and Prevention. This rate has remained relatively constant since 1986, ranging from 0.18 case per 100,000 population in 1993 (456 cases) and 1994 (465 cases) to 0.32 case per 100,000 population in 1986 (760 cases). However, RMSF has undergone cyclic changes in prevalence with a nadir in the early 1960s and a peak around 1980; yet another nadir appears to have occurred in 1993 to 1994 because the rate in 1995 represents a substantial increase.

The name is misleading because most cases are recognized in the central and southeastern regions of the United States. For example, in 1995, 280 (47%) of the cases occurred in the South Atlantic states, and North Carolina alone reported 150 (54%) of those. Other geographic regions with significant numbers of RMSF cases include the West South Central states (86 cases), especially Oklahoma and Arkansas, and the East South Central states (83 cases), especially Mississippi and

Tennessee. In spite of this more typical geographic distribution, cases have been identified in nearly every state in the United States, including urban areas such as the South Bronx, New York. Cases occur predominantly during summer months, with 80% of cases in 1995 reported between April and October, correlating with periods of peak tick activity and outdoor recreational activity.

RMSF has been considered chiefly a disease of children in the past, with high frequency in 5- to 9-year-old children. In 1995, the rate of RMSF was highest among 5- to 14-year-old children (0.30 case per 100,000), but it was also high in the 25- to 44-year age group (0.25 case per 100,000), the group younger than 5 years (0.24 case per 100,000), and the 45- to 64-year age group (0.22 case per 100,000).[1] Whether these changing epidemiologic statistics reflect changes in life style habits, increased awareness of tick-borne infections among parents of younger children, or other factors is not known. In general, most of the patients described in the past have been male (55%) and white (85%).[10] However, RMSF in patients older than 60 years can have particularly grave consequences. Thus, a febrile illness in a child or adolescent or in men older than 60 years that occurs during May through September with the potential for tick exposure should warrant the inclusion of RMSF in the differential diagnosis. In spite of the availability of effective therapy, the rate of death due to RMSF had been relatively steady since the 1980s, ranging from 1.1% to 4.1%.

Pathogenesis and Pathophysiology

After inoculation of *R. rickettsii* into the dermis of a susceptible patient, there is an incubation period that averages approximately 7 days (range, 3 to 12 days) during which the initial proliferation and dissemination of the bacteria occur. The rickettsiae that are inoculated into the pool of blood created in the dermis at the site of tick bite apparently gain entrance to endothelium in the adjacent dermal capillaries and venules. Dissemination from this site must occur rapidly, because eschars and necrotic lesions at the tick bite site are rare.[10] Dissemination probably occurs by hematogenous spread, and the vascular beds of any or all tissues and organs can then become infected.

As the rickettsiae are spread, attachment to a surface receptor of vascular endothelium occurs. This process appears to be mediated by the 190-kDa protein of *R. rickettsii*, because attachment and entry can be inhibited in vitro by monoclonal antibodies that react with this protein.[12] Once within the endothelial cell, the rickettsiae multiply and damage the cell by the accumulated effects of phospholipase A_2, phospholipase C,[13] and free radical–mediated membrane damage.[14] In vitro, infected endothelial cells are up-regulated to express cell surface selectins and procoagulant tissue factor and to release von Willebrand factor and interleukin-1α.[15–18] If analogous circumstances occur in vivo, these events would lead to enhanced recruitment of inflammatory cells and deposition of fibrin and platelets on the surface of affected cells. In fact, the hallmark lesion of *R. rickettsii* infection is vasculitis characterized predominantly by an influx of lymphocytes and histiocytes, except where rickettsia-mediated necrosis has occurred that in addition elicits neutrophil influx.[19] Similarly, thrombosis is a relatively infrequent finding in most vasculitic lesions in vivo. The more frequent histopathologic lesion detected in patients with RMSF is a perivascular infiltrate of lymphohistiocytic inflammatory cells that may occur in almost any tissue. Whether the E-selectins expressed in vitro that typically bind neutrophils predominantly and the up-regulated in vitro tissue factor expression that predisposes to thrombosis are important for in vivo pathogenesis is still not clear. Regardless of whether vasculitis has compromised local perfusion, significant vascular injury can occur. The net result of this vascular injury is vascular leakage, leading to hypoperfusion, ischemia, and interstitial edema.

The septic shock–like course of RMSF might suggest a pathologic role for cytokines.[20] However, experimental evidence now seems to indicate that the cytokines produced as an inflammatory and immune initiating response to the presence of *R. rickettsii* are, in the balance, beneficial and lead to a decrease in rickettsial load and elimination of rickettsia-infected cells that cannot be affected by antibody.[21–24] Animal models of spotted fever group rickettsiosis show that cytokines are an essential part of the protective immune and inflammatory responses and recovery from RMSF. Guinea pigs made deficient of interferon-γ have more severe and fatal infections.[21] Mice produce tumor necrosis factor, interleukin-1, and interleukin-6 early in the infectious process.[22] As the infection becomes lethal in mice, levels of these cytokines become undetectable. In murine endothelial cells, the protective effects of interferon-γ and tumor necrosis factor-α are synergistic and act by apparently inducing endothelial nitric oxide synthase.[23] The increased production of nitric oxide that results then leads to tryptophan sequestration and production of membrane-damaging hydrogen peroxide.[24] The net result is a reduction in the numbers of rickettsiae and of rickettsia-infected cells.

Pathologic studies show a typical sequence of events that explain the clinical and laboratory findings at various times in the course of RMSF.[19, 25] As the rickettsial vasculitis and endothelial injury accrue, a significant increase begins in vascular permeability manifested by edema, decreases in plasma volume, hypoproteinemia, hypoalbuminemia, reduced serum oncotic pressure, and the resultant effects of hypovolemia and hypotension that are present in 17% of patients. The clinical manifestations often depend on the systemic degree of vascular compromise and the specific organs that are indirectly damaged by hypoperfusion or direct rickettsia-mediated vascular damage. The frequent occurrence of acute renal insufficiency is best explained by this hypotension. As the rickettsial proliferation diminishes, either by specific antimicrobial therapy or by waxing immunity, microvascular integrity and tissue perfusion are reestablished, intravascular blood volume normalizes, and edema resolves.

At the time that illness begins, the initial findings include fever, headache, malaise, and myalgias.[3, 26, 27] After the initial signs and symptoms begin, some patients will develop other findings including chills or rigors, stiff neck, nausea, vomiting, diarrhea, abdominal pain and tenderness, conjunctival suffusion, photophobia, cough, facial or pedal edema, neurologic signs (meningismus, confusion, convulsions, coma), occasional cardiac abnormalities (e.g., arrhythmias, heart failure), hepatomegaly, splenomegaly, gangrene of digits or extremities, and hypotension (Table 178–1). Likewise, RMSF is often associated with a spectrum of clinical laboratory findings that suggest a systemic process.[3, 26, 27] Frequently encountered abnormalities in a patient who appears clinically infected, if not septic, include a normal leukocyte count or slight leukopenia with an increased number of bands, thrombocytopenia, hyponatremia, mild to moderate elevations in serum aspartate and alanine aminotransferase activities, and acute elevations in serum urea nitrogen and creatinine levels (Table 178–2). As expected, hypoproteinemia, hypoalbuminemia, and associated abnormalities in serum electrolyte concentrations (such as hypocalcemia) are also often detected.

The involvement of the coagulation system in RMSF is greatly misunderstood. It is often assumed that much of the pathologic injury associated with the vasculitis results from thrombosis, vascular occlusion, and tissue infarction; how-

TABLE 178–1 ■ Frequent Clinical Features of Rocky Mountain Spotted Fever in Three Case Series*

HISTORY, SIGNS, OR SYMPTOMS	HELMICK ET AL[3] (N = 262)	KAPLOWITZ ET AL[27] (N = 131)	SEXTON AND BURGDORFER[76] (N = 75)
Tick bite	60	NR	68
Fever	99	100	100
Rash	88	90	100
Rash on palms and soles	74	82	NR
Headache	91	79	92
Myalgia	83	72	67
Nausea or vomiting	60	63	39
Abdominal pain	52	23	33
Conjunctivitis	30	30	15
Edema	18	20	17
Pneumonitis	12	17	NR
Any severe neurologic complication†	26	23	48

*Data are expressed as a percentage of total cases in each series. NR, Not reported.
†Neurologic complications include stupor, delirium, seizures, ataxia, papilledema, focal neurologic deficits, and coma.

ever, these situations are infrequent events that do not often influence the course of disease.[10, 28] Necrosis of the skin is seen in only 4% of patients and probably results from hypoperfusion rather than thrombosis in most patients.[27] The data that support this notion are derived from extensive experience with autopsy and biopsy specimens from patients with RMSF, in which thrombosis is infrequent but evidence of nonocclusive vascular injury is the norm.[19] Small, nonocclusive thrombi that attach to sites of rickettsia-mediated vascular damage are more protective than damaging and preclude significant ischemic necrosis and hemorrhage by maintaining patency.[10] The development of concurrent hypotension, leukopenia with a leftward shift, and thrombocytopenia suggests a clinical picture consistent with disseminated intravascular coagulation; however, true disseminated intravascular coagulation due to systemic cytokine induction of leukocyte-endothelial adherence and damage is infrequent.[3, 27] Most of the consumptive coagulopathy can be explained by the widespread rickettsia-mediated vasculitis and increased vascular permeability.[3, 10, 27]

Clinical Manifestations and Pathology

Rash

Cutaneous manifestations occur in only 14% of patients on the first day of illness and in 49% during the first 3 days.[3, 27] Rash appears between days 3 and 5 of illness in most patients and later than day 6 in 20% of patients; 9% to 16% of patients do not have a rash detected at any time.[3, 11, 27] The absence of rash should not be taken as a sign of relatively mild illness because there is a clear association with an increased risk for a severe or fatal outcome when rash is not detected.[3, 4, 29]

Rash often occurs in several stages, and an evolution toward petechiae and hemorrhagic lesions may be observed if treatment is not appropriate.[3, 10, 30] The initial appearance is that of erythematous macules that often occur first on the ankles or wrists and may subsequently be found on the trunk, palms, or soles.[3, 27] These lesions blanch with pressure and become papular as local edema and perivascular mononuclear inflammatory cell infiltrates accrue.[19] As the rickett-

TABLE 178–2 ■ Selected Laboratory Abnormalities Reported in Patients with Rocky Mountain Spotted Fever, North Carolina Memorial Hospital, 1970 Through 1979

LABORATORY FINDING	PATIENTS TESTED (N)	PATIENTS WITH FINDING N	PATIENTS WITH FINDING %
White cell count			
<10,000/mm³	129	93	72
>10% bands	121	83	69
Platelet count			
<150,000/mm³	117	61	52
<99,000/mm³	117	38	32
Serum sodium value < 132 mEq/L	131	72	56
Aspartate aminotransferase ≥ twice normal value	71	44	62
Alanine aminotransferase ≥ twice normal value	66	26	39
Bilirubin value > 1.4 mg/dL	53	16	30
Cerebrospinal fluid*			
Opening pressure ≥ 250 mm H_2O	35	5	14
Glucose value ≤ 50 mg/dL	52	5	8
Protein value ≥ 50 mg/dL	62	22	35
White cell count ≥ 5/mm³	63	24	38
Mononuclear cell predominance	24	11	46
Polymorphonuclear cell predominance	24	12	50

*Lumbar puncture was performed in 63 of 131 patients before therapy was started.
Data from Kaplowitz LG, Fischer JJ, Sparling PF: Rocky Mountain spotted fever: A clinical dilemma. *In* Remington JS, Swartz MN (eds): Current Clinical Topics in Infectious Diseases, Vol 2. New York, McGraw-Hill, 1981, pp 89–108.

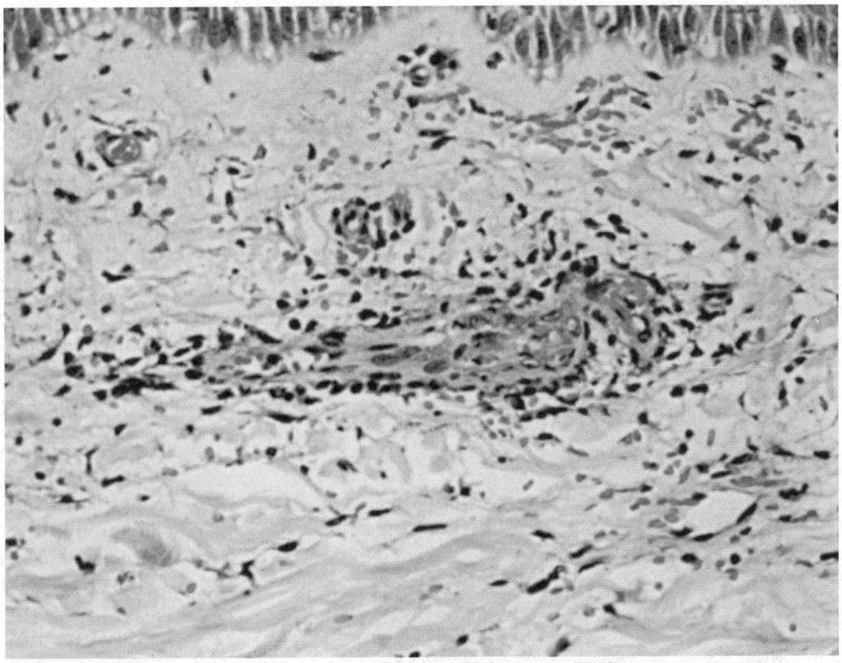

FIGURE 178–1 □ Rocky Mountain spotted fever. Skin biopsy specimen of a petechial lesion shows a moderate lymphohistiocytic perivascular infiltrate and lymphohistiocytic vasculitis. Note the endothelial cell necrosis, erythrocyte extravasation into the dermis, and minimal nonocclusive thrombosis in this dermal venule. (H&E, × 250.)

siae continue to proliferate, lymphohistiocytic or leukocytoclastic vasculitis with infiltration of the vascular wall and endothelial injury may be present[19] (Fig. 178–1). The irreversible endothelial injury caused by *R. rickettsii* results in extravasation of blood into the surrounding dermal tissues and the development of nonblanching petechiae, hemorrhagic lesions, or palpable purpura (Fig. 178–2). Petechiae are observed in 41% to 59% of patients and often appear after the sixth day of illness.[3, 4, 27] The petechial rash on the soles and palms that is often considered most typical of RMSF in fact occurs in only 43% of patients with a rash and after day 5 of illness in 36% to 82% of patients.[3, 4, 27] Thus, at the typical time of presentation, around day 3 of illness, many patients lack the findings most often considered critical to render an accurate diagnosis of RMSF.[3, 4] In later disease, especially in severe cases with extensive vascular injury, many of the lesions may coalesce and become ecchymotic (Fig. 178–3).

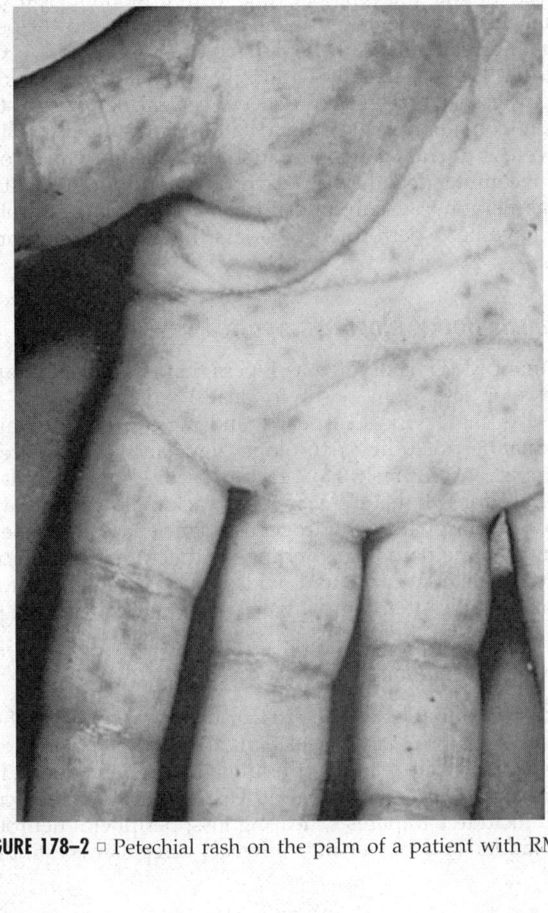

FIGURE 178–2 □ Petechial rash on the palm of a patient with RMSF.

Gastrointestinal System

The frequent occurrence of gastrointestinal abnormalities in RMSF sometimes leads to the erroneous diagnosis of an acute abdomen.[3, 27, 31, 32] These findings may be present early during the illness and involve between 39% and 63% of patients.[3, 33] The underlying pathologic lesion that accounts for these frequent abnormalities is vasculitis and rickettsia-mediated endothelial damage of the visceral wall and lamina propria vasculature.[19, 31] Several reports documented surgical intervention in cases in which appendicitis and acute cholecystitis were clinically suspected.[31, 32, 34] Involvement of other gastrointestinal structures, such as the pancreas, may similarly result in presentations that are atypical for RMSF and are likely to be misdiagnosed.[34] Liver involvement is frequent with RMSF and is manifested mostly by mild to moderate elevations in serum hepatic aminotransferase activities.[3, 26, 27, 35] However, jaundice may occasionally develop and, when present, is a risk factor for fatal disease.[3] Rickettsiae may infect the endothelium lining the liver sinusoids and the portal vascular structures but not hepatocytes, which will lead to mild focal hepatitis and periportal inflammation that indirectly lead to the mild liver injury.[19] More severe liver injury is seen with fulminant RMSF as vast regions of the hepatic microvasculature are destroyed by the actively growing rickettsiae with or without significant vasculitis.[36]

Cardiopulmonary System

Among the most worrisome complications with RMSF is the diffuse injury that occurs in the pulmonary vascular beds. The pathologic lesion is characterized by widespread intersti-

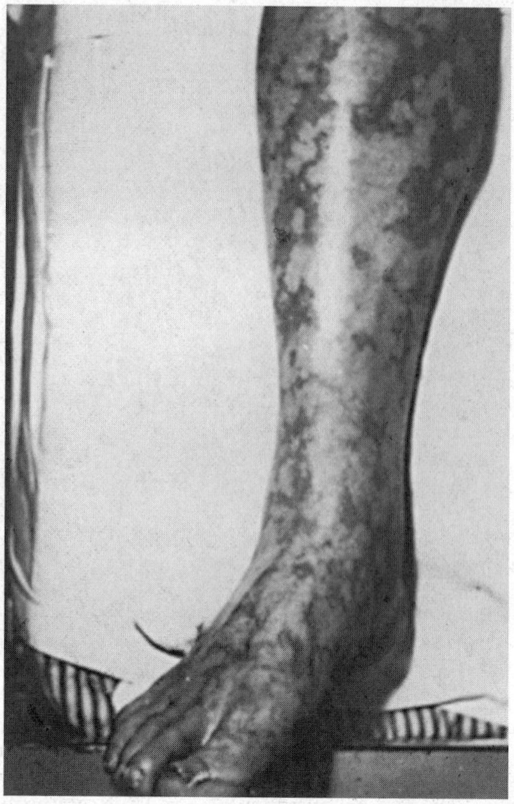

FIGURE 178–3 □ Purpuric rash in a patient with RMSF complicated by widespread *R. rickettsii*–mediated vascular injury. (From Woodward TE: Rickettsial diseases in the United States. Med Clin North Am 43:1516, 1959.)

tial pneumonitis and capillary endothelial injury.[19] Interstitial pneumonitis results from recruitment of lymphoid and histiocytic cells into the alveolar septal interstitial spaces adjacent to infected pulmonary capillaries. The resulting severe vascular permeability leads to exudation into the interstitial and alveolar spaces to cause noncardiogenic pulmonary edema, which may be partly precipitated by excessive intravenous fluid therapy for hypotension.[10, 25, 37, 38] Pulmonary involvement occurs in 17% of patients and is manifested by cough, rales, hypoxemia, or infiltrates on chest radiographs.[27, 39] Of these patients, 12% will have severe respiratory dysfunction and 8% will require intubation and mechanical ventilation. Cardiopulmonary hemodynamic monitoring often shows relatively normal pulmonary capillary wedge pressures and left ventricular function, and careful monitoring will help effectively manage fluid volume and hypotension to preclude worsening pulmonary function. When diffuse infiltrates are present, the mortality rate can be as high as 50%.[39]

Cardiac involvement in RMSF is relatively infrequent and often clinically insignificant.[37] Congestive heart failure in the elderly may occur, particularly if there is volume overload with therapy for hypotension. The principal evidence for myocardial involvement is the demonstration of arrhythmias that occur in 7% to 16% of patients,[3, 27] but gallops, murmurs, cardiac enlargement, and electrocardiographic abnormalities (low voltage, ST-T changes, and atrioventricular conduction disturbances) have been reported.[3, 27, 40, 41] The arrhythmias result from focal rickettsial lymphohistiocytic myocarditis with insignificant myocardial necrosis that involves the conduction tracts or nodes. Significant clinical sequelae from these lesions are rare.

Renal System

Although renal involvement with rickettsia-mediated interstitial nephritis is well documented in autopsies,[19, 31] the predominant renal abnormality in RMSF is prerenal azotemia that accounts for elevations in serum urea nitrogen and creatinine values; however, continued hypoperfusion secondary to hypotensive shock can cause acute tubular necrosis and acute renal failure.[10, 31] Glomerulonephritis due to active rickettsial infection of the glomerulus may occur[42] but is infrequently the cause of renal dysfunction. Urinalysis will sometimes show proteinuria and hematuria, but an active urine sediment as evidence of nephritis is infrequent.

Neurologic System

Next to pulmonary involvement, central nervous system infection is the most significant cause of severe and fatal outcome for RMSF.[3, 25, 27, 43–45] The rickettsiae invade endothelial cells within the brain parenchyma to cause focal vasculitis or perivascular infiltrates called microglial or typhus nodules.[19] Clinically evident encephalitis, manifested as confusion or lethargy, is present in 26% to 28% of patients, and more severe manifestations such as stupor and delirium occur almost as frequently, in 21% to 26% of patients.[3, 27] Ataxia (18%), coma (9% to 10%), and convulsions (8%) also occur at alarmingly frequent rates.[3, 45] Other evidence of neurologic involvement includes cranial nerve palsies, unilateral corticospinal signs, hearing loss, vertigo, dysarthria, aphasia, hemiplegia, paraplegia, paralysis, ankle clonus, nystagmus, hyperreflexia, spasticity, fasciculations, athetosis, and neurogenic bladder.

In the meninges, the presence of rickettsiae elicits a lymphohistiocytic meningitis. A cerebrospinal fluid (CSF) pleocytosis and an elevated CSF protein level are present in about one third of patients.[3, 26, 27] The cellular content is usually between 10 and 100 cells per mm^3 with a mononuclear predominance; however, occasional patients with mostly polymorphonuclear cells in the CSF have been observed.[26, 27] CSF glucose values are usually within the normal range. There is a strong association between severe central nervous system disease (coma and seizures) and fatality, presumably related to severe intracranial inflammation and edema. Thus, some have recommended the use of corticosteroids for rickettsial central nervous system infections, although no controlled trials have been performed to assess the utility of this practice.

Fulminant Rocky Mountain Spotted Fever

Fulminant RMSF is defined as illness that is unusually rapid (5 days or less from onset to death).[46] This form of the disease is characterized by early and rapid onset of clinical abnormalities including neurologic signs and the absence or late appearance of rash. Host factors seem to be particularly important for fulminant RMSF, and black male patients with glucose-6-phosphate dehydrogenase deficiency are prone to this form.[36] The pathologic findings in this rare manifestation of RMSF include early and widespread vascular necrosis without significant accompanying inflammation.

Long-term Sequelae

Nearly 50% of patients who recover from severe RMSF (hospitalized for more than 2 weeks) are likely to have long-term complications that relate to the initial acute infection.[29] The abnormalities that are present at least 1 year after the acute illness include paraparesis; hearing loss; peripheral neuropathy; bladder and bowel incontinence; cerebellar, vestibular, and motor dysfunction; language disorders; limb amputation; and scrotal pain after cutaneous necrosis.

Laboratory Findings

The results of clinical laboratory tests sometimes provide helpful clues for the diagnosis of RMSF. These findings vary depending on organ system involvement, severity of involvement, and duration of infection. Table 178–2 shows some of the frequent laboratory abnormalities associated with RMSF.

Hematologic Findings

One of the early findings (during the first week) is a normal leukocyte count or a slight leukopenia, accompanied by a high proportion of bands in the peripheral blood in a patient who appears seriously ill or septic.[3, 26, 27, 47] The mean high leukocyte count during the overall course of RMSF is 14,900/mm^3, and the mean lowest value is 7700/mm^3, with a range from 3800 to 16,800/mm^3. An increased proportion of bands (greater than 10%) is seen in nearly three fourths of patients; thrombocytopenia (less than 150,000 platelets per mm^3), a sensitive early marker, is present in half. The mean platelet count is generally around the limits of low-normal (143,000/mm^3), but profound thrombocytopenia may occasionally be present. After the first week of illness, leukocytosis and worsening thrombocytopenia occur more frequently.

Coagulation System

Evidence for activation of the coagulation system and other abnormalities of coagulation in RMSF is represented in several publications.[26, 48–52] About half of all patients have slight elevations in prothrombin time and activated partial thromboplastin time; hypofibrinogenemia and evidence for fibrin deposition (fibrin degradation products) may be detected in 36% to 67% of patients.[26] Factor inhibitors may also be identified as the cause of the abnormal coagulation test results.[53] These findings indicate that intravascular coagulation is occurring, most likely at sites of rickettsia-infected endothelium, but not as a result of true disseminated intravascular coagulation. Severe clinical hemorrhage is an infrequent finding with RMSF.[3, 26, 27]

Serum Electrolytes and Chemistry

Increased vascular permeability probably results in a net efflux of sodium ions from the serum, perhaps related to appropriate antidiuretic hormone secretion in response to hypovolemia.[54] Laboratory evaluation shows that hyponatremia is frequent with RMSF, occurring in between 56% and 91% of patients.[3, 26, 27] As the disease and accompanying hypotension progress, hyponatremia becomes more profound.[11]

Liver function test abnormalities occur early and late in disease and are best reflected by elevations in serum aspartate or alanine aminotransferase activities.[3, 26, 27, 33] These values are elevated more than twice the high-normal result in 40% to 80% of patients.[3, 26, 27] Marked elevations with levels above 1000 units/L are sometimes identified in severely affected individuals.[26, 33] Bilirubin levels are similarly elevated in 30% to 54% of patients at any time during the course of illness.[3, 26, 27] With more severe illness and injury to other organs, aminotransferase and creatine kinase isozyme activities may also be demonstrated in the serum.[19, 33] Serum urea nitrogen and serum creatinine levels may be elevated, but this effect is usually secondary to prerenal mechanisms.[10]

Cerebrospinal Fluid

With central nervous system involvement, a CSF pleocytosis is sometimes identified. The opening pressure and glucose concentrations are usually within normal limits, whereas the protein concentration is slightly elevated in about half of all cases.[26, 27] When examined, the CSF may have a small number of cells (0 to 184 cells per mm^3), of which approximately 70% are mononuclear cells. Electroencephalograms show diffusely slow cortical activity, and brain scans are normal.[25, 27]

Diagnosis

Delay in recognition and treatment of RMSF is the most significant factor in severe morbidity, development of long-term sequelae, and fatality.[3, 4] The risk for death due to RMSF is five times greater for patients treated after day 5 of illness, and the majority of patients eventually diagnosed with RMSF are not treated with an antirickettsial antibiotic until after 5 days of illness in spite of being examined before that time by a physician.[4] Three major factors contribute to the ineffective diagnosis and delayed therapy: absence of rash, presentation during nonpeak season for tick activity, and presentation during the first 3 days of illness. Unfortunately, timely and highly sensitive laboratory-based diagnostic methods are not widely available, and serologic assays can be used safely only for retrospective diagnostic confirmation. Thus, all patients with a presumptive diagnosis of RMSF on the basis of clinical and epidemiologic history should be empirically treated.

The factors important to know for rendering an appropriate clinical diagnosis of RMSF are the specific tick association and the presence of *D. variabilis* (American dog tick) or other appropriate vectors in the region; the seasonality of these tick vectors; the human factors that predispose to tick exposure and tick bites; and the various clinical presentations, both typical and atypical.[4, 10] Tick vectors have specific seasons but may emerge and maintain activity for a longer season in warm climates or when local weather conditions are conducive. Although individual cases of RMSF have been acquired by aerosols and wound or conjunctival contamination, transmission must be assumed to be through a tick bite in all cases. Thus, exposure to ticks and tick bites during occupational or recreational activities are important clues. However, not all patients report tick bites or exposure; thus, the lack of definite tick association should not exclude the diagnosis in suspected cases.

Given that the epidemiologic hallmarks for RMSF are not always present, the diagnosis of RMSF should be considered in any patient who presents with an acute febrile illness with headache and myalgia, especially if the patient is presenting during a season with tick activity or with relevant tick exposure or bite.[10] If a rash appears, RMSF must be considered in the differential diagnosis. Unfortunately, the clinical triad of fever, rash, and tick exposure is identified in only 3% of patients during the first 3 days of illness,[3] an interval within which 73% of patients will first seek medical attention.[4] This same triad occurs in only two thirds of patients with RMSF during the entire course of illness[3] and is thus not a highly reliable diagnostic feature.

Differential Diagnosis

The differential diagnosis of RMSF is broad and modified by the presentation and degree of organ involvement. Within the first 3 days of illness, when rash is absent or inconspicuous, the list of potential diagnoses includes influenza A, enteroviral infection, typhoid fever, leptospirosis, infectious mononucleosis, viral hepatitis, bacterial sepsis, and monocytic and granulocytic ehrlichiosis. Most of these entities have undifferentiated signs and symptoms; however, patients with RMSF often complain of severe headache, a finding that might lead one to favor the diagnosis of RMSF. With manifestations that focus attention to a single organ system, such as nausea, vomiting, diarrhea, and abdominal pain, viral or bacterial gastroenteritis or perhaps a perforated viscus would be considered. Patients with a prominent cough and chest radiographic infiltrates or opacities might be considered to have an exacerbation of chronic bronchitis or acute bronchopneumonia.

When a rash develops, the differential list extends to include meningococcemia, disseminated gonococcal infection, secondary syphilis, bacterial endocarditis, toxic shock syndrome, scarlet fever, rheumatic fever, measles, rubella, murine typhus, rickettsialpox, recrudescent typhus, Lyme disease, drug hypersensitivity reactions, idiopathic thrombocytopenic purpura, thrombotic thrombocytopenic purpura, Kawasaki disease, immune complex vasculitis, or other connective tissue disorders.

Etiologic Laboratory Diagnosis

Most clinical laboratories have little to offer as objective diagnostic assays for RMSF. Several useful diagnostic methods include serology; culture; immunohistologic or immunofluorescent demonstration of *R. rickettsii* organisms in skin biopsy specimens, tissue samples, or circulating endothelial cells; and polymerase chain reaction demonstration of *R. rickettsii* nucleic acids in blood.[10, 19, 55–63] The routine and standard confirmatory diagnostic measure is the demonstration of an increase in antibody titer to *R. rickettsii* during convalescence. Serologic reactivity is rarely present at the time of the acute infectious process; thus, withholding therapy while awaiting diagnostic serologic confirmation is a dangerous practice. A serologic diagnosis may be rendered when a fourfold increase in antibody titer to *R. rickettsii* is demonstrated between acute and convalescent serum samples obtained at least 2 weeks apart.

Current serologic methods cannot distinguish *R. rickettsii* antibodies from those elicited by infection with other spotted fever group rickettsiae. Several highly sensitive and specific serologic assays have been developed, including the indirect fluorescent antibody test,[55] enzyme-linked immunosorbent assay,[64] solid-phase enzyme immunoassays, and latex agglutination assays.[56] Reliable serologic testing can usually be obtained by reference to state, federal, or territorial health laboratories. Reagents and kits for these assays may be purchased from commercial suppliers, or samples may be sent to commercial laboratories to have these tests performed. The standard serodiagnostic assay is the indirect fluorescent antibody test, in which a titer of 1:64 or greater is generally first detected between days 7 and 10 of illness; confirmation requires a fourfold increase in titer. A single convalescent titer of 1:128 or greater is considered probable evidence of infection in the setting of a recent clinically compatible illness. This assay has been widely used and has a sensitivity that ranges between 94% and 100% with a specificity of nearly 100%.[65, 66] The latex agglutination test detects predominantly immunoglobulin M antibodies and is most useful after 7 to 9 days and within the first several weeks of RMSF.[56] The sensitivity of the latex agglutination methods has been reported between 71% and 94%, with a specificity of 96% to 99%.[56] The archaic Weil-Felix reaction, a part of the febrile agglutinins panel of many laboratories, is a relic of a previous serologic age and is based on cross-reactivity of *Proteus* species antigens with those of *Rickettsia* species. The sensitivity and specificity of the OX-19 agglutination test are 70% and 78%, respectively; for the OX-2 antigen, the sensitivity is even lower, 47%.[57]

The only test that may currently give a timely diagnosis during the acute phase of infection is the immunohistologic or immunofluorescent demonstration of *R. rickettsii* organisms in tissue biopsy specimens from rash lesions.[59–61] The test may be performed on fresh tissue; on tissue stored in Michel transport medium; or on formalin-fixed, paraffin-embedded tissues. The method is useful only for those patients with a rash and thus is less useful during the first few days of illness.[10, 19] An appropriate rash lesion is selected, preferably a petechia. After preparation of the site, a 3- or 4-mm punch biopsy is performed, allowing the lesion to be centrally located within the biopsy specimen. With frozen sections, *R. rickettsii* organisms may be demonstrated as early as 3 hours after biopsy; if the tissue is fixed and paraffin embedded, a longer interval is required. This test and service are available at only a few hospital laboratories but may be obtained through many public health laboratories or reference laboratories. The additional delay and expense incurred in the shipment of samples must be weighed against the value of the potential diagnostic information. Despite the consideration by many that this test is invasive, skin biopsy is a simple, relatively painless procedure that can provide reassuring diagnostic information.

Immunohistologic and immunofluorescent demonstration of *R. rickettsii* organisms in biopsy tissues has a specificity of 100%; the sensitivity is 70%.[27, 61, 67] Thus, a negative result should not dissuade the physician from continuing the antirickettsial therapy while other diagnostic considerations are being evaluated. The skin biopsy should be performed before initiation of therapy because sensitivity diminishes thereafter.[59]

Other new diagnostic modalities have been developed but are incompletely evaluated and generally not available except in research laboratories. Two novel methods are the isolation of circulating endothelial cells with monoclonal antibodies followed by immunofluorescent demonstration of *R. rickettsii* organisms within the endothelial cells[62] and polymerase chain reaction amplification of *R. rickettsii* nucleic acids in acute-phase blood samples.[63] The former method has not been evaluated for RMSF, but the latter appears to lack sensitivity.[63] Culture in embryonated chicken egg yolk sacs and animal inoculations are no longer viable diagnostic methods except in rare circumstances. Many consider rickettsial cultures to be hazardous; however, a modification of culture methods using shell vials with early demonstration of spotted fever group antigens has proved to be a rapid, sensitive, and useful diagnostic method for boutonneuse fever (*Rickettsia conorii* infection).[58]

Treatment

RMSF can be treated effectively with doxycycline or tetracycline, except in pregnant and allergic patients. Chloramphenicol has been used extensively in the treatment of RMSF, particularly in patients younger than 9 years to preclude the potential for tooth staining observed with tetracyclines. Whereas chloramphenicol would be considered an appropriate choice for therapy, especially in pregnant or allergic patients, a cogent argument for the use of doxycycline in young patients at risk for a life-threatening infection should be considered.[2, 68] The reason underlying this argument is that staining of teeth is dose dependent. One study showed that in children younger than 5 years after five courses of therapy for 6 days each, there was no tooth staining.[69] Doxycycline, now the drug of choice for treatment of RMSF, binds less to calcium than previous preparations of tetracyclines do and is less likely to discolor teeth. Regardless of the choice of antibiotic, it would be advisable to document in the medical record a thorough discussion of the therapeutic choices and attendant complications.

Minimal inhibitory concentrations of antibiotics have been determined by several methods, which have shown values of 0.06 to 0.1 μg/mL for doxycycline and 0.3 to 0.5 μg/mL for chloramphenicol.[70, 71] These antirickettsial drugs are bacteriostatic. Thus, recovery relies on effective induction of appropriate immunity. Moreover, therapy should not be administered for a tick bite only, because the course of prophylactic therapy would only delay the onset of illness and confound the epidemiologic history.[72] The current recommended dosages are (1) oral or intravenous doxycycline, 200 mg/d in two divided doses; (2) oral tetracycline, 25 to 50 mg/kg per day in four divided doses; and (3) chloramphenicol, 50 to 75 mg/kg per day in four divided doses. Therapy is continued for at least 2 days after defervescence.

Evaluations of fluoroquinolone antibiotics for RMSF have not been performed. In vitro testing suggests that ciprofloxacin and ofloxacin may have activity against *R. rickettsii*.[73] Both have been used successfully to treat boutonneuse fever, but lack of data for their use prevents recommending these as therapy for RMSF. Rifampin is of unproven in vivo efficacy but has an in vitro minimal inhibitory concentration of 0.5 μg/mL.[71] The use of sulfonamides is contraindicated in RMSF.[25]

Response to therapy is usually prompt, within 48 to 72 hours. However, patients with severe complications may require a longer interval before recovery. Relapse may occur on occasion, especially in those treated early in the course of disease before an effective immune response has occurred.[72, 74] Patients who are treated late in the course of disease or have significant vascular damage may on occasion have irreversible injury and a lack of therapeutic response to the antirickettsial drugs.

Mildly ill patients can often be managed effectively as outpatients. However, moderately to severely ill patients will require admission to the hospital and potentially to an intensive care unit.[10] Those patients with a particularly severe illness will require careful administration of intravenous fluids for depletion of intravascular volume and are best managed by hemodynamic monitoring procedures to detect and diminish the risk for noncardiogenic pulmonary edema, even if some degree of prerenal azotemia is present. Likewise, fluid replacement should not be restricted in those patients with hyponatremia because it is usually not life threatening and responds to appropriate and judicious volume management.[10, 54]

Other types of therapies may be required for specific indications, such as mechanical ventilators for severe hypoxemia, hemodialysis for renal failure due to acute tubular necrosis, anticonvulsants for tonic-clonic seizures, packed red blood cells for anemia and hemorrhage, and platelet transfusions for severe thrombocytopenia and bleeding. Because the disseminated intravascular coagulation–like appearance of RMSF is due to rickettsia-damaged endothelium, heparin therapy is contraindicated. Corticosteroid therapy may be administered to patients with rickettsial meningoencephalitis, but controlled trials to prove the benefit of this measure have not been performed.

Prevention

There is currently no vaccine for RMSF. Prophylactic antirickettsial therapy for tick bites only delays the onset of disease. Thus, prevention of tick bites is the major preventive measure. This requires the avoidance of tick habitats, such as environments with wooded or grassy terrains. Protective light-colored clothing helps in the identification of ticks before they reach skin surfaces and presents a physical barrier. Tick repellents on clothing and skin may offer limited benefits. A careful search for ticks after potential exposure, including inspection of the scalp, axillae, and groin, will identify hidden sites of attachment. Similar inspection of pets will prevent animals from acting as vehicles that transport ticks into human environments.

Prompt removal of embedded ticks before exchange of salivary secretions will often prevent infection even if the tick contains the pathogenic rickettsiae. Unengorged, flat ticks are unlikely to have achieved significant exchange of infectious salivary secretions. If attached, ticks are removed by gentle but firm retraction of the mouthparts from the skin with forceps. This will often result in the additional removal of a small tag of skin, but complete removal of all potentially infected tick parts will interrupt any transmission. In general, folklore remedies such as petroleum jelly or hot matches do little to encourage a tick to disattach and should be avoided.[75] Crushing or handling of ticks that are potentially infectious should also be avoided to preclude mechanical transmission into conjunctivae or other mucous membranes.

References

1. Centers for Disease Control and Prevention: Summary of notifiable diseases, United States, 1995. MMWR Morbid Mortal Wkly Rep 44:1, 1996.
2. Dalton MJ, Clarke MJ, Holman RC, et al: National surveillance for Rocky Mountain spotted fever, 1981–1992: Epidemiologic summary and evaluation of risk factors for fatal outcome. Am J Trop Med Hyg 52:405, 1995.
3. Helmick CG, Bernard KW, D'Angelo LJ: Rocky Mountain spotted fever: Clinical, laboratory, and epidemiological features of 262 cases. J Infect Dis 150:480, 1984.
4. Kirkland KB, Wilkinson WE, Sexton DJ: Therapeutic delay and mortality in cases of Rocky Mountain spotted fever. Clin Infect Dis 20:1118, 1995.
5. McDade JE, Newhouse VF: Natural history of *Rickettsia rickettsii*. Annu Rev Microbiol 40:287, 1986.
6. Burgdorfer W: The spotted fever–group diseases. *In* Steele JH (ed): CRC Handbook Series in Zoonoses, Section A, Vol 2. Boca Raton, FL, CRC Press, 1980, pp 279–301.
7. Burgdorfer W, Hayes SF, Mavros AJ: Nonpathogenic rickettsiae in *Dermacentor andersoni*: A limiting factor for the distribution of *Rickettsia rickettsii*. *In* Burgdorfer W, Anacker RL (eds): Rickettsiae and Rickettsial Diseases. New York, Academic Press, 1981, pp 585–594.
8. Hayes SF, Burgdorfer W: Reactivation of *Rickettsia rickettsii* in *Dermacentor andersoni* ticks: An ultrastructural analysis. Infect Immun 37:779, 1982.
9. Gage KL, Burgdorfer W, Hopla CE: Hispid cotton rats *(Sigmodon hispidus)* as a source for infecting immature *Dermacentor variabilis* (Acari: Ixodidae) with *Rickettsia rickettsii*. J Med Entomol 27:615, 1990.
10. Walker DH: Rocky Mountain spotted fever: A seasonal alert. Clin Infect Dis 20:1111, 1995.
11. Wilfert CM, MacCormack JN, Kleeman K, et al: Epidemiology of Rocky Mountain spotted fever as determined by active surveillance. J Infect Dis 150:469, 1984.
12. Li H, Walker DH: Characterization of rickettsial attachment to host cells by flow cyotmetry. Infect Immun 60:2030, 1992.
13. Manor E, Carbonetti NH, Silverman DJ: *Rickettsia rickettsii* has proteins with cross-reacting epitopes to eukaryotic phospholipase A_2 and phospholipase C. Microb Pathog 17:99, 1994.
14. Silverman DJ, Santucci L: Potential for free radical–induced lipid peroxidation as a cause of endothelial cell injury in Rocky Mountain spotted fever. Infect Immun 56:3110, 1988.
15. Sporn LA, Lawrence SO, Silverman DJ, Marder VJ: E-selectin–dependent neutrophil adhesion to *Rickettsia rickettsii*–infected endothelial cells. Blood 81:2406, 1993.

16. Sporn LA, Haidaris PJ, Rui-Jin S, et al: *Rickettsia rickettsii* infection of cultured human endothelial cells induces tissue factor expression. Blood 83:1527, 1994.
17. Sporn LA, Rui-Jin S, Lawrence SO, et al: *Rickettsia rickettsii* infection of cultured endothelial cells induces release of large von Willebrand factor multimers from Weibel-Palade bodies. Blood 78:2595, 1991.
18. Sporn LA, Marder VJ: Interleukin-1α production during *Rickettsia rickettsii* infection of cultured endothelial cells: Potential role in autocrine cell stimulation. Infect Immun 64:1609, 1996.
19. Walker DH: Diagnosis of rickettsial diseases. Pathol Annu 23:69, 1988.
20. Sessler CN, Schwartz M, Windsor A, et al: Increased serum cytokines and intercellular adhesion molecule-1 in fulminant Rocky Mountain spotted fever. Crit Care Med 23:973, 1995.
21. Li H, Jerrells TR, Spitalny GL, Walker DH: Gamma interferon as a crucial host defense against *Rickettsia conorii* in vivo. Infect Immun 55:1252, 1987.
22. Feng H-M, Wen J, Walker DH: *Rickettsia australis* infection: A murine model of a highly invasive vasculopathic rickettsiosis. Am J Pathol 142:1471, 1993.
23. Feng H-M, Walker DH: Interferon-γ and tumor necrosis factor-α exert their antirickettsial effect via induction of synthesis of nitric oxide. Am J Pathol 143:1016, 1993.
24. Walker DH, Popov VL, Welsh JR, Feng H-M: Mechanisms of rickettsial killing within cytokine-stimulated endothelial cells. *In* Kazár J, Toman R (eds): Rickettsiae and Rickettsial Diseases, Proceedings of the Vth International Symposium. Bratislava, Slovak Republic, Slovak Academy of Sciences, Institute of Virology, 1996, pp 51–56.
25. Harrell GT: Rocky Mountain spotted fever. Medicine (Baltimore) 28:333, 1949.
26. Kirk JL, Fine DP, Sexton DJ, Muchmore HG: Rocky Mountain spotted fever. A clinical review based on 48 confirmed cases, 1943–1986. Medicine (Baltimore) 69:35, 1990.
27. Kaplowitz LG, Fischer JJ, Sparling PF: Rocky Mountain spotted fever: A clinical dilemma. *In* Remington JS, Swartz MN (eds): Current Clinical Topics in Infectious Diseases, Vol 2. New York, McGraw-Hill, 1981, pp 89–108.
28. Kirkland KB, Marcom PK, Sexton DJ, et al: Rocky Mountain spotted fever complicated by gangrene: Report of six cases and review. Clin Infect Dis 16:629, 1993.
29. Archibald LK, Sexton DJ: Long-term sequelae of Rocky Mountain spotted fever. Clin Infect Dis 20:1122, 1995.
30. Hattwick MA, O'Brien RJ, Hanson BF: Rocky Mountain spotted fever: Epidemiology of an increasing problem. Ann Intern Med 84:732, 1976.
31. Walker DH, Mattern WD: Acute renal failure in Rocky Mountain spotted fever. Arch Intern Med 139:443, 1979.
32. Davis AE, Bradford WD: Abdominal pain resembling acute appendicitis in Rocky Mountain spotted fever. JAMA 247:2811, 1982.
33. Middleton DB: Rocky Mountain spotted fever: Gastrointestinal and laboratory manifestations. South Med J 71:629, 1978.
34. Randall MB, Walker DH: Rocky Mountain spotted fever. Gastrointestinal and pancreatic lesions and rickettsial infection. Arch Pathol Lab Med 108:963, 1984.
35. Adams JS, Walker DH: The liver in Rocky Mountain spotted fever. Am J Clin Pathol 75:156, 1981.
36. Walker DH, Hawkins HK, Hudson P: Fulminant Rocky Mountain spotted fever. Its pathologic characteristics associated with glucose-6-dehydrogenase deficiency. Arch Pathol Lab Med 107:121, 1983.
37. Walker DH, Mattern WD: Rickettsial vasculitis. Am Heart J 100:896, 1980.
38. Donohue JF: Lower respiratory tract involvement in Rocky Mountain spotted fever. Arch Intern Med 140:223, 1980.
39. Martin W, Choplin RH, Shertzer ME: The chest radiograph in Rocky Mountain spotted fever. Am J Radiol 139:889, 1982.
40. Marin-Garcia J, Gooch WM, Coury DL: Cardiac manifestation of Rocky Mountain spotted fever. Pediatrics 67:358, 1981.
41. Marin GJ, Mirvis DM: Myocardial disease in Rocky Mountain spotted fever: Clinical, functional, and pathologic findings. Pediatr Cardiol 5:149, 1984.
42. Bradford WD, Croker BP, Tisher CC: Kidney lesions in Rocky Mountain spotted fever: A light, immunofluorescence, and electron microscopic study. Am J Pathol 97:381, 1979.
43. Miller JQ, Price TR: The nervous system in Rocky Mountain spotted fever. Neurology 22:561, 1972.
44. Massey EW, Thames T, Coffey CE, Gallis HA: Neurologic complications of Rocky Mountain spotted fever. South Med J 78:1288, 1985.
45. Haynes RE, Sanders DY, Cramblett HG: Rocky Mountain spotted fever in children. J Pediatr 76:685, 1970.
46. Parker RR: Rocky Mountain spotted fever. JAMA 110:1185, 1938.
47. Hall GW, Schwartz RP: White blood cell count and differential in Rocky Mountain spotted fever. N C Med J 40:212, 1971.
48. Rao AK, Shapira M, Clements ML, et al: A prospective study of platelets and plasma proteolytic systems during the early stages of Rocky Mountain spotted fever. N Engl J Med 318:1021, 1988.
49. Graybill JR, Hawiger J, Des Prez RM: Complement and coagulation in Rocky Mountain spotted fever. South Med J 66:410, 1973.
50. Kurnick JE, Malinow SH, Snyderman MC: Disseminated intravascular coagulation in Rocky Mountain spotted fever. South Med J 67:623, 1974.
51. Mosher DF, Fine DP, Moe JB, et al: Studies of the coagulation and complement systems during experimental Rocky Mountain spotted fever in rhesus monkeys. J Infect Dis 135:985, 1977.
52. Yamada T, Harber P, Petit GW, et al: Activation of the kallikrein-kinin system in Rocky Mountain spotted fever. Ann Intern Med 88:764, 1978.
53. Scimeca PG, Weinblatt ME, Kochen JA: Acquired coagulation inhibitor in association with Rocky Mountain spotted fever: With review of other acquired coagulation inhibitors. Clin Pediatr 26:459, 1987.
54. Kaplowitz LG, Robertson GL: Hyponatremia in Rocky Mountain spotted fever: Role of antidiuretic hormone. Ann Intern Med 98:334, 1983.
55. Philip RN, Casper EA, Ormsbee RA, et al: Microimmunofluorescence test for the serological study of Rocky Mountain spotted fever and typhus. J Clin Microbiol 3:51, 1976.
56. Hechemy KE, Michaelson EE, Anacker RL, et al: Evaluation of latex–*Rickettsia rickettsii* test for Rocky Mountain spotted fever in 11 laboratories. J Clin Microbiol 18:938, 1983.
57. Hechemy KE, Stevens RW, Sasowski S, et al: Discrepancies in Weil-Felix and microimmunofluorescence test results for Rocky Mountain spotted fever. J Clin Microbiol 9:292, 1979.
58. Marrero M, Raoult D: Centrifugation–shell vial technique for rapid detection of Mediterranean spotted fever rickettsiae in blood culture. Am J Trop Med Hyg 40:197, 1989.
59. Walker DH, Cain BG, Olmstead PM: Laboratory diagnosis of Rocky Mountain spotted fever by immunofluorescent demonstration of *Rickettsia rickettsii* in cutaneous lesions. Am J Clin Pathol 69:619, 1978.
60. Woodward TE, Pedersen CE Jr, Oster CN, et al: Prompt confirmation of Rocky Mountain spotted fever: Identification of rickettsiae in skin tissues. J Infect Dis 134:297, 1976.
61. Dumler JS, Gage WR, Pettis GL, et al: Rapid immunoperoxidase demonstration of *Rickettsia rickettsii* in fixed cutaneous specimens from patients with Rocky Mountain spotted fever. Am J Clin Pathol 93:410, 1990.
62. Drancourt M, George F, Brouqui P, et al: Diagnosis of Mediterranean spotted fever by indirect immunofluorescence of *Rickettsia conorii* in circulating endothelial cells isolated with monoclonal antibody–coated immunomagnetic beads. J Infect Dis 166:660, 1992.
63. Sexton DJ, Kanj SS, Wilson K, et al: The use of polymerase chain reaction as a diagnostic test for Rocky Mountain spotted fever. Am J Trop Med Hyg 50:59, 1994.
64. Clements ML, Dumler JS, Fiset P, et al: Serodiagnosis of Rocky Mountain spotted fever: Comparison of IgM and IgG enzyme-linked immunosorbent assays and indirect fluorescent antibody test. J Infect Dis 148:876, 1983.
65. Philip RN, Casper EA, MacCormack JN, et al: A comparison of serologic methods for diagnosis of Rocky Mountain spotted fever. Am J Epidemiol 105:56, 1977.
66. Kaplan JE, Schonberger LB: The sensitivity of various serologic tests in the diagnosis of Rocky Mountain spotted fever. Am J Trop Med Hyg 35:840, 1986.
67. Walker DH, Burday MS, Folds JD: Laboratory diagnosis of Rocky Mountain spotted fever. South Med J 73:1443, 1980.
68. Abramson JS, Givner LB: Should tetracycline be contraindicated for therapy of presumed Rocky Mountain spotted fever in children less than 9 years of age? Pediatrics 86:123, 1990.

69. Grossman ER, Walchek A, Freedman H: Tetracyclines and permanent teeth: The relation between dose and tooth color. Pediatrics 47:567, 1971.
70. Wisseman CL Jr, Waddell A: In vitro sensitivity of *Rickettsia rickettsii* to doxycycline. J Infect Dis 145:584, 1982.
71. Raoult D, Rousellier P, Bestris G, Tamalet J: In vitro susceptibility of *Rickettsia rickettsii* and *Rickettsia conorii*: Plaque assay and microplaque colorimetric assay. J Infect Dis 155:1059, 1987.
72. DuPont HL, Hornick RB, Dawkins AT, et al: Rocky Mountain spotted fever: A comparative study of the active immunity induced by inactivated and viable pathogenic *Rickettsia rickettsii*. J Infect Dis 128:340, 1973.
73. Jabarit-Aldighieri N, Torres H, Raoult D: Susceptibility of *Rickettsia conorii, R. rickettsii,* and *Coxiella burnetii* to PD 127,391, PD 131,628, pefloxacin, ofloxacin, and ciprofloxacin. Antimicrob Agents Chemother 36:2529, 1992.
74. Clements ML, Wisseman CL Jr, Woodward TE, et al: Reactogenicity, immunogenicity, and efficacy of a chick embryo cell–derived vaccine for Rocky Mountain spotted fever. J Infect Dis 148:922, 1983.
75. Needham GR: Evaluation of five popular methods for tick removal. Pediatrics 75:997, 1985.

179

Ehrlichiosis, Q Fever, Typhus, Rickettsialpox, and Other Rickettsioses

Joseph E. McDade
James G. Olson

Ehrlichiosis

History of Disease and Microorganisms

Ehrlichia canis, the type species of the genus, was first recognized in 1935, as a pathogen of dogs. It was assigned to the genus *Rickettsia* at the time, and the disease was called canine rickettsiosis.[1] Subsequently, members of the genus were found to cause acute and chronic diseases in a wide range of animal species.[2] Canine ehrlichiosis was studied intensively in Vietnam in 1968 to 1970, when tropical canine pancytopenia, a severe hemorrhagic disease that caused extensive morbidity and mortality in military working dogs, was found to be due to *E. canis.*[3, 4] *E. canis* is now a well-recognized pathogen of dogs worldwide, especially in tropical and other warm climates where its vector, *Rhipicephalus sanguineus,* flourishes.

The first human pathogen of the genus, *Ehrlichia sennetsu,* was isolated in Japan in 1954.[5] Two additional forms of human ehrlichiosis were recognized in the United States. In 1986,[6] human monocytic ehrlichiosis (HME) was described and shown to be caused by *Ehrlichia chaffeensis.*[7, 8] In 1994,[9] a similar disease was described that is known as human granulocytic ehrlichiosis (HGE). Sennetsu rickettsiosis (sennetsu fever, caused by *E. sennetsu)* is believed to be limited to western Japan.[5]

Characteristics of the Pathogen

Ehrlichia is a genus in the family Rickettsiaceae; microorganisms in the genus are characterized by a life cycle that takes place primarily within the cytoplasm of circulating leukocytes or platelets.[10] The gram-negative pleomorphic organisms appear as compact inclusions and proceed through elementary body, initial body, and morula stages[1, 2] (Fig. 179–1). Some *Ehrlichia* organisms can be cultivated on primary monocyte cultures and in continuous cell lines,[11] but they do not grow in chick embryos or cell-free media.

Serologically and morphologically, *E. chaffeensis* seems to be closely related but not identical to *E. canis.*[6] The agent of HGE is closely related serologically, morphologically, and by genomic sequencing to *Ehrlichia phagocytophila* and *Ehrlichia equi,* which are pathogenic for sheep, goats, dogs, horses, and deer.[9] In addition to the human diseases described in this chapter, *Ehrlichia* species cause a number of diseases of veterinary importance: Potomac horse fever *(Ehrlichia risticii),* equine ehrlichiosis *(E. equi),* tick-borne fever in sheep *(E. phagocytophila),* infectious cyclic thrombocytopenia of dogs *(Ehrlichia platys),* and canine granulocytic ehrlichiosis of dogs *(Ehrlichia ewingii).*

Epidemiology

Since the recognition of HME in the United States in 1986, more than 400 cases, including several fatalities, have been identified in 30 states, principally those where Rocky Mountain spotted fever (RMSF) is also found. Most cases have been reported from the south central states (especially Missouri, Tennessee, Oklahoma, Texas, and Arkansas) and the south Atlantic states (Virginia and Georgia)[12–15]; however, surveillance outside this region has detected a limited number of cases in other states.[11, 15] Data on incidence rates are limited,

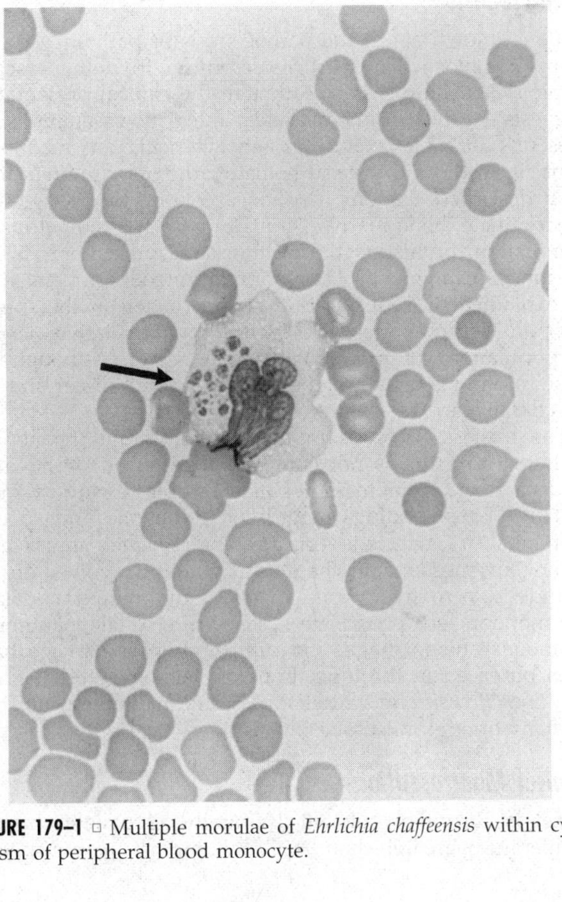

FIGURE 179–1 □ Multiple morulae of *Ehrlichia chaffeensis* within cytoplasm of peripheral blood monocyte.

but surveillance in Oklahoma in 1987 revealed that ehrlichiosis was as common as RMSF[16]; surveillance for both diseases in southeast Georgia revealed eight cases of ehrlichiosis and only one case of RMSF. The incidences of ehrlichiosis in these two areas were 3.3 and 5.3 per 100,000, respectively.[17] Although most cases have been sporadic, one outbreak of human ehrlichiosis occurred in a group of army reservists camping in a tick-infested field in New Jersey,[18] and another occurred in a golfing retirement community in Tennessee.[19] The highest incidence of infection with *E. chaffeensis* was noted among military recruits exposed to training areas infested with ticks.[20] Of 1194 soldiers exposed during their 6-week training, 15 persons (1.3%) were infected; 5 (33%) of these reported symptoms.

Most confirmed cases of HGE have occurred in Wisconsin and Minnesota,[9, 21] but cases have also been documented in Connecticut[22] and Massachusetts.[23]

About 68% of HME patients report a tick bite and 83% report having had an exposure to ticks 7 to 21 days before onset of illness.[15] Among HGE patients, 67% reported a tick bite and virtually all have had exposure to ticks.[21] Although the reservoir and the exact vectors are unknown, available data suggest that HME is transmitted by *Amblyomma americanum*. The geographic distribution of HME cases is coincident with the distribution of *A. americanum*,[14] and *E. chaffeensis* has been detected in this species.[24] The vector of HGE is probably *Ixodes scapularis*, the black-legged or deer tick, or *Dermacentor variabilis*, the brown dog tick.[21] The white-tailed deer, *Odocoilus virginianus*, has been shown to be a potential reservoir of *E. chaffeensis*.[25–27] No studies of the potential reservoir of the agent that causes HGE have been completed, but epidemiologic evidence suggests that dogs, horses, goats, sheep, or deer may have a role.[21]

Clinical and epidemiologic features of rickettsial diseases found in the United States are given in Table 179–1.

Pathogenesis

Little is known about the pathogenesis or pathology of human ehrlichiosis. The ehrlichioses differ from the vasculotropic rickettsial diseases. Although the clinical presentation suggests a defect in microvascular integrity, vasculitis is not present. Leukopenia and thrombocytopenia are manifestations of HME, and several hematopathologic findings have been described. Lesions involving mononuclear phagocytes predominate; bone marrow granulomata, granulomatous inflammation, or histiocytic infiltrates are present in 75% of specimens examined.[28] The peripheral blood cytopenias can be explained by sequestration or destruction in the spleen, liver, and lymph nodes, as evidenced by the relative increase in populations of mononuclear phagocytes. Although the bone marrow is usually hypercellular, normocellular and hypocellular marrows occur.[22]

The liver is involved in most patients, but the hepatic pathologic picture is not completely described. Lesions include a range from focal hepatic necroses to ring granulomata.[28, 29] These findings suggest the induction of nonspecific mononuclear phagocyte– or cytokine-mediated injury as a pathogenic mechanism. The most commonly involved organs include spleen, liver, bone marrow, and lymph nodes of the mononuclear phagocyte system. Interstitial pneumonia, pulmonary hemorrhage, and diffuse alveolar damage have been observed in the lung. Immunohistologic studies show that *E. chaffeensis* and the agent of HGE can establish infection in many organs and tissues.

Clinical Manifestations

Onset is abrupt or subacute. Virtually all patients have a temperature greater than 38°C. Symptoms are nonspecific and resemble those of RMSF. Symptoms common to both diseases include malaise, headaches, myalgia, rigors or chills, anorexia, and nausea or vomiting. Rash is less common in ehrlichiosis than in RMSF,[15, 16] and a rash, usually macular or papular but occasionally petechial or erythematous, occurs on the trunk, legs, arms, or face. Rash on the palms or the soles is found in less than 10% of cases.[16, 30] The patient may be confused, but the results of the physical examination are usually otherwise normal. Ehrlichiosis is a severe illness, with more than 60% of patients requiring hospitalization.[15] The case-fatality ratio is 2%.

Laboratory evaluation reveals leukopenia in about 60% of patients and thrombocytopenia in 68%.[15] In one study, the median white cell count at admission to the hospital was 4450/mm^3, and the median platelet count was 133,000/mm^3.[18] Elevated hepatic transaminase values are found in more than 75% of hospitalized patients, but the degree of elevation is usually relatively mild at the time of admission (median aspartate aminotransferase value of 68 units/L and median alanine aminotransferase value of 62 units/L), becoming most marked later in the clinical course.[14, 17] A few patients with a clinical picture suggestive of aseptic meningitis have been found to have cerebrospinal fluid pleocytosis. Complications include gastrointestinal hemorrhage[32] and fungal superinfection[6]; nine patients have died.

A milder form of illness was noted during investigations of outbreaks of ehrlichiosis in military personnel.[19, 21] In one study, seven of the nine infected had sought medical care; only three missed more than a day of work because of illness, and none was hospitalized.[19] In the other study, 5 (33%) of 15 soldiers who were infected with *E. chaffeensis* recalled being ill during the 6 weeks of the study.[21]

HGE is clinically similar to HME. All of the 12 HGE patients for whom data are available had fever, malaise, myalgia, headache, and rigors. Rash is seen in only 8% of patients.[23] Thrombocytopenia and elevated serum aspartate aminotransferase and creatine values occur in most patients. The case-fatality ratio is 7% to 10%. Risk of death and severity of disease are clearly associated with patients of older age. Cause of death has been difficult to establish, but secondary infections with opportunistic pathogens or nosocomial agents include bacterial and fungal pneumonias, disseminated candidiasis, and candidal esophagitis. Death occurs after pulmonary or gastrointestinal hemorrhage that may have been secondary to thrombocytopenia and concurrent intravascular coagulation.

Sennetsu ehrlichiosis is also an acute febrile illness. Besides a number of nonspecific symptoms, patients often have generalized lymphadenopathy, most prominent in the postcervical and postauricular regions, and some have hepatosplenomegaly.[5]

Diagnosis

Recognizing a case of ehrlichiosis is dependent on laboratory confirmation of infection with *Ehrlichia* spp. The case definition depends on either a positive serologic test result or positive polymerase chain reaction assay. A positive serologic test result shows a fourfold or greater change in antibody titer in serum samples collected at different intervals after onset of symptoms. Confirmation of HME requires a minimal antibody titer of 1:64 when tested by indirect immunofluorescence using *E. chaffeensis*–infected DH82 cells as the antigen. Testing of single serum specimens is not recommended; however, patients who have antibody titers greater than 128 may be considered presumptive cases and followed up for confirmation. Serologic confirmation of HGE requires the use of surrogate antigens. Because these agents have not been adapted to cell culture, production of infected cells for sero-

TABLE 179–1 ■ Clinical and Epidemiologic Features of Rickettsial Diseases Found in the United States

FEATURES	FLYING SQUIRREL–ASSOCIATED TYPHUS	MURINE TYPHUS	ROCKY MOUNTAIN SPOTTED FEVER	HUMAN MONOCYTIC EHRLICHIOSIS	HUMAN GRANULOCYTIC EHRLICHIOSIS	Q FEVER	RICKETTSIALPOX
Pathogen	*Rickettsia prowazekii*	*Rickettsia typhi*	*Rickettsia rickettsii*	*Ehrlichia chaffeensis*	*Ehrlichia equi* or *Ehrlichia phagocytophila?*	*Coxiella burnetii*	*Rickettsia akari*
Severity	Moderate to severe	Moderate to severe	Moderate to severe	Asymptomatic to severe	Moderate to severe	Asymptomatic to moderate	Mild to moderate
Hospitalization (%)	100 (?)	67	60–80	60	100 (?)	5	10
Case-fatality ratio (%)	No reported fatalities	<1	3–5	2–5	7–10	<<1	No reported fatalities
Vector	Flying squirrels' lice or fleas	Primarily rat flea; also cat flea	Tick	Tick *(Amblyomma americanum?)*	Tick *(Ixodes scapularis?)*	Infectious aerosols	Mouse mite
Animal reservoir	Eastern flying squirrels	Rat; opossum (?)	Various small wild animals	Unknown	Unknown	Ungulates, expecially sheep, cattle; cats	House mouse
Distribution	Principally eastern states	Primarily Florida, Texas, California, Hawaii	Primarily south central and south Atlantic states	Primarily south central and south Atlantic States	Wisconsin, Minnesota, Connecticut, Massachusetts	Corresponds to distribution of reservoir	Primarily New York City
Habitat	Rural to suburban	Urban	Rural to suburban, occasionally urban	Rural	Rural, suburban	Abattoirs, farms, research facilities	Urban
Seasonality	Late fall to early spring	Summer and fall	Spring (primarily) to fall	Spring (primarily) to fall	Spring to fall	Primarily at parturition	Spring
Household clustering	No	Occasional	Occasional	No	No	Occasional	Occasional

logic testing depends on maintaining infections in susceptible hosts and harvesting infected neutrophils for use as antigen in an indirect immunofluorescent test. A positive test result requires a minimal titer of 1:80.[22]

Polymerase chain reaction has shown great promise as an alternative for confirming infection with *Ehrlichia* spp. The assay is done on a single specimen of blood collected when the patient is first suspected of having ehrlichiosis, before the initiation of antibiotic therapy. Anderson and coworkers[32] identified *E. chaffeensis* infections by amplifying the 16S ribosomal RNA gene using a polymerase chain reaction. Similar approaches using genetic sequences specific for *E. equi* and *E. phagocytophila* were used to identify cases of HGE.[9, 21]

Cases of ehrlichiosis resemble a number of other tick-borne diseases, especially "spotless" RMSF. When a tick-borne infection is suspected, RMSF, tularemia, relapsing fever, Lyme disease, Colorado tick fever, and babesiosis should also be considered. Ehrlichiosis has been mistaken for pyelonephritis, non-A, non-B hepatitis, gastroenteritis, and unexplained febrile illnesses with leukopenia or thrombocytopenia.

Treatment

Data suggest that human ehrlichiosis responds to treatment with doses of tetracycline similar to those used for other rickettsial diseases. The recommended therapy for adults or children is oral or intravenous doxycycline, 100 mg twice daily for adults or 3 mg/kg body weight per day divided in two doses for children. The total dose for children should be minimized to prevent staining of teeth. A short course of doxycycline therapy continued for 3 days after defervescence for a minimum of 5 to 7 days has been reported useful in treating RMSF.[22] Patients suspected of having ehrlichiosis should be treated before laboratory confirmation is made. The disease is potentially life threatening. The case-fatality ratios are approximately 2% for HME[15] and between 7% and 10% for HGE.[22]

Prevention

All evidence suggests that ehrlichiosis is transmitted by ticks. Recommendations for prevention are similar to those for RMSF. The wearing of permethrin-treated clothing has clearly reduced the frequency of tick bites in experimental settings[33, 34] and reduced the risk of *E. chaffeensis* infections among occupationally exposed soldiers.[20]

Epidemic, Recrudescent (Brill-Zinsser Disease), and Flying Squirrel–Associated Typhus

History of Disease

Epidemic (louse-borne) typhus is one of the oldest diseases of humans. Although the first accurate clinical description of typhus can be traced back only to Hieronymus Fracastorius in 1546,[35] brief references to a compatible illness can be found in the ancient writings of Greek and Arab physicians. Epidemic typhus has had a major effect on the history of civilization, periodically ravaging cities and decimating armies from antiquity to the present day.[36]

After World War II, after the introduction of antibiotics and insecticides (especially DDT) that were effective against lice vectors, epidemic typhus became much less common in areas where millions of cases formerly occurred, including parts of Europe, Asia, and Africa.[37] The number of cases reported to the World Health Organization declined further in the early 1980s, from 18,359 in 1979 to 3036 in 1982; in each of these years, more than 90% of the reported cases were from Ethiopia.[38–40] However, typhus surveillance is limited, and the disease is believed to occur in Africa and the highland areas of Latin America, from Mexico through South America.[41] In the United States, the last outbreak of classic epidemic typhus occurred in 1922 and the last diagnosed case in 1950; it was contracted in Mexico.[38]

As epidemic typhus has become rare, so has the recrudescent form of the disease. Although hundreds of cases occurred in the United States[41, 42] in this century among persons who had emigrated from southeastern Europe about 10 years before, few cases have been reported in the last several decades.

Another variety of infection caused by *Rickettsia prowazekii* was reported in the United States in the 1970s and 1980s.[43–45] Onset was usually during the winter months, and many cases had reported contact with the eastern flying squirrel (*Glaucomys volans*). *R. prowazekii* has been isolated from flying squirrels[46] and transmitted experimentally between flying squirrels by their ectoparasites.[47]

Epidemiology

Epidemic typhus usually occurs in association with war, famine, and other factors that inflict poor living conditions on a given population. It is transmitted among humans by body lice (*Pediculus humanus corporis*). Lice acquire *R. prowazekii* when they imbibe a blood meal from a rickettsemic typhus patient. Typhus rickettsiae infect the midgut epithelial cells of the louse, where they grow profusely and spill over into the louse feces.[48] As many as 10^8 *R. prowazekii* organisms are present in an infected louse.[49] Louse secretions irritate the bite site, prompting scratching; humans become infected when contaminated louse feces are rubbed into abraded skin. Typhus rickettsiae have also been shown to be infectious for head lice (*Pediculus humanus capitis*), but head lice have not proved to be a significant vector of disease.

Body lice are usually found in the folds of clothing, where the ambient temperature ranges from about 20°C to 30°C. Lice leave dead hosts or persons with body temperatures greater than 40°C, practices that improve their efficiency as vectors of epidemic typhus. Body lice usually die within 1 to 2 weeks of the time they become infected with *R. prowazekii*, however, and they do not transmit infection to their progeny. Thus, lice are vectors but not reservoirs of typhus rickettsiae.

Humans are the principal interepidemic reservoir of *R. prowazekii*. Patients who recover from epidemic typhus develop a state of premunition, and viable typhus rickettsiae remain sequestered in their bodies. Years, perhaps even decades later, some of these individuals develop recrudescent infections, and depending on the prevalence of lice and immunity in the population, another epidemic may occur and repeat the infectious cycle (Fig. 179–2).

Recrudescent typhus was first identified as a distinct clinical entity by Nathan Brill in 1898. Working in New York, he observed 17 patients who had a mild febrile illness similar to typhoid fever but whose Widal tests were negative. During the next decade he saw 221 patients with the disease, and although he was aware of its similarity to typhus, he concluded that it was a different illness because the cases occurred sporadically, the fatality rate was low, and none of the patients were infested with body lice.[41] It was not until 25 years later that Hans Zinsser recognized the significance of Brill's disease. Zinsser analyzed the epidemiologic features of 538 cases of Brill's disease that occurred in Boston and New York. Noting that 93% of the patients had emigrated from typhus zones of Europe, he concluded that Brill's disease was a recrudescent form of louse-borne typhus and postulated that humans were the interepidemic reservoirs of

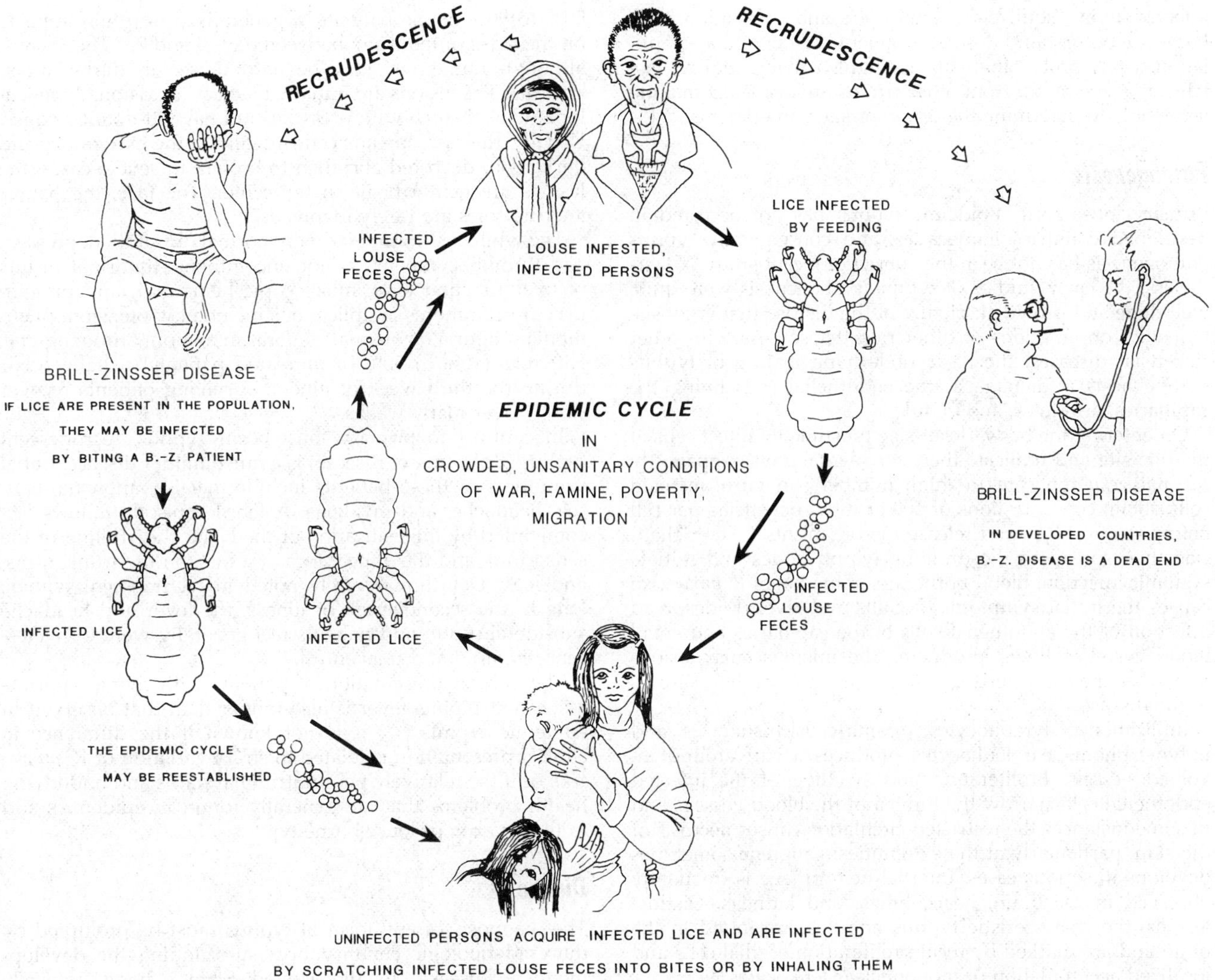

FIGURE 179–2 □ Transmission cycle of epidemic typhus by the body louse *(Pediculus humanus)*.

R. prowazekii.[42] Recrudescent typhus is usually called Brill-Zinsser disease in honor of both scientists.

Zinsser's concepts of the epidemiology of the disease were subsequently proved by others. After World War II, Murray and colleagues[50, 51] isolated seven strains of *R. prowazekii* from 14 patients with Brill-Zinsser disease and observed that each of the isolates was indistinguishable from classic strains of *R. prowazekii*. Furthermore, normal body lice became infected with *R. prowazekii* after taking a blood meal from patients with Brill-Zinsser disease.[50, 51] Several years later, Price[52] reported the isolation of *R. prowazekii* from the lymph nodes of former typhus patients who were undergoing elective surgery for other conditions. The latter observation, however, has not been independently verified.

Although the fundamental concepts of the epidemiology of epidemic typhus have withstood the test of time, various investigators have considered the possibility that wild or domestic animals are also interepidemic reservoirs of *R. prowazekii* and can transmit infection to humans. Serosurveys of domestic animals, conducted primarily in the 1950s and 1960s, suggested that, among others, cattle and donkeys were reservoirs of *R. prowazekii*.[53] Critical reevaluations of those studies, however, showed that a substantial portion of the previously reported positive results were likely due to serologic artifact.[54]

Studies conducted in the 1970s and 1980s revealed that the eastern flying squirrel *(G. volans)* is a bona fide reservoir of *R. prowazekii* and a likely source of infection in humans. In 1975, Bozeman and colleagues[46] reported the isolation of six strains of *R. prowazekii* from flying squirrels and their ectoparasites obtained in Florida and Virginia. Subsequent biologic and biochemical characterization of these isolates showed that they were virtually identical to strains of *R. prowazekii* that had been isolated from patients with louse-borne epidemic typhus.[55, 56] Sporadic cases of human *R. prowazekii* infection, which were clinically compatible with typhus and occurred after the patients had contact with flying squirrels, were subsequently reported in various parts of the United States.[43, 44] The mechanism by which disease is transmitted to humans is unclear. Squirrel lice *(Neohaematopinus sciuropteri)* and fleas *(Orchopeas howardi)* have been found to be infected with *R. prowazekii*, and squirrel fleas occasionally bite humans. It is also possible that humans become infected by inhalation of contaminated feces from ectoparasites.

It is not known whether humans who develop sporadic cases of flying squirrel–associated typhus could initiate an epidemic of human louse-borne typhus. Theoretically this would be possible because flying squirrel isolates of *R. prowazekii* grow quite well in human body lice.[47] Presumably, such an outbreak could occur only in an area of the world where infected flying squirrels are enzootic and infestation with body lice occurs among some segments of the human population. DNA probes that can distinguish flying squirrel isolates of *R. prowazekii* from other strains are available, making it possible to determine the origin of such an epidemic.[57]

Pathogenesis

Primary louse-borne epidemic typhus has not occurred in developed countries in decades, and consequently typhus pathogenesis has not been the subject of recent study. Nevertheless, the early studies of typhus pathogenesis were quite well done and provide a picture of the disease that is consistent with observations of other rickettsioses. As with other rickettsial diseases, the basic underlying feature of typhus pathogenesis is damage to the endothelial cells lining the capillaries, arterioles, and venules.

On entering the body, rickettsiae presumably infect cells at the bite site and replicate there for several days. Apparently *R. prowazekii* replicates to high numbers; in vitro, infected cells obtain concentrations of 100 or more rickettsiae per cell before they rupture and release the organisms.[58] The rickettsiae then spread to the draining lymph nodes and initiate systemic infection. Blood-borne dissemination of *R. prowazekii* causes the initial symptoms of chills and fever. Widespread infection of the endothelial cells of the capillaries and small blood vessels follows, producing the microvascular lesions that cause the characteristic rash and the many other features of the disease.

Infiltration of lymphocytes, plasma cells, histiocytes, and polymorphonuclear leukocytes produces a cuff around involved vessels. Proliferation and swelling of the infected endothelial cells narrow the lumina of the blood vessels, and in some instances the restricted circulation causes necrosis of the skin, particularly at the extremities; gangrene sometimes develops in serious cases. Internal hemorrhage is frequently observed in the brain, heart, lungs, and kidneys. Distinct lesions, the characteristic typhus nodules, are found in the brain and are marked by focal proliferation of glial cells and localized accumulation of mononuclear leukocytes.[59]

It is generally accepted, primarily on the basis of laboratory studies, that humoral and cellular immunity is important in the recovery from epidemic typhus. In studies conducted during World War II, the administration of hyperimmune rabbit serum ameliorated the symptoms of epidemic typhus, when administered during the second or third day of illness.[60] In subsequent laboratory investigations, immune serum enhanced the destruction of *R. prowazekii* in human and mouse macrophages in vitro.[61] Cellular immunity is also vital to recovery. Lymphokine-activated (primarily $OKT8^+$) killer cells, obtained from typhus immune donors, lyse target cells infected with *R. prowazekii* in vitro.[62] Other laboratory studies have shown that pretreatment of fibroblasts or macrophage-like cells with interferon makes them unsuitable hosts for *R. prowazekii*.[63, 64]

Clinical Manifestations

Primary louse-borne typhus is the most serious type of typhus infection, particularly when it occurs in epidemic form among undernourished populations. The onset of symptoms is usually abrupt and includes fever (a temperature higher than 39.5°C), chills, frontal headache, and myalgias; many patients report generalized weakness. Other symptoms include some that are constitutional (rigors, arthralgia, or generalized pain) and others referable to the central nervous system (deafness, tinnitus, vertigo, drowsiness, disorientation, delirium) and the gastrointestinal system (anorexia, nausea, constipation, diarrhea, vomiting, abdominal pain). In 50% to 90% of the patients, a generalized eruption appears on the sides of the trunk between days 4 and 7.[65] The lesions, although numerous, may be hard to see in dark-skinned patients. The lesions are initially macular (occasionally maculopapular), blanch with pressure, and have ill-defined edges. Usually, the rash spreads centrifugally to the extremities and darkens to deep red and then to brown. In severe cases, the lesions are hemorrhagic in the center. The face, the palms, and the soles are rarely involved.

The white cell count is usually normal or mildly depressed, and thrombocytopenia is not uncommon. Abnormal results of liver function tests, microscopic hematuria, and proteinuria are common. Complications include hypotension, pneumonia, oliguria, azotemia, cerebral infarction, and gangrene. Fatalities (10% to 50% in untreated patients) usually occur during the third week of illness. Surviving patients recover slowly over many weeks.

In contrast to primary louse-borne typhus, recrudescent typhus (Brill-Zinsser disease) is a much milder disease. Initial symptoms of these patients include malaise, anorexia, nausea, headache, and myalgias. A febrile episode follows, accompanied by intensification of the headache, dulling of the sensorium, and the appearance of a rash on the trunk, arms, and legs. Delirium is rarely noted in recrudescent typhus. Late in the second week of illness, the fever and headache subside abruptly and patients feel generally well. Convalescence is rapid and uneventful.[41]

The clinical presentation of patients with flying squirrel–associated typhus fever is also milder than that observed in epidemic typhus.[43, 44] It is not known if the difference in clinical presentation is related to strain variation of *R. prowazekii* or if the relatively poor nutritional status and underlying health problems that are generally found in epidemics add to the severity of louse-borne typhus.

Diagnosis

The diagnosis of any form of typhus must be prompted by the epidemiologic circumstances surrounding the development of disease. In the United States, flying squirrel–associated typhus should be suspected in the winter months in patients with a history of contact with flying squirrels. In developing countries, classic louse-borne typhus should be considered in persons who have been exposed to war, poverty, and famine and who are infested with lice and among dislocated persons who are arriving from areas where the disease is endemic. Under such conditions the differential diagnosis of febrile illnesses includes malaria, meningitis, influenza, and viral encephalitis. Recrudescent typhus should be suspected when refugees from countries with endemic typhus have unexplained febrile illnesses years after emigration.

Definitive diagnosis can be accomplished by visualizing rickettsiae in tissues, isolating rickettsiae, detecting rickettsiae by polymerase chain reaction technology,[66] or testing acute- and convalescent-phase serum specimens. Serum can be tested for antibodies to typhus rickettsiae by any of several established procedures; the indirect immunofluorescent technique is currently the method most commonly employed, but the enzyme-linked immunosorbent assay, microagglutination, latex agglutination, and other procedures have been used successfully. Because *R. prowazekii* and *Rickettsia typhi* possess common antigens, serum specimens from epidemic or murine typhus patients frequently react at equivalent titers with both organisms.

A positive result (a fourfold rise in titer, a positive immunoglobulin M titer, or a single high titer in a clinically compatible case) indicates recent infection with either *R. prowazekii* or *R. typhi*. Epidemiologic criteria can then be used to distinguish between epidemic and murine typhus infections. Antibody absorption[67] or toxin neutralization[68] tests are necessary to determine the specificity of serologic reactions. Such tests are usually available only from reference laboratories. Rickettsial isolation is hazardous and should be attempted only in a biosafety level 3 facility by experienced microbiologists. The Weil-Felix test, used widely in the past, lacks both sensitivity and specificity and is not recommended.[69]

Brill-Zinsser disease has occurred infrequently in more recent years because the major source of patients with prior epidemic typhus infections, that is, survivors of epidemics during World War II, becomes smaller each year. A history of earlier typhus infection is crucial to the diagnosis. Serologic testing is performed as recommended for louse-borne typhus, except that specific immunoglobulin G and immunoglobulin M titers are also determined. Patients with Brill-Zinsser disease have immunoglobulin G but not immunoglobulin M antibodies to typhus rickettsiae.

Flying squirrel–associated typhus is a rare disease that has been reported only in the United States.[43, 44] Available epidemiologic data suggest that, in contrast to RMSF and murine typhus, most cases occur in the winter months and among patients with documented or presumed contact with flying squirrels. Patients with a compatible clinical presentation and epidemiologic history should be tested for antibodies to typhus rickettsiae as indicated earlier.

Treatment

Because no rapid diagnostic test is available, treatment must be instituted before the diagnosis is confirmed. Tetracycline and chloramphenicol are both effective against typhus infections. Patients are normally given tetracycline at 20 to 40 mg/kg per 24 hours in four doses when the drug is administered orally; 10 to 20 mg/kg per 24 hours is recommended when the patient must be treated intravenously. Single-dose (100 mg) doxycycline treatment has also been shown to be effective in treating patients with louse-borne typhus[70] and may be the most practical approach in situations in which large numbers of patients must be managed. Chloramphenicol (50 mg/kg per 24 hours in four doses) is also effective. The temperature should begin to fall within 24 hours; patients should be treated until they remain afebrile for 48 to 72 hours. Other symptoms may persist for a week or more after treatment is begun.[65, 71]

Prevention

Typhus vaccines are not available. Production of killed typhus vaccines was discontinued years ago because the vaccine lacked efficacy. A live attenuated vaccine, made from the Madrid E strain of *R. prowazekii*, proved to be efficacious,[72] but it did not gain widespread acceptance because of the possible fear of reversion to virulence.

Cases of epidemic typhus can be reduced in endemic areas by delousing campaigns and institution of hygienic measures that preclude reinfestation. Travelers to areas with endemic typhus are unlikely to contract epidemic typhus unless they are in constant, close association with louse-infested individuals. In the latter situation, maintenance of strict personal hygiene and frequent washing of clothing are recommended.

Risk factors for contracting flying squirrel–associated typhus fever have not been firmly identified, so it is not possible to recommend prevention strategies for that particular illness.

Murine Typhus

"Murine typhus is a good example of a disease whose importance is inadequately appreciated—except by the patient, and even today, in most parts of the world, he will never know what ails him because the diagnosis will not be made."[73]

History of Disease

Murine typhus was first reported in 1913 by a physician in Atlanta, who described the clinical features of six cases.[74] Definitive identification of murine typhus as a distinct clinical entity was quite difficult at that time because murine typhus is clinically similar to Brill-Zinsser disease, and techniques for distinguishing the respective etiologic agents were not yet available. Mooser[75] and Neill[76] provided a methodologic advance that allowed the first differentiation of murine and epidemic typhus infection. They noted that rickettsial strains that were isolated from patients with Mexican typhus fever (tabardillo, later identified as murine typhus) developed a characteristic swelling of the scrotum that did not occur in animals infected with *R. prowazekii*.[75, 76] The most important breakthrough, however, came in 1929, when Maxcy[77] reported his studies of typhus patients in the southeastern United States. With remarkable foresight, he postulated that (1) the disease was distinct from louse-borne typhus and had a different etiologic agent, (2) the reservoir was probably rats or mice, and (3) a bloodsucking ectoparasite was the likely vector. Shortly thereafter, Mooser and colleagues[78] isolated a new species of typhus rickettsiae from rats and Dyer and coworkers[79] isolated the same species from rat fleas, verifying Maxcy's hypothesis.

Epidemiology

Commensal rats of the genus *Rattus* are the primary reservoirs of *R. typhi* and are the common factor associated with the transmission of murine typhus to humans. The oriental rat flea, *Xenopsylla cheopis*, is the principal vector. In all, six genera and seven species of flea, including the cat flea (*Ctenocephalides felis*), have been found to be naturally infected with *R. typhi*. Cats and peridomestic opossums infested with cat fleas have been implicated in the transmission of murine typhus in the United States.[80–83] *X. cheopis* transmits *R. typhi* transovarially to some of its progeny, indicating that this flea may also be a reservoir of *R. typhi* in nature.[84] There are no good data to implicate human lice, ticks, or mites as vectors of murine typhus.[73]

X. cheopis fleas become infected with *R. typhi* when they feed on rickettsemic rodents. Fleas remain infected for life and apparently are not harmed by the infection. Experimental infectivity studies have shown that the lining and lumen of the flea gut contain large numbers of *R. typhi* (approximately 10^4 to 10^6 plaque-forming units per flea) beginning about 10 days after infectious feeding; 67% of rats seroconverted to *R. typhi* when inoculated with as little as 0.2 μg of contaminated flea feces. Temperature has a pronounced effect on the rickettsial titers of infected fleas. Fleas maintained at 24°C to 30°C contain two to three times more *R. typhi* than fleas maintained at 18°C. In the same studies, rats became infected under circumstances that precluded the involvement of contaminated feces, indicating that fleas can transmit murine typhus directly during the feeding process.[85] Humans become infected when they intrude on these natural cycles of infection, usually by rubbing contaminated flea feces into scarified skin, inhaling infectious aerosols containing contaminated flea feces, or contaminating their mucous membranes with infectious excreta.

Murine typhus exists on all continents, but its distribution is usually limited to areas where large numbers of *Rattus* are found. Typically, seaports, coastal areas, and the major commercial arteries are sites of endemic disease. Although sporadic cases may occur anywhere within an area in which the disease is endemic, murine typhus frequently occurs in small outbreaks, so-called minifoci of infection.

Murine typhus became a reportable disease in the United States in 1920, but it was not until 1931, when the fundamental concepts of the epidemiology of typhus were developed, that surveillance gained impetus. For example, 333 cases of murine typhus were reported in the United States in 1931, but more than 2000 cases were reported in 1933, and by World War II, more than 5000 cases were documented annually. Even then, it was estimated that only one third of the actual number of cases were reported.[86] After World War II, flea and rodent control programs caused a precipitous drop in the number of reported cases. By 1955, only 155 cases were reported,[87] and in the 1980s fewer than 50 cases were reported each year. Currently, murine typhus is most frequently reported from Texas and California. Murine typhus cases are no longer notifiable to the Centers for Disease Control and Prevention.

During the peak incidence years from 1941 through 1956, 82% to 93% of all cases were reported from seven states—South Carolina, Georgia, Florida, Alabama, Mississippi, Louisiana, and Texas. Presumably, this is attributable to the higher indices of infestation of rodents with *X. cheopis* in warmer temperatures. Epidemiologic data suggest that murine typhus cases that occur in colder areas of the world are restricted to urban areas where *Rattus* species occupy warm indoor harborages. In contrast, murine typhus in southern areas occurs in both rural and urban areas, presumably because rodents and their fleas can thrive equally well indoors and outdoors in the relatively warm climate.[73] Epidemiologic principles of cat- or opossum-associated murine typhus are not yet well defined.

Pathogenesis and Clinical Manifestations

Murine typhus is clinically similar to epidemic typhus and virtually identical to Brill-Zinsser disease. Murine typhus is usually much milder than epidemic typhus, but there are enough exceptions to the rule to confound the diagnosis of individual patients. Damage to the central nervous system is generally much less extensive in murine typhus, and fatalities are rare.

Onset is usually abrupt, but occasionally a mild prodrome is present for a few days. Symptoms are usually severe enough to warrant hospitalization. Fever, usually a temperature greater than 39°C, is almost always present; headache, myalgia, and rash are noted in more than half of the cases, and chills, anorexia, nausea, and photophobia are usually reported less frequently.[88–90] The rash, which appears an average of 5 to 6 days after symptoms begin, is usually macular (less often maculopapular or papular) and most often is found on the trunk, legs, or arms. Physical examination may reveal splenomegaly or hepatomegaly. Complications, including pneumonia and encephalitis, are rare; the case-fatality ratio is about 1%.

Leukocyte and erythrocyte sedimentation rates are usually normal; most patients have mild thrombocytopenia and mildly elevated hepatic transaminase levels. Leukocytosis, mild leukopenia, and anemia have been reported.[90]

As with other rickettsial infections, humoral immunity and cellular immunity both contribute to recovery. In vitro studies have shown that *R. typhi* antigens appear on the surface of infected cells and are the targets for cytotoxic effector cells.[91, 92]

Diagnosis

The nonspecific clinical manifestations of murine typhus preclude a clinical diagnosis. Epidemiologic considerations are, therefore, essential for identifying the cause of the disease. In the United States, residence in a endemic area and possible exposure to rodents provide important clues. A history of travel to a foreign country where the disease is endemic should also alert the physician to the possibility of murine typhus infection. The differential diagnosis is particularly confusing to the physician working in areas of the world where louse-borne typhus and murine typhus are both endemic. Both diseases can occur sporadically and in small outbreaks. Moreover, in otherwise healthy individuals, the clinical presentations are similar. Serologic testing with typhus group antigens provides preliminary confirmation, and epidemiologic data may be useful in differentiating the two diseases. Routine serologic tests do not differentiate *R. prowazekii* infections from *R. typhi* infections.

Treatment

The regimens for suspected *R. typhi* infections are the same as those for *R. prowazekii* infections, and prompt treatment shortens the duration of fever. Relapses have been reported in patients treated with chloramphenicol but not those treated with tetracycline, suggesting that tetracycline or tetracycline analogs may be preferable.[89]

Prevention

Avoidance of rodent-infested areas is the best method of preventing murine typhus infection. Rodent and flea eradication programs are recommended for areas where harborages already exist. However, the latter programs should not be initiated until the relative potential environmental effect of poisons or insecticides has been considered. No vaccine is available. Risk factors for acquiring murine typhus from other sources (e.g., cats, opossums, and cat fleas) are not sufficiently defined to allow firm recommendations for prevention.

Rickettsialpox

History

Rickettsia akari is the etiologic agent of rickettsialpox. It was first isolated in 1946 in association with an outbreak of rickettsialpox at a housing development in New York City. *R. akari* was isolated from the blood of two patients, from a house mouse *(Mus musculus)* trapped on the premises, and from two pools of rodent mites *(Liponyssoides sanguineus)* that were collected at the same site. The investigation also revealed a strong association between mite exposure and rickettsialpox, further incriminating mites as vectors of the disease.[93–96]

Epidemiology

Neither the distribution of *R. akari* nor its natural history is well described. After the initial description of rickettsialpox, additional cases were reported in Massachusetts, Pennsylvania, Connecticut, and Ohio. *R. akari* was also isolated from a wild rodent *(Microtus fortis pelliceus)* in Korea and from a mite collected in Russia.[97] Rickettsialpox apparently occurs infrequently; 13 patients were reported in a New York City hospital from 1980 to 1989.[98]

R. akari is thought to exist in urban and sylvan cycles throughout the world; mites are the vector and principal reservoir. *R. akari* is maintained in successive generations of mites by transovarial transmission. Mice and other susceptible rodents become transient reservoirs of *R. akari* during periods of peak rickettsemia, and uninfected mites can become infected with *R. akari* if they imbibe infectious blood. However, it is uncertain if infectious feeding contributes significantly to the establishment of new lines of persistently infected mites. Humans become infected when they intrude on these natural cycles of infection. *R. akari* is transmitted to humans by mites when they feed.

Clinical Manifestations

Compared with most rickettsioses, rickettsialpox is a relatively mild illness that is rarely fatal. A clinical triad—an initial lesion (eschar), fever, and, usually 1 to 2 days later, a generalized rash—characterizes the disease.[99] The eschar, which occurs in almost all patients, may be located anywhere on the body.[99–101] It begins as an asymptomatic or pruritic erythematous papule 24 to 48 hours after the mite bite.[102] A fluid-filled vesicle appears. As it dries, it leaves a brown to black eschar surrounded by a 0.5- to 3-cm area of induration.[99, 102] Between 7 and 14 (occasionally as long as 24) days after the exposure, chills, fever, sweats, and myalgia begin fairly suddenly. The peak temperature is usually 39°C to 40°C; without treatment, fever persists for about 1 week. Other common symptoms include profuse diaphoresis and headache (usually frontal) and photophobia; occasionally vertigo, rhinorrhea, cough, sore throat, nausea, and vomiting are present.[99, 100] Within 1 to 3 days after the onset of systemic symptoms, a sparse rash appears, with 5 to 100 discrete, firm erythematous papules on the face, trunk, and extremities.[85] Less often the lesions are maculopapular or are found on the palms and soles. In most cases, a vesicle develops at the summit of the papule, and the lesions then resolve by crusting. Except for toxicity, the rash, and some regional lymphadenopathy, the findings of the physical examination are normal.[100] Rickettsialpox usually resolves uneventfully in 2 to 3 weeks.

Leukopenia (2400 to 4000 cells per mm^3) with relative lymphocytosis is usually present. Hematocrit, hemoglobin, erythrocyte sedimentation rate, and electrolyte and liver function values are normal; urinalysis may detect mild proteinuria.[100]

Diagnosis

Diagnosis of rickettsialpox typically requires a combination of clinical and epidemiologic findings in conjunction with group-specific serologic tests. Patients with a compatible illness and known or possible mite exposure should be tested for antibodies to spotted fever group rickettsiae. *R. rickettsii* is typically used as a surrogate antigen because it is antigenically related to *R. akari* and is more readily available. Seroconversion in a clinically compatible case would provide good evidence of rickettsialpox. Direct fluorescent antibody tests of punch biopsies taken from skin lesions have also been used to confirm the diagnosis.[98]

Although the foregoing criteria are sufficient to diagnose cases of rickettsialpox, definitive confirmation requires the isolation of *R. akari* from the patient's blood. Mice inoculated intraperitoneally with infected blood develop symptoms (ruffled fur, rapid breathing) within 3 to 14 days. Spleen, liver, and lymph nodes become enlarged during infection and serve as excellent tissues for cultivation of potential isolates. *R. akari* isolates can be propagated in any of a variety of cell cultures, provided that no antibiotics are added to supplement the medium. The identity of presumed isolates should be confirmed with monoclonal antibodies or by cross-neutralization tests in experiments with animals.[103]

Differential diagnosis includes the other rickettsial diseases that may be accompanied by an eschar (scrub typhus and tick typhus), varicella, and infections caused by coxsackievirus (types A9, A16, and B5). In contrast to rickettsialpox, the vesicles of varicella do not have a papular base or eschar.[100]

Treatment

Although no fatalities have been reported, uncontrolled studies show that treatment hastens defervescence.[104] Tetracycline and chloramphenicol (in doses of 250 mg every 6 hours) for 2 to 5 days seem equally effective. As in other rickettsial infections, a response should occur within 48 hours; continued fever suggests another cause for the illness.

Prevention

Because rickettsialpox routinely occurs after exposure to mouse mites, the disease can best be prevented by enforcing sanitary measures that preclude the development of rodent harborages. Rodent eradication programs may be necessary to eliminate existing infestation problems.

Scrub Typhus

History of Disease

Scrub typhus gained prominence in World War II, when tens of thousands of soldiers in the Asiatic-Pacific theaters contracted the disease: case-fatality ratios were as high as 35%.[105] It was a serious problem in U.S. military personnel in Vietnam in the 1960s.[106] Thousands of cases still occur each year in certain areas and may be important causes of fever among hospitalized patients and outpatients. The disease is endemic to an extremely large geographic area, ranging from the coastal portions of northern Australia to Asia and the Indian subcontinent and including, among others, Japan, Korea, southern China and Tibet, Indochina, the Philippines, New Guinea, Sri Lanka, and islands of the Chagos archipelago (Fig. 179–3). Proven habitats of *Rickettsia tsutsugamushi* range from sandy beaches and mountain deserts to equatorial rain forests. Thus, the term scrub typhus is a misnomer; chigger-borne rickettsiosis has been suggested as a more accurate term.[107]

Epidemiology

Despite their apparent diversity, scrub typhus habitats do have one thing in common: they have experienced ecologic modifications by humans or nature that have resulted in transitional, nonclimactic vegetation.[107] Such areas bring together the classic scrub typhus triad, *Rattus* rats, *Leptotrombidium* mites, and *R. tsutsugamushi*. Chiggers (larval mites) of the *Leptotrombidium deliense* group are the principal vectors to humans, but other mite species are also vectors.[107] *R. tsutsugamushi* is maintained in mites primarily by transovarial transmission. Although rats are hosts for the chiggers, they are not thought to contribute significantly to the maintenance of *R. tsutsugamushi*, except perhaps to occasionally infect a previously uninfected female mite that could pass the infection to its progeny.

Incidence figures for scrub typhus are generally unavailable because adequate surveillance systems are lacking. One study in Malaysia estimated the incidence there to be 3% to 4% per month.[108] In a related study,[109] 19.3% of all diagnosed febrile illnesses in a rural area of Malaysia were due to scrub typhus. Such a high incidence is not surprising, particularly when one realizes that infection with a given strain of *R. tsutsugamushi* does not confer immunity to all infecting strains. Multiple scrub typhus infections are common among occupationally exposed persons.

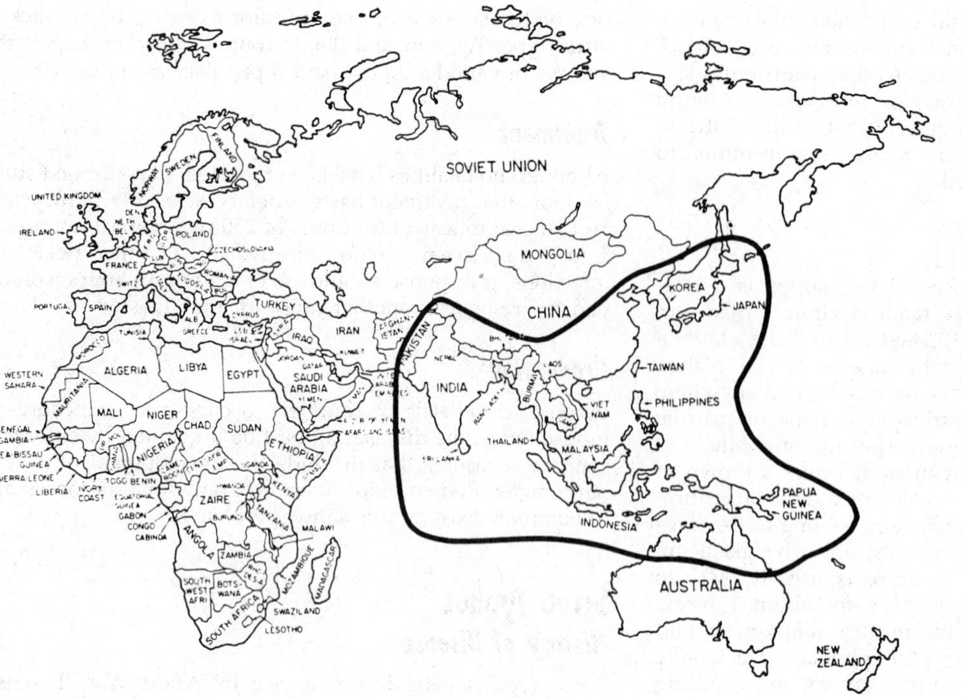

FIGURE 179–3 ▫ Partial map of the Eastern Hemisphere showing the area endemic for scrub typhus.

Clinical Manifestations and Pathogenesis

Scrub typhus patients usually have nonspecific clinical manifestations (chills, fever, and headache). Other symptoms include cough, myalgias, arthralgias, retroorbital pain, and gastrointestinal abnormalities. Eschars are observed at the site of mite attachment in many patients. A macular rash frequently appears on the patient's trunk during the first week of illness and subsequently progresses to the face and extremities, sparing the palms and soles. Hepatomegaly and splenomegaly are common. Respiratory, neurologic, cardiovascular, and hematologic abnormalities develop during the second week of illness, usually as a result of generalized vasculitis.[110] Documentation of scrub typhus resistant to doxycycline and chloramphenicol[111] raises serious questions for treatment.

Diagnosis

Scrub typhus is usually diagnosed by serologic tests, performed with the three prototype strains of *R. tsutsugamushi* (Karp, Gilliam, and Kato) as antigens. Currently, the indirect immunofluorescent technique is the method of choice,[68] but the immunoperoxidase test,[112] enzyme immunoassays,[113, 114] and passive hemagglutination assay[115] have also been employed successfully. Minimal titers have not been established with certainty, and, therefore, tests of paired serum specimens are recommended so a rise in antibody titer can be demonstrated. Polymerase chain reaction assays have confirmed *R. tsutsugamushi* infections in acute-phase blood of patients and may be of great potential use as a diagnostic tool.[116–118] Isolation attempts are performed only by specialty laboratories.

Treatment

Chloramphenicol and the tetracyclines are both effective for treating scrub typhus patients; however, symptoms abate more quickly with tetracycline therapy. Relapses are common with short therapeutic courses[119] or when therapy is begun before 5 days after onset of symptoms.

Prevention

Chloramphenicol and tetracyclines are also effective for the chemoprophylaxis of scrub typhus.[120–122] In one of these studies,[122] 9 of 10 volunteers who were exposed to infected chiggers developed scrub typhus, whereas only 1 of 10 similarly exposed individuals who received weekly (200 mg orally) doxycycline prophylaxis developed the disease. Eight of nine of the doxycycline-treated individuals developed minor symptoms after the chemoprophylactic regimen was completed.

References

1. Ewing SA: Canine ehrlichiosis. Adv Vet Sci Comp Med 13:331, 1969.
2. Ristic M: Pertinent characteristics of leukocytic rickettsiae of humans and animals. *In* Leive L (ed): Microbiology—1986. Washington, DC, American Society for Microbiology, 1986, pp 182–187.
3. Kelch WJ: The canine ehrlichiosis (tropical canine pancytopenia) epizootic in Vietnam and its implications for the veterinary care. Mil Med 149:327, 1984.
4. Buhles WCJ, Huxsoll DL, Ristic M: Tropical canine pancytopenia: Clinical, hematologic, and serological response of dogs to *Ehrlichia canis* infection, tetracycline therapy, and challenge inoculation. J Infect Dis 130:357, 1974.
5. Tachibana N: Sennetsu fever: The disease, diagnosis, and treatment. *In* Leive L (ed): Microbiology—1986. Washington, DC, American Society for Microbiology, 1986, pp 205–208.
6. Maeda K, Markowitz N, Hawley RC, et al: Human infection with *Ehrlichia canis*, a leukocytic rickettsia. N Engl J Med 316:853, 1987.
7. Anderson BE, Dawson JE, Jones DC, Wilson KH: *Ehrlichia chaffeensis*, a new species assocciated with human ehrlichiosis. J Clin Microbiol 29:2838, 1991.
8. Dawson JE, Anderson BE, Fishbein DB, et al: Isolation and characterization of an *Ehrlichia* sp. from a patient diagnosed with human ehrlichiosis. J Clin Microbiol 29:2741, 1991.
9. Chen S, Dumler JS, Bakken JS, Walker DH: Identification of a granulocytotropic *Ehrlichia* species as the etiologic agent of human disease. J Clin Microbiol 32:589, 1994.

10. Ristic M, Huxsoll DL: Ehrlichiae. *In* Krieg NR, Holt JG (eds): Bergey's Manual of Systematic Bacteriology. Baltimore, Williams & Wilkins, 1984, pp 704–709.
11. Dawson JE, Candal FJ, George VG, Ades EW: Human endothelial cells as an alternative to DH82 cells for the isolation of *Ehrlichia chaffeensis, E. canis* and *Rickettsia rickettsii.* Pathobiology 61:293, 1993.
12. Rohrbach BW, Harkess JR, Ewing SA, et al: Epidemiologic and clinical characteristics of persons with serologic evidence of *E. canis* infection. Am J Public Health 80:442, 1990.
13. Fishbein DB, Sawyer LA, Holland CJ, et al: Unexplained febrile illnesses after exposure to ticks: Infection with an *Ehrlichia?* JAMA 257:3100, 1987.
14. Harkess JR: Ehrlichiosis. Infect Dis Clin North Am 5:37, 1991.
15. Fishbein DB, Dawson JE, Robinson LE: Human ehrlichiosis in the United States, 1985 to 1990. Ann Intern Med 120:736, 1994.
16. Harkess JR, Ewing SA, Crutcher JM, et al: Human ehrlichiosis in Oklahoma. J Infect Dis 159:576, 1989.
17. Fishbein DB, Kemp A, Dawson JE, et al: Human ehrlichiosis: Prospective active surveillance in febrile hospitalized patients. J Infect Dis 160:803, 1989.
18. Petersen LR, Sawyer LA, Fishbein DB, et al: An outbreak of ehrlichiosis in members of an army reserve unit exposed to ticks. J Infect Dis 159:562, 1989.
19. Standaert SM, Dawson JE, Schaffner W, et al. A hyperendemic focus of human ehrlichiosis at a golf-oriented retirement community. N Engl J Med 333:420, 1995.
20. Yevich SJ, Sanchez JL, DeFraites RF, et al. Seroepidemiology of infections due to spotted fever group Rickettsiae and *Ehrlichia* species in military personnel exposed in areas of the United States where such infections are endemic. J Infect Dis 171:1266, 1994.
21. Bakken JS, Dumler JS, Chen S-M, et al: Human granulocytic ehrlichiosis in the upper Midwest. A new species emerging? JAMA 272:212, 1994.
22. Dumler JS, Bakken JS: Ehrlichial diseases of humans: Emerging tick-borne infections. Clin Infect Dis 20:1102, 1995.
23. Telford SR 3rd, Lepore TJ, Snow P, et al: Human granulocytic ehrlichiosis in Massachusetts. Ann Intern Med 123:277, 1995.
24. Anderson BE, Sims KG, Olson JG, et al: *Amblyomma americanum*: A potential vector of human ehrlichiosis. Am J Trop Med Hyg 49:239, 1993.
25. Dawson JE, Childs JE, Biggie KL, et al: White-tailed deer as a potential reservoir of *Ehrlichia* spp. J Wildl Dis 30:162, 1994.
26. Dawson JE, Stallknecht DE, Howereth EW, et al: Susceptibilty of white-tailed deer *(Odocoilus virginianus)* to infection with *Ehrlichia chaffeensis*, the etiologic agent of human ehrlichiosis. J Clin Microbiol 32:2725, 1994.
27. Ewing SA, Dawson JE, Kocan AA, et al: Experimental transmission of *Ehrlichia chaffeensis* (Rickettsiales: Ehrlichieae) among white-tailed deer by *Amblyomma americanum* (Acari: Ixodidae). J Med Entomol 32:368, 1995.
28. Moskovitz M, Fadden R, Min T: Human ehrlichiosis: A rickettsial disease associated with severe cholestasis and multisystemic disease. J Clin Gastoenterol 13:86, 1991.
29. Dumler JS, Sutker WL, Walker DH: Persistent infection with *Ehrlichia chaffeensis.* Clin Infect Dis 17:903, 1993.
30. Edwards MS, Jones JE, Leass DL, et al: Childhood infection caused by *Ehrlichia canis* or a closely related organism. Pediatr Infect Dis J 7:651, 1988.
31. Eng TR, Harkess JR, Fishbein DB, et al: Epidemiologic, clinical, and laboratory findings of human ehrlichiosis in the United States, 1988. JAMA 264:2251, 1990.
32. Anderson BE, Sumner JW, Dawson JE, et al: Detection of the etiologic agent of human ehrlichiosis by polymerase chain reaction. J Clin Microbiol 30:775, 1992.
33. Evans SR, Korch GW, Lawson MA: Comparative field evaluation of permethrin and DEET-treated military uniforms for personal protection against ticks (Acari). J Med Entomol 27:829, 1990.
34. Mount GA, Snoddy EL: Pressurized sprays of permethrin and DEET on clothing for personal protection against the Lone Star tick and the American dog tick (Acari: Ixodidae). J Econ Entomol 76:529, 1983.
35. Hahon N: Selected Papers on the Pathogenic Rickettsiae. Cambridge, MA, Harvard University Press, 1968, p 369.
36. Woodward TE: A historical account of the rickettsial diseases with a discussion of unsolved problems. J Infect Dis 127:583, 1973.
37. Weyer F: Progress in ecology and epidemiology of rickettsioses: A review. Acta Trop 35:5, 1978.
38. World Health Organization: Louse-borne typhus in 1979. Wkly Epidemiol Rec 56:129, 1981.
39. World Health Organization: Louse-borne typhus 1981–1982. Wkly Epidemiol Rec 59:29, 1984.
40. Centers for Disease Control: Production of typhus vaccine discontinued in the United States. MMWR Morbid Mortal Wkly Rep 29:465, 1980.
41. Brill NE: An acute infectious disease of unknown origin. A clinical study based on 221 cases. Am J Med Sci 139:484, 1910.
42. Zinsser H: Varieties of typhus virus and the epidemiology of the American form of European typhus fever (Brill's disease). Am J Hyg 20:513, 1934.
43. McDade JE, Shepard CC, Redus MA, et al: Evidence of *Rickettsia prowazekii* infections in the United States. Am J Trop Med Hyg 29:277, 1980.
44. Duma RJ, Sonenshine DE, Bozeman FM, et al: Epidemic typhus in the United States associated with flying squirrels. JAMA 245:2318, 1981.
45. Russo PK, Mendelson DC, Etkind PH, et al: Epidemic typhus *Rickettsia prowazekii* in Massachusetts: Evidence. N Engl J Med 304:1166, 1981.
46. Bozeman MF, Masiello SA, Williams MS, et al: Epidemic typhus rickettsiae isolated from flying squirrels. Nature 255:545, 1975.
47. Bozeman MF, Sonenshine DE, Williams MS, et al: Experimental infection of ectoparasitic arthropods with *Rickettsia prowazekii* (GvF-16 strain) and transmission to flying squirrels. Am J Trop Med Hyg 30:253, 1981.
48. Silverman DJ, Boese JL, Wisseman CL Jr: Ultrastructural studies of *Rickettsia prowazekii* from louse midgut cells to feces: Search for "dormant" forms. Infect Immun 10:257, 1974.
49. Boese JL, Wisseman CL Jr, Walsh WT, et al: Antibody and antibiotic action on *Rickettsia prowazekii* in body lice across the host-vector interface, with observations on strain virulence and retrieval mechanisms. Am J Epidemiol 98:262, 1973.
50. Murray ES, Baehr G, Schwartzman G, et al: Brill's disease. I. Clinical and laboratory diagnosis. JAMA 142:1059, 1950.
51. Murray ES, Snyder JC: Brill's disease. II. Etiology. Am J Hyg 53:22, 1951.
52. Price WH: Studies of the interepidemic survival of louse-borne epidemic typhus fever. J Bacteriol 69:105, 1955.
53. Philip CB: A review of growing evidence that domestic animals may be involved in cycles of rickettsial zoonoses. Zentralbl Bakteriol Parasitenkd Infektionskr Hyg Abt Orig 206:343, 1968.
54. McDade JE, Wisseman CL Jr: Studies of proposed extrahuman reservoirs of epidemic typhus. *In* International Symposium on the Control of Lice and Louse-Borne Diseases. Washington, DC, Pan-American Health Organization, 1973, p 113. Scientific publication 263.
55. Woodman DR, Weiss E, Dasch GA, et al: Biological properties of *Rickettsia prowazekii* strains isolated from flying squirrels. Infect Immun 16:853, 1977.
56. Dasch GA, Samms JR, Weiss E: Biochemical characteristics of typhus group rickettsiae with special attention to the *Rickettsia prowazekii* strains isolated from flying squirrels. Infect Immun 19:676, 1978.
57. Regnery RL, Fu ZY, Spruill CL: Flying squirrel–associated *Rickettsia prowazekii* (epidemic typhus rickettsiae) characterized by a specific DNA fragment produced by restriction endonuclease digestion. J Clin Microbiol 23:189, 1986.
58. Silverman DJ, Wisseman CL Jr, Waddell A: In vitro studies of rickettsia–host cell interactions: Ultrastructural study of *Rickettsia prowazekii*–infected chicken embryo fibroblasts. Infect Immun 29:778, 1980.
59. von Lichtenberg F: Rickettsial diseases. *In* Cotran RS, Kumar V, Robbins SL (eds): The Pathologic Basis of Disease, ed 4. Philadelphia, WB Saunders, 1989, pp 328–333.
60. Yeomans A, Snyder JC, Gilliam AG: The effects of concentrated hyperimmune rabbit serum in louse-borne typhus. JAMA 129:19, 1945.
61. Beaman L, Wisseman CL Jr: Mechanisms of immunity in typhus infections. VI. Differential opsonizing and neutralizing action

of human typhus rickettsia–specific cytophilic antibodies in cultures of human macrophages. Infect Immun 14:1071, 1976.
62. Carl M, Dasch GA: Characterization of human cytotoxic lymphocytes directed against cells infected with typhus group rickettsiae: Evidence for lymphokine activation of effectors. J Immunol 136:2654, 1986.
63. Turco J, Winkler HH: Effect of mouse lymphokines and cloned mouse interferon-γ on the interaction of *Rickettsia prowazekii* with mouse macrophage-like RAW264.7 cells. Infect Immun 45:303, 1984.
64. Turco J, Winkler HH: Cloned mouse interferon-γ inhibits the growth of *Rickettsia prowazekii* in cultured mouse fibroblasts. J Exp Med 158:2159, 1983.
65. Kamal AM, Messih GA: Typhus fever: Review of 11,410 cases. Symptomatology, laboratory investigations and treatment. J Egypt Public Health Assoc 1:125, 1943.
66. Carl M, Tibbs CW, Dobson ME, et al: Diagnosis of acute typhus infection using the polymerase chain reaction. Ann N Y Acad Sci 590:439, 1990.
67. Goldwasser RA, Shepard CC: Fluorescent antibody methods in the differentiation of murine and epidemic typhus sera: Specificity changes resulting from previous immunization. J Immunol 82:373, 1959.
68. Elisberg BL, Bozeman FM: The rickettsiae. *In* Lennette EH, Schmidt NJ (eds): Diagnostic Procedures for Viral, Rickettsial, and Chlamydial Infections. Washington, DC, American Public Health Association, 1979, pp 1061–1108.
69. Zuerіein TJ, Smith PW: The diagnostic utility of the febrile agglutinin tests. JAMA 254:1211, 1985.
70. Perine PL, Krause DW, Awoke S, et al: Single-dose doxycycline treatment of louse-borne relapsing fever and epidemic typhus. Lancet 2:742, 1974.
71. Krause DW, Perine PL, McDade JE, et al: Treatment of louseborne typhus fever with chloramphenicol, tetracycline, or doxycycline. East Afr Med J 52:421, 1975.
72. Fox JP, Jordan ME, Conwell DP, et al: Immunization of man against epidemic typhus by infection with avirulent *Rickettsia prowazekii* (strain E). II. The seroimmune state and resistance to virulent challenge two years after immunization and a note as to the nature of immediate postvaccination reactions. Am J Hyg 61:174, 1955.
73. Traub R, Wisseman CL Jr, Farhang-Azad A: The ecology of murine typhus—A critical review. Trop Dis Bull 75:237, 1978.
74. Paullin JE: Typhus fever with a report of cases. South Med J 6:36, 1913.
75. Mooser H: Reaction of guinea pigs to Mexican typhus (tabardillo). JAMA 91:19, 1928.
76. Neill MH: Experimental typhus fever in guinea pigs. Public Health Rep 32:1105, 1917.
77. Maxcy KF: Typhus fever in the United States. Public Health Rep 44:1735, 1929.
78. Mooser H, Castaneda MR, Zinsser H: Rats as carriers of Mexican typhus fever. JAMA 97:231, 1931.
79. Dyer RE, Rumreich A, Badger LF: Typhus fever. A virus of the typhus type derived from fleas collected from wild rats. Public Health Rep 46:334, 1931.
80. Adams WJ, Emmons RW, Brooks JE: The changing ecology of murine (endemic) typhus in southern California. Am J Trop Med Hyg 19:311, 1970.
81. Williams SG, Sacci JB Jr, Schriefer ME, et al: Typhus and typhuslike rickettsiae associated with opossums and their fleas in Los Angeles County, California. J Clin Microbiol 30:1758, 1992.
82. Schriefer ME, Sacci JB Jr, Taylor JP, et al: Murine typhus: Updated role of multiple urban components and a second typhuslike rickettsia. J Med Entomol 31:681, 1994.
83. Sorvillo FJ, Gondo B, Emmons R, et al: A suburban focus of endemic typhus in Los Angeles County: Association with seropositive domestic cats and opossums. Am J Trop Med Hyg 48:269, 1993.
84. Farhang-Azad A, Traub R, Baqar S: Transovarial transmission of murine typhus rickettsiae in *Xenopsylla cheopis* fleas. Science 227:543, 1985.
85. Farhang-Azad A, Traub R: Transmission of murine typhus rickettsiae by *Xenopsylla cheopis,* with notes on experimental infection and effects of temperature. Am J Trop Med Hyg 34:555, 1985.
86. Pratt HD: The changing picture of murine typhus in the United States. Ann N Y Acad Sci 70:517, 1958.
87. White PC Jr: Murine typhus in the United States. Mil Med 130:469, 1965.
88. Taylor JP, Betz TG, Rawlings JA: Epidemiology of murine typhus in Texas, 1980 through 1984. JAMA 255:2173, 1986.
89. Shaked Y, Samra Y, Maeir MK, et al: Murine typhus and spotted fever in Israel in the eighties: Retrospective analysis. Infection 16:283, 1988.
90. Dumler JS, Taylor JP, Walker DH: Clinical and laboratory features of murine typhus in south Texas, 1980 through 1987. JAMA 266:1365, 1991.
91. Rollwagen FM, Bakun AJ, Dorsey CH, et al: Mechanisms of immunity to infection with typhus rickettsiae: Infected fibroblasts bear rickettsial antigens on their surfaces. Infect Immun 50:911, 1985.
92. Rollwagen FM, Dasch GA, Jerrells TR: Mechanisms of immunity to rickettsial infection: Characterization of a cytotoxic effector cell. J Immunol 136:1418, 1986.
93. Huebner RJ, Jellison WL, Armstrong C: Rickettsialpox—A newly recognized rickettsial disease. V. Recovery of *Rickettsia akari* from a house mouse *(Mus musculus).* Public Health Rep 62:777, 1947.
94. Huebner RJ, Jellison WL, Pomerantz C: Rickettsialpox—A newly recognized rickettsial disease. IV. Isolation of a rickettsia apparently identical with the causative agent of rickettsialpox from *Allodermanyssus sanguineus,* a rodent mite. Public Health Rep 61:1677, 1946.
95. Huebner RJ, Stamps P, Armstrong C: Rickettsialpox—A newly recognized rickettsial disease: I. Isolation of the etiologic agent. Public Health Rep 61:1605, 1946.
96. Greenberg M, Pellitteri OJ, Jellison WL: Rickettsialpox—A newly recognized rickettsial disease. III. Epidemiology. Am J Public Health 37:860, 1947.
97. Jackson EB, Danauskas JX, Coale MC, et al: Recovery of *Rickettsia akari* from the Korean vole *Microtus fortis pelliceus.* Am J Hyg 66:301, 1957.
98. Kass EM, Szaniawski WK, Levy H, et al: Rickettsialpox in a New York City hospital, 1980 to 1989. N Engl J Med 331:1612, 1994.
99. Greenberg M, Pellitteri OJ: Rickettsialpox. Bull N Y Acad Sci 23:338, 1947.
100. Barker LP: Rickettsialpox. Clinical and laboratory study of twelve hospitalized cases. JAMA 141:1119, 1949.
101. Greenberg M, Pellittari O, Klein IF, et al: Rickettsialpox—A newly recognized rickettsial disease: II. Clinical observations. JAMA 133:901, 1947.
102. Brettman LR, Lewin S, Holzman RS, et al: Rickettsialpox: Report of an outbreak and a contemporary review. Medicine (Baltimore) 60:363, 1981.
103. Bell EJ, Stoenner HG: Immunologic relationships among the spotted fever group of rickettsias determined by toxin neutralization tests in mice with convalescent animal serums. J Immunol 84:171, 1960.
104. Rose HM: The treatment of rickettsialpox with antibiotics. Ann N Y Acad Sci 55:1019, 1952.
105. Farner DS, Katsampes CP: Tsutsugamushi disease. U S Nav Med Bull 43:800, 1944.
106. Berman SJ, Kundin WD: Scrub typhus in South Vietnam: A study of 87 cases. Ann Intern Med 79:26, 1973.
107. Traub R, Wisseman CL Jr: The ecology of chigger-borne rickettsiosis (scrub typhus). J Med Entomol 11:237, 1974.
108. Brown GW, Robinson DM, Huxsoll DL: Serological evidence for a high incidence of transmission of *Rickettsia tsutsugamushi* in two Orang Asli settlements in penisular Malaysia. Am J Trop Med Hyg 27:121, 1978.
109. Brown GW, Shirai A, Jegathesan M, et al: Febrile illness in Malaysia—An analysis of 1,629 hospitalized patients. Am J Trop Med Hyg 33:311, 1984.
110. Sheehy TW, Hazlett D, Turk RE: Scrub typhus. A comparison of chloramphenicol and tetracycline in its treatment. Arch Intern Med 132:77, 1973.
111. Watt G, Chouriyagune C, Ruangweerayud R, et al: Scrub typhus infections poorly responsive to antibiotics in Northern Thailand. Lancet 348:86, 1996.
112. Suto T: A ten years experience on diagnosis of rickettsial dis-

eases using the indirect immunoperoxidase methods. Acta Virol 35:580, 1991.
113. Furiya Y, Yamamoto S, Otu M, et al: Use of monoclonal antibodies against *Rickettsia tsutsugamushi* Kawasaki for serodiagnosis by enzyme-linked immunosorbent assay. J Clin Microbiol 29:340, 1991.
114. Kim I-K, Seong S-Y, Woo S-G, et al: High level expression of a 56-kilodalton protein gene *(bor56)* of *Rickettsia tsutsugamushi* Boryong and its application to enzyme-linked immunosorbent assays. J Clin Microbiol 31:598, 1993.
115. Kim I-K, Seong S-Y, Woo S-G, et al: Rapid diagnosis of scrub typhus by passive hemagglutination assay using recombinant 56-kilodalton polypeptides. J Clin Microbiol 31:2057, 1993.
116. Kawamori F, Akiyama M, Sugeida M, et al: Two-step polymerase chain reaction for diagnosis of scrub typhus and identification of antigenic variants of *Rickettsia tsutsugamushi.* J Vet Med Sci 55:749, 1993.
117. Murai K, Tachibana N, Okayama A, et al: Sensitivity of polymerase chain reaction assay for *Rickettsia tsutsugamushi* in patients' blood samples. Microbiol Immunol 36:1145, 1992.
118. Sugita Y, Yamankawa Y, Takahashi K, et al: A polymerase chain reaction system for rapid diagnosis of scrub typhus within six hours. Am J Trop Med Hyg 49:636, 1993.
119. Olson JG, Bourgeois AL, Fang RCY, et al: Prevention of scrub typhus. Prophylactic administration of doxycycline in a randomized double blind trial. Am J Trop Med Hyg 29:989, 1980.
120. Smadel JE, Traub R, Frick LP, et al: Chloramphenicol (chloromycetin) in the chemoprophylaxis of scrub typhus (tsutsugamushi disease). III. Suppression of overt disease. Am J Hyg 51:216, 1950.
121. Twartz JC, Shirai A, Selvaraju G, et al: Doxycycline prophylaxis for human scrub typhus. J Infect Dis 146:811, 1982.

180

Cat-Scratch Disease

Jennifer S. Daly

History

Cat-scratch disease (CSD) was first diagnosed in 1931 by Debré and Semelaigne, and since that time this disorder has been a microbiologic, diagnostic, and therapeutic challenge to the medical community (Table 180–1). The first patient recognized with CSD was a 10-year-old boy with multiple cat scratches, epitrochlear lymphadenitis, and a draining fistula.[1] Debré and Semelaigne at the University of Paris recognized the disease after the fistula and the adenitis resolved spontaneously, the skin test for tuberculosis was negative, and the patient's mother maintained that the disease was related to the boy's close contact with cats. Years later when Debré visited Cincinnati he discussed his findings with Foshay, who had recognized the syndrome himself while studying patients thought to have tularemia. Foshay developed the first skin test antigen and it was used by Rose and Hanger in New York. These U.S. physicians did not publish their work,[1] but Debré and coworkers[2] published the first report on CSD in 1950, naming the syndrome "la maladie des griffes de chat."

Rapidly the literature expanded with case reports by Mollaret from the Institut Pasteur and Greer in the United States.[1] By 1954, Daniels and MacMurray[3] had collected 160 cases from the Washington, DC area and published a review. Later, Margileth, Carithers, and their colleagues[4–7] independently published their findings on more than 1000 cases collected by each author for decades and contributed extensively to the understanding and recognition of the disease. They have used the skin test extensively and have provided skin test material to other physicians. They have helped develop standard criteria for the diagnosis of CSD, but these criteria may now become less important as culture techniques and serologic testing become more reliable and available.

The infectious nature of the disorder was recognized soon after the disease was first seen, but the isolation of the etiologic agent or agents and pathogenesis of the disease continue to provoke controversy. In 1983, Wear and coworkers[8] related finding delicate pleomorphic gram-negative bacilli in 34 of 39 lymph nodes from patients with CSD. The organisms were best seen with the Warthin-Starry silver stain within the walls of capillaries and microabscesses and appeared as single organisms or in chains or clumps. Convalescent serum from patients who had reacted to the antigen skin test also reacted with the bacteria (using an immunoperoxidase stain) seen in the lymph nodes. The following year, Margileth and colleagues[9] reported finding the Warthin-Starry–staining bacteria at the primary inoculation site in three patients. The organisms were similar to those seen in 1913 when Verhoff first described a filamentous organism in the conjunctiva of patients with Parinaud ocular glandular syndrome,[10] a syndrome later recognized as a rare manifestation of CSD. These silver-staining organisms were found more consistently than the miscellaneous agents implicated in other studies that suggested a viral, mycobacterial, chlamydial, or bacterial etiology for CSD.[10, 11] Finally, in 1988, English and others[12] at the same institution (Armed Forces Institute of Pathology) as Wear isolated and propagated a gram-negative bacterium from one patient with CSD. This isolate and three isolates from another patient were characterized more extensively and named *Afipia felis* by Brenner and colleagues.[13] English and colleagues[12] described what they called delicate pleomorphic forms in nine other patients; the forms were reported to grow in culture in biphasic brain-heart infusion medium incubated at 30°C to 32°C. Electron microscopy revealed that the delicate pleomorphic forms lacked a portion of their cell walls, which the authors thought helped explain the inability to subculture the unusual forms. The one patient

TABLE 180–1 ■ Cat-Scratch Disease History

YEAR	EVENT
1931	Debré and Semelaigne recognize the first case of CSD.
1946	Foshay, Rose, and Hanger use cat-scratch antigen as a skin test.
1950	Debré and colleagues publish first report (in French) on CSD.
1954	Daniels and MacMurray report findings for 160 cases in the United States.
1983	Wear and colleagues discover bacilli using the Warthin-Starry stain.
1988	English and coworkers culture *A. felis*.
1990	Slater, Welch, and colleagues culture *B. henselae* from the blood of immunocompromised patients with fever and bacteremia. Relman and others find *B. henselae* DNA in tissue specimens from patients with peliosis hepatis.
1992	Regnery and others find that patients with CSD have a serologic response to *B. henselae* and culture the organism from the blood of a cat.
1993	Dolan and colleagues recover *B. henselae* from lymph nodes of patients with CSD.
1995	Laboratories culture both *B. henselae* and *A. felis* from patients with CSD.

whose lymph node grew *A. felis* had an antibody titer of 1:512 by immunofluorescence assay with antigen derived from the cultured organism. English and coworkers were able to produce lesions histologically similar to those of CSD by injecting the organism in the skin of an armadillo and, like others before them, thought they had isolated the etiologic agent of CSD. Several other laboratories have isolated *A. felis* from patients with CSD, but most patients with CSD do not demonstrate a serologic reaction to this organism.

In the 1990s, several investigators brought a new pathogen, distinct from *A. felis*, to the attention of medical scientists. As the epidemic of acquired immunodeficiency syndrome progressed, patients with human immunodeficiency virus infection were diagnosed with severe, disseminated CSD.[10, 14–16] About the same time, a new entity was recognized, bacillary angiomatosis, consisting of skin lesions similar histologically to those in CSD and containing organisms that stained with the Warthin-Starry silver stain preparation.[15, 17] Comparable organisms were found in the liver of patients with peliosis hepatis, and eventually the diseases bacillary angiomatosis and peliosis of the liver and spleen were linked. In 1990, Slater and colleagues[18] reported a new pathogen, later named *Bartonella henselae*,[19, 20] from the blood of immunocompromised individuals with fever and bacteremia, and Relman and coworkers[21] detected *B. henselae* in tissue from patients with the acquired immunodeficiency syndrome who had bacillary angiomatosis or peliosis hepatis. Because of the similarities between CSD and bacillary angiomatosis, Regnery and colleagues[22] undertook a study using serum from patients with suspected CSD. By an indirect immunofluorescent antibody test, 88% of 41 patients with clinically suspected CSD had antibodies to *Bartonella* antigens.[22] In the same year they cultured *B. henselae* from the blood of a domestic cat.[23] In 1993, Zangwill and coworkers[24] studied 60 persons with suspected CSD and found that 84% of cases had antibody to the *Bartonella* antigen versus 3.6% of healthy control subjects. Eighty-one percent of the cats from households of patients with the disease also had antibody.[24] Although these serologic studies showed that 84% to 96% of patients had antibody titers greater than or equal to 1:64 to *B. henselae*, these authors and other investigators have postulated that cross-reactions occur between some strains of *Bartonella quintana* (the agent of trench fever and some of the cases of bacillary angiomatosis) and *B. henselae*.[25, 26] Waldvogel and colleagues[25] have reported that the originally developed immunofluorescent antibody test should be regarded as genus rather than species specific. In my practice I have seen a patient with classic symptoms who developed a fourfold rise in antibody to *B. quintana* with no antibody response to *B. henselae*, consistent with the concept that the relative importance of cross-reacting antibody has not been determined.

The evidence for the role of *B. henselae* in CSD goes beyond serologic studies. *B. henselae* DNA was detected in several preparations of CSD skin test antigen by using species-specific polymerase chain reaction primers.[27] In 1993, Dolan and colleagues[28] isolated *B. henselae* from the lymph nodes of two patients with CSD. Once laboratories had become aware of culture and serologic techniques necessary to detect infection with *Bartonella* species, other investigators confirmed a role for *B. henselae* in CSD. However, this story has not concluded. French investigators cultured *B. quintana* from a cat owner with chronic lymphadenopathy[29] but not classic CSD, and Alkan and colleagues[30] have isolated both *B. henselae* and *A. felis* from the nodes of several patients with CSD. There continues to be a small group of patients (5% to 15%) with negative skin tests, serology, and culture for *Bartonella*, in whom CSD may be due to other pathogens, including *A. felis*. The story of CSD continues to unfold. With careful study using molecular techniques and defined culture methods, clinical syndromes and pathologic features of patients with CSD should be further defined. Most likely, a majority of the patients have infection with *B. henselae* and a few may have *A. felis* or other organisms.

Characteristics of the Pathogen

Bartonella henselae

This organism was first cultured by using a lysis-centrifugation blood culture system and was originally named *Rochalimaea henselae*, after Diane Hensel, a microbiologist who first isolated the organism from the blood of a patient at the University of Oklahoma.[19, 20] In 1993, the genera *Bartonella* and *Rochalimaea* were unified after DNA relatedness data, base content, and phenotypic similarities were recognized, with the result that the organism is now known as *B. henselae*.[31] It is a member of the α-2 subgroup of the class Proteobacteria but is distinct from the branch that contains *A. felis*. *B. henselae* is a small, curved gram-negative bacillus that grows best on fresh chocolate agar plates or heart infusion agar with 5% rabbit blood, incubated at 35°C to 37°C in 5% to 10% carbon dioxide with high humidity. Primary isolation usually requires 5 to 15 days from blood and 7 to 60 days from tissue. The whitish colonies are dry, adherent, and embedded in the agar, and with multiple passages they become less dry and larger and the time to visualization decreases. The organism is motile by the wet mount method and utilization of carbohydrates is undetectable. The organism is catalase- and urease-negative and does not reduce nitrate or hydrolyze esculin. It is weakly oxidase-positive when tested using the Kovacs method for the oxidase tests.[19, 20] A MicroScan Rapid Anaerobe Identification Panel can be used along with phenotypic characteristics to suggest to the technologist that *Bartonella* species have been isolated, but currently molecular techniques or analysis of cellular fatty acids is needed to confirm the identification.[32] A chemically defined liquid medium containing hemin, developed by Wong and associates,[33] allows recovery of *B. henselae* (and theoretically *A. felis*) from tissue after only 10 to 16 days of incubation. *B. henselae* has been cultured from cats,[23, 34] but a serologic response to *B. quintana* alone has been found in some cats.[35] Other species of *Bartonella* may have a role in patients with findings similar to those of CSD (see Chapter 228).

Afipia felis

The organism is a gram-negative, oxidase-positive rod in the α-2 subgroup of the class Proteobacteria. It was first cultured using brain-heart infusion biphasic medium incubated 1 to 6 days at 32°C aerobically. It is motile and grows on buffered charcoal–yeast extract agar and in nutrient broth. It grows best at 32°C and poorly at 35°C. Colonies are gray-white, glistening, convex, and opaque. It reduces nitrate and produces acid oxidatively from D-xylose in a delayed, weak reaction. It is catalase-, citrate-, and D-mannitol–negative and urease-positive.[13] It reportedly exists in a cell wall–defective form, but observations on *B. henselae* cast doubt on this finding. The genus name is taken from the initials of the Armed Forces Institute of Pathology (AFIP), where it was first cultured, and the species designation after *felis* for cat.[13]

Epidemiology

CSD occurs throughout the world where humans have contact with cats. It has been reported from many different countries and throughout the United States. Some authors have suggested that the disease is more common between August and December, and others have observed that the disease is seasonal only in temperate climates and occurs in the seasons when cats spend more time indoors, such as during the winter in the northern climates and during the summer and fall in the southern states.[6, 10, 36] Seasonal patterns may reflect variations in the flea population parasitizing the cats, if transmission of the organism parallels transmission of other *Bartonella* species in small mammals. There do not appear to be epidemics of the disease, although there are periods during which physicians are more aware of the disease and thus report it more often. Accurate epidemiologic studies are difficult because the disease is not easily recognized or diagnosed definitively, and most patients with a diagnosis of CSD rarely require admission to the hospital. It has been estimated that 22,000 cases occur each year in the United States and that 2000 patients are hospitalized.[36] Thus, studies of hospital discharge data are not adequate to map the disease.

Traditionally, CSD is a disease of children who have had contact with a kitten. Studies by Margileth and Carithers suggest that about 80% of the cases occur in children, with the highest number occurring in children between 3 and 12 years old.[4, 5] The incidence of the disease is suspected to be between 6 and 9 cases per 100,000 people.[36, 37] It is slightly more common in boys than girls[4, 5] and is seen in households with kittens (a cat younger than 1 year) more often than households with older cats. In most series 90% to 95% of the patients have a history of a contact with a cat; 75% report a scratch or a bite and the disease may be transmitted by any close contact with a cat. It is thought that cases occurring after traumatic injury such as a splinter of wood or an insect bite are due to contact of the cat with the open wound, but proof is lacking. About 4% of the cases in one series occurred after contact with dogs[4] and a few cases have no history of animal contact. When considering the diagnosis in patients without animal contact the clinician should consider doing the skin test, serology, and/or a biopsy as these patients may have lymphadenopathy of another cause. Serologic reactivity or skin test reactivity is more likely to occur in cat owners, households of families of patients with CSD, and veterinary workers.[4, 5, 10] In a case-control study in Connecticut, CSD was strongly associated with owning a kitten, owning a kitten with fleas, and being scratched or bitten by a kitten.[24] The organism has been cultured from and can be transmitted by fleas.[36, 38]

B. henselae has been cultured from the blood of cats, who may remain bacteremic for long periods (several months) without showing any ill effects or disease.[34, 35, 37, 38] The method of acquisition of the organism by the cats is thought to be via the cat flea.[38] Experimental infection has been established in cats by inoculation of blood from an infected kitten.[37] Cats also mount an immune response to *B. henselae*.[24, 35] In general, only one case occurs per family, yet studies using the skin test showed that 18% of family members were positive, with a difference between family members who liked cats (19% reacted) and those who disliked cats (1.5% reacted to the skin test).

Pathogenesis

The organism of CSD invades the human by way of a cat scratch, bite, or lick. Silver-staining organisms can be seen on biopsy of a primary papule that forms within 3 to 10 days at the inoculation site.[9] Within about 2 to 3 weeks, patients develop regional lymphadenopathy involving one or multiple lymph nodes.[4] The histology of the lesions reflects the host response to the organism. Initially there is a neutrophilic response and bacteria can be seen around vessels and in microabscesses. Later in the disease, as the node enlarges, lymphoid hyperplasia occurs with stellate necrotizing granulomata.[4, 8] Some lymph nodes have caseous necrosis. Few organisms are found with the silver stain in the tissue in the later stages. The pathologic findings are nonspecific, and without the finding of the organism on Warthin-Starry staining or probing of the tissue with a *Bartonella*-specific primer, the diagnosis can only be suggested by the pathologist. About 10% of the nodes suppurate and a fistulous tract may form. The disease usually remits spontaneously in normal hosts but may involve the central nervous system, or other organs.[7, 39–45] In the immunocompromised patient, the clinical and pathologic manifestations of the disease are much different, and they are described in Chapter 228; in general, the organism density is greater and the patients are frequently bacteremic.

Clinical Manifestations

The most common presenting symptom of a patient with CSD is lymphadenopathy in the region draining the primary inoculation. Sites usually involved (in order of frequency) are the upper extremity, head and neck, and groin.[4, 6, 24] See Table 180–2. The papule at the inoculation site is often unrecognized by physicians not used to dealing with the disease or may disappear by the time the lymphadenopathy is recognized. In a study from Connecticut, only 25% of patients' charts indicated the presence of a primary papule.[24] This study was done using a survey mailed to physicians and may represent an atypical group of patients. In Carithers' study[4] of 1200 patients (including more than 250 he had seen as a primary care physician), 93% had a history of a lesion at the inoculation site. The lymphadenopathy develops during 2 to 3 weeks but sometimes is not noticed for up to 8 weeks. Approximately 30% to 50% of the patients have fever and as many as 9% have temperatures as high as 102°F to 105°F.[4, 5, 6, 24] In more than three quarters of the patients the disease is mild, although these patients may have generalized achiness, malaise, and anorexia. The lymphadenopathy usually disappears within 2 to 4 months. About 10% of the nodes suppurate and may require drainage or drain spontaneously. A few patients exhibit more unusual presentations, including

TABLE 180–2 ■ Presenting Features of Cat-Scratch Disease in Immunocompetent Patients

FEATURE	FREQUENCY (%)
Adenopathy	95–100
Upper extremity	46–65
Head and neck	26–28
Groin	15–18
Other	8
Inoculation lesion	25–93
Fever	25–48
Malaise or fatigue	20–45
Headache	13
Anorexia	10–14
Splenomegaly	8–12
Parinaud oculoglandular symptoms	3–6
Sore throat	3–9
Rash	3–4
Arthralgia	3
Conjunctivitis	2–7

Compiled from references 4–6 and 24.

Parinaud ocular glandular fever, central nervous system manifestations, fever of unknown origin, granulomatous hepatitis, pulmonary symptoms, or persistent fatigue.[39–49] The spectrum of neurologic symptoms and the list of unusual manifestations are given in Table 180–3. In some patients who present with meningoencephalitis, seizures (including status epilepticus) are the first recognized feature of CSD. Patients who are immunocompromised may develop widespread disease including the skin lesions of bacillary angiomatosis, peliosis or microabscesses of the liver and spleen, lytic bone lesions, lymphadenopathy, or persistent bacteremia.[10, 16, 41, 46] A review of these infections is given in Chapter 228.

Diagnosis

Diagnosis of CSD has traditionally relied on certain diagnostic criteria. These included (1) a history of animal contact with the presence of a scratch or primary skin or eye lesion, (2) regional lymphadenopathy developing about 2 weeks after contact, (3) negative studies for other causes, (4) a positive CSD skin test, and (5) a node biopsy revealing histopathologic features consistent with CSD.[4, 6] The difficulty with these criteria has been that only a few physicians use the cat-scratch antigen skin test, a serologic assay was not available until 1992, and most patients are not ill enough to warrant lymph node biopsy or require hospital admission.

In primary care practice today, the diagnosis of CSD is generally made clinically when a patient presents with lymphadenopathy after contact with a cat. The presence or history of a papule or pustule at the inoculation site in the absence of other causes of lymphadenopathy supports the diagnosis, and the clinician must rule out other causes of lymphadenopathy. A complete blood count with differential, a rapid plasma reagin test for syphilis, a Monospot or heterophile test for mononucleosis, and a purified protein derivative skin test rule out some more common or treatable causes of lymphadenopathy. Often physicians treat the patient with antibiotics active against usual suppurative bacteria, and in most series 50% to 75% of patients have received antibiotics before their lymph node biopsy or referral to a specialist.[4, 5, 24] When available, the cat-scratch skin test suggests the diagnosis if it is positive and results are available in 24 to 36 hours. Unfortunately, the test is not widely available, is not licensed by the U.S. Food and Drug Administration, is not standardized, and is prepared using material from infected human lymph nodes (after heating the prepared antigen to 56°C for 72 hours). False-negative results may be noted early in the illness. Serologic tests are available[22, 26, 50, 51] and should be positive by the time a lymph node biopsy would be required, but the timing of the immunoglobulin M or immunoglobulin G antibody response has not been studied conclusively.

One of the best clues to the diagnosis of CSD is the history of contact with cats. A careful history and consideration of the disease for every patient with chronic regional lymphadenopathy are required. If diagnostic needle aspiration is done, cultures for routine bacteria, mycobacteria, and fungi and cultures to detect *Bartonella* or *Afipia* species should be performed. If the clinical course is atypical and the lymphadenopathy does not resolve, biopsy should be considered to rule out malignancy or infectious causes other than CSD. Details of the microbiology of these species may be found in Chapter 228.

TABLE 180–3 ■ Cat-Scratch Disease: Unusual Clinical Manifestations

Neurologic involvement	Other
Meningoencephalitis	Granulomatous hepatitis
Combative behavior	Splenic granuloma or splenomegaly
Seizures, including status epilepticus	Fever of unknown origin
Coma	Lytic bone lesions
Neuroretinitis	Prolonged or recurrent bacteremia
Aseptic meningitis	Erythema nodosum
Facial nerve paralysis	Pleural effusion
Myelopathy	Atypical pneumonia
Radiculitis	Synovitis
Cerebral arteritis	Pancytopenia
	Chronic malaise or fatigue
	Thrombocytopenic purpura

Treatment

No treatment is required or has been proved effective in most of the cases of CSD. In the normal host with suspected CSD, the most important aspect of treatment is careful follow-up to ensure that the disease resolves spontaneously in 2 to 4 months. If fatigue is present, bed rest may be required, and the patient should avoid trauma to the involved nodes and to the abdomen if the spleen is enlarged. Sometimes analgesics such as aspirin, acetaminophen, or ibuprofen may be used for relief of tender nodes. Warm compresses may provide local relief. Incision and drainage of nodes are not recommended because a chronic sinus tract may develop and persist for months. Needle aspiration of a markedly enlarged lymph node may relieve pain as well as provide material for culture. Biopsy may be indicated to rule out neoplasm.

Systemic antibiotics have not been uniformly successful in normal hosts with CSD.[6, 10, 52–54] Although Collipp[55] reported oral trimethoprim-sulfamethoxazole effective, other investigators have found little improvement with this agent.[56] Rifampin and ciprofloxacin have been reported to be effective.[53] For immunocompromised patients, including those with human immunodeficiency virus infection, erythromycin has been successful in clearing the bacteremia and skin lesions associated with bacillary angiomatosis[10, 14, 57] (see Chapter 228). In vitro, *B. henselae* is susceptible to many agents including macrolides, tetracyclines, rifampin, amoxicillin, ceftriaxone, trimethoprim-sulfamethoxazole, and aminoglycosides.[58]

Prevention

The best way to prevent CSD is to avoid all contact with cats, especially kittens. Because there are more than 60 million cats in the United States, including one in up to 46% of American households,[59] CSD is difficult to prevent. The disease seems to occur more often in young cats, suggesting that protective immunity may occur in felines. It is possible that a vaccine could be developed that could be given to cats at birth to prevent the prolonged bacteremia with *B. henselae*.[60] A vaccine for humans could also be feasible.[24, 28] If fleas or ticks are found on cats, ridding pets of these vectors may decrease the disease in the animals and decrease the transmission to humans.

References

1. Carithers HA: Cat-scratch disease: Notes on its history. Am J Dis Child 119:200, 1970.
2. Debré R, Lany M, Jammet M-L, et al: La maladie des griffes de chat. Bull Mem Soc Med Hop Paris 66:76, 1950.

3. Daniels WB, MacMurray FG: Cat scratch disease: Report of 160 cases. JAMA 154:1247, 1954.
4. Carithers HA: Cat-scratch disease: An overview based on a study of 1,200 patients. Am J Dis Child 139:1124, 1985.
5. Margileth AM, Wear DJ, English CK: Systemic cat scratch disease: Report of 23 patients with prolonged or recurrent severe bacterial infection. J Infect Dis 155:390, 1987.
6. Margileth AM: Cat scratch disease: etiology, diagnosis, and therapy. Infect Med 10:38, 1993.
7. Carithers HA, Margileth AM: Cat-scratch disease: Acute encephalopathy and other neurologic manifestations. Am J Dis Child 145:98, 1991.
8. Wear DJ, Margileth AM, Hadfield TL, et al: Cat scratch disease: A bacterial infection. Science 221:1403, 1983.
9. Margileth AW, Wear DJ, Hadfield TL, et al: Cat-scratch disease: Bacteria in skin at the primary inoculation site. JAMA 252:928, 1984.
10. Adal KA, Cockerell CJ, Petri WA Jr: Cat scratch disease, bacillary angiomatosis, and other infections due to *Rochalimaea*. N Engl J Med 330:1509, 1994.
11. Gerber MA, MacAlister TJ, Ballow M, et al: The aetiological agent of cat scratch disease. Lancet 1:1236, 1985.
12. English CK, Wear DJ, Margileth AM, et al: Cat-scratch disease: Isolation and culture of the bacterial agent. JAMA 259:1347, 1988.
13. Brenner DJ, Hollis DG, Moss CW, et al: Proposal of *Afipia* gen. nov., with *Afipia felis* sp. nov. (formerly the cat scratch disease bacillus), *Afipia clevelandensis* sp. nov. (formerly the Cleveland Clinic Foundation strain), *Afipia broomeae* sp. nov., and three unnamed genospecies. J Clin Microbiol 29:2450, 1991.
14. Koehler JE, LeBoit PE, Egbert BM, et al: Cutaneous vascular lesions and disseminated cat-scratch disease in patients with the acquired immunodeficiency syndrome (AIDS) and AIDS-related complex. Ann Intern Med 109:449, 1988.
15. Kemper CA, Lombard CM, Deresinski SC, et al: Visceral bacillary epithelioid angiomatosis: Possible manifestations of disseminated cat scratch disease in the immunocompromised host: A report of two cases. Am J Med 89:216, 1990.
16. Schlossberg D, Morad Y, Krouse TB, et al: Culture-proved disseminated cat-scratch disease in acquired immunodeficiency syndrome. Arch Intern Med 149:1437, 1989.
17. Stoler MH, Bonfiglio TA, Steigbigel RT, et al: An atypical subcutaneous infection associated with acquired immune deficiency syndrome. Am J Clin Pathol 80:714, 1983.
18. Slater LN, Welch DF, Hensel D, Coody DW: A newly recognized fastidious gram-negative pathogen as a cause of fever and bacteremia. N Engl J Med 323:1587, 1990.
19. Welch DF, Pickett DA, Slater LN, et al: *Rochalimaea henselae* sp. nov., a cause of septicemia, bacillary angiomatosis, and parenchymal bacillary peliosis. J Clin Microbiol 30:275, 1992.
20. Regnery RL, Anderson BE, Clarridge JE III, et al: Characterization of a novel *Rochalimaea* species, *R. henselae* sp. nov., isolated from blood of a febrile, human immunodeficiency virus–positive patient. J Clin Microbiol 30:265, 1992.
21. Relman DA, Loutit JS, Schmidt TM, et al: The agent of bacillary angiomatosis: An approach to the identification of uncultured pathogens. N Engl J Med 323:1573, 1990.
22. Regnery RL, Olson JG, Perkins BA, et al: Serological response to "*Rochalimaea henselae*" antigen in suspected cat-scratch disease. Lancet 339:1443, 1992.
23. Regnery R, Martin M, Olson J: Naturally occurring "*Rochalimaea henselae*" infection in domestic cat. Lancet 340:557, 1992.
24. Zangwill KM, Hamilton DH, Perkins BA, et al: Cat scratch disease in Connecticut. N Engl J Med 329:8, 1993.
25. Waldvogel K, Regnery RL, Anderson BE, et al: Disseminated cat-scratch disease: Detection of *Rochalimaea henselae* in affected tissue. Eur J Pediatr 153:23, 1994.
26. Drancourt M, Birtles R, Chaumentin G, et al: New serotype of *Bartonella henselae* in endocarditis and cat-scratch disease. Lancet 347:441, 1996.
27. Anderson B, Sims K, Regnery R, et al: Detection of *Rochalimaea henselae* DNA in specimens from cat-scratch disease patients by PCR. J Clin Microbiol 32:942, 1994.
28. Dolan MJ, Wong MT, Regnery RL, et al: Syndrome of *Rochalimaea henselae* adenitis suggesting cat scratch disease. Ann Intern Med 118:331, 1993.
29. Raoult D, Drancourt M, Carta A, et al: *Bartonella (Rochalimaea) quintana* isolation in patient with chronic adenopathy, lymphopenia, and a cat. Lancet 343:977, 1994.
30. Alkan S, Morgan MB, Sandin RL, et al: Dual role for *Afipia felis* and *Rochalimaea henselae* in cat-scratch disease. Lancet 345:385, 1995.
31. Brenner DJ, O'Connor SP, Winkler HH, et al: Proposals to unify the genera *Bartonella* and *Rochalimaea*, with descriptions of *Bartonella quintana* comb. nov., *Bartonella vinsonii* comb. nov., *Bartonella henselae* comb. nov., and *Bartonella elizabethae* comb. nov., and to remove the family Bartonellaceae from the order Rickettsiales. Int J Syst Bacteriol 43:777, 1993.
32. Welch DF, Hensel DM, Pickett DA, et al: Bacteremia due to *Rochalimaea henselae* in a child: Practical identification of isolates in the clinical laboratory. J Clin Microbiol 31:2381, 1993.
33. Wong MT, Thornton DC, Kennedy RC, et al: A chemically defined liquid medium that supports primary isolation of *Rochalimaea (Bartonella) henselae* from blood and tissue specimens. J Clin Microbiol 33:742, 1995.
34. Kordick DL, Wilson KH, Sexton DJ, et al: Prolonged *Bartonella* bacteremia in cats associated with cat-scratch disease patients. J Clin Microbiol 33:3245, 1995.
35. Childs JE, Rooney JA, Cooper JL, et al: Epidemiologic observations on infection with *Rochalimaea* species among cats living in Baltimore, Md. J Am Vet Med Assoc 204:1775, 1994.
36. Jackson LA, Perkins BA, Wenger JD: Cat scratch disease in the United States: An analysis of three national databases. Am J Public Health 83:1707, 1993.
37. Koehler JE, Glaser CA, Tappero JW: *Rochalimaea henselae* infection: A new zoonosis with the domestic cat as reservoir. JAMA 271:531, 1994.
38. Chomel BB, Kasten RW, Floyd-Hawkins K, et al: Experimental transmission of *Bartonella henselae* by the cat flea. J Clin Microbiol 34:1952, 1996.
39. Lucey D, Dolan MJ, Moss CW, et al: Relapsing illness due to *Rochalimaea henselae* in immunocompetent hosts: Implication for therapy and new epidemiological associations. Clin Infect Dis 14:683, 1992.
40. Torres JR, Sanders CV, Strub RL, et al: Cat-scratch disease causing reversible encephalopathy. JAMA 240:1628, 1978.
41. Chrousos GA, Drack AV, Young M, et al: Neuroretinitis in cat scratch disease. J Clin Neuroophthalmol 10:92, 1990.
42. Hadley S, Albrecht MA, Tarsy D: Cat-scratch encephalopathy: A cause of status epilepticus and coma in a healthy young adult. Neurology 45:196, 1995.
43. Drancourt M, Donnet A, Pelletier J, et al: Acute meningoencephalitis associated with seroconversion to "*Afipia felis.*" Lancet 340:558, 1992.
44. Golnik KC, Marotto ME, Fanous MM, et al: Ophthalmic manifestations of *Rochalimaea* species. Am J Ophthalmol 118:145, 1994.
45. Sweeney VP, Drance SM: Optic neuritis and compressive neuropathy associated with cat scratch disease. Can Med Assoc J 103:1380, 1970.
46. Dangman BC, Albanese BA, Kacica MA: Cat scratch disease in two children presenting with fever of unknown origin: Imaging features and association with a new causative agent, *Rochalimaea henselae*. Pediatrics 95:767, 1995.
47. Koranyi K: Fever, back pain and pleural effusion in a four-year-old-boy. Pediatr Infect Dis J 13:657, 1994.
48. Abbasi S, Chesney PJ: Pulmonary manifestations of cat-scratch disease; a case report and review of the literature. Pediatr Infect Dis J 14:547, 1995.
49. Malatack JJ, Jaffe R: Granulomatous hepatitis in three children due to cat-scratch disease without peripheral adenopathy. Am J Dis Child 147:949, 1993.
50. Barka NE, Hadfield T, Patnaik M, et al: EIA for detection of *Rochalimaea henselae*–reactive IgG, IgM, and IgA antibodies in patients with suspected cat-scratch disease. J Infect Dis 167:1503, 1993.
51. Schwartzman WA, Patnaik M, Barka NE, et al: *Rochalimaea* antibodies in HIV-associated neurologic disease. Neurology 44:1312, 1994.
52. Holley HP: Successful treatment of cat-scratch disease with ciprofloxacin. JAMA 265:1563, 1991.
53. Mui BSK, Mulligan ME, George WL: Response of HIV-associated disseminated cat scratch disease to treatment with doxycycline. Am J Med 89:229, 1990.

54. Bogue CW, Wise JD, Gray GF, et al: Antibiotic therapy for cat-scratch disease? JAMA 262:813, 1989.
55. Collipp PJ: Cat-scratch disease therapy. Am J Dis Child 143:1261, 1989.
56. Margileth AM: Antibiotic therapy for cat-scratch disease: Clinical study of therapeutic outcome in 268 patients and a review of the literature. Pediatr Infect Dis J 11:474, 1992.
57. Tompkins DC, Steigbigel RT: *Rochalimaea's* role in cat scratch disease and bacillary angiomatosis. Ann Intern Med 118:388, 1993.
58. Maurin M, Raoult D: Antimicrobial susceptibility of *Rochalimaea quintana, Rochalimaea vinsonii*, and the newly recognized *Rochalimaea henselae*. J Antimicrob Chemother 32:587, 1993.
59. Margileth AM, Hayden GF: Cat scratch disease: From feline affection to human infection. N Engl J Med 329:53, 1993.
60. Anderson B, Lu E, Jones D, Regnery R: Characterization of a 17-kilodalton antigen of *Bartonella henselae* reactive with sera from patients with cat scratch disease. J Clin Microbiol 33:2358, 1995.

181

Trichinosis

Peter M. Schantz
Marco K. Michelson

History

Trichinella cysts were first recognized in 1835 when, in the midst of an anatomic dissection, Paget noted distinct white flecks distributed throughout a muscle specimen. Microscopic examination of this material revealed what was to become recognized as the typical trichina cyst containing a dormant larva. However, the association between the encysted organism and the ingestion of contaminated meat products was not realized until 1850, when Herbst demonstrated that the carcass of a badger fed trichinous meat could transfer cysts to the musculature of dogs that ate meat from the carcass. The first recognized fatality associated with this organism was documented by Zenker in 1860, when postmortem examination of a young woman dying of presumed typhoid fever revealed a heavy infection with *Trichinella* larvae. In 1862, Friedreich diagnosed and described the first clinical case of acute trichinosis.[1] Current knowledge of the nematode parasites and the diseases they cause have been reviewed.[2]

Etiology

Trichinosis is an infection caused by tissue-dwelling nematodes of the genus complex *Trichinella*. Formerly, the etiologic agent was considered a monotypic nematode species, *Trichinella spiralis*. However, accumulating evidence of variation in transmission cycles, infectivity to experimental hosts, and biochemical and genetic characteristics has led to taxonomic revision. At least five genetically distinct species exist that vary according to major reservoir hosts and geographic distribution; all are capable of infecting humans.[2, 3] *T. spiralis*, acquired through the domestic pig, is responsible for most of the infections in the United States and Europe. *Trichinella nelsoni*, transmitted to humans through wild pigs, is found in Africa and southern Europe. *Trichinella nativa* is contracted by eating Arctic game (e.g., bear, walrus, fox). *Trichinella britovi* occurs in a variety of carnivores but not domestic swine in northern Europe. *Trichinella pseudospiralis* primarily infects birds and has not yet been implicated in human disease.[2, 3]

Epidemiology

Human outbreaks of trichinosis were documented as early as 1845. Outbreaks occurring in 1849, 1862, and 1865 in Germany were associated with mortalities of 19%, 17%, and 30%, respectively. Clinical trichinosis was first recognized in the United States by Krombein in 1864. By the 1880s this disease was recognized worldwide.[1] In the United States, numerous outbreaks involving hundreds of cases were subsequently reported in the literature.

Studies conducted on samples of diaphragmatic muscle obtained from hospitals throughout the United States from 1936 to 1941 revealed the magnitude of trichinosis. Of 5113 cadavers examined, one of every six samples tested (16.7%) had *Trichinella* organisms.[4] National reporting of trichinosis, however, did not begin until 1947, at which time 451 cases and 14 related deaths were documented.[5] The incidence of this disease has declined (Fig. 181–1) as a result of legislation prohibiting the feeding of raw garbage to swine (Federal Swine Health Protection Act of 1980), widespread commercial and home freezing of pork, and increased public awareness of the dangers of eating inadequately cooked pork products.[5] From 1982 to 1986, an annual average of only 57 cases was reported, along with three associated fatalities.[6]

Currently, most infections are outbreak associated,[6] which accounts for the great variability in total case numbers from year to year. Outbreaks are commonly associated with ethnic groups that prefer pork raw, partially cooked, or lightly processed. Immigrants from Southeast Asia appear to be especially at risk because of their preference for raw spiced pork. The greater incidence of human trichinosis in the northeastern United States (Table 181–1) probably results, in part, from the greater concentration of ethnic groups (e.g., German, Italian, Eastern European) that have a fondness for lightly cooked sausage dishes.

Gender does not seem to be a factor; 60% of patients are 20 to 49 years old. Case reporting from December through March consistently increases, probably a result of homemade pork products eaten during the holiday season.[6]

Although the decline in cases is related to a decrease in infections acquired from commercial pork, pork products continue to be the major source of trichinosis in the United States (Table 181–2). As the number of cases caused by commercial pork products has decreased, the percentage of cases associated with noncommercial pork (purchased directly from the farm) and wild game (bear, walrus) has increased (see Table 181–2). These will probably continue to be important sources of infection.[6]

Pathogenesis

Trichinosis is acquired by eating raw or inadequately cooked meat products containing encysted larvae (Fig. 181–2). Larvae are released after gastric digestion of the cyst wall and lodge in the mucosa of the small bowel. Within 48 hours, female worms mature and are fertilized. Larval deposition begins within days. Each female worm is capable of producting up to 1500 larvae during its lifetime. Larviposition generally continues for approximately 5 weeks.[7] Newborn

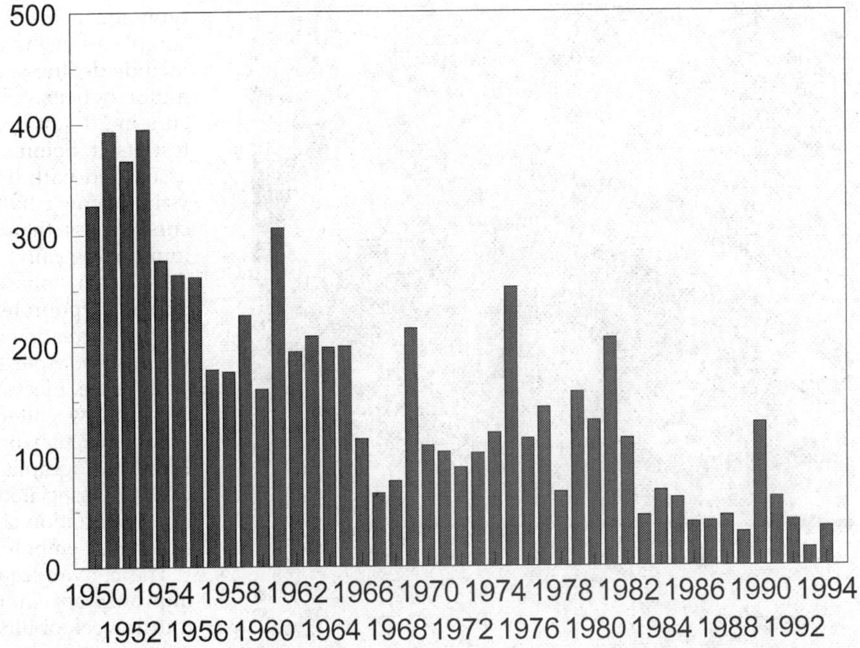

FIGURE 181–1 ▫ Decline in reported trichinosis cases in the United States, 1950 to 1994. (Data from Division of Parasitic Diseases, National Center for Infectious Diseases, Centers for Disease Control and Prevention, Atlanta.)

larvae penetrate the mucosa to enter the capillaries and lymphatics of the small intestine, from which they are distributed systemically. Immature larvae that reach striated muscle will enter and induce the myocyte to differentiate into a "nurse-cell" unit, which subsequently contributes to and supports the process of encystation. These cystic structures may begin to calcify as early as 6 months after the initial infection. However, larvae may remain viable within cysts for several years. If infection occurs in wild game or animals destined for slaughter, the cycle may be reinitiated when a human eats the infected meat. Larvae that reach nonstriated muscles or other tissues do not encyst. These larvae continue to migrate within the tissues, which results in marked inflammation and local tissue necrosis. Although this process is usually self-limited, severe multiorgan disease and chronic sequelae may develop.

TABLE 181–1 ▪ Regional Cases of Trichinosis in the United States, 1975 to 1986

REGION	NUMBER OF CASES (% OF TOTAL) IN INDICATED REGION 1975–1981	1982–1986
Northeast*	589 (55.3)	163 (56.8)
Midwest†	166 (15.6)	17 (5.9)
South‡	131 (12.3)	47 (16.4)
Mountain West§	79 (7.4)	37 (12.9)
Alaska	101 (9.5)	23 (8.0)
Total	1066	287

*Includes Maine, New Hampshire, Vermont, Massachusetts, Rhode Island, Connecticut, New York, New Jersey, and Pennsylvania.

†Includes Ohio, Indiana, Illinois, Michigan, Wisconsin, Minnesota, Iowa, Missouri, North Dakota, South Dakota, Nebraska, and Kansas.

‡Includes Delaware; Maryland; Washington, DC; Virginia; West Virginia; North Carolina; South Carolina; Georgia; Florida; Kentucky; Tennessee; Alabama; Mississippi; Arkansas; Louisiana; Oklahoma; and Texas.

§Includes Montana, Idaho, Wyoming, Colorado, New Mexico, Arizona, Utah, Nevada, Washington, Oregon, California, and Hawaii.

From Bailey TM, Schantz PM: Trends in the incidence and transmission patterns of human trichinellosis in the United States, 1982–1986. Rev Infect Dis 12:5–11, 1990.

Immunology

Murine models of trichinosis suggest that humoral and cellular mechanisms both play a role in host defense. Several stage-specific parasite antigens have been isolated and shown to induce antibody responses in infected animals.[8] Specific antibodies generated against these determinants may act in concert with granulocyte or macrophage effector cells to destroy the worm.[9, 10] In addition, challenging a previously infected animal with an oral dose of *Trichinella* larvae results in more rapid mucosal expulsion of worms than occurs in naive controls. This process may depend on the interaction of worm antigens and mucosal mast cells that have been sensitized with immunoglobulin E. Mast cell degranulation and the associated release of proinflammatory mediators produce a local reaction consisting of increased vascular permeability; mucosal edema; increased movement of fluid from tissue to lumen; and influx of cellular constituents, such as

TABLE 181–2 ▪ Cases of Trichinosis by Reported Food Source

FOOD SOURCE	NUMBER OF CASES (% OF TOTAL) FROM INDICATED FOOD SOURCE 1975–1981	1982–1986
Pork products		
Domestic pig	740 (69.4)	172 (59.9)
Wild pig	9 (0.8)	22 (7.7)
Subtotal	749	194
Nonpork products		
Bear meat	64 (6.0)	42 (14.6)
Other wild animal	68 (6.4)	2 (0.7)
Ground beef*	67 (6.3)	12 (4.2)
Subtotal	199	56
Unknown	118 (11.1)	37 (12.9)
Total	1066	287

*Mixed with pork during processing.

From Bailey TM, Schantz PM: Trends in the incidence and transmission patterns of human trichinellosis in the United States, 1982–1986. Rev Infect Dis 12:5–11, 1990.

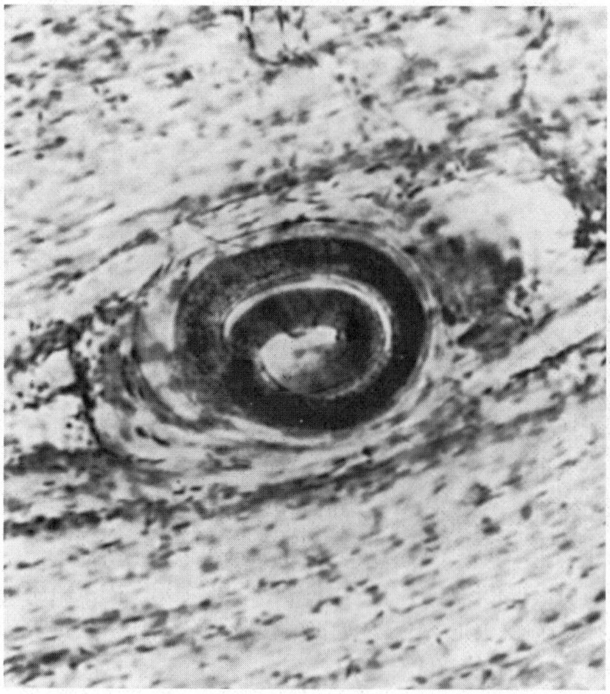

FIGURE 181–2 □ Section of striated muscle demonstrating encysted *Trichinella* larva.

eosinophils, that are capable of eliminating this organism.[11, 12] Cellular mechanisms of immunity that may become operative in the later phases of infection are still poorly understood. However, work has suggested that lymphocyte populations are important in both modulating immunologic reactivity to *Trichinella*[12] and modifying the surface composition of enterocyte membranes, which may affect parasite attachment.[13] Little is known about the mechanism of encystation or the factors that maintain the nurse-cell unit in an immunocompetent host.

Clinical Manifestations

Most *Trichinella* infections are asymptomatic or mildly symptomatic and are therefore undiagnosed. Clinical symptoms often correlate with the number of infective larvae ingested and parallel the developmental stages of the organism in the human host. Thus, the predominant clinical features of trichinosis are frequently grouped into intestinal, visceral (muscular), and convalescent phases. The intestinal phase corresponds to the period of larval penetration of intestinal mucosa and generally begins within 7 days of the ingestion of infected food. Symptoms during this phase include malaise, nausea, vomiting, epigastric or right lower quadrant pain, diarrhea, constipation, and low-grade fever.

Visceral involvement manifests itself as early as the second week or as late as the eighth week of illness and represents newborn larval dissemination to striated musculature and other organs. Initial findings include headache, intermittent or remittent fever, chills, cough, diaphoresis, muscle pain and tenderness, periorbital or facial edema, conjunctivitis, subconjuctival hemorrhages, splinter hemorrhages, peripheral edema, diarrhea, constipation, and pruritus. The various types of rashes that occur shortly after the onset of muscular symptoms include folliculitis, furunculosis, herpes labialis, herpes zoster, urticaria, dermatographia, petechiae, and maculopapular eruptions resembling those seen in scarlet fever, typhoid, measles, and secondary syphilis. Major neurologic complications, which develop in 10% to 24% of serious cases, include deafness, encephalitis, generalized seizures, and focal motor deficits. Clinically significant myocarditis, which occurs in 20% of hospitalized patients, usually does not manifest itself before the fourth week of illness. This may be associated with hypotension, congestive heart failure, paroxysmal tachyarrhythmias, and sudden death. Pneumonitis occurs in less than 5% of hospitalized patients and may be immunologically mediated.[1, 14, 15] Laboratory abnormalities during this phase of illness include leukocytosis, eosinophilia, hypoproteinemia, hypoalbuminemia, hypokalemia, elevated creatine kinase and aldolase levels, and mild elevations in aspartate aminotransferase and alanine aminotransferase. Electrocardiographic changes are nonspecific and include low voltage, flattening or inversion of T waves, and atrioventricular or intraventricular conduction disturbances. Chest radiographs may reveal transient pulmonary infiltrates with an associated pleural reaction or, rarely, multiple areas of consolidation characteristic of pulmonary vasculitis or disseminated emboli.[1, 14]

The convalescent phase is heralded by lysis of fever and improvement in muscular symptoms during the third to fourth week of illness. Although recovery is usually complete within a few months, fatigue, weakness, and diarrhea may persist for months after the initial infection.[14, 16] It has been suggested that chronic allergic symptoms, myalgias, fever, and a variety of nonspecific complaints may recur for months to years after the primary syndrome resolves.[17–19] However, other studies indicate that this is a rare phenomenon and dispute the notion of a distinct chronic process.[20–23]

Diagnosis

The syndrome of myositis, periorbital edema, fever, and eosinophilia in a person who has recently eaten undercooked meat products suggests the diagnosis of trichinosis.

A variety of serologic tests have been developed to detect the human antibody response to antigens from infective muscle stage larvae. The most commonly used is the bentonite flocculation test. A colloidal suspension of aluminum silicate particles (bentonite), to which *Trichinella* antigen is bound, is incubated with serial dilutions of serum from a suspected case. Agglutination of these particles at a dilution of 1:5 or greater represents the presence of specific antibody and denotes a positive test.[24] Alternative methods of detection include indirect hemagglutination, larval precipitin, enzyme-linked immunosorbent assay, and counterimmunoelectrophoresis. With the exception of the enzyme-linked immunosorbent assay, however, lack of standardization, expense, and complexity have limited the general availability of these techniques. All serologic tests are limited by their inability to detect infection until approximately the third to fourth week of infection. Moreover, the frequent persistence of circulating antibody for months or years complicates the interpretation of a single positive test. Thus, serologic testing is most useful in conjunction with a thorough clinical evaluation.[7]

A definitive diagnosis of acute trichinosis can be made by demonstrating encysted, uncalcified larvae in muscle tissue. Unfortunately, encystation is not evident in biopsy specimens until at least the third to fourth week of infection. Preferred sampling sites include the deltoid and the gastrocnemius muscles.

Skin testing is considered unreliable for the diagnosis of acute trichinosis and has been supplanted by more sensitive serologic tests.

Ova and parasite examination of stool specimens is a low-yield procedure. This is because adult *Trichinella* organisms do not produce eggs, newborn larvae are rapidly disseminated systemically from their submucosal location, and adult worms are rarely found in feces.

Differential Diagnosis

The nonspecificity of many of the symptoms associated with trichinosis results in frequent misdiagnosis. This is particularly true during the intestinal phase, when the symptoms are often confused with those of viral gastroenteritis or food poisoning. Components of the visceral phase should be distinguished from serum sickness, dermatomyositis, periarteritis nodosa, angioneurotic edema, periorbital cellulitis, periorbital abscess, cavernous sinus thrombosis, typhoid fever, rheumatic fever, trypanosomiasis, hypothyroidism, and congestive heart failure. Myositis associated with eosinophilia may also occur in the setting of visceral larva migrans and, rarely, cysticercosis. Neurologic involvement may be confused with meningitis, encephalitis, cerebral infarct, or polyneuritis. Cardiac involvement may mimic viral or bacterial myocarditis, endocarditis, or ischemic cardiomyopathy. Pulmonary findings may suggest the diagnosis of pneumonia or congestive heart failure.[1, 14, 25–27]

Treatment

The most effective agents yet developed for the treatment of trichinosis are the benzimidazole compounds.

Murine models suggest that infection detected during the intestinal phase of infection may be treated with mebendazole, 7.5 mg/kg by mouth (PO) twice a day (bid) for 3 days.[28] Pyrantel pamoate has also shown promise in animal models and may prove to be an alternative agent (10 mg/kg as a single dose, PO every day [qd] for 4 days) in this setting.[14] Prophylaxis with these agents may effectively prevent evolution of disease if they are taken within a few days of eating contaminated food.[18, 29]

During the visceral phase of infection, mebendazole, 5 mg/kg PO bid for 10 to 13 days, is more active against encysted muscle larva and it is better tolerated.[30, 31] Thiabendazole, 25 mg/kg PO bid for 5 days,[31] may also be used, although the effectiveness of this agent against the encysted phase of the parasite is not clearly established and adverse reactions are common and sometimes life threatening. Albendazole, given in a dose of 400 mg PO bid for 14 days, is probably the most effective drug. Concurrent administration of corticosteroids (prednisone, 40 to 60 mg PO qd) is indicated in severe disease characterized by incapacitating symptoms; prolonged or recurrent fever; intense hypersensitivity reactions occurring during the course of the illness or as a complication of therapy; and cardiac, pulmonary, or neurologic involvement.

Infection acquired during pregnancy has resulted in spontaneous abortion, fetal death, placental parasitism, and transplacental passage of larvae.[14, 32] However, use of the benzimidazole preparations during pregnancy can cause significant toxicity to the embryo and should be undertaken with caution.[31]

Rarely, this infection occurs in an unusual location[33] or as a solitary mass[34] that is incidentally diagnosed as trichinosis only after surgical exploration. These lesions most often result from inflammation associated with old or calcified muscle cysts and do not necessarily require additional drug therapy after surgical excision.

Prevention

Reliable methods of killing *T. spiralis* larvae in meat up to 6 inches thick include cooking to 170°F (77°C) or freezing at 5°F (−15°C) for a minimum of 20 days. Shorter periods of freezing may be effective at lower temperatures. Thus, freezing at −10°F (−23.3°C) would be required for only 10 days, and a temperature of −20°F (−28.9°C) would be effective after only 6 days. The larvae of *T. nativa*, however, are more resistant to freezing temperatures and may not be completely inactivated.[35, 36]

Curing (salting), drying, and smoking, except under rigidly defined conditions, may not be consistently effective in removing infective larvae. In addition, microwave cooking may not maintain meat at a sufficiently uniform temperature to guarantee elimination of all larvae.[35, 36] Low levels of ionizing radiation (0.15 kGy) applied to infected pork prevents development of the parasites.[37] Although this process is now approved by the U.S. Food and Drug Administration, its application for control of trichinosis requires acceptance by consumers and the industry.

The complete elimination of trichinosis in the United States ultimately depends on the active enforcement of the Federal Swine Health Protection Act, proper hog management practices, detection and elimination of infected herds, continued public education on the most reliable methods of preparing pork products, and increasing public awareness of the risk of contracting trichinosis from noncommercial sources of pork and wild game.[38]

References

1. Gould SE: Trichinosis in Man and Animals. Springfield, IL, Charles C Thomas, 1970.
2. Murrell KD, Bruschi F: Clinical trichinosis. Prog Clin Parasitol 4:117, 1994.
3. Pozio E, La Rosa G, Murrell KD, Lichtenfels R: Taxonomic revision of the genus *Trichinella*. J Parasitol 78:654, 1992.
4. Wright WH, Kerr KB, Jacobs L: Studies on trichinosis. XV. Summary of the findings of *Trichinella spiralis* in a random sampling and other samplings of the population of the United States. Public Health Rep 58:1293, 1943.
5. Schantz PM: Trichinosis in the United States, 1947–1981. Food Technol March:83, 1983.
6. Bailey TM, Schantz PM: Trends in the incidence and transmission patterns of human trichinellosis in the United States, 1982–1986. Rev Infect Dis 12:5, 1990.
7. Despommier DD: Trichinellosis. *In* Walls KW, Schantz PM (eds): Immunodiagnosis of Parasitic Diseases, Vol 1, Helminthic Diseases. Orlando, FL, Academic Press, 1986, pp 163–181.
8. Despommier DD: Antigens of *Trichinella spiralis*. *In* Kim CW (ed): Trichinellosis: Proceedings of the Sixth International Conference on Trichinosis, July 8–12, 1984, Quebec, Canada. Albany, NY, State University of New York Press, 1985, pp 8–16.
9. Gansmuller A, Anteunis A, Venturiello SM, et al: Nature of the cells involved in the "in vitro" immune cytotoxicity of newborn *Trichinella spiralis* larvae. *In* Kim CW (ed): Trichinellosis: Proceedings of the Sixth International Conference on Trichinosis, July 8–12, 1984, Quebec, Canada. Albany, NY, State University of New York Press, 1985, pp 47–51.
10. Kazura JW: Host defense mechanisms against nematode parasites: Destruction of newborn *Trichinella spiralis* larvae by human antibodies and granulocytes. J Infect Dis 143:712, 1981.
11. Wakelin D, Denham DA: The immune response. *In* Campbell WC (ed): *Trichinella* and Trichinosis. New York, Plenum Publishing, 1983, pp 265–308.
12. Castro GA, Russell DA: Immunopathology of enteric phase of trichinellosis. *In* Kim CW (ed): Trichinellosis: Proceedings of the Sixth International Conference on Trichinosis, July 8–12, 1984, Quebec, Canada. Albany, NY, State University of New York Press, 1985, pp 17–25.
13. Grencis RK, Wakelin D: Analysis of lymphocyte subsets involved in mediation of intestinal immunity to *Trichinella spiralis* in the mouse. *In* Kim CW (ed): Trichinellosis: Proceedings of the Sixth International Conference on Trichinosis, July 8–12, 1984, Quebec, Canada. Albany, NY, State University of New York Press, 1985, pp 26–30.

14. Pawlowski ZS: Clinical aspects in man. *In* Campbell WC (ed): *Trichinella* and Trichinosis. New York, Plenum Publishing, 1983, pp 367–401.
15. Januszkiewicz J: Participation of the respiratory system in trichinosis. Epidemiol Rev 21:169, 1967.
16. MacLean JD, Viallet J, Law C, Staudt M: Trichinosis in the Canadian Arctic: Report of five outbreaks and a new clinical syndrome. J Infect Dis 160:513, 1989.
17. Kozar Z, Sladki E, Zolnierkowa D: Clinical aspects of chronic trichinellosis in people. Parts 1–3. Wiad Parazytol 10:651, 1964.
18. Ozeretskovskaya NN, Pereverzeva EV, Tumolskaya NI, et al: Benzimidazoles in the treatment and prophylaxis of synanthropic and sylvatic trichinellosis. *In* Kim CW, Pawlowski ZS (eds): Trichinellosis. Hanover, NH, University Press of New England, 1978, pp 381–393.
19. Froscher W, Gullotta F, Saathoff M, Tackmann W: Chronic trichinosis: Clinical, bioptic, serological, and electromyographic observations. Eur Neurol 28:221, 1988.
20. Cox PM, Schultz MG, Kagan IG, Preizler J: Trichinosis: Five-year serologic and clinical follow-up. Am J Epidemiol 89:651, 1969.
21. Kassur B, Januszkiewicz J: On the inappropriateness of the idea of chronic trichinellosis. Epidemiol Rev 24:68, 1970.
22. Chodera L, Gerwel C, Kociecka W, Pawlowski Z: On the problem of late clinical sequelae of human trichinellosis. Wiad Parazytol 20:125, 1974.
23. Harms G, Binz P, Feldmeier H, et al: Trichinosis: A prospective controlled study of patients ten years after acute infection. Clin Infect Dis 17:637, 1993.
24. Kagan IG: Diagnostic, epidemiologic, and experimental parasitology: Immunologic aspects. Am J Trop Med Hyg 28:429, 1979.
25. Frayha RA: Trichinosis-related polyarteritis nodosa. Am J Med 71:307, 1981.
26. Herrera R, Varela E, Morales G, et al: Dermatomyositis-like syndrome caused by trichinae—Report of two cases. J Rheumatol 12:782, 1985.
27. Bia FJ, Barry M: Parasitic infections of the central nervous system. Neurol Clin 4:171, 1986.
28. McCracken RO, Garcia A, Robins HG: Mebendazole therapy of enteral trichinellosis. J Parasitol 68:259, 1982.
29. Gerwel C, Pawlowski Z, Mochecka W, Chodera L: Probable sterilization of *Trichinella spiralis* by thiabendazole: Further clinical observations of human infections. *In* Kim CW (ed): Trichinellosis. New York, Intext, 1974, pp 471–475.
30. Campbell WC, Denham DA: Chemotherapy. *In* Campbell WC (ed): *Trichinella* and Trichinosis. New York, Plenum Publishing, 1983, pp 335–366.
31. Drugs for parasitic infections. Med Lett 36:104, 1994.
32. Bourns TKT: The discovery of trichina cysts in the diaphragm of a six-week-old child. J Parasitol 38:367, 1952.
33. Hansen LS, Allard RHB: Encysted parasitic larvae in the mouth. J Am Dent Assoc 108:632, 1984.
34. Snyderman NL: Trichinosis presenting as a neck mass. Laryngoscope 97:353, 1987.
35. Kagan IG: Trichinosis in the United States. Public Health Rep 74:159, 1959.
36. World Health Organization: Prevention of trichinellosis by meat hygiene and other measures. *In* Campbell WC, Griffiths RB, Mantovani A, et al (eds): Guidelines on Surveillance, Prevention, and Control of Trichinellosis. Rome, Collaborating Centre for Research and Training in Veterinary Public Health, Instituto Superiore di Sanita, 1988, pp 85–98.
37. Loaharanu P, Murrell D: A role for irradiation in the control of foodborne parasites. Trends Food Sci Technol 5:190, 1994.
38. Leighty JC: Control I: Public-health aspects (with special reference to the United States). *In* Campbell WC (ed): *Trichinella* and Trichinosis. New York, Plenum Publishing, 1983, pp 501–513.

182

Toxoplasmosis

Jack S. Remington
Rima McLeod

The term toxoplasmosis has been used, imprecisely, to refer to both infection and disease caused by *Toxoplasma gondii.* The distinction between infection and disease caused by this organism is important, clinically and epidemiologically.[1, 2] *Toxoplasma* infection refers to the presence of the protozoan in persons regardless of whether they have clinical manifestations. Toxoplasmosis refers to the disease caused by the organism. *Toxoplasma* infection is usually asymptomatic in older children and adults, but when signs and symptoms are present, they are usually of short duration (acute) and self-limited. Chronic *Toxoplasma* infection describes persistence of the organism in the cyst form without clinical manifestations. The term chronic toxoplasmosis is best reserved to describe the disease in which active *Toxoplasma* infection is the proven cause of persistent or recrudescent clinical manifestations (e.g., encephalitis in infants, myocarditis, chorioretinitis, lymphadenopathy). Throughout the world, *Toxoplasma* infection occurs with significantly greater frequency than toxoplasmosis.

Characteristics of the Pathogen

Classification of the Organism

T. gondii is an obligate intracellular protozoan. It has an enteroepithelial and extraintestinal cycle in members of the cat family and only an extraintestinal cycle in all other mammalian and avian hosts. The organism is classified among the Sporozoa and exists in three forms: tachyzoite, bradyzoites in cysts, and oocyst[3–7] (Fig. 182–1). The tachyzoite (see Fig. 182–1*A* to *C*) is crescent or oval shaped, one end pointed and the other rounded. It measures approximately 3 by 7 μm. It stains well with either Wright or Giemsa stain. The nucleus is centrally located, and there are no flagella, cilia, or pseudopodia. Tachyzoites are found in tissues during the acute stage of infection and invade all mammalian cells except nonnucleated erythrocytes. Multiplication is by endodyogeny (i.e., two *Toxoplasma* organisms form within each parent cell). Division continues until the host cell ruptures or a tissue cyst forms. Desiccation, freezing and thawing, and gastric secretions kill tachyzoites.

Tachyzoites can be propagated in the peritoneum of mice, in tissue culture, and in eggs. Antigens of tachyzoites are used in complement fixation and hemagglutination tests for diagnosis of *Toxoplasma* infection, and whole tachyzoites are used in the Sabin-Feldman dye test, the agglutination test, and the fluorescent antibody method.

Bradyzoites in Cysts

The tissue cyst (see Fig. 182–1*D* to *F*) develops within host cells and may contain thousands of organisms. Cysts range in size from 10 to 100 μm and stain well with periodic acid–Schiff stain. The cyst wall also stains with silver. Be-

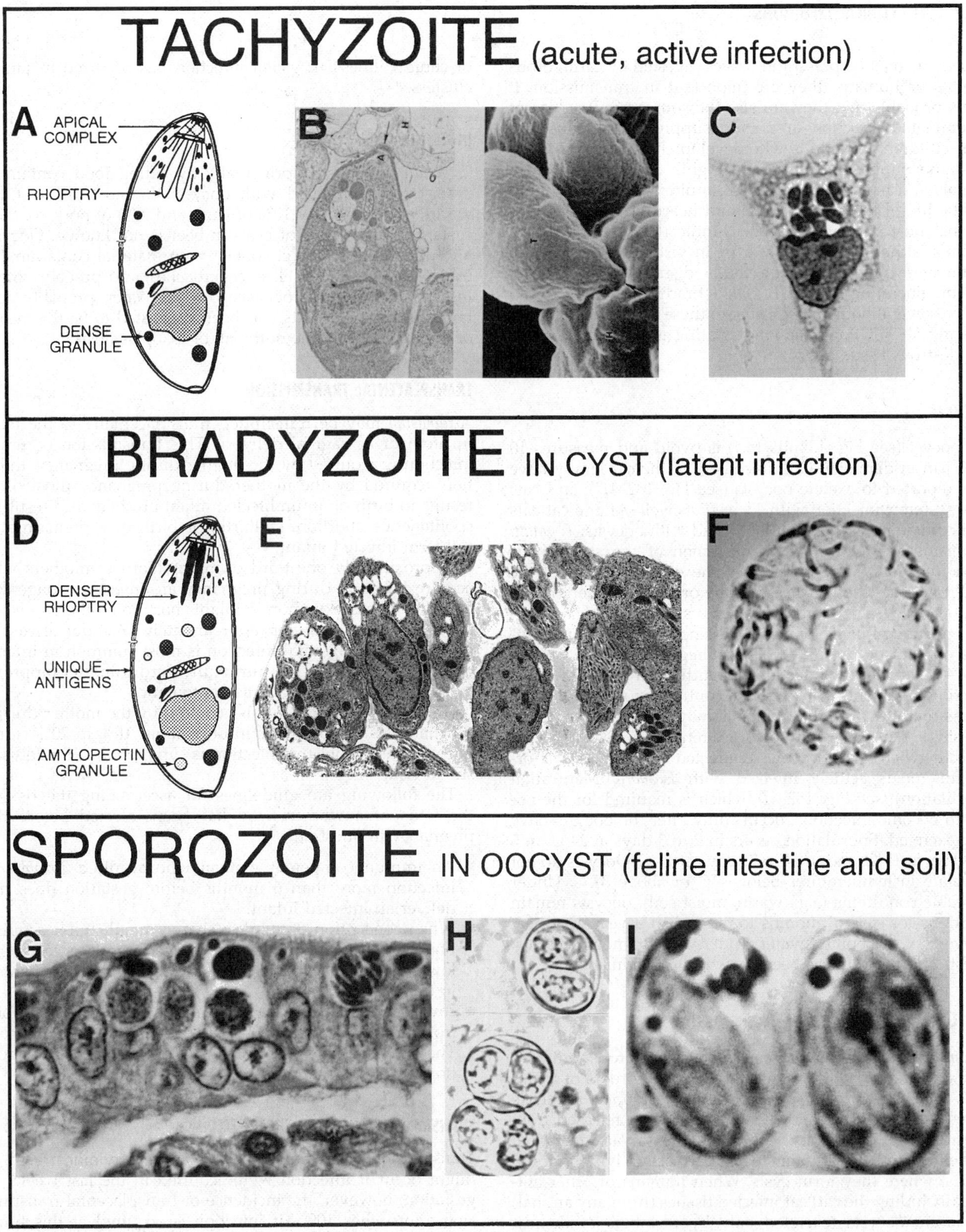

FIGURE 182–1 ▫ Stages of *Toxoplasma gondii.* Tachyzoites: *A,* schematic diagram; *B,* transmission and scanning electron micrographs of tachyzoite invading a host cell; *C,* light micrograph of tachyzoites replicating within a parasitophorous vacuole in the host cell cytoplasm. Bradyzoites: *D,* schematic diagram; *E,* transmission electron micrograph of cyst containing bradyzoites, with the arrow indicating amylopectin granules; *F,* light micrograph of cyst containing bradyzoites. Sporozoites: *G,* development of oocysts in cat intestine; *H,* oocysts in lumen of cat intestine; *I,* sporulating oocysts that contain sporozoites. (From Boyer K, McLeod R: *Toxoplasma gondii* [toxoplasmosis]. *In* Long SS, Proeber GC, Pickering LK [eds]: Principles and Practice of Pediatric Infectious Diseases. New York, Churchill Livingstone, 1996, pp 645–672. *A* from McLeod R, Mack D, Brown C: New advances in cellular and molecular biology of *Toxoplasma gondii.* Exp Parasitol 72:109–121, 1991; *B* and *C* from Aikawa M, Komata Y, Asai T, Midorikawa O: Transmission and scanning electron microscopy of host cell entry by *Toxoplasma gondii.* Am J Pathol 87:285–296, 1977; *F* from Weiss L, LaPlace D: Bradyzoite development in vitro. J Eukaryot Microbiol 42:150–157, 1995; *G* from Remington JS: In discussion, Lainson R: Observations on the nature and transmission of *Toxoplasma gondii* in light of its wide host and geographical range. Toxoplasmosis. Surv Ophthalmol 6:721–758, 1961; *H* and *J* from Dubey JP, Miller NL, Frenkel JK: The *Toxoplasma gondii* oocyst from cat feces. J Exp Med 132:636–662, 1970; *I* from Dubey JP, unpublished.)

cause cysts may be present in tissues ingested by carnivorous animals or humans, they are important in transmission. It seems probable that they are also the source of recrudescent disseminated infection in immunosuppressed persons and older children and adults who develop chorioretinitis. Cysts are demonstrable as early as the eighth day of infection in animals and may remain viable in multiple tissues throughout the life of the host. Skeletal and heart muscle and brain are the most common sites of chronic (latent) infection in humans, although cysts may exist in virtually every organ. Peptic and tryptic digestive fluids disrupt the cyst wall, thereby liberating viable *T. gondii* bradyzoites, which can survive several hours of exposure to these digestive enzymes. Freezing (−20°C) and thawing, heating to 60°C, or desiccation destroys tissue cysts.

Oocysts

The oocyst (see Fig. 182–1*G* to *I*) is ovoid and measures 10 to 12 μm in diameter. Only members of the cat family have been reported to excrete oocysts (see Fig. 182–1*H*), and cats have systemic infection with *T. gondii* as well. After a cat eats food containing cysts or contaminated with oocysts, *T. gondii* organisms are released into the lumen of the stomach or small intestine. After invasion of the epithelial cells of the small intestine (see Fig. 182–1*G*), the organism undergoes an asexual cycle (schizogony) and then a sexual cycle (gametogony), resulting in development of the noninfectious, unsporulated oocyst (see Fig. 182–1*H*). A cat begins to excrete oocysts 3 to 24 days after the infection, depending on the form of the infecting organism. This excretion continues for 7 to 20 days, and as many as 10 million oocysts may be shed in the feces in a single day. Renewed oocyst excretion has been reported to occur when a cat becomes reinfected with *Toxoplasma* organisms or is acutely infected with *Isospora*. Maturation (sporulation) (see Fig. 182–1*I*), which is required for the oocyst to become infectious, occurs only after the oocysts have been excreted. Sporulation occurs in 2 to 3 days at 24°C, in 5 to 8 days at 15°C, and in 14 to 21 days at 11°C. Oocysts do not sporulate in temperatures below 4°C or above 37°C. Under favorable conditions (e.g., warm, moist soil), oocysts remain infectious for several months to more than a year. Dry heat (above 66°C) or boiling water renders oocysts noninfectious. Ingestion of oocysts has been shown to cause infection.

Life Cycle and Modes of Transmission

T. gondii is ubiquitous and can infect herbivorous, omnivorous, and carnivorous animals, including all orders of mammals, some birds, and some reptiles. Most often it infects humans or other animals when organisms are released from ingested cysts or oocysts. The tachyzoites invade intestinal epithelium and spread hematogenously or via lymphatics to tissues, where they form cysts. When humans or other animals (including the cat) eat infected tissues (from any animal) or mature oocysts (excreted only by members of the cat family), the life cycle is completed. Members of the family Felidae, including both domestic and feral cats, appear to be the definitive hosts in this life cycle, because they are the only animals that are known to shed oocysts. Oocysts have been found in the feces of approximately 1% of cats in diverse areas of the world (including Costa Rica, Germany, Japan, and the United States).

Toxoplasma organisms are acquired mainly by ingestion and transplacental transmission, and less commonly through blood or leukocyte transfusion, organ transplantation,[8] and laboratory accident[9] (Fig. 182–2). Reinfection from an exogenous source occurs but has not been recognized as a cause of clinical illness. *T. gondii* infection has occurred in family clusters.[10]

INGESTION

T. gondii is acquired principally by eating food containing cysts or contaminated with oocysts. In most areas of the world, approximately 10% of lamb and 25% of pork contains cysts; the prevalence of cysts in beef is not known. Oocysts are ingested after direct contact with material contaminated by infected cat feces. Flies, cockroaches, and probably other insects can transport oocysts to food. Water, probably contaminated with oocysts, has been suggested to be the means of transmission in one outbreak of toxoplasmosis.[11]

TRANSPLACENTAL TRANSMISSION

Toxoplasma may be transmitted transplacentally to the fetus in utero or at vaginal delivery. This transmission occurs if infection is acquired by the mother during pregnancy. Infection acquired by the mother during pregnancy most often results in birth of an uninfected infant but may also result in spontaneous abortion, stillbirth, or birth of a premature or full-term infected infant.

Approximately one third of infants born to mothers who acquire infection during pregnancy are infected. Congenital infection is least common in infants born to mothers infected during the first trimester (approximately 17%) but disease is most severe; congenital infection is most common in infants born to mothers infected during the third trimester (approximately 65%) but is usually asymptomatic.

Toxoplasma infection that is acquired by the mother during pregnancy is symptomatic in only about 10% to 20% cases, but whether or not the infection is symptomatic, the fetus is still at risk.

The following are guidelines for ascertaining the risk to the fetus of a woman who has been infected before the pregnancy in question:

- An immunocompetent woman who acquired *Toxoplasma* infection more than 6 months before gestation does not deliver an infected infant.
- When conception occurs less than 6 months after acquisition of the infection, the risk to the fetus is exceedingly low, but transplacental transmission has been documented in this setting.
- *Toxoplasma* organisms have been isolated on rare occasions from abortuses of women with chronic (latent) infection. The frequency of *Toxoplasma* infection as a cause of abortion is unknown and is a controversial subject.

TRANSMISSION THROUGH BREAST-FEEDING

Transmission by human milk has not been demonstrated. It might occur if infection were acquired in the last weeks of gestation; however, the incidence of transplacental transmission approaches 100% if infection is acquired at this time, so the possible additional risk of breast-feeding would be insignificant.

TRANSMISSION BY BLOOD OR LEUKOCYTE TRANSFUSION OR ORGAN TRANSPLANTATION

Parasitemia has been reported to persist in otherwise normal persons for up to 1 year after acquisition of infection, and *Toxoplasma* organisms have been recovered from leukocytes of persons who have no recognized clinical evidence of *Toxoplasma* infection. The organism can survive for up to 50 days in whole citrated blood stored at 4°C. This poses a particular

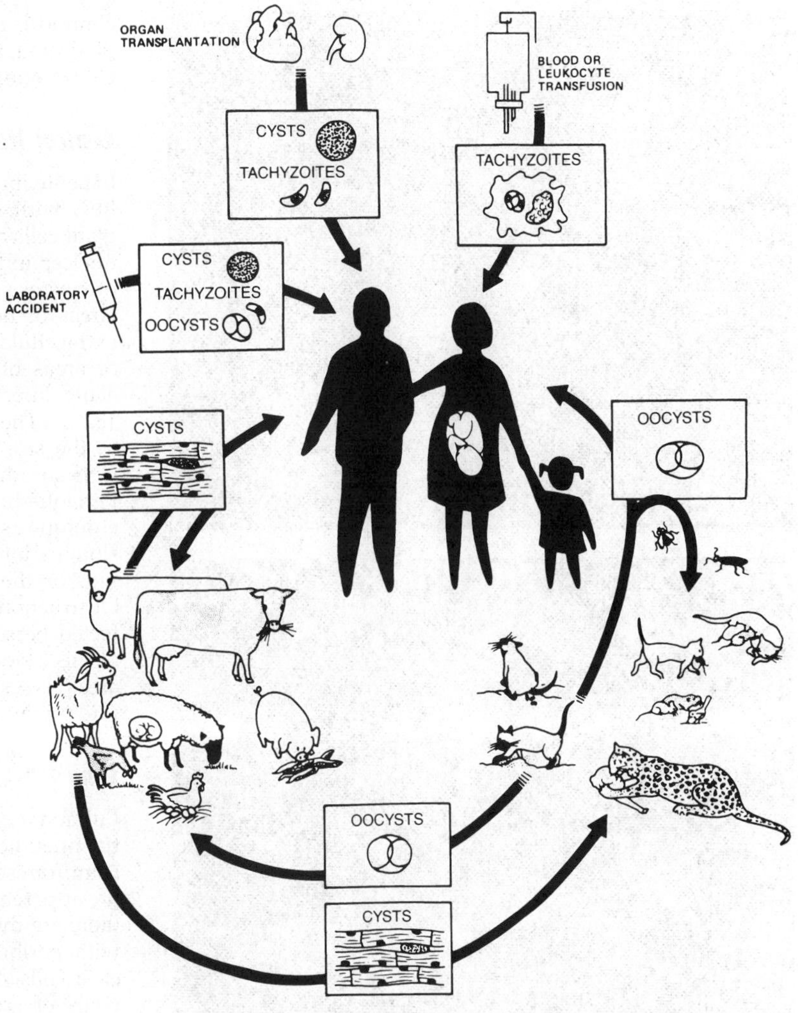

FIGURE 182–2 □ Life cycle and modes of transmission of *T. gondii.* Infection in humans and other animals occurs primarily after ingestion of either the cyst or the oocyst. Released organisms invade the intestinal epithelium, spread to tissues (either hematogenously or via lymphatics), and form cysts. When humans or other animals (including the cat) eat infected tissues (from any animal) or mature oocysts (excreted only by members of the cat family), the life cycle is completed. Laboratory accidents, organ transplantation, and blood and white blood cell transfusion have also been implicated in transmission of the organism. (From Remington JS, McLeod R: Toxoplasmosis. *In* Braude AI [ed]: International Textbook of Medicine, Vol II, Medical Microbiology and Infectious Diseases. Philadelphia, WB Saunders, 1981, pp 1816–1832.)

threat to immunodeficient patients who require multiple blood transfusions. *Toxoplasma* has been transmitted by heart, bone marrow, liver, and kidney transplantation from acutely infected donors to recipients who were not previously infected with *Toxoplasma* and has caused morbidity and death.

Pathogenesis

After their release from cysts or oocysts, the organisms enter gastrointestinal cells, where they multiply, disrupt cells, and infect contiguous cells. Extracellular organisms or organisms within leukocytes may be transported via the lymphatics and blood stream to every organ and tissue. Proliferating tachyzoites usually produce necrotic foci of invaded cells surrounded by an intense cellular reaction. The outcome of the acute process depends on both humoral and cell-mediated immunity. In some apparently normal people, and especially in immunodeficient persons, the acute infection may progress and cause potentially lethal lesions, such as acute necrotizing encephalitis, pneumonitis, or myocarditis. With development of the normal immune response, tachyzoites disappear from the tissues.

A unique aspect of the infection is that organisms persist as cysts in multiple organs for the life span of the host. The tissue cysts, which are characteristic of chronic infection, provoke little or no inflammatory response. Either rupture of cysts or persistence of viable tachyzoites within monocytes and macrophages may be the source of recurrent parasitemia in some asymptomatic persons who have chronic infection. Cysts are the likely source of organisms that cause recrudescent disease in immunocompromised patients or chorioretinitis in older children and adults with congenital toxoplasmosis.

Pathology

The meager information on the pathologic changes of toxoplasmosis in immunologically normal persons is derived largely from lymph node biopsy, because most of these infections are asymptomatic and self-limited. Limited information is available concerning changes in other organs. Pathology has been defined most clearly in congenitally infected infants and in immunosuppressed patients with disseminated infection.

The degree of organ and tissue involvement of infants with congenital infection varies considerably. In some, autopsy reveals only central nervous system (CNS) and eye involvement, whereas in others there is wide dissemination of lesions and organisms. The CNS is never spared. In extraneural organs, whose tissues can regenerate, residual lesions may be so slight that they are easily overlooked. In the CNS and eye, on the other hand, the inability of nerve cells to regenerate leads to more severe, permanent damage.

The pathologic changes described in the following are the same in adults and in congenitally infected infants unless otherwise specified.

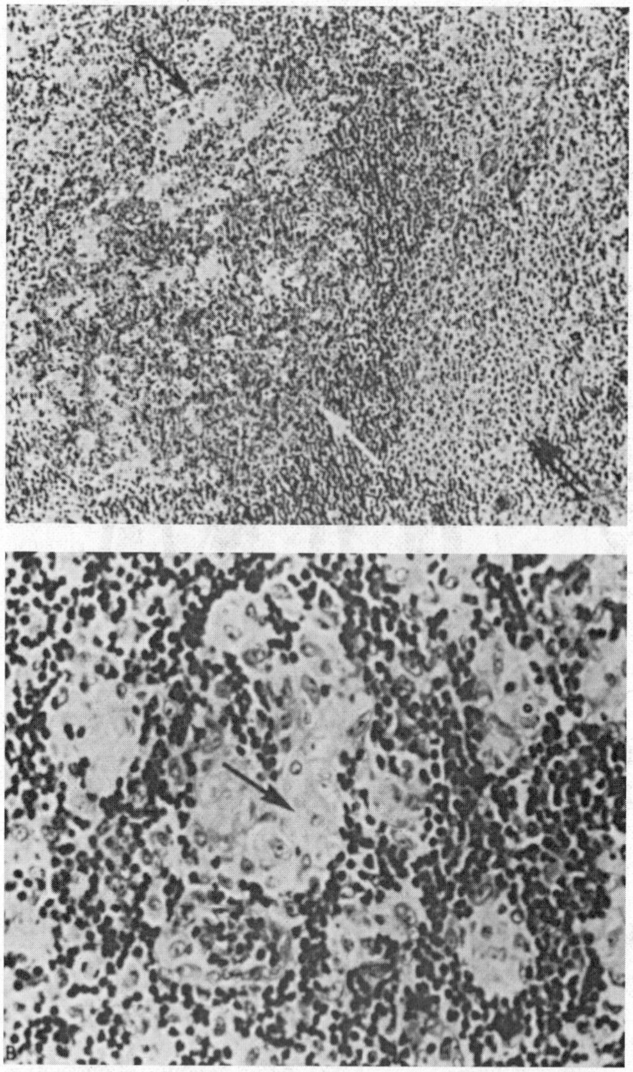

FIGURE 182–3 □ Characteristic lymph node pathology in lymphadenitis caused by *Toxoplasma*. *A*, Epithelioid cells *(black arrow)* encroach on and blur margins of germinal center *(white arrow)*, and there is focal distension of subcapsular and trabecular sinuses by monocytoid cells *(double black arrows)*. *B*, Irregular clusters of epithelioid cells *(arrow)* scattered throughout paracortical lymphoid stroma. (*A* and *B* from Dorfman RF, Remington JS: Value of lymph-node biopsy in the diagnosis of acute acquired toxoplasmosis. N Engl J Med 289:878–881, 1973.)

Lymph Node

In older children and adults, the histopathologic changes in toxoplasmic lymphadenitis are distinctive[12] (Fig. 182–3). The characteristic lesion is a reactive follicular hyperplasia, with irregular clusters of epithelioid histiocytes that encroach on and blur the margins of germinal centers. There is also an associated focal distension of sinuses with monocytoid cells. Giant cells are absent, and *T. gondii* can be demonstrated only rarely.

Eye

The earliest changes in the eye are single or multiple foci of necrosis. The infiltrate consists largely of lymphocytes, plasma cells, and mononuclear phagocytes. Intra- and extracellular tachyzoites and numerous cysts may be found in the retinal lesions. It has been suggested that the retinitis originates from cyst rupture. Granulomatous inflammation of the choroid is secondary to the necrotizing retinitis. Iridocyclitis, glaucoma, and cataracts may occur as complications of the chorioretinitis.

Central Nervous System

In acute infection, there is a focal or diffuse meningoencephalitis, with necrosis and microglial nodules. Multinucleated giant cells are not a characteristic feature. Perivascular mononuclear inflammation is frequent and is contiguous to areas of necrosis. Occasionally there is necrosis of vessel walls. Areas of necrosis may mimic mass lesions, and intra- and extracellular tachyzoites are usually found at the periphery of areas of necrosis. Cysts in the brain may occur during acute infection or reflect infection of long duration[13] (Fig. 182–4). The extent and location of CNS involvement, as well as the size of lesions, vary considerably. The lesions in the CNS in adults and congenitally infected infants are similar. Periaqueductal or periventricular vasculitis with necrosis is a unique aspect of severe congenital infection. Necrotic tissue sloughs into the ventricles, obstructing the aqueduct of Sylvius or the foramen of Monro and causing hydrocephalus. Obstruction of the aqueduct of Sylvius in congenitally infected persons may also occur later in life. The pathogenesis of this lesion has not been delineated. Calcification of necrotic areas is especially prominent in congenital infection but rarely may also occur in older children or adults.

Lung

Pulmonary infection may cause clinically significant interstitial pneumonitis in congenitally infected infants, in immunocompromised patients, and sometimes, in persons who have no apparent underlying disease. In each of these settings, there are thickened and edematous alveolar septa that, along with peribronchial areas, may be infiltrated with mononuclear cells, occasional plasma cells, and rare eosinophils. The walls of small blood vessels may also be infiltrated with lymphocytes and mononuclear cells, and *Toxoplasma* may be present in endothelial cells. Both tachyzoites and cysts have been seen within alveolar lining cells. Necrosis within granu-

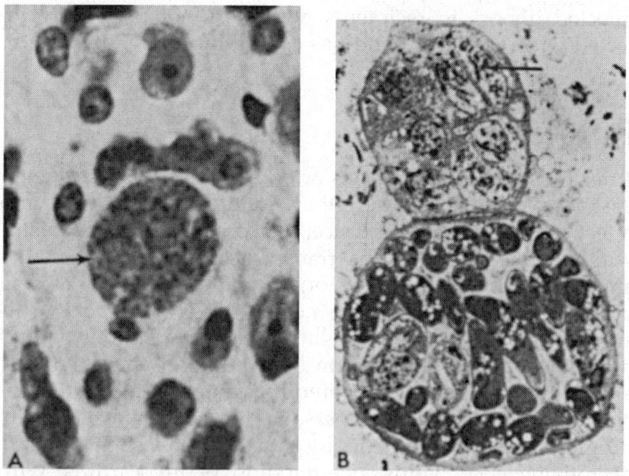

FIGURE 182–4 □ Infection of the CNS with *Toxoplasma*. *A*, Cyst in brain *(arrow)* is seen in acute infection as early as 8 days, or in chronic (latent) infection. *B*, Electron micrograph of CNS *Toxoplasma* infection. The diagnosis may be established by electron microscopic identification of organism *(arrow)* when light microscopic examination is not definitive. (*A* and *B* from Ghatak NR, Poon TP, Zimmerman HM: Toxoplasmosis of the central nervous system in the adult. A light and electron microscopic study of three cases. Arch Pathol 89:337–348, 1970.)

lomatous foci is prominent in some patients with disseminated toxoplasmosis and malignancy but is rarely seen in infants or in patients without malignancy. In many cases, there is some bronchopneumonia, often caused by superimposed infection with other organisms.

Heart

Myocarditis is associated with congenital infection, infection of immunocompromised persons, and, rarely, severe acute infection of apparently otherwise healthy persons. In patients with acquired immunodeficiency syndrome (AIDS) who die with toxoplasmosis, autopsies have revealed involvement of the heart and lung in 40% to 70%. Cysts and large aggregates of tachyzoites occur within muscle fibers (see Fig. 182–1C). Single organisms are found adjacent to and within areas of necrotic tissue. Foci of inflammatory cells (lymphocytes, plasma cells, mononuclear cells, and occasionally eosinophils) are associated with hyaline necrosis and fragmentation of myocardial cells, usually without organisms. Hemorrhagic pericarditis has also been reported in some patients with toxoplasmosis.

Kidney

In congenital toxoplasmosis and disseminated infection in older children and adults, the pathologic changes in the kidney resemble those in other organs (i.e., necrosis and the presence of cysts, tachyzoites, and inflammatory cells). Necrosis may occur in both glomeruli and tubules. In addition, glomerulonephritis with deposits of immunoglobulin M (IgM), fibrinogen, and *Toxoplasma* antigen and antibody has been reported.

Other Sites

The organisms and foci of necrosis have been found in the adrenal cortex, testes, and ovaries of infected infants; and *Toxoplasma* organisms, usually without inflammation, have been found in the pituitary. In infected infants and adults, cysts or tachyzoites, with or without inflammation, have been reported in multiple organs, including liver, spleen, bone marrow, thyroid, pancreas, adipose tissue, and skin. Involvement of pancreas, stomach, and intestine in patients with AIDS and toxoplasmosis is striking. Involvement of skeletal muscles varies from parasitized fibers without pathologic changes to focal areas of infiltration or widespread myositis with necrosis.

Immunologic Abnormalities

Monoclonal gammopathy of the immunoglobulin G (IgG) class has been described in infants with congenital toxoplasmosis. IgM levels may be elevated in newborns with congenital toxoplasmosis. Circulating immune complexes have been detected by C1q-binding assay in sera from adults with the systemic, febrile, and lymphadenopathic forms of toxoplasmosis and in an infant with congenital toxoplasmosis but not after signs and symptoms resolved. Reversible immunoglobulin A (IgA) deficiency has been reported in infants with congenital toxoplasmosis.

Marked and prolonged alterations in T-lymphocyte subpopulations are associated with *T. gondii* infection, which can be correlated with disease syndromes but not necessarily with disease outcome. Some patients with prolonged fever and malaise exhibit lymphocytosis, increased numbers of suppressor T cells, and a depressed helper/suppressor cell ratio. Some patients have fewer helper cells even when they are asymptomatic. Sometimes, with lymphadenopathy, the number of helper cells diminishes for longer than 6 months after onset of infection. Asymptomatic patients have abnormal T-cell subpopulations. Some patients with disseminated disease have a markedly reduced number of T cells and a markedly depressed ratio of helper to suppressor lymphocytes.

Clinical Manifestations

Lymphadenopathy and Other Manifestations

The most commonly recognized clinical manifestation of acute acquired toxoplasmosis is lymphadenopathy.[14, 15] The cervical nodes (either a single posterior one or multiple nodes) are involved most frequently, and discovery of their involvement is often incidental. Asymptomatic lymphadenopathy may mimic lymphoma. Involvement of a pectoral node may be mistaken for carcinoma of the breast in females. Suboccipital, supraclavicular, axillary, and inguinal nodes are involved frequently. It is important to recognize that mediastinal, mesenteric, and retroperitoneal nodes may also be involved. With infection of the mesenteric or retroperitoneal nodes there may be abdominal pain and fever, with a temperature to 40°C. Involved lymph nodes are usually discrete and vary in firmness; they may be tender but do not suppurate. Confusion, malaise, fever, stiff neck, myalgias, arthralgias, headache, sore throat, maculopapular rash (which spares the palms and soles), urticaria, hepatosplenomegaly, hepatitis, or reactive lymphocytes may occur. In one epidemic, 35 of 37 persons who had serologic evidence of acute acquired *Toxoplasma* infection had signs or symptoms of infection. Although 25 persons consulted physicians, toxoplasmosis was correctly diagnosed in only three. The lymphadenopathic form of toxoplasmosis is self-limited, but lymphadenopathy or malaise may persist or recur for months. If toxoplasmosis is in the differential diagnosis in a patient with lymphadenopathy, serologic studies to exclude acute *T. gondii* infection should be performed before lymph node biopsy to exclude lymphoma.

Rarely, someone whose immune system seems to be normal may develop any of the following, alone or in combination: myocarditis, pericarditis, pericardial effusion, polymyositis, hepatitis, pneumonitis, encephalitis, or meningoencephalitis. None of the signs or symptoms resulting from involvement of these organs is specific for infection with *T. gondii*. Some of these patients have died.

Ocular Involvement

Toxoplasma has been estimated to cause approximately 35% of the cases of chorioretinitis in the United States and in Central and Western Europe. In older children and adults, ocular disease is most frequently a consequence of congenital *Toxoplasma* infection, but chorioretinitis does occur in patients with acute acquired *Toxoplasma* infection. The frequency of *Toxoplasma* chorioretinitis is lower than that of cytomegalovirus retinitis in patients with AIDS, but it does occur, usually in conjunction with CNS and/or systemic infection. Active chorioretinitis may produce blurred vision, scotomata, pain, photophobia, or epiphora. Central vision may be impaired or lost if the macula is involved. Strabismus may be an early sign of chorioretinitis in children. In congenital toxoplasmosis, microophthalmia, small cornea, posterior cortical cataract, anisometropia, strabismus, nystagmus, and leukocoria also occur. Nystagmus may result either from poor fixation related to the chorioretinitis or from involvement of the CNS. Convergent or divergent strabismus may be caused by involvement of extraocular muscles or the brain. Associated systemic signs of infection are uncommon. Because ocular involvement may cause the only clinical sign of infection in newborns, newborn infants suspected to have congenital toxoplasmosis require ophthalmologic examination to exclude toxoplasmosis. As inflammation subsides, vision improves but often incompletely. Episodic flares of chorioretinitis are common and destroy retinal tissue. Such multiple recurrences may result in glaucoma.

On ophthalmoscopic examination, the acute lesions appear as yellowish white, cottony patches that have elevated, indistinct margins surrounded by a zone of hyperemia. The inflammatory exudate in the vitreous may obscure the fundus. Older lesions are atrophic, whitish gray plaques with distinct borders and black spots of choroidal pigment. The lesions may be single or, more commonly, multiple and are usually located near the posterior pole of the retina, although they may be peripheral. Lesions of varying age may be seen simultaneously[16] (Fig. 182–5*A*). Less common are panuveitis and papillitis with optic atrophy. Isolated anterior uveitis related to toxoplasmosis has never been proved. Infants with congenital toxoplasmosis may have (1) unilateral or bilateral macular involvement, (2) other unilateral or bilateral lesions, (3) peripheral involvement in one or more quadrants of the retina and choroid, (4) punched-out lesions in the late phase, (5) massive chorioretinal degeneration, (6) extensive fibrosis and heavy pigmentation (in contrast to the dissociation of these changes in other chorioretinal lesions), (7) normal retina and vasculature surrounding the lesions throughout the infection, (8) rapid development of sequential optic nerve atrophy, and (9) clarity of the media despite severe chorioretinitis. In patients with AIDS, *Toxoplasma* retinal lesions are often large, and there is diffuse necrosis of the retina with substantial numbers of encysted organisms and free tachyzoites. They usually do not have well-developed granulomatous chorioiditis, significant inflammatory, cell infiltrate, or preexisting chorioretinal scar formation (Fig. 182–5*B*).

Toxoplasmosis in Immunocompromised Patients

All forms of toxoplasmosis that occur in normal persons also occur in those whose immune system is compromised.[17–19] Acute toxoplasmosis in an immunocompromised patient may be due to reactivation of latent infection or to acquisition of infection from exogenous sources, including organ transplants and blood or leukocyte transfusion.[20] Immunosuppressed patients with the greatest predilection for life-threatening toxoplasmosis are those with AIDS and those receiving immunosuppressive therapy for lymphoproliferative disorders (especially Hodgkin's disease), hematologic malignancy, or prevention of organ graft rejection. Disease is often fulminant and rapidly fatal in immunocompromised patients, and because effective therapy is available, it is incumbent on clinicians to be aware of the clinical presentation in this type of patient. An emerging problem is infants born with both human immunodeficiency virus and *T. gondii* infection. This results from reactivation of toxoplasmosis in the human immunodeficiency virus–infected mother.

The most characteristic clinical manifestations of toxoplasmosis in immunocompromised patients result from brain involvement, which is present in more than 50% of documented cases. The symptoms and signs are manifestations of diffuse encephalopathy, meningoencephalitis, or cerebral mass lesions and include changes in mental status, headache, seizures, and focal neurologic deficits. Toxoplasmosis in patients with AIDS is described in detail in Chapter 125. Briefly, in AIDS patients, *Toxoplasma* encephalitis is fatal without treatment. It is the major cause of focal intracerebral lesions in AIDS. At least 30% of persons who have human immunodeficiency virus infection and antibodies to *T. gondii* will develop *Toxoplasma* encephalitis if they are not receiving prophylaxis. It may be the presenting manifestation of AIDS. Geographic origin (e.g., residence in Germany and France, where meat is consumed raw or undercooked), proximity to cats that may be excreting oocysts, and dietary habits (e.g., exposure to undercooked meat) may suggest that *T. gondii* infection is likely. Typical findings include fever (in 10% to 74% of patients), headache (56%), altered mental status, psychosis, cognitive impairment, seizures (33%), and focal neurologic defects (60%), including hemiparesis, aphasia, ataxia; visual field loss, cranial nerve palsies, dysmetria, or movement disorders. Uncommon findings include meningis-

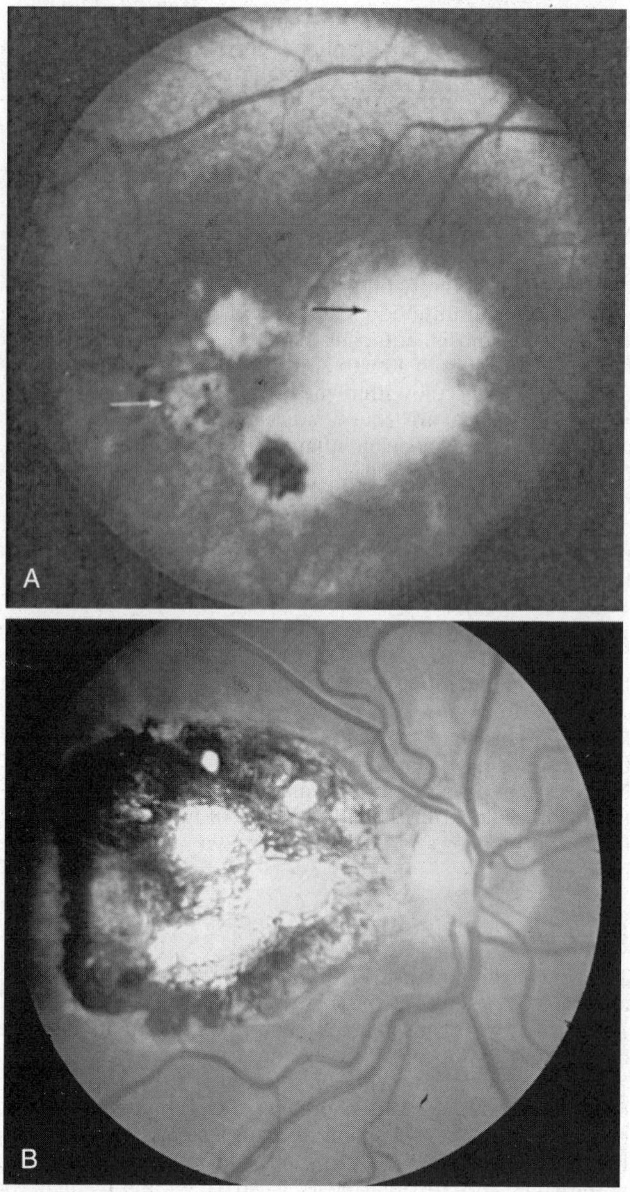

FIGURE 182–5 □ *A*, Chorioretinitis caused by *Toxoplasma*. The characteristic lesion is a focal necrotizing retinitis with cotton-like patches in the fundus. Note that the acute lesions *(black arrow)* have indistinct borders and appear soft and white, whereas older lesions *(white arrow)* are whitish gray, sharply outlined, and spotted by accumulations of choroidal pigment. (From O'Connor GR: Ocular toxoplasmosis. *In* Locatcher-Khorazo D, Seegal BC [eds]: Microbiology of the Eye. St. Louis, CV Mosby, 1972, p 199.) *B*, Toxoplasmic chorioretinitis in a patient with AIDS. (From Polis MA: Differential diagnosis of retinal lesions in persons with HIV infection. Opportunistic Infect Interaction 3:1, 1994.)

mus; involvement of heart, abdomen, or testes; panhypopituitarism; and the syndrome of inappropriate secretion of antidiuretic hormone. Between 97% and 99% of patients with AIDS and *Toxoplasma* encephalitis have IgG antibody to *T. gondii* in serum; however, *Toxoplasma* IgM antibodies are usually not demonstrable. Intrathecal antibody production may be present. A therapeutic trial of antitoxoplasma medications in AIDS patients who have characteristic findings on neuroradiologic imaging studies is often used to help establish this diagnosis. Alternative causes are sought by brain biopsy if the patient fails to respond clinically or "radiographically." Time to resolution at computed tomography (CT) usually varies between 20 days and 6 months. Positron emission tomographic scans appear to be useful in differentiating toxoplasmic encephalitis (hypometabolic lesions) and lymphoma (hypermetabolic lesions).[21]

Areas of predilection for CNS toxoplasmosis in patients with AIDS are the basal ganglia and corticomedullary junction. Lesions may occur anywhere and are generally enhanced when contrast is administered. Magnetic resonance imaging is significantly more sensitive than CT and frequently reveals multiple focal lesions in patients with toxoplasmic encephalitis who have only a single lesion at CT.

Persons who have not been infected previously with *Toxoplasma* and receive a heart transplant from an infected person often develop signs and symptoms of toxoplasmosis. The diagnosis of brain involvement can be made by finding tachyzoites in a biopsy specimen or in material aspirated from mass lesions that resemble a brain abscess at CT. The cerebrospinal fluid (CSF) typically shows mononuclear pleocytosis, a moderate elevation in protein concentration, and a normal glucose level. In any immunosuppressed patient with symptoms or signs of brain involvement, the diagnosis of toxoplasmosis must be excluded. Other manifestations of the disease in immunocompromised patients may be nonspecific or reflect inflammation and necrosis of the organs involved, particularly the heart and lungs.

T. gondii infection has also been transmitted by liver transplantation and resulted in multiorgan failure in the early period after liver transplantation. We recommend serologic testing to detect acute acquired *T. gondii* infection in the evaluations of all organ donors and recipients because, in a number of instances, disseminated infection has resulted from transplantation of an organ from an individual with acute acquired infection into a seronegative recipient.

Toxoplasmosis and Toxoplasma Infection in Pregnant Women

Toxoplasma infection acquired in pregnancy causes symptoms in only about 10% to 20% of mothers, but the fetus is at risk whether symptoms are present or not. Guidelines on toxoplasmosis and *Toxoplasma* infection in pregnant women were offered earlier (in the section on transplacental transmission).

Congenital Toxoplasmosis

Most infected newborns have no symptoms at birth and may suffer untoward sequelae of the infection: without treatment most develop chorioretinitis, about half with impairment of vision, by the time they reach adolescence.[22–24] Less frequent manifestations of infection include strabismus, blindness, epilepsy, and psychomotor or mental retardation, which may occur weeks, months, or even years later. Those with clinically apparent infection at birth may have all or any combination of the following signs: mild nonspecific illness, fever, hypothermia, vomiting, diarrhea, jaundice, rash (most commonly petechiae caused by thrombocytopenia), hydrocephalus, microcephaly, cerebral calcifications, microphthalmia, strabismus, cataracts, glaucoma, chorioretinitis, optic atrophy, deafness, lymphadenopathy, pneumonitis, myocarditis, hepatosplenomegaly, convulsions, psychomotor retardation, other CNS signs, anemia, abnormal bleeding, thrombocytopenia, eosinophilia, monocytosis, and abnormal CSF with xanthochromia, mononuclear pleocytosis, and high protein value (grams per deciliter). Although they are not specific for toxoplasmosis in infants, these CSF changes should prompt consideration of toxoplasmosis even in subclinical cases. *Toxoplasma* infection does not cause fetal malformation.

Complications and Sequelae

The lymphadenopathic form of acquired toxoplasmosis is usually self-limited but may persist or recur for months, in the presence or absence of constitutional symptoms.

When clinical signs of infection are present at birth, mental retardation, epilepsy, spasticity, palsies, and severe vision impairment sometimes develop in children who are treated, and they are common sequelae for untreated children. Prompt treatment induces resolution of signs of active infection, and many treated children function normally. Deafness has been reported in untreated children. Microcephaly has been reported in approximately 13% and hydrocephalus in approximately 28% of untreated infants with signs or symptoms of toxoplasmosis involving the CNS. These serious sequelae are a threat to all congenitally infected infants, whether or not they exhibit signs in the perinatal period.

Ocular toxoplasmosis is characterized by frequent relapses. It may result in glaucoma or loss of vision and ultimately may necessitate enucleation.

Acute infection is extremely serious in immunodeficient patients. Although the mortality rate is high, the actual death rate is not known. Relapse is frequent in patients with AIDS who do not receive chronic suppressive therapy.

Geographic Variations in Disease and Infection

There are considerable geographic variations in prevalence of infection with *Toxoplasma*[25] (Fig. 182–6). In all areas surveyed, the prevalence of positive serologic reactions increases with age. Generally, there are fewer human infections in cold regions, in hot and arid areas, and at high elevations. Exceptions do exist: Eskimos, once thought to be free of this infection, have been found to have prevalence rates of 13% to 46%, whereas some isolated tropical communities have little or no *Toxoplasma* infection. It is interesting that these tropical communities have no known exposure to domestic or feral cats. However, there are also populations who are infected with *T. gondii* and who have no known exposure to cats. Most of the variations in prevalence and incidence of infections from area to area have not been explained, but personal habits and exposure to cat feces are important in transmission. For example in the United States and Europe ingestion of undercooked meat is common and is probably important in transmission. In Costa Rica, proximity of the area where cats defecate to human habitation is important in transmission.

The actual incidence of congenital toxoplasmosis is unknown. Approximations, per 1000 live births, are as follows: Vienna, 6 to 7; Paris, 3; New York City, 1.3; and Mexico City, 2.

Association of certain major histocompatibility complex haplotypes and susceptibility has been documented for humans. Epidemics of toxoplasmosis have been documented in humans and in domestic animals in several countries, includ-

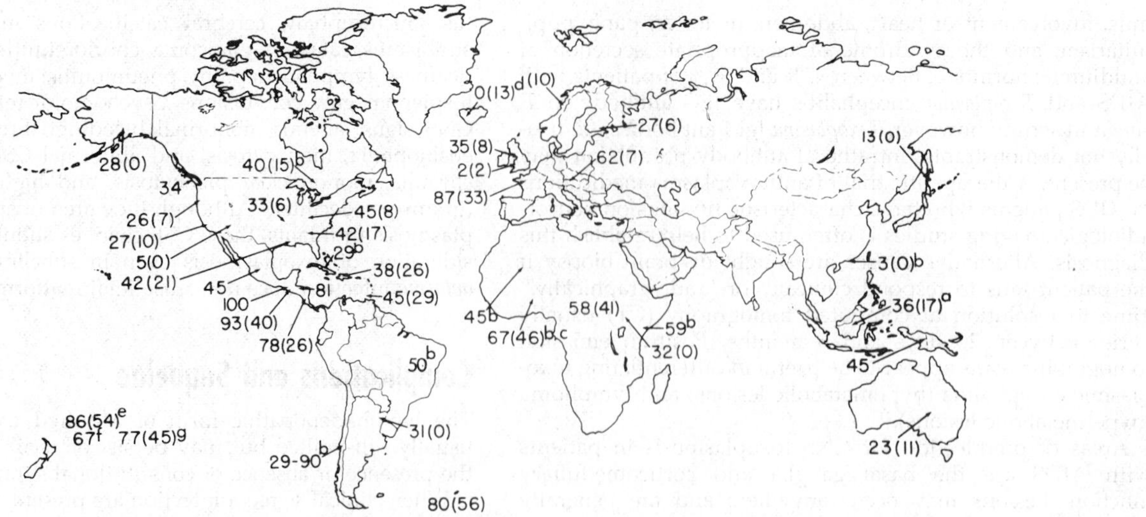

FIGURE 182–6 ▫ Prevalence of antibodies against *T. gondii* in persons in selected locales. Unless otherwise specified, figures outside parentheses represent the percentage of seropositive adults approximately 30 to 40 years of age; figures inside parentheses are the percentage of seropositive children younger than 10 years. Notes: *a,* IHA antibodies; others were IFA or dye test. *b,* Adults with either age range not clearly specified or wider age range than approximately 30 to 40 years. *c,* "Juveniles." *d,* Although 14 individuals 30 to 39 years old had no *Toxoplasma* antibody, 29% of 14 individuals 40 to 49 years old did have *Toxoplasma* antibody. *e,* Society island. *f,* American Samoa. *g,* Tahiti. (From Remington JS, McLeod R: Toxoplasmosis. *In* Braude AI [ed]: International Textbook of Medicine, Vol II, Medical Microbiology and Infectious Diseases. Philadelphia, WB Saunders, 1981, pp 1816–1832.)

ing the United States, Canada, Brazil, and Spain. Simultaneous infections in multiple members of the same family who cohabit have been reported.

Diagnosis

The diagnosis of acute infection with *Toxoplasma* is made by isolation of *T. gondii* from blood or body fluids. It is also made by demonstration of tachyzoites in sections or preparations of tissues and body fluids; of cysts in the placenta or tissues of a fetus or newborn; and of characteristic lymph node histology. Serologic tests are also useful for diagnosis.

The organism can be isolated by inoculation of body fluids, leukocytes, or tissue specimens into the peritoneal cavity of mice or into tissue cultures. Body fluids should be processed and inoculated immediately; tissues and blood may be stored overnight at 4°C. Freezing or treating specimens with formalin kills the organism.

Mice should be examined for *Toxoplasma* in their peritoneal fluid 6 to 10 days after inoculation or earlier if they die. Mice that survive 6 weeks should be tested for *Toxoplasma* antibody in serum. If antibody is present, definitive diagnosis is made by visualization of *Toxoplasma* cysts in the mouse's brain. If no cysts are seen in mice with *Toxoplasma* antibody, portions of brain, liver, and spleen from the mice should be inoculated into other mice. *T. gondii* organisms can be isolated using tissue cultures by diagnostic microbiology or virology laboratories. When examined microscopically, plaques stained with Wright or Giemsa stain show necrotic, heavily infected cells with numerous extracellular tachyzoites. They may form as early as 4 days (Fig. 182–7).

Isolation of *T. gondii* from body fluids reflects acute infection, as does isolation from the blood in most patients. Persistent parasitemia in asymptomatic people with latent infection appears to be rare, except perhaps in chronic myelogenous leukemia. Isolation from tissues (e.g., skeletal muscle, lung, brain, eye) obtained by biopsy or at autopsy may reflect the presence of tissue cysts and thus is not proof of acute infection.

Histologic Diagnosis

Demonstration of tachyzoites in tissue sections (e.g., endomyocardial biopsy in heart transplant recipients), smears (e.g., brain biopsy, bone marrow aspirate, bronchoalveolar lavage), or in body fluids (e.g., CSF, amniotic fluid) establishes the diagnosis of acute toxoplasmosis. Although it is

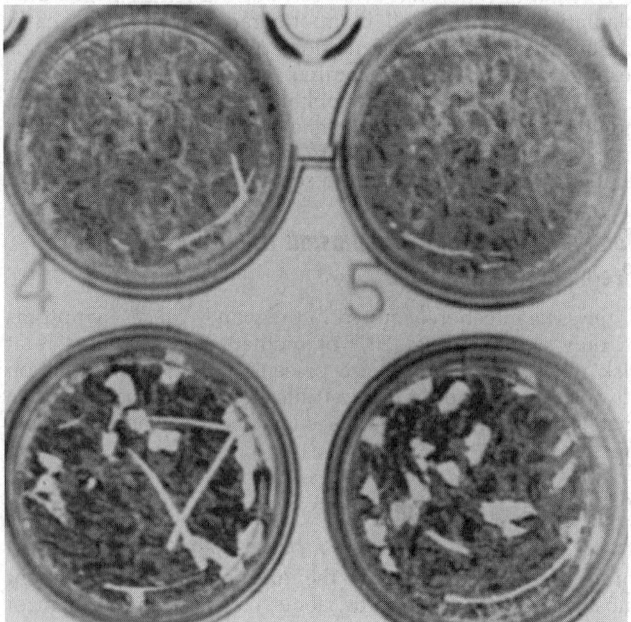

FIGURE 182–7 ▫ Plaque formation by *T. gondii:* 100 RH strain *Toxoplasma* tachyzoites were inoculated onto semiconfluent monolayers of human foreskin fibroblasts. Plaques *(bottom row)* were observed at 96 hours. Top row are uninfected (control) monolayers. (Adapted from Israelski DM, Remington JS: Toxoplasmic encephalitis in patients with AIDS. *In* Sande MA, Volberding PA [eds]: The Medical Management of AIDS. Philadelphia, WB Saunders, 1988, p 193.)

difficult to see the tachyzoite with ordinary stains, immunofluorescent antibody techniques and a peroxidase-antiperoxidase immunohistochemical staining technique have been successful.[26] Demonstration of the tissue cyst is diagnostic of *Toxoplasma* infection but does not differentiate between acute and chronic infection. Numerous cysts in any organ usually indicate recent acute infection. The presence of cysts in the placenta or tissues of the newborn infant establishes the diagnosis of congenital infection. The characteristic histologic criteria are sufficient to establish the diagnosis of *Toxoplasma* lymphadenitis[12] (see Fig. 182–3).

Serologic Tests

It is important to understand that the diagnosis of toxoplasmosis usually requires results from more than one serologic test. The titers in such tests may vary when performed by different laboratories or with different commercial test kits. Thus, it is the responsibility of each laboratory to provide adequate standardization and interpretation with its test results. Results that affect therapy should be confirmed in a reference laboratory.

The Sabin-Feldman dye, indirect fluorescent antibody (IFA), and indirect hemagglutination (IHA) tests are the methods most widely used for diagnosis of acute toxoplasmosis. Tests for antigenemia are particularly promising (although experimental) for diagnosis in newborns and in immunocompromised persons. Immunosorbent assays and radioimmunoassay are potentially valuable because they allow automation.

The dye test is sensitive and specific and measures principally IgG antibodies.[27] The World Health Organization has recommended that dye test titers be expressed in international units per milliliter. An international standard reference serum for this purpose is available on request from the World Health Organization.

The IFA test appears to measure the same antibodies as the dye test. In both tests, the titers tend to be parallel. Dye test and IFA test antibodies usually appear 1 to 2 weeks after infection, reach high titers in 6 to 8 weeks, and then gradually decline over months to years; low titers (1:4 to 1:64) commonly persist for life. Magnitude of antibody titer does not correlate with severity of illness. Commercially available kits produce significant numbers of false-positive or false-negative results.

The agglutination test[28] is available commercially (BioMerieux, Lyon, France). It employs formalin-preserved whole parasites and detects IgG. This method should not be used to measure IgM antibodies. It is accurate, simple to perform, and inexpensive. The agglutination test has special usefulness for serologic screening to diagnose acute infection in pregnant women. Because it takes 2 to 6 months for IgG antibodies detected with the whole-cell agglutination test to reach a steady high titer,[28] the existence of a steady high titer signifies that the infection was acquired more than 2 months earlier. As a consequence, if the first sample of serum has been obtained during the first 2 months of pregnancy, a stable agglutination test titer demonstrates that the infection occurred before the time of conception and that there is little risk to the baby of congenital infection.

The differential agglutination test (AC/HS [acetone-fixed parasites/formalin-fixed parasites]) has proved useful in the differentiation of recent infection in contrast to more distant infection.[27, 29, 30] (Table 182–1).

The IgM fluorescent antibody (IgM-IFA) test is useful for the diagnosis of acute infection with *T. gondii* because IgM antibodies appear faster (as early as 5 days after infection) and disappear sooner than IgG antibodies. In most cases, IgM-IFA test antibody levels rise rapidly (to levels of 1:80 to 1:1000) and fall to low titers (1:10 or 1:20) or disappear within a few weeks or months[31] (Fig. 182–8). In some patients, they remain positive at low titers for as long as several years. IgM antibodies in neonates represent synthesis in utero by the infected fetus because IgM does not normally pass the placental barrier. IgM *Toxoplasma* antibodies may not be demonstrable in some immunodeficient patients with acute toxoplasmosis and in most patients with active toxoplasmosis limited to the eye and are demonstrable in only approximately 25% of newborns with congenital toxoplasmosis. Antinuclear antibodies may cause false-positive reactions in both the IFA and IgM-IFA tests; rheumatoid factor may cause false-positive reactions in the IgM-IFA test.

Detection of IgM antibodies by the double-sandwich enzyme-linked immunosorbent assay[32] (DS-IgM-ELISA) is more sensitive and specific than the IgM-IFA test. Rheumatoid factor and antinuclear antibodies do not cause false-positive test results. The DS-IgM-ELISA detects approximately 75% of infants with proven congenital infection, whereas the IgM-IFA detects only 25% of such cases. The DS-IgM-ELISA avoids false-positive results associated with rheumatoid factor, which the infant can produce in utero, and false-negatives related to competition from high levels of maternal IgG antibody, which occur in the IgM-IFA test. IgM antibodies are detected by the IgM-IFA test for a shorter time than by

TABLE 182–1 ■ Criteria Used for Interpretation of AC/HS Test Results*

HS TEST RESULT (IU/mL)	INTERPRETATION WITH THE FOLLOWING AC TEST RESULT (IU/mL)†							
	<50	50	100	200	400	800	1600	>1600
<100	NA‡	NA‡	A	A	A§	A§	A§	A§
100	NA	NA	A	A	A	A	A§	A§
200	NA	NA	A	A	A	A	A	A§
400	NA	NA	A	A	A	A	A	A
800	NA	NA	NA	A	A	A	A	A
1600	NA	NA	NA	NA	A	A	A	A
3200	NA	NA	NA	NA	NA	A	A	A
>3200	NA	NA	NA	NA	NA	NA	A	A

*The AC/HS test was performed as described in Dannemann et al: J Clin Microbiol 28:1928–1933, 1990.
†A, Acute pattern; NA, not acute pattern.
‡HS titer of >0 but <100; this pattern may be seen in the earliest stages of infection. Follow-up serum samples are necessary to clarify whether the infection is acute.
§Results were not observed in routine use of the test.
From Dannemann BR, Vaughn WC, Thulliez P, Remington JS: Differential agglutination test for diagnosis of recently acquired infection with *Toxoplasma gondii*. J Clin Microbiol 28:1928–1933, 1990.

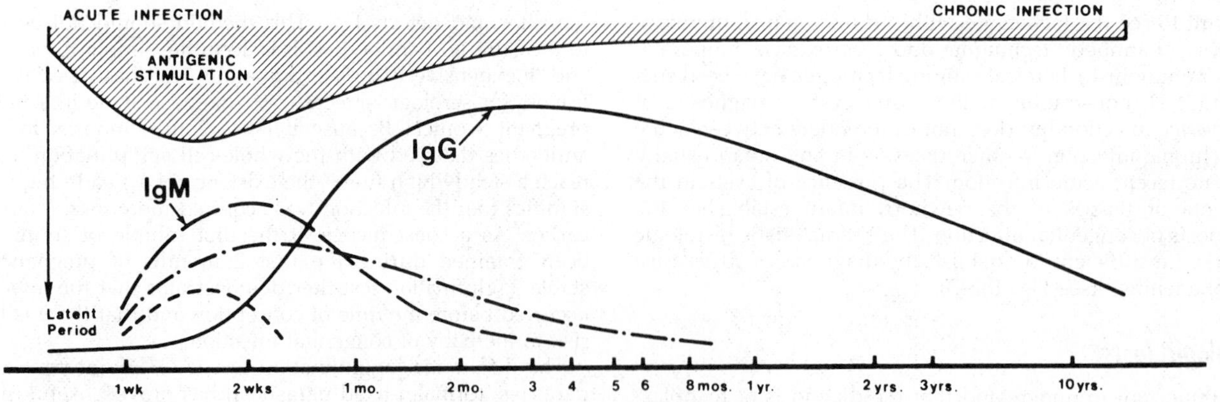

FIGURE 182–8 □ Antibody response of humans to *Toxoplasma* infection. IgM antibodies (— —), detectable by the IgM-IFA test, reach their maximal titer within the first weeks after infection and may decline within a few weeks (- -) or persist for months (—•—•). IgG antibodies (———), detectable by either the Sabin-Feldman dye test or the conventional IFA test, reach their maximal titer within 2 months, maintain a plateau for months or years, and then decline, but usually persist at a low titer for life. (Data from Desmonts G: Sérodiagnostic de la toxoplasmose. Feuill Biol 16:61, 1975.)

the DS-IgM-ELISA. The IgM-ISAGA is more sensitive than the IgM-ELISA and may detect specific IgM antibodies before and for a longer time than the IgM-ELISA.

The IgM immunosorbent agglutination assay (IgM-ISAGA), which combines trapping of a patient's IgM to a solid surface and formalin-fixed organisms or antigen-coated latex particles to detect the IgM antibodies, is specific and sensitive. The test is read as an agglutination test. It avoids false-positive results caused by rheumatoid factor or antinuclear antibodies and is more sensitive and specific than the IgM-IFA test. We use it routinely in the newborn. The IgA and IgE-ELISA and IgE-ISAGA are also useful tests in establishing the diagnosis of newly acquired or congenital toxoplasmosis.[33, 34]

The antibodies measured in the IHA test are different from those measured in the IFA and dye tests and may persist for years. Because IHA titers rise later than IFA or dye test titers, the IHA test may be helpful when these titers have stabilized. The IHA test should not be used for infants with suspected congenital infection or to screen for infection acquired during pregnancy, because the result may be negative for too long a period early in the infection. There is a great need for proper standardization of methodology for this and all other serologic tests and particularly for quality control of commercial kits that are often used by laboratories inexperienced in performing these serologic tests.

The level of *Toxoplasma* antibody in CSF or aqueous humor may be used to demonstrate local production of antibody in active ocular or CNS toxoplasmosis. Local antibody production is assessed by application of the following equation:

$$c = \frac{\text{antibody titer in body fluid}}{\text{antibody titer in serum}} \times \frac{\text{concentration of } \gamma\text{-globulin in serum}}{\text{concentration of } \gamma\text{-globulin in body fluid}}$$

A significant correlation coefficient (c) is 8 and reflects local antibody production related to active infection of the CNS or eye. If the dye test serum titer is 1:1000 or more, it is usually not possible to demonstrate significant local antibody production by application of this formula. The formula has been applied by using dye test titers and IgM-IFA test titers.

Toxoplasma antigen has been detected in serum of adults with the lymphadenopathic form of toxoplasmosis or with other acute *Toxoplasma* infection but not in serum of uninfected or chronically infected persons. It was detected in serum, amniotic fluid, and CSF from the few congenitally infected infants tested.

More avid *T. gondii*–specific IgG antibody (using an avidity ELISA) was described in association with recently acquired (and not chronic) infection. Additional experience with this test is needed to determine its clinical utility in differentiating recently and remotely acquired infection.

Comparative Western blots of serum samples from a mother and her baby demonstrating that both contain antibodies that react with different antigens have been reported as a means of diagnosing congenital toxoplasmosis.

Enzyme-linked immunofiltration assay is carried out on a micropore membrane and permits simultaneous study of antibody specificity by immunoprecipitation and characterization of antibody isotypes by immunofiltration with enzyme-labeled antibodies. The authors reported that this method detects 85% of cases of congenital infection in the first few days of life. Although the method has not been used in sufficient numbers of laboratories to define its usefulness, it appears promising. It is interesting that by this method IgE may by found at birth in the infant's CSF or serum. IgA antibodies were present in 5% of cases of congenital infection after the fifth month of life and were found in the CSF.

Polymerase chain reaction (PCR) can be used to amplify DNA of *T. gondii*, which can then be detected using a DNA probe.[35] This is a useful technique for detecting *T. gondii* DNA in CSF and amniotic fluid.

The lymphocyte blastogenic response to *Toxoplasma* antigens has also been useful in the diagnosis of congenital toxoplasmosis.

ACUTE ACQUIRED *TOXOPLASMA* INFECTION IN THE IMMUNOCOMPETENT PERSON

In settings in which acute acquired *Toxoplasma* infection is suspected in an immunocompetent person, a negative dye test or IFA test virtually excludes the diagnosis. The diagnosis of recent acute acquired infection is confirmed if there is seroconversion from a negative to a positive titer (in the absence of transfer of antibody by transfusion) or if there is a serial two-tube rise in titer when serum samples drawn at 3-week intervals are run in parallel. Although suggestive of active infection, one high titer in any test is not diagnostic.

Titers obtained using each kit and results as performed by each laboratory may vary. It is the responsibility of each laboratory to provide reliable information concerning results they consider to be indicative of recently or remotely acquired infection for each clinical illness. Some representative guidelines are based on results from the laboratory of one of the authors (JSR). Tables 182–2 and 182–3 (see Table 182–1) are helpful in interpreting test results, but exceptions may occur.[36, 37] A dye test or IFA test titer of 1:1000 or greater in the presence of a high IgM-IFA test titer (1:80 or greater) or DS-IgM-ELISA or IgM-ISAGA titer is probably diagnostic of recent acute infection, with or without symptoms. In immunologically normal people with positive titers in the dye test or IFA test, the absence of IgM-IFA test or DS-IgM-ELISA or IgM-ISAGA antibodies almost always excludes the diagnosis of acute infection.

Ocular Toxoplasmosis

The diagnosis of ocular toxoplasmosis in older children and adults is difficult because the titer of antibody in the serum does not necessarily correlate with presence of active lesions in the fundus. Indeed, low serologic test titers (1:4 to 1:64) are usual in older children and adults with active *Toxoplasma* chorioretinitis. For practical purposes, *Toxoplasma* chorioretinitis is probably excluded if results of serologic tests are negative when performed on undiluted serum. If retinal lesions are characteristic and serologic test results are positive, the diagnosis can be made with a high degree of confidence. If the retinal lesion is atypical and the result is positive, the diagnosis of toxoplasmosis is only presumptive; a high prevalence of antibodies in the normal population precludes the assumption of a causal relationship in this situation.

Active Infection in the Immunocompromised Individual

The available diagnostic techniques, including the IgM-IFA test, DS-IgM-ELISA, and IgM-ISAGA are at times insufficient for detection of active infection in immunocompromised patients because antibody responses may be abnormal. Serologic tests in immunocompromised persons can identify those at risk for primary infection or reactivation of latent infection (see also prophylaxis later).

Kinetics of serologic responses in heart transplant recipients who receive a heart donated by a seropositive person are variable. Seronegative patients who received hearts donated by seropositive persons exhibited seroconversion 4 to 7 weeks later and severe illness 1 week to 9 months after transplantation. Approximately 50% of patients who were seropositive before transplantation demonstrated a significant rise in IgG and IgM antibodies, although all remained asymptomatic.

Detection of *Toxoplasma* antigen in blood and CSF, by PCR, seems promising for identifying disseminated *Toxoplasma* infection in immunocompromised persons.

Toxoplasmosis and Toxoplasma *Infection in Pregnant Women*

Any woman who is considering becoming pregnant should have a *Toxoplasma* serologic test to determine whether she has *Toxoplasma* infection before pregnancy. (See the section on transplacental transmission for a complete discussion of risks to the fetus in relation to *Toxoplasma* infection acquired by the mother before pregnancy versus during pregnancy.)

In systematic monthly screening of pregnant women, serum IgM antibodies usually appear first, but low titers of IgG antibodies as measured in the dye test also appear early. Sera in which only IgM antibodies are detectable are uncommon. Because IgM antibodies measured by ELISA or ISAGA can persist for many months or even years, their greatest value is for determining that a pregnant woman has not recently been infected. A negative result virtually rules out recently acquired infection, unless serum samples are tested so early after acute infection that the antibody response has not yet occurred. In this case, acute infection would be identified in a screening program in which follow-up serology is performed in seronegative pregnant women. IgM antibodies that are measured by the IFA test may disappear earlier than those measured by IgM-ELISA or ISAGA. Thus, a negative IgM-IFA test late in gestation may not necessarily exclude recent acute infection. A positive IgM test is more difficult to evaluate unless it is possible to demonstrate a significant rise in IgG or IgM titer when serum samples are run in parallel or when other tests (e.g., tests for IgA and IgE antibody and the AC/HS test) suggest recent infection. A high IgM titer is more likely to reflect recent infection, but such high titers may persist for months. Such positive serum samples should be tested with additional methods, such as the AC/HS test and tests that detect IgE antibodies. Usually, this requires use of and consultation with a reference laboratory. A rise in IgM antibody titer is infrequent, suggesting that the rise was steep and reached its peak in 1 or 2 weeks. In contrast, the rise in IgG antibody is initially slow. The dye test titer usually remains relatively low (2 to 50 IU/mL or 1:10 to 1:200) for 3 to 6 weeks. Thus, acute infection cannot be ruled out when two samples collected 2 or even 3 weeks apart show no significant rise in titer, especially if the dye test is performed with fourfold dilutions of the sera, which would require an eightfold (two-tube) rise in titer to be considered significant. For this reason, twofold dilutions are imperative. A fourfold rise is often difficult to detect in the IgG-IFA test. After the initial 3 to 6 weeks, the rise in IgG antibody becomes steeper, and high titers (400 IU/mL or 1:1000) are usually reached within an additional 3 weeks. Thereafter, the rise is slower but still detectable over an additional 3 to 6 weeks by careful methodology avoiding fourfold dilutions of serum. Thus, although the rise in IgG antibody in the dye test differs from case to case, it lasts more than 2 months and sometimes 3 months. In the agglutination test with 2-mercaptoethanol, the IgG antibody value may parallel exactly the dye test response or may rise more slowly, reaching the peak no earlier than 6 months after infection. By 6 months, the IgM-IFA test result is negative in most cases, whereas the DS-IgM-ELISA and the IgM-ISAGA results usually remain positive; in women who become infected during pregnancy, the latter two tests are usually positive at the time of parturition.

When *Toxoplasma* infection is treated during the initial antibody response (when the IgG titer is low), the rise in IgG antibody titer slows and the titer (e.g., in the dye test or conventional IFA test) may remain low as long as treatment is continued. A late (delayed) rise often occurs after cessation of treatment.

In the absence of a routine screening program in which *Toxoplasma* serologic tests are performed each month in pregnant women, an IgM-IFA or DS-IgM-ELISA or IgM-ISAGA test should be performed if any other serologic test result is positive at any titer. If the IgM-IFA or DS-IgM-ELISA or IgM-ISAGA test is unavailable, the serologic test should be repeated in 3 or 4 weeks with serial twofold dilutions, to determine whether the titer is stable or rising. If the IgM-IFA test or DS-IgM-ELISA or IgM-ISAGA is negative and an IFA or dye test titer is stable and less than 1:1000 (300 IU), no further evaluation is necessary. Because titers in the dye test or IFA test usually stabilize at high levels (1:1000 6 to 8 weeks after acquisition of infection or longer, if the dye test or IFA test titer is 1:1000 [300 IU] IU and stable regardless of titer in the IgM-IFA test or DS-IgM-ELISA or IgM-ISAGA), the infection was acquired at least 4 weeks earlier and probably more than 8 weeks before the serum was obtained. Thus, for practical purposes, if the dye test or IFA test titer is 1:1000

Table 182–2 ■ Approach to Serologic Diagnosis of Toxoplasmosis*

	T. GONDII–SPECIFIC IgG†				*T. GONDII*–SPECIFIC IgM‡				*T. GONDII*–SPECIFIC IgA	*T. GONDII*–SPECIFIC IgE	*T. GONDII*–SPECIFIC IgE	OTHER TESTS		
PATIENT AND SPECIMEN	Dye Test	IFA	IgG ELISA	Direct Agglutination	DS-IgM-ELISA	IgM-ISAGA	ELISA for IgM to P30	IFA	IgA ELISA	IgE ELISA	IgE ISAGA	PCR	Isolation	AC/HS
Newborn congenital toxoplasmosis														
Serum	C	C	C	C	C	C	C	Do not use	C	C	C		C	
CSF	C				C							R	C	
Peripheral blood clot or peripheral blood cells													C	
Placenta												R	C	
Pregnant woman														
Maternal serum	C	C	C	C	C	C	C	C	C	C	C			C
Amniotic fluid												C	C	
Immunologically normal patient														
Serum	C	C	C	C	C	C	C	C						C
CSF	C				C									
Immunologically deficient patient														
Serum	C	C	C	C	C§	C§	C§	C§						
CSF	C	C	C	C	C§	C§	C§	C§				R	C	

*IFA, Indirect fluorescent antibody; Ig, immunoglobulin; ELISA, enzyme-linked immunosorbent assay; IgM-ISAGA, immunosorbent test for IgM; PCR, polymerase chain reaction; AC/HS, differential agglutination test; CSF, cerebrospinal fluid; C, commercially available; R, research test at present in reference laboratories.

†When properly standardized, any one of these tests is useful for demonstration of IgG antibody.

‡ISAGA is usually most sensitive; IFA is least sensitive (do not use for congenital infection).

§Rarely positive.

Adapted from Roberts F, Boyer KM, McLeod R: Toxoplasmosis. *In* Krugman S, Gershon AA, Katz SL, et al (eds): Infectious Diseases of Children, ed 10. St. Louis, Mosby–Year Book, 1997.

TABLE 182–3 ■ Guidelines for Interpretation of Serologic Tests for Toxoplasmosis*

TEST	POSITIVE TITER	TITER IN CONGENITAL INFECTION (INFANT) OR ACUTE INFECTION (OLDER CHILD, ADULT)	TITER IN CHRONIC INFECTION	DURATION OF ELEVATION OF TITER
IgG				
Sabin-Feldman dye test	Undiluted	NC: S OCA: 1:4 to ≥1:1000 (usual)	1:4 to 1:2000	Years
Direct agglutination test	≥1:20	NC: S OCA: Rises slowly from negative to low to high titer (1:512)	Stable (≥1:1000) or slowly decreasing titer	≥1 y
Indirect fluorescent IgG antibody	≥1:10	NC: S OCA: ≥1:1000	1:8 to 1:2000	Years
Indirect hemagglutination test	≥1:16	NC: S OCA: ≥1:1000	1:16 to 1:256	Years
Complement fixation	≥1:4	NC: S OCA: varies among laboratories	Negative to 1:8	Years
IgM				
Indirect fluorescent for IgM	≥1:10, adults	OCA: ≥1:80 (use only for OCA, not NC)	Negative to 1:20	Weeks to months, occasionally years
Double-sandwich IgM-ELISA	≥0.2, newborn, fetus; ≥1.7, older children, adults	NC: ≥0.2 OCA: ≥1.7	Negative to 1.7 (OCA)	Can be ≥1 y
Immunosorbent test for IgM	≥3, infant; 8, adult	NC: ≥3 OCA: >8	Negative to 1	Unknown, can be ≥1 y
IgA				
IgA, ELISA	≥1.0, infants; ≥2.1, adults	NC: ≥1.0 OCA: >2.1	Negative to <1.0 Negative to ≤2.1	Weeks to months, occasionally longer
IgE				
IgE, ELISA	≥1.9, infants and adults	NC and OCA: ≥1.9	Negative	Weeks to months, occasionally longer
Immunosorbent test for IgE	≥4, infants and adults	NC and OCA: ≥4	Negative	Weeks to months, occasionally longer
AC/HS	See Table 182–1	See Table 182–1	See Table 182–1	Usually <9 mo
PCR (amniotic fluid; CSF)	Positive	Positive	Negative	Only when *Toxoplasma* DNA present during active infection

*Ig, Immunoglobulin; NC, titer in newborn with congenital infection; OCA, titer in older child or adult with acute, acquired infection; S, usually the same as the mother; ELISA, enzyme-linked immunosorbent assay; AC/HS, differential agglutination test; PCR, polymerase chain reaction; CSF, cerebrospinal fluid. Note: values are those of one reference laboratory; each laboratory must provide its own standards and interpretation of results in each clinical setting.

Adapted from McLeod R, Remington JS: Toxoplasmosis. *In* Braunwald E, Isselbacher K, Petersdorf R, et al (eds): Harrison's Principles of Internal Medicine, ed 11. New York, McGraw-Hill, 1987, pp 791–797. Reproduced by permission of The McGraw-Hill Companies.

and stable when measured in the first 2 months of pregnancy, risk to the fetus is low.

Whereas titers in the dye test or IFA test may have stabilized and peaked by 8 weeks after onset of infection, titers in the complement fixation or IHA test may continue to rise for 4 to 6 months or longer after acquisition of infection. Therefore, rises in the last two test results may not be helpful in defining when the infection occurred relative to conception. The AC/HS test is also useful in determining that an infection was recently acquired. If the AC/HS test has an acute pattern (see Table 182–1), infection has usually been acquired in the preceding 9 months.

A common problem is the interpretation of serologic test results in an asymptomatic woman who is tested for *Toxoplasma* antibody late in the first trimester or in the second trimester of pregnancy. If her IFA or dye test titer is found to be in the range of 1:2000, her IgM-IFA test titer or DS-IgM-ELISA or IgM-ISAGA test is negative, and no significant rise in titer in any test is demonstrable, it is impossible to determine whether her infection occurred before, at, or after conception.

Detection of the *Taxoplasma B1* gene in amniotic fluid is useful in establishing the diagnosis of congenital toxoplasmosis in the fetus.

Congenital Toxoplasmosis

Guidelines for evaluation of a neonate when serology of the mother or illness in the neonate indicates that the diagnosis of congenital toxoplasmosis is suspected or likely are presented in Table 182–4. When the diagnosis of toxoplasmosis is suspected in a neonate, evaluation should proceed as outlined in Table 182–4. Representative results of specific serologic tests indicative of congenital infection are shown in Table 182–2. Persistent or rising titers in the dye test or a positive IgM, IgA, or IgE test specific for *T. gondii* in the absence of placental leak indicates infection. Repeating these tests on the 7th to 10th day of life may help to establish the

TABLE 182–4 ■ Evaluation of Neonate When Serology of Mother or Illness of Neonate Indicates That Diagnosis of Congenital Toxoplasmosis Is Suspected or Likely

In addition to a careful examination, the infant is examined by the following:

Clinical Evaluation and Nonspecific Tests
- A pediatric ophthalmologist
- A pediatric neurologist
- Brain computed tomography
- Blood tests
  - Complete blood count with differential and platelet counts
  - Serum total IgM, IgG, IgA, and albumin
  - Serum alanine aminotransferase, total and direct bilirubin
  - Cerebrospinal fluid (CSF) cell count, glucose, protein, and total IgG

***T. gondii*–Specific Tests**
- Newborn serum analyzed for antibody detected by the Sabin-Feldman dye test, IgM-ISAGA, IgA-ELISA, IgE-ELISA/ISAGA (0.5 mL of serum to Toxoplasma Serology Laboratory, Palo Alto Medical Foundation, 860 Bryant Street, Palo Alto, CA 94301, 415-326-8120); if value for IgA-ELISA measured in the first day of life is borderline, another sample on the 7th to 10th day of life may be useful in establishment of the diagnosis
- Newborn blood for inoculation into mice (1–2 mL of clotted whole blood in red-topped tube to Toxoplasma Serology Laboratory, address above)
- Lumbar puncture: CSF dye test and IGM-ELISA (0.5 mL of CSF to Toxoplasma Serology Laboratory, address above); consider PCR (1 mL of frozen CSF to Toxoplasma Serology Laboratory, address above)
- Sterile placental tissue (100 g in saline, from fetal side near insertion of cord, no formalin) to Toxoplasma Serology Laboratory for subinoculation
- Maternal serum analyzed for antibody detected by dye test, IgM-ELISA, IgA-ELISA, IgE-ELISA/ISAGA, and AC/HS

Adapted from Roberts F, Boyer KM, McLeod R: Toxoplasmosis. *In* Krugman S, Gershon AA, Katz SL, et al (eds): Infectious Diseases of Children, ed 10. St. Louis, Mosby–Year Book, 1997.

significance of a borderline or indeterminate value obtained initially at birth. It may be necessary to utilize multiple diagnostic tests, as none is positive in all infected infants. Because rheumatoid factor may be present in a newborn with congenital infection, it is important to exclude the presence of this antibody in an infant with a positive IgM-IFA test. If a placental leak of maternal blood has occurred, an elevated level of human chorionic gonadotropin-β may be present in the infant's serum and the IgM test titer in the neonate drops significantly within a week, because the half-life of IgM is approximately 3 to 5 days. IgM synthesis by the infant could also have stopped at this time, resulting in the fall in titer, however. Passively transferred maternal antibodies may require 6 to 12 months or longer to disappear from the infant's serum, depending on the original titer. The serum half-life of IgG is approximately 1 month. Synthesis of *Toxoplasma* antibody by the infected infant is usually demonstrable by the third month of life if the infant is not treated, but it may be delayed until the sixth or ninth month if the infant is treated. Infrequently, it may not occur at all. Thus, at the time the infant begins to synthesize antibody, infection may be documented serologically, even when IgM antibodies are not demonstrable. This may be accomplished by computation of the specific antibody "load" (i.e., the ratio of specific serum antibody titer to the level of serum IgG in mother and infant). For example, in an uninfected infant with only maternal antibody there is no change in antibody load because, as the titer of antibody decreases in the infant's serum, total IgG decreases in a similar manner. During the second and third months, the amount of IgG synthesized by the infant increases. Because this newly synthesized IgG does not contain *Toxoplasma* antibodies, the antibody load decreases and continues to decrease as IgG synthesis in the child progresses. In congenitally infected infants, the production of antibody may vary considerably from one case to another. Early and delayed antibody production can be demonstrated by increases in antibody load. The diagnosis of congenital toxoplasmosis has also been established as follows: demonstration of *Toxoplasma* DNA in the infant's blood or CSF; demonstration of antibodies to unique *T. gondii* epitopes in the infant's serum not present in the mother's serum; lymphocyte blastogenic response of the infant to lymphocyte *T. gondii* antigens; isolation of *T. gondii* from placenta, blood, or CSF of the infant. The approach to serologic diagnosis of toxoplasmosis in each of these clinical settings is summarized in Table 182–2.

Therapy

Therapy in Specific Clinical Settings

The need for and duration of therapy are determined by the clinical severity of the illness and by the person who is infected.

Immunologically normal patients with the lymphadenopathic form of acute toxoplasmosis do not require specific treatment unless there are severe and persistent symptoms or evidence of damage to vital organs.[38] Infections acquired in laboratory accidents or via transfusions may be more severe than naturally acquired infections and probably should be treated.

Patients with active chorioretinitis should be treated with specific drug therapy.[39, 40] Patients with active ocular toxoplasmosis should receive pyrimethamine and sulfadiazine 7 days beyond the time that active lesions resolve. Within 10 days of initiation of treatment, the borders of retinal lesions should sharpen and the vitreous haze (caused by inflammatory cells) should disappear. A favorable clinical response is seen in most cases; if unfavorable, the courses of pyrimethamine and sulfadiazine are repeated. Systemic corticosteroids are administered if vision is endangered by lesions involving the macula, optic nerve head, or papillomacular bundle. Occasionally, vitrectomy and removal of the lens may be necessary to restore visual acuity.

Toxoplasmosis should be treated in a patient whose resistance to infection is compromised by an underlying disease or by therapy (e.g., corticosteroids or cytotoxic drugs).[18, 20, 41, 42] Either serologic evidence of acute infection in an immunocompromised patient, whether or not signs and symptoms of infection are present, or the demonstration of tachyzoites in tissue, regardless of serologic test titers, is an indication for therapy. In 80% of immunocompromised patients in whom the diagnosis was established ante mortem, improvement occurred when specific therapy was administered. The major problem lies in making the diagnosis early enough to institute treatment.

Treatment of toxoplasmosis in patients with AIDS[43, 44] is discussed in depth in Chapter 125. Briefly, at present the dosage of pyrimethamine used is 75 to 100 mg/d after a 100- to 200-mg loading dose. This is given with 4 to 6 g of sulfadiazine or triple sulfonamides. Ten to 15 mg of leucovorin daily is also administered. Alternative treatment regimens are listed in Table 182–5.[45] AIDS patients who complete a primary course of therapy must receive a lifelong suppressive regimen. Pyrimethamine (25 to 50 mg) and sulfadiazine (2 to 4 g) each day have been used. Other potentially effective regimens are listed in Table 182–6.

TABLE 182–5 ■ Guidelines for Acute or Primary Therapy of Toxoplasmic Encephalitis in Patients with Acquired Immunodeficiency Syndrome*

DRUG	DOSAGE SCHEDULE
Standard regimens	
Pyrimethamine	Oral 200 mg loading dose, then 50 to 75 mg/d
Folinic acid (leucovorin)†	Oral, intravenous, or intramuscular 10–20 mg/d (up to 50 mg/d)
plus	
Sulfadiazine	Oral 1–1.5 g q 6 h
or	
Clindamycin	Oral or intravenous 600 mg q 6 h (up to intravenous 1200 mg q 6 h)
Possible alternative regimens‡	
a. Trimethoprim-sulfamethoxazole§	Oral or intravenous 5 mg (trimethoprim component) per kg q 6 h
b. Pyrimethamine and folinic acid	As in standard regimens plus one of the following:
Clarithromycin	Oral 1 g q 12 h
Azithromycin‖	Oral 1200–1500 mg/d
Atovaquone	Oral 750 mg q 6 h
Dapsone	Oral 100 mg/d

*This table is intended as a guide only and readers are referred to detailed reviews for individual regimens.[57–72]

†The dose of folinic acid can be titrated on the basis of the hemogram to reduce pyrimethamine-associated myelotoxicity. Up to 50 mg/d has been used.

‡These agents have been used in clinical studies with small numbers of patients and have response rates lower than those of the standard regimens. They should be used only in patients who are intolerant of the standard regimens. Alternative agents must be used in combination with another antimicrobial agent (most frequently, pyrimethamine with folinic acid) that has proven clinical activity against *T. gondii*.

§In a small study, trimethoprim-sulfamethoxazole at a dose of 6.6 mg (trimethoprim component) per kg per day has been reported to have similar efficacy to 20 mg of trimethoprim per kg per day. Further studies are required to determine the optimal dosage schedule (see text).

‖The optimal dose of azithromycin for the treatment of toxoplasmic encephalitis is being investigated in a dose escalation trial conducted by the AIDS Clinical Trials Group. The dosages given here are those that appear to have been effective in a small number of patients.

Adapted from Wong SY, Remington JS: Toxoplasmosis in the setting of AIDS. *In* Broder S, Merigan TC Jr, Bolognesi D (eds): Textbook of AIDS Medicine. Baltimore, Williams & Wilkins, 1994, pp 223–257. © by Samuel Broder, MD.

If a woman who acquires infection at any time during pregnancy is treated, the chance of congenital infection in her infant is decreased but not eliminated. In one series, the incidence of infection was decreased from 17% to 5%, and in another series it was decreased from 60% to 23%. The drugs effective in the only two reported studies were spiramycin in France[46] and pyrimethamine plus sulfonamide in Germany.[47] Because of the potential teratogenicity of pyrimethamine, sulfadiazine (which is highly effective in animal models when used alone) should be used alone if treatment is to be given in the first trimester of pregnancy. Spiramycin (available in the United States through the U.S. Food and Drug Administration [telephone 302-443-7580]) has also been used safely for prevention during the first trimester of pregnancy.

An approach, with apparent good outcome, for prevention, diagnosis, and treatment of congenital toxoplasmosis during a fetus' gestation is utilized in France and in part has been described by Hohfeld and coworkers as outlined in Table 182–7.[34, 47–49] In France, the methods for prevention include education about methods to avoid acquisition of *T. gondii* (Table 182–8). In one study, in one hospital, little or no information was given to pregnant women about how they might avoid acquisition of infection. The observed incidence of 59 per 1000 per year remained essentially identical to the incidence observed before the mode of transmission of the infection was discovered. In another hospital, the observed incidence was 37 per 1000 per year in 1973, when verbal instructions about hygienic measures were given to seronegative women, and 11 per 1000 per year in 1974, when explanatory drawings were given to patients. From these results, health education appears to be moderately effective in reduc-

TABLE 182–6 ■ Primary Prophylaxis and Suppressive Treatment

- Medications with documented efficacy for primary prophylaxis for seropositive patients with CD4+ cell counts <200/mm³
  - Trimethoprim-sulfamethoxazole (same as doses for *Pneumocystis carinii* pneumonia [PCP])
  - Pyrimethamine-dapsone (same as doses for PCP)
  - Sulfadoxine-pyrimethamine (Fansidar)
- Suppressive regimens
  - Pyrimethamine (25 mg/d) plus sulfadiazine (500 mg qid)—lowest relapse rate
  - Pyrimethamine (25 mg/d) plus clindamycin (1200 mg/d); often unacceptable gastrointestinal toxicity
  - Pyrimethamine-dapsone two or three times per week
  - Fansidar

TABLE 182–7 ■ French Approach to Prenatal Prevention, Diagnosis, and Treatment

- Diagnosis of mother: systematic serologic screening, before conception and intrapartum
- Treatment of mother: if acute serology, spiramycin reduces transmission. Untreated 94 (60%) of 154 versus treated 91 (23%) of 388.*
- Diagnosis of fetus: ultrasound examinations; amniocentesis, PCR at ≥18 wk of gestation. Sensitivity 37 (97%) of 38; specificity 301 of 301.†
- Treatment of fetus: pyrimethamine, sulfadiazine, or termination. $N = 54$ live births; 34 terminations.†‡
- Outcome: all 54 had normal development; 10 (19%) subtle findings; 7 (13%) intracranial calcifications; 3 (6%) chorioretinal scars§

*From Desmonts G, Couvreur J: Congenital toxoplasmosis. A prospective study of 378 pregnancies. N Engl J Med 290:1110–1116, 1974.

†From Hohlfeld P, Daffos F, Costa JM, et al: Prenatal diagnosis of congenital toxoplasmosis with a polymerase-chain-reaction test on amniotic fluid. N Engl J Med 331:695–699, 1994.

‡From Daffos F, Forestier F, Capella-Pavlovsky M, et al: Prenatal management of 746 pregnancies at risk for congenital toxoplasmosis. N Engl J Med 318:271–275, 1988.

§From Hohlfeld P, Daffos F, Thulliez P, et al: Fetal toxoplasmosis: Outcome of prenancy and infant follow-up after in utero treatment. J Pediatr 115:765–769, 1989.

TABLE 182–8 ■ Effect of Attempts at Health Education on the Incidence Rate of *Toxoplasma* Infection in Selected Populations of Pregnant Women in the Paris Area

HOSPITAL	PERIOD	INSTRUCTION	SEROCONVERSION	INCIDENCE PER 1000 PER YEAR
Hospitals Pinard and Baudelocque	Pre-1960	None	11 of 356	60
Centres Medico-Sociaux CPCAM	1961–1970	None	73 of 2496	64
Hospital X	1973–1975	None	18 of 710	59
Saint Antoine	1973	Verbal drawings	7 of 463	37
	1974		3 of 658	11
Longjumeau	1974–1981	Verbal	20 of 1938	22

Adapted from Remington JS, McLeod R, Desmonts G: Toxoplasmosis. *In* Remington JS, Klein JO (eds): Infectious Diseases of the Fetus and Newborn Infant, ed 4. Philadelphia, WB Saunders, 1995, pp 140–263.

ing incidence rates, and pictures and graphics appear to be more effective than the written word for such education.

In addition, acquisition of *T. gondii* by mothers during gestation is detected in a systematic serologic screening program[46, 48–50] (see Table 182–7). An acutely infected woman receives oral spiramycin (1 g three times a day), which reduces the incidence of transmission to the fetus. Fetal ultrasonography is performed every 2 weeks, with special attention to whether there are cerebral calcifications, hydrocephalus, hepatic calcification, hepatomegaly, or ascites. Amniocentesis is performed at approximately 18 weeks' gestation or later until term, as described before and PCR is performed to determine whether DNA of *T. gondii* is present. The cell pellet from a separate aliquot of amniotic fluid is inoculated into mice. If an infant is found to be infected using these tests, the well-informed pregnant patient can choose either to treat the fetus in utero with pyrimethamine, sulfadiazine, and leucovorin or to terminate the pregnancy. In the description of this method by Daffos and colleagues,[49] 28 such pregnancies were terminated and 15 infants of women who acquired *T. gondii* between the 16th and 25th weeks of gestation were treated in utero (i.e., their mothers received 3-week courses of spiramycin alternating with 3-week courses of 50 mg of pyrimethamine daily and 3 g of sulfadiazine daily until term) and then during their first year of life, beginning at birth. All the children are functioning normally at 2 years of age. Four had cerebral calcifications demonstrated during the first year of life, and two had peripheral retinal lesions.

Hohlfeld and colleagues[50] described their experience in detail. They presented results of treatment of 54 infants, 43 of whom were treated in utero with a mean follow-up of 19 months. Forty-one infants had subclinical infection, 12 had isolated asymptomatic signs (intracerebral calcifications and normal neurologic status, chorioretinal scar without visual impairment), and 1 had severe congenital toxoplasmosis. This outcome is considerably better than that found for historical controls without treatment in utero.

In Austria, Aspock and coworkers[47] treated all pregnant women with evidence of acquisition of *T. gondii* during their gestation with spiramycin until the 17th week of gestation and then pyrimethamine and sulfonamide until the infant is born. Studies are needed to determine the best approach. There are no carefully controlled studies to support the contention that a pregnant woman who has *Toxoplasma* antibody and a history of habitual abortion benefits from treatment.

We suggest that pregnant women who have depressed cell-mediated immunity (e.g., a pregnant woman with systemic lupus erythematosus who is receiving corticosteroids) and with serologic or other clinical evidence of *Toxoplasma* infection receive antitoxoplasma therapy in an attempt to prevent transmission to the fetus, whether the infection is newly acquired or chronic.

Both symptomatic and asymptomatic infants with congenital toxoplasmosis should be treated in an effort to prevent further destruction of vital organs.[40, 51–54] Guidelines for treatment of congenitally infected infants in whom the diagnosis is strongly suspected are outlined in Table 182–9.[36] Data from Europe and the United States suggest that early institution of specific treatment in these infants may prevent some sequelae and that it corrects manifestations of this infection such as active chorioretinitis, meningitis, encephalitis, hepatitis, splenomegaly, and thrombocytopenia. Hydrocephalus caused by aqueductal obstruction may develop or worsen during therapy. Such treatment also may reduce the incidence of some sequelae, such as chorioretinitis. Children with extensive involvement at birth may function normally later in life. Treatment does not eradicate the parasite in most children.[51]

Therapeutic Agents

Pyrimethamine plus Sulfadiazine or Trisulfapyrimidines. Pyrimethamine and sulfadiazine act synergistically against *Toxoplasma* in vivo with a combined activity that is eight times the amount expected if their effects were merely additive. Clinical experience confirms their efficacy. There is evidence that treatment of an acutely infected pregnant woman may prevent infection of her fetus (see the earlier section on therapy in specific clinical settings). The simultaneous use of both drugs is indicated except during the first trimester of pregnancy. Comparative tests have shown that sulfapyrazine, sulfamethazine, and sulfamerazine are about as effective as sulfadiazine. All the other sulfonamides tested (sulfathiazole, sulfapyridine, sulfadimetine, and sulfisoxazole) are much less effective.

Pyrimethamine. For adults, a loading dose of 100 to 200 mg of pyrimethamine should be given orally in two divided doses on the first day of treatment. For young children, a loading dose of 2 mg/kg body weight should be given for the first 2 days of treatment. Infants are given 2 mg/kg body weight for the first 2 days of treatment as a loading dose. Thereafter, a usual dosage for an immunologically normal adult is 25 mg/d in one dose. Higher dosages (e.g., 50 to 70 mg/d have been used for adults with AIDS to treat toxoplasmosis.[44, 55] Dosages in young children should not exceed 1 mg/kg body weight to a maximum of 25 mg/d. Because there are no data on absorption of the drug in patients who are quite ill, daily administration is recommended. Daily therapy is recommended for active ocular infection. Pyrimethamine is available only in tablet form. For infants, it may be crushed and administered with food or fluid.[51]

Pyrimethamine is a folic acid antagonist and therefore produces a dose-related, reversible, and usually gradual depres-

TABLE 182–9 ■ Treatment of Toxoplasmosis

MANIFESTATION OF INFECTION	MEDICATION	DOSAGE	DURATION OF THERAPY
Pregnant women with acute toxoplasmosis First 18 wk of gestation or until term if fetus not infected	Spiramycin*	1 g q 8 h without food	Until fetal infection is documented or excluded at 18–20 wk; if documented, has been used in France in alternate months with pyrimethamine, sulfadiazine, and leucovorin until term†
Fetal infection confirmed after 17th wk of gestation or if maternal infection acquired in last few weeks of gestation	Pyrimethamine	Loading dose: 100 mg/d in two divided doses for 2 d, then 50 mg/d	Until term (leucovorin is continued 1 wk after pyrimethamine is discontinued)
(after amniocentesis and PCR to determine whether there is *Toxoplasma* infection in the fetus)	Sulfadiazine	Loading dose: 75 mg/kg/d in two divided doses (maximum 4 g/d) for 2 d, then 100 mg/kg/d in two or four divided doses (maximum 4 g/d)	
	Leucovorin (folinic acid)	5–20 mg/d‡	
Congenital *Toxoplasma* infection in infants	Pyrimethamine§	Loading dose: 2 mg/kg/d for 2 d, then 1 mg/kg/d for 2 or 6 mo,‖ then this dose every Monday, Wednesday, and Friday	1 y¶ (leucovorin is continued 1 wk after pyrimethamine is discontinued)
	Sulfadiazine§	100 mg/kg/d in two divided doses	
	Leucovorin§	5–10 mg three times weekly‡	
CSF protein value ≥ 1 g/dL or active chorioretinitis that threatens vision	Corticosteroids (prednisone)	1 mg/kg/d in two divided doses**	Until resolution of elevated CSF protein level or active chorioretinitis
Active chorioretinitis in older children	Pyrimethamine	Loading dose: 2 mg/kg/d (maximum 50 mg) for 2 d, then maintenance, 1 mg/kg/d (maximum 25 mg)	Usually 1–2 wk beyond resolution of signs and symptoms (leucovorin is continued 1 wk after pyrimethamine is discontinued)
	Sulfadiazine	Loading dose: 75 mg/kg, then maintenance, 50 mg/kg every 12 h or 6 h	
	Leucovorin	5–20 mg three times weekly‡	
	Corticosteroids	1 mg/kg/d of prednisone in two divided doses**	Until resolution**
Immunologically normal children Lymphadenopathy	No therapy		
Significant organ damage that is life threatening	Pyrimethamine, sulfadiazine, leucovorin	Same as above for active chorioretinitis in older children; no corticosteroids	Usually 4–6 wk or 2 wk beyond resolution of signs and symptoms
Immunocompromised children Non-AIDS	Pyrimethamine, sulfadiazine, leucovorin	Same as above for active chorioretinitis in older children; no corticosteroids	Usually 4–6 wk beyond complete resolution of signs and symptoms
AIDS	Pyrimethamine, sulfadiazine, leucovorin	Same as above for active chorioretinitis in older children; no corticosteroids	Lifetime
	Clindamycin in place of sulfadiazine	Reported trials for adults, but not infants and children	

*Available only on request from the U.S. Food and Drug Administration; telephone 301-443-5680.
†The only studies are those of Hohlfeld et al.[48] However, because Hohlfeld and colleagues found pyrimethamine-sulfadiazine therapy to be superior to spiramycin for treatment of the fetus, continuous therapy with pyrimethamine, sulfadiazine, and leucovorin should be considered in the third trimester.
‡Adjusted for megaloblastic anemia, granulocytopenia, or thrombocytopenia; blood counts, including platelets, should be monitored as described in text.
§Optimal dosage, feasibility, and toxicity are currently being evaluated or planned in ongoing Chicago-based National Collaborative Treatment Trial; telephone 312-791-4152.
‖These two regimens are currently being compared in a randomized National Collaborative Treatment Trial. Data are not yet available to determine which, if either, is superior. Both regimens appear to be feasible and relatively safe.
¶In infants with AIDS. The duration of therapy is unknown. Please see discussion in section on congenital toxoplasmosis and AIDS.
**Corticosteroids should be continued until signs of inflammation (high CSF protein value ≥ 1 g/dL) or active chorioretinitis that threatens vision have subsided; dosage can then be tapered and discontinued; use only with pyrimethamine, sulfadiazine, and leucovorin.
From Roberts F, Boyer KM, McLeod R: Toxoplasmosis. *In* Krugman S, Gershon AA, Katz SL, et al (eds): Infectious Diseases of Children, ed 10. St. Louis, Mosby–Year Book, 1997.

sion of the bone marrow. Thrombocytopenia, leukopenia, and anemia may occur. All patients treated with pyrimethamine should have platelet and peripheral blood cell counts twice weekly.

Leucovorin calcium (folinic acid) should be administered with pyrimethamine to prevent suppression of the bone marrow. The optimal frequency for administration of folinic acid is unknown. An oral dose of 10 mg or more is recommended daily for older children and adults, or 10 mg three times weekly or more frequently for infants.

Sulfadiazine or Trisulfapyrimidine. Sulfadiazine or trisulfapyrimidine is administered to older children and adults in a loading dose of 50 to 75 mg/kg body weight; thereafter, 75 to 100 mg/kg body weight is administered daily in two doses 12 hours apart or four doses 6 hours apart. In infants, the loading dose is 100 mg/kg body weight; therefore, a total daily dose of 100 mg/kg is administered in two doses every 12 hours. Only a tablet form is available.

The potential toxic effects of sulfonamides (e.g., crystalluria, hematuria, rash) must be carefully monitored. Hypersensitivity reactions to sulfonamides may be a particular problem for patients with AIDS.[56]

Other Drugs. Treatment of pregnant women with spiramycin to reduce transplacental transmission of *T. gondii* has been with 3 g daily (i.e., 1.0 g morning, noon, and evening). Food impairs absorption of spiramycin. Toxicity is infrequent and has included paresthesia, allergic rash, nausea, vomiting, and diarrhea.

In a small number of patients with AIDS, high doses of pyrimethamine and large doses of clindamycin appeared as efficient as sulfonamides and high doses of pyrimethamine.[44] Azithromycin or clarithromycin and pyrimethamine have also been used in this setting.[57]

Other agents that have had some success when used in combination with pyrimethamine for treatment of toxoplasmosis in immunocompromised patients are azithromycin, clarithromycin, atovaquone, and interferon-γ. Because of potential interactions between zidovudine and pyrimethamine and possible additive bone marrow toxocity, when possible zidovudine therapy should be discontinued during treatment with pyrimethamine. Concomitant therapy with phenobarbital may reduce the half-life of pyrimethamine by induction of hepatic enzymes that degrade pyrimethamine.[58] Usual therapeutic doses of sulfadiazine interfere with metabolism of other agents such as phenytoin and warfarin by hepatic microsomal enzymes.

Duration of Therapy. The optimal duration of specific therapy of toxoplasmosis is not known. Patients who appear to be immunologically normal but have severe and persistent symptoms or damage to vital organs (e.g., chorioretinitis, myocarditis) require specific therapy until these specific symptoms resolve followed by therapy for an additional 2 weeks. This is usually for at least 4 to 6 weeks and sometimes longer.

For immunocompromised patients, therapy should continue for at least 4 to 6 weeks beyond complete resolution of all signs and symptoms of active disease. Careful follow-up of these patients is imperative because relapse requires prompt reinstitution of therapy.

Relapse is frequent in patients with AIDS. Prolonged prophylaxis should be given.[41, 43, 59–70] Although therapy may be effective against *T. gondii* tachyzoites and may induce a beneficial response clinically, it does not eradicate the cyst form from the CNS and perhaps not from other tissues. Patients infected with human immunodeficiency virus who have neurologic signs or symptoms, $CD4^+$ cell counts less than 100/mm^3, and radiographic scans consistent with toxoplamic encephalitis are treated empirically with pyrimethamine plus either clindamycin or sulfadiazine. Clinical response to treatment is noted in 1 to 2 weeks and radiographic resolution in 3 to 6 weeks. Relapse occurs after this treatment in more than 50% of such individuals if treatment is discontinued. Daily pyrimethamine (25 mg) and sulfadiazine (2 g) prophylaxis reduced the relapse rate to 6% in one study, and tolerance of this regimen was reasonable. In this study, twice-weekly prophylaxis with the same dosages of medications resulted in a 30% relapse rate. Other suppressive regimens for individuals who cannot tolerate sulfadiazine, the efficacy of which has not been proved are listed in Table 182–6.

Desmonts and Couvreur[46] treated acutely infected pregnant women with 3 g of spiramycin daily, administered orally in three doses, from the time of diagnosis until term. Aspoch[47] in Germany gave a course of sulfonamide and pyrimethamine followed by one to two courses of sulfonamide administered alone or in combination with pyrimethamine. Each course was given for approximately 2 weeks. The courses of treatment were separated by 3- to 4-week intervals of no treatment. Pyrimethamine was not given in the first trimester of pregnancy.

Infants with congenital toxoplasmosis should be treated as outlined in Table 182–9.

Prophylaxis

Prophylaxis against *Toxoplasma* involves intervention in the cycle of transmission[71, 72] (Table 182–10). Prevention of infection by *T. gondii* is most important in immunodeficient patients and seronegative pregnant women.[71–73]

Meat and eggs should be heated to 60°C to kill cysts. Freezing to −20°C kills cysts in meat, but commercial freezers in most areas of the world do not reach or maintain this temperature reliably. Hands should be washed after touching uncooked meat. Fruits and vegetables may be contaminated with oocysts and should be washed. Contact with cat feces should be avoided.

Although there are no definitive data on the risks of using seropositive donors, the following are our recommendations: blood or blood products donated by people with *Toxoplasma* antibody should not be given to immunosuppressed recipi-

TABLE 182–10 ▪ Methods for Preventing Congenital Toxoplasmosis

PREVENTION OF INFECTION IN ADULTS
Cook meat to 66°C (well done), smoke it, or cure it in brine.
Cook eggs and do not drink unpasteurized milk.
Avoid touching mucous membranes of mouth and eyes while handling raw meat.
Wash hands thoroughly after handling raw meat.
Wash kitchen surfaces that come into contact with raw meat.
Wash fruits and vegetables before consumption.
Prevent access of flies, cockroaches, and so on to fruits and vegetables.
Avoid contact with materials that are potentially contaminated with cat feces (e.g., cat litter boxes) or wear gloves when handling such materials or when gardening or playing with children in a sandbox.
Disinfect cat litter box for 5 min with nearly boiling water.
PREVENTION OF INFECTION IN FETUS
Identify women at risk by serologic testing.
Treatment during pregnancy results in ≈50% reduction in infected infants and can treat manifestations of infection in the fetus.
Therapeutic abortion prevents birth of infected infant; used only when women acquire infection in first or second trimester (50% of cases).

Adapted from Wilson CB, Remington JS: What can be done to prevent congenital toxoplasmosis? Am J Obstet Gynecol 138:357–363, 1980.

ents, and organs of those with *Toxoplasma* antibody should not be given to seronegative recipients.

A nontoxic drug that eliminates the organism in the tissue cyst form as well as in the tachyzoite form is needed to prevent the devastating complications of recrudescent infection in immunocompromised patients.

For prevention of transmission of *Toxoplasma* to the fetus, see the section on therapy in specific clinical settings. There is no effective vaccine to prevent *Toxoplasma* infection. Because maternal immunity appears to prevent congenital transmission of *T. gondii,* development of a vaccine should be explored. Vaccines that prevent oocyst development in household cats could interrupt the life cycle of *T. gondii.*

References

1. Boyer K, McLeod R: *Toxoplasma gondii* (toxoplasmosis). *In* Long SS, Prober CG, Pickering LK (eds): Principles and Practice of Pediatric Infectious Diseases. New York, Churchill Livingstone, 1996, pp 645–672.
2. Remington JS, McLeod R, Desmonts G: Toxoplasmosis. *In* Remington JS, Klein JO (eds): Infectious Diseases of the Fetus and Newborn Infant, ed 4. Philadelphia, WB Saunders, 1995, pp 140–268.
3. McLeod R, Mack D, Brown C: New advances in cellular and molecular biology of *Toxoplasma gondii.* Exp Parasitol 72:109, 1991.
4. Aikawa M, Komata Y, Asai T, Midorikawa O: Transmission and scanning electron microscopy of host cell entry by *Toxoplasma gondii.* Am J Pathol 87:285, 1977.
5. Weiss LM, Laplace D, Takvorian PM, et al: Development of bradyzoites of *Toxoplasma gondii* in vitro. J Eukaryol Microbiol 41:18S, 1994.
6. Remington JS: In Discussion, Lainson R: Observations on the nature and transmission of *Toxoplasma gondii* in light of its wide host and geographical range. Toxoplasmosis. Surv Ophthalmol 6:721, 1961.
7. Dubey JP, Miller NL, Frenkel JK: The *Toxoplasma gondii* oocyst from cat feces. J Exp Med 132:636, 1970.
8. Mayes JT, O'Connor BJ, Avery R, et al: Transmission of *Toxoplasma gondii* infection by liver transplantation. Clin Infect Dis 21:511, 1995.
9. Remington JS, McLeod R: Toxoplasmosis. *In* Braude AI (ed): International Textbook of Medicine, Vol II, Medical Microbiology and Infectious Diseases. Philadelphia, WB Saunders, 1981, pp 1816–1832.
10. Luft BJ, Remington JS: Acute *Toxoplasma* infection among family members of patients with acute lymphadenopathic toxoplasmosis. Arch Intern Med 144:53, 1984.
11. Bennenson MW, Takafuji ET, Lemon SM, et al: Oocyst-transmitted toxoplasmosis associated with ingestion of contaminated water. N Engl J Med 307:666, 1982.
12. Dorfman RF, Remington JS: Value of lymph-node biopsy in the diagnosis of acute acquired toxoplasmosis. N Engl J Med 289:878, 1973.
13. Ghatak NR, Poon TP, Zimmerman HM: Toxoplasmosis of the central nervous system in the adult. A light and electron microscopic study of three cases. Arch Pathol 89:337, 1970.
14. Brooks RG, McCabe RE, Remington JS: Role of serology in the diagnosis of toxoplasmic lymphadenopathy. Rev Infect Dis 9:1055, 1987.
15. McCabe RE, Brooks RG, Dorfman RF, Remington JS: Clinical spectrum in 107 cases of toxoplasmic lymphadenopathy. Rev Infect Dis 9:754, 1987.
16. O'Connor GR: Ocular toxoplasmosis. *In* Locatcher-Khorazo D, Seegal BC (eds): Microbiology of the Eye. St. Louis, CV Mosby, 1972, p 199.
17. Polis MA: Differential diagnosis of retinal lesions in persons with HIV infection. Opportunistic Infect Interaction 3:1, 1994.
18. Ruskin J, Remington JS: Toxoplasmosis in the compromised host. Ann Intern Med 84:193, 1976.
19. Israelski DM, Remington JS: Toxoplasmic encephalitis in patients with AIDS. *In* Sande MA, Volberding PA (eds): The Medical Management of AIDS. Philadelphia, WB Saunders, 1988, pp 193–211.
20. Luft BJ, Naot Y, Araujo FG, et al: Primary and reactivated toxoplasma infection in patients with cardiac transplants. Clinical spectrum and problems in diagnosis in a defined population. Ann Intern Med 99:27, 1983.
21. Pierce M, Johnson M, Maciunas R, et al: Evaluating contrast-enhancing brain lesions in patients with AIDS by using positron emission tomography. Ann Intern Med 123:594, 1995.
22. Desmonts G, Couvreur J: Natural history of congenital toxoplasmosis. Ann Pediatr 31:799, 1984.
23. Koppe JG, Loewer-Sieger DH, De Roever-Bonnet H: Results of 20-year follow-up of congenital toxoplasmosis. Lancet 1:254, 1986.
24. Wilson CB, Remington JS, Stagno S, Reynolds DW: Development of adverse sequelae in children born with subclinical congenital *Toxoplasma* infection. Pediatrics 66:767, 1980.
25. Frenkel JK, Ruiz A: Endemicity of toxoplasmosis in Costa Rica. Am J Epidemiol 113:254, 1981.
26. Conley FK, Remington JS: *Toxoplasma gondii* infection of the central nervous system. Use of the PAP method to demonstrate *Toxoplasma* in formalin-fixed paraffin-embedded tissue sections. Hum Pathol 12:690, 1981.
27. Montoya JG, Remington J: Studies on the serodiagnosis of toxoplasmic lymphadenopathy. Clin Infect Dis 20:781, 1995.
28. Desmonts G, Remington JS: Direct agglutination test for diagnosis of *Toxoplasma* infection: Method for increasing sensitivity and specificity. J Clin Microbiol 11:562, 1980.
29. Dannemann BR, Vaughan WC, Thulliez P, et al: The differential agglutination test for diagnosis of recently acquired infection with *Toxoplasma gondii.* J Clin Microbiol 28:1928, 1990.
30. Thulliez P, Remington JS, Santoro F, et al: Une nouvelle réaction d'agglutination pour le diagnostic du stade évolutif de la toxoplasmose acquise. Pathol Biol 34:173, 1986.
31. Desmonts G: Sérodiagnostic de la toxoplasmose. Feuill Biol 16:61, 1975.
32. Naot Y, Remington JS: An enzyme-linked immunosorbent assay for detection of IgM antibodies to *Toxoplasma gondii:* Use for diagnosis of acute acquired toxoplasmosis. J Infect Dis 142:757, 1980.
33. Decoster A, Darcy F, Caron A, et al: IgA antibodies against P30 as markers of congenital and acute toxoplasmosis. Lancet 2:1104, 1988.
34. Stepick-Biek P, Thulliez P, Araujo FG, et al: IgA antibodies for diagnosis of acute congenital and acquired toxoplasmosis. J Infect Dis 162:270, 1990.
35. Grover CM, Thulliez P, Remington JS, et al: Rapid prenatal diagnosis of congenital *Toxoplasma* infection by using polymerase chain reaction and amniotic fluid. J Clin Microbiol 28:2297, 1990.
36. Roberts F, Boyer KM, McLeod R: Toxoplasmosis. *In* Krugman S, Gershon AA, Katz SL, et al (eds): Infectious Diseases of Children, ed 10. St. Louis, Mosby–Year Book, 1997.
37. McLeod R, Remington JS: Toxoplasmosis. *In* Braunwald E, Isselbacher K, Petersdorf R, et al (eds): Harrison's Principles of Internal Medicine, ed 11. New York, McGraw-Hill, 1987, pp 791–797.
38. Townsend JJ, Wolinsky JS, Baringer JR, Johnson PC: Acquired toxoplasmosis. Arch Neurol 32:335, 1975.
39. O'Connor GR: Manifestations and management of ocular toxoplasmosis. Bull N Y Acad Med 50:192, 1974.
40. Mets M, Holfels E, Boyer KM, et al: Eye manifestations of congenital toxoplasmosis. Am J Ophthamol 122:309, 1996.
41. Kovacs JA: Efficacy of atovaquone in treatment of toxoplasmosis in patients with AIDS. The NIAID–Clinical Center Intramural AIDS Program. Lancet 340:637, 1992.
42. Luft BJ, Hafner R, Korzun AH, et al: Toxoplasmic encephalitis in patients with the acquired immunodeficiency syndrome. Members of the ACTG 077p/ANRS 009 Study Team. N Engl J Med 329:995, 1993.
43. Consensus recommendations: Disease-specific recommendations; toxoplasmic encephalitis. Clin Infect Dis 21(Suppl 1), 1995.
44. Dannemann BR, McCutchan JA, Israelski D, et al: Treatment of toxoplasmic encephalitis in patients with AIDS. A randomized trial comparing pyrimethamine plus clindamycin to pyrimethamine plus sulfadiazine. Ann Intern Med 116:33, 1992.
45. Wong SY, Remington JS: Toxoplasmosis in the setting of AIDS. *In* Broder S, Merigan TC Jr, Bolognesi D (eds): Textbook of AIDS Medicine. Baltimore, Williams & Wilkins, 1994, pp 223–257.

46. Desmonts G, Couvreur J: Congenital toxoplasmosis. A prospective study of 378 pregnancies. N Engl J Med 290:1110, 1974.
47. Aspock H: Prevention of congenital toxoplasmosis by serological surveillance during pregnancy: Current strategies and future perspectives. *In* Marget W, Lang W, Gabler-Sandberger E (eds): Parasitic Infections, Immunology, Mycotic Infections, General Topics, Vol 3. Munich, MMV Medizin Verlag, 1986, pp 69–72.
48. Hohlfeld P, Daffos F, Costa JM, et al: Prenatal diagnosis of congenital toxoplasmosis with a polymerase-chain-reaction test on amniotic fluid. N Engl J Med 331:695, 1994.
49. Daffos F, Forestier F, Capella-Paviovsky M, et al: Prenatal management of 746 pregnancies at risk for congenital toxoplasmosis. N Engl J Med 318:271, 1988.
50. Hohlfeld P, Daffos F, Thulliez P, et al: Fetal toxoplasmosis outcome of pregnancy and infant follow-up after in utero treatment. J Pediatr 115:765, 1989.
51. McAuley J, Boyer K, Patel D, et al: Early and longitudinal evaluations of treated infants and children and untreated historical patients with congenital toxoplasmosis: The Chicago Collaborative Treatment Trial. Clin Infect Dis 18:38, 1994.
52. Swisher, CN, Boyer K, McLeod R: Congenital toxoplasmosis. Semin Pediatr Neurol 1:4, 1994.
53. Roizen N, Swisher C, Stein M, et al: Developmental and neurologic outcome in treated congenital toxoplasmosis. Pediatrics 95:11, 1995.
54. Patel D, Holfels EM, Vogel NP, et al: Resolution of intracerebral calcifications in children with treated congenital toxoplasmosis. Radiology 199:433, 1996.
55. Weiss LM, Harris C, Berger M, et al: Pyrimethamine concentrations in serum and cerebrospinal fluid during treatment of acute *Toxoplasma* encephalitis in patients with AIDS. J Infect Dis 157:580, 1988.
56. Moreno JN, Poblete RB, Maggio C, et al: Rapid oral desensitization for sulfonamides in patients with the acquired immunodeficiency syndrome. Ann Allergy Asthma Immunol 74:140, 1995.
57. Fernandez-Martin J, Leport C, Morlat P, et al: Pyrimethamine-clarithromycin combination for therapy of acute *Toxoplasma* encephalitis in patients with AIDS. Antimicrob Agents Chemother 35:2049, 1991.
58. McLeod R, Mack D, Foss R, et al: Levels of pyrimethamine in sera and cerebrospinal and ventricular fluids from infants treated for congenital toxoplasmosis. Antimicrob Agents Chemother 36:1040, 1992.
59. de Gans J, Portegies P, Reiss P, et al: Pyrimethamine alone as maintenance therapy for central nervous system toxoplasmosis in 38 patients with AIDS. J Acquir Immune Defic Syndr 5:137, 1992.
60. Kovacs JA: Toxoplasmosis in AIDS: Keeping the lid on. Ann Intern Med 123:230, 1995.
61. Leport C, Chene G, Morlat P, et al: Pyrimethamine for primary prophylaxis of toxoplasmic encephalitis in patients with human immunodeficiency virus infection: A double-blind, randomized trial. J Infect Dis 173:91, 1996.
62. Katlama C, De Wit S, O'Doherty E, et al: Pyrimethamine-clindamycin vs. pyrimethamine-sulfadiazine as acute and long-term therapy for toxoplasmic encephalitis in patients with AIDS. Clin Infect Dis 22:268, 1996.
63. Heald A, Flepp M, Chave JP, et al: Treatment for cerebral toxoplasmosis protects against *Pneumocystis carinii* pneumonia in patients with AIDS. The Swiss HIV Cohort Study. Ann Intern Med 155:760, 1991.
64. Pedrol E, Gonzalez-Clemente JM, Gatell JM, et al: Central nervous system toxoplasmosis in AIDS patients: Efficacy of an intermittent maintenance therapy. AIDS 4:511, 1990.
65. Podzamczer D, Salazar A, Jimenez J, et al: Intermittent trimethoprim-sulfamethoxazole compared with dapsone-pyrimethamine for the simultaneous primary prophylaxis of *Pneumocystis* pneumonia and toxoplasmosis in patients infected with HIV. Ann Intern Med 122:755, 1995.
66. Podzamczer D, Miro JM, Bolao F, et al: Twice weekly maintenance therapy with sulfadiazine-pyrimethamine to prevent recurrent toxoplasmic encephalitis in patients with AIDS. Ann Intern Med 123:175, 1995.
67. Porter SB, Sande MA: Toxoplasmosis of the central nervous system in the acquired immunodeficiency syndrome. N Engl J Med 327:1643, 1992.
68. Richards F Jr, Kovacs J, Luft B: Preventing toxoplasmic encephalitis in persons infected with human immunodeficiency virus. Clin Infect Dis 21(Suppl 1):S49, 1995.
69. Ruf B, Schurmann D, Bergmann F, et al: Efficacy of pyrimethamine/sulfadoxine in the prevention of toxoplasmic encephalitis relapses and *Pneumocystis carinii* pneumonia in HIV-infected patients. Eur J Clin Microbiol Infect Dis 12:325, 1993.
70. Saba J, Morlat P, Raffi F, et al: Pyrimethamine plus azithromycin for treatment of acute toxoplasmic encephalitis in patients with AIDS. Eur J Clin Microbiol Infect Dis 12:853, 1993.
71. McCabe R, Remington JS: Toxoplasmosis: The time has come. N Engl J Med 318:313, 1988.
72. Wilson CB, Remington JS: What can be done to prevent congenital toxoplasmosis? Am J Obstet Gynecol 138:357, 1980.
73. Wong SY, Remington JS: State of the art clinical article: Toxoplasmosis in pregnancy. Clin Infect Dis 18:853, 1994.

183

Larva Migrans Syndromes Caused by *Toxocara* Species and Other Nematodes

Peter M. Schantz

History

Certain parasitic helminths of lower animals can infect a variety of mammals that are not their definitive hosts. Under such conditions the invading larvae usually do not develop further but survive indefinitely in the tissues. If these animals, called paratenic or transport hosts, form part of the food chain of the definitive host, the parasite's life cycle is eventually completed. In the first half of this century, several parasitologists speculated that such animal parasites might cause disease in human beings. However, it was not until 1952 that Beaver and colleagues[1] described larvae of *Toxocara canis*, an intestinal roundworm of dogs, in the tissues of children with eosinophilia-hepatomegaly, which is a common clinical syndrome of previously unknown cause. The authors proposed the term visceral larva migrans (VLM) to describe the syndrome. Wilder[2] observed nematode larvae in 24 of 46 eyes that had been enucleated, in most instances after a clinical diagnosis of retinoblastoma. She identified the worms as third-stage hookworm larvae, but Nichols[3] reexamined the specimens and identified the larvae as *T. canis*. The concept of larva migrans was redefined by Beaver[4] to describe the prolonged migration and long persistence of larvae whose behavior reflects the behavior of paratenic hosts. Subsequently, Sprent[5] described the complex life cycles of *Toxocara* spp. The development of a sensitive and specific serologic test greatly stimulated clinical and epidemiologic research.[6] Toxocaral larva migrans syndromes are now recognized as common zoonotic infections in all countries.[7] In developed countries, toxocariasis ranks with pinworm among the most frequent human helminth infections.[8]

Other species of helminth larvae have been reported to infect human beings and cause larva migrans syndromes

TABLE 183–1 ■ Some Animal Helminth Agents of Larva Migrans Syndromes and Their Hosts and Modes of Transmission to Humans

HELMINTH AGENT	NATURAL DEFINITIVE HOSTS	SOURCE AND MODE OF TRANSMISSION TO HUMANS
Toxocara canis	Dogs, other canids	Ingestion of eggs
Toxocara cati	Cats, other felids	Ingestion of eggs
Ancylostoma spp.	Dogs, cats	Direct skin penetration by larvae
Baylisascaris spp.	Raccoons and other wild mammals	Ingestion of infective eggs
Gnathostoma spp.	Cats, other carnivores	Ingestion of larvae in uncooked flesh of fish, amphibian, avian, or mammalian transport hosts
Spirometra spp.	Cats	Ingestion of larvae in aquatic crustaceans or vertebrate transport hosts

(Table 183–1). The clinical manifestations of the larva migrans syndromes vary according to the helminth species, number of infective larvae, mode of transmission, migration of larvae to critical locations, and other factors.

Toxocara Species

Characteristics of the Pathogen

Toxocara species (family Ascaridae) are large (8 to 18 cm long), heavy-bodied nematodes, the adult stages of which reside in the small intestine of their final host. Two species infect dogs and cats: *T. canis* of dogs and other canids and *Toxocara cati* of cats and other felids. Clinical and epidemiologic evidence indicates that the majority of human infections are caused by *T. canis*. The infective stage for humans is the third-stage larva in the egg (75 to 90 × 65 to 75 μm). When released by hatching, the larva measures 350 to 450 × 16 to 20 μm and is capable of penetrating and migrating extensively in tissues (Fig. 183–1).

Epidemiology

Toxocara species are well adapted for transmission and survival. Dogs can become infected with *T. canis* by ingestion of infective eggs, ingestion of larvae in tissues of paratenic hosts (mice, birds, pigs, earthworms), transplacental migration of larvae from a pregnant bitch to her developing pups, transmammary passage of larvae in milk from a lactating bitch to nursing pups, and ingestion of late-stage larvae or immature adults in the vomitus or feces of infected pups.[9] The transplacental route of infection is so efficient that, unless heroic measures have been taken to eliminate larvae from bitches, nearly all pups from infected mothers are born with *Toxocara* larvae in migration. By the fourth postpartum week, these larvae have matured in the pups' intestines and are producing eggs. The life cycle of *T. cati* in cats is similar to that of *T. canis* in dogs, except that there is no placental transfer of larvae. The life span of adult *Toxocara* organisms averages 4 months. Individual female *T. canis* organisms can produce 200,000 eggs per day; because intestinal worm burdens range from one to several hundred worms, infected animals can contaminate the environment daily with millions of eggs. Fertilized eggs passed in dog or cat feces require a minimum of 14 to 21 days in optimal temperature and humidity to molt and develop to the infective larval stage. Direct sunlight and desiccation are rapidly lethal to eggs; in humid soil, however, they may survive for months or even years.

The immense popularity of pets (more than 50% of U.S. households have dogs or cats), the high prevalence of toxocariasis in puppies and kittens, and the intimate association of dogs and children favor widespread environmental contamination and transmission to children.[7] Almost all cases of severe VLM are diagnosed in children 18 months to 3 years old. In the United States, studies have implicated household dogs, particularly puppies, in combination with pica as the principal risk factors for infection.[7] Children with geophagic pica (compulsion to eat dirt), a behavior disorder noted in 2% to 10% of children 1 to 6 years old,[10] are extremely vulnerable to infection if they are in a contaminated environment. Older children and adults exposed to the same environments may avoid infection altogether or ingest fewer eggs. Ocular larva migrans (OLM) and milder signs and symptoms of VLM are seen more frequently in older children and adults than in extremely young children.[7] Most children with toxocariasis have kept a dog in the house or yard within 1 year of onset of symptoms. However, numerous surveys have verified that soil in parks and other public places is frequently contaminated by *Toxocara* eggs.

Although underrecognized and underreported, *Toxocara* larva migrans is a relatively common infection. Serosurveys in the United States suggest that many thousands of persons are infected every year[7]; the great majority of new infections are apparently asymptomatic. One indication of the number of clinical cases is the number of serum specimens submitted every year to state health laboratories for serodiagnosis of toxocariasis. From 1978 through 1987, this number varied from 2500 to 3500 samples, of which 25% to 30% tested positive.[8] Approximately two thirds of the patients had presumptive cases of OLM.

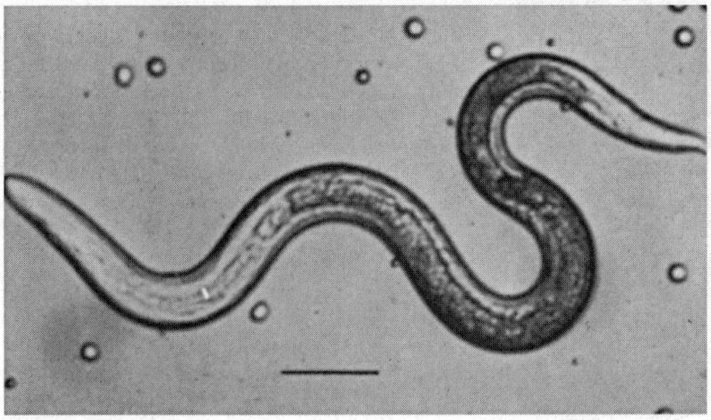

FIGURE 183–1 □ Infective-stage larva of *Toxocara canis* after artificial hatching from egg. Bar = 50 μm.

Pathogenesis

Toxocariasis in humans is acquired by ingestion of the eggs of *Toxocara* spp. that contain the infective-stage larvae. The eggs hatch in the proximal small intestine, and the released larvae penetrate the mucosa, migrate to the liver via the portal circulation, follow vascular channels to the lungs, and then enter the systemic circulation. When the size of the larvae exceeds the diameter of the blood vessel, they are impeded and actively bore through the vessel wall and migrate in the surrounding tissue. Larvae migrate extensively through the body and have been found in every tissue and organ system, including liver, lungs, heart, and brain.[1] The distribution and survival of larvae are determined by the size of the inoculum and the frequency of reinfection. In *Toxocara*-naive animals, the total number of recoverable larvae, especially in the liver and lungs, is reduced markedly after the first week post infection.[11] Thereafter, however, most larvae survive for many months or even years, although the distribution in the host's tissues may continue to shift. Larvae accumulate progressively in the brain while disappearing from other tissues.[12] Larvae in the brain may be relatively free from the harmful effects of the host immunologic response. The number of larvae in the liver is greater with superinfection and reinfection than with lower doses or single infections. The migrating larvae leave tracks of hemorrhage, necrosis, and inflammatory cells. In early infections (e.g., 2 weeks), the earliest response is an acute inflammatory reaction consisting of aggregates of eosinophils, neutrophils, and some monocytes.[11] As a result of rapid migration, most larvae visualized at this time in tissues are not associated with inflammatory cells (Fig. 183–2). By 1 month, larvae and larval tracks are surrounded by rudimentary collagenous capsules. In chronic infections, most larvae are encapsulated by mature granulomata composed of a central core of multinucleated cells and leukocytes. A narrow zone of fibroblastic tissue may delineate the granuloma from the adjacent hepatic parenchyma (Fig. 183–3). Although larvae are not seen in most granulomata, those that are seen usually appear intact and are presumably viable. The remarkable capacity of *Toxocara* larvae to survive and continue migrating in host tissues despite vigorous immunologic responses seems to be associated with the larvae's capacity to shield themselves from host antibody and cells by producing and shedding substances from the larval surface.[13–15]

Clinical Manifestations

Most people with *Toxocara* infection do not develop overt clinical disease. The spectrum of clinical manifestations reflects the numbers of larvae ingested, the frequency of reinfection, the distribution of larvae in the tissues, and the intensity of the inflammatory response.

Two syndromes caused by *Toxocara* infection, VLM and OLM, are well defined.[7, 16] VLM, usually diagnosed in quite young children (average age 2 years), is a marked inflammatory immune response to numerous larvae migrating in the liver and other tissues. VLM is characterized by persistent eosinophilia, leukocytosis, fever, hepatomegaly, hypergammaglobulinemia, and elevated titers of blood group isohemagglutinins. Clinical signs often include wheezing or coughing, and pulmonary infiltration is evident in one third of patients.[16, 17] Asthma and recurrent bronchitis have been associated with *Toxocara* antibody reactivity.[18] Neurologic manifestations, including focal or generalized seizures and behavior disorders, have been reported in as many as 28% of VLM patients.[17] The term covert toxocariasis has been suggested to describe the signs and symptoms of patients with clinical features that singly are nonspecific but together form a recognizable symptom complex.[19] Such signs include abdominal pain, anorexia, sleep and behavior disturbances, cervical adenitis, wheezing, limb pains, and fever. VLM is ordinarily self-resolving once patients are prevented from reinfecting themselves. Rare fatal cases have resulted from larval migration through the myocardium or the central nervous system.

Larval invasion of the eye, typically unilateral, is not uncommon. Common complaints include visual loss, strabismus, and, more rarely, eye pain. On funduscopic examination, the lesion may range from a solitary posterior pole or peripheral granuloma in a "quiet" eye to severe exudative endophthalmitis with retinal detachment. In addition, *Toxocara* infection may cause posterior and peripheral retinochoroiditis, optic papillitis, uveitis, and other lesions.[20] The average age of patients with OLM is approximately 8 years, but the condition is often diagnosed in adults as well.[16]

Clinical and epidemiologic differences between VLM and OLM suggest distinct pathogenetic mechanisms.[7, 16] These differences seem to be related to the number of infective larvae ingested.[7] Lower doses of *Toxocara* are associated with a higher probability of OLM than VLM. As the number of ingested larvae increases, the probability of OLM decreases and the chance of VLM increases. As the parasite load increases further, the likelihood of OLM (concurrent with VLM) once again increases, as does the severity of systemic signs. This may explain why most children with VLM have a his-

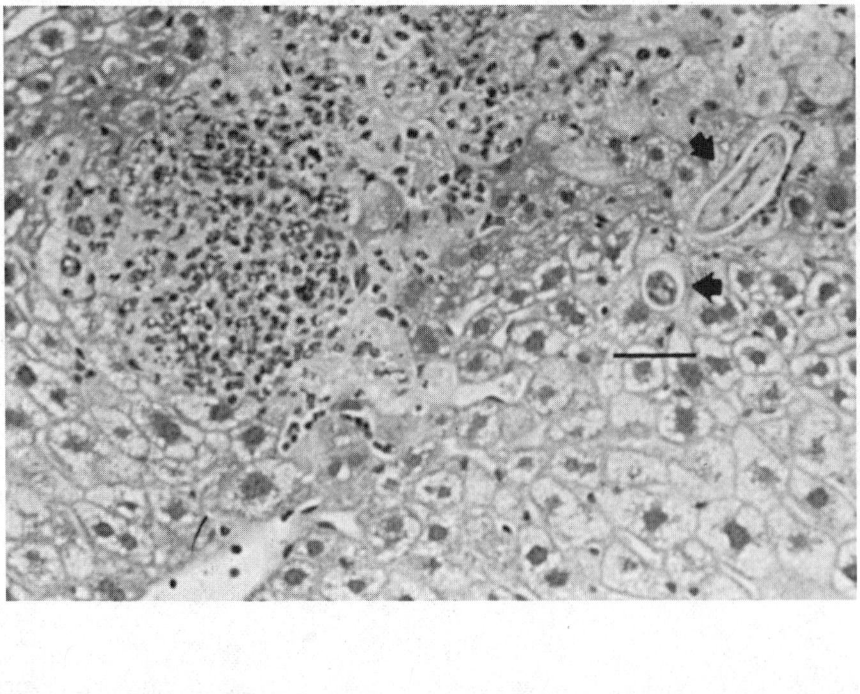

FIGURE 183–2 □ Section of mouse liver 2 days after experimental infection with 5000 eggs of *T. canis.* Areas of hepatocellular necrosis and infiltration of neutrophils associated with a *T. canis* larva *(arrows).* Note that larva is free of inflammatory cells. Hematoxylin-eosin; bar = 50 μm. (Courtesy of Dr. Jim C. Parsons, Victorian Institute of Animal Sciences, Victoria, Australia.)

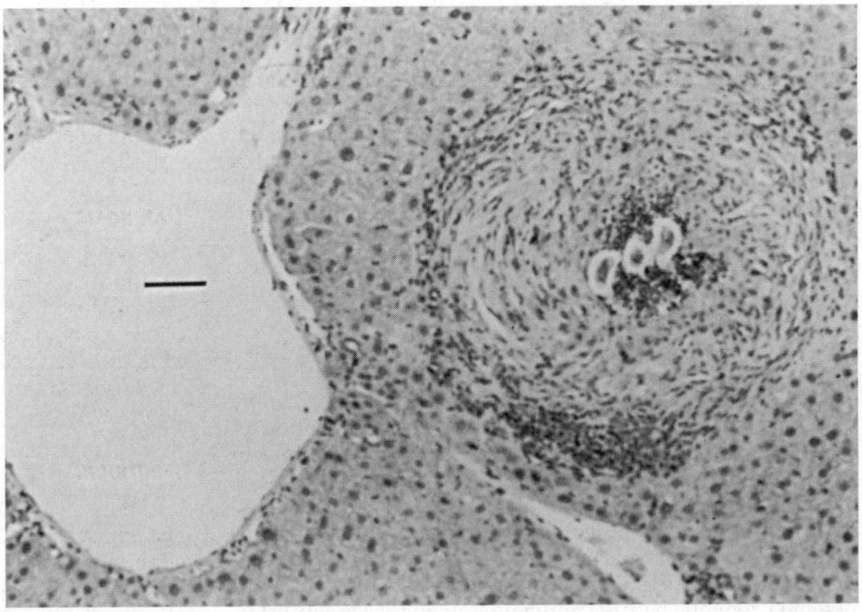

FIGURE 183–3 □ Section of mouse liver 5 months after experimental infection with 500 eggs of *T. canis*. Note granuloma containing a coiled larva within a central core of eosinophils surrounded by epithelioid cells and a collagenous capsule. Hematoxylin-eosin; bar = 100 μm. (Courtesy of Dr. Jim C. Parsons, Victorian Institute of Animal Sciences, Victoria, Australia.)

tory of pica and recent exposure to puppies, both of which indicate exposure to large numbers of *Toxocara* eggs. In contrast, patients with OLM are usually older, lack systemic signs, and do not have pica. In these persons, infection with only a small number of eggs is more likely. This may explain why *Toxocara* serum antibody titers are generally lower in persons with OLM than in those with VLM.

Diagnosis

The diagnosis of toxocaral VLM should be considered in any person with persistent hypereosinophilia. A history of geophagia and association with dogs or cats is helpful. The clinical and laboratory findings (other than serologic tests) are nondiagnostic and do not help to differentiate VLM from other conditions associated with eosinophilia. As the parasite does not mature beyond the larval stage in human tissues, adult worms do not develop in the intestine and diagnosis by egg detection in feces is not possible.

OLM should be considered in any patients who have raised, unilateral, whitish or gray lesions in the fundus.

Identification of larvae in biopsy tissue permits the definitive diagnosis of *Toxocara* infection; other larval nematodes can be differentiated on the basis of characteristic morphologic features.[3] Biopsy is often unrewarding, however. Even in the liver, biopsy specimens may not yield larvae unless the infection is massive.

The enzyme-linked immunosorbent assay (ELISA), using excretory-secretory antigens from infective-stage larvae, is the best diagnostic test for VLM and OLM.[6] In the patient whose clinical signs and history suggest VLM, a toxocaral ELISA titer of 1:32 or more should be considered positive. A rising or a falling titer of at least twofold in a recently ill patient is consistent with VLM infection. Because toxocaral antibody titers may remain elevated for years after infection, a measurable titer is not proof of a causative relationship between *T. canis* and the current illness. Surveys have shown that as many as 1% to 10% of asymptomatic children have ELISA titers of 1:32 or more. In patients with ocular lesions compatible with OLM, ELISA titers of 1:8 or more support the diagnosis but do not rule out retinoblastoma. Toxocaral ELISA testing is available at the Centers for Disease Control and Prevention and several of the larger clinical laboratories in the United States.

Toxocaral VLM must be differentiated from signs and symptoms caused by other tissue-migrating helminths (ascarids, hookworm, filariae, *Strongyloides stercoralis*, and *Trichinella spiralis*) and hypereosinophilic syndromes. Ocular disease may be confused with retinoblastoma, ocular tumors, developmental anomalies, exudative retinitis (Coats disease), trauma, and other childhood uveitides.[20]

Treatment

Asymptomatic toxocariasis does not require the institution of anthelmintic therapy. Although there are isolated reports of ocular disease occurring years after an episode of VLM, available data suggest that asymptomatic individuals have spontaneous resolution of their eosinophilia and seroreactivity without adverse sequelae.[21]

Treatment of patients with symptoms of VLM is primarily supportive. Anthelmintics, diethylcarbamazine, 50 to 150 mg by mouth (PO) three times a day for 1 to 3 weeks, and thiabendazole, 25 to 50 mg/kg per day PO for 1 to 3 weeks, have been used in the management of VLM but have not been consistently effective. Although the efficacy of treatment remains controversial and the decision to treat must be individualized for each patient, the newer benzimidazole compounds, mebendazole (20 to 25 mg/kg per day PO for 21 days) and albendazole (10 mg/kg per day PO for 5 days), are preferable to other anthelmintics because of their greater safety.[22, 23] Severe pulmonary, myocardial, or central nervous system involvement may warrant corticosteroid therapy.

Treatment of acute ocular toxocariasis is directed toward suppressing the inflammatory response associated with larval migration or worm death.[20] Systemic and intraocular corticosteroids (prednisone, 30 to 60 mg PO each day for 2 to 4 weeks; triamcinolone acetonide, 40 mg sub-Tenon weekly for 2 weeks; or topical prednisolone acetate) are the most consistently effective form of intervention if instituted within the first 4 weeks of illness. The concurrent use of anthelmintic drugs has not been shown to be of any additive benefit in managing OLM. If visualization of the nematode is made possible by clearing of the vitreal inflammatory reaction, laser photocoagulation becomes an effective means of destroying the migrating larva.

The management of patients with long-standing ocular *Toxocara* infection (longer than 8 weeks) is more problematic. Corticosteroids may be effective in treating exacerbations of ocular inflammation; however, relapse and progression of ocular disease are common. Intraocular fibrous adhesions, retinal traction and detachment, retrolental plaques, and chronic vitreal inflammation are most effectively managed by surgical intervention. Commonly employed procedures include pars plana vitrectomy and scleral buckling.[24]

Prevention

Most cases of human toxocariasis can be prevented by simple measures, such as careful personal hygiene, elimination of intestinal parasites from pets, and not allowing children to play in potentially contaminated environments. Unfortunately, few people are aware of the health hazards associated with pets and therefore lack motivation to inquire about or to take the necessary precautions. Efforts must be directed at increasing awareness, especially among pet owners, about potential zoonotic hazards and how to minimize them. Veterinarians are uniquely suited to provide pet owners with sound advice: they have the knowledge, they have established rapport with clients, and a high proportion of pet owners use veterinary services.[8]

All pet dogs and cats should receive anthelmintics periodically to prevent the dissemination of infectious eggs. It is particularly important to treat puppies and bitches shortly after whelping and several times during the first year to prevent passage of infectious eggs. Laws prohibiting puppies and dogs from running free and defecating in public areas, particularly areas used by children, are neither strictly followed nor strictly enforced. Therefore, parents should not allow children, especially those with pica, to play unattended outdoors where they are likely to have access to infectious eggs.

Ancylostoma Species

Characteristics of the Pathogen

Ancylostoma braziliense, a hookworm of dogs and cats, and *Ancylostoma caninum*, a common hookworm of dogs, are found throughout North, Central, and South America, most commonly in tropical and subtropical areas. Other *Ancylostoma* spp. are found in animal hosts in other parts of the world. Some species of animal *Strongyloides* can cause cutaneous larva migrans syndromes.

Epidemiology

Cutaneous larva migrans is a disease of utility workers, gardeners, children, sea bathers, and others who come in contact with damp sandy soil that is contaminated by cat and dog feces. Humans become infected when the infective larvae enter the skin by direct penetration.[25] *A. caninum* can also infect when the larvae are ingested. The euteric form of infection by *A. caninum* is seen relatively commonly in northern Australia[26] and has been diagnosed in the United States.[27]

Pathogenesis and Disease

In humans these larvae cause a dermatitis called creeping eruption. The larvae, which enter the skin, migrate intracutaneously for long periods but eventually penetrate to deeper tissues.[25] Each larva causes a serpiginous tract, advancing 1 mm to a few centimeters a day, with intense itching that becomes more marked at night. The disease is self-limited; cure is spontaneous after several weeks or months. *A. caninum* may occasionally enter and partially mature in the small intestine and has been causally associated with eosinophilic enteritis.[26]

Diagnosis

Cutaneous larva migrans is diagnosed from the clinical appearance and history of possible exposure.[25] Eosinophilic enteritis caused by *A. caninum* is diagnosed on the basis of obscure abdominal pain and blood eosinophilia. Serologic tests, not yet widely available, do not distinguish infection by *A. caninum* from that caused by human-adapted forms of hookworm.

Treatment

Albendazole (200 mg PO twice a day for 1 to 3 days)[28] and ivermectin (200 μg/kg PO for 1 day)[29] are effective in eliminating signs and symptoms of cutaneous larval migration. Mebendazole (100 mg twice a day PO for 3 days) is effective for eliminating hookworms that reach the intestinal lumen.

Baylisascaris Species

Characteristics of the Pathogen

Baylisascaris procyonis, an intestinal roundworm of raccoons, is prevalent throughout North America. Other species of *Baylisascaris*, which are found in skunks, bears, and other hosts, may also be capable of infecting human beings.

Epidemiology

Humans and other aberrant hosts are infected when they ingest infective eggs in soil or other contaminated materials. Although few human cases have been documented, the potential for exposure is widespread and growing as the numbers of raccoons in suburban areas increase.

Pathogenesis and Disease

Ingested eggs hatch in the intestine, penetrate the gut wall, and are carried throughout the body by the circulatory system. Pathogenesis is similar to that of *Toxocara* infection, but the disease seems to be more severe. The larvae increase in size by several factors and have a predilection for the heart and central nervous system. Consequently, the disease is a severe or fatal cerebrospinal nematodiasis.[30, 31] Ocular invasion may occur, causing an OLM syndrome.[32, 33]

Diagnosis

In most human cases the specific cause was not suspected before the patients died and the *Baylisascaris* larvae were identified at autopsy. Specific serologic tests have been described but are not yet widely available.[31, 33]

Treatment

No effective anthelmintic treatment is known.

Gnathostoma Species

Characteristics of the Pathogen

Gnathostoma spinigerum is an intestinal nematode parasite of cats and dogs. Human infection is common in Thailand and elsewhere in Southeast Asia, Japan, and South America.[34]

Epidemiology

Humans become infected when they ingest undercooked fish, frogs, snakes, or other intermediate hosts containing third-stage larvae.

Pathogenesis and Disease

After ingestion the parasites migrate through the tissues, forming transient inflammatory lesions or abscesses in various parts of the body. The disease is characterized systemically by eosinophilia and locally by migratory swelling of the skin and various visceral organs.[34] Larvae may invade the brain, producing focal cerebral lesions associated with eosinophilic pleocytosis.

Diagnosis

Serologic tests available in Asia are reportedly specific. Diagnosis is usually by biopsy of lesions.

Treatment

Albendazole (400 mg twice a day PO for 28 days) has been reported effective.[35]

Spirometra Species (Sparganosis)

Characteristics of the Pathogen

Sparganosis is infection by the second-stage larvae (plerocercoid or sparganum) of pseudophyllidean cestodes, usually assumed to be of the genus *Spirometra*. The sparganum is a fleshy, motile, elongated larva (3 to 40 cm in length) that is flattened dorsoentrally and has a broad evaginated anterior end, which is the future scolex.

Epidemiology

The adult tapeworms occur in the intestines of domestic and wild carnivores. Intermediate hosts for the larval stages include aquatic crustaceans and a variety of amphibians, reptiles, birds, and mammals. People become infected by (1) drinking water infested by copepods; (2) ingesting tissues of an amphibian, reptilian, mammalian, or avian host of second-stage larvae; or (3) applying the flesh of an infected intermediate host as a poultice to the eye or an open wound. Human sparganosis has been reported worldwide but is more common in Japan, China, Korea, and Southeast Asia. In the United States, approximately 60 cases have been confirmed, but many more cases go undescribed.[36]

Pathogenesis and Disease

Larvae migrate from the human intestine to peripheral tissues, where they coil or remain elongated. Manifestation is by palpation of a firm mass or nodule (2 to 3 cm), which may be inflamed, tender, painful, or pruritic. Spargana are most commonly localized in subcutaneous connective tissue and in superficial muscles, but infection can develop anywhere on the body. Sparganum can migrate to internal organs or brain, giving rise to the rare visceral and cerebral forms of the disease.[37] An infrequent but serious form is proliferative sparganosis, caused by *Spirometra proliferum*. This form, which can proliferate throughout the body, is ultimately fatal.[38]

Diagnosis

The diagnosis may be suggested by the clinical manifestations but is usually not confirmed until sparganum is identified in a biopsy specimen.

Treatment

Treatment is surgical removal of the subcutaneous nodules. Chemotherapy of the proliferative form has not been successful.

References

Toxocara

1. Beaver PC, Snyder MD, Carrera GM, et al: Chronic eosinophilia due to visceral larva migrans. Pediatrics 9:7, 1952.
2. Wilder HC: Nematode endophthalmitis. Trans Am Acad Ophthalmol 55:99, 1951.
3. Nichols RL: The etiology of visceral larva migrans. 1. The diagnostic morphology of infective second-stage *Toxocara* larvae. J Parasitol 42:349, 1956.
4. Beaver PC: The nature of visceral larval migrans. J Parasitol 55:3, 1969.
5. Sprent JFA: Observations on the development of *Toxocara canis* (Werner, 1782) in the dog. Parasitology 48:184, 1958.
6. Glickman LT, Schantz PM, Grieve RB: Toxocariasis. *In* Walls KW, Schantz PM (eds): Immunodiagnosis of Parasitic Diseases, Vol 1, Helminthic Diseases. New York, Academic Press, 1986, pp 201–231.
7. Glickman LT, Schantz PM: Epidemiology and pathogenesis of zoonotic toxocariasis. Epidemiol Rev 3:230, 1981.
8. Schantz PM: Toxocaral larva migrans now. Am J Trop Med Hyg 41(Suppl):21, 1989.
9. Parsons JC: Ascarid infections of cats and dogs. Vet Clin North Am Small Anim Pract 17:1307, 1987.
10. Bicknell J: Pica: A Childhood Symptom. London, Butterworth, 1975, pp 4–25.
11. Kayes SG, Oaks JA: Effect of inoculum size and length of infection on the distribution of *Toxocara canis* larvae in the mouse. Am J Trop Med Hyg 25:573, 1976.
12. Dunsmore JD, Thompson RCA, Bates IA: The accumulation of *Toxocara canis* larvae in the brains of mice. Int J Parasitol 13:517, 1983.
13. Parsons JC, Bowman DD, Grieve RB: Tissue localization of excretory-secretory antigens of larval *Toxocara canis* in acute and chronic murine toxocariasis. Am J Trop Med Hyg 35:974, 1986.
14. Maizels RM, de Savigny D, Ogilvie BM: Characterization of surface and excretory-secretory antigens of *Toxocara canis* infective larvae. Parasite Immunol 6:23, 1984.
15. Badley JE, Grieve RB, Rockey JH, Glickman LT: Immune-mediated adherence of eosinophils to *Toxocara canis* infective larvae: The role of excretory-secretory antigens. Parasite Immunol 9:133, 1987.
16. Zinkham WH: Visceral larva migrans. A review and reassessment indicating two forms of clinical expression: Visceral and ocular. Am J Dis Child 132:627, 1978.
17. Huntley CC, Costas MC, Lyerly A: Visceral larval migrans syndrome: Clinical characteristics and immunologic studies in 51 patients. Pediatrics 36:523, 1965.
18. Buijs J, Borsboom G, van Gemond JJ, et al: *Toxocara* seroprevalence in 5-year-old elementary school children: Relation with allergic asthma. Am J Epidemiol 140:839, 1994.
19. Taylor MRH, Keane CT, O'Connor P, et al: The expanded spectrum of toxocaral disease. Lancet 1:692, 1988.
20. Shields JA: Ocular toxocariasis: A review. Surv Ophthalmol 28:361, 1984.
21. Bass JL, Mehta KA, Glickman LT, et al: Asymptomatic toxocariasis in children. Clin Pediatr 26:441, 1987.
22. Sturchler D, Schubarth P, Gualzata M, et al: Thiabendazole vs. albendazole in treatment of toxocariasis: A clinical trial. Ann Trop Med Parasitol 83:473, 1989.
23. Magnaval J-F: Comparative efficacy of diethylcarbamazine and

mebendazole for the treatment of human toxocariasis. Parasitology 110:529, 1995.
24. Hagler WS, Pollard ZF, Jarrett WH, Donnelly EH: Results of surgery for ocular *Toxocara canis*. Ophthalmology 88:1081, 1981.

Ancylostoma

25. Enander MW, Adam RC: Cutaneous larva migrans: A literature review and case report. J Am Podiatr Assoc 79:83, 1988.
26. Croese J, Lookas A, Opdebeeck J, Prociv P: Occoltenteric infection by *Ancylostoma caninum*: A previously unrecognized zoonosis. Gastroenterology 106:3, 1994.
27. Khoshoo V, Schantz P, Craver R, et al: Dog hookworm: A cause of eosinophilic enterocolitis in humans. J Pediatr Gastroenterol Nutr 19:448, 1994.
28. Orihuela AR, Torres JR: Single dose of albendazole in the treatment of cutaneous larva migrans. Arch Dermatol 126:396, 1990.
29. Caumes E, Datry A, Paris L, et al: Efficacy of ivermectin in the therapy of cutaneous larva migrans. Arch Dermatol 128:994, 1992.

Baylisascaris

30. Fox AS, Kazacos KR, Gould NS, et al: Fatal eosinophilic meningoencephalitis and visceral larva migrans caused by the raccoon ascarid *Baylisascaris procyonis*. N Engl J Med 312:1619, 1985.
31. Cunningham CR, Kazacos KR, McMillan JA, et al: Diagnosis and management of *Baylisascaris procyonis* infection in an infant with nonfatal meningoencephalitis. Clin Infect Dis 18:868, 1994.
32. Kazacos KR, Raymond LA, Kazacos EA, Vestre WA: The raccoon ascarid: A probable cause of human ocular larva migrans. Ophthalmology 92:1735, 1985.
33. Goldberg MA, Kazacos KR, Boyce WM, et al: Diffuse unilateral subacute neuroretinitis. Ophthalmology 100:1695, 1993.

Gnathostoma

34. Rosnak JM, Locey DR: Clinical gnathostomiasis: Case report and review of the English-language literature. Clin Infect Dis 16:33, 1993.
35. Southarasamai P, Riganti M, Chittamas S, Desakorn V: Albendazole stimulates outward migration of *Gnathostoma spinigerum* to the dermis in man. Southeast Asian J Trop Med Public Health 23:716, 1992.

Spirometra

36. Norman SH, Kreutner A Jr: Sparganosis: Clinical and pathologic observations in ten cases. South Med J 73:297, 1980.
37. Chang KH: Cerebral sparganosis: CT characteristics. Radiology 165:505, 1987.
38. Beaver PC, Rolon FA: Proliferating larval cestodes in a man in Paraguay: A case report and review. Am J Trop Med Hyg 30:625, 1981.

LYMPH NODE SYNDROMES

184

Epstein-Barr Virus Infection and Infectious Mononucleosis

Kenneth M. Kaye
Elliott Kieff

History

The initial descriptions of infectious mononucleosis (IM) are attributed to Filatov[1] and Pfeiffer[2] who independently described clinical syndromes of lymphadenopathy with fever in the 1880s. Sprunt and Evans[3] first used the term infectious mononucleosis in 1920 when they described six cases of fever, lymphadenopathy, and atypical lymphocytosis in healthy adults. In 1932, Paul and Bunnell[4] first described the presence of heterophile antibodies in IM, and Davidsohn[5] later devised a more specific heterophile test using differential absorption of patients' serum with guinea pig kidney and beef erythrocytes. After the description by Dennis Burkitt of a lymphoma occurring in Africa, a previously undescribed herpesvirus was described by Epstein, Achong, and Barr from electron microscopic studies of cell lines derived from such tumors.[6, 7] This virus was subsequently termed Epstein-Barr virus (EBV) by Gertrude Henle and Werner Henle. They developed an indirect immunofluorescent assay for EBV and found that 90% of U.S. adults had antibody directed against it.[8] Under fortuitous circumstances, Henle and colleagues[9] described seroconversion to EBV positivity in a laboratory technician with IM and generated an EBV-infected lymphoblastoid cell line from the patient. Subsequent epidemiologic studies went on to demonstrate that EBV causes heterophile-positive IM.[10–13]

This chapter describes the epidemiology, pathogenesis, clinical manifestations, diagnosis, and treatment of EBV-induced IM.

Epidemiology

EBV infection is usually transmitted through contact of saliva of an infected person with oropharyngeal epithelium of an uninfected person. Primary EBV infection in children often occurs by sharing food with infected family members; adolescents or adults usually are infected by salivary transfer during kissing (thus IM as the kissing disease).[14–17] Little is known regarding transmission among children during play. EBV most likely does not survive long on fomites, and there is little evidence that EBV infection spreads readily among roommates.

After exposure via infected saliva, EBV replicates in epithelial cells in the oropharynx. Although EBV is shed most consistently into saliva during primary infection, virus shedding from the oropharynx into saliva occurs intermittently over years and likely occurs throughout life. Immunocompromised persons have higher rates of oropharyngeal shedding of EBV compared with immunocompetent persons.[18–21] After infecting oropharyngeal epithelium, EBV infects B lymphocytes, and virus persists indefinitely in a small fraction of circulating B lymphocytes. Therefore, transfusion of blood products that contain white blood cells to susceptible (nonimmune) persons can result in primary infection.[22] In patients who have undergone allogeneic bone marrow transplantation, EBV shed from the oropharynx can be traced to the donor, indicating that infected B cells may serve as a source of EBV that can infect pharyngeal epithelium. EBV may also be shed in salivary gland secretions and secretions from the cervix,[23] indicating that epithelial tissues other than that of the oropharynx may serve as infectious sites.

In less industrialized societies and in lower socioeconomic groups in industrialized societies, children are usually infected with EBV in the first decade of life,[24, 25] whereas it is more common for those in higher socioeconomic groups to remain uninfected until adolescence or adulthood. Primary EBV infection during adolescence or adulthood often causes the syndrome of IM.[26] IM accounts for approximately 5% of hospitalizations in the university setting.[27, 28] More than 90% of adults worldwide have serologic evidence of EBV infection and remain latently infected with EBV.[24, 29]

Pathogenesis

Because primary EBV infection usually occurs during the first 3 years of life and is usually asymptomatic in this age group, little is known about the pathogenesis of infection in this population.[24, 25] EBV pathogenesis is best studied in the less common circumstance in which infection occurs during adolescence or adulthood, because these patients often have symptomatic disease that can be readily identified.[26] It is believed that EBV initially infects oropharyngeal epithelial cells. EBV most likely subsequently infects circulating B lymphyocytes as they pass near the infected oropharyngeal cells. In two studies,[30, 31] EBV-infected lymphoblastoid cell lines were established from the blood of patients during the incubation period of IM, before the onset of symptoms and the onset of an EBV-specific immune response. Therefore, EBV infection of B cells precedes the symptoms of IM. Immunofluorescent staining of circulating B-cell lymphocytes from patients with IM has shown that 0.1% to 1.0% of cells are usually EBV infected, although more than 10% of cells may be infected with EBV in some cases.[31–34] The numbers of EBV-infected cells fall rapidly with disease progression and the mounting of an immune response. Histologic analysis of lymphoid tissue from patients in the acute phase of IM reveals considerable numbers of EBV-infected B cells in extrafollicular areas.[35]

The most commonly used serologic tests of EBV infection measure antibody responses to EBV nuclear antigen expressed in latently infected cells[36]; early antigen, which is divisible into diffuse (EA-D, methanol-resistant) and restricted (EA-R, methanol-sensitive) components, which are expressed in early lytic infection[37]; and virus capsid antigen (VCA), which is expressed in late lytic infection.[8] Typically, such tests are done using indirect immunofluorescence microscopy or enzyme-linked immunosorbent assay. Each of these "antigens" is actually a composite of distinct viral proteins that can be further identified with more specific testing. However, attempts to replace these older assays with more specific tests have largely been unsuccessful, and most clinical testing is still done with the original assays.[38–41]

At the onset of IM symptoms, immunoglobulin M antibodies to early antigen and VCA are usually present and immunoglobulin G titers to both VCA and early antigen (most frequently to the D component) are rising. Immunoglobulin M antibodies to VCA are diagnostic of IM and disappear within several months of illness in most patients.[42–46] Patients in the recovery phase of IM have low EBV nuclear antigen titers, which then rise and persist for years. Documentation of EBV nuclear antigen seroconversion is diagnostic of IM. Immunoglobulin G anti-VCA titers reach a peak after illness and then slowly fall during months to a steady-state level. Immunoglobulin G anti–early antigen titers fall faster and further than immunoglobulin G anti-VCA and become undetectable or stabilize at low levels.[47] Low-titer virus-neutralizing antibodies directed at the gp350 antigen are present in acute IM and later increase to relatively stable levels.[48] This antibody response is summarized in Figure 184–1.

There is usually a polyclonal increase in total immunoglobulins in IM, which is most likely related to EBV activation of B cells.[47] As part of this nonspecific antibody response, heterophile antibodies appear in 90% of patients with IM.[49] The Paul-Bunnell-Davidsohn test for heterophile antibodies is positive when antibodies are present that agglutinate sheep or horse erythrocytes. However, serum must first be absorbed with guinea pig kidney to increase specificity because only heterophile antibodies and not antibodies of serum sickness or naturally occurring Forssman antibodies will agglutinate the erythrocytes after such absorption.[4] The Monospot test assays for the ability of serum to agglutinate horse red blood cells after absorption with guinea pig kidney. A further control for this test includes absorption of serum with beef red blood cells, which reduces or eliminates agglutination of horse erythrocytes when heterophile antibodies are present. Horse erythrocyte agglutination tends to be somewhat more sensitive and specific than sheep erythrocyte agglutination (approximately 7% false-positives versus approximately 12% false-positives, respectively). Horse erythrocyte agglutinins also persist longer than do sheep erythrocyte agglutinins (75% versus 30%, respectively, present 1 year after infection).[42] In young children, particularly those younger than age 4 years, the heterophile test result is often negative in primary EBV infection.[50] When IM is suspected and the heterophile test result is negative, specific EBV antibody titers can distinguish EBV-induced IM from other causes of IM-like illness (e.g., cytomegalovirus or *Toxoplasma*).[47]

In addition to specific and nonspecific antibody responses, IM causes a strong cell-mediated immune response. The "atypical" lymphocytes seen in IM are predominantly $CD8^+$ cells but also $CD4^+$ T cells and not the EBV-infected B lymphocytes.[51, 52] During IM, delayed-type hypersensitivity responses are suppressed.[53]

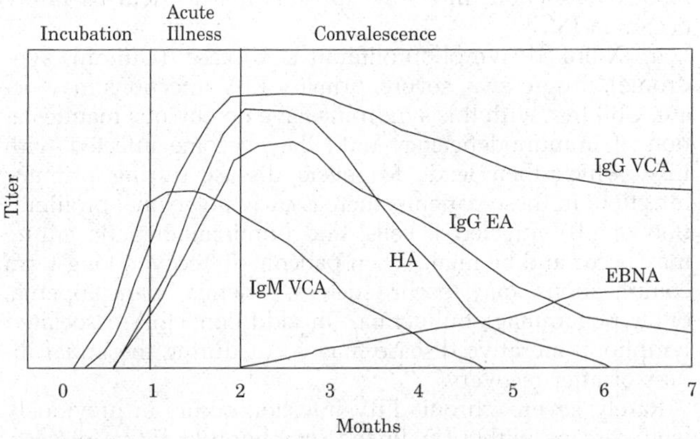

FIGURE 184–1 □ Antibody response to acute infection with EBV. VCA, Virus capsid antigen; HA, heterophile antibody; EA, early antigen; EBNA, EBV nuclear antigen. (Adapted from Henle W, Henle G: Seroepidemiology of the virus. *In* Epstein M, Achong B [eds]: The Epstein-Barr Virus. Berlin, Springer-Verlag, 1979, pp 61–78 © by Springer-Verlag; and Tomkinson B, Sullivan J: Epstein-Barr virus infection and mononucleosis. *In* Gorbach S, Bartlett J, Blacklow N [eds]: Infectious Diseases. Philadelphia, WB Saunders, 1992, pp 1348–1356.)

Clinical Manifestations

After exposure to EBV, there is a 2- to 5-week incubation period before the onset of IM. Symptoms include pharyngitis, lymphadenopathy, fever, headache, and malaise, which may last from 1 week to several weeks. The presenting complaint of IM is often pharyngitis, which is exudative in about 50% of patients. Cervical lymph nodes (posterior more often than anterior) may be significantly enlarged and are usually moderately tender. The range of elevated temperature is generally between 38°C and 40°C.[54, 55] Tonsils may enlarge dramatically and may meet at the midline of the oropharynx. Other findings may include splenomegaly (50%), hepatitis (20% to 90%), palatal petechiae (11% to 33%), periorbital or facial edema (33%), vomiting (5% to 20%), and jaundice (5% to 9%).[54–58] Rash occurs in about 10% of IM cases and may be maculopapular, urticarial, petechial, or erythema multiforme–like. However, if ampicillin or amoxicillin is administered, a distinctive, diffuse maculopapular rash develops in about 90% of patients.[58] Intermittent malaise or weakness may persist during a period of several months after IM.

Complications occur rarely in IM and occasionally result in fatal outcomes. At times, a complication of IM may present as the predominant or only clinical finding and may occur without an atypical lymphocytosis or heterophile antibodies. A variety of neurologic complications may occur with IM. These include encephalitis (cerebellar dysfunction often predominates), aseptic meningitis, mono- or polyneuritis, transverse myelitis, Guillain-Barré syndrome, uveitis, optic neuritis, seizures, and cranial nerve palsies.[59–68] Hematologic complications include autoimmune hemolytic anemia due to anti-i antibodies,[69] thrombocytopenia likely due to antiplatelet antibodies,[70] neutropenia, pancytopenia, and a hemophagocytic syndrome.[71] Splenic rupture occurs in about 0.2% of patients with IM, and it is important to note that these patients may have no clinical evidence of splenomegaly. Splenic rupture occurs most commonly at the height of illness or early in the convalescent stage of IM. Signs of splenic rupture include abdominal pain, pain referred to the left shoulder, and signs of hypovolemia. Because of the possibility of splenic rupture, contact sports should be avoided during IM.[72, 73] Cardiac complications of IM include myocarditis, pericarditis, and cardiac conduction abnormalities. Renal complications of IM may include nephrotic syndrome and renal dysfunction. Interstitial pneumonia or pleuritis rarely occurs in IM.[74, 75]

In X-linked lymphoproliferative disease (Duncan syndrome), progressive, severe, primary EBV infections may occur. Children with this syndrome have no obvious manifestation of immunodeficiency until they become infected with EBV, which then leads to severe disease during primary infection. In these patients, there is early polyclonal proliferation of EBV-infected B cells, and fulminant hepatic failure may occur and be fatal. When patients do recover, long-term complications may occur such as anemia, pancytopenia, or hypogammaglobulinemia. In addition, EBV-associated lymphoproliferative disease may occur during the initial illness or after recovery.[76–79]

Rarely, severe, chronic EBV infection occurs in previously well persons without X-linked lymphoproliferative disease. Clinical findings may include lymphadenopathy, uveitis, hepatosplenomegaly, and polyneuropathy.[80, 81] These patients usually have antibody titers directed against EBV replicative proteins that are 10- to 100-fold higher than titers typically found in IM.

HIV-infected patients may manifest oral hairy leukoplakia, which causes white, corrugated lesions on the inferolateral surfaces of the tongue and typically occurs once the $CD4^+$ cell count drops below 150/mm^3. The lesions of oral hairy leukoplakia contain replicating EBV in epithelial cells.[82–84]

Chronic fatigue syndrome is characterized by recurrent malaise, weakness, myalgias, arthralgias, pharyngitis, lymphadenitis, and low-grade fever. Initially, EBV was believed to be the etiologic agent of chronic fatigue syndrome. However, after extensive study, this hypothesis has been disproved because it has been found that titers of antibodies directed against EBV in patients with the chronic fatigue syndrome are not significantly different from those in control subjects.[85, 86]

Diagnosis

Laboratory findings in IM include a relative or absolute lymphocytosis, and lymphocytes may account for more than 50% of the total leukocyte count. Atypical lymphocytes often constitute more than 10% of the total white cell count. Atypical lymphocytes are large cells with abundant, basophilic, vacuolated cytoplasm. Relatively mild neutropenia with an absolute neutrophil count less than 2000/mm^3 may occur during the second week of illness. Mild thrombocytopenia with platelet counts of 100,000 to 140,000/mm^3 occur in about 50% of patients. Hepatic transaminase, alkaline phosphatase, and bilirubin levels are elevated two- to threefold in up to 90% of IM patients, and levels usually peak in the second or third week of illness.[54, 87–91]

Typically, the diagnosis of IM is made when patients present with fever, pharyngitis, lymphadenopathy, and an atypical lymphocytosis, and the heterophile titer is found to be positive. Specific serology for EBV (see Fig. 184–1) is helpful diagnostically in cases with negative heterophile tests. Direct culturing of EBV involves infecting and immortalizing primary human B lymphocytes with EBV and is not available commercially.

The differential diagnosis of EBV-induced IM includes other diseases that can cause pharyngitis or atypical lymphocytosis. Group A streptococcal pharyngitis presents with an exudative pharyngitis, cervical lymphadenopathy, and fever and can be diagnosed with a throat culture or rapid streptococcal antigen test. Because 3% to 30% of IM patients have positive results of throat cultures for group A streptococcus, these patients should be given penicillin (or erythromycin if allergic to penicillin) to avoid amoxicillin- or ampicillin-induced rash.[55] Cytomegalovirus-induced IM can present similarly to EBV-induced IM with fever and lymphocytosis with atypical lymphocytes, but pharyngitis and lymphadenopathy are usually absent and the heterophile test is negative. Acute viral hepatitis caused by hepatitis A, B, or C can also cause an atypical lymphocytosis, but the level of atypical lymphocytes is usually less than 10% of the total white cell count. More significantly, transaminase levels rise substantially higher in acute viral hepatitis than the mild two- to threefold elevation seen in IM. Acute toxoplasmosis can cause a mononucleosis syndrome with cervical lymphadenopathy and fever, but the atypical lymphocytosis is usually less than 10% and the heterophile test is negative. Other causes of atypical lymphocytosis include rubella, acute human immunodeficiency virus infection, mumps, other herpesvirus infections, rickettsial infections, and drug hypersensitivity reactions.[92–96]

Treatment

Therapy for IM is primarily supportive. Aspirin or acetaminophen may help alleviate fever and symptoms of pharyngitis. It is generally recommended that patients rest during the initial phase of disease and then slowly resume normal activities, but firm data are lacking. Owing to the risk of splenic rupture, sports (especially contact) or strenuous activity such as heavy lifting should be avoided for at least 1 month, and patients with enlarged or tender spleens should avoid such activity until splenomegaly and tenderness have resolved. Ultrasonography can be used to ensure normal spleen size before resuming strenuous activity.[54, 55]

The therapeutic use of corticosteroids for IM is controversial. Although corticosteroids enhance the rapidity of resolution of pharyngitis and fever in uncomplicated IM, their routine use is not recommended. It is possible that corticosteroids might enhance EBV infection as a result of immunosuppression, and there have been rare reports of an association between corticosteroids and encephalitis or myocarditis in IM.[55] The least controversial role for corticosteroids is for impending airway obstruction due to enlarged tonsils meeting at the midline. Short courses of corticosteroids (i.e., 60 mg of prednisone per day for about 4 days followed by a rapid taper) usually result in significant improvement in the obstruction with shrinkage of the tonsils within 24 hours.[54, 55, 97] Corticosteroids may be beneficial in cases of severe hemolytic anemia or thrombocytopenia.[98–101] The efficacy of corticosteroids for other complications of IM is less clear.

Acyclovir has activity against EBV in vitro and in vivo but is not approved for use in EBV infection and has not been shown to alter the course of IM.[55, 102–104] Acyclovir can be effective for oral hairy leukoplakia because EBV is primarily actively replicating in this illness. Neither acyclovir nor corticosteroids appear to be effective in treating EBV infection in X-linked lymphoproliferative disease. Instead, these patients may partially respond to interferon-γ or interferon-α plus immune globulin.[55, 105, 106] Patients with well-documented severe, progressive EBV infection may respond to acyclovir. Corticosteroids plus a cytotoxic agent induced responses in three of five patients with progressive EBV infection.[55, 80] Acyclovir does not improve outcome in EBV-associated lymphoproliferative syndromes. Partial restoration of immune function by decreasing immunosuppression when possible has been beneficial in treating EBV-associated lymphoproliferative disease. There have been reports of responses of EBV-associated lymphoproliferative disease to interferon-α plus immune globulin or to the use of monoclonal antibodies directed against B cells.[55]

References

1. Filatov N: Lektuse ob ostrikh infektsion Nikj Lolieznyak [Lectures on acute infectious diseases of children]. Moscow, U Deitel, 1885.
2. Pfeiffer EE: Drüsenfieber. Jahrb Kinderheilkd Phys Erzieh 29:257–267, 1889.
3. Sprunt T, Evans F: Mononuclear leukocytosis in reaction to acute infections ("infectious mononucleosis"). Johns Hopkins Hosp Bull 31:410, 1920.
4. Paul J, Bunnell W: The presence of heterophile antibodies in infectious mononucleosis. Am J Med Sci 183:91, 1932.
5. Davidsohn I, Walker P: The nature of the heterophilic antibodies in infectious mononucleosis. Am J Clin Pathol 5:455, 1935.
6. Epstein MA, Achong BG: Discovery and general biology of the virus. *In* Epstein M, Achong B (eds): The Epstein-Barr Virus. Berlin, Springer-Verlag, 1979, pp 1–22.
7. Rickinson AB, Kieff E: Epstein-Barr virus. *In* Fields BN, Knipe DM, Howley PM (eds): Fields Virology, ed 3. Philadelphia, Lippincott-Raven, 1996, pp 2397–2446.
8. Henle G, Henle W: Immunofluorescence in cells derived from Burkitt lymphoma. J Bacteriol 91:1248–1256, 1966.
9. Henle G, Henle W, Diehl V: Relation of Burkitt's tumor-associated herpes-type virus to infectious mononucleosis. Proc Natl Acad Sci USA 59:94–101, 1968.
10. Niederman J, McCollum R, Henle G, et al: Infectious mononucleosis: Clinical manifestations in relation to EB virus antibodies. JAMA 203:205–209, 1968.
11. Evans A, Niderman J, McCollum R: Seroepidemiologic studies of infectious mononucleosis with EB virus. N Engl J Med 279:1121–1127, 1968.
12. Sawyer R, Evans A, Niederman J, et al: Prospective studies of a group of Yale University freshmen. I. Occurrence of infectious mononucleosis. J Infect Dis 123:263–279, 1971.
13. A joint investigation of infectious mononucleosis and its relationship to EB virus antibody. Br Med J 4:643–646, 1971.
14. Lipman M, Andrews L, Niederman J, Miller G: Direct visualization of enveloped Epstein-Barr herpesvirus in throat washing with leukocyte-transforming activity. J Infect Dis 132:520–523, 1975.
15. Hoagland R: The transmission of infectious mononucleosis. Am J Med Sci 229:262–272, 1955.
16. Fleisher GR, Pasquariello PS, Warren WS, et al: Intrafamilial transmission of Epstein-Barr virus infections. J Pediatr 98:16–19, 1981.
17. Larsson BO, Linde A: Intrafamilial transmission of symptomatic Epstein-Barr virus infection among six adult members of one family. Scand J Infect Dis 22:363–366, 1990.
18. Miller G, Niederman JC, Andrews LL: Prolonged oropharyngeal excretion of Epstein-Barr virus after infectious mononucleosis. N Engl J Med 288:229–232, 1973.
19. Strauch B, Andrews LL, Siegel N, Miller G: Oropharyngeal excretion of Epstein-Barr virus by renal transplant recipients and other patients treated with immunosuppressive drugs. Lancet 1:234–237, 1974.
20. Chang RS, Lewis JP, Reynolds RD, et al: Oropharyngeal excretion of Epstein-Barr virus by patients with lymphoproliferative disorders and by recipients of renal homografts. Ann Intern Med 88:34–40, 1978.
21. Chang R, Lewis J, Abildgaard C: Prevalence of oropharyngeal excreters of leukocyte transforming agents among a human population. N Engl J Med 289:1325–1329, 1973.
22. Gerber P, Walsh J, Rosenblum E, et al: Association of EB virus infection with the post perfusion syndrome. Lancet 1:593–595, 1969.
23. Sixbey JW, Lemon SM, Pagano JS: A second site for Epstein-Barr virus shedding: The uterine cervix. Lancet 2:1122–1124, 1986.
24. Henle G, Henle W, Clifford P, et al.: Antibodies to Epstein-Barr virus in Burkitt's lymphoma and control groups. J Natl Cancer Inst 43:1147–1157, 1969.
25. Lang DJ, Garruto RM, Gajdusek DC: Early acquisition of cytomegalovirus and Epstein-Barr virus antibody in several isolated Melanesian populations. Am J Epidemiol 105:480–487, 1977.
26. Henle G, Henle W: Observations on childhood infections with the Epstein-Barr virus. J Infect Dis 121:303–310, 1970.
27. Evans A: Infectious mononucleosis in University of Wisconsin students. Report of a 5 year investigation. Am J Hyg 71:342–362, 1960.
28. Evans A: Epidemiology and pathogenesis of infectious mononucleosis. International Infectious Mononucleosis Symposium; 1967; Evanston, IL.
29. Pereira M, Blake J, Macrae A: EB virus antibody at different ages. Br Med J 4:526–527, 1969.
30. Diehl V, Henle G, Henle W, Kohn G: Demonstration of a herpes group virus in cultures of peripheral leukocytes from patients with infectious mononucleosis. J Virol 2:663–669, 1968.
31. Svedmyr E, Ernberg I, Seeley J, et al: Virologic, immunologic, and clinical observations on a patient during the incubation, acute, and convalescent phases of infectious mononucleosis. Clin Immunol Immunopathol 30:437–450, 1984.
32. Robinson JE, Smith D, Niederman J: Plasmacytic differentiation of circulating Epstein-Barr virus–infected B lymphocytes during acute infectious mononucleosis. J Exp Med 153:235–244, 1981.
33. Katsuki T, Hinuma Y, Saito T, et al: Simultaneous presence of EBNA positive and colony-forming cells in peripheral blood of patients with infectious mononucleosis. Int J Cancer 23:746–750, 1979.
34. Klein G, Svedmyr E, Jondal M, Persson PO: EBV-determined nuclear antigen (EBNA)–positive cells in the peripheral blood of infectious mononucleosis patients. Int J Cancer 17:21–26, 1976.
35. Niedobitek G, Herbst H, Young LS, et al: Patterns of Epstein-Barr virus infection in non-neoplastic lymphoid tissue. Blood 79:2520–2526, 1992.

36. Reedman BM, Klein G: Cellular localization of an Epstein-Barr virus (EBV)–associated complement-fixing antigen in producer and non-producer lymphoblastoid cell lines. Int J Cancer 11:499–520, 1973.
37. Henle W, Henle G, Zajac BA, et al: Differential reactivity of human serums with early antigens induced by Epstein-Barr virus. Science 169:188–190, 1970.
38. Henle W, Henle G, Andersson J, et al: Antibody responses to Epstein-Barr virus–determined nuclear antigen (EBNA)-1 and EBNA-2 in acute and chronic Epstein-Barr virus infection. Proc Natl Acad Sci USA 84:570–574, 1987.
39. Hille A, Klein K, Baumler S, et al: Expression of Epstein-Barr virus nuclear antigen 1, 2A and 2B in the baculovirus expression system: Serological evaluation of human antibodies to these proteins. J Med Virol 39:233–241, 1993.
40. Pearson G, Luka J: Characterisation of the virus-determined antigens. *In* Epstein M, Achong B (eds): The Epstein-Barr Virus: Recent Advances. London, Heinemann, 1986, pp 47–73.
41. van Grunsven WM, Spaan WJ, Middeldorp JM: Localization and diagnostic application of immunodominant domains of the BFRF3-encoded Epstein-Barr virus capsid protein. J Infect Dis 170:13–19, 1994.
42. Evans AS, Niederman JC, Cenabre LC, et al. A prospective evaluation of heterophile and Epstein-Barr virus–specific IgM antibody tests in clinical and subclinical infectious mononucleosis: Specificity and sensitivity of the tests and persistence of antibody. J Infect Dis 132:546–554, 1975.
43. Schimitz H, Scherer M: IgM antibodies to Epstein-Barr virus in infectious mononucleosis. Arch Gesamte Virusforsch 37:332–339, 1972.
44. Henle W, Henle GE, Horwitz CA: Epstein-Barr virus specific diagnostic tests in infectious mononucleosis. Hum Pathol 5:551–565, 1974.
45. Horwitz CA, Henle W, Henle G, et al: Clinical and laboratory evaluation of infants and children with Epstein-Barr virus–induced infectious mononucleosis: Report of 32 patients (aged 10–48 months). Blood 57:933–938, 1981.
46. Wahren B: Diagnosis of infectious mononucleosis by the Monospot test. Am J Clin Pathol 52:303–308, 1968.
47. Henle G, Henle W: The virus as the etiologic agent of infectious mononucleosis. *In* Epstein M, Achong B (eds): The Epstein-Barr Virus. Berlin, Springer-Verlag, 1979, pp 279–320.
48. Pearson GR, Qualtiere LF, Klein G, et al. Epstein-Barr virus–specific antibody-dependent cellular cytotoxicity in patients with Burkitt's lymphoma. Int J Cancer 24:402–406, 1979.
49. Garzelli C, Taub FE, Scharff JE, et al. Epstein-Barr virus–transformed lymphocytes produce monoclonal autoantibodies that react with antigens in multiple organs. J Virol 52:722–725, 1984.
50. Sumaya CV, Ench Y: Epstein-Barr virus infectious mononucleosis in children. II. Heterophil antibody and viral-specific responses. Pediatrics 75:1011–1019, 1985.
51. Reinherz EL, O'Brien C, Rosenthal P, Schlossman SF: The cellular basis for viral-induced immunodeficiency: Analysis by monoclonal antibodies. J Immunol 125:1269–1274, 1980.
52. Sheldon P, Papamichael M, Hemsted E, et al: Thymic origin of atypical lymphoid cells in infectious mononucleosis. Lancet 1:1153–1155, 1973.
53. Mangi R, Niederman J, Kelleher J, et al: Depression of cell-mediated immunity during acute infectious mononucleosis. N Engl J Med 291:1149–1153, 1974.
54. Chetham M, Roberts K: Infectious mononucleosis in adolescents. Pediatr Ann 20:206–213, 1991.
55. Straus SE, Cohen JI, Tosato G, Meier J: NIH conference. Epstein-Barr virus infections: Biology, pathogenesis, and management. Ann Intern Med 118:45–58, 1993.
56. Decker GR, Berberian BJ, Sulica VI: Periorbital and eyelid edema: The initial manifestation of acute infectious mononucleosis. Cutis 47:323–324, 1991.
57. Halevy J: Clinical presentation and course of infectious mononucleosis in older patients. Intern Med 10:48–57, 1989.
58. Finkel M, Parker G, Fanselau H: The hepatitis of infectious mononucleosis: Experience with 235 cases. Milit Med 129:533–538, 1964.
59. Silverstein A, Steinberg G, Nathanson M: Nervous system involvement in infectious mononucleosis. The heralding and-or major manifestation. Arch Neurol 26:353–358, 1972.
60. Bennett D, Peter H: Acute cerebellar syndrome secondary to infectious mononucleosis in a 52 year old man. Ann Intern Med 55:147–149, 1961.
61. Gilbert JW, Culebras A: Cerebellitis in infectious mononucleosis. JAMA 220:727, 1972.
62. Bajada S: Cerebellitis in glandular fever. Med J Aust 1:153–156, 1976.
63. Joncas JH, Chicoine L, Thivierge F, Bertrand M: Epstein-Barr virus antibodies in the cerebrospinal fluid. A case of infectious mononucleosis with encephalitis. Am J Dis Child 127:282–285, 1974.
64. Grose C, Henle W, Henle G, Feorino PM: Primary Epstein-Barr-virus infections in acute neurologic diseases. N Engl J Med 292:392–395, 1975.
65. Tanner O: Ocular manifestations of infectious mononucleosis. Arch Ophthalmol 51:229–241, 1954.
66. Schechter F, Lipsius E, Rasansky H: Retrobulbar neuritis. Am J Dis Child 89:58–61, 1955.
67. Gautier-Smith PC: Neurological complications of glandular fever (infectious mononucleosis). Brain 88:323–334, 1965.
68. Cotton PB, Webb-Peploe MM: Acute transverse myelitis as a complication of glandular fever. Br Med J 5488:654–655, 1966.
69. Capra JD, Dowling P, Cook S, Kunkel HG: An incomplete cold-reactive gamma G antibody with i specificity in infectious mononucleosis. Vox Sang 16:10–17, 1969.
70. Ellman L, Carvalho A, Jacobson BM, Colman RW: Platelet autoantibody in a case of infectious mononucleosis presenting as thrombocytopenic purpura. Am J Med 55:723–726, 1973.
71. Mroczek E, Weisenburger D, Grierson H, et al: Fatal infectious mononucleosis and virus-associated hemophagocytic syndrome. Arch Pathol Lab Med 111:530–535, 1987.
72. Farley D, Zietlow S, Bannon M, et al: Spontaneous rupture of the spleen due to infectious mononucleosis. Mayo Clin Proc 67:846–853, 1992.
73. Aldrete J: Spontaneous rupture of the spleen in patients with infectious mononucleosis (Editorial). Mayo Clin Proc 67:910–912, 1992.
74. Mundy GR: Infectious mononucleosis with pulmonary parenchymal involvement. Br Med J 1:219–220, 1972.
75. Offit PA, Fleisher GR, Koven NL, Plotkin SA: Severe Epstein-Barr virus pulmonary involvement. J Adolesc Health Care 2:121–125, 1981.
76. Purtilo DT, Szymanski I, Bhawan J, et al: Epstein-Barr virus infections in the X-linked recessive lymphoproliferative syndrome. Lancet 1:798–801, 1978.
77. Purtilo DT, Cassel CK, Yang JP, Harper R: X-linked recessive progressive combined variable immunodeficiency (Duncan's disease). Lancet 1:935–940, 1975.
78. Purtilo DT, Cassel C, Yang JP: Fatal infectious mononucleosis in familial lymphohistiocytosis (Letter). N Engl J Med 291:736, 1974.
79. Provisor AJ, Iacuone JJ, Chilcote RR, et al: Acquired agammaglobulinemia after a life-threatening illness with clinical and laboratory features of infectious mononucleosis in three related male children. N Engl J Med 293:62–65, 1975.
80. Schooley RT, Carey RW, Miller G, et al: Chronic Epstein-Barr virus infection associated with fever and interstitial pneumonitis. Clinical and serologic features and response to antiviral chemotherapy. Ann Intern Med 104:636–643, 1986.
81. Straus S: The chronic mononucleosis syndrome. J Infect Dis 157:405–412, 1988.
82. Resnick L, Herbst JS, Raab-Traub N: Oral hairy leukoplakia. J Am Acad Dermatol 22:1278–1282, 1990.
83. Greenspan D, Greenspan JS, Hearst NG, et al: Relation of oral hairy leukoplakia to infection with the human immunodeficiency virus and the risk of developing AIDS. J Infect Dis 155:475–481, 1987.
84. Greenspan JS, Greenspan D: Oral hairy leukoplakia: Diagnosis and management. Oral Surg Oral Med Oral Pathol 67:396–403, 1989.
85. Holmes G, Kaplan J, Gantz N, et al: Chronic fatigue syndrome: A working case definition. Ann Intern Med 108: 387–389, 1988.
86. Holmes G: Defining the chronic fatigue syndrome. Rev Infect Dis 13:S53–S55, 1991.
87. Hoagland R: Infectious mononucleosis. Am J Med 13:158–171, 1952.

88. Mason WJ, Adams E: Infectious mononucleosis. An analysis of 100 cases with particular attention to diagnosis, liver function tests, and treatment of selected cases with prednisone. Am J Med Sci 236:447–459, 1958.
89. Carter R: Granulocyte changes in infectious mononucleosis. J Clin Pathol 19:279–283, 1966.
90. Cantow E, Kostinas J: Studies on infectious mononucleosis. iv. Changes in the granulocytic series. Am J Clin Pathol 46:43–47, 1966.
91. Carter R: Platelet levels in infectious mononucleosis. Blood 25:817–821, 1965.
92. Wood TA, Frenkel EP: The atypical lymphocyte. Am J Med 42:923–936, 1967.
93. Chin TD: Diagnosis of infectious mononucleosis. South Med J 69:654–658, 1976.
94. Horwitz CA, Henle W, Henle G, et al: Heterophile negative infectious mononucleosis and mononucleosis-like illnesses. Laboratory confirmation of 43 cases. Am J Med 63:947–957, 1977.
95. Cooper DA, Gold J, Maclean P, et al: Acute AIDS retrovirus infection. Definition of a clinical illness associated with seroconversion. Lancet 1:537–540, 1985.
96. Goudsmit J, de Wolf F, Paul DA, et al: Expression of human immunodeficiency virus antigen (HIV-Ag) in serum and cerebrospinal fluid during acute and chronic infection. Lancet 2:177–180, 1986.
97. Bender CE: The value of corticosteroids in the treatment of infectious mononucleosis. JAMA 199:529–531, 1967.
98. Clark B, Davies S: Severe thrombocytopenia in infectious mononucleosis. Am J Med Sci 248:703–708, 1964.
99. Radel E, Schorr J: Thrombocytopenic purpura with infectious mononucleosis. J Pediatr 63:46–60, 1963.
100. Goldstein E, Porter DY: Fatal thrombocytopenia with cerebral hemorrhage in mononucleosis. Arch Neurol 20:533–535, 1969.
101. Grossman L, Wolff S: Acute thrombocytopenic purpura in infectious mononucleosis. JAMA 171:2208–2210, 1959.
102. van der Horst C, Joncas J, Ahronheim G, et al: Lack of effect of peroral acyclovir for the treatment of acute infectious mononucleosis. J Infect Dis 164:788–792, 1991.
103. Andersson J, Britton S, Ernberg I, et al: Effect of acyclovir on infectious mononucleosis: A double-blind, placebo-controlled study. J Infect Dis 153:283–290, 1986.
104. Andersson J, Skoldenberg B, Henle W, et al: Acyclovir treatment in infectious mononucleosis: A clinical and virological study. Infection 15(Suppl 1):S14–S20, 1987.
105. Okana M, Pirruccelo S, Grierson H, et al: Immunovirological studies of fatal infectious mononucleosis in a patient with X-linked lymphoproliferative syndrome treated with intravenous immunoglobulin and interferon-alpha. Clin Immun Immunopathol 54:410–418, 1990.
106. Okana M, Thiele G, Kobayashi R, et al: Interferon-gamma in a family with X-linked lymphoproliferative syndrome with acute Epstein-Barr virus infection. J Clin Immunol 9:48–54, 1989.
107. Henle W, Henle G: Seroepidemiology of the virus. *In* Epstein M, Achong B (eds): The Epstein-Barr Virus. Berlin, Springer-Verlag, 1979, pp 61–78.
108. Tomkinson B, Sullivan J: Epstein-Barr virus infection and mononucleosis. *In* Gorbach S, Bartlett J, Blacklow N (eds): Infectious Diseases. Philadelphia, WB Saunders, 1992, pp 1348–1356.

185

Chronic Fatigue Syndrome

Stephen E. Straus

History

The chronic fatigue syndrome is a new name for what is, in all likelihood, an ancient condition. As currently defined, it comprises a subset of heterogeneous disorders of uncertain pathogenesis that are associated with chronic fatigue and a variety of other physical, constitutional, and neuropsychologic symptoms[1–3] (Fig. 185–1).

An early, clear reference to chronic fatigue was made by Manningham, who in 1750 described an illness, known at the time as febricula, as exhibiting "low, continued fever . . . transient chilliness . . . listlessness with great lassitude and weariness . . . and little flying pains."[4]

In 1869, Beard[5] postulated that an acquired weakness of the nerves, or neurasthenia, causes severe exhaustion. His contemporary, DaCosta, disagreed. Extensive assessments of battle-worn soldiers of the U.S. Civil War led DaCosta[6] to conclude that the condition resulted from an irritable heart. Beard's concept of neurasthenia was widely acknowledged; the term persisted as a veritable neuropsychiatric diagnosis for about a century. Among cardiologists, in turn, DaCosta's hypothesis was well entrenched until World War II, when detailed investigations failed to identify defects in cardiac physiology.[7]

Discussion of chronic fatigue syndrome in this book is warranted because of its alleged causal relationship, in many instances, with infections. In the 1930s, Evans[8] argued that chronic brucellosis ranges from osteomyelitis, endocarditis, and other highly morbid infections to a syndrome of chronic fatigue with other vague but unsettling complaints. Spink, Cluff, and their colleagues discerned in well-conducted stud-

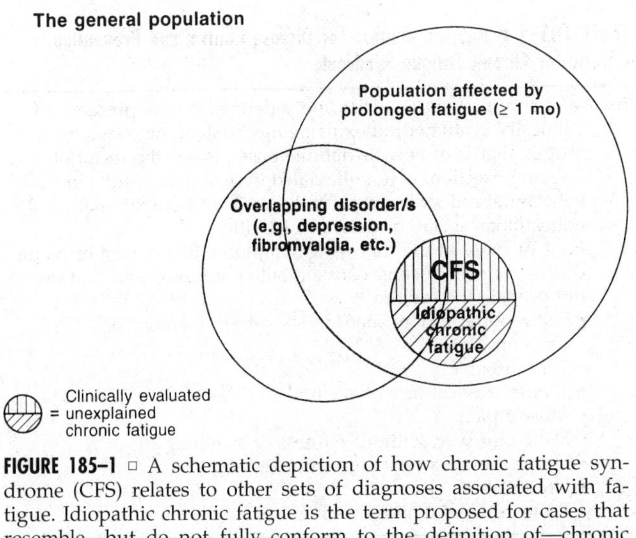

FIGURE 185–1 □ A schematic depiction of how chronic fatigue syndrome (CFS) relates to other sets of diagnoses associated with fatigue. Idiopathic chronic fatigue is the term proposed for cases that resemble—but do not fully conform to the definition of—chronic fatigue syndrome. (From Fukuda K, Straus SE, Hickie I, et al: The chronic fatigue syndrome: A comprehensive approach to its definition and study. Ann Intern Med 121:953–959, 1994.)

ies that active infection could not be verified in many of the patients with the fatiguing form of chronic brucellosis. They found, instead, that such patients exhibited evidence of psychoneurosis.[9, 10]

These findings induced Cluff's group and several others to explore reasons for delayed convalescence from a variety of infections. The most compelling work involved influenza and infectious mononucleosis.[11–13] In each instance, evidence was accumulated that patients who experienced prolonged symptoms after the acute illness tended to differ in premorbid personality from patients who recovered promptly.

Epstein-Barr virus has been postulated to cause chronic fatigue.[14–17] The hypothesis was based on three observations. First, the virus persists for life and reactivates frequently, thus affording the virus the biologic potential for chronic infection. Second, patients were often found to possess higher than expected titers of antibodies to Epstein-Barr virus capsid and early antigens, or to lack antibodies to the viral nuclear antigens, each suggesting recent or active infection. Third, some patients clearly attributed the onset of their illness to a mononucleosis-like infection.

Thoughtful examination of this hypothesis verified that chronic Epstein-Barr virus infection is a rare, moderate to severe illness of the compromised host, but it is not the cause of chronic fatigue syndrome. The serologic profiles of patients with chronic fatigue syndrome prove to be nonspecific.[17, 18] Moreover, most cases of chronic fatigue syndrome either evolve insidiously or follow influenza-like or gastroenteric-type illnesses rather than mononucleosis.

In 1988, the Centers for Disease Control recommended that the disorder be named chronic fatigue syndrome, rather than chronic Epstein-Barr virus infection or other terms then in vogue, to move beyond the idea of a unitary infectious cause.[19] Tentative criteria for the syndrome were field tested for several years and proved lacking in several regards. A number of the elements were vague and redundant, and so many symptoms were required for diagnosis as to bias selection toward patients with somatization disorder. Revised criteria were formulated in 1994 and are now under study[3] (Table 185–1).

Epidemiology

Chronic fatigue is an extremely common complaint. One study of patients in a primary care setting reported 24% to have fatigue for more than 1 month.[20] In many such persons, the fatigue persists 6 months or longer.[21] What proportion of these meet the revised Centers for Disease Control and Prevention case definition awaits completion of a surveillance study being conducted in four U.S. cities. Estimates based on the original definition range from 2.0 to 7.3 cases per 100,000 population.[22] The revised case definition is more inclusive and may yield estimates closer to those obtained earlier with a similar Australian case definition, namely, 37 cases per 100,000.[23]

Chronic fatigue syndrome is primarily a disorder of young to middle-aged adults, but cases in children have been recognized. It may also occur in the elderly, but coexisting medical conditions usually preclude its consideration. Most reports since Manningham's attest that chronic fatigue syndrome is more common in women than in men by a ratio of about 2:1.[4, 14–17] Few cases are seen in minorities or among lower socioeconomic groups. Because such groups lack equivalent access to health care institutions in which chronic fatigue syndrome is studied, the incidence of the disorder in these groups may be underestimated.

Cases of chronic fatigue syndrome usually arise in a sporadic manner, but closely related, if not identical, illnesses occur in outbreaks. The first recorded outbreak led to the temporary closure of Los Angeles County Hospital in 1934; more than 1000 people, including many staff members, fell ill. Other well-known outbreaks occurred in Iceland in 1948, in the Royal Free Hospital of London in 1955, and in Lake Tahoe, Nevada, in 1985.[18, 24–27] The name epidemic neuromyasthenia is often attached to these outbreaks.[26] Myalgic encephalomyelitis is another term for epidemic illnesses such as these, particularly when neurologic features are prominent.[27]

TABLE 185–1 ■ Revised Centers for Disease Control and Prevention Criteria for Chronic Fatigue Syndrome

A case of chronic fatigue syndrome is defined by the presence of
1. Clinically evaluated, unexplained, persistent, or relapsing fatigue that is of new or definite onset; is not the result of ongoing exertion; is not alleviated by rest; and results in substantial reduction in previous levels of occupational, educational, social, or personal activities
2. Four or more of the following symptoms that persist or recur during 6 or more consecutive months of illness and that do not predate the fatigue:
   - Self-reported impairment in short-term memory or concentration
   - Sore throat
   - Tender cervical or axillary nodes
   - Muscle pain
   - Multijoint pain without redness or swelling
   - Headaches of a new pattern or severity
   - Unrefreshing sleep
   - Postexertional malaise lasting ≥24 h

From Fukuda K, Straus SE, Hickie I, et al: The chronic fatigue syndrome: A comprehensive approach to its definition and study. Ann Intern Med 121:953–959, 1994.

Pathogenesis

Little more light can be shed on the pathophysiology of chronic fatigue syndrome than on its epidemiology. As indicated previously, chronic fatigue syndrome often has its onset in the context of an acute infection. Therefore, the possibility of chronic infection cannot be totally dismissed. *Brucella* species and Epstein-Barr virus no longer seem likely to cause a large proportion of cases.

Other agents have also been considered: human herpesvirus type 6, retroviruses, and enteroviruses. Antibodies to these and other viruses were initially found to be more prevalent in chronic fatigue syndrome patients than in control subjects. Subsequent studies revealed only higher titers or irreproducible results in patients with chronic fatigue syndrome.[18, 28] Investigators in the United Kingdom reported detection of enteroviral RNA and proteins in the muscle of chronic fatigue syndrome patients with pronounced myalgias.[29] A U.S. group reported detection of retroviral sequences in chronic fatigue syndrome patients using polymerase chain reaction.[30] Neither of these reports could be confirmed in other laboratories.[31]

Other than virologic investigations, the research on the pathogenesis of chronic fatigue syndrome focuses on two primary areas: immunology and neuropsychiatry. Several studies have shown immunologic abnormalities in chronic fatigue syndrome.[17, 32–35] The most consistent findings entail minor reductions in number and activity of a subset of natural killer cells and increases in the proportion of circulating lymphocytes displaying activation or adhesion markers.

The immunologic features of chronic fatigue syndrome led to the speculation that many of the disease symptoms are caused by dysregulation of lymphokines or interleukins, substances that induce fever, myalgias, and fatigue.[17] Unfortunately, the degree of immune abnormalities has not yet been correlated with the severity of complaints, nor do these abnormalities appear to be specific for chronic fatigue syndrome. Patients with depression also possess natural killer cell deficiencies and other abnormalities similar to those reported in chronic fatigue syndrome.

Depression is a theme that has pervaded chronic fatigue syndrome literature for years. It is obviously a charged issue that patients prefer to dismiss because of the personal and societal stigma attached to psychiatric diagnoses. Three studies verified that two thirds or more of patients with chronic fatigue syndrome meet existing psychiatric criteria for anxiety disorders, dysthymia, or depression.[36–38] Some interpret these findings as implying that the fatigue results from a psychiatric disorder; others argue that the psychiatric problems arise from the chronic fatigue and disability.

A prospective study of patients with an acute viral-type illness found that psychiatric morbidity, the patient's belief about viruses as the cause of his or her complaints, and how the physician reinforced those beliefs conspire to predict chronic fatigue. The infective symptoms predicted fatigue initially, but not 6 months later.[39]

Clinical Manifestations

Besides fatigue, there are numerous other subjective features of chronic fatigue syndrome that fluctuate with time but do not appear to progress[14–17] (Table 185–2). Once the inciting illness, if any, is resolved, the physical examination is typically normal. Although patients commonly feel febrile, few ever demonstrate elevated temperatures. Joints ache, but there is no erythema, effusion, or limitation of motion. Although the muscles are easily fatigued, strength is normal, as are biopsy results and electromyograms. Mild lymphadenitis is occasionally noted but not true lymphadenopathy. Biopsied lymph nodes show only reactive hyperplasia.

All routine hematologic and chemical tests are typically normal. Patients may have intermittent low positive titers of antinuclear antibodies, slightly elevated levels of circulating immune complexes, or partial hypogammaglobulinemia.[15, 16]

Many patients with chronic fatigue syndrome are partially or totally disabled by its manifestations. Their outward, healthy appearance belies the internal sense of ill health. It is common for relatives and colleagues to accuse them of malingering. A vicious circle of frustration, anger, and depression commonly ensues.

Although chronic fatigue syndrome does not seem to progress, spontaneous remissions seem to diminish in rate with time. The clinician can predict a high rate of prolonged debility. In one prospective study, 4 of 27 patients achieved significant sustained remissions during a 3-year observation period.[40]

TABLE 185–2 ▪ Patients with Chronic Fatigue Syndrome Reporting the Indicated Symptoms

SYMPTOM	PERCENTAGE*
Easy fatigability	100
Difficulty concentrating	90
Headache	90
Sore throat	85
Tender lymph nodes	80
Muscle aches	80
Joint aches	75
Feverishness	75
Difficulty sleeping	70
Psychiatric problems	65
Allergies	55
Abdominal cramps	40
Weight loss	20
Rash	10
Rapid pulse	10
Weight gain	5
Chest pain	5
Night sweats	5

*Percentages are approximate.

From Straus SE: The chronic mononucleosis syndrome. J Infect Dis 157:405–412, 1988. © by The University of Chicago.

Diagnosis

Chronic fatigue syndrome remains a diagnosis of exclusion.[3] As such, there is a temptation to conduct an exhaustive laboratory evaluation. Such a work-up is expensive and does not add measurably to management.

Although the chronic fatigue syndrome may have numerous somatic and psychosomatic causes, it is useful for family practitioners, pediatricians, and internists to recognize its common features and its prognosis, which are distinct from those of many other chronic conditions.[41]

Treatment

There are no proven or specific treatments for chronic fatigue syndrome. Commonsense recommendations to patients include a balanced diet, reduction in stress, attention to sleep habits, and regular exercise below the threshold at which further exhaustion is induced. Symptomatic therapies help reduce pain and feverishness.

Claims for other treatments abound. Few have been seriously tested. Anecdotes regarding amantadine, doxycycline, magnesium, evening primrose oil, vitamin B_{12}, and cimetidine are but a few that do not hold up in clinical studies.[42] Intramuscular immunoglobulin injections were found beneficial in a small, controlled trial, somewhat in contrast to the more general experience.[43] Controlled trials of intravenous immunoglobulins, at best, yielded conflicting and unimpressive results.[44]

Because Epstein-Barr virus was associated with chronic fatigue syndrome, a controlled trial of intravenous and oral acyclovir was conducted.[40] The outcome clearly showed no benefit of treatment. More important, the study revealed the wide, natural fluctuations in severity of illness and the close linkage of mood to the perception of symptoms.

Antidepressants appear to benefit certain patients with chronic fatigue syndrome. Not only does mood improve but fatigue, aches, and other symptoms often ease as well. The broad somatic effects of antidepressants in the syndrome are similar to those proved in controlled trials to occur in a closely related disorder, fibrositis.[45] The choice of antidepressants is empirical. Patients tolerate relatively low doses of drugs such as doxepin or fluoxetine. Empirical drug trials should be accompanied by education and counseling. Because the patient's beliefs are at the heart of chronic fatigue syndrome, cognitive-behavioral therapies can help.[46]

References

1. Bock GR, Whelan J (eds): Chronic Fatigue Syndrome. Ciba Foundation Symposium 173. West Sussex, England, John Wiley & Sons, 1993.
2. Straus SE (ed): Chronic Fatigue Syndrome. New York, Marcel Dekker, 1994.
3. Fukuda K, Straus SE, Hickie I, et al: The chronic fatigue syn-

drome: A comprehensive approach to its definition and study. Ann Intern Med 121:953, 1994.
4. Manningham R: The Symptoms, Nature, Causes and Cure of the Febricula or Little Fever: Commonly Called the Nervous or Hysteric Fever; the Fever on the Spirits; Vapours, Hypo, or Spleen, ed 2. London, J Robinson, 1750.
5. Beard G: Neurasthenia, or nervous exhaustion. Boston Med Surg J 3(new series):217, 1869.
6. DaCosta JM: On irritable heart: A clinical study of a form of functional cardiac disorder and its consequences. Am J Med Sci 121:17, 1871.
7. Wood P: DaCosta's syndrome (or effort syndrome). Br Med J 1:767, 805, 845, 1941.
8. Evans AC: Brucellosis in the United States. Am J Public Health 37:139, 1947.
9. Spink WW: What is chronic brucellosis? Ann Intern Med 35:358, 1951.
10. Imboden JB, Canter A, Cluff LE, Trever RW: Brucellosis. III. Psychologic aspects of delayed convalescence. Arch Intern Med 103:406, 1959.
11. Imboden JB, Canter A, Cluff LE: Convalescence from influenza: A study of the psychological and clinical determinants. Arch Intern Med 108:393, 1961.
12. Greenfield NS, Roessler R, Crosley AP: Ego strength and length of recovery from infectious mononucleosis. J Nerv Ment Dis 128:125, 1959.
13. Kasl SV, Evans AS, Niederman JC: Psychological risk factors in the development of infectious mononucleosis. Psychosom Med 41:445, 1979.
14. DuBois RE, Seeley JK, Brus I, et al: Chronic mononucleosis syndrome. South Med J 77:1376, 1984.
15. Jones JF, Ray CF, Minnich LL, et al: Evidence for active Epstein-Barr virus infection in patients with persistent, unexplained illnesses: Elevated anti-early antigen antibodies. Ann Intern Med 102:1, 1985.
16. Straus SE, Tosato G, Armstrong G, et al: Persisting illness and fatigue in adults and evidence of Epstein-Barr virus infection. Ann Intern Med 102:7, 1985.
17. Straus SE: The chronic mononucleosis syndrome. J Infect Dis 157:405, 1988.
18. Holmes GP, Kaplan JE, Steward JA, et al: A cluster of patients with a chronic mononucleosis-like syndrome: Is Epstein-Barr virus the cause? JAMA 257:2297, 1987.
19. Holmes GP, Kaplan JE, Gantz NM, et al: Chronic fatigue syndrome: A working case definition. Ann Intern Med 108:387, 1988.
20. Kroenke K, Wood DR, Mangelsdorf AD, et al: Chronic fatigue is primary care. Prevalence, patient characteristics, and outcome. JAMA 206:929, 1988.
21. Sharpe M, Hawton K, Seagroatt V, Pasvol G: Follow up of patients presenting with fatigue to an infectious diseases clinic. BMJ 305:147, 1992.
22. Gunn WJ, Connell DB, Randall B: Epidemiology of chronic fatigue syndrome: The Centers for Disease Control study. *In* Bock GR, Whelan J (eds): Chronic Fatigue Syndrome. Ciba Foundation Symposium 173. West Sussex, England, John Wiley & Sons, 1993, pp 83–93.
23. Lloyd A, Hickie I, Boughton CR, et al: Prevalence of chronic fatigue syndrome in an Australian population. Med J Aust 153:522, 1990.
24. Gilliam AG: Epidemiologic Study of an Epidemic Diagnosed as Poliomyelitis, Occurring Among Personnel of Los Angeles County General Hospital During the Summer of 1934. Washington, DC, US Public Health Service, Division of Infectious Diseases, Institute of Health, 1938. Bulletin 240.
25. Acheson ED: The clinical syndrome variously called benign myalgic encephalomyelitis, Iceland disease and epidemic neuromyasthenia. Am J Med 26:569, 1959.
26. Henderson DA, Shelokov A: Epidemic neuromyasthenia: Clinical syndrome? N Engl J Med 260:757, 1959.
27. Medical Staff of the Royal Free Hospital: An outbreak of encephalomyelitis in the Royal Free Hospital Group, London, in 1955. Br Med J 3:895, 1957.
28. Ablashi DV, Josephs SF, Buchbinder A, et al: Human B-lymphotropic virus (human herpesvirus-6). J Virol Methods 21:29, 1988.
29. Archard LC, Bowles NE, Behan PO, et al: Postviral fatigue syndrome: Persistence of enterovirus RNA in muscle and elevated creatine kinase. J R Soc Med 81:326, 1988.
30. DeFreitas E, Hilliard B, Cheney PR, et al: Retroviral sequences related to human T-lymphotropic virus type II in patients with chronic fatigue immune dysfunction syndrome. Proc Natl Acad Sci USA 88:2922, 1991.
31. Khan AS, Heneine WM, Chapman LE, et al: Assessment of a retrovirus sequence and other possible risk factors for the chronic fatigue syndrome in adults. Ann Intern Med 118:241, 1993.
32. Borysiewicz LK, Haworth SJ, Cohen J, et al: Epstein-Barr virus-specific immune defects in patients with persistent symptoms following infectious mononucleosis. Q J Med 58:111, 1986.
33. Califuri M, Murray C, Buchwald D, et al: Phenotypic and functional deficiency of natural killer cells in patients with chronic fatigue syndrome. J Immunol 139:3306, 1987.
34. Lloyd A, Wakefield D, Boughton C, Dwyer J: Immunological abnormalities in the chronic fatigue syndrome. Med J Aust 151:122, 1989.
35. Strober W: Immunological function in chronic fatigue syndrome *In* Straus SE (ed): Chronic Fatigue Syndrome. New York, Marcel Dekker, 1994, pp 207–237.
36. Taerk GS, Toner BB, Salit IE, et al: Depression in patients with neuromyasthenia (benign myalgic encephalomyelitis). Int J Psychiatry Med 17:49, 1987.
37. Kruesi MJP, Dale JK, Straus SE: Psychiatric diagnoses in patients who have the chronic fatigue syndrome. J Clin Psychiatry 50:53, 1989.
38. Manu P, Lane TJ, Matthews DA: The frequency of the chronic fatigue syndrome in patients with symptoms of persistent fatigue. Ann Intern Med 109:554, 1988.
39. Cope H, David A, Pelosi A, Mann A: Predictors of chronic "postviral" fatigue. Lancet 344:864, 1994.
40. Straus SE, Dale JK, Tobi M, et al: Acyclovir treatment of the chronic fatigue syndrome: Lack of efficacy in a placebo-controlled trial. N Engl J Med 319:1692, 1988.
41. Swartz MN: The chronic fatigue syndrome: One entity or many? (Editorial). N Engl J Med 319:1726, 1988.
42. McCluskey DR: Pharmacological approaches to the therapy of chronic fatigue syndrome. *In* Bock GR, Whelan J (eds): Chronic Fatigue Syndrome. Ciba Foundation Symposium 173. West Sussex, England, John Wiley & Sons, 1993, pp 280–287.
43. DuBois RE: Gamma globulin therapy for chronic mononucleosis syndrome. AIDS Res 2(Suppl 1):S191, 1986.
44. Peterson PK, Shepard J, Macres M, et al: A controlled trial of intravenous immunoglobulin G in chronic fatigue syndrome. Am J Med 89:554, 1990.
45. Yunus MB: Diagnosis, etiology, and management of fibromyalgia syndrome: An update. Compr Ther 14:8, 1988.
46. Sharp M: Cognitive-behavioral therapy and the treatment of chronic fatigue syndrome. *In* Straus SE (ed): Chronic Fatigue Syndrome. New York, Marcel Dekker, 1994, pp 435–453.

186

Cytomegalovirus Infections

Sarah H. Cheeseman

History

The clinical importance of cytomegalovirus (CMV) was first recognized in the cytomegalic inclusion disease of infants. Transplant and postperfusion syndromes were defined in the 1960s. CMV was one of the candidate viruses considered as a cause of acquired immunodeficiency syndrome (AIDS) when the disease appeared in the early 1980s. Its current clinical prominence, and perhaps some progress in therapy, reflect its frequent and severe manifestations in AIDS patients, as well as the increasing frequency of organ transplantation.

Characteristics of the Pathogen

Molecular methods to identify strains of CMV have been useful for epidemiologic purposes but have not shown any genetic correlates with virulence.[1] Human CMV is not known to replicate in any other species, although various animal herpesviruses are called CMVs because they induce similar histopathologic changes. Some of these viruses are useful models for certain aspects of human CMV infection, such as guinea pig CMV for congenital infection and murine CMV for infection associated with transplantation. However, the model must be carefully chosen to replicate the aspects of the human infection one wants to study. In general, the animal CMVs replicate far more rapidly in tissue culture than does human CMV.

For details on CMV, see Chapter 244.

Epidemiology

About 1% of mothers infected with CMV before conception transmit virus to their children in utero. For primary maternal infection during pregnancy, the transmission rate is nearly 50%.[2–4] Virtually all of the severe disease and major neurologic sequelae occur in those infected as a result of maternal primary infection,[2, 5–8] although there are isolated case reports of mothers who have had more than one child with cytomegalic inclusion disease.[9, 10] The relative role of reinfection versus true reactivation in congenital infection as well as the site of reactivation responsible for fetal infection, has yet to be defined. Viremia, long suspected, has been difficult to prove by culture[11] but has now been documented by polymerase chain reaction.[12] It occurs more commonly, although not exclusively, in women with recent acquisition of CMV and in those who subsequently give birth to congenitally infected infants. Postnatal CMV may be derived from maternal cervical secretions,[11] but the most common source is breast milk.[13–15]

Young children appear to be effective vectors of CMV transmission, both in daycare and at home. In families with young children, the introduction of CMV results in infection of 50% of the remaining susceptible family members within 6 months.[16] This is probably the result of close contact with virus-containing urine and saliva characteristic of this age group, as occurs with diaper changing and sharing of toys that have been mouthed.[17] By contrast, health care workers, even in pediatric and transplantation settings, have not generally been found to have higher seroconversion rates than the general population,[18–24] nor have they been shown by genomic analysis to have the same virus as their patients.[23, 25–27] This suggests that the norms of professional hygiene are sufficient to protect against what might seem to be equally close contact with urine and other infected secretions.[22, 28]

Sexual transmission is the other major route of spread of CMV.[29] Twelve of 34 seronegative homosexual men in San Francisco in the early 1980s became infected during an average follow-up period of 13.6 months.[30] All women older than 30 years seen in a sexually transmitted disease clinic in Kansas City, Missouri, in 1970 were seropositive, compared with only 45% of 30-year-old nuns working as nurses or school teachers.[31]

Transfusion-transmitted CMV disease occurs in both seronegative and seropositive adults[32] and in preterm infants who require transfusion as part of neonatal intensive care.[33] In the case of newborns, molecular methods have confirmed transfusion as the source of infection[34, 35] and demonstrated the absence of nosocomial transmission by other routes.[35] The risk of infection is related both to total number of units transfused and to the number of units from seropositive donors.[36–38] Overall, the risk has been estimated at 2.5 to 7.0 cases per 100 units transfused[32] and may be as high as 25% for seronegative persons receiving 30 or more units.[39] The rate of CMV infection can be reduced to zero by the use of seronegative blood products for seronegative recipients or by filtration to remove contaminating white blood cells.[40]

The serologic status of the blood product donor, organ donor, and recipient all contribute to the risk of CMV infection after transplantation. In kidney transplantation, which does not require massive blood product support, the kidney plays the dominant role, with organs from seropositive donors conferring a high rate of CMV infection.[41, 42] A seropositive donor organ is also the major risk for CMV infection in liver transplantation.[43, 44] In heart transplantation, the donor heart can be shown to transmit virus, but its effect is overwhelmed by that of transfusion unless CMV-seronegative blood is used for seronegative recipients.[45]

In all three types of solid organ transplantation, the highest risk of CMV disease occurs in the recipient who acquires a primary infection.[43–51] However, severe, even fatal, CMV disease is occasionally seen in patients with pretransplant antibody. A study that distinguished between reinfection and reactivation in kidney transplantation identified the same spectrum of illness in reinfection as in primary infection, albeit at a somewhat lower rate of occurrence, whereas reactivation appeared clinically benign.[52]

By contrast, in bone marrow transplantation the major risk for CMV infection derives from the recipient's seropositivity before transplantation.[53] In a few instances, the identity of a patient's pretransplant and posttransplant CMV isolates has been confirmed by genomic analysis.[54] However, if the recipient is seronegative, the infection rate is the same for recipients of either seropositive marrow or seropositive granulocyte transfusions.[53]

Immunity and Pathogenesis

Severe CMV infection has not been reported among persons with isolated immunoglobulin deficiency. However, it is common in patients with cell-mediated immunodeficiency associated with transplantation or human immunodeficiency virus infection, indicating the importance of cell-mediated response in controlling this infection.

Our understanding of the mechanisms of the clinical manifestations of CMV infection is fragmentary. The atypical lymphocyte in CMV mononucleosis has been identified as a killer cell,[55] as in classic infectious mononucleosis induced by Epstein-Barr virus. Also like Epstein-Barr virus, CMV induces broad-spectrum helper cell activity,[56] but CMV infection of a monocyte may render it capable of suppressing natural killer cell activity.[57] An explanation for the frequent association of leukopenia with CMV infection may lie in the capability of even abortive infection of bone marrow monocytes to suppress both granulocyte-macrophage and erythroid colony-forming activity.[58] Vasculitis, perhaps due to CMV infection of endothelial cells, may underlie ulcerative and necrotizing lesions.[59]

Clinical Manifestations

More than 90% of congenitally infected infants appear normal at birth.[60, 61] CMV syndromes are rarely recognized in early childhood. Even in prospectively followed adults, only about 10% of seroconvertors have any clinical syndrome.[8] The most common feature of CMV disease at any age is a nonspecific illness. The signs and symptoms seen in infants with symptomatic congenital CMV infection do not differ greatly from those of other congenital infections or even acquired bacterial sepsis in the newborn.

Cytomegalic Inclusion Disease of the Newborn

Infants with cytomegalic inclusion disease are recognizably ill within the first few days of birth. Hepatosplenomegaly is nearly universal, petechiae and thrombocytopenia are quite common, and there may be a "blueberry muffin" appearance due to cutaneous islands of extramedullary erythropoiesis. Although congenital anomalies have been reported in association with congenital CMV infection, none are particularly characteristic and causation has not been established.[60] Intrauterine growth retardation and postnatal failure to thrive may occur. Encephalitis is an invariable part of this process and is of a progressive and ongoing nature, because the active phase of the infection does not cease until some time after birth. In fact, these infants are quite slow to mount a cell-mediated immune response to the infection[61] and continue to shed large quantities of virus in urine for up to 8 years.[62] Thus, microcephaly may not be present at birth, but as a result of impaired head growth it is found in a majority of surviving children by the end of the first year,[63–68] often in association with periventricular calcifications. The neurologic outcome of this form of CMV infection is usually devastating. Severe mental and motor retardation may occur in up to 90% of patients,[60–68] although one report suggests a slightly better prognosis.[69]

This form of CMV disease affects approximately 3000 to 4000 infants in the United States each year.[70] As stated previously, it results almost exclusively from primary infection of the mother during pregnancy, which is a major impetus for the development of an effective preventive strategy.

Subclinical Congenital Infection

The dire outcome of overt congenital CMV infection has led to scrutiny of asymptomatic congenitally infected infants and their development. Occasional instances of severe mental retardation and motor impairment have been reported, but the most consistent finding has been an 11% to 25% risk of profound sensorineural hearing loss.[71–73] A battery of neuropsychologic tests predicted school failure in CMV-infected children 2.8 times more often than in control subjects in lower socioeconomic groups.[72]

Acquired Cytomegalovirus in Neonates

Preterm infants who acquire CMV often have an episode of "gray baby" syndrome, with pallor and hypotension, and may have renewed respiratory distress requiring reintubation and ventilatory support.[36] CMV infection increases the duration of hospital stay in infants of seronegative mothers and may be the direct cause of death in very small infants (<1200 g).[74] Reports have documented a declining rate of this complication, probably because of screening for other blood-borne pathogens, and also established that significant CMV disease is more common among premature infants of seropositive than of seronegative mothers.[75]

Cytomegalovirus Mononucleosis

CMV mononucleosis is exemplified by the spontaneously occurring disease resulting from acute primary CMV infection. It also occurs as a result of transfusion-transmitted infection, perhaps the most famous case of which is that of Pope John Paul II, in whom it complicated recovery from an assassination attempt.[76] Burn victims, who may be slightly immunocompromised by their injury, have the same clinical manifestations.[77, 78] Heterophile-negative mononucleosis and postperfusion syndrome, the latter named for its occurrence after heart-lung bypass for cardiac surgery, are other terms for the same illness, which may be due to either primary acquisition of CMV or recurrence (whether reinfection or reactivation is not yet established).

Table 186–1 compares the frequency of signs and symptoms of this condition in two series[79, 80] with summary data for primary infection in kidney[81] and heart transplant recipients[50, 51] to demonstrate the common features. The most frequent finding is fever, usually accompanied by profound fatigue and malaise. In classic (Epstein-Barr virus) infectious mononucleosis, sore throat and lymphadenopathy are the next most common symptoms, but they occur in a much smaller proportion of patients with CMV disease: pharyngitis in 30% to 40% and lymphadenopathy in 17% to 27%. The laboratory features of the two forms of mononucleosis are nearly identical: atypical lymphocytosis and mild elevation of serum transaminase values are seen in the vast majority of patients. Approximately 15% to 20% of these patients have more severe abnormalities of liver function tests, and a hepatitis-like presentation of CMV can certainly occur in the normal host. In summary, in a patient who "feels ill" and has fever but no real localizing signs by history and physical examination, the finding of abnormal liver function or atypical lymphocytosis points in the direction of CMV or Epstein-Barr virus mononucleosis.

The peripheral white cell count may be either elevated or depressed; one series reported leukocytosis in most patients,[79] but another recorded it in only 3.8%.[80] Leukopenia is clearly a frequent part of the syndrome in transplant recipients and may be seen in normal hosts as well. Infrequent but recurrently reported sequelae of CMV mononucleosis are Guillain-Barré syndrome and Bell palsy.[79, 80, 82] Other specific organ syndromes are rare but reported in the normal host, including interstitial pneumonia, colitis, and even encephalitis. Many of these cases rest primarily on serologic evidence and have not been confirmed histologically. Nonetheless, the fact that the same syndromes are well-established expressions of CMV in the immunosuppressed patient lends credence to their relation to the virus in the ostensibly normal host.

Transplant Syndromes

The CMV syndrome after kidney transplantation was once called 40-day fever.[83] The time of onset and the nature of CMV disease after heart transplantation are similar.[50, 84] There may be transient and benign fever without localizing signs, or the patient may become progressively more ill with hepatitis, leukopenia, and pneumonitis constituting a "deadly triad."[85] Significant superinfection, either bacterial or opportunistic, is common in these latter patients, particularly in the lung. Although viral damage to the lung, as in influenza, and low numbers of circulating granulocytes may both predispose to bacterial infection, the reason for the high attack rate of *Pneumocystis carinii* and fungi in these patients appears to be a CMV-related inversion of the helper/suppressor T-cell ratio.[86] Thus, the finding of CMV makes it more imperative, rather than less, to exclude other pathogens in this setting. However, in some patients CMV infection is the only demonstrable pathologic process, even at autopsy.

Isolated involvement of specific organs may also occur. CMV is the most common cause of esophagitis in bone mar-

TABLE 186–1 ■ Symptoms of Primary Cytomegalovirus Infection

	NORMAL HOSTS*		TRANSPLANT RECIPIENTS†		
	Literature Review	Consecutive Cases	Renal	Heart or Lung	
SYMPTOM	(N = 62)[79]	(N = 82)[80]	(N = 31–51)[81]	(N = 12)[50]	(N = 16)[51]
Fever	98	94	84	90	69
Leukopenia	0		57	50	
Pneumonia			25	44	31
Pharyngitis	38	31			
Atypical lymphocytes	88	100‡	70	67	
Elevated liver function tests	91	92	46	75	

*Percentage of reported or recognized patients (all symptomatic).
†Percentage of all pretransplant seronegative patients with CMV infection documented after transplantation.
‡Required for inclusion in series.

row transplant recipients.[87] In these patients, the disease has its onset at 50 to 70 days after grafting,[53, 87, 88] later than in solid organ transplantation. CMV chorioretinitis can be a late complication, occurring as a result of prolonged viremia.[89, 90]

More rarely seen is a progressive wasting syndrome associated with failure to mount a complement-fixing antibody response to the CMV infection.[91] This illness progresses inexorably to death over several weeks, and disseminated CMV is found at autopsy.

Another phenomenon associated with CMV infection is graft rejection. Although renal dysfunction during active CMV infection seems to be due to glomerulitis rather than rejection,[92] epidemiologic evidence associates graft rejection with primary CMV infection.[46, 93–97] Furthermore, decreased rejection and improved graft survival are the most striking results of the use of a candidate CMV vaccine in patients awaiting kidney transplantation[98] (see Chapter 244). In heart transplantation, both rejection and accelerated atherosclerosis are associated with CMV infection,[99, 100] and CMV hepatitis figures prominently in liver transplantation.

The interaction between CMV infection and the allogeneic response comes to the fore in bone marrow transplantation, in which CMV and graft-versus-host disease contribute jointly to the pathogenesis of a devastating form of interstitial pneumonitis.[53, 101, 102] This complication affects 15% to 20% of patients and carried an 87% mortality[53] until reports of successful treatment with the combination of ganciclovir and CMV hyperimmune globulin.[103, 104] The failure of antiviral therapy alone to affect clinical outcome despite 1000-fold reduction in lung viral titers[105] demonstrates the important role of the allogeneic reaction in this syndrome; the contribution of the immune globulin may well be to the immunopathologic part of the process rather than its anti-CMV properties.

Cytomegalovirus Syndromes in Acquired Immunodeficiency Syndrome

Although a large majority of persons infected with the human immunodeficiency virus type 1 are coinfected with CMV, disease attributable to CMV is usually restricted to those with the most severe levels of immunodeficiency. In fact, most studies of CMV syndromes in AIDS report median $CD4^+$ cell counts of $25/mm^3$ or less at diagnosis,[106–108] although an occasional patient may present with CMV disease with a higher number of $CD4^+$ cells. The most frequent form of CMV disease in AIDS is retinitis, with characteristic funduscopic findings of yellow-white exudate, often accompanied by hemorrhage. Alternatively, a white granular lesion may occur.[109] CMV retinitis is painless; the symptoms are floaters, blurring of vision, and loss of portions of the visual field, sometimes described as though a veil were covering the area. These symptoms in a person at risk demand prompt ophthalmologic evaluation, even if recent routine ophthalmologic examination showed no evidence of disease. In the absence of treatment, CMV retinitis progresses rapidly[110] and eventually leads to blindness. Retinal detachment frequently complicates CMV retinitis and should be suspected whenever sudden visual loss occurs in the course of treatment.

Among patients with disease limited to one eye at presentation who were treated with an intravitreal implant releasing ganciclovir into the eye but not the systemic circulation, 50% developed CMV retinitis in the other eye within 6 months, and 11 of 26 eventually had CMV disease in other organs diagnosed either by biopsy or at autopsy.[107] As many as one third to one half of patients with CMV retinitis may have coexisting encephalitis, and half of those ultimately diagnosed with CMV encephalitis at autopsy had CMV retinitis during life.[111]

The gastrointestinal tract is the next most frequently recognized site of CMV involvement in AIDS. Colitis, characterized by diarrhea, bleeding, and abdominal pain, may progress to perforation. Some patients have macroscopically normal colonic mucosa with typical cytomegalic inclusions on biopsy, but patchy erythematous lesions are more common; ulcers may also occur.[112] CMV esophagitis typically presents with odynophagia; endoscopy demonstrates large, usually solitary, ulcers. Biopsies taken at the edge of the lesions show CMV inclusions in endothelial cells.[113]

In the past, it was more difficult to attribute specific neurologic syndromes in AIDS to CMV because of a lack of diagnostic tools, although response to ganciclovir therapy strongly suggested a role for CMV in some patients with encephalitis who had not improved with zidovudine.[114] Several distinct clinical entities have now been described, and the development of polymerase chain reaction for CMV DNA in cerebrospinal fluid offers a firm basis for diagnosis in the future.[111] A polyradiculopathy or cauda equina syndrome associated with CMV causes lower extremity weakness associated with bowel and bladder dysfunction, most commonly urinary retention.[115, 116] Cerebrospinal fluid of persons with this syndrome shows a predominantly polymorphonuclear pleocytosis,[111, 117] somewhat surprising for a viral etiology, and hypoglycorrhachia may occur relatively frequently.[118] Another syndrome that may coexist with polyradiculopathy or occur independently has been recognized by a pattern of periventricular enhancement at magnetic resonance imaging of the brain corresponding to necrotizing ependymitis.[119] Interestingly, this is the same anatomic distribution as the intracranial calcification that occurs in infants with severe congenital cytomegalic inclusion disease. Oculomotor and other cranial nerve palsies and nystagmus are frequent clues to this syndrome, as are elevated cerebrospinal fluid protein level and depressed glucose values.[111, 119] Progression from lethargy and confusion to coma and death is rapid, usually within 1 to 2 months.

CMV encephalitis in the absence of these relatively characteristic features is difficult to distinguish clinically from that caused by human immunodeficiency virus, but necropsy-verified cases point to associations with CMV retinitis (despite treatment); quasi-psychiatric symptoms such as delirium, confusion, apathy, and withdrawal; and electrolyte abnormalities.[120] Coexisting CMV adrenalitis was found in nearly all cases in this autopsy series, but the electrolyte abnormalities at the time of presentation were not always related to adrenal insufficiency.

CMV adrenalitis may be the cause of postural hypotension in some AIDS patients,[121–123] and biliary tract disease may be related to the virus as well.[124] CMV pneumonia is believed to be much less common than isolation of virus from bronchoalveolar lavage specimens[125, 126] and probably constitutes only about 4% of pneumonias in AIDS patients.[123]

Diagnosis

Mere detection of CMV is not sufficient evidence of a causative role in the syndrome in question. For example, CMV is frequently isolated from bronchoalveolar lavage specimens in patients with AIDS who have other diagnosed pulmonary infections (usually *P. carinii* pneumonia) and respond to treatment directed solely at the other pathogen.[126] Isolation of CMV from urine of a newborn within the first week of life unequivocally establishes congenital infection (virus acquired postnatally is not shed until after 3 to 4 weeks) but does not distinguish symptomatic from asymptomatic infants. Virus shedding can persist for up to 8 years from congenitally infected children[62] and last for an average of 18 months when children are infected in daycare.[127] One fourth of patients studied 2 to 14 years after kidney transplantation excreted CMV in urine.[90]

The presence of the typical enlarged cell with "owl's eye" basophilic nuclear inclusion in tissue is the standard criterion for accepting a causal role for the virus in a specific organ syndrome. An exception is the isolation of virus from buffy coat leukocytes, which has a high correlation with the presence of disease but is not highly sensitive.[128, 129] Detection of pp65 in circulating leukocytes by fluorescent antibody or immunoperoxidase staining has improved sensitivity without loss of specificity; these are valuable techniques for the identification of immunosuppressed patients with clinically significant CMV infection.[130–134] Although molecular techniques may be more sensitive, they remain positive longer and have lower predictive value for active symptomatic illness in kidney transplant recipients.[135]

Polymerase chain reaction identifies CMV DNA in the cerebrospinal fluid of both AIDS patients and congenitally infected infants with central nervous system disease.[136–138] Detection of CMV DNA in plasma has a high predictive value for the development of disease in bone marrow transplant recipients.[118] Both this assay and enumeration of DNA copy number in peripheral blood cells may prove useful in identifying AIDS patients at imminent risk of CMV retinitis.[139, 140]

In adults, the presence of serum antibody establishes a diagnosis of CMV infection but not disease. Conversion from seronegative to seropositive status defines the time of acquisition and could confirm CMV as the cause of an episode of heterophile-negative mononucleosis. However, most patients will already have detectable or peak antibody levels by the time they are investigated for this possibility. A fourfold rise in antibody titer is accepted as evidence of active infection, although it may occur in the absence of symptoms—and presumably in the presence of symptoms of other causes. Theoretically, a test for serum immunoglobulin M antibody should solve these problems, but the difficulties with CMV-specific immunoglobulin M assays are numerous, as discussed in Chapter 244. A commercially available immunoglobulin M test identified 73% of pregnant women undergoing documented primary CMV infection and 69% of congenitally infected infants. However, the false-positive rate was 11% among pregnant women known not to be undergoing primary infection and 5.7% among uninfected newborns.[141] In the presence of a compatible clinical syndrome such as CMV mononucleosis, this test might be useful supporting evidence because it does not require collection of a second serum sample after adequate time for further antibody rise. Clearly, this test should not be used as a sole means of identifying primary infection in a pregnant woman.

Assay for CMV antibody of the immunoglobulin G class can be extremely useful in excluding the diagnosis. Absence of antibody in a newborn excludes congenital infection except in rare circumstances, because maternal antibody should be present even if the child has failed to make any response. In a patient with a puzzling febrile illness of several weeks' duration, absence of CMV antibody would exclude the diagnosis. If a serum sample obtained early in illness is negative or has a low antibody titer or an indeterminate reaction, that serum sample should be saved to be retested at the same time as subsequent specimens.

Treatment

At the time of this writing, two drugs are approved for use in CMV infections of immunocompromised hosts: ganciclovir and foscarnet. They differ markedly in their toxicity profiles, with ganciclovir being a myelosuppressive agent and foscarnet producing nephrotoxicity and electrolyte disorders, specifically hypocalcemia and hypomagnesemia, presumably due to urinary cation wasting. Seizures and cardiac arrhythmias may occur, particularly during rapid infusion of foscarnet, and are thought to be a result of abrupt decrease in levels of ionized calcium. Much of the nephrotoxicity of foscarnet may be abrogated by vigorous hydration with normal saline.

A period of 2 to 3 weeks of intensive induction therapy is usual with both agents; AIDS patients with CMV retinitis require lifelong maintenance therapy and even with that can expect periodic episodes of disease progression requiring reintensification or change of therapy. The need for maintenance has not been as rigorously established in other syndromes but may be inferred from the tendency of nearly every late-stage opportunistic infection to relapse with cessation of specific therapy in AIDS. Reasonable disease-free intervals have been reported in CMV esophagitis after cessation of induction therapy.[108] By contrast, transplant recipients appear to recover sufficient host defense to permit limited duration of antiviral therapy, although they may suffer relapses after the first attempt at discontinuation.

A trial in previously untreated persons with AIDS and CMV retinitis is the only direct comparison of the therapeutic efficacy of ganciclovir and foscarnet. Time to first progression of retinitis and final visual outcome did not differ significantly,[142] but the foscarnet group had a median survival of 12.5 months, whereas that for ganciclovir-treated patients was only 8.5 months.[106] The source of this difference has never been adequately explained, although the anti–human immunodeficiency virus effect of foscarnet and protocol constraints on the management of concomitant antiretroviral therapy (mostly zidovudine at the time the study took place) are suspected. This study did not lead to overwhelming acceptance of foscarnet as the therapy of first choice because of its toxicity, the time required for infusions, and the introduction of new antiretroviral drugs with less overlapping toxicity with ganciclovir. An oral formulation of ganciclovir became available for maintenance therapy in early 1995; the time to progression of retinitis appears slightly shorter than with intravenous maintenance, but reductions in leukopenia and episodes of catheter sepsis, as well as freedom from daily intravenous infusions, may offset this detriment for many patients.

The desire to achieve better control of retinitis with less impairment of quality of life impelled development of an intravitreal sustained-release device for ganciclovir. Early studies suggest a much longer interval to progression of retinitis, probably attributable to higher intraocular concentrations of ganciclovir, but the study was limited to persons with peripheral retinitis and no extraocular disease.[107] Median survival for intraocular therapy was 8.5 months, similar to that on the ganciclovir arm of the comparative trial[106] and to the 8.2 months observed in patients with CMV esophagitis not maintained after an initial course of therapy.[108] A potent systemic drug given by infrequent intravenous infusion, cidofovir, is currently undergoing a trial for CMV retinitis as well.[143]

Ganciclovir therapy alone is inadequate for the treatment of interstitial pneumonitis in bone marrow transplant recipients, but combined with immune globulin ganciclovir has reduced mortality to 30% to 48%.[103, 104, 144] Monitoring high-risk transplant recipients virologically and initiating antiviral therapy (usually ganciclovir) at the time of positive culture or leukocyte antigen detection reduce the rate of CMV disease and improve survival.[145–147]

Prevention

Intravenous CMV immune globulin does not prevent CMV infection but does modify disease in seronegative recipients of seropositive kidneys.[148] In liver transplantation, seronegative recipients with seropositive donors did not benefit from this therapy, but there was a modest overall reduction in serious CMV-related disease, including fungal superinfection.[149] Hyperimmune globulin did not protect premature infants of seronegative mothers from either CMV infection or disease.[75]

Although some studies have suggested prophylactic efficacy for high-dose acyclovir against CMV,[150–154] many have not.[154] In particular, a study of patients with AIDS showed no reduction in the occurrence of CMV retinitis.[155] The prophylactic use of intravenous ganciclovir in bone marrow transplantation starting either before transplantation or at engraftment reduces the incidence of CMV disease but at a cost because of neutropenia and sepsis.[156, 157] Prophylactic intravenous ganciclovir has proved both safe and effective in heart transplantation.[158] Oral ganciclovir halved the rate of CMV disease in AIDS patients in a placebo-controlled trial.[159] Its role in transplantation is under investigation.

References

1. Grillner L, Ahlfors K, Ivarsson SA, et al: Endonuclease cleavage pattern of cytomegalovirus DNA of strains isolated from congenitally infected infants with neurologic sequelae. Pediatrics 81:27, 1988.
2. Stagno S, Pass RF, Dworsky ME, et al: The relative importance of primary and recurrent maternal infection. N Engl J Med 306:945, 1982.
3. Kumar ML, Gold E, Jacobs IB, et al: Primary cytomegalovirus infection in adolescent pregnancy. Pediatrics 74:493, 1984.
4. Stagno S, Pass RF, Cloud G, et al: Primary cytomegalovirus infection in pregnancy. JAMA 256:1904, 1986.
5. Monif GRG, Egan EA, Held B, Eitzman DV: The correlation of maternal cytomegalovirus infection during varying stages in gestation with neonatal involvement. J Pediatr 80:17, 1972.
6. Stern H, Tucker SM: Prospective study of cytomegalovirus infection in pregnancy. Br Med J 2:268, 1973.
7. Griffiths PD, Campbell-Benzie A, Heath RB: A prospective study of primary cytomegalovirus infection in pregnant women. Br J Obstet Gynaecol 87:308, 1980.
8. Ahlfors K, Forsgen M, Ivarsson S, et al: Congenital cytomegalovirus infection: On the relation between type and time of maternal infection and infant's symptoms. Scand J Infect Dis 15:129, 1983.
9. Embil JA, Ozere RL, Haldane EV: Congenital cytomegalovirus infection in two siblings from consecutive pregnancies. J Pediatr 77:417, 1970.
10. Ahlfors K, Harris S, Ivarsson S, Svanberg L: Secondary maternal cytomegalovirus infection causing symptomatic congenital infection. N Engl J Med 305:284, 1981.
11. Reynolds DW, Stagno S, Hosty TS, et al: Maternal cytomegalovirus excretion and perinatal infection. N Engl J Med 289:1, 1973.
12. Balcarek KB, Oh MK, Pass RF: Maternal viremia and congenital CMV infection. *In* Michelson S, Plotkin SA (eds): Multidisciplinary Approach to Understanding Cytomegalovirus Disease. Amsterdam, Elsevier Science Publishers, 1993, pp 169–173.
13. Hayes K, Danks DM, Gibas H, Jack I: Cytomegalovirus in human milk. N Engl J Med 287:177, 1972.
14. Cheeseman SH, McGraw BR: Studies on cytomegalovirus in human milk. J Infect Dis 148:615, 1983.
15. Dworsky M, Yow M, Stagno S, et al: Cytomegalovirus infection of breast milk and transmission in infancy. Pediatrics 72:295, 1983.
16. Taber LH, Frank AL, Yow MD, Bagley A: Acquisition of cytomegaloviral infections in families with young children: A serological study. J Infect Dis 151:948, 1985.
17. Hutto C, Little EA, Ricks R, et al: Isolation of cytomegalovirus from toys and hands in a day care center. J Infect Dis 154:527, 1986.
18. Tolkoff-Rubin NE, Rubin RH, Keller EE, et al: Cytomegalovirus infection in dialysis patients and personnel. Ann Intern Med 89:625, 1978.
19. Betts RF, Cestero RVM, Freeman RB, Douglas RG: Epidemiology of cytomegalovirus infection in end stage renal disease. J Med Virol 4:89, 1979.
20. Dworsky ME, Welch K, Cassady G, Stagno S: Occupational risk for primary cytomegalovirus infection among pediatric health-care workers. N Engl J Med 390:950, 1983.
21. Hatherley LI: Is primary cytomegalovirus infection an occupational hazard for obstetrics nurses? Infect Control 7:452, 1986.
22. Balfour CL, Balfour HH Jr: Cytomegalovirus is not an occupational risk for nurses in renal transplant and neonatal units. JAMA 256:1909, 1986.
23. Demmler GJ, Yow MD, Spector SA, et al: Nosocomial cytomegalovirus infections within two hospitals caring for infants and children. J Infect Dis 156:9, 1987.
24. Gerberding JL: Incidence and prevalence of human immunodeficiency virus, hepatitis B virus, hepatitis C virus, and cytomegalovirus among health care personnel at risk for blood exposure: Final report from a longitudinal study. J Infect Dis 170:1410, 1994.
25. Yow MD, Lakeman AD, Stagno S, et al: Use of restriction enzymes to investigate the source of a primary cytomegalovirus infection in a pregnant nurse. Pediatrics 70:713, 1982.
26. Wilfert CM, Eng-Shang H, Stagno S: Restriction endonuclease analysis of cytomegalovirus deoxyribonucleic acid as an epidemiologic tool. Pediatrics 70:717, 1982.
27. Dworsky ME, Lakeman A, Stagno S: Cytomegalovirus transmission within a family. Pediatr Infect Dis 3:286, 1984.
28. Haneberg B, Bertnes, E, Haukenes G: Antibodies to cytomegalovirus among personnel at a children's hospital. Acta Paediatr Scand 69:407, 1980.
29. Forbes BA: Acquisition of cytomegalovirus infection: An update. Clin Microbiol Rev 2:204, 1989.

30. Drew WL, Mills J, Levy J, et al: Cytomegalovirus infection and abnormal T-lymphocyte subset ratios in homosexual men. Ann Intern Med 103:61, 1985.
31. Davis LE, Stewart JA, Garvin S: Cytomegalovirus infection: A seroepidemiologic comparison of nuns and women from a venereal disease clinic. Am J Epidemiol 102:327, 1975.
32. Adler SP: Transfusion-associated cytomegalovirus infections. Rev Infect Dis 5:977, 1983.
33. Yeager AS: Transfusion-acquired cytomegalovirus infection in newborn infants. Am J Dis Child 128:478, 1974.
34. Tolpin MD, Stewart JA, Warren D, et al: Transfusion transmission of cytomegalovirus confirmed by restriction endonuclease analysis. J Pediatr 107:953, 1985.
35. Adler SP, Baggett J, Wilson M, et al: Molecular epidemiology of cytomegalovirus in a nursery: Lack of evidence for nosocomial transmission. J Pediatr 108:117, 1986.
36. Ballard RA, Drew WL, Hufnagle KG, Riedel PA: Acquired cytomegalovirus infection in preterm infants. Am J Dis Child 133:482, 1979.
37. Spector SA, Schmidt K, Ticknor W, Grossman M: Cytomegalovirus in older infants in intensive care nurseries. J Pediatr 95:444, 1979.
38. Beneke JS, Tegtmeier GE, Alter HJ, et al: Relation of titers of antibodies to CMV in blood donors to the transmission of cytomegalovirus infection. J Infect Dis 150:883, 1984.
39. Preiksaitis JK, Brown L, McKenzie M: The risk of cytomegalovirus infection in seronegative transfusion recipients not receiving exogenous immunosuppression. J Infect Dis 157:523, 1988.
40. Hillyer CD, Emmens RK, Zago-Novaretti M, Berkman EM: Methods for the reduction of transfusion-transmitted cytomegalovirus infection: Filtration versus the use of seronegative donor units. Transfusion 34:929, 1994.
41. Ho M, Suwansirikul S, Dowling JN, et al: The transplanted kidney as a source of cytomegalovirus infection. N Engl J Med 293:1109, 1975.
42. Betts RF, Freeman RB, Douglas RG, Jr., et al: Transmission of cytomegalovirus infection with renal allograft. Kidney Int 8:385, 1975.
43. Rakela J, Wiesner RH, Taswell HF, et al: Incidence of cytomegalovirus infection and its relationship to donor-recipient serologic status in liver transplantation. Transplant Proc 19:2399, 1987.
44. Gorensek MJ, Carey WD, Vogt D, Goormastic M: A multivariate analysis of risk factors for cytomegalovirus infection in liver transplant recipients. Gastroenterology 98:1326, 1990.
45. Preiksaitis JK, Rosno S, Grumet C, Merigan TC: Infections due to herpesviruses in cardiac transplant recipients: Role of the donor heart and immunosuppressive therapy. J Infect Dis 147:974, 1983.
46. Betts RF, Freeman RB, Douglas RJ Jr, Talley TE: Clinical manifestations of renal allograft derived primary cytomegalovirus infection. Am J Dis Child 131:759, 1977.
47. Naraqi S, Jackson GG, Jonasson O, Yamashiroya HM: Prospective study of prevalence, incidence, and source of herpes-virus infections in patients with renal allografts. J Infect Dis 136:531, 1977.
48. Pass RF, Long WK, Whitley RJ, et al: Productive infection with cytomegalovirus and herpes simplex virus in renal transplant recipients: Role of source of kidney. J Infect Dis 137:556, 1978.
49. Suwansirikul S, Rao N, Dowling JN, Ho M: Primary and secondary cytomegalovirus infection. Arch Intern Med 137:1026, 1977.
50. Pollard RB, Rand KH, Arvin AM, Merigan TC: Cell-mediated immunity to cytomegalovirus infection in normal subjects and cardiac transplant recipients. J Infect Dis 137:541, 1978.
51. Dummer JS, White LT, Ho M, et al: Morbidity of cytomegalovirus infection in recipients of heart or heart-lung transplants who received cyclosporine. J Infect Dis 152:1182, 1985.
52. Grundy JE, Super M, Sweny P, et al: Symptomatic cytomegalovirus infection in seropositive kidney recipient: Reinfection with donor virus rather than reactivation of recipients virus. Lancet 2:132, 1988.
53. Meyers JD, Fluornoy N, Thomas ED: Risk factors for cytomegalovirus infection after human marrow transplantation. J Infect Dis 153:478, 1986.
54. Winston DJ, Huang ES, Miller MJ, et al: Molecular epidemiology of cytomegalovirus infections associated with bone marrow transplantation. Ann Intern Med 102:16, 1985.
55. Lemon SM, Hutt LM, Huang YT: Cytotoxicity of circulating leukocytes in cytomegalovirus mononucleosis. Clin Microbiol Immunopathol 8:513, 1977.
56. Yachie A, Tosato G, Straus SE, Blaese RM: Immunostimulation by cytomegalovirus: Helper T cell–dependent activation of immunoglobulin production in vitro by lymphocytes from CMV-immune donors. J Immunol 135:1305, 1985.
57. Kapasi K, Rice GPA: Role of the monocyte in cytomegalovirus-mediated immunosuppression in vitro. J Infect Dis 154:881, 1986.
58. Rakusan TA, Juneja HS, Fleischmann WR: Inhibition of hemopoietic colony formation by human cytomegalovirus in vitro. J Infect Dis 159:127, 1989.
59. Golden MP, Hammer SM, Wanke CA, Albrecht MA: Cytomegalovirus vasculitis. Medicine (Baltimore) 73:246, 1994.
60. Hanshaw JB, Dudgeon JA, Marshall WC: Viral Diseases of the Fetus and Newborn, ed 2. Philadelphia, WB Saunders, 1985, pp 92–131.
61. Stagno S, Whitley RJ: Herpesvirus infections of pregnancy. Part I. Cytomegalovirus and Epstein-Barr virus infection. N Engl J Med 313:1270, 1985.
62. Hanshaw JB: Congenital cytomegalovirus infection: A fifteen year perspective. J Infect Dis 123:555, 1971.
63. Weller TH, Hanshaw JB: Virological and clinical observations on cytomegalic inclusion disease. N Engl J Med 266:1233, 1964.
64. Medearis DN Jr: Observation concerning human cytomegalovirus infection and disease. Bull Johns Hopkins Hosp 114:181, 1964.
65. McCracken GH Jr, Shinefield HR, Cobb K, et al: Congenital cytomegalic inclusion disease a longitudinal study of 20 patients. Am J Dis Child 117:522, 1969.
66. Berenberg W, Nankervis G: Long-term follow-up of cytomegalic inclusion disease of infancy. Pediatrics 46:403, 1970.
67. Pass RF, Stagno S, Meyers GJ, Alford CA: Outcome of symptomatic congenital cytomegalovirus infection: Results of long-term longitudinal follow-up. Pediatrics 66:758, 1980.
68. Williamson WD, Desmond MM, LaFevers N, et al: Symptomatic congenital cytomegalovirus: Disorders of language, learning and hearing. Am J Dis Child 136:902, 1982.
69. Conboy TJ, Pass RF, Stagno S, et al: Early clinical manifestations and intellectual outcome in children with symptomatic congenital cytomegalovirus infection. J Pediatr 111:343, 1987.
70. Yow MD: Congenital cytomegalovirus disease: A NOW problem. J Infect Dis 159:163, 1989.
71. Reynolds DW, Stagno S, Stubbs KG, et al: Inapparent congenital cytomegalovirus infection with elevated cord IgM levels: Causal relation with auditory and mental deficiency. N Engl J Med 2290:291, 1974.
72. Hanshaw JB, Scheiner AP, Moxley AW, et al: School failure and deafness after "silent" congenital cytomegalovirus infection. N Engl J Med 295:468, 1976.
73. Saigal S, Lunyk O, Larke RPB, Chernesky MA: The outcome in children with congenital cytomegalovirus infection: A longitudinal follow-up study. Am J Dis Child 136:896, 1982.
74. Yeager AS, Grumet FC, Hafleigh EB, et al: Prevention of transfusion-acquired cytomegalovirus infections in newborn infants. J Pediatr 98:281, 1981.
75. Snydman DR, Werner BG, Meissner HC, et al: Use of cytomegalovirus immunoglobulin in multiply transfused premature neonates. Pediatr Infect Dis J 14:34, 1995.
76. CMV: Pathogenesis and prevention of human infection. Birth Defects Orig Artic Ser 20:1, 1984.
77. Linnemann CC, MacMillan BG: Viral infections in pediatric burn patients. Am J Dis Child 135:750, 1981.
78. Deepe G, MacMillan BG, Linnemann CC: Unexplained fever in burn patients due to cytomegalovirus infection. JAMA 248:2299, 1982.
79. Cohen JI, Corey GRE: Cytomegalovirus infection in the normal host. Medicine (Baltimore) 64:100, 1985.
80. Horwitz CA, Henle W, Henle G, et al: Clinical and laboratory evaluation of cytomegalovirus-induced mononucleosis in previously healthy individuals: Report of 82 cases. Medicine (Baltimore) 65:124, 1986.
81. Hirsch MS, Cheeseman SH, Hammer SM: Human herpesvirus infections: Pathogenesis and clinical implications. *In* Weinstein L, Fields BN (eds): Seminars in Infectious Diseases. New York, Stratton Intercontinental Medical Book, 1979, pp 217–264.

82. Kaplan JE, Greenspan JR, Bomgarrs M, et al: Simultaneous outbreaks of Guillain-Barré syndrome and Bell's palsy in Hawaii in 1981. JAMA 250:2635, 1983.
83. Coulson AS, Lucas ZJ, Condy M, Cohn R: Forty-day fever: An epidemic of cytomegalovirus disease in a renal transplant population. West J Med 120:1, 1974.
84. Gorensek MJ, Stewart RW, Keys TF, et al: A multivariate analysis of the risk of cytomegalovirus infection in heart transplant recipients. J Infect Dis 157:515, 1988.
85. Rubin RH, Cosimi AB, Tolkoff-Rubin NE, et al: Infectious disease syndromes attributable to cytomegalovirus and their significance among renal transplant recipients. Transplantation 24:458, 1977.
86. Schooley RT, Hirsch MS, Colvin RB, et al: Association of herpesvirus infections with T-lymphocyte subset alterations, glomerulopathy, and opportunistic infections after renal transplantation. N Engl J Med 308:307, 1983.
87. McDonald GB, Sharma PJ, Hackman RC, et al: Esophageal infections in immunosuppressed patients after marrow transplantation. Gastroenterology 88:1111, 1985.
88. Miller W, Flynn P, McCullough J, et al: Cytomegalovirus infection after bone marrow transplantation: An association with acute graft-v-host disease. Blood 4:1162, 1986.
89. Fiala M, Payne JE, Berne TV, et al: Epidemiology of cytomegalovirus after transplantation and immunosuppression. J Infect Dis 132:421, 1975.
90. Cheeseman SH, Stewart JA, Winkle S, et al: Cytomegalovirus excretion 2–14 years after renal transplantation. Transplant Proc 11:71, 1979.
91. Simmons RL, Matas AJ, Rattazzi LC, et al: Clinical characteristics of the lethal cytomegalovirus infection following renal transplantation. Surgery 82:537, 1977.
92. Richardson WP, Colvin RB, Cheeseman SH, et al: Glomerulopathy associated with cytomegalovirus viremia in renal allografts. N Engl J Med 305:57, 1981.
93. David DS, Millian SJ, Whitsell JC, et al: Viral syndromes and renal homograft rejection. Ann Surg 175:257, 1972.
94. Lopez C, Simmons RL, Mauer SM, et al: Association of renal allograft rejection with virus infections. Am J Med 56:280, 1974.
95. Simmons RL, Lopez C, Balfour HH, et al: Cytomegalovirus: Clinical virological correlations in renal transplant recipients. Ann Surg 180:623, 1974.
96. May AG, Betts RF, Freeman RB, Andrus CH: An analysis of cytomegalovirus infection and HLA antigen matching on the outcome of renal transplantation. Ann Surg 187:110, 1978.
97. Rubin RH, Tolkoff-Rubin NE, Oliver D, et al: Multicenter seroepidemiologic study of the impact of cytomegalovirus infection on renal transplantation. Transplantation 40:243, 1985.
98. Brayman KL, Dafoe DC, Smythe WR, et al: Prophylaxis of serious cytomegalovirus infection in renal transplant candidates using live human cytomegalovirus vaccine: Interim results of a randomized controlled trial. Arch Surg 123:1502, 1988.
99. Grattan MT, Moreno-Cabral CE, Starnes VA, et al: Cytomegalovirus infection is associated with cardiac allograft rejection and atherosclerosis. JAMA 261:3561, 1989.
100. Speir E, Modali R, Huang E, et al: Potential role of human cytomegalovirus and p53 interaction in coronary restenosis. Science 265:391, 1994.
101. Meyers JD, Spencer HC, Watts JC, et al: Cytomegalovirus pneumonia after human marrow transplantation. Ann Intern Med 82:181, 1975.
102. Thomas ED, Buckner CD, Banaji M, et al: One hundred patients with acute leukemia treated by chemotherapy, total body irradiation, and allogeneic marrow transplantation. Blood 49:511, 1977.
103. Emanuel D, Cunningham I, Jules-Elysee K, et al: Cytomegalovirus pneumonia after bone marrow transplantation successfully treated with the combination of ganciclovir and high-dose intravenous immune globulin. Ann Intern Med 109:777, 1988.
104. Reed EC, Bowden RA, Dandliker PS, et al: Treatment of cytomegalovirus pneumonia with ganciclovir and intravenous cytomegalovirus immunoglobin in patients with bone marrow transplants. Ann Intern Med 109:783, 1988.
105. Shepp DH, Dandliker PS, de Miranda P, et al: Activity of 9-[2-hydroxy-1-(hydroxymethyl)ethoxymethyl]guanine in the treatment of cytomegalovirus pneumonia. Ann Intern Med 103:368, 1985.
106. Studies of Ocular Complications of AIDS Research Group in Collaboration with the AIDS Clinical Studies Group: Mortality in patients with the acquired immunodeficiency syndrome treated with either foscarnet or ganciclovir for cytomegalovirus retinitis. N Engl J Med 326:213, 1992.
107. Martin DF, Parks DJ, Mellow SD, et al: Treatment of cytomegalovirus retinitis with an intraocular sustained-release ganciclovir implant. Arch Ophthalmol 112:1531, 1994.
108. Wilcox CM, Straub RF, Schwartz DA: Cytomegalovirus esophagitis in AIDS: A prospective evaluation of clinical responses to ganciclovir therapy, relapse rate, and long-term outcome. Am J Med 98:169, 1995.
109. Bloom JN, Palestine AG: The diagnosis of cytomegalovirus retinitis. Ann Intern Med 109:963, 1988.
110. Spector SA, Weingeist T, Pollard RB, et al: A randomized, controlled study of intravenous ganciclovir therapy for cytomegalovirus peripheral retinitis in patients with AIDS. AIDS Clinical Trials Group and Cytomegalovirus Cooperative Study Group. J Infect Dis 168:557, 1993.
111. McCutchan JA: Cytomegalovirus infections of the nervous system in patients with AIDS. Clin Infect Dis 30:747, 1995.
112. Dieterich DT, Rahmin M: Cytomegalovirus colitis in AIDS: Presentation in 44 patients and a review of the literature. J Acquir Immune Defic Syndr Hum Retrovirol 4(Suppl 1):S29, 1991.
113. Wilcox CM, Diehl DL, Cello JP, et al: Cytomegalovirus esophagitis in patients with AIDS. A clinical, endoscopic, and pathologic correlation. Ann Intern Med 113:589, 1990.
114. Fiala M, Cone LA, Cohen N, et al: Responses of neurologic complications of AIDS to 3′-azido-3′-deoxythymidine and 9-(1,3-dihydroxy-2-propoxymethyl) guanine. I. Clinical features. Rev Infect Dis 10:250, 1988.
115. Behar R, Wiley C, McCutchan A: Cytomegalovirus polyradiculoneuropathy in acquired immune deficiency syndrome. Neurology 37:557, 1987.
116. Kim YS, Hollander H: Polyradiculopathy due to cytomegalovirus: Report of two cases in which improvement occurred after prolonged therapy and review of the literature. Clin Infect Dis 17:32, 1993.
117. de Gans J, Tiessens G, Portegies P, et al: Predominance of polymorphonuclear leukocytes in cerebrospinal fluid of AIDS patients with cytomegalovirus polyradiculomyelitis. J Acquir Immune Defic Syndr 3:1155, 1990.
118. Wolf DG, Spector SA: Early diagnosis of human cytomegalovirus disease in transplant recipients by DNA amplification in plasma. Transplantation 56:330, 1993.
119. Kalayjian RC, Cohen ML, Bonomo RA, Flanigan TP: Cytomegalovirus ventriculoencephalitis in AIDS. Medicine (Baltimore) 72:67, 1993.
120. Holland N, Power C, Mathews V, et al: Cytomegalovirus encephalitis in acquired immunodeficiency syndrome (AIDS). Neurology 44:507, 1994.
121. Tapper ML, Rotterdam HZ, Lerner CW, et al: Adrenal necrosis in the acquired immunodeficiency syndrome. Ann Intern Med 100:239, 1984.
122. Greene LW, Cole W, Greene LB, et al: Adrenal insufficiency as a complication of the acquired immunodeficiency syndrome. Ann Intern Med 101:497, 1984.
123. Jacobson MA, Mills J: Serious cytomegalovirus disease in the acquired immunodeficiency syndrome (AIDS): Clinical findings, diagnosis and treatment. Ann Intern Med 108:585, 1988.
124. Schneiderman DJ, Cello JP, Laing FC: Papillary stenosis and sclerosing cholangitis in patients with the acquired immunodeficiency syndrome. Ann Intern Med 106:546, 1987.
125. Drew WL: Cytomegalovirus infection in patients with AIDS. J Infect Dis 158:449, 1988.
126. Bozzette SA, Arcia J, Bartok AE, et al: Impact of *Pneumocystis carinii* and cytomegalovirus on the course and outcome of atypical pneumonia in advanced human immunodeficiency virus disease. J Infect Dis 165:93, 1992.
127. Adler SP, Starr SF, Plotkin SA, et al: Immunity induced by primary cytomegalovirus infection protects against secondary infection in women of childbearing age. J Infect Dis 171:26, 1995.
128. Cheeseman SH, Rubin RH, Stewart JA, et al: Controlled clinical trial of prophylactic human-leukocyte interferon in renal transplantation: Effects on cytomegalovirus and herpes simplex virus infection. N Engl J Med 300:1345, 1979.

129. Meyers JD, Ljungman P, Fisher LD: Cytomegalovirus excretion as a predictor of cytomegalovirus disease after marrow transplantation: Importance of cytomegalovirus viremia. J Infect Dis 162:373, 1990.
130. van der Bij W, Torensma R, van Son W, et al: Rapid immunodiagnosis of active cytomegalovirus infection by monoclonal antibody staining of blood leukocytes. J Med Virol 25:179, 1988.
131. Erice A, Holm MA, Gill PC, et al: Cytomegalovirus (CMV) antigenemia assay is more sensitive than shell vial cultures for rapid detection of CMV in polymorphonuclear blood leukocytes. J Clin Microbiol 30:2822, 1992.
132. Mazzulli T, Rubin RH, Ferraro MJ, et al: Cytomegalovirus antigenemia: Clinical correlations in transplant recipients and in persons with AIDS. J Clin Microbiol 31:2824, 1993.
133. Landry ML, Ferguson D: Comparison of quantitative cytomegalovirus antigenemia assay with culture methods and correlation with clinical disease. J Clin Microbiol 31:2851, 1993.
134. Storch GA, Buller RS, Bailey TC, et al: Comparison of PCR and pp65 antigenemia assay with quantitative shell vial culture for detection of cytomegalovirus in blood leukocytes from solid-organ transplant recipients. J Clin Microbiol 32:997, 1994.
135. Meyers-Konig U, Serr A, von Laer D, et al: Human cytomegalovirus immediate early and late transcripts in peripheral blood leukocytes: Diagnostic value in renal transplant recipients. J Infect Dis 171:705, 1995.
136. Wolf DG, Spector SA: Diagnosis of human cytomegalovirus central nervous system disease in AIDS patients by DNA amplification from cerebrospinal fluid. J Infect Dis 166:1412, 1992.
137. Anque P, Vago L, Brytting M, et al: Cytomegalovirus infection of the central nervous system in patients with AIDS: Diagnosis by DNA amplification from cerebrospinal fluid. J Infect Dis 166:1408, 1992.
138. Atkins J, Demmler GJ, Williamson WD, et al: Polymerase chain reaction to detect cytomegalovirus DNA in the cerebrospinal fluid of neonates with congenital infection. J Infect Dis 169:1334, 1994.
139. Spector SA, Wolf D, Salunga K: Human cytomegalovirus (HCMV) DNA detected in plasma by PCR predicts development of HCMV disease in patients with AIDS or following transplantation. *In* Michelson S, Plotkin SA (eds): Multidisciplinary Approach to Understanding Cytomegalovirus Disease. Amsterdam, Elsevier Science Publishers, 1993, pp 225–230.
140. Rasmussen S, Morris S, Zipeto D, et al: Quantitation of human cytomegalovirus DNA from peripheral blood cells of human immunodeficiency virus-infected patients could predict cytomegalovirus retinitis. J Infect Dis 171:177, 1995.
141. Stagno S, Tinker MK, Elrod C, et al: Immunoglobulin M antibodies detected by enzyme-linked immunosorbent assay and radioimmunoassay in the diagnosis of cytomegalovirus infections in pregnant women and newborn infants. J Clin Microbiol 21:930, 1985.
142. Studies of Ocular Complications of AIDS Research in Collaboration with the AIDS Clinical Study Group: Foscarnet-ganciclovir cytomegalovirus retinitis trial. Ophthalmology 101:1250, 1994.
143. Lalezari JP, Drew WL, Glutzer E, et al: (*S*)-1-[3-Hydroxy-2-(phosphonylmethoxy)propyl]cytosine (cidofovir): Results of a phase I/II study of a novel antiviral nucleotide analogue. J Infect Dis 171:788, 1995.
144. Schmidt GM, Kovacs A, Zaia JA, et al: Ganciclovir/immunoglobulin combination therapy for the treatment of human cytomegalovirus-associated interstitial pneumonia in bone marrow allograft recipients. Transplantation 46:905, 1988.
145. Schmidt GM, Horak DA, Niland JC, et al: A randomized controlled trial of prophylactic ganciclovir for cytomegalovirus pulmonary infection in recipients of allogeneic bone marrow transplants. N Engl J Med 324:1005, 1991.
146. Goodrich JM, Mori M, Gleaves CA, et al: Early treatment with ganciclovir to prevent cytomegalovirus disease after bone marrow transplantation. N Engl J Med 325:1601, 1991.
147. Singh N, Yu UL, Mieles L, et al: High-dose acyclovir compared with short-course preemptive ganciclovir to prevent cytomegalovirus disease in liver transplant recipients: A randomized trial. Ann Intern Med 120:375, 1994.
148. Snydman DR, Werner BG, Heinze-Lacey B, et al: Use of cytomegalovirus immune globulin to prevent cytomegalovirus disease in renal-transplant recipients. N Engl J Med 317:1049, 1987.
149. Snydman DR, Werner BG, Dougherty NN, et al: Cytomegalovirus immune globulin prophylaxis in liver transplantation. Ann Intern Med 119:984, 1993.
150. Meyers JD, Reed EC, Shepp DH, et al: Acyclovir for prevention of cytomegalovirus infection and disease after allogeneic marrow transplantation. N Engl J Med 318:70, 1988.
151. Balfour HH, Chace BA, Stapleton JT, et al: A randomized, placebo-controlled trial of oral acyclovir for the prevention of cytomegalovirus disease in recipients of renal allografts. N Engl J Med 320:1381, 1989.
152. Goodrich JM, Boeckh M, Bowden R: Strategies for the prevention of cytomegalovirus disease after marrow transplantation. Clin Infect Dis 19:287, 1994.
153. Prentice HG, Gluckman E, Powles RL, et al: Impact of long-term acyclovir on cytomegalovirus infection and survival after allogeneic bone marrow transplantation. Lancet 343:749, 1994.
154. Baily TC, Ettinger NA, Starch GA, et al: Failure of high-dose oral acyclovir with or without immune globulin to prevent primary cytomegalovirus disease in recipients of solid organ transplants. Am J Med 95:273, 1993.
155. Youle MS, Gazzard BG, Johnson MA, et al: Effects of high-dose oral acyclovir on herpesvirus disease and survival in patients with advanced HIV disease: A double-blind, placebo-controlled study. AIDS 8:641, 1994.
156. Winston DJ, Ho WG, Bartoni K, et al: Ganciclovir prophylaxis of cytomegalovirus infection and disease in allogeneic bone marrow transplant recipients. Ann Intern Med 118:179, 1993.
157. Goodrich JM, Bowden RA, Fisher L, et al: Ganciclovir prophylaxis to prevent cytomegalovirus disease after allogeneic marrow transplant. Ann Intern Med 118:173, 1993.
158. Merigan TC, Renlund DG, Keay S, et al: A controlled trial of ganciclovir to prevent cytomegalovirus disease after heart transplantation. N Engl J Med 326:1182, 1992.
159. Spector SA, McKinley GF, Lalezari JP, et al: Oral ganciclovir for the prevention of cytomegalovirus disease in persons with AIDS. N Engl J Med 334:1491, 1996.

187

Kawasaki Syndrome

H. Cody Meissner
Donald Y. M. Leung

Kawasaki syndrome (KS) is an acute, generalized vasculitis of childhood that was first described by Tomisaku Kawasaki[1] in 1967 in the Japanese medical literature. Although the etiology remains incompletely understood, effective therapy is well defined.[2] The most serious complication is coronary arteritis that can lead to aneurysm formation in up to 25% of untreated children.[3] KS has emerged as one of the two major causes of acquired heart disease in childhood, surpassing rheumatic fever in many geographic areas.[4]

Epidemiology

KS has been reported from countries throughout the world, although the highest incidence rates are found in children with Japanese and Korean ancestry. In Japan, the annual incidence rate during nonepidemic years approximates 90 cases per 100,000 children younger than 5 years, a figure that is about 10 times higher than the endemic rate in the United

States and Europe.[5] In the United States, the incidence rate in black persons is about twice that of white. During epidemic periods, incidence rates may increase 10-fold or more.[6] The disease is approximately 1.5 times more common in boys than in girls. Both epidemic disease and nonepidemic disease are most common in the winter and spring; the lowest seasonal occurrence is in the summer and autumn.[7]

KS is almost exclusively an illness of childhood. The peak frequency of occurrence is between 10 and 18 months of age. Eighty percent of cases occur before 5 years of age.[5] Reports of KS in teenagers and adults probably represent other diseases that closely mimic KS. Several risk factors for KS have been proposed: preceding upper respiratory tract infection,[6] exposure to recently shampooed carpets,[8, 9] exposure to dust mites, and living within 200 yards of an open body of water.[10] However, it has not been possible to confirm a role for any of these factors. The overall case-fatality rate due to KS in Japan is 0.35%. This figure is four times higher among children younger than 12 months than in older children.

Three epidemics of KS have been identified in Japan in 1979, 1982, and 1985 to 1986. There have been no new outbreaks in the last 10 years. Outbreaks have occurred in several geographic sites within the United States.[6] Even in outbreaks, evidence of person-to-person spread such as transmission among family members or close contacts is rare.

Etiology and Pathogenesis

It is widely believed that KS represents an infectious disease despite the fact that exhaustive efforts using culture and serologic analysis have failed to conclusively identify an etiologic microbe.[11] The evidence supporting an infectious cause includes seasonal clustering of outbreaks; the acute self-limited nature of the disease; the young age distribution, which suggests that immunity develops in the first decade of life after loss of maternal antibody; and the clinical symptoms of fever and rash, which mimic bacterial toxin–mediated diseases such as scarlet fever and toxic shock syndrome.

Whereas a number of factors are likely to be involved in the pathogenesis of KS, several observations suggest an unusual degree of immune activation in this syndrome.[12–14] Study of autopsy tissue from patients who died of KS shows marked inflammation of coronary arteries as well as of other small- and medium-sized vessels. The mononuclear cells infiltrating vessel walls include both $CD4^+$ and $CD8^+$ T cells as well as monocyte/macrophages. The acute stage is associated with polyclonal activation of B cells as well as an increased number of circulating activated T lymphocytes and monocytes. During the early stages of KS, mononuclear cells produce high levels of circulating cytokines interleukin-1β, tumor necrosis factor-α, and interleukin-6, which are reversed after intravenous immune globulin (IVIG) therapy.[15] Acute KS serum is associated with antibodies that are cytotoxic to cytokine-pretreated endothelial cells in vitro.[16, 17] Such immunologic changes are unusual in response to a conventional antigen and are not seen in association with most infectious diseases of childhood.

The marked T-cell and monocyte activation that characterizes the early phase of KS has been described in certain toxin-mediated bacterial diseases. Staphylococcal exotoxins (toxic shock syndrome toxin 1) and streptococcal pyrogenic exotoxins B and C have been classified as superantigens, a distinct class of antigens that induce the massive immune stimulation similar to that seen in KS.[18] These bacterial toxins bind directly to conserved amino acid residues outside of the antigen binding groove on class II major histocompatibility complex molecules and selectively stimulate T cells expressing specific T-cell receptor β-chain variable gene segments. This results in the stimulation of an uncharacteristically large number of T lymphocytes. Two reports analyzing T lymphocytes from patients in the acute stage of KS demonstrated a selective skewing of T lymphocytes bearing Vβ2 T-cell receptors.[19, 20] Other T-cell subpopulations show no such elevation. Normal subjects and patients with other febrile illnesses show no evidence of T-cell receptor Vβ skewing. These observations support the role of a superantigen as a stimulus for KS. During convalescence, the distribution of T cells returns to normal, indicating that the T-cell imbalance is due to KS. A similar selective expansion of Vβ2 T cells is found in peripheral blood T cells from patients with staphylococcal toxic shock syndrome, a superantigen mediated–illness with many clinical similarities to KS.[21]

A report describing a search for superantigen-producing bacteria on the skin or mucous membranes of KS patients provides additional data supporting a role for bacterial superantigens in KS. In a "blinded" study, bacteria that produce superantigens were found in 13 of 16 acute KS patients but in only 1 of 15 control patients.[22] On the basis of the role of superantigens, the following sequence of events has been proposed. Colonization occurs on the mucous membranes (especially the lower gastrointestinal tract) of a susceptible host by superantigen-producing bacteria. Absorption of the toxin stimulates mononuclear cells with production of proinflammatory cytokines in those patients who lack sufficient antibody to neutralize the superantigen. Elevated cytokine levels result in fever and tissue inflammation, with elevation of acute-phase reactants. Cytokines result in neoantigen expression on the surface of endothelial cells, which makes them more thrombogenic as well as more susceptible to attack and infiltration by cytotoxic antibodies and T lymphocytes, causing vasculitis. IVIG therapy is likely to modify inflammation by more than one mechanism, but one critical factor may be the administration of antibodies to superantigens, resulting in the rapid elimination of the stimulus for cytokine production.[23]

Clinical Features

The decision to treat a patient is based on the history and physical examination findings because no laboratory test is available to confirm the diagnosis of KS. Not every child with KS will manifest each symptom. Furthermore, the symptoms are nonspecific, and it is important to rule out other disorders that may present with similar findings. There is no specific prodrome to KS. A diagnosis of KS is determined by the presence of fever for 5 days and at least four of five established criteria in the absence of another more likely diagnosis[2] (Table 187–1). Fever is almost always the first symptom, with the temperature often exceeding 40°C. Children who present with typical symptoms of KS before 5 days of fever should be treated with IVIG and aspirin if no other diagnosis appears more likely. Treatment with IVIG

TABLE 187–1 ■ Criteria and Diagnostic Features of Kawasaki Syndrome

Exclusion of other diagnoses
Fever for 5 d without explanation
At least four of the following five criteria
Extremity changes including erythema, induration, or desquamation
Polymorphous rash
Nonexudative bulbar conjunctivitis
Oral cavity changes including hyperemia, lip changes, or strawberry tongue
Cervical lymphadenopathy

generally results in rapid defervescence. In untreated children, spiking fevers may continue for 2 to 3 weeks or longer. KS has become an important consideration in children who present with fever of unknown origin.

Changes in the extremities may be the most unique feature of KS. Erythema develops in the palms and soles with or without induration. Induration may evolve to the point of limiting fine motor function. By the end of the second week or the beginning of the third week after onset of fever, periungual desquamation begins, often extending to involve the fingers and toes. Desquamation may occur in other areas, particularly in the perineal area after a severe rash. The rash of KS typically appears within 5 days of onset of fever and may assume a number of forms. Involvement of the face, trunk, and extremities varies from extensive to relatively minimal. Most often the eruption is a morbilliform, maculopapular eruption. Bullae, vesicles, or pustules are distinctly unusual. Oral cavity changes may include dryness, fissuring, cracking, and bleeding of the lips. A strawberry tongue may occur with prominence of the papillae identical to that seen with streptococcal infections. A generalized erythema of the oropharynx is common. Eye changes appear soon after onset of fever. Vascular injection of the bulbar conjunctiva is common, whereas follicular palpebral conjunctivitis is rare. Differentiation from Stevens-Johnson syndrome is suggested by the lack of exudative discharge or corneal ulcerations, both of which are unusual in KS. The acute stage of KS may be associated with anterior uveitis. Generalized lymphadenopathy is the least consistent finding among the diagnostic criteria, occurring in 50% to 75% of patients. At least one lymph node greater than 1.5 cm in diameter is necessary to satisfy this criterion. Adenopathy may be unilateral or bilateral; the nodes are typically firm, nonfluctuant, and either nontender or only mildly tender. Aspiration of the node does not produce pus. An occasional child with KS will present with torticollis secondary to cervical lymphadenopathy.

KS is a multisystem disease, and a number of organ systems may be involved. Joint involvement is common early in the disease, generally manifested as a polyarticular involvement of the smaller joints. A pauciarticular involvement of the larger, weight-bearing joints may be seen later in the illness. Central nervous system involvement is characterized by extreme irritability, especially in younger patients, and may be associated with cerebrospinal fluid pleocytosis. The degree of inconsolability is more severe than that seen in other febrile exanthems of young children, at times suggesting an encephalopathy. Gastrointestinal findings include diarrhea, vomiting, mild elevations of hepatic enzyme levels, and hydrops of the gallbladder. Tympanitis is often present. Hearing deficits range from mild to complete, although this is a rare complication.

Some patients present with fever and fewer than four diagnostic criteria only to later develop coronary artery aneurysms. Such children are diagnosed as having atypical KS and provide evidence that fully developed KS represents only one end of the clinical spectrum. Children who present with a syndrome that does not fulfill sufficient criteria for diagnosis pose a difficult dilemma. To reduce the risk for coronary artery abnormalities, it is important to identify and treat patients presenting with "incomplete" KS with IVIG and aspirin when this diagnosis cannot be excluded.

Recurrent cases of KS have been reported in North America as well as in Japan. Despite a frequently cited figure of approximately 1%, it has been difficult to confirm this rate of recurrence because convincing evidence of both episodes is often not available. It has been noted that second episodes tend to be less severe than the initial illness, suggesting that partial immunity may attenuate disease expression. It has also been suggested that recurrent disease is more likely to be associated with the development of abnormalities of the coronary arteries than is the first episode. This discrepancy cannot be easily resolved because of the rarity of recurrent cases.

Differential Diagnosis

A firm diagnosis of KS is often difficult because the symptoms of KS are not unique to this disease and because not all symptoms are seen in all patients. Because therapy within the first 10 days of onset of fever is clearly desirable in terms of reducing the risk for cardiac complications, rapid diagnosis and treatment are important. In many patients, differentiation of KS from other illnesses that resemble this syndrome may be difficult. Table 187–2 lists the most common illnesses that confound the diagnosis of KS. When measles is common in the community, this diagnosis may be among the most difficult to exclude. Considerations that may eliminate measles from the differential diagnosis include local epidemiology, vaccination history, and culture results. Other viral illnesses that may enter the differential diagnosis include Epstein-Barr virus, adenovirus, and influenza virus infections. Nasal secretions should be cultured in a patient whose symptoms include evidence of an upper respiratory tract infection, especially to rule out adenovirus infection. Group A β-hemolytic streptococcus and *Staphylococcus aureus* infections may also mimic KS. Noninfectious diseases that frequently appear in the differential diagnosis include drug reactions and juvenile rheumatoid arthritis. Findings at physical examination that are not typical of KS include discrete intraoral ulcerations, exudative conjunctivitis, and generalized lymphadenopathy.

Cardiac Involvement

The greatest concern for patients with KS is the development of cardiac involvement and particularly involvement of the coronary arteries.[24, 25] During the acute stage, myocarditis is suggested by echocardiographic evidence of decreased left ventricular contractility; tachycardia out of proportion to the temperature elevation; a gallop rhythm; and an abnormal electrocardiogram showing ST segment depression, T wave changes, and QT interval prolongation. Congestive heart failure and atrial or ventricular arrhythmia may also occur. Transient mitral insufficiency is common, whereas aortic insufficiency is rare. Pericardial effusion is present in the majority of children with KS and usually resolves promptly after IVIG and aspirin therapy.

About 25% of untreated children with KS develop aneu-

TABLE 187–2 ■ Differential Diagnoses

Viral illnesses
Measles
Adenovirus infection
Epstein-Barr virus infection
Bacterial illness
Streptococcal
Scarlet fever
Staphylococcal
Toxic shock syndrome
Staphylococcal scalded skin syndrome
Rocky Mountain spotted fever
Leptospirosis
Juvenile rheumatoid arthritis
Drug reaction

rysms of the coronary arteries. Typically, aneurysms can be detected by echocardiography after the first week and before the fourth week of illness. Rarely, they may occur during the first week of fever. Peripheral aneurysms of the brachial, renal, and iliac arteries are infrequent and usually occur in association with coronary artery involvement.

Factors associated with an increased risk for coronary artery involvement include male sex, age younger than 12 months, and prolonged signs of inflammation such as fever lasting longer than 10 days. The major complication of aneurysms includes thrombosis and stenosis leading to myocardial infarction. Aneurysms greater than 8 mm in diameter (giant aneurysms) pose the greatest risk for myocardial infarction and sudden death. Infarction most commonly occurs within 1 year after onset of disease. Approximately 50% of aneurysms regress within 1 year because of intimal proliferation as assessed by angiography. In those children with aneurysms that do not regress, long-term studies suggest that most will continue to show normal blood flow and normal myocardial function during stress testing.[26]

During the acute stage, two-dimensional echocardiography should be performed as soon as possible in an appropriately sedated child to assess ventricular function, coronary artery structure, valvular function, and the presence of pericardial effusion. Follow-up echocardiography is generally performed 6 to 8 weeks later if the initial study shows no aneurysm formation and inflammation promptly subsides with treatment. The next echocardiogram should be performed 12 months later if the earlier studies remain normal. If the initial echocardiogram is abnormal, management involves therapy to reduce the risk for thrombosis, restrictions on physical activity, and consideration of cardiac catheterization. Such management should be conducted by a physician experienced in pediatric cardiology.[27]

Laboratory Abnormalities

Although there are no specific laboratory changes in patients with KS, certain abnormalities may be useful in supporting the diagnosis and in ruling out other possibilities. Acute-phase reactants (erythrocyte sedimentation rate, C-reactive protein, and α_1-antitrypsin) are elevated at the time of presentation. A leukocytosis with an increased number of immature granulocytes is usually present. Mild anemia and hypoalbuminemia are common. Thrombocytosis is generally present by the second week of illness, with platelet counts as high as 1 million/mm^3 or greater. Abnormalities in the urine include pyuria (a reflection of generalized mucosal inflammation that involves the urethra) and proteinuria.

Abnormalities in plasma lipid profiles have been observed in patients with acute KS. Plasma concentrations of both total cholesterol and high-density lipoprotein cholesterol are reduced; triglyceride concentrations are elevated.[28] Cholesterol levels quickly return to normal, whereas high-density lipoprotein levels may remain elevated for several years.[29]

Treatment

The goal of therapy during the acute stage is to reduce inflammation in the myocardium and in the wall of arteries, particularly the coronary arteries. The use of both salicylate therapy and IVIG therapy is directed at this objective.[2] Since the beneficial effect of IVIG was first noted in a report from Japan in 1984, two multiinstitutional trials conducted in the United States have confirmed and extended observations on the beneficial effects of IVIG.[3, 30, 31] The current recommendation is for aspirin plus IVIG administered as a single dose of 2 g/kg in 8 to 12 hours, usually while the patient is hospitalized (Table 187–3). Children who receive a single infusion of 2 g/kg IVIG appear to have a lower frequency of coronary artery abnormalities than do children treated with four daily doses of 400 mg/kg, the treatment regimen that was first studied in the United States.[31] More rapid normalization of acute-phase reactants as well as more rapid defervescence is seen in children treated with a single dose of IVIG in comparison to four daily infusions. The beneficial effect of IVIG in reducing signs of inflammation is frequently apparent before the end of the IVIG infusion. Symptomatic children who are first diagnosed beyond 10 days of fever should receive treatment even though clinical trials demonstrating IVIG efficacy in this group have not been conducted.

TABLE 187–3 ■ Therapy for Acute Kawasaki Syndrome

Intravenous immune globulin, 2 g/kg in 12 h as single infusion
Aspirin, 80–100 mg/kg/d in four divided doses until afebrile, then 3–5 mg/kg once daily for 6–8 wk

Aspirin is used for both its antiinflammatory and antithrombotic actions, although convincing data that aspirin reduces coronary artery abnormalities are not available. Aspirin shortens the duration of fever and the manifestations of acute disease when it is used in conjunction with IVIG. The current recommendations from the American Heart Association include aspirin at 80 to 100 mg/kg per day in four doses until the patient is afebrile. In a patient who has no coronary artery abnormalities at echocardiography, low-dose aspirin should be continued at a dose of 3 to 5 mg/kg per day for 6 to 8 weeks.

Two abnormalities of aspirin metabolism have been described in patients with KS. First, patients may have reduced absorption of salicylate from the gastrointestinal tract and enhanced plasma clearance rates leading to low serum salicylate levels.[32] Second, during the acute stage, there is decreased protein binding of salicylate owing to low serum albumin levels, leading to an increase in free salicylate levels despite a low total salicylate concentration.[33] Because toxicity is a function of free salicylate level, low serum albumin levels may necessitate adjustment of the aspirin dose to avoid toxic effects.

A small number of children may remain febrile with unabating signs of inflammation at 48 to 72 hours after treatment with a standard regimen of aspirin and IVIG. Retreatment of such children may be undertaken out of concern that persistent fever correlates with elevated levels of proinflammatory cytokines, which in turn correlate with an ongoing risk for coronary artery involvement. Clinical trials suggest that there may be a threshold level of immunoglobulin G that is necessary to reduce the clinical signs of inflammation. Although there are no specific recommendations for retreatment, some children benefit from a second dose of IVIG. Failure to respond to IVIG should always prompt consideration of other possible diagnoses.

References

1. Kawasaki T: Acute febrile mucocutaneous syndrome with lymphoid involvement with specific desquamation of the fingers and toes in children: Clinical observations of 50 cases. Jpn J Allergol 16:178, 1967.
2. Dajani AS, Taubert KA, Gerber MA, et al: Diagnosis and therapy of Kawasaki disease in children. Circulation 87:1776, 1993.
3. Newburger JW, Takahashi M, Burns JC, et al: The treatment of Kawasaki syndrome with intravenous gamma globulin. N Engl J Med 315:341, 1986.

4. Taubert KA, Rowley AH, Shulman ST: Nationwide survey of Kawasaki disease and acute rheumatic fever. J Pediatr 119:279, 1991.
5. Yanagawa H, Nakamura Y, Yashiro M, et al: A nationwide survey of Kawasaki disease in 1985–1986 in Japan. J Infect Dis 158:1296, 1988.
6. Bell DM, Brink EW, Nitzkin JL, et al: Kawasaki syndrome: Description of two outbreaks in the United States. N Engl J Med 304:1568, 1981.
7. Rauch AM: Kawasaki syndrome: Review of new epidemiologic and laboratory developments. Pediatr Infect Dis J 6:1016, 1987.
8. Patriarca P, Rogers M, Morens D, et al: Kawasaki syndrome: Association with application of rug shampoo. Lancet 2:578, 1982.
9. Rogers M, Kochel R, Hurwitz E, et al: Kawasaki syndrome: Is exposure to rug shampoo important? Am J Dis Child 139:777, 1985.
10. Rauch AM, Kaplan SL, Nihill MR, et al: Kawasaki syndrome clusters in Harris County, Texas, and eastern North Carolina. Am J Dis Child 142:441, 1988.
11. Meissner HC, Schlievert PM, Leung DY: Mechanisms of immunoglobulin action: Observations on Kawasaki syndrome and RSV prophylaxis. Immunol Rev 139:109, 1994.
12. Leung DYM: Immunologic aspects of Kawasaki syndrome. J Rheumatol Suppl 24:15, 1990.
13. Leung DYM: Overview of disease mechanisms. *In* Takahashi M, Taubert K (eds): Proceedings of the Fourth International Symposium of Kawasaki Disease. Dallas, American Heart Association, 1993, pp 155–159.
14. Leung DYM, Chu ET, Wood N, et al: Immunoregulatory T cell abnormalities in mucocutaneous lymph node syndrome. J Immunol 130:2002, 1983.
15. Leung DYM, Burns J, Newburger J, et al: Reversal of immunoregulatory abnormalities in Kawasaki syndrome by intravenous gammaglobulin. J Clin Invest 79:468, 1987.
16. Leung DYM, Collins T, LaPierre LA, et al: IgM antibodies present in the acute phase of Kawasaki syndrome lyse cultured vascular endothelial cells stimulated by gamma interferon. J Clin Invest 77:1428, 1986.
17. Leung DYM, Cotran RS, Kurt-Jones EZ, et al: Endothelial cell activation and increased interleukin 1 secretion in the pathogenesis of acute Kawasaki disease. Lancet 2:1298, 1989.
18. Kotzin BL, Leung DYM, Kappler J, et al: Superantigens and human disease. Adv Immunol 54:99, 1993.
19. Abe J, Kotzin BL, Jujo K, et al: Selective expansion of T cells expressing T cell receptor variable regions Vββ8 in Kawasaki disease. Proc Natl Acad Sci USA 89:4066, 1992.
20. Curtis N, Zheng R, Lamb JR, et al: Evidence for a superantigen mediated process in Kawasaki disease. Arch Dis Child 72:308, 1995.
21. Choi Y, Lafferty JA, Clements JR, et al: Selective expansion of T cells expressing Vβ2 in toxic shock syndrome. J Exp Med 172:981, 1990.
22. Leung DYM, Meissner HC, Fulton DR, et al: Toxic shock syndrome toxin–secreting *Staphylococcus aureus* in Kawasaki syndrome. Lancet 342:1385, 1993.
23. Takei S, Arora YK, Walder SM: Intravenous immunoglobulin contains specific antibodies inhibitory to activation of T cells by staphylococcal toxin superantigens. J Clin Invest 91:602, 1993.
24. Suzuki A, Kamiya T, Kuwahara N, et al: Coronary arterial lesions of Kawasaki disease: Cardiac catheterization findings of 1100 cases. Pediatr Cardiol 7:3, 1986.
25. Nakamura Y, Fujita Y, Nagai M, et al: Cardiac sequelae of Kawasaki disease in Japan: Statistical analysis. Pediatrics 88:1144, 1991.
26. Hijazi ZM, Udelson JE, Snapper H, et al: Physiologic significance of chronic coronary aneurysms in patients with Kawasaki disease. J Am Coll Cardiol 24:1633, 1994.
27. Dajani AS, Taubert KA, Takahashi M, et al: Guidelines for long-term management of patients with Kawasaki disease. Circulation 89:916, 1994.
28. Newburger JW, Burns JC, Beiser AS, et al: Altered lipid profile after Kawasaki disease. Circulation 84:625, 1991.
29. Salo E, Pesonen E, Viikari J: Serum cholesterol levels during and after Kawasaki disease. J Pediatr 119:557, 1991.
30. Furusho K, Kamiya T, Nakano H, et al: High dose intravenous gamma globulin for Kawasaki disease. Lancet 2:1055, 1984.
31. Newburger JW, Takahashi M, Beiser AS, et al: A single intravenous infusion of gamma globulin as compared with four infusions in the treatment of acute Kawasaki syndrome. N Engl J Med 324:1633, 1991.
32. Koren G, Schaffer F, Silverman E, et al: Determinants of low serum concentration of salicylates in Kawasaki disease. J Pediatr 112:663, 1988.
33. Koren G, Silverman E, Sundel R, et al: Decreased protein binding of salicylates in Kawasaki disease. J Pediatr 118:456, 1991.

OTHER INFECTIONS

188

Infections in a Prosthetic Device

Adolf W. Karchmer

Insertion of prosthetic devices to provide relief for an increasing array of symptoms is a major advance in medical therapeutics, but it has created diseases of medical progress—infections of prosthetic devices (Table 188–1). Although infection is a rare complication with the devices that are completely implanted, it is not unusual with those that traverse a cutaneous or mucosal surface. Nevertheless, infections of both partially and fully implanted devices produce major morbidity, mortality, and expense.

Prosthetic devices are always vulnerable to infection. Whenever a patient with a prosthesis presents with systemic symptoms or signs of infection or evidence of prosthesis dysfunction or periprosthesis inflammation, the possibility of an infected device must be entertained. When a prosthesis is found to be infected, the clinical importance of both the infection and the device must be considered. The patient's life may be threatened acutely by systemic infection or prosthesis dysfunction or merely inconvenienced by the loss of a cosmetic device or the need for antimicrobial therapy. Formulating a diagnostic and therapeutic plan for an infected prosthesis requires an understanding of the pathogenesis of infection of the specific device and of foreign bodies in general, as well as the pathologic physiology that arises with a dysfunctional device. The infecting organism must be recovered in order that appropriate antimicrobial therapy can be selected. The limitations of host defenses and antimicrobial therapy in eradicating infection associated with foreign material must be understood. In addition, detailed knowledge of prior experience treating infections of the device must be considered, particularly those caused by the specific patho-

TABLE 188–1 ■ Infections of Prosthetic Devices

DEVICE*	PREVALENCE OF INFECTION	COMMON PATHOGENS	MAJOR SYNDROMES
Heart valve	3% at 1 y 4%–6% at 4–5 y	*Staphylococcus epidermidis* *Staphylococcus aureus* Streptococci	Endocarditis
Joints	Hip 0.5%–1.3% Knee 1.3%–2.9%	*S. aureus* *S. epidermidis*	Indolent, progressively painful joint, acute septic arthritis
Transvenous permanent pacemaker	Pocket sepsis 1%–7% Lead only <1%	*S. aureus* *S. epidermidis*	Localized pocket infection, bacteremia (infected intravascular wire)
Arterial graft	Aortoiliac <1%–1.5% Femoropopliteal 2%–7%	*S. aureus* *S. epidermidis*	Bacteremia, false aneurysm, occlusion, anastomotic rupture
Intraocular lens	<1%	*S. epidermidis* *S. aureus*	Endophthalmitis
CSF shunt	1.5%–15%	*S. epidermidis* *S. aureus*	Ventriculitis, meningitis, hydrocephalus, bacteremia
CAPD catheter	60% first year; 0.5–1.0 episodes/patient/y	*S. epidermidis* *S. aureus* Streptococci	Mild peritonitis, catheter track wound infection
Breast implant	Augmentation 2%–3% Reconstruction >3%	*S. aureus* *S. epidermidis*	Wound infection
Penile prosthesis	1%–5%	*S. epidermidis* Enterobacteriaceae	Indolent or purulent wound infection

*CSF, Cerebrospinal fluid; CAPD, continuous ambulatory peritoneal dialysis.

gen. In selecting therapy, the morbidity and mortality risks of the treatment required to eradicate infection, to salvage or replace the device, and to correct infection-induced pathologic physiology must be balanced against the hazards of the infection itself, the role of the device, and the alternatives to the device. The device may be essential for life (prosthetic heart valve), essential for life but with convenient alternatives (hemodialysis shunt), necessary for important activities (prosthetic hip joint), an aid in performing nonessential activities (penile prosthesis), or primarily cosmetic (breast prosthesis). Thus, salvaging, replacing, and eliminating the device are fundamental considerations in designing therapy.

Pathogenesis

The introduction of foreign material into the complex interaction between a microorganism and the host and its defenses increases the likelihood of infection. Elek and Conen[1] demonstrated that the minimal number of staphylococci required to induce infection could be reduced from 10^6 to 10^2 by the presence of a braided silk suture. Foreign material not only enhances the pathogenicity of known virulent microorganisms by reducing the inoculum necessary to initiate infection but also allows organisms that are typically not pathogenic to establish infection. The latter is illustrated by the striking frequency with which usually avirulent *Staphylococcus epidermidis* organisms cause prosthetic device infection. Foreign material was required in order for subcutaneously injected *S. epidermidis* or *Staphylococcus aureus* Wood 46 strain organisms to cause infection in mice and guinea pigs.[2, 3]

Adherence of an organism to a device is the initial step in establishing an infection. Physiochemical interactions between the device and the microorganism promote adherence, but studies suggest that more selective binding occurs.[4, 5] Host proteins, including fibrinogen and fibronectin, promptly coat foreign materials. Complex dynamic interactions occur between specific bacterial surface receptors and foreign body–bound adhesions derived from host proteins, glycoproteins, and cellular elements.[4] Studies suggest that fibronectin and its active fragments promote greater adherence of laboratory strains and clinical isolates of *S. aureus* to chronically implanted intravascular catheters than do fibrinogen and fibrin, which undergo in situ degradation.[5, 6] In contrast, fibrinogen, acting as receptor-specific adhesin, promotes greater adherence of *S. aureus* to catheters after a short-term interaction with blood.[7] The interaction of coagulase-negative staphylococci and host proteins coating foreign devices (adhesins) is less well defined at a molecular level. Not only is this interaction less vigorous but also the proteins and glycoproteins facilitating adherence of these organisms differ from those that are adhesins for *S. aureus*. For example, fibronectin promotes adherence of both coagulase-positive and coagulase-negative staphylococci, whereas fibrinogen facilitates adherence primarily of *S. aureus*.[4]

The extracellular substance produced by bacteria, called slime or glycocalyx, has been associated with coagulase-negative staphylococci that infect foreign bodies, particularly *S. epidermidis*.[8–13] Slime has been postulated to function by facilitating the adherence of coagulase-negative staphylococci to foreign materials. Slime, however, did not facilitate adherence of coagulase-negative staphylococci to fibrinogen- or fibronectin-coated polymethyl methacrylate, so its role as an adhesin in vivo remains controversial.[5, 14] Alternatively, slime may facilitate foreign body infection by promoting the accumulation of bacteria as they multiply, thus creating a microcolony on the device.[14] A capsular polysaccharide adhesin, distinct from slime, facilitates adherence of coagulase-negative staphylococci to foreign material and functions as an antiphagocytic capsule.[15–17] This material may facilitate the infection of foreign bodies by coagulase-negative staphylococci.

Foreign body infection is difficult to eradicate without removing the foreign material. This difficulty results, in part, from impairment of host defenses in the immediate environment of the foreign body. The opsonizing capability of fluid surrounding foreign materials is reduced relative to that of serum and deteriorates further during local infection. Nevertheless, preopsonizing *S. aureus* organisms before inoculating them into an implanted foreign body fails to prevent infection. Thus, although it may contribute to the pathogenesis of foreign body infection, the opsonization defect is not the dominant abnormality.[3] The bactericidal activity of polymorphonuclear leukocytes (PMNs) that have been in contact with foreign materials is significantly weaker than that of PMNs from acute and chronic inflammatory exudates and from peripheral blood.[3] This abnormality is associated with defective oxygen-dependent PMN killing mechanisms, deficient PMN superoxide production, and evidence of prior degranulation by the defective PMNs.[18] Defective PMNs appear to play an important role in the initiation of foreign body infection by small inocula of bacteria. Functional PMNs infused locally before or shortly after a bacterial challenge prevent infection of a subcutaneously implanted foreign body.[18] Other host-parasite–foreign body interactions make eradication of these infections difficult. For example, the ability of fully effective PMNs to phagocytose and kill *S. aureus* organisms that are adherent to polymethyl methacrylate is reduced[19]; alteration in the production of cytokines, for example, tumor necrosis factor, in the immediate vicinity of foreign devices may impair PMN bactericidal activity[20]; and extracellular slime impairs the ability of PMNs to phagocytose *S. epidermidis* adherent to a plastic surface.[21] Bacteria recovered from infected foreign bodies and from glycocalyx biofilms and those adherent to foreign materials are less susceptible to killing by selected antibiotics when studied immediately after recovery from the foreign material than are the same strains grown in a planktonic fashion.[22–24]

The clinical events that lead to infection of a prosthesis provide important clues to the time of presentation and the infecting organism. Intraoperative or perioperative contamination, which accounts for a large portion of infections involving fully implanted devices, results in infections clustered in the initial months after surgery. Often these are indolent infections caused by coagulase-negative staphylococci or other components of normal skin flora. Foreign body infections that present within the early weeks after surgery as typical wound infections are caused by more virulent bacteria. In a review of 205 vascular graft infections, Bunt[25] noted that early infections were often caused by *S. aureus* and occurred in association with inguinal wound infection. Small epidemics result from contamination of the devices or materials used during surgery. In these epidemics, the infections share clinical and epidemiologic features and a pathogen and cluster in time according to the virulence of the contaminating microorganism. Endocarditis caused by *Mycobacterium chelonae* contaminating porcine bioprosthetic valves typifies this process.[26] Occasionally, infections resulting from perioperative contamination of a prosthesis by avirulent organisms remain asymptomatic for many months. This sequence has been postulated for coagulase-negative staphylococcal and other bacterial infections of prosthetic heart valves,[27, 28] joint replacements,[29–31] and synthetic vascular grafts.[32] Usually, infection beginning a year or more after surgery results from proximate seeding of a device. This seeding may occur hematogenously, by extension of adjacent infection to the device, or by erosion of the device into a contaminated area as seen with the development of an aortoenteric fistula or erosion of a pacemaker generator through the skin. The virulence of the causative organism determines the toxicity associated with these late-onset infections. Toxicity can range from the subacute presentations of viridans streptococcal prosthetic valve endocarditis (PVE)[33] to highly febrile presentations of acute septic arthritis involving a joint prosthesis.[29] Devices placed transcutaneously and manipulated regularly (e.g., Tenckhoff peritoneal dialysis catheters) are infected repeatedly by organisms that are part of the patient's flora.[34, 35] In addition, contamination of medical materials or machines used with a device can lead to epidemic infection. *Pseudomonas cepacia* peritonitis in patients undergoing chronic intermittent peritoneal dialysis has been linked to contaminated automatic dialysis machines.[36] As a consequence of the transcutaneous drive line required to power the implantable total artificial heart, infection caused by skin flora and nosocomial organisms is almost universal and limits the time during which this prosthesis can be used.[37]

Clinical Manifestations

The diversity of clinical presentations among patients with infected prosthetic devices exceeds that attributable to the spectrum of devices in use. Typical clinical syndromes are associated with infection involving some prostheses (e.g., acute or subacute endocarditis with prosthetic valve infection,[33] endophthalmitis with infection of an intraocular lens implant[38, 39]), but infections in a given prosthesis may present variably. Signs and symptoms may be localized, systemic, or both and may range in severity from dramatic to minimal. These extremes are contingent in part on the location of the device—depth of implantation, surrounding tissue or space, intravascular position—and on the pathogen. For example, infection involving a total hip prosthesis may manifest as an early postoperative wound infection with local and systemic symptoms, delayed onset of progressive postoperative pain on weight bearing without local or systemic signs of infection, or an acute septic arthritis with marked systemic toxicity and local pain. Infection of cerebrospinal fluid (CSF) shunts developing shortly after surgery may present as fever and inflammation along the subcutaneous path of the shunt.[40] Approximately a third of patients with CSF shunt infections have clinical features characteristic of meningitis,[40–42] although, among patients with infected ventriculoperitoneal CSF shunts, 33% present primarily with abdominal pain and tenderness.[41]

The predominant signs provoked by prosthesis infection are not always those of inflammation. Instead, they may reflect physiologic alterations caused by prosthesis dysfunction or the immune consequences of chronic infection. These symptoms can be dramatic, masking those of inflammation, or can be subtle and indolent. Patients with PVE with minimal symptoms of infection may present with severe congestive heart failure caused by acute aortic valve regurgitation or with neurologic symptoms resulting from a massive cerebrovascular event. Nonspecific symptoms and signs of increased intracranial pressure may indicate CSF shunt dysfunction due to infection.[42, 43] With infection of a ventriculoatrial CSF shunt with immune complex–induced vasculitis and glomerulonephritis, presenting manifestations may be palpable purpuric skin lesions and azotemia with proteinuria and hematuria.[44–46] Infection involving a synthetic vascular graft may present with signs of local incisional infection or septicemia, or with graft dysfunction, including occlusion, hemorrhage, or with formation of a false aneurysm.[47] Infection of the artery-graft anastomosis eventually produces suture line breakdown. When this occurs at the aorta-graft anastomosis, the presentations include a painful abdominal mass, hydronephrosis due to ureteral compression, or low-grade fever and intermittent gastrointestinal tract bleeding due to an aortoenteric fistula.[32, 48] If the diagnosis of aortoenteric fistula is not made promptly, the initial sign may be brisk gastrointestinal bleeding as the false aneurysm or fistula drains more freely into the bowel lumen.[32, 48]

Microbiology

An awareness of the unusually broad array and variable virulence of microorganisms that infect prosthetic devices is important in approaching the patient with a possibly infected prosthesis. It is crucial, however, to realize that staphylococci commonly cause these infections (see Table 188–1) and that often the identity of the pathogen can be predicted from the clinical circumstances. The microbiology of device infections is the consequence of interrelated circumstances: (1) the presence of the foreign body; (2) the placement of the device entirely within the body or across a skin or mucosal surface; (3) the anatomic location of the prosthesis; (4) the clinical events leading to contamination. The clinical circumstances that lead to an infection are often a strong predictor of the infecting microorganism. Placement of a foreign body across an external surface affords microorganisms continuous access along the insertion route to the implanted portion. Similarly, repeated manipulation of a totally implanted device affords increased opportunity for direct seeding. Until it is covered with a pseudoendothelium, a prosthesis implanted in the circulatory system is vulnerable to organisms in the blood. Unless there is a major break in sterile technique, perioperative contamination of a prosthesis favors infection with skin flora, particularly *S. aureus* and coagulase-negative staphylococci, and occasionally streptococci and diphtheroids. The prominent role of *S. aureus* and coagulase-negative staphylococci, which are usually *S. epidermidis,* is more than a chance occurrence; it reflects, in addition to the likelihood that they contaminate wounds by virtue of their presence on the skin, biologic properties that facilitate their adherence to and proliferation on foreign materials. The result of perioperative contamination is reflected in the microbiology of PVE that occurs within the year after valve surgery,[33] in early and delayed-onset prosthetic joint infections,[29] in CSF shunt infections,[40, 42] and in infections of intraocular lenses,[38, 39] prosthetic arterial grafts,[25, 47] and penile prostheses.[49, 50] As for native valve endocarditis, transient bacteremia is the predominant clinical event that leads to PVE with onset a year or more after surgery. Consequently, the microbiology of late-onset PVE resembles that of native valve endocarditis.[33] The location of a prosthesis renders it vulnerable to invasion by microorganisms that are resident in contiguous areas. Thus, transmural spread of enterobacteria from the bowel causes peritoneal dialysis–associated peritonitis,[34] and gram-negative bacteria, as part of perineal skin flora[50] are important causes of infection of penile prostheses. Peripheral infections give rise to bacteremia that seeds prosthetic devices; thus, the presence of a distant infection provides an important clue to the organism causing device infection. *S. aureus,* β-hemolytic streptococci, or enteric, gram-negative bacilli have spread via the blood from skin or urinary tract infection to well-established, functioning prosthetic joints.[29, 51] Similarly, the prevalence of primary bacteremic meningitis is increased in patients with CSF shunts and leads to secondary infection of the shunt by the bacteria that commonly cause meningitis.[42] In contrast, the unanticipated discovery of bacteremia due to an avirulent organism (e.g., *S. epidermidis,* diphtheroids) should prompt consideration of infection of an intravascular device such as a prosthetic valve, vascular graft, ventriculoatrial CSF shunt, or transvenous pacemaker.[28, 44–46]

Diagnosis

A prosthesis exposed in the base of an unhealed surgical wound or at the end of a sinus track is obviously infected. Typically, however, the impetus to pursue this diagnosis hinges on recognizing subtle findings. Prosthesis dysfunction, particularly as a new development or one that progresses over a brief interval, is an important clue to potential infection. Occasionally the inflammatory process is subclinical or minimal and the dysfunction itself is the major manifestation of infection. Mild local inflammation adjacent to a device, although appearing more consistent with a sterile reaction to the foreign body, may be indicative of infection. Ultimately, the diagnosis of device infection hinges on demonstrating microorganisms on the prosthesis or in the area immediately surrounding it.

Documentation of local inflammation and infection is difficult. Leukocytosis and an accelerated erythrocyte sedimentation rate are rarely noted, but even when they are, at best they are nonspecific. The discriminatory capacity of radiography, nuclear imaging, and sonography is often reduced by the presence of implanted devices. Frequently these modalities cannot distinguish between changes produced by infection and those induced by the disease that necessitated placement of the prosthesis, by local tissue reaction to the prosthesis itself, or by the implant insertion procedure. For example, when persistent hip pain develops 6 months after insertion of a joint prosthesis, none of these signs—lucency at the bone-cement interface, periosteal reaction on radiographs, uptake of technetium Tc 99m diphosphonate–labeled or gallium 111–labeled PMNs—is specific enough to distinguish between changes related to recent surgery, infection, or aseptic loosening (the major alternative diagnosis to low-grade infection).[29] The capability of other modalities may also be limited; device-induced artifacts in computed tomography and magnetic resonance imaging and prominent reflective properties in sonography compromise their utility, although, with careful interpretation of results in the context of the clinical problem, selected noninvasive studies can provide important information even if they are not diagnostic. Echocardiography, with Doppler, particularly using a transesophageal approach, may detect perivalvular abscess formation, fistulae, or transvalvular pressure gradients indicative of prosthetic valve dysfunction, which in the context of fever, bacteremia, or clinical signs of endocarditis is highly suggestive of PVE.[52] Similarly, even if ultrasonography, computed tomography, magnetic resonance imaging, and arteriography cannot provide direct evidence of inflammation or infection, they may disclose a false aneurysm arising at the artery-graft anastomosis, perigraft air or fluid collection, or graft occlusion.[47] Negative findings may be of importance also—no increase in uptake of technetium 99m around a joint prosthesis argues against local infection. Failure to demonstrate dysfunction or local inflammation of a prosthesis does not always rule out infection. For example, radionuclide scans are not sufficiently sensitive to eliminate the possible diagnosis of vascular graft infection.[47]

If infection is suspected, it is necessary to attempt to recover microorganisms from the device or adjacent tissues before initiating antibiotic therapy, even if treatment is delayed briefly. Empirical antimicrobial therapy is rarely justifiable before optimal cultures are obtained. With devices that are intravascular (at least in part), such as prosthetic heart valves, transvenous cardiac pacers, synthetic arterial grafts, and ventriculoatrial CSF shunts, repeated isolation of an organism from blood establishes the pathogen. If blood cultures fail to demonstrate the organism and an extravascular or partially extravascular device is in place, material for culture must be obtained, where feasible, by direct aspiration of fluid in the device or of adjacent fluid. For example, aspiration of the intraarticular space, the pacemaker generator pocket, the subcutaneous space adjacent to a CSF shunt, or the CSF shunt valve reservoir may be necessary. Scrupulous sterile technique must be used to avoid contaminating the device and the aspirated material.

Even with diligent efforts it may be difficult to recover organisms from an infected device or to conclude that an isolated organism is responsible for an infection. The density of organisms at the site of infection may be low, which would reduce the sensitivity of cultures, especially when the inoculum is small. In addition, organisms infecting prosthetic devices may be fastidious and difficult to recover. Anticipating these problems and using generous inocula, multiple media, and in selected situations, special culture techniques to recover anaerobic bacteria, fungi, mycobacteria, *Legionella* species, or mycoplasmas enhance the yield of cultures. Foreign body infection characterized by organisms embedded in surface biofilms may be difficult to document microbiologically. The recovery of organisms in cultures, especially coagulase-negative staphylococci, is increased by culturing a fragment of the device and its attached biofilm. Similarly, organisms can be recovered from surface biofilms that have been mechanically disrupted by ultrasonic oscillations or grinding tissue.[47]

Concluding that an isolate is the cause of infection and not a contaminant can be problematic. This quandary arises because organisms that are usually dismissed as contaminants, such as coagulase-negative staphylococci, α-hemolytic streptococci, and diphtheroids, often cause these infections. Such organisms are implicated when they are present in large numbers. If material is cultured promptly, recovering the organism in at least moderate amounts on one or more solid media, rather than only in broth media, indicates that large numbers of organisms are present. In addition, when inflammatory cells and the organism are seen at microscopic examination of the specimen, or when identical organisms are recovered from sequential aspirates or from preoperative and intraoperative specimens, it is likely that the organism is the pathogen. Organisms commonly viewed as contaminants must not be disregarded when they are recovered from a prosthetic device. When the significance of an organism is not clear, efforts to recover it from additional specimens are warranted. Determining that coagulase-negative staphylococci isolated sporadically from a device are identical increases the likelihood that the unique organism is causing the infection. Because most coagulase-negative staphylococci isolated are *S. epidermidis* and possess similar antibiotic susceptibility profiles, special tests such as biotyping, phage typing, DNA karyotype pattern, and plasmid pattern analysis are required to establish the uniqueness of isolates from sequential cultures.[9, 27, 53] Thus, determining that an organism isolated from a foreign body is causing infection may require semiquantitative assessment of specimens, repeated cultures, or special tests to establish the uniqueness of a sporadically isolated organism.

Differential Diagnosis

The presence of fever or of signs and symptoms of inflammation in the patient with an indwelling medical device invariably raises the possibility that the device is infected. In seeking an explanation for these signs and symptoms, the temporal relationship of the febrile episode to the insertion of the device helps to focus the investigation, as do symptoms suggestive of a remote infection. Shortly after surgery, the usual causes of early postoperative fever, including infections and noninfectious entities, are sought. In addition, during the early postoperative period, causes of fever that are peculiar to the specific device must be considered. For example, fever after prosthetic valve placement may be due to the postpericardiotomy syndrome, and that after neurosurgery that included placement of a CSF shunt may be due to surgically induced aseptic meningitis. When surgical placement of the prosthesis is more distant, the number of possible explanations is greatly increased; in the evaluation of fever of unknown origin a device infection is simply one consideration. If there is inflammation around a recently inserted device but no fever, infection must still be excluded; however, alternative causes, including reactions to the trauma of surgery, to the device itself, and materials used in the insertion, and hematoma, must be considered also. Inflammation of the eye after cataract extraction and intraocular lens implantation results from infection, surgical trauma, toxicity due to residual polishing compounds or sterilizing agents on the lens implant, or allergic reactions to crystalline lens cortical remnants.[39]

Prosthesis dysfunction, a possible clue to infection, may also result from noninfectious problems. Technical problems can account for persistently elevated intracranial pressure after placement of a CSF shunt or a murmur of valvular incompetence after insertion of a prosthetic heart valve. Interactions between the device and surrounding tissues can result in the late appearance of prosthesis dysfunction. For example, aseptic loosening of the femoral component of a total hip replacement causes late onset of pain on weight bearing. Inflammatory signs and symptoms in the area of the prosthesis can be caused by unrelated diseases that coincidentally involve that anatomic region. Distinguishing a ventriculoperitoneal CSF shunt infection from acute appendicitis may be difficult. Similarly, diverticulitis, cholecystitis, and the many other causes of abdominal pain must be considered in the differential diagnosis of peritonitis associated with continuous ambulatory peritoneal dialysis (CAPD).

Treatment

Effective treatment of an infected prosthesis must achieve two objectives: eradication of the infection and maintenance of a functioning device or provision of a functional alternative. Failure to achieve both objectives is less than optimal. The clinical dictum that an infected device must be removed to eliminate infection is inaccurate and oversimplified. Some foreign body infections can be eradicated with aggressive antimicrobial therapy. Furthermore, the ultimate goal of eradicating infection and maintaining function, while limiting the risks of therapy itself, is not always best served by removing the prosthesis.

The fundamentals of effective antimicrobial therapy include identifying the infecting organism or organisms and their antimicrobial susceptibility profiles, designing a bactericidal antimicrobial regimen with minimal toxicity, and adminstering the antimicrobial so as to produce an adequate concentration at the site of infection. The bactericidal activity of antibiotics against stationary-phase organisms and those that are adherent to foreign material correlates directly with the eradication of infection involving foreign bodies.[54] Rifampin possesses this type of bactericidal activity against susceptible staphylococci. Furthermore, when used in combination with one or two additional antibiotics to prevent the emergence of rifampin resistance during therapy, treatment with rifampin-containing regimens eradicated infections caused by *S. epidermidis* and *S. aureus* in animal models without removing the foreign body.[54–56] These studies suggest a specific important role for rifampin in combination therapy for foreign body infection. Also, combination antibiotic therapy may be necessary to achieve bactericidal activity, to provide a synergistic or enhanced bactericidal effect, or to broaden the spectrum of antimicrobial activity when treating a polymicrobial infection. The duration and route of antibiotic administration are based on experience with analogous infections. Prolonged courses of intravenous antibiotics are used for PVE and infected orthopedic devices; more abbreviated courses are used for peritonitis complicating CAPD and soft tissue infections that persist after a device has been removed. Direct instillation of antibiotics at the infection site is used to treat selected infections. Because systemically administered antibiotics penetrate the anterior and posterior chambers of the eye poorly, infected intraocular lens replacements are treated by local injections of antibiotics.[38, 39] Although the benefit has not been clearly documented, local treatment with antibiotic-impregnated cement has been used in conjunction with systemic antibiotics in the replacement of an infected orthopedic prosthesis with a new device.[29, 57] Occasionally, device-related infection that is totally confined to a closed body space (e.g., peritonitis associated with CAPD) can be treated by instillation of antimicrobials directly into the infected area.[34, 58, 59]

The essential considerations in deciding whether an infection can be successfully treated without removing the device are the initial and continued functional status of the prosthesis, prior experience in treating the specific infection, and the infecting organism. PVE occurring a year or more after valve placement and caused by avirulent, antibiotic-susceptible organisms, such as viridans streptococci or fastidious gram-negative coccobacilli, can usually be cured by intensive antibiotic therapy; however, if there are initial or subsequent valve dysfunction and congestive heart failure, cardiac surgery is necessary to remove the infected valve and to implant a new prosthesis.[33, 60–62] Often, removal of the prosthesis is necessary to eradicate infection by highly virulent, destructive, antibiotic-resistant organisms, such as *S. aureus*, enteric and nonenteric gram-negative bacilli, and fungi. Intraperitoneal antibiotic treatment without removing a functioning Tenckhoff catheter often eradicates CAPD-associated peritonitis caused by coagulase-negative staphylococci or enteric gram-negative bacilli,[34, 59] but peritonitis due to *S. aureus*, *Pseudomonas aeruginosa*, or fungi, particularly if there is tunnel infection or dialysis catheter dysfunction, usually requires catheter removal.[59, 63–66] In selected clinical settings, the device and the associated function are most likely to be salvaged with aggressive antibiotic treatment. Because of the hazards of hemorrhage and retinal tears when operating on an inflamed eye, eradication of infection with maintenance of visual function is best achieved by antibiotic treatment of infected intraocular lens implants without lens removal.[38, 39]

Although marked virulence or antibiotic resistance of an infecting organism suggests the need to remove a device to eliminate infection, the clinical setting and other characteristics of the infecting agent are important considerations. Infection of a prosthetic joint by a highly virulent organism can be cured by surgical débridement and intensive antibiotic therapy without removal of the prosthesis, if the infection is recognized early, before the bone-cement-prosthesis interface is involved and the prosthesis becomes loosened, painful, and dysfunctional.[67, 68] In contrast, successful treatment of smoldering infection of a painful, loosened, joint prosthesis, even though the infection is caused by an avirulent organism, requires removal of the device.[69–71] Slime or glycocalyx formation by avirulent coagulase-negative staphylococci has been associated with a decreased likelihood of eradicating infection from CSF shunts[13, 72] and other devices[12] without removing the infected foreign material.

In planning therapy, the role of a prosthetic device in sustaining a patient's well-being must be considered as well as the patient's general health and prognosis. Attempting to salvage a device by antibiotic therapy must be weighed against the consequences of further injury to periprosthetic tissue if the infection does not respond. If additional damage during attempted salvage would compromise survival or functional outcome, optimal therapy includes early prosthesis removal and either reinsertion of another device or provision of a functional alternative. For example, in patients with PVE, prolonged antibiotic therapy and delay of surgery in spite of persistent fever, progressive destruction of the valve anulus, or worsening congestive heart failure results in higher mortality rates than prompt valve replacement.[33, 73] Infection involving synthetic arterial grafts in the lower extremity, wherein the anastomoses are intact and the grafts are fully functional, may be treated effectively without graft removal. Treatment includes not only intensive antibiotic therapy but also aggressive wound drainage and débridement and often rotational muscle flaps to cover the exposed synthetic graft.[74–77] In contrast, attempted cure with antibiotic therapy of an infected dysfunctional synthetic arterial graft (leaking anastomosis, partial occlusion), particularly one in a body cavity where further deterioration in function cannot be continuously monitored, is likely to be associated with increased morbidity and mortality due to graft occlusion or rupture of the anastamosis.[32, 33, 47, 48] In this latter setting, better results are obtained with antibiotic therapy in combination with graft resection and vascular reconstruction through an uninfected extraanatomic route.[33, 47, 77] Failure to eradicate infection involving a breast implant and the need to subsequently remove the device are unlikely to jeopardize the patient's life or the potential for reconstructive surgery.[78] Finally, aggressive surgical intervention may be unfeasible because of the patient's poor general health or refusal to allow removal of the infected prosthesis. Attempted medical therapy, including long-term antibiotic suppression, may be the sole option. To be successful or at least to temporize using this approach, the prosthesis must function adequately and the infecting organism must be highly susceptible to antibiotics.

Specific Prosthetic Device Infections

Prostheses and medical devices can be categorized by their position: (1) intravascular (prosthetic valve); (2) partially intravascular (transvenous pacemaker, synthetic vascular graft); (3) extravascular (prosthetic joint, ventriculoperitoneal shunt); and (4) partially implanted (Tenckhoff catheter, artificial heart). An examination of infections involving a prosthesis from each category illustrates features that are common to device-related infections as well as some that are unique to the category and the prosthesis. In addition, the principles that guide the evaluation and treatment of patients with device-related infection are demonstrated.

Prosthetic Valve Endocarditis

The hazard of prosthetic valve infection, while it continues indefinitely, is greatest in the first year after surgery. By actuarial analysis, the cumulative rate of PVE is 1.5% to 3.0% 1 year after valve surgery and increases to 3.2% to 5.7% after 4 to 5 years.[28, 79, 80] Thus, PVE must be considered when any valve recipient has unexplained fever, but particularly during the first year after surgery. The cause of prosthetic valve infection at various times after surgery is relatively predictable (Table 188–2). Coagulase-negative staphylococci, which are almost exclusively methicillin-resistant *S. epidermidis*, had been recognized as the predominant agent of PVE during the initial 2 months after surgery; they have since been noted to be the major cause of infection during the entire initial postoperative year.[28, 81] Thereafter, although they are still an important cause of PVE, organisms that are commonly associated with native valve endocarditis become prominent: viridans streptococci, enterococci, *S. aureus*, and fastidious gram-negative coccobacilli.[28, 79] The coagulase-negative staphylococci that cause these later onset cases are often species other than *S. epidermidis*, and less than 30% of the isolates are resistant to methicillin.[33, 53] In spite of the relative predictability of the microbiology of PVE, a vast array of organisms have caused sporadic cases, including unusual bacteria (*Legionella pneumophila, Listeria monocytogenes, Nocardia asteroides, Achromobacter xylosoxidans, Flavobacterium* species, *Moraxella* species), fungi (*Histoplasma capsulatum, Mucor, Curvularia,*

TABLE 188–2 ■ Microbiology of Prosthetic Valve Endocarditis, 1975 to 1989

	NO. OF CASES (%) AT TIME OF ONSET AFTER CARDIAC SURGERY		
ORGANISM	<2 Months N = 73	2–12 Months N = 38	>12 Months N = 94
Coagulase-negative staphylococci	28 (38)	19 (50)	14 (15)
Staphylococcus aureus	10 (14)	4 (11)	12 (13)
Gram-negative bacilli	8 (11)	2 (5)	1 (1)
Streptococci	0	1 (3)	31 (33)
Enterococci	5 (7)	2 (5)	10 (11)
Diphtheroids	9 (12)	1 (3)	2 (2)
Fastidious gram-negative coccobacilli	0	1 (3)	11 (12)
Fungi	7 (10)	2 (5)	3 (3)
Miscellaneous	3 (4)	2 (5)	1 (1)
Culture-negative	3 (4)	4 (11)	9 (10)

Adapted from Karchmer AW: Infective endocarditis. *In* Braunwald E (ed): Heart Disease, ed 5. Philadelphia, WB Saunders, 1997, pp 1077–1104.

Paecilomyces), Mycobacterium, Rickettsia (Coxiella burnetii), and *Mycoplasma* organisms.[33, 82] If an optimal antimicrobial regimen is to be selected, the specific cause of PVE must be identified. This may necessitate blood cultures in special media, serologic testing, microbiologic and histologic examination of embolic vegetations, or judicious delay of antimicrobial therapy for patients who recently received inadequate antibiotic therapy. If empirical therapy is used unsuccessfully, the infected prosthesis should be removed and analyzed to establish the cause.

PVE is a highly invasive disease. Anulus infection and myocardial abscess occur in at least 40% and 14% of patients with mechanical valve PVE, respectively.[83–86] Partial dehiscence of the prosthesis from the infected anulus results in paravalvular regurgitant blood flow. Vegetations on the mitral valve occasionally encroach on the valve orifice and cause functional stenosis.[83, 84] Infection involving porcine bioprosthetic valves is highly invasive during the first year after surgery and thereafter is more frequently confined to the leaflets.[33, 87, 88] Infection may destroy the porcine leaflets or render them stiff and immobile, resulting in regurgitation and stenosis, respectively.[33, 89]

The clinical features of PVE resemble those of acute or subacute native valve infection, except that new murmurs indicative of valve dysfunction are more frequent among patients with infected prosthetic valves. Although recent surgery, hemodynamic instability, or neurologic complications may obscure the clinical features, the diagnosis is suggested by the endocarditis syndrome or by unexplained fever. Persistent bacteremia in the absence of an obvious alternative focus of infection, coupled with either the typical endocarditis syndrome or evidence of new prosthesis dysfunction, allows a clinical diagnosis. Echocardiographic detection of paravalvular infection and vegetations provides anatomic evidence of the diagnosis. In detecting these abnormalities, studies performed transesophageally are more sensitive and specific than are those done transthoracically.[52] Valve dysfunction or an embolus, although either is suggestive of PVE, may also result from technical problems or bland thromboemboli, respectively.

Antibiotic therapy for patients with PVE, although more prolonged in duration, is similar to that used for the analogous organism causing native valve endocarditis. One difference, however, is the recommended treatment of patients with staphylococcal PVE with combination regimens that contain rifampin. This recommendation is based on animal model as well as clinical experience.[33, 51, 54–56, 90] For 50% to 65% of patients with PVE, valve replacement surgery will be necessary to eliminate infection and maintain effective valve function.[33, 91] This requirement is the consequence of invasive disease causing valve dysfunction or infection by destructive antibiotic-resistant organisms. Surgical intervention is necessary for patients with valve dysfunction (with or without congestive heart failure), fever unresponsive to appropriate antibiotic therapy, evidence of invasive perivalvular disease by echocardiogram or new-onset electrocardiographic conduction abnormalities, or fungal PVE.[26, 33, 87, 91, 92] Valve replacement is usually indicated for patients with PVE caused by *S. aureus, S. epidermidis,* and antibiotic-resistant gram-negative bacilli, as well as for patients whose infection has relapsed after appropriate therapy.[26, 33, 68, 87, 91, 92] Increasingly, aggressive surgical treatment of patients with PVE, including surgery early during antibiotic therapy, extensive reconstruction using prosthetic devices, and reconstruction of the aortic outflow tract using cryopreserved allografts, has significantly enhanced the survival rate of patients with PVE complicated by perivalvular invasion and valve dysfunction.[33, 61, 93–95]

Infected Transvenous Pacemakers. From 1% to 7% of permanently implanted transvenous cardiac pacemakers become infected, and the rate is higher after placement of new generators in existing subcutaneous pockets. The infection can involve one or more sites along the pacemaker, including the pocket containing the generator, the subcutaneous tissue along the electrode, and the intravascular space, including the right side of the heart, along the electrode. Generator pocket infections often occur shortly after pacemaker insertion, suggesting contamination of the wound at the time of surgery, and are frequently associated with septicemia.[96, 97] Erosion of a pacemaker component through the overlying skin occasionally results in late infection.[97] The intravascular portion of the electrode usually becomes infected as disease extends from the generator or extravascular electrode; occasionally the intravascular electrode is seeded via the blood.[97–99] Although a variety of organisms have caused pacemaker infections, including gram-negative bacilli, viridans streptococci, *Corynebacterium* species, and *Candida* species, staphylococci are the most common cause.[96–99] *S. aureus* is the predominant cause of bacteremia and generator site infections that occur within weeks of surgery.[97, 98] Polybacterial infections are generally confined to the generator site.[97]

Infection is documented by recovery of organisms from an inflamed area or sinus tracks associated with the pacer or from blood cultures. Occasionally, cultures are required to distinguish infection from a generator pocket hematoma, a sterile inflammatory reaction to pacemaker components, or sterile erosion of the pacing unit. In the absence of infection at a remote site, sustained staphylococcal bacteremia strongly suggests infection involving the intravascular electrode. In contrast, gram-negative bacillus bacteremia, particularly if remote sites of infection are noted, does not necessarily indicate infection of the intravascular lead.[96, 99] Echocardiography demonstrating vegetations on the pacing leads or involving the right side of the heart helps to confirm infection of the intravascular electrode.[96, 98, 99]

Conservative therapy—débridement, local irrigation, and systemic antibiotics for generator pocket infection and intensive intravenous antibiotic therapy for intravascular electrode infection—has occasionally eradicated these infections. Failure of conservative therapy, however, hazards septicemia that may be life threatening. Prompt eradication of subcutaneous or intravascular infection is almost universal when the entire pacing unit is removed in conjunction with intravenous antimicrobial therapy; hence, this approach is preferred.[96–101] If the infection is suppressed by antibiotic therapy, insertion of a replacement pacemaker at a new site while the infected unit is removed does not increase the risk of recurrent infection.[97] If infection cannot be controlled before the infected device is removed, placement of a new permanent unit should be delayed. A temporary pacer is used until the infection is controlled. Technical considerations and the degree to which an infection is under control determine whether a new transvenous or epicardial electrode is used.

Although recently placed generators and electrodes are easily removed, electrodes that have been in place for an extended period, particularly those with tines and wire mesh tips, are often bound by fibrous tissue to the venous and intracardiac endothelium.[102] They may be impossible to remove without disrupting endothelial and intracardiac structures. Electrodes that cannot be removed with firm but gentle traction should be removed surgically with the patient on cardiopulmonary bypass support. If surgical removal of an entrapped infected intravascular electrode entails unacceptable risks, 4 to 6 weeks of intravenous antibiotic therapy can be administered. Occasionally this is successful.[96–98] If infection is confined to the generator pocket, the intravascular portion of the electrode is interrupted proximally, the distal electrode and generator are removed through the infected pocket, and an electrode extender that has been spliced to the proximal portion of the original electrode is tunneled to a new generator at a sterile site.[103] The original pocket is packed open until the infection is eliminated. This partial revision is effective if the original electrode was not infected at the point where it was interrupted.

Prosthetic Joint Infection

The cumulative rate (hazard) of infection involving total hip and knee arthroplasty during the initial year after surgery is 6.5 infections per 1000 joint-years and is 3.2 and 1.4 infections per 1000 joint-years during the second year and during the third year and beyond, respectively.[29] Infection rates in carefully studied populations with other joints replaced are not available. Perioperative wound infection that extends to the device and intraoperative contamination of the prosthesis with delay in onset and diagnosis of infection result in the high rate noted during the initial year after hip and knee replacement. Late hematogenous seeding and extension from adjacent soft tissue infection are the mechanisms whereby these joint prostheses become infected in year 3 and thereafter. Rheumatoid arthritis, prior joint surgery, reoperation in the early postimplantation period, early discharge from the operative wound, and the presence of metal-on-metal prostheses are factors associated with increased risk for arthroplasty infection.[29, 67, 68, 104]

The presentation of a patient with an infected arthroplasty depends on the time and route of infection and the virulence of the pathogen. Local inflammation or joint pain should always raise the question of infection. From 35% to 50% of patients with an infected prosthesis present within 3 months of surgery with joint pain and clinical evidence of wound infection, although systemic toxicity often is absent.[68, 69, 104] The challenge for the physician is to distinguish mechanical complications and superficial infections from infections that involve the prosthesis. In some patients these questions can be answered only by aspirating or reexploring the wound in the operating room. Another 30% to 45% of patients with infected arthroplasties present from 3 to 24 months postoperatively with joint pain as the predominant symptom.[68, 69, 104] Signs of local inflammation, fever, and sinus tracks are uncommon. The white cell count and erythrocyte sedimentation rate are usually normal. Although radiographs, radionuclide scans, and arthrographs occasionally suggest infection, these studies often fail to distinguish low-grade infection from aseptic loosening of the prosthesis, and, most important, they do not identify the infecting organism.[57] Consequently, to diagnose infection, antibiotics are omitted for at least 2 weeks, and, by using sterile technique, fluid is aspirated from the joint for microscopic examination and culture.[105, 106] The fluid usually contains inflammatory cells; organisms are visible on Gram stain in 30% and are recovered by culture in 85% to 98%. The joint fluid should be promptly delivered to the microbiology laboratory where it should be cultured anaerobically and aerobically using multiple media, quantitative cultures should also be performed when possible. Recovery of large numbers of an organism or the organism on multiple media strongly suggests infection. To diagnose infection when only scant numbers of an organism are isolated, it is necessary to repeat the aspiration and reconfirm the presence of the organism, using careful speciation or molecular techniques in the case of organisms such as coagulase-negative staphylococci whose identity is difficult to establish. Infection can be confirmed by microscopic examination and culture of periprosthetic tissue obtained at surgery. Inflammatory changes are found in 55% of specimens, and if antimicrobial therapy has not been administered, the infecting organism is recovered in almost every case.[57] Approximately 10% to 15% of patients with infected prostheses present with acute septic arthritis due to hematogenous seeding from a remote infection.[67–69, 104, 107] These infections, which are characterized by systemic toxicity and local inflammation, usually develop in patients whose prosthesis has been functioning normally. The diagnosis is established by examination of periprosthetic fluid.

Staphylococci are isolated from 55% of the infected arthroplasties (Table 188–3). Gram-negative bacilli are involved when arthroplasty infection results from acute wound complications or late hematogenous seeding. Indolent infections presenting 3 to 24 months after surgery are caused by avirulent organisms such as coagulase-negative staphylococci, viridans streptococci, anaerobic gram-positive cocci,

TABLE 188–3 ■ Microbiology of Infected Hip, Knee, or Elbow Prostheses

ORGANISM	ALL INFECTIONS (314 JOINTS)	HEMATOGENOUS INFECTIONS (54 JOINTS)
Staphylococcus aureus	109	20
Coagulase-negative staphylococci	79	4
Enterococci	17	5
β-Hemolytic streptococci	12	4
Group B streptococci	5	1
Other streptococci	15	5
Corynebacteria	9	1
Other gram-positive bacteria	8	1*
Escherichia coli	13	5
Klebsiella spp.	4	—
Enterobacter spp.	7	1
Pseudomonas spp.	20	3
Proteus spp.	9	2
Other gram-negative bacilli	10	6†
Peptostreptococci	3	
Peptococci	9	
Bacteroides spp.	6	2
Propionibacterium acnes	2	
Clostridium spp.	1	
Mycobacterium fortuitum	1	

**Listeria monocytogenes.*
†*Pasteurella multocida* (two infections).

and corynebacteria. *Candida* organisms that contaminated the wound perioperatively cause rare episodes of indolent prosthetic joint infection.[108] Hematogenous infections of arthroplasties are caused by virulent organisms such as *S. aureus*, β-hemolytic streptococci, and gram-negative bacilli[29, 107] (see Table 188–3).

To eradicate infection and maintain a pain-free, fully functional joint usually requires removal of the prosthesis, meticulous débridement of all infected bone and cement, and intensive antimicrobial therapy targeted to the specific pathogen. In nonpurulent arthroplasty infections caused by highly antibiotic susceptible, avirulent organisms, satisfactory results can be achieved with removal of the infected device, débridement, and immediate reinsertion of a new prosthesis using antibiotic-impregnated cement followed by prolonged antibiotic therapy.[57, 109] More often, a two-stage procedure is used whereby the new prosthesis is implanted after 6 weeks of intensive antibiotic therapy.[29, 57, 69–71] More than 85% of infections in hip and knee prostheses treated with the two-stage procedure are cured.[29, 70–72] When a hip arthroplasty is infected by virulent, antibiotic-resistant organisms, some authors advise a delay of 1 year before implanting a new prosthesis. If a knee prosthesis is to be reimplanted, technical considerations prohibit delays beyond six weeks.[29, 71] Antibiotic-impregnated cement is often used when cemented prostheses are reimplanted.[29, 57] In approximately 20% of patients, the original prosthesis can be salvaged by débridement and intensive antibiotic therapy. This approach is successful only when infection is diagnosed early, the prosthesis remains securely fixed, and the bone-cement interface is not disrupted by infection.[67–69, 104] Resection arthroplasty, including arthrodesis when the knee is involved, is recommended for patients who are not candidates for reinsertion of a prosthesis because of inability to tolerate extensive surgery, incomplete débridement, or other technical reasons.[29, 68, 69, 104, 110] When removal of an infected prosthesis is not possible, chronic suppressive oral antibiotic therapy has permitted satisfactory retention of the arthroplasty if the pathogen is avirulent and exquisitely susceptible to the antibiotic and the prosthesis is not loose or painful.[29] Salvage of nonpainful, appropriately functioning prostheses infected by staphylococci has been achieved with prolonged administration of antimicrobial therapy that included rifampin.[111, 112]

Peritonitis Associated with Continuous Ambulatory Peritoneal Dialysis

The Tenckhoff catheter used for dialysis is typical of devices that are not totally implanted. Because it traverses the skin and is repeatedly manipulated it is continuously at risk of infection. In contrast to the low incidence of infection with totally implanted devices, the rate of infection with partially implanted devices is high. Approximately 60% of patients who undergo CAPD develop peritonitis during the first 12 months, and 80% have had peritoneal infection by 30 months of CAPD.[58] Infection occurs, although less frequently, at the exit site and subcutaneous tunnel of the catheter. Most often the peritoneum is infected by organisms that invade along the transcutaneous catheter track or contaminate the dialysis fluid delivery system.[34, 58] Sterile technique and compliance with dialysis regimens are important risk factors for peritonitis.[113] Organisms from the gastrointestinal tract infect the peritoneum as a consequence of transmural migration in the absence of disease, as well as at sites of disease or trauma.[34, 58] Occasionally, the peritoneum is seeded hematogenously.[34, 58] Although macrophages in uninfected CAPD effluent phagocytose and kill opsonized staphylococci and *Escherichia coli*, repetitive large-volume dialysis exchanges render the effluent quantitatively deficient in opsonins (immunoglobulin G and complement C3) and macrophages, deficits that may facilitate progression to peritonitis after peritoneal contamination.[114, 115] A large number of bacterial species, yeast, and fungi have caused sporadic cases of CAPD peritonitis, but a few organisms, particularly staphylococci, represent the major causes of these infections[34, 58, 59] (Table 188–4). Catheter tunnel infection often complicates *S. aureus* peritonitis.[63] Of the coagulase-negative staphylococci, at least 70% are *S. epidermidis;* many are resistant to semisynthetic penicillinase-resistant penicillins and cephalosporins.[63, 116, 117] CAPD peritonitis caused by anaerobes or by multiple bacteria, especially if the organisms are fecal flora, is likely to have resulted from spontaneous or catheter-induced intestinal perforation.[59] Fungal peritonitis, which can be distinguished from bacterial infection only by microscopy and culture, is associated with recent bacterial peritonitis, hospitalization, or antibiotic therapy.[64] Culture-negative dialysate from patients with peritonitis most likely results from less than optimal culture techniques or concurrent antimicrobial therapy. Occasionally these culture-negative episodes are caused by organisms that are fastidious or require specific culture media, such as *Mycobacterium* species. Last, eosinophilic peritonitis (eosinophils at least 15% of the total dialysate white cell count), which may result from an allergic response to dialysis materials, presents as sterile peritonitis.

Patients with CAPD peritonitis present with cloudy dialysis effluent (98%), abdominal pain (78%), tenderness (70%), and nausea and vomiting (25%).[34, 58] Less than 50% have fever, and most have a mild illness.[34, 58, 59] Systemic toxicity or hypotension is more likely if the mechanism of peritonitis is intestinal perforation or the agent is *S. aureus*. The diagnosis of peritonitis is established by two of the following: (1) symptoms of peritoneal inflammation; (2) cloudy dialysis effluent containing more than 100 PMNs per mm^3; (3) demonstration of organisms in the effluent. Although the sensitivity of Gram stain of the effluent is less than 30%, the potential to partially categorize the infecting organism supports its use.[58, 59] Organisms should be recovered from dialysate in 80% to 90% of patients with peritonitis in spite of the low concentration of organisms in the effluent. This is achieved by culturing the filtered sediment of large volumes of dialysate or a large volume itself: 10 to 20 mL inoculated into blood culture flasks; 10 mL inoculated into Isolator tubes; culture of a 0.45-μm (pore size) filter after passage of 100 to 250 mL of dialysate.[59, 118–120] Cultures of effluent using small volumes or sediment after low-speed centrifugation are insensitive. Because bacteremia is unusual, blood cultures are not obtained routinely but are reserved for patients with

TABLE 188–4 ■ Principal Organisms Causing Continuous Ambulatory Peritoneal Dialysis–Associated Peritonitis

ORGANISM	EPISODES (%)
Coagulase-negative staphylococci	30–45
Staphylococcus aureus	10–20
Streptococcus spp.	5–15
Enterococcus spp.	2–6
Diphtheroids	1–2
Escherichia coli	5–10
Pseudomonas spp.	5–10
Proteus spp.	2–4
Other gram-negative bacilli	2–4
Anaerobic bacteria	2–6
Fungi, yeast	<5
Mycobacteria	≤5
None demonstrated	10–20

Data from Vas,[34] Peterson et al,[58] and Bint et al.[59]

signs of systemic toxicity.[58, 59] Screening clear CAPD effluent with routine cultures or cell counts does not predict peritonitis and is not recommended.[58, 59] Before the diagnosis of CAPD-associated peritonitis is accepted, the many causes of abdominal pain, with or without peritoneal inflammation, must be considered and the patient evaluated for any suspected problem.

After CAPD-associated peritonitis is diagnosed clinically, dialysis effluent should be cultured and empirical antimicrobial therapy instituted. Because the infection is confined to the abdominal cavity and symptoms are generally mild, most patients are treated as outpatients. Antibiotics selected to cover the majority of the anticipated pathogens are mixed with dialysis fluid for intraperitoneal administration. CAPD dialysis with antibiotic-containing fluid is continued as usual. Compared with systemic therapy this is a more efficient and predictable technique for delivering antibiotics to the peritoneal cavity. Because antibiotics administered intraperitoneally achieve therapeutic systemic concentrations slowly, patients with symptoms that suggest disseminated infection should be hospitalized and treated with both intravenous and intraperitoneal antibiotics.

Antibiotic treatment of CAPD-associated peritonitis and related antibiotic pharmacokinetics have been reviewed.[34, 58, 59, 121] The antibiotic selected must be effective in vitro against the infecting organism at concentrations that are achievable intraperitoneally. Thus, cephalosporins are not as effective as vancomycin in treating peritonitis caused by coagulase-negative staphylococci, many of which are methicillin and cephalosporin resistant.[116, 122] The antibacterial activity of antibiotics in peritoneal dialysis effluent, however, is not always equivalent to that seen in standard culture media.[115, 123] The activity of tobramycin against *P. aeruginosa* is comparable in cation-supplemented Mueller-Hinton broth and in dialysate effluent. On the other hand, the activity of piperacillin or ceftazidime against this organism is markedly reduced in dialysis effluent.[123] Antibiotics that are effective against the infecting organism in the dialysis effluent should be used to treat CAPD peritonitis.[58] Initial empirical therapy with vancomycin plus an aminoglycoside has been recommended[34, 59, 122]; thereafter, specific therapy is based on the antimicrobial susceptibility of the isolate. The antibiotic regimen must minimize the risk of adverse effects. In particular, the risk of eighth cranial nerve toxicity from aminoglycosides demands that those agents be used judiciously. If dialysate cultures fail to propagate a pathogen, empirical therapy should be continued until its inefficacy is apparent, whereupon efforts to establish a microbiologic diagnosis should be reinstituted. CAPD-associated peritonitis responds to treatment with abatement of symptoms in 2 to 3 days and clearing of cloudy dialysis fluid shortly thereafter. Treatment is continued for at least 5 days after the effluent clears, although longer courses are sometimes advocated for infection caused by gram-negative bacilli.[58, 59]

Most episodes of peritonitis can be eradicated and CAPD continued without removing the infected Tenckhoff catheter.[34, 58, 59] Persisting or relapsing peritonitis in the face of appropriate antibiotic therapy is often a sign of catheter tunnel infection or an intraabdominal abscess and warrants catheter removal. Prompt removal of the Tenckhoff catheter is generally recommended when peritonitis is caused by fungi, yeasts, mycobacteria, or *P. aeruginosa* or is due to a perforated or gangrenous viscus.[28, 34, 58, 59, 64–66] Relapsing *S. aureus* peritonitis in the absence of tunnel infection has been attributed to intraleukocyte sequestration of organisms; this infection can be eradicated without removing the catheter by combining rifampin, which kills intracellular organisms, with standard therapy.[124] Reinsertion of a catheter and resumption of CAPD is usually feasible after eradication of infection. Occasionally, however, injury to the peritoneal membrane or the presence of adhesions prevents resumption of CAPD, forcing the use of alternative strategies.

References

1. Elek SD, Conen PE: Virulence of *Staphylococcus pyogenes* for man: A study of the problems of wound infection. Br J Exp Pathol 38:573, 1957.
2. Christensen GD, Simpson WA, Bisno AL, et al: Experimental foreign body infections in mice challenged with slime-producing *Staphylococcus epidermidis.* Infect Immun 40:407, 1983.
3. Zimmerli W, Waldvogel F, Vaudaux P, et al: Pathogenesis of foreign body infection: Description and characteristics of an animal model. J Infect Dis 146:487, 1982.
4. Vaudaux PE, Lew DP, Waldvogel FA: Host factors predisposing to and influencing therapy of foreign body infections. *In* Bisno AL, Waldvogel FA (eds): Infections Associated with Indwelling Medical Devices. Washington, DC, American Society for Microbiology, 1994, pp 1–29.
5. Hermann M, Vaudaux PE, Pittet D, et al: Fibronectin, fibrinogen and laminin act as mediators of adherence of clinical staphylococcal isolates to foreign material. J Infect Dis 158:693, 1988.
6. Vaudaux P, Pittet D, Hacberli A, et al: Fibronectin is more active than fibrin or fibrinogen in promoting *Staphylococcus aureus* adherence to inserted intravascular catheters. J Infect Dis 167:633, 1993.
7. Vaudaux PE, Francois P, Proctor RA, et al: Use of adhesion-defective mutants of *Staphylococcus aureus* to define the role of specific plasma proteins in promoting bacterial adhesion to canine arteriovenous shunts. Infect Immun 63:585, 1995.
8. Bayston R, Penny SR: Excessive production of mucoid substance in staphylococcus SIIA: A possible factor in colonization of Holter shunts. Dev Med Child Neurol 14(Suppl 27):25, 1972.
9. Christensen GD, Parisi JT, Bisno AL, et al: Characterization of clinically significant strains of coagulase-negative staphylococci. J Clin Microbiol 18:258, 1983.
10. Christensen GD, Bisno AL, Parisi JT, et al: Nosocomial septicemia due to multiply antibiotic-resistant *Staphylococcus epidermidis.* Ann Intern Med 96:1, 1982.
11. Ishak MA, Groschel DHM, Mandell GL, et al: Association of slime with pathogenicity of coagulase-negative staphylococci causing nosocomial septicemia. J Clin Microbiol 22:1025, 1985.
12. Davenport DS, Massanari RM, Pfaller MA, et al: Usefulness of a test for slime production as a marker for clinically significant infections with coagulase-negative staphylococci. J Infect Dis 153:332, 1986.
13. Diaz-Mitoma F, Harding GKM, Hoban DJ, et al: Clinical significance of a test for slime production in ventriculoperitoneal shunt infections caused by coagulase-negative staphylococci. J Infect Dis 156:555, 1987.
14. Christensen GD, Baldassarri L, Simpson WA: Colonization of medical devices by coagulase-negative staphylococci. *In* Bisno AL, Waldvogel FA (eds): Infections Associated with Indwelling Medical Devices. Washington, DC, American Society for Microbiology, 1994, pp 45–78.
15. Tojo M, Yamashita N, Goldmann DA, et al: Isolation and characterization of a capsular polysaccharide adhesin from *Staphylococcus epidermidis.* J Infect Dis 157:713, 1988.
16. Muller E, Takeda S, Shiro H, et al: Occurrence of capsular polysaccharide/adhesin among clinical isolates of coagulase-negative staphylococci. J Infect Dis 168:1211, 1993.
17. Shiro H, Muller E, Gutierrez N, et al: Transposon mutants of *Staphylococcus epidermidis* deficient in elaboration of capsular polysaccharide/adhesin and slime are avirulent in a rabbit model of endocarditis. J Infect Dis 169:1042, 1994.
18. Zimmerli W, Lew PD, Waldvogel FA: Pathogenesis of foreign body infection. Evidence for a local granulocyte defect. J Clin Invest 73:1191, 1984.
19. Vaudaux PE, Zulian G, Huggler E, et al: Attachment of *Staphylococcus aureus* to polymethylmethacrylate increases its resistance to phagocytosis in foreign body infection. Infect Immun 50:472, 1985.
20. Vaudaux P, Grau GE, Huggler E, et al: Contribution of tumor

necrosis factor to host defense against staphylococci in a guinea pig model of foreign body infections. J Infect Dis 166:58, 1992.
21. Johnson GM, Lee DA, Regelmann WE, et al: Interference with granulocyte function by *Staphylococcus epidermidis* slime. Infect Immun 54:13, 1986.
22. Gilbert P, Collier PJ, Brown MRW: Influence of growth rate on susceptibility to antimicrobial agents: Biofilms, cell cycle, dormancy, and stringent response. Antimicrob Agents Chemother 34:1865, 1990.
23. Chuard C, Lucet JC, Rohner P, et al: Resistance of *Staphylococcus aureus* recovered from infected foreign body in vivo to killing by antimicrobials. J Infect Dis 163:1369, 1991.
24. Chuard C, Vaudaux P, Waldvogel FA, Lew DP: Susceptibility of *Staphylococcus aureus* growing on fibronectin-coated surfaces to bactericidal antibiotics. Antimicrob Agents Chemother 37:625, 1993.
25. Bunt TJ: Synthetic vascular graft infections. I. Graft infections. Surgery 93:733, 1983.
26. Rumisek JD, Albus RA, Clarke JS: Late *Mycobacterium chelonei* bioprosthetic valve endocarditis: Activation of implanted contaminant? Ann Thorac Surg 39:277, 1985.
27. Archer GL, Vishniavsky N, Stiver HG: Plasmid pattern analysis of *Staphylococcus epidermidis* isolates from patients with prosthetic valve endocarditis. Infect Immun 35:627, 1982.
28. Calderwood SB, Swinski LA, Waternaux CM, et al: Risk factors for the development of prosthetic valve endocarditis. Circulation 72:31, 1985.
29. Steckelberg JM, Osmon DR: Prosthetic joint infections. *In* Bisno AL, Waldvogel FA (eds): Infections Associated with Indwelling Medical Devices. Washington, DC, American Society for Microbiology, 1994, pp 259–290.
30. Lidwell OM, Lowbury EJL, Whyte W, et al: Effect of ultraclean air in operating rooms on deep sepsis in the joint after total hip or knee replacement: A randomised study. Br Med J 285:10, 1982.
31. Glynn MK, Sheehan JM: An analysis of causes of deep infection after hip and knee arthroplasties. Clin Orthop 178:202, 1983.
32. Bandyk DF, Berni GA, Thiele BL, et al: Aortofemoral graft infection due to *Staphylococcus epidermidis.* Arch Surg 119:102, 1984.
33. Karchmer AW, Gibbons GW: Infections of prosthetic heart valves and vascular grafts. *In* Bisno AL, Waldvogel FA (eds): Infections Associated with Indwelling Devices. Washington, DC, American Society for Microbiology, 1994, pp 213–249.
34. Vas SI: Infections associated with the peritoneum and hemodialysis. *In* Bisno AL, Waldvogel FA (eds): Infections Associated with Indwelling Medical Devices. Washington, DC, American Society for Microbiology, 1994, pp 309–346.
35. Luzar MA, Coles GA, Faller B, et al: *Staphylococcus aureus* nasal carriage and infection in patients on continuous ambulatory peritoneal dialysis. N Engl J Med 322:505, 1990.
36. Berkelman RL, Godley J, Weber JA, et al: *Pseudomonas cepacia* peritonitis associated with contamination of automatic peritoneal dialysis machines. Ann Intern Med 96:456, 1982.
37. Kunin CM, Dobbins JJ, Melo JC, et al: Infectious complications in four long-term recipients of the Jarvik-7 artificial heart. JAMA 259:860, 1988.
38. Baker AS, Schein OD: Ocular infections. *In* Bisno AL, Waldvogel FA (eds): Infections Associated with Indwelling Medical Devices. Washington, DC, American Society for Microbiology, 1994, pp 111–134.
39. Carlson AN, Fetz MR, Apple DJ: Infectious complications of modern cataract surgery and intraocular lens implantation. Infect Dis Clin North Am 3:339, 1989.
40. Gardner P, Leipzig T, Phillips P: Infections of central nervous system shunts. Med Clin North Am 69:297, 1985.
41. Forward KP, Fewer HD, Stiver HG: Cerebrospinal fluid shunt infections. A review of 35 infections in 32 patients. J Neurosurg 59:389, 1983.
42. Schoenbaum SC, Gardner P, Shillito J: Infections of cerebrospinal fluid shunts: Epidemiology, clinical manifestations and therapy. J Infect Dis 131:543, 1975.
43. Myers MG, Schoenbaum SC: Shunt fluid aspiration: An adjunct in the diagnosis of cerebrospinal fluid shunt infection. Am J Dis Child 129:220, 1975.
44. Rames L, Wise B, Goodman JR, et al: Renal disease with *Staphylococcus albus* bacteremia. JAMA 8:212:1671, 1970.
45. Becker BA, Crowder JG, Smith JW: *Propionibacterium acnes*: Pathogen in central nervous system shunt infection. Report of three cases including immune complex glomerulonephritis. Am J Med 61:935, 1976.
46. Bolton WK, Sande MA, Normansell DE, et al: Ventriculojugular shunt nephritis with *Corynebacterium bovis.* Am J Med 59:417, 1975.
47. Bandyk DF: Diagnosis and treatment of biomaterial-associated vascular infections. Infect Dis Clin North Amer 6:719, 1992.
48. Champion MC, Sullivan SN, Coles JC, et al: Aortoenteric fistula. Incidence, presentation, recognition, and management. Ann Surg 195:314, 1982.
49. Blum MD: Infections in genitourinary prostheses. Infect Dis Clin North Am 3:259, 1989.
50. Moul JW, Carson CC: Infectious complications of penile prostheses. Infect Urol 97, 1989.
51. Stinchfield FE, Bigliani LU, Neu HC, et al: Late hematogenous infection of total joint replacement. J Bone Joint Surg Am 62:1345, 1980.
52. Daniel WG, Mugge A, Grote J, et al: Comparison of transthoracic and transesophageal echocardiography for detection of abnormalities of prosthetic and bioprosthetic valves in the mitral and aortic positions. Am J Cardiol 71:210, 1993.
53. Archer GL, Karchmer AW, Vishniavsky N, et al: Plasmid-pattern analysis for differentiation of infecting from noninfecting *Staphylococcus epidermidis.* J Infect Dis 149:913, 1984.
54. Widmer AF, Frei R, Rajacic Z, et al: Correlation between in vivo and in vitro efficacy of antimicrobial agents against foreign body infections. J Infect Dis 162:96, 1990.
55. Lucet JC, Herrmann M, Rohner P, et al: Treatment of experimental foreign body infection caused by methicillin-resistant *Staphylococcus aureus.* Antimicrob Agents Chemother 34:2312, 1990.
56. Chuard C, Herrmann M, Vaudaux P, et al: Successful therapy of experimental chronic foreign-body infection due to methicillin-resistant *Staphylococcus aureus* by antimicrobial combinations. Antimicrob Agents Chemother 35:2611, 1991.
57. Hanssen AD, Rand JA, Osmon DR: Treatment of the infected total knee arthroplasty with insertion of another prosthesis: The effect of antibiotic-impregnated bone cement. Clin Orthop 309:44, 1994.
58. Peterson PK, Matzke G, Keane WF: Current concepts in the management of peritonitis in patients undergoing continuous ambulatory peritoneal dialysis. Rev Infect Dis 9:604, 1987.
59. Bint AJ, Finch RG, Gokal R, et al: Diagnosis and management of peritonitis in continuous ambulatory peritoneal dialysis. Lancet 1:845, 1987.
60. Meyer DJ, Gerding DN: Favorable prognosis of patients with prosthetic valve endocarditis caused by gram-negative bacilli of the HACEK group. Am J Med 85:104, 1988.
61. Lytle BW, Priest BP, Taylor PC, et al: Surgery for acquired heart disease: Surgical treatment of prosthetic valve endocarditis. J Thorac Cardiovasc Surg 111:198, 1996.
62. Grace CJ, Levitz RE, Katz-Pollak H, et al: *Actinobacillus actinomycetemomitans* prosthetic valve endocarditis. Rev Infect Dis 10:922, 1988.
63. West TE, Walshe JJ, Krol CP, et al: Staphyloccal peritonitis in patients on continuous peritoneal dialysis. J Clin Microbiol 23:809, 1986.
64. Eisenberg ES, Leviton I, Soeiro R: Fungal peritonitis in patients receiving peritoneal dialysis: Experience with 11 patients and review of the literature. Rev Infect Dis 8:309, 1986.
65. Krothapalli R, Duffy WB, Lacke C, et al: *Pseudomonas* peritonitis and continuous ambulatory peritoneal dialysis. Arch Intern Med 142:1862, 1982.
66. Bernardini J, Piraino B, Sorkin M: Analysis of continuous ambulatory peritoneal dialysis–related *Pseudomonas aeruginosa* infections. Am J Med 83:829, 1987.
67. Poss R, Thornhill TS, Ewald FC, et al: Factors influencing the incidence and outcome of infection following total joint arthroplasty. Clin Orthop 182:117, 1984.
68. Grogan TJ, Dorey F, Rollins J, et al: Deep sepsis following total knee arthroplasty. J Bone Joint Surg Am 68:226, 1986.
69. Canner GC, Steinberg ME, Heppenstall RB, et al: The infected hip after total hip arthroplasty. J Bone Joint Surg Am 66:1393, 1984.
70. Lieberman JR, Callaway GH, Salvati EA, et al: Treatment of the

infected total hip arthroplasty with a two-stage reimplantation protocol. Clin Orthop 301:205, 1994.

71. Insall JN, Thompson FM, Brause BD: Two-stage reimplantation for the salvage of infected total knee arthroplasty. J Bone Joint Surg Am 65:1087, 1983.
72. Jounger JJ, Christensen GD, Bartley DL, et al: Coagulase-negative staphylococci isolated from cerebrospinal fluid shunts: Importance of slime production, species identification, and shunt removal to clinical outcome. J Infect Dis 156:548, 1987.
73. Boyd AD, Spencer FC, Isom DW, et al: Infective endocarditis: An analysis of 54 surgically treated patients. J Thorac Cardiovasc Surg 73:23, 1977.
74. Cherry JJ Jr, Roland CF, Pairolero PC, et al: Infected femorodistal bypass: Is graft removal mandatory? J Vasc Surg 15:295, 1992.
75. Perler BA, Vander Kolk CA, Manson PM, et al: Rotational muscle flaps to treat localized prosthetic graft infection: Long-term follow-up. J Vasc Surg 18:358, 1993.
76. Calligaro KD, Veith FJ, Sales CM, et al: Comparison of muscle flaps and delayed secondary intention wound healing for infected lower extremity arterial grafts. Ann Vasc Surg 8:32, 1994.
77. Calligaro KD, Veith FJ, Schwartz ML, et al: Selective preservation of infected prosthetic arterial grafts: Analysis of a 20-year experience with 120 extracavitary-infected grafts. Ann Surg 220:461, 1994.
78. Freedman AM, Jackson IT: Infections of breast implants. Infect Dis Clin North Am 3:275, 1989.
79. Ivert TSA, Dismukes WE, Cobbs CG, et al: Prosthetic valve endocarditis. Circulation 69:223, 1984.
80. Rutledge R, Kim J, Applebaum RE: Actuarial analysis of the risk of prosthetic valve endocarditis in 1,598 patients with mechanical and bioprosthetic valves. Arch Surg 120:469, 1985.
81. Karchmer AW, Archer GL, Dismukes WE: *Staphylococcus epidermidis* causing prosthetic valve endocarditis: Microbiologic and clinical observations as guides to therapy. Ann Intern Med 98:447, 1983.
82. Tompkins LS, Roessler BJ, Redd SC, et al: *Legionella* prosthetic valve endocarditis. N Engl J Med 318:530, 1988.
83. Arnett EN, Roberts WC: Prosthetic valve endocarditis. Am J Cardiol 38:281, 1976.
84. Anderson DJ, Bulkley BH, Hutchins GM: A clinicopathologic study of prosthetic valve endocarditis in 22 patients: Morphologic basis for diagnosis and therapy. Am Heart J 94:325, 1977.
85. Dismukes WE, Karchmer AW, Buckley MJ, et al: Prosthetic valve endocarditis: Analysis of 38 cases. Circulation 43:365, 1973.
86. Richardson JV, Karp RB, Kirklin JW, et al: Treatment of infective endocarditis: A 10 year comparative analysis. Circulation 58:589, 1978.
87. Cortina JM, Martinell J, Artiz V, et al: Surgical treatment of active prosthetic valve endocarditis: Results in 66 patients. Thorac Cardiovasc Surg 35:209, 1987.
88. Fernicola DJ, Roberts WC: Frequency of ring abscess and cuspal infection in active infective endocarditis involving bioprosthetic valves. Am J Cardiol 72:314, 1993.
89. Magilligan DJ Jr: Bioprosthetic valve endocarditis. *In* Magilligan DJ Jr, Quinn EL (eds): Endocarditis: Medical and Surgical Management. New York, Marcel Decker, 1986, pp 253–263.
90. Wilson WR, Karchmer AW, Bisno AL, et al: Antibiotic treatment of adults with infective endocarditis due to viridans streptococci, enterococci, other steptococci, staphylococci, and HACEK microorganisms. JAMA 274:1706, 1995.
91. Calderwood SB, Swinski LA, Karchmer AW, et al: Prosthetic valve endocarditis: Analysis of factors affecting outcome of therapy. J Thorac Cardiovasc Surg 92:776, 1986.
92. Wolff M, Witchitz S, Chastang C, et al: Prosthetic valve endocarditis in the ICU: Prognosis factors of overall survival in a series of 122 cases and consequences for treatment decision. Chest 108:688, 1995.
93. Ross D: Allograft root replacement for prosthetic endocarditis. J Cardiac Surg 5:68, 1990.
94. Jault F, Gandjbakhch I, Chastre JC, et al: Prosthetic valve endocarditis with ring abscesses: Surgical management and long-term results. J Thorac Cardiovasc Surg 105:1106, 1993.
95. Nataf P, Jault F, Dorent R, et al: Extra-annular procedures in the surgical management of prosthetic valve endocarditis. Eur Heart J 16(Suppl B):99, 1995.
96. Waldvogel F: Pacemaker infections. *In* Bisno AL, Waldvogel FA (eds): Infections Associated with Indwelling Mechanical Devices. Washington, DC, American Society for Microbiology, 1994, pp 251–258.
97. Lewis AB, Hayes DL, Holmes DR Jr, et al: Update on infections involving permanent pacemakers: Characterization and management. J Thorac Cardiovasc Surg 89:758, 1985.
98. Arber N, Pras E, Copperman Y, et al: Pacemaker endocarditis: Report of 44 cases and review of the literature. Medicine (Baltimore) 73:299, 1994.
99. Camus C, Leport C, Raffi F, et al: Sustained bacteremia in 26 patients with a permanent endocardial pacemaker: Assessment of wire removal. Clin Infect Dis 17:46, 1993.
100. Beeler BA: Infections of permanent transvenous and epicardial pacemakers in adults. Heart Lung 11:152, 1982.
101. Phibbs B, Marriott HJL: Complications of permanent transvenous pacing. N Engl J Med 312:1428, 1985.
102. Huang T-Y, Baba N: Cardiac pathology of transvenous pacemakers. Am Heart J 83:469, 1972.
103. Hawthorne JW, Eisenhauer AC, Steinhaus DM: Cardiac pacing. *In* Eagle KA, Haber E, DeSanctis RW, Austen WG (eds): The Practice of Cardiology. Boston, Little, Brown, 1989, pp 287–336.
104. Morrey BF, Bryan RS: Infection after total elbow arthroplasty. J Bone Joint Surg Am 65:330, 1983.
105. Tigges S, Stiles RG, Meli RJ, Roberson JR: Hip aspiration: A cost-effective and accurate method of evaluating the potentially infected hip prosthesis. Radiology 189:485, 1993.
106. Roberts P, Walters AJ, McMinn DJW: Diagnosing infection in hip replacements: The use of fine-needle aspiration and radiometric culture. J Bone Joint Surg Br 74:265, 1992.
107. Inman RD, Gallegos KV, Brause BD, et al: Clinical and microbial features of prosthetic joint infection. Am J Med 77:47, 1984.
108. Lambertus M, Thordarson D, Goetz MB: Fungal prosthetic arthritis: Presentation of two cases and review of the literature. Rev Infect Dis 10:1038, 1988.
109. Jupiter JB, Karchmer AW, Lowell JD, et al: Total hip arthroplasty in the treatment of adult hips with current or quiescent sepsis. J Bone Joint Surg Am 63:194, 1981.
110. Bliss DG, McBride GG: Infected total knee arthroplasties. Clin Orthop 199:207, 1985.
111. Drancourt M, Stein A, Argenson JN, et al: Oral rifampin plus ofloxacin for treatment of *Staphylococcus*-infected orthopedic implants. Antimicrob Agents Chemother 37:1214, 1993.
112. Widmer AF, Gaechter A, Ochsner PE, Zimmerli W: Antimicrobial treatment of orthopedic implant-related infections with rifampin combinations. Clin Infect Dis 14:1251, 1992.
113. Oreopoulos DG, Williams P, Khanna R, et al: Treatment of peritoneal dialysis. Peritoneal Dialysis Bull 1(Suppl):17, 1981.
114. Verbrugh HA, Keane WF, Hoidal JR, et al: Peritoneal macrophages and opsonins: Antibacterial defense in patients undergoing chronic peritoneal dialysis. J Infect Dis 147:1018, 1983.
115. Verbrugh HA, Keane WF, Conroy WE, et al: Bacterial growth and killing in chronic ambulatory peritoneal dialysis fluids. J Clin Microbiol 20:199, 1984.
116. Gruer LD, Bartlett R, Ayliffe GAJ: Species identification and antibiotic sensitivity of coagulase-negative staphylococci from CAPD peritonitis. J Antimicrob Chemother 13:577, 1984.
117. Holley JL, Bernardini J, Johnston JR, Piraino B: Methicillin-resistant staphylococcal infections in an outpatient peritoneal dialysis program. Am J Kidney Dis 15:142, 1990.
118. Doyle PW, Crichton EP, Mathias RG, et al: Clinical and microbiological evaluation of four culture methods for the diagnosis of peritonitis in patients on continuous ambulatory peritoneal dialysis. J Clin Microbiol 27:1206, 1989.
119. Ryan S, Fessia S: Improved method for recovery of peritonitis-causing microorganisms from peritoneal dialysate. J Clin Microbiol 25:383, 1987.
120. Woods GL, Washington JA II: Comparison of methods for processing dialysate in suspected continuous ambulatory peritoneal dialysis–associated peritonitis. Diagn Microbiol Infect Dis 7:155, 1987.
121. Johnson CA, Zimmerman SW, Rogge M: The pharmacokinetics of antibiotics used to treat peritoneal dialysis–associated peritonitis. Am J Kidney Dis 4:3, 1984.
122. Gruer LD, Turney JH, Curley J, et al: Vancomycin and tobra-

mycin in the treatment of CAPD peritonitis. Nephron 41:279, 1985.
123. Shalit I, Welch DF, SanJoaquin VH, et al: In vitro antibacterial activities of antibiotics against *Pseudomonas aeruginosa* in peritoneal dialysis fluid. Antimicrob Agents Chemother 27:908, 1985.
124. Buggy BP, Schaberg DR, Swartz RD: Intraleukocytic sequestration as a cause of persistent *Staphylococcus aureus* peritonitis in continuous ambulatory peritoneal dialysis. Am J Med 76:1035, 1984.

189

Fever of Unknown Origin

Burke A. Cunha

A standard definition of fever of unknown origin (FUO) was established by Petersdorf and Beeson[1] in their classic article in 1961. During the past several decades, FUOs have been reported and reviewed extensively in the literature.[1–30] Although prolonged or perplexing fevers have been diagnostic problems for decades, many previously reported cases do not fit the current definition of FUO and would no longer be considered causes of FUO. FUO is defined as prolonged febrile illness lasting 3 weeks, with temperature of 101°F (38.3°C) or higher, that defies diagnosis after 1 week of in-hospital evaluation. Infections were traditionally the most common cause of FUO, followed by collagen-vascular diseases and malignant neoplasms. FUOs without diagnoses were also common.

The relative representation of diseases diagnosed as FUOs has changed because of improved diagnostic methods. Malignant neoplasms and infectious diseases remain the most common causes of FUO. Rheumatologic diseases, particularly rheumatoid arthritis and systemic lupus erythematosus, are now rare causes of FUO, but adult Still disease and temporal arteritis remain important causes. Tuberculosis and subacute bacterial endocarditis are less common causes of FUO because of improved scanning methods and blood culture processing techniques.

FUO etiology varies somewhat with age. Infections in children are a more common cause of FUO than are neoplasms, and viral illnesses are common causes of FUO in children. Some diseases presenting as FUO are seen almost exclusively in the pediatric age group (e.g., cat-scratch fever), whereas other diseases are conspicuously absent (e.g., subacute bacterial endocarditis). FUOs due to regional arteritis, systemic lupus erythematosus, cytomegalovirus infection, and lymphomas are particularly common in young adults; elderly patients more frequently have subacute bacterial endocarditis, tuberculosis, carcinomas, alcoholic hepatitis, pulmonary emboli, or temporal arteritis. The more prolonged the period of undiagnosed fever in a patient with FUO, the more likely it is due to a recently recognized noninfectious cause. Two new causes of FUO are Kikuchi disease and the hyperimmunoglobulinemia D syndrome[29, 81] (Table 189–1).

Causes of Fever of Unknown Origin

Malignant Neoplasms

LYMPHOMAS

Occult lymphomas located in the retroperitoneal area are a common cause of neoplastic FUOs. Retroperitoneal lymphomas are common in the elderly and present with few symptoms or clinical clues. On occasion, lymphomas present with a Pel-Epstein type of intermittent fever or a hectic-septic fever curve, which suggests an infection or abscess.[17] Retroperitoneal lymphomas may be associated with systemic symptoms (e.g., weight loss, decreased appetite, malaise), suggesting disseminated tuberculosis. Abdominal hepatosplenomegaly is not present with these lymphomas, and the only clue may be an unexpectedly elevated erythrocyte sedimentation rate (ESR), eosinophilia, or basophilia. The presumptive diagnosis is suggested by finding retroperitoneal node involvement by computed tomography (CT) or magnetic resonance imaging (MRI). Definitive diagnosis is by node biopsy.[10, 18]

METASTATIC MALIGNANT NEOPLASMS

Fever may be the sole presenting sign of early metastatic disease to the liver or central nervous system (CNS) in elderly patients. Small metastatic infiltrations in the liver are frequently clinically silent and present only with low-grade fevers. Physical findings are usually absent early, and an unexplained elevation of the alkaline phosphatase value, especially if it is accompanied by an increase in the ESR, should suggest the hepatic involvement. Metastatic disease to the CNS resulting in meningeal carcinomatosis or basilar infiltration of the brain, with or without hypothalamic involvement, occurs secondary to neoplasms that frequently metastasize to the brain. These may be difficult to diagnose in the early stage in the absence of definite neurologic abnormalities.[12, 16]

HYPERNEPHROMAS

Another common malignant neoplasm that presents as FUO is renal cell carcinoma (hypernephroma). Fever is an important feature of both the primary tumor and its metastases. Metastatic hypernephroma with multisystem involvement is a difficult diagnostic challenge because most patients with hypernephroma do not have hematuria. A left varicocele, thrombocytosis, elevated alkaline phosphatase value, and eosinophilia are diagnostic clues. Diagnosis is by tissue biopsy.[10, 28]

COLON CARCINOMA

Adenocarcinomas of the colon were represented in the early FUO literature presenting as mass lesions or with associated septic complications. Right-sided colon carcinomas without symptoms of tarry stools may present as FUO. Colon cancer may be missed by colonoscopy and CT.

HEPATIC AND PANCREATIC CARCINOMA

Pancreatic carcinoma remains a difficult diagnosis and may be suggested by vague changes in mental status, hyperglycemia, vague abdominal discomfort, or abnormalities on gallium and indium scanning or CT and MRI.[16, 18]

Hepatomas often manifest with hepatomegaly and hepatic bruit or rub: the diagnosis is usually made by liver biopsy. Hepatomas are indistinguishable from metastatic liver disease with current imaging techniques. Laboratory clues include an elevated alkaline phosphatase value, ESR, or α-fetoprotein level. Definitive diagnosis is by liver biopsy.[28]

PRELEUKEMIAS

Preleukemic monocytic leukemia is the most frequent cause of FUO among the acute and chronic leukemias. Patients

TABLE 189–1 ■ Diseases Causing Fever of Unknown Origin

TYPE OF DISORDER	COMMON	UNCOMMON	RARE
Malignant neoplasms	Lymphoma Metastasis to liver or central nervous system Hypernephromas	Hepatoma Pancreatic carcinoma Preleukemia Colon carcinoma	Atrial myxoma Central nervous system tumor Myelodysplastic disease
Infections	Extrapulmonary tuberculosis Renal tuberculosis Tuberculous meningitis Miliary tuberculosis Intraabdominal abscess Subdiaphragmatic abscess Periappendiceal Pericolonic Hepatic Pelvic abscess	Subacute bacterial endocarditis Cytomegalovirus infection Toxoplasmosis *Salmonella* enteric fever Intrarenal or perinephric abscess Splenic abscess	Periapical dental abscess Small brain abscess Chronic sinusitis Subacute vertebral osteomyelitis Chronic meningitis-encephalitis *Listeria* infection *Yersinia* infection Brucellosis Relapsing fever Rat-bite fever Chronic Q fever Cat-scratch fever Human immunodeficiency virus infection Epstein-Barr virus mononucleosis (elderly) Malaria Leptospirosis Blastomycosis Histoplasmosis Coccidioidomycosis Cryptococcosis Infected aortic aneurysm Infected vascular grafts Rocky Mountain spotted fever Lyme disease Leishmaniasis Trypanosomiasis Lymphogranuloma venereum Permanently placed central intravenous line infections Trichinosis Prosthetic device infection Relapsing mastoiditis Septic jugular phlebitis
Rheumatologic causes	Adult Still disease (juvenile rheumatoid arthritis) Temporal arteritis (elderly)	Periarteritis nodosa Rheumatoid arthritis (elderly)	Systemic lupus erythematosus Vasculitis (e.g., Takayasu arteritis, hypersensitivity vasculitis) Felty syndrome Pseudogout (calcium pyrophosphate deposition disease) Acute rheumatic fever Sjögren syndrome Behçet disease Familial Mediterranean fever
Miscellaneous causes	Drug fever Cirrhosis Alcoholic hepatitis	Granulomatous hepatitis	Regional enteritis Whipple's disease Fabry disease Hyperthyroidism Hyperparathyroidism Pheochromocytoma Addison disease Subacute thyroiditis Cyclic neutropenia Polymyositis Wegener granulomatosis Occult hematoma Subacute aortic dissecting aneurysm Weber-Christian disease Sarcoidosis (e.g., basilar meningitis, hepatic granulomata) Pulmonary emboli (multiple, recurrent) Hypothalamic dysfunction Habitual hyperthermia Factitious fever Giant hepatic hemangioma Mesenteric fibromatosis Pseudolymphoma Idiopathic granulomatosis Kikuchi disease Malacoplakia Hyperimmunoglobulinemia D syndrome

usually have vague and nonspecific symptoms in addition to prolonged fevers. On physical examination, sternal tenderness may be the only finding. Blast cells are not present in the peripheral blood smear, and diagnosis is by bone marrow aspirate.[19]

ATRIAL MYXOMAS

Atrial myxomas may present with low-grade fevers, embolic phenomena, or heart murmur that may or may not be influenced by changes in position. Atrial myxomas mimic and are most frequently confused with subacute bacterial endocarditis. Although renal involvement is not a feature of atrial myxomas, the clinical presentation closely resembles subacute bacterial endocarditis in many respects. Polyclonal gammopathy on serum protein electrophoresis suggests atrial myxoma versus subacute bacterial endocarditis, and an intracardiac mass is diagnostic by echocardiography.[10, 17]

Infectious Diseases

EXTRAPULMONARY TUBERCULOSIS

Disseminated tuberculosis is less commonly a cause of FUO than it was previously, but tuberculous meningitis and miliary tuberculosis are not uncommon and remain difficult diagnostic problems. Renal tuberculosis may present with sterile pyuria, microscopic hematuria, slowly progressive renal failure, or epididymal orchitis in men. Diagnosis is suggested by microscopic hematuria or sterile pyuria in patients with simultaneous upper and lower tract involvement by intravenous pyelography, CT, or MRI. Renal tuberculosis is one of the few diseases that simultaneously affects the upper and lower urinary tracts. The upper tract changes resemble chronic pyelonephritis; the ureters are frequently scalloped or kinked or have a corkscrew configuration. Diagnosis is by recovery of the organism in the urine.[14, 21]

Early tuberculous meningitis presents with subtle neurologic abnormalities (cognitive difficulties, mild headaches, difficulties in concentration) with intermittent low-grade fevers. Cranial nerve abnormalities and unilateral or bilateral abducens nerve palsies are late findings in basilar meningitis due to tuberculosis. Early CT or MRI results are frequently unremarkable, and cerebrospinal fluid abnormalities may not be present. As tuberculous meningitis progresses without treatment, the cerebrospinal fluid glucose level will fall in concert with a rise in the cerebrospinal fluid protein level. The need for serial lumbar punctures cannot be underestimated in making the diagnosis of tuberculous meningitis to detect the protein-glucose dissociation. Definitive diagnosis is by culture of the organism from the cerebrospinal fluid. Not infrequently, the chest radiograph is unremarkable in patients with CNS tuberculosis.[10, 32]

Miliary tuberculosis remains an important cause of FUO. Elderly patients and those receiving corticosteroids may have silent dissemination of previously quiescent disease and slowly become chronically ill with disseminated tuberculosis. Miliary tuberculosis has no localizing signs, and the diagnosis may be made retrospectively by analysis of serial chest radiographs to appreciate the gradual appearance of miliary infiltrates. Because miliary tuberculosis involves the reticular endothelial system, the diagnosis may be made by biopsy of the liver or bone marrow. Not infrequently, the only way to make a definite diagnosis is by empirical trial of antituberculous agents in a rapidly deteriorating patient with presumed miliary tuberculosis.[1, 20, 32, 33]

INTRAABDOMINAL AND PELVIC ABSCESSES

Perforation of the pelvic or gastrointestinal organs by procedures, surgery, or disease may result in abscess formation in various parts of the pelvis or abdomen. Location of the abscess depends on the degree of intraabdominal spillage and the position of the patient after organ perforation. Most commonly, periappendiceal or pericolonic collections are responsible for prolonged fevers. Subdiaphragmatic collections and intrahepatic abscesses are also responsible for prolonged fevers. The majority of these patients will have some, albeit subtle, physical findings suggesting intraabdominal or pelvic disease. Trapezius tenderness may be the only manifestation of a subdiaphragmatic abscess. CT and MRI can reveal pelvic and intraabdominal abscesses, less common causes of obscure and prolonged fevers. Splenic abscesses associated with endocarditis, typhoid fever, or brucellosis are invariably part of multisystem infection. Perinephric abscesses may result from hematogenous dissemination from a distant source or from previous pyelonephritis. If there is not communication between the collecting system, urine may show only sterile pyuria. Intrarenal abscesses associated with medullary sponge kidney, medullary polycystic kidneys, or stone disease rarely cause diagnostic confusion as renal causes of FUO.[2–4, 15, 18]

SALMONELLA ENTERIC FEVERS

Enteric fever due to *Salmonella typhi* or other invasive *Salmonella* strains is associated with infection of the reticuloendothelial system and multisystem involvement. Established typhoid fever may present with splenomegaly or spinal tenderness, but frequently there are no localizing signs with typhoid fever. The white cell count is normally decreased; the ESR is minimally elevated, if at all; and the only clue may be a sustained fever with a pulse-temperature deficit. Eosinophilia is not a feature of the *Salmonella* enteric fevers. Febrile agglutinins to *Salmonella* may suggest the diagnosis, which may be confirmed by recovery of the organism from body fluids or bone marrow aspirate.[10, 34]

TOXOPLASMOSIS

Toxoplasmosis in the immunocompetent adult with FUO may present with a prolonged mononucleosis-like illness or isolated lymphadenopathy. Except for adenopathy, there is a paucity of physical findings, sometimes with atypical lymphocytosis and mild liver abnormalities. Biopsy of the affected node is characteristic. A serologic diagnosis is made by demonstrating increased immunoglobulin M antitoxoplasma titers on indirect fluorescent antibody assay.[35]

EPSTEIN-BARR VIRUS

Epstein-Barr virus, except in elderly patients, is a rare cause of FUO. Elderly patients with Epstein-Barr virus infection usually present without prominent posterior cervical adenopathy or pharyngitis. Such patients may have hepatic tenderness or enlargement, but they usually have mildly abnormal liver function test results. The combination of mild "hepatitis" in an elderly patient with atypical lymphocytosis should suggest Epstein-Barr virus infection, and a positive serologic response is diagnostic.[20, 33]

SUBACUTE BACTERIAL ENDOCARDITIS

Subacute bacterial endocarditis is less common than it was previously as a cause of FUO because of the widespread practice of obtaining blood cultures in patients with prolonged fevers. Fastidious or unculturable organisms produce prolonged unexplained fevers. Brucellosis and Q fever are the most common causes of culture-negative endocarditis presenting as FUO.[1, 18, 24]

Other Infectious Causes

Virtually any chronic infectious disease capable of producing prolonged fevers has been reported as a cause of FUO. Certain diseases such as malaria, Rocky Mountain spotted fever, Q fever, visceral leishmaniasis, or histoplasmosis may present as FUOs in nonendemic areas where clinicians are not familiar with their protean manifestations. Cytomegalovirus mononucleosis may be a difficult diagnosis months after disease onset when atypical lymphocytes are no longer present, and the only diagnostic clue is a mild serum transaminase elevation. HIV infection may present with prolonged fevers, but with improved serologic tests and increased index of suspicion, HIV should be considered an important cause of prolonged fevers even without opportunistic infections or neoplasms. Cat-scratch fever occurs primarily in children but may occur in adults and is frequently manifested by adenopathy of the affected lymph node area. Tissue biopsy is needed to rule out other causes of infectious or neoplastic node enlargement. Leptospirosis is a biphasic illness characterized by an infectious phase and an immune phase, and prolonged fevers are only rarely associated with leptospirosis. Leptospirosis is suggested by the hepatic, renal, or CNS involvement and a history of appropriate animal contact. Disseminated histoplasmosis and, to a lesser extent, disseminated cryptococcosis may mimic miliary tuberculosis. In general, parasitic diseases, fungi, and rickettsiae are rare causes of FUO. Amebic liver abscesses were mentioned in the early FUO literature, but current imaging techniques and high index of suspicion even in nonendemic areas make this a rare cause of FUO. Subacute vertebral osteomyelitis in male patients is a difficult diagnosis to make if the preceding history of urinary tract infection is not appreciated. The organisms ascend from the urinary tract through Batson plexus to the spine. Such patients may have fever and nonspecific low back pain, or they may complain of symptoms of disk disease or sciatica. A variety of other infections including chronic sinusitis, brain abscesses, and periapical dental abscesses have infrequently been associated with FUO. Periapical dental abscesses are particularly difficult to diagnose because there is no local tenderness or pyorrhea and the jaws appear normal on panoramic film of the jaw. Diagnosis may be made by doing a local gallium scan of the jaws, which may reveal the periapical collection. Dental abscesses may metastasize to the brain, presenting as a brain tumor that at craniotomy proves to be a brain abscess.

Arthritis of the knee and vertebral osteomyelitis are typical findings in chronic brucellosis, but often there are no hard findings. Unexplained headache, unusual affect, or cognitive difficulties complicate the clinical picture. Renal and genitourinary involvement is not uncommon.[33, 36]

The constellation of headache, often accompanied by photophobia or meningismus, with abdominal and joint pain is suggestive of relapsing fever. Hepatosplenomegaly and thrombocytic pain are also diagnostic features of relapsing fever.[33] The other unusual infections causing FUO are presented in Table 189–1.[10, 16, 21, 24, 33]

Rheumatologic Causes

ADULT STILL DISEASE

Juvenile rheumatoid arthritis (adult Still disease) remains an important cause of FUO in adults. Patients usually present with hepatosplenomegaly and evanescent truncal "salmon-colored" rash, with or without the Koebner phenomenon, and minimal joint or eye findings. Rheumatoid factors are absent, and the only clue to the diagnosis may be double quotidian fever.[37]

TEMPORAL ARTERITIS

Granulomatous arteritis of the temporal arteries is a common cause of FUO in the elderly. Patients often complain of visual disturbances, vague headache, or stiffness and myalgias. Tenderness over the temporal arteries is not unusual, but complaints of pain over the angle of the jaw, when present, may provide a clue to the diagnosis, and the ESR is characteristically rapid (100 mm/h and above). Definitive diagnosis is by temporal artery biopsy of the involved segments.[12, 15, 19, 38]

PERIARTERITIS NODOSA

Periarteritis nodosa is a midsize vasculitis characterized by multisystem involvement. Abdominal pain, headache, and arthritic complaints are common. The constellation of hypertension and peripheral eosinophilia with a history of acalculous cholecystitis, or epididymoorchitis, should suggest the diagnosis. Renal insufficiency, heart failure, or stroke in someone with hepatitis B surface antigenemia should suggest periarteritis nodosa.[7, 39]

RHEUMATOID ARTHRITIS

Rheumatoid arthritis presenting as FUO in the elderly can be a difficult diagnosis because of the absence of joint involvement or elevated rheumatoid factors. Prolonged fevers and rheumatic complaints may be the only manifestations of late-onset rheumatoid arthritis in aged individuals. Systemic lupus erythematosus is only a rare cause of FUO today.[10, 39]

VASCULITIS

Many vasculitides produce intermittent or prolonged fevers. Hypersensitivity vasculitis and Takayasu arteritis are infrequent but important causes of FUO. Multisystem organ involvement is characteristic, and diagnosis is made by tissue biopsy.[40, 41]

LYME DISEASE

Lyme disease has been reported as a rare cause of FUO. However, Lyme disease with its musculoskeletal and neurologic manifestations is not characterized by high or prolonged fevers.[30, 33]

KIKUCHI DISEASE

Kikuchi disease is necrotizing adenitis with fever and leukopenia that usually occurs in young women. Necrotizing mediastinal and retroperitoneal adenopathy has been reported, as has splenomegaly in Kikuchi disease presenting as FUO.[42–45]

Miscellaneous Causes

A variety of other diseases rarely present as FUOs, including dissecting aortic aneurysms, occult hematomas, subacute thyroiditis, hyperthyroidism, hyperparathyroidism, Fabry disease, and cyclic neutropenia. In addition, multiple recurrent pulmonary emboli may present a difficult diagnostic problem in the patient with prolonged obscure fevers. The diagnosis is suggested by the appropriate setting, such as an immobilized patient which may or may not have wheezing. The diagnosis may be suspected by vague chest discomfort or shortness of breath, and the only laboratory clues may be an increase in the ESR or fibrin split products.[7, 8, 10, 33]

DRUG FEVER

An important cause of FUO is drug fever. Most drugs are potentially sensitizing and therefore may cause fever as the sole manifestation of their hypersensitivity reaction. It is a popular misconception that antibiotics are primarily responsible for drug fevers. Although antibiotics, particularly sulfonamides and the β-lactam antibiotics, remain important causes of drug fevers, antiarrhythmics, pain medications, diuretics, sulfa-containing stool softeners, sleep medications, antiseizure medications, antithyroid medications, and tranquilizers are more frequent causes of drug fevers. The temperature range with a drug fever is variable, but if the temperature is higher than 102°F, a pulse-temperature deficit is usually apparent. Patients with drug fever often have low-grade eosinophilia, usually within the normal ranges. Eosinophils are commonly present, but eosinophils are infrequently present at above-normal elevations of serum transaminase or alkaline phosphatase.[46]

The diagnosis of drug fever is made on the basis of excluding other causes of fever and withdrawing the potentially offending drug. The patient with drug fever does not necessarily give a history of allergic reactions to medications and appears to be surprisingly well. Patients may have been taking medications for many years without development of hypersensitivity reactions to their medications. It should never be assumed that because the patient has been receiving a particular medication for an extended time that it is not the cause of the drug fever. Patients occasionally develop hypersensitivity reactions to fumes or toxin exposures. Fume fevers are exceedingly rare but have been reported to cause FUO.[10, 46, 47]

ALCOHOLIC LIVER DISEASE

Alcoholic liver disease is a common cause of prolonged fevers. Cirrhosis and particularly alcoholic hepatitis are frequently missed causes of prolonged fevers in the patient with alcoholic liver disease. Alcoholic hepatitis is suggested by mildly abnormal liver function test results and a white cell count greater than 10,000/mm^3. Definitive diagnosis is by liver biopsy.[48, 49]

GRANULOMATOUS HEPATITIS

Granulomatous hepatitis is a diagnosis of exclusion and is characterized by normochromic normocytic anemia, occasional liver enlargement, and mildly abnormal liver function test results. Liver biopsy shows granuloma formation, which also occurs with regional enteritis, sarcoidosis, lymphoma, histoplasmosis, or tuberculosis in the FUO differential diagnosis.[10, 50, 51]

SARCOIDOSIS

Sarcoidosis is a disease not characterized by fever. However, sarcoidosis may be associated with fever if there is bilateral hilar adenopathy with or without erythema nodosum, uveal tract and parotid involvement (Heerfordt syndrome), or hepatic granuloma infiltration. On liver biopsy specimens, sarcoid granulomata are numerous and accompanied by many giant cells. This is in contrast to tuberculosis, in which giant cells and granulomata are few. If sarcoidosis is accompanied by fevers in the absence of these clinical conditions, coexisting tuberculosis should be suspected.[33]

FAMILIAL MEDITERRANEAN FEVER

Familial Mediterranean fever is characterized by intermittent pleuritic or abdominal pain, with or without joint pain or headache. Unexplained persistent chest pain or abdominal pain with fever in individuals of western European Mediterranean ancestry should suggest the diagnosis.[33, 39]

REGIONAL ENTERITIS

Vague abdominal pain and persistent low-grade fevers are the usual presentations of FUO in patients with regional enteritis. Malabsorption and a right lower quadrant mass are late features. Fever may precede gastrointestinal symptoms, and the ESR is usually elevated.

WHIPPLE'S DISEASE

Patients with Whipple's disease usually have knee or ankle joint symptoms, and changes in mentation are also common. Skin hyperpigmentation and adenopathy are variably present. The majority of patients have low carotene serum levels, and diagnosis is by periodic acid–Schiff–positive material on small intestine biopsy.[33]

HYPERIMMUNOGLOBULINEMIA D PERIODIC FEVER SYNDROME

Hyperimmunoglobulinemia D syndrome presents as periodic prolonged febrile episodes with hepatitis A, abdominal pain, arthralgias, cervical adenopathy, and splenomegaly (children). Large joints are usually affected, and some patients have an erythematous extremity rash. The ESR and white cell count are elevated in addition to serum immunoglobulin D and A levels. Serum immunoglobulin D levels are elevated in sarcoidosis, Hodgkin's lymphoma, human immunodeficiency virus (HIV) infection, and tuberculosis but are highly elevated in the hyperimmunoglobulinemia D syndrome (100 units/mL and greater). This syndrome is benign and is a problem of clinical recognition because it may be confused with many diseases.

FACTITIOUS FEVER

Patients with factitious fever may present with FUO, but with the advent of electronic thermometers, factitious temperature elevations are less common. Patients with factitious fevers are usually young women in the medical field. Factitious fevers are usually high and are not accompanied by an appropriate pulse response. The single best way to determine the true temperature of a patient with a suspected factitious fever is to measure the temperature of a recently voided urine specimen, which closely approximates core temperature. Some individuals have higher core temperatures that are 1° to 2° above normal without any physical or laboratory abnormalities, just as some individuals have lower than normal temperatures. Individuals with higher than normal temperatures should not be regarded as abnormal. Such individuals should be reassured, because they are usually preoccupied with their apparent fevers.[8, 50, 52]

Diagnostic Approach

Clinical Aspects

Excluding isolated case reports, historical, physical, and laboratory clues should be used to determine the pattern of organ involvement. The pattern of abnormalities is more likely to suggest a diagnosis than are isolated findings. For example, splenomegaly alone suggests cirrhosis, subacute endocarditis, psittacosis, Q fever, typhoid fever, tuberculosis, brucellosis, or systemic lupus erythematosus. With the added findings of relative bradycardia and abnormal liver function test results, the differential diagnosis is quickly narrowed to psittacosis. Diagnostic tests should be directed at the organs likely to contain diagnostic material.[2, 6, 16]

Common diseases responsible for prolonged febrile illnesses should be considered, taking into account clues from the patient's history, physical examination, and appropriate laboratory tests. The diagnostic approach should not include every conceivable cause of FUO but should be specifically directed by the clinical presentation or specific organ involvement. The clinician should use the clues to get an appreciation of what sort of disease behavior is suggested by the patient's presentation. Is it likely to be neoplastic, infectious, rheumatologic, or some other miscellaneous cause? Because common diseases frequently present atypically, a statistical approach toward the patient should always be used unless there are specific clues suggesting alternative diagnoses. In adults, care should be taken to consider malignant neoplasm as a cause of fever because it is so common. If an infectious cause is entertained, then a previous intraabdominal or pelvic infection or surgery would suggest the possibility of an abscess. Tuberculosis presenting as FUO is extrapulmonary and usually presents as tuberculous meningitis, renal tuberculosis, or disseminated miliary tuberculosis. Particular effort should be made to diagnose infectious and collagen-vascular diseases because most are treatable, albeit less common than malignant neoplasms.

The miscellaneous causes of FUO, particularly drug fevers and fevers associated with cirrhosis or alcoholic hepatitis, are commonly overlooked causes of FUO. Because nearly all medications are potentially sensitizing and may result in prolonged febrile reactions, drug fevers should always be considered in FUO patients without localizing signs. The various causes of FUO by frequency of occurrence are listed in Table 189–1.

Although fever patterns are infrequently helpful diagnostically, they may provide the only clue to the diagnosis in the FUO patient with no localizing signs. Most patients with FUO present with low-grade fevers (temperatures less than 102°F). Temperature of 102°F or higher suggests an infectious cause, lymphoma, or vasculitis. More important, a temperature above 102°F excludes certain diseases that rarely, if ever, are associated with high fevers (e.g., recurrent pulmonary emboli). Drug fevers may be high or low grade, but drug fevers presenting as FUOs usually have temperatures below 102°F. Relative bradycardia is an important diagnostic clue suggesting typhoid fever, psittacosis, leptospirosis, lymphoma, or drug fever. A reversal of diurnal temperature rhythm with a morning temperature spike may suggest periarteritis nodosa, tuberculosis, or factitious fever. The most specific temperature pattern in the patient with FUO is a double quotidian fever (two fever spikes within a 24-hour period) not induced by antipyretics. Double quotidian fever may be the only clue to adult Still disease (adult juvenile rheumatoid arthritis), leishmaniasis, malaria, or miliary tuberculosis. Periodic or relapsing fevers point to cyclic neutropenias, malaria, lymphoma, or one of the relapsing fevers due to *Borrelia, Spirillum,* or *Streptobacillus.* Intermittent hectic-septic fevers suggest abscess, miliary tuberculosis, or lymphoma.

The history from the patient is usually more important than the physical examination in providing clues to the possible cause of prolonged fevers. Headache or mental confusion focuses the work-up on a CNS source; a history of a heart murmur, previous surgery, animal contact, or medication ingestion suggests specific diagnoses. Complaints of myalgias or fatigue suggest many diagnostic possibilities and are less helpful unless they are considered in concert with other findings. Of particular importance are complaints that limit diagnostic possibilities and are therefore more specific or useful in suggesting a diagnosis. For example, back pain over the spine suggests subacute vertebral osteomyelitis, typhoid fever, brucellosis, or enterococcal endocarditis. Historical clues are presented in Tables 189–2 to 189–4.

Physical examination of the patient with FUO is important, particularly with respect to the cardiac and abdominal examination. A heart murmur might suggest subacute endocarditis or an atrial myxoma; hepatomegaly points to lymphoma, metastatic carcinoma, or alcoholic liver disease. Frequently overlooked areas on the physical examination include the eyes, muscles, lymph nodes, sternum, and spine. Trapezial tenderness may be the only subtle expression of an occult subdiaphragmatic abscess. Epididymal or testicular tenderness may be the only clue to renal tuberculosis, lymphoma, brucellosis, leptospirosis, periarteritis nodosa, or infectious mononucleosis. Adenopathy should be carefully looked for in the epitrochlear, supraclavicular, axillary, and posterior cervical areas. Adenopathy is an important finding in FUO patients with lymphomas, rheumatoid arthritis, systemic lupus erythematosus, disseminated tuberculosis, infectious mononucleosis, cytomegalovirus infection, toxoplasmosis, or HIV infection. Physical examination is unhelpful in retroperitoneal lymphomas, intraabdominal abscess, bacterial infections without localization, and drug reactions. Physical

TABLE 189–2 ■ Historical Clues to Fever of Unknown Origin

MEDICATION OR TOXIC SUBSTANCES Drug fever Fume fever	**CARDIOVASCULAR ACCIDENT** Subacute bacterial endocarditis Takayasu arteritis Periarteritis nodosa Rocky Mountain spotted fever
TICK EXPOSURE Relapsing fever Rocky Mountain spotted fever Lyme disease	**NONPRODUCTIVE COUGH** Tuberculosis Q fever Psittacosis Typhoid fever Pulmonary neoplasms Rocky Mountain spotted fever Acute rheumatic fever
ANIMAL CONTACT Psittacosis Leptospirosis Brucellosis Toxoplasmosis Cat-scratch disease Q fever Rat-bite fever	**VISION DISORDERS OR EYE PAIN** Temporal arteritis (emboli) Subacute bacterial endocarditis Relapsing fever Brain abscess Takayasu arteritis
MYALGIAS Trichinosis Subacute bacterial endocarditis Periarteritis nodosa Rheumatoid arthritis Familial Mediterranean fever Polymyositis	**FATIGUE** Carcinoma Lymphoma Cytomegalovirus mononucleosis Typhoid fever Systemic lupus erythematosus Rheumatoid arthritis Toxoplasmosis
HEADACHE Relapsing fever Rat-bite fever Chronic meningitis-encephalitis Malaria Brucellosis Central nervous system neoplasm Rocky Mountain spotted fever	**ABDOMINAL PAIN** Periarteritis nodosa Familial Mediterranean fever Relapsing fever
MENTAL CONFUSION Sarcoid meningitis Tuberculous meningitis Cryptococcal meningitis Carcinomatous meningitis Central nervous system neoplasm Brucellosis Typhoid fever Human immunodeficiency virus infection	**BACK PAIN** Brucellosis Subacute bacterial endocarditis **NECK PAIN** Subacute thyroiditis Adult Still disease Temporal arteritis (angle of jaw) Relapsing mastoiditis Septic jugular phlebitis

TABLE 189–3 ■ Physical Clues to Fever of Unknown Origin

SKIN HYPERPIGMENTATION
Whipple's disease
Hypersensitivity vasculitis

BAND KERATOPATHY
Adult Still disease

DRY EYES
Rheumatoid arthritis
Systemic lupus erythematosus
Sjögren syndrome

WATERY EYES
Periarteritis nodosa

EPISTAXIS
Relapsing fever
Psittacosis

CONJUNCTIVITIS
Tuberculosis
Cat-scratch fever
Systemic lupus erythematosus

CONJUNCTIVAL SUFFUSION
Leptospirosis
Relapsing fever
Rocky Mountain spotted fever

SUBCONJUNCTIVAL HEMORRHAGE
Subacute bacterial endocarditis
Trichinosis

UVEITIS
Tuberculosis
Adult Still disease
Sarcoidosis
Systemic lupus erythematosus

LYMPHADENOPATHY
Lymphoma
Cat-scratch fever
Tuberculosis
Lymphogranuloma venereum
Epstein-Barr virus mononucleosis
Cytomegalovirus infection
Toxoplasmosis
Human immunodeficiency virus infection
Adult Still disease
Brucellosis
Whipple's disease
Pseudolymphoma
Kikuchi disease

STERNAL TENDERNESS
Metastatic carcinoma
Preleukemia

HEART MURMUR
Subacute bacterial endocarditis
Atrial myxoma

HEPATOMEGALY
Hepatoma
Relapsing fever
Lymphoma
Metastatic carcinoma
Alcoholic liver disease
Granulomatous hepatitis
Q fever
Typhoid fever

SPLENOMEGALY
Leukemia
Lymphoma
Tuberculosis
Brucellosis
Subacute bacterial endocarditis
Cytomegalovirus infection
Epstein-Barr virus mononucleosis
Rheumatoid arthritis
Sarcoidosis
Psittacosis
Relapsing fever
Alcoholic liver disease
Typhoid fever
Rocky Mountain spotted fever
Kikuchi disease

TRAPEZIUS TENDERNESS
Subdiaphragmatic abscess

THIGH TENDERNESS
Brucellosis
Polymyositis

RELATIVE BRADYCARDIA
Typhoid fever
Malaria
Leptospirosis
Psittacosis
Central fever
Drug fever

SPLENIC ABSCESS
Subacute bacterial endocarditis
Brucellosis
Salmonella enteric fevers

EPIDIDYMOORCHITIS
Tuberculosis
Lymphoma
Brucellosis
Leptospirosis
Periarteritis nodosa
Epstein-Barr virus mononucleosis

SPINAL TENDERNESS
Subacute vertebral osteomyelitis
Subacute bacterial endocarditis
Brucellosis
Typhoid fever

ARTHRITIS/JOINT PAIN
Familial Mediterranean fever
Pseudogout
Rat-bite fever
Rheumatoid arthritis
Systemic lupus erythematosus
Lyme disease
Lymphogranuloma venereum
Whipple's disease
Brucellosis
Hyperimmunoglobulinemia D syndrome

CALF TENDERNESS
Rocky Mountain spotted fever
Polymyositis

TONGUE TENDERNESS
Relapsing fever

THROMBOPHLEBITIS
Psittacosis

examination is most helpful in detecting nonmalignant intraabdominal disease. Physical clues are given in Table 189–5.

Laboratory Tests

The history and physical examination should suggest the appropriate diagnostic direction of laboratory testing. Routine laboratory tests may provide important clues and should be obtained for all patients with FUO. The hemogram should include a complete white cell count with differential and platelet count. Leukopenia may suggest miliary tuberculosis, brucellosis, lupus, or lymphoma. A monocytosis may be the initial clue to cytomegalovirus infection, tuberculosis, brucellosis, lymphoma, regional enteritis, or carcinoma. Eosinophilia in a patient with FUO suggests lymphoma, trichinosis, drug fever, or periarteritis nodosa; basophilia almost invariably points to carcinoma or lymphoma in patients with prolonged fevers. Chronic lymphocytosis suggests cytomegalovirus infection, infectious mononucleosis, tuberculosis, or toxoplasmosis.

The ESR is a sensitive although nonspecific test, but it is diagnostically useful in combination with other clinical or laboratory abnormalities. In a patient with FUO and eosinophilia, an ESR of 2 mm/h would immediately suggest the possibility of trichinosis. A rapid ESR (i.e., 100 mm/h or greater) in a patient with FUO suggests drug fever, adult Still disease, giant cell arteritis, subacute endocarditis, abscess, osteomyelitis, carcinoma, lymphoma, or hyperimmunoglobulinemia D syndrome. Moderate elevations of ESR are seen with most disease entities causing FUO. The absence of an elevated ESR does not rule out the presence of infectious, rheumatic, or neoplastic disease as a cause of prolonged fever.

Liver function tests are particularly important as part of the work-up in the patient with FUO because so many of the diseases causing FUO are characterized by hepatic involvement. Elevation of the alkaline phosphatase value out of proportion to serum transaminases suggests an infiltrative or obstructive process and may be the only clue to adult Still disease, subacute thyroiditis, giant cell arteritis, or periarteritis nodosa. An isolated, modest elevation of the alkaline

TABLE 189–4 ■ Laboratory Clues to Fever of Unknown Origin

MONOCYTOSIS
- Tuberculosis
- Periarteritis nodosa
- Temporal arteritis
- Cytomegalovirus infection
- Sarcoidosis
- Brucellosis
- Subacute bacterial endocarditis
- Systemic lupus erythematosus
- Lymphoma
- Carcinoma
- Regional enteritis
- Myeloproliferative disease

EOSINOPHILIA
- Trichinosis
- Lymphomas
- Drug fever
- Addison disease
- Periarteritis nodosa
- Hypersensitivity vasculitis
- Hypernephroma
- Myeloproliferative disease

LEUKOPENIA
- Miliary tuberculosis
- Brucellosis
- Systemic lupus erythematosus
- Lymphoma
- Preleukemia
- Typhoid fever
- Kikuchi disease

BASOPHILIA
- Carcinoma
- Lymphoma
- Preleukemia
- Myeloproliferative disease

LYMPHOCYTOSIS
- Tuberculosis
- Epstein-Barr virus mononucleosis
- Cytomegalovirus infection
- Toxoplasmosis
- Non-Hodgkin's lymphoma

LYMPHOCYTOPENIA
- Human immunodeficiency virus infection
- Whipple's disease
- Miliary tuberculosis
- Systemic lupus erythematosus
- Sarcoidosis

ATYPICAL LYMPHOCYTOSIS
- Epstein-Barr virus mononucleosis
- Cytomegalovirus infection
- Brucellosis
- Toxoplasmosis
- Drug fever

THROMBOCYTOSIS
- Myeloproliferative disease
- Tuberculosis
- Carcinoma
- Lymphoma
- Sarcoidosis
- Vasculitis
- Temporal arteritis
- Subacute osteomyelitis
- Hypernephroma

THROMBOCYTOPENIA
- Leukemia
- Lymphoma
- Myeloproliferative disease
- Relapsing fever
- Epstein-Barr virus mononucleosis
- Drug fever
- Vasculitis
- Systemic lupus erythematosus
- Human immunodeficiency virus infection

RHEUMATOID FACTOR
- Subacute bacterial endocarditis
- Chronic active hepatitis
- Rheumatoid arthritis
- Malaria
- Hypersensitivity vasculitis

ERYTHROCYTE SEDIMENTATION RATE (>100 mm/h)
- Adult Still disease
- Temporal arteritis
- Hypernephroma
- Subacute bacterial endocarditis
- Drug fever
- Carcinoma
- Lymphoma
- Myeloproliferative disease
- Abscess
- Subacute osteomyelitis
- Polymyositis
- Hyperimmunoglobulinemia D syndrome

INCREASED ALKALINE PHOSPHATASE LEVEL
- Hepatoma
- Miliary tuberculosis
- Lymphoma
- Epstein-Barr virus mononucleosis
- Cytomegalovirus infection
- Adult Still disease
- Subacute thyroiditis
- Temporal arteritis
- Hypernephroma
- Periarteritis nodosa
- Liver metastasis
- Granulomatous hepatitis

INCREASED SERUM TRANSAMINASE LEVEL
- Epstein-Barr virus mononucleosis
- Cytomegalovirus infection
- Q fever
- Psittacosis
- Drug fever
- Leptospirosis
- Toxoplasmosis
- Brucellosis
- Relapsing fever
- Kikuchi disease

SERUM PROTEIN ELECTROPHORESIS (POLYCLONAL GAMMOPATHY)
- Atrial myxoma
- Alcoholic cirrhosis
- Sarcoidosis
- Lymphoma
- Periarteritis nodosa
- Human immunodeficiency virus infection
- Takayasu arteritis
- Idiopathic granulomatosis

ABNORMAL RENAL TEST RESULTS
- Subacute bacterial endocarditis
- Renal tuberculosis
- Periarteritis nodosa
- Fabry disease
- Leptospirosis
- Brucellosis
- Lymphomas
- Systemic lupus erythematosus
- Hypernephroma
- Human immunodeficiency virus infection
- Malacoplakia

QUANTITATIVE IMMUNOGLOBULINS
- Hyperimmunoglobulinemia D syndrome

phosphatase is a normal finding in healthy elderly adults. Elevation of the serum transaminase values, with minimal or no elevation of the serum alkaline phosphatase level, suggests infectious disease of the liver, particularly cytomegalovirus infection, Epstein-Barr virus mononucleosis, Q fever, or psittacosis, but it is also common with drug fever. The serum protein electrophoresis may provide a clue to lymphoma with an isolated elevation of the α_2-globulin fraction. A diffuse polyclonal gammopathy in a patient with FUO would suggest atrial myxoma, sarcoidosis, lymphoma, or HIV infection. Fibrin split products may be the only clue to multiple recurrent pulmonary emboli, not detectable by scanning methods or angiography. Laboratory clues are shown in Table 189–4.

Other Diagnostic Tests

Therapeutic agents can be used diagnostically in selected cases to support or confirm the diagnosis when diagnosis is not possible by other means. Patients with drug fevers can be diagnosed with certainty only by discontinuation of the drug. Temperature elevations due to drug fever will return to nearly normal within 72 hours if the sensitizing medication is discontinued. The naproxen (Naprosyn) test has been em-

TABLE 189–5 ■ Organ System Involvement in Fever of Unknown Origin by Symptoms, Physical Signs, or Laboratory Abnormalities

CENTRAL NERVOUS SYSTEM
- Tuberculous meningitis
- Sarcoid meningitis
- Tumors, hemorrhage
- Chronic encephalitis
- Brain abscess
- Subacute bacterial endocarditis
- Takayasu arteritis

NECK
- Subacute thyroiditis
- Adult Still disease
- Dental abscess
- Relapsing mastoiditis
- Septic jugular phlebitis
- Kikuchi disease

LYMPH NODES
- Lymphoma
- Cat-scratch disease
- Tuberculosis
- Lymphogranuloma venereum
- Epstein-Barr virus mononucleosis
- Cytomegalovirus infection
- Toxoplasmosis
- Human immunodeficiency virus infection
- Adult Still disease
- Brucellosis
- Whipple's disease
- Kikuchi disease

JOINTS
- Whipple's disease
- Rat-bite fever
- Brucellosis
- Familial Mediterranean fever
- Acute rheumatic fever
- Lymphogranuloma venereum
- Hyperimmunoglobulinemia D syndrome

SMALL INTESTINE
- Familial Mediterranean fever
- Lymphoma
- Regional enteritis
- Whipple's disease

PELVIS
- Pelvic abscess
- Pelvic tumors

NO LOCALIZING SIGNS
- Infected aortic aneurysm
- Dissecting aortic aneurysm
- Subacute bacterial endocarditis
- Miliary tuberculosis
- Brucellosis
- Q fever
- Colon cancer
- Human immunodeficiency virus infection
- Lymphomas
- Typhoid fever
- Drug fever
- Factitious fever
- Preleukemia
- Myeloproliferative disease

HEART
- Subacute bacterial endocarditis
- Atrial myxoma
- Takayasu arteritis

KIDNEYS
- Subacute endocarditis
- Hypernephroma
- Intrarenal or perinephric abscess
- Periarteritis nodosa
- Renal tuberculosis
- Human immunodeficiency virus infection
- Fabry disease
- Lymphoma
- Systemic lupus erythematosus
- Leptospirosis
- Brucellosis
- Malacoplakia

SPLEEN
- Subacute bacterial endocarditis
- Splenic abscess
- Lymphomas
- Cytomegalovirus infection
- Human immunodeficiency virus infection

LIVER
- Metastatic carcinoma
- Hepatoma
- Cirrhosis
- Alcoholic hepatitis
- Liver abscess
- Miliary tuberculosis
- Sarcoidosis
- Giant hemangioma
- Granulomatous hepatitis
- Brucellosis
- Q fever
- Epstein-Barr virus mononucleosis
- Cytomegalovirus mononucleosis
- Rat-bite fever
- Adult Still disease
- Drug fever
- Kikuchi disease
- Idiopathic granulomatosis

BILIARY TRACT
- Subactue cholangitis
- Periarteritis nodosa
- Gallbladder wall abscess

BONE MARROW
- Lymphomas
- Carcinomas
- Miliary tuberculosis
- Histoplasmosis
- Brucellosis
- Typhoid fever

ployed to differentiate malignant from benign fevers. The mechanism of action is obscure, but nevertheless experience suggests that this simple and safe noninvasive test differentiates neoplastic from infectious fever. This test should be used because this is a frequently difficult diagnostic problem, but results should be interpreted with caution, as is the case with all laboratory test results.[51, 52]

Imaging Tests

Noninvasive imaging techniques have made the diagnosis of many cryptic processes presenting with prolonged fevers possible. Abdominal ultrasonography has been useful in detecting intrahepatic, intrasplenic, intrarenal, and perinephric mass lesions. Percutaneous or transesophageal echocardiography has been useful in detecting vegetations and intracardiac myxomas. CT and MRI have been most sensitive in detecting intracranial, intraabdominal, and pelvic pathologic processes. CT and MRI are the best way to detect retroperitoneal lymphomas or subacute vertebral osteomyelitis. The diagnosis of intraabdominal and pelvic abscesses has been greatly improved by CT and MRI, and fewer of these diseases present now as FUOs. Gallium and indium scans are useful in detecting abscesses or malignant neoplasms, but these scans are associated with problems of false-positive and false-negative findings and should be interpreted with caution. Gallium scans should be employed early in the diagnostic work-up, and abnormal findings should be confirmed by CT and MRI. Steroids and a variety of antibiotics may cause false-negative results of gallium scans.[53–56]

Invasive techniques usually provide the definitive diagnosis in many patients with FUO. Because most of the neoplastic and infectious diseases that result in FUO invade the reticuloendothelial system, liver biopsy and bone marrow biopsy are important diagnostic procedures in patients with clinical or laboratory involvement of these organ systems. Liver biopsy may be the only way to make a diagnosis of miliary tuberculosis, or metastatic carcinoma, if the deposits are small and below the resolution of liver or spleen on gallium and indium scanning.[57] Bone marrow biopsy may provide the diagnosis in patients with lymphoma, miliary tuberculosis, or typhoid fever. Small bowel biopsy is indicated in patients with the possibility of intestinal lymphoma or Whipple's disease. Patients with findings suggesting a CNS source should have a lumbar puncture, which may provide clues to the presence of meningeal carcinomatosis, lymphocytic choriomeningitis, HIV infection, CNS lymphoma, or basilar meningitis due to tuberculosis or sarcoidosis. If temporal arteritis is a reasonable diagnostic possibility, biopsy of the affected segments of the artery is usually diagnostic. A trial of low-dose steroids would support the diagnosis of giant cell arteritis when there is shoulder stiffness and rapid ESR, when temporal biopsy is not possible.[58]

Prolonged Fevers in Special Populations

The classic definition of FUO has stood the test of time. Petersdorf and Beeson's original inclusion criteria remain valid and eliminate the many infectious and noninfectious diseases that present with prolonged fever but are diagnosed and treated before 3 weeks of clinical illness. Acute FUO, a newer category, is a contradiction in terms and should not be used. Similarly, FUO in special populations (e.g., the elderly, pediatric patients, neutropenic patients, hospitalized patients, and HIV-infected patients) has been proposed. The causes of FUOs in these subgroups reflect the usual diseases causing prolonged fevers in these settings, but the reclassification of FUOs by specific subgroup population offers no advantage in diagnosis or understanding and has no useful clinical purpose or advantage.[29, 59, 60]

Because the pathogens in HIV-infected patients with FUO are different from those in the non–HIV-infected population, it may be helpful to consider this subgroup separately[61] (Table 189–6).

Episodic or Recurrent Fevers of Unknown Origin

Fevers lasting months or years limit diagnostic possibilities to a relatively small number of diseases, which should be used to guide the diagnostic approach.[62]

TABLE 189–6 ■ Fever of Unknown Origin in Human Immunodeficiency Virus Infection

INFECTIOUS CAUSES

Common*
Human immunodeficiency virus
Mycobacterium tuberculosis
Mycobacterium avium-intracellulare
Cytomegalovirus
Pneumocystis carinii pneumonia

Uncommon
Sinusitis
Toxoplasmosis
Mycobacteria other than *M. tuberculosis* and *M. avium-intracellulare*

NONINFECTIOUS CAUSES
Drug fever

*Leishmaniasis and histoplasmosis in patients from endemic areas.

An interesting subgroup of FUO patients are those with episodic or recurrent fevers. These patients have bona fide FUOs and in addition have prolonged fever of the episodic or recurrent type. FUOs with prolonged fever are usually noninfectious, multisystem, relapsing diseases. The diagnostic approach should reflect the predominant noninfectious disease entities in this subgroup of patients[62] (Table 189–7).

Therapy for Fevers of Unknown Origin

Therapeutic trials of antibiotics for FUOs are to be discouraged and are rarely justifiable. True culture-negative endocarditis is uncommon, and an empirical trial of antimicrobial therapy should not be applied to patients with a fever and heart murmur in lieu of a thorough search of another cause of the prolonged elevated temperatures. Extrapulmonary tuberculosis may be difficult to diagnose, and clinically silent dissemination may occur in patients taking steroids or in

TABLE 189–7 ■ Recurrent or Episodic Fevers of Unknown Origin

INFECTIOUS CAUSES	NONINFECTIOUS CAUSES
Common	**Common**
Chronic prostatitis	Adult Still disease
Subacute cholangitis	Familial Mediterranean fever
	Crohn disease
	Drug fever
	Hodgkin's lymphoma
	Hyperimmunoglobulinemia D syndrome
Uncommon	**Uncommon**
Fever, aphthous ulcers, pharyngitis, and adenopathy (FAPA) syndrome	Ankylosing spondylitis
Dental abscess	Factitious fever
	Granulomatous hepatitis
	Carcinoma
	Atrial myxoma
	Fabry disease
	Gaucher disease
	Castleman disease
	Fume fever
	Hypersensitivity pneumonitis
	Deafness, urticaria, amyloidosis
	Hypertriglyceridemia (type V)
	Cholesterol emboli

elderly patients. Therefore, because miliary tuberculosis and CNS tuberculosis are frequently difficult to diagnose, an empirical trial of antituberculosis treatment is not unreasonable and may be lifesaving.[33, 58]

References

1. Petersdorf RO, Beeson PB: Fever of unexplained origin: Report on 100 cases. Medicine (Baltimore) 40:1, 1961.
2. Keefer CS: The diagnosis of the causes of obscure fever. Tex State J Med 35:203, 1939.
3. Hamman L, Wainwright CW: The diagnosis of obscure fever. I. The diagnosis of unexplained, long-continued, low-grade fever. Bull Johns Hopkins Hosp 58:109, 1936.
4. Gleckman R, Crowley M, Esposito A: Fever of unknown origin: A view from the community hospital. Am J Med Sci 274:21, 1977.
5. Esposito AL, Gleckman RA: Fever of unknown origin in the elderly. J Am Geriatr Soc 26:498, 1978.
6. Tumulty PA: The patient with fever of undetermined origin. A diagnostic approach. Johns Hopkins Med J 95:120, 1967.
7. Wolff SM, Fauci SS, Dale DC: Unusual etiologies of fever and their evaluation. Annu Rev Med 26:277, 1975.
8. Weinstein L: Clinically benign fever of unknown origin: A personal retrospective. Rev Infect Dis 7:692, 1985.
9. Hurley DL: Fever in adults. What to do when the cause is not obvious. Postgrad Med J 74:232, 1983.
10. Brusch JL, Weinstein L: Fever of unknown origin. Med Clin North Am 72:1247, 1988.
11. Smith JW: Southwestern Internal Medicine Conference: Fever of undetermined origin: Not what it used to be. Am J Med Sci 292:56, 1986.
12. Kauffman CA, Jones PG: Diagnosing fever of unknown origin in older patients. Geriatrics 39:46, 1984.
13. Welsby PD: Pyrexia of unknown origin sixty years on. Postgrad Med J 61:887, 1985.
14. Kerttula V, Hirvonen P, Pettersson T: Fever of unknown origin: A follow-up investigation. Scand J Infect Dis 15:185, 1983.
15. Cunha BA: Fever of unknown origin in the elderly. Geriatrics 37:30, 1982.
16. Louria DB: Fever of unknown etiology. Del Med J 43:343, 1971.
17. Larsen EB, Feathersone HJ, Petersdorf RG: Fever of undetermined origin: Diagnosis and follow-up of 105 cases, 1970–1980. Medicine (Baltimore) 61:269, 1982.
18. Petersdorf RG: FUO: How it has changed in 20 years. Hosp Pract 20:84, 1985.
19. Gleckman RA, Esposito AL: Fever of unknown origin in the elderly: Diagnosis and treatment. Geriatrics 41:45, 1986.
20. Greenberg SB, Taber L: Fever of unknown origin. *In* Mackowiak P (ed): Fever: Basic Mechanisms and Management. New York, Raven Press, 1991, pp 183–193.
21. Kernbaum S: Miscellaneous causes of unexplained fever. *In* Isaac B, Kernbaum S, Burke M (eds): Unexplained Fever. Boca Raton, FL, CRC Press, 1991, pp 393–404.
22. Barbado FJ, Vazquez JJ, Pena JM, et al: Pyrexia of unknown origin: Changing spectrum of diseases in two consecutive series. Postgrad Med J 68:884, 1992.
23. Gartner JC Jr: Fever of unknown origin. Adv Pediatr Infect Dis 7:1, 1992.
24. Knockaert DC: Fever of unknown origin: A literature survey. Acta Clin Belg 47:42, 1992.
25. Knockaert DC, Vanneste LJ, Vanneste SB, et al: Fever of unknown origin in the 1980s. An update of the diagnostic spectrum. Arch Intern Med 152:51, 1992.
26. Shoji S, Imamura A, Imai Y, et al: Fever of unknown origin: A review of 80 patients from the Shin'etsu area of Japan from 1986–1992. Intern Med 33:74, 1994.
27. Iikuni Y, Okada J, Kondo H, et al: Current fever of unknown origin 1982–1992. Intern Med 33:67, 1994.
28. Dinarello CA, Wolff SM: Pathogenesis of fever and the acute phase response. *In* Mandel GL, Bennett JE, Dolin R (eds): Principles and Practice of Infectious Diseases, ed 4. New York, John Wiley & Sons, 1995, pp 530–561.
29. Durack DT, Street AC: Fever of unknown origin—Reexamined and redefined. *In* Remington JS, Swartz MN (eds): Current Clinical Topics in Infectious Diseases, Vol II. Boston, Blackwell Scientific Publications, 1991, pp 35–51.
30. Kazanjian PH: Fever of unknown origin: Review of 86 patients treated in community hospitals. Clin Infect Dis 15:968, 1992.
31. Drenth JPH, Haagsma CJ, van der Meer JWM, et al: Hyperimmunoglobulinemia D and periodic fever syndrome. Medicine (Baltimore) 73:133, 1994.
32. Cunha BA: Clinical implications of fever. Postgrad Med 85:188, 1989.
33. Harris HW, Menitove S: Miliary tuberculosis. *In* Schlossberg D (ed): Tuberculosis, ed 3. New York, Springer-Verlag, 1994, pp 233–245.
34. Rubin RH, Weinstein L: Salmonellosis: Microbiologic, Pathologic and Clinical Features. New York, Stratton International Medical Book Corporation, 1977.
35. Krick JA, Remington JA: Toxoplasmosis in the adult—An overview. N Engl J Med 298:550, 1978.
36. Monir Madkour M: Brucellosis. London, Butterworth, 1989.
37. Calabro JJ, Marchesano JM: Juvenile rheumatoid arthritis. N Engl J Med 277:696, 1967.
38. Fauchald P, Rygvold O, Oipstese B: Temporal arteritis and polymyalgia rheumatica. Ann Intern Med 77:845, 1972.
39. Weinberger A, Kessler A, Pinkhas J: Fever in various rheumatic diseases. Clin Rheumatol 4:258, 1985.
40. Fauci AS, Haynes B, Katz P: The spectrum of vasculitis. Ann Intern Med 89:660, 1978.
41. Wu YJJ, Martin BR, Ong K, et al: Takayasu's arteritis presenting as a cause of fever of unknown origin. Am J Med 87:476, 1989.
42. Bailey EM, Klein NC, Cunha BA: Kikuchi's disease with liver dysfunction presenting as fever of unknown origin. Lancet 2:986, 1989.
43. Kapadia V, Robinson BA, Angus HB: Kikuchi's disease presenting as fever of unknown origin. Lancet 2:1519, 1989.
44. Pearl D, Strauchen JA: Kikuchi's disease as a cause of fever of unknown origin. N Engl J Med 320:1147, 1989.
45. Rudniki C, Kessler E, Zarfati M, et al: Kikuchi's necrotizing lymphadenitis: A cause of fever of unknown origin and splenomegaly. Acta Haematol 79:99, 1988.
46. Cunha BA: Drug fever. Postgrad Med 80:123, 1986.
47. Mackowiak PA: Southwestern Internal Medicine Conference: Drug fever: Mechanisms, maxims and misconceptions. Am J Med Sci 294:275, 1987.
48. Tisdale WA, Klatskin G: The fever of Laennec's cirrhosis. Yale J Biol Med 33:94, 1960.
49. Lischner MW, Alexander JF, Galambos JT: Natural history of alcoholic hepatitis. The acute disease. Am J Dig Dis 16:181, 1971.
50. Simon HB, Wolff SM: Granulomatous hepatitis and prolonged fever of unknown origin. A study of 13 patients. Medicine (Baltimore) 52:1, 1973.
51. Telente A, Hermans PE: Idiopathic granulomatosis manifesting as fever of unknown origin. Mayo Clin Proc 64:44, 1989.
52. Murray HW: Factitious or fraudulent fever. *In* Murray HW (ed): FUO: Fever of Undetermined Origin. Mount Kisco, NY, Futura Publishing, 1983, pp 87–108.
53. Knockaert DC: Diagnostic strategy for fever of unknown origin in the ultrasonography and computed tomography era. Acta Clin Belg 47:100, 1992.
54. Palestro CJ: The current role of gallium imaging in infection. Semin Nucl Med 24:128, 1994.
55. Sen P, Louria DB: Non-invasive and diagnostic procedures and laboratory methods. *In* Murray HW (ed): FUO: Fever of Undetermined Origin. Mount Kisco, NY, Futura Publishing, 1983, pp 159–190.
56. Knockaert D, Mortelmans LA, De Roo MC, et al: Clinical value of gallium-67 scintigraphy in evaluation of fever of unknown origin. Clin Infect Dis 18:60, 1994.
57. Holtz T, Moseley RH, Scheiman JM: Liver biopsy in fever of unknown origin. A reappraisal. J Clin Gastroenterol 17:29, 1993.
58. Klein NC, Cunha BA: Treatment of fever of unknown origin. *In* Schlossberg D (ed): Current Therapy of Infectious Disease. Philadelphia, CV Mosby, 1996, pp 1–3.
59. Anceno-Reyes RI: Acute fevers of unknown origin. Arch Intern Med 154:2253, 1994.

60. DiNubile MJ: Acute fevers of unknown origin. A plea for restraint. Arch Intern Med 153:2525, 1993.
61. Bissuel F, Leport C, Perronne C, et al: Fever of unknown origin in HIV-infected patients: A critical analysis of a retrospective series of 57 cases. J Intern Med 236:529, 1994.
62. Knockaert DC, Vanneste LJ, Bobbaers HJ: Recurrent or episodic fever of unknown origin. Review of 45 cases and review of the literature. Medicine (Baltimore) 72:184, 1993.

190

Toxic Shock Syndrome

Patrick M. Schlievert
Kristine L. MacDonald

History

Staphylococcal toxic shock syndrome (TSS) is an acute multisystem illness characterized by fever, hypotension, erythematous rash, desquamation of the skin on recovery, and a variable multiorgan component. The illness has been reported in the literature sporadically since 1927, principally as staphylococcal scarlet fever, but it was brought to the attention of the medical community as a major entity in 1978 by Todd and coworkers,[1] who also renamed the illness. These investigators noted the association with *Staphylococcus aureus*, mainly of phage group I. Since their article was published, a large number of articles have provided additional clinical information, epidemiologic risk factors, and determinants of pathogenicity in a relatively short time. A TSS-like illness has also been described that is associated with group A streptococcal infection.[2, 3] Both staphylococcal TSS and streptococcal TSS are discussed in this chapter.

Characteristics of the Pathogen

S. aureus is a gram-positive coccus that grows in clusters and causes more infections than perhaps any other bacterium, ranging from mild or subclinical to life threatening. The organisms are facultative anaerobes and are categorized into five major groups, designated lytic groups I, II, III, IV, and "not allotted," on the basis of lysis by bacteriophages. In addition, a large number of nontypeable organisms occur.

It is now generally accepted that staphylococcal TSS is caused by certain strains of *S. aureus*; coagulase-negative strains do not appear to be associated with TSS. Numerous studies indicate that TSS toxin 1 (TSST-1) is the cause of all or nearly all menstrual cases[4, 5] and approximately half of nonmenstrual cases.[6] The toxin, which was formerly known as pyrogenic exotoxin type C, or enterotoxin F, is capable of inducing TSS symptoms in experimental animals, notably rabbits.[7] It has been shown that enterotoxins B and C are the causes of nearly 50% of nonmenstrual cases, approximately 47% and 1% to 3%, respectively.[6] Other enterotoxins may also rarely cause the illness.

S. aureus strains that make TSST-1 do not make enterotoxin B but may simultaneously express enterotoxin A or C. The mechanism for this toxin exclusion is not known. The role of enterotoxins A and C in TSS, made by TSST-1–positive strains, is unknown, because TSST-1 clearly can induce severe illness in their absence. Other unique characteristics of TSS-associated *S. aureus* are listed in Table 190–1.

A large number of coagulase-negative staphylococci isolated from TSS patients and unused tampons have been examined for TSS toxins; none has been found to make toxins, and all were negative when tested for the TSST-1 gene *(tst)*.[8]

The majority of streptococcal TSS is caused by group A streptococcal strains, but groups B, C, F, and G occasionally cause the illness. Most of the group A streptococcal strains associated with TSS belong to M protein types 1 and 3, but other M types may also be associated.[9, 10] Group A streptococci *(Streptococcus pyogenes)* are β-hemolytic, catalase-negative, gram-positive cocci that grow in chains and cause large numbers of mucous membrane (pharyngitis) and skin (impetigo) acute inflammatory infections. The organisms also cause invasive infections (including streptococcal TSS) and delayed sequelae, including rheumatic fever, acute glomerulonephritis, and erythema nodosum. Group A streptococci are aerotolerant anaerobes and are serotyped on the basis of surface, antiphagocytic M protein, of which 80 types have been identified. Large numbers of nontypeable organisms also occur; these organisms presumably have M proteins, but they have not been characterized. Immunity against group A streptococci depends on development of opsonic antibody against M protein.

Group A streptococci that cause TSS have been associated with production of streptococcal pyrogenic exotoxin (SPE, scarlet fever toxins) superantigens, notably types A and C but also type B (which has been characterized as a cysteine protease) and type F (mitogenic factor) and streptococcal superantigen.[9–13]

Pyrogenic toxin superantigens are a large family of proteins, secreted by *S. aureus* and group A streptococci, that share biologic activity and in many instances amino acid sequence similarity.[14] All these toxins (TSST-1; the staphylococcal enterotoxin serotypes A, B, C1, C2, C3, D, E, G, and H; and the SPE serotypes A, B, C, and F and streptococcal superantigen) are relatively low molecular weight (20,000 to 30,000), simple proteins that are secreted into the culture medium primarily in the late logarithmic phase of growth (SPE-B is primarily made during late stationary phase). The toxins induce fever, enhance host susceptibility to lethal endotoxin shock, nonspecifically stimulate T-lymphocyte proliferation, and induce sustained release of cytokines from both macrophages and T lymphocytes. The T-lymphocyte proliferation results in interferon-γ release sufficient to suppress immunoglobulin synthesis in experimental animals and amplify delayed hypersensitivity, which may explain the erythematous rash and erythrophagocytosis seen in TSS ill-

TABLE 190–1 ■ Phenotypic Characteristics of Toxic Shock Syndrome–Associated *Staphylococcus aureus*

Approximately 75% are positive for toxic shock syndrome toxin 1 (TSST-1), 23% are positive for enterotoxin B, and 2% are positive for enterotoxin C or another enterotoxin type.
Most do not express α-hemolysin.
Most belong to phage group I or are not typeable; not associated with phage group II.
Most lack plasmids.
TSST-1–positive strains are typically resistant to cadmium, arsenate, penicillin, and ampicillin.
Most strains are susceptible to antibiotics other than penicillin and ampicillin.
Many strains that make enterotoxins B or C, although not making TSST-1, are methacillin resistant.
Most express large amounts of protease.

nesses.[15] The shared properties of the toxins are summarized in Table 190–2. The staphylococcal enterotoxins have the additional capacity, not shared with other pyrogenic toxin superantigens, to induce vomiting and diarrhea after oral administration; this property may depend in part on the ability of the toxins to resist proteolysis in the gut. The scarlet fever toxins are also more capable than other pyrogenic toxins of inducing myocardial damage. Finally, TSST-1 has the unique property of being able to reactivate arthritis in experimental animals.

Because the pyrogenic toxin superantigens have in common many biologic activities, it may be expected that they share structural similarities. This is not obvious from primary sequence determination in which TSST-1 and SPE-C have little if any similarity with enterotoxins or other SPEs. However, SPE-A shares highly significant sequence similarity with enterotoxins B and C. Furthermore, enterotoxins A, D, and E share highly significant primary sequence similarity. The crystal structures of TSST-1[16] and of enterotoxins A,[17] B,[18] and C[19] and the modeled structure of SPE-A indicate that the three-dimensional structures of the toxins are highly similar (Fig. 190–1). All of the toxins have a short N-terminal α-helix of amino acids followed by a barrel (or claw) of β-strands that compose domain B. Domain B is connected to a wall of β-strands in domain A by a central diagonal α-helix. The enterotoxins have a loop of amino acids (referred to as a cystine loop) that is not present in TSST-1. Minor other differences in structure are seen in some of the toxins.

All of the toxins have been cloned and sequenced.[20–31] The toxin genes are variable traits, being present in some strains and not in others. SPE-A and SPE-C and staphylococcal enterotoxin A are phage encoded, whereas the remainder of the toxins appear to be present mainly in the bacterial genome on mobile elements. In the majority of strains expressing phage-encoded toxins, the phages are defective and thus are incapable of being excised from the chromosome.

Several animal models for the study of TSS have been developed, most in rabbits, and observations indicate that pyrogenic toxin superantigens have the ability to induce TSS illness. In one type of experiment, isogenic pairs of *Staphylococcus* strains that differ only in ability to express pyrogenic toxin superantigen were used to examine toxin role in TSS.[32] Only the toxin-positive organism was capable of inducing TSS symptoms. In another set of experiments, several members of the pyrogenic toxin family (TSST-1; enterotoxins A, B, and C1; and SPE-A and SPE-C) were implanted subcutaneously in miniosmotic pumps designed to release toxin during a 7-day period.[7, 33] On administration of approximately 100 μg of toxin to a 1- to 2-kg rabbit, typical TSS symptoms were seen, which culminated in death. It appears that continuous exposure to the toxins for a period of days is necessary for the development of TSS symptoms, because single injections of up to 1 mg per animal often do not produce TSS manifestations. The need for continuous exposure to toxin is consistent with the observation that menstrual TSS most often begins on the third or fourth day of menstruation, in spite of the fact that numbers of *S. aureus* grow in the vagina early in menstruation. Finally, studies with viable group A streptococci administered to rabbits indicate that immunity against SPE-A can protect the animals from both streptococcal TSS and necrotizing fasciitis due to M1 and M3 organisms.[34] However, SPE-A alone does not have the ability to cause necrotizing fasciitis despite having the capacity to cause TSS. It appeared that other streptococcal factors were required to induce soft tissue necrosis.

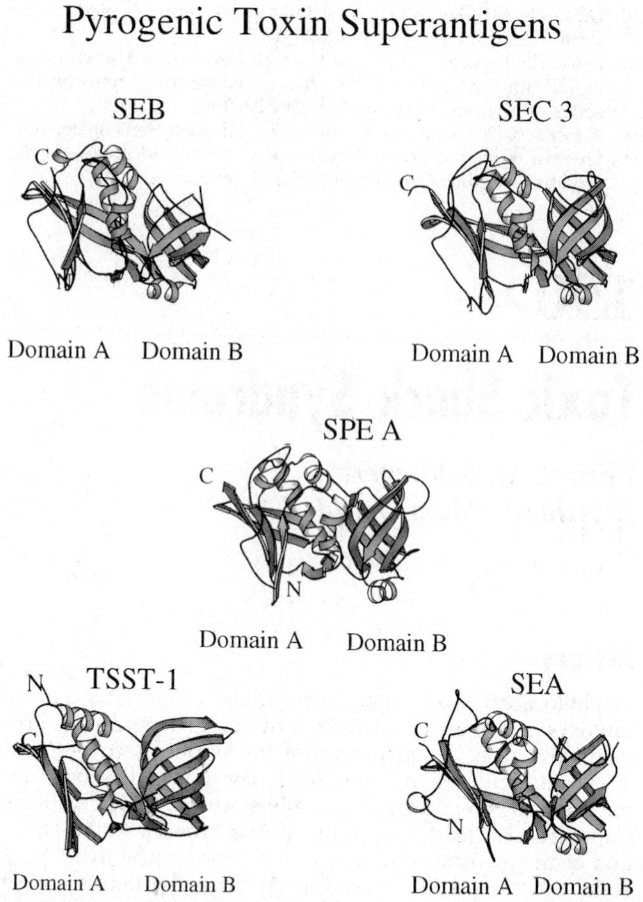

FIGURE 190–1 □ Ribbon diagrams of the three-dimensional structures of toxic shock syndrome–associated toxins, including enterotoxins (SEs) A, B, and C; toxic shock syndrome toxin 1 (TSST-1); and streptococcal pyrogenic exotoxin (SPE) A.

TABLE 190–2 ■ Shared Properties of Toxic Shock Syndrome–Associated Pyrogenic Toxin Superantigens

BIOCHEMICAL

Relatively low molecular weight (20,000–30,000), simple proteins, secreted mainly in late logarithmic phase of growth

Relatively resistant to heat and protease treatment

BIOLOGIC

Pyrogenicity

Enhancement of susceptibility to endotoxin shock and cellular killing

Nonspecific T-lymphocyte mitogenicity (superantigenicity) results in
- B-cell immunosuppression
- Rash
- Erythrophagocytosis
- Lymphokine release (tumor necrosis factor-β, interferon-γ, interleukin-2)

Induction of monokine release from macrophages (tumor necrosis factor-α, interleukin-1)

Alteration of liver clearance function

Epidemiology

The epidemiology of TSS can best be examined by reviewing available studies on disease caused by *S. aureus* and *S. pyogenes* separately. Most of the major epidemiologic studies on TSS caused by *S. aureus* infection were conducted in the 1980s. Although TSS caused by *S. aureus* was first described by Todd and coworkers in 1987, interest in TSS caused by *S. aureus* increased dramatically with publication of a report from the Centers for Disease Control and Prevention (CDC) describing cases in healthy young women.[35] Numerous studies were subsequently conducted to determine the incidence of disease and risk factors for its occurrence. Cases of TSS caused by *S. aureus* can be broken down into menstruation-associated cases and nonmenstrual cases. A large proportion of cases recognized in the early 1980s were menstruation associated and related to use of high-absorbency tampons. With changes in the tampon industry, the number of menstrual cases has declined significantly, and thus the total incidence has decreased substantially as well. In contrast, cases of TSS associated with *S. pyogenes* in the United States first received a high level of attention after a report of 20 patients published by Stevens and coworkers[3] in 1989. Most patients in that case series presented with soft tissue streptococcal infections, and all except one developed TSS.

Trends in Disease Occurrence of Toxic Shock Syndrome Caused by Staphylococcus aureus Infection

In the early 1980s, three states conducted active surveillance to ascertain the incidence of TSS in their respective areas.[36–38] Results of these surveillance projects demonstrated the following: the incidence was 9.0 cases per 100,000 women aged 12 to 45 years in Minnesota, 12.3 per 100,000 women aged 12 to 49 years in Utah, and 6.2 per 100,000 women aged 12 to 49 years in Wisconsin. In 1986, the CDC conducted an active surveillance project for TSS in Los Angeles County and in the states of Missouri, New Jersey, Oklahoma, Tennessee, and Washington.[39] The overall incidence of TSS detected in this surveillance project was 0.53 case per 100,000 persons with an incidence of 1.05 cases per 100,000 women aged 15 to 44 years. The cumulative incidence varied by geographic region and ranged from 1.23 per 100,000 in Oklahoma to 0.22 per 100,000 in New Jersey. The highest incidence in women aged 15 to 44 years was 2.04 per 100,000 and also occurred in Oklahoma. Results of these different surveillance projects indicate that the incidence of TSS declined during the 1980s.

In addition to active surveillance projects conducted in selected geographic areas, several studies have examined hospital discharge data as a method to ascertain valid estimates for the incidence of TSS. To date, three major studies have been conducted.[40–42] Results of a study performed in Colorado demonstrated that the incidence in selected counties was relatively high between 1974 and 1982, with 16 cases per 100,000 women 10 to 30 years of age.[40] A second study conducted in California demonstrated that the incidence of TSS was 2.4 cases per 100,000 women 15 to 34 years of age during the time interval 1972 through 1983.[41] Because these two studies used similar case definitions and methods of identifying cases, these data suggest that geographic variations in the incidence of TSS can occur. A third study evaluated data from the Commission on Professional and Hospital Activities, Professional Activities Study.[42] The data were used to project the incidence for the U.S. population in 1981 and 1982; results were 0.78 cases per 100,000 and 0.84 cases per 100,000, respectively.

A third mechanism for obtaining surveillance data is through passive surveillance. The CDC has conducted national passive surveillance for TSS since 1980. This system demonstrated a peak in the incidence of cases in mid-1980, with a consistent decline in incidence since that time. The peak in 1980 was in part due to publicity about the syndrome and enhanced surveillance activities that occurred at that time. Approximately 325 menstruation-associated cases meeting the strict case definition were identified in 1980. Since 1986, fewer than 50 menstrual cases have been reported each year.[43] Although the decline may in part reflect a decrease in reporting, it is consistent with active surveillance data that also demonstrated a decline in incidence from 1980 to 1986.[43, 44]

In the CDC passive surveillance system, 93% of cases have occurred in women.[44] These data are similar to results from the three studies involving hospital record reviews, in which the proportion of cases occurring in women ranged from 92% in the California study to 77% in the Colorado study.[40, 41] Available studies have indicated that the highest age-specific incidence rates have consistently occurred in young adult women (between the ages of 15 and 19 years).

Menstruation-Associated Toxic Shock Syndrome Caused by Staphylococcus aureus Infection

When TSS was first widely recognized in 1980, multiple studies confirmed the association between use of tampons and onset of TSS in menstruating women.[36–38, 45, 46] In addition, early studies demonstrated elevated odds ratios for the use of Rely tampons compared with the use of other brands.[36, 37, 46] As a result of these studies, Rely tampons were taken off the market in September 1980. One of the early studies demonstrated not only an increased risk related to the use of these particular tampons but also an increased risk related to the use of all tampons with high absorbency.[36] Two subsequent studies confirmed these findings and demonstrated that the risk for TSS increased proportionately to the absorbency of tampon brand used.[47, 48] In one of these studies, the odds ratio was 1.34 per g of increase in absorbency.[48]

In 1985, polyacrylate was removed from tampons. Because tampons containing polyacrylate were generally of high absorbency, this led to a decrease in availability of high-absorbency tampons in the United States. Data from the CDC passive surveillance system suggest that the incidence of TSS decreased after the withdrawal of polyacrylate-containing products from the market.[43, 44] This finding lends further support to other studies that have demonstrated an increased risk for menstruation-associated TSS among users of high-absorbency tampons. Although the number of reported menstrual cases of TSS has declined substantially since the peak was identified in the early 1980s, menstruation-associated cases still occur and account for more than 50% of TSS cases in women of reproductive age.[49]

Women who have had a single episode of TSS are at increased risk for developing a second episode.[50] Women who are not treated with antibiotics and continue to use tampons are at highest risk for recurrence, and women who are treated with antibiotics and discontinue tampon use are at lowest risk for recurrence.[50] The high recurrence rate indicates that some women remain susceptible to TSS after an initial episode. This may be related to an absence of or delay in immunologic response to TSST-1.

Nonmenstrual Toxic Shock Syndrome Caused by Staphylococcus aureus Infection

Nonmenstrual cases of TSS caused by *S. aureus* have been reported in a variety of settings, including skin and soft tissue infections, such as periodontal abscesses; superinfection of existing skin lesions caused by varicella-zoster virus and burns; primary staphylococcal soft tissue infections; and postoperatively.[51–54] TSS has also been associated with a variety of respiratory tract infections, including sinusitis, pharyngitis, tracheitis, and rhinoplasty with nasal packing.[55–60] Cases have also been described after infection with influenza virus.[61–63] Some of the postinfluenza cases have occurred in the absence of overt clinical evidence of *S. aureus* pneumonia or purulent bacterial tracheitis, suggesting that TSS resulted from colonization of the respiratory tract with a toxigenic strain of *S. aureus*.

Postpartum cases of TSS have been recognized after both vaginal and cesarean deliveries.[51] Use of barrier contraceptives has also been demonstrated to be a risk factor for nonmenstrual TSS.[64, 65] Of 383 nonmenstrual TSS cases reported through 1986 to the CDC passive surveillance system, 26 occurred in women using the contraceptive sponge and 33 occurred in women using the contraceptive diaphragm.[44]

Toxic Shock Syndrome Caused by Streptococcus pyogenes

TSS caused by *S. pyogenes* was first described by Cone and coworkers[2] in 1987. Subsequently, streptococcal TSS was further characterized by a report of 20 patients identified in the Rocky Mountain region.[3] Of the 20 patients described by Stevens and coworkers,[3] 19 had shock and most had associated soft tissue infections. Seven (35%) had underlying risk factors for disease, including diabetes, obesity, alcoholism, cerebellar ataxia, or intravenous drug use. The median age of patients was 35 years, and 16 of the patients were younger than 60 years.

Few data are available on the incidence of streptococcal TSS. Two studies have assessed incidence rates for invasive group A streptococcal disease, but neither study specifically reported the incidence of disease caused by streptococcal TSS. The first incidence study was a retrospective medical record review of cases of invasive group A streptococcal disease occurring between April 1985 and March 1990 in hospitals located in Pima County, Arizona.[66] In that study, the overall incidence rate of invasive group A streptococcal disease was 4.3 per 100,000 population. TSS occurred in 6 (8%) of 74 patients identified during 1988, 1989, and the first 3 months of 1990. However, TSS did not occur in any of 54 patients with invasive disease occurring between April 1985 and December 1987. On the basis of this finding, the authors concluded that the incidence of streptococcal TSS had increased in Pima County during the 5 years under observation. A single prospective population-based study on the incidence of invasive group A streptococcal infections has been published.[67] During 1992 and 1993, these investigators conducted active surveillance of invasive group A streptococcal disease in Ontario, Canada. Three hundred twenty-three patients were identified, for an annual incidence rate of 1.5 cases per 100,000 population; 42 (13%) of these patients were classified as having streptococcal TSS. The patients with TSS were older than other patients (median age of 61 years compared with a median age of 38 years), more likely to have underlying chronic illnesses (71% compared with 51%), and less likely to have nosocomial disease (2% compared with 15%). The overall case-fatality rate for patients with streptococcal TSS was 81% compared with 5% of invasive group A streptococcal cases without TSS. Streptococcal TSS occurred in 11 (55%) of 20 patients with necrotizing fasciitis compared with 31 (10%) of 303 patients who had invasive group A streptococcal disease with a diagnosis other than necrotizing fasciitis.

The population-based surveillance project in Ontario also involved follow-up of household members to identify subsequent cases in households.[68] The authors estimated that the risk for developing invasive group A streptococcal infection (not specifically limited to TSS) was 2.9 per 100,000 among household members, almost 200 times the risk in the general population. These data suggest that the use of chemoprophylaxis among household contacts of patients with severe invasive group A streptococcal disease, including streptococcal TSS, may be warranted. However, the level of risk to household members needs to be clarified by additional surveillance studies. Furthermore, the efficacy of chemoprophylaxis in actually preventing subsequent disease in household contacts remains unknown. Therefore, no public health recommendations on this issue have yet been made.

Two community-based outbreaks of invasive group A streptococcal infection, including TSS, have been reported.[68, 69] One outbreak involved seven cases of severe invasive group A streptococcal disease, including four with TSS. All cases occurred in three adjacent southeastern Minnesota counties during a 3-month period. Epidemiologic investigation demonstrated a high rate of carriage of the outbreak clone of group A streptococcus among children attending an elementary school in the outbreak area.[68] The other outbreak involved 13 cases, 5 with streptococcal TSS, in the Shenandoah Valley of Virginia between December 1, 1994, and the end of February 1995.[69]

Pathogenesis

A model for the production of TSS symptoms by pyrogenic toxins is presented in Figure 190–2. The model depends primarily on the toxins' ability to alter immune system function. Several of the toxins have been shown to cause sustained release of monokines, tumor necrosis factor, and interleukin-1 from macrophages.[70–72] The effect of these two endogenous pyrogens or, in some cases, the direct action of the toxins on the hypothalamus probably explains the production of fever. In addition, monokine release has also been proposed to explain many of the other TSS symptoms, most notably hypotension and shock.

All of the pyrogenic toxin superantigens are potent nonspecific T-lymphocyte mitogens. This activity depends on two properties of the toxins: (1) the ability of the toxins to interact directly with class II major histocompatibility complex products (without the need for processing) on the surface of antigen-presenting cells[73, 74] and to be presented to T lymphocytes; and (2) the toxins' ability to bind to subsets of the variable part of the β-chain of the T-cell–receptor complex.[75, 76] Because the toxins stimulate only a subset, although without regard for antigen specificity, they have been referred to as superantigens. Both $CD4^+$ and $CD8^+$ cells are induced to proliferate.

Toxin stimulation of $CD4^+$ cells leads to production of high levels of interferon-γ, which activates macrophages and thus has been proposed to explain the TSS-associated rash as a manifestation of amplified delayed hypersensitivity. This activity may also result from release of high levels of interleukin-2. Macrophage activation also explains the erythrophagocytosis seen on autopsy in staphylococcal TSS. The high levels of interferon-γ released have been shown in experimental animals to lead to suppression of B-cell function[15] and may, therefore, explain the failure of approximately 85% of patients to develop neutralizing antibody against TSST-1 in TSST-1–associated illness. Thus, most TSS patients remain susceptible to the illness on recovery. Indeed, large numbers of recurrences have been reported, particularly in menstrual cases. Interestingly, treatment of animals with cyclosporine to prevent T-cell proliferation induced by toxins does not prevent the hypotension, shock, and death associated with the illness.

The most dramatic and potentially important biologic property of the toxins is their capacity to enhance host susceptibility to lethal endotoxin shock.[15, 77] Thus, an animal may show up to 100,000-fold enhanced susceptibility to the lethal effects of endotoxin, and this may represent picogram amounts in humans. Although it is still controversial, there is evidence to suggest that this activity plays a role in the

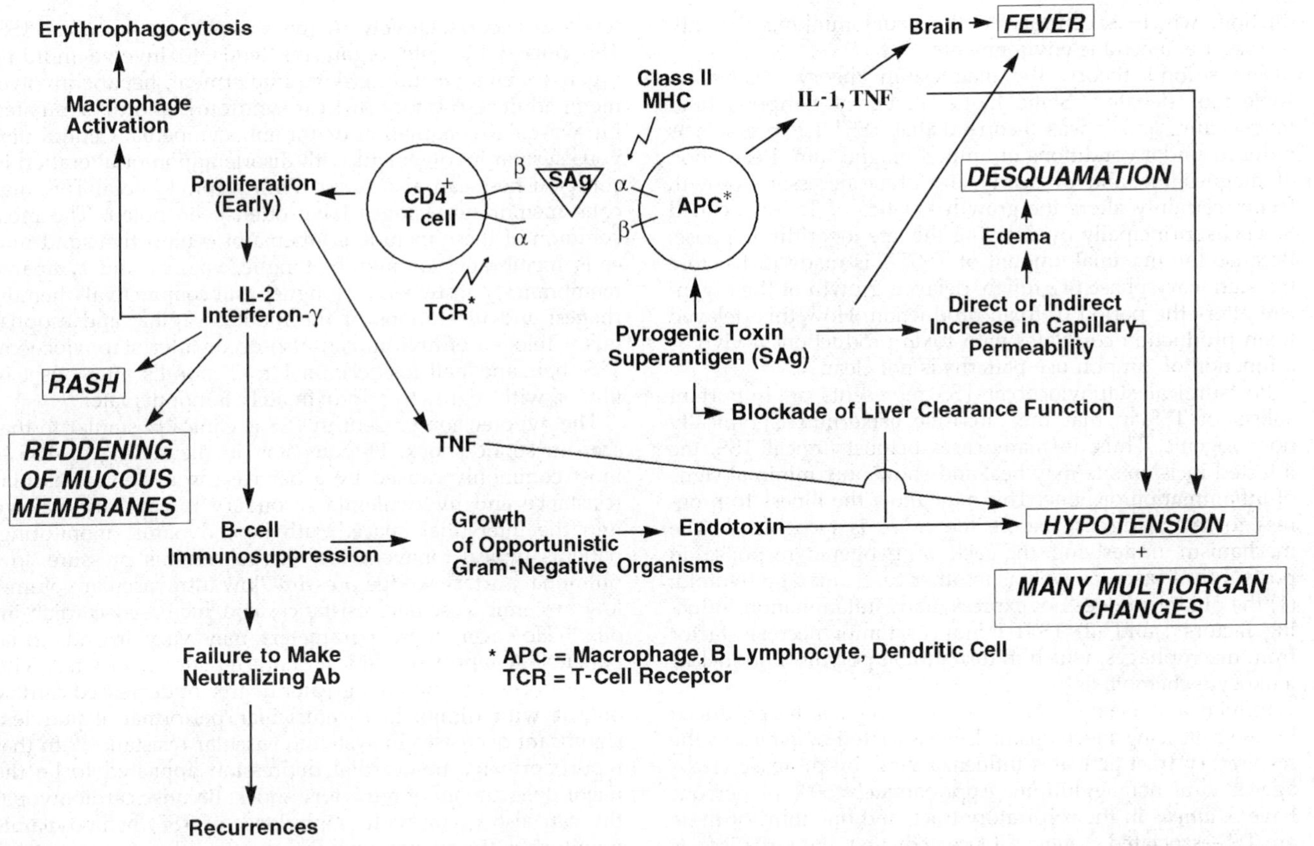

FIGURE 190–2 □ Model for the development of toxic shock syndrome and related illnesses. Ab, Antibody; IL1, interleukin-1; IL2, interleukin-2; MHC, major histocompatibility complex; SAg, superantigen; TNF, tumor necrosis factor.

most severe manifestations of TSS or at least increases the severity of illness. Studies have shown that when rabbits are given pyrogenic toxin superantigens, endotoxin appears in the circulation.[77] Also, polymyxin B blocks the lethal effect of the toxins.[77, 78] This antibiotic binds and neutralizes the active lipid A part of endotoxin. Germ-free piglets are relatively resistant to pyrogenic toxin superantigens compared with conventional animals.[79] Finally, endotoxins amplify monokine release from macrophages.[80] TSST-1 has been shown to enhance the susceptibility of rat renal tubule cells to the lethal effect of endotoxin, and this may in part explain kidney effects seen in TSS.[81]

A final noteworthy property of at least TSST-1 is its capacity to bind endothelial cells.[82] Clearly, capillary leak is a major cause of hypotension and shock in TSS, and it is possible that this results directly from toxin actions on endothelial cells and indirectly through the actions of monokines and lymphokines.

A major difference between staphylococcal and streptococcal TSS is the association of streptococcal TSS with necrotizing fasciitis, whereas soft tissue necrosis is not often associated with staphylococcal TSS. Studies in experimental animals suggest that necrotizing fasciitis depends on production of high levels of tumor necrosis factor, which appears to down-regulate chemotactic receptors on polymorphonuclear leukocytes, thus delaying phagocytosis.[34, 83] The consequence of this delay is growth of the streptococci and production of other virulence factors such as streptolysins, nucleases, and proteases (notably SPE-B) that are likely to cause the soft tissue necrosis. The reason that staphylococcal TSS is not associated with necrotizing fasciitis is unclear, but most staphylococci associated with TSS do not produce α-toxin, a major dermonecrotic virulence factor.

One of the most controversial and publicized aspects of staphylococcal TSS is the role of certain tampons in the illness. Several theories have been put forward, but only two remain as viable possibilities. Investigators have identified the physicochemical factors necessary to promote TSST-1 production (Table 190–3). Toxin production occurs in protein (or amino acid)–containing media, at 37°C to 40°C, in a pH range of 6.5 to 8, and in the presence of oxygen; the toxin is susceptible to catabolite repression by glucose.[84] With the exception of oxygen, these conditions are present in the human vagina at times of menstruation or of trauma that causes bleeding. It has been shown that tampons increase the oxygen content of the vagina to an extent that toxin can be induced.[85] These data, combined with the observation that nearly 5% of menstruating women have TSST-1–positive *S. aureus* in the vagina, have given rise to the oxygen theory for the role of tampons in TSS. Interestingly, data obtained by Todd and colleagues[86] showed that the oxygen content of staphylococcal abscesses is sufficient to permit TSST-1 pro-

TABLE 190–3 ■ Physicochemical Factors That Affect Production of Staphylococcal Toxic Shock Syndrome–Associated Toxins

Animal protein stimulates toxin production; high levels of glucose inhibit
pH 6.5–8 required for toxin production
Temperature of 37°C–40°C required for toxin production
Oxygen required for production of staphylococcal but not streptococcal toxins; carbon dioxide has variable effects, depending on medium used, sometimes stimulating toxin production and sometimes having no effect

duction, which is contrary to the usual thinking that abscesses are anaerobic environments.

The second theory, the magnesium theory, remains a subject of debate.[87] Some high-absorbency tampons bind magnesium, and it was theorized that TSST-1 expression is induced under conditions of limited magnesium. Restriction of magnesium, and of nearly any other necessary growth factor, certainly alters the growth kinetics of TSS-associated *S. aureus*, principally by delaying the late logarithmic phase. Because the maximal amount of TSST-1 is made just before the stationary phase of growth, delayed growth of the organism alters the period of toxin production. How this delayed toxin production correlates with toxin production in vivo as a function of tampon use patterns is not clear.

Postsurgical staphylococcal TSS represents an important subset of TSS in that the causative bacterium is typically nonpyogenic. Thus, in many cases of postsurgical TSS, the infected incision site may heal and show only minimal signs of inflammation or none. This may allow the illness to progress to severe disease before the cause is recognized. The mechanism underlying the lack of pyogenic response in postsurgical cases, as well as in other cases, may be twofold: (1) the organism does not express many inflammation-inducing factors[88]; and (2) TSST-1 induces tumor necrosis factor from macrophages, which in turn inhibit polymorphonuclear leukocyte chemotaxis.

Influenza-associated staphylococcal TSS *may* be produced by the following mechanism: TSS-associated *S. aureus* in the respiratory tract activates influenza virus by protease cleavage of viral hemagglutinin. Approximately 50% of persons have *S. aureus* in the respiratory tract, and one third of these are TSS-associated *S. aureus*. Once activated, the virus infects and damages cells of the respiratory tract. Finally, superinfection of the traumatized tissue by TSS-associated *S. aureus* then gives rise to toxin production and consequent TSS.

It has been shown that upper respiratory tract colonization by TSS-associated *S. aureus* is insufficient to give rise to TSS, possibly because the pH is below that required for optimal toxin production. However, after nasal surgery or influenza virus infection, sufficient traumatized tissue or blood may be present to allow toxin production. It is our experience that the majority of influenza-associated cases occur in the months of January and February and that the illness may have a case-fatality rate as high as 50%, the most severe cases occurring in children.

The physicochemical factors that influence production of the streptococcal pyrogenic toxin superantigens are similar to those required for production of staphylococcal toxins except that SPE production is independent of oxygen levels (as would be expected because streptococci are aerotolerant anaerobes) and is not as susceptible to catabolite repression by glucose (again as expected because streptococci are fermentative).

Clinical Features

The CDC has developed case definitions for TSS caused by both *S. aureus* and *S. pyogenes*.[35, 89] Both case definitions include hypotension (systolic blood pressure less than or equal to 90 mm Hg in adults or less than the fifth percentile by age for children). The case definition for TSS caused by *S. aureus* also requires fever, presence of a diffuse macular rash, and desquamation (particularly of palms and soles) 1 to 2 weeks after onset of illness. Whereas a generalized erythematous rash followed by desquamation can occur with streptococcal TSS, it is less common than with staphylococcal TSS and not an essential feature of the case definition. Conversely, soft tissue necrosis, including necrotizing fasciitis or myositis, tends to occur relatively frequently with streptococcal TSS. TSS caused by both organisms tends to involve multiple organ systems, including renal impairment, hepatic involvement, adult respiratory distress syndrome, and disseminated intravascular coagulation or thrombocytopenia. Central nervous system involvement with disorientation or alteration in consciousness can also occur. With staphylococcal TSS, mucous membrane changes have often been noted. The most common of these include erythema of conjunctivae and mucous membranes of mouth, tongue, vagina, and tympanic membranes; strawberry tongue; subconjunctival hemorrhages; and ulcerations of the mouth, vagina, and esophagus.[90] Telogen effluvium can also occur after staphylococcal TSS; hair and nail loss occurs 1 to 2 months after onset of illness, with regrowth approximately 6 months later.[91]

The hypotension present in TSS is clinically similar to that seen in septic shock. Hypotension in the setting of TSS is most commonly caused by a decrease in systemic vascular resistance and hypovolemia secondary to capillary leakage into the interstitial space. With hemodynamic monitoring, patients typically have a low central venous pressure, low pulmonary artery wedge pressure, low intravascular volume, low systemic vascular resistance, and increased cardiac index.[92] However, these parameters may vary in individual patients. A report of clinical characteristics associated with streptococcal TSS noted a greater degree of decreased cardiac output with diminished ventricular performance and less significant decreases in systemic vascular resistance.[93] In that report, primary myocardial depression appeared to be the major determinant of refractory shock. Because cardiomyopathy can also occur with staphylococcal TSS, hemodynamic monitoring of patients with TSS due to either *S. aureus* or *S. pyogenes* is particularly important to ensure that therapy is appropriate.

Diagnosis

The diagnosis of TSS can be strongly suspected on the basis of clinical presentation. However, isolation of toxin-producing *S. aureus* or *S. pyogenes* from a normally sterile body site in patients with a compatible illness is the most definitive way to make the diagnosis. Similarly, isolation of toxin-producing *S. aureus* or *S. pyogenes* from a nonsterile site (e.g., throat, sputum, vagina, superficial skin lesion, or wound) is strongly supportive of a diagnosis.

Therapy

In treating staphylococcal or streptococcal TSS, aggressive management of shock and organ system complications is essential. Correction of hypovolemia, appropriate plasma expanders, inotropic agents to improve myocardial contractility, and pressor agents to raise peripheral resistance may all be needed. Second, appropriate antibiotic therapy must be administered. For staphylococcal TSS, agents effective against coagulase-positive staphylococci should be used. Isolates of *S. pyogenes* are generally susceptible to penicillin; clindamycin has also been recommended for treatment of these infections because of the ability to inhibit toxin production even at antibiotic doses that do not inhibit bacterial growth. Third, surgical débridement and removal of any foreign bodies may be necessary, particularly for streptococcal TSS. Fourth, intravenous immunoglobulin may inhibit activation of T cells and may be useful in the treatment of staphylococcal or streptococcal TSS.[94, 95]

References

1. Todd J, Fishaut M, Kapral F, Welch T: Toxic shock syndrome associated with phage group I staphylococci. Lancet 2:1116, 1978.
2. Cone LA, Woodard DR, Schlievert PM, Tomory GS: Clinical and bacteriologic observations of a toxic shock–like syndrome due to *Streptococcus pyogenes*. N Engl J Med 317:146, 1987.
3. Stevens DL, Tanner MH, Winship J, et al: Severe group A streptococcal infections associated with a toxic shock–like syndrome and scarlet fever toxin A. N Engl J Med 321:1, 1989.
4. Schlievert PM, Shands KN, Dan BB, et al: Identification and characterization of an exotoxin from *Staphylococcus aureus* associated with toxic-shock syndrome. J Infect Dis 143:509, 1981.
5. Bergdoll MS, Crass B, Reiser RF, et al: A new staphylococcal enterotoxin, enterotoxin F, associated with toxic shock syndrome *Staphylococcus aureus* isolates. Lancet 1:1017, 1981.
6. Schlievert PM: Staphylococcal enterotoxin B and toxic-shock syndrome toxin-1 are significantly associated with nonmenstrual TSS. Lancet 1:1149, 1986.
7. Parsonnet J, Gillis ZA, Richter AG, Pier GB: A rabbit model of toxic shock syndrome that uses a constant, subcutaneous infusion of toxic shock syndrome toxin-1. Infect Immun 55:1070, 1987.
8. Kreiswirth BN, Schlievert PM, Novick RP: Evaluation of coagulase-negative staphylococci for ability to produce toxic shock syndrome toxin-1. J Clin Microbiol 25:2028, 1987.
9. Hauser AR, Stevens DL, Kaplan EL, Schlievert PM: Molecular analysis of pyrogenic exotoxins from *Streptococcus pyogenes* isolates associated with toxic shock–like syndrome. J Clin Microbiol 29:1562, 1991.
10. Musser JM, Hauser AR, Kim M, et al: *Streptococcus pyogenes* causing toxic shock–like syndrome and other invasive diseases: Clonal diversity and pyrogenic exotoxin expression. Proc Natl Acad Sci USA 88:2668, 1991.
11. Reda KB, Kapur V, Mollick JA, et al: Molecular characterization and phylogenetic distribution of the streptococcal superantigen gene (SSA) from *Streptococcus pyogenes*. Infect Immun 62:1867, 1994.
12. Wheeler MC, Roe MH, Kaplan EL, et al: Clinical, epidemiological, and microbiological correlates of an outbreak of group A streptococcal septicemia in children. JAMA 266:533, 1991.
13. Iwasaki M, Igarashi H, Hinuma Y, Yutsudo T: Cloning, characterization and overexpression of a *Streptococcus pyogenes* gene encoding a new type of mitogenic factor. FEBS Lett 331:187, 1993.
14. Bohach GA, Fast DJ, Nelson RD, Schlievert PM: Staphylococcal and streptococcal pyrogenic toxins involved in toxic shock syndrome and related illnesses. Crit Rev Microbiol 17:251, 1989.
15. Schlievert PM: Alteration of immune function by staphylococcal pyrogenic exotoxin type C: Possible role in toxic-shock syndrome. J Infect Dis 147:391, 1983.
16. Prasad GS, Earhart CA, Murray DL, et al: Structure of toxic shock syndrome toxin-1. Biochemistry 32:13761, 1993.
17. Schad EM, Zaitseva I, Vaitsev VN, et al: Crystal structure of the superantigen, staphylococcal enterotoxin type A. EMBO J 14:3292, 1995.
18. Swaminathan S, Furrey W, Pletcher J, Sax M: Crystal structure of staphylococcal enterotoxin B, a superantigen. Nature 359:801, 1993.
19. Hoffmann ML, Jablonski LM, Crum KK, et al: Predictions of T-cell receptor– and major histocompatibility complex–binding sites on staphylococcal enterotoxin C1. Infect Immun 62:3396, 1994.
20. Goshorn SC, Schlievert PM: Nucleotide sequence of streptococcal pyrogenic exotoxin type C. Infect Immun 56:2518, 1988.
21. Bohach GA, Schlievert PM: Nucleotide sequence of the staphylococcal enterotoxin C1 gene and relatedness to other pyrogenic toxin genes. Mol Gen Genet 209:15, 1987.
22. Bohach GA, Handley JP, Schlievert PM: Biological and immunological properties of the carboxyl terminus of staphylococcal enterotoxin C1. Infect Immun 57:23, 1989.
23. Betley MJ, Mekalanos JJ: Nucleotide sequence of the type A staphylococcal enterotoxin gene. J Bacteriol 170:34, 1988.
24. Jones CL, Khan SA: Nucleotide sequence of the enterotoxin B gene from *Staphylococcus aureus*. J Bacteriol 166:29, 1986.
25. Bohach GA, Schlievert PM: Conservation of the biologically-active portions of staphylococcal enterotoxins C1 and C2. Infect Immun 57:2249, 1989.
26. Bayles KW, Iandolo JJ: Genetic and molecular analyses of the gene encoding staphylococcal enterotoxin B. J Bacteriol 171:4799, 1989.
27. Blomster-Hautamaa DA, Kreiswirth BN, Kornblum JS, et al: The nucleotide and partial amino acid sequence of toxic-shock syndrome toxin-1. J Biol Chem 261:15783, 1986.
28. Couch JL, Soltis MT, Betley MJ: Cloning and nucleotide sequence of the type E staphylococcal enterotoxin gene. J Bacteriol 170:2954, 1988.
29. Weeks CR, Ferretti JJ: Nucleotide sequence of the type A streptococcal exotoxin (erythrogenic toxin) gene from *Streptococcal pyogenes* bacteriophage T12. Infect Immun 52:144, 1986.
30. Hauser AR, Schlievert PM: Nucleotide sequence of the streptococcal pyrogenic exotoxin type B gene and toxin relationship to streptococcal proteinase precursor. J Bacteriol 172:4536, 1990.
31. Ren K, Bannan JD, Pancholi V, et al: Characterization and biological properties of a new staphylococcal exotoxin. J Exp Med 180:1675, 1994.
32. de Azavedo JCS, Foster TJ, Hartigan PJ, et al: Expression of the cloned toxic shock syndrome toxin-1 gene *(tst)* in vivo with a rabbit uterine model. Infect Immun 50:304, 1985.
33. Lee PK, Schlievert PM: Group A streptococcal pyrogenic exotoxins: Quantification and toxicity in an animal model of toxic shock syndrome–like illness. J Clin Microbiol 27:1890, 1989.
34. Schlievert PM, Assimacopoulos AP, Cleary PP: Severe invasive group A streptococcal disease: Clinical description and mechanisms of pathogenesis. J Lab Clin Med 127:13, 1996.
35. Centers for Disease Control: Toxic-shock syndrome—United States. MMWR Morbid Mortal Wkly Rep 29:229, 1980.
36. Osterholm MT, Davis JP, Gibson RW, et al: Tri-state toxic-shock syndrome study. I. Epidemiologic findings. J Infect Dis 145:431, 1982.
37. Latham RH, Kehrberg MW, Jacobson JA, Smith CB: Toxic shock syndrome in Utah: A case-control and surveillance study. Ann Intern Med 96:906, 1982.
38. Davis JP, Chesney PJ, Wand PJ, La Venture M, the Investigation and Laboratory Team: Toxic shock syndrome: Epidemiologic features, recurrence, risk factors, and prevention. N Engl J Med 303:1429, 1980.
39. Gaventa S, Reingold AL, Hightower AW, et al: Active surveillance for toxic shock syndrome in the United States, 1986. Rev Infect Dis 2(Suppl 1):S28, 1989.
40. Todd JK, Wiesenthal AM, Ressman M, et al: Toxic shock syndrome. II. Estimated occurrence in Colorado as influenced by case ascertainment methods. Am J Epidemiol 122:857, 1985.
41. Petitti DB, Reingold AL, Chin J: The incidence of toxic shock syndrome in northern California: 1972 through 1983. JAMA 255:368, 1986.
42. Markowitz LE, Hightower AW, Broome CV, Reingold AL: Toxic shock syndrome: Evaluation of national surveillance data using a hospital discharge survey. JAMA 258:75, 1987.
43. Schuchat A, Broome CV: Toxic shock syndrome and tampons. Epidemiol Rev 13:99, 1991.
44. Broome CV: Epidemiology of toxic shock syndrome in the United States: Overview. Rev Infect Dis 2(Suppl 1):S14, 1989.
45. Shands KN, Schmid GP, Dan BB, et al: Toxic shock syndrome in menstruating women. N Engl J Med 303:1436, 1980.
46. Schlech WF, Shands KN, Reingold AL, et al: Risk factors for development of toxic shock syndrome: Association with a tampon brand. JAMA 248:835, 1982.
47. Berkley SF, Hightower AW, Broome CV, Reingold AL: The relationship of tampon characteristics to menstrual toxic shock syndrome. JAMA 258:917, 1987.
48. Reingold AL, Broome CV, Gaventa S, Hightower AW, the Toxic Shock Syndrome Study Group: Risk factors for menstrual toxic shock syndrome: Results of a multistate case-control study. Rev Infect Dis 2(Suppl 1):S35, 1989.
49. Reingold AL: Toxic shock syndrome: An update. Am J Obstet Gynecol 165:1236, 1991.
50. Davis JP, Osterholm MT, Helms CM, et al: Tri-state toxic-shock syndrome study. II. Clinical and laboratory findings. J Infect Dis 145:441, 1982.
51. Reingold AL, Hargrett NT, Dan BB, et al: Nonmenstrual toxic shock syndrome: A review of 130 cases. Ann Intern Med 96(pt 2):871, 1982.
52. Parsonnet J: Nonmenstrual toxic shock syndrome: New insights

into diagnosis, pathogenesis, and treatment. Curr Clin Top Infect Dis 16:1, 1996.
53. Navazesh M, Mulligan R, Sobel S: Toxic shock and Down syndromes in a dental patient: A case report and review of the literature. Spec Care Dent 14:246, 1994.
54. Bartlett P, Reingold AL, Graham DR, et al: Toxic shock syndrome associated with surgical wound infections. JAMA 247:1448, 1982.
55. Solomon R, Truman T, Murray DL: Toxic shock syndrome as a complication of bacterial tracheitis. Pediatr Infect Dis 4:298, 1985.
56. Surh L, Read SE: Staphylococcal tracheitis and toxic shock syndrome in a young child. J Pediatr 105:585, 1984.
57. Hirsch B, Stair T, Horowitz Z, et al: Toxic shock syndrome from staphylococcal pharyngitis. Ear Nose Throat J 63:494, 1984.
58. Wilkins EGL, Nye F, Roberts C, et al: Case report: Probable toxic shock syndrome with primary staphylococcal pneumonia. J Infect 11:231, 1985.
59. Barbour SD, Shlaes DM, Guertin SR: Toxic shock syndrome associated with nasal packing: Analogy to tampon-associated illness. Pediatrics 73:163, 1984.
60. Hull HF, Mann JM, Sands CH, et al: Toxic shock syndrome related to nasal packing. Arch Otolaryngol Head Neck Surg 109:624, 1983.
61. MacDonald KL, Osterholm MT, Hedberg CW, et al: Toxic shock syndrome: A newly recognized complication of influenza and influenzalike illness. JAMA 257:1053, 1987.
62. Sperber SJ, Francis JB: Toxic shock syndrome during an influenza outbreak. JAMA 257:1086, 1987.
63. Tolan RW Jr: Toxic shock syndrome complicating influenza A in a child: Case report and review. Clin Infect Dis 17:43, 1993.
64. Faich G, Pearson K, Fleming D, et al: Toxic shock syndrome and the vaginal contraceptive sponge. JAMA 255:216, 1986.
65. Schwartz B, Gaventa S, Broome CV, et al: Nonmenstrual toxic shock syndrome associated with barrier contraceptives: Report of a case-control study. Rev Infect Dis 2(Suppl 1):S43, 1989.
66. Hoge CW, Schwartz B, Talkington DF, et al: The changing epidemiology of invasive group A streptococcal toxic shock–like syndrome. JAMA 269:384, 1993.
67. Davis HD, McGeer A, Schwartz B, et al: Invasive group A streptococcal infections in Ontario, Canada. N Engl J Med 335:547, 1996.
68. Cockerill FR, MacDonald KL, Thompson RL, et al: An outbreak of invasive group A streptococcal disease associated with high carriage rates of the invasive clone among school-age children. JAMA 277:38, 1997.
69. Levine OS, Turf E, Ginsberg R, et al: An outbreak of invasive group A streptococcal (GAS) disease in the Shenandoah Valley of Virginia (Abstr K134). Presented at the 35th Interscience Conference on Antimicrobial Agents and Chemotherapy; September 17–20, 1995; San Francisco, CA; p 312.
70. Parsonnet J, Hickman RK, Eardley DD, Pier GB: Induction of human interleukin 1 toxic shock syndrome toxin-1. J Infect Dis 151:514, 1985.
71. Fast DJ, Schlievert PM, Nelson RD: Nonpurulent response to toxic shock syndrome toxin-1 producing *Staphylococcus aureus*: Relationship to toxin-stimulated production of tumor necrosis factor. J Immunol 140:949, 1988.
72. Fast DJ, Schlievert PM, Nelson RD: Toxic shock syndrome–associated staphylococcal and streptococcal pyrogenic toxins are potent inducers of tumor necrosis factor production. Infect Immun 57:291, 1989.
73. Norton SD, Schlievert PM, Novick RP, Jenkins MK: Molecular requirements for T cell activation by the staphylococcal toxic shock syndrome toxin-1. J Immunol 144:2089, 1990.
74. Scholl P, Diez A, Mourad W, et al: Toxic shock syndrome toxin-1 binds to MHC class II molecules. Proc Natl Acad Sci USA 86:4210, 1989.
75. Kappler J, Kotzin B, Herron L, et al: VB-specific stimulation of human T cells by staphylococcal toxins. Science 244:811, 1989.
76. White J, Herman A, Pullen AM, et al: The VB-specific superantigen staphylococcal enterotoxin B: Stimulation of mature T cells and clonal deletion in neonatal mice. Cell 56:27, 1989.
77. Stone RL, Schlievert PM: Evidence for the involvement of endotoxin in toxic-shock syndrome. J Infect Dis 155:682, 1987.
78. de Azavedo JCS, Arbuthnott JP: Toxicity of staphylococcal toxic shock syndrome toxin-1 in rabbits. Infect Immun 46:314, 1984.
79. Bulanda M, Zaleska M, Mandel L, et al: Toxicity of staphylococcal toxic shock syndrome toxin 1 for germ-free and conventional piglets. Rev Infect Dis 11(Suppl 1):S248, 1989.
80. Beezhold DH, Best GK, Bonventre PF, Thompson M: Endotoxin enhancement of toxic shock syndrome toxin-1–induced secretion of interleukin 1 by murine macrophages. Rev Infect Dis 11(Suppl 1):S289, 1989.
81. Keane WF, Gekker G, Schlievert PM, Peterson PK: Toxic-shock syndrome-1 sensitizes renal tubular cells to lipopolysaccharide induced necrosis. Am J Pathol 122:169, 1986.
82. Kusnaryov VM, MacDonald HS, Reiser RF, Bergdoll MS: Reaction of toxic shock syndrome toxin-1 with endothelium of human umbilical cord vein. Rev Infect Dis 11(Suppl 1):S282, 1989.
83. Nelson RD, Fast DJ, Schlievert PM: Pyrogenic toxin stimulation of TNF production by human mononuclear leukocytes and effect of TNF on neutrophil chemotaxis. *In* Bonavida B, Granger G (eds): Tumor Necrosis Factor: Structure, Mechanism of Action, Role in Disease and Therapy. Basel, S Karger, 1990, p 177.
84. Schlievert PM, Blomster DA: Production of staphylococcal pyrogenic exotoxin type C: Influence of physical and chemical factors. J Infect Dis 146:236, 1983.
85. Wagner G, Bohr L, Wagner P: Tampon-induced changes in vaginal oxygen and carbon dioxide tension. Am J Obstet Gynecol 148:147, 1984.
86. Todd JK, Todd BH, Franco-Fuff A, et al: Influence of focal growth conditions on the pathogenesis of toxic shock syndrome. J Infect Dis 155:673, 1987.
87. Kass EH, Schlievert PM, Parsonnet J, Mills JT: Effect of magnesium on production of toxic shock syndrome toxin-1: A collaborative study. J Infect Dis 158:44, 1988.
88. Schlievert PM, Osterholm MT, Kelly JA, Nishimura RD: Toxin and enzyme characterization of *Staphylococcus aureus* isolates from patients with and without toxic-shock syndrome. Ann Intern Med 96(pt 2):937, 1982.
89. The Working Group on Severe Streptococcal Infections: Defining the group A streptococcal toxic shock syndrome. JAMA 269:390, 1993.
90. Tofte RW, Williams DN: Clinical and laboratory manifestations of toxic shock syndrome. Ann Intern Med 96:843, 1982.
91. Bernstein GM, Crollick JS, Hassett JM Jr: Post febrile telogen effluvium in critically ill patients. Crit Care Med 16:98, 1988.
92. Chesney PJ: Clinical aspects and spectrum of illness of toxic shock syndrome: Overview. Rev Infect Dis 11:1, 1989.
93. Forni AL, Kaplan EL, Schlievert PM, Roberts RB: Clinical and microbiological characteristics of severe group A streptococcus infections and streptococcal toxic shock sydrome. Clin Infect Dis 21:333, 1995.
94. DeSimone C, Delogu G, Corbetta G: Intravenous immunoglobulin in association with antibiotics: A therapeutic trial in septic intensive care unit patients. Crit Care Med 16:23, 1988.
95. Lamothe F, D'Amico P, Ghosn P, et al: Clinical usefulness of intravenous human immunoglobulins in invasive group A streptococcal infections: Case report and review. Clin Infect Dis 21:1469, 1995.

GRAM-POSITIVE COCCI

191

Staphylococci

John N. Sheagren
Dennis R. Schaberg

History

A summary of the history of staphylococci was provided by A. C. Baird-Parker.[1] Briefly, cocci were first associated with human diseases when they were observed in purulent material obtained from human abscesses. The Scottish surgeon Sir Alexander Ogston demonstrated conclusively in 1880 that "a cluster-forming coccus was the cause of certain pyogenous abscesses in man." Louis Pasteur had reached similar conclusions at approximately the same time in Paris. Ogston named the cluster-forming coccus "staphylococcus" in 1882, deriving the name from the Greek nouns *staphyle* ("a bunch of grapes") and *kokkus* ("berry"). Morphologically, Ogston proposed the term staphylococcus for the cluster-forming cocci to distinguish them from the chain-forming streptococci. Ogston showed that injection of pus containing staphylococci into mice produced the same disease symptoms observed in humans. He also observed that when the pus was heated or treated with phenol, infection was prevented.

Characteristics of the Pathogen

The two genera of the Micrococcaceae family are *Staphylococcus* and *Micrococcus* (Table 191–1). The genus *Staphylococcus* contains at least 13 species, several of which have been classified into subspecies or biotypes.[2] Three species, however, are responsible for almost all recognized human infections: *Staphylococcus aureus*, the agent of most acute pyogenic and toxin-related staphylococcal infections in humans; *Staphylococcus epidermidis*, a major component of the normal flora of the skin and mucous membranes but increasingly a pathogen of infections of skin and skin structures, of foreign bodies, and of deep infections in immunocompromised patients; and *Staphylococcus saprophyticus*, which produces lower urinary tract infections in young women.

TABLE 191–1 ■ Microbiologic Characteristics of Staphylococci and Micrococci

CHARACTERISTIC	*STAPHYLOCOCCUS* SPECIES	*MICROCOCCUS* SPECIES
Anaerobic acid production from glucose	+	−
Anaerobic acid production from glycerol (in presence of erythromycin, 0.4 mg/mL)	+	−
Selective media		
SK medium	+	−
FTO medium	−	+
Modified oxidase and benzidine tests (to identify presence of cytochrome *c*)	− (most)	+
Sensitivity to lysostaphin, 200 mg or less	+	−

Structure

The staphylococci are gram-positive organisms with a diameter between 0.7 and 1.2 μm. The organisms divide randomly in three planes, and because the daughter cells do not separate completely, they form grapelike clusters (Fig. 191–1) that, when viable, are densely stained by Gram stain. When present in purulent material or infected body fluids, the organisms' morphology may vary: occasionally they pair up or form chains, and as they succumb to host defenses, they may lose some of their avidity for Gram stain. In electron micrographs of thin sections, the cell wall of staphylococci usually consists of a thick (up to 80 nm) layer that is more or less homogeneous. The cell envelope is surrounded by a unit membrane (cytoplasmic membrane), and the cell wall outside the plasma membrane is thick, rather homogeneous, and less electron dense. Some strains also have a capsule surrounding the cell wall. Overall, however, the fine structure of staphylococci is not much different from that of other typical prokaryotic cells.

Biologic and Biochemical Properties

The appearance of staphylococci as they grow in the laboratory provides the initial clues to identification. Typical *S. aureus* isolates growing on blood agar usually produce opaque, golden-yellow (*aureus* is Latin for "golden") colonies, approximately 2 to 3 mm in diameter, that usually produce beta hemolysis on blood agar plates. When encapsulated, *S. aureus* colonies may appear mucoid and sticky. Small-colony variants of *S. aureus* produce small, nonpigmented, nonhemolytic colonies, which can be misidentified in the microbiology laboratory.[3] These organisms revert to normal growth in the presence of menadione, hemin, or a carbon dioxide supplement. They are usually resistant to aminoglycosides. Their importance lies in the fact that they may play a role in chronic relapsing infections characterized by long periods of quiescence, especially osteomyelitis. In contrast, coagulase-negative colonies (e.g., *S. epidermidis*, *S. saprophyticus*) are usually white and nonhemolytic. Unfortunately, pigment production, as well as hemolytic characteristics, may vary.

The pathogenic genus *Staphylococcus*, with its three species of major significance, *S. aureus*, *S. epidermidis*, and *S. saprophyticus*, is differentiated in the standard laboratory by a number of tests. The most important is that for coagulase, which distinguishes *S. aureus* from all the other species, which, not surprisingly, are designated as coagulase-negative. Other tests that differentiate *S. aureus* from the coagulase-negative species include mannitol fermentation (positive in *S. aureus* and only rarely positive in coagulase-negative strains) and the deoxyribonuclease test (positive in *S. aureus* and negative in coagulase-negative species). An additional test, usually performed only on urine isolates of staphylococci, is the

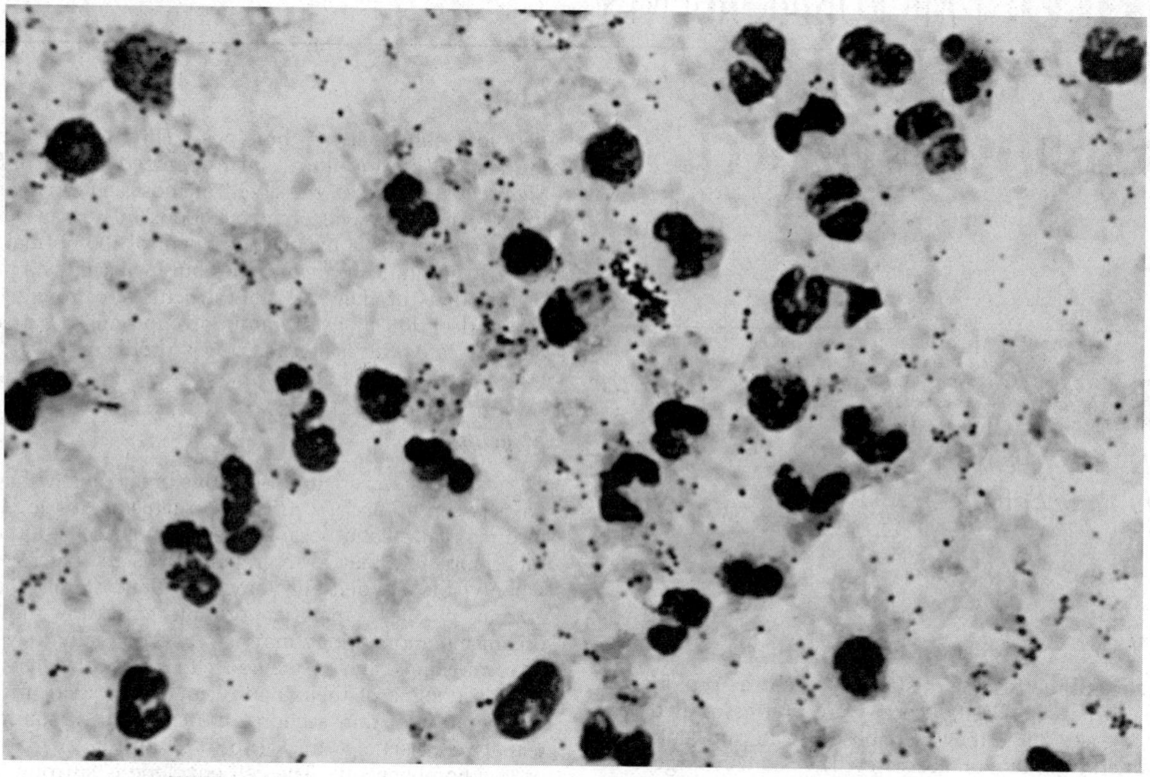

FIGURE 191–1 □ Gram stain of pus from a typical abscess caused by *Staphylococcus aureus.*

ability to grow in the presence of concentrations of 1.6 μg/mL or more of novobiocin. Staphylococci that are found to be novobiocin resistant and coagulase-negative can be identified presumptively as *S. saprophyticus*, an important urinary pathogen in young women.

Rapid screening tests are becoming more readily available that identify staphylococci in general and *S. aureus* in particular. These tests quickly identify organisms presumptively as *S. aureus* if protein A is detected on the surface.

THE CELL WALL

The cell wall structure of staphylococci is important for a number of reasons.[4] First, the actions of many of the effective classes of antibiotics involve inhibition of the synthesis of the cell wall; second, a number of diagnostic tests that are potentially useful in the management of staphylococcal disease (including the measurement of antibody to a component of the cell wall, teichoic acid), depend on cell wall characteristics. The Gram stain examination depends on the ability of the bacterial cell when washed with ethanol to retain the basic dye crystal violet. Gram-positive bacteria retain the stain principally because their cell walls contain large quantities of peptidoglycan, the most important material for maintaining the shape and structure of the staphylococci. Surrounding the entire cell is a huge macromolecule consisting of glycan chains composed of alternating β-1,4–linked units of the amino sugars *N*-acetylglucosamine and *N*-acetylmuramic acid, all of which are cross-linked through short peptide chains (usually tetrapeptides of L-alanine, D-isoglutamine, L-lysine, and D-alanine). These tetrapeptides are further cross-linked (in a second dimension) by interpeptide bridges consisting, usually, of penta- or hexaglycine peptides extending from the C-terminal D-alanine in position 4 of one peptide to the amino group of L-lysine in position 3 of an adjacent peptide. In the coagulase-negative species of staphylococci, the peptidoglycan differs mainly in the interpeptide bridges (some of the glycines are replaced by L-serines).

The other major cell wall component of staphylococci is teichoic acid. Teichoic acids are water-soluble polymers of glycerol or ribitol phosphate, sugars, and sometimes D-alanine. They are linked covalently to the peptidoglycan backbone. *S. aureus* contains predominantly ribitol teichoic acid, whereas most of the other coagulase-negative staphylococci contain glycerol teichoic acid. Antibodies are generated against ribitol teichoic acid in many patients with deep, invasive *S. aureus* infections, and the presence of such antibodies may be helpful in diagnosing and guiding the duration of therapy for patients who have suffered *S. aureus* bacteremia.[5, 6]

Capsule formation is variable among staphylococci but may be important pathogenically. For example, strains of *S. epidermidis* that produce a slimelike glycocalyx adhere much more avidly to foreign bodies and so are more important pathogens in infections of prosthetic implants of all types.[7] The few strains of *S. aureus* that are encapsulated in vitro seem to be more pathogenic in animal models; however, the role of the capsule in *S. aureus* foreign body infections, for example, is not clear. It is tempting to speculate that the same relationship to capsule or slime production in *S. epidermidis* holds for *S. aureus.*

The adherence of *S. aureus* to heart valves and foreign bodies appears to be mediated in part by receptors for fibronectin on the surface of *S. aureus.* Fibronectin is a large glycoprotein important in various adhesive functions, including clot stabilization. *S. aureus* strains that express large numbers of receptors for fibronectin appear to be more invasive and better able to adhere.[8] The role of surface-associated proteins of *S. aureus* and their possible roles in virulence have been reviewed.[9] These substances include not only fibronectin binding proteins but protein A, collagen, and fibrinogen binding proteins as well.[9]

ENZYMES AND TOXINS

Enzymes and toxins[10, 11] have been strongly implicated as potential pathogenic factors in diseases produced by *S. aureus*. Among the more important enzymes is catalase, which inactivates potentially bactericidal hydrogen peroxide. Thus, catalase production creates a healthier milieu for invading staphylococci, which effect some investigators believe contributes to its pathogenicity. Other enzymes that may be important in the pathogenicity of *S. aureus* by permitting the organism to spread through tissues include hyaluronidase (which hydrolyzes hyaluronic acids, part of the connective tissue matrix) and lipase (which breaks down lipid components of tissue).

In addition to the extracellular enzymes, a number of extracellular protein products of *S. aureus* have been identified. These have been called toxins because of their adverse effects on cell function or the production of cell lysis. The α-toxin is a protein that acts on a wide variety of cell membranes and, when injected parenterally, rapidly produces an area of necrosis. Most pathogenic strains of *S. aureus* elaborate α-toxin, but its exact role in the clinical manifestation of human disease is not clear. Data may implicate it more forcibly in human disease, as human platelets are highly susceptible to α-toxin[12] and human monocytes are also vulnerable, releasing interleukin-2 and tumor necrosis factor on exposure to α-toxin.[13] The β-toxin is another enzyme-like protein, which breaks down sphingomyelin, a substance present in many cells and tissues throughout the body. The γ- and δ-toxins may also lyse cells or stimulate intestinal secretion. Leukocidin has a dramatic effect on granulocytes, resulting in degranulation and lysis. Finally, three toxins are related specifically to human diseases caused by *S. aureus*: exfoliatin (responsible for the staphylococcal scalded skin syndrome), enterotoxin (an important cause of food poisoning), and the toxic shock syndrome toxin 1 (the agent of a potentially lethal multisystem disorder that mimics bacteremic septic shock). The most important new concept with regard to toxin-associated diseases is that these protein toxins (especially toxic shock syndrome toxin 1) function as "superantigens."[14] Superantigens interact simultaneously with immune receptors on macrophages and lymphocytes, resulting in release of inflammatory cytokines.

Replication

The staphylococci are nonmotile and do not form spores, and most species are facultative anaerobes. With the exception of an occasional strain of *S. aureus*, growth is more rapid and abundant under aerobic conditions; however, some strains may require the carbon dioxide for optimal growth. Cell wall–deficient forms have been described; these require a hypertonic environment. Small-colony variants of *S. aureus* were discussed earlier.[3] Staphylococcal cell division takes place in successive, perpendicular planes; incomplete separation of the daughter cells results in irregular aggregates or clusters (see Fig. 191–1).

Antigenic Characteristics

The antigenic components of staphylococci have been studied extensively. The cell wall of *S. aureus* contains a ribitol teichoic acid and that of *S. epidermidis*, a glycerol teichoic acid. *S. saprophyticus*, although it is coagulase-negative, contains predominantly ribitol teichoic acid of two types: one has *N*-acetylglucosamine residues and the other, glucose residues, and both may be contained in a single strain. The immunologic effect or diagnostic usefulness of these staphylococcal antigens is not clear. Classification of staphylococci by using serotyping has not been successful. Strains of staphylococci within individual species have been best delineated by their biochemical characteristics (biotyping), by phage typing, or by plasmid profile typing (see later). Clinically, antibiotic sensitivity patterns can occasionally help identify an epidemic strain of *Staphylococcus* involved in a hospital-acquired outbreak.

Epidemiology

Transmission

The central event in diseases caused by all types of staphylococci seems to be the carrier state. Coagulase-negative staphylococci are important components of the normal flora of the body, and it is presumed that virtually all humans carry *S. epidermidis* on the skin and in and around body orifices. Contamination by coagulase-negative staphylococci carried by the patient is believed to be the most important event in infections associated with foreign bodies (intravascular devices, heart valves, prosthetic joints), although some studies have demonstrated hospital acquisition of strains that are resistant to several antibiotics.[15]

Human carriers of *S. aureus* are at risk not only of transmitting the organism to others but of inoculating their own portals of entry, which could result in self-infection.[16] Approximately 25% of adults are asymptomatic carriers of *S. aureus* in the anterior nares or the intertriginous regions (axillae, groin, perineum), and they may experience recurrent staphylococcal infections of the skin and mucous membranes and are at substantially higher risk than noncarriers of developing a more serious *S. aureus* infection (e.g., intravenous line infection, wound infection, pneumonia).[17, 18] This concept is now coming to clinical fruition in that preidentification of *S. aureus* carriers can help prevent nosocomial infections (see the later section on treatment of the *S. aureus* carrier state).

The carrier state of *S. aureus* is still poorly understood, but it probably combines certain host characteristics (which may be genetic or related to human leukocyte antigens) with the important phenomenon of control by the normal flora of the body. Genetic factors may control certain receptors or tissue components, to which *S. aureus* may attach.

In addition to the 25% of otherwise healthy persons who carry *S. aureus*, certain subgroups of patients are more likely to be *S. aureus* carriers[16]: patients with chronic dermatologic conditions (up to 100% are carriers); patients who regularly undergo hemodialysis (approximately 75%); diabetic patients who take insulin (approximately 50%); patients receiving allergy shots (up to 50%); and intravenous drug abusers (approximately 40%). Such persons may also have other immune deficits that predispose them to more frequent and more serious infections with *S. aureus*. Another group of patients at extremely high risk are those receiving interleukin-2.[19, 20]

Human immunodeficiency virus–infected patients have a significantly increased carriage rate of *S. aureus*, which increases as patients progress to full-blown acquired immunodeficiency syndrome.[21, 22] Such patients are at particularly high risk for symptomatic infections, especially if patients are neutropenic and require an indwelling line.[22] Colonization of patients who have acquired immunodeficiency syndrome with strains of *S. aureus* that produce toxic shock syndrome toxin 1 may result in what has been described as a recalcitrant, erythematous desquamating disorder,[23] thought to be due to low-grade, toxic shock syndrome toxin 1–induced systemic inflammatory cytokine activation.[24, 25]

Distribution and Prevalence

S. aureus is ubiquitous not only in humans but also in a number of animal species. It is now the single most frequently identified isolate from true-positive blood cultures in the hospital setting, according to data from the Centers for Disease Control and Prevention.[26] *S. aureus* is the most common cause of postsurgical wound infections and of other traumatic infections of the skin and skin structures. It is the leading cause of both soft tissue and bone and joint infections. *S. epidermidis* is a frequent (25% to 50%) cause of infections of foreign bodies such as prosthetic heart valves and prosthetic joints of all types; like *S. aureus*, it may infect intravascular lines, becoming increasingly important in infections of indwelling central lines such as those used for chemotherapy of patients with neoplastic disease, for parenteral hyperalimentation, or for vascular monitoring devices and pacemakers. *S. saprophyticus* accounts for approximately 10% of urinary tract infections in otherwise healthy young women[27] and is often called simply a coagulase-negative staphylococcus or is misidentified as *S. epidermidis*.

Typing systems for studying the epidemiology of staphylococcal infections have been investigated intensively, for it is important to be able to distinguish one strain from another, especially in the hospital setting. Cowan developed a slide agglutination test based on antiserum raised in rabbits[2]; however, the complexity of the technique and lack of agreement on which reagents to use have limited the usefulness of serotyping. Phage typing of *S. aureus* has been in use since the 1940s, and it has been quite valuable in investigating the epidemiology of staphylococcal infections, especially in hospital outbreaks.[28] Because of problems with the interpretation of phage-typing data, such information is far more useful in *excluding* possible epidemiologic relationships than it is in defining groups of related staphylococcal strains in an epidemic situation. Still, the persistence of certain phage-typeable strains of staphylococci has led to their recognition as virulent strains in the hospital setting.

Because as many as 50% of strains have not been phage typeable, continued attempts to identify relationships between isolated organisms have been undertaken. Plasmid profile analysis has been used to identify the reservoir and mode of transmission of *S. aureus* infections, especially in hospitals.[29] Plasmid profile analyses now appear to be most useful in investigating outbreaks, although the stability of strains over a long time has not been completely clarified. The technique of the arbitrarily primed polymerase chain reaction combined with plasmid profile analysis has provided complementary epidemiologic information in several nosocomial *S. aureus* outbreaks.[30]

TABLE 191–2 ■ Infections Produced by *Staphylococcus aureus*

Direct invasion
Superficial
Pyodermas, including impetigo, paronychia
Skin and soft tissue infections—boils, furuncles, carbuncles, cellulitis, lymphangitis, lymphadenitis
Deep
Septic arthritis
Osteomyelitis
Pyomyositis
Dissemination via the blood stream
Bacteremia (sometimes accompanied by bacterial vasculitis), with or without septic shock or multiple organ system failure
Metastatic abscess formation (brain, lung, liver, spleen, retroperitoneum, kidney, genital tract)
Toxin mediated
Skin disease: staphylococcal scalded skin syndrome
Gastrointestinal disease: gastroenteritis (staphylococcal food poisoning)
Multisystem disease: toxic shock syndrome

TABLE 191–3 ■ Virulence Factors of Coagulase-Producing *Staphylococcus aureus* Species

Enzymes	Catalase, hyaluronidase, lipase
Toxins	α-, β-, γ-, δ-toxins, leukocidin, exfoliatin, enterotoxin, toxic shock syndrome toxin 1
Immune system factors	Antigen-antibody complexes, pseudoimmune complexes, superantigens
Cell wall components	Activated complement, tumor necrosis factor, interleukin-1, and other cytokines and mediator systems

Pathogenesis

Staphylococci produce disease in two ways: directly, by invasion and subsequent tissue destruction, whether locally or after having spread via the blood stream,[16] and through the effects of toxins.[11, 16] Table 191–2 lists the types of infections produced by *S. aureus*; Table 191–3, the various virulence factors the organisms produce; and Table 191–4, the sequence of pathogenic events associated with serious infections.

Invasive Staphylococcal Infections

In invasive infections, the primary event is the presence of staphylococci as colonizing organisms, which then invade, usually through breaches in the barrier systems of the skin and mucous membranes. The sine qua non of staphylococcal infections is the abscess, presenting on the skin as a boil or furuncle. This lesion is an exquisitely tender, erythematous, warm lesion that, during the course of 24 to 48 hours, develops a central white pustule. The purulent material is creamy, yellowish, and often contains a "core" (the follicle and its debris) at the site where the infection was initiated. Around foreign bodies, the inoculum of staphylococci necessary to produce disease is quite small and antibiotic therapy is much less successful. Some persons develop *S. aureus* bacteremia "spontaneously" (i.e., they have no identifiable primary focus of infection), and it is assumed either that they had subclinical infection of the skin and skin structures or that the organism arises from a nasopharyngeal—or even, possibly, a gastrointestinal—source. Most infections, however, are related directly to traumatic breaks in the skin and mucous membranes and often involve the presence of a foreign body. Once through the barrier systems and into the subcutaneous

TABLE 191–4 ■ Sequence of Pathogenic Events in Serious *Staphylococcus aureus* Infections

Colonization → carriage → toxin production
Barrier breach or break
Invasion (all are enhanced by the presence of a foreign body)
Cellulitis, lymphangitis
Abscess formation
Blood stream invasion
Bacteremia or septicemia
Syndrome of severe sepsis
Cell wall components
Toxic shock syndrome toxin 1
Role of triggered mediators
Complications
Suppurative: metastatic abscesses, endocarditis, and others
Inflammatory: septic shock or multiple organ system failure syndromes
Death

or submucous tissues, *S. aureus* organisms spread quickly, forming abscesses and seeking deep, chronically inflamed or avascular areas. Once in and around bones and other support structures or sequestered in blood clots, the organisms become quite resistant to attack and eradication by host defenses, the most important host defense cell being the polymorphonuclear leukocyte. The bacteria frequently enter the blood stream, through which they can spread around the body, sometimes forming multiple metastatic abscesses. From venous foci (e.g., septic thrombophlebitis), they can seed the lungs, causing bacteremic pneumonia with or without the presence of septic thrombi. Once into the arterial circulation, they can adhere directly to damaged endothelial surfaces (deformed valves, arterial aneurysms) and can, of course, seed to the major organ systems served by the arterial circulation (central nervous system, kidneys). In the course of an overwhelming infection, bacterial vasculitis may develop. In such cases, the patient often develops coagulopathy, and the combined vasculitis and coagulopathy produce a petechial rash that is difficult to distinguish from those of meningococcemia, Rocky Mountain spotted fever, and other septicemic, coagulopathic states.[31, 32]

The sequence of events during fulminant *S. aureus* bacteremia is still not entirely clear, but it probably duplicates that which has been studied more extensively in gram-negative bacteremic infections. Specifically, in the latter situation, endotoxin from the gram-negative cell wall triggers a series of "mediators," which together produce the manifestations of both hemodynamic instability (septic shock) and end organ failure. We assume that the same sequence is occurring in gram-positive infections (see Table 191–4). In the case of gram-positive microbes, it is the cell wall peptidoglycan or the teichoic acid complex, or both, that trigger the release of mediators, in much the same way as endotoxin does in gram-negative bacteremic states. In almost every assay system developed for endotoxin, the peptidoglycan or teichoic acid residues can produce similar biologic effects (fever, lipidemia, septic shock, or multiple organ system failure), but amounts 10 to 100 times greater are required.[33] Clinically, septic shock or multiple organ system failure is more common with gram-negative infections, but the same sequence can transpire in gram-positive bacteremia. On the other hand, peripheral seeding of the microbe (e.g., into organs and tissues to cause metastatic abscesses, endocarditis) is much more common with gram-positive infections, especially staphylococcal infections, than with gram-negative ones.[16] The probable reason for this phenomenon is that gram-positive microbes have receptors (surface-associated proteins[9]) on their cell walls for subendothelial vascular components (fibronectin, laminen) and for components of clots, whereas gram-negative microbes have none (or have fewer or less avid ones) and so are much less likely to seed throughout the body. Seeding of bacteria around the body and a propensity to cause secondary abscess formation are hallmarks of *S. aureus* bacteremia. From an initial focus (e.g., infected intravascular line, furuncle, urinary tract infection), *S. aureus* can seed secondarily to heart valves, bones, joints, and back to the kidneys and other retroperitoneal tissues. Occasionally, liver, brain, and meninges are also sites of secondary infections. All such specific infections are discussed at length in other chapters of this book.

S. epidermidis, even though it is frequently a cause of low-grade bacteremia (usually from intravenous lines or infected prostheses), rarely produces a septic shock–like picture and does not seed as frequently as *S. aureus* to deep organs and tissues. Immunocompromised hosts with high-grade *S. epidermidis* bacteremia, however, can look quite septic and develop secondary foci of infection. *S. saprophyticus* seems quite specifically to affect only the urinary tract, usually of young women,[27] and it seems to have an unusual propensity to adhere to uroepithelial cells. It hardly ever causes urinary tract infection in men.[34]

Toxigenic Staphylococcus *Infections*

The classic syndromes associated with toxin-producing strains of *S. aureus* are the staphylococcal scalded skin syndrome (see Chapter 140), gastroenteritis (see Chapter 82) and the toxic shock syndrome (see Chapter 190). None of the coagulase-negative strains of staphylococci produce clinically significant toxins.

Clinical Manifestations

Invasive Infections

Patients with peripheral, localized infections caused by staphylococci (and especially those who develop bacteremia) may exhibit the usual manifestations of sepsis. Initially, patients are usually afebrile. Later, they may develop fever, and experience a chill, and a few develop confusion, tachypnea, tachycardia, and ultimately signs of peripheral organ hyperperfusion. Some patients with septicemia may develop a vasculitic rash consisting of palpable purpuric lesions, which eventually develop small pustules.[32] These small pustules are the key to differentiating the petechial rash of *S. aureus* bacteremia from that of meningococcal infection, Rocky Mountain spotted fever, and idiopathic thrombocytopenic purpura, among others. Patients with severe but localized organ infections—for example, pneumonia, urinary tract infection, septic arthritis, or osteomyelitis—usually present as does any such patient, with symptoms and signs relevant to the involved organ.

Toxigenic Staphylococcus aureus *Infections*

See Chapters 82, 140, and 190.

Diagnosis

Specific Laboratory Diagnostic Procedures

On Gram stain examination, purulent material from staphylococcal infections exhibits clusters of large gram-positive cocci (see Fig. 191–1). Interpretation of results of cultures is complicated by the need to discriminate colonization from infection, as both *S. aureus* and *S. epidermidis* can be part of the normal flora. Careful specimen collection and communication between clinician and laboratory personnel are vital for accurate assessment. Initially, the laboratory will report from blood cultures only the presence of "gram-positive cocci," and empirical therapy to cover staphylococci usually will already have been initiated. Later, the laboratory will be able to determine whether the organism produces coagulase and so differentiate *S. aureus* from coagulase-negative staphylococci. At that point, *S. aureus* is generally considered to be a true pathogen until proved otherwise; *S. epidermidis* is rarely (15% or less) a true bacteremic pathogen and is usually a skin contaminant from the site where blood was taken for culture. True *S. epidermidis* bacteremia is identified by the findings of multiple positive blood cultures for a brief period in the presence of an appropriate clinical syndrome and epidemiologic setting.[35]

Treatment

Specific treatment of all staphylococcal infections is one or more antibiotics. *S. saprophyticus* continues to be sensitive to all the β-lactam antibiotics, including penicillin. A brief course of large doses of penicillin (or for penicillin-allergic patients, a cephalosporin or trimethoprim-sulfamethoxazole) suffices to treat most *S. saprophyticus* urinary tract infections in young women.

Treatment of *S. aureus* and *S. epidermidis* infections is now becoming much more difficult because an increasingly large percentage of strains have become resistant to all of the β-lactam antibiotics.[36–38] Detection of β-lactam antibiotic–resistant staphylococci is a complicated procedure, often requiring special testing conditions to ensure that resistance is not overlooked.[39–41] Thus, whenever the clinical setting is such that a resistant strain cannot be ruled out, vancomycin must be added to the initial antibiotic regimen. Vancomycin resistance has not yet been reported in strains of *S. aureus* or *S. epidermidis*. Other glycopeptide antibiotics are under development, the most promising of which is teicoplanin. The quinolone group of antibiotics has been effective initially against many resistant strains of *S. aureus* and *S. epidermidis*; however, with increasing use, resistance is becoming a more significant problem. Data have been presented suggesting that the glycopeptide antibiotics (e.g., vancomycin and teicoplanin) are not as effective in controlling complicated *S. aureus* infections as are the β-lactam antibiotics, especially the penicillinase-resistant penicillins (e.g., nafcillin or oxacillin).[42, 43] These data have been well summarized by Mortara and Bayer.[44] Thus, whenever a β-lactam antibiotic–susceptible strain of staphylococcus is found to be the cause of an infection, nafcillin or oxacillin should be used long term. Note that every effort should be made to reduce vancomycin usage, as continued use is a major factor in selecting for vancomycin-resistant enterococci, which in vitro can transmit vancomycin resistance to other gram-positive microbes. Although teicoplanin resistance has been described in clinical isolates of *S. aureus*[45] and can readily be produced in the laboratory,[46] thus far no clinical isolate of *S. aureus* has developed vancomycin resistance.

Prevention

Immunization

Despite the multiple immune sequelae of staphylococcal infections and exerted attempts to develop vaccines, no type of immunization has been shown to be effective in ameliorating *S. aureus* infections in humans.

Treatment of the Staphylococcus aureus Carrier State

In day-to-day practice, patients with recurrent staphylococcal infections of the skin (e.g., boils, furuncles) benefit from having the strain of *S. aureus* they harbor eliminated from the nose. Oral therapy with rifampin, 600 mg daily for 5 days, combined with either a topical antistaphylococcal agent or concurrent treatment with an oral antistaphylococcal drug such as dicloxacillin or, for penicillin-allergic patients, trimethoprim-sulfamethoxazole, eradicates the carrier state for the vast majority of persons with "positive nasal secretion cultures."[47] Yu and colleagues[48] have shown that rifampin prophylaxis significantly reduced the frequency of *S. aureus* infections in hemodialysis patients. Repeated treatment is usually necessary anywhere from 6 to 12 weeks later, and individual patients have different cycles of recurrence. Mupirocin (Bactroban) also seems to be highly effective at eliminating *S. aureus* carried in the nose. The agent is available in a 2% ointment, which, when applied to the anterior nares four times daily for 5 days, eradicates the pathogen.[49] Again, repeated treatment may be necessary in 6 to 12 weeks, depending on the individual patient.

General Preventive Measures

Because the agent of most staphylococcal infections is one of the patient's own colonizing organisms, eradication of the carried microbe may be prophylactic. The colonization rate of hemodialysis patients is approximately 75% for *S. aureus*[48, 50]; prospective treatment of colonized patients with rifampin has been shown to reduce the number of subsequent infections.[48] As anticipated, nasal carriage of *S. aureus* has been shown to be a major risk factor for post–cardiac surgery sternotomy wound infections.[51] Thus, it seems reasonable to recommend identification of nasal *S. aureus* carriers before major surgical procedures wherein postoperative *S. aureus* wound and prosthesis infections are known to be common (e.g., cardiac, orthopedic, neurosurgical, ear-nose-throat). Treatment of carriers with a 5-day course of mupirocin (as just described) would permit the operation to occur during the subsequent carriage-free period. Prospective, randomized, "blinded" studies would document the validity of this approach as well as identify any potential risks (e.g., an increase in nonstaphylococcal infections).

Identification and treatment of carriers among hospital personnel has occasionally been found to be helpful in outbreaks of staphylococcal infections. In day-to-day medical practice, simply washing the hands *before and after* interacting with each patient essentially *stops* the spread of organisms. Strict adherence to standard protocols for the placement and maintenance of intravascular lines can substantially reduce the rate of line infections. Mupirocin applied intranasally has been found to eliminate *S. aureus* nasal carriage in healthy persons for up to 3 months and appears to decrease hand carriage at 72 hours after therapy. Thus, mupirocin may have a role in decreasing hand carriage of colonized medical personnel.[52, 53]

References

1. Baird-Parker AC: Classification of staphylococci and their resistance to physical agents. *In* Cohen JO (ed): The Staphylococci. New York, Wiley Interscience, 1972, pp 1–20.
2. Oeding P: Taxonomy and identification. *In* Easmon CSF, Adlam C (eds): Staphylococci and Staphylococcal Infections. New York, Academic Press, 1983, pp 1–31.
3. Proctor RA, van Langeveld P, Kristjansson M, et al: Persistent and relapsing infections associated with small-colony variants of *Staphylococcus aureus*. Clin Infect Dis 20:95, 1995.
4. Schleifer KH: The cell envelope. *In* Easmon CSF, Adlam C (eds): Staphylococci and Staphylococcal Infections. New York, Academic Press, 1983, pp 385–428.
5. Tuazon CU, Sheagren JN, Choa MS, et al: *Staphylococcus aureus* bacteremia: Relationship between teichoic acid antibody formation and the development of metastatic abscesses. J Infect Dis 131:57, 1978.
6. Sheagren JN: Guidelines for the use of the teichoic acid antibody assay. Arch Intern Med 144:250, 1984.
7. Christensen GD, Simpson WA, Bisno AL, et al: Experimental foreign body infections in mice challenged with slime-producing *Staphylococcus epidermidis*. Infect Immun 40:407, 1983.
8. Proctor RA: The staphylococcal fibronectin receptor: Evidence for its importance in invasive infections. Rev Infect Dis 9(Suppl):S317, 1987.
9. Foster TJ, McDevitt D: Surface-associated proteins of *Staphylococcus aureus*: Their possible roles in virulence. FEMS Microbiol Lett 118:199, 1994.
10. Arvidson SO: Extracellular enzymes from *Staphylococcus aureus*. *In* Easmon CSF, Adlam C (eds): Staphylococci and Staphylococcal Infections. New York, Academic Press, 1983, pp 745–808.
11. Wadstrom T: Biological effects of cell-damaging toxins. *In* Easmon CSF, Adlam C (eds): Staphylococci and Staphylococcal Infections. New York, Academic Press, 1983, pp 671–704.
12. Bhakdi S, Muhly M, Mannhardt U, et al: Staphylococcal α toxin

promotes blood coagulation via attack on human platelets. J Exp Med 168:527, 1988.
13. Bhakdi S, Mannhardt U, Muhly M, et al: Human hyperimmune globulin protects against the cytotoxic action of staphylococcal α toxin in vitro and in vivo. Infect Immun 57:3214, 1989.
14. Kotb M: Bacterial pyrogenic exotoxins as superantigens. Clin Microbiol Rev 8:411, 1995.
15. Archer GL, Tenenbaum MJ: Antibiotic-resistant *S. epidermidis* in patients undergoing cardiac surgery. Antimicrob Agents Chemother 17:269, 1980.
16. Sheagren JN: *Staphylococcus aureus*: The persistent pathogen. N Engl J Med 310:1368, 1437, 1984.
17. Weinstein HJ: The relation between the nasal staphylococcal carrier state and the incidence of postoperative complications. N Engl J Med 260:1303, 1959.
18. Calia FM, Wokinsky E, Mortimer EA Jr, et al: Importance of the carrier state as a source of *Staphylococcus aureus* in wound sepsis. J Hyg (Lond) 67:49, 1969.
19. Snydman DR, Sullivan B, Gould JA, et al: Nosocomial sepsis associated with interleukin 2. Ann Intern Med 112:102, 1990.
20. Pockaj BA, Topalian SL, Steinberg SM, et al: Infectious complications associated with interleukin 2 administration: A retrospective review of 935 treatment courses. J Clin Oncol 11:136, 1993.
21. Raviglione MC, Mariuz P, Pablos-Mendez A, et al: High *Staphylococcus aureus* nasal carriage rate in patients with acquired immunodeficiency syndrome of AIDS-related complex. Am J Infect Control 18:64, 1990.
22. Weinke T, Schiller R, Ferenbach FJ, et al: Association between *Staphylococcus aureus* nasopharyngeal colonization and septicemia in patients infected with the human immunodeficiency virus. Eur J Clin Microbiol Infect Dis 11:985, 1992.
23. Cone LA, Woodward DR, Byrd RG, et al: A recalcitrant erythematous desquamating disorder associated with toxin-producing staphylococci in patients with AIDS. J Infect Dis 165:638, 1992.
24. Dondorp AM, Veenstra J, van der Poll T, et al: Activation of the cytokine network in a patient with AIDS and the recalcitrant erythematous desquamating disorder. Clin Infect Dis 18:942, 1994.
25. Fast DJ, Schlievert PM, Nelson RD: Toxic shock syndrome–associated staphylococcal and streptococcal pyrogenic toxins are potent inducers of tumor necrosis factor production. Infect Immun 57:291, 1989.
26. Horan TC, White JW, Jarvis WR, et al: Nosocomial infection surveillance, 1984. MMWR CDC Surveill Summ 35:17SS, 1986.
27. Hovelius B, Mardh PA, Bygren P: Urinary tract infections caused by *Staphylococcus saprophyticus*. J Urol 122:645, 1979.
28. Parker MT: The significance of phage-typing patterns in *Staphylococcus aureus*. *In* Easmon CSF, Adlam C (eds): Staphylococci and Staphylococcal Infections. New York, Academic Press, 1983, pp 33–62.
29. Cohen ML, Wong ES, Falkow S: Common R plasmids in *Staphylococcus aureus* during a nosocomial *Staphylococcus aureus* outbreak. Antimicrob Agents Chemother 21:210, 1982.
30. Fang FC, McClelland M, Guiney DG, et al: Value of molecular epidemiologic analysis in a nosocomial methicillin resistant *Staphylococcus aureus* outbreak. JAMA 270:1323, 1993.
31. Murray HW, Tuazon CU, Sheagren JN: Staphylococcal septicemia and disseminated intravascular coagulation: *S. aureus* endocarditis mimicking meningococcemia. Arch Intern Med 137:844, 1977.
32. Milunski MR, Gallis HA, Fuekerson WJ: *Staphylococcus aureus* septicemia mimicking fulminant Rocky Mountain spotted fever. Am J Med 83:801, 1987.
33. Sheagren JN: Inflammation induced by *Staphylococcus aureus*. *In* Gallin JI, Goldstein IM, Synderman R (eds): Inflammation: Basic Principles and Clinical Correlates. New York, Raven Press, 1988, pp 829–840.
34. Kauffman CA, Hertz CS, Sheagren JN: *Staphylococcus saprophyticus*: Role in urinary tract infections in men. J Urol 130:493, 1983.
35. Kirchhoff LV, Sheagren JN: Epidemiology and clinical significance of blood cultures positive for coagulase-negative *Staphylococcus*. Infect Control 6:479, 1985.
36. Brumfitt W, Hamilton-Miller J: Methicillin-resistant *Staphylococcus aureus*. N Engl J Med 320:1188, 1989.
37. Mulligan ME, Murray-Leisure KA, Ribner BS, et al: Methicillin resistant *Staphylococcus aureus*: A consensus review of the microbiology, pathogenesis and epidemiology with implications for prevention and management. Am J Med 94:313, 1993.
38. Martin MA: Methicillin-resistant *Staphylococcus aureus*: The persistent, resistant pathogen. Curr Clin Top Infect Dis 14:170, 1994.
39. McDougal LK, Thornsberry C: The role of β-lactamase in staphylococcal resistance to penicillinase penicillins and cephalosporins. J Clin Microbiol 23:832, 1986.
40. Hackbarth CJ, Chambers HF: Methicillin-resistant staphylococci: Genetics and mechanisms of resistance. Antimicrob Agents Chemother 33:991, 1989.
41. Kloos WE, Jorgensen JH: Staphylococci. *In* Lennette EM (ed): Manual of Clinical Microbiology. Washington, DC, American Society for Microbiology, 1985, pp 143–153.
42. Small PM, Chambers HF: Vancomycin for *Staphylococcus aureus* endocarditis in intravenous drug users. Antimicrob Agents Chemother 34:1227, 1990.
43. Levine DP, Fromm BS, Reddy BR: Slow response to vancomycin or vancomycin plus rifampin in methicillin resistant *Staphylococcus aureus* endocarditis. Ann Intern Med 115:674, 1991.
44. Mortara LA, Bayer AS: *Staphylococcus aureus* bacteremia and endocarditis: New diagnostic and therapeutic concepts. Infect Dis Clin North Am 7:53, 1993.
45. Kaatz GW, Seo SM, Dorman NJ, et al: Emergence of teicoplanin resistance during therapy of *Staphylococcus aureus* endocarditis. J Infect Dis 162:103, 1990.
46. Daum RS, Gupta S, Sabbagh R, et al: Characterization of *Staphylococcus aureus* isolates with decreased susceptibility to vancomycin and teicoplanin: Isolation and purification of a constitutively produced protein associated with decreased susceptibility. J Infect Dis 166:1066, 1992.
47. Wheat LJ, Kohler RB, Shite AL, et al: Effect of rifampin on nasal carriers of coagulase-positive staphylococci. J Infect Dis 144:177, 1984.
48. Yu VL, Goetz A, Wagener M, et al: *Staphylococcus aureus* nasal carriage and infection in patients on hemodialysis: Efficacy of antibiotic prophylaxis. N Engl J Med 315:91, 1986.
49. Parenti MA, Hatfield SM, Leyden JJ: Mupirocin: A topical antibiotic with a unique structure and mechanism of action. Clin Pharm 6:761, 1987.
50. Kirmani N, Tuazon CU, Murray HW, et al: *Staphylococcus aureus* carriage rate among patients on chronic hemodialysis. Arch Intern Med 138:1657, 1978.
51. Kluytmans JAJW, Mouton JW, Ijzerman EPF, et al: Nasal carriage of *Staphylococcus aureus* as a major risk factor for wound infections after cardiac surgery. J Infect Dis 171:216, 1995.
52. Reagan DR, Doebbeling BN, Pfaller MA, et al: Elimination of coincident *Staphylococcus aureus* nasal and hand carriage with intranasal application of mupirocin calcium ointment. Ann Intern Med 114:101, 1991.
53. Doebling BN, Breneman DL, Neu HC, et al: Elimination of *Staphylococcus aureus* nasal carriage in health care workers: Analysis of six clinical trials with calcium mupirocin ointment. Clin Infect Dis 17:466, 1993.

192

Streptococcus pyogenes (Group A Streptococci)

Gene H. Stollerman

As a result of the great variety of clinical syndromes it causes, *Streptococcus pyogenes* (group A streptococcus) has been studied more extensively than most other bacterial pathogens by clinicians and microbiologists. *S. pyogenes* owes its species name to its role in causing pyogenic infections, either as a primary invader of the throat (pharyngitis) and lower respiratory tract (pneumonia) or as a secondary invader of the skin (pyoderma, erysipelas), of the endometrium (puerperal sepsis), or of wounds (cellulitis, lymphangitis, and necrotizing fasciitis). It is, however, the postinfectious sequelae of acute rheumatic fever (ARF) and acute glomerulonephritis (AGN), especially the former, that make it a particularly dreaded infection. Moreover, some of its toxin-producing properties result in scarlet fever and toxic shock syndrome (TSS).

The diversity of these clinical syndromes, their geographic variation, and the secular changes in their epidemiology within the relatively short history of their discovery speak for the diversity of the strains that are found within this single streptococcal species, which is only 1 among 29 others in the genus *Streptococcus.*

Characteristics of the Pathogen

Microscopic Appearance

Streptococci are gram-positive organisms, spherical or ovoid, and no larger than 2 μm in diameter. Cell division occurs in one plane by the formation of an equatorial plate, which results in the formation of chains of varied length, usually 6 to 12 cocci but fewer for encapsulated strains. Chain length diminishes under optimal growth conditions.

Colonial Morphology

Growth on blood agar was the earliest basis for classifying streptococci according to hemolytic properties. Beta hemolysis is that resulting from complete lysis of red blood cells in the agar, which accounts for the clear zone around colonies. Alpha hemolysis is the result of conversion of hemoglobin to a greenish pigment and incomplete lysis of red blood cells in the surrounding medium. Streptococcal γ colonies are nonhemolytic. The great majority of group A streptococci are β-hemolytic, although some strains lack both streptolysin S (SLS) and streptolysin O (SLO) production (see later) and so are nonhemolytic. Sheep blood is ideal for primary isolation of cultures on blood agar because it is inhibitory to the growth of *Haemophilus haemolyticus,* a common throat commensal organism that may be confused with hemolytic streptococcal colonies. Human blood should not be used for diagnostic throat cultures because it may be inhibitory to streptococcal growth and because beta hemolysis is not as clearly visible as on sheep blood.

Strains of group A streptococci that are encapsulated form large mucoid colonies, which on fresh growth have the appearance of a drop of oil.[1] When dehydration of the colony occurs, however, its surface becomes roughened (matte). Nonencapsulated or slightly encapsulated colonies have an opaque, pearly appearance. Dissociating encapsulated strains may show variations in colony morphology, and the mucoid properties of such strains may be restored by mouse passage. The instability of virulent, M-rich, mucoid strains requires preservation of such strains in a fully virulent phase by frequent passage through noninhibiting fresh human blood or through mice. Preservation of freshly isolated strains by prompt lyophilization is necessary if virulence properties are to be studied adequately.

Cultural Characteristics

Group A streptococci are facultative anaerobes. They do not produce catalase or oxidase and do not contain heme compounds. They are sensitive to heat, requiring but 30 minutes at 60°C for sterilization. The cultures are optimally made in blood-enriched media at pH 7.4 to 7.6 incubated at 37°C under reduced oxygen tension and in a carbon dioxide–enriched (e.g., 10%) atmosphere. Under anaerobic conditions, hemolysis is enhanced. Reducing substances such as thioglycollate shorten the lag period of growth.

Antigenic Structure

THE CELL WALL MEMBRANE

The cell wall membrane of group A streptococci contains an epitope that has received considerable attention because it cross-reacts with a component of cardiac myosin that is also present in a non–type-specific epitope of M protein that has similar cross-reactions (see later). Its extension to the surface of the streptococcus is still uncertain, but if it surrounds fimbriae, as expected, it is certainly closely associated with M protein and the hyaluronate capsule.

MURAMYL PEPTIDE PEPTIDOGLYCANS

These basic cell wall components are particularly interesting because they are potent immunologic adjuvants capable of amplifying host antibody responses.[2] Indeed, coupled with protective peptide epitopes they have been used to produce synthetic vaccines. The peptidoglycan consists of *N*-acetyl-D-glucosamine, *N*-acetyl-D-muramic acid, and a tripeptide, D-glutamic acid, L-lysine, and D- and L-alanine.

GROUP A CARBOHYDRATE

In the 1920s and early 1930s, Lancefield[3] classified streptococci serologically on the basis of their carbohydrate cell wall antigens extracted from whole cells. Precipitin tests made with cross-absorbed antisera specific for the carbohydrate in these extracts are the most accurate method for defining the major streptococcal serologic groups. The group A carbohydrate is composed of a branched polymer of L-rhamnose, *N*-acetyl-D-glucosamine in a 2:1 ratio, the latter composing the antigenic determinant. The group A polysaccharide is linked in the cell wall to the peptidoglycan.

M PROTEINS

Historically, group A streptococci were first serotyped in agglutinin tests by Griffith.[4] Later, Lancefield subserotyped group A streptococci, identifying subtypes by three protein antigens, M, T, and R. More than 90% of strains may be classified by using M and T antigens. It is M protein, however, that is the major surface antigen of virulent strains and by which their identification should be made. More than 90 M serotypes have been identified to date.

T antigens, which are resistant to pepsin and trypsin and to hot-acid extraction, are useful in the epidemiologic identification of strains because of their stability. Strains that have dissociated and lost virulence factors may still be identified by their T antigens. For this reason, the T-typing system is often employed along with the M-typing system in epidemiologic studies. Some T antigens are restricted to a single M type, whereas others may be shared by several M types.

R antigens are surface proteins that are destroyed by pepsin but not by trypsin. They are not commonly used, except to identify some unusual serotypes that are not otherwise identifiable by M- and T-typing systems.

M protein has been most intensively researched because it is primarily responsible for resistance to phagocytosis, only homologous M antibodies are protective, it contains the immunologic potential for a streptococcal vaccine, and it con-

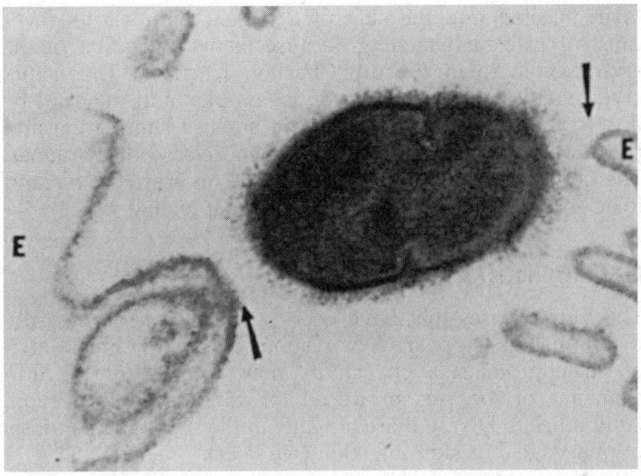

FIGURE 192–1 □ Electron micrograph of group A streptococci adhering to the surface of a buccal mucosal cell. Prominent surface projections (fimbriae) contain both M protein and lipoteichoic acid. (From Beachey EH, Ofek I: Epithelial cell binding of group A streptococci by lipoteichoic acid on fimbriae denuded of M protein. Reproduced from The Journal of Experimental Medicine, 1976, vol 143, pp 759–771 by copyright permission of The Rockefeller University Press.)

tains some epitopes that are cross-reactive with host tissues, especially in the myocardium (see later).

At electron microscopy, virulent streptococci show prominent fimbriae, surface projections that appear as a fuzz and that are removed with the M protein by hot-acid extraction[5] (Fig. 192–1). Research of the past two decades has led to a remarkably complete characterization of the M protein molecule.[6–17] Gentle extraction from the organism's surface by dilute pepsin has yielded the terminal peptide, pep M, of an extremely long M protein molecule[6] that is a particular feature of the virulent throat strains that cause rheumatic fever (see later). The surface structures of group A streptococci determine not only their virulence properties but also their primary tropism for either the throat or the skin. The molecular composition of the M-associated surface protein extractable from virulent throat strains of M serotypes associated with rheumatic fever has an epitope distinguishable from that of the M-associated proteins of nonrheumatogenic serotypes. The former strains have been referred to as class I and the latter as class II group A streptococci.[12] Patients with rheumatic fever display elevated levels of serum immunoglobulin G directed toward the class I–specific epitope and lack immunoreactivity to the class II–specific epitope.[15] Moreover, the genes of M protein *(emm)* have been identified as four subfamilies of nucleotide sequences arranged in five distinctive chromosomal patterns, labeled A to E. Impetigo strains are virtually all of the D,E gene pattern, whereas rheumatic fever throat strains are almost all of the A,B,C pattern (Fig. 192–2). Nonrheumatogenic throat strains appear to be distributed between both of these groupings.[16]

The structure of pep M is that of a coiled coil consisting of a series of repeating peptides.[9] The N-terminal of pep M contains the isotope that confers type-specific immunity.[6] This epitope is separable from the proximal portion of the molecule where the isotopes that cross-react with host tissues, heart, skin, synovia, and brain[8, 10, 11, 13, 14] are localized. The pep M peptide has proved to be immunogenic in animals and humans and seems to be free of the toxic properties of the former crude M protein hot-acid extracts that produced unacceptable local inflammatory reactions in earlier studies. This "toxic" portion of the M molecule has typical superantigen properties that have been described for pyrogenic toxins (see later), that is, the capacity to activate T lymphocytes nonspecifically at sites other than that of the T-cell antigen receptor (Vβ specificity).[17] As discussed later, this property may be responsible for the intense antigenicity of rheumatogenic streptococci.

The possible role of M protein in the pathogenesis of rheumatic fever and its potential use in a vaccine against this disease are discussed later. Surface properties related to resistance to phagocytosis and virulence are discussed further later.

LIPOTEICHOIC ACID

The adherence of group A streptococci to host epithelium involves a highly regulated and complex interplay of multiple bacterial adhesins and their specific receptors. M protein constitutes one of these adhesins. However, when M protein is gently extracted by pepsin the remaining tiny projecting fimbriae that extend from the bacterial cell surface contain another surface adhesin composed of lipoteichoic acid.[18] The terminal fatty acids of this phosphoglycerol polymer bind avidly to fibronectin on buccal mucosal cells. Other non-A serologic groups of streptococci also possess this adhesin, which may have a role in the colonization of the throat with various species of streptococci.[19]

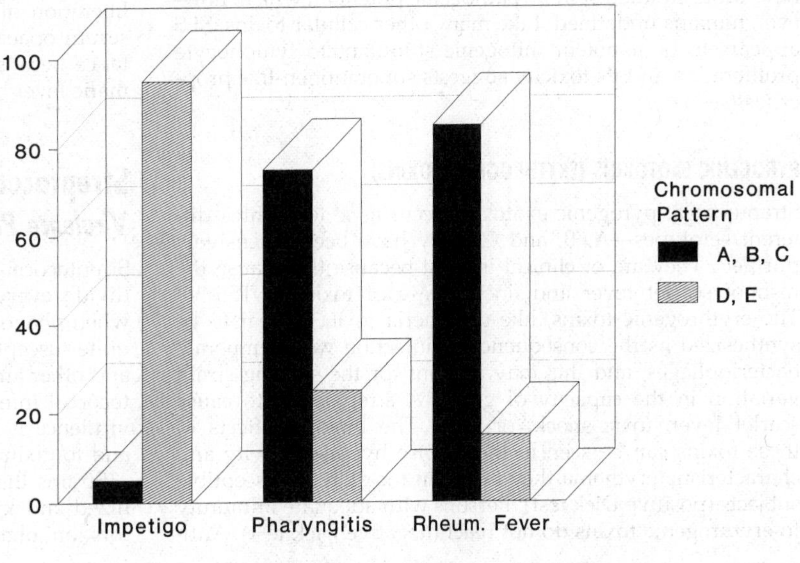

FIGURE 192–2 □ Relationship between group A streptococcal disease and chromosomal patterns (A to E) of M protein genes *(emm)* in 105 strains obtained from several worldwide locations during a period of more than 50 years. The 26 rheumatic fever strains studied were collected from patients during an acute attack. Rheumatic fever strains were almost all the A,B,C gene pattern, whereas impetigo strains were almost all D,E. Other nonrheumatogenic pharyngeal strains were less sharply divided. (From Bessen DE, Sotir CM, Readdy TL, Hollingshead SK: Genetic correlates of throat and skin isolates of group A streptococci. J Infect Dis 173:896–900, 1996. Copyright by University of Chicago.)

THE HYALURONATE CAPSULE

Encapsulation is a feature of the strains of *S. pyogenes* that are usually richest in M protein and most resistant to phagocytosis. Such encapsulation is best demonstrated after 1 or 2 hours of log-phase growth in media rich in protein (e.g., blood broth). Strains with the largest capsules produce the shortest chains, often no more than two to four cocci.[20] Large capsule formation is characteristic of rheumatogenic streptococci, but encapsulation is not limited to strains that possess this property. The precise structure of the capsule is not known. Earlier reports of the demonstration of antibodies to streptococcal hyaluronate[21] were considered controversial because contaminating antigens in the media could not be excluded as the source of antigenic stimulation. Streptococcal hyaluronate is chemically identical to that of the human host, and highly polymerized, intact hyaluronate did not appear to be immunogenic in mammals in early experimental studies. However, more sensitive immunologic methods (enzyme-linked immunosorbent assay) have revealed that antibodies can be raised to hyaluronate that has been partially denatured.[22] The finding may be significant for the possible molecular mimicry of hyaluronate with host tissues and is therefore of theoretical interest.

Extracellular Products

S. pyogenes releases a great variety of extracellular products into the culture medium during growth, many of which are biologically active.

HEMOLYSINS

Beta hemolysis is caused by either or both of two hemolysins, SLO and SLS. SLO is produced by most group A strains and by streptococci belonging to groups C and G as well. SLO is so named because of its sensitivity to oxygen, by which it is reversibly inactivated; SLO is inhibited by cholesterol and by serum lipoproteins. It cross-reacts immunologically with other oxygen-labile hemolysins of pneumococci and clostridia. SLO is a potent cardiac toxin and is highly antigenic.

SLS is an oxygen-stable, nonantigenic toxin that is bound to the surface of streptococci. It is extractable from the cells by serum (hence its name) or by albumin, RNA, or detergents. SLS is a potent cellular toxin of relatively low molecular weight. It is inhibited by phospholipids; hence its inhibition by human serum is due to serum lipoproteins and not to antibodies.[23] Its cardiac toxicity and its lack of antigenicity have aroused interest in its pathogenic potential, which, however, remains undefined. Like many other cellular toxins, SLS appears to be a potent mitogenic stimulant to lymphocyte proliferation and its toxicity suggests superantigen-like properties (see later).

PYROGENIC EXOTOXINS (ERYTHROGENIC TOXINS)

Streptococcal pyrogenic exotoxins occur as at least three different serotypes—A, B, and C. They have been extensively purified. They are of clinical interest because they cause the rash of scarlet fever and, in the case of toxin A, TSS.[24–28] The erythrogenic toxins, like diphtheria toxin, appear to be synthesized as the consequence of infection with temperate bacteriophages, and this may account for the striking strain variation in the capacity of group A streptococci to cause scarlet fever, toxic shock, or both. The biologic effects of these toxins can be seen in the intense hypersensitivity and characteristic erythema they evoke in the skin of susceptible subjects (positive Dick test). Persons with adequate immunity to erythrogenic toxins do not react (negative Dick test). Antitoxin injected into the skin of a patient with scarlet fever causes localized blanching because of neutralization of the erythrogenic toxin (Schultz-Charlton reaction). The actual erythrogenic reaction, however, is complex and may not be due to the toxin directly but to its intense stimulation and recruitment of lymphocytes and their release of cytokines. The clinical role of toxins A, B, and C in scarlet fever and toxic shock is described later and in Chapter 190.

DEOXYRIBONUCLEASES A, B, C, AND D

The four DNases that have been purified and serologically distinguished[29] appear to be responsible for the breakdown of nucleoproteins. Such activity may account for the thin character of the pus produced by streptococcal infection. Antibodies to DNase B are of value in the serologic diagnosis of pharyngeal or skin infection (see later).

STREPTOKINASE

Two different streptokinases are produced by group A streptococci. These enzymes are antigenically distinct from group C streptokinase, the source of the commercial streptokinase used in therapeutic thrombolysis. Streptokinase forms complexes with plasminogen activator and catalyzes the conversion of plasminogen to plasmin. Plasmin in turn digests fibrinogen and fibrin. It also cleaves the third component of complement into the chemotactic factor C3a. Streptokinase antibodies are raised after most streptococcal infections, and these can be measured by the antistreptokinase serologic test.[30, 31] Streptokinase probably contributes to the thinning of streptococcal pus and with hyaluronidase may facilitate the rapid spread of streptococci through the skin and lymphatics that is seen in cellulitis.

Streptococcal hyaluronidase hydrolyzes hyaluronic acid, present in the streptococcal capsule, and also that found in animal tissues. Known as a spreading factor in the skin, this enzyme appears to be produced readily in the infected host, because, like streptokinase, in patients with streptococcal pharyngitis it produces antibodies with virtually the same frequency as SLO and DNase B.[32]

Other enzymes produced by many strains include proteinases, NADase, adenosinetriphosphatase, phosphatases, esterases, amylase, and neuraminidase. Special note should be made of a lipoproteinase called serum opacity factor. Strains that produce this enzyme can be identified by their growth in human serum and production of a clouding or "creaming" of the serum caused by the cleaving of lipoprotein, with the liberation of fatty acids, cholesterol, and other lipids. Such serum opacity factor–producing strains have clinical importance because they are rarely if ever associated with rheumatic fever but are closely associated with skin infections.[33, 34]

Streptococcal Infections

Virulence Properties of Infecting Strains

Streptococci grow rapidly under ideal conditions. They can divide every 20 minutes in the log phase of growth, but when phagocytosed they are rapidly killed because they are quite susceptible to the antibacterial action of oxygen radicals and other antibacterial substances within phagosomes. Streptococcal infection, therefore, is principally extracellular, and virulence is related primarily to resistance to phagocytosis and to toxin production.

Strains that lack M protein and capsules are easily recognized and killed. Such avirulent strains interact with receptors on phagocytes and activate complement components through the alternative and classical complement pathways.[35] M protein–rich strains that resist phagocytosis were demonstrated by Todd[36] using a bactericidal test. This test was first employed to measure type-specific M antibodies in whole fresh human blood. These antibodies opsonize homologous M serotypes, which are then rapidly phagocytosed.[37] The bactericidal test is also a measure of the virulence of streptococcal strains, as it tests their ability to evade phagocytes and grow rapidly in whole human blood that is free of homologous type-specific antibody.

M protein precipitates fibrinogen from human plasma, which further blocks surface interactions with complement components and phagocytic receptors.[37] There is some evidence to suggest that M protein may have active as well as passive antiphagocytic effects.[8] In addition, a cell surface–bound group A streptococcal component that inactivates phagocytosis has been isolated in M protein–containing strains. By cleaving a six-peptide residue from human C5 it inactivates this potent chemoattractant.[38]

Clinical Syndromes and Infecting Strains

Group A streptococci may be classified clinically as the agents of pharyngitis (throat strains), pyoderma (skin strains), rheumatic fever (throat only), glomerulonephritis (skin or throat), and scarlet fever and toxic shock (throat or skin strains). Invasive infections of skin and soft tissues may be produced by any of these strains that contain the relevant virulence factors. As noted earlier, the M protein gene *emm* patterns on chromosomes are distinctive for either impetigo strains (pattern D,E) or rheumatogenic throat strains (A,B,C), whereas nonrheumatogenic strains isolated from the throat may belong to either or both patterns[16] (see Fig. 192–2). Some of the strains isolated from the throat may have spread there secondarily from skin lesions. Of special interest is the difference between rheumatogenic and nonrheumatogenic strains of the A,B,C pattern (see later).

STREPTOCOCCAL PHARYNGITIS (Fig. 192–3)

Group A streptococcal pharyngitis is one of the most common bacterial infections of humans. It differs much in frequency, severity, and clinical characteristics, depending on the patient's age, the character of the infecting strains, and the epidemiologic circumstances that affect their transmission. Thus, the high attack rate in military recruits is the result of contact among susceptible persons close enough to ensure spread of infection by droplets. Organisms with the greatest virulence produce the most rapid spread and the most severe epidemics of streptococcal pharyngitis. On the other hand, mildly virulent strains of group A streptococci may cause asymptomatic colonization and spread through populations that are in intimate contact. For this reason, throat culture of material from asymptomatic schoolchildren who have endemic sporadic infections isolates group A streptococci with high frequency, whether or not sequelae (rheumatic fever, AGN, or another) occur.[39] Streptococci that contaminate fomites and dust do not cause pharyngeal infection, even though the organisms are viable and can be propagated readily on blood agar cultures. Untreated patients spread the infection principally during the period of acute pharyngitis and for a week or so during convalescence. The organisms may dissociate rapidly during convalescent carriage. Except in epidemics, they are usually not a significant problem to contacts, even though the patient may carry the organisms for weeks or months.

In the setting of epidemic group A streptococcal pharyngitis, however, it may be necessary to treat asymptomatic carriers of freshly acquired virulent strains. Moreover, acquisition of such virulent strains may produce asymptomatic infection in some persons and can lead to rheumatic fever. For this reason, it is not uncommon for patients with rheumatic fever or AGN not to recall antecedent infection.

The urgency of diagnosis and treatment of streptococcal pharyngitis therefore depends on the epidemiologic setting.[40] A negative throat culture in a patient with pharyngitis has great predictive value, but the confidence of the clinician in such negative results depends on the prevalence in the community of epidemic strains, especially of rheumatogenic or nephritogenic strains.

Factors that influence the spread of streptococcal pharyngitis are socioeconomic only insofar as crowded living quarters foster close contact.[41] Host susceptibility to streptococcal pharyngitis does not appear to be influenced by race, ethnic group, climate, geography, or nutrition alone. Age is important in that infants and quite young children who have not yet developed hyperimmunity may express only mild rhinorrhea rather than acute local symptoms and signs of pharyngitis. On the other hand, infants are prone to develop secondary suppurative complications of otitis media, sinusitis, cervical adenitis, and even bacteremia. Contrariwise, by school age, pharyngeal infection becomes explosive, with

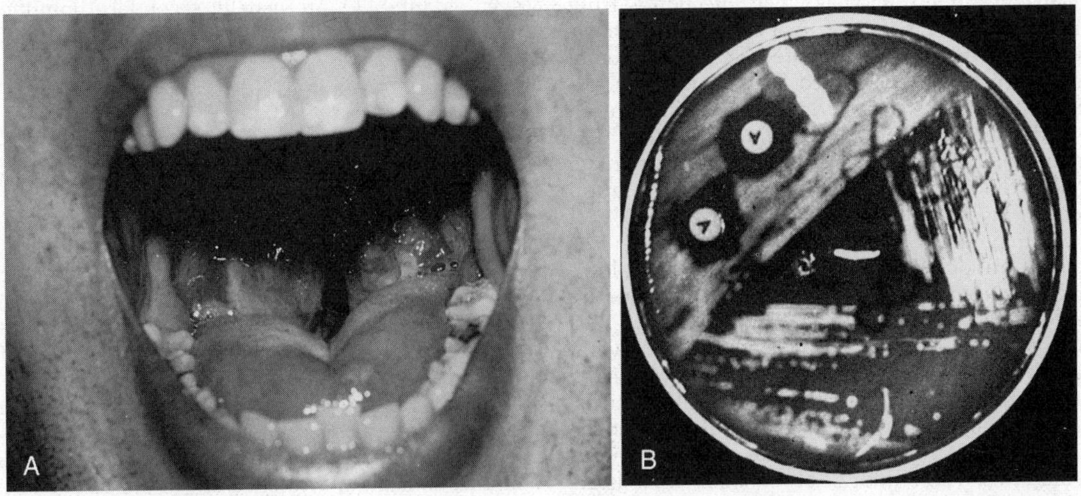

FIGURE 192–3 □ *A,* Patient with group A streptococcal pharyngitis. *B,* Throat culture from patient in *A* showing colonies of β-hemolytic streptoccocci growing on sheep's blood agar. Bacitracin disks marked A show zone of inhibition of growth.

intense local and systemic responses. Although older patients may have acquired immunity to many M types, in the absence of such type-specific immunity, adults acquire infection at a rate similar to that for children.[41]

For these reasons, the streptococcal pharyngitis attack rate within a family is greatest in siblings nearest in age to the index patient, next in frequency in the mother, and less frequent in the father. Peak rates of streptococcal pharyngitis and streptococcal carrier state occur in the school-age population between 5 and 15 years.

Clinical Features. The incubation period is brief: 2 to 4 days. Onset of sore throat and fever is sudden. Pain on swallowing may be severe. Rhinitis, laryngitis, and bronchitis are not associated symptoms as they are in viral respiratory infections. Systemic symptoms include fever, headache, malaise, anorexia, and, especially in younger children, abdominal pain and vomiting. Chilliness is common but not rigors. Examination of the throat reveals diffuse erythema, edema, and hypertrophy of the lymphoid tissues of the posterior pharynx. In the most characteristic cases the tonsils are covered with a punctate or confluent yellow-gray exudate (see Fig. 192–3). The anterior cervical nodes are typically enlarged and tender. The white cell count is usually greater than 12,000/mm^3. If specimens are properly taken the throat culture propagates large numbers of group A β-hemolytic streptococci in patients with these symptoms and signs. The course of the infection is relatively brief. Fever abates within several days, and sore throat and constitutional symptoms rarely last more than a week. Indeed, in controlled studies in military recruits, significant differences in duration of fever were not observed in patients treated with penicillin compared with those treated symptomatically.[42]

The clinical features just described are typical for relatively severe streptococcal pharyngeal infection confirmed by unequivocal immune responses. Milder infections, however, may not show these classic findings.

Laboratory Diagnosis

Culture of Throat Secretions. To obtain culture material from the throat, swabs should be passed under direct vision over the pharyngeal tonsils and posterior pharynx. The swab should then be streaked directly, as soon as possible, on a sheep's blood agar plate of low dextrose content. Stabbing through the agar with the inoculating loop is recommended to grow some colonies below the surface at low oxygen tension. The culture is best incubated at 10% carbon dioxide tension. Colonies of hemolytic streptococci should be recorded in a semiquantitative manner. If that is properly done, these organisms are quite numerous when infection is truly caused by the streptococcus. When organisms are few, however, the culture is more likely to represent a streptococcal carrier state. Colonies should be noted for mucoid characteristics (see earlier). It has become fairly routine to implant on the surface of the agar a paper disk containing less than 0.02 units of bacitracin. Hemolytic colonies that are resistant to such low concentrations of bacitracin are unlikely to be group A streptococci. On the other hand, approximately 5% of non–group A streptococci are also sensitive to such a low bacitracin concentration. For more definitive epidemiologic studies, serologic grouping and typing should be done by reference laboratories.

As an alternative to conventional throat culture, several methods have been developed for rapid detection of group A streptococcal antigen on throat swabs. Other alternatives, such as fluorescent antibody techniques for detection of the group-specific streptococcal polysaccharide, have been used in some laboratories. These fluorescent antibody tests, however, have not increased the practicality or efficiency of culture isolation of throat secretions and now are rarely performed. To meet a perceived need for a faster laboratory diagnosis, rapid tests for identifying minute amounts of group A polysaccharide extracted from the swab have been developed, resulting in the availability of numerous commercial kits.[43–45] Whereas the specificity of some products has been greater than 95%, the sensitivity has been less than 90%. The significance of a false-negative result depends on whether the epidemiologic prevalence of serious infections supports this degree of false negativity. The test may therefore be useful in sporadic streptococcal pharyngitis when the prevalence of rheumatic fever and other sequelae in the population is low, particularly in controlling the overuse of antibiotics for the relatively "benign" sore throats that are associated with negative antigen test results.

Streptococcal Antibodies. Extensive studies have established the behavior and usefulness of antibodies to streptococcal extracellular products such as SLO, DNase B, hyaluronidase, streptokinase, and NADase, among others.[35, 46] The first two have become the most commonly available commercially. Repeated streptococcal infections set the expected mean level of "normalcy" of antibody titers in a given population, and such values therefore relate to both the age groups studied and the epidemiologic setting. The curve of the rate of decline of elevated streptococcal antibody titers has been established in patients with ARF who received monthly injections of benzathine penicillin G to prevent intercurrent streptococcal infection.[31] When such patients receive penicillin prophylaxis, the decline in titer is rapid for the first 2 to 3 months. Anti-SLO titers, for example, fall much more slowly when levels decline to approximately 200 units/mL. After streptococcal pharyngitis (except in quite young children) the increase in titer is rapid, consistent with secondary antigenic stimulation, and peak titers are usually observed within a few weeks. When titers are initially increased above 300 units/mL in serum samples obtained during the acute phase of infection, further increases may be more difficult to demonstrate. Given an initial titer of less than 200 units/mL, approximately 80% of patients demonstrate a twofold or greater increase between acute- and convalescent-phase values. When two different antibodies are tested with the same serum, a boost in titer is observed in one or the other in at least 90% of patients who have streptococcal pharyngitis.[31]

Type-specific antibodies to M protein can be detected by several methods,[47–50] but the methodology is technically complex and is used principally for investigative and epidemiologic purposes. Prompt and effective antibiotic therapy suppresses anti-M immune responses, which are primary. In contrast, other streptococcal antibodies commonly measured, such as anti-SLO, are usually secondary immune responses and therefore much less readily suppressed by antibacterial therapy.

SCARLET FEVER

The epidemiology of scarlet fever is closely related to that of streptococcal pharyngitis and also to that of streptococcal pyoderma because it depends on the capability of any strain to produce one or more of the erythrogenic toxins A, B, and C. Scarlet fever may be produced by rheumatogenic strains as well, and the epidemiology of the two diseases was superimposable in the preantibiotic era. In the 19th century, the severe toxicity of scarlet fever in industrializing nations made it a dreaded, and sometimes fatal, disease.[51] By the 1920s, however, its severity and frequency waned,[52] and by the 1950s the prevalence of scarlet fever dramatically declined.[53] It was noted by then to be no more than a dermatologic marker indicating a recent bout of streptococcal pharyngitis or pyoderma. The TSS associated with staphylococcal infections has been clearly shown to be related to the production of *Staphylococcus* pyrogenic toxins, notably TSS toxin 1. Pyrogenic toxins are a large family of proteins secreted by *Staphylococcus aureus* and group A streptococci. These toxins share biologic activity and in many instances amino acid sequence homology (see later and Chapter 190). Streptococcal toxin A–producing strains have been reappearing in the United States, principally as a result of soft tissue infections.[26] Most of these infections are relatively mild but paradoxically result in severe systemic symptoms, frequently associated with shock or severe organ damage, particularly of the kidneys and myocardium.[54–56] Streptococcal strains, therefore, can produce any one of the erythrogenic toxins in any kind of streptococcal disease, and this independent expression of the three toxins may account for the vagaries of scarlatina throughout modern medical history.

Clinical Manifestations. The clinical picture of scarlet fever may include the classic enanthema, strawberry tongue (one that is coated with red, protruding papillae) or raspberry tongue (bright red with large papillae). Within a day or two of the sore throat, the scarlatinal rash appears on the face, sparing the area around the lips (circumoral pallor) and spreading to the neck, chest, back, and remainder of the trunk and extremities. The rash is a diffuse erythema, blanching on pressure, and may have punctate elevations that roughen the skin. The inner aspects of the trunk, arms, and thighs are most intensely affected. Pastia lines are linear striations of confluent petechiae and petechiae related to capillary fragility induced by the erythrogenic toxin, which may be demonstrated by an applied tourniquet (the Rumpel-Leede sign). The erythema abates in 6 to 9 days, followed by a characteristic desquamation of the skin during the second week, most often affecting the palms and soles. Striking eosinophilia often occurs during this stage of desquamation. The scarlatinal rash must be differentiated from the rashes of viral exanthems, Kawasaki disease, staphylococcal TSS, and drug eruptions.

Diagnosis. Group A streptococcal pharyngitis must be differentiated from sore throat produced by other bacterial and viral agents. Of the former, group C and G streptococcal infections may be most confusing, but these are milder, do not often cause suppurative complications, and do not cause nonsuppurative sequelae. Gonococcal pharyngitis must be considered in populations in which fellatio is practiced, and its clinical appearance may be readily confused with that of group A streptococcal infection. Although diphtheria is now rare, it should be considered in vulnerable, nonimmunized populations. *Myocoplasma* pharyngitis has been proved to cause sore throat, but the infection usually involves some other part of the respiratory tract as well.

The major confusion in differential diagnosis stems from the common viral respiratory infections, some of which cause pharyngeal and tonsillar exudate, particularly adenovirus infections and infectious mononucleosis. Adenovirus causes herpangina. Herpes simplex virus stomatitis can produce sore throat and painful pharyngeal vesicles. Both add to the confusion when group A streptococci are also carried in the throat of populations in which these infections are common. Indeed, failure to respond to a trial of penicillin therapy should alert the clinician to the fact that in such cases culture isolation of streptococci from throat secretions represents an intercurrent earlier state and is not the cause of the infection[46] (see later).

Suppurative Complications. Suppurative complications most frequently affect contiguous pharyngeal cavities, such as the middle ear and paranasal sinuses. Mastoiditis and meningitis caused by *S. pyogenes* are now quite rare. Bacteremia leading to metastatic involvement of joints, bones, and other sites and group A streptococcal pneumonia also now occur mostly in epidemics caused by highly virulent strains, as has been observed in military recruit camp epidemics (see later).[57–59] Streptococcal pneumonia also occurs in economically depressed populations where medical care is inadequate and living conditions are crowded.

Peritonsillar abscess, or quinsy, is not usually caused by group A streptococcal infection alone but is due, rather, to the formation of a polymicrobial abscess in which anaerobic throat flora predominate. Aerobic cultures of aspirate from such abscesses therefore do not isolate a pathogen, but the infecting anaerobic throat flora are exquisitely sensitive to penicillin treatment, which, with adequate drainage, produces a dramatic response. Peritonsillar abscess must be suspected when an abrupt increase in pain and dysphagia, swelling of the neck, and fever arise after a primary pharyngitis. Displacement of the tonsil can be seen on the affected side, and a fluctuant mass can be readily palpated with a gloved finger. Early diagnosis and prompt penicillin therapy are essential to prevent the development of necrotizing fasciitis of the neck, which can be a fatal complication (Ludwig angina).[60]

INVASIVE STREPTOCOCCAL INFECTIONS: CHANGING EPIDEMIOLOGY

The changing epidemiology of group A streptococcal infection in the past several years deserves special comment.[25] First noted in the mid-1980s were focal outbreaks of ARF in military and civilian populations in the United States (see later). These were associated with the reappearance of highly virulent, rheumatogenic, M protein serotypes. Shortly thereafter, unusually severe invasive streptococcal infections began to be reported, both in the United States and abroad,[26, 55–58] especially life-threatening infections caused by M types 1 and 3. The portal of entry for these infections was usually the skin and soft tissues. Some of these gave rise to shock and multiorgan failure, with manifestations similar to those of the staphylococcal TSS, and therefore were named streptococcal TSSs.[56] Clinical features of serious streptococcal skin and soft tissue infection and TSS are described later.

Streptococcal Cellulitis. Rapid spread of group A streptococci through the skin and subcutaneous tissues with lymphangitis and bacteremia is a distictive feature of infection with virulent group A streptococci. It may occur as a complication of burns and traumatic and surgical wounds but may also follow mild trauma. It is differentiated from erysipelas in that the lesion is not raised; the demarcation between involved and uninvolved skin is indistinct (long red streaks rather than an advancing border of intradermal swelling). Parenteral injection of illicit drugs into extremities with impaired lymphatic drainage resulting from previous episodes of cellulitis has made this streptococcal infection increasingly common. A strong predisposing factor is impaired lymphatic drainage such as that seen after radical mastectomy, saphenous vein removal for coronary bypass grafting,[61] and recurrent lymphangitis caused by chronic tinea pedis.

Streptococcal cellulitis responds brilliantly to intravenous or repository intramuscular penicillin G therapy. Semisynthetic penicillinase-resistant penicillin may be used when staphylococcal infection cannot be excluded on initial presentation. In the absence of a positive blood culture, a clear distinction between streptococcal and staphylococcal infection may not be made because aspirate or biopsy results are often negative or because surface skin contamination by staphylococci is quite common and may confuse the diagnosis.[62]

Pyoderma. As noted earlier (see the section on M protein), the M protein genes of impetigo strains have a distinct chromosomal pattern.

Necrotizing Fasciitis (Streptococcal Gangrene). This terrifying and often fatal fulminating infection has received much publicity. Notwithstanding the high index of suspicion caused by sensational media coverage (a "flesh-eating" organism), the incidence of this infection is definitely increasing.[63] Necrotizing fasciitis is an infection of the deeper subcutaneous tissues and fascia, characterized by rapidly spreading necrosis and gangrene of the skin and underlying structures. The infection may be polymicrobial with both aerobic and anaerobic microorganisms. That caused by the group A streptococcus, called streptococcal gangrene by Meleney,[64] characteristically begins at the site of a trivial or inapparent trauma as a mild erythema. It progresses rapidly in 24 to 72 hours to an extensive, dusky bluish swelling. Bullae containing yellowish or hemorrhagic fluid may appear. Bacteremia and frank gangrene follow within a few days. Mortality is high even with appropriate medical and surgical intervention.

A biopsy with frozen sections may aid in diagnosis.[65] Prompt surgical intervention is necessary when the diagnosis is confirmed.

Streptococcal Toxic Shock Syndrome (see Chapter 190). Most cases of streptococcal TSS reported from North America, Europe, and Australia have occurred in healthy patients with an initial focal infection of the skin and soft tissue.[66] Severe puerperal infections associated with disseminated intravascular coagulation are also well documented.[67, 68]

Athough most cases of TSS, even in children, are a consequence of soft tissue infections, TSS has also occurred in association with pharyngeal infection alone.[69–71] Streptococcal strains causing TSS are readily transmitted from person to person and tend to initiate invasive disease in contacts.[72, 73]

Clinical features of TSS are often complicated by the associated features of a soft tissue infection. The clue to the presence of the superimposed toxic effect is the suddeness of local pain, intensification, swelling, arrhythmia, high fever, and prostration. The subsequent hypotension, disseminated intravascular coagulation, and multiorgan failure duplicate findings in other TSSs produced by staphylococci, meningococci, and gram-negative endotoxemia. Delirium, renal failure, acute respiratory distress syndrome, toxic cardiomyopathy, and hepatic failure are common clinical pathways for toxins that act as superantigens and massively activate cells that produce cytokines, such as tumor necrosis factor and interleukin-1, which mediate acute inflammation and tissue necrosis.[74–76]

In contrast to staphylococcal TSS, in which positive blood culture results are unusual, blood culture results are positive in approximately 60% of cases of streptococcal TSS. Criteria for the clinical diagnosis of streptococcal TSS have been proposed by an ad hoc working group.[77]

The management of streptococcal TSS in its severe form requires support of vital functions and hemodynamic abnormalities provided by intensive care units. Mechanical ventilators, renal dialysis, management of disseminated intravascular coagulation, and surgical intervention are usually needed. Empirical broad-spectrum antibiotic coverage appropriate for septic shock is usually instituted initially. Once the streptococcal etiology is confirmed, high-dose intravenous penicillin G therapy is the treatment of choice. Mortality rates, despite such management, may be at least 30%.[26]

STREPTOCOCCAL SKIN INFECTIONS

Pyoderma. Skin wounds or burns can be secondarily infected by any virulent group A streptococcus, but certain streptococcal strains have particular tropism for the skin. They are the strains that cause the common pyodermas usually referred to as streptococcal impetigo or impetigo contagiosa.[78, 79] In temperate climates, impetigo is most common during summer months, when children frequently sustain insect bites and trauma to exposed skin, particularly in populations whose poor hygiene and sanitation promote transmission, as do flies and other insects.

Streptococci responsible for pyoderma can adhere to and colonize intact skin, so insect bites and minor abrasions and trauma can initiate the superficial lesions. Washing and proper hygiene are therefore major preventive measures. Skin strains find their way within a few weeks to the mucosa of the nose and throat, where they may cause mild pharyngitis and acute glomerulonephritis but not rheumatic fever.

Skin strains of streptococci are distinguished by certain features. In general, they belong to certain M types, the ones that have the highest numbers because of their historically later identification (see the earlier section on M protein, class II). Such strains rarely form mucoid colonies and have low virulence for mice. They do not resist phagocytosis in human blood as strikingly as encapsulated, M-rich throat strains. The skin infections they cause are associated with blunted anti-SLO but brisk anti–DNase B responses. Type-specific anti-M responses are also relatively weak.[78, 79] Skin strains usually produce SOR (see earlier).[28]

The lesions of pyoderma begin as papules, usually on an exposed area of the body that is traumatized by an abrasion or an insect bite. They are often multiple, and within a few days they form thick crusts that heal slowly and leave depigmented areas. Systemic symptoms are absent but regional lymphadenitis may occur. Culture of material from the surface of these lesions yields staphylococci much more often than streptococci. The latter are easily overgrown by the former on surfaces exposed to air. When crusts and scabs are removed, however, and the deeper exudate is propagated in culture, virtually pure isolates of group A streptococci result. The association of certain pyoderma-producing strains with epidemic acute glomerulonephritis is well recognized (see later). A more serious form of pyoderma is the deeper ulcerated lesion known as ecthyma. These lesions caused by skin irritation and maceration by footwear (especially in tropical climates) are often located on the ankle or dorsum of the foot and may be complicated by cellulitis and lymphangitis. *S. aureus,* either alone or in combination with *S. pyogenes,* has been shown to be associated with a penicillin-resistant form of pyoderma, apparently related to the ability of the colonizing staphylococcal strain to produce penicillinase.[80] What was once an infection easily treated with oral penicillin G now often requires a β-lactamase–resistant penicillin, such as cloxacillin, or a cephalosporin such as cephalexin, cefadroxil, or cefaclor given orally for 10 days. Erythromycin's effectiveness is limited in areas in which erythromycin-resistant strains are prevalent.[81] Mupirocin ointment is an effective but expensive alternative therapy.[82, 83]

Erysipelas. The features of erysipelas make it unique clinically because of its explosive onset. Unlike the indolent pyoderma lesions described earlier, this infection spreads rapidly through skin lymphatics from a small abrasion, particularly around the nares. Erysipelas often erupts across the cheeks and nose and affects the eyelids, which may become edematous or shut, so that the presentation may resemble angioneurotic edema. The lesion is intensely painful and erythematous, has a characteristic elevated advancing margin, and may vesiculate and even form bullae that rupture and crust. Erysipelas can lead to bacteremia and death, particularly in infants and in frail elders. Attempts at culture isolation of material from the lesions are usually frustrated because bacteria are not numerous locally, suggesting hypersensitivity or toxin-producing features. Management, therefore, depends on prompt clinical recognition and penicillin therapy, which is curative.

Postinfectious Sequelae

Acute Rheumatic Fever

The most important complication of *S. pyogenes* infections is ARF because of the resultant rheumatic heart disease. The reader is referred to other texts for details of the cardiac,[84] rheumatic,[85] and immune[46] features of ARF. Its history, pathology, and global significance are also described extensively elsewhere.[46, 86–88] In this chapter I am concerned mainly with the diagnosis and management of ARF as an infectious disease, because the group A streptococcus has been established as its sole agent.

The syndrome of rheumatic fever is predominantly one of polyarthritis and pancarditis, Sydenham chorea being a less common, but no less clinically striking and characteristic, manifestation. Erythema marginatum and subcutaneous nodules, the other two major manifestations, are important only because they improve diagnostic accuracy. Because rheumatic fever appears well after the subsidence of the antecedent pharyngitis, usually after a latent period of 10 to 30 days, residual clinical evidence of such infection is not observed and may not be recalled at all by approximately 30% of patients. Because the lesions of rheumatic fever are sterile, it has been called a nonsuppurative sequela.

ETIOLOGY AND PATHOGENESIS

Infecting Strain and Site of Infection

The epidemiology of ARF is superimposable on that of streptococcal pharyngitis—and even on that of scarlet fever in the preantibiotic era. The most confusing aspect of streptococcal epidemiology, however, as already noted, is related to the variation in streptococcal strain virulence[40] and sites of infection.[89] M protein–associated epitopes distinguish throat strains (class I) from skin strains (class II)[12] (see earlier).

Clearly, to initiate ARF the site of infection must be pharyngeal, but not all strains that infect the pharynx cause ARF. This fact has been clearly demonstrated in settings in which seasonal changes completely dissociate ARF related to pharyngitis from AGN related to pyoderma.[90] Throat carriage with the "skin" strains is common and actual pharyngeal infection may be milder. This may contribute to their nonrheumatogenicity. On the other hand, it has long been recognized that ARF has not been observed to follow pharyngeal infection with strains belonging to certain common pharyngeal[91] serotypes, notably types 2, 4, and 28. An outbreak of M type 4 pharyngitis, for example, failed to reactivate ARF during a well-studied epidemic among convalescent children.[92]

The strains that clearly cause epidemics of ARF, however, have shown consistently the virulence features described earlier. Not all strains within a given M serotype are necessarily rheumatogenic. Some strains that can be M serotyped may already have lost much of their virulence potential. Epidemiologic studies of M and T serotypes that are random surveys of throat cultures of a population and that are not carefully related to clinical and epidemiologic observations have been confusing rather than helpful. The new potential for identifying rheumatogenic strains by their genome may further clarify their identification in the future (see the earlier M protein section).

Although the prevalence of ARF declined dramatically after World War II and precipitously in the 1970s in the developed countries of the world, it has been growing in the industrializing slums of developing countries. Contemporary physicians of the developed countries of the world, for whom rheumatic fever is now a disease that they rarely encounter, may find it difficult to conceive of the magnitude of the prevalence of this disease in other parts of the world. It is rampant in the industrialized slums of South Africa,[93] the Indian subcontinent, the Middle East, and certain areas of South America and Africa,[94, 95] and French and American Polynesia, and in the Maori communities of New Zealand; perhaps the highest recorded point prevalence has been seen among aborigines of northern and central Australia.[94, 95] Nutritional or other exogenous factors do not seem to play a primary role. The attack rate of streptococcal pharyngitis has been observed to be constant and relatively predictable among healthy, well-nourished military recruits.[41] Indeed, the dramatic reappearance in the 1980s of outbreaks of rheumatic fever in the United States among such military recruits[57, 58] (Fig. 192–4) and in communities from Utah[96, 97] to Ohio and Pennsylvania involved middle-class populations that observed relatively high health care standards.[98, 99] Moreover, the strains that were associated with these epidemics were shown to have all of the original characteristics that were noted in the carefully studied military epidemics of the 1940s and 1950s: they are rich in M protein, belong to certain notorious rheumatogenic M types, and are heavily encapsulated, forming mucoid colonies.[40, 100, 101] As noted earlier, they possess the class I rather than class II epitope and the chromosomal patterns of the subfamilies of the nucleotide sequences of their M protein genes belong to the A,B,C rather than D,E pattern. In addition, they contain epitopes cross-reactive with host tissues and their M-associated proteins have potent superantigenic properties (see the section on M protein). As noted earlier, the resurgence of rheumatic fever in the 1980s was followed by the appearance in North America and Europe of invasive streptococcal infections of unusual virulence. These were associated with pyrogenic toxin–producing strains and TSS. Despite such toxicity, these infections (of the skin and soft tissues) were not associated with rheumatic fever. Rheumatogenic pharyngeal infections,

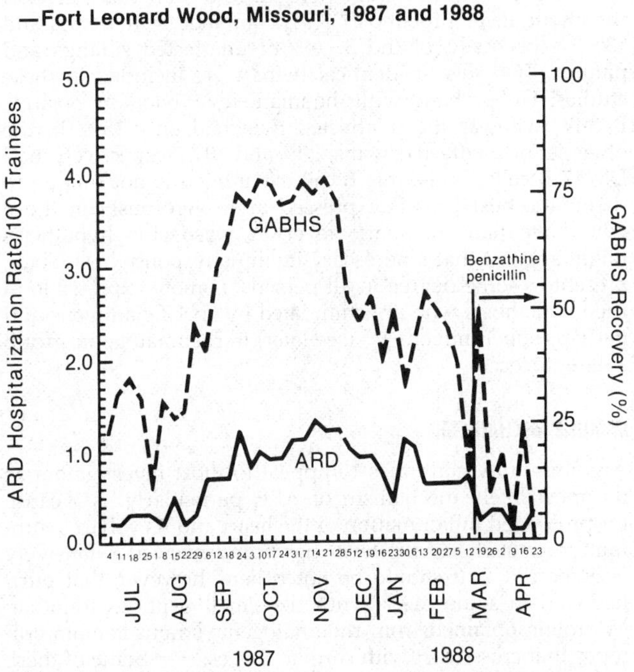

FIGURE 192–4 □ Epidemic of streptococcal pharyngitis associated with an outbreak of rheumatic fever and terminated by mass prophylaxis with intramuscular benzathine penicillin G. (From Centers for Disease Control: Acute rheumatic fever among Army trainees—Fort Leonard Wood, Missouri, 1987–1988. MMWR Morbid Mortal Wkly Rep 37:519–522, 1988.)

however, may or may not be associated with strains capable of producing pyrogenic toxin (e.g., as in scarlet fever). Thus, the relation of pyrogenic toxin to rheumatic fever remains moot.[25, 59]

HOST FACTORS

The gradual acquisition of susceptibility to ARF by schoolchildren after repeated infections suggests that rheumatic hosts have acquired increased potential for a streptococcal hyperimmune response. Every streptococcal antibody response that has been studied in ARF patients has been exaggerated compared with those of populations of patients with acute streptococcal pharyngitis that is not complicated by rheumatic fever. Both hyperimmunity and the intensity of antigenic stimulation by the initiating infection (perhaps by the superantigen effects of M protein described before) have been considered important in the pathogenesis of rheumatic fever.[46]

The relatively low attack rate of ARF (approximately 3%) even in epidemics, however, has focused attention on immune response genes of the host. No association of class I human leukocyte antigens (HLAs) with rheumatic fever has been found. The trend toward an association of HLA-B5 may be related to an increased response to streptococcal antigens produced by these persons.[102] HLA-DR2, -3, and -4 have been detected with increased frequency in black, white, and Indian patients, respectively,[103, 104] principally those who developed carditis. HLA-DR1 and -DRw6 were observed with increased frequency in South African black persons.[105] In contrast to the lack of a definitive association with HLA-DR antigens, a strong relationship has been detected with a non-HLA B-cell antigen designated 883 and detected in widely distributed populations from New York to Bogota, Colombia, and New Mexico to India.[106, 107] Studies with a series of monoclonal antibodies directed against B cells from rheumatic fever patients have identified another B-cell alloantigen labeled D8/17.[108] It is present in a large percentage of the total B cells of rheumatic fever probands: 33.5% compared with 14.6% and 13%, respectively, of the B cells of unaffected siblings and parents. Two sets of identical twins were included in these studies. The proband with rheumatic fever had 43% positive B cells, whereas the unaffected twin had only 15%. In the other set of unaffected twins, 20% and 10%, respectively, had D8/17 B cells. Thus, this B-cell alloantigen is not unique to rheumatic hosts but is expressed more vigorously in those who have had rheumatic fever. A reasonable hypothesis might suggest that a necessary immune response host factor, present to some degree in all persons, is more expressible in rheumatic hosts who are stimulated by specific antigens and perhaps superantigens[74, 75] (see later) in rheumatogenic group A streptococci.

IMMUNE MECHANISMS

Autoimmunity continues to appeal to most investigators as the most likely mechanism of ARF, particularly as a cause for prolonged inflammation of the heart and its valves. Autoimmunity in rheumatic fever has been reviewed extensively elsewhere.[109–111] It should be noted here, however, that purified–and in some cases synthetic—small peptides found in M protein obtained from rheumatogenic strains contain epitopes that cross-react with cardiac tissues.[5, 13, 14] Some of these react with myosin and keratin, coiled proteins of primary and secondary (and perhaps tertiary) molecular structure similar to that of M protein.[11] It is noteworthy that some of these peptides may be separated from other epitopes of M protein that raise type-specific M antibodies without cross-reacting with heart tissues and thus may be important as potential streptococcal vaccines.[9] Other streptococcal antibodies have been shown to be cross-reactive with cardiac elements such as valve glycoproteins and fibroblasts, synovia and articular cartilage, brain tissues and skeletal muscles, smooth muscle, liver, lymphocytes, thymus, skin, and kidney.[110, 111]

CLINICAL FEATURES

ARF is remarkable for the unity and diversity of the syndrome. The major manifestations of rheumatic fever may sometimes appear as isolated findings, but more impressive is the relative consistency of their association. For example, in the outbreak of ARF in Utah,[96, 97] polyarthritis, carditis, and chorea occurred with the same frequency as they did many years ago in the cities of the temperate zone of the United States, before the great decline of ARF began (Table 192–1). Moreover, when careful prospective observations were made in a pediatric population served by a general medical clinic in New Delhi, India, the relative respective frequencies of these manifestations were similar to those reported in the Western world.[112]

The migratory polyarthritis of rheumatic fever is its least specific although most common manifestation. Its latent period from the antecedent streptococcal pharyngitis is readily measured because of the dramatic and painful onset. Latency is rarely less than 10 days or more than a month. Maximal streptococcal antibody titers, therefore, should be observed at the onset of polyarthritis. These help to support the diagnosis of rheumatic fever. Because polyarthritis of causes other than rheumatic fever may also occur coincidentally with streptococcal pharyngitis, an increased streptococcal antibody titer may be a false-positive finding. The diagnosis of ARF polyarthritis can be virtually excluded by negative streptococcal antibody titers, which therefore have strong negative predictive value.

Rheumatic polyarthritis does not respond to penicillin or other antibiotics. A therapeutic trial of penicillin may be necessary to rule out a highly responsive pyogenic polyarthritis such as acute gonococcal polyarthritis. Rheumatic polyarthritis is readily suppressed by salicylates and related compounds and its duration may be relatively brief, usually less than 2 weeks. Particularly in medically underserved populations, failure to seek medical attention may create a false perception of low prevalence.

RHEUMATIC CARDITIS

Rheumatic carditis is symptomatic only when cardiac insufficiency is expressed as fatigue or shortness of breath or when pericarditis is painful. Most cases of carditis are not

TABLE 192–1 ■ Acute Rheumatic Fever as Defined by Three Major Manifestations of Jones Criteria in Utah, 1985 to 1986

MAJOR MANIFESTATIONS*	NUMBER	PERCENTAGE
Carditis	14	14
Polyarthritis	14	14
Chorea	4	4
Carditis and polyarthritis	43	44
Carditis and chorea	14	14
Carditis, chorea, and polyarthritis	6	6
Polyarthritis and chorea	4	4
Total	99	100

*Categories are mutually exclusive.

From Centers for Disease Control: Acute rheumatic fever—Utah. MMWR Morbid Mortal Wkly Rep 36:108–110, 1987.

severe enough to produce such symptoms and therefore carditis is usually diagnosed by auscultation of the heart alone. These facts account for the frequency of the discovery of rheumatic valvular disease in patients who do not recall having ARF, particularly in populations who do not receive adequate medical attention. Mild, sporadic bouts of ARF can therefore lead to a confusing global epidemiologic pattern of rheumatic heart disease in populations wherein overt ARF is claimed to be rare despite the high prevalence of rheumatic heart disease. Where Doppler echocardiography is available, so-called silent rheumatic carditis has been identified by slight degrees of valvular regurgitation in the mildest cases of rheumatic fever.[112a] Right ventricular encodardial biopsy does not ordinarily yield useful diagnostic information because of its relatively low sensitivity and specificity.[112b] A full discussion of the clinical features of rheumatic carditis can be found elsewhere.[46, 84]

SYDENHAM CHOREA

Sydenham chorea has features that have caused confusion and controversy as to its prevalence and its specificity for rheumatic fever. The sex distribution of chorea is noteworthy. Before puberty, it is equally common in both sexes. Thereafter, chorea disappears in mature men, accounting for its absence in military epidemics. On the other hand, pregnancy aggravates and exacerbates chorea (chorea gravidarum). The latent period between streptococcal pharyngitis and chorea is prolonged, often to 2 to 3 months or more, by which time evidence of antecedent streptococcal infection may be absent if streptococcal antibody titers have returned to relatively low levels by the time they are measured.[113] At such time, all evidence of rheumatic inflammation, including C-reactive protein and erythrocyte sedimentation rate elevation, may also have abated. If polyarthritis was not noted in the initial phase of the disease and carditis was also either transient or absent, the syndrome of "pure" chorea may emerge. Such patients suffer frequent recurrences of chorea with intercurrent and often asymptomatic streptococcal infections.[114]

ERYTHEMA MARGINATUM

Erythema marginatum is a vasohumoral, focal, evanescent erythema localized mostly to parts of the body usually covered by clothes (trunk and proximal extremities). Its pink color is not readily seen except on fair skin and with the aid of natural light. Although it is less frequently expressed as part of the rheumatic syndrome and is often difficult to recognize, it is a characteristic, if nonspecific, manifestation of ARF.

Subcutaneous nodules are also easily overlooked because they are pea sized, painless, and movable and appear transitorily over bony prominences. They are most often associated with rheumatic carditis.

DIAGNOSIS

The modified Jones criteria continue to be a useful standard for the diagnosis of ARF.[115] They require for diagnosis the presence of either one major and two minor or two major manifestations supported by evidence of antecedent streptococcal infection. The latter relies heavily on evidence of increased levels of streptococcal antibodies, but an understanding of the behavior of such antibodies after streptococcal infection is necessary to appreciate their limitations.

TREATMENT OF RHEUMATIC FEVER

Treatment of streptococcal infections including primary and secondary prevention of rheumatic fever is discussed in the following. Once ARF has appeared, however, treatment with penicillin does not shorten or alter the course of the disease, and therapy is only antiinflammatory and supportive, as discussed fully elsewhere.[84] Both salicylates and corticosteroids are highly effective in suppressing inflammation but do not prevent cardiac damage.[116] Corticosteroids are often given priority over salicylates by many physicians when overt carditis is present because they are more potent antiinflammatory agents for the symptomatic relief of the acute manifestations of rheumatic fever, regardless of whether they diminish the frequency of valvular heart disease.[117]

Recurrences of Rheumatic Fever

In the general population, the attack rate of recurrences of ARF (secondary attacks) after streptococcal pharyngitis is many times that of primary attacks. The latent period between pharyngitis and recurrent ARF does not become shorter, even with repeated attacks, and this observation continues to challenge conventional pathogenic theories of streptococcal hypersensitivity.

The factors that affect the attack rate of recurrences of ARF after rheumatogenic streptococcal pharyngitis have been studied extensively.[118] They include the magnitude of the immune response, the presence or absence of rheumatic heart disease, the number of previous attacks, and the interval since the previous attack (Table 192–2).

The dramatic decline in primary attacks of ARF has been paralleled by a similar decline in secondary attacks. Studies in the late 1970s showed that streptococcal infections detected by the increases in streptococcal antibodies in patients with rheumatic heart disease, which in an earlier era would have been associated with a high rate of secondary rheumatic attacks, failed to reactivate the disease.[119] Such studies also suggested the disappearance of rheumatogenic strains. In a Chilean study,[120] penicillin prophylaxis against recurrent attacks of rheumatic fever was discontinued in a local cohort after several years when the recurrence rate in the cohort had become quite low (0.7 per 100 patient-years) and rheumatogenic strains of streptococci seemed to have disappeared (only 7% were M typeable, compared with the former rate of 52%). Yet pockets of rheumatic fever still persisted in other sections of the area, producing a situation similar to that in other places in the world where focal populations are heavily affected by ARF, whereas nearby populations are almost completely spared.[88] In view of such findings, the indications for continuous prophylaxis of rheumatic heart disease are being reevaluated (vide infra).

TABLE 192–2 ■ Ratio of Rheumatic Recurrences to Streptococcal Infections in Patients Stratified for Heart Disease and for Anti–Streptolysin O Rise

ANTI-SLO (TUBE DILUTIONS)	HEART DISEASE		NO HEART DISEASE	
	Ratio	%	Ratio	%
0–1	3/24	13	1/72	1
2	10/36	28	2/46	4
3	6/16	37	4/32	13
4	9/14	65	9/25	36

From Taranta A, Wood HF, Feinstein AR, et al: Rheumatic fever in children and adolescents. A long-term epidemiologic study of subsequent prophylaxis, streptococcal infections, and clinical sequelae. IV. Relation of the rheumatic fever recurrence rate per streptococcal antibodies to the titers of streptococcal antibodies. Ann Intern Med 60(Suppl 5):47–57, 1964.

Acute Glomerulonephritis

EPIDEMIOLOGY AND PATHOGENESIS

AGN follows infection with specific nephritogenic strains of *S. pyogenes.*[121] These may be either pharyngeal or skin strains. Unlike rheumatic fever, however, the clinical syndrome of AGN is not specific for *S. pyogenes* alone. It can be initiated as well by a variety of infections capable of causing immune complexes to deposit in glomeruli, particularly when persistent antigenemia continues in the presence of a sustained antibody reponse and thus leads to the formation of insoluble antigen-antibody complexes.[122]

The possible role of autoimmunity resulting from shared components among glomerular and streptococcal membranes continues to be explored. Autoantibodies to glomerular connective tissue components have been identified in patients with poststreptococcal AGN.[123] The putative nephritogenic factor in nephritogenic strains of *S. pyogenes,* however, has not been identified. Renal glomerular autoimmune epitopes have also been identified in a tetrapeptide of type 1 streptococcal M protein.[124] Epitopes have also been isolated from the streptococcal plasma membrane that have been purified and shown to react with antibodies present in convalescent serum of patients with AGN.[125, 126]

Nephritogenic strains have been associated with a well-defined group of M serotypes: 1, 2, 3, 4, 12, 15, 49, 55, 56, 59, 60, 61, and probably others. Type 12 is most frequent among the pharyngeal strains that have caused AGN, but this serotype is a common one and most strains of it are not nephritogenic. Thus, M serotype alone is not an adequate marker for nephritogenicity. Seasonal peaks of AGN have been clearly dissociated from those of ARF in climates and populations in which both diseases are endemic, such as the southern United States.[90] In the Caribbean island of Trinidad, the epidemiologic patterns of AGN and ARF are clearly distinct—ARF is present year-round and AGN occurs in approximately 6-year cycles[127]—and the streptococcal strains that cause each sequela appear to be distinct as well.[128]

The attack rate of AGN after throat or skin infection with a nephritogenic strain may be high (10% to 15%). Unlike the case of ARF, however, recurrences are quite rare, presumably because of the relatively limited number of M serotypes harboring nephritogenic strains and because of the acquisition of type-specific immunity. In addition, patients who contract AGN do not appear to be susceptible to recurrent attacks. More common is the propensity for streptococcal infection to exacerbate chronic glomerulonephritis. Because the development of chronic glomerulonephritis after AGN has been documented prospectively in few patients, the opportunity to study the effect of recurrent streptococcal infection on its course has been quite limited. It is often difficult or impossible to differentiate an acute exacerbation of chronic glomerulonephritis, such as may be precipitated by streptococci or by a variety of other intercurrent infections, from a true attack of poststreptococcal AGN.

CLINICAL FEATURES AND COURSE

The latent period between streptococcal infection and the appearance of AGN is 1 to 2 weeks after pharyngitis and perhaps 2 to 3 weeks after skin infection, although the exact onset of the latter is more difficult to establish. Microscopic proteinuria, hematuria, and cylindruria are often present without causing symptoms, even when they are associated with hypertension, azotemia, and decline in serum complement value. AGN is therefore usually underdiagnosed except when edema, noticeable darkening of the urine by red blood cells, or more severe symptoms such as heart failure secondary to fluid overload occur. Establishing that the pathogen is *Streptococcus* by immunohistochemical techniques may be more difficult when pyoderma is the cause of antecedent infection, because the ASO titer in skin infections is blunted whereas the DNase antibody titer is more consistently increased.[78, 79]

The coexistence of ARF and AGN in the same patient presumably from the same antecedent infection is extremely rare. When acute polyarthritis and glomerulonephritis occur in a patient at the same time, some other multiorgan vasculitis, such as systemic lupus erythematosus, is a much more likely diagnosis.

Because of the generally benign prognosis of AGN, renal biopsy is usually performed only when the course of the disease becomes subacute or chronic. That, however, is a relatively rare development. Renal biopsy specimens that have been collected in the early stages of AGN show edema and hypercellularity of the glomerular tuft (proliferative AGN). Except in rare cases, however, scarring or adhesion of the tuft to the Bowman capsule (crescents) does not occur. Immunofluorescence studies identify complement components and/or immunoglobulins (immunoglobulin G and C3) deposited in a granular pattern. Such deposits can be shown by electron microscopy to be subepithelial on the glomerular basement membrane.[122]

As in the case of ARF, the incidence of AGN has declined greatly where cleanliness and good hygiene prevail and adequate medical facilities exist. Reports from areas as distant from each other as Memphis, Tennessee,[129] and Singapore[130] indicate a marked decline in the disease during the 1980s.

Treatment of Streptococcal Infections

Group A streptococci are uniformly highly sensitive to the action of penicillin, which is rapidly bactericidal in a concentration of 0.01 to 0.04 units/mL in a standard broth culture. No penicillin-resistant strains have emerged despite almost half a century of intense clinical use. Sustained bactericidal blood levels, however low, eradicate proliferating group A streptococci. Treatment of streptococcal pharyngitis adequate to prevent primary attacks of rheumatic fever should ensure penicillin levels for at least 10 days.[42] Because this can be achieved by a single intramuscular injection of 1.2 million units of benzathine penicillin G, or 600,000 units for children who weigh less than 27 kg or 60 pounds,[131, 132] this regimen is a favored one. Intramuscular injections of repository penicillins, however, produce some local pain and discomfort, and they must be administered by physicians or nurses. Injectable benzathine penicillin G for pharyngitis, therefore, has declined in popularity, especially in populations in which the fear of ARF has virtually disappeared. Because oral penicillin regimens must extend to a full 10 days, long after symptoms have abated, compliance is quite poor. Oral absorption of penicillin compounds may also be erratic. The oral regimens appear to be adequate, however, to provide rapid symptomatic relief and to prevent suppurative complication of pharyngitis. Penicillin V given orally twice daily in 1.0-g doses has been shown to be at least as effective as 0.5 g four times daily, with greater compliance seen with a twice-daily regimen.[133] Oral cephalosporins are also highly effective in the treatment of streptococcal pharyngitis, and some reports show even a slightly higher rate of clinical cure and eradication of convalescent carriage than that achieved with penicillin therapy.[134] Despite these observations, penicillin remains the drug of choice because of its proven efficacy in preventing rheumatic attacks, its low cost, and its relatively narrow spectrum.[135]

If penicillin allergy is suspected or known to exist, erythromycin has been the drug of choice, 20 mg/pound per day (not to exceed 1 g/d) for a period of 10 days. Although erythromycin resistance is not a serious problem in the United States, the drug has caused resistance with striking frequency in Japan, where it was once considered the drug of choice because of fear of penicillin allergy. However, with a change of policy favoring penicillin, erythromycin resistance of Japanese strains of *S. pyogenes* has returned to its expected low frequency.[86] Treating streptococcal pharyngitis with sulfonamides does not prevent rheumatic fever. Sulfonamides are quite effective, however, as prophylactic agents (see later).

Treatment of sore throat should be started promptly, although a delay of a few days while awaiting culture results does not seem to interfere with prevention of attacks of ARF.[136] Secondary attacks are not as readily prevented by treating pharyngitis, however prompt such treatment may be. Despite the clinical efficacy of penicillin G in the treatment of streptococcal sore throat, some 10% to 15% of patients continue to carry the original strain of group A streptococci, without relapse of symptoms or signs of pharyngitis, for days, weeks, or months after the recommended course of penicillin. Such failure of eradication is more common when the subject is a streptococcal carrier rather than acutely infected. It has long been appreciated that virulent streptococci dissociate during convalescence, losing M protein and becoming avirulent. Repeated treatment of such asymptomatic patients with persistent throat carriage is not recommended because such carriage has not caused problems.[137] The reappearance of rheumatogenic streptococci in many widely separated areas of the United States may reflect less assiduous diagnosis and therapy of streptococcal pharyngitis in current years.[96, 100]

The prevention of AGN by the treatment of streptococcal pharyngitis or pyoderma caused by a nephritogenic strain has not been systematically studied, but isolated reports of failure of such treatment suggest that treating the antecedent infection prevents AGN less often than it does ARF. In an outbreak of poststreptococcal AGN, however, the use of benzathine penicillin G prevents spread of such strains throughout the family and community and terminates the epidemic if used extensively in the affected population. The lesions of streptococcal pyoderma usually respond well to penicillin therapy. As noted earlier, however, in the presence of colonization of the surface of the lesions of streptococcal pyoderma with a β-lactamase–producing *S. aureus,* oral therapy with penicillins resistant to this enzyme, such as oxacillin, cloxacillin, or cephalosporin, may be required.[81] Impetigo, however, is readily prevented with good personal hygiene and adequate cleansing of the skin.

More severe suppurative streptococcal infections respond well to intramuscular injections of procaine penicillin G, 600,000 units once or twice daily. For life-threatening infections in hospitalized patients, intravenous penicillin may be employed and is recommended in larger doses.

Prophylaxis of Streptococcal Infections

An outbreak of streptococcal pharyngitis may call for mass prophylaxis—treatment of an entire population—when sequelae are associated with the epidemic. Such events are rare now except in military populations or in institutions. A single injection of 1.2 million units of benzathine penicillin G to each person in the population affected has terminated such epidemics promptly.[138]

Primary rheumatic fever prophylaxis is also highly effective when benzathine penicillin G is used widely for the treatment of acute pharyngitis in settings where acute rheumatic fever is highly endemic. Less stringent oral regimens

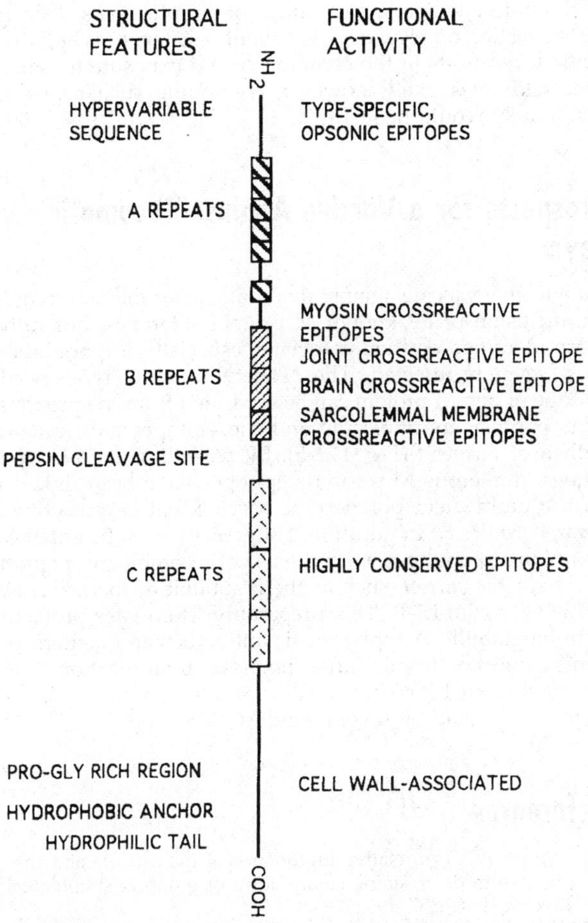

FIGURE 192–5 □ Schema depicting the location on the M protein molecule of the epitopes cross-reactive with myocardium, synovia, and brain. They are shown located within and flanking the repeats of the M5 molecule, well proximal to the type-specific epitopes within the N-terminal of M5. (From Dale JB: Type-specific multivalent group A streptococcal M protein vaccines. *In* Stevens DL, Kaplan [eds]: Streptococcal Infectious Disease. Oxford, Oxford University Press, 1997. By permission of Oxford University Press.)

have been suggested in settings where ARF has disappeared, as discussed earlier.[88]

Secondary attacks of ARF are best prevented by monthly injections of 1.2 million units of intramuscular benzathine penicillin G.[135, 137, 139] Oral prophylactic regimens are less reliable. Daily doses of either sulfadiazine or buffered penicillin G are effective, however, if low risk of recurrences makes the requirement for prophylaxis less stringent.[119, 120] The recommended dose of oral sulfadiazine is 0.5 g once daily for patients who weigh less than 27 kg (60 pounds) and 1 g daily for heavier persons. Penicillin G or V may be given by mouth in doses of 200,000 to 250,000 units/d. Even when oral penicillin is given twice daily, no superiority over sulfadiazine has been demonstrated in the prevention of rheumatic recurrences.[139] For the rare patient who is sensitive to both penicillin and sulfonamides, erythromycin may be substituted in a dose of 250 mg twice daily.

The duration of continuous prophylaxis for rheumatic subjects cannot be stated arbitrarily because of the number of variables influencing the rate of recurrences.[118–120] Such variables include the presence or absence of rheumatic heart disease, the duration from the previous attack, the number of previous attacks, and the severity of the antecedent infection. To these should now be added variation in the nature of the antecedent infecting strain of streptococcus. (See the earlier section on recurrences of rheumatic fever.) When rheumatic fever exists in the community and exposure to school-age children is likely, however, continuing such protection indefinitely would be justified.

Prospects for a Vaccine Against Rheumatic Fever

An effective vaccine against rheumatic fever may not require the inclusion of all known M protein serotypes, but rather those identified as rheumatogenic, especially in populations most severely affected. The *N*-acetyl-terminal type-specific epitope of pep M protein can be separated from the proximal, toxic parts of the molecule and the epitopes cross-reactive with host tissues[13] (Fig. 192–5). By recombinant DNA techniques, numerous M serotype epitopes have been linked to form a multivalent polypeptide vaccine that is protective in animal studies.[140] In addition, antigenicity may be enhanced by linking M epitopes, with the use of recombinant methods, to a haptenic carrier, such as the B subunit of the *Escherichia coli* labile toxin, LT-B. This preparation stimulates protective immunoglobulin A type-specific antibodies and confers systemic protection in mice after *intranasal* immunization.[141] The potential of such preparations for oral human immunization is now suggested by several studies.[142, 143]

References

1. Wilson AT: The relative importance of the capsule and the M antigen in determining colony form of group A streptococci. J Exp Med 109:257, 1959.
2. Bahr GM, Majeed HA, Yousof AM, et al: Detection of antibodies to muramyl dipeptide (MDP), the adjuvant of streptococcal cell wall, in patients with rheumatic fever. J Infect Dis 154:1012, 1986.
3. Lancefield RC: Specific relationship of cell composition to biological activity of hemolytic streptococci. Harvey Lect (1940–1941) 35:251, 1941.
4. Griffith F: Types of haemolytic streptococci in relation to scarlet fever. J Hyg 25:385, 1926.
5. Swanson J, Hsu KC, Gotschlich EC: Electron microscopic studies on streptococci. I. M antigen. J Exp Med 130:1063, 1969.
6. Beachey EH, Stollerman GH, Chiang EY, et al: Purification and properties of M protein extracted from group A streptococci with pepsin. Covalent structure of the amino terminal region of type 24 M antigen. J Exp Med 145:1469, 1977.
7. Manjula BN, Fischetti VA: Studies on group A streptococcal M proteins: Purification of type 5 M protein and comparison of its amino terminal sequence with two immunologically unrelated M protein molecules. J Immunol 124:261, 1980.
8. Manjula BN, Fischetti VA: Tropomyosin-like seven residue periodicity in three immunologically distinct streptococcal M proteins and its implications for the antiphagocytic property of the molecule. J Exp Med 151:695, 1980.
9. Phillips GN Jr, Flicker PF, Cohen C, et al: Streptococcal M protein: Alpha-helical coiled-coil structure and arrangement on the cell surface. Proc Natl Acad Sci USA 78:4689, 1981.
10. Dale JB, Beachey EH: Sequence of myosin cross-reactive epitopes of streptococcal M protein. J Exp Med 164:1785, 1986.
11. Bronze MS, Beachey EH, Dale JB: Protective and heart cross-reactive epitopes located within the NH_2 terminus of type 19 streptococcal M protein. J Exp Med 167:1849, 1988.
12. Bessen D, Jones KF, Fischetti VA: Evidence for two distinct classes of streptococcal M-protein and their relationship to rheumatic fever. J Exp Med 169:269, 1989.
13. Dale JB: Type-specific multivalent group A streptococcal M protein vaccines. *In* Stevens DL, Kaplan (eds): Streptococcal Infections. London, Oxford Univesity Press (in press).
14. Cunningham MW, Swerlich RA: Polyspecificity of antistreptococcal monoclonal antibodies and their implications in autoimmunity. J Exp Med 164:998, 1986.
15. Bessen DE, Veasy LG, Hill HR, et al: Serologic evidence for a class I group A streptococcal infection among rheumatic fever patients. J Infect Dis 172:1608, 1995.
16. Bessen DE, Sotir CM, Readdy TL, Hollingshead SK: Genetic correlates of throat and skin isolates of group A streptococci. J Infect Dis 173:896, 1996.
17. Watanabe-Ohnishi R, Aelion J, LeGros L, et al: Characterization of unique human TCR V-beta specificities for a family of streptococcal superantigens represented by rheumatogenic serotypes of M protein. J Immunol 152:2066, 1994.
18. Beachey EH, Ofek I: Epithelial cell binding of group A streptococci by lipoteichoic acid on fimbriae denuded of M protein. J Exp Med 143:759, 1976.
19. Hasty DL Ofek I, Courtney HS, et al: Multiple adhesins of streptococci. Infect Immunol 69:2147, 1992.
20. Eckstedt RD, Stollerman GH: Factors affecting the chain length of group A streptococci. I. Demonstration of a metabolically active chain splitting system. J Exp Med 112:671, 1960.
21. Sandson J, Hamerman D, Janis R, Rojkind M: Immunologic chemical similarities between the streptococcus and human connective tissue. Trans Assoc Am Physicians 81:249, 1968.
22. Fillit HM, Blake M, MacDonald C, McCarty M: Immunogenicity of liposome-bound hyaluronate in mice. J Exp Med 168:971, 1988.
23. Stollerman GH, Bernheimer AW, MacLeod CM: The association of lipoproteins with the inhibition of streptolysin S by serum. J Clin Invest 29:1636, 1950.
24. Johnson LP, L'Italier JJ, Schlievert PM: Streptococcal pyrogenic exotoxin type A (scarlet fever toxin) is related to *Staphylococcus aureus* enterotoxin B. Mol Gen Genet 203:354, 1986.
25. Stollerman GH: Changing group A streptococci. The reappearance of streptococcal 'toxic shock' (Editorial). Arch Intern Med 148:1268, 1988.
26. Stevens DL, Tanner MH, Winship J, et al: Severe group A streptococcal infections associated with a toxic shock-like syndrome and scarlet fever toxin A. N Engl J Med 321:1, 1989.
27. Nelson K, Schlievert PM, Selader RK, Musser JM: Characterization and clonal distribution of four alleles of the *speA* gene encoding pyrogenic exotoxin A (scarlet fever toxin). J Exp Med 154:1271, 1991.
28. Alkington DF, Schwartz B, Black CM, et al: Association of phenotypic and genotypic characteristics of invasive *Streptococcus pyogenes* isolates with clinical components of streptococcal toxic shock syndrome. Infect Immunol 61:3369, 1993.
29. Wannamaker LW: The differentiation of three distinct deoxyribonucleases of group A streptococci. J Exp Med 107:797, 1958.
30. Christensen LR: Methods for measuring the activity of components of the streptococcal fibrinolytic system and streptococcal deoxyribonuclease. J Clin Invest 28:163, 1949.
31. Stollerman GH, Lewis AJ, Schultz I, et al: Relationship of the immune response to group A streptococci to the course of acute, chronic and recurrent rheumatic fever. Am J Med 20:163, 1956.
32. Ayoub EM, Wannamaker LW: Evaluation of the streptococcal deoxyribonuclease B and diphosphopyridine nucleotidase antibody tests in acute rheumatic fever and acute glomerulonephritis. Pediatrics 29:527, 1962.
33. Widdowson JP, Maxted WR, Grant DL: The production of opacity in serum by group A streptococci and its relationship with the presence of M antigen. J Gen Microbiol 61:343, 1970.
34. Widdowson JP, Maxted WR, Grant DL, et al: The relationship between M antigen and opacity factor in group A streptococci. J Gen Microbiol 65:69, 1971.
35. Whitnack E, Stollerman GH: Antistreptococcal antibodies in the diagnosis of rheumatic fever. *In* Cohen AS (ed): Laboratory Diagnostic Procedures in Rheumatic Diseases, ed 3. Boston, Little, Brown, 1985, pp 273–292.
36. Todd EW: A method of measuring the increase or decrease of the population of haemolytic streptococci in blood. Br J Exp Pathol 8:1, 1927.
37. Whitnack E, Beachey EH: Inhibition of complement mediated opsonization and phagocytosis of *Streptococcus pyogenes* by D fragments of fibrinogen and fibrin bound to cell surface M protein. J Exp Med 162:1983, 1985.
38. O'Connor SP, Cleary PD: Localization of the streptococcal C_{5a}

peptidase to the surface of the group A streptococci. Infect Immun 53:432, 1986.
39. Kaplan EL, Top FH, Dudding BA, Wannamaker LW: Diagnosis of streptococcal pharyngitis: Differentiation of active infection from the carrier state in the symptomatic child. J Infect Dis 123:490, 1971.
40. Stollerman GH: The relative rheumatogenicity of strains of group A streptococci. Mod Concepts Cardiovasc Dis 44:35, 1975.
41. Rammelkamp CH, Denny FW, Wannamaker LW: Studies on the epidemiology of rheumatic fever in the armed services. *In* Thomas L (ed): Rheumatic Fever. Minneapolis, Minnesota, University of Minnesota Press, 1952, pp 72–89.
42. Denny FW Jr, Wannamaker LW, Brink WR, et al: Prevention of rheumatic fever. Treatment of the preceding streptococcal infection. JAMA 143:151, 1950.
43. Facklam RR: Specificity study of kits for detection of group A streptococci directly from throat swabs. J Clin Microbiol 25:504, 1987.
44. Tenjarla G, Kumar A, Dyke JW: TestPak strep A kit for the rapid detection of group A streptococci on 11,088 throat swabs in the clinical pathology laboratory. Am J Clin Pathol 96:759, 1991.
45. Petts DN: Evaluation of a modified nitrous acid extraction latex agglutination kit for grouping beta hemolytic streptococci and enterococci. J Clin Microbiol 33:4, 1995.
46. Stollerman GH: Rheumatic Fever and Streptococcal Infection. New York, Grune & Stratton, 1975.
47. Rothbard S: Bacteriostatic effect of human sera on group A streptococci. I. Type-specific antibodies in sera of patients convalescing from group A streptococcal pharyngitis. J Exp Med 82:93, 1945.
48. Rothbard S: Bacteriostatic effect of human sera on group A streptococci. II. Comparative bacteriostatic effect of normal whole blood from different animal species in presence of human convalescent sera. J Exp Med 82:107, 1945.
49. Rothbard S: Bacteriostatic effect of human sera on group A streptococci. III. Interference with bacteriostatic activity by blockage of leukocytes. J Exp Med 82:119, 1945.
50. Stollerman GH, Siegel AC, Johnson EE: Evaluation of the "long chain reaction" as a means for detecting type specific antibody to group A streptococci in human sera. J Exp Med 110:887, 1959.
51. Bloomfield AL: A bibliography of internal medicine. Scarlet fever. Stanford Med Bull 10:114, 1952.
52. Dochez AR: Etiology of scarlet fever. Harvey Lect 20:131, 1926.
53. Stollerman GH: The historical role of the Dick test. JAMA 250:22, 1983.
54. Nathan L, Peters MT, Ahmed AM, et al: The return of life-threatening puerperal sepsis caused by group A streptococci. Am J Obstet Gynecol 169:571, 1993.
55. Cone LA, Woodard DR, Schlievert PM, et al: Clinical and bacteriologic observations of a toxic shock–like syndrome due to *Streptococcus pyogenes*. N Engl J Med 317:146, 1987.
56. Bartter T, Doscal A, Carroll K, et al: "Toxic strep syndrome": Manifestation of group A streptococcal infection. Arch Intern Med 148:1421, 1988.
57. Centers for Disease Control: Acute rheumatic fever at a Navy training center—San Diego, California. MMWR Morbid Mortal Wkly Rep 37:101, 1988.
58. Centers for Disease Control: Acute rheumatic fever among Army trainees—Fort Leonard Wood, Missouri, 1987–1988. MMWR Morbid Mortal Wkly Rep 37:519, 1988.
59. Johnson DR, Stevens DL, Kaplan EL: Epidemiologic analysis of group A streptococcal serotypes associated with severe systemic infections, rheumatic fever or uncomplicated pharyngitis. J Infect Dis 166:374, 1992.
60. Steinberg DG, Stollerman GH: Dangerous pyogenic skin infections. Hosp Pract 24:101, 1989.
61. Bisno AL: Cutaneous infections: Microbiologic and epidemiologic considerations. Am J Med 76:172, 1984.
62. Stevens DL: Invasive group A strep infections. Clin Infect Dis 14:2, 1991.
63. Chelsom J, Halstensen A, Haga T, Hoiby EA: Necrotising fasciitis due to group A streptococci in western Norway: Incidence and clinical features. Lancet 344:1111, 1994.
64. Meleney FL: Hemolytic streptococcus gangrene. Arch Surg 9:317, 1924.
65. Stamenkovic I, Lew PD: Early recognition of potentially fatal necrotizing fasciitis: The use of frozen-section biopsy. N Engl J Med 312:1689, 1984.
66. Wolf JE, Rabinowitz LG: Streptococcal toxic shock–like syndrome. Arch Dermatol 131:73, 1995.
67. Silver RM, Heddleston LN, McGregor JA, et al: Life-threatening puerperal infection due to group A strepococci. Obstet Gynecol 79:894, 1992.
68. Dotters DJ, Katz VL: Streptococcal toxic shock associated with septic abortion. Obstet Gynecol 78:549, 1991.
69. Herold AH: Group A beta-hemolytic streptococcal toxic shock from a mild pharyngitis. J Fam Pract 31:549, 1990.
70. Bradley JS, Schlievert PM, Petum BM: Toxic shock–like syndrome; a complication of strep throat. Pediatr Infect Dis J 10:790, 1991.
71. Chapnick CK, Graden JD, Leitwich LI, et al: Streptococcal toxic shock syndrome due to noninvasive pharyngitis. Clin Infect Dis 14:1074, 1992.
72. Schwartz B, Elliott JA, Butler JC, et al: Clusters of invasive group A infections in family, hospital and nursing home settings. Clin Infect Dis 15:277, 1992.
73. Hoge CW, Schwartz B, Talkington DF, et al: The changing epidemiology of invasive group A streptococcal infections and the consequence of streptococcal toxic shock–like syndrome. A retrospective population-based study. JAMA 269:384, 1993.
74. Mollick JA, Miller GG, Musser JM, et al: A novel superantigen isolated from pathogenic strain of *Streptococcus pyogenes* with aminoterminal homology to staphylococcal enterotoxin B and C. J Clin Invest 92:710, 1993.
75. Bisno AL, Stevens DL: Streptococcal infections of skin and soft tissues. N Engl J Med 334:240, 1995.
76. Hackett SP, Stevens DL: Superantigens associated with staphylococcal and streptococcal toxic-shock syndrome are potent inducers of tumor necrosis factor beta synthesis. J Infect Dis 168:232, 1993.
77. The Working Group on Severe Streptococcal Infections: Defining the group A streptococcal toxic shock syndrome. Rationale and consensus definition. JAMA 269:390, 1993.
78. Wannamaker LW: Differences between streptococcal infections of the throat and of the skin. I. N Engl J Med 282:23, 1970.
79. Wannamaker LW: Differences between streptococcal infections of the throat and of the skin (second of two parts). N Engl J Med 282:78, 1970.
80. Demidovich CW, Wittler RR, Ruff ME, et al: Impetigo. Current etiology and comparison of penicillin, erythromycin and cephalexin therapies. Am J Dis Child 144:1313, 1990.
81. Rasmussen JE: The changing nature of impetigo. Patient Care (July 15):233, 1992.
82. Barton LL, Friedman AD, Sharkey AM, et al: Impetigo contagioso. III. Comparative efficacy of oral erythromycin and topical mupirocin. Pediatr Dermatol 6:134, 1989.
83. Mertz PM, Marshall DA, Eagelstein WH, et al: Topical mupirocin treatment of impetigo is equal to oral erythromycin therapy. Arch Dermatol 125:1069, 1989.
84. Stollerman GH: Rheumatic fever and other rheumatic diseases of the heart. *In* Braunwald E (ed): Heart Disease. A Textbook of Cardiovascular Medicine, ed 4. Philadelphia, WB Saunders, 1992, pp 1721–1741.
85. Stollerman GH: Rheumatic fever. *In* Kelley WN, Harris ED, Ruddy S, et al (eds): Textbook of Rheumatology, ed 3. Philadelphia, WB Saunders, 1988.
86. Stollerman GH: Global changes in group A streptococcal diseases and strategies for their prevention. Adv Intern Med 27:373, 1982.
87. Ferguson GW, Schultz JM, Bisno AL: Epidemiology of acute rheumatic fever in a multi-ethnic, multi-racial U.S. urban community. The Miami-Dade experience. J Infect Dis 164:720, 1991.
88. Stollerman GH: Rheumatogenic group A streptococci and the return of rheumatic fever. Adv Intern Med 35:1, 1990.
89. Wannamaker LW: The chain that links the heart to the throat. Circulation 48:9, 1973.
90. Bisno AL, Pearce IA, Wall HP, et al: Contrasting epidemiology of acute rheumatic fever and acute glomerulonephritis. Nature of the antecedent streptococcal infection. N Engl J Med 283:561, 1970.
91. Coburn AF, Pauli RH: Studies on the immune response of the

rheumatic subject and its relationship to activity of the rheumatic process. IV. Characteristics of strains of hemolytic streptococcus, effective and noneffective in initiating rheumatic activity. J Clin Invest 14:755, 1935.
92. Kuttner AG, Krumwiede E: Observations on the effect of streptococcal upper respiratory infections on rheumatic children. A three-year study. J Clin Invest 20:273, 1941.
93. McLaren MJ, Markowitz M, Gerber MA: Rheumatic heart disease in developing countries: The consequence of inadequate prevention. Ann Intern Med 120:243, 1994.
94. World Health Organization: WHO programme for the prevention of rheumatic fever/rheumatic heart disease in 16 developing countries: Report from phase I (1986–90). Bull World Health Organ 70:213, 1992.
95. Carapetis JR, Wolff DR, Currie BJ: Acute rheumatic fever and rheumatic heart disease in the top end of Australia's northern territory. Med J Aust 164:146, 1996.
96. Veasy LG, Wiedmeier SE, Garth SO, et al: Resurgence of acute rheumatic fever in the intermountain area of the United States. N Engl J Med 316:421, 1987.
97. Centers for Disease Control: Acute rheumatic fever—Utah. MMWR Morbid Mortal Wkly Rep 36:108, 1987.
98. Congeni B, Rizzo C, Congeni J, Screenivasan VV: Outbreak of acute rheumatic fever in northeast Ohio. J Pediatr 111:176, 1987.
99. Wald ER, Dashefsky B, Feidt C, et al: Acute rheumatic fever in western Pennsylvania and the tristate area. Pediatrics 80:371, 1987.
100. Kaplan EL, Johnson DR, Cleary PP: Group A streptococcal serotypes isolated from patients and sibling contacts during the resurgence of rheumatic fever in the United States in the mid-1980's. J Infect Dis 159:101, 1989.
101. Macron MJ, Hribar MM, Hosier DM, et al: Occurrence of mucoid M-18 *Streptococcus pyogenes* in a central Ohio pediatric population. J Clin Microbiol 26:1539, 1988.
102. Yoshimoya S, Pope RM: Detection of immune complexes in acute rheumatic fever and their relationship to HLA-B5. J Clin Invest 65:136, 1980.
103. Jhinghan B, Mehra VK, Reddy KS, et al: HLA blood groups and secretor status in patients with established rheumatic fever and rheumatic heart disease. Tissue Antigens 27:172, 1986.
104. Ayoub EM, Barrett DJ, Maclain MC, et al: Association of class II human histocompatibility leukocyte antigens with rheumatic fever. J Clin Invest 77:2019, 1986.
105. Maharaj B, Hammond MG, Appadoo B, et al: HLA-A, B, DR and DQ antigens in black patients with severe chronic rheumatic heart disease. Circulation 76:259, 1987.
106. Patarroyo ME, Winchester RJ, Vejerano A, et al: Association of a B-cell alloantigen with susceptibility to rheumatic fever. Nature 278:173, 1979.
107. Zabriskie JB, Lavenchy D, Williams RC Jr, et al: Rheumatic fever–associated B cell alloantigens as identified by monoclonal antibodies. Arthritis Rheum 28:1047, 1985.
108. Khanna AK, Buskirk DR, Williams RC Jr, et al: Presence of a non-HLA B cell antigen in rheumatic fever patients and their families as defined by a monoclonal antibody. J Clin Invest 83:1710, 1989.
109. Stollerman GH: Rheumatogenic streptococci and autoimmunity. Clin Immunol Immunopathol 61:131, 1991.
110. Cairns LM: Immunological studies in rheumatic fever. The immunology of rheumatic fever. N Z Med J 101:388, 1987.
111. Baird RW, Bronze MS, Kraus W, et al: Epitopes of group A streptococcal M protein shared with antigens of articular cartilage and synovium. J Immunol 146:3132, 1991.
112. Sanyal SK, Thapar MK, Ahmed SH, et al: The initial attack of acute rheumatic fever during childhood in north India. A prospective study of the clinical profile. Circulation 49:7, 1974.
112a. Wilson NJ, Neutze JM: Echocardiographic diagnosis of subclinical carditis in acute rheumatic fever (Editorial). Int J Cardiol 50:1, 1995.
112b. Narula J, Chopra P, Talwar KK, et al: Does endomyocardial biopsy aid in the diagnosis of active myocarditis? Circulation 88:2198, 1996.
113. Taranta A, Stollerman GH: The relationship of Sydenham's chorea to infection with group A streptococci. Am J Med 20:170, 1956.
114. Taranta A: Relation of isolated recurrences of Sydenham's chorea to preceding streptococcal infections. N Engl J Med 260:1204, 1959.
115. Jones criteria (revised) for guidance in the diagnosis of rheumatic fever, updated 1992. Circulation 87:302, 1993.
116. Albert DA, Harel L, Karrison T: The treatment of rheumatic carditis: A review and meta-analysis. Medicine (Baltimore) 74:1, 1995.
117. Stollerman GH: Rheumatic carditis. Lancet 346:390, 1995.
118. Taranta A, Wood HF, Feinstein AR, et al: Rheumatic fever in children and adolescents. A long-term epidemiologic study of subsequent prophylaxis, streptococcal infections, and clinical sequelae. IV. Relation of the rheumatic fever recurrence rate per streptococcal antibodies to the titers of streptococcal antibodies. Ann Intern Med 60(Suppl 5):47, 1964.
119. Bisno AL, Pearce IA, Stollerman GH: Streptococcal infections that fail to cause recurrences of rheumatic fever. J Infect Dis 136:278, 1977.
120. Berrios X, delCampo E, Guzman B, Bisno AL: Discontinuing rheumatic fever prophylaxis in selected adolescents and young adults: A prospective study. Ann Intern Med 118:401, 1993.
121. Rammelkamp CH Jr, Weaver RS: Acute glomerulonephritis. The significance of the variations in the incidence of the disease. J Clin Invest 32:345, 1953.
122. Culpepper RM, Andreoli TE: The pathophysiology of the glomerulopathies. Adv Intern Med 28:161, 1983.
123. Fillit H, Damle SP, Gregory JD, et al: Sera from patients with poststreptococcal glomerulonephritis contain antibodies to glomerular heparan sulfate proteoglycan. J Exp Med 161:277, 1985.
124. Kraus W, Beachey EH: Renal autoimmune epitope of group A streptococci specified by M protein tetrapeptide Ile-Arg-Leu-Arg. Proc Natl Acad Sci USA 85:4516, 1988.
125. Kefalides NA, Pegg MT, Ohmo N, et al: Antibodies to basement membrane collagen and to laminin are present in sera from patients with poststreptococcal glomerulonephritis. J Exp Med 163:588, 1986.
126. Yoshizawa N, Oshima S, Sagel I, et al: Role of a streptococcal antigen in the pathogenesis of acute poststreptococcal glomerulonephritis. J Immunol 148:3110, 1992.
127. Poon-King T, Mohammed I, Cox R, et al: Recurrent epidemic nephritis in south Trinidad. N Engl J Med 277:728, 1967.
128. Potter EV, Svartman M, Mohammed I, et al: Tropical acute rheumatic fever and associated streptococcal infections compared with concurrent acute glomerulonephritis. J Pediatr 92: 325, 1978.
129. Roy S, Stapleton FB: Changing perspectives in children hospitalized with post-streptococcal glomerulonephritis. Pediatr Nephrol 4:585, 1990.
130. Yap HK, Chia KS, Murugasu B, et al: Acute glomerulonephritis—Changing patterns in Singapore children. Pediatr Nephrol 4:482, 1990.
131. Stollerman GH, Rusoff JR: Prophylaxis against group A streptococcal infections in rheumatic fever patients. Use of a new repository penicillin. JAMA 150:1571, 1952.
132. Stollerman GH, Rusoff JH, Hirshfield I: Prophylaxis against group A streptococci in rheumatic fever. The use of single monthly injections of benzathine penicillin G. N Engl J Med 252:787, 1955.
133. Raz R, Elchanan G, Colodner R, et al: Penicillin V twice daily vs four times daily in the treatment of streptococcal pharyngitis. Infect Dis Clin Pract 4:50, 1995.
134. Picherero ME: Cephalosporins are superior to penicillin for the treatment of tonsillopharyngitis: Is the difference worth it? Pediatr Infect Dis J 123:268, 1993.
135. Dajani AS, Bisno AL, Chung KJ, et al: Treatment of acute streptococcal pharyngitis and prevention of rheumatic fever. Pediatrics 96:758, 1995.
136. Catanzaro FJ, Stetson CA, Morris AJ, et al: The role of the streptococcus in the pathogenesis of rheumatic fever. Am J Med 17:749, 1954.
137. Stollerman GH: Commentary: Penicillin therapy for streptococcal pharyngitis—What have we learned in 50 years? Infect Dis Clin Pract 4:54, 1995.
138. Frank PF, Stollerman GH, Miller LF: Protection of a military population from rheumatic fever. JAMA 193:775, 1965.
139. Wood HF, Stollerman GH, Feinstein AR, et al: A controlled study of three methods of prophylaxis against streptococcal

infection in a population of rheumatic children. N Engl J Med 257:394, 1957.
140. Dale JB, Simmons M, Chiang EC, Chiang EY: Recombinant octavalent group A streptococcal vaccine. Vaccine 14:944, 1996.
141. Dale JB, Chiang EC: Intranasal immunization with recombinant group A streptococcal M protein fragment fused to the B subunit of *Escherichia coli* labile toxin protects mice against systemic challenge infections. J Infect Dis 171:1038, 1995.
142. Stollerman GH: The nature of rheumatogenic streptococci. Mt Sinai J Med 63:144, 1996.
143. Stollerman GH: Rheumatic fever: 1997. Lancet (in press).

193

Streptococcus pneumoniae

Robert Austrian

History

The pneumococcus, *Streptococcus pneumoniae,* was isolated first in 1880 from carriers of the organism by Sternberg and by Pasteur. Its role as the principal cause of community-acquired bacterial pneumonia was established by Fraenkel and by Weichselbaum in the 1880s,[1] as was its ability to cause otitis media, meningitis, and arthritis.

Characteristics of the Pathogen

The pneumococcus is a member of the genus *Streptococcus,* bacteria characterized by a lack of cytochromes and catalase.[2] Absence of catalase prevents degradation of hydrogen peroxide formed by the cells and necessitates an exogenous source of the enzyme, such as intact erythrocytes, to prevent the death of cultures. Pneumococci are gram-positive and grow as single cells, diplococci, and in chains of variable length. They are α-hemolytic. Their nutritional requirements are complex and include choline, which is incorporated into the teichoic acid of the cell wall. Pneumococci produce an autolytic enzyme, L-alanine-muramyl amidase, which hydrolyzes the cell wall[3] and is activated by detergents, including bile, resulting in lysis of the cell. The growth of most strains of pneumococci is inhibited by ethylhydrocupreine hydrochloride (optochin), but resistant strains occur.[4]

Several well-characterized surface antigens of *S. pneumoniae* are known: the C polysaccharide of the cell wall; type-specific M proteins with chemical properties similar to those of *Streptococcus pyogenes* and related to, if not identical to, another group of type-specific surface proteins known as PspA[5]; and type-specific capsular polysaccharides. Ninety distinct capsular polysaccharides have been identified.[5a] These polymers, although nontoxic, exert an antiphagocytic effect, and their presence is essential to the virulence of the organism and its ability to cause infection.[6, 7]

Epidemiology

S. pneumoniae is an obligate parasite of humans, although occasionally it may be isolated from other mammalian species. Colonization of the human upper respiratory tract may occur on the first day of life.[8] As many as four distinct capsular types may be carried simultaneously, although colonization with one or two capsular types is more usual. Children are more likely to be carriers of pneumococci than are adults, but the latter are colonized frequently. Antibodies to pneumococcal capsular polysaccharides do not eliminate established carriage of organisms of the homologous type but reduce by approximately half the likelihood of becoming colonized with the same organism.[9] Pneumococci are spread from person to person by direct contact with secretions bearing the organism. Infection is thought to result most frequently after acquisition of a previously unencountered capsular type.

Not all pneumococcal types are equally invasive. In childhood, capsular types 4, 6A, 6B, 9V, 12F, 14, 18C, 19F, 19A, and 23F account for 85% of bacteremic pneumococcal infection. In adults, capsular types 1, 3, 4, 6A, 6B, 7F, 8, 9N, 9V, 10A, 11A, 12F, 14, 15B, 17F, 19F, 19A, 20, 22F, 23F, and 33F cause approximately 90% of bacteremic pneumococcal infections in the United States.

At present, *S. pneumoniae* causes approximately 500,000 cases of otitis media in the United States annually.[10] The minimum annual attack rate of pneumococcal bacteremia, determined retrospectively, is 30 per 100,000[11]; that of pneumococcal pneumonia is 1 to 2 per 1000 and that of pneumococcal meningitis, 1 to 1.5 per 100,000.[12]

Pathogenesis

Pneumococci are a component of the normal bacterial flora of the human nasopharynx and, in the absence of injury to the epithelial lining of the upper and lower respiratory tract, live in a commensal state with humans. Anatomic alterations in the cells lining the respiratory tract, be they viral, mechanical, or chemical, predispose to bacterial infection of the affected region.[13] Viral infections of the upper respiratory tract causing edema of the eustachian tube and negative pressure in the middle ear predispose to bacterial otitis media, of which pneumococci are the most common cause.[14, 15] Any disturbance of the complex and coordinated neuromuscular reflexes protecting the lower respiratory tract from aspiration of foreign material may be followed by infection of the lungs. Bacteria reaching the alveoli of the normal lung are usually cleared rapidly. Injury to the alveolar lining cells by viral infection such as that caused by influenza virus or rhinoviruses or by chemical agents, trauma, or aspirated material delays clearance of bacteria and allows the establishment of progressive infection furthered by the inflammatory properties of fragments of the pneumococcal cell wall[16] and the oxygen-labile intracellular hemolysin pneumolysin.[17] Pharmacologically active substances retarding the migration of polymorphonuclear leukocytes, including alcohol, anesthetics, and corticosteroids, facilitate the establishment and spread of pneumonia. Failure of the host's defensive mechanisms to limit infection to the lung results in extension of bacteria to hilar lymph nodes and, in cases developing bacteremia, from the latter site to the systemic circulation via the thoracic duct. Pneumococci in infants, and less commonly in adults, like meningococci and *Haemophilus influenzae,* appear capable of penetrating the nasopharyngeal mucosa and gaining access to the systemic circulation via the cervical lymphatic vessels in the absence of a demonstrable focus of infection.[18] Bacteremia, once established, may be followed by metastatic foci of infection, notably of serous cavities such as the meninges, joints, and peritoneum. Meningitis may also arise by extension of infection from the middle ear or paranasal sinuses and pleural empyema or pericarditis by direct extension from the lung. Pneumococcal endocarditis, a complication of bacteremic infection, occurs most commonly in persons older than 40 years.

Spontaneous recovery from pneumococcal infection is mediated by the development of type-specific anticapsular antibodies that, acting with complement,[19] combine with the polysaccharide capsule surrounding the infecting pneumococci, causing them to adhere to one another and to alveolar walls and to be phagocytosed with increased efficiency. Antibodies of both the immunoglobulin M and immunoglobulin G classes are formed. Reinfection with the same pneumococcal capsular type is rare in the absence of agammaglobulinemia or dysgammaglobulinemia, and immunity to reinfection with a given pneumococcal type is usually lifelong. Congenital or acquired deficiency of the early components of complement also predisposes to pneumococcal bacteremia[20] and to infection of soft tissues.[21]

Clinical Manifestations

The prototypic clinical picture of lobar pneumonia in the adult is characterized by an antecedent history of a common cold or influenza marked by a sudden worsening of the patient's condition manifested by a shaking chill and rise in body temperature, development of cough productive of rusty sputum, pleural pain, dyspnea, anorexia, and prostration.[22] With the illness unmodified by therapy, signs of segmental or lobar pulmonary consolidation evolve in the next 24 to 48 hours. Elevation of temperature persists for 5 to 10 days and may fall abruptly in one third of patients ("crisis") or by lysis. Defervescence frequently coincides with the demonstrable presence of circulating anticapsular antibody. In infants and the elderly, the clinical picture may deviate significantly from that described and mimic that of pneumonia of any cause. The clinical manifestations of otitis media, meningitis, arthritis, pleural empyema, pericarditis, peritonitis, and endocarditis caused by *S. pneumoniae* do not differ significantly from those of infections of these sites by other pyogenic bacteria, and diagnosis rests on isolation and identification of the infecting organism. Patients who have anatomic or functional asplenia are at risk of fulminant pneumococcal sepsis manifesting itself not infrequently with a clinical picture resembling that of the Waterhouse-Friderichsen syndrome and running its course from onset to death in 24 to 48 hours. The incidence of bacteremic pneumococcal infection in children and in adults infected with human immunodeficiency virus is greatly increased both before and after the development of the acquired immunodeficiency syndrome, approximating 10 times that in the uninfected population, and results apparently from multiple disturbances of host defenses.[23] In other respects, pneumococcal infection in persons infected with human immunodeficiency virus resembles clinically that seen in immunocompetent hosts.

Laboratory investigation should include determination of the concentration of hemoglobin and of polymorphonuclear leukocytes in the blood, measurement of arterial blood gas levels in the more seriously ill, and both posteroanterior and lateral radiographs of the chest.

Diagnosis

Although differences exist among the historical and clinical manifestations of pneumonias caused by different infectious agents, identification of the cause of a given illness rests on the proper use and interpretation of the appropriate microbiologic and immunologic tests in relation to that illness.

Diagnosis of pneumococcal infection with certainty rests on isolation of the organism from a normally sterile body site such as the blood, middle ear, subarachnoid space, or other serous cavity. A strongly presumptive diagnosis of pneumococcal pneumonia can be made from microscopic and cultural examination of expectorated respiratory secretions (sputum), but, because pneumococci are normal inhabitants of the upper respiratory tract, isolation of the organism from material passing through it does not establish absolutely its role in infection of the lung. In the absence of bacteremia, the causal role of pneumococci in pneumonia can be demonstrated by recovery of the organism from material obtained by transtracheal or transthoracic lung puncture; however, because both procedures are accompanied by small but finite morbidity, their use should be limited to situations in which they are deemed necessary for the patient's welfare.

Because pneumococci may be highly sensitive to most antimicrobial drugs, it is essential that material for culture be obtained before the administration of such therapeutic agents. Sputum should be collected in a sterile container by the physician to ensure that it is expectorated from the lung. After microscopic examination, sputum should be plated on nutrient blood agar and incubated in an atmospheric concentration of 5% carbon dioxide (candle jar). Characteristic colonies of pneumococci are depicted in Figures 193–1 and 193–2.

Most strains of pneumococci lyse in the presence of bile, bile salts, or other detergents and their growth is inhibited by ethylhydrocupreine hydrochloride (optochin). The most useful test for identification of pneumococci in the diagnostic laboratory is the quellung or capsular precipitin reaction.[24] The test can be carried out either directly with sputum or other body fluids such as cerebrospinal fluid or with organisms isolated from cultures. When type-specific anticapsular antibodies combine with capsular polysaccharide of the same type surrounding the pneumococcal cell, a refractile gel is formed that can be seen readily in the light microscope (Fig. 193–3). Visualization of the reaction is facilitated by the use of a substage concave mirror and oblique illumination. The test is performed by allowing a loopful of a suspension of the material to be examined to dry on a glass slide. A loopful of 1% methylene blue is deposited on a coverslip, and a loopful of anticapsular antiserum is placed on the dried suspension on the slide. The residual serum in the loop is

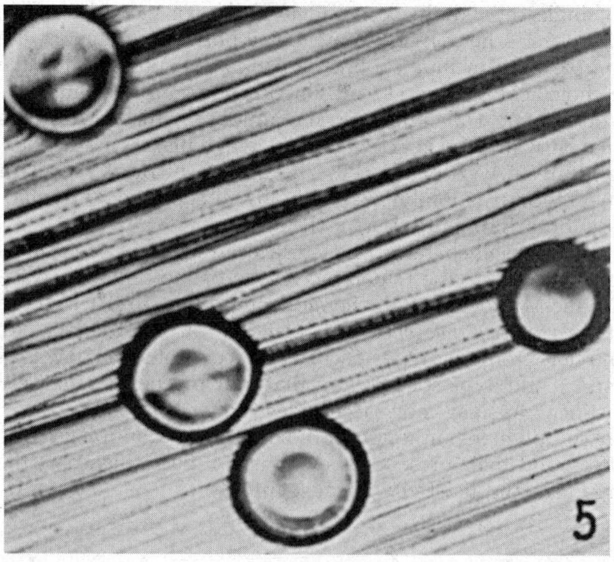

FIGURE 193–1 □ Typical colonies of *Streptococcus pneumoniae* on the surface of a blood agar plate. Central autolysis gives the colony the appearance of a checker (× 18). (Reproduced from The Journal of Experimental Medicine, 1953, vol 98, pp 21–34, by copyright permission of The Rockefeller University Press.)

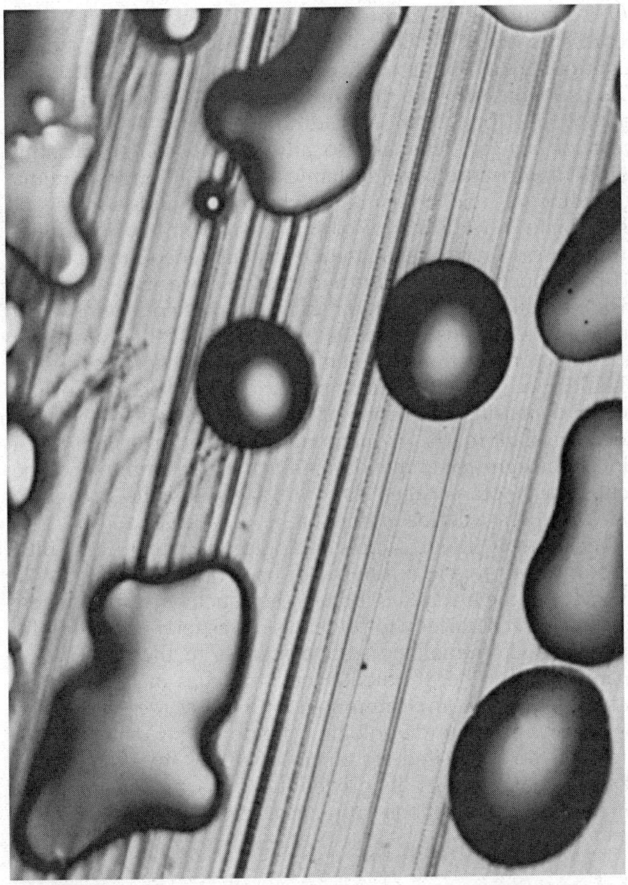

FIGURE 193–2 □ Typical mucoid colonies of *S. pneumoniae* type 3 (× 21). (Reproduced from The Journal of Experimental Medicine, 1953, vol 98, pp 21–34, by copyright permission of The Rockefeller University Press.)

then mixed sequentially with the methylene blue on the coverslip and then with the serum on the slide. The coverslip is placed over the suspension, and the preparation is examined under the oil immersion lens of the microscope. To avoid interference by excess antigen (prozone), no more than 50 to 100 pneumococci should be present in a single microscopic field. Sera for identifying all the pneumococcal types known currently are available commercially, including a preparation from the Danish Statens Seruminstitut designated Omniserum, which contains antibodies to 84 pneumococcal capsular polysaccharides and is an invaluable reagent for the rapid presumptive identification of pneumococcal infection.

Cocci suspected of being pneumococci may now also be identified with the use of a chemiluminescent labeled single-stranded DNA probe that is complementary to the ribosomal RNA of the bacterium. For this purpose, a pure culture of the organism to be tested, grown on solid or in liquid medium, must be employed.[25] Methods using the polymerase chain reaction to identify pneumococcal DNA in body fluids of presumptively infected patients are currently under investigation.[26]

Treatment

Since recognition of *S. pneumoniae* as a pathogen of humans, treatment of pneumococcal infection has undergone continual change, the result of better understanding of the biology of such infection and of pharmacologic advances. The case-fatality rate of pneumococcal pneumonia of 30% to 35%, affected little if at all by symptomatic therapy, fell to 20% to 25% among the infections for which serum therapy became available after recognition of the diversity of pneumococcal types in 1910. A further decline in case-fatality rate to 12% to 15% followed the introduction of sulfapyridine and its congeners, and the case-fatality rate reached its present nadir of 5% to 8% when penicillin and other comparably effective antibiotics became the accepted therapeutic agents.[27]

Although mutants of pneumococci resistant to penicillin G (benzylpenicillin) were recovered from experimentally infected animals treated with the drug a year before the report in 1944 of its efficacy in the management of both nonbacteremic and bacteremic pneumococcal pneumonia in humans, penicillin G became the unquestioned drug of first choice in the management of such infections in those not hypersensitive to it. Two decades were to elapse before resistant mutants similar to those described earlier were isolated from humans; since their initial recovery, both their frequency and the degree of resistance manifested by them have increased steadily. In addition, strains of pneumococci resistant to cephalosporins (ceftriaxone, cefotaxime), macrolides (e.g., erythromycin, clindamycin), tetracyclines, chloramphenicol, co-trimoxazole, and aminoglycosides have been recognized, posing potential problems in the treatment of pneumococcal disease. The sole antimicrobial drug to which pneumococci remain uniformly susceptible to date is vancomycin. If alternative therapy is used, it is now mandatory that the susceptibility of the infecting strain to the drug(s) employed be determined. For such determinations of drug sensitivity or

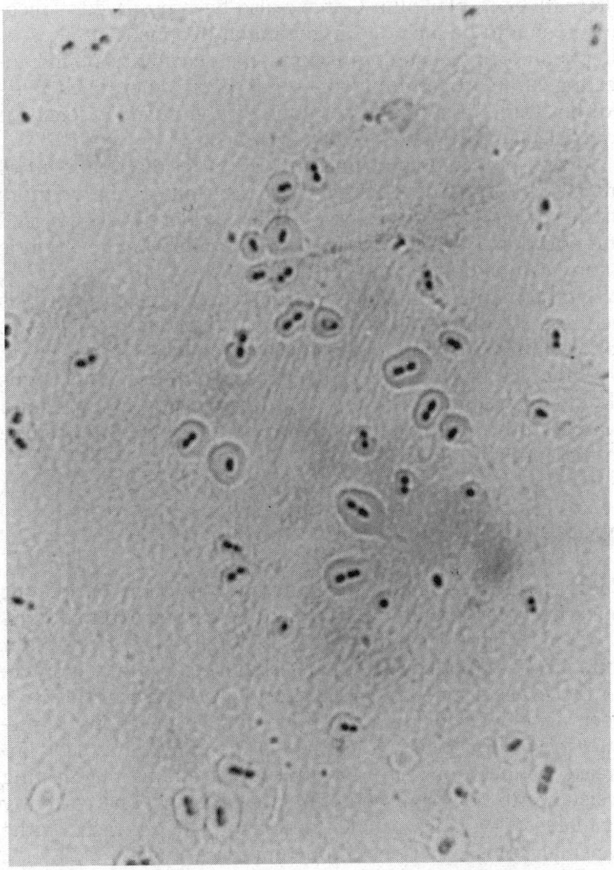

FIGURE 193–3 □ Quellung preparation of pneumococcal cells showing the refractile halo surrounding the bacterial cell (× 1100). (Reproduced from The Journal of Experimental Medicine, 1953, vol 98, pp 21–34, by copyright permission of The Rockefeller University Press.)

resistance, the E test shows significant promise for the rapid quantification of such drug effects.[28]

Resistance of pneumococci to penicillin is the result of mutations in one or more of the penicillin binding proteins concerned with the synthesis of the pneumococcal cell wall.[29, 30] Strains sensitive to 0.1 μg/mL or less are classified as sensitive, those inhibited by concentrations between 0.1 and 2 μg/mL are said to manifest intermediate resistance, and those inhibited only by concentrations greater than 2 μg/mL are considered to be fully resistant.[31] Resistance of any degree to penicillin is independent of capsular type but is observed most frequently among the types that most often affect children, types 6A, 6B, 9V, 14, 18C, 19F, 19A, and 23F. The proportion of penicillin-resistant pneumococcal strains varies with time and place, and knowledge of its extent may play an ancillary role in the choice of therapy. In some geographic areas, pneumococcal strains fully resistant to penicillin constitute more than 20% of the total isolated from blood cultures.[27, 32–34]

For treatment of pneumococcal pneumonia caused by normally sensitive organisms, conventional doses of penicillin G of 300,000 to 600,000 units administered parenterally every 6 hours are adequate. For those gravely ill or with complications, especially where strains manifesting increased resistance to penicillin are known to exist, penicillin in parenteral doses of 1,200,000 units every 2 hours result in serum levels of penicillin of approximately 5 μg/mL[35] while the sensitivity of the infecting organism is being determined. This regimen, however, is not adequate for the treatment of pneumococcal meningitis caused by strains of the organism that manifest increased resistance to penicillin. Because strains of pneumococci with increased resistance to ceftriaxone and cefotaxime, alternatives to penicillin G, have also been observed, vancomycin should be included in the initial treatment of all cases of pneumococcal meningitis until the sensitivity of the infecting strain to antimicrobials has been determined.[36] Its administration may be discontinued if the isolate is sensitive to a β-lactam drug.

Several new agents of potential utility in the treatment of infections caused by pneumococci resistant to one or more of the drugs currently employed are under investigation,[37] but additional clinical experience is required before the role of any can be determined.

Symptomatic treatment of pneumococcal infections entails bed rest, a liquid or light diet, adequate hydration, analgesics for pleural pain, and oxygen when cyanosis is present in pneumonia. During the acute phase of illness, vital signs should be recorded no less often than every 4 hours, and temperature should be measured rectally or by thermocouple in the auditory canal.

Prophylaxis

Because the case-fatality rate of uncomplicated bacteremic pneumococcal pneumonia in adults treated optimally is 17%[38] and that of pneumococcal meningitis in persons older than 40 years treated in similar fashion exceeds 40%, polyvalent vaccines of pneumococcal capsular polysaccharides have been developed for the prevention of such infections. A second reason for their availability is the slow but steady increase of the number of pneumococcal strains manifesting resistance to one or more antimicrobial drugs. The currently available 23-valent vaccine, containing 25 μg each of the capsular polysaccharides of pneumococcal types 1, 2, 3, 4, 5, 6B, 7F, 8, 9N, 9V, 10A, 11A, 12F, 14, 15B, 17F, 18C, 19F, 19A, 20, 22F, 23F, and 33F, has been shown to be safe, immunogenic, and effective. It has an aggregate efficacy of 60% to 70% in both young and elderly adults in preventing infection with any of the 23 immunologically distinct capsular types represented in it.[39–41] It was recommended by the Advisory Committee on Immunization Practices of the Centers for Disease Control[42] and by the American College of Physicians[43] that the vaccine be administered to all persons 65 years of age or older and to any immunocompetent adult with chronic underlying systemic illness. Although agammaglobulinemic and dysgammaglobulinemic individuals and those with other forms of compromised immunity resulting from illness or treatment manifest heightened susceptibility to pneumococcal infection and may be vaccinated without risk, the likelihood of their being protected against such infection is, in most instances, reduced. All individuals with anatomic or functional asplenia, however, regardless of age, should receive the 23-valent pneumococcal vaccine. In light of the increasing frequency of infection caused by pneumococci resistant to one or more antimicrobial drugs, modification of current recommendations to include immunocompetent adults of all ages as candidates for the receipt of pneumococcal vaccine is now highly desirable.

The human infant is immunologically immature at birth and unresponsive to a number of bacterial capsular polysaccharides in the first years if life. When such bacterial antigens are coupled chemically to protein, such as tetanus or diphtheria toxoid, immunologic responsiveness to the conjugate is manifested by the production of antibodies of both the immunoglobulin M and immunoglobulin G classes and by the development of immunologic "memory."[44] Conjugate vaccines of the kind cited are currently under investigation for their potential utility in preventing otitis media and other pneumococcal infections in infancy and early childhood.[45, 46]

References

1. Austrian R: The Gram stain and the etiology of lobar pneumonia, an historical note. Bacteriol Rev 24:261, 1960.
2. Austrian R: Pneumococci. *In* Davis BD, Dulbecco R, Eisen HN, Ginsberg HS (eds): Microbiology, ed 4. Philadelphia, JB Lippincott, 1990, pp 515–524.
3. Mosser JL, Tomasz A: Choline-containing teichoic acid as a structural component of pneumococcal cell wall and its role in sensitivity to lysis by an autolytic enzyme. J Biol Chem 245:287, 1970.
4. Ragsdale AR, Sanford JP: Interfering effect of incubation in carbon dioxide on the identification of pneumococci by optochin discs. Appl Microbiol 22:854, 1971.
5. Boulnois GJ: Pneumococcal proteins and pathogenesis of disease caused by *Streptococcus pneumoniae.* J Gen Microbiol 138:249, 1992.

5a. Henrichsen J: Six newly recognized types of *Streptococcus pneumoniae.* J Clin Microbiol 33:2759, 1995.

6. Avery OT, Dubos R: Protective action of a specific enzyme against type III pneumococcus in mice. J Exp Med 54:73, 1931.
7. Rich AR, McKee CM: The pathogenicity of avirulent pneumococci for animals deprived of leukocytes. Bull Johns Hopkins Hosp 64:434, 1939.
8. Austrian R: Some aspects of the pneumococcal carrier state. J Antimicrob Chemother 18(Suppl A):35, 1986.
9. MacLeod CM, Hodges RG, Heidelberger M, Bernhard WG: Prevention of pneumococcal pneumonia by vaccination. J Exp Med 82:445, 1945.
10. Austrian R, Howie VM, Ploussard JH: The bacteriology of pneumococcal otitis media. Johns Hopkins Med J 141:104, 1977.
11. Austrian R: Pneumococcal pneumonia: Diagnostic, epidemiologic, therapeutic and prophylactic considerations. Chest 90:738, 1986.
12. Fraser DW, Geil CC, Feldman RA: Bacterial meningitis in Bernalillo County, New Mexico: A comparison with three other American populations. Am J Epidemiol 100:29, 1974.
13. Harford CG, Hara M: Pulmonary edema in influenzal pneumonia of the mouse and the relation of fluid in the lung to the inception of pneumococcal pneumonia. J Exp Med 91:245, 1950.
14. Giebink GS: The pathogenesis of pneumococcal otitis media in

chinchillas and the efficacy of vaccination in prophylaxis. Rev Infect Dis 3:342, 1981.
15. Klein JO: Otitis media. Clin Infect Dis 19:823, 1994.
16. Tuomanen EI, Austrian R, Masure HR: Pathogenesis of pneumococcal infection. N Engl J Med 332:1280, 1995.
17. Boulnois GJ, Paton JC, Mitchell TJ, et al: Structure and function of pneumolysin, the multifunctional, thiol-activated toxin of *Streptococcus pneumoniae.* Mol Microbiol 5:2611, 1991.
18. Austrian R: Untreated pneumococcal bacteraemia of cryptic origin in the human adult with spontaneous recovery. S Afr Med J 70(Suppl):46, 1986.
19. Hosea SW, Brown EJ, Frank MM: The critical role of complement in experimental pneumococcal sepsis. J Clin Invest 142:903, 1980.
20. Ross SC, Densen P: Complement deficiency states and infection: Epidemiology, pathogenesis and consequences of neisserial and other infections in an immune deficiency. Medicine (Baltimore) 63:243, 1984.
21. Patel M, Ahrens JC, Moyer DV, et al: Pneumococcal soft-tissue infections: A problem deserving more recognition. Clin Infect Dis 19:149, 1994.
22. Heffron R: Pneumonia with Special Reference to Pneumococcus Lobar Pneumonia, 2nd printing. Boston, Harvard University Press, 1979.
23. Janoff EN, Breiman RF, Daley CL, et al: Pneumococcal disease during HIV infection. Epidemiologic, clinical, and immunologic perspectives. Ann Intern Med 117:314, 1992.
24. Austrian R: The quellung reaction, a neglected microbiologic technique. Mt Sinai J Med 43:699, 1976.
25. Denys GA, Carey RB: Identification of *Streptococcus pneumoniae* with a DNA probe. J Clin Microbiol 30:2725, 1992.
26. Zhang Y, Isaacman DJ, Wadowsky RM, et al: Detection of *Streptococcus pneumoniae* in whole blood by PCR. J Clin Microbiol 33:596, 1995.
27. Austrian R: Confronting drug-resistant pneumococci (Editorial). Ann Intern Med 121:807, 1994.
28. Jacobs MR, Bajaksouzian S, Applebaum PC, et al: Evaluation of the E-test for susceptibility testing of pneumococci. Diagn Microbiol Infect Dis 15:473, 1992.
29. Shockley TE, Hotchkiss RD: Stepwise introduction of transformable penicillin resistance in pneumococcus. Genetics 64:397, 1970.
30. Zighelboim S, Tomasz A: Penicillin-binding proteins of multiply-resistant South African strains of *Streptococcus pneumoniae.* Antimicrob Agents Chemother 17:434, 1980.
31. Klugman KP: Pneumococcal resistance to antibiotics. J Clin Microbiol 3:171, 1990.
32. Doern GV, Brueggemann A, Holley AP Jr, et al: Antimicrobial resistance of *Streptococcus pneumoniae* recovered from outpatients in the United States during the winter months of 1994 to 1995: Results of a 30-center national surveillance study. Antimicrob Agents Chemother 40:1208, 1996.
33. Hofmann J, Cetron MS, Farley MM, et al: The prevalence of drug-resistant *Streptococcus pneumoniae* in Atlanta. N Engl J Med 333:481, 1995.
34. Pallares R, Liñares J, Vadillo M, et al: Resistance to penicillin and cephalosporin and mortality from severe pneumococcal pneumonia in Barcelona, Spain. N Engl J Med 333:474, 1995.
35. Tucker HA, Eagle H: Serum concentrations of penicillin G in man following intramuscular injections in aqueous solution and in peanut oil–beeswax. Am J Med 4:343, 1948.
36. Viladrich PF, Gudiol F, Liñares J, et al: Evaluation of vancomycin for therapy of adult pneumococcal meningitis. Antimicrob Agents Chemother 35:2467, 1991.
37. Applebaum PC: New prospects for antibacterial agents against multidrug-resistant pneumococci. Microb Drug Resist 1:43, 1995.
38. Austrian R, Gold J: Pneumococcal bacteremia with especial reference to bacteremic pneumococcal pneumonia. Ann Intern Med 60:759, 1964.
39. Shapiro ED, Clemens JD: A controlled evaluation of the protective efficacy of pneumococcal vaccine for patients at high risk of serious pneumococcal infections. Ann Intern Med 101:325, 1984.
40. Bolan G, Broome CV, Facklam RR, et al: Pneumococcal vaccine efficacy in selected populations in the United States. Ann Intern Med 104:1, 1986.
41. Shapiro ED, Berg AT, Austrian R, et al: The protective effect of polyvalent pneumococcal polysaccharide vaccine. N Engl J Med 325:1453, 1991.
42. Immunization Practices Advisory Committee: Pneumococcal polysaccharide vaccine. MMWR Morb Mortal Wkly Rep 38:64, 1989.
43. American College of Physicians: Guide for Adult Immunization, ed 3. Philadelphia, American College of Physicians, 1994, pp 108–114.
44. Beuvery EC, van Rossum F, Nagel J: Comparison of induction of immunoglobulin M and G antibodies in mice with purified pneumococcal type 3 and meningococcal group C polysaccharides and their protein conjugates. Infect Immun 37:15, 1982.
45. Vella PP, Marburg S, Staub JM, et al: Immunogenicity of conjugate vaccines consisting of pneumococcal capsular types 6B, 14, 19F and 23F and a meningococcal membrane protein complex. Infect Immun 60:4977, 1992.
46. Klein DL: Pneumococcal conjugate vaccines: Review and update. Microb Drug Resist 1:49, 1995.

194

Enterococci

Barbara E. Murray

The name enterococcus derives from a paper in France published in 1899 that described an "entérocoque," a new gram-positive coccus of intestinal origin.[1] The name *Streptococcus faecalis* (faecalis, related to feces) was given in 1906 to an organism isolated from the blood of a patient with endocarditis.[2] Probably the first description of *Streptococcus faecium* was in 1919, but this organism was not formally recognized as a separate species for several decades.[3] Through the years, a number of other types of enterococci were recognized, including *Streptococcus durans* and *Streptococcus avium*; motile enterococci, which were also known as *S. faecium* var. *mobilis*; and organisms producing a yellow pigment, referred to as *S. faecium* var. *casseliflavus*.

More than a decade ago, DNA-DNA and DNA–ribosomal RNA hybridization studies showed that enterococci, contrary to their long-standing classification, are not actually members of the genus *Streptococcus*.[4, 5] With foresight and consideration not always typical of taxonomists, the common name enterococcus became the new genus, that is, *Enterococcus*. In addition to *Enterococcus faecalis, Enterococcus faecium, Enterococcus durans,* and *Enterococcus avium*, a number of other organisms have been classified in this genus,[6, 7] a current list of which is shown in Table 194–1.

Identification

For a number of years, enterococci have been presumptively identified by their morphologic appearance in culture and on Gram stain together with their ability to hydrolyze esculin in the presence of bile and to grow in the presence of 6.5% NaCl. Many laboratories also test organisms with group D antiserum. It is now clear that a number of other, less often encountered organisms may have most or all of these characteristics. For example, most pediococci and a number of leuconostocs test positive with group D antiserum. Lactococci, pediococci, and leuconostocs are often bile esculin–positive and able to grow in high salt concentrations.[8, 9] Leuconostocs and pediococci are characteristically resistant to

TABLE 194–1 ■ List of Generally Recognized *Enterococcus* Species

Predominant human isolates	No known reports of human infections
*E. faecalis**	*E. malodoratus*
*E. faecium**	*E. pseudoavium*
Occasional human isolates	*E. sulfureus*
E. casseliflavus†	*E. cecorum*§
E. gallinarum†	*E. columbae*§
E. flavescens†‡	*E. saccharolyticus*§
E. avium	
E. raffinosus	
E. mundtii	
E. durans	
E. hirae	

*The ratio of *E. faecalis* to *E. faecium* among clinical specimens is typically 8:1 to 9:1, unless organisms are vancomycin resistant.
†May express vancomycin resistance because of VanC phenotype.
‡Some evidence suggests that this species is the same as *E. casseliflavus*.[90]
§These species have less genetic similarity to other enterococcal species.[91]

vancomycin, which formerly was useful for distinguishing these organisms from enterococci.[9] Other helpful tests include the demonstration of pyrrolidonyl arylamidase (the PYRase test), growth at 45°C, and leucine aminopeptidase, which are characteristic of enterococci but not leuconostocs, and the production of gas from glucose, which is characteristic of leuconostocs but not enterococci.[8, 9] This topic has been reviewed, and the reader is referred to these articles for more details.[6, 10] It is important to note that some of the rapid kit identification systems for species identification of enterococci were evaluated before some of the newer species were recognized and may not be accurate, particularly for species other than *E. faecalis*.

Habitat and Typing Schemes

As the names of the two most common species suggest, *E. faecalis* and *E. faecium* are commonly found in the feces of normal individuals. In most studies, *E. faecalis* has been more common than other enterococcal species and is usually present in higher numbers, often 10^5 to 10^7 colony-forming units per gram of stool.[3, 9, 11, 12] Enterococci are also found at other sites, although much less frequently than in fecal contents.[13, 14]

Epidemiologic studies of enterococcal infections have been difficult in the past because of the lack of convenient and reliable subspecies typing schemes. Although phage and bacteriocin typing have been described for enterococci for at least two decades, this system has not gained widespread use.[15] Total plasmid content analysis, a technique used with a variety of other organisms, has also been used to compare strains of enterococci,[16] although plasmid analysis has not been as convenient or reproducible, at least in our hands, with enterococci as with other organisms. Pulsed-field gel electrophoresis of enterococcal chromosomal DNA has shown that enterococci, like other nosocomial pathogens, can be spread within and even between hospitals.[17–19]

Clinical Infections (Table 194–2)

Endocarditis

It is estimated that enterococci cause between 5% and 15% of cases of bacterial endocarditis. The first report of this disease was probably in 1899; although the organism was called *Micrococcus zymogenes*, it was probably a β-hemolytic enterococcus.[3] The authors who first coined the name *S. faecalis* in 1906 isolated the organism from a patient with endocarditis.[2] Although most enterococcal endocarditis isolates are *E. faecalis*, *E. faecium* is also seen and, with the emergence of vancomycin resistance, may be increasing. Enterococcal endocarditis occurs rarely in infants, occasionally in children, and more often in older individuals; the average age in one study was 65 years.[20] Risk factors include genitourinary and biliary tract infections; in one study, 50% of men had had genitourinary instrumentation or urinary tract infection and 38% of women had a genitourinary source, including instrumentation or abortion.[20–22] The disease can occur on valves that are apparently normal as well as on those with underlying disease. In drug addicts, enterococci are estimated to cause between 5% and 10% of cases, although in one study 53% of 20 cases of endocarditis were caused by enterococci.[3, 23] The valves most often involved in drug addicts are the mitral and aortic valves.

Bacteremia

Bacteremia caused by enterococci is much more common than enterococcal endocarditis and appears to be increasing in frequency.[3, 23–25] The rates reported for endocarditis versus bacteremia differ widely from study to study depending on whether all positive blood cultures or a selected subset was evaluated.[3] For example, Maki and Agger[24] found 13 patients with enterococcal endocarditis among 153 episodes of enterococcal bacteremia (8%). Among those with community-acquired bacteremias, however, 36% of enterococcemias were thought to be due to endocarditis, whereas only 1 of 120 nosocomially acquired enterococcemias (0.8%) was associated with endocarditis.[24] Nosocomial enterococcemia, but not endocarditis, is often associated with concurrent or temporally associated polymicrobial bacteremia.[3, 24]

Urinary Tract Infections

Enterococci are also a common cause of urinary tract infections. Perinephric abscesses and prostatitis are occasionally

TABLE 194–2 ■ Clinical Infections Caused by Enterococci

TYPE OF INFECTION	% OF CASES CAUSED BY ENTEROCOCCI
Endocarditis	5–15
Urinary tract infections	<5 in young otherwise healthy women; ~15 of nosocomial infections
Intraabdominal pelvic and wound infections	15; frequently isolated, but other organisms are more important
Spontaneous peritonitis (cirrhosis)	5–10
Nosocomial bacteremia	5–10 (often polymicrobial)
Neonatal sepsis	Unusual
Central nervous system infections	Rare
Osteomyelitis	Rare
Pneumonia	Rare

seen. Enterococcal urinary tract infections are more common among hospitalized individuals, those who have had instrumentation, those who have structural abnormalities or recurrent urinary tract infections, and those who have received antibiotics.[3] In one study from a Veterans Administration hospital, for example, enterococci were found in 21% of urinary tract infections.[26] In a 1986 report, the Centers for Disease Control listed the enterococcus as the third most common cause of nosocomial urinary tract infections, causing 14.7% of urinary tract infections.[27] In contrast, enterococci cause less than 5% of urinary tract infections in young, healthy women with cystitis who do not have structural abnormalities and have not had instrumentation or recurrent infections.

Intraabdominal and Pelvic Infections

As discussed previously, enterococci are found in the feces of most normal adults; they are also found in approximately 17% of routine vaginal cultures.[13] Enterococci have been reported to cause salpingitis, endometritis with bacteremia, abscess formation after cesarean section, and bacteremia in obstetric and gynecologic patients.[3, 28, 29] Enterococci can also cause spontaneous peritonitis in cirrhotic patients, those with the nephrotic syndrome, and those receiving chronic peritoneal dialysis.[30, 31] Intraabdominal abscesses and biliary infections with bacteremia have also occurred.[24, 32–34]

The problem with intraabdominal and pelvic infections is not in deciding whether enterococci can contribute to these infections but in deciding who is likely to become infected and who should receive antienterococcal therapy. It is well established that antibiotic regimens that have little or no in vitro enterococcal activity but are active against *Escherichia coli* and anaerobes can be used successfully in animal models and in most patients with peritoneal contamination by fecal contents.[35–38] It has not been established which patients should receive antienterococcal therapy, but it is suggested for use in patients with persistent or recurrent intraabdominal sepsis, in those who have been hospitalized for a long time with abdominal infection, and possibly in those who are immunodepressed with the potential of developing enterococcal infection.[39] Unfortunately, enterococcal intraabdominal infection has occurred even in patients who were receiving appropriate antienterococcal therapy.[34]

Miscellaneous Infections

Enterococci can also cause neonatal infections. In a study of more than 30,000 live births at Parkland Memorial Hospital in Dallas in the 1970s, enterococci caused between 0.6 and 2.0 infections per 1000 live births in a 4-year period, compared with the rates for *E. coli* of 0.4 to 1.4 infections per 1000 live births.[40] Infection can occur in apparently normal infants, but those with severe underlying disease, intravascular devices, nasogastric endotracheal intubation, and prematurity appear to be more susceptible.[41, 42] Some of these risk factors are also thought to predispose adults to enterococcal infection.

Enterococcal infections of the central nervous system are uncommon but have been described in all age groups. The predisposing factors are thought to be underlying long-term primary disease, invasive procedures of the central nervous system, and prior therapy with antimicrobial agents. For example, case reports have included the development of enterococcal meningitis in patients with underlying meningeal leukemia while receiving intrathecal chemotherapy; after basilar skull fracture; and after intracranial surgery. Enterococcal meningitis has also occurred in patients with central nervous system shunts, particularly ventriculoperitoneal and lumboureteral shunts.[3, 43, 44]

Nosocomial Infections and Superinfections, Including Those with Vancomycin-Resistant Enterococci

The Centers for Disease Control and Prevention's National Nosocomial Infection Surveillance survey listed the enterococcus as the third most common organism recovered from nosocomial infections in 1990 to 1992,[45] following *E. coli* and staphylococci. Enterococci were found in about 10% of all nosocomial infections, 9% of bacteremias, and approximately 16% of urinary tract infections.[45] In the past, it was assumed that nosocomial enterococcal disease resulted from the endogenous flora with which the patient was admitted, but, as stated earlier, it is now clear that nosocomial spread of these organisms can occur.[16–19, 41] Several factors appear to be involved in the emergence of enterococci as important nosocomial pathogens, including the multiple resistances characteristic of these organisms, heavy use of antimicrobial agents to which these organisms are resistant, use of mechanically compromising devices such as intravascular lines and urinary catheters, and increasing numbers of seriously ill and debilitated patients in hospitals. For example, enterococcal superinfection was reported in 2.1% of more than 2000 patients treated with moxalactam, has occurred after the use of polymyxin aerosol for prevention of gram-negative pneumonia, and has been reported in patients receiving aztreonam, cephalosporins, ciprofloxacin, and vancomycin.[3, 16, 46, 47] Many of these patients not only had received an antibiotic to which enterococci are resistant but also had one or more of the mechanically compromising devices mentioned previously.

Enterococci have become even more important in the hospital setting because of the emergence of strains resistant to vancomycin. In the United States, vancomycin-resistant enterococci (VRE) were first a problem in the northeastern part of the country but have now spread into most states.[48] The Centers for Disease Control and Prevention, in the National Nosocomial Infections Surveillance survey, has found VRE in about 14% of intensive care unit isolates of enterococci. Many published outbreaks of VRE from the United States have reported finding a predominant strain or "clone," and one report found the same strain in three hospitals in two states, indicating spread of specific organisms between patients. Most of these reports have also identified some distinctly different strains, indicating that horizontal spread of the vancomycin resistance gene cluster(s) has also occurred. Of interest, although *E. faecalis* has traditionally outnumbered *E. faecium* among clinical isolates of enterococci by about 10:1, among VRE, isolates of *E. faecium* outnumber those of *E. faecalis* by 10:1.

A number of studies have indicated that prior receipt of vancomycin is a risk factor for acquisition of VRE. This and the clear evidence by genetic fingerprinting of patient-to-patient spread of VRE form the basis for recommendations by the Hospital Infection Control Practices Advisory Committee that appeared in a preliminary form in the Federal Register[49] and in medical journals.[50, 51] These recommendations focus on the two factors most often blamed for the general problem of antibiotic resistance, that is, antibiotic use and ease of spread of bacteria from person to person. One recommendation is that all hospitals develop a policy regarding the prudent use of vancomycin, including using oral vancomycin for antibiotic-associated colitis only if the patient has failed to respond to primary therapy with metronidazole, a recommendation previously made in the *Medical Letter on Drugs and Therapeutics*.[52] A long list of other circumstances in which the use of intravenous vancomycin would be considered inappropriate was also presented.

To control transmission of VRE within the hospital, the Hospital Infection Control Practices Advisory Committee recommended that a VRE-infected or -colonized patient be placed in a private room or with other culture-positive patients; that gloves be worn when entering a room with a VRE-positive patient; that gowns be worn if contact with environmental surfaces (which have frequently been contaminated with VRE) is anticipated; that gowns and gloves be removed, before exiting the room; and that hands be washed with an antiseptic soap (e.g., chlorhexidine). It should be kept in mind that enterococci are hardy organisms and may persist on environmental surfaces, so rooms previously inhabited by VRE culture-positive individuals should be thoroughly disinfected. A number of other recommendations were also made including possible fecal screening for VRE in high-risk areas, even in hospitals without prior known VRE.

An unexpected and interesting twist in the epidemiology of VRE is that in Europe, but apparently not in the United States, VRE have been found as part of the normal flora of animals and normal community volunteers.[53] This may be related to the frequent administration of *E. faecium* as well as the frequent administration of the glycopeptide antibiotic avoparcin to animals in Europe (but not the United States or Canada) as a food supplement for growth promotion.[53, 54]

Resistance

With the emergence of resistance to vancomycin, enterococci have displayed resistance to essentially every antimicrobial agent used to treat them, making them some of our most troublesome and difficult to treat pathogens. Resistance to antimicrobial agents can be divided into that which is an intrinsic or natural property of the species and that which is acquired (Table 194–3).

Intrinsic Resistance

Enterococci are intrinsically resistant or at least relatively resistant to β-lactams. The most effective agents in this group include penicillin, ampicillin, ureidopenicillins, and imipenem. Minimal inhibitory concentrations (MICs) of these agents typically range between 0.5 and 8 μg/mL for *E. faecalis* but are higher for *E. faecium*[3, 55]; occasional strains of *E. faecium* have quite high MICs.[3] Enterococci are less susceptible to ticarcillin and carbenicillin and are more resistant to the penicillinase-resistant semisynthetic penicillins, such as methicillin, and the cephalosporins, including the third-generation compounds.[3, 56, 57] In addition to the high MICs of β-lactams displayed by enterococci, these organisms often have high minimal bactericidal concentrations, greater than 100 μg/mL for β-lactams, and are thus a natural example of β-lactam–"tolerant" organisms.[3] As discussed later, the high minimal bactericidal concentrations presumably explain why endocarditis (a disease for which bactericidal activity is required for optimal results) caused by enterococci has an unacceptably low cure rate when treated with β-lactams alone.

Enterococci frequently show intrinsic low-level resistance to clindamycin and aminoglycosides.[3, 55, 56, 58] However, when strains with low-level aminoglycoside resistance (typically, MICs of 8 to 250 μg/mL) are treated with penicillin or ampicillin plus the aminoglycoside, there is markedly enhanced killing or synergism (which is described in more detail later). *E. faecium* has an additional problem not seen with *E. faecalis*. For these organisms, MICs of certain aminoglycosides, namely tobramycin, kanamycin, netilmicin, and sisomicin, are higher than for *E. faecalis* although still less than 2000 μg/mL, and combinations of penicillin or ampicillin plus these aminoglycosides fail to show synergism against *E. faecium*; this appears to be true of all members of this species.[55] These organisms normally produce an aminoglycoside-modifying enzyme (a 6′-acetyltransferase) that is an inherent species characteristic.[59]

Problems are also seen with enterococci and other antimicrobial agents. Currently available fluoroquinolones are only moderately active against enterococci, and true resistance has emerged in isolates, apparently as a result of mutations.[60] The value of trimethoprim-sulfamethoxazole for enterococcal infections is also debatable. This is related partially to the ability of enterococci to use both thymidine and thymine (unlike most other bacteria) and to use preformed dihydrofolate and tetrahydrofolate.[56, 61, 62] The MICs of trimethoprim-sulfamethoxazole are increased in media containing these compounds and in urine, which raises the question of in vivo efficacy.[63] Unless clinical data are published to indicate in vivo efficacy, this compound should be considered for therapy only as a last possible resort. The potential problem is illustrated by a report of two patients who developed enterococcal bacteremia during or shortly after therapy with trimethoprim-sulfamethoxazole for enterococcal urinary tract infections and by poor results in some animal models.[64–66]

TABLE 194–3 ■ Resistances Found in Enterococci

Intrinsic (naturally occurring) resistances
Aminoglycosides (low level)
β-Lactams, particularly semisynthetic penicillinase-resistant penicillins, cephalosporins, and aztreonam
Clindamycin (low level)
Acquired resistances
Aminoglycosides (high level; minimal inhibitory concentration usually greater than 2000 μg/mL)
Chloramphenicol
Erythromycin and high levels of clindamycin
Fluoroquinolones
Penicillins via penicillinase or low-affinity penicillin binding proteins
Rifampin
Tetracycline
Trimethoprim
Vancomycin

Acquired Resistance

In addition to the intrinsic resistance just described, enterococci may acquire resistance to antimicrobial agents. This can occur either by mutation in existing DNA or by the acquisition of new DNA, such as a plasmid or a transposon. Resistance to chloramphenicol, erythromycin, high levels of clindamycin, tetracycline, high levels of aminoglycosides, and vancomycin is common and often plasmid and/or transposon mediated,[59] whereas resistance to rifampin and fluoroquinolones arises via mutations.

Resistance to Aminoglycosides and β-Lactams

As mentioned previously, enterococci with low-level aminoglycoside resistance are usually killed by the combination of an agent that inhibits cell wall synthesis, such as vancomycin or penicillin, with an aminoglycoside. There is characteristically a greater than or equal to 2 $\log_{10}$ increase in killing versus the effect of the cell wall–active agent alone, even when the aminoglycoside is used in a subinhibitory concentration.[67] The first description of high-level resistance (MIC $\geq$ 2000 μg/mL) to aminoglycosides involved streptomycin. High-level resistance to streptomycin can occur because of a mutation leading to ribosomal resistance or via the acquisition of new DNA, which encodes an enzyme that adenylates streptomycin.[68] High-level resistance to kanamycin has also been recognized for some years; when not accompanied by high-level gentamicin resistance, this trait is due to the production of a 3′-phosphotransferase.[69] Although high-level resistance to kanamycin is per se of little clinical significance, the 3′-phosphotransferase also modifies amikacin. The MICs for amikacin may not be elevated (i.e., no high-level resistance), but the 3′-phosphotransferase eliminates the synergistic effect that would otherwise be seen with a cell wall–active agent plus amikacin.[69] High-level resistance to gentamicin is due to the presence of a bifunctional fusion protein that has both acetyltransferase and phosphotransferase activities.[16, 58, 70, 71] This enzyme confers high-level resistance and/or resistance to synergism for all commercially available aminoglycosides (gentamicin, sisomicin, netilmicin, tobramycin, kanamycin, and amikacin) except streptomycin. Some strains have acquired high-level resistance to all aminoglycosides by a combination of mechanisms; for such strains, there is no synergism with any aminoglycoside and thus no value in adding an aminoglycoside to a therapeutic regimen.[58, 71]

A β-lactamase–producing strain of *E. faecalis* was first reported in the early 1980s.[72] Currently, such strains are still apparently rare but have been reported from a variety of locations, including multiple isolates found in a pediatric unit in Boston.[73–75] The structural gene for the enterococcal β-lactamase enzyme is the same as the gene for the common β-lactamase of staphylococci, strongly suggesting spread from these organisms[76]; as expected, the enzyme is highly active against penicillin, ampicillin, and the ureidopenicillins. It is important to note that the amount of β-lactamase produced by enterococci is low, and thus the resistance of strains may not be detected by routine susceptibility testing.[73] At higher inocula and in animal model studies, the resistance of β-lactamase–producing strains to penicillin and ampicillin is obvious.[77] Although the enzyme is not active against the semisynthetic penicillinase-resistant penicillins or cephalosporins, these agents have little intrinsic activity against enterococci and are not useful for such strains. Imipenem and vancomycin remain active against β-lactamase–producing *E. faecalis*, but, as with other cell wall–active agents, are not bactericidal.[73, 78]

In addition to β-lactamase production as a mechanism of penicillin resistance, many enterococci, particularly *E. faecium*, are resistant to penicillin by a nonpenicillinase mechanism. *E. faecium* are typically more resistant than *E. faecalis* to penicillins, and this appears to be related to the fact that their cell wall synthesis enzymes are less inhibitable by (i.e., have lower affinity for) penicillin. Higher levels of penicillin resistance have been reported to arise from either increased production of these low-affinity cell wall synthesis enzymes (referred to as penicillin binding proteins) or a further reduction in the affinity of these penicillin binding proteins for penicillin.

Resistance to Vancomycin

The latest and most disturbing resistance to appear in enterococci is resistance to vancomycin, which was first reported in 1988.[79, 80] In at least some instances, the resistance has been found to be plasmid and transposon mediated and has been transferable by conjugation to other species, including *Staphylococcus aureus*.[81] The mechanism of vancomycin resistance has been best defined for the VanA phenotype, which is associated with the *vanA* gene cluster. This cluster has been shown to be part of a transposon named Tn*1546*. On the basis of polymerase chain reaction and hybridization data, this transposon or related elements have a wide geographic distribution and appear to account for much of the VanA type resistance. Two genes on this transposon encode proteins associated with transposition function, and at least six of the other seven genes (*vanS, vanR, vanA, vanH, vanX, vanY,* and *vanZ*) encode proteins involved with the vancomycin resistance phenotype. The genes *vanR* and *vanS* encode two proteins that function as part of a two-component regulatory system that somehow senses (VanS, the sensor) the presence (or the effect) of vancomycin and then regulates (VanR, the response regulator) the response of other genes of this cluster. VanH (encoded by *vanH*) is a dehydrogenase that generates D-lactate; VanA (encoded by *vanA*) is a ligase that ligates D-alanine with D-lactate to form the depsipeptide, D-alanine-D-lactate; VanX is a dipeptidase that cleaves the dipeptide D-alanine-D-alanine; VanY is a carboxypeptidase that can cleave the terminal unit (e.g., D-alanine or D-lactate) from the pentapeptide part of cell wall precursors; and VanZ is of unknown function.

To understand the mechanism of resistance to vancomycin, it is necessary to understand how vancomycin inhibits cell wall synthesis. It does this by binding to the terminal two amino acids (D-alanine-D-alanine) of *N*-acetylmuramyl-*N*-acetylglucosamine pentapeptide, which is a precursor unit for cell wall peptidoglycan synthesis. Once vancomycin binds to this pentapeptide-containing precursor, it blocks the rest of cell wall peptidoglycan synthesis and thus leads to inhibition of cell growth. Resistance to vancomycin associated with the VanA phenotype and, by analogy, the VanB phenotype occurs when the cell wall pentapeptide precursor ends in something to which vancomycin cannot bind. This is accomplished through a complex system of steps that involves the generation of a new peptidoglycan pentadepsipeptide precursor, as well as the destruction of the cell's normal pentapeptide-containing precursor. Vancomycin resistance is normally inducible; that is, the presence of vancomycin leads to the synthesis of the resistance-associated proteins. As just mentioned, VanH generates D-lactate, which is the substrate for the ligase, VanA. After generation, by VanA, of D-alanine-D-lactate, the cell's own enzymes apparently add D-alanine-D-lactate to the peptidoglycan precursor tripeptide, resulting in the pentadepsipeptide precursor containing a terminal D-alanine-D-lactate. The action of VanX, the dipeptidase, results in cleavage of the normally present D-alanine-D-alanine, thus preventing the formation of normal, vancomycin-susceptible pentapeptide precursor. Should any D-alanine-D-alanine escape cleavage and end up in cell wall subunits, the carboxypeptidase VanY can cleave the terminal D-alanine, resulting in a tetrapeptide chain to which vancomycin does not bind. The purpose of the remaining gene, *vanZ*, in the *van* cluster is unknown.

Although the VanB phenotype has been less well studied, there are homologs of each of the genes of the *vanA* cluster and presumably the mechanism of resistance is similar. Cell wall precursor units of strains expressing the VanB phenotype also end in D-alanine-D-lactate.

The VanC phenotype is a naturally occurring trait of *Enterococcus gallinarum* and *Enterococcus casseliflavus* and confers low to moderate levels of resistance (MICs $\leq$ 32 μg/mL), although most strains have MICs of 8 μg/mL or less. Two genes, *vanC-1* and *vanC-2*, are found in *E. gallinarum* and *E. casseliflavus*, respectively. Cell wall peptidoglycan of *E. gallinarum* has been shown to end in D-alanine-D-serine, which appears to have lower affinity for vancomycin than does D-alanine-D-alanine.

In addition to the remarkable complexity of the vancomycin resistance mechanism, two additional interesting phenomena related to this resistance are vancomycin dependence and penicillin-vancomycin synergy. Enterococci dependent on vancomycin for growth have been isolated from patients who have been treated with vancomycin. In cases described, cultures were negative but patients were strongly suspected of being infected. Organisms were eventually recovered either by using vancomycin-containing media or by noting growth around vancomycin disks. It appears that these vancomycin-dependent cells turned off their normal production of D-alanine-D-alanine, which, in the presence of vancomycin, was being destroyed by VanX and/or VanY. In the presence of vancomycin, the cells make D-alanine-D-lactate, and D-alanine-D-alanine is unnecessary for survival. However, when cells are removed from vancomycin, no VanA or VanB ligase is made, so no D-alanine-D-lactate is made. If neither D-alanine-D-alanine nor D-alanine-D-lactate is made, the cell cannot survive. Revertants can survive independent of vancomycin by either turning back on the production of its normal D-alanine-D-alanine ligase (to make once again the dipeptide D-alanine-D-alanine) or by mutating to constitutive production of the VanA or VanB ligase, to make D-alanine-D-lactate independent of the presence of vancomycin.

The phenomenon of penicillin-vancomycin synergy refers to the fact that some strains of VRE, in the presence of vancomycin, have a lower MIC of penicillin. The proposed mechanism for this enhanced activity is that not all of the cell wall synthesis enzymes are able to use D-alanine-D-lactate pentadepsipeptide precursor to make cell wall and that when this precursor is present and D-alanine-D-alanine–ending pentapeptide is not, the cell must shift to enzymes that can use D-alanine-D-lactate–containing precursor to survive. If these enzymes are more susceptible to inhibition by penicillin, the MIC of penicillin is decreased in the presence of vancomycin. Unfortunately, many VRE do not display this phenomenon and even for those that do, mutants arise frequently, in vitro as well as in animal models, that no longer show this beneficial interaction, so the clinical usefulness of this phenomenon appears to be limited.

Susceptibility Testing

In most instances, susceptibility of enterococci to penicillin, ampicillin, and vancomycin should be determined; for urinary isolates, a fluoroquinolone and/or nitrofurantoin may be considered. Because routine testing may not detect β-lactamase–producing strains, the possible presence of this enzyme should be determined with nitrocefin for isolates from patients with serious enterococcal infections; nitrocefin is a chromogenic cephalosporin that changes color when hydrolyzed by penicillinase.[72, 82, 83] Isolates from patients with endocarditis and possibly those with other serious infections, including meningitis, should also be tested for the presence of high-level aminoglycoside resistance. This resistance can be detected by several methods, including a plate screening method with plates containing streptomycin at 2000 μg/mL or gentamicin at 500 μg/mL, a single-concentration broth test with 1000 μg/mL streptomycin or 500 μg/mL gentamicin (it should be noted that discrepancies have arisen with some commercial microdilution susceptibility methods), or use of disks impregnated with a high concentration of aminoglycosides (120 mg of gentamicin and 300 mg of streptomycin).[82, 83] Some isolates with low to moderate levels of vancomycin resistance have been missed by routine tests,[84, 85] which led to revised criteria for interpretation of disk diffusion results (from ≥12 mm as defining susceptible to ≥17 mm)[82] and to the recommendation of an agar screening test employing brain-heart infusion agar with 6 μg/mL vancomycin.[83]

Management of Enterococcal Infection

Formerly, most enterococcal soft tissue and urinary tract infections could be treated with single-drug therapy such as penicillin, ampicillin, or vancomycin. Although the MICs of penicillin are approximately twice those of ampicillin, adequate concentrations are normally achieved. Ureidopenicillins such as piperacillin and mezlocillin also appear adequate, but these drugs have a broader spectrum of activity than is needed, unless mixed infection is suspected. Ticarcillin and carbenicillin are only moderately active in vitro and probably have little role in therapy for enterococcal infections. For the occasional isolates of *E. faecalis* that produce penicillinase, vancomycin, imipenem, ampicillin-sulbactam, and amoxicillin-clavulanate all appear active.[72, 86] The fluoroquinolones have been successful in enterococcal urinary tract infections, but susceptibility is marginal. Rifampin, like other agents, lacks bactericidal activity against enterococci, does not appear to enhance the efficacy of other agents, and is associated with rapid emergence of resistant strains.[87]

Enterococcal endocarditis, and probably meningitis and other serious enterococcal infections, should be treated with a combination of a cell wall–active agent such as penicillin or vancomycin plus an aminoglycoside to which the strain is not highly resistant.[88] The rationale for this therapy dates back to the early antibacterial chemotherapeutic era, when it was observed that therapy with penicillin alone was associated with an unacceptably high relapse rate and that the empirical combination of streptomycin with penicillin was much more likely to produce cure.[3] Unfortunately, high-level resistance to streptomycin has become quite common, and high-level resistance to gentamicin (and all other aminoglycosides) is increasing.[16, 58, 71] Optimal therapy for patients with serious infections caused by strains with high-level resistance to all aminoglycosides is unknown, but it is clear that adding an aminoglycoside to the cell wall–active agent adds nothing to the therapy except for toxicity.[58, 89] No current clinical data suggest that any single-drug regimen reliably produces cure. However, animal model studies with one strain showed that continuous infusion ampicillin was more effective than intermittent ampicillin in therapy for enterococcal endocarditis caused by a single strain that was highly resistant to gentamicin.[89]

For infections caused by VRE, susceptibility to ampicillin should be determined. Most *E. faecalis* organisms are susceptible to ampicillin and a number of *E. faecium* organisms, although reported as resistant to ampicillin, may be sufficiently inhibited by ampicillin to warrant its use; clinical data are lacking, but MICs of 16 to 32 μg/mL ampicillin are readily exceeded by high-dose parenteral ampicillin therapy. For vancomycin-resistant *E. faecium* with high-level resistance to ampicillin, therapy is even more problematic. Nitrofurantoin may be effective for lower urinary tract infections caused by nitrofurantoin-susceptible organisms. Chloramphenicol and tetracycline have been active in vitro against some strains and have been used in some infected patients; clinical efficacy, however, has been difficult to evaluate because of the presence of other variables (e.g., resolution of neutropenia). Regimens that have shown some promise in vitro and/or in animal models include vancomycin plus ampicillin plus gentamicin (for *E. faecium* that lack high-level resistance to gentamicin and for which there is a reduction in the MIC of ampicillin in the presence of vancomycin), ciprofloxacin plus rifampin plus gentamicin (for organisms susceptible to the first two drugs and lacking high-level gentamicin resistance), tetracycline plus novobiocin, and ciprofloxacin plus novobiocin. Experimental agents that offer some promise include newer fluoroquinolones with enhanced gram-positive activity (clinafloxacin, sparfloxacin, and trovafloxacin), the glycopeptide teicoplanin with or without an aminoglycoside (for teicoplanin-susceptible, VanB-type strains), and the pristinamycin combination RP 59500; the last two agents have been used on a compassionate basis and are in clinical trials for infections caused by VRE.

Conclusion

The enterococcus is an old pathogen with a new classification and a newly recognized role as a nosocomially transmitted pathogen. Although the organism is normally of relatively low virulence, its remarkable antibiotic resistance more than compensates. The addition of high-level aminoglycoside resistance, β-lactamase, and vancomycin resistance to the enterococcal armamentarium indicates that enterococci will cause therapeutic problems for years to come.

References

1. Thiercelin ME: Sur un diplocoque saprophyte de l'intestin susceptible de devenir pathogène. C R Seances Soc Biol Paris 5:269, 1899.
2. Andrewes FW, Horder TJ: A study of the streptococci pathogenic for man. Lancet 2:708, 1906.
3. Murray BE: The life and times of the enterococcus. Clin Microbiol Rev 3:46, 1990.
4. Farrow JAE, Jones D, Phillips BA, Collins MD: Taxonomic studies on some group D streptococci. J Gen Microbiol 129:1423, 1983.
5. Schleifer KH, Kilpper-Balz R: Transfer of *Streptococcus faecalis* and *Streptococcus faecium* to the genus *Enterococcus* nom. rev. as *Enterococcus faecalis* comb. nov. and *Enterococcus faecium* comb. nov. Int J Syst Bacteriol 34:31, 1984.
6. Facklam RR, Hollis D, Collins MD: Identification of gram-positive coccal and coccobacillary vancomycin-resistant bacteria. J Clin Microbiol 27:724, 1989.
7. Collins MD, Facklam RR, Farrow JAE, Williamson R: *Enterococcus raffinosus* sp. nov., *Enterococcus solitarius* sp. nov. and *Enterococcus pseudoavium* sp. nov. FEMS Microbiol Lett 57:283, 1989.
8. Facklam RR, Collins MD: Identification of *Enterococcus* species isolated from human infections by a conventional test scheme. J Clin Microbiol 27:731, 1989.
9. Benno Y, Suzuki K, Suzuki K, et al: Comparison of the fecal microflora in rural Japanese and urban Canadians. Microbiol Immunol 30:521, 1986.
10. Facklam RR, Sahm DA: *Enterococcus*. *In* Murray PR. Baron EJ, Pfaller MA, et al (eds): Manual of Clinical Microbiology, ed 6. Washington, DC, American Society for Microbiology, 1995, pp 308–314.
11. Mead GC: Streptococci in the intestinal flora of man and other non-ruminant animals. *In* Skinner FA, Quesnel LB (eds): Streptococci. London, Academic Press, 1978, pp 245–261.
12. Noble CJ: Carriage of group D streptococci in the human bowel. J Clin Pathol 31:1182, 1978.
13. Beargie R, Lynd P, Tucker E, Duhring J: Perinatal infection and vaginal flora. Am J Obstet Gynecol 122:31, 1975.
14. Kurrie E, Bhaduri S, Krieger D, et al: Risk factors for infections of the oropharynx and the respiratory tract in patients with acute leukemia. J Infect Dis 144:128, 1981.
15. Kuhnen E, Richter F, Richter K, Andries L: Establishment of a typing system for group D streptococci. Zentralbl Bakteriol Mikrobiol Hyg A 267:322, 1988.
16. Zervos MJ, Kauffman CA, Therasse PM, et al: Nosocomial infection by gentamicin-resistant *Streptococcus faecalis*: An epidemiologic study. Ann Intern Med 106:687, 1987.
17. Chow JW, Kuritza A, Shlaes DM, et al: Clonal spread of vancomycin-resistant *Enterococcus faecium* between patients in three hospitals in two states. J Clin Microbiol 31:1609, 1993.
18. Handwerger S, Raucher B, Altarac D, et al: Nosocomial outbreak due to *Enterococcus faecium* highly resistant to vancomycin, penicillin and gentamicin. Clin Infect Dis 16:750, 1993.
19. Murray BE, Singh KV, Markowitz SM, et al: Evidence for clonal spread of a single strain of β-lactamase–producing *Enterococcus faecalis* to six hospitals in five states. J Infect Dis 163:780, 1991.
20. Wilson WR, Wilkowske CJ, Wright AJ, et al: Treatment of streptomycin-susceptible and streptomycin-resistant enterococcal endocarditis. Ann Intern Med 100:816, 1984.
21. Koenig MG, Kaye D: Enterococcal endocarditis: Report of nineteen cases with long-term follow-up data. N Engl J Med 264:257, 1961.
22. Mandell GL, Kaye D, Levison ME, Hook EW: Enterococcal endocarditis: An analysis of 38 patients observed at the New York Hospital–Cornell Medical Center. Arch Intern Med 125:258, 1970.
23. Reiner NE, Gopalakrishna KV, Lerner PI: Enterococcal endocarditis in heroin addicts. JAMA 235:1861, 1976.
24. Maki DG, Agger WA: Enterococcal bacteremia: Clinical features, the risk of endocarditis, and management. Medicine (Baltimore) 67:248, 1988.
25. Gullberg RM, Homann SR, Phair JP: Enterococcal bacteremia: Analysis of 75 episodes. Rev Infect Dis 11:74, 1989.
26. Gross PA, Harkavy LM, Barden GE, Flower MF: The epidemiology of nosocomial enterococcal urinary tract infection. Am J Med Sci 272:75, 1976.
27. Horan TC, White JW, Jarvis WR, et al: Nosocomial infection surveillance, 1984. MMWR CDC Surveill Summ 35:17SS, 1986.
28. Ledger WJ, Norman M, Gee C, Lewis W: Bacteremia on an obstretric-gynecologic service. Am J Obstet Gynecol 121:205, 1975.
29. Odendaal H, DeKock M: Acute salpingitis in pregnancy. S Afr Med J 47:21, 1973.
30. Gorensek MJ, Lebel MH, Nelson JD: Peritonitis in children with nephrotic syndrome. Pediatrics 81:849, 1988.
31. Leigh DA: Peritoneal infections in patients on long-term peritoneal dialysis before and after human cadaveric renal transplantation. J Clin Pathol 22:539, 1969.
32. Dougherty SH, Flahr AB, Simmons RL: Breakthrough enterococcal septicemia in surgical patients. 19 cases and a review of the literature. Arch Surg 118:232, 1983.
33. Garrison RN, Fry DE, Berberich S, Polk HC: Enterococcal bacteremia: Clinical implications and determinants of death. Ann Surg 196:43, 1982.
34. Zervos MJ, Bacon AE, Patterson JE, et al: Enterococcal superinfection in patients treated with ciprofloxacin. J Antimicrob Chemother 21:113, 1988.
35. Bartlett JG, Onderdonk AB, Louis T, et al: A review: Lessons from an animal model of intra-abdominal sepsis. Arch Surg 113:850, 1978.
36. Canadian Metronidazole Study Group: Prospective, randomized comparison of metronidazole and clindamycin, each with gentamicin, for the treatment of serious intraabdominal infection. Surgery 93:221, 1983.
37. Hemsell DW, Wendel GD, Gall SA, et al: Multicenter comparison of cefotetan and cefoxitin in the treatment of acute obstetric and gynecologic infections. Am J Obstet Gynecol 158:722, 1988.
38. Stone HH, Morris ES, Geheber CE, et al: Clinical comparison of cefotaxime with gentamicin plus clindamycin in the treatment of peritonitis and other soft tissue infections. Rev Infect Dis 4(Suppl):439, 1982.
39. Dougherty SH: Role of enterococcus in intraabdominal sepsis. Am J Surg 148:308, 1984.
40. Siegel JD, McCracken GH Jr: Group D streptococcal infections. J Pediatr 93:542, 1978.
41. Luginbuhl LM, Rotbart HA, Facklam RR, et al: Neonatal enterococcal sepsis: Case-control study and description of an outbreak. Pediatr Infect Dis 6:1022, 1987.
42. Coudron PE, Mayhall CG, Facklam RR, et al: *Streptococcus faecium* outbreak in a neonatal intensive care unit. J Clin Microbiol 20:1044, 1984.
43. Bayer AS, Seidel JS, Yoshikawa TT, et al: Group D enterococcal meningitis: Clinical and therapeutic considerations with report of three cases and review of the literature. Arch Intern Med 136:883, 1976.
44. Schoenbaum SC, Gardner P, Shillito J: Infections of cerebrospinal fluid shunts: Epidemiology, clinical manifestations, and therapy. J Infect Dis 131:543, 1975.
45. Centers for Disease Control: Nosocomial enterococci resistant to vancomycin—United States 1989–1993. MMWR Morbid Mortal Wkly Rep 42:597, 1993.
46. Moellering RC Jr: Enterococcal infections in patients treated with moxalactam. Rev Infect Dis 4:S708, 1982.
47. Chandrasekar PH, Smith BR, LeFrock JL, Carr B: Enterococcal superinfection and colonization with aztreonam therapy. Antimicrob Agents Chemother 26:280, 1984.

48. Jones RN, Sader HS, Erwin ME, et al: Emerging multiply resistant enterococci among clinical isolates. I. Prevalence data from 97 medical center surveillance study in the United States. Diagn Microbiol Infect Dis 21:85, 1995.
49. Centers for Disease Control and Prevention: Preventing the spread of vancomycin resistance—Report from the Hospital Infection Control Practices Advisory Committee. Fed Regist 59:25757, 1994.
50. Centers for Disease Control and Prevention: Recommendations for preventing the spread of vancomycin resistance. Infect Control Hosp Epidemiol 16:105, 1995.
51. Shay DK, Goldmann DA, Jarvis WR: Reducing the spread of antimicrobial-resistant microorganisms. Control of vancomycin-resistant enterococci. Pediatr Clin North Am 42:703, 1995.
52. The choice of antibacterial drugs. Med Lett Drugs Ther 36:53, 1994.
53. Murray BE: Editorial response: What can we do about vancomycin-resistant enterococci? Clin Infect Dis 20:1134, 1995.
54. Klare I, Heier H, Claus H, et al: *vanA*-mediated high-level glycopeptide resistance in *Enterococcus faecium* from animal husbandry. FEMS Microbiol Lett 125:165, 1995.
55. Moellering RC Jr, Korzeniowski OM, Sande MA, Wennersten CB: Species-specific resistance to antimicrobial synergism in *Streptococcus faecium* and *Streptococcus faecalis*. J Infect Dis 140:203, 1979.
56. Tofte RW, Solliday J, Crossley KB: Susceptibilities of enterococci to twelve antibiotics. Antimicrob Agents Chemother 25:532, 1984.
57. Fass RJ: In vitro activities of β-lactam and aminoglycoside antibiotics: A comparative study of 20 parenterally administered drugs. Arch Intern Med 140:766, 1988.
58. Mederski-Samoraj BD, Murray BE: High-level resistance to gentamicin in clinical isolates of enterococci. J Infect Dis 147:751, 1983.
59. Costa Y, Galimand M, Leclercq R, et al: Characterization of the chromosomal *aac(6')-Ii* gene specific for *Enterococcus faecium*. Antimicrob Agents Chemother 37:1896, 1993.
60. Korten V, Huang WM, Murray BE: Analysis by PCR and direct DNA sequencing of *gyrA* mutations associated with fluoroquinolone resistance in *Enterococcus faecalis*. Antimicrob Agents Chemother 38:2091, 1994.
61. Hamilton-Miller JMT: Reversal of activity of trimethoprim against gram-positive cocci by thymidine, thymine and "folates." J Antimicrob Chemother 22:35, 1988.
62. Crider SR, Colby SD: Susceptibility of enterococci to trimethoprim and trimethoprim-sulfamethoxazole. Antimicrob Agents Chemother 27:71, 1985.
63. Zervos MJ, Schaberg DS: Reversal of the in vitro susceptibility of enterococci to trimethoprim-sulfamethoxazole by folinic acid. Antimicrob Agents Chemother 28:446, 1985.
64. Chenoweth CE, Robinson KA, Schaberg DR: Efficacy of ampicillin versus trimethoprim-sulfamethoxazole in a mouse model of lethal enterococcal peritonitis. Antimicrob Agents Chemother 34:1800, 1990.
65. Goodhart GL: In vivo v in vitro susceptibility of enterococcus to trimethoprim-sulfamethoxazole. A pitfall. JAMA 252:2748, 1984.
66. Grayson ML, Thauvin-Eliopoulos C, Eliopoulos GM, et al: Failure of trimethoprim-sulfamethoxazole therapy in experimental enterococcal endocarditis. Antimicrob Agents Chemother 34:1792, 1990.
67. Calderwood SA, Wennersten C, Moellering RC Jr, et al: Resistance to six aminoglycoside aminocyclitol antibiotics among enterococci: Prevalence, evolution, and relationship to synergism with penicillin. Antimicrob Agents Chemother 12:401, 1977.
68. Eliopoulos GM, Farber BF, Murray BE, et al: Ribosomal resistance of clinical enterococcal isolates to streptomycin. Antimicrob Agents Chemother 25:398, 1984.
69. Krogstad DJ, Korfhagen TR, Moellering RC Jr, et al: Aminoglycoside-inactivating enzymes in clinical isolates of *Streptococcus faecalis*: An explanation for antibiotic synergism. J Clin Invest 62:480, 1978.
70. Horodniceanu T, Bougueleret T, El-Solh N, et al: High-level, plasmid-borne resistance to gentamicin in *Streptococcus faecalis* subsp. *zymogenes*. Antimicrob Agents Chemother 16:686, 1979.
71. Murray BE, Tsao J, Panida J: Enterococci from Bangkok, Thailand, with high-level resistance to currently available aminoglycosides. Antimicrob Agents Chemother 23:799, 1983.
72. Murray BE, Mederski-Samoraj B: Transferable β-lactamase: A new mechanism for in vitro penicillin resistance in *Streptococcus faecalis*. J Clin Invest 72:1168, 1983.
73. Murray BE, Church DA, Wanger A, et al: Comparison of two β-lactamase–producing strains of *Streptococcus faecalis*. Antimicrob Agents Chemother 30:861, 1986.
74. Patterson JE, Masecar BL, Zervos MJ: Characterization and comparison of two penicillinase producing strains of *Streptococcus (Enterococcus) faecalis*. Antimicrob Agents Chemother 32:122, 1988.
75. Rhinehart E, Smith NE, Wennersten C, et al: Rapid dissemination of β-lactamase–producing, aminoglycoside-resistant *Enterococcus faecalis* among patients and staff on an infant-toddler surgical ward. N Engl J Med 323:1814, 1990.
76. Zscheck K, Murray BE: Nucleotide sequence of the β-lactamase gene from *Enterococcus faecalis* HH22 and its similarity to staphylococcal β-lactamase genes. Antimicrob Agents Chemother 35:1736, 1991.
77. Ingerman M, Pitsakis PG, Rosenberg A, et al: β-Lactamase production in experimental endocarditis due to aminoglycoside-resistant *Streptococcus faecalis*. J Infect Dis 155:1226, 1987.
78. Scheld WM, Keeley JM: Imipenem therapy of experimental *Staphylococcus aureus* and *Streptococcus faecalis* endocarditis. J Antimicrob Chemother 12(Suppl D):65, 1983.
79. Leclercq R, Deriot E, Duval J, Courvalin P: Plasmid-mediated resistance to vancomycin and teicoplanin in *Enterococcus faecium*. N Engl J Med 319:157, 1988.
80. Uttley AHC, Collins CH, Naidoo J, George RC: Vancomycin-resistant enterococci. Lancet 1:57, 1988.
81. Noble WD, Virani Z, Cree RGA: Co-transfer of vancomycin and other resistance genes from *Enterococcus faecalis* NCTC 12201 to *Staphylococcus aureus*. FEMS Microbiol Lett 93:195, 1992.
82. National Committee for Clinical Laboratory Standards: Performance Standards for Antimicrobial Disk Susceptibility Tests, ed 5, Approved Standard. Villanova, PA, National Committee for Clinical Laboratory Standards, 1993. NCCLS document M2-A5.
83. National Committee for Clinical Laboratory Standards: Methods for Dilution Antimicrobial Susceptibility Tests for Bacteria That Grow Aerobically, ed 3, Approved Standard. Villanova, PA, National Committee for Clinical Laboratory Standards, 1993. NCCLS document M7-A3.
84. Swenson JM, Hill BC, Thornsberry C: Problems with the disk diffusion test for detection of vancomycin resistance in enterococci. J Clin Microbiol 27:2140, 1989.
85. Sahm DF, Olsen L: In vitro detection of enterococcal vancomycin resistance. Antimicrob Agents Chemother 34:1846, 1990.
86. Murray BE, Mederski-Samoraj B, Foster SK, et al: In vitro studies of plasmid-mediated penicillinase from *Streptococcus faecalis* suggest a staphylococcal origin. J Clin Invest 77:289, 1986.
87. Moellering RC Jr, Wennersten CB: Therapeutic potential of rifampin in enterococcal infections. Rev Infect Dis 5(Suppl):528, 1983.
88. Bisno AL, Dismukes WE, Durack DT, et al: Antimicrobial treatment of infective endocarditis due to viridans streptococci, enterococci, and staphylococci. JAMA 261:1471, 1989.
89. Thauvin C, Eliopoulos GM, Willey S, et al: Continuous-infusion ampicillin therapy of enterococcal endocardidtis in rats. Antimicrob Agents Chemother 31:139, 1987.
90. Navarro F, Courvalin P: Analysis of genes encoding D-alanine-D-alanine ligase–related enzymes in *Enterococcus casseliflavus* and *Enterococcus flavescens*. Antimicrob Agents Chemother 38:1788, 1994.
91. Woodford N, Morrison D, Johnson AP, et al: Application of DNA probes for rRNA and VanA genes to investigation of a nosocomial cluster of vancomycin-resistant enterococci. J Clin Microbiol 31:653, 1993.

195

Group B *Streptococcus*

Michael R. Wessels
Dennis L. Kasper

History

The bacterial species now known as *Streptococcus agalactiae*, or group B *Streptococcus*, was recognized in the dairy industry for many years as an important cause of mastitis in cows. Definition of the organism as distinct from other hemolytic streptococci, however, did not come until the 1930s, when Rebecca Lancefield developed a classification scheme for streptococci based on serologic reactions of specific antisera with hot hydrochloric acid extracts of the organisms. On the basis of antigenic differences among strains, Lancefield[1] distinguished several groups of streptococci as distinct from *Streptococcus pyogenes*. The strains she classified as belonging to group B came from bovine sources, although within a few years group B streptococci were also isolated from the vaginas of postpartum women.[2] Although vaginal colonization appeared, in most women, not to be associated with clinical disease, occasional cases of postpartum fever were noted, and in 1938 Fry[3] reported three cases of fatal postpartum sepsis related to group B *Streptococcus*, demonstrating the potential of the organism to cause invasive disease in humans. Multiple subsequent reports documented the role of group B streptococci as occasional causes of serious infections in adults, most commonly postpartum sepsis, and also as a cause of neonatal bacteremia and meningitis. Beginning in the early 1960s, reports appeared implicating group B *Streptococcus* as a more important cause of neonatal septicemia than had been appreciated previously.[4, 5] By the early 1970s, group B *Streptococcus* had been clearly established as a major cause of neonatal sepsis and meningitis; it continues to be the leading cause of serious bacterial infection among neonates in the United States.

Characteristics of the Pathogen

When cultured on sheep blood agar, group B streptococci form glistening gray-white colonies surrounded by a narrow zone of beta hemolysis. The colonies of group B *Streptococcus* are usually somewhat larger, more definitely gray in color, and surrounded by a narrower hemolytic zone than those of group A *Streptococcus*. Although definitive identification of a strain as group B *Streptococcus* is based on serologic reaction with specific antiserum, clinical laboratory identification can be done quite reliably on the basis of biochemical reactions. Helpful tests for presumptive identification of group B *Streptococcus* include hydrolysis of sodium hippurate (99% of strains are positive),[6] bile-esculin hydrolysis (99% to 100% of strains are negative),[6] bacitracin sensitivity (>90% of strains are resistant),[6, 7] and production of CAMP factor (>98% of strains are positive). CAMP factor, named after the authors of its description,[8] is a product of group B streptococci that produces synergistic hemolysis on blood agar with the β-lysin of *Staphylococcus aureus*. A reasonable combination of tests for presumptive identification of streptococci as belonging to group B includes bacitracin sensitivity, CAMP factor production, and bile-esculin hydrolysis.[9] Definitive identification of a strain as group B *Streptococcus* is made serologically, using group-specific antiserum. Commercially available kits utilizing latex agglutination or staphylococcal coagglutination compare favorably with the standard Lancefield microprecipitin method for identification of the organisms in culture.

Surface Antigens

In Lancefield's early studies,[1] the acid-extractable antigen that gave a positive precipitin reaction with group B–specific antiserum was found to be a complex carbohydrate associated with the cell wall of the organisms. Subsequent studies have shown the common group B antigen to be a complex polysaccharide of rhamnose, *N*-acetylglucosamine, and glycerol phosphate.[10–12] The group B carbohydrate molecule appears to be anchored in the cell wall, with a tetraantennary branching structure extending outward from the cell surface, each branch terminating in an $\alpha(1\rightarrow2)$-linked rhamnose trisaccharide.[13] Lancefield[14, 15] also found that strains of group B *Streptococcus* could be divided into serotypes based on antigenic differences in a carbohydrate antigen distinct from the group B carbohydrate, the type-specific antigen. The type-specific antigen has been shown to represent the polysaccharide capsule of the organisms[16] (Figure 195–1). The capsular polysaccharides from the four serotypes described by Lancefield (Ia, Ib, II, and III) have been isolated and their

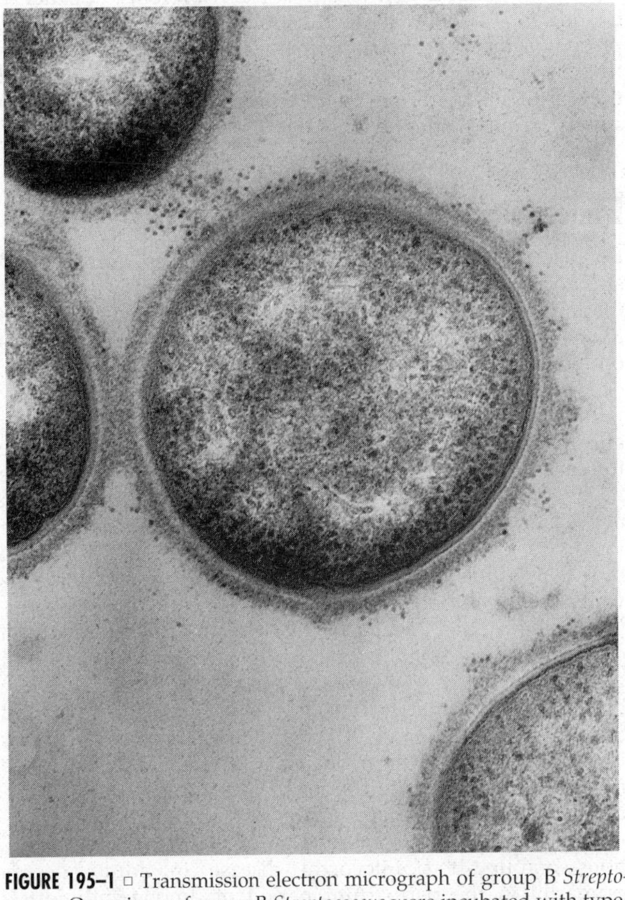

FIGURE 195–1 □ Transmission electron micrograph of group B *Streptococcus*. Organisms of group B *Streptococcus* were incubated with type-specific antiserum followed by ferritin-labeled anti–immunoglobulin G. An irregular layer of capsular polysaccharide is visible exterior to the cell wall, decorated by ferritin particles. (Original magnification, × 55,000.)

structures determined.[17–19] Additional capsular types IV, V, VI, VII, and VIII (also called JM9) were subsequently identified. Each of the group B *Streptococcus* capsular polysaccharides is a high-molecular-weight (100,000 to 500,000) polymer made up of a linear backbone with short side chains. The type Ia, Ib, II, III, IV, and V polysaccharides contain galactose, glucose, *N*-acetylglucosamine, and *N*-acetylneuraminic acid (sialic acid) as exclusive sugars. The component sugars of the capsular polysaccharides are similar, with minor variations: types VI, VII, and VIII lack *N*-acetylglucosamine and type VIII contains rhamnose.[20–25] Although types IV, VI, VII, and VIII appear to be uncommon among human disease isolates in the United States, data suggest that type V is relatively frequent among isolates associated with infant infections and may be the predominant serotype in adult disease.[26, 27]

Group B streptococci also express cell surface protein antigens. A serologically defined protein antigen, originally called the Ibc antigen, is present on all strains of capsular type Ib and many strains of capsular type Ia (>90%), type II (50%), and type IV (>90%) and is seen infrequently on type III strains (<5%).[28–30] According to a proposed convention for classification of group B *Streptococcus* strains, the presence of the Ibc antigen (now termed C protein) is indicated by /C after the capsular type designation, for example, Ia/C (formerly termed Ic).[31] At least two distinct types of C proteins have been defined, the alpha and beta C proteins, one or both of which may be present on an individual strain. Other protein antigens, termed R and X, have been identified on some strains of various capsular types, but their functional importance has not been defined. A protein termed Rib, which may be identical to one of the R proteins, appears to be present on many type III strains.[32] Evidence has been presented that the two C proteins and Rib can elicit protective antibodies in animals, suggesting that one or more of these proteins might be useful as a component of a vaccine against group B streptococci.[28, 29, 32–34]

Epidemiology

Because there is no uniform reporting system for group B streptococcal infections, precise incidence data for large populations are not available. Neonatal infections with group B *Streptococcus* have been divided into two clinical syndromes on the basis of time of onset after delivery: early-onset sepsis, occurring within the first 5 to 7 days of life and usually within the first 24 hours; and late-onset sepsis, occurring after the first week but rarely after 3 months. The attack rate for early-onset disease was estimated to be 1.4 per 1000 live births, on the basis of 1990 incidence data from a multistate active surveillance system[35]; the same study estimated the incidence of late-onset disease at 0.3 to 0.4 per 1000 live births. A population-based study of metropolitan Atlanta, as well as several smaller hospital-based surveys, reported similar or slightly higher rates of neonatal group B streptococcal disease.[36–38] The combined incidence (early and late onset) of group B *Streptococcus* neonatal sepsis is about 2 per 1000 live births or approximately 10,000 cases per year in the United States. Although the rate of group B *Streptococcus* infection is lower in adults than in neonates, a number of reports have indicated that serious infections in adults may be more common than previously appreciated, accounting for approximately one half of all invasive group B streptococcal infections. Group B streptococcal disease in adults occurs primarily in the peripartum period or among individuals with underlying chronic conditions, particularly diabetes mellitus or a malignancy.[35, 39, 40]

Asymptomatic colonization of the vagina and lower gastrointestinal tract occurs commonly and of the upper respiratory tract occasionally. Surveys of pregnant and nonpregnant women have indicated carriage rates of 10% to 25% in both groups, with higher rates for sexually active women and in teenagers. Vertical transmission of group B *Streptococcus* from mother to infant at the time of vaginal delivery occurs with a frequency of approximately 60%[37, 41]; of infants who are colonized at birth, only 1% to 3% develop symptomatic infection. Neonatal acquisition of the organism at or shortly before birth has been shown to be the source of infection in early-onset neonatal disease; in late-onset infection, the organism may be acquired in this manner, or may be transmitted to the infant after birth from the mother, from nursery personnel, or from other contacts. Maternal risk factors for neonatal group B *Streptococcus* infection include black race, maternal age younger than 20 years, and obstetric complications including prematurity, prolonged rupture of membranes, and peripartum fever.[36, 38]

Pathogenesis

The observation that colonization of both adults and neonates with group B *Streptococcus* is common whereas clinical infection is relatively uncommon indicates that particular strain characteristics of the organisms and/or differences in host susceptibility must play a role in the development of invasive disease. Studies by Baker and Kasper[42] and coworkers in the 1970s demonstrated that the presence of antibodies directed against the capsular polysaccharide was a key factor in human immunity to group B *Streptococcus*. Cord blood of infants with type III group B *Streptococcus* bacteremia and meningitis invariably contained low or undetectable levels of specific antibody against the type III capsule. In vitro studies have shown that virulent strains of group B *Streptococcus* require serum complement for opsonophagocytic killing by peripheral blood leukocytes, and opsonophagocytosis is more efficient in the presence of specific antibody.[43, 44] The importance of the capsule in pathogenesis has been borne out by studies of genetically manipulated strains of type III group B *Streptococcus*. Unencapsulated mutants derived from type III strains by transposon mutagenesis had reduced virulence in a neonatal rat model of lethal group B *Streptococcus* infection.[45, 46] Resistance to opsonophagocytosis appears to be conferred by the capsular polysaccharide, with more highly encapsulated strains being more resistant than those with only a thin capsular layer.[47] The presence of capsular sialic acid residues may play a role in pathogenesis by inhibiting complement activation, as has been suggested for the sialic acid–containing capsules of *Neisseria meningitidis* groups B and C and for *Escherichia coli* K1.[48, 49] The importance of capsular sialic acid was supported by studies showing reduced virulence of type III group B *Streptococcus* mutants that elaborated a sialic acid–deficient capsular polysaccharide.[50, 51]

Group B streptococci elaborate a variety of other potential virulence factors including hemolysin, CAMP factor, C5a peptidase, and an enzyme, previously called neuraminidase, but later shown to be a hyaluronidase.[52, 53] Each of these products might play a role in pathogenesis, but none has been clearly shown to be a virulence factor during infection.

Clinical Manifestations (Table 195–1)

Early-onset neonatal sepsis with group B *Streptococcus* typically presents with the same manifestations as other types of bacterial sepsis in the newborn: respiratory distress, apnea, hypothermia or fever, lethargy, and hypotension. The risk of early-onset disease is increased in premature infants and in those born after prolonged rupture of membranes or mater-

TABLE 195–1 ■ Characteristics of Early- and Late-Onset Neonatal Sepsis Caused by Group B *Streptococcus*

CHARACTERISTIC	EARLY ONSET	LATE ONSET
Mean age (range)	20 h (0–7 d)	24 d (7–90 d)
Signs	Respiratory distress Apnea Fever or hypothermia Hypotension	Fever Lethargy Irritability
Affected sites	Bacteremia Pneumonia (40%) Meningitis (5%–10%)	Bacteremia Meningitis (30%) Focal infections (especially bone and joint)
Serotypes	All types	Type III (70%)

nal peripartum fever.[38] Premature rupture of membranes with infection of the infant in utero probably accounts for the fact that approximately half of infants with early-onset infection are symptomatic at birth. Respiratory symptoms are common and often constitute the initial clinical indication of infection. Radiographic evidence of pneumonia, often indistinguishable from hyaline membrane disease, is present in 40% of cases. Autopsies of infants dying of early-onset disease have shown pathologic findings in the lungs resembling those in hyaline membrane disease in patients with group B *Streptococcus* pneumonia.[54] Meningitis is present in about 5% to 10% of early-onset cases. Because there are rarely distinctive clinical features to suggest the presence of meningitis, all patients with suspected sepsis should undergo lumbar puncture before initiation of antibiotic therapy.

The mean age at presentation of infants with late-onset infection is 24 days, with a range of 7 days to 3 months and rarely later.[42] Usual manifestations are nonspecific and include fever, poor feeding, lethargy or irritability, and respiratory distress. In contrast to early-onset infection, in which the distribution of serotypes closely parallels that of colonizing strains, approximately two thirds of late-onset infections are caused by type III strains.[26, 37] Type III strains appear to have a predilection for meningeal invasion, and meningitis is more common in late-onset disease, occurring in about one third of cases. Although bacteremia and meningitis are the usual manifestations of late-onset infection, a variety of other infections have been described, including septic arthritis, osteomyelitis, endocarditis, cellulitis, sinusitis, and pyelonephritis. Except for bone and joint infections, focal infections are uncommon. Osteomyelitis caused by group B *Streptococcus* generally has an indolent onset and most often occurs in the proximal humerus or, less commonly, in other long bones. Septic arthritis may occur in association with osteomyelitis or as an isolated entity, usually in the lower extremity.

Group B streptococcal infections in adults may be divided into two groups: those occurring in peripartum women and those occurring in patients with underlying predisposing conditions. Peripartum infections are often manifested by fever and bacteremia. Although these infections typically produce only mild symptoms, occasional patients have severe and sometimes rapidly fatal sepsis. Symptoms and signs of chorioamnionitis and/or endometritis are often, but not always, present. Less common manifestations include meningitis and endocarditis. Outside the peripartum period, group B *Streptococcus* infections in otherwise healthy adults are unusual. Most adult patients with group B *Streptococcus* have some underlying condition, diabetes mellitus and malignancy being the most common. Skin and soft tissue are the most frequent sites of infection, particularly in association with diabetic foot ulcers.[39] A variety of other infections in adults have been described, including endocarditis, pneumonia, pyelonephritis, osteomyelitis, and septic arthritis.[55–57] Group B streptococcal endocarditis often has an acute presentation and is frequently associated with embolization and metastatic infection.[55, 57]

Diagnosis

The clinical manifestations of neonatal sepsis caused by group B *Streptococcus* are nonspecific and do not distinguish group B *Streptococcus* disease from sepsis caused by other agents. Suggestive findings include respiratory distress, apnea, lethargy, disturbed thermoregulation, and hypotension. Laboratory findings are also nonspecific; the presence of metabolic acidosis and leukopenia are signs of poor prognosis. Diagnosis generally depends on identification of the organism in blood cultures (positive in essentially all cases of untreated neonatal group B *Streptococcus* sepsis), in cultures of cerebrospinal fluid (positive in 5% to 10% of early-onset cases and in 30% of late-onset disease), or in cultures of other normally sterile sites. Rapid diagnostic tests are available for detection of group B antigen in cerebrospinal fluid and urine; these assays employ antibodies against the group B carbohydrate to detect antigen shed from the organisms during bacteremic infections. The latex agglutination assays currently available have a sensitivity of approximately 90% in cases of neonatal sepsis when both cerebrospinal fluid and concentrated urine samples are tested. The occasional false-negative results of the antigen detection tests mean that empirical therapy must often be initiated on the basis of clinical suspicion of infection while culture results are awaited. Although rapid antigen detection tests are useful for detecting group B *Streptococcus* antigen in body fluids of infected neonates, these tests lack sufficient sensitivity to be reliable for detection of the organism in maternal vaginal or anorectal swab specimens.

Treatment

Penicillin is the drug of choice for treatment of all forms of group B *Streptococcus* infection. All strains are sensitive, although the minimal inhibitory concentrations are higher than for group A *Streptococcus*, ranging from 0.01 to 0.4 μg/mL.[5] Although in vitro synergy with aminoglycosides has been demonstrated, no adequate data exist to evaluate the role of combination therapy in human infection. However, it is common practice to initiate therapy for suspected neonatal sepsis and meningitis (in infants <7 days of age) with ampicillin (200 to 300 mg/kg per day) and gentamicin (5 mg/kg per day), changing to high-dose penicillin (150,000 units/kg per day for bacteremia, 300,000 units/kg per day for meningitis) alone after culture results are back and clinical improvement is evident. Infants older than 7 days of age should receive penicillin at 200,000 units/kg per day for group B *Streptococcus* bacteremia or 400,000 units/kg per day for meningitis. Adults should receive penicillin G 12 to 18 million units/d in divided doses for bacteremia or serious local infection or 24 million units/d for meningitis or endocarditis. For patients allergic to penicillin, vancomycin or clindamycin may be used.

Prevention

Even with prompt institution of antibiotic therapy and other supportive measures, neonatal group B *Streptococcus* disease carries a 5% to 15% mortality and substantial morbidity in the form of persistent neurologic sequelae in approximately 30% of survivors of group B streptococcal meningitis. Therefore, considerable attention has been focused on strategies to prevent neonatal infection. Attempts to eradicate maternal carriage by antibiotic treatment during pregnancy have had an unacceptably high failure rate; 30% or more of women treated during pregnancy had positive cultures at the time of delivery. Presumptive antibiotic treatment of high-risk infants was also unsuccessful, with no effect on mortality. Therefore, newer approaches to prevention have focused on three strategies: (1) prophylactic antibiotic treatment of colonized pregnant women during delivery; (2) passive immunization of mother (with transplacental transfer of antibody to the infant *in utero*) or of the infant after delivery, using intravenous immune globulin (IVIG); (3) active immunization of women with a group B *Streptococcus* vaccine containing purified components of one or more antigens to elicit maternal antibodies that would cross the placenta and persist in the neonate through the first several weeks of life. Although each of these approaches has its theoretical advantages and disadvantages, only the first (antibiotic prophylaxis) has had sufficient clinical testing to permit evaluation of efficacy. Several trials have shown that intrapartum administration of antibiotics reduces transmission of group B *Streptococcus* to the infants and prevents group B *Streptococcus* disease.[38, 58–60] In a well-designed, randomized trial, Boyer and Gotoff[58] administered ampicillin intrapartum to 83 prenatally colonized women with risk factors for early-onset group B *Streptococcus* disease (premature labor or prolonged rupture of membranes). No cases of group B *Streptococcus* disease occurred in the infants of these women, but five cases of early-onset sepsis occurred among infants of 76 untreated control women ($P = .02$).[58] In this study, ampicillin was given to the infants in the treatment group for 36 hours after delivery.

Although maternal chemoprophylaxis of high-risk carriers has been shown to reduce the incidence of neonatal group B *Streptococcus* infection, it has been difficult to define the optimal approach to identifying and treating women at risk for having affected infants for several reasons: maternal cultures early in pregnancy may not reliably predict carriage at delivery; cultures may not be done or the results may not be available for some patients; approximately 25% of early-onset cases occur in infants of women without risk factors. On the basis of the conclusions of a 1995 consensus conference on group B *Streptococcus* disease prevention, the Centers for Disease Control and Prevention has recommended the following interim strategy for maternal chemoprophylaxis to prevent neonatal infection:

1. All pregnant women should be screened at 35 to 37 weeks of gestation for anogenital group B *Streptococcus* colonization or sooner if membrane rupture occurs. The likelihood of recovering group B *Streptococcus* is increased substantially by using a selective culture method: a standard culture swab of the lower vagina and anorectum, specifically identified to the laboratory as a group B *Streptococcus* culture, should be placed in transport medium until it can be inoculated into selective broth medium (Lim or SBM broth) and then subcultured onto solid medium.
2. Intrapartum chemoprophylaxis should be offered to group B *Streptococcus* carriers, that is, those with a positive screening culture. Prophylaxis should be recommended to women with risk factors for development of group B *Streptococcus* disease in the newborn (premature labor, preterm or prolonged rupture of membranes, intrapartum fever, multiple birth, or history of delivering an infant with group B streptococcal infection) if they are group B *Streptococcus* carriers or if carrier status is unknown.
3. The recommended regimen is penicillin G, 5 million units initially, then 2.5 million units every 4 hours until delivery. Clindamycin or erythromycin may be substituted for women allergic to penicillin.
4. Infants of mothers receiving intrapartum chemoprophylaxis for group B *Streptococcus* should be observed for at least 24 hours. Those with signs of sepsis should have a full diagnostic evaluation and receive empirical treatment for neonatal sepsis (e.g., ampicillin and gentamicin).

There is some controversy about whether to administer peripartum antibiotic prophylaxis to women colonized with group B *Streptococcus* without other risk factors. The risk of group B *Streptococcus* disease is relatively low in this population (1 in 300, versus 1 in 35 in infants of colonized women with risk factors), and antibiotic treatment of the 15% to 25% of pregnant women who are group B *Streptococcus* carriers entails not only enormous expense but also the risks of allergic reactions in the mother and potential drug sensitization of the infant. Empirical administration of antibiotics intrapartum also complicates management of the infant in cases of suspected neonatal sepsis, because cultures of the infant are likely to be negative. In addition, large-scale maternal prophylaxis may lead to emergence of antibiotic resistance among group B streptococci or selective pressure for colonization and infection of infants with other antibiotic-resistant organisms.

The observation that antibodies directed against the capsular polysaccharide of group B *Streptococcus* are protective in animal models and appear to correlate with human immunity has led to efforts to prevent neonatal group B *Streptococcus* disease by passive or active immunization. Administration of IVIG has been shown to protect neonatal rats against experimental group B *Streptococcus* infection.[61, 62] However, no adequate clinical trials in human neonates have shown IVIG to be effective in preventing group B *Streptococcus* neonatal sepsis. Individual lots of IVIG vary considerably in specific antibody levels, so standard IVIG preparations may not contain sufficient quantities of antibodies to group B *Streptococcus*. Until data from larger randomized trials are available, routine use of IVIG for prevention or treatment of neonatal group B *Streptococcus* disease is not recommended.

Another strategy for prevention of neonatal group B *Streptococcus* disease is the immunization of pregnant women with a vaccine based on the purified group B *Streptococcus* capsular polysaccharide(s). Purified capsular polysaccharides from three of the major serotypes (Ia, II, and III) have been tested in human subjects; immunogenicity rates in nonimmune volunteers range from 40% for type Ia to 88% for type II.[63–67] Baker and colleagues[65] showed that the type III polysaccharide vaccine elicited protective levels of antibody in 57% of pregnant women and that comparable levels of antibody were detectable in the infants' sera after delivery, establishing the feasibility of this approach for preventing neonatal group B *Streptococcus* infection. Because the purified polysaccharides are not immunogenic in all recipients, efforts are under way to develop a polysaccharide or oligosaccharide-protein conjugate vaccine to increase the immunogenicity of these antigens. Conjugate vaccines based on the type Ia, Ib, II, III, and V group B streptococcal capsular polysaccharides have been synthesized by coupling the polysaccharide to tetanus toxoid.[68–73] These polysaccharide-protein conjugate vaccines have been highly immunogenic in experimental animals, and vaccines of similar design are currently being tested in volunteers. Phase I testing of a vaccine consisting of group B *Streptococcus* type III polysaccharide coupled to tetanus toxoid indicated that the vaccine was safe, well tolerated, and highly immunogenic.[74] Encouraging results have also been obtained in animal testing of a vaccine consisting of type III polysaccharide coupled to the group B streptococcal beta C protein.[75] A vaccine for clinical use would probably consist of several group B streptococcal polysaccharides, representing the prevalent serotypes, coupled to carrier protein(s), one or more of which may also be derived from group B streptococci. Although still in the investigational stage, active immunization of childbearing women may ultimately prove an effective approach for prevention of neonatal group B *Streptococcus* infection.

References

1. Lancefield RC: A serological differentiation of human and other groups of hemolytic streptococci. J Exp Med 57:571, 1933.
2. Lancefield RC: The serological differentiation of pathogenic and nonpathogenic strains of hemolytic streptococci from parturient women. J Exp Med 61:335, 1935.
3. Fry RM: Fatal infection by haemolytic streptococcus group B. Lancet 1:199, 1938.
4. Hood M, Janney A, Dameron G: Beta hemolytic streptococcus group B associated with problems of perinatal period. Am J Obstet Gynecol 82:809, 1961.
5. Eickhoff TC, Klein JO, Daly AL, et al: Neonatal sepsis and other infections due to group B beta-hemolytic streptococci. N Engl J Med 271:1221, 1964.
6. Facklam RR, Padula JR, Thacker LG, et al: Presumptive identification of group A, B, and D streptococci. Appl Microbiol 27:107, 1974.
7. Pollack HM, Dahlgren BJ: Distribution of streptococcal groups in clinical specimens with evaluation of bacitracin screening. Appl Microbiol 27:141, 1974.
8. Christie R, Atkins NE, Munch-Petersen E: A note on a lytic phenomenon shown by group B streptococci. Aust J Exp Biol Med Sci 22:197, 1944.
9. Facklam RR, Padula JR, Wortham EC, et al: Presumptive identification of group A, B and D streptococci on agar plate medium. J Clin Microbiol 9:665, 1979.
10. Kane JA, Karakawa WW: Multiple polysaccharide antigens of group B *Streptococcus,* type Ia: Emphasis on a sialic acid type-specific polysaccharide. J Immunol 118:2155, 1977.
11. Carey RB, Eisenstein TK, Shockman GD, et al: Soluble group- and type-specific antigens from type III group B *Streptococcus.* Infect Immun 28:195, 1980.
12. Pritchard DG: Characterization of the group-specific polysaccharide of group B *Streptococcus.* Arch Biochem Biophys 235:385, 1984.
13. Michon F, Brisson JR, Dell A, et al: Multiantennary group-specific polysaccharide of group B *Streptococcus.* Biochemistry 27:5341, 1988.
14. Lancefield RC: A serological differentiation of specific types of bovine hemolytic streptococci (group B). J Exp Med 59:441, 1934.
15. Lancefield RC: Two serological types of group B hemolytic streptococci with related, but not identical, type-specific substances. J Exp Med 67:25, 1938.
16. Kasper DL, Baker CJ: Electron microscopic definition of surface antigens of group B *Streptococcus.* J Infect Dis 139:147, 1979.
17. Jennings HJ, Rosell K-G, Katzenellenbogen E, Kasper DL: Structural determination of the capsular polysaccharide antigen of type II group B streptococci. J Biol Chem 258:1793, 1983.
18. Jennings HJ, Katzenellenbogen E, Lugowski C, Kasper DL: Structure of the native polysaccharide antigens of type Ia and type Ib group B *Streptococcus.* Biochemistry 22:1258, 1983.
19. Wessels MR, Pozsgay V, Kasper DL, Jennings HJ: Structure and immunochemistry of an oligosaccharide repeating unit of the capsular polysaccharide of type III group B *Streptococcus.* J Biol Chem 262:8262, 1987.
20. Jelinkova J, Motlova J: Worldwide distribution of two new serotypes of group B streptococci: Type IV and provisional type V. J Clin Microbiol 21:361, 1985.
21. Wessels MR, Benedi V-J, Jennings HJ, et al: Isolation and characterization of type IV group B *Streptococcus* capsular polysaccharide. Infect Immun 57:1089, 1989.
22. DiFabio JL, Michon F, Brisson J-R, et al: Structure of the capsular polysaccharide antigen of type IV group B *Streptococcus.* Can J Chem 67:877, 1989.
23. Wessels MR, DiFabio JL, Benedi V-J, et al: Structural determination and immunochemical characterization of the type V group B *Streptococcus* capsular polysaccharide. J Biol Chem 266:6714, 1991.
24. von Hunolstein C, d'Ascenzi S, Wagner B, et al: Immunochemistry of capsular type polysaccharide and virulence properties of type VI *Streptococcus agalactiae* (group B streptococci). Infect Immun 61:1272, 1993.
25. Kogan G, Uhrin D, Brisson J-R, et al: Structure of the type VI group B *Streptococcus* capsular polysaccharide determined by high resolution NMR spectroscopy. J Carbohydr Chem 13:1071, 1994.
26. Wenger JD, Hightower AW, Facklam RR, et al: Bacterial meningitis in the United States, 1986: Report of a multistate surveillance study. J Infect Dis 162:1316, 1990.
27. Blumberg HM, Modansky M, Stephens DS, et al: Emergence of invasive serotype V group B streptococcal disease. Clin Res 42:298, 1994.
28. Wilkinson HW, Eagon RG: Type-specific antigens of group B type Ic streptococci. Infect Immun 4:596, 1971.
29. Lancefield RC, McCarty M, Everly WN: Multiple mouse-protective antibodies directed against group B streptococci. Special reference to antibodies effective against protein antigens. J Exp Med 142:165, 1975.
30. Johnson DR, Ferrieri P: Group B streptococcal Ibc protein antigen: Distribution of two determinants in wild-type strains of common serotypes. J Clin Microbiol 19:506, 1984.
31. Henrichsen J, Ferrieri P, Jelinkova J, et al: Nomenclature of antigens of group B streptococci. Int J Syst Bacteriol 34:500, 1984.
32. Stalhammer-Carlemalm M, Stenberg L, Lindahl G: Protein Rib: A novel group B streptococcal cell surface protein that confers protective immunity and is expressed by most strains causing invasive infections. J Exp Med 177:1593, 1993.
33. Michel JL, Madoff LC, Kling DE, et al: Cloned alpha and beta C-protein antigens of group B streptococci elicit protective immunity. Infect Immun 59:2023, 1991.
34. Madoff LC, Michel JL, Gong EW, et al: Protection of neonatal mice from group B streptococcal infection by maternal immunization with beta C protein. Infect Immun 60:4989, 1992.
35. Zangwill KM, Schuchat A, Wenger JD: Group B streptococcal disease in the United States, 1990: Report from a multistate active surveillance system. MMWR CDC Surveill Summ 41:25, 1992.
36. Schuchat A, Oxtoby M, Cochi S, et al: Population-based risk factors for neonatal group B streptococcal disease: Results of a cohort study in metropolitan Atlanta. J Infect Dis 162:672, 1990.
37. Dillon HC Jr, Khare S, Gray BM: Group B streptococcal carriage and disease: A 6-year prospective study. J Pediatr 110:31, 1987.
38. Boyer KM, Gadzala CA, Burd LI, et al: Selective intrapartum chemoprophylaxis of neonatal group B streptococcal early-onset disease. I. Epidemiologic rationale. J Infect Dis 148:795, 1983.
39. Schwartz B, Schuchat A, Oxtoby MJ, et al: Invasive group B streptococcal disease in adults, a population-based study in metropolitan Atlanta. JAMA 266:1112, 1991.
40. Farley MM, Harvey RC, Stull T, et al: A population-based assessment of invasive disease due to group B *Streptococcus* in nonpregnant adults. N Engl J Med 328:1807, 1993.
41. Hoogkamp-Korstanje JAA, Gerards LJ, Cats BP: Maternal carriage and neonatal acquisition of group B streptococci. J Infect Dis 145:800, 1982.
42. Baker CJ, Kasper DL: Correlation of maternal antibody deficiency with susceptibility to neonatal group B streptococcal infection. N Engl J Med 294:753, 1976.
43. Shigeoka AO, Hall RT, Hemming VG, et al: Role of antibody and complement in opsonization of group B streptococci. Infect Immun 21:34, 1978.

44. Baltimore RS, Kasper DL, Baker CJ, Goroff DK: Antigenic specificity of opsonophagocytic antibodies in rabbit anti-sera to group B streptococci. J Immunol 118:673, 1977.
45. Rubens CE, Wessels MR, Heggen LM, Kasper DL: Transposon mutagenesis of group B streptococcal type III capsular polysaccharide: Correlation of capsule expression with virulence. Proc Natl Acad Sci USA 84:7208, 1987.
46. Rubens CE, Heggen LM, Haft RF, Wessels MR: Identification of *cpsD*, a gene essential for type III capsule expression in group B streptococci. Mol Microbiol 8:843, 1993.
47. Marques MB, Kasper DL, Pangburn MK, Wessels MR: Prevention of C3 deposition is a virulence mechanism of type III group B *Streptococcus* capsular polysaccharide. Infect Immun 60:3986, 1992.
48. Edwards MS, Nicholson-Weller A, Baker CJ, Kasper DL: The role of specific antibody in alternative pathway–mediated opsonophagocytosis of type III, group B *Streptococcus*. J Exp Med 151:1275,1980.
49. Edwards MS, Kasper DL, Jennings HJ, et al: Capsular sialic acid prevents activation of the alternative complement pathway by type III, group B streptococci. J Immunol 128:1278, 1982.
50. Wessels MR, Rubens CE, Benedi V-J, Kasper DL: Definition of a bacterial virulence factor: Sialylation of the group B streptococcal capsule. Proc Natl Acad Sci USA 86:8983, 1989.
51. Wessels MR, Haft RF, Heggen LM, Rubens CE: Identification of a genetic locus essential for capsule sialylation in type III group B streptococci. Infect Immun 60:392, 1992.
52. Bohnsack JF, Mollison KW, Buko AM, et al: Group B streptococci inactivate complement component C5a by enzymic cleavage at the C-terminus. Biochem J 273:635, 1991.
53. Pritchard DG, Lin B: Group B streptococcal neuraminidase is actually a hyaluronidase. Infect Immun 61:3234, 1993.
54. Katzenstein A, Davis C, Braude A: Pulmonary changes in neonatal sepsis due to group B beta-hemolytic streptococcus: Relation to hyaline membrane disease. J Infect Dis 133:430, 1976.
55. Lerner PI, Gopalakrishna KV, Wolinsky E, et al: Group B streptococcus *(S. agalactiae)* bacteremia in adults: Analysis of 32 cases and review of the literature. Medicine (Baltimore) 56:457, 1977.
56. Verghese A, Mireault K, Arbeit R: Group B streptococcal bacteremia in men. Rev Infect Dis 8:912, 1986.
57. Gallagher PG, Watanakunakorn C: Group B streptococcal endocarditis: Report of seven cases and review of the literature. Rev Infect Dis 8:175, 1986.
58. Boyer KM, Gotoff SP: Prevention of early-onset neonatal group B streptococcal disease with selective intrapartum chemoprophylaxis. N Engl J Med 314:1665, 1986.
59. Easmon CSF, Hastings MJG, Deeley J, et al: The effect of intrapartum chemoprophylaxis on the vertical transmission of group B streptococci. Br J Obstet Gynaecol 90:633, 1983.
60. Morales WJ, Lim DV, Walsh AF: Prevention of neonatal group B streptococcal sepsis by the use of a rapid screening test and selective intrapartum chemoprophylaxis. Am J Obstet Gynecol 155:979, 1986.
61. Fischer GW, Hunter KW, Wilson SR: Modified human immune serum globulin for intravenous administration: *In vitro* protection against group B streptococcal disease in suckling rats. Acta Paediatr Scand 71:639, 1982.
62. Santos JI, Shigeoka AO, Rote NS, Hill HR: Protective efficacy of a modified immune serum globulin in experimental group B streptococcal infection. J Pediatr 99:873, 1981.
63. Baker CJ, Edwards MS, Kasper DL: Immunogenicity of polysaccharides from type III, group B *Streptococcus*. J Clin Invest 61:1107, 1978.
64. Baker CJ, Kasper DL: Group B streptococcal vaccines. Rev Infect Dis 7:458, 1985.
65. Baker CJ, Rench MA, Edwards MS, et al: Immunization of pregnant women with a polysaccharide vaccine of group B *Streptococcus*. N Engl J Med 319:1180, 1988.
66. Eisenstein TK, De Cueninck BJ, Resavy D, et al: Quantitative determination in human sera of vaccine-induced antibody to type-specific polysaccharides of group B streptococci using an enzyme-linked immunosorbent assay. J Infect Dis 147:847, 1983.
67. Kasper L, Baker CJ, Galdes B, et al: Immunochemical analysis and immunogenicity of the type II group B streptococcal capsular polysaccharide. J Clin Invest 72:260, 1983.
68. Wessels MR, Paoletti LC, Rodewald AK, et al: Stimulation of protective antibodies against type Ia and Ib group B streptococci by a type Ia polysaccharide–tetanus toxoid conjugate vaccine. Infect Immun 61:4760, 1993.
69. Paoletti LC, Wessels MR, Michon F, et al: Group B *Streptococcus* type II polysaccharide–tetanus toxoid conjugate vaccine. Infect Immun 60:4009, 1992.
70. Wessels MR, Paoletti LC, Kasper DL, et al: Immunonogenicity in animals of a polysaccharide-protein conjugate vaccine against type III group B *Streptococcus*. J Clin Invest 86:1428, 1990.
71. Lagergard T, Shiloach J, Robbins JB, Schneerson R: Synthesis and immunological properties of conjugates composed of group B streptococcus type III capsular polysaccharide covalently bound to tetanus toxoid. Infect Immun 58:687, 1990.
72. Paoletti LC, Wessels MR, Rodewald AK, et al: Neonatal mouse protection against infection with multiple group B streptococcal serotypes by maternal immunization with a tetravalent GBS polysaccharide–tetanus toxoid conjugate vaccine. Infect Immun 62:3236, 1994.
73. Wessels MR, Paoletti LC, Pinel J, Kasper DL: Immunogenicity and protective activity in animals of a group B *Streptococcus* type V polysaccharide–tetanus toxoid conjugate vaccine. J Infect Dis 171:879, 1995.
74. Kasper DL, Paoletti LC, Wessels MR, et al: Immune response to type III group B streptococcal polysaccharide-tetanus toxoid conjugate vaccine. J Clin Invest 98:2308, 1996.
75. Madoff LC, Paoletti LC, Tai JY, Kasper DL: Maternal immunization of mice with group B streptococcal type III polysaccharide–beta C protein conjugate elicits protective antibody to multiple serotypes. J Clin Invest 94:286, 1994.

196

Miscellaneous Streptococci

David M. Shlaes
Ronald J. Zabransky

In this chapter we discuss the β-hemolytic streptococci that form small colonies; the pyogenes-like β-hemolytic streptococci belonging to the Lancefield groups F, C, and G and the nongroupable strains; and the viridans streptococci, which are not β-hemolytic. This heterogeneous group of bacteria requires division into several categories for a more complete understanding of the organisms and their associated disease syndromes. These groupings are based on specific, well-recognized, phenotypic and pathogenic characteristics.

Taxonomy and Laboratory Identification

The streptococci were first divided on the basis of the type of hemolysis they produce on blood agar medium. The literature describes the use of human, horse, sheep, rabbit, and guinea pig blood, among others. Over the years this became problematic because of the varied source of the red blood cells, different conditions of incubation, presence or absence of carbohydrate in the medium, and lack of agreement on the interpretation of the results. A major advance occurred when Rebecca Lancefield and coworkers identified specific capsular antigens of the β-hemolytic streptococci. These antigens became important taxonomic tools that allowed the characterization of clinical syndromes caused by the various taxa. We know today that a taxonomy based solely on the

Lancefield serologic groups is not completely valid because unrelated species may produce the same Lancefield antigen[1] and because genetically related strains possess heterogeneous Lancefield antigens.[2] Thus, the current taxonomic status and relationship of the species of streptococci are based primarily on DNA homology.

Nevertheless, Lancefield grouping and other phenotypic characteristics serve as an important part of our understanding of streptococcal disease. The first division of the streptococci should probably remain at the level of hemolysis as defined on 5% sheep blood agar, a medium without carbohydrate, incubated in the presence of 5% carbon dioxide at 35°C to 37°C for 16 to 24 hours. Beta hemolysis is indicated by a clear zone around the colony; thus colonies should be considered either β-hemolytic or not. β-Hemolytic isolates can then be further divided into two large groups: formers of large colonies (pyogenes-like) and formers of small colonies (*Streptococcus intermedius* group).[3, 4] About 75% of the β-hemolytic streptococci carry a Lancefield antigen. Large-colony types usually have colonies at least 0.5 mm in diameter under the conditions described earlier. The taxonomy of these streptococci is illustrated in Table 196–1. Note that the β-hemolytic small-colony formers are classified as being in a single taxon, which also includes all members of the non–β-hemolytic *S. intermedius* group. All of group F, 75% of group C, 15% of group G, less than 5% of group A, and virtually all nongroupable stains fall into this small-colony taxon.[5]

Streptococci Forming Large Colonies

These strains are in taxa that are defined first by the Lancefield grouping. For example, strains of group C are divided into *Streptococcus equi* (including *zooepidemicus*) and *Streptococcus dysgalactiae* (including *Streptococcus equisimilis* and some group G strains).[6] Group G species (not *S. dysgalactiae*) are simply labeled group G streptococci or *Streptococcus canis*, a denotation representing its ecology rather than taxonomy.[7] Group A strains are called *Streptococcus pyogenes* (see Chapter 192).

Streptococci Forming Small Colonies

The taxonomy of the small- or minute-colony streptococci is still being debated. These organisms have been referred to as *Streptococcus* MG, *Streptococcus anginosus* group,[8] or more commonly the *Streptococcus milleri* group.[9, 10] In the 1986 edition of *Bergey's Manual of Systematic Bacteriology*, Hardie[11] stated that the name *S. anginosus* had priority, and it is now accepted that *S. milleri* was an illegal epithet for the group or any one species. Hardie also stated that it would be more sensible to group these organisms in a single species; however, taxonomists have now assigned members of this collective group to separate species status: *S. intermedius*, *Streptococcus constellatus*, and *S. anginosus*.[12] For purposes of this discussion, we refer to the these organisms as the *S. intermedius* group and discuss the individual species only when they are associated with the incidence of infections in certain locations.

The division between large- and small-colony formers is key to understanding the disease syndromes likely to be caused by these organisms. Most laboratories do not provide this distinction for the clinician. They usually identify only groups A and B versus others using presumptive and nonserologic tests that do not separate the *S. intermedius* group from the pyogenes-like group. The presumptive test most frequently used is the bacitracin disk, sometimes in combination with a trimethoprim-sulfamethoxazole disk. Table 196–1 shows the expected results for the presumptive disk test when performed on trypticase soy agar supplemented with 5% sheep blood and incubated in 5% carbon dioxide at 37°C for 18 hours. The trimethoprim-sulfamethoxazole disk separates the bacitracin-susceptible non–group A strains from the bona fide group A strains.[6, 7] When used in conjunction with the trimethoprim-sulfamethoxazole disk, the CAMP (Christie, Atkins, and Munch-Petersen) test differentiates *Streptococcus agalactiae* (group B) from group C or G. Group B streptococci produce a proteinaceous extracellular substance (CAMP factor) that acts synergistically with the β-toxin produced by some strains of *Staphylococcus aureus* to produce a characteristic arrow-shaped zone of enhanced hemolysis. The Lancefield groups or identifications can be confirmed by any of a number of commercially available kits. These may involve either latex particles coated with antibody against the appropriate capsular polysaccharide or antibodies fixed to protein A of the walls of a specific strain of *S. aureus*. The latex particles or bacterial cells agglutinate in the presence of the appropriate antigen. The latter, termed coagglutination, has the advantage of not requiring that the antigen be extracted from the cell wall of the test organism.

Viridans Streptococci

The viridans streptococci are, taxonomically, the most difficult group to deal with in the laboratory.[4, 13] They are non–β-hemolytic but may cause a greening of the agar (alpha hemolysis) or be nonhemolytic (gamma hemolysis); the former phenomenon is due to an enzyme not related to the hemolysin responsible for beta hemolysis. The greening effect was the original derivation of the term viridans, but the viridans group now includes strains that produce no discoloration as well. The group consists of at least 12 species, some of which appear to be relatively unimportant clinically. The taxonomy of the viridans group has been and continues to be a subject of study and debate, nationally and internationally.[14–17] This is further complicated by the transfer of several previous members of this group into different or entirely new genera.[15, 18]

A summary of the current classification of the more commonly seen viridans and small-colony streptococci is presented in Table 196–2. *Streptococcus bovis* is also included,

TABLE 196–1 ■ Characteristics and Presumptive Identification of β-Hemolytic Streptococci*

SPECIES	HEMOLYSIS	COLONY TYPE	LANCEFIELD GROUP	CAMP REACTION	BACITRACIN	TMP-SMX
Streptococcus agalactiae	Beta	Large	B	+	R	R
Streptococcus canis	Beta	Large	G	–	R	S
Streptococcus equi	Beta	Large	C	–	R	S
Streptococcus dysgalactiae or *equisimilis*	Beta	Large	C or G	–	R	S
Streptococcus intermedius group	Alpha, beta, gamma	Minute	A, C, F, G, or none	–	R	V
Streptococcus pyogenes	Beta	Large	A	–	S	R

* See text for information on the CAMP reaction and bacitracin or trimethoprim-sulfamethoxazole (TMP-SMX) susceptibility tests. R, Resistant; S, sensitive; V, variable.

TABLE 196–2 ■ Identification of the Major Groups of Viridans and Small-Colony Streptococci[a]

SPECIES[b]	HEMOLYSIS	FERMENTATION			PYR	BE	VP	ESC	ARG	ECP
		Man	Sor	Inu						
Streptococcus acidominimus	Alpha	+	+	−	−	−	+	−	−	N
Streptococcus bovis	Gamma	±[c]	±	±	−	+	+	+	−	L[c]
Streptococcus defectivus group[d]	Alpha	−	−	−	+	−	ND	ND	−	ND
Streptococcus intermedius group[e]	Alpha, beta, or gamma	−	−	±	−	−	±	±	±	N
Streptococcus mitis group	Gamma	−	−	−	−	−	−	−	−	D
Streptococcus mutans group	Beta or gamma	+	+	+	−	±	+	+	−[f]	D
Streptococcus sanguis group	Gamma	−	−	±	−	−	−	±[g]	±[h]	N
Streptococcus salivarius group	Gamma	−	−	+	−	−	±	±[i]	−	L
Streptococcus uberis	Alpha	+	+	+	−	−	+	+	+	N

[a] Man, Mannitol; Sor, sorbitol; Inu, inulin; PYR, production of pyrrolidonyl arylamidase; BE, growth in bile-esculin; VP, Voges-Proskauer; ESC, hydrolysis of esculin; ARG, arginine dihydrolase; ECP, production of extracellular polysaccharides: N indicates none, D indicates dextrans, L indicates levans; + or −, > 90% reactions are positive or negative; ±, variable results or exceptions occur; ND, no data.
[b] Groups contain two or more recognized species.
[c] A variant of *S. bovis* is mannitol-negative and usually does not produce extracellular polysaccharides (see text).
[d] *S. adjacens* and *S. defectivus* are pyridoxal dependent (see text).
[e] *S. intermedius* may be listed as *S. milleri* or *S. anginosus* by others (see text).
[f] *S. rattus* is arginine-positive.
[g] *S. crista* is esculin-negative; *S. parasanguis* may be esculin-negative.
[h] *S. crista* may be arginine-negative.
[i] *S. vestibularis* is hemolytic and may be esculin-negative.
Data from references 4, 15, 16, 20, and 21.

although it is more often discussed with the enterococci, because it carries the Lancefield group D antigen (glycerol teichoic acid) and is able to hydrolyze esculin in the presence of bile. Unlike *Enterococcus* spp. it does not grow in 6.5% NaCl. *S. bovis* more appropriately belongs within the viridans division because of its clinical behavior and other biochemical and growth characteristics. In the laboratory *S. bovis* can be easily confused with other viridans species such as the *S. intermedius* group, *Streptococcus salivarius,* and *Streptococcus mutans.* These species may be bile-esculin–positive and they do not grow in high concentrations of NaCl. The latter species are discussed in more detail later. A variant of *S. bovis* has been shown to be biochemically distinct but nevertheless belongs to the species.[19] *S. bovis* variants would be difficult for clinical laboratories to recognize if the test for group D antigen was not included in the testing scheme. We recommend that before reporting an *S. bovis,* laboratories confirm the presence of group D antigen. The other viridans species listed in Table 196–2 represent a combination of taxonomic considerations from Ruoff[4] and others,[16] Janda,[15] Facklam and Sahm,[20] and Holt and colleagues.[21] Thus, although this description is not official it represents the current approach to the taxonomy of this group in the United States. Gram-positive cocci previously classified as *Streptococcus morbillorum* and a hemolytic variant, *Streptococcus haemolysans,* have been transferred to the genus *Gemella.*[15]

Other phenotypically similar organisms that make identification difficult in the clinical laboratory include the genera *Aerococcus, Leuconostoc, Pediococcus, Stomatococcus, Lactococcus, Globicatella,* and *Helcococcus,* all of which have been isolated from clinical specimens and may be part of the indigenous flora of humans.[18] Some of these genera existed and were just expanded to accept newly transferred species; in other cases, the ability to recognize phenotypic differences revealed the presence of previously described species in infections; and in still other situations new genera were described to accommodate the new isolates from clinical material. The major basis for these revisions is the advance in molecular techniques.

Finally, one additional group of pathogenic viridans streptococci should be mentioned, the pyridoxal (vitamin B_6)-dependent or nutritionally deficient streptococci (NDS).[22, 23] These organisms may be recognized in the laboratory by their "satelliting" growth around colonies of other bacteria that produce pyridoxal, most often staphyloccci and yeast. Evidence indicates that all the NDS fall within a single taxon, as opposed to being mutants of strains belonging to a variety of species, as was once thought. These can be distinguished from the other viridans streptococci by their production of pyrrolidonyl arylamidase. They have been further subdivided into two distinct species, *Streptococcus defectivus* and *Streptococcus adjacens,* on the basis of their α- and β-galactosidase and fermentation activities.[24] These organisms pose problems in recognition and identification, because they do not grow well on media not supplemented with vitamin B_6. They do grow in most liquid media supplemented with blood and incubated in carbon dioxide but not on subculture to ordinary trypticase soy agar, which is commonly used in clinical laboratories. They also grow on many of the highly supplemented media such as those used for the cultivation of anaerobes, and because they are facultatively anaerobic or microaerophilic in their oxygen requirements, they are frequently mistaken for anaerobic cocci such as peptostreptococci. It should be noted here that the *Gemella* species, which are also pyrrolidonyl arylamidase–positive, can be confused with NDS as well.

The problem the clinical microbiology laboratory has to face is how much effort should go into identifying a given streptococcal isolate. In many cases, laboratory information alone is sufficient to determine the significance of an isolate. This includes the source, repeated isolation from the same specimen source, presence of other organisms, and numbers present in culture. When the issue is not clear, the laboratory staff must consult the ordering clinician. The immune status of the patient, presence of malignancy, concurrent antimicrobial therapy, and correlation with the clinical syndrome and findings are issues to be evaluated. If an organism is determined significant enough to identify, it should also be tested for antimicrobial susceptibility using accepted standard methods.[25] Most of the organisms discussed in this chapter are susceptible to a variety of antimicrobial agents, including the β-lactams; nevertheless, there have been reports of penicillin-resistant and high-level aminoglycoside–resistant strains.[26, 27] Not all drugs need to be tested and reported, but it is critical to include vancomycin to rule out vancomycin-resistant genera or species that closely resemble the viridans and other streptococci.[18]

Ruoff[4] described a minimal battery of conventional tests than can be used to identify these streptococci to the group level. To go further may be beyond the resources of many clinical laboratories. A number of commercially available kit systems have been described for this purpose, but the resultant identifications do not always agree with each other or conventional approaches, and different systems use different approaches to nomenclature. As a result, various levels of agreement have been reported, ranging from 50% to 75%,[28] and additional tests are frequently required. Therefore, the task of identifying this heterogeneous group of streptococci for routine clinical purposes should be undertaken prudently.

Virulence

Little is known about the potential virulence of the large-colony β-hemolytic streptococci. Although they have an array of toxins, enzymes, and adhesins similar to those produced by *S. pyogenes*, they do not produce the pyrogenic enterotoxins associated with streptococcal toxic shock syndrome and *S. pyogenes*.[29] They are also not associated with the development of rheumatic fever. Some of the large-colony β-hemolytic streptococci, especially the group G strains, have been shown to encode M protein sequences in their chromosome similar to those of *S. pyogenes*.[7] *S. equisimilis* (group C) strains carry human Fc (immunoglobulin G) receptors, whereas group C *S. intermedius* strains do not[30]; the former can cause pharyngitis and the latter do not. These observations are consistent with the hypothesis that the pyogenes-like β-hemolytic streptococci resemble *S. pyogenes* in some of their virulence characteristics and in pathogenesis of disease as well as morphologically and biochemically. Unfortunately, little is known about the virulence of the small-colony formers. This should be an area of considerable interest given the frequency with which these infections occur and their frequently morbid consequences.

The viridans strains, aside from the *S. intermedius* group, can be divided into those that are frequently associated with endocarditis and those that are not. Those that produce dextrans, specific forms of exopolysaccharide, appear most likely to cause endocarditis. The latter strains include *S. bovis*, *S. mutans*, *Streptococcus sanguis*, and the *Streptococcus mitis* group. The *S. mitis* group includes strains that were previously called *Streptococcus mitior* and *Streptococcus sanguis II*. Isogenic strains of *S. mutans* proficient or defective in their ability to produce sucrose-derived exopolymers have been compared in vitro and in vivo for their ability to adhere to fibrin plates, their resistance to phagocytic killing, and their ability to provoke endocarditis. Wild-type strains grown in the absence of sucrose bound to fibrin plates less efficiently, were susceptible to phagocytic killing, and were less efficient at producing endocarditis in vivo.[31, 32] Strains with transposon insertions in genes responsible for exopolymer synthesis grown in the presence of sucrose had the same phenotype as wild-type strains grown in the absence of sucrose.[31, 32] Similar evidence has been developed for *Streptococcus gordonii*.[33] In addition, evidence supporting a role for binding of fibronectin in the pathogenesis of streptococcal endocarditis has been described.[34] However, other factors are probably also important, as *S. mitis* has been described to cause infections other than endocarditis.[36] *S. salivarius*, in comparison, produces levan as its exopolysaccharide, is only a rare cause of endocarditis, and when found in blood cultures is often a contaminant.

Clinical Manifestations and Epidemiology

Infections with S. intermedius Group, Including β-Hemolytic Streptococci Forming Small Colonies

Small-colony β-hemolytic streptococci are normally carried in the oropharynx and upper gastrointestinal tract of humans.[5, 35] They are found in about 11% of normal appendixes. Although little is known about the epidemiology of infections caused by these strains, they are thought to arise from endogenous flora, even when they occur nosocomially. *S. intermedius* (group) tends to cause abscesses either by hematogenous spread or by direct extension from visceral injury. The most frequent infections caused by these organisms include primary bacteremia, brain abscess, purulent pleuropulmonary infections, bone and joint infections, and intraabdominal abscesses. Interestingly, *S. intermedius* is more commonly associated with tooth and brain abscesses and *S. anginosus* is found more frequently in abdominal and pelvic organ abscesses.[36] Skin and soft tissue infections and endocarditis occur but are less frequent. Endocarditis, rarely associated with these strains, is, however, frequently complicated by metastatic purulent infections. Puerperal sepsis and urinary tract infections are rare.

Infections with β-Hemolytic Streptococci Forming Large Colonies

These streptococci have an epidemiology and clinical spectrum similar to those described for *S. pyogenes*.[6, 7] Pharyngitis is common and well described, followed by skin and soft tissue infections. Rheumatic fever is not associated with non–group A streptococcal infections, although glomerulonephritis after these infections is well recognized. Primary bacteremia, pleuropulmonary infections, and endocarditis are common and puerperal sepsis, bone and joint infections, and ophthalmologic infections also occur. Urinary tract and central nervous system infections are rare.

Viridans Streptococcal Infection

The clinical spectrum of infection and epidemiology of the viridans streptococci varies somewhat by species. In general, they appear capable of causing, or at least participating in, infections other than endocarditis. These include bacteremias, including those involving intravascular devices. Because the normal habitat for many species of viridans streptococci, including the NDS, is the oropharynx, they have been associated with respiratory infections, such as pneumonia, empyema, and lung abscess, as well as mediastinitis. These streptococci also reside in the upper gastrointestinal tract and can therefore be involved in intraabdominal abscess, liver abscess, cholecystitis, and pancreatic abscess. Bone and joint, skin, and soft tissue infections in patients other than diabetic patients and urinary tract infections are rare but do occur. Some species, such as *Streptococcus uberis* and *Streptococcus acidominimus*, are poorly understood and are considered to be predominantly animal pathogens even though they can be isolated from human clinical material. Their epidemiologic picture appears to resemble that of endogenous flora infections in general. *S. sanguis*, *S. salivarius*, *S. mitis*, and *S. mutans*, the exopolysaccharide-producing strains, are normally carried in the mouth and oropharynx. *S. mutans* binds tightly to tooth surfaces and plays an important role in the formation of dental caries. There is some evidence for the spread of cariogenic strains of *S. mutans* within families. *S. sanguis* and *S. mitis* may play an important role in infections resulting from trauma to viscera in which they normally reside, whereas *S. mutans* appears not to be important in such situations. In a small series[37] of *S. mitis* infections, two of five cases involved the mediastinum by direct extension from a ruptured esophagus; only one of five was an endovascular infection. *S. mutans, S. mitis,* and *S. sanguis* all appear capable of establishing infection by hematogenous spread. Infections with *S. mutans* appear to be limited to endocarditis, whereas endocarditis is a major part of the spectrum of infections caused by *S. mitis* and *S. sanguis.* When *S. mutans* is isolated from the blood stream, it almost always signifies endocarditis, but *S. sanguis* and *S. mitis* are frequent contaminants in blood cultures (about two thirds of cases), although they can cause endocarditis.[38] *S. salivarius* is an infrequent pathogen.[38]

Streptococcus bovis *Infections*

S. bovis strains are nonenterococcal and carry the Lancefield group D antigen. The pitfalls in their laboratory identification were discussed earlier. It is not clear whether associations noted for *S. bovis* are true for the *S. bovis* variant strains, but until further data are available and because both belong within a single species as determined by DNA homology,[19] it is prudent to assume that all *S. bovis* strains produce the same clinical syndromes. These organisms cause bacteremia and endocarditis, which are highly associated with gastrointestinal neoplasm.[39] Because of this association, the isolation of *S. bovis* from blood cultures obligates the physician to search carefully for such a tumor, and it is imperative that the microbiology laboratory provide accurate identification (discussed previously).

Infections with Nutritionally Deficient Streptococci

Clinically, the NDS have been associated with culture-negative endocarditis and "sterile" abscesses. Interestingly, in vitro testing has revealed both resistance to and tolerance for penicillin in some strains of NDS.[22] The NDS have been mainly identified as causing bacteremia and endocarditis. However, this may be a laboratory artifact related to their fastidious growth requirements as manifested by the specimen source (blood) and use of liquid blood culture media.

Therapy

The miscellaneous streptococci are all highly susceptible to penicillin and other cell wall synthesis inhibitors, although not all are killed by these agents at concentrations within 32-fold of those that inhibit growth (tolerance). The clinical importance of tolerance as it occurs among the streptococci has yet to be established. The semisynthetic penicillinase-resistant penicillins such as oxacillin or nafcillin and oral phenoxymethylpenicillin are not as active as penicillin G or ampicillin; however, sufficiently high levels of these agents can be achieved in the blood stream to treat most infections. Other agents that appear to be active in vitro include the glycopeptides vancomycin and teicoplanin, the macrolides erythromycin and its newer analogs, and the lincosamides such as clindamycin. Cell wall–active agents with limited activities against the streptococci include some of the extended-spectrum cephalosporins such as ceftazidime and the cephamycins including cefoxitin, cefotetan, and moxalactam. Some have argued that for serious infections combination therapy with penicillin and an aminoglycoside should be the therapy of choice.[40, 41] These recommendations are based on in vitro observations of the occasionally poor bactericidal activity of penicillin alone, in conjunction with anecdotal observations of clinical failure of single-agent therapy. Many of the reported failures could be explained by problems related to the host rather than the antibiotic. In the case of endocarditis caused by the viridans streptococci, it appears that 2 weeks of combined therapy may be able to substitute for 4 weeks of single-agent (penicillin) therapy in some cases (see Chapter 68). The major exception to this guideline appears to be endocarditis caused by the NDS, which respond less well to penicillin as a single agent.[11] In these cases a combination of penicillin and an aminoglycoside for 4 to 6 weeks appears to be the prudent choice.

References

1. Lawrence J, Yajko DM, Hadley WK: Incidence and characterization of beta-hemolytic *Streptococcus milleri* and differentiation from *S. pyogenes* (group A), *S. equisimilis* (group C) and large-colony group G streptococci. J Clin Microbiol 22:772, 1985.
2. Farrow JAE, Collins MD: Taxonomic studies on streptococci of serological groups C, G, and L and possibly related taxa. Syst Appl Microbiol 5:483, 1984.
3. Ezaki T, Facklam R, Takeuchi N, Yabuuchi E: Genetic relatedness between the type strain of *Streptococcus anginosus* and minute colony forming beta-hemolytic streptococci carrying different Lancefield group antigens. Int J Syst Bacteriol 36:345, 1986.
4. Ruoff KL: Streptococcus. *In* Murray PR, Baron EJ, Pfaller MA, et al (eds): Manual of Clinical Microbiology, ed 6. Washington, DC, ASM Press, 1995, p 299.
5. Ruoff KL, Kunz LJ, Ferraro MJ: Occurrence of *Streptococcus milleri* among beta-hemolytic streptococci isolated from clinical specimens. J Clin Microbiol 22:149, 1985.
6. Salata, RA, Lerner PI, Shlaes DM, et al: Infections due to Lancefield group C streptococci. Medicine (Baltimore) 68:225, 1989.
7. Vartian C, Lerner PI, Shlaes DM, Goplalkrishna KV: Infections due to Lancefield group C streptococci. Medicine (Baltimore) 64:75, 1988.
8. Coykendall AL, Wesbecher PM, Gustafson KB: "*Streptococcus milleri,*" *Streptococcus constellatus,* and *Streptococcus intermedius* are later synonyms of *Streptococcus anginosus.* Int J Syst Bacteriol 37:222, 1987.
9. Gossling, J: Occurrence and pathogenicity of the *Streptococcus milleri* group. Rev Infect Dis 10:257, 1988.
10. Ruoff KL: *Streptococcus anginosus* ("*Streptococcus milleri*"): The unrecognized pathogen. Clin Microbiol Rev 1:102, 1988.
11. Hardie JM: Genus *Streptococcus* Rosenbach 1884, 22. *In* Sneath PHA, Mair NS, Sharpe ME (eds): Bergey's Manual of Systematic Bacteriology, Vol 2. Baltimore, Williams & Wilkins, 1986, p 1043.
12. Whiley RA, Beighton D: Emended descriptions and recognition of *Streptococcus constellatus, Streptococcus intermedius,* and *Streptococcus anginosus* as distinct species. Int J Syst Bacteriol 41:1, 1991.
13. Colman G, Williams REO: Taxonomy of some human viridans streptococci. *In* Wannamaker LW, Matsen JM (eds): Streptococci and Streptococcal Diseases: Recognition, Understanding and Management. New York, Academic Press, 1972, p 288.
14. Facklam RR: The major differences in the American and British *Streptococcus* taxonomy schemes with special reference to *Streptococcus milleri.* Eur J Clin Microbiol Infect Dis 3:91, 1984.
15. Janda WM: Streptococci and "*Streptococcus*-like" bacteria: Old friends and new species. Clin Microbiol Newslett 16:161, 1994.
16. Kilpper-Balz R, Williams BL, Lutticken R, Schleifer KH: Relatedness of *Streptococcus milleri* with *Streptococcus anginosus* and *Streptococcus constellatus.* Syst Appl Microbiol 5:494, 1984.
17. Ruoff, KL: Dealing with viridans streptococci in the clinical laboratory: The continuing challenge. Clin Microbiol Newslett 15:73, 1993.
18. Ruoff KL: The "new" catalase-negative, gram-positive cocci. Clin Microbiol Newslett 6:153, 1994.
19. Knight RG, Shlaes DM: Physiological characteristics and deoxyribonucleic acid relatedness of human isolates of *Streptococcus bovis* and *Streptococcus bovis* (var.). Int J Syst Bacteriol 35:357, 1985.
20. Facklam RR, Sahm DF: *Enterococcus. In* Murray PR, Baron EJ, Pfaller MA, et al (eds): Manual of Clinical Microbiology, ed 6. Washington, DC, ASM Press, 1995, p 308.
21. Holt JG, Krieg NR, Sneath PHA, et al (eds): Bergey's Manual of Determinative Bacteriology, ed 9. Baltimore, Williams & Wilkins, 1994, p 552.

22. Carey RB, Brause BD, Roberts RB: Antimicrobial therapy of vitamin B_6–dependent streptococcal endocarditis. Ann Intern Med 87:150, 1977.
23. Ruoff KL: Update on nutritionally variant streptococci *(Streptococcus defectivus* and *Streptococcus adjacens).* Clin Microbiol Newslett 12:97, 1990.
24. Bouvet A, Grimont F, Grimont AD: *Streptococcus defectivus* sp. nov. and *Streptococcus adjacens* sp. nov., nutritionally variant streptococci from human clinical specimens. Int J Syst Bacteriol 39:290, 1989.
25. National Committee for Clinical Laboratory Standards: M7–A3. Methods for Dilution Antimicrobial Susceptibility Tests for Bacteria That Grow Aerobically, ed 3, Approved Standard. Villanova, PA, National Committee for Clinical Laboratory Standards, 1993.
26. Farber BF, Eliopoulos GM, Ward JJ, et al: Multiply resistant viridans streptococci: Susceptibility to beta-lactam antibiotics and comparison of penicillin-binding protein patterns. Antimicrob Agents Chemother 24:702, 1983.
27. Horodniceanu T, Buu-Hoi A, Delbos F, Bieth G: High-level aminoglycoside resistance in group A, B, G, D *(Streptococcus bovis)* and viridans streptococci. Antimicrob Agents Chemother 21:176, 1982.
28. Hinnebusch CJ, Nikolai DM, Bruckner DA: Comparison of API Rapid Strep, Baxter MicroScan Rapid Pos ID Panel, BBL Minitek Differential Identification System, IDS RapID STR System, and Vitek GPI to conventional biochemical tests used for identification of viridans streptococci. Am J Clin Pathol 96:459, 1991.
29. Schlievert PM, Bettin KM, Watson DW: Production of pyrogenic exotoxin by groups of streptococci: Association with group A. J Infect Dis 140:676, 1979.
30. Lebrun L, Guibert M, Wallet P, et al: Human Fc(G) receptors for differentiation in throat cultures of group C *"Streptococcus equisimilis"* and group C *"Streptococcus milleri."* J Clin Microbiol 24:705, 1986.
31. Munro C, Michalek SM, Macrina FL: Cariogenicity of *Streptococcus mutans* V403 glucosyltransferase and fructosyltransferase mutants constructed by allelic exchange. Infect Immun 59:2316, 1991.
32. Munro CF, Macrina FL: Sucrose-derived exopolysaccharides of *Streptococcus mutans* V403 contribute to infectivity in endocarditis. Mol Microbiol 8:133, 1993.
33. Wells VD, Munro CL, Sulavik MC, et al: Infectivity of a glucan-synthesis defective mutant of *Streptococcus gordonii* (Challis) in a rat endocarditis model. FEMS Microbiol Lett 112:301, 1993.
34. Lowrance JH, Baddour LM, Simpson WA: The role of fibronectin binding in the rat model of experimental endocarditis caused by *Streptococcus sanguis.* J Clin Invest 86:7, 1990.
35. Shlaes DM, Lerner PI, Wolinsky E, Gopalakrishna KV: Infections due to Lancefield group F and related streptococci *(S. milleri, S. anginosus).* Medicine (Baltimore) 60:197, 1981.
36. Whiley RA, Beighton D, Winstanley TG, et al: *Streptococcus intermedius, Streptococcus constellatus,* and *Streptococcus anginosus* (the *Streptococcus milleri* group): Association with different body sites and clinical infections. J Clin Microbiol 30:243, 1992.
37. Catto BA, Jacobs MR, Shlaes DM: *Streptococcus mitis:* A cause of serious infections in adults. Arch Intern Med 147:885, 1987.
38. Parker MT, Ball LC: Streptococci and aerococci associated with systemic infection in man. J Med Microbiol 9:275, 1976.
39. Klein RS, Catalano MT, Edberg SC, et al: Association of *Streptococcus bovis* with carcinoma of the colon. N Engl J Med 297:800, 1977.
40. Lam K, Bayer AS: Serious infections due to group G streptococci: Report of 15 cases with in-vitro–in-vivo correlations. Am J Med 75:561, 1983.
41. Lam K, Bayer AS: In vitro bactericidal synergy of gentamicin combined with penicillin G, vancomycin or cefotaxime against group G streptococci. Antimicrob Agents Chemother 26:260, 1984.

GRAM-POSITIVE BACILLI

197

Corynebacteria

Neal Halsey

Characteristics of the Pathogen

The genus *Corynebacterium* contains one important pathogen of normal hosts, *Corynebacterium diphtheriae,* and nondiphtheria corynebacteria, often referred to as diphtheroids, which cause disease principally in persons whose host defenses are altered.[1] The genus has been substantially revised in more recent years with many species reclassified on the basis of ribosomal RNA sequencing.[2, 3] Some organisms formerly classified as corynebacteria have been reclassified as belonging in the *Arcanobacterium* or *Actinomyces* genus. Other species are under consideration for reclassification.[3a, 3b]

Corynebacteria are nonmotile unencapsulated bacilli. The organisms stain gram-positive, but decolorization occurs readily, and they are tapered or slightly curved. Methylene blue stains are particularly useful and bring out the characteristic purple-red metachromatic granules of *C. diphtheriae.* On Gram stains of colonies, many corynebacteria are club shaped, owing to a weakness in one side of the cell wall. The organisms frequently remain attached after division and form sharp angles, resulting in a "Chinese letter" configuration. Biochemical testing is essential for proper identification of individual species. Corynebacteria are generally catalase-positive and do not hydrolyze esculin or gelatin; clinically relevant strains are negative for lactose, xylose, and mannitol utilization.[2]

C. diphtheriae strains are divided into three biotypes *(mitis, gravis, intermedius)* on the basis of colony morphology and biochemical characteristics. Tentative differentiation may be made by colony morphology and the formulation of starch and glycogen in heart infusion broth.[3] The use of antibiotic susceptibility patterns and phage typing has largely been replaced by phage-DNA restriction enzyme patterns, bacterial polypeptide analysis, and DNA probes as epidemiologic markers.[4–8] Although *C. diphtheriae* is not a spore-forming organism, it survives drying and can be transported in silica gel packs at room temperature.[9]

Diphtheria toxin is produced by lysogenized strains of *C. diphtheriae, Corynebacterium ulcerans,* and occasionally other strains; however, toxin-mediated disease is caused primarily by *C. diphtheriae.* The gene sequence of this 62,000-dalton protein has been identified, and the receptor site on the organism for the phage can be identified with molecular techniques.[10, 11]

Epidemiology

Corynebacteria have been identified in all climates and regions of the world. Nondiphtheria corynebacteria, normal inhabitants of the skin and respiratory tract, often produce disease by entering the blood stream through breaks in the skin and seeding of foreign material such as valves, patches, and catheters in the vascular tree or central nervous system. Other specific disease entities are described later. Disease caused by *C. diphtheriae* has been identified in all countries where laboratory facilities are available. *C. diphtheriae* is transmitted from person to person by respiratory secretions or droplets, by direct skin-to-skin contact, and from skin to respiratory tract via hands. Silent carriers of the organisms on skin and in the pharynx are common sources of transmission in outbreaks. In crowded impoverished urban settings and in tropical climates, skin diphtheria has been more common than have respiratory infections.[12–16] Contaminated cow's milk has been identified as a source of *C. diphtheriae* infections and has been a common mode of transmission for *Corynebacterium pseudotuberculosis.* The latter organism has also been acquired by humans in close contact with animals, especially livestock.[17–19] *Corynebacterium aquaticum* is found in freshwater and has been recovered from distilled water.[1, 20, 21]

Diphtheria has occurred principally during the winter months in temperate zones.[22] In tropical climates, infections occur throughout the year, but peaks in disease have been observed in some but not all countries during the rainy season.[23, 24] Cutaneous disease is also less frequent during summer in temperate climates, presumably owing to decreased contact among impoverished persons.[12]

Infants born to immune mothers are protected against toxin-mediated disease for several months by passively acquired maternal immunoglobulin G antibodies.[25] Before routine immunization with diphtheria toxoid, the peak incidence of respiratory disease was in school-age children. After widespread immunization of young children became a reality, the peak incidence shifted to older persons.[26, 27] In most tropical countries, persons often acquire antibodies to toxin through repeated low-grade skin infections.[27a] In the United States, the peak incidence of skin infections has been in persons older than 30 years, and the highest incidence of skin disease has been in coastal regions.[12, 17, 27] Outbreaks have occurred among the homeless populations in urban centers, especially Seattle.[12]

Higher attack rates of both skin and respiratory disease have occurred in populations of lower socioeconomic status in all areas of the world. Contributing factors probably include crowding, skin abrasions, use of less clothing in warm climates, decreased availability of water for hand washing, and lower immunization rates. In the United States and Canada, the incidence of diphtheria has been higher among the native populations.[12, 17, 27] However, the case-fatality rate has been lower in these populations, presumably owing to a high incidence of skin disease. The incidence of the nasopharyngeal carrier state of toxigenic *C. diphtheriae* strains has been similar for males and females, but the incidence of respiratory disease and case-fatality rates have been higher for males. The occurrence of skin infections in persons older than 19 years has been eight times higher for men than for women, presumably because of the larger numbers of homeless men in the population.

The incidence of diphtheria in the United States has diminished to only a few cases per year during the past 25 years (Fig. 197–1); however, many persons have suboptimal immunity and additional outbreaks could occur, especially among homeless persons in coastal cities[12] (see the later prevention section). An epidemic of diphtheria affecting primarily adults involving more than 125,000 cases and 4000 deaths has taken place in the Newly Independent States of the former Soviet Union since 1990[27a] (Fig. 197–2). Factors contributing to this epidemic have included decreased immunization rates in children, the use of adult tetanus and diphtheria toxoid preparations for primary immunization in children in place of full-strength diphtheria-tetanus-pertussis vaccine in some areas, waning immunity among adults who did not receive booster doses, and increased movement of the population after the breaking up of the Soviet Union.[27b] The epidemic appears to have peaked in 1995 in response to intensive efforts to improve immunization of children and adults.

Pathogenesis

Nondiphtheria corynebacteria produce disease principally by colonizing foreign bodies introduced into host tissue (catheters, shunts, prosthetic valves), by attaching to damaged cardiac valves, or by producing systemic infections (e.g., sepsis, abscess, meningitis) in immunocompromised hosts after disruption of the skin.[1, 28–31] Several nondiphtheria corynebacteria cause skin and soft tissue infections and lymphadenitis by direct extension from local breaks in the skin (see the later section on clinical manifestations).

Most disease caused by *C. diphtheriae* is related to toxin

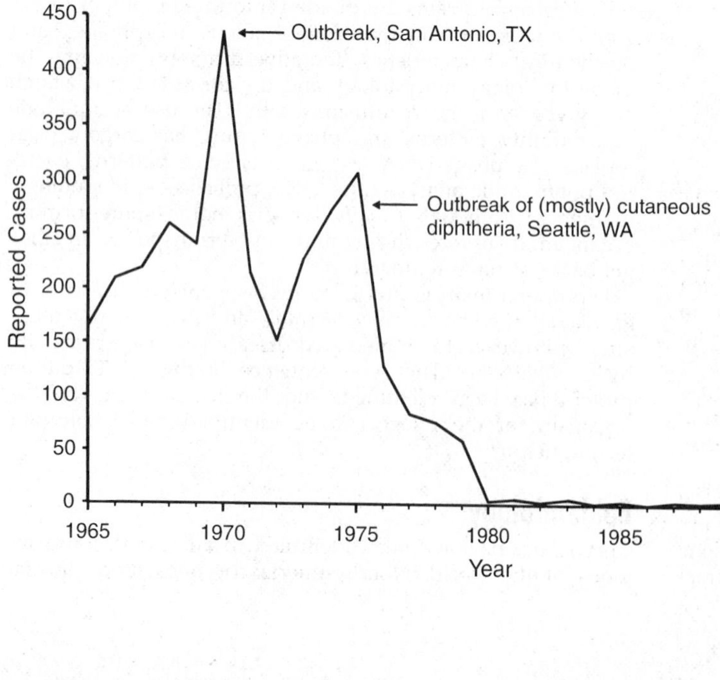

FIGURE 197–1 □ Diphtheria by year in the United States, 1965 to 1995. (From Centers for Disease Control and Prevention: Summary of notifiable diseases, United States 1995. MMWR Morbid Mortal Wkly Rep 44:1–87, 1995.)

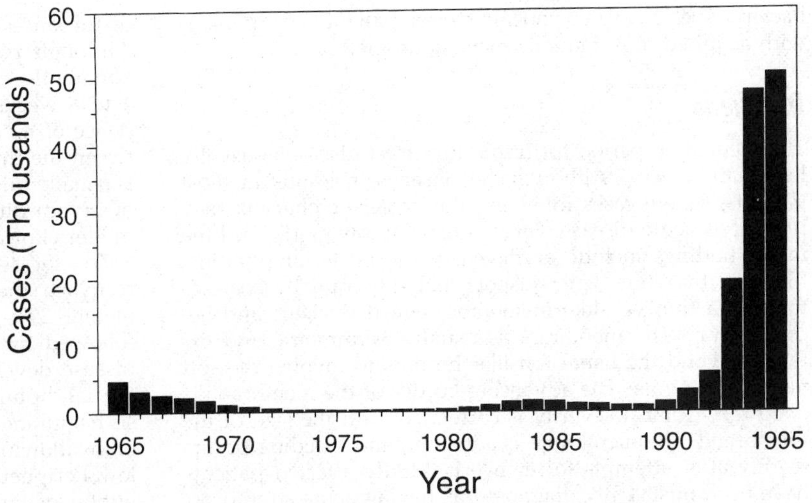

FIGURE 197–2 □ Number of reported cases of diphtheria in the former Soviet Union, 1965 to 1995. (From Centers for Disease Control and Prevention: Update: Diphtheria epidemic—New Independent States of the Former Soviet Union, January 1995–March 1996. MMWR Morbid Mortal Wkly Rep 45:693–697, 1996.)

production and excretion. Diphtheria toxin is a 62,000-dalton protein produced by strains that have been lysogenized by phages containing the genetic material for toxin production.[11, 32] *C. diphtheriae* replicates on the mucous membrane of the respiratory tract or in superficial skin infections and the toxin is disseminated via the blood stream. Toxin induces local cell death, producing more favorable growth conditions for the organism and increased toxin production.[11] The toxin is composed of two fragments. Attachment to specific receptors on host cells is via the B fragment. All cells of the body are susceptible to the action of the active A fragment, but differential effects are noted in tissues, depending on the availability of specific receptor sites.[32] Proteolytic cleavage, usually by trypsin, results in the breaking of two disulfide bonds and release of the A fragment, which enters the host cell by endocytosis. The A fragment catalyzes an enzymatic reaction, binding elongation factor 2 to adenosine diphosphate, and the product becomes irreversibly bound to the surface of ribosomes. Bacteria do not have elongation factor 2 and therefore are not affected by the toxin. The production of protein is stopped by preventing the addition of further amino acids into polypeptide chains. Chang and coworkers[33] found evidence for nuclease activity as an alternative mechanism of cell killing by diphtheria toxin. However, several investigators[34–36] questioned those findings and presented evidence that the nuclease activity was a contaminant in the studies of Chang and colleagues. One molecule of fragment A can produce cell death within a few hours. The fatal dose for humans has been estimated to be 13 μg/kg.[10, 32]

Local tissue necrosis in the respiratory tract results in the formation of a thin gray membrane composed of necrotic cell material, exudative fluid, bacteria, and red and white blood cells. The surrounding tissues become edematous, and local and regional lymph nodes are usually enlarged. Circulating toxin affects all tissues but the organs most affected are heart muscle, kidneys, and peripheral nervous system. Pathologic changes in muscle tissue include lipid accumulation, hyaline degeneration, edema, and mononuclear cell infiltration.[37–39] Muscle regeneration is observed in survivors, but fibrosis is evident in biopsy specimens. Neuronal changes consist primarily of demyelination and tubular necrosis and are found in kidneys.[39] The A subunit of diphtheria toxin has been purified, placed inside microcarriers, and selectively targeted to cancer cells, resulting in clinical responses in animals.[40, 41]

Clinical Manifestations

Disease Caused by Nondiphtheria Corynebacteria

Because nondiphtheria corynebacteria colonize the skin, they are frequently found as contaminants in blood cultures, but septicemia, endocarditis, and other serious diseases are being seen with increasing frequency owing to the growing population of immunocompromised patients and large numbers of patients with catheters and prosthetic devices in vessels and the central nervous system. Neutropenia appears to be the most important predisposing factor for severe systemic diseases, but patients with breaks in the skin who have received prolonged courses of antibiotics are at increased risk for disease.

Species identified lately have been assigned to groups rather than being given specific names. Some organisms have been associated with specific disease entities. Erythrasma, caused by *Corynebacterium minutissimum,* is a commonly diagnosed skin infection.[1] Pruritic reddish brown macular lesions that fluoresce coral-red under a Wood lamp occur in intertriginous areas.

C. ulcerans, formerly thought to be a separate species, is now considered to be a variant of *C. diphtheriae* and causes clinical disease with cardiac and nervous system involvement.[3, 42–44] This organism also causes disease in horses and cattle.

C. pseudotuberculosis produces a dermonecrotic toxin and has been identified as the agent of suppurative granulomatous lymphadenitis in several patients.[3, 18, 19, 45] The organism is a common cause of infections in farm animals, and most affected humans have been persons exposed to cattle or horses or who are consumers of raw milk.[45] Therapy requires a several weeks' course of erythromycin or tetracycline.

Many nondiphtheria corynebacteria species have been shown to cause endocarditis or intravenous line sepsis.[1, 3, 46, 47] *C. diphtheriae* can also cause endocarditis, septic arthritis, and septicemia.[3, 47a, 47b, 47c] Patients with artificial cardiac valves or indwelling vascular catheters are at particular risk and intraocular lenses have been contaminated, leading to endophthalmitis.[48]

Corynebacterium bovis has been associated with meningitis and an epidural abscess.[1, 3, 49] Several species have been associated with ventriculojugular or ventriculoperitoneal shunt infections.[1, 29–31]

Pneumonia has been found to be associated with *Corynebacterium pseudodiphtheriticum, Corynebacterium striatum,* and group JK corynebacteria.[1, 3, 29, 30, 50, 51] Reports of the association with *C. pseudodiphtheriticum* are convincing as sputum cultures have revealed heavy ($\geq 10^7$ colony-forming units/mL) growth, intracellular organisms have been found in neutrophils on Gram stain and by electron microscopy, and responses to appropriate antibiotic therapy have been noted.[50, 51]

Sepsis and abscesses have been caused by several corynebacteria species in neutropenic cancer patients and persons with acquired immunodeficiency syndrome.[3]

Diphtheria

The incubation period for respiratory tract disease is usually less than 1 week. Although the onset is insidious in most patients, severe cases involving the posterior pharynx may present as acute disease. Fever is usually low grade, and the initial findings include erythema of the posterior pharynx, followed by white or gray spots that subsequently coalesce to form a thin veil-like membrane, which thickens and becomes gray. The membrane is usually asymmetric and extends beyond the usual tonsillar borders to involve the soft palate and uvula. The advancing border of the membrane is deep red. Clinical severity is correlated with the size of the membrane. The membrane is adherent, and bleeding occurs readily after attempts to remove it. Mildly affected patients have been mistakenly diagnosed as having acute streptococcal pharyngitis, and simultaneous infections with group A streptococci do occur. The submandibular and anterior cervical lymph nodes are usually enlarged, and soft tissue edema may be present. Severely affected persons have a bull-necked appearance and are at high risk of airway obstruction and sudden death. Severe cases may be complicated by bleeding secondary to thrombocytopenia or disseminated intravascular coagulation.[38, 52] Laryngeal and tracheal involvement may occur primarily or by extension from the pharynx. Hoarseness, respiratory stridor, and dyspnea develop and progress to respiratory obstruction and death in young children unless an artificial airway is provided. Older children and adults are less likely to have complete obstruction because of the larger size of the airway. The membrane may form a cast of the trachea and upper bronchi in severe cases. Nasal diphtheria presents with purulent and often serosanguineous discharge. Nasal diphtheria can be chronic, and patients are efficient transmitters during outbreaks. Otitis media can occur primarily or by extension from the pharynx, and conjunctivitis has been reported. Corneal involvement can be severe, resulting in severe scarring, blindness, and loss of the eye. Cutaneous lesions may resemble a variety of dermatologic conditions, including impetigo, pyoderma, ecthyma, insect bites, and deep, punched-out lesions with a leathery eschar.[12, 53, 54] Underlying conditions that predispose to skin lesions include eczema, psoriasis, scabies, insect bites, human bites, trauma, and surgical wounds.[12] Coinfection with β-hemolytic streptococci and staphylococci is common. Most lesions occur on the extremities, but the trunk and genitals are also affected. Endocarditis has been reported, but bacteremia is exceedingly rare, and almost all systemic complications are due to circulating toxin. Myocarditis and neuropathies are much more common in patients with symptomatic nasopharyngeal diphtheria than in patients with only cutaneous infections; however, the rate of systemic complications from cutaneous infections with toxigenic strains of *C. diphtheriae* is sufficient to warrant antitoxin therapy in most instances.[12]

Myocarditis presents during the second week of clinical symptoms in 20% to 65% of patients. The presentation may be insidious, with progressive weakness and dyspnea, but acute congestive heart failure and circulatory collapse do occur. Physical examination reveals muffled heart sounds and loss of the difference in the first and second heart sounds with progression to cardiac dilatation and a gallop rhythm. Endocardial thrombi may be dislodged, with resultant embolic phenomena. Conduction disturbances are common, ranging from prolongation of the PR interval to bundle branch blocks or complete atrioventricular block. High mortality rates occur in patients with atrioventricular conduction disturbances, and many are left with permanent damage. Although patients often recover completely, cardiac arrest, apparently caused by conduction disturbances, has occurred 4 to 8 weeks after onset. In cutaneous diphtheria the incidence of myocarditis is lower, the onset is usually later (between the third and eighth week of illness), and the disease is usually milder than in pharyngeal diphtheria.[12] A late form of myocarditis with onset in the fourth to sixth week and milder clinical findings is less common.

The incidence of neurologic complications is related directly to the severity of respiratory symptoms. Approximately 20% of all symptomatic respiratory infections are followed by polyneuritis, but 75% of patients with severe disease develop some form of neuropathy. In patients with faucial diphtheria the initial finding is usually palatal paralysis beginning 1 to 2 weeks after onset of symptoms. Paralysis of swallowing and involvement of other cranial nerves follow. Peripheral polyneuritis, with a glove-and-stocking distribution of motor and sensory loss, may resemble Guillain-Barré syndrome. The neuropathy can progress for 1 to 3 months and may take up to 6 months for complete recovery. Residual pharyngeal paralysis occurred in approximately 3% of patients in the preantibiotic era, and rare cases of partial paralysis may present with swallowing disorders.[38, 55, 56]

Diagnosis

In severe cases of pharyngeal diphtheria the clinical diagnosis is not difficult. The presence of an asymmetric gray, adherent membrane with lymph node enlargement and soft tissue swelling in a toxic-looking person should be easily identified as diphtheria. The presence of hoarseness and stridor helps to suggest laryngeal disease. Unilateral palatal paralysis with an exudate is most likely diphtheria.

Laboratory confirmation should be sought for all cases, especially mild ones. Interpretation of Gram stains of scabs from lesions has been discouraged, but some institutions with extensive clinical and laboratory experience have found methylene blue stains of pharyngeal and skin lesions to be sensitive and specific.[12] These stains have allowed rapid decision-making in suspect cases. Cultures should be obtained from under the membrane if possible or by rubbing the surface of the membrane. Because the nasopharynx is usually colonized, culture material should be collected from every patient's nose. In cutaneous disease, cultures should be obtained from more than one skin lesion and from the nasopharynx. Selective media should be utilized to avoid overgrowth by normal respiratory and skin flora.

Corynebacteria grow on the media routinely used to culture organisms from skin, wounds, and throats, but the colonies resemble the abundant normal flora and selective media are needed to distinguish *C. diphtheriae* from other organisms. Suspect infections should be cultured on tellurite-containing agar. Because cystine-tellurite agar may inhibit some *C. diphtheriae* strains, blood agar cultures should also be propagated and colonies should be examined as possible *C. diphtheriae* in suspect cases when no characteristic colonies grow on selective media. Tinsdale medium has been useful in outbreak situations, but its short shelf life precludes routine use. Also, some commercial preparations have been too inhibitory. If selective media are not available, blood agar with a fosfomycin disk can be inoculated.[3] Coryneforms growing in the zone of inhibition should be selected for identification.

Presumptive identification can be made rapidly by examining immunofluorescent-stained specimens from 4- to 8-hour cultures. Classification is based on colony morphology and biochemical profiles, but definitive identification can be difficult.[3]

Toxin production can be demonstrated in vivo by the guinea pig lethality test, and some laboratories use the more rapid Elek test in vitro.[3] Filter paper strips or circles soaked in diphtheria antitoxin (100 units/mL) are allowed to dry on supplemental Elek agar containing 2% sterile rabbit serum and 0.3% potassium tellurite. Suspect colonies are streaked up to the filter paper with appropriate known toxigenic and nontoxigenic control strains on the same plate. Toxigenic strains produce an arrow-shaped line of precipitation pointing toward the filter paper.

Polymerase chain reaction methods have allowed rapid probing of suspect isolates for genetic sequences responsible for producing the B subunit of diphtheria toxin.[57, 57a] Commercial application of these methods would simplify laboratory procedures. Other causes of pharyngeal disease that could cause confusion include group A β-hemolytic streptococcal infections. Although group A streptococci are found in up to one third of pharyngeal diphtheria cases, the appearance of the diphtheria membrane is not changed. The asymmetric appearance of the membrane and involvement of the soft palate and uvula are helpful diagnostic signs. Other causes of exudative lesions include Vincent angina, Epstein-Barr virus, adenovirus, and herpes simplex virus or *Candida* (severe infections) in immunocompromised hosts. A foreign body in the nose of a child results in profuse, foul-smelling nasal discharge. Epiglottitis caused by *Haemophilus influenzae* type b can present in a similar manner, and Ludwig angina, with severe soft tissue infection of the neck, can be caused by mixed mouth flora. The clinical manifestations of retropharyngeal and peritonsillar abscesses can resemble those of diphtheria, and the presence of exudative streptococcal pharyngitis could be confusing. Ulcerative lesions have been seen with chemical or thermal burns of the posterior pharynx.

Treatment

Treatment of nondiphtheria corynebacteria depends on susceptibility testing. Although some species are highly susceptible to penicillins, many corynebacteria are resistant to multiple antibiotics. Initial therapy with vancomycin is encouraged for serious systemic infections, and combination therapy may be necessary.[57b]

Diphtheria

For patients with moderate to severe respiratory disease, initial management must be based on the clinical impression, because delays in therapy can increase the rates of complications and mortality. When antitoxin was administered on the first day of illness, mortality was less than 1%, as compared with 30% when treatment was initiated after 6 days' illness.[38] Diphtheria antitoxin neutralizes circulating toxin but is ineffective against intracellular toxin and toxin that has been bound to cells for more than a short time. There is no effective specific therapy to reverse toxin-mediated neurologic or cardiac disease. Only horse serum antitoxin is available commercially and approved for treatment of diphtheria. Patients should be tested for hypersensitivity before the full dose is administered.

The conjunctival test involves administering 1 drop of antitoxin diluted 1:10 in one eye. Saline is placed in the other eye. Skin testing with a 1:1000 dilution of antitoxin in normal saline can be used for uncooperative infants or adults. If the result is negative after 20 minutes, the full dose of antitoxin is administered intravenously. Desensitization is required for allergic patients. Antitoxin should be diluted 1:20 in physiologic saline and administered at a rate not to exceed 1 mL/min. The dose is dependent on the location and severity of disease and the duration of disease before therapy rather than on the age or weight of the patient. For pharyngeal or laryngeal disease of less than 48 hours' duration, the dose is 20,000 to 40,000 units; nasopharyngeal disease, 40,000 to 60,000 units; extensive disease of 3 or more days' duration, 80,000 to 100,000 units.

Antitoxin has no proven value in cutaneous disease, but toxin-mediated illness occurs and some experts advise administering 20,000 to 40,000 units of antitoxin. Serum sickness occurs in 5% to 20% of patients who receive antitoxin. Intravenous preparations of human immune globulin contain diphtheria antitoxin, but the products have not been evaluated or approved for use in clinical diphtheria.

Antibiotics are administered to prevent further toxin formation, to treat local infection, and to prevent transmission of *C. diphtheriae* to contacts.[57c] Treated patients are usually infectious for less than 4 days, although some remain carriers. Erythromycin, 40 to 50 mg/kg per day (maximum, 2 g/d), is the drug of choice unless large proportions of resistant organisms have been identified in the area.[12] Procaine penicillin G, 600,000 units per day for patients who weigh more than 10 kg, is an acceptable alternative. Severely affected patients should be treated with intravenous penicillin initially. Treatment should continue for 14 days, and elimination of the organism should be confirmed by three consecutive negative cultures after completion of therapy. Rifampin, 600 mg/d for 7 days, has been used successfully to eliminate the carrier state of erythromycin-resistant strains.[12] Recurrent infections have been reported to be associated with erythromycin resistance and chronic dermatoses.[12] It is not known whether these patients had suffered relapse because of inadequate therapy or repeated infection. Material for respiratory tract cultures should be collected 7 days after completion of erythromycin therapy, as up to 20% of patients are colonized at this time.[58] There is a need for clinical trials to determine whether rifampin is more effective than erythromycin for eliminating the carrier state.

Supportive care and management of complications, especially maintenance of an airway, are essential to minimize mortality. Tracheostomy or intubation should be undertaken early in moderate to severe laryngeal disease, and equipment for suction must be available at all times. Sudden obstruction of the respiratory tract by sloughing of tracheal membranes may occur with little notice 48 to 96 hours after initiation of therapy.

Strict bed rest is recommended during the acute phase of pharyngeal diphtheria, to minimize the risks of arrhythmias and exacerbation of myocarditis. Severe cardiac failure can develop rapidly. Digitalis and monitoring for cardiac arrhythmias are indicated for patients with myocarditis. Cardiac pacing may be necessary. Steroids are not effective for the prevention of neuropathy or carditis.[59] Patients with neuropathies require intensive nursing care similar to that provided for quadriplegic patients. Pharyngeal paralysis can lead to difficulty in swallowing. Elevation of the foot of the bed and keeping the patient on his or her side should minimize the risk of aspiration. Because clinical diphtheria does not reliably induce an antitoxin immune response adequate to prevent recurrent disease, all patients should be immunized with diphtheria toxoid.

Prevention

Three doses of diphtheria toxoid are recommended in infancy as part of routine childhood immunization. Diphtheria and tetanus toxoid combined with pertussis vaccine contains 5 to 25 limit flocculation units (Lf) per dose. Three doses are given in the first year of life and boosters at ages 15 to 18 months and 4 to 6 years. Immunity wanes with age, and 10% to 60% of persons older than 30 years have antitoxin levels below the protective level (0.01 IU/mL).[27a, 60–66] Booster doses of tetanus–diphtheria toxoid contain only 1 to 2 Lf diphtheria toxoid and should be administered every 10 years. Unfortunately, many practitioners administer tetanus toxoid alone, contributing to the high rates of inadequate protection in older individuals. Preparations containing 5 Lf diphtheria toxoid induce higher antitoxin levels and are utilized in some Scandinavian countries. Preparations containing less than 6 Lf diphtheria toxoid are less effective for primary immunization of persons who did not receive diphtheria-tetanus-pertussis vaccine during infancy. Immunization does not protect against becoming a carrier during outbreaks, but immune persons do not become ill and harbor small numbers of organisms. In populations with high rates of immunization coverage, reduced rates of carriage are seen and shifts toward nontoxigenic strains have occurred.[67]

Contacts of patients with diphtheria should be observed closely for 7 days, and they should receive erythromycin, 40 to 50 mg/kg per day (maximum, 2 g) for 7 days, or benzathine penicillin intramuscularly, 600,000 units if they weigh less than 30 kg and 1.2 million units for larger patients. Benzathine penicillin is preferred for patients who cannot be depended on for close surveillance. Antitoxin is not indicated for contacts because of the risk of serum sickness. Individuals with inadequate or uncertain immunization status should receive a dose of diphtheria toxoid at the first visit and complete the immunization series with the appropriate product (diphtheria-tetanus-pertussis or tetanus and diphtheria toxoid).

References

1. Lipsky BA, Goldberger AC, Tompkins LS, et al: Infections caused by nondiphtheria corynebacteria. Rev Infect Dis 4:1220, 1982.
2. Colins MD, Jones D, Scholfield GM: Reclassification of *Corynebacterium haemolyticum* (MacLean, Liebow & Rosenberg) in the genus *Arcanobacterium* gen. nov. as *Arcanobacterium haemolyticum* nom. rev., comb, nov. J Gen Microbiol 128:1279, 1982.
3. Clarridge JE, Spiegel CA: *Corynebacterium* and miscellaneous irregular gram-positive rods, *Erysipelothrix*, and *Gardnerella*. *In* Murray PR, Baron EJ, Pfaller MA, et al (eds): Manual of Clinical Microbiology, ed 6. Washington, DC, ASM Press, 1995, pp 357–378.

3a. Funke G, Lawson PA, Bernard KA, et al: Most *Corynebacterium xerosis* strains identified in the routine clinical laboratory correspond to *Corynebacterium amycolatum*. J Clin Microbiol 34:1124, 1996.

3b. Riegel P, Ruimy R, de Briel D, et al: Taxonomy of *Corynebacterium diphtheriae* and related taxa, with recognition of *Corynebacterium ulcerans* sp. nov. nom. rev. FEMS Microbiol Lett 126:271, 1995.

4. Rappuoli R, Perugini M, Falsen E: Molecular epidemiology of the 1984–1986 outbreak of diphtheria in Sweden. N Engl J Med 318:12, 1988.
5. Gruner E, Opravil M, Altwegg M, et al: Nontoxigenic *Corynebacterium diphtheriae* isolated from intravenous drug users. Clin Infect Dis 18:94, 1994.
6. De Zoysa A, Efstratiou A, George RC, et al: Molecular epidemiology of *Corynebacterium diphtheriae* from northwestern Russia and surrounding countries studied by using ribotyping and pulsed-field gel electrophoresis. J Clin Microbiol 33:1080, 1995.
7. Coyle MB, Groman NB, Russell JQ, et al: The molecular epidemiology of three biotypes of *Corynebacterium diphtheriae* in the Seattle outbreak, 1972–1982. J Infect Dis 159:670, 1989.
8. Sacchi CT, de Lemos AP, Casagrande ST, et al: Genetic relationships of *Corynebacterium diphtheriae* strains isolated from a diphtheria case and carriers by restriction fragment length polymorphism of rRNA genes. Rev Inst Med Trop Sao Paulo 37:291, 1995.
9. Kim-Farley RJ, Soewarso TI, Rejeki S, et al: Silica gel as transport medium for *Corynebacterium diphtheriae* under tropical conditions (Indonesia). J Clin Microbiol 25:964, 1987.
10. Uchida T: Diphtheria toxin. Pharmacol Ther 19:107, 1983.
11. Pappenheimer A: The diphtheria bacillus and its toxin: A model system. J Hyg (Lond) 93:397, 1984.
12. Harnisch JP, Tronca E, Nolan CM, et al: Diphtheria among alcoholic urban adults: A decade of experience in Seattle. Clinical review. Ann Intern Med 111:71, 1989.
13. Liebow AA, MacLean PD, Bumstead JH, et al: Tropical ulcers and cutaneous diphtheria. Arch Intern Med 78:225, 1946.
14. Bacon DF, Marples MJ: Researches in western Samoa. II. Lesions of the skin and their bacteriology. Trans R Soc Trop Med Hyg 49:76, 1955.
15. Galazka AM, Robertson SE: Diphtheria: Changing patterns in the developing world and the industrialized world. Eur J Epidemiol 11:107–117, 1995.
16. Bray JP, Burt EG, Potter EV, et al: Epidemic diphtheria and skin infections in Trinidad. J Infect Dis 126:34, 1972.
17. Dixon JMS: Diphtheria in North America. J Hyg (Lond) 93:419, 1984.
18. Richards M, Hurse A: *Corynebacterium pseudotuberculosis* abscesses in a young butcher. Aust N Z J Med 15:85, 1985.
19. House RW, Schousboe M, Allen JP, et al: *Corynebacterium bovis* (pseudotuberculosis) lymphadenitis in a sheep farmer: A new occupational disease in New Zealand. N Z Med J 99:659, 1986.
20. Casella P, Bosoni MA, Tommasi A: Recurrent *Corynebacterium aquaticum* peritonitis in a patient undergoing continuous ambulatory peritoneal dialysis. Clin Microbiol Newslett 10:62, 1988.
21. Moore C, Norton R: *Corynebacterium aquaticum* septicaemia in a neutropenic patient. J Clin Pathol 48:971, 1995.
22. Brooks GF, Bennett JV, Feldman RA: Diphtheria in the United States, 1959–1970. J Infect Dis 129:172, 1974.
23. Chakraborty SM: The incidence and treatment of faucial diphtheria in a rural West Bengal population. J Indian Med Assoc 55:371, 1970.
24. Bennett SW: Investigation of tropical pattern of diphtheria in Buenaventura, Colombia. *In* Proceedings of the International Symposium of Tropical Dermatoses in the Pacific Region; 1966; Tokyo; p 38.
25. Halsey N, Galazka A: The efficacy of DPT and oral poliomyelitis immunization schedules initiated from birth to 12 weeks of age. Bull World Health Organ 63:1151, 1985.
26. Khuri-Bulos N, Hamzah Y, Sammerrai SM, et al: The changing epidemiology of diphtheria in Jordan. Bull World Health Organ 66:65, 1988.
27. Diphtheria Surveillance. Report No 12. Atlanta, Centers for Disease Control, July 1978.

27a. Centers for Disease Control and Prevention: Update: Diphtheria epidemic—New Independent States of the Former Soviet Union, January 1995–March 1996. MMWR Morbid Mortal Wkly Rep 45:693, 1996.

27b. Galazka AM, Robertson SE, Oblapenko GP: Resurgence of diphtheria. Eur J Epidemiol 11:95, 1995.

28. Murray BA, Karchmer AW, Moellering RC: Diphtheroid prosthetic valve endocarditis. Am J Med 69:838, 1980.
29. Johnson WD, Kaye D: Serious infections caused by diphtheroids. Ann N Y Acad Sci 174:568, 1970.
30. Kaplan K, Weinstein L: Diphtheroid infections of man. Ann Intern Med 70:919, 1969.
31. Washington JA II: Bacteriology, clinical spectrum of disease, and therapeutic aspects in coryneform bacterial infection. Curr Clin Top Infect Dis 2:68, 1981.
32. Pappenheimer AM, Harper AA, Moynihan M, et al: Diphtheria toxin and related proteins: Effect of route of injection of toxicity and the determination of cytotoxicity for various cultured cells. J Infect Dis 145:94, 1982.
33. Chang MP, Baldwin RL, Bruce C, Wisnieski BJ: Second cytotoxic pathway of diphtheria toxin suggested by nuclease activity. Science 246:1165, 1989.
34. Bodley JW: Does diphtheria toxin have nuclease activity? Science 250:832, 1990.
35. Johnson VG: Does diphtheria toxin have nuclease activity? Science 250:834, 1990.
36. Wilson BA, Blanke SR, Murphy JR, et al: Does diphtheria toxin have nuclease activity? Science 250:835, 1990.

37. Boyer NH, Weinstein L: Diphtheritic myocarditis. N Engl J Med 239:913, 1948.
38. Naiditch MJ, Bower AG: Diphtheria: A study of 1,433 cases observed during a ten year period at the Los Angeles County Hospital. Am J Med 17:229, 1954.
39. Solders G, Nennesmo I, Persson A: Diphtheritic neuropathy, an analysis based on muscle and nerve biopsy and repeated neurophysiological and autonomic function tests. J Neurol Neurosurg Psychiatry 52:876, 1989.
40. Carroll SF, Barbieri JT, Collier RJ: Diphtheria toxin: Purification and properties. Methods Enzymol 165:68, 1988.
41. Maxwell IH, Maxwell F, Glode LM: Regulated expression of a diphtheria toxin A-chain gene transfected into human cells: Possible strategy for inducing cancer cells suicide. Cancer Res 46:4660, 1986.
42. Meers PD: A case of classical diphtheria and other infections due to *Corynebacterium ulcerans*. J Infect 1:139, 1979.
43. Hadfield TL, Monson MH: *Corynebacterium ulcerans* infection. Clin Microbiol Newslett 5:104, 1983.
44. Siegel SM, Haile CA: *Corynebacterium ulcerans* pneumonia. South Med J 78:1267, 1985.
45. Augustine JL, Renshaw HW: Survival of *Corynebacterium pseudotuberculosis* in axenic purulent exudate on common barnyard fomites. Am J Vet Res 47:713, 1986.
46. Wilson AP: The return of *Corynebacterium diphtheriae*: The rise of non-toxigenic strains. J Hosp Infect 30(Suppl):306, 1995.
47. Claeys G, Vanhouteghem H, Riegel P, et al: Endocarditis of native aortic and mitral valves due to *Corynebacterium accolens*: Report of a case and application of phenotypic and genotypic techniques for identification. J Clin Microbiol 34:1290, 1996.
47a. Pennie RA, Malik AS, Wilcox L: Misidentification of toxigenic *Corynebacterium diphtheriae* as a *Corynebacterium* species with low virulence in a child with endocarditis. J Clin Microbiol 34:1275, 1996.
47b. Tiley SM, Kociuba KR, Heron LG, et al: Infective endocarditis due to nontoxigenic *Corynebacterium diphtheriae*: Report of seven cases and review [see comments]. Clin Infect Dis 16:271, 1993.
47c. Damade R, Pouchot J, Delacroix I, et al: Septic arthritis due to *Corynebacterium diphtheriae*. Clin Infect Dis 16:446, 1993.
48. Doyle A, Beigi B, Early A, et al: Adherence of bacteria to intraocular lenses: A prospective study. Br J Ophthalmol 79:347, 1995.
49. Vale JA, Scott GW: *Corynebacterium bovis* as a cause of human disease. Lancet 2:682, 1977.
50. Andavolu RH, Jagadha V, Lue Y, et al: Lung abscess involving *Corynebacterium pseudodiphtheriticum* in a patient with AIDS-related complex. N Y State J Med 86:594, 1986.
51. Ahmed K, Kawakami K, Watanabe KX, Mitsushima H, et al: *Corynebacterium pseudodiphtheriticum*: A respiratory tract pathogen. Clin Infect Dis 20:41, 1995.
51a. Manzella JP, Kellogg JA, Parsey KS: *Corynebacterium pseudodiphtheriticum*: A respiratory tract pathogen in adults. Clin Infect Dis 20:37, 1995.
52. Wesley AG, Pather M, Chrystol V: The haemorrhagic diathesis in diphtheria with special reference to disseminated intravascular coagulation. Ann Trop Pediatr 1:51, 1981.
53. Belsey MA, Sinclair M, Roder MR, et al: *Corynebacterium diphtheriae* skin infections in Alabama and Louisiana. A factor in the epidemiology of diphtheria. N Engl J Med 176:273, 1969.
54. Liebow AA, MacLean PD, Bumstead JH, et al: Tropical ulcers and cutaneous diphtheria. Arch Intern Med 78:255, 1946.
55. Scheid W: Diphtheria paralysis: An analysis of 2292 cases of diphtheria which include 174 cases of polyneuritis. J Nerv Ment Dis 116:1095, 1952.
56. Obana KK, Fee WE: Unusual pharyngeal lesion causing dysphagia. Ann Otol Rhinol Laryngol 96:527, 1987.
57. Aravena-Roman M, Bowman R, O'Neill G: Polymerase chain reaction for the detection of toxigenic *Corynebacterium diphtheriae*. Pathology 27:71, 1995.
57a. Mikhailovich VM, Melnikov VG, Mazurova IK, et al: Application of PCR for detection of toxigenic *Corynebacterium diphtheriae* strains isolated during the Russian diphtheria epidemic, 1990 through 1994. J Clin Microbiol 33:3061, 1995.
57b. Wilson AP: Treatment of infection caused by toxigenic and non-toxigenic strains of *Corynebacterium diphtheriae*. J Antimicrob Chemother 35:717, 1995.
57c. Farizo KM, Strebel PM, Chen RT, et al: Fatal respiratory disease due to *Corynebacterium diphtheriae*: Case report and review of guidelines for management, investigation, and control. Clin Infect Dis 16:59, 1993.
58. Miller LW, Bickham S, Jones WL, et al: Diphtheria carriers and the effect of erythromycin therapy. Antimicrob Agents Chemother 6:166, 1974.
59. Thisyakorn USA, Wongvanich J, Kumpeng V: Failure of corticosteroid therapy to prevent diphtheritic myocarditis or neuritis. Pediatr Infect Dis 3:126, 1984.
60. Koblin BA, Townsend TR: Immunity to diphtheria and tetanus in inner-city women of childbearing age. Am J Public Health 79:1297, 1989.
61. Bjorkholm B, Wahl M, Granstrom M, Hagberg L: Immune status and booster effects of low doses of diphtheria toxoid in Swedish medical personnel. Scand J Infect Dis 21:429, 1989.
62. Simonsen O, Kjeldsen K, Vendborg HA, Heron I: Revaccination of adults against diphtheria I: Responses and reactions to different doses of diphtheria toxoid in 30 to 70 year old persons with low serum antitoxin levels. Acta Pathol Microbiol Immunol Scand [C] 94:213, 1986.
63. Simonsen O, Klaerke M, Klaerke A, et al: Revaccination of adults against diphtheria. II: Combined diphtheria and tetanus revaccination with different doses of diphtheria toxoid 20 years after primary vaccination. Acta Pathol Microbiol Immunol Scand [C] 94:219, 1986.
64. Jones AE, Johns A, Magrath DI, et al: Durability of immunity to diphtheria, tetanus and poliomyelitis after a three dose immunization schedule completed in the first eight months of life. Vaccine 7:300, 1989.
65. Cellesi C, Zanchi A, Michelangeli C, et al: Immunity to diphtheria in a sample of adult population from central Italy. Vaccine 7:417, 1989.
66. Kjeldsen K, Simonsen O, Heron I: Immunity against diphtheria and tetanus in the age group 30–70 years. Scand J Infect Dis 20:177, 1988.
67. Pappenheimer AM Jr: Diphtheria: Studies on the biology of an infectious disease. Harvey Lect 76:45, 1982.

198

Bacillus anthracis and Other Aerobic Spore Formers

Christopher C. Penn
Stephen A. Klotz

Bacillus anthracis, the agent of anthrax, has been recognized as a pathogen since the work of Davaine, Koch, and Pasteur in the 19th century. The other species of *Bacillus,* with the exception of *Bacillus cereus,* have not been fully appreciated as pathogens in their own right. The genus *Bacillus* is a member of Bacillaceae, a family of aerobic and facultatively anaerobic bacilli. The bacteria are motile by means of peritrichous flagella with the exception of *B. anthracis,* which is nonmotile. Characteristic of the genus is the ability of vegetative cells to form spores (Fig. 198–1). The spores are central, subterminal, or terminal in location and are oval or round. They may cause swelling of the cell in some species but not in *B. anthracis.* The size of vegetative cells varies from a width of 0.4 μm and length of 3 μm in small species to a width of 2.0 μm and length of 9.0 μm in the large species (Fig. 198–2; see Fig. 198–1). Although the majority of species

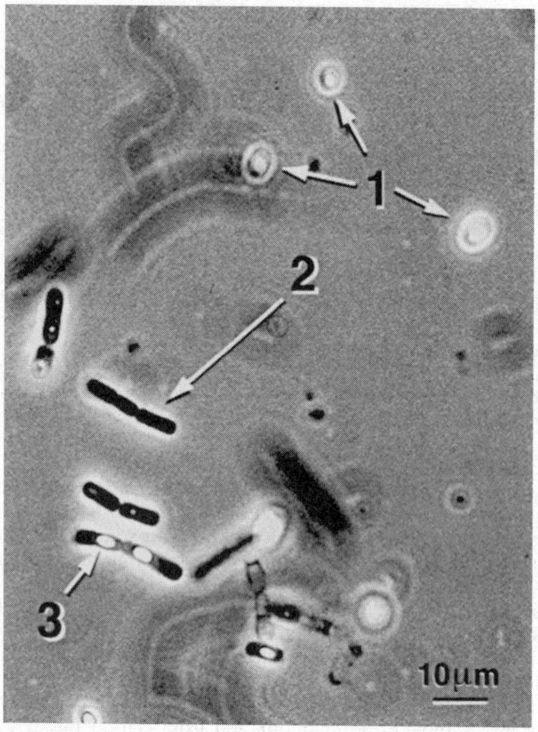

FIGURE 198–1 □ Morphologic forms of *Bacillus anthracis*. Arrow 1, Spores; arrow 2, vegetative forms; arrow 3, spores forming subterminally. (Sterne strain, isolate courtesy of Dr. Max Glass, Bayer, Lenexa, KS.)

are gram-positive, some species are characteristically gram variable on staining.

Bacillus anthracis

Characteristics of the Pathogen

B. anthracis can be provisionally identified by finding large gram-positive rods in cutaneous lesions (see Fig. 198–2). Capsules are always present in tissue specimens. Giemsa, polychrome methylene blue, and India ink stains demonstrate the presence of the capsule. The production of the capsule is mediated by a 60-kDa plasmid. *B. anthracis* grows in extended chains on solid medium, giving rise to the formation of a Medusa head recognized by finger-like projections from the edge of the colonies. It is not encapsulated on a solid medium unless it is grown on nutrient agar containing 0.7% bicarbonate in the presence of increased carbon dioxide. Under these growth conditions it exhibits exuberant capsule formation. Furthermore, in the presence of increased carbon dioxide and bicarbonate, colonies are smooth and mucoid, but in their absence colonies are rough. If grown in a liquid medium containing bicarbonate, *B. anthracis* produces an aromatic acid that colors the medium from brown to red.

The spore of *B. anthracis* is central to subterminal in location and does not swell the vegetative cell. Some strains are asporogenous, but the ability to form spores is independent of virulence. The bacterium is nonmotile, unlike the majority of members of the *Bacillus* genus. It is catalase-positive and almost never causes hemolysis on blood agar. Typical virulent strains of *B. anthracis* can be differentiated from other *Bacillus* species with accuracy by determining the reaction pattern to a battery of preformed substrates, the API 50CH strip (Analytab Products, Plainview, New York) in conjunction with the API 20E strip (Analytab Products). This test can identify 38 species and subspecies of the genus *Bacillus*.[1]

Virulence and Immunity

The capsule is composed of poly-γ-D-glutamic acid, is antigenic but not protective, and can be visualized when stained with polychrome methylene blue (M'Fadyean reaction). *Bacillus subtilis, Bacillus licheniformis,* and *Bacillus megaterium* can also produce capsules in the presence of bicarbonate. *B. anthracis* produces an antigenic exotoxin that is believed to be responsible for many of the clinical symptoms in anthrax. The toxin is tripartite, consisting of edema factor, lethal factor, and protective antigen. The production of each factor occurs in response to the presence of bicarbonate and is sensitive to temperature.[2] Edema factor is an adenylate cyclase, dependent on host cell calmodulin for its activation.[3] The toxin is closely related to, but distinct from, *Bordetella pertussis* toxin, which is also an adenylate cyclase. Protective antigen is required for the effects of both edema and lethal factors to be expressed toward host cells, because edema and lethal factors are biologically inactive in the absence of protective antigen. Toxin production is mediated by a 110-kDa plasmid. Edema toxin is composed of edema factor plus protective antigen and causes edema of the skin in experimental animals. Lethal toxin is composed of lethal factor plus protective antigen and causes pulmonary edema and death in some experimental animals, lyses macrophages, and inhibits growth of cultured cells. Lethal toxin causes a release of numerous cytokines including interleukin-1, and its effects can be negated by the use of interleukin-1 receptor antagonists. Both edema and lethal toxins inhibit superoxide anion release by polymorphonuclear leukocytes. After infection, antibodies are detectable to all four virulence factors (i.e., capsule, edema factor, lethal factor, and protective antigen).

Prevention

Greenfield in London[4] and later Pasteur at Pouilly-le-Fort demonstrated that anthrax could be prevented in livestock by the use of a vaccine containing *B. anthracis* attenuated

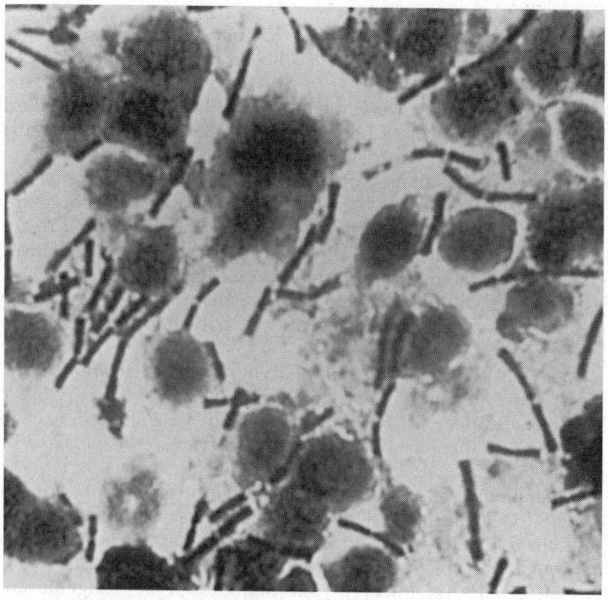

FIGURE 198–2 □ Gram stain of mouse tissue infected with *B. anthracis* demonstrates large, gram-positive bacilli in short chains. (Courtesy of Dr. Gene Luther, Louisiana State University, Baton Rouge, LA.)

through in vitro cultivation.[5] The current, highly effective animal vaccine (Sterne vaccine) is a live spore vaccine derived from an isolate cured of the plasmid required for encapsulation (pXO2$^-$). The human vaccines used in the Western Hemisphere are cell-free filtrate vaccines composed principally of protective antigen. Annual booster injections of both vaccines are required. A live spore vaccine (pXO2$^-$ strain) has been developed and used extensively in the former Soviet Union. This vaccine has been shown to be effective in challenge experiments with humans and in large field trials but has not yet found favor in the Western world.

Infected animals should be quarantined and carcasses burned or buried after being covered with quicklime (calcium oxide). Buildings, work sites, and soil have all been successfully decontaminated. The most effective and widely used decontaminant is formalin.

Care should be taken in handling anthrax bacilli. A biologic hood should be used, as well as gloves. The organism and contaminated containers should be autoclaved or treated with dilute hypochlorite (Clorox) solutions. Laboratory personnel should be alerted by clinicians to the possibility of isolating this microorganism.

Other *Bacillus* Species

Bergey's Manual of Systematic Bacteriology lists 33 other species in genus *Bacillus* in addition to *B. anthracis*.[6] These saprophytic species, in common with *B. anthracis,* form endospores, presumably as a maneuver to survive unfavorable conditions. *B. cereus* and *B. subtilis* are the best known to clinicians among these soil microorganisms, which are thought to play a major role in the natural cycling of carbon and nitrogen. Five *Bacillus* species are primarily insect pathogens, yet even two of these species have caused disease in humans.

The clinical epidemiology and clinical findings usually alert physicians to the possibility of isolating *B. anthracis.* On the other hand, the isolation of one of the other *Bacillus* species is often unexpected, and the laboratorian and clinician must determine whether or not it is a contaminant. The finding of aerobic gram-positive rods that hemolyze blood agar is characteristic of many of the *Bacillus* species. A combination of morphology and special tests is usually sufficient to allow speciation of the isolate. Morphologic features that help to distinguish one species from another are the size of the vegetative cells, the location of spores, and whether or not spores swell the vegetative cells. Special biochemical tests of value in differentiating the species are casein hydrolysis, sugar fermentation reactions, production of lecithinase (phospholipase), nitrate reduction, and the Voges-Proskauer reaction. Vitek (Hazelwood, Missouri), which has one of the automated microbial identification systems, has developed a *Bacillus* card for industry that identifies the more common *Bacillus* species. Further data about the determination of a *Bacillus* isolate to the specific level can be found in *Bergey's Manual of Systematic Bacteriology*[6] or the *Manual of Clinical Microbiology*.[1]

The *Bacillus* species, in particular *B. cereus,* are equipped with an armamentarium of extracellular products such as collagenase, phospholipase C, a hemolysin, and a soluble toxin lethal for mice. In light of these facts it is interesting to note that some authorities consider *B. anthracis* to be only a variant of *B. cereus.* Whether or not *B. anthracis* and *B. cereus* are one and the same species, *B. anthracis* is closely related to *B. cereus, Bacillus mycoides,* and *Bacillus thuringiensis,* which poses difficulties in identification.

In the appropriate circumstances, all *Bacillus* species should be regarded as pathogenic, especially when associated with traumatic wounds (particularly to the eye) and when isolates are obtained from blood culture of intravenous drug abusers. In addition, isolation of these bacteria from febrile, immunocompromised patients should prompt empirical antibiotic coverage and determination by further diagnostic tests, whether or not the isolates are responsible for disease. *B. cereus* is the species most often encountered in these circumstances. The *Bacillus* species can clearly cause nosocomial

TABLE 198–1 ■ Clinical Problems Associated with Gram-Positive Bacilli

CLINICAL PRESENTATION	ASSOCIATED PROBLEMS	GRAM STAIN RESULTS	MOST LIKELY GRAM-POSITIVE ROD	EMPIRICAL THERAPY	REFERENCE
Pneumonia	Ventilator	Gram stain of aspirated material may be positive.	*Bacillus* spp.	Clindamycin or vancomycin plus gentamicin	7
			Corynebacterium spp.	Vancomycin	
Endophthalmitis	Posttraumatic or intravenous drug use	Smears of vitreous humor are positive.	*B. cereus* *B. subtilis*	Clindamycin or vancomycin plus gentamicin (these should be coupled with intravitreal and subconjunctival injection with vitrectomy)	8, 9
	Postoperative	Smears of aqueous humor are positive after lens implantation.	*Propionibacterium acnes* or *Corynebacterium* spp.	Vancomycin	
Keratitis	Contact lens wear or trauma	Scrapings of cornea are positive.	*B. cereus*	Clindamycin plus gentamicin (topical vancomycin)	
Bacteremia	Immunosuppression with central venous lines; intravenous drug abuse	Stain of tip of central venous catheter may be positive (?).	*Corynebacterium, B. cereus, Bacillus* spp.	Vancomycin plus aminoglycoside	10, 11
Skin wound	Posttraumatic	Stain of touch preparation is often positive.	*B. cereus*	Clindamycin or vancomycin plus gentamicin	12
	Postoperative	Stain of touch preparation is often positive.	*Clostridium* spp.	Penicillin	

pneumonia in patients undergoing ventilation and patients with postoperative wound infections as well.

Differential points that aid in determining the role of *Bacillus* species in infections are shown in Table 198–1. This table presents only the more commonly encountered clinical problems. The *Bacillus* species have been reported to cause pneumonia, peritonitis, urinary tract infection, and meningitis.[13, 14]

Drug Susceptibility

Almost all isolates of *B. anthracis* are susceptible to penicillin, and this antibiotic is still considered the drug of choice for treating anthrax (see Chapter 174). Almost all isolates of *B. cereus* and many of the other species are resistant to penicillin but sensitive to numerous other antibiotics. Clindamycin, vancomycin, and gentamicin have had the widest clinical use and the most apparent success, so it appears prudent to include one or more of these three drugs in any empirical regimen. In serious infections it is probably prudent to administer an aminoglycoside in addition to clindamycin or vancomycin. Combination regimens may be synergistic against *B. cereus* ocular isolates.[15] Clindamycin penetrates the vitreous reasonably well and it is probably the current drug of choice for the empirical treatment of *B. cereus* endophthalmitis; however, resistant *Bacillus* species have been reported. Imipenem penetrates the vitreous and aqueous humor to significant levels, and this drug and ciprofloxacin may represent major additions to effective drugs for treatment of *Bacillus* infections.

References

1. Turnbull PCB, Kramer JM: *Bacillus. In* Balows A, Hausler WJ Jr, Herrmann KL, et al (eds): Manual of Clinical Microbiology, ed 5. Washington, DC, American Society for Microbiology, 1991, pp 296–303.
2. Sirard JC, Mock M, Fouet A: The three *Bacillus anthracis* toxin genes are coordinately regulated by bicarbonate and temperature. J Bacteriol 176:5188, 1994.
3. Masure HR, Shattuck RL, Storm DR: Mechanisms of bacterial pathogenicity that involve production of calmodulin-sensitive adenylate cyclases. Microbiol Rev 51:60, 1987.
4. Tigertt WD: Anthrax. William Smith Greenfield, M.D., F.R.C.P., Professor Superintendent, the Brown Animal Sanatory Institution (1978–81). Concerning the priority due to him for the production of the first vaccine against anthrax. J Hyg (Lond) 85:415, 1980.
5. Turnbull PCB: Anthrax vaccines: Past, present and future. Vaccine 9:533, 1991.
6. Claus D, Berkeley RCW: Genus *Bacillus. In* Sneath PHA, Mair NS, Sharpe ME, Holt JG (eds): Bergey's Manual of Systematic Bacteriology, Vol 2. Baltimore, Williams & Wilkins, 1986, pp 1105–1139.
7. Bryce EA, Smith JA, Tweeddale M, et al: Dissemination of *Bacillus cereus* in an intensive care unit. Infect Control Hosp Epidemiol 14:459, 1993.
8. Davey RT Jr, Tauber WB: Posttraumatic endophthalmitis: The emerging role of *Bacillus cereus* infection. Rev Infect Dis 9:110, 1987.
9. Pulido JS, Hyndiuk RA: *Bacillus* species infections. *In* Fraunfelder FT, Roy FH, Grove J (eds): Current Ocular Therapy. Philadelphia, WB Saunders, 1995, pp 9–11.
10. Cotton DJ, Gill VJ, Marshall DJ, et al: Clinical features and therapeutic interventions in 17 cases of *Bacillus* bacteremia in an immunosuppressed patient population. J Clin Microbiol 25:672, 1987.
11. Banerjee C, Bustamante CI, Wharton R, et al: *Bacillus* infections in patients with cancer. Arch Intern Med 148:1769, 1988.
12. Wong MT, Dolan MJ: Significant infections due to *Bacillus* species following abrasions associated with motor vehicle–related trauma. Clin Infect Dis 15:855, 1992.
13. Tauzon CU, Murray HW, Levy C, et al: Serious infections from *Bacillus* sp. JAMA 241:1137, 1979.
14. Drobniewski FA: *Bacillus cereus* and related species. Clin Microbiol Rev 6:324, 1993.
15. Gignatelli JW, Gomez JT, Osato MS: In vitro susceptibilities of ocular *Bacillus cereus* isolates to clindamycin, gentamicin, and vancomycin alone or in combination. Antimicrob Agents Chemother 35:201, 1991.

Suggested Reference Source for *Bacillus anthracis*

- Turnbull PCB (ed): Proceedings of the International Workshop on Anthrax. Wiltshire, England, Salisbury Printing, 1990.

199

Listeria monocytogenes

Claire Broome
Robert Pinner
Anne Schuchat

Listeria monocytogenes has been recognized as a human pathogen since 1929, but food-borne outbreaks and ensuing concern about food safety have brought this bacterium into the spotlight. An intracellular pathogen, *L. monocytogenes* has provided a classic model for investigating cell-mediated immunity. Comprehensive reviews of the epidemiology[1] and pathogenesis[2] of listeriosis have been published.

Characteristics of the Pathogen

Taxonomic work has demonstrated that the genus *Listeria* is located in the *Clostridium* subbranch, which also includes the genera *Staphylococcus, Streptococcus,* and *Lactobacillus.*[3] The genus *Listeria* comprises six species: *L. monocytogenes, Listeria innocua, Listeria ivanovii* (subspecies *ivanovii* and *londoniensis*), *Listeria welshimeri,* and *Listeria seeligeri* are genetically closely related to one another, whereas *Listeria grayii* stands apart. Virtually all human disease is caused by *L. monocytogenes;* rare cases of human disease caused by *L. ivanovii, L. seeligeri,* and *L. welshimeri* have been reported.

Listeria organisms are gram-positive, non–spore-forming rods that are aerobic and facultatively anaerobic. The organisms are 0.4 to 0.5 μm in diameter and 0.5 to 2.0 μm long. In older cultures, filaments up to 20 μm or more may develop; some cells in older cultures may lose the ability to retain the Gram stain. *Listeria* organisms have one to five peritrichous flagella, which produce a "tumbling" motility in cultures grown at 20°C to 25°C and a characteristic "umbrella" below the surface of motility medium. The organisms grow readily on the usual bacteriologic media for isolations from sterile sites, although they do not grow on selective media typically used to isolate agents causing diarrhea from stool cultures, which inhibit growth of gram-positive bacteria such as *Listeria.* They grow best at neutral to slightly alkaline pH but die at pH below 5.5. *Listeria* species grow optimally between

30°C and 37°C but are capable of growth at the wide range of 1°C to 45°C. The ability of these bacteria to grow better than other bacteria at low temperatures formed the basis for cold enrichment, a method now mainly of historic interest for isolating *Listeria* from nonsterile sites, foods, or environmental specimens. A variety of selective media and techniques have been developed and are currently used to enhance the yield of *Listeria* from nonsterile sites.[3]

Colonies of *L. monocytogenes* on blood-free agar have a characteristic blue-green sheen when viewed in obliquely transmitted light. On blood agar, *L. monocytogenes*, as well as *L. ivanovii* and *L. seeligeri*, shows beta hemolysis.

Biochemical features of *L. monocytogenes* include catalase positivity, oxidase negativity, fermentative metabolism, methyl red positivity, and Voges-Proskauer reaction positivity. The CAMP test (named after the original investigators who described the test: Christie, Atkins, and Munch-Petersen) can be used to distinguish among the hemolysis patterns produced by the various species of *Listeria*.[4] Table 199–1 lists biochemical characteristics of the species of *Listeria*.[3]

Strains of *L. monocytogenes* can be classified by several methods. A serotyping scheme based on both cellular O and flagellar H antigens defines 13 different serotypes; however, because only three of these (1/2a, 1/2b, and 4b) account for about 95% of all human cases of listeriosis, serotyping is of limited value for epidemiologic studies. Other, more discriminating methods have been devised to further classify *Listeria*, including phage typing, multilocus enzyme electrophoretic analysis, subtyping based on patterns of endonuclease restriction of chromosomal or ribosomal DNA, and polymerase chain reaction–based typing. Because many *L. monocytogenes* isolates were not typeable, phage typing has been of limited utility for epidemiologic studies. Several studies that illuminated the role of foods in outbreaks and sporadic cases of listeriosis have used multilocus enzyme electrophoretic analysis to compare clinical and food isolates of *L. monocytogenes*.[1, 5]

Ecology

L. monocytogenes is distributed widely in the environment. It is a well-known cause of disease among sheep and cattle, in which it causes septic abortion and "circling" disease (basilar meningoencephalitis). Many mammalian and avian species can harbor the organism, and it has been recovered from dust, soil, water, sewage, animal feed, and silage. *L. monocytogenes* has been isolated from many different foods, including meats, vegetables, seafood, and dairy products. In addition, the organism inhabits the gastrointestinal tract of 1% to 5% or more of asymptomatic humans.[6, 7]

Epidemiology

Listeriosis tends to occur in well-defined risk groups—pregnant women, neonates, and immunocompromised adults—but the disease also occasionally occurs in persons who have no predisposing underlying condition.

A multistate active surveillance project conducted by the Centers for Disease Control and Prevention has provided information on trends in listeriosis in the United States.[8] Through regular contact with all acute care hospital laboratories in an aggregate population of 19 million to 34 million to identify bacteriologically confirmed cases, this investigation estimated that the annual incidence of listeriosis in the United States declined from 7.9 cases per million in 1989—or 1965 cases and 481 deaths—to 4.4 cases per million in 1993—or 1092 cases and 248 deaths. Of more than 600 invasive listeriosis cases identified through this surveillance system, 32% occurred in association with pregnancy, affecting pregnant women, newborns, or both. No pregnant women died from listeriosis, but 22% of pregnancy-associated cases resulted in either fetal loss or neonatal death. Among nonperinatal cases, 28% were fatal.

Large studies in the United States, Europe, and Australia demonstrated that the vast majority of patients with nonperinatal listeriosis have immunosuppressive conditions.[9–11] The most common predisposing conditions include immunosuppressive therapy, malignancy, diabetes mellitus, organ transplantation, and in some populations acquired immunodeficiency syndrome. Although listeriosis is not common among patients with acquired immunodeficiency syndrome, such

TABLE 199–1 ■ Characteristics of *Listeria* Species*

CHARACTERISTIC	*L. GRAYI*	*L. INNOCUA*	*L. IVANOVII* SUBSP. *IVANOVII*	*L. IVANOVII* SUBSP. *LONDONIENSIS*	*L. MONOCYTOGENES*	*L. SEELIGERI*	*L. WELSHIMERI*
Beta hemolysis	−	−	++†	++	+	+	−
CAMP test reaction							
Staphylococcus aureus	−	−	−	−	+	+	−
Rhodococcus equi	−	−	+	+	−	−	−
Acid production from							
Mannitol	+	−	−	−	−	−	−
α-Methyl-D-mannoside	+	+	−	−	+	−	+
L-Rhamnose	V	V	−	−	+	−	V
Soluble starch	+	−	−	−	−	ND	ND
D-Xylose	−	−	+	+	−	+	+
Ribose	V	−	+	−	−	−	−
N-Acetyl-β-D-mannosamine			−	+			
Hippurate hydrolysis	−	+	+	+	+	ND	ND
Reduction of nitrate	−	−	−	−	−	ND	ND
Pathogenicity for mice	−	−	+	?	+	−	−
Serotype	S	4ab, US, 6a, 6b	5	5	1/2a, 1/2b, 1/2c, 3a, 3b, 3c, 4a, 4ab, 4b, 4c, 4d, 4e, 7	1/2a, 1/2b, 1/2c, US, 4b, 4d, 6b	1/2b, 4c, 6a, 6b, US

*+, ≥90% of strains are positive; −, ≥90% of strains are negative; ND, not determined; V, variable; US, undesignated serotype; S, specific.
†Usually a wide zone or multiple zones.
Adapted from Swaminathan B, Rocourt J, Bille J: *Listeria. In* Murray PR, Baron EJ, Pfaller MA, et al (eds): Manual of Clinical Microbiology, ed 6. Washington, DC, ASM Press, 1995, p 344.

persons have approximately 280 times the risk of listeriosis of the general population.[9]

Geographic differences have been observed in the incidence of perinatal listeriosis within the United States.[8, 9] The rate of perinatal listeriosis in Los Angeles County has been consistently higher than the rate in other surveillance areas. This geographic variation may reflect differences in dietary habits, host susceptibility, or enhanced diagnosis by obstetric providers in Los Angeles. The Centers for Disease Control and Prevention surveillance project did not find clear evidence of a seasonal pattern, although other reports have observed a peak of listeriosis during the summer months.

Investigations of several outbreaks of listeriosis have enhanced understanding of the epidemiology of this disease (Table 199–2). In 1981, an outbreak in Nova Scotia, Canada, was caused by locally produced coleslaw. Investigation of this outbreak first established listeriosis as a food-borne illness.[12] The epidemiologic investigation of a 1983 outbreak of listeriosis in Massachusetts implicated a particular brand of pasteurized milk.[13] This controversial finding prompted several studies that concluded that properly performed pasteurization is adequate to kill *L. monocytogenes*, but products can be contaminated after pasteurization or if pasteurization is not done properly. The largest outbreak in the United States involved 142 cases in Los Angeles in 1985, the result of consumption of Mexican-style cheese made from contaminated milk that was not adequately pasteurized. Recall of the implicated product ended the epidemic.[14] Several large outbreaks in Europe were associated with ready-to-eat foods—soft cheese, pâté, and pork tongue in jelly.[15–17]

These investigations confirmed that *L. monocytogenes* organisms can cause epidemic food-borne disease, but the role of foods in sporadic listeriosis has been of considerable interest. Epidemiologic and microbiologic studies implicated uncooked hot dogs, undercooked chicken, soft cheeses, and food purchased from delicatessen counters as causes of sporadic listeriosis.[5, 9, 18] Further evidence was provided by a report documenting the isolation of the same rare enzyme type of *L. monocytogenes* from the blood of a patient, an opened package of turkey franks in her refrigerator, and an unopened package of the same brand of turkey franks purchased at a local store.[19] Evaluation of foods collected from patients with listeriosis suggested that foods that are ready to eat, heavily contaminated, or contaminated with serotype 4b are more often associated with cases than are other contaminated foods.[5]

On the basis of well-documented cases of food-borne listeriosis, the incubation period between ingestion of contaminated food and bacteremia is much longer than that for other food-borne illnesses (median of 3 weeks, range of 11 to 70 days).[14, 20] The long incubation period has made it difficult to identify specific food vehicles responsible for sporadic cases. The infectious dose for this organism is not known, and host susceptibility probably alters the number of organisms necessary to produce symptoms. Human feeding experiments are not appropriate for *L. monocytogenes*, given the high mortality associated with infection.

A substantial proportion of listeriosis is due to food-borne transmission, but other modes of transmission occur. Newborns can acquire the organism transplacentally from bacteremic mothers or during passage through an infected birth canal. Some reports have suggested cross-infection in neonatal nurseries,[21] and one common-source nosocomial outbreak was caused by contaminated mineral oil used for infant baths.[22] Cutaneous, nonsystemic infections have occurred in veterinarians and ranchers who have delivered infected and aborted calves and in workers who have handled infected poultry.

Pathogenesis

The pathogenesis of listeriosis involves a complex interaction of host immunologic response, organism factors, and dose. The association of listeriosis with underlying malignancies and immunosuppressive therapy such as corticosteroids implies that cell-mediated immune function plays a key role in the immune response to *L. monocytogenes*. Mackaness[23] used a mouse model of listeriosis in an early demonstration of the phenomenon of cell-mediated immunity to this intracellular pathogen, and later experiments suggested that helper T cells, suppressor cells, and macrophages all figure in the cell-mediated immune response to *Listeria*. Other murine experiments have shown that genetically determined characteristics, age, nutritional status, and pregnancy all affect susceptibility to *L. monocytogenes*.

Listeriosis is one of several diseases that are more common or more severe during pregnancy. The phenomenon may represent an immune compromise that permits tolerance of the fetus and diminishes cell-mediated resistance to certain infections. Whether this immunologic alteration is systemic, local, or both remains uncertain.

Humoral immunity plays a limited role in establishing immunity to *Listeria*. Both immunoglobulin M (absent in newborns) and classical complement activity (low in newborns) appear to be necessary for efficient opsonization of *L. monocytogenes*, suggesting possible mechanisms for the susceptibility of newborns to this infection.[24]

Experimental evidence supports the epidemiologic conclusion that *Listeria* organisms are transmitted by the food-borne route. Listeriosis can be induced in laboratory animals by oral feeding of pathogenic *L. monocytogenes*.[25] Experiments using a rat model of food-borne *Listeria* infection found that cimetidine significantly lowered the infective dose of *L. monocytogenes*, supporting an association found in a few epidemiologic studies of listeriosis and decreased gastric acidity.[26] *Listeria* has also been shown to invade and even multiply in enterocytes, supporting its role as an enteroinvasive pathogen.

Applications of newer technology, particularly transposon

TABLE 199–2 ■ Major Food-Borne Outbreaks of Invasive Listeriosis

DATE	PLACE	NUMBER OF CASES (DEATHS)*	IMPLICATED VEHICLE	REFERENCE
1981	Nova Scotia, Canada	41 (18)	Coleslaw	12
1983	Massachusetts, United States	49 (14)	Pasteurized milk	13
1985	Los Angeles, California, United States	142 (48)	Soft Mexican-style cheese	14
1983–1987	Switzerland	122 (34)	Soft cheese	15
1988–1989	United Kingdom	NA	Pâté	16
1992	France	279 (86)	Pork tongue in jelly	17

*Total number of listeriosis deaths includes stillbirths and spontaneous abortions. NA, Not available.

mutagenesis and tissue culture models of infection, have enhanced understanding of the cell biology of *Listeria* infections and identified several potential virulence factors.[2] After entry into host cells, *Listeria* organisms escape from host cell vacuoles and multiply in the cytoplasm. Listeriolysin O, the best characterized of the molecular virulence determinants of *L. monocytogenes*, appears to participate in the dissolution of host vacuoles. Once free in the cell cytoplasm, the bacteria are soon surrounded by actin filaments, which mediate intracytoplasmic movement and propel them toward the cell surface, where they protrude in pseudopod-like structures. These structures are apparently recognized and phagocytosed by a neighboring cell; this direct cell-to-cell spread reflects at the cellular level the limited role humoral factors play in immunity to *Listeria* infection.

Clinical Manifestations

Listeriosis During Pregnancy

Pregnant women generally have mild clinical illness, but maternal infection can result in intrauterine infection, spontaneous abortion, and neonatal infection (Table 199–3). The most common clinical picture in pregnant women is an influenza-like illness with fever and myalgias, sometimes accompanied by gastrointestinal symptoms. The organism may grow in blood cultures. Listeriosis during pregnancy can cause amnionitis, premature labor, premature rupture of membranes, and stillbirth. Infants with no clinical infection have been born to women treated for listeriosis during pregnancy, suggesting that listeriosis does not invariably affect the fetus and that treatment of maternal cases may prevent adverse pregnancy outcomes.

Listeriosis in Neonates

In contrast to the mild clinical syndrome that usually occurs in pregnant women, in neonates listeriosis can be a serious and often fatal illness. As with disease caused by group B streptococci, two clinical forms of neonatal listeriosis are recognized: early-onset and late-onset disease. Early-onset disease generally occurs in infants infected in utero from bacteremic mothers, whereas infection in late-onset disease may result from passage through an infected birth canal or nosocomial transmission. Early-onset disease usually presents as sepsis rather than meningitis. It often occurs in preterm infants, perhaps causing prematurity. Classically, widely disseminated microabscesses are noted, to which the term granulomatosis infantisepticum has been applied. No findings are specific for neonatal sepsis caused by *Listeria*, but papular skin lesions may occur. Late-onset disease tends to occur in full-term infants of uncomplicated pregnancies. These infants are usually healthy at birth, and symptoms develop several days to weeks after birth. In late neonatal listeriosis, the clinical syndrome is more likely to be meningitis than sepsis. The mortality rate is lower than for early-onset disease.

Nonperinatal Listeriosis

Nonperinatal listeriosis is generally an infection of patients immunocompromised by underlying illness or immunosuppressive therapy,[9, 10] but some patients who develop listeriosis have no apparent immunocompromising conditions. Sepsis and meningitis are the usual clinical presentations of nonperinatal listeriosis. Although meningitis has been reported to be the most common form of listeriosis in adults, bacteremia without meningitis was more common in the Centers for Disease Control and Prevention active surveillance project.[27] Patients with bacteremia generally have fever but may have a variety of symptoms, including myalgias and gastrointestinal complaints. No symptoms or findings are specific for *L. monocytogenes* bacteremia. Central nervous system findings such as tremors, seizures, ataxia, and fluctuating consciousness seem to be characteristic of *Listeria* meningitis, however. In *Listeria* meningitis, the cerebrospinal fluid is abnormal, but a wide range of values may occur for the cerebrospinal fluid white cell count and differential, glucose value, and protein level. Gram stain frequently demonstrates no organisms, so the cerebrospinal fluid profile cannot be used to distinguish *Listeria* meningitis from meningitis caused by other bacteria. Monocytosis is not a characteristic feature of listeriosis. In addition to meningitis, *Listeria* causes other infections of the central nervous system, such as meningoencephalitis, cerebritis, brain stem abscesses, and spinal cord abscesses. Brain stem encephalitis (rhombencephalitis) is characterized by asymmetric cranial nerve palsies, cerebellar signs, motor or sensory loss, and impaired consciousness.[28] *Listeria* endocarditis resembles other forms of subacute endocarditis; it usually occurs in patients who previously had valvular disease. A variety of focal infections with *L. monocytogenes* have been reported, including endophthalmitis, septic arthritis, osteomyelitis, liver abscesses, cholecystitis, hepatitis, peritonitis, pleuropulmonary infection, and arterial infections.

Mild Gastrointestinal Illness

Investigators have speculated that *L. monocytogenes*, like other food-borne pathogens, may cause a mild gastrointestinal syndrome, distinct from the well-documented invasive disease syndromes. However, the role of *L. monocytogenes* in acute

TABLE 199–3 ■ Syndromes Associated with Infection with *Listeria monocytogenes*

POPULATION	CLINICAL PRESENTATION	DIAGNOSIS	PREDISPOSING CONDITIONS OR CIRCUMSTANCES
Pregnant women	Fever, ± myalgias ± diarrhea	Blood culture ± amniotic fluid culture	
	Preterm delivery Abortion/stillbirth		
Newborns			
<7 d old	Sepsis, pneumonia	Blood, cerebrospinal fluid cultures	Prematurity
≥7 d old	Meningitis, sepsis		
Nonpregnant adults	Sepsis, meningitis, encephalitis, focal infections	Culture of blood, cerebrospinal fluid, or other normally sterile site	Immunosuppressed, elderly
Healthy adults	? Diarrhea and fever	Stool culture in selective enrichment broth	? High inoculum ? Unusual strains

gastrointestinal illness has been difficult to define. Routine stool cultures, which use selective media that inhibit the growth of gram-positive organisms such as *Listeria*, are not adequate for isolation of the organism. In addition, asymptomatic gastrointestinal carriage is well described.[6, 7] However, investigations of outbreaks of gastrointestinal disease have strengthened the hypothesis that *L. monocytogenes* causes diarrheal illness in normal hosts. Diarrheal illness occurred in healthy adults within 2 days of exposure to heavily contaminated foods, and the same strain of *L. monocytogenes* was isolated from stool specimens and food in one of these outbreaks (Dalton C, personal communication, 1996).

Diagnosis

The diagnosis of listeriosis depends on isolation of the organism from a normally sterile site such as blood or cerebrospinal fluid. Because *L. monocytogenes* may be mistaken for diphtheroid contaminants with Gram stain, complete bacteriologic evaluation is important. From specimens collected from normally sterile sites, *Listeria* grow readily in routine media, and culture results are usually positive within 36 hours. Isolation of *L. monocytogenes* from sites containing other flora may pose problems, however. Selective enrichment media permit isolation of *L. monocytogenes* from stool cultures. Methods using fluorescent antibody reagents and DNA probes coupled with polymerase chain reaction technology may prove useful in identifying *L. monocytogenes* in some specimens. Serologic tests have been neither sufficiently sensitive nor specific to be useful for routine diagnosis in clinical practice. However, serologic assays for antibody to listeriolysin O[29] may be useful in some epidemiologic investigations and have been used to suggest the diagnosis in culture-negative central nervous system infection.[30]

Treatment

The optimal antibiotic therapy of human listeriosis has not been defined by controlled clinical trials. The most commonly recommended therapy is ampicillin; some evidence suggests synergy with the addition of an aminoglycoside, and this combination is often used. Penicillin may be comparably effective.[31–33] Treatment failures are common with cephalosporins, which should not be used to treat listeriosis. *Listeria* organisms are susceptible in vitro to a number of commonly available antibiotics, except cephalosporins, but clinical experience is limited.[34] For penicillin-allergic patients, trimethoprim-sulfamethoxazole may be useful; this combination demonstrates bactericidal activity against *Listeria*, and there have been reports of its effectiveness. Other drugs, including erythromycin, tetracycline, and rifampin, have been suggested. Information is inadequate to judge the use of the newer macrolide antibiotics in listeriosis. Case reports on the use of vancomycin in listeriosis have included both treatment successes and failures. The outcome of antibiotic therapy depends on the severity of the infection; therapy is made difficult because listeriosis often occurs in immunocompromised hosts and because, as an intracellular pathogen, the organism may be relatively inaccessible to antibiotics.

Optimal duration of therapy also remains uncertain. A prudent treatment course is 2 weeks for listeriosis in pregnancy; 2 to 3 weeks for neonatal listeriosis; 2 to 4 weeks for adults with bacteremia; and longer for complicated infections such as meningitis, parenchymal central nervous system infections, or endocarditis.

Prevention

Because *L. monocytogenes* is commonly found in the environment, avoiding exposure to the organism is difficult. For persons at increased risk, however (including those who are pregnant or immunocompromised), several dietary measures can be taken to minimize risk. Such measures include thorough cooking of foods of animal origin, avoiding foods made from unpasteurized milk, and avoiding cross-contamination when handling raw foods of animal origin and foods that are ready to eat without further cooking. Pregnant women and immunosuppressed persons may also choose to avoid soft cheeses, pâté, and other foods that have been epidemiologically linked with listeriosis, such as ready-to-eat processed meats with long shelf lives. Currently, U.S. regulatory agencies recommend recalls when *L. monocytogenes* is detected in processed foods that are available for consumption without further cooking. Food industry approaches to minimizing the risk of food-borne listeriosis, introduced in response to regulatory policy, are temporally related to a decline in the incidence of listeriosis in the United States.[8]

References

1. Schuchat A, Swaminathan B, Broome CV: Epidemiology of human listeriosis. Clin Microbiol Rev 4:169–183, 1991.
2. Portnoy DA, Chakraborty T, Goebel W, Cossart P: Molecular determinants of *Listeria monocytogenes* pathogenesis. Infect Immun 60:1263–1267, 1992.
3. Swaminathan B, Rocourt J, Bille J: *Listeria*. *In* Murray PR, Baron EJ, Pfaller MA, et al (eds): Manual of Clinical Microbiology, ed 6. Washington, DC, ASM Press, 1995, pp 341–348.
4. Seeliger HPR, Jones D: Genus *Listeria* Pirie 1940, 383. *In* Sneath PHA, Mair NS, Sharpe ME, Holt JKF (eds): Bergey's Manual of Systematic Bacteriology, Vol 2. Baltimore, Williams & Wilkins, 1986, pp 1235–1245.
5. Pinner RW, Schuchat A, Swaminathan B, et al: Role of foods in sporadic listeriosis. II: Microbiologic and epidemiologic investigation. JAMA 267:2046–2050, 1992.
6. Kampelmacher EH, van Noorle Jansen LM: Isolation of *Listeria monocytogenes* from feces of clinically healthy humans and animals. Zentralbl Bakteriol Mikrobiol Hyg Abt I 211:353–359, 1969.
7. Schuchat A, Deaver KA, Hayes PS, et al: Gastrointestinal carriage of *Listeria monocytogenes* in household contacts of patients with listeriosis. J Infect Dis 167:1261–1262, 1993.
8. Tappero JW, Schuchat A, Deaver KA, et al: Reduction in the incidence of human listeriosis in the United States: Effectiveness of prevention efforts. JAMA 273:1118–1122, 1995.
9. Schuchat A, Deaver K, Wenger JD, et al: Role of foods in sporadic listeriosis. I: Case-control study of dietary risk factors. JAMA 267:2041–2045, 1992.
10. Skogberg K, Syrjanen J, Jahkola M, et al: Clinical presentation and outcome of listeriosis in patients with and without immunosuppressive therapy. Clin Infect Dis 14:815–821, 1992.
11. Paul ML, Dwyer DE, Chow C, et al: Listeriosis—A review of eighty-four cases. Med J Aust 160:489–493, 1994.
12. Schlech WF, Lavigne PM, Bortolussi RA, et al: Epidemic listeriosis—Evidence for transmission by food. N Engl J Med 308:203–206, 1983.
13. Fleming DW, Cochi SL, MacDonald KL, et al: Pasteurized milk as a vehicle of infection in an outbreak of listeriosis. N Engl J Med 312:404–407, 1985.
14. Linnan MJ, Mascola L, Lou XD, et al: Epidemic listeriosis associated with Mexican-style cheese. N Engl J Med 319:823–828, 1988.
15. Bille J: Epidemiology of human listeriosis in Europe, with special reference to the Swiss outbreak. *In* Miller AJ, Smith JL, Somkuti GA (eds): Foodborne Listeriosis. Amsterdam, Elsevier Science Publishing, 1990, pp 71–74.
16. McLauchlin J, Hall SM, Velani SK, Gilbert RJ: Human listeriosis and pâté: A possible association. BMJ 303:773–775, 1991.
17. Goulet V, Lepoutre A, Rocourt J, et al: Épidémie de listeriose en France: Bilan final et résultats de l'enquête épidémiologique. Bull Epidemiol Hebd 39:13–14, 1993.

18. Schwartz B, Ciesielski CA, Broome CV, et al: Association of sporadic listeriosis with consumption of uncooked hotdogs and undercooked chicken. Lancet 2:779–782, 1988.
19. Centers for Disease Control: Listeriosis associated with consumption of turkey franks. MMWR Morbid Mortal Wkly Rep 38:267–268, 1989.
20. Riedo FX, Pinner RW, Tosca ML, et al: A point-source foodborne listeriosis outbreak: Documented incubation period and possible mild illness. J Infect Dis 170:693–696, 1994.
21. McLauchlin J, Audurier A, Taylor AG: Aspects of the epidemiology of human *Listeria monocytogenes* infections in Britain 1967–1984; the use of serotyping and phage typing. J Med Microbiol 22:367–377, 1986.
22. Schuchat A, Lizano C, Broome CV, et al: Outbreak of neonatal listeriosis associated with mineral oil. Pediatr Infect Dis J 10:183–189, 1991.
23. Mackaness GB: Cellular resistance to infection. J Exp Med 116:381–406, 1962.
24. Bortolussi R, Issekutz A, Faulkner G: Opsonization of *Listeria monocytogenes* type 4b by human adult and newborn sera. Infect Immun 52:493–498, 1986.
25. Schlech WF 3d: New perspectives on the gastrointestinal mode of transmission in invasive *Listeria monocytogenes* infection. Clin Invest Med 7:321–324, 1984.
26. Schlech WF III, Chase DP, Badley A: A model of food-borne *Listeria monocytogenes* infection in the Sprague-Dawley rat using gastric inoculation: Development and effect of gastric acidity on infective dose. Int J Food Microbiol 18:15–24, 1993.
27. Gellin BG, Broome CV, Bibb WF, et al: The epidemiology of listeriosis in the United States—1986. Am J Epidemiol 133:392–401, 1991.
28. Armstrong RW, Fung PC: Brainstem encephalitis (rhombencephalitis) due to *Listeria monocytogenes*: Case report and review. Clin Infect Dis 16:689–702, 1993.
29. Berche P, Reich KA, Bonnichon M, et al: Detection of anti-listeriolysin O for serodiagnosis of human listeriosis. Lancet 335:624–627, 1990.
30. Gaillard JL, Beretti JL, Boulot-Tolle M, et al: Serological evidence for culture-negative listeriosis of central nervous system (Letter). Lancet 340:560, 1992.
31. McLauchlin J, Audurier A, Taylor AG: Treatment failure and recurrent human listeriosis. J Antimicrob Chemother 27:851–857, 1991.
32. Trautmann M, Wagner J, Chahin M, et al: *Listeria* meningitis: Report of ten recent cases and review of current therapeutic recommendations. J Infect 10:107–114, 1985.
33. Cherubin CE, Appleman MD, Heseltine PNR, et al: Epidemiological spectrum and current treatment of listeriosis. Rev Infect Dis 13:1108–1114, 1991.
34. Hof H: Therapeutic activities of antibiotics in listeriosis. Infection 19:229–233, 1991.

200

Erysipelothrix rhusiopathiae

Judith L. Nerad
David R. Snydman

Erysipelothrix rhusiopathiae is a gram-positive bacillus that causes occupationally related skin infections (erysipeloid) and, rarely, septicemia in humans. It is a significant cause of swine morbidity (swine erysipelas). The disease was first clinically described in butchers in 1873 by Fox and Baker, who named it erythema serpens.[1] In 1880, Koch first isolated the organism from infected mouse blood and named it *Erysipelothrix muriseptica*. A few years later, in 1883, Pasteur and Thullier demonstrated that swine could be immunized with a strain of *E. muriseptica,* which would prevent erysipelas in swine. Löffler in 1886 definitively identified *Erysipelothrix* as the causative agent of erysipelas in swine. Rosenbach in 1909 was the first to identify *E. muriseptica* as the pathogen responsible for the human skin disease and named it erysipeloid. He made the association among the human, swine, and mouse diseases, stating, however, that the organisms were different strains. Rickman, at the same time (1909), did not concur but thought that the strains were not sufficiently different on morphologic, cultural, or serologic grounds. This was later confirmed by Kohl in 1940.[2]

Characteristics of the Pathogen

E. rhusiopathiae is a gram-positive, non–spore-forming bacillus that is nonmotile, is facultatively anaerobic, and has no capsule.[3, 4] However, evidence in mice suggests that a capsule may play a role in virulence.[5] It is easily decolorized with Gram stain and may appear gram-negative with gram-positive granules or beads. Rods are usually 0.2 to 0.4 μm in diameter and 0.8 to 2.5 μm long. They can occur singly or in short chains and may form filaments up to 60 μm long. Colonies grow on sheep blood agar (not human blood agar) and form small, nonpigmented, transparent colonies that may be smooth or rough. Smooth colonies are often more coccobacillary or coryneform, whereas rough colonies are often larger, more beaded, and associated with long filaments. *E. rhusiopathiae* causes narrow zones of alpha hemolysis on blood agar. Optimal growth temperature is 30°C to 37°C. The organisms are killed by heating for 15 minutes at 60°C but tolerate cold (35 days at 3°C). The organisms prefer alkaline pH; are able to be grown aerobically or anaerobically; and grow better in 5% serum, low oxygen tension, and enhanced carbon dioxide environments. *E. rhusiopathiae* tolerates a high salt environment and can survive in seawater. Specific nutrients (riboflavin and oleic acid, several amino acids, and glucose) are necessary for growth. On gelatin stab culture at 22°C to 28°C, *E. rhusiopathiae* forms a characteristic "pipe cleaner" or "test-tube brush" growth pattern.

E. rhusiopathiae is catalase-negative, oxidase-negative, and weakly fermentative (Table 200–1). The organisms produce acid from glucose and lactose within 48 hours, but not galactose and fructose. They do not ferment xylose, mannitol, or sucrose. Most strains produce hydrogen sulfide on triple sugar iron agar, a differentiating characteristic from other gram-positive rods. They do not reduce nitrates and are indole-negative.

Serologically, there are heat- and acid-stable type-specific antigens and heat-labile antigens. Twenty-three serotypes are described, types 1 and 2 being most common in swine erysipelas.[6] These antigens are thought to be peptidoglycans.[7]

There are two species in the genus, *E. rhusiopathiae* and *Erysipelothrix tonsillarum*, and strains can be heterogeneous.[6, 8–11] Thus far, only *E. rhusiopathiae* has been reported as a pathogen in humans.

E. rhusiopathiae can easily be confused with *Bacillus, Corynebacterium, Lactobacillus, Listeria,* and *Streptococcus*.[3, 12] Major differentiating factors can be found in Table 200–1.

Epidemiology

E. rhusiopathiae is ubiquitous in nature.[1, 2, 13] It is associated with many types of animals (mammals, birds, fish, insects), organic matter, and water. It causes disease most commonly

TABLE 200–1 ■ Major Morphologic and Biochemical Differentiating Factors Among Gram-Positive Rods

FACTOR	BACILLUS	CORYNEBACTERIUM	ERYSIPELOTHRIX	LACTOBACILLUS	LISTERIA
Quality					
Gram stain	Large rods, square ends, with spores	Pleomorphic	Slender with filaments	Straight rods, few coccobacilli	Short rods with short chains
Rod diameter	1–1.3 by 3–10 μm	0.5–1 by 2–3 μm in palisades	0.2–0.5 by 0.5–2.5 μm	0.5–1.1 by 2–3 μm	0.4–0.5 by 1–2 μm
Colony size	2 mm to several	0.5–1 mm	Rough >1 mm, or smooth 0.5–1 mm	<0.5 mm	0.5–1 mm
Spores	Yes	No	No	No	No
Motility	Usually	Usually	No	No	Yes (20°C–25°C)
Hemolysis	Large zone of beta	Variable	Alpha	Usually alpha	Beta
Atmosphere requirement	Aerobic	Usually aerobic	Facultatively aerobic	Microaerophilic	Aerobic
Biochemistry					
Catalase	Positive	Variable	Negative	Negative	Positive
Oxidase	Positive	Negative	Negative	Negative	Negative
Hydrogen sulfide from triple sugar iron agar	Negative (usually)	Negative	Positive	Negative	Negative
Nitrate reduction	Variable	Variable	Negative	Negative	Positive
Neomycin	Resistant	Variable	Resistant	Resistant	Sensitive
Vancomycin	Sensitive	Sensitive (JK diphtheroids)	Resistant	Variable	Sensitive

in pigs, and its prevention and treatment have a major economic impact on industry relevant to hog marketing.[7] In humans, the major manifestation of *E. rhusiopathiae* infection is erysipeloid; however, septicemia and endocarditis are also seen. More common names for erysipeloid include whale finger, seal finger,[14] speck finger, blubber finger, and fish-handler's disease.[15] The general route of transmission in humans is thought to be by direct contact with contaminated animals, animal products including leather,[16] or soil with a break in the skin. Veterinarians, abattoir workers, fish handlers, farmers, butchers, poultry workers, and housewives handling infected meat or fish are most commonly exposed, but cases have been described in people without known exposures; males predominate over females, probably because of the occupational exposure. Reports of two patients suggest oral transmission: (1) a woman with *E. rhusiopathiae* endocarditis whose consumption of infected pork was her only exposure risk,[2] and (2) a woman with a history of ethanol abuse and subsequent pancreatitis with persistent *E. rhusiopathiae* bacteremia whose consumption of shellfish was her only exposure risk.[17] In humans, the incubation period is 1 to 4 days, rarely up to 1 week.[18]

The organism can persist in the environment,[3, 19] remaining viable for 5 to 15 days in water and for weeks to 3 months in salted or pickled bacon or smoked ham; it has been grown after 9 months in a buried carcass. One study from Lund, Sweden, reported isolation of *E. rhusiopathiae* from 30% to 60% of retail samples of pork, cod, and herring.[20]

Clinical Manifestations

In humans, *E. rhusiopathiae* manifests itself primarily as a skin disease. However, systemic disease has also been reported.[1, 2, 13, 14, 21]

Erysipeloid of Rosenbach[22]

These skin lesions are the most common clinical presentation of *E. rhusiopathiae* infection. They are characterized by a purplish red, indurated lesion usually on the hands or fingers that probably represents the site of inoculation 1 to 3 days prior. The margins are slightly raised and sharp and spread peripherally with central clearing. The area can be swollen, and contiguous lesions may occur despite improvement in the initial area. Hemorrhagic vesicles may be present. Pitting edema and suppuration are rare, and their presence serves to differentiate *E. rhusiopathiae* infection from other cutaneous lesions (cellulitis, erythema multiforme, diphtheria, and anthrax). Lesions may be pruritic or burning and painful. Arthralgia in the area of the lesion occurs. Arthritis may occur concomitantly. Systemic symptoms, diffuse arthralgias, fever, lymphangitis, and regional lymphadenopathy are seen approximately 10% of the time.

A severe, diffuse cutaneous form occurs rarely. This is manifested by similar spreading violaceous lesions with central pallor.[22] Diffuse vesicobullous lesions have also occurred.[22] Patients have systemic symptoms (e.g., fever and lymphadenopathy); however, blood cultures are negative.

Septicemia and Endocarditis[14, 21, 23–25]

These are rare complications of *E. rhusiopathiae* infection occurring less than 1% of the time. Most cases of endocarditis have a documented history of appropriate contact with an infected animal (89%) or an erysipeloid lesion (36%). Bacteremia and septic shock without endocarditis have also been reported.[17, 26–30]

In more than 75% of septicemic cases, acute or subacute bacterial endocarditis develops. Factors predisposing to this condition include a chronic debilitating disease, ethanol abuse (33%), an immunocompromised state (17%),[21] or intravenous drug abuse.[31] The presence of valvular heart disease is less commonly a predisposing factor. Only 40% of *E. rhusiopathiae* endocarditis cases have preexisting valvular disease compared with 60% to 80% of all cases of endocarditis. The aortic valve is affected in about 60% of cases of *E. rhusiopathiae* endocarditis. The disease tends to be virulent, with complications such as aortic valve perforation, myocardial abscess, and heart failure. It is not uncommon for patients with *E. rhusiopathiae* endocarditis to require valve replacement. *E. rhusiopathiae* is the most common cause of native valve endocarditis caused by gram-positive bacilli. Prosthetic valve endocarditis with *E. rhusiopathiae* has also been reported.[32, 33]

Rare Complications

Other complications of *E. rhusiopathiae* infection include diffuse cerebral involvement[34]; intracranial brain abscess[35]; optic neuritis[22]; pulmonary infarction, probably from an infected intravascular source[36]; pericarditis[37]; septic bursitis[38]; osseous necrosis[39]; and chronic arthritis[18, 22] and osteomyelitis.[22]

Diagnosis

Most cases of *E. rhusiopathiae* are diagnosed on the basis of clinical presentation and a history of exposure. Gram stain and culture of skin biopsy specimens yield a definitive diagnosis. Gram-positive rods growing in blood cultures may not be diphtheroids and should be further identified given the appropriate epidemiologic setting. The same can be said for small α-hemolytic colonies growing on blood agar; they could be confused with *Streptococcus viridans.* Besides culturing techniques, identification of *E. rhusiopathiae* DNA by polymerase chain reaction techniques has allowed rapid detection of the organism, especially in commercial slaughterhouses.[40]

Treatment and Prophylaxis

Penicillin is the drug of choice for treating *E. rhusiopathiae* infections.[1, 13, 21] Minimal inhibitory concentrations and minimal bactericidal concentrations to penicillin are in the range of 0.0025 to 0.75 μg/mL. *E. rhusiopathiae* is generally susceptible to all classes of the penicillin family, cephalosporins, and clindamycin. It has variable sensitivity to erythromycin, chloramphenicol, and tetracycline. It is notably resistant to vancomycin (minimal inhibitory concentration greater than 25 μg/mL), aminoglycosides, sulfa derivatives, neomycin, and polymyxin.[21, 41] The minimal inhibitory concentrations of teicoplanin and daptomycin are better than that of vancomycin; however, the activity in vitro is poor.[41] Although clinical data on the quinolones and *E. rhusiopathiae* infections are minimal, ofloxacin (200 mg orally twice daily) was successful in eradicating soft tissue infections,[42] and ciprofloxacin has successfully been used to treat tricuspid valve endocarditis and pneumonia.[23] Studies of in vitro susceptibility of veterinary strains have shown ciprofloxacin to have more activity than norfloxacin.[43]

Uncomplicated skin infections may be treated with either oral penicillin (1 g/d for 5 to 10 days) or intramuscular procaine or benzathine penicillin. The disease is usually self-limited. However, treatment decreases the duration of symptoms and potentially reduces the development of complications.

The recommended antibiotic therapy for endocarditis is 12 to 20 million units of penicillin per day in divided doses for 4 to 6 weeks. Synergy with streptomycin has not been demonstrated. Shorter courses of intravenous penicillin (2 weeks) followed by 2 to 4 weeks of oral penicillin therapy have been reported to be successful. Surgery has been necessary in 36% of cases with *E. rhusiopathiae* endocarditis[21] and should be determined on the basis of general criteria for valve replacement in endocarditis. Despite seemingly appropriate antibiotic therapy, the mortality rate for treated *E. rhusiopathiae* endocarditis is 38%.

In patients who are allergic to penicillin, clindamycin or erythromycin plus rifampin may be the drugs of choice. Two cases of septicemia in penicillin-allergic immunocompromised hosts have been successfully treated with either clindamycin alone for 2 weeks[44] or erythromycin (6 weeks) and rifampin (3 weeks).[38]

At present, there is no effective vaccine against *E. rhusiopathiae* in humans. Protective clothing (gloves, aprons, boots) is helpful in preventing occupational exposure.

References

1. Freland C: Erysipeloid. *In* Braude AI, Davis CE, Fierer J (eds): Infectious Diseases and Medical Microbiology, ed 2. Philadelphia, WB Saunders, 1986, pp 1512–1514.
2. Woodbine M: *Erysipelothrix rhusiopathiae.* Bacteriology and chemotherapy. Bacteriol Rev 14–15:161–178, 1950–1951.
3. Jones D: Genus *Erysipelothrix* Rosenbach 1909, 367. *In* Sneath PHA, Mair NS, Sharpe ME, Holt JG (eds): Bergey's Manual of Systematic Bacteriology, Vol 2. Baltimore, Williams & Wilkins, 1986, pp 1245–1249.
4. Bille J, Doyle MP: *Listeria* and *Erysipelothrix. In* Balows A, Hausler WJ Jr, Herrmann KL, et al (eds): Manual of Clinical Microbiology, ed 5. Washington, DC, American Society for Microbiology, 1991, pp 287–295.
5. Shimoji Y, Yokomizo Y Sekizaki T, et al: Presence of a capsule in *Erysipelothrix rhusiopathiae* and its relationship to virulence for mice. Infect Immun 62:2806–2810, 1994.
6. Takahashi T, Fujisawa T, Tamura Y, et al: DNA relatedness among *Erysipelothrix rhusiopathiae* strains representing all twenty-three serovars and *Erysipelothrix tonsillarum.* Int J Syst Bacteriol 42:469–473, 1992.
7. Wood RL: Swine erysipelas—A review of prevalence and research. J Am Vet Med Assoc 184:944–949, 1984.
8. Feresu SB, Jones D: Taxonomic studies on *Brochothrix, Erysipelothrix, Listeria* and atypical lactobacilli. J Gen Microbiol 134:1165–1183, 1988.
9. Takahashi T, Fujisawa T, Benno Y, et al: *Erysipelothrix tonsillarum* sp. nov. isolated from tonsils of apparently healthy pigs. Int J Syst Bacteriol 37:166–168, 1987.
10. Tamura Y, Takahashi T, Zarkasie K, et al: Differentiation of *Erysipelothrix rhusiopathiae* and *Erysipelothrix tonsillarum* by sodium dodecyl sulfate–polyacrylamide gel electrophoresis of cell proteins. Int J Syst Bacteriol 43:111–114, 1993.
11. Chooromoney K, Hampson D, Eamens G, et al: Analysis of *Erysipelothrix rhusiopathiae* and *Erysipelothrix tonsillarum* by multilocus enzyme electrophoresis. J Clin Microbiol 32:371–376, 1994.
12. Yu PKW, Washington JA II: Identification of aerobic and facultatively anaerobic bacteria. *In* Washington JA II (ed): Laboratory Procedures in Clinical Microbiology. New York, Springer-Verlag, 1985, pp 164–179.
13. Grieco MH, Sheldon C: *Erysipelothrix rhusiopathiae.* Ann N Y Acad Sci 174:523–532, 1970.
14. Proctor WI: Subacute bacterial endocarditis due to *Erysipelothrix rhusiopathiae.* Am J Med 38:820–824, 1965.
15. Auerbach PS: Natural microbiologic hazards of the aquatic environment. Clin Dermatol 5:52–61, 1987.
16. Popugailo VM, Podkin IUA, Gurvich VB, et al: Erysipeloid as an occupational disease of workers in shoe enterprises [in Russian]. Zh Microbiol Epidemiol Immunobiol (10):46–49, 1983.
17. Shuster M, Brennan P, Edelstein P: Persistent bacteremia with *Erysipelothrix rhusiopathiae* in a hospitalized patient. Clin Infect Dis 17:783–784, 1993.
18. Klauder JV: Erysipeloid as an occupational disease. JAMA 111:1345–1348, 1938.
19. David CE: *Erysipelothrix rhusiopathiae. In* Braude AI, Davis CE, Fierer J (eds): Infectious Diseases and Medical Microbiology, ed 2. Philadelphia, WB Saunders, 1986, pp 310–315.
20. Stenstrom I, Norrung V, Ternstrom A, et al: Occurrence of different serotypes of *Erysipelothrix rhusiopathiae* in retail pork and fish. Acta Vet Scand 33:169-173, 1992.
21. Gorby GL, Peacock JE Jr: *Erysipelothrix rhusiopathiae* endocarditis: Microbiologic, epidemiologic, and clinical features of an occupational disease. Rev Infect Dis 10:317–325, 1988.
22. Ehrlich JC: *Erysipelothrix rhusiopathiae* infection in man. Arch Intern Med 78:565–577, 1946.
23. MacGowan A, Reeves D, Wright C, et al: Tricuspid valve infective endocarditis and pulmonary sepsis due to *Erysipelothrix rhusiopathiae* fully treated with high doses of ciprofloxacin but complicated by gynaecomastia (Letter). J Infect 22:100–101, 1991.

24. Venditti M, Gelfusa V, Castelli F, et al: *Erysipelothrix rhusiopathiae* endocarditis. Eur J Clin Microbiol Infect Dis 9:50–52, 1990.
25. Bibler M: *Erysipelothrix rhusiopathiae* endocarditis (Letter). Rev Infect Dis 10:1062–1063, 1988.
26. Ognibene FP, Cunnion RE, Gill V, et al: *Erysipelothrix rhusiopathiae* bacteremia presenting as septic shock. Am J Med 78:861–864, 1985.
27. Fakoya A, Bendall R, Churchill D, et al: *Erysipelothrix rhusiopathiae* bacteraemia in a patient without endocarditis. J Infect 30:180–181, 1995.
28. Asnis D, Bresciani A: Bacteremia due to *Erysipelothrix rhusiopathiae* (Letter). South Med J 85:332–333, 1992.
29. Callon R Jr, Brady P: Toothpick perforation of the sigmoid colon: An unusual case associated with *Erysipelothrix rhusiopathiae* septicemia. Gastrointest Endosc 36:141–143, 1990.
30. Garcia-Restoy E, Espejo E, Bella F, et al: Bacteremia due to *Erysipelothrix rhusiopathiae* in immunocompromised hosts without endocarditis (Letter). Rev Infect Dis 13:1252–1253, 1991.
31. Kramer Mr, Gombert ME, Corrado ML, et al: *Erysipelothrix rhusiopathiae* endocarditis. South Med J 75:892, 1982.
32. Gransden WR, Eykyn SJ: *Erysipelothrix rhusiopathiae* endocarditis (Letter). Rev Infect Dis 10:1228, 1988.
33. Hayek LF: *Erysipelothrix rhusiopathiae* endocarditis affecting a porcine xenograft heart valve (Letter). J Infect 27:203–204, 1993.
34. Silberstein EB: *Erysipelothrix* endocarditis. JAMA 191:862–864, 1965.
35. Torkildsen A: Intracranial erysipeloid (swine-erysipelas) abscess: A variety of abscess not hitherto observed. Bull Hyg 18:1013, 1943.
36. Townshend RH, Jephcott AE, Yekta MH: *Erysipelothrix* septicaemia without endocarditis. Br Med J 1:464, 1973.
37. Quabeck K, Muller J, Wendt F, et al: Pericarditis in *Erysipelothrix rhusiopathiae* septicemia (Letter). Infection 14:301, 1986.
38. Shumack SL, McDonald S, Baer P, et al: *Erysipelothrix* septicemia in an immunocompromised host. Can Med Assoc J 136:273–274, 1987.
39. Klauder JV, Kramer DW, Nicholas L: *Erysipelothrix rhusiopathiae* septicemia: Diagnosis and treatment. JAMA 122:938–943, 1943.
40. Makino S, Ikada Y, Maruyama T, et al: Direct and rapid detection of *Erysipelothrix rhusiopathiae* DNA in animals by PCR. J Clin Microbiol 32:1526–1531, 1994.
41. Venditti M, Gelfusa V, Tarasi A, et al: Antimicrobial susceptibilities of *Erysipelothrix rhusiopathiae*. Antimicrob Agents Chemother 34:2038–2040, 1990.
42. Fritzen T, Marx E, Uy J: Treatment of surgical infections with a modern quinolone: Therapy of soft tissue infections and pneumonia with ofloxacin. Infection 14(Suppl 4):S293–S296, 1986.
43. Prescott J, Yielding K: In vitro susceptibility of selected veterinary bacterial pathogens to ciprofloxacin, enrofloxacin and norfloxacin. Can J Vet Res 54:195-197, 1990.
44. Berg RA: *Erysipelothrix rhusiopathiae* (Letter). South Med J 77:1614, 1984.

GRAM-NEGATIVE COCCI

201

Neisseria gonorrhoeae

Edmund C. Tramont
John W. Boslego

History

Urethritis and its association with copulation was known to biblical authors, thus suggesting that gonorrhea is one of the oldest diseases known. The word gonorrhea comes from the Greek words *gene* ("seed") and *rhoia* ("flow"). *Neisseria gonorrhoeae* was first described in urethral pus by Albert Neisser in 1879. It was soon thereafter isolated on artificial culture media and definitively recognized as the agent causing the clinical disease gonorrhea. Because of the famed British surgeon John Hunter's unfortunate self-inoculation with urethral pus containing both *N. gonorrhoeae* and *Treponema pallidum*, clinical gonorrhea was previously believed to be a variant of syphilis.

Early treatment modalities were rather disparate and included such drastic measures as intraurethral inoculation of heavy metals and other disinfectants. Successful therapy was introduced with the advent of the sulfa drugs during the 1930s, but widespread resistance developed in less than 6 years. In contrast, penicillin's dramatic impact lasted for more than 40 years. In 1944, as little as 50,000 units of penicillin cured gonorrhea and reduced the duration of treatment, which had often required hospitalization,[1] to the few hours of outpatient therapy that we have come to expect.

In 1976, plasmid-mediated penicillinase-producing *N. gonorrhoeae* (PPNG) emerged and quickly rendered penicillin inadequate in some parts of the world. The United States was relatively spared of PPNG, but by 1983 chromosomally mediated penicillin resistance had become widespread enough to render it inadequate in many parts of the United States. The utility of spectinomycin, the first antibiotic to replace penicillin, lasted barely 5 years.[2] Increasing resistance to ceftriaxone and the quinolones, the currently recommended treatments for gonorrhea, have also been demonstrated, although it is not yet clinically relevant.

Characteristics of the Pathogen

N. gonorrhoeae belongs to the family Neisseriaceae, which includes another recognized pathogen, *Neisseria meningitidis* (see Chapter 202) and many nonpathogenic species such as *Neisseria sicca*, *Neisseria subflava*, and *Neisseria flava*.[3]

On Gram stain, *N. gonorrhoeae* characteristically appears as a gram-negative diplococcus (Fig. 201–1). It is a fastidious organism with complex growth requirements that include enriched media, a 3% to 5% carbon dioxide atmosphere (candle jar), and an incubation temperature of 35°C to 37°C. It can be maintained for 5 to 7 days in special transport media,[4] a characteristic that is a boon to outlying clinics with limited access to a nearby laboratory. Gonococci grow in vivo under relatively anaerobic conditions and are capable of growing anaerobically in vitro. As with other bacteria, the growth conditions alter the antigenic makeup of the microorganism.

N. gonorrhoeae produces unusually high levels of catalase, an enzyme that converts hydrogen peroxide into oxygen and water. Hydrogen peroxide is produced by most lactobacilli, which are part of the normal flora of the vagina, and catalase production is likely an important survival mechanism for gonococci.[5]

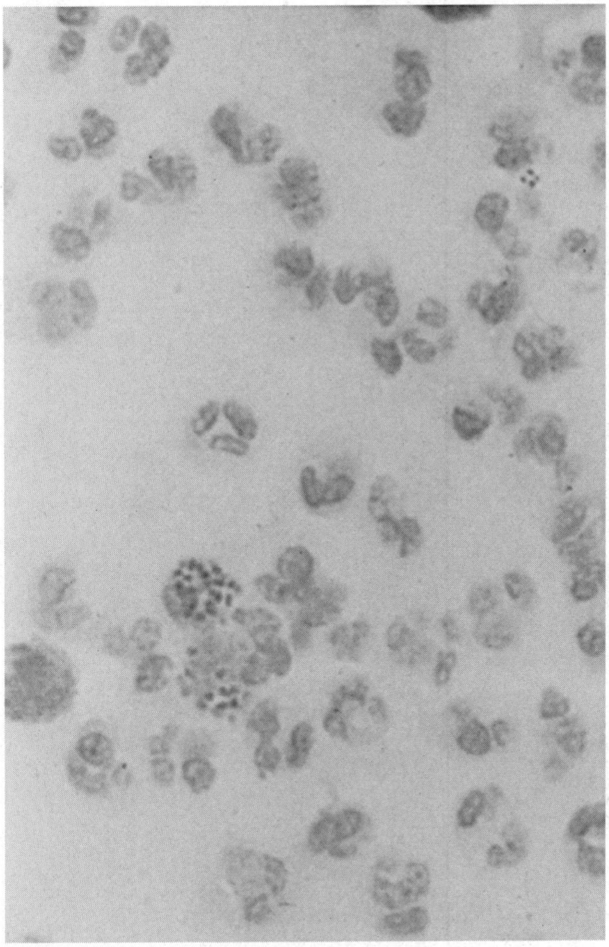

FIGURE 201–1 □ Urethral exudate with gram-negative diplococci.

N. gonorrhoeae also produces an oxidase. Because this characteristic can be easily and quickly identified in the laboratory, gram-negative diplococci obtained from appropriate clinical specimens (e.g., urethral exudate) that are "oxidase-positive" and grow on selective media (supplemented with antimicrobials such as vancomycin, colistin, and nystatin to suppress commensal organisms) are presumed to be *N. gonorrhoeae* by the vast majority of clinical laboratories. Species verification is usually reserved for problem cases (e.g., blood isolates), antibiotic sensitivity testing, and research endeavors.

The "gold standard" for distinguishing *N. gonorrhoeae* from other *Neisseria* species is sugar fermentation patterns (Table 201–1). *N. gonorrhoeae* organisms utilize only glucose, pyruvate, and lactate as carbon sources. Newer and more rapid techniques (see later) have occasionally resulted in misdiagnosis, a potential problem because of the social and medicolegal consequences of infections that are sexually transmitted. Besides other *Neisseria* species, *Kingella denitrificans, Moraxella* species, and *Branhamella (Moraxella) catarrhalis* may be mistaken for *N. gonorrhoeae.*

Colonies examined from cultures of fresh clinical specimens within 16 to 20 hours contain organisms that are piliated (see later) and are designated P^+, P^{++} or T_1, T_2. As colonies incubate longer in vitro or are passed blindly on artificial media, there is a loss of pilus expression and these organisms and colonies are labeled P^- or T_3, T_4). Any colonial type (P^+, P^{++}, or P^-) may also differ in opacity (O^-, O^+, O^{++}, O^{+++}, O^{++++}), owing to the presence of an outer membrane protein termed Opa protein or protein II (see later).

The antigenic characteristics and molecular biology of *N. gonorrhoeae* have been extensively studied. The cell wall (Fig. 201–2) consists of pili, a putative capsule, a number of distinctive outer membrane proteins known as protein I, Opa protein (protein II), protein III (Rmp), iron-regulating proteins, lipooligosaccharide (LOS), and H.8 (Lip), as well as a series of other unnamed proteins induced by varying growth or stress conditions such as reduced or increased oxygen tension[6] and heat.[7] As discussed later, the gonococcus has an impressive array of dynamic mechanisms that it can utilize to adjust to changing environments, including antibiotic pressure and immune pressure.

Pili and Pilin

The pili of *N. gonorrhoeae* are hairlike filamentous appendages about 7 nm in diameter and up to 2.5 μm in length that extend from the cell surface as individual fibrils or fibrillar aggregates. They consist of protein subunits of approximately 160 amino acids,[8] called pilin, which are encoded by the chromosomal gene *pilE.*[9] They are collectively called type IV fimbriae.

Pili are an important virulence factor. In human challenge studies in men, piliate organisms produced classic gonococcal urethritis, but nonpiliate organisms did not.[10, 11] Their primary function is mediating adherence of the gonococcus to the host cell, especially to microvilli of nonciliate columnar cells.[12] It is believed that pili enable the organism to overcome the normal repulsive electrostatic barrier due to the negative charge that exists on most bacteria and host cells.[13]

The gonococcus can switch between a piliate and a nonpiliate state (phase variation), depending on whether pilin genes are being expressed. This expression may also be regulated by proteins that regulate other functions.[14] Obviously, when pilin genes are deleted (a common consequence of prolonged blind passage in vitro) the organism cannot revert to a piliate state.

In addition to this phase variation there is extensive antigenic interstrain and intrastrain variation in pilin, predominantly in the C-terminal portion of the pilin, which can be mediated by many mechanisms. The genes responsible for these tremendous antigenic variations appear to be distributed in a random fashion along the gonococcal chromosome. Antigenic variation may be mediated by insertions and deletions of one to four amino acid residues,[15] or conversion of pilin gene copies into an expression site may give rise to expressed pilin of different antigenic types.[9, 16–20] Furthermore, this variable portion is immunodominant with regard to the primary humoral immune response. As with other organisms, DNA transformation of pilin genes between organisms may also occur.[21] Thus, the gonococcal pilus is engineered for altering the antigenic nature of this important virulence factor and likely represents a major escape mechanism of the organism for evading immune-mediated control by the host. It also appears to be important for selective individual strain tropisms necessary to colonize different hosts and host cells.[22]

In contrast to the C-terminal, the N-terminal region is highly conserved and is homologous to pilin of many other species, including *N. meningitidis, Pseudomonas aeruginosa, Vibrio cholerae,* enteropathogenic *Escherichia coli,* and *Moraxella* and *Bacteroides* species. Expression of these proteinaceous appendages is also associated with a phenomenon known as twitching mobility. This property is due to a protein located in the cytoplasmic membrane encoded by the gene *pilT.*[23]

Because of the demonstrated pivotal role of gonococcal pili in the pathogenesis of clinical gonorrhea, pili were investigated as a potential vaccine candidate. However, despite the

TABLE 201–1 ■ Differentiation of *Neisseria gonorrhoeae* from Related Species That May Be Isolated on Gonococcal Selective Media*

SPECIES	PRODUCES ACID FROM				SUPEROXOL	HYDROXYPROLYL AMINOPEPTIDASE	γ-GLUTAMYL-AMINOPEPTIDASE	NITRATE REDUCTION	DEOXYRIBO-NUCLEASES	COLISTIN SUSCEPTIBILITY
	Glucose	Maltose	Lactose	Sucrose						
Neisseria gonorrhoeae	+	−	−	−	+	+	−	−	−	R
Neisseria meningitidis†	+	+	−	−	−	NA	+	−	−	R
Neisseria cinerea	+‡	−	−	−	−	+	−	−	−	S
Branhamella (Moraxella) catarrhalis	−	−	−	−	−	−	−	+§	+	R‖
Kingella denitrificans	+	−	−	−	−	+	−	+	−	R
Neisseria lactamica	+	+	+	−	−	NA	−	−	−	R
Neisseria polysaccharea	+	+	−	+	−	+	−	−	−	R
Neisseria kochii¶	+	−	−	−	+	NA	−	−	−	R
Neisseria flavescens	−	−	−	−	−	+	−	−	−	R

*R, Resistant; S, susceptible; some strains of *N. cinerea* grow on selective media that do not contain colistin; NA, not available.
†Maltose-negative strains.
‡Some strains produce weak acid reactions that are not delayed and are not glucose-positive in all test systems.
§Reaction is weak or delayed; cannot be performed reliably as a rapid test (unpublished observations).
‖Some strains are colistin resistant and grow on selective media.
¶*N. kochii* grows without CO_2 and at 35°C.
Adapted from Knapp JS: Historical perspectives and identification of *Neisseria* and related species. Clin Microbiol Rev 1:415–431, 1988.

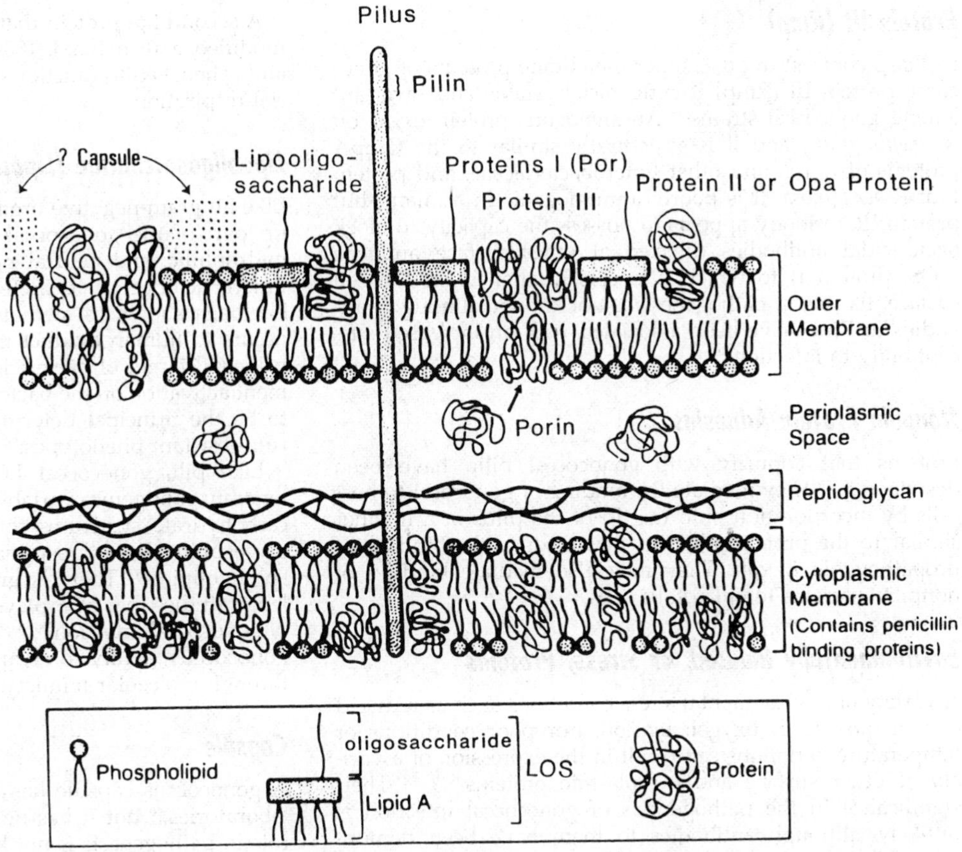

FIGURE 201–2 □ Cell wall of *Neisseria gonorrhoeae.* (Adapted from Hook EW III, Holmes KK: Gonococcal infections. Ann Intern Med 102:229–243, 1985.)

limited success of a pilus vaccine in a human challenge study,[24] and the demonstration of an immune response that blocked pilus function,[25] a phase II field trial failed to demonstrate broad protection,[26] probably because of the extreme degree of pilin antigenic diversity.

Protein I

Protein I, the most prominent outer membrane protein of *N. gonorrhoeae,* ranges in molecular mass from 32 to 37 kDa.[27] It functions as a porin, forming a hydrophilic channel through the outer membrane; it appears to trigger endocytosis of the organism by the host mucosal cell[27, 28] and it may inhibit neutrophil function[28] or moderate attachment to host cells,[27] each of which is an important step in the pathogenesis of gonorrhea (see later). It is located on the cell wall proximate to LOS and protein III, thus making up a unique antigenic constellation.

Unlike most other proteins in the outer membrane surface, protein I is always expressed, and because a single strain produces only one antigenically stable protein I, it has proved to be a useful tool for classifying gonococci. There are two principal subclasses of protein I, known as protein IA and protein IB, that respectively represent a family of structurally related proteins.[29] The most commonly used coagglutination assay employs six protein IA monoclonal antibodies and six protein IB monoclonal antibodies. On the basis of a reaction pattern to a panel of these antibodies, a given strain can be classified into a serovar.[3, 27] At least 24 protein IA and 32 protein IB serovars have been recognized. In any given geographic region, the vast majority of strains belong to a small number of serovars.

Antibodies to protein I develop in both serum and genital secretions.[30–32] Serum antibodies exhibit both bactericidal and opsonic properties.[33, 34] Furthermore, in women this antibody appears to be protective against infection of the same protein I type[35] and serovar.[36]

In addition, organisms with protein IA are more often associated with disseminated gonococcal infection and resistance to the bactericidal action of normal (uninfected) human serum.[37] Conversely, protein IB organisms are more closely associated with urethritis, cervicitis, and increased antibiotic resistance.[38]

Opa Protein, or Protein II

Opa protein, or protein II, is a family of 24- to 30-kDa heat-modifiable outer membrane proteins that manifest extensive intrastrain and interstrain antigenic and phase variation analogous to pilus variation. Opa protein is not always expressed. It imparts to an organism the capability of forming opaque colonies in vitro, a property associated with isolates obtained from the male urethra[39] and from the cervix about midway in the menstrual cycle (day 15). Functionally, Opa protein allows greater gonococcal cell-to-cell adhesion,[40] thus encouraging the formation of an infectious unit, which is possibly an important virulence factor.[41] It appears to enhance adhesion to human conjunctival cells, epithelial cells, and, in particular, neutrophils.[42, 43] When Opa protein is not expressed, the organism forms "transparent" colonies, a characteristic more often found in isolates obtained from asymptomatic and disseminated gonococcal infections,[44] and is associated with increased resistance to killing by normal (uninfected) human serum as well as trypsin. It predominates in cervical cultures obtained at times other than midcycle and in isolates from blood, synovial fluid, and fallopian tubes. Expression is clearly related to environmental growth conditions. The role of these proteins in the pathogenesis of gonococcal infections, especially in determining clinical manifestations, is strongly suggested but not understood.

Protein III (Rmp)

In sharp contrast to other outer membrane proteins of gonococci, protein III (Rmp) is antigenically stable and invariant among gonococcal strains.[45] An analogous protein exists on *N. meningitidis,* and it is structurally similar to the OmpA proteins of *E. coli* and other Enterobacteriaceae, and protein F of *P. aeruginosa.* It is poorly immunogenic in humans, but protein III antibody appears to possess the capacity to block bactericidal antibodies directed at other surface antigens (LOS, protein I) to which it is closely aligned on the cell surface. Its role in pathogenesis is not known, although antibodies to Rmp have been associated with an increased susceptibility to infection.[45a]

Nonpilin Protein Adhesins

Proteins that copurify with gonococcal pilin have been described.[46, 47] They mediate the binding of gonococci to host cells by incorporation onto the tip of the pilus in a manner similar to the protein adhesins that mediate the binding of uropathogenic *E. coli.* They may also mediate binding of nonpiliate strains to eukaryotic cells.

Environmentally Induced, or Stress, Proteins

A variety of environmental stress conditions such as reduced carbon dioxide or oxygen tension, iron-poor conditions or temperature variations can result in the expression of a variety of other surface and cytoplasmic proteins.[6, 48, 49] Their significance in the pathogenesis of gonococcal infection is unlikely, although antibodies to them have been demonstrated in women with pelvic inflammatory disease.[50]

Major Iron-Regulated Protein

Most bacteria, especially those that reside on mucous membranes, must acquire iron from their environment. The major iron-regulated protein of gonococci is a unique 37 kDa protein that scavenges iron directly from the specific host iron binding proteins lactoferrin and transferrin rather than the more common means of other bacteria utilizing siderophores.[51] Antibodies to the major iron-regulated protein have been demonstrated in patients with gonococcal infection. This protein is obviously important for the organism's survival, but its role in pathogenesis remains speculative.

Immunoglobulin A Protease

Many bacteria that normally reside on a mucosal surface, such as the *Neisseria* species, *Haemophilus influenzae,* or *Streptococcus pneumoniae,* produce a protease that cleaves human immunoglobulin A1 (IgA1) at the hinge region.[52] Secretory IgA, significant for its predominance in local mucosal secretions, can thus be rendered inactive. The role of IgA protease in the pathogenesis of gonococcal infections is only speculative at this time. Antibody to IgA protease is uncommon in patients with gonococcal infections.

H.8 Outer Membrane Protein

H.8 (Lip) refers to a conserved and stable epitope contained on two different lipoproteins. H.8 outer membrane protein is present on *N. gonorrhoeae, N. meningitidis, Neisseria lactamica,* and *Neisseria cinerea,* but not on other nonpathogenic *Neisseria* species.[53] The protein consists of a repeating heptapeptide of 22 to 30 kDa. Its exact function is not known. The presence of serum antibody to the H.8 epitope does not protect against a subsequent infection.[54]

A second lipoprotein that contains the H.8 epitope is lipid-modified azurin (Laz). It is present on all *Neisseria* species and is believed to function in electron transport during bacterial respiration.

Lipooligosaccharide (Lipopolysaccharide)

Like all gram-negative organisms, lipopolysaccharide makes up part of the gonococcal cell wall. Because it lacks long, hydrophilic, and neutral polysaccharides that are found in Enterobacteriaceae, it is referred to as LOS.[55] Gonococcal LOS has been shown to mediate most of the toxic damage that occurs to human oviduct mucosa in organ culture. It is the principal target of bactericidal antibodies, regulates complement activation on the bacterial cell surface, and thus appears to be the principal determinant of serum-sensitive and serum-resistant phenotypes.[56]

Like pili, gonococcal LOS exhibits both intra- and interstrain antigenic variability. Some LOS moieties have carbohydrate structures that are analogous to mammalian glycosphingolipids, especially human erythrocyte glycosphingolipids.[57] There is growing evidence in human challenge studies that LOS plays a a key role in the pathogenesis of gonococcal infection[58, 58a, 58b] and may be responsible for the gonococcus' ability to escape an effective immune response through molecular mimicry.[59]

Capsule

A gonococcus capsule has been described by two different laboratories,[60] but it has never been isolated or purified. Its role in pathogenesis is not known.

Plasmids

Most gonococci possess a 2.6-MDa cryptic plasmid.[61] A number of β-lactamase plasmids have been described that independently result in PPNG strains: 4.4 MDa (Asia), 3.2 MDa (Africa), 2.9 MDa (Rio de Janeiro), 3.05 MDa (Toronto), 4.0 MDa (Nîmes, France), and 6.0 MDa (New Zealand). A conjugative plasmid that mediates high-level tetracycline resistance has also been described, 25.2-MDa Tet M. These plasmids have become more prevalent. New plasmids carrying antibiotic resistance determinants are also being found with increased frequency among commensal *Neisseria* species, a precursor of their eventual appearance in pathogenic species.

Epidemiology

Gonorrhea is a sexually transmitted disease and remains a frequently reported infectious disease in the United States (estimated 1 million cases in 1995). Its overall incidence has decreased (Fig. 201–3), in large part because of the decreasing proportion of the population who are between 15 and 30 years of age, behavioral changes coincident with the threat of human immunodeficiency virus, and perhaps decreased transmissibility associated with increasing antibiotic resistance. There is a disproportionately high occurrence of cases among urban minority groups and those caused by penicillin, tetracyclines, and spectinomycin drug-resistant strains, which have rendered these antibiotics inadequate. In some developing countries, the morbidity caused by gonorrhea rivals that of the more traditional tropical diseases. As with all sexually transmitted diseases, the principal risk factor is unprotected sex with many partners or with someone who has had multiple sexual partners.

The need to (1) characterize gonococcal isolates to gain a

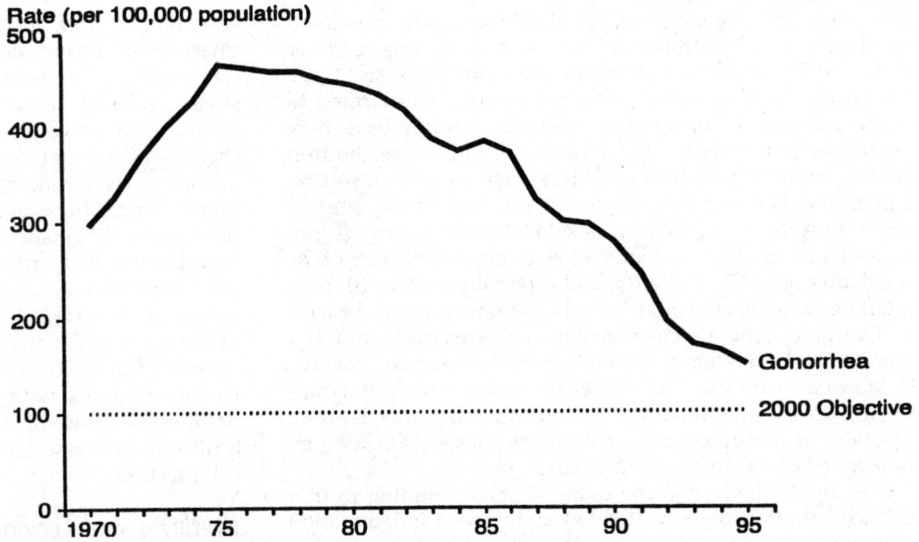

FIGURE 201–3 □ Gonorrhea. Reported rates: United States, 1970 to 1995 and the year 2000 objective. (Data from STD Surveillance, 1995. Atlanta, Centers for Disease Control and Prevention.)

greater understanding of the spread of disease; (2) devise and evaluate strategies to control outbreaks caused by a single strain or a limited number of strains; (3) determine epidemiologic correlates of pathogenicity; and (4) study reinfection versus treatment failure, coinfection, and forensics has resulted in numerous classification strategies (Table 201–2). Antibiograms, the characterization of gonococcal strains by susceptibility to various antibodies and plasmid profiles, are not discriminating enough for most epidemiologic studies. Auxotyping, the characterization of gonococcal strains according to nutritional requirements, also has limited discriminatory utility but has offered some interesting insights. For example, arginine-dependent isolates are rare in the Far East; isolates that require arginine, hypoxanthine, and uracil (AXU), rare before 1950, appear to be predisposed to cause asymptomatic urethral infections in men and disseminated

TABLE 201–2 ■ Characterization of *Neisseria gonorrhoeae* for Epidemiologic Purposes

TEST	COMMENT
Antimicrobial susceptibility patterns (antibiograms)	Quick, easy, broad categories; limited utility, with resistant strains
Auxotyping (nutritional requirements)	Broad categories; certain auxotypes more often associated with certain clinical states; cluster in certain geographic areas
Serologic tests	Historical interest only
Polyclonal antibody	
Monoclonal antibody (utilizes protein I; stable, flexible, destined to be continuously refined and expanded)	
Combined auxotyping plus serotyping (A/S) antibiograms plus auxotyping, or any combination thereof	Provides greater discrimination of gonococcal isolates; can be specifically tailored (e.g., to monitor antimicrobial resistance patterns); method most likely to be used in future
Pulsed-field gel electrophoresis	Stable, reproducible, sensitive

gonococcal infection in both sexes, are susceptible to lower doses of penicillin G, produce type 1 IgA1 protease and *dam* methylase (DNA adenine methyltransferase, EC 2.1.1), grow atypically as small colonies, are normally serum bactericidal resistant, and because they are sensitive to vancomycin at 4 μg/mL they may not grow on selective culture media. Isolates that require proline, citrulline, and uracil (PCU) do not contain the 2.6-MDa plasmid found in most other gonococci.

Pulsed-field gel electrophoresis, utilizing enzymes that cleave the chromosome at rare restriction sites, is the most recently developed technique.[62] It is stable, reproducible, and sensitive. As noted earlier, protein I (Por) serotyping, utilizing a standard panel of protein IA–specific and protein IB–specific monoclonal antibody reagents, has been widely used. The auxotype/serotype (A/S) classification utilizes auxotypes and Por serotyping. The most useful serologic typing system at present utilizes a standard panel of protein IA–specific and protein IB–specific monoclonal antibody reagents[63] alone or in conjunction with other tests.[62] Because no single antigen has yet to be correlated with protective immunity, new, more sophisticated typing systems are continuously being devised.[63a]

Pathogenesis

N. gonorrhoeae is a uniquely human pathogen. It is spread from person to person by contact with infected secretions, most often by sexual contact. Once the pathogen is deposited on a mucosal surface, a complex series of molecular interactions ensue that result in invasion of mucosal columnar cells.[63b] The steps include distant attachment mediated by pili; close attachment, which is most likely mediated by protein I and Opa protein (protein II); ingestion by the host mucosal cell, which is probably also mediated by protein I; transportation through the cell in phagosomes and possible egestion into the submucosa; and, on rare occasions, blood stream invasion (see Fig. 201–3). In organ culture models, the integrity of the epithelial lining is markedly affected, with loss of ciliary motility (mediated by LOS) and extrusion of ciliated cells.

Attachment is the critical first step in establishing infection. Human challenge studies have clearly established the importance of pili and Opa proteins (protein II) in this event,[10, 40] and the rapid selection in vivo of new types of these proteins.[11, 40] It is speculated that these latter events are an adaptation by the gonococcus to selective pressures mediated by diverse host cell tropisms[22, 64, 65] or immune pressures, or both.[64, 65] Pili may also interfere with phagocytosis. Once colonization is established, the gonococcus is well armed to evade mucosal defenses. For example, IgA protease may degrade secretory IgA,[52] the gonococcus can utilize the iron binding proteins transferrin and lactoferrin as an iron source, and bactericidal antibody, the critical protective host immune response to *N. meningitidis,* a close relative of gonococci, can be overcome by blocking antibodies to protein III (Rmp)[45] or sialylation of LOS.[56] Protein I, and especially protein III, may interfere with bactericidal activity. Serum-resistant isolates and variants generate chemotaxins at a slower rate and at a quantitatively smaller concentration than do serum-sensitive isolates and variants. The former is more common in symptomatic (brisk inflammatory) disease and the latter is more common in asymptomatic urethral infection.[57] LOS may be directly cytotoxic to some host cells.

It is highly likely that the tissue damage resulting from a gonococcal infection is related to the degree of inflammation (leukorrhea), making this interaction critical in the pathogenesis. However, despite extensive study, the molecular interaction between the gonococcus and human phagocytes remains elusive.[65] For example, the factors responsible for evoking the intensity of the inflammatory response are only partially understood and the probability and extent of bacterial survival in phagocytes are largely unknown.[65] The induction of leukorrhea correlates well with the expression of LOS, which closely mimics mammalian cell glycosphingolipid.[59] Also, sialylation of the LOS, which can occur during active infection,[56] renders the organism resistant to bactericidal activity.

The host's response is usually inflammatory and brisk,[59a] producing the classic exudate that contains host inflammatory cells (principally polymorphonuclear leukocytes [PMNs]), epithelial cells, and gonococci, most of which have been ingested by PMNs (see Fig. 201–1). However, a mild or even quiescent infection may ensue. The reasons for the modulation of the host response are only partially known and include both host and microbial factors. For example, gonococcal strains isolated from patients with a milder inflammatory response are quite sensitive to antibiotics, have unique nutritional requirements, are more resistant to bactericidal activity, or have limited ability to generate neutrophil chemotactic activity.[64] IgA protease may inactivate secretory IgA, which can block attachment of gonococci to host mucosal cells.[66]

A variety of tests for gonococcal antibodies (serologic tests) that have been developed have repeatedly demonstrated the following: (1) a humoral antibody response is directed at a wide variety of antigens, principally pili, Opa protein, and LOS; (2) a local genital antibody response is less intense; (3) neither the type nor the level of antibody has been correlated with protection; (4) the magnitude and character of the response are not predictable but tend to be more pronounced in women and those with invasive disease (salpingitis, epididymitis, bacteremia); (5) so-called naturally occurring antibody resulting from colonization or infection by other bacterial species is common.[30, 54, 64, 65]

Because repeated gonococcal infections are not unusual, it has been suggested that humans do not develop immunity to gonorrhea. However, a relative resistance to infection has been correlated with a history of previous infection[35, 36] and protein I.[35] Serovar-specific protection has been described,[36] suggesting that at least some modulation of the infection does occur.

Clinical Manifestations

A more complete discussion of the clinical manifestations of gonorrhea is presented in Chapter 110. The spectrum of disease ranges from local infection (urethritis, cervicitis, oropharyngitis) to invasion restricted to sex organs (pelvic inflammatory disease, epididymitis), to invasion of the blood stream, with or without dissemination to distant organs (e.g., joints, heart valves, pericardium) (Table 201–3). Like other organisms that may colonize the oropharynx, gonococci have a tropism for serous membranes such as the synovial membrane, pericardium, aortic valve, and conjunctiva. When the peritoneum is invaded, the gonococcus can cause perihepatitis (Fitz-Hugh–Curtis syndrome). Systemic invasion is usually characterized by a subacute course and a relatively small antigen load, attested to by the difficulty often experienced in attempts to isolate the causative organism from blood or synovial fluid. Gonococcal endocarditis is an exception and usually presents with florid symptoms because there is a predilection to involve the aortic valve. Premature and low birth rates are associated in particular with genital gonococcal infection.[67]

Urethritis and Cervicitis (Urogenital Gonorrhea)

Symptomatic urethritis in men and cervicitis in women are the most common clinical manifestations of gonorrhea. In men, a purulent urethral discharge and dysuria usually develop after a 2- to 5-day incubation period. For women the signs and symptoms of primary gonococcal infection are less specific: vaginal discharge (cervicitis), dysuria and frequency of urination (skenitis or urethritis), and, less frequently, labial pain and swelling (acute bartholinitis) or lower abdominal pain (pelvic inflammatory disease). Symptoms in women are usually most prominent during menses, probably as a result of the increased availability of iron and other nutrients that afford the gonococcus a selective advantage. An asymptomatic infection develops in about 15% of men and 50% of women. Local extension in men most often involves the epididymis (pain, swelling, tenderness, redness). The signs and symptoms of repeated episodes of gonorrhea are almost always less dramatic, especially if treatment of a previous episode has not been prompt, thus allowing more time for a host immune response to develop.

Pelvic Inflammatory Disease

Extension of the gonococcal infection "upward" to involve the endometrium, fallopian tubes, and peritoneum is the most common cause of morbidity (sterility, ectopic pregnancy) due to gonorrhea. It occurs most often with the initial episode, but once it has developed, it occurs more frequently after subsequent episodes. At least 40% of cases of salpingitis in the United States are caused, at least in part, by *N. gonorrhoeae.* Coinfection with *Chlamydia trachomatis* is common.[68] Hence, empirical treatment must include antibiotics capable of eradicating both of these organisms.

Asymptomatic Carrier State

Asymptomatic carriage is most common in women (at least 50% of cases). It occurs in approximately 15% of men with

TABLE 201–3 ■ Clinical Manifestations of Gonorrhea

Urethritis (urogenital gonorrhea)
Cervicitis (urogenital gonorrhea)
Epididymitis
Pelvic inflammatory disease
Asymptomatic carriage
Rectal gonorrhea (proctitis)
Oropharyngitis
Conjunctivitis
Disseminated gonococcal infection

gonorrhea. Asymptomatic carriage has been associated more often with transparent colony types and certain auxotypes, and serovars, but these same "types" have often been associated with pelvic inflammatory disease. Thus, they are an important reservoir for the most common significant sequelae of gonococcal infections, namely salpingitis, sterility, and ectopic pregnancy.[69] Whether this reflects a predisposition of the infecting organism to involve the fallopian tubes or the reluctance of asymptomatic men to seek medical consultation is not known.

Rectal Gonorrhea

Gonococcal proctitis, a consequence of anal intercourse, usually presents with a discharge, bleeding, rectal pain, tenesmus, constipation, or rectal abscess, singly or severally. The causative gonococci are more likely to carry the *mtr* locus that confers a selective advantage for survival in the relatively hydrophobic rectal environment.[70]

Oropharyngitis

Gonococci colonize the oropharynx of about 5% of persons who have a urethral or cervical infection. Orogenital sex is the usual predisposing event. It may be asymptomatic but most often presents as a symptomatic oropharyngitis. In the appropriate setting, a Gram stain examination of the exudate that reveals PMNs with gram-negative intracellular gonococci is suggestive of the infection. The clinical microbiology laboratory must be advised to plate the throat specimen on appropriate selective media to isolate the gonococcus and verify the diagnosis. Gonococcal oropharyngitis is more difficult to treat with antibiotics than the usual genital infection and often requires larger doses and more prolonged treatment.

Conjunctivitis

Gonococcal conjunctivitis may develop whenever the gonococcus comes in contact with the conjunctiva. (Most *Neisseria* species share tropisms for the genital mucosa, oropharynx, and conjunctiva.) It is most often contracted by neonates passing through an infected birth canal, although adults can also be infected. Silver nitrate and antibiotic eyedrops have significantly reduced the incidence of neonatal gonococcal conjunctivitis in the United States.

Disseminated Gonococcal Infection

Disseminated gonococcal infection occurs most frequently in women, especially during menses. It also occurs more frequently during the later stages of pregnancy. Whether this increased virulence is innately due to the increased utilization of iron or to an increased antigen load is not known. In the United States, strains isolated from patients with disseminated gonococcal infection tend to be quite sensitive to penicillin and resistant to the lytic activity of normal human serum[71] and of the AXU auxotype, which suggests a genetic predilection of certain strains to disseminate.

Tenosynovitis and septic arthritis are the most common complications of disseminated gonococcal infection. The usual course is manifested by fever, asymmetric arthralgias, and "migrating" tenosynovitis that later "settles" in one joint—usually the knee, elbow, ankle, wrist, or small joints of the hands and feet, in that order. Skin lesions secondary to a microscopic septic arteritis often develop, usually on the extremities. They range from macular lesions to discrete pustules, which may become hemorrhagic and necrotic. Endocarditis, meningitis, and pericarditis are unusual complications. The diagnosis is made by isolation of *N. gonorrhoeae* from blood, synovial fluid, urogenital tract, oropharynx, or rectum or from a sexual partner of a patient who has typical joint and cutaneous manifestations. Isolation from blood and joint fluid is often difficult and may require culturing relatively large amounts of blood, synovial fluid, and cerebrospinal fluid, and using osmotically stabilized (hypertonic) media. Disseminated gonococcal infection occurs most frequently in persons with a concomitant asymptomatic genital infection.

Diagnosis

Gram Stain Examination

The diagnosis of gonococcal urethritis or conjunctivitis is usually made by a Gram stain examination of the exudate (see Fig. 201–1). The characteristic finding of intracellular (PMN) gram-negative diplococci is as sensitive as culture isolation. The examination is considered negative if no gram-negative diplococci are seen, equivocal if only extracellular gram-negative diplococci are present or if atypical gram-negative cocci are seen within PMNs.[72] Thus, because of its simplicity and cost, it is the diagnostic test of choice. Obviously, the diagnosis is presumptive unless verified by a culture or another antigen-specific technique.

In contrast to specimens obtained from the urethra or conjunctiva, Gram stain examination cannot be relied on to make a presumptive diagnosis of gonococcal infection involving other mucosal sites such as the cervix, rectum, or oropharynx. In these instances, culture isolation or an antigen detection system must be used. Nevertheless, in the appropriate setting, a characteristic Gram stain in a patient with cervicitis will be positive in up to 60% of infected women. Quick nonspecific tests such as measuring urinary esterase have not proved useful.[73]

Cultures

Specimens from normally sterile sites (blood, joint fluid, cerebrospinal fluid) should be inoculated onto nonselective media, in hypertonic liquid media, and large inocula should be cultured.[74] Specimens from potentially contaminated sites (culdocentesis, endocervical aspirate) should be inoculated onto both selective and nonselective media. Specimens from any mucosal surface should be inoculated onto selective media to inhibit the growth of less fastidious organisms. The selective medium usually contains a combination of vancomycin or lincomycin (inhibits gram-positive organisms), colistimethate or trimethoprim (inhibits gram-negative organisms), and nystatin, amphotericin B, or anisomycin (inhibits fungi, especially *Candida* species). Some gonococci, especially those that have a predilection to disseminate, may be inhibited by the low concentration of vancomycin or trimethoprim used in selective culture media, hence the necessity to culture specimens from other than mucosal surfaces onto nonselective media. The most popular commercial selective media are Thayer-Martin, Martin-Lewis, and NYC (New York City) media.[75] Other *Neisseria* species may also be isolated[76] but because antibiotic treatment is the same, specific identification is not usually of practical importance.

Ideally, specimens should be inoculated and incubated promptly. When this is not possible, inoculation onto a medium held in a carbon dioxide atmosphere in a candle jar or in a reduced nonnutrient transport medium up to 6 hours limits loss of viability to an acceptable degree. Longer delay requires the use of a transport medium (usually with a carbon dioxide–generating system).[4] Because antibiotic sensitivity is not required as a guide to therapy, antimicrobial susceptibility testing is usually restricted to specialized laboratories.

Other Diagnostic Methods

Because culture isolation takes at least 24 hours, a number of antigen detection systems utilizing clinical specimens have been developed (monoclonal antibody assays, enzyme immunoassays, genetic transformation, DNA hybridization, DNA amplification[76a]). As yet, these tests offer no advantage of sensitivity, specificity, or cost over Gram stain examination for men with urethritis. Their greatest utility would be rapidly diagnosing a genital infection in women and gonococcal oropharyngitis in both sexes. The GenProbe Pau-2 system utilizing chemiluminescence (GenProbe, San Diego, California) has proved to be about as sensitive and specific as culture.[77] Similar preliminary results were obtained with a ligase chain reaction utilizing Opa and pilin gene probes.[78]

Laboratory Specification

Species verification requires biochemical characterization, principally sugar fermentation (see Table 201–1), and takes an additional 24 to 48 hours. Newer techniques to reduce the waiting period are available.[3] For clinical purposes, they are in general quite acceptable. These include rapid acid production tests, tagged monoclonal antibody tests, and nucleic acid probes.

Acid production tests detect fermentation of prepackaged carbohydrates (glucose, maltose, lactose, sucrose) that have been suspended in buffers and dehydrated. The results have sometimes been equivocal when the gonococcal strain is a weak acid producer. Care must be taken to use only pure cultures.

Enzyme substrate tests utilize chromogenic substrates such as *O*-nitrophenyl-β-D-galactopyranoside to indicate the production of hydroxyprolyl aminopeptidase. In essence, this is another of a battery of tests (see Table 201–1) that can be used to distinguish species that are oxidase-producing gram-negative diplococci. It offers a quick turnaround time. Pure cultures must be used. Serologic tests utilizing a "cocktail" of enzymatically tagged monoclonal antibodies to proteins IA and IB offer the advantage that pure cultures are not absolutely necessary. DNA probes have proved to be specific and sensitive but are relatively expensive.

Because all of these newer techniques require close attention to the manufacturer's instructions and good quality assurance, their practicality and expense have been questioned. Furthermore, specimens from the oropharynx and rectum can be particularly troublesome, exactly the settings for which diagnostic improvements are most needed. As noted before, isolating *N. gonorrhoeae* from blood can be difficult and often requires multiple cultures and osmotically stabilized culture media.

Treatment

Antibiotic Resistance

Penicillin remained the drug of choice for more than 40 years. Nevertheless, slowly increasing resistance to penicillin steadily progressed over time as a result of chromosomal mutations at multiple sites, each of which produced a small increment in resistance. Thus far, the loci identified have been designated *penA, penB, mtr, tem, pem, ampA, ampB, ampC, ampD,* and *mom.* Because the effects are additive, resistance at 2 μg/mL, the level associated with an unacceptable failure rate in patients treated with a standard course of penicillin, has increased in prevalence to the point at which penicillin is no longer the antibiotic of choice. Resistance is conferred by decreasing the affinity of penicillin binding proteins for β-lactam antibiotics, decreasing the permeability of the gonococcal outer membrane, and altering the concentration of penicillin binding proteins.[79–81] Resistance to other antibiotics (spectinomycin, tetracycline, streptomycin) is mediated by other chromosomal mutations. Although resistance capabilities are often shared,[82] mutation at the *env* locus confers increased antibiotic susceptibility by suppression of the *mtr* locus.[83]

Penicillin resistance may also be mediated enzymatically. PPNG was first reported in 1976. By 1982, the prevalence was as high as 60% of isolates in some areas.[83, 84] The first antibiotic to replace penicillin as the treatment of choice was spectinomycin, but its usefulness lasted barely 5 years.[2, 84] Resistance in vitro has been reported to ceftriaxone, ciprofloxacin, and ofloxacin, the present antibiotics of choice. Although the level of antibiotic resistance to these antibiotics is not yet clinically relevant, it is reminiscent of the inexorable accretion of penicillin resistance and it appears a safe bet that they will eventually need to be replaced.

The frequency (40%) of intercurrent *C. trachomatis* with *N. gonorrhoeae* infections makes it imperative that patients be treated for both organisms at the same time (see Chapter 111). The effectiveness of routine screening for gonorrhea depends on the population being evaluated. It is cost-effective when the prevalence of infection is at least 1.5 per 100 persons.

In general, urogenital gonococcal infections require smaller total doses of antibiotics than infections that occur elsewhere in the body, such as salpingitis or oropharyngitis, and the doses used or length of therapy should be adjusted accordingly.[85]

Prevention

Immunization

The quest for a gonococcal vaccine has been ongoing for many years. Unfortunately, none has so far proved efficacious.[86] The three most recent attempts have included vaccines consisting of killed autolyzed piliate gonococci,[87] purified pili,[26, 88] and protein I (Hook EW, personal communication, 1990). One of the issues with regard to gonococcal vaccines is philosophical: should the aim be to protect against the local infection (e.g., urethritis or cervicitis) or is it sufficient to protect only against the systemic complications associated with greater morbidity, such as pelvic inflammatory disease? Would a vaccine result in more asymptomatic disease and thus a broader epidemic?

General Measures

As with any sexually transmitted disease, abstinence and preexposure and postexposure antibiotic prophylaxis have been used successfully.[89–91] Most spermicides are toxic to gonococci, and some findings have suggested that they reduce the incidence of infection. The effectiveness of a number of home remedies, such as washing the genitals or urinating after sexual intercourse, has been asserted to be effective anecdotally through the years, but none has been evaluated clinically.

Epidemiologic Treatment

Epidemiologic treatment refers to the treatment of sexual partners after high-risk exposure and before culture verification. Its effectiveness has been proved, and it is recommended because of the great probability of acquired secondary infections. High-risk exposure is contact with prostitutes, promiscuous homosexual men, or a named contact.

Acknowledgment

The authors express their appreciation and thanks to Ms. Sandra Boyd for her superb assistance.

References

1. Sternberg TH, Howard EB, Dewey LA, et al: Venereal disease. *In* Preventive Medicine in World War II, Vol V. Washington, DC, U.S. Government Printing Office, 1961, pp 139–332.
2. Boslego JW, Tramont EC, Takafuji ET, et al: Effect of spectinomycin on the prevalence of spectinomycin-resistant and penicillinase-producing *Neisseria gonorrhoeae.* N Engl J Med 517:27, 1987.
3. Knapp JS: Historical perspectives and identification of *Neisseria* and related species. Clin Microbiol Rev 1:415, 1988.
4. Carlson BL, Haley MS, Tisei NA, et al: Evaluation of four methods for isolation of *Neisseria gonorrhoeae.* J Clin Microbiol 12:301, 1980.
5. Zheng H, Alcor TM, Cohen MS: Effects of H_2O_2-producing lactobacilli or *Neisseria gonorrhoeae* growth and catalase activity. J Infect Dis 170:1209, 1994.
6. Clark VL, Campbell LA, Palmero DA, et al: Induction and repression of outer membrane proteins by anaerobic growth of *Neisseria gonorrhoeae.* Infect Immun 55:1359, 1987.
7. Woods ML, Bonfiglioli, McGee ZA, et al: Synthesis of a select group of proteins by *Neisseria gonorrhoeae* in response to thermal stress. Infect Immun 58:719, 1990.
8. Schoolnik GK, Fernandez R, Tay JY, et al: Gonococcal pili: Primary structure and receptor binding domain. J Exp Med 159:1351, 1984.
9. Meyer TF, Billyard E, Haas R, et al: Pilus gene of *Neisseria gonorrhoeae*: Chromosomal organization and DNA sequence. Proc Natl Acad Sci USA 81:6110, 1984.
10. Kellogg DS, Cohen IR, Norins LC, et al: *Neisseria gonorrhoeae.* II. Colonial variation and pathogenicity during 35 months in vitro. J Bacteriol 96:596, 1968.
11. Swanson J, Robbins K, Barrera O, et al: Gonococcal pilin variants in experimental gonorrhea. J Exp Med 165:1344, 1987.
12. Heckels JE: Structure and function of pili of *Neisseria* species. Clin Microbiol Rev 2:S66, 1989.
13. Heckels JE: Molecular studies on the pathogenesis of gonorrhea. J Med Microbiol 18:293, 1984.
14. Taha M, Marchal C: Conservation of *Neisseria gonorrhoeae* pilus expression regulatory genes *pilA* and *pilB* in the genus *Neisseria.* Infect Immun 58:4145, 1990.
15. Hagblom P, Segal E, Billyard E, et al: Intragenic recombination leads to pilus antigenic variation in *Neisseria gonorrhoeae.* Nature 315:156, 1985.
16. Meyer TF, Mlawer N, So M: Pilus expression in *Neisseria gonorrhoeae* involves chromosomal rearrangement. Cell 30:45, 1982.
17. Potts WJ, Saunders JR: Nucleotide sequence of the structural gene for class I pilin from *Neisseria meningitidis.* Mol Microbiol 2:647, 1988.
18. Bergström S, Robbins K, Koomey JM, et al: Piliation control mechanisms in *Neisseria gonorrhoeae.* Proc Natl Acad Sci USA 83:3890, 1986.
19. Haas R, Meyer TF: The repertoire of silent pilus genes in *Neisseria gonorrhoeae*: Evidence for gene conversion. Cell 44:107, 1986.
20. Meyer TF, Haas R: Phase and antigenic variation by DNA rearrangements in procaryotes. Symp Soc Gen Microbiol 43:193, 1988.
21. Seifert HS, Ajioka R, So M: Alternative model for *Neisseria gonorrhoeae* pilin variation. Vaccine 6:107, 1988.
22. Tramont EC, Hodge WC, Gilbreath MJ, Ciak J: Differences in attached antigens of gonococci in reinfection. J Lab Clin Med 93:730, 1979.
23. Brossay L, Paradis G, Fox R, et al: Identification, localization, and distribution of the PilT protein in *Neisseria gonorrhoeae.* Infect Immun 62:2302, 1994.
24. Brinton CC, Wood Sw, Brown A, et al: The development of a neisserial pilus vaccine for gonorrhea and meningococcal meningitis. *In* Robbins JB, Hill JC, Sadoff JC (eds): Seminars in Infectious Diseases, Vol IV, Bacterial Vaccines. New York, Thieme-Stratton, 1982, pp 140–159.
25. Tramont EC, Boslego JW, Chung R, et al: Parenteral gonococcal pilus vaccine. *In* Schoolnik GK, Brooks GF, Falkow S, et al (eds): The Pathogenic Neisseriae. Washington DC, American Society for Microbiology, 1985, pp 316–322.
26. Boslego JW, Tramont EC, Chung R, et al: Efficacy trial of a parenteral gonococcal pilus vaccine. Vaccine 9:154, 1991.
27. Judd RC: Protein I: Structure, function, and genetics. Clin Microbiol Rev 2:S41, 1989.
28. Bjerknes R, Guttormsen HK, Solberg CO, Wetzler LM: Neisserial porins inhibit human neutrophil actin polymerization, degranulation, opsonin receptor expression, and phagocytosis but prime the neutrophils to increase their oxidative burst. Infect Immun 63:160, 1995.
29. Carbonetti NH, Simnad VI, Seifert HS, et al: Genetics of protein I of *Neisseria gonorrhoeae*: Construction of hybrid porins. Proc Natl Acad Sci USA 85:6841, 1988.
30. Hicks CB, Boslego JW, Brandt B: Evidence of serum antibodies to *Neisseria gonorrhoeae* before gonococcal infection. J Infect Dis 155:1276, 1987.
31. Hook EW III, Olsen DA, Buchanan TM: Analysis of antigen specificity of the human sera immunoglobulin G immune response to complicated gonococcal infection. Infect Immun 43:706, 1984.
32. Ison CA, Hadfield SG, Bellinger CM, et al: The specificity of serum and local antibodies in female gonorrhea. Clin Exp Immunol 65:198, 1986.
33. Sarafian SK, Tam MR, Morse SA: Gonococcal protein I-specific opsonic IgG in normal human serum. J Infect Dis 148:1025, 1983.
34. Heckels JE, Virji M, Zak K, et al: Immunobiology of gonococcal outer membrane protein I. Antonie Van Leeuwenhoek 53:461, 1987.
35. Buchanan T, Eschenbach D, Knapp J, et al: Gonococcal salpingitis is less likely to recur with *Neisseria gonorrhoeae* of the same principal outer membrane protein antigenic type. Am J Obstet Gynecol 138:978, 1981.
36. Plummer FA, Simonsen JN, Chubb H, et al: Epidemiologic evidence for the development of serovar-specific immunity after gonococcal infection. J Clin Invest 83:1472, 1989.
37. Brunham RC, Plummer F, Slaney L, et al: Correlation of auxotype and protein I type with expression of disease due to *Neisseria gonorrhoeae.* J Infect Dis 152:339, 1985.
38. Rice RJ, Biddle JW, JeanLouise YA, et al: Chromosomally mediated resistance in *Neisseria gonorrhoeae* in the United States: Results of surveillance and reporting, 1983–1984. J Infect Dis 153:340, 1986.
39. Swanson J, Barrera O, Sela J, et al: Expression of outer membrane protein II by gonococci in experimental gonorrhea. J Exp Med 168:221, 1988.
40. Blake MS, Blake CM, Apicella MA, et al: Gonococcal opacity: Lectin-like interactions between Opa proteins and lipooligosaccharide. Infect Immun 63:1434, 1995.
41. Novotry P, Caronley K: Immunological anatomy of *Neisseria gonorrhoeae. In* Brooks GE, Gotschlich EC, Holmes KK, et al (eds): Immunobiology of *Neisseria gonorrhoeae.* Washington, DC, American Society for Microbiology, 1978, pp 263–271.
42. Naids FL, Belisle B, Lee N, et al: Interactions of *Neisseria gonorrhoeae* with human neutrophils: Studies with purified PII (Opa) outer membrane proteins and synthetic Opa peptides. Infect Immun 59:4628, 1991.
43. Elkins C, Rest RF: Monoclonal antibodies to outer membranes protein PII block interactions of *Neisseria gonorrhoeae* with human neutrophils. Infect Immun 58:1078, 1990.
44. James JF, Swanson J: Studies on gonococcus infection. XIII. Occurrence of color/opacity colonial variants in clinical cultures. Infect Immun 19:332, 1978.
45. Blake MS, Wetzler LM, Gotschlich C, et al: Protein III: Structure, function and genetics. Clin Microbiol Rev 2(Suppl):S60, 1989.

45a. Plummer FA, Chubb H, Simonsen JN, et al: Antibody to Rmp (outer membrane protein 3) increases susceptibility to gonococcal infection. J Clin Invest 91:339, 1993.

46. Muir LL, Strugnell RA, Davies JK: Proteins that appear to be

associated with pili in *Neisseria gonorrhoeae.* Infect Immun 56:1743, 1988.
47. Rudel T, Scheuerpflug I, Meyer TF: *Neisseria* PilC protein identified as type-4 pilus tip-located adhesin. Nature 373:357, 1995.
48. Frangipane JV, Rest R: Anaerobic growth and cytidine 5′-monophospho-*N*-acetylneuraminic acid act synergistically to induce high-level serum resistance in *Neisseria gonorrhoeae.* Infect Immun 61:1657, 1993.
49. Hoehn GT, Clark VL: Distribution of a protein antigenically related to the major anaerobically induced gonococcal outer membrane protein among other *Neisseria* species. Infect Immun 38:3929, 1990.
50. Clark VL, Knapp JS, Thompson S, et al: Presence of antibodies to the major anaerobically induced gonococcal outer membrane protein in sera from patients with gonococcal infections. Microb Pathog 5:381, 1988.
51. Morse SA, Chen CY, LeFaou A, et al: A potential role for the major iron-regulated protein expressed by pathogenic *Neisseria* species. Rev Infect Dis 10(Suppl 2):S306, 1988.
52. Lomholt H, Mogens K: Antigenic relationships among immunoglobulin A1 proteases from *Haemophilus, Neisseria,* and *Streptococcus* species. Infect Immun 62:3178, 1994.
53. Cannon JG, Black W, Nachamkin I, et al: Monoclonal antibody that recognizes an outer membrane antigen common to pathogenic *Neisseria* species but not to most nonpathogenic *Neisseria* species. Infect Immun 43:994, 1985.
54. Chow AW, Malkasian KL, Marshall JR, Guze LB: The bacteriology of acute pelvic inflammatory disease. Am J Obstet Gynecol 122:876, 1975.
55. Griffiss JM, Schneider H, Mandrell RE, et al: Lipooligosaccharides: The principal glycolipids of the neisserial outer membrane. Rev Infect Dis 10(Suppl):S287, 1988.
56. Mandrell RE, Lesse AJ, Sugai JV, et al: In vitro and in vivo modification of *Neisseria gonorrhoeae* lipooligosaccharide epitope structure by sialylation. J Exp Med 171:1649, 1990.
57. Mandrell RE, Griffiss JM, Macher BA: Lipooligosaccharides (LOS) of *Neisseria gonorrhoeae* and *Neisseria meningitidis* have components that are immunochemically similar to precursors of human blood group antigens: Carbohydrate sequence specificity of the mouse monoclonal antibodies that recognize cross-reacting antigens on LOS and human erythrocytes. J Exp Med 168:107, 1988.
58. Schneider H, Griffiss JM, Boslego JW, et al: Expression of paragloboside-like lipooligosaccharides may be a necessary component of gonococcal pathogenesis in men. J Exp Med 174:1601, 1991.
58a. Schneider H, Schmidt KA, Skillman D, et al: Sialylation lessens the infectivity of *Neisseria gonorrhoeae* MS11mkC. J Infect Dis 173:1422, 1996.
58b. Smith H, Parsons NJ, Cole JA: Sialylation of neisserial lipopolysaccharide: A major influence on pathogenicity. Microb Pathog 19:365, 1995.
59. Mandrell RE: Further antigenic similarities of *Neisseria gonorrhoeae* lipooligosaccharides and human glycosphingolipids. Infect Immun 60:3017, 1992.
59a. Ramsey KH, Schneider H, Cross AS, et al: Inflammatory cytokines produced in response to experimental human gonorrhea. J Infect Dis 172:186, 1995.
60. Richardson WP, Sadoff JC: Production of a capsule by *Neisseria gonorrhoeae.* Infect Immun 15:663, 1977.
61. Roberts MC: Plasmids of *Neisseria gonorrhoeae* and other *Neisseria* species. Clin Microbiol Rev 2(Suppl):S18, 1989.
62. Xia M, Whittinghan WL, Holmes KK, et al: Pulsed-field gel electrophoresis for genomic analysis of *Neisseria gonorrhoeae.* J Infect Dis 17:455, 1995.
63. Gill MJ: Serotyping *Neisseria gonorrhoeae,* a report of the Fourth International Workshop. Genitourin Med 67:53, 1991.
63a. O'Rourke M, Ison CA, Renton AM, Spratt BG: Opa-typing: A high-resolution tool for studying the epidemiology of gonorrhoea. Mol Microbiol 17:865, 1995.
63b. Apicella MA, Ketterer M, Lee FKN, et al: The pathogenesis of gonococcal urethritis in men: Confocal and immunoelectron microscopic analysis of urethral exudates from men infected with *Neisseria gonorrhoeae.* J Infect Dis 173:636, 1996.
64. Cohen MS, Sparling PF: Mucosal infection with *Neisseria gonorrhoeae.* Bacterial adaption and mucosal defenses. J Clin Invest 89:1699, 1992.
65. Britigan BE, Cohen MS, Sparling PF: Gonococcal infection: A model of molecular pathogenesis. N Engl J Med 312:1683, 1985.
66. Tramont EC: Inhibition of adherence of *Neisseria gonorrhoeae* by genital secretions. J Clin Invest 59:117, 1977.
67. Elliott B, Brunham RC, Laga M, et al: Maternal gonococcal infection as a preventable risk factor for low birth weight. J Infect Dis 161:531, 1990.
68. Tubal infertility: Serologic relationship of past chlamydial and gonococcal infection. WHO Task Force on the Prevention and Management of Infertility. Sex Transm Dis 22:71, 1995.
69. Sarafian SK, Knapp JC: Molecular epidemiology of gonorrhea. Clin Microbiol Rev 2(Suppl):S49, 1989.
70. Morse SA, Lysko PG, McFarland L, et al: Gonococcal strains from homosexual men have outer membranes with reduced permeability to hydrophobic molecules. Infect Immun 37:432, 1982.
71. Rice PA: Molecular basis for serum resistance in *Neisseria gonorrhoeae.* Clin Microbiol Rev 2(Suppl):S112, 1989.
72. Jacobs NF, Kraus SF: Gonococcal and nongonococcal urethritis in men: Clinical and laboratory differentiation. Ann Intern Med 82:7, 1975.
73. McNagny SE, Parker RM, Zenilman JM, et al: Urinary leukocyte esterase test: A screening method for the detection of asymptomatic chlamydial and gonococcal infection in men. J Infect Dis 165:573, 1992.
74. Martinez E, Domingo P, Verger G, et al: Difficulties in diagnosing gonococcemia. Clin Infect Dis 20:19, 1995.
75. Bonin P, Tanino TT, Handsfield HH: Isolation of *Neisseria gonorrhoeae* on selective and nonselective media in a sexually transmitted disease clinic. J Clin Microbiol 19:218, 1984.
76. Hagman M, Forslin L, Moi H, Danielsson D: *Neisseria meningitidis* in specimens from urogenital sites. Is increased awareness necessary? Sex Transm Dis 18:228, 1991.
76a. Camarena JJ, Nogueira JM, Dasi MA, et al: DNA amplification fingerprinting for subtyping *Neisseria gonorrhoeae* strains. Sex Transm Dis 22:128, 1995.
77. Stary A, Kopp W, Zahel B, et al: Comparison of DNA-probe test and culture for the detection of *Neisseria gonorrhoeae* in genital samples. Sex Transm Dis 20:243, 1993.
78. Birkenmeyer L, Armstrong AS: Preliminary evaluation of the ligase chain reaction for specific detection of *Neisseria gonorrhoeae.* J Clin Microbiol 30:3089, 1992.
79. Dougherty TJ: Peptidoglycan biosynthesis in *Neisseria gonorrhoeae* strains sensitive and intrinsically resistant to β-lactam antibiotics. J Bacteriol 153:429, 1983.
80. Dillon JR, Yeung K: β-Lactamase plasmids and chromosomally mediated antibiotic resistance in pathogenic *Neisseria* species. Clin Microbiol Rev 2(Suppl):S125, 1989.
81. Dougherty TJ, Koller AE, Tomasz A: Competition of β-lactam antibiotics for the penicillin-binding proteins of *Neisseria gonorrhoeae.* Antimicrob Agents Chemother 20:109, 1981.
82. De La Fuente L, Vazquez JA: Genetic structures of non-penicillinase producing *Neisseria gonorrhoeae* strains in relation to auxotype and serovar class. J Infect Dis 170:696, 1994.
83. Handsfield HH, Sandström EG, Knapp JS, et al: Epidemiology of penicillinase-producing *Neisseria gonorrhoeae* infections: Analysis of auxotyping and serogrouping. N Engl J Med 306:950, 1982.
84. Berg WS, Harrison WO: Spectinomycin as primary treatment of gonorrhea in areas of high prevalence of penicillinase-producing *Neisseria gonorrhoeae.* Sex Transm Dis 8:38, 1981.
85. Moran JS: Treating uncomplicated *Neisseria gonorrhoeae* infections: Is the anatomic site of infection important? Sex Transm Dis 22:39, 1995.
86. Tramont EC: Gonococcal vaccines. Clin Microbiol Rev 2(Suppl):S74, 1989.
87. Greenberg L, Diena FA, Ashton FA, et al: Gonococcal vaccine studies in Inuvik. Can J Public Health 65:29, 1974.
88. Johnson S, Chung RCY, Deal CD, et al: Human immunization with Pgh 3-2 gonococcal pilus results in cross-reactive antibody to the cyanogen bromide fragment-2 of pilin. J Infect Dis 163:128, 1991.
89. Darrow WW, Weisner PJ: Personal prophylaxis for venereal disease. JAMA 233:444, 1975.
90. Harrison WO, Hooper RR, Weisner PJ, et al: A trial of microcycline given after exposure to prevent gonorrhea. N Engl J Med 300:1074, 1979.
91. Jick H, Hannan MT, Stergachis A, et al: Vaginal spermicides and gonorrhea. JAMA 248:1619, 1982.

202

Neisseria meningitidis

John W. Boslego
Edmund C. Tramont

History

The history of meningococcal disease is both fascinating and humbling, fascinating when one reflects on what we have learned over the years about the epidemiology, pathogenesis, pathophysiology, and the principal determinant of host susceptibility (the lack of bactericidal antibody)[1] but humbling from the standpoint of how little we understand about the virulence properties of the organism or the dynamics involved in epidemic disease.

From 1805 to 1810, *Neisseria meningitidis* was the likely cause of a series of epidemics of meningitis that ravaged the Napoleonic and Persian armies ("meningitic de congélation") as well as an epidemic in New England known as "spotted fever." The next 150 years were marked by a peculiar pattern of periodic outbreaks occurring every 8 to 15 years interspersed with sporadic cases. At first, high rates of meningococcal disease predominated in Europe and North America, but over time, the disease spread throughout the world, especially to sub-Saharan Africa, leaving in its wake milder and less explosive outbreaks with each successive epidemic wave.

The first description of the etiologic agent appeared in 1886 when Anton Weichselbaum demonstrated gram-negative diplococci in the cerebrospinal fluid (CSF) of a young Viennese patient who had died of purulent meningitis. Five years later, Quincke introduced the lumbar puncture as a therapeutic measure to reduce the increased pressure associated with meningitis. But its major impact was diagnostic: the isolation of *N. meningitidis* (and other bacteria) in pure culture. Armed with the knowledge of the etiologic agent of epidemic "cerebrospinal meningitis," numerous investigative studies quickly elucidated basic information concerning (1) epidemiology—the episodic nature of epidemics interspersed with sporadic cases, the difficulty in linking cases with one another, the propensity for higher attack rates during the winter months, the predilection to occur in young children and young adults, and the asymptomatic carrier state; (2) bacteriology—serogrouping and characterization of strains; (3) clinical aspects—a bacterium that is usually a normal saprophyte but that can become one of the quickest killers of humans; and (4) immunology—the lack of serum bactericidal activity predisposing to invasive disease. Such studies set the stage for attempts at innovative treatments such as passive immunotherapy and eventually vaccine development.

Meningococcal Disease and the Military

Meningococcal disease has had a long and special relationship with the military.[2] The collection of a large number of young adults from disparate localities who train, eat, and sleep in proximity creates an ecologic setting highly favorable for the spread of meningococci. Indeed, some of the most dramatic outbreaks of meningococcal meningitis have occurred in military training camps.

The introduction of sulfa drugs successfully controlled such outbreaks when it became routine practice to give prophylaxis to entire units after the occurrence of a single case. This approach was highly effective until sulfadiazine-resistant strains emerged in the early 1960s.

Against this backdrop, the classic studies of Goldschneider and coworkers[3] on the natural history of meningococcal infections firmly established that the absence of bactericidal antibody against the infecting strain predisposed an individual to develop invasive meningococcal disease soon after colonization of the oropharynx. They further demonstrated that bactericidal antibody could be elicited by purified, high-molecular-weight meningococcal capsular polysaccharides. Their studies quickly led to the development of the highly effective group C meningococcal vaccine.[4]

Antimicrobial Therapy and Prophylaxis

The introduction of antimicrobial agents dramatically transformed this highly fatal disease into a usually curable one, particularly when the diagnosis is made early.

Antimicrobial prophylaxis continues to play a role in the management of meningococcal outbreaks. With the inevitable advent of antimicrobial resistance, however, the effectiveness of routine prophylaxis of contacts has become less predictable.[5]

Characteristics of the Pathogen

The genus *Neisseria* is a member of the family Neisseriaceae, which also includes *Moraxella, Acinetobacter,* and *Kingella*[6] (Table 202–1). Although 12 species of *Neisseria* have been isolated from humans, only *N. meningitidis* and *Neisseria gonorrhoeae* are regularly pathogenic. The other species are usually part of the normal flora and only rarely cause disease.

N. meningitidis is an aerobic, oxidase-positive, gram-nega-

TABLE 202–1 ■ Taxonomy of Neisseriaceae

Genus: *Neisseria*
*N. meningitidis**
*N. gonorrhoeae** (includes subspecies *kochii**)
*N. subflava** (includes biovars *perflava,* flava**)
*N. flavescens**
N. caviae
*N. mucosa**
N. canis
*N. cinerea**
N. cuniculi
N. denitrificans
N. elongata
*N. lactamica**
N. ovis
*N. polysaccharea**
Genus: *Acinetobacter*
A. calcoaceticus
Genus: *Kingella*
K. kingae
K. indologenes
K. denitrificans
Genus: *Moraxella*
M. lacunata
M. bovis
M. nonliquefaciens
M. phenylpyruvica
M. osloensis
Branhamella (Moraxella) catarrhalis

**Neisseria* strains that have been isolated from humans.

tive diplococcus. Under culture conditions, it grows best at 35°C to 37°C in a moist 5% to 7% CO_2 environment (candle jar).

The optimal isolation medium depends on the source of the specimen. Antibiotic-containing medium (such as modified Thayer-Martin or New York City medium) is necessary when the culture specimen is obtained from a nonsterile site such as the oropharynx. When a normally sterile site such as blood or CSF is cultured, nonselective chocolate agar is preferable.

Oxidative metabolism of specific carbohydrates with resultant acid production is the major means for differentiating *Neisseria* species (see Table 201–1). *N. meningitidis* produces acid from glucose and maltose but not sucrose, lactose, or fructose. A pure subculture of the organism is required for proper evaluation.

A wide array of tests has been developed to provide a more rapid, specific identification of *N. meningitidis*. Such tests utilize acid production, enzyme elaboration, and serologic specificity.[6] These tests have greatly aided quick and accurate diagnosis in the laboratory but can occasionally result in misidentification. Acid fermentation reactions by an occasional strain may not be easily interpreted. Likewise, enzyme identification may sometimes be difficult to interpret. For example, *N. meningitidis* produces γ-glutamylaminopeptidase, but so does an occasional nonpathogenic *Neisseria* species. Therefore, the combined use of biochemical and enzyme tests is necessary to obtain the greatest diagnostic precision.

Structurally, the meningococcus resembles other gram-negative bacteria. The organism is surrounded by a polysaccharide capsule. Beneath it, the cell envelope consists of a lipid bilayer, outer membrane proteins (OMPs), lipooligosaccharide (LOS), pili (filamentous projections that extend through the capsule), and a dense peptidoglycan layer. A cytoplasmic membrane encloses the cytoplasm and nucleus.

The capsule is composed of an anionic polysaccharide. This serves as the basis for categorizing the organism into serogroups. To date, 13 serogroups have been identified: A, B, C, D, 29E, H, I, K, L, W135, X, Y, and Z. Serogroups A, B, C, W135, and Y are the serogroups responsible for the overwhelming majority of cases of invasive disease. All serogroups except D have been chemically and structurally defined.[7–11] The presence of a capsule is associated with virulence. Invasive meningococci are almost always encapsulated, whereas meningococci colonizing mucous membranes frequently are not.

Subcapsular antigens are used to classify meningococci further into serotypes, subtypes, and immunotypes.[12] There are five classes of major OMPs, designated class 1 to class 5 and differentiated on the basis of molecular weight, peptide maps, and electrophoretic behavior.[13] The serotype is based on serologic (monoclonal antibody) reactivity to the class 2 or 3 OMP (a strain has either a class 2 or a class 3 OMP but not both). The subtype is based on serologic reactivity to the class 1 OMP. The LOS immunotype is based on serologic reactivity to LOS. Each serogroup contains strains with a variety of types, subtypes, and LOS immunotypes, and each type is not restricted to a given serogroup. For example, approximately 15 serotypes, 13 subtypes, and 13 LOS immunotypes have been identified among group B strains, but many strains remain nontypable. According to convention, a strain can be designated as B:15:P1.3:L3,8, which means serogroup B, serotype 15, subtype 3, immunotypes 3 and 8.

These grouping and typing schemes have been quite useful for epidemiologic studies and for vaccine development, but continued studies are required to develop a more complete, standardized, and universally accepted set of typing reagents.

Another method of classifying meningococci is based on the electrophoretic mobilities of metabolic enzymes produced by *N. meningitidis*.[14] Multilocus enzyme electrophoresis provides a mechanism for characterizing the chromosomal genome and grouping strains by their genetic relatedness. Analysis of hundreds of isolates from around the world has yielded 78 electrophoretic types representing multilocus genotypes. Only a small number of electrophoretic types are responsible for most of the invasive disease cases. Preliminary studies indicate that strains that colonize the throat are usually from clones different from those that cause invasive disease.[15] With continued experience, this enzyme typing system should provide a better understanding of the virulence determinants of meningococci.

Epidemiology

Meningococcal infections are a worldwide health problem. The vast majority of cases occur in childhood. Attack rates are highest in infants 6 months to 1 year old and then decrease over time. A minor secondary peak occurs in the late teens and early 20s and reflects outbreaks in military recruits and college populations. In temperate climates, disease rates peak during the winter months. Even with the introduction of effective antibiotics, the fatality rate remains high at 5% to 15%. In the United States, *N. meningitidis* causes approximately 3000 cases a year and has replaced *Haemophilus influenzae* type b as the most frequent cause of bacterial meningitis in children. This is the result of a substantial reduction in the incidence of *H. influenzae* type b infections because of the high effectiveness and widespread use of protein-polysaccharide conjugate vaccines in infants.

The sub-Saharan "meningitis belt" in Africa is one of the areas most severely affected. Major epidemics have occurred in that region every 8 to 12 years during the past century, resulting in an estimated 500,000 deaths in the past 50 years. One of the largest more recent epidemics occurred in China between 1963 and 1970.[16] The peak year was 1967, when there was an attack rate of 400 cases per 100,000 persons per year, resulting in more than 3 million cases and 166,000 deaths.

N. meningitidis is a uniquely human pathogen. Humans are the only reservoir, and the organism is carried on the nasopharyngeal mucosa. Transmission occurs from person to person, presumably through passage of respiratory secretions or aerosolized droplets.

Carrier rates of meningococci among cohorts vary tremendously. The bacteria serogroup and strain, age and socioeconomic status of the person, prevalence of disease activity, and crowded living conditions are all factors.[17] However, there is no critical "carrier rate" that accurately predicts an epidemic or outbreak.

In an individual person, the virulence of a particular strain, host susceptibility (immunity), and environmental influences all play a role in the development of invasive disease. These interrelationships have not yet been fully defined. Often, a preceding respiratory infection such as influenza occurs and may facilitate entry of meningococci through respiratory mucosa. Additional precipitating factors are probably needed for an epidemic to occur, such as exceptional climatic conditions, an infectious cofactor, or the introduction of a new virulent strain to which many individuals lack immunity.

Epidemics of meningococcal disease normally result from a single dominant strain or clone. Specific combinations of serotype and subtype have been found to be associated with epidemic group B and group C disease. Conversely, endemic disease is caused by diverse serogroups, serotypes, and subtypes.

Serogroups A, B, and C have been responsible for practically all known epidemics. Serogroup A has been most often associated with explosive widespread epidemics. In sub-Saharan Africa, outbreaks generally occur during the dry season, terminate at the onset of the rainy season, and generally occur in cycles with an interval of 8 to 12 years. The large epidemics in China have been due exclusively to group A as well and have also followed an 8- to 10-year cyclic pattern. Group A outbreaks in industrialized countries are now rare and, when they occur, are generally small and affect those of the lowest socioeconomic status.

Although serogroup C can cause large outbreaks, it is more often associated with smaller outbreaks and endemic disease. São Paulo, Brazil, experienced a large group C outbreak in the early 1970s, but the responsible serogroup later shifted to group A.[18] Subsequently, Los Angeles, California, experienced clusters of group C cases.[17, 19]

Serogroup B does not generally cause the extraordinarily high attack rates of meningitis common with group A or C disease. However, this serogroup is now the major cause of endemic disease and small outbreaks in industrialized countries.[17, 20] During the 1970s, group B disease emerged in northwest Europe and caused sustained outbreaks in Norway, Iceland, the Faeroe Islands, Great Britain, Denmark, and the Netherlands. Clonally related group B strains (electrophoretic type 5 [ET5] complex) have also spread to the Western Hemisphere, causing outbreaks in Cuba, Chile, and Brazil.[17]

As noted earlier, the diverse patterns of disease imply differences in virulence determinants, host immunity, and efficiency of transmission. Unfortunately, little is understood about these differences.

Pathogenesis

Although the organism may cause an oropharyngitis, it is primarily a saprophyte that asymptomatically colonizes the majority of human beings sometime during their lives. As with other neisserial species, it can sometimes colonize the genital tract or conjunctiva. Rarely, the organism escapes from its customarily benign ecologic niche and invades the blood stream. The frequency or reasons why this occurs are poorly understood. On the basis of studies in military recruits, invasion probably takes place within hours or days after colonization. Once the organism has disseminated, an overlapping array of clinical outcomes may ensue (Fig. 202–1). The host's immune status plays a critical role in the ultimate course.[3, 21]

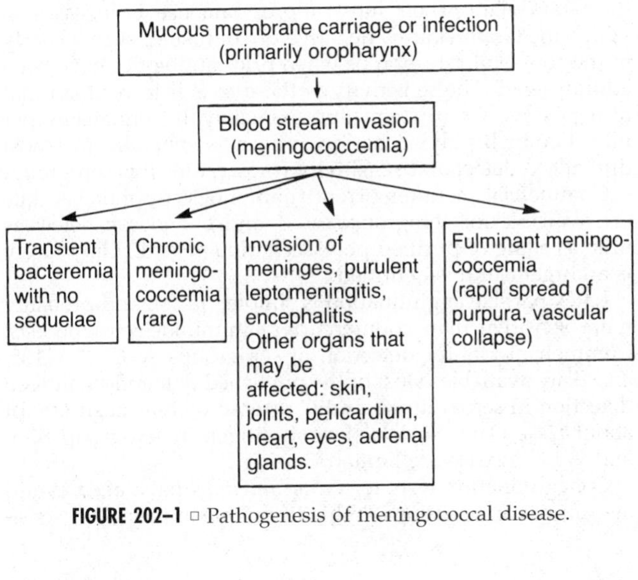

FIGURE 202–1 □ Pathogenesis of meningococcal disease.

Host Immunity

Serum bactericidal antibody is the cornerstone of an effective host defense against meningococcal disease.[1, 3] Protective antibody may be acquired transplacentally or actively, as a result of colonization or infection with meningococci or other organisms possessing cross-reactive antigens (i.e., other neisserial species and/or commensal organisms in the oropharynx or gut) or by vaccination. Transplacental (maternal) antibodies protect newborn infants up to 6 months of age, after which susceptibility increases until age 2. It then wanes over time as the child's immune experience broadens, reflected by the acquisition of serum bactericidal activity against *N. meningitidis* species. Apparently, the development of antibody protective against invasion by colonizing strains of *N. meningitidis* is commonplace because in military recruits, the oropharyngeal carriage rate can be as high as 95%, yet the incidence of systemic disease remains well under 1%.[3]

Meningococcal Disease

When bactericidal antibody is present in the serum, the meningococcus appears to be rapidly destroyed on entry into the blood stream. If bactericidal antibody is absent, the organism multiplies and disseminates. If inadequate amounts and/or low-affinity antibody is present, the disease process may be modulated, but the factors that determine the clinical presentation (transient bacteremia, chronic meningococcemia, meningococcal meningitis, fulminant meningococcemia, or any combination thereof) are unknown (see Fig. 202–1).

At least three host factors can influence the efficiency of bactericidal antibody: complement deficiency, blocking immunoglobulin (Ig) A antibody, and IgM deficiency. Meningococcal disease is a common infection experienced by complement-deficient individuals. Inherited deficiencies of properdin, early complement components (C1, C4, C2), or late complement components (C6, C7, C8) all predispose to invasive meningococcal disease.[22] Specific antibody can partially overcome deficiencies of properdin and early complement components. But patients with late component complement deficiencies exhibit a striking susceptibility to initial and recurrent infections, emphasizing the importance of serum bactericidal activity in the control of this infection. Some persons may also develop transient blocking IgA antibody. Because IgA does not effectively bind complement, the organisms are not killed.[23] Removing the IgA experimentally restores the serum's ability to lyse the bacterium. Because the IgM class of antibody readily binds complement, persons with an IgM deficiency lyse meningococci less efficiently.[24]

Like many other encapsulated organisms, *N. meningitidis* has a predilection to invade the meninges (pia and arachnoid) and cause a leptomeningitis. In most instances, acute infection is common and is probably the result of rapid multiplication of meningococci and the release of endotoxin (LOS), which in turn invokes an intense, acute inflammatory response characterized by an exudate consisting primarily of polymorphonuclear cells. Direct invasion of brain parenchyma is rare, but encephalitis commonly results from swelling secondary to impeded venous drainage. However, the ultimate outcome in appropriately treated patients is not related to the intensity of the inflammatory response.

In the blood stream, endotoxin from propagating organisms reacts with macrophages to release cytokines (e.g., tumor necrosis factor), prostaglandins, and free radicals. These vasoactive substances disrupt vascular endothelium and cause petechiae, ecchymoses, and disseminated intravascular coagulation. Occasionally, shock and multiorgan system failure ensue and presage a morbid outcome.[25]

Clinical Manifestations

The clinical manifestations of meningococcal disease have already been alluded to. An oropharyngitis may occur. Rarely, a pneumonia may develop, usually with serogroup Y or B strains.[26] The cultural diagnosis of these infections is often missed unless the clinical microbiology laboratory has been alerted to use selective media. Occasionally, a person can develop a meningococcal genital tract infection, proctitis, or conjunctivitis.

Once the blood stream is invaded, a spectrum of clinical manifestations may ensue (see Fig. 202–1). The mildest form is a transient bacteremia that usually begins insidiously with fever and malaise. Only a few, if any, petechial skin lesions occur. No meningeal signs develop. The symptoms spontaneously resolve in 24 to 48 hours. Blood cultures subsequently grow *N. meningitidis.*

In rare instances, a chronic meningococcemia develops. This curious clinical entity is similar to the gonococcal dermatitis-arthritis syndrome and consists of intermittent febrile episodes lasting 2 to 10 days associated with a variety of skin lesions (macular, maculopapular, pustular) and migratory arthralgias and myalgias. Blood cultures may be continuously or intermittently positive. Sometimes multiple blood cultures are required to isolate the organism. The infection may last months and may resolve spontaneously; the effect of appropriate antibiotic treatment is dramatic.[27]

Acute meningococcemia occurs most often after several days of upper respiratory symptoms. The patient's temperature rises abruptly followed by chills and malaise. Weakness, myalgias, arthralgias, nausea, vomiting, and headache usually develop quickly, but the most remarkable manifestation is the development of characteristic petechial skin lesions. They are the most common type of skin lesion occurring with meningococcal disease, usually appearing in crops on the ankles, wrists, and armpits, but may progress to involve any part of the body. The palms, soles, and head are usually spared. The number of lesions can advance rapidly within a few hours, and new lesions may continue to develop for up to 24 hours after appropriate treatment. Other skin manifestations include macular and maculopapular lesions. The patients tend to have only a moderate fever (39.5°C) but a marked leukocytosis. Signs of vascular collapse are infrequent.

Fulminant meningococcemia, also referred to as the Waterhouse-Friderichsen syndrome or purpura fulminans, is the toxic extension of acute meningococcemia. It occurs in 5% to 15% of cases and is characterized by apprehension, restlessness, and delirium developing in a few hours. The skin lesions rapidly become widespread, purpuric, and ecchymotic. Vascular collapse eventually ensues.[28] Acute renal failure, pulmonary insufficiency, and cardiac insufficiency, the most frequently reported autopsy finding,[29] are secondary complications. High fever is usually present, but sometimes a febrile response fails to develop, which represents a poor prognostic sign. The white cell count can be high, normal, or low (neutropenia), and thrombocytopenia is frequent. Evidence of intravascular coagulation is common. Mortality rates remain high despite appropriate antibiotic treatment.

With the exception of mild transient bacteremia, all of the foregoing syndromes can be associated with acute meningitis (see Chapter 158). Clinically, meningococcal meningitis resembles acute bacterial meningitis of any etiology.

Diagnosis

Clinical diagnosis rests on a high index of suspicion and, in a patient presenting with a febrile illness, a rapid and thorough search for petechiae and purpura. Evidence of meningeal irritation is helpful but may be absent early in the disease course. Diagnostic specimens should be collected as rapidly as possible but should not delay initiation of treatment.

The laboratory diagnosis of meningococcal disease is based on the isolation of the organism from blood, CSF, or skin lesions.

Blood cultures are positive in up to 75% of patients with proven meningococcal disease.[30] They may be positive when CSF cultures are not, even in the setting of inflamed meninges.

An abnormal CSF demonstrating an elevated white cell count consisting of predominantly polymorphonuclear cells, associated with a low glucose level, is highly suggestive of bacterial meningitis. A CSF Gram stain is positive in about 70% of cases, but meningococci may sometimes be confused with pneumococci or *H. influenzae,* particularly when few organisms are seen. Culture of the CSF is the most reliable diagnostic test and is positive in about 70% of cases. Because of the organism's fragility, efforts must be made to plate the CSF on chocolate agar as soon as possible (within minutes) and place it in a 5% to 7% carbon dioxide environment (candle jar). This usually allows the culture to remain viable for up to 8 hours before incubation at 35°C to 37°C. Rarely, the culture of an otherwise normal CSF specimen may yield *N. meningitidis.*[31]

Petechial skin lesions also represent a potential diagnostic specimen. Meningococci are often present in petechiae, and Gram-stained smears of needle aspirates or punch biopsies from skin lesions are positive in up to 75% of cases.[30] This can be particularly useful when antibiotics were started before cultures were obtained.

Nasopharyngeal cultures for *N. meningitidis* must be interpreted with caution. A positive throat culture may reveal serogroupable *N. meningitidis* in patients with invasive disease. However, a positive throat culture alone should not be considered proof of meningococcal infection because patients with other forms of meningitis may be coincident carriers of *N. meningitidis.*

Newer techniques for the rapid identification of *N. meningitidis* capsular polysaccharide in blood and CSF are available. Countercurrent immunoelectrophoresis, latex particle agglutination, and coagglutination techniques have been developed.[32] CSF is the optimal specimen for analysis by these techniques. Although antigen can be detected in serum, urine, and other body fluids, the sensitivity is lower than with CSF. The main advantage of these tests is to provide a rapid identification (minutes to hours) of the specific bacterium responsible for infection. These tests should not replace the Gram stain. Their most appropriate use is in cases in which the Gram stain is negative or confusing, such as early in the course of infection or when prior antibiotics have been administered. The sensitivity of these tests is lower than that of a positive Gram stain (approximately 10^5 organisms per mL). Group B polysaccharide antigen is generally the most difficult to detect and sensitivity is lowest for this serogroup.

Commercial countercurrent immunoelectrophoresis kits are available for serogroups A, B, and C and can detect as little as 50 ng of purified polysaccharide per mL. Only rarely is an organism misidentified.

Latex particle agglutination is simpler, faster, and probably more sensitive than countercurrent immunoelectrophoresis. Commercial kits for detection of serogroups A, C, Y, W135, and B are available. Most of the published data reflect antigen detection in serogroup A and C disease with a sensitivity of about 80%. Data on detection of antigen in serogroup B, Y, and W135 disease are limited.

Coagglutination tests for *N. meningitidis* have been evaluated in research settings.[32] This technique appears less sensitive than countercurrent immunoelectrophoresis or latex particle agglutination.

Preliminary data on the use of the polymerase chain reaction for the diagnosis of meningococcal meningitis are promising. In one study, the sensitivity and specificity of this technique were both 91%.[33] Moreover, sensitivity was not affected by prior antibiotic treatment. As the polymerase chain reaction technology becomes more widely available in clinical laboratories, additional studies will be needed to define its utility in various demographic populations.

Treatment

Few infections progress with the rapidity of those caused by *N. meningitidis*, and a successful outcome is highly dependent on early, appropriate antibiotic administration.

Penicillin G has remained the treatment of choice for more than 50 years. In infants and children, 300,000 units/kg per day (in divided doses every 4 hours) should be given intravenously for at least 7 days, longer in more serious cases. In adults, 24 million units/d intravenously (in divided doses every 2 to 4 hours) should be given initially; the dose can be reduced after a few days depending on the clinical status of the patient. Treatment duration is usually 10 to 14 days, depending on the clinical response.

The antibiotic armamentarium for bacterial meningitis has greatly expanded. Unlike the first-generation cephalosporins (e.g., cephalothin), the third-generation cephalosporins exhibit excellent CSF penetration.[34] This feature, combined with their excellent in vitro activity against common meningeal pathogens, makes them an attractive selection in cases in which the etiologic diagnosis is uncertain or for patients with a nonanaphylactic history of penicillin intolerance. Clinical experience with cefotaxime and ceftriaxone has verified the pharmacologic data. Chloramphenicol (75 to 100 mg/kg per day [up to 4 g/d] intravenously in divided doses every 6 hours) also remains an alternative regimen. Ciprofloxacin, a carboxyquinolone, has excellent in vitro activity against *N. meningitidis* and excellent CSF penetration.[35] Its role in the treatment of meningococcal meningitis must await the results of clinical trials.

Occasional isolates of *N. meningitidis* from clinical cases have demonstrated a relative resistance to penicillin.[36–38] These isolates are termed penRR and are defined by a minimal inhibitory concentration of penicillin of 0.1 to 1.0 mg/L. These isolates do not produce β-lactamase, and the mechanism of resistance is related to a decreased affinity of one of the organism's penicillin binding proteins to penicillin. The penRR isolates have been reported from Spain, South Africa, the United Kingdom, Canada, Greece, Switzerland, Romania, Belgium, and the United States. In Spain, penRR *N. meningitidis* strains account for up to 50% of isolates, but the incidence is much lower in other regions.

The clinical significance of this relative resistance is not established. Patients infected with penRR strains recover when treated with penicillin or ampicillin, although there are suggestions of a higher rate of complications or a slightly prolonged clinical course.

Third-generation cephalosporins continue to demonstrate low minimal inhibitory concentrations for penRR strains. Until more information is available, clinical cases caused by penRR meningococci should be treated with a third-generation cephalosporin. In addition, continued surveillance for penRR isolates and β-lactamase–producing isolates is warranted.

As in other patients with vascular collapse, supportive therapy is vitally important for a successful outcome (see Chapter 67). Monitoring of fluid replacement and renal and cardiovascular function is essential. The value of steroid therapy in meningococcal infections is still unknown. Short-term administration of high-dose dexamethasone decreased the likelihood of moderate to severe hearing loss in infants and children with bacterial meningitis primarily caused by *H. influenzae*. Although an effect is probable, there were too few cases of meningococcal meningitis in the study to document a beneficial effect for this subgroup.[39] Obviously, steroid replacement is essential in patients with acute adrenal insufficiency secondary to adrenal gland infarction. Heparin therapy for an accompanying intravascular coagulopathy has not proved beneficial.

Prevention

Immunoprophylaxis

Currently licensed meningococcal vaccines consist of mixtures of purified, high-molecular-weight capsular polysaccharides from serogroups A, C, Y, and W135. Serogroup A and C vaccines were developed in the late 1960s and were shown to be remarkably safe and highly effective.[4, 40] Serogroup Y and W135 polysaccharides were never subjected to efficacy field studies, but licensure was based on their molecular size, chemical purity, ability to elicit a high titer of bactericidal antibodies in humans, and safety. In 1982, serogroups Y and W135 were added to serogroup A and C polysaccharides to form a single tetravalent vaccine. Use of this vaccine in all U.S. military recruits has virtually eliminated meningococcal disease except for serogroup B in this cohort.[2]

The tetravalent vaccine is indicated for all intimate contacts of meningococcal cases, except for those known to be caused by group B organisms. The vaccine can also be used in institutional settings when one or more cases occur. Travelers to regions experiencing epidemics or high rates of endemic disease should be immunized before departure. All patients with meningococcal disease should be evaluated for inherited complement deficiencies after their recovery from acute infection. Patients and their family members with properdin and early component deficiencies respond well to vaccination and should be immunized. Patients with late complement component deficiencies respond less well, but periodic immunization should be considered as part of their management strategy.

Despite their safety and effectiveness, there remain several important limitations of the current meningococcal vaccines. In addition to cost and distribution difficulties similar to those for other vaccines in worldwide use, the duration of immunity of capsular polysaccharide vaccines is unknown but estimated to be 2 to 3 years.[41] Consequently, disease unpredictability, logistic difficulties, and cost considerations often delay the initiation of immunization until the onset of an outbreak or epidemic. More important, these vaccines, particularly the group C component, are poorly immunogenic in children younger than 2 years,[42] the age group at highest risk of infection. Lastly, no licensed vaccine is currently available for serogroup B.

Efforts to improve the immunogenicity of capsular polysaccharide vaccines in infants and young children have focused on the conjugation of polysaccharides to carrier proteins. This approach has been used successfully with *H. influenzae* polysaccharide vaccine, with resultant improved immunogenicity and protection in children younger than 1 year.[43] Improvements in the immunogenicity of meningococcal polysaccharides conjugated to proteins bode well for an effective vaccine for infants.[44]

Unlike those of the other major serogroups, purified group B meningococcal capsular polysaccharide is not immunogenic in humans.[45] Efforts to enhance its immunogenicity have been generally unsuccessful. These results, coupled with the shared antigenicity of B polysaccharide and determinants on gangliosides of animal and human cells, have dampened enthusiasm for purified B polysaccharide as a vaccine component.[46]

Emphasis for serogroup B vaccine development has shifted to subcapsular antigens. OMP preparations are quite insoluble. When complexed to capsular polysaccharide, however, they become more soluble and immunogenic.[47] Numerous prototype vaccines consisting of mixtures of LOS-depleted proteins have been produced and tested. These vaccines are safe and cause only mild local and/or systemic side effects. They elicit a bactericidal antibody response that is generally serotype specific.

An initial efficacy study of a serotype 2a–group B polysaccharide vaccine provided encouragement, but the number of cases was too small for conclusive results.[48] Subsequently, large efficacy trials were conducted in Chile, Cuba, and Norway.[49–51] Protection rates of approximately 50% were demonstrated in Norway and Chile. The Cuban trial reported efficacy of about 80%. However, a case-control evaluation of this vaccine during a mass immunization campaign in Brazil demonstrated lower protective efficacy, particularly in children younger than 4 years.[52, 53]

Although encouraging, these OMP-based vaccines have yet to demonstrate that they can generate high sustained levels of bactericidal antibodies and acceptable rates of protection, particularly in infants.

Alternative approaches to development of a group B vaccine rest on the identification of the important virulence determinants of the meningococcus and specific antigens capable of eliciting bactericidal antibody. Other potential meningococcal vaccine candidates include detoxified LOS, the H.8 antigen, iron-regulated proteins, IgA protease, and pili.[54–58]

Chemoprophylaxis

Antibiotic administration for the prevention of invasive meningococcal disease is based on the premise that close contacts (e.g., defined as living and sleeping in the same household, dormitory, or barracks) of meningococcal disease cases are at a considerably higher risk than the normal population for development of disease. Although close contacts are at a 500- to 1000-fold higher risk than are control subjects, the risk of invasive disease in an individual contact is still quite low.[30] Nonetheless, the standard practice is to prescribe an antibiotic course designed to eradicate meningococcal throat carriage in all close contacts. Nonimmunized contacts should also receive the tetravalent meningococcal vaccine in all situations except group B outbreaks because protective antibody develops quickly after immunization. Time does not permit bacteriologic screening to determine an individual's carrier status, because those who develop invasive disease usually do so within a few days of exposure to the index case.

Because chemoprophylaxis is not uniformly successful or sufficient for treatment of invasive disease, patients must be advised to seek prompt evaluation in the event of symptoms even remotely suggestive of meningococcal infection.

Sulfadiazine was employed as chemoprophylaxis with great success in the 1940s and 1950s. But the emergence and high prevalence of sulfadiazine-resistant meningococci in the 1960s rendered it inadequate. Although the prevalence of sulfadiazine resistance has waned, sulfadiazine prophylaxis is rarely practical because of the time involved in determining sulfadiazine susceptibility.

Despite their efficacy in the treatment of invasive disease, penicillins do not predictably eradicate carriage and consequently are not used.[30]

Rifampin and minocycline are the mainstays of chemoprophylaxis. Rifampin, given twice daily for 2 days in a dose of 10 mg/kg (up to 600 mg per dose), eradicates meningococci from 75% to 98% of carriers.[41, 59] Side effects are few, but treatment failure has been associated with rifampin resistance.[60] Minocycline can also be used in patients older than 8 years in an oral dose of 100 mg twice daily for 5 days. Eradication rates approximate those seen with rifampin, and resistance does not readily emerge.[61] However, vestibular side effects are common.

Early reports using third-generation cephalosporins or carboxyquinolones are encouraging. A single intramuscular injection of ceftriaxone was 97% effective in eradicating meningococci from patients with throat carriage.[62] However, the cost, availability, and route of administration complicate its worldwide use. Ciprofloxacin has an efficacy of 89% to 100%.[59, 63] The last two antibiotics offer the important additional advantage that they achieve good central nervous system levels.

Acknowledgment

The authors would like to express their appreciation and thanks to Ms. Lyn Heskett for her superb assistance.

References

1. Heist GD, Solis-Cohen S, Solis-Cohen M: A study of the virulence of meningococci for man and of human susceptibility of meningococcic infection. J Immunol 7:1, 1922.
2. Brundage JF, Zollinger WD: Evolution of meningococcal disease epidemiology in the US Army. *In* Vedros NA (ed): Evolution of Meningococcal Disease, Vol I. Boca Raton, FL, CRC Press, 1987, pp 6–25.
3. Goldschneider I, Gotschlich EC, Artenstein MS: Human immunity to the meningococcus. I. The role of humoral antibodies. J Exp Med 129:1307, 1969.
4. Artenstein MS, Gold R, Zimmerly JG, et al: Prevention of meningococcal disease by group C polysaccharide vaccine. N Engl J Med 282:417, 1970.
5. Artenstein MS: Chemoprophylaxis of meningococcal carriers. N Engl J Med 281:678, 1969.
6. Knapp JS: Historical perspectives and identification of *Neisseria* and related species. Clin Microbiol Rev 1:415, 1988.
7. Jenning HJ: Capsular polysaccharides as human vaccines. Adv Carbohydr Chem Biochem 41:155, 1983.
8. Michon F, Roy R, Jennings HJ, et al: Structural elucidation of the capsular polysaccharide of *Neisseria meningitidis* group H. Can J Chem 62:1519, 1984.
9. Michon F, Brisson JR, Roy R, et al: Structural determination of the capsular polysaccharide of *Neisseria meningitidis* group I: A two-dimensional NMR analysis. Biochemistry 24:5592, 1985.
10. Michon F, Brisson JR, Roy R, et al: Structural determination of the group K capsular polysaccharide of *Neisseria meningitidis:* A 2D-NMR analysis. Can J Chem 63:2781, 1985.
11. Jenning HJ: The structure of the capsular polysaccharide obtained from a new serogroup (L) of *Neisseria meningitidis*. Carbohydr Res 112:105, 1983.
12. Frasch CE, Zollinger WD, Poolman JT: A proposed nomenclature for designation of serotypes within *Neisseria meningitidis*. Rev Infect Dis 7:504, 1985.
13. Tsai CM, Frasch CE, Mocca LF: Five structural classes of major outer membrane proteins in *Neisseria meningitidis*. J Bacteriol 146:69, 1981.
14. Caugant DA, Froholm LO, Borre K, et al: Intercontinental spread of a genetically distinctive complex of clones of *Neisseria meningitidis* causing epidemic disease. Proc Natl Acad Sci USA 83:4927, 1986.
15. Caugant DA, Kristiansen BE, Froholm LO, et al: Clonal diversity of *Neisseria meningitidis* from a population of asymptomatic carriers. Infect Immun 56:2060, 1988.

16. Zhen H: Epidemiology of meningococcal disease in China. *In* Vedros NA (ed): Evolution of Meningococcal Disease, Vol II. Boca Raton, FL, CRC Press, 1987, pp 19–32.
17. Schwartz B, Moore PS, Broome CV: Global epidemiology of meningococcal disease. Clin Microbiol Rev 2(Suppl):S118, 1989.
18. Centers for Disease Control: Follow up on meningococcal meningitis—Brazil. MMWR Morb Mortal Wkly Rep 23:349, 1974.
19. Tappero JW, Reporter R, Wenger JD, et al: Meningococcal disease in Los Angeles County, California, and among men in the county jails. N Engl J Med 335:833, 1996.
20. Peltola H: Meningococcal disease: Still with us. Rev Infect Dis 5:71, 1983.
21. DeVoe IW: The meningococcus and mechanisms of pathogenicity. Microbiol Rev 46:162, 1982.
22. Densen P: Interaction of complement with *Neisseria meningitidis* and *Neisseria gonorrhoeae*. Clin Microbiol Rev 2(Suppl):S11, 1989.
23. Griffiss JM, Bertram MA: Immuno-epidemiology of meningococcal disease in military recruits. II. Blocking of serum bactericidal activity by circulating IgA early in the course of invasive disease. J Infect Dis 136:733, 1977.
24. Hobbs JR, Milner RDG, Watt PJ: Gamma M deficiency predisposing to meningococcal septicaemia. Br Med J 4:583, 1967.
25. Brandtzaeg P, Ovstebo R, Kierrulf P: Compartmentalization of lipopolysaccharide production correlates with clinical presentation in meningococcal disease. J Infect Dis 166:650, 1992.
26. Irwin RS, Woelk WK, Condon WL: Primary meningococcal penumonia. Ann Intern Med 82:493, 1975.
27. Benoit FL: Chronic meningococcemia. Am J Med 35:103, 1963.
28. Waage A, Brandizag P, Holstensen A, et al: The complex pattern of cytokines in serum from patients with meningococcal septic shock. J Exp Med 169:333, 1989.
29. Hardman JM: Fatal meningococcal infections: The changing pathologic picture in the '60's. Mil Med 12:951, 1968.
30. Gold R: Clinical aspects of meningococcal disease. *In* Vedros NA (ed): Evolution of Meningococcal Disease, Vol II. Boca Raton, FL, CRC Press, 1987, pp 69–97.
31. Rosenthal J, Golan A, Dagan R: Bacterial meningitis with initial normal cerebrospinal fluid findings. Isr J Med Sci 25:186, 1989.
32. Wilson CB, Smith AL: Rapid tests for the diagnosis of bacterial meningitis. *In* Remington J, Swartz MN (eds): Current Clinical Topics in Infectious Diseases, Vol XII. New York, McGraw-Hill, 1986, pp 134–156.
33. Ni H, Knight AI, Cartwright K, et al: Polymerase chain reaction for diagnosis of meningococcal meningitis. Lancet 340:1432, 1992.
34. Cherubin CE, Eng RHK, Norrby R, et al: Penetration of newer cephalosporins into cerebrospinal fluid. Rev Infect Dis 11:526, 1989.
35. Scheld NM: Quinolone therapy for infections of the central nervous system. Rev Infect Dis 11(Suppl):S1194, 1989.
36. Jackson LA, Tenover FC, Baker C, et al: Prevalence of *Neisseria meningitidis* relatively resistant to penicillin in the United States, 1991. J Infect Dis 169:438, 1994.
37. Berron S, Vazquez JA: Increase in moderate penicillin resistance and serogroup C in meningococcal strains isolated in Spain. Is there any relationship? Clin Infect Dis 18:161, 1994.
38. Woods CR, Smith AL, Wasilauskas BL, et al: Invasive disease caused by *Neisseria meningitidis* relatively resistant to penicillin in North Carolina. J Infect Dis 170:453, 1994.
39. Lebel MH, Freig BJ, Syrogiannopoulos A, et al: Dexamethasone therapy for bacterial meningitis: Results of two double-blind, placebo-controlled trials. N Engl J Med 319:964, 1988.
40. Wahdan MH, Rizk F, El-Addad AM, et al: A controlled field trial of a serogroup A meningococcal polysaccharide vaccine. Bull WHO 48:667, 1973.
41. Centers for Disease Control: Meningococcal vaccines. MMWR Morbid Mortal Wkly Rep 34:255, 1985.
42. Lepow ML, Gold R: Meningococcal A and other polysaccharide vaccines: A five year progress report. N Engl J Med 308:1158, 1983.
43. Eskola J, Peltola H, Takala AK, et al: Efficacy of *Haemophilus influenzae* type b polysaccharide–diphtheria toxoid conjugate vaccine in infancy. N Engl J Med 317:717, 1987.
44. Twumasi PA Jr, Kumah S, Leach A, et al: A trial of a group A plus group C meningococcal polysaccharide–protein conjugate vaccine in African infants. J Infect Dis 171:632, 1995.
45. Wyle FA, Artenstein MS, Brandt BL, et al: Immunologic response of man to group B meningococcal polysaccharide vaccines. J Infect Dis 126:514, 1972.
46. Finne J, Leinonen M, Makela PH: Antigenic similarities between brain components and bacteria causing meningitis: Implications for vaccine development and pathogenesis. Lancet 2:355, 1983.
47. Zollinger WD, Boslego JW, Brandt B, et al: Safety and antigenicity studies of a polyvalent meningococcal protein–polysaccharide vaccine. Antonie Van Leeuwenhoek 52:225, 1985.
48. Frash CE, Coetzee G, Zahradnik JM, et al: Development and evaluation of group B serotype 2 protein vaccines: Report of a group B field trial. Med Trop (Mars) 43:177, 1983.
49. Boslego J, Garcia J, Cruz C, et al: Efficacy, safety, and immunogenicity of a meningococcal group B (15:P1.3) outer membrane protein vaccine in Iquique, Chile. Vaccine 13:821, 1995.
50. Sierra GVG, Campa HCC, Garcia IL, et al: Efficacy evaluation of the Cuban vaccine VA-MENGOC-BC® against disease caused by serogroup B *Neisseria meningitidis*. *In* Atchtman M (ed): *Neisseria*. Berlin, Walter de Gruyter, 1990, pp 129–134.
51. Bjune G, Hoiby EA, Gronnesby JK, et al: Effect of outer membrane vesicle vaccine against group B meningococcal disease in Norway. Lancet 338:1093, 1991.
52. De Moraes JC, Perkins BA, Camargo MCC, et al: Protective efficacy of a serogroup B meningococcal vaccine in São Paulo, Brazil. Lancet 340:1074, 1992.
53. Milagres LG, Ramos SR, Sacchi CT, et al: Immune response of Brazilian children to a *Neisseria meningitidis* serogroup B outer membrane protein vaccine: Comparison with efficacy. Infect Immun 62:4419, 1994.
54. Jennings HJ, Lugowski C, Ashton FE: Conjugation of meningococcal lipopolysaccharide R type oligosaccharides to tetanus toxoid as route to potential vaccine against group B *Neisseria meningitidis*. Infect Immun 43:407, 1984.
55. Bhattachaujee AK, Moran EE, Ray JS, et al: Purification and characterization of H.8 antigen from group B *Neisseria meningitidis*. Infect Immun 56:773, 1988.
56. Mietzner TA, Bolan G, Schoolnik GK, Morse SA: Purification and characterization of the major iron-regulated protein expressed by pathogenic *Neisseriae*. J Exp Med 165:1041, 1987.
57. Koomey JM, Falkow S: Nucleotide sequence homology between the immunoglobulin A1 protease genes of *Neisseria gonorrhoeae*, *Neisseria meningitidis*, and *Haemophilus influenzae*. Infect Immun 43:101, 1984.
58. Stephens DS, Whitney AM, Rothbard J, et al: Pili of *Neisseria meningitidis*: Analysis of structure and investigation of antigenic relationships to gonococcal pili. J Exp Med 161:1539, 1985.
59. Cuevas LE, Kazembe P, Mughogho GK, et al: Eradication of nasopharyngeal carriage of *Neisseria meningitidis* in children and adults in rural Africa: A comparison of ciprofloxacin and rifampicin. J Infect Dis 171:728, 1995.
60. Cooper ER, Ellison RT, Smith GS, et al: Rifampin-resistant meningococcal disease in a contact patient given prophylactic rifampin. J Pediatr 108:93, 1986.
61. Guttler RB, Beaty HN: Minocycline in the chemoprophylaxis of meningococcal disease. Antimicrob Agents Chemother 1:397, 1972.
62. Schwartz B, Al-Tobaiqi A, Al-Ruwais A, et al: Comparative efficacy of ceftriaxone and rifampicin in eradicating pharyngeal carriage of group A *Neisseria meningitidis*. Lancet 1:1239, 1988.
63. Gaunt PN, Lambert BE: Single dose ciprofloxacin for the eradication of pharyngeal carriage of *Neisseria meningitidis*. J Antimicrob Chemother 21:489, 1988.

203

Miscellaneous Gram-Negative Cocci: Other *Neisseria, Branhamella, Moraxella,* and *Kingella* Species

Timothy F. Murphy

The family Neisseriaceae is composed of six genera: *Neisseria, Branhamella, Moraxella, Acinetobacter, Kingella,* and *Oligella.* Table 203–1 lists some of the characteristics that are used to differentiate the genera of the family.

In this chapter, *Neisseria* species other than *Neisseria gonorrhoeae* and *Neisseria meningitidis* are discussed. *N. gonorrhoeae* and *N. meningitidis* are discussed in Chapters 201 and 202, respectively. *Acinetobacter* is discussed in Chapter 216.

Other *Neisseria* Species

N. meningitidis and *N. gonorrhoeae* have long been recognized as the pathogenic *Neisseria,* whereas other *Neisseria* species have been regarded as the nonpathogenic or commensal. These other *Neisseria* species, listed in Table 203–2, are unusual causes of disease in humans. DNA hybridization studies have demonstrated that these other *Neisseria* species lack several markers associated with virulence in the meningococcus and gonococcus. These include pili, the protein II outer membrane protein, and the H.8 antigen.[1]

Neisseria species can be distinguished from one another by a variety of methods, which are based on carbohydrate utilization, colorimetry involving chromogenic substrates, monoclonal antibody reactivity, and isoenzyme electrophoresis.[2–4] Several kits are commercially available.

Other *Neisseria* species are common inhabitants of the normal upper respiratory tract.[5, 6] Asymptomatic carriage of *Neisseria lactamica* induces antibody that cross-reacts with lipooligosaccharide (LOS) of *N. meningitidis;* this antibody may be important in protection from meningococcal infection.[6, 7] *N. lactamica* has rarely been recovered from the female genital tract.[8]

Other *Neisseria* species are unusual causes of human disease. Infections that are caused by these organisms are documented primarily by small series and case reports. These infections include meningitis,[9, 10] endocarditis,[11–18] bacteremia,[19, 20] ocular infections,[21–23] pericarditis,[24] empyema,[25] septic arthritis,[26] bursitis,[27, 28] osteomyelitis,[20, 29] otitis media,[19, 30] and Bartholin gland abscess.[31] The former Centers for Disease Control and Prevention group M5 strains have been characterized as the species *Neisseria weaveri.*[32] These strains are strongly associated with dog bite wounds in humans.[32, 33]

Many of these infections have been treated successfully with penicillin or ampicillin. However, isolates of *Neisseria* species showing increased resistance to penicillin have emerged in more recent years.[34, 35] One mechanism of resistance in *Neisseria* species is an alteration of penicillin binding protein 2 genes *(penA).*[36] Interspecies transfer of *penA* genes by genetic transformation from commensal *Neisseria* species to pathogenic *Neisseria* is an important mechanism of acquisition of penicillin resistance of *N. gonorrhoeae* and *N. meningitidis.*[36–39] Susceptibility testing should be performed on all isolates associated with invasive infections.

Branhamella

Branhamella (Moraxella) catarrhalis was previously known as *Neisseria catarrhalis* and had been regarded as a harmless saprophyte of the upper respiratory tract. During the past 15 years, *B. catarrhalis* has emerged as an important human respiratory tract pathogen.

The taxonomic relationship of *B. catarrhalis* to *Moraxella* and other related genera is controversial. *B. catarrhalis* was transferred to the new genus, *Branhamella,* in 1970 on the basis of differences in fatty acid content and DNA hybridization studies compared with other Neisseriaceae.[40] An alternative scheme has *Branhamella* as a subgenus of *Moraxella.*[41] Experimental data to support both schemes exist.[42] The changing and unstable nomenclature of the bacterium has been a frustration for practicing physicians and investigators working on the organism. Placement in the genus *Branhamella* is most rational at this time for two reasons: (1) this nomenclature serves to place rod-shaped organisms *(Moraxella)* in one species and cocci *(Branhamella)* in a separate species. (2) *B. catarrhalis* is an important and common human respiratory tract pathogen, whereas *Moraxella* species are unusual human pathogens. This distinction is highlighted by classifying them

TABLE 203–1 ■ Differential Characteristics of the Genera of the Family Neisseriaceae*

CHARACTERISTIC	*NEISSERIA*	*MORAXELLA*	*BRANHAMELLA*	*ACINETOBACTER*	*KINGELLA*	*OLIGELLA*[133]
Cell morphology						
Cocci	+	−	+	−	−	−
Rods	+	+	−	+	+	+
Oxidase test	+	+	+	−	+	+
Catalase test	+	+	+	+	−	+
Presence of carbonic anhydrase	+	−	−			
Acid from glucose	[+]	−	−	D	+	−
Nitrite reduction	+	−	D	−	+	+
Mol% G + C of DNA	46.5–53.5	40–47.5	40–47.5	38–47	47–55	46–47

*+, Positive for the majority of strains and some strains of each species; [+], positive for all strains of the majority of species (only one species uniformly negative); D, positive and negative species (or strains of *Acinetobacter*) about equally represented; −, all strains negative; G, guanine; C, cytosine.

Adapted from Bøvre K: Family VIII. Neisseriaceae Prévot 1933, 119. *In* Krieg NR, Holt JG (eds): Bergey's Manual of Systematic Bacteriology, Vol 1. Baltimore, Williams & Wilkins, 1984, p 289.

TABLE 203–2 ■ Genera and Species of the Family Neisseriaceae

Neisseria	*Moraxella*
N. gonorrhoeae	*M. lacunata*
N. meningitidis	*M. liquefaciens*
N. lactamica	*M. nonliquefaciens*
N. sicca	*M. osloensis*
N. subflava	*M. phenylpyruvica*
N. mucosa	*M. atlantae*
N. flavescens	*M. bovis*
N. cinerea	*M. lincolnii*
N. perflava	*Kingella*
N. flava	*K. kingae*
N. weaveri	*K. indologenes*
N. elongata	*K. denitrificans*
Branhamella	*Acinetobacter*
B. catarrhalis	*A. calcoaceticus (anitratus)*
B. caviae	*A. lwoffi*
B. ovis	*Oligella*
B. cuniculi	*O. urethralis*
	O. ureolytica

as separate species. The nomenclature of these bacteria continues to be a matter of debate and additional changes may occur.

B. catarrhalis has generated investigative interest because of its importance as a human pathogen in certain clinical settings. It is predominantly a mucosal pathogen. It is a common cause of otitis media in children, sinusitis in children and adults, and lower respiratory tract infection in the elderly and in the setting of chronic bronchitis.

Characteristics of the Pathogen

Growth and Identification. *B. catarrhalis* is morphologically indistinguishable from *Neisseria* species. Therefore, for the bacterium to be identified in respiratory tract secretions, the clinical microbiology laboratory must specifically test colonies to distinguish *Branhamella* from commensal *Neisseria. B. catarrhalis* is a gram-negative diplococcus with kidney-shaped cells. The organism grows well on blood agar, chocolate agar, and a variety of media. Isolates of *B. catarrhalis* produce cytochrome oxidase, catalase, and DNase. They are unable to utilize maltose, glucose, lactose, and sucrose as carbohydrate sources. Several kits to speciate strains of *B. catarrhalis* are commercially available.

Surface Antigens. The surface of *B. catarrhalis* is composed of outer membrane proteins, LOS, and pili. Preliminary observations suggest that *B. catarrhalis* may have a small capsule.[43] However, these observations are limited to electron microscopic observations; further work is needed to determine definitively whether *B. catarrhalis* has a capsule.

The outer membrane proteins of *B. catarrhalis* have generated substantial interest in the past 10 years. Analysis of strains of *B. catarrhalis* from diverse clinical and geographic sources reveals that the molecular weights of eight major outer membrane proteins are nearly identical from strain to strain.[44] This contrasts with other species of nonenteric gram-negative bacteria for which differences in outer membrane protein patterns among isolates are generally observed. Table 203–3 summarizes information on five outer membrane proteins that are of particular interest. Current lines of investigation are evaluating these outer membrane proteins as potential virulence factors for the organism and as potential vaccine antigens.

The LOS of *B. catarrhalis* consists of a lipid A core coupled to oligosaccharides. The molecule lacks the long O-polysaccharide side chains observed in enteric gram-negative bacteria. The molecular mass is approximately 5500 daltons, and the molecule shares many structural features with the LOS of other nonenteric gram-negative bacteria that colonize mucosal surfaces.[45, 46] A serotyping system based on antigenic differences in the LOS molecule has been developed. Three antigenic types have been identified by using adsorbed antisera in an inhibition enzyme-linked immunosorbent assay.[47] The LOS of *B. catarrhalis* exhibits biologic activity that is characteristic of endotoxin.[48] Although specific studies have not yet been performed, LOS is likely an important virulence factor in *B. catarrhalis* infections.

Clinical isolates of *B. catarrhalis* express pili, which are lost with progressive passage in vitro.[49] Preliminary studies suggest a role for pili in adherence,[50, 51] but elucidation of the precise of role of pili in adherence awaits the development of appropriate model systems for the study of *B. catarrhalis* adherence.

Typing Systems. A variety of approaches have been used to develop methods for typing strains of *B. catarrhalis*. Table 203–4 lists seven systems that have been used to help elucidate the epidemiology of colonization and infection. Each system has advantages and limitations. An ideal serotyping system for *B. catarrhalis* has not yet been developed. This system would divide strains into several groups based on antigenic differences in important surface antigens, be convenient and reproducible, and be capable of placing all strains into a serotype. Such a system would be a powerful tool for understanding the epidemiology, pathogenesis, and protection from infection by *B. catarrhalis*.

Epidemiology

B. catarrhalis colonizes primarily the upper respiratory tract, although it has occasionally been recovered from genital mucosa. Nasopharyngeal colonization with *B. catarrhalis* is common throughout infancy.[52–55] A prospective study in which nasopharyngeal cultures were obtained monthly showed that 66% of infants were colonized at some time during the first year of life and 78% were colonized by the age of 2 years.[53] A high rate of colonization with *B. catarrhalis* is associated

TABLE 203–3 ■ Characteristics of Selected Outer Membrane Proteins of *Branhamella catarrhalis*

OUTER MEMBRANE PROTEIN*	MOLECULAR MASS (kDa)	PROPOSED FUNCTION	OTHER OBSERVATIONS	REFERENCES
HMW-OMP (UspA)	350–700	Adhesin	Oligomer; antibodies enhance clearance in mice; mediates complement resistance	134, 135
OMP B1	84	Iron acquisition	Major target of human antibody	136, 137
OMP B2 (CopB)	80	Iron acquisition	Antibodies enhance clearance in mice	138, 139
OMP CD	46	Porin	Highly conserved; homology with *Pseudomonas* OprF	44, 140, 141
OMP E	50	Porin	Highly conserved	142, 143

*HMW, High molecular weight; OMP, outer membrane protein.

TABLE 203–4 ■ Typing Systems for *Branhamella catarrhalis*

TYPING SYSTEM	REFERENCE
SDS-PAGE and immunoblot assays*	75
Esterase electrophoretic polymorphism	144, 145
LOS serotyping	47
Restriction enzyme analysis	72–77, 146
Southern blot assays with DNA probes	72
Ribotyping	144
Pulsed-field gel electrophoresis of genomic DNA	56, 147

*SDS-PAGE, Sodium dodecyl sulfate–polyacrylamide gel electrophoresis.

with an increased incidence of otitis media.[53] Healthy adults have a low rate of respiratory tract colonization by *B. catarrhalis*.[54] A subset of patients with bronchiectasis is colonized with *B. catarrhalis*.[56] Analysis of prospectively collected strains from the sputum of patients with bronchiectasis has shown that one strain colonizes for a mean duration of 2.3 months.[56] These observations indicate that colonization by *B. catarrhalis* is a dynamic process.

B. catarrhalis is an important cause of otitis media. Studies from several centers in the 1990s have established that *B. catarrhalis* is the third most common cause of otitis media (Table 203–5). In all of the series in Table 203–5, cultures of middle-ear aspirates were performed; this is the most reliable method of establishing the cause of otitis media. Two additional lines of evidence that *B. catarrhalis* is a middle-ear pathogen exist. First, the cellular nature of middle-ear fluid containing *B. catarrhalis* is generally indistinguishable from that of middle-ear fluid obtained from patients with pneumococcal otitis media.[57] Second, antibodies specific for *B. catarrhalis* develop after otitis media in which a pure culture of *B. catarrhalis* is obtained from middle-ear fluid.[58] As strategies for preventing otitis media caused by pneumococcus and nontypeable *Haemophilus influenzae* are developed, the relative importance of *B. catarrhalis* as a cause of otitis media will increase in the next decade.

B. catarrhalis causes sinusitis in adults and children.[59, 60] The organism can be recovered alone or in combination with other bacteria from direct sinus aspirates from patients with clinical and radiographic evidence of acute bacterial sinusitis. In addition, serologic data provide evidence for *B. catarrhalis* as a cause of sinusitis.[59]

B. catarrhalis causes lower respiratory tract infections, particularly in the setting of chronic bronchitis and chronic obstructive pulmonary disease (COPD).[61] Four sets of observations indicate that *B. catarrhalis* is a lower respiratory tract pathogen. (1) Some patients with COPD have exacerbations in which a sputum Gram stain shows a predominance of intracellular and extracellular gram-negative diplococci and culture reveals *B. catarrhalis*. (2) *B. catarrhalis* can be obtained from transtracheal aspirates in pure culture from patients with clinical evidence of respiratory infection.[62, 63] (3) Administration of specific antimicrobial therapy directed at β-lactamase–producing *B. catarrhalis* results in clinical improvement in these patients after failure of therapy with β-lactams. (4) Patients with clinical, Gram stain, and culture evidence of respiratory infection with *B. catarrhalis* develop bactericidal antibodies specific for their own isolate.[64]

In addition to causing purulent exacerbations of COPD, which are generally not associated with infiltrates on chest films, *B. catarrhalis* causes pneumonia, particularly in the elderly.[65–70] A highly characteristic feature is a predominance of gram-negative diplococci on the sputum Gram stain. When *B. catarrhalis* is the etiologic agent of pneumonia or causes an exacerbation of COPD, the organism is usually present in large numbers in the sputum.

Nosocomial outbreaks of lower respiratory tract infections caused by *B. catarrhalis* have been recognized since the mid-1980s. Reports from several centers indicate that clusters of *B. catarrhalis* infections occur in hospitals.[71–77] The reservoir of infection and the mode of transmission are largely unknown. Several of these outbreaks have occurred in respiratory units, suggesting that the presence of a susceptible population contributed to the clusters. The availability of a serotyping system will be important in elucidating the factors responsible for nosocomial outbreaks so that rational strategies for preventing them can be developed.

In addition to the relatively common clinical manifestations just noted, *B. catarrhalis* is a rare cause of invasive infections. These are documented predominantly by case reports. Invasive infections rarely caused by *B. catarrhalis* include meningitis,[78] endocarditis,[79, 80] bacteremia,[81–83] septic arthritis,[84, 85] osteomyelitis,[86] epiglottitis,[87] cellulitis,[88] shunt-associated ventriculitis,[89] peritonitis,[90] pericarditis,[91] wound infection,[92] and others. In addition, *B. catarrhalis* is an unusual cause of acute urethritis[93, 94] and can also cause conjunctivitis.[95, 96]

Clinical Manifestations and Diagnosis

The clinical manifestations of otitis media and sinusitis caused by *B. catarrhalis* are indistinguishable from those of infection by other organisms. Otitis and sinusitis caused by *B. catarrhalis* may be associated with less fever and fewer constitutional symptoms of infection compared with pneumococcus and nontypable *H. influenzae*, but substantial overlap exists. The diagnosis of otitis media is best made by pneumatic otoscopy. A compatible clinical picture and radiograph suggest a diagnosis of sinusitis. Tympanocentesis is required to establish an etiologic diagnosis of otitis media, and sinus aspiration is necessary to establish the cause of

TABLE 203–5 ■ Causes of Otitis Media: Results of Tympanocentesis

			% OF CASES CAUSED BY		
REFERENCE	YEAR	LOCATION	*Streptococcus pneumoniae*	*Haemophilus influenzae*	*Branhamella catarrhalis*
148	1990	Norway and Finland	28	16	16
149	1991	Dallas, Texas	29	30	15
150	1991	Cleveland, Ohio	25	27	11
151	1992	Buffalo, New York	19	35	18
152	1992	Philadelphia, Pennsylvania	48	20	23
153	1992	Galveston, Texas	39	34	18
154	1993	Galveston, Texas	29	37	15
155	1994	United States—five centers	39	27	14

sinusitis, but these are not routinely performed. Nasopharyngeal and throat cultures are not helpful in establishing a cause of either otitis media or sinusitis because bacteria colonize the nasopharynx and throat in the absence of infection.

The clinical manifestations of lower respiratory tract infection caused by *B. catarrhalis* are similar to those of infection by other bacteria such as nontypeable *H. influenzae*. Exacerbations of COPD are characterized by cough; purulent sputum, which is sometimes copious; and shortness of breath. When fever is present, it is usually low grade. Pneumonia caused by *B. catarrhalis* occurs almost exclusively in the elderly and in patients with COPD. It is characterized by temperature as high as 103°F, cough, purulent sputum, and shortness of breath. Auscultation sometimes reveals signs of consolidation. The chest film shows either patchy or lobar alveolar infiltrates. Pleural effusion and empyema are uncommon. The most practical method for making a diagnosis is a sputum Gram stain. A Gram-stained sputum sample that shows a predominance of intracellular and extracellular gram-negative diplococci is a rapid, simple, and reliable indicator for making a diagnosis.[64]

Treatment

Approximately 90% of strains of *B. catarrhalis* produce β-lactamase.[97, 98] The β-lactamase of *B. catarrhalis* is inducible, remains cell associated, and is more active against penicillins than against cephalosporins, and its activity is inhibited by β-lactamase inhibitors such as clavulanic acid and sulbactam. β-Lactamase–producing strains show an inoculum-dependent susceptibility to ampicillin. Therefore, ampicillin should not be used for β-lactamase–producing strains regardless of the results of susceptibility testing. One study showed persistently positive middle-ear cultures during ampicillin therapy for *B. catarrhalis* otitis media caused by a β-lactamase–producing strain.[52] Most *B. catarrhalis* infections can be treated with orally administered antimicrobial agents. Oral agents active against *B. catarrhalis* include erythromycin, trimethoprim-sulfamethoxazole, tetracycline, ciprofloxacin, azithromycin, clarithromycin, and the combination of amoxicillin and clavulanate.[97–99] *B. catarrhalis* is also uniformly susceptible to ticarcillin, piperacillin, mezlocillin, azlocillin, most cephalosporins, chloramphenicol, and aminoglycosides. *B. catarrhalis* is resistant to penicillin, ampicillin, vancomycin, clindamycin, and methicillin.[100, 101]

Moraxella

Moraxella organisms are normal inhabitants of the upper respiratory tract and can occasionally be recovered from the skin and genital tract. Species can be differentiated biochemically, but genetic transformation assays are useful for identification of some species.[102–104] The taxonomy of *Moraxella* species is an active area of research and is constantly changing as more is learned about these bacteria.[105–108] Indeed, the classification of some of these bacteria is controversial.[42, 109, 110] Some species of *Moraxella* are listed in Table 203–2.

Moraxella bovis causes bovine keratoconjunctivitis, the most common ocular disease of cattle throughout the world. *Moraxella* species are unusual pathogens in humans, although certain studies have emphasized the role of these bacteria as ocular pathogens.[111–113] *Moraxella* is often overlooked as a causative agent of conjunctival infection; *Moraxella nonliquefaciens* is the most common *Moraxella* species associated with eye infection, and in one study represented the fourth most common cause of corneal infection after pneumococcus, staphylococcus, and *Pseudomonas* species.[111] *Moraxella* is susceptible to all conventional topical ocular antibiotics. Topical treatment of these infections should continue for 7 to 10 days.

Moraxella species are uncommon causes of invasive infection in humans. *Moraxella* is an important cause of endophthalmitis, a serious ocular infection associated with a high likelihood of vision loss.[112, 113] Other invasive infections include endocarditis,[80, 114, 115] bacteremia,[33, 116, 117] septic arthritis,[118, 119] pneumonia,[120] purulent pericarditis,[121] and meningitis.[33, 122] A high frequency of inherited or acquired complement deficiency exists in patients with meningitis due to *Moraxella* species; therefore, such patients should be studied for complement deficiency.[122] *Moraxella* species are generally susceptible to penicillins and cephalosporins.

Kingella

In 1976, *Moraxella kingae* was transferred to the new genus *Kingella*.[123, 124] *Kingella* has three species: *Kingella kingae*, *Kingella indologenes*, and *Kingella denitrificans*. *Kingella* species are recovered from the human upper respiratory tract and are rare human pathogens. Case reports have described *Kingella* as a cause of endocarditis,[125–127] epiglottitis,[128] bacteremia,[129] and intervertebral diskitis.[130] Reports have noted a surprising increase in the incidence of invasive *K. kingae* infections in infants and children.[33, 131] Septic arthritis and osteomyelitis were the most common infections.[131] *Kingella* species are generally susceptible to a wide variety of antimicrobial agents, including penicillins and cephalosporins.[132]

References

1. Aho EL, Murphy GL, Cannon JG: Distribution of specific DNA sequences among pathogenic and commensal *Neisseria* species. Infect Immun 55:1009–1013, 1987.
2. Dillon JR, Carballo M, Pauze M: Evaluation of eight methods for identification of pathogenic *Neisseria* species: *Neisseria*-Kwik, RIM-N, Gonobio-Test, Minitek, Gonochek II, GonoGen, Phadebact Monoclonal GC OMNI Test, and Syva MicroTrak Test. J Clin Microbiol; 26:493–497, 1988.
3. Hosmer MA, Cohenford MA, Ellner PD: Preliminary evaluation of a rapid colorimetric method for identification of pathogenic *Neisseria*. J Clin Microbiol 24:141–142, 1986.
4. Braude AI, McCutchan JA, Ison C, et al: Differentiation of Nesseriaceae by isoenzyme electrophoresis. J Infect Dis 147:247–251, 1983.
5. Knapp JS, Hook EW III: Prevalence and persistence of *Neisseria cinerea* and other *Neisseria* spp. in adults. J Clin Microbiol 26:896–900, 1988.
6. Gold R, Goldschneider I, Lepow ML, et al: Carriage of *Neisseria meningitidis* and *Neisseria lactamica* in infants and children. J Infect Dis 137:112–121, 1978.
7. Kim JJ, Mandrell RE, Griffis JM: *Neisseria lactamica* and *Neisseria meningitidis* share lipooligosaccharide epitopes but lack common capsular and class 1, 2, and 3 protein epitopes. Infect Immun 57:602–608, 1989.
8. Brunton WAT, Young H, Fraser DRK: Isolation of *Neisseria lactamica* from the female genital tract. Br J Vener Dis 56:325–326, 1980.
9. Denning DW, Gill SS: *Neisseria lactamica* meningitis following skull trauma. Rev Infect Dis 13:216–218, 1991.
10. Stotka JL, Rupp ME, Meier FA, et al: Meningitis due to *Neisseria mucosa:* Case report and review. Rev Infect Dis 13:837–841, 1991.
11. Clark H, Patton RD: Postcardiotomy endocarditis due to *Neisseria perflava* on a prosthetic aortic valve. Ann Intern Med 68:386–389, 1968.
12. Anderson MD, Miller LK: Endocarditis due to *Neisseria mucosa* (Letter). Clin Infect Dis 16:184, 1993.
13. Deger R, Ludmir J: *Neisseria sicca* endocarditis complicating pregnancy. A case report. J Reprod Med 37:473–475, 1992.
14. Valenzuela GA, Davis TD, Pizzani E, McGroarty D: Infective

endocarditis due to *Neisseria sicca* and associated with intravenous drug abuse. South Med J 85:929, 1992.
15. Struillou L, Raffi F, Barrier JH: Endocarditis caused by *Neisseria elongata* subspecies *nitroreducens:* Case report and literature review. Eur J Clin Microbiol Infect Dis 12:625–627, 1993.
16. Lopez-Velez R, Fortun J, de Pablo C, et al: Native-valve endocarditis due to *Neisseria sicca.* Clin Infect Dis 18:660–661, 1994.
17. Heiddal S, Sverrisson JT, Yngvason FE, et al: Native-valve endocarditis due to *Neisseria sicca*: Case report and review. Clin Infect Dis 16:667–670, 1993.
18. Ingram RJH, Cornere B, Ellis-Pegler RB: Endocarditis due to *Neisseria mucosa*: Two case reports and review. Clin Infect Dis 15:321–324, 1992.
19. Wilson HD, Overman TL: Septicemia due to *Neisseria lactamica.* J Clin Microbiol 4:214–215, 1976.
20. Wong JD, Janda JM: Association of an important *Neisseria* species, *Neisseria elongata* subsp. *nitroreducens,* with bacteremia, endocarditis, and osteomyelitis. J Clin Microbiol 30:719–720, 1992.
21. Gini GA: Ocular infection in a newborn caused by *Neisseria mucosa.* J Clin Microbiol 25:1574–1575, 1987.
22. Au Y-K, Reynolds MD, Rambin ED, et al: *Neisseria cinerea* acute purulent conjunctivitis. Am J Ophthalmol 109:96–97, 1990.
23. Bourbeau P, Holla V, Piemontese S: Ophthalmia neonatorum caused by *Neisseria cinerea.* J Clin Microbiol 28:1640–1641, 1990.
24. Fainstein V, Musher DM, Young EJ: Purulent pericarditis due to *Neisseria mucosa.* Chest 74:476–477, 1978.
25. Thorsteinsson SB, Minuth JN, Musher DM: Postpneumonectomy empyema due to *Neisseria mucosa.* Am J Clin Pathol 64:534–536, 1975.
26. Obeid EMH: *Neisseria subflava* causing septic arthritis of the ankle in a child. J Infect 27:100–101, 1993.
27. Linquist PR, Linquist JA: *Neisseria mucosa* bursitis. A rare cause of gas in soft tissue. Clin Orthop 231:222–224, 1988.
28. Halla JT: Septic olecranon bursitis caused by *Neisseria sicca.* J Rheumatol 17:1240–1241, 1990.
29. Doern GV, Blacklow NR, Gantz NM, et al: *Neisseria sicca* osteomyelitis. J Clin Microbiol 16:595–597, 1982.
30. Orden B, Amerigo MA: Acute otitis media caused by *Neisseria lactamica.* Eur J Clin Microbiol Infect Dis 10:986–987, 1991.
31. Berger SA, Gorea A, Peyser MR, Edberg SC: Bartholin's gland abscess caused by *Neisseria sicca.* J Clin Microbiol 26:1589, 1988.
32. Holmes B, Costas M, On SLW, et al: *Neisseria weaveri* sp. nov. (formerly CDC group M-5), from dog bite wounds of humans. Int J Syst Bacteriol 43:687–693, 1993.
33. Graham DR, Band JD, Thornsberry C, et al: Infections caused by *Moraxella, Moraxella urethralis, Moraxella*-like groups M-5 and M-6, and *Kingella kingae* in the United States, 1953–1980. Rev Infect Dis 12:423–431, 1990.
34. Roberts MC, Moncla BJ: Tetracycline resistance and TetM in oral anaerobic bacteria and *Neisseria perflava–N. sicca.* Antimicrob Agents Chemother 32:1271–1273, 1988.
35. Piot P, Roberts M, Ninane G: β-lactamase production in commensal Neisseriaceae. Lancet 1:619, 1979.
36. Lujan R, Zhang Q-Y, Saez-Nieto JA, et al: Penicillin-resistant isolates of *Neisseria lactamica* produce altered forms of penicillin-binding protein 2 that arose by interspecies horizontal gene transfer. Antimicrob Agents Chemother 35:300–304, 1991.
37. Frosch M, Meyer TF: Transformation-mediated exchange of virulence determinants by co-cultivation of pathogenic *Neisseria.* FEMS Microbiol Lett 100:345–350, 1992.
38. Spratt BG, Bowler LD, Zhang Q-Y, et al: Role of interspecies transfer of chromosomal genes in the evolution of penicillin resistance in pathogenic and commensal *Neisseria* species. J Mol Evol 34:115–125, 1992.
39. Bowler LD, Zhang Q-Y, Riou J-Y, et al: Interspecies recombination between the *penA* genes of *Neisseria meningitidis* and commensal *Neisseria* species during the emergence of penicillin resistance of *N. meningitidis:* Natural events and laboratory simulation. J Bacteriol 176:333–337, 1994.
40. Catlin BW: Transfer of the organism named *Neisseria catarrhalis* to *Branhamella* genus. Int J Syst Bacteriol 20:155–159, 1970.
41. Bovre K: Proposal to divide the genus *Moraxella* into two subgenera, subgenus *Moraxella* and subgenus *Branhamella.* Int J Syst Bacteriol 29:403–406, 1979.
42. Catlin BW: Branhamaceae fam. nov., a proposed family to accommodate the genera *Branhamella* and *Moraxella.* Int J Syst Bacteriol 41:320–323, 1991.
43. Ahmed K, Rikitomi N, Ichinose A, et al: Possible presence of a capsule in *Branhamella catarrhalis.* Microbiol Immunol 35:361–366, 1991.
44. Bartos LC, Murphy TF: Comparison of the outer membrane proteins of 50 strains of *Branhamella catarrhalis.* J Infect Dis 158:761–765, 1988.
45. Edebrink P, Jansson P-E, Rahman MM, et al: Structural studies of the O-polysaccharide from the lipopolysaccharide of *Moraxella (Branhamella) catarrhalis* serotype A (strain ATCC 25238). Carbohydr Res 257:269–284, 1994.
46. Masoud H, Perry MB, Richards JC: Characterization of the lipopolysaccharide of *Moraxella catarrhalis.* Structural analysis of the lipid A from *M. catarrhalis* serotype A lipopolysaccharide. Eur J Biochem 220:209–216, 1994.
47. Vaneechoutte M, Verschraegen G, Claeys G, et al: Serological typing of *Branhamella catarrhalis* strains on the basis of lipopolysaccharide antigens. J Clin Microbiol 28:182–187, 1990.
48. Fomsgaard JS, Fomsgaard A, Hoiby N, et al: Comparative immunochemistry of lipopolysaccharides from *Branhamella catarrhalis* strains. Infect Immun 59:3346–3349, 1991.
49. Ahmed K, Rikitomi N, Matsumoto K: Fimbriation, hemagglutination and adherence properties of fresh clinical isolates of *Branhamella catarrhalis.* Microbiol Immunol 36:1009–1017, 1992.
50. Rikitomi N, Andersson B, Matsumoto K, et al: Mechanism of adherence of *Moraxella (Branhamella) catarrhalis.* Scand J Infect Dis 23:559–567, 1991.
51. Ahmed K: Fimbriae of *Branhamella catarrhalis* as possible mediators of adherence to pharyngeal epithelial cells. APMIS 100:1066–1072, 1992.
52. Van Hare GF, Shurin PA, Marchant CD, et al: Acute otitis media caused by *Branhamella catarrhalis*: Biology and therapy. Rev Infect Dis 9:16–27, 1987.
53. Faden H, Harabuchi Y, Hong JJ, et al: Epidemiology of *Moraxella catarrhalis* in children during the first 2 years of life: Relationship to otitis media. J Infect Dis 169:1312–1317, 1994.
54. Vaneechoutte M, Verschraegen G, Claeys G, et al: Respiratory tract carrier rates of *Moraxella (Branhamella) catarrhalis* in adults and children and interpretation of the isolation of *M. catarrhalis* from sputum. J Clin Microbiol 28:2674–2680, 1990.
55. Aniansson G, Alm B, Andersson B, et al: Nasopharyngeal colonization during the first year of life. J Infect Dis 165(Suppl1): S38–S42, 1992
56. Klingman KL, Pye A, Murphy TF, Hill SL: Dynamics of respiratory tract colonization by *Branhamella catarrhalis* in bronchiectasis. Am J Respir Crit Care Med 152:1072–1078, 1995.
57. Luotonen J, Herva E, Karma P, et al: The bacteriology of acute otitis media in children with special reference to *Streptococcus pneumoniae* as studied by bacteriological and antigen detection method. Scand J Infect Dis 13:177–183, 1981.
58. Leinonen M, Luotonen J, Herva E, et al: Preliminary serologic evidence for a pathogenic role of *Branhamella catarrhalis.* J Infect Dis 144:570–574, 1981.
59. Brorson J-E, Axelsson A, Holm SE: Studies on *Branhamella catarrhalis (Neisseria catarrhalis)* with special reference to maxillary sinusitis. Scand J Infect Dis 8:151–155, 1976.
60. Wald ER, Reilly JS, Casselbrant M, et al: Treatment of acute maxillary sinusitis in childhood: A comparative study of amoxicillin and cefaclor. J Pediatr 104:297–302, 1984.
61. Murphy TF, Sethi S: Bacterial infection in chronic obstructive pulmonary disease. Am Rev Respir Dis 146:1067–1083, 1992.
62. West M, Berk SL, Smith JK: *Branhamella catarrhalis* pneumonia. South Med J 75:1021–1023, 1982.
63. Ninane G, Joly J, Kraytman M: Bronchopulmonary infection due to *Branhamella catarrhalis*: 11 cases assessed by transtracheal puncture. Br Med J 1:276–278, 1978.
64. Chapman AJ, Musher DM, Jonsson S, et al: Development of bactericidal antibody during *Branhamella catarrhalis* infection. J Infect Dis 151:878–882, 1985.
65. Carr B, Walsh JB, Coakley D, et al: Prospective hospital study of community acquired lower respiratory tract infection in the elderly. Respir Med 85:185–187, 1991.
66. Collazos J, de Miguel J, Ayarza R: *Moraxella catarrhalis* bacteremic pneumonia in adults: Two cases and review of the literature. Eur J Clin Microbiol Infect Dis 11:237–240, 1992.
67. Barreiro B, Esteban L, Prats E, et al: *Branhamella catarrhalis* respiratory infections. Eur Respir J 5:675–679, 1992.

68. Nicotra B, Rivera M, Luman JI, et al: *Branhamella catarrhalis* as a lower respiratory tract pathogen in patients with chronic lung disease. Arch Intern Med 146:890–893, 1986.
69. Choo PW, Gantz NM: *Branhamella catarrhalis* pneumonia with bacteremia. South Med J 82:1317–1318, 1989.
70. Verghese A, Berk SL: *Moraxella (Branhamella) catarrhalis*. Infect Dis Clin North Am 5:523–538, 1991.
71. Cook PP, Hecht DW, Snydman DR: Nosocomial *Branhamella catarrhalis* in a paediatric intensive care unit: Risk factors for disease. J Hosp Infect 13:299–307, 1989.
72. Beaulieu D, Scriver S, Bergeron MG, et al: Epidemiological typing of *Moraxella catarrhalis* by using DNA probes. J Clin Microbiol 31:736–739, 1993.
73. Patterson JE, Patterson TF, Farrel P, et al: Evaluation of restriction endonuclease analysis as an epidemiologic typing system for *Branhamella catarrhalis*. J Clin Microbiol 27:944–946, 1989.
74. Patterson TF, Patterson JE, Masecar BL, et al: A nosocomial outbreak of *Branhamella catarrhalis* confirmed by restriction endonuclease analysis. J Infect Dis 157:996–1001, 1988.
75. McKenzie H, Morgan MG, Jordens JZ, et al: Characterisation of hospital isolates of *Moraxella (Branhamella) catarrhalis* by SDS-PAGE of whole-cell proteins, immunoblotting and restriction-endonuclease analysis. J Med Microbiol 37:70–76, 1992.
76. Morgan MG, McKenzie H, Enright MC, et al: Use of molecular methods to characterize *Moraxella catarrhalis* strains in a suspected outbreak of nosocomial infection. Eur J Clin Microbiol Infect Dis 11:305–312, 1992.
77. Richards SJ, Greening AP, Enright MC, et al: Outbreak of *Moraxella catarrhalis* in a respiratory unit. Thorax 48:91–92, 1993.
78. Newing WJ, Christie R: Meningitis: isolation of an organism resembling *Neisseria catarrhalis* from cerebrospinal fluid: Report of a case. Med J Aust 1:306, 1947.
79. Douer D, Danziger Y, Pinkhas J: *Neisseria catarrhalis* endocarditis (Letter). Ann Intern Med 86:116, 1977.
80. Sanyal SK, Wilson N, Twum-Danso K, et al: *Moraxella* endocarditis following balloon angioplasty of aortic coarctation. Am Heart J 119:1421–1423, 1990.
81. Wallace MR, Oldfield EC, III: *Moraxella (Branhamella) catarrhalis* bacteremia. Arch Intern Med 150:1332–1334, 1990.
82. Alaeus A, Stiernstedt G: *Branhamella catarrhalis* septicemia in an immunocompetent adult. Scand J Infect Dis 23:115–116, 1991.
83. Cimolai N, Adderley RJ: *Branhamella catarrhalis* bacteremia in children. Acta Paediatr Scand 78:465–468, 1989.
84. Craig DB, Wehrle PA: *Branhamella catarrhalis* septic arthritis. J Rheumatol 10:985–986, 1983.
85. Melendez PR, Johnson RH: Bacteremia and septic arthritis caused by *Moraxella catarrhalis*. Rev Infect Dis 13:428–429, 1991.
86. Prallet B, Lucht F, Alexandre C: Vertebral osteomyelitis due to *Branhamella catarrhalis* (Letter). Rev Infect Dis 13:769, 1991.
87. Vernham GA, Crowther JA: Acute myeloid leukaemia presenting with acute *Branhamella catarrhalis* epiglottitis. J Infect 26:93–95, 1993.
88. Rotta AT, Asmar BI: *Moraxella catarrhalis* bacteremia and preseptal cellulitis. South Med J 87:541–542, 1994.
89. Cooke RPD, Williams R, Bannister CM: Shunt-associated ventriculitis caused by *Branhamella catarrhalis*. J Hosp Infect 15:197–198, 1990.
90. Contreras MR, Ash SR, Swick SD, et al: Peritonitis due to *Moraxella (Branhamella) catarrhalis* in a diabetic patient receiving peritoneal dialysis. South Med J 86:589–590, 1993.
91. Kostiala AAI, Honkanen T: *Branhamella catarrhalis* as a cause of acute purulent pericarditis. J Infect 19:291–292, 1989.
92. Gray LD, Van Scoy RE, Anhalt JP, et al: Wound infection caused by *Branhamella catarrhalis*. J Clin Microbiol 27:818–820, 1989.
93. Smith GL: *Branhamella catarrhalis* infection imitating gonorrhea in a man (Letter). N Engl J Med 316:1277, 1987.
94. Doern GV, Gantz NM: Isolation of *Branhamella (Neisseria) catarrhalis* from men with urethritis. Sex Transm Dis 9:202–204, 1982.
95. Lue YA, Simms DH, Ubriani R, et al: Ophthalmia neonatorum caused by penicillin-resistant *Branhamella catarrhalis*. N Y State J Med 81:1775–1776, 1981.
96. Kawakami Y, Segawa K, Kandi M: A case of acute catarrhal conjunctivitis due to *Branhamella catarrhalis*. Microbiol Immunol 27:641–642, 1983.
97. Barry AL, Pfaller MA, Fuchs PC, et al: In vitro activities of 12 orally administered antimicrobial agents against four species of bacterial respiratory pathogens from U.S. medical centers in 1992 and 1993. Antimicrob Agents Chemother 38:2419–2425, 1994.
98. Fung CP, Powell M, Seymour A, et al: The antimicrobial susceptibility of *Moraxella catarrhalis* isolated in England and Scotland in 1991. J Antimicrob Chemother 30:47–55, 1992.
99. Powell M, McVey D, Kassim MH, et al: Antimicrobial susceptibility of *Streptococcus pneumoniae, Haemophilus influenzae* and *Moraxella (Branhamella) catarrhalis* isolated in the UK from sputa. J Antimicrob Chemother 28:249–259, 1991.
100. Doern GV, Siebers KG, Hallick LM: Antibiotic susceptibility of β-lactamase–producing strains of *Branhamella (Neisseria) catarrhalis*. Antimicrob Agents Chemother 26:424–425, 1984.
101. Fung C-P, Yeo S-F, Livermore DM: Susceptibility of *Moraxella catarrhalis* isolates to β-lactam antibiotics in relation to β-lactamase pattern. J Antimicrob Chemother 33:215–222, 1994.
102. Juni E, Heym GA, Maurer MJ, et al: Combined genetic transformation and nutritional assay for identification of *Moraxella nonliquefaciens*. J Clin Microbiol 25:1691–1694, 1987.
103. Henriksen SD: *Moraxella, Neisseria, Branhamella,* and *Acinetobacter*. Annu Rev Microbiol 30:63–83, 1976.
104. Henriksen SD: *Moraxella, Acinetobacter*, and the *Mimeae*. Bacteriol Rev 37:522–561, 1973.
105. Tonjum T, Caugant DA, Bovre K: Differentiation of *Moraxella nonliquefaciens, M. lacunata*, and *M. bovis* by using multilocus enzyme electrophoresis and hybridization with pilin-specific DNA probes. J Clin Microbiol 30:3099–3107, 1992.
106. Veron M, Lenvoise-Furet A, Coustere C, et al: Relatedness of three species of "false *Neisseria*," *Neisseria caviae, Neisseria cuniculi*, and *Neisseria ovis*, by DNA-DNA hybridizations and fatty acid analysis. Int J Syst Bacteriol 43:210–220, 1993.
107. Jannes G, Vaneechoutte M, Lannoo M, et al: Polyphasic taxonomy leading to the proposal of *Moraxella canis* sp. nov. for *Moraxella catarrhalis*–like strains. Int J Syst Bacteriol 43:438–449, 1993.
108. Van damme P, Gillis M, Van Canneyt M, et al: *Moraxella lincolnii* sp. nov., isolated from the human respiratory tract, and reevaluation of the taxonomic position of *Moraxella osloensis*. Int J Syst Bacteriol 43:474–481, 1993.
109. Rossau R, Van Landschoot A, Gillis M, et al: Taxonomy of *Moraxellaceae* fam. nov., a new bacterial family to accommodate the genera *Moraxella, Acinetobacter*, and *Psychrobacter* and related organisms. Int J Syst Bacteriol 41:310–319, 1991.
110. Catlin BW: *Branhamella catarrhalis*: An organism gaining respect as a pathogen. Clin Microbiol Rev 3:293–320, 1990.
111. Cobo LM, Coster DJ, Peacock J: *Moraxella* keratitis in a nonalcoholic population. Br J Ophthalmol 65:683–686, 1981.
112. Schmidt ME, Smith MA, Levy CS: Endophthalmitis caused by unusual gram-negative bacilli: Three case reports and review. Clin Infect Dis 17:686–690, 1993.
113. Sherman MD, York M, Irvine AR, et al: Endophthalmitis caused by β-lactamase-positive *Moraxella nonliquefaciens*. Am J Ophthalmol 115:674–676, 1993.
114. Perez RE: Endocarditis with *Moraxella*-like M-6 after cardiac catheterization. J Clin Microbiol 24:501–502, 1986.
115. Silberfarb PM, Lawe JE: Endocarditis due to *Moraxella liquefaciens*. Arch Intern Med 122:512–513, 1968.
116. Buchman AL, Pickett MJ: *Moraxella atlantae* bacteraemia in a patient with systemic lupus erythematosus. J Infect 23:197–199, 1991.
117. Phillips G, Patterson D, Montieth P, et al: Septicaemia caused by a penicillin-resistant *Moraxella*-like organism in a neutropenic patient. Eur J Clin Microbiol Infect Dis 10:947–948, 1991.
118. Feigin RD, San Joaquin V, Middelkamp JN: Septic arthritis due to *Moraxella osloensis*. J Pediatr 75:116–117, 1969.
119. Juvin Ph, Boulot-Telle M, Triller R, et al: *Moraxella lacunata* infectious arthritis. J R Soc Med 84:629–630, 1991.
120. Goetz MB, Jones J: Pneumonia and bacteremia caused by a previously undescribed *Moraxella*-like bacterium. J Clin Microbiol 15:720–722, 1982.
121. Appelbaum A, Giladi A, Borman JB: *Moraxella* purulent pericarditis. J Cardiovasc Surg 15:479–481, 1974.
122. Fijen CAP, Kuijper EJ, Tjia HG, et al: Complement deficiency predisposes for meningitis due to nongroupable meningococci and *Neisseria*-related bacteria. Clin Infect Dis 18:780–784, 1994.

123. Snell JJS, Lapage SP: Transfer of some saccharolytic *Moraxella* species to *Kingella* Henriksen and Bovre 1976, with descriptions of *Kingella indologenes* sp. nov. and *Kingella denitrificans* sp. nov. Int J Syst Bacteriol 26:451–458, 1976.
124. Henriksen SD, Bovre K: Transfer of *Moraxella kingae* Henriksen and Bovre to the genus *Kingella* gen. nov. in the family Neisseriaceae Int J Syst Bacteriol 26:447–450, 1976.
125. Jenny DB, Letendre PW, Iverson G: Endocarditis caused by *Kingella indologenes*. Rev Infect Dis 9:787–789, 1987.
126. Verbruggen A-M, Hauglustaine D, Schildermans F, et al: Infections caused by *Kingella kingae*: Report of four cases and review. J Infect 13:133–142, 1986.
127. Hassan IJ, Hayek L: Endocarditis caused by *Kingella denitrificans*. J Infect 27:291–295, 1993.
128. Kennedy CA, Rosen H: *Kingella kingae* bacteremia and adult epiglottitis in a granulocytopenic host. Am J Med 85:701–702, 1988.
129. Redfield DC, Overturf GD, Ewing N, et al: Bacteremia, arthritis, and skin lesions due to *Kingella kingae*. Arch Dis Child 55:411–414, 1980.
130. Amir J, Schockelford PG: *Kingella kingae* intervertebral disk infection. J Clin Microbiol 29:1083–1086, 1991.
131. Yagupsky P, Dagan R, Howard CB, et al: Clinical features and epidemiology of invasive *Kingella kingae* infections in southern Israel. Pediatrics 92:800–804, 1993.
132. Jensen KT, Schonheyder H, Thomsen VF: In-vitro activity of β-lactam and other antimicrobial agents against *Kingella kingae*. J Antimicrob Chemother 33:635–640, 1994.
133. Rossau R, Kersters K, Falsen E, et al: *Oligella*, a new genus including *Oligella urethralis* comb. nov. (formerly *Moraxella urethralis*) and *Oligella ureolytica* sp. nov. (formerly CDC group IVe): Relationship to *Taylorella equigenitalis* and related taxa. Int J Syst Bacteriol 37:198–210, 1987.
134. Klingman KL, Murphy TF: Purification and characterization of a high-molecular-weight outer membrane protein of *Moraxella (Branhamella) catarrhalis*. Infect Immun 62:1150–1155, 1994.
135. Helminen ME, Maciver I, Latimer JL, et al: A large, antigenically conserved protein on the surface of *Moraxella catarrhalis* is a target for protective antibodies. J Infect Dis 170:867–872, 1994.
136. Sethi S, Hill SL, Murphy TF: Serum antibodies to outer membrane proteins of *Moraxella (Branhamella) catarrhalis* in patients with bronchiectasis: Identification of OMP B1 as an important antigen. Infect Immun 63:1516–1520, 1995.
137. Campagnari AA, Shanks KL, Dyer DW: Growth of *Moraxella catarrhalis* with human transferrin and lactoferrin: expression of iron-repressible proteins without siderophore production. Infect Immun 62:4909–4914, 1994.
138. Helminen ME, Maciver I, Latimer JL, et al: A major outer membrane protein of *Moraxella catarrhalis* is a target for antibodies that enhance pulmonary clearance of the pathogen in an animal model. Infect Immun 61:2003–2010, 1993.
139. Helminen ME, Maciver I, Paris M, et al: A mutation affecting expression of a major outer membrane protein of *Moraxella catarrhalis* alters serum resistance and survival in vivo. J Infect Dis 168:1194–1201, 1993.
140. Sarwar J, Campagnari AA, Kirkham C, et al: Characterization of an antigenically conserved heat-modifiable major outer membrane protein of *Branhamella catarrhalis*. Infect Immun 60:804–809, 1992.
141. Murphy TF, Kirkham C, Lesse AJ: The major heat-modifiable outer membrane protein CD is highly conserved among strains of *Branhamella catarrhalis*. Mol Microbiol 10:87–98, 1993.
142. Bhushan R, Craigie R, Murphy TF: Molecular cloning and characterization of outer membrane protein E of *Moraxella (Branhamella) catarrhalis*. J Bacteriol 176:6636–6643, 1994.
143. Murphy TF, Bartos LC: Surface-exposed and antigenically conserved determinants of outer membrane proteins of *Branhamella catarrhalis*. Infect Immun 57:2938–2941, 1989.
144. Denamur E, Picard-Pasquier N, Mura C, et al: Comparison of molecular epidemiological tools for *Branhamella catarrhalis* typing. Res Microbiol 142:585–589, 1991.
145. Picard B, Goullet P, Denamur E, et al: Esterase electrophoresis: A molecular tool for studying the epidemiology of *Branhamella catarrhalis* nosocomial infection. Epidemiol Infect 103:547–554, 1989.
146. Dickinson DP, Loos BG, Dryja DM, et al: Restriction fragment mapping of *Branhamella catarrhalis*: A new tool for studying the epidemiology of this middle ear pathogen. J Infect Dis 158:205–208, 1988.
147. Robert MC, Pang Y, Spencer RC, et al: Tetracycline resistance in *Moraxella (Branhamella) catarrhalis*: Demonstration of two clonal outbreaks by using pulsed-field gel electrophoresis. Antimicrob Agents Chemother 35:2453–2455, 1991.
148. Stenfors L-E, Raisanen S: Quantitative analysis of the bacterial findings in otitis media. J Laryngol Otol 104:749–757, 1990.
149. Gan VN, Kusmiesz H, Shelton S, et al: Comparative evaluation of loracarbef and amoxicillin-clavulanate for acute otitis media. Antimicrob Agents Chemother 35:967–971, 1991.
150. Johnson CE, Carlin SA, Super DM, et al: Cefixime compared with amoxicillin for treatment of acute otitis media. J Pediatr 119:117–122, 1991.
151. Faden H, Bernstein J, Stanievich J, et al: Effect of prior antibiotic treatment on middle ear disease in children. Ann Otol Rhinol Laryngol 101:87–91, 1992.
152. DelBeccaro MA, Mendelman PM, Inglis AF, et al: Bacteriology of acute otitis media: A new perspective. J Pediatr 120:81–84, 1992.
153. Chonmaitree T, Owen MJ, Patel JA, et al: Effect of viral respiratory tract infection on outcome of acute otitis media. J Pediatr 120:856–862, 1992.
154. Owen MJ, Anwar R, Nguyen HK, et al: Efficacy of cefixime in the treatment of acute otitis media in children. Am J Dis Child 147:81–86, 1993.
155. Aspin MM, Hoberman A, McCarty J, et al: Comparative study of the safety and efficacy of clarithromycin and amoxicillin-clavulanate in the treatment of acute otitis media in children. J Pediatr 125:135s–141s, 1994.

GRAM-NEGATIVE BACILLI

204

Enterobacteriaceae

Henry D. Isenberg
Richard F. D'Amato

The family of Enterobacteriaceae—obviously mislabeled in view of its numerous, diverse, extraintestinal habitats—is a fitting example of the mastery exerted by the microbial world over all living forms. Their very ubiquity and the beneficial and harmful effects of these straight gram-negative bacteria have contributed to their role as favorite test objects. The haploid nature of the prokaryotic chromosome has complicated the application of Linnaean taxonomy to all "primitive" organisms, requiring special definitions of species and genera, based lately on the degree of DNA homology achieved under the most stringent environmental conditions. Fortunately, many of the accepted classifications within the family, based on biochemical and immunologic characteristics, have been confirmed by this approach. Still, new genera and species have emerged: in 1972, 11 genera and 26 species made up the family; in 1995, there were 28 genera, 115 species, and 7 enteric groups.[1]

This expansion, based on ongoing analyses, continues unabated, and it is complicated still further by the discovery that variants within a species represent a spectrum of interactions, some of which are injurious to the host, others of which are beneficial, and some of which have no effect, all depending on the individual host.[2, 3] The references[4–8] should be consulted for detailed scientific treatments of this significant family.

All members of Enterobacteriaceae are straight gram-negative rods. When motile, they possess peritrichous flagella. except for organisms of the genus *Tatumella,* which display polar, subpolar, or lateral flagella at 25°C and are nonmotile at 36°C.[4] The cellular organization of these bacteria is typical of gram-negative organisms: an outer membrane overlies the murein sacculus, and there is a periplasmic space between the peptidoglycan cell wall and the cytoplasmic membrane. The outer membrane, in contact with the environment, displays protective properties such as hydrophilic, mostly negatively charged carbohydrate chains and acidic proteins to prevent phagocytosis. Enterobacteriaceae organisms display in their somatic (O) and capsular (K) polysaccharides incredible structural variations that may prevent interactions with preexisting host antibodies or enzymes. This outer membrane[9] contains lipids, proteins, and various polysaccharides arranged in concert with the peptidoglycan layer in a hexagonal lattice that ionically links the outer membrane and cell wall. In addition, a small lipoprotein in the outer membrane anchors to the C-terminal of the several diaminopimelic acid constituents of the peptidoglycan.

The Enterobacteriaceae lipopolysaccharides that are so fascinating to investigators are composed of three distinct regions: lipid A, closest to the cell wall; core antigen; and the polysaccharide chains responsible for the O or somatic antigenicity of species and subspecies variants (Fig. 204–1). Lipid A consists of a phosphorylated glucosamine sequence linked by β-1,4- or β-1,6-glycosidic bonds. Generally, the amino group of the glucosamine is substituted by D-3-hydroxy fatty acids; the hydroxyl groups of the molecule are esterified with various long chain saturated fatty acids. The core polysaccharide unites the outer O polysaccharide with the lipid A moiety. This core is usually composed of glucosamine, heptose, 3-deoxy-D-manooctulosonic acid (also known as 2-keto-3-deoxyoctonate, or KDO), galactose, and other hexoses and pentoses. It is attached through a ketocytic link of 2-keto-3-deoxyoctonate to glucosamines of lipid A. The complex somatic antigens consist of various polysaccharides, many of them peculiar to Enterobacteriaceae, in addition to a "common" antigen, an acidic polysaccharide composed of *N*-acetyl-D-glucosamine, *N*-acetylmannosaminuronic acid, and 4-acetamido-4,6-dideoxygalactose. The presence, absence, linkage types, and sequences of glucose, galactose, and acetylglucosamine, 3-deoxy-D-manooctulosonic acid, mannose, ribose, xylose, rhamnose, fucose, and 2,6-dideoxyhexoses such as abequose, colitose, and tyvelose account for the display of antigenic diversity observed in the outermost hydrophilic polysaccharide chains.

Several members of the family express additional antigenic polysaccharides in the form of capsules or envelopes (K antigens) as well as fimbriae, structures useful for adhesion of bacteria to environmental surfaces, including mammalian cells. The K antigens are specific polysaccharides that are found in *Escherichia coli;* specific polysaccharides are also found as Vi and M antigens among *Salmonella* species and as capsular antigens of *Klebsiella* species. These polysaccharides are acidic, always containing different uronic acids in addition to hexoses, deoxyhexoses, and hexosamines. Considerable variation in the expressions of all antigens must be expected. Although the antigenicity of various outer membrane proteins and polypeptides has not been exploited for laboratory recognition of these bacteria, more than 20 different representatives have been recognized, including matrix proteins, proteins in combination with lipid moieties, and the proteins of the porin channels. The explanation of the significance of these molecules in the reaction of bacteria to antibiotics and other environmental challenges is in its infancy; the molecules may function as receptors for bacteriophage attachments, transporters of selected nutrients, and barriers to hydrophobic substances such as dyes or detergents.

Bacterial survival depends on the organism's ability to adhere to surfaces and to form microcolonies on them. The latter is accomplished by exopolysaccharide production that forms a protective cement that is rarely penetrated by host immune defenses or antibiotics. These exopolysaccharides probably serve also as reservoirs for nutrients required by the constituents of the microbial mats that are not necessarily monomicrobial.[10] Adherence mechanisms determined by fimbriae and other structures are described and discussed in other chapters of this book, as are the mechanisms of bacterial responses to environmental and host challenges resulting from conjugation and extrachromosomal DNA in the form of plasmids.

The widespread distribution of the family in nature complicates the interpretation of laboratory results with respect to significance of an isolate. The sources listed in Table 204–1 do not necessarily constitute permanent habitats; they may reflect contamination of these environments by animals or humans. Traditionally, the major diseases attributed to the members of the family are intestinal disorders, ranging from diarrhea and food poisoning to dysentery and typhoid-like

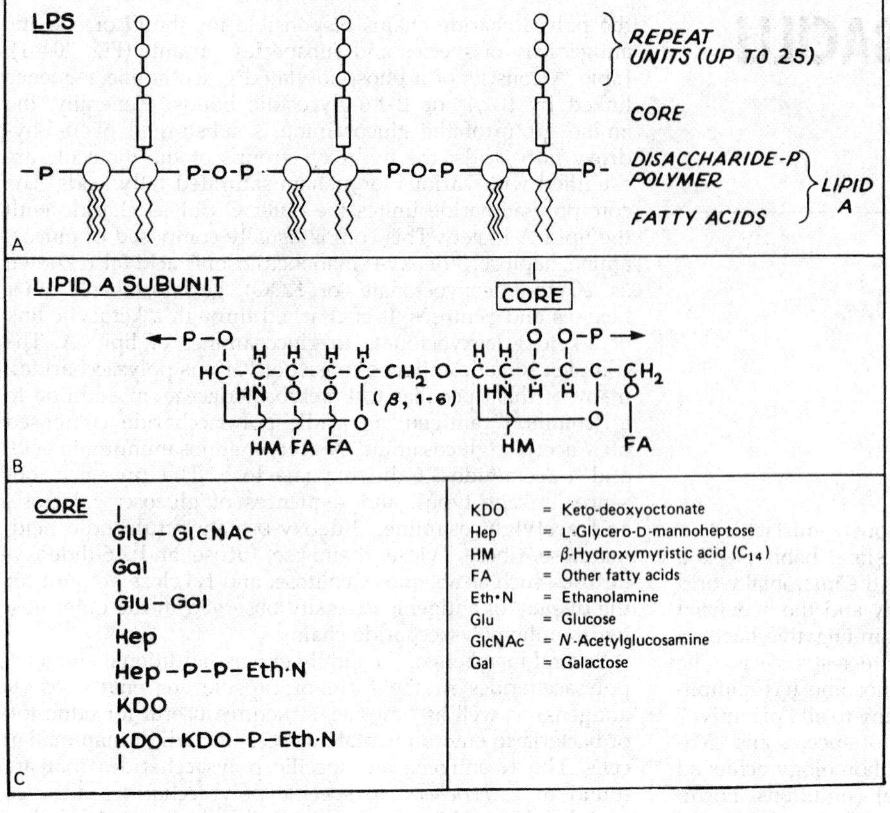

FIGURE 204–1 ▫ The outer membrane of Enterobacteriaceae. LPS, Lipopolysaccharide.

TABLE 204–1 ■ Environmental Sources of Enterobacteriaceae*

GENUS	ANIMALS	WATER	SOIL	ENVIRONMENT (NOT SPECIFIED)	FOOD	UNKNOWN†	HUMAN
Budvicia		+					+
Cedecea						+	+
Citrobacter	+	+	+		+	+	+
Edwardsiella	+	+			+	+	+
Enterobacter	+	+		+	+	+	+
Escherichia	+	+	+	+	+	+	+
Ewingella					+	+	+
Hafnia						+	+
Klebsiella	+	+		+	*	+	+
Kluyvera	+	+	+	+	+	+	+
Leclercia	+	+		+	+		+
Leminorella	+						+
Moellerella		+					+
Morganella							+
Pragia		+					+
Proteus	+					+	+
Providencia						+	+
Rhanella		+					+
Salmonella	+	+	+	+	+	+	+
Serratia	+	+	+	+	+	+	+
Shigella	Primates						+
Tatumella						+	+
Trabulsiella							+
Yersinia	+	+	+	+	+	+	+
Yokenella							+
Xenorhabdus	+						+

*Different species of each genus are recovered from different environmental sources.
†The exact source of all species has not been determined.

fever. The inclusion of *Yersinia* in the family now warrants consideration of plague and other yersinioses.

In addition to urinary tract infections, the major role of Enterobacteriaceae representatives in developed countries is in extraintestinal infections as agents of enteric bacterioses, which are acquired through colonization of prostheses or lesions in patients whose immunity is impaired.[11] Enteric bacteriosis manifests as bacteremia; pneumonia; urinary tract, wound, or central nervous system infections; abscess formation; and colonization of implants, prostheses, and catheters, these last-named devices serving as niches for the spread of infection. The various clinical consequences of these bacteria are described in the relevant chapters of this book. Still, it is worth remembering the assertion of Farmer and colleagues[12] that in the United States as many as 90% of Enterobacteriaceae isolates from clinical specimens are composed of three species: *E. coli*, *Klebsiella pneumoniae*, and *Proteus mirabilis*.[12]

Specimen Collection

Appropriate specimens for laboratory analysis should be collected in suitable transport media that ensure the preservation of the organisms, and for polymicrobial infections, that preserve the proportions of representative bacteria. Special neutralizing buffers are recommended when salmonellae, and especially shigellae, are sought in stool specimens, because room temperature lowers the pH to levels that most of these bacteria cannot tolerate.[13]

Isolation and Identification

All Enterobacteriaceae species grow readily on nutrient media. In most instances laboratorians use, besides general media, selective agars that allow presumptive identification of the organisms in the specimen after 18 to 24 hours' incubation. Media such as MacConkey, deoxycholate, and eosin–methylene blue agar are used[13–16] for their isolation in general. Only *Yersinia pestis* and *Yersinia pseudotuberculosis* may not grow on selective media. The isolation and separation of the so-called enteric pathogens, *Salmonella* and *Shigella* organisms, are aided by the use of an entire array of selective agars supplemented by enrichment broths that enhance the detection of these organisms in the presence of many other bacteria. For this purpose, *Salmonella-Shigella* agar, bismuth sulfite agar (for the isolation of *Salmonella*), brilliant green agar (for the isolation of *Salmonella*), Hektoen enteric agar, lysine-deoxycholate agar, and many others are used widely.[14–16] Separation on the basis of lactose fermentation is still a widely accepted tool for sequestering the diarrheogenic salmonellae and shigellae; however, not all of the genera designated as lactose fermenters do so invariably. The next level of identification tests usually involves soliciting fermentation reactions on various carbohydrate substrates and the detection of enzymes. Many commercial systems are available and have been incorporated into automated devices linked to computers. Identification on the basis of 12 to 30 substrates can be provided in this manner. Most such methods require that a lack of oxidase be demonstrated. These biochemical examinations usually allow identification of the species. For certain isolates, further identifications are required; usually they involve serologic classifications. Although molecular tools are useful taxonomically and epidemiologically and for the recognition of plasmid-associated so-called virulence factors, routine applications of these markers are not yet practical.

Separation of Enterobacteriaceae into Genera and Species

Taxonomists and clinical microbiologists, aware that they always deal with enormous populations of organisms, prefer to score bacterial action on individual substrates in percentages (Table 204–2). Aversion to dichotomous keys[17] must be tempered by the utility of this approach as a rough guide to the separation of the genera of the family (Fig. 204–2). This approach is useful as an index of suspicion to suggest the genus of an isolate with ordinary, readily determined reactions. Therefore, the latest additions to the named genera of the family have been omitted because their role in human disease production requires elucidation. Not indicated in Figure 204–2 is the necessity to test all motile representatives for oxidase production to avoid confusion with aeromonad-like bacteria.

Once the genus has been designated, identification at the species level may be indicated, but this step may be expensive and not clinically warranted. Laboratorians must decide whether more information will affect the choice of therapy as well as determine the epidemiologic implications of the isolate. Antibiotic profiles, the patient's history, the anatomic source of the clinical specimen, and the desires of the responsible clinician are factors in the decision.

Escherichia

E. coli, the best-known and most common member of Enterobacteriaceae, shares with other members of the family the characteristic shape and tinctorial properties—and when motile, peritrichous flagella. *Escherichia* organisms may have capsules or extracellular slime. These chemoorganotrophic bacteria can attack carbohydrates fermentatively or oxidatively, producing pyruvate that may lead to lactic, acetic, and formic acids. These acids can be attacked by a complex hydrogenlyase enzyme system, leading to the liberation of carbon dioxide and hydrogen, one of the earliest clues used to detect *E. coli* in water and clinical specimens. The characteristic biochemical activities that distinguish the less active *E. coli* strains are presented in Table 204–2. *E. coli* is a common inhabitant of the human and animal large intestine. It is easily recognized by a few salient tests: indole production, a positive result on methyl red tests, negative Voges-Proskauer reaction, and inability to utilize citrate.

The serologic analysis of *E. coli* has established the antigens previously discussed. At present, there are 171 O antigens, approximately 80 K antigens, and 56 H antigens of *E. coli*. The outermost border of *E. coli* displays fimbrae, fibrils, or colonizing factors now classified as F antigens. The more recently recognized members of the genus *Escherichia* are rarely encountered in clinical specimens. *Escherichia blattae*, a cockroach resident, has not as yet been discovered in the intimate human biosphere. *Escherichia fergusonii* and *Escherichia hermannii* have been isolated from stool and extraintestinal sources, whereas *Escherichia vulneris* has been recovered from extraintestinal specimens, mostly wounds. The differences between the various *Escherichia* and *Shigella* species are shown in Table 204–3. *E. coli*, always suspect when encountered in appropriate quantity extraintestinally, has now been recognized for the diarrheogenic potential of certain variants. Those capable of producing intestinal disease are much more prevalent in developing countries; extraintestinal involvement of *E. coli* in disease complications is more common in developed areas. One group of *E. coli* serotypes, the enterotoxigenic *E. coli*, associated with traveler's diarrhea in developing countries, are characterized by the production of en-

TABLE 204–2 ■ Biochemical Reactions of the Named Species, Biogroups, and Enteric Groups of the Family Enterobacteriaceae*†

ORGANISM	INDOLE PRODUCTION	METHYL RED	VOGES-PROSKAUER	CITRATE (SIMMONS)	HYDROGEN SULFIDE (TSI)	UREA HYDROLYSIS	PHENYLALANINE DEAMINASE	LYSINE DECARBOXYLASE	ARGININE DIHYDROLASE	ORNITHINE DECARBOXYLASE	MOTILITY (36°C)	GELATIN HYDROLYSIS (22°C)	GROWTH IN KCN	MALONATE UTILIZATION	D-GLUCOSE, ACID	D-GLUCOSE, GAS	LACTOSE FERMENTATION	SUCROSE FERMENTATION	D-MANNITOL FERMENTATION	DULCITOL FERMENTATION	SALICIN FERMENTATION	ADONITOL FERMENTATION	*MYO*-INOSITOL FERMENTATION
Budvicia																							
B. aquatica‡	0	93	0	0	80	33	0	0	0	0	27	0	0	0	100	53	87	0	60	0	0	0	0
Buttiauxella																							
B. agrestis	0	100	0	100	0	0	0	0	0	100	100	0	80	60	100	100	100	0	100	0	100	0	0
Cedecea‡																							
C. davisae	0	100	50	95	0	0	0	0	50	95	95	0	86	91	100	70	19	100	100	0	99	0	0
C. lapagei	0	40	80	99	0	0	0	0	80	0	80	0	100	99	100	100	60	0	100	0	100	0	0
C. neteri	0	100	50	100	0	0	0	0	100	0	100	0	65	100	100	100	35	100	100	0	100	0	0
Cedecea sp. 3	0	100	50	100	0	0	0	0	100	0	100	0	100	0	100	100	0	50	100	0	100	0	0
Cedecea sp. 5	0	100	50	100	0	0	0	0	50	50	100	0	100	0	100	100	0	100	100	0	100	0	0
Citrobacter‡																							
C. freundii	33	100	0	78	78	44	0	0	67	0	89	0	89	11	100	89	78	89	100	11	0	0	0
C. diversus (koseri)	99	100	0	99	0	75	0	0	80	99	95	0	0	95	100	98	50	40	99	40	15	99	0
C. amalonaticus	100	100	0	95	5	85	0	0	85	95	95	0	99	1	100	97	35	9	100	1	30	0	0
C. farmeri	100	100	0	10	0	59	0	0	85	100	97	0	93	0	100	96	15	100	100	2	9	0	0
C. youngae	15	100	0	75	65	80	0	0	50	5	95	0	95	5	100	75	25	20	100	85	10	0	5
C. braakii	33	100	0	87	60	47	0	0	67	93	87	0	100	0	100	93	80	7	100	33	0	0	0
C. werkmanii	0	100	0	100	100	100	0	0	100	0	100	0	100	100	100	100	17	0	100	0	0	0	0
C. sedlakii	83	100	0	83	0	100	0	0	100	100	100	0	100	100	100	100	100	0	100	100	17	0	0
Citrobacter sp. 9	0	100	0	0	0	100	0	0	0	100	0	0	0	100	100	100	100	0	100	0	0	0	0
Citrobacter sp. 10	0	100	0	33	67	0	0	0	33	0	67	0	100	100	100	100	67	33	100	0	0	0	0
Citrobacter sp. 11	100	100	0	100	67	67	0	0	67	0	100	0	100	0	100	100	67	33	100	100	33	0	0
Edwardsiella																							
E. tarda‡	99	100	0	1	100	0	0	100	0	100	98	0	0	0	100	100	0	0	0	0	0	0	0
E. tarda biogroup‡	100	100	0	0	0	0	0	100	0	100	100	0	0	0	100	50	0	100	100	0	0	0	0
E. hoshinae‡	50	100	0	0	0	0	0	100	0	95	100	0	0	100	100	35	0	100	100	0	50	0	0
E. ictaluri	0	0	0	0	0	0	0	100	0	65	0	0	0	0	100	50	0	0	0	0	0	0	0
Enterobacter																							
E. aerogenes‡	0	5	98	95	0	2	0	98	0	98	97	0	98	95	100	100	95	100	100	5	100	98	95
E. cloacae‡	0	5	100	100	0	65	0	0	97	96	95	0	98	75	100	100	93	97	100	15	75	25	15
E. agglomerans group‡	20	50	70	50	0	20	20	0	0	0	85	2	35	65	100	20	40	75	100	15	65	7	15
E. gergoviae	0	5	100	99	0	93	0	90	0	100	90	0	0	96	100	98	55	98	99	0	99	0	0
E. sakazakii‡	11	5	100	99	0	1	50	0	99	91	96	0	99	18	100	98	99	100	100	5	99	0	75
E. taylorae‡	0	5	100	100	0	1	0	0	94	99	99	0	98	100	100	100	10	0	100	0	92	0	0
E. amnigenus biogroup 1‡	0	7	100	70	0	0	0	0	9	55	92	0	100	91	100	100	70	100	100	0	91	0	0
E. amnigenus biogroup 2‡	0	65	100	100	0	0	0	0	35	100	100	0	100	100	100	100	35	0	100	0	100	0	0
E. asburiae‡	0	100	2	100	0	60	0	0	21	95	0	0	97	3	100	95	75	100	100	0	100	0	0
E. hormaechei‡	0	57	100	96	0	87	4	0	78	91	52	0	100	100	100	83	9	100	100	87	44	0	0
E. intermedium	0	100	100	65	0	0	0	0	0	89	89	0	65	100	100	100	100	65	100	100	100	0	0
E. cancerogenus	0	0	100	100	0	0	0	0	100	100	100	0	100	100	100	100	0	0	100	0	100	0	0
E. dissolvens	0	0	100	100	0	100	0	0	100	100	0	0	100	100	100	100	0	100	100	0	100	0	0
E. nimipressuralis	0	100	100	0	0	0	0	0	0	100	0	0	100	100	100	100	0	0	100	0	100	0	0
Escherichia-Shigella																							
E. coli‡	98	99	0	1	1	1	0	90	17	65	95	0	3	0	100	95	95	50	98	60	40	5	1
E. coli, inactive‡	80	95	0	1	1	1	0	40	3	20	5	0	1	0	100	5	25	15	93	40	10	3	1
Shigella, O groups A, B, C‡	50	100	0	0	0	0	0	0	5	1	0	0	0	0	100	2	0	0	93	2	0	0	0
S. sonnei‡	0	100	0	0	0	0	0	0	2	98	0	0	0	0	100	0	2	1	99	0	0	0	0
E. fergusonii‡	98	100	0	17	0	0	0	95	5	100	93	0	0	35	100	95	0	0	98	60	65	98	0
E. hermannii‡	99	100	0	1	0	0	0	6	0	100	99	0	94	0	100	97	45	45	100	19	40	0	0
E. vulneris‡	0	100	0	0	0	0	0	85	30	0	100	0	15	85	100	97	15	8	100	0	30	0	0
E. blattae	0	100	0	50	0	0	0	100	0	100	0	0	0	100	100	100	0	0	0	0	0	0	0

ORGANISM	D-SORBITOL FERMENTATION	L-ARABINOSE FERMENTATION	RAFFINOSE FERMENTATION	L-RHAMNOSE FERMENTATION	MALTOSE FERMENTATION	D-XYLOSE FERMENTATION	TREHALOSE FERMENTATION	CELLOBIOSE FERMENTATION	α-METHYL-D-GLUCOSIDE FERMENTATION	ERYTHRITOL FERMENTATION	ESCULIN HYDROLYSIS	MELIBIOSE FERMENTATION	D-ARABITOL FERMENTATION	GLYCEROL FERMENTATION	MUCATE FERMENTATION	TARTRATE, JORDAN	ACETATE UTILIZATION	LIPASE (CORN OIL)	DNASE AT 25°C	NITRATE → NITRITE	OXIDASE, KOVACS	ONPG TEST	YELLOW PIGMENT	D-MANNOSE FERMENTATION
Budvicia																								
B. aquatica‡	0	80	0	100	0	93	0	0	0	0	0	0	27	0	20	27	0	0	0	100	0	93	0	0
Buttiauxella																								
B. agrestis	0	100	100	100	100	100	100	100	0	0	100	100	0	60	100	60	0	0	0	100	0	100	0	100
Cedecea‡																								
C. davisae	0	0	10	0	100	100	100	100	5	0	45	0	100	0	0	0	0	91	0	100	0	90	0	100
C. lapagei	0	0	0	0	100	0	100	100	0	0	100	0	100	0	0	0	60	100	0	100	0	99	0	100
C. neteri	100	0	0	0	100	100	100	100	0	0	100	0	100	0	0	0	0	100	0	100	0	100	0	100
Cedecea sp. 3	0	0	100	0	100	100	100	100	50	0	100	100	100	0	0	0	50	100	0	100	0	100	0	100
Cedecea sp. 5	100	0	100	0	100	100	100	100	0	0	100	100	100	0	0	0	50	50	0	100	0	100	0	100
Citrobacter‡																								
C. freundii	100	100	44	100	100	89	100	44	11	0	0	100	0	100	100	100	44	0	0	100	0	89	0	100
C. diversus (koseri)	99	99	0	99	100	100	100	99	40	0	1	0	98	99	95	90	75	0	0	100	0	99	0	100
C. amalonaticus	99	99	5	100	99	99	100	100	2	0	5	0	0	60	96	96	86	0	0	99	0	97	0	100
C. farmeri	98	100	100	100	100	100	100	100	75	0	0	100	0	65	100	93	80	0	0	100	0	100	0	100
C. youngae	100	100	10	100	95	100	100	45	0	0	5	10	5	90	100	100	65	0	0	85	0	90	0	100
C. braakii	100	100	7	100	100	100	100	73	33	0	0	80	0	87	100	93	53	0	0	100	0	80	0	100
C. werkmanii	100	100	0	100	100	100	100	0	0	0	0	0	0	100	100	100	100	0	0	100	0	100	0	100
C. sedlakii	100	100	0	100	100	100	100	100	0	0	17	100	0	83	100	100	83	0	0	100	0	100	0	100
Citrobacter sp. 9	100	100	0	100	100	100	100	100	0	0	0	0	0	0	100	100	0	0	0	100	0	100	0	100
Citrobacter sp. 10	100	100	0	100	100	100	100	67	0	0	0	67	0	67	67	100	0	0	0	100	0	67	0	100
Citrobacter sp. 11	100	100	33	100	100	100	100	100	0	0	0	33	0	100	100	100	33	0	0	100	0	100	0	100
Edwardsiella																								
E. tarda‡	0	9	0	0	100	0	0	0	0	0	0	0	0	30	0	25	0	0	0	100	0	0	0	100
E. tarda biogroup‡	0	100	0	0	100	0	0	0	0	0	0	0	0	0	0	0	0	0	0	100	0	0	0	100
E. hoshinae‡	0	13	0	0	100	0	100	0	0	0	0	0	0	65	0	0	0	0	0	100	0	0	0	100
E. ictaluri	0	0	0	0	100	0	0	0	0	0	0	0	0	0	0	0	0	0	0	100	0	0	0	100
Enterobacter																								
E. aerogenes‡	100	100	96	99	99	100	100	100	95	0	98	99	100	98	90	95	50	0	0	100	0	100	0	95
E. cloacae‡	95	100	97	92	100	99	100	99	85	0	30	90	15	40	75	30	75	0	0	99	0	99	0	100
E. agglomerans group‡	30	95	30	85	89	93	97	55	7	0	60	50	50	30	40	25	30	0	0	85	0	90	75	98
E. gergoviae	0	99	97	99	100	99	100	99	2	0	97	97	97	100	2	97	93	0	0	99	0	97	0	100
E. sakazakii‡	0	100	99	100	100	100	100	100	96	0	100	100	0	15	1	1	96	0	0	99	0	100	98	100
E. taylorae‡	1	100	0	100	99	100	100	100	1	0	90	0	0	1	75	0	35	0	0	100	0	100	0	100
E. amnigenus biogroup 1‡	9	100	100	100	100	100	100	100	55	0	91	100	0	0	35	9	0	0	0	100	0	91	0	100
E. amnigenus biogroup 2‡	100	100	0	100	100	100	100	100	100	0	100	100	0	0	100	0	0	0	0	100	0	100	0	100
E. asburiae‡	100	100	70	5	100	97	100	100	95	0	95	0	0	11	21	30	87	0	0	100	0	100	0	100
E. hormaechei‡	0	100	0	100	100	96	100	100	83	0	0	0	0	4	96	13	74	0	0	100	0	95	0	100
E. intermedium	100	100	100	100	100	100	100	100	100	0	100	100	0	100	100	100	0	0	0	100	0	100	0	100
E. cancerogenus	0	100	0	100	100	100	100	100	0	0	100	0	0	0	100	0	33	0	0	100	0	100	0	100
E. dissolvens	100	100	100	100	100	100	100	100	100	0	100	100	0	0	100	0	100	0	0	100	0	100	0	100
E. nimipressuralis	100	100	0	100	100	100	100	100	100	0	100	100	0	0	100	0	0	0	0	100	0	100	0	100
Escherichia-Shigella																								
E. coli‡	94	99	50	80	95	95	98	2	0	0	35	75	5	75	95	95	90	0	0	100	0	95	0	98
E. coli, inactive‡	75	85	15	65	80	70	90	2	0	0	5	40	5	65	30	85	40	0	0	98	0	45	0	97
Shigella, O groups A, B, C‡	30	60	50	5	30	2	80	0	0	0	0	50	0	10	0	30	2	0	0	100	0	2	0	100
S. sonnei‡	2	95	3	75	90	2	100	5	0	0	0	25	0	15	10	90	0	0	0	100	0	90	0	100
E. fergusonii‡	0	98	0	92	96	96	96	96	0	0	46	0	100	20	0	96	96	0	0	100	0	83	0	100
E. hermannii‡	0	100	40	97	100	100	100	97	0	0	40	0	8	3	97	35	78	0	0	100	0	98	98	100
E. vulneris‡	1	100	99	93	100	100	100	100	25	0	20	100	0	25	78	2	30	0	0	100	0	100	50	100
E. blattae	0	100	0	100	100	100	75	0	0	0	0	0	0	100	50	50	0	0	0	100	0	0	0	100

Ewingella																																															
E. americana‡	0	84	95	95	0	0	0	0	0	0	60	0	5	0	100	0	70	0	100	0	80	0	0	0	0	0	23	16	13	99	10	0	0	50	0	99	24	0	35	10	0	0	97	0	85	0	99
Hafnia																																															
H. alvei‡	0	40	85	10	0	4	0	100	6	98	85	0	95	50	100	98	5	10	99	0	13	0	0	0	95	2	97	100	98	95	15	0	0	7	0	0	95	0	70	15	0	0	100	0	90	0	100
H. alvei biogroup 1	0	85	70	0	0	0	0	100	0	45	0	0	0	45	100	0	0	0.	55	0	55	0	0	0	0	0	0	0	0	70	0	0	0	0	0	0	0	0	30	0	0	0	100	0	30	0	100
Klebsiella																																															
K. pneumoniae‡	0	10	98	98	0	95	0	98	0	0	0	0	98	93	100	97	98	99	99	30	99	90	95	99	99	99	99	98	99	99	98	90	0	99	99	98	97	90	95	75	0	0	99	0	99	0	00
K. oxytoca‡	99	20	95	95	0	90	1	99	0	0	0	0	97	98	100	97	100	100	99	55	100	99	98	99	98	100	100	100	100	100	100	98	2	100	99	98	99	93	98	90	0	0	100	0	100	0	100
K. ornithinolytica‡	100	96	70	100	0	100	0	100	0	100	0	0	100	100	100	100	100	100	100	10	100	100	95	100	100	100	100	100	100	100	100	100	0	100	100	100	100	96	100	95	0	0	100	0	100	0	100
K. planticola‡	20	100	98	100	0	98	0	100	0	0	0	0	100	100	100	100	100	100	100	15	100	100	100	92	100	100	100	100	100	100	100	100	0	100	100	100	100	100	100	62	0	0	100	0	100	0	100
K. ozaenae‡	0	98	0	30	0	10	0	40	6	3	0	0	88	3	100	50	30	20	100	2	97	97	55	65	98	90	55	95	95	98	92	70	0	80	97	95	65	25	50	2	0	0	80	0	80	0	100
K. rhinoscleromatis‡	0	100	0	0	0	0	0	0	0	0	0	0	80	95	100	0	0	75	100	0	98	100	95	100	100	90	96	100	100	100	100	0	0	30	100	100	50	0	50	0	0	0	100	0	0	0	100
K. terrigena	0	60	100	40	0	0	0	100	0	20	0	0	100	100	100	80	100	100	100	20	100	100	80	100	100	100	100	100	100	100	100	100	0	100	100	100	100	100	100	20	0	0	100	0	100	0	100
Kluyvera																																															
K. ascorbata	92	100	0	96	0	0	0	97	0	100	98	0	92	96	100	93	98	98	100	25	100	0	0	40	100	98	100	100	99	100	100	98	0	99	99	0	40	90	35	50	0	0	100	0	100	0	100
K. cryocrescens‡	90	100	0	80	0	0	0	23	0	100	90	0	86	86	100	95	95	81	95	0	100	0	0	45	100	100	100	100	91	100	100	95	0	100	100	0	5	81	19	86	0	0	100	0	100	0	100
Leclercia																																															
L. adecarboxylata‡	100	100	0	0	0	48	0	0	0	0	79	0	97	93	100	97	93	66	100	86	100	93	0	0	100	66	100	100	100	100	100	0	0	100	100	96	3	93	83	28	0	0	100	0	100	37	100
Leminorella																																															
L. grimontii	0	100	0	100	100	0	0	0	0	0	0	0	0	0	100	33	0	0	0	83	0	0	0	0	100	0	0	0	83	0	0	0	0	0	0	0	17	100	100	0	0	0	100	0	0	0	0
L. richardii	0	0	0	0	100	0	0	0	0	0	0	0	0	0	100	0	0	0	0	0	0	0	0	0	100	0	0	0	100	0	0	0	0	0	0	0	0	50	100	0	0	0	100	0	0	0	0
Moellerella																																															
M. wisconsensis‡	0	100	0	80	0	0	0	0	0	0	0	0	70	0	100	0	100	100	60	0	0	100	0	0	0	100	0	30	0	0	0	0	0	0	100	75	10	0	30	10	0	0	90	0	90	0	100
Morganella																																															
M. morganii subsp. *morganii*‡	95	95	0	0	20	95	95	1	0	95	95	0	98	1	99	90	1	0	0	0	0	0	0	0	0	0	0	0	0	0	0	0	0	0	0	0	5	0	95	0	0	0	90	0	10	0	98
M. morganii biogroup 1‡	100	95	0	0	15	100	100	100	0	80	0	0	90	5	100	93	0	0	0	0	0	0	0	0	0	0	0	0	0	0	0	0	0	0	0	0	100	0	100	0	0	0	90	0	20	0	100
M. morganii subsp. *sibonii* 1‡	50	86	0	0	7	100	93	29	0	64	79	0	79	0	100	86	0	7	0	0	0	0	0	0	0	0	0	0	0	100	0	0	0	0	0	0	7	7	100	0	0	0	100	0	0	0	100
Obesumbacterium																																															
O. proteus biogroup 2	0	15	0	0	0	0	0	100	0	100	0	0	0	0	100	0	0	0	0	0	0	0	0	0	0	0	15	50	15	85	0	0	0	0	0	0	0	0	15	0	0	0	100	0	0	0	85
Pragia																																															
P. fontium	0	100	0	89	89	0	22	0	0	0	100	0	0	0	100	0	0	0	0	0	78	0	0	0	0	0	0	0	0	0	0	0	0	78	0	0	0	0	0	0	0	0	100	0	0	0	0
Proteus																																															
P. mirabilis‡	2	97	50	65	98	98	98	0	0	99	95	90	98	2	100	96	2	15	0	0	0	0	0	0	0	1	1	0	98	98	1	0	0	0	0	0	70	0	87	20	92	50	95	0	0	0	0
P. vulgaris‡	98	95	0	15	95	95	99	0	0	0	95	91	99	0	100	85	2	97	0	0	50	0	0	0	0	1	5	97	95	30	0	60	1	50	0	0	60	0	80	25	80	80	98	0	1	0	0
P. penneri‡	0	100	0	0	30	100	99	0	0	0	85	50	99	0	100	45	1	100	0	0	0	0	0	0	0	1	0	100	100	55	0	80	0	0	0	0	55	0	85	5	45	40	90	0	1	0	0
P. myxofaciens	0	100	100	50	0	100	100	0	0	0	100	100	100	0	100	100	0	100	0	0	0	0	0	0	0	0	0	100	0	100	0	100	0	0	0	0	100	0	100	0	100	50	100	0	0	0	0
Providencia																																															
P. rettgeri‡	99	93	0	95	0	98	98	0	0	0	94	0	97	0	100	10	5	15	100	0	50	100	90	1	0	5	70	2	10	0	3	2	75	35	5	100	60	0	95	60	0	0	100	0	5	0	100
P. stuartii‡	98	100	0	93	0	30	95	0	0	0	85	0	100	0	100	0	2	50	10	0	2	5	95	1	1	7	0	1	7	98	5	0	0	0	0	0	50	0	90	75	0	10	100	0	10	0	100
P. alcalifaciens‡	99	99	0	98	0	0	98	0	0	1	96	0	100	0	100	85	0	15	2	0	1	98	1	1	1	1	0	1	1	2	0	0	0	0	0	0	15	0	90	40	0	0	100	0	1	0	100
P. rustigianii‡	98	65	0	15	0	0	100	0	0	0	30	0	100	0	100	35	0	35	0	0	0	0	0	0	0	0	0	0	0	0	0	0	0	0	0	0	5	0	50	25	0	0	100	0	0	0	100
P. heimbachae	0	85	0	0	0	0	100	0	0	0	46	0	8	0	100	0	0	0	0	0	0	92	46	0	0	0	100	54	8	0	0	0	0	0	0	92	0	0	69	0	0	0	100	0	0	0	100
Rhanella																																															
R. aquatalis‡	0	88	100	94	0	0	95	0	0	0	6	0	0	100	100	98	100	100	100	88	100	0	0	94	100	94	94	94	94	100	100	0	0	100	100	0	13	30	6	6	0	0	100	0	100	0	100
Salmonella‡																																															
DNA group 1 strains																																															
Most serotypes	1	100	0	95	95	1	0	98	70	97	95	0	0	0	100	96	1	1	100	96	0	0	35	95	99	2	95	97	97	99	5	2	0	5	95	0	5	90	90	90	0	2	100	0	2	0	100
S. typhi	0	100	0	0	97	0	0	98	3	0	97	0	0	0	100	0	1	0	100	0	0	0	0	99	2	0	0	97	82	100	0	0	0	0	100	0	20	0	100	0	0	0	100	0	0	0	100
S. choleraesuis	0	100	0	25	50	0	0	95	55	100	95	0	0	0	100	95	0	0	98	5	0	0	0	90	0	1	100	95	98	0	0	0	1	0	45	1	0	0	85	1	0	0	98	0	0	0	95
S. paratyphi A	0	100	0	0	10	0	0	0	15	95	95	0	0	0	100	99	0	0	100	90	0	0	0	95	100	0	100	95	0	100	5	0	0	0	95	0	10	0	0	0	0	0	100	0	0	0	100
S. gallinarum	0	100	0	0	100	0	0	90	10	1	0	0	0	0	100	0	0	0	100	90	0	0	0	1	80	10	10	90	70	50	10	0	1	0	0	0	0	50	100	0	0	10	100	0	0	0	100
S. pullorum	0	90	0	0	90	0	0	100	10	95	0	0	0	0	100	90	0	0	100	0	0	0	0	10	100	1	100	5	90	90	5	0	0	0	0	0	0	0	0	0	0	0	100	0	0	0	100
DNA group 2 strains	2	100	0	100	100	0	0	100	90	100	98	2	0	95	100	100	1	1	100	90	5	0	5	100	100	0	100	100	100	100	0	8	0	15	8	0	25	96	50	95	0	0	100	0	15	0	95
DNA group 3a strains	1	100	0	99	99	0	0	99	70	99	99	0	1	95	100	99	15	1	100	0	0	0	0	99	99	1	99	98	100	99	1	1	0	1	95	1	10	90	5	90	0	2	100	0	100	0	100
DNA group 3b strains	2	100	0	98	99	0	0	99	70	99	99	0	1	95	100	99	85	5	100	1	0	0	0	99	99	1	99	98	100	99	1	1	0	1	95	1	10	30	20	75	0	2	100	0	92	0	100
DNA group 4 strains	0	100	0	98	100	2	0	100	70	100	98	0	95	0	100	100	0	0	98	0	60	5	0	100	100	0	98	100	100	100	50	0	0	0	100	5	0	0	65	70	0	0	100	0	0	0	100
DNA group 5 strains	0	100	0	94	100	0	0	100	94	100	100	0	100	0	100	94	0	0	100	94	0	0	0	100	94	0	88	100	100	100	0	0	0	0	94	0	0	88	0	100	0	0	100	0	94	0	100
DNA group 6 strains	0	100	0	89	100	0	0	100	67	100	100	0	0	0	100	100	22	0	100	67	0	0	0	0	100	0	100	100	100	100	0	0	0	0	89	0	33	89	100	98	0	0	100	0	44	0	100

Table continued on following page

TABLE 204–2 ■ Biochemical Reactions of the Named Species, Biogroups, and Enteric Groups of the Family Enterobacteriaceae*† *Continued*

ORGANISM	INDOLE PRODUCTION	METHYL RED	VOGES-PROSKAUER	CITRATE (SIMMONS)	HYDROGEN SULFIDE (TSI)	UREA HYDROLYSIS	PHENYLALANINE DEAMINASE	LYSINE DECARBOXYLASE	ARGININE DIHYDROLASE	ORNITHINE DECARBOXYLASE	MOTILITY (36°C)	GELATIN HYDROLYSIS (22°C)	GROWTH IN KCN	MALONATE UTILIZATION	D-GLUCOSE, ACID	D-GLUCOSE, GAS	LACTOSE FERMENTATION	SUCROSE FERMENTATION	D-MANNITOL FERMENTATION	DULCITOL FERMENTATION	SALICIN FERMENTATION	ADONITOL FERMENTATION	*MYO*-INOSITOL FERMENTATION	D-SORBITOL FERMENTATION	L-ARABINOSE FERMENTATION	RAFFINOSE FERMENTATION	L-RHAMNOSE FERMENTATION	MALTOSE FERMENTATION	D-XYLOSE FERMENTATION	TREHALOSE FERMENTATION	CELLOBIOSE FERMENTATION	α-METHYL-D-GLUCOSIDE FERMENTATION	ERYTHRITOL FERMENTATION	ESCULIN HYDROLYSIS	MELIBIOSE FERMENTATION	D-ARABITOL FERMENTATION	GLYCEROL FERMENTATION	MUCATE FERMENTATION	TARTRATE, JORDAN	ACETATE UTILIZATION	LIPASE (CORN OIL)	DNASE AT 25°C	NITRATE → NITRITE	OXIDASE, KOVACS	ONPG TEST	YELLOW PIGMENT	D-MANNOSE FERMENTATION
Serratia																																															
S. marcescens‡	1	20	98	98	0	15	0	99	0	99	97	90	95	3	100	55	2	99	99	0	95	40	75	99	0	2	0	96	7	99	5	0	1	95	0	0	95	0	75	50	98	98	98	0	95	0	99
S. marcescens biogroup 1‡	0	100	60	30	0	0	0	55	4	65	17	30	70	0	100	0	4	100	96	0	92	30	30	92	0	0	0	70	0	100	4	0	0	96	0	0	92	0	50	4	75	82	83	0	75	0	100
S. liquefaciens group‡	1	93	93	90	0	3	0	95	0	95	95	90	90	2	100	75	10	98	100	0	97	5	60	95	98	85	15	98	100	100	5	5	0	97	75	0	95	0	75	40	85	85	100	0	93	0	100
S. rubidaea‡	0	20	100	95	0	2	0	55	0	0	85	90	25	94	100	30	100	99	100	0	99	99	20	1	100	99	1	99	99	100	94	1	0	94	99	85	20	0	70	80	99	99	100	0	100	0	100
S. odorifera biogroup 1‡	60	100	50	100	0	5	0	100	0	100	100	95	60	0	100	0	70	100	100	0	98	50	100	100	100	100	95	100	100	100	100	0	0	95	100	0	40	5	100	60	35	100	100	0	100	0	100
S. odorifera biogroup 2‡	50	60	100	97	0	0	0	94	0	0	100	94	19	0	100	13	97	0	97	0	45	55	100	100	100	7	94	100	100	100	100	0	7	40	96	0	50	0	100	65	65	100	100	0	100	0	100
S. plymuthica‡	0	94	80	75	0	0	0	0	0	0	50	60	30	0	100	40	80	100	100	0	94	0	50	65	100	94	0	94	94	100	88	70	0	81	93	0	50	0	100	55	70	100	100	0	70	0	100
S. ficaria‡	0	75	75	100	0	0	0	0	0	0	100	100	55	0	100	0	15	100	100	0	100	0	55	100	100	70	35	100	100	100	100	8	0	100	40	100	0	0	17	40	77	100	92	8	100	0	100
S. entomophila	0	20	100	100	0	0	0	0	0	0	100	100	100	0	100	0	0	100	100	0	100	0	0	0	0	0	0	100	40	100	0	0	0	100	0	60	0	0	100	80	20	100	100	0	100	0	100
"*Serratia*" *fonticola*‡	0	100	9	91	0	13	0	100	0	97	91	0	70	88	100	79	97	21	100	91	100	100	30	100	100	100	76	97	85	100	6	91	0	100	98	100	88	0	58	15	0	0	100	0	100	0	100
Tatumella																																															
T. ptyseos‡	0	0	5	2	0	0	90	0	0	0	0	0	0	0	100	0	0	98	0	0	55	0	0	0	0	11	0	0	9	93	0	0	0	0	25	0	7	0	0	0	0	0	98	0	0	0	100
Trabulsiella																																															
T. guamensis	40	100	0	88	100	0	0	100	50	100	100	0	100	0	100	100	0	0	100	0	13	0	0	100	100	0	100	100	100	100	100	0	0	40	0	0	0	100	50	88	0	0	100	0	100	0	100
Xenorhabdus																																															
X. luminescens (25°C)	50	0	0	50	0	25	0	0	0	0	100	50	0	0	75	0	0	0	0	0	0	0	0	0	0	0	0	25	0	0	0	0	0	0	0	0	0	0	50	0	0	0	0	0	0	50	100
X. luminescens DNA group 5‡	0	0	0	20	0	60	0	0	0	0	100	80	20	0	100	0	0	0	0	0	0	0	0	0	0	0	0	0	0	0	0	0	0	0	0	0	0	0	60	20	0	0	0	0	0	60	100
X. nematophilus (25°C)	40	0	0	0	0	0	0	0	0	0	100	80	0	0	80	0	0	0	0	0	0	0	0	0	0	0	0	0	0	0	0	0	0	0	0	0	0	0	60	0	0	20	20	0	0	60	80
Yersinia																																															
Y. enterocolitica‡	50	97	2	0	0	75	0	0	0	95	2	0	2	0	100	5	5	95	98	0	20	0	30	99	98	5	1	75	70	98	75	0	0	25	1	40	90	0	85	15	55	5	98	0	95	0	100
Y. frederiksenii‡	100	100	0	15	0	70	0	0	0	95	5	0	0	0	100	40	40	100	100	0	92	0	20	100	100	30	99	100	100	100	100	0	0	85	0	100	85	5	55	15	55	0	100	0	100	0	100
Y. intermedia‡	100	100	5	5	0	80	0	0	0	100	5	0	10	5	100	18	35	100	100	0	100	0	15	100	100	45	100	100	100	100	96	77	0	100	80	45	60	6	88	18	12	0	94	0	90	0	100
Y. kristensenii‡	30	92	0	0	0	77	0	0	0	92	5	0	0	0	100	23	8	0	100	0	15	0	15	100	77	0	0	100	85	100	100	0	0	0	0	45	70	0	40	8	0	0	100	0	70	0	100
Y. rohdei‡	0	62	0	0	0	62	0	0	0	25	0	0	0	0	100	0	0	100	100	0	0	0	0	100	100	62	0	0	38	100	25	0	0	0	50	0	38	0	100	0	0	0	88	0	50	0	100
Y. aldovae	0	80	0	0	0	60	0	0	0	40	0	0	0	0	100	0	0	20	80	0	0	0	0	60	60	0	0	0	40	80	0	0	0	0	0	0	0	0	100	0	0	0	100	0	0	0	100
Y. bercovieri‡	0	100	0	0	0	60	0	0	0	80	0	0	0	0	100	0	20	100	100	0	20	0	0	100	100	0	0	100	100	100	100	0	0	20	0	0	0	0	100	0	0	0	100	0	80	0	100
Y. mollaretii‡	0	100	0	0	0	20	0	0	0	80	0	0	0	0	100	0	40	100	100	0	20	0	0	100	100	0	0	60	60	100	100	0	0	0	0	0	20	0	100	0	0	0	100	0	20	0	100
Y. pestis‡	0	80	0	0	0	5	0	0	0	0	0	0	0	0	100	0	0	0	97	0	70	0	0	50	100	0	1	80	90	100	0	0	0	50	20	0	50	0	0	0	0	0	85	0	50	0	100
Y. pseudotuberculosis‡	0	100	0	0	0	95	0	0	0	0	0	0	0	0	100	0	0	0	100	0	25	0	0	0	50	15	70	95	100	100	0	0	0	95	70	0	50	0	50	0	0	0	95	0	70	0	100
"*Yersinia*" *ruckeri*‡	0	97	10	0	0	0	0	50	5	100	0	30	15	0	100	5	0	0	100	0	0	0	0	50	5	5	0	95	0	95	5	0	0	0	0	0	30	0	30	0	30	0	75	0	50	0	100
Yokenella (Koserella)																																															
Y. regensburgei‡	0	100	0	92	0	0	0	100	8	100	100	0	92	0	100	100	0	0	100	0	8	0	0	0	100	25	100	100	100	100	100	0	0	67	92	0	0	0	0	25	0	0	100	0	100	0	100
Enteric group 58‡	0	100	0	85	0	70	0	100	0	85	100	0	100	85	100	85	30	0	100	85	100	0	0	100	100	0	100	100	100	100	100	55	0	0	0	0	30	0	60	45	0	0	100	0	100	0	100
Enteric group 59‡	10	100	0	100	0	0	30	0	60	0	100	0	80	90	100	100	80	0	100	0	100	0	0	0	100	0	100	100	100	100	100	10	0	100	0	10	10	60	50	50	0	0	100	0	100	25	100
Enteric group 60‡	0	100	0	0	0	50	0	0	0	100	75	0	0	100	100	100	0	0	50	0	0	0	0	0	25	0	75	0	0	100	0	0	0	0	0	0	75	0	75	0	0	0	100	0	100	0	100
Enteric group 63	0	100	0	0	0	0	0	100	0	100	65	0	0	0	100	100	0	0	100	0	100	0	0	100	100	0	100	100	100	100	100	65	0	100	0	0	0	65	0	0	0	0	100	0	100	0	100
Enteric group 64	0	100	0	50	0	0	0	0	50	0	100	0	100	100	100	50	100	0	100	0	100	100	0	0	100	0	100	100	100	100	100	0	0	100	0	100	0	100	50	0	0	0	100	0	100	0	100
Enteric group 68‡	0	100	50	0	0	0	0	0	0	0	0	0	100	0	100	0	0	100	100	0	50	0	0	0	0	0	0	50	0	100	0	0	0	0	0	0	50	0	0	0	0	100	100	0	0	0	100
Enteric group 69‡	0	0	100	100	0	0	0	0	100	100	100	0	100	100	100	100	100	25	100	100	100	0	0	100	100	100	100	100	100	100	100	100	0	100	100	0	0	100	0	25	0	0	100	0	100	0	100

*TSI, Triple sugar iron agar; ONPG, *o*-nitrophenyl-β-D-galactopyranoside.
†Each number gives the percentage of positive reactions after 2 d of incubation at 36°C (unless a different temperature is indicated). The vast majority of these positive reactions occur within 24 h. Reactions that become positive after 2 d are not considered.
‡Known to occur in clinical specimens.
Modified from Farmer JJ III: Enterobacteriaceae. Introduction and identification. *In* Murray PR, Baron EJ, Pfaller MA, et al (eds): Manual of Clinical Microbiology, ed 6. Washington, DC, ASM Press, 1995, pp 438–449.

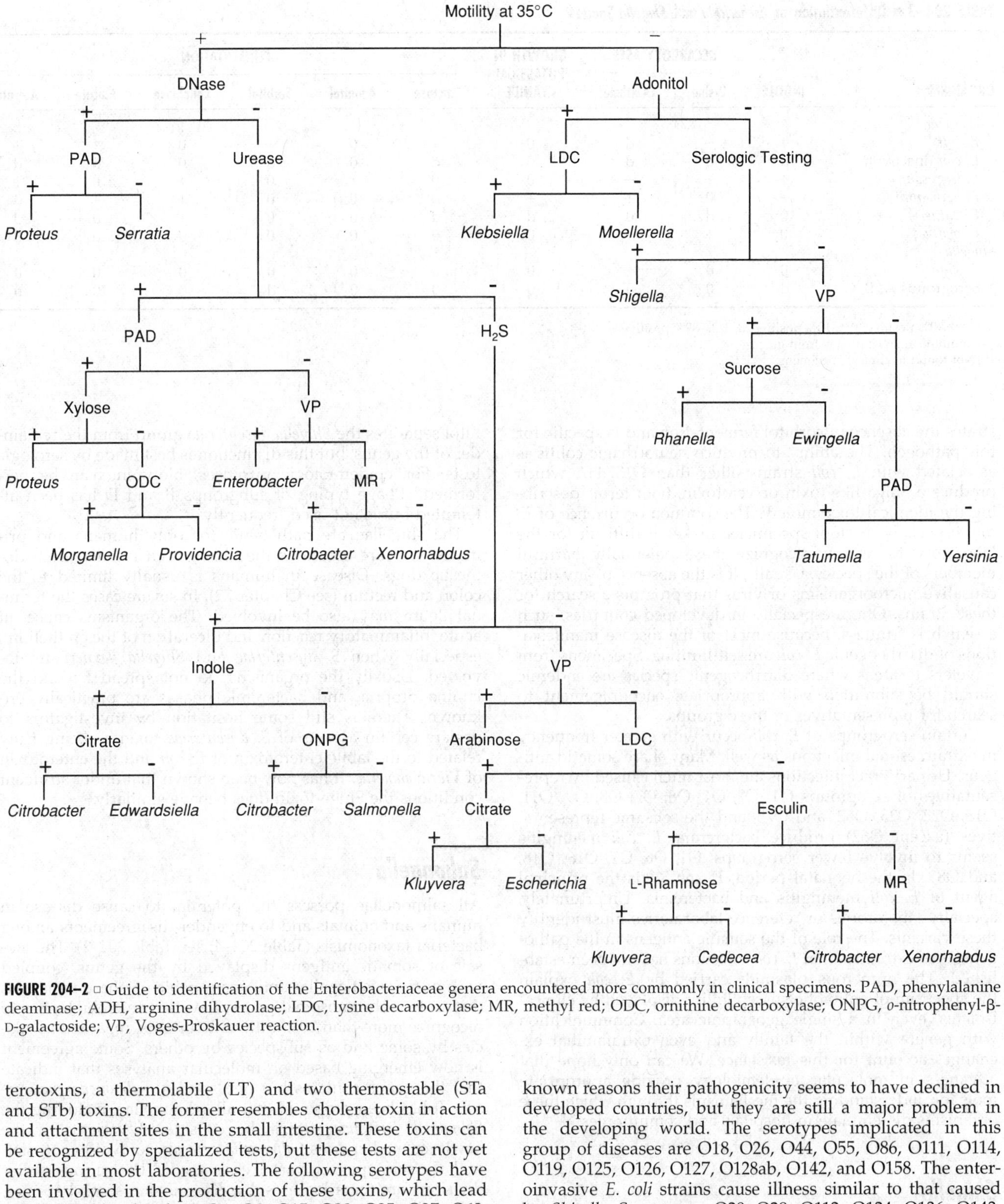

FIGURE 204–2 ☐ Guide to identification of the Enterobacteriaceae genera encountered more commonly in clinical specimens. PAD, phenylalanine deaminase; ADH, arginine dihydrolase; LDC, lysine decarboxylase; MR, methyl red; ODC, ornithine decarboxylase; ONPG, *o*-nitrophenyl-β-D-galactoside; VP, Voges-Proskauer reaction.

terotoxins, a thermolabile (LT) and two thermostable (STa and STb) toxins. The former resembles cholera toxin in action and attachment sites in the small intestine. These toxins can be recognized by specialized tests, but these tests are not yet available in most laboratories. The following serotypes have been involved in the production of these toxins, which lead to cholera-like diarrhea: O6, O8, O15, O20, O25, O27, O63, O78, O80, O85, O114, O115, O128ac, O148, O153, O159, and O167. However, the genetic determinants for the production of enterotoxins reside on transmissible plasmids that can be lost. Thus, typing of isolates by biochemical or serologic methods may be unreliable for detecting enterotoxigenic *E. coli.*

Another group of *E. coli* strains, the enteropathogenic group, were prominent causes of neonatal diarrhea in Europe and the United States during the 1950s and 1960s. For unknown reasons their pathogenicity seems to have declined in developed countries, but they are still a major problem in the developing world. The serotypes implicated in this group of diseases are O18, O26, O44, O55, O86, O111, O114, O119, O125, O126, O127, O128ab, O142, and O158. The enteroinvasive *E. coli* strains cause illness similar to that caused by *Shigella*. Serogroups O28, O29, O112, O124, O136, O143, O144, O152, O164, and O167 can cause ulceration of the intestine and symptoms resembling those of bacterial dysentery. The enterohemorrhagic *E. coli* O157:H7 causes a range of illnesses, from mild diarrhea to hemorrhagic colitis and hemolytic-uremic syndrome. Asymptomatic colonization may also occur. A cardinal feature of *E. coli* O157:H7 is its inability to ferment sorbitol in 24 hours, which allows it to be detected in the stool microbiota through the use of a selective medium, a modified MacConkey agar, that demon-

TABLE 204–3 ■ Differentiation of *Escherichia* and *Shigella* Species*

ORGANISM	INDOLE	DECARBOXYLASES		GROWTH IN POTASSIUM CYANIDE	FERMENTATION					
		Lysine	Ornithine		Lactose	Adonitol	Sorbitol	Cellobiose	Mucate	Acetate
Escherichia										
E. coli	+	+	d	0	+	0	+	0	+	+
E. coli (inactive)†	d	d	d	0	d	0	d	0	d	d
E. fergusonii	+	+	+	0	0	+	0	+	0	+
E. hermannii	+	0	+	+	d	0	0	+	+	d
E. vulneris	0	d	0	d	d	0	0	+	d	d
E. blattae‡	0	+	+	0	0	0	0	0	d	0
Shigella										
S. sonnei†	0	0	+	0	0	0	0	0	0	0
Serogroups A, B, C	d	0	0	0	0	0	d	0	0	0

*+, ≥90% positive; 0, ≤10% positive; d, 11%–89% positive.
†Immotile at 36°C; no gas from glucose.
‡Not found in clinical specimens.

strates the absence of sorbitol fermentation and is specific for this pathogen. The ability to produce hemorrhagic colitis is associated with *E. coli* strains other than O157:H7, which produce a Shiga-like toxin or verotoxin, both terms describing the identical toxic moiety. The common occurrence of *E. coli,* especially in stool specimens, makes it difficult for the laboratory to readily recognize these potentially harmful members of the species. Usually, it is the absence of any other causative microorganisms or virus that prompts a search for these strains. Often, especially in developed countries, such a search is fruitless, because most of the disease manifestations of diarrheogenic *E. coli* are self-limiting. Specimens from travelers to areas where diarrheogenic species are endemic should be submitted with appropriate encouragement to search for representatives of these groups.

Certain serogroups of *E. coli* occur with greater frequency in extraintestinal infections as well. Many share somatic antigens. Urinary tract infections are most often caused by representatives of serogroups O1, O2, O4, O6, O7, O8, O9, O11, O18, O22, O25, O62, and O75, and the selfsame representatives (except O62) produce bacteremia. *E. coli* meningitis seems to involve fewer serogroups: O1, O6, O7, O16, O18, and O83. In the neonatal period, *E. coli* K1 is the principal agent of *E. coli* meningitis and bacteremia. Unfortunately, specialty laboratories or reference laboratories must identify these variants. The role of the somatic antigens in the pathogenesis of extraintestinal *E. coli* infections has not been established. The numerous plasmids carried by *E. coli* explain the spectrum of antibiotic susceptibility displayed by clinical isolates, even in a single geographic area. Communication with genera within the family and even extrafamilial exchanges account for this resistance. We can only hope that advances in molecular epidemiology provide appropriate tools for understanding the mechanisms through which these organisms disseminate in hospitals and communities.[4, 8, 18]

Shigella

Genetically, shigellae are *E. coli.* They may be separated from classically reacting *E. coli* by a variety of tests (see Table 204–3). Inability to grow on acetate is the most useful characteristic of *Shigella* species, which separates them from the nonmotile, nonaerogenic groups of *E. coli,* especially the alkalescens-dispar group. For convenience, the genus *Shigella* is divided into four "species" with 32 serotypes and more subserotypes. Biochemical reactions are not helpful or conclusive in separating the four species. Inability to ferment mannitol separates the *Shigella dysenteriae* group from the remainder of the genus, but this distinction is best made by serologic tests. For epidemiologic purposes, biotyping can be performed.[7] Phage typing of subgroups B and D has been attempted but is not used frequently.

The shigellae are pathogenic for only humans and primates. On rare occasions they have been isolated from domestic dogs. Disease in humans is usually limited to the colon and rectum (see Chapter 72). In severe cases the terminal ileum may also be involved. The organisms cause an acute inflammatory reaction and ulceration of the epithelium, especially when *S. dysenteriae* and *Shigella flexneri* are involved. Usually the organisms do not spread beyond the lamina propria, and bacteremic phases are practically unknown. There is still some hesitation by investigators to declare certain aspects of *S. dysenteriae* toxin as being truly related to the labile enterotoxin of *E. coli* and the enterotoxin of *Vibrio cholerae.* It has now been shown that under stringent conditions the Shiga toxin does behave similarly.[19]

Salmonella

All salmonellae possess the potential to cause disease in humans and animals and to engender disagreements among bacterial taxonomists (Table 204–4; see Table 204–2). The mosaic of somatic antigens displayed by the genus, coupled with numerous flagellar antigens capable of phase variations due to two chromosomal genes, have led microbiologists to recognize more than 2000 different variants, regarded as species by some and as subspecies by others. Some agreement is now emerging based on molecular analyses that indicate that the genus contains but one species, *Salmonella choleraesuis.* It has been proposed that all salmonellae, including the *Salmonella arizonae* strains, be considered variants of the newly created species *Salmonella enterica,* to avoid confusion with the serotype (serovar) *S. choleraesuis.*[7] The various earlier divisions are regarded as subspecies, and a second species, *Salmonella bongor,* has been proposed for those errant salmonellae that may occasionally display confusing biochemical reactions.

Salmonellae have selected the intestinal tract of humans and warm- and cold-blooded wild and domestic animals as their habitat. They may be present as colonizers, but all can cause infections in humans, usually after ingestion of food or water. Two major disease manifestations characterize *Salmonella* infections: enteric fever and food poisoning. The former is characterized by headache, malaise, anorexia, and

TABLE 204–4 ■ Differences Between the Major Subgroups of *Salmonella* Organisms

	DNA SUBGROUP*						
PROPERTY OR TEST	1	2	3a	3b	4	5	6
DNA hybridization group	1	2	3	4	5	?	?
Fermentation							
Dulcitol	+	+	0	0	0	+	d
Lactose	0	0	d	d	0	0	d
Mucate	+	+	+	d	0	+	d
o-Nitrophenyl-β-galactoside	0	d	+	+	0	+	d
Malonate utilization	0	+	+	+	0	0	0
Growth in potassium cyanide	0	0	0	0	+	+	0
Gelatin hydrolysis	0	+	0	+	+	+	0

*+, ≥90% positive; 0, ≤10% positive; d, 11%–89% positive.
Modified from Farmer JJ III: Enterobacteriaceae. Introduction and identification. *In* Murray PR, Baron EJ, Pfaller MA, et al (eds): Manual of Clinical Microbiology, ed 6. Washington, DC, ASM Press, 1995, pp 438–449.

symptoms not referable to the gastrointestinal tract, as well as fever. Food poisoning presents with diarrhea, abdominal cramps, and vomiting, often accompanied by fever. The salmonellae invade the small bowel lumen, penetrate the ileum (more rarely the colonic epithelium), and induce an inflammatory reaction. After the bacteria reach the lymph nodes, the follicles enlarge and many ulcerate. The bacteria finally enter the blood stream and produce enteric fever, of which typhoid fever is the classic example. In food poisoning, *Salmonella* organisms remain confined to the intestine (see Chapter 73).

The isolation of salmonellae from clinical specimens can be accomplished with differential media grouped on the basis of their selectivity for the genus.[14, 16] Salmonellae grow readily on all routine media, including those selected for members of the Enterobacteriaceae. Moderately selective media, such as *Salmonella-Shigella* agar, Hektoen enteric agar, and xylose-deoxycholate agar, are also helpful in their isolation and produce a high degree of suspicion for the presence of the genus. Highly selective media, such as bismuth sulfite and brilliant green agar, should be used when salmonellae are suspected on clinical grounds; many laboratories use them routinely for stool culture. Enrichment broths are helpful, especially for investigating food-borne outbreaks or ruling out the carrier state.[14–16] Members of the genus *Salmonella* are usually recognized by their biochemical reactions. Simple laboratory-prepared media may be used, such as triple sugar iron agar supplemented with lysine-iron agar and certain other reactions.[7] Commercial manual and automated systems approaches have gained favor in most clinical laboratories to achieve this level of identification. Commercially available antisera permit the clinical laboratory to group isolates. The capability to type to the serotype (serovar) level is the province of specialty or reference laboratories. *Salmonella typhi* can be recognized by biochemical reactions producing minimal amounts of hydrogen sulfide and fermenting glucose without producing gas. Such isolates may not group readily with group D antisera until the blocking Vi antigen has been removed by boiling for 30 minutes. Vi antiserum is part of the commercially available battery.

Recognition of a serogroup is based on the presence of shared somatic antigens. More than 90% of clinically encountered salmonellae belong to DNA group 1 (see Table 204–2). Serotypes of group B share O antigen 4; group C1, 7; C2, 6, 8; C3, 8; D, 9; E1, 10; E2, 15; E3, 34; E4, 19; F, 11; and G, 13. The somatic antigens can occur among other bacteria, but the flagellar antigens are highly specific for the individual salmonellae. Fimbriae, other antigens such as M and the aforementioned Vi antigens, antigenic polysaccharide changes induced by bacteriophages, and other findings may confound identification of an isolate.[7] Bacteriophage typing has helped epidemiologic analyses.[20]

The salmonellae and shigellae are the traditional enteric pathogens of the Enterobacteriaceae. *K. pneumoniae* and *P. mirabilis* are second only to *E. coli* in the frequency with which they are isolated from clinical specimens. Both organisms may be involved in community-acquired urinary tract infections, and *K. pneumoniae* can be found in lower respiratory tract specimens of older persons who have a history of ethanol abuse or chronic obstructive pulmonary disease. *Klebsiella* and *Proteus* species and most other members of the family have attained significance as agents of nosocomial infections called enteric bacterioses.[11] The ability of Enterobacteriaceae to meet environmental challenges has brought into the intimate human biosphere genera and species that were unknown there only a few years ago. The introduction of these organisms reflects the selective pressures in communities and medical facilities. Most of the genera and species were considered commensal organisms in the past but have now been shown to participate in complicating the recovery of patients in medical facilities.[3] The one characteristic that these diverse species share is their almost exclusive involvement with immunocompromised patients. Rarely are these bacteria isolated from patients in the community, and when they are it is often from persons who have an underlying disease that is in remission. In the hospital setting, where many procedures, therapies, and devices permit colonization of patients with microorganisms residing in the institution, the Enterobacteriaceae bacteria behave as infectious agents. Antimicrobial agents may well have been the most influential factor leading to their ubiquitous presence in hospitals, where their inherent and plasmid-mediated antibiotic resistance capabilities allow them to replace susceptible members of the institutional microbiota and to complicate patients' recovery. They may enter the intimate human biosphere from the sources listed in Table 204–1 (to which plants should be added for *Klebsiella, Enterobacter,* and *Serratia* species). Practically all clinical specimens may harbor these organisms. It bears repeating that these bacteria are involved in all types of infections that plague patients whose immunity is compromised by disease or therapy or who may require a prosthesis. All these bacteria grow well on ordinary laboratory media, including those designed specifically to isolate all Enterobacteriaceae, such as MacConkey and eosin–methylene blue agars.

Klebsiella

Klebsiella species (see Table 204–2) are characteristically nonmotile; attack most carbohydrates; do not, except for *Klebsiella ornithinolytica,* produce ornithine decarboxylase; and display few somatic antigens but numerous capsular ones. Most representatives produce acetylmethylcarbinol, utilize citrate growing on potassium cyanide medium, and utilize malonate. *Klebsiella oxytoca* is isolated with increasing frequency from blood, urine, and respiratory tract specimens, but stool remains its principal source. *Klebsiella planticola* is a plant organism that has intruded into drinking water and into occasional clinical specimens; *Klebsiella terrigena* has not yet

TABLE 204–5 ■ Differentiation of *Klebsiella pneumoniae* Subspecies*

TEST	SUBSP. *PNEUMONIAE*	SUBSP. *OZAENAE*	SUBSP. *RHINOSCLEROMATIS*
Acid from lactose	+	+	0
Acid from dulcitol	d	0	0
Voges-Proskauer	+	0	0
Urease	+	d	0
Mucate	+	d	0
Lysine decarboxylase	+	d	0

*+, ≥90% positive; 0, ≤10% positive; d, 11%–89% positive.

been found in clinical specimens. *K. pneumoniae* is now divided into three subspecies, which are differentiated by certain tests (Table 204–5). *Klebsiella ozaenae* and *Klebsiella rhinoscleromatis* are inactive variants of *K. pneumoniae* that have adapted to specific disease manifestations[21] rarely encountered in the United States.

The Tribe Proteae

Members of the tribe Proteae are distinguished by their ability to elaborate phenylalanine deaminase; they may be separated from one another by DNase production (some *Proteus* species), swarming, and xylose fermentation by DNase-negative *Proteus* species that separates them from *Morganella* and *Providencia,* members of Ewing's tribe Proteae.[7] These genera may be distinguished from one another as shown in Figure 204–2. The species of *Proteus* are separated by reactions given in Table 204–6. Clinical laboratories have no difficulty in recognizing *P. mirabilis* and *Proteus vulgaris* organisms. Certain variants of the latter display variation, especially in esculin hydrolysis and salicin fermentation[1]; this suggests a need for taxonomic investigation but is of no consequence in the clinical setting. The epidemiology of cluster outbreaks may require that these variations be used and may lead to the establishment of new species, as was the case for *Proteus penneri,*[22] a bacterium of increasing significance in infections of agranulocytic patients. Another species, *Proteus myxofaciens,*[1] has not yet been observed in clinical specimens. *Providencia rettgeri* and *Providencia stuartii* have caused an appreciable number of nosocomial urinary tract infections. The natural habitat and means by which these organisms gain access to patients are not known. *Providencia rustigianii* and *Providencia alcalifaciens* have been isolated occasionally from diarrheal stools of infants and children, but their role in producing disease has not been clearly defined (Table 204–7). A newly described species, *Providencia heimbachae,* has not yet been isolated from humans.

Morganella morganii may be distinguished from *Proteus* organisms by an absence of swarming; hydrogen sulfide production; absence of gelatinase, lipase, and citrate utilization; but production of acid from mannose. *Morganella* species differ from *Providencia* species by producing ornithine decarboxylase and by their inability to produce acid from inositol, D-mannitol, adonitol, D-arabitol, and erythritol. *M. morganii* is suspected to be the agent of summer diarrhea,[23] and it is isolated with considerable frequency from wounds, urine, and respiratory tract specimens of hospitalized patients. Species of *Morganella* may be differentiated as shown in Table 204–2.

TABLE 204–6 ■ Differentiation of *Proteus* Species

TEST	*P. MIRABILIS*	*P. VULGARIS*	*P. PENNERI*
Indole	0	+	+
Ornithine decarboxylase	+	0	0
Acid from maltose	0	+	+
Esculin hydrolysis	0	d	0
Chloramphenicol susceptibility†	+	d	0

*+, ≥90% positive; 0, ≤10% positive; d, 11%–89% positive.
†Usual clinical isolates; exceptions can be encountered.

Serratia

The several *Serratia* species (see Table 204–1) are widely distributed in nature—in freshwater and saltwater and on leaves, shrubs, fruits, vegetables, herbs, mushrooms, and mosses. They are also recovered from a considerable number of insects, and some may be pathogenic for the insect species from which they have been isolated. Several of the *Serratia* species have become established in hospitals, where they complicate the recovery of immunocompromised patients. The frequency with which these bacteria are involved in nosocomial disease varies from hospital to hospital in a given geographic area and may reflect the antibiotic use patterns of the institution. Ingestion of raw vegetables and salads by patients and flowers in patients' rooms may play a role in colonization of patients who subsequently develop disease manifestations caused by *Serratia* species.

Serratia species (Table 204–8) produce extracellular DNase at 25°C and gelatinase at 22°C. They also elaborate lipase and are resistant to colistin and cephalothin. The combination of these biochemical activities and the responses to the two antimicrobial agents do not characterize any other Enterobacteriaceae.

The only *Serratia* species isolated frequently is *Serratia marcescens.* The inability to ferment L-arabinose is an important biochemical feature, because not all *S. marcescens* organisms produce the typical red pigment prodigiosin (2-methyl-3-amyl-6-methoxyprodigiosene). Even pigment production does not clinch the identification of *S. marcescens,* as *Serratia rubidaea* and *Serratia plymuthica* elaborate the same water-insoluble compound or a similar one. Epidemiologic differentiation of *S. marcescens* can be achieved by biotyping based primarily on carbon sources. Of the 19 biogroups established, only six produced the pigment; however, the nonpigmented representatives are most frequently involved in disease, most often biogroups A5, A8, A8b, A8c, and TCT. A variant group, *S. marcescens* biogroup 1, has been isolated almost exclusively from urine specimens.[1] Serologic identification of *S. marcescens* is difficult, because the 20 somatic and 20 flagellar antigens recognized to date cross-react. In the hospital setting, *S. marcescens* is characterized by its ability to resist antimicrobial challenges.[24]

Serratia liquefaciens, a common inhabitant of water, plants, insects, and foods, is encountered less frequently in human specimens than is *S. marcescens,* but it can become established as a nosocomial bacterium with antimicrobial resistance patterns similar to those of *S. marcescens.* This organism has been reported more frequently in England than in other countries. In the United Kingdom especially, it has been recovered from blood cultures. *S. liquefaciens* may represent a group of phenotypically related bacteria that eventually might be separated into distinct species.

S. rubidaea and *S. plymuthica* are rarely isolated from hospitalized patients. *Serratia odorifera* and *Serratia ficaria* are even rarer. All the *Serratia* species may display susceptibility to cephalosporins and aminocyclitols initially but manifest resistance during therapy.

TABLE 204–7 ■ Differentiation of *Providencia* Species

TEST	P. ALCALIFACIENS	P. RETTGERI	P. RUSTIGIANII	P. STUARTII	P. HEIMBACHAE
Urease	0	+	0	d	0
Produces acid from					
myo-Inositol	0	+	0	+	d
Adonitol	+	+	0	0	+
Arabitol	0	+	0	0	+
Trehalose	0	0	0	+	0
Indole	+	+	+	+	0

*+, >90% positive; 0, <10% positive; d, 11%–89% positive.

Citrobacter

Citrobacter organisms, comprising 11 different species, are easily differentiated from other members of the family by their ability to utilize citrate as the sole carbon source, by not producing acetylmethylcarbinol, and especially by their inability to produce lysine decarboxylase.[1] These bacteria are considered normal inhabitants of the intestinal tract of humans and animals, including mammals, birds, reptiles, and some insects. They are also encountered in soil, water, sewage, food, and industrial wastewater. Disease production is once again opportunistic, as the bacteria take advantage of the underlying disease of hospitalized patients. Organisms are recovered from clinical specimens such as urine, sputum, blood, cerebrospinal fluid, and otitis media exudates, and from surgical and traumatic wounds, abscesses, and postmortem specimens. *Citrobacter freundii* is by far the most common isolate, but the others have been isolated from nosocomial infections, at times from cluster epidemics. *C. freundii* representatives possess 42 somatic antigens and more than 70 flagellar ones. These antigens are closely related to those of *Salmonella* and *Escherichia. Citrobacter diversus* has displayed some 6 to 17 O antigens and at least 7 flagellar antigens. Investigations of *Citrobacter amalonaticus* reveal to date 13 somatic antigens, some of which seem to be related to those of *S. dysenteriae* and *Shigella boydii.*

Enterobacter and Hafnia

These two genera are considered together because the similarity of *Hafnia alvei* to *Enterobacter* organisms is considerable. The former designation of the organism was *Enterobacter hafnia.* The organisms share many biochemical characteristics (Table 204–9; see Fig. 204–2 and Table 204–2). These bacteria are widely distributed in nature. They are found in human and animal feces, quite probably as transients. They are encountered in soil, sewage, milk and dairy products, animal hides, meat, and fish from contaminated waters, and on grasses, feed, corn, sugar cane, and bananas. *Enterobacter sakazakii* and *Enterobacter gergoviae,* comparatively recently described, have been encountered only in clinical specimens; their natural habitats are not known. In addition, *Enterobacter intermedium, Enterobacter cancerogenus, Enterobacter dissolvens,* biogroup 1 of *H. alvei,* and *Enterobacter nimipressuralis* have not yet been isolated from human specimens.

These organisms represent typical examples of opportunistic enteric bacteriosis. They constitute approximately 5% of nosocomial infections and have been isolated from blood, urinary tract, surgical wound infections, lungs, and burn wounds. The frequency with which they are encountered reflects their ability to resist an appreciable number of antibiotic agents. The resistance mechanisms involve constitutive and inducible chromosomal mechanisms as well as plasmid-mediated ones. They are thought to contribute to the resistance plasmid pools in institutions by their ability to transfer extrachromosomal resistance factors to susceptible bacteria.

Although they can be recognized fairly readily on routine media in the microbiology laboratory, the biochemical activities of *Enterobacter agglomerans* are a challenge to clinical microbiologists. This bacterium, recognized by agricultural microbiologists as *Erwinia herbicola,* may be divided into two major groups that are distinguished by their ability to form gas from glucose. Ewing[7] described 11 biogroups that can be differentiated on the basis of indole production, Voges-Proskauer reaction, and nitrate reduction. *E. agglomerans* can be recognized by its failure to decarboxylate lysine and ornithine and the inability to hydrolize arginine. In addition, many strains produce a yellow pigment after several days' incubation; they ferment arabinose and rhamnose. This bacte-

TABLE 204–8 ■ Differentiation of *Serratia* Species*

TEST	S. MARCESCENS	S. LIQUEFACIENS	S. RUBIDAEA	S. PLYMUTHICA	S. ODORIFERA	S. FICARIA
DNase 25°C	+	+	+	+	+	+
Lipase	+	+	+	d	d	+
Gelatinase 22°C	+	+	+	d	+	+
Lysine decarboxylase	+	+	d	0	+	0
Ornithine decarboxylase	+	+	0	0	d	0
Distinct odor	0	0	0	0	+	+
Prodigiosin production	d	0	0	0	0	0
Fermentation						
L-Arabinose	0	+	+	+	+	+
D-Arabitol	0	0	+	0	0	+
D-Sorbitol	+	+	0	d	+	+
Adonitol	d	0	+	0	d	0

*+, ≥90% positive; 0, ≤10% positive; d, 11%–89% positive.

TABLE 204–9 ■ Differentiation of *Enterobacter* and *Hafnia* species*

TEST	*E. AEROGENES*	*E. CLOACAE*	*E. AGGLOMERANS*	*E. GERGOVIAE*	*E. SAKAZAKII*	*E. TAYLORAE*	*E. AMNIGENUS*	*E. ASBURIAE*	*E. HORMAECHEI*	*HAFNIA ALVEI*
Indole	0	0	d	0	0	0	0	0	0	0
Methyl red	0	0	d	0	0	0	0	+	d	d
Urease	0	d	d	+	0	0	0	d	d	0
Lysine decarboxylase	+	0	0	+	0	0	0	0	0	+
Ornithine decarboxylase	+	+	0	+	+	+	d	+	+	+
Arginine dihydrolase	+	0	0	+	0	0	0	d	d	0
Growth in potassium cyanide	+	+	d	0	+	+	+	+	+	+
Gas from glucose	+	+	d	+	+	+	+	+	d	+
Fermentation	+	+	d	d	+	0	d	d		0
Lactose	+	+	d	+	+	0	+	+	0	0
Sucrose	+	+	d	+	+	0	+	+	+	0
Dulcitol	0	d	d	0	0	0	0	0	d	0
Adonitol	+	d	0	0	0	0	0	0	0	0
D-Arabitol	+	d	d	+	0	0	0	0	0	0

*+, ≥90% positive; 0, ≤10% positive; d, 11%–89% positive.

rium is readily confused with other Enterobacteriaceae; several tests are required to identify *E. agglomerans* with some degree of certainty.

The somatic and capsular antigens of the genus are presently under intensive investigation for epidemiologic purposes, as are bacteriocins, plasmids, and bacteriophages. Molecular and immunochemical probes may aid in the detection of *Enterobacter* species in clinical specimens.

The versatility of *Enterobacter* and *Hafnia* in their response to antimicrobial agents requires the caveat that each clinically significant isolate be tested for its antibiotic susceptibility. Whereas laboratory tests may indicate susceptibility to ampicillin and the first-generation cephalosporins, clinical experience has not supported the use of these agents in the treatment of patients. The problem of inducible β-lactamase resistance of many *Enterobacter* species must be kept in mind when their laboratory response is evaluated, especially because second- and third-generation cephalosporins and the broad-spectrum penicillins are powerful β-lactamase inducers.

H. alvei, separated from *Enterobacter* species on the basis of DNA evaluations, has been implicated as a possible agent of diarrhea and gastroenteritis; it has been recovered from normal stool. As an opportunistic pathogen, it has been found in feces, sputum, urine, wounds, abscesses, peritonitis, and upper respiratory tract infections. Rarely has it been isolated in pure culture from these patients, except from ones who had severe underlying disease. The cardinal laboratory characteristic that separates it from *Enterobacter* species is the inability of *Hafnia* to ferment melibiose and cellobiose.

Edwardsiella

Edwardsiella tarda organisms have been isolated from a wide variety of animals. They have been recovered on occasion in stool specimens of healthy persons. They are regarded as opportunistic pathogens that have been involved in wound infections and implicated in some cases of diarrhea. Of the two remaining species in the genus, *Edwardsiella ictaluri* has not yet intruded into the human environment, whereas *Edwardsiella hoshinae* has been isolated from normal human feces. To date, *E. ictaluri* has been recognized only as a pathogen of catfish.[25] The members of the genus grow more slowly than do other Enterobacteriaceae on ordinary media. *E. tarda* may be differentiated by its motility, inability to produce DNase and urease, production of hydrogen sulfide and indole, and inability to ferment lactose or utilize citrate. (See Fig. 204–2 and Table 204–2.)

Ewingella

Ewingella americana is the only species in this genus[1] (see Fig. 204–2 and Table 204–2). Little is known about its normal habitat; to date it has been isolated only from food. The organism has been recovered from various clinical specimens, including blood, wounds, respiratory tract specimens, and stools. The bacterium is a nonmotile member of Enterobacteriaceae that does not ferment adonitol and has a positive Voges-Proskauer reaction. It may thus present problems of separation from *Yersinia* species.

Kluyvera

Kluyvera ascorbata is distinguished from *Kluyvera cryocrescens* by the fact that it uses D-ascorbate and by the ability of *K. cryocrescens* to ferment glucose at 5°C after 21 days. The precise habitat of these organisms has not been established; they have been found in water, sewage, soil, and food. These bacteria have complicated the recovery of hospitalized patients and have been isolated from blood, urine, wounds, respiratory tract, and feces. Both rapidly acquire resistance to antimicrobial agents. The bacteria are motile and do not produce DNase, urease, hydrogen sulfide, or acetylmethylcarbinol. Both may or may not produce lysine decarboxylase–negative variants and attack esculin, which helps to distinguish them from *Citrobacter.* A significant isolation of the organisms should lead to a reexamination of their antibiotic profile during therapy to avoid the emergence of resistant variants. (See Table 204–2 and Fig. 204–2.)

Cedecea

The five species of the newly described genus *Cedecea* (see Table 204–2) can be differentiated by their reaction with ornithine decarboxylase; malonate utilization; and fermentation of sucrose, D-sorbitol, raffinose, D-xylose, and melibiose.[1] The natural habitat of the members of the genus has not been discovered. They were identified as isolates from blood, urine, wound, respiratory tract, and stool specimens. *Cedecea* organisms produce lipase and are resistant to colistin and cephalothin, properties they share with *Serratia. Cedecea davisae* has been isolated principally from the respiratory tract. *Cedecea lapagei* was derived from sputum and the throat, but no real clinical significance has been attributed to it. *Cedecea neteri* may have been involved in complicating the recovery of a few patients, but it has not been encountered with any frequency in the clinical setting to date. The two unnamed species, *Cedecea* species 3 and 5, are rarely isolated in the clinical setting. Their significance in nosocomial infections depends on the ability of clinical laboratories to identify them.

Yersinia

The genus *Yersinia* has been included in the family of Enterobacteriaceae as the result of DNA hybridization findings, the presence of common enterobacterial antigens in all representatives, its biochemical activities, and its antibiotic susceptibility profiles (see Table 204–2 and Chapter 209). With the exception of *Yersinia ruckeri,* DNA hybridization studies indicate a close relationship between the remaining members of the genus. Molecular analysis of *Y. pestis* and *Y. pseudotuberculosis* indicates that they are so closely related as to probably constitute two subspecies of one species.[26] *Yersinia* is nonmotile at 37°C, but all species except *Y. pestis* move with peritrichous flagella when grown at temperatures below 30°C. The organisms are widely distributed in nature. All members of the genus grow on the usual laboratory media, although they form smaller colonies and often require a longer period of incubation, especially at temperatures above 30°C, than other members of the Enterobacteriaceae. Their slow growth is not accelerated by the incorporation of enrichments such as serum, blood, or yeast extracts. These observations are especially true for *Y. pestis.* The organisms also grow more slowly in broth. The following four species have been added to the genus: *Yersinia aldovae, Yersinia bercovieri, Yersinia mollaretii,* and *Yersinia rohdei;* all except *Y. aldovae* have been recovered from clinical material.

Plasmids in *Yersinia* species may be rare, but metabolic plasmids that enable the organisms to ferment lactose and raffinose have been observed in *Yersinia enterocolitica* and appear to be the result of 40- to 48-kD DNA. The antigens of *Yersinia* represent a complex group of carbohydrate and protein antigens. Their use in classification has not been studied sufficiently. Epidemiologically significant serogrouping of *Y. enterocolitica* depends on 34 different O antigens and 20 different H antigens.

Yersinia species are susceptible in vitro to drugs such as tetracycline, chloramphenicol, streptomycin, gentamicin, kanamycin, neomycin, sulfonamides, and nalidixic acid. They are not susceptible to β-lactam antibiotics, and the more modern agents have not been studied.

Six different factors are involved in the ability of *Y. pestis* to produce disease, of which the production of V and W antigens is probably the most significant. *Y. pestis* causes disease in rodents. The disease is transmitted when fleas regurgitate bacteria while taking a blood meal from animals—or from humans when no other hosts are readily available. Bubonic, septicemic, or pneumonic plague follows. The organisms are phagocytosed and killed in polymorphonuclear neutrophils, but those ingested by macrophages survive and multiply, acquiring resistance to further phagocytosis. Invasion of other organs leads to the usual presentation of the disease. Plague is enzootic in North and South America, Africa, the Middle East, and Asia. In the United States, wild rodents and similar animals are the reservoir. Several methods are available for testing the virulence of a *Y. pestis* strain (see also Chapter 209).

Y. pseudotuberculosis causes epizootics in many animal species, especially rodents. It involves primarily the lymphatic system. On occasion, humans acquire *Y. pseudotuberculosis* infection and may develop mesenteric adenititis that mimics acute appendicitis; immunocompromised patients can develop severe septicemia. *Y. enterocolitica,* on the other hand, is pathogenic for hares, monkeys, and humans. In animals, the disease caused by this organism resembles *Y. pseudotuberculosis* infection. In children, *Y. enterocolitica* is introduced via the oral route and the bacteria gain access to and multiply in Peyer patches. The serogroup and the presence of certain virulence-associated plasmids determine the subsequent manifestations of human disease. *Yersinia* organisms may remain localized and cause ileitis, or they may invade the lymphatics, producing mysenteric adenitis. When they reach the circulation, septicemia ensues. *Yersinia* arthritis is caused by *Y. enterocolitica* serogroup O9, which organisms share an antigen with *Brucella.* Patients who have human leukocyte antigen type 27 seem especially prone to this type of infection. The role in human disease of the remaining *Yersinia* species has not been clearly established. Many behave as opportunistic pathogens.[27] *Y. ruckeri,* an organism suspected of belonging to a different group of bacteria, is the agent of red-mouth disease of fish. Only one case of human disease has been reported.[1]

New Enterobacteriaceae Genera

Rhanella aquatalis has been isolated principally from water and rarely from human sources. It is difficult to distinguish from other Enterobacteriaceae, especially *E. agglomerans.*[1]

Tatumella ptyseos has occasionally been isolated from clinical specimens—blood, urine, stool, and mostly respiratory tract specimens. Its habitat is not known. The organism has been shown to be related to Enterobacteriaceae on the basis of DNA hybridization, including relatedness to the genus *Escherichia.* However, it differs from other Enterobacteriaceae by its inability to survive on agar or on semisolid culture media. Preservation requires storage in rabbit blood at −40°C. It also displays large zones of inhibition around a 10-unit penicillin G disk. The strains are nonmotile at 35°C and many do not move at 25°C. Flagella are usually not seen in most strains, but when they are they are polar, subpolar, or lateral.[1] This bacterium is more active biochemically at 25°C.

Xenorhabdus, a new member of the Enterobacteriaceae, is divided into two species, *Xenorhabdus nematophilus* and *Xenorhabdus luminescens* (see Fig. 204–2 and Table 204–2), that are pathogenic for nematodes and were believed to be incapable of intruding into the human biosphere because they do not grow at 35°C. They have been isolated from clinical specimens, however, and eventually they may become occasional nosocomial bacteria.

A number of other genera have been added to Enterobacteriaceae. *Budvicia, Leclercia, Leminorella,* and *Yokenella* have been recovered from clinical material. *Trabulsiella* and *Pragia* are genera as yet unknown in the human biosphere.

Table 204–2 suggests that the family Enterobacteriaceae continues to grow. The various enteric groups will eventually receive genus and species designations. In addition, the application of molecular biology methods to understanding relationships among microorganisms may lead to the creation of more genera. The continued advances in medicine may also make it possible for organisms hitherto unknown in the intimate human biosphere to gain access and to complicate the recovery of patients receiving therapy. That some of these organisms may be members of the family Enterobacteriaceae is not unlikely, although there seems to be little chance that the predominance of *E. coli, K. pneumoniae,* and *P. mirabilis* will be challenged by newcomers to the human environment. However, these bacteria are significant for the care of hospitalized—and especially of immunocompromised—patients. We need to recognize them to control cluster epidemics. The Enterobacteriaceae that are established, albeit not necessarily autochthonous residents, will continue to dominate in the economy of human health and disease.

References

1. Farmer JJ III: Enterobacteriaceae: Introduction and identification. *In* Murray PR, Baron EJ, Pfaller MA, et al (eds): Manual of Clinical Microbiology, ed 6. Washington, DC, ASM Press, 1995, pp 438–449.
2. Isenberg HD, Balows A: Bacterial pathogenicity in man and animals. *In* Starr MP, Stolp H, Truper HG, et al (eds): The Prokaryotes—A Handbook on Habitats, Isolation and Identification of Bacteria. Berlin, Springer-Verlag, 1981, pp 83–122.
3. Isenberg HD: Pathogenicity and virulence: Another view. Clin Microbiol Rev 1:40, 1988.
4. Brenner DJ: Family Enterobacteriaceae. *In* Krieg NR, Holt JG (eds): Bergey's Manual of Systematic Bacteriology, Vol 1. Baltimore, Williams & Wilkins, 1984, pp 408–420.
5. Krieg NR, Holt JG (eds): Bergey's Manual of Systemic Bacteriology, Vol 1. Baltimore, Williams & Wilkins, 1984.
6. Kauffman F: The Bacteriology of Enterobacteriaceae. Baltimore, Williams & Wilkins, 1966.
7. Ewing WH: Edwards and Ewing's Identification of Enterobacteriaceae, ed 4. New York, Elsevier Science Publishing, 1986.
8. Neidhardt FC, Ingraham JL, Low KB, et al (eds): *Escherichia coli* and *Salmonella typhimurium:* Cellular and Molecular Biology. Washington, DC, American Society for Microbiology, 1987.
9. Nikaido H, Vaara M: 1987. Outer membrane. *In* Neidhardt FC, Ingraham JL, Low KB, et al (eds): *Escherichia coli* and *Salmonella typhimurium:* Cellular and Molecular Biology, Vol 1. Washington, DC, American Society for Microbiology, 1987, pp 7–22.
10. Costerton JW, Cheng KJ, Geesay, GG, et al: Bacterial biofilms in nature and disease. Annu Rev Microbiol 41:435, 1987.
11. D'Amato RF, Isenberg HD: Enteric bacteriosis. *In* Balows A, Hausler WJ Jr, Ohashi M, Turano A (eds): Laboratory Diagnosis of Infectious Disease: Principles and Practice, Vol 1. New York, Springer-Verlag, 1988, pp 217–231.
12. Farmer JJ II, Davis Br, Hickman-Brenner FW, et al: Biochemical identification of new species and biogroups of Enterobacteriaceae isolated from clinical specimens. J Clin Microbiol 21:46, 1985.
13. Miller JM, Holmes HT. Specimen collection, transport and storage. *In* Murray PR, Baron EJ, Pfaller MA, et al (eds): Manual of Clinical Microbiology, ed 6. Washington, DC, ASM Press, 1995, pp 19–32.
14. Isenberg HD: Clinical Microbiology Procedures Handbook. Washington, DC, American Society for Microbiology, 1992.
15. McFaddin JF: Media for Isolation, Cultivation, Identification, Maintenance of Medical Bacteria. Baltimore, Williams & Wilkins, 1985.
16. Baron EJ, Peterson LR, Finegold SM: Bailey and Scott's Diagnostic Microbiology, ed 9. St. Louis, Mosby–Year Book, 1994.
17. Isenberg HD, MacLowry JC: Automated methods and data handling in bacteriology. Annu Rev Microbiol 30:483, 1976.
18. Smith GR (ed): Topley and Wilson's Principles of Bacteriology, Virology and Immunity, ed 7. Baltimore, Williams & Wilkins, 1984.
19. Rowe B, Gross RJ: *Shigella. In* Krieg NR, Holt JG (eds): Bergey's Manual of Systematic Bacteriology, Vol 1. Baltimore, Williams & Wilkins, 1984, pp 423–427.
20. Parker MT: *Salmonella. In* Smith GR (ed): Topley and Wilson's Principles of Bacteriology, Virology and Immunity, ed 7, Vol 2. Baltimore, Williams & Wilkins, 1984, pp 337–355.
21. Orskov I: *Klebsiella. In* Krieg NR, Holt JG (eds): Bergey's Manual of Systematic Bacteriology, Vol 1. Baltimore, Williams & Wilkins, 1984, pp 461–465.
22. Hickman FW, Steigerwalt AG, Farmer JJ III, Brenner DJ: Identification of *Proteus penneri,* sp. nov., formerly known as *Proteus vulgaris* indole negative or as *Proteus vulgaris* biogroup 1. J Clin Microbiol 15:1097, 1982.
23. Penner JL: The tribe Proteae. *In* Starr MP, Stolp H, Truper HG, et al (eds): The Prokaryotes—A Handbook on Habitats, Isolation and Identification of Bacteria. Berlin, Springer-Verlag, 1981, pp 1204–1244.
24. Grimont PAD, Grimont F: *Serratia. In* Krieg NR, Holt JG (eds): Bergey's Manual of Systematic Bacteriology, Vol 1. Baltimore, Williams & Wilkins, 1984, pp 477–484.
25. Farmer JJ III, McWhorter AC: *Edwardsiella. In* Krieg NR, Holt JG (eds): Bergey's Manual of Systematic Bacteriology, Vol 1. Baltimore, Williams & Wilkins, 1984, pp 486–491.
26. Bercovier H, Mollaret HH: *Yersinia. In* Krieg NR, Holt JG (eds): Bergey's Manual of Systematic Bacteriology, Vol 1. Baltimore, Williams & Wilkins, 1984, pp 498–506.
27. Bottone EJ: *Yersinia enterocolitica:* A panoramic view of a charismatic microorganism. Crit Rev Microbiol 5:211, 1977.

205

Salmonella

Sandra Sallustio
Robert H. Rubin
Marcia B. Goldberg

The pathogenic characteristics of *Salmonella* species are as varied as their natural habitats. *Salmonella* species are distributed worldwide, adapted to a wide spectrum of ecologic niches. They are found throughout the animal kingdom and cause a broad spectrum of diseases in their various hosts.

Serotyping and Bacteriology

More than 2000 serotypes of salmonellae are found in nature. They can be categorized simply according to their habitats: *Salmonella typhi* and *Salmonella paratyphi* are highly adapted to human hosts; others are highly adapted to nonhuman hosts; and still others are not adapted to any specific host. Serotypes in the first category cause a large number of infections in developing countries. Serotypes in the second category rarely produce disease in humans, with the exception of the equine pathogen *Salmonella dublin* and the swine pathogen *Salmonella choleraesuis.* The third category contains more than 1800 serotypes, which cause more than 80% of *Salmonella* infections in the United States and Europe.[1]

Salmonellae are aerobic or facultatively anaerobic, usually motile, flagellated, non-spore-forming, gram-negative bacilli. They grow well on rich media, such as blood agar, chocolate agar, and nutrient broth. These nonselective media are appropriate for culture of normally sterile body fluids.

Growth of salmonellae and shigellae is less inhibited by citrate than is growth of coliform organisms. *Salmonella-Shigella* agar, which contains citrate and bile salts, therefore selects for growth of either of these two pathogens. Normally, nonsterile body fluids such as stool should be plated on such selective media. If *S. typhi* is suspected, the specimen should also be plated on bismuth sulfite agar, which is the most efficient medium for its isolation. On this medium, *S. typhi* forms black colonies.

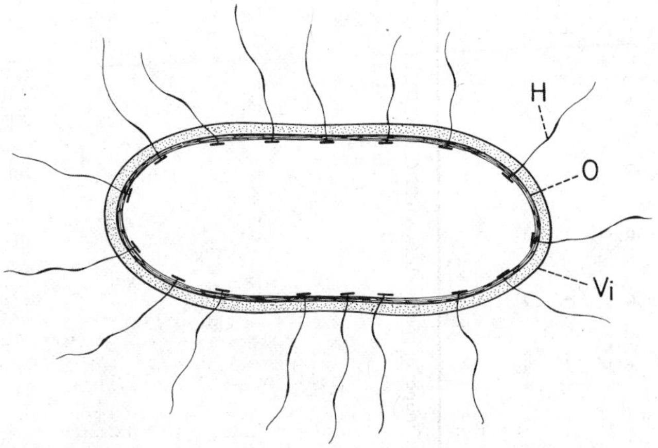

FIGURE 205–1 □ Schematic representation of the *Salmonella* bacterium. Surface antigens are indicated: somatic O-specific chains (O), flagellar H antigens (H), and virulence antigen (Vi).

In the laboratory, *Salmonella* species are distinguished from other Enterobacteriaceae by biochemical reactions (Table 205–1). Like *Shigella, Proteus,* and *Yersinia* species, they are unable to ferment lactose and thus give rise to white colonies on solid media containing lactose and the color indicator neutral red (e.g., MacConkey or *Salmonella-Shigella* agar). Most salmonellae produce abundant hydrogen sulfide, form gas in glucose media, decarboxylate lysine and ornithine, and do not ferment sucrose. Hydrogen sulfide production results in the green color of these colonies on blood agar. *Salmonella* species are distinguished from several *Proteus* species by their inability to metabolize urea. An important exception to these rules is *S. typhi,* which produces little or no hydrogen sulfide, does not form gas in glucose media, and does not decarboxylate ornithine. Lactose-fermenting strains of *S. typhi* have also been reported rarely.

Salmonella serotypes are traditionally classified on the basis of two surface antigens, somatic O antigens and flagellar H antigens (Fig. 205–1). Lipopolysaccharide, a major component of the outer leaflet of the outer membrane of gram-negative bacteria, consists of O antigens covalently linked to a basal core polysaccharide, which in turn is covalently linked to the membrane-anchoring moiety lipid A. The core polysaccharide is structurally similar in all salmonellae. The O antigens are linear polymers of repeating oligosaccharide units that vary structurally among salmonellae; these structural variations form the primary basis of serotype classification. H antigens are flagellar proteins that also vary structurally, forming the secondary basis of serotype classification.

According to the Kauffmann-White classification system, nine serogroups (A through I) are defined by O antigens. (Table 205–2). All members of a serogroup carry the same major O antigen, and individual members of a serogroup may carry different minor O antigens. Serotypes within the serogroups are defined by H antigens. At different times, an individual serotype may carry one or more types of H antigen, referred to as phase 1 or phase 2.[1] Ninety percent of human isolates are from serogroups A through E, which contain fewer than 40 serotypes. Certain serotypes are linked with particular clinical syndromes. For example, within serogroup D, the *S. typhi* serotypes commonly cause enteric fever, the *Salmonella enteritidis* serotypes result in gastroenteritides, and the *S. dublin* serotypes often result in bacteremias.[2] Moreover, the serotyping of clinical isolates is important in the characterization and control of epidemics. Only a few highly specialized laboratories have collections of specific antisera adequate to type strains precisely. Most clinical laboratories group their *Salmonella* isolates both by agglutination reactions using group-specific antisera and by biochemical tests. In the United States, all *Salmonella* isolates confirmed by appropriate biochemical tests should be forwarded to reference laboratories in state health departments for more exhaustive serotyping as part of the national *Salmonella* surveillance system.[3]

The Widal agglutination test for the detection of serum antibodies against the O and H antigens is in common use but lacks adequate sensitivity and specificity in most clinical settings. For a nonimmune person, a positive test is one in which either the anti-O antibody rises fourfold or a titer of greater than 1:50 or 1:100 is present in a single sample drawn during the initial 2 to 3 weeks of disease.[4] The test is potentially useful only in typhoid fever or some chronic infections such as osteomyelitis, because the antibody response to gastroenteritis and to the chronic carrier state is minimal. Nevertheless, not all cases of typhoid fever, treated or untreated, produce diagnostic titers. Moreover, the specificity of the test is low, as both anti-O and anti-H antibodies are acute-phase reactants, often rising in response to nonspecific inflammatory processes. After immunization, the anti-O antibody titer may remain elevated for months, and that of anti-H antibody for years, making interpretation of the test difficult.[2] Finally, some cross-reactivity occurs with non-*typhi* salmonellae.[5]

A third type of antigen, the virulence or Vi antigen, is present on *S. typhi* and occasionally on *S. paratyphi* C. This virulence factor is a capsular polysaccharide (a polymer of *N*-acetylgalactosaminic acid[6]) that appears to protect the organisms from the actions of complement (see Fig. 205–1).

For epidemiologic characterization of outbreaks, it is frequently useful to define *Salmonella* strains or subtypes within a single serotype. The two techniques that have been useful in these evaluations are phage typing and plasmid profile analysis. Phage typing serves to characterize strains by their differential susceptibility to lysis by specific bacteriophages. Plasmid profile analysis serves to characterize strains by the size and restriction enzyme fragment patterns of their plasmid DNA. Both techniques have been useful in tracing outbreaks due to single serotypes. Additional molecular techniques for serotype identification, such as ribotyping (a method for comparing ribosomal RNA genes and associated sequences of bacteria), are currently being developed.

Immunology

A large body of information, including vaccine studies, demonstrates that protective immunity to *S. typhi* is possible and that it requires both cell-mediated and humoral immune responses.[7–9] Assays of antibody titers and lymphocyte responses demonstrate that typhoid fever or *S. typhi* vaccination induces both immune responses[10, 11]; in spite of a prodigious body of work, however, all of the antigens responsible for these responses have not been characterized. Little is known about the immune response to non-*typhi Salmonella.*[12] In studies of murine infection with *Salmonella typhimurium,* antibodies to the outer membrane lipopolysaccharide and its O-antigen side chain, along with cell-mediated immune responses, have been shown to be important to host survival.[13–22]

After *Salmonella* infection in humans, significant elevations occur in antilipopolysaccharide and anti-O antigen antibody titers. However, the protection against subsequent infection conferred by the normal antibody response is at best only partial. Specific immunoglobulin M, immunoglobulin G, and secretory immunoglobulin A antibodies persist for only 16 weeks, 2 years, and 48 weeks, respectively, after an episode of typhoid fever.[23] Recurrences of typhoid fever have been

TABLE 205–1 ■ Useful Biochemical Reactions for Distinguishing *Salmonella* from Other Enterobacteriaceae and *Aeromonas* and *Vibrio* Organisms*

REACTION	*ESCHERICHIA* SPP.	*SHIGELLA* SPP.	*EDWARDSIELLA* SPP.	*SALMONELLA* SPP.	*ARIZONA* SPP.	*CITROBACTER FREUNDII*	*CITROBACTER DIVERSUS*	*KLEBSIELLA PNEUMONIAE*	*ENTEROBACTER CLOACAE*	*ENTEROBACTER AEROGENES*	*ENTEROBACTER HAFNIAE*	*ENTEROBACTER AGGLOMERANS*	*SERRATIA MARCESCENS*
Hydrogen sulfide	−	−	+	+	+	+/−	−	−	−	−	−	−	−
Urease	−	−	−	−	−	a	a	+	+/−	−	−	a	a
Motility	+/−	−	+	+	+	+	+	−	+	+	+	+/−	+
Lysine decarboxylase	a	−	+	+	+	−	−	+	−	+	+	−	+
Ornithine decarboxylase	a	a	+	+	+	a	+	−	+	+	+	−	+
Gas production from glucose	+	−	+	+	+	+	+	+	+	+	+	−/+	+/−
Lactose	+	−	−	−	a	c	a	+	c	+	a	a	−
Sucrose	a	−	−	−	−	a	−/+	+	+	+	a	a	+

REACTION	*SERRATIA LIQUEFACIENS*	*SERRATIA RUBIDAEA*	*PROTEUS VULGARIS*	*PROTEUS MIRABILIS*	*PROTEUS MORGANII*	*PROTEUS RETTGERI*	*PROVIDENCIA ALCALIFACIENS*	*PROVIDENCIA STUARTII*	*YERSINIA ENTEROCOLITICA*	*YERSINIA PSEUDOTUBERCULOSIS*	*YERSINIA PESTIS*	*AEROMONAS HYDROPHILA*	*VIBRIO CHOLERAE*
Hydrogen sulfide	−	−	+	+	−	−	−	−	−	−	−	−	−
Urease	a	a	+	+	+	+	−	−	+	+	−/a	−	−
Motility	+	+/−	+	+	+/−	+	+	+	b	b	b	+	+
Lysine decarboxylase	c	c	−	− +	−	−	−	−	−	−	−	−	+
Ornithine decarboxylase	+	−	−	+ −	+	−	−	−	+	−	−	−	+
Gas production from glucose	+/−	a	+/−	a	+/−	−/+	+/−	−	−	−	−	+/−	−
Lactose	a	+	−		−	−	−	−	−	−	−	−/+	d
Sucrose	+	+	+		−	a	a	c	+	−	−	+	+

*+, 90% or more are positive in 1 to 2 days; −, 90% or more are negative; +/−, majority are positive; −/+, majority are negative; a, different biochemical types are found; b, positive between 22°C and 37°C; c, positive or delayed positive; d, positive reaction delayed.

Modified from Holt JG, Krieg NR, Sneath PHA, et al: Bergey's Manual of Determinative Bacteriology, ed 9. Baltimore, Williams & Wilkins, 1994, pp 203–222.

TABLE 205–2 ■ Kauffmann-White Classification of Common *Salmonella* Serotypes*

SEROTYPE	GROUP	O ANTIGENS	H ANTIGENS Phase 1	H ANTIGENS Phase 2
S. paratyphi A	A	1,2,12	a	(1),(5)
S. paratyphi B†	B	1,4,(5),12	b	1,2
S. typhimurium	B	1,4,(5),12	i	1,2
S. heidelberg	B	1,4,(5),12	r	1,2
S. canada	B	4,12	b	1,6
S. saintpaul	B	1,4,(5),12	e, h	1,2
S. paratyphi C‡	C1	6,7,(Vi)	e	1,5
S. bareilly	C1	6,7	y	1,5
S. choleraesuis	C1	6,7	(c)	1,5
S. montevideo	C1	6,7	g,m,(p),s	(1),(2),(7)
S. oranienburg	C1	6,7	m,t	—
S. newport	C2	6,8	e,h	1,2
S. typhi	D1	9,12,(Vi)	d	—
S. enteritidis	D1	1,9,12	g,m	(1),(7)
S. gallinarum-pullorum	D1	1,9,12	—	—
S. anatum	E1	3,10	e,h	1,6
S. vancouver	I	16	c	1,5

*Parentheses indicate that the antigenic determinant may be absent or difficult to detect.
†Also designated *S. schottmülleri*.
‡Also designated *S. hirschfeldii*.
Adapted from Le Minor L: Genus III. *Salmonella* Lignières 1900, 389. *In* Krieg NR, Holt JG (eds): Bergey's Manual of Systematic Bacteriology, Vol 1. Baltimore, Williams & Wilkins, 1984, pp 427–458.

reported[24]; however, these have been in the setting of prior immunization or rapid antibiotic administration, which may reduce immunity acquired from natural, untreated infection.

For *S. typhi*, several observations suggest that the Vi antigen plays a role in both the pathogenesis of infection and the acquisition of protective immunity: (1) 75% of asymptomatic carriers of *S. typhi* have high serum antibody titers to Vi antigen[25]; (2) purification methods that partially depolymerize the Vi polysaccharide and remove the *O*-acetyl and *N*-acetyl moieties also reduce the immunogenicity of the resulting material[26–28]; (3) intramuscular vaccination with Vi antigen caused a significant rise in serum antibody levels to Vi antigen[29–32] and conferred 65% to 75% protection against subsequent infections with *S. typhi*.[30, 31] Interestingly, in a comparative trial of single versus combined vaccination against yellow fever and typhoid fever, the immune response to yellow fever was moderately higher in volunteers injected with a combined vaccine preparation versus volunteers injected with yellow fever vaccine alone, implying that the Vi antigen preparation may have mild adjuvant properties.[29]

In the pathogenesis of typhoid fever, *S. typhi* traverses the intestinal mucosa and localizes in regional and distal lymphoid tissue. Organisms appear to replicate within cells of the reticuloendothelial system. The ability of host macrophages to kill intracellular *Salmonella* organisms likely plays a key role in the generation of an effective immune response.[2, 33] Clinically, this is borne out by the increased frequency and virulence of salmonellosis in persons with impaired immunity. Thus, patients with impaired intracellular killing have difficulty eradicating infection, as is described for a woman heterozygous for chronic granulomatous disease.[34] Patients with altered splenic and reticuloendothelial function, such as those with sickle cell anemia or those suffering from malaria, disseminated histoplasmosis, louse-borne relapsing fever, or bartonellosis, develop more systemic *Salmonella* infections.[2, 35, 36] In certain patients with dysgammaglobulinemias, salmonellosis occurs with increased frequency and may be persistent or recurrent.[37, 38] Transplant recipients,[39, 40] persons with neoplasia,[41, 42] and persons with acquired immunodeficiency syndrome[43–46] also manifest an increase in the frequency and severity of infection. Patients with acquired immunodeficiency syndrome are usually unable to eradicate the infection and require long-term antimicrobial suppressive therapy. Conversely, mutant strains of *S. typhimurium* that are unable to survive in macrophages have reduced virulence in mice.[47]

Molecular Pathogenesis of *Salmonella* Infections

In spite of extensive investigations of the pathogenesis of *Salmonella* infections, in both humans and several animal hosts, the actual mechanisms underlying the various disease manifestations are still incompletely understood. The molecular events surrounding the invasion of and replication within eukaryotic cells by these organisms have been detailed to a much greater extent than have macromolecular pathogenic processes. The latter have been studied using a murine model, which does not directly reflect the pathogenic process in humans: *S. typhi* strains are avirulent in mice, whereas infection of these animals with *S. typhimurium* produces a syndrome that closely mirrors typhoid fever in humans.[48] Consequently, *S. typhimurium* infection has served as the model for most laboratory investigations of salmonellosis.

After oral ingestion by the host, *Salmonella* organisms make their way to the small bowel, where they interact with enterocytes lining the intestinal wall. As the microorganism makes contact with the enterocyte, there is disruption of brush border microvilli, followed by morphologic alterations in the apical membranes, with subsequent internalization of the bacteria in membrane-bound vesicles.[49] A major intestinal target cell for *Salmonella* is likely the class of specialized epithelial cell known as M cells, which overlie the mucosal lymphoid tissues of Peyer patches. These polarized cells lack an apical brush border and are characterized by a basolateral invagination that contains antigen-presenting cells as well as lymphocytes.[50] The internalized organisms, still within endosomes, traverse, or transcytose, the M cell and are exocytosed into the subepithelial region, where they interact with the lymphoid cells. Alternatively, it has been proposed that endocytosed bacteria eventually kill the M cells and thereby acquire access to the underlying lymphoid tissue,[51] resulting in the stimulation of an immune response. At the tissue level, this stimulation is reflected in marked enlargement of Peyer patches shortly after infection.[2]

M cells, however, are likely not the sole intestinal cell type that participates in uptake of *Salmonella* during infection. Further, the ability of these organisms to invade and replicate within both macrophages and nonprofessional phagocytes is thought to contribute to the tissue and blood stream dissemination seen in syndromes such as typhoid fever. Progress on the elucidation of the molecular basis for invasion and replication of *Salmonella* within eukaryotic cells has been achieved through in vitro studies of the interaction of *Salmonella* strains (predominantly *S. typhimurium*) with epithelial cells and, to a lesser extent, macrophages (reviewed in Finlay[52]). These studies have contributed to the identification of many host and bacterial factors that participate in infection.

Thus, on exposure to bacteria, epithelial cell membranes undergo distinct morphologic changes (a process described as "membrane ruffling"),[53–57] which are accompanied by host cytoskeletal protein rearrangements[58] and capping of host proteins that interact with the cytoskeleton.[59] Uptake of bacteria in membrane-bound vesicles is an energy-requiring process that is affected by incompletely characterized bacterial virulence factors. For *S. typhimurium*, these virulence determinants include members of the *inv* locus as well as the *prg* gene products.[60–66] Within the infected cell, bacteria remain in membrane-bound structures, or phagosomes. Live organisms are able to slow the acidification of these phagosomes,[67] which is thought to contribute to intracellular survival via effects on the PhoP-PhoQ regulatory system. (The PhoP-PhoQ proteins regulate transcription of *Salmonella* genes in response to environmental stimuli.[68, 69]) Additional bacterial factors thought to affect survival of *Salmonella* within eukaryotic cells include a cytolysin[70] and an outer membrane protein that appears to protect bacteria from oxidative killing within human polymorphonuclear leukocytes.[71] Replication of *Salmonella* within phagosomes of nonprofessional phagocytes has been demonstrated[72–75]; virulent, replicating *Salmonella* organisms localized within phagosomes of epithelial cells have been specifically reported to induce formation of lysosomal glycoprotein-rich filamentous aggregates that appear to be connected to the phagosome and are of uncertain significance.[76]

As stated earlier, the ability of *Salmonella* to survive within phagocytes and epithelial cells likely plays an important role in the pathogenesis of typhoid fever. Bacteria that escape killing and invade the intestinal wall can subsequently disseminate to various body sites via both the blood stream and the lymphatic circulation. Pathogenic characteristics typical of typhoid fever, such as hepatosplenomegaly, likely reflect the interplay of bacterial virulence factors and the host immune response to these factors. Understanding the molecular mechanisms that underlie virulence will lead to improved strategies for preventing morbidity and mortality due to *Salmonella* species.

Vaccines

An ideal *Salmonella* vaccine should fulfill five criteria. First, the vaccine should induce lasting and protective immune responses both locally, that is, in the intestinal tract, and systemically. Vaccines prepared from live attenuated strains are more apt to meet this requirement than are vaccines prepared from killed or inactivated organisms, as has been demonstrated in a comparison of immune responses to volunteers given oral formulations of *S. typhi* Ty21a.[77] Second, an ideal vaccine should provide adequate immunity after only a single dose. Third, the vaccine should be administered orally. Fourth, vaccine preparations should be stable under field conditions; for example, they should not require refrigeration. Finally, an ideal vaccine strain should have an extremely low rate of reversion to a virulent strain. None of the currently available vaccines meet all of these criteria.

To date, the *Salmonella* vaccines that have been developed provide protection against single serotypes only. Three vaccines for *S. typhi* are currently approved for use in the United States (Table 205–3). A fourth vaccine is now available only to members of the United States armed forces.[78]

Typhoid vaccine, manufactured by Wyeth-Ayerst, is a heat-phenol–killed parenteral vaccine that is administered in a primary series as two sequential doses (0.5 mL subcutaneously) separated by an interval of at least 4 weeks. Field trials of a heat-phenol–killed vaccine similar to this vaccine demonstrated an efficacy ranging from 51% to 77% in a 2.5- to 3-year follow-up period.[79–81] This vaccine is not recommended for children younger than 6 months. Adverse effects are common and include systemic reactions such as fever and malaise as well as local reactions, such as pain or swelling at the injection site.[80, 81] The high incidence of adverse effects renders this vaccine a poor candidate for prophylaxis of large populations.

The second *S. typhi* vaccine available in the United States is a live attenuated form of strain Ty21a. The primary immunization series consists of ingestion of an enteric-coated capsule containing 2 to 6 $\times$ 10^9 viable and 5 to 50 $\times$ 10^9 nonviable *S. typhi* Ty21a organisms every other day for a total of four doses. Field trials conducted with this vaccine among schoolchildren in Chile have demonstrated variable levels of efficacy, ranging from 66% protection during a period of 5 years[82, 83] to only a 33% reduction in cases of typhoid fever in a 3-year period.[84] In these trials, the vaccine was administered as an enteric-coated capsule in three doses in a 1-week period. In a follow-up trial, also in Chile, designed to test the protective effect of one or two doses of the enteric-coated formulation among school-age children, efficacies of 29% and 59% were obtained in the first 2 years after vaccination with one or two doses, respectively; ominously, no protective efficacy was demonstrable with either dosing regimen 3 to 5 years after vaccination.[85] An earlier clinical trial conducted in Egypt among children who received a liquid formulation of the oral Ty21a vaccine reported a 96% efficacy in a 3-year period.[86] A direct comparison of the oral formulations in two trials demonstrated higher efficacy for the liquid versus the enteric-coated preparation (77% versus 33% efficacy in a 3-year period for the Chilean study and 53% versus 42% efficacy for an Indonesian study, respectively).[84, 87] The liquid formulation may be available for routine use in the near future.[88] In the United States, this vaccine is not recommended for children younger than 6 years. In addition, the vaccine is contraindicated in immunocompromised persons or those receiving antimicrobial agents.[78] The Ty21a vaccine produces no significant adverse reactions.

The third typhoid vaccine available in the United States is a parenteral vaccine that consists of the Vi capsular polysaccharide of *S. typhi*. The vaccine is administered in the primary series as a single intramuscular injection of 25 μg of antigen in 0.5 mL. The efficacy of this antigen has been evaluated in two field trials: one large clinical trial in Nepal demonstrated 75% protection for 17 months or longer,[30] and a trial in South Africa reported 65% protection during a 2-year period.[31] The Vi capsular polysaccharide vaccine is not approved for children younger than 2 years. Adverse reactions included fever, headache, and erythema or induration at the site of injec-

TABLE 205–3 ■ Currently Available *Salmonella typhi* Vaccines

VACCINE	EFFICACY	ADMINISTRATION	ADVERSE REACTIONS
Heat-phenol killed, parenteral	51%–77% for 2.5–3.0 y[79–81]	Two 0.5-mL subcutaneous injections >4 wk apart*; booster every 3 y	Fever, malaise, pain, or swelling at injection site[80, 81]
Live attenuated, oral Ty21a	29%–96% for 2 y or longer[82–87]	Four doses of capsule	None
Vi capsular polysaccharide, parenteral†	65%–75% for 17 mo or longer[30, 31]	One 0.5-mL intramuscular dose; booster every 2 y	Fever, headache, and erythema or induration at injection site[31, 32, 89]

*For children younger than 10 y, each injection should be 0.25 mL.
†Not approved for children younger than 2 y.

tion.[31, 32, 89] Advantages of this vaccine include the single-dose administration schedule as well as its stability at ambient temperature, precluding the need for refrigeration. In the United States, vaccination is recommended for travel to regions where there is a recognized risk of exposure to *S. typhi,* especially to developing countries in Latin America, Asia, and Africa. The recommendations apply to persons who expect to be exposed to potentially contaminated food or water for prolonged periods. For less prolonged or significant exposure, as might apply to tourists lodging in international hotels in developing countries, many physicians advocate dietary precautions rather than vaccination. Vaccination against *S. typhi* is also advocated for persons with intimate exposure to documented carriers of this organism, as well as for laboratory personnel who work with virulent strains of *S. typhi.*[78]

Newer vaccines for *S. typhi* are on the horizon. Several *Salmonella* strains containing genetically defined mutations are currently under study. These include strains that are auxotrophic for chorismic acid biosynthesis (the *aro* mutants),[90–97] that have deletions in genes encoding adenylate cyclase *(cya)* or cyclic 3′,5′-adenosine monophosphate receptor protein *(crp)*,[98] that carry mutations in the regulatory locus involved in the protection of *Salmonella* from microbicidal host proteins,[68] and that harbor mutations in the gene encoding the regulatory histidine kinase inner membrane protein, *ompR.*[99] More recent candidates for potential vaccine strains include *hemA* (deficient in functional transfer RNA reductase) and *htrA* (deficient in a serine protease that degrades aberrant periplasmic proteins) *S. typhimurium,*[100, 101] as well as the doubly auxotrophic *(his-pur) S. typhimurium* strains 1771 and 3334.[102] All of these are attenuated, yet highly immunogenic in murine models, and several show promise or are under study in human volunteers.

Live attenuated strains of *Salmonella* have the exciting ability to serve as carriers of heterologous antigens of human pathogens.[103] Genes encoding such antigens can be inserted on plasmids and introduced into the vaccine strain. Hosts challenged with these recombinant strains can be expected to manifest an immune response to both the foreign protein and the vaccine strain. Several experimental difficulties must be overcome before there can be widespread use of this antigen delivery system. Specifically, the foreign proteins must be expressed at levels that simultaneously have negligible effects on carrier strain physiology yet are sufficient to elicit the desired immune response. In addition, the plasmids carrying the heterologous gene must segregate equally among progeny bacteria after division. In routine molecular biology work, this requirement is met by propagating such plasmid-carrying strains in the presence of substances (usually antibiotics) that allow survival only of organisms maintaining plasmids (encoding resistance to these substances). As the use of antibiotic resistance genes is obviously precluded in candidate vaccine strains, investigators have either placed foreign genes on plasmids that complement auxotrophic mutations in recipient strains (and hence must be carried by the bacteria to allow their survival in the host) or engineered such heterologous genes on so-called suicide vectors, which cannot replicate permissively in transformants. In the latter case, homologous recombination of the suicide vector with the bacterial chromosome yields a stably integrated, chromosomal copy of the foreign gene and, advantageously, can result in an additional attenuating mutation in the vaccine strain.

References

1. Goldberg MB, Rubin RH: The spectrum of *Salmonella* infection. Infect Dis Clin North Am 2:571, 1988.
2. Rubin RH, Weinstein L: Salmonellosis: Microbiologic, Pathologic and Clinical Features. New York, Stratton Intercontinental, 1977.
3. Farmer JJ, Kelly MT: Enterobacteriaceae. *In* Manual of Clinical Microbiology, ed 5. Washington, DC, American Society for Microbiology, 1991, pp 371–373.
4. Schroeder SA: Interpretation of serologic tests for typhoid fever. JAMA 206:839, 1968.
5. Reynolds DW, Carpenter RL, Simon WH: Diagnostic specificity of Widal's reaction for typhoid fever. JAMA 214:2192, 1970.
6. Heyns K, Kiessling G: Strukturaufklärung des Vi-antigens aus *Citrobacter freundii (E. coli)* 5396/38. Carbohydr Res 3:340, 1967.
7. Forrest BD, LaBrooy JT, Beyer L, et al: The human humoral immune response to *Salmonella typhi* Ty21a. J Infect Dis 163:336, 1991.
8. Levine MM, Ferreccio C, Black RE, et al: Progress in vaccines against typhoid fever. Rev Infect Dis 11:S552, 1989.
9. Nencione L, Villa L, DeMagistris MT: Cellular immunity against *Salmonella typhi* after live oral vaccine. Adv Exp Med Biol 216B:1669, 1987.
10. Murphy JR, Baqar S, Munoz C, et al: Characteristics of humoral and cellular immunity to *Salmonella typhi* in residents of typhoid-endemic and typhoid-free regions. J Infect Dis 156:1005, 1987.
11. Murphy J, Wasserman S, Baqar S, et al: Immunity to *Salmonella typhi:* Considerations relevant to measurement of cellular immunity in typhoid-endemic regions. Clin Exp Immunol 75:228, 1989.
12. Robbins JB, Chu C, Schneerson R: Hypothesis for vaccine development: Protective immunity to enteric diseases caused by nontyphoidal salmonellae and shigellae may be conferred by serum IgG antibodies to the O-specific polysaccharide of their lipopolysaccharides. Clin Infect Dis 15:346, 1992.
13. Hsu HS: Pathogenesis and immunity in murine salmonellosis. Microbiol Rev 53:390, 1989.
14. Ding HF, Nakoneczna I, Hsu HS: Protective immunity induced in mice by detoxified *Salmonella* lipopolysaccharide. J Med Microbiol 31:95, 1990.
15. Hormaeche CE, Joysey HS, Desilva L, et al: Immunity conferred by Aro-*Salmonella* live vaccines. Microb Pathog 10:149, 1991.
16. O'Callaghan D, Maskell D, Tite J, Dougan G: Immune responses in BALB/c mice following immunization with aromatic com-

pound or purine-dependent *Salmonella typhimurium* strains. Immunology 69:184, 1990.
17. Mastroeni P, Villareal-Ramos B, Hormaeche CE: Adoptive transfer of immunity to oral challenge with virulent salmonellae in innately susceptible BALB/c mice requires both immune serum and T cells. Infect Immun 61:3981, 1993.
18. Mastroeni P, Villareal-Ramos B, Hormaeche CE: Role of T cells, TNF-alpha and IFN-gamma in recall of immunity to oral challenge with virulent salmonellae in mice vaccinated with live attenuated aro-*Salmonella* vaccines. Microb Pathog 13:477, 1992.
19. Villareal B, Mastroeni P, Demarco de Hormaeche R, Hormaeche CE: Proliferative and T-cell specific interleukin (IL-2/IL-4) production responses in spleen cells from mice vaccinated with *aroA* live *Salmonella* vaccines. Microb Pathog 13:305, 1992.
20. Muotiala A, Makela PH: Role of gamma interferon in late stages of murine salmonellosis. Infect Immun 61:4248, 1993.
21. Blanden RV, Mackaness MB, Collins FM: Mechanisms of acquired resistance in mouse typhoid. J Exp Med 124:585, 1966.
22. Udhayakumar V, Muthukkaruppan VR: Protective immunity induced by outer membrane proteins of *Salmonella typhimurium* in mice. Infect Immun 55:816, 1987.
23. Sarasombath S, Banchuin N, Sukosol T, et al: Systemic and intestinal immunities after natural typhoid infection. J Clin Microbiol 25:1088, 1987.
24. Marmion DE, Naylor GRE, Stewart IO: Second attacks of typhoid fever. J Hyg 51:260, 1953.
25. Lanata CF, Levine MM, Ristori C, et al: Vi serology in detection of chronic *Salmonella typhi* carriers in an epidemic area. Lancet 2:441, 1983.
26. Landy M: Studies on Vi antigen: VI. Immunization of human beings with purified Vi antigen. Am J Hyg 60:52, 1954.
27. Robbins JD, Robbins JB: Reexamination of the protective role of the capsular polysaccharide (Vi antigen) of *Salmonella typhi.* J Infect Dis 150:436, 1984.
28. Tacket CO, Ferreccio C, Robbins JB, et al: Safety and immunogenicity of two *Salmonella typhi* Vi capsular polysaccharide vaccines. J Infect Dis 154:342, 1986.
29. Ambrosch F, Fritzell B, Gregor J, et al: Combined vaccination against yellow fever and typhoid fever: A comparative trial. Vaccine 12:625, 1994.
30. Acharya IL, Lowe CU, Thapa R, et al: Prevention of typhoid fever in Nepal with the Vi capsular polysaccharide of *Salmonella typhi.* N Engl J Med 317:1101, 1987.
31. Klugman KP, Gilbertson IT, Koornhof HJ, et al: Protective activity of Vi capsular polysaccharide vaccine against typhoid fever. Lancet 330:1165, 1987.
32. Keitel WA, Bond NL, Zahradnik JM, et al: Clinical and serological responses following primary and booster immunization with *Salmonella typhi* Vi capsular polysaccharide vaccines. Vaccine 12:195, 1994.
33. Hornick RB, Greisman SE, Woodward TE, et al: Typhoid fever: Pathogenesis and immunologic control. N Engl J Med 283:686, 1970.
34. Moellering RC, Weinberg AN: Persistent *Salmonella* infection in a female carrier for chronic granulomatous disease. Ann Intern Med 73:595, 1970.
35. Wheat LJ, Rubin RH, Harris NL, et al: Systemic salmonellosis in patients with disseminated histoplasmosis. Arch Intern Med 147:561, 1987.
36. Barrett-Connor E: Bacterial infection and sickle cell anemia: An analysis of 250 infections in 166 patients and a review of the literature. Medicine (Baltimore) 50:97, 1971.
37. Douglas SD, Goldberg LS, Fudenberg HH: Clinical, serologic and leukocyte function studies on patients with idiopathic "acquired" agammaglobulinemia and their families. Am J Med 48:48, 1970.
38. Stites DP, Levin AS, Lauer BA, et al: Selective "dysgammaglobulinemia" with elevated serum IgA levels and chronic salmonellosis. Am J Med 54:260, 1973.
39. Mussche MM, Lameire NH, Ringoir SMG: *Salmonella typhimurium* infections in renal transplant patients. Nephron 15:143, 1975.
40. Rubin RH: Infection in the renal and liver transplant patients. *In* Rubin RH, Young LS (eds): Clinical Approach to Infection in the Compromised Host, ed 2. New York, Plenum Publishing, 1988, pp 557–621.
41. Han T, Sokal JE, Neter E: Salmonellosis in disseminated malignant diseases: A seven year review 1959–1965. N Engl J Med 276:1045, 1967.
42. Wolfe MS, Armstrong D, Louria DB, et al: Salmonellosis in patients with neoplastic diseases. A review of 100 episodes at Memorial Cancer Center over a 13 year period. Arch Intern Med 128:546, 1971.
43. Chaisson RE: Infections due to encapsulated bacteria, *Salmonella, Shigella,* and *Campylobacter.* Infect Dis Clin North Am 2:474, 1988.
44. Sperber SJ, Schleupner CJ: Salmonellosis during infection with human immunodeficiency virus. Rev Infect Dis 9:925, 1987.
45. Celum CL, Chaisson RE, Rutherford GW, et al: Incidence of salmonellosis in patients with AIDS. J Infect Dis 156:998, 1987.
46. Gotuzzo E, Frisancho O, Liendo G, et al: Association between the acquired immunodeficiency syndrome and infection with *Salmonella typhi* or *Salmonella paratyphi* in an area endemic for typhoid fever. Arch Intern Med 151:381, 1991.
47. Fields PI, Swanson RV, Haidaris CG, et al: Mutants of *Salmonella typhimurium* that cannot survive within the macrophage are avirulent. Proc Natl Acad Sci USA 83:5189, 1986.
48. Hormaeche, CE: Natural resistance to *Salmonella typhimurium* in different inbred mouse strains. Immunology 37:311, 1979.
49. Takeuchi A: Electron microscope studies of experimental *Salmonella* infection. I. Penetration into the intestinal epithelium by *Salmonella typhimurium.* Am J Pathol 50:109, 1967.
50. Neutra MR, Phillips TL, Mayer EI, Fishkind DJ: Transport of membrane-bound macromolecules by M cells in follicle-associated epithelium of rabbit Peyer's patch. Cell Tissue Res 247:537, 1987.
51. Jones, JBD, Ghori N, Falkow S: *Salmonella typhimurium* initiates murine infection by penetrating and destroying the specialized epithelial M cells of the Peyer's patches. J Exp Med 180:15, 1994.
52. Finlay BB: Cell biology of *Salmonella* pathogenesis. *In* Miller VL, Kaper JB, Portnoy DA, Isberg RR (eds): Molecular Genetics of Bacterial Pathogenesis. Washington, DC, ASM Press, 1994, pp 249–261.
53. Alpuche-Aranda CM, Racoonsin EI, Swanson JA, Miller SI: *Salmonella* stimulate macrophage macropinocytosis and persist within spacious phagosomes. J Exp Med 179:601, 1994.
54. Finlay BB, Falkow S: *Salmonella* interactions with polarized human intestinal Caco-2 epithelial cells. J Infect Dis 162:1096, 1990.
55. Francis CL, Ryan TA, Jones BD, et al: Ruffles induced by *Salmonella* and other stimuli direct macropinocytosis of bacteria. Nature 364:639, 1993.
56. Jones BD, Paterson HF, Hall A, Falkow S: *Salmonella typhimurium* induces membrane ruffling by a growth factor-receptor–independent mechanism. Proc Natl Acad Sci USA 90:10390, 1993.
57. Ginocchio CG, Olmsted SB, Wells CI, Galan JE: Contact with epithelial cells induces the formation of surface appendages on *Salmonella typhimurium.* Cell 76:717, 1994.
58. Finlay BB, Ruschkowski S, Dedhar S: Cytoskeletal rearrangements accompanying *Salmonella* entry into epithelial cells. J Cell Sci 99:283, 1991.
59. Garcia-del Portillo F, Pucciarelli MG, Jefferies WA, Finlay BB: *Salmonella typhimurium* induces selective aggregation and internalization of host cell surface proteins during invasion of epithelial cells. J Cell Sci 107:2005, 1994.
60. Belden WJ, Miller SI: Further characterization of the PhoP regulon: Identification of new PhoP-activated virulence loci. Infect Immun 62:5095, 1994.
61. Galan JE, Curtiss R: Cloning and molecular characterization of genes whose products allow *Salmonella typhimurium* to penetrate tissue culture cells. Proc Natl Acad Sci USA 86:6383, 1989.
62. Galan JE, Ginocchio C, Costeas P: Molecular and functional characterization of the *Salmonella* invasion gene *invA:* Homology of InvA to members of a new protein family. J Bacteriol 174:4338, 1992.
63. Galan JE, Pace J, Hayman MJ: Involvement of the epidermal growth factor receptor in the invasion of cultured mammalian cells by *Salmonella typhimurium.* Nature 357:588, 1992.
64. Altmeyer RM, McNern JK, Bossio JC, et al: Cloning and molecular characterization of a gene involved in *Salmonella* adherence and invasion of cultured epithelial cells. Mol Microbiol 7:89, 1993.

65. Ginocchio CG, Pace J, Galan JE: Identification and molecular characterization of a *Salmonella typhimurium* gene involved in triggering the internalization of salmonellae into cultured epithelial cells. Proc Natl Acad Sci USA 89:5976, 1992.
66. Galan JE, Curtiss R: Distribution of the *invA, -B, -C,* and *-D* genes of *Salmonella typhimurium* among other *Salmonella* serovars: *invA* mutants of *Salmonella typhi* are deficient for entry into mammalian cells. Infect Immun 59:2901, 1991.
67. Alpuche-Aranda CM, Swanson JA, Loomis WP, Miller SI: *Salmonella typhimurium* activates virulence gene transcription within acidified macrophage phagosomes. Proc Natl Acad Sci USA 89:10079, 1992.
68. Miller SI, Kukral AM, Mekalanos JJ: A two-component regulatory system *(phoPphoQ)* controls *Salmonella typhimurium* virulence. Proc Natl Acad Sci USA 86:5054, 1989.
69. Miller SI: PhoP/PhoQ: Macrophage-specific modulators of *Salmonella* virulence? Mol Microbiol 5:2073, 1991.
70. Libby SJ, Goebel W, Ludwig A, et al: A cytolysin encoded by *Salmonella* is required for survival within macrophages. Proc Natl Acad Sci USA 91:489, 1994.
71. Stinavage PS, Martin LE, Spitznagel JK: A 59 kilodalton outer membrane protein of *Salmonella typhimurium* protects against oxidative intraleukocytic killing due to human neutrophils. Mol Microbiol 4:283, 1990.
72. Conlan JW, North RJ: Early pathogenesis of infection in the liver with the facultative intracellular bacteria *Listeria monocytogenes, Francisella tularensis,* and *Salmonella typhimurium* involves lysis of infected hepatocytes by leukocytes. Infect Immun 60:5164, 1992.
73. Finlay BB, Falkow S: Comparison of the invasion strategies used by *Salmonella cholerae-suis, Shigella flexneri,* and *Yersinia enterocolitica* to enter cultured animal cells: Endosome acidification is not required for bacterial invasion or intracellular replication. Biochimie 70:1089, 1988.
74. Gahring LC, Heffron F, Finlay BB, Falkow S: Invasion and replication of *Salmonella typhimurium* in animal cells. Infect Immun 58:443, 1990.
75. Yokoyama H, Ikedo M, Kohbata S, et al: An ultrastructural study of HeLa cell invasion with *Salmonella typhi* GIFU 10007. Microbiol Immunol 31:1, 1987.
76. Garcia-del Portillo F, Zwick MB, Leung KY, Finlay BB: *Salmonella* induces the formation of filamentous structures containing lysosomal membrane glycoproteins in epithelial cells. Proc Natl Acad Sci USA 90:10544, 1993.
77. Kantele A, Arvilommi H., Kantele JM, et al: Comparison of the human immune response to live oral, killed oral or killed parenteral *Salmonella typhi* Ty21a vaccines. Microb Pathog 10:117, 1991.
78. Centers for Disease Control and Prevention: Typhoid immunization: Recommendations of the Advisory Committee on Immunization Practices (ACIP). MMWR Morbid Mortal Wkly Rep 43(RR-14):1, 1994.
79. Aschroft MT, Singh B, Nicholson CC, et al: A 7 year field trial of two typhoid vaccines in Guyana. Lancet 2:1056, 1967.
80. Hejfec LB, Salmin LV, Lejtman MZ, et al: A controlled field trial and laboratory study of five typhoid vaccines in the USSR. Bull WHO 34:321, 1966.
81. Yugoslav Typhoid Committee: A controlled trial of the effectiveness of acetone-dried and inactivated and heat-phenol-inactivated typhoid vaccines in Yugoslavia. Bull WHO 30:623, 1964.
82. Levine MM, Ferreccio C, Black RE, Germanier R, et al: Large-scale field trials of Ty21a live oral typhoid vaccine in enteric-coated capsule formulation. Lancet 1:1049, 1987.
83. Levine MM, Taylor DN, Ferreccio C: Typhoid vaccines come of age. Pediatr Infect Dis J 8:374, 1989.
84. Levine MM, Ferreccio C, Cryz S, Ortiz E: Comparison of enteric-coated capsules and liquid formulation Ty21a typhoid vaccine in randomised controlled field trial. Lancet 336:891, 1990.
85. Black RE, Levine MM, Ferreccio C, et al: Efficacy of one or two doses of Ty21a *Salmonella typhi* vaccine in enteric-coated capsules in a controlled field trial. Vaccine 8:81, 1990.
86. Wahdan MH, Serie C, Cerisier Y, et al: A controlled field trial of live *Salmonella typhi* strain Ty21a oral vaccine against typhoid: Three-year results. J Infect Dis 145:292, 1982.
87. Simanjuntak CH, Paleolog FP, Punhabi NH, et al: Oral immunisation against typhoid fever in Indonesia with Ty21a vaccine. Lancet 338:1055, 1991.
88. Levine MM: Vaccines and milk immunoglobulin concentrates for prevention of infectious diarrhea. J Pediatr 118:S129, 1991.
89. Cumberland NS, Roberts JS, Arnold WSG, et al: Typhoid Vi: A less reactogenic vaccine. J Int Med Res 20:247, 1992.
90. Hoiseth SK, Stocker BAD: Aromatic-dependent *Salmonella typhimurium* are non-virulent and effective as live vaccines. Nature 291:238, 1981.
91. Dougan G, Maskell D, Pickard D, Hormaeche CE: Isolation of stable *aroA* mutants of *Salmonella typhi* Ty2: Properties and preliminary characterization in mice. Mol Gen Genet 207:402, 1987.
92. Nnalue NA, Stocker BA: Test of the virulence and live-vaccine efficacy of auxotrophic and ga1E derivatives of *Salmonella choleraesuis.* Infect Immun 55:955, 1987.
93. Dougan G, Chatfield S, Pickard D, et al: Construction and characterization of vaccine strains of *Salmonella* harboring mutations in two different *aro* genes. J Infect Dis 156:1329, 1988.
94. Miller IA, Chatfield S, Dougan G, et al: Bacteriophage P22 as a vehicle for transducing cosmid gene banks between smooth strains of *Salmonella typhimurium:* Use in identifying a role for *aroD* in attenuating virulent *Salmonella* strains. Mol Gen Genet 215:312, 1989.
95. Jones PW, Dougan G, Hayward C, et al: Oral vaccination of calves against experimental salmonellosis using a double *aro* mutant of *Salmonella typhimurium.* Vaccine 9:29, 1991.
96. Chatfield SN, Fairweather N, Charles I, et al: Construction of a genetically defined *Salmonella typhi* Ty2 *aroA aroC* mutant for the engineering of a candidate typhoid-tetanus vaccine. Vaccine 10:53, 1992.
97. Hone DM, Harris AM, Chatfield S, et al: Construction of genetically-defined double *aro* mutants of *Salmonella typhi.* Vaccine 9:810, 1991.
98. Curtiss R, Kelly SM: *Salmonella typhimurium* deletion mutants lacking adenylate cyclase and cyclic AMP receptor protein are avirulent and immunogenic. Infect Immun 55:3035, 1987.
99. Dorman CJ, Chatfield S, Higgins CF, et al: Characterisation of porin and *ompR* mutants of a virulent strain of *Salmonella typhimurium: ompR* mutants are attenuated *in vivo.* Infect Immun 57:2136, 1989.
100. Benjamin WH, Hall P, Briles DE: A *hemA* mutation renders *Salmonella typhimurium* avirulent in mice, yet capable of eliciting protection against intravenous infection with *S. typhimurium.* Microb Pathog 11:289, 1991.
101. Chatfield SN, Strahan K, Pickard D, et al: Evaluation of *Salmonella typhimurium* strains harbouring defined mutations in *htrA* and *aroA* in the murine salmonellosis model. Microbial Pathog 12:145, 1992.
102. Mitov I, Denchev V, Linde K: Humoral and cell-mediated immunity in mice after immunization with live oral vaccines of *Salmonella typhimurium:* Auxotrophic mutants with two attenuating markers. Vaccine 10:61, 1992.
103. Chatfield SN, Strugnell RA, Dougan G: Live salmonellae as vaccines and carriers of foreign antigenic determinants. Vaccine 7:495, 1989.

206

Shigella

Gerald T. Keusch

The genus *Shigella* is probably best considered as an end stage of differentiation of *Escherichia coli,* achieved by acquisition of virulence attributes to the point where *Shigella* species are almost always pathogens rather than usually being a commensal in the normal gut flora. It is because the genus *Shigella* is so closely related to *E. coli* that the two actually cannot be distinguished by DNA hybridization methods.[1] It is not surprising that the majority of microbiologic properties of the four *Shigella* species are also identical to those of *E. coli.* Like *E. coli,* they are also classified in the family Enterobacteriaceae and belong to the tribe Escherichieae. Their common evolutionary path is further suggested by the striking frequency with which they share surface carbohydrate antigens[2] and specific virulence factors, including plasmid-mediated invasion determinants[3] and cytotoxins closely related to Shiga toxin.[4] Nonetheless, *Shigella* species are highly host adapted to humans, whereas *E. coli* strains are widely distributed among animals.

The genus *Shigella* was discovered because of its association with the clinical picture of epidemic dysentery,[5] resulting in a severe, febrile, inflammatory colitis characterized by a triad of clinical findings, including (1) a characteristic small volume of stool composed primarily of blood, mucus, and inflammatory cells; (2) abdominal cramps and pain; and (3) tenesmus (painful straining to pass stool).[6] The discovery of *Entamoeba histolytica* in 1875 and the description of histologic criteria for its diagnosis in humans in 1891 set the stage for the subsequent identification of *Shigella.*[7] Although the first isolation can probably be attributed to Chantemesse and Widal in 1888, a much more complete description was provided by Kiyoshi Shiga during an epidemic of dysentery in Japan in the late 1890s.[5] Not only did Shiga isolate a distinct non–lactose-fermenting organism from the stool of patients that was not present in healthy subjects or in patients with other clinical entities, but also he proved its importance by demonstrating the development of agglutinating antibodies during the course of the infection. For this classic work, Shiga's name ultimately was honored in the genus designation, *Shigella,* and the organism he reported and called *Bacillus dysenteriae* is now known as *Shigella dysenteriae* type 1.

Three years after Shiga's report on *B. dysenteriae,* Kruse isolated a similar organism from dysenteric cases except that it was mannitol fermenting (in contrast to the mannitol-negative *B. dysenteriae*) and serologically distinct, that is, it would not agglutinate in convalescent serum from patients with *B. dysenteriae.*[7] This bacterium was designated *Bacillus pseudodysenteriae* and was quickly confirmed by Flexner and by Castellani in Ceylon. Others referred to these isolates as *B. dysenteriae* Flexner, and when the genus name was formally established, these organisms were designated *Shigella flexneri.* Boyd, working somewhat later in Bangalore, India, identified a common isolate biochemically resembling *S. flexneri* except for its inability to agglutinate in group- or type-specific antiserum to *S. flexneri.* The nonagglutinable organisms could, of course, be agglutinated by homologous antiserum.[7] These strains were ultimately defined as a third *Shigella* species, *Shigella boydii.* The fourth species was described by Kruse, Castellani, and Duval as a late lactose-fermenting variant that was serologically distinct from the other known dysentery bacilli.[7] Kruse first called this organism *B. pseudodysenteriae* type E, but because of the extensive work on these organisms carried out by Sonne, it became known as *B. pseudodysenteriae* Sonne, and ultimately as *Shigella sonnei.*

Thus, during the 40 years from 1898 to 1938, the four clinically virulent species of *Shigella* were biochemically and serologically distinguished by group- and type-specific antigens. These include *S. dysenteriae* (serogroup A, 12 serotypes), *S. flexneri* (serogroup B, 14 serotypes), *S. boydii* (serogroup C, 15 serotypes), and *S. sonnei* (serogroup D, 1 serotype, but multiple colicin types).

Characteristics of the Pathogen

Shigella organisms are gram-negative, facultatively anaerobic rod-shaped bacilli that are devoid of flagella. Although they share major biochemical properties with *E. coli* (Table 206–1), *Shigella* species can be distinguished from nearly all *E. coli* species by their failure to ferment lactose within 24 hours, their inability to produce gas from glucose (with rare exceptions), and, of course, their lack of motility. In fact, diagnostic microbiology schemata utilize these characteristics to quickly separate putative *Shigella* species from *E. coli* within the first 24 hours of culture (see later). *S. sonnei,* which is positive for *o*-nitrophenyl-β-D-galactopyranoside, can utilize lactose, but only after a delay of several days. Biochemical characteristics that differentiate *E. coli* and *Shigella* are shown in Table 206–2. It should be noted that *Shigella* is one of the least biochemically active members of the Enterobacteriaceae family.

The four *Shigella* species are also biochemically similar to one another, except for the inability of *S. dysenteriae* to ferment mannitol, positive ornithine utilization by *S. sonnei,* and the ability of most *S. sonnei* strains to ferment lactose after several days in culture. In practice, differentiation among species is usually accomplished by serologic methods, and group- and type-specific antisera can be used to identify the four serogroups and different serotypes.

Virulence Attributes

LIPOPOLYSACCHARIDE O ANTIGENS

Considerable information has been obtained about the specific structures of the O antigens of the most clinically relevant *Shigella* species and the structural basis for the known serologic cross-reactivity with certain *E. coli.*[8] For example,

TABLE 206–1 ■ Shared Biochemical Characteristics of *Shigella* and *Escherichia coli*

TEST OR SUBSTRATE USED	RESULT
Adonitol	Negative
DNase	Negative
Hydrogen sulfide on triple sugar iron agar	Negative
Inositol	Negative
Potassium cyanide	Negative
Malonate	Negative
Mannitol	Positive (except *S. dysenteriae*)
Methyl red	Positive
Mucate	Variable
Phenylalanine deaminase	Negative
Urease	Negative
Voges-Proskauer	Negative

TABLE 206–2 ■ Differentiation of *Shigella* and *Escherichia coli*

TEST OR SUBSTRATE	*SHIGELLA* (%)*	*E. COLI* (%)
Acetate	Negative (0)	Positive (84)
Arginine decarboxylase	Negative (8)	Variable (17)
Citrate	Negative (0)	Variable (24)
Esculin	Negative (0)	Variable (31)
Gas from glucose†	Negative (<2)	Positive (91)
Indole	Variable (38)	Positive (99)
Lactose fermentation‡	Negative (<1)	Positive (91)
Lysine decarboxylase	Negative (0)	Positive (90)
Motility	Negative (0)	Positive (80)
Mucate	Negative (0)	Positive (92)
Ornithine decarboxylase§	Variable (20)	Positive (63)
Salicin	Negative (0)	Positive (40)
Sucrose	Negative (<1)	Positive (50)
Xylose	Negative (2–5)	Positive (95)

*Percent positive are in parentheses.
†Some *S. flexneri* type 6 organisms produce gas from glucose.
‡*S. sonnei* usually ferments lactose or sucrose after several days in culture.
§Some *S. sonnei* organisms decarboxylate ornithine.

S. dysenteriae type 1 has a unique repeating unit (→3α-D-GlcNAc1→3-α-L-Rha1→3-α-L-Rha1→2-α-D-Gal1→), which is shared only with *E. coli* O1 and O120 and not with other species of *Shigella*. The somatic antigens of two other group A serotypes, *S. dysenteriae* types 2 and 3, are also known to be identical to the O antigens of *E. coli* O112 and O124, respectively, but distinct from that of *S. dysenteriae* type 1.

All *S. flexneri* serotypes except *S. flexneri* type 6 have a common repeating unit of four sugars (→2α-L-Rha1→2-α-L-Rha1→3-α-L-Rha1→3-β-D-GlcNac→), which constitutes the serologic specificity termed group Y.[8] The more frequently found 1a-5b seroreactivities of *S. flexneri* result from the attachment of α-D-glucopyranosyl and *O*-acetyl groups to various sites on the basic repeat unit. These sorts of antigens are relatively common among Enterobacteriaceae; as a result there are many cross-reactions between *S. flexneri* and *E. coli.*[8] In addition to possessing unique sequences, *S. flexneri* type 6 shares the α-L-Rha1→2-α-L-Rha1→ disaccharide with *S. flexneri* 1-5, so that it is recognized by convalescent sera from patients with the latter infections.

S. sonnei has a disaccharide of unusual nature in common with *Plesiomonas shigelloides*, consisting of 2-acetamido-2-deoxy-L-altruronic acid-α1→4-2-acetamido-4-amino-2,4,6-trideoxy-D-Gal, linked to one another in a β1→6 linkage.[8]

The rest of the lipopolysaccharide molecule is similar among all gram-negative organisms.[9] The 2-keto-3-deoxyoctonate inner core region of the *Shigella* lipopolysaccharide resembles that of *Salmonella* or *E. coli*, whereas the short outer core region is markedly similar in all *Shigella* species. There is no evidence of significant variation in lipid A structure or biologic activity from *Shigella* to *E. coli.*[10]

Although it is known that rough mutants are avirulent, the actual role of lipopolysaccharide in virulence of *Shigella* is unclear. Evidence suggests that this may be related to a requirement for O antigens in the transport and insertion of IcsA, a critical virulence determinant involved in intra- and intercellular spread of an organism, within the outer membrane of the organism.[11] Further evidence of the role of lipopolysaccharide comes from Tn5 mutagenesis experiments in which insertional inactivation of the *rfa* locus involved in the synthesis of lipopolysaccharide basal core structures results in inefficient cell-to-cell spread in in vitro models and reduced inflammatory lesions in in vivo models.[12] Previous speculations that O antigens were helpful to the organisms by blocking the complement-dependent serum bacteriolytic system appear to be incorrect. The invasive strains most frequently causing shigellemia, *S. dysenteriae* type 1 and *S. flexneri*, are sensitive to complement-mediated lysis; rather, it is a host serum bactericidal activity that is lacking.[13] This explains why patients with bacteremic shigellosis are usually younger than 1 year and are significantly malnourished.[14] Endotoxemia has been described in patients with hemolytic-uremic syndrome due to *S. dysenteriae* type 1, and, as described later, circulating endotoxin may play a role in pathogenesis.[15]

CELL INVASION

There is little doubt that the ability to invade epithelial cells is central to the virulence of *Shigella* species.[16] Creation of noninvasive *Shigella* variants renders those organisms avirulent.[17] Invasiveness is now known to be a complex process dependent on gene products and regulatory elements present on both chromosomal and plasmid DNA (Fig. 206–1). In vivo, invasion occurs predominantly in the human colon; however, most of our information comes from either animal models or in vitro studies of HeLa or other extraenteric cells in tissue culture. Early studies utilizing conjugal transfer or transduction of *E. coli* chromosomal DNA from the *xyl-rha, his,* or *purE* loci to virulent *Shigella flexneri* type 2a recipients resulted in hybrids that were able to invade but not survive within cells.[18] The *xyl-rha* region of *S. flexneri* codes for iron-binding hydroxymate proteins and several iron-regulated outer membrane proteins,[19] which may directly affect intracellular survival of the organisms, although no effect on survival in HeLa cells of a Tn10-induced aerobactin mutation

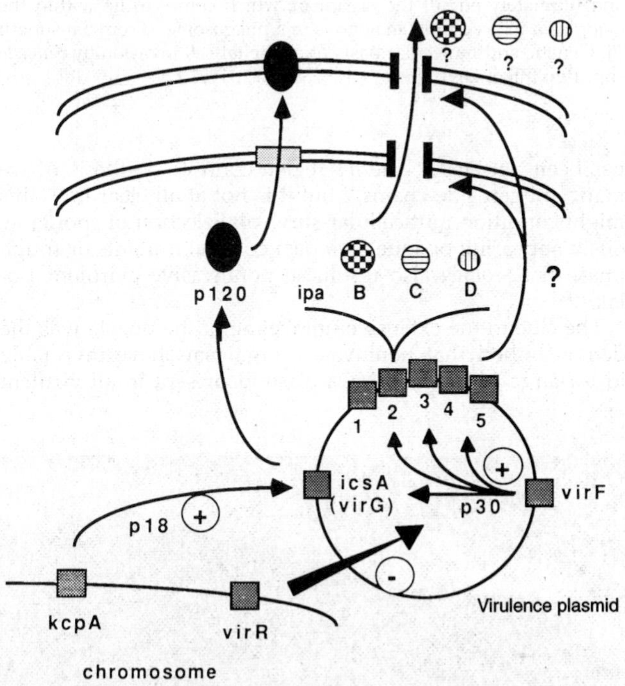

FIGURE 206–1 □ Location of some virulence determinant genes and regulatory elements in *Shigella flexneri.* Structural genes for the invasion plasmid antigens (Ipas) are present on the large 140-kDa *S. flexneri* plasmid and are positively regulated by the nearby *virF* locus at the transcriptional level. *virF* encodes a 30-kDa protein, which also positively regulates the *icsA* gene (formerly known as *virG*), along with the chromosomal locus *kcpA*. The *icsA* product, a 120-kDa protein, which is inserted in the outer membrane of the organism, is necessary for intracellular spread of the organism. *virR* is a chromosomal negative regulator of the *ipa* genes. (From Sansonetti PJ: Genetic and molecular basis of epithelial cell invasion by *Shigella* spp. Rev Infect Dis 13[Suppl 4]:S285–S291, 1991.)

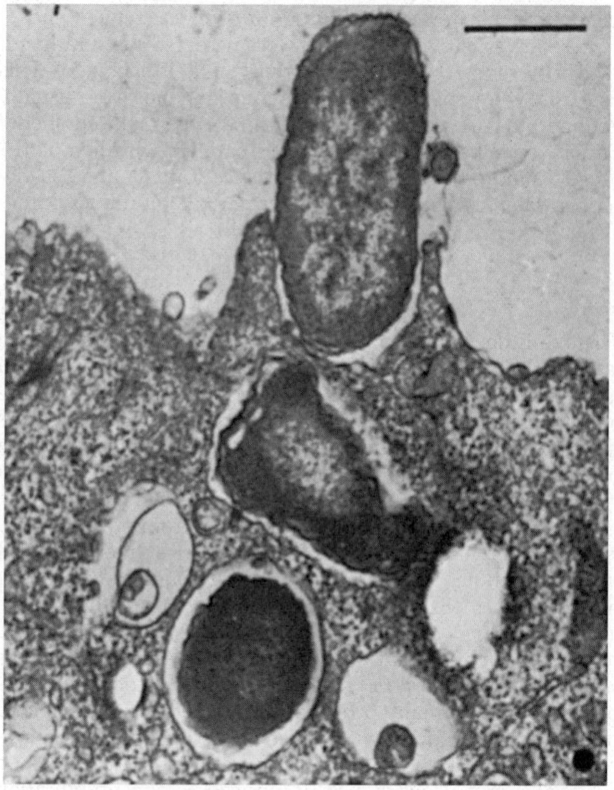

FIGURE 206–2 ▫ Entry of *S. flexneri* into a HeLa cell. Pseudopods extend from the surface of the nonprofessional phagocytic HeLa cell and ultimately engulf the organism, which comes to lie within the cytoplasm in a vacuole analogous to a phagosome. (From Sansonetti PJ: Genetic and molecular basis of epithelial cell invasion by *Shigella* spp. Rev Infect Dis 13[Suppl 4]:S285–S291, 1991.)

has been detected.[20] The *his* region controls synthesis of somatic antigen side chains,[14] but it is not at all clear how this might condition intracellular survival. Selection of spontaneously appearing opaque *S. flexneri* colonial mutants or rough phase II *S. sonnei* also results in noninvasive avirulent isolates.[17]

The clue to the extensive unraveling of the puzzle was the demonstration that noninvasive organisms have invariably lost a large 140- to 160-MDa plasmid present in all virulent *Shigella* strains and enteroinvasive *E. coli*.[21–23] These plasmids contain certain highly conserved regions common to all, constituting an operon that encodes a group of outer membrane proteins termed invasion plasmid antigens (Ipas).[24, 25] Of the multiple Ipas, IpaA to IpaD (polypeptides of 78, 62, 43, and 38 kDa, respectively) are usually recognized by convalescent human serum.[25] Tn5 insertions in the genes for IpaB, IpaC, and IpaD, but not IpaA, have been found to impair *Shigella* invasiveness, indicating their importance in the process.[24] These essential virulence factors are transported and inserted in the bacterial surface membrane under the control of two regulatory gene sets known as *mxi* (membrane export of Ipa)[26] and *spa* (surface presentation of Ipas).[27] Growth of *Shigella* on cultured epithelial cells leads to release of Ipa proteins.[28] In response, host cells respond with complex changes in the cytoskeleton that result in formation of phagocytic vesicles and bacterial uptake.[29]

Significant insights into invasion have resulted from the realization that it is essentially analogous to phagocytosis of bacteria by neutrophils or macrophages[30] (Fig. 206–2). This followed from observations that internalization of *Shigella* by tissue culture or intestinal cells occurs within membrane-bounded vesicles and that the process requires polymerization of actin filaments.[31–33] Sansonetti and colleagues[33] have effectively used transposon mutagenesis to define the further functions and antigens of importance to virulence. Electron microscopy has demonstrated that virulent *Shigella* organisms are able to lyse the phagocytic vacuole within a few minutes and gain rapid entry to the cytoplasm (Fig. 206–3). This has been correlated with a plasmid-mediated acid-activated contact hemolysin, activated at a pH known to occur in phagocytic vesicles. Hemolysin-negative isolates are invasive but avirulent. Tn5 mutants, which delete the hemolysin function, also eliminate the ability to invade cells and escape from vesicles. Ipa proteins are also required for vesicle lysis, because nonpolar inactivation mutants of IpaB, IpaC, or IpaD are inhibited in both entry and vesicle lysis.[34]

Another characteristic of intracellular *Shigella* organisms is their impressive ability to multiply.[33] The basis for this is, however, uncertain. Intracellular multiplication is necessary for virulence, because mutants defective in folic acid synthesis via the aromatic pathway, or bearing mutations of the porins OmpC and OmpF, or their regulatory gene, *ompB*,[35, 36] are unable to do so and are avirulent as well. The reason may be related to events during cell division that assist the organism in spreading from cell to cell (see later).

An avirulent Tn*phoA* mutant, SC557, has helped delineate

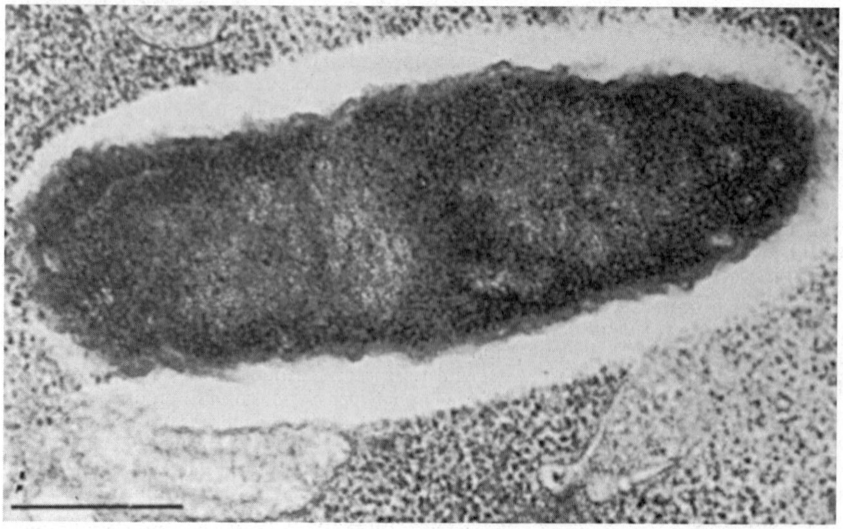

FIGURE 206–3 ▫ Shortly after invasion of a HeLa cell, *S. flexneri* lyses the phagosomal membrane and lies freely within the cytoplasm of the cell. Note the lack of host cell membrane surrounding the bacterium. (From Sansonetti PJ: Genetic and molecular basis of epithelial cell invasion by *Shigella* spp. Rev Infect Dis 13[Suppl 4]:S285–S291, 1991.)

the mechanism of intracellular spread, the next step in pathogenesis.[37] This strain invades cells and rapidly lyses the vacuole but it fails to spread within the cytoplasm or to spread from cell to cell, forming plaques in HeLa cell monolayers. This strain fails to synthesize an immunogenic 120-kDa outer membrane protein named IcsA and coded for by a plasmid gene, *icsA* (intra-intercellular spread). This same gene locus was previously identified as *virG* and defined as a plasmid gene needed for continuing reinfection of adjacent cells in culture.[38] It turns out that expression of IcsA occurs during bacterial division at the back pole of the organism (which is defined with respect to the direction of subsequent motion of the bacterial cell).[39] Expression of IcsA is associated with actin polymerization at the site, forming an actin tail just behind the organism. An actin-binding host protein, plastin, is present in the same location, and actin cross-linking causes a sphincter-like contraction and generation of a forward propulsive force. This is referred to as the actin "motor," which apparently uses energy derived from adenosine triphosphate by the adenosine triphosphatase activity of IcsA itself.[40] By this means, the organisms create and utilize an intracellular network of polymerized actin to spread throughout the cell interior to reach the plasma membrane,[41] where they utilize the propulsive force of the actin motor to protrude beyond the plane of the host cell and extend into the adjacent cell, still within the plasma membrane of the first host cell (Fig. 206–4). Addition of cytochalasins after initial invasion to block the polymerization of actin filaments also inhibits spread of the organism within the cell.[37] IcsA functions are regulated via phosphorylation mediated by cyclic nucleotide–dependent host cell protein kinases.[42] Because phosphorylation mutations lead to enhanced microbial spread, it is possible that the host cell modulates bacterial virulence through its own protein kinases.

Shigella organisms also move to the cell periphery along actin stress fibers, following the architecture of the cytoskeleton. This has been termed organelle-like movement (Olm).[43] Although Olm is distinct from IcsA-mediated propulsion, the former could act together with the latter in a complementary manner.[44] Once at the host cell surface, membrane-bounded organisms spread to the adjacent cell by fusion of the two host cell membranes, permitting the bacterium to enter the second cell within a vesicle to begin the process again. An important host target for this membrane fusion event appears to be a calcium-dependent adhesin, L-CAM.[45] When L-CAM is altered, bacteria containing protrusions fail to complete the intercellular microbial transfer process. A second gene within the *ics* operon, *icsB*, is required for this final stage of microbial spread.[41] If *icsB* is mutationally inactivated, the double host membrane–bounded vesicle cannot lyse and the organism cannot spread. Such mutants are also avirulent.

Both in vitro and in vivo, invasion and cell-to-cell spread of *Shigella* are accompanied by host cell death by an as yet unknown mechanism. Some evidence suggests that apoptosis is involved, at least when macrophages are used as targets for invasion by *Shigella flexneri*.[46] Ipa proteins may be required as well, because when these are mutationally inactivated in a strain engineered to still express low levels of a cloned *E. coli* hemolysin to allow lysis of the phagocytic vesicle, apoptosis is not observed.[47]

Just as there are several genes involved in invasion, there are also several levels of regulation of these genes (see Fig. 206–1). One such locus, termed *virF*, is located on the invasion plasmid and acts in trans as a positive inducer.[48] It codes for a 30-kDa protein that up-regulates production of Ipas and also of the *icsA* gene product. A second locus, termed *virR*, is located on the chromosome at 27 minutes between *trp* and *galU*.[49] It is a temperature-dependent repressor of the plasmid invasion genes, and it acts in trans at 30°C but not at 37°C. Another chromosomal gene, *kcpA*, located at 12 minutes near the *purE* gene, originally defined as a necessary locus for induction of keratoconjunctivitis in guinea pigs,[50] has been shown to positively regulate expression of *icsA*.[51]

TOXINS

S. dysenteriae type 1 was first shown in 1903 to produce a lethal toxin that became known as Shiga neurotoxin because

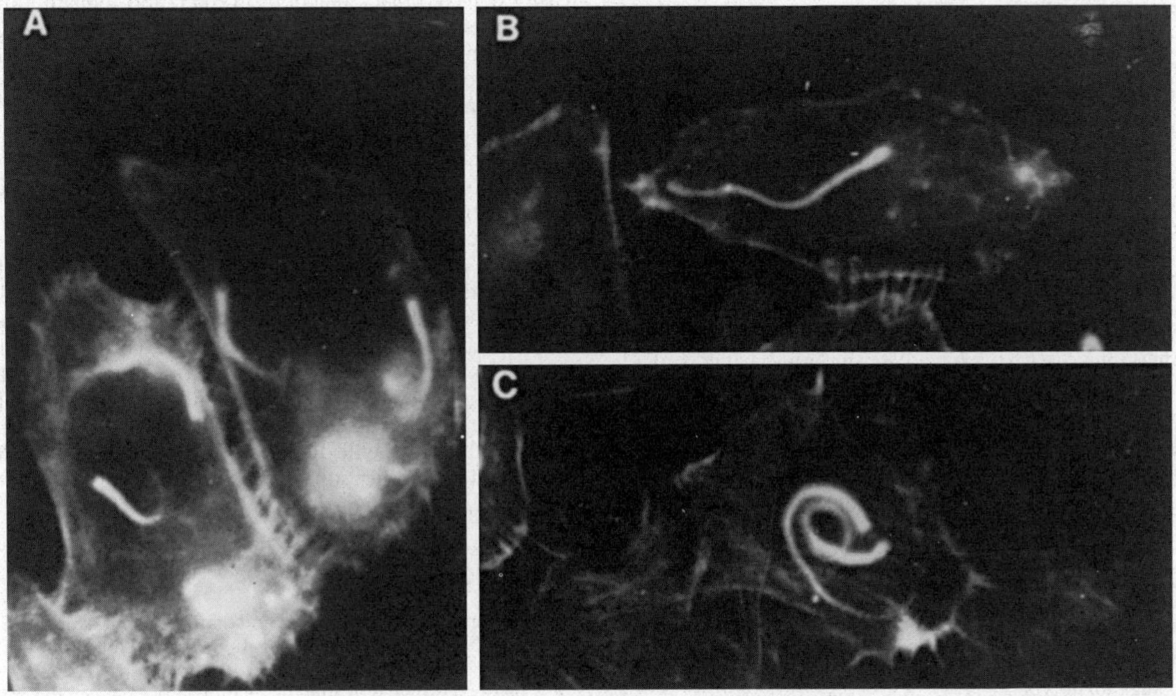

FIGURE 206–4 □ Intracellular spread of *S. flexneri* within HeLa cells is detected by the trail of polymerized F-actin it produces. *A* to *C* show three views of actin trails in an experimental tissue culture system. In this figure, F-actin is brightly stained with fluorescein-tagged NBD-phallacidin, a fungal product that reacts specifically with F-actin. (*A* to *C* from Sansonetti PJ: Genetic and molecular basis of epithelial cell invasion by *Shigella* spp. Rev Infect Dis 13[Suppl 4]:S285–S291, 1991.)

it resulted first in limb paralysis in animals.[52] Since then, this toxin has been found to cause fluid accumulation in rabbit gut and to be cytotoxic for cells in culture.[53, 54] Shiga toxin is the prototype of a family of enzymatically and structurally similar toxins, known as Shiga-like toxins, that are produced by other members of the genus and by certain *E. coli* serotypes.[4] On the basis of these common features, the toxin nomenclature has changed (Table 206–3). Although the *E. coli*–produced Shiga toxins, Stx-1 and Stx-2, are encoded by genes present in transforming phage, the Shiga toxin gene in Shigella, *stx,* is uniquely present on the chromosome of *S. dysenteriae* type 1, near the *pyrF* locus.[55]

The toxin is composed of two different peptide subunits, an enzymatically active 32-kDa A subunit and a complex of five identical 7.8-kDa B subunits responsible for binding to the host cell receptor,[56] a glycolipid containing a terminal disaccharide composed of galactose-linked $\alpha 1 \rightarrow 4$ to galactose.[57] The A subunit is an *N*-glycosidase identical in action to the plant toxin ricin, which cleaves a specific adenine base in the 28S ribosomal RNA of the 60S ribosomal subunit and permanently inactivates the ribosome in protein synthesis.[58] The active site of the A subunit has not been fully characterized; however, glutamic acid 167 appears to be a critical residue, and even a conservative change to aspartic acid reduces the A subunit enzymic activity by more than 1000-fold.[59] The x-ray crystallographic structure of the B subunit of *E. coli* Stx-1, which is identical to Shiga toxin itself, has been solved.[60] The three-dimensional view suggests that a conserved carbohydrate binding site is formed by β-sheet interactions between adjacent B monomers, which are arranged in a pentameric structure, producing five potential binding sites per holo-B subunit. Site-directed mutagenesis of aspartate residues at positions 16 and 17, which are within the potential binding cleft noted in the crystal structure,[60] alters the toxin's binding capability.[61]

The structural genes for the A and B subunits form an operon that is organized in tandem and translated in-frame, with the open reading frame for *stxA* 5′ to *stxB* and separated from one another by 12 nucleotides.[55] Shiga toxin production is regulated by iron concentration through the *fur* locus,[62] an iron-dependent negative regulator of a number of iron-regulated genes, including those controlling the synthesis of iron-binding siderophores and inner and outer membrane proteins involved in the uptake of the iron-siderophore complex. The *fur* gene also appears to control the *E. coli* Stx-1 gene but not the Stx-2 gene.[63] A binding site for the *fur* gene product has been found 5′ to *stxA* in *S. dysenteriae* type 1 and in a region of dyad symmetry within the *stx* promoter.[64] When iron is present in sufficient quantities, it complexes with the Fur protein, enabling Fur to bind to sites near or within the promoters of iron-regulated genes, which serves to down-regulate these genes at the transcriptional level.

Two new *Shigella* toxins have been reported, called ShET1 and ShET2 (for *Shigella* enterotoxin) because they increase net electrolyte transport by rabbit small bowel tissue in vitro and cause net fluid secretion in vivo in ligated rabbit ileal loops.[65,66] These toxins are much less active on a weight basis than is Shiga toxin, which causes the same physiologic response by intestinal tissue. Humans infected with *Shigella* develop neutralizing antibody to ShET1 and ShET2, indicating that they are produced in vivo. The former is encoded by a chromosomal gene, whereas the latter is controlled by an iron-regulated plasmid gene and is homologous with a previously described enteroinvasive *E. coli* enterotoxin.[67] Although the role of the ShET toxins in disease pathogenesis remains uncertain, the potential importance of ShET1 is limited by the observation that the gene is found predominantly in *S. flexneri* type 2 and not other *S. flexneri* serotypes or *Shigella* species.[68]

TABLE 206–3 ■ Nomenclature for Shiga Family Toxins

NEW NAME (OLD NAME)	NOMENCLATURE Gene	Gene Product
Shiga toxin (Shiga toxin)	*stx*	Stx
Shiga toxin type 1 (SLT-1, VT-1)	*stx1*	Stx-1
Shiga toxin type 2* (SLT-2, VT-2)	*stx2*	Stx-2

*Variant Stx-2 toxins, such as the toxin associated with porcine edema disease, are designated Stx-2e (formerly SLT-2e or VT-2e).

Diagnostic Microbiology

Diagnostic microbiology depends first on screening agar plates inoculated with stool samples for the presence of lactose-negative bacterial colonies. For this purpose, stool is streaked onto selective media such as MacConkey, Hektoen enteric, *Shigella-Salmonella,* or other agars that contain inhibitors of the growth of gram-positive organisms and a dye indicator to show acid production resulting from lactose fermentation. Lactose-negative colonies are then picked and streaked onto the slant of triple sugar iron agar or Kligler iron agar and stabbed into the butt to create anaerobic conditions. These media are designed to show several typical features of the genus, the failure of *Shigella* to ferment lactose aerobically on the slant and its ability to anaerobically utilize glucose in the butt, which results in a drop of pH and a local color change of the pH dye indicator from red to yellow. *Salmonella* species also produce a red slant and yellow butt but can be distinguished from *Shigella* because the organisms characteristically produce hydrogen sulfide, which forms an easily detected black reaction product, and their motility can often be seen on the slant. In the clinical laboratory, rapid presumptive identification can be made by agglutination of suspect colonies in group-specific antisera, which are available commercially. Further tests can be performed to distinguish the presumptive *Shigella* from other organisms, but this is rarely necessary in the clinical laboratory.

Modern molecular and immunologic diagnosis is also possible with the use of gene probes and polymerase chain reaction primers to identify virulence genes of *Shigella* or virulence gene products such as Ipa proteins or Shiga toxin. Some of these assays can be carried out directly on clinical samples such as stool or may serve a useful purpose after the initial isolation of organisms by more conventional bacteriologic methods. However, except for experimental studies of pathogenesis and molecular epidemiology, DNA-based tests and immunoassays are not in clinical use and it is unlikely that they will displace the time-honored traditional culture and identification methods in the near future.

References

1. Brenner DJ: Characterization and clinical identification of Enterobacteriaceae by DNA-hybridization. Progr Clin Pathol 7:71–117, 1978.
2. Cheasty T, Rowe B: Antigenic relationships between the enteroinvasive *Escherichia coli* O-antigen O28ac, O112ac, O124, O136, O143, O144, O152, and O164 and *Shigella* O-antigens. J Clin Microbiol 17:681–684, 1983.
3. Sansonetti PJ, d'Hauteville H, Ecobichon C, Pourcel C: Molecular

expression of virulence plasmids in *Shigella* and enteroinvasive *E. coli.* Ann Microbiol (Paris) 134A:295–318, 1983.

4. Acheson DWK, Donohue-Rolfe A, Keusch GT: The family of Shiga and Shiga-like toxins. *In* Alouf JE, Freer JH (eds): Sourcebook of Bacterial Protein Toxins. London, Academic Press, 1991, pp 415–433.
5. Shiga K: Ueber den Dysenterie-bacillus *(Bacillus dysenteriae).* Zentralbl Bakteriol Orig 24:913–918, 1898.
6. Keusch GT: *Shigella* infections. Clin Gastroenterol 8:645–662, 1979.
7. Keusch GT, Bennish ML: Shigellosis. *In* Evans AE, Brachman P (eds): Bacterial Infections of Humans, ed 3. New York, Plenum Publishing (in press).
8. Ewing WH, Lindberg AA: Serology of *Shigella. In* Bergan T (ed): Methods in Microbiology, Vol 14. London, Academic Press, 1984, pp 113–142.
9. Galanos C, Luderitz O, Rietschel ET, Westphal O: Newer aspects on the chemistry and biology of bacterial lipopolysaccharides with special reference to the lipid A component. *In* Goodwin KW (ed): International Review of Biochemistry, Vol 2, Biochemistry of Lipids. Baltimore, University Park Press, 1977, pp 239–335.
10. Hase S, Rietschel ET: Isolation and analysis of the lipid A backbone. Lipid A structure of lipopolysaccharides from various bacterial groups. Eur J Biochem 63:101–107, 1976.
11. Sandlin RC, Lampel KA, Keasler SP, et al: Avirulence of rough mutants of *Shigella flexneri:* Requirement of O antigen for correct unipolar localization of IcsA in the bacterial outer membrane. Infect Immun 63:229–237, 1995.
12. Okada N, Sasakawa C, Tobe T, et al: Virulence-associated chromosomal loci of *Shigella flexneri* identified by random Tn5 insertion mutagenesis. Mol Microbiol 5:187–195, 1991.
13. Struelens MJ, Mondal G, Roberts M, Williams PH: Role of bacterial and host factors in the pathogenesis of *Shigella* septicemia. Eur J Clin Microbiol Infect Dis 9:337–344, 1990.
14. Struelens MJ, Patte D, Kabir I, et al: *Shigella* septicemia: Prevalence, presentation, risk factors and outcome. J Infect Dis 152:784–790, 1985.
15. Koster F, Levin J, Walker L, et al: Hemolytic-uremic syndrome after shigellosis: Relation to endotoxin and circulating immune complexes. N Engl J Med 298:927–933, 1978.
16. LaBrec EH, Schneider H, Magnani TJ, Formal SB: Epithelial cell penetration is an essential step in the pathogenesis of bacillary dysentery. J Bacteriol 88:1503–1518, 1964.
17. Formal SB, Hale TL, Sansonetti PJ: Invasive enteric pathogens. Rev Infect Dis 5:S702–S707, 1983.
18. Formal SB, LaBrec EH, Kent TH, Falkow S: Abortive intestinal infection with an *Escherichia coli–Shigella flexneri* hybrid strain. J Bacteriol 89:1374–1382, 1965.
19. Griffiths E, Stevenson P, Hale TL, Formal SB: Synthesis of aerobactin and a 76,000 dalton iron-regulated outer membrane protein by *Escherichia coli* K-12–*Shigella flexneri* hybrids and by enteroinvasive strains of *Escherichia coli.* Infect Immun 49:67–71, 1985.
20. Nassif X, Mazert M-C, Mounier J, Sansonetti P: Evaluation with an iuc::Tn10 mutant of the role of aerobactin production in the virulence of *Shigella flexneri.* Infect Immun 55:1963–1969, 1987.
21. Kopecko DJ, Washington O, Formal SB: Genetic and physical evidence for plasmid control of *Shigella sonnei* form I cell surface antigen. Infect Immun 29:207–214, 1980.
22. Sansonetti PJ, Kopecko DJ, Formal SB: *Shigella sonnei* plasmids: Evidence that a large plasmid is necessary for virulence. Infect Immun 34:75–83, 1981.
23. Sansonetti PJ, Kopecko DJ, Formal SB: Involvement of a plasmid in the invasive ability of *Shigella flexneri.* Infect Immun 35:852–860, 1982.
24. Baudry B, Maurelli AT, Clerc P, et al: Localization of plasmid loci necessary for the entry of *Shigella flexneri* into HeLa cells, and characterization of one locus encoding four immunogenic polypeptides. J Gen Microbiol 133:3409–3413, 1987.
25. Hale TL, Oaks EV, Formal SB: Identification and antigenic characterization of virulence-associated, plasmid-coded proteins of *Shigella* spp. and enteroinvasive *Escherichia coli.* Infect Immun 50:620–629, 1985.
26. Andrews GP, Hromockyj AE, Coker C, Maurelli AT: Two novel virulence loci, *mxiA* and *mxiB,* in *Shigella flexneri* 2a facilitate excretion of invasion plasmid antigens. Infect Immun 59:1997–2005, 1991.
27. Venkatesan MM, Buysse JM, Oaks EV: Surface presentation of *Shigella flexneri* invasion plasmid antigens requires the products of the *spa* locus. J Bacteriol 174:1990–2001, 1992.
28. Menard R, Sansonetti P, Parsot C: The secretion of the *Shigella flexneri* Ipa invasins is activated by epithelial cells and controlled by IpaB and IpaD. EMBO J 13:5293–5302, 1994.
29. Goldberg MB, Sansonetti PJ: *Shigella* subversion of the cellular cytoskeleton: A strategy for epithelial colonization. Infect Immun 61:4941–4946, 1993.
30. Clerc P, Sansonetti PJ: Entry of *Shigella flexneri* into HeLa cells: Evidence for directed phagocytosis involving actin polymerization and myosin accumulation. Infect Immun 55:2681–2688, 1987.
31. Hale TL, Bonventre PF: *Shigella* infection of Henle intestinal epithelial cells: Role of the bacteria. Infect Immun 24:879–886, 1979.
32. Hale TL, Morris RE, Bonventre PF: *Shigella* infection of Henle intestinal epithelial cells: Role of the host cell. Infect Immun 24:887–894, 1979.
33. Sansonetti PJ, Ryter A, Clerc P, et al: Multiplication of *Shigella flexneri* within HeLa cells: Lysis of the phagocytic vacuole and plasmid mediated contact hemolysis. Infect Immun 55:521–527, 1986.
34. Menard R, Sansonetti PJ, Parsot C: Nonpolar mutagenesis of the ipa genes defines IpaB, IpaC, and IpaD as effectors of *Shigella flexneri* entry into epithelial cells. J Bacteriol 175:5899–5906, 1993.
35. Sansonetti PJ, Arondel J, Fontaine A, et al: OmpB (osmo-regulation) and *icsA* mutants of *Shigella flexneri:* Vaccine candidates and probes to study the pathogenesis of shigellosis. Vaccine 9:416–422, 1991.
36. Bernardini ML, Sanna MG, Fontaine A, Sansonetti PJ. OmpC is involved in invasion of epithelial cells by *Shigella flexneri.* Infect Immun 61:3625–3635, 1993.
37. Bernardini ML, Mounier J, d'Hauteville H, et al: Identification of icsA, a plasmid locus of *Shigella flexneri* that governs bacterial intra- and intercellular spread through interactions with F-actin. Proc Natl Acad Sci USA 86:3867–3871, 1989.
38. Makino S, Sasakawa C, Kamata K, et al: A genetic determinant required for continuous reinfection of adjacent cells on a large plasmid in *Shigella flexneri* 2a. Cell 46:551–555, 1986.
39. Goldberg MB, Theriot JA, Sansonetti PJ: Regulation of surface presentation of IcsA, a *Shigella* protein essential to intracellular movement and spread, is growth phase dependent. Infect Immun 62:5664–5668, 1994.
40. Goldberg MB, Barzu O, Parsot C, Sansonetti PJ: Unipolar localization and ATPase activity of IcsA, a *Shigella flexneri* protein involved in intracellular movement. J Bacteriol 175:2189–2196, 1993.
41. Allaoui A, Mounier J, Prevost MC, et al: *icsB:* A *Shigella flexneri* virulence gene necessary for the lysis of protrusions during intercellular spread. Mol Microbiol 6:1605–1616, 1992.
42. d'Hauteville H, Sansonetti PJ: Phosphorylation of IcsA by cAMP-dependent protein kinase and its effect on intercellular spread of *Shigella flexneri.* Mol Microbiol 6:833–841, 1992.
43. Vasselon T, Mounier J, Prevost MC, et al: A stress fiber-based movement of *Shigella flexneri* within cells. Infect Immun 59:1723–1732, 1991.
44. Vasselon T, Mounier J, Hellio R, Sansonetti PJ: Movement along actin filaments of the perijunctional area and de novo polymerization of cellular actin are required for *Shigella flexneri* colonization of epithelial Caco-2 cell monolayers. Infect Immun 60:1031–1040, 1992.
45. Sansonetti PJ, Mounier J, Prevost MC, Mege R-M: Cadherin expression required for formation and internalization of *Shigella flexneri*–induced intercellular protrusions involved in spread between epithelial cells. Cell 76:829–839, 1994.
46. Zychlinsky A, Prevost MC, Sansonetti PJ: *Shigella flexneri* induces apoptosis in infected macrophages. Nature 358:167–169, 1992.
47. Zychlinsky A, Kenny B, Menard R, et al: IpaB mediates macrophage apoptosis induced by *Shigella flexneri.* Mol Microbiol 11:619–627, 1994.
48. Sakai T, Sasakawa C, Makino S, Yoshikawa M: DNA sequence and product analysis of the *virF* locus responsible for Congo red binding and cell invasion in *Shigella flexneri* 2a. Infect Immun 54:395–402, 1986.
49. Maurelli AT, Sansonetti PJ: Identification of a chromosomal gene controlling temperature regulated expression of *Shigella* virulence. Proc Natl Acad Sci USA 85:2820–2824, 1988.

50. Formal SB, Gemski P Jr, Baron LS, LaBrec EH: A chromosomal locus which controls the ability of *Shigella flexneri* to evoke keratoconjunctivitis. Infect Immun 3:73–79, 1971.
51. Pal TL, Newland JW, Tall BD, et al: Intracellular spread of *Shigella flexneri* associated with the kcpA locus and a 140-kilodalton protein. Infect Immun 57:477–486, 1989.
52. Conradi H: Ueber lösliche durch aseptische Autolyse erhalten Giftstoffe von Ruhr und Typhusbazillen. Dtsch Med Wochenschr 29:26–28, 1903.
53. Keusch GT, Grady GF, Mata LJ, McIver JM: The pathogenesis of *Shigella* diarrhea. 1. Enterotoxin production by *Shigella dysenteriae* 1. J Clin Invest 51:1212–1218, 1972.
54. Vicari G, Olitzki AL, Olitzki Z: The action of the thermolabile toxin of *Shigella dysenteriae* on cells cultivated in vitro. Br J Exp Pathol 41:179–189, 1960.
55. Strockbine NA, Jackson MP, Sung LM, et al: Cloning and sequencing of the genes for Shiga toxin from *Shigella dysenteriae* type 1. J Bacteriol 170:1116–1122, 1988.
56. Donohue-Rolfe A, Jacewicz M, Keusch GT: Isolation and characterization of functional Shiga toxin subunits and renatured holotoxin. Mol Microbiol 3:1231–1236, 1989.
57. Jacewicz M, Clausen H, Nudelman E, et al: Pathogenesis of shigella diarrhea. XI. Isolation of a shigella toxin–binding glycolipid from rabbit jejunum and HeLa cells and its identification as globotriaosylceramide. J Exp Med 163:1391–1404, 1986.
58. Endo Y, Tsurugi K, Yutsudo T, et al: Site of action of a Vero toxin (VT2) from *Escherichia coli* O157:H7 and of Shiga toxin on eukaryotic ribosomes. Eur J Biochem 171:45–50, 1988.
59. Hovde CJ, Calderwood SB, Mekalanos JJ, Collier RJ: Evidence that glutamic acid 167 is an active-site residue of Shiga-like toxin I. Proc Natl Acad Sci USA 85:2568–2572, 1988.
60. Stein PE, Boodhoo A, Tyrrell GJ, et al: Crystal structure of the cell-binding B oligomer of verotoxin-1 from *E. coli.* Nature 355:748–750, 1992.
61. Jackson MP, Wadolkowski EA, Weinstein DL, et al: Functional analysis of the Shiga toxin and Shiga-like toxin type II variant binding subunits by using site-directed mutagenesis. J Bacteriol 172:653–658, 1990.
62. Calderwood SB, Mekalanos JJ: Iron regulation of Shiga-like toxin expression is *Escherichia coli* is mediated by the *fur* locus. J Bacteriol 169:4759–4764, 1987.
63. Weinstein DL, Jackson MP, Samuel JE, et al: Cloning and sequencing of a Shiga-like toxin type II variant from an *Escherichia coli* strain responsible for edema disease of swine. J Bacteriol 170:4223–4230, 1988.
64. de Lorenzo V, Wee S, Herrero M, Neilands JB: Operator sequences of the aerobactin operon of plasmid ColV-K30 binding site of the ferric uptake regulation *(fur)* repressor. J Bacteriol 169:2624–2630, 1987.
65. Fasano A, Noriega FR, Maneval DR Jr, et al: *Shigella* enterotoxin 1: An enterotoxin of *Shigella flexneri* 2a active in rabbit small intestine in vivo and in vitro. J Clin Invest 95:2853–2861, 1995.
66. Nataro JP, Seriwatana J, Fasano A, et al: Cloning a sequencing of a new plasmid-encoded enterotoxin in enteroinvasive *E. coli* and *Shigella. In* Program and Abstracts of the 29th Joint Conference on Cholera and Related Diseases. Bethesda, MD, National Institutes of Health, 1993, pp 144–147.
67. Fasano A, Kay BA, Russell RG, et al: Enterotoxin and cytotoxin production by enteroinvasive *Escherichia coli.* Infect Immun 58:3717–3723, 1990.
68. Noriega FR, Liao FM, Formal SB, et al: Prevalence of *Shigella* enterotoxin 1 (ShET1) among *Shigella* clinical isolates of diverse serotypes. J Infect Dis 172:1408–1411, 1995.

207

Campylobacter

Ban Mishu Allos

Campylobacter species are relatively recently recognized human pathogens that cause more diarrhea than almost all other bacteria. In addition, *Campylobacter jejuni* and *Campylobacter coli* are the most common causes of food-borne bacterial illness. Although *Campylobacter* species were first identified in stools in 1957, the wide scope and importance of the organisms as a cause of diarrhea were not appreciated until the 1980s. *C. jejuni* and *C. coli* are closely related species; *C. jejuni,* however, is predominant and the name is commonly used to refer to both organisms.[1] In this chapter, *C. jejuni* refers to both species unless otherwise indicated. Other *Campylobacter* species are discussed in Chapter 76.

Microbiology and Isolation

Campylobacter organisms are slender, curved, or spiral gram-negative rods; they are motile via a single polar flagellum at one or both ends.[2] *Campylobacter* species are microaerophilic, requiring 3% to 15% oxygen for growth. *C. jejuni* grows best at 42°C, unlike other *Campylobacter* species, which grow best at 37°C. *C. jejuni* grows slowly; up to 2 weeks may be required for primary isolation from blood.[3] The organism may be isolated from stools within 72 hours.[1] If more than 2 hours is anticipated before arrival of the specimen at the laboratory, a transport medium such as Cary-Blair should be used.[4] Because most *C. jejuni* strains are resistant to cephalothin, they may be isolated from stools by using a medium that contains cephalothin or another antibiotic to which the organism is resistant. These *Campylobacter*-selective media inhibit the growth of more rapidly growing components of the enteric flora. However, some *Campylobacter* species are susceptible to cephalothin; culture techniques using antibiotic-free media are needed to isolate these organisms (see Chapter 76).

When *Campylobacter*-selective media are used, colonies that appear after 24 to 48 hours and that are gray, mucoid, or wet appearing should be suspected of being *Campylobacter.* The organism may be identified using standard biochemical tests.[5] A rapid presumptive identification can be made by the following characteristics: (1) typical colonial morphology, (2) Gram stain showing gram-negative curved rods, (3) oxidase and catalase positivity, and (4) motility.

The two most widely used serotyping systems for *C. jejuni* and *C. coli* are the Penner system, which identifies heat-stable (somatic, O) antigens, and the Lior system, which measures heat-labile (flagellar, H) antigens.[6] There are more than 90 reference serotypes defined by the Penner system and 112 by the Lior system. Both systems identify more than 90% of *Campylobacter* species isolated from human and nonhuman sources.[7, 8] The Lior system is quicker and easier to use and consequently more applicable for outside reference laboratories.[9]

Epidemiology

Incidence and Seasonality

Campylobacter infections occur everywhere in the world. Isolations have been made in tropical, temperate, and arctic climates.[10] The incidence of *C. jejuni* infections in the United States peaks in the late summer and early fall.[11] Infants have the highest rate of infections, but a second surge occurs in young adulthood. Not surprisingly, *C. jejuni* infections are the most common cause of diarrheal disease at U.S. universities.[12, 13] In developing countries too, the highest isolation rate occurs in young children; however, no second peak occurs in the early adult years.[10] Isolation rates for *C. jejuni* in males are higher than in females from infancy through age 40 years; no explanation for this phenomenon is available.

The incidence of *Campylobacter* infections in developed countries is difficult to estimate. Many hospital microbiology laboratories do not routinely culture diarrheal stools for *Campylobacter* as they might for *Salmonella* or *Shigella*. Furthermore, many patients with *Campylobacter* infection may experience illness so mild they might not seek medical attention and, therefore, their infections would remain undiagnosed. Nevertheless, the Centers for Disease Control and Prevention, using the best data available, estimates that the annual incidence of *Campylobacter* infections is 1000 per 100,000 population.[14] Similarly, in England, studies at the level of community-based physicians show that the true annual incidence is 1100 per 100,000 population.[15]

In developing countries, *Campylobacter* species are ubiquitous in the environment and infection is hyperendemic among young children. Breast-fed children have a lower risk of infection, but once weaned, a high proportion develop symptomatic infection. *Campylobacter* infection is an important cause of morbidity from watery diarrhea in this age group. In adults and in children older than 3 years, infections are usually asymptomatic,[16, 17] suggesting that acquired immunity is protective.

Sources and Mechanisms of Infection

The principal route of infection with *C. jejuni* in developed countries is through preparation and consumption of chicken. Indeed, case-control studies of sporadic cases of *C. jejuni* infection show that more than 70% of cases are associated with eating chicken.[18, 19] Other foods of animal origin (e.g., beef, pork) may occasionally be related to *C. jejuni* infection.[20] In contrast to sporadic cases, outbreaks of *C. jejuni* infection are associated most commonly not with eating chicken but with drinking raw milk.[11] From 1981 to 1990, 20 raw milk–associated outbreaks of *C. jejuni* occurred in the United States, involving 458 teenagers and children.[21] In the United Kingdom, pasteurized, bottled milk may be a source of *Campylobacter* infections because of contamination of the milk by birds pecking the bottle tops.[22, 23]

Water-borne outbreaks of *C. jejuni* infection have been reported in the United States, Europe, and Israel.[24–26] Contamination of drinking water with feces from birds or animals is usually the cause. In Colorado, ingestion of untreated water from rivers or streams is an important cause of *C. jejuni* infections.[27] Indeed, in the Rocky Mountain states, diarrhea occurring after drinking untreated surface water is more often caused by *C. jejuni* than by *Giardia*.[28]

C. jejuni infections have been associated with foreign travel and with exposure to dogs and cats.[19, 29] Person-to-person transmission of *C. jejuni* infection has been reported[30, 31] but rarely occurs. Unlike *Shigella, Giardia,* or hepatitis A virus infections, there have been no outbreaks of *C. jejuni* infection reported in daycare centers or institutions for the mentally retarded. Likewise, transmission via infected food handlers or health care workers has not been described.

Clinical Features

The consequences of *C. jejuni* infection range from complete absence of symptoms to fulminant sepsis and death (Table 207–1). The proportion of asymptomatic infected persons depends on the population studied but can be greater than 50%.[32, 33] Alternatively, a high proportion of infected persons may become severely ill and require hospitalization.[34, 35] The case-fatality rate for *Campylobacter* infections is 0.05 per 1000 infections.[36]

Signs and Symptoms of Gastrointestinal Illness

The typical infection with *C. jejuni* is characterized by an acute diarrheal illness, which is indistinguishable from gastroenteritis caused by *Salmonella, Shigella,* or other enteric bacterial pathogens. Usually, the illness has an abrupt onset with abdominal cramps and diarrhea. Some patients, however, have an influenza-like prodrome consisting of fever, headache, myalgias, and dizziness. Nevertheless, the most common symptom experienced by most patients with *C. jejuni* infection is diarrhea. The diarrhea may be severe, and many patients have at least 1 day with 8 or more stools; 20% report more than 15 stools on at least 1 day.[37] Almost half describe grossly bloody diarrhea. Occasionally, the diarrhea is minimal or absent and the abdominal pain (which can be quite intense) may be mistakenly attributed to appendicitis. Exploratory laparotomy and appendectomy are not unusual in *C. jejuni*–infected persons whose infections have not yet been diagnosed.[35, 38–40] Although nausea is frequently reported, vomiting is uncommon. Subjective fever is reported by more than 90% of infected persons. Resolution of symptoms in most patients occurs within 1 week; however, 20% experience more prolonged or relapsing illness lasting several weeks.[35, 41] Rarely, *C. jejuni* infection may cause mild, chronic diarrhea lasting many months.[42–44]

The signs and laboratory findings associated with *C. jejuni* infection are also not distinguishable from those produced by other enteric bacterial pathogens. Almost two thirds of persons with documented infection have a temperature higher than 37.5°C.[45] However, temperatures higher than 40°C are unusual. Fecal leukocytes are found in 75% of cases; gross or occult blood is seen in 50%. Sigmoidoscopic examination reveals diffuse colonic inflammation; *Campylobacter* enteritis may be confused with early inflammatory bowel disease. Although the peripheral white cell count may be mildly elevated, other laboratory findings, including liver function tests, serum electrolyte values, and hematocrit, are normal.

Local and Systemic Complications

Gastrointestinal complications of *C. jejuni* infection are relatively rare and are the result of local invasion. Massive gas-

TABLE 207–1 ■ Consequences of Infection by *Campylobacter jejuni*

Asymptomatic	Systemic complications
Gastrointestinal symptoms	Bacteremia
Diarrhea	Meningitis
Fever	Purulent arthritis
Abdominal cramps	Osteomyelitis
Nausea	Neonatal sepsis
Vomiting	Death
Malaise	Postinfectious complications
Myalgias	Guillain-Barré syndrome
Local complications	Reactive arthritis
Cholecystitis	Uveitis
Pancreatitis	Encephalopathy
Peritonitis	Hemolytic-uremic syndrome
Gastrointestinal hemorrhage	Hemolytic anemia
Pseudoappendicitis	Carditis
Toxic megacolon	

trointestinal hemorrhage may occur. Infection of the biliary tract may lead to cholecystitis, pancreatitis, or obstructive hepatitis.[40, 46, 47] Eleven (6%) of 188 patients hospitalized with *C. jejuni* enteritis developed pancreatitis—a far higher rate than that seen with *Salmonella* or *Shigella* infections.[40] In patients undergoing peritoneal dialysis, *C. jejuni* infection may cause peritonitis.[48] Spontaneous bacterial peritonitis due to *C. jejuni* infection may occur in patients with cirrhosis. *C. jejuni* infection has been reported to cause splenic rupture.[49] *Campylobacter* infection may exacerbate inflammatory colitis, but there are no data to suggest that it causes the disease. Infections in pregnant women are likely to be mild and self-limited; however, neonatal sepsis and death can occur if the woman is infected during her third trimester.[50]

Extraintestinal complications of *C. jejuni* infection such as bacteremia, meningitis, and purulent arthritis are usually the result of systemic spread. *C. jejuni* bacteremia occurs in approximately 1.5 per 1000 intestinal infections.[51] The rate is higher in elderly individuals and in immunodeficient persons.[52] It is possible that transient bacteremia occurs in many cases of *C. jejuni* enteritis but is not detected because blood cultures are not routinely done in healthy patients with uncomplicated diarrheal illness. Clinically significant bacteremia is infrequent because most *C. jejuni* strains are susceptible to killing by normal human serum. In contrast, *Campylobacter fetus* is intrinsically serum resistant, and *C. fetus* infection is less likely to be contained within the gastrointestinal tract. Although a far higher proportion of *C. fetus* infections are bacteremias, *C. jejuni* still accounts for most (89%) *Campylobacter* isolates from blood.[51] One minor extraintestinal manifestation of infection is urticaria.[53, 54] *C. jejuni* has occasionally been isolated from the urinary tract in women.

Postinfectious Complications

The most important postinfectious complication of *C. jejuni* infection is Guillain-Barré syndrome (GBS). GBS is an infrequent complication of *C. jejuni* infection; approximately 1 in 2000 to 5000 infections is followed by GBS. However, because these infections are common, they account for 30% of cases of GBS occurring in the United States each year.[55] Furthermore, GBS occurring after *C. jejuni* infection may be more severe, with a greater likelihood of irreversible neurologic damage. The likelihood of developing GBS after *C. jejuni* infection does not appear to be related to the severity of gastroenteritis. Indeed, GBS may follow asymptomatic infections. GBS is more likely to occur after infection with *C. jejuni* Penner serotype O:19.

The pathogenic mechanism of *C. jejuni*–associated GBS is not known precisely. However, because neurologic symptoms usually begin 1 to 3 weeks after onset of diarrhea,[56, 57] a humoral immunopathogenic mechanism is likely. Studies suggest possible antibody cross-reactivity between structures on the cell surface of *Campylobacter* and peripheral nerve glycolipids or myelin proteins.[58]

Another postinfectious complication of *C. jejuni* infection, reactive arthritis, is most likely in persons who carry the human leukocyte antigen B27 phenotype. Like GBS, it may follow symptomatic or asymptomatic *C. jejuni* infection.[59, 60] Reactive arthritis also occurs after *Salmonella, Shigella,* and *Yersinia* infections. The rate of this postinfectious complication of *C. jejuni* infection is not known but is likely low. In Scandinavia, 1% to 2% of patients with *Campylobacter* enteritis develop arthritis 4 days to 4 weeks after the onset of diarrhea.[61] Interestingly, in another Scandinavian study, 32 patients in a hospital for rheumatic diseases developed culture-confirmed *C. jejuni* infection during a hospital outbreak; none of these patients had exacerbations of their existing conditions.[62]

Uveitis without arthritis has been reported in two patients with *Campylobacter* enteritis[63, 64]; erythema nodosum has been reported in five.[65–69] Nine reports of hemolytic-uremic syndrome developing during the course of *C. jejuni* enteritis have been reported[70–77]; however, the presence of *Escherichia coli* O157:H7 was not excluded in these patients. Other reported but rare postinfectious complications of *C. jejuni* infection include nephritis, carditis, hemolytic anemia, and encephalopathy.

Campylobacter jejuni *Infections in Immunodeficient Persons*

Among persons with acquired immunodeficiency syndrome, *C. jejuni* infections are detected almost 40 times as frequently as in the general population.[78] This excess of infections affects patients with the lowest $CD4^+$ cell counts; patients with early human immunodeficiency virus infection are not especially likely to develop *C. jejuni* infections.[79] *C. jejuni* infections in patients with acquired immunodeficiency syndrome are generally more persistent and more severe than in immunocompetent persons.[79–84] Hypogammaglobulinemic patients develop severe persistent and relapsing infections caused by *C. jejuni*.[85, 86] Asplenic patients or others who lack opsonizing activity are predisposed to extraintestinal spread of infection, including meningitis, osteomyelitis, and cellulitis.[87–89] Immunodeficient persons with even mild *C. jejuni* infections should receive prompt antibiotic treatment.

Pathogenesis and Immunity

Despite the ubiquity of *C. jejuni* and the frequency of both symptomatic and asymptomatic infections, the pathogenesis of *C. jejuni* enteritis remains poorly understood. The organism's motility, conferred by its flagella, enables it to directly invade and proliferate within the intestinal epithelium. The virulence of individual strains may depend on the activity of their flagella,[90, 91] as well as their ability to adhere to intestinal cells.[92, 93]

The incubation period depends on the number of organisms ingested but can range from 1 day to 1 week.[94] The attack rate is also dose dependent; infection may be induced with as few as 500 organisms.[94, 95] Serum and mucosal serum responses are elicited in both natural and experimental infections.[96] Serum immunoglobulin A, G, and M responses peak within 2 to 4 weeks, then decline rapidly.[97, 98] The increased frequency and severity of *C. jejuni* infections in human immunodeficiency virus–infected persons suggest that cellular immunity also plays a protective role.

Enterotoxins are unlikely to play a role in the pathogenesis of *C. jejuni* infections. Toxins were once thought to play an important role because some isolates were reported to be enterotoxigenic[99, 100] and because infection frequently produces watery diarrhea. It appears clear now that enterotoxins are not involved in *C. jejuni* pathogenesis. First, enterotoxin production by *C. jejuni* cannot be demonstrated in vivo. Second, infected patients do not form antibodies against toxin.[101] Finally, the clinical picture of *C. jejuni* enteritis (fever, bloody stools, fecal leukocytes) is not consistent with illness produced by enterotoxins.

Infection with *C. jejuni* produces an acute inflammatory enteritis affecting the small intestine and the colon. Acute exudative and hemorrhagic inflammation may be seen; the appendix, mesenteric lymph nodes, and gallbladder may also be affected.[39, 102] Histopathologically, epithelial cell injury, edema, and infiltration of the lamina propria by mononuclear cells and neutrophils may be seen; eosinophils may also be present.[103] In general, the findings of *C. jejuni* enteritis are

TABLE 207–2 ■ Groups of Patients in Whom Diagnosis of *Campylobacter* Infection Should Be Considered

Nonhospitalized persons with acute onset of fever and diarrhea
Persons with symptoms of appendicitis
Persons having a work-up for inflammatory bowel disease
Immunocompromised patients with chronic diarrhea
Travelers to developing countries who develop diarrhea

nonspecific; there are no pathognomonic features.[104] A trained pathologist will recognize that *C. jejuni* enteritis may produce crypt abscesses (which can look like ulcerative colitis) and granulomata (which can look like Crohn disease).[103–105]

Diagnosis

Because the signs, symptoms, and laboratory findings associated with *C. jejuni* infection are not distinct from those of other bacterial enteric pathogens, diagnosis depends on isolation of the organism from stool or another infected site (Table 207–2). Cultures for *Campylobacter* are indicated in nonhospitalized patients with acute onset of fever and diarrhea. The suspicion of *C. jejuni* gastroenteritis is even higher if the stools contain blood or fecal leukocytes. Stool cultures should not be routinely ordered for patients who develop fever and diarrhea after being hospitalized longer than 3 days. However, hospitalized patients with appendicitis should have cultures done for *C. jejuni,* as infection may mimic appendicitis. Identification of *C. jejuni* in stools could eliminate the need for surgery, although culture results may not be available in time to prevent many laparotomies. Persons suspected of having inflammatory bowel disease should have cultures for *C. jejuni* and other *Campylobacter* species and related organisms as part of their diagnostic work-up. Other persons who are at high risk for *C. jejuni* infection include travelers to developing countries and persons with possible occupational or recreational exposure to *Campylobacter* in whom an acute diarrheal illness develops. Immunocompromised persons should have stool cultures for *Campylobacter* even if their diarrhea is chronic.

Treatment

The most important intervention in treatment of patients with acute gastroenteritis caused by *C. jejuni* or any other organism is maintenance of proper hydration and electrolyte balance. In almost all cases, this can be accomplished by encouraging proper oral intake of liquids; occasionally, intravenous fluids are required, especially in the very young and very old.

C. jejuni is susceptible to a number of antimicrobial agents; however, not all infected patients require such treatment. Many infections result in mild illness, and only rest and rehydration are required. Some studies show shortened duration of symptoms and *Campylobacter* excretion in patients who receive antibiotics at the onset of their illness.[106, 107] However, most healthy persons do not seek medical care until they have been ill a few days and therefore would not benefit from antibiotics. Patients in whom antimicrobial therapy is indicated include those with persistent or severe illness, temperature greater than 38.5°C, or bloody diarrhea. Because immunocompromised persons, elderly persons, and pregnant women may have more dire consequences of infection, these patients should also receive prompt antibiotic therapy.

Most *C. jejuni* organisms are still susceptible to erythromycin. Because this drug is safe, inexpensive, and easy to administer and has less of an inhibitory effect on fecal flora than do other antibiotics, it remains the treatment of choice for *C. jejuni* infections (Table 207–3). The newer macrolides (azithromycin, clarithromycin) are also effective in the treatment of *C. jejuni* infections; however, they are more expensive and have no proven advantage over erythromycin. At one time, it appeared that fluoroquinolones such as ofloxacin and ciprofloxacin were becoming the best agents to use in the treatment of acute diarrheal illness caused by *C. jejuni* and other bacterial enteric pathogens. However, the emerging resistance of organisms to these agents has diminished their usefulness.[106–109] Nevertheless, fluroquinolones have retained the advantage of being effective against a wide range of enteric pathogens. Because *Campylobacter* infections are clinically indistinguishable from infections caused by other enteric bacteria, fluoroquinolones may yet be the best choice when a bacterial gastroenteritis is suspected but no organisms have yet been isolated.

C. jejuni strains are almost universally resistant to cephalosporins, vancomycin, and rifampin; 25% are resistant to tetracycline. Susceptibility to ampicillin and trimethoprim-sulfa-

TABLE 207–3 ■ Oral Antimicrobial Agents Effective in Treatment of *Campylobacter* Infections

	DOSES*	
AGENT	**Adults**	**Children**
Macrolides		
Erythromycin stearate†	500 mg PO bid × 5 d	10–15 mg/kg PO tid × 5 d
Azithromycin	500 mg PO on day 1; 250 mg/d on days 2–5	Not recommended for children <16 y
Clarithromycin	250 mg PO q 12 h × 5 d	Safe doses not established
Quinolones		
Ciprofloxacin	500 mg PO bid × 5 d	Safe doses not established
Ofloxacin	200–400 mg PO q 12 h × 5 d	Safe doses not established
Nitrofurans		
Furazolidone	100 mg PO qid × 5 d	1.25 mg/kg PO qid × 5 d
Alternatives		
Clindamycin	150–300 mg PO q 6 h × 5 d	2–4 mg/kg q 6 h × 5 d
Tetracycline	250–500 mg PO qid	6–12 mg/kg PO qid for children >8 y

*PO, By mouth; bid, twice daily; tid, three times daily; qid, four times daily.
†Treatment of choice.

methoxazole is variable. Less than 1% of *C. jejuni* strains are resistant to aminoglycosides and imipenem. Aminoglycosides may be used in extraintestinal *C. jejuni* infections, but oral therapy must also be given as they are ineffective against gut infections.

Prevention

Because most *C. jejuni* infections are transmitted via eating chicken, ultimately, the most effective way to control *C. jejuni* enteritis is to control infections in broiler flocks. *Campylobacter* infection of chickens is nearly universal. One raw chicken carcass may contain a million *Campylobacter* organisms.[97] Current mass processing and distribution of chicken may amplify the bacterial load; perhaps future work will devise a system that will produce chickens that are free of, or only lightly colonized with, *Campylobacter.* Observing careful food preparation habits in the kitchen is also important in preventing infections. Chicken should be adequately cooked—not charred on the outside and left pink near the bone. Cutting boards and utensils used in handling uncooked poultry or other meats should be washed with hot, soapy water before being used for preparation of salads or other foods eaten raw.

Although person-to-person transmission of *C. jejuni* infection is unusual, persons with any acute diarrheal illness should avoid preparation and handling of food until their illness resolves. Of course, as part of good general hygiene, all people should wash their hands after using the bathroom, especially if they have diarrhea. Similarly, all people, but especially those who handle pets or other animals, should wash their hands before eating. Prevention of many outbreaks of *C. jejuni* infection could be accomplished by avoiding consumption of unpasteurized milk; this should be emphasized to pregnant women, elderly people, immunocompromised persons, or other persons in whom *C. jejuni* infection may have serious consequences. Travelers to developing countries and campers should be cautioned against drinking untreated water. Routine use of antibiotic prophylaxis to prevent *Campylobacter* infections is not recommended.

References

1. Nachamkin I: *Campylobacter and Arcobacter. In* Murray PR, Baron EJ, Pfaller MA, et al (eds): Manual of Clinical Microbiology, ed 6. Washington, DC, American Society for Microbiology, 1995, pp 483–491.
2. Vandamme P, De Ley J: Proposal for a new family, Campylobacteraceae. Int J Syst Bacteriol 41:451–455, 1991.
3. Wang WL, Blaser MJ: Detection of pathogenic *Campylobacter* species in blood culture systems. J Clin Microbiol 23:709–714, 1986.
4. Wang WL, Reller LB, Smallwood B, et al: Evaluation of transport media and filtration for the isolation of *Campylobacter* in human fecal specimens. J Clin Microbiol 18:803–807, 1983.
5. Smibert RM: Genus *Campylobacter* Sebald and Véron 1963, 907. *In* Krieg NR, Holt JG (eds): Bergey's Manual of Systematic Bacteriology, Vol 1. Baltimore, Williams & Wilkins, 1984, pp 111–118.
6. Lior H, Woodward DL, Edgar JA, et al: Serotyping of *Campylobacter jejuni* by slide agglutination based on heat-labile antigenic factors. J Clin Microbiol 15:761–768, 1982.
7. Jones DM, Sutcliffe EM, Abbott JD: Serotyping of *Campylobacter* species by combined use of two methods. Eur J Clin Microbiol 4:562–565, 1985.
8. Patton CM, Barrett TJ, Morris GK: Comparison of the Penner and Lior methods for serotyping *Campylobacter* spp. J Clin Microbiol 22:558–565, 1985.
9. Nicholson MA, Patton CM: Application of Lior biotyping by use of genetically identified *Campylobacter* strains. J Clin Microbiol 31:3348–3350, 1993.
10. Taylor DN, Blaser MJ: *Campylobacter* infections. *In* Evans A, Brachman P (eds): Bacterial Infections of Humans. New York, Plenum Publishing, 1991, pp 151–172.
11. Tauxe RV, Hargrett-Bean N, Patton CM, Wacchsmuth IK: *Campylobacter* isolates in the United States, 1982–1986. MMWR CDC Surveill Summ 37:1–14, 1988.
12. Murray BJ: *Campylobacter* enteritis: A college campus average incidence and a prospective study of the risk factors for exposure. West J Med 145:341–342, 1986.
13. Tauxe RV, Deming MS, Blake PA: *Campylobacter jejuni* infections on college campuses: A national survey. Am J Public Health 75:659–660, 1985.
14. Tauxe RV: Epidemiology of *Campylobacter jejuni* infections in the United States and other industrialized nations. *In* Nachamkin I, Blaser MJ, Tompkins LS (eds): *Campylobacter jejuni*—Current Strategy and Future Trends. Washington, DC, American Society for Microbiology, 1992, pp 9–19.
15. Kendall EJ, Tanner EI: *Campylobacter* enteritis in general practice. J Hyg 88:155–163, 1982.
16. Taylor DN, Echeverria P, Pitarangsi C, et al: The influence of strain characteristics and immunity on the epidemiology of *Campylobacter* infections in Thailand. J Clin Microbiol 26:863–868, 1988.
17. Glass RI, Stoll BJ, Huq MI, et al: Epidemiology and clinical features of endemic *Campylobacter jejuni* infection in Bangladesh. J Infect Dis 148:292–296, 1983.
18. Seattle–King County Department of Public Health: Surveillance of the flow of *Salmonella* and *Campylobacter* in a community. Seattle, Communicable Disease Control Section, Seattle–King County Department of Public Health, 1984.
19. Deming MS, Tauxe RV, Blake PA, et al: *Campylobacter* enteritis at a university: Transmission from eating chicken and from cats. Am J Epidemiol 126:526–534, 1984.
20. Harris NV, Thomson D, Martin DC, Nolan CM: A survey of *Campylobacter* and other bacterial contaminants of pre-market chicken and retail poultry and meats, King County, Washington. Am J Public Health 76:401–406, 1986.
21. Wood RC, MacDonald KL, Osterholm MT: *Campylobacter* enteritis outbreaks associated with drinking raw milk during youth activities. JAMA 268:3228–3230, 1992.
22. Palmer SR, McGuirk SM: Bird attacks on milk bottles and *Campylobacter* infections (Letter). Lancet 35:326–327, 1995.
23. Lighton LL, Kaczmarski EB, Jones DM: A study of risk factors for *Campylobacter* infections in late spring. Public Health 105:199–203, 1991.
24. Mentzing LO: Waterborne outbreaks of *Campylobacter* enteritis in central Sweden. Lancet 2:352–354, 1981.
25. Vogt RL, Sours HE, Barrett T, et al: *Campylobacter* enteritis associated with contaminated water. Ann Intern Med 96:292–296, 1982.
26. Melby K, Dahl OP, Crisp L, Penner JL: Clinical and serological manifestations in patients during a waterborne epidemic due to *Campylobacter jejuni.* J Infect 21:309–316, 1990.
27. Hopkins RS, Olmsted R, Istre GR: Endemic *Campylobacter jejuni* infection in Colorado: Identified risk factors. Am J Public Health 74:249–250, 1984.
28. Taylor DN, McDermott KT, Little JR, et al: *Campylobacter* enteritis from untreated water in the Rocky Mountains. Ann Intern Med 99:38–40, 1983.
29. Kapperud G, Skjerve E, Bean NH, et al: Risk factors for sporadic *Campylobacter* infections: Results of a case-control study in southeastern Norway. J Clin Microbiol 30:3117–3121, 1992.
30. Blaser MJ, Waldman RJ, Barrett T, Erlandson AL: Outbreaks of *Campylobacter* enteritis in two extended families: Evidence for person-to-person transmission. J Pediatr 98:254–257, 1981.
31. Oosterom J, den Uyl CH, Banffer JR, Huisman J: Epidemiological investigations on *Campylobacter jejuni* in households with a primary infection. J Hyg 93:325–332, 1984.
32. Riordan T: Intestinal infection with *Campylobacter* in children (Letter). Lancet 1:992, 1988.
33. Calva JJ, Ruiz-Palacioz GM, Lopez-Vidal AB, et al: Cohort study of intestinal infection with *Campylobacter* in Mexican children. Lancet 1:503–506, 1988.
34. Walder M: Epidemiology of *Campylobacter* enteritis. Scand J Infect Dis 14:27–33, 1982.
35. Kapperud G, Lassen J, Ostroff SM, Aasen S: Clinical features of

sporadic *Campylobacter* infections in Norway. Scand J Infect Dis 24:741–749, 1992.
36. Smith GS, Blaser MJ: Fatalities associated with *Campylobacter jejuni* infections. JAMA 253:2873–2875, 1985.
37. Blaser MJ, Wells JG, Feldman RA, et al: *Campylobacter* enteritis in the United States: A multicenter study. Ann Intern Med 98:360–365, 1983.
38. Ponka A, Pitkanen T, Kosunen TU: *Campylobacter* enteritis mimicking acute abdominal emergency. Acta Chir Scand 147:663–666, 1981.
39. Skirrow MB: *Campylobacter* enteritis: A "new" disease. Br Med J 2:9–11, 1977.
40. Pitkanen T, Ponka A, Pettersson T, Kosunen TU: *Campylobacter* enteritis in 188 hospitalized patients. Arch Intern Med 143:215–219, 1983.
41. Blaser MJ, Reller LB, Leuchtefeld NW, Wang WLL: *Campylobacter* enteritis in Denver. West J Med 136:287–290, 1982.
42. Paulet P, Coffernils M: Very long-term diarrhea due to *Campylobacter jejuni.* Postgrad Med J 66:410–411, 1990.
43. Richardson NJ, Koornhof HJ, Bokkenheuser VD: Long-term infections with *Campylobacter fetus* subsp. *jejuni.* J Clin Biol 13:846–849, 1981.
44. Berezin S, Newman LJ: Prolonged mild diarrhea caused by *Campylobacter* (Letter). N Y State J Med 86:29, 1986.
45. Blaser MJ, Berkowitz ID, LaForce M, et al: *Campylobacter* enteritis: Clinical and epidemiologic features. Ann Intern Med 91:179–185, 1979.
46. van der Hoop Ag, Veringa EM: Cholecystitis caused by *Campylobacter jejuni.* Clin Infect Dis 17:133, 1993.
47. Ezpeleta C, de Ursa PR, Obregon F, et al: Acute pancreatitis associated with *Campylobacter jejuni* bacteremia. Clin Infect Dis 15:1050, 1992.
48. Wood CJ, Fleming V, Turridge J, et al: *Campylobacter* peritonitis in continuous ambulatory peritoneal dialysis: Report of eight cases and a review of the literature. Am J Kidney Dis 19:257–263, 1992.
49. Frizelle FA, Rietveld JA: Spontaneous splenic rupture associated with *Campylobacter jejuni* infection. Br J Surg 81:718, 1994.
50. Simor AE, Ferro S: *Campylobacter jejuni* infection occurring during pregnancy. Eur J Clin Microbiol Infect Dis 9:142–144, 1990.
51. Skirrow MB, Jones DM, Sutcliffe E, Benjamin J: *Campylobacter* bacteremia in England and Wales, 1981–91. Epidemiol Infect 110:567–573, 1993.
52. de Guevara CL, Gonzalez J, Pena P: Bacteraemia caused by *Campylobacter* spp. J Clin Pathol 47:174–175, 1994.
53. Bretag AH, Archer RS, Atkinson HM, Woods WH: Circadian urticaria: Another campylobacter association (Letter). Lancet 1:954, 1984.
54. Lopez-Brea M, Fontelos PM, Baquero M, Aragon L: Urticaria associated with campylobacter enteritis (Letter). Lancet 1:1354, 1984.
55. Mishu B, Blaser MJ: Role of infection due to *Campylobacter jejuni* in the initiation of Guillain-Barré syndrome. Clin Infect Dis 17:104–108, 1993.
56. Mishu B, Amjad AA, Koski CL, et al: Serologic evidence of previous *Campylobacter jejuni* infection in patients with the Guillain-Barré syndrome. Ann Intern Med 118:947–953, 1993.
57. Kuroki S, Saida T, Nukina M, et al: *Campylobacter jejuni* strains from patients with Guillain-Barré syndrome belong mostly to Penner serogroup 19 and contain β-*N*-acetylglucosamine. Ann Neurol 22:243–247, 1993.
58. Yuki N, Taki T, Inagaki F, et al: A bacterium lipopolysaccharide that elicits Guillain-Barré syndrome has a GM1 ganglioside-like structure. J Exp Med 178:1771–1775, 1993.
59. Gumpel JM, Martin C, Sanderson PJ: Reactive arthritis associated with *Campylobacter* enteritis. Ann Rheum Dis 40:64–65, 1981.
60. Bremell T, Bjelle A, Svedhem A: Rheumatic symptoms following an outbreak of campylobacter enteritis: A five year follow up. Ann Rheum Dis 50:934–938, 1991.
61. Eastmond CJ, Rennie JA, Reid TM: An outbreak of *Campylobacter* enteritis: A rheumatological follow-up survey. J Rheumatol 10:107–108, 1983.
62. Rautelin H, Koota K, von Essen R, et al: Waterborne *Campylobacter jejuni* epidemic in a Finnish hospital for rheumatic diseases. Scand J Infect Dis 22:321–326, 1990.
63. Lever AML, Dolby JM, Webster ADB, Price AB: Chronic campylobacter colitis and uveitis in patient with hypogammaglobulinaemia. Br Med J 288:531, 1984.
64. Howard RS, Sarkies NJC, Sanders MD: Anterior uveitis associated with *Campylobacter jejuni* infection. J Infect 14:186–187, 1987.
65. Wilson PG, Davies JR, Hoskins TW, et al: Epidemiology of an outbreak of milk-borne enteritis in a residential school. *In* Pearson AD, Skirrow MB, Rowe B, et al (eds): *Campylobacter* II: Proceedings of the Second International Workshop on *Campylobacter* Infections. London, Public Health Laboratory Service, 1983, p 143.
66. Lambert M, Marion E, Coche E, Butzler JP: *Campylobacter* enteritis and erythema nodosum. Lancet 1:1409, 1982.
67. Ellis ME, Pope J, Mokashi A, Dunbar E: *Campylobacter* colitis associated with erythema nodosum. Br Med J 285:937, 1982.
68. Eastmond CJ, Reid TMS: *Campylobacter* enteritis and erythema nodosum. Br Med J 285:1421–1422, 1982.
69. Ashworth J, English JSC: Recurrent erythema nodosum and prolonged *Campylobacter jejuni* excretion. Br Med J 288:830, 1984.
70. Denneberg T, Freidberg M, Holmberg L, et al: Combined plasmapheresis and hemodialysis treatment for severe hemolytic-uremic syndrome following *Campylobacter* colitis. Acta Paediatr Scand 71:243–245, 1982.
71. Chamovitz BN, Hartstein AI, Alexander SR, et al: *Campylobacter jejuni*–associated hemolytic-uremic syndrome in a mother and daughter. Pediatrics 71:253–256, 1983.
72. Shulman ST, Moel D: *Campylobacter* infection (Letter). Pediatrics 72:437, 1983.
73. Dickgiesser A: Campylobakterinfektion und hämolytisch-uramisches Syndrom. Immun Infect 11:71–74, 1983.
74. Delans RJ, Biuso JD, Saba SR, Ramirez G: Hemolytic uremic syndrome after *Campylobacter*-induced diarrhea in an adult. Arch Intern Med 144:1074–1076, 1984.
75. Haq JA, Rahman KM, Akbar MS: Haemolytic-uraemic syndrome and campylobacter. Med J Aust 142:662–663, 1985.
76. Morton AR, Yu R, Waldek S, et al: *Campylobacter* induced thrombocytopenic purpura. Lancet 2:1133–1134, 1985.
77. May TH, Gerard A, Voiriot P, et al: Entérite à *Campylobacter jejuni* associée à un syndrome hémolytique et urémique. Presse Med 15:803–804, 1986.
78. Sorvillo FJ, Lieb LE, Waterman SH: Incidence of campylobacteriosis among patients with AIDS in Los Angeles County. J Acquir Immune Defic Syndr 4:598–602, 1991.
79. Nelson MR, Shanson DC, Hawkins DA, Gazzard BG: *Salmonella, Campylobacter* and *Shigella* on HIV-seropositive patients. AIDS 6:1495–1498, 1992.
80. Johnson RJ, Nolan C, Wang SP, et al: Persistent *Campylobacter jejuni* infection in an immunocompromised patient. Ann Intern Med 100:832–834, 1984.
81. Wheeler AP, Gregg CR: *Campylobacter* bacteremia, cholecystitis, and the acquired immunodeficiency syndrome (Letter). Ann Intern Med 105:804, 1986.
82. Bernard E, Roger PM, Bonaldi CV, et al: Diarrhea and *Campylobacter* infections in patients infected with human immunodeficiency virus. J Infect Dis 159:143–144, 1989.
83. Peterson MC, Farr RW, Castiglia M: Prosthetic hip infections and bacteremia due to *Campylobacter jejuni* in a patient with AIDS. Clin Infect Dis 16:439–440, 1993.
84. Perlman DM, Ampel NM, Schifman RB, et al: Persistent *Campylobacter jejuni* infections in patients infected with human immunodeficiency virus (HIV). Ann Intern Med 108:540–546, 1988.
85. Melamed I, Bujanover Y, Igra YS, et al: *Campylobacter* enteritis in normal and immunodeficient children. Am J Dis Child 137:752–753, 1983.
86. Van der Meer JWM, Mouton RP, Daha MR, Schuurman RKB: *Campylobacter jejuni* bacteraemia as a cause of recurrent fever in a patient with hypogammaglobulinaemia. J Infect 12:235–239, 1986.
87. Melamed A, Zakuth V, Schwartz D, Spirer Z: The immune system response to *Campylobacter* infection. Microbiol Immunol 32:75–82, 1988.
88. Kerstens PJSM, Endtz HP, Meis JFGM, et al: Erysipelas-like skin lesions associated with *Campylobacter jejuni* septicemia in patients with hypogammaglobulinemia. Eur J Clin Microbiol Infect Dis 11:842–847, 1992.

89. Hammarstrom V, Smith CIE, Hammarstrom L: Oral immunoglobulin treatment in *Campylobacter jejuni* enteritis (Letter). Lancet 341:1036, 1993.
90. Guerry P, Logan SM, Thornton S, Trust TJ: Genomic organization and expression of *Campylobacter* flagellin genes. J Bacteriol 172:1853–1860, 1990.
91. Alm RA, Guerry P, Trust TJ: Distribution and polymorphism of the flagellin genes from isolates of *Campylobacter coli* and *Campylobacter jejuni.* J Bacteriol 175:3051–3057, 1993.
92. McSweegan E, Walker RI: Identification and characterization of two *Campylobacter jejuni* adhesins for cellular and mucous substrates. Infect Immun 53:141–148, 1986.
93. Lindblom GB, Cervantes LE, Sjogren E, et al: Adherence, enterotoxigenicity, invasiveness, and serogroups in *Campylobacter jejuni* and *Campylobacter coli* strains from adult humans with acute enterocolitis. APMIS 98:179–184, 1990.
94. Black RE, Levine MM, Clements ML, et al: Experimental *Campylobacter jejuni* infection in humans. J Infect Dis 157:472–479, 1988.
95. Robinson DA: Infective dose of *Campylobacter jejuni* in milk. Br Med J 282:1584, 1981.
96. Black RE, Perlman D, Clements ML, et al: Human volunteer studies with *Campylobacter jejuni. In* Nachamkin I, Blaser MJ, Tompkins LS (eds): *Campylobacter jejuni*—Current Strategy and Future Trends. Washington, DC, American Society for Microbiology, 1992, pp 207–215.
97. Hood AM, Pearson AD, Shahamat M: The extent of surface contamination of retailed chickens with *Campylobacter jejuni* serogroups. Epidemiol Infect 100:17–25, 1988.
98. Blaser MJ, Duncan D: Human serum antibody response to *Campylobacter jejuni* infection as measured in an enzyme-linked immunosorbent assay. Infect Immun 44:292–298, 1984.
99. Goossens H, Butzler JP, Takeda Y: Demonstration of cholera-like enterotoxin production by *Campylobacter jejuni.* FEMS Microbiol Lett 29:73–76, 1985.
100. Lindblom GB, Johny M, Khalil K, et al: Enterotoxigenicity and frequency of *Campylobacter jejuni, C. coli,* and *C. laridis* in human and animal stool isolates from different countries. FEMS Microbiol Lett 54:163–168, 1990.
101. Perez-Perez GI, Taylor DN, Echeverria PD, Blaser MJ: Lack of evidence of enterotoxin involvement in pathogenesis of *Campylobacter* diarrhea. *In* Nachamkin I, Blaser MJ, Tompkins LS (eds): *Campylobacter jejuni*—Current Strategy and Future Trends. Washington, DC, American Society for Microbiology, 1992, pp 184–192.
102. Bayerdorffer E, Hochter W, Schwarzkopf-Steinhauser G, et al: Bioptic microbiology in the differential diagnosis of enterocolitis. Endoscopy 18:177–181, 1986.
103. Blaser MJ, Parsons RB, Wang WLL: Acute colitis caused by *Campylobacter fetus* ssp. *jejuni.* Gastroenterology 78:448–453, 1980.
104. Surawicz CM, Belic L: Rectal biopsy helps to distinguish acute self-limited colitis from idiopathic inflammatory bowel disease. Gastroenterology 86:104–113, 1984.
105. Price AB, Jewkes J, Sanderson PJ: Acute diarrhoea: *Campylobacter* colitis and the role of rectal biopsy. J Clin Pathol 32:990–997, 1979.
106. Goodman LJ, Trenholme GM, Kaplan RL, et al: Empiric antimicrobial therapy of domestically acquired acute diarrhea in urban adults. Arch Intern Med 150:541–546, 1990.
107. Petruccelli BP, Murphy GS, Sanchez JL, et al: Treatment of traveler's diarrhea with ciprofloxacin and loperamide. J Infect Dis 165:557–560, 1992.
108. Wistrom J, Jertborn M, Ekwall E, et al: Empiric treatment of acute diarrheal disease with norfloxacin. Ann Intern Med 117:202–208, 1992.
109. Rautelin H, Renkonen OV, Kosunen TU: Emergence of fluoroquinolone resistance in *Campylobacter jejuni* and *Campylobacter coli* in subjects from Finland. Antimicrob Agents Chemother 35:2065–2069, 1991.

208

Vibrios

David A. Sack

The family Vibrionaceae includes the medically important vibrios, aeromonads, and *Plesiomonas shigelloides.* These are a group of gram-negative, curved or straight motile rods that normally inhabit the environmental waters. Humans become infected either through the gastrointestinal tract (e.g., ingestion of contaminated water or food) or through a wound exposed to contaminated water. Many of the strains have specific virulence factors, such as toxins, capsules, or colonization factors, that increase virulence or explain the mechanism of the symptoms that the organisms produce. Also, certain host factors, especially hypochlorhydria, immunodeficiency, cirrhosis, hemochromatosis, and diabetes, increase susceptibility to or severity of the infection. Finally, being environmental organisms, their concentration in the environment varies with the season, and the infections, at least in temperate climates, are much more common in the warmer months. The biochemical characteristics of the clinically important vibrios that are useful for their laboratory identification are shown in Table 208–1.

Vibrio cholerae O1 and O139

V. cholerae is of special interest because it includes the serogroups that cause pandemic cholera, serogroups O1 and O139. Strains belonging to other serogroups (e.g., serogroups O2 to O138) and strains that are not toxin producing (even if they are serogroup O1 or O139) may cause sporadic illnesses, but they have never caused widespread epidemics and thus are of less public health importance.

Cholera is an illness characterized by severe watery diarrhea. In suspected cases of cholera, fecal specimens should be cultured for vibrios. Cholera is more likely in patients who live in cholera endemic areas or have recently (within the last week) traveled to a cholera area or eaten seafood from a cholera area (including the Gulf Coast of the United States) during the warm months. *V. cholerae* survives well in fecal specimens en route to the laboratory if kept moist, but if there is a delay of more than a few hours, Cary-Blair transport medium should be used. The feces (either fresh or in the transport medium) should then be plated onto thiosulfate citrate bile salts sucrose (TCBS) agar, a medium that inhibits most normal flora but supports the growth of the vibrios. In addition, the specimen should be inoculated into alkaline peptone water, a high-pH enrichment broth, which preferentially supports the growth of vibrios. After 6 to 12 hours of incubation, a second TCBS plate is inoculated. The TCBS plates are incubated for 18 to 24 hours, and *V. cholerae* colonies appear as smooth yellow colonies. Presumptive identification of *V. cholerae* O1 can be made on the basis of typical colonies, which are oxidase-positive and agglutinate with O1 or O139 antiserum. If such colonies are recovered, they should be reported immediately to the state health department and sent to the appropriate referral laboratory for confirmation. Agglutination should be carried out after subculture onto a nonselective agar (e.g., nutrient or trypticase

TABLE 208–1 ■ Key Differential Tests* for Clinically Important *Vibrio* Species

SPECIES	GROWTH IN NUTRIENT BROTH		OXIDASE	NITRATE TO NITRITE	MYOINOSITOL FERMENTATION	ARGININE DIHYDROLASE	LYSINE DECARBOXYLASE	ORNITHINE DECARBOXYLASE
	0% NaCl	1% NaCl						
V. cholerae	+	+	+	+	−	−	+	+
V. mimicus	+	+	+	+	−	−	+	+
V. metschnikovii	−	+	−	−	V	V	V	−
V. cincinnatiensis	−	+	+	+	+	−	V	−
V. hollisae	−	+	+	+	−	−	−	−
V. damsela	−	+	+	+	−	+	V	−
V. fluvialis	−	+	+	+	−	+	−	−
V. furnissii	−	+	+	+	−	+	−	−
V. alginolyticus	−	+	+	+	−	−	+	V
V. parahaemolyticus	−	+	+	+	−	−	+	+
V. vulnificus	−	+	+	+	−	−	+	V

*+, More than 90% positive; −, less than 10% positive; V, 10%–90% positive.
Adapted from Bopp CA, Kay BA, Wells JG: Laboratory Methods for the Diagnosis of *Vibrio cholerae*. Atlanta, National Center for Infectious Diseases, Centers for Disease Control and Prevention, 1994.

soy agar) because colonies from TCBS may give atypical agglutination results.

V. cholerae organisms are short, curved rods (hence their historic name, the comma bacillus). They are oxidase-positive; have a single polar flagellum; ferment glucose, sucrose, and mannitol; and produce lysine and ornithine decarboxylase. Strains associated with epidemics produce a potent enterotoxin, but not all strains of *V. cholerae* O1 produce the toxin. Isolates, especially from surface water, may be serogroup O1 but not produce the toxin, and these nontoxigenic strains do not represent a cholera threat.

V. cholerae serogroup O1 is divided into two serotypes (Ogawa and Inaba) and two biotypes (classical and *eltor*). Classical strains predominated until they were replaced by the *eltor* strains during the seventh pandemic, which began in the 1960s. Currently, classical strains are found only in southern Bangladesh, but *eltor* strains are found throughout Asia, Africa, and South America. The *eltor* strains appear better suited to the environmental waters and persist there once established. Fewer of those infected with *eltor* strains develop severe cholera, and there are more asymptomatic infections. Among patients with severe cholera, however, the clinical illness is identical regardless of biotype. The *eltor* strains are distinguished from classical strains by agglutination with chicken red blood cells and their resistance to polymyxin B.

The serotype, defined by agglutination with monovalent antiserum, is a useful marker for strains, but the clinical illness of Ogawa and Inaba strains is identical. Also, strains occasionally switch between the two serotypes during an epidemic season, so this marker is not altogether stable. A few unusual strains agglutinate with both Inaba and Ogawa monospecific antiserum and are designated Hikojima strains.

The major virulence factor for *V. cholerae* O1 and O139 is the cholera toxin, but additional properties include the colonization pili (mannose-sensitive hemagglutinin and toxin-coregulated pilus).[1] Additional toxins that may play some role in the disease include Zot toxin (zonula occludens toxin), which increases permeability of the mucosa, and the Ace toxin (accessory cholera toxin).[2] The flagellum can also be considered a virulence factor because motility increases virulence.

The nature of the persistence of *V. cholerae* between epidemic seasons has been of great interest because, in many locations, cases completely disappear and the bacterium cannot be cultured from surface waters. It now appears that *V. cholerae* (and other vibrios) may enter a viable but nonculturable survival form—a form in which the bacterium metabolizes slowly but is not detectable with use of usual culture media.[3] Under certain conditions, it can then revert to the normal form.

Molecular methods (e.g., plasmid profiles, ribotyping, restriction fragment length polymorphisms, multilocus enzyme electrophoresis, DNA sequencing of selected genes, and others) have become useful in characterizing strains of *V. cholerae*. By use of these molecular techniques, strains can be characterized as belonging to clusters associated with certain geographic regions.[4] Further, by using polymerase chain reaction techniques, specimens can be screened for both culturable and nonculturable forms. These methods provide a greatly improved understanding of the molecular epidemiology of the organism and improve the sensitivity of detecting the bacterium.

Clinically useful rapid methods are now also available to detect cases of cholera. The most practical of the rapid tests include darkfield examination of stool specimens; coagglutination tests using antibody-coated *Staphylococcus aureus* cells (Cowan 1 strain); and the sensitive membrane antigen rapid test,[5] a membrane-bound monoclonal antibody–based test that uses a gold label to detect the O antigen in the specimen in about 5 minutes. If the case is the first in a geographic area, the results of the rapid test must be confirmed with culture.

In the past, most strains of *V. cholerae* were sensitive to the clinically useful antibiotics, but in more recent years, many epidemics have been due to plasmid-containing strains, which renders them resistant to multiple antibiotics including tetracycline (which was the drug of choice), ampicillin, chloramphenicol, trimethoprim, and others. Thus, antibiotic sensitivity patterns of local strains must be determined to establish optimal antibiotic therapy.

Other Vibrios

***Vibrio cholerae* Non-O1.** Strains of *V. cholerae* that do not agglutinate with O1 or O139 antisera are known as non-O1 *V. cholerae* (formerly called nonagglutinating vibrios); otherwise, they give the same reactions in microbiologic tests. They occasionally produce cholera toxin, but even then, they have not caused epidemics. Few laboratories carry out serotyping for these strains, and from a clinical perspective, knowing the specific serotype is not important; hence, except in unusual outbreaks, sending these strains to a reference laboratory for serotyping is not needed. These bacteria most often cause watery diarrhea, but they may rarely cause systemic infections (bacteremia or meningitis) and wound infections, especially in patients with increased susceptibility due to immunodeficiency, cirrhosis, or hemochromatosis.

Vibrio mimicus. *V. mimicus* is similar to *V. cholerae* in that it may produce cholera-like illness, and many strains produce cholera toxin nearly identical to that produced by *V. cholerae.*[6] It differs from *V. cholerae* epidemiologically in not being associated with epidemics and microbiologically in being sucrose-negative and Voges-Proskauer–negative. Cases occur mostly in patients in the Indian subcontinent but are occasionally seen in other areas.

Vibrio parahaemolyticus. *V. parahaemolyticus* is a common halophilic (salt-loving) vibrio that has been an especially common cause of acute diarrhea among people who eat raw or undercooked seafood. It was commonly isolated in Japan, but it is now recognized as a pathogen in all parts of the world including both industrialized and developing countries. Outbreaks do occur and are nearly always due to consumption of seafood.

Fecal specimens of patients with a suspected vibrio infection should be cultured with use of TCBS agar because these organisms may not be recognized on the routine media used for isolation of *Salmonella* and *Shigella*, unless oxidase-positive colonies are identified. On TCBS agar, colonies appear as green (sucrose-negative) colonies. Once isolated, the colonies can be identified by use of biochemical tests. *V. parahaemolyticus* is a halophilic vibrio (e.g., the organisms grow in nutrient broth containing 1% sodium chloride, but not in the same broth without salt). Other biochemical tests useful in differentiating this from other vibrios are shown in Table 208–1. If there is a delay in transporting the specimen to the laboratory, Cary-Blair transport medium should be used to preserve the strains en route.

Most strains from patients produce thermostable direct hemolysin (TDH) or a related hemolysin, TDH-related hemolysin.[7] The TDH strains are hemolytic on Wagatsuma agar and are known as Kanagawa-positive strains, but those that produce TDH-related hemolysin may be Kanagawa-negative; however, these factors can now best be detected with use of gene probe techniques. Because most environmental strains, as well as other vibrios, are negative for both TDH and TDH-related hemolysin, detection of these markers helps in differentiating pathogenic from nonpathogenic strains.

Most patients with *V. parahaemolyticus* infection have acute watery diarrhea, but occasionally systemic infections (e.g., sepsis and wound infections) may occur,[8] especially in patients at increased risk because of immunodeficiency or liver cirrhosis.

Vibrio vulnificus. *V. vulnificus* has become the most common vibrio causing serious morbidity and mortality in the United States[9, 10] and is associated primarily with systemic infections. Rarely, it causes diarrhea. When persons with an underlying illness (e.g., immunodeficiency, cirrhosis, hemochromatosis, diabetes) ingest foods contaminated with the bacteria, the bacteria can invade and cause severe sepsis associated with high case-fatality rates (about 50%). The organism may also infect wounds, leading to severe necrotic wound infections and sepsis, also associated with high case-fatality rates (about 25%). The wound infections frequently have bullous lesions, which provide a clue to the etiology, and the organism can often be identified in the bullous fluid. Among the survivors of the wound infection, disability is common because the infections are so destructive to the tissue.

V. vulnificus produces several enzymes (e.g., lipase, hyaluronidase, mucinase, DNase); however, the primary virulence factor appears to be its capsule.[11] Encapsulated strains predominate among clinical isolates but are unusual in environmental specimens.

In the United States, there is a marked seasonality of *V. vulnificus* infections, with most occurring during the warm months of the year. Persons with a predisposing risk factor should be warned against consumption of raw or undercooked seafood (especially raw oysters), especially during the summer.

Other Halophilic Vibrios. *Vibrio fluvialis* is closely related to *Aeromonas* and is commonly found in brackish waters. It can cause severe diarrhea.[12] *Vibrio hollisae* and *Vibrio furnissii* similarly are causes of diarrhea. Like *V. vulnificus, V. hollisae* may rarely cause sepsis in susceptible hosts. Unlike other vibrios, *V. hollisae* does not grow well on TCBS agar.

Vibrio alginolyticus and *Vibrio damsela* are rare causes of sepsis or wound infections and are associated with exposure to seawater or seafood. The other vibrios listed in Table 208–1 (*Vibrio metschnikovii, Vibrio cincinnatiensis*) are extremely rare causes of systemic illness in humans.

Aeromonas Species

Aeromonads are gram-negative rods in the family Vibrionaceae. Like other members of this family, they are frequently found in water, although their normal habitat is freshwater. Persons living in developing countries who drink untreated water thus consume *Aeromonas* daily, and these organisms are found in a high proportion of fecal samples in these people. Whereas *Aeromonas* may cause diarrhea in some individuals,[13, 14] studies comparing rates of isolation of this organism in diarrhea patients and control subjects without diarrhea are complicated by the high background excretion rates in normal people. Also, volunteers challenged with *Aeromonas* did not develop diarrhea consistently; hence, the relative importance of *Aeromonas* as a pathogen causing diarrhea remains unsettled.[15]

Aeromonas species can cause severe systemic infections (wound infection, bacteremia, meningitis[16]) in some individuals, especially those with underlying illnesses such as immunodeficiency, liver cirrhosis, and diabetes.

On the basis of biochemical tests, the genus is divided into three species, *Aeromonas hydrophila, Aeromonas sobria,* and *Aeromonas caviae.* So far, however, no clinically relevant patterns have emerged that relate these species to specific clinical syndromes. Several potent toxins and lectins have been described from *Aeromonas* species,[13] but these potential virulence factors have not correlated with specific syndromes.

Because *Aeromonas* survives and multiplies in cold temperatures and is relatively resistant to chlorine, there are concerns about the safety of refrigerated foods and drinks,[17] but so far there have been no large common-source outbreaks.

Because *Aeromonas* species are usually resistant to ampicillin, an ampicillin-containing medium is frequently used for detecting these strains in fecal specimens.[18]

Plesiomonas shigelloides

Like *Aeromonas, P. shigelloides* is an oxidase-positive, gram-negative rod frequently inhabiting freshwater. Some think that *P. shigelloides* may be a cause of diarrhea; however, the evidence is not clear because the rates of isolation have been similar in patients with diarrhea and in control subjects, and volunteers challenged with *P. shigelloides* did not develop diarrhea.[19, 20] Its name was derived from the cross-agglutination of one serotype (type 17) of *P. shigelloides* with *Shigella sonnei* due to an identical O antigen between the two strains. Because of this cross-reacting antigen and the frequency of *P.*

shigelloides in surface waters, it seems probable that drinking surface water may provide a degree of natural immunity against *S. sonnei* infection to residents of developing countries.[21]

P. shigelloides rarely causes severe systemic infections (e.g., sepsis) in persons with underlying illnesses such as immunodeficiency, liver cirrhosis, and diabetes.

References

1. Herrington DA, Hall RH, Losonsky G, et al: Toxin, toxin-coregulated pili, and the *toxR* regulon are essential for *Vibrio cholerae* pathogenesis in humans. J Exp Med 168:1487–1492, 1988.
2. Tacket CO, Losonsky G, Nataro JP, et al: Safety and immunogenicity of live oral cholera vaccine candidate CVD 110, a δ *ctxA* δ *zot* δ *ace* derivative of El Tor Ogawa *Vibrio cholerae*. J Infect Dis 168:1536–1540, 1993.
3. Linder K, Oliver JD: Membrane fatty acid and virulence changes in the viable but nonculturable state of *Vibrio vulnificus*. Appl Environ Microbiol 55:2837–2842, 1989.
4. Wachsmuth IK, Evins GM, Fields PI, et al: The molecular epidemiology of cholera in Latin America. J Infect Dis 167:621–626, 1993.
5. Hasan JA, Huq A, Tamplin ML, et al: A novel kit for rapid detection of *Vibrio cholerae* O1. J Clin Microbiol 32:249–252, 1994.
6. Chowdhury MA, Aziz KM, Kay BA, Rahim Z: Toxin production by *Vibrio mimicus* strains isolated from human and environmental sources in Bangladesh. J Clin Microbiol 25:2200–2203, 1987.
7. Shirai H, Ito H, Hirayama T, et al: Molecular epidemiologic evidence for association of thermostable direct hemolysin (TDH) and TDH-related hemolysin of *Vibrio parahaemolyticus* with gastroenteritis. Infect Immun 58:3568–3573, 1990.
8. Klontz KC: Fatalities associated with *Vibrio parahaemolyticus* and *Vibrio cholerae* non-O1 infections in Florida (1981 to 1988). South Med J 83:500–502, 1990.
9. Hlady WG, Mullen RC, Hopkin RS: *Vibrio vulnificus* from raw oysters. Leading cause of reported deaths from foodborne illness in Florida. J Fla Med Assoc 80:536–538, 1993.
10. Morris JG Jr: *Vibrio vulnificus*—A new monster of the deep? Ann Intern Med 109:261–263, 1988.
11. Hayat U, Reddy GP, Bush CA, et al: Capsular types of *Vibrio vulnificus*: An analysis of strains from clinical and environmental sources. J Infect Dis 168:758–762, 1993.
12. Klontz KC, Desenclos JC: Clinical and epidemiological features of sporadic infections with *Vibrio fluvialis* in Florida, USA. J Diarrhoeal Dis Res 8:24–26, 1990.
13. Wadstrom T, Ljungh A: *Aeromonas* and *Plesiomonas* as food- and waterborne pathogens. Int J Food Microbiol 12:303–311, 1991.
14. Holmberg SD, Schell WL, Fanning GR, et al: *Aeromonas* intestinal infections in the United States. Ann Intern Med 105:683–689, 1986.
15. Morgan DR, Johnson PC, DuPont HL, et al: Lack of correlation between known virulence properties of *Aeromonas hydrophila* and enteropathogenicity for humans. Infect Immun 50:62–65, 1985.
16. Parras F, Diaz MD, Reina J, et al: Meningitis due to *Aeromonas* species: Case report and review. Clin Infect Dis 17:1058–1060, 1993.
17. Kirov SM: The public health significance of *Aeromonas* spp. in foods. Int J Food Microbiol 20:179–198, 1993.
18. Kay BA, Guerrero CE, Sack RB: Media for the isolation of *Aeromonas hydrophila*. J Clin Microbiol 22:888–890, 1985.
19. Sack DA, Chowdhury KA, Huq A, et al: Epidemiology of *Aeromonas* and *Plesiomonas* diarrhoea. J Diarrhoeal Dis Res 6:107–112, 1988.
20. Herrington DA, Tzipori S, Robins-Browne RM, et al: In vitro and in vivo pathogenicity of *Plesiomonas shigelloides*. Infect Immun 55:979–985, 1987.
21. Sack DA, Hoque AT, Huq A, Etheridge M: Is protection against shigellosis induced by natural infection with *Plesiomonas shigelloides?* Lancet 343:1413–1415, 1994.

209

Francisella tularensis, Pasteurella, and Yersinia pestis

Edward J. Bottone

Francisella tularensis

F. tularensis, the causative agent of a human zoonosis affecting skin and internal organs, and *Francisella novicida*, a nonhuman pathogen, compose the genus *Francisella*. *F. tularensis* is widely distributed geographically, with cases of the disease reported in North America, the Middle East, Russia, and Japan.[1, 2] In the United States, the disease occurs in the central, southern, and southwestern parts of the country. A tick-borne outbreak involving 50 soldiers occurred in Tennessee in 1943.[3] Although the disease is rare in New England states,[4] 47 cases linked to contact with muskrats occurred in Vermont.[5]

F. tularensis is a minute, nonmotile and non–spore-forming, faintly staining gram-negative coccobacillus. Capsules may be discerned in clinical material. Although uniform morphologic features are observed in vivo and in young cultures, marked pleomorphism, manifested by swollen oval bodies and teardrop-shaped bacillary forms, may prevail in older cultures. Bipolar morphology is particularly evident with Giemsa stain.

Growth occurs optimally under aerobic conditions at 37°C in media supplemented with cystine or cysteine and defibrinated rabbit blood or human packed red blood cells.[4, 6] Antibiotic-containing media such as Thayer-Martin chocolate agar may also be used for isolation,[7] especially from contaminated clinical specimens (e.g., skin, sputum, gastric lavage fluid). It is stressed, however, because of the highly infectious nature of *F. tularensis*, that attempts at cultivation be undertaken only under meticulous laboratory conditions and aseptic technique.[6] Once isolated, *F. tularensis* may be confirmed serologically through agglutination with specific antisera. Differentiation of the virulent *F. tularensis* biotype *tularensis* from the serologically identical but less virulent *F. tularensis* biotype *palaearctica*[8] and the virulent animal pathogen *F. novicida* may be achieved through comparison of biochemical characteristics.[9] *F. tularensis* biotype *tularensis* (type A) is the predominant isolate in North America, whereas *F. tularensis* biotype *palaearctica* (type B) occurs mainly in Asia, in Europe, and to a lesser extent in North America.

The clinical manifestations of tularemia and their categorization into glandular, ulceroglandular, oculoglandular, oropharyngeal, typhoidal, and pneumonic depend on the route of acquisition or portal of entry of the organism (Table 209–1). Infection is initiated by as few as 10 biotype *tularensis* organisms inoculated subcutaneously[10] or 25 aerosolized cells.[11] General symptoms accompanying infection include fever, chills, headache, cough, and myalgias.[1] Infection with *F. tularensis* induces serum agglutinin titers of 1:160 or greater, which usually develop during the second week of infection.[12] Natural infection confers lifelong immunity.

Virulence of *F. tularensis* is associated with the presence of

TABLE 209–1 ■ Clinical Presentation and Route of Acquisition of *Francisella tularensis* Infection

CLINICAL FORM	ROUTE OF ACQUISITION	CLINICAL SIGNS AND SYMPTOMS
Ulceroglandular-glandular	Direct contact by skinning and dressing infected animals—rabbits, squirrels, muskrats Animal bites, scratches Bites of ticks, deerflies, mosquitoes	Cutaneous ulcers Predominantly on hands Lymphadenopathy Autoinoculation to other sites possible Ulcers: head, neck, back Absence of primary lesion at site of inoculation Regional lymphadenopathy
Oculoglandular	Rubbing of eyes after handling infected animals	Conjunctivitis with discrete ulcers Periauricular, parotid, submaxillary lymphadenopathy Erythema and edema of eyelids
Oropharyngeal	Inhalation of large infected droplets Ingestion of contaminated food or water	Exudative pharyngitis Anterior-posterior cervical lymphadenopathy Enteritis, peritonitis, and appendicitis rare complications
Typhoidal	Unclear	Local signs possibly absent Fever, shaking chills; meningitis rare
Pneumonic	Inhalation of contaminated aerosols, dust Hematogenous spread Pulmonary involvement possible regardless of route of transmission	Bronchopneumonia Pleural effusion Hilar lymphadenopathy

a capsule composed of lipid, protein, and carbohydrate.[13] In contrast to the attenuated live vaccine strain, which is poorly encapsulated, or a capsule-deficient mutant of the live vaccine strain that shows decreased virulence,[14] wild-type encapsulated strains are slowly phagocytosed[15] and are able to withstand the lethal effect of polymorphonuclear lysosomal oxidants including hypochlorous acid.[16] Although the capsules of wild-type *F. tularensis* may protect against hypochlorous acid, the exact mechanism underscoring resistance to polymorphonuclear oxidants by wild-type *F. tularensis* is unknown. The capsule, however, seems to protect *F. tularensis* against complement-mediated serum bactericidal activity.[17]

F. tularensis is a facultative intracellular pathogen that survives and grows in macrophages.[18] Host defense against this species, therefore, depends on cell-mediated immunity propelled by cytokines, especially interferon-γ, produced by antigen-specific T lymphocytes to enhance the microbicidal activity of inflammatory macrophages; the effector molecule generated to toxic levels by activated macrophages that inhibits intracellular growth of *F. tularensis* has been identified as nitric oxide.[19] T-cell ($CD4^+$, $CD8^+$)–independent host defense mechanisms may also be operative in resolving *F. tularensis* infection.[20]

Antimicrobial treatment of *F. tularensis* infection centers on streptomycin, the recommended drug of choice.[1] Cure rates of 97% have been achieved with this agent with no relapses.[21] On the basis of an extensive review of the literature, Enderlin and colleagues[21] concluded that gentamicin is an acceptable alternative to streptomycin, with a reported 86% cure rate and 6% relapse rate. Prophylaxis against tularemia is mediated through the use of an attenuated live vaccine strain developed in 1961 by Eigelsbach and Downs.[22]

Pasteurella

Members of the genus *Pasteurella* of the family Pasteurellaceae are enjoined by their small coccobacillary form, which they share with *Actinobacillus* and *Haemophilus* species.[6]

Considered zoonotic agents, pasteurellae, especially *Pasteurella multocida,* colonize the mucous membranes of the upper respiratory tract of a wide variety of wild and domesticated animals including livestock, poultry, and especially dogs and cats.[6] It is predominantly from these last sources that most human infections with *P. multocida* ensue as a consequence of direct contact (bites and scratches) and indirect contact (e.g., biting or scratching by domestic cats of catheters in use during peritoneal dialysis[23, 24] or adjuvant chemotherapy[25]). In some instances of *P. multocida* infection, an association with animal exposure cannot be established.[26] Furthermore, a nosocomial outbreak of *P. multocida* infection occurred among seven patients in a chronic care facility without a definitive source identified.[27]

Pasteurella species are gram-negative, non–spore-forming minute coccobacilli with a tendency toward pleomorphism. Bipolar staining may be observed and heightened with Wright, Giemsa, or Wayson stains. *P. multocida* is encapsulated, especially when it is seen directly in purulent exudates.[6]

When grown on 5% sheep blood agar, *Pasteurella* species produce small convex colonies with a glistening consistency. Isolates of *P. multocida* derived from respiratory secretions of patients with underlying chronic pulmonary diseases, such as bronchitis, emphysema, or bronchietasis, are often mucoid and watery.[6] With the exception of *Pasteurella haemolytica,* which produces β-hemolytic colonies, *Pasteurella* species are nonhemolytic; growth of *P. multocida* on blood agar is accompanied by a distinct musty odor, possibly attributed to indole production from tryptone in the blood agar.

Pasteurellae are fermentative and, with the exception of *Pasteurella aerogenes*, anaerogenic (Table 209–2). All species are oxidase-, catalase-, and nitrate reductase–positive. Several species are urease-positive (see Table 209–2). Biotyping of *P. multocida* may be achieved through assessment of sugar fermentation reactions.[6]

P. multocida is the most frequently encountered *Pasteurella* species incriminated in human infections. Localized infections surrounding a dog or cat bite represent the majority of infectious complications. Traumatic introduction of *P. multocida* may result in cellulitis, abscess formation, and osteomyelitis of bone underlying the penetrating bite. Because *P. multocida* is not geographically restricted in the human body, it may cause a spectrum of infections mimicking those produced by *Haemophilus influenzae*, including chronic pulmo-

TABLE 209–2 ■ Salient Characteristics Differentiating *Pasteurella* Species*

	PASTEURELLA SPECIES					
CHARACTERISTIC	*multocida*	*haemolytica*	*pneumotropica*	*ureae*	*dagmatis*	*aerogenes*
Fermentation						
Glucose	+	+	+	+	+ (gas)	+ (gas)
Xylose	V	V	(+)	0	0	V
Lactose	V	V	V	0	0	V
Production of						
Urease	0	0	+	+	V	+
Indole	+	0	+	0	+	0
Ornithine decarboxylase	+	0	+	0	0	V
Growth						
MacConkey agar	0	V	V	0	0	+
Beta hemolysis	0	+	0	0	0	0

*All species are oxidase- and catalase-positive, reduce nitrates, and are nonmotile; +, positive; 0, negative; V, variable; (+), delayed positive.

nary infections, in which *P. multocida* is able to colonize devitalized pulmonary tissue, and systemic disease including septicemia and meningitis[28] (Table 209–3). *P. multocida* bacteremia associated with hepatic cirrhosis and peritonitis is an unusual manifestation,[28, 29] as is sepsis or peritonitis after a cat bite or scratch to an indwelling vascular or peritoneal catheter. Chronic otitis media may also be caused by *P. multocida*.[26] Infections caused by *Pasteurella* species other than *P. multocida* are listed in Table 209–4.

Virulence factors of *P. multocida* include an antiphagocytic capsule that allows classification into six serotypes[30] and confers resistance to complement-mediated lysis,[31] an outer membrane protein also with antiphagocytic activity,[32] and iron-scavenging capacity.[33]

Depending on the nature of the infectious process (e.g., abscess, septicemia), treatment of *P. multocida* infection may require surgery or antimicrobial therapy, usually with penicillin (drug of choice), cephalosporins, tetracyclines, or chloramphenicol. Data referable to 318 bovine respiratory isolates of *P. multocida* have shown overall resistance to ampicillin, tetracycline, erythromycin, and sulfamethazine but 100% susceptibility to ceftiofur, an extended-spectrum cephalosporin.[34] Because of emerging resistance among zoonotic isolates of *P. multocida*, the antibiotic susceptibility pattern of individual human isolates should be determined.

TABLE 209–3 ■ Spectrum of Human *Pasteurella multocida* Infections

LOCAL	RESPIRATORY
Skin and bone infections	Pneumonia
Cellulitis	Empyema
Subcutaneous abscesses	Epiglottitis
Osteomyelitis	Pharyngitis
Septic arthritis	Sinusitis
	Lung abscess
SYSTEMIC	**RARE**
Blood and vascular	Abdominal
Septicemia	Peritonitis
Endocarditis	Appendicitis
Mycotic aneurysm	Hepatosplenic abscesses
Infected vascular graft	Renal abscess
Pericarditis	Upper genitourinary tract
Central nervous system	Ocular
Meningitis	Corneal ulcer
Cerebral abscesses	Conjunctivitis
	Endophthalmitis

Yersinia pestis

The genus *Yersinia* is composed of 10 species, of which three, *Y. pestis*, *Yersinia enterocolitica*, and *Yersinia pseudotuberculosis*, are major human pathogens. Because the last two species are predominantly gastrointestinal tract pathogens, they are dealt with separately from *Y. pestis*, which causes mainly a systemic disease.

Y. pestis, the causative agent of human plague, is primarily an infectious agent of rodents transmitted to humans by the bite of a flea carrying *Y. pestis* or through the handling of *Y. pestis*–infected carcasses of rodents and rabbits or other infected animals, including dogs and cats.[49–52] In flea vectors, the bacterium multiplies in the esophagus and is transmitted by the flea during the course of a blood meal. *Y. pestis* may also be transmitted by aerosols generated by humans or animals with pneumonic plague. Interestingly, both forms of plague, bubonic[49, 50] and pneumonic,[51, 52] have been transmitted to humans by the domestic cat in plague endemic areas of the southwestern United States—the bubonic form through a scratch and bite from an infected cat, the pneumonic form through face-to-face exposure to a cat with pneumonic plague.

Y. pestis is a gram-negative encapsulated coccobacillus with distinct bipolar staining when it is viewed directly in clinical material after Wayson or Giemsa staining.[53] As do other pathogenic *Yersinia* species, *Y. pestis* grows on most bacteriologic media, albeit slowly, producing pinpoint colonies

TABLE 209–4 ■ Human Infections Associated with *Pasteurella* Species Other Than *Pasteurella multocida*

SPECIES	INFECTION	REFERENCE
Pasteurella haemolytica	Cutaneous infection	35
	Endocarditis	36
	Septicemia, shock	37
Pasteurella dagmatis	Endocarditis	38
	Wound infection	6
Pasteurella pneumotropica	Wound infection	39–41
	Bone and joint infection	42
	Septicemia	43
Pasteurella ureae	Meningitis	44, 45
	Peritonitis	46
	Septicemia	47
	Pneumonia	48

TABLE 209–5 ■ Differential Characteristics of Pathogenic *Yersinia* Species*

	YERSINIA SPECIES		
CHARACTERISTIC	*pestis*	*pseudotuberculosis*	*enterocolitica*
Motility (25°C)	0	+	+
Urease production	0	+	+
Ornithine decarboxylase production	0	0	+
Voges-Proskauer test	0	0	+ (25°C)
Indole production	0	0	V
Fermentation			
Glucose	+	+	+
Rhamnose	0	V	0
Melibiose	V	V	0
Sucrose	0	0	+

*+, Positive; 0, negative; V, variable.

within 24 hours of incubation. Hemolysis is absent on blood agar, but colonies of fully virulent *Y. pestis* have a "hammered copper" or "fried egg" appearance after 48 hours of incubation at 37°C.[54] On nutrient agar, colonies may become mucoid and glistening, an attribute associated with the proteinaceous capsular material. In liquid media, *Y. pestis*, in contrast to *Y. enterocolitica* and *Y. pseudotuberculosis*, produces granular growth at the bottom of the tube with streaking of growth upward along the inner aspect of the tube.[54] Smears of such cultures show chains of bacilli.

Like other yersiniae, *Y. pestis* is oxidase-negative and fermentative, producing acid without gas from a variety of carbohydrates (Table 209–5). Unlike *Y. pseudotuberculosis*, with which it may easily be confused,[52] *Y. pestis* is nonmotile regardless of incubation temperature (25°C or 37°C), does not produce urease, and fails to ferment melibiose and rhamnose (see Table 209–5). Suspected *Y. pestis* isolates can be confirmed at plague reference laboratories by bacteriophage sensitivity testing at 20°C to 22°C and agglutination with *Y. pestis*–specific antisera.[54]

Fully virulent wild-type *Y. pestis* possesses several plasmid species ranging from 70 to 75 kb that it shares with *Y. enterocolitica* and *Y. pseudotuberculosis* and that encode a number of virulence determinants.[55] In addition, *Y. pestis* has two distinct plasmids, a 110-kb plasmid and a 9.5-kb plasmid, that also encode virulence determinants. Expression of the 70- to 75-kb plasmid-encoded virulence attributes is under exquisite control of temperature and calcium concentration.[55] At 37°C, in the absence of Ca^{2+}, several virulence determinants (e.g., V and W antigens, outer membrane proteins) are produced; in the presence of millimolar concentrations of Ca^{2+} at 37°C, plasmid function is down-regulated but still higher than at 25°C. The 70- to 75-kb (45-MDa) plasmid encodes a series of outer membrane proteins (Yops) involved in adherence, invasion, and antiphagocytic activity and a set of Ca^{2+} and temperature-sensitive regulatory genes *(lcr)* that control synthesis of other plasmid genes; the 110-kb plasmid encodes an antiphagocytic protein capsule termed fraction 1 (Fra); the 9.5-kb plasmid encodes an outer membrane protease (Pla) that activates plasminogen, which aids in systemic spread of *Y. pestis* (Table 209–6). This plasmid also encodes coagulase activity and pesticin synthesis. *Y. pestis* also contains a chromosomally encoded surface antigen that is expressed at 37°C and acidic pH, termed pH6 antigen.[56] This outer membrane protein may serve as an epithelial cell adhesin and function maximally in the acid environment induced by an inflammatory response. This antigen is also produced intracellularly in macrophage phagolysosomes and may aid intracellular survival.[57] Chromosomally controlled virulence factors also include purine synthesis (Pur^+) and production of surface structures involved in absorption and storage of hemin.[54]

Virulent plague strains produce two phage-encoded toxins: one a soluble heat-labile exotoxin that is highly toxic for rats and mice (murine toxin), the other a lipopolysaccharide endotoxin lethal for guinea pigs and rabbits. The role of these toxins in human plague is still uncertain,[58] although endotoxin shock and disseminated intravascular coagulation can occur in plague.

Plague ensues clinically subsequent to a bite of a flea or infected animal or by inhalation of infected aerosols from individuals with pneumonic plague. The flea bite introduces *Y. pestis* into the victim's blood stream, from which the nearest lymph node sequesters the injected bacteria. At this site, *Y. pestis* is phagocytosed by local macrophages but survives intracellular killing and multiplies in the regional lymph node. Proliferation produces swelling (bubo) of the lymph node, and organisms gain access to the blood stream after 5 to 10 days, causing septicemia. Subsequently, the lung becomes involved, and pneumonic plague develops. Aerosols from such individuals are highly infectious and lead to a form of plague more rapidly progressive than that after a flea bite; this may be attributed to the release of fully virulent bacilli expressing all virulence factors, subsequent to host passage.

Plague is linked epidemiologically to rodent and flea populations and climatic conditions, with warm areas predominating, especially the southwestern part of the United States. Interestingly, a warm climate may actually favor development of virulence factors in the flea by *Y. pestis*, such as plasminogen activator, which would enhance spread of the bacillus subsequent to a flea bite. Plague endemic areas also

TABLE 209–6 ■ Virulence Factors of *Yersinia pestis*

FACTOR	DETERMINANT	ROLE IN PATHOGENESIS
Serum resistance	Chromosome	Resistance to complement-mediated lysis
Fraction 1 (Fra) (protein capsule)	110-kb plasmid	Antiphagocytic
V antigen (LcrV) (protein)	72-kb plasmid	Unknown; essential for virulence; neutralized by antibody; intracellular survival and multiplication
W antigen (envelope lipoprotein)	72-kb plasmid	Unknown; essential for virulence; intracellular survival and multiplication
pH6 antigen	Chromosome	Epithelial cell adherence; intracellular survival?
Plasminogen activator	9.5-kb plasmid	Dissolves fibrin clots; enhances systemic spread; degrades C3b, C5a
Coagulase	9.5-kb plasmid	Dissolves fibrin clots
Hemin absorption	Chromosome	Iron source masks bacterial surface
Pesticin	9.5-kb plasmid	Unknown

include Southeast Asia (Myanmar, China), South America (Bolivia, Brazil, Ecuador, Peru), Africa, and the Middle East (Saudi Arabia, Afghanistan).[59]

Treatment of plague is through administration of antibiotics (streptomycin, tetracycline, chloramphenicol)[60]; prevention is achieved through a formalin-inactivated vaccine. Control entails curtailing wild rodent and flea populations and instituting quarantine measures.

References

1. Evans ME, Gregory DW, Schaffner W, et al: Tularemia: A 30-year experience with 88 cases. Medicine (Baltimore) 64:251, 1985.
2. Ohara Y, Sato T, Fugita H, et al: Clinical manifestations of tularemia in Japan—Analysis of 1,355 cases observed between 1924 and 1987. Infection 19:14, 1991.
3. Warring WB, Ruffin JS Jr.: A tick-borne epidemic of tularemia. N Engl J Med 234:137, 1946.
4. Francis E: A summary of present knowledge of tularemia. Medicine (Baltimore) 7:411, 1928.
5. Young LS, Bickwell DS, Archer BG, et al: Tularemia epidemic: Vermont, 1968. Forty-seven cases linked to contact with muskrats. N Engl J Med 280:1253, 1969.
6. Weaver RE, Hollis DG, Bottone EJ: Gram-negative fermentative bacteria and *Francisella tularensis*. *In* Lennette E, Balows A, Hausler WJ Jr, Shadomy HJ (eds): Manual of Clinical Microbiology, ed 4. Washington, DC, American Society for Microbiology, 1985, pp 305–329.
7. Berdal BP, Soderlund E: Cultivation and isolation of *Francisella tularensis* on selective chocolate agar as used routinely for the isolation of gonococci. Acta Pathol Microbiol Scand B 85:108, 1977.
8. Schmid GP, Kornblatt AN, Connors CA, et al: Clinically mild tularemia associated with tick-borne *Francisella tularensis*. J Infect Dis 148:63, 1983.
9. Holt JG, Krieg NR, Sneath PHA, et al: Gram-negative aerobic microaerophilic rods and cells. *In* Holt JG, Krieg NR, Sneath PHA, et al (eds): Bergey's Manual of Determinative Bacteriology, ed 9. Baltimore, Williams & Wilkins, 1994, pp 83, 141.
10. Saslaw S, Eigelsbach HT, Wilson HE, et al: Tularemia vaccine study. I. Intracutaneous challenge. Arch Intern Med 107:689, 1961.
11. Saslaw S, Eigelsbach HT, Prior JA, et al: Tularemia vaccine study. II Respiratory challenge. Arch Intern Med 107:702, 1961.
12. Tärnvik A: Nature of protective immunity to *Francisella tularensis*. Rev Infect Dis 11:440, 1989.
13. Hood AM: Virulence factors of *Francisella tularensis*. J Hyg 79:47, 1977.
14. Cherwonogrodzky JW, Knodel MH, Spence MR: Increased encapsulation and virulence of *Francisella tularensis* live vaccine strain (LVS) by subculturing on synthetic medium. Vaccine 12:773, 1994.
15. Lofgren S, Tärnvik A, Blood GD, et al: Phagocytosis and killing of *Francisella tularensis* by human polymorphonuclear leukocytes. Infect Immun 39:715, 1983.
16. Lofgren S, Tärnvik A, Thore M, et al: A wild and an attenuated strain of *Francisella tularensis* differ in susceptibility to hypochlorous acid: A possible explanation to their different handling by polymorphonuclear leukocytes. Infect Immun 43:730, 1984.
17. Sandstrom G, Lofgren S, Tärnvik A: A capsule-deficient mutant of *Francisella tularensis* LVS exhibits enhanced sensitivity to killing by serum but diminished sensitivity to killing by polymorphonuclear leukocytes. Infect Immun 56:1194, 1988.
18. Anthony LSD, Burke RD, Nano FE: Growth of *Francisella* spp. in rodent macrophages. Infect Immun 59:3291, 1991.
19. Fortier AH, Polsinelli T, Green SJ, et al: Activation of macrophages for destruction of *Francisella tularensis*: Identification of cytokines, effector cells, and effector molecules. Infect Immun 60:817, 1992.
20. Conlan JW, Sjöstedt A, North RJ: $CD4^+$ and $CD8^+$ T-cell–dependent and –independent host defense mechanisms can operate to control and resolve primary and secondary *Francisella tularensis* LVS infection in mice. Infect Immun 62:5603, 1994.
21. Enderlin G, Morales L, Jacobs RF, et al: Streptomycin and alternative agents for the treatment of tularemia: Review of the literature. Clin Infect Dis 19:42, 1994.
22. Eigelsbach HT, Downs CM: Prophylactic effectiveness of live and killed tularemia vaccines 1. Production of vaccine and evaluation in the white mouse and guinea pig. J Immunol 87:415, 1961.
23. Paul RV, Rostand SG: Cat-bite peritonitis: *Pasteurella multocida* peritonitis following feline contamination of peritoneal dialysis tubing. Am J Kidney Dis 10:318, 1987.
24. London RD, Bottone EJ: *Pasteurella multocida*: Zoonotic cause of peritonitis in a patient undergoing peritoneal dialysis. Am J Med 91:202, 1991.
25. Majeed H, Verghese A, Rivera RR: The cat and the catheter (Letter). N Engl J Med 332:338, 1995.
26. Hubbert WT, Rosen MN: *Pasteurella multocida* infection in man unrelated to animal bites. Am J Public Health 60:1109, 1970.
27. Itoh M, Tierno PM, Milstoc M, et al: A unique outbreak of *Pasteurella multocida* in a chronic disease hospital. Am J Public Health 70:1170, 1983.
28. Weber DJ, Wolfson JS, Swartz MN, Hooper DC: *Pasteurella multocida* infections. Report of 34 cases and review of the literature. Medicine (Baltimore) 63:133, 1984.
29. Jacobson JA, Miner P, Duffy O: *Pasteurella multocida* bacteremia associated with peritonitis and cirrhosis. Am J Gastroenterol 68:489, 1977.
30. Rimler RB, Rhoades KR: Serogroup F, a new capsule serogroup of *Pasteurella multocida*. J Clin Microbiol 25:615, 1987.
31. Snides KP, Hirsch DC: Association of complement sensitivity with virulence of *Pasteurella multocida* isolated from turkeys. Avian Dis 30:500, 1986.
32. Truscott WM, Hirsch DC: Demonstration of an outer membrane protein with antiphagocytic activity from *Pasteurella multocida* of avian origin. Infect Immun 56:1538, 1988.
33. Snipes KP, Hansen LM, Hirsch DC: Plasma and iron-regulated expression of high molecular weight outer membrane proteins by *Pasteurella multocida*. Am J Vet Res 49:1336, 1988.
34. Watts JL, Yancey RJ, Salmon SA, et al: A 4-year survey of antimicrobial susceptibility trends for isolates from cattle with bovine respiratory disease in North America. J Clin Microbiol 32:725, 1994.
35. Muraski TF, Smith CK, Miller JK: Primary cutaneous (ulceroglandular) infection due to *Pasteurella hemolytica*. N Y State J Med 62:3137, 1962.
36. Doty GL, Loomus GN, Wolf PL: *Pasteurella* endocarditis. N Engl J Med 268:830, 1963.
37. Bitterman H, Shmilovitz M, Rotfeld M, Cohen L: Septic shock due to *Pasteurella hemolytica*. Isr J Med Sci 21:397, 1985.
38. Gump DW, Holden RA: Endocarditis caused by a new species of *Pasteurella*. Ann Intern Med 76:275, 1972.
39. Olson JR, Meadows TR: *Pasteurella pneumotropica* infection resulting from a cat bite. Am J Clin Pathol 51:709, 1969.
40. Medley S: A dog bite wound infected with *Pasteurella pneumotropica*. Med J Aust 2:224, 1977.
41. Winton FW, Mair NS: *Pasteurella pneumotropica* isolated from a dog bite wound. Microbios 2:155, 1969.
42. Gadberry JL, Zipper R, Taylor JA, et al: *Pasteurella pneumotropica* isolated from bone and joint infections. J Clin Microbiol 19:926, 1984.
43. Rogers BT, Anderson JC, Palmer A, et al: Septicemia due to *Pasteurella pneumotropica*. J Clin Pathol 26:396, 1973.
44. Wang WLL, Haiby G: Meningitis caused by *Pasteurella ureae*. Am J Clin Pathol 45:562, 1966.
45. Brass EP, Wray LM, McDuff T: *Pasteurella ureae* meningitis associated with endocarditis. Report of a case and review of the literature. Eur Neurol 22:138, 1983.
46. Noble RC, Marek BJ, Overman SB: Spontaneous bacterial peritonitis caused by *Pasteurella ureae*. J Clin Microbiol 25:442, 1987.
47. Gatti F, Seynhaeve V, Weaver R: First description of a case of human septicemia due to *Pasteurella ureae*. Ann Soc Belg Med Trop 48:463, 1968.
48. Starkebaum GA, Plorde JJ: *Pasteurella* pneumonia: Report of a case and review of the literature. J Clin Microbiol 5:332, 1977.
49. Weniger BG, Warren AJ, Forseth V, et al: Human bubonic plague transmitted by a domestic scratch. JAMA 251:927, 1984.
50. Thornton DJ, Tustin RC, Pienaar BJ, et al: Cat bite transmission of *Yersinia pestis* infection to man. J S Afr Vet Assoc 46:165, 1975.
51. Werner SB, Weidmer CE, Nelson BC, et al: Primary plague pneu-

monia contracted from a domestic cat at South Lake Tahoe, CA. JAMA 251:929, 1984.
52. Doll JM, Zeitz DS, Ettestad P, et al: Cat-transmitted fatal pneumonic plague in a person who traveled from Colorado to Arizona. Am J Trop Med Hyg 51:109, 1994.
53. Mann JD, Hull HF, Schmid GP, et al: Plague and the peripheral smear. JAMA 251:953, 1984.
54. Quan TJ: *Yersinia pestis. In* Balows A (ed): The Prokaryotes: A Handbook on the Biology of Bacteria: Ecophysiology, Isolation, Identification, Applications, ed 2. New York, Springer-Verlag, 1992, pp 2888–2898.
55. Straley SS, Skrzypek E, Plano GV, et al: Yops of *Yersinia* species pathogenic for humans. Infect Immun 61:3105, 1993.
56. Ben-Efrain S, Aronson M, Bichowsky-Slomnicki L: New antigen component of *Pasteurella pestis* formed under specific conditions of pH and temperature. J Bacteriol 81:704, 1961.
57. Linder LE, Tall B: *Y. pestis* pH6 antigen forms fimbriae and is induced by intracellular association with macrophages. Mol Microbiol 8:311, 1993.
58. Ferber DM, Brubaker JR: Plasmids in *Yersinia pestis*. Infect Immun 31:839, 1981.
59. World Health Organization: Weekly Epidemiologic Record. Plague in 1973, 49:253; Plague in 1974, 59:317; Plague in 1975, 51:237; Plague in 1976, 53:229; Human plague in 1986, 40:299, 1974–1987.
60. Barnes AM, Quan TJ: Plague. *In* Gorbach SL, Bartlett JG, Blacklow NR (eds): Infectious Diseases. Philadelphia, WB Saunders, 1992, pp 1285–1291.

210

Pseudomonas aeruginosa and Related Bacteria

Matthew Pollack

Pseudomonas aeruginosa and other *Pseudomonas* species, *Burkholderia* (formerly *Pseudomonas*) *cepacia*, and *Stenotrophomonas* (formerly *Xanthomonas*) *maltophilia* are aerobic, nonfermentative, nonenterobacterial gram-negative bacilli.[1] These bacteria are cosmopolitan in their distribution, inhabiting soil, water, plants, and animals. Their medical importance derives principally from their being opportunistic pathogens, and the clinical diseases they cause are usually nosocomial in origin. Approximately 15% of all gram-negative clinical isolates are non–glucose-fermenting gram-negative rods; of these, more than two thirds are *P. aeruginosa*.

P. aeruginosa and related bacteria share many epidemiologic and clinical characteristics. They are hearty, free-living organisms with minimal nutritional requirements and a predilection for wet environments. They are widely distributed in nature, despite the absence of a discrete natural reservoir, and they abound in hospitals. They rarely infect normal persons but are capable of producing serious, sometimes life-threatening disease in immunocompromised persons. They exhibit innate resistance to many commonly used antibiotics and are capable of developing new resistance on exposure to antimicrobial agents. They are found in the inanimate hospital environment, particularly in association with moisture. They may be spread from patient to patient on the hands of hospital personnel or by other fomites. Patients with serious underlying illnesses who are exposed to the hospital environment, subjected to invasive procedures, immunosuppressed, or treated with broad-spectrum antibiotics are more likely to become colonized with *P. aeruginosa* or related bacteria and are more susceptible to subsequent infection.

The opinions or assertions contained herein are the private ones of the author and are not to be construed as official or reflecting the views of the Department of Defense or the Uniformed Services University of the Health Sciences.

Pseudomonas aeruginosa

Microbiologic Characteristics of the Pathogen

P. aeruginosa is isolated from clinical sources more often than all other *Pseudomonas* species combined and is more often associated with clinical disease. Most *P. aeruginosa* strains are identifiable on the basis of their grapelike odor and production of pyocyanin, a blue-green, nonfluorescent, phenazine pigment. Apyocyanogenic strains are identified on the basis of their polar monotrichous flagella, motility, acid production from glucose but not lactose or sucrose on open oxidation-fermentation medium, positive indophenol oxidase and L-arginine dihydrolase reactions, and growth at 42°C.[2] *P. aeruginosa* is usually identifiable by computer-based, automated gram-negative identification systems. However, differentiation of pyocyanin-negative *P. aeruginosa* strains from non-*aeruginosa* species may require further testing for differential growth at 42°C, oxidation of various sugars, and flagellar morphologic characteristics.

Epidemiology

P. aeruginosa frequents moist microenvironments in hospitals, such as sinks, disinfectant solutions, inhalation equipment, medicines, and food. Although not usually part of normal human bacterial flora, *P. aeruginosa* does colonize hospitalized patients. The frequency of colonization is increased by underlying disease or injury and by invasive procedures that breach, circumvent, or impair normal physical barriers to bacterial invasion or other host defense mechanisms. Nosocomial infections with *P. aeruginosa* are often preceded by colonization by the infecting strain. Although discrete sources for these infections are rarely identified, occasional epidemics are traced to a single source, such as an operating room suction apparatus, respiratory equipment, transvenous pacemaker, endoscope, or physiotherapy pool.

According to data from the Centers for Disease Control and Prevention National Nosocomial Infections Surveillance System covering the period 1986 to 1996,[3, 4] *P. aeruginosa* was the fifth most common hospital pathogen and second leading gram-negative organism after *Escherichia coli*, accounting for 9% of all nosocomial bacterial and fungal isolates. It was the second most common cause of hospital-acquired pneumonia and the leading cause of intensive care unit–related pneumonia (17% of isolates), the third most common urinary tract isolate (11%), the fourth most common cause of surgical site infection (8%), and the eighth most common blood stream isolate (3%).

Pathogenesis

The pathogenesis of *Pseudomonas* infections is complex. A classic opportunistic pathogen, *P. aeruginosa* is a rare cause of disease in normal persons but is highly virulent in patients with impaired host defense mechanisms. The broad spectrum of disease produced by *Pseudomonas* suggests pathogenic versatility based on use of multiple virulence factors. The opportunistic virulence of *P. aeruginosa* is related to its ability to colonize a variety of anatomic sites (owing to effective adherence mechanisms, minimal nutritional requirements, and antibiotic resistance), its capacity for local tissue invasion and damage, and its propensity for blood stream invasion with resulting systemic disease.

The colonization by *Pseudomonas* of mucosal surfaces such as respiratory epithelium is facilitated by its attachment to epithelial cells by means of pili or fimbriae. Adherence is enhanced by prior tissue injury, such as that produced in the respiratory tract by influenza virus infection or endotracheal intubation.[5] So-called mucoid exopolysaccharide (MEP) elaborated by mucoid strains of *P. aeruginosa* isolated from the respiratory secretions of cystic fibrosis (CF) patients also acts as an "adhesin" for tracheal epithelial cells and for tracheobronchial mucin. The putative receptors for pili and MEP appear to contain *N*-acetylneuraminic acid (sialic acid) and *N*-acetylglucosamine, respectively.[6,7]

The MEP produced by mucoid *Pseudomonas* contains a polymer of mannuronic and guluronic acid called alginate. MEP serves a virulence function by protecting mucoid CF respiratory isolates from mucociliary and opsonophagocytic clearance mechanisms. MEP may also protect *Pseudomonas* against the antibacterial activity of aminoglycoside antibiotics. Like MEP, lipopolysaccharide contained in the outer membrane of *Pseudomonas* organisms appears to protect the organism from antibody- and complement-mediated clearance.

The locally invasive and destructive properties of *Pseudomonas* appear to be interrelated. *P. aeruginosa* elaborates a number of extracellular enzymes or toxins that act selectively on various host tissues. Alkaline protease and elastase, for example, produce necrosis in lung, cornea, and skin.[8] Elastase dissolves the internal elastic lamina of blood vessels and is in part responsible for the hemorrhage and necrosis observed in certain locally invasive *Pseudomonas* infections. More specifically, *Pseudomonas* proteases appear to contribute to the characteristic necrotic skin lesions referred to as ecthyma gangrenosum (see later). These enzymes are not cytotoxic but disrupt connections between cells. They cleave human collagen, degrade the laminin component of basement membranes, and solubilize lung elastin. Proteases potentiate the invasive properties of *Pseudomonas* through tissue breakdown and the proteolysis of immunoglobulins and complement.

P. aeruginosa produces heat-labile and heat-stable hemolysins; the heat-labile hemolysin is referred to as phospholipase C, which breaks down lipids and lecithin.[9,10] Like protease, these enzymes produce tissue necrosis and contribute to the invasive properties of the organism. Another toxin produced by *P. aeruginosa*, leukocidin or cytotoxin, is cytopathic for polymorphonuclear leukocytes and other eukaryotic cells. It has been implicated in microvascular injury commonly associated with *Pseudomonas* disease.[11]

Pseudomonas lipopolysaccharide (endotoxin) and exotoxin A appear to be responsible for many of the systemic manifestations of *Pseudomonas* disease. Endotoxin causes fever, leukocytosis or leukopenia, hypotension, and oliguria and is a direct participant in events leading to disseminated intravascular coagulation and adult respiratory distress syndrome. These and other physiologic abnormalities associated with gram-negative sepsis are largely produced by endotoxin acting indirectly through mediators such as tumor necrosis factor, interleukin-1, and interleukin-6; arachidonic acid metabolites; and components of the complement, kinin, clotting, and fibrinolytic systems. Whereas endotoxin is common to all gram-negative bacteria, exotoxin A is specific for *P. aeruginosa.* A single polypeptide chain of 613 amino acids, exotoxin A is a potent inhibitor of protein synthesis by a mechanism involving adenosine diphosphate ribosylation of elongation factor-2, which is inactivated by this reaction and is no longer capable of catalyzing polypeptide biosynthesis.[12,13] Exotoxin A has direct cytopathic effects on a wide variety of mammalian cells and appears to mediate systemic toxic effects as well. Exotoxin A is lethal in exceedingly small quantities for animals, including subhuman primates. Toxin-positive *P. aeruginosa* blood isolates have been associated with greater virulence in *Pseudomonas* septicemia compared with toxin-negative strains.[14] Moreover, enhanced survival has been noted in patients with high preexisting levels of toxin A–specific serum antibodies at the onset of *Pseudomonas* septicemia.[15] These data suggest a lethal pathogenic role for toxin A in septicemic *Pseudomonas* infections and a protective role for toxin A–specific antibodies.

Clinical Manifestations and Treatment

GENERAL PRINCIPLES

Because *P. aeruginosa* is a common human saprophyte and is ubiquitous in the hospital environment, it may be difficult to distinguish infection from colonization, particularly in the case of specimens obtained from superficial sites such as wounds, sinus drainage, or respiratory secretions. Clinical evidence of infection must therefore accompany simple demonstration of the organism at a potential infection site.

P. aeruginosa is responsible for a broad spectrum of disease in a variety of clinical settings (Table 210–1). Some *P. aeruginosa* infections are acute, even fulminant; others are subacute or chronic and more indolent. The protean manifestations of *Pseudomonas* disease, as well as the varying levels of severity

TABLE 210–1 ■ Infections Caused by *Pseudomonas aeruginosa*

Acquired immunodeficiency syndrome–related infections
Bacteremia
Primary
Secondary
Bone and joint infections
Sternoarticular pyarthrosis
Vertebral osteomyelitis
Symphysis pubis infection
Osteochondritis of the foot
Chronic contiguous osteomyelitis
Central nervous system infections
Meningitis
Brain abscess
Ear infections
Otitis externa
Malignant external otitis
Chronic suppurative otitis media
Endocarditis
Native heart valve infection in intravenous drug users
Prosthetic heart valve infection
Eye infections
Keratitis (corneal ulcer)
Endophthalmitis
Gastrointestinal infections
Necrotizing enterocolitis
Epidemic diarrhea
Shanghai fever
Respiratory infections
Pneumonia
Nonbacteremic
Bacteremic
Lower respiratory tract infection in cystic fibrosis
Skin and soft tissue infections
Ecthyma gangrenosum
Pyoderma
Wound infection
Dermatitis
Burn wound sepsis
Urinary tract infections
Acute
Chronic (frequently with sites of persistence or obstruction)

and acuteness, dictate different therapies and signal different prognoses.

The nature and severity of a patient's underlying disease and the immune status determine both the likelihood of *Pseudomonas* infection and the level of associated morbidity and mortality. Persistent neutropenia is an especially critical predisposing factor as well as an indicator of unfavorable prognosis. *P. aeruginosa* infections involving the lower respiratory tract or blood stream are associated with inordinately high mortality, reflecting the poor clinical status of susceptible patients in addition to the inherent virulence of the organism. The anatomic location of infection and overall clinical status of the infected patient thus dictate appropriate therapy.

P. aeruginosa exhibits innate or acquired resistance to many commonly used antibiotics, thus complicating therapy. This and other mechanisms of bacterial persistence at sites of infection make *P. aeruginosa* infections particularly difficult to treat and the organism difficult to eradicate. These factors often necessitate aggressive therapy employing maximal safe antibiotic doses, synergistic antimicrobial combinations, and prolonged treatment.

On the other hand, many *P. aeruginosa* clinical isolates remain sensitive to the aminoglycosides (e.g., gentamicin, tobramycin, amikacin, netilmicin), selected extended-spectrum penicillins (e.g., ticarcillin, ticarcillin-clavulanate, piperacillin, piperacillin-tazobactam, mezlocillin, azlocillin), cephalosporins (e.g., ceftazidime, cefoperazone, cefepime), carbapenems (e.g., imipenem, meropenem), monobactams (aztreonam), and fluoroquinolones (e.g., ciprofloxacin, ofloxacin, enoxacin, lomefloxacin, norfloxacin). Two of the newer broad-spectrum agents, meropenem[16–19] and cefepime,[20, 21] may prove particularly useful in treating infections due to multidrug-resistant strains of *P. aeruginosa* because of their favorable microbial susceptibility profiles, pharmacokinetic properties, and safety characteristics. The therapeutic efficacy of these newer agents against *P. aeruginosa* requires further confirmation in clinical practice.

BACTEREMIA

P. aeruginosa is the fourth leading cause of hospital-acquired gram-negative rod bacteremia[3] and possibly that associated with the highest mortality rate.[22] *Pseudomonas* bacteremia may result from identifiable focal infections but is described as primary when no other infection site is discernible. Primary *Pseudomonas* bacteremia is particularly common in patients with hematologic malignant neoplasms who suffer from chemotherapy-induced neutropenia. Secondary bacteremias are most commonly associated with respiratory, gastrointestinal, urinary tract, or skin and soft tissue infections. Infected intravascular devices are also common sources of *Pseudomonas* bacteremia.

Most of the clinical signs and symptoms of *Pseudomonas* bacteremia are indistinguishable from those associated with gram-negative sepsis caused by other bacteria. Exceptions are the greater likelihood of respiratory failure associated with bacteremic *Pseudomonas* pneumonia; more frequent jaundice; and ecthyma gangrenosum skin lesions, which, although found in a minority of bacteremic patients, are virtually pathognomonic when they are present.[23] Other types of skin lesions have also been reported in association with *Pseudomonas* bacteremia, including small painful vesicles that occur in clusters on an erythematous base; flat, sharply demarcated areas of cellulitis, which may expand rapidly, becoming hemorrhagic and necrotic; diffuse maculopapular eruptions concentrated on the trunk; and metastatic abscesses on the extremities, which occasionally are seen late in the disease.[24]

Like most other invasive *Pseudomonas* infections, bacteremia should be treated with an antibiotic combination, such as an aminoglycoside and β-lactam agent with antipseudomonal activity. The choice of particular agents should be dictated by local antibiotic susceptibility patterns and prescribing practices. Care should be exercised, however, in choosing a third-generation cephalosporin, because moxalactam and cefotaxime exhibit unpredictable efficacy against *P. aeruginosa*. The use of synergistic antibiotic combinations is most critical in immunocompromised patients, particularly those with severe or persistent neutropenia. In such patients, synergy between the antimicrobial agents employed increases the likelihood of survival.[25–27] Maximal safe doses of both agents should be used. The proper duration of therapy is dictated by the severity of the infection, therapeutic response, and presence or persistence of neutropenia.

BONE AND JOINT INFECTIONS

Pseudomonas infections of the bones and joints result from direct inoculation, contiguous spread, or hematogenous dissemination from distant sites. *Pseudomonas* bone and joint infections occur in the face of underlying diseases such as diabetes mellitus or other predisposing factors such as chronic debilitation, intravenous drug abuse, and penetrating trauma. *Pseudomonas* has a particular affinity for fibrocartilaginous joints of the axial skeleton, involving cartilage, synovium, joint space, and contiguous bone. *Pseudomonas* osteomyelitis tends to be more indolent and less destructive than bone infections caused by *Staphylococcus aureus*.[28]

Pseudomonas pyarthrosis of the sternoclavicular or sternochondral joints occurs principally in intravenous drug users.[29] The most common symptoms, which may begin months before diagnosis, are anterior chest pain at the site of involvement and restriction of movement of the ipsilateral shoulder. Swelling, erythema, and tenderness occur over the affected joint; range of motion of the shoulder may be limited on the affected side; and fever is usually present. There is typically an accompanying leukocytosis, and the erythrocyte sedimentation rate is almost always elevated. Aspiration of synovial fluid reveals characteristics of a pyogenic infection, and cultures propagate *Pseudomonas* despite the frequent difficulty in identifying organisms on Gram stain of joint fluid. Blood cultures are also occasionally positive. Radiographs reveal soft tissue swelling; demineralization or lytic lesions of adjacent bone; and periosteal elevation of the sternum, rib, or clavicular head. Arthrotomy may be required to débride contiguous areas of involved bone, and perisynovial or retrosternal abscesses may necessitate surgical drainage. An aminoglycoside and extended-spectrum penicillin should be administered for a minimum of 6 weeks.

P. aeruginosa produces vertebral osteomyelitis in elderly patients in association with complicated urinary tract infections and genitourinary instrumentation or surgery.[30] The lumbosacral spine is most commonly involved. *Pseudomonas* vertebral osteomyelitis also occurs in intravenous drug users.[31] The cervical spine is most frequently affected in these patients. Symptoms, including neck or back pain, may last weeks or months. Fever and other systemic symptoms are relatively uncommon. Local tenderness and decreased range of motion of the spine are found on physical examination, whereas neurologic signs are observed in approximately 15% of patients. Fever, when present, is usually low grade. Leukocytosis is variable, and the erythrocyte sedimentation rate is almost always elevated. Radiographs of the affected spine may demonstrate loss of bone density, lytic lesions of vertebral bodies, sclerosis, a narrowed interspace, destruction of adjacent vertebral end plates, and osteophyte formation. Computed tomography (CT) or magnetic resonance imaging (MRI) reveals changes in bone density or soft tissue densities and may be the most sensitive means for defining the extent of disease. Technetium- and gallium-enhanced scans are also useful for this purpose. The diagnosis of *Pseudomonas* vertebral osteomyelitis can often be established through needle biopsy or aspiration under fluoroscopic guidance. Surgery is sometimes necessary for adequate exploration and bone biopsy or for decompression of a rare associated epidural or paravertebral abscess. An aminoglycoside antibiotic should be administered for at least 4 weeks, preferably in combination with a second agent to which the infecting strain is susceptible. The need for antibiotic combinations in this disease is not well documented, however. A longer course of therapy may be advisable if the area of involvement is extensive, the erythrocyte sedimentation rate remains elevated, or a single antibiotic is employed.

Pseudomonas infections of the symphysis pubis are associated with pelvic surgery and intravenous drug abuse.[32] Symptoms include groin, thigh, hip, and lower abdominal pain, which is made worse by walking. There is typically exquisite tenderness over the symphysis pubis, and the patient may be febrile. Symptoms may be present for weeks or months before the patient seeks medical attention. Leukocytosis is variable, whereas an elevated erythrocyte sedimentation rate is common. Radiography shows irregularity of the pubic margins, separation of the symphysis pubis, and involvement of the pubic rami, in most cases. Findings of bone scans are usually abnormal. Biopsy or needle aspiration of the symphysis pubis is necessary to make the diagnosis and to distinguish osteomyelitis from osteitis pubis, a presumably noninfectious disease. Most *Pseudomonas* infections of the symphysis pubis are curable with antibiotics alone and do not require surgical débridement. An aminoglycoside should be used, alone or in combination with a semisynthetic penicillin active against *Pseudomonas,* and therapy is continued at least 4 weeks.

P. aeruginosa is the most common cause of osteochondritis after puncture wounds of the foot.[33] This infection is seen primarily in children but also occurs occasionally in adults. It involves cartilage and bone surrounding small joints and bones of the foot, reflecting the peculiar predilection of *Pseudomonas* for fibrocartilaginous joints. Pain and swelling may develop a number of days after a puncture wound of the foot, and weeks may pass before the patient seeks medical attention. Fever and other systemic signs are usually absent. Tenderness or frank cellulitis is discernible over the affected joint. Possible areas of involvement include the proximal phalanges, metatarsals, metatarsophalangeal joints, tarsal bones, and calcaneus. Radiography and bone scan findings are usually abnormal, and aspiration of the infected joint may yield a small amount of purulent, culture-positive fluid. Treatment consists of surgical débridement and antibiotics, which are continued for a minimum of 4 weeks.

Chronic contiguous osteomyelitis[34] arises by direct extension from infected overlying soft tissue or direct inoculation rather than by hematogenous spread. *P. aeruginosa* is frequently implicated in this type of infection, which may follow a compound fracture, penetrating trauma, or surgery involving bone. These infections may also complicate peripheral neuropathy or peripheral vascular disease associated with pressure necrosis of skin and soft tissue or ischemic ulcers overlying bone. The heterogeneity of these infections makes it difficult to establish general therapeutic guidelines. The immediate goal of therapy is to achieve and sustain effective antibiotic levels in blood and bone. An aminoglycoside and antipseudomonal penicillin can be administered parenterally for 4 to 6 weeks; complicated infections may require longer treatment, however. Surgical removal of necrotic or prosthetic material or drainage of loculated pus may also be necessary. Single agents such as ceftazidime, imipenem, and ciprofloxacin have been employed successfully in the treatment of chronic *Pseudomonas* osteomyelitis. Treatment failures have occurred with these single-drug regimens, however, necessitating repeated treatment with different antibiotic combinations.[35, 36]

CENTRAL NERVOUS SYSTEM INFECTIONS

P. aeruginosa central nervous system infections (meningitis or brain abscess) may result from (1) direct inoculation of the subarachnoid space or brain secondary to penetrating head trauma or surgery; (2) extension from a contiguous focus, such as infected paranasal sinus or mastoid; or (3) blood stream infection. Other predisposing factors or conditions include previous lumbar puncture, spinal anesthesia, intraventricular shunt or reservoir, cerebrospinal fluid leak, and cancer involving the head or subarachnoid space. *P. aeruginosa* is the second most common cause of meningitis and brain abscess in patients with cancer.[37]

Pseudomonas meningitis presents, as do other forms of meningitis, with fever, headache, irritability, and obtundation. The onset of meningitis symptoms may be acute, or even fulminant, particularly in association with bacteremia. The clinical course may be compressed into several hours or days and may be accompanied by septic shock. In contrast, *Pseudomonas* meningitis may develop insidiously, especially when it is associated with a contiguous site of infection or cancer involving the subarachnoid space.

Appropriate antibiotic therapy for *Pseudomonas* meningitis is dictated by the relative bactericidal activity of various agents and their ability to penetrate the subarachnoid space.[38] Ceftazidime has generally been dependable in vitro and in vivo against *Pseudomonas* and achieves cerebrospinal fluid concentrations well in excess of the mean inhibitory concentration for most strains. Ceftazidime may therefore be considered the drug of first choice for the treatment of *Pseudomonas* meningitis.[39–41] The need for combination therapy with a second agent is unclear, but it is probably wise to include an aminoglycoside with initial therapy, particularly if the infection is rapidly progressive or life threatening. Because ceftazidime crosses the blood-brain barrier efficiently, there is ordinarily no need for intrathecal administration of either it or an accompanying aminoglycoside. When there is obstruction of the subarachnoid space or ventriculitis is present, the aminoglycoside may have to be instilled directly into the ventricular system through a catheter or reservoir.[42, 43] The proper duration of antibiotic treatment of *Pseudomonas* meningitis is determined by the extent of disease, structural integrity of the involved central nervous system, and initial response to therapy. A minimum of 2 weeks' treatment is usually appropriate. Relapses are common and must be managed aggressively.

Pseudomonas brain abscess is treated with surgical drainage and prolonged antibiotic therapy. The choice of antimicrobial agents should be determined as it is for meningitis. Intrathecal therapy is not indicated unless persistent meningitis or ventriculitis is present. Abscess size is monitored by CT or MRI, and antibiotic therapy is continued until a marked diminution in abscess size or closure is achieved. Failure of initial therapy may necessitate surgical reexploration and drainage, with additional antibiotic treatment.

EAR INFECTIONS

P. aeruginosa is isolated from the external auditory canal of most patients with external otitis,[44] a superficial, self-limited infection that usually resolves spontaneously or responds to local measures. On occasion, however, *Pseudomonas* penetrates the epithelium at the junction between cartilage and bone in the floor of the lateral portion of the external auditory canal and invades underlying soft tissue, cartilage, and bone.

This invasive, necrotizing process is commonly referred to as malignant external otitis.[45–48] It is principally a disease of elderly diabetic patients but occasionally affects young infants with serious underlying diseases.[49, 50] Once the infection enters the parotid space or retromandibular area, bypassing the tympanic membrane and middle ear, it enters the mastoid airspaces and temporal bone. It may spread through the temporal bone and the base of the skull, involving the 7th cranial nerve at the stylomastoid foramen; the 9th, 10th, and 11th cranial nerves at the jugular foramen; and the 12th cranial nerve at the hypoglossal canal. The lateral and sigmoid sinuses may also become involved, with further extension through vascular channels across the base of the skull. Meningitis and brain abscess are infrequent complications.

The most common symptoms of malignant external otitis are otalgia and otorrhea. Facial nerve paralysis occurs early, and other nerve palsies are observed later in the disease. The pinna of the involved ear may be tender; trismus may be present; and diminished hearing is sometimes reported. Fever and weight loss are uncommon. Physical examination reveals a swollen, erythematous external auditory canal with purulent discharge. The tympanic membrane is intact in some patients, perforated in others, or hidden from view by edema, granulation tissue, and debris. Pain and tenderness are often noted in the pinna and soft tissue adjacent to the ear.

Leukocytosis and cerebrospinal fluid pleocytosis are occasional laboratory findings in malignant external otitis. A marked elevation in the erythrocyte sedimentation rate is almost always observed. CT may reveal bony erosions and new bone formation in the mastoid and temporal bone. Soft tissue densities are associated with areas of cellulitis involving the floor of the skull. MRI is superior to CT in defining the extent of disease and soft tissue involvement.[51] Technetium Tc 99m–enhanced bone scans may document early bone involvement, whereas gallium Ga 67 scans help distinguish infection from neoplastic disease. *P. aeruginosa* is isolated from the external auditory canal or from surgical specimens in virtually all cases of malignant external otitis. Although other bacteria may also be present, *P. aeruginosa* should be considered the primary agent of this disease.

Malignant external otitis is treated with antibiotics in conjunction with surgical débridement and drainage. Surgical drainage, dictated by sites of involvement and the presence of pus or devitalized tissue, might include débridement of necrotic bone or cartilage, mastoidectomy, or facial nerve decompression. Current thinking favors more limited surgery in conjunction with aggressive antibiotic therapy,[48] which usually entails use of an aminoglycoside in combination with a β-lactam agent with good antipseudomonal activity. The duration of therapy should be a minimum of 4 weeks in the case of relatively limited disease and 6 to 8 weeks when the infection is more extensive. Although single agents have been used successfully in some cases, published data suggest the greater efficacy of combination therapy in more severe disease.[47, 52] Because malignant external otitis is difficult to eradicate and relapse is common, optimal management entails the prolonged use of two agents. Even in the face of optimal therapy, the mortality from malignant external otitis remains as high as 15% to 20%. Long-term follow-up, necessitated by the risk for relapse, should include the monitoring of pain, erythrocyte sedimentation rate, and serial CT or MRI studies.

Chronic suppurative otitis media is most often caused by *P. aeruginosa*, sometimes in combination with other organisms. Tympanomastoid surgery is frequently employed when medical treatment alone is unsuccessful; however, evidence suggests that aggressive antibiotic therapy, in conjunction with daily otic toilet, may be curative, precluding surgery in cases in which cholesteatoma is not present.[53]

ENDOCARDITIS

P. aeruginosa causes infections of native heart valves in intravenous drug abusers as well as infections of prosthetic heart valves.[54–57] The tricuspid valve is most frequently involved in drug addicts, but the pulmonic, aortic, or mitral valve and mural endocardium of either atrium may also be affected. Right-sided involvement is often subacute in onset, whereas left-sided disease tends to be more acute. Septic pulmonary emboli occur in tricuspid valve endocarditis and may be associated with productive cough, pleuritic chest pain, and pulmonary infiltrates. Left-sided disease, on the other hand, may be accompanied by large systemic arterial embolization and intractable congestive heart failure. Cardiac murmurs are usual. Diagnosis is based on positive blood cultures and appropriate clinical signs. Abnormal two-dimensional echocardiographic findings are often confirmatory. Tricuspid insufficiency may be documented by cardiac catheterization or cineangiography.

Medical therapy for tricuspid endocarditis should include an aminoglycoside (e.g., tobramycin, 8 mg/kg per day) plus an antipseudomonal penicillin (e.g., ticarcillin, 18 g/d). If bacteremia persists beyond 2 weeks' therapy or recurs after 6 weeks' therapy, tricuspid valvulectomy should be undertaken, without valve replacement.[55–57] The pulmonic valve should be inspected at the time of surgery and also removed if it is involved. Left-sided *Pseudomonas* endocarditis represents a medical and surgical emergency. Antibiotic therapy, as described for right-sided disease, should be started and the involved aortic or mitral valve replaced immediately. CT should be performed before surgery, and if splenic abscesses are found, splenectomy should be accomplished before cardiac surgery. Antibiotic therapy should be continued for at least 6 weeks, with peak gentamicin or tobramycin serum levels maintained at 12 to 20 μg/mL or at least 10 times the mean bactericidal concentration. The prognosis for cure of tricuspid endocarditis, with valvulectomy if necessary, is approximately 80%. The success rate for treatment of left-sided disease is as low as 11%,[54] but higher cure rates may be achieved with early surgery.[58]

EYE INFECTIONS

P. aeruginosa causes keratitis (corneal ulcer) and endophthalmitis. When introduced by direct inoculation or hematogenous spread into the avascular, immunologically sequestered environment of the eye, *P. aeruginosa* can produce rapidly destructive and sometimes sight-threatening disease. Treatment is complicated by the existence of the so-called blood-eye barrier, which limits the delivery of antibiotics to infected intraocular structures.

Eye trauma, sometimes extremely minor, predisposes to *P. aeruginosa* corneal infections by causing a break in the epithelial surface and allowing access of bacteria to the underlying stroma. *Pseudomonas* keratitis appears to be more common in warm, humid environments such as those found in the southeastern United States. It is also associated with contact lens use, particularly the soft extended-wear type.[59] There is a higher frequency of *Pseudomonas* keratitis in patients with underlying ocular conditions and in those treated with topical steroids or contaminated eye medications.[60] Other predisposing conditions include coma, tracheostomy or endotracheal intubation, extensive burns, intensive care, and ocular irradiation.[61–63]

Pseudomonas keratitis often starts as a small central ulcer that spreads centrifugally to involve the entire cornea and portions of the surrounding sclera. The infection may also penetrate more deeply into underlying stroma, causing corneal perforation in some instances. Typical clinical signs of

Pseudomonas keratitis include a rapidly evolving grayish, necrotic stromal infiltrate in the bed of an epithelial injury; tenacious mucopurulent discharge; surrounding epithelial edema; and severe anterior chamber reaction. The lesion may spread rapidly in 24 to 48 hours to involve the entire cornea, leading in some cases to perforation, or it may evolve more gradually during several days. Systemic symptoms, including low-grade fever, are somewhat unusual.

Pseudomonas corneal ulcer should be considered a medical emergency because of the chance of perforation into the anterior chamber, leading to a rapidly destructive intraocular infection and possibly blindness. Scrapings from the floor of the ulcer are examined by Gram stain and cultured. The presence of gram-negative rods, or even a negative Gram stain, requires the institution of combined topical and subconjunctival or subtenon therapy with an aminoglycoside antibiotic such as gentamicin. An ophthalmic solution containing 8 mg/mL of aminoglycoside should be instilled hourly in the affected eye.[64] A quinolone-containing ophthalmic solution (e.g., enoxacin) may be an effective alternative for topical therapy.[65] Although small ulcers can often be treated effectively with topical therapy alone, more advanced lesions require simultaneous treatment with subconjunctival or subtenon injections of an aminoglycoside.[66] This is particularly critical if perforation into the anterior chamber appears imminent. Gentamicin can be used at a dose of 20 mg, administered once or twice daily for 3 days or until cultures are negative. Subconjunctival ceftazidime may represent an effective alternative to gentamicin, although clinical data are limited.

Pseudomonas endophthalmitis may occur as a complication of perforating corneal ulcer, penetrating injuries, intraocular surgery, or bacteremia originating outside the eye.[67–69] It is an acute, fulminant disease that can lead rapidly to the loss of sight. This characteristic of *Pseudomonas* endophthalmitis distinguishes it from other less severe forms of endophthalmitis caused by less virulent bacteria. Clinical features include pain, decreased visual acuity, conjunctival chemosis and hyperemia, lid edema, hypopyon, and anterior uveitis. These are followed by involvement of the vitreous and panophthalmitis. Proper management of *Pseudomonas* endophthalmitis begins with aspiration of the anterior chamber or vitreous cavity to obtain material for Gram stain and culture. Wound drainage after intraocular surgery may be cultured in lieu of aspirated material from the eye, although superficial conjunctival cultures are undependable. Appropriate antibiotic therapy includes an aminoglycoside administered by the topical, subconjunctival (or subtenon), intraocular, and parenteral routes as well as an antipseudomonal penicillin given subconjunctivally. Ceftazidime may provide effective alternative therapy. Vitrectomy is frequently useful to clear areas of loculated infection, dispose of necrotic material, and enhance antibiotic penetration into the eye. Antibiotic therapy should be continued until clinical improvement occurs and signs of infection in the eye have subsided. The prognosis for *Pseudomonas* endophthalmitis diagnosed early and treated aggressively has improved markedly compared with that in the past.

GASTROINTESTINAL INFECTIONS

The gastrointestinal tract represents a common portal of entry for *Pseudomonas* blood stream infections as well as a frequent site of primary infection. *Pseudomonas* is one of the most common causes of necrotizing enterocolitis in young infants.[70, 71] Affected patients present with irritability, vomiting, diarrhea, and dehydration. Physical findings include fever, abdominal distention, and signs of peritonitis. A similar disease occurs in neutropenic cancer patients.[72, 73] The most common sites of involvement are the distal ileum, cecum, and colon. Localized lesions of the cecum associated with necrosis and gangrene (typhlitis), sometimes leading to perforation with resultant peritonitis, are most often seen in patients with acute leukemia. On pathologic examination, necrotizing enterocolitis is similar in young infants and adults. Ulcerating lesions begin in the bowel mucosa and extend into the submucosa. The ulcers are hemorrhagic as well as necrotic and contain *Pseudomonas* on culture. Bacteria may invade submucosal blood vessels, spread to involve the muscularis and serosa, and cause bowel perforation with associated peritonitis. Necrotizing enterocolitis is best treated with an aminoglycoside antibiotic combined with a second agent active against *P. aeruginosa*. Surgical intervention may be necessary in the event of bowel gangrene or perforation. Death is common despite aggressive therapy.

Epidemic diarrhea due to *P. aeruginosa* has been reported in children.[74, 75] The seriousness of diarrheal disease associated with such outbreaks varies from mild to severe; the severe type is sometimes accompanied by vascular collapse and even death. *P. aeruginosa* has also been associated with a syndrome that resembles enteric fever. So-called Shanghai fever[76, 77] presents with constipation or diarrhea, rash, and fever lasting 1 to 2 weeks. *Pseudomonas* is isolated from stool, but its causal role is unclear, and the curative action of antibiotics is not known. Even less clear is the pathogenic role of a putative enterotoxin produced by selected *P. aeruginosa* strains associated with cases of secretory diarrhea.[78]

RESPIRATORY INFECTIONS

P. aeruginosa causes acute, life-threatening, bacteremic[79–81] or nonbacteremic pneumonia[82] in immunocompromised patients, including those with acquired immunodeficiency syndrome (AIDS),[83] as well as chronic lower respiratory tract disease in patients with CF. Patients exposed to the hospital environment, particularly in an intensive care setting, are subject to upper respiratory tract colonization by *P. aeruginosa*. Previous antibiotic administration and respirator therapy, as well as underlying chronic lung disease and congestive heart failure, predispose colonized patients to lower respiratory tract infection through aspiration of upper respiratory secretions. *Pseudomonas* pneumonia may present as a fulminant infection accompanied by chills, fever, dyspnea, productive cough, cyanosis, and signs of severe systemic toxic effects.[82] Chest radiographs may show a diffuse bronchopneumonia, often bilateral, with distinctive nodular infiltrates, sometimes associated with areas of radiolucency. Lobar consolidation is sometimes seen, pleural effusions are common, but empyema is rare. Microabscesses occur in *Pseudomonas* pneumonia, and necrosis of alveolar septa is observed, but blood vessels are not involved in nonbacteremic infections.

Bacteremic *Pseudomonas* pneumonia occurs principally in neutropenic patients.[79–81] It begins in the lower respiratory tract, is accompanied by blood stream invasion, and often spreads to metastatic sites of infection. Small, nodular, hemorrhagic (and sometimes necrotic) lesions form diffusely in both lung fields. On microscopic examination, these lesions involve small blood vessels and contain many bacteria but lack a leukocytic reaction. They represent the pulmonary counterpart of ecthyma gangrenosum involving the skin (see later). The radiographic picture of bacteremic *Pseudomonas* pneumonia is typified by rapid progression from pulmonary vascular congestion to pulmonary edema to necrotizing bronchopneumonia.[81] The course of this disease is usually compressed into 2 to 3 days and ends fatally.

Most patients with CF suffer from chronic lower respiratory tract infection by mucoid strains of *P. aeruginosa* beginning between the ages of 5 and 18 years.[84] Once established, these infections usually persist for life and follow a progressive, waxing and waning course punctuated by frequent acute exacerbations. Although cause and effect are difficult to separate, genetically determined defects in CF respiratory defense mechanisms clearly predispose to *Pseudomonas* lung infections. Conversely, lower respiratory tract infection by *Pseudomonas* contributes substantially to acute exacerbations and chronic progression of CF lung disease.

The clinical signs and symptoms of *Pseudomonas* pulmonary infection in CF patients vary considerably as a function of the extent of underlying lung disease and the frequency and severity of acute exacerbations.[85] Patients develop a chronic productive cough, decreased appetite, weight loss, and diminished activity, particularly during acute episodes. Wheezing and tachypnea may be present, and low-grade fever is usually documented during acute exacerbations. Physical signs include evidence of undernutrition, clubbing, increased anteroposterior diameter, retractions, cyanosis, wheezing, moist rales and rhonchi, and abdominal distention. Leukocytosis with a leftward shift is usual. Blood gas values demonstrate hypoxemia with or without hypercapnia. Results of pulmonary function tests indicate an obstructive defect and restriction in the presence of chronic fibrosis. Radiographs of the chest show overaeration, peribronchial thickening, patchy atelectasis, and pneumonia.

The treatment of life-threatening *Pseudomonas* lower respiratory tract infections requires the aggressive use of antibiotics. An aminoglycoside and a β-lactam agent, for example, can be combined in maximal tolerable doses to attain optimal bactericidal activity in lung tissue, pulmonary secretions, and blood. Such combination therapy is meant to achieve synergistic killing and to minimize the emergence of resistant strains bearing inducible β-lactamases. The duration of therapy, dictated by the severity of disease and clinical response, should be no less than 10 days in most cases. Maintenance of good pulmonary toilet, respiratory support as required, and appropriate measures to counter septic complications are critical elements of treatment.

The treatment of acute exacerbations of *Pseudomonas* lower respiratory tract infections in CF follows the same principles as those just outlined.[86–89] Antibiotics may be expected to produce temporary improvement in both respiratory symptoms and pulmonary function. *P. aeruginosa* may disappear temporarily from the patient's sputum or persist, sometimes developing resistance to the antibiotic used.[88, 89] After cessation of treatment, however, *P. aeruginosa* usually returns to the sputum or reverts to its original antibiotic susceptibility pattern. Moreover, the clinical improvement associated with antibiotic treatment appears to bear little relation to the microbiology of sputum. Acute exacerbations of *Pseudomonas* lung disease are treated with antibiotics until clinical improvement is noted, customarily 1 to 2 weeks. Larger than usual doses of aminoglycosides and β-lactam agents are frequently required by CF patients because of altered antibiotic pharmacokinetics.[90] Although antibiotic combinations are often used, monotherapy with agents such as piperacillin, ceftazidime, and meropenem has been successfully employed.[91–94] Another promising strategy entails intermittent antibiotic therapy for chronic *Pseudomonas* lung disease aimed at preventing acute exacerbations. This approach, employed in Denmark and facilitated by the availability of quinolone antibiotics, may be responsible in part for improvements in mortality rates.[95–97] Intermittent aerosolization of antibiotics into the lower respiratory tract of CF patients has also apparently resulted in symptomatic improvement and reduced number of hospitalizations.[97–99] Finally, lung transplantation has been employed successfully in CF patients with end-stage *P. aeruginosa*–associated lower respiratory tract disease.[100–103]

SKIN AND SOFT TISSUE INFECTIONS

Ecthyma gangrenosum is a focal skin lesion characterized by hemorrhage, necrosis, surrounding erythema, and vascular invasion by bacteria.[23, 104, 105] Ecthyma lesions are usually associated with *Pseudomonas* bacteremia, although they occur in a minority of such cases. Whereas it is sometimes claimed that ecthyma gangrenosum is pathognomonic for *P. aeruginosa* infections, it has been reported, albeit rarely, in association with *S. maltophilia* sepsis[106, 107] and other forms of gram-negative sepsis.[108] *P. aeruginosa* septicemia, on the other hand, has also been associated with vesicular or pustular skin lesions, subcutaneous nodules, deep abscesses, cellulitis, and bullae.[109–112] Large, destructive lesions of the skin or mucous membranes can complicate *Pseudomonas* sepsis, particularly in neutropenic patients.[113–115] These lesions may produce frank gangrene involving the face, oropharynx, perineum, or extremities. Primary *Pseudomonas* skin lesions may be focal or diffuse. Predisposition to such infections results from skin breakdown secondary to severe burns, trauma, dermatitis, or local ulcerations; moisture involving the perineum, diaper area of small infants, swimmers' ears, soldiers' feet in the tropics, or the skin of spa users; and neutropenia secondary to cancer chemotherapy. Primary *Pseudomonas* pyoderma looks much like ecthyma lesions associated with *Pseudomonas* bacteremia.[114] Both lesions appear hemorrhagic and necrotic, and both are likely to demonstrate vascular invasion by bacteria. Primary and metastatic skin lesions may coexist in septic patients.

Pseudomonas wound infections usually do not have a characteristic appearance that distinguishes them from those caused by other bacteria. However, *Pseudomonas* wound infections or pyoderma may occasionally give rise to a blue-green exudate resulting from the production by *P. aeruginosa* of pyocyanin pigment,[116] and a characteristic fruity odor may be noted. The pyocyanin pigment produced by *Pseudomonas* may be seen more readily on wound dressings or bandages than within the wound itself. Virtually any nonoperative or postoperative wound infection may be caused by *P. aeruginosa,* but the organism should be seriously considered in any wound, such as a compound fracture, that is contaminated with soil, water, or plant material.

P. aeruginosa causes diffuse, pruritic, maculopapular or vesiculopustular rashes in association with exposure to contaminated hot tubs, spas, or whirlpools.[117–119] Many cases are reported as a part of a common-source outbreak. Rashes tend to be more pronounced in the area covered by the bathing suit but can be diffuse. Other clinical manifestations may include headache, dizziness, sore eyes, earache, sore nose, sore throat, breast tenderness, and abdominal pain. Fever is absent or low grade. *Pseudomonas* rashes occurring in this setting are usually self-limited and require no specific therapy. Possible exceptions are immunocompromised patients, including those with neutropenia and AIDS, whose skin involvement may be more invasive and require systemic antimicrobial therapy.[120, 121] The source of exposure should be identified, if possible, and reexposure prevented.

P. aeruginosa was the second most common cause of hospital-acquired burn wound infection, after *S. aureus*, according to a National Nosocomial Infections Surveillance study carried out between 1980 and 1993.[122] This was not the universal experience, however, because the rate of *Pseudomonas*-related burn infections fell dramatically during a similar period at some burn centers.[122] This situation has been largely unaffected by advances in antimicrobial and supportive therapy. *Pseudomonas* burn wound infections typically occur at least 1 to 2 weeks after severe thermal injury. During the lag period, the patient's normal skin flora may be replaced by hospital flora, including *Pseudomonas,* particularly under the selective pressure of antibiotics. Sepsis results from colonization of the burn eschar, invasion of the subeschar space and underlying dermis, and blood stream invasion leading to septicemia. Clinical manifestations include multifocal discoloration of the burn eschar, degeneration of underlying granulation tissue leading to premature eschar separation and hemorrhage, edema or hemorrhagic necrosis of tissue adjacent to the infected burn site, and brown or black neoeschar formation. Systemic symptoms may include fever or hypothermia, disorientation, hypotension, oliguria, and abdominal distention. Ecthyma gangrenosum lesions may appear at sites distant from the infected burn wound, and pneumonia may be present, especially if inhalation injury has occurred.

Early recognition of *Pseudomonas* burn wound sepsis is essential for successful treatment. Daily surveillance of burn sites should focus on signs of inflammation or fresh tissue damage, as described before. Systemic symptoms should also be monitored closely. Biopsy of suspicious skin sites should be accomplished emergently and specimens evaluated by quantitative culture and histologic examination. Diagnostic features include greater than 10^5 organisms per gram of tissue, bacteria in unburned tissue, masses of organisms in the subeschar space, perivascular inflammation, hemorrhage, and an inflammatory reaction at the burn wound margin.[123, 124] If *Pseudomonas* burn wound sepsis is suspected, it should be treated presumptively and immediately with at least two antibiotics to which the infecting strain is likely to be susceptible. The specific choice of antibiotics, which ordinarily includes an aminoglycoside and a β-lactam agent, is dictated by local susceptibility patterns and complicated by the fact that burn centers tend to harbor highly resistant strains of *P. aeruginosa*.[125] Single-agent antimicrobial therapy should not ordinarily be used for *Pseudomonas* burn wound sepsis because of the huge populations of bacteria present in burned tissues, the accompanying possibility of emerging antibiotic resistance, and the limited access of antibiotics to poorly perfused burn sites. An absorbable topical agent such as mafenide acetate (Sulfamylon) should be applied to burn sites colonized or infected by *Pseudomonas* organisms to reduce the population of bacteria present. In addition, subeschar antibiotic injections have been advocated in the case of infections that do not extend beneath the investing fascia.[126] Finally, surgical débridement of necrotic tissue, eschar removal, or even amputation may be necessary in addition to systemic and local antibiotic therapy.

URINARY TRACT INFECTIONS

Many *Pseudomonas* urinary tract infections are hospital acquired, and some are iatrogenic. Common predisposing factors are urinary tract catheterization, instrumentation, and surgery, including renal transplantation.[127–130] *Pseudomonas* urinary tract infections are frequently associated with persistent sites of infection (such as chronic prostatitis or stones), obstruction, or previous antibiotic therapy. Recurrences are common, and chronic *Pseudomonas* urinary tract infections are often seen. In contrast, *Pseudomonas* urinary tract infections sometimes occur in ostensibly normal women or girls who have neither sites of persistence nor stones.[131] *Pseudomonas* urinary tract infections are usually the same clinically as those caused by other bacterial pathogens. Rarely seen are ulcerative mucosal lesions of the bladder, ureters, and renal pelvis, which may become necrotic and slough into the urine.[132] Another form of urinary tract disease peculiar to *Pseudomonas* occurs in bacteremic patients when bacteria invade small and medium-sized renal arteries, causing multiple renal infarcts.[133] These lesions appear to be similar in pathogenesis to ecthyma gangrenosum lesions of skin.

Proper therapy for *Pseudomonas* urinary tract infections is governed by the area of involvement, extent of infection, association with bacteremia, chronicity, presence of a persistent focus or obstruction, and antibiotic susceptibility of the infecting strain. Most symptomatic *Pseudomonas* urinary tract infections should be treated. Sites of persistence (such as an indwelling Foley catheter or stone) should be removed if possible, obstruction relieved, or abscess drained. Aminoglycosides are first-line drugs in the treatment of *Pseudomonas* urinary tract infections, although antipseudomonal penicillins, extended-spectrum cephalosporins, imipenem, aztreonam, and the oral fluoroquinolones are all possible alternatives. Ciprofloxacin has been widely evaluated for treatment of *Pseudomonas* urinary tract infections because of its superior activity against *P. aeruginosa* and good systemic distribution.[134–136] Oral ciprofloxacin has been used effectively in acute, complicated, and chronic *Pseudomonas* urinary tract infections, even in the presence of a persistent focus. The emergence of ciprofloxacin-resistant strains has been noted, however, and relapse is common. Treatment failure and relapse rates are high generally in complicated *Pseudomonas* urinary tract infections, and there are insufficient data on which to base an accurate assessment of the comparative efficacy of various antimicrobial agents with antipseudomonal activity in this setting. Parenteral therapy for *Pseudomonas* urinary tract infections limited to the bladder should be administered for 3 to 5 days; urosepsis should be treated for at least 10 days; and documented or suspected upper tract involvement associated with obstruction or abscess formation is best treated for 2 to 3 weeks. Although optimal dosing schedules for oral quinolones have not been firmly established, ciprofloxacin may be administered at a dose of 250 to 500 mg twice daily for 5 to 14 days, depending on the extent and severity of a particular infection; the upper limits of dose and duration of therapy would normally be employed for complicated infections. Longer courses of treatment using ciprofloxacin have been employed for certain chronic *Pseudomonas* urinary tract infections, especially those associated with a persistent focus, and chronic suppression has been attempted in some instances, with varying success. The long-term benefits of such therapy are difficult to assess.

PSEUDOMONAS AERUGINOSA INFECTIONS IN PATIENTS WITH ACQUIRED IMMUNODEFICIENCY SYNDROME

P. aeruginosa infections have been reported with increasing frequency in patients with advanced stages of AIDS.[83, 137–139] These infections have been documented in the presence or absence of traditional risk factors for the development of *Pseudomonas* disease, such as hospitalization, previous antibiotic therapy, neutropenia, indwelling vascular catheters, or other factors associated with the interruption of normal anatomic barriers to infection. The majority of such infections occur in human immunodeficiency virus (HIV)–infected individuals with profoundly low $CD4^+$ T cell counts and a history of opportunistic infections. In rare instances, *P. aeruginosa* infections have been reported in previously asymptomatic individuals seropositive for HIV, and there has been at least one documented case[140] in which community-acquired *P. aeruginosa* pneumonia and bacteremia represented a patient's initial AIDS-defining illness.

Although earlier reports suggested that *P. aeruginosa* infections in AIDS patients were primarily nosocomial, later studies have documented that the majority of such infections are actually community acquired, albeit associated, in some instances, with previous hospitalization or antibiotic therapy.

The immunologic factors in AIDS that predispose patients

to *Pseudomonas* disease have not been specifically identified or prioritized. It has been speculated, nonetheless, that compromised host defense mechanisms, including loss of mucosal integrity, defects in humoral and cellular immunity, and leukocyte abnormalities, may render HIV-infected patients more susceptible to life-threatening *P. aeruginosa* infections.[138]

Bacteremic and nonbacteremic AIDS-related *P. aeruginosa* infections have been reported. Bacteremic disease has been associated with central venous catheters and pneumonia as well as with skin and soft tissue and urinary tract sites. Nonbacteremic infections have occurred most frequently in conjunction with pulmonary involvement, soft tissue sites, and sinusitis.[83] Morbidity and mortality are high, and relapse or recurrence is common.

P. aeruginosa bronchopulmonary infections account for a substantial proportion of *Pseudomonas* disease observed in patients with late-stage HIV infections.[141–147] Most of these infections are community acquired, many are recurrent or chronic despite appropriate antibiotic therapy, and a substantial proportion are associated with cavitary pulmonary lesions. It has been suggested that more fulminant cases of *P. aeruginosa* pneumonia, accompanied by sepsis and high mortality, are associated with hospitalization and other traditional risk factors, whereas more indolent community-acquired lower respiratory tract infections are associated with fewer traditional risk factors and lower acute mortality.[144] Survivors of the initial episode of nonfatal *Pseudomonas* infection, however, are likely to relapse and may die as a result of recurrent disease. This pattern of recurrent or chronic *Pseudomonas* lower respiratory tract infection has been compared with that observed in patients with CF.[144]

AIDS-related *P. aeruginosa* lung infections have been reported to produce bronchopneumonia,[144] lobar pneumonia,[145] diffuse interstitial involvement,[146] cavitary lesions,[141, 142] empyema,[138] acute and chronic bronchitis, and bronchiectasis.[143]

P. aeruginosa bacteremia occurs in children[148, 149] as well as in adults[150] with AIDS. It can be either community or hospital acquired and may be associated with a primary site of infection involving the lungs, upper respiratory tract, ear, or indwelling vascular catheter.[150] Bacteremic infections are often fulminant, particularly in children, and may be associated with signs of sepsis as well as with skin manifestations. Mortality rates are high, relapse is common, and death after relapse is particularly likely.[150] On the other hand, bacteremic infections are not necessarily associated with a fatal outcome, especially when the correct diagnosis is established or at least suspected early and appropriate antimicrobial therapy is instituted promptly.[149]

Bacterial infections of the paranasal sinuses are a common complication of advanced HIV disease,[151, 152] and *P. aeruginosa* is a frequent cause of these infections.[151, 153–155] Like AIDS-associated *Pseudomonas* infections at other sites, *P. aeruginosa* sinus infections are usually community acquired although sometimes associated with previous hospitalization or antibiotic therapy. These infections may be accompanied by involvement of other respiratory sites and by blood stream invasion. Multiple sinuses are typically involved, and infections tend to be recurrent or chronic. Therapy includes antibiotics with antipseudomonal activity and appropriate irrigation or drainage procedures.[152] Repeated courses of treatment or chronic suppressive therapy is often indicated.

Skin manifestations of *Pseudomonas* disease in AIDS patients include classic ecthyma gangrenosum,[121, 156] subcutaneous abscesses or nodules,[157] skin papules, and folliculitis evolving into cellulitis after exposure in a hot tub.[121]

Other AIDS-associated *Pseudomonas* soft tissue infections have included breast abscess,[158, 159] parapharyngeal abscess,[160] orbital cellulitis,[161] rectovaginal abscess,[162] and polymicrobial pyomyositis.[163]

Osteitis pubis due to *P. aeruginosa* has been reported after a first-trimester abortion in an HIV-seropositive patient.[164]

Malignant external otitis due to *P. aeruginosa* has also been reported in AIDS patients, unassociated with diabetes mellitus.[165–167]

The treatment of *P. aeruginosa* infections in AIDS patients relies on antimicrobial agents and ancillary measures similar to those employed in treating *Pseudomonas* infections in other immunocompromised patients. In AIDS-related infections, however, repeated or longer term therapy is often required to control or prevent recurrent or chronic *Pseudomonas* disease, exemplified by that found in the lower respiratory tract or paranasal sinuses. Moreover, therapeutic end points are often unclear, and the appropriate duration of therapy is largely empirical and sometimes open-ended.

Stenotrophomonas maltophilia

S. maltophilia, like *P. aeruginosa*, is a ubiquitous free-living organism. It colonizes various body sites of hospitalized patients and occasionally acts as an opportunistic pathogen. Among the documented infections caused by this organism are bacteremia, pneumonia, endocarditis, urinary tract infection, meningitis, wound infection, and cholangitis.[107, 168–171] A salient characteristic of *S. maltophilia* is its resistance to antibiotics, including agents such as the aminoglycosides and imipenem, which are active against *P. aeruginosa*. *S. maltophilia* is resistant, or develops resistance, to many β-lactam agents because of low outer membrane permeability and at least two inducible broad-spectrum β-lactamases.[172] The antibiotic resistance of *S. maltophilia* has contributed to its emergence as a nosocomial pathogen in areas, such as the intensive care unit, where patients are severely ill and broad-spectrum antibiotic use is commonplace.

S. maltophilia is sometimes associated with pseudoinfection, particularly pseudobacteremia, as a result of contamination of blood-drawing materials. Care must be taken, therefore, to interpret culture results in the context of appropriate clinical evidence of infection. Authentic intravenous line–related sepsis has also been reported, as have bacteremias associated with a number of different primary sites of infection. *S. maltophilia* urosepsis occurs in the setting of chronic indwelling urinary catheterization or urologic procedures. It is generally indistinguishable from urinary tract sepsis caused by other organisms. *S. maltophilia* peritonitis has been reported in patients undergoing chronic ambulatory peritoneal dialysis. Pneumonia, although relatively uncommon, is seen increasingly among critically ill or debilitated intensive care unit patients; positive blood cultures may accompany as many as 75% of such cases.[169] *S. maltophilia* has been reported as a cause of native valve endocarditis among intravenous drug abusers[107] and of prosthetic valve infections.[170] *S. maltophilia* endocarditis is usually subacute, although extensive abscess and fistula formation has been reported. Ecthyma gangrenosum skin lesions, apparently identical to those associated with *P. aeruginosa* infections, have been observed in two leukemia patients with *S. maltophilia* bacteremia.[106, 107] Extracellular enzymes produced by *S. maltophilia* were thought to be responsible for the necrotic character of these lesions.[106] Postoperative *S. maltophilia* meningitis has also been reported.[107]

S. maltophilia infections have been treated successfully with trimethoprim-sulfamethoxazole, to which the organism is usually sensitive, alone or in combination with an antipseudomonal penicillin[170] or rifampin. Third-generation cephalosporins such as cefoperazone or ceftazidime may also be used, although susceptibility must be documented initially and monitored during therapy. Long-acting tetracyclines such as doxycycline also have activity against most *S. maltophilia* strains; first- and second-generation cephalosporins, aminoglycosides, and imipenem have little or no activity.

Burkholderia cepacia

B. cepacia has been identified as both an endemic and an epidemic nosocomial pathogen.[173–175] Outbreaks are usually traced to a contaminated liquid reservoir or moist environmental surface. It is often difficult to distinguish between *B. cepacia* colonization and infection, and pseudoinfections are common because of the capacity of the organism to contaminate liquids of all kinds, including antiseptics and disinfectants.[176] At least two outbreaks of *B. cepacia* pseudobacteremia (and bacteremia) have been traced to contaminated blood gas analyzers.[177] *B. cepacia* colonization of various body sites is relatively common in the hospital setting. On occasion, this leads to serious infections, including surgical and burn wound infections, bacteremia, urinary tract infections, pneumonia, meningitis, and peritonitis. In addition, *B. cepacia* endocarditis has been reported as a complication of intravenous drug abuse.[178]

The increasing frequency of *B. cepacia* lower respiratory tract infections in CF patients is a trend of growing concern.[175, 179, 180] *B. cepacia* is being isolated, alone or in combination with *P. aeruginosa,* from respiratory secretions of patients from many CF centers. Isolation of *B. cepacia* correlates, in a general way, with clinical deterioration. Of special concern is a subgroup of such patients who, when colonized with *B. cepacia,* exhibit a fulminant downhill disease course. These patients suffer extensive necrotizing pneumonia, sometimes accompanied by *B. cepacia* bacteremia.[181] The factors responsible for this particularly severe form of pneumonia are poorly understood.

Therapy for *B. cepacia* infections is complicated by the resistance of the organism to many β-lactam agents as well as to the aminoglycosides.[182] Although they are traditionally susceptible to trimethoprim-sulfamethoxazole and chloramphenicol, some *B. cepacia* strains have developed resistance to these agents as well. Third-generation cephalosporins have variable activity against *B. cepacia,* as do the quinolones, including ciprofloxacin. The aminoglycosides are generally inactive against *B. cepacia.* Synergy against *B. cepacia* in vitro has been demonstrated for various antibiotic combinations such as tobramycin or gentamicin and aztreonam[183] or ciprofloxacin, imipenem, and rifampin.[184] The clinical significance of these interactions in vitro is unknown. Finally, meropenem shows some promise against *B. cepacia* on the basis of generally favorable in vitro antibiotic susceptibilities.[175]

Other Related Bacteria

Pseudomonas fluorescens, together with *P. aeruginosa* and *Pseudomonas putida,* composes the so-called fluorescent group of pseudomonads; it is a rare cause of iatrogenic human infections. Although it has been implicated in bacteremia, pneumonia, urinary tract infection, and soft tissue infection, its best known association is with blood transfusion–induced bacteremia.[185, 186] The ability of psychrophilic *P. fluorescens* to grow, multiply, and survive in blood at 4°C is the primary basis for its causative role in bacteremia associated with the administration of contaminated blood products. Transfusion-associated *P. fluorescens* bacteremia can be fatal, even when it is suspected and treated promptly. *P. fluorescens* pseudobacteremia has also been reported, attributed in one case to cross-contamination of blood cultures after inoculation of contaminated citrated collection tubes.[187]

Rare infections have been associated with *P. putida, Pseudomonas stutzeri, Pseudomonas alcaligenes,* and *Pseudomonas pseudoalcaligenes; Burkholderia pickettii; Comomonas acidovorans* and *Comomonas testosteroni; Brevundimonas diminuta* and *Brevundimonas vesicularis;* and other related species.[2] Although unusual human pathogens, the aforementioned species share common features with *P. aeruginosa:* wide distribution in nature, primarily saprophytic or commensal relationship to humans, and occasional emergence as opportunistic pathogens in the face of impaired host defenses.

References

1. Bruckner DA, Colonna P: Nomenclature for aerobic and facultative bacteria. Clin Infect Dis 21:263, 1995.
2. Gilardi GL: *Pseudomonas. In* Lennette EH, Balows L, Hausler WJ Jr, Shadomy HJ (eds): Manual of Clinical Microbiology. Washington, DC, American Society for Microbiology, 1985, pp 350–372.
3. National Nosocomial Infections Surveillance (NNIS) System, Centers for Disease Control and Prevention: National Nosocomial Infections Surveillance (NNIS) report, data summary from October 1986–April 1996, issued May 1996. Am J Infect Control 24:380, 1996.
4. Edwards JR: Results from the NNIS intensive care unit surveillance component. Presented at the National Nosocomial Infections Surveillance Conference; October 24, 1996; Atlanta.
5. Ramphal R, Small PM, Shands JW Jr, et al: Adherence of *Pseudomonas aeruginosa* to tracheal cells injured by influenza infection or by endotracheal intubation. Infect Immun 27:614, 1980.
6. Ramphal R, Pyle M: Evidence for mucins and sialic acid as receptors for *Pseudomonas aeruginosa* in the lower respiratory tract. Infect Immun 41:339, 1983.
7. Vishwanath S, Ramphal R: Tracheobronchial mucin receptor for *Pseudomonas aeruginosa*: Predominance of amino sugars in binding sites. Infect Immun 48:331, 1985.
8. Morihara K: Production of elastase and proteinase by *Pseudomonas aeruginosa.* J Bacteriol 88:745, 1964.
9. Berka RM, Vasil ML: Phospholipase C (heat-labile hemolysin) of *Pseudomonas aeruginosa*: Purification and preliminary characterization. J Bacteriol 152:239, 1981.
10. Johnson MK, Boese-Marrazzo D: Production and properties of heat-stable extracellular hemolysin from *Pseudomonas aeruginosa.* Infect Immun 29:1028, 1980.
11. Seeger W, Walmrath D, Neuhof H, et al: Pulmonary microvascular injury induced by *Pseudomonas aeruginosa* cytotoxin in isolated rabbit lungs. Infect Immun 52:846, 1986.
12. Iglewski BH, Kabat D: NAD-dependent inhibition of protein synthesis by *Pseudomonas aeruginosa* toxin. Proc Natl Acad Sci USA 22:2284, 1975.
13. Allured VS, Collier RJ, Carroll SF, et al: Structure of exotoxin A of *Pseudomonas aeruginosa* at 3.0 Ångstrom resolution. Proc Natl Acad Sci USA 83:1320, 1986.
14. Cross AS, Sadoff JC, Iglewski BH, et al: Evidence for the role of toxin A in the pathogenesis of infection with *Pseudomonas aeruginosa* in humans. J Infect Dis 142:538, 1980.
15. Pollack M, Young LS: Protective activity of antibodies to exotoxin A and lipopolysaccharide at the onset of *Pseudomonas aeruginosa* septicemia in man. J Clin Invest 63:276, 1979.
16. Edwards JR, Turner PJ: Laboratory data which differentiate meropenem and imipenem. Scand J Infect Dis Suppl 96:5, 1995.
17. Chen HY, Livermore DM: In-vitro activity of biapenem, compared with imipenem and meropenem, against *Pseudomonas aeruginosa* strains and mutants with known resistance mechanisms. J Antimicrob Chemother 33:949, 1994.
18. Edwards JR: Meropenem: A microbiological overview. J Antimicrob Chemother 36(Suppl A):1, 1995.
19. Giamarellos-Bourboulis EJ, Grecka P, Giamarellou H: Comparative in vitro killing activity of meropenem versus imipenem against multiresistant nosocomial *Pseudomonas aeruginosa.* J Chemother 7:179, 1995.
20. Holloway WJ, Palmer D: Clinical applications of a new parenteral antibiotic in the treatment of severe bacterial infections. Am J Med 100(Suppl 6A):52, 1996.

21. Sanders CC: Cefepime: The next generation? Clin Infect Dis 17:369, 1993.
22. Kreger BE, Craven DE, Carling PC, et al: Gram-negative bacteremia. III. Reassessment of etiology, epidemiology and ecology in 612 patients. Am J Med 68:332, 1980.
23. Dorff GJ, Geimer NF, Rosenthal DR, et al: *Pseudomonas* septicemia. Illustrated evolution of its skin lesions. Arch Intern Med 128:591, 1971.
24. Forkner CE Jr, Frei E III, Edgcomb JH, et al: *Pseudomonas* septicemia. Observations on twenty-three cases. Am J Med 25:877, 1958.
25. Love LJ, Schimpff SC, Schriffer CA, et al: Improved prognosis for granulocytopenic patients with gram-negative bacteremia. Am J Med 68:643, 1980.
26. DeJongh CA, Joshi JH, Newman KA, et al: Antibiotic synergism and response in gram-negative bacteremia in granulocytopenic cancer patients. Am J Med 80(Suppl 5C):96, 1986.
27. Hilf M, Yu VL, Sharp J, et al: Antibiotic therapy for *Pseudomonas aeruginosa* bacteremia: Outcome correlations in a prospective study of 200 patients. Am J Med 87:540, 1989.
28. Norden CW, Myerowitz RL, Keleti E: Experimental osteomyelitis due to *Staphylococcus aureus* or *Pseudomonas aeruginosa*: A radiographic-pathological correlative analysis. Br J Exp Pathol 61:451, 1980.
29. Bayer AS, Chow AW, Louie JS, et al: Sternoclavicular pyarthrosis due to gram-negative bacilli. Report of eight cases. Arch Intern Med 137:1036, 1977.
30. Forkner CE: *Pseudomonas aeruginosa* Infections. New York, Grune & Stratton, 1960, p 6.
31. Sapico FL, Montgomerie JZ: Vertebral osteomyelitis in intravenous drug abusers: Report of three cases and review of the literature. Rev Infect Dis 2:196, 1980.
32. Sequeira W, Jones E, Siegel ME, et al: Pyogenic infections of the pubic symphysis. Ann Intern Med 96:604, 1982.
33. Jacobs RF, Adelman L, Sack CM, et al: Management of *Pseudomonas* osteochondritis complicating puncture wounds of the foot. Pediatrics 69:432, 1982.
34. Gilbert DN, Tice AD, Marsh PK, et al: Oral ciprofloxacin therapy for chronic contiguous osteomyelitis caused by aerobic gram-negative bacilli. Am J Med 82(Suppl 4A):254, 1987.
35. Bach MC, Cocchetto DM: Ceftazidime as single-agent therapy for gram-negative aerobic bacillary osteomyelitis. Antimicrob Agents Chemother 31:1605, 1987.
36. Greenberg RN, Tice AD, Marsh PK, et al: Randomized trial of ciprofloxacin compared with other antimicrobial therapy in the treatment of osteomyelitis. Am J Med 82(Suppl 4A):266, 1987.
37. Stanley MM: *Bacillus pyocyaneus* infections. A review, report of cases and discussion of newer therapy including streptomycin (concluded). Am J Med 2:347, 1947.
38. Rahal JJ, Simberkoff MS: Host defense and antimicrobial therapy in gram-negative bacillary meningitis. Ann Intern Med 96:468, 1982.
39. Norrby SR: Role of cephalosporins in the treatment of bacterial meningitis in adults. Overview with special emphasis on ceftazidime. Am J Med 79:56, 1985.
40. Fong IW, Tomkins KB: Review of *Pseudomonas aeruginosa* meningitis with special emphasis on treatment with ceftazidime. Rev Infect Dis 7:604, 1985.
41. Marone P, Concia E, Maserati R, et al: Ceftazidime in the therapy of *Pseudomonas* meningitis. Chemioterapia 4:289, 1985.
42. Wright DF, Kaiser AB, Bowman CM, et al: The pharmacokinetics and efficacy of an aminoglycoside administered into the cerebral ventricles in neonates: Implications for further evaluation of this route of therapy in meningitis. J Infect Dis 143:141, 1981.
43. Swartz MN: Intraventricular use of aminoglycosides in the treatment of gram-negative bacillary meningitis: Conflicting views. J Infect Dis 143:293, 1981.
44. Feinmesser R, Wiesel YM, Argaman M, et al: Otitis externa—Bacteriological survey. ORL J Otorhinolaryngol Relat Spec 44:121, 1982.
45. Chandler JR: Malignant external otitis. Laryngoscope 78:1257, 1968.
46. Zaky DA, Bentley DW, Lowy K, et al: Malignant external otitis: A severe form of otitis in diabetic patients. Am J Med 61:298, 1976.
47. Doroghazi RM, Nadol JB Jr, Hyslop NE Jr, et al: Invasive external otitis. Report of 21 cases and review of the literature. Am J Med 71:603, 1981.
48. Rubin J, Yu VL: Malignant external otitis: Insights into pathogenesis, clinical manifestations, diagnosis, and therapy. Am J Med 85:391, 1988.
49. Cóser PL, Stamm AE, Lobo RC, et al: Malignant external otitis in infants. Laryngoscope 90:312, 1980.
50. Sherman P, Black S, Grossman M: Malignant external otitis due to *Pseudomonas aeruginosa* in childhood. Pediatrics 66:782, 1980.
51. Gherini SG, Brackmann DE, Bradley WG: Magnetic resonance imaging and computerized tomography in malignant external otitis. Laryngoscope 96:542, 1986.
52. Meyers BR, Mendelson MH, Parisier SC, et al: Malignant external otitis: Comparison of monotherapy vs. combination therapy. Arch Otolaryngol Head Neck Surg 113:974, 1987.
53. Kenna MA, Bluestone CD, Reilly JS, et al: Medical management of chronic suppurative otitis media without cholesteatoma in children. Laryngoscope 96:146, 1986.
54. Wieland M, Lederman MM, Kline-King C, et al: Left-sided endocarditis due to *Pseudomonas aeruginosa*. A report of 10 cases and review of the literature. Medicine (Baltimore) 65:180, 1986.
55. Reyes MP, Lerner AM: Current problems in the treatment of infective endocarditis due to *Pseudomonas aeruginosa*. Rev Infect Dis 5:314, 1983.
56. Levine DP, Crane LR, Zervos MJ: Bacteremia in narcotic addicts and the Detroit Medical Center. II. Infectious endocarditis: A prospective comparative study. Rev Infect Dis 8:374, 1986.
57. Reyes MP, Brown WJ, Lerner AM: Treatment of patients with *Pseudomonas* endocarditis with high dose aminoglycoside and carbenicillin therapy. Medicine (Baltimore) 57:57, 1978.
58. Myerowitz PD, Gardner R, Campbell C, et al: Earlier operation for left-sided *Pseudomonas* endocarditis in drug addicts. J Thorac Cardiovasc Surg 77:577, 1979.
59. Butrus SI, Klotz SA, Misra RP: The adherence of *Pseudomonas aeruginosa* to soft contact lenses. Ophthalmology 94:1310, 1987.
60. Schein OD, Wasson PJ, Boruchoff SA, et al: Microbial keratitis associated with contaminated ocular medications. Am J Ophthalmol 105:361, 1988.
61. Hansen KD, Meyer RF: Amikacin treatment of *Pseudomonas*-caused corneal ulcer. Arch Ophthalmol 98:1991, 1980.
62. Hutton WL, Sexton RS: Atypical *Pseudomonas* corneal ulcers in semicomatose patients. Am J Ophthalmol 73:37, 1972.
63. Tarr KH, Constable IJ: *Pseudomonas* endophthalmitis associated with scleral necrosis. Br J Ophthalmol 64:676, 1980.
64. Davis SD, Sarff LD, Hyndfink RA: Relative efficacy of the topical use of amikacin, gentamicin, and tobramycin in experimental *Pseudomonas* keratitis. Can J Ophthalmol 15:28, 1980.
65. Sugar A, Cohen MA, Bien PA, et al: Treatment of experimental *Pseudomonas* corneal ulcers with enoxacin, a quinolone antibiotic. Arch Ophthalmol 104:1230, 1986.
66. Golden B: Subtenon injection of gentamicin for bacterial infections of the eye. J Infect Dis 124(Suppl):S271, 1971.
67. Forster RK: Endophthalmitis. *In* Duane TD (ed): Clinical Ophthalmology. New York, Harper & Row, 1978, pp 1–20.
68. Ayliffe GAJ, Barry DR, Lowbury EJL, et al: Postoperative infection with *Pseudomonas aeruginosa* in an eye hospital. Lancet 1:1113, 1966.
69. Yannis RA, Rissing JP, Buxton TB, et al: Multistrain comparison of three antimicrobial prophylaxis regimens in experimental postoperative *Pseudomonas* endophthalmitis. Am J Ophthalmol 100:404, 1985.
70. Geppert LJ, Baker HJ, Copple BI, et al: *Pseudomonas* infections in infants and children. J Pediatr 141:555, 1952.
71. Stone HH, Kolb LD, Geheber CE: Bacteriologic considerations in perforated necrotizing enterocolitis. South Med J 72:1540, 1979.
72. Amromin GD, Solomon RD: Necrotizing enteropathy. A complication of treated leukemia and lymphoma patients. JAMA 182:23, 1962.
73. Sherman NJ, Woolley MM: The ileocecal syndrome in acute childhood leukemia. Arch Surg 107:39, 1973.
74. Ensign PR, Hunter CA: An epidemic of diarrhea in the newborn nursery caused by a milk-borne epidemic in the community. J Pediatr 29:620, 1946.
75. Florman AL, Schifrin N: Observations on a small outbreak of infantile diarrhea associated with *Pseudomonas aeruginosa*. J Pediatr 36:758, 1950.

76. Dold H: On *pyocyaneus* sepsis and intestinal infections in Shanghai due to *Bacillus pyocyaneus*. Chin Med J 32:435, 1918.
77. Chakravarti DN, Tyagi NN: Pyrexia simulating that of enteric fever caused by *Pseudomonas pyocyaneus* in children. Indian Med Gaz 72:367, 1937.
78. Kubota Y, Liu PV: An enterotoxin of *Pseudomonas aeruginosa*. J Infect Dis 123:97, 1971.
79. Pennington JE, Reynolds HY, Carbone PP: *Pseudomonas* pneumonia: A retrospective study of 36 cases. Am J Med 55:155, 1973.
80. Rose HD, Heckman MG, Unger JD: *Pseudomonas aeruginosa* pneumonia in adults. Am Rev Respir Dis 107:416, 1973.
81. Iannini PB, Claffey T, Quintiliani R: Bacteremic *Pseudomonas* pneumonia. JAMA 230:558, 1974.
82. Tillotston JR, Lerner AM: Characteristics of nonbacteremic *Pseudomonas* pneumonia. Ann Intern Med 68:295, 1968.
83. Dropulic LK, Leslie JM, Eldred LJ, et al: Clinical manifestations and risk factors of *Pseudomonas aeruginosa* infection in patients with AIDS. J Infect Dis 171:930, 1995.
84. Huang NN, Doggett RG: Antibiotic therapy of *Pseudomonas* infection in patients with cystic fibrosis. *In* Doggett RG (ed): *Pseudomonas aeruginosa*. New York, Academic Press, 1979, pp 409–444.
85. Reynolds HY, Fick RB: *Pseudomonas aeruginosa* pulmonary infections (emphasizing nosocomial pneumonia and respiratory infections in cystic fibrosis). *In* Sabath LD (ed): *Pseudomonas aeruginosa:* The Organism, Diseases It Causes, and Their Treatment. Bern, Switzerland, Hans Huber Publishers, 1980, pp 71–88.
86. Wientzen R, Prestidge CB, Kramer RI, et al: Acute pulmonary exacerbations in cystic fibrosis. A double-blind trial of tobramycin and placebo therapy. Am J Dis Child 134:1134, 1980.
87. Beaudry PH, Marks MI, McDougall D, et al: Is anti-*Pseudomonas* therapy warranted in acute respiratory exacerbations in children with cystic fibrosis? J Pediatr 97:144, 1980.
88. Møller NE, Høiby N: Antibiotic treatment of chronic *Pseudomonas aeruginosa* infection in cystic fibrosis patients. Scand J Infect Dis Suppl 29:87, 1981.
89. Hyatt AC, Chipps BE, Kumor KM, et al: A double-blind controlled trial of anti-*Pseudomonas* chemotherapy of acute respiratory exacerbations in patients with cystic fibrosis. J Pediatr 99:307, 1981.
90. de Groot R, Smith AL: Antibiotic pharmacokinetics in cystic fibrosis. Differences and clinical significance. Clin Pharmacokinet 13:228, 1987.
91. Jackson MA, Kusmiesz H, Shelton S, et al: Comparison of piperacillin vs. ticarcillin plus tobramycin in the treatment of acute pulmonary exacerbations of cystic fibrosis. Pediatr Infect Dis J 5:440, 1986.
92. Gold R, Overmeyer A, Knie B, et al: Controlled trial of ceftazidime vs. ticarcillin and tobramycin in the treatment of acute respiratory exacerbations in patients with cystic fibrosis. Pediatr Infect Dis J 4:172, 1985.
93. Bosso JA, Black PG, Matsen JM: Efficacy of aztreonam in pulmonary exacerbations of cystic fibrosis. Pediatr Infect Dis J 6:393, 1987.
94. Webb AK: The treatment of pulmonary infection in cystic fibrosis. Scand J Infect Dis Suppl 96:24, 1995.
95. Pedersen SS, Jensen T, Høiby N, et al: Management of *Pseudomonas aeruginosa* lung infection in Danish cystic fibrosis patients. Acta Paediatr Scand 76:955, 1987.
96. Jensen T, Pedersen SS, Nielsen CH, et al: The efficacy and safety of ciprofloxacin and ofloxacin in chronic *Pseudomonas aeruginosa* infection in cystic fibrosis. J Antimicrob Chemother 20:585, 1987.
97. Høiby N: Antibiotic therapy for chronic infection of *Pseudomonas* in the lung. Annu Rev Med 44:1, 1993.
98. Stead RJ, Hodson ME, Batten JC: Inhaled ceftazidime compared with gentamicin and carbenicillin in older patients with cystic fibrosis infected with *Pseudomonas aeruginosa*. Br J Dis Chest 81:272, 1987.
99. Mukhopadhyay S, Singh M, Cater JI, et al: Nebulised antipseudomonal antibiotic therapy in cystic fibrosis: A meta-analysis of benefits and risks. Thorax 51:364, 1996.
100. Whitehead B, Helms P, Goodwin M, et al: Heart-lung transplantation for cystic fibrosis. 2: Outcome. Arch Dis Child 66:1022, 1991.
101. Ramirez JC, Patterson GA, Winton TL, et al: Bilateral lung transplantation for cystic fibrosis. J Thorac Cardiovasc Surg 103:287, 1992.
102. Massard G, Shennib H, Metras D, et al: Double-lung transplantation in mechanically ventilated patients with cystic fibrosis. Ann Thorac Surg 55:1087, 1993.
103. Couetil JPA, Houssin DP, Soubrane O, et al: Combined lung and liver transplantation in patients with cystic fibrosis. A 4½-year experience. J Thorac Cardiovasc Surg 110:1415, 1995.
104. Teplitz C: Pathogenesis of *Pseudomonas* vasculitis and septic lesions. Arch Pathol 80:297, 1965.
105. Greene SL, Wu WP, Muller SA: Ecthyma gangrenosum: Report of clinical, histopathologic, and bacteriologic aspects of eight cases. J Am Acad Dermatol 11(pt 1):781, 1984.
106. Bottone EJ, Reitano M, Janda JM, et al: *Pseudomonas maltophilia* exoenzyme activity as correlate in pathogenesis of ecthyma gangrenosum. J Clin Microbiol 24:995, 1986.
107. Muder RR, Yu VL, Dummer JS, et al: Infections caused by *Pseudomonas maltophilia*. Arch Intern Med 147:1672, 1987.
108. Rajan RK: Spontaneous bacterial peritonitis with ecthyma gangrenosum due to *Escherichia coli*. J Clin Gastroenterol 4:145, 1982.
109. Schlossberg D: Multiple erythematous nodules as a manifestation of *Pseudomonas aeruginosa* septicemia. Arch Dermatol 116:446, 1980.
110. Bagel J, Grossman ME: Subcutaneous nodules in *Pseudomonas* sepsis. Am J Med 80:528, 1986.
111. Fleming MG, Milburn PB, Prose NS: *Pseudomonas* septicemia with nodules and bullae. Pediatr Dermatol 4:18, 1987.
112. Roberts R, Tarpay MM, Marks MI, et al: Erysipelas-like lesions and hyperesthesia as manifestations of *Pseudomonas aeruginosa* sepsis. JAMA 248:2156, 1982.
113. Koopmann CF, Coulthard SW: Infectious facial and nasal cutaneous necrosis: Evaluation and diagnosis. Laryngoscope 92:1130, 1982.
114. Berg A, Armitage JO, Burns CP: Fournier's gangrene complicating aggressive therapy for hematologic malignancy. Cancer 57:2291, 1986.
115. Schuster DI: Palatopharyngeal and lower extremity soft tissue loss in an infant secondary to *Pseudomonas* gangrenous cellulitis. Ann Plast Surg 6:138, 1981.
116. Hall JH, Callaway JL, Tindal JP, et al: *Pseudomonas aeruginosa* in dermatology. Arch Dermatol 97:312, 1968.
117. Washburn J, Jacobson JA, Marston E, et al: *Pseudomonas aeruginosa* rash associated with a whirlpool. JAMA 235:2205, 1976.
118. Thomas P, Moore M, Bell E, et al: *Pseudomonas* dermatitis associated with a swimming pool. JAMA 253:1156, 1985.
119. Schlech WF 3rd, Simonsen N, Sumarah R, et al: Nosocomial outbreak of *Pseudomonas aeruginosa* folliculitis associated with a physiotherapy pool. Can Med Assoc J 134:909, 1986.
120. el Baze P, Thyss A, Caldani C, et al: *Pseudomonas aeruginosa* O-11 folliculitis. Development into ecthyma gangrenosum in immunosuppressed patients. Arch Dermatol 121:873, 1985.
121. Berger TG, Kaveh S, Becker D, et al: Cutaneous manifestations of *Pseudomonas* infections in AIDS. J Am Acad Dermatol 32:279, 1995.
122. Mayhall CG: Nosocomial burn wound infections. *In* Mayhall CG (ed): Hospital Epidemiology and Infection Control. Baltimore, Williams & Wilkins, 1996, pp 225–236.
123. Pruitt BA Jr: Infections of burns and other wounds caused by *Pseudomonas aeruginosa*. *In* Sabath LD (ed): *Pseudomonas aeruginosa:* The Organism, Diseases It Causes, and Their Treatment. Bern, Switzerland, Hans Huber Publishers, 1980, pp 55–70.
124. Pruitt BA Jr, Foley FD: The use of biopsies in burn patient care. Surgery 73:887, 1973.
125. Hansbrough JF, Carroll WB, Zapata-Sirvent RL, et al: Identification and antibiotic susceptibility of bacterial isolates from burned patients. Burns Incl Therm Inj 11:393, 1985.
126. McManus WF, Goodwin CW Jr, Pruitt BA Jr: Subeschar treatment of burn wound infection. Arch Surg 118:291, 1983.
127. Marrie TJ, Major H, Gurwith M, et al: Prolonged outbreak of nosocomial urinary tract infection with a single strain of *Pseudomonas aeruginosa*. Can Med Assoc J 119:593, 1978.
128. Moore B, Forman A: An outbreak of urinary *Pseudomonas aeruginosa* infection acquired during urological operations. Lancet 2:929, 1966.
129. Anderson RJ, Schafer LA, Olin DB, et al: Septicemia in renal transplant recipients. Arch Surg 106:692, 1973.
130. Krieger JN, Brem AS, Kaplan MR: Urinary tract infection in pediatric renal transplantation. Urology 15:362, 1980.

131. Kunin CM: A ten-year study of bacteriuria in school girls: Final report of bacteriologic, urologic and epidemiologic findings. J Infect Dis 122:382, 1970.
132. Carroll G, Allen HN, Doubly EK: Study of bacillary infections of the urinary tract. JAMA 135:683, 1947.
133. Fraenkel E: Weitere Untersuchungen über die Menschenpathogenität des *Bacillus pyocyaneus*. Z Hyg Infekt 84:369, 1917.
134. Leigh DA, Emmanuel FXS, Petch VJ: Ciprofloxacin therapy in complicated urinary tract infections caused by *Pseudomonas aeruginosa* and other resistant bacteria. J Antimicrob Chemother 18(Suppl D):117, 1986.
135. Brown EM, Morris R, Stephenson TP: The efficacy and safety of ciprofloxacin in the treatment of chronic *Pseudomonas aeruginosa* urinary tract infection. J Antimicrob Chemother 18(Suppl D):123, 1986.
136. Malinverni R, Glauser MP: Comparative studies of fluoroquinolones in the treatment of urinary tract infections. Rev Infect Dis 10(Suppl 1):S153, 1988.
137. Fichtenbaum CJ, Woeltje KF, Powderly WG: Serious *Pseudomonas aeruginosa* infections in patients infected with human immunodeficiency virus: A case-control study. Clin Infect Dis 19:417, 1994.
138. Kielhofner M, Atmar RL, Hamill RJ, et al: Life-threatening *Pseudomonas aeruginosa* infections in patients with human immunodeficiency virus infection. Clin Infect Dis 14:403, 1992.
139. Shepp DH, Tang IT-L, Ramundo MB, et al: Serious *Pseudomonas aeruginosa* infection in AIDS. J Acquir Immune Defic Syndr 7:823, 1994.
140. Amundson DE, Mancini SA: *Pseudomonas aeruginosa* pneumonia/sepsis as an initial opportunistic infection in an HIV patient. Mil Med 3:179, 1996.
141. Schuster MG, Norris AH: Community-acquired *Pseudomonas aeruginosa* pneumonia in patients with HIV infection. AIDS 8:1437, 1994.
142. Gallant JE, Ko AH: Cavitary pulmonary lesions in patients infected with human immunodeficiency virus. Clin Infect Dis 22:671, 1996.
143. Verghese A, Al-Samman M, Nabhan D, et al: Bacterial bronchitis and bronchiectasis in human immunodeficiency virus infection. Arch Intern Med 154:2086, 1994.
144. Baron AD, Hollander H: *Pseudomonas aeruginosa* bronchopulmonary infection in late human immunodeficiency virus disease. Am Rev Respir Dis 148:992, 1993.
145. Miller RF, Foley NM, Kessel D, et al: Community acquired lobar pneumonia in patients with HIV infection and AIDS. Thorax 49:367, 1994.
146. Ali NJ, Kessel D, Miller RF: Bronchopulmonary infection with *Pseudomonas aeruginosa* in patients infected with human immunodeficiency virus. Genitourin Med 71:73, 1995.
147. Ainsworth JG, Mitchell D, Harris JRW: Successful prevention of recurrent pneumonia caused by *Pseudomonas aeruginosa* in a patient with AIDS. Int J STD AIDS 6:123, 1995.
148. Flores G, Stavola JJ, Noel GJ: Bacteremia due to *Pseudomonas aeruginosa* in children with AIDS. Clin Infect Dis 16:706, 1993.
149. Roilides E, Butler KM, Husson RN, et al: *Pseudomonas* infections in children with human immunodeficiency virus infection. Pediatr Infect Dis J 11:547, 1992.
150. Mendelson MH, Gurtman A, Szabo S, et al: *Pseudomonas aeruginosa* bacteremia in patients with AIDS. Clin Infect Dis 18:886, 1994.
151. Godofsky EW, Zinreich J, Armstrong M, et al: Sinusitis in HIV-infected patients: A clinical and radiographic review. Am J Med 93:163, 1992.
152. Tami TA: The management of sinusitis in patients infected with the human immunodeficiency virus (HIV). Ear Nose Throat J 74:360, 1995.
153. O'Donnell JG, Sorbello AF, Condoluci DC, et al: Sinusitis due to *Pseudomonas aeruginosa* in patients with human immunodeficiency virus infection. Clin Infect Dis 16:404, 1993.
154. Farr RW, Ramadan HH: Report of *Pseudomonas aeruginosa* sinusitis in a patient with AIDS. W V Med J 89:284, 1993.
155. Grant A, von Schoenberg M, Grant HR, et al: Paranasal sinus disease in HIV antibody positive patients. Genitourin Med 69:208, 1993.
156. Nelson MR, Barton SE, Langtrey JAA, et al: Ecthyma gangrenosum without bacteraemia in an HIV seropositive male. Int J STD AIDS 2:295, 1991.
157. Sangeorzan JA, Bradley SF, Kauffman CA: Cutaneous manifestations of *Pseudomonas* infection in the acquired immunodeficiency syndrome. Arch Dermatol 126:832, 1990.
158. Higgins SP, Stedman YF, Bundred NJ, et al: Periareolar breast abscess due to *Pseudomonas aeruginosa* in an HIV antibody positive male. Genitourin Med 70:147, 1994.
159. Roca B, Vilar C, Pérez EV, et al: Breast abscess with lethal septicemia due to *Pseudomonas aeruginosa* in a patient with AIDS. Presse Med 25:803, 1996.
160. Sanderson RJ, Anstey ST: Parapharyngeal abscess from *Pseudomonas aeruginosa* infection in an HIV positive patient. J Infect 31:174, 1995.
161. Cano-Parra J, España E, Esteban M, et al: *Pseudomonas* conjunctival ulcer and secondary orbital cellulitis in a patient with AIDS. Br J Ophthalmol 78:72, 1994.
162. Sharland M, Peake J, Davies EG: Pseudomonal rectovaginal abscesses in HIV infection. Arch Dis Child 72:275, 1995.
163. Lortholary O, Jehl F, Petitjean O, et al: Polymicrobial pyomyositis and bacteremia in a patient with AIDS. Clin Infect Dis 19:552, 1994.
164. Desmond N, Bignardi GE, Coker RJ, et al: Infectious osteitis pubis in an HIV seropositive female. Genitourin Med 70:127, 1994.
165. McElroy EA Jr, Marks GL: Fatal necrotizing otitis externa in a patient with AIDS (Letter). Rev Infect Dis 13:1246, 1991.
166. Daniels DG, Nelson MR, Barton SE, et al: Malignant otitis externa in a patient with AIDS. Int J STD AIDS 3:214, 1992.
167. Weinroth SE, Schessel D, Tuazon CU: Malignant otitis externa in AIDS patients: Case report and review of the literature. Ear Nose Throat J 73:772, 1994.
168. Schoch PE, Cunha BA: *Pseudomonas maltophilia*. Infect Control 8:169, 1987.
169. Morrison AJ Jr, Hoffmann KK, Wenzel RP: Associated mortality and clinical characteristics of nosocomial *Pseudomonas maltophilia* in a university hospital. J Clin Microbiol 24:52, 1986.
170. Gutiérrez Rodero F, del Mar Masía M, Cortés J, et al: Endocarditis caused by *Stenotrophomonas maltophilia*: Case report and review. Clin Infect Dis 23:1261, 1996.
171. Elting LS, Bodey GP: Septicemia due to *Xanthomonas* species and non-*aeruginosa Pseudomonas* species. Increasing incidence of catheter-related infections. Medicine (Baltimore) 69:296, 1990.
172. Mett H, Rosta S, Schacher B, et al: Outer membrane permeability and β-lactamase content in *Pseudomonas maltophilia* clinical isolates and laboratory mutants. Rev Infect Dis 10:765, 1988.
173. Martone WJ, Tablan OC, Jarvis WR: The epidemiology of nosocomial epidemic *Pseudomonas cepacia* infections. Eur J Epidemiol 3:222, 1987.
174. Yamagishi Y, Fujita J, Takigawa K, et al: Clinical features of *Pseudomonas cepacia* pneumonia in an epidemic among immunocompromised patients. Chest 103:1706, 1993.
175. Pitt TL, Kaufmann ME, Patel PS, et al: Type characterisation and antibiotic susceptibility of *Burkholderia (Pseudomonas) cepacia* isolates from patients with cystic fibrosis in the United Kingdom and the Republic of Ireland. J Med Microbiol 44:203, 1996.
176. Goldmann DA, Klinger JD: *Pseudomonas cepacia*: Biology, mechanisms of virulence, epidemiology. J Pediatr 108:806, 1986.
177. Henderson DK, Baptiste R, Parrillo J, et al: Indolent epidemic of *Pseudomonas cepacia* bacteremia and pseudobacteremia in an intensive care unit traced to a contaminated blood gas analyzer. Am J Med 84:75, 1988.
178. Mandell IN, Feiner HD, Price NM, et al: *Pseudomonas cepacia* endocarditis and ecthyma gangrenosum. Arch Dermatol 113:119, 1977.
179. Tablan OC, Martone WJ, Jarvis WR: The epidemiology of *Pseudomonas cepacia* in patients with cystic fibrosis. Eur J Epidemiol 3:336, 1987.
180. Taylor RFH, Gaya H, Hodson ME: *Pseudomonas cepacia*: Pulmonary infection in patients with cystic fibrosis. Respir Med 87:187, 1993.
181. Tomashefski JF, Thomassen MJ, Bruce MC, et al: *Pseudomonas cepacia*–associated pneumonia in cystic fibrosis. Arch Pathol Lab Med 112:166, 1988.
182. Aronoff SC: Outer membrane permeability in *Pseudomonas cepacia*: Diminished porin content in a β-lactam–resistant mutant and in resistant cystic fibrosis isolates. Antimicrob Agents Chemother 32:1636, 1988.

183. Bosso JA, Saxon BA, Matsen JM: In vitro activity of aztreonam combined with tobramycin and gentamicin against clinical isolates of *Pseudomonas aeruginosa* and *Pseudomonas cepacia* from patients with cystic fibrosis. Antimicrob Agents Chemother 31:1403, 1987.
184. Kumar A, Wofford-McQueen R, Gordon RC: Ciprofloxacin, imipenem and rifampicin: In-vitro synergy of two and three drug combinations against *Pseudomonas cepacia.* J Antimicrob Chemother 23:831, 1989.
185. Murray AE, Bartzokas CA, Shepherd AJN, et al: Blood transfusion–associated *Pseudomonas fluorescens* septicaemia: Is this an increasing problem? J Hosp Infect 9:243, 1987.
186. Scott J, Boulton FE, Govan JRW, et al: A fatal tranfusion reaction associated with blood contaminated with *Pseudomonas fluorescens.* Vox Sang 54:201, 1988.
187. Simor AE, Ricci J, Lau A, et al: Pseudobacteremia due to *Pseudomonas fluorescens.* Pediatr Infect Dis 4:508, 1985.

211

Brucella

Eduardo Gotuzzo
Carlos Carrillo

Brucellosis is an anthropozoonosis and an important cause of morbidity in humans and animals, with an estimated half-million new cases every year.[1] Some nations such as Peru and Mexico in Latin America, Spain and Greece in Europe, and Iraq, Iran, Jordan, and Kuwait in the Middle East[2] are defined as hyperendemic areas with more than 4000 cases per year, caused mainly by *Brucella melitensis.* In the United States, with the implementation of bovine brucellosis eradication programs and the pasteurization of milk, the number of cases dropped to only 172 in 1978; these were found mainly in Iowa, California, and Texas.[3] Because the incidence is small (0.1 case per 100,000 inhabitants per year in 1985), the Centers for Disease Control and Prevention has listed brucellosis as a notifiable disease of low frequency.[4] In the past 10 years, fewer than 100 cases a year have been reported, usually associated with dairy products from endemic areas.

Historical Aspects

In 1885, Sir David Bruce[5] described "a disease of long duration, clinically characterized by fever, profuse perspiration, splenomegaly, frequent relapses, rheumatoid or neuralgic pain, swelling of the joints and orchitis." He isolated the pathogen from the spleen of soldiers who died as a consequence of "Malta disease."

In 1905, Zammit[6] discovered that the goat was the reservoir of *B. melitensis* and produced an immediate decrease in deaths and infection in members of the army by prohibiting the use of untreated goat milk.

Brucella abortus was isolated in Denmark by Bang[7] from intrauterine membranes of aborting cows. *Brucella suis* is a cause of enzootic disease in swine. Carmichael[7a] described *Brucella canis* as epidemic in beagle dogs and their trainers.

Bacteriologic Aspects

Brucellae are small coccoid or rodlike aerobic, gram-negative bacteria 0.5 to 1.5 μm in length. The genus *Brucella* comprises six species that can be distinguished by their oxidative utilization and by their sensitivity to bacteriophages. *B. melitensis* has three biotypes, *B. abortus* has nine, *B. suis* has four, and other species have one.[8] Brucellae are parasites of mammalian cells and have a facultative intracellular reproduction.

Brucella organisms can survive in soil for up to 10 weeks, in liquid manure for up to 2 years, in goat cheese for up to 180 days at 4°C to 8°C, and in tap water for up to 60 days.[9, 10] They are quite sensitive to heat, to ionizing radiation, and to the most commonly used disinfectants, and they are killed by pasteurization.

Epidemiology (Table 211–1)

Brucellosis is a disease affecting various domesticated animals, including cattle *(B. abortus),* goats *(B. melitensis),* swine *(B. suis),* and dogs *(B. canis).* The disease incidence worldwide is estimated as 500,000 cases a year. In developed countries, brucellosis is considered to be an occupational hazard, especially among farmers, veterinarians, and butchers, who may become infected through the skin or conjunctiva.[11–14] Ingestion of unpasteurized dairy products is another common mechanism, especially in Texas and Florida, which account for 50% of reported cases in the United States. *Brucella* is also one of the most infectious bacteria to laboratory personnel, probably by means of aerosols.[15, 16] Human-to-human transmission of brucellosis does not exist.

Internationally, the most important mechanism of transmission is the consumption of fresh, nonpasteurized goat cheese and untreated milk.[1, 17, 18] *B. melitensis* produces a more severe disease, and the attack rate is high, especially in family infections.[19] *B. abortus* has been the most frequent cause of brucellosis in the United States and produces a mild clinical disease. It has a low rate of clinical disease, with more subclinical infections; there are only rare family outbreaks.[20]

TABLE 211–1 ■ Species of *Brucella* and Animal Reservoirs

SPECIES	RESERVOIR	OTHER HOSTS	HUMAN CASES (WORLDWIDE)
B. melitensis	Goat, sheep	Cattle or antelope	+ + + + + (70% of cases)
B. abortus	Cattle, water buffalo, jackal, and hyena	Horse	+ + + (25% of cases)
B. suis	Pig, wolf, and fox	Cattle or caribou	+ + (5% of cases)
B. ovis	Sheep	—	No
B. canis	Dog	—	Few
B. neotomae	Desert wood rat	—	No

Clinical Manifestations

Brucellosis has been recognized as a disease of great clinical polymorphism.[21]

In our experience, which includes observation of nearly 2000 patients with brucellosis caused by *B. melitensis*, we have classified the disease as acute, subacute or undulant, and chronic (Table 211–2).

Acute Form

This is the typical form, with a temperature of 100°F to 104°F, especially in the evenings. It is accompanied by general discomfort, weakness, headache, and profuse diaphoresis, arthralgias, and myalgias. Back pain is frequent. Anorexia, constipation, and weight loss in the first 3 to 4 weeks are commonly seen. Physical examination shows fever and hepatomegaly (two thirds of cases) and splenomegaly (50% in children and young adults). In other types of *Brucella* infection, hepatomegaly is infrequent.

Subacute (Undulant) Form

At present, we recognize patients who have relapsed because of incomplete or partial antibiotic treatment and patients who have received incorrect antibiotic treatment owing to erroneous diagnoses. The clinical pattern is more protean and may be an important cause of fever of unknown origin.[22] The symptoms are milder; arthritis is more frequent,[23] and orchiepididymitis is more common among young male patients.

Chronic Form

This includes patients who have had the disease for more than 1 year. It is extremely rare in children but frequent in older people, with a cyclic course of depressive episodes and a reappearance of sweating. Fever is rare. Chronic brucellosis is similar to chronic fatigue syndrome. Hepatic and hematologic complications are rare; however, ocular damage, such as cyclic episcleritis and uveitis,[24] is frequent. Spondylitis can be present in this form.[23]

Complications

Liver

The most frequent manifestation is granulomatous hepatitis. Authors from Mediterranean countries and Latin America highlight the frequency of granulomatous hepatitis.[25–27] In our group, a review of 59 liver biopsies showed that more than 95% had granulomata and the liver function tests showed a mild increase of aminotransferase and a substantial increase in alkaline phosphatase. With electron microscopy,[28] we observed a cell-mediated immune response with epithelioid histiocytes and typical granulomata. Other more severe hepatic lesions were described in 1951 by Arias Stella,[29] who showed subacute atrophy of the liver in six patients who had died from brucellosis.

Arthritis

Huddleson,[30] in his classic book, indicated a low frequency of articular involvement related to *B. abortus*, but Debono[31] showed a high frequency with brucellosis caused by *B. melitensis* in Malta. In an extensive retrospective revision[32] we pointed out sacroiliitis, the most frequent articular lesion, as shown by Debono.[31] This complication appears in 33.6% of our patients, and the published range of articular involvement is between 9% and 57%.[14, 33–36] Most cases are unilateral and are usually accompanied by a positive Lasègue sign and night pain. Radiographs in a Ferguson view showed blurring with erosions; a bone scan may be helpful for early detection.[37]

In our prospective series, peripheral arthritis is the most common finding, present in 40% to 45% of those with the articular form.[32] It primarily affects young adults and children, especially during relapse, and is rare in persons older than 55 years. Most cases are monarticular, involving a large lower extremity joint such as the knee, hip, or ankle. But one quarter of patients have polyarthritis with pauciarticular involvement, some of them having a rheumatoid-like sydrome.

We propose two pathogenic patterns: the first is infectious arthritis with monarticular involvement and isolation of *Brucella* organisms in synovial fluid using a Ruiz-Castañeda medium modified by Gotuzzo and coworkers.[38] The second form is reactive arthritis, with polyarticular involvement and failure to isolate *Brucella* organisms from the joint. This type affects the ankles, wrists, elbows, and both knees. Joint fluid analysis does not distinguish between the groups; the white cell count is usually 300 to 10,000/mm^3 and protein level exceeds 3 g/dL.[23] Low levels of lactate in joint fluid have been reported in infectious arthritis[39] when the biopsy does not show the difference between these two forms. In our hospital, the main cause of sternoclavicular arthritis is brucellosis and not *Staphylococcus aureus* as has been reported in intravenous drug abusers.[40] Extraarticular rheumatism is seen in about 10% to 15% of our patients, mainly in women between 30 and 55 years of age. Tendinitis, bursitis, and fibrositis are frequent.

Spondylitis occurs in 3% to 15% of cases, is age dependent, and usually involves the lumbar spine. About 20% of the

TABLE 211–2 ■ Clinical Differences Between Various Forms of Brucellosis

OBSERVATION	ACUTE FORM (BACTEREMIA, <8 wk)	UNDULANT FORM (<52 wk)	CHRONIC FORM (>52 wk)
Age	Young adults, children	Young adults	Adults older than 40 y
Arthralgia	Frequent, + +	Frequent, + + +	Quite frequent, + + +
High fever	95%	50%–70%	No
Hepatomegaly	66%	50%	Only occasional
Splenomegaly	50%–70%	<40%	Rare
Hematologic involvement	Occasional	Frequent	Rare
Psychiatric disorders	No	Occasional	Frequent depression, neurasthenia
Ocular damage (uveitis)	No	Rare, 1%–2%	Frequent, 5%–10%

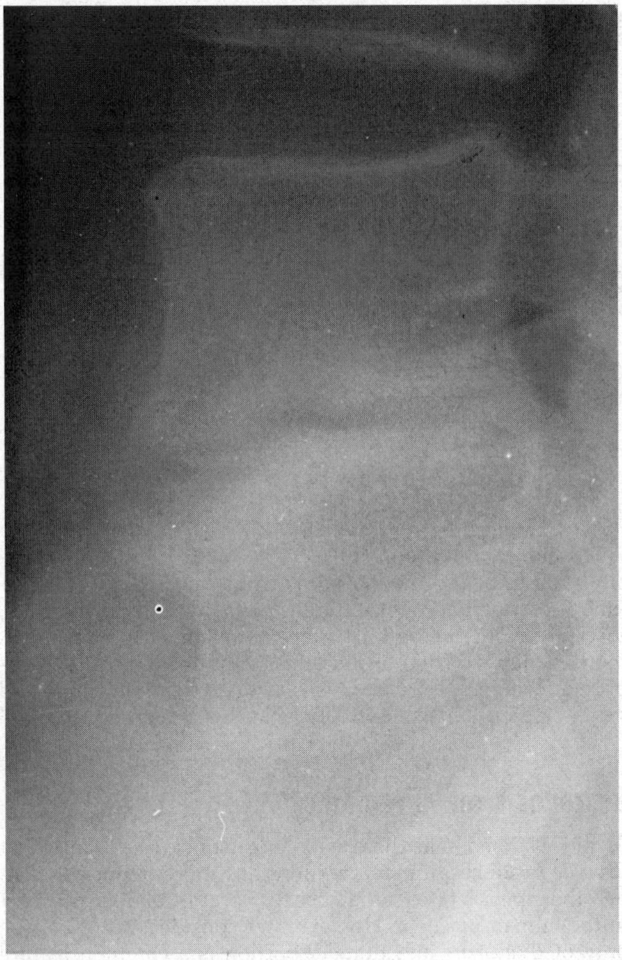

FIGURE 211–1 □ Narrowing of the disk space, epiphysitis, and erosion of the anterosuperior margin of the vertebrae with blastic reaction.

spondylitis cases show involvement of two or more vertebrae. The narrowing of the disk space and epiphysitis are the earliest signs, but the erosions of the anterosuperior margin of the vertebral body (Pons sign) with a rounding off of the corner and narrowing of the intervertebral disk are the most characteristic radiographic manifestations. The distinction from Pott disease (or spinal tuberculosis) is early bone repair with dense sclerosis and syndesmophytes resulting in "parrot peak."[41] The combination of lytic and blastic lesions is rare in tuberculosis but frequent in *Brucella* infections (Fig. 211–1).

Spondylitis may occur in the course of systemic brucellosis with fever, sweating, and back pain[42] but may also occur without systemic symptoms,[32, 43] as in chronic brucellosis. High suspicion based on clinical, radiologic, and epidemiologic clues may enable the diagnosis to be made. Computed tomography has been shown to be effective in the detection of paravertebral abscess and in guided needle aspiration of abscess or vertebral bone. Between 10% and 20% of spondylitis patients have paravertebral abscess.[42, 44]

In summary, brucellar arthritis is frequent, but the different clinical patterns are primarily associated with age (Fig. 211–2).

Hematologic Involvement

Anemia, leukopenia, and thrombocytopenia were frequently found. Bleeding complications were significantly associated with clotting abnormalities, and lymphopenia was significantly correlated with the severity of clinical manifestations.[45] In our study of 60 patients, the evaluation of bone marrow aspirate showed iron deficiency in 34.5% of the patients.[46] Pancytopenia has been described, caused by granulomata in the bone marrow,[47, 48] although cytophagocytosis is an important mechanism in the pathogenesis of these abnormalities[46, 49] and sometimes suggests the diagnosis of medullary malignant histiocytosis (Robb-Smith syndrome).[50]

Thrombocytopenic purpura has been described in 1% of adults and 4% of children with brucellosis. Thrombocytopenia can be severe and some patients need steroids or splenectomy.[51] In our series, we detected 2.5% of patients with severe thrombocytopenia; 6 of 485 were males and 21 of 606 females ($P < .05$). In these cases, bone marrow showed absence of iron in 59.1%, and 12 of 13 of the patients with iron absence were women.

In most infectious diseases, thrombocytopenia is transitory and disappears when the infection is under control. In brucellosis, an important number of cases have severe thrombocytopenia persisting for several weeks despite administration of corticosteroid and having the infection controlled with appropriate antibiotics. As shown in Figure 211–3, it is an important cause of death (rarely observed in brucellosis). An adequate response is obtained in 52.6%, but 37% require prolongation of corticosteroid treatment for more than 2 months, and in some cases after 4 to 6 months, if thrombocytopenia was not controlled, we had to use splenectomy to control it.[52]

Neurologic Involvement

The incidence of neurobrucellosis is reported to be 3% to 5%,[53, 54] although Spink[14] estimated that 10% of patients suffered neuropsychiatric complications. In children, neurobrucellosis has been reported as a rare complication.[55] Lubani and colleagues[56] reported nine children with neurobrucellosis: six with meningitis, one with encephalitis, one with meningoencephalitis, and one with meningomyeloencephalitis. *B. melitensis* was recovered from the cerebrospinal fluid in three patients. Mousa and coworkers[57] described acute *Brucella* meningitis characterized by fever, headache, nuchal rigidity, and altered consciousness. We have sometimes seen Guillain-Barré syndrome, as has been reported by Bashir and colleagues.[58]

The cerebrospinal fluid analysis in *Brucella* meningitis is similar to that for other chronic meningitides, with lymphocytic pleocytosis, an increase in protein content, and a slight decrease in glucose level; the cerebrospinal fluid culture may also be useful (but the organism has been isolated in only a few cases), as may the finding of *Brucella* antibodies in cerebrospinal fluid.[59]

In chronic brucellosis, psychiatric disorders are frequent, including depression, chronic fatigue, amnesia, and even suicide.[21]

Eye Involvement

Uveitis, optic neuritis, papilledema, and corneal involvement have been reported.[60–63] Woods[64] reinforced the role of *Brucella* as an etiologic agent of uveitis; in Peru it is one of the most frequent causes of uveitis.[65]

Circulating immune complexes in brucellosis may have a role in the physiopathology of the uveal damage as in reactive arthritis of brucellosis.[66, 67] Uveitis was present in 14 of 71 cases (20%) with chronic brucellosis. All these cases showed circulating immune complexes by the Raji cell assay and solid-phase C1q assay.[68, 69] In our series, the uveal syndrome occurred as follows: anterior uveitis, six; posterior uveitis, nine; and total uveitis, eight. The evolution showed the fol-

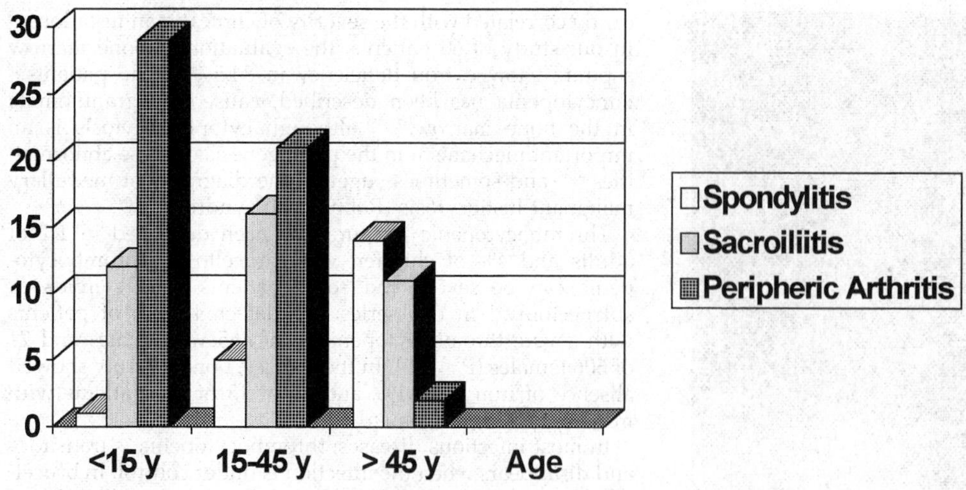

FIGURE 211-2 □ Brucellosis: arthritis by age. Variances among brucellar arthritis patterns according to age groups, showing important differences.

lowing complications: cataract, detachment of the macula, phthisis bulbi, and secondary glaucoma. The prognosis was poor for those with total uveitis compared with those with posterior or anterior involvement, who had a good visual prognosis.[70] A rare case of retinal detachment in chronic brucellosis has been reported.[68, 69]

Other Complications

Unilateral epididymoorchitis occurs in approximately 10% of men and is rare in children. With treatment, most patients recover without sequelae.

Brucella endocarditis occurs mainly on the aortic valve; 50% of the patients have had preexisting valvular abnormalities. In some series, 85% of the deaths occur as a consequence of infective endocarditis,[21] and the majority of patients require valve replacement with 8 to 12 weeks of systemic antibiotic therapy.[70a]

Brucellosis in Childhood

In endemic *B. melitensis* areas, children represent 20% to 25% of cases.[71] Reports of sporadic outbreaks[72] and some reviews of brucellosis in children have been published.[73–78] The infection occurs more frequently in school-age children and in familial outbreaks; the attack rate in children younger than 5 years is significantly less ($P < .05$) than that in older children and adults.[19]

The clinical disease in children is usually mild and moderate (progression to the chronic form is rare), and it is sometimes described as a self-limiting infection.[79] In our hospital, cases are moderate and articular involvement is frequent. A monarticular arthritis of the knee is the most frequently reported form.[23, 32, 80] Spondylitis is rare. Liver involvement and hematologic changes are frequent in this age group.

Brucellosis and Pregnancy

Spink[14] claimed that there was "no definitive evidence that *Brucella* produces human abortions any more frequently than do other species of bacteria" because erythritol does not exist in the human placenta. However, we consider this to be true only of *B. abortus* infection.[81] Abortion is a common feature in animals with brucellosis and appears to be related to high concentrations of erythritol in placental tissues.[81, 82] Nevertheless, in areas where brucellosis *(B. melitensis)* is endemic, there is an increased rate of abortion in asymptomatic women with serologic evidence of brucellosis.[83] Asymptomatic women with agglutination titers greater than 1:160 had significantly more frequent abortions than women with low or negative titers.

In our series, among 75 pregnant women with clinical evidence of brucellosis, we observed increased rates of abortion, premature delivery, miscarriage, and intrauterine infection with fetal death. These complications were especially common in patients with several weeks of untreated disease.

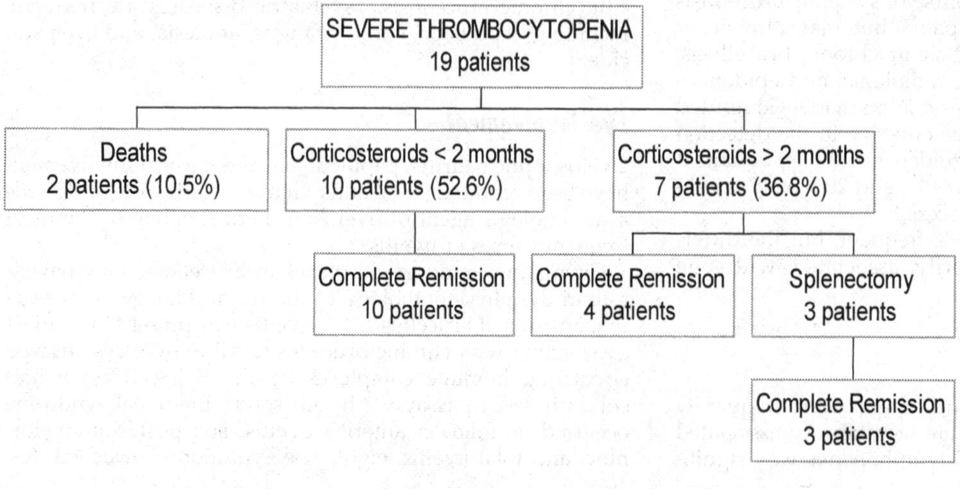

FIGURE 211-3 □ Severe thrombocytopenia complicating brucellosis: treatment and evolution. Evolution of severe thrombocytopenia purpura (<50,000 platelets per mm³) after patients received standard anti-*Brucella* treatment. (From Ulloa V, Rojas J, Gotuzzo E: Púrpura thrombocitopénica asociada a brucelosis. Rev Med Hered 3:87–93, 1992.)

Women with early diagnosis and adequate treatment had a good maternal and fetal outcome.

Tetracyclines, the drug of choice for the treatment of brucellosis, should not be administered during pregnancy; for this reason, the tendency of pregnant women is to have relapses 2 to 4 months after having completed treatment.

Family Studies in Brucellosis

Several outbreaks of brucellosis have been reported in individuals infected through contaminated edible products,[84–87] but brucellosis occurring within family groups has been reported only rarely.[88, 89] Spink[89a] studied several family groups over a period of 16 years in an endemic area for *B. abortus* and emphasized the relatively low rate of symptomatic infection in family members. In our study of 39 families with a family member infected with *B. melitensis*,[19] with a follow-up period of 6 months, half of those affected became symptomatic, confirming the high degree of infectivity of *B. melitensis*.[90] The attack rate was lowest in children younger than 10 years. The clinical manifestations were more severe in women. Articular involvement was also more frequent in women—34.5% versus only 8.1% in men ($P < .01$).[87] Genetically determined susceptibility factors may also play a role in this arthritis; however, immunogenetic studies have not shown any association between a given human leukocyte antigen (HLA) type and osteoarticular involvement,[91, 92] even in Peruvian family studies.[93] Only Hodinka and coworkers[94] in Hungary have published a relationship between HLA-B27 and brucellar spondylitis.

Diagnosis

Worldwide, the diagnosis of brucellosis is usually made by serology,[95, 96] with the agglutination assay, rose bengal test, immunofluorescence, enzyme-linked immunosorbent assay, or counterimmunoelectrophoresis.[97–99]

In Spain, the rose bengal test is extensively used, especially in acute brucellosis; it is easily and rapidly performed, with a low rate of false-positive results.[97, 98] A titer of 1:160 or more in any of the agglutination tests could be interpreted as positive. False-positive results may be caused by *Francisella tularensis* infection, *Yersinia enterocolitica* infection, and *Vibrio cholerae* vaccine,[100] and, in our experience, rare cases of lymphoma and tuberculosis.[101]

With the cholera pandemic in Latin America, where brucellosis is endemic, there was a restriction caused by the cross-reaction detected in cholera patients. We studied 44 patients with cholera, and of those, 7 had titers greater than 1:80, which decreased at the fourth week.[102] Another Peruvian publication also indicated this cross-reaction.[103]

In patients with relapses, in this clinical situation, we prefer the addition of 2-mercaptoethanol, permitting detection of immunoglobulin G. Any titer higher than 1:40 with 2-mercaptoethanol indicates active infection.

The main problem in chronic brucellosis is its diagnosis. In this case we recommend the Coombs test[97, 104] and/or blocking antibodies,[101, 105] and we recommend, in addition, bone marrow culture as routine.

Bacteriologic Diagnosis

The diagnosis of brucellosis is established with certainty by the isolation of *Brucella*. Blood culture in 10% carbon dioxide is the simplest and most frequently used method, and the yield is 50% to 80%, even in afebrile patients.[105a]

The original medium of Ruiz-Castañeda[106] was useful; however, a modification by Gotuzzo and colleagues,[38] with the addition of 0.025% sodium polyethylene sulfonate and 0.05% cysteine, increased the yield of organisms, especially in patients with the acute form of disease.[38] The yield with blood cultures decreases significantly with chronic and subacute forms of brucellosis.

Bone marrow aspirates from the iliac crest (0.5 to 1.0 mL) showed a yield of 92% in comparison with a 70% yield for two blood cultures ($P < .001$). Bacteria multiplied significantly faster in bone marrow culture.

We recommend the bone marrow culture for patients for whom there is clinical and/or epidemiologic suspicion of brucellosis but whose serologic tests are negative in the diagnostic evaluation of fever of unknown origin, unexplained arthritis, unexplained hematologic abnormalities and relapsing or severe uveitis, and suspicion of chronic brucellosis.

Immune Response and Physiopathology

The immune response induced by *Brucella* is complex and results are sometimes contradictory. The response involves humoral and cellular immunity. In the humoral response, antibodies appear early in the infection and may persist for months, especially immunoglobulin M.[104, 107]

Some clinical manifestations such as glomerulonephritis, uveitis, arthritis, and hepatitis are highly suggestive of immune complex disease (circulating immune complexes). We showed high levels of circulating immune complexes by Raji cell C1q assay in a group of patients with acute brucellosis[67]; the level was decreased several months after therapy. Also, 25% of patients had antinuclear antibodies and 37.5% had rheumatoid factors positive during the acute phase. Impaired cell-mediated immune response was studied extensively by Spink and colleagues.[108] The classic pathologic response is the granuloma.

Brucella infection has some analogies to infections with other intracellular pathogens such as *Listeria*. The role of macrophages in resistance to these intracellular pathogens was described by Mackaness (see reference 109). A genetic susceptibility to brucellosis was described by Serre and coworkers,[109a] although the influencing factors appear to be more complex than those described in the *Listeria* model. A Hungarian group suggested that brucellosis, like yersiniosis and salmonellosis, can be associated with HLA-B27 with spondyloarthritis.[94] However, in our studies with arthritis, spondylitis, and familial infection we found no relation between HLA haplotypes and *Brucella*-induced arthritis in Peruvians.[8, 90–92]

Treatment

Antibiotics should have in vitro activity and adequate intracellular concentrations. Tetracyclines are drugs that have shown excellent in vitro activity against *Brucella*.[110–112] In our experience, tetracyclines, mainly doxycycline, had excellent activity, and during the past 25 years the pattern has not changed. The minimal inhibitory concentration for 90% of the strains (MIC_{90}) is 0.125 μg/mL for doxycycline and 2.0 μg/mL for tetracyclines. The MIC and the minimal bactericidal concentration are 1 μg/mL; this means that tetracyclines are bactericidal to *Brucella*.[113] These features and the worldwide experience indicate that tetracyclines are the "gold standard" drug (Table 211–3).

Another therapeutic aspect in brucellosis is the necessity to combine antibiotics to reduce relapse rates and chronicity of the disease.[114, 115]

Other drugs for which there is substantial experience in the treatment of brucellosis are aminoglycosides, which maintain excellent in vitro activity. The MIC_{90} for streptomycin was 8.0 μg/mL but for gentamicin, netilmicin, and amikacin was less than 4.0 μg/mL, in our strains. The largest experience was with streptomycin; sometimes other intravenous aminoglycosides are required because of the presence of purpura. Aminoglycosides have moderate activity against *Brucella*.[11–13, 111, 116] With streptomycin, there is more clinical experience, especially in synergic activity[117]; most authors use 1 g/d intramuscularly for 2 weeks.[14, 18, 21, 115, 118] Prolonging treatment with streptomycin for more than 2 weeks has not proved more effective.[38] Other aminoglycosides have documented activity in vitro, especially gentamicin,[116, 119] but there is limited clinical information.[120] We showed good in vitro activity for netilmicin, gentamicin, spectinomycin, and amikacin.[113] Solera and colleagues,[121] in a prospective study of 64 patients with the administration of doxycycline, 100 mg twice a day for 45 days, plus netilmicin, 300 mg intramuscularly once a day for 7 days, showed a cure rate of 92.3%; the relapse rate was 12.5% (confidence interval 5.6% to 23.2%). For children, Lubani and coworkers[80] recommended therapy for 5 to 10 days with gentamicin in association with co-trimoxazole,[80] for 4 weeks.

Rifampin is also considered one of the first-line drugs because of its excellent in vitro activity and good intracellular penetration. In Peruvian strains it has maintained an MIC_{90} of 4.0 μg/mL in the past 15 years; however, lately an MIC_{90} of 16.0 μg/mL has been found.[113] The World Health Organization recommendation is for doxycycline, 200 mg/d, combined with rifampin, 600 to 900 mg/d for 6 weeks. In a metaanalysis of five comparative studies done in Spain with doxycycline plus rifampin versus doxycycline plus streptomycin, both schedules showed high cure rates, but doxycycline plus rifampin was associated with a significantly higher relapse rate ($P < .01$).[121]

Colmenero and coworkers[122] in Spain presented an interaction between doxycycline and rifampin. Results were found in rapid acetylators with high clearance of doxycycline. In addition, the area under the curve and half-life of doxycycline were significantly lower with the use of rifampin compared with the doxycycline-streptomycin association. They assumed that this interaction would explain the high rate of relapses, nearly 40%, in Spain; however, the results of this experience are not the same as those in other countries, where the relapse rate with this combination is between 5% and 15%.

In spondylitis, some authors prolong therapy for several months. We recommend standard treatment during 6 weeks, followed by low-dose oxytetracyclines for 2 to 4 months (i.e., 100 mg of doxycycline daily) to reduce relapse.

Doxycycline is preferred because it is used twice a day and is little affected when administered with meals. There is high gastrointestinal intolerance for tetracyclines, because four to eight capsules are required daily, resulting in an important interaction with meals and antacids. Our standard treatment in adults is doxycycline (or minocycline), 100 mg twice a day, plus aminoglycoside for 10 to 14 days or rifampin for 6 weeks could be used.

In children 7 years of age or younger, tetracyclines are contraindicated because these agents are deposited in bones and on teeth enamel. The treatment is only for 4 weeks because the relapse rate is low and the chronic form is rare in children.

Rifampin for 4 weeks plus 10 days of aminoglycosides is highly effective in this age. Lubani and colleagues[122a] in Kuwait, in a large series, used co-trimoxazole for 4 weeks plus 5 to 10 days of gentamicin and obtained excellent results.

Different antibiotics, such as chloramphenicol, ampicillin, erythromycin, and cephalosporins, show moderate in vitro activity, but despite the fall in fever with most of the antibiotics, the rate of cure is low and the relapse rate is high.

In some studies, including our in vitro study,[113] good in vitro activity was found for ciprofloxacin, lomefloxacin, and fleroxacin and only mild susceptibility for norfloxacin. The clinical response in a few patients with norfloxacin or ciprofloxacin was poor; however, fluoroquinolones have good intracellular penetration. Akova and colleagues[123] in Ankara published a comparative trial of ofloxacin, 400 mg/d, plus rifampin, 600 mg/d, for 6 weeks in comparison with doxycycline, 200 mg/d, plus rifampin for 6 weeks; both regimens resulted in greater than 95% cure but gastric discomfort or intolerance was more frequent with doxycycline (43.3%), whereas only 6.5% of patients were affected with ofloxacin (see Table 211–3).

García-Rodríguez and coworkers[124] in Spain studied the lack of bactericidal activity of fluoroquinolones against *Brucella*,[123] and in experimental murine brucellosis, fluoroquinolones yielded poor therapeutic results.[125]

A special problem is brucellosis in pregnant women, because the best treatment, tetracyclines or doxycycline, is contraindicated. In these cases, we recommend rifampin for 4 weeks plus streptomycin for 2 weeks, or 4 weeks of rifampin plus trimethoprim-sulfamethoxazole for 4 weeks with close follow-up.

Rifampin is safe in leprosy and in tubercular pregnant women without fetal problems associated with the drug. Short treatments with aminoglycosides—14 days or less—are

TABLE 211–3 ■ Brucellosis: Treatment*

PATIENTS	TREATMENT		
Adults	Doxycycline, 100 mg twice a day for 6 wk	*plus*	Rifampin, 600–900 mg/d (in 2 doses) for 6 wk *or* Streptomycin or netilmicin, once a day for 14 d
Children older than 7 y	Same treatment as adults for 4 wk		
Children younger than 7 y	Rifampin, 10 mg/kg/d (in 2 doses) for 4 wk	*plus*	Streptomycin, once a day for 14 d *or* Co-trimoxazole for 4 wk
Pregnancy	Rifampin, 600 mg/d for 4 wk	*plus*	Streptomycin, once a day for 14 d *or* Co-trimoxazole for 4 wk

*Treatment schedules recommended according to age.

safe. The information about co-trimoxazole is still controversial because of trimethoprim restriction; however, worldwide experience with trimethoprim-sulfamethoxazole in pregnant women with urinary tract infection shows no side effects.

Early diagnosis and proper treatment can improve maternal and fetal prognosis. Women who had the disease for less than 3 weeks and who had proper treatment had newborns at term, healthy, with normal weight.

References

1. Thimm BM: Brucellosis: Distribution in Man, Domestic and Wild Animals. Berlin, Springer-Verlag, 1982.
2. Lulu AR, Braj GF, Khateeb MI, et al: Human brucellosis in Kuwait: A prospective study of 400 cases. Q J Med 66:39, 1988.
3. Centers for Disease Control: Brucellosis Surveillance Annual Summary 1978. Atlanta, Centers for Disease Control, 1979.
4. Centers for Disease Control: Annual summary 1984. MMWR Morbid Mortal Wkly Rep 32:54, 1986.
5. Bruce D: Note on discovery of a micrococcus in Malta fever. Practitioner 39:161, 1887.
6. Zammit T: A Preliminary Note of Examination of the Blood of Goats Suffering from Mediterranean Fever in Reports of the Royal Society of London. Mediterranean Fever Commission, Part III. London, Harrison Sons, 1905, p 83.
7. Bang BF: Die Actiologie des Sevchenhattern (Infectiosen). Verwerfens Z Tiormed 1: 241, 1897.

7a. Carmichael LE: Canine brucellosis: Isolation, diagnosis, transmission. Proc US Livestock Sanit Assoc 71:517, 1967.

8. Alton GG, Elberg SS: Rev. 1 *Brucella melitensis* vaccine: A review of ten years of study. Vet Bull 37:793, 1967.
9. Corbel MJ: Microbiology of the genus *Brucella*. *In* Young EJ, Corbel MJ (eds): Brucellosis: Clinical and Laboratory Aspects. Boca Raton, FL, CRC Press, 1989, pp 53–72.
10. Daminova LF: Survival of brucella in soil, water and animal buildings. Veterneriya (Moscow) 44:103, 1967.
11. Buchanan TM, Feber LC, Feldman RA: Brucellosis in the United States, 1960–1972, an abbatoir-associated disease. Part I. Clinical features and therapy. Medicine (Baltimore) 53:402, 1974.
12. Buchanan TM, Hendricks SI, Patton DM, et al: Brucellosis in the United States 1960–1972, an abbatoir-associated disease. Part III. Epidemiology and evidence for acquired immunity. Medicine (Baltimore) 53:427, 1974.
13. Buchanan TM, Sulzeir CR, Frix MK, et al: Brucellosis in the United States, 1960–1972, an abbatoir-associated disease. Part II. Diagnostic aspects. Medicine (Baltimore) 53:415, 1974.
14. Spink WW: The Nature of Brucellosis. Minneapolis, MN, University of Minnesota Press, 1956, pp 207–208.
15. Pike RM: Laboratory associated infections. Incidence, fatalities, causes and prevention. Annu Rev Microbiol 33:41, 1979.
16. Pike RM: Laboratory associated infections. Summary and analysis of 3921 cases. Health Lab Sci 13:105–114, 1976.
17. Roux J: Epidémiologie et prévention de la brucellose. Bull WHO 57:179, 1979.
18. Elberg SS (ed): A Guide to the Diagnosis, Treatment and Prevention of Human Brucellosis. Geneva, World Health Organization, 1981.
19. Gotuzzo E, Carrillo C, Seas C, et al: Características epidemiológicas y clínicas de la brucelosis en 39 grupos familiares. Rev Esp Enferm Infecc Microbiol Clin 7:519, 1989.
20. Jordan CF, Borths IH: Brucellosis and infections caused by three species of *Brucella*: Clinical, laboratory and epidemiological observations. Am J Med 2:156, 1947.
21. Pacheco G, Thiago de Mello M: Brucellose Monograph del Instituto Brasileiro de Geografia y Estadísticas. Rio de Janeiro, Instituto "Oswaldo Cruz," 1956.
22. Farid Z, Trabolsi B, Yassin W, et al: Acute brucellosis presenting as fever of unknown origin (FUO). Trans R Soc Trop Med Hyg 74:402, 1980.
23. Gotuzzo E, Alarcón G, Bocanegra T, et al: Articular involvement in human brucellosis. A retrospective analysis of 304 cases. Semin Arthritis Rheum 12:245, 1982.
24. Carbone A, Rolando I, Gotuzzo E, Tobaru L: La brucelosis lesiones oftalmológicas. Diagnostico 12:196, 1983.
25. Fernández-Guerrero ML, Días-Curiel, Cortez-Cansino JM: Hepatic granulomas in brucellosis (Letter). Ann Intern Med 92: 572, 1980.
26. Jordans HGM, De Bruin KD: Granulomas in *Brucella melitensis* infection (Letter). Ann Intern Med 92:264, 1980.
27. Lang R, Raz R, Sacks T, Shapiro M: Failure of prolonged treatment with ciprofloxacin in acute brucellosis (Abstr 386). *In* Program and Abstracts of the 28th Interscience Conference on Antimicrobial Agents and Chemotherapy. Washington, DC, American Society for Microbiology, 1988.
28. Recavarren S, Gotuzzo E: Patogenesis de la hepatitis granulomatosa por *Brucella*; estudios ultraestructurales. Acta Med Peru 4:39, 1975.
29. Arias Stella J: Brucellosis. Contribución al conocimiento patológico. Ann Fac Med (Peru) 34:429, 1951.
30. Huddleson IF: Brucellosis in Man and Animals. New York, The Commonwealth Fund, 1943.
31. Debono JE: Brucellosis in Malta. *In* Huddleson IF (ed): Brucellosis in Man and Animals. New York, The Commonwealth Fund, 1943, pp 115–143.
32. Gotuzzo E, Carrillo C: *Brucella* arthritis. *In* Espinoza L, Goldberg D, Arnett F, Alarcón G (eds): Infections in the Rheumatic Disease. Orlando, FL, Grune & Stratton, 1988.
33. Brito M, Gonzales-Díaz J, Marques J, et al: Brucelosis osteoarticular. Revisión de 20 casos observados recientemente. Rev Esp Reum Enferm Osteoartic 15:219, 1972.
34. Feldman JL, Menkes GJ, Weil B, et al: Les sacro-ileites infectieuses. Étude multicentrique sur 214 observations. Rev Rheum Mal Osteartic 48:83, 1981.
35. Norton WL: Brucellosis and rheumatic syndromes in Saudi Arabia. J Rheumatol 43:810, 1984.
36. Porat S, Shapiro M: *Brucella* arthritis of the sacro-iliac joint. Infection 12:205, 1984.
37. Cano R, Falcon S, Gotuzzo E, et al: La gamagrafía ósea: Un procedimiento diagnóstico de valor en la artritis brucelar (Abstr). Presented at IV Jornadas Científicas; September 1986; Universidad Peruana Cayetano Heredia, Lima, Peru.
38. Gotuzzo E, Carrillo C, Guerra J, Llosa L: Evaluation of diagnostic methods in brucellosis. Value of bone marrow culture. J Infect Dis 153:122, 1986.
39. Mavidris AK, Drossos AA, Tsolas O, et al: Lactate levels in *Brucella* arthritis. Rheumatol Int 4:169, 1984.
40. Berrocal A, Gotuzzo E, Calvo A, et al: Sternoclavicular brucellar arthritis: A report of seven cases and a review of the literature. J Rheumatol 20:1184, 1993.
41. Pons P: Le spondylitis melitoccocita. Ann Med 5:227, 1929.
42. Ariza J, Gudiol F, Valverde J, et al: Brucellar spondylitis: A detailed analysis based on current findings. Rev Infect Dis 7:656, 1985.
43. Martin WJ, Nichols DR, Beahrs OH: Chronic localized brucellosis. Arch Intern Med 107:143, 1961.
44. Rotes-Querol J: Osteo-articular sites of brucellosis. Ann Rheum Dis 16:63, 1957.
45. Crosby E, Llosa L, Miroquesada M, et al: Hematologic changes in human brucellosis. J Infect Dis 150:419, 1984.
46. García P, Yrivarren JL, Argumans C, et al: Evaluación de la médula ósea en pacientes con brucelosis. Correlación clinicopatológica. Rev Esp Enferm Infecc Microbiol Clin 8:37, 1990.
47. Lynch EC, McKechnie JC, Alfrey CP Jr: Brucellosis with pancytopenia. Ann Intern Med 69:319, 1968.
48. Stoll DB, Blum S, Pasquale D, Murphy S: Thrombocytopenia with decreased megakaryocytes. Ann Intern Med 94:170, 1981.
49. Martín-Moreno S, Soto-Guzmán O, Bernardo-de-Quiros J, et al: Pancytopenia due to hemophagocytosis in patients with brucellosis; a report of four cases. J Infect Dis 147:445, 1983.
50. Zuazu J, Duran J, Julia A: Hemofagocitosis en brucelosis aguda. Rev Clin Esp 152:231, 1981.
51. McGaraty WC, Serafin D: Brucellosis, indications for splenectomy. Am J Surg 115:355, 1968.
52. Ulloa V, Rojas J, Gotuzzo E: Púrpura trombocitopénica asociada a brucelosis. Rev Med Hered 3(3):87, 1992.
53. Bouza E, García de la Torre M, Parras F, et al: Brucellar meningitis. Rev Infect Dis 9:810, 1987.
54. Shakir RA, Al-Din ASN, Araj GF, et al: Clinical categories of neurobrucellosis. A report on 19 cases. Brain 110:213, 1987.
55. Swick HM: *Brucella* meningoencephalitis in childhood. Neuropediatrics 12:330, 1981.

56. Lubani MM, Dudin KI, Araj GF, et al: Neurobrucellosis in children. Pediatr Infect Dis 8:779, 1989.
57. Mousa AR, Koshy TS, Araj GF, et al: *Brucella* meningitis: Presentation, diagnosis and treatment, a prospective study of ten cases. Q J Med 60:873, 1986.
58. Bashir R, Al-Kawl Z, Harder EJ, Jinkins J: Nervous system brucellosis: Diagnosis and treatment. Neurology 35:1576, 1985.
59. Bouza E: Brucelosis crónica. *In* Baquero F, Buzon L (eds): Encuentro Internacional sobre Brucellosis. Madrid, 1985, pp 57–60.
60. Corrado A, Toselli C: Contributo clinico alto studio delle complicanze ocularinella brucellosis. Rass Ital Oftalmol 18:163, 1979.
61. Lyall M: Ocular brucellosis. Trans Ophthalmol Soc U K 93:689, 1973.
62. Oppermann A, Royer I, Joubert L, et al: La brucellose oculaire. Ann Anat Pathol 3:499, 1969.
63. Pichon A: L'Uvéite Brucelliene. Tours, Faculté de Médecine de Tours, 1976. Thesis.
64. Woods A: Endogenous Uveitis. Baltimore, Williams & Wilkins, 1960.
65. Tobaru L: Uveitis: Aspectos Clinicos y Etiologicos. Estudio Prospectivo. Lima, Universidad Peruona Cayetano Heredia 1983. Thesis Especialidad.
66. Bocanegra T, Gotuzzo E, Alarcón G, et al: Circulating immune complexes in acute fever and brucellosis. Clin Res 29:381, 1981.
67. Gotuzzo E, Bocanegra T, Carrillo C, et al: Immunological abnormalities in human brucellosis. Allergol Immunopathol (Madr) 13:417, 1985.
68. Rolando I, Carbone O, Gotuzzo E, Carrillo C: Circulating immune complexes in the pathogenesis of human brucellar uveitis. Chilbret Int J Ophthalmol 3:30, 1985.
69. Rolando I, Carbone O, Haro D, et al: Retinal detachment in chronic brucellosis. Am J Ophthalmol 99:733, 1985.
70. Rolando I, Tobaru L, Hinostroza S, et al: Clinical manifestations of 25 *Brucella* uveitis. Ophthalmic Pract 5:12, 1987.
70a. Jacobs F, Abramowicz D, Vereerstraeten P, et al: Brucella endocarditis: The role of combined medical and surgical treatment. Rev Infect Dis 12:740, 1990.
71. Burgio R: Brucellosis. *In* Sala Ginebra JD (ed): Tratado de las Enfermedades Infecciosas en la Infancia, Vol II. Barcelona, Editorial Cientifico-Medico, 1962, pp 873–900.
72. Chattas A, Ramaccio HF, Zamar R, et al: Brucelosis en el niño. Gaceta Sanit (Argent) 6:69, 1963.
73. Gorbar JP: Brucelosis en el niño. El Dia Mex 3(2):21, 1961.
74. Llorens-Terol J, Busquets RM: Brucellosis treated with rifampicin. Arch Dis Child 55:486, 1980.
75. Martín-Fontelos P, Barreiro Casal B, Pérez Jurado M, et al: Brucelosis en la infancia (Abstr 12/4). Presented at II Congreso Sociedad Española de Enfermedad Infecciosas y Microbiologia Clínico (SEIMC); May 1986; Palma de Mallorca, Spain.
76. McCullough NB: Brucellosis in children. Symposium of unusual infections in childhood. Pediatr Clin North Am 2:73, 1955.
77. Sattarov AI, Ambeev SA: Characteristics of brucellosis epidemiology in children in the Kasakh SSR. Zh Microbiol Epidemiol Immunobiol 9:92, 1983.
78. Shan PM, Joshi VG: Brucellosis in children. Indian Pediatr 4:226, 1967.
79. Hagebusch OE, Frei CF: Undulant fever in children. Am J Clin Pathol 11:497, 1947.
80. Lubani MM, Dudin KI, Sharda DC, et al: A multicenter therapeutic study of 1100 children with brucellosis. Pediatr Infect Dis J 8:75, 1989.
81. Keppie J, Williams AE, Witt K, Smith H: The role of erythritol in the tissue localization of the brucellae. Br J Exp Pathol 46:104, 1965.
82. Smith H, Williams AE, Pearce JH, et al: Foetal erythritol: A cause of the localization of *Brucella abortus* in bovine contagious abortion. Nature 193:47, 1962.
83. Criscuolo E, DiCarlo FB: El aborto y otras manifestaciones ginecobstétricas en el curso de la brucelosis humana. Rev Fac Cienc Min Educ Univ Cordoba 12:321, 1954.
84. Arnow PM, Smaron M, Ormiste V: Brucellosis in a group of travelers to Spain. JAMA 251:505, 1984.
85. Eckman MR: Brucellosis linked to Mexican cheese. JAMA 232:636, 1975.
86. Galbraith NS, Ross MS, De Mowbray RR, Payne DJH: Outbreak of *Brucella melitensis* type 2 infection in London. Br Med J 1:612, 1969.
87. Gotuzzo E, Seas C, Guerra J, et al: Brucellar arthritis—Study of 39 Peruvian families. Ann Rheum Dis 46:506, 1987.
88. Dalrymple-Champneys W: Undulant fever, a neglected problem. Lancet 1:429, 1950.
89. Damdhere M, Bhagwat R, Sainini G: Outbreak of brucellosis in family. Indian J Med Sci 18:145, 1964.
89a. Spink WW: Family studies in brucellosis. Am J Med Sci 227:128, 1954.
90. Williams E: Brucellosis. Practitioner 226:1507, 1982.
91. Alarcón GS, Bocanegra T, Gotuzzo E, et al: Reactive arthritis associated with brucellosis: HLA studies. J Rheumatol 8:621, 1981.
92. Alarcón GS, Gotuzzo E, Hinostroza SA, et al: HLA studies in brucellar spondylitis. Clin Rheumatol 4:312, 1985.
93. Alarcón GS, Gotuzzo E, Hinostroza TS, et al: Familial studies in human brucellosis. Tissue Antigens 26:77, 1985.
94. Hodinka L, Gomor B, Meretey K, et al: HLA-B27 associated spondyloarthritis in chronic brucellosis. Lancet 1:499, 1978.
95. Elberg SS: Rev 1. *Brucella melitensis*. Part II 1968–1980. Vet Bull 51:67, 1981.
96. Spink WW, Cullough NB, Hutchings LM, Mingle CK: Diagnostic criteria for human brucellosis: Report No. 2 of the National Research Council, Committee of Public Health Aspects of Brucellosis. JAMA 149:805, 1952.
97. Díaz R, Moriyón I: Laboratory techniques in the diagnosis of human brucellosis. *In* Young EJ, Corbel MI (eds): Brucellosis: Clinical and Laboratory Aspects. Boca Raton, FL, CRC Press, 1989, pp 73–83.
98. Díaz RE, Maraví-Poma E, Rivero A: Comparison of counterimmunoelectrophoresis with other serological tests in the diagnosis of human brucellosis. Bull WHO 53:417, 1976.
99. Sippel JE, El-Masry NA, Farid Z: Diagnosis of human brucellosis with ELISA. Lancet 2:19, 1982.
100. Ahvonen P, Sievers K: *Yersinia enterocolitica* infection associated with brucella agglutinins. Clinical features of 24 patients. Acta Med Scand 185:121, 1969.
101. Carrillo C, Sanchez-Griñan E, Guerra J, Gotuzzo E: Evaluación de las metodologías diagnósticas en brucellosis, según las diferentes formas clínicas. *In* Libro de Resúmenes del 3rd Congreso Peruano de Medicina Interna. Lima, Peruvian Society of Internal Medicine, 1984, p 102.
102. Goicochea C, Gotuzzo E, Carrillo C: Cholera-*Brucella* cross-reaction: A new potential diagnostic problem for travelers to Latin America. J Travel Med 3:37, 1996.
103. Begue R, Guillen A, Meza R: *Brucella* antibodies and oral cholera vaccination (Letter). Lancet 346:115, 1995.
104. Foz A, Garriga S: Relation entre la fixation de complément et les anticorps incomplets (test de Coombs) dans la brucellose humaine. Rev Immunol 18:288, 1954.
105. Ruiz-Castañeda M, Tovar R, Velez R: Studies on brucellosis in Mexico. Comparative study of various diagnostic tests and classification of the isolated bacteria. J Infect Dis 70:97, 1942.
105a. Rodriguez-Torres A, Fermoso J, Landinez A: Brucellosis. Medicina 48:3126, 1983.
106. Ruiz-Castañeda MA: Equipo perfeccionado para el aislamiento de *Brucella, Salmonella*, etc, por hemocultivo. Bol Sanit Panam 42:564, 1957.
107. Bradstreet PCM, Tannahill AJ, Pollack TM, Mogford HE: Intradermal test and serological tests in suspected brucella infection in man. Lancet 26:653, 1970.
108. Spink WW, Hoffbauer FW, Walker WW, Green RA: Histopathology of the liver in human brucellosis. J Lab Clin 34:40, 1949.
109. Young EJ: Clinical manifestations of human brucellosis. *In* Young EJ, Corbel MI (eds): Brucellosis. Clinical and Laboratory Aspects. Boca Raton, FL, CRC Press, 1989, pp 97–126.
109a. Serre H, Kalfa G, Brousson A, et al: Manifestations osteoarticulaires de la brucellose. Aspects actuels. Rev Rheum Mal Osteoartic 48:143, 1981.
110. Bertrand A, Roux J, Jonquet O: Place de la rifampicine dans le traitement de la brucellose. *In* Baquero F (ed): Proceedings of the First Mediterranean Congress of Chemotherapy. Madrid, 1978, pp 785–791.
111. Hall WH, Mannion RE: In vitro susceptibility of brucella to various antibiotics. Appl Microbiol 20:600, 1970.
112. Spink WW, Braude AI, Castañeda MR, Goytia RS: Aureomycin therapy in human brucellosis due to *Brucella melitensis*. JAMA 138:1145, 1948.

113. Carrillo C, Gotuzzo E, Adachi J, Tolmos J: Sensibilidad antimicrobiana in vitro de cepas de Brucella melitensis aisladas en un área endémica (Lima, Perú). Rev Esp Quimioter 6:309, 1993.
114. Al-Majed SA, Al-Aska AK, Al-Mitwalli A, et al: Use of antibiotics in the treatment of human brucellosis. Curr Ther Res 57:175, 1986.
115. Young EJ: Human brucellosis. Rev Infect Dis 15:821, 1983.
116. Robertson L, Farell ID, Hinchliffe PM: The sensitivity of *Br. abortus* to chemotherapeutic agents. J Med Microbiol 6:549, 1973.
117. Richardson M, Holt JN: Synergist action of streptomycin with other antibiotics on intracellular *Br. abortus* in vitro. J Bacteriol 84:638, 1962.
118. Schirger A, Nichols DR, Martin WJ, et al: Brucellosis, experiences with 224 patients. Ann Intern Med 52:827, 1960.
119. Waitz JA, Weinstein MJ: Recent microbiological studies with gentamicin. J Infect Dis 119:355, 1969.
120. Novotny A, Moeschlin S: Klinische Erfahrung mit dem Breitspektrumantibisti kum Gentamizin. Schweiz Med Wochenschr 102:24, 1972.
121. Solera J, Martínez-Alfaro E, Saez L: Meta-análisis sobre la eficacia de la combinación de rifampicina y doxiciclina en el tratamiento de la brucelosis humana. Med Clin (Barc) 102:731, 1994.
122. Colmenero JD, Fernández-Gallardo LC, Agundez JAG, et al: Possible implication of doxycycline-rifampicin interaction for treatment of brucellosis. Antimicrob Agents Chemother 38:2798, 1994.
122a. Lubani MM, Dudin KI, Sharda DC, et al: A multicenter therapeutic study of 1100 children with brucellosis. Pediatr Infect Dis 8:75, 1989.
123. Akova M, Uzun O, Akalin HE, et al: Quinolones in treatment of human brucellosis: Comparative trial of ofloxacin-rifampicin versus doxycycline-rifampicin. Antimicrob Agents Chemother 37:1831, 1993.
124. García-Rodríguez JA, García-Sánchez JE, Trujillano I: Lack of bactericidal activity of new quinolones against *Brucella* spp. Antimicrob Agents Chemother 35:756, 1991.
125. Shasha B, Lang R, Rubinstein E: Therapy of experimental murine brucellosis with streptomycin, co-trimoxazole, ciprofloxacin, ofloxacin, pefloxacin, doxycyclines, and rifampicin. Antimicrob Agents Chemother 36:973, 1992.

212

Haemophilus

Timothy F. Murphy

Haemophilus influenzae

Characteristics of the Pathogen

H. influenzae is a small nonmotile, non–spore-forming, gram-negative bacterium. The bacterium was first recognized in 1892 by Pfeiffer, who erroneously concluded that the bacterium was the cause of influenza. On microscopic examination, *H. influenzae* is a small (approximately 1 × 0.3 μm) gram-negative organism whose shape is variable; hence, it is often described as a pleomorphic coccobacillary form. In clinical specimens such as cerebrospinal fluid and sputum, it frequently stains faintly with safranin dye and therefore can easily be overlooked.

H. influenzae is capable of both aerobic and anaerobic growth. Aerobic growth requires two factors: hemin (X factor) and nicotinamide adenine dinucleotide (V factor). The growth requirement for these two factors is used in the clinical laboratory to identify the bacterium.[1]

CAPSULAR SEROTYPES

Six major serotypes of *H. influenzae* have been identified.[2] These serotypes, designated a through f, are based on antigenically distinct polysaccharide capsules. In addition, some strains lack a polysaccharide capsule, and these strains are referred to as nontypeable strains. Type b and nontypeable strains are the clinically relevant strains of *H. influenzae.*

Slide agglutination using serotype-specific antiserum has been the most widely used method to determine the serotype of a strain of *H. influenzae.* The accuracy of this method is variable, and the results must be interpreted cautiously. The most common error is that a nontypeable strain is misidentified as a typeable strain.[3] Counterimmunoelectophoresis using serotype-specific antiserum is a more accurate and reproducible method for determining the capsular serotype of a strain of *H. influenzae.*[3]

HAEMOPHILUS INFLUENZAE: TYPE B AND NONTYPEABLE STRAINS

Type b strains are distinguished by their antigenically distinct capsule consisting of a linear polymer of ribosylribitol phosphate (polyribosylribitolphosphate [PRP]). *H. influenzae* type b strains cause disease primarily in infants and children younger than 6 years. These strains are an important cause of meningitis in children and also cause a variety of other serious invasive infections, including epiglottitis, pneumonia, septic arthritis, cellulitis, and others.

As a result of difficulty in defining disease due to nontypeable *H. influenzae,* these unencapsulated organisms have been overlooked in the past. However, nontypeable strains have gained increasing attention in the past decade.[3–7] These strains are important human pathogens but differ from type b strains in several respects. Nontypeable strains lack a polysaccharide capsule. They are primarily mucosal pathogens, although the frequency of invasive disease caused by nontypeable strains is increasing.[6] The most common clinical manifestations of infection with nontypeable *H. influenzae* are otitis media in children and respiratory infections in adults with chronic bronchitis and in children in developing countries. Therefore, clear distinctions exist between type b and nontypeable strains. These organisms affect different populations of patients, cause different infections, and present different surface antigens to the host. In addition, type b and nontypeable strains are genetically different. Type b strains represent a restricted subset of genotypes of the species as a whole, suggesting a clonal origin for type b strains.[8] By contrast, nontypeable strains are genetically diverse.[9, 10] Table 212–1 summarizes these differences.

TYPING SYSTEMS

In addition to determining the capsular serotype of strains of *H. influenzae,* it is now possible to subtype strains by a variety of methods. These typing methods make it possible to discriminate among strains of the same capsular serotype, allowing studies of pathogenesis and epidemiology of infections by both type b and nontypeable strains. Table 212–2 lists the typing systems that have been developed and the basis of strain differentiation for each system. Subtyping systems based on outer membrane protein patterns in sodium dodecyl sulfate–polyacrylamide gel electrophoresis have been a practical and useful means for clinical and epidemiologic studies involving both type b and nontypeable isolates.[11–13]

TABLE 212–1 ■ Characteristics of *Haemophilus influenzae* Type b Versus Nontypeable Strains

CHARACTERISTIC	TYPE B	NONTYPEABLE
Capsule	Ribosylribitol phosphate polysaccharide capsule	Unencapsulated
Pathogenesis	Invasive infections	Mucosal infections
Clinical manifestations	Meningitis in infants	Otitis media in infants and children
	Invasive disease in infants and children	Respiratory infection in adults with chronic obstructive pulmonary disease
Immunity	Primarily antibody to capsule	Antibody to noncapsular somatic antigens
Evolutionary history	Basically clonal	Genetically diverse

Epidemiology and Transmission

H. influenzae is an exclusively human pathogen. The bacterium resides on the upper respiratory mucosa of adults and children. Nontypeable strains are common inhabitants of the normal human upper respiratory tract, being present in up to three fourths of healthy adults.[14–17] Colonization with nontypeable *H. influenzae* is a dynamic process, with new strains being acquired and replacing old strains periodically.[18] Children colonized with nontypeable *H. influenzae* in the first year of life are at increased risk for otitis media compared with children who remain free of nontypeable *H. influenzae*.[19] Otitis media occurs earlier in colonized children and is directly related to age at the initial time of colonization. A direct relationship exists between the number of times a child is colonized with nontypeable *H. influenzae* and the number of episodes of otitis media.[19]

Type b strains colonize the nasopharynx of children at a rate of 3% to 5%, with higher rates seen in settings such as daycare centers. The rate of nasopharyngeal colonization by type b strains is decreasing with the widespread use of conjugate vaccines to prevent invasive infections caused by *H. influenzae* type b.

H. influenzae is spread by airborne droplets or by direct contact with secretions or fomites.[20] Young children in the same household as a child with *H. influenzae* meningitis are at an increased risk for secondary disease; the risk is estimated at 2% to 4%.[21–23] A controversy exists regarding the secondary attack rate in nonhousehold settings such as daycare centers.[24–27]

Studies of siblings with otitis media caused by nontypeable *H. influenzae* indicate that person-to-person transmission of nontypeable strains occurs among children in the same household.[11] The epidemiology and transmission of nontypeable strains in patients with chronic bronchitis are yet to be defined.

Certain populations have a higher frequency of invasive type b disease than that of the general population. Black children had a three to four times higher rate of meningitis due to *H. influenzae* type b than did white children in several studies.[28, 29] This might be related to the effect of different immunoglobulin allotypes in the populations on susceptibility to infection by encapsulated bacteria.[30, 31] Certain Native American groups have a markedly increased frequency of invasive type b disease. These include Apache[32] and Navajo[33] and Alaskan Eskimos,[34, 35] who have a rate that is 10 times greater than that of the general population. Although the precise explanation for this increased occurrence is not yet defined, several factors might explain the observation. These include early age at exposure to the bacterium and genetic differences in the populations with regard to ability to mount an immune response.

Pathogenesis

COLONIZATION AND INVASION

H. influenzae resides predominantly on the human upper respiratory mucosal surface. Many strains that are recovered from the mucosal surface are piliated, including both type b and nontypeable strains. Pili probably play an important role in colonization of the upper respiratory mucosa by *H. influenzae*.[36–41] Other surface molecules in addition to pili are involved in adherence to human respiratory epithelial cells and are likely to play a role in the ability of *H. influenzae* to colonize the human respiratory tract.[42–46]

Type b strains cause systemic disease after invasion and hematogenous spread to distant sites such as meninges and

TABLE 212–2 ■ Typing Systems for *Haemophilus influenzae**

TYPING SYSTEM	ASSAY	BASIS OF STRAIN DIFFERENTIATION
Capsular serotype	Counterimmunoelectrophoresis with type-specific antiserum[2, 3]	Antigenically distinct polysaccharide capsule
OMP subtype	SDS-PAGE of outer membranes[58]	Molecular weights of major OMPs
LOS serotype	Western blot assay of LOS with adsorbed antisera[78]	Antigenic heterogeneity of LOS
OMP serotype	Kinetic ELISA of OMPs with polyclonal antiserum[247]	Antigenic heterogeneity of OMPs
Biotype	Tests for ornithine, indole, and urease[248, 249]	Biochemical differences among strains
Electrophoretic type	Starch gel electrophoresis and selective enzyme stains[8, 250]	Genetic diversity among strains
Restriction endonuclease analysis of genomic DNA	Agarose gel electrophoresis of restriction enzyme–digested genomic DNA[251–253]	Genetic diversity among strains
PCR	PCR using primers with common sequences[254, 255]	Genetic diversity among strains

*OMP, Outer membrane protein; LOS, lipooligosaccharide; PCR, polymerase chain reaction; SDS-PAGE, sodium dodecyl sulfate–polyacrylamide gel electrophoresis; ELISA, enzyme-linked immunosorbent assay.

epiglottis. The type b polysaccharide capsule is an important virulence factor in the bacterium's ability to invade and cause systemic disease. Isolates recovered from blood and cerebrospinal fluid are invariably nonpiliated, indicating that the bacterium turns off expression of these structures after invasion.

Nontypeable strains cause disease by local invasion of mucosal surfaces. Otitis media results when bacteria migrate from the nasopharynx to the middle ear by way of the eustachian tube.[11] Lower respiratory infection in adults with chronic bronchitis results when nontypeable strains gain access to and colonize the lower respiratory tract of these patients. Nontypeable strains cause invasive disease infrequently, although the incidence is increasing.[6]

ANIMAL MODELS OF INFECTION

An infant rat model of meningitis and bacteremia due to *H. influenzae* type b strains has provided useful information regarding pathogenesis of infection and preliminary identification of potentially protective antigenic determinants. Bacteria are inoculated intraperitoneally into infant rats, and blood is obtained for quantitative culture 24 hours later.[47] *H. influenzae* type b causes bacteremia in most infant rats thus inoculated. In a somewhat different version of the model, infant rats are infected in their nasopharynx, and the bacteria disseminate from there.[48] This model has allowed the study of virulence factors and the investigation of the potential protective effect of antibodies to specific bacterial antigens.

An experimental model of otitis media caused by nontypeable *H. influenzae* has been developed in chinchillas.[49, 50] Bacteria are directly inoculated into the middle ear of the animal. This model has provided insight into the pathogenesis of and immune response to infection, although one must be cautious in applying the results to humans in view of differences in the immune response.[51, 52] In a modification of this model, intranasal inoculation of nontypeable *H. influenzae* causes otitis media in animals that have previously been infected with adenovirus type 1.[53] This model offers the advantage of studying pathogenesis of mucosal infection and avoids direct inoculation of bacteria into the middle ear.

SURFACE ANTIGENS

Type b strains express on their surface a polysaccharide capsule that is a linear polymer of ribose, ribitol, and phosphate. Serum antibody to type b capsule is bactericidal in vitro,[54] confers protection from bacteremia in experimental animals,[55] and protects against disease in humans.[56, 57] The capsule is an important virulence factor in the ability of type b strains to cause invasive disease.

The outer membrane protein composition of *H. influenzae* is typical for that of nonenteric gram-negative bacteria in that approximately 20 proteins are present, with 4 to 6 proteins predominating. The sodium dodecyl sulfate–polyacrylamide gel electrophoresis patterns of outer membrane proteins are the basis of subtyping systems for both type b and nontypeable strains.[11, 58, 59] In general, outer membrane proteins are similar for type b and nontypeable strains except that nontypeable *H. influenzae* shows more diversity in outer membrane proteins from strain to strain.

The outer membrane of *H. influenzae* has a single major porin protein called P2 or b/c; its molecular mass varies among strains from 36,000 to 42,000 daltons.[60–63] P2 exists as a trimer in the outer membrane, and its molecular mass exclusion limit is approximately 1400 daltons.[64, 65] Outer membrane protein P6 is a peptidoglycan-associated lipoprotein that has a molecular mass of 16,000 daltons. Antigenic and molecular studies show that P6 is highly conserved among strains.[66–70] Several other outer membrane proteins are the focus of antigenic and molecular studies in an effort to identify virulence factors and mediators of the human immune response to infection.[71–76]

The *H. influenzae* outer membrane contains lipooligosaccharide. It is similar to that of other nonenteric gram-negative bacteria in that it lacks the repeating polysaccharide side chains and demonstrates all the biologic activity characteristic of endotoxins.[77] The lipooligosaccharide of *H. influenzae* demonstrates marked antigenic heterogeneity and undergoes phase variation.[78–81] Approximately half of strains of *H. influenzae* have sialylated lipooligosaccharide.[82] Sialylation of lipooligosaccharide may represent a form of molecular mimicry because its structure mimics host cell membrane glycosphingolipids.[82, 83] The precise role of lipooligosaccharide in pathogenesis is an area of active investigation.[81, 84, 85]

IMMUNE RESPONSE

Antibody to capsule is important in protection from infection. The age-related susceptibility to *H. influenzae* type b disease is inversely related to the presence of serum bactericidal antibody.[86] Much of this serum bactericidal antibody is directed at capsular polysaccharide.[54] After the level of serum antibody to PRP declines from birth to 6 months of age (maternal antibody), the titer stays low until around 2 to 3 years of age in the absence of vaccination. The antibody nadir correlates with the peak age incidence of type b disease. Antibody to PRP then appears partly as a result of exposure to *H. influenzae* type b or other cross-reacting antigens and partly as a result of the ability of older children to respond to polysaccharide antigens. Systemic type b disease is unusual after the age of 6 years because of the presence of protective antibody. Vaccines in which PRP is conjugated to diphtheria toxoid, tetanus toxoid, and meningococcal outer membrane protein complex have been developed in an effort to stimulate an antibody response to the polysaccharide antigen in young infants. These vaccines generate an antibody response to PRP in infants and are effective in preventing invasive infections in infants and children.[87–97]

Noncapsular antigens of *H. influenzae* have generated considerable interest as targets of the human immune response and as potential vaccine components. Nontypeable strains lack a capsule, so the immune response to infection is to noncapsular antigens. Antibodies to outer membrane proteins P1 (molecular weight approximately 50,000), P2, and P6 protect infant rats from bacteremia by type b strains.[61, 70, 72] In addition, P2 and P6 of nontypeable strains are targets of human bactericidal antibody.[98, 99] These observations suggest that antibodies to these outer membrane proteins might be protective. Indeed, secretory immunoglobulin A in the nasopharynx to P6 is associated with a lower rate of colonization by nontypeable *H. influenzae*.[19, 100]

Studies indicate that the human immune response to the P2 protein of nontypeable strains is important in patients with chronic bronchitis. The P2 protein contains immunodominant epitopes that are abundantly expressed on the surface of the organism.[101, 102] Potentially protective bactericidal and opsonic antibodies are directed against these regions of the molecule.[102, 103] The P2 genes of strains recovered longitudinally from chronic bronchitics show point mutations that have occurred under immune selective pressure.[104–107] The resultant variants have alterations in the immunodominant surface epitopes of the P2 molecule, providing these variants with a selective advantage for survival in the host.

Clinical Manifestations

HAEMOPHILUS INFLUENZAE TYPE B

The most serious manifestation of infection with *H. influenzae* type b is meningitis. The peak age incidence of disease varies somewhat among populations, but this is primarily an infection of infants younger than 2 years. There is little distinctive about the clinical manifestations of meningitis caused by *H. influenzae* type b compared with meningitis caused by other bacterial pathogens. Fever and altered central nervous system function are the most common presentation. Nuchal rigidity may or may not be present. Subdural effusion is the most common complication. One suspects this complication when the infant has seizures, hemiparesis, or continued obtundation in spite of 2 or 3 days of appropriate antibiotic therapy. The overall mortality of meningitis caused by *H. influenzae* type b is approximately 5%, and the rate of morbidity is high. Six percent of survivors have permanent sensorineural hearing loss, and about one fourth of survivors have significant handicap. If more subtle handicaps are sought, up to half of survivors have some neurologic sequelae such as partial hearing loss and delay in language development.[108–110]

Epiglottitis is a life-threatening infection involving cellulitis of the epiglottis and supraglottic tissues.[111] It can lead to acute upper airway obstruction. Unique epidemiologic features are that it occurs in an older age group (2 to 7 years) compared with other *H. influenzae* type b infections and that it is not seen in Navajos and Alaskan Eskimos. Sore throat and fever rapidly progress to dysphagia, drooling, and airway obstruction.

Cellulitis due to *H. influenzae* type b occurs in young children. The most common location is on the face or neck, and the involved area sometimes has a characteristic bluish red color. Bacteremia is usually present, and 10% of patients will have an additional focus of infection.[112]

H. influenzae type b causes pneumonia in infants with an age distribution similar to that of meningitis. The infection is clinically indistinguishable from other bacterial pneumonias, such as pneumococcal pneumonia, except that *H. influenzae* is more likely to involve the pleura.

Several less common invasive infections are seen as important clinical manifestations of *H. influenzae* type b infection in children. These include osteomyelitis, septic arthritis, pericarditis, orbital cellulitis, endophthalmitis, urinary tract infection, abscesses, and bacteremia without an identifiable focus.[113–125] Historically, it was unusual to see *H. influenzae* type b infections in patients older than 6 years. Since the recommendation for routine use of *H. influenzae* type b conjugate vaccine in infant vaccinations in 1990, invasive infections by *H. influenzae* type b have become rare in the United States in any age group.[96]

NONTYPEABLE *HAEMOPHILUS INFLUENZAE*

Nontypeable *H. influenzae* is the second most common cause of community-acquired bacterial pneumonia in adults after the pneumococcus.[126–128] It is especially common in the setting of chronic obstructive pulmonary disease and in patients with the acquired immunodeficiency syndrome.[129, 130] The clinical features of pneumonia due to *H. influenzae* are indistinguishable from those of other bacterial pneumonias including pneumococcal pneumonia. Patients present with fever, cough, and purulent sputum, usually of several days' duration. The chest radiograph shows alveolar infiltrates in a patchy or lobar distribution. The sputum Gram stain shows a predominance of small, pleomorphic, coccobacillary gram-negative bacteria.

Exacerbations of chronic obstructive pulmonary disease caused by nontypeable *H. influenzae* are characterized by increased cough, sputum production, and shortness of breath. Fever is low grade, and infiltrates are not present on the chest film. It is frequently difficult to establish the specific microbial etiology of exacerbations of chronic obstructive pulmonary disease in individual patients.

Nontypeable *H. influenzae* is one of the three most common causes of childhood otitis media along with *Streptococcus pneumoniae* and *Branhamella (Moraxella) catarrhalis*.[131–133] There is nothing distinctive about the clinical presentation of otitis media due to nontypeable *H. influenzae* compared with other middle-ear pathogens such as *S. pneumoniae* and *B. catarrhalis.* Infants present with fever and irritability, whereas older children complain of ear pain. Symptoms of viral upper respiratory infection often precede otitis media. The diagnosis is established by pneumatic otoscopy. An etiologic diagnosis can be established by tympanocentesis and culture of middle-ear fluid, but this is not routinely done. Nontypeable *H. influenzae* is also an obstetric pathogen. It causes puerperal sepsis and is now an important cause of neonatal bacteremia. These strains tend to be biotype IV and cause invasive disease after colonizing the female genital tract.[134, 135]

Nontypeable *H. influenzae* causes sinusitis in adults and children.[136, 137] In addition, the bacterium is a less common cause of a variety of invasive infections that are documented primarily by small series and case reports. These include empyema, adult epiglottitis, pericarditis, cellulitis, septic arthritis, osteomyelitis, endocarditis, cholecystitis, intraabdominal infections, urinary tract infections, mastoiditis, aortic graft infection, and bacteremia without a detectable focus of infection.[138–150] In studies performed before the early 1980s, nontypeable strains were frequently misidentified as type b strains.

Diagnosis

The most reliable method for establishing a diagnosis of *H. influenzae* type b infection depends on recovery of the organism in culture. The cerebrospinal fluid of a patient with suspected meningitis should be subjected to Gram stain and culture. The presence of gram-negative coccobacilli in Gram-stained cerebrospinal fluid is strong evidence for *H. influenzae* type b meningitis. Recovery of the organism from cerebrospinal fluid confirms the diagnosis. Cultures of other normally sterile body fluids such as blood, joint fluid, pleural fluid, pericardial fluid, and subdural effusion are confirmatory in other infections.

Detection of capsular antigen (PRP) is an important adjunct to culture in reaching a diagnosis. Several methods have been effective, and these include immunoelectrophoresis, latex agglutination, coagglutination, and enzyme-linked immunosorbent assay.[151–153] PRP can be detected in cerebrospinal fluid, serum, and sterile body fluids of patients, and this is specific for *H. influenzae* type b infection. Antigen detection can provide a rapid diagnosis before culture results are available. In addition, these assays are particularly helpful in patients who have received prior antimicrobial therapy and are, therefore, more likely to have negative cultures.

Because nontypeable *H. influenzae* is primarily a mucosal pathogen, the organism is present as part of a mixed flora, making it challenging to establish an etiologic diagnosis. A Gram-stained sputum specimen from a patient with suspected pneumonia or tracheobronchitis is highly suggestive of nontypeable *H. influenzae* infection when a predominance of gram-negative coccobacilli are seen among abundant polymorphonuclear leukocytes.[126] A sputum culture is helpful when it is interpreted along with results of the Gram stain.

A diagnosis of otitis media is made by demonstrating the presence of fluid in the middle ear by pneumatic otoscopy. An etiologic diagnosis requires a tympanocentesis, but this is not routinely performed. Treatment is generally empirical, based on the pathogens known to be the most likely to cause otitis media. These include *S. pneumoniae,* nontypeable *H. influenzae,* and *B. catarrhalis.* As is the case with otitis media, it is necessary to perform an invasive procedure to determine the cause of sinusitis, so that treatment is often empirical once a diagnosis is suspected from clinical symptoms and sinus radiographs.

Treatment

Initial therapy for meningitis due to *H. influenzae* type b should be one of the new cephalosporins, such as ceftriaxone, cefuroxime, or cefotaxime.[154–156] An alternative regimen for initial therapy is ampicillin plus chloramphenicol.[154]

Approximately 25% of strains produce β-lactamase and are ampicillin resistant.[157] Therefore, when ampicillin is administered, it should be given initially in combination with chloramphenicol. If the isolate is ampicillin sensitive on susceptibility testing, chloramphenicol can be discontinued. If the isolate is ampicillin resistant, the patient should receive chloramphenicol alone. Chloramphenicol resistance is rare. Because chloramphenicol levels are unpredictable, serum levels should be determined and doses adjusted accordingly. Therapy should continue for a total of 1 to 2 weeks.

Studies have provided evidence that administration of corticosteroids to patients with *H. influenzae* meningitis is beneficial with regard to reducing the frequency of subsequent neurologic sequelae.[158–162] The presumed mechanism is that steroids reduce the inflammation induced by bacterial cell wall mediators of inflammation when cells are killed by antimicrobial agents. Dexamethasone therapy is recommended for infants and children 2 months and older with *H. influenzae* type b meningitis.[154]

Invasive infections other than meningitis are treated with the same antimicrobial agents. Epiglottitis is a medical emergency, and maintenance of an airway is critical. Duration of therapy is determined by the clinical response. One to 2 weeks of therapy is usually appropriate.

Many infections caused by nontypeable strains of *H. influenzae* can be treated with oral antimicrobial agents. These include otitis media, sinusitis, and exacerbations of chronic obstructive pulmonary disease. Approximately 25% of nontypeable strains produce β-lactamase and are resistant to ampicillin. Infections caused by ampicillin-resistant strains can be treated with a variety of agents, including sulfonamides, trimethoprim-sulfamethoxazole, erythromycin-sulfisoxazole, cefaclor, amoxicillin-clavulanate, fluoroquinolones, and clarithromycin.[163–165]

Prevention

VACCINES

The development of conjugate vaccines to prevent invasive infections by *H. influenzae* type b in infants and children represents a dramatic success in the prevention of an infectious disease. Conjugating the PRP capsular polysaccharide to protein carriers has resulted in vaccine formulations that effectively induce protection from invasive *H. influenzae* type b infections in infants. Four such vaccines are licensed in the United States (Table 212–3). Studies from several centers in the United States and Europe have established that conjugate vaccines are highly effective in preventing disease.[92, 94–97, 166, 167] Indeed, invasive *H. influenzae* type b disease was nearly eradicated in a fully immunized population.[92] One mechanism by which these vaccines prevent disease is by reducing pharyngeal colonization by *H. influenzae* type b.[168–172] The reduction of pharyngeal colonization in infants may delay the age at initial acquisition of *H. influenzae* type b in a population.[173] It will be important to monitor colonization patterns and disease incidence now that conjugate vaccines are in widespread use in many countries.

All children should be immunized with an *H. influenzae* type b conjugate vaccine beginning at approximately 2 months of age. Infants should receive a primary series of immunizations between 2 and 6 months of age and a booster vaccination at 12 to 15 months of age. Specific recommendations vary for the different conjugate vaccines. The reader is referred to the recommendations by the American Academy of Pediatrics for specific details.[154]

No vaccines are currently available for prevention of disease caused by nontypeable *H. influenzae.* The PRP conjugates discussed before will not elicit antibody that is protective against nontypeable strains, because none of the conjugate vaccines contains noncapsular antigens of *H. influenzae.* Work is under way to identify somatic antigens that will elicit protective antibodies. Such a vaccine would be useful in preventing otitis media caused by nontypeable *H. influenzae.*

PASSIVE IMMUNIZATION

Human hyperimmune globulin (bacterial polysaccharide immune globulin) prepared from the plasma of immunized adult donors reduced the incidence of *H. influenzae* type b infections in Apache infants, a group with a high frequency of infections caused by *H. influenzae* type b.[32] Administration of bacterial polysaccharide immune globulin at 3-month intervals to infants at high risk for infection with *H. influenzae* type b might reduce the frequency of these infections.

CHEMOPROPHYLAXIS

An increased risk for secondary disease is seen in household contacts of patients with *H. influenzae* type b disease.[21–23] The attack rate can be as high as 4% of susceptible infants. Therefore, in households where there are contacts younger than 4 years, rifampin prophylaxis should be administered.[154] All members (children and adults) of a household with a child in the susceptible age group should receive oral rifampin. On the basis of the high rate of efficacy of conjugate vaccines, rifampin prophylaxis is not required when all of the household contacts younger than 4 years have completed their immunization. Children younger than 12 years should receive 20 mg/kg once daily for 4 days, and adults should receive 600 mg daily for 4 days. The index case should receive rifampin before or at the time of discharge from the hospital because antimicrobial agents used to treat meningitis do not reliably eradicate the organism from the nasopharynx.

The data regarding secondary cases among nonhousehold

TABLE 212–3 ■ Conjugate Vaccines for *Haemophilus influenzae* Type b

VACCINE	CARRIER	PRP	TRADE NAME
PRP-T	Tetanus toxoid	Polysaccharide	ActHIB/OmniHIB
PRP-D	Diphtheria toxoid	Heat-sized polysaccharide	ProHIBiT
HbOC	CRM_{197}, a mutant diphtheria toxin	Oligosaccharide	HibTITER
PRP-OMP	Group B *Neisseria meningitidis* outer membrane complex	Polysaccharide	PedvaxHIB

contacts, such as in daycare settings, are conflicting.[24–27] Some studies show a substantially increased risk among contacts, whereas other studies show a risk for infection similar to the background rate seen among children in daycare centers. Consideration should be given to administering rifampin prophylaxis to contacts in daycare centers, but the decision should be individualized on the basis of the size of the center, extent of contact, exposure to single or multiple cases, and other factors. In addition, consideration should be given to administering a dose of conjugate vaccine to contacts younger than 4 years who are unvaccinated or incompletely vaccinated.

Haemophilus influenzae Biogroup *aegyptius*

H. influenzae biogroup *aegyptius* was formerly called *Haemophilus aegyptius* because of phenotypic characteristics distinct from *H. influenzae.* These include a distinct rod shape, susceptibility to troleandomycin, inability to grow on trypticase soy agar with added hemin and nicotinamide adenine dinucleotide, agglutination of human erythrocytes, and inability to ferment xylose. However, more studies involving DNA hybridization and DNA transformation have demonstrated that *H. aegyptius* and *H. influenzae* are members of the same species.[174–176] Therefore, strains that were previously called *H. aegyptius* are now referred to as *H. influenzae* biogroup *aegyptius*.

H. influenzae biogroup *aegyptius* has long been associated with conjunctivitis. This strain is now also known to be the cause of Brazilian purpuric fever (BPF), first recognized in 1984 in the rural Brazilian town of Promissao.[177] The peak age incidence of BPF is 1 to 4 years, with a range of 3 months to 8 years. The illness can occur sporadically or in outbreaks. Typically, after an episode of purulent conjunctivitis, high fever is seen initially in association with vomiting and abdominal pain. Within 12 to 48 hours from onset, the patient experiences petechiae, purpura, peripheral necrosis, and vascular collapse. The laboratory features of the illness are characterized by thrombocytopenia, prolonged prothrombin time, a uniformly unrevealing cerebrospinal fluid, and positive blood cultures for *H. influenzae* biogroup *aegyptius*.[177, 178] The mortality in initial reports was high (about 70%), but subsequent studies have indicated that milder forms of the illness exist. Most patients have resolved or resolving purulent conjunctivitis, and culture of the conjunctiva is positive in approximately one third of patients with BPF. The illness has been seen in several towns in Brazil and on two occasions in Australia.[179, 180]

Strains of *H. influenzae* biogroup *aegyptius* that cause BPF are of a clonal origin.[181] Case clone strains share the following characteristics: (1) a 24-MDa plasmid that has a characteristic restriction digest pattern; (2) a typical banding pattern in sodium dodecyl sulfate–polyacrylamide gel electrophoresis of whole-organism lysates; (3) identical electrophoretic type in multilocus enzyme typing; (4) typical ribosomal DNA restriction patterns; (5) trimethoprim-sulfamethoxazole resistance; (6) a highly conserved surface epitope on the P1 outer membrane protein[182]; and (7) a unique immunoglobulin A1 protease.[183] Of interest, the Australian strains do not share these characteristics and represent a second clone.[184] Strains recovered from Valparaiso, Brazil, lack the 24-MDa plasmid typical of case clone strains yet are capable of causing BPF.[185]

Several potentially useful model systems have been developed to study the pathogenesis of BPF. Case clone strains (1) are relatively serum resistant in spite of the absence of capsular genes,[186, 187] (2) show increased virulence in an infant rat model of bacteremia,[183, 188, 189] and (3) are cytotoxic in an in vitro model using a human microvascular endothelial cell line.[190, 191] These models distinguish strains of *H. influenzae* biogroup *aegyptius* capable of causing BPF from strains not associated with the fulminant syndrome. They hold promise in facilitating the identification of virulence factors that enable these strains to cause invasive disease.

Several surface structures on BPF case clone strains have been identified and characterized. A unique surface-exposed epitope on the P1 outer membrane protein is highly predictive of disease-causing strains.[182] The pilus gene has been sequenced and shares extensive homology with pili of other strains of *H. influenzae*.[192, 193] A phase-variable 145-kDa surface protein is present in case clone strains.[194] Lipooligosaccharide phenotype is related to virulence in the infant rat model.[195] Identifying the virulence factors expressed by case clone strains is important in understanding BPF. In addition, the identification and characterization of factors that enable a clone of an otherwise noninvasive bacterium (nontypeable *H. influenzae*) to become invasive are of general importance in understanding the pathogenesis of invasive bacterial infections.

Haemophilus ducreyi (Chancroid)

H. ducreyi is the etiologic agent of chancroid, a sexually transmitted disease characterized by genital ulceration and inguinal adenitis. *H. ducreyi* is a major health problem in developing countries. Although chancroid is less common in the United States, the incidence of infection has increased dramatically in the past several years. In 1993, 1399 cases of chancroid were reported, compared with 788 cases in 1980.[196] In addition to morbidity associated with chancroid itself, it is associated with human immunodeficiency virus positivity by virtue of the role of genital ulceration in transmission of human immunodeficiency virus.[197, 198]

Characteristics of the Pathogen

H. ducreyi is a coccobacillary gram-negative bacterium that has a growth requirement for X factor (hemin). Therefore, the bacterium is placed within the genus *Haemophilus.* However, studies of DNA homology[199] and chemotaxonomic studies established major differences between *H. ducreyi* and other *Haemophilus* species. Transfer in taxonomic assignment of the organism is likely in the future, but this awaits further study.[200]

H. ducreyi is highly fastidious in its growth requirements. It is inert to most standard biochemical tests. There is not yet an established method for typing strains. Several methods have been studied. These include sodium dodecyl sulfate–polyacrylamide gel electrophoresis of outer membrane proteins,[201] indirect immunofluorescence using absorbed polyclonal antiserum,[202] and specific aminopeptidase activities.[203] More recently, plasmid analysis and restriction fragment length polymorphism of genomic DNA have provided information on the epidemiology of *H. ducreyi* infection.[204]

The classic test for virulence of *H. ducreyi* strains was the rabbit intradermal test.[205, 206] More recent work has resulted in the development of better model systems to study pathogenesis.[207] A temperature-dependent rabbit model of experimental chancroid has been developed. Lesion development requires both a viable inoculum of *H. ducreyi* and housing of animals at reduced ambient temperatures (15°C to 17°C).[208] Immunization with killed whole bacteria induces protection on rechallenge.[209] Experimental infections that produce lesions similar to those in humans have been established in macaques.[210] Experimental human infections with *H. ducreyi* resulted in dermal infiltration with macrophages and activated T cells.[211] In addition to these in vivo systems, several in vitro cultured cells are being used to study adherence, invasion, and cytopathic effect of *H. ducreyi*.[212–215] Use of these experimental models promises to provide important insights into the pathogenesis and immune response in chancroid in the next several years.

H. ducreyi expresses hemolysins, and these are likely to be involved in pathogenesis.[215–217] Several surface structures, including lipooligosaccharide,[218] pili,[219] and outer membrane proteins,[220, 221] have been identified; their role in pathogenesis is being investigated.

Epidemiology and Prevalence

The epidemiology of *H. ducreyi* infections is not well defined because of difficulty in reliable cultures of chancroid lesions. Most studies have relied on the clinical picture to establish a diagnosis. A clinical diagnosis based on the appearance of the ulcer is often inaccurate, particularly in areas where the incidence of chancroid is low. Chancroid is a common cause of genital ulcers in developing countries. Several large outbreaks of chancroid have been identified in the United States since 1981.[204, 222] Recurring epidemiologic themes in these outbreaks are apparent: (1) affected patients were primarily black and Hispanic, (2) transmission was predominantly heterosexual, (3) men outnumbered women 3:1 to 25:1, and (4) prostitutes were important in transmission of the infection. The incidence of chancroid in the United States will undoubtedly increase in the coming years, and chancroid will continue to be important in the transmission of human immunodeficiency virus because of production of genital ulcers.

Clinical Manifestations

Infection occurs as a result of a break in the epithelium during sexual contact with an infected individual. After an incubation period of 4 to 7 days, the initial lesion is a papule with surrounding erythema. In 2 to 3 days, the papule evolves into a pustule that spontaneously ruptures and forms a sharply circumscribed ulcer that is generally not indurated. The ulcers are painful and bleed easily, and little or no inflammation of the surrounding skin is seen. Approximately half of the patients develop enlarged tender inguinal lymph nodes, which frequently become fluctuant and spontaneously rupture.

Chancroid does not usually present with all of the typical clinical features and sometimes manifests atypically. Multiple ulcers can coalesce to form giant ulcers. Ulcers can appear and then resolve, followed by inguinal adenitis with suppuration 1 to 3 weeks later. This can be confused with lymphogranuloma venereum. Multiple small ulcers can look like folliculitis. Other differential diagnostic considerations include the causes of genital ulceration, such as primary syphilis, condyloma latum of secondary syphilis, genital herpes, and donovanosis. Rarely, chancroid lesions can become secondarily infected with bacteria, leading to extensive inflammation.

Diagnosis

Clinical diagnosis is often inaccurate, and laboratory confirmation should be attempted in suspected cases.[200] Gram stain of a swab of the lesion can show a predominance of characteristic gram-negative coccobacilli, but the presence of other bacteria can often confuse the interpretation. Immunofluorescence assays using monoclonal antibodies specific for *H. ducreyi* have been developed, but these are not widely available.[223] An accurate diagnosis of chancroid relies on cultures of *H. ducreyi* from the lesion. The organism can be difficult to grow, and the use of selective and supplemented media is necessary. The highest rate of recovery from clinical samples has been obtained with GC agar base containing 1% to 2% hemoglobin, 5% fetal bovine serum, and 3 μg/mL of vancomycin. Media containing a variety of other supplements have been used. The use of more than one medium will enhance the likelihood of obtaining a positive culture because of different growth requirements of strains of *H. ducreyi*. Colonies are pinpoint at 24 hours and grow to 1 to 2 mm in diameter at 48 hours. Laboratory strains tend to grow more readily than clinical strains.

Treatment

Clinical isolates often have plasmid-mediated resistance to ampicillin, chloramphenicol, tetracyclines, and sulfonamides. *H. ducreyi* can acquire resistance determinants and can exchange plasmids with other human pathogens such as *H. influenzae* and *Neisseria gonorrhoeae*. Chancroid can be treated effectively with several regimens.[224, 225] These include (1) ceftriaxone, 250 mg intramuscularly as a single dose; (2) erythromycin, 500 mg orally four times daily for 7 days; (3) ampicillin-clavulanate, three times daily for 7 days; (4) trimethoprim-sulfamethoxazole, one double-strength tablet two times daily for 7 days in regions where resistant strains are not prevalent; and (5) ciprofloxacin, 500 mg orally twice daily for 3 days. Susceptibility testing of isolates for patients who do not respond promptly to treatment should be performed.

Other *Haemophilus* Species

Haemophilus species are frequently recovered as part of the normal upper respiratory tract flora in humans.[226, 227] However, these bacteria are infrequent causes of infection because of their low pathogenic potential. *Haemophilus* species have fastidious growth requirements and generally grow slowly. The species implicated in human infections are noted in Table 212–4. *Haemophilus* species are differentiated by several characteristics. Requirements for X and V factors are the primary means. Species designated *para* require V factor only for growth, whereas others require either X and V or X only. Other tests to differentiate species include hemolysis; the porphyrin test; nitrate reduction; lysine decarboxylase activity; and acid production from glucose, sucrose, lactose, and xylose.[228, 229]

Haemophilus species, particularly *Haemophilus parainfluenzae*, are an increasingly recognized cause of infective endocarditis.[230–245] Several series indicate that *H. parainfluenzae* must be considered a cause of endocarditis, especially when initial blood cultures are negative but when the clinical suspicion of endocarditis is present. It is likely that some cases of what has been called culture-negative endocarditis are actually caused by fastidious, slow-growing bacteria such as *H. parainfluenzae* and *Haemophilus paraphrophilus*. To increase the chances of recovering the organisms, blood cultures should be subcultured onto chocolate agar and incubated in 5% carbon dioxide.

Endocarditis caused by *Haemophilus* species usually presents with a subacute course, but variability in the presenta-

TABLE 212–4 ■ Other *Haemophilus* Species* Associated with Human Disease

Haemophilus parainfluenzae	*Haemophilus parahaemolyticus*
Haemophilus aphrophilus	*Haemophilus haemolyticus*
Haemophilus paraphrophilus	*Haemophilus segnis*

*Not including *H. influenzae* and *H. ducreyi*.

TABLE 212–5 ■ Human Infections Caused by Other *Haemophilus* Species*

INFECTION	REFERENCE
Endocarditis	230–245, 256, 257
Pulmonary infection	230, 235, 237, 258, 259
Epiglottitis	230, 260, 261
Meningitis	230, 262
Bacteremia without an identifiable focus	235, 237, 244
Intraabdominal infection	235, 259, 263, 264
Septic arthritis	230, 265–267
Soft tissue infection or abscess	235, 237
Neonatal sepsis	268
Otitis media	242
Brain abscess	235
Sinusitis	235
Necrotizing fasciitis	269
Hepatic abscess	270
Urinary tract infection	271

*Not including *H. influenzae* and *H. ducreyi*.

tion is seen. The diagnosis is often delayed because of the difficulty in recovering the organism from blood cultures, which is a result of fastidious growth requirements and the intermittent nature of the bacteremia seen with these organisms. Preexisting valvular heart disease and other underlying conditions can be seen, but these are not constant features. Several series have noted a propensity for large-vessel embolization; this might be a result of large vegetations seen in the face of a frequently delayed diagnosis.

A variety of other infections in addition to endocarditis can be caused by *Haemophilus* species, and these are listed in Table 212–5. These are unusual manifestations of infection with these bacteria, and most are documented by case reports and small series.

The antimicrobial susceptibility characteristics of *Haemophilus* species are similar to those of *H. influenzae.* Some strains produce β-lactamase, and these are resistant to ampicillin.[246] Other strains are sensitive to ampicillin, and this has been used successfully to treat many of these infections. Alternative agents with good activity against most *Haemophilus* species include chloramphenicol, trimethoprim-sulfamethoxazole, third-generation cephalosporins, tetracycline, and aminoglycosides. Endocarditis caused by ampicillin-sensitive strains should be treated with ampicillin plus aminoglycoside. In addition, careful observation is required because surgical intervention is sometimes necessary because of the large size of vegetations and their propensity for embolization.

References

1. Evans MN, Smith DD, Wicken AJ: Haemin and nicotinamide adenine dinucleotide requirement of *Haemophilus influenzae* and *Haemophilus parainfluenzae.* J Med Microbiol 7:359–365, 1974.
2. Pittman M: Variation and type specificity in the bacterial species *Haemophilus influenzae.* J Exp Med 53:471–492, 1931.
3. Wallace RJ Jr, Musher DM, Septimus EJ, et al: *Haemophilus influenzae* infections in adults: Characterization of strains by serotypes, biotypes, and beta-lactamase production. J Infect Dis 144:101–106, 1981.
4. Murphy TF, Apicella MA: Nontypable *Haemophilus influenzae:* A review of clinical aspects, surface antigens, and the human immune response to infection. Rev Infect Dis 9:1–15, 1987.
5. Murphy TF, Sethi S: Bacterial infection in chronic obstructive pulmonary disease. Am Rev Respir Dis 146:1067–1083, 1992.
6. Farley MM, Stephens DS, Brachman PS Jr, et al: Invasive *Haemophilus influenzae* disease in adults. Ann Intern Med 116:806–812, 1992.
7. Falla TJ, Dobson SRM, Crook DWM, et al: Population-based study of non-typable *Haemophilus influenzae* invasive disease in children and neonates. Lancet 341:851–854, 1993.
8. Musser JM, Granoff DM, Pattison PE, Selander RK: A population genetic framework for the study of invasive diseases caused by serotype b strains of *Haemophilus influenzae.* Proc Natl Acad Sci USA 82:5078–5082, 1985.
9. Musser JM, Barenkamp SJ, Granoff DM, Selander RK: Genetic relationships of serologically nontypable and serotype b strains of *Haemophilus influenzae.* Infect Immun 52:183–191, 1986.
10. Porras O, Caugant DA, Gray B, et al: Difference in structure between type b and nontypable *Haemophilus influenzae* populations. Infect Immun 53:79–89, 1986.
11. Murphy TF, Bernstein JM, Dryja DD, et al: Outer membrane protein and lipooligosaccharide analysis of paired nasopharyngeal and middle ear isolates in otitis media due to nontypable *Haemophilus influenzae:* Pathogenetic and epidemiological observations. J Infect Dis 156:723–731, 1987.
12. Barenkamp SJ, Granoff DM, Munson RS Jr: Outer-membrane protein subtypes of *Haemophilus influenzae* type b and spread of disease in day-care centers. J Infect Dis 144:210–217, 1981.
13. Edmonson MB, Granoff DM, Barenkamp SJ, Chesney PJ: Outer membrane protein subtypes and investigation of recurrent *Haemophilus influenzae* type b disease. J Pediatr 100:202–208, 1982.
14. Lees AW, McNaught W: Bacteriology of lower-respiratory-tract secretions, sputum, and upper-respiratory-tract secretions in "normals" and chronic bronchitics. Lancet 1112–1115, 1959.
15. Laurenzi GA, Potter RT, Kass EH: Bacteriologic flora of the lower respiratory tract. N Engl J Med 265:1273–1278, 1961.
16. Miller DL, Jones R: The bacterial flora of the upper respiratory tract and sputum of working men. J Pathol Bacteriol 87:182–186, 1964.
17. Masters PL, Brumfitt W, Mendez RL, Likar M: Bacterial flora of the upper respiratory tract in Paddington families, 1952–4. Br Med J 1:1200–1205, 1958.
18. Spinola SM, Peacock J, Denny FW, et al: Epidemiology of colonization of nontypable *Haemophilus influenzae* in children: A longitudinal study. J Infect Dis 154:100–109, 1986.
19. Harabuchi Y, Faden H, Yamanaka N, et al: Nasopharyngeal colonization with nontypeable *Haemophilus influenzae* and recurrent otitis media. J Infect Dis 170:862–866, 1994.
20. Glode MP, Daum RS, Goldmann DA, et al: *Haemophilus influenzae* type B meningitis: A contagious disease of children. Br Med J 280:899–901, 1980.
21. Ward JI, Fraser DW, Baraff LJ, Plikaytis BD: *Haemophilus influenzae* meningitis: A national study of secondary spread in household contacts. N Engl J Med 301:122–126, 1979.
22. Filice GA, Andrews JS Jr, Hudgins MP, Fraser DW: Spread of *Haemophilus influenzae:* Secondary illness in household contacts of patients with *H. influenzae* meningitis. Am J Dis Child 132:757–759, 1978.
23. Campbell LR, Zedd AJ, Michaels RH: Household spread of infection due to *Haemophilus influenzae* type b. Pediatrics 66:115–117, 1980.
24. Makintubee S, Istre GR, Ward JI: Transmission of invasive *Haemophilus influenzae* type b disease in day care settings. J Pediatr 111:180–186, 1987.
25. Osterholm MT, Pierson LM, White KE, et al: The risk of subsequent transmission of *Hemophilus influenzae* type b disease among children in day care. N Engl J Med 316:1–5, 1987.
26. Murphy TV, Clements JF, Breedlove JA, et al: Risk of subsequent disease among day-care contacts of patients with systemic *Hemophilus influenzae* type b disease. N Engl J Med 316:5–10, 1987.
27. Broome CV, Mortimer EA, Katz SL, et al: Use of chemoprophylaxis to prevent the spread of *Hemophilus influenzae* b in day-care facilities. N Engl J Med 316:1226–1228, 1987.
28. Granoff DM, Basden M: *Haemophilus influenzae* infections in Fresno County, California: A prospective study of the effects of age, race, and contact with a case on incidence of disease. J Infect Dis 141:40–46, 1980.
29. Parke JC, Schneerson R, Robbins JB: The attack rate, age, incidence, social distribution, and case fatality rate of *Haemophilus influenzae* type b meningitis in Mecklenburg County, North Carolina. J Pediatr 81:765–769, 1972.
30. Ambrosino DM, Schiffman G, Gotschlich EC, et al: Correlation

between G2m(n) immunoglobulin allotype and human antibody response and susceptibility to polysaccharide encapsulated bacteria. J Clin Invest 75:1935–1942, 1985.
31. Granoff DM, Pandey JP, Boies E, et al: Response to immunization with *Haemophilus influenzae* type b polysaccharide–pertussis vaccine and risk of *Haemophilus* meningitis in children with Km(1) immunoglobulin allotype. J Clin Invest 74:1708–1714, 1984.
32. Santosham M, Reid R, Ambrosino DM, et al: Prevention of *Haemophilus influenzae* type b infections in high-risk infants treated with bacterial polysaccharide immune globulin. N Engl J Med 317:923–929, 1987.
33. Coulehan JL, Michaels RH, Williams KE, et al: Bacterial meningitis in Navajo Indians. Public Health Rep 91:464–468, 1976.
34. Ward JI, Lum MKW, Bender TR: *Haemophilus influenzae* disease in Alaska: Epidemiologic, clinical and serologic studies of a population at high risk of invasive disease. *In* Sell SH, Wright (eds): *Haemophilus influenzae:* Epidemiology, Immunology and Prevention of Disease. New York, Elsevier Science Publishing, 1982, pp 23–34.
35. Ward JI, Margolis HS, Lum MKW, et al: *Haemophilus influenzae* disease in Alaskan Eskimos: Characteristics of a population with an unusual incidence of invasive disease. Lancet 1:1281–1285, 1981.
36. Apicella MA, Shero M, Dudas KC, et al: Fimbriation of *Haemophilus* species isolated from the respiratory tract of adults. J Infect Dis 150:40–43, 1984.
37. Stull TL, Mendelman PM, Haas JE, et al: Characterization of *Haemophilus influenzae* type b fimbriae. Infect Immun 46:787–796, 1984.
38. Guerina NG, Langermann S, Schoolnik GK, et al: Purification and characterization of *Haemophilus influenzae* pili, and their structural and serological relatedness to *Escherichia coli* P and mannose-sensitive pili. J Exp Med 161:145–159, 1985.
39. Guerina NG, Langermann S, Clegg HW, et al: Adherence of piliated *Haemophilus influenzae* type b to human oropharyngeal cells. J Infect Dis 146:564, 1982.
40. Van Alphen L, Levene C, Geelen-van den Broek L, et al: Combined inheritance of epithelial and erythrocyte receptors for *Haemophilus influenzae.* Infect Immun 58:3807–3809, 1990.
41. Van Alphen L, Geelen-van den Broek L, Blaas L, et al: Blocking of fimbria-mediated adherence of *Haemophilus influenzae* by sialyl gangliosides. Infect Immun 59:4473–4477, 1991.
42. Noel GJ, Barenkamp SJ, St. Geme JW III, et al: High-molecular-weight surface-exposed proteins of *Haemophilus influenzae* mediate binding to macrophages. J Infect Dis 169:425–429, 1994.
43. Bakaletz LO, Barenkamp SJ: Localization of high-molecular-weight adhesion proteins of nontypeable *Haemophilus influenzae* by immunoelectron microscopy. Infect Immun 62:4460–4468, 1994.
44. Noel GJ, Love DC, Mosser DM: High-molecular-weight proteins of nontypeable *Haemophilus influenzae* mediate bacterial adhesion to cellular proteoglycans. Infect Immun 62:4028–4033, 1994.
45. St. Geme JW III: The HMW1 adhesin of nontypeable *Haemophilus influenzae* recognizes sialylated glycoprotein receptors on cultured human epithelial cells. Infect Immun 62:3881–3889, 1994.
46. St. Geme JW III, de la Morena ML, Falkow S: A *Haemophilus influenzae* IgA protease-like protein promotes intimate interaction with human epithelial cells. Mol Microbiol 14:217–233, 1994.
47. Granoff DM, Rockwell R: Experimental *Haemophilus influenzae* type b meningitis: Immunological investigation of the infant rat model. Infect Immun 20:705–713, 1978.
48. Moxon ER, Smith AL, Averill DR, Smith DH: *Haemophilus influenzae* meningitis in infant rats after intranasal inoculation. J Infect Dis 129:154–162, 1974.
49. Giebink GS: Experimental otitis media due to *Haemophilus influenzae* in the chinchilla. *In* Sell SH, Wright PF (eds): *Haemophilus influenzae:* Epidemiology, Immunology and Prevention of Disease. New York, Elsevier Science Publishing, 1982, pp 73–80.
50. Doyle WJ, Supance JS, Marshack G, et al: An animal model of acute otitis media consequent to beta lactamase–producing nontypable *Haemophilus influenzae.* Otolaryngol Head Neck Surg 90:831–836, 1982.
51. Karasic RB, Trumpp CE, Gnehm H, et al: Modification of otitis media in chinchillas rechallenged with nontypable *Haemophilus influenzae* and serological response to outer membrane antigens. J Infect Dis 151:273–279, 1985.
52. Green BA, Vazquez ME, Zlotnick GW, et al: Evaluation of mixtures of purified *Haemophilus influenzae* outer membrane proteins in protection against challenge with nontypeable *H. influenzae* in the chinchilla otitis media model. Infect Immun 61:1950–1957, 1993.
53. Suzuki K, Bakaletz LO: Synergistic effect of adenovirus type 1 and nontypeable *Haemophilus influenzae* in a chinchilla model of experimental otitis media. Infect Immun 62:1710–1718, 1994.
54. Anderson P, Johnston RB, Smith DH: Human serum activities against *Haemophilus influenzae* type b. J Clin Invest 51:31–38, 1972.
55. Gigliotti F, Insall RA: Protection from infection with *Haemophilus influenzae* type b by monoclonal antibody to the capsule. J Infect Dis 146:249–254, 1983.
56. Peltola H, Kayhty H, Sivonen A, Makela PH: *Haemophilus influenzae* type b capsular polysaccharide vaccine in children: A double-blind field study of 100,000 vaccinees 3 months to 5 years of age in Finland. Pediatrics 60:730–737, 1977.
57. Peltola H, Kayhty H, Virtanen M, Makela PH: Prevention of *Hemophilus influenzae* type b bacteremic infections with the capsular polysaccharide vaccine. N Engl J Med 310:1561–1566, 1984.
58. Murphy TF, Dudas KC, Mylotte JM, Apicella MA: A subtyping system for nontypable *Haemophilus influenzae* based on outer-membrane proteins. J Infect Dis 147:838–846, 1983.
59. Barenkamp SJ, Munson RS Jr, Granoff DM: Subtyping isolates of *Haemophilus influenzae* type b by outer-membrane protein profiles. J Infect Dis 143:668–676, 1981.
60. Vachon V, Lyew DJ, Coulton JW: Transmembrane permeability channels across the outer membrane of *Haemophilus influenzae* type b. J Bacteriol 162:918–924, 1985.
61. Munson RS Jr, Shenep JL, Barenkamp SJ, Granoff DM: Purification and comparison of outer membrane protein P2 from *Haemophilus influenzae* type b isolates. J Clin Invest 72:677–684, 1983.
62. Murphy TF, Bartos LC: Purification and analysis with monoclonal antibodies of P2, the major outer membrane protein of nontypable *Haemophilus influenzae.* Infect Immun 56:1084–1089, 1988.
63. Munson R Jr, Tolan RW Jr: Molecular cloning, expression, and primary sequence of outer membrane protein P2 of *Haemophilus influenzae* type b. Infect Immun 57:88–94, 1989.
64. Klingman KL, Jansen EM, Murphy TF: Nearest neighbor analysis of outer membrane proteins of nontypeable *Haemophilus influenzae.* Infect Immun 56:3058–3063, 1988.
65. Vachon V, Kristjanson DN, Coulton JW: Outer membrane porin protein of *Haemophilus influenzae* type b pore size and subunit structure. Can J Microbiol 34:134–140, 1988.
66. Deich RA, Metcalf BJ, Finn CW, et al: Cloning of genes encoding a 15,000-dalton peptidoglycan-associated outer membrane lipoprotein and an antigenically related 15,000-dalton protein from *Haemophilus influenzae.* J Bacteriol 170:489–498, 1988.
67. Murphy TF, Bartos LC, Campagnari AA, et al: Antigenic characterization of the P6 protein of nontypable *Haemophilus influenzae.* Infect Immun 54:774–779, 1986.
68. Murphy TF, Nelson MB, Dudas KC, et al: Identification of a specific epitope of *Haemophilus influenzae* on a 16,600-dalton outer membrane protein. J Infect Dis 152:1300–1307, 1985.
69. Nelson MB, Apicella MA, Murphy TF, et al: Cloning and sequencing of *Haemophilus influenzae* outer membrane protein P6. Infect Immun 56:128–134, 1988.
70. Nelson MB, Munson RS Jr, Apicella MA, et al: Molecular conservation of the P6 outer membrane protein among strains of *Haemophilus influenzae:* Analysis of antigenic determinants, gene sequences, and restriction fragment length polymorphisms. Infect Immun 59:2658–2663, 1991.
71. Kimura A, Gulig PA, McCracken GH Jr, et al: A minor high-molecular-weight outer membrane protein of *Haemophilus influenzae* type b is a protective antigen. Infect Immun 47:253–259, 1985.
72. Loeb MR: Protection of infant rats from *Haemophilus influenzae* type b infection by antiserum to purified outer membrane protein a. Infect Immun 55:2612–2618, 1987.
73. Munson R Jr, Grass S: Purification, cloning, and sequence of outer membrane protein P1 of *Haemophilus influenzae* type b. Infect Immun 56:2235–2242, 1988.

74. Janson H, Ruan M, Forsgren A: Limited diversity of the protein D gene *(hpd)* among encapsulated and nonencapsulated *Haemophilus influenzae* strains. Infect Immun 61:4546–4552, 1993.
75. Janson H, Melhus A, Hermansson A, Forsgren A: Protein D, the glycerophosphodiester phosphodiesterase from *Haemophilus influenzae* with affinity for human immunoglobulin D, influences virulence in a rat otitis model. Infect Immun 62:4848–4854, 1994.
76. Song X-M, Forsgren A, Janson H: The gene encoding protein D *(hpd)* is highly conserved among *Haemophilus influenzae* type b and nontypeable strains. Infect Immun 63:696–699, 1995.
77. Flesher AR, Insel RA: Characterization of lipopolysaccharide of *Haemophilus influenzae.* J Infect Dis 138:719–730, 1978.
78. Campagnari AA, Gupta MR, Dudas KC, et al: Antigenic diversity of lipooligosaccharides of nontypable *Haemophilus influenzae.* Infect Immun 55:882–887, 1987.
79. Apicella MA, Dudas KC, Campagnari A, et al: Antigenic heterogeneity of lipid A of *Haemophilus influenzae.* Infect Immun 50:9–14, 1985.
80. Weiser JN: Relationship between colony morphology and the life cycle of *Haemophilus influenzae:* The contribution of lipopolysaccharide phase variation to pathogenesis. J Infect Dis 168:672–680, 1993.
81. Weiser JN: The oligosaccharide of *Haemophilus influenzae.* Microb Pathog 13:335–342, 1992.
82. Mandrell RE, McLaughlin R, Abu Kwaik Y, et al: Lipooligosaccharides (LOS) of some *Haemophilus* species mimic human glycosphingolipids, and some LOS are sialylated. Infect Immun 60:1322–1328, 1992.
83. Phillips NJ, Apicella MA, Griffis JM, Gibson BW: Structural characterization of the cell surface lipooligosaccharides from a nontypable strain of *Haemophilus influenzae.* Biochemistry 31:4515–4526, 1992.
84. Zwahlen A, Rubin LG, Connelly CJ, et al: Alteration of the cell wall of *Haemophilus influenzae* type b by transformation with cloned DNA: Association with attenuated virulence. J Infect Dis 152:485–492, 1985.
85. Kaplan SL, Hawkins EP, Inzana TJ, et al: Contribution of *Haemophilus influenzae* type b lipopolysaccharide to pathogenesis of infection. Microb Pathog 5:55–62, 1988.
86. Fothergill LD, Wright J: Influenzal meningitis: The relation of age incidence to the bactericidal power of blood against the causal organism. J Immunol 24:273–284, 1933.
87. Black SB, Shinefield HR, Lampert D, et al: Safety and immunogenicity of oligosaccharide conjugate *Haemophilus influenzae* type b (HbOC) vaccine in infancy. Pediatr Infect Dis J 10:92–96, 1991.
88. Eskola J, Peltola H, Takala AK, et al: Efficacy of *Haemophilus influenzae* type b polysaccharide–diphtheria toxoid conjugate vaccine in infancy. N Engl J Med 317:717–722, 1987.
89. Centers for Disease Control and Prevention: FDA approval of use of a new *Haemophilus* b conjugate vaccine and a combined diphtheria-tetanus-pertussis and *Haemophilus* b conjugate vaccine for infants and children. JAMA 269:2359, 1993.
90. Eskola J, Peltola H, Kayhty H, et al: Finnish efficacy trials with *Haemophilus influenzae* type b vaccines. J Infect Dis 165 (Suppl):S137–S138, 1992.
91. Rathore MH, Dick M, Buckner P, Ayoub EM: *Haemophilus influenzae* type B invasive disease in urban and rural children: Immunization patterns and prevalence of disease. South Med J 87:1083–1087, 1994.
92. Vadheim CM, Greenberg DP, Eriksen E, et al, and The Kaiser-UCLA Vaccine Study Group: Eradication of *Haemophilus influenzae* type b disease in Southern California. Arch Pediatr Adolesc Med 148:51–56, 1994.
93. Black SB, Shinefield HR, Fireman B, et al: Efficacy in infancy of oligosaccharide conjugate *Haemophilus influenzae* type b (HbOC) vaccine in a United States population of 61,080 children. Pediatr Infect Dis J 10:97–104, 1991.
94. Peltola H, Kilpi T, Anttila M: Rapid disappearance of *Haemophilus influenzae* type b meningitis after routine childhood immunisation with conjugate vaccines. Lancet 340:592–594, 1992.
95. Singleton RJ, Davidson NM, Desmet IJ, et al: Decline of *Haemophilus influenzae* type b disease in a region of high risk: Impact of passive and active immunization. Pediatr Infect Dis J 13:362–367, 1994.
96. Murphy TV, White KE, Pastor P, et al: Declining incidence of *Haemophilus influenzae* type b disease since introduction of vaccination. JAMA 269:246–248, 1993.
97. Santosham M, Wolff M, Reid R, et al: The efficacy in Navajo infants of a conjugate vaccine consisting of *Haemophilus influenzae* type b polysaccharide and *Neisseria meningitidis* outer membrane protein complex. N Engl J Med 324:1767–1772, 1991.
98. Murphy TF, Bartos LC: Human bactericidal antibody response to outer membrane protein P2 of nontypeable *Haemophilus influenzae.* Infect Immun 56:2673–2679, 1988.
99. Murphy TF, Bartos LC, Rice PA, et al: Identification of a 16,600-dalton outer membrane protein on nontypable *Haemophilus influenzae* as a target for human serum bactericidal antibody. J Clin Invest 78:1020–1027, 1986.
100. Harabuchi Y, Faden H, Yamanaka N, et al: Human milk secretory IgA antibody to nontypeable *Haemophilus influenzae:* Possible protective effects against nasopharyngeal colonization. J Pediatr 124:193–198, 1994.
101. Haase EM, Campagnari AA, Sarwar J, et al: Strain-specific and immunodominant surface epitopes of the P2 porin protein of nontypeable *Haemophilus influenzae.* Infect Immun 59:1278–1284, 1991.
102. Haase EM, Yi K, Morse GD, Murphy TF: Mapping of bactericidal epitopes on the P2 porin protein of nontypeable *Haemophilus influenzae.* Infect Immun 62:3712–3722, 1994.
103. Troelstra A, Vogel L, Van Alphen L, et al: Opsonic antibodies to outer membrane protein P2 of nonencapsulated *Haemophilus influenzae* are strain specific. Infect Immun 62:779–784, 1994.
104. Groeneveld K, Van Alphen L, Voorter C, et al: Antigenic drift of *Haemophilus influenzae* in patients with chronic obstructive pulmonary disease. Infect Immun 57:3038–3044, 1989.
105. Van Alphen L, Eijk P, Geelen-van den Broek L, Dankert J: Immunochemical characterization of variable epitopes of outer membrane protein P2 of nontypeable *Haemophilus influenzae.* Infect Immun 59:247–252, 1991.
106. Duim B, Dankert J, Jansen HM, Van Alphen L: Genetic analysis of the diversity in outer membrane protein P2 of non-encapsulated *Haemophilus influenzae.* Microb Pathog 14:451–462, 1993.
107. Duim B, Van Alphen L, Eijk P, et al: Antigenic drift of non-encapsulated *Haemophilus influenzae* major outer membrane protein P2 in patients with chronic bronchitis is caused by point mutations. Mol Microbiol 11:1181–1189, 1994.
108. Sell SH, Merrill RE, Doyne EO: Long term sequelae of *Haemophilus influenzae* meningitis. Pediatrics 49:206–211, 1972.
109. Feigin RD, Stechenberg BW, Chaig MJ: Prospective evaluation of treatment of *Haemophilus influenzae* meningitis. J Pediatr 88:542–548, 1976.
110. Ferry PC, Culbertson JL, Cooper JA, et al: Sequelae of *Haemophilus influenzae* meningitis: Preliminary report of a long-term follow-up study. *In* Sell SH, Wright PF (eds): *Haemophilus influenzae:* Epidemiology, Immunology and Prevention of Disease. New York, Elsevier Science Publishing, 1982, pp 111–117.
111. Bottenfield GW, Arcinue EL, Sarnaik A: Diagnosis and management of acute epiglottitis. Report of 90 consecutive cases. Laryngoscope 90:822–825, 1980.
112. Fleisher G, Ludwig S, Campos J: Cellulitis: Bacterial etiology, clinical features, and laboratory findings. J Pediatr 97:591–592, 1980.
113. Ricketts RR, Ilbawi MN, Idriss FS: Management of *Haemophilus influenzae* pericarditis. J Pediatr Surg 17:285–289, 1982.
114. Leggiadro RJ, Balsam D: *Haemophilus influenzae* sepsis leading to pericarditis despite antimicrobial therapy. Johns Hopkins Med J 146:133–136, 1980.
115. Cheatham JE. Jr, Grantham RN, Peyton MD: *Haemophilus influenzae* purulent pericarditis in children. J Thorac Cardiovasc Surg 79:933–936, 1980.
116. Morgan RJ, Stephenson LW, Woolf PK: Surgical treatment of purulent pericarditis in children. J Thorac Cardiovasc Surg 85:527–531, 1983.
117. Boomla K, Quilliam RP: *Haemophilus influenzae* endophthalmitis. Br Med J 2828:989–990, 1981.
118. Taylor JRW, Cibis GW, Hamtil LW: Endophthalmitis complicating *Haemophilus influenzae* type b meningitis. Arch Ophthalmol 98:324–326, 1980.
119. Sastry RV, Baker CJ: Endophthalmitis associated with *Haemophilus influenzae* type b bacteremia and meningitis. Am J Dis Child 133:606–608, 1979.

120. Liechty E, Kleiman MB, Ballantine TVN: Primary *Haemophilus influenzae* lung abscesses with bronchial obstruction. J Pediatr Surg 17:281–284, 1982.
121. Feldman WE, Schwartz J: *Haemophilus influenzae* type b brain abscess complicating meningitis: Case report. Pediatrics 72:473–475, 1983.
122. Sugita J, Kawamura S, Icikawa G: Microorganisms isolated from peritonsillar abscess and indicated chemotherapy. Arch Otolaryngol 108:655–658, 1982.
123. McCarthy LG: *Haemophilus influenzae* associated with periappendiceal abscess. Am J Gastroenterol 76:157–159, 1981.
124. Broughton RA, Edwards MS, Taber LH: Systemic *Haemophilus influenzae* type b infection presenting as fever of unknown origin. J Pediatr 98:925–928, 1981.
125. Marshall R, Teele DW, Klein JO: Unsuspected bacteremia due to *Haemophilus influenzae:* Outcome in children not initially admitted to hospital. J Pediatr 95:690–695, 1979.
126. Musher DM, Kubitschek KR, Crennan J, Baughn RE: Pneumonia and acute febrile tracheobronchitis due to *Haemophilus influenzae.* Ann Intern Med 99:444–450, 1983.
127. Berk SL, Holtsclaw SA, Wiener SL, Smith JK: Nontypeable *Haemophilus influenzae* in the elderly. Arch Intern Med 142:537–539, 1982.
128. Musher DM: *Haemophilus influenzae* infections. Hosp Pract 18:158–170, 1983.
129. Steinhart R, Reingold AL, Taylor F, et al: Invasive *Haemophilus influenzae* infections in men with HIV infection. JAMA 268:3350–3352, 1992.
130. Schlamm HT, Yancovitz SR: *Haemophilus influenzae* pneumonia in young adults with AIDS, ARC, or risk of AIDS. Am J Med 86:11–14, 1989.
131. Mortimer EA Jr, Watterson RL Jr: A bacteriologic investigation of otitis media in infancy. Pediatrics 17:359–367, 1956.
132. Feingold M, Klein JO, Haslam GE, et al: Acute otitis media in children. Am J Dis Child 111:361–365, 1966.
133. DelBeccaro MA, Mendelman PM, Inglis AF, et al: Bacteriology of acute otitis media: A new perspective. J Pediatr 120:81–84, 1992.
134. Wallace RJ Jr, Baker CJ, Quinones FJ, et al: Nontypable *Haemophilus influenzae* (biotype 4) as a neonatal, maternal, and genital pathogen. Rev Infect Dis 5:123–135, 1983.
135. Quentin R, Goudeau A, Wallace RJ Jr, et al: Urogenital, maternal and neonatal isolates of *Haemophilus influenzae:* Identification of unusually virulent serologically non-typeable clone families and evidence for a new *Haemophilus* species. J Gen Microbiol 136:1203–1209, 1990.
136. Wald ER, Milmoe GJ, Bowen A, et al: Acute maxillary sinusitis in children. N Engl J Med 304:749–754, 1981.
137. Evans FO Jr, Sydnor JB, Moore WEC, et al: Sinusitis of the maxillary antrum. N Engl J Med 293:735–739, 1975.
138. Spagnuolo PJ, Ellner JJ, Lerner PI, et al: *Haemophilus influenzae* meningitis: The spectrum of disease in adults. Medicine (Baltimore) 61:74–85, 1982.
139. Snyder SN, Brunjes S: *Hemophilus influenzae* meningitis in adults. Review of the literature and report of 18 cases. Am J Med Sci 250:658–667, 1965.
140. Hirschmann JV, Everett ED: *Haemophilus influenzae* infections in adults: Report of nine cases and a review of the literature. Medicine (Baltimore) 58:80–94, 1979.
141. McGowan JE Jr, Klein JO, Bratton L, et al: Meningitis and bacteremia due to *Haemophilus influenzae:* Occurrence and mortality at Boston City Hospital in 12 selected years, 1935–1972. J Infect Dis 130:119–124, 1974.
142. Eykyn SJ, Thomas RD, Phillips I: *Haemophilus influenzae* meningitis in adults. Br Med J 2:463–465, 1974.
143. Addy MG, Ellis PDM, Turk DC: *Haemophilus* epiglottitis: Nine recent cases in Oxford. Br Med J 1:40–42, 1972.
144. Williams NFR, Achong MR, Ruff T: Acute epiglottitis and systemic infection with *Hemophilus influenzae.* Can Med Assoc J 118:63–64, 1978.
145. Black MJ, Harbour J, Remsen KA, Baxter JD: Acute epiglottitis in adults. J Otolaryngol 10:23–27, 1981.
146. Ossoff RH, Wolff AP, Ballenger JJ: Acute epiglottitis in adults: Experience with fifteen cases. Laryngoscope 90:1155–1161, 1980.
147. Alsever RN, Stiver HG, Dinerman N, et al: *Haemophilus influenzae* pericarditis and empyema and thyroiditis in an adult. JAMA 230:1426–1427, 1974.
148. Crossley K, Bigos T, Joffe CD: *Hemophilus influenzae* pericarditis. Am Heart J 230:1426–1427, 1973.
149. Duke M, Donovan TJ: *Hemophilus influenzae* pericarditis with cardiac tamponade. Am J Cardiol 31:778–780, 1973.
150. Borenstein DG, Simon GL: *Hemophilus influenzae* septic arthritis in adults. Medicine (Baltimore) 65:191–201, 1986.
151. McGraw TP, Bruckner DA: Sensitivity of commercial agglutination and counterimmunoelectrophoresis methods for the detection of *Haemophilus influenzae* type b capsular polysaccharide. Am J Clin Pathol 80:703–706, 1983.
152. Kaplan SL: Antigen detection in cerebrospinal fluid—Pros and cons. Am J Med 75:109–118, 1983.
153. Tiller FW, and Diener E: *Haemophilus influenzae* type b capsular polysaccharide detection and measurement by an enzyme-linked immunosorbent assay (ELISA). Zentralbl Bakteriol Hyg A 248:488–493, 1981.
154. Committee on Infectious Diseases: *Haemophilus influenzae* infections. *In* Peter G, Hall CB, Lepow ML, Phillips CF (eds): 1994 Red Book. Report of the Committee on Infectious Diseases. Elk Grove Village, IL, American Academy of Pediatrics, 1994, pp 203–216.
155. Barson WJ, Miller MA, Brady MT, Powell DA: Prospective comparative trial of ceftriaxone vs. conventional therapy for treatment of bacterial meningitis in children. Pediatr Infect Dis 4:362–367, 1985.
156. Marks WA, Stutman HR, Marks MI, et al: Cefuroxime versus ampicillin plus chloramphenicol in childhood bacterial meningitis: A multicenter randomized controlled trial. J Pediatr 109:123–130, 1986.
157. Smith AL: Antibiotic resistance in *Haemophilus influenzae.* Pediatr Infect Dis 2:352–355, 1983.
158. McCracken GH Jr, Lebel M: Dexamethasone therapy for bacterial meningitis in infants and children. Am J Dis Child 143:287–289, 1989.
159. Lebel MH, Hoyt MJ, Waagner DC, et al: Magnetic resonance imaging and dexamethasone therapy for bacterial meningitis. Am J Dis Child 143:301–306, 1989.
160. Tuomanen E: Partner drugs: A new outlook for bacterial meningitis. Ann Intern Med 109:690–692, 1988.
161. Smith AL: Neurologic sequelae of meningitis. N Engl J Med 319:1012–1014, 1988.
162. Lebel MH, Freij BJ, Syrogiannopoulos GA, et al: Dexamethasone therapy for bacteria meningitis. Results of two double-blind, placebo-controlled trials. N Engl J Med 319:964–971, 1988.
163. Barry AL, Pfaller MA, Fuchs PC, Packer RR: In vitro activities of 12 orally administered antimicrobial agents against four species of bacterial respiratory pathogens from U.S. medical centers in 1992 and 1993. Antimicrob Agents Chemother 38:2419–2425, 1994.
164. Jorgensen JH, Doern GV, Maher LA, et al: Antimicrobial resistance among respiratory isolates of *Haemophilus influenzae, Moraxella catarrhalis,* and *Streptococcus pneumoniae* in the United States. Antimicrob Agents Chemother 34:2075–2080, 1990.
165. Scriver SR, Walmsley SL, Kau CL, et al: Canadian *Haemophilus* Study Group: Determination of antimicrobial susceptibilities of Canadian isolates of *Haemophilus influenzae* and characterization of their β-lactamases. Antimicrob. Agents Chemother 38:1678–1680, 1994.
166. Shapiro ED: Infections caused by *Haemophilus influenzae* type b. The beginning of the end? JAMA 269:264–266, 1993.
167. Santosham M: Prevention of *Haemophilus influenzae* type b disease. Vaccine 11(Suppl 1):S52–S57, 1993.
168. Takala AK, Eskola J, Leinonen M, et al: Reduction of oropharyngeal carriage of *Haemophilus influenzae* type b (Hib) in children immunized with an Hib conjugate vaccine. J Infect Dis 164:982–986, 1991.
169. Kauppi M, Saarinen L, Kayhty H: Anti-capsular polysaccharide antibodies reduce nasopharyngeal colonization by *Haemophilus influenzae* type b in infant rats. J Infect Dis 167:365–371, 1993.
170. Takala AK, Santosham M, Almeido-Hill J, et al: Vaccination with *Haemophilus influenzae* type b meningococcal protein conjugate vaccine reduces oropharyngeal carriage of *Haemophilus influenzae* type b among American Indian children. Pediatr Infect Dis J 12:593–599, 1993.
171. Murphy TV, Pastor P, Medley F, et al: Decreased *Haemophilus* colonization in children vaccinated with *Haemophilus influenzae* type b conjugate vaccine. J Pediatr 122:517–523, 1993.

172. Mohle-Boetani JC, Ajello G, Breneman E, et al: Carriage of *Haemophilus influenzae* type b in children after widespread vaccination with conjugate *Haemophilus influenzae* type b vaccines. Pediatr Infect Dis J 12:589–593, 1993.
173. Barbour ML, Mayon-White RT, Coles C, et al: The impact of conjugate vaccine on carriage of *Haemophilus influenzae* type b. J Infect Dis 171:93–98, 1995.
174. Albritton WL, Setlow JK, Thomas M, et al: Heterospecific transformation in the genus *Haemophilus.* Mol Gen Genet 193:358–363, 1984.
175. Casin L, Grimont F, Grimont PAD: Deoxyribonucleic acid relatedness between *Haemophilus aegyptius* and *Haemophilus influenzae.* Ann Microbiol (Paris) 137B:155–163, 1986.
176. Leidy G, Jaffee I, Alexander HE: Further evidence of a high degree of genetic homology between *H. influenzae* and *H. aegyptius.* Proc Soc Exp Biol Med 118:671–679, 1965.
177. Brazilian Purpuric Fever Study Group: Brazilian purpuric fever: Epidemic purpura fulminans associated with antecedent purulent conjunctivitis. Lancet 2:757–761, 1987.
178. Brazilian Purpuric Fever Study Group: *Haemophilus aegyptius* bacteraemia in Brazilian purpuric fever. Lancet 2:761–763, 1987.
179. McIntyre P, Wheaton G, Erlich J, Hansman D: Brasilian purpuric fever in central Australia (Letter). Lancet 2:112, 1987.
180. Wild BE, Pearman JW, Campbell PB, et al: Brazilian purpuric fever in Western Australia (Letter). Med J Aust 150:344, 346, 1989.
181. Brenner DJ, Mayer LW, Carlone GM, et al: Biochemical, genetic, and epidemiologic characterization of *Haemophilus influenzae* biogroup *aegyptius (Haemophilus aegyptius)* strains associated with Brazilian purpuric fever. J Clin Microbiol 26:1524–1534, 1988.
182. Lesse AJ, Gheesling LL, Bittner WE, et al: Stable, conserved outer membrane epitope of strains of *Haemophilus influenzae* biogroup *aegyptius* associated with Brazilian purpuric fever. Infect Immun 60:1351–1357, 1992.
183. Carlone GM, Gorelkin L, Gheesling LL, et al: Potential virulence factors of *Haemophilus influenzae* biogroup *aegyptius* in Brazilian purpuric fever. Pediatr Infect Dis J 8:245–247, 1989.
184. Mayer LW, Bibb WF, Birkness KA, et al: Distinguishing clonal characteristics of the Brazilian purpuric fever–producing strain. Pediatr Infect Dis J 8:241–243, 1989.
185. Tondella MLC, Quinn FD, Perkins BA: Brazilian purpuric fever caused by *Haemophilus influenzae* biogroup *aegyptius* strains lacking the 3031 plasmid. J Infect Dis 171:209–212, 1995.
186. Porto MH, Noel GJ, Edelson PJ, and the Brazilian Purpuric Fever Study Group: Resistance to serum bactericidal activity distinguishes Brazilian purpuric fever (BPF) case strains of *Haemophilus influenzae* biogroup *aegyptius (H. aegyptius)* from non-BPF strains. J Clin Microbiol 27:792–794, 1989.
187. Dobson SRM, Kroll JS, Moxon ER: Insertion sequence IS1016 and absence of *Haemophilus* capsulation genes in the Brazilian purpuric fever clone of *Haemophilus influenzae* biogroup *aegyptius.* Infect Immun 60:618–622, 1992.
188. Rubin LG, Gloster ES, Carlone GM, et al: An infant rat model of bacteremia with Brazilian purpuric fever isolates of *Haemophilus influenzae* biogroup *aegyptius.* J Infect Dis 160:476–482, 1989.
189. Rubin LG, Carlone GM, et al: An infant rat model of bacteremia with Brazilian purpuric fever isolates of *Haemophilus influenzae* biogroup *aegyptius (Haemophilus aegyptius).* Pediatr Infect Dis J 8:247–248, 1989.
190. Weyant RS, Quinn FD, Utt EA, et al: Human microvascular endothelial cell toxicity caused by Brazilian purpuric fever–associated strains of *Haemophilus influenzae* biogroup *aegyptius.* J Infect Dis 169:430–433, 1994.
191. Quinn FD, Weyant RS, Candal FJ, Ades EW: Destruction of human microvascular endothelial cell capillary–like microtubules by Brazilian purpuric fever–associated *Haemophilus influenzae* biogroup *aegyptius.* Pathobiology 62:109–112, 1994.
192. Whitney AM, Farley MM: Cloning and sequence analysis of the structural pilin gene of Brazilian purpuric fever–associated *Haemophilus influenzae* biogroup *aegyptius.* Infect Immun 61:1559–1562, 1993.
193. St. Geme JW III, Falkow S: Isolation, expression, and nucleotide sequencing of the pilin structural gene of the Brazilian purpuric fever clone of *Haemophilus influenzae* biogroup *aegyptius.* Infect Immun 61:2233–2237, 1993.
194. Rubin LG: Phase-variable expression of the 145-kDa surface protein of Brazilian purpuric fever case-clone strains of *Haemophilus influenzae* biogroup *aegyptius.* J Infect Dis 171:713–717, 1995.
195. Rubin LG, St. Geme JW III: Role of lipooligosaccharide in virulence of the Brazilian purpuric fever clone of *Haemophilus influenzae* biogroup *aegyptius* in infant rats. Infect Immun 61:650–655, 1993.
196. Centers for Disease Control and Prevention: Summary of notifiable diseases, United States 1994. MMWR Morbid Mortal Wkly Rep 43:1–80, 1994.
197. Kreiss JK, Koech D, Plummer FA, et al: AIDS virus infection in Nairobi prostitutes. Spread of the epidemic to East Africa. N Engl J Med 314:414–418, 1986.
198. Quinn TC, Mann JM, Curran JW, Piot P: AIDS in Africa: An epidemiologic paradigm. Science 234:955–963, 1986.
199. Casin I, Grimont F, Grimont PAD, Sanson-Le Pors MJ: Lack of deoxyribonucleic acid relatedness between *Haemophilus ducreyi* and other *Haemophilus* species. Int J Syst Bacteriol 35:23–25, 1985.
200. Morse SA: Chancroid and *Haemophilus ducreyi.* Clin Microbiol Rev 2:137–157, 1989.
201. Odumeru JA, Ronald AR, Albritton WL: Characterization of cell proteins of *Haemophilus ducreyi* by polyacrylamide gel electrophoresis. J Infect Dis 148:710–714, 1983.
202. Slootmans L, Vanden Berghe DA, Piot P: Typing *Haemophilus ducreyi* by indirect immunofluorescence assay. Genitourin Med 61:123–126, 1985.
203. Van Dyck E, Piot P: Enzyme profile of *Haemophilus ducreyi* strains isolated on different continents. Eur J Clin Microbiol 6:40–43, 1987.
204. Flood JM, Sarafian SK, Bolan GA, et al: Multistrain outbreak of chancroid in San Francisco, 1989–91. J Infect Dis 167:1106–1111, 1993.
205. Dienst RB: Virulence and antigenicity of *Haemophilus ducreyi.* Am J Syph Gonorrhea Vener Dis 32:289–291, 1948.
206. Feiner RR, Mortara F: Infectivity of *Haemophilus ducreyi* for the rabbit and the development of skin hypersensitivity. Am J Syph Gonorrhea Vener Dis 29:71–79, 1945.
207. Lagergard T: *Haemophilus ducreyi:* Pathogenesis and protective immunity. Trends Microbiol 3:87–92, 1995.
208. Purcell BK, Richardson JA, Radolf JD, Hansen EJ: A temperature-dependent rabbit model for production of dermal lesions by *Haemophilus ducreyi.* J Infect Dis 164:359–367, 1991.
209. Hansen EJ, Lumbley SR, Richardson JA, et al: Induction of protective immunity to *Haemophilus ducreyi* in the temperature-dependent rabbit model of experimental chancroid. J Immunol 152:184–192, 1994.
210. Totten PA, Morton WR, Knitter GH, et al: A primate model for chancroid. J Infect Dis 169:1284–1290, 1994.
211. Spinola SM, Wild LM, Apicella MA, et al: Experimental human infection with *Haemophilus ducreyi.* J Infect Dis 169:1146–1150, 1994.
212. Alfa MJ: Cytopathic effect of *Haemophilus ducreyi* for human foreskin cell culture. J Med Microbiol 37:43–50, 1992.
213. Lammel CJ, Dekker NP, Palefsky J, Brooks GF: In vitro model of *Haemophilus ducreyi* adherence to and entry into eukaryotic cells of genital origin. J Infect Dis 167:642–650, 1993.
214. Brentjens RJ, Spinola SM, Campagnari AA: *Haemophilus ducreyi* adheres to human keratinocytes. Microb Pathog 16:243–247, 1994.
215. Lagergard T, Purven M, Frisk A: Evidence of *Haemophilus ducreyi* adherence to and cytotoxin destruction of human epithelial cells. Microb Pathog 14:417–431, 1993.
216. Palmer KL, Grass S, Munson RS Jr: Identification of a hemolytic activity elaborated by *Haemophilus ducreyi.* Infect Immun 62:3041–3043, 1994.
217. Lagergard T: The role of *Haemophilus ducreyi* bacteria, cytotoxin, endotoxin and antibodies in animal models for study of chancroid. Microb Pathog 13:203–217, 1992.
218. Campagnari AA, Wild LM, Griffiths GE, et al: Role of lipooligosaccharides in experimental dermal lesions caused by *Haemophilus ducreyi.* Infect Immun 59:2601–2608, 1991.
219. Spinola SM, Castellazzo A, Shero M, Apicella MA: Characterization of pili expressed by *Haemophilus ducreyi.* Microb Pathog 9:417–426, 1990.

220. Spinola SM, Griffiths GE, Bogdan J, Menegus MA: Characterization of an 18,000-molecular-weight outer membrane protein of *Haemophilus ducreyi* that contains a conserved surface-exposed epitope. Infect Immun 60:385–391, 1992.
221. Spinola SM, Griffiths GE, Shanks KL, Blake MS: The major outer membrane protein of *Haemophilus ducreyi* is a member of the OmpA family of proteins. Infect Immun 61:1346–1351, 1993.
222. Schmid GP, Sanders LL Jr, Blount JH, Alexander ER: Chancroid in the United States. Reestablishment of an old disease. JAMA 258:3265–3268, 1987.
223. Hansen EJ, Loftus TA: Monoclonal antibodies reactive with all strains of *Haemophilus ducreyi*. Infect Immun 44:196–198, 1984.
224. Schmid GP: The treatment of chancroid. JAMA 255:1757–1762, 1986.
225. Aldridge KE, Cammarata C, Martin DH: Comparison of the in vitro activities of various parenteral and oral antimicrobial agents against endemic *Haemophilus ducreyi*. Antimicrob Agents Chemother 37:1986–1988, 1993.
226. Kraut MS, Attebery HR, Finegold SM, Sutter VL: Detection of *Haemophilus aphrophilus* in the human oral flora with a selective medium. J Infect Dis 126:189–192, 1972.
227. Kilian M, Heine-Jensen J, Bulow P: *Haemophilus* in the upper respiratory tract of children. Acta Pathol Microbiol Scand B 80:571–578, 1972.
228. Brondz I, Olsen I: Chemotaxonomy of selected species of the *Actinobacillus-Haemophilus-Pasteurella* group by means of gas chromatography, gas chromatography–mass spectrometry and bioenzymatic methods. J Chromatogr 380:1–17, 1986.
229. Albritton WL: Species identification in *Haemophilus* infection (Letter). Rev Infect Dis 6:1226, 1988.
230. Oill PA, Chow AW, Guze LB: Adult bacteremic *Haemophilus parainfluenzae* infections. Arch Intern Med 139:985–988, 1979.
231. Jemsek JG, Greenberg SB, Gentry LO, et al: *Haemophilus parainfluenzae* endocarditis. Two cases and review of the literature in the past decade. Am J Med 66:51–57, 1979.
232. Blair DC, Weiner LB: Prosthetic valve endocarditis due to *Haemophilus parainfluenzae* biotype II. Am J Dis Child 133:617–618, 1979.
233. Chunn CJ, Jones SR, McCutchan JA, et al: *Haemophilus parainfluenzae* infective endocarditis. Medicine (Baltimore) 56:99–113, 1977.
234. Lynn DJ, Kane JG, Parker RH: *Haemophilus parainfluenzae* and *influenzae* endocarditis: A review of forty cases. Medicine (Baltimore) 56:115–128, 1977.
235. Bieger RC, Brewer NS, Washington JA II: *Haemophilus aphrophilus:* A microbiologic and clinical review and report of 42 cases. Medicine (Baltimore) 57:345–355, 1978.
236. Hammond GW, Richardson H, Lian CJ, Ronald AR: Two cases of *Hemophilus* endocarditis of prolapsed mitral valves—*Hemophilus paraphrophilus* or *parainfluenzae?* Am J Med 65:537–541, 1978.
237. Hable KA, Logan GB, Washington JA II: Three *Hemophilus* species. Am J Dis Child 121:35–37, 1971.
238. Parker SW, Apicella MA, Fuller CM: *Hemophilus* endocarditis. Two patients with complications. Arch Intern Med 143:48–51, 1983.
239. Geraci JE, Wilkowske CJ, Wilson WR, Washington JA II: *Haemophilus* endocarditis. Report of 14 patients. Mayo Clin Proc 52:209–215, 1977.
240. Geraci JE, Wilson WR: Endocarditis due to gram-negative bacteria. Report of 56 cases. Mayo Clin Proc 57:145–148, 1982.
241. Elster SK, Mattes LM, Meyers BR, Jurado RA: *Hemophilus aphrophilus* endocarditis: Review of 23 cases. Am J Cardiol 35:72–79, 1975.
242. Sutter VL, Finegold SM: *Haemophilus aphrophilus* infections: Clinical and bacteriologic studies. Ann N Y Acad Sci 174:468–487, 1970.
243. Bangsborg JM, Tvede M, Skinhoj P: *Haemophilus segnis* endocarditis. J Infect 16:81–85, 1988.
244. Julander I, Lindberg AA, Svanbon M: *Haemophilus parainfluenzae*—An uncommon cause of septicemia and endocarditis. Scand J Infect Dis 12:85–89, 1980.
245. Raucher B, Dobkin J, Mandel L, et al: Occult polymicrobial endocarditis with *Haemophilus parainfluenzae* in intravenous drug abusers. Am J Med 86:169–172, 1989.
246. Brunton J, Clare D, Meier MA: Molecular epidemiology of antibiotic resistance plasmids of *Haemophilus* species and *Neisseria gonorrhoeae*. Rev Infect Dis 8:713–724, 1986.
247. Murphy TF, Apicella MA: Antigenic heterogeneity of outer membrane proteins of nontypable *Haemophilus influenzae* is a basis for a serotyping system. Infect Immun 50:15–21, 1985.
248. Kilian M: A rapid method for the differentiation of *Haemophilus* strains: The porphyrin test. Acta Pathol Microbiol Scand B 82:835–842, 1974.
249. Oberhofer TR, Back AB: Biotypes of *Haemophilus* encountered in clinical laboratories. J Clin Microbiol 10:168–174, 1979.
250. Porras O, Caugant DA, Lagergard T, Svanborg-Eden C: Application of multilocus enzyme gel electrophoresis to *Haemophilus influenzae*. Infect Immun 53:71–78, 1986.
251. Groeneveld K, Van Alphen L, Eijk PP, et al: Changes in outer membrane proteins of nontypable *Haemophilus influenzae* in patients with chronic obstructive pulmonary disease. J Infect Dis 158:360–365, 1988.
252. Loos BG, Bernstein JM, Dryja DM, et al: Determination of the epidemiology and transmission of nontypeable *Haemophilus influenzae* in children with otitis media by comparison of total genomic DNA restriction fingerprints. Infect Immun 57:2751–2757, 1989.
253. Bruce KD, Jordens JZ: Characterization of noncapsulate *Haemophilus influenzae* by whole-cell polypeptide profiles, restriction endonuclease analysis, and rRNA gene restriction patterns. J Clin Microbiol 29:291–296, 1991.
254. Jordens JZ, Leaves NI, Anderson EC, Slack MPE: Polymerase chain reaction–based strain characterization of noncapsulate *Haemophilus influenzae*. J Clin Microbiol 31:2981–2987, 1993.
255. Van Belkum A, Duim B, Regelink A, et al: Genomic DNA fingerprinting of clinical *Haemophilus influenzae* isolates by polymerase chain reaction amplification: Comparison with major outer-membrane protein and restriction fragment length polymorphism. J Med Microbiol 41:63–68, 1994.
256. Coll-Vinent B, Suris X, Lopez-Soto A, et al: *Haemophilus paraphrophilus* endocarditis: Case report and review. Clin Infect Dis 20:1381–1383, 1995.
257. Hamed KA, Dormitzer PR, Su CK, Relman DA: *Haemophilus parainfluenzae* endocarditis: Application of a molecular approach for identification of pathogenic bacterial species. Clin Infect Dis 19:677–683, 1994.
258. Cooney TG, Harwood BR, Meisner DJ: *Haemophilus parainfluenzae* thoracic empyema. Arch Intern Med 141:940–941, 1981.
259. Kiddy K, Webberley J: *Haemophilus aphrophilus* as a cause of chronic suppurative pulmonary infection and intra-abdominal abscesses. J Infect 15:161–163, 1987.
260. Jones RN, Slepack J, Bigelow J: Ampicillin-resistant *Haemophilus paraphrophilus* laryngo-epiglottitis. J Clin Microbiol 4:405–407, 1976.
261. Dudley JP: Supraglottitis and *Hemophilus parainfluenzae:* Pathogenic potential of the organism. Ann Otol Rhinol Laryngol 96:400–402, 1987.
262. Bachman DS: *Hemophilus* meningitis: Comparison of *H. influenzae* and *H. parainfluenzae.* Pediatrics 55:526–530, 1975.
263. Welch WD, Southern PM Jr, Schneider NR: Five cases of *Haemophilus segnis* appendicitis. J Clin Microbiol 24:851–852, 1986.
264. Gallant TE, Malinak LR, Gump DW, Mead PB: *Hemophilus parainfluenzae* peritonitis associated with an intrauterine contraceptive device. Am J Obstet Gynecol 129:702–703, 1977.
265. Warman ST, Reinitz E, Klein RS: *Haemophilus parainfluenzae* septic arthritis in an adult. JAMA 246:868–869, 1981.
266. von Essen R, Kostiala AA, Anttolainen I, et al: Arthritis caused by *Haemophilus paraphrophilus* and isolation of the organism by using an improved culture protocol. J Clin Microbiol 25:2447–2448, 1987.
267. Merino D, Saavedra J, Pujol E, et al: *Haemophilus aphrophilus* as a rare cause of arthritis. Clin Infect Dis 19:320–322, 1994.
268. Milne LM, Isaacs D, Crook PJ: Neonatal infections with *Haemophilus* species. Arch Dis Child 63:83–85, 1988.
269. Crawford SA, Evans JA, Crawford GE: Necrotizing fasciitis associated with *Haemophilus aphrophilus*. Arch Intern Med 138:1714–1715, 1978.
270. Black CT, Kupferschmid JP, West KW, Grosfeld JL: *Haemophilus parainfluenzae* infections in children, with the report of a unique case. Rev Infect Dis 10:342–346, 1988.
271. Blaylock BL, Baber S: Urinary tract infection caused by *Haemophilus parainfluenzae.* Am J Clin Pathol 73:285–287, 1980.

213

Streptobacillus moniliformis

Gary Doern

Microbiology

Streptobacillus moniliformis, one of the causative agents of rat-bite fever, is a facultatively anaerobic, pleomorphic, nonmotile, gram-negative bacillus. Its general dimensions are approximately 0.3 × 3.0 μm; however, one of the principal distinguishing attributes of this organism is its morphologic variability. Depending on age, condition of culture, and composition of growth media, single bacillary forms, many with central round enlargements, may be observed, or chains of bacilli may be seen. The filamentous forms, when found to possess the central swellings, resemble a string of beads. In addition, stable cell wall–defective L-phase variants often arise both in vivo and in vitro.

S. moniliformis may be visualized with Gram, Wayson, Giemsa, or acridine orange stain; Gram stain yields the least consistent results. The organism is readily propagated on or within standard microbiologic agar and broth media, assuming the media are supplemented with blood, serum, or ascites fluid from practically any animal source.[1, 2] Indeed, the patient's blood will act as a satisfactory supplement, which perhaps explains the relatively frequent isolation of *S. moniliformis* from broth-based blood cultures. One concern with respect to detecting *S. moniliformis* bacteremia is the relative sensitivity of this organism to sodium polyanetholesulfonate (Liquoid). Sodium polyanetholesulfonate is an anticoagulant that is added to most broth-based blood culture bottles at a concentration of 0.025%, a concentration inhibitory to many strains of *S. moniliformis.*[3] Therefore, sodium polyanetholesulfonate should probably be eliminated from broth blood culture media or neutralized by the addition of 1.5% sterile gelatin when an effort is made to document *S. moniliformis* bacteremia. Finally, supplementation of blood culture broth with papain digest of ox liver (Panmede) has been shown to yield early growth of small inocula of *S. moniliformis.*[4]

Cultures should be incubated at 35°C to 37°C in an atmosphere of 5% to 8% carbon dioxide. In broth, *S. moniliformis* forms characteristic puffball aggregates. On solid media, 1- to 2-mm, grayish, round, glistening colonies appear after 2 to 6 days' incubation. L-phase variants pit the agar and resemble a fried egg. Positive biochemical reactions useful in the identification of *S. moniliformis* include starch and esculin hydrolysis; production of oxidase, catalase, and alkaline phosphatase; reduction of 2,3,5-triphenyltetrazolium chloride, potassium tellurite, and nitrate; and use of glucose, maltose, fructose, galactose, mannose, dextrin, and glycogen. Gas is not produced from carbohydrate fermentation.[5, 6] Last, gas-liquid chromatography has been used to achieve rapid identification of *S. moniliformis.* The characteristic fatty acid profile of this organism includes palmitic, linoleic, oleic, and stearic acids.[7]

Epidemiology and Pathogenesis

The primary reservoir of *S. moniliformis* is the respiratory tract of rodents. More than 50% of wild and laboratory rats harbor this organism in the nasopharynx or oral cavity.[8] The organism has also been isolated from various respiratory sources from wild and laboratory mice, turkeys, and guinea pigs.[9, 10] Furthermore, rat-bite fever is reported to have occurred after close contact with cats, dogs, pigs, and squirrels.[3, 11]

Human infections usually arise after one of two distinct modes of transmission: traumatic implantation of the organism through the skin, or ingestion of contaminated food with subsequent penetration of the organism through the mucosal epithelium of the gastrointestinal tract. In the first case, the most common trauma is the bite of a rat or another rodent. It is clear, however, that handling a colonized animal without incurring a bite wound can lead to infection. In the second case, the most common vehicle has been raw milk, presumably contaminated by rodents harboring *S. moniliformis.*[12–14] Water has also been incriminated.[15] *S. moniliformis* infection that occurs as a consequence of ingesting contaminated food or water has been termed Haverhill fever; it typically arises in the setting of a common-source outbreak.

After the organism penetrates the skin or the gastrointestinal tract mucosa, it presumably multiplies locally and then is disseminated throughout the host by the blood stream. Hematogenous seeding of any organ may result; however, joints are most often involved.

Infection due to *S. moniliformis* is relatively uncommon. Thirteen cases were reported between 1958 and 1983 in the United States.[16] Approximately half of cases occur in laboratory workers who have extensive contact with laboratory rats and mice.[17] The majority of cases among persons who do not work in laboratories occur in children, presumably because they suffer more rodent bites.[11]

Clinical Manifestations

Infection due to *S. moniliformis* characteristically manifests with fever, rash, and constitutional symptoms. Patients usually experience abrupt onset of fever and shaking chills. The incubation period is extremely variable (1 day to 3 weeks, mean of 10 days). Constitutional symptoms (headache, malaise, myalgias) are prominent. A characteristic rash occurs in 90% of cases within 1 week of the onset of symptoms, usually an erythematous macular eruption that is widely distributed but most prominent on the soles and palms.[18] Skin lesions may be discrete or confluent, petechial or purpuric. In cases in which infection arises after a rodent bite, the bite wound is often initially conspicuous; however, it heals rapidly and is inapparent by the time the rash appears. Half of all patients suffer arthralgias.[11, 18] Knees, wrists, and elbows are most often affected. Joint involvement may be monarticular or polyarticular and may progress to frank arthritis with purulent effusion. Without treatment, symptoms usually abate within 2 weeks; however, episodic relapses have been described at intervals of weeks to months.

Rat-bite fever can also be due to infection with another commensal organism of the respiratory tract of rodents, *Spirillum minus. S. minus* infection, also referred to as sodoku, differs clinically from that caused by *S. moniliformis* insofar as the disease usually has a more insidious onset, there is rarely any evidence of the bite entry wound, and joints are not involved. Only a single case of *S. minus* infection has been reported in the United States in the past 31 years. Most infections due to this bacterium occur in Asia.[9]

Treatment

When a patient is seen soon after a rodent bite, the lesion should be cleaned thoroughly and tetanus immunization administered. There is no proven benefit of antimicrobial prophylaxis for rat-bite fever.

Recommended therapy of uncomplicated rat-bite fever and Haverhill fever for penicillin-tolerant patients consists of intravenous procaine penicillin G, 600,000 units every 12 hours.[11] Therapy should be continued for 10 to 14 days. It is possible to switch to oral therapy (penicillin, 2 g/d) after 1 week of parenteral therapy if a favorable clinical response is achieved. Systemic focal infections such as endocarditis require larger doses of antimicrobial agent administered for a longer period.[19] For penicillin-allergic patients, tetracycline, 500 mg orally every 6 hours, is the therapy of choice.[10]

Prevention

The only measure effective in preventing rat-bite fever and Haverhill fever in the general public is the elimination of rodent reservoirs (i.e., rats and mice) from environments in which humans live, work, and play. Disease among laboratory workers can be prevented by exercising care in handling laboratory animals, especially mice, rats, and guinea pigs, so that the risk for bites and scratches is minimized.

References

1. Faro S, Walker C, Pierson RL: Amnionitis with intact amniotic membranes involving *Streptobacillus moniliformis.* Obstet Gynecol 55:9S, 1980.
2. Portnoy BL, Satterwhite TK, Dyckman JD: Rat-bite fever misdiagnosed as Rocky Mountain spotted fever. South Med J 72:607, 1979.
3. Lambe DW, McPhedran AM, Mertz JA, Stewart P: *Streptobacillus moniliformis* from a case of Haverhill fever. Am J Clin Pathol 60:854, 1973.
4. Shanson DC, Pratt J, Greene P: Comparison of media with and without Panmede for the isolation of *Streptobacillus moniliformis* from blood cultures and observations on the inhibitory effect of sodium polyanethol sulphonate. J Med Microbiol 19:181, 1985.
5. Rogesa M: *Streptobacillus moniliformis* and *Spirillum minor. In* Linnete EH, Balows A, Hausler WJ, Shadomy HJ (eds): Manual of Clinical Microbiology, ed 4. Washington, DC, American Society for Microbiology, 1985, pp 400–406.
6. Edwards R, Finch RG: Characterization and antibiotic susceptibility of *Streptobacillus moniliformis.* J Med Microbiol 21:39, 1986.
7. Rowbotham TJ: Rapid identification of *Streptobacillus moniliformis.* Lancet 2:567, 1983.
8. Strangeways WI: Rats as carriers of *Streptobacillus moniliformis.* J Pathol Bacteriol 37:45, 1933.
9. Josephson SL: Rat-bite fever. *In* Balows A, Hausler WJ, Lennette EH (eds): Laboratory Diagnosis of Infectious Disease: Principles and Practices, Vol 1. New York, Springer-Verlag, 1988, pp 443–447.
10. Murray HW: *Streptobacillus moniliformis* (rat-bite fever). *In* Mandell GL, Douglas RG, Bennett JE (eds): Principles and Practice of Infectious Diseases, ed 2. New York, John Wiley & Sons, 1985, pp 1305–1306.
11. Roughgarden JW: Antimicrobial therapy of rat-bite fever. Arch Intern Med 116:39, 1965.
12. Parker F, Hudson NP: The etiology of Haverhill fever. Am J Pathol 2:357, 1926.
13. Place EH, Sutton LE: Erythema arthriticum epidemicum (Haverhill fever). Arch Intern Med 54:659, 1934.
14. Shanson DC, Midgley J, Gazzard BG, et al: *Streptobacillus moniliformis* isolated from blood in four cases of Haverhill fever. Lancet 1:92, 1983.
15. McEvoy MB, Noak ND, Pilsworth R: Outbreak of fever caused by *Streptobacillus moniliformis.* Lancet 2:1361, 1987.
16. Hadfield TL: Bartonellosis, cat-scratch disease and rat-bite fever. *In* Wentworth BB (ed): Diagnostic Procedures for Bacterial Infections, ed 7. Washington, DC, American Public Health Association, 1987, pp 147–154.
17. Anderson LC, Leary SL, Manning PJ: Rat-bite fever in animal research laboratory personnel. Lab Anim Sci 33:292, 1983.
18. Raffin BJ, Freemark M: Streptobacillary rat-bite fever: A pediatric problem. Pediatrics 64:214, 1979.
19. McCormack RC, Kaye D, Hook EW: Endocarditis due to *Streptobacillus moniliformis.* JAMA 200:77, 1967.

214

Legionella

Janet E. Stout

Nearly 6 months after the dramatic outbreak of pneumonia at the American Legion Convention in Philadelphia in 1976, the causative agent was isolated by investigators at the Centers for Disease Control and Prevention in Atlanta, Georgia. The newly discovered bacterium was assigned to the family Legionellaceae, the genus *Legionella,* and the species *pneumophila.* There are now 39 named species, of which at least 20 have been implicated in human disease (Table 214–1); the remainder have been isolated from environmental water sources.[1, 2] There are more than 60 serogroups among the numerous species; however, most cases of legionellosis are caused by *Legionella pneumophila* serogroups 1, 4, and 6.[3]

Classification

Members of the family Legionellaceae are obligate aerobic slow-growing nonfermenters and are distinguished from other saccharolytic bacteria by their requirement for L-cysteine and iron salts for primary isolation on solid media and by their unique cellular fatty acids and ubiquinones. Gas-liquid chromatography demonstrates unusually large amounts of cellular branched chain fatty acids and respiratory ubiquinones with 10 or more isoprene units.[4]

DNA relatedness as measured by DNA-DNA hybridization, guanine plus cytosine content, and 16S ribosomal RNA–encoding (ribosomal DNA) sequencing analysis can definitively identify these organisms and have also been used to delineate phylogeny within the Legionellaceae family.[5, 6] Differences among species have also been assessed by chemotaxonomic study of lipopolysaccharide,[7] electrophoretic protein profiles,[8] monoclonal antibodies,[9] and gas chromatography–mass spectrophotometry.[10]

Laboratory Diagnosis and Identification

Legionella species are small (0.3 to 0.9 μm in width and 2 to 20 μm in length) gram-negative rods with polar flagella (except *Legionella oakridgensis*).[5] They generally appear as small coccobacilli in infected tissue or secretions, whereas long filamentous forms can be seen when they are grown in culture media.

Neither Gram stain nor Gimenez stain is particularly useful for respiratory specimens, because *Legionella* organisms are not notably different morphologically from other oropharyngeal flora. Silver impregnation stains, including the Dieterle stain and Warthin-Starry stain, allow visualization in

TABLE 214–1 ■ *Legionella* Species Implicated in Infections*

SPECIES	GROWTH ON TYROSINE-SUPPLEMENTED AGAR	GELATINASE PRODUCTION	HIPPURATE HYDROLYSIS	OXIDASE	β-LACTAMASE PRODUCTION	AUTOFLUORESCENCE (365-NM UV LIGHT)	FLAGELLA
L. pneumophila	+	+	+	±	+	−	+
L. micdadei	−	−	−	+	−	−	+
L. bozemanii	+	+	−	±	±	+ (BW)	+
L. dumoffii	−	+	−	−	+	+ (BW)	+
L. longbeachae	+	+	−	±	±	−	+
L. jordanis	+	+	−	+	+	−	+
L. rubrilucens	+	+	−	−	+	+ (R)	+
L. feeleii	+	−	±	−	−	−	+
L. gormanii	−	+	−	−	+	+ (BW)	+
L. wadsworthii	−	+	−	−	+	−	+
L. hackeliae	+	+	−	±	+	−	+
L. maceachernii	−	−	−	+	−	−	+
L. oakridgensis	+	+	−	−	±	−	−
L. birminghamensis	+	+	−	±	+	−	+
L. cherrii	+	+	−	−	+	+ (BW)	+
L. sainthelensi	+	+	−	+	+	−	+
L. cincinnatiensis	+	+	−	−	ND	−	+
L. tucsonensis	ND	+	−	−	+	+ (BW)	+
L. anisa	+	+	−	−	+	+ (BW)	+
L. lansingensis	−	−	−	+	−	−	+

*+, Positive; −, negative; ±, weak reaction; ND, not done; UV, ultraviolet; BW, blue-white autofluorescence; R, red autofluorescence.

From Hookey JV, Saunders NA, Fry NK, et al: Phylogeny of Legionellaceae based on small-subunit ribosomal DNA sequences and proposal of *Legionella lytica* comb. nov. for *Legionella*-like amoebal pathogens. Int J Syst Bateriol 46:526–531, 1996.

paraffin-fixed tissue sections. *Legionella micdadei* can stain weakly acid-fast in tissue with the Kinyoun and Fite stains and in smears with the modified Ziehl-Neelsen stain from tissue or sputum specimens.[11] Interestingly, the acid-fastness is rarely seen in *L. micdadei* grown from culture. The direct fluorescent antibody stain is specific for *Legionella,* but viewing stained specimens requires a fluorescence microscope.

Culture remains the definitive method for diagnosis. Buffered charcoal–yeast extract agar, buffered with *N*-(2-acetamido)-2-aminoethanesulfonic acid and supplemented with α-ketoglutarate, L-cysteine, and ferric pyrophosphate (pH 6.9), is the primary medium for isolation of *Legionella* by culture. Both α-ketoglutarate and charcoal stimulate *Legionella* growth by decreasing production of toxic peroxides: α-ketoglutarate indirectly by inhibiting cysteine oxidation,[12] and charcoal directly by promoting decomposition of peroxides.[13] Addition of albumin, which blocks the toxic effects of starch products, also increases the yield of *L. micdadei, Legionella bozemanii,* and *Legionella anisa* in culture.[14] Optimal recovery of legionellae from respiratory specimens requires the use of multiple dye-containing selective media with acid (pH 2.2 hydrochloric acid and potassium chloride buffer) or heat pretreatment to minimize overgrowth of competing microorganisms.[15] Colonies may be visible after 2 to 5 days' incubation at 35°C (with or without carbon dioxide) in a moist chamber. When viewed through a dissecting microscope, the colonies are convex and circular with a characteristic ground-glass surface texture and speckled green or pinkish purple iridescent edges (Fig. 214–1).

Other diagnostic tests include visualization of *Legionella* in respiratory secretions by the direct fluorescent antibody stain, *Legionella* urinary antigen test by radioimmunoassay or enzyme immunoassay, serologic testing by the indirect fluorescent antibody stain or the enzyme-linked immunosorbent assay, and the polymerase chain reaction (PCR). For detecting *L. pneumophila* in respiratory specimens, I have found the direct fluorescent monoclonal antibody reagent (Genetic Systems, Sanofi Diagnostics Pasteur, Chaska, Minnesota) to be superior to polyclonal reagents because background fluorescence is reduced and cross-reactivity with non-*Legionella* bacteria does not occur. The *Legionella* urinary antigen test detects antigens of *L. pneumophila* serogroup 1 in urine (Binax, Portland, Maine). The radioimmunoassay test appears to be slightly more sensitive than the enzyme immunoassay test.[16] Serologic tests are most useful for epidemiologic studies and are of lesser diagnostic value given the requirement for a convalescent titer. Although PCR-based assays for detection of *Legionella* in clinical samples have been shown to be highly specific, they have not been shown to be more sensitive than culture.[17, 18] The primary advantage of this technique is the ability to detect *Legionella* rapidly and to detect species other than *L. pneumophila*.

The Legionellaceae share a number of phenotypic characteristics (see Table 214–1). These characteristics are of limited value in species identification but include the following: absence of growth on blood agar, nonfermentive metabolism, weakly catalase- and peroxidase-positive, production of a β-lactamase (eight species including *L. micdadei* are negative for this trait), gelatinase-positive (except *Legionella feeleii, Legionella lansingensis, Legionella fairfieldensis, Legionella maceachernii,* and *L. micdadei*), production of a soluble brown pigment from tyrosine, and variable oxidase reaction.[6] All *Legionella* species produce a water-soluble, extracellular fluorescing compound when they are grown on buffered charcoal–yeast extract agar. On exposure to long-wave ultraviolet light (365 nm), the organisms and surrounding medium show a yellow-green fluorescence. The brightness of the fluorescence can be intensified by alkalinization or quenched by acidification.[19] Some species also exhibit a blue-white *(L. bozemanii, Legionella dumoffii, Legionella gormanii, L. anisa, Legionella cherrii, Legionella tucsonensis, Legionella parisiensis, Legionella steigerwaltii)* or red *(Legionella erythra, Legionella rubrilucens)* intracellular fluorescence within the colonies when they are viewed under ultraviolet light. This finding can be useful in preliminary identification.[19] *L. micdadei* and *L. maceachernii* demonstrate red fluorescence with the bromocresol purple spot test, whereas the other 27 species demonstrate blue fluorescence.[19] *L. maceachernii* and *L. micdadei* also produce blue colonies on media containing bromocresol purple and bromothymol blue dyes, whereas the other members produce yellow-

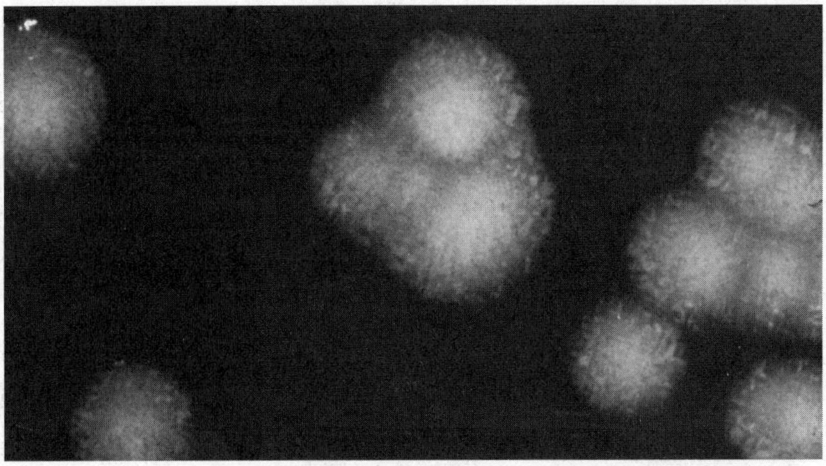

FIGURE 214–1 □ Colonies of *Legionella pneumophila* with characteristic ground-glass surface texture. (Magnification approximately × 10.)

green to apple-green colonies.[19] Combinations of phenotypic traits (pigment, fluorescence, biochemical reactions) have been used with variable degrees of accuracy in distinguishing between the numerous *Legionella* species.[20–22]

Specific antibody reactions as detected by indirect immunofluorescence, direct immunofluorescence, crossed immunoelectrophoresis,[23] slide agglutination,[24] and immunodiffusion[25] can also be used for identification of *Legionella* species.

Both phenotypic and genotypic differences among strains of *L. pneumophila* have been used in epidemiologic investigations to link isolates from patients to an environmental reservoir.[26] These include serotyping, monoclonal antibody subtyping, isoenzyme analysis, protein and carbohydrate profiling, plasmid analysis, restriction endonuclease analysis, restriction fragment length polymorphism of ribosomal RNA (ribotyping)[27] or chromosomal DNA, amplified fragment length polymorphism,[28] restriction endonuclease analysis of whole-cell DNA with or without pulsed-field gel electrophoresis,[29] arbitrarily primed PCR,[30] and repetitive element PCR.[31]

Antigenic Properties

As with other gram-negative bacteria, lipopolysaccharide is a major constituent of the outer membrane of *L. pneumophila.* Lipopolysaccharide is the predominant antigen recognized by human antisera and is the serogroup-specific antigen.[32, 33] Preliminary identification of *L. pneumophila* can be achieved by use of a monoclonal antibody that recognizes a lipopolysaccharide antigenic determinant in the outer membrane.[34] A study of protein profiles of *L. pneumophila,* serogroup 1, revealed two major immunoreactive proteins of 24 and 43 kDa.[35, 36] The 24-kDa protein forms ion-permeable channels in contact with lipid membranes, as is characteristic for porins.[33] A 38-kDa exoprotease termed the zinc metalloprotease, or major secretory protein, has been shown to induce cell-mediated immune responses and protective immunity against lethal aerosol challenge with *L. pneumophila* in a guinea pig model.[37, 38] The major secretory protein was considered to be a candidate for a vaccine; however, it was not capable of producing protective immunity for all *Legionella* species. Another immunodominant antigen, the major cytoplasmic membrane protein, is a heat shock protein and a genus common antigen of the Legionellaceae.[39, 40] This protein has also been shown to induce protective immunity in a guinea pig model.[41]

Pathogenesis and Virulence Factors

Cell-mediated immunity is the primary host defense against *Legionella.* Human mononuclear, polymorphonuclear, and alveolar macrophages readily phagocytose *Legionella.* Phagocytosis occurs by a coiling mechanism mediated by complement receptors that bind to the outer membrane protein of *Legionella.*[42] Interferon-γ activation of macrophages limits internalization of the bacterium and intracellular multiplication by restricting complement receptors and limiting the availability of iron. Polymorphonuclear leukocytes are the predominant cells seen on histologic smears from the lungs of infected patients; however, these cells do not support intracellular replication of *Legionella.*

Epidemiologic and genetic studies have revealed a number of factors that affect the virulence of *Legionella.*[43] Multiple strains of *L. pneumophila* may colonize a water system, but only a few strains cause disease in patients exposed to the water. Although 40 different *Legionella* species have been identified, less than half of these have been liked to disease in humans. *L. pneumophila* is the most pathogenic, accounting for 90% of the cases of legionellosis, followed by *L. micdadei* and *Legionella longbeachae.*[3] Whereas more than 15 serogroups of *L. pneumophila* have been identified, serogroup 1 accounts for more than 80% of the reported cases of legionellosis caused by *L. pneumophila.*

The presence of flagella is one phenotypic difference between virulent and avirulent *L. pneumophila;* isogeneic avirulent strains obtained by laboratory passage lose their flagella.[44] A surface antigen of *L. pneumophila,* serogroup 1, that is recognized by one particular monoclonal antibody (MAB2) may be associated with virulence.[45–47] Regulation of *Legionella* virulence has been ascribed to several genetic loci that appear to direct intracellular infection.[48–50] Cianciotto and colleagues[51] cloned and sequenced the gene encoding the 24-kDa protein and, using site-specific mutagenesis and allelic exchange, found that the expression of this protein was necessary for optimal intracellular infectivity. The protein was designated Mip, for macrophage infectivity potentiator, and the gene encoding the protein was similarly named *mip.* The *mip* gene sequence is specific for *L. pneumophila.* An *L. pneumophila mip* mutant has been shown to infect alveolar epithelial cells.[52] Furthermore, virulent strains of *L. pneumophila* were more toxic to alveolar macrophages when ingested[53] and more suppressive of oxidative burst in human polymorphonuclear leukocytes compared with avirulent strains.[54]

Tissue-destructive proteases may also play a role in the pathogenicity of *Legionella* by causing cytolysis and destruction of pulmonary tissue. One such exoprotease is the 38-kDa zinc metalloprotease. This enzyme has been shown to be cytolytic for tissue culture cells. The gene encoding this protein was cloned and shown to encode a trifunctional polypeptide responsible for cytotoxic, hemolytic, and proteolytic activities.[55]

It has been suggested that the virulence of *Legionella* may be increased by replication in amoebae.[56, 57] Avirulent strains of *Legionella* were unable to multiply intracellularly in a ciliated protozoan.[58]

Environmental Ecology

Pathogens that are able to survive in the environment for an extended time tend to be relatively virulent.[59] *Legionella* organisms are readily found in natural aquatic bodies, and some species have been recovered from soil.[60] The organisms can survive in a wide range of conditions, including temperatures of 0°C to 63°C, pH of 5.0 to 8.5, and dissolved oxygen concentrations of 0.2 to 15 parts per million in water.[61] In addition, commensal organisms such as bacteria *(Flavobacterium, Pseudomonas, Alcaligenes, Acinetobacter)* and blue-green algae (cyanobacteria) can stimulate the growth of *Legionella* in the aquatic environment.[62–65] *L. pneumophila* can also infect and multiply within soil and aquatic species of amoebae *(Hartmannella, Acanthamoeba)* and ciliated protozoa *(Tetrahymena, Naegleria)*, including amoebae isolated from hot-water tanks.[66] This intracellular parasitism parallels that seen in humans, except that mononuclear cells are the targets in humans.

The aquatic environment of *Legionella* also includes artificial habitats such as cooling towers, evaporative condensers, and potable water distribution systems.[67] The reservoir for nosocomial and community-acquired Legionnaires' disease has been linked to the contamination of potable water distribution systems by *Legionella* species.[68, 69] Thus, control of nosocomial Legionnaires' disease has been achieved by disinfection of the hospital water system.[70] Three primary disinfection methods have been used with variable success: superheat and flush, hyperchlorination, and copper-silver ionization (Liqui-Tech, Willowbrook, Illinois).

Temperature is a critical determinant for *Legionella* proliferation. The organism has appeared in higher concentrations in thermally enriched rivers[71] and hot-water systems in buildings.[72] Colonization of hot-water tanks is more likely if tank temperatures are between 40°C and 50°C (104°F to 122°F).[72, 73]

Legionella and other microorganisms become attached to surfaces in an aquatic environment, forming a slimelike substance known as biofilm. *Legionella* has been shown to attach to and colonize various materials found in water systems, including plastics, rubber, and wood.[74, 75] Particulates such as sediments or scale and inorganic precipitates provide *Legionella* with a surface for attachment and a protective barrier.[75] Interestingly, the growth of other environmental organisms is stimulated by sediment, which in turn leads to the formation of by-products that stimulate the growth of *Legionella*.[64]

Culture is the method of choice for detecting *Legionella* in environmental samples. Optimal recovery of *Legionella* can be accomplished by combining acid pretreatment and culture on antibiotic-containing media.[76] A widely used agar medium for environmental isolation contains glycine, vancomycin, polymyxin B, and α-ketoglutarate in buffered charcoal–yeast extract agar with dyes.[15] The glycine, vancomycin, and polymyxin B inhibit competing microflora. Some *Legionella* species other than *L. pneumophila* are inhibited by glycine and some antibiotics, so it is recommended that multiple selective and nonselective buffered charcoal–yeast extract media be used to optimize recovery.[76]

A potentially sensitive method for the detection of *Legionella* in water samples is PCR.[77] A *Legionella* PCR kit has been developed for detection of *Legionella* in water samples (EnviroAmp, Perkin-Elmer Corp., Branchburg, New Jersey). Two primers are used to detect and amplify gene sequences of legionellae; one is genus specific and detects the 5S ribosomal RNA, and the other is species specific and detects the *mip* gene sequence of *L. pneumophila*. PCR does not appear to be more sensitive than culture, particularly with respect to detecting *L. pneumophila*.

Antibiotic Susceptibility

Legionella species are facultative intracellular pathogens that can avoid the effects of antimicrobial agents that cannot penetrate the host-cell membranes. For example, agents that cannot penetrate macrophages, such as penicillins and cephalosporins, demonstrate activity in minimal inhibitory concentration assays but are clinically ineffective.[78] In vitro antibiotic susceptibility studies have been a problem owing to lack of standardized methodology, variable susceptibility results according to the type of medium employed, and poor correlation with clinical observations. Three methods are generally used for susceptibility testing: extracellular testing in broth or agar, intracellular testing in tissue culture, and studies using infected guinea pigs.[78]

Erythromycin, rifampin, tetracycline, fluoroquinolones, and newer macrolide-azalide antimicrobial agents are considered to be effective agents in the treatment of Legionnaires' disease.[79] In vitro and in vivo results have shown the following agents to be highly active: azithromycin, clarithromycin, ciprofloxacin, pefloxacin, levofloxacin, fleroxacin, trovafloxacin, minocycline, and doxycycline.[78, 80, 81] Synergy in vitro has also been shown for trimethoprim and sulfamethoxazole, erythromycin and rifampin, and macrolide-quinolone combinations.[82, 83] Variable results (including antagonism) have been reported for quinolones and rifampin.[82, 84] *Legionella* species that lack β-lactamase may presumably be susceptible to β-lactam agents, but clinical experience indicates a high likelihood of failure. However, as the intravenous formulations of the newer macrolides become available and there is more clinical experience with the quinolones, these agents are likely to displace erythromycin as the drug of choice.

References

1. Harris TG, Saunders NA: Taxonomy and typing of legionellae. Rev Med Microbiol 5:79–90, 1994.
2. Thacker WL, Dyke JW, Benson RF, et al: *Legionella lansingensis* sp. nov. isolated from a patient with pneumonia and underlying chronic lymphocytic leukemia. J Clin Microbiol 30:2398–2401, 1992.
3. Marston BJ, Lipman HB, Breiman RF: Surveillance for Legionnaires' disease. Risk factors for morbidity and mortality. Arch Intern Med 154:2417–2422, 1994.
4. Waite R: Confirmation of identity of legionellae by whole cell fatty-acid and isoprenoid quinone profiles. *In* Harrison TG, Taylor AG (eds): A Laboratory Manual for *Legionella*. Chichester, UK, John Wiley & Sons, 1988, p 69.
5. Brenner DJ: Classification of legionellae. Semin Respir Infect 2:190–205, 1987.
6. Hookey JV, Saunders NA, Fry NK, et al: Phylogeny of Legionellaceae based on small-subunit ribosomal DNA sequences and proposal of *Legionella lytica* comb. nov. for *Legionella*-like amoebal pathogens. Int J Syst Bacteriol 46:526–531, 1996.
7. Sonesson A, Jantzen E, Bryn K, et al: Composition of 2,3-dihydroxy fatty acid–containing lipopolysaccharides from *Legionella israelensis, Legionella maceachernii*, and *Legionella micdadei*. Microbiology 140:1261–1271, 1994.

8. Lema M, Brown A: Electrophoretic characteristic of soluble protein extracts of *Legionella pneumophila* and other members of the family Legionellaceae. J Clin Microbiol 17:1132–1140, 1983.
9. Brindle RJ, Bryant TN, Draper PW: Taxonomic investigation of *Legionella pneumophila* using monoclonal antibodies. J Clin Microbiol 27:536–539, 1989.
10. Fox A, Lau PY, Brown A, et al: Capillary gas chromatographic analysis of carbohydrates of *Legionella pneumophila* and other members of the family Legionellaceae. J Clin Microbiol 19:326–332, 1984.
11. Hilton E, Freedman RA, Cintron F, et al: Acid-fast bacilli in sputum: A case of *Legionella micdadei* pneumonia. J Clin Microbiol 24:1102–1103, 1986.
12. Pine L, Hoffman PS, Malcolm G, et al: Role of keto acids and reduced oxygen-scavenging enzymes in the growth of *Legionella* species. J Clin Microbiol 23:33–42, 1986.
13. Hoffman PS, Pine L, Bell S: Production of superoxide and hydrogen peroxide in medium used to culture *L. pneumophila:* Catalytic composition by charcoal. Appl Environ Microbiol 45:784–791, 1983.
14. Morrill WE, Barbaree JM, Fields BS, et al: Increased recovery of *Legionella micdadei* and *Legionella bozemanii* on buffered charcoal yeast extract agar supplemented with albumin. J Clin Microbiol 28:616–618, 1990.
15. Vickers RM, Stout JE, Yu VL, Rihs JD: Culture methodology for the isolation of *Legionella pneumophila* and other Legionellaceae from clinical and environmental specimens. Semin Respir Infect 2:274–279, 1987.
16. Plouffe JF, File TM, Breiman RF: Reevaluation of the definition of Legionnaires' disease: Use of the urinary antigen assay. Clin Infect Dis 20:1286–1291, 1995.
17. Kessler HH, Reinthaler FF, Pschaid A, et al: Rapid detection of *Legionella* species in bronchoalveolar lavage fluids with the EnviroAmp *Legionella* PCR amplification and detection kit. J Clin Microbiol 31:3325–3328, 1993.
18. Matsiota-Bernard P, Pitsouni E, Legakis N, Nauciel C: Evaluation of commercial amplification kit for detection of *Legionella pneumophila* in clinical samples. J Clin Microbiol 32:1503–1505, 1994.
19. Fang GD, Yu VL, Vickers RM: Disease due to Legionellaceae (other than *Legionella pneumophila*): Historical, microbiological, clinical and epidemiological review. Medicine (Baltimore) 68:116–139, 1989.
20. Vickers RM, Yu VL: Clinical laboratory differentiation of Legionellaceae family members with pigment production and fluorescence on media supplemented with aromatic substrates. J Clin Microbiol 19:583–587, 1984.
21. Fox KF, Brown A: Application of numerical systematics to the phenotypic differentiation of legionellae. J Clin Microbiol 27:1952–1955, 1989.
22. Vesey G, Dennis PJ, Lee J, West A: Further development of simple tests to differentiate the legionellas. J Appl Bacteriol 65:339–345, 1988.
23. Bangsborg JM, Shand G, Pearlman E, Hoiby N: Cross-reactive *Legionella* antigens and the antibody response during infection. APMIS 99:854–865, 1991.
24. Wilkinson HW, Fikes BJ: Slide agglutination tests for serogrouping *Legionella pneumophila* and atypical *Legionella*-like organisms. J Clin Microbiol 11:99–101, 1980.
25. Orrison LH, Bibb WF, Cherry WB, Thacker L: Determination of antigenic relationships among legionellae and non-legionellae by direct fluorescent-antibody and immunodiffusion tests. J Clin Microbiol 17:332–337, 1983.
26. Barbaree JM: Selecting a subtyping technique for use in investigations of legionellosis epidemics. *In* Barbaree JM, Breiman RF, Dufour AP (eds): *Legionella:* Current Status and Emerging Perspectives. Washington, DC, American Society for Microbiology, 1993, p 169.
27. Bangsborg JM, Gerner-Smidt P, Colding H, et al: Restriction fragment length polymorphism of rRNA genes for molecular typing of members of the family Legionellaceae. J Clin Microbiol 33:402–406, 1995.
28. Valsangiacomo C, Baggi F, Gaia V, et al: Use of amplified fragment length polymorphisms in molecular typing of *Legionella pneumophila* and application to epidemiological studies. J Clin Microbiol 33:1716–1719, 1995.
29. Schoonmaker D, Heimberger T, Birkhead G: Comparison of ribotyping and restriction enzyme analysis using pulsed-field gel electrophoresis for distinguishing *Legionella pneumophila* isolates obtained during a nosocomial outbreak. J Clin Microbiol 30:1491–1498, 1992.
30. Pruckler JM, Mermel LA, Benson RF: Comparison of *Legionella pneumophila* isolates by arbitrarily primed PCR and pulsed-field gel electrophoresis: Analysis from seven epidemic investigations. J Clin Microbiol 33:2872–2875, 1995.
31. Georghiou PR, Doggett AM, Kielhofner MA, et al: Molecular fingerprinting of *Legionella* species by repetitive element PCR. J Clin Microbiol 32:2989–2994, 1994.
32. Ciesielski CA, Blaser MJ, Wang WLL: Serogroup specificity of *Legionella pneumophila* is related to lipopolysaccharide characteristics. Infect Immun 51:397–404, 1986.
33. Gabay J, Blake M, Niles W, et al: Purification of *Legionella pneumophila* major outer membrane protein and demonstration that it is a porin. J Bacteriol 162:85–91, 1985.
34. Barth C, Joly JR, Ramsay D, et al: Common epitope on the lipopolysaccharide of *Legionella pneumophila* recognized by monoclonal antibody. J Clin Microbiol 26:1016–1023, 1988.
35. Pearlman E, Engleberg NC, Eisenstein BI: Identification of protein antigens of *Legionella pneumophila* serogroup 1. Infect Immun 47:74–79, 1985.
36. Engleberg NC, Drutz DJ, Eisenstein BI: Cloning and expression of *Legionella pneumophila* antigens in *Escherichia coli.* Infect Immun 44:222–227, 1984.
37. Szeto L, Shuman HA: The *Legionella pneumophila* major secretory protein, a protease, is not required for intracellular growth or cell killing. Infect Immun 58:2585–2592, 1990.
38. Blander SJ, Breiman R, Horwitz MA: A live avirulent mutant *L. pneumophila* vaccine induces protective immunity against lethal aerosol challenge. J Clin Invest 83:810–815, 1989.
39. Lema MW, Brown A, Butler CA, Hoffman PS: Heat-shock response in *Legionella pneumophila.* Can J Microbiol 34:1148–1153, 1988.
40. Sampson JS, Plikaytis BB, Wilkinson HW: Immunologic response of patients with legionellosis against major protein-containing antigens of *Legionella pneumophila* serogroup 1 as shown by immunoblot analysis. J Clin Microbiol 23:92–99, 1986.
41. Blander SJ, Horwitz MA: Major cytoplasmic membrane protein of *Legionella pneumophila,* a genus common antigen and member of hsp 60 family of heat shock proteins, induces protective immunity in a guinea pig model of Legionnaires' disease. J Clin Invest 91:717–723, 1993.
42. Horwitz MA: Toward an understanding of host and bacterial molecules mediating *L. pneumophila* pathogenesis. *In* Barbaree JM, Breiman RF, Dufour AP (eds): *Legionella:* Current Status and Emerging Perspectives. Washington, DC, American Society for Microbiology, 1993, p 55.
43. Dowling JN, Saha AK, Glew RH: Virulence factors of the family Legionellaceae. Microbiol Rev 56:32–60, 1992.
44. Pruckler J, Benson R, Martin W, Fields B: Association of flagella and intracellular growth of *L. pneumophila* (Abstr). Annual Meeting of the American Society for Microbiology; May 1995; Washington, DC.
45. Stout JE, Joly J, Para M, et al: Comparison of molecular methods for subtyping patients and epidemiologically-linked environmental isolates of *L. pneumophila.* J Infect Dis 157:486–494, 1988.
46. Dournon E, Bibb WF, Rajagopalan P, et al: Monoclonal antibody reactivity as a virulence marker for *Legionella pneumophila* serogroup 1 strains. J Infect Dis 157:496–501, 1988.
47. Joly JR, McKinney RM, Tobin J, et al: Development of a standardized subtyping scheme for *L. pneumophila,* serogroup 1, using monoclonal antibodies. J Clin Microbiol 23:768–771, 1986.
48. Berger KH, Isberg RR: Two distinct defects in intracellular growth complemented by a single genetic locus in *Legionella pneumophila.* Mol Microbiol 7:7–19, 1993.
49. Marra A, Shuman HA: Genetics of *Legionella pneumophila* virulence. Annu Rev Genet 26:51–69, 1992.
50. Engleberg CN: Genetic studies of *Legionella* pathogenesis. *In* Barbaree JM, Breiman RF, Dufour AP (eds): *Legionella:* Current Status and Emerging Perspectives. Washington, DC, American Society for Microbiology, 1993, p 63.
51. Cianciotto NP, Eisenstein BI, Mody CH, et al: A *Legionella pneumophila* gene encoding a species-specific surface protein potentiates initiation of intracellular infection. Infect Immun 57:1255–1262, 1989.

52. Cianciotto NP, Stamos JK, Kamp DW: Infectivity of *Legionella pneumophila mip* mutant for alveolar epithelial cells. Curr Microbiol 30:247–250, 1995.
53. Caparon M, Johnson W: Macrophage toxicity and complement sensitivity of virulent and avirulent strains of *Legionella pneumophila.* Rev Infect Dis 10:S377–S384, 1988.
54. Summersgill JT, Raff MJ, Miller RD: Interactions of virulent and avirulent *Legionella pneumophila* with human polymorphonuclear leukocytes. Microb Pathog 4:41–47, 1988.
55. Quinn FD, Keen MG, Tompkins LS: Genetic, immunological, and cytotoxic comparisons of *Legionella* proteolytic activities. Infect Immun 57:2719–2725, 1989.
56. Cirillo JD, Falkow S, Tompkins LS: Growth of *Legionella pneumophila* in *Acanthamoeba castellanii* enhances invasion. Infect Immun 62:3254–3261, 1994.
57. Moffat JF, Tompkins LS: A quantitative model of intracellular growth of *Legionella pneumophila* in *Acanthamoeba castellanii.* Infect Immun 60:296–301, 1992.
58. Fields BS, Barbaree JM, Shotts EB, et al: Comparison of guinea pig and protozoan models for determining virulence of *Legionella* species. Infect Immun 53:553–559, 1986.
59. Ewald PW: The evolution of virulence. Sci Am 268:86–93, 1993.
60. Steele TW, Moore CY, Sangster N: Distribution of *Legionella longbeachae* serogroup 1 and other legionellae in potting soil in Australia. Appl Environ Microbiol 56:2984–2988, 1990.
61. Fliermans CB: Philosophical ecology: *Legionella* in historical perspective. *In* Thornsberry C, Balows A, Feeley JC, et al (eds): *Legionella*—Proceedings of the 2nd International Symposium. Washington, DC, American Society for Microbiology, 1984, p 285.
62. Wadowsky RM, Yee RB: Effect of non-Legionellaceae bacteria on the multiplication of *Legionella pneumophila* in potable water. Appl Environ Microbiol 49:1206–1210, 1985.
63. Wadowsky RM, Yee RB: Satellite growth of *Legionella pneumophila* with an environmental isolate of *Flavobacterium breve.* Appl Environ Microbiol 46:1147–1149, 1983.
64. Stout JE, Yu VL, Best M: Ecology of *Legionella pneumophila* within water distribution systems. Appl Environ Microbiol 49:221–228, 1985.
65. Tison DL, Pope DH, Cherry WB, Fliermans CB: Growth of *Legionella pneumophila* in association with blue-green algae (cyanobacteria). Appl Environ Microbiol 39:456–459, 1980.
66. Fields BS: *Legionella* and protozoa: Interaction of a pathogen and its natural host. *In* Barbaree JM, Breiman RF, Dufour AP (eds): *Legionella:* Current Status and Emerging Perspectives. Washington, DC, American Society for Microbiology, 1993, p 129.
67. Muraca PW, Stout JE, Yu VL: Environmental aspects of Legionnaires' disease. J Am Water Works Assoc 80:78–86, 1988.
68. Stout JE, Yu VL, Muraca P, et al: Potable water as the cause of sporadic cases of community-acquired Legionnaires' disease. N Engl J Med 326:151–154, 1992.
69. Best M, Yu VL, Stout J, et al: Legionellaceae in the hospital water supply—Epidemiological link with disease and evaluation of a method of control of nosocomial Legionnaires' disease and Pittsburgh pneumonia. Lancet 2:307–310, 1983.
70. Freije MR: Legionellae Control in Health Care Facilities, A Guide for Minimizing Risk. Indianapolis, IN, HC Information Resources, 1996.
71. Tyndall RL, Christensen SW, Solomon J, et al: Thermally altered habitats as a source of known and new *Legionella* species. *In* Thornsberry C, Balows A, Feeley JC, et al (eds): *Legionella*—Proceedings of the 2nd International Symposium. Washington, DC, American Society for Microbiology, 1984, p 311.
72. Vickers RM, Yu VL, Hanna SS, et al: Determinants of *Legionella pneumophila* contamination of water distribution systems: 15-hospital prospective study. Infect Control 8:357–363, 1987.
73. Plouffe JF, Webster LR, Hackman B: Relationship between colonization of hospital buildings with *Legionella pneumophila* and hot water temperatures. Appl Environ Microbiol 46:769–770, 1983.
74. Rogers J, Dowsett AB, Dennis PJ, et al: Influence of temperature and plumbing material selection on biofilm formation and growth of *Legionella pneumophila* in a model potable water system containing complex microbial flora. Appl Environ Microbiol 60:1585–1592, 1994.
75. Wright JB, Ruseska I, Athar M, et al: *Legionella pneumophila* grows adherent to surfaces in vitro and in situ. Infect Control Hosp Epidemiol 10:408–415, 1989.
76. Ta AC, Stout JE, Yu VL, Wagener MM: Comparison of culture methods for monitoring *Legionella* species in hospital potable water systems and recommendations for standardization of such methods. J Clin Microbiol 33:2118–2123, 1995.
77. Bej AK, Mahbubani MD, Atlas RM: Detection of viable *Legionella pneumophila* in water by polymerase chain reaction and gene probe methods. Appl Environ Microbiol 57:597–600, 1991.
78. Edelstein PH: Antimicrobial chemotherapy for Legionnaires' disease: A review. Clin Infect Dis 21(Suppl 3):S265–S276, 1995.
79. Yu VL: *Legionella* infections. *In* Neu HD, Young LS, Zinner SH (eds): The New Macrolides, Azalides, and Streptogramins. New York, Marcel Dekker, 1993, p 141.
80. Edelstein PH, Edelstein MAC, Lehr KH, Ren J: In-vitro activity of levofloxacin against clinical isolates of *Legionella* spp., its pharmacokinetics in guinea pigs, and use in experimental *Legionella pneumophila* pneumonia. J Antimicrob Chemother 37:117–126, 1996.
81. Edelstein PH, Edelstein MAC, Ren J, et al: Activity of trovafloxacin (CP-99, 219) against *Legionella* isolates: In vitro activity, intracellular accumulation, and killing in macrophages, and pharmacokinetics and treatment of guinea pigs with *L. pneumophila* pneumonia. Antimicrob Agents Chemother 40:314–331, 1996.
82. Moffie BG, Mouton RP: Sensitivity and resistance of *L. pneumophila* to some antibiotics and combination of antibiotics. J Antimicrob Chemother 22:457–462, 1988.
83. Martin SJ, Pendland SL, Chen C, et al: In vitro synergy testing of macrolide-quinolone combinations against 41 clinical isolates of *Legionella.* Antimicrob Agents Chemother 40:1419–1421, 1996.
84. Havlichek D, Saravolatz L, Pohlod D: Effect of quinolones and other antimicrobial agents on cell-associated *Legionella pneumophila.* Antimicrob Agents Chemother 31:1529–1534, 1987.

215

Bordetella

William A. Durbin, Jr.

History

Pertussis (literally, intensive cough) is a highly contagious disease caused by organisms of the genus *Bordetella,* which have a highly selective tropism for the ciliated epithelium of the respiratory tract. The name is an apt general description and more appropriate than the familiar term whooping cough, because coughing paroxysms in small infants and older persons with pertussis are often not associated with a whoop. Surprisingly, despite its distinctive clinical presentation, pertussis was not described until 1578, when an epidemic occurred in Paris.[1] The term pertussis was introduced a century later. As recently as the 1940s in the United States, pertussis accounted for more deaths in infants younger than 1 year than meningitis, measles, diphtheria, poliomyelitis, and scarlet fever combined.[2] Even now, on a worldwide basis, pertussis is estimated to cause more than 300,000 deaths each year, mostly in unimmunized infants.[3]

Characteristics of the Pathogen

Bordetella species are small (0.2 to 1 mm) gram-negative coccobacilli that are obligate aerobes, have many nutritional requirements, and grow slowly in vitro, even on enriched media.[4] Four species are recognized. *Bordetella pertussis* is the agent responsible for most human pertussis. Less fastidious than *B. pertussis* are *Bordetella parapertussis*, associated with a mild pertussis-like illness in humans, and *Bordetella bronchiseptica*, an agent that rarely causes human respiratory or systemic disease but is more often associated with respiratory illness in horses, rabbits (snuffles), dogs (kennel cough), and pigs (atrophic rhinitis).[5] A fourth species, *Bordetella avium*, which grows readily on MacConkey agar, causes turkey rhinotracheitis but has not been associated with human disease.[6] Phenotypic characteristics distinguish *Bordetella* species, but their genetic composition is similar.[7]

B. pertussis was first cultured by Bordet and Gengou in 1906, in a medium of potato starch infusion, glycerol, and defibrinated blood. This medium, freshly made up, is still used today. Also used are Regan-Lowe agar (a more stable agar consisting of charcoal, horse blood, and cephalexin), Jones-Kendrick charcoal agar, and a modified Stainer-Scholte medium.[4] All *Bordetella* species require either niacin or nicotinamide for growth, whereas unsaturated fatty acids (such as those potentially found on glassware or on cotton swabs) inhibit their growth. On Bordet-Gengou medium, *B. pertussis* forms tiny, glistening, translucent colonies with a hazy zone of hemolysis; in charcoal–horse blood agar, they are small, shiny, round, and mercury-silver in color. The colonies generally take at least 3 days to appear. Other *Bordetella* species having fewer growth requirements are recovered more quickly and are distinguished from *B. pertussis* by colonial morphologic features, biochemical testing, and agglutination reactions.

A number of biologically active components of *B. pertussis* have been identified that appear to contribute to pathogenicity.[8, 9] Unlike diphtheria, tetanus, and botulism, pertussis is not a single-toxin disease.[10] Filamentous hemagglutinin (FHA) is a surface protein of *B. pertussis* that is an important mediator of attachment of the organism to ciliated epithelial cells. Antibody to FHA may play a role in protecting against infection. Pertussis agglutinogens are also protein surface antigens that may play a role in bacterial attachment; agglutinating antibodies have provided serologic markers for epidemiologic studies and may contribute to protection. Lymphocytosis-promoting factor (LPF), also referred to as pertussis toxin, histamine-sensitizing factor, islet-activating protein, and pertussigen, is composed of a hemagglutinin envelope protein and has many important biologic functions,[11] including the induction of leukocytosis, anaphylaxis, and histamine sensitivity.[4] Antibody to LPF may play a role in protection from disease. Other recognized antigenic components of *B. pertussis* for which potential biologic roles have been described include adenylate cyclase, heat-labile toxin, endotoxin (*Bordetella* lipopolysaccharide), tracheal cytotoxin, hemolysin, and an outer membrane protein (pertactin).

From observations in animal studies, the pathogenesis of pertussis has been divided arbitrarily into four steps: attachment, evasion of host defenses, local tissue damage, and systemic disease.[12] *B. pertussis* has a striking tropism in humans for ciliated cells of the respiratory epithelium. Attachment by *B. pertussis* to the cilia of epithelial cells is enhanced by FHA and LPF and possibly by pertussis agglutinogens or other factors. Persons who are immune to pertussis have secretory immunoglobulin A that appears to inhibit bacterial attachment. Once attachment occurs, LPF, adenylate cyclase, and tracheal cytotoxin appear to disrupt normal host clearance mechanisms and promote bacterial proliferation. Subsequent local tissue damage, with sloughing of the respiratory mucosal surface and inhibition of phagocytic function, is mediated by tracheal cytotoxin, heat-labile toxin, adenylate cyclase, and hemolysin. Of the various toxins, only LPF and lipopolysaccharide have a clear role in the systemic manifestations of pertussis. However, pertussis toxin alone is not responsible for disease manifestations, and similar disease caused by *B. parapertussis* occurs despite the absence of pertussis toxin. The mechanism of the most important systemic complication of pertussis, encephalopathy, is unclear. Anoxia related to coughing paroxysms with obstructive apnea probably accounts for most of the central nervous system insult; whether metabolic disturbances, hypoglycemia, hemorrhage, or toxins play a role is unclear.[13, 14]

Epidemiology

Pertussis demonstrates a number of striking epidemiologic features. *B. pertussis* and *B. parapertussis* are strictly human pathogens that have no animal reservoir. Pertussis occurs in all parts of the world, with no clear seasonal pattern, although some regions may have a higher frequency during certain times of the year. Both endemic disease and epidemic disease occur, the latter every 2 to 5 years.[15–17] Unlike the case with most other infections, female patients account for more than half of reported cases.[2] Attack rates do not vary appreciably by race.

Pertussis is highly contagious. Person-to-person transmission occurs through aerosolized respiratory droplets. Transmission occurs during the catarrhal stage and during the first 2 to 3 weeks of the paroxysmal phase. The attack rate ranges from 70% to 100% in susceptible household contacts, whereas it is about 25% to 50% in schools.[8] Hospital outbreaks have been reported,[18–20] as have outbreaks in communities with high immunization rates.[21] Asymptomatic carriage is infrequent and does not represent a source of spread.[22] Disease transmission usually occurs in settings in which mildly symptomatic adults (with intermittent paroxysmal coughs) spread infection to inadequately immunized infants, who in turn become dramatically ill, prompting recognition of pertussis.[23–25] Immunity after natural infection is thought to be lifelong, with second symptomatic episodes being uncommon.[2] On the other hand, vaccine-induced immunity is not durable; by 5 to 10 years after immunization, most people are again at risk for infection.[26–28] Serologic surveys demonstrate a high frequency of nondiagnosed infection in young men,[29] and studies of adults with cough lasting more than 1 to 2 weeks demonstrate evidence of recent pertussis infection in more than 20%.[30, 31]

Before a vaccine was introduced, more than 90% of persons in the United States developed clinical pertussis.[2] Attack rates started to decline in the early 1900s, and a more precipitous drop followed introduction of vaccine in the 1940s.[32, 33] Before introduction of the vaccine, there were approximately 150 cases per 100,000 population in the United States, with 115,000 to 270,000 cases per year and 5000 to 10,000 deaths. By the mid-1970s, the incidence dropped to its lowest point, about 1 case per 100,000 per year with 5 to 10 deaths reported annually.[16] However, since the late 1970s and 1980s, more pertussis cases have been reported, two thirds of them in infants and children[34–37] (Fig. 215–1). Furthermore, it is estimated that only about 10% of cases are formally reported in the United States.[38] The highest incidence of disease, with virtually all the mortality, is in infants younger than 6 months, who represent more than two thirds of hospital days for pertussis.[16, 39, 40] Newborns do not necessarily gain transplacental protection even when mothers are immune because of natural infection.[2] Currently, children between ages 1 and 9 years (the population with the highest vaccination rate) make up a much smaller percentage of reported pertussis cases than in prevaccination days[35, 41] (Fig. 215–2). The population of pertussis-susceptible teenagers and young adults is increasing because of waning vaccine protection,

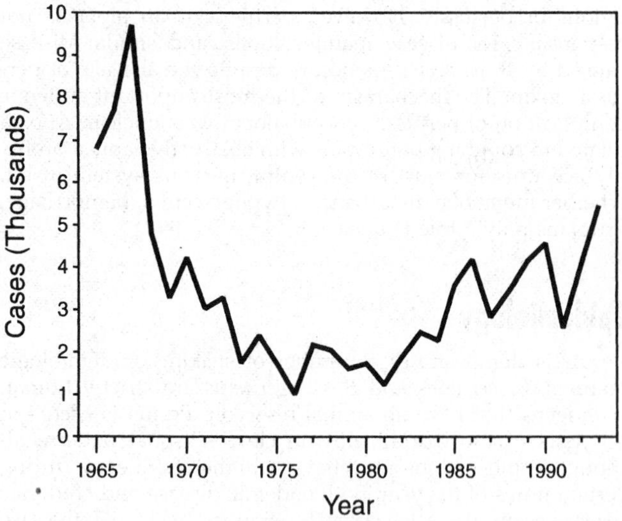

FIGURE 215–1 ▫ Reported cases of pertussis in the United States, 1965 to 1993. (From Centers for Disease Control and Prevention: Resurgence of pertussis—United States, 1993. MMWR Morbid Mortal Wkly Rep 42:952–953, 959–960, 1993.)

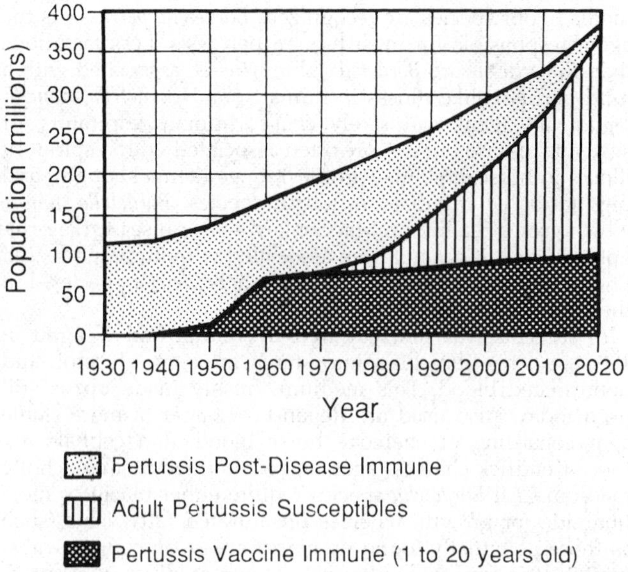

FIGURE 215–3 ▫ Projected pertussis epidemiology in the United States through the year 2020 with continued use of present-day whole-cell pertussis vaccines. (Adapted from Bass JW, Stephenson SR: The return of pertussis. Pediatr Infect Dis J 6:141–144, 1987.)

whereas the population of older persons who have lifelong immunity as a consequence of natural disease is declining[42] (Fig. 215–3). This trend is worrisome, because young, susceptible infants will probably continue to have more exposure to adults with pertussis. Thus, even with widespread use of an effective vaccine, pertussis outbreaks will continue to occur until adults, like children, receive booster immunizations.

Clinical Manifestations

Traditionally, pertussis has been arbitrarily divided into catarrhal, paroxysmal, and convalescent stages, the entire duration of illness usually being 6 to 10 weeks. Illness is most severe in young children, in those who were never immunized or were immunized years earlier, and in persons with *B. pertussis* infection as opposed to *B. parapertussis* infection. After an average incubation period of 7 days (range, 6 to 20 days), the patient develops mild upper respiratory tract symptoms with coryza, conjunctival injection, tearing, sneezing, and mild cough. During the first week to 10 days, the cough, usually dry and hacking, becomes more intense and frequent and may be triggered by such stimuli as exercise, eating, or drinking. Fever is usually low grade or absent, and patients generally feel well. Except in outbreak situations, the disease generally goes unrecognized and untreated at this catarrhal stage; unfortunately, this is also the period of greatest contagiousness.

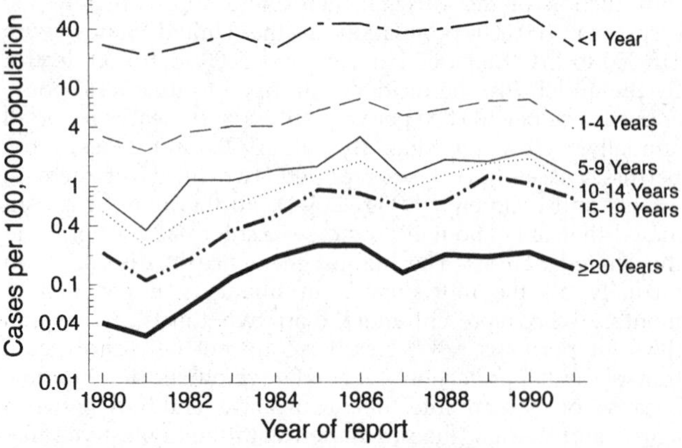

FIGURE 215–2 ▫ Incidence rates of reported pertussis cases per 100,000 population by age group in the United States, 1980 to 1991. (From Davis SF, Strebel PM, Cochi SL, et al: Pertussis surveillance—United States, 1989–1991. MMWR CDC Surveill Summ 41[SS–8]:11–19, 1992.)

After the first week or so, the illness enters the paroxysmal stage, which generally lasts 2 to 4 weeks. The cough becomes more pronounced, with increasingly severe attacks that become debilitating. A paroxysm consists of a long series of forceful, staccato coughs during a single expiration. During these attacks, there may be protruding of the tongue and drooling, tearing, bulging of the eyes, facial cyanosis, and bulging of the head and neck veins. At the end of the violent expiration, during which the patient is trying to clear the tenacious secretions from the upper airway, there is a last sudden inspiratory gasp; air is forcefully inhaled through the glottic opening, producing the characteristic stridorous whoop.[43]

A whoop is usually heard in children, although generally not in infants in the first few months of life, and is often absent or less pronounced in adolescents and adults. Paroxysms may be triggered by a number of events, including eating, drinking, yawning, sneezing, or being examined, and even by suggestion. Vomiting of clear fluid often accompanies or follows the attacks, and patients often become exhausted, apathetic, and anorectic. On the other hand, between paroxysms, patients generally appear well and are comfortable with no fever and a normal respiratory rate. The physical examination may show entirely normal findings between attacks or reveal some manifestations of the increased pressure generated during the violent cough and vomiting, such as facial or eyelid edema, petechiae, subconjunctival hemorrhages, or erosion of the lingual frenulum. The chest examination shows normal findings or may reveal scattered rhonchi; wheezing and signs of consolidation are generally absent.

During the convalescent stage (usually lasting 2 weeks to 2 months), the coughing spells gradually decrease in number and severity. Mild cough may persist for several months, and coughing paroxysms may be triggered by subsequent respiratory infections.

Pertussis-related morbidity and mortality are greatest for small infants. For children younger than 3 to 6 months, a whoop is usually absent, and *B. pertussis* is often not considered among the numerous respiratory pathogens that commonly cause illness in this age group.[44, 45] In *B. pertussis*–infected infants, feeding difficulties, choking spells, and apnea may be seen, with or without apparent coughing paroxysms. Because the less effective cough mechanism of small infants leads to inability to clear upper airway secretions, respiratory tract obstruction with apnea and resultant hypoxemia and asphyxia may occur.[46] Older children and adults tend to have milder disease, especially those who have been immunized. Typically, adults with pertussis simply have an intermittent paroxysmal cough that lasts several weeks. The coughing spells may be striking, with affected individuals gasping, choking, and even collapsing because of difficulty getting their breaths but feeling well between attacks. Unless there are unusual epidemiologic circumstances, pertussis is unlikely to be considered in adults.[47]

Complications of pertussis are usually confined to the respiratory tract and central nervous system or are related to the intense mechanical forces generated during coughing paroxysms. In the respiratory tract, otitis media is a common complication. In addition, pneumonia, usually secondary to bacterial superinfection rather than primary infection caused by *Bordetella*, may result from the damaged respiratory epithelium. Childhood pathogens such as *Streptococcus pneumoniae*, group A streptococci, *Staphylococcus aureus*, or *Haemophilus influenzae* are usually responsible. Such patients usually develop fever, tachypnea, and focal infiltrates, features that distinguish their condition from uncomplicated pertussis. In addition, patients with pertussis may develop atelectasis, particularly of the right upper lobe, which may persist for months. Bronchiectasis has also been reported. Longitudinal studies are inconclusive about long-term impairment of pulmonary function in children who have recovered from pertussis.[48, 49]

Central nervous system dysfunction is unusual during pertussis but can be severe. It may be manifested by seizures; by encephalopathy with development of gradual coma (with or without seizures); or by specific abnormalities such as hemiplegia, paraplegia, blindness, or deafness. In some cases, the manifestations are thought to be secondary to anoxia; in others, there is evidence of cerebral hemorrhage and thrombosis.[50] In addition, toxins may play a role in some cases.[13] The cerebrospinal fluid is usually normal; mild pleocytosis (less than 100 cells per mm^3) and protein elevation (less than 100 mg/dL) are occasionally seen. Long-term follow-up of children with pertussis suggests that those with uncomplicated disease have normal intelligence and reading performance,[51] whereas those with apnea or seizures may sustain long-term intellectual and school impairment.[52]

The high pressures generated by the explosive cough of pertussis have resulted in a number of hemorrhagic events ranging from subconjunctival hemorrhages, petechiae, and epistaxis to melena and subdural and spinal epidural hematomas. Other mechanical consequences of the violent cough and vomiting include ulceration of the frenulum, umbilical and inguinal hernias, rectal prolapse, pneumothorax, mediastinal and subcutaneous emphysema, and diaphragmatic rupture.

Diagnosis

The diagnosis of pertussis can often be made readily on clinical grounds, especially during outbreaks, because of the distinctive findings during the paroxysmal stage. Laboratory tests may be helpful. During the late catarrhal and paroxysmal stages, the white cell count is typically elevated, often in the range of 20,000 to 30,000/mm^3, with a predominance of small, mature lymphocytes. However, the white cell count may be normal, especially in small infants and in older persons. The erythrocyte sedimentation rate is generally normal or even low.[53] The chest radiograph is usually normal; on occasion, it may demonstrate dense markings that fan out from the heart borders, the so-called shaggy heart sign.[54] These densities reflect peribronchial thickening rather than pneumonic infiltrates.

The differential diagnosis of severe paroxysmal coughing includes infection by other agents that may be associated with a pertussis syndrome. *B. parapertussis* and *B. bronchiseptica* cause a similar illness that is generally milder than that caused by *B. pertussis*. A number of adenovirus serotypes have been recovered from patients with clinical pertussis, but usually from those who have concurrent *B. pertussis* infection; thus, an independent role for adenoviruses in causing a pertussis syndrome has not been conclusively established.[55] Respiratory syncytial virus may also be isolated from patients with proven *B. pertussis* infection, but it does not appear to cause the pertussis syndrome by itself.[56] *Chlamydia trachomatis* respiratory tract infection in infants, which generally occurs between 4 and 8 weeks of life, is also associated with a prominent cough, but that of chlamydial disease is described as a series of staccato coughs, each followed by an inspiration (as opposed to pertussis, in which the inspiration comes only at the end of the paroxysm).[57] In addition, infants with chlamydial respiratory tract disease, unlike those with pertussis, usually have resting tachypnea and hypoxemia, with rales on auscultation and infiltrates at chest radiography; laboratory studies may demonstrate peripheral eosinophilia and hypergammaglobulinemia. Noninfectious considerations include diseases associated with severe coughing, such as cystic fibrosis, foreign body aspiration, tracheoesophageal fistula, gastroesophageal reflux, and mass lesions compressing the trachea.

Definitive diagnosis of pertussis requires recovery of the organism in culture; demonstration of its presence by DNA detection techniques, direct fluorescein-labeled immunofluorescense antibody (DFA) stains, or other immunohistochemical technique; or the demonstrated development of specific antibody responses. The most definitive means for making a diagnosis of pertussis is recovery of the organism from nasopharyngeal specimens, but *B. pertussis* is fastidious and grows slowly, and attempts to isolate it may fail up to 50% of the time (compared with seroconversion).[4] Selective media containing antibiotics are generally used for transport and isolation. Highest rates of recovery are achieved by collecting nasopharyngeal secretions with calcium alginate or Dacron-tipped swabs on a flexible wire and inoculating them directly onto suitable selective media at the patient's bedside. Use of cotton-tipped swabs or delayed inoculation of media decreases the likelihood of successful isolation. Recovery rates may also be increased by obtaining both a nasopharyngeal swab and a nasal suction aspirate.[58] The recovery rate for *B. pertussis* is highest during the first 2 to 3 weeks of illness and declines thereafter, even in the absence of antibiotic administration. Specimens from patients who have received antimicrobial therapy or who were previously immunized are less likely to yield the organism.

A DFA staining technique has been used in an attempt to circumvent some of the difficulties of culture. Some investigators have found this method to be less sensitive than culture; others have found it to be more sensitive.[59] The discrepancy may be related to quality control issues as well as to the time in the disease process at which specimens are obtained; the DFA test is less sensitive than culture early in the illness and more sensitive in later stages. In addition, false-positive and false-negative results are potential problems with DFA, and the microscopist's experience may influence interpretation. Unfortunately, culture is an insensitive "gold standard" for comparison. In experienced hands, a positive DFA determination is useful in making a presumptive diagnosis of pertussis; in general, this result should be confirmed by culture, DNA detection, or serologic studies. The most promising new technique is the polymerase chain reaction, which is coming into routine clinical use and could ultimately replace culture techniques.[60–62]

Several different antibody responses to *B. pertussis* have been described.[59] A frequently used and well-studied response has been the agglutination reaction; however, owing to the absence of a standardized method, the test's poor sensitivity, and the lack of commercially available test reagents, it has a limited role in the diagnosis of pertussis. Enzyme-linked immunosorbent assays[59] as well as immunoblotting techniques[63] have been described, using both whole-cell sonicates and more specific antigens such as LPF and FHA. Unfortunately, methods vary widely, as do the reported sensitivity and specificity of these techniques, and a reliable, sensitive, specific, and readily available test is lacking.[4, 64] Determination of serum immunoglobulin A[65] and immunoglobulin M[66] and nasopharyngeal immunoglobulin A[67] also shows promise as a way of diagnosing pertussis. Other techniques under investigation include the measurement of adenylate cyclase[68] and direct detection of *B. pertussis* antigens by counterimmunoelectrophoresis.[69]

Clinical case definitions that do not depend on laboratory confirmation (e.g., cough longer than 2 weeks or paroxysmal cough longer than 1 week) have been used in monitoring community outbreaks.[70]

Treatment

The most important aspect of treatment of patients with pertussis is the provision of general supportive care. Infants younger than 3 to 6 months are at greatest risk for serious complications and generally should be hospitalized, monitored closely, and supported until coughing paroxysms, apnea, cyanosis, and feeding problems have diminished or resolved and can be managed safely at home. Such support includes the use of oxygen, suctioning, and airway maintenance; avoidance of unnecessary stimuli; and fluid and nutritional support. In terms of pharmacologic support, the few data available on corticosteroids suggest that these drugs are safe in children and may ultimately reduce the number of coughing paroxysms if they are administered for more than a few days.[71–73] Similarly, inhaled salbutamol (albuterol) is safe and may reduce coughing.[74, 75] Administration of specific antipertussis immunoglobulin may also be beneficial in reducing cough frequency and duration.[76]

Because of the contagiousness of *B. pertussis*, respiratory isolation of patients is necessary until the index case has received antibiotic therapy for 5 days[77, 78] to prevent intrafamily transmission[79] and hospital outbreaks.[18–20] In vitro and in vivo, erythromycin has been demonstrated to be the most efficacious antimicrobial agent,[80] although resistance has been reported.[81] The most important role of antibiotic therapy is to reduce infectivity and contagiousness by eliminating the organism from the nasopharyngeal secretions of the index patient. If erythromycin is given during the incubation period or catarrhal stage, it may also prevent or ameliorate clinical disease.[82] Therapy begun during the paroxysmal stage is generally thought to have little or no impact on the clinical course, although in two studies, whoop frequency was ultimately believed to be reduced in treated groups, even though therapy was not started until the paroxysmal stage.[83, 84] Erythromycin therapy should be continued 2 weeks, because bacterial relapse may occur with a shorter course.[80] Erythromycin estolate may be the preferred form of the drug, especially for children.[83] Trimethoprim-sulfamethoxazole is generally considered to be the second drug of choice for persons who are allergic to or intolerant of erythromycin, but efficacy data are much more limited.[84] The fluoroquinolones clarithromycin and azithromycin also demonstrate in vitro activity, but clinical data are limited.

Intimate contacts of pertussis-infected persons, including household, daycare, and classroom contacts, and health care providers who did not use respiratory precautions should also receive a prophylactic 14-day course of erythromycin, regardless of their immunization status. Contacts younger than 7 years should also generally receive diphtheria and tetanus toxoids and pertussis vaccine (DTP) if they are inadequately immunized or have not received vaccine in longer than 3 years.[77] Because of the potential for adverse reactions,[19] routine whole-cell pertussis vaccine immunization for adults is generally not recommended.

Prevention

Vaccines for pertussis were first studied in the 1920s and came into widespread use in the late 1940s and early 1950s. The whole-cell vaccine long available in the United States is composed of a suspension of inactivated *B. pertussis* combined with diphtheria and tetanus toxoids and adsorbed onto an aluminum salt adjuvant. The protective efficacy in fully immunized children is 80% to 90%. Durability of protection, however, is limited to about a decade, as previously discussed. Five doses of DTP are recommended.[77] The primary series consists of a dose administered at 2 months of age; two additional doses given at intervals of 2 months; and a fourth dose given 6 to 12 months later, generally at 12 to 18 months of age. A fifth dose is given as a kindergarten booster at age 4 to 6 years. In outbreak situations, immunizations may be started as early as 2 weeks of age, and doses may be scheduled at intervals as short as 1 month. Minor adverse reactions to vaccine are common: erythema, swelling, or pain at the injection site and fever, drowsiness, fretfulness, anorexia, and vomiting. These reactions generally occur on the day of administration and subside uneventfully. Although such reactions may be more likely to recur with subsequent injections, they do not represent a contraindication to further DTP dosing. Acetaminophen is usually effective in reducing their frequency and severity.

More serious sequelae of pertussis immunization include convulsions (usually associated with fever); persistent uncontrollable screaming or an unusual, high-pitched cry; collapse or shocklike state (hypotonic-hyporesponsive episode); and temperature greater than 40.5°C. These are uncommon reactions, but the possibility of recurrence of these reactions justifies caution in repeating doses of whole-cell pertussis vaccine. In outbreak situations, further immunizations may be warranted. Immediate anaphylaxis represents the only true contraindication to further DTP administration but is exceedingly rare. No causal relationship between pertussis immunization and sudden infant death syndrome or infantile spasms is recognized,[8] and a family history of seizures does not constitute a contraindication to pertussis immunization.

Complacency about the seriousness of pertussis combined with concerns about whole-cell pertussis vaccine toxicity led to a marked decline in use of the vaccine in many countries during the 1970s and, subsequently, a large increase in the number of reported cases of pertussis in England, Japan, and

Sweden. Careful analysis of the available data suggests that most of the serious neurologic illness associated with DTP is probably not actually caused by the vaccine. Rather, DTP immunization may unmask (i.e., accelerate the onset of) a neurologic disorder that would eventually become manifest anyway. Results of numerous careful risk/benefit analyses indicate that the benefits of vaccination far outweigh the risk,[8] and most experts including the American Academy of Pediatrics have concluded that pertussis vaccine has not been proved to cause brain damage.[77]

The ultimate goal of eliminating pertussis requires a vaccine with a high efficacy rate that provides durable immunity (by booster doses if necessary), prevents colonization as well as infection, and is safe for children and adults, including pregnant women. It is hoped that acellular pertussis vaccines may help fill this role.[85–88] These vaccines, which have been universally used in Japan since 1981 and have been studied in the United States and Europe, consist of *B. pertussis* components rather than whole-cell sonicates.[8] Various combinations of pertussis toxin (LPF), FHA, and pertactin agglutinogens have been used.[9] Evidence to date demonstrates that these vaccines cause significantly fewer adverse minor reactions than do whole-cell vaccines in children and adults. Because serious adverse reactions are uncommon with any of the vaccines, it has not been possible to compare whole-cell vaccines and acellular ones in this regard. Efficacy data from Japan and Sweden are encouraging,[89, 90] although whether these vaccines are as effective as whole-cell vaccine is not clear. They were initially licensed for use in the United States just for the fourth and fifth dose, given after 15 months of age.[77] In 1996, they became available for use for the primary immunizing series. Studies of their use in adults are under way.[91, 92] If these vaccines fulfill their potential of being both safe and efficacious, pertussis could join diphtheria and tetanus as diseases for which booster immunizations throughout life could potentially reduce disease incidence to a low level.

References

1. Cone TE: Whooping cough is first described as a disease *sui generis* by Baillou in 1640. Pediatrics 46:522, 1970.
2. Gordon JE, Hood RL: Whooping cough and its epidemiological anomalies. Am J Med Sci 222:333, 1951.
3. Galazka A: Control of pertussis in the world. World Health Stat Q 45:238, 1992.
4. Marion MJ: *Bordetella*. *In* Murray PR (ed): Manual of Clinical Microbiology, ed 5. Washington, DC, American Society for Microbiology, 1995, pp 566–576.
5. Goodnow RA: Biology of *Bordetella bronchiseptica*. Microbiol Rev 44:722, 1980.
6. Kersters K, Hinz KH, Hertle A: *Bordetella avium* sp. nov. isolated from the respiratory tracts of turkeys and other birds. Int J Syst Bacteriol 34:56, 1984.
7. Musser JM, Heulett EL, Peppler MJ: Genetic diversity and relationships in populations of *Bordetella* spp. J Bacteriol 166:230, 1986.
8. Cherry JD, Brunnel PA, Golden GJ, et al: Report of the task force on pertussis and pertussis immunization—1988. Pediatrics 81(Suppl):939, 1988.
9. Cattaneo L, Edwards K: *Bordetella pertussis* (whooping cough). Semin Pediatr Infect Dis 6:107, 1995.
10. Pittman M: The concept of pertussis as a toxin-mediated disease. Pediatr Infect Dis 3:467, 1984.
11. Monack D, Munoz JJ, Peacock MG, et al: Expression of pertussis toxin correlates with pathogenesis in *Bordetella* species. J Infect Dis 159:205, 1989.
12. Weiss AA, Hewlett EL: Virulence factors of *Bordetella pertussis*. Annu Rev Microbiol 40:661, 1986.
13. Davis LE, Burstyn DG, Manclark CR: Pertussis encephalopathy with a normal brain biopsy and elevated lymphocytosis-promoting factor antibodies. Pediatr Infect Dis 3:448, 1984.
14. Halperin SA, Marrie TJ: Pertussis encephalopathy in an adult: Case report and review. Rev Infect Dis 13:1043, 1991.
15. Thomas M: Epidemiology of pertussis. Rev Infect Dis 11:255, 1989.
16. Farizo KM, Cochi SL, Zell ER, et al: Epidemiologic features of pertussis in the United States, 1980–1989. Clin Infect Dis 14:708, 1992.
17. Wright PF: Pertussis in developing countries: Definition of the problem and prospects for control. Rev Infect Dis 13(Suppl 6):5528, 1991.
18. Kurt TL, Yeager AS, Guenette S, et al: Spread of pertussis by hospital staff. JAMA 221:264, 1972.
19. Linnemann CC, Ramundo N, Perlstein PH, et al: Use of pertussis vaccine in an epidemic involving hospital staff. Lancet 2:540, 1975.
20. Shefer A, Dales L, Nelson M, et al: Use and safety of acellular pertussis vaccine among adult hospital staff during an outbreak of pertussis. J Infect Dis 171:1053, 1995.
21. Hardy IRB, Strobel PM, Wharton M: The 1993 pertussis epidemic in Cincinnati. N Engl J Med 331:1455, 1994.
22. Bass JW: Is there a carrier state in pertussis? Lancet 1:98, 1987.
23. Nelson JD: The changing epidemiology of pertussis in young infants. The role of adults as reservoirs of infection. Am J Dis Child 132:371, 1978.
24. Herwaldt L: Pertussis in adults—What physicians need to know. Arch Intern Med 151:1510, 1991.
25. Centers for Disease Control and Prevention: Transmission of pertussis from adult to infant—Michigan, 1993. MMWR Morbid Mortal Wkly Rep 44:74, 1995.
26. Lambert H: Epidemiology of a small pertussis outbreak in Kent County, Michigan. Public Health Rep 80:365, 1965.
27. Jenkinson D: Duration of effectiveness of pertussis vaccine: Evidence from a 10 year community study. Br Med J 296:612, 1988.
28. Mink CM, Sirota NM, Nugent S: Outbreak of pertussis in a fully immunized adolescent and adult population. Arch Pediatr Adolesc Med 148:153, 1994.
29. Cherry J, Beer T, Chartrand S, et al: Comparison of values of antibody to *Bordetella pertussis* antigens in young German and American men. Clin Infect Dis 20:1271, 1995.
30. Mink CM, Cherry JD, Christenson P, et al: A search for *Bordetella pertussis* in university students. Clin Infect Dis 14:464, 1992.
31. Wright SW, Edwards KM, Decker MD, et al: Pertussis infection in adults with persistent cough. JAMA 273:1044, 1995.
32. Cherry JD: The epidemiology of pertussis and pertussis immunization in the United Kingdom and the United States: A comparative study. Curr Probl Pediatr 14:1, 1984.
33. Hodder S, Mortimer E: Epidemiology of pertussis and reactions to pertussis vaccine. Epidemiol Rev 14:243, 1992.
34. Centers for Disease Control: Pertussis surveillance—United States, 1984 and 1985. MMWR Morbid Mortal Wkly Rep 36:168, 1987.
35. Davis SF, Strebel PM, Cochi SL, et al: Pertussis surveillance—United States, 1989–1991. MMWR CDC Surveill Summ 41(SS-8):11, 1992.
36. Centers for Disease Control and Prevention: Resurgence of pertussis—United States, 1993. MMWR Morbid Mortal Wkly Rep 42:952, 1993.
37. Bass J, Wittler R: Return of epidemic pertussis in the United States. Pediatr Infect Dis J 13:343, 1994.
38. Sutter RW, Cochi SL: Pertussis hospitalizations and mortality in the United States, 1985–1988: Evaluation of the completeness of national reporting. JAMA 267:386, 1992.
39. Marchant C, Loughlin A, Lett S, et al: Pertussis in Massachusetts, 1981–1991: Incidence, serologic diagnosis, and vaccine effectiveness. J Infect Dis 169:1297, 1994.
40. Gordon M, David HD, Gold R: Clinical and microbiologic features of children presenting with pertussis to a Canadian pediatric hospital during an eleven-year period. Pediatr Infect Dis J 13:617, 1994.
41. Onorato M, Wassilak S, Meade B: Efficacy of whole-cell pertussis vaccine in preschool children in the United States. JAMA 267:2745, 1992.
42. Bass JW, Stephenson SR: The return of pertussis. Pediatr Infect Dis J 6:141, 1987.

43. Olson LC: Pertussis. Medicine (Baltimore) 54:427, 1975.
44. Sotomayor J, Wiener LB, McMillan JA: Inaccurate diagnosis in infants with pertussis: An 8 year experience. Am J Dis Child 139:724, 1985.
45. Congeni BL, Orenstein DM, Nankervis GA: Three infants with neonatal pertussis. Clin Pediatr 17:115, 1978.
46. Southall DP, Thomas MG, Lambert HP: Severe hypoxemia in pertussis. Arch Dis Child 163:598, 1988.
47. Cherry JD, Baraff LJ, Hewlett E: The past, present, and future of pertussis—The role of adults in epidemiology and future control. West J Med 150:319, 1989.
48. Johnston IDA, Bland JM, Ingram D, et al: Effect of whooping cough in infancy on subsequent lung infection. Am Rev Respir Dis 134:270, 1986.
49. Howenstine M, Eigen H, Tepper R: Pulmonary function in infants after pertussis. J Pediatr 118:563, 1991.
50. Zellweger H: Pertussis encephalopathy. Arch Pediatr 76:381, 1959.
51. Johnston IDA: Reading attainment and physical development after whooping cough. J Epidemiol Community Health 39:314, 1985.
52. Swansea Research Unit of the Royal College of General Practitioners: Study of intellectual performance of children in ordinary school after certain serious complications of whooping cough. Br Med J 295:1044, 1987.
53. Lagergren G: The white blood cell count and the erythrocyte sedimentation rate in pertussis. Acta Paediatr 52:405, 1963.
54. Barnhard HJ, Kniker WT: Roentgenologic findings in pertussis with particular emphasis on the "shaggy heart" sign. AJR 84:445, 1960.
55. Keller MA, Affandelians R, Connor JD: Etiology of pertussis syndrome. Pediatrics 66:50, 1980.
56. Nelson WL, Hopkins RS, Roe MH, et al: Simultaneous infection with *Bordetella pertussis* and respiratory syncytial virus in hospitalized children. Pediatr Infect Dis 5:540, 1986.
57. Beem MO, Saxon EM: Respiratory-tract colonization and a distinctive pneumonia syndrome in infants infected with *Chlamydia trachomatis*. N Engl J Med 296:306, 1977.
58. Bejuk D, Beguvac J, Buce A, et al: Culture of *Bordetella pertussis* from three upper respiratory tract specimens. Pediatr Infect Dis J 14:64, 1995.
59. Onorato IM, Wassilak SGF: Laboratory diagnosis of pertussis: The state of the art. Pediatr Infect Dis J 6:145, 1987.
60. Meade B, Bollen A: Recommendations for use of the polymerase chain reaction in the diagnosis of *Bordetella pertussis* infections. J Med Microbiol 41:51, 1994.
61. He Q, Mertsola J, Soini H, et al: Sensitive and specific polymerase chain reaction assays for detection of *Bordetella pertussis* in nasopharyngeal specimens. Pediatrics 124:421, 1994.
62. Li Z, Jansen DL, Finn TM, et al: Identification of *Bordetella pertussis* infections by shared-primer PCR. J Clin Microbiol 32:783, 1994.
63. Thomas M, Redhead K, Lamber HP: Human serum antibody responses to *Bordetella pertussis* infection and pertussis vaccination. J Infect Dis 159:211, 1989.
64. Halperin SA: Interpretation of pertussis serologic tests. Pediatr Infect Dis J 10:791, 1991.
65. Nagel J, Poot-Scholtens EJ: Serum IgA antibody to *Bordetella pertussis* as an indicator of infection. J Med Microbiol 16:417, 1983.
66. Conway SP, Balfour AH, Ross H: Serologic diagnosis of whooping cough by enzyme-linked immunosorbent assay. Pediatr Infect Dis J 7:570, 1988.
67. Grunstrom G, Askelof P, Grunstrom M: Specific immunoglobulin A to *Bordetella pertussis* antigens in mucosal secretions for rapid diagnosis of whooping cough. J Clin Microbiol 26:869, 1988.
68. Confer DL, Eaton IW: *Bordetella* adenylate cyclase: Host toxicity and diagnostic utility. Dev Biol Stand 61:3, 1985.
69. Borland PC, Gillespie SH, Ashworth LA: Rapid diagnosis of whooping cough using monoclonal antibody. J Clin Pathol 41:573, 1988.
70. Strebel PM, Cochi SL, Farizo KM, et al: Pertussis in Missouri: Evaluation of nasopharyngeal culture, direct fluorescent antibody testing, and clinical case definitions in the diagnosis of pertussis. Clin Infect Dis 16:276, 1993.
71. Bass JW: Pertussis: Current status and prevention and treatment. Pediatr Infect Dis 4:624, 1985.
72. Torre D, Tambini R, Ferrario G, et al: Treatment with steroids in children with pertussis. Pediatr Infect Dis J 12:419, 1993.
73. Roberts I, Gavin R, Lennon D: Randomized controlled trial of steroids in pertussis. Pediatr Infect Dis J 11:982, 1992.
74. Krantz I, Norrby JR, Trollfors B: Salbutamol vs. placebo for treatment of pertussis. Pediatr Infect Dis J 4:638, 1985.
75. Mertsula J, Viljaned MK, Ruuskanen O: Salbutamol in the treatment of whooping cough. J Infect Dis 18:593, 1986.
76. Granstrom M, Olinder-Nielsen, Holmblad P: Specific immunoglobulin for treatment of whooping cough. Lancet 338:1230, 1991.
77. American Academy of Pediatrics: Pertussis. *In* Peter G (ed): Report of the Committee on Infectious Diseases, ed 23. Elk Grove Village, IL, American Academy of Pediatrics, 1994, pp 355–367.
78. Weber DJ, Rutula WA: Management of health care workers exposed to pertussis. Infect Control Hosp Epidemiol 15:411, 1994.
79. Sprauer M, Cochi S, Zell E, et al: Prevention of secondary transmission of pertussis in households with early use of erythromycin. Am J Dis Child 146:177, 1992.
80. Bass JW: Erythromycin for treatment and prevention of pertussis. Pediatr Infect Dis 5:154, 1986.
81. Lewis K, Soubolle MA, Tenover FC, et al: Pertussis caused by an erythromycin-resistant strain of *Bordetella pertussis*. Pediatr Infect Dis J 14:388, 1995.
82. Bergquist S-O, Bernander S, Dahnsjo H, et al: Erythromycin in the treatment of pertussis: A study of bacteriologic and clinical effects. Pediatr Infect Dis J 6:458, 1987.
83. Hoppe R: Comparison of erythromycin estolate and erythromycin ethylsuccinate for treatment of pertussis. Pediatr Infect Dis J 11:189, 1991.
84. Hoppe JE, Haug A: Treatment and prevention of pertussis by antimicrobial agents (Part II). Infection 16:148, 1988.
85. Cherry J: Acellular pertussis vaccines—A solution to the pertussis problem. J Infect Dis 168:21, 1993.
86. Wintermeyer S, Nahata M, Kyllonen K: Whole-cell and acellular pertussis vaccines. Ann Pharmacother 28:925, 1994.
87. Robbins J, Pittman M, Trollfors B, et al: *Primum non nocere:* A pharmacologically inert pertussis toxoid alone should be the next pertussis vaccine. Pediatr Infect Dis J 12:795, 1993.
88. Edwards KM: Acellular pertussis vaccines—A solution to the pertussis problem? J Infect Dis 168:15, 1993.
89. Aoyama T, Iwata T, Iwai H, et al: Efficacy of acellular pertussis vaccine in young infants. J Infect Dis 167:483, 1993.
90. Ad Hoc Group for the Study of Pertussis Vaccines: Placebo-controlled trial of two acellular pertussis vaccines in Sweden—Protective efficacy and adverse effects. Lancet 1:955, 1988.
91. Herwaldt L: Pertussis and pertussis vaccines in adults. JAMA 269:93, 1993.
92. Edwards K, Decker M, Graham B, et al: Adult immunization with acellular pertussis vaccine. JAMA 269:53, 1993.

216

Miscellaneous Gram-Negative Bacilli: *Acinetobacter, Cardiobacterium, Actinobacillus, Chromobacterium, Capnocytophaga,* and Others

Judith L. Nerad
Maria Teresa Seville
David R. Snydman

Although most gram-negative infections that are clinically significant are caused by members of the Enterobacteriaceae and Pseudomonadaceae, a small percentage of infections are caused by a variety of uncommon gram-negative organisms. These are usually identified by Gram stain and growth characteristics, biochemical reactions, and appropriate epidemiologic circumstances. Patients infected with these more unusual gram-negative organisms present with both localized and systemic infections, may be normal or immunocompromised hosts, and may present with acute or chronic disease. These infections may arise from endogenous or environmental exposures.

These heterogeneous organisms are often grouped according to their ability to ferment glucose (produce acid from carbohydrate in the absence of oxygen). Therefore, they are considered here as such and are discussed in the groupings glucose fermenters and nonfermenters, as found in Table 216–1. See subsequent tables for other general characteristics regarding natural reservoirs (Table 216–2), clinical manifestations of infection (Table 216–3), antimicrobial susceptibilities (Table 216–4), and host immune defects (Table 216–5).

Glucose Fermenters

Actinobacillus

The genus *Actinobacillus* consists of several species: *Actinobacillus lignieresii* (type species), *Actinobacillus equuli, Actinobacillus suis, Actinobacillus hominis, Actinobacillus pleuropneumoniae,* and *Actinobacillus actinomycetemcomitans.*[1] The last affects only humans; the others have rarely been associated with disease in humans and more often infect domestic animals. *A. pleuropneumoniae*[2] is a significant pathogen in pigs; however, only *A. actinomycetemcomitans* is discussed here.

A. actinomycetemcomitans was initially described in 1912. For 50 years the organism was thought to be a contaminant and not a pathogen. This was because of its frequency of isolation in infections with *Actinomyces israelii.*[1] There is some debate whether *A. actinomycetemcomitans* should be classified in the genus *Haemophilus.*[2]

A. actinomycetemcomitans refers to a bacillus in ray form

TABLE 216–1 ■ Growth and Biochemical Characteristics of Selected Gram-Negative Organisms

	GROWTH CHARACTERISTICS				BIOCHEMICAL CHARACTERISTICS			
ORGANISM	Gram Stain Morphology	CO_2 Requirement	Growth on MacConkey Agar	Growth on Blood Agar	Oxidase	Catalase	Indole	Reduce Nitrates
Glucose fermenters								
Actinobacillus	Coccobacilli	↑ CO_2	–	Slow (3–6 d)	Weak +	+	–	+
Capnocytophaga	Long, thin rods, fusiform	↑ CO_2	–	Slow (2–4 d), gliding	–	–	–	+
Capnocytophaga canimorsus	Long, thin rods (curved)	↑ CO_2	–	Slow (2–3 d), gliding	+	+	–	+
DF-3	Coccobacilli	Facultative anaerobe	–	Slow (2–3 d), fruity odor	–	–	+	–
Cardiobacterium	Pleomorphic rods	↑ CO_2	–	Slow (>2 d)	+	–	+	–
Chromobacterium	Small to medium curved rod	Facultative anaerobe	+	Violet pigment	+	+	–	+
Glucose nonfermenters								
Acinetobacter	Diplococci-coccobacilli	Aerobe	+	Within 1 d	–	+	–	–
Achromobacter	Medium straight rods	Aerobe	+	Within 1 d	+	+	–	+
Alcaligenes	Medium straight rods	Obligate aerobe	+	Within 1 d	+	+	–	(+)*
Eikenella	Coccobacilli	Facultative anaerobe and hemin required with ↑ CO_2	–	Pitting (2–3 d)	+	–	–	+
Ochrobactrum	Rods	Aerobe	+	Within 1 d	+	+	–	+
Flavobacterium	Long, thin rods, occasionally filamentous	Aerobe	+	Within 1 d, yellow pigment	+	+	+/–*	–

*Species dependent.

TABLE 216–2 ■ Natural Reservoirs of Selected Gram-Negative Organisms

Environmental sources	Endogenous sources
Soil, water	Normal oral flora
Achromobacter	*Acinetobacter*
Acinetobacter	*Actinobacillus*
Alcaligenes	*Capnocytophaga*
Chromobacterium	*Cardiobacterium*
Flavobacterium	*Eikenella*
Hospital equipment	Skin
Achromobacter	*Acinetobacter*
Acinetobacter	*Alcaligenes*
Alcaligenes	Stool
Flavobacterium	*Achromobacter*
Ochrobactrum	*Alcaligenes*
	Chromobacterium
	Eikenella
	DF-3
	Ochrobactrum

that accompanies an actinomycete. It is a gram-negative bacillus predominantly but is found in both coccobacillary and filamentous forms. Biochemically, it is oxidase variable and catalase-positive, does not hydrolyze urea or form indole, and does reduce nitrates. It is nonmotile and does not grow on MacConkey agar. It ferments glucose, not lactose or sucrose. Growth in blood culture media may not be seen until 3 to 6 days of incubation, and cultures should be held for 2 to 3 weeks. Early growth is manifested by discrete floccules in sedimented blood or adherence to the wall of the bottle. *A. actinomycetemcomitans* organisms are facultatively anaerobic or aerobic and require carbon dioxide for growth. Colonies are smooth, translucent, and slightly domed with a corrugated surface. They are quite "sticky" and, with further incubation, about 3 to 5 days, a four- to six-pointed star shape forms with the colony or "crossed cigars" form. *A. actinomycetemcomitans* has eight biotypes depending on sugar fermentation and serotype, although these are not clinically relevant. Local and serum antibodies develop to *A. actinomycetemcomitans*, but it has not been established that they are protective.[1, 3–5] *A. actinomycetemcomitans* are easily confused with *Pasteurella*, *Haemophilus*, and *Yersinia*. None of these forms sticky colonies, however.

TABLE 216–3 ■ Common Clinical Syndromes Associated with Selected Gram-Negative Bacteria

Sepsis
- *Achromobacter*
- *Acinetobacter*
- *Capnocytophaga*
- *Chromobacterium*
- DF-3
- *Ochrobactrum*
- *Flavobacterium*

Associated with bites (human or animal)
- *Acinetobacter*
- *Actinobacillus*
- *Capnocytophaga*
- *Eikenella*

Soft tissue infection
- *Acinetobacter*
- *Achromobacter*
- *Actinobacillus*
- *Alcaligenes*
- *Chromobacterium*
- *Eikenella* (often mixed infections)

Endocarditis
- *Actinobacillus*
- *Alcaligenes*
- *Cardiobacterium*
- *Eikenella*

Meningitis
- *Achromobacter*
- *Acinetobacter*
- *Capnocytophaga*
- *Flavobacterium*

Abscess formation
- *Acinetobacter*
- *Actinobacillus*
- *Capnocytophaga*
- *Chromobacterium*
- *Eikenella*

Chronic diarrhea
- DF-3

Virulence properties possessed by actinobacilli include endotoxin[6] and leukotoxin,[7, 8] which may be significant in the development of periodontal disease.[9] Endotoxin may indirectly enhance collagen breakdown (via prostaglandin E_2 or interleukin-1 involvement) and interfere with monocyte defenses recruited against the bacteria. Leukotoxin may lyse polymorphonuclear cells and inhibit chemotaxis. Interference with lymphocyte function either directly or indirectly, via altered monocyte integrity, occurs. There is no evidence that *A. actinomycetemcomitans* degrades fibronectin.[10] Because it grows in environments with low oxygen tension (e.g., tissues), neutrophil myeloperoxidase systems may not be effective in killing *A. actinomycetemcomitans*.

A. actinomycetemcomitans has been isolated from oral flora of about 20% of healthy adults and children.[5, 11] It has been found in dental plaque, buccal mucosa, tonsils, and the gastrointestinal and genital tracts of humans and animals.[1, 5] Clinical isolates include food, oral pharynx (especially in young adults with localized juvenile periodontitis), abscesses,

TABLE 216–4 ■ Antibiotic Sensitivities of Miscellaneous Gram-Negative Bacilli*

ORGANISM	PENICILLINS	EXPANDED-SPECTRUM PENICILLINS	CEPHALOSPORINS 1°, 2°	CEPHALOSPORINS 3°	VANCOMYCIN	ERYTHROMYCIN	TETRACYCLINE	CLINDAMYCIN	AMINOGLYCOSIDES
Glucose fermenters									
Actinobacillus	R, V	S	V	S	R	R	S	R	S
Capnocytophaga	V	S	V	S	R		S	S	R
Capnocytophaga canimorsus	S	S		S	S	S		S	S[a]
DF-3	R		R		R	V	S	S	R
Cardiobacterium	S	S	S	S	V	V	S		S
Chromobacterium	R	R, V	R	R		R	S		S
Glucose nonfermenters									
Acinetobacter	R	V+	R	S			V		V
Achromobacter	R	V+	R	V			V		R
Alcaligenes	V	V	V	V					V
Eikenella	S	S	V	S	R		V	R	R
Ochrobactrum	R	R	R	R			V		S
Flavobacterium	R	R	R	R	S	V		S	

*R, Most strains are resistant in vitro; V, variable resistance; S, most strains are sensitive; [a], not sensitive in older literature because of different techniques of evaluation; +, imipenem is a consistently effective agent against these organisms; 1°, 2°, first- and second-generation cephalosporins; 3°, third-generation cephalosporins; T-S, trimethoprim-sulfamethoxazole.

sinus tracts, and pleural fluid. Sites distant from the oral cavity are thought to be infected through hematogenous spread.

Common clinical syndromes include endocarditis, periodontal disease, and soft tissue abscesses either alone or in association with *Actinomyces*.

ENDOCARDITIS

Endocarditis is the most common serious infection associated with *A. actinomycetemcomitans*. In a review by Kaplan and coworkers,[11] 60% of patients had underlying valvular heart disease and 46% of patients had periodontal disease or recent dental manipulation. Of those with valvular heart disease, roughly 40% had prosthetic valves. The majority of patients were male, presenting with subacute disease (after 1 to 16 weeks). One third had presenting manifestations of classic endocarditis (hepatosplenomegaly, peripheral manifestations). Anemia and elevated erythrocyte sedimentation rate were seen in 90% or more of patients. Emboli occurred in 39% of patients and were associated with a poor prognosis. Similar findings were reported by Chen and coworkers[12] in a much smaller series.

The presentation of symptoms can occur during a prolonged time period. In patients with prosthetic valve endocarditis caused by *A. actinomycetemcomitans*, presentation generally occurred more than a year after surgery. Of 13 patients reviewed, all but 1 were treated medically and only 1 died.[11, 13] There is one reported case of pulmonary valve endocarditis related to *A. actinomycetemcomitans* with a presenting course during 18 months.[14] In addition, persistent bacteremia for more than 1 year in a patient with an infected pacemaker and positive dental cultures has been reported.[15]

Most patients were treated with penicillin or ampicillin and an aminoglycoside. The overall mortality rate was about 23% and was the same for native valve versus prosthetic valve involvement. Valve replacement was generally required in about 25%. Patients with prosthetic valve endocarditis caused by gram-negative bacilli of the HACEK group (*Haemophilus aphrophilus*, *A. actinomycetemcomitans*, *Cardiobacterium hominis*, *Eikenella corrodens*, and *Kingella kingae*) generally have a more favorable outcome than patients with a non-HACEK gram-negative bacillus infection on a prosthetic or native valve. Specifically, they have less mortality and do not require valve replacement as often.[16]

TABLE 216–5 ■ Host Immune Status Related to Infecting Organisms

ORGANISM	HOST IMMUNE DEFECT
Acinetobacter	Debilitation, prolonged hospital stay, after surgery, trauma
Achromobacter	As for *Acinetobacter*
Actinobacillus	Neutrophil chemotactic defect
Alcaligenes	Neutrophil chemotactic defect and IVDU*
Eikenella	IVDU
Capnocytophaga	Neutropenia, periodontal disease
Capnocytophaga canimorsus	Splenectomy, alcohol abuse
Chromobacterium	Chronic granulomatous disease
DF-3	Malignancy, human immunodeficiency virus infection, common variable hypogammaglobulinemia, chronic illness
Ochrobactrum	Immunosuppressive therapy
Flavobacterium	Premature and small-for-gestational-age infants, immunocompromised status, debilitation

*IVDU, Intravenous drug user.

LOCALIZED JUVENILE PERIODONTITIS OR ACUTE NECROTIZING ULCERATIVE GINGIVITIS

A. actinomycetemcomitans is thought to be involved in the pathogenesis of localized juvenile periodontitis or acute necrotizing ulcerative gingivitis. Predisposing factors include a neutrophil chemotactic defect that is either familial or acquired, perhaps from infection with *A. actinomycetemcomitans*.[17, 18] More than 90% of patients with localized juvenile periodontitis have had *A. actinomycetemcomitans* identified from plaque samples or gingival tissue. Most cases are successfully treated with penicillin. Pavicic and coworkers[19] reported success in treating patients with chronic periodontitis with mechanical débridement and oral amoxicillin and metronidazole.

OTHER CLINICAL PRESENTATIONS

A. actinomycetemcomitans infections have included pericarditis,[20] parotitis, endophthalmitis,[21, 22] tenosynovitis,[23] arthritis,[24]

QUINOLONES	CHLORAMPHENICOL	T-S	METRONIDAZOLE	RIFAMPIN	AZTREONAM	IMIPENEM
S	S			S		
S	S	R	S		R	S
S	S	S		S	R	S
S	R	S			R	S
	S					
	S	S				
S	R	S			V	S
V	V	S				S
V	S	S				
S	S		R	V		
S	R	S			R	S
S	V	S		S	R	R

osteomyelitis (vertebral), urinary tract infections, pneumonia,[25, 26] empyema, synovitis, mycetoma,[27] lymphadenitis,[28] and abscess formation.[11, 29] Abscesses in the brain, thyroid gland, chest wall, hand, and head and neck have all been described,[11] including coinfection with *Actinomyces*.[30–32] *A. lignieresii, A. suis,* and *A. equuli*–like bacteria have been isolated from infected horse and sheep bite wounds in humans.[33, 34]

On the basis of data from the review by Kaplan and coworkers,[11] *A. actinomycetemcomitans* is generally susceptible to chloramphenicol, tetracycline, streptomycin, aminoglycosides, and cephalosporins. More than 90% of isolates are also susceptible to mezlocillin and carbenicillin. About 80% of isolates are susceptible to ampicillin and penicillin.[11] *Actinobacillus* is generally resistant (less than 30% of isolates sensitive) to erythromycin, clindamycin, vancomycin,[35] and methicillin. Goldstein and Citron[36] have demonstrated excellent in vitro activity by the new quinolones azithromycin and amoxicillin-clavulanate on clinical isolates from bite wounds.

Topical potassium iodide may be beneficial in chronic periodontal infections. Reviews studying in vitro susceptibilities of periodontal isolates have found 100% susceptibility to cefaclor, cefuroxime, cefixime,[37] tetracycline, doxycycline, trimethoprim-sulfamethoxazole, and ciprofloxacin.[37, 38] Amoxicillin or ciprofloxacin synergy with metronidazole has been demonstrated and has been successfully used in combination with mechanical débridement for therapy of periodontitis.[37]

Conservative therapy for endocarditis would dictate 4 to 6 weeks of therapy with a cephalosporin and aminoglycoside. Reports show that penicillin, erythromycin, and vancomycin have all failed as prophylaxis against endocarditis with *A. actinomycetemcomitans* after dental procedures.[11] It has been suggested that patients with valvular disease and severe periodontitis who are undergoing dental work have prophylaxis 14 days before the procedure with tetracycline.

Capnocytophaga

Capnocytophaga species were first described in the 1950s and were known as a variant of *Fusobacterium nucleatum* or *Bacteroides oralis*. King, of the Centers for Disease Control (CDC; now the Centers for Disease Control and Prevention), named the strain DF-1 (dysgonic fermenter 1) in the 1960s. In 1972, the earlier strains of capnophilic, fastidious gram-negative bacteria were recognized as the same organism and named *Bacteroides ochraceus*. In 1979, the genus *Capnocytophaga* was described to include the DF-1 and *Bacteroides* species.[39, 40]

There are five clinically relevant species: *Capnocytophaga ochracea, Capnocytophaga sputigena, Capnocytophaga gingivalis*,[41] *Capnocytophaga canimorsus* (formerly dysgonic fermenter 2 [DF-2]), and *Capnocytophaga cynodegmi* (DF-2–like organisms). *C. canimorsus* and *C. cynodegmi* were established later as *Capnocytophaga* species[42] and are discussed separately.

Capnocytophaga organisms are gram-negative long, thin rods, often fusiform, that are "gliding" or spreading on agar. They grow slowly, during at least 2 to 4 days, require carbon dioxide under either aerobic or anaerobic growth conditions, and have the capacity to ferment glucose. Colonies leave a yellow pigment on the agar. Special selective media[43, 44] are required for optimal growth because the organisms do not grow on MacConkey agar. Biochemically, they are oxidase-, catalase-, and indole-negative, and reduction of nitrates is variable between species. Each species also ferments a different profile of carbohydrates.[41] Of note, *C. ochracea* has been reported to cause a false-positive *Legionella* latex agglutination test.[45]

Virulence factors are important regarding pathogenesis.[41] Endotoxin is biologically active and contains a unique C_{15} branched chain fatty acid. Endotoxin, a peptidoglycan, and a slime layer may be immunomodulators. Patients with neutrophil dysfunction or deficiency are predisposed to developing periodontitis[46] and septicemia in granulocytopenic hosts caused by *Capnocytophaga*.[47] *Capnocytophaga* may induce a chemotactic defect in polymorphonuclear leukocytes by elaborating a dialyzable substance that interferes with neutrophil migration. Other *Capnocytophaga* species have been shown to enhance (B-cell activation, lymphocyte, and macrophage proliferation) or inhibit (fibroblast proliferation) various immunologic functions that may interfere with optimal host response to infection. *Capnocytophaga* species also synthesize trypsin and an immunoglobulin A protease. β-Lactamase production has been described.[48] A review of clinical isolates from oral and nonoral lesions demonstrated a reduced ability to activate complement by nonoral isolates and hence reduced serum bactericidal capacity.[49]

The major site of *Capnocytophaga* colonization is the oral cavity; however, organisms have been isolated from the vagina as well as upper and lower respiratory tract sources (nose and throat, sputum, trachea, bronchial specimens, pleural fluid).[50, 51] Clinical isolates have been obtained from blood, cerebrospinal fluid, wounds (especially bite wounds), eyes (both the corneal ulcers and vitreous fluid), vagina,[52] and amniotic fluid.[51]

Clinically important infections are most commonly seen with cases of juvenile periodontitis[53] or systemic disease in granulocytopenic cancer patients with oral lesions. A variety of infections have been reported in nonimmunocompromised hosts as well. The cases of juvenile periodontitis are thought to be related to an acquired neutrophil defect secondary to *Capnocytophaga* infection[46]; the defect resolves as the infection is treated. Other local immunosuppressive actions may occur, including immunoglobulin A protease activity.

Immunocompromised patients with *Capnocytophaga* infection tend to be young, mostly children with malignancies, have low neutrophil counts (e.g., chemotherapy-induced granulocytopenia), and have significant oral disease[51] (oral ulcers[50] or glossitis[54]). Clinical presentations include bacteremia and septicemia.[50, 51, 55]

Nonimmunocompromised patients have had a variety of clinically significant infections with *Capnocytophaga* species. These include ocular infections[51, 56] (keratitis,[57, 58] conjunctivitis, endophthalmitis,[59] corneal ulcer[60]), cardiothoracic infections (endocarditis,[61] pericardial abscess,[62] mediastinitis,[63] lung and subphrenic abscess, empyema[51]), septic arthritis,[64] cervical[65] and inguinal[66] lymphadenitis, sinusitis,[67] thyroiditis,[68] osteomyelitis,[69] peritonitis[70] and abdominal abscess, and traumatic hand wounds.[51] Cases of peripartum infections[71] including amniotic fluid infection associated with premature delivery[72, 73] and congenital bacteremia[74, 75] have been described. Endometritis secondary to an intrauterine device has also been reported.[76] Like *Actinobacillus* infection, *Capnocytophaga* infection has been reported in association with *A. israelii* infection.[77]

Capnocytophaga species are sensitive to clindamycin, third-generation cephalosporins, newer penicillins, imipenem, and the quinolones (ciprofloxacin, ofloxacin).[78–82] Chloramphenicol, tetracycline, and metronidazole also have activity against *Capnocytophaga*. Penicillin, ampicillin, amoxicillin, and first- and second-generation cephalosporins have variable activity against these organisms. β-Lactamase production has been reported in as many as 32% of strains.[83] In general, *Capnocytophaga* organisms are resistant to aztreonam, aminoglycosides, vancomycin, trimethoprim, and polymyxin B. Resistance may be plasmid mediated. Special media are usually required to assess in vitro susceptibility. Susceptibility testing using the E-test showed good agreement with results using agar dilution[84] and may provide an easier method for testing antimicrobial susceptibility of *Capnocytophaga* strains.

CAPNOCYTOPHAGA CANIMORSUS (FORMERLY GROUP DF-2)

In 1976, the first case report of a "previously undescribed Gram negative bacillus causing septicemia and meningitis" was published. This was followed by further reports and reviews of similar cases, and the gram-negative bacilli were classified as CDC group DF-2. Later, on the basis of DNA hybridization studies, DF-2 was classified as a new species, *C. canimorsus*, and DF-2–like organisms as *C. cynodegmi*.[42]

Both species are long filamentous gram-negative rods, often curved, that grow slowly on blood or chocolate agar and not on MacConkey agar. Optimal growth is on brain-heart infusion agar supplemented with 5% rabbit or sheep blood incubated at 37°C in a candle extinction jar (carbon dioxide present). Neither species has flagella, but both exhibit gliding motility. As opposed to the other *Capnocytophaga* species, *C. canimorsus* and *C. cynodegmi* are oxidase- and catalase-positive. Both species are indole-negative and reduce nitrates and show variable reduction of nitrites. They all differ from each other in the pattern of sugar fermentation; however, they all ferment glucose.[4, 42]

Virulence factors are not well defined. *C. canimorsus* is thought to have low virulence as it has been demonstrated to be serum sensitive and immunocompromised hosts are more commonly affected. Studies evaluating the humoral aspects of DF-2 infection suggested that the early response may be immunoglobulin G mediated as the immunoglobulin M response does not occur or thus far has not been observed.[85]

Sources of *C. canimorsus* in nature include oral flora of dogs and cats.[86] Clinical isolates have included blood and cerebrospinal fluid most frequently but also wounds from dog bites and cat scratches, heart valve, petechiae, adrenal gland, and cornea (DF-2–like organism).[42] Of note is that a false-positive cryptococcal latex agglutination result was obtained from the cerebrospinal fluid of an immunocompetent patient with septicemia caused by DF-2. Blood and cerebrospinal fluid cultures were positive and the cerebrospinal fluid Gram stain, white cell differential, and biochemistry values were negative.[87]

Infection with *C. cynodegmi* has been reported only in wound infections after dog bites or cat scratches; however, *C. canimorsus* has been reported with similar exposure or as a severe systemic infection, without known exposure, particularly in splenectomized individuals.[42] In 1977, Butler and coworkers[88] described 17 patients with systemic infection, 13 with bacteremia, 3 with meningitis, and 1 with both. Hicklin and coworkers[85] reviewed 41 cases reported in the English literature by 1987 (including Butler and coworkers' cases). Of these 41 cases, 34 had either septicemia or bacteremia, 4 had meningitis, and 3 had both presentations. Other clinical manifestations included endocarditis, renal failure, disseminated intravascular coagulation, adrenal hemorrhage (Waterhouse-Friderichsen syndrome), rash[87] (urticarial, petechial, macular), joint effusion and arthritis, cellulitis, pneumonia, empyema,[89] and mononeuropathy.[90] Predisposing factors to infection include splenectomy for any reason (35%), alcohol abuse (35%), and evidence for immune dysfunction (steroids, hematologic malignancies, autoimmune disease) (17%). Four patients had no known predisposing factors for infection. More than 75% of cases involved previous exposure to a dog either through ownership or direct bite.

In 50% of splenectomized patients, the clinical course was fulminant, that is, hypotension, renal failure, disseminated intravascular coagulation, gangrene, pulmonary infiltrates, and death. Gram stain of the buffy coat demonstrated the organism in all splenectomized patients examined and may prove helpful in early diagnosis. The overall mortality rate was 27% in these 41 cases.[85]

Antimicrobial susceptibility studies in vitro must utilize appropriate techniques for fastidious organisms. For *Capnocytophaga* isolates, longer incubation times and carbon dioxide are required for optimal growth. Broth dilution techniques in a carbon dioxide–enriched atmosphere are desirable. On this basis, Verghese and coworkers[91] examined eight clinical isolates. With the exception of aztreonam, all eight isolates were sensitive to penicillin, piperacillin, imipenem, erythromycin, vancomycin, clindamycin, third-generation cephalosporins, gentamicin, amikacin, chloramphenicol, rifampin, trimethoprim-sulfamethoxazole, and ciprofloxacin. Previous studies[82, 87] using disk diffusion or agar dilution assays have demonstrated resistance to aminoglycosides.

An organism thought to be closely related to *Capnocytophaga* is CDC DF-3. It is a facultatively anaerobic gram-negative coccobacillus that does not grow on MacConkey, *Salmonella-Shigella*, xylose-lysine-deoxycholate agars or most *Campylobacter* media incubated at 42°C[92] and thus is not detected on routine stool culture. It grows well on blood agar, chocolate agar, and cefoperazone-vancomycin–amphotericin B agar incubated at 35°C within 48 to 72 hours. Colonies are usually nonhemolytic and have a unique fruity odor. This organism is catalase- and oxidase-negative, like the DF-1 organisms, but can be distinguished by being indole-positive and fermenting different sugars. The presence of 12-methyltetradecanoate in cell wall fatty acid analysis assists in identification.[93]

DF-3 has been isolated from multiple sites,[94] the most frequent being stools, blood, and wounds. It has been isolated from asymptomatic persons and is rarely pathogenic. The most common clinical presentation is chronic diarrhea, which is usually not bloody and not accompanied by fever. It has also been reported to cause bacteremia with sepsis,[95] urinary tract infection,[96] and abscess.[97] The majority of those infected are immunocompromised (malignancy, human immunodeficiency virus infection, common variable hypogammaglobulinemia, corticosteroid therapy) or have chronic illness (diabetes mellitus, cirrhosis).

Most strains of DF-3 are susceptible to clindamycin, trimethoprim-sulfamethoxazole, tetracycline, and chloramphenicol. They are variably susceptible to erythromycin and imipenem but are generally resistant to penicillin, ampicillin, cephalosporins, aminoglycosides, ciprofloxacin, aztreonam, and vancomycin. Patients with diarrhea usually show clinical improvement within a few days to a week into a 2-week course of antibiotics. Of note, in human immunodeficiency virus–infected patients with diarrhea believed to be due to DF-3, therapy has been associated with clinical improvement and clearance of infection maintained months after therapy was discontinued.

Cardiobacterium

The only species in the genus *Cardiobacterium* is *C. hominis*. It is a gram-negative rod occurring in pleomorphic form including rosette clusters, teardrops, and enlargement of one or both ends. Retention of crystal violet may occur, resulting in a gram-positive appearance. Biochemically, *C. hominis* is oxidase-positive, catalase-negative, and nitrate reduction–negative. It forms indole in small amounts, a major identifying characteristic, but usually after 24 to 48 hours and extraction with xylene. *C. hominis* ferments glucose to lactic acid and oxidizes a variety of other sugars. It is nonmotile and requires 5% to 10% carbon dioxide for growth. On blood agar after 48 hours, colonies are 1 to 2 mm, circular, convex, smooth, and moist without hemolysis. It does not grow well aerobically, unless air is humidified, or anaerobically, accounting for its fastidious nature. Cultures must be held for 2 to 3 weeks.[5, 98]

Virulence properties of *C. hominis* have not been documented. The organisms do not produce exotoxins or cause disease in laboratory animals.[5] There are both antigenic similarity and heterogeneity between strains. *C. hominis* has been isolated from normal nasal and pharyngeal flora of 68% of humans as well as cervical and vaginal cultures. *C. hominis* has *not* been isolated from animals, soil, water, or hospital equipment.[3–5]

Clinical isolates have been obtained from blood, cerebrospinal fluid, and valve tissue.[99] The major clinical syndromes are subacute endocarditis and late prosthetic valve endocarditis, including endocarditis after endoscopic procedures.[100] One case each of meningitis[101] and mycotic aneurysm,[102] probably secondary to endocarditis, has been described. The best estimate of prevalence of *C. hominis* infective endocarditis is 0.1% of all cases of endocarditis.[103] To date, fewer than 50 cases of *C. hominis* endocarditis have been reported in the literature.[99, 104–107] The course is generally insidious (mean duration of symptoms is 169 days), with many of the classic features of subacute bacterial endocarditis (fever, splenomegaly, petechiae, anemia, elevated erythrocyte sedimentation rate, hematuria) occurring in more than 40% of the cases. Seventy-five percent of the cases occur in patients with abnormal valves. Emboli and congestive heart failure occur in 44% of cases. The mitral and aortic valves most often are affected. A high proportion (87%) of patients can be cured, most (70%) with antimicrobial therapy alone.[105, 108, 109] Bacteremia without endocarditis has been reported in a patient with an abdominal abscess caused by *C. hominis* and *Clostridium bifermentans*.[110]

C. hominis is generally quite sensitive to penicillin and ampicillin, as well as cephalothin, chloramphenicol, tetracycline, and aminoglycosides. Susceptibility to vancomycin and erythromycin is variable. Results of tests in vitro are difficult to interpret, given the slow-growing nature of the organism. Most cases have been treated with either penicillin or ampicillin, with or without an aminoglycoside for bacteriologic and clinical cure. Second- and third-generation cephalosporins also have excellent activity in vitro and have been used clinically.[111] Endocarditis successfully treated with ciprofloxacin has been reported.[112]

Chromobacterium

Chromobacterium violaceum is the type species for the genus *Chromobacterium*. It is the only known pathogenic member of the genus and the only violet-colored pathogenic bacterium.[113] Other names have included *Bacillus violaceous* and *Chromobacterium janthinum*. *Chromobacterium lividum* is a nonpathogenic species that can be differentiated by its lack of violet color and growth at 4°C but not at 37°C.[3, 4, 114] *Chromobacterium typhiflavium* is now classified as CDC group Ve-1, which may soon be grouped as a *Pseudomonas* species.[115]

C. violaceum is a gram-negative, sometimes slightly curved, rod, facultatively anaerobic, that produces a violet-colored tryptophan metabolite (violacein) that is insoluble in water. The pigment is not produced when the organism is grown anaerobically, and not all strains produce the pigment. The organisms grow within 24 hours on conventional media (blood and MacConkey agar) and media containing tryptophan. *C. violaceum* organisms are motile with both polar and lateral flagella (antigenically distinct). They are usually oxidase-positive, but the pigment may interfere with the reading and they can be confused with *Aeromonas* species. They are catalase-positive, are generally indole-negative, and reduce nitrates and nitrites. They ferment glucose to acid, sometimes produce gas (20%), and produce hydrogen cyanide. *C. violaceum* organisms also produce substances that are inhibitory to gram-positive and some gram-negative bacteria. Two such agents that have antibacterial properties, aerocavin[116] and aerocyanidin,[117] have been described.

Virulence properties include production of a biologically active endotoxin, chromosomally mediated β-lactamase,[113] and possibly an extracellular slime layer. A report comparing a virulent clinical isolate and an avirulent soil isolate demonstrated greater superoxide dismutase and catalase production from the virulent isolate.[118] There is evidence that humans with neutrophil defects may be more susceptible to infections with *C. violaceum*.

Chromobacterium is generally found in the environment; sources include soil, freshwater, stagnant water, and food (refrigerated food grows only *C. lividum*).[119, 120] Because *C. violaceum* grows optimally at 20°C to 37°C, most infections have been documented in tropical or subtropical climates between the latitudes 35 degrees north and 35 degrees south. In the United States, most infections are reported from Florida and Louisiana between the months of June and September,[121] although one case has been reported from Ohio (after exposure in New England)[122] and one case (in Florida)[123] during January.

C. violaceum is an uncommon to rare cause of infection in that fewer than 40 cases have been reported in the world literature.[124] Clinical isolates have included visceral and skin abscesses, blood, cerebrospinal fluid, brain, eye and ear specimens, urine, feces, sputum, throat, bone, and joint fluid.[113, 121] Clinically, the portal of entry of *C. violaceum* is thought to be a break in the skin, although ingestion of contaminated food or water may also play a role because it has been isolated from feces when near-drowning[125] has been the only source of exposure.

Typically, the infection begins around a break in the skin followed by local cellulitis, regional or diffuse lymphadenitis, and then hematologic dissemination. Septicemia, acute respiratory distress syndrome, disseminated intravascular coagulation, and multiorgan system failure subsequently occur. Multiple liver abscesses develop and can be seen by hepatic imaging. The mortality rate is 60% to 70% and is probably related to underlying disease (e.g., neutrophil defects), appropriateness of antibiotic therapy, and accuracy of diagnosis. Autopsy specimens have frequently demonstrated multiple liver, lung, and spleen abscesses. Other clinical presentations besides septicemia include fever, cutaneous[126, 127] lesions (minor abrasions, rashes, cellulitis), lymphadenitis, abdominal pain, osteomyelitis, arthritis, meningitis,[128, 129] ocular infections[130, 131] (necrotizing conjunctivitis, periorbital cellulitis), and pneumonia.[121, 123–125]

Multiple reports suggest an association with chronic granulomatous disease and *C. violaceum* infection.[121, 122, 126, 130, 132] Most patients with overwhelming infection are younger than 28 years. *C. violaceum* infection in patients with other neutrophil defects such as glucose-6-phosphate dehydrogenase deficiency[133] of the polymorphonuclear leukocyte (and red blood cell) and leukemia[127, 134] has been described. Normal hosts with overwhelming exposure (near-drowning) and minimal exposure (barefoot in mud) have been described; however, formal leukocyte testing has not been performed in these cases.[125]

C. violaceum is generally quite susceptible to chloramphenicol, gentamicin, and tetracycline. It is uniformly resistant to cephalosporins and is generally resistant to most penicillins. It has variable sensitivity to some of the carboxy- and ureidopenicillins.[113, 121, 134] Treatment failure and relapse have occurred with the use of erythromycin.[122] Trimethoprim-sulfamethoxazole has been used successfully as outpatient therapy after prolonged (4 week) intravenous therapy with other agents.[113, 123, 135]

Glucose Nonfermenters

Acinetobacter

The first descriptions of *Acinetobacter* species were made by DeBord in 1939 when he isolated gram-negative coccobacilli from urethral specimens.[136] The classification has changed frequently during the past 50 years. *Acinetobacter* is a member of the family Neisseriaceae and according to *Bergey's Manual of Systematic Bacteriology*[137] has only one species, *Acinetobacter calcoaceticus. Acinetobacter* derives from the Greek for nonmotile rod and *calcoaceticus* (from Latin) for its ability to use calcium acetate as a carbon source. Previously, the most common isolates involved in human disease included *A. calcoaceticus* var. *anitratus* (formerly *Herellea vaginicola, Bacterium anitratum, Achromobacter anitratum, Micrococcus calcoaceticus*), which oxidizes carbohydrates to acid, and *A. calcoaceticus* var. *lwoffi* (formerly *Mima polymorpha* var. *nonoxidans, Moraxella lwoffi*, B5W organism), which does not form acid. Subsequently, four major biotypes of *Acinetobacter* were described: *A. calcoaceticus* var. *anitratus* and var. *hemolyticus* both oxidize glucose to acid, whereas var. *lwoffi* and var. *alcaligenes* do not. *A. calcoaceticus* var. *anitratus* and var. *lwoffi* are not hemolytic, whereas var. *haemolyticus* and var. *alcaligenes* are.

The taxonomy of *Acinetobacter* has been evolving during the past several years. It was redefined by Bouvet and Grimont[138] in 1986 on the basis of DNA hybridization techniques in which they have distinguished 17 genospecies of *Acinetobacter*, including *A. calcoaceticus, Acinetobacter baumannii, Acinetobacter haemolyticus, Acinetobacter junii, Acinetobacter johnsonii, Acinetobacter lwoffi, Acinetobacter radioresistens,* and 10 undesignated species.[3, 139–141] These are the currently accepted taxonomic definitions. Because *A. calcoaceticus, A. baumannii,* and DNA groups 3 and 13 are genotypically and phenotypically similar, they are often referred to as *A. calcoaceticus-baumannii* complex.[140, 141] Speciation versus subspeciation may not be clinically relevant to the individual patient; however, it may be useful in epidemiologic investigations of outbreaks.

Acinetobacter is a gram-negative rod, predominantly coccobacillary or diplococcoid.[137, 142, 143] It looks more rodlike in the exponential phase of growth and more coccoid in the stationary phase, which makes it easily confused with *Neisseria* and *Haemophilus* on Gram stain. *Acinetobacter* may also be difficult to decolorize on Gram stain, hence appearing gram-positive. It is nonmotile but may exhibit twitching motility as a result of polar fimbriae. *Acinetobacter* organisms are oxidase-negative, catalase-positive, and indole-negative and do not reduce nitrates. Some strains may be encapsulated. Capsules consist of a polysaccharide and, at least from one strain, have cross-reacted with antisera made to group B and G streptococci and pneumococcus. Some strains cross-react with antichlamydial antibodies.[144, 145] More than 28 serotypes of the acid-forming strains have been described.

Acinetobacter organisms grow well on complex media and selective media including MacConkey agar. They grow aerobically and produce gray-white colonies 2 to 3 mm in diameter after 18 to 24 hours at 33°C to 35°C.[142] *Acinetobacter* species differ from Enterobacteriaceae in that they cannot grow anaerobically or reduce nitrates. They are distinguished from *Neisseria* and *Moraxella* in their reaction to the oxidase test.[137]

Acinetobacter is thought to have a low potential for virulence. Most infections are nosocomial and occur in severely ill patients who have had previous antibiotics, surgery, trauma, or instrumentation. Potential virulence factors include a polysaccharide capsule, which may prevent phagocytosis, fimbriae that potentiate adherence to epithelial cells, and a lipopolysaccharide known to be biologically active.[143] In addition, human serum resistance is more common among *A. anitratus* than *A. lwoffi* strains.[146]

Acinetobacter is widely distributed in the environment. It is found in soil, food,[147] water,[121] and sewage[137] and has been transmitted by contact with these sources. Infections in foundry workers[148] and others[149, 150] have suggested airborne transmission. Chickens,[151] septic hens,[152, 153] rubber and stainless steel milk pipelines,[154] and bottled uncarbonated mineral drinking water[155] have also been sources in nature. Typically, moist environments including hospital equipment such as ventilator tubing and resuscitation bags,[156] peak flowmeters,[157] humidifiers,[158] sinks,[159] mist tents,[160] dialysis baths[161] and dialysis hardware (O-rings),[162] duodenoscopes,[163] angiography catheters,[164] intravenous catheters,[165] pressure transducers,[166] caloric testing water tanks,[167] and latex gloves[168] or pharmacologic solutions such as plasma protein solutions,[169] intravenous anesthetics,[170] and enteral feeding solutions[171] contain this organism or have been associated with outbreaks. It is found on the skin of many animal species and humans, usually as a commensal organism. From 2% to 25% of humans carry it on their skin,[172, 173] including the hands of hospital personnel.[174] It is also found as part of normal oral flora (up to 7% of healthy people carry it)[172] and in the upper respiratory tract, genitourinary tract, and lower gastrointestinal tract. *Acinetobacter* has been isolated from tracheostomy sites in adults, sputum, urine, feces,[175] vaginal secretions, saliva, conjunctiva,[172] frozen human milk,[176] wound sites, and blood.[177–179] It has been identified in the pharyngeal flora of normal healthy infants[180] older than 1 week as one of the five most common gram-negative rods isolated.

Acinetobacter accounted for 0.6% of all nosocomial infections reported to the CDC by participating hospitals in 1984[181] and 1% in 1990 to 1992.[182] The prevalence may have regional or institutional variation because some studies have reported 1.4% of hospital-acquired infections (Seattle)[183] and 2% of bacteremias (Denver).[178] In the 1990 to 1992 National Nosocomial Infections Surveillance data, 2% of blood stream infections and 4% of nosocomial pneumonia cases were due to *Acinetobacter*.[182] Inexplicably, a seasonal peak incidence in the late summer has also been noted.[184]

Predisposing factors include debilitating conditions (e.g., alcoholism, advanced age, chronic disease, acute and severe illness), major surgery, major trauma and burn injury, previous antibiotic therapy, intensive care unit stay, and prior instrumentation in the hospital.[136] These procedures include endotracheal tube intubation, tracheostomy, urinary tract catheterization, peripheral and central intravenous catheter placement, and chest tube insertion.

Acinetobacter infections have been reported for almost all organ systems. It is usually an opportunistic pathogen as evidenced by the fact that 14% to 62% of infections are mixed infections.[136, 174, 181] The most common sites involved are the respiratory and urinary tracts. The mortality rate can be up to 36% depending on the site and the presence of factors indicating poor prognosis such as polymicrobial sepsis and shock.

Nosocomial infections include septicemia in adults[136, 174, 185, 186] and neonates,[187] which can be associated with vascular catheters,[188] oral or nasopharyngeal intubation,[189] or transhepatic cholangiography,[190] and endocarditis, including prosthetic valve endocarditis.[191] Meningitis, often associated with neurosurgical procedures,[192–194] and brain abscesses have been reported. Respiratory tract infections include pneumonia, usually multilobar, occasionally with associated pleural effusion, cavity formation, and rarely bronchopulmonary fistula[136] and are associated with increased morbidity and mortality rates compared with those for other gram-negative organisms.[195] Pneumonia may be chronic.[196] Empyema, lung abscess, and tracheobronchitis have also been reported. Upper and lower urinary tract infections occur, upper tract infections being associated with renal calculi. Wound infections, cellulitis, skin abscess, phlebitis, an infected abdominal aortic aneurysm,[197] and intraabdominal abscess have been described. Peritonitis associated with continuous ambulatory peritoneal dialysis has also been reported and can be successfully treated with intraperitoneal, intravenous, or oral antibiotics often without removal of the catheter.[198–201] Musculoskeletal infections including pyarthrosis and osteomyelitis[202] may occur. Conjunctivitis, exposure keratitis,[203] endophthalmitis[204] and corneal ulcer[205] secondary to trauma, and blepharitis[206] have been reported.

Community-acquired infections with *Acinetobacter* are not uncommon. Pneumonia has been reported infrequently in the United States (Texas,[173] foundry workers in Connecticut,[148] Chicago[207]) and in Papua New Guinea[208] and Australia.[209] The community-acquired pneumonia tends to be more fulminant, associated with bacteremia and higher mortality rate (43%).[173] Predisposing factors in patients include chronic pulmonary disease, cigarette smoking, alcohol abuse, diabetes mellitus, and non-Hodgkin's lymphoma. Community-acquired meningitis[210] is rarely reported. Native valve endocarditis[211] can be more aggressive than prosthetic valve endocarditis in this setting. Long-term indwelling tunneled catheters used for home intravenous therapy have also been associated with *Acinetobacter* infections.[212] *Acinetobacter* infection has been reported after a dog bite.[213]

Acinetobacter organisms are commonly multidrug-resistant organisms,[214, 215] and isolated pathogens must be evaluated for specific sensitivity patterns within each hospital. They are generally resistant to penicillin, ampicillin, most first- and second-generation cephalosporins, gentamicin, chloramphenicol, and nalidixic acid.[143, 216, 217] They are variably resistant to tetracycline, tobramycin, kanamycin, ureidopenicillins, and aztreonam. Most strains are still sensitive to imipenem, ceftazidime, cefotaxime, amikacin, trimethoprim-sulfamethoxazole,[218] and minocycline. Imipenem is the most reliable agent against *Acinetobacter*; however, imipenem-resistant strains have been reported. In those cases, the addition of sulbactam in vitro killed the *Acinetobacter* and treating the patients with ampicillin-sulbactam resulted in clinical improvement in 9 of 10 cases.[219] The new quinolones, including ciprofloxacin, ofloxacin, pefloxacin, and enoxacin,[220,221] are effective against *Acinetobacter,* although resistance has been reported.

Antibacterial resistance is greater among *A. baumannii* strains than among other *Acinetobacter* species. In a review of antimicrobial susceptibility testing by *Acinetobacter* species,[222] *A. baumannii* biotype 9 was resistant to all antibiotics except imipenem and amoxicillin-clavulanate (>90% susceptible at National Committee for Clinical Laboratory Standards [NCCLS] breakpoints), and *A. baumannii* biotype 6 was sensitive to amoxicillin-clavulanate, cefotaxime, ceftazidime, ceftriaxone, imipenem, amikacin, tobramycin, and ciprofloxacin (>90% susceptible at NCCLS breakpoints). Other *Acinetobacter* species showed sensitivity patterns similar to those of biotype 6 but with more susceptibility to the expanded-spectrum penicillins. Newer antibiotics, biapenem, piperacillin-tazobactam, cefpirome, and cefepime, were all active against *A. baumannii* in in vitro studies against 149 clinical isolates from hospitalized patients in Toronto, Canada.[223] Similar results have been seen with meropenem.[224]

Many mechanisms of resistance to antibiotics have been reported for *Acinetobacter.* Resistance to β-lactam antibiotics (including resistance to imipenem) is mediated by altered penicillin binding proteins,[225, 226] reduced outer membrane permeability,[225, 227] and both constitutive and plasmid-mediated β-lactamases.[228, 229] *Acinetobacter* exhibits high-level resistance to aminoglycosides by producing acetylating and phosphorylating enzymes to inactivate these agents.[228, 229] The particular chromosomal resistance gene against amikacin may be species specific.[230, 231]

Depending on the severity of infection and the sensitivities of the clinical isolate, conservative therapy dictates combination therapy for *Acinetobacter* infections, for example, imipenem or a third-generation cephalosporin with or without amikacin. For imipenem-resistant strains, ampicillin-sulbactam and piperacillin-tazobactam may be better alternatives.

Alcaligenes

The taxonomy of the *Alcaligenes* genus is controversial. The clinically relevant species include *Alcaligenes faecalis, Alcaligenes denitrificans* (subsp. *denitrificans* and subsp. *xylosoxidans*), *Alcaligenes odorans*, and a newly described species, *Alcaligenes piechaudii. Bergey's Manual of Systematic Bacteriology* lists *A. faecalis* and *A. odorans* as members of the same species. Two subspecies under the species *A. denitrificans* are, as just listed, in *Bergey's Manual of Systematic Bacteriology*[232]; however, the CDC has recognized *A. dentrificans* subsp. *xylosoxidans* as its own species, *Achromobacter xylosoxidans* (see the next section).[142] Species differentiation occurs on the basis of ability to grow with 6% NaCl, reduce nitrates, and use carbohydrates.

The name *Alcaligenes* means alkali-producing bacteria. Organisms are gram-negative rods or cocci on Gram stain and are motile with peritrichous flagella, and most are obligately aerobic (i.e., *A. faecalis).* Some strains grow anaerobically, reducing nitrate or nitrite to nitrogen gas (i.e., *A. denitrificans). Alcaligenes* are oxidase- and catalase-positive and indole-negative. They grow utilizing a variety of organic acids, including amino acids, but generally not carbohydrates, for energy. Strains grow on blood and selective media (MacConkey). Virulence factors include production of bacteriocins and resistance via β-lactamase production.[142, 232]

Sources of *Alcaligenes* include soil and water[121] as well as part of normal human flora, especially the skin and gastrointestinal tract. Dairy products and rotten eggs have been sources for *Alcaligenes.* Clinical isolates include blood, sputum, urine, feces, chronic ear discharge, material from wounds, cerebrospinal fluid, pleural fluid, eye and throat swabs, and bronchial washings. Isolation is not always associated with infections, especially respiratory and urinary isolates. *Alcaligenes* have been isolated from hospital equipment including respirators, hemodialysis systems, intravenous solution, and disinfectants.[233]

Clinically important infections are found in patients with severe underlying illnesses. *A. faecalis* isolated from the urine is often considered to be a contaminant. Blood isolates from patients with septicemia are thought to be associated with contaminated hospital equipment, although blood isolates have also been obtained from patients without clinical evidence of sepsis. Clinical syndromes are varied,[233] including endocarditis (late prosthetic valve endocarditis[108] and native valve endocarditis[234]), meningitis,[235] chronic purulent otitis,[236] meibomianitis,[237] corneal ulcer,[238] pyelonephritis, hepatitis, appendicitis, and diarrhea. Many infections are mixed with other flora.

Alcaligenes organisms are generally susceptible to trimethoprim-sulfamethoxazole and chloramphenicol. Sensitivity to β-lactams and aminoglycosides is variable; however, *A. faecalis* is more likely to be sensitive to these than are the other species. Greater resistance is seen in the hospital setting especially with *A. denitrificans* subsp. *denitrificans* and *A. xylosoxidans* subsp. *xylosoxidans.* Piperacillin and ciprofloxacin may be reasonable alternatives.[220, 239–241]

Achromobacter

Achromobacter (*Alcaligenes xylosoxidans* subsp. *xylosoxidans*) taxonomy remains controversial. The CDC and most clinical microbiologists recognized it as its own genus; however, it is classified as *A. denitrificans* biotype *xylosoxidans* in

Bergey's Manual of Systematic Bacteriology.[232] It differs from *Alcaligenes* (see preceding section) by its ability to reduce nitrate to nitrite and grow anaerobically in the presence of nitrate. Yabuuchi and Yano[242] published a revised classification in 1981 of *Achromobacter* as its own genus. The CDC recognized two species of *Achromobacter*: *A. xylosoxidans* and CDC group Vd.[142] Currently, *Achromobacter xylosoxidans* is classified in the *Alcaligenes* genus as *A. xylosoxidans* subsp. *xylosoxidans* and *Achromobacter* sp. group Vd is *Ochrobactrum anthropi*.[3]

Achromobacter organisms are gram-negative rods that are oxidase- and catalase-positive, exhibit motility related to peritrichous flagella, and do not produce indole. They can be easily confused with *Pseudomonas* species unless a stain for flagella is done. They can grow in the presence of a variety of sugars including glucose, xylose, and gluconate, whereas other *Alcaligenes* do not. Colonies grow well on blood and MacConkey agar.

Achromobacter is found widely distributed in nature, including soil and water[121] (swimming pools, well water).[243] It may be part of the normal flora of the lower gastrointestinal tract. *Achromobacter* has been isolated from pharyngeal swabs, sputum, skin, feces, and vaginal secretions. Clinical isolates include blood, urine, wounds, abscesses, orbital swabs, purulent ear discharge, cerebrospinal fluid and brain tissue, and pleural and peritoneal fluids.[137, 232, 244, 245] The organisms have been found as contaminants in disinfectants (chlorhexidine),[245] diagnostic tracer solution[246] (presumably in nonbacteriostatic saline), intravenous computed tomography contrast solution,[247] and hemodialysis solutions. *Achromobacter* has been isolated from hospital equipment[245] including ventilators, humidifiers, and pressure transducers[248] and hand-washing machines.[249]

Yabuuchi and Oyama[250] first described *A. xylosoxidans* in 1971 from the purulent discharge from the ears of seven patients with chronic otitis media. Subsequently, it has been reported as an uncommon causative agent in a variety of nosocomial and community-acquired infections. Community-acquired infections include a case of bacteremia in a 79-year-old woman with metastatic breast cancer in whom the only identifiable source was well water that she had ingested.[243] A second case resulted in meningitis in a young male after a gunshot wound to the chest,[251] presumably the source of contamination. This patient underwent spinal surgery within 24 hours of hospital admission and did not develop meningitis until 2 weeks into the hospital course, however. In other reports of *Achromobacter* meningitis, almost all cases were related to previous neurosurgical manipulation.[252, 253] Maternal-fetal transmission has been reported in a case of a mother with chorioamnionitis and neonate with fatal meningitis caused by *A. xylosoxidans*.[254]

Achromobacter has been described in nosocomial outbreaks.[245, 255] Clinical presentations include meningitis,[256, 257] ventriculitis (related to neurosurgical procedures), septicemia and bacteremia[258–261] (including prosthetic valve endocarditis and catheter-associated infections), pseudobacteremia,[262] otitis, endophthalmitis,[263] corneal ulcer,[264] keratitis,[265] pharyngitis, pneumonia,[244] wounds (skin, burns, ulcers), peritonitis, urinary tract infection, arthritis (native[266, 267] and prosthetic[268] joint), osteomyelitis,[269–271] and abscesses (lung,[272] skin). Mandell and coworkers[244] have reviewed cases of bacteremia with *A. xylosoxidans* and described the major predisposing factor as severe underlying disease. The mortality rate was approximately 52% in the seven well-documented cases of bacteremia.

A. xylosoxidans is generally resistant to penicillin, ampicillin, first- and second-generation cephalosporins, and aminoglycosides. Resistance may occur via β-lactamases and either plasmid-mediated[255] or constitutively expressed cephalosporinases or penicillinases.[239, 257, 273] Trimethoprim-sulfamethoxazole, chloramphenicol, tetracycline, and the new quinolones exhibit variable activity[239]; however, trimethoprim-sulfamethoxazole is active for most strains.[239, 241, 273] Imipenem was the most consistently active agent in vitro against 37 clinical isolates.[274] Piperacillin, carbenicillin, ticarcillin-clavulanate, and ceftazidime were active against at least 50% of strains. Clinical isolates should be tested for their sensitivity to these antibiotics. For severe infections, more than one drug may be necessary; however, synergistic combination therapy has not been established.

Ochrobactrum anthropi

O. anthropi (formerly CDC group Vd) is another organism previously included under the genus *Achromobacter*.[275] In contrast to *A. xylosoxidans*, *O. anthropi* is urease-positive, does not utilize the same carbon sources, and does not grow on cetrimide agar.[121, 232, 276] *O. anthropi* is also oxidase-positive, non–lactose fermenting, and motile by peritrichous flagella. *Ochrobactrum* is gram-negative, although it can stain gram-positive even after the agar or broth is boiled.[277]

Ochrobactrum has been isolated from blood, wounds, stool, urine, throat, and vaginal secretions. It has also been isolated from the hospital environment. In general, infections are rare; however, the most common clinical presentation is bacteremia associated with a central venous catheter.[278–284] It has caused an outbreak of bacteremia in organ transplant patients associated with contaminated vials of rabbit antithymocyte globulin.[285] Another outbreak of meningitis was reported in children receiving pericardial allograft transplant tissue for dural defect repair.[285a] Other reported cases include pancreatic abscess,[286] osteochondritis of the foot secondary to a puncture wound,[287] wound infection and cellulitis,[288] empyema,[288] and a case of necrotizing fasciitis in which the tissue grew group G streptococci but blood cultures grew *Ochrobactrum*.[289] The majority of the patients are immunocompromised (resulting from malignancy) or receiving immunosuppressive therapy.

Ochrobactrum is typically resistant to the penicillins, cephalosporins, aztreonam, and chloramphenicol. The drugs most frequently active are ciprofloxacin, trimethoprim-sulfamethoxazole, imipenem, and amikacin.[278–284] Therapy should be guided by in vitro susceptibility testing, although there have been reports of treatment failure using drugs active in vitro,[278] and likewise, clinical response with inactive drugs based on susceptibility tests.[279] The recommendations are contradictory regarding the removal of central venous catheters. Catheter removal may be necessary only for patients not responding to antimicrobial therapy alone.

Eikenella

E. corrodens is a gram-negative, pleomorphic coccobacillus that, after 48 to 72 hours, has the characteristic colonial morphology of "corroding" or pitting the agar surface on which it is grown. It was formerly known as bacillus HB-1 of King and *Bacteroides corrodens*. The genus was established in 1972 by Jackson and Goodman,[290] who differentiated the genus from *Bacteroides ureolyticus* by genetic analysis and growth characteristics. *E. corrodens* is a facultative anaerobe, whereas *B. ureolyticus* is an obligate anaerobe. *Eikenella* is nonmotile but exhibits twitching motility on agar. About half of the strains corrode; those that do not also do not exhibit twitching motility. There is a characteristic musty odor on agar similar to "hypochlorite bleach, crackers, or musty mouse cages."[291] It is often grown from mixed cultures but can easily be overgrown. Clindamycin disks on media can be used to select for *E. corrodens* because it is resistant to this drug. Aerobic, but not anaerobic, growth requires the presence of hemin (blood or chocolate agar); 3% to 10% carbon dioxide also enhances growth. It does not grow on MacConkey agar. It is oxidase-positive and catalase-, indole-, and urease-negative. It reduces nitrate to nitrite and does not utilize carbohydrate as a carbon source.[137, 290, 291] A species-specific DNA probe has been used to detect *E. corrodens* in advanced periodontitis[292] and may provide an alternative means of diagnosis.

Virulence properties include a slime layer that may be immunosuppressive and a biologically active lipopolysaccharide. A number of hydrolytic enzymes, particularly proline aminopeptidase and a thiol-dependent hemolysin, may also be important virulence factors.[293] Isolation of *E. corrodens* has been associated with mixed infections with α-hemolytic or nonhemolytic streptococci and Enterobacteriaceae as well as *Actinomyces* infection, although pure cultures have been obtained. These other organisms may enhance the virulence of *E. corrodens*.[137, 290, 291]

E. corrodens is found in normal human oral flora, dental plaques, and gastrointestinal and genitourinary flora. It may be an opportunistic pathogen in that breaks in the mucosal surface or trauma contaminated by oral flora may lead to hematogenous dissemination. Treatment with inappropriate antibiotics may select for *E. corrodens* growth. It is well documented that drug abusers who use methylphenidate have subcutaneous abscesses with *E. corrodens* near the site of injection, probably from chewing the tablets before injection.[294]

Clinical manifestations are varied but most often are associated with a history of abnormal exposure to oral flora contamination, for example, human bites, dental extractions, trauma. In a review by Stoloff and Gillies,[295] 22 of 33 infections with *E. corrodens* occurring in an 18-month period were related to human bites, fist fights, or trauma. These included face or hand abscesses, septic arthritis, and osteomyelitis. Other infections, either pure or mixed, involving *E. corrodens* include abscess formation (cellulitis,[296] tooth, wound,[297] brain,[298, 299] liver, spleen,[300] appendix,[295] intraabdominal,[301, 302] Brodie abscess,[303] intervertebral diskitis[304]), intrathoracic infections[305] (empyema,[306, 307] pneumonia,[308–310] lung abscess,[311] mediastinitis and pericarditis[312]), head and neck infections (dacryocystitis, conjunctivitis, keratitis,[313] orbital cellulitis,[314] canaliculitis,[315] otitis externa, gingivitis,[53, 316] parotitis,[317] thyroiditis,[318] and thyroid abscess[319, 320]), meningitis and subdural empyema,[294] and obstetric and gynecologic infections (chorioamnionitis,[321] endometritis associated with an intrauterine device,[322] and Bartholin abscess[323]). Cardiovascular involvement has been described including endocarditis[16, 108, 234, 324, 325] (native and prosthetic valve), mycotic aneurysm,[326] intravascular space infections,[325] and septic pulmonary emboli from internal jugular vein phlebitis.[327]

E. corrodens is generally susceptible to penicillin, ampicillin, carbenicillin, ticarcillin, piperacillin, mezlocillin, second- and third-generation cephalosporins, chloramphenicol, and the quinolones.[328–330] *E. corrodens* is variably sensitive to tetracycline and rifampin[331] and uniformly resistant to clindamycin and metronidazole.[295] Aminoglycosides and vancomycin are relatively inactive, as are first-generation cephalosporins and isoxazolyl penicillins.[328–330] β-Lactamase production[301] and tetracycline resistance[331] have been reported.

In the review by Stoloff and Gillies,[295] 25 of 32 strains were resistant to penicillin as tested by the disk diffusion method. This is quite misleading, because the only reliable way to evaluate in vitro sensitivity of *E. corrodens* is by agar dilution techniques. This is because of the slow rate of growth of *E. corrodens* as well as the higher minimal inhibitory concentration (1 to 4 μg/mL) needed to be effective.[329]

Flavobacterium

Organisms belonging to the genus *Flavobacterium* are common inhabitants of soil and water that occasionally cause human disease. *Flavobacterium meningosepticum* is the species most commonly isolated, but *Flavobacterium odoratum, Flavobacterium balustinum,* and other *Flavobacterium* species have also been reported to cause human infections.

Flavobacterium organisms are long, thin, slightly curved, occasionally filamentous gram-negative rods. They are nonmotile and are catalase-, oxidase-, gelatinase-, and phosphatase-positive.[332] They are weakly fermentative but are usually strongly proteolytic, with diffuse beta hemolysis on blood agar plates.[3] They grow on blood agar and MacConkey agar under aerobic conditions, and colonies are visible in 1 to 2 days. Colonies are translucent, circular, convex, smooth, and typically pigmented (yellow to orange), although nonpigmented strains occur. DNA amplification using universal polymerase chain reaction primers along with a specific *Bacteroides-Flavobacterium* probe was used to identify *F. meningosepticum*; this may provide an alternative to culture for diagnosis of *Flavobacterium* infections.[333]

The pathogenicity of *Flavobacterium* may be derived from production of an elastase. This elastase is structurally similar to that produced by *Pseudomonas* species; however, it has been shown to be less proteolytic than the latter in animal studies.[334]

Flavobacterium species are generally of low virulence. They are uncommon pathogens in adults, rarely causing infections beyond the newborn period. In neonates, infections present as sepsis and meningitis. Premature and small-for-gestational-age infants seem to be at particular risk. The development of meningitis may be insidious. The prognosis is extremely poor with mortality rates of more than 60%. Half of the survivors develop significant neurologic complications, often with hydrocephalus.

In adults, infections with *Flavobacterium* are seen among immunocompromised or debilitated patients. Meningitis has been reported in adults. Other clinical presentations include bacteremia, endocarditis,[335, 336] pneumonia,[337] sinusitis,[338] peritonitis,[339] keratitis,[340] and cellulitis.[337, 341] Most of the described cases are nosocomial and some are associated with prolonged antibiotic use.

In hospitals, *Flavobacterium* organisms have been isolated from ice machines,[342] sinks, humidifiers, drinking fountain bubblers,[343] nebulizers, and contaminated disinfectants.[344] They have also been isolated from tap water, sink traps, tube feedings,[345] the hands of hospital personnel, the air in the operating room,[346] and pasteurization tanks.[347] There is evidence to suggest that *Flavobacterium* organisms enter the hospital through the municipal water supply.[345] These organisms have been shown to survive chlorination, resisting levels of chlorine as high as 100 ppm.[343] It has been suggested that susceptible patients acquire *Flavobacterium* through contaminated water or ice. Colonized patients could then serve as secondary reservoirs, with bacterial transmission to noncolonized patients occurring through hand carriage by contaminated hospital personnel.

Flavobacterium species have an unusual antimicrobial susceptibility pattern in that they are resistant to most drugs but are usually susceptible to antibiotics used for gram-positive bacteria. Antimicrobial susceptibilities vary depending on the method used, with dilution methods being more reliable than the agar disk diffusion method.[348, 349] Most *Flavobacterium* species produce β-lactamases and carbapenemases and are thus resistant to β-lactam drugs, including aztreonam[339] and imipenem.[339, 350] Clindamycin, trimethoprim-sulfamethoxazole, rifampin, and ciprofloxacin are active in vitro against most strains. Other drugs that have been used alone or in combination with some success include erythromycin, chloramphenicol, and vancomycin. Erythromycin and rifampin have both been given concurrently intravenously and intrathecally with some success. Development of resistance during therapy has been documented with erythromycin, rifampin, trimethoprim-sulfamethoxazole, and ciprofloxacin; this should be considered in case of persistence of infection.

Recovery is the rule in immunocompetent older patients infected with contaminated materials. There have been reports of patients with bacteremia that resolved spontaneously without sequelae.[351] In immunocompromised patients and neonates, however, prognosis is poor, with mortality rates up to 75% and development of neurologic sequelae.

References

Actinobacillus

1. Phillips JE: Genus III. *Actinobacillus* Brumpt 1910, 849. *In* Krieg NR, Holt JG (eds): Bergey's Manual of Systematic Bacteriology, Vol 1. Baltimore, Williams & Wilkins, 1984, pp 570–575.
2. Negrete-Abascal E, Tenorio V, Garcia C, et al: *Actinobacillus pleuropneumoniae*: Virulence and gene cloning. Arch Med Res 25:229–233, 1994.
3. Pickett M, Hollis D, Bottone E: Miscellaneous gram-negative bacteria. *In* Balows A, Hausler W Jr, Herrmann K, et al (eds): Manual of Clinical Microbiology. Washington, DC, American Society for Microbiology, 1991, pp 410–428.
4. Weaver RE, Hollis DG, Bottone EJ: Gram-negative fermentative bacteria and *Francisella tularensis*. *In* Lennette EH, Balows A, Hausler WJ Jr, et al (eds): Manual of Clinical Microbiology. Washington, DC, American Society for Microbiology, 1985, pp 309–329.
5. Slotnick IJ: *Actinobacillus* and *Cardiobacterium*. *In* Braude AI (ed): Infectious Diseases and Medical Microbiology, ed 2. Philadelphia, WB Saunders, 1986, pp 348-352.
6. Heath JK, Atkinson SJ, Hembry RM, et al: Bacterial antigens induce collagenase and prostaglandin E_2 synthesis in human gingival fibroblasts through a primary effect on circulating mononuclear cells. Infect Immun 55:2148–2154, 1987.
7. Rabie G, Lally ET, Shenker BJ: Immunosuppressive properties of *Actinobacillus actinomycetemcomitans* leukotoxin. Infect Immun 56:122–127, 1988.
8. Simpson DL, Berthold P, Taichman NS: Killing of human myelomonocytic leukemia and lymphocytic cell lines by *Actinobacillus actinomycetemcomitans* leukotoxin. Infect Immun 56:1162–1166, 1988.
9. Loesche W: Bacterial mediators in periodontal disease. Clin Infect Dis 16(Suppl 4):S203–S210, 1993.
10. Wikstrom M, Linde A: Ability of oral bacteria to degrade fibronectin. Infect Immun 51:707–711, 1986.
11. Kaplan AH, Weber DJ, Oddone EZ, Perfect JR: Infection due to *Actinobacillus actinomycetemcomitans*: 15 cases and review. Rev Infect Dis 11:46–63, 1989.
12. Chen Y, Chang S, Luh K, et al: *Actinobacillus actinomycetemcomitans* endocarditis: A report of four cases and review of the literature. Q J Med 81:871–878, 1991.
13. Grace CJ, Levitz RE, Katz-Pollak H, et al: *Actinobacillus actinomycetemcomitans* prosthetic valve endocarditis. Rev Infect Dis 10:922–929, 1988.
14. Collazos J, Diaz F, Ayarza R, et al: *Actinobacillus actinomycetemcomitans*: A cause of pulmonary-valve endocarditis of 18 months duration with unusual manifestations (Letter). Clin Infect Dis 18:115-116, 1994.
15. van Winkelhoff A, Overbeek B, Pavicic M, et al: Long-standing bacteremia caused by oral *Actinobacillus actinomycetemcomitans* in a patient with a pacemaker. Clin Infect Dis 16:216–218, 1993.
16. Meyer DJ, Gerding DN: Favorable prognosis of patients with prosthetic valve endocarditis caused by gram-negative bacilli of the HACEK group. Am J Med 85:104–107, 1988.
17. Wilson ME, Genco RJ: The role of antibody, complement and neutrophils in host defense against *Actinobacillus actinomycetemcomitans*. Immunol Invest 18:187–209, 1989.
18. Genco RJ, Van-Dyke TE, Levine MJ, et al: 1985 Kreshover Lecture. Molecular factors influencing neutrophil defects in periodontal disease. J Dent Res 65:1379–1391, 1986.
19. Pavicic M, van Winkelhoff A, Douque N, et al: Microbiological and clinical effects of metronidazole and amoxicillin in *Actinobacillus actinomycetemcomitans*--associated periodontitis. A 2-year evaluation. J Clin Periodontol 21:107–112, 1994.
20. Horowitz EA, Pugsley MP, Turbes PG, et al: Pericarditis caused by *Actinobacillus actinomycetemcomitans*. J Infect Dis 155:152–153, 1987.
21. Ishak MA, Zablit KV, Duman J: Endogenous endophthalmitis caused by *Actinobacillus actinomycetemcomitans*. Can J Ophthalmol 21:284–286, 1986.
22. Schmidt M, Smith M, Levy C: Endophthalmitis caused by unusual gram-negative bacilli: Three case reports and review. Clin Infect Dis 17:686–690, 1993.
23. Burgess RC: Chronic tenosynovitis caused by *Actinobacillus actinomycetemcomitans*. J Hand Surg 12:294–295, 1987.
24. Molina F, Echaniz A, Duran M, et al: Infectious arthritis of the knee due to *Actinobacillus actinomycetemcomitans* (Letter). Eur J Clin Microbiol Infect Dis 13:687–689, 1994.
25. Morris J, Sewell D: Necrotizing pneumonia caused by mixed infection with *Actinobacillus actinomycetemcomitans* and *Actinomyces israelii*: Case report and review. Clin Infect Dis 18:450–452, 1994.
26. Yuan A, Yand P, Lee L, et al: *Actinobacillus actinomycetemcomitans* pneumonia with chest wall involvement and rib destruction. Chest 101:1450–1452, 1992.
27. Dommann S, Widmer M, Dommann-Scherrer C, et al: *Actinobacillus actinomycetemcomitans* isolated from a mycetoma (of the forearm) [in German]. Hautarzt 45:402–405, 1994.
28. Hammerberg O, Gregson D, Gopaul D, et al: Recurrent cervical and submandibular lymphadenitis due to *Actinobacillus actinomycetemcomitans* (Letter). Clin Infect Dis 17:1077–1078, 1993.
29. Page MI, King EO: Infection due to *Actinobacillus actinomycetemcomitans* and *Haemophilus aphrophilus*. N Engl J Med 275:181–188, 1966.
30. Kuijper E, Wiggerts H, Jonker G, et al: Disseminated actinomycosis due to *Actinomyces meyeri* and *Actinobacillus actinomycetemcomitans*. Scand J Infect Dis 24:667–672, 1992.
31. Tyrrell J, Noone P, Prichard J: Thoracic actinomycosis complicated by *Actinobacillus actinomycetemcomitans*: Case report and review of literature. Respir Med 86:341–343, 1992.
32. Zijlstra E, Swart G, Godfroy F, et al: Pericarditis, pneumonia and brain abscess due to a combined *Actinomyces–Actinobacillus actinomycetemcomitans* infection. J Infect 25:83–87, 1992.
33. Benaoudia F, Escande F, Simonet M: Infection due to *Actinobacillus lignieresii* after a horse bite (Letter). Eur J Clin Microbiol Infect Dis 13:439–440, 1994.
34. Peel M, Hornidge K, Luppino M, et al: *Actinobacillus* spp. and related bacteria in infected wounds of humans bitten by horses and sheep. J Clin Microbiol 29:2535–2538, 1991.
35. Baker PJ, Wilson ME: Effect of clindamycin on neutrophil killing of gram-negative periodontal bacteria. Antimicrob Agents Chemother 32:1521–1527, 1988.
36. Goldstein EJC, Citron DM: Comparative activities of cefuroxime, amoxicillin–clavulanic acid, ciprofloxacin, enoxacin, and ofloxacin against aerobic and anaerobic bacteria isolated from bite wounds. Antimicrob Agents Chemother 32:1143–1148, 1988.
37. Pavicic M, van Winkelhoff A, de Graaf J: In vitro susceptibilities of *Actinobacillus actinomycetemcomitans* to a number of antimicrobial combinations. Antimicrob Agents Chemother 36:2634–2638, 1992.
38. Pajukanta R, Asikainen S, Saarela M, et al: In vitro antimicrobial susceptibility of different serotypes of *Actinobacillus actinomycetemcomitans*. Scand J Dent Res 101:299–303, 1993.

Capnocytophaga

39. Williams BL, Hollis D, Holdeman LV: Synonymy of strains of Centers for Disease Control group DF-1 with species of *Capnocytophaga*. J Clin Microbiol 10:550–556, 1979.
40. Newman MG, Sutter VL, Pickett MJ, et al: Detection, identification, and comparison of *Capnocytophaga*, *Bacteroides ochraceus*, and DF-1. J Clin Microbiol 10:557–562, 1979.
41. Davis CE: *Capnocytophaga*. *In* Braude AI (ed): Infectious Diseases and Medical Microbiology, ed 2. Philadelphia, WB Saunders, 1986, pp 361–364.
42. Brenner DJ, Hollis DG, Fanning R, et al: *Capnocytophaga canimorsus* sp. nov. (formerly CDC group DF-2), a cause of septicemia following dog bite, and *C. cynodegmi* sp. nov., a cause of local-

ized wound infection following dog bite. J Clin Microbiol 27:231–235, 1989.
43. Rummens JL, Fossepre JM, De Gruyter M, et al: Isolation of *Capnocytophaga* species with a new selective medium. J Clin Microbiol 22:375–378, 1985.
44. Mashimo PA, Yamamoto Y, Nakamura M, et al: Selective recovery of oral *Capnocytophaga* spp. with sheep blood agar containing bacitracin and polymyxin B. J Clin Microbiol 17:187–191, 1983.
45. Chen S, Hicks L, Mitchell D, et al: Serological cross-reaction between *Legionella* spp. and *Capnocytophaga ochracea* by using latex agglutination test. J Clin Microbiol 32:3054–3055, 1994.
46. Shurin SB, Socransky SS, Sweeney E, et al: A neutrophil disorder induced by *Capnocytophaga*, a dental micro-organism. N Engl J Med 301:849–854, 1979.
47. Forlenza SW, Newman MG, Lipsey AI, et al: *Capnocytophaga* sepsis: A newly recognised clinical entity in granulocytopenic patients. Lancet 1:567–568, 1980.
48. Arlet G, Sanson-Le Pors MJ, Castaigne S, et al: Isolation of a strain of β-lactamase–producing *Capnocytophaga ochracea* (Letter). J Infect Dis 155:1346, 1987.
49. Wilson ME, Jonak-Urbanczyk JT, Bronson PM, et al: *Capnocytophaga* species: Increased resistance of clinical isolates to serum bactericidal action. J Infect Dis 156:99–106, 1987.
50. Warren JS, Allen SD: Clinical, pathogenetic, and laboratory features of *Capnocytophaga* infections. Am J Clin Pathol 86:513–518, 1986.
51. Parenti DM, Snydman DR: *Capnocytophaga* species: Infections in nonimmunocompromised and immunocompromised hosts. J Infect Dis 151:140–147, 1985.
52. Miller K, Hansen W, Labbe M, et al: Isolation of *Neisseria elongata* and of *Capnocytophaga ochracea* from vaginal specimens (Letter). J Infect 10:174–175, 1985.
53. Newman MG, Socransky SS, Savitt ED, et al: Studies of the microbiology of periodontosis. J Periodontol 47:373–379, 1976.
54. Gandola C, Butler T, Badger S, et al: Septicemia caused by *Capnocytophaga* in a granulocytopenic patient with glossitis. Arch Intern Med 140:851–852, 1980.
55. Applebaum PC, Ballard JO, Eyster ME: Septicemia due to *Capnocytophaga (Bacteroides ochraceus)* in Hodgkin's disease. Ann Intern Med 90:716–717, 1979.
56. Ormerod LD, Foster CS, Paton BG, et al: Ocular *Capnocytophaga* infection in an edentulous, immunocompetent host. Cornea 7:218–222, 1988.
57. Roussel TJ, Osato MS, Wilhelmus KR: *Capnocytophaga* keratitis. Br J Ophthalmol 69:187–188, 1985.
58. Heidemann DG, Pflugfelder SC, Kronish J, et al: Necrotizing keratitis caused by *Capnocytophaga ochracea.* Am J Ophthalmol 105:655–660, 1988.
59. Rubsamen PE, McLeish WM, Pflugfelder S, et al: *Capnocytophaga* endophthalmitis. Ophthalmology 100:456–459, 1993.
60. Eiferman RA, Levartovsky S, Box JD: Anaerobic *Capnocytophaga* corneal ulcer. Am J Ophthalmol 105:427, 1988.
61. Buu-Hoi AY, Joundy S, Acar JF: Endocarditis caused by *Capnocytophaga ochracea*. J Clin Microbiol 26:1061–1062, 1988.
62. Matlow A, Vellend H: *Capnocytophaga*: A pathogen in immunocompetent hosts. J Infect Dis 152:233–234, 1985.
63. Mosher CB, Corp R: Mediastinal abscess with *Capnocytophaga* spp. in a competent host. J Clin Microbiol 24:161–162, 1986.
64. Winn RE, Chase WF, Lauderdale PW, et al: Septic arthritis involving *Capnocytophaga ochracea*. J Clin Microbiol 19:538–540, 1984.
65. Seger R, Kloeti J, Von Graevenitz A, et al: Cervical abscess due to *Capnocytophaga ochracea*. Pediatr Infect Dis 1:170–172, 1982.
66. Johnson CC, Poupard J: Inguinal lymphadenitis associated with *Capnocytophaga* bacilli. J Clin Microbiol 29:832–833, 1991.
67. Brown R, McCann MP: *Capnocytophaga* bacteremia in a neutropenic patient with sinusitis. Ala Med 54:33–35, 1985.
68. Goudreau E, Comtois R, Bayardelle P, et al: *Capnocytophaga ochracea* and group F beta-hemolytic *Streptococcus* suppurative thyroiditis. J Otolaryngol 15:59–61, 1986.
69. Elster AD, Macone AB, Kasser JR: Osteomyelitis caused by *Capnocytophaga ochracea*. J Pediatr Orthop 3:613–615, 1983.
70. Tarrero MT, Baranda MM, Arizaga JI, et al: Peritonitis involving *Capnocytophaga ochracea*. Am J Gastroenterol 84:206–207, 1989.
71. Hager H, DeLasho G, Zenn R: Peripartum infections with *Capnocytophaga*. A case report. J Reprod Med 33:657–660, 1988.
72. Ernest JM, Wasilauskas B: *Capnocytophaga* in the amniotic fluid of a woman in preterm labor with intact membranes. Am J Obstet Gynecol 153:648-649, 1985.
73. McDonald H, Gordon DL: *Capnocytophaga* species: A cause of amniotic fluid infection and preterm labour. Pathology 20:74–76, 1988.
74. Mercer LJ: *Capnocytophaga* isolated from the endometrium as a cause of neonatal sepsis: A case report. J Reprod Med 30:67–68, 1985.
75. Feldman JD, Kontaxis EN, Sherman MP: Congenital bacteremia due to *Capnocytophaga*. Pediatr Infect Dis 4:415–416, 1985.
76. Arlet G, Sanson-Le-Pors MJ, Ortenberg M, et al: Infections à *Capnocytophaga*. À propos de huit observations. Ann Biol Clin (Paris) 44:373–379, 1986.
77. Juhl G, Brzezinski WA: Disseminated actinomycosis associated with infection by *Capnocytophaga* species. J Infect Dis 149:654, 1984.
78. Forlenza SW, Newman MG, Horikoshi AL, et al: Antimicrobial susceptibility of *Capnocytophaga*. Antimicrob Agents Chemother 19:144–146, 1981.
79. Sutter VL, Pyeatt D, Kwok YY: In vitro susceptibility of *Capnocytophaga* strains to 18 antimicrobial agents. Antimicrob Agents Chemother 20:270–271, 1981.
80. Rummens JL, Gordts B, Van Landuyt HW: In vitro susceptibility of *Capnocytophaga* species to 29 antimicrobial agents. Antimicrob Agents Chemother 30:739–742, 1986.
81. Hawkey PM, Smith SD, Haynes J, et al: In vitro susceptibility of *Capnocytophaga* species to antimicrobial agents. Antimicrob Agents Chemother 31:331–332, 1987.
82. Fuchs PC: In vitro antimicrobial activity and susceptibility testing of ofloxacin. Am J Med 87(Suppl 6C):10S–13S, 1989.
83. Roscoe DL, Zemcov SJV, Thornber D, et al: Antimicrobial susceptibilities and β-lactamase characterization of *Capnocytophaga* species. Antimicrob Agents Chemother 36:2197–2200, 1992.
84. Nachnani S, Scuteri A, Newman MG, et al: E-test: A new technique for antimicrobial susceptibility testing for periodontal microorganisms. J Periodontol 63:576–583, 1992.
85. Hicklin H, Verghese A, Alvarez S: Dysgonic fermenter 2 septicemia. Rev Infect Dis 9:884–890, 1987.
86. Bailie WE, Stowe EC, Schmitt AM: Aerobic bacterial flora of oral and nasal fluids of canines with reference to bacteria associated with bites. J Clin Microbiol 7:223–234, 1978.
87. Westerink MAJ, Amsterdam D, Petell RJ, et al: Septicemia due to DF-2. Am J Med 83:155–158, 1987.
88. Butler T, Weaver RE, Ramani TKV, et al: Unidentified gram-negative rod infection: A new disease of man. Ann Intern Med 86:1–5, 1977.
89. Chambers GW, Westblom TU: Pleural infection caused by *Capnocytophaga canimorsus*, formerly CDC group DF-2. Clin Infect Dis 15:325–326, 1992.
90. Banerjee TK, Grubb W, Otero C, et al: Musculocutaneous mononeuropathy complicating *Capnocytophaga canimorsus* infection. Neurology 43:2411–2412, 1993.
91. Verghese A, Fawwaz H, Berk S, et al: Susceptibility of dysgonic fermenter 2 to antimicrobial agents in vitro. Antimicrob Agents Chemother 32:78–80, 1988.
92. Blum RN, Berry CD, Phillips MG: Clinical illnesses associated with isolation of dysgonic fermenter 3 from stool samples. J Clin Microbiol 30:396–400, 1992.
93. Gill VJ, Travis LB, Williams DY: Clinical and microbiological observations on CDC group DF-3, a gram-negative coccobacillus. J Clin Microbiol 29:1589–1592, 1991.
94. Wagner DK, Wright JJ, Ansher AF, et al: Dysgonic fermenter 3–associated gastrointestinal disease in a patient with common variable hypogammaglobulinemia. Am J Med 84:315–318, 1988.
95. Aronson NE, Zbick CJ: Dysgonic fermenter 3 bacteremia in a neutropenic patient with acute lymphocytic leukemia. J Clin Microbiol 26:2213–2215, 1988.
96. Schonheyder H, Ejlertsen T, Frederiksen W: Isolation of a dysgonic fermenter (DF-3) from urine of a patient. Eur J Clin Microbiol Infect Dis 10:530–531, 1991.
97. Bangsborg JM, Frederiksen W, Bruun B: Dysgonic fermenter 3–associated abscess in a diabetic patient. J Infect 20:237–240, 1990.

Cardiobacterium

98. Weaver RE: Genus *Cardiobacterium* Slotnick and Dougherty 1964, 271. *In* Krieg NR, Holt JG (eds): Bergey's Manual of

Systematic Bacteriology, Vol 1. Baltimore, Williams & Wilkins, 1984, pp 583-585.

99. Taveras J 3d, Campo R, Segal N, et al: Apparent culture-negative endocarditis of the prosthetic valve caused by *Cardiobacterium hominis*. South Med J 86:1439–1440, 1993.
100. Pritchard T, Foust R, Cantely J, et al: Prosthetic valve endocarditis due to *Cardiobacterium hominis* occurring after upper gastrointestinal endoscopy. Am J Med 90:516–518, 1991.
101. Francioli PB, Roussianos D, Glauser MP: *Cardiobacterium hominis* endocarditis manifesting as bacterial meningitis. Arch Intern Med 143:1483–1484, 1983.
102. Lin B, Vieco P: Intracranial mycotic aneurysm in a patient with endocarditis caused by *Cardiobacterium hominis*. Can Assoc Radiol J 46:40–42, 1995.
103. Ben-Chetrit E, Nashif M, Levo Y: Infective endocarditis caused by uncommon bacteria. Scand J Infect Dis 15:179–183, 1983.
104. Kiwan Y, Shuhaiber H, Chungh T: *Cardiobacterium hominis* endocarditis. J Cardiovasc Surg 39:281–283, 1989.
105. Wormser GP, Bottone EJ: *Cardiobacterium hominis*: Review of microbiologic and clinical features. Rev Infect Dis 5:680–691, 1983.
106. Zehnter E, Seifert H, Petit M, et al: A protracted course in *Cardiobacterium hominis* endocarditis [in German]. Dtsch Med Wochenschr 116:768–771, 1991.
107. Lecluse E, Scanu P, Saloux E, et al: Endocarditis caused by *Cardiobacterium hominis* [in French]. Presse Med 23:325–328, 1994.
108. Geraci JE, Wilson WR: Endocarditis due to gram-negative bacteria: Report of 56 cases. Mayo Clin Proc 57:145–148, 1982.
109. Ellner JJ, Rosenthal MS, Lerner PI, et al: Infective endocarditis caused by slow-growing, fastidious, gram-negative bacteria. Medicine (Baltimore) 58:145–158, 1979.
110. Rechtman D, Nadler J: Abdominal abscess due to *Cardiobacterium hominis* and *Clostridium bifermentans*. Rev Infect Dis 13:418–419, 1991.
111. Watanakunakorn C: The use of beta-lactam antibiotics in the treatment of septicaemia and endocarditis. Scand J Infect Dis Suppl 42:110–116, 1984.
112. Vogt K, Klefisch F, Hahn H, et al: Antibacterial efficacy of ciprofloxacin in a case of endocarditis due to *Cardiobacterium hominis*. Int J Med Microbiol Virol Parasitol Infect Dis 28:80–84, 1994.

Chromobacterium

113. Davis CE: *Chromobacterium. In* Braude AI (ed): Infectious Diseases and Medical Microbiology, ed 2. Philadelphia, WB Saunders, 1986, pp 358–361.
114. Peter HAS: Genus *Chromobacterium* Bergonzini 1881, 153. *In* Krieg NR, Holt JG (eds): Bergey's Manual of Systematic Bacteriology, Vol 1. Baltimore, Williams & Wilkins, 1984, pp 580–582.
115. Engel JM, Alexander FS, Pachucki CT: Bacteremia caused by CDC group Ve-1 in previously healthy patient with granulomatous hepatitis. J Clin Microbiol 25:2023–2024, 1987.
116. Singh PD, Liu WC, Gougoutas JZ, et al: Aerocavin, a new antibiotic produced by *Chromobacterium violaceum*. J Antibiot (Tokyo) 41:446–453, 1988.
117. Parker WL, Rathnum ML, Johnson JH, et al: Aerocyanidin, a new antibiotic produced by *Chromobacterium violaceum*. J Antibiot (Tokyo) 41:454–463, 1988.
118. Miller DP, Blevins WT, Steele DB, et al: A comparative study of virulent and avirulent strains of *Chromobacterium violaceum*. Can J Microbiol 34:249–255, 1988.
119. Ponte R, Jenkins S: Fatal *Chromobacterium violaceum* infections associated with exposure to stagnant waters. Pediatric Infect Dis J 11:583–586, 1992.
120. Koburger JA, May SO: Isolation of *Chromobacterium* spp. from foods, soil, and water. Appl Environ Microbiol 44:1463–1465, 1982.
121. Auerbach PS: Natural microbiologic hazards of the aquatic environment. Clin Dermatol 5:52–61, 1987.
122. Macher AM, Casale TB, Fauci AS: Chronic granulomatous disease in childhood and *Chromobacterium violaceum* infections in the southeastern United States. Ann Intern Med 97:51–55, 1982.
123. Sorensen RU, Jacobs MR, Shurin SB: *Chromobacterium violaceum* adenitis acquired in the northern United States as a complication of chronic granulomatous disease. Pediatr Infect Dis 4:701–702, 1985.
124. Suarez AE, Wenokur B, Johnson JM, et al: Nonfatal chromobacterial sepsis. South Med J 79:1146–1148, 1986.
125. Kaufman SC, Ceraso D, Schugurensky A: First case report from Argentina of fatal septicemia caused by *Chromobacterium violaceum*. J Clin Microbiol 23:956–958, 1986.
126. Centers for Disease Control: Chromobacteriosis—Florida. MMWR Morbid Mortal Wkly Rep 29:613–615, 1981.
127. Ti T, Tan W, Chong A, et al: Nonfatal and fatal infections caused by *Chromobacterium violaceum*. Clin Infect Dis 17:505–507, 1993.
128. Hassan H, Suntharalingam S, Dhillon K: Fatal *Chromobacterium violaceum* septicaemia. Singapore Med J 34:456–458, 1993.
129. Shetty M, Venkatesh A, Shenoy S, Shivananda PG: *Chromobacterium violaceum* meningitis—A case report. Indian J Med Sci 41:275–276, 1987.
130. Martin J, Brimacombe J: *Chromobacterium violaceum* septicaemia: The intensive care management of two cases. Anaesth Intensive Care 20:88–90, 1992.
131. Feldman RB, Stern GA, Hood CI: *Chromobacterium violaceum* infection of the eye. A report of two cases. Arch Ophthalmol 102:711–713, 1984.
132. Macher AM, Casale TB, Gallin JI, et al: *Chromobacterium violaceum* infections and chronic granulomatous disease (Letter). Ann Intern Med 98:259, 1983.
133. Mamlok RJ, Mamlok V, Mills GC, et al: Glucose-6-phosphate dehydrogenase deficiency, neutrophil dysfunction and *Chromobacterium violaceum* sepsis. J Pediatr 111:852–854, 1987.
134. Dreizen S, McCredie KB, Bodey GP, et al: Unusual mucocutaneous infections in immunosuppressed patients with leukemia—Expansion of an earlier study. Postgrad Med 79:287–294, 1986.
135. Aldridge KE, Valainis GT, Sanders CV: Comparison of the in-vitro activity of ciprofloxacin and 24 other antimicrobial agents against clinical strains of *Chromobacterium violaceum*. Diagn Microbiol Infect Dis 10:31–39, 1988.

Acinetobacter

136. Glew RH, Moellering RC, Kunz LJ: Infections with *Acinetobacter calcoaceticus (Herellea vaginicola)*: Clinical and laboratory studies. Medicine (Baltimore) 56:79–97, 1977.
137. Juni E: Genus III. *Acinetobacter* Brisou and Prevot 1954, 727. *In* Krieg NR, Holt JG (eds): Bergey's Manual of Systematic Bacteriology, Vol 1. Baltimore, Williams & Wilkins, 1984, pp 303–307.
138. Bouvet PJM, Grimont PAO: Taxonomy of the genus *Acinetobacter* with the recognition of *Acinetobacter baumannii* sp. nov., *Acinetobacter haemolyticus* sp. nov., *Acinetobacter johnsonii* sp. nov., and *Acinetobacter junii* sp. nov. and extended descriptions of *Acinetobacter calcoaceticus* and *Acinetobacter lwoffii*. Int J Syst Bacteriol 36:228–240, 1986.
139. Traub WH: *Acinetobacter baumannii* serotyping for delineation of outbreaks of nosocomial cross-infection. J Clin Microbiol 27:2713–2716, 1989.
140. Gerner-Smidt P, Frederiksen W: *Acinetobacter* in Denmark: I. Taxonomy, antibiotic susceptibility, and pathogenicity of 112 clinical strains. APMIS 101:815–825, 1993.
141. Dijkshoorn L, van der Toorn J: *Acinetobacter* species: Which do we mean (Letter)? Clin Infect Dis 15:748–749, 1992.
142. Rubin SJ, Granato PA, Wasilauskas BL: Glucose-nonfermenting gram-negative bacteria. *In* Lennette EH, Balows A, Housler NJ (eds): Manual of Clinical Microbiology. Washington, DC, American Society for Microbiology, 1985, pp 330–349.
143. Davis CE, Baer H: *Moraxella, Kingella* and *Acinetobacter. In* Braude AI (ed): Infectious Diseases and Medical Microbiology, ed 2. Philadelphia, WB Saunders, 1986, pp 287–292.
144. Saikku P, Puolakkainen M, Leiononen M, et al: Cross-reactivity between Chlamydiazyme and *Acinetobacter* strains (Letter). N Engl J Med 314:922–923, 1986.
145. Brade H, Brunner H: Serological cross-reactions between *Acinetobacter calcoaceticus* and chlamydiae. J Clin Microbiol 10:819–822, 1979.
146. Jankowski S, Grzybek-Hryncewicz K, Fleischer M, et al: Susceptibility of isolates of *Acinetobacter anitratus* and *Acinetobacter lwoffii* to the bactericidal activity of normal human serum. FEMS Microbiol Immunol 4:255–260, 1992.
147. Gennari M, Lombardi P: Comparative characterization of *Aci-*

netobacter strains isolated from different foods and clinical sources. Int J Med Microbiol Virol Parasitol Infect Dis 279:553–564, 1993.
148. Cordes LG, Brink EW, Checko PJ, et al: A cluster of *Acinetobacter* pneumonia in foundry workers. Ann Intern Med 95:688–693, 1981.
149. Allen KD, Green HT: Hospital outbreak of multi-resistant *Acinetobacter anitratus*: An airborne mode of spread? J Hosp Infect 9:110–119, 1987.
150. Daschner FD, Habel H: Hospital outbreak of multi-resistant *Acinetobacter anitratus*: An airborne mode of spread? J Hosp Infect 10:211–212, 1987.
151. Vivian A, Hinchliffe E, Fewson CA: *Acinetobacter calcoaceticus*: Some approaches to a problem. J Hosp Infect 2:199–203, 1981.
152. Erganis O, Corlu M, Kaya O, Ates M: Isolation of *Acinetobacter calcoaceticus* from septicaemic hens. Vet Rec 123:374, 1988.
153. Kaya O, Ates M, Erganis O, et al: Isolation of *Acinetobacter lwoffi* from hens with septicemia. Zentralbl Veterinarmed [B] 36:157–158, 1989.
154. Lewis SJ, Gilmour A: Microflora associated with the internal surfaces of rubber and stainless steel milk transfer pipeline. J Appl Bacteriol 62:327–333, 1987.
155. Gonzalez C, Gutierrez C, Grande T: Bacterial flora in bottled uncarbonated mineral drinking water. Can J Microbiol 33:1120–1125, 1987.
156. Hartstein AI, Rashad AL, Liebler JM, et al: Multiple intensive care unit outbreak of *Acinetobacter calcoaceticus* subspecies *anitratus* respiratory infection and colonization associated with contaminated, reusable ventilator circuits and resuscitation bags. Am J Med 85:624–631, 1988.
157. Ahmed J, Brutus A, D'Amato R, et al: *Acinetobacter calcoaceticus anitratus* outbreak in the intensive care unit traced to a peak flow meter. Am J Infect Control 22:319–321, 1994.
158. Smith RW, Masanari M: Room humidifiers as the source of *Acinetobacter* infection. JAMA 237:795–797, 1977.
159. Van-Saene HK, Van-Putte JC, Van-Saene JJ, et al: Sink flora in a long-stay hospital is determined by the patients' oral and rectal flora. Epidemiol Infect 102:231–238, 1989.
160. Snydman DR, Mallow MF, Brock SM, et al: Pseudobacteremia: False-positive blood cultures from mist tent contamination. Am J Epidemiol 106:154–159, 1977.
161. Abrutyn E, Goodhard GL, Roos K, et al: *Acinetobacter calcoaceticus* outbreak associated with peritoneal dialysis. Am J Epidemiol 107:328–335, 1978.
162. Flaherty J, Garcia-Houchins S, Chudy R, et al: An outbreak of gram-negative bacteremia traced to contaminated O-rings in reprocessed dialyzers. Ann Intern Med 119:1072–1078, 1993.
163. Alfa M, Sitter D: In-hospital evaluation of contamination of duodenoscopes: A quantitative assessment of the effect of drying. J Hosp Infect 19:89–98, 1991.
164. Shawker TH, Kluge RM, Ayella RJ: Bacteremia associated with angiography. JAMA 229:1090–1092, 1974.
165. Haslett TM, Isenberg HD, Hilton E, et al: Microbiology of indwelling central intravascular catheters. J Clin Microbiol 26:696–701, 1988.
166. Beck-Sague CM, Jarvis WR: Epidemic bloodstream infections associated with pressure transducers: A persistent problem. Infect Control Hosp Epidemiol 10:54–59, 1989.
167. Baguley D, Whipp J, Farrington M: A microbiological hazard in caloric testing. Br J Audiol 25:427–428, 1991.
168. Patterson J, Vecchio J, Pantelick E, et al: Association of contaminated gloves with transmission of *Acinetobacter calcoaceticus* var. *anitratus* in an intensive care unit. Am J Med 91:479–483, 1991.
169. Matsen JM: The source of hospital infection. Medicine (Baltimore) 52:271–277, 1973.
170. Arduino M, Bland L, McAllister S, et al: Microbial growth and endotoxin production in the intravenous anesthetic propofol. Infect Control Hosp Epidemiol 12:535–539, 1991.
171. Oie S, Kamiya A, Hironaga K, et al: Microbial contamination of enteral feeding solution and its prevention. Am J Infect Control 21:34–38, 1993.
172. Rosenthal SL: Sources of *Pseudomonas* and *Acinetobacter* species found in human culture materials. Am J Clin Pathol 62:807–811, 1974.
173. Rudin ML, Michael JR, Huxley EJ: Community-acquired *Acinetobacter* pneumonia. Am J Med 67:39–43, 1979.
174. Smego RA: Endemic nosocomial *Acinetobacter calcoaceticus* bacteremia: Clinical significance, treatment, and prognosis. Arch Intern Med 145:2174–2179, 1985.
175. Timsit J, Garrait V, Misset B, et al: The digestive tract is a major site for *Acinetobacter baumannii* colonization in intensive care unit patients (Letter). J Infect Dis 168:1336–1337, 1993.
176. el-Mohandes A, Schatz V, Keiser J, et al: Bacterial contaminants of collected and frozen human milk used in an intensive care nursery. Am J Infect Control 21:226–230, 1993.
177. Henriksen SD: *Moraxella*, *Acinetobacter* and the Mimeae. Bacteriol Rev 37:522–561, 1973.
178. Weinstein MP, Reller LB, Murphy JR, et al: The clinical significance of positive blood cultures: A comprehensive analysis of 500 episodes of bacteremia and fungemia in adults. I. Laboratory and epidemiologic observations. Rev Infect Dis 5:35–53, 1983.
179. Seifert H, Baginski R, Schulze A, et al: The distribution of *Acinetobacter* species in clinical culture materials. Int J Med Microbiol Virol Parasitol Infect Dis 279:544–552, 1993.
180. Baltimore RS, Duncan RL, Shapiro ED, et al: Epidemiology of pharyngeal colonization of infants with aerobic gram-negative rod bacteria. J Clin Microbiol 27:91–95, 1989.
181. Horan TC, White JW, Jarvis WR, et al: Nosocomial infection surveillance, 1984. MMWR CDC Surveill Summ 35:17SS–29SS, 1986.
182. Emori TG, Gaynes RP: An overview of nosocomial infections, including the role of the microbiology laboratory. Clin Microbiol Rev 6:428–442, 1993.
183. Larson E: A decade of nosocomial *Acinetobacter*. Am J Infect Control 12:14–18, 1984.
184. Retailliau HF, Hightower AW, Dixon RE, et al: *Acinetobacter calcoaceticus*: A nosocomial pathogen with an unusual seasonal pattern. J Infect Dis 139:371–375, 1979.
185. Tilley P, Roberts F: Bacteremia with *Acinetobacter* species: Risk factors and prognosis in different clinical settings. Clin Infect Dis 18:896–900, 1994.
186. Chen Y, Chang S, Hsieh W, et al: *Acinetobacter calcoaceticus* bacteremia: Analysis of 48 cases. J Formos Medic Assoc 90:958–963, 1991.
187. Regev R, Dolfin T, Zelig I, et al: *Acinetobacter* septicemia: A threat to neonates? Special aspects in a neonatal intensive care unit. Infection 21:394–396, 1993.
188. Seifert H, Strate A, Schulze A, et al: Vascular catheter–related bloodstream infection due to *Acinetobacter johnsonii* (formerly *Acinetobacter calcoaceticus* var. *lwoffi*): Report of 13 cases. Clin Infect Dis 17:632–636, 1993.
189. Ali M, Tremewen D, Hay A, et al: The occurrence of bacteremia associated with the use of oral and nasopharyngeal airways. Anaesthesia 47:153–155, 1992.
190. Sacks-Berg A, Calubiran O, Epstein H, et al: Sepsis associated with transhepatic cholangiography. J Hosp Infect 20:43–50, 1992.
191. Weinberger I, Davidson E, Rotenberg Z, et al: Prosthetic valve endocarditis caused by *Acinetobacter calcoaceticus* subsp. *lwoffi*. J Clin Microbiol 25:955–957, 1987.
192. Nguyen M, Harris S, Muder R, et al: Antibiotic-resistant *Acinetobacter* meningitis in neurosurgical patients. Neurosurgery 35:851–855, 1994.
193. Seigman-Igra Y, Bar-Yosef S, Gorea A, et al: Nosocomial *Acinetobacter* meningitis secondary to invasive procedures: Report of 25 cases and review. Clin Infect Dis 17:843–849, 1993.
194. Baltas I, Tsoulfa S, Sakellariou P, et al: Posttraumatic meningitis: Bacteriology, hydrocephalus, and outcome. Neurosurgery 35:422–426, 1994.
195. Fagon J, Chastre J, Hance A, et al: Nosocomial pneumonia in ventilated patients: A cohort study evaluating attributable mortality and hospital stay. Am J Med 94:281–288, 1993.
196. Suchyta MR, Peters JI, Black RD: Chronic *Acinetobacter calcoaceticus* var *anitratus* pneumonia. Am J Med Sci 294:117–119, 1987.
197. Ishihara H, Yamamori Y, Ihaya A, et al: Successful management of abdominal aortic aneurysm due to bacterial infection: Report of a case. Nippon Geka Gakkai Zasshi 88:907–911, 1987.
198. Galvao C, Swartz R, Rocher L, et al.: *Acinetobacter* peritonitis during chronic peritoneal dialysis. Am J Kidney Dis 14:101–104, 1989.
199. Benzakour M, Lagarde C, Benevent D, et al: Peritonitis during continuous ambulatory peritoneal dialysis. Nephron 50:175–176, 1988.

200. Lye W, Lee E, Ang K: *Acinetobacter* peritonitis in patients on CAPD: Characteristics and outcome. Adv Perit Dial 7:176–179, 1991.
201. Valdez J, Asperilla M, Smego R Jr: *Acinetobacter* peritonitis in patients receiving continuous ambulatory peritoneal dialysis. South Med J 84:607–610, 1991.
202. Volpin G, Krivoy N, Stein H: *Acinetobacter* sp. osteomyelitis of the femur: A late sequel of unrecognized foreign body implantation. Injury 24:345–346, 1993.
203. Marcovoch A, Levartovsky S: *Acinetobacter* exposure keratitis. Br J Ophthalmol 78:489–490, 1994.
204. Melki T, Sramek S: Trauma-induced *Acinetobacter lwoffi* endophthalmitis (Letter). Am J Ophthalmol 113:598–599, 1992.
205. Zabel RW, Winegarden T, Holland EJ, et al: *Acinetobacter* corneal ulcer after penetrating keratoplasty. Am J Ophthalmol 107:677–678, 1989.
206. Groden L, Murphy B, Rodnite J, et al: Lid flora in blepharitis. Cornea 10:50–53, 1991.
207. Bick J, Semel J: Fulminant community-acquired *Acinetobacter* pneumonia in a healthy woman. Clin Infect Dis 17:820–821, 1993.
208. Barnes DJ, Naraqi S, Igo JD: Community-acquired *Acinetobacter* pneumonia in adults in Papua New Guinea. Rev Infect Dis 10:636–639, 1988.
209. Anstey N, Currie B, Withnall K: Community-acquired *Acinetobacter* pneumonia in the Northern Territory of Australia. Clin Infect Dis 14:83–91, 1992.
210. Reindersma P, Nohlmans L, Korten J: *Acinetobacter*, an infrequent cause of community acquired bacterial meningitis. Clin Neurol Neurosurg 95:71–73, 1993.
211. Gradon J, Chapnick E, Lutwick L, et al: Infective endocarditis of a native valve due to *Acinetobacter*: Case report and review. Clin Infect Dis 14:1145–1148, 1992.
212. Brown R, Cipriani D, Schulte M, et al: Community-acquired bacteremias from tunneled central intravenous lines: Results from studies of a single vendor. Am J Infect Control 22:149–151, 1994.
213. Auerbach PS, Morris JA Jr: *Acinetobacter calcoaceticus* infection following a dog bite. J Emerg Med 5:363–366, 1987.
214. Vila J, Almela M, Jimenez de Anta MT: Laboratory investigation of hospital outbreak caused by two different multiresistant *Acinetobacter calcoaceticus* subsp. *anitratus* strains. J Clin Microbiol 27:1086–1089, 1989.
215. Muller-Serieys C, Lesquoy JB, Perez E, et al: Nosocomial infections caused by *Acinetobacter*. Epidemiology and therapeutic difficulties. Presse Med 18:107–110, 1989.
216. Rolston KVI, Bodey GP: In vitro susceptibility of *Acinetobacter* species to various antimicrobial agents. Antimicrob Agents Chemother 30:769–770, 1986.
217. Bergogne-Berezin E, Joly-Guillou ML: Comparative activity of imipenem, ceftazidime and cefotaxime against *Acinetobacter calcoaceticus*. J Antimicrob Chemother 18(Suppl E):35–39, 1986.
218. Overturf GD: Use of trimethoprim-sulfamethoxazole in pediatric infections: Relative merits of intravenous administration. Rev Infect Dis 9(Suppl 2):S168–S176, 1987.
219. Urban C, Go E, Mariano N, et al: Effect of sulbactam on infections caused by imipenem-resistant *Acinetobacter calcoaceticus* biotype *anitratus*. J Infect Dis 167:448–451, 1993.
220. Sanders CC: Ciprofloxacin: In vitro activity, mechanism of action, and resistance. Rev Infect Dis 10:516–527, 1988.
221. Phillips I, King A: Comparative activity of the 4-quinolones. Rev Infect Dis 10(Suppl 1):S70–S76, 1988.
222. Seifert H, Baginski R, Schulze A, et al: Antimicrobial susceptibility of *Acinetobacter* species. Antimicrob Agents Chemother 37:750–753, 1993.
223. Simor A, Louie L, Louie M: In vitro susceptibility of *Acinetobacter baumannii* to biapenem, piperacillin/tazobactam and thirteen other antimicrobial agents. Eur J Clin Microbiol Infect Dis 13:521–523, 1994.
224. Lang C, Beuth J, Ko H, et al: Antibacterial in vitro-activity of meropenem against 200 clinical isolates in comparison to 11 selected antibiotics. Int J Med Microbiol Virol Parasitol Infect Dis 277:485–492, 1992.
225. Obaraa M, Nakae T: Mechanisms of resistance to beta-lactam antibiotics in *Acinetobacter calcoaceticus*. J Antimicrob Chemother 28:791–800, 1991.
226. Gehrlein M, Leying H, Cullmann W, et al: Imipenem resistance in *Acinetobacter baumannii* is due to altered penicillin-binding proteins. Chemotherapy 37:405–412, 1991.
227. Sato K, Nakae T: Outer membrane permeability of *Acinetobacter calcoaceticus* and its implication in antibiotic resistance. J Antimicrob Chemother 28:35–45, 1991.
228. Joly-Guillou ML, Bergogne-Berezin E, Moreau N: Enzymatic resistance to beta-lactams and aminoglycosides in *Acinetobacter calcoaceticus*. J Antimicrob Chemother 20:773–776, 1987.
229. Vila J, Marcos A, Marco F, et al: In vitro antimicrobial production of beta-lactamases, aminoglycoside-modifying enzymes, and chloramphenicol acetyltransferase by and susceptibility of clinical isolates of *Acinetobacter baumannii*. Antimicrob Agents Chemother 37:138–141, 1993.
230. Lambert T, Gerbaud G, Courvalin P: Characterization of the chromosomal *AAC(6')-IJ* gene of *Acinetobacter* sp 13 and the *AAC(6')-IH* plasmid gene of *Acinetobacter baumannii*. Antimicrob Agents Chemother 38:1883–1889, 1994.
231. Lambert T, Gerbaud G, Galimand M, et al: Characterization of *Acinetobacter haemolyticus AAC(6')-IG* gene encoding an aminoglycoside 6'-*N*-acetyltransferase which modifies amikacin. Antimicrob Agents Chemother 37:2093–2100, 1993.

Alcaligenes

232. Kersters K, De Ley J: Genus *Alcaligenes* Castellani and Chalmece 1919, 936. *In* Krieg NR, Holt JG (eds): Bergey's Manual of Systematic Bacteriology, Vol 1. Baltimore, Williams & Wilkins, 1984, pp 361–373.
233. Gardner P, Griffin WB, Swartz MN, et al: Nonfermentative gram-negative bacilli of nosocomial interest. Am J Med 48:735–749, 1970.
234. Cohen PS, Maguire JH, Weinstein L: Infective endocarditis caused by gram-negative bacteria: A review of the literature, 1945–1977. Prog Cardiovasc Dis 22:205–242, 1980.
235. Kishan J, Elzouki AY, Mir NA: Bacillus *Alcaligenes faecalis* septicemia and meningitis in the newborn. Indian J Pediatr 55:443–444, 1988.
236. Peel MM, Hibberd AJ, King BM, et al: *Alcaligenes piechaudii* from chronic ear discharge. J Clin Microbiol 26:1580–1581, 1988.
237. Ooishi M, Miyao M: A clinical evaluation of sultamicillin fine granules in the treatment of meibomianitis. Jpn J Antibiot 41:2059–2064, 1988.
238. Tayeri T, Kelly L: *Alcaligenes faecalis* corneal ulcer in a patient with cicatricial pemphigoid (Letter). Am J Ophthalmol 115:255–256, 1993.
239. Auckenthaler R, Michea-Hamzehpour M, Pechere JC: In-vitro activity of newer quinolones against aerobic bacteria. J Antimicrob Chemother 17(Suppl B):29–39, 1986.
240. Schell RF, Francisco M, Bihl JA, LeFrock JL: The activity of ceftazidime compared with those of aztreonam, newer cephalosporins, and Sch 29482 against nonfermentative gram-negative bacilli. Chemotherapy 31:181–190, 1985.
241. Bizet C, Tekaia F, Philippon A: In-vitro susceptibility of *Alcaligenes faecalis* compared with those of other *Alcaligenes* spp. to antimicrobial agents including seven beta-lactams (Letter). J Antimicrob Chemother 32:907–910, 1993.

Achromobacter

242. Yabuuchi E, Yano I: *Achromobacter* gen. nov. and *Achromobacter xylosoxidans* nom. rev. Int J Syst Bacteriol 31:477–478, 1981.
243. Spear JB, Fuhrer J, Kirby BD: *Achromobacter xylosoxidans* (*Alcaligenes xylosoxidans* subsp. *xylosoxidans*) bacteremia associated with a well-water source: Case report and review of the literature. J Clin Microbiol 26:598–599, 1988.
244. Mandell WF, Garvey GJ, Neu HC: *Achromobacter xylosoxidans* bacteremia. Rev Infect Dis 9:1001–1005, 1987.
245. Reverdy ME, Freney J, Fleurette J, et al: Nosocomial colonization and infection by *Achromobacter xylosoxidans*. J Clin Microbiol 19:140–143, 1984.
246. McGuckin MB, Thorpe RJ, Koch KM, et al: An outbreak of *Achromobacter xylosoxidans* related to diagnostic tracer procedures. Am J Epidemiol 115:785–793, 1982.
247. Reina J, Antich M, Siquier B, et al: Nosocomial outbreak of *Achromobacter xylosoxidans* associated with a diagnostic contrast solution. J Clin Pathol 41:920–921, 1988.

248. Gahrn-Hansen B, Alstrup P, Dessau R, et al: Outbreak of infection with *Achromobacter xylosoxidans* from contaminated intravascular pressure transducers. J Hosp Infect 12:1–6, 1988.
249. Wurtz R, Moye G, Jovanovic B: Handwashing machines, handwashing compliance, and potential for cross-contamination. Am J Infect Control 22:228–230, 1994.
250. Yabuuchi E, Oyama A: *Achromobacter xylosoxidans* n. sp. from human ear discharge. Jpn J Microbiol 15:477–481, 1971.
251. D'Amato RF, Salemi M, Mathews A, et al: *Achromobacter xylosoxidans* (*Alcaligenes xylosoxidans* subsp. *xylosoxidans*) meningitis associated with a gunshot wound. J Clin Microbiol 26:2425–2426, 1988.
252. Sepkowitz DV, Bostic DE, Maslow MJ: *Achromobacter xylosoxidans* meningitis: Case report and review of the literature. Clin Pediatr 26:483–485, 1987.
253. Namnyak SS, Holmes B, Fathalla SE: Neonatal meningitis caused by *Achromobacter xylosoxidans*. J Clin Microbiol 22:470–471, 1985.
254. Hearn Y, Gander R: *Achromobacter xylosoxidans*. An unusual neonatal pathogen. Am J Clin Pathol 96:211–214, 1991.
255. Arroyo JC, Jordan W, Lema MW, et al: Diversity of plasmids in *Achromobacter xylosoxidans* isolates responsible for a seemingly common-source nosocomial outbreak. J Clin Microbiol 25:1952–1955, 1987.
256. Boukadida J, Monastiri K, Snoussi N, et al: Nosocomial neonatal meningitis by *Alcaligenes xylosoxidans* transmitted by aqueous eosin. Pediatr Infect Dis J 12:696–697, 1993.
257. Decre D, Arlet G, Danglot C, et al: A beta-lactamase–overproducing strain of *Alcaligenes dentrificans* subsp. *xylosoxidans* isolated from a case of meningitis. J Antimicrob Chemother 30:769–779, 1992.
258. Legrand C, Anaissie E: Bacteremia due to *Achromobacter xylosoxidans* in patients with cancer. Clin Infect Dis 14:479–484, 1992.
259. Dupon M, Winnock S, Rogues A, et al: *Achromobacter xylosoxidans* (*Alcaligenes xylosoxidans* subsp. *xylosoxidans*) bacteremia after liver transplantation (Letter). Intensive Care Med 19:480, 1993.
260. Cieslak T, Robb M, Drabick, et al: Catheter-associated sepsis caused by *Ochrobactrum anthropi*: Report of a case and review of related nonfermentative bacteria. Clin Infect Dis 14:902–907, 1992.
261. Cieslak T, Raszka W: Catheter-associated sepsis due to *Alcaligenes xylosoxidans* in a child with AIDS (Letter). Clin Infect Dis 16:592–593, 1993.
262. Kerr J, Webb C: Five cases of *Alcaligenes* pseudobacteraemia. Ulster Med J 61:163–165, 1992.
263. Ficker L, Meredith, TA, Wilson LA, et al: Chronic bacterial endophthalmitis. Am J Ophthalmol 103:745–748, 1987.
264. Newman PE, Hider P, Waring GO, et al: Corneal ulcer due to *Achromobacter xylosoxidans*. Br J Ophthalmol 68:472–474, 1984.
265. Siganos D, Tselentis I, Papatzanaki M, et al: *Achromobacter xylosoxidans* keratitis following penetrating keratoplasty. Refractive Corneal Surg 9:71–73, 1993.
266. San Miguel V, Lavery J, York J, et al: *Achromobacter xylosoxidans* septic arthritis in a patient with systemic lupus erythematosus. Arthritis Rheum 34:1484–1485, 1991.
267. Taylor P, Fischbein L: Septic arthritis in Waldenström's macroglobulinemia (Letter). J Rheumatol 21:776–777, 1994.
268. Taylor P, Fischbein L: Prosthetic knee infection due to *Achromobacter xylosoxidans*. J Rheumatol 19:992–993, 1992.
269. Barton LL, Hoddy DM: Osteomyelitis due to *Achromobacter xylosoxidans* (Letter). Clin Infect Dis 17:296–297, 1993.
270. Hoddy D, Barton L: Puncture wound–induced *Achromobacter xylosoxidans* osteomyelitis of the foot (Letter). Am J Dis Child 145:599–600, 1991.
271. Walsh R, Klein N, Cunha B: *Achromobacter xylosoxidans* osteomyelitis (Letter). Clin Infect Dis 16:176–178, 1993.
272. Gradon J, Mayrer A, Hayes J: Pulmonary abscess associated with *Alcaligenes xylosoxidans* in a patient with AIDS (Letter). Clin Infect Dis 17:1071–1072, 1993.
273. Rolston K, Messer M: The in-vitro susceptibility of *Alcaligenes dentrificans* subsp. *xylosoxidans* to 40 antimicrobial agents. J Antimicrob Chemother 26:857–859, 1990.
274. Glupczynski Y, Hansen W, Freney J, et al: In vitro susceptibility of *Alcaligenes denitrificans* subsp. *xylosoxidans* to 24 antimicrobial agents. Antimicrob Agents Chemother 32:276–278, 1988.

Ochrobactrum anthropi

275. Holmes B, Popoff M, Kiredjian M, et al: *Ochrobactrum anthropi* gen. nov., sp. nov. from human clinical specimens and previously known as group Vd. Int J Syst Bacteriol 38:406–416, 1988.
276. Chester B, Cooper LH. *Achromobacter* species (CDC group Vd): Morphological and biochemical characterization. J Clin Microbiol 9:425–436, 1979.
277. Van Horn KG, Gedris CA, Ahmed T, et al: Bacteremia and urinary tract infection associated with CDC group Vd biovar 2. J Clin Microbiol 27:201–202, 1989.
278. Kern WV, Oethinger M, Kaufhold A, et al: *Ochrobactrum anthropi* bacteremia: Report of four cases and short review. Infection 21:306–310, 1993.
279. Haditsch M, Binder L, Tschurtschenthaler G, et al: Bacteremia caused by *Ochrobactrum anthropi* in an immunocompromised child. Infection 22:291–292, 1994.
280. Klein JD, Eppes SC: *Ochrobactrum anthropi* bacteremia in a child. Del Med J 65:493–495, 1993.
281. Kish MA, Buggy BP, Forbes BA: Bacteremia caused by *Achromobacter* species in an immunocompromised host. J Clin Microbiol 19:947–948, 1984.
282. Cieslak TJ, Robb ML, Drabick CJ, et al: Catheter-associated sepsis caused by *Ochrobactrum anthropi*: Report of a case and review of related nonfermentative bacteria. Clin Infect Dis 14:902–907, 1992.
283. Gransden WR, Eykyn SJ: Seven cases of bacteremia due to *Ochrobactrum anthropi* (Letter). Clin Infect Dis 15:1068–1069, 1992.
284. Alnor D, Frimodt-Moller N, Espersen F, et al: Infections with the unusual human pathogens *Agrobacterium* species and *Ochrobactrum anthropi*. Clin Infect Dis 18:914–920.
285. Ezzedine H, Mourad M, Van Ossel C, et al: An outbreak of *Ochrobactrum anthropi* bacteraemia in five organ transplant patients. J Hosp Infect 27:35–42, 1994.
285a. Chang HJ, Christenson JC, Pavia AT, et al: *Ochrobactrum anthropi* meningitis in pediatric pericardial allograft transplant recipients. J Infect Dis 173:656–669, 1996.
286. Applebaum PC, Campbell DB: Pancreatic abscess associated with *Achromobacter* group Vd biovar 1. J Clin Microbiol 12:282–283, 1980.
287. Barson WJ, Cromer BA, Marcon MJ: Puncture wound osteochondritis of the foot caused by CDC group Vd. J Clin Microbiol 25:2014–2016, 1987.
288. Cieslak TJ, Drabick CJ, Robb ML: Pyogenic infections due to *Ochrobactrum anthropi*. Clin Infect Dis 22:845–847, 1996.
289. Brivet F, Guibert M, Kiredjian M, et al: Necrotizing fasciitis, bacteremia, and multiorgan failure caused by *Ochrobactrum anthropi*. Clin Infect Dis 17:516–518, 1993.

Eikenella

290. Jackson FL, Goodman Y: Genus *Eikenella* Jackson and Goodman 1972, 74. *In* Krieg NR, Holt JG (eds): Bergey's Manual of Systematic Bacteriology, Vol 1. Baltimore, Williams & Wilkins, 1984, pp 591–597.
291. Brooks GF: *Eikenella corrodens*. *In* Braude AI (ed): Infectious Diseases and Medical Microbiology, ed 2. Philadelphia, WB Saunders, 1986, pp 346–348.
292. Soder P-O, Jin LJ, Soder B: DNA probe detection of periodontopathogens in advanced periodontitis. Scand J Dent Res 101:363–370, 1993.
293. Alkaler RP, Young KA, Hardie JM: Production of hydrolytic enzymes by oral isolates of *Eikenella corrodens*. FEMS Microbiol Lett 123:69–74, 1994.
294. Brooks GF, O'Donoghue JM, Rissing JP, et al: *Eikenella corrodens*, a recently recognized pathogen: Infections in medical-surgical patients and in association with methylphenidate abuse. Medicine (Baltimore) 53:325–342, 1974.
295. Stoloff AL, Gillies ML: Infections with *Eikenella corrodens* in a general hospital: A report of 33 cases. Rev Infect Dis 8:50–53, 1986.
296. Datar SD, Shafran SD: Cellulitis of the foot due to *Eikenella corrodens* (Letter). Arch Dermatol 125:849–850, 1989.
297. Rayan GM, Putnam JL, Cahill SL, et al: *Eikenella corrodens* in human mouth flora. J Hand Surg 13:953–956, 1988.

298. Cheng AF, South JR, French GL: *Eikenella corrodens* as a cause of brain abscess. Scand J Infect Dis 20:667–671, 1988.
299. Burdick CO, Erasmus D, Jayaram A, et al: *Eikenella* brain abscess (Letter). JAMA 248:1972–1973, 1982.
300. Ramos JM, Pacho E, Garcia-Valle B, et al: Splenic abscess due to *Eikenella corrodens*. Postgrad Med J 70:848–849, 1994.
301. Perez Trallero E, Garcia Arenzana JM, Cilla Eguiluz G, Tovar Larrucea J: β-Lactamase–producing *Eikenella corrodens* in an intraabdominal abscess (Letter). J Infect Dis 153:379–380, 1986.
302. Danziger LH, Schoonover LL, Kale P, et al: *Eikenella corrodens* as an intraabdominal pathogen. Am Surg 60:296–299, 1994.
303. Kyi MS, Al Wali W, Gillespie SH, et al: Brodie's abscess caused by *Eikenella corrodens*. J Infect 23:213–214, 1991.
304. Noordeen MHH, Godfrey LW: Case report of an unusual cause of low back pain: Intervertebral diskitis caused by *Eikenella corrodens*. Clin Orthop 280:175–178, 1992.
305. Allen MB: Intrathoracic infections due to *Eikenella corrodens* (Letter). Thorax 43:344, 1988.
306. Harcombe A, Allen M: Empyema due to *Eikenella corrodens* (Letter). J Infect 17:86–87, 1988.
307. St. John MA, Belda AA, Matlow A, et al: *Eikenella corrodens* empyema in children. Am J Dis Child 135:415–417, 1981.
308. Goldstein EJ, Kirby BD, Finegold SM: *Eikenella corrodens* and pulmonary infections (Letter). Am Rev Respir Dis 120:217, 1979.
309. Goldstein EJ, Kirby BD, Finegold SM: Isolation of *Eikenella corrodens* from pulmonary infections. Am Rev Respir Dis 119:55–58, 1979.
310. Green SL, Oster SE, Tillman TJ: Pneumonia due to *Eikenella corrodens*: Case report. VA Med 110:257–259, 1983.
311. Kentos A, De Vuyst P, Struelens MJ, et al: Lung abscess due to *Eikenella corrodens*: Three cases and review. Eur J Clin Microbiol Infect Dis 14:146–148, 1995.
312. Hardy CC, Roza SN, Isalska B, et al: A traumatic suppurative mediastinitis and pericarditis due to *Eikenella corrodens*. Thorax 43:494–495, 1988.
313. Kelly L, Eliason J: *Eikenella corrodens* keratitis: Case report. Br J Ophthalmol 73:22–24, 1989.
314. Hemady R, Zimmerman A, Katzen BW, et al: Orbital cellulitis caused by *Eikenella corrodens*. Am J Ophthalmol 114:584–588, 1992.
315. Jordan DR, Agapitos RJ, McCunn PD: *Eikenella corrodens* canaliculitis. Am J Ophthalmol 115:823–824, 1993.
316. Page RC: Gingitivis. J Clin Periodontol 13:345–359, 1986.
317. Bissell P, Glew RH, Liland JB: Parotitis associated with *Eikenella corrodens* in a healthy adult. Arch Otolaryngol 109:772–773, 1983.
318. Queen JS, Clegg HW, Council JC, et al: Acute suppurative thyroiditis caused by *Eikenella corrodens*. J Pediatr Surg 23:359–361, 1988.
319. Cheng AF, Man DW, French GL: Thyroid abscess caused by *Eikenella corrodens*. J Infect 16:181–185, 1988.
320. Vichyanond P, Howard CP, Olson LC: *Eikenella corrodens* as a cause of thyroid abscess. Am J Dis Child 137:971–973, 1983.
321. Jeppson KG, Reimer LG: *Eikenella corrodens* chorioamnionitis. Obstet Gynecol 78:503–505, 1991.
322. Drouet E, De Montclos H, Boude M, Denoyel GA: *Eikenella corrodens* and intrauterine contraceptive device (Letter). Lancet 2:1089, 1987.
323. Riche O, Vernet V, Megier P: Bartholin's abscess associated with *Eikenella corrodens* (Letter). Lancet 2:1089, 1987.
324. Landis SJ, Korver J: *Eikenella corrodens* endocarditis: Case report and review of the literature. Can Med Assoc J 128:822–824, 1983.
325. Decker MD, Graham BS, Hunter EB, et al: Endocarditis and infections of intravascular devices due to *Eikenella corrodens*. Am J Med Sci 292:209–212, 1986.
326. Burger AJ, Messineo FC, Schulman P, et al: Mycotic aneurysm of the sinus of Valsalva due to *Eikenella corrodens* bacterial endocarditis. Cardiology 71:220–228, 1984.
327. Celikel TH, Muthuswamy PP: Septic pulmonary emboli secondary to internal jugular vein phlebitis (postanginal sepsis) caused by *Eikenella corrodens*. Am Rev Respir Dis 130:510–513, 1984.
328. Goldstein EJ, Cherubin CE, Corrado ML, et al: Comparative susceptibility of *Yersinia enterocolitica, Eikenella corrodens*, and penicillin-resistant and penicillin-susceptible *Streptococcus pneumoniae* to beta-lactam and alternative antimicrobial agents. Rev Infect Dis 4(Sept–Oct Suppl):S406–S410, 1982.
329. Goldstein EJC, Citron DM: Susceptibility of *Eikenella corrodens* to penicillin, apalcillin, and twelve new cephalosporins. Antimicrob Agents Chemother 26:947–948, 1984.
330. Goldstein EJC, Citron DM, Vagvolgyi AE, et al: Susceptibility of *Eikenella corrodens* to newer and older quinolones. Antimicrob Agents Chemother 30:172–173, 1986.
331. Knapp JS, Johnson SR, Zenilman JM, et al: High-level tetracycline resistance resulting from TetM in strains of *Neisseria* spp., *Kingella denitrificans*, and *Eikenella corrodens*. Antimicrob Agents Chemother 32:765–767, 1988.

Flavobacterium

332. Holmes B, Owen RJ, McMeekin TA: Genus *Flavobacterium* Bergey, Harrison, Breed, Hammer and Huntoon 1923, 97. *In* Krieg NR, Holt JG (eds): Bergey's Manual of Systematic Bacteriology, Vol 1. Baltimore, Williams & Wilkins, 1984, pp 353–360.
333. Greisen K, Loeffelholz M, Purohit A, et al: PCR primers and probes for the 16S rRNA gene of most species of pathogenic bacteria, including bacteria found in cerebrospinal fluid. J Clin Microbiol 32:335–351, 1994.
334. Miyazaki S: Biological activities of partially purified elastase produced by *Flavobacterium meningosepticum*. Microbiol Immunol 28:1083–1092, 1984.
335. Schiff J, Suter LS, Gourley RD, et al: *Flavobacterium* infection as a cause of bacterial endocarditis. Ann Intern Med 55:499–506, 1961.
336. Ferrer C, Jakob E, Pastorino G, et al: Right-sided bacterial endocarditis due to *Flavobacterium odoratum* in a patient on chronic hemodialysis. Am J Nephrol 15:82–84, 1995.
337. Ashdown LR, Previtera S: Community-acquired *Flavobacterium meningosepticum* pneumonia and septicemia. Med J Aust 156:69–70, 1992.
338. Skapek SX, Jones WS, Hoffman KM, Kaskie MR: Sinusitis and bacteremia caused by *Flavobacterium meningosepticum* in a sixteen-year-old with Shwachman Diamond syndrome. Pediatr Infect Dis 11:411–413, 1992.
339. Marnejon T, Watanakunakorn C: *Flavobacterium meningosepticum* septicemia and peritonitis complicating CAPD. Clin Nephrol 38:176–177, 1992.
340. Bucci FA, Holland EJ: *Flavobacterium meningosepticum* keratitis successfully treated with topical trimethoprim/sulfamethoxazole. Am J Ophthalmol 111:116–118, 1991.
341. Abter EIM, Lutwick LI, Torrey MJ, et al: Cellulitis associated with bacteremia due to *Flavobacterium meningosepticum*. Clin Infect Dis 17:929–930, 1993.
342. Stamm WE, Colella JJ, Anderson LL, et al: Indwelling arterial catheters as a source of nosocomial bacteremia: An outbreak caused by *Flavobacterium* species. N Engl J Med 292:1099–1102, 1975.
343. Herman LG, Himmelsbach CK: Detection and control of hospital sources of flavobacteria. Hospitals 39:72–76, 1965.
344. Coyle-Gilchrist MM, Crewe P, Roberts G: *Flavobacterium meningosepticum* in the hospital environment. J Clin Pathol 29:824–826, 1976.
345. du Moulin GC: Airway colonization by *Flavobacterium* in an intensive care unit. J Clin Microbiol 10:155–160, 1979.
346. Olsen H: An epidemiological study of hospital infection with *Flavobacterium meningosepticum*. Dan Med Bull 14:6–9, 1967.
347. Pokrywka M, Viazanko K, Medvick J, et al: A *Flavobacterium meningosepticum* outbreak among intensive care patients. Am J Infect Control 21:139–145, 1993.
348. Aber RC, Wennersten C, Moellering RC: Antimicrobial susceptibility of flavobacteria. Antimicrob Agents Chemother 14:483–487, 1978.
349. Von Graevenitz A, Grehn M: Susceptibility studies on *Flavobacterium* II-b. FEMS Microbiol Lett 2:289–292, 1977.
350. Blahova J, Hupkova M, Krcmery V, Kubonova K: Resistance to and hydrolysis of imipenem in nosocomial strains of *Flavobacterium meningosepticum* (Letter). Eur J Clin Microbiol Infect Dis 13:833, 1994.
351. Olsen H: *Flavobacterium meningosepticum*: A bacteriological, epidemiological and clinical study. Dan Med Bull 17:171–172, 1970.

ANAEROBIC BACTERIA

217

Anaerobic Bacteria

John G. Bartlett

Anaerobic bacteria are the predominant components of the abundant microbial flora of the human body. The role of these microbes as pathogens was well established at the turn of the century, but fastidious growth requirements often limit recovery, and ubiquity on mucocutaneous surfaces often raised doubts about pathogenic potential. During the past three decades, there has been renewed interest in anaerobic infections, particularly with regard to the definition of virulence factors and response to antimicrobial therapy.

Definition of Anaerobes

Anaerobic bacteria are defined as bacteria that grow in the absence of oxygen and fail to show surface growth in 10% carbon dioxide in air. Anaerobes may be further classified by aerotolerance: strict anaerobes cannot tolerate 0.5% oxygen; most clinically important anaerobes (*Bacteroides fragilis, Prevotella melaninogenica* [formerly classified as *Bacteroides melaninogenicus*], and *Fusobacterium nucleatum*) are moderate anaerobes that tolerate 2% to 8% oxygen.

Historical Perspective

Louis Pasteur is credited with the discovery of anaerobes with the successful cultivation of *Clostridium butyricum* in the absence of atmospheric oxygen.[1] Veillon, and subsequently Veillon and Zuber, from the Faculty of Medicine of Paris, published a series of important contributions in the 1890s concerning the role of anaerobic bacteria as the cause of putrid discharge and of infections at multiple anatomic sites, including pelvic infections, purulent arthritis, brain abscess, lung gangrene, and appendicitis.[2]

The classic histotoxic clostridial syndromes, botulism and tetanus, were also well recognized by the end of the 19th century. In fact, by 1890, *Clostridium tetani* organisms were recovered in pure culture, and studies of immunization had begun.[1]

Around the turn of the century, numerous papers in the French and German literature reviewed the role of anaerobic bacteria in diverse types of infections. Many were described as "fusospirochetal infections" characterized by the appearance of fusiform gram-negative rods (presumably *F. nucleatum*) and anaerobic spirochetes. In retrospect, it seems that these infections were probably analogous to those encountered in present-day practice, but the organisms identified generated considerable interest owing to the unique morphologic character of *F. nucleatum* and to the special interest in spirochetes because of the importance at that time of syphilis.

Among the major contributions was the observation by Schottmueller[3] that anaerobic streptococci, rather than group A β-hemolytic streptococci, were actually the predominant pathogens in puerperal sepsis. He postulated that the infection was acquired endogenously from the normal genital flora; this suggested an unconventional pathophysiologic mechanism at a time when contagion was a dominant thesis in the field of infectious diseases.

Contributions by British and American investigators in the early 1900s were modest, but hallmark studies were provided by David Smith[4, 5] from Duke, who studied the bacteriology and pathophysiology of lung abscess in the late 1920s. This investigator noted that the organisms in the abscess walls obtained at autopsy resembled the organisms seen in the gingival crevice, leading to the postulate that aspiration was the mechanism of infection. He subsequently supported this notion by intratracheal inoculation of pyorrhea pus into experimental animals to demonstrate the sequential progression from pneumonitis ("aspiration pneumonia") to lung abscess. In a tedious series of subsequent experiments, he isolated 17 different organisms from the inoculum; he challenged animals with each component alone and then with various microbes in combination. Eventually he showed that four microbial species were required to reproduce lung abscess: anaerobic streptococci, an anaerobic spirochete, an anaerobic vibrio, and the fusiform bacillus. This was one of the first studies of synergy, the demonstration that two or more organisms could produce a pathologic event that could not be reproduced with a simpler inoculum.

Additional important contributions were noted by two American surgeons—Meleney and subsequently Altemeier. Meleney made many important observations about anaerobic bacteria and their role in soft tissue infections and surgical infections. Especially noteworthy is his work with the condition subsequently known as Meleney synergistic gangrene. Altemeier[6] examined the bacteriology of appendicitis in the late 1930s and was able to isolate anaerobic bacteria from 96 of 100 patients. He also noted that putrid discharge was found exclusively in the presence of infections involving anaerobic bacteria and that these were also the only organisms to produce the characteristic odor in vitro.[7]

Interest in anaerobic infections seemed to subside during the first two decades of the antibiotic era. This was the period when there were relatively few clinical reports; most important, clinical laboratories either made no attempt to recover anaerobes or used only a broth culture, which was a problem because anaerobic bacteria were readily overgrown by aerobic bacteria that were also present. When anaerobes were recovered, there was often confusion about their role owing to the multiplicity of bacterial species at the infection site, the failure to use standard methods of identification and classification, and the lack of demonstrable benefit from antimicrobial treatment directed against anaerobes.

Renewed interest in anaerobic infections in the middle and late 1960s reflected three simultaneous developments. First, and most important, was the availability of the GasPak system, in which anaerobiosis could be easily produced with a sealed jar and a commercial packet to which one simply added water. This made isolation of anaerobes relatively easy for most microbiology laboratories. The second important development was that the taxonomic classification of anaerobic bacteria was finally put in order by the outstanding work of many contributors but especially workers from the Virginia Polytechnic Institute. Third, the therapeutic implication of infections involving anaerobes was the subject of many studies in vitro and clinical trials by Sydney Finegold and others; this work initially highlighted the potential role of lincomycin, and subsequent reports dealt with clindamycin, metronidazole, cefoxitin, and then a host of others.[8]

Later work has shown that anaerobic bacteria account for a relatively large number of infections, although the frequency is profoundly influenced by the anatomic site of infection, the mechanism of disease acquisition (exogenous versus endogenous), and clinical features. Detection of anaerobes in the laboratory is also highly variable, depending on the methods used to collect, transport, and process specimens. Martin[9] reviewed the experience at the Mayo Clinic in the early 1970s and found that anaerobic bacteria could be recovered from 49% of 14,839 clinical specimens that were deemed appropriate for anaerobic culture. At that time, *B. fragilis* was second only to *Escherichia coli* as a cause of gram-negative bacillary bacteremia at the Mayo Clinic.[10] Brook[11] reported that anaerobes accounted for 28% of positive blood cultures in two military hospitals from 1973 to 1985. These results have been translated into practical application by the use of drugs directed specifically at anaerobic bacteria. Among the most frequently used drugs in hospital practice are three whose raison d'être is largely anaerobic infections: clindamycin, metronidazole, and cefoxitin. The extensive publicity accorded anaerobic bacteria and anaerobic infections in the 1960s and 1970s resulted in widespread acceptance of these organisms as major pathogens in selected types of infections. This was accompanied by widespread use of appropriate antimicrobials. Anaerobes are neither gone nor forgotten, but their role as major agents of mortality and morbidity is notably reduced by what must be viewed as one of the most successful education campaigns in the history of modern medicine. In 1995, the *B. fragilis* group accounted for only 10 of 510 clinically significant bacteremias at the Johns Hopkins Hospital.

Normal Flora

Most mucocutaneous surfaces of humans harbor a rich indigenous flora composed of aerobic and anaerobic bacteria, the microbial species and concentrations of which vary at different anatomic sites (Table 217–1). Anaerobic bacteria are the dominant forms, often accounting for 99% to 99.9% of the culturable flora.[12] The total number of bacterial species in a single individual probably exceeds 500.

The upper airways, including the oral cavity, nasal passages, oropharynx, and nasopharynx, harbor a complex flora that differs at various sites known as ecologic niches.[12] Concentrations of bacteria in saliva are approximately 10^8 per mL, of which approximately 90% are anaerobic bacteria, the predominant organism being *Veillonella parvula*. Dental plaque includes a complicated matrix of bacteria, including *Streptococcus mutans*, the principal organism implicated in dental caries, but also anaerobic bacteria that have been similarly implicated. The gingival crevice may be likened to the colon in that the oxidation-reduction potential is as low as −300 mV, concentrations of bacteria reach 10^{12} per mL (the geometric limits with which bacteria may occupy space), and anaerobic bacteria account for 99% of the culturable flora. In healthy persons, the sinuses, eustachian tubes, and respiratory passages below the level of the glottis are generally sterile.

TABLE 217–1 ■ Bacteriology of the Normal Flora

ANATOMIC SITE	TOTAL BACTERIA (per mL or g)	ANAEROBE/AEROBE RATIO
Upper airways		
Nasal washings	10^3–10^4	3–5:1
Saliva	10^8–10^9	1:1
Tooth surface	10^{10}–10^{11}	1:1
Gingival crevice	10^{11}–10^{12}	1000:1
Gastrointestinal tract		
Stomach	0–10^5	1:1
Small bowel	10^2–10^4	1:1
Ileum	10^4–10^7	1:1
Colon	10^{11}–10^{12}	1000:1
Female genital tract		
Endocervix	10^7–10^9	1–5:1
Vagina	10^7–10^9	1–5:1

The most important anaerobic potential pathogens found in the upper airways include *Fusobacterium* species, especially *F. nucleatum*; *P. melaninogenica*; the *Prevotella oralis* group; the *Bacteroides ureolyticus* group; and *Peptostreptococcus* species. These are the predominant organisms in anaerobic infections of the oral cavity and anaerobic pleuropulmonary infections.

The gastrointestinal tract shows marked variations in bacteriologic patterns in concentrations at different levels.[13–16] The stomach is protected by gastric acidity (the "gastric barrier") and consequently harbors relatively small numbers of bacteria derived from swallowed salivary bacteria that are predominately gram-positive. The number and types of bacteria increase with loss of gastric acidity (histamine H_2 blockers, antacids, aging), gastric bleeding, gastric obstruction, or gastric carcinoma. In the small bowel, the major mechanism of population control is intestinal motility, so the organisms commonly found are simply passing through. Interruption of this flow, as with a stagnant segment (stricture, obstruction, diverticulum, blind loop), may result in high concentrations of bacteria with a predominance of anaerobes, similar to the flora of the colon.[13] This bacterial overgrowth pattern may be responsible for malabsorption and is best treated with antibiotics directed against anaerobes.

The largest concentrations of anaerobic bacteria are found in the relatively stagnant terminal ileum and colon, where concentrations reach $10^{11.7}$ per g and anaerobic bacteria account for approximately 99.9%.[14, 15] The total number of microbial species is estimated at 300 to 400, but the most important anaerobic bacteria with respect to frequency of isolation from infected sites of intraabdominal sepsis are *Bacteroides* species (principally members of the *B. fragilis* group), *Prevotella* species, *Clostridium* species, and *Peptostreptococcus* species.

The colon flora becomes established after weaning and is thought to remain relatively stable throughout life unless it is disrupted by antibiotic treatment. The role of the flora in health is debated, but many believe that it is important in maintaining an ecologic balance by preventing colonization with exogenous organisms. This protection, known as colonization resistance, is compromised with antibiotic treatment, which presumably enhances the potential for infection with enteric pathogens and colonization by gram-negative bacilli that eventually are the agents of many or most nosocomial infections and bacteremia complicating neutropenia. A logical extension of this thesis is "selective modulation of the fecal flora" by use of antibiotics that are directed against aerobic gram-negative bacilli but preserve the anaerobic component of the flora in an effort to prevent colonization by resistant strains.[17] Antibiotics may have a major impact in the normal colonic flora on the basis of multiple contributing factors, including activity versus components of the flora, concentrations (reflecting enterohepatic circulation or failed absorption), susceptibility to inactivating enzymes such as β-lactamases, and activity in the environmental conditions of the gut.

The flora of the female genital tract is far less stable than that of the gastrointestinal tract. Concentrations of bacteria in the vagina or cervix average approximately 10^8 per mL during reproductive years.[18–20] There is considerable variation (10^5 to 10^{11} per mL); simultaneous cultures of material from the cervix and vagina show unique bacteriologic patterns, and sequential cultures show considerable shifts at various stages of the menstrual cycle that may be hormonally influenced.[18–21] Approximately 50% are anaerobic bacteria, but there is considerable variation, and approximately 20% of women have no detectable anaerobes or at least low concentrations. The dominant organisms are aerobic, microaerobic, and anaerobic lactobacilli; the dominant anaerobes are *Lactobacillus, Peptostreptococcus*, and *Bacteroides* species, including *Prevotella bivia* (formerly *Bacteroides bivius*). *B. fragilis* is found in only 2% to 10%. Studies of premenarchal or postmenopausal genital tract flora show a substantial difference in the flora, with an especially high yield of coliforms.[22] Other factors that appear to influence the bacteriologic findings in the genital tract include pregnancy, antibiotic therapy, and gynecologic surgery.[23–26] The role of the genital tract flora in maintaining homeostasis is not well studied, although antibiotic treatment clearly predisposes to vaginal candidiasis; bacterial vaginosis (*Gardnerella* vaginitis or nonspecific vaginitis) appears to reflect dysbiosis of the genital tract flora in which concentrations of lactobacilli are notably reduced, the dominant organisms are anaerobic bacteria, vaginal effluent contains a predominance of the short chain volatile fatty acids produced by anaerobes, and current therapeutic recommendations are restricted to drugs directed against anaerobes (metronidazole and clindamycin).[19, 27]

The skin flora contains large numbers of anaerobic bacteria, the predominant organisms being *Propionibacterium acnes* and to a lesser extent other species of *Propionibacterium* and *Peptostreptococcus* species.[27] The skin flora of the perineum, and to some extent of the lower extremities, often contains the usual components of the colon flora. *P. acnes* and *Propionibacterium granulosum* colonize hair follicles and sebaceous glands, where concentrations correlate with sebum content.

Pathophysiology

Anaerobic infections are usually endogenous, meaning that they originate from the host's own flora. The only important exceptions are some of the histotoxic clostridial syndromes, such as botulism, *Clostridium perfringens* food poisoning, enteritis necroticans, tetanus, and gas gangrene. Even this tabulation is somewhat deceptive, because many or most cases of *Clostridium difficile*–associated diarrhea or colitis, most cases of gas gangrene, and some cases of tetanus appear to involve clostridia that are residents of the host's normal colonic flora.

The usual pathophysiologic mechanism for anaerobic infection is a breach in the mucocutaneous defense barrier resulting in displacement of the normal flora. This simplistic mechanism applies to the great majority of anaerobic infections encountered in clinical practice. Host defense mechanisms are obviously important, but patients with neutropenia, defective complement systems, previous splenectomy, congenital or acquired defects in humoral immunity, defective cell-mediated immunity, advanced human immunodeficiency virus infection, cancer chemotherapy, or corticosteroid treatment infrequently acquire infections involving anaerobic bacteria. The exception is infections associated with defects of mucocutaneous barriers, such as carcinoma with obstruction, mucositis, perirectal lesions, or compromised consciousness with aspiration.

Virulence Factors

One of the most important observations to lend credibility to microbes as pathogens is the identification of specific mechanisms or virulence factors that account for pathologic events. Such studies have been applied to anaerobes with use of traditional methods to detect capsules, toxins, and other virulence factors in vitro and in vivo.

One of the more common approaches to the study of anaerobes has been investigations of the concept of synergy, reflecting the fact that most such infections are polymicrobial. The work of David Smith was alluded to earlier; this showed that four anaerobic species were necessary to produce lung abscess in experimental animals.[4, 5] Meleney's studies of synergistic gangrene are another good example of the interaction between microbial species, in this case *Staphylococcus aureus* and an anaerobic or microaerophilic streptococcus.[28] These organisms were frequently found at the infection site, but inoculation of either in pure culture failed to reproduce typical lesions; the disease known as Meleney synergistic gangrene could be reproduced only when both microbes were injected. Subsequent studies showed that *S. aureus* produced a collagenase that permitted the anaerobic streptococcus to invade tissue as an explanation of in vivo observations. Altemeier[29] also demonstrated that multiple microbial species produced more extensive disease with intraabdominal challenge. Despite these studies suggesting synergy, results of other investigations in experimental animals have not always supported the concept. More important, the identification of specific virulence factors has increased interest in these organisms as legitimate pathogens without the necessity for multiple bacterial species.

The most clearly identified virulence factors for anaerobic bacteria are the exotoxins produced by clostridial species: that of *Clostridium botulinum* and *C. tetani*, the most potent microbial toxin known; the two toxins of *C. difficile* that are only about 100 times less active according to mouse lethality tests; and the 11 toxins produced by *C. perfringens* (as well as many other clostridial species), including 5 that are lethal to experimental animals. Clinical expression of these histotoxic clostridia syndromes depends on the site of toxin production and the physiologic effects of the toxin.

Anaerobic gram-negative bacteria, like all gram-negative bacteria, contain lipopolysaccharide that can be extracted from the envelope, but the biologic activity of this endotoxin (mouse lethality assays, the chick embryo death test, and the Shwartzman reaction) is 100 to 1000 times less than that of lipopolysaccharide from Enterobacteriaceae.[30] The lipopolysaccharide of *B. fragilis* is structurally similar to the lipid A of *E. coli* but lacks a phosphate group on the C-4 of the nonreducing amino sugar and has a limited number of monosaccharides. These structural differences appear to explain the weak endotoxicity.[30] Other anaerobic gram-negative bacteria, such as fusobacteria, are thought to contain endotoxin with more biologic activity.

One of the most extensively studied virulence properties of *B. fragilis* is the capsular polysaccharide that promotes abscess formation by resistance to opsonophagocytosis. This polysaccharide is capable of inducing abscesses in the absence of viable bacteria.[31–33] There are actually a family of *B. fragilis* polysaccharides composed of oligosaccharide repeating units possessing sugars with positively charged free amino groups and negatively charged carboxyl or phosphonate groups. These positively and negatively charged groups mediate the capacity to induce abscess formation.[34] The capsule also serves as an immunogen that confers protection to experimental animals on repeated challenge, a protective effect that appears to rely on cellular rather than humoral mechanisms.[33, 35]

Another virulence factor of *B. fragilis* that is shared by many other anaerobic bacteria is the production of short chain fatty acids that inhibit phagocytic killing at low pH values.[36, 37] Short chain volatile fatty acids are metabolic products of anaerobic bacteria that are used to classify these organisms, and some, such as butyric or succinic acid, are probably responsible for the putrid odor noted at the bedside and in the laboratory with growth of anaerobic bacteria. The best studied as a possible virulence factor is succinic acid, which inhibits phagocytic killing, an effect that is pH dependent (increased inhibition in acid conditions as found in abscesses) and nonselective in the sense that all microbial species are protected.[36, 37]

Host Defenses

Studies of host resistance to *B. fragilis* began in the mid-1970s with the observation that fecal isolates were susceptible to killing by serum. Subsequent work indicated that clinical isolates of *B. fragilis* were substantially more resistant, and heat inactivation suggested that this effect was mediated by complement.[38, 39] Of the various species of the *B. fragilis* group, *B. fragilis* is the most resistant to the bactericidal action of serum.[39, 40] Clinical isolates require opsonization with serum before ingestion and killing by neutrophils[41]; the alternative pathway is the major complement mechanism for opsonization by all species of the *B. fragilis* group.[42] Natural antibodies in serum directed against these bacteria belong primarily to the immunoglobulin M class[43] and are directed against strain-specific antigenic determinants in the outer membrane complex.[44] The polysaccharide capsule, as expected, influences opsonization and phagocytosis so that natural variants lacking capsules are more susceptible.[45]

Biphasic Disease Model

Numerous animal models have been used to examine the pathophysiologic mechanism of anaerobic infections, but one of the most extensively studied during the past three decades has been the rat model of intraabdominal sepsis.[31, 46] Rats are challenged with an intraperitoneal implant of fecal contents with an adjuvant in an effort to simulate the septic complications of colonic perforation. The initial phase of the infection is characterized by generalized peritonitis, followed by the second phase characterized by abscess formation. Initial work showed a 43% mortality rate, all deaths occurring during the first 4 days after challenge. Abscesses were defined as loculated collections with the characteristic outer collagen wall, an interface of polymorphonuclear cells, and a central area of necrotic debris and bacteria. Lesions satisfying this definition were initially detected 5 days after challenge, and all animals sacrificed 7 days or more after challenge had typical abscesses; follow-up evaluations of untreated animals at 3 months showed that some developed large abscesses and others had spontaneous resolution.

Studies of this animal model were designed to distinguish the role of various bacteria by use of quantitative cultures, antimicrobial probes (such as gentamicin for its selective activity against coliforms and clindamycin for its selective activity against anaerobes), and monomicrobial challenge with the organisms recovered from infected sites. This work supported the role of *E. coli* as the major pathogen in the initial phase of infection characterized by generalized peritonitis, bacteremia, and death. Supporting evidence was the presence of *E. coli* in 95% of blood cultures obtained during the first 5 days after challenge; this organism was the numerically dominant one in peritoneal exudate; gentamicin prevented the early mortality; and this was the only isolate that reproduced acute mortality with monomicrobial challenge. *B. fragilis* assumed unique importance in the second phase of the infection characterized by abscess formation. The role of this microbe in abscess formation was supported by evidence that it was the numerically dominant microbe in abscesses, clindamycin prevented this complication, and it was the only organism that caused abscesses with monomicrobial challenge. Further testimony to the "abscessogenic potential" of *B. fragilis* was the demonstration of typical abscesses after challenge with the capsular polysaccharide of *B. fragilis*.[31–33]

The conclusion is that both coliforms and anaerobic bacteria represent pathogens in this model of intraabdominal sepsis, although they appear to be responsible for different biologic events as the infection evolves through its two stages. Although *E. coli* was the principal coliform in the inoculum in this work, other coliforms could be equally devastating—effects that may well reflect the biologic activity of endotoxin shared by these organisms. Similarly, it is now known that many members of the *B. fragilis* group, as well as some in the *P. melaninogenica* group, also possess polysaccharide capsules and produce short chain fatty acids. The practical application of these data is that antimicrobial therapy should be directed against both coliforms and anaerobes, a thesis that is well supported in clinical studies.[47, 48]

Clues to Anaerobic Infections

Clinical clues to the probable presence of anaerobic bacteria at infected sites are summarized in Table 217–2. Infections that occur in continuity with mucosal surfaces where anaerobic bacteria compose the normal flora often involve these microbes. In most cases, an associated condition—oral or dental infection, intraabdominal sepsis, infections of the female genital tract—has caused a breach in the barrier defense mechanisms.

Infections associated with tissue necrosis and abscess formation are often due to anaerobic bacteria. The specific role of virulence factors such as capsular polysaccharide and short chain fatty acids to possibly account for this association is summarized previously. Thus, anaerobic bacteria are reported as the dominant isolates in abscesses at virtually all anatomic sites, including cerebral, dental, peritonsillar, lung, intraabdominal, tuboovarian, prostatic, and cutaneous abscess.

The putrid odor of infections or discharges is considered diagnostic of anaerobic infection. This tends to be a relatively late feature of most anaerobic infections and is seen in approximately a third to half of patients. The chemical basis for the odor is not well established, but it presumably reflects the metabolic products of anaerobic bacteria, including volatile fatty acids such as succinic and butyric acid, and methylmercaptan. As noted, these short chain fatty acids are used

TABLE 217–2 ■ Clues to Probability of Anaerobic Bacteria at Infection Site

Infection adjacent to surfaces that normally harbor anaerobes as normal flora
Infections characterized by abscess formation or tissue necrosis
Infections associated with putrid odor
Infections characterized by gas formation
Gram stain or exudate showing polymicrobial flora or organisms with morphologic features of anaerobes
Failure to cultivate likely pathogens from infected site, possibly because of failure to perform anaerobic cultures, suboptimal anaerobic microbiologic technique, or prior use of antimicrobial agents active against anaerobes
Classic features of toxins produced by histotoxic clostridia: tetanus, botulism, *Clostridium perfringens* food poisoning, gas gangrene, *Clostridium difficile*–induced diarrhea or colitis, enteritis necroticans
Infections that, by prior experience, usually involve anaerobic bacteria

to identify anaerobic bacteria; they may represent virulence factors, and direct detection of these acids in exudate by gas-liquid chromatography may be used as an early clue to the presence of anaerobes.[49]

Gas in the tissue is another clue to the presence of anaerobic bacteria, but it is not considered diagnostic because occasional aerobic bacteria produce gas.[50] Gas may be detected by palpation, radiography, or scanning techniques. This may reflect not only gas production by microbes but also air introduced during irrigations or other manipulations, such as the release of carbon dioxide with hydrogen peroxide.

Infections involving a polymicrobial flora are often anaerobic or represent mixtures of both obligate and facultative anaerobic bacteria. This may be easily suspected when Gram stain examination of exudate shows multiple different morphotypes at infected sites. This examination may also indicate the unique morphologic features of many anaerobes, especially *Bacteroides* species, *Fusobacterium* species, and clostridia; by contrast, *Peptostreptococcus*, the other major genus of clinically significant anaerobes, cannot be distinguished from aerobic or microaerophilic gram-positive cocci on the basis of Gram stain appearance.

The failure to grow likely pathogens in the laboratory often serves as a clue to the presence of relatively fastidious bacteria, including anaerobes. This may reflect failure to obtain an appropriate specimen for anaerobic culture, failure of the laboratory to use appropriate microbiologic techniques, or the impact of prior antimicrobial therapy. With regard to the last, it is well established that treatment with clindamycin, metronidazole, and possibly other antimicrobial agents rapidly modifies the culturable flora from infection sites. Perhaps the best clue to the presence of anaerobic bacteria is simply the clinical features of the infection based on a century of published data to document microbial associations.

Microbiologic Methods

Microbiologist and clinician must work together to achieve optimal recovery of anaerobic bacteria, giving proper attention to collection, transport, and processing of specimens.[51] Anaerobic bacteriology is relatively expensive because of the often tedious and technically demanding additional laboratory work required and the multiplicity of bacteria found at infected sites. In an era of cost restraint, it is likely that emphasis on anaerobic bacteriology will be reduced, technical expertise will decrease, and management strategies ("clinical pathways") including antibiotic decisions will be increasingly empirical.

Specimen Selection

Specimens appropriate for anaerobic culture must be devoid of the normal flora. Optimal specimens are normally sterile body fluids and aspirates or biopsy material from normally sterile sites (Table 217–3). On occasion, the problem of contamination may be obviated by quantitative cultures, al-

TABLE 217–3 ■ Specimens Appropriate for Anaerobic Culture

SPECIMEN AND COLLECTION METHOD	COMMENT
Normally sterile body fluids	Includes blood, pleural fluid, peritoneal fluid, bile, cerebrospinal fluid.
Abscess contents	Needle aspirates are preferred.
Wound*	Exudate, preferably collected by syringe aspiration using care to decontaminate surface areas.
Pulmonary	
Pleural fluid	Results of growth in broth cultures only are difficult to interpret.
Transtracheal aspirate*	
Transthoracic needle aspirate	
Thoracotomy specimen	
Bronchoscopic aspirate*	Requires double-lumen catheter brush with distal occluding plug or bronchoalveolar lavage, each combined with quantitative culture.
Tracheostomy aspirate*	Validity is not well established; one third of patients without evidence of infection yield anaerobes, and quantitative cultures may be required.
Urinary tract	Rare source of anaerobic infections.
Suprapubic aspirate	
Female genital tract	
Culdocentesis	Experience is varied, seldom done.
Specimens obtained above pelvic reflection at surgery or laparoscopy	
Transabdominal needle aspirates of uterus	
Intrauterine brush using double catheter with a distal occluding plug*	Requires quantitative culture.
Intraabdominal	
Aspirates, biopsy specimens	Specimen must be devoid of the gastrointestinal flora.
Small bowel aspirate	Quantitative culture is necessary to detect overgrowth syndromes.
Oral-dental	
Aspirate of closed spaces	Collected from endodontal canal and preferably transported in conditions that preserve hydration and anaerobiosis.
Paper point specimen	
Paranasal sinuses	
Aspirate using catheter or syringe*	Plastic catheter inserted into depths of sinus track is preferred.
Middle-ear aspirate	Optimal specimens are obtained with intact tympanic membrane.
Soft tissue	
Aspirate of closed spaces, e.g., abscesses	
Biopsies using 3-mm dermal punch*	

*Because contamination with normal flora is common, broth cultures are inappropriate and interpretation is facilitated with quantitative or semiquantitative culture.

though most laboratories do not provide this service. As a general rule, liquid or tissue specimens are preferred; swab specimens should be avoided.

Specimen Transport

The optimal way to transport specimens is immediate delivery to permit prompt microbiologic processing. A variety of specialized transport devices are available that provide an oxygen-free environment, including commercially available anaerobic transport vials. These generally contain an atmosphere of oxygen-free gas, such as a mixture of carbon dioxide, hydrogen, and nitrogen; also included in most is an indicator such as resazurin, to document anaerobic conditions, and a reducing agent, such as cysteine, to eliminate small amounts of oxygen that are inadvertently introduced. Tissue specimens may be placed in a sterile tube flushed with carbon dioxide; if the tube is held upright with the stopper removed, the heavier carbon dioxide will exclude oxygen until the stopper is replaced. Although they are theoretically attractive, there is little evidence that such techniques are actually necessary. A study of survival of anaerobic bacteria in clinical specimens using quantitated culture techniques of exudate left for various periods showed nearly complete qualitative and quantitative recovery of anaerobic bacteria with exposure to room air for periods of up to 48 to 72 hours.[52] A possible limitation of this study is that the specimens contained relatively large volumes of exudate, but the experiment does suggest that most clinically significant anaerobes survive for extended periods despite exposure to air. Swabs represent an important exception, although here it appears that drying may be more important than oxygen sensitivity. When swab specimens are necessary, the clinician is advised to place the swab in a specially prepared prereduced and anaerobically sterilized semisolid medium such as Cary-Blair medium.

Laboratory Processing

Direct microscopic examination is an important clue to the probable presence of anaerobic bacteria and an important method of quality assurance of microbiology culture technique. Three systems are generally advocated for anaerobic culture: the anaerobic jar (GasPak, evacuation-replacement, and Bio-Bags); the anaerobic glovebox; and prereduced, anaerobically sterilized roll tubes (the Virginia Polytechnic Institute system). Several studies indicate comparable results in the yield of anaerobes from clinical specimens with these various systems.[51] Consequently, the decision of which system to use depends on previous training of personnel, the volume of specimens, and the resources of the laboratory. Many clinical laboratories have found the GasPak jar method particularly convenient, although the jar should remain inviolate for at least 48 hours after the GasPak has been generated. An alternative, more convenient method for one or two plates is Bio-Bags. Anaerobic chambers may be preferred when a large number of specimens are processed. Quality assurance with anaerobic technology indicates that the major discrepancies in most clinical laboratories are (1) failure to use the initial Gram-stained specimen to ensure that culture results account for all recognized morphotypes; (2) improper use of anaerobic jars, especially by opening before 48 hours has elapsed; (3) failure to use plate media that have not been maintained in a reduced environment; (4) premature discarding of plates; (5) inadequate picking of colonies from primary isolation plates; and (6) inadequate selective and nonselective plate media or excessive dependence on broth cultures.

Identification

The major clinically significant anaerobes are summarized in Table 217–4. This includes reference to prior taxonomic classification. Most clinical laboratories should be able to identify a majority of these organisms; however, peptostreptococci, which account for approximately 25% of all anaerobic isolates in most microbiology laboratories, rarely merit speciation, except for research studies, because these organisms lack distinctive virulence properties and appear to be susceptible to the same antimicrobial agents. The non–spore-forming gram-positive bacilli require chromatographic analysis for genus designation and extensive biochemical testing for speciation. With the exception of *Actinomyces*, these organisms have minimal documented pathogenic potential, and cursory identification is generally adequate. A rational approach is to separate *Propionibacterium*, a common contaminant, from the others simply by a catalase test and indole reaction. Clostridia are identified by spores seen on Gram stain examination or by survival with exposure to ethanol for 30 minutes or to 80°C for 10 minutes. Extensive biochemical testing is required for speciation, which generally is unnecessary but desirable in selected cases and for detection of the most clinically significant and common isolates, *C. perfringens, Clostridium ramosum*, and occasionally others such as *C. difficile*. The *B. fragilis* group (*B. fragilis, B. thetaiotaomicron, B. distasonis, B. ovatus*, and *B. vulgatus*) is distinguished by the ability to grow in the presence of 20% bile, and most are catalase-positive. Pigmented *Prevotella* species (*P. melaninogenica, P. corporis, P. denticola, P. intermedia, P. loescheii*, and *P. nigrescens*) are distinguished by the production of brown or black pigment, although this may take a week or more and may require rabbit blood agar medium; this is a clinically important group of anaerobes that are relatively fastidious, and frequency of recovery provides testimony to anaerobic expertise. Fusobacteria are also relatively fastidious, are distinguished from *Bacteroides* species by susceptibility to the 1000-μg kanamycin disk, are indole-positive, are nonmotile, produce butyric acid, and show distinctive morphologic features on Gram stain. The major anaerobic gram-positive cocci of clinical importance are peptostreptococci.

TABLE 217–4 ■ Clinically Important Anaerobes Seen with Greatest Frequency

GRAM-NEGATIVE BACTERIA

Bacteroides fragilis group: *B. fragilis, B. thetaiotaomicron, B. distasonis, B. ovatus, B. vulgatus*
Pigmented *Prevotella* (formerly *Bacteroides*): *P. intermedia, P. melaninogenica, P. corporis, P. denticola, P. loescheii, P. nigrescens*
Prevotella (other): *P. bivia* (formerly *B. bivius*), *P. disiens* (formerly *B. disiens*), *P. oralis* (formerly *B. oralis*)
Porphyromonas asaccharolytica (formerly *B. asaccharolyticus*)
Fusobacterium: F. nucleatum, F. necrophorum, F. varium
Bilophila: B. wadsworthia

GRAM-POSITIVE COCCI

Peptostreptococcus: P. intermedius, P. micros, P. anaerobius, P. magnus, P. asaccharolyticus, P. prevotii

GRAM-POSITIVE SPORE-FORMING BACILLI

Clostridium: C. perfringens, C. difficile, C. sporogenes, C. sordellii, C. septicum, C. tertium, C. ramosum, C. novyi, C. histolyticum, C. bifermentans, C. innocuum, C. tetani, C. botulinum

GRAM-POSITIVE NON–SPORE-FORMING BACILLI

Propionibacterium: P. acnes
Eubacterium: E. lentum
Bifidobacterium: B. dentium
Actinomyces: A. israelii, A. naeslundii, A. odontolyticus, A. viscosus

Anaerobic Bacteria at Infection Sites

Anaerobes have been encountered in infections at virtually all anatomic sites, although the frequency of recovery is highly variable and the bacteriologic patterns depend largely on the flora at adjacent mucocutaneous sites (Table 217–5).

Central Nervous System Infections

Pyogenic intracranial infections that commonly involve anaerobic bacteria include cerebral and epidural abscess and subdural empyema. Meningitis rarely involves these bacteria.

TABLE 217–5 ■ Recovery Rates of Anaerobic Bacteria in Infectious Disease

DISEASE CATEGORY	CASES STUDIED (NO.)	ANAEROBES RECOVERED Number	%
Head and neck			
Nontraumatic brain abscess[53]	18	16	89
Subdural empyema[54]	84	24	29
Chronic sinusitis[55]	83	44	53
Chronic otitis[56]	68	35	51
Perimandibular space infection[57, 58]	31	29	94
	21	21	100
Peritonsillar abscess[59, 60]	30	23	76
	45	38	84
Dental abscess[61]	10	9	90
Chest infections			
Aspiration pneumonia[62, 63]	70	61	87
	47	29	62
Lung abscess[64, 65]	57	53	93
	26	22	85
Empyema[66, 67]	83	63	76
	37	23	62
Bronchiectasis[68]	18	17	94
Unselected patients[69, 70]	89	29	33
	74	16	22
Hospital-acquired pneumonia[71]	159	56	35
Intraabdominal sepsis[72]	759	627	83
Abscess or peritonitis[73, 74]	72	68	94
	64	52	81
Appendiceal abscess[6]	100	96	96
Liver abscess[75]	40	21	52
Female genital tract			
Miscellaneous types[76–78]	33	33	100
	91	67	74
	50	36	72
Pelvic abscess[79]	25	22	88
Pelvic inflammatory disease[80–82]	54	13	25
	74	57	77
	70	53	78
Septic abortion[83]	29	20	69
Postpartum endometritis[84]	128	49	38
Soft tissue			
Wound infection after elective colon surgery[85]	19	18	95
Postappendectomy wound[86]	65	15	79
Cutaneous abscess[87]	135	81	60
Pilonidal abscess[88]	41	36	88
Perirectal abscess[88]	74	57	77
Diabetic foot ulcer[89]	19	12	63
Nonclostridial crepitant cellulitis[90]	57	9	75
Pilonidal sinus[91]	45	33	73
Breast abscess[92, 93]	52	41	79
Necrotizing synergistic cellulitis[94]	57	51	89
Paronychia[95]	32	23	72
Bite wound infections[96]	34	18	53
Bacteremia			
All blood cultures[97]	4659	296	6
Intraabdominal sepsis[85]	8	7	88
Septic abortion[98]	76	48	63
Decubitus ulcers[99]	62	10	16
Endometritis[84]	28	15	54

The most extensively studied is cerebral abscess, which is usually a polymicrobial infection with some variation in bacteriologic patterns, depending on the associated condition. One of the first careful bacteriologic studies of nontraumatic brain abscesses in which anaerobic cultures were performed systematically showed anaerobes in 16 of 18 cases.[53] *B. fragilis* is usually present when the associated condition is a middle-ear or mastoid infection with local extension, usually to the temporal lobe; coliforms, *Pseudomonas aeruginosa*, various streptococci, and other anaerobic bacteria are often present as well.[100] When sinusitis is the source of the infection, the usual bacteriologic pattern includes a variety of anaerobic bacteria other than *B. fragilis* and streptococci, especially *Streptococcus milleri*. Metastatic abscesses tend to involve polymicrobial flora like that at the site of origin, most often a pulmonary infection and less frequently intraabdominal sepsis. The exception is cerebral abscess associated with endocarditis or cyanotic heart disease, in which there is usually a single microbe, either *Staphylococcus* or an anaerobic or microaerophilic *Streptococcus*. Occasional cerebral abscesses involve *Actinomyces* species. Brain abscess associated with neurosurgery or head trauma is usually due to a diverse array of predominantly aerobic bacteria. Other central nervous system infections likely to involve anaerobes are subdural empyema and epidural empyema.[54]

Antibiotic recommendations reflect these bacteriologic patterns. In cases in which anaerobes are suspected or established pathogens, good results have been achieved with metronidazole, which produces demonstrably high levels within the cerebral abscess, and clinical outcome is good.[100] However, metronidazole is ill-advised as a single agent owing to its inactivity against aerobic streptococci, especially *S. milleri*, gram-negative aerobes, and *Actinomyces* species. For this reason, metronidazole is often combined with penicillin or a third-generation cephalosporin. Neurosurgical drainage, once the mainstay of treatment for cerebral abscess, has now been largely supplanted by medical management owing to improved evaluation techniques using computed tomography and magnetic resonance imaging and by more appropriate selection of antimicrobial agents.[101]

Infections of the Upper Airways

Anaerobic bacteria are involved in a variety of infections of the oral cavity and adjacent structures. Bacteriologic patterns reflect the flora at these sites, with the dominant isolates being the *Bacteroides oralis* group, the pigmented *Prevotella* (formerly *B. melaninogenicus* group), *Porphyromonas asaccharolytica*, *Fusobacterium* species, *Peptostreptococcus*, microaerophilic streptococci, and aerobic streptococci.

Nearly all clinically important dental infections are likely to involve anaerobes, including pulpitis (endodontal infection),[102] periapical or dental abscess, and perimandibular space infections.[57, 58] These three infections usually represent a continuum. The initial lesion is endodontal; the infection progresses to the periapical region, and then it may extend through the mandible to involve the potential spaces created by insertions of fascia along the mandible. The perimandibular spaces are contiguous, although infections are usually localized to specific anatomic sites adjacent to the portal of entry. The usual presentation is pain and swelling, and the mainstay of therapy is surgical drainage. Life-threatening forms of perimandibular infections that are important to recognize clinically include Ludwig angina and Lemierre syndrome. Ludwig angina is an infection characterized by bilateral involvement of the sublingual and submandibular spaces that causes swelling of the base of the tongue and potential airway compromise. Lemierre syndrome is an infection involving the posterior compartment of the lateral pharyngeal space complicated by suppurative thrombophlebitis of the jugular vein with *Fusobacterium* bacteremia and metastatic abscesses, primarily to the lung.[103, 104]

Infections of the gingival crevice and gums, including gingivitis, periodontitis, and pyorrhea, usually involve anaerobic bacteria.[105] An infrequent but distinct form is necrotizing ulcerative gingivitis, sometimes known as Vincent angina or trench mouth. This is a relatively fulminant infection associated with severe pain, tissue destruction, pseudomembrane formation, and putrid discharge. The bacterial agent is not well established, although anaerobic spirochetes have been detected within tissue at the advanced edge of inflammation, and antibiotic treatment directed against anaerobes is necessary. A possibly related necrotizing infection of the oral mucous membranes is cancrum oris, or noma, characterized by destruction of soft tissue and bone. It occurs most frequently in children with malnutrition or systemic disease; this is usually fatal in the absence of intensive antibiotic therapy.

Anaerobic bacteria are also frequently implicated in chronic sinusitis,[55] chronic otitis media,[56] and mastoiditis but play a minimal role in acute otitis media or acute sinusitis. Peritonsillar abscesses are frequently caused by anaerobic bacteria, especially *Peptostreptococcus* species, which appear to be more common than *Streptococcus pyogenes*.[59, 60] Human bites—and, to a lesser extent, animal bites—often involve anaerobic bacteria.[96] These include the clenched fist injury that is the equivalent of a human bite. Also important are *Eikenella corrodens* and aerobic and microaerophilic streptococci from the oral flora; *S. aureus* from the recipient's skin may also be involved.

Penicillin was previously regarded as the drug of choice for oral and dental infections involving anaerobic bacteria[106]; however, increasing resistance has been noted among these organisms, principally with β-lactamase production by *Bacteroides, Prevotella*, and *Fusobacterium* species.[107] Many authorities continue to believe that penicillins, such as penicillin G, penicillin V, ampicillin, or amoxicillin, are preferred agents, especially for oral treatment of less serious infections. For infections that are more serious or prove refractory to penicillin, the alternative oral regimens include clindamycin, metronidazole, metronidazole plus penicillin, and amoxicillin-clavulanate. Macrolides, fluoroquinolones, trimethoprim-sulfamethoxazole, tetracyclines, oral cephalosporins, and antistaphylococcal penicillin are not active or are less predictably active.[106]

Pleuropulmonary Infections

Anaerobic bacteria are relatively common—and frequently overlooked—pathogens in the lower airways. The usual mechanism is aspiration of oral and dental secretions, which results in aspiration pneumonitis, which may be an indolent form of pneumonia but may also simulate other forms of acute bacterial pneumonia, including pneumococcal pneumonia.[108] Patients seen at this early or pneumonitis stage of infection rarely have putrid sputum and may well be classified as having atypical pneumonia, because no likely pathogen is recovered with routine aerobic culture of the expectorated specimen. The usual clues to the likelihood of anaerobes are the features seen in the later stages of disease, when there is likely to be putrid discharge and necrosis of tissue with abscess formation or empyema. Another clue to anaerobic involvement with chronic infections is the indolent course of many of these infections. Patients often present with weight loss, anemia, and chronic pulmonary complaints, all features that are relatively uncommon in pneumonia due to most aerobic bacteria other than mycobacteria.[108]

The frequency of anaerobic pulmonary infections was studied most extensively in the period from 1970 through the early 1980s, when transtracheal aspiration was a common method of obtaining uncontaminated specimens from the lower airways. This work showed that 60% to 90% of cases of aspiration pneumonia, lung abscess, and empyema involved anaerobic bacteria.[62–67, 108] Studies of nosocomial pneumonia also showed a 35% frequency of anaerobes, although in contrast to community-acquired cases, these tended to be mixed infections involving aerobic gram-negative bacilli or *S. aureus* as well.[71] There are two studies in which an attempt was made to define the role of anaerobes in unselected patients with community-acquired pneumonia; one used transtracheal aspiration with a yield of 33%,[69] and the other used fiberoptic bronchoscopy with quantitative cultures and showed a yield of 22%.[70] These studies suggest that anaerobic pulmonary infections are substantially more common than is generally appreciated.

Bacteriologic patterns in anaerobic pulmonary infection are similar to those described for oral and dental infections (Table 217–6). Many reports from the 1970s showed that *B. fragilis* was recovered in 15% to 20% of cases.[62–67, 108] This finding was somewhat surprising, because studies of the oral flora, the presumed source of the inoculum, have not observed *B. fragilis*. More recent findings suggest that *B. fragilis* was identified erroneously and that other penicillin-resistant *Bacteroides* species presumably account for the discrepancies.[108, 109]

With regard to therapeutic recommendations, clinicians from the 1950s and 1960s often did not know what pathogen was involved in aspiration pneumonia or lung abscess, but penicillin became widely recognized as the drug of choice for both conditions.[110–114] Somewhat paradoxically, when the pathogens were identified by the combination of transtracheal aspiration and meticulous anaerobic bacteriologic tests, considerable controversy developed about the preferred

TABLE 217–6 ■ Bacteriology of Anaerobic Infections of the Lung

MEASURE	BARTLETT[108]	MARINA ET AL[109]
Period reviewed	1968–1975	1976–1991
Cases	193	110
Total anaerobic isolates	461	404
Average anaerobic isolates per case	2.4	3.5
Former *Bacteroides* species		
B. fragilis group	38*	18
Pigmented *Prevotella*	76*	63
Nonpigmented *Prevotella*	—	40
B. ureolyticus	—	23
Other	37	38
Fusobacterium nucleatum	56	34
Fusobacterium necrophorum	2	6
Peptostreptococci	87	39
Peptococci	39*	—
Gram-positive bacilli		
Clostridium species	18	12
Eubacterium species	18	22
Actinomyces	5	19
Lactobacillus species	8	22
Propionibacterium species	10	9
Bifidobacterium species	9	4
Veillonella	23	18

*Numbers refer to the number of isolates. Differences in the two series reflect, in part, taxonomic changes and variations in microbiologic methods. In the earlier series,[108] the "black-pigmented *Bacteroides* species" were reported as *B. melaninogenicus*, whereas the later series reported these according to reclassification as *B. melaninogenicus, B. intermedius*, and *B. asaccharolyticus*. These organisms are now classified as pigmented *Prevotella*, including *P. melaninogenica* and *P. intermedia*. For gram-positive cocci, the clinically important organisms formerly classified as *Peptococcus* have been reclassified as *Peptostreptococcus*.

treatment, because 20% to 25% of patients harbored penicillin-resistant anaerobes. Two comparative trials of large doses of intravenous penicillin versus clindamycin for patients with anaerobic lung abscesses have subsequently shown clear superiority for clindamycin in terms of clinical response rates, time to defervescence, and time to elimination of putrid sputum.[112, 113] Most authorities now consider clindamycin to be the drug of choice for lung abscess and aspiration pneumonia. Another option sometimes advocated is metronidazole plus penicillin, although metronidazole as a single agent is ill-advised in view of results of clinical trials showing a therapeutic failure rate of approximately 50%, presumably due to inactivity against aerobic and microaerophilic streptococci.[108, 115] β-Lactam–β-lactamase inhibitor combinations are likely to be effective, although the published experience is limited.

Intraabdominal Sepsis

Infections within the abdominal cavity may be classified as monomicrobial or polymicrobial, depending on the number of bacterial species at the infection site. Infections likely to involve a single species include biliary tract infections, primary or "spontaneous" peritonitis, and pancreatic infections (pancreatic abscess, infected pseudocyst). In each instance, the dominant organism is a coliform, especially *E. coli*, followed by various streptococci and *Enterococcus* species. Anaerobic bacteria are relatively uncommon in these monomicrobial infections. Polymicrobial infections include peritonitis, which may be generalized or localized (phlegmon), and intraabdominal abscess. The predominant bacteria in these cases are combinations of coliforms and anaerobic bacteria. There is an average of four to six microbial species per specimen, and the dominant isolates in most series are *B. fragilis* and *E. coli*[72–75] (Table 217–7).

In most cases of intraabdominal sepsis, the pathophysiologic mechanism is a breach in the mucosal defense barrier that affords entry for an inoculum composed of the normal intestinal flora. Colonic flora is especially common, reflecting the frequency of associated diseases at this anatomic site, including appendicitis, diverticulitis, carcinoma of the colon, inflammatory bowel disease, and previous colon surgery. In such cases, the inoculum of bacteria presumably involves the approximately 400 species that compose the normal flora. Thus, the pathogens at the infection site, an average of four to six species, represent a distillate of the inoculum in which the organisms presumably survive owing to virulence factors and their ability to accommodate to the new environmental conditions. Perforation of the proximal bowel, as with perforated peptic ulcer, results in an infection that is microbiologically distinct, reflecting the flora of the upper gastrointestinal tract; the predominant microbial species in such cases often include aerobic and anaerobic gram-positive bacteria or *Candida* species.

TABLE 217–7 ■ Bacteriology of Intraabdominal Sepsis

Cases studied	759
Period reviewed	1979–1982
Bacteriology	
Aerobes only	132 (17%)
Anaerobes only	7 (1%)
Anaerobes + aerobes	620 (82%)
Bacterial isolates	
Aerobes	1256
Escherichia coli	306
Pseudomonas aeruginosa	121
Klebsiella	119
Proteus species	89
Enterobacter	46
Citrobacter	40
Serratia marcescens	16
Other gram-negative bacilli	79
Enterococcus	277
Staphylococcus aureus	111
Other gram-positive cocci	62
Anaerobes	1187
Bacteroides species	443
Bacteroides fragilis	133
Clostridium species	256
Clostridium perfringens	50
Peptostreptococcus	220
Fusobacterium	35
Eubacterium	60
Miscellaneous	116

Adapted from Stone HH, Strom PR, Fabian TC, Dunlop WE: Third-generation cephalosporins for polymicrobial surgical sepsis. Arch Surg 118:193–200, 1983.

The outcome of intraabdominal sepsis is highly variable, depending on multiple factors, the most important of which is the condition of the patient as measured by the Acute Physiology and Chronic Health Evaluation (APACHE) score.[116] This appears to be a better prognostic indicator than the level of the gastrointestinal tract at which the perforation took place, the bacteriology at the infected site, or the antibiotic regimen selected for treatment. The most important facet of treatment is usually surgical intervention or percutaneous drainage. With regard to antibiotic decisions, most patients are treated empirically without benefit of bacteriologic studies. The traditional standard is a two-drug regimen using one agent for coliforms (such as an aminoglycoside) and a second for anaerobes (such as clindamycin, cefoxitin, or metronidazole). Newer agents with expanded spectra of activity against both coliforms and anaerobes (e.g., imipenem or ticarcillin-clavulanate) appear to be as successful as the usual two-drug regimens.[117] In fact, findings of numerous comparative clinical trials suggest that multiple antimicrobial regimens are equally effective so long as they provide activity against both coliforms and anaerobes.[118–124] Controversies in the field concerning management of intraabdominal sepsis include the following issues.

Treatment of Enterococcal Infection. *Enterococcus* is encountered in 15% to 20% of cases, and some of these, primarily in nosocomial cases, may be vancomycin-resistant *Enterococcus faecium*.[125, 126] Prior studies suggested that *Enterococcus* species in mixed infections were of doubtful clinical significance. The animal model failed to show virulence of *Enterococcus* with intraperitoneal challenge, clinical studies showed that use of antibiotics active against *Enterococcus* did not improve outcome, and enterococci were rarely recovered in blood cultures.[127] The issue, once seemingly resolved, is increasingly controversial because of increased rates of enterococcal bacteremia and concern for vancomycin-resistant enterococci.[126] Some authorities advocate adding a third drug (ampicillin or vancomycin) to counter the enterococcus, although clinical and experimental animal studies do not support this tactic.

Percutaneous Drainage Under Ultrasonographic or Computed Tomographic Guidance. Experts agree that most intraabdominal abscesses require drainage, but the best means of accomplishing this is a matter of controversy. The initial experience suggests that most abscesses, especially those that are unilocular and accessible, should be drained percutaneously in an effort to avoid general anesthesia and common postoperative complications.[128, 129]

Bowel Preparation for Colon Surgery. Many authorities prefer the erythromycin plus neomycin oral preparation because of its extensive track record of excellent results, relatively low cost, ease of administration, and lack of impact on the therapeutic options for postoperative infections in the event that resistance emerges.[130] Others prefer a parenteral preparation such as cefoxitin or metronidazole plus tobramycin. Despite the controversy about the relative merits of oral versus parenteral administration, market surveys show that most surgeons use both—regimens such as oral neomycin and erythromycin combined with parenteral cefoxitin or cefotetan.[131]

Single-Agent Antimicrobial Therapy. Clinicians are accustomed to a two-drug regimen for intraabdominal sepsis (one agent for coliforms and another for anaerobes), and some include ampicillin for *Enterococcus* organisms, the triple-drug regimen. Single-drug therapy appears to be equally effective with imipenem; alternative single-drug treatments are β-lactam–β-lactamase inhibitor combinations, such as ticarcillin-clavulanate (Timentin), ampicillin-sulbactam (Unasyn), and piperacillin-tazobactam (Zosyn).[118, 119]

Infections of the Female Genital Tract

Nearly all infections of the female genital tract that are not caused by sexually transmitted pathogens are likely to involve anaerobic bacteria. Early investigators emphasized the role of *Peptostreptococcus* species in these infections.[7, 79] Later work suggested that anaerobic gram-negative bacilli are common and often dominant. Reports during the 1970s emphasized the frequency of *B. fragilis*, coliforms, and *Enterococcus* organisms, drawing an analogy to the bacteriologic patterns of intraabdominal sepsis.[76–78] The recovery of *B. fragilis* in these infections was mysterious. Studies of genital tract flora identify this organism in less than 2% of women. Subsequent work showed that *B. fragilis* was probably erroneously identified in the earlier studies and that far more common were other penicillin-resistant anaerobes, especially *P. bivia* and, to a lesser extent, *Prevotella disiens* (formerly *Bacteroides disiens*)[81–84] (Table 217–8).

Infections likely to involve anaerobic bacteria include Bartholin gland abscess, tuboovarian abscess, pyometra, endometritis, adnexal abscess, salpingitis, pelvic cellulitis, amnionitis, septic thrombophlebitis of the pelvic veins, and wound infections after gynecologic surgery or obstetric procedures. One of the great difficulties encountered in many of these infections is obtaining appropriate material for meaningful anaerobic culture. The problem of contamination by the normal genital tract flora may be obviated by using culdocentesis, laparoscopy, or quantitative cultures with telescoping catheters for transcervical sampling of the endometrium.[80–84]

TABLE 217–8 ■ Bacteria Recovered from the Upper Genital Tract of 188 Women Hospitalized with Acute Pelvic Inflammatory Disease

BACTERIA	NUMBER OF ISOLATES
Anaerobes	
Prevotella sp.	88
Prevotella bivia	72
Prevotella disiens	25
Bacteroides sp.	99
Peptostreptococcus asaccharolyticus	93
Peptostreptococcus anaerobius	72
Facultative Bacteria	
Gardnerella vaginalis	121
Escherichia coli	25
Group B streptococcus	29
α-Hemolytic streptococcus	45
Nonhemolytic streptococcus	49
Coagulase-negative staphylococcus	72

From Sweet RL: Role of bacterial vaginosis in pelvic inflammatory disease. Clin Infect Dis 20(Suppl 2):S271–S275, 1995. © by University of Chicago.

Pelvic inflammatory disease deserves emphasis owing to its prevalence, new insights into the microbiology, and the extensive associated morbidity (high rates of infertility and ectopic pregnancy). Studies using culdocentesis or laparoscopy to sample the fallopian tube implicate anaerobic bacteria, often combined with aerobic bacteria, in 27% to 61% of cases.[81] Infections associated with intrauterine devices often involve *Actinomyces*.[132] Another infection that presumably involves anaerobic bacteria is bacterial vaginosis, sometimes referred to as anaerobic vaginosis and formerly known as nonspecific vaginitis.[26, 133–135] Early studies implicated *Gardnerella vaginalis* as the agent of this disease, but later work suggested that it is an anaerobic infection on the basis of the putrid discharge, the large concentrations of anaerobes with quantitative cultures, the large concentration of succinic acid in the discharge, and the response to antimicrobial agents directed against anaerobes (clindamycin and metronidazole). No specific pathogen has been implicated, although some have suggested *Mobiluncus* species; others postulate dysbiosis—a secretory response to an altered microbial flora reflecting loss of lactobacilli and an altered pH.[133]

Choosing antimicrobial agents for mixed aerobic-anaerobic infections of the pelvis follows many of the principles noted for intraabdominal sepsis.[136] Recommendations for patients with pelvic inflammatory disease require regimens active against the usual aerobic and anaerobic flora, *Chlamydia trachomatis*, and *Neisseria gonorrhoeae*; these include doxycycline combined with cefoxitin, cefotetan, clindamycin, or ampicillin-sulbactam. Clinical trials indicate that these regimens are equally effective.[81, 137] Infections of the female pelvis that do not represent sexually transmitted diseases are usually complications of pregnancy or gynecologic surgery. The major anaerobic pathogens are *P. bivia*, *P. disiens*, and *Peptostreptococcus*.

Infections of Soft Tissue

Anaerobic bacteria are common pathogens in a diverse array of skin and soft tissue infections. Most involve the cutaneous flora, especially *Peptostreptococcus*, or the flora of adjacent mucosal surfaces.

S. aureus and *S. pyogenes* are commonly viewed as the dominant pathogens in soft tissue infections, although anaerobic bacteria account for a major portion. With regard to superficial soft tissue infections, cutaneous abscesses above the waist usually involve *S. aureus* or *Peptostreptococcus* species; abscesses below the waist are more likely to involve anaerobic bacteria and often reflect the organisms in the colon.[87] Similarly, anaerobes are the predominant isolates in breast abscesses.[92, 93] Other superficial infections that usually involve anaerobes include infected sebaceous cysts, infected pilonidal cysts, and paronychia.[91, 95] Soft tissue infections that result from a breach in the cutaneous barrier also show a high yield of anaerobes. Examples are wound infections after surgery, bite wounds, diabetic foot ulcers, and decubitus ulcers.[85, 86, 89, 96, 99] Quantitative cultures of diabetic foot ulcers show anaerobes to be the numerically dominant microbes[138]; osteomyelitis secondary to decubitus ulcers or diabetic foot ulcer is also likely to involve anaerobes.[139, 140]

Deep soft tissue infections likely to involve anaerobic bacteria include necrotizing fasciitis, necrotizing synergistic cellulitis, crepitant cellulitis, and gas gangrene. These infections involve the fascia, the muscle compartment formed by the enveloping fascia, or both. Major pathogens in these deep infections are group A β-hemolytic streptococci, clostridia, and combinations of aerobic and anaerobic bacteria. The most common is synergistic necrotizing cellulitis, a deep soft tissue infection involving both the fascial plane and muscle compartment caused by a mixed aerobic-anaerobic flora. Clinical features are severe pain, gas in the soft tissue, and surgical drainage yielding putrid "dishwater" pus (thin, grayish discharge).[94] Clinical clues in these and other deep soft tissue infections that specifically suggest anaerobic bacteria include the putrid discharge; Gram stains showing a mixed factor; and gas in the soft tissue as detected by palpation, radiography, or scans.

Bacteremia

Anaerobes account for 2% to 5% of blood culture isolates from patients with clinically significant bacteremia.[91, 141] This excludes *Propionibacterium*, which almost invariably represents a skin contaminant. The yield of anaerobes was substantially higher 20 to 30 years ago when recognition was less and commonly used antibiotics in hospital practice showed poor activity against anaerobes. The use of metronidazole, clindamycin, cefoxitin, cefotetan, and β-lactam–β-lactamase inhibitors for infections involving anaerobes is largely based on studies done in the 1970s and 1980s. Before this, there was little appreciation of the pathogenic role of anaerobes, and the major potentially useful antibiotics were penicillin, ampicillin, tetracycline, and chloramphenicol. The most common blood culture isolates among anaerobes are the *B. fragilis* group, which account for 60% to 80%.[141] A review of the suspected portal of entry for 855 episodes of bacteremia involving anaerobes indicated an intraabdominal source in 52%, the female genital tract in 20%, the lower respiratory tract in 6%, the upper respiratory tract in 5%, and soft tissue infections in 8%.[141] Anaerobes account for the majority of blood culture isolates in patients with bacteremia complicating infections of the female genital tract,[84, 98] intraabdominal sepsis,[85] decubitus ulcers,[99] and synergistic necrotizing cellulitis.[94] The usual clinical features are those that would be expected—fever, chills, and leukocytosis as well as signs of infection at the site of entry. Hypotension is relatively common, but disseminated intravascular coagulation is rare. This may reflect the fact that most anaerobic gram-negative bacilli do not contain biologically active endotoxin. Nevertheless, the mortality rate is reported to be 15% to 35%; as expected, it is lower when appropriate antimicrobial agents are used.[142]

Antibiotic Selection

A unique feature of anaerobic infections is that the decision regarding antimicrobial agents is usually made empirically, without the benefit of in vitro susceptibility tests. This reflects the difficulty in obtaining test results within a useful time frame, the difficulty with interpretation of culture results, the difficulty of performing sensitivity tests in vitro, the cost of testing multiple isolates from an infected site (surveys show that most clinicians ignore these results even when they are promptly reported), and generally favorable results with empirical decisions. Consequently, the National Committee for Clinical Laboratory Standards Working Group on Anaerobic Susceptibility Testing has recommended this type of testing for four settings: (1) to monitor susceptibility patterns in various geographic areas to determine changing sensitivity profiles; (2) to determine the activity of newly introduced

TABLE 217–9 ■ Activity of Antimicrobial Agents Versus Anaerobes

AGENTS	COMMENTS
Nearly Always Active	
Metronidazole	Inactive versus *Propionibacterium* and *Actinomyces* species in vitro; bactericidal versus most strains[107, 143–149]
Chloramphenicol	Good activity versus virtually all clinically significant anaerobes, but published clinical experience is limited[143–149]
Imipenem	Resistant to most *Bacteroides* β-lactamases, although a novel β-lactamase that inhibits imipenem was found in 2 of 350 *B. fragilis* strains[144, 149]
β-Lactam plus β-lactamase inhibitor	Only carbapenems (imipenem) and cefamycins (cefoxitin) are resistant to hydrolysis by the β-lactams produced by most *B. fragilis* strains. The addition of a β-lactamase inhibitor dramatically increases activity in vitro.[107, 143, 144, 149]
Usually Active	
Clindamycin	*B. fragilis* group: 5%–10% of strains resistant; some clostridia other than *C. perfringens* are resistant[143–149]
Cefoxitin	*B. fragilis* group: 5%–15% of strains resistant with considerable institutional variation at least partly reflecting use patterns[143–149]; poor activity versus clostridia
Antipseudomonad penicillins	Relatively resistant to β-lactamases of *Bacteroides* sp.; large doses usually employed[143–149]
Variable Activity	
Penicillin	Inactive versus some or most penicillinase-producing anaerobes, including most of the *B. fragilis* group and many strains of *Prevotella melaninogenica, P. intermedia, P. bivia, P. disiens,* and some clostridia[107, 143–149]
Cephalosporins other than cefotetan, cefoxitin, and cefmetazole	Less activity in vitro than penicillin G versus most anaerobes and limited published clinical experience to document efficacy[143–149]
Tetracycline	Inactive versus many anaerobes and most strains of *B. fragilis*; doxycycline and minocycline are somewhat more active than tetracycline
Vancomycin	Active against gram-positive anaerobes; inactive versus gram-negative anaerobes
Macrolides	Inactive versus many *Fusobacterium* spp. and *B. fragilis* spp.
Poor Activity	
Aminoglycosides	
Quinolones	
Monobactams (aztreonam)	

antibiotics; (3) to monitor sensitivity patterns in local hospitals as a reflection of local antimicrobial pressure; and (4) to assist in the management of infections in selected patients.[143] The last recommendation applies to infections in which intensive—and often prolonged—pathogen-directed treatment is generally required. Specific examples are cerebral abscess, joint infections, osteomyelitis, endocarditis, infections associated with prosthetic devices, and refractory or recurrent bacteremia. Most clinical laboratories will not do susceptibility tests unless they are specifically requested; many hospitals do not offer this service, and those that do often use techniques that are not considered reliable.

A common adage in the past was that infections above the diaphragm infrequently involve *B. fragilis*, so penicillin was usually regarded as the drug of choice. By contrast, because subdiaphragmatic infections were likely to involve *B. fragilis*, other drugs were preferred, especially chloramphenicol, metronidazole, cefoxitin, and clindamycin. The issue of drug selection has been complicated by the recognition of increasing resistance, geographic variation in resistance profiles that may reflect drug use patterns within hospitals, and a continual supply of new drugs.[107, 143–149] Many anaerobes are resistant to penicillins because of β-lactamase production. This includes most strains of the *B. fragilis* group, *P. bivia, P. disiens*, and *Bilophila wadsworthia*; many strains of the pigmented *Prevotella*; and occasional strains of *Porphyromonas, Fusobacterium*, and *Clostridium*. Cephalosporins other than cefoxitin, cefotetan, and cefmetazole are considered inferior versus anaerobes on the basis of in vitro activity and limited clinical experience. Drugs that are active against nearly all anaerobes, especially anaerobic gram-negative bacteria, are chloramphenicol, metronidazole, imipenem, and any combination of a β-lactam–β-lactamase inhibitor (Table 217–9). Clindamycin and cefoxitin have been used extensively for anaerobic infections for 25 and 15 years, respectively; many report that 10% to 15% of *B. fragilis* strains are resistant to one or both agents, although the clinical significance of this observation is unknown.

References

1. Finegold SM, George WL, Mulligan ME: Anaerobic infections, Part 1. Dis Mon 31:1, 1985.
2. Veillon A, Zuber A: Sur quelques microbes strictment anaerobies et leur role dans la pathologie humaine. C R Soc Biol (Paris) 49:253, 1897.
3. Schottmueller H: Allgemeinen Krankenhaus Hamburg-Eppendorf. Mitt Grenzt Med Chir 21:450, 1910.
4. Smith DT: Fusospirochetal disease of the lungs, its bacteriology, pathology and experimental reproduction. Am Rev Tuberc 16:584, 1927.
5. Smith DT: Fusospirochetal disease of the lungs produced with cultures from Vincent's angina. J Infect Dis 46:303, 1930.
6. Altemeier WA: Bacterial flora of acute perforated appendicitis with peritonitis: Bacteriologic study based upon 100 cases. Ann Surg 107:517, 1938.
7. Altemeier WA: The cause of the putrid odor of perforated appendicitis with peritonitis. Ann Surg 107:634, 1938.
8. Gorbach SL, Bartlett JG: Anaerobic infections. N Engl J Med 290:1177, 1974.
9. Martin WJ: Isolation and identification of anaerobic bacteria in the clinical laboratory. Mayo Clin Proc 49:300, 1974.
10. Wilson WR, Martin WJ, Wilkowske CJ, et al: Anaerobic bacteremia. Mayo Clin Proc 47:639, 1972.
11. Brook I: Recovery of anaerobic bacteria from clinical specimens in 12 years at two military hospitals. J Clin Microbiol 26:1181, 1988.
12. Sutter VL: Anaerobes as normal oral flora. Rev Infect Dis 6(Suppl):S62, 1984.
13. Broido PW, Gorbach SL, Condon RE, et al: Upper intestinal microflora control. Arch Surg 106:90, 1973.
14. Finegold SM, Attebery HR, Sutter V: Effect of diet on human fecal flora. Am J Clin Nutr 27:1456, 1974.
15. Moore WEC, Holdeman LV: Human fecal flora: The normal flora of 20 Japanese-Hawaiians. Appl Microbiol 27:961, 1974.
16. Mackowiak PA: The normal microbial flora. N Engl J Med 307:83, 1982.
17. Van der Waaij D: Colonization resistance of the digestive tract: Clinical consequences and implications. J Antimicrob Chemother 10:263, 1982.
18. Bartlett JG, Polk BF: Bacterial flora of the vagina: Quantitative study. Rev Infect Dis 6(Suppl 1):S67, 1984.
19. Rendondo-Lopez V, Cook R, Sobel JD: Emerging role of lactobacilli in the control and maintenance of the vaginal bacterial microflora. Rev Infect Dis 12:856, 1990.
20. Hillier S, Krohn MA, Klebanoff SJ, Eschenbach DA: The relationship of hydrogen peroxide–producing lactobacilli to bacterial vaginosis and genital microflora in pregnant women. Obstet Gynecol 79:369, 1992.
21. Sautter RL, Brown WJ: Sequential vaginal cultures from normal young women. J Clin Microbiol 11:479, 1980.
22. Hammerschlag MR, Alpert S, Rosner I, et al: Microbiology of the vagina in children: Normal and potentially pathogenic organisms. Pediatrics 62:57, 1978.
23. Goplerud CP, Ohm MJ, Galask RP: Aerobic and anaerobic flora of the cervix during pregnancy and the puerperium. Am J Obstet Gynecol 126:858, 1976.
24. Ohm MJ, Galask RP: Bacterial flora of the cervix from 100 prehysterectomy patients. Am J Obstet Gynecol 122:683, 1975.
25. Ohm MJ, Galask RP: The effect of antibiotic prophylaxis on patients undergoing vaginal operations. Am J Obstet Gynecol 123:597, 1975.
26. Spiegel CA: Bacterial vaginosis. Clin Microbial Rev 4:485, 1991.
27. Nielsen ML, Raahave D, Stage JG, et al: Anaerobic and aerobic skin bacteria before and after skin disinfection with chlorhexidine: An experimental study in volunteers. J Clin Pathol 28:793, 1975.
28. Meleney FL: Clinical Aspects and Treatment of Surgical Infections. Philadelphia, WB Saunders, 1949.
29. Altemeier WA: The pathogenicity of the bacteria of appendicitis peritonitis. Surgery 11:374, 1942.
30. Lindberg AA, Weintraub A, Zahringer U, Rietschel ET: Structure-activity relationships in lipopolysaccharides of *Bacteroides fragilis*. Rev Infect Dis 12:S133, 1990.
31. Onderdonk AB, Cisneros RL, Finberg R, et al: Animal model system for studying virulence of and host response to *Bacteroides fragilis*. Rev Infect Dis 12:S169, 1990.
32. Pantosti A, Tzianabos AO, Onderdonk AB, Kasper DL: Immunochemical characterization of two surface polysaccharides of *Bacteroides fragilis*. Infect Immun 59:2075, 1991.
33. Pantosti A, Tzianabos AO, Reinap BG, et al: *Bacteroides fragilis* strains express multiple capsular polysaccharides. J Clin Microbiol 31:1850, 1993.
34. Tzianabos AO, Onderdonk AB, Zaleznik DF, et al: Structural characteristics of polysaccharides that induce protection against intra-abdominal abscess formation. Infect Immun 62:4881, 1994.
35. Tzianabos AO, Kasper DL, Cisneros RL, et al: Polysaccharide-mediated protection against abscess formation in experimental intra-abdominal sepsis. J Clin Invest 96:2727, 1995.
36. Rotstein OD, Nasmith PE, Grinstein S: The *Bacteroides* by-product succinic acid inhibits neutrophil respiratory burst by reducing intracellular pH. Infect Immun 55:864, 1987.
37. Rotstein OD, Vittorini T, Kao J, et al: A soluble *Bacteroides* by-product impairs phagocytic killing of *Escherichia coli* by neutrophils. Infect Immun 57:745, 1989.
38. Casciato DA, Rosenblatt JE, Goldberg LS, Bluestone R: In vitro interaction of *Bacteroides fragilis* with polymorphonuclear leukocytes and serum factors. Infect Immun 11:337, 1975.
39. Casciato DA, Rosenblatt JE, Bluestone R, et al: Susceptibility of isolates of *Bacteroides* to the bactericidal activity of normal human sera. J Infect Dis 140:109, 1979.
40. Rotimi VO, Eke PI: The bactericidal action of human serum on *Bacteroides* species. J Med Microbiol 18:355, 1984.
41. Bjornson AB, Bjornson HS: Participation of immunoglobulin and alternative complement pathway in opsonization of *Bacteroides fragilis* and *Bacteroides thetaiotaomicron*. J Infect Dis 138:351, 1978.

42. Dahlen G, Nygren H: An electron microscopic study of surface polysaccharides in *Bacteroides*. Microbios 35:119, 1982.
43. Sonnenwirth AC: Antibody response to anaerobic bacteria. Rev Infect Dis 1:337, 1979.
44. Bjornson AB, Bjornson HS, Kitko BP: Specificity of immunoglobulin M antibodies in normal human serum that participate in opsonophagocytosis and intracellular killing of *Bacteroides fragilis* and *Bacteroides thetaiotaomicron* by human polymorphonuclear leukocytes. Infect Immun 30:263, 1980.
45. Reid JH, Patrick S: Phagocytic and serum killing of capsulate and noncapsulate *Bacteroides fragilis*. J Med Microbiol 17:247, 1984.
46. Bartlett JG, Onderdonk AB, Louie T, et al: A review: Lessons from an animal model of intra-abdominal sepsis. Arch Surg 113:853, 1978.
47. Thadepalli H, Gorbach SL, Broido PW, et al: Abdominal trauma, anaerobes and antibiotics. Surg Gynecol Ostet 137:270, 1973.
48. diZerega GS, Yonekura ML, Roy S, et al: A comparison of clindamycin-gentamicin and penicillin-gentamicin in the treatment of postcesarean endomyometritis. Am J Obstet Gynecol 134:238, 1979.
49. Gorbach SL, Mayhew JW, Bartlett JG, et al: Rapid diagnosis of anaerobic infections by direct gas-liquid chromatography of clinical specimens. J Clin Invest 57:478, 1976.
50. Gorbach SL, Proppe KH: Fulminant illness with subcutaneous crepitance: Case records of the Massachusetts General Hospital. N Engl J Med 301:1276, 1979.
51. Citron DM: Specimen collection and transport, anaerobic culture techniques and identification of anaerobes. Rev Infect Dis 6:S51, 1984.
52. Bartlett JG, Sullivan-Sigler N, Louie TJ, Gorbach SL: Anaerobes survive in clinical specimens despite delayed processing. J Clin Microbiol 3:133, 1976.
53. Heineman HS, Braude AL: Anaerobic infection of the brain: Observations on eighteen consecutive cases of brain abscess. Am J Med 35:682, 1963.
54. Swartz MN: Central nervous infections. *In* Finegold SM, George WL (eds): Anaerobic Infections in Humans. San Diego, CA, Academic Press, 1989, pp 156–232.
55. Frederick J, Braude AL: Anaerobic infection of the paranasal sinuses. N Engl J Med 290:135, 1974.
56. Brook I: The role of anaerobic bacteria in otitis media: Microbiology, pathogenesis, and implications on therapy. Am J Otolaryngol 8:109, 1987.
57. Bartlett JG, O'Keefe P: The bacteriology of perimandibular space infections. J Oral Surg 37:407, 1979.
58. Chow AW, Roser AM, Brady FA: Orofacial odontogenic infections. Ann Intern Med 88:392, 1978.
59. Flodstrom A, Hallander HO: Microbiological aspects on peritonsillar abscesses. Scand J Infect Dis 8:157, 1976.
60. Mitchelmore IJ, Prior AJ, Montgomery PQ, Tabaqchali S: Microbiological features and pathogenesis of peritonsillar abscesses. Eur J Clin Microbiol Infect Dis 14:870, 1995.
61. Williams BL, McCann GF, Schoenknecht FD: Bacteriology of dental abscesses of endodontic origin. J Clin Microbiol 18:770, 1983.
62. Bartlett JG, Finegold SM: Anaerobic infections of the lung and pleural space. Am Rev Respir Dis 110:56, 1974.
63. Lorber B, Swenson RM: Bacteriology of aspiration pneumonia. A prospective study of community and hospital acquired cases. Ann Intern Med 81:329, 1974.
64. Bartlett JG, Gorbach SL, Tally FP, Finegold SM: Bacteriology and treatment of primary lung abscess. Am Rev Respir Dis 109:510, 1974.
65. Beerens H, Tahon-Castel M: Infections Humaines à Bactéries Anaérobies Nontoxigènes. Bruxelles, Presses Académiques Européenes, 1965, pp 91–114.
66. Bartlett JG, Gorbach SL, Thadepalli H, Finegold SM: The bacteriology of empyema. Lancet 1:338, 1974.
67. Varkey B, Rose H, Kutty K, et al: Empyema thoracis during a ten-year period. Arch Intern Med 141:1771, 1981.
68. Greey PH: The bacteriology of bronchiectasis. An analysis based on nine cases in which lobectomy was done. J Infect Dis 50:203, 1932.
69. Ries K, Levison ME, Kaye D: Transtracheal aspiration in pulmonary infection. Arch Intern Med 133:453, 1974.
70. Pollack HM, Hawkins EL, Bonner JR, et al: Diagnosis of bacterial pulmonary infections and quantitative protected catheter cultures obtained during bronchoscopy. J Clin Microbiol 17:255, 1983.
71. Bartlett JG, O'Keere P, Tally FP, et al: The bacteriology of hospital-acquired pneumonia. Arch Intern Med 146:868, 1986.
72. Stone HH, Strom PR, Fabian TC, Dunlop WE: Third-generation cephalosporins for polymicrobial surgical sepsis. Arch Surg 118:193, 1983.
73. Gorbach SL: Management of anaerobic infections: Intra-abdominal sepsis. Ann Intern Med 83:377, 1975.
74. Swenson RM, Lorber B, Michaelson TC, et al: The bacteriology of intra-abdominal infections. Arch Surg 109:398, 1974.
75. Sabbaj J, Sutter VL, Finegold SM: Anaerobic pyogenic liver abscess. Ann Intern Med 77:629, 1972.
76. Thadepalli H, Gorbach SL, Keith L: Anaerobic infections of the female genital tract: Bacteriologic and therapeutic aspects. Am J Obstet Gynecol 117:1034, 1973.
77. Swenson RM, Michaelson TC, Daly MJ, et al: Anaerobic bacterial infections of the female genital tract. Obstet Gynecol 42:538, 1973.
78. Ledger WJ, Gee CL, Pollin P, et al: The use of prereduced media and a portable jar for the collection of anaerobic organisms from clinical sites of infection. Am J Obstet Gynecol 125:677, 1976.
79. Altemeier WA: The anaerobic streptococci in tuboovarian abscess. Am J Obstet Gynecol 39:1038, 1940.
80. Eschenbach DA, Buchanan TM, Pollock HM: Polymicrobial etiology of acute pelvic inflammatory disease. N Engl J Med 193:166, 1975.
81. Sweet RL: Role of bacterial vaginosis in pelvic inflammatory disease. Clin Infect Dis 20(Suppl 2):S271, 1995.
82. Sweet RL, Schachter J, Landers DV, et al: Treatment of hospitalized patients with acute pelvic inflammatory disease: Comparison of cefotetan plus doxycycline and cefoxitin plus doxycycline. Am J Obstet Gynecol 158:736, 1988.
83. Chow AW, Marshall JR, Guze LB: A double-blind comparison of clindamycin with penicillin plus chloramphenicol in treatment of septic abortion. J Infect Dis 135:S35, 1977.
84. Rosene K, Eschenbach DA, Tompkins LS, et al: Polymicrobial early postpartum endometritis with facultative and anaerobic bacteria, genital mycoplasmas, and *Chlamydia trachomatis*: Treatment with piperacillin or cefoxitin. J Infect Dis 153:1028, 1986.
85. Bartlett JG, Condon RE, Gorbach SL, et al: Veterans Administration Cooperative study on bowel preparation for elective colon surgery. Ann Surg 188:126, 1978.
86. Sanderson PJ, Wren MWD, Baldwin AWF: Anaerobic organisms in postoperative wounds. J Clin Pathol 32:143, 1979.
87. Meislin HW, Lerner SA, Graves MH, et al: Cutaneous abscesses. Ann Intern Med 87:145, 1977.
88. Whitehead SM, Leach RD, Eykyn SJ, et al: The aetiology of perirectal sepsis. Br J Surg 69:166, 1982.
89. Louie TJ, Bartlett JG, Tally FP, Gorbach SL: The microbiology of diabetic foot ulcers. Ann Intern Med 85:461, 1976.
90. MacLennan JD: The histotoxic clostridial infections of man. Bacteriol Rev 26:232, 1962.
91. Pearson HE, Smiley DF: *Bacteroides* in pilonidal sinuses. Am J Surg 115:336, 1968.
92. Edmiston CE Jr, Walker AP, Krepel CJ, Gohr C: The nonpuerperal breast infection: Aerobic and anaerobic microbial recovery from acute and chronic disease. J Infect Dis 162:695, 1990.
93. Brook I: Microbiology of non-puerperal breast abscesses. J Infect Dis 157:377, 1988.
94. Stone HH, Martin JD Jr: Synergistic necrotizing cellulitis. Ann Surg 175:702, 1972.
95. Brook I: Bacteriologic study of paronychia in children. Am J Surg 141:703, 1981.
96. Goldstein EJC, Citron DM, Finegold SM: Role of anaerobic bacteria in bite-wound infections. Rev Infect Dis 6:S177, 1984.
97. Brook I: Anaerobic bacterial bacteremia: 12 year experience in two military hospitals. J Infect Dis 160:1071, 1989.
98. Smith JW, Southern PM Jr, Lehmann JD: Bacteremia in septic abortion: Complications and treatment. Obstet Gynecol 35:404, 1970.
99. Bryan CS, Dew CE, Reynolds KL: Bacteremia associated with decubitus ulcers. Arch Intern Med 143:2093, 1983.
100. Ingham HR, Selkon JB, Roxby CM: Bacteriological study of

otogenic cerebral abscesses: Chemotherapeutic role of metronidazole. Br Med J 2:991, 1977.
101. Boom WH, Tuazon CU: Successful treatment of multiple brain abscesses with antibiotics alone. Rev Infect Dis 7:189, 1985.
102. Zavistoski J, Dzink JA, Onderdonk AB, Bartlett JG: Quantitative bacteriology of endodontic infections. Oral Surg Oral Med Oral Pathol 1:46, 1980.
103. Lemierre A: On certain septicaemias. Lancet 1:701, 1936.
104. Sinave CP, Hardy GJ, Fardy PW: The Lemierre syndrome: Suppurative thrombophlebitis of the internal jugular vein secondary to oropharyngeal infection. Medicine (Baltimore) 68:85, 1989.
105. Loesche WJ, Syed SA, Laughon BE, et al: The bacteriology of acute necrotizing ulcerative gingivitis. J Periodontol 53:223, 1982.
106. Sutter VL, Jones MJ, Ghoneim ATM: Antimicrobial susceptibilities of bacteria associated with periodontal disease. Antimicrob Agents Chemother 23:483, 1983.
107. Appelbaum PC, Spangler SK, Jacobs MR: β-Lactamase production and susceptibilities to amoxicillin, amoxicillin-clavulanate, ticarcillin, ticarcillin-clavulanate, cefoxitin, imipenem, and metronidazole of 320 non–*Bacteroides fragilis Bacteroides* isolates and 129 fusobacteria from 28 U.S. centers. Antimicrob Agents Chemother 34:1546, 1990.
108. Bartlett JG: Anaerobic bacterial infections of the lung and pleural space. Clin Infect Dis 16(Suppl 4):S248, 1993.
109. Marina M, Strong CA, Civen R, et al: Bacteriology of anaerobic pleuropulmonary infections: Preliminary report. Clin Infect Dis 16(Suppl 4):S256, 1993.
110. Bartlett JG: Treatment of anaerobic pleuropulmonary infections. Ann Intern Med 83:376, 1975.
111. Weiss W: Oral antibiotic therapy of acute primary lung abscess: Comparison of penicillin and tetracycline. Curr Ther Res 12:154, 1970.
112. Levison ME, Mangura CT, Lorber B, et al: Clindamycin compared with penicillin for the treatment of anaerobic lung abscess. Ann Intern Med 98:466, 1983.
113. Gudiol F, Manresa F, Pallares R, et al: Clindamycin vs. penicillin for anaerobic lung infections: High rate of penicillin failures associated with penicillin-resistant *Bacteroides melaninogenicus*. Arch Intern Med 150:2525, 1990.
114. Drugs for anaerobic infections. Med Lett 26:87, 1984.
115. Sanders CV, Hanna BJ, Lewis AC: Metronidazole in the treatment of anaerobic infections. Am Rev Respir Dis 120:337, 1979.
116. Knaus WA, Wagner DP, Draper EA: Relationship between acute physiologic derangement and risk of death. J Chronic Dis 38:295, 1985.
117. Malangoni MA, Condon RE, Spiegel CA: Treatment of intra-abdominal infections is appropriate with single-agent or combination antibiotic therapy. Surgery 98:648, 1985.
118. Malangoni MA, Condon RE, Spiegel CA: Treatment of intra-abdominal infections is appropriate with single-agent or combination antibiotic therapy. Surgery 98:648, 1985.
119. Nichols RL, Smith JW, Klein DB, et al: Risk of infection after penetrating abdominal trauma. N Engl J Med 311:1065, 1984.
120. Harding GKM, Buckwold FJ, Ronald AR, et al: Prospective, randomized comparative study of clindamycin, chloramphenicol, and ticarcillin, each in combination with gentamicin, in therapy for intraabdominal and female genital tract sepsis. J Infect Dis 142:384, 1980.
121. Smith JA, Skidmore AG, Forward AD, et al: Prospective, randomized, double-blind comparison of metronidazole and tobramycin with clindamycin and tobramycin in the treatment of intraabdominal sepsis. Ann Surg 192:213, 1980.
122. Tally FP, McGowan K, Kellum JM, et al: A randomized comparison of cefoxitin with or without amikacin and clindamycin plus amikacin in surgical sepsis. Ann Surg 193:318, 1981.
123. Heseltine PNR, Yellin AE, Appleman MD, et al: Perforated and gangrenous appendicitis: An analysis of antibiotic failures. J Infect Dis 148:322, 1983.
124. Wilson SE, Boswick JA Jr, Duma RJ, et al: Cephalosporin therapy in intraabdominal infections. Am J Surg 155(5A):61, 1988.
125. Centers for Disease Control and Prevention: Recommendation for preventing the spread of vancomycin resistance. MMWR Morbid Mortal Wkly Rep 44(RR-12):1, 1995.
126. Frieden TR, Munsiff SS, Low DE, et al: Emergence of vancomycin-resistant enterococci in New York City. Lancet 342:76, 1993.
127. Barie PS, Christou NV, Dellinger EP, et al: Pathogenicity of the enterococcus in surgical infections. Ann Surg 212:155, 1990.
128. Gerzof SG, Johnson WC, Robbins AH, Nabseth DC: Expanded criteria for percutaneous abscess drainage. Arch Surg 120:227, 1985.
129. Olak J, Christou NV, Stein LA, et al: Operative vs percutaneous drainage of intraabdominal abscesses: Comparison of morbidity and mortality. Arch Surg 121:141, 1986.
130. Condon RE, Bartlett JG, Greenlee H, et al: Efficacy of oral and systemic antibiotic prophylaxis in colorectal operations. Arch Surg 118:496, 1983.
131. Solla JA, Rothenberger DA: Preoperative bowel preparation: A Survey of colon and rectal surgeons. Dis Colon Rectum 33:154, 1990.
132. Burkman R, Schlesselman S, McCaffrey L, et al: The relationship of genital tract actinomycetes and the development of pelvic inflammatory disease. Am J Gynecol 143:585, 1982.
133. Spiegel CA, Roberts M: *Mobiluncus* gen. nov., *Mobiluncus curtisii* subsp. *curtisii* sp. nov., *Mobiluncus curtisii* subsp. *holmesii* subsp. nov., and *Mobiluncus mulieris* sp. nov., curved rods from human vagina. Int J Syst Bacteriol 34:177, 1984.
134. Spiegel CA, Eschenbach DA, Amsel R, et al: Curved anaerobic bacteria in bacterial (nonspecific) vaginosis and their response to antimicrobial therapy. J Infect Dis 148:817, 1983.
135. Hillier SL, Nugent RP, Eschenbach DA, et al: Association between bacterial vaginosis and preterm delivery of a low-birth-weight infant. N Engl J Med 333:1737, 1995.
136. Ledger WJ: Selection of antimicrobial agents for treatment of infections of the female genital tract. Rev Infect Dis 5:S98, 1983.
137. Hemsell DL, Little BB, Faro S, et al: Comparison of three regimens recommended by the Centers for Disease Control and Prevention for the treatment of women hospitalized with acute pelvic inflammatory disease. Clin Infect Dis 19:720, 1994.
138. Sapico FL, Canawati HN, Witte JL, et al: Quantitative aerobic and anaerobic bacteriology of infected diabetic feet. J Clin Microbiol 12:413, 1980.
139. Templeton WC III, Wawrukiewicz A, Melo JC, et al: Anaerobic osteomyelitis of long bones. Rev Infect Dis 5:692, 1983.
140. Nakata MM, Lewis RP: Anaerobic bacteria in bone and joint infections. Rev Infect Dis 6(Suppl):S165, 1984.
141. Finegold SM, George WL, Mulligan ME: Anaerobic infections. Dis Mon 31:4, 1988.
142. Condo RE: *Bacteroides* bacteremia. Arch Surg 119:897, 1984.
143. Finegold SM: Susceptibility testing of anaerobic bacteria. J Clin Microbiol 26:1253, 1988.
144. Cuchural GJ, Tally FP, Jacobus NV, et al: Comparative activities of newer β-lactam agents against members of the *Bacteroides fragilis* group. Antimicrob Agents Chemother 34:479, 1990.
145. Wexler HM, Harris B, Carter WT, et al: Six year retrospective survey of the resistance of *Bacteroides fragilis* group species to clindamycin and cefoxitin. Diagn Microbiol Infect Dis 4:247, 1986.
146. Cuchural GJ, Tally FP, Jacobus NY, et al: Susceptibility of the *Bacteroides fragilis* group in the United States: Analysis by site of isolation. Antimicrob Agents Chemother 32:717, 1988.
147. Edson RS, Rosenblatt JE, Lee DT, et al: Recent experience with antimicrobial susceptibility of anaerobic bacteria. Mayo Clin Proc 57:737, 1982.
148. Cuchural GJ, Malamy MH, Tally FP: β-Lactamase–mediated imipenem resistance in *Bacteroides fragilis*. Antimicrob Agents Chemother 30:645, 1986.
149. Grollier G, Mory F, Quentin C, et al: Susceptibility of strict anaerobic bacteria to antibiotics in France: A multicenter study. Pathol Biol 42:498, 1994.

218

Anaerobic Cocci

John G. Bartlett

Anaerobic cocci are prominent components of the normal flora on virtually all mucocutaneous surfaces in humans, and they are common clinical isolates in endogenous infections, usually as components of a polymicrobial flora. The organisms most frequently isolated and considered clinically important are in the genus *Peptostreptococcus.*

Taxonomy

Anaerobic gram-positive cocci include the genera *Peptostreptococcus, Streptococcus,* and *Gemella* (previously *Streptococcus morbillorum*). Other anaerobic cocci that are less important clinically include *Coprococcus, Peptococcus, Ruminococcus, Sarcina,* and *Staphylococcus saccharolyticus.* Older studies showed high yields of *Peptococcus* in various types of specimens, but most of the former species in the genus have now been transferred to *Peptostreptococcus* on the basis of DNA content of guanine plus cytosine.[1, 2] *Peptococcus niger* is retained in the *Peptococcus* genus but is an infrequent clinical isolate. Another taxonomic change has been gram-positive cocci that produce abundant lactic acid and were formerly considered anaerobic but are now classified as *Streptococcus* on the basis of aerotolerance. These include *Streptococcus intermedius, Streptococcus constellatus,* and *Gemella morbillorum.* These organisms produce lactic acid as the sole major end product and show morphologic characteristics of variable size and form in chains and pairs. *S. intermedius* and *S. constellatus* usually grow initially on anaerobic plate media but become aerotolerant after subculturing. *S. intermedius, S. constellatus,* and *Streptococcus anginosus* were formerly classified as *Streptococcus anginosus* or *Streptococcus milleri.* They are common isolates in infectious diseases and abscesses, and they are often found in polymicrobial infections that include anaerobic bacteria.[3, 4] Unlike true anaerobes, these species of *Streptococcus* are resistant to metronidazole.[5]

Of the peptostreptococci, the most common isolates are *Peptostreptococcus magnus* and *Peptostreptococcus asaccharolyticus;* less common are *Peptostreptococcus micros* and *Peptostreptococcus anaerobius.*[6–8] More recently described species are *Peptostreptococcus vaginalis, Peptostreptococcus lactolyticus,* and *Peptostreptococcus pydrogenalis.* With regard to anatomic site, *P. magnus* is usually associated with skin and soft tissue infections and is infrequently found with other anaerobes. *P. asaccharolyticus* is found at widely distributed sites, and *P. anaerobius* is usually found in subdiaphragmatic locations.[6]

The anaerobic gram-negative cocci include *Veillonella, Acidaminococcus,* and *Megasphaera. Veillonella* is virtually always found as indigenous flora of the mouth and is common in the gastrointestinal tract and vaginal flora as well. *Megasphaera* and *Acidaminococcus* are common components of the intestinal flora. The pathogenic role of these organisms is unclear, but they are usually considered nonpathogens or contaminants.

Microbiologic Characteristics

The anaerobic cocci grow well on nonselective plate and broth media that are commonly recommended for recovering anaerobic bacteria.[9] These include Schaedler agar, *Brucella* agar, brain-heart infusion agar, and CDC anaerobic blood agar. Selective media include blood agar plates containing phenylethyl alcohol or neomycin. Growth is generally slow, usually requiring 48 hours or longer. Gram stain does not distinguish among anaerobic, microaerophilic, and aerotolerant gram-positive cocci. Exposure of strict anaerobes to oxygen may result in loss of integrity of cell walls, causing Gram stain variability.[10] Sensitivity to vancomycin with use of a 5-μg disk on *Brucella* blood agar will confirm Gram stain results. *Peptostreptococcus productus* and *P. anaerobius* may appear as coccobacilli. Identification at the genus and species levels is based on fermentation reaction and product of metabolism detected by gas-liquid chromatography; rapid tests such as RapID-ANA II and ID32A have been useful for rapid identification of *P. micros, P. anaerobius,* and *P. asaccharolyticus* but are unreliable for other species such as *Peptostreptococcus prevotii.*[11] Nevertheless, the utility of speciation is often questioned on the basis of the time and resources required. Differences between these organisms based on virulence and in vitro sensitivity test results are minimal.

Normal Flora

Anaerobic cocci are found at virtually all mucocutaneous surfaces that harbor a normal flora. *Veillonella* species, primarily *Veillonella parvula,* are universally present in saliva and may be used as a marker of salivary contamination of respiratory specimens.[12] In addition, numerous anaerobic gram-positive cocci are found in the normal flora of the upper airways.[13] Concentrations are often on the order of 10^7 to 10^9 bacteria per mL of saliva.[12] Quantitative studies of the vaginal and cervical flora indicate anaerobic gram-positive cocci in 60% to 80% of women of childbearing age in mean concentrations of $10^{8.7}$ per g of secretions.[14, 15] The dominant species are *P. anaerobius, P. asaccharolyticus, P. magnus,* and *P. micros.*[11] The fecal flora shows anaerobic gram-positive cocci usually present in mean concentrations of approximately 10^{10} per g.[16, 17] The most common species are *P. productus, P. magnus, P. prevotii, P. micros,* and *P. asaccharolyticus.* This flora also commonly includes *Veillonella, Ruminococcus, Acidaminococcus fermentans,* and *Megasphaera elsdenii.* Anaerobic gram-positive cocci are also constituents of the normal flora of skin, urethra, stomach, and small bowel.

Clinical Infections

Anaerobic gram-positive cocci are frequently found in clinical specimens with appropriate culture techniques (Table 218–1). They are usually found as components of mixed infections. The experience at the Mayo Clinic indicates that these bacteria are present in 17% to 31% of all specimens that yield anaerobic bacteria.[9, 18, 19]

Bacteremia

Peptostreptococci account for 4% to 7% of blood culture isolates involving anaerobic bacteria.[9, 18–20] Transient bacteremia is common with dental procedures.[21] Anaerobic or microaerophilic streptococci account for 5% to 10% of endocarditis cases, but a relatively small portion of these organisms are now classified as *Peptostreptococcus.* These organisms con-

TABLE 218–1 ■ Recovery of *Peptostreptococcus* from Clinical Specimens

CLINICAL SETTING	REFERENCE	NUMBER OF PATIENTS	TOTAL NUMBER OF ANAEROBIC ISOLATES	TOTAL NUMBER OF PEPTOSTREPTOCOCCAL ISOLATES
Anaerobic infections of the lung	29	193	461	136 (29.5%)
Intraabdominal sepsis	37	759	1187	220 (18.5%)
Infections of the female genital tract	35	188	449	165 (36.7%)

stitute normal skin flora, and their appearance in blood may often represent contaminants.

Respiratory Tract Infections

Peptostreptococci constitute a major component of the flora of upper airways[22, 23] and are commonly noted in dental infections, perimandibular space infections, chronic sinusitis, and chronic otitis[24–27]; they are the most common isolates in peritonsillar abscesses.[28] These organisms are found in 10% to 20% of anaerobic infections of the lung.[20, 29, 30]

Genital Tract Infections

Peptostreptococci have been reported in 25% to 40% of infections of the female pelvis, including pelvic abscess, Bartholin gland abscess, endometritis, puerperal sepsis, infections after gynecologic surgery, and pelvic inflammatory disease.[31–36]

Intraabdominal Sepsis

Peptostreptococci account for 10% to 30% of bacteria recovered in intraabdominal sepsis.[20, 37–41] These organisms, including microaerophilic streptococci, are common and are considered clinically important in pyogenic liver abscess and ascending cholangitis.[38]

Skin and Soft Tissue Infections

Peptostreptococci are common isolates in infections of skin and soft tissue, including cutaneous abscesses below the waist, diabetic foot ulcers, infected decubitus ulcers, necrotizing fasciitis, necrotizing synergistic gangrene, and infected sebaceous cysts. They are also common in wound infections after intestinal or gynecologic surgery.[42–45] Infections involving human bites and animal bites often involve these organisms.[20] Streptococcal myositis is often attributed to *Streptococcus pyogenes*, but *Peptostreptococcus* species appear to cause the same syndrome.

Osteomyelitis

P. magnus appears to play a prominent role in septic arthritis and osteomyelitis among patients who have orthopedic surgical implants.[19] The clinical course in these cases is typically chronic and indolent; removal of the prosthesis is eventually necessary in most.

Treatment

Peptostreptococci are usually recovered as part of a mixed flora so that a pathogenic role is difficult to determine. Many of these organisms are relatively fastidious, and they may be readily apparent on Gram stain but difficult to recover in culture. They usually have predictable sensitivity patterns, making empirical treatment relatively easy. For these reasons, most authorities do not recommend routine sensitivity testing except in selected clinical settings such as endocarditis, cerebral abscess, osteomyelitis, and septic arthritis.[46]

Penicillin G is usually considered the preferred agent for infections involving peptostreptococci. Because these organisms are usually present in polymicrobial infections, therapeutic decisions are often dictated by other components that may be more resistant. Other drugs that are usually effective in vitro are other penicillins (except nafcillin or oxacillin), vancomycin, imipenem, chloramphenicol, macrolides, many cephalosporins (other than ceftazidime), and any combination of a β-lactam–β-lactamase inhibitor.[47–51] Drugs that are not active include monobactams (aztreonam), aminoglycosides, and many fluoroquinolones; some of the newer fluoroquinolones appear to be active in vitro.[49] Metronidazole and clindamycin are somewhat unpredictable because 12% to 15% of peptostreptococci are resistant. Some strains that are initially clindamycin sensitive but erythromycin resistant often have inducible clindamycin resistance.[52] Strains belonging to the "*S. milleri*" group, more frequently *S. anginosus* than *S. constellatus*, show occasional resistance to penicillin.[53]

References

1. Ezaki T, Yamamoto N, Ninomiya K, et al: Transfer of *Peptococcus indolicus*, *Peptococcus asaccharolyticus*, *Peptococcus prevotii*, and *Peptococcus magnus* to the genus *Peptostreptococcus* and proposal of *Peptostreptococcus tetradius* sp. nov. Int J Syst Bacteriol 33:683, 1983.
2. Huss VAR, Festl H, Schleifer KH: Nucleic acid hybridization studies and deoxyribonucleic acid base compositions of anaerobic gram-positive cocci. Int J Syst Bacteriol 34:95, 1984.
3. Cato EP: Transfer of *Peptostreptococcus parvulus* (Weinberg, Nativelle, and Prevot 1937) Smith 1957 to the genus *Streptococcus: Streptococcus parvulus* (Weinberg, Nativelle, and Prevot 1937) comb. nov., rev., emend. Int J Syst Bacteriol 33:82, 1983.
4. Gossling J: Occurrence and pathogenicity of the *Streptococcus milleri* group. Rev Infect Dis 10:257, 1988.
5. Madinger NE, McGregor JA, McKinney PJ, et al: Comparative antibiotic susceptibilities of anaerobes associated with infection of the female reproductive tract. Clin Infect Dis 16(Suppl 4):S349, 1993.
6. Murdoch DA, Mitchelmore IJ, Tabaqchali S: The clinical importance of gram-positive anaerobic cocci isolated at St. Bartholomew's Hospital, London, in 1987. J Med Microbiol 41:36, 1994.
7. Murdoch DA, Magee T: A numerical taxonomic study of the gram-positive anaerobic cocci. J Med Microbiol 43:148, 1995.
8. Brook I: Peptostreptococcal infection in children (Review). Scand J Infect Dis 26:503, 1994.
9. Rosenblatt J: Anaerobic cocci. *In* Lennette EH (ed): Manual of Clinical Microbiology, ed 4. Washington, DC, American Society for Microbiology, 1985, pp 445–449.
10. Johnson MJ, Thatcher E, Cox ME: Techniques for controlling variability in Gram staining of obligate anaerobes. J Clin Microbiol 33:755, 1995.
11. Ng J, Ng LK, Chow AW, Dillon JA: Identification of five *Peptostreptococcus* species isolated predominantly from the female genital tract by using the rapid ID32A system. J Clin Microbiol 32:1302, 1994.

12. Bartlett JG, Finegold SM: Bacteriology of expectorated sputum with quantitative culture and wash technique compared to transtracheal aspiration. Am Rev Respir Dis 117:1010, 1978.
13. Socransky SS, Manganiello SD: The oral microbiota of man from birth to senility. J Periodontol 42:485, 1971.
14. Bartlett JG, Onderdonk AB, Drude E, et al: Quantitative bacteriology of the vaginal flora. J Infect Dis 136:271, 1977.
15. Ohm MJ, Galask RP: Bacterial flora of the cervix from 100 prehysterectomy patients. Am J Obstet Gynecol 122:683, 1975.
16. Finegold SM, Attebery HR, Sutter VL: Effect of diet on human fecal flora: Comparison of Japanese and American diets. Am J Clin Nutr 27:1456, 1974.
17. Hentges DJ: The anaerobic microflora on the human body. Clin Infect Dis 16(Suppl 4):S175, 1993.
18. Martin WJ: Isolation and identification of anaerobic bacteria in the clinical laboratory: A 2-year experience. Mayo Clin Proc 49:300, 1974.
19. Bourgault A-M, Rosenblatt JE, Fitzgerald RH: *Peptococcus magnus:* A significant human pathogen. Ann Intern Med 93:244, 1980.
20. Finegold SM, George WL, Mulligan ME: Anaerobic infections. Dis Mon 31:8, 1985.
21. Montejo M, Ruiz-Irastorza G, Aguirrebengoa K, et al: Prosthetic-valve endocarditis caused by *Peptostreptococcus anaerobius* (Letter). Clin Infect Dis 20:1431, 1995.
22. von Troil-Linden B, Torkko H, Alaluusua S, et al: Salivary levels of suspected periodontal pathogens in relation to periodontal status and treatment. J Dent Res 74:1789, 1995.
23. Gomes BP, Lilley JD, Drucker DB: Clinical significance of dental root canal microflora. J Dent 24:47, 1996.
24. Bartlett JG, O'Keefe P: The bacteriology of perimandibular space infections. J Oral Surg 37:407, 1979.
25. Frederick J, Braude AI: Anaerobic infection of the paranasal sinuses. N Engl J Med 290:135, 1974.
26. Brook I: The role of anaerobic bacteria in otitis media: Microbiology, pathogenesis, and implications on therapy. Am J Otolaryngol 8:109, 1987.
27. Ito K, Ito Y, Mizuta K, et al: Bacteriology of chronic otitis media, chronic sinusitis, and paranasal mucopyocele in Japan. Clin Infect Dis 20(Suppl 2):S214, 1995.
28. Mitchelmore IJ, Prior AJ, Montgomery PQ, Tabaqchali S: Microbiological features and pathogenesis of peritonsillar abscesses. Eur J Clin Microbiol Infect Dis 14:870, 1995.
29. Bartlett JG: Systemic infection involving anaerobes: Anaerobic bacterial infections of the lung and pleural space. Clin Infect Dis 16(Suppl 4):S248, 1993.
30. Civen R, Jousimies-Somer H, Marina M, et al: A retrospective review of cases of anaerobic empyema and update of bacteriology. Clin Infect Dis 20(Suppl 2):S224, 1995.
31. Rotheram EB Jr, Schick SF: Nonclostridial anaerobic bacteria in septic abortion. Am J Med 46:80, 1969.
32. Smith JW, Southern PM Jr, Lehmann JD: Bacteremia in septic abortion: Complications and treatment. Obstet Gynecol 35:704, 1970.
33. Chow AW, Malkasian KL, Marshall JR, et al: The bacteriology of acute pelvic inflammatory disease. Am J Obstet Gynecol 122:876, 1975.
34. Eschenbach DA, Buchanan TM, Pollock HM, et al: Polymicrobial etiology of acute pelvic inflammatory disease. N Engl J Med 293:166, 1975.
35. Sweet R, Schachter J, Landers DV, et al: Treatment of hospitalized patients with acute pelvic inflammatory disease: Comparison of cefotetan plus doxycycline and cefoxitin plus doxycycline. Am J Obstet Gynecol 158:736, 1988.
36. Sweet R: Role of bacterial vaginosis in pelvic inflammatory disease. Clin Infect Dis 20(Suppl 2):S271, 1995.
37. Stone HH, Strom PR, Fabian TC, et al: Third-generation cephalosporins for polymicrobial surgical sepsis. Arch Surg 118:193, 1983.
38. Sabbaj J, Sutter VL, Finegold SM: Anaerobic pyogenic liver abscess. Ann Intern Med 77:629, 1972.
39. Gorbach SL: Management of anaerobic infections: Intra-abdominal sepsis. Ann Intern Med 83:377, 1975.
40. Moore WEC, Cato EP, Holdeman LV: Anaerobic bacteria of the gastrointestinal flora and their occurrence of clinical infections. J Infect Dis 119:641, 1969.
41. Swenson RM, Lorber B, Michaelson TC, et al: The bacteriology of intra-abdominal infections. Arch Surg 109:398, 1974.
42. Gerding DN: Foot infections in diabetic patients: The role of anaerobes (Review). Clin Infect Dis 20(Suppl 2):S283, 1995.
43. MacLennan JD: The histotoxic clostridial infections of man. Bacteriol Rev 26:232, 1962.
44. Summanen PH, Talan DA, Strong C, et al: Bacteriology of skin and soft-tissue infections: Comparison of infections in intravenous drug users and individuals with no history of intravenous drug use. Clin Infect Dis 20(Suppl 2):S279, 1995.
45. Brook I, Frazier EH: Clinical and microbiological features of necrotizing fasciitis. J Clin Microbiol 33:2382, 1995.
46. Finegold SM, and the National Committee for Clinical Laboratory Standards Working Group on Anaerobic Susceptibility Testing: Susceptibility testing of anaerobic bacteria. J Clin Microbiol 26:1253, 1988.
47. Edson RS, Rosenblatt JE, Lee DT, McVey EA III: Recent experience with antimicrobial susceptibility of anaerobic bacteria. Mayo Clin Proc 57:737, 1982.
48. Bourgault A-M, Harding GK, Smith JA, et al: Survey of anaerobic susceptibility patterns in Canada. Antimicrob Agents Chemother 30:798, 1986.
49. Garcia-Rodriguez JA, Garcia-Sanchez JE, Trujillano-Martin I, et al: In vitro activity of BAY y3118 and nine other antimicrobial agents against anaerobic bacteria. J Chemother 7:189, 1995.
50. Krepel CJ, Gohr CM, Edmiston CE, Condon RE: Surgical sepsis: Constancy of antibiotic susceptibility of causative organisms. Surgery 117:505, 1995.
51. Aldridge KE, Morice N, Schiro DD: Increased in vitro activity of ceftriaxone by addition of tazobactam against clinical isolates of anaerobes. Diagn Microbiol Infect Dis 19:227, 1994.
52. Reig M, Moreno A, Baquero F: Resistance of *Peptostreptococcus* spp to macrolides and lincosamides: Inducible and constitutive phenotypes. Antimicrob Agents Chemother 36:662, 1992.
53. Bantar C, Canigia LF, Relloso S, et al: Species belonging to the *"Streptococcus milleri"* group: Antimicrobial susceptibility and comparative prevalence in significant clinical specimens. J Clin Microbiol 34:2020, 1996.

219

Anaerobic Gram-Negative Rods: *Bacteroides, Prevotella, Porphyromonas, Fusobacterium, Bilophila, Sutterella*

Sydney M. Finegold

In this chapter I describe members of the genera *Anaerobiospirillum, Anaerorhabdus, Anaerovibrio, Bacteroides, Bilophila, Butyrivibrio, Campylobacter, Centipeda, Desulfomonas, Desulfovibrio, Fibrobacter, Fusobacterium, Leptotrichia, Megamonas, Porphyromonas, Prevotella, Rikenella, Ruminobacter, Sebaldella, Selenomonas, Succinimonas, Succinivibrio,* and *Sutterella*. These organisms are part of the normal flora of the mouth and upper respiratory, intestinal, and urogenital tracts of humans and animals.

Characteristics of the Pathogens

The initial differentiation of these genera is based on motility, flagellar arrangement, cellular morphology, and gas-liquid chromatographic analysis of cellular fatty acids and metabolic end products[1–19] (Table 219–1). Species definition is based on biochemical characteristics, nucleic acid base composition, and homology.[20, 21] For the majority of clinical specimens, only the genera *Bacteroides*, *Prevotella*, *Porphyromonas*, and *Fusobacterium* need to be considered. However, *Bilophila* and *Sutterella* do occur fairly commonly in intraabdominal and other infections.[5, 11] The taxonomy of anaerobic gram-negative bacilli has been in a state of great change in recent years, and the trend will continue. It has been proposed that only the present *Bacteroides fragilis* group (including *Bacteroides eggerthii*) should be included in the genus *Bacteroides* and that other species that have not yet been reclassified should be.[22] A new genus, *Prevotella*, includes the moderately saccharolytic organisms previously in the genus *Bacteroides*[6]; this includes the *Prevotella* species *P. oris*, *P. buccae*, the *P. oralis* group, *P. melaninogenica*, *P. denticola*, *P. loescheii*, *P. intermedia*, *P. nigrescens*,[23] *P. corporis*, *P. bivia*, and *P. disiens*. Nonsaccharolytic pigmented rods are placed in the genus *Porphyromonas*[7]; this includes the species *Porphyromonas asaccharolytica*, *Porphyromonas gingivalis*, *Porphyromonas endodontalis*, and *Porphyromonas macacae*. For more recent taxonomic changes, see Table 219–2.[24–33] The most common gram-negative anaerobic rods are listed in Table 219–3.[34, 35]

B. fragilis (Fig. 219–1), one of the most important of all anaerobes because of its frequency in clinical infection and its resistance to antimicrobial agents, is a gram-negative bacillus 0.5 to 0.8 μm in diameter and 1.5 to 4.5 μm long with rounded ends. Most strains are encapsulated. Vacuolization, irregular staining, and pleomorphism are common, particularly in broth media. The ultrastructure of *B. fragilis* is similar to that of other gram-negative bacteria. The guanine plus cytosine content is 42%. *P. melaninogenica* and *P. asaccharolytica* are short to coccoid gram-negative rods that produce a distinctive brown to black pigment, which is a heme derivative (Figs. 219–2 and 219–3). *P. asaccharolytica* is encapsulated. Many strains of *P. melaninogenica* require vitamin K or similar compounds as well as heme. Other anaerobic gram-negative rods are much less common.

TABLE 219–1 ■ Differentiation of the Genera of Gram-Negative Anaerobic Bacilli

CHARACTERISTIC	GENUS
Nonmotile or peritrichous flagella	
Produce butyric acid (without isobutyric and isovaleric acids)	*Fusobacterium*
Produce major lactic acid	*Leptotrichia*
Produce acetic acid and hydrogen sulfide, reduce sulfate	*Desulfomonas*
Not as above	*Anaerorhabdus* *Bacteroides* *Bilophila* *Fibrobacter* *Megamonas* *Porphyromonas* *Prevotella* *Rikenella* *Ruminobacter* *Sebaldella* *Sutterella*
Polar flagella	
Fermentative	
Produce butyric acid	*Butyrivibrio*
Produce succinic acid	
Spiral-shaped cells	*Succinivibrio*
Ovoid cells	*Succinimonas*
Produce propionic and acetic acids	*Anaerovibrio*
Nonfermentative, produce succinic acid from fumarate	*Campylobacter*
Tufts of flagella on concave side of curved cells, fermentative	*Selenomonas*
Flagella in a spiral arrangement along cell body, fermentative	*Centipeda*
Bipolar tufts of flagella	*Anaerobiospirillum*

TABLE 219–2 ■ Recent Taxonomic Changes

NEW NOMENCLATURE	PREVIOUS NOMENCLATURE
Anaerorhabdus furcosus	*Bacteroides furcosus*
Bacteroides	
B. caccae	*Bacteroides* "3452A"
B. forsythus	New species
B. galacturonicus	New species
B. merdae	New species
B. pectinophilus	New species
B. stercoris	New species
B. tectum	New species
Bilophila wadsworthia	New genus and species
Campylobacter	
C. concisus	New species
C. curvus	*Wolinella curva*
C. gracilis	*Bacteroides gracilis*
C. rectus	*Wolinella recta*
C. showae	New species
Centipeda periodontii	New genus and species
Fibrobacter intestinalis	New species
Fusobacterium	
F. alocis	New species
F. periodonticum	New species
F. pseudonecrophorum	New species
F. sulci	New species
F. ulcerans	New species
Megamonas hypermegas	*Bacteroides hypermegas*
Porphyromonas	
P. asaccharolytica	*Bacteroides asaccharolyticus*
P. catoniae	New species
P. circumdentaria	New species
P. endodontalis	*Bacteroides endodontalis*
P. gingivalis	*Bacteroides gingivalis*
P. levii	*Bacteroides levii*
P. macacae	*Bacteroides macacae, Bacteroides salivosus*
Prevotella	
P. bivia	*Bacteroides bivius*
P. buccae	*Bacteroides buccae*
P. buccalis	*Bacteroides buccalis*
P. corporis	*Bacteroides corporis*
P. dentalis	*Mitsuokella dentalis*
P. denticola	*Bacteroides denticola*
P. disiens	*Bacteroides disiens*
P. enoeca	New species
P. heparinolytica	*Bacteroides heparinolyticus*
P. intermedia	*Bacteroides intermedius*
P. loescheii	*Bacteroides loescheii*
P. melaninogenica	*Bacteroides melaninogenicus*
P. nigrescens	New species
P. oralis	*Bacteroides oralis*
P. oris	*Bacteroides oris*
P. oulora	*Bacteroides oulorum*
P. ruminicola	*Bacteroides ruminicola*
P. tannerae	New species
P. veroralis	*Bacteroides veroralis*
P. zoogleoformans	*Bacteroides zoogleoformans*
Rikenella microfusus	*Bacteroides microfusus*
Ruminobacter amylophilus	*Bacteroides amylophilus*
Sebaldella termitidis	*Bacteroides termitidis*
Selenomonas	
S. artemidis	New species
S. dianae	New species
S. flueggei	New species
S. infelix	New species
S. noxia	New species
Sutterella wadsworthensis	New genus and species
Wolinella succinogenes	*Bacteroides succinogenes*

TABLE 219–3 ■ Common Gram-Negative Anaerobic Rods

***BACTEROIDES FRAGILIS* GROUP**	**NONPIGMENTED BILE-SENSITIVE *PREVOTELLA* AND *BACTEROIDES***
B. fragilis	*Prevotella*
B. thetaiotaomicron	*P. oris*
B. distasonis	*P. buccae*
B. ovatus	*P. oralis*
B. vulgatus	*P. buccalis*
B. uniformis	*P. veroralis*
B. caccae	*P. oulora*
B. merdae	*P. disiens*
B. stercoris	*P. tannerae*
B. eggerthii	*Bacteroides*
B. splanchnicus	*B. capillosus*
PIGMENTED *PORPHYROMONAS* AND *PREVOTELLA*	*B. putredinis*
Porphyromonas	*B. forsythus*
P. asaccharolytica	***FUSOBACTERIUM* SPECIES**
P. gingivalis	*F. nucleatum*
P. endodontalis	*F. necrophorum*
P. macacae	*F. gonidiaformans*
Prevotella	*F. naviforme*
P. intermedia	*F. necrogenes*
P. nigrescens	*F. varium*
P. corporis	*F. mortiferum*
P. melaninogenica	*F. russii*
P. denticola	*F. alocis*
P. loescheii	*F. periodonticum*
P. bivia	*F. sulci*
P. heparinolytica	***BILOPHILA WADSWORTHIA***
P. zoogleoformans	***SUTTERELLA WADSWORTHENSIS***

Modified from Finegold SM: Classification and taxonomy of anaerobes. *In* Finegold SM, George WL (eds): Anaerobic Infections in Humans. San Diego, CA, Academic Press, 1989, p 23–36.

Numerous studies of the endotoxin of gram-negative anaerobic bacilli have determined that in *B. fragilis,* the endotoxin contains little or no lipid A, 2-ketodeoxyoctonate, or heptose. It also lacks β-hydroxymyristic acid. This endotoxin exhibits little biologic activity.[36] Poor biologic activity of endotoxin has also been demonstrated for *B. fragilis* group members, *P. melaninogenica,* and *P. asaccharolytica.*

Members of the genus *Fusobacterium* (Fig. 219–4) may be spindle shaped or may have parallel sides and rounded ends. Guanine plus cytosine content ranges from 26% to 34%. Cells of *Fusobacterium mortiferum* (and sometimes *Fusobacterium ne-*

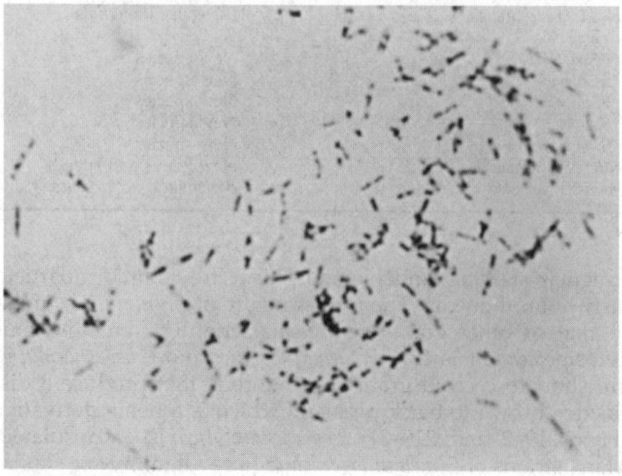

FIGURE 219–1 ▫ Microscopic morphology of *Bacteroides fragilis.* Note the irregularity of the staining.

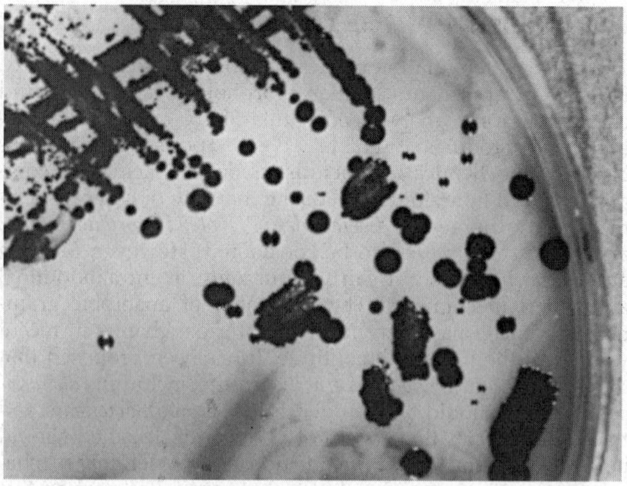

FIGURE 219–2 ▫ Colonial morphology of pigmented *Prevotella.* Pigment varies from brown to black.

crophorum) are often elongated or filamentous and curved and possess spherical enlargements and large, free, round bodies. *Fusobacterium nucleatum,* although it does not usually produce infections as serious as those caused by *F. necrophorum,* is encountered clinically much more often. The cells of this species are usually spindle shaped, 5 to 10 μm long, and are often seen in pairs, end to end.

The 2-ketodeoxyoctonate and sugar content of lipopolysaccharide of *F. necrophorum* varies from strain to strain. Although biologic activity varies, many or most strains do show strong biologic activity comparable to that of *Salmonella enteritidis.*[36] The biologic activity of the endotoxin of *F. nucleatum* is also variable but often strong.

Bilophila wadsworthia (Fig. 219–5) is a large, pale-staining, gram-negative bacillus with some pleomorphism and irregular staining. Its guanine plus cytosine content is 33% to 34%.

Plasmids have been found in about half of the *Bacteroides* strains studied. For the most part, their biologic and clinical significance is not known; however, some have been found to code for resistance to antimicrobial agents.

Most strains of the *B. fragilis* group can deconjugate bile acids.[37] *P. melaninogenica, P. oralis,* and *F. nucleatum* are inhib-

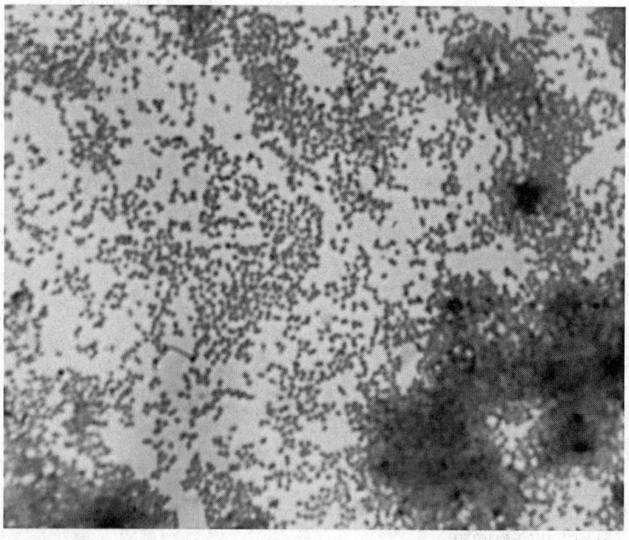

FIGURE 219–3 ▫ Microscopic morphology of pigmented *Prevotella.* The organisms are coccobacilli.

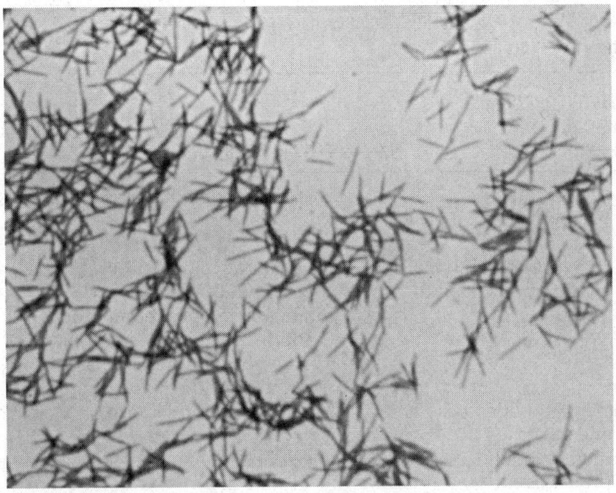

FIGURE 219–4 □ Microscopic morphology of *Fusobacterium nucleatum*. Note the delicate rods with tapered ends.

ited by bile. *Bilophila* and *Sutterella*, as well as the *B. fragilis* group, are resistant to bile.[5, 11] *F. necrophorum* deconjugates bile acids, primarily taurine conjugates.[37] Some *Bacteroides* species can convert primary bile acids to secondary ones. Glucuronidase produced by anaerobic gram-negative bacilli may be of special significance in deconjugating compounds that had previously been detoxified in the liver by combination with glucuronide.[13]

Certain *Bacteroides* species possess distinguishing enzymes. Superoxide dismutase has been found in *B. fragilis*, *Bacteroides thetaiotaomicron*, *Bacteroides vulgatus*, and *Bacteroides ovatus*.[38] In general, a good correlation exists between superoxide dismutase activity and oxygen tolerance. β-Lactamase activity has been demonstrated in several species of anaerobic gram-negative rods; it accounts for most of the resistance to various β-lactam antibiotics, such as certain penicillins and cephalosporins, although other mechanisms are occasionally responsible.[39, 40] Urease is produced by *B. wadsworthia*[5] and by *Bacteroides ureolyticus*. *B. ureolyticus* also produces an agarase, which accounts for pitting of the agar by the colonies. A related pitting organism, *Sutterella wadsworthensis*,[11] is much more pathogenic and relatively resistant to antimicrobial drugs.

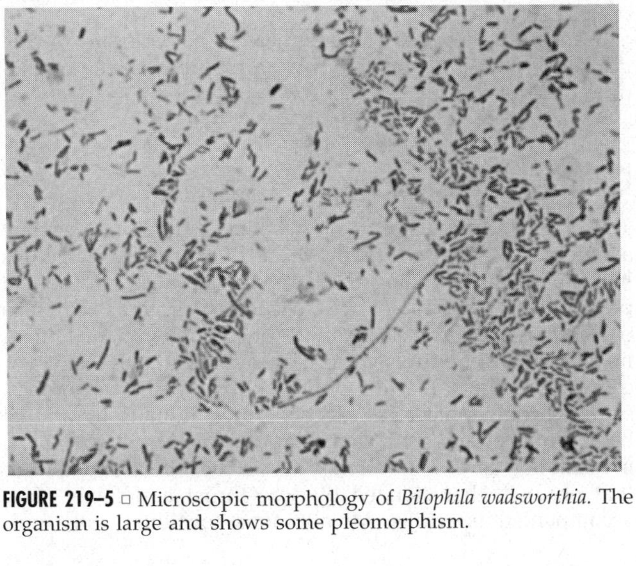

FIGURE 219–5 □ Microscopic morphology of *Bilophila wadsworthia*. The organism is large and shows some pleomorphism.

Epidemiology

All anaerobic, gram-negative bacillary infections arise when mucosal damage related to surgery, trauma, or disease permits indigenous flora to penetrate tissue. Knowledge of the indigenous flora at various sites under different circumstances permits the clinician to anticipate the likely infecting flora in acute infections. The pathogenicity of various species must also be considered. Ecologic determinants include oxygen sensitivity, ability of organisms to adhere, and microbial interrelationships.

At birth, an infant's oral cavity is usually sterile, but by age 12 months, *Fusobacterium* species can be cultured from 50% of infants and *Bacteroides* from a smaller percentage. In the human gingival crevice area, gram-negative anaerobic rods account for 16% to 20% of the total cultivatable flora. *P. melaninogenica* is seldom isolated before age 6 years, but this organism can be isolated from the gingival crevice area of most humans by the early teens. In the presence of acute ulcerative gingivitis or advanced chronic periodontal disease, *Fusobacterium* counts in saliva are higher than the usual 10^4 to 10^6 per mL. Gram-negative anaerobic rods usually constitute 8% to 17% of the cultivatable flora of human dental plaque. Selective localization is illustrated by the fact that *P. melaninogenica* is routinely found in the gingival crevice but only rarely on the tongue, cheek, or coronal tooth surface.[41, 42]

The normal stomach has few organisms and, as a rule, no anaerobic bacteria; however, in the presence of pathologic conditions such as duodenal ulcer with bleeding or obstruction, abnormal colonization with *B. fragilis* can occur in the stomach.[43] The terminal ileum has approximately equal numbers of facultative aerobes and anaerobes, *Bacteroides* being one of the major anaerobes. Almost invariably, *Bacteroides* organisms are found in the feces of adult subjects; the mean count is 10^{11} per g. *Fusobacterium* species are found in 18% of adults (mean 10^8 per g). *B. thetaiotaomicron* and *B. vulgatus* are the dominant species of *Bacteroides* in feces, followed by *Bacteroides distasonis*, *B. ovatus*, and *B. fragilis*. It has been found in animal studies that *Bacteroides* species protect against intestinal infections due to *Salmonella* and *Shigella* organisms.[41]

Bacteroides, *Prevotella*, and *Fusobacterium* organisms have often been found in the vaginal flora. Vaginal and cervical flora studies show that *Bacteroides* species are recovered from half of patients; mean concentrations are 10^6 per g. Species of *Bacteroides* and *Prevotella* recovered from the normal cervical flora of healthy women include *P. oralis*, *B. fragilis*, *Bacteroides capillosus*, *P. bivia*, *P. disiens*, *P. oris*, *P. buccae*, and *B. ureolyticus*.[41, 44]

Studies of normal urethral flora are relatively limited, but various *Fusobacterium* and *Bacteroides* species have been isolated. Fusiform bacilli and *P. melaninogenica* are found regularly on the external genitalia.

Bilophila organisms are found in about half of normal stool specimens, usually in counts of 10^5 to 10^6 per g of dry feces. They are part of the normal oral or vaginal flora in 2% of subjects.

Pathogenesis

Bacteroides, *Prevotella*, *Porphyromonas*, and *Fusobacterium* organisms are prevalent as indigenous flora on all mucosal surfaces. Under circumstances such as surgical or other trauma or when tumors arise or other diseases occur at the mucosal surface, they may penetrate tissues and produce an infection. In certain cases, for example, aspiration pneumonia, anaerobic bacteria from a site of normal carriage may move into one that is normally free of them and infect that site. Tissue necrosis and poor blood supply lower the oxidation-reduction potential, favoring the growth of anaerobes; accordingly, vascular disease, cold, shock, trauma, surgery, foreign bodies, malignant neoplasm, edema, and gas production by bacteria may significantly predispose tissue to infection with anaerobes, as may prior infection with aerobic or facultative bacteria. Antimicrobial agents, such as aminoglycosides, trimethoprim-sulfamethoxazole, or the earlier quinolones, to which anaerobes are notably resistant, may facilitate anaerobic infection. The relatively aerotolerant anaerobes are more likely to survive after the normally protective mucosal barrier is broken until conditions are satisfactory for their multiplication and invasion. Once anaerobes begin to multiply, they can maintain their own reduced environment by excreting end products of fermentative metabolism. Infections involving gram-negative anaerobic bacilli are often characterized by abscess formation and tissue destruction, as are most anaerobic infections. Table 219–4 lists common infections that involve gram-negative anaerobic bacilli.

Bacteroides, *Prevotella*, *Porphyromonas*, and *Fusobacterium* produce enzymes that may play a pathogenic role: collagenase, trypsin-like enzymes, various proteinases, neuraminidase, deoxyribonuclease, phosphatase, heparinase, and phospholipase.[36] Fibrinolysin is produced by many *P. melaninogenica* group strains and by a few of the *B. fragilis* group strains. Strains of *Bacteroides*, *Prevotella*, and *Porphyromonas* have been shown to degrade complement factors and immunoglobulins G and M. The lipopolysaccharides of *B. fragilis*, *B. vulgatus*, and *F. mortiferum* activate Hageman factor and thereby initiate the intrinsic pathway of coagulation. *F. necrophorum* produces a leukocidin, hemolysin, and a hemagglutinin.

Other factors may be involved in pathogenicity of certain anaerobes[44] (Table 219–5). *P. melaninogenica* may inhibit phagocytosis and killing of other organisms in mixed infections. Constituents of the cell envelope and cell surface may contribute to pathogenicity. The capsule of organisms such as *B. fragilis* may be an important virulence factor, as may fimbriae, pili, and lectin-like adhesins. Butyrate and succinate produced by *Bacteroides* are cytotoxic.

Polymorphonuclear leukocytes have oxygen-dependent and oxygen-independent microbicidal systems. Polymorphonuclear leukocytes normally kill *B. fragilis* under anaerobic and aerobic conditions. In response to factors generated by bacteria in plasma, however, chemotaxis is depressed markedly under anaerobic conditions, and products of *Bacteroides* may suppress neutrophil chemotaxis and phagocytic killing.[45, 46]

Studies of host defenses indicate that various other interactions may occur between the bacteria and the host cells. *B. fragilis* is more resistant to the normal bactericidal activity of serum than are other members of the *B. fragilis* group.

Immunoglobulin and components of the classical and alternative complement pathways participate in chemotaxis, bacteriolysis, and opsonophagocytic killing of various gram-negative anaerobic bacilli. Antibody to the capsular polysaccharide of *B. fragilis* confers significant protection against subsequent abscess development from *B. fragilis* strains[36]; furthermore, a study of women with acute pelvic inflammatory disease whose infecting flora contained *B. fragilis* demonstrated antibody to its capsular antigen.[47]

F. necrophorum has been demonstrated to persist for an extended period in the liver, where its proliferation in Kupffer cells impairs macrophage function. T cells are involved in immunity to *B. fragilis*, specifically linked to early stages of abscess formation.[36, 48]

Sears and colleagues[49] have indicated that enterotoxin-producing *B. fragilis* strains may play a role in diarrhea in children on occasion.

TABLE 219–4 ■ Common Syndromes of Gram-Negative Anaerobic Rod Infection

Bite infection
Oral or dental infection
Aspiration pneumonia, lung abscess, empyema
Postabortion and puerperal infections
Infection after bowel, gallbladder, or gynecologic surgery
Appendicitis, diverticulitis
Septicemia with malignant neoplasm, diabetes, corticosteroid therapy, negative blood cultures
Septic thrombophlebitis
Gas-forming infection
Putrid infection

TABLE 219–5 ■ Potential Virulence Factors of Gram-Negative Anaerobic Bacilli

PUTATIVE VIRULENCE FACTOR OR PROPERTY	POSSIBLE SIGNIFICANCE
Adherence to peritoneal mesothelium	Factor in development of peritonitis
Adherence to gingival crevicular epithelium	Factor in development of periodontal disease
Capsule	Inhibits macrophage migration, antiphagocytic for aerobes and anaerobes, promotes abscess formation
Superoxide dismutase and catalase	Confer oxygen tolerance
Immunoglobulin proteases	Resist host defenses
Hyaluronidase, collagenase, chondroitin sulfatase, neuraminidase, fibrinolysin	Tissue digestion or dissolution (i.e., spreading factors)
Heparinase and other coagulation-promoting factors	Impair blood supply to infected area
Lipopolysaccharide	Causes inflammation and bone resorption in periodontal disease
"Leukotoxin"	Cytopathic for a variety of mammalian cell types
Butyrate	Cytotoxic substance
Soluble inhibitors of chemotaxis	Blunting of inflammatory response

Clinical Manifestations

The clinical characteristics of infection with gram-negative anaerobic rods are primarily those of anaerobic infections in general: foul-smelling discharge, location of infection in proximity to mucosal surfaces, tissue necrosis, gas in tissues or discharge fluid, association of infection with malignant neoplasm, infection related to the use of aminoglycosides or other antimicrobials with poor activity against anaerobes, septic thrombophlebitis, infection after human or animal bites, and certain distinctive clinical features. The clinical presentation of *F. necrophorum* sepsis may be distinctive in that onset is characterized by sore throat and fever, often accompanied by chills. Membranous tonsillitis with foul-smelling breath may be noted, and in the absence of effective therapy, bacteremia and widespread metastatic infection may occur.[50, 51] Black discoloration of bloody exudates or red fluorescence of such exudates under ultraviolet light indicates infection with a pigmented anaerobic gram-negative rod.

Table 219–4 lists common syndromes of infection involving gram-negative anaerobic rods; in addition, there are infections, such as brain abscess, that are uncommon but that usually involve anaerobic gram-negative rods and other anaerobes. The frequency of occurrence of specific gram-negative anaerobic rods in various infections is noted in Table 219–6.

Gram-negative anaerobic bacilli, the most common anaerobes in clinical infections, are found in more than half of specimens yielding anaerobes.[52–54] *B. fragilis* and *B. thetaiotaomicron* are the members of the *B. fragilis* group that have the greatest clinical significance. They are recovered from most intraabdominal infections and may be found in infections at other sites.

The pigmented anaerobic gram-negative bacilli are composed of saccharolytic and asaccharolytic species of the genera *Prevotella* and *Porphyromonas*, respectively. At least 10 species of these genera are found in human clinical material.[55] *P. corporis, P. denticola, P. intermedia, P. nigrescens, P. loescheii, P. melaninogenica, P. endodontalis, P. asaccharolytica,* and *P. gingivalis* are found in the human oral cavity. Some are important pathogens in oral, dental, and bite wound infections and may produce infections of the head, neck, and lower respiratory tract. *P. asaccharolytica* and some of the pigmented organisms already mentioned are also prevalent in the urogenital and intestinal tract and are important in various infections. Other pigmented species—*Porphyromonas levii* and *P. macacae*—are of animal origin and may be found in humans with infected animal bite wounds.

The bile-sensitive, saccharolytic, gram-negative bacilli are found in the same setting as the pigmented gram-negative rods.[56] *P. bivia* and *P. disiens*, particularly, are found in female genital tract infections and less frequently in oral infections. It is important that they be recognized, because these strains are often resistant to the β-lactam antibiotics, including penicillin, aminopenicillins, and most cephalosporins. *P. oris* and *P. buccae* are found in a variety of oral[24] and other infections. The *P. oralis* group is now represented by *P. oralis, P. veroralis, P. buccalis,* and *P. oulora*.[1, 2, 25, 26]

Strains that produce a viscous material in broth are represented by (indole-negative) *Prevotella zoogleoformans* and (indole-positive) *Prevotella heparinolytica*[34, 35]; they are found in the oral cavity and in related infections. *Prevotella dentalis* has been isolated from infected dental root canals.[10, 57]

The bile-sensitive asaccharolytic species *B. capillosus* and *Bacteroides putredinis* inhabit the intestinal tract and have occasionally been recovered from various infections.[56] *Bacteroides forsythus*,[27] a fusiform, gram-negative rod, has been recovered from subgingival sites in patients with periodontitis.

The asaccharolytic, formate- and fumarate-requiring, nitrate- or nitrite-reducing gram-negative rods include *B. ureolyticus, Campylobacter gracilis* (formerly *Bacteroides gracilis*), *Campylobacter curvus* (formerly *Wolinella curva*), *Campylobacter rectus* (formerly *Wolinella recta*), and *Campylobacter succinogenes. S. wadsworthensis* has been recovered from a variety of infections including infections of the lungs, head and neck, abdomen, urogenital tract, bone, soft tissue, and others. Almost half of *Sutterella* strains produce β-lactamase, and *Sutterella* is resistant to metronidazole about one third of the time.[11] *Wolinella succinogenes* is also an oral isolate found primarily in periodontitis and periodontosis.[8] *B. wadsworthia* resembles *B. ureolyticus* and *Desulfomonas* species but is stimulated by bile, is strongly catalase-positive, and does not reduce sulfate. It is frequently recovered from inflamed and noninflamed appendices and related abscesses. *Bilophila* is also found in a variety of significant infections, including bacteremia.[58] About 95% of *Bilophila* strains are resistant to penicillin by virtue of β-lactamase production.[7]

F. nucleatum is often found in clinical infections. The organism is found in the mouth and in the genital, gastrointestinal, and upper respiratory tracts. It is often involved in the same types of infection as the pigmented *Prevotella* species and *Porphyromonas* species.[59] *F. nucleatum* was isolated more often in pure culture from cases of pleural empyema than any other organism, an indication of its virulence.[60] *Fusobacterium alocis, Fusobacterium sulci*,[28] and *Fusobacterium periodonticum* (all new species) are primarily isolated from subgingival sites in gingivitis and periodontitis. *F. necrophorum* is a virulent anaerobe that may cause severe infection originating from pharyngotonsillitis, usually in children or young adults. Local complications include peritonsillar abscess and jugular vein septic thrombophlebitis. There may also be multiple metastatic abscesses (most frequently in the lungs, pleural space, liver, and large joints) related to bacteremia (postanginal sepsis syndrome or Lemierre disease).[51, 59] *F. necrophorum* is found less often now than in the era before antimicrobial agents. *Fusobacterium ulcerans* is found in tropical ulcer.[29]

Leptotrichia buccalis is a common mouth organism that may also be found in the vagina and intestinal tract. It has caused septicemia in immunocompromised patients with oral mucosal infections.[61]

Selenomonas sputigena and the new species *Selenomonas artemidis, Selenomonas dianae, Selenomonas flueggei, Selenomonas infelix,* and *Selenomonas noxia*[30] are all oral organisms, as is *Centipeda periodontii*,[1, 2] which is found in subgingival sites in patients with periodontitis.

Desulfomonas pigra, Desulfovibrio species, *Succinimonas amylolytica, Succinivibrio dextrinosolvens,* and *Butyrivibrio fibrisolvens*, all normal colon flora, may occasionally be encountered in clinical infections as well.[62] The normal sites of carriage of *Anaerobiospirillum succiniciproducens* in humans are not known at present, but *Anaerobiospirillum* species are common in the fecal flora of cats and dogs.[63] Strains have been isolated from blood cultures of immunocompromised patients[62, 64] and from feces of patients with diarrhea.[63] In one report,[63] a role was proposed for *Anaerobiospirillum* species in zoonotic infections.

Specific clinical entities involving anaerobic gram-negative rods are discussed elsewhere in this text and are described in numerous reports.[39, 52, 53, 60, 65–74] Most gram-negative bacillary anaerobic infections are characterized by a prolonged course, significant tissue destruction, and abscess formation. Virtually all of these infections are mixed, containing other anaerobes and aerobic and facultative organisms as well.

Diagnosis

Anaerobic culture is the major method for specific laboratory diagnosis. Relatively good educated guesses about the involvement of certain specific anaerobic gram-negative rods can be made from examination of Gram stain of clinical specimens; however, different species can resemble one another. A limited number of fluorescent antibody reagents are available commercially, but they are not as specific as one might wish. Although gas chromatographic analysis of clinical specimens (or blood cultures) may provide definitive identification of an anaerobe, principally at the genus level (e.g., *Fusobacterium* organisms produce large amounts of butyric acid without isoacids), there are many potential pitfalls. DNA probes have been developed for a few gram-negative anaerobic rods, but none is yet available commercially except for diagnosis of periodontal disease.

TABLE 219–6 ■ Frequency of Specific Anaerobes in Various Infections (Wadsworth Veterans Administration Medical Center Experience, 1984 to 1990)

	BLOOD	CENTRAL NERVOUS SYSTEM	HEAD AND NECK INFECTIONS	DENTAL	HUMAN BITES	ANIMAL BITES	TRANSTRACHEAL ASPIRATION AND PLEURAL FLUID	LUNG
Number of specimens	161	50	60	12	7	21	90	32
Number of specimens yielding anaerobes	147	19	37	11	3	10	38	11
Bacteroides fragilis	41	2	5	3	0	0	2	0
Bacteroides thetaiotaomicron	7	0	3	0	0	0	1	0
Other *B. fragilis* group	14	0	7	0	0	1	4	1
Bilophila wadsworthia	0	0	0	0	0	0	1	0
Prevotella melaninogenica group	0	3	10	5	0	0	18	5
Prevotella intermedia-corporis	3	2	4	10	1	0	9	2
Other pigmented *Prevotella*	1	3	8	8	0	0	11	0
Porphyromonas asaccharolytica	1	0	0	0	0	0	0	0
Porphyromonas sp.	1	2	4	2	0	1	0	1
Campylobacter gracilis	1	1	2	0	0	0	1	1
Other *Bacteroides ureolyticus* group	2	0	6	6	0	1	4	1
Prevotella oralis group	0	2	8	8	0	0	13	1
Other *Bacteroides/Prevotella* sp.	3	0	5	0	1	0	10	0
Fusobacterium nucleatum	4	3	3	5	1	1	8	2
Fusobacterium necrophorum	1	0	0	0	0	0	0	0
Fusobacterium mortiferum-varium	0	0	0	0	0	0	0	
Other *Fusobacterium* sp.	4	3	5	5	1	2	0	0
Other gram-negative bacilli	2	2	2	3	0	1	5	1

*Designations stated on culture requisition.
†Mostly from appendiceal infections.
Modified from Summanen P, Baron EJ, Citron DM, et al: Wadsworth Anaerobic Bacteriology Manual, ed 5. Belmont, CA, Star Publishing, 1993, pp 11–13.

Optimal culture requires prereduced or fresh media. It is probably desirable to use an anaerobic chamber at least for the initial culture; obviously, it is critical that optimal specimen collection and transport techniques be used. Collection must avoid sources of indigenous flora; tissue and pus collected in a syringe are the best specimens. A variety of good transport setups are available commercially.

Species are identified presumptively on the basis of a few observations: colonial and cellular morphology, pigment production, fluorescence under long-wave ultraviolet light, susceptibility to special-potency antibiotic disks, and certain rapidly determined biochemical characteristics.[3] Definitive identification requires the determination of multiple characteristics with a battery of biochemical tests.[1–3, 21, 75] Cellular fatty acid determination is particularly helpful.[18] Definitive identification is not feasible for all anaerobic isolates because of financial constraints and is not ordinarily important for clinical purposes. Such detailed bacteriologic tests should be available in certain teaching centers or reference laboratories for special circumstances, such as unusual clinical cases, organisms never before encountered, and publication and teaching purposes. For clinical purposes, it is commonly sufficient to know the broad groupings of isolates, whether they produce β-lactamase, and their usual patterns of susceptibility to antimicrobial agents. Details on definitive identification may be found in anaerobic laboratory manuals.[1–3]

Treatment

Surgical or percutaneous computed tomography–guided or ultrasonography-guided drainage of abscesses and surgical débridement or excision of necrotic tissue are crucial to successful treatment. Hyperbaric oxygen is of doubtful value in infections with non–spore-forming anaerobic organisms.

Mixed infections involving anaerobic and aerobic or facultative bacteria typically involve a complex flora, so results of cultures do not become available for some time; accordingly, initial therapy for such infections must be empirical, although information such as that derived from examination of a Gram-stained specimen may be used effectively to assist in the choice of drug. The physician should base the initial choice of therapeutic agents on the nature and location of the infection, the usual flora anticipated in infections of the type being treated, factors that might have modified such flora, Gram stain results, and severity of the infection.

Most anaerobic infections are mixed; if the agent chosen for the anaerobes does not provide adequate coverage for the nonanaerobes, an additional agent may be needed. Other factors to be considered in certain circumstances include central nervous system penetration and bactericidal effect. Clearly, the toxicity of various agents under consideration for therapy is important, as is their impact on the normal flora. Agents that produce relatively little disturbance of indigenous flora are less likely to lead to significant superinfection. One major superinfection to be kept in mind is pseudomembranous colitis, which is usually caused by *Clostridium difficile*, although other clostridia and *Staphylococcus aureus* may cause it on occasion. Agents that suppress normal colon flora significantly and have relatively poor activity against *C. difficile*, of course, are more likely to lead to this complication. The cost of the various antimicrobial agents that may be suitable in terms of activity is certainly an important consideration, and pharmacokinetic characteristics that may permit less frequent dosing must be factored into the decision.

The breakpoint is the concentration of drug in the body at

				MISCELLANEOUS SOFT TISSUE INFECTIONS					
OSTEOMYELITIS*	FOOT ULCER*	DECUBITUS ULCER	PERIRECTAL ABSCESS	Below the Waist	Above the Waist	APPENDICEAL TISSUE OR ABSCESS	PERITONEAL FLUID†	GALLBLADDER	ABDOMINAL, OTHER
72	278	15	15	80	33	70	126	20	15
20	148	8	12	32	9	66	74	17	5
2	17	2	8	9	0	35	37	3	3
2	1	0	1	4	0	25	34	0	2
4	15	7	10	19	0	60	93	3	8
0	0	0	0	0	1	29	30	0	0
1	15	0	0	3	2	3	3	0	1
2	6	0	1	4	1	7	16	0	1
3	15	2	3	11	0	3	5	1	1
0	3	0	0	8	0	2	1	0	0
3	5	0	2	3	0	6	3	0	0
1	1	0	2	0	1	6	9	0	0
4	10	0	3	8	0	3	3	0	0
0	10	0	1	1	0	0	7	0	0
5	22	1	4	15	3	29	24	1	2
0	9	0	1	1	1	10	14	0	0
0	1	0	0	0	0	2	2	0	0
0	0	0	0	0	0	3	2	0	0
1	5	0	2	1	0	3	7	0	0
0	3	0	1	7	0	8	12	0	0

or below which infection with the organism in question will generally respond to therapy; this is usually equivalent to peak levels achievable in serum with the maximal approved dosage in the case of anaerobes.

Finally, the severity of infection should be considered. The most potent agents should not be used for relatively mild infections. This practice is likely to lead eventually to the development of resistance and to the consequent loss of important agents for treating serious infections. Less powerful agents may be perfectly adequate for milder infections in patients with good host defense mechanisms; indeed, it may be impossible to demonstrate any advantage for a more potent agent in such a setting. Young, otherwise healthy patients with a community-acquired infection (such as appendicitis without generalized peritonitis or with pelvic inflammatory disease) will usually respond well to less potent agents if needed surgical management is provided. If the less effective agents have other advantages (e.g., low toxicity, low cost), it makes good sense to use them. On the other hand, an elderly diabetic patient in an intensive care unit with a hospital-acquired, intraabdominal infection needs the best antimicrobial agents available.

Antimicrobial resistance is as much a problem with anaerobic gram-negative rods as with most other bacteria. Various major mechanisms of resistance are noted in Table 219–7, and gram-negative anaerobic rods known to produce β-lactamases are listed in Table 219–8. Susceptibility data are given in Table 219–9 for various anaerobic gram-negative rods isolated at the Wadsworth Veterans Hospital (VA Medical Center, West Los Angeles); in Table 219–10 for motile, anaerobic, gram-negative rods (mostly from reports in the literature); and in Table 219–11 for isolates from bite wounds.

Details of therapy for anaerobic infections are found in specific chapters.

TABLE 219–7 ■ Mechanisms of Resistance in Anaerobes

MECHANISMS

- Drug inactivation
- Failure of drug to get into bacterial cells
- Pumping drug out of bacterial cells
- Changes in targets for drugs
- Failure to reduce drug to active form

FACILITATORS

- Inducibility
- Conjugation
- Plasmid transfer

Susceptibility Testing

A number of problems are encountered in susceptibility testing of anaerobic bacteria: lack of standardized techniques, failure to use recent clinical isolates, testing too few strains, use of nonrepresentative species, clustering at the breakpoint, difficulty in reading end points, poor growth of certain anaerobes, and need for clinical correlation. Interlaboratory varia-

TABLE 219–8 ■ β-Lactamase–Producing Gram-Negative Anaerobic Rods

Bacteroides fragilis group	*Prevotella buccae*
Bacteroides splanchnicus	*Fusobacterium nucleatum*
Bacteroides coagulans	*Fusobacterium mortiferum*
Pigmented *Prevotella* and *Porphyromonas*	*Fusobacterium varium*
Prevotella oralis group	*Bilophila wadsworthia*
Prevotella disiens	*Sutterella wadsworthensis*
Prevotella oris	*Megamonas hypermegas*

TABLE 219–9 ■ Activity of Various Drugs* Versus Gram-Negative Anaerobes (Wadsworth Agar Dilution Procedure)

PERCENTAGE SUSCEPTIBLE†	*BACTEROIDES FRAGILIS*	OTHER *BACTEROIDES FRAGILIS* GROUP‡	*CAMPYLOBACTER GRACILIS*	OTHER *BACTEROIDES*	*PREVOTELLA*	*PORPHYROMONAS*	*SUTTERELLA WADSWORTHENSIS*	*FUSOBACTERIUM NUCLEATUM*	*FUSOBACTERIUM MORTIFERUM-VARIUM*	OTHER *FUSOBACTERIUM*	*BILOPHILA WADSWORTHIA*
>95	Ampicillin-sulbactam Piperacillin-tazobactam Ticarcillin-clavulanate Cefoperazone-sulbactam Imipenem Chloramphenicol Clinafloxacin Metronidazole	Ampicillin-sulbactam Cefoperazone-sulbactam Piperacillin-tazobactam Ticarcillin-clavulanate Imipenem Chloramphenicol Clinafloxacin Metronidazole Minocycline	Piperacillin Amoxicillin-clavulanate Piperacillin-tazobactam Ticarcillin-clavulanate Cefoxitin Ceftizoxime Ceftriaxone Imipenem Meropenem Ciprofloxacin Fleroxacin Clindamycin Metronidazole Minocycline Tetracycline	Ampicillin-sulbactam Piperacillin Ticarcillin-clavulanate Cefoperazone Cefoperazone-sulbactam Cefotaxime Cefoxitin Imipenem Chloramphenicol Clinafloxacin Clindamycin	Amoxicillin-clavulanate Ceftizoxime Imipenem Chloramphenicol Clinafloxacin Clindamycin Metronidazole	Amoxicillin-clavulanate Ceftizoxime Imipenem Chloramphenicol Clinafloxacin Metronidazole Minocycline	Amoxicillin-clavulanate Ticarcillin-clavulanate Cefoxitin Ceftizoxime Ceftriaxone Clindamycin	Amoxicillin-clavulanate Ceftizoxime Imipenem Chloramphenicol Clinafloxacin Clindamycin Metronidazole Minocycline Tetracycline	Imipenem Chloramphenicol Clinafloxacin Metronidazole Minocycline	Ampicillin-sulbactam Ceftizoxime Penicillin G Piperacillin Piperacillin-tazobactam Imipenem Chloramphenicol Clinafloxacin Clindamycin Minocycline Metronidazole	Amoxicillin-clavulanate Ampicillin-sulbactam Penicillin G Piperacillin Ticarcillin Cefoxitin Ceftizoxime Imipenem Chloramphenicol Ciprofloxacin Clindamycin Metronidazole Minocycline Tetracycline
85–95	Cefotetan Cefoxitin Ceftizoxime Piperacillin Clindamycin Minocycline	Piperacillin Ceftizoxime		Cefotetan Ceftazidime Ceftizoxime Ceftriaxone Minocycline		Ciprofloxacin Clindamycin	Piperacillin Piperacillin-tazobactam		Amoxicillin-clavulanate	Ticarcillin-clavulanate Cefoperazone Cefoperazone-sulbactam Cefotaxime Cefotetan Cefoxitin	
70–84	Moxalactam	Cefoxitin Clindamycin		Penicillin G Moxalactam	Minocycline			Ciprofloxacin	Clindamycin Tetracycline	Ceftazidime Moxalactam	
50–69	Cefoperazone Cefotaxime Ceftazidime Ceftriaxone	Cefoperazone Cefotetan Moxalactam		Ciprofloxacin Tetracycline	Ciprofloxacin Tetracycline	Tetracycline	Metronidazole		Ciprofloxacin		
<50	Penicillin G Ciprofloxacin Tetracycline	Penicillin G Cefotaxime Ceftazidime Ceftriaxone							Ceftizoxime		Amoxicillin Ampicillin

*The order of listing of drugs within percentage susceptible categories is not significant.
†According to the National Committee for Clinical Laboratory Standards–approved breakpoints (M11-A3), using the intermediate category as susceptible.
‡Excluding *B. fragilis*.
Modified from Finegold SM: Aspiration pneumonia. Semin Respir Crit Care Med 16:475–483, 1995.

TABLE 219–10 ■ Antimicrobial Susceptibility of Motile, Anaerobic Gram-Negative Bacilli in Vitro

	DRUGS ELICITING INDICATED RESULT IN SUSCEPTIBILITY TESTS*		
ORGANISM	**Susceptible**	**Variable**	**Resistant**
Butyrivibrio (1)†	Penicillin G, chloramphenicol, erythromycin, tetracyclines	—	Bacitracin, streptomycin, kanamycin, lincomycin, sulfonamides
Succinimonas‡ (1)	Bacitracin, oxytetracycline, penicillin G	—	Kanamycin, streptomycin, erythromycin
Succinivibrio (2)	Penicillin G, tetracycline, erythromycin, chloramphenicol	Clindamycin	—
Wolinella§ (19)	Metronidazole, clindamycin, chloramphenicol, tetracycline, erythromycin, imipenem, ciprofloxacin	Penicillin G, piperacillin, cephalosporins, gentamicin, rifampin, polymyxins	Vancomycin, bacitracin, nalidixic acid
Campylobacter (7)	Clindamycin, chloramphenicol, metronidazole, penicillin G, tetracycline, erythromycin	—	Vancomycin, bacitracin, rifampin
Desulfovibrio (1)	Penicillin G, clindamycin, chloramphenicol, tetracycline, erythromycin	—	Vancomycin, colistin
Selenomonas (32)	Clindamycin, chloramphenicol, metronidazole	Penicillin G, ampicillin, erythromycin, tetracycline	Vancomycin, colistin
Anaerobiospirillum (17)	Cephalothin, chloramphenicol, tetracycline, rifampin	Ampicillin, erythromycin, metronidazole, nalidixic acid	Vancomycin, trimethoprim, penicillin G

*Strains are reported as susceptible if more than 90% of tested isolates were susceptible, as variable if 50% to 90% of tested isolates were susceptible, and as resistant if less than 50% of tested isolates were susceptible. The susceptibility of all isolates was not reported for all antimicrobial agents.

†Approximate number of isolates is given in parentheses.

‡Susceptibility data are for a strain isolated from an animal rumen. (From Johnson CC, Finegold SM: Uncommonly encountered, motile, anaerobic gram-negative bacilli associated with infection. Rev Infect Dis 9:1150, 1987.)

§Now reclassified as *Campylobacter*; various species are involved.

From Finegold SM: Therapy of anaerobic infections. *In* Finegold SM, George WL (eds): Anaerobic Infections in Humans. San Diego, CA, Academic Press, 1989, pp 793–818.

tions in testing procedures have produced confusion about the extent of resistance among anaerobes. The current National Committee for Clinical Laboratory Standards reference method is unsatisfactory because the medium does not support the growth of a number of strains of clinically important anaerobes, such as pigmented anaerobic bacilli, *F. nucleatum*, and anaerobic cocci. The phenomenon of clustering of end points within one dilution of the breakpoint is relatively common with certain β-lactam agents, clindamycin, and chloramphenicol.[40] Because the error factor common to most of the procedures used is one twofold dilution, this clustering effect may lead to significant variability, even within one laboratory. The broth disk elution procedure, a simple test preferred by many clinical laboratories, has given undependable results with a number of antimicrobial agents and is no longer approved by the National Committee for Clinical Laboratory Standards. However, gradient end point procedures such as the E test are easy to use and useful.

Susceptibility testing of anaerobes should be done to determine the activity of new agents, to monitor susceptibility patterns periodically in various centers and in a particular hospital or community, and to guide the management of infections in individual patients. In the last case, indications include treatment failure, relapse, persistence of infection despite empirical therapy, and serious illness (brain abscess, endocarditis, osteomyelitis, infection of prosthetic device or vascular graft) requiring prolonged therapy.

These problems notwithstanding, a great deal of valuable information has been accumulated on the activity of various drugs against different anaerobic pathogens. There are no simple answers, unfortunately, as to the best or correct test in vitro for susceptibility. The most practical tests available for studying small numbers of isolates in clinical laboratories are the broth microdilution test (available commercially in frozen or lyophilized form in trays already containing serial twofold dilutions of various antimicrobial agents) and the E

TABLE 219–11 ■ Activity of Selected Oral Antimicrobials Against Anaerobic Bite Wound Isolates

	MIC_{90} (μg/mL)*		
DRUG	**Pigmented *Prevotella* or *Porphyromonas***	**Other *Bacteroides, Prevotella,* and *Porphyromonas***	***Fusobacterium***
Penicillin G	1 (≤0.06–8)	8 (≤0.06–16)	0.5 (≤0.06–1)
Oxacillin	16 (<0.06–16)	32 (≤0.06–32)	2 (≤0.06–4)
Cephalexin	2 (≤0.06–4)	8 (0.5–16)	1 (≤0.06–1)
Minocycline	1 (≤0.06–32)	4 (≤0.06–8)	0.12 (≤0.06–0.25)
Erythromycin	1 (≤0.06–1)	1 (≤0.06–1)	32 (2–64)
Trimethoprim-sulfamethoxazole	32 (≤0.06–32)	64 (1–>64)	64 (1–≥64)

*Minimal inhibitory concentration for 90% of strains; range is given in parentheses.

Adapted from Goldstein EJ, Citron DM, Vagvolgyi AE, Finegold SM: Susceptibility of bite wound bacteria to seven oral antimicrobial agents, including RU-985, a new erythromycin: Considerations in choosing empiric therapy. Antimicrob Agents Chemother 29:556–559, 1986.

test strips containing gradients of antibiotic concentrations. Agar plate dilution procedures and the spiral gradient agar procedure are preferred for larger numbers of strains.

The information gleaned from susceptibility studies provides us with good guidance for empirical therapy. There is a considerable mass of clinical data that shows a good correlation with data from in vitro tests, although more correlative studies are clearly needed, particularly with certain newer agents and with older agents to which significant resistance has developed.

References

1. Holdeman LV, Cato EP, Moore WEC (eds): Anaerobe Laboratory Manual, ed 4. Blacksburg, VA, Virginia Polytechnic Institute and State University, 1977.
2. Moore LVH, Cato EP, Moore WEC: Anaerobe Laboratory Manual Update. Blacksburg, VA, Virginia Polytechnic Institute and State University, 1987. (Published as a supplement to the VPI Anaerobe Laboratory Manual, ed 4.)
3. Summanen P, Baron EJ, Citron DM, et al: Wadsworth Anaerobic Bacteriology Manual, ed 5. Belmont, CA, Star Publishing, 1993.
4. Shah HN, Collins MD: Reclassification of *Bacteroides furcosus* Veillon and Zuber (Hauduroy, Ehringer, Urbain, Guillot and Magrou) in a new genus *Anaerorhabdus*, as *Anaerorhabdus furcosus* comb. nov. Syst Appl Microbiol 8:86, 1986.
5. Baron EJ, Summanen P, Downes J, et al: *Bilophila wadsworthia*, a unique gram-negative anaerobic rod recovered from appendicitis specimens and human feces. J Gen Microbiol 135:3405, 1989.
6. Shah HN, Collins MD: *Prevotella*, a new genus to include *Bacteroides melaninogenicus* and related species formerly classified in the genus *Bacteroides*. Int J Syst Bacteriol 40:205, 1990.
7. Shah HN, Collins MD: Proposal for reclassification of *Bacteroides asaccharolyticus*, *Bacteroides gingivalis*, and *Bacteroides endodontalis* in a new genus, *Porphyromonas*. Int J Syst Bacteriol 38:128, 1988.
8. Tanner ACR, Badger S, Lai C-H, et al: *Wolinella* gen. nov., *Wolinella succinogenes* (*Vibrio succinogenes* Wolin et al.) comb. nov., and description of *Bacteroides gracilis* sp. nov., *Wolinella recta* sp. nov., *Campylobacter concisus* sp. nov., and *Eikenella corrodens* from humans with periodontal disease. Int J Syst Bacteriol 31:432, 1981.
9. Gharbia SE, Shah HN: Characteristics of glutamate dehydrogenase, a new diagnostic marker for the genus *Fusobacterium*. J Gen Microbiol 134:327, 1988.
10. Willems A, Collins MD: 16S rRNA gene similarities indicate that *Hallella seregens* (Moore and Moore) and *Mitsuokella dentalis* (Haapasalo et al.) are genealogically highly related and are members of the genus *Prevotella*: Emended description of the genus *Prevotella* (Shah and Collins) and description of *Prevotella dentalis* comb. nov. Int J Syst Bacteriol 45:832, 1995.
11. Wexler HM, Reeves D, Summanen PH, et al: *Sutterella wadsworthensis* gen. nov., sp. nov., bile-resistant microaerophilic *Campylobacter gracilis*–like clinical isolates. Int J Syst Bacteriol 46:252, 1996.
12. Vandamme P, Daneshvar MI, Dewhirst FE, et al: Chemotaxonomic analyses of *Bacteroides gracilis* and *Bacteroides ureolyticus* and reclassification of *B. gracilis* as *Campylobacter gracilis* comb. nov. Int J Syst Bacteriol 45:145, 1995.
13. Vandamme P, Falsen E, Rossau R, et al: Revision of *Campylobacter*, *Helicobacter*, and *Wolinella* taxonomy: Emendation of generic descriptions and proposal of *Arcobacter* gen. nov. Int J Syst Bacteriol 41:88, 1991.
14. Willems A, Collins MD: Reclassification of *Oribaculum catoniae* (Moore and Moore 1994) as *Porphyromonas catoniae* comb. nov. and emendation of the genus *Porphyromonas*. Int J Syst Bacteriol 45:578, 1995.
15. Love D: *Porphyromonas macacae* comb. nov., a consequence of *Bacteroides macacae* being a senior synonym of *Porphyromonas salivosa*. Int J Syst Bacteriol 45:90, 1995.
16. Love DN, Bailey GD, Collings S, Briscoe DA: Description of *Porphyromonas circumdentaria* sp. nov. and reassignment of *Bacteroides salivosus* (Love, Johnson, Jones, and Calverley 1987) as *Porphyromonas* (Shah and Collins 1988) *salivosa* comb. nov. Int J Syst Bacteriol 42:434, 1992.
17. Tanner A, Maiden MFJ, Paster BJ, Dewhirst FE: The impact of 16S ribosomal RNA–based phylogeny on the taxonomy of oral bacteria. Periodontology 2000 5:26, 1994.
18. Moore LVH, Bourne DM, Moore WEC: Comparative distribution and taxonomic value of cellular fatty acids in thirty-three genera of anaerobic gram-negative bacilli. Int J Syst Bacteriol 44:338, 1994.
19. Farrow JAE, Lawson PA, Hippe H, et al: Phylogenetic evidence that the gram-negative nonsporulating bacterium *Tissierella (Bacteroides) praeacuta* is a member of the *Clostridium* subphylum of the gram-positive bacteria and description of *Tissierella creatini* sp. nov. Int J Syst Bacteriol 45:436, 1995.
20. Wayne LG, Brenner DJ, Colwell RR, et al: Report of the ad hoc committee on reconciliation of approaches to bacterial systematics. Int J Syst Bacteriol 37:463, 1987.
21. Jousimies-Somer HR, Summanen PH, Finegold SM: *Bacteroides*, *Porphyromonas*, *Prevotella*, *Fusobacterium*, and other anaerobic gram-negative bacteria. *In* Baron EJ, Pfaller MA, Tenover FC, Yolken RH (eds): Manual of Clinical Microbiology. Washington, DC, ASM Press, 1995, p 603.
22. Shah HN, Collins MD: Proposal to restrict the genus *Bacteroides* (Castellani and Chalmers) to *Bacteroides fragilis* and closely related species. Int J Syst Bacteriol 39:85, 1989.
23. Shah HN, Gharbia SE: Biochemical and chemical studies on strains designated *Prevotella intermedia* and proposal of a new pigmented species, *Prevotella nigrescens* sp. nov. Int J Syst Bacteriol 42:542, 1992.
24. Haapasalo M: *Bacteroides buccae* and related taxa in necrotic root canal infections. J Clin Microbiol 24:940, 1986.
25. Shah HN, Collins MD, Watabe J, Mitsuoka T: *Bacteroides oulorum* sp. nov., a nonpigmented saccharolytic species from the oral cavity. Int J Syst Bacteriol 35:193, 1985.
26. Watabe J, Benno Y, Mitsuoka T: Taxonomic study of *Bacteroides oralis* and related organisms and proposal of *Bacteroides veroralis* sp. nov. Int J Syst Bacteriol 33:57, 1983.
27. Tanner ACR, Listgarten MA, Ebersole JL, Strzempko MN: *Bacteroides forsythus* sp. nov., a slow-growing, fusiform *Bacteroides* sp. from the human oral cavity. Int J Syst Bacteriol 36:213, 1986.
28. Cato EP, Moore LVH, Moore WEC: *Fusobacterium alocis* sp. nov. and *Fusobacterium sulci* sp. nov. from the human gingival sulcus. Int J Syst Bacteriol 35:475, 1985.
29. Adriaans B, Shah H: *Fusobacterium ulcerans* sp. nov. from tropical ulcers. Int J Syst Bacteriol 38:447, 1988.
30. Moore LVH, Johnson JL, Moore WEC: *Selenomonas noxia* sp. nov., *Selenomonas flueggei* sp. nov., *Selenomonas infelix* sp. nov., *Selenomonas dianae* sp. nov., and *Selenomonas artemidis* sp. nov., from the human gingival crevice. Int J Syst Bacteriol 36:271, 1987.
31. Love DN, Bailey GD: Chromosomal DNA probes for the identification of *Bacteroides tectum* and *Bacteroides fragilis* from the oral cavity of cats. Vet Microbiol 34:89, 1993.
32. Moore LV, Johnson JL, Moore WE: Descriptions of *Prevotella tannerae* sp. nov. and *Prevotella enoeca* sp. nov. from the human gingival crevice and emendation of the description of *Prevotella zoogleoformans*. Int J Syst Bacteriol 44:599, 1994.
33. Bolstad AI, Jensen HB: Polymerase chain reaction–amplified nonradioactive probes for identification of *Fusobacterium nucleatum*. J Clin Microbiol 31:528, 1993.
34. Bailey GD, Moore LVH, Love DN, Johnson JL: *Bacteroides heparinolyticus*: Deoxyribonucleic acid relatedness of strains from the oral cavity and oral-associated disease conditions of horses, cats, and humans. Int J Syst Bacteriol 38:42, 1988.
35. Okuda K, Kato T, Shiozu J, et al: *Bacteroides heparinolyticus* sp. nov. isolated from humans with periodontitis. Int J Syst Bacteriol 35:438, 1985.
36. Zaleznik DF, Kasper DL: Role of bacterial virulence factors in pathogenesis of anaerobic infections. *In* Finegold SM, George WL (eds): Anaerobic Infections in Humans. San Diego, CA, Academic Press, 1989, pp 81–95.
37. Shimada K, Sutter VL, Finegold SM: Effect of bile and desoxycholate on gram-negative anaerobic bacteria. Appl Microbiol 20:737, 1970.
38. Goldin BR, Gorbach SL: Impact of anaerobic bowel flora on metabolism of endogenous and exogenous compounds. *In* Finegold SM, George WL (eds): Anaerobic Infections in Humans. San Diego, CA, Academic Press, 1989, pp 691–714.
39. Nord CE: The role of anaerobic bacteria in recurrent episodes of sinusitis and tonsillitis. Clin Infect Dis 20:1512, 1995.

40. Wexler HM, Finegold SM: Antimicrobial resistance in *Bacteroides*. J Antimicrob Chemother 19:143, 1987.
41. Hentges DJ: Anaerobes as normal flora. *In* Finegold SM, George WL (eds): Anaerobic Infections in Humans. San Diego, CA, Academic Press, 1989, pp 37–53.
42. Hentges DJ: The anaerobic microflora of the human body. Clin Infect Dis 16(Suppl 4):S175, 1993.
43. Nichols RL, Smith JW: Intragastric microbial colonization in common disease states of the stomach and duodenum. Ann Surg 182:557, 1975.
44. Hillier SL, Krohn MA, Rabe LK, et al: The normal vaginal flora, H_2O_2-producing lactobacilli, and bacterial vaginosis in pregnant women. Clin Infect Dis 16(Suppl 4):S273, 1993.
45. Rotstein OD: Interactions between leukocytes and anaerobic bacteria in polymicrobial surgical infections. Clin Infect Dis 16(Suppl 4):S190, 1993.
46. Bjornson AB: Host defense mechanisms against non–spore-forming anaerobic bacteria. *In* Finegold SM, George WL (eds): Anaerobic Infections in Humans. San Diego, CA, Academic Press, 1989, pp 97–110.
47. Eschenbach DA, Holmes KK: The etiology of acute pelvic inflammatory disease. Sex Transm Dis 6:224, 1979.
48. Tzianabos AO, Kasper DL, Onderdonk AB: Structure and function of *Bacteroides fragilis* capsular polysaccharides: Relationship to induction and prevention of abscesses. Clin Infect Dis 20(Suppl 2):S132, 1995.
49. Sears CL, Myers LL, Lazenby A, Van Tassell RL: Enterotoxigenic *Bacteroides fragilis*. Clin Infect Dis 20(Suppl 2):S142, 1995.
50. Mulligan ME: Ear, nose, throat, and head and neck infections. *In* Finegold SM, George WL (eds): Anaerobic Infections in Humans. San Diego, CA, Academic Press, 1989, pp 263–288.
51. Moreno S, Altozano JG, Pinilla B, et al: Lemierre's disease: Postanginal bacteremia and pulmonary involvement caused by *Fusobacterium necrophorum*. Rev Infect Dis 11:319, 1989.
52. Finegold SM: Anaerobic Bacteria in Human Disease. New York, Academic Press, 1977.
53. Finegold SM, George WL (eds): Anaerobic Infections in Humans. San Diego, CA, Academic Press, 1989.
54. Finegold SM: Overview of clinically important anaerobes. Clin Infect Dis 20(Suppl 2):S205, 1995.
55. Finegold SM, Strong CA, McTeague M, Marina M: The importance of black-pigmented gram-negative anaerobes in human infections. FEMS Immunol Med Microbiol 6:77, 1993.
56. Kirby BD, George WL, Sutter VL, et al: Gram-negative anaerobic bacilli: Their role in infection and patterns of susceptibility to antimicrobial agents. I. Little-known *Bacteroides* species. Rev Infect Dis 2:914, 1980.
57. Haapasalo M, Ranta H, Shah H, et al: *Mitsuokella dentalis* sp. nov. from dental root canals. Int J Syst Bacteriol 36:566, 1986.
58. Summanen PH, Jousimies-Somer H, Manley S, et al: *Bilophila wadsworthia* isolates from clinical specimens. Clin Infect Dis 20(Suppl 2):S210, 1995.
59. Bennett KW, Eley A: Fusobacteria: New taxonomy and related diseases. J Med Microbiol 39:246, 1993.
60. Civen R, Jousimies-Somer H, Marina M, et al: A retrospective review of cases of anaerobic empyema and update of bacteriology. Clin Infect Dis 20(Suppl 2):S224, 1995.
61. Baquero F, Fernández J, Dronda F, et al: Capnophilic and anaerobic bacteremia in neutropenic patients: An oral source. Rev Infect Dis 12(Suppl 2):S157, 1990.
62. Johnson CC, Finegold SM: Uncommonly encountered, motile, anaerobic gram-negative bacilli associated with infection. Rev Infect Dis 9:1150, 1987.
63. Malnick H, Jones A, Vickers JC: *Anaerobiospirillum*: Cause of a "new" zoonosis? (Letter) Lancet 1:1145, 1989.
64. McNeil MM, Martone WJ, Dowell VR Jr: Bacteremia with *Anaerobiospirillum succiniciproducens*. Rev Infect Dis 9:737, 1987.
65. Tanner A, Stillman N: Oral and dental infections with anaerobic bacteria: Clinical features, predominant pathogens, and treatment. Clin Infect Dis 16(Suppl 4):S304, 1993.
66. Gharbia SE, Haapasalo M, Shah HN, et al: Characterization of *Prevotella intermedia* and *Prevotella nigrescens* isolates from periodontic and endodontic infections. J Periodontol 65:56, 1994.
67. Tabaqchali S: Anaerobic infections in the head and neck region. Scand J Infect Dis Suppl 57:24, 1988.
68. Jousimies-Somer H, Savolainen S, Makitie A, Ylikoski J: Bacteriologic findings in peritonsillar abscess in young adults. Clin Infect Dis 16(Suppl 4):S292, 1993.
69. Bennion RS, Baron EJ, Thompson JE Jr, et al: The bacteriology of gangrenous and perforated appendicitis—Revisited. Ann Surg 211:165, 1990.
70. Vandamme P, Falsen E, Pot B, et al: Identification of EF group 22 campylobacters from gastroenteritis cases as *Campylobacter concisus*. J Clin Microbiol 27:1775, 1989.
71. Germain M, Krohn MA, Hillier SL, Eschenbach DA: Genital flora in pregnancy and its association with intrauterine growth retardation. J Clin Microbiol 32:2162, 1994.
72. Hillier SL, Krohn MA, Cassen E, et al: The role of bacterial vaginosis and vaginal bacteria in amniotic fluid infection in women in preterm labor with intact fetal membranes. Clin Infect Dis 20(Suppl 2):S276, 1995.
73. McGregor JA, French JI, Bloom BS, et al: Bacterial vaginosis and preterm birth (Letter). N Engl J Med 334:1337, 1996.
74. Summanen PH, Talan DA, Strong C, et al: Bacteriology of skin and soft-tissue infections: Comparison of infections in intravenous drug users and individuals with no history of intravenous drug use. Clin Infect Dis 20(Suppl 2):S279, 1995.
75. Jousimies-Somer HR: Update on the taxonomy and the clinical and laboratory characteristics of pigmented anaerobic gram-negative rods. Clin Infect Dis 20(Suppl 2):S187, 1995.

220

Clostridium tetani

John G. Bartlett

Tetanus (lockjaw) is a neurologic syndrome caused by a neurotoxin elaborated by *Clostridium tetani* at a site of injury. This disease is relatively uncommon in the United States and the developed world, but the estimated worldwide annual mortality exceeds 1 million, owing largely to the failure of immunization programs in developing countries.

Pathogenesis

C. tetani is an anaerobic, gram-positive, slender, motile bacillus. The spore form has a characteristic drumstick or tennis-racket shape (Fig. 220–1). Vegetative forms of *C. tetani* are highly susceptible to heat and disinfectants, but the spores are highly resistant, and killing them requires boiling for at least 4 hours or autoclaving for 12 minutes at 121°C.

Tetanospasmin is the neurotoxin responsible for tetanus. This is a protein with a molecular mass of about 150 kDa that may be proteolytically cleaved to a light chain and a heavy chain linked by a disulfide bond.[1] The heavy chain (100 kDa) is responsible for binding to eukaryotic cells, and the light chain (50 kDa) is responsible for blocking the release of neurotransmitters. The entire amino acid sequence has been defined[2] and shows considerable homology with botulinum toxin.[3] Tetanospasmin ranks with botulinum toxin as the most potent known microbial toxins. One milligram is capable of killing 50 million to 70 million mice.

The clinical syndrome requires a source of the organism, local tissue conditions that promote production by vegetative forms, and immune system naiveté. The organism is introduced at the site of injury. The prevalence of *C. tetani* spores in soil samples is 2% to 23%.[4] Local factors that are important

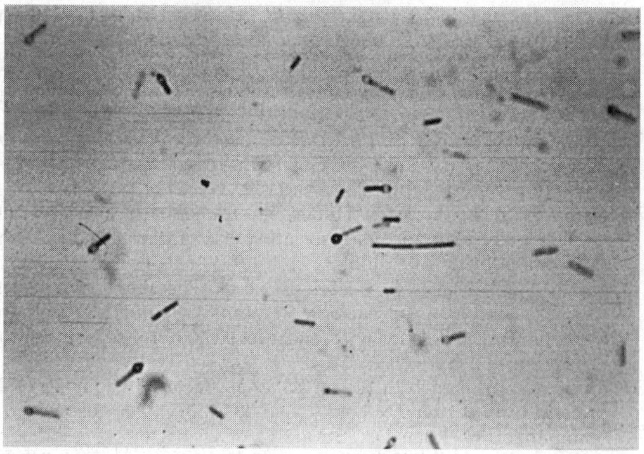

FIGURE 220–1 ▫ Gram stain of *Clostridium tetani* showing typical "drumstick" forms.

at the site of injury in promoting toxin elaboration by vegetative forms are necrotic tissue, suppuration, and the presence of a foreign body. The toxin is produced as a protoplasmic protein and is released with lysis of bacilli. Tetanospasmin is taken up by peripheral nerve terminals and then transported intraaxonally within membrane-bound vesicles to spinal neurons at a transport rate of 75 to 250 mm/d.[5] Large amounts of the toxin may spread by blood and lymphatics to myoneural junctions throughout the body. After retrograde transport the neurotoxin reaches the perikarya of the motor neuron and passes to the presynaptic terminals, where it blocks release of neurotransmitters, including glycine and γ-aminobutyric acid, the neurotransmitters used by group 1A inhibitory afferent motor neurons.[6] The absence of inhibition results in unrestrained firing with sustained muscle contraction of both agonist and antagonist muscles. Toxin binding is irreversible, so recovery requires the generation of new axonal terminals. In severe cases there is also involvement of the sympathetic chain, resulting in autonomic dysfunction.

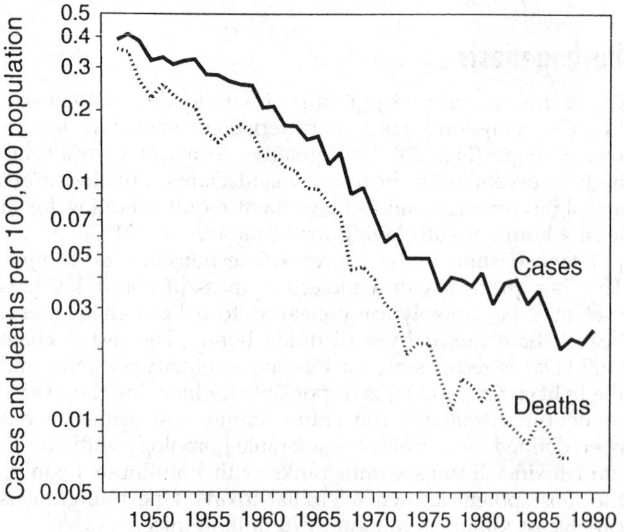

FIGURE 220–2 ▫ Reported incidence of tetanus and tetanus-related deaths—United States, 1947 to 1990. (From Prevots R, Sutter RW, Strebel PM, et al: Tetanus surveillance—United States, 1989–1990. MMWR CDC Surveill Summ 41[8]:1–9, 1992).

Epidemiology

Tetanus is most common in warm climates and heavily cultivated rural areas.[7–9] The greatest problem is in economically deprived countries, reflecting poor immunization standards and poor hygiene.[8] The greatest toll is in neonates, reflecting the prevalent practices of dressing the umbilical wound with animal dung and performing circumcision without aseptic technique on children born to unimmunized mothers. Neonatal tetanus accounts for more than half of all lethal cases of tetanus in the world; only two cases were reported in the United States from 1984 to 1990.

The rate of tetanus in the United States decreased approximately 20-fold since immunization became generally available in the early 1940s. The tetanus rate was 0.39 per 100,000 population when reporting began in 1947 and is now 0.02 per 100,000[9] (Fig. 220–2). About 50 to 100 cases of tetanus are reported annually in the United States; reporting efficiency is estimated at 40%. The reported experience with tetanus for the United States is summarized in Table 220–1, which shows that the majority are patients older than 60 years (Fig. 220–3), reflecting declining immunity that is observed in patients older than 40 years.[10] Most of the patients had puncture wounds with sharp objects, most did not seek medical attention, and none received prophylaxis with tetanus immune globulin.

Clinical Features

The forms of tetanus are generalized, localized, cephalic, and neonatal. Generalized tetanus is most common.[11–15] The usual incubation period from the time of injury is 4 to 14 days,

TABLE 220–1 ■ Experience with Tetanus in the United States for 1989 and 1990

Reported cases (1989, 1990): 110
Demographic data
Female: 57 (52%)
Age >60 y: 63 (58%)
<20 y: 7 (6%)
Portal of entry
Acute injury: 86 (78%)
Puncture wound: 45 (52%)
Lacerations: 20 (23%)
Abrasion: 15 (17%)
Chronic wound: 14* (9%)
Intravenous drug abuse: 5 (5%)
Neonatal tetanus: 1 (1%)
No portal of entry or associated condition: 10 (9%)
Persons who sought medical care for initial injury: 27/86 (32%)
Persons treated with tetanus toxoid: 15 (58%)
Persons treated with tetanus immunoglobulin (TIG): 0†
Persons who had received primary immunization: 12/57 (21%)‡
Type of tetanus (90 patients)
Generalized: 79 (88%)
Localized: 8 (9%)
Cephalic: 3 (3%)
Outcome of tetanus
Length of hospitalization (median): 17 d
No. requiring assisted ventilation: 55/94 (58%)
TIG dosage (median): 3000 IU
Mortality rate: 24%

*Skin ulcers, abscesses, or gangrene (three diabetic patients).
†Seven were considered candidates for tetanus and diphtheria toxoids absorbed for adult use (Td) and TIG, of whom four received Td and none received TIG.
‡Vaccination status was unknown for 53 patients.
From Prevots R, Sutter RW, Strebel PM, et al: Tetanus surveillance—United States, 1989–1990. MMWR CDC Surveill Summ 41(8):1–9, 1992.

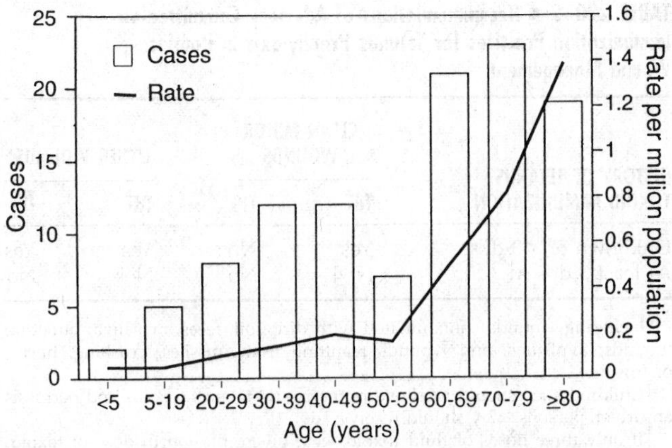

FIGURE 220–3 ▫ Reported tetanus cases and incidence rates, by age group—United States, 1989 and 1990. (From Prevots R, Sutter RW, Strebel PM, et al: Tetanus surveillance—United States, 1989–1990. MMWR CDC Surveill Summ 41[8]:1–9, 1992.)

depending to some extent on the distance of the site of injury from the central nervous system. The onset period refers to the interval between the first symptoms of tetanus and the first generalized spasm. An incubation period of less than 9 days and an onset period of less than 48 hours are associated with more severe disease.

The initial symptoms of tetanus may include localized or generalized weakness and difficulty in swallowing or chewing. Muscles served by nerves with the shortest neural pathways are usually the first to be affected, including cervical, facial, and masticatory muscles. Trismus, the presenting complaint in about 75% of patients, reflects increased tone in the masseter muscle, accounting for the term lockjaw. Muscle rigidity then increases progressively, in a descending or ascending pattern. Other early features include irritability, diaphoresis, listlessness, dysphagia, and drooling. Sustained contracture of the orbicularis oris may result in a characteristic sardonic smile, risus sardonicus; persistent spasm of the back musculature may result in opisthotonos. Reflex spasms are a common feature of the disease, with waves of tonic contractions of various muscle groups that are often triggered by sensory stimuli. The spasms may cause waves of opisthotonos, flexion and adduction of the arms with clenched fists over the lower part of the chest, and extension of the legs resulting in a characteristic posturing. The autonomic nervous system is often involved with arrhythmias, extreme oscillation in blood pressure, diaphoresis, rhabdomyolysis, laryngeal spasms, hyperthermia, and urinary retention.[13] The patient generally remains lucid and suffers intense pain with the spasms, which may be precipitated by noise, light, or touch. Generalized tetanus often progresses over 2 weeks, representing the time required for completion of toxin transport, which is intraaxonal when antitoxin is given. Complications include fractures resulting from the sustained contractions and convulsions, aspiration, pulmonary emboli, bacterial superinfections, dehydration, respiratory failure, and cardiac arrest.

Localized tetanus refers to involvement of an extremity with a contaminated wound.[5, 11, 12] There is considerable variation in severity. There may be muscle weakness and diminished tone that resolves spontaneously or may persist in a chronic form. More severe cases are characterized by intense, painful spasms, and most cases progress to generalized tetanus. This is a relatively unusual form of tetanus, and the prognosis for survival is excellent.

Cephalic tetanus usually occurs in association with a head injury or with *C. tetani* infection of the middle ear.[11, 12, 16, 17] Clinical features consist of an isolated or combined cranial motor nerve dysfunction, most often the seventh cranial nerve. This also may remain localized or progress to generalized tetanus. Cephalic tetanus is an unusual form of the disease; the incubation period is only 1 or 2 days and the prognosis variable.[16, 17]

Tetanus neonatorum is generalized tetanus in neonates that occurs almost exclusively in underdeveloped countries.[8, 18, 19] The incubation period after birth is 3 to 10 days, and it is sometimes referred to as the "disease of the seventh day." The child typically shows facial grimacing, irritability, and severe spasms in response to being touched. The mortality rate is about 90%, and this disease accounted for an estimated 515,000 neonatal deaths in 1993.[19]

Diagnosis

The diagnosis is usually established by clinical observation. The organism is rarely recovered from cultures of wound material. A confirmed history of immunization or a serum antitoxin level of 0.01 unit/mL or higher makes tetanus unlikely but does not exclude the diagnosis. Cerebrospinal fluid analysis findings are normal, imaging studies of the brain are normal, and the electroencephalogram usually shows a sleep pattern. Electrophysiologic studies of the masseter muscle show a characteristic absence or shortening of the silent period ascribed to the failure of Renshaw cell inhibition.[20] This may also show exaggerated F responses, indicating hyperexcitability. The differential diagnosis depends to some extent on the dominant clinical features and includes dental infection with trismus, seizure disorder, oculogyric crisis secondary to phenothiazine toxicity, subarachnoid hemorrhage, meningitis, hypocalcemic or alkalotic tetany, alcohol withdrawal, stiff-man syndrome,[21] and strychnine poisoning. The last produces similar symptoms, but patients usually recover rapidly with supportive care. Strychnine poisoning can be excluded with toxicologic studies of serum and urine.

Treatment

Patients with tetanus are usually cared for in intensive care units, where appropriate measures are taken to avoid noxious stimuli. Benzodiazepines such as diazepam, which enhance γ-aminobutyric acid–mediated central inhibition, are advocated to control spasms, reduce anxiety, promote muscle relaxation, and prevent seizures.[12, 22–25] The usual doses of diazepam are 10 to 30 mg every 1 to 8 hours, but doses up to 40 mg/h may be required. A possible complication is lactic acidosis from the vehicle, propylene glycol.[15] Alternatives are midazolam by constant intravenous infusion (5 to 15 mg/h) or infusions of propofol.[25–27] If muscle spasms are severe or interfere with ventilation, therapeutic paralysis is rarely indicated using pancuronium bromide or metocurine combined with mechanical ventilation. Dantrolene has been used for relaxation of peripheral muscles, but prolonged use in large doses may cause hepatic dysfunction.

Pulmonary complications are common and most worrisome. Trismus, laryngeal spasm, respiratory muscle spasm, dysphagia, and sedatives all compound the difficulty of maintaining effective ventilation. Intubation followed by tracheostomy is usually necessary. These patients may be sustained with mechanical ventilation with diazepam given intravenously in doses adequate to relieve rigidity without excessive sedation. Other measures of supportive care may include nasogastric feedings and intravenous fluids with careful attention to fluid balance, because there may be large losses owing to the profuse sweating. Other supportive measures to consider are anticoagulation to prevent pulmonary emboli, sucralfate for gastrointestinal bleeding, a cooling blanket for hyperthermia, antibiotics for established infections, and dialysis for renal failure secondary to rhabdomyolysis with myoglobinuria.

Autonomic nervous system involvement may cause hypertension and tachycardia, increased cardiac output, and arrhythmias. With the ventilatory support that is currently available in intensive care units, autonomic instability now represents the major cause of lethality. This may be treated with combined α- and β-adrenergic blocking agents using intravenous labetalol. Additional therapeutic modalities include morphine sulfate, esmolol, epidural blockage, and infusions of magnesium sulfate.[25, 28–31]

Local wounds should be débrided, and metronidazole is the preferred antibiotic, with 2 g/d given orally or parenterally. Penicillin G is often advocated but, like tetanus toxin, is a γ-aminobutyric acid antagonist and was inferior to metronidazole in a therapeutic trial.[32] Alternative agents include erythromycin, tetracycline, and chloramphenicol. Human tetanus immunoglobulin (TIG) should be given quickly to neutralize any toxin that has not entered neurons. The dose is 500 units; higher doses and intrathecal administration do not appear advantageous.[33, 34] An alternative to TIG is pooled intravenous immunoglobulin.[35] Active immunization should also be initiated.

Prognosis

The overall mortality rate for generalized tetanus in industrialized countries is 20% to 25%.[9–12, 36] Prognostic indicators are the form of tetanus, the incubation period, the onset period, and the patient's age.[37] Some patients have only trismus with minor muscle spasms and do quite well. Moderately severe disease is often characterized by trismus, dysphagia, rigidity, and intermittent muscle spasms. Severe tetanus is associated with generalized convulsions and respiratory failure. Patients with moderate or severe generalized tetanus usually require 3 to 6 weeks to recover, and most of this time is usually spent in the intensive care unit. The most common causes of death are pneumonia and autonomic instability.[38]

Prevention

Tetanus is a preventable disease: virtually all victims are not immunized or inadequately immunized. The Immunization Practices Advisory Committee recommends active immunization for infants and children with diphtheria and tetanus toxoids and pertussis absorbed at ages 2 months, 4 months, 6 months, 15 months, and 4 to 6 years.[10, 15, 39] Tetanus toxoid is an excellent antigen, and protective levels among persons who complete the primary series persist for a minimum of 10 years. Tetanus and diphtheria toxoids absorbed for adult use (Td) are recommended every 10 years at middecade (ages 15 years, 25 years, and so on).

Nearly all states now require diphtheria, pertussis, and tetanus immunization for school enrollment, but booster vaccinations after the primary series are often neglected. Serosurveys indicate that 28% of persons older than 70 years in the United States lack protective levels of 0.15 IU/mL (enzyme immunoassay) or higher.[10] These observations account for the frequency of tetanus in older persons in the United States. Some authorities advocate hospital-based Td immunization programs for adults unless there is proof of immunization within 10 years or a convincing history of a severe reaction to the toxoid.[40] On a global scale, the World Health Organization has adopted a resolution for worldwide elimination of neonatal tetanus. To achieve this goal it will be necessary to protect 80% or more of infants through maternal vaccination with at least two doses of toxoid or through clean delivery and cord care practices.

TABLE 220–2 ■ Recommendations of Advisory Committee on Immunization Practices for Tetanus Prophylaxis in Routine Wound Management

HISTORY OF TETANUS TOXOID IMMUNIZATION	CLEAN MINOR WOUNDS		OTHER WOUNDS*	
	Td†	TIG	Td†	TIG
Unknown or <3 doses	Yes	No	Yes	Yes
At least 3 doses‡	No§	No	No‖	No

*Including wounds contaminated with dirt, soil, feces, or saliva; puncture wounds; avulsions; and wounds resulting from missiles, crushing, burns, or frostbite.

†Children <7 y should receive diphtheria and tetanus toxoids and pertussis absorbed; persons ≥7 y should receive Td.

‡If only three doses of fluid toxoid were given, the fourth dose of toxoid, preferably an absorbed toxoid, should be given.

§Yes, if >10 y since last dose.

‖Yes, if >5 y since last dose.

From Advisory Committee on Immunization Practices: Adult immunization. MMWR Morbid Mortal Wkly Rep 39:37, 1990.

Also important for preventing tetanus is appropriate management of patients with wounds, especially in emergency departments, where mistakes are common.[9, 41, 42] The goal is to provide adequate wound management, ensure adequate immunity, and consider antibiotic prophylaxis. The goal of surgery is to remove necrotic tissue, drain purulent collections, and remove foreign bodies that promote the environmental conditions necessary for the germination of spores.

Guidelines for immunoprophylaxis are based on the immunization status and characteristics of the wound (Table 220–2). Passive immunization with TIG is recommended for wounds described as tetanus prone if the patient has not been immunized. Tetanus prone is defined as having wounds contaminated with dirt, soil, stool, or saliva; puncture wounds; avulsions; and wounds resulting from missiles, crush injuries, burns, or frostbite. The definition of a tetanus-prone wound also depends on the interval between injury and treatment, the severity of contamination, the extent of devitalized tissue or foreign bodies at the site of the wounding, and the depth of the injury. The usual dose of TIG is 250 units intramuscularly, but up to 500 units is given for highly tetanus prone wounds. Active immunization is done simultaneously using separate syringes for TIG and tetanus toxoid. Simultaneous administration does not appear to blunt the immune response to the toxoid.

Antimicrobial agents, including penicillin, erythromycin, and metronidazole, may be given to prevent replication of vegetative forms of *C. tetani;* however, the local management of the wound and immunoprophylaxis are considered much more important.

References

1. Habermann E, Dreyer F: Clostridial neurotoxins: Handling and action at the cellular and molecular level. Curr Top Microbiol Immunol 129:93, 1986.
2. Fairweather NF, Lyness VA: The complete amino acid sequence of tetanus toxin. Nucleic Acids Res 14:7809, 1986.
3. Halpern JL, Smith LA, Seamon KB, et al: Sequence homology between tetanus and botulinum toxins detected by an antipeptide antibody. Infect Immun 57:18, 1989.
4. Boyd JSK, MacLennan JD: Tetanus in the Middle East: Effect of active immunization. Lancet 2:745, 1942.

5. Griffin JW: Local tetanus. Johns Hopkins Med J 149:84, 1981.
6. Dowell VR Jr: Botulism and tetanus: Selected epidemiologic and microbiologic aspects. Rev Infect Dis 6(Suppl 1):202, 1984.
7. Schiavo G, Benfenati B, Poulain B, et al: Tetanus and botulinum-B neurotoxins block neurotransmitter release by proteolytic cleavage of synaptobrevin. Nature 359:832, 1992.
8. Schofield F: Selective primary health care: Strategies for control of disease in the developing world. XXII. Tetanus: A preventable problem. Rev Infect Dis 8:144, 1986.
9. Prevots R, Sutter RW, Strebel PM, et al: Tetanus surveillance—United States, 1989–1990. MMWR CDC Surveill Summ 41(8):1, 1992.
10. Gergen PJ, McQuillan GM, Kiely M, et al: A population-based serologic survey of immunity to tetanus in the United States. N Engl J Med 332:761, 1995.
11. Weinstein L: Tetanus. N Engl J Med 289:1293, 1973.
12. Bleck TP: Tetanus: Dealing with the continuing clinical challenge. J Crit Illness 2:41, 1987.
13. Kerr JH, Corbett JL, Prys-Roberts C, et al: Involvement of the sympathetic nervous system in tetanus: Studies on 82 cases. Lancet 2:236, 1968.
14. LaForce FM, Young LS, Bennett JV: Tetanus in the United States (1965–1966): Epidemiologic and clinical features. N Engl J Med 280:569, 1969.
15. Sanford JP: Tetanus—Forgotten but not gone. N Engl J Med 332:812, 1995.
16. Abde VW, Dekate MP: Cephalic tetanus. J Indian Med Assoc 74:111, 1980.
17. Mayo J, Berciano J: Cephalic tetanus presenting with Bell's palsy. J Neurol Neurosurg Psychiatry 48:290, 1985.
18. Salimpour R: Cause of death in tetanus neonatorum: Study of 233 cases with 54 necropsies. Arch Dis Child 52:587, 1977.
19. Progress towards the global elimination of neonatal tetanus, 1989–1993. MMWR Morbid Mortal Wkly Rep 43:885, 1994.
20. Risk WS, Bosch EP, Kimura J, et al: Chronic tetanus: Clinical report and histochemistry of muscle. Muscle Nerve 4:363, 1981.
21. Solimena M, Folli F, Denis-Donini S, et al: Autoantibodies to glutamic acid decarboxylase in a patient with stiff-man syndrome, epilepsy, and type I diabetes mellitus. N Engl J Med 318:1012, 1988.
22. Olsen KM, Hiller FC: Management of tetanus. Clin Pharm 6:570, 1987.
23. Trujillo MH, Castillo A, Espana J, et al: Impact of intensive care management on the prognosis of tetanus: Analysis of 641 cases. Chest 92:63, 1987.
24. Bleck TP: Tetanus. Dis Mon 37:547, 1991.
25. Bleck TP: *Clostridium tetani. In* Mandell GL, Bennett JE, Dolin R (eds): Principles and Practice of Infectious Diseases, ed 4, Vol 2. New York, Churchill Livingstone, 1995, pp 2173–2178.
26. Orko R, Rosenberg PH, Himberg JJ: Intravenous infusion of midazolam, propofol and vercuronium in a patient with severe tetanus. Acta Anaesthesiol Scand 32:590, 1988.
27. Borgeat A, Dessibourg C, Rochani M, et al: Sedation by propofol in tetanus—Is it a muscular relaxant? Intensive Care Med 17:427, 1991.
28. King WW, Cave DR: Use of esmolol to control autonomic instability of tetanus. Am J Med 91:425, 1991.
29. Rocke DA, Wasley AG, Pather M, et al: Morphine in tetanus: The management of sympathetic nervous system overactivity. S Afr Med J 70:666, 1986.
30. Lipman J, James MFM, Erskine J, et al: Autonomic dysfunction in severe tetanus: Magnesium sulfate as an adjunct to deep sedation. Crit Care Med 15:987, 1987.
31. Southorn PA, Blaise GA: Treatment of tetanus-induced autonomic dysfunction with continuous epidural blockade. Crit Care Med 14:251, 1986.
32. Ahmadsyah I, Salim A: Treatment of tetanus: An open study to compare the efficacy of procaine penicillin and metronidazole. Br Med J 291:648, 1985.
33. Gupta PS, Kapoor R, Goyal S, et al: Intrathecal human tetanus immunoglobulin in early tetanus. Lancet 2:439, 1980.
34. Begue RE, Lindo-Soriano I: Failure of intrathecal antitoxin in the treatment of neonatal tetanus. J Infect Dis 164:619, 1991.
35. Lee DC, Lederman HM: Anti-tetanus toxoid antibodies in intravenous gamma globulin: An alternative to tetanus immune globulin. J Infect Dis 166:642, 1992.
36. Armitage P, Clifford R: Prognosis in tetanus: Use of data from therapeutic trials. J Infect Dis 138:1, 1978.
37. Nolla-Salas M, Garces-Bruses J: Severity of tetanus in patients older than 80 years: Comparative study with younger patients. Clin Infect Dis 16:591, 1993.
38. Edmondson RS, Flowers MWW: Intensive care in tetanus: Management, complications and mortality in 100 patients. Br Med J 1:1401, 1979.
39. Advisory Committee on Immunization Practices: Adult immunization. MMWR Morbid Mortal Wkly Rep 39:37, 1990.
40. Thorley JD, Holmes RK, Sanford JP: Tetanus and diphtheria antitoxin levels following a hospital-based adult immunization program. Am J Epidemiol 101:438, 1975.
41. Brand DA, Acampora D, Gotlieb LD, et al: Adequacy of antitetanus prophylaxis in six hospital emergency rooms. N Engl J Med 309:636, 1983.
42. Giangrosso J, Smith RK: Misuse of tetanus immunoprophylaxis in wound care. Ann Emerg Med 14:573, 1985.

221

Clostridium botulinum

Charles L. Hatheway

History

Botulism has long been recognized as a food-borne illness. The name is derived from the Latin word *botulus,* which means "sausage," because of the association of the illness with the consumption of sausages and other preserved meat products over the centuries in Europe.[1] The bacterial etiology and toxicologic mechanism of the illness were elucidated by van Ermengem[2] in 1895 in the investigation of a large outbreak in Belgium. The name *Bacillus botulinus* was given to the toxigenic organism that was responsible for the outbreak. Investigations of subsequent incidents repeatedly confirmed van Ermengem's findings, but they also revealed that the toxins in different outbreaks might have different serologic specificities and that the implicated toxigenic organisms could have various physiologic and cultural characteristics. Foods other than meat products were encountered as vehicles. Botulism was seen to occur also in cattle[3] and chickens[4] as well as in other mammalian and avian species.[1] A second form of human botulism (wound botulism) was found on rare occasions to result from growth of toxigenic organisms in infected wounds.[5, 6] A third form, resulting from colonization of the intestinal tract of infants (infant botulism) was recognized in 1976.[7–9] In 1978, a fourth category of human botulism was established by the Centers for Disease Control and Prevention (CDC) for single-case incidents involving adults and noninfant children for which there was no apparent food vehicle[10]; this provided a classification for cases that might actually have been due to intestinal colonization.

Because the organisms that cause botulism are anaerobic spore formers, they were placed in the genus *Clostridium* on the recommendation of the Committee on Classification of the Society of American Bacteriologists.[11] The name *Clostridium botulinum* is applied to four diverse groups of organisms that produce potent neurotoxins that can cause botulism.

Characteristics of the Pathogen

The most distinguishing characteristic of the organisms is their ability to produce botulism neurotoxin. All the organisms noted to date clearly fit into the genus *Clostridium.* They are all anaerobic, spore-forming bacilli that are usually referred to as gram-positive, although the Gram reaction is variable, often appearing as positive in young cultures but changing to negative in cultures after 18 hours.

Toxin Types

The first differential characteristic among the toxin-producing organisms is the serologic specificity of the neurotoxins. There are seven toxin types, each designated by a letter of the alphabet, A through G.[1] The biologic activity of each type of toxin is specifically neutralized by its corresponding antitoxin. There is no cross-neutralization except for a low-level reciprocal cross-reactivity between types E and F.[12]

Early investigators noticed a difference among organisms that produce type C neurotoxin. An antitoxin prepared against the Bengtson strain[4] isolated from a chicken outbreak neutralized both the homologous toxin and the toxin from the Seddon strain,[3] implicated as the cause of botulism in cattle, whereas antitoxin against the latter strain neutralized only its homologous toxin. The distinctions Cα and Cβ were established to identify the two subtypes.[13] It was found that Cα produces two toxins, C_1 and C_2, whereas Cβ produces only C_2. C_1 toxin is a true botulinal neurotoxin, whereas C_2 toxin is not. C_2 toxin has a binary structure, that is, it consists of two separate peptide molecules, C_2I (50 kDa) and C_2II (105 kDa)[14]; it elicits vascular permeability and enterotoxic activities as well as lethality by the cooperative effect of the two components. C_2I acts as an enzyme that catalyzes adenosine diphosphate–ribosylation of actin inside the cell.[15] C_2 toxin does not appear to play any direct role in botulism. In addition to C_1 and C_2, type C organisms may also produce a minimal amount of type D neurotoxin; on the other hand, type D organisms also produce C_2 toxin and in some cases a minimal amount of C_1 neurotoxin.[16] Because of this, a low level of cross-neutralization may be demonstrable with the toxins and antitoxins of types C and D.

Types C and D neurotoxins are phage mediated, that is, the genes that code for them are carried by bacteriophages with which the toxigenic organisms are infected.[17] Studies with toxigenic (type E) *C. botulinum* have provided evidence that the toxin gene in that organism is phage associated.[18] There is evidence that the gene for type G toxin is present on a plasmid.[19, 20] Because all attempts so far have failed to show evidence of phage or plasmid association with toxigenicity of types A, B, or F, the genes for those types are presumed to be present on the chromosome.

Physiologic Groups

C. botulinum is divided into four groups[17] on the basis of different metabolic characteristics. The differences are sufficient to designate a separate species name for each group. Group I consists of "proteolytic" organisms, that is, those that can digest complex proteins such as casein or coagulated serum or egg albumin. At one time these were classified under the name of *Clostridium parabotulinum.*[11] All organisms that produce type A toxin and certain strains that produce type B or type F toxin belong in this group. Group II includes all type E strains, some type B strains (notably those implicated in botulism outbreaks associated with meat products in Europe), and some type F strains. These organisms have a notably lower optimal growth temperature; they do not digest complex proteins and are referred to as nonproteolytic. These (in particular the ones that produce type B toxin) conform to the organism described by van Ermengem.[2] Group III consists of the organisms that produce type C or type D toxin. They have been reported alternatively as proteolytic[21] and as nonproteolytic[11] but have shown cultural and metabolic characteristics, for example, production of propionic acid, that distinguish them from both group I and group II.[22] All three of these groups are saccharolytic and produce lipase.[17] Group IV was established to classify the organism isolated from soil in Argentina that produces type G toxin, because its characteristics are so different from those of any of the other groups.[23] The organisms are proteolytic, asaccharolytic, and lipase-negative.

The four groups are clearly distinguishable by DNA relatedness studies.[24–27] Analysis of the phylogeny of the clostridia by 16S ribosomal RNA gene sequences has reinforced these groupings.[28] Some nonneurotoxigenic organisms known by other clostridial species names are phenotypically and genetically related to group I *(Clostridium sporogenes)* and group III *(Clostridium novyi).* Thus, in essence, there are toxigenic and nontoxigenic members of the same "species." Because neurotoxigenic organisms identifiable as *Clostridium baratii* and *Clostridium butyricum*[29] have been implicated in human botulism, it is difficult to insist that all organisms that produce the neurotoxin be called *C. botulinum.* In view of this, and because of the disparate characteristics of the organisms that produce type G toxin and the fact that they do not seem to cause botulism in nature, the name *Clostridium argentinense* has been proposed for those organisms, as well as for their genetically related nontoxigenic counterparts.[27] It would be taxonomically sound to allow a distinct species name for

TABLE 221–1 ■ Groups of *Clostridium botulinum* and Other Species Capable of Producing Botulism Neurotoxin: Differential Characteristics and Related Nontoxigenic Species

GROUP OR SPECIES	TYPE OF TOXIN	FERMENT GLUCOSE	DIGEST CASEIN	LIQUEFY GELATIN	REACTIONS ON EGG YOLK AGAR		METABOLIC ACIDS*	RELATED SPECIES
					Lipase	Lecithinase		
I	A, B, F	+	+	+	+	−	A, iB, B, iV	*Clostridium sporogenes*
II	B, E, F	+	−	+	+	−	A, B	
III	C, D	+	±	+	+	±	A, P, B	*Clostridium novyi*
Clostridium argentinense†	G	−	+	+	−	−	A, iB, B, iV	
Clostridium baratii	F	+	−	−	−	+	A, B	
Clostridium butyricum	E	+	−	−	−	−	A, B	

*Volatile metabolic acids produced in peptone–yeast extract–glucose, analyzed by gas-liquid chromatography. A, Acetic; iB, isobutyric; B, butyric; iV, isovaleric.
†Also commonly known as *C. botulinum* type G.

TABLE 221–2 ■ Incidence of Food-Borne, Wound, and Infant Botulism in the United States Since 1950*

		TOXIN TYPE						
DISEASE FORM	YEARS	A	B	E	F	Unknown	TOTAL	CASE-FATALITY RATE (%)
Food-borne	1950–1993	436	183	196	3	303†	1126	17.9
Wound	1950–1993	37	15	0	0	6‡	58	10.3
Infant	1975–1993	575	603	0	2	10§	1190	1.1
Other	1978–1993	17	6	0	4	4	31	29.0

*Numbers of cases of botulism; unpublished data, Centers for Disease Control and Prevention.
†Toxin type not determined.
‡Botulism diagnosed on clinical evidence; no confirmatory laboratory evidence.
§Three cases without report of toxin type, two due to single organism producing two types of toxin (B, F), and one due to colonization by two organisms (A, B).

each of the other three groups, although each specific epithet should convey the relationship to the disease botulism. The groups of organisms identified to date that produce botulism neurotoxin and their characteristics are listed in Table 221–1.

Toxin Types in Human Botulism

Human botulism is essentially restricted to toxin types A, B, and E.[1] The occurrence of botulism in the United States since 1950 is summarized in Table 221–2 by disease form and toxin type. Of the more than 2000 cases whose types are known, all are type A, B, or E, except for nine cases identified as type F.

Type F botulism was first recognized in a food-borne outbreak in Denmark in 1958.[30] It has since been recognized in the United States in eight instances involving nine patients (Table 221–3); two food-borne incidents were caused by *C. botulinum*,[31] and two infant cases[32] and three adult cases (probably due to intestinal colonization[33]) were caused by toxigenic *C. baratii* (see Table 221–3). One case, confirmed on the basis of detection of type F toxin in the blood,[34] was of undetermined classification; no toxigenic organism was isolated because no stool was submitted. One type F food-borne outbreak was reported in Norway.[35]

Although toxin type C is frequently associated with botulism in birds and in domestic and wild mammals,[1] only one type C human food-borne outbreak, reported from France, has been documented in the literature.[36] One type D outbreak was reported from Chad.[37] The type C outbreak was confirmed only on the basis of recovery of a toxigenic organism from a food sample in which no toxin was detected. The type D outbreak was confirmed after finding type D toxin in the epidemiologically incriminated salted ham. The occurrence of type G botulism is controversial. Although one laboratory has reported isolating type G organisms from autopsy specimens,[38] there was no convincing evidence that botulism had occurred in those cases. The report of frequent isolation of toxin types C, D, and F in those same studies also casts doubt on the reliability of the type G findings. There were no reports of persons hospitalized with botulism of any toxin type associated with the time and locale of the study. During a 17-year period encompassing that time, five outbreaks of botulism had been reported for the country, and only types A and B had been involved.[35]

Epidemiology

Food-Borne Botulism

Food-borne botulism remains the most common form of botulism worldwide, although in the United States infant cases have become the most frequent. Hauschild[35] reviewed the incidence of food-borne botulism in 1993. Poland, China, the United States, and France lead in the number of reported food-borne cases. The foods are largely home processed. In Europe they are most often meat products and the toxin is largely type B; the general opinion is that the organisms conform to the one isolated by van Ermengem,[2] that is, they are nonproteolytic. In China the vehicle is more commonly a vegetable (or cereal grain) product and type A toxin predominates.[1, 35]

Food-borne botulism in the continental United States is typically due to inadequately processed home-preserved vegetables. In these cases, the causative organism is almost always type A or B (group I), and the incidence of each type correlates with the toxin type distribution in the soil of the region of origin of the food. Type A predominates in the western part of the country, and type B in the eastern part.[39] Type E food-borne botulism, associated with fish and other marine foods, is common in Alaska[40] and is enhanced by some of the traditional food preparation and preservation

TABLE 221–3 ■ Type F Botulism in Humans in the United States

YEAR	STATE	FORM	NO. OF CASES	*CLOSTRIDIUM* SPECIES	REFERENCE
1966	California	Food-borne	2	*C. botulinum*	31
1979	New Mexico	Infant	1	*C. baratii*	32
1981	Florida	Undetermined	1	Not isolated	34
1986	California	Food-borne	1	*C. botulinum*	CDC*
1987	Georgia	Undetermined	1	*C. baratii*	33
1992	District of Columbia	Undetermined	1	*C. baratii*	CDC*
1992	Oregon	Infant	1	*C. baratii*	CDC*
1993	Pennsylvania	Undetermined	1	*C. baratii*	CDC*

*Unpublished records, Centers for Disease Control and Prevention.

methods used by the Alaska Native populations.[41] Type E *C. botulinum* is well represented in the soil and beach flora in areas where those foods are obtained, processed, and consumed.[42] Between 1976 and 1995, the case-fatality rate for food-borne botulism in the United States has been 6.6%.

Wound Botulism

The first case of wound botulism was documented in 1943.[43] Weber and colleagues[6] reviewed 47 cases of laboratory-confirmed wound botulism that occurred between 1943 and 1990 in the United States. Through 1993, 58 cases were reported to the CDC (see Table 221–2); the toxin types have been either A or B, and the causative organisms, when identified, are always group I strains. Of the known types of associated wounds listed by Weber and colleagues, 30 were traumatic, 5 were surgical, and 9 were associated with illicit drug abuse. The case-fatality rate for wound botulism is about 10%.

Infant Botulism

Infant botulism (due to colonization of infants younger than 1 year) was first recognized in 1976 as distinct from food-borne botulism.[7, 8] It has been documented in at least 14 countries[44] and since 1980 has become the most frequently recognized form of botulism in the United States[45] (see Table 221–2). Approximately 50% of the U.S. cases are found in California. The usual source of the organisms is most likely the soil, but honey has been implicated in 26 instances.[45] The case-fatality rate for infant botulism is about 1%.

The organisms that cause infant botulism are almost exclusively group I strains of *C. botulinum* of toxin type A or B. One case in Japan was identified by Oguma and colleagues[46] as type C, two type F cases in the United States were caused by *C. baratii*[32] (see Table 221–3), and two type E cases in Italy were caused by *C. butyricum*.[47]

Undetermined Classification

Single cases of botulism for which there are no plausible food sources for botulism toxin nor any wound site for possible infection with *C. botulinum* are sometimes confirmed on the basis of detection of toxin in serum or feces or both and isolation of the organism from the feces. This suggests the possibility of botulism due to intestinal colonization, which, although quite rare, has been documented.[48] Several cases of botulism were confirmed among patients who had had surgical alteration of the bowel.[49–51] The altered environment of the intestinal lumen appears to be conducive to germination and outgrowth of spores of toxigenic organisms. The occurrence of botulism immediately after surgery[52] might be due to infection of the surgical wound rather than colonization of the lumen. One case of botulism associated with Crohn disease has been documented[52a]; it is not clear if this was due to colonization or to infection of the lesions associated with the disease.

Three cases of adult type F botulism caused by toxigenic *C. baratii* (see Table 221–3) are suggestive of intestinal colonization. The 1981 type F case from Florida might have also been caused by the same agent, but the organism was not isolated. It appears that *C. baratii* is adept at colonizing the gut, because it has also been seen in two infant cases, but it has not been implicated in botulism caused by preformed toxin in foods.

Pathogenesis

Botulism is a neuroparalytic disease caused by blockage of acetylcholine release by the nerves that activate skeletal muscles.[53] Botulism neurotoxin may also interfere with certain autonomic nervous system functions, as has been evidenced by abnormal heart rate and blood pressure responses to cardiovascular reflex tests.[54] Botulism neurotoxins, regardless of toxin type, consist of a dichain peptide molecule with a molecular mass of about 150,000.[55] They exist in the native state as complexes with nontoxic proteins, which greatly enhance their stability. Toxin absorbed from the intestine or produced in an infected wound is carried throughout the body in the circulating blood. The toxin molecules bind to specific receptors on the nerve endings, and a portion of the molecule gains entrance into the nerve cell.[53] The fragment has endopeptidase activity and cleaves membrane proteins essential for exocytosis of the neurotransmitter.[56] The paralytic signs of the disease reflect the specific nerve fibers to which the toxin binds. Death from botulism in the absence of intensive supportive care is usually due to respiratory failure.

Clinical Manifestations

Botulism is characterized by symmetric impairment of cranial nerves, followed by a descending paralysis of the muscles of the limbs and trunk.[57] Respiratory impairment occurs in the more severe cases. The signs and symptoms observed in food-borne botulism are listed by toxin type in Table 221–4.[58] Time of onset of signs and symptoms ranges from 6 hours to as late as 10 days after exposure; the incubation period varies inversely with the amount of toxin consumed. The incubation period is shortest for type E botulism, but type A botulism is more severe, as indicated by a greater number of patients requiring intubation (67%, 52%, and 39% for types A, B, and E, respectively).[59] The signs observed in a study of infant botulism[60] are summarized in Table 221–5. Wound botulism patients show the same paralytic signs as those with food-borne disease, but the initial gastrointestinal features are absent.

Diagnosis

Botulism is first recognized or suspected on the basis of the clinical signs and symptoms. Epidemiologic evidence in multipatient outbreaks can make the diagnosis rather easy. In single-case noninfant incidents, recognition may be difficult when there is no obvious suggestive food history. Diseases sometimes confused with botulism are Guillain-Barré syndrome, myasthenia gravis, stroke, and chemical poisoning. Confirmation of botulism requires detection of toxin in the patient's serum or stool or in the suspected food vehicle.[61] Finding *C. botulinum* in the stool of a patient exhibiting signs consistent with botulism is fairly good confirmatory evidence because it is rarely ever recovered in the absence of botulism.[62, 63] Wound botulism is confirmed by detecting toxin in the serum or by culturing *C. botulinum* from the wound. Failure to find toxin or the organism in a noninfant patient does not rule out the diagnosis. In infants, however, botulism can generally be ruled out if two or more stools obtained during the acute phase of the illness are toxin- and culture-negative. Serum is usually negative in infant botulism.[64] Antitoxin has not been detected in postrecovery serum, except in the unusual case associated with Crohn disease mentioned earlier.[52a] Rubin and coworkers[65] reported that convalescent serum from two infants gave positive reactions in enzyme-linked immunosorbent assays against botulism toxin.

At present, the only reliable diagnostic test for identifying the toxin is the mouse bioassay. Many in vitro tests have been proposed, but none have been adequately evaluated as

TABLE 221–4 ■ Symptoms and Signs of Illness Observed in Food-Borne Botulism Outbreaks Occurring 1953 to 1973 Expressed as Number of Outbreaks in Which One or More Patients Experienced Symptoms or Exhibited Signs

SYMPTOMS AND SIGNS	TYPE A, 34 OUTBREAKS, 97 CASES	TYPE B, 15 OUTBREAKS, 46 CASES	TYPE E, 10 OUTBREAKS, 36 CASES	TYPE F, 1 OUTBREAK, 3 CASES	UND,* 44 OUTBREAKS, 90 CASES	TOTAL, 104 OUTBREAKS, 272 CASES	WITH SIGNS OR SYMPTOMS (%)
Symptoms							
Blurred vision, diplopia, photophobia	31	13	9	1	40	94	90.4
Dysphagia	27	14	3		35	79	76.0
Generalized weakness	22	12	4		22	60	57.7
Nausea and/or vomiting	15	13	10	1	19	58	55.8
Dysphonia	25	8	5		19	57	54.8
Dizziness or vertigo	8	4	5		15	32	30.8
Abdominal pain, cramps, fullness	5	6	3		7	21	20.2
Diarrhea	5	6			5	16	15.4
Urinary retention or incontinence	2	2	1		2	7	6.7
Sore throat	4	2	1			7	6.7
Constipation	2	2		1	3	6	5.8
Paresthesias	1					1	1.0
Signs							
Respiratory impairment	32	7	7		30	76	73.1
Specific muscle weakness or paralysis	23	9	3		13	48	46.2
Eye muscle involvement, including ptosis	16	9	3	1	17	46	44.2
Dry mouth, throat, or tongue	7	6	2		7	22	21.2
Dilated, fixed pupils	3	4	2		8	16	15.4
Ataxia	3	1		1	4	9	8.7
Postural hypotension			1		2	3	2.9
Nystagmus	1		1		1	3	2.9
Somnolence			1			1	1.0

*Toxin type undetermined or unspecified.
Data from Centers for Disease Control: Botulism in the United States, 1899–1977. Handbook for Epidemiologists, Clinicians, and Laboratory Workers. Atlanta, Public Health Service, US Department of Health, Education, and Welfare, 1979.

yet.[66] Because botulism is so rare, and because even a single case may represent a public health emergency, emergency diagnostic services should be obtained through state public health departments or the CDC. Consultation on the diagnosis and arranging for therapeutic antitoxin laboratory testing may be obtained through one of these facilities. Outside the United States, appropriate local and national health departments should be consulted. Detailed laboratory procedures for toxin testing and culturing for *C. botulinum* are described elsewhere.[58, 61]

Electrophysiologic studies are sometimes used in the diagnosis of botulism.[67] They may be more successful for diagnosis of infant botulism,[68] but for this form of the disease, fecal analysis is reliable and virtually conclusive.[64]

TABLE 221–5 ■ Physical Findings in 44 Cases of Infant Botulism in Pennsylvania

FINDING*	% OF INFANTS
Weakness	100
Hypotonia	95
Constipation	95
Failure of oral feeding	93
Diminished gagging or sucking reflex	91
Respiratory failure	89
Facial diparesis or ptosis	84
Decreased spontaneous movement	82
Decreased deep tendon reflexes	57

*Findings in more than 50% of cases.
From Long SS, Gajewski JL, Brown LW, Gilligan PH: Clinical, laboratory, and environmental features of infant botulism in southeastern Pennsylvania. Pediatrics 75:935–941, 1985.

Treatment

Intensive supportive care is most important in treating persons with botulism. Improvements in mechanical ventilatory support have been the most important factor in lowering the case-fatality rate for food-borne botulism from about 70% in 1910 to about 12% in more recent years.[69] Therapeutic antitoxin (trivalent, types A, B, E) is available for specific treatment of adult (but not infant) botulism in the United States through the CDC. Antitoxin of human origin for use in infant botulism is currently being evaluated.[70, 71] An analysis of 132 cases of type A food-borne botulism in which 115 of the patients received antitoxin therapy suggests that it is beneficial.[72] Animal studies, however, show that unless antitoxin is given early, usually before the onset of signs of illness, the protective effect is questionable.[73] Antitoxin will not reverse paralysis or the binding of toxin to nerve endings. It will, however, neutralize any unbound toxin in the circulation and prevent further paralysis. Because the antitoxin is of equine origin, hypersensitive reactions occur in about 9% of treated patients; serum sickness was notably more frequent in those receiving more than four vials.[74] Treatment with two vials can provide serum antitoxin levels more than sufficient to neutralize unbound toxin, and residual circulating antitoxins have half-lives of about 1 week.[75] Paralysis may progress for a while after antitoxin administration because of the effects of the bound toxin. If two vials fail to stabilize the patient's condition, the failure is unlikely to be due to insufficient antitoxin.[75]

There has been little experience with treatment of botulism with guanidine and little evidence to support its use.[69] For wound botulism, antibiotic treatment is generally accepted. However, it is not recommended in the treatment of infant botulism because it might result in lysis of intraintestinal organisms, thus liberating more neurotoxin into the gut.[45]

Prevention

Food-borne botulism is prevented by careful food preservation and handling practices. Careful surveillance, immediate reporting, and swift public health investigation of suspected incidents to determine the source can prevent further cases in an outbreak. If commercial food products or food sources are involved, a single case may herald the beginning of a large outbreak. Therefore, close coordination with local and state public health epidemiologists is critical to management of even apparently isolated cases of botulism. Good sterile practice in surgery and wound management may lessen the rare incidence of wound botulism. Because honey has been implicated as a vehicle for spores in infant botulism, it should not be fed to infants younger than 1 year.[45, 76] Pentavalent (A, B, C, D, E) botulism toxoid[77] is available from the CDC for immunization of laboratory workers who work with the neurotoxins or neurotoxigenic organisms.

References

1. Smith LDS, Sugiyama H. Botulism: The Organism, Its Toxins, the Disease, ed 2. Springfield, IL, Charles C Thomas, 1988.
2. Van Ermengem E: Ueber einen neuen anaeroben Bacillus and seine Beziehungen zum Botulismus. Z Hyg Infektionskr 26:1, 1897.
3. Seddon HR: Bulbar paralysis in cattle due to the action of a toxicogenic bacillus with a discussion of the relationship of the condition to forage poisoning (botulism). J Comp Pathol Ther 35:147, 1922.
4. Bengtson IA: Preliminary note on a toxin-producing anaerobe isolated from the larvae of *Lucilia caesar.* Public Health Rep 37:164, 1922.
5. Merson MH, Dowell VR Jr: Epidemiologic, clinical and laboratory aspects of wound botulism. N Engl J Med 289:1105, 1973.
6. Weber JT, Goodpasture HC, Alexander H, et al: Wound botulism in a patient with a tooth abscess: Case report and review. Clin Infect Dis 16:635, 1993.
7. Pickett J, Berg B, Chaplin E, et al: Syndrome of botulism in infancy: Clinical and electrophysiologic study. N Engl J Med 295:770, 1976.
8. Midura TF, Arnon SS: Infant botulism: Identification of *Clostridium botulinum* and its toxin in faeces. Lancet 2:934, 1976.
9. Arnon SS: Infant botulism. *In* Borriello SP (ed): Clostridia in Gastrointestinal Disease. Boca Raton, FL, CRC Press, 1985, pp 39–57.
10. Centers for Disease Control: Botulism—United States, 1978. MMWR Morbid Mortal Wkly Rep 28:73, 1979.
11. Bengtson IA: Studies on organisms concerned as causative factors in botulism. Hyg Lab Bull 136:101, 1924.
12. Yang KH, Sugiyama H: Purification and properties of *Clostridium botulinum* type F toxin. Appl Microbiol 29:598, 1975.
13. Gunnison JB, Meyer KF: Cultural study of an international collection of *Clostridium botulinum* and *parabotulinum.* J Infect Dis 45:119, 1929.
14. Ohishi I, DasGupta BR: Molecular structure and biological activities of *Clostridium botulinum* C2 toxin. *In* Eklund MW, Dowell VR Jr (eds): Avian Botulism. Springfield, IL, Charles C Thomas, 1987, pp 223–247.
15. Aktories K, Wegner A: ADP-ribosylation of actin by clostridial toxins. J Cell Biol 109:1385, 1989.
16. Jansen BC: *Clostridium botulinum* type C, its isolation and taxonomic position. *In* Eklund MW, Dowell VR Jr (eds): Avian Botulism. Springfield, IL, Charles C Thomas, 1987, pp 123–132.
17. Cato EP, George WL, Finegold SM: Genus *Clostridium* Prazmuwski 1880, 23. *In* Sneath PHA, Mair NS, Sharpe ME, Holt JG (eds): Bergey's Manual of Systematic Bacteriology, Vol 2. Baltimore, Williams & Wilkins, 1986, pp 1141–1200.
18. Zhou Y, Sugiyama H, Johnson EA: Transfer of neurotoxigenicity from *Clostridium butyricum* to a nontoxigenic *Clostridium botulinum* type E–like strain. Appl Environ Microbiol 59:3825, 1993.
19. Eklund MW, Poysky FT, Mseitif LM, et al: Evidence for plasmid-mediated toxin and bacteriocin production in *Clostridium botulinum* type G. Appl Environ Microbiol 54:1405, 1988.
20. Zhou Y, Sugiyama H, Nakano H, et al: The genes for the *Clostridium botulinum* type G toxin complex are on a plasmid. Infect Immun 63:2087, 1995.
21. Eklund MW, Poysky F, Oguma K, et al: Relationship of bacteriophages to toxin and hemagglutinin production and its significance in avian botulism outbreaks. *In* Eklund MW, Dowell VR Jr (eds): Avian Botulism. Springfield, IL, Charles C Thomas, 1987, pp 191–222.
22. Holdeman LV, Cato EP, Moore WEC: Anaerobe Laboratory Manual, ed 4. Blacksburg, VA, Department of Anaerobic Microbiology, Virginia Polytechnic Institute and State University, 1977.
23. Giménéz DF, Ciccarelli AS: Another type of *Clostridium botulinum.* Zentralbl Bakteriol [Orig A] 215:221, 1970.
24. Schroeder K, Tollefsrud A: Botulism fra rekorret. Tidsskr Nors Laegeforen 82:1084, 1962.
25. Lee WH, Riemann H: The genetic relatedness of proteolytic *Clostridium botulinum* strains. J Gen Microbiol 64:85, 1970.
26. Nakamura S, Okado I, Nakashio S, et al: *Clostridium sporogenes* isolates and their relationship to *C. botulinum* based on deoxyribonucleic acid reassociation. J Gen Microbiol 100:395, 1977.
27. Suen JC, Hatheway CL, Steigerwalt AG, et al: *Clostridium argentinense,* sp. nov: A genetically homogenous group composed of all strains of *Clostridium botulinum* toxin type G and some nontoxigenic strains previously identified as *Clostridium subterminale* or *Clostridium hastiforme.* Int J Syst Bacteriol 38:375, 1988.
28. Collins MD, Lawson PA, Willems A, et al: The phylogeny of the genus *Clostridium:* Proposal of five new genera and eleven new species combinations. Int J Syst Bacteriol 44:812, 1994.
29. Hatheway CL, McCroskey LM: Unusual neurotoxigenic clostridia recovered from human fecal specimens in the investigation of botulism. *In* Hattori T, Ishida Y, Maruyama Y, et al (eds): Recent Advances in Microbial Ecology. Tokyo, Japan Scientific Societies Press, 1989, pp 477–481.
30. Moller V, Scheibel I: Preliminary report on the isolation of an apparently new type of *Cl. botulinum.* Acta Pathol Microbiol Scand 48:80, 1960.
31. Midura TF, Nygaard GS, Wood RM, et al: *Clostridium botulinum* type F: Isolation from venison jerky. Appl Microbiol 24:165, 1972.
32. Hall JD, McCroskey LM, Pincomb BJ, et al: Isolation of an organism resembling *Clostridium barati* which produces type F botulinal toxin from an infant with botulism. J Clin Microbiol 21:654, 1985.
33. McCroskey LM, Hatheway CL, Woodruff BA, et al: Type F botulism due to neurotoxigenic *Clostridium baratii* from an unknown source in an adult. J Clin Microbiol 29:2618, 1991.
34. Green J, Spear H, Brinson RR: Human botulism type F—A rare type. Am J Med 75:893, 1983.
35. Hauschild AHW: Epidemiology of human foodborne botulism. *In* Hauschild AHW, Dodds KL (eds): *Clostridium botulinum:* Ecology and Control in Foods. New York, Marcel Dekker, 1993, pp 69–104.
36. Prevot AR, Terrasse J, Daumail J, et al: Existence en France du botulisme humain de type C. Bull Acad Natl Med Paris 139:355, 1955.
37. Demarchi J, Mourgues C, Orio J, et al: Existence du botulisme humain de type D. Bull Acad Natl Med Paris 142:580, 1958.
38. Sonnabend OA, Sonnabend WF, Krech U, et al: Continuous microbiological study of 70 sudden and unexpected infant deaths: Toxigenic intestinal *Clostridium botulinum* infection in 9 cases of sudden infant death syndrome. Lancet 2:237, 1985.
39. Smith LDS: The occurrence of *Clostridium botulinum* and *Clostridium tetani* in the soil of the United States. Health Lab Sci 15:74, 1978.
40. Wainwright RB, Heyward WL, Middaugh JP, et al: Foodborne botulism in Alaska, 1947–1985: Epidemiology and clinical findings. J Infect Dis 157:1158, 1988.
41. Shaffer N, Wainwright RB, Middaugh JP, Tauxe RV: Botulism among Alaskan Natives. The role of changing food preparation and consumption practices. West J Med 153:390, 1990.
42. Miller LG, Clark PS, Kunkle GA: Possible origin of *Clostridium botulinum* contamination of Eskimo foods in northwestern Alaska. Appl Microbiol 23:427, 1972.
43. Davis JB, Mattman LH, Wiley M: *Clostridium botulinum* in a fatal wound infection. JAMA 146:646, 1951.

44. Dodds KL: Worldwide incidence and ecology of infant botulism. *In* Hauschild AHW, Dodds KL (eds): *Clostridium botulinum:* Ecology and Control in Foods. New York, Marcel Dekker, 1993, pp 105–117.
45. Arnon SS: Infant botulism. *In* Feigen RD, Cherry JD (eds): Textbook of Pediatric Infectious Diseases, ed 3. Philadelphia, WB Saunders, 1992, pp 1095–1102.
46. Oguma K, Yokota K, Hayashi S, et al: Infant botulism due to *Clostridium botulinum* type C toxin. Lancet 336:1449, 1990.
47. Aureli P, Fenicia L, Pasolini B, et al: Two cases of type E infant botulism caused by neurotoxigenic *Clostridium butyricum* in Italy. J Infect Dis 154:201, 1986.
48. McCroskey LM, Hatheway CL: Laboratory findings in four cases of adult botulism suggest colonization of the intestinal tract. J Clin Microbiol 26:1052, 1988.
49. English WL, Williams LP, Bryant RE, et al: Case 48-1980: Botulism (Letter). N Engl J Med 304:789, 1981.
50. Freedman M, Armstrong RM, Killian JM, et al: Botulism in a patient with jejunoileal bypass. Ann Neurol 20:641, 1986.
51. Chia JK, Clark JB, Ryan CA, et al: Botulism in an adult associated with food-borne intestinal infection with *Clostridium botulinum.* N Engl J Med 315:239, 1986.
52. Isacsohn M, Cohen A, Steiner A, et al: Botulism intoxication after surgery in the gut. Isr J Med Sci 21:150, 1985.
52a. Griffin PM, Hatheway CL, Rosenbaum RB, et al: Endogenous antibody production to botulinum toxin in an adult with intestinal colonization botulism and underlying Crohn's disease. J Infect Dis 175:633, 1997.
53. Simpson LL: Peripheral actions of the botulinum toxins. *In* Simpson LL (ed): Botulinum Neurotoxin and Tetanus Toxin. San Diego, CA, Academic Press, 1989, pp 153–178.
54. Vita G, Girlanda P, Puglisi RM, et al: Cardiovascular-reflex testing and single-fiber electromyography in botulism. Arch Neurol 44:202, 1987.
55. Hatheway CL: Toxigenic clostridia. Clin Microbiol Rev 3:67, 1990.
56. Montecucco C, Schiavo G: Mechanism of action of tetanus and botulinum neurotoxins. Mol Microbiol 13:1, 1994.
57. Weber JT, Hatheway CL, St Louis ME: Botulism. *In* Hoeprich PD, Jordan MC, Ronald AR (eds): Infectious Diseases: A Treatise of Infectious Processes, ed 5. Philadelphia, JB Lippincott, 1994, pp 1185–1194.
58. Centers for Disease Control: Botulism in the United States, 1899–1977. Handbook for Epidemiologists, Clinicians, and Laboratory Workers. Atlanta, Public Health Service, US Department of Health, Education, and Welfare, 1979.
59. Woodruff BA, Griffin PM, McCroskey LM, et al: Clinical and laboratory comparison of botulism from toxin types A, B, and E in the United States, 1975–1988. J Infect Dis 166:1281, 1992.
60. Long SS, Gajewski JL, Brown LW, Gilligan PH: Clinical, laboratory, and environmental features of infant botulism in southeastern Pennsylvania. Pediatrics 75:935, 1985.
61. Hatheway CL: Botulism. *In* Balows A, Hausler WH Jr, Ohashi M, et al (eds): Laboratory Diagnosis of Infectious Diseases: Principles and Practice, Vol. 1. New York, Springer-Verlag, 1988, pp 111–133.
62. Dowell VR Jr, McCroskey LM, Hatheway CL, et al: Coproexamination for botulinal toxin and *Clostridium botulinum.* A new procedure for laboratory diagnosis of botulism. JAMA 238:1829, 1977.
63. Easton EJ, Meyer KF: Occurrence of *Bacillus botulinus* in human and animal excreta. J Infect Dis 35:207, 1924.
64. Hatheway CL, McCroskey LM: Examination of feces and serum for diagnosis of infant botulism in 336 patients. J Clin Microbiol 25:2334, 1987.
65. Rubin LG, Dezfulian M, Yolkin RH: Serum antibody response to *Clostridium botulinum* toxin in infant botulism. J Clin Microbiol 16:770, 1982.
66. Hatheway CL, Ferreira JL: Detection and identification of *Clostridium botulinum* neurotoxins. Adv Exp Med Biol 391:481, 1996.
67. Cherrington M: Electrophysiologic methods as an aid in diagnosis of botulism: A review. Muscle Nerve 5:S28, 1982.
68. Cornblath DR, Sladky JT, Sumner AJ: Clinical electrophysiology of infantile botulism. Muscle Nerve 6:448, 1983.
69. Morris JG: Current trends in therapy of botulism in the United States. *In* Lewis GE Jr (ed): Biomedical Aspects of Botulism. New York, Academic Press, 1981, pp 317–326.
70. Schwartz PJ, Arnon SS: Botulism immune globulin for infant botulism arrives—One year and a Gulf War later. West J Med 156:197, 1992.
71. Arnon SS: Clinical trial of human botulism immune globulin. *In* DasGupta BR (ed): Botulinum and Tetanus Neurotoxins: Neurotransmission and Biomedical Aspects. New York, Plenum Publishing, 1992, pp 483–488.
72. Tacket CO, Shandera WX, Mann JM, et al: Equine antitoxin use and other factors that predict outcome in type A foodborne botulism. Am J Med 76:794, 1984.
73. Lewis GE Jr, Metzger JF: Studies on the prophylaxis and treatment of botulism. *In* Eaker D, Wadström T (eds): Natural Toxins. Oxford, UK, Pergamon Press, 1980, pp 601–606.
74. Black RE, Gunn RA: Hypersensitivity reactions associated with botulinal antitoxin. Am J Med 69:567, 1980.
75. Hatheway CL, Snyder JD, Seals JE, et al: Antitoxin levels in botulism patients treated with trivalent equine botulism antitoxin to toxin types A, B, and E. J Infect Dis 150:407, 1984.
76. Arnon SS, Midura TF, Damus K, et al: Honey and other environmental risk factors for infant botulism. J Pediatr 94:331, 1979.
77. Cardella MA: Botulinum toxoids. *In* Lewis KH, Cassel K Jr (eds): Botulism: Proceedings of a Symposium. Cincinnati, OH, US Department of Health, Education, and Welfare, 1964, pp 113–130. Public Health Service publication 999 FP-1.

222

Clostridium perfringens and Other Clostridia

Sherwood L. Gorbach

The genus *Clostridium* is composed of gram-positive, spore-forming, anaerobic rods that live in soil and in animals. To date, more than 80 species have been defined biochemically and metabolically, and numerous others await characterization.[1, 2] Usually, these organisms reside in peaceful coexistence with their human or animal host, but given the proper circumstances their pathogenic potential can be realized. Various clostridia are capable of endogenous and exogenous infection, producing disease that is either toxin mediated or suppurative.[3–5]

Characteristics of the Pathogen

Clostridia are ubiquitous throughout nature in animals and soil. All species grow better under anaerobic conditions, but some—*Clostridium perfringens, Clostridium septicum, Clostridium histolyticum*, and *Clostridium tertium*—are remarkably aerotolerant. Clostridia can be distinguished from *Bacillus* species by the absence of catalase, peroxidase, and cytochrome oxidase. Spore formation, a trait that is useful in species identification, may be either terminal or subterminal, but it is not noted in all clinical isolates, particularly *C. perfringens* and *Clostridium ramosum*, and it may be necessary to use ethanol or heat shock to induce sporulation. By electron microscopy, most clostridia appear as fat, boxcar-shaped rods with a typical gram-positive cell wall. Because many species seem to be gram-negative in clinical material or in late cultures, the tinctorial characteristics should not be an absolute criterion for classification.

Approximately 30 of the 83 clostridial strains described in *Bergey's Manual of Systematic Bacteriology*[6] are involved in infection in humans (Table 222–1). Production of protein toxins has been noted in 14 species, and these species have been associated with certain classic infections such as botulism, tetanus, gas gangrene, pseudomembranous colitis, and food poisoning (Table 222–2).

Normal Flora

Clostridia are present in the normal intestinal flora of humans and of many animal species.[1, 7–9] The organisms can be isolated from the feces of 70% of humans, at a concentration of 10^8 to 10^9 per g.[9, 10] Clostridia are cultured from the vagina of 4% to 10% of healthy women[11–13] and from 19% to 29% after unsanitary abortion.[14] A variety of *Clostridium* species are present in the fecal flora, *C. ramosum* being the most common, followed by *C. perfringens* and, in smaller numbers, 30 or more other species. Occasionally the organisms can be isolated from the skin of the perineum and other cutaneous sites.

Clostridium perfringens

C. perfringens is the species most frequently isolated from clinical material. It has been recovered from virtually every organ site, including infections in the abdomen, female pelvis, skin and soft tissues, and blood stream.[3, 15, 16] The organism is relatively aerotolerant, and it exhibits "stormy fermentation" when cultured in milk. It is the fastest growing clostridial species: generation time is 8 minutes under ideal conditions.[6] *C. perfringens* can be recognized by its gray, spreading colonies, which often produce a double zone of hemolysis on blood agar, depending on the isolate and culture medium. The organism is known to produce 12 toxins: four major toxins (α, β, ϵ, and ι) and eight minor toxins, including the enterotoxin[1, 2] (see Table 222–2). On the basis of the distribution of the four major toxins, the species has been divided into five types, A through E (Table 222–3). The α-toxin is a zinc metallophospholipase, which interacts with eukaryotic cell membranes and hydrolyzes phosphatidycholine and sphingomyelin, leading to cell death.[17] Its activity, as measured in medium containing egg yoke (Nagler), can be inhibited by specific antitoxin. The α-toxin has been purified and crystallized, and its C-terminal domain has been expressed in *Escherichia coli*.[18, 19] This toxin plays an essential role in the causation of gas gangrene; α-toxin causes muscle inflammation and necrosis, platelet aggregation, hemolysis, lethality in animals, vasodilatation, and increased vascular permeability.[17, 20, 21]

C. perfringens type A is responsible for virtually all the infections of humans caused by this species. Types B, D, and E cannot be isolated from soil samples and only rarely are associated with human disease. *C. perfringens* type C is found in pigs. It causes enteritis necroticans (EN; also known as *Darmbrand*,[22] and pig-bel[23]) (see later).

TABLE 222–1 ■ *Clostridium* Species Isolated from Clinical Specimens

SPECIES	BLOOD CULTURES	SOFT TISSUE INFECTIONS	INTRAABDOMINAL SEPSIS	TOTAL
C. perfringens	37	20	4	61
C. ramosum	3	15	5	23
C. bifermentans	2	5	4	11
C. sphenoides	2	4	1	7
C. sporogenes	—	3	3	6
C. innocuum	1	3	2	6
C. difficile	1	3	1	5
C. butyricum	—	3	2	5
C. septicum	2	2	—	4
C. tertium	2	1	—	3
C. sordellii	—	3	—	3
C. limosum	2	—	1	3
C. baratii	1	1	1	3
C. pseudotetanicum	1	1	—	2
C. beijerinckii	—	1	—	2
C. fallax	—	1	1	2
C. ghoni	—	1	1	2
C. carnis	—	1	1	2
C. subterminale	—	2	—	2
C. novyi	—	2	—	1
C. putrificum	1	—	—	1
C. hastiforme	1	—	—	1
C. cadaveris	—	1	1	1
C. paraputrificum	—	—	1	1
Clostridium (unclassified)	11	12	13	36
Total	65	87	43	195

Data from Gorbach SL, Thadepalli H: Isolation of *Clostridium* in human infections: Evaluation of 114 cases. J Infect Dis 131:S81–S85, 1975; and Gorbach SL, Thadepalli H, Norsen J: Anaerobic microorganisms in intraabdominal infections. *In* Balows A, DeHann RM, Dowell VR Jr, Guze LB (eds): Anaerobic Bacteria: Role in Disease. Springfield, IL, Charles C Thomas, 1974, pp 399–407.

Clostridium septicum

This species distinguished itself in early reports by causing generalized edema and bacteremia in animals,[1] and it was the second or third most common cause of gas gangrene in wartime.[24] More recently, it has been associated with bacteremia and neutropenic enterocolitis seen in conjunction with malignancy (see later). *C. septicum* is unusually aerotolerant, perhaps accounting for its ability to survive in the blood stream. Four major toxins and neuraminidase are produced by *C. septicum*; the lethal, necrotizing α-toxin and the oxygen-labile hemolysin (δ-toxin) seem to be responsible for pathogenicity.[25, 26]

Clinical Conditions

A wide range of clostridial species can be isolated from soft tissues (see Table 222–1). *C. perfringens* is the most common, although it represents only one fourth of all isolates. *C. ramosum* is nearly as common in soft tissues, and a host of other species are seen with regularity. Clostridia can be recovered from suppurative processes without local or systemic signs of toxin activity. Indeed, it is often impossible to separate the role of clostridia from the roles of multiple other organisms at the same site. In one study, 84% of soft tissue infections that harbored clostridia also contained other bacteria, often as many as 5 to 10 different types.[3]

Simple contamination by clostridia, without clinical signs or symptoms, is by all accounts the most frequent setting for isolating clostridial species from clinical material.[5] Before antibiotics came into widespread use, clostridia could be isolated from 10% to 30% of wounds in civilians and from up to 80% of war wounds. Even with antibiotic treatment, such as with cephalothin and kanamycin, clostridia were isolated from 16% of penetrating abdominal wounds.[27] Clostridia are isolated with similar frequency from suppurating wounds and from well-healing wounds. Indeed, recovery of clostridia from a wound does not determine its clinical status, nor does it dictate specific therapeutic decisions. Clostridial infections (as opposed to contamination) are clinical entities, not bacteriologic diagnoses.

Gas production, detected by palpation or radiologic studies, has been noted in infections caused by clostridia such as

TABLE 222–2 ■ Toxigenic Clostridia and Their Toxins*

SPECIES	TOXINS	SIZE OF MOLECULE (kDa)	ACTIVITY OR DISEASE
C. botulinum	Neurotoxin	150	Botulism
	C_2 (binary)		Permease
	Component I	50	ADP-ribosylation
	Component II	105	Binding
	C_3	25	ADP-ribosylation
C. argentinense (*C. botulinum* type G)	Neurotoxin	ND†	Botulism (experimental)
C. tetani	Neurotoxin	150	Tetanus
	Tetanolysin	48	Oxygen-labile hemolysin
C. perfringens	Major		
	α	43	Phospholipase C/myonecrosis
	β	40	Lethal, necrotic/enterotoxemia
	ε	34	Lethal, permease/enterotoxemia
	ι (binary)		Enterotoxemia
	Component a	48	ADP-ribosylation
	Component b	72	Binding
	Other		
	Enterotoxin	35	Food-borne diarrhea
	δ	42	Hemolysin
	θ	51	Oxygen-labile hemolysin
	κ	80	Collagenase
	λ	ND	Protease
	μ	ND	Hyaluronidase
	ν	ND	DNase
	Neuraminidase	43, 64, 105, 310	*N*-Acetylneuraminic acid glycohydrolase
C. difficile	Toxin A	400–500	Enterotoxin/AAPMC
	Toxin B	360–470	Cytotoxin/AAPMC
	CDT	43	ADP-ribosylation
C. sordellii (*C. bifermentans*)	α	43	Phospholipase C
	β		Lethal
	HT	525	Equivalent to *C. difficile* toxin A
	LT	250	Equivalent to *C. difficile* toxin B
	Hemolysin	43	Oxygen-labile hemolysin
C. novyi, C. haemolyticum	α	260–280	Lethal
	β	32	Phospholipase C
	γ	30	Phospholipase C
	δ	ND	Oxygen-labile hemolysin
	ε	ND	Lipase
C. chauvoei, C. septicum	α	27	Lethal, necrotizing
	β	45	DNase
	γ	ND	Hyaluronidase
	δ	ND	Oxygen-labile hemolysin
C. histolyticum	α	ND	Necrotizing
	β		Collagenases
	Class I	68, 115, 79, 130	
	Class II	100, 110, 125	
	γ	>10, <50	Proteinase, thiol activated
	δ	ND	Proteinase
	ε		Oxygen-labile hemolysin
C. spiroforme	ι (binary)		Diarrhea in rabbits
	Component a	43–47	ADP-ribosylation
	Component b	ND	Binding
C. butyricum	Neurotoxin	145	Botulism, type E
C. baratii	Neurotoxin	ND	Botulism, type F

*ND, Not determined; AAPMC, antibiotic-associated pseudomembranous colitis.
†For neurotoxin of *C. argentinense,* a 16S complex of 500 kDa has been purified, but the size of its toxic subcomponent has not been determined.
From Hatheway CL: Toxigenic clostridia. Clin Microbiol Rev 3:66–98, 1990.

gas gangrene, crepitant cellulitis,[28] emphysematous cholecystitis,[29, 30] emphysematous gastritis,[31] and emphysematous cystitis.[32–34] Yet, gas production is not unique to clostridial infections: it can be associated with infections by coliforms, streptococci, staphylococci, and *Bacteroides* species,[28, 35] and even in noninfectious settings such as trauma (air hose injuries, penetrating wounds of the airway or thorax), benzine injection, wound irrigation with hydrogen peroxide, and tracking along an intravascular catheter.

The histotoxic clostridial syndromes include neurologic diseases, botulism (Chapter 221), and tetanus (Chapter 220); enteric diseases such as food poisoning (Chapter 82); EN, pseudomembranous colitis (Chapter 79); and soft tissue infections (gas gangrene, spontaneous [nontraumatic] myonecrosis, Chapter 102).

Intraabdominal infections, especially those caused by bowel perforation, are associated with clostridia in 30% to 50% of cases.[36–39] In a study of 67 patients with intraabdominal infection,[27] 43 clostridial strains were isolated, including 16 known species and a number of nontypeable ones. *C. ramosum* was the most common isolate, followed by *C. perfringens* and *Clostridium bifermentans*. None of these patients

TABLE 222-3 ■ Distribution of the Major Lethal Toxins Among the Types of *Clostridium perfringens*

TYPE	TOXIN			
	α	β	ε	ι
A	+	−	−	−
B	+	+	+	−
C	+	+	−	−
D	+	−	+	−
E	+	−	−	+

From Smith L, Williams BL: The Pathogenic Anaerobic Bacteria, ed 3. Springfield, IL, Charles C Thomas, 1984.

had gas gangrene, and it was impossible to differentiate on clinical grounds those whose specimens yielded *Clostridium* organisms in culture.

The diseased gallbladder is contaminated by clostridia in 10% to 20% of cases sampled at surgery.[40–43] A particularly virulent form of cholangitis, termed emphysematous cholecystitis because of gas formation in the biliary tract radicles and the wall of the gallbladder, is caused in at least 50% of cases by clostridial species.[29, 44–47] More common in male diabetic patients, this complication has a higher mortality rate than other biliary tract infections. There is, however, no evidence of muscle invasion or systemic signs of clostridial toxin; rather, patients succumb to severe sepsis.

Female pelvic infections are associated with clostridia in 4% to 20% of cases, and they are particularly common in patients with tuboovarian or pelvic abscess.[48–52] In the era before antibiotic therapy, clostridia were often isolated from discharges of women with septic abortions, indeed, with such frequency in women with mild infection that Ramsey[53] referred to *Clostridium welchii (perfringens)* as a harmless saprophyte. Nevertheless, this organism continues to cause severe postpartum infection in the modern era, even in uncomplicated deliveries.[54] (For discussion of uterine gas gangrene, see Chapter 102.)

Pulmonary infections can be caused by clostridia, but usually they are mixed infections. Clostridia have been isolated from approximately 10% of patients with various aspiration syndromes, either from empyema fluid or from transtracheal aspirates, and *C. perfringens* is the most frequent isolate.[55] There are scattered reports in the older literature of pure *C. perfringens* pulmonary infections.[56–63] Clostridia have also been associated with infection after chest injury or thoracotomy.[64, 65] Like other suppurative clostridial infections, these typically show no signs of local or systemic toxin production; they are indistinguishable from pulmonary infections that do not involve clostridia, notwithstanding the rare case of myonecrosis with gas formation.[58, 61]

Central nervous system infections involving clostridia are relatively rare, consisting mostly of case reports of penetrating head wounds,[66] brain abscess,[67–70] or purulent meningitis.[71, 72] Seventeen cases of clostridial bacterial endocarditis have been reported, including the case of an intravenous drug user who was infected with *C. bifermentans*[73] and a patient with colon cancer who developed endocarditis caused by *C. septicum*.[74] When clostridia cause suppurative arthritis the isolate is usually *C. perfringens* and the setting is penetrating trauma to the joint, an immunocompromised host, or knee arthroplasty.[75–77] A miscellany of chronic wound infections have been associated with clostridia as part of a mixed flora, including diabetic foot ulcers, stump infections, decubitus ulcers, and perirectal infections.[4, 78]

Intestinal Disorders

Clostridia are known to cause three types of intestinal illness: food poisoning, related to *C. perfringens* type A; EN, caused by *C. perfringens* type C; and pseudomembranous colitis (PMC) and its milder form, antibiotic-associated diarrhea, caused by *Clostridium difficile*. These toxin diseases are entirely distinct, and each has its own epidemiology and pathogenesis. (*C. difficile* is discussed in Chapter 79; the epidemiology of food poisoning, in Chapter 82.)

EN is a severe, necrotizing disease of the small intestine caused by β-toxin–producing strains of *C. perfringens* type C. Known originally by its German name, *Darmbrand*, EN was described in malnourished people in Germany and Norway after World War II.[22] Subsequently, the same condition, with the name pig-bel, was recognized in the highlands of Papua New Guinea.[23, 79] Scattered reports of EN have come from Africa, Southeast Asia, Nepal, China, and most recently Thailand.[79, 80] In New Guinea, pig-bel accounts for 10% of deaths of children between the ages of 1 and 15 years. It is the most common cause of death in children 6 to 10 years of age, the mortality rate being as high as 30 in 10,000 in some districts.[81] Pork consumption is the mode of transmission, either in ritual pig feasting or in a family setting (now the more common venue).[82]

The major pathologic focus of EN is the small intestine, particularly the jejunum, where a spotty coagulative necrosis causes transmural destruction of the intestinal wall.[83] The result is a friable mucosa, which often sloughs, leaving deep ulcers that are liable to perforate.

In Papua New Guinea, the disease is said to occur when a specific set of cultural and epidemiologic circumstances coincide.[79] The organism, usually acquired by eating undercooked pork, colonizes the host's intestine.[84] The basic requirement for disease is a disturbance of the fine balance in the intestinal lumen between toxin production by the organism and toxin destruction by intestinal proteases such as trypsin. Because the unfortunate hosts habitually consume a low-protein diet, the concentration of trypsin in their intestine is low. Trypsin activity is further reduced during the pork meal by simultaneous consumption of sweet potatoes, which contain trypsin inhibitors. In addition, many people are infected with *Ascaris* worms, which produce protein inhibitors. The result is low proteolytic activity in the intestine, with failure to degrade the toxin elaborated by the clostridia that are now attached to the intestinal surface.[85] This hypothesis is supported by experiments in which pig-bel developed in guinea pigs given *C. perfringens* type C only when sweet potatoes were fed concomitantly.[86]

In view of the high mortality rate and the frequent need for surgery (pig-bel is the most common indication for laparotomy in the highland hospitals of Papua New Guinea), it is most encouraging to learn of the successful development of a vaccine based on the β-toxin. In a field trial, the vaccine conferred significant protection, and subsequent studies in Papua New Guinea have shown a marked reduction in pig-bel incidence and mortality.[79, 87]

Clostridial food poisoning, caused by enterotoxin-producing strains of *C. perfringens* type A, ranks second or third on the list of types of food poisoning in the United States[88, 89] (see Chapter 82). Such strains are responsible for about 10% of the diagnosed outbreaks; about 25 epidemics are reported each year, each involving an average of 24 persons.[90, 91] Hospital outbreaks of clostridial food poisoning have also been reported.[92] The usual vehicle is meat or meat products, and there is a high attack rate, often greater than 50%. The organisms are more likely to be heat resistant in outbreaks reported in England, but they tend to be heat sensitive in the United States.[2, 93] The optimal temperature for *C. perfringens* is 43°C to 47°C.[94] Although it was originally thought that the toxin was ingested preformed in food, it is now believed that the organism is ingested in its vegetative state and the toxin is elaborated in the intestinal tract. Approximately 10^8 colony-forming units are required to initiate infection in volunteers; the viable forms cause disease, but spores and cell-free fluid cannot induce clinical symptoms.[95, 96] The toxin was believed to be related to sporulation, but subsequently it has been shown that nonsporulating cultures can elaborate toxin.[97] Enterotoxin-producing strains are isolated from most ill patients; when sensitive methods are employed they can also be recovered from the stools of about 30% of healthy persons.[98]

The clinical illness is caused by a heat-labile protein enterotoxin with a molecular mass of approximately 35,000.[99] Clostridial enterotoxin induces fluid production in the rabbit ileal loop model.[100] It also causes vomiting in monkeys, death in mice, and cytotoxicity in Vero cells.[101–103] The toxin differs from cholera toxin in the following respects: clostridial toxin has its maximal activity in the ileum and minimal activity in the duodenum, just the opposite of cholera toxin. Clostridial enterotoxin inhibits glucose transport, damages the intestinal epithelium, and causes protein loss into the intestinal lumen, none of which are observed with cholera toxin.[100] *C. perfringens* enterotoxin has a unique mechanism for disturbing cell membrane permeability of eukaryotic cells.[104] It binds to a protein receptor on the plasma membrane and inserts into the membrane. The plasma membrane becomes freely permeable to small molecules such as ions and amino acids. The toxin causes cytoskeleton collapse and inhibition of cell metabolism, with resulting cell death and loss of the ability of the intestinal cell to secrete fluid and electrolytes.[103, 105–107]

The most prominent symptoms of clostridial food poisoning are diarrhea (90% of cases) and moderate to severe mid-epigastric pain (80%); additional findings include nausea (25%), vomiting (9%), and fever (24%), but the entire illness generally lasts less than 24 hours.[91, 108, 109]

An outbreak of clostridial food poisoning should be suspected when the incubation period is short (8 to 12 hours), a meat product is incriminated, the attack rate is 50% or greater, and the illness lasts less than 24 hours.

Three criteria are used to establish the diagnosis of *C. perfringens* food poisoning: more than 10^5 *C. perfringens* organisms per gram of incriminated food; a median spore count of more than 10^6 *C. perfringens* organisms per gram of stool from ill persons; or isolation of the same serotype of *C. perfringens* from stools and suspected food.[110, 111]

For *C. perfringens* type A, serotyping has limited value in the United States because only 40% of strains are typeable[90]; nevertheless, this method may be useful in some epidemics, especially when tests of food items fail to demonstrate clostridia.[112] Plasmid profiles can be a helpful typing system, but their role is limited because not all enterotoxin strains have detectable plasmids.[113] The fecal spore count can also be unreliable, because in an outbreak ill and healthy people can have the same count. Alternative methods of enterotoxin detection in stool are enzyme-linked assay,[114] Vero cell assay,[115] and the preferred test, reverse passive latex agglutination assay.[116, 117]

Enterotoxigenic *C. perfringens* has been implicated in sporadic cases of diarrhea in the absence of an identified food vehicle. In these cases, free enterotoxin was detected in stool, along with large numbers (10^7 to 10^9 per g) of enterotoxin-producing *C. perfringens* organisms. Most of the serotypes were not those commonly associated with food poisoning. Some cases were sporadic, but most were associated with antibiotic use or with a chronic care facility. In contrast to classic *C. perfringens* food poisoning, these cases have a more prolonged course, generally lasting longer than 1 week, and many patients experience relapses.[115, 118–120]

Bacteremia

In a large general hospital, in which good anaerobic technique was used, clostridia were found in 0.3% of all blood cultures and represented 2.6% of the positive isolates.[3] *C. perfringens* accounts for 60% of the blood cultures that grow clostridia; the prevalence of *C. perfringens* in soft tissues is approximately 25% of all clostridia isolated in culture (see Table 222–1). Yet clostridia bacteremia often represents an intriguing paradox, in that a "positive" blood culture is not necessarily associated with serious illness—and in some cases cannot be correlated with the patient's clinical condition. For patients who had a septic abortion, for example, positive clostridial blood cultures were noted in 18% to 27%, most of whom had a benign disease course, even without antibiotics, and none of whom had evidence of gas gangrene.[53, 121–123] In another series of 29 patients with clostridial bacteremia, only 12 had a concurrent infection involving clostridia, whereas the others had "spontaneous" clostridial bacteremia documented at the time of admission to the hospital for a variety of unrelated medical conditions.[3] These patients recovered from their primary illness, and the source of the *Clostridium* in the blood stream was never uncovered. On the other hand, two studies reported that more than 95% of cases of clostridial bacteremia were clinically significant. These patients' mortality rate was 43% to 48%, nearly all attributable to the clostridial infection.[124, 125] Two thirds of these infections were related to intraabdominal sources; half were associated with malignancy, mostly colon cancer. Several studies have shown that anaerobic bacteremia has decreased, probably as a result of early and appropriate use of antimicrobial drugs in suspected cases. Nevertheless, clostridia accounted for 31% of significant anaerobic bacteremias in one series, with an attributable mortality of 45%. *C. perfringens* and *C. septicum* were present in equal frequencies, 38% each.[126] Thus, clostridial bacteremia must be treated with respect, and colon cancer should be suspected, but the experience in at least some hospitals is that many such cases are in fact benign or spontaneous.

Several clostridial species have been associated with malignancy, including *C. perfringens*,[1, 127, 128] *C. ramosum*,[3] *C. difficile*,[3] *Clostridium sordellii*,[129] *C. histolyticum*,[130] *C. tertium*,[131] and *Clostridium sporogenes*.[132] Yet, when cases of clostridial bacteremia were reviewed in a general hospital, only 3% to 4% were, in fact, associated with malignancy.[3, 133]

C. septicum bacteremia represents a special case. Under healthy conditions, *C. septicum* is a rather rare inhabitant of the normal intestinal flora,[9, 127, 134–136] although it has been isolated from the ileum and appendix, especially from patients with leukemia.[137] In a review of 162 bacteremia cases in the world literature, 89% were related to malignancy[138]; this percentage is nearly identical to that cited in the initial review of *C. septicum* bacteremia published some 20 years earlier.[139] Approximately half of the patients with bacteremia had colon cancer, whereas most of the others had hematologic malignancies and a few had some other tumor. Nearly 20% of the subjects had diabetes. Remarkably, 37% of patients presenting with *C. septicum* bacteremia were found at a later examination to have an occult malignancy, of which 84% were located in the large bowel.

Besides the usual signs of sepsis, *C. septicum* bacteremia often has findings related to the abdomen—abdominal pain, tenderness, vomiting, diarrhea. Approximately one fourth of patients have metastatic infection and myonecrosis at a distant site (see Chapter 102). Although the clinical picture is often dramatic, such cases are relatively rare, and *C. septicum* is responsible for only 1% to 3% of all clostridial bacteremias.[3, 140, 141]

Neutropenia, associated with leukemia or lymphoproliferative disorders or with cyclic neutropenia, has also been correlated with *C. septicum* bacteremia.[3, 133, 142–144] The intestinal mucosa of the terminal ileum and cecum in such patients is often involved with neutropenic enterocolitis, a condition characterized by mucosal infiltrates of leukemic deposits and necrosis.[145] *C. septicum* can be seen penetrating the bowel wall at sites of mucosal damage. Many patients with leukemia, especially those with neutropenia secondary to disease or to chemotherapy, have inflamed, necrotic areas in the ileum and colon, even without evidence of infection.[146–149] It is likely that *C. septicum* makes its way through an intestinal mucosa damaged by the underlying disease, aided and abetted by toxin production and its relative aerotolerance[138, 147]; the absence of neutrophils, which is almost universal in leukemia patients with clostridial bacteremia, facilitates dissemination of the organism into the blood stream and to other parts of the body.[150]

Approximately 20% of patients with *C. septicum* bacteremia have diabetes.[138, 151] Complications of diabetes, such as foot ulcers and amputation stumps, may be contaminated with this species and other clostridia.[78, 152]

C. tertium bacteremia is also associated with neutropenia.[153–155] This species is somewhat unusual in that it is resistant to β-lactam antibiotics as well as to clindamycin and metronidazole, but it is sensitive to vancomycin, trimethoprim-sulfamethoxazole, and ciprofloxacin. Presenting symptoms are often related to the abdomen or perirectal area. In contrast to *C. septicum* bacteremia, the outcome with *C. tertium* bacteremia is often favorable when appropriate antibiotics are employed.

Treatment

The therapeutic approach, whether medical or surgical, must be tailored to the specific clinical condition and the incriminated *Clostridium* strain. Simple contamination of open wounds by clostridia is managed with good wound care and calculated avoidance of antibiotics. Judicious surgical débridement may be necessary, depending on clinical circumstances. Suppurative infections that involve clostridia—for example, in the abdomen or female pelvis—should be treated with broad-spectrum antibiotics to suppress the aerobic and anaerobic bacteria that are invariable components of this infection. Patients with benign clostridial bacteremia generally should not be treated with antibiotics, although the incriminated pathogen may dictate otherwise (e.g., patients with *C. septicum* or *C. tertium* bacteremia require early and aggressive treatment). Obviously, when bacteremia is associated with organ site involvement or soft tissue infection, therapy is indicated. Clostridial infections that are related to toxin production may, in some circumstances, be treated with immunotherapy. Tetanus and botulism should be managed with passive antibodies in the form of specific immunoglobulin. Vaccines can be used for tetanus and EN. On the other hand, immunotherapy is not indicated for *C. difficile* diarrhea, *C. perfringens* food poisoning, or gas gangrene (see Chapter 102).

Antibiotic therapy should be used in clinically significant clostridial infections (with the notable exception of *C. perfringens* food poisoning). Antimicrobial susceptibility tests in vitro have shown a somewhat variable pattern[156–163] (Table 222–4). Most strains of *C. perfringens* are sensitive to β-lactam antibiotics, although some resistance to penicillin at low concentrations has been encountered. Clindamycin is also active against this species, but resistance has been noted in *C. ramosum* and *C. tertium*. In general, antibiotic resistance has been seen most often in strains of *C. ramosum, C. sporogenes*, and *C. tertium* (which is resistant to β-lactam antibiotics, clindamycin, and metronidazole).[153–155]

Resistance of clostridia to β-lactam antibiotics can be explained by β-lactamase production or decreased affinity of penicillin binding proteins (PBPs).[164] Three species, *Clostridium butyricum, Clostridium clostridioforme*, and *C. ramosum*, produce β-lactamase[164–168]; the enzymes are usually inducible, and some of the strains can be inhibited by cefoxitin and sulbactam. Plasmid-mediated β-lactamase has been found only in *C. ramosum*,[169] and most of the other enzyme-producing strains are thought to be chromosomally mediated. PBPs have been found in *C. perfringens*: β-lactam affinity is greatest for PBP 3 and PBP 4.[170] Reduced affinity to PBP 1 of *C. perfringens* has been associated with increased resistance to penicillin.[171]

Animal models of clostridial infections, mostly *C. perfringens*, have shown that antibiotics that inhibit protein synthesis (clindamycin, tetracycline, chloramphenicol) produce higher survival rates than cell wall drugs such as penicillin, and this may be related to inhibition of toxin production.[172, 173] Metronidazole and rifampin are also superior to penicillin in animal models.[172, 174, 175] Yet, animal models are artificial, especially because surgery and adjunctive therapy are not used. Furthermore, penicillin can be given in large doses to humans because it is not toxic, whereas most other drugs have a limited safe dose range.

Penicillin therapy for *C. perfringens* infections has enjoyed a long and largely untarnished record,[4, 176–179] although it must be conceded that this experience is based on anecdotal observation rather than controlled trials. With regard to *C. septicum*, data from studies in vitro[163, 180] and clinical experience establish its extreme sensitivity to penicillin as well as to other antibiotics. Resistance to penicillin may be encountered with *C. tertium, C. ramosum*, and *C. sporogenes*, and infections with these organisms should be treated with other antibiotics, according to their sensitivity.

TABLE 222–4 ■ Susceptibility (%) of Clostridial Species to Antimicrobial Agents

ANTIMICROBIAL DRUG (μg/mL)	C. PERFRINGENS	C. DIFFICILE	C. SEPTICUM	C. BOTULINUM	C. RAMOSUM	C. BIFERMENTANS
Penicillin (1)	93	92	100	95	49	100
Metronidazole (4)	73	99	100	100	50	—
Clindamycin (4)	99	77	100	94	30	100
Cephalothin (16)	100	49	100	98	—	—
Cefoxitin (16)	100	15	100	99	—	—
Cefotaxime (16)	—	—	100	—	—	—
Imipenem (4)	100	0	—	—	—	—
Vancomycin (4)	—	99	100	88	49	—
Chloramphenicol (16)	99	93	100	100	100	100

Data from references 156–163.

References

1. Smith LD, Williams BL: The Pathogenic Anaerobic Bacteria, ed 3. Springfield, IL, Charles C Thomas, 1984.
2. Hatheway CL: Toxigenic clostridia. Clin Microbiol Rev 3:66, 1990.
3. Gorbach SL, Thadepalli H: Isolation of *Clostridium* in human infections: Evaluation of 114 cases. J Infect Dis 131:S81, 1975.
4. Finegold SM: Anaerobic Bacteria in Human Disease. New York, Academic Press, 1977.
5. MacLennan JD: The histotoxic clostridial infections of man. Bacteriol Rev 26:177, 1962.
6. Cato EP, George WL, Finegold SM: Genus *Clostridium* Prazmowski 1880, 23. *In* Sneath PHA, Mair NS, Sharpe ME, Holt JG (eds): Bergey's Manual of Systematic Bacteriology, Vol 2. Baltimore, Williams & Wilkins, 1986, pp 1141–1200.
7. Smith LDS, Gardner VM: Vegetative cells of *Clostridium perfringens* in soil. J Bacteriol 58:407, 1949.
8. Beerens H, Delcourte F: Caractère différential entre *Clostridium perfringens* fécal et tellurique. Ann Inst Pasteur 195:739, 1958.
9. Finegold SM, Attebery HR, Sutter VL: Effect of diet on human fecal flora: Comparison of Japanese and American diets. Am J Clin Nutr 27:1456, 1974.
10. Stringer MF, Watson GN, Gilbert RJ, et al: Fecal carriage of *Clostridium perfringens*. J Hyg 95:277, 1985.
11. Gorbach SL, Menda KB, Thadepalli H, Keith L: Anaerobic microflora of the cervix in healthy women. Am J Obstet Gynecol 117:1053, 1973.
12. Ohm MJ, Galask RP: The effect of antibiotic prophylaxis on patients undergoing vaginal operations. Am J Obstet Gynecol 123:597, 1975.
13. Bartlett JG, Onderdonk AB, Drude E, et al: Quantitative bacteriology of the vaginal flora. J Infect Dis 136:271, 1977.
14. Holtz F, Mauch EW: Gas gangrene of uterus. Survival following hysterectomy. Obstet Gynecol 19:545, 1962.
15. Martin WJ: Isolation and identification of anaerobic bacteria in the clinical laboratory. A 2-year experience. Mayo Clin Proc 49:300, 1974.
16. Finegold SM, George WL, Mulligan ME: Anaerobic infections. Dis Mon 31:10, 1985.
17. Titball RW: Bacterial phospholipases C. Microbiol Rev 57:347, 1993.
18. Basak AK, Stuart DI, Nikura T, et al: Purification, crystallization and preliminary X-ray diffraction studies of alpha-toxin of *Clostridium perfringens*. J Mol Biol 244:648, 1994.
19. Titball RW, Fearn AM, Williamson ED: Biochemical and immunological properties of the C-terminal domain of the alpha-toxin of *Clostridium perfringens*. FEMS Microbiol Lett 110:45, 1993.
20. Williamson ED, Titball RW: A genetically engineered vaccine against the alpha-toxin of *Clostridium perfringens* protects mice against experimental gas gangrene. Vaccine 11:1253, 1993.
21. Awad MM, Bryant AE, Stevens DL, Rood JI: Virulence studies on chromosomal alpha-toxin and theta-toxin mutants constructed by allelic exchange provide genetic evidence for the essential role of alpha-toxin in *Clostridium perfringens*–mediated gas gangrene. Mol Microbiol 15:191, 1995.
22. Zeissler J, Rassfeld-Sternberg L: Enteritis necroticans due to *Clostridium welchii* type F. Br Med J 1:267, 1949.
23. Murrell TCG, Egerton JR, Rampling A, et al: The ecology and epidemiology of the pig bel syndrome in New Guinea. J Hyg 64:375, 1966.
24. MacLennan JD: Anaerobic infections of war wounds in the Middle East. Lancet 2:94, 1943.
25. Bernheimer AW: Parallelism in the lethal and hemolytic activity of the toxin of *Cl. septicum*. J Exp Med 80:309, 1944.
26. Moussa RS: Complexity of toxins from *Clostridium septicum* and *Clostridium chauvoei*. J Bacteriol 76:538, 1958.
27. Thadepalli H, Gorbach SL, Broido PW, et al: Abdominal trauma, anaerobes, and antibiotics. Surg Gynecol Obstet 137:270, 1973.
28. Nichols RL, Smith JW: Gas in the wound: What does it mean? Surg Clin North Am 55:1289, 1975.
29. Ram MD, Ghavari MA: Biliary infections and the choice of antibiotics. Am J Gastroenterol 62:134, 1974.
30. Mentzer RM Jr, Golden GT, Chandler JG, et al: Emphysematous cholecystitis: An important clinical variant of acute cholecystitis. Rev Surg 31:454, 1974.
31. Stephenson SE Jr, Yasrebi H, Rhatigan R, et al: Acute phlegmasia of the stomach. Am Surg 36:225, 1970.
32. Lazurus JA: *Bacillus welchii* infections complicating surgical procedures upon the upper urinary tract. J Urol 51:315, 1944.
33. Greene MH: Emphysematous cystitis due to *Clostridium perfringens* and *Candida albicans* in two patients with hematologic malignant conditions. Cancer 70:2658, 1992.
34. Katz DS, Aksoy E, Cunha BA: *Clostridium perfringens* emphysematous cystitis. Urology 41:458, 1993.
35. Bessman AN, Wagner W: Nonclostridial gas gangrene: Report of 48 cases and review of the literature. JAMA 182:23, 1962.
36. Gorbach SL, Thadepalli H, Norsen J: Anaerobic microorganisms in intraabdominal infections. *In* Balows A, DeHann RM, Dowell VR Jr, Guze LB (eds): Anaerobic Bacteria: Role in Disease. Springfield, IL, Charles C Thomas, 1974, pp 399–407.
37. Dunn DL, Simmons RL: The role of anaerobic bacteria in intraabdominal infections. Rev Infect Dis 6:S139, 1984.
38. Moore WEC, Cato EP, Holdeman LV: Anaerobic bacteria of the gastrointestinal flora and their occurrence in clinical infections. J Infect Dis 119:641, 1969.
39. Stone HH, Kolb LD, Geheber CE: Incidence and significance of intraperitoneal anaerobic bacteria. Ann Surg 181:705, 1975.
40. Gordon-Taylor G, Whitby LEK: The incidence of anaerobic infections in the gallbladder. Br J Surg 19:619, 1932.
41. England DM, Rosenblatt JE: Anaerobes in human biliary tract. J Clin Microbiol 6:494, 1977.
42. Lykkegaard NM, Justesen T: Anaerobic and aerobic bacteriological studies in biliary tract disease. Scand J Gastroenterol 11:437, 1976.
43. Shimada K, Inamatsu R, Yamashiro M: Anaerobic bacteria in biliary disease in elderly patients. J Infect Dis 135:850, 1977.
44. Sarmiento RV: Emphysematous cholecystitis: Report of four cases and review of the literature. Arch Surg 93:1099, 1966.
45. Edinburgh A, Geffen A: Acute emphysematous cholecystitis. Am J Surg 96:66, 1958.
46. Mentzer RM Jr, Golden GT, Chandler JG, et al: A comparative appraisal of emphysematous cholecystitis. Am J Surg 129:11, 1975.
47. Hegner CF: Gaseous pericholecystitis with cholecystitis and cholelithiasis. Arch Surg 22:993, 1931.
48. Thadepalli H, Gorbach SL, Keith L: Anaerobic infections of the female genital tract: Bacteriologic and therapeutic aspects. Am J Obstet Gynecol 117:103, 1973.
49. Swenson RM, Michaelson TC, Daly MJ, et al: Anaerobic bacterial infections of the female genital tract. Obstet Gynecol 42:538, 1973.
50. DiZerega GS, Yonekura ML, Keegan K, et al: Bacteremia in postcesarean section endomyometritis: Differential response to therapy. Obstet Gynecol 55:587, 1980.
51. Sweet RL: Anaerobic infections of the female genital tract. Am J Obstet Gynecol 122:891, 1975.
52. Ledger WJ, Norman M, Gee C, et al: Bacteremia on an obstetric-gynecologic service. Am J Obstet Gynecol 121:205, 1975.
53. Ramsay AM: The significance of *Clostridium welchii* in the cervical swab and blood stream in postpartum and postabortum sepsis. J Obstet Gynaecol Br Commonw 56:247, 1949.
54. Dylewski J, Wiesenfeld H, Latour A: Postpartum uterine infection with *Clostridium perfringens*. Rev Infect Dis 11:470, 1989.
55. Bartlett JG: Anaerobic bacterial infections of the lung. Chest 91:901, 1987.
56. Bayer AS, Nelson SC, Galpin JE, et al: Necrotizing pneumonia and empyema due to *Clostridium perfringens*. Am J Med 59:851, 1975.
57. O'Donnell AE: Primary clostridial pneumonia—Report of a case. Lancet 2:367, 1952.
58. Sweeting J, Rosenberg L: Primary clostridial pneumonia. Ann Intern Med 151:805, 1959.
59. Jacox R: A case report of an unusual lung abscess due to *Clostridium perfringens (B. welchii)*. Ann Intern Med 34:479, 1951.
60. Glaser LF, Glynn R, Ernest HB: Gas bacillus gangrene of lung. JAMA 116:827, 1941.
61. Goldberg NM, Rifkind D: Clostridial empyema. Arch Intern Med 116:421, 1941.
62. Mamborg AS, Rylander M, Selander H: Primary thoracic empyema caused by *Clostridium sporogenes*. Scand J Infect Dis 2:155, 1970.
63. Hardison JE: Primary clostridial pneumonia and empyema. Chest 57:390, 1970.

64. Elliot TR, Henry H: Infections of hemothorax by anaerobic gas-producing bacilli. Br Med J 1:413, 1917.
65. Lynch JF, Strieder J: Hemothorax complicated by infection with *Clostridium welchii*. N Engl J Med 226:685, 1942.
66. Cairns H, Calbert CA, Daniel P, et al: Complications of head wounds with special reference to infection. Br J Surg (War Surg Suppl):198, 1947.
67. Keogh AJ: Clostridial brain abscess and hyperbaric oxygen. Postgrad Med J 49:64, 1973.
68. Russell JA, Taylor JC: Circumscribed gas gangrene abscess of the brain. Case report together with an account of the literature. Br J Surg 50:434, 1963.
69. Clark PR: Gas gangrene abscess of the brain. J Neurol Neurosurg Psychiatry 31:391, 1958.
70. Gilbert AI, Tolmach RS, Farrell JJ: Gas gangrene of the brain. Am J Surg 101:366, 1961.
71. Colwell FG, Sullivan J, Shuman HH, et al: Acute purulent meningitis due to *Clostridium perfringens*. N Engl J Med 262:618, 1960.
72. Heidemann SM, Meert KL, Perrin E, Sarnaik AP: Primary clostridial meningitis in infancy. Pediatr Infect Dis J 8:126, 1989.
73. Kolander SA, Cosgrove EM, Molavi A: Clostridial endocarditis. Report of a case caused by *Clostridium bifermentans* and review of the literature. Arch Intern Med 149:455, 1989.
74. Ridgway EJ, Grech ED: Clostridial endocarditis: Report of a case caused by *Clostridium septicum* and review of the literature. J Infect 26:309, 1993.
75. Fauser DJ, Zuckerman JD: Clostridial septic arthritis: Case report and review of the literature. Arthritis Rheum 31:295, 1988.
76. Wilde AH, Sweeney RS, Borden LS: Hematogenously acquired infection of a total knee arthroplasty by *Clostridium perfringens*. Clin Orthop 229:228, 1988.
77. Stern SH, Sculco TP: *Clostridium perfringens* infection in a total knee arthroplasty. A case report. J Arthroplasty 3(Suppl):S37, 1988.
78. George WL: Other infections of skin, soft tissue, and muscle. *In* Finegold SM, George WL (eds): Anaerobic Infections in Humans. San Diego, CA, Academic Press, 1989, pp 485–506.
79. Murrell TGC: Enteritis necroticans. *In* Finegold SM, George LW (eds): Anaerobic Infections in Humans. San Diego, CA, Academic Press, 1989, pp 639–659.
80. Johnson S, Escheverria P, Taylor DN, et al: Enteritis necroticans among Khmer children at an evacuation site in Thailand. Lancet 2:496, 1987.
81. Smith D: Mortality from pig-bel (enteritis necroticans) in children in Tari 1971 to 1976. Papua New Guinea Med J 22:24, 1979.
82. Millar JS, Smellie S: Antecedent nutritional status of children with enteritis necroticans. *In* MW Davis (ed): Pig Bel—Necrotizing Enteritis in Papua New Guinea. Goroka, Papua New Guinea Institute of Medical Research, 1984, pp 47–49.
83. Cooke R: The pathology of pig bel. Papua New Guinea Med J 22:35, 1979.
84. Murrell TGC, Walker PD: Pig bel—A zoonosis? J Trop Med Hyg 81:231, 1978.
85. Lawrence G: Necrotizing enteritis and *Clostridium perfringens*. J Infect Dis 153:803, 1986.
86. Lawrence G, Cooke R: Experimental pigbel: The production and pathology of necrotizing enteritis due to *Clostridium welchii* type C in the guinea pig. Br J Exp Pathol 61:261, 1980.
87. Lawrence G, Shann F, Freestone DS, Walker PD: Prevention of necrotising enteritis in Papua New Guinea by active immunisation. Lancet 1:227, 1979.
88. MacDonald KL, Griffin PM: Foodborne disease outbreaks, annual summary, 1982. MMWR 35:7SS, 1985.
89. Johnson CC: *Clostridium perfringens* food poisoning. *In* Finegold SM, George WL (eds): Anaerobic Infections in Humans. San Diego, CA, Academic Press, 1989, pp 629–638.
90. Hatheway CL, Whaley DN, Dowell VR Jr: Epidemiological aspects of *Clostridium perfringens* foodborne illness. Food Technol 34:77, 90, 1980.
91. Shandera WX, Tacker CO, Blake PA: Food poisoning due to *Clostridium perfringens* in the United States. J Infect Dis 147:167, 1983.
92. Regan CM, Syed Q, Tunstall PJ: A hospital outbreak of *Clostridium perfringens* food poisoning—Implications for food hygiene review in hospitals. J Hosp Infect 29:69, 1995.
93. Hall HE, Angelotti R: *Clostridium perfringens* in meat and meat products. Appl Microbiol 13:353, 1965.
94. Hobbs BC: *Clostridium welchii* and *Bacillus cereus* infection and intoxication. Postgrad Med J 50:597, 1974.
95. Dische FE, Elek SD: Experimental food poisoning by *Clostridium welchii*. Lancet 2:71, 1957.
96. Hauschild AHW, Thatcher FS: Experimental food poisoning with heat-susceptible *Clostridium perfringens* type A. J Food Sci 32:467, 1967.
97. Goldner SB, Solberg M, Jones S, Post LS: Enterotoxin synthesis by nonsporulating cultures of *Clostridium perfringens*. Appl Environ Microbiol 52:407, 1986.
98. Uemura T: Incidence of enterogenic *Clostridium perfringens* in healthy humans in relation to the enhancement of enterotoxin production by heat treatment. J Appl Bacteriol 44:411, 1978.
99. Stark RL, Duncan CL: Biological characteristics of *Clostridium perfringens* type A enterotoxin. Infect Immun 4:89, 1971.
100. McDonel JL, Duncan CL: Regional localization of activity of *Clostridium perfringens* type A enterotoxin in the rabbit ileum, jejunum and duodenum. J Infect Dis 136:661, 1977.
101. Niilo L: Measurement of biological activities of purified and crude enterotoxin of *Clostridium perfringens*. Infect Immun 12:440, 1975.
102. Granum PE, Skjelkvale R: Chemical modification and characterization of enterotoxin from *Clostridium perfringens* type A. Acta Pathol Microbiol Scand 95:89, 1977.
103. McDonel JL, McClane BA: Binding versus biologic activity of *Clostridium perfringens* enterotoxin in Vero cells. Biochem Biophys Res Commun 87:497, 1979.
104. McClane BA: *Clostridium perfringens* enterotoxin acts by producing small molecule permeability alterations in plasma membranes. Toxicology 87:43, 1994.
105. McDonel JL: Binding of *Clostridium perfringens* enterotoxin to rabbit intestinal cells. Biochemistry 21:4801, 1980.
106. McClane BA, McDonel JL: The effects of *Clostridium perfringens* enterotoxin on morphology, viability and macromolecular synthesis in Vero cells. J Cell Physiol 99:191, 1979.
107. McClane BA, Hanna PC, Wnek AP: *Clostridium perfringens* enterotoxin. Microb Pathog 5:317, 1988.
108. Finegold SM: Anaerobic Bacteria in Human Disease. New York, Academic Press, 1977, pp 511–512.
109. Skjelkvale R, Uemura R: Experimental diarrhoea in human volunteers following oral administration of *Clostridium perfringens* enterotoxin. J Appl Bacteriol 43:281, 1977.
110. Hauschild AHW: Criteria and procedures for implicating *Clostridium perfringens* in foodborne outbreaks. Can J Public Health 66:388, 1975.
111. Birkhead G, Vogt RL, Heum EM, et al: Characterization of an outbreak of *Clostridium perfringens* food poisoning by quantitative fecal culture and fecal enterotoxin measurement. J Clin Microbiol 26:471, 1988.
112. Gross TP, Kamara LB, Hathaway CL, et al: *Clostridium perfringens* food poisoning: Use of serotyping in an outbreak setting. J Clin Microbiol 4:660, 1989.
113. Eisgruber H, Wiedmann M, Stolle A: Use of plasmid profiling as a typing method for epidemiologically related *Clostridium perfringens* isolates from food poisoning cases and outbreaks. Lett Appl Microbiol 20:290, 1995.
114. McClane BA, Strouse RJ: Rapid detection of *Clostridium perfringens* type A enterotoxin by enzyme-linked immunosorbent assay. J Clin Microbiol 19:112, 1984.
115. Larson HE, Borriello SP: Infectious diarrhea due to *Clostridium perfringens*. J Infect Dis 157:390, 1988.
116. Harmon SM, Kautter DA: Evaluation of a reverse passive latex agglutination test kit for *Clostridium perfringens* enterotoxin. J Food Prot 49:523, 1986.
117. Harmon SM, Kautter DA: Evaluation of reverse passive latex agglutination test kit for *Clostridium perfringens*. J Food Prot 49:523, 1986.
118. Borriello SP, Larson HE, Welch AR, et al: Enterotoxigenic *Clostridium perfringens*: A possible cause of antibiotic-associated diarrhoea. Lancet 1:305, 1984.
119. Jackson SG, Yip-Chuck DA, Clark JB, et al: Diagnostic importance of *Clostridium perfringens* enterotoxin analysis in recurring enteritis among elderly chronic care psychiatric patients. J Clin Microbiol 49:523, 1986.
120. Luzzi I, Caprioli A, Bisicchia R, et al: A sporadic case of diarrhoea due to enterotoxigenic *Clostridium perfringens*. Microbiol Ecol Health Dis 1:69, 1988.

121. Decker WH, Hall W: Treatment of abortion infected with *Clostridium welchii*. Am J Obstet Gynecol 95:394, 1966.
122. Smith LP, McLean AP, Maughan GB: *Clostridium welchii* septicotoxemia. Am J Obstet Gynecol 110:135, 1971.
123. Pritchard JA, Whalley PJ: Abortion complicated by *Clostridium perfringens* infection. Am J Obstet Gynecol 111:484, 1971.
124. Chu DZ, Fainstein V, Bodey GP, et al: Necrotizing gas-forming infections in cancer patients. South Med J 82:860, 1989.
125. Tanable KK, Jones WG, Barie PS: Clostridial sepsis and malignant disease. Surg Gynecol Obstet 169:423, 1989.
126. Lombardi DP, Engleberg NC: Anaerobic bacteremia: Incidence, patient characteristics, and clinical significance [see comments]. Am J Med 92:53, 1992.
127. Cabrera A, Tsukada Y, Pickren JW: Clostridial gas gangrene and septicemia in malignant disease. Cancer 18:800, 1965.
128. Burrell MI, Hyson EA, Walker-Smith GI: Spontaneous clostridial infection and malignancy. AJR 134:1153, 1980.
129. Thys JP, Ectors P, Noel P: Nontraumatic clostridial myositis. An unusual feature of brain death. Postgrad Med J 56:501, 1980.
130. Kaiser CW, Milgrom ML, Lynch JA: Distant nontraumatic clostridial myonecrosis and malignancy. Cancer 57:885, 1986.
131. Mzabi R, Himal HS, MacLean LD: Gas gangrene of the extremity: The presenting clinical picture in perforating carcinoma of the caecum. Br J Surg 62:373, 1975.
132. Jones LE, Wirth WA, Farrow CC: Clostridial gas gangrene and septicemia complicating leukemia. South Med J 53:863, 1960.
133. Epidemiological Research Laboratory of the Public Health Service: *Clostridium welchii* from blood culture. Br Med J 1:845, 1976.
134. Draser BS, Goddard P, Heaton S, et al: Clostridia isolated from faeces. J Med Microbiol 9:63, 1976.
135. Moore WEC, Holdeman LV: Human fecal flora: The normal flora of 20 Japanese-Hawaiians. Appl Microbiol 27:961, 1974.
136. Holdeman LV, Good IJ, Moore WEC: Human fecal flora: Variations in bacterial composition with individuals and a possible effect of emotional stress. Appl Environ Microbiol 31:359, 1974.
137. Borriello SP: Newly described clostridial diseases of the gastrointestinal tract: *Clostridium perfringens* enterotoxin–associated diarrhea and neutropenic enterocolitis due to *Clostridium septicum*. *In* Borriello SP (ed): Clostridia in Gastrointestinal Disease. Boca Raton, FL, CRC Press, 1985, pp 223–229.
138. Kornbluth AA, Danzig JB, Bernstein LH: *Clostridium septicum* infection and associated malignancy. Medicine (Baltimore) 68:30, 1989.
139. Alpern RJ, Dowell VR: *Clostridium septicum* infections and malignancy. JAMA 209:385, 1969.
140. Wilson WR, Martin WJ, Wilkowske CJ, Washington JA: Anaerobic bacteremia. Mayo Clin Proc 47:639, 1972.
141. Lewis JF, Mullins N, Johnson P: Isolation and evaluation of clostridia from clinical sources. South Med J 73:427, 1980.
142. Gazzaniga AB: Nontraumatic, clostridial gas gangrene of the right arm and adenocarcinoma of the cecum: Report of a case. Dis Colon Rectum 10:298, 1967.
143. Graham BS, Johnson AC, Sawyers JL: Clostridial infection of renal cell carcinoma. J Urol 135:354, 1986.
144. Bretzke ML, Bubrick MP, Hitchcock CR: Diffuse spreading *Clostridium septicum* infections, malignant disease and immune suppression. Surg Gynecol Obstet 166:197, 1988.
145. Lev R, Sweeney KG: Neutropenic enterocolitis. Two unusual cases with review of the literature. Arch Pathol Lab Med 117:524, 1993.
146. Amromin GD, Solomon RD: Necrotizing enteropathy: A complication of treated leukemia or lymphoma patients. JAMA 182:23, 1962.
147. Prolla JC, Kirsner JB: The gastrointestinal lesion and complication of the leukemias. Ann Intern Med 61:1084, 1964.
148. Moir DH, Bale PM: Necropsy findings in childhood leukemia emphasizing neutropenic colitis and cerebral calcification. Pathology 8:247, 1976.
149. Dosik GM, Luna M, Valdivieso M, et al: Necrotizing colitis in patients with cancer. Am J Med 67:646, 1979.
150. Caya JG, Farmer SG, Ritch PS, et al: Clostridial septicemia complicating the course of leukemia. Cancer 57:2045, 1986.
151. Koransky JR, Stargel MD, Dowell VR: *Clostridium septicum* bacteremia: Its clinical significance. Am J Med 66:63, 1979.
152. Louie TJ, Bartlett JG, Tally FB, Gorbach SL: Aerobic and anaerobic bacteria in diabetic foot ulcers. Ann Intern Med 85:461, 1976.
153. Thaler M, Gill V, Pizzo PA: Emergence of *Clostridium tertium* as a pathogen in neutropenic patients. Am J Med 81:596, 1986.
154. Spiers G, Warren RE, Rampling A: *Clostridium tertium* septicemia in patients with neutropenia. J Infect Dis 158:1336, 1988.
155. Valtonen M, Sivonen A, Elonen E: A cluster of seven cases of *Clostridium tertium* septicemia in neutropenic patients. Eur J Clin Microbiol Infect Dis 9:40, 1990.
156. Tally FP, Armfield AY, Dowell VR, et al: Susceptibility of *Clostridium ramosum* to antimicrobial agents. Antimicrob Agents Chemother 5:589, 1974.
157. Sutter VL, Finegold SM: Susceptibility of anaerobic bacteria to 23 antimicrobial agents. Antimicrob Agents Chemother 10:736, 1976.
158. Scheartzman JD, Reller LB, Wang WL: Susceptibility of *Clostridium perfringens* isolated from human infections to twenty antibiotics. Antimicrob Agents Chemother 11:695, 1977.
159. Applebaum PC, Chatterton SA: Susceptibility of anaerobic bacteria to ten antimicrobial agents. Antimicrob Agents Chemother 14:271, 1978.
160. Brown WJ, Waatti PE: Susceptibility testing of clinically isolated anaerobic bacteria by an agar dilution technique. Antimicrob Agents Chemother 17:629, 1980.
161. Dzink J, Bartlett JG: In vitro susceptibility of *Clostridium difficile* isolates from patients with antibiotic-associated diarrhea or colitis. Antimicrob Agents Chemother 17:695, 1980.
162. Swenson JM, Thornsberry C, McCroskey LM, et al: Susceptibility of *Clostridium botulinum* to thirteen antimicrobial agents. Antimicrob Agents Chemother 18:13, 1980.
163. Gabey EL, Rolfe RD, Finegold SM: Susceptibility of *Clostridium septicum* to 23 antimicrobial agents. Antimicrob Agents Chemother 20:852, 1981.
164. Nord CE, Hedberg M: Clinical infections and treatment. Resistance to β-lactam antibiotics in anaerobic bacteria. Rev Infect Dis 12(Suppl 2):S231, 1990.
165. Blandino G, Olsson-Liljequist B, Nord CE: Characterization of β-lactamase from *Clostridium butyricum*. Chemioterapia 2:95, 1983.
166. Hart CA, Barr K, Makin T, et al: Characteristics of a β-lactamase produced by *Clostridium butyricum*. J Antimicrob Chemother 10:31, 1982.
167. Magot M: Some properties of the *Clostridium butyricum* group β-lactamase. J Gen Microbiol 127:113, 1981.
168. Weinrich AE, Del Bene VE: β-Lactamase activity in anaerobic bacteria. Antimicrob Agents Chemother 10:106, 1976.
169. Matthew M: Plasmid-mediated β-lactamases of gram-negative bacteria: Properties and distribution. J Antimicrob Chemother 5:349, 1979.
170. Murphy TF, Barza M, Park JT: Penicillin-binding proteins in *Clostridium perfringens*. Antimicrob Agents Chemother 20:809, 1981.
171. Williamson R: Resistance of *Clostridium perfringens* to β-lactam antibiotics mediated by a decreased affinity of a single essential penicillin-binding protein. J Gen Microbiol 129:2339, 1983.
172. Stevens DL, Maier KA, Laine BM, Mitten JE: Comparison of clindamycin, rifampin, tetracycline, metronidazole, and penicillin for efficacy in prevention of experimental gas gangrene due to *Clostridium perfringens*. J Infect Dis 155:220, 1987.
173. Stevens DL, Maier KA, Mitten JE: Effect of antibiotics on toxin production and viability of *Clostridium perfringens*. Antimicrob Agents Chemother 31:213, 1987.
174. Altemeier WA, Furste WL: Gas gangrene. Surg Gynecol Obstet 84:507, 1947.
175. Altemeier WA, McMurrin JA, Alt AP: Chloromycetin and aureomycin in experimental gas gangrene. Surgery 28:621, 1950.
176. Altemeier WA, Fullen WD: Prevention and treatment of gas gangrene. JAMA 217:806, 1971.
177. Knight RJ: Reception and resuscitation of casualties in South Vietnam. Experience at the first Australian Field Hospital. Lancet 2:29, 1972.
178. Darke SG, King AM, Slack WK: Gas gangrene and related infection: Classification, clinical features and aetiology, management and mortality. A report of 88 cases. Br J Surg 64:104, 1977.
179. Weinstein L, Barza MA: Gas gangrene. N Engl J Med 289:1129, 1973.
180. Brazier JS, Levett PN, Stannard AJ, et al: Antibiotic susceptibility of clinical isolates of clostridia. J Antimicrob Chemother 15:181, 1985.

SPIROCHETES

223

Treponemes: Microbiology

Robert E. Baughn
Daniel M. Musher

The treponemes within the order Spirochaetales compose one of the four genera of the family Spirochaetaceae; two species, *Treponema pallidum* and *Treponema carateum*, are known to be pathogenic for humans. By known morphologic, chemical, and immunochemical methods, *T. pallidum* subsp. *pallidum*, the agent of syphilis, is indistinguishable from *T. carateum*, which causes pinta, and the other two *T. pallidum* subspecies, *T. pallidum* subsp. *pertenue*, the etiologic agent of yaws, and *T. pallidum* subsp. *endemicum*, the etiologic agent of endemic syphilis.[1, 2] *Treponema paraluiscuniculi*, which infects lagomorphs, morphologically resembles the other species, although it has not been subjected to extensive DNA hybridization studies.[3] *T. pallidum* subsp. *pallidum* shares less than 5% DNA homology with the avirulent species *Treponema phagedenis* and *Treponema refringens* and with *Serpulina hyodysenteriae* (formerly *Treponema hyodysenteriae*).

Structure

T. pallidum, being 10 to 13 μm long but only 0.15 μm wide, is below the limits of resolution of light microscopy. These organisms can be observed with use of a darkfield microscope, which is important in clinical practice; they are seen under these conditions to be helical and to have a characteristic pattern of motility. By electron microscopy,[4] organisms appear wavelike ("wavelength" of 1.1 μm, "amplitude" of 0.2 to 0.3 μm). The two ends of the organism are identical. *T. pallidum* organisms have outer and cytoplasmic membranes, an electron-dense peptidoglycan layer, and periplasmic flagella (endoflagella). The flagellar filament, which consists of a sheath and core structure, is assumed to play a role in locomotion, although its location within the outer membrane and the failure of antiflagellar antibodies to immobilize certain culturable spirochetes raise questions about this assumption. The outer membrane includes a number of different proteins that have been characterized by polyacrylamide gel electrophoresis,[5] and many have been shown to participate in immune responses to infection.[6] In vivo, *T. pallidum* may surround itself with an amorphous outer layer, perhaps resulting from production of mucopolysaccharides.[7]

The inability to readily propagate this organism in vitro has hindered study of the metabolism and the antigenic composition of T. *pallidum* and has also made it difficult to examine components that cause tissue damage, dose-response relationships, and induction of immunity. Limited replication has been observed in vitro in the presence of mammalian cells at 34°C to 35°C with 3% to 5% oxygen and 5% carbon dioxide[8]; under these conditions, treponemal replication time is similar to that reported in vivo, about 30 hours. *T. pallidum* metabolizes glucose and pyruvate aerobically, has a cytochrome system, and has superoxide dismutase and catalase activity.[9]

Animal Models

Animal models for the study of syphilis have been a problem.[1] Rabbits develop chancres at sites of intradermal injection and develop widespread cutaneous lesions after intravenous injection, provided that their fur is shaved. A limited form of infection characterized by a transient rash appears analogous to secondary infection. Hamsters and guinea pigs develop atypical lesions at injection sites, and infection may also be produced in mice, but only after vigorous immunosuppression. In discussing the pathogenesis of syphilis, it is generally assumed that there is no essential difference between experimentally induced infection in rabbits and naturally acquired infection in humans, at least in the early, active phase of infection. There is no known parallel in rabbits or in any other animal, including subhuman primates, for any of the forms of tertiary syphilis. (The evolution of syphilitic infection and its various stages are discussed in Chapter 112.)

Virulence Factors

T. pallidum probably does not have the ability to penetrate unbroken skin, despite the conjecture that its rotatory motion enables it to do so. Rather, implantation of treponemes subcutaneously (intradermally) is thought to occur at sites of macroscopically invisible abrasions in the skin. Intradermal injection of 50 to 100 organisms produces a syphilitic chancre in rabbits. The dividing time is said to be 24 to 30 hours[10]; thus, these slowly replicating organisms have the capability to resist normal host defense mechanisms, although the basis for this resistance is not known. *T. pallidum* does not have a capsule and produces no recognized toxins that might repel or damage polymorphonuclear leukocytes. Nevertheless, replication occurs and some organisms escape the local area, leading to spread through lymphatics or the blood stream.

Viable *T. pallidum* organisms attach by one or both ends to mammalian cells in vitro, although they rarely if ever penetrate these cells.[11] Adherence can be inhibited by antitreponemal antibody. A specialized receptor site on the end of the treponeme has not been documented by electron microscopy. Some studies have suggested that adherent *T. pallidum* organisms damage tissues[12] despite the absence of recognized toxins or lipopolysaccharide (endotoxin).

Host Defense Mechanisms

Local Responses

Once treponemes find their way into dermal sites, normal serum constituents may have an antitreponemal effect,[13] perhaps resulting from antigenic cross-reactivity between *T. pallidum* and other gram-negative nonpathogenic treponemes that colonize the alimentary tract. The complement cascade is triggered by *T. pallidum*, although the interaction with components of the membrane attack complex (C5b,6,7,8,9) has not been studied. Normal human serum has been shown to exert low-grade treponemicidal activity in vitro.[14] As is the case with many other infections, factors that govern natural resistance of certain species to syphilis are not known. Serum bactericidal activity does not appear to be an important contributing factor to the ability of mice or guinea pigs to resist infection, and a variety of other factors, ranging from the role of natural killer cells to the availability of receptor sites on host cells, need to be considered.

The first cells attracted to an area of invasion by *T. pallidum* are polymorphonuclear leukocytes.[15] Incubation of polymorphonuclear leukocytes with *T. pallidum* stimulates a chemoluminescent response that is rapidly followed by phagocytosis, as documented by the electron microscopic finding of treponemes within phagocytic vacuoles. Phagocytosis of *T. pallidum* without additional opsonization is consistent with the presence of host immunoglobulin G (the only way to obtain these organisms is to extract them from infected mammalian tissue) and perhaps complement on the surface of the organism. In light of these observations, it remains unclear why inoculation with a small number of organisms so regularly causes disease.

Within a few days of an injection of a large inoculum of *T. pallidum,* T lymphocytes accumulate[16]; in natural transmission, this tissue reaction occurs more slowly, but it presumably follows the same pattern. Lymphocytes predominate, but macrophages and occasional polymorphonuclear leukocytes are also noted. B lymphocytes that contain surface antibody to *T. pallidum* may also be attracted to the infected area. The primary site of inoculation contains mucoid material consisting mainly of hyaluronic acid and chondroitin sulfate; the exact origin and properties of this substance are not fully understood, but some authorities believe that it may modulate or alter immune responses. The syphilitic chancre, the initial lesion that arises at a site of treponemal infection, thus contains a mucoid center and is surrounded by a cellular infiltrate that is chiefly lymphocytic; infiltrating cells are found most prominently in a perivascular location.

Cell-Mediated Immunity

Syphilitic infection also induces cell-mediated immunity. A line of sensitized thymus-dependent lymphocytes appears in primary syphilitic lesions,[16] and generalized activation of macrophages has been demonstrated on the basis of enhanced ability to ingest and kill *Listeria monocytogenes*.[17] An initial treponeme-macrophage interaction presumably allows processing of antigens, followed by proliferation of a clone of T lymphocytes, which in the presence of treponemal antigen produce lymphokines that attract or activate macrophages. Activated macrophages have been shown to ingest *T. pallidum* in vitro in the presence of exogenous antibody.[18] Ingestion in vivo has also been said to occur,[19] correlating with a decline in the number of detectable treponemal forms and demonstration of degenerating treponemes in phagocytic vacuoles. It is not certain whether killing by macrophages or ingestion of damaged treponemal forms is responsible. The antigens involved in the sensitization reaction have not been identified.

Humoral Responses

SPECIFIC TREPONEMAL ANTIBODIES

That *T. pallidum* infection stimulates a vigorous cell response may be inferred from the variety of antibodies present in the serum of most patients by the time they seek medical attention for a syphilitic chancre. Antibodies directed against treponemal antigens are detected in 90% of cases of primary syphilis by the fluorescent treponemal antibody test after absorption of serum with the nonvirulent *T. phagedenis* or by the newer *T. pallidum*–hemagglutinating antibody tests, which can be done without a fluorescence microscope. The *T. pallidum* immobilization test, which detects immobilization and inactivation of *T. pallidum* by serum antibody in vitro in the presence of exogenous complement, is now performed only by research laboratories. It is still not known whether these antibodies are directed against the same or different antigens or, in the case of the *T. pallidum* immobilization test, whether immunoglobulin G or immunoglobulin M is chiefly involved. Studies have documented the sequential emergence of immunoglobulin M and immunoglobulin G reactive with individual outer membrane proteins of *T. pallidum* during the course of syphilis.[10, 20]

NONTREPONEMAL (ANTICARDIOLIPIN) ANTIBODIES

Antibody against cardiolipin is also present in primary syphilis and is detected in about two thirds of cases by the Venereal Disease Research Laboratory (VDRL) test or the rapid plasma reagin test, which are modifications of the initial Wassermann reaction. Cardiolipin constitutes about 13% of treponemal lipids and is also present in mammalian tissue.[21] Treponemes do not synthesize this material but, rather, incorporate it from the mammalian host. An interesting and unanswered question is whether VDRL antibody is directed against human tissue cardiolipin that is altered by syphilitic infection, thus representing an autoimmune reaction, or against treponeme-incorporated mammalian lipids, normal or altered.

CIRCULATING IMMUNE COMPLEXES

Circulating complexes may be detected in some patients with primary syphilis and in the majority of those with secondary syphilis.[22] These complexes contain immunoglobulin (mainly immunoglobulin G and immunoglobulin G3), complement, and identifiable outer membrane proteins of *T. pallidum* as well as human proteins such as fibronectin and creatine kinase and antibody to these substances,[23] suggesting a further link between syphilis and autoimmune events associated with the disease.

MOLECULAR MIMICRY AND AUTOIMMUNE EVENTS

Although the significance of the various autoantibodies in the early stages of syphilis is not clear, their existence suggests that host-derived responses may be operational in disseminated infection. Epitope mapping studies of one of the organism's immunodominant lipoproteins (Tpp47)[24] suggested that molecular mimicry plays a pivotal role in triggering antifibronectin and anticollagen responses associated with disseminated syphilis. Those studies also suggested that expansion of the autoimmune responses may be due to other self-epitopes by intramolecular and intermolecular epitope spreading once tolerance is abrogated.

Evidence for Aberrant Immune Responses

A variety of aberrant immune responses have been demonstrated in syphilis, which may contribute to the unusual nature of the infection. The response of human peripheral blood lymphocytes to nontreponemal or treponemal antigens appears to be depressed during syphilis. There have been different opinions as to whether serum factors or abnormalities in the lymphocytes themselves are responsible.[25] In experimental studies in rabbits, early syphilitic infection has been shown to powerfully suppress immunoglobulin G responses to a nontreponemal T-lymphocyte–dependent antigen.[26] Immunoglobulin M responses were found to be increased. Technical problems precluded this same kind of observation with use of treponemal antigen. These findings are analogous to those in some chronic parasitic infections in which the host controls but fails to eradicate the infecting organisms. In the rabbit model, evidence suggests that resolution of acute infection may occur through a helper T cell type 1 response, whereas the persistence of a chronic infection is associated with a helper T cell type 2 response.[27]

Evolution of Infection: Immunologic Aspects

By the time the primary syphilitic chancre appears, both humoral and cell-mediated immune mechanisms have been activated. Treponeme-sensitized lymphocytes and activated macrophages are present in lesions, and antitreponemal humoral antibody is detectable in serum. The number of treponemes has begun to decrease, although extracellular organisms are still present. All these observations suggest that the infection is being controlled, especially in the case of this relatively slow-growing and nontoxigenic organism. The proof of the effectiveness of this immune response at this point would be spontaneous resolution of infection.

Secondary Syphilis

The phenomenon of secondary syphilis indicates that the host response to this unusual infection is incomplete. For reasons that are poorly understood, as the local immune process brings the primary lesion under control, generalized infection appears. Widespread, small, individual lesions are seen in naturally infected human subjects 3 to 6 weeks after the primary chancre appears. Their characteristics and timing reflect several processes: (1) hematogenous spread of treponemes throughout the body; (2) establishment of lesions in the skin, an area that may offer better growth conditions for *T. pallidum* because of reduced temperature; and (3) development of some degree of systemic immunity that modifies the appearance of these disseminated lesions. If not for this third feature, these lesions would all look like primary chancres, which is exactly what happens when previously uninfected rabbits are infected intravenously with *T. pallidum.* In rare cases of syphilis in humans, a florid form of infection (called lues maligna) resembles that which follows intravenous challenge in rabbits.

Latency

Eventually, the host suppresses the infection sufficiently so that no lesions are clinically apparent. This stage is called latency. Delayed-type hypersensitivity to *T. pallidum* is uniformly present at this time and may be important, together with humoral antibody, in finally controlling infection.[28] For example, it has not been possible to demonstrate a fully protective role for humoral immunity despite the presence of *T. pallidum* immobilization antibody, which immobilizes and inactivates *T. pallidum* in vitro. Infusion of large amounts of globulin at the time of treponemal inoculation delays the onset of lesions and attenuates them but does not prevent them from appearing.[29] Similarly, transfusing lymphocytes from syphilis-immune rabbits into normal rabbits does not transfer immunity to syphilis,[30] although immunity to *T. pallidum* (strain Bosnia A) has been transferred in hamsters by use of this same approach,[31] and there is a report that local infusion of immune lymphocytes at a site of treponemal infection provides protection.[32]

The absence of a fully immune state can be shown both clinically and experimentally. In the pretreatment era, after the host's immune response had seemingly controlled the infection (as evidenced by onset of latency), relapse of disseminated secondary lesions still occurred in up to one fourth of cases.[33] Moreover, lymph nodes from human or animal subjects can be shown to harbor infective treponemes during latency or even after seemingly adequate antibiotic therapy.[34] Finally, infection progresses to a tertiary stage, which may be due to the host's response in some manifestations but certainly reflects the presence of active treponemes in others.

Tertiary Syphilis (See Chapter 112 for Clinical Aspects)

Gummata that characterize tertiary syphilis may appear in soft tissue or viscera. These large granulomatous lesions suggest an immune response, presumably to treponemal antigens; however, treponemes demonstrated by a silver stain may have been artifactual. One report has used immunofluorescent technique to demonstrate treponemes in a single and somewhat atypical case.[35] Neurosyphilis is associated with a variety of histologic appearances; some lesions contain treponemes, others do not. Perhaps the immunologically privileged nature of the central nervous system has something to do with this.

References

1. Turner TB, Hollander DH: Biology of the treponematoses. WHO Monogr Ser 35:1, 1957.
2. Canale-Parola E: Family I. Spirochaetaceae Swellengrebel 1907, 581. *In* Krieg NR, Holt JG (eds): Bergey's Manual of Systematic Bacteriology, Vol 1. Baltimore, Williams & Wilkins, 1984, pp 39–62.
3. Miao RH, Fieldsteel AH: Genetic relationship between *Treponema pallidum* and five cultivable treponemes. J Bacteriol 133:101, 1978.
4. Hovind-Hougen K: Determination by means of electron microscopy of morphological criteria of value for classification of some spirochetes, in particular treponemes. Acta Pathol Microbiol Scand B 255(Suppl):1, 1976.
5. Norris SJ, Alderete JF, Baker-Zander SA, et al: Identity of *Treponema pallidum* polypeptides: Correlation of sodium dodecyl sulfate–polyacrylamide gel electrophoresis results from different laboratories. Electrophoresis 8:77, 1987.
6. Hanff PA, Fehniger TE, Miller JN, Lovett MA: Humoral immune response in human syphilis to polypeptides of *Treponema pallidum.* J Immunol 129:1287, 1982.
7. Fitzgerald TJ, Johnson RC, Sykes JA, et al: Relationship of *Treponema pallidum* to acidic mucopolysaccharides. Infect Immun 24:252, 1979.
8. Fieldsteel AH, Cox DL, Moeckli RA: Cultivation of virulent *Treponema pallidum* in tissue culture. Infect Immun 32:908, 1981.
9. Austin FE, Barbier JT, Corin RE, et al: Distribution of superoxide dismutase, catalase, and peroxidase activities among *Treponema pallidum* and other spirochetes. Infect Immun 33:372, 1981.
10. Cumberland MC, Turner TB: The rate of multiplication of *Treponema pallidum* in normal and immune rabbits. Am J Syphilol Gonorr Vener Dis 33:201, 1949.
11. Hayes NS, Muse KE, Collier AM, et al: Parasitism by virulent *Treponema pallidum* of host cell surfaces. Infect Immun 17:174, 1977.
12. Fitzgerald TJ, Repesh LA: Toxic activities of *Treponema pallidum.* *In* Schell RF, Musher DM (eds): Pathogenesis and Immunology of Treponemal Infection. New York, Marcel Dekker, 1982, pp 173–193.
13. Hederstedt B: Studies on the *Treponema pallidum* immobilizing activity in normal human serum: 2. Serum factors participating in the normal serum immobilization reaction. Acta Pathol Microbiol Scand C 84:135, 1976.
14. Bishop NH, Miller JN: Humoral immune mechanisms in acquired syphilis. *In* Schell RF, Musher DM (eds): Pathogenesis and Immunology of Treponemal Infections. New York, Marcel Dekker, 1982, pp 241–269.
15. Musher DM, Hague-Park M, Gyorkey F, et al: The interaction between *Treponema pallidum* and human polymorphonuclear leukocytes. J Infect Dis 147:77, 1983.
16. Baker-Zander S, Sell S: A histopathologic and immunologic study of the course of syphilis in the experimentally infected rabbit:

Demonstration of long-lasting cellular immunity. Am J Pathol 101:387, 1980.
17. Schell R, Musher DM, Jacobson K, et al: Induction of acquired cellular resistance following transfer of thymus-dependent lymphocytes from syphilitic rabbits. J Immunol 114:550, 1975.
18. Lukehart SA, Miller JN: Demonstration of the in vitro phagocytosis of *Treponema pallidum* by rabbit peritoneal macrophages. J Immunol 121:2014, 1978.
19. Hardy PH, Graham DL, Nell EE, et al: Macrophages in immunity to syphilis: Suppressive effect of concurrent infection with *Mycobacterium bovis* BCG on the development of syphilitic lesions and growth of *Treponema pallidum* in tuberculin-positive rabbits. Infect Immun 26:751, 1979.
20. Lukehart SA, Baker-Zander SA, Gubish ER: Identification of *Treponema pallidum* antigens: Comparisons with a nonpathogenic treponeme. J Immunol 129:833, 1982.
21. Matthews HM, Yang T-K, Jenkin HM: Unique lipid composition of *Treponema pallidum* (Nichols virulent strain). Infect Immun 24:713, 1979.
22. Engel S, Diezel W: Persistent serum immune complexes in syphilis. Br J Vener Dis 56:221, 1980.
23. Baughn RE, McNeeley MC, Jonzzo IL, et al: Characterization of the antigenic determinants and host components in immune complexes from patients with secondary syphilis. J Immunol 136:1406, 1986.
24. Baughn RE, Jiang A, Abraham R, et al: Molecular mimicry between an immunodominant amino acid motif on the 47-kDa lipoprotein of *Treponema pallidum* (Tpp47) and multiple repeats of analogous sequences in fibronectin. J Immunol 157:720, 1996.
25. Musher DM, Schell RF, Jones RH, et al: Lymphocyte transformation in syphilis: An in vitro correlate of immune suppression in vivo? Infect Immun 11:1261, 1975.
26. Baughn RE, Musher DM: Altered immune responsiveness associated with experimental syphilis in the rabbit: Elevated IgM and depressed IgG response to sheep erythrocytes. J Immunol 120:1691, 1978.
27. Fitzgerald TJ: The Th1/Th2-like switch in syphilitic infection. Is it detrimental? Infect Immun 60:3475, 1992.
28. Musher DM, Baughn RE: Syphilis. *In* Samter M (ed): Immunological Diseases, ed 3. Boston, Little, Brown, 1978, p 639.
29. Weiser RS, Erickson D, Perine PL, et al: Immunity to syphilis: Passive transfer in rabbits using serial doses of immune serum. Infect Immun 13:1402, 1976.
30. Baughn RE, Musher DM, Simmons CB: Inability of spleen cells from chancre-immune rabbits to confer immunity to challenge with *Treponema pallidum*. Infect Immun 17:535, 1977.
31. Schell RF, Chan JK, LeFrock IL, Bagasra O: Endemic syphilis: Transfer of resistance to *Treponema pallidum* strain Bosnia A in hamsters with cell suspension enriched in thymus-derived cells. J Infect Dis 141:752, 1980.
32. Metzger M: The role of immunologic responses in protection against syphilis. *In* Johnson RC (ed): The Biology of Parasitic Spirochetes. New York, Academic Press, 1976, pp 327–337.
33. Clark EG, Danbolt N: The Oslo study of the natural course of untreated syphilis: An epidemiologic investigation based on a re-study of the Boeck-Bruusgaard material. Med Clin North Am 48:613, 1964.
34. Yobs AR, Clark JW, Mothershed SE, et al: Further observations on persistence of *Treponema pallidum* after treatment in rabbits and humans. Br J Vener Dis 44:116, 1968.
35. Handsfield HH, Lukehart SA, Sell S, et al: Demonstration of *Treponema pallidum* in a cutaneous gumma by indirect immunofluorescence. Arch Dermatol 719:677, 1983.

224

Borrelia burgdorferi

Raymond J. Dattwyler
Benjamin J. Luft

History

In 1981, Burgdorfer and colleagues[1] isolated a new *Borrelia* species as the etiologic agent of Lyme disease. As a result of their finding, it was concluded soon thereafter that several distinct clinical syndromes described in both the European and the U.S. medical literature since the early 20th century were caused by infection with this pathogen. The newly identified spirochete was named *Borrelia burgdorferi,* in 1984, in honor of Burgdorfer's discovery. To fully appreciate the multiplicity of manifestations associated with *B. burgdorferi* infection, a historical perspective regarding the evolution of our understanding of this particular borreliosis is important.

Erythema migrans (EM), the earliest sign of Lyme borreliosis, was first appreciated by Afzelius in 1909.[2] He hypothesized that this cutaneous lesion was the result of a tick bite by which the causative agent could be transmitted to humans from an animal source. Subsequently, in 1921, Lipshitz identified an *Ixodes* tick as the vector for this disease.[3] By the 1940s, European investigators had demonstrated that EM could be associated with the subsequent development of several neurologic syndromes, including acute meningitis, meningopolyneuritis, meningoencephalitis and chronic lymphocytic meningitis, musculoskeletal complaints, and a number of dermatologic conditions, including acrodermatitis chronica atrophicans (ACA), lymphadenosis benigna cutis, and lymphocytoma.[4–9] In 1948, Lenhoff, a Swedish pathologist, observed spirochete-like structures in skin biopsy specimens from EM lesions.[3] By 1950, European investigators had demonstrated the efficacy of penicillin in the treatment of EM.[10, 11]

The first well-documented case of EM acquired in the United States was reported in 1970 by Scrimenti, a Wisconsin dermatologist.[12] Mast and Burrows[13] reported a cluster of cases of EM in southeastern Connecticut in 1976. Subsequently, Steere and colleagues[14] reported an association between EM and arthritis in a small group of patients living around the town of Old Lyme, Connecticut. They coined the name Lyme arthritis for this entity. Once it was realized that organs such as the heart and nervous system could also be involved in Lyme arthritis, the name was changed to Lyme disease.[15] Since the late 1980s, Lyme borreliosis established itself as another acceptable term for this infectious disease.

With the identification of *B. burgdorferi,* it has become increasingly obvious that the differences between the United States and Europe in the description of this illness are more apparent than real, and that there was an overemphasis on the rheumatologic aspects by some U.S. authors.

Characteristics of the Pathogen

B. burgdorferi belongs to the family Spirochaetaceae, genus *Borrelia.* This loosely coiled spirochete is motile with a flexible helix structure and measures approximately 10 to 30 μm in length and 0.18 to 0.25 μm in width. Like most spirochetes,

B. burgdorferi is difficult to visualize under brightfield conditions, but it is readily visible by phase-contrast or darkfield microscopy. It can be identified with acridine orange, Giemsa, or silver stains, such as the Dieterle and Warthin-Starry stains, and by immunohistochemical techniques.[16] Demonstration of the spirochete in tissue sections is difficult, especially in chronic disease; therefore, histopathologic identification of the organism cannot be used routinely to diagnose this infection. The organism is microaerophilic and can be grown in a modified Kelly medium (Barbour-Stoener-Kelly) at 33°C.[17] *B. burgdorferi* is easily isolated from the tick vector. However, culture from the human host has proved to be more difficult and is not a routine diagnostic tool at this time. Although yields from cultures of skin biopsy specimens of EM lesions are as high as 85%, *B. burgdorferi* has only rarely been cultured from blood, cerebrospinal fluid (CSF), or synovial tissue.[18]

Three genospecies, *Borrelia burgdorferi sensu stricto, Borrelia garinii,* and *Borrelia afzelii,* are known to cause disease in humans. Collectively, these three genospecies are referred to as *B. burgdorferi sensu lato.* However, the full scope of the diversity of this pathogen is still being defined. There are at least eight genospecies in the *B. burgdorferi* species complex[19] and an unknown number of substrains. The *B. burgdorferi* species complex evolves by differentiation of lineages (asexually) and is consequently composed of an array of clones. Sequence analysis of chromosomal genes and outer surface protein A genes *(ospA)* from a number of variant strains shows that there has been no horizontal transfer of chromosomal genes and little plasmid transfer within or between species.[20] In the United States, *B. burgdorferi sensu stricto* and three additional genospecies have been isolated; in Europe, all three known pathogenic genospecies and at least two other genospecies have been isolated.[19, 21] In addition, another genospecies, *Borrelia japonica,* has been found in Japan.[22] *B. burgdorferi sensu stricto* is the only species found on two different continents, Europe and North America, suggesting that *B. burgdorferi* may have been introduced to North America from Europe relatively recently.[20]

European studies have demonstrated that humans can be multiply infected with spirochetes representing each of the three predominant genospecies of *Borrelia burgdorferi sensu lato.*[21] By using polymerase chain reaction with primers specific for the *ospA* gene from each of the three genospecies, it was possible to detect multiple species in clinical specimens obtained from patients exhibiting neurologic Lyme disease. The results were corroborated by immunoblot analyses with antibodies that could also differentiate the three phylogenetic groups. It is not known if pluriinfection is the result of consecutive infections or simultaneous infection from a single tick. It has been shown that *Ixodes ricinus* can carry more than one kind of *B. burgdorferi sensu lato.* By using polymerase chain reaction along with single-stranded conformational polymorphism, we found that *Ixodes scapularis* ticks from North America can harbor more than one variant of *B. burgdorferi sensu stricto.* Taken together, these data are consistent with the hypothesis that the multisystem nature of Lyme disease may, in part, be the result of infection with multiple strains of *B. burgdorferi sensu lato,* which vary in their antigenic properties, their tropisms, and the types of clinical symptoms they elicit. If this hypothesis holds true, it could help explain the wide array of clinical manifestations associated with this infection.

Structurally, these spirochetes possess outer cell and cytoplasmic membranes. Between these membranes, 7 to 11 flagella are inserted at the ends of the spirochete.[23] The antigenic structure of *B. burgdorferi* is only partially characterized (Table 224–1). Two major outer surface proteins, OspA and OspB, encoded on a 49-kb linear plasmid,[24] are not found on all strains. Although quantitatively OspA is the major surface protein expressed in cultured organisms and in the tick, the immune response to OspA develops in only a minority of individuals and then only later in the course of infection.[25] Evidence has shown that there is a rapid change from OspA expression to OspC expression as the spirochete is transferred to the skin by the feeding tick. Three additional outer surface lipoproteins have been identified (OspD, OspE, and OspF). OspD is expressed in low-passage strains of *B. burgdorferi* and may therefore function as a virulence factor.[26] OspE and OspF form a plasmid-encoded operon.[27] As with OspC, OspF can elicit protective immune responses in rodents; however, this response is less pronounced than the response to OspA. In contrast to the structure of the outer surface proteins, the structure of the 41-kDa flagellar antigen is consistent among strains. The immune responses to the flagellar antigen are elicited early in the course of infection.[28] This 41-kDa protein is highly cross-reactive with similar flagellar antigens of both *Borrelia* and *Treponema* species. The 60-kDa protein is a common heat shock antigen; similar proteins are found in a variety of bacteria.[29]

TABLE 224–1 ■ Major Antigens of *Borrelia burgdorferi*

MOLECULAR MASS (kDa)	CHARACTERISTICS
93	Protoplasmic cylinder antigen; immunodominant
73	Common bacterial antigen of the HSP 70 family
60–66	Common bacterial antigen of the HSP 60 family
41	Flagellar antigen; immunodominant; high degree of homology with other flagellar antigens
39	Membrane associated
37	Not localized
34	OspB; plasmid encoded
31	OspA; plasmid encoded
23	OspC; plasmid encoded
18	Not localized

Epidemiology

Lyme borreliosis has been recognized as the most prevalent vector-borne illness in the United States and Europe.[3, 30] *Ixodes* ticks are the principal vector of this infection throughout the world (Table 224–2); cases are limited to areas where this species is endemic.[31–33] Although Lyme borreliosis has been reported in most states in the United States, the vast majority of these cases occur in three regions: coastal areas in the Northeast from Maryland to Massachusetts; in the upper Midwest, predominantly in Wisconsin and Minnesota; and

TABLE 224–2 ■ Tick Vectors of Lyme Borreliosis

SPECIES	LOCATION	PERCENT INFECTED
Ixodes scapularis	Northeast, upper midwestern, southeastern United States	0–70+
Ixodes pacificus	West Coast of United States	2–5
Ixodes ricinus	Europe	Unknown
Ixodes persulcatus	Asia	10–70+
Amblyomma americanum	South and eastern United States	Unknown

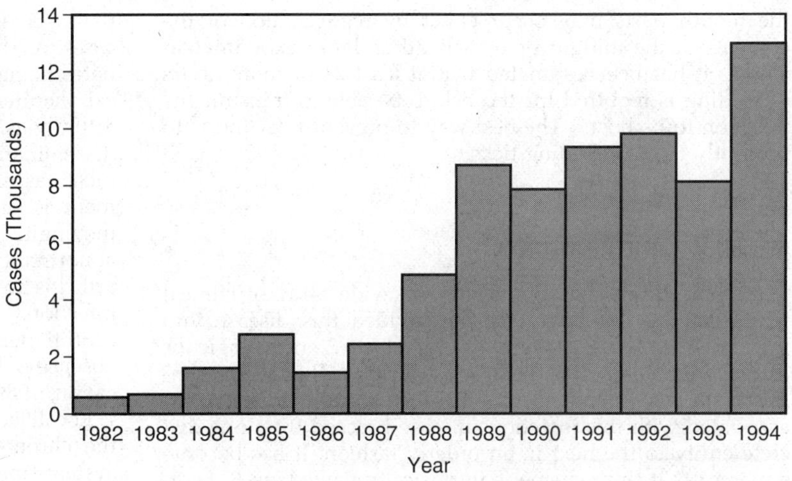

FIGURE 224–1 ▫ Number of reported Lyme disease cases, by year, in the United States, 1982 to 1994. (From Centers for Disease Control and Prevention: Lyme disease—United States, 1994. MMWR Morbid Mortal Wkly Rep 44:459–462, 1995.)

in the far West, in California and western Nevada[34] (Figs. 224–1 and 224–2). These geographic areas correspond to the distribution of the primary tick vectors of Lyme borreliosis in North America: *I. scapularis* (the black-legged tick [shoulder tick in the South]; the deer tick [formerly *Ixodes dammini*] in the Northeast and Midwest) and *Ixodes pacificus* (western black-legged tick).[35] Small numbers of Lyme borreliosis cases have been reported in the South, especially in eastern Texas and Arkansas.[34] In Europe, Lyme borreliosis is transmitted by *I. ricinus* (sheep tick), and in central-northern Asia *Ixodes persulcatus* (taiga tick) is the vector. Because the *Ixodes* tick requires a relative surface humidity of approximately 85%, this infection is commonly acquired along river valleys, lakeshores, and coastal areas.

Small mammals, such as the white-footed mouse *Peromyscus leucopus,* and other small rodents act as primary reservoirs of *B. burgdorferi.*[35] Tick feeding patterns influence the distribution of this disease in the wild. *Ixodes* ticks are three-stage ticks: larval, nymphal, and adult. Larval ticks are usually born uninfected and become infected with the spirochete only after feeding on an infected animal. Although all tick stages can be found in various species, not all animals are equally favored as hosts.[35] *I. scapularis,* the major vector in the eastern and midwestern United States, is the best studied vector. The larvae of *I. scapularis,* which peak in number during the late summer and early fall, feed preferentially on small rodents. Each successive stage tends to feed on larger mammals. Peaking in numbers during the spring and summer, nymphs feed on medium-sized mammals such as raccoons and squirrels but also feed on small rodents. The adult tick feeds mainly on larger animals, in particular the white-tailed deer. In contrast to *I. scapularis* larvae, the larvae of *I. pacificus* tend to feed on reptiles. Reptiles do not harbor the pathogen, and this may be one of the reasons why the prevalence of *B. burgdorferi* in *I. pacificus* (approximately 5%) is so much less than that in *I. scapularis* (50% to 70% in endemic areas). The nymphal form is the most frequent vehicle for transmission of the infection to humans.

Within the tick, spirochetes can be found in the midgut diverticulum and to a lesser extent, systemically. Shortly after onset of feeding, spirochetal cell division accelerates in the midgut diverticulum. Transmission of the spirochete through

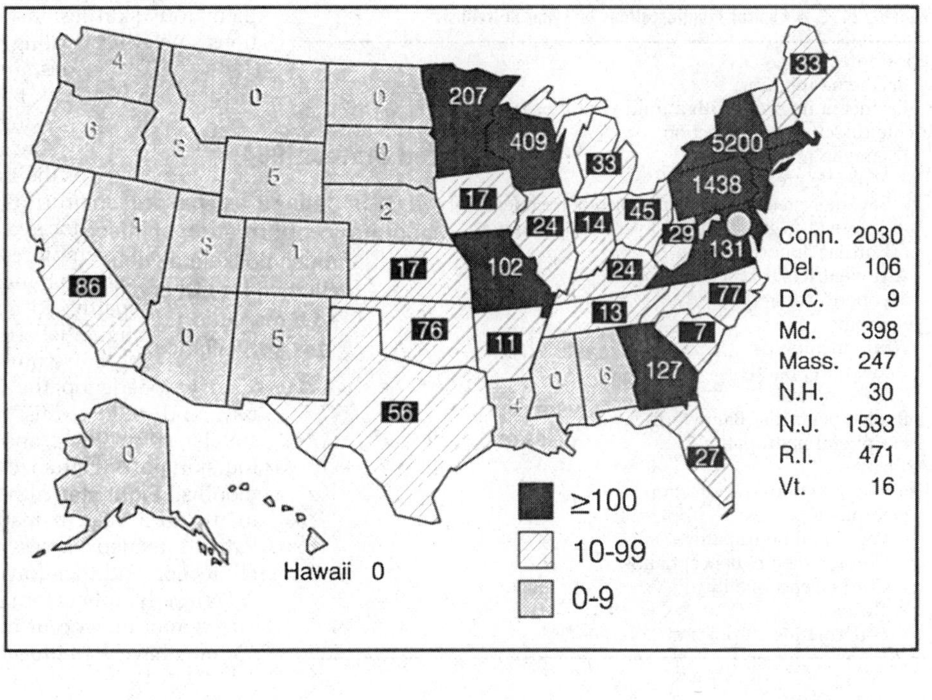

FIGURE 224–2 ▫ Number of reported Lyme disease cases, by state, in the United States, 1994. (From Centers for Disease Control and Prevention: Lyme disease—United States, 1994. MMWR Morbid Mortal Wkly Rep 44:459–462, 1995.)

the mouth parts may occur either by regurgitation of the contents of the midgut or by salivation. From experimental studies it has been estimated that at least 24 or more hours of feeding is required for the tick to be able to transmit the infection to its host.[31] The best way to prevent infection is to promptly remove feeding ticks.

Clinical Manifestations

Lyme borreliosis is associated with a wide array of clinical manifestations. An early scheme divided this disease into three distinct stages: stage 1, EM; stage 2, neurologic or cardiac involvement; and stage 3, arthritis.[36] This overly simplistic staging scheme implies that the clinical manifestations associated with this infectious disease proceed from one discrete entity to the next in an orderly fashion. It has become apparent that this scheme is intrinsically flawed, as *B. burgdorferi* infection is a progressive infectious disease that may disseminate to multiple organs and tissues early in its course. As such, in electing the best therapeutic approach for a given patient one must consider whether this infection is localized or disseminated, and whether it is acute or chronic (Table 224–3).

Between the time of acute dissemination to the onset of the manifestations of chronic disease, there is usually a disease-free interval in which the infection remains latent. The earliest and most easily recognized manifestation of *B. burgdorferi* infection is EM, a characteristic skin lesion observed in 50% to 75% of patients. EM usually develops 2 days to 2 weeks after a painless and often unnoticed tick bite. One or more systemic signs or symptoms, including fever, malaise, headache, stiff neck, and fatigue, occur concurrently with EM in the majority of patients.[37–39] The development of these systemic signs and symptoms often heralds the hematogenous spread of the spirochete. Multiple EM lesions are clear indicators of hematogenous spread, and most series report an 8% to 15% incidence of multiple lesions. Rates as high as 50% have been reported.[39] In some patients, there may be a nonspecific influenza-like illness with no obvious rash. The infectious load in this early phase increases rapidly, and the pathogen is demonstrable in skin lesions in up to 50% of cases. As the spirochete load increases, the organism disseminates hematogenously, producing a broad spectrum of clinical manifestations, including multifocal EM lesions, fever, arthralgias, myalgias, conjunctivitis, and meningismus. This dissemination occurs in the first few weeks of infection in most cases. Acute or subacute major organ system involvement is often associated with acute dissemination. Acute meningitis, myocarditis with or without conduction block abnormalities, hepatitis, myositis, and less commonly frank arthritis are the most dramatic manifestations of this phase of infection.[39, 40] In patients with systemic signs and symptoms, central nervous system (CNS) infection may occur in the absence of localizing findings (Asbrink E, personal communication, 1989).

TABLE 224–3 ■ Clinical Manifestations of Lyme Borreliosis

Local infection
Erythema migrans
Erythema migrans with a mild viral illness
Acute disseminated infection
Erythema migrans
Multiple areas
Severe systemic symptoms, or other evidence of systemic spread (e.g., abnormal liver function tests)
Cardiac abnormalities
Atrioventricular block
Myopericarditis
Neurologic
Acute meningitis
Acute encephalitis
Cranial neuritis
Radiculoneuritis (Bannwarth syndrome)
Peripheral neuropathy
Arthritis
Chronic disseminated infection
Neurologic
Peripheral neuropathy
Chronic meningoencephalitis
Chronic encephalitis
Arthritis
Acrodermatitis chronica atrophicans

Localized inflammatory processes tend to predominate in the chronic phase of the illness, although multiple organ systems may also be involved. There tend to be few constitutional signs and symptoms. Three organ systems (skin, nervous system, and musculoskeletal system) are predominantly involved during this phase. It is important to know the chronicity of the infection because the pathogenesis of the disease and the response to therapy may be different in patients with acute compared with chronic disease.

In assessing the clinical manifestations of this disease, it is important to be aware that *Ixodes* ticks are also the vector for various other infectious diseases, including babesiosis, flavivirus infections,[41, 42] and ehrlichiosis.[30] A much-cited fatal case of babesiosis, for instance, was found to have concomitant fulminant myocarditis secondary to *B. burgdorferi* infection.[43] Previously, Russian investigators noticed a relationship between tick-borne encephalitis caused by flavivirus and EM.[44, 45] Because Lyme borreliosis may be associated with meningitis, meningoencephalitis, or encephalitis, it is not clear whether these particular cases of tick-borne encephalitis associated with EM were due to flavivirus infection or not. Furthermore, *B. burgdorferi* infection should also be considered in all patients suspected of having arbovirus encephalitis in regions where *Ixodes* ticks are endemic, as well as in patients with a history of travel to such regions.

Dermatologic Manifestations

EM is most often characterized as an expanding anular erythematous skin lesion that clears centrally. However, variations, including scaling, vesicular, purpuric, and uniformly erythematous lesions, are common. The skin lesion develops at the site of the tick bite, which is painless. After 24 to 48 hours of the tick's taking its blood meal, it generally falls off spontaneously. In more than half of the cases, the patient is totally unaware of the tick bite. Lesions are often associated with mild, local pruritus or dysesthesia but are seldom painful. EM may be located anywhere on the body. Associated constitutional symptoms may vary from none; to mild and transitory, including malaise, fatigue, headache, chills, and lymphadenopathy; to a debilitating illness associated with profound fatigue, lethargy, mild encephalopathy, meningeal irritation, migratory musculoskeletal pain, hepatitis, generalized lymphadenopathy or splenomegaly, pharyngitis, pleurisy, and myocarditis.[39, 40] Secondary lesions tend to be smaller, migrate less, and lack an indurated center. Untreated, the skin lesions often clear spontaneously within weeks to months after onset, although in rare cases they may persist for up to a year. If inadequately treated, EM may relapse. Patients treated successfully for EM may be susceptible to reinfection and therefore to recurrent episodes.

Borrelia lymphocytoma may occur concurrently with acute infection or may occur months later.[46] The solitary, bluish red nodules have a predilection for occurring in the earlobes of children and on the nipple areas of adults. Other manifestations of infection such as meningitis, choroiditis, arthritis, or ACA can be present along with the lymphocytoma. The clinical appearance of this lesion may be confused with breast malignancy. Histopathologically, *Borrelia* lymphocytoma is characterized by a dense lymphocytic infiltrate in the dermis or subcutaneous tissue, and at times it can be difficult to differentiate the lymphocytoma from lymphoma. *B. burgdorferi* has been isolated from lymphocytoma in only one instance.[46]

ACA is a chronic and insidious skin infection occurring predominantly in elderly women.[47] It is well described throughout northern, central, and eastern Europe but is rarely reported in the United States. ACA usually develops 10 years after the onset of infection. The characteristic skin lesions are described as violaceous to bluish discolored areas with a doughy consistency. The lesions eventually become atrophic or sclerotic. Most commonly, these lesions are found on the distal extremities, and in most cases they spare the face, palms, and soles. The trunk, however, may also be the initial site. Concomitant with ACA, neurologic and rheumatologic evidence of *B. burgdorferi* infection may be present.[47, 48] Polyneuropathy, small joint arthritis with subluxation, arthritis of the large joints, and periosteal thickening of the bones frequently occur in the same extremity as does ACA. Bursitis, epicondylitis, and tendonitis have also been reported.

Musculoskeletal Manifestations

Within days to weeks after *B. burgdorferi* infection, a majority of untreated patients develop musculoskeletal manifestations of Lyme borreliosis. During the acute infection, arthralgias are the most common sign of disease. Some patients develop acute arthritis, often involving large joints such as the knee. Musculoskeletal involvement early in the course of the infection is most frequently manifested as pain in joints, tendons, bursae, muscles, or bones. Usually, however, there is no joint swelling or other signs of active inflammation. One or two sites at a time are affected, and symptoms may last from a few hours to several days.

If untreated, approximately half of those infected in North America develop arthritis as the infection progresses.[36] This arthritis is primarily a large joint arthritis and is characteristically episodic. Only 10% of those with arthritis develop chronic arthritis, and even those who develop it tend to remit spontaneously. The knee is the most commonly affected joint; other large joints can be affected. Although it was once believed that arthritis was not associated with Lyme borreliosis in Europe, heightened awareness of the infection has led to the realization that arthritis is also observed in all parts of Europe where the disease is endemic. Overall, the incidence of frank arthritis has dramatically decreased because of earlier diagnosis and treatment, which significantly reduce the incidence of this late complication. Thus, Lyme arthritis has become an uncommon presentation. In patients with symmetric polyarthritis, especially if small joints are involved, diagnoses other than Lyme disease should be considered.

There have been attempts to link the development of arthritis with certain human leukocyte antigen haplotypes, but associations between specific haplotypes have not been consistent. Early reports of an association of arthritis and the haplotype DR2[49] have not been substantiated, and the linkage of the DR4 haplotype to a poor response to antibiotic therapy remains to be confirmed. Although there are instances in which *B. burgdorferi* is cultured from affected joints, some patients may have an autoreactive process and may not have infection as the cause of continued arthritis. DNA detection by polymerase chain reaction assays can be used to determine which patients have ongoing infection and which may have other causes of their continued arthritis.

Nervous System Manifestations

Clinical data support the hypothesis that in most individuals *B. burgdorferi* invades the CNS early in the course of infection. The most compelling evidence is the frequency of complaints referable to the nervous system in patients with EM. In one study, 80% of all patients with EM had malaise, fatigue, and lethargy; 64% had headaches; and 48% had neck stiffness.[39] The high frequency of early invasion of the CNS was confirmed by polymerase chain reaction detection of borrelial DNA in the CSF of two thirds of patients with acute disseminated infection.[50]

Within the first 3 months after infection, approximately 15% of patients develop one or more of these three acute disorders: meningitis, cranial neuritis, and painful radiculitis. The distinguishing feature in patients in whom meningitis occurs is the presence of CSF abnormalities, pleocytosis, moderate elevations of CSF protein, and a normal CSF glucose level.[51] Papilledema and increased CSF pressure may occur, resulting in a syndrome indistinguishable from pseudotumor cerebri. Acute meningitis presents as the most acute and dramatic CNS manifestation of this infectious process. Cranial neuropathies are commonly associated with acute disseminated infection. These may occur with or without clinical evidence of meningitis. A significant number of patients with cranial nerve abnormalities may have asymptomatic meningitis. Lumbar puncture and examination of the CSF are required to evaluate these patients appropriately. Seventh cranial nerve involvement, both unilateral and bilateral, is by far the most common cranial nerve abnormality. Additional involvement of the second, third, fourth, fifth, sixth, and eighth cranial nerves, along with the optic and recurrent laryngeal nerves, has been reported.[52] These cranial nerve abnormalities can occur alone or with other evidence of polyneuritis. Optic disk edema can occur as a result of optic neuritis or increased intracranial pressure. Pupillary changes can occur including the development of an Argyll Robertson pupil.[53]

Chronic disseminated *B. burgdorferi* infection is frequently associated with symptoms of nervous system dysfunction, but proving that any symptom is directly related to active *B. burgdorferi* infection is difficult. At present, the most commonly used test for making the initial diagnosis of nervous system infection is the measurement of anti–*B. burgdorferi* antibody in the CSF.[54] The use of polymerase chain reaction to demonstrate borrelial DNA in the CSF may prove to be an important new diagnostic technique; however, its role remains to be defined.

B. burgdorferi can cause unifocal or multifocal areas of inflammation in the brain and spinal cord. Whether this neurologic complication is due to vasculitis, direct infection, or immune-mediated mechanisms has yet to be determined. The clinical manifestations of this process range from prominent focal CNS abnormalities to more subtle alterations of cognitive function. Although some reports have confused the more dramatic focal form of the disorder with multiple sclerosis, these two disorders can usually be easily differentiated. Neuroborreliosis is less likely to follow a relapsing and remitting course, does not usually cause abnormal evoked responses, and is associated with intrathecal production of specific antibody against *B. burgdorferi*. Other patients with apparent *B. burgdorferi* infection have an alteration of cognitive function but lack clinical or laboratory evidence of CNS infection. Whether these patients represent the coincidental occurrence of other disorders in patients with anti–*B. burgdorferi* immunoreactivity or whether this situation represents a remote noninfectious CNS manifestation of neuroborreliosis remains to be clarified. There is no clear documentation that *B. burgdorferi* infection directly causes any specific psychiatric disorder. Patients with well-documented Lyme borreliosis given the Beck Depression Inventory test did not demonstrate significant levels of depression.[55]

The peripheral nervous system is also frequently involved in patients with *B. burgdorferi* infection.[55] A spectrum of disease severity has been noted, ranging from severe, painful, and debilitating meningopolyneuritis (Garin-Bujadoux-Bannwarth syndrome) to a milder, but much more common, neuropathy in patients with chronic infection. Meningopolyneuritis, the most dramatic of the peripheral nervous system abnormalities, occurs early in the course of the infection. This syndrome is characterized by intense reticular pain, paresthesias, and hyperesthesias.[56, 57] The CSF may reveal lymphocytic pleocytosis with this syndrome.[56] Concomitant encephalitis and myelitis occur in more than 20% of the patients. In these patients, long-term sequelae such as spastic paraparesis and neurogenic bladder may persist after appropriate therapy.[56, 57] Peripheral neuropathies may be distributed symmetrically or asymmetrically and may resemble polyneuritis multiplex. Paresis of involved extremities may be associated with neuritis. Many patients with chronic infection complain of paresthesia and hyperesthesias.[58] Sensitive neurologic techniques reveal that the abnormalities due to axonopathy of the peripheral nerves are common in disseminated disease. Although the literature has repeatedly emphasized the rather protean neurologic manifestations of this disorder, it is now becoming possible to be more restrictive in the disorders considered causally linked to *B. burgdorferi* infection. As the common threads unifying these different disorders are elucidated, it should become possible to design more specific studies to clarify the pathogenetic mechanisms underlying them.

Cardiac Manifestations

Acute cardiac involvement has been reported in up to 8% of adult patients,[59] although in our experience it occurs in only 1% to 2% of patients with acute disseminated infection. Approximately 90% of patients with cardiac involvement develop varying degrees of atrioventricular block, including complete heart block. Heart block is almost always reversible.[60] Atrioventricular block can fluctuate rapidly. In the majority of cases, the dysfunction is proximal to the bundle of His, and only rarely is it diffuse. Syncope can occur. Third-degree heart block can persist but is usually self-limited even without treatment. Myocarditis or pericarditis is observed in approximately 65% of patients with cardiac involvement, and although left ventricular dysfunction can be documented in almost 50% of these patients, it is usually not severe.[59, 61–64] When left ventricular dysfunction occurs, it does not usually significantly compromise cardiac function. However, in rare instances congestive heart failure has been reported. Electrocardiogram abnormalities, including T wave changes and ST segment depression, are frequently observed. In addition, Lyme myocarditis may be detected by gallium scan.[62, 63] Myopericarditis can be associated with chest pain or shortness of breath. Endomyocardial biopsy can also be used to document cardiac involvement and may show spirochetes.[61] There has been only one report of cardiac death in association with this disease.[43] However, it is possible that the incidence of sudden cardiac death secondary to acute ventricular arrhythmias is higher, but this issue has not been studied. Late cardiac manifestations associated with *B. burgdorferi* infection have not been well defined. Stanek and associates[64a] reported in European patients that chronic infection can be associated with a chronic carditis and the development of cardiomyopathy. Similar cases are found in the United States. Nonetheless, the incidence of Lyme-associated cardiomyopathy is quite low.

Involvement of Other Organs

B. burgdorferi has been localized in other organs and systems during acute infection. Hepatitis with mild to moderate elevation of transaminase levels simulating acute viral hepatitis has occurred in early Lyme disease.[39] Cases of myositis, osteomyelitis, and pneumonitis have also been reported. One patient with pneumonitis ultimately died of respiratory failure, and *B. burgdorferi* was demonstrated in lymph nodes.[65]

Diagnosis

EM is the classic marker for Lyme borreliosis, and its presence is virtually diagnostic. Unfortunately, this characteristic skin lesion is recognized in only about 75% of patients with *B. burgdorferi* infection, and it is typically seen only early in the course of infection. In the absence of EM, definitively diagnosing Lyme borreliosis can be troublesome. *B. burgdorferi* is difficult to culture, and in the chronic phase of the disease it is rarely observed in clinical samples. Therefore, unlike most bacterial diseases, which can be defined microbiologically by direct observation or culture of the pathogen, Lyme borreliosis is defined indirectly. In the absence of EM, the basis for diagnosis is the demonstration of an immune response against *B. burgdorferi* in an appropriate clinical setting. This is not optimal, especially in view of the lack of agreement on a precise clinical definition for this illness and the lack of standardization of serologic assays.

Antibody responses to *B. burgdorferi* in the infected host follow the usual pattern. Immunoglobulin (Ig) M antibody appears first, followed by IgG and IgA responses.[66] Within 2 to 3 weeks after the onset of infection, a rise in antibody against two or more spirochetal antigens can be detected in most patients. During the second and third months of infection, specific IgG and IgA responses gradually increase, and once established, may remain detectable for years. In most humans, the earliest immune response to *B. burgdorferi* is directed to the protein antigens, flagellin (p41), and OspC (25 kDa),[67, 68] with 37- and 39-kDa protein antigens also eliciting an early response in many persons. Sensitive techniques can detect some response to OspA in early infection, but large amounts of antibodies to the major outer surface lipoproteins, OspA and OspB, generally appear only much later in the course of infection, if at all. The delayed immune response to OspA with respect to OspC may be the result of host-dependent differential expression of these surface proteins.[69] OspA is adapted to the tick, whereas OspC predominates in the mammal.

In the clinical laboratory, antibodies against *B. burgdorferi* are usually detected by either indirect immunofluorescence assay (IFA) or enzyme-linked immunosorbent assay (ELISA). Whole *B. burgdorferi* preparations are generally used for these assays. For the IFA, fixed *B. burgdorferi* organisms are used as the antigen substrate; for most ELISAs, crude fractions of sonicated organisms are utilized. None of these assays are standardized. Consequently, there is wide variability among laboratories as to how assays are performed and reported. The sensitivity, specificity, and normal values are not comparable, and each laboratory must establish its own criteria. The positive predictive value of current IFA and ELISA assays is poor. Spirochetes make up part of the normal human flora, and most patients have circulating antibodies that cross-react with one or more *B. burgdorferi* antigens (see Table 224–2). This is especially true for the 41-kDa and some of the common bacterial antigens expressed by this pathogen.[25, 54, 70]

Further complicating the assessment of the humoral response is that, as for syphilis, prompt antimicrobial therapy can abort the development of a mature humoral response, and patients treated before they develop a mature humoral response often lack diagnostic levels of *Borrelia*-specific antibodies.[25, 59, 70]

We have found that using highly sensitive immunoblots, more than 50% of normal healthy adults with no history of *B. burgdorferi* infection had circulating anti–41-kDa IgG antibody.[70] Many also had antibodies against other spirochetal antigens, most commonly the 60-kDa common bacterial antigen and the 66-kDa antigen. This high level of cross-reactive antibodies is the reason that most laboratories performing IFA have established negative cutoff points between 1:64 and 1:256. ELISAs can be more easily used to screen large numbers of serum samples and do not have the problem of observer error intrinsic to IFA. Most laboratories utilizing ELISAs have established normal and negative cutoff points statistically. Absorbency values of 3 SD or more above the mean of healthy control subjects are used by most laboratories to establish the cutoff point.

Although IFA can be as useful as ELISA for the detection of antibodies against *B. burgdorferi* in the peripheral blood, to measure anti–*B. burgdorferi* antibody concentrations in CSF the superior sensitivity of ELISA offers a marked advantage. With the exception of demonstrating local antibody production in the CNS, the positive predictive value of a positive assay by itself is low, no matter which test is used, IFA or ELISA. To improve the specificity of serology, the Centers for Disease Control and Prevention has proposed that all positive ELISA and IFA results be confirmed by Western blot analysis. The IgM blot is believed to be helpful only early in the course of infection, whereas the IgG Western blot is useful at any point. For a result to be considered positive, there should be IgM reactivity against any two of the following proteins: 23 kDa (OspC), 39 kDa, and 41 kDa. The criteria proposed by Dressler and colleagues[71] are recommended for IgG blot. It is recognized that the apparent molecular mass of individual proteins can vary among strains or under different growth conditions; therefore, a standardized panel of monoclonal antibodies against key bacterial proteins is being developed to more clearly characterize Western blots.

It should be remembered that the finding that an individual has significant amounts of anti–*B. burgdorferi* antibodies can be interpreted only in the context of the clinical setting. Simply demonstrating that the patient has an immune response against the organism does not mean that he or she is actively infected, or that any symptoms have anything to do with *B. burgdorferi* infection. To make a diagnosis of Lyme borreliosis requires that objective clinical abnormalities be documented. Likewise, if an individual has objective abnormalities clinically compatible with Lyme borreliosis, the diagnosis of *B. burgdorferi* infection should be pursued even if the peripheral antibody titer is below diagnostic levels. Some antibiotic regimens (e.g., low-dose oral penicillin or tetracycline) fail to provide adequate levels within the CNS and perhaps other sites. Examination of CSF should be carried out in all patients suspected of having CNS disease. Some patients with negative peripheral serologic test results have evidence of local antibody production in the CNS.[72] These patients can also have a peripheral T-cell response to *B. burgdorferi*. Patients without diagnostic levels of antibody in either serum or CSF are highly unlikely to have active *B. burgdorferi* infection, and other reasons for their signs and symptoms should be sought.

Treatment

The optimal antibiotic, dose, and duration of treatment of Lyme borreliosis remain areas of controversy. There are a number of reasons for this:

1. There have been few randomized prospective studies of the treatment of Lyme borreliosis.
2. For all studies published so far, the diagnosis of Lyme borreliosis was primarily based on clinical grounds, not on microbiologic criteria.
3. Treatment has also been based on clinical grounds and not on microbiologic criteria.
4. The natural history of untreated Lyme disease is that in most persons the disease will spontaneously remit.
5. The mechanisms producing persistent signs and symptoms are not well defined and may be due to a number of factors: continued infection, permanent tissue damage, or some undefined immune mechanism. Thus, suggestions as to the treatment of this infection should be taken with some reservations.

In general, β-lactam antibiotics and tetracyclines are effective against *B. burgdorferi.* Although the response to treatment with various tetracyclines and penicillins is good in patients with local infection or uncomplicated EM, studies of early infection must be interpreted with caution. Initial studies of patients with EM failed to recognize that *B. burgdorferi* can spread to the CNS and other sites early in the course of infection. In one study, low-dose oral tetracycline (250 mg) was judged to be the drug of choice for early disease,[38] despite the fact that approximately half of the patients continued to have recurrent episodes of headache, chronic lethargy, arthralgias, or Bell palsy. Well-documented failures of low-dose oral tetracycline were reported subsequently.[73] Nonetheless, tetracyclines have an established place in the treatment of Lyme borreliosis. There has been a trend toward the use of semisynthetic tetracyclines (doxycycline or minocycline) because of their better absorption and better tissue penetration, especially into the CNS.[74] Although no study has clearly defined the optimal treatment of early *B. burgdorferi* infection, there are retrospective clinical studies and in vitro sensitivity data to suggest that in addition to the semisynthetic tetracyclines, amoxicillin and cefuroxime are effective.[75] The role of macrolides in this infection needs further study.

In the absence of being able to define microbiologically the patients in whom this infection has disseminated, we treat patients with acute infection with amoxicillin at 500 mg three times daily, doxycycline at 100 mg twice daily, or minocycline at 100 mg twice daily. These regimens provide sustained serum levels. We do not recommend tetracycline, but if it is used, we believe that the dose should be increased to at least 500 mg four times daily.

Penicillin and ceftriaxone are the most widely used antibiotics in the treatment of severe *B. burgdorferi* infection.[76–79] Acute meningitis or meningoencephalitis caused by *B. burgdorferi* is usually quite responsive to high-dose penicillin therapy. However, there are several instances in which acute CNS infection has progressed despite penicillin therapy.[80, 81] Meningopolyradiculitis, or Bannwarth syndrome, is more difficult to treat.[48, 56, 82] Although therapy usually halts the progression of the disease, as many as 50% of patients continue to have severe neurologic signs such as spastic paraparesis after treatment.[48, 56, 82] Similarly, approximately 50% or more of patients with arthritis secondary to *B. burgdorferi* fail to respond to intravenous penicillin therapy.[78] Treatment of ACA with penicillin is successful in about 50% of patients, with a similar percentage experiencing continued extracutaneous manifestations.[40] Thus, failure rates as high as 50% or more are commonly reported with penicillin treatment of chronic rheumatologic, dermatologic, or neurologic disease caused by *B. burgdorferi.* It is not clear whether these treatment failures are due to persistent, smoldering infection, to immune autoreactivity triggered by the infection, to the pathologic changes that occurred before treatment, or to some combination of the three possible causes.

In our experience, ceftriaxone is superior to penicillin in the treatment of late Lyme borreliosis.[76, 77] However, larger long-term studies are required to determine the precise role of this and other third-generation cephalosporins in the treatment of *B. burgdorferi* infection. Even though ceftriaxone appears to be promising, it is still associated with a failure rate of 15% to 20%. We currently treat patients with disseminated infection and significant CNS or cardiac involvement with 21 to 28 days of ceftriaxone 2 g once a day. The treatment of Lyme arthritis is more problematic. Lyme arthritis can be treated with oral regimens. One study of Lyme arthritis compared two oral regimens: doxycycline versus amoxicillin plus probenecid.[32] In that study, 18 of 20 patients treated with doxycycline and 16 of 18 patients treated with amoxicillin plus probenecid had resolution of their arthritis. However, neuroborreliosis later developed in five patients, one in the doxycycline group and four in the group receiving amoxicillin plus probenecid. All five patients who developed neurologic manifestations recovered after intravenous ceftriaxone. Although Lyme arthritis may respond to oral regimens, Lyme borreliosis is a systemic infectious disease, and any patient with evidence of disseminated infection is at risk for neurologic manifestations. Further studies are needed to establish the optimal duration of therapy and the efficacy of various antimicrobial agents in the treatment of both early and chronic Lyme borreliosis.

Prevention

Although a number of possibilities are being investigated, there is no proven method to totally eliminate *Ixodes* ticks from the environment. *I. scapularis* has been associated with deer, and it has been postulated that by limiting the number of deer the number of ticks could be controlled. Unfortunately, short of the complete eradication of all deer, this method is unlikely to prove successful. The Great Island study where virtually all the deer were killed off demonstrated a slow decline in the number of ticks.[83] However, other studies, in which the numbers of deer were merely reduced, failed to demonstrate significant reductions in the tick population. The use of chemical insecticide sprays may reduce the number of ticks, but total eradication seems unlikely. Moreover, the use of long-acting sprays may cause unacceptable damage to the environment.

On an individual level, it is difficult to avoid some exposure to ticks in most endemic areas without a major disruption of one's daily activities. However, an individual can take a number of measures to limit tick exposure and the risk of developing Lyme borreliosis.[1] Permethrin, an agent cidal to ticks, can be applied to clothing. Repellents such as DEET (*N,N*-diethyl-*m*-toluamide), Indalone (butyl 3,4-dihydro-2,2-dimethyl-4-oxo-2*H*-pyran-6-carboxylate), dimethyl carbate, dimethyl phthalate, benzyl benzoate, and M-1960 (2-butyl-2-ethyl-1,2-propanediol; *N*-butylacetanilide; benzyl benzoate) can be applied. Wearing light-colored clothing makes the dark-colored ticks easier to spot, so that they can be brushed away. Even if a person is bitten, the prompt removal of ticks markedly reduces the risk of infection with *B. burgdorferi.* Spirochetes are inoculated into the skin as the tick salivates and by regurgitation of midgut contents as the tick feeds. Most infections occur after the 24 or more hours of feeding, and the prompt removal of ticks significantly reduces the risk of infection.

In murine models of infection, passively transferred anti-OspA monoclonal antibodies have been shown to be protective, and vaccination with recombinant protein has induced protective immunity against subsequent infection with the homologous strain of *B. burgdorferi*.[68, 84–88] Our studies indicate that there are common epitopes in the C-terminal of the protein that are shared among genospecies and that may have immunoprotective potential,[89, 90] but additional work is needed to further define this observation. At present, clinical trials are in progress of at least three recombinant vaccines for Lyme disease based on OspA. The overall efficacy of a recombinant OspA vaccine derived from a single strain will depend on the frequency of genetic variation of OspA, and how these changes alter the antigenicity of the protective epitopes of the outer surface proteins.

We have demonstrated that the variability of the protective epitope of OspA is dependent, at least in part, on the alteration of six amino acids in a hypervariable portion of the C-terminal of the protein.[91] In a study by Norris and colleagues,[92] vaccination with OspB from strain B31 did not protect mice from challenge with strain N40, a member of the same genospecies. In a gerbil model of infection, active immunization with a recombinant form of OspC afforded protection against the homologous strain from which the vaccine was derived. However, protection against heterologous strains has been erratic.[93]

References

1. Burgdorfer W, Barbour AG, Hayes SF, et al: Lyme disease—A tick-borne spirochetosis? Science 216:1317–1319, 1982.
2. Afzelius A: Verhandlungen der dermatologischen Gesellschaft zu Stockholm. Arch Dermatol Syphilol 101:104, 1910.
3. Burgdorfer W: Discovery of the Lyme disease spirochete: A historical review. Zentralbl Bakteriol Mikrobiol Hyg [A] 263:7–10, 1986.
4. Garin C, Bujadoux C: Paralysie par les tiques. J Med Lyon 3:765–767, 1922.
5. Hellerstrom S: Erythema chronicum migrans Afzelii. Acta Derm Venereol 11:315–321, 1930.
6. Bannwarth A: Zur Klinik und Pathogenese der "chronischen lymphocytären Meningitis." Arch Psychiatr Nervenkr 117:161–185, 1944.
7. Bannwarth A: Chronische lymphocytäre Meningitis entzündliche Polyneuritis und Rheumatismus. Arch Psychiatr Nervenkr 113:284–376, 1941.
8. Herxheimer K, Hartman K: Über Acrodermatitis chronica atrophicans. Arch Dermatol Syph 61:57–76, 255–300, 1902.
9. Bafverstedt B: Über Lymphadenosis benigna cutis. Eine klinische und pathologisch-anatomische Studie. Stockholm, PA Norstedt, 1943.
10. Bianchi G: Penicillinbehandlung der Lymphozytome. Dermatologia 100:270–273, 1950.
11. Hollstrom E: Successful treatment of erythema migrans Afzelius. Acta Dermatol Venereol (Stockh) 31:325, 1951.
12. Scrimenti R: Erythema chronicum migrans. Arch Dermatol 236:859–860, 1970.
13. Mast WE, Burrows WM: Erythema chronicum migrans and "lyme arthritis" (Letter). JAMA 236:2392, 1976.
14. Steere AC, Malawista SE, Snydman DR, et al: Lyme arthritis: An epidemic of oligoarticular arthritis in children and adults in three Connecticut communities. Arthritis Rheum 20:7–17, 1977.
15. Steere AC, Malawista SE: Cases of Lyme disease in the United States: Locations correlated with distribution of *Ixodes dammini.* Ann Intern Med 91:730–733, 1979.
16. de Koning J, Hoogkamp KJ: Diagnosis of Lyme disease by demonstration of spirochetes in tissue biopsies. Zentralbl Bakteriol Mikrobiol Hyg [A] 263:179–188, 1986.
17. Barbour AG: Isolation and cultivation of Lyme disease spirochetes. Yale J Biol Med 57:521–525, 1984.
18. Berger BW, Johnson RC, Kodner C, Coleman L: Cultivation of *Borrelia burgdorferi* from human tick bite sites: A guide to the risk of infection. J Am Acad Dermatol 32:184–187, 1995.
19. Postic D, Assous MV, Grimont PAD, Baranton G: Diversity of *Borrelia burgdorferi sensu lato* evidenced by restriction fragment length polymorphism of rrf (5S)-rrl (23S) intergenic spacer amplicons. Int J Syst Bacteriol 44:743–752, 1994.
20. Dykhuizen DE, Polin DS, Dunn JJ, et al: *Borrelia burgdorferi* is

clonal: Implications for taxonomy and vaccine development. Proc Natl Acad Sci USA 90:10163–10167, 1993.
21. Marconi RT, Garon CF: Phylogenetic analysis of the genus *Borrelia*—A comparison of North American and European isolates of *Borrelia burgdorferi.* J Bacteriol 174:241–244, 1992.
22. Postic D, Belfazia J, Isogai E, et al: A new genomic species of *Borrelia burgdorferi sensu lato* isolated from Japanese ticks. Res Microbiol 144:467–473, 1993.
23. Hovind HK, Asbrink E, Stiernstedt G, et al: Ultrastructural differences among spirochetes isolated from patients with Lyme disease and related disorders, and from *Ixodes ricinus.* Zentralbl Bakteriol Mikrobiol Hyg [A] 263:103–111, 1986.
24. Howe TR, LaQuier FW, Barbour AG: Organization of genes encoding two outer membrane proteins of the Lyme disease agent *Borrelia burgdorferi* within a single transcriptional unit. Infect Immun 54:207–212, 1986.
25. Craft JE, Fischer DK, Shimamoto GT, Steere AC: Antigens of *Borrelia burgdorferi* recognized during Lyme disease. Appearance of a new immunoglobulin M response and expansion of the immunoglobulin G response late in the illness. J Clin Invest 78:934–939, 1986.
26. Nguyen TK, Lam TT, Bartold SW, et al: Destruction of *Borrelia burgdorferi* in ticks engorging on OspE and OspF. Infect Immun 62:2079–2085, 1994.
27. Probert WS, Lefebvre RB: Protection of C3H/HeN mice from challenge with *Borrelia burgdorferi* through active immunization with OspA, OspB or OspC, but not OspD or the 83 kilodalton antigen. Infect Immun 62:1920–1926, 1994.
28. Wilske B, Preac MV, Schierz G, et al: Antigenic variability of *Borrelia burgdorferi.* Ann N Y Acad Sci 539:126–143, 1988.
29. Hansen K, Bangsborg JM, Fjordvang H, et al: Immunochemical characterization of and isolation of the gene for a *Borrelia burgdorferi* immunodominant 60-kilodalton antigen common to a wide range of bacteria. Infect Immun 56:2047–2053, 1988.
30. Fishbein DB, Dennis DT: Tick-borne diseases—A growing risk (Editorial). N Engl J Med 333:452–453, 1995.
31. Benach JL, Coleman JL, Skinner RA, Bosler EM: Adult *Ixodes dammini* on rabbits: A hypothesis for the development and transmission of *Borrelia burgdorferi.* J Infect Dis 155:1300–1306, 1987.
32. Kawabata M, Baba S, Iguchi K, et al: Lyme disease in Japan and its possible incriminated tick vector, *Ixodes persulcatus* (Letter). J Infect Dis 156:854, 1987.
33. Lane R, Burgdorfer W: Transovarial and transstadial passage of *Borrelia burgdorferi* in the Western black-legged tick, *Ixodes pacificus.* Am J Trop Med Hyg 37:188–192, 1987.
34. Centers for Disease Control and Prevention: Lyme disease—United States, 1994. MMWR Morbid Mortal Wkly Rep 44:459–462, 1995.
35. Bosler E, Coleman J, Benach JL, et al: Natural distribution of the *Ixodes scapularus* spirochete. Science 220:321–322, 1983.
36. Steere AC, Schoen RT, Taylor E: The clinical evolution of Lyme arthritis. Ann Intern Med 107:725–731, 1987.
37. Stiernstedt G: Tick-borne *Borrelia* infection in Sweden. Scand J Infect Dis Suppl 45:1–70, 1985.
38. Steere AC, Hutchinson GJ, Rahn DW, et al: Treatment of the early manifestations of Lyme disease. Ann Intern Med 99:22–26, 1983.
39. Steere AC, Bartenhagen NH, Craft JE, et al: The early clinical manifestations of Lyme disease. Ann Intern Med 99:76–82, 1983.
40. Asbrink E, Hovmark A: Early and late cutaneous manifestations in *Ixodes*-borne borreliosis (erythema migrans borreliosis, Lyme borreliosis). Ann N Y Acad Sci 539:4–15, 1988.
41. Piesman J, Mather T, Dammin GJ, et al: Seasonal variation of transmission risk of Lyme disease and human babesiosis. Am J Epidemiol 126:1187–1189, 1987.
42. Piesman J, Hicks TC, Sinsky RJ, Obiri G: Simultaneous transmission of *Borrelia burgdorferi* and *Babesia microti* by individual nymphal *Ixodes dammini* ticks. J Clin Microbiol 25:2012–2013, 1987.
43. Marcus LC, Steere AC, Duray PH, et al: Fatal pancarditis in a patient with coexistent Lyme disease and babesiosis. Demonstration of spirochetes in the myocardium. Ann Intern Med 103:374–376, 1985.
44. Edlinger E, Rodhain F, Perez C: Lyme disease in patients previously suspected of arbovirus infection (Letter). Lancet 2:93, 1985.
45. Rodhain F, Edlinger E: Serodiagnostic of erythema chronicum migrans (Lyme disease) in cases initially suspected as caused by arboviruses. Zentralbl Bakteriol Mikrobiol Hyg [A] 263:425–426, 1987.
46. Hovmark A, Asbrink E, Olsson I: The spirochetal etiology of lymphadenosis benigna cutis solitaria. Acta Derm Venereol 66:479–484, 1986.
47. Asbrink E, Brehmer-Andersson E, Hovmark A: Acrodermatitis chronica atrophicans—A spirochetosis. Clinical and histopathological picture based on 32 patients; course and relationship to erythema chronicum migrans Afzelius. Am J Dermatopathol 8:209–219, 1986.
48. Kristoferitsch W, Sluga E, Graf M, et al: Neuropathy associated with acrodermatitis chronica atrophicans. Clinical and morphological features. Ann N Y Acad Sci 539:35–45, 1988.
49. Steere AC, Gibofsky A, Patarroyo ME, et al: Chronic Lyme arthritis: Clinical and immunogenetic differentiation from rheumatoid arthritis. Ann Intern Med 90:896–901, 1979.
50. Luft BJ, Steinman CR, Neimark HC, et al: Invasion of the central nervous system by *Borrelia burgdorferi* in acute disseminated infection [published erratum in JAMA 268:872, 1992]. JAMA 267:1364–1367, 1992.
51. Halperin JJ, Luft BJ, Anand AK, et al: Lyme neuroborreliosis: Central nervous system manifestations. Neurology 39:753–759, 1989.
52. Schmutzhard E, Stanek G, Pohl P: Polyneuritis cranialis associated with *Borrelia burgdorferi.* J Neurol Neurosurg Psychiatry 48:1182–1184, 1985.
53. Koudstaal PJ, Vermeulen M, Wokke JH: Argyll Robertson pupils in lymphocytic meningoradiculitis (Bannwarth's syndrome) (Letter). J Neurol Neurosurg Psychiatry 50:363–365, 1987.
54. Stiernstedt G, Gustafsson R, Karlsson M, et al: Clinical manifestations and diagnosis of neuroborreliosis. Ann N Y Acad Sci 539:46–55, 1988.
55. Halperin JJ, Pass HL, Anand AK, et al: Nervous system abnormalities in Lyme disease. Ann N Y Acad Sci 539:24–34, 1988.
56. Kamper AL, Andersen JT: Reversible bladder denervation in acute polyradiculitis. Scand J Urol Nephrol 16:291–293, 1982.
57. Maida E, Kristoferitsch W, Spiel G: Cerebrospinal fluid changes in Garin-Bujadoux-Bannwarth meningoradiculitis. Nervenarzt 57:149–152, 1986.
58. Halperin JJ, Little BW, Coyle PK, et al: Lyme disease: Cause of a treatable peripheral neuropathy. Neurology 37:1700–1706, 1987.
59. Steere A, Batsford WP, Weinberg M, et al: Lyme carditis: Cardiac abnormalities of Lyme disease. Ann Intern Med 93:8–16, 1980.
60. McAlister HF, Klementowicz PT, Andrews C, et al: Lyme carditis: An important cause of reversible heart block. Ann Intern Med 110:339–345, 1989.
61. Reznick JW, Braunstein DB, Walsh RL, et al: Lyme carditis: Electrophysiologic and histopathologic study. Am J Med 81:923–927, 1986.
62. Ponsonnaille J, Citron B, Karsenty B, et al: Acute myocarditis in Lyme's syndrome. Value of myocardial scintigraphy with gallium 67 [in French]. Arch Mal Coeur Vaiss 79:1946–1950, 1986.
63. Rienzo RJ, Morel DE, Prager D, et al: Gallium avid Lyme myocarditis. Clin Nucl Med 12:475–476, 1987.
64. Lorcerie B, Boutron MC, Portier H, et al: Pericardial manifestations of Lyme disease. Ann Med Interne (Paris) 138:601–603, 1987.
64a. Stanek G, Klein J, Bittner R, Glogar D: Isolation of *Borrelia burgdorferi* from the myocardium of a patient with longstanding cardiomyopathy. N Engl J Med 322:249–252, 1990.
65. Kirsch M, Ruben FL, Steere AC, et al: Fatal adult respiratory distress syndrome in a patient with Lyme disease. JAMA 259:2737–2739, 1988.
66. Craft JE, Fischer DK, Shimamoto GT, Steere AC: Antigens of *Borrelia burgdorferi* recognized during Lyme disease. Appearance of a new immunoglobulin M response and expansion of the immunoglobulin G response late in the illness. J Clin Invest 78:934–939, 1986.
67. Schaible UE, Kramer MD, Eichmann K, et al: Monoclonal antibodies specific for the outer surface protein A (OspA) of *Borrelia burgdorferi* prevent Lyme borreliosis in severe combined immunodeficiency (scid) mice. Proc Natl Acad Sci USA 87:3768–3772, 1990.
68. Wilske B, Preac-Mursic V, Schierz G, Busch KV: Immunochemical

and immunological analysis of European *Borrelia burgdorferi* strains. Zentralbl Bakteriol Parasitenkd Infektionskr Hyg Abt 1 Orig Reihe A 263:92–102, 1986.
69. Margolis N, Hogan D, Tilly K, Rosa PA: Plasmid location of *Borrelia* purine biosynthesis gene homologs. J Bacteriol 176:6427–6432, 1994.
70. Dattwyler RJ, Volkman DJ, Luft BJ, et al: Seronegative Lyme disease: Dissociation of specific T- and B-lymphocyte responses to *Borrelia burgdorferi.* N Engl J Med 319:1441–1446, 1988.
71. Dressler F, Whalen JA, Reinhardt BN, Steere AC: Western blotting in the serodiagnosis of Lyme disease. J Infect Dis 167:392–400, 1993.
72. Hansen K, Hindersson P, Pedersen NS: Measurement of antibodies to the *Borrelia burgdorferi* flagellum improves serodiagnosis in Lyme disease. J Clin Microbiol 26:338–346, 1988.
73. Dattwyler RJ, Halperin JJ: Failure of tetracycline in early Lyme disease. Arthritis Rheum 30:448–450, 1987.
74. Dotevall L, Alestig K, Hanner P, et al: The use of doxycycline in nervous system *Borrelia burgdorferi* infection. Scand J Infect Dis Suppl 53:74–79, 1988.
75. Berger BW: Treatment of erythema chronicum migrans of Lyme disease. Ann N Y Acad Sci 539:346–351, 1988.
76. Dattwyler RJ, Halperin JJ, Pass H, Luft BJ: Ceftriaxone as effective therapy in refractory Lyme disease. J Infect Dis 155:1322–1325, 1987.
77. Dattwyler RJ, Halperin JJ, Volkman DJ, Luft BJ: Treatment of late Lyme borreliosis—Randomised comparison of ceftriaxone and penicillin. Lancet 2:1191–1194, 1988.
78. Steere AC, Green J, Schoen RT, et al: Successful parenteral penicillin therapy of established Lyme arthritis. N Engl J Med 312:869–874, 1985.
79. Kristoferitsch W, Baumhackl U, Sluga E, et al: High-dose penicillin therapy in meningopolyneuritis Garin-Bujadoux-Bannwarth. Clinical and cerebrospinal fluid data. Zentralbl Bakteriol Mikrobiol Hyg A 263:357–364, 1987.
80. Pal G, Baker JT, Wright DJ: Penicillin-resistant *Borrelia* encephalitis responding to cefotaxime (Letter). Lancet 1:50–51, 1988.
81. Diringer MN, Halperin JJ, Dattwyler RJ: Lyme meningoencephalitis: Report of a severe, penicillin-resistant case. Arthritis Rheum 30:705–708, 1987.
82. Kristoferitsch W: Lyme borreliosis in Europe. Neurologic disorders. Rheum Dis Clin North Am 15:767–774, 1989.
83. Spielman A: Prospects for suppressing transmission of Lyme disease. Ann N Y Acad Sci 539:212–220, 1988.
84. Erdile LF, Brandt M, Warakomski D, et al: Role of attached lipid in immunogenicity of *Borrelia burgdorferi* OspA. Infect Immun 61:81–90, 1993.
85. Stover CK, Bansal GP, Hanson MS, et al: Protective immunity elicited by recombinant bacille Calmette-Guérin (BCG) expressing outer surface protein A (OspA) lipoprotein: A candidate Lyme disease vaccine. J Exp Med 178:197–209, 1993.
86. Schaible UE, Wallich R, Kramer MD, et al: Immune sera to individual *Borrelia burgdorferi* isolates or recombinant OspA thereof protect SCID mice against infection with homologous strains, but only partially or not at all against those of different OspA/OspB genotypes. Vaccine 11:1049–1054, 1993.
87. Luft BJ, Jiang W, Munoz P, et al: Biochemical and immunological characterization of the surface proteins of *Borrelia burgdorferi.* Infect Immun 57:3637–3645, 1989.
88. Schubach WH, Mudri S, Dattwyler RJ, Luft BJ: Mapping antibody binding domains of the major outer surface protein (OspA) of *Borrelia burgdorferi.* Infect Immun 59:1911–1915, 1991.
89. McGrath BC, Dunn JJ, Gorgone G, et al: Identification of an immunologically important hyervariable domain of the major outer surface protein A of *Borrelia burgdorferi.* Infect Immun 63:1356–1361, 1995.
90. Fikrig E, Bartold SW, Marcantonio N, et al: Roles of OspA, OspB and flagellin in protective immunity to Lyme borreliosis in laboratory mice. Infect Immun 59:553–559, 1992.
91. Preac-Mursic V, Wilske B, Patsouris E, et al: Active immunization with pC protein of *Borrelia burgdorferi* protects gerbils against *Borrelia burgdorferi* infection. Infection 20:342–349, 1992.
92. Norris SJ, Carter CJ, Howell JK, Barbour AG: Low-passage associated proteins of *Borrelia burgdorferi* B31—Characterization and molecular cloning of OspD, a surface-exposed plasmid-encoded lipoprotein. Infect Immun 60:4662–4672, 1992.
93. Lam TT, Nguyen TK, Montgomery RR, et al: Outer surface proteins E and F of *Borrelia burgdorferi,* the Lyme disease agent. Infect Immun 62:290–298, 1994.

225

Borrelia Species and *Spirillum minus*

Thomas Butler

The genus *Borrelia* comprises spirochetal bacteria that cause the human diseases relapsing fever and Lyme disease. *Borrelia recurrentis* causes louse-borne relapsing fever and *Borrelia hermsii, Borrelia turicatae, Borrelia parkeri,* and other species cause tick-borne relapsing fever. *Borrelia burgdorferi* is the cause of Lyme disease and is described in Chapter 224. Animal borrelioses include bovine borreliosis *(Borrelia thelleri),* epizootic bovine abortion *(Borrelia coriaceae),* and avian borreliosis *(Borrelia anserma).* Another pathogenic spirochete that is considered in this chapter is *Spirillum minus,* a cause of rat-bite fever.

History

Borrelia organisms were discovered in 1873 by Obermeier, who observed them with a microscope in the blood of a person with relapsing fever. The transmission of *Borrelia* spirochetes by arthropod vectors was suggested in 1891 by Flugge, who postulated the body louse as a vector. In 1905, Dutton and Todd demonstrated the infection in the *Ornithodoros* ticks of Africa. The genus name *Borrelia* was proposed in 1907, to honor the French bacteriologist Borrel. Successful cultivation of *Borrelia* in vitro was reported by Kelly in 1971. The discovery of *B. burgdorferi* as the cause of Lyme disease was made in 1982. A spiral organism, later named *S. minor,* and subsequently *S. minus,* was shown to be a cause of rat-bite fever (*sodoku* in Japanese) in 1908.

Characteristics of the Pathogen

Borrelia organisms are spiral shaped and vary in length from 5 to 40 μm and in width from 0.2 to 0.5 μm. Like other bacteria, these organisms possess an outer cell wall (outer envelope) and an inner cytoplasmic membrane that contains muramic acid. Between the cell wall and cytoplasmic membrane are 7 to 20 flagella, which are anchored to the ends of the spirochete and wrap around its body until they meet near the middle. In three dimensions the spirochetes have a helical configuration consisting of about 4 to 10 coils with "amplitudes" of about 1 to 4 μm. Under darkfield or phase-contrast microscopy, *Borrelia* spirochetes display an active corkscrew-like motility. Inside the cytoplasmic membrane are ribosomes, DNA, and RNA. These prokaryotic organisms divide by transverse binary fission.

Borrelia organisms are microaerophilic and fermentative in their growth characteristics. Like other pathogenic spirochetes, they require long chain fatty acids for growth They are cultivatable in Kelly medium,[1] a complex broth containing proteose peptone, tryptone, bovine serum albumin, rabbit serum, *N*-acetylglucosamine, citric acid, and pyruvate, in addition to glucose and salts. *B. recurrentis* is more fastidious than the tick-borne *Borrelia* species and requires the further addition of asparagine and choline to Kelly medium. *Borrelia* organisms grow slowly in Kelly medium (doubling time 18 to 26 hours).

Antigenic variation of *Borrelia* occurs in the course of relapsing fever, giving rise to relapse strains that are not recognized by antibody that develops against the initial infecting serotype. In *B. hermsii* infection, 25 different serotypes have been identified with different outer membrane proteins. Barbour[2] showed that switches among serotypes follow from recombination between linear plasmids that carry the genes for these antigens.

S. minus is fundamentally different from *Borrelia* spirochetes in structure, being a tightly coiled gram-negative rod with external polar flagella. The organisms are 2 to 5 μm long and have two to six spirals. They cannot be propagated in artificial culture media.

Epidemiology

In louse-borne relapsing fever, the vector for *B. recurrentis* is the human body louse, *Pediculus humanus humanus,* and the only known natural reservoir is humans. Thus, the cycle of infection is simply from person to person via the louse. Body lice acquire the infection by feeding on a spirochetemic person, and they remain infected for their entire life span, 10 to 61 days under laboratory conditions.[3] The ingested spirochetes pass through the esophagus to the midgut, where they penetrate the gut epithelium to reach the hemolymph, in which they will multiply. Infection is believed to be transmitted to humans after lice are crushed on the skin, which allows liberated spirochetes to penetrate through a bite site or through intact skin. Body lice prefer the normal human body temperature of 37°C over higher temperatures, so lice are likely to leave the skin of a febrile person to go to another person. This may in part explain the rapid transmission of infection during epidemics.

The vectors of tick-borne relapsing fever are argasid ticks of the genus *Ornithodoros.* The major reservoirs of the tick-borne relapsing fevers are wild rodents The infection is passed between the reservoir animals by tick bites, and humans are accidental hosts when they come into contact with infected animal ticks. The exception to the animal reservoirs may be *Borrelia duttonii* in East Africa, which is carried by the domestic tick *Ornithodoros moubata,* for which humans appear to be the reservoir. Neonates have acquired infection from their mother's blood by either transplacental infection or exchange of blood at the time of birth.[4]

Ticks acquire the infection by biting and sucking blood from a spirochetemic animal. After entering the hemocele, the spirochetes invade other tissues of the tick, including the salivary glands, coxal glands on the legs, and the ovaries. Transmission of the infection to animals or humans follows either injection of infected saliva or coxal fluid through the bite site or intact skin. Ticks are more durable vectors than are body lice, being able to survive as long as 15 years between blood meals and to harbor viable spirochetes for years. In addition, female ticks can pass *Borrelia* spirochetes transovarially to their offspring, so ticks can be infective without having bitten an infected host.

Infections with *S. minus* are rare because of the rarity of rodent bites in the general population. *S. minus* is one cause of rat-bite fever; the other is *Streptobacillus moniliformis,* which can also cause a febrile illness without antecedent rat bites, known as Haverhill fever.

Pathogenesis and Clinical Manifestations

After a bite by a *Borrelia*-infected tick or louse, during an incubation period of 3 to 32 days, the spirochetes migrate outward in the skin and multiply. They are also disseminated via the lymph and blood to other skin sites and to other organs, including the heart and brain. The number of spirochetes that circulate in the blood is small in Lyme disease compared with relapsing fever.

In relapsing fever, the fever is caused by a nonendotoxic pyrogen in the spirochete that elicits interleukin-1 production by mononuclear phagocytes. Disseminated intravascular coagulation with thrombocytopenia leads to a petechial rash in some patients. The relapsing nature of the disease has been attributed to antigenic variation in the infecting population of spirochetes. In experimental infections of rats with *B. hermsii,* separate serotypes emerged sequentially during relapses with the appearance of specific antibody in response to each of the antigenic variants.

The majority of patients with relapsing fever recover from their illness with or without antibiotic treatment. (For a more clinical description, see Chapter 177.) Patients develop antibodies against *Borrelia,* which can agglutinate, kill, or opsonize the spirochetes. In the presence of opsonizing antibody, spirochetes are rapidly phagocytosed and digested by polymorphonuclear leukocytes.[5] These antibodies also participate in rendering patients immune to future infection with *Borrelia* of the same serotype.

In rat-bite fever, there is an incubation period of 1 to 4 weeks from the bite to the appearance of inflammation at the bite site. The disease starts with fever. A red-brown macular rash spreads outward on the skin and has been described to recede and sometimes to relapse. A purulent ulcer at the bite site is common, and patients may develop lymphangitis and regional lymphadenitis. The disease resolves spontaneously in 1 to 2 months. Antibodies against *S. minus* arise during the disease and may cause a false-positive Venereal Disease Research Laboratory test result.

Diagnosis

Culture of the causative spirochetes in these diseases is not feasible in routine laboratories. The diagnosis of relapsing fever is made by demonstrating spirochetemia using Wright-stained blood smears. In *S. minus* infections, the spirochetes may be visualized by darkfield microscopy of skin lesion or lymph node specimens and, sometimes, blood. Intraperitoneal inoculation of clinical specimens into guinea pigs or mice has been used to demonstrate the organism in the animal's blood.

Treatment

Antibiotic treatment is effective against these infections. For relapsing fever, a single dose of tetracycline or erythromycin is recommended. Procaine penicillin G is also effective but results in relapses more often than does tetracycline (see Chapter 177). *S. minus* infections are treatable with intramuscular procaine penicillin G for 10 days or oral ampicillin or penicillin V for 10 days.[6]

Prevention

No vaccine is available against *Borrelia* spirochetes and *S. minus*. Prevention of these infections can be achieved by avoiding exposure to ticks and lice in endemic areas. Useful measures include wearing garments that cover arms and legs completely and applying tick repellants to the skin.

References

1. Kelly R: Cultivation of *Borrelia hermsii*. Science 17:433, 1971.
2. Barbour AG: Antigenic variation of a relapsing fever *Borrelia* species. Annu Rev Microbiol 44:155, 1990.
3. Burgdorfer W: The epidemiology of the relapsing fevers *In* Johnson RC (ed): The Biology of Parasitic Spirochetes. New York, Academic Press, 1976, pp 191–200.
4. Yagupsky P, Moses S: Neonatal *Borrelia* species infection (relapsing fever). Am J Dis Child 139:74, 1985.
5. Butler T, Aikawa M, Hable-Michael A, et al: Phagocytosis of *Borrelia recurrentis* by polymorphonuclear leukocytes is enhanced by antibiotic treatment. Infect Immun 28:1009, 1980.
6. Roughgarden JW: Antimicrobial treatment of rat bite fever Arch Intern Med 116:39, 1965.

226

Leptospira

Patrick W. Kelley

Human infections with pathogenic members of the genus *Leptospira* can cause clinical manifestations—jaundice, hemorrhage, renal failure, and death—or no symptoms. Among domestic animals, *Leptospira* organisms are economically important causes of morbidity and mortality; the acute and long-term manifestations of infection can include loss of milk production, abortion, stillbirth, infertility, death, and chronic urinary shedding of viable organisms. Leptospiral infections are among the most widespread zoonoses, being transmitted by both wild and domestic animals through direct or indirect contact with their urine. Humans are accidental hosts in the transmission cycle.

Characteristics of the Pathogen

Classification and Antigenic Characteristics

Traditionally, members of the genus *Leptospira* have been classified as one of three species: *Leptospira interrogans*, the pathogenic strains, or *Leptospira biflexa* and *Leptospira parva*, the free-living, saprophytic strains. Except where otherwise noted, this chapter is confined to a discussion of the pathogenic strains. The basic taxon for serologically distinct strains within species is the serovar. The standard method for categorizing *Leptospira* organisms in one of the serovar categories is the microagglutination test with cross-agglutinin absorption. Two strains are said to belong to different serovars if, after cross-absorption with adequate amounts of heterologous antigen, more than 10% of the homologous titer regularly remains in at least one of the two antiserum samples in repeated tests.[1] This technique is time-consuming and exacting. There are more than 200 serovars of *L. interrogans* grouped into approximately 23 serogroups on the basis of shared major agglutinogens; *L. biflexa* contains about 65 serovars divided into about 38 serogroups.[2] *L. parva* has one serovar. Serogroups have no taxonomic status but are useful for defining the composition of screening batteries used to test sera or identify isolates. This approach to classification is not fully satisfactory for defining epidemiologically important entities and is laborious to perform. Various molecular biologic methods are now being investigated that can use antigenic or genetic approaches to classification. DNA hybridization techniques demonstrate extreme heterogeneity within the two currently defined species. This heterogeneity is independent of the grouping of serovars into serogroups, in that serovars from antigenically defined serogroups may belong to different genetically defined categories.[3,4] Restriction endonuclease analysis has also been applied to *Leptospira*.[5–7] Monoclonal antibody techniques may eventually find applications not only in classification but also in diagnosis and immunization.[1] Polymerase chain reaction methods are also being used to classify leptospires.[8]

Structure

Leptospira organisms are motile, flexible, tightly coiled (18 or more coils per cell) helicoid rods 0.1 to 0.2 μm in diameter and 6 to 20 μm in length (Fig. 226–1). Their narrow diameters allow them to pass through 0.2-μm membrane filters. One or both ends of the cell are usually hooked. Morphologically, *L. interrogans* and *L. biflexa* are indistinguishable. Like other members of the order Spirochaetales, *Leptospira* organisms have two independent, periplasmic, axial filaments that are attached subterminally at each end of the cell; the filaments' free ends extend down the axis of the coil toward the middle, where they may overlap a bit. The helicoid body has a cytoplasmic membrane–cell wall complex similar to that of gram-negative bacteria. A three- to five-layered outer envelope or sheath surrounds the protoplasmic cylinder and axial filaments. Even with staining, owing to the thinness of the organism and its motility, darkfield microscopy is necessary for optimal visualization. The motion of *Leptospira* is characteristic and appears in liquid environments as an alternating

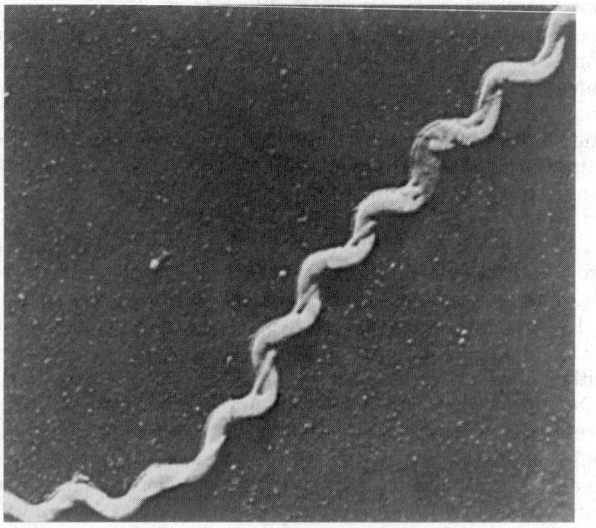

FIGURE 226–1 □ Electron micrograph of *Leptospira interrogans* (serovar *canicola*) showing the tightly coiled helicoid rod with the periplasmic axial filament. (Armed Forces Institute of Pathology, AFIP No. 60–10941.)

---

rotation around the long axis and translation in the direction of the unhooked cell end. In environments of higher viscosity, flexing, boring, and serpentine movements have also been described. There are a few strains without hooked ends, which have little or no translational motility.[2]

Biologic and Biochemical Properties

Leptospira organisms are obligate aerobes. Their nutritional requirements are simple but unique. They use long-chain fatty acids or fatty alcohols (15 carbons or more) rather than carbohydrates or amino acids as a source of energy and carbon. Because they cannot synthesize fatty acids, exogenous supplies are also the source of cellular lipids. Because free fatty acids are inherently toxic, in artificial media they are usually supplied bound to albumin or in a detoxified, esterified form. Nitrogen requirements can be met by urea or ammonium salts but not by amino acids. Unlike other spirochetes, *Leptospira* can use exogenous purines but not pyrimidines for DNA synthesis. This fact permits the use in culture media of the pyrimidine analog 5-fluorouracil as a means of selectively preventing the overgrowth of potential contaminants. *Leptospira* organisms also differ from other spirochetes in their ability to synthesize whatever amino acids they require.[9] In addition to the fatty acids, vitamin B_1 (thiamine), vitamin B_{12} (cyanocobalamin), iron, and other trace elements are absolute nutritional requirements. Pyruvate enhances the growth of *Leptospira,* particularly the *hardjo* and *ballum* serovars. *Leptospira* organisms have been shown to possess cytochrome enzymes and catalase as well as enzymes of the citric acid cycle and glycolytic and pentose pathways; they also have an acyl coenzyme A dehydrogenase for the β-oxidation of fatty acids.[10] They are oxidase-positive. Hyaluronidase produced by pathogenic *Leptospira* species may account for their invasive capability (e.g., into the cerebrospinal fluid). Potentially toxic components or products of *Leptospira* have been identified, but their role in the pathogenesis of the disease remains to be established.

Leptospira organisms can live free or in association with human and animal hosts. A key characteristic of *L. interrogans,* the parasitic species, is its ability to survive for long periods in the proximal convoluted tubules of the kidney of some animals. On being shed, *L. interrogans* can survive under favorable conditions in the environment as long as 6 months. The optimal temperature for survival is 28°C to 32°C, although they can also survive subzero temperatures, including freezing in liquid nitrogen.[11] Acid environments or concentrated acid urine significantly reduces survival. Tropical, unpolluted, nonsaline waters that are slightly alkaline (pH 7.2 to 8.0) provide an ideal environment. Survival is less favored in tropical areas, where rainfall is low to moderate and seasonal. Under dry conditions, *Leptospira* may die within minutes.[11] The free-living species *(L. biflexa)* can be found in soil or surface waters; several *L. biflexa* strains have also been isolated from seawater. Survival of *L. interrogans* in seawater is short.[12] Serovars of *L. biflexa* rarely, if ever, appear to cause disease in animals or humans, although they can be isolated from animals.[2]

In addition to its pathogenicity and its more fastidious growth requirements, *L. interrogans* can be differentiated from *L. biflexa* in other ways. Unlike *L. biflexa, L. interrogans* does not grow at 13°C or in the presence of 8-azaguanine (225 μg/mL). All *L. interrogans* cells convert to spherical forms in the presence of 1 M sodium chloride; *L. biflexa* serovars do not. There is no genetic homology between *L. interrogans* and *L. biflexa.*[2]

Replication

Pathogenic *Leptospira* organisms can be isolated from water, blood, urine, cerebrospinal fluid, anterior chamber of the eye, peritoneal fluid, amniotic fluid, and various tissues. Successful isolation from a particular human source depends on the phase of the infection. The optimal time to isolate *Leptospira* from blood and cerebrospinal fluid is during the first week of symptoms; isolation from urine is best after the first week. *Leptospira* organisms are effectively cultivated in a variety of media that meet the essential nutritional and other conditions. Modifications of the formulations of Ellinghausen-McCullough-Johnson-Harris (EMJH or Tween 80 albumin) or Fletcher are especially effective.[12; 13] When properly inoculated with a minimal amount of material, kept in the dark, and aerated at 28°C to 30°C, these media can support generation times of about 7 to 12 hours and yield 6 to 8 × 10^9 cells per mL.[12] Cultures should be kept for 6 to 8 weeks and examined weekly for growth by darkfield microscopy. When growth is observed, subcultures of fresh media should be made because primary cultures may become nonviable.

Liquid media are used for cultures employed in serodiagnostic techniques and for typing isolates. For the purpose of obtaining isolates from body fluids or tissues, a semisolid medium is made by incorporating 0.2% agar. Growth may be visualized as one or more dense rings several millimeters to centimeters below the surface of the medium.[12] Absence of rings does not preclude the presence of *Leptospira.* Solid media (made by adding 1% or 2% agar to the liquid) are useful for making isolations from contaminated sources or for cloning leptospires. Colonies on 1% agar solid media are diffuse to discrete and are usually subsurface. Colonies grown on 2% agar are usually turbid to clear and are located on the surface. Some strains on 1% and 2% agar can be either surface or subsurface.[2] Some pathogenic strains tend to lose their virulence and immunogenicity after a series of passages in media. Animal passage is better for maintaining these characteristics, and weanling hamsters are best for this purpose.[2] Baby guinea pigs, baby rabbits, or gerbils are acceptable although inferior alternatives, as they are comparatively less susceptible to *Leptospira.*

Epidemiology

Transmission

Human beings, accidental hosts in the transmission cycle, usually become infected when, in the course of occupational or recreational activities, pathogens in animal urine or urine-contaminated water or soil enter through the skin or mucous membranes (Fig. 226–2). Through urination and consequent contamination of soil and surface waters, animals that shed *Leptospira* can also infect their offspring, others of their species, and other species. Animals may shed *Leptospira* for months or even years, continuously or sporadically. Pigs and other herbivores that have alkaline urine tend to excrete greater numbers of organisms and consequently may pose a greater risk than animals with more acid urine, such as dogs. The infection in animals can be transmitted to offspring transplacentally, venereally, or through milk.[12, 14, 15] As in humans, infection in animals may be asymptomatic or it may be fatal.

Distribution

Leptospira organisms can be found in virtually all tropical and temperate areas of the world. Their density in the environment depends on the presence of suitable domestic and wild animal carriers and on environmental variables, including season and moisture conditions. If carrier animals come into close contact with humans and other animals, even relatively arid regions can develop endemic foci of lep-

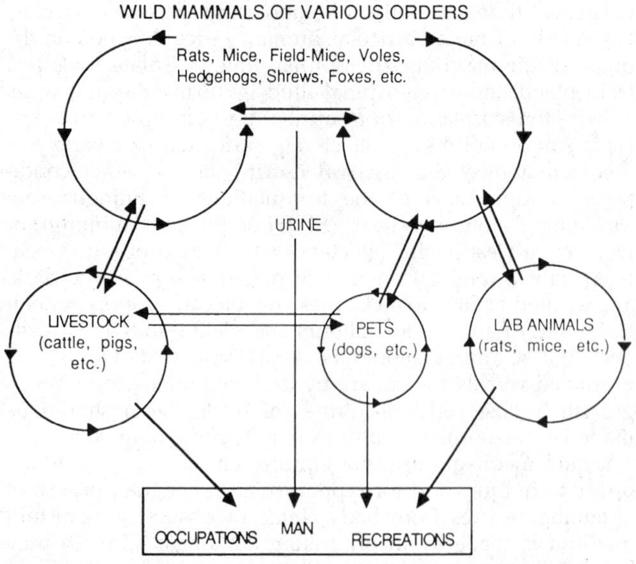

FIGURE 226–2 □ The leptospiral transmission cycle. (From Turner LH: Leptospirosis. I. Trans R Soc Trop Med Hyg 61:842–855, 1967.)

tospirosis. The number of serovars tends to be greater in wet tropical regions than in temperate areas. This may reflect the variety and density of animals in the tropics. Classically, specific serovars have been associated with specific animal species (e.g., rats and *Leptospira icterohaemorrhagiae* or dogs and *Leptospira canicola*), although host-serovar associations are dynamic and can vary between geographic areas and over time. Surveillance can show previously "alien" serovars adapting for carriage in a particular species.[16] Virulence or transmissibility of a specific serovar for animals and humans is not necessarily constant either and may be influenced by intermediate host factors.[11, 14] The changing dynamics of animal-serovar relationships are not fully understood. Alterations in the local ecology (e.g., increased contact between farm animals and rodents) probably contribute to some alterations of distribution and risk to humans. Although one should assume that any pathogenic species of *Leptospira* can produce the full spectrum of clinical disease in humans and animals, knowledge of the prevailing serovars and their hosts is important so that evolving transmission patterns may be documented and appropriate preventive interventions employed. Also, animal vaccines against leptospirosis are serovar specific and so must periodically be reevaluated.

Prevalence

Evidence of past or current leptospiral infection in both animals and humans may be quite high in various subpopulations. The chronic carrier state is a common finding in animals, including asymptomatic ones. In 1977, Thiermann[17] found that more than 90% of Norway rats *(Rattus norvegicus)* collected in Detroit were carriers of *Leptospira*. A 1984 survey of six small-mammal species that live in an area of Panamanian jungle and that are associated with many cases of leptospirosis in U.S. troops there showed that 42% of 139 animals caught carried leptospires (Takafuji ET, unpublished data). Alston and Broom[18] reviewed 19 *Leptospira* prevalence studies in dogs and noted that 30% to 40% of the apparently healthy dogs in some areas of the world showed infection. Traditionally, leptospirosis has been described as an occupationally transmitted infection. Occupational groups with a high incidence of infection include agriculture and aquaculture workers; abattoir workers; persons employed in rat-infested environments such as various fish or poultry processors; those involved in animal husbandry or veterinary medicine; sewer, construction, and mine workers; certain laboratory workers; and military personnel. Over time, a greater proportion of leptospirosis cases have been attributed to recreational activities that bring people into contact with leptospiruric animals or with contaminated soil or bodies of water.[19]

Pathogenesis

After *Leptospira* organisms enter humans via breaks in the skin or through mucous membranes, they circulate in the blood stream and spread to various target organs. The primary pathologic lesion is damage to the endothelium of small blood vessels. This is associated with localized ischemic damage to the renal tubules, liver, meninges, muscle, and placenta. The mechanism by which *Leptospira* organisms cause vascular damage is not fully understood, although elaborated toxins may play a role with at least some serovars. The immune response to leptospirosis depends on the production of specific antibody, opsonization, and subsequent phagocytosis. The immunoglobulin M antibody becomes detectable late in the first week of illness. Titers reach maximum by the third or fourth week. Low agglutinin titers may be measurable for months or years. Secondary infections with an unrelated serovar are possible. Among survivors of leptospirosis, target organ damage usually resolves and chronic sequelae are uncommon.

Clinical Manifestations

Human infections by the pathogenic *Leptospira* species usually present as mild influenza-like illness characterized by sudden onset of fever, headache, profound myalgias, chills, back pain, joint pain, neck stiffness, conjunctival suffusion, and prostration. Most cases with this presentation are self-limited and last less than 10 days. Some patients experience relapse after a brief asymptomatic period, with fever and frequently headache. The relapse tends to last only a few days. A minority of patients with leptospirosis develop severe disease associated with a variety of manifestations, which can include renal failure, jaundice, skin and mucosal hemorrhage, hemoptysis, myocarditis, liver failure, and death. The renal failure appears to be most highly correlated with a fatal outcome; dialysis is frequently lifesaving. Recovery is usually complete, even in severe cases. Leptospirosis in pregnancy has been associated with fetal death. Asymptomatic infections with pathogenic *Leptospira* are uncommon. The clinical manifestations of human leptospiral infections are described in more detail in Chapter 176.

Leptospiral infections in animals can also vary significantly within and between species.[12] Typically, animal leptospirosis is also associated with symptoms of an acute febrile illness, including malaise, depression, anorexia, and conjunctivitis. Signs of bleeding, jaundice, central nervous system involvement, and liver and renal failure may also be noted. Acute leptospirosis in animals may also result in abortion, stillbirth, and mastitis. Some species of animals may develop a chronic kidney infection and shed *Leptospira* intermittently or continuously for months or years. These animals may or may not have had a detectable clinical illness.

Diagnosis

The diagnosis of leptospirosis in humans is typically based on clinical, epidemiologic, and serologic grounds. The initial test customarily employed to evaluate suspect cases of leptospirosis is the macroscopic slide agglutination test. Slides for this test are available commercially. The serovar pool or pools used in this test should represent the serovars endemic to the area where the patient may have been infected. Human sera cross-react between serovars to a greater extent than do sera from domestic animals. This allows some of the macroagglutination tests for the screening of humans to use serovars of *L. biflexa* as the antigen. The sensitivity and specificity of either approach to macroagglutination screening are limited. Determination of the pathogenic serovar often requires a more specific procedure, such as the microagglutination test.[12] The microagglutination test, which is the traditional method used for serologic confirmation, is complicated and time-consuming, requires a darkfield microscope, and is somewhat hazardous; unlike the macroagglutination test, it usually employs a battery of live *Leptospira* for antigen. Again, it is best when the organisms in the battery are fresh and represent the serovars that are endemic in the area of possible transmission. In general, three weekly serum specimens should be collected for serologic testing. A serologically confirmed case of leptospirosis is defined by a microagglutination test that shows either seroconversion from a titer of less than 1:50 to at least 1:200 or a fourfold or greater change in the titer between acute- and convalescent-phase serum specimens studied at the same laboratory. A presumptive case of leptospirosis can be defined by a microagglutination titer of at least 1:200 on a single specimen obtained after the onset of symptoms or a stable titer of at least 1:100 on consecutive specimens. A titer of at least 1:800 in the presence of compatible symptoms is strong evidence of recent or current leptospirosis.[14, 20] A variety of other testing methods have been used, including enzyme-linked immunosorbent assay tests.[21] Dot enyme-linked immunosorbent assays that are genus specific, simple, sensitive, specific, and easily adaptable for use in the field are being developed,[22, 23] along with indirect hemagglutination and immunofluorescent antibody tests and gold immunoblot and polymerase chain reaction assays.[8, 24–26] False-negative serologic results may reflect antibiotic treatment, suboptimal timing of specimen collection, or suboptimal composition of the antigen pool used in the various tests.

Vigorous attempts should be made to culture the organism from blood, urine, and (when indicated) cerebrospinal fluid or tissue specimens. One reason for this is that the highest microagglutination titer observed among individual serovars in the test panel does not necessarily indicate the infecting serovar. As early as possible during the first week of symptoms (and before antibiotic administration), patients who have an appropriate clinical and epidemiologic history should have multiple blood specimens taken aseptically for culture on Fletcher, EMJH, or a similar, commercially prepared semisolid medium.[12] Cultures should be inoculated at the bedside. If special media are not immediately available, blood should be collected aseptically in a tube containing either sodium oxalate or sodium heparin as the anticoagulant, held at room temperature, and inoculated onto media as soon as possible. Because large amounts of blood can inhibit leptospiral growth, serial dilutions are essential. Impressive recovery rates have been achieved by adding 1 mL of fresh, unclotted blood to 10 mL of medium in a tube and then serially diluting the cultures to yield three cultures with concentrations of 1:10, 1:100, and 1:1000. Several more blood specimens for culture should be taken during the first week of illness.

After the first several days of illness, *Leptospira* may be recoverable from the urine of infected humans and may persist for 30 days or longer. Because leptospiral shedding may be intermittent, several urine specimens for culture should be obtained. Patients whose urine is not alkaline should be given an alkalinizing regimen. Aseptically collected midstream urine should be inoculated promptly, as just described, to produce three tubes with 1:10, 1:100, and 1:1000 dilutions. The addition of 5-fluorouracil (100 to 200 μg/mL of media) to each tube can help control bacterial contamination. Tubes are incubated in the dark at 28°C to 30°C for up to 8 weeks. Cultures should be examined every few days by inspection and, if necessary, by darkfield examination of a loopful of medium.

Under certain conditions, it is possible to visualize *Leptospira* organisms in tissues by darkfield or phase-contrast (but not brightfield) microscopy. Silver-deposition techniques can enhance visualization of organisms; aniline dyes cannot. Nevertheless, failure to visualize the pathogen is never conclusive evidence. Fluorescent antibody staining techniques are useful if cultural or serologic techniques are not possible.[12] In some cases, differential centrifugation of body fluids is useful for removing cellular fibrils, extrusions, or fibrin strains that can resemble *Leptospira.* Close microscopic observation for both the characteristic morphology and mobility is necessary, but confirmation of the diagnosis requires serologic proof or isolation in culture. Direct microscopic examination of blood or tissues is most useful in situations in which the concentration of pathogens is high (e.g., in blood or liver suspensions from animals used for passage or in the examination of urine or kidney suspensions from natural animal hosts).

Treatment

Both penicillin and doxycycline are effective for the early treatment of leptospirosis, but the efficacy of these antibiotics after the first 4 or 5 days of illness has been controversial.[27–31] Details on relevant treatment studies are provided in Chapter 176. Animal studies suggest that some of the newer penicillins and cephalosporins may also be useful in treating leptospirosis.[32]

Prevention

Implementation of specific approaches to the prevention of leptospirosis in a particular area requires an understanding of the transmission factors that are important locally. A good medical surveillance program for both humans and animals is invaluable in providing this sort of information. Preventive measures can include techniques to reduce wild animal contact with humans and domestic animals; use, when practical, of protective clothing and other equipment; and avoiding contact with water or soil in potentially contaminated areas, such as the land near farm ponds or slowly moving streams. Annual immunizations can significantly reduce the risk of disease in domestic animals. Secondarily, immunized animals may be less likely to infect their human caretakers. Animal vaccines do not necessarily prevent infection and subsequent shedding of viable *Leptospira* organisms. Laboratory workers should be cognizant of the risk associated with handling leptospiral isolates and infectious tissues. Appropriate measures are indicated to disinfect contaminated surfaces and to prevent mucous membrane or needlestick exposures to the agent. In certain groups of people with short-term exposure to *Leptospira,* 200 mg of doxycycline weekly may be used for prophylaxis.[33] In the United States, there are no licensed human vaccines against leptospirosis, but in some other countries human vaccines against leptospirosis have been reported to be useful.[34]

References

1. Stallman ND: International Committee on Systematic Bacteriology: Subcommittee on the Taxonomy of Leptospira. Int J Syst Bacteriol 37:472, 1987.
2. Johnson RC, Faine S: Family II. Leptospiraceae Hovind-Hougen *In* Krieg NR, Holt JG (eds): Bergey's Manual of Systematic Bacteriology, Vol 1. Baltimore, Williams & Wilkins, 1984, pp 62–67.
3. Yasuda PH, Steigerwalt AG, Sulzer KR, et al: Deoxyribonucleic acid relatedness between serogroups and serovars in the family Leptospiraceae with proposals for seven new *Leptospira* species. Int J Syst Bacteriol 37:407, 1987.
4. Brendel JJ, Rogul M, Alexander AD: Deoxyribonucleic acid hybridization among selected leptospiral serotypes. Int J Syst Bacteriol 24:205, 1974.
5. Terpstra WJ: Serodiagnosis of bacterial diseases: Problems and developments. Scand J Immunol 36(Suppl) 11:91, 1992.
6. Hookey JV: Characterization of Leptospiraceae by 16S DNA restriction fragment length polymorphisms. J Gen Microbiol 139:1681, 1993.
7. Hookey JV, Bryden J, Gatehouse L: The use of 16S rDNA sequence analysis to investigate the phylogeny of Leptospiraceae and related spirochaetes. J Gen Microbiol 139:2585, 1993.
8. Merien F, Amouriaux P, Perolat P, et al: Polymerase chain reaction for detection of *Leptospira* spp. in clinical samples. J Clin Microbiol 30:2219, 1992.
9. Johnson RC: Comparative spirochete physiology and cellular composition. *In* Johnson RC (ed): The Biology of Parasitic Spirochetes. New York, Academic Press, 1976, pp 39–48.
10. Smibert RM: Spirochaetales, a review. Crit Rev Microbiol 2:491, 1973.
11. Torten M: Leptospirosis. *In* Steele JH (ed): Handbook Series in Zoonoses, Vol 1. Boca Raton, FL, CRC Press, 1979, pp 363–421.
12. Faine S (ed): Guidelines for the Control of Leptospirosis. Geneva, World Health Organization, 1982.
13. Ellinghausen HC, McCullough WG: Nutrition of *Leptospira pomona* and growth of 13 other serotypes. Fractionation of oleic albumin complex and a medium of bovine albumin and polysorbate 80. Am J Vet Res 26:45, 1965.
14. Feigin RD, Anderson DC: Human leptospirosis. Crit Rev Clin Lab Sci 5–413, 1975.
15. Bolin CA, Koellner P: Human-to-human transmission of *Leptospira interrogans* by milk. J Infect Dis 158:246, 1988.
16. Shenberg E, Birnbaum S, Rodrig E, et al: Dynamic changes in the epidemiology of canicola fever in Israel: Natural adaptation of an established serotype to a new reservoir host. Am J Epidemiol 105:42, 1977.
17. Thiermann AB: Incidence of leptospirosis in the Detroit rat population. Am J Trop Med Hyg 26:970, 1977.
18. Alston JM, Broom JC: Leptospirosis in Man and Animals. Edinburgh, E & S Livingstone, 1958.
19. Kaufmann AF: Epidemiologic trends of leptospirosis in the United States, 1965–1974. *In* Johnson RC (ed): The Biology of Parasitic Spirochetes. New York, Academic Press, 1976, pp 177–190.
20. Faine S: Leptospirosis. *In* Balows A, Hausler WA, Ohashi M, Turano A (eds): Laboratory Diagnosis of Infectious Diseases—Principles and Practice, Vol 1. New York, Springer-Verlag, 1988, pp 344–352.
21. Terpstra WJ, Lighart GS, Schoone GJ: Serodiagnosis of human leptospirosis by enzyme-linked immunosorbent assay (ELISA). Zentralbl Bakteriol Hyg 247:400, 1980.
22. Pappas MG, Ballou WR, Gray MR, et al: Rapid serodiagnosis of leptospirosis using the IgM-specific dot ELISA: Comparison with the microscopic agglutination test. Am J Trop Med Hyg 34:346, 1985.
23. Watt G, Alquiza LM, Padre LP, et al: The rapid diagnosis of leptospirosis: A prospective comparison of the dot enzyme-linked immunosorbent assay and the genus-specific microscopic agglutination test at different stages of illness. J Infect Dis 157:840, 1988.
24. Petchclai B, Hiranras S, Kunakorn M, et al: Enzyme-linked immunosorbent assay for leptospirosis immunoglobulin M specific antibody using surface antigen from a pathogenic *Leptospira:* A comparison with indirect hemagglutination and microagglutination tests. J Med Assoc Thai 75:203, 1992.
25. Appassakij H, Silpapojakul K, Wansit R, Woodtayakorn J: Evaluation of the immunofluorescent antibody test for the diagnosis of human leptospirosis. Am J Trop Med Hyg 52:340, 1995.
26. Petchclai B, Hiranras S, Potha U: Gold immunoblot analysis of IgM-specific antibody in the diagnosis of human leptospirosis. Am J Trop Med Hyg 45:672, 1991.
27. McClain JB, Ballou WR, Harrison SM, Steinweg DL: Doxycycline therapy for leptospirosis. Ann Intern Med 100:696, 1984.
28. Kocen RS: Leptospirosis: A comparison of symptomatic and penicillin therapy. Br Med J 1:1181, 1962.
29. Russell RW: Treatment of leptospires with oxytetracycline. Lancet 2:1143, 1958.
30. Watt G, Padre LP, Tuazon ML, et al: Placebo-controlled trial of intravenous penicillin for severe and late leptospirosis. Lancet 1:433, 1988.
31. Edwards CN, Nicholson GD, Hassell TA, et al: Penicillin therapy in icteric leptospirosis. Am J Trop Med Hyg 39:388, 1988.
32. Alexander AD, Rule PL: Penicillins, cephalosporins, and tetracyclines in treatment of hamsters with fatal leptospirosis. Antimicrob Agents Chemother 30:835, 1986.
33. Takafuji ET, Kirkpatrick JW, Miller RN, et al: An efficacy trial of doxycycline chemoprophylaxis against leptospirosis. N Engl J Med 310:497, 1984.
34. Alexander AD: Immunity in leptospirosis. *In* Johnson RC (ed): The Biology of Parasitic Spirochetes. New York, Academic Press, 1976, pp 339–349.

227

Helicobacter

Julie Parsonnet

Spiral gastric bacteria have been recognized in the human stomach since 1906.[1] It was not until 1982, however, that *Helicobacter pylori* was isolated and speciated for the first time. Today, *Helicobacter* is a rapidly expanding genus of bacteria that encompasses numerous species, four of which infect humans. The *Helicobacter* species that infect humans can be divided into two types: the gastric, urease producers (*H. pylori* and *Helicobacter heilmannii* [also known as *Gastrospirillum hominis*]) and the enteric non–urease producers (*Helicobacter cinaedi* and *Helicobacter fennelliae* [formerly *Campylobacter cinaedi* and *Campylobacter fennelliae*]). Case reports of human infection with three *Helicobacter* species that infect animals (*Helicobacter pullorum, Helicobacter felis,* and *Helicobacter canis*) have not been fully enough substantiated to classify them definitively as human pathogens.[2, 3] With the exception of *H. pylori, Helicobacter* infections of humans are unusual. *H. pylori*, on the other hand, is one of the most common bacterial infections of humans. Moreover, the diseases attributed to *H. pylori* infection, peptic ulcer disease and gastric malignancy, are major causes of morbidity and mortality worldwide. Consequently, the past decade has witnessed intense research into diagnosis, treatment, and prevention of this infection. Because of its clinical importance relative to other *Helicobacter* species, this chapter focuses predominantly on *H. pylori.*

Microbiology

Helicobacter organisms are microaerophilic, spiral, gram-negative rods that are phylogenetically closest to *Wolinella, Arco-*

bacter, and *Campylobacter*.[3, 4] Under stress, such as prolonged culture, *Helicobacter* may lose their spiral morphologic characteristic and first become more simply curved and eventually coccoid.[5, 6] In the case of *H. pylori*, these coccoid forms appear to be metabolically active and transmissible but noncultivatable.[5, 7, 8] *Helicobacter* are motile and typically have multiple flagella. *H. pylori* is 2.5 to 5.0 μm long with four to eight unipolar flagella providing a corkscrew motility. *H. fennelliae* and *H. cinaedi*, in contrast, have only one monopolar or two bipolar flagella. Chemical characteristics of the *Helicobacter* species can be seen in Table 227–1. The chemical characteristics of *H. heilmannii* are largely unknown because it has not yet been cultured in vitro. These gastric organisms, which are longer (3.5 to 7.5 μm) and much more tightly coiled than *H. pylori*, may represent several genetically distinct species.

Helicobacter organisms are relatively fastidious. To culture *H. pylori* from the stomach, biopsy specimens should be immediately placed in transport medium to prevent desiccation. As soon as possible, the ground specimens should be plated on solid agar.[9] Recovery of enteric *Helicobacter* from stool or blood is conducted in much the same way as culture of *Campylobacter* except at 37°C instead of 42°C. Many agar bases sustain *Helicobacter* if supplemented with blood or serum; antimicrobial supplements in the medium minimize overgrowth of competing organisms and increase culture sensitivity.[9] Plates should be incubated under microaerophilic conditions at 37°C. *Helicobacter* organisms grow slowly, and plates and BACTEC bottles may require incubation for 7 days to develop recognizable colonies. Because of their indolent growth, positive results of blood cultures may be missed unless an automated growth detection system is used. Presumptive identification can be made if organisms have typical gram-negative, curved morphologic characteristics on Gram stain and produce both catalase and oxidase.

Helicobacter pylori

Pathology, Pathogenesis, and Immunity

H. pylori resides beneath the mucous layer, adjacent to the surface and pit epithelial cells of the gastric antrum and body. Aside from ectopic gastric mucosa (e.g., Meckel's diverticula), no other tissue besides the stomach is known to be infectable with *H. pylori*. Motility appears to be critical for this colonization.[10] Approximately one fifth of the organisms are adherent to the mucosal surface, whereas the remainder appear to be free-living within the mucus layer.[11] Adherence is species specific and is related to features of both the host (e.g., blood group type) and the bacterium (e.g., production of adhesins such as pili and hemagglutinins).[12–14]

H. pylori produces urease at a constitutively high level. This enzyme, a 300- to 625-kDa nickel-containing hexamer, is located on the cell membrane and is also actively excreted into the gastric lumen.[11] Urease is essential for *H. pylori* colonization of the stomach but is not required for survival after colonization.[11, 15] The precise physiologic role of urease has not been definitively established.[16, 17] By hydrolyzing urea to carbon dioxide and ammonia, urease may surround the organism with a cloud of ammonia, protecting it from the stomach's acid environment.[18] Damage to the gastric mucosa induced by urease and ammonia may also provide the organism with the necessary nutrients and/or an appropriate environment for attachment and growth. Alternatively, urease activity may facilitate nitrogen assimilation by the organism.

H. pylori exhibits enormous genetic diversity. By using molecular typing methods (restriction fragment length polymorphisms, arbitrary primer polymerase chain reaction, or gene sequencing), it is unusual to find identical strains in different subjects.[19–21] Two biotypes, however, are currently recognized: types I and II.[22] Type I, but not type II, *H. pylori* strains produce a vacuolating cytotoxin that induces vacuole formation in tissue culture cells.[23] In mouse models, oral administration of purified cytotoxin results in vacuolization, inflammation, and gastric ulceration.[24] Expression of the vacuolating cytotoxin occurs in only 50% to 60% of strains, although all possess the *vacA* gene.[25] A second gene (the cytotoxin-associated gene [*cagA*]) is an excellent marker for cytotoxin expression. Although the function of the 128-kDa surface-exposed CagA protein remains unknown (it is not actually involved in cytotoxin expression), its detection by enzyme-linked immunosorbent assay has proved an excellent serologic tool for diagnosis of type I strains.

Infection with *H. pylori* is virtually always accompanied by acute and chronic inflammatory cells in the submucosa. The characteristic polymorphonuclear and mononuclear infiltrate has been termed superficial active gastritis, chronic superficial gastritis, type B gastritis, or *H. pylori*–associated chronic gastritis with polymorphonuclear cell activity.[26] In most patients, lymphoid follicles (mucosa-associated lymphoid tissue) are also evident.[27] These follicles may be particularly prominent in children. Gastric inflammation is accompanied by elevations in serum immunoglobulin G against several *H. pylori* antigens including the urease subunits and, when expressed by the bacterium, the vacuolating cytotoxin and the CagA protein. Two thirds of infected persons also mount an opsonizing immunoglobulin A response.[28]

H. pylori–related inflammation is thought to be mediated

TABLE 227–1 ■ Bacteriologic Characteristics of Human *Helicobacter* Infections*

	ENTERIC *HELICOBACTER*		GASTRIC *HELICOBACTER*	
CHARACTERISTIC	*H. cinaedi*	*H. fennelliae*	*H. heilmannii*	*H. pylori*
Urease production	−	−	+	+
Oxidase production	+	+	NA	+
Catalase production	+	+	NA	+
Nitrate reduction	+	−	NA	−
Alkaline phosphatase hydrolysis	−	+	NA	+
Indoxyl acetate hydrolysis	−	+	NA	−
Growth at 42°C	−	−	NA	−
Susceptibility to				
Nalidixic acid	S	S	NA	R
Cephalothin	I	S	NA	S

*S, Sensitive; I, intermediate; R, resistant; NA, not available.
Data from references 3 and 139.

by several pathogenic factors. Soluble surface proteins from *H. pylori,* including urease, cause activation of monocytes, polymorphonuclear chemotaxis, and induction of inflammatory cytokines.[29] The vacuolating cytotoxin also enhances cytokine expression. Increased interleukin-8 expression has been particularly well documented.[30, 31] The in vitro cytokine response to cytotoxin corresponds to the clinical observation that persons with type I strains of *H. pylori* have more severe inflammatory changes than those without.[32] *H. pylori* can also directly or indirectly cause cell damage and death. Urease and ammonia have both been implicated in this cell destruction.[33, 34]

Little is known about host or bacterial factors required for establishing infection. Given the high, but not universal, prevalence of *H. pylori* throughout the world, it seems likely that many exposures do not result in chronic infection. Windows of opportunity (such as periods of hypochlorhydria) may exist when the stomach permits infection. In vivo experiments support this finding; in two human inoculation experiments, infection could not be established without altering the gastric pH with histamine antagonists.[35, 36] Without treatment, infection with *H. pylori* persists as long as normal gastric epithelial cells remain lining the stomach (*H. pylori* cannot live in an epithelium replaced by atrophy or intestinal metaplasia). For many people, this probably means that the organism remains for a lifetime. Restriction fragment length polymorphism analyses demonstrated persistence of specific strains of *Helicobacter* in individuals for years.[37] Repeated serologic testing of infected individuals over time also demonstrated that the serum titers do not change in the absence of specific eradication therapy.[38, 39]

Persons with *H. pylori*–related gastritis can progress to a variety of clinical diseases. The pathogenic mechanisms for the variable outcome of infection, that is, asymptomatic, ulcer, or cancer, are largely unknown. It is assumed that differences in outcome can be explained by a combination of bacterial, environmental, and host factors. One popular model for peptic ulcer pathogenesis holds that, in some people, *H. pylori* infection increases postprandial gastrin production. This, in turn, increases acid production and predisposes the host to develop gastric metaplasia in the duodenum. Development of gastric metaplasia may be enhanced by smoking or use of nonsteroidal antiinflammatory agents. Gastric metaplasia allows *H. pylori* to colonize the duodenal mucosa, where its mucinases weaken the mucous barrier, fostering ulceration.[29, 40, 41] This process is particularly likely in persons with cytotoxin-producing strains of *H. pylori.*[23]

The pathogenesis of gastric malignancy differs from that of peptic ulcer disease (Fig. 227–1). Superficial gastritis progresses not to ulcers but to chronic atrophic gastritis, a condition characterized by destruction of the acid-secreting gastric glands.[42] In monkey models, chronic atrophic gastritis can be induced by sustaining *H. pylori* infection in the animal for several years.[43] Persons with atrophic gastritis are at increased risk for gastric cancer but are largely protected from peptic ulcer disease by virtue of their high gastric pH.[44, 45] It has been suggested that, in persons predisposed to cancer, loss of acid production is enhanced by a bacterial inhibitor of acid secretion.[46]

Chronic inflammation secondary to infection has long been known to predispose to malignancy at the inflamed site. Inflammation typically results in increased cell proliferation, enhancing the likelihood of random mutation. Inflammation also induces oxidative bursts of free radicals that can potentially damage DNA. Both enhanced cell proliferation and free radical formation have been observed in patients with *H. pylori*–associated gastritis.[47, 48] Given these factors, the likelihood for a carcinogenic combination of mutations to occur would almost certainly be higher in infected than in uninfected hosts. Undoubtedly, environmental, bacterial, and host factors can augment or minimize cancer risk attributable to *H. pylori* infection.[49, 50]

Epidemiology

H. pylori infection is common worldwide. Between and within population groups, however, prevalence can vary widely (Fig. 227–2). In some developing countries, most of the population is infected by age 10 years and infection is universal by midlife.[51] In industrialized countries, on the other hand, prevalence of infection is considerably lower although still far from rare. In the United States, at least one

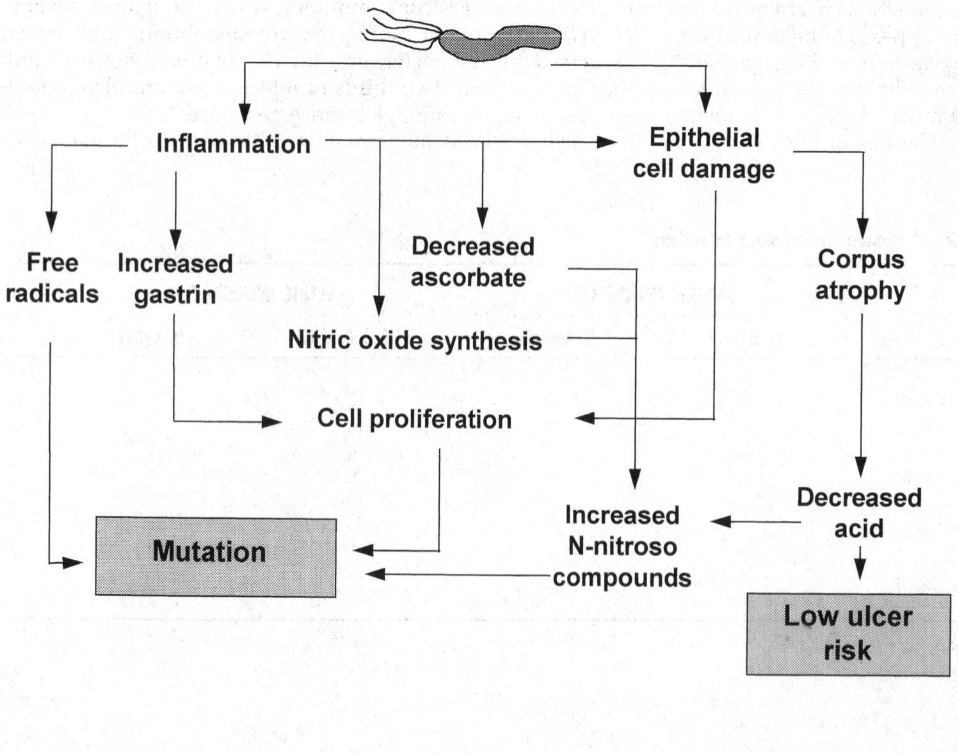

FIGURE 227–1 □ Hypothetic mechanism of *H. pylori*–related carcinogenesis. Chronic inflammation leads to mutation by inducing free radical formation, cell proliferation, and production of mutagens such as *N*-nitrosamines.

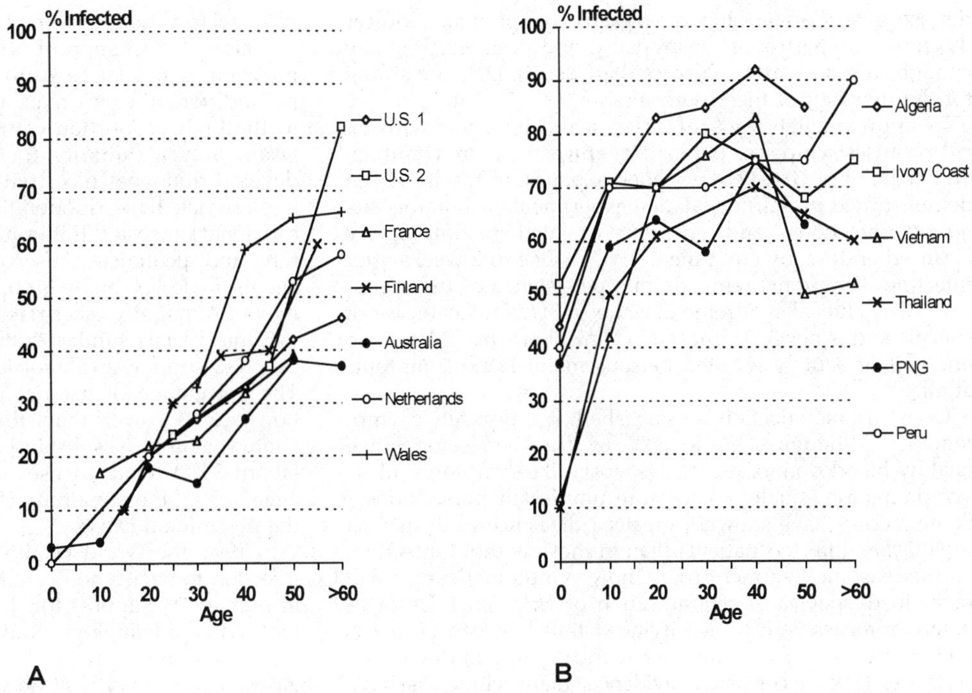

FIGURE 227–2 ▫ Prevalence of *H. pylori* infection by age in *(A)* industrialized countries and *(B)* developing countries. In industrialized countries, prevalence increases approximately 1% for each year of life. In developing countries, infection is much more common, particularly in childhood. (From Taylor DN, Blaser MJ: The epidemiology of *Helicobacter pylori* infection. Epidemiol Rev 13:50–51, 1991.)

third of the population is likely to be infected. This figure increases with advancing age. Frequently, a disproportionately high prevalence of *H. pylori* infection is observed in the elderly. This appears to reflect a birth cohort effect. In other words, older individuals have more infection because they were born at times when infection was more common than it is today.[38, 52, 53] Overall, *H. pylori* incidence is decreasing in industrialized countries with time. Seroconversion studies indicate that only 0.4% of uninfected adults acquire *H. pylori* each year.[54] In children, however, the incidence of infection may be higher than in adults. Thus, many now consider *H. pylori* a predominantly childhood infection that persists throughout life.

Virtually all studies to date have shown an inverse relationship between *H. pylori* infection and socioeconomic status.[55, 56] Socioeconomic status during childhood may serve as a particularly good indicator of *H. pylori* risk.[57] In the United States, African-American and Hispanic persons exhibit higher rates of infection than do non-Hispanic whites.[56, 58, 59] Outside the United States, racial and ethnic variations in *H. pylori* prevalence have also been observed.[60, 61] The reasons for racial and ethnic differences are not understood. Poor socioeconomic conditions during childhood, as measured by household crowding and parental income, are thought to play an important role. These cannot, however, completely explain observed differences, and a genetic component to infection cannot be excluded.[59] A comparison of *H. pylori* concordance in monozygotic and dizygotic twins suggested that a proportion of infection may be attributable to genetic factors.[62]

Person-to-person spread is widely considered to be the most prevalent means of *H. pylori* transmission. Infection is most likely to occur in populations in which fecal-oral disease transmission is common, such as in institutions for the disabled or families with young children.[63–68] Infection with *H. pylori* has also been related to other markers of fecal-oral transmission such as sibship size, birth order, and current number of children in the family.[60] Household crowding particularly engenders greater risk for infection, with sharing of beds during childhood an especially hazardous practice.[57, 69, 70] *H. pylori* is substantially more common among first-degree relatives of infected persons than in the general population, and strains of *H. pylori* among family members may, on occasion, be identical.[71–73] *H. pylori* has been cultured from feces of both children and adults, demonstrating that *H. pylori* can pass through the gastrointestinal tract and remain viable.[74, 75]

An oral-oral route of *H. pylori* transmission is supported by microbiologic but not epidemiologic studies. *H. pylori* DNA has frequently been recovered by polymerase chain reaction from both saliva and dental plaque; only on rare occasions, however, has *H. pylori* been cultured from the mouth.[76–78] Iatrogenic transmission of *H. pylori* via endoscopy has been well documented through the isolation of identical strains of *H. pylori* from patients undergoing endoscopy in the same suite. Transmission has been estimated to occur in 0.3% of endoscopy procedures when the endoscope is mechanically cleaned with detergent and ethanol alone.[79] More rigorous cleansing methods, however, prevent transmission.[80, 81] Endoscopists and endoscopy nurses appear to be at particularly high risk for infection, leading some to call *H. pylori* an occupational hazard.[82, 83]

Although the preponderance of evidence supports direct person-to-person spread of infection, some data suggest other transmission modalities. In particular, two epidemiologic studies from Latin America suggested that water and water-contaminated food might be vehicles for *H. pylori*.[84, 85] Similarities in the epidemiology of *H. pylori* infection and that of the hepatitis A virus have also been touted to support fecal-oral transmission through infected water.[86, 87] These correlations may well reflect common socioeconomic conditions, however, rather than common vectors.[88] To date, *H. pylori* has not been cultured from suspected water sources, although *H. pylori* DNA can be amplified from drinking water by using the polymerase chain reaction. Identification of naturally acquired *H. pylori* in laboratory cats (but not pet cats) suggests that domestic animals may carry infection, but transmission to humans is not yet supported by epidemiologic data.[89]

Clinical Disease

H. pylori infection has been linked to numerous diseases or syndromes including duodenal ulcer disease, gastric ulcer disease, gastric adenocarcinoma, gastric lymphoma, nonulcer dyspepsia, hypertrophic gastropathy, and even, surprisingly enough, coronary artery disease (Fig. 227–3). Data are strong for the first four of these outcomes.

In approximately 50% of cases, acute infection with *H. pylori* causes symptoms of bloating, epigastric pain, vomiting, and irritability 3 to 7 days after exposure. This has been demonstrated by self-inoculation experiments, laboratory-acquired infections, and epidemics related to improperly cleansed endoscopy equipment.[35, 36, 90–92] One to 2 weeks after infection, symptoms remit despite persistence of the organism.[36] The clinical syndrome of acute *H. pylori* infection is not specific and is never diagnosed in clinical practice. Moreover, one half of acutely infected persons manifest no symptoms at all.

Once chronic infection is established, it is typically asymptomatic. Although 20% to 30% of *H. pylori*–seropositive healthy blood donors report dyspepsia-like symptoms, these symptoms are equally common in uninfected populations.[93] Some studies have shown a greater prevalence of dyspepsia in *H. pylori*–infected patients than in those without infection. Similarly, some treatment trials show symptomatic improvement in dyspepsia after eradication of *H. pylori*.[94] Unfortunately, for each study identifying a link between *H. pylori* and dyspepsia, there is another with negative findings. Despite the lack of consistent evidence, many clinicians have observed cases of seemingly miraculous improvement in refractory, nonulcer dyspepsia after *H. pylori* eradication. Thus, *H. pylori* treatment may alleviate symptoms in some individuals, but it remains impossible to pinpoint a priori those who will benefit from such treatment.

H. pylori is the single most important cause of both duodenal and gastric ulcer diseases. Duodenal ulcers should now be assumed to be *H. pylori* related unless other predisposing conditions such as use of nonsteroidal antiinflammatory drugs, Zollinger-Ellison syndrome, or Crohn disease are present.[95] More than 90% of persons with duodenal ulcer disease have concomitant *H. pylori* infection. Moreover, persons treated with antimicrobial agents have much lower rates of

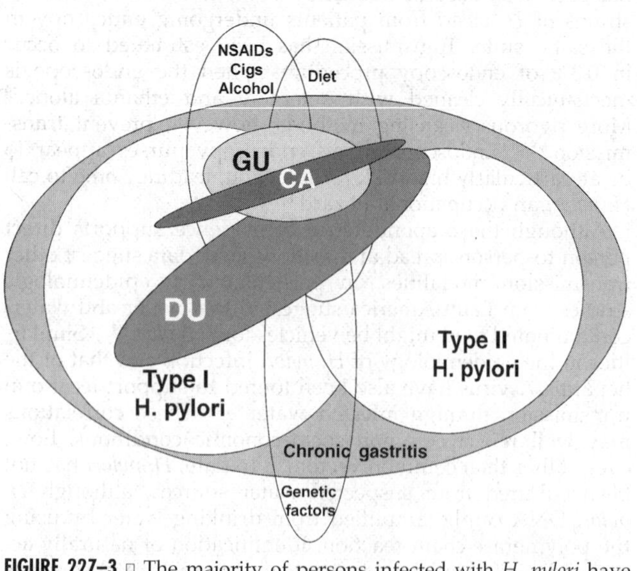

FIGURE 227–3 ▫ The majority of persons infected with *H. pylori* have asymptomatic chronic gastritis (outer oval). Approximately 20% eventually develop duodenal ulcer (DU) and a smaller percentage, gastric ulcer (GU) and/or gastric cancer (CA). Reasons for different clinical outcomes are not completely known. Important factors include biotype of *H. pylori* (type I strains are more virulent and more closely associated with ulcers and with cancer), host genetics, diet, and other environmental cofactors.

ulcer relapse than persons treated with acid inhibitory therapy alone.[96, 97] In support of a causal relationship, if *H. pylori* infection is not successfully eradicated, antibiotics provide no additional benefit over acid inhibition alone. In contrast to the high proportion of ulcers that are attributable to *H. pylori*, only a minority (perhaps 20%) of infected persons develop duodenal ulcer within a 10-year period.[42] Those at highest risk have duodenitis and gastric metaplasia of the duodenal mucosa.[98] Environmental cofactors, including cigarette and alcohol use, use of nonsteroidal antiinflammatory agents, male sex, blood group O, and other hereditary factors, may also magnify ulcer risk.[99]

Clinical trials similar to those conducted for duodenal ulcers also support a role for *H. pylori* in gastric ulcer disease.[96] The percentage of gastric disease attributable to *H. pylori*, however, is lower than that for duodenal ulcers. In the United States, a substantial proportion of gastric ulcers (about 35%) relate to use of nonsteroidal antiinflammatory agents.[100] Of the remaining 65%, *H. pylori* must be considered the preeminent cause.

In 1994, the World Health Organization declared *H. pylori* infection to be a type I carcinogen, a definite cause of cancer in humans.[101] Support for this declaration came from pathologic and epidemiologic studies. Together, these studies show that (1) chronic gastritis is an important cancer precursor, (2) gastric cancer occurs at an increased rate in regions with a high prevalence of *H. pylori* infection, (3) persons with *H. pylori* infection are at three- to eightfold higher risk for cancer than those without infection, and (4) *H. pylori* infection precedes cancer by many years.[102–104] It is estimated that 40% to 50% of malignancies in the gastric body and antrum (but not the gastroesophageal junction) are directly related to *H. pylori* infection. Yet despite this high attributable risk, less than 1% of infected persons can be expected to develop malignancy. The progression of mucosal changes from superficial gastritis to carcinoma probably requires decades. Therefore, individuals who acquire *H. pylori* infection early in life have the highest risk of malignancy, whereas those infected later in life are unlikely to develop cancer.[105] Other factors influencing the development of cancer include dietary exposures (nitrates and salts increase risk, fruits and vegetables decrease risk), genetic predisposition, and infection with cytotoxin-producing strains.[106, 107]

Gastric lymphoma is a rare disease; there are only seven cases per million population per year.[108] Because lymphocytes would probably not be in the stomach were *H. pylori* not present (the normal stomach contains few, if any, lymphocytes), it seems intuitive that infection would be linked to lymphoma. In epidemiologic studies, *H. pylori* infection has been found to increase the risk of developing diffuse histiocytic gastric lymphomas sixfold.[109] A particularly strong association of infection has been observed for mucosa-associated lymphoid tissue lymphoma, a type of low-grade lymphoma that arises from lymphoid follicles.[110, 111] The remarkable feature of these mucosa-associated lymphoid tissue lymphomas is that they may completely regress if *H. pylori* infection is eradicated with antibiotics.[79, 112] Why a few people with *H. pylori* infection develop these rare lymphomas is at present unknown.

Diagnosis

For patients undergoing endoscopy, a rapid urease test is the diagnostic test of choice (Table 227–2). A biopsy specimen of the stomach is obtained and placed in a urea-containing medium with a pH indicator. Production of ammonia turns the indicator red and confirms the presence of the organism. The rapid urease test can often be interpreted in less than 1 hour and is substantially less expensive than histology. It has

TABLE 227–2 ■ Diagnostic Tests for *Helicobacter pylori* Infection

TEST	SENSITIVITY (%)	SPECIFICITY (%)	COMMENTS	COST
Endoscopic				
Histology	93–99	95–99	Based on at least two antral biopsies	$$$
Culture	77–92	100	Technically demanding; best reserved for research	$$$
Rapid urease test	89–98	93–98	Endoscopic method of choice for diagnosis	$
Nonendoscopic				
Carbon 13 or carbon 14 breath test	90–100	89–100	Good for children and for follow-up; currently not widely available	$$
Serology	88–99	86–95	Nonendoscopic method of choice for initial diagnosis; not good for short-term follow-up	$

Adapted from Brown KE, Peura DA: Diagnosis of *Helicobacter pylori* infection. Gastroenterol Clin North Am 22:105–115, 1993.

90% sensitivity with even greater specificity for *H. pylori* infection.[113–115] For patients in whom evaluation of underlying gastric disease is essential, histologic examination may be preferable to the rapid urease test. Because *H. pylori* is not evenly distributed throughout the gastric mucosa, however, at least two biopsies need to be performed to diagnose infection sensitively.[116, 117] Routine hematoxylin-eosin or Giemsa staining usually reveals the organism; the more sensitive but more expensive silver stains should be reserved for inconclusive examinations.[118] Culture is the least sensitive but most specific endoscopic method for diagnosis of *H. pylori*. Because other diagnostic tests are cheaper and more widely available, however, culture is best reserved for research laboratories.

For patients for whom endoscopy is not necessary, serology is currently the simplest option for diagnosis. Most currently available assays are quantitative enzyme-linked immunosorbent assays that measure serum immunoglobulin G titers against *H. pylori*--specific antigens. In untreated patients, the immunoglobulin G response to *H. pylori* infection is stable for years, reflecting the chronic nature of infection even in the presence of routine antibiotic use.[38] Six months after successful eradication therapy against *H. pylori* infection, antibody titers typically decrease by at least 50%.[28, 119] This drop in titer appears to be quite sensitive and specific for successful treatment. Numerous commercial enzyme-linked immunosorbent assays with variable accuracy are currently available.[120] At their best, these assays have sensitivity and specificity for active infection exceeding 90% and sometimes exceeding 95%. Unfortunately, a serum sample obtained after successful therapy is not necessarily quantitatively negative. Thus, comparison of pre- and posttreatment titers is necessary for treatment follow-up. In-office, qualitative serologic assays are also now available. Like the commercial enzyme-linked immunosorbent assays, these appear to have excellent accuracy in the untreated patient.

Carbon-labeled urea breath tests hold much promise for *H. pylori* diagnosis and for treatment follow-up.[118, 121, 122] In these tests, the subject ingests either carbon 13– or carbon 14–labeled urea. If *H. pylori* is present in the stomach, the labeled urea is hydrolyzed by the urease enzyme into ammonia and labeled carbon dioxide. Using mass spectroscopy (carbon 13) or scintillography (carbon 14), labeled carbon dioxide is then measured in exhaled air. Although extensively used in research settings because of their high sensitivity, specificity, and ease of administration, breath tests are not yet readily available to clinicians. In the future, however, the breath test is expected to provide the "gold standard" for determining the success of *H. pylori* eradication therapy.

Treatment

H. pylori infection is curable with antimicrobial therapy. The three most widely used regimens are 2 weeks of metronidazole, tetracycline, and bismuth (70% to 90% cure); 2 weeks of omeprazole with either clarithromycin or amoxicillin (50% to 85% cure); and 1 week of omeprazole with clarithromycin and either metronidazole or amoxicillin (>90% cure). Because of the shorter duration of the last treatment, this combination seems to engender the best compliance and fewest side effects.[123, 124] Reinfection after successful treatment is rare (less than 1% per year in industrialized countries).[54] Eradication of the *H. pylori* is associated with slow improvement in submucosal inflammation. One year after successful treatment, neutrophil infiltration resolves; lymphocyte infiltration and lymphoid follicles improve but persist.[125]

The National Institutes of Health recommends treating only persons with active ulcer disease (gastric or duodenal) or persons receiving maintenance antihistamine therapy for recurrent ulcer disease.[95] Some investigators, however, have reported that treatment could be a cost-effective approach to preventing ulcer disease, dyspepsia, and cancer in populations at high risk.[126] Still others maintain that eradicating infection in all infected persons, regardless of symptoms, is the correct approach.[127] As new information accumulates, it is likely that diagnosis and therapy will be offered to a wider segment of the population to prevent adverse outcomes of infection. For now, however, there are no recommendations for diagnostic testing or treatment in asymptomatic persons or persons with dyspepsia of unknown etiology.

Helicobacter heilmannii

H. heilmannii, like *H. pylori,* is thought to cause acute and chronic gastritis. It has also been anecdotally reported in scattered cases of gastric cancer and gastric erosion. It is as yet unclear, however, whether *H. heilmannii* causes significant human disease. It is considerably rarer than *H. pylori.* In one Swiss series, *H. heilmannii* was identified endoscopically in only 2 (1.1%) of 175 asymptomatic adults.[128] It may be somewhat more common (up to 8% prevalence) in Asia.[129] Some data suggest direct transmission of *H. heilmannii* to humans from domestic animals, although this is not firmly established.[130, 131]

Unlike *H. pylori* infection, colonization and inflammation with *H. heilmannii* appear to be restricted to the acid-secreting portion of the mucosa.[129] Pathogenic mechanisms are unknown. Because *H. heilmannii,* like *H. pylori,* does produce urease, some tissue destruction may be similarly related to this enzyme and its toxic metabolites.

Helicobacter fennelliae and *Helicobacter cinaedi*

H. fennelliae and *H. cinaedi* are unusual pathogens that cause a varied spectrum of clinical disease. Both were identified in the mid-1980s in homosexual men with proctitis and colitis.[132, 133] Subsequent data indicated that these organisms more typically cause mild noninflammatory diarrhea. This diarrhea is self-limited in normal hosts but prolonged in immunocompromised patients.[134] These species have also been reported to cause recurrent bacteremia in immunocompromised patients.[135, 136] Persons with bacteremia are typically febrile with temperatures of 38.5°C or higher without a leukocytosis. They do not typically appear septic. Accompanying cellulitis, which is frequent with *H. cinaedi* bacteremia, may be multifocal with a distinctive copper or red-brown color and absence of warmth. Endocarditis and arthritis have also been reported.

The most common predisposing factor for *H. cinaedi* or *H. fennelliae* infection is human immunodeficiency virus infection (at least 60% of cases), although *H. cinaedi* and *H. fennelliae* have also been observed in alcoholics as well as in immunocompetent hosts. Sexual transmission of both *H. fennelliae* and *H. cinaedi* seems likely because these infections occur predominantly in homosexual men.[132, 135] Sixteen percent of homosexual men with intestinal symptoms and 8% of those without symptoms have been found to harbor these organisms.[133] The reservoir for enteric *Helicobacter* is unknown. *H. cinaedi* has been recovered from hamsters, but it is far from clear that this has any role as a disease vector.[137]

Pathogenic mechanisms for *H. fennelliae* and *H. cinaedi* have not yet been identified. In experiments performed in monkeys, oral inoculation of *H. fennelliae* or *H. cinaedi* caused noninflammatory diarrhea invariably associated with bacteremia. No mucosal disruption was observed, suggesting that the colitis seen in humans reflects coinfection with other enteric pathogens.[138] Carriage of enteric *Helicobacter* in monkeys was sustained well after resolution of symptoms despite a brisk serologic response to organism-specific antigens.[138] Humans, too, develop specific immunoglobulin G against the enteric *Helicobacter* after either bacteremia or enteric infection.[6]

H. cinaedi and *H. fennelliae* should be considered in patients with human immunodeficiency virus infection, diarrhea, and unexplained fever. Clinical laboratories should be informed if suspicion is high, so that blood and stool cultures are appropriately processed. As yet, there have been no clinical series addressing treatment. Case reports suggest that penicillin, tetracycline, or aminoglycosides are effective for bacteremic disease.[135] Cephalosporins and quinolones appear to be less successful, and bacteremia may recur.

Acknowledgments

This work was supported by a Clinical Fellowship in Epidemiology from Merck and the Society for Epidemiologic Research.

References

1. Goodwin CS, Worsley BW: The *Helicobacter* genus: The history of *H. pylori* and toxonomy of current species. *In* Goodwin CS, Worsley BW (eds): *Helicobacter pylori*: Biology and Clinical Practice. Boca Raton, FL, CRC Press, 1993, pp 2–13.
2. Stanley J, Linton D, Burnens AP, et al: *Helicobacter canis* sp. nov., a new species from dogs: An integrated study of phenotype and genotype. J Gen Microbiol 139:2495–2504, 1993.
3. Stanley J, Linton D, Burnens AP, et al: *Helicobacter pullorum* sp. nov.—Genotype and phenotype of a new species isolated from poultry and from human patients with gastroenteritis. Microbiology 140:3441–3449, 1994.
4. Fox JG, Yan LL, Dewhirst FE, et al: *Helicobacter bilis* sp. nov., a novel *Helicobacter* species isolated from bile, livers, and intestines of aged, inbred mice. J Clin Microbiol 33:445–454, 1995.
5. Eaton KA, Catrenich CE, Makin KM, Krakowka S: Virulence of coccoid and bacillary forms of *Helicobacter pylori* in gnotobiotic piglets. J Infect Dis 171:459–462, 1995.
6. Flores BM, Fennell CL, Stamm WE: Characterization of *Campylobacter cinaedi* and *C. fennelliae* antigens and analysis of the human immune response. J Infect Dis 159:635–640, 1989.
7. Bode G, Mauch F, Malfertheiner P: The coccoid forms of *Helicobacter pylori*. Criteria for their viability. Epidemiol Infect 111:483–490, 1993.
8. Cellini L, Allocati N, Angelucci D, et al: Coccoid *Helicobacter pylori* not culturable in vitro reverts in mice. Microbiol Immunol 38:843–850, 1994.
9. Hazell SL: Cultural techniques for the growth and isolation of *Helicobacter pylori*. *In* Goodwin CS, Worsley BW (eds): *Helicobacter pylori*: Biology and Clinical Practice. Boca Raton, FL, CRC Press, 1993, pp 273–283.
10. Eaton KA, Morgan DR, Krakowka S: Motility as a factor in the colonisation of gnotobiotic piglets by *Helicobacter pylori*. J Med Microbiol 37:123–127, 1992.
11. Lee A, Fox J, Hazell S: Pathogenicity of *Helicobacter pylori*: A perspective. Infect Immun 61:1601–1610, 1993.
12. Boren T, Falk P, Roth KA, et al: Attachment of *Helicobacter pylori* to human gastric epithelium mediated by blood group antigens. Science 262:1892–1895, 1993.
13. Valkonen KH, Wadstrom T, Moran AP: Interaction of lipopolysaccharides of *Helicobacter pylori* with basement membrane protein laminin. Infect Immun 62:3640–3648, 1994.
14. Lingwood CA, Wasfy G, Han H, Huesca M: Receptor affinity purification of a lipid-binding adhesin from *Helicobacter pylori*. Infect Immun 61:2474–2478, 1993.
15. Eaton KA, Brooks CL, Morgan DR, Krakowka S: Essential role of urease in pathogenesis of gastritis induced by *Helicobacter pylori* in gnotobiotic piglets. Infect Immun 59:2470–2475, 1991.
16. Ferrero RL, Labigne A: The organization and expression of the *Helicobacter pylori* urease gene cluster. *In* Goodwin CS, Worsley BW (eds): *Helicobacter pylori*: Biology and Clinical Practice. Boca Raton, FL, CRC Press, 1993, pp 171–190.
17. Hazell SL, Mendz GL: The metabolism and enzymes of *Helicobacter pylori*: Function and potential virulence effects. *In* Goodwin CS, Worsley BW (eds): *Helicobacter pylori*: Biology and Clinical Practice. Boca Raton, FL, CRC Press, 1993, pp 115–142.
18. Marshall BJ, Barrett LJ, Prakash C, et al: Urea protects *Helicobacter (Campylobacter) pylori* from the bactericidal effect of acid. Gastroenterology 99:697–702, 1990.
19. Akopyanz N, Bukanov NO, Westblom TU, Berg DE: PCR-based RFLP analysis of DNA sequence diversity in the gastric pathogen *Helicobacter pylori*. Nucleic Acids Res 20:6221–6225, 1992.
20. Hurtado A, Chahal B, Owen RJ, Smith AW: Genetic diversity of the *Helicobacter pylori* haemagglutinin/protease *(hap)* gene. FEMS Microbiol Lett 123:173–178, 1994.
21. Taylor DE, Eaton M, Chang N, Salama SM: Construction of a *Helicobacter pylori* genome map and demonstration of diversity at the genome level. J Bacteriol 174:6800–6806, 1992.
22. Xiang Z, Censini S, Bayeli PF, et al: Analysis of expression of CagA and VacA virulence factors in 43 strains. Infect Immun 63:94–98, 1995.
23. Cover TL, Dooley CP, Blaser MJ: Characterization of and human serologic response to proteins in *Helicobacter pylori* broth culture supernatants with vacuolizing cytotoxin activity. Infect Immun 58:603–610, 1990.
24. Telford JL, Ghiara P, Dell'Orco M, et al: Gene structure of the *Helicobacter pylori* cytotoxin and evidence of its key role in gastric disease. J Exp Med 179:1653–1658, 1994.
25. Cover TL, Cao P, Murthy UK, et al: Serum neutralizing antibody response to the vacuolating cytotoxin of *Helicobacter pylori*. J Clin Invest 90:913–918, 1992.
26. Price A: The Sydney system: Histological division. J Gastroenterol Hepatol 6:209–222, 1991.
27. Genta RM, Hamner HW, Graham DY: Gastric lymphoid follicles in *Helicobacter pylori* infection: Frequency, distribution, and response to triple therapy. Hum Pathol 24:577–583, 1993.
28. Kosunen TU, Seppala K, Sarna S, Sipponen P: Diagnostic value of decreasing IgG, IgA, and IgM antibody titres after eradication of *Helicobacter pylori*. Lancet 339:893–895, 1992.
29. Blaser MJ, Parsonnet J: Parasitism by the "slow" bacterium *Helicobacter pylori* leads to altered gastric homeostasis and neoplasia. J Clin Invest 94:4–8, 1994.

30. Crabtree JE, Farmery SM, Lindley IJ, et al: CagA/cytotoxic strains of *Helicobacter pylori* and interleukin-8 in gastric epithelial cell lines. J Clin Pathol 47:945–950, 1994.
31. Sharma SA, Tummuru MK, Miller GG, Blaser MJ: Interleukin-8 response of gastric epithelial cell lines to *Helicobacter pylori* stimulation in vitro. Infect Immun 63:1681–1687, 1995.
32. Phadnis SH, Ilver D, Janzon L, et al: Pathological significance and molecular characterization of the vacuolating toxin gene of *Helicobacter pylori*. Infect Immun 62:1557–1565, 1994.
33. Tsujii M, Kawano S, Tsuji S, et al: Mechanism of gastric mucosal damage induced by ammonia. Gastroenterology 102:1881–1888, 1992.
34. Smoot DT, Mobley HL, Chippendale GR, et al: *Helicobacter pylori* urease activity is toxic to human gastric epithelial cells. Infect Immun 58:1992–1994, 1990.
35. Marshall BJ, Armstrong JA, McGeche DB, Glancy RJ: Attempt to fulfill Koch's postulates for pyloric *Campylobacter*. Med J Aust 142:436–439, 1985.
36. Morris A, Nicholson G: Ingestion of *Campylobacter pyloridis* causes gastritis and raised fasting gastric pH. Am J Gastroenterol 82:192–194, 1987.
37. Langenberg W, Rauws EA, Widjojokusumo A, et al: Identification of *Campylobacter pyloridis* isolates by restriction endonuclease DNA analysis. J Clin Microbiol 24:414–417, 1986.
38. Parsonnet J, Blaser MJ, Perez-Perez GI, et al: Symptoms and risk factors of *Helicobacter pylori* infection in a cohort of epidemiologists. Gastroenterology 102:41–46, 1992.
39. Langenberg W, Rauws EA, Houthoff HJ, et al: Follow-up study of individuals with untreated *Campylobacter pylori*–associated gastritis and of noninfected persons with non-ulcer dyspepsia. J Infect Dis 157:1245–1249, 1988.
40. Goodwin CS: Duodenal ulcer, *Campylobacter pylori*, and the "leaking roof" concept. Lancet 2:1467–1469, 1988.
41. Tarnasky PR, Kovacs TOG, Sytnik B, Walsh JH: Asymptomatic *H. pylori* infection impairs pH inhibition of gastrin and acid secretion during second hour of peptone meal stimulation. Dig Dis Sci 38:1681–1687, 1993.
42. Sipponen P: Natural history of gastritis and its relationship to peptic ulcer disease. Digestion 5:70–75, 1992.
43. Shuto R, Fujioka T, Kodama R, Nasu M: Experimental study in Japanese monkeys with *Helicobacter pylori* infection. Nippon Rinsho 51:3132–3137, 1993.
44. Sipponen P, Kekki M, Haapakoski J, et al: Gastric cancer risk in chronic atrophic gastritis: Statistical calculations on cross-sectional data. Cancer 35:173–177, 1985.
45. Sipponen P, Seppala K: Gastric carcinoma: Failed adaptation to *Helicobacter pylori*. Scand J Gastroenterol 27(Suppl):33–38, 1992.
46. Vargas M, Lee A, Fox JG, Cave DR: Inhibition of acid secretion from parietal cells by non–human infecting *Helicobacter* species—A factor in colonization of gastric mucosa. Infect Immun 59:3694–3699, 1991.
47. Davies GR, Simmonds NJ, Stevens TRJ, et al: *Helicobacter pylori* stimulates antral mucosal reactive oxygen metabolite production in vivo. Gut 35:179–185, 1994.
48. Lynch DAF, Mapstone NP, Clarke AMT, et al: Cell proliferation in *Helicobacter pylori* associated gastritis and the effect of eradication therapy. Gut 36:345–350, 1995.
49. Hirai M, Azuma T, Ito S, et al: High prevalence of neutralizing activity to *Helicobacter pylori* cytotoxin in serum of gastric-carcinoma patients. Int J Cancer 56:56–60, 1994.
50. Fox JG, Correa P, Taylor NS, et al: High prevalence and persistence of cytotoxin-positive *Helicobacter pylori* strains in a population with high prevalence of atrophic gastritis. Am J Gastroenterol 87:1554–1560, 1992.
51. Taylor DN, Parsonnet J: The epidemiology and natural history of *Helicobacter pylori* infection. *In* Blaser MJ, Smith PD, Ravdin JI, et al (eds): Infections of the Gastrointestinal Tract. New York, Raven Press, 1995, pp 551–564.
52. Banatvala N, Mayo K, Megraud F, et al: The cohort effect and *Helicobacter pylori*. J Infect Dis 168:219–221, 1993.
53. Cullen DJE, Collins BJ, Christiansen KJ, et al: When is *Helicobacter pylori* infection acquired? Gut 34:1681–1682, 1993.
54. Parsonnet J: The incidence of *Helicobacter pylori* infection. Aliment Pharamacol Ther 9(Suppl 2):45–51, 1995.
55. Eurogast Study Group: Epidemiology of, and risk factors for, *Helicobacter pylori* infection among 3194 asymptomatic subjects in 17 populations. Gut 34:1672–1676, 1993.
56. Hopkins RJ, Russell RG, O'Donnoghue JM, et al: Seroprevalence of *Helicobacter pylori* in Seventh-Day Adventists and other groups in Maryland. Lack of association with diet. Arch Intern Med 150:2347–2348, 1990.
57. Malaty HM, Graham DY: Importance of childhood socioeconomic status on the current prevalence of *Helicobacter pylori* infection. Gut 35:742–745, 1994.
58. Smoak B, Kelley P, Taylor DN: Seroprevalence of *Helicobacter pylori* infections in a cohort of US Army recruits. Am J Epidemiol 139:513–519, 1994.
59. Replogle ML, Glaser SL, Hiatt RA, Parsonnet J: Biologic sex as a risk factor for *Helicobacter pylori* infection in young healthy adults. Am J Epidemiol 142:856–863, 1995.
60. Teh BH, Lin JT, Pan WH, et al: Seroprevalence and associated risk factors of *Helicobacter pylori* infection in Taiwan. Anticancer Res 14:1389–1392, 1994.
61. Blecker U, Hauser B, Lanciers S, et al: The prevalence of *Helicobacter pylori*–positive serology in asymptomatic children. J Pediatr Gastroenterol Nutr 16:252–256, 1993.
62. Malaty HM, Engstrand L, Pedersen NL, Graham DY: *Helicobacter pylori* infection: Genetic and environmental influences. A study of twins. Ann Intern Med 120:982–986, 1994.
63. Perez-Perez GI, Taylor DN, Bodhidatta L, et al: Seroprevalence of *Helicobacter pylori* infections in Thailand. J Infect Dis 161:1237–1241, 1990.
64. Berkowicz J, Lee A: Person-to-person transmission of *Campylobacter pylori* (Letter). Lancet 2:680–681, 1987.
65. Reiff A, Jacobs E, Kist M: Seroepidemiological study of the immune response to *Campylobacter pylori* in potential risk groups. Eur J Clin Microbiol Infect Dis 8:592–596, 1989.
66. Drumm B, Perez-Perez GI, Blaser MJ, Sherman PM: Intrafamilial clustering of *Helicobacter pylori* infection. N Engl J Med 322:359–364, 1990.
67. Mitchell JD, Mitchell HM, Tobias V: Acute *Helicobacter pylori* infection in an infant, associated with gastric ulceration and serological evidence of intra-familial transmission. Am J Gastroenterol 87:382–386, 1992.
68. Malaty HM, Graham DY, Klein PD, et al: Transmission of *Helicobacter pylori* infection. Studies in families of healthy individuals. Scand J Gastroenterol 26:927–932, 1991.
69. Webb PM, Knight T, Greaves S, et al: Relation between infection with *Helicobacter pylori* and living conditions in childhood: Evidence for person to person transmission in early life. BMJ 308:750–753, 1994.
70. Mendall MA, Goggin PM, Molineaux N, et al: Childhood living conditions and *Helicobacter pylori* seropositivity in adult life. Lancet 339:896–897, 1992.
71. Blecker U, Lanciers S, Mehta DI, Vandenplas Y: Familial clustering of *Helicobacter pylori* infection. Clin Pediatr (Phila) 33:307–308, 1994.
72. Mitchell HM, Bohane T, Hawkes RA, Lee A: *Helicobacter pylori* infection within families. Int J Med Microbiol Virol Parasitol Infect Dis 280:128–136, 1993.
73. Wang JT, Sheu JC, Lin JT, et al: Direct DNA amplification and restriction pattern analysis of *Helicobacter pylori* in patients with duodenal ulcer and their families. J Infect Dis 168:1544–1548, 1993.
74. Thomas JE, Gibson GR, Darboe MK, et al: Isolation of *Helicobacter pylori* from human faeces. Lancet 340:1194–1195, 1992.
75. Kelly SM, Pitcher MC, Farmery SM, Gibson GR: Isolation of *Helicobacter pylori* from feces of patients with dyspepsia in the United Kingdom. Gastroenterology 107:1671–1674, 1994.
76. Krajden S, Fuksa M, Anderson J, et al: Examination of human stomach biopsies, saliva, and dental plaque for *Campylobacter pylori*. J Clin Microbiol 27:1397–1398, 1989.
77. Mapstone NP, Lynch DA, Lewis FA, et al: Identification of *Helicobacter pylori* DNA in the mouths and stomachs of patients with gastritis using PCR. J Clin Pathol 46:540–543, 1993.
78. Ferguson DA, Li C, Patel NR, et al: Isolation of *Helicobacter pylori* from saliva. J Clin Microbiol 31:2802–2804, 1993.
79. Langenberg W, Rauws EA, Oudbier JH, Tytgat GN: Patient-to-patient transmission of *Campylobacter pylori* infection by fiberoptic gastroduodenoscopy and biopsy. J Infect Dis 161:507–511, 1990.
80. Fantry GT, Zheng QX, James SP: Conventional cleaning and disinfection techniques eliminate the risk of endoscopic trans-

mission of *Helicobacter pylori.* Am J Gastroenterol 90:227–232, 1995.
81. Katoh M, Saito D, Noda T, et al: *Helicobacter pylori* may be transmitted through gastrofiberscope even after manual Hyamine washing. Jpn J Cancer Res 84:117–119, 1993.
82. Chong J, Marshall BJ, Barkin JS, et al: Occupational exposure to *Helicobacter pylori* for the endoscopy professional: A sera epidemiological study. Am J Gastroenterol 89:1987–1992, 1994.
83. Lin SK, Lambert JR, Schembri MA, et al: *Helicobacter pylori* prevalence in endoscopy and medical staff. J Gastroenterol Hepatol 9:319–324, 1994.
84. Klein PD, Graham DY, Gaillour A, et al: Water source as risk factor for *Helicobacter pylori* infection in Peruvian children. Lancet 337:1503–1506, 1991.
85. Hopkins RJ, Vial PA, Ferreccio C, et al: Seroprevalence of *Helicobacter pylori* in Chile: Vegetables may serve as one route of transmission. J Infect Dis 168:222–226, 1993.
86. Gill HH, Desai HG, Majmudar P, et al: Epidemiology of *Helicobacter pylori*: The Indian scenario. Indian J Gastroenterol 12:9–11, 1993.
87. Gill HH, Majmudar P, Shankaran K, Desai HG: Age-related prevalence of *Helicobacter pylori* antibodies in Indian subjects. Indian J Gastroenterol 13:92–94, 1994.
88. Hazell SL, Mitchell HM, Hedges M, et al: Hepatitis A and evidence against the community dissemination of *Helicobacter pylori* via feces. J Infect Dis 170:686–689, 1994.
89. Handt LK, Fox JG, Dewhirst FE, et al: *Helicobacter pylori* isolated from the domestic cat: Public health implications. Infect Immun 62:2367–2374, 1994.
90. Sobala GM, Crabtree JE, Dixon MF, et al: Acute *Helicobacter pylori* infection: Clinical features, local and systemic immune response, gastric mucosal histology and gastric juice ascorbic acid concentrations. Gut 32:1415–1418, 1991.
91. Gledhill T, Leicester RJ, Addis B, et al: Epidemic hypochlorhydria. Br Med J (Clin Res) 290:1383–1386, 1985.
92. Ramsey EJ, Carey KV, Peterson WL, et al: Epidemic gastritis with hypochlorhydria. Gastroenterology 76:1449–1457, 1979.
93. Holtmann G, Goebell H, Holtmann M, Talley NJ: Dyspepsia in healthy blood donors. Pattern of symptoms and association with *Helicobacter pylori.* Dig Dis Sci 39:1090–1098, 1994.
94. Lambert JR: The role of *Helicobacter pylori* in nonulcer dyspepsia. A debate—For. Gastroenterol Clin North Am 22:141–151, 1993.
95. NIH Consensus Development Panel on *Helicobacter pylori* in Peptic Ulcer Disease: *Helicobacter pylori* in peptic ulcer disease. JAMA 272:65–69, 1994.
96. Graham DY, Lew GM, Klein PD, et al: Effect of treatment of *Helicobacter pylori* infection on the long-term recurrence of gastric or duodenal ulcer. A randomized, controlled study. Ann Intern Med 116:705–708, 1992.
97. Hentschel E, Brandstatter G, Dragosics B, et al: Effect of ranitidine and amoxicillin plus metronidazole on the eradication of *Helicobacter pylori* and the recurrence of duodenal ulcer. N Engl J Med 328:308–312, 1993.
98. Graham DY: Treatment of peptic ulcers caused by *Helicobacter pylori.* N Engl J Med 328:349–350, 1993.
99. Sipponen P, Aarynen M, Kaariainen I, et al: Chronic antral gastritis, Lewis(a+) phenotype, and male sex as factors in predicting coexisting duodenal ulcer. Scand J Gastroenterol 24:581–588, 1989.
100. Marshall BJ: *Helicobacter pylori.* Am J Gastroenterol 89:S116–S128, 1994.
101. IARC Working Group on the Evaluation of Carcinogenic Risks to Humans: *Helicobacter pylori. In* Schistosomes, Liver Flukes and *Helicobacter pylori:* Views and Expert Opinions of an IARC Working Group on the Evaluation of Carcinogenic Risks to Humans. Lyon, France, International Agency for Research on Cancer, 1994, pp 177–240.
102. Parsonnet J, Friedman GD, Vandersteen DP, et al: *Helicobacter pylori* infection and the risk of gastric carcinoma. N Engl J Med 325:1127–1131, 1991.
103. Nomura AMY, Stemmerman GN, Chyou P, et al: *Helicobacter pylori* infection and gastric carcinoma in a population of Japanese-Americans in Hawaii. N Engl J Med 325:1132–1136, 1991.
104. Eurogast Study Group: An international association between *Helicobacter pylori* infection and gastric cancer. Lancet 341:1359–1362, 1993.
105. Blaser MJ, Chyou PH, Nomura A: Age at establishment of *Helicobacter pylori* infection and gastric carcinoma, gastric ulcer, and duodenal ulcer risk. Cancer Res 55:562–565, 1995.
106. Howson C, Hiyama T, Wynder E: The decline in gastric cancer: Epidemiology of an unplanned triumph. Epidemiol Rev 8:1–27, 1986.
107. Blaser MJ, Perez-Perez GI, Kleanthous H, et al: Infection with *Helicobacter pylori* strains possessing cagA is associated with an increased risk of developing adenocarcinoma of the stomach. Cancer Res 55:2111–2115, 1995.
108. Severson RK, Davis S: Increasing incidence of primary gastric lymphoma. Cancer 66:1283–1287, 1990.
109. Parsonnet J, Hansen S, Rodriguez L, et al: *Helicobacter pylori* infection and gastric lymphoma. N Engl J Med 330:1267–1271, 1994.
110. Talley NJ, Zinsmeister AR, Weaver A, et al: Gastric adenocarcinoma and *Helicobacter pylori* infection. J Natl Cancer Inst 83:1734–1739, 1991.
111. Wotherspoon AC, Ortiz-Hidalgo C, Falzon MR, Isaacson PG: *Helicobacter pylori*–associated gastritis and primary B-cell gastric lymphoma. Lancet 338:1175–1176, 1991.
112. Hussell T, Isaacson PG, Crabtree JE, Spencer J: The response of cells from low-grade B-cell gastric lymphomas of mucosa-associated lymphoid tissue to *Helicobacter pylori.* Lancet 342:571–574, 1993.
113. McNulty CA, Dent JC, Uff JS, et al: Detection of *Campylobacter pylori* by the biopsy urease test: An assessment of 1445 patients. Gut 30:1058–1062, 1989.
114. Marshall BJ, Warren JR, Francis GJ, et al: Rapid urease test in the management of *Campylobacter pyloridis*–associated gastritis. Am J Gastroenterol 82:200–210, 1987.
115. Lee N, Lee TT, Fang KM: Assessment of four rapid urease test systems for detection of *Helicobacter pylori* in gastric biopsy specimens. Diagn Microbiol Infect Dis 18:69–74, 1994.
116. Nedenskov-Sorensen P, Aase S, Bjorneklett A, et al: Sampling efficiency in the diagnosis of *Helicobacter pylori* infection and chronic active gastritis. J Clin Microbiol 29:672–675, 1991.
117. Morris A, Ali MR, Brown P, et al: *Campylobacter pylori* infection in biopsy specimens of gastric antrum: Laboratory diagnosis and estimation of sampling error. J Clin Pathol 42:727–732, 1989.
118. Brown KE, Peura DA: Diagnosis of *Helicobacter pylori* infection. Gastroenterol Clin North Am 22:105–115, 1993.
119. Cutler A, Schubert A, Schubert T: Role of *Helicobacter pylori* serology in evaluating treatment success. Dig Dis Sci 38:2262–2266, 1993.
120. Andersen LP: The antibody response to *Helicobacter pylori* infection, and the value of serologic tests to detect *H. pylori* and for post-treatment monitoring. *In* Goodwin CS, Worsley BW (eds): *Helicobacter pylori:* Biology and Clinical Practice. Boca Raton, FL, CRC Press, 1993, pp 285–305.
121. Atherton JC, Spiller RC: The urea breath test for *Helicobacter pylori.* Gut 35:723–725, 1994.
122. Dill S, Payne-James JJ, Misiewicz JJ, et al: Evaluation of ^{13}C-urea breath test in the detection of *Helicobacter pylori* and in monitoring the effect of tripotassium dicitratobismuthate. Gut 31:1237–1241, 1990.
123. Jaup BH, Norrby A: Low dose, short-term triple therapy for cure of *Helicobacter pylori* infection and healing of peptic ulcers. Am J Gastroenterol 90:943–945, 1995.
124. Labenz J, Stolte M, Ruhl GH, et al: One-week low-dose triple therapy for the eradication of *Helicobacter pylori* infection. Eur J Gastroenterol Hepatol 7:9–11, 1995.
125. Genta RM, Lew GM, Graham DY: Changes in the gastric mucosa following eradication of *Helicobacter pylori.* Mod Pathol 6:281–289, 1993.
126. Hack HM, Harris R, Owens DK, Parsonnet J: Prevention of gastric cancer: A cost-effectiveness analysis of screening for *H. pylori* (Abstr). Clin Res 42:23A, 1994.
127. Graham DY: Benefits from elimination of *Helicobacter pylori* infection include major reduction in the incidence of peptic ulcer disease, gastric cancer, and primary gastric lymphoma. Prev Med 23:712–716, 1994.
128. Mazzucchelli L, Wilder-Smith CH, Ruchti C, et al: *Gastrospirillum hominis* in asymptomatic, healthy individuals. Dig Dis Sci 38:2087–2089, 1993.
129. Dubois A: Spiral bacteria in the human stomach: The gastric helicobacters. Emerging Infect Dis 1:79–85, 1995.

130. Thomson MA, Storey P, Greer R, Cleghorn GJ: Canine-human transmission of *Gastrospirillum hominis.* Lancet 343:1605–1607, 1994.
131. Stolte M, Wellens E, Bethke B, et al: *Helicobacter heilmannii* (formerly *Gastrospirillum hominis)* gastritis: An infection transmitted by animals? Scand J Gastroenterol 29:1061–1064, 1995.
132. Totten PA, Fennell CL, Tenover FC, et al: *Campylobacter cinaedi* (sp. nov.) and *Campylobacter fennelliae* (sp. nov.): Two new *Campylobacter* species associated with enteric disease in homosexual men. J Infect Dis 151:131–139, 1985.
133. Quinn TC, Goodell SG, Fennell C, et al: Infections with *Campylobacter jejuni* and *Campylobacter*-like infections in homosexual men. Ann Intern Med 101:187–192, 1985.
134. Mishu Allos B, Lastovica AJ, Blaser MJ: Atypical campylobacters and related organisms. *In* Blaser MJ, Smith PD, Ravdin JI, et al (eds): Infections of the Gastrointestinal Tract. New York, Raven Press, 1995, pp 849–866.
135. Kiehlbauch JA, Tauxe RV, Baker CN, Wachsmuth IK: *Helicobacter cinaedi*–associated bacteremia and cellulitis in immunocompromised patients. Ann Intern Med 121:90–93, 1994.
136. Kemper CA, Mickelsen P, Morton A, et al: *Helicobacter (Campylobacter) fennelliae*–like organisms as an important but occult cause of bacteraemia in a patient with AIDS. J Infect 26:97–101, 1993.
137. Gebhart CJ, Fennell CL, Murtaugh MP, Stamm WE: *Campylobacter cinaedi* is normal intestinal flora in hamsters. J Clin Microbiol 27:1692–1694, 1989.
138. Flores BM, Fennell CL, Kuller L, et al: Experimental infection of pig-tailed macaques *(Macaca nemestrina)* with *Campylobacter cinaedi* and *Campylobacter fennelliae.* Infect Immun 58:3947–3953, 1990.
139. Dewhirst FE, Seymour C, Fraser GJ, et al: Phylogeny of *Helicobacter* isolates from bird and swine feces and description of *Helicobacter pametensis* sp. nov. Int J Syst Bacteriol 44:553–560, 1994.

MISCELLANEOUS MICROORGANISMS

228

Bartonella Species

Jennifer S. Daly

History

The genus *Bartonella* contains not only its original member, *Bartonella bacilliformis,* the etiologic agent of Oroya fever and verruga peruana, but now includes the organisms previously classified as *Rochalimaea* and *Grahamella* species. The new members of the genus are cultivatable on cell-free blood- or hemin-containing bacteriologic media and have been determined by 16S ribosomal RNA sequencing studies, DNA-relatedness data, content of guanine plus cytosine, and phenotypic characteristics to be closely related to *B. bacilliformis.* Not only are these organisms related in the laboratory but the clinical characteristics of the diseases produced in humans and the prolonged asymptomatic bacteremia occurring in animals are similar within the genus (Table 228–1). With the inclusion of the *Rochalimaea* and *Grahamella* species, there are now 11 species in the genus *Bartonella: B. bacilliformis, Bartonella quintana, Bartonella henselae, Bartonella elizabethae, Bartonella vinsonii, Bartonella clarridgeiae, Bartonella talpae, Bartonella peromysci, Bartonella grahamii, Bartonella taylorii,* and *Bartonella doshiae*[1–3] (Table 228–2). Although the genus *Bartonella* has been classified in the family Bartonellaceae within the order Rickettsiales,[2] the closest relatives to the expanded genus *Bartonella* are the *Brucella* species rather than any of the *Rickettsia* species, a fact that has prompted taxonomists to propose that the family Bartonellaceae be removed from the order Rickettsiales.[1, 2]

B. bacilliformis causes two distinct syndromes. The chronic form of bartonellosis is verruga peruana, or warts of the Andes. The first records of these verrucous lesions are represented on ceramic pottery from the pre-Inca era, and medical description of these lesions can be traced back to the year 1630.[4] In 1871, an epidemic of bartonellosis occurred in workers building a railroad line between Lima and La Oroya, Peru. Nearly 7000 workers developed fever, massive hemolysis, and died, and the disease was given the name Oroya fever, a misnomer because transmission occurs only in the mountainous area near La Oroya and not in the city at its lower elevation. In 1885, a Peruvian medical student, Daniel Carrión, showed that the indolent skin disease, verruga peruana, and highly lethal Oroya fever were caused by the same pathogen when he performed a foolhardy experiment.[5] In an attempt to study the skin disease, he inoculated himself with material from the verruga of a patient. He was assisted by a classmate despite the warnings of the older clinicians, and developed fever, followed by massive hemolysis. Before he died, he recognized that he was suffering from Oroya fever and the disease has been known as Carrión disease since that time.[5] In 1909, Barton demonstrated the organism in red blood cells,[6] and it was cultured in 1925 by Noguchi.[7] *B. bacilliformis* was the sole member of this genus until 1993 when the agent of trench fever and related organisms were added.

Trench fever, caused by *B. quintana,* first recognized during World War I, affected more than 1 million soldiers involved

TABLE 228–1 ■ *Bartonella* Species Causing Human Disease

ORGANISM	MAJOR HUMAN DISEASES	VECTOR
B. bacilliformis	Verruga peruana Oroya fever (Carrión disease)	Sandfly
B. quintana	Trench fever Bacillary angiomatosis Visceral peliosis Fever and bacteremia Endocarditis Lymphadenopathy	Body louse
B. henselae	Fever and bacteremia Bacillary angiomatosis Visceral peliosis Cat-scratch disease Endocarditis	Cats
B. elizabethae	Endocarditis	Unknown

TABLE 228–2 ■ Nomenclature of *Bartonella* Species

CURRENT NAME	PREVIOUS DESIGNATIONS
Human Pathogens	
B. bacilliformis	
B. quintana	*Rochalimaea quintana* *Rickettsia quintana* *Rickettsia pediculi*
B. henselae	*Rochalimaea henselae*
B. elizabethae	*Rochalimaea elizabethae*
Animal Isolates	
B. vinsonii	Vole agent *Rochalimaea vinsonii*
B. talpae	*Grahamella talpae*
B. peromysci	*Grahamella peromysci*
B. grahamii	—
B. taylorii	—
B. doshiae	—
B. clarridgeiae	—

in trench warfare in Europe. Transmitted by the body louse, the disease reappeared in epidemic form in World War II, particularly in Germany, and the eastern front. The organism was originally designated *Rickettsia quintana* by Schmincke[8] in 1917 when he isolated it in cell culture. Sikora, who propagated the organism on human blood agar in 1921,[9] did not realize he had grown the pathogen of trench fever and thought it to be a harmless parasite of lice. He called it *Rickettsia pediculi.* In 1948, *B. quintana* was cultured from the blood of a patient in Yugoslavia[10] and in 1961 it was propagated by Vinson and Fuller[11]; the Fuller strain currently is in use in immunologic studies. In 1969, Varela and colleagues[11a] showed that the organism could be propagated from the blood of patients with trench fever and could be inoculated into volunteers and produce the disease. Volunteer patients had prolonged bacteremia with the organism, and the lice that fed on these patients would exhibit organisms in their feces. The organism was initially named *Rochalimaea* to honor Henrique da Rocha-Lima and five-day or quintan fever (quintana), which is seen frequently with the disease. Trench fever had been known as Wolhynia fever, His-Werner disease, shin bone fever, and shank fever. After World War II, small epidemics and sporadic cases were noted in Europe, but epidemics were not recognized in the United States until 1994 when eight cases were reported in homeless men in Seattle.[12] In addition to its role as etiologic agent in cases of trench fever, *B. quintana* has been isolated from skin lesions of patients with bacillary angiomatosis,[13] detected in the liver of patients with peliosis hepatis,[14] and cultured from the blood of patients with endocarditis.[15, 16]

The other species found in patients with bacillary angiomatosis, *B. henselae,* was first isolated in 1986 by Slater and colleagues[17] from the blood of two patients with fever and symptomatic human immunodeficiency virus type 1 (HIV-1) infection.[17] They determined that the organism resembled *B. quintana* or *Brucella* species and reported their findings in 1990. At the same time, Relman and colleagues[18] reported identification of the agent of bacillary angiomatosis by using polymerase chain reaction amplification of the 16S ribosomal RNA gene from tissue specimens. The organism remained unnamed until 1992 when Welch and colleagues[19] and Regnery and colleagues[20] formally described the species and proposed the name *Rochalimaea henselae.* Included in the report by Welch and colleagues were patients with prolonged fever and bacteremia and, in some, vascular proliferative lesions, including bacillary peliosis hepatis and bacillary angiomatosis. In 1992, Koehler and coworkers[13] cultured *B. henselae* and *B. quintana* directly from the skin lesions of patients with bacillary angiomatosis. The organism was named *R. henselae* and in 1993 was transferred to the genus *Bartonella.*[2] It has been recognized as an etiologic agent in many cases of cat-scratch disease (CSD) (see Chapter 180), in immunocompetent patients with fever and relapsing bacteremia, and as a cause of endocarditis.[21]

In 1986, another species of *Bartonella, B. elizabethae,* was cultured from a patient with endocarditis.[22] This organism grew from a subculture taken from a BACTEC (Becton-Dickinson Microbiology Systems, Cockeysville, MD) blood culture bottle inoculated on blood and chocolate agar plates that were incubated for 14 days in 5% to 10% carbon dioxide. The organism was unidentifiable at that time but was reexamined in 1992 after the microbiologic and molecular characteristics of *B. henselae* had been reported. It was found to be a unique organism related to the *Bartonella* species by phenotypic characteristics, cellular fatty acid contents, DNA-relatedness data, and 16S ribosomal RNA sequence analysis. No other isolates of this species have been found to date, but serologic responses to this organism have been detected in patients whose serum has been submitted for serologic testing for *Bartonella* antibody with the immunofluorescent assay available from the Centers for Disease Control and Prevention.

B. vinsonii, a species also previously classified with the *Rochalimaea* group, has not been shown to be associated with disease in humans. The organism was isolated by Baker[23] from voles on Grosse Isle, Quebec, Canada. During World War II, Baker, a captain in the veterinary corps of the U.S. Army, was stationed at the War Disease Control Station on this small island that had served one century earlier as a quarantine station and mass graveyard for thousands of Irish immigrants who had died of typhus. On the island, Baker had the company of U.S. and Canadian scientists, a few species of small animals, two families who were caretakers, and their domestic cats. Baker trapped and performed autopsies on voles living on the island and found that many had enlarged spleens. Baker attempted to isolate a member of the Rickettsiaceae family to determine if the agent of typhus had persisted in the small rodents. He grew an organism in yolk sac cultures from multiple animals and found that almost all of the wild voles were infected. He inoculated hamsters, mice, and guinea pigs intraperitoneally and was able to recover the organism from their blood. The organism, when examined later by researchers, was found to grow on cell-free media and was related to *B. quintana.*[24] It was formally described in 1982 and named after J. William Vinson who had done extensive work with the agent of trench fever.[25] In 1995, Breitschwerdt and colleagues[26] cultured a subspecies of *B. vinsonii* from the blood of a dog in North Carolina.

Like *B. vinsonii* (previously *Rochalimaea vinsonii*), the organisms originally classified as *Grahamella* species (*B. talpae, B. peromysci, B. grahamii, B. taylorii,* and *B. doshiae*) have been found only in animals and in the past were named for the animal host.[1, 27] These organisms are erythrocyte-associated bacteria that were first observed in 1905 by G. S. Graham-Smith in moles. They have been found most commonly in rodents, were first cultured in 1932, and were poorly characterized until 1994 when Birtles and coworkers[28] reported isolation of several species from the blood of two thirds of small mammals trapped in Shropshire, United Kingdom. The authors found the same species, *B. grahamii,* in five different small woodland mammals. They found only one species in each individual animal. These organisms are related genetically but are distinct from the *Bartonella* species that have been isolated from humans up to the present time,[28, 29] although erythrocyte-associated organisms have been found in humans.[30] They were not cultured and therefore had not been identified at the species level. The newest member of the genus, *B. clarridgeiae,* was isolated in Texas from the blood of a cat. Although the owner of the cat had lymphadenopathy, the patient's sample of blood grew only *B. henselae.*[3]

Characteristics of the Pathogen

The members of this genus are thin, gram-negative, aerobic, slightly curved rods that stain weakly with safranin but can be stained with the Warthin-Starry, Giemsa, and Gimenez stains. For primary isolation they require prolonged (7 to 14 days) incubation on fresh media containing blood or hemin and grow optimally in 5% to 10% carbon dioxide and high humidity. *B. bacilliformis* grows best at 25°C to 32°C, and the other species grow at 35°C to 37°C.[1, 29] The organisms do not utilize carbohydrates but can be identified by the characteristic content of guanine plus cytosine of their DNA (38.5% to 41%)[1, 2] and cellular fatty acids. The organisms are hemotrophic, parasitizing the erythrocytes of their hosts (*B. bacilliformis* and animal species).[28, 30, 31] *B. bacilliformis* and *B. clarridgeiae* are motile by means of polar flagella but *B. henselae* and *B. quintana* exhibit twitching motility. If the Kovacs method for the standard oxidase test is employed, some of the species *(B. quintana, B. vinsonii)* may have a weakly positive reaction. All *Bartonella* species are catalase-, urea-, and indole-negative.[2, 22] The previously classified *Grahamella* species are Voges-Proskauer (acetoin from glucose) test–positive, and several species may be distinguished from one another using commercial tests to detect specific preformed enzymes.[20, 32–34] Four species have been found to be pathogenic for humans. *B. henselae* can cause prolonged bacteremia in humans and cats, and *B. quintana* and *B. bacilliformis* have been cultured from their insect vectors and from humans. The other species have been grown only in animals, including rats, voles, moles, mice, cats, cows, and dogs.[6, 28] Genetic variability in *Bartonella* species, especially *B. henselae* (which may possess bacteriophage-like particles), allows differentiation of isolates for epidemiologic analyses.[35]

Epidemiology

A number of epidemiologic associations with insect vectors and animals are known. *B. bacilliformis* infection is associated with transmission by the bite of the sandfly,[4] *B. quintana* is associated with the presence of body lice,[11] and *B. henselae* and CSD appear to be more common in people owning cats and in one study owning cats with fleas.[36] An association with cats is common in many HIV-infected patients with *B. henselae* but is not apparent in all reported cases of bacteremia, bacillary angiomatosis, or peliosis of the liver or spleen.[37, 38] There may be more than one vector for each species. Five of the 10 patients bacteremic with *B. quintana* in the report by Spach and coworkers[12] had scabies and 1 had lice. In the report by Koehler and coworkers,[13] one patient with *B. quintana*–associated bacillary angiomatosis owned a pet rat. Voles were common in the trenches in World War I,[39] and evidence for the transmission of *Grahamella* species in mammals by fleas has been reported.[29] The prevalence of *Bartonella* bacteremia in animals is greatest in late summer and early autumn when flea infestations are heaviest,[27, 29] and there seems to be a parallel seasonal increase in the incidence of CSD in humans. CSD is associated with the acquisition of young cats (less commonly dogs) in the household (see Chapter 180). In 1995, Lucey and colleagues[40] reported two immunocompetent patients who acquired persistent *B. henselae* bacteremia and who had experienced tick bites before their illnesses. *B. vinsonii* has been cultured only from voles and the blood of a dog.[26] There is no known vector for *B. elizabethae. B. bacilliformis* is found in a limited geographic region, whereas *B. quintana* and *B. henselae* are found worldwide, with *B. quintana* being more common in Europe and *B. henselae* in the United States.[35] It is not known if asymptomatic, chronically infected humans serve as a reservoir for some of these organisms.

Clinical Manifestations

B. bacilliformis produces a biphasic illness transmitted by phlebotomine sandflies of the genus *Lutzomyia verrugarum* and is limited geographically to the western slopes of the Andes Mountains at elevations between 500 and 3375 m in Colombia, Ecuador, Peru, Chile, Bolivia, and probably Guatemala.[4, 41, 42] Chronic bartonellosis is characterized by vascular proliferation (verruga peruana) histologically similar to bacillary angiomatosis, an illness caused by *B. quintana* and *B. henselae.*[21, 38, 43] The organism grows in the vascular epithelium of the skin. Skin lesions consist of nodules exhibiting active proliferation of newly formed capillaries, dilated venules, and precapillary vessels with endothelial hyperplasia[43] and may be found in bones, mucous membranes, lungs, liver, spleen, brain, and lymph nodes. Lesions may undergo spontaneous regression. The acute phase illness (Oroya fever) is characterized by high fever and intravascular hemolysis.[41] The organism is associated with erythrocytes and infiltrates the reticuloendothelial system. In the preantibiotic era, mortality was high, with 40% of patients dying of bacterial superinfection, particularly bacteremic salmonellosis. During an epidemic in 1987 in Peru, Gray and coworkers[42] observed a case-fatality rate of 88% (14 of 16 patients) in patients not treated with antibiotics and noted the survival of at least 10 patients who were treated with chloramphenicol. The chronic form of the disease may be preceded by the acute febrile phase, with skin lesions appearing weeks to months later. Some patients, especially those from an endemic area, may have a mild illness, and up to 15% may exhibit prolonged, asymptomatic bacteremia. Travelers may develop a biphasic illness and present to physicians outside an endemic area, with a resultant delay in diagnosis. Soon after returning from a visit to an area of Peru with an elevation of 3100 feet, an Italian woman suffered a brief febrile illness, followed by the development of skin lesions, that was clinically and pathologically consistent with verruga peruana. She responded to treatment with chloramphenicol.[44]

B. quintana is the organism that produces trench fever, initially recognized during World War I.[21, 39] Although it resulted in significant loss of personnel, with soldiers frequently ill for 5 to 6 weeks, mortality was uncommon. Occasionally, soldiers developed a relapsing or prolonged fever. The agent of trench fever is transmitted by the body louse and has been recognized in nonepidemic situations. The organism has been found in several different geographic areas, including Europe, North America, Ethiopia, and China. The most recent description of this illness was reported from Seattle by Spach and coworkers,[12] who described eight patients with *B. quintana* bacteremia who had febrile illnesses compatible with trench fever, and two patients with endocarditis. Many of these patients were homeless, used alcoholic beverages, and had lice or scabies. *B. quintana* has been cultured from the lymph node of a patient with chronic lymphadenopathy who had contact with cats but has not been isolated from patients with the classic findings of CSD.[45]

Bacillary angiomatosis is a relatively new disease affecting primarily immunocompromised patients. This disease was first diagnosed in 1983 in an HIV-infected man with subcutaneous nodules, fever, and weight loss.[46] *B. quintana* and *B. henselae* are known to cause both cutaneous and systemic disease. Clinical manifestations of the illness are similar to those seen in patients with *B. bacilliformis* infection and those with CSD. Patients most commonly present with multiple, angiomatous, tender papules or subcutaneous nodules consisting of proliferating endothelial and histiocytic cells in a framework of weakly formed capillaries.[21, 38, 47] The lesions contain bacteria that stain with the Warthin-Starry stain and may be few or widely disseminated. Some patients may have only skin mucosal lesions, and others have histologically similar lesions in bone, lung, liver, spleen, lymph nodes, and central nervous system. Lesions in the liver and spleen have been termed bacillary peliosis hepatis or bacillary peliosis splenitis. Histologic examination of this type of lesion shows cystic, blood-filled spaces, foci of necrosis or granulation-like tissue, and bacteria by Warthin-Starry stain.[48] Patients with peliosis often complain of fever, abdominal pain, and weight loss and exhibit hepatomegaly or splenomegaly, or both. Surgery or abdominal imaging studies may demonstrate perihepatic or abdominal lymph nodes, and laboratory evaluation characteristically reveals a markedly elevated alkaline phosphatase level and mild to moderate elevation of hepatocellular enzyme levels.[38, 48] Peliotic lesions also have been found in patients with wasting due to pulmonary tuberculosis, advanced cancer, anabolic steroids, and other drugs and have been seen in immunocompromised patients such as renal transplant patients and in a child undergoing chemotherapy for leukemia.[48, 49]

Bacillary angiomatosis, in patients with or without skin lesions, may involve areas other than the skin and abdominal viscera. Bone lesions, which are lytic in nature, are often extremely painful and most frequently involve the long bones. Lesions may occur in mucosal sites, including the mouth, stomach, large or small intestine, and the respiratory tract. Central nervous system and retinal lesions have been documented.[21, 48, 50] In one patient, a cerebral lesion resembled an abscess, bacteria were seen on brain biopsy, and the patient responded to oral erythromycin. Cures have been described of neuroretinitis, or Leber stellate neuroretinitis, a form of optic neuropathy manifested as optic nerve swelling with a macular star of exudate, similar to that seen in CSD.[50] These patients had serologic evidence of *Bartonella* infection, and the retinitis resolved with or without therapy and often with little visual damage. Patients with bacillary angiomatosis may have prolonged bacteremia, which can be documented by processing the blood cultures to detect *Bartonella* species.[51] Systemic signs and symptoms include fever, chills, malaise, headache, anorexia, and weight loss and may be present weeks to months before the diagnosis is made. Most of the clinical manifestations of bacillary angiomatosis respond to treatment with erythromycin or doxycycline, and immunocompromised patients may require treatment indefinitely.[13, 21, 38, 47] Occasional patients relapse with fever, bacteremia, or skin lesions when treatment is stopped.

B. henselae appears to be a cause of the majority of the cases of CSD.[52–55] Although *Afipia felis* causes occasional cases of CSD,[56] certain studies (microbiologic and serologic) indicate that most cases are caused by *B. henselae.* Because both *A. felis* and *Bartonella* species stain with the Warthin-Starry stain, some of the unidentified organisms initially described in cases of CSD were probably *B. henselae* rather than *A. felis.* The similarity between bacillary angiomatosis and CSD was first noted in HIV-infected patients, and serologic studies provided confirmation of this association. Regnery and coworkers,[52] using an indirect fluorescent antibody test for detection of antibodies to *B. henselae,* found that 88% of patients with suspected CSD had serum titers of 1:64 or higher. Subsequently, Dolan and coworkers[53] cultured the organism from the lymph nodes of two patients with CSD, and Anderson and colleagues,[54] using polymerase chain reaction techniques, detected *B. henselae* DNA in specimens from patients with CSD. In addition, *Bartonella*-specific sequences have been detected in the material used for the CSD skin test. *B. henselae* has been isolated from the blood of cats,[57] and antibody to *B. henselae* has been found in cats owned by patients with CSD (see Chapter 180). Some patients have presented with fever of unknown origin.[58]

Diagnosis

Microbiology

Isolation of these nutritionally fastidious organisms from the blood of patients can be accomplished using commercially available blood culture systems and prolonged incubation of subculture plates in an atmosphere of 5% carbon dioxide with high humidity.[34] Both a lysis-centrifugation technique (Isolator, Wampole, Cranberry, New Jersey) and the BACTEC system have been used to isolate these organisms[17, 22, 34] as long as subculture plates are incubated for up to 45 days. One successful technique involves routine acridine orange staining of broth blood cultures after 8 days.[51] This method enabled Arson and coworkers[51] to identify 10 patients with *Bartonella* bacteremia whose blood was inoculated into BACTEC nonradiometric aerobic resin blood culture bottles. Subcultured plates with chocolate agar, anaerobic blood agar, and freshly prepared brain-heart infusion agar with 5% rabbit blood allow the best growth and recovery. The organisms are not detected reliably by the BACTEC radiometric or infrared carbon dioxide detection system because they do not produce sufficient carbon dioxide and are not detected by traditional broth cultures as they produce little or no visible growth. After initial isolation, the organisms will grow in *Haemophilus* test media and specially prepared blood-free media.[59]

Isolation of the organism from tissue is more difficult. Koehler and Tappero[38] initially isolated *B. quintana* and *B. henselae* from biopsy specimens of skin lesions in patients with bacillary angiomatosis using cocultivation with an endothelial cell monolayer. Length of time to recovery was about 21 days. Direct plating of tissue has yielded *B. henselae* but in some cases only after up to 60 days' incubation. A chemically defined liquid medium containing hemin, developed by Wong and coworkers,[33] allows recovery of *B. henselae* from tissue after only 10 to 16 days of incubation. Fresh chocolate plates and heart infusion agar with 5% rabbit blood permit the best growth on solid media for recovery from tissue as well as from blood. Growth of *B. bacilliformis* is enhanced at 25°C to 32°C, but this lower temperature does not seem to be necessary for the other species.

Identification to the species level by the clinical microbiology laboratory is difficult.[34, 35] All species are catalase- and urease-negative. The oxidase reaction, when tested by the Kovacs procedure, is weakly positive for strains of *B. quintana* and *B. vinsonii* but negative for most strains of *B. henselae* and for *B. elizabethae. B. elizabethae,* the type strains of *R. quintana* and *R. vinsonii,* and one of three *R. henselae* strains grew within 72 hours on heart infusion agar around an X (hemin) strip.[22] The colonies are tiny, white, heterogeneous in size, adherent to the agar, and weakly gram-negative on staining. After several passages, incubation time decreases, and colonies become larger and less adherent. Drancourt and Raoult[32] used media supplemented with hemin and observed biochemical reactivity in a commercial identification system. A MicroScan rapid anaerobe identification panel can be used along with phenotypic characteristics to suggest to the technologist that *Bartonella* species have been isolated, but determination of cellular fatty acids or molecular techniques are needed to confirm the identification.[34] Techniques available in research laboratories include reactivity with specific antiserum, cellular fatty acid analysis, 16S ribosomal RNA gene sequencing, restriction fragment length polymorphism after polymerase chain reaction amplification of the citrate synthase gene or the 16S to 23S ribosomal RNA gene intergenic spacer region, and pulsed-field gel electrophoresis.[2, 21, 34, 35]

Serology

Serologic tests are available to aid in the diagnosis of infection with these organisms and have been used in patients with bacillary angiomatosis, fever and bacteremia, and CSD. Indirect fluorescent antibody tests for *B. henselae, B. quintana,* and *B. elizabethae* are available from the Centers for Disease Control and Prevention. An enzyme immunoassay for the detection of immunoglobulin G antibodies to *B. henselae* is available from Specialty Laboratories, Santa Monica, California,[60] and an immunoblot technique that can detect both immunoglobulins M and G to *B. henselae* has been developed by Welch and colleagues[34] in Oklahoma. The enzyme immunoassay study also can separate immunoglobulins M and G. In their initial report, Regnery and colleagues[57] found that 36 (88%) of 41 patients with suspected CSD had titers of 1:64 or greater to the *B. henselae* antigen, but it appears that a cross-reaction between antibodies against *B. quintana* and *B. henselae* occurs. Further epidemiologic study, including studies of the rate of antibody response to these organisms, is needed. Several patients I have treated with CSD had low levels of antibodies initially, often to both *B. henselae* and *B. quintana,* but during 2 to 4 weeks developed titers as high as 1:1048. A similar finding was noted in a patient with hepatic granulomata.[55] The patient described by Waldvogel and colleagues[55] had an antibody titer of 1:16,384 to *B. quintana* and only 1:1024 to *B. henselae.* Problems persist with serologic testing, including cross-reactions within the genus[61] and with other genera (especially *Chlamydia* species),[16, 62] the need for a specific immunoglobulin M assay, and elucidation of antibody response in the clinical setting over time.

The diagnosis can be suggested by histologic findings in tissue from skin lesions, lymph nodes, spleen, or liver. Clinical findings consistent with CSD or neuroretinitis in an HIV-infected patient should lead the physician to perform the serologic tests. Bartonellosis caused by *B. bacilliformis* should be considered in patients living in or traveling to endemic areas. Physicians should consider *Bartonella* species in patients with endocarditis and negative routine cultures of blood after 3 to 5 days' incubation. As laboratories become aware of the growth characteristics of *Bartonella* species and physicians better understand the illnesses caused by these pathogens, it is likely that more cases will be recognized. With the increase in detection, more in vitro information about antimicrobial susceptibility and in vivo data about clinical risk factors for infection will emerge to help clinicians correctly diagnose and treat patients with infection with these organisms.

Treatment

Antibiotics are known to reduce mortality in Oroya fever. Chloramphenicol, penicillins, and aminoglycosides have been used, but it is not known whether the improved outcome has been due to therapy of the *Bartonella* infection or because of efficacy against secondary pathogens such as *Salmonella* species. Antibiotics appear to be beneficial in patients with bacillary angiomatosis, peliosis hepatis, and bacteremia and fever but not in most patients with CSD. Erythromycin, 500 mg four times daily, is the drug of choice for infection with *B. quintana* or *B. henselae;* doxycycline or other tetracyclines are alternatives. Other agents have appeared to be successful, although β-lactam agents appear to be the least active.[63, 64] Immunocompromised patients with typical or disseminated CSD do not clearly respond to antibiotic treatment, making the value of treatment in this illness unclear, although various agents have been tried in patients with CSD, including trimethoprim-sulfamethoxazole, rifampin, ciprofloxacin, and gentamicin (see Chapter 180).

The optimal duration of therapy is not known, but prolonged treatment from weeks to months, even lifelong, may be needed for HIV-infected patients. The number of reports of infection with *B. henselae* continues to increase, and the course of the illness and response to treatment in various groups of patients are variable. Fever and bacteremia in immunocompetent persons initially appeared to be cured after relatively brief courses (7 to 10 days) of antibiotics. However, Lucey and coworkers[40] reported two immunocompetent patients (one with aseptic meningitis) with clinical relapses after treatment who were cured after retreatment. This spectrum of clinical disease is similar to that seen in patients with trench fever and infection with *B. bacilliformis,* and the influence of antibiotic treatment on the course and duration of chronic disease is not well understood. In vitro testing reveals that the organisms are susceptible to several classes of antimicrobials[63, 64] and does not clearly reflect clinical experience. It is thought that the intracellular growth of bacteria and perhaps inhibitory rather than bactericidal activity of the agents may explain clinical relapses and treatment failure.

Prevention

Infection with these organisms can be prevented by avoidance of contact with the vectors. Insecticide spraying of an area inhabited by sandflies, the use of insect netting and repellents, and avoidance of outdoor activities at night have been useful in reducing the incidence of disease in areas endemic for *B. bacilliformis.* The issuance of new clothing to British soldiers returning from the trenches is credited with preventing spread of *B. quintana* to the civilian population after World War I. Programs to rid people of lice and to provide better nourishment to homeless people might decrease transmission in settings such as that described in the report from Seattle.[12] Avoidance of contact with cats, a recommendation that cannot be made generally because of the large number of cat owners and cat fanciers, might be considered for individuals infected with HIV.

References

1. Birtles RJ, Harrison TG, Saunders NA: Proposals to unify the genera *Grahamella* and *Bartonella,* with descriptions of *Bartonella talpae* comb. nov., *Bartonella peromysci* sp. nov., *Bartonella taylorii* sp. nov., and *Bartonella doshiae* sp. nov. Int J Syst Bacteriol 45:1, 1995.
2. Brenner DJ, O'Connor SP, Winkler HH, et al: Proposals to unify the genera *Bartonella* and *Rochalimaea,* with descriptions of *Bartonella quintana* comb. nov., *Bartonella vinsonii* comb. nov., *Bartonella henselae* comb. nov., and *Bartonella elizabethae* comb. nov., and to remove the family *Bartonellaceae* from the order Rickettsiales. Int J Syst Bacteriol 43:777, 1993.
3. Lawson PA, Collins MD: Description of *Bartonella clarridgeiae* sp. nov. isolated from the cat of a patient with *Bartonella henselae* septicemia. Med Microbiol Lett 5:64, 1996.
4. Alexander B: A review of bartonellosis in Ecuador and Colombia. Am J Trop Med Hyg 52:354, 1995.
5. Schultz MG: Special article: Daniel Carrion's experiment. N Engl J Med 278:1323, 1968.
6. Weiman D, Kreier JP: *Bartonella* and *Grahamella. In* Kreier JP

(ed): Parasitic Protozoa, Vol 4. New York, Academic Press, 1977, pp 197–233.
7. Noguchi, H: Etiology of Oroya fever, I. Cultivation of *Bartonella bacilliformis*. J Exp Med 4:851, 1926.
8. Schmincke A: Histopathologischer Befund in Roseolen der Haut bei Wolhynischem Feiber. Munch Med Wochenschr 64:91, 1917.
9. Sikora H: Uber die Züchtung der *Rickettsia pediculi*. Arch Schiffs Trop Hyg 25:123, 1921.
10. Mooser H, Leeman A, Chao SH, et al: Beobachtungen an Funftagefieber. Schweiz Z Allgemeine Pathol Bakteriol 11:513, 1948.
11. Vinson JW, Fuller HS: Studies on trench fever. I. Propagation of rickettsia-like microorganisms from a patient's blood. Path Microbiol 24(Suppl):152, 1961.
11a. Varela G, Vinson JW, Molina-Pasquel C: Trench fever II. Propagation of *Rickettsia quintana* on cell-free medium from the blood of two patients. Am J Trop Med Hyg 18:708, 1969.
12. Spach DO, Candor AS, Dougherty MJ, et al: *Bartonella (Rochalimaea) quintana* bacteremia in inner-city patients with chronic alcoholism. N Engl J Med 332:424, 1995.
13. Koehler JE, Quinn FD, Berger TG, et al: Isolation of *Rochalimaea* species from cutaneous and osseous lesions of bacillary angiomatosis. N Engl J Med 327:1625, 1992.
14. Slater LN, Welch DF, Min K: *Rochalimaea henselae* causes bacillary angiomatosis and peliosis hepatis. Arch Intern Med 152:602, 1992.
15. Spach DO, Callis KP, Paauw DS, et al: Endocarditis caused by *Rochalimaea quintana* in a patient infected with the human immunodeficiency virus. J Clin Microbiol 31:692, 1993.
16. Drancourt M, Mainardi JL, Brouqui P, et al: *Bartonella (Rochalimaea) quintana* endocarditis in three homeless men. N Engl J Med 332:419, 1995.
17. Slater LN, Welch DF, Hensel D, et al: A newly recognized fastidious gram-negative pathogen as a cause of fever and bacteremia. N Engl J Med 323:1587, 1990.
18. Relman DA, Loutit JS, Schmidt TM, et al: The agent of bacillary angiomatosis: An approach to the identification of uncultured pathogens. N Engl J Med 323:1573, 1990.
19. Welch DF, Pickett DA, Slater LN, et al: *Rochalimaea henselae* sp. nov., a cause of septicemia, bacillary angiomatosis, and parenchymal bacillary peliosis. J Clin Microbiol 30:275, 1992.
20. Regnery RL. Anderson BE, Clarridge JE III, et al: Characterization of a novel *Rochalimaea* species, *R. henselae* sp. nov., isolated from blood of a febrile, human immunodeficiency virus–positive patient. J Clin Microbiol 30:265, 1992.
21. Adal KA, Cockerell CJ, Petri WA: Cat scratch disease, bacillary angiomatosis, and other infections due to *Rochalimaea*. N Engl J Med 330:1509, 1994.
22. Daly JS, Worthington MG, Brenner DJ, et al: *Rochalimaea elizabethae* sp. nov. isolated from a patient with endocarditis. J Clin Microbiol 31:872, 1993.
23. Baker JA: A rickettsial infection in Canadian voles. J Exp Med 84:37, 1946.
24. Weiss E, Dasch GA, Woodman GR, et al: Vole agent identified as a strain of the trench fever rickettsia, *Rochalimaea quintana*. Infect Immun 19:1013, 1978.
25. Weiss E, Dasch GA: Differential characteristics of strains of *Rochalimaea: Rochalimaea vinsonii* sp. nov., the Canadian vole agent. Int J Syst Bacteriol 32:305, 1982.
26. Breitschwerdt EB, Kordick DL, Malarkey DE, et al: Endocarditis in a dog due to infection with a novel *Bartonella* subspecies. J Clin Microbiol 33:154, 1995.
27. Hoyte HMD: *Grahamella* (Rickettsiales) in the common shrew *Sorex araneus*. Parasitology 46:224, 1954.
28. Birtles RJ, Harrison TG: *Grahamella* in small woodland mammals in the U.K.: Isolation, prevalence and host specificity. Ann Trop Med Parasitol 88:317, 1994.
29. Brenner DJ, O'Connor SP, Hollis DG, et al: Molecular characterization and proposal of a neotype strain for *Bartonella bacilliformis*. J Clin Microbiol 29:1299, 1991.
30. Dooley JR: Occasional survey: Haemotropic bacteria in man. Lancet 2:1237, 1980.
31. Peters D, Wigand R: Bartonellaceae. Bacteriol Rev 19:150, 1954.
32. Drancourt M, Raoult D: Proposed test for the routine identification of *Rochalimaea* species. Eur J Clin Microbiol Infect Dis 12:710, 1994.
33. Wong MT, Thornton DC, Kennedy RC, Dolan MJ: A chemically defined liquid medium that supports primary isolation of *Rochalimaea (Bartonella) henselae* from blood and tissue specimens. J Clin Microbiol 33:742, 1995.
34. Welch DF, Hensel DM, Pickett DA, et al: Bacteremia due to *Rochalimaea henselae* in a child: Practical identification of isolates in the clinical laboratory. J Clin Microbiol 31:2381, 1993.
35. Roux V, Raoult D: Inter- and intraspecies identification of *Bartonella (Rochalimaea)* species. J Clin Microbiol 33:1573, 1995.
36. Zangwill KM, Hamilton DH, Perkins BA, et al: Cat scratch disease in Connecticut. N Engl J Med 329:8, 1993.
37. Tappero JW, Mohle-Boetani J, Koehler J, et al: The epidemiology of bacillary angiomatosis and bacillary peliosis. JAMA 269:770, 1993.
38. Koehler JE, Tappero JW: Bacillary angiomatosis and bacillary peliosis in patients infected with human immunodeficiency virus. Clin Infect Dis 17:612, 1993.
39. Weiss E, Moulder JW: Genus II *Rochalimaea* (Macchiavello 1947) Krieg 1961, 162. *In* Krieg NR, Holt JG (eds): Bergey's Manual of Systematic Bacteriology, Vol 1. Baltimore: Williams & Wilkins; 1984, pp 698–701.
40. Lucey D, Dolan MJ, Moss CW, et al: Relapsing illness due to *Rochalimaea henselae* in immunocompetent hosts: Implication for therapy and new epidemiological associations. Clin Infect Dis 14:683, 1992.
41. Ricketts WE: Clinical manifestations of Carrion's disease. Arch Intern Med 84:751, 1949.
42. Gray GC, Johnson AA, Thornton SA, et al: An epidemic of Oroya fever in the Peruvian Andes. Am J Trop Med Hyg 42:215, 1990.
43. Arias-Stella J, Lieberman PH, Erlandson RA, et al: Histology, immunohistochemistry, and ultrastructure of the verruga in Carrion's disease. Am J Surg Pathol 10:595, 1986.
44. Matteelli A, Castelli F, Spinetti A, et al: Short report: Verruga peruana in an Italian traveler from Peru. Am J Trop Med Hyg 50:143, 1994.
45. Raoult D, Drancourt M, Carta A, Gastaut JA: *Bartonella (Rochalimaea) quintana* isolation in patient with chronic adenopathy, lymphopenia, and a cat (Letter). Lancet 343:977, 1994.
46. Stoler MH, Bonfiglio TA, Steigbigel RT, et al: Case reports: An atypical subcutaneous infection associated with acquired immune deficiency syndrome. Am J Clin Pathol 80:714, 1983.
47. Cotell SL, Noskin GA: Bacillary angiomatosis: Clinical and histologic features, diagnosis, and treatment. Arch Intern Med 154:524, 1994.
48. Perkocha LA, Geaghan SM, Benedict Yen TS, et al: Clinical and pathological features of bacillary peliosis hepatis in association with human immunodeficiency virus infection. N Engl J Med 323:1581, 1990.
49. Myers SA, Prose NS, Garcia JA, et al: Bacillary angiomatosis in a child undergoing chemotherapy. J Pediatr 121:574, 1992.
50. Golnik KC, Marotto ME, Fanous MM, et al: Ophthalmic manifestations of *Rochalimaea* species. Am J Ophthalmol 118:145, 1994.
51. Arson AM, Dougherty MJ, Nowowiejski DJ, et al: Detection of *Bartonella (Rochalimaea) quintana* by routine acridine orange staining of broth blood cultures. J Clin Microbiol 32:1492, 1994.
52. Regnery RL, Olson JG, Perkins BA, et al: Serological response to "*Rochalimaea henselae*" antigen in suspected cat-scratch disease. Lancet 339:1443, 1992.
53. Dolan MJ, Wong MT, Regnery RL, et al: Syndrome of *Rochalimaea henselae* adenitis suggesting cat scratch disease. Ann Intern Med 118:331, 1993.
54. Anderson B, Sims K, Regnery R, et al: Detection of *Rochalimaea henselae* DNA in specimens from cat-scratch disease patients by PCR. J Clin Microbiol 32:942, 1994.
55. Waldvogel K, Regnery RL, Anderson BE, et al: Disseminated cat-scratch disease: Detection of *Rochalimaea henselae* in affected tissue. Eur J Pediatr 153:23, 1994.
56. Alkan S, Morgan MB, Sandin RL, et al: Dual role for *Afipia felis* and *Rochalimaea henselae* in cat-scratch disease. Lancet 345:385, 1995.
57. Regnery R, Martin M, Olson J: Naturally occurring "*Rochalimaea henselae*" infection in domestic cat. Lancet 340:557, 1992.
58. Dangman BC, Albanese BA, Kacica MA: Cat scratch disease in two children presenting with fever of unknown origin: Imaging features and association with a new causative agent, *Rochalimaea henselae*. Pediatrics 95:767, 1995.
59. Schwartzman WA, Nesbit CA, Baron EJ: Development and evalu-

ation of a blood-free medium for determining growth curves and optimizing growth of *Rochalimaea henselae.* J Clin Microbiol 31:1882, 1993.
60. Barka NE, Hadfield T, Patnaik M, et al: EIA for detection of *Rochalimaea henselae*–reactive IgG, IgM, and IgA antibodies in patients with suspected cat-scratch disease. J Infect Dis 167:1503, 1993.
61. Golden SE: Hepatosplenic cat-scratch disease associated with elevated anti–*Rochalimaea* antibody titers. Pediatr Infect Dis J 12:868, 1993.
62. Drancourt M, Birtles R, Chaumentin G, et al: New serotype of *Bartonella henselae* in endocarditis and cat-scratch disease. Lancet 347:441, 1996.
63. Maurin M, Raoult D: Antimicrobial susceptibility of *Rochalimaea quintana, Rochalimaea vinsonii,* and the newly recognized *Rochalimaea henselae.* J Antimicrob Chemother 32:587, 1993.
64. Maurin M, Raoult D: *Bartonella (Rochalimaea)* quintana infections. Clin Microbiol Rev 9:273, 1996.

229

Calymmatobacterium granulomatis

Gary Doern

History

Donovanosis, or granuloma inguinale, was first described by McLeod[1] in 1882, when he noted "serpiginous ulcerations associated with more or less thickening of tissues" in patients living in Calcutta, India. The causative agent of the disease was initially recognized by Donovan in 1905.[2] Microscopic examination of tissue biopsy specimens revealed intracellular organisms originally thought to be protozoa, which were named Donovan bodies. Subsequently, the agent of donovanosis was determined to be a bacterium and was named *Donovania granulomatis.*[3] It is now referred to as *Calymmatobacterium granulomatis.*

Characteristics of the Pathogen

C. granulomatis is a gram-negative, nonmotile, non–spore-forming coccobacillus that measures 0.5 to 1.0 × 1.5 to 20 μm. It is generally categorized as a bacterium of uncertain affiliation; however, it bears many similarities to members of the family Enterobacteriaceae, in particular *Klebsiella rhinoscleromatis* and *Enterobacter aerogenes.*[4] The organism possesses a cytoplasmic membrane, a typical gram-negative cell wall, and in many instances, a sharply delineated capsule.[5] Surface projections, which appear to be fimbriae or pili, have been observed by electron microscopy.[6]

C. granulomatis has been propagated in yolk sacs of chick embryos.[3] Growing the organisms in cell-free, defined media has been more difficult. Although there have been sporadic reports of propagation, or at least maintenance, using specialized media[7] and on slants composed of coagulated egg yolk,[8] for practical purposes the organism cannot be grown on standard laboratory media. Indeed, currently, there are no cultures of this organism in existence.

Epidemiology

Donovanosis is often referred to as one of the classic ulcerative sexually transmitted diseases, along with syphilis, herpes simplex virus infection, chancroid, and lymphogranuloma venereum. In reality, the role of sexual transmission remains controversial. The high frequency of infection in persons between 20 and 40 years old, the years of greatest sexual activity; the fact that rectal lesions are found in male homosexuals who engage in anal intercourse and whose partners have penile lesions; and the predilection for lesions to occur on the genitalia support the notion of venereal transmission.[9] Conversely, in certain parts of the world donovanosis occurs with great frequency in young children who have no history of sexual contact.[10] Furthermore, it is uncommon to find evidence of infection in the heterosexual partners of patients with well-defined genital lesions of *C. granulomatis* infection.[11, 12] Finally, although infrequently, primary donovanian lesions have been described on skin surfaces such as the trunk and proximal upper extremities, for which sexual contact is an implausible explanation for transmission. It is likely, therefore, that *C. granulomatis* can be transmitted via direct sexual contact as well as by indirect means. An example of the latter mode of transmission is the frequently cited but largely unproven assertion that fecal soilage of the perineal skin and vagina can lead to infection of these sites, presumably by traumatic inoculation of organisms normally present in stool.[13] This, of course, presupposes that *C. granulomatis* is a commensal organism in stool, something that also has not been proved.

Donovanosis occurs primarily in tropical and subtropical areas of the world. It used to be more common in the United States, particularly among black persons in the southeastern Atlantic coast region. Today fewer than 100 cases occur annually. Autochthonous infection by *C. granulomatis* is also nearly unheard of in the developed countries of Western Europe and in Japan. At present, donovanosis is endemic in parts of India; the arid and semiarid regions of central, northern, and western Australia; western New Guinea; southern China; and parts of southwest Asia and Africa. In the Western Hemisphere, endemic donovanosis may be found in Brazil and in some of the Caribbean islands.[6, 9]

In endemic areas, the prevalence of donovanosis may be quite high. For instance, a 1971 surveillance study performed in Papua New Guinea revealed overall infection rates of nearly 5%.[10] In male patients attending a venereal disease clinic, the prevalence of donovanosis was 23.5%.[14] Men are more often found to be infected than are women (2.5:1).[15] Historically, a preponderance of cases of donovanosis has been observed in black persons. This is probably explained by socioeconomic factors and the geography of endemicity rather than a racial predisposition.

Pathogenesis and Clinical Manifestations

Organisms gain entrance into infected tissue by direct traumatic inoculation through the skin. The incubation period is extremely variable, ranging from 8 to 80 days (mean, 17 days).[9] A dense accumulation of mononuclear cells forms within the affected dermis. Occasional clusters of neutrophils and histiocytes are also found. Acanthosis may be present in the surrounding epithelium. In addition, areas of pseudoepitheliomatous hyperplasia may be found to envelop the granulomatous lesion. The pathognomonic cells of donovanosis are found scattered throughout the lesion but are usually more numerous and conspicuous at the margins. These cells consist of enlarged histocytes with intracytoplasmic vacuoles containing variable numbers of the infectious agent, *C. granu-*

lomatis. More than one cytoplasmic inclusion may be found per histiocyte. As noted later, the appearance of the organism within what are apparently phagocytic vacuoles is quite characteristic. These inclusions have been termed Donovan bodies.

Grossly, the lesions usually begin as solitary, superficial, small, firm papules, which eventually evolve into ulcers as the overlying skin breaks down. Although the actual appearance of the ulcer may be variable, the most common form is a painless, fleshy, beefy-red granulomatous lesion that is neither tender nor indurated and that bleeds profusely when touched. Lesions may take on a verrucous appearance at the periphery when epithelial hyperplasia has occurred. Secondarily infected lesions may become tender and necrotic and show evidence of a purulent exudate. Surrounding cellulitis is rare. Multiple adjacent lesions may coalesce as they enlarge, forming large single lesions. Although there is little tendency to spread locally or disseminate systemically, secondary donovanian lesions have been noted in the uterus, fallopian tubes, ovaries, and epididymis (contiguous spread),[9, 16] and in the liver and skeletal system (systemic spread).[17] Systemic dissemination is most likely the result of hematogenous seeding.

Ninety percent of primary lesions are found on the skin of the genitalia[10]: in men, on the prepuce, coronal sulcus, shaft, glans, and frenum[9]; in women, usually on the labia minora and majora and the fourchette.[16] In 10% of cases, lesions appear on the inguinal skin.[10] The perianal skin is involved in 5% to 10% of cases.[17] Primary lesions do occur in other sites such as the rectum and oral cavity, but much less frequently. Inguinal lymphadenopathy, a common finding in patients with syphilis, chancroid, herpes simplex virus infection, or lymphogranuloma venereum, is typically absent in patients with donovanosis unless lesions become superinfected. "Pseudobuboes" may occur, but rather than representing enlarged inguinal lymph nodes, they are subcutaneous granulation tissue that arises as a result of secondary foci of infection formed from local extension.

There are two major consequences of untreated infections: fibrosis and scarring of involved tissue can result in loss of function, and, if the lymphatics are involved, lymph stasis and lymphedema are possible. A second concern pertains to the relationship between donovanosis and squamous cell carcinoma of the penis and vulva.[18] This relationship is supported by the following observations. The incidence of genital carcinoma is greater than normal in areas where donovanosis is endemic. Squamous cell carcinomas have been observed within healed *C. granulomatis* lesions. The two conditions have often been found to occur concurrently. Finally, in one investigation, 9 of 62 patients with squamous cell carcinoma of the penis were noted to have circulating antibody reactive with *C. granulomatis.*[18] These observations certainly do not prove a role for *C. granulomatis* as a cause of genital carcinoma, but they do justify further investigation of this possibility.

Diagnosis

An accurate clinical diagnosis of donovanosis can be achieved in approximately 63% of men and 83% of women by experienced clinicians working in an endemic area.[19] A definitive diagnosis of *C. granulomatis* infections, however, is best accomplished by microscopic visualization of characteristic Donovan bodies in tissue biopsy material. Biopsies should be obtained from the advancing margins of the base of ulcers. A portion of the specimen should be fixed in formalin and submitted for sectioning and histologic examination. The remainder should be placed between two cleaned glass microscope slides and then crushed and smeared across the slides to produce a thin film of macerated tissue.[20] The slides are air-dried, and then one is stained with either Wright[21] or Giemsa[20] stain and the other is processed with either the Dieterle silver impregnation stain or Warthin-Starry stain.[22]

A diagnosis of donovanosis is made when clusters of coccobacillus-shaped organisms are observed within phagocytic vacuoles in histiocytes. The organisms possess a distinct bipolar staining characteristic that gives the appearance of two adjacent coccal forms (i.e., a closed safety pin appearance). This results from the accumulation of condensed chromatin material at the poles of the cell. All four of the stains just noted stain the organisms dark blue to black. Organisms examined with the Wright or Giemsa stain may be surrounded by pink capsular material.[23]

Crush preparations are usually more rewarding than histologic sections. Culture is of no practical value because of the difficulties of propagating the organism. Similarly, no serologic procedures of proven utility in diagnosing donovanosis are currently available.

Treatment

Numerous antimicrobial agents have been used to successfully treat donovanosis: antimony salts, tetracyclines, streptomycin, trimethoprim-sulfamethoxazole, chloramphenicol, erythromycin, various penicillins, ceftriaxone, and aminoglycosides. Because no controlled comparative clinical trials have been performed, there is little objective basis for defining optimal therapy. In view of this, tetracycline appears to be the drug of first choice; it is certainly the agent with which the greatest clinical experience treating donovanosis has been accumulated.[24] Tetracycline should be administered orally in 500-mg doses every 6 hours.[25] A clinical response should be evident within approximately 1 week, as lesions begin to regress. Therapy should be continued until the lesions disappear completely. In some cases, this takes 2 to 3 months. Discontinuing therapy before lesions have healed completely often results in recrudescence of disease. For pregnant women and children with deciduous teeth, trimethoprim-sulfamethoxazole, two single-strength tablets every 12 hours, is adequate alternative therapy.[26]

Prevention

Preventive measures for reducing the incidence of donovanosis include prompt treatment of recognized cases and improving the personal hygiene and sanitation facilities of persons in areas where the disease is endemic.

References

1. McLeod K: Precis of operations by Major McLeod. Indian Med Gaz 15:113, 1882.
2. Donovan C: Medical cases from Madras General Hospital: Ulcerating granuloma of the pudenda. Indian Med Gaz 40:414, 1905.
3. Anderson K, DeMonbreaun WA, Goodpasture EW: An etiologic consideration of *Donovania granulomatis* cultivated from granuloma inguinale (three cases) in embryonic yolk. J Exp Med 81:25, 1943.
4. Goldberg J: Studies on granuloma inguinale IV. Growth requirements of *Donovania granulomatis* and its relationship to the natural habitat of the organism. Br J Vener Dis 35:266, 1959.
5. Davis CM, Collins C: An ultrastructural study of *Calymmatobacterium granulomatis.* J Invest Dermatol 53:315, 1969.
6. Hart G: Donovanosis. *In* Holmes KK, Mardh P-A, Sparling PF,

Weisner PJ (eds): Sexually Transmitted Disease. New York, McGraw-Hill, 1984, pp 393–395.
7. Dunham W, Rake G: Cultural and serologic studies on granuloma inguinale. Am J Syphilol 32:145, 1948.
8. Goldberg J, Weaver RH, Packer H: Studies on granuloma inguinale: I. Bacteriologic behavior of *Donovania granulomatis.* Am J Syphilol 12:57, 1953.
9. Sehgal VN, Shyan Prasad AL: Donovanosis: Current concepts. Int J Dermatol 25:8, 1986.
10. Zigas V: Medicine from the past: Donovanosis project in Goilala (1951–1954). Papua New Guinea Med J 14:148, 1971.
11. Hart G: Chancroid, Donovanosis, Lymphogranuloma Venereum. Washington, DC, US Department of Health Education and Welfare publication (CDC) 75-8302, 1975.
12. O'Farrell N: Clinico-epidemiological study of donovanosis in Durban, South Africa. Genitourin Med 69:108, 1993.
13. Goldberg J: Studies on granuloma inguinale: VII. Some epidemiological considerations of the disease. Br J Vener Dis 40:140, 1964.
14. Hart G: Psychological and social aspects of venereal disease in Papua New Guinea. Br J Vener Dis 50:453, 1974.
15. Canizares O: Nontreponemal veneral infections. *In* Moschella SL, Pillsbury DM, Hurley HJ (eds): Dermatology, Vol 1. Philadelphia, WB Saunders, 1975, pp 741–744.
16. Wysoki RS, Majmudar B, Willis D: Granuloma inguinale (donovanosis) in women. J Reprod Med 33:709, 1988.
17. Kirkpatrick DJ: Donovanosis (granuloma inguinale): A rare cause of osteolytic bone lesions. Clin Radiol 21:101, 1970.
18. Goldberg J, Annamunthodo H: Studies on granuloma inguinale. VIII. Serologic reactivity of sera from patients with carcinoma of the penis when tested with *Donovania* antigens. Br J Vener Dis 42:205, 1966.
19. O'Farrell N, Hoosen AA, Coetzee KD, van den Ende J: Genital ulcer disease: Accuracy of clinical diagnosis and strategies to improve control in Durban, South Africa. Genitourin Med 70:7, 1994.
20. Cannefax GR: The technic of tissue spread method for demonstrating Donovan bodies. J Vener Dis Inf 29:201, 1948.
21. Greenblatt RB, Dienst RD, West RM: A simple stain for Donovan bodies in diagnosis of granuloma inguinale. Am J Syphilol 35:291, 1951.
22. Greenblatt RF, Barfield WE: Newer methods in diagnosis and treatment of granuloma inguinale. Br J Vener Dis 28:123, 1952.
23. Sehgal VN, Prasad ALS, Beohar PC: The histopathology of donovanosis. Br J Vener Dis 60:145, 1984.
24. Nongonococcal urethritis and other sexually transmitted diseases of public health importance. Report of a WHO Scientific Group. World Health Organ Tech Rep Ser 660:1, 1981.
25. Robinson HM: The treatment of granuloma inguinale, lymphogranuloma venereum, chancroid and gonorrhea. Arch Dermatol Syphilol 64:284, 1951.
26. Lal S, Garg BR: Further evidence of the efficacy of co-trimoxazole in granuloma venereum. Br J Vener Dis 56:412, 1980.

230

Nocardia

Michael C. Bach

History

Nocardia was first described by Nocard in 1889 after he investigated an outbreak of a granulomatous disease in cattle on the island of Guadeloupe. These animals developed multiple draining abscesses with cutaneous sinuses and eventually pneumonia followed by death. Nocard isolated an aerobic actinomycete, which he named *Streptothrix farcini,* as the cause of this bovine farcy. The organism was formally reclassified in 1896 by Blanchard. The first human isolate was described by Eppinger in 1891 in a patient with pneumonia and brain abscess.

Subsequently, *Nocardia* was implicated in the complications of a wide variety of diseases (Table 230–1) and was found to cause infection in normal hosts.[1,2] It has been estimated that there are between 500 and 1000 new cases diagnosed annually in the United States.[1] More recently, the organism has caused infection in patients suffering from the acquired immunodeficiency syndrome.

TABLE 230–1 ■ Conditions Associated with *Nocardia*

Pulmonary alveolar proteinosis
Malignancy
Acquired immunodeficiency syndrome
Corticosteroid therapy
Cushing's syndrome
Organ transplantation
Chronic granulomatous disease of childhood
Congenital immunodeficiency diseases

Classification

Nocardia is classified in the order Actinomycetales along with *Actinomyces* and *Streptomyces* (Table 230–2). It is in the family Nocardiaceae with the non–acid-fast *Actinomadura* that is a cause of chronically draining sinuses of the extremities. Although *Nocardia* exhibits the classic fungal characteristics of true aerial hyphae, it is considered a higher bacterium rather than a fungus because its cell wall consists of peptidoglycans and does not contain either chitin or cellulose.

Structurally, it appears as a thin (0.5 to 1.0 μm), branching, often beaded, gram-positive rod (Fig. 230–1). Although not acid-fast in the standard acid-alcohol decolorization of the Ziehl-Neelsen method, it is weakly acid-fast when decolorized with 1% sulfuric acid (Kinyoun method) (Fig. 230–2). This helps distinguish *Nocardia* from the anaerobic *Actinomyces* group of organisms.

Nocardia is a hardy aerobe. It can be cultivated on simple

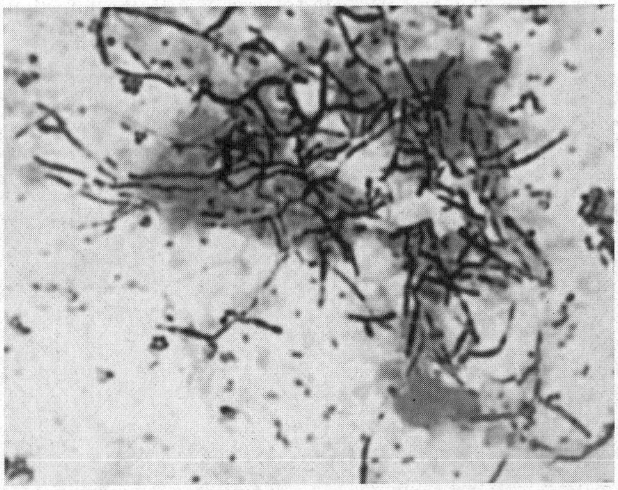

FIGURE 230–1 □ Gram stain of sputum from a patient with *Nocardia* pneumonia (× 1000). (From Bach MC: Nocardial infection. *In* Kass EH, Platt R [eds]: Current Therapy in Infectious Disease—3. Philadelphia, BC Decker, 1990, pp 326–328.)

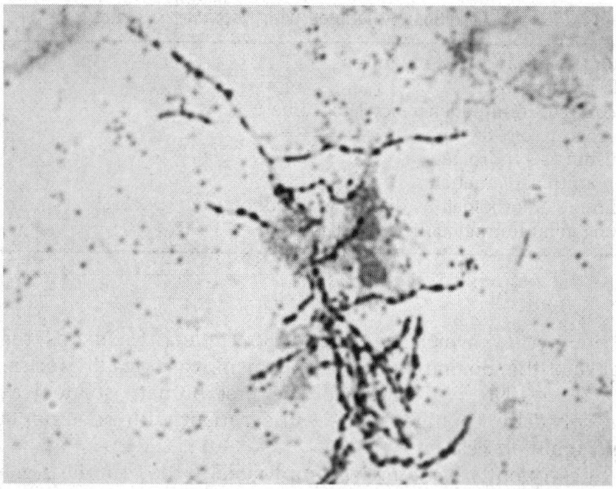

FIGURE 230–2 □ Specimen now stained by the Kinyoun method showing acid-fast characteristics (× 1000).

media and can tolerate temperatures up to 50°C. Ten percent carbon dioxide will encourage growth. It is a slow grower, however, and sometimes 4 to 5 days elapse before visible colonies appear on the culture medium.

Epidemiology

Nocardia is ubiquitous and is found primarily in soil and organic matter. There is no evidence for person-to-person transmission, and these infections should therefore be considered environmentally acquired. The aerosol route is the major portal of entry into the body, the lung being the most common site of infection. The gastrointestinal tract may be an alternative route, organisms entering the blood stream or lymphatics through breaks in the gut mucosa. Traumatic inoculation through the skin or eye is also a mechanism for implantation.

Pathogenesis

Nocardia elicits a brisk inflammatory response in the host. Both polymorphonuclear leukocytes and activated lymphocytes are involved in the cellular response to the infection.

TABLE 230–2 ■ Characteristics of Actinomycetales

CHARACTERISTIC	*ACTINOMYCES*	*NOCARDIA*	*STREPTOMYCES*
Requires oxygen	No	Yes	Yes
Acid-fast (Ziehl-Neelsen)	No	No	No
Weakly acid-fast (Kinyoun)	No	Yes	No

Histologically, necrosis and abscess formation are common (Fig. 230–3).

Immunology

Work has begun to clarify the host response to infection by *Nocardia.* Polymorphonuclear leukocytes alone are not sufficient to eradicate the organisms despite the fact that histologic examination of infected tissues reveals large numbers of them. Evidence now suggests that the neutrophil may delay the growth of *Nocardia,* allowing time for recruitment and activation of macrophages. This delay involves both phagocytosis and temporary inhibition of filament formation.[4] Although the oxidative metabolic burst has not been shown to inhibit filament formation in vitro, the observation that patients with chronic granulomatous disease appear to be more susceptible to *Nocardia* suggests that some other mechanism may be operative.[5]

Cell-mediated immunity appears to be the most important host defense mechanism against *Nocardia.* It begins with phagocytosis by macrophages and then lysosomal enzyme release, with resulting destruction of the organism. Virulent organisms appear to be more resistant to phagocytosis and better able to inhibit phagosome-lysosome fusion.[6]

Clinical Manifestations

Infection is most commonly seen in the lung, where the organism causes an acute, often necrotizing pneumonia, commonly associated with cavitation (Fig. 230–4). Other presentations may include a slowly enlarging pulmonary nodule or pneumonia with an associated empyema. Patients are usually systemically ill with fever, cough, and weight loss. Pleuritic chest pain often precedes or accompanies development of

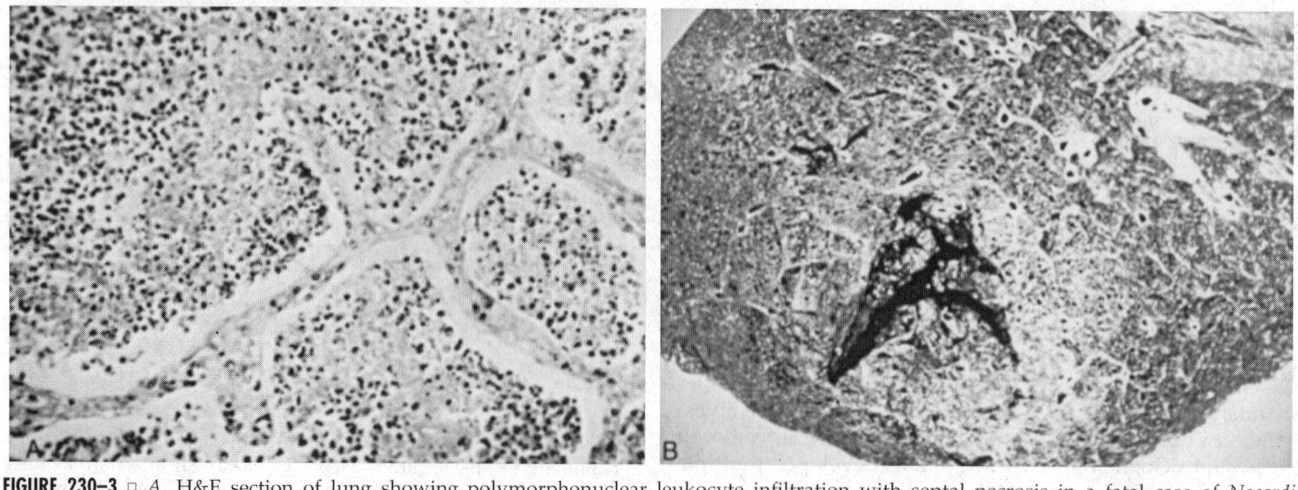

FIGURE 230–3 □ *A,* H&E section of lung showing polymorphonuclear leukocyte infiltration with septal necrosis in a fatal case of *Nocardia* pneumonia. *B,* Gross appearance of the lung showed a *Nocardia* lung abscess.

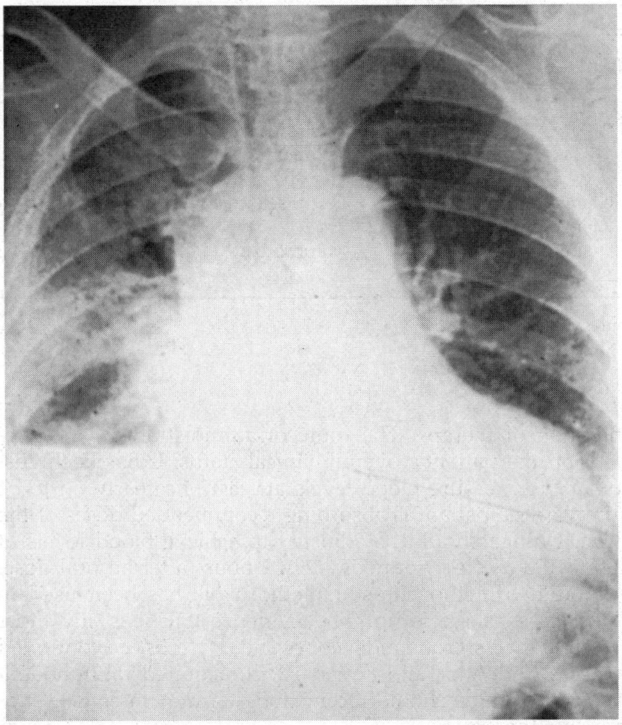

FIGURE 230–4 □ Right lower lobe *Nocardia* pneumonia in a renal transplant recipient.

empyema. The progress of the infection may be slow, thus mimicking chronic granulomatous infections such as tuberculosis or neoplastic diseases such as bronchogenic carcinoma. The organisms can also spread to involve the pericardium, resulting in suppurative pericarditis. Because of its propensity for hematogenous dissemination, *Nocardia* often produces metastatic spread, most commonly to the brain (Fig. 230–5) but also to the kidney, spleen, liver, thyroid, adrenal, prostate, and rarely, bone. The metastatic foci may be clinically silent early on, and patients may develop neurologic signs while receiving therapy for their pulmonary infection.

Infection as a result of inoculation can occur through the skin or the eye. On the skin this is seen most commonly with *Nocardia brasiliensis.* Clinically this appears as a chronically draining ulcerative lesion or a slowly expanding nodule. The infection may present as a mycetoma with sinus tracts; occasionally, even sulfur granules can be observed in the exudate. One should not attribute a cutaneous lesion always to inoculation, because occasionally disseminated disease can result in secondary seeding of the skin. Thus, all patients with cutaneous nocardiosis should initially be evaluated for disseminated disease.

Diagnosis

A Gram stain of secretions from the infected area provides a useful clue, because it will alert one early to the possibility

TABLE 230–3 ■ Identification of *Nocardia* Species

PROCEDURE	*N. ASTEROIDES* COMPLEX	*N. BRASILINSIS*	*N. OTITIDISCAVIARUM*
Gram stain	Positive	Positive	Positive
Kinyoun stain	Acid-fast	Acid-fast	Acid-fast
Kasein hydrolysis	–	+	–
Tyrosine (decomposes)	–	+	+
Xanthine (decomposes)	–	–	–

TABLE 230–4 ■ In Vitro Antimicrobial Susceptibility of *Nocardia asteroides* Complex*

DRUG	*N. ASTEROIDES*	*N. FARCINICA*	*N. NOVA*
Cefotaxime	S	R	S
Imipenem	S	R	S
Erythromycin	R	R	S
Ampicillin	V	R	S
Amikacin	S	S	S
Minocycline	S	V	S

*S, Sensitive; V, variable sensitivity; R, resistant.

of infection due to *Nocardia.* Because the organism grows slowly, the microbiology laboratory should be alerted to the possible presence of the organism so that the culture plates will be held for 7 to 10 days. Species identification can be accomplished with a variety of biochemical tests (Table 230–3). Additional species have been characterized by antimicrobial resistance patterns, thus giving rise to the use of the term *Nocardia asteroides* complex (Table 230–4). This consists of *Nocardia farcinica,* which appears to be a highly virulent species, often seen with disseminated infection and characteristically resistant to cefotaxime, tobramycin, and erythromycin.[7] Another species, *Nocardia nova,* appears to be quite sensitive to ampicillin and erythromycin.[8] Both of these species are similar in terms of biochemical tests and are therefore all classified as *N. asteroides* by the standard testing. They may make up 10% to 20% of the *N. asteroides* complex. In culture, the colonies are chalky and raised, with colors varying from white to pink to orange (Fig. 230–6). They are crumbly and have a characteristic odor. Both Brown-Brenn and Grocott-Gomori methenamine silver stains show the organisms well histologically; hematoxylin-eosin and the periodic acid–Schiff techniques do not.

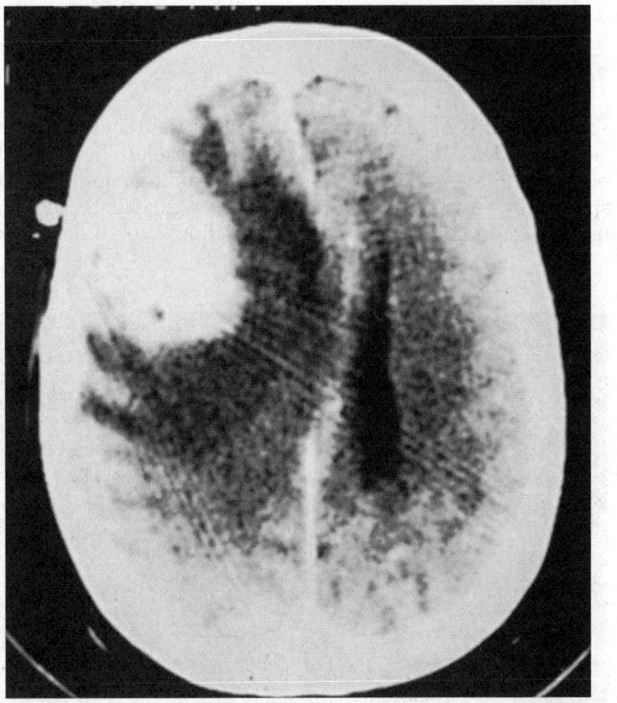

FIGURE 230–5 □ Computed tomographic scan of the brain showing a large parietal lobe abscess with surrounding edema. (From Bach MC: Nocardial infection. *In* Kass EH, Platt R [eds]: Current Therapy in Infectious Disease—3. Philadelphia, BC Decker, 1990, pp 326–328.)

TABLE 230–5 ■ Therapy of *Nocardia* Infection

DRUG	DOSAGE	DURATION*	SIDE EFFECTS
Sulfisoxazole	2 g q 6 h	6 mo	Rash, fever, leukopenia, crystalluria
Trimethoprim-sulfamethoxazole	1 double-strength tablet twice daily	6 mo	Rash, fever, leukopenia, *Candida* infection
Minocycline	200 mg twice daily	6 mo	Dizziness, rash
Imipenem-cilastatin†	500 mg intravenously q 6 h	Until change to oral therapy	Rash, seizures with high blood levels
Cefotaxime†	1 g intravenously q 8 h	Until change to oral therapy	Rash
Amikacin	7.5 mg/kg intravenously q 12 h	Until change to oral therapy	Nephrotoxic, eighth cranial nerve toxicity

*Patients with acquired immunodeficiency syndrome should receive long-term suppression.
†Shows in vitro synergism.

Serologic diagnosis has been hampered by a lack of suitable antigens and by cross-reactivity with other related organisms, such as actinomycetes and the mycobacteria. However, a 55 kDa protein subunit obtained from a culture filtrate has been characterized and appears to have good specificity for *N. asteroides*. In one study, 91% of patients with either systemic nocardiosis or localized cutaneous disease demonstrated an immunoglobulin G response to the specific subunit protein.[9, 10] This test is not yet commercially available.

Differential Diagnosis

Because nocardiosis can progress rapidly in immunocompromised patients, it should be considered in the differential diagnosis of acute pulmonary infections in these patients. Nocardial infection can also result in a gradually progressive indolent process and may mimic tuberculosis, fungal disease, sarcoidosis, and neoplasia. *Nocardia* may also be mistaken for agents such as *Mycobacterium fortuitum* when presenting as a skin or bone lesion,[11] *Gordona bronchialis* in postcardiac surgical sternotomy infections, or *Rhodococcus equi* in pulmonary infections.

Therapy

The mainstay of therapy up to the present has been the sulfonamides.[12] Despite poor in vitro correlation (probably because of the vagaries of media-drug interaction), the response of *Nocardia* to sulfonamides is excellent. There is usually good clinical improvement within 7 to 10 days after initiation of therapy. The route of administration is dependent on the patient's overall clinical status. It has been customary to measure blood levels at least once early on to be sure that the patient is absorbing recommended doses of the drug. Dosage should be adjusted to achieve blood levels of 100 to 150 μg/mL approximately 2 hours after an oral dose. Although trimethoprim-sulfamethoxazole has been used in many cases, there is no good evidence that it is any more effective than sulfonamide alone. Therapy must be continued for 4 to 6 months, and patients with acquired immunodeficiency syndrome should receive long-term maintenance suppressive therapy.

There are indications that some *Nocardia* strains are clinically resistant to the sulfonamides, and a number of acceptable alternative therapies are available (Table 230–5). Minocycline, a potent tetracycline analog, has excellent in vitro efficacy against the majority of strains and has been shown to be clinically effective.[13, 14] If patients do not develop dizziness or vertigo, it has been a good alternative form of therapy.

For patients who are acutely ill and toxic or who are severely immunocompromised and require bactericidal therapy for rapid control of their infection, imipenem-cilastatin and cefotaxime have been shown to be effective.[15, 16] Synergism has been shown in vitro when these two agents are used together.[17] Amikacin, an aminoglycoside, has shown excellent activity against *Nocardia* in vitro and could be used in combination with imipenem-cilastatin or cefotaxime until the patient shows clinical improvement.[17, 18] It is important to remember the varying susceptibility of the *N. asteroides* complex, and the response to therapy should be watched carefully (see Table 242–4).

Should the patient remain febrile while receiving therapy, the possible causes include drug fever, a sequestered abscess that may require drainage, or even a second opportunistic pathogen. Primary drug resistance is another important reason for treatment failure; thus, all significant clinical isolates should be tested for antibiotic susceptibility, preferably at a specialized reference laboratory, thus allowing rational alternative drug selection. Susceptibility testing is also important because of the expected long duration of therapy and the possibility of complications resulting from the initial drug chosen.

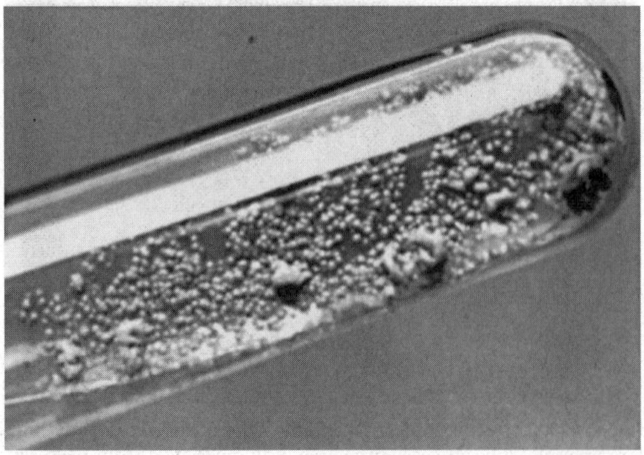

FIGURE 230–6 □ *Nocardia* growing in culture showing orange colonies after 7 days' growth.

References

1. Beauman BL, Burnside J, Edwards B, Causey W: Nocardial infections in the United States, 1972–74. J Infect Dis 134:286, 1976.
2. Wilson JP, Turner HR, Kirchner KA, Chapman SW: Nocardial infections in renal transplant recipients. Medicine (Baltimore) 68:38, 1989.
3. McNeil MM, Brown JM: The medically important aerobic actino-

mycetes: Epidemiology and microbiology. Clin Microbiol Rev 7:357, 1994.
4. Filice GA: Inhibition of *Nocardia asteroides* by neutrophils. J Infect Dis 151:47, 1985.
5. Idriss ZH, Cunningham RJ, Wilfert CM: Nocardiosis in children: Report of three cases and review of the literature. Pediatrics 55:479, 1975.
6. Black CM, Beauman BL, Donovan RM, Goldstein E: Effect of virulent and less virulent strains of *Nocardia asteroides* on acid-phosphatase activity in alveolar and peritoneal macrophages maintained in vitro. J Infect Dis 148:117, 1983.
7. Wallace RJ Jr, Tsukamura M, Brown BA, et al: Cefotazime-resistant *Nocardia asteroides* strains are isolates of the controversial species *Nocardia farcinica.* J Clin Microbiol 28:2726, 1990.
8. Wallace RJ Jr, Brown BA, Tsukamura M, et al: Clinical and laboratory features of *Nocardia nova.* J Clin Microbiol 29:2407, 1991.
9. Sugar AM, Schoolnik GK, Stevens DA: Antibody response in human nocardiosis: Identification of two immunodominant culture-filtrate antigens derived from *Nocardia asteroides.* J Infect Dis 151:895, 1985.
10. Beaman BL, Beaman L: *Nocardia* species: Host-parasite relationships. Clin Microbiol Rev 7:213, 1994.
11. Staneck JL, Frame PT, Altemeier WA, Miller EH: Infection of bone by *Mycobacterium fortuitum* masquerading as *Nocardia asteroides.* Am J Clin Pathol 76:216, 1981.
12. Bach MC, Sabath LD, Finland M: Susceptibility of *Nocardia asteroides* to 45 antimicrobial agents in vitro. Antimicrob Agents Chemother 3:1, 1973.
13. Bach MC, Gold O, Finland M: Activity of minocycline against *Nocardia asteroides:* V. Comparison with tetracycline in agar-dilution and standard disc diffusion tests and with sulfadiazine in an experimental infection of mice. J Lab Clin Med 81:787, 1973.
14. Petersen EA, Nash ML, Mammana RB, Copeland JG: Minocycline treatment of pulmonary nocardiosis. JAMA 250:930, 1983.
15. Gombert ME: Susceptibility of *Nocardia asteroides* to various antibiotics, including newer β-lactams, trimethoprim-sulfamethoxazole, amikacin and *N*-formimidoyl thienamycin. Antimicrob Agents Chemother 21:1011, 1982.
16. Gutmann L, Goldstein FW, Kitzis MD, et al: Susceptibility of *Nocardia asteroides* to 46 antibiotics including 22 β-lactams. Antimicrob Agents Chemother 23:248, 1983.
17. Gombert ME, Aulicino TM: Synergism of imipenem and amikacin in combination with other antibiotics against *Nocardia asteroides.* Antimicrob Agents Chemother 24:810, 1983.
18. Wallace RJ, Septimus E, Musher DM, et al: Treatment of experimental nocardiosis in mice: Comparison of amikacin and sulfonamide. J Infect Dis 140:244, 1979.

231

Agents of Actinomycosis

John G. Bartlett

Actinomycosis is a relatively unusual infection caused primarily by bacteria from the genus *Actinomyces.* The most commonly recognized form is cervicofacial actinomycosis, but multiple other anatomic sites may be involved as well. Clinical features include a chronic, often woody hard induration that forms external sinuses that drain characteristic "sulfur granules" (grains) and as the infection spreads to contiguous sites without regard to anatomic barriers. The term actinomycosis is derived from the Greek *aktinos,* in reference to radiating organisms in the sulfur granule, and *mykes,* indicating fungus. Thus, the term indicates "ray fungus" on the basis of the erroneous impression that this was a mycotic infection. Actinomycetes are anaerobic bacteria found primarily as part of the endogenous flora of the mouth. Infection involving any of the six agents of actinomycosis is characterized by terms based on anatomic location: cervicofacial, thoracic, abdominal, pelvic, musculoskeletal, central nervous system, or disseminated. Nearly all infections involve companion bacteria to the agents of actinomycosis, especially *Actinobacillus actinomycetemcomitans* (so named because of this association), oral *Bacteroides* and *Prevotella* species, fusobacteria, streptococci, and *Eikenella corrodens.* The specific associated organisms depend to a large extent on the anatomic site of the lesion and the normal flora of the adjacent mucosal surface.

History

The first possible case is traced to circa AD 230,[1, 2] but the best descriptions begin with Bollinger,[3] who reported *Actinomyces bovis* as the cause of "lumpy jaw" in cattle in 1877. This investigator was responsible for the appellation actinomyces (ray fungus) based on the microscopic appearance of granules from tongue lesions.[4] Actinomycosis in patients was first described by Israel[5] in 1878. In 1891, Wolff and Israel successfully cultivated the anaerobe that was subsequently named *Actinomyces israelii.* For a long time, *A. bovis* and *A. israelii* were considered identical bacteria isolated from two different host species, but it is now recognized that they are distinctive.[6] *A. bovis* has not been found in humans, although *A. israelii* has been found in cattle.[7] Wolff and Israel[8] postulated the endogenous infection theory on the basis of the observation that the putative agent was a delicate anaerobe found only in animals or humans and never in nature. The opposing theory postulated by Bostroem in 1890 was that *Actinomyces* was found in nature, primarily on grass and grains.[7] This led to the misconception that chewing grass or straw was the cause of cervicofacial actinomycosis, and this represented an occupational hazard to farmers. The evidence in favor of an endogenous source of *Actinomyces* was well supported, especially with the work by Wright[9] in 1905, and is now generally accepted.

Epidemiology

Actinomycosis is a relatively rare infection. The number of annual reported deaths from the disease in the United States from 1930 to 1936 was approximately 60.[10] The annual incidence during the antibiotic era has been estimated at 1 per 100,000 population in the Netherlands[11] and 1 per 300,000 population in Cleveland.[12] The disease is worldwide in distribution with equal frequency in urban and rural dwellers. There is an unexplained 3:1 ratio for men versus women[12–18]; the obvious exception is pelvic actinomycosis. Most cases are seen in adolescents and middle-aged adults. *Actinomyces* becomes a component of the normal oral flora at about 3 years of age, and *Actinomyces* in younger children is rare.[19] The most common form of actinomycosis is cervicofacial, followed by thoracic and abdominal.[1, 7, 13–18] The frequency of pelvic actinomycosis is related to usage rates of intrauterine contraceptive devices (IUDs), and its frequency depends to a large extent on criteria used for this diagnosis.

Microbial Agents of Actinomycosis

The agents of actinomycosis include *A. israelii, Actinomyces naeslundii, Actinomyces odontolyticus, Actinomyces viscosus, Ac-*

tinomyces meyeri, and *Propionibacterium propionicum* (previously classified as *Arachnia propionica*).[1, 19–24] *Actinomyces pyogenes (Corynebacterium pyogenes)* has also been proposed as an agent of actinomycosis.[25] The most frequent is *A. israelii;* less frequent in rank order are *P. propionicum, A. naeslundii, A. viscosus, A. odontolyticus,* and *A. meyeri.*[26] All grow best in anaerobic conditions at 37°C with the exception of *A. viscosus,* which grows aerobically. These organisms are slow-growing, gram-positive, branching bacilli (Fig. 231–1*A*). A selective medium containing mupirocin and metronidazole facilitates recovery of *Actinomyces* species from specimens with a mixed flora.[27] All are normally present in the oral flora including the gingival crevice, dental plaque, and tonsillar crypts; they are less frequently found as a component of the colonic flora and are found in the vaginal flora of 5% of women without an IUD.[7]

A. israelii grows optimally under anaerobic conditions, but many strains are microaerophilic. Mature colonies, after 5 to 10 days of incubation, show large, white, rough colonies giving a characteristic "molar tooth" appearance (Fig. 231–1*B*). The organisms appear as gram-positive filaments, sometimes with branching, in early lesions. Late lesions usually show the characteristic features of sulfur granules. *P. propionicum* appears identical to *A. israelii* on Gram stain, resembles this organism biochemically, and was originally named *Actinomyces propionicus.* Colonies are smoother and not molar tooth in character. This organism was assigned to a distinct genus, *Arachnia,* in 1969[26] and has more recently been reclassified as *P. propionicum.*[1] *A. naeslundii* is found in virtually all forms of actinomycosis; it grows both anaerobically and in microaerophilic conditions and is more likely to show free filamentous forms in tissue.[26] *A. viscosus* grows well aerobically, is a prominent component of dental plaque, and has primarily been associated with orodental and thoracic infections. *A. odontolyticus* has been involved in all forms of actinomycosis but less frequently than the other species noted. *A. meyeri* is a relatively recent addition to the agents of actinomycosis and is a relatively infrequent cause of disease.[23] *A. pyogenes* is a proposed agent,[25] but this is not yet clearly accepted.[1]

Pathology and Pathogenesis

The characteristic feature of actinomycosis is disruption of the mucosal barrier to permit entry of normal flora. Common associated conditions for cervicofacial lesions are dental disease, jaw trauma, and oral surgery; for abdominal infections, the usual associated conditions are surgery, other inflammatory conditions of the gut, and foreign bodies. In thoracic actinomycosis, the presumed pathogenic mechanism is aspiration. With pelvic infections, the usual associated condition is IUD use. In many cases, the predisposing event is in the remote past because of the indolent nature of actinomycosis. One of the most striking examples illustrating this point is the case of abdominal actinomycosis in Jerry Kramer, the all-pro guard of the national champion Green Bay Packers football team. As related in his autobiography, *Instant Replay,* he presented to training camp with enigmatic fevers, abdominal pain, and an abdominal mass; laparotomy showed an indurated, inflammatory mass with a wood splinter in the center that was traced to penetrating abdominal trauma 20 years previously.[28]

Nearly all cases are polymicrobial, and some think that synergy is an essential component of pathogenesis.[11, 29, 30] This issue is not trivial because of the implications regarding selection of antimicrobial agents. The most frequent companions reflect, to a large extent, the site of infection. Most frequent are *A. actinomycetemcomitans,* various anaerobic bacteria *(Bacteroides, Prevotella, Fusobacterium, and Peptostreptococcus), E. corrodens, Haemophilus* species, aerobic and microaerophilic streptococci, staphylococci, and (in abdominal actinomycosis) Enterobacteriaceae.

Although the association with a breach in the mucosal integrity is common, there may be an important role for foreign bodies. This is most striking with the IUD-associated form of actinomycosis but has also been seen with fish bones in the abdomen,[12] root fillings,[31, 32] and wire sutures.[33]

Actinomycosis is not clearly associated with the immunocompromised state. Occasional cases are reported in patients with human immunodeficiency virus infection[34, 35] or in patients receiving corticosteroids,[17] but these are unusual. This is in distinct contrast to *Nocardia,* which resembles the agents of actinomycosis morphologically. The family Actinomycetaceae previously included both aerobic and anaerobic strains. The aerobic nocardioform actinomycetes have subsequently been placed in the genus *Nocardia* and now constitute the family Nocardiaceae.[36] Nocardiosis resembles actinomycosis, but the putative agent is aerobic; the infection is clearly associated with the immunocompromised state, is usually exogenously acquired, is usually monomicrobial, and is treated with completely different antimicrobial agents (Table 231–1).

Actinomycosis is characterized by an acute inflammatory phase of infection that may be associated with pain, erythema, edema, and tenderness as with other common infec-

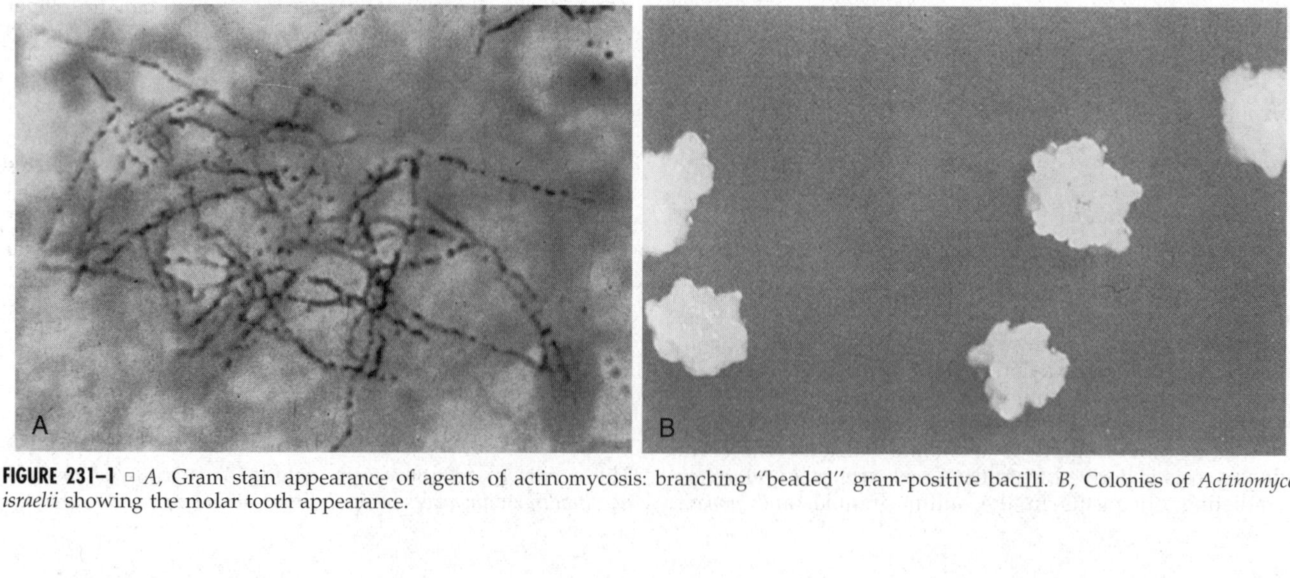

FIGURE 231–1 □ *A,* Gram stain appearance of agents of actinomycosis: branching "beaded" gram-positive bacilli. *B,* Colonies of *Actinomyces israelii* showing the molar tooth appearance.

TABLE 231–1 ■ Comparison of Actinomycosis and Nocardiosis

PARAMETER	ACTINOMYCOSIS	NOCARDIOSIS
Agents	*Actinomyces israelii, Actinomyces naeslundii, Actinomyces odontolyticus, Actinomyces viscosus, Actinomyces meyeri, Propionibacterium propionicum*	*Nocardia asteroides*
Culture	Anaerobic (except *A. viscosus*)	Aerobic
Gram stain	Thin, branching, gram-positive bacilli	Thin, branching, gram-positive bacilli
Modified acid-fast stain	Negative	Positive
Source	Mouth, colon, genital tract	Soil
Host	Usually previously healthy young adult	Immunocompromised, especially reduced cell-mediated immunity
Pathophysiologic process	Endogenous infection starting in oral cavity, lung (aspiration), abdomen, or genital tract	Pneumonia presumably by inhalation; dissemination to extrapulmonary sites
Characteristic of infection	Indurated, draining sinuses, sulfur granules, penetration through tissue	No sulfur granules, penetration through tissue is unusual
Course	Indolent, chronic	Acute, subacute, or asymptomatic

tions of soft tissue. More frequently, the disease is indolent with gradual evolution for a period of weeks, months, or even years. The early lesion may be soft and fluctuant with central suppuration (see Fig. 231–1). With maturation, the lesion becomes extremely fibrous, which gives it a "wooden" character. With cervicofacial actinomycosis, the acute inflammatory phase of the disease may appear similar to other types of acute soft tissue infections along the mandible. The more characteristic indurated, woody hard lesion is often mistaken for a neoplasm. Highly characteristic is the formation of sinus tracts that often drain sulfur granules (in reference to the macroscopic, hard, yellow particles that resemble elemental sulfur particles previously used in pharmaceuticals).[7] Microscopic examination of typical lesions shows an outer zone of fibrous tissue and central foci of acute inflammation with polymorphonuclear cells. The sulfur granules consist of an amorphic central area surrounded with a rosette of filamentous organisms that often show branching (Fig. 231–2). Most lesions show multiple loculations of suppuration with intervening granulation tissue that shows collagen fibers, fibroblasts, lymphocytes, and occasionally multinucleated giant cells.[37]

Diagnosis

The diagnosis of actinomycosis is based on the typical clinical features of this disease, preferably combined with recovery

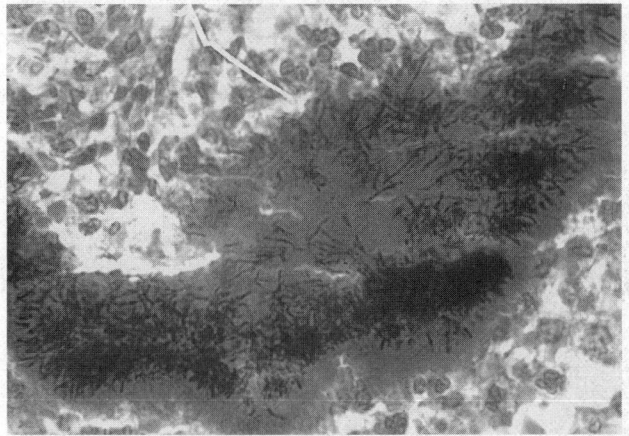

FIGURE 231–2 □ Sulfur granule or grain showing amorphous material with a rosette of filamentous radiating gram-positive bacilli.

of an agent of actinomycosis. Clinical features include an indolent progressive inflammatory mass with sinus tracts, fistulae, fever, leukocytosis, weight loss, and elevated erythrocyte sedimentation rate. The recovery of an agent of actinomycosis may be difficult to achieve owing to the fastidious growth requirements of actinomycetes and *P. propionica*. These organisms may be particularly difficult to recover in the presence of antibiotic exposure. An alternative is identification of the specific species by immunofluorescent stains. Species-specific antisera conjugated with fluorescein are available for the four major species of *Actinomyces* and for *P. propionicum*.[38, 39] Cultivation of an agent of actinomycosis or its detection with fluorescent antibody stain is most meaningful with sulfur granules or in a specimen from a normally sterile site.[40] These organisms are components of the normal flora so that recovery from specimens subject to contamination, such as expectorated sputum, bronchoscopy aspirates, genital tract specimens, and swabs from the oral cavity, is meaningless.[41] Gram stains of lesions show filamentous, gram-positive bacilli that often show branching. Among gram-positive bacilli, *Actinomyces* and *Nocardia* are the only organisms that show branching in tissue.

Sulfur granules are pathognomonic when they are recovered from a typical lesion other than on tonsils.[1] These may be microscopic or macroscopic concretions consisting of a mineralized mass with calcium phosphate and radiating filamentous organisms on the surface.[42] The granules may drain through sinus tracts and may be seen on covering bandages. Exudate placed on a vertical glass often shows granules adherent to the glass. Sulfur granules may also be seen in microabscesses.

Other infections that may be associated with the production of granules are mycetoma and botryomycosis. Botryomycosis is a chronic bacterial infection of soft tissue caused by *Staphylococcus aureus*, streptococcus, and selected gram-negative bacilli. These organisms and the fungal agents of mycetoma show distinctive morphologic characteristics with Gram stain. A possible exception is *Nocardia* when it is responsible for mycetoma because this organism may be indistinguishable from *Actinomyces* with Gram stain. The distinction may be made with immunofluorescent staining for the agents of actinomycosis or by the Fite-modified acid-fast stain to detect *Nocardia*.

Nocardiosis may resemble actinomycosis with clinical features that include an indolent course with indurated lesions, that progresses without respect to anatomic boundaries. Tuberculosis may occasionally show these features as well. Visceral forms of nocardiosis do not have granules, but these may be seen with the mycetoma form of nocardiosis. Other characteristic features of nocardiosis are summarized in Table 231–1.

Granules, when identified, should be washed and crushed between slides for examination using Gram stain and immunofluorescent stains.

Cervicofacial and Oral Actinomycosis

This is the most frequently recognized form of actinomycosis and accounts for approximately 50% of reported cases.[1] Cervicofacial actinomycosis should be considered in any acute, subacute, or chronic infection involving the head and neck. The most frequent presentation is a soft tissue swelling that progresses slowly without regard to tissue planes and without involvement of adjacent lymph nodes (Fig. 231–3). Polar extremes include, at one end, a painless, indurated, slowly expanding lesion, often with a bluish hue, along the mandible or neck that may suggest neoplasm; the other extreme resembles an acute pyogenic infection along the mandible that may seem like parotitis, a perimandibular space infection, or cervical adenitis. The infection at the portal of entry may no longer be obvious, and the initial presentation may be at a relatively distant site such as the scalp, orbit, tongue, larynx, or sinuses. Many patients are treated for more common types of bacterial infection, and actinomycosis will often respond temporarily but recur when antibiotics are discontinued.[43] Fever and leukocytosis are variable.[18, 43] Most cases are restricted to soft tissue, although there may be osteomyelitis. Dental infections often involve actinomycetes, especially periapical abscesses[44]; these are often treated sufficiently early in the course to preclude advancement to the more characteristic, indurated form. Infection at sites of tooth extraction is common, especially at third molars. A dental portal of entry is implicated even with sites that are distant, and most patients show periodontal disease or gingivitis.[45] When bone is involved, it is usually the mandible rather than the maxilla.[46] Other forms of actinomycosis in the head and neck region include lacrimal canaliculitis,[47] postoperative endophthalmitis,[48] sinusitis,[49] parotitis,[50] thyroid infection,[51] and middle-ear infections.[52]

Thoracic Actinomycosis

This accounts for about 15% of cases of actinomycosis.[53] There may be involvement of the lungs, pleura, mediastinum, and chest wall. The presumed mechanism in most cases is aspiration, and many patients have suggestive dental disease. Less frequent are direct extension from oral infections, hematogenous dissemination, and extension from an abdominal site.

The diagnosis is often not made until relatively late in the course. The usual presentation is a slowly progressive pneumonia with fever, chest pain, weight loss, and cough.[53–55] Pleural involvement is common. There may be hemoptysis, hilar adenopathy, bone involvement, pulmonary cavities, cardiac involvement, or mediastinal involvement.[53, 55–59]

The classic presentation is extension to the chest wall with the development of a soft tissue mass or a draining sinus, although this late form has become uncommon in the antibiotic era (Fig. 231–4). Radiographic changes and computed tomographic findings are often nonspecific but may be highly suggestive with pulmonary lesions that extend to and through the chest wall, often with pleural involvement and destruction of adjacent bones.[60, 61] One or more small cavities are found in about half of cases, but large cavities are unusual.[60] Cardiac involvement is common, especially of the pericardium; nevertheless, clinical features of pericarditis are rarely seen.[62] Endocarditis is rare.

The diagnosis is infrequently suspected except for patients with the classic presentation of a penetrating chest infection with a chest wall mass or draining sinus, which is found in less than 2% of cases.[7] Occasional cases are detected with cytologic examination showing sulfur granules.[63] Agents of actinomycosis are not usually recovered from expectorated sputum or bronchoscopy aspirates because these specimens should not be cultured anaerobically and the aerotolerant forms are often too fastidious; even with recovery from these specimens, these results are considered nondiagnostic. Recovery of these agents from pleural fluid or a transthoracic needle aspirate would be considered diagnostic in the presence of an appropriate clinical presentation. In many cases, the diagnosis is made histologically after resection for a suspected neoplasm. This is a chronic, indolent disease with involvement of the pulmonary parenchyma so that the usual diagnostic considerations are tuberculosis, nocardiosis, endemic fungal infection, cryptococcosis, anaerobic pulmonary infection, lymphoma, and bronchogenic cancer.

Abdominal Actinomycosis

This form accounts for about 20% of all cases of actinomycosis.[14, 15, 20, 64–70] The usual mechanism is entry through the gut

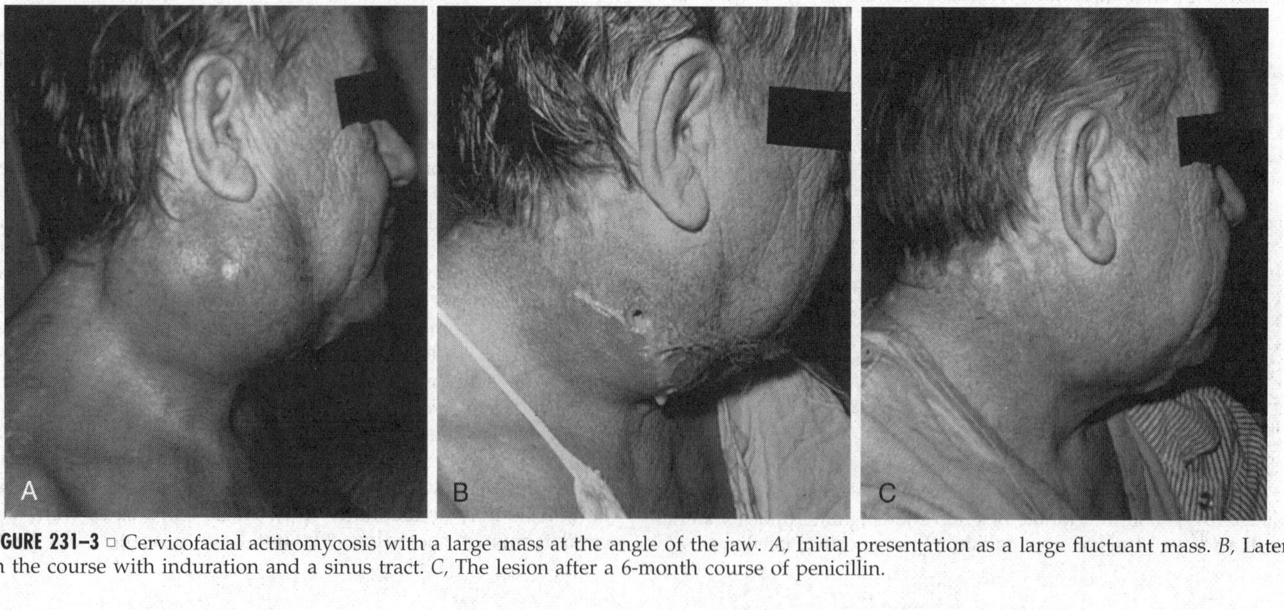

FIGURE 231–3 ▫ Cervicofacial actinomycosis with a large mass at the angle of the jaw. *A*, Initial presentation as a large fluctuant mass. *B*, Later in the course with induration and a sinus tract. *C*, The lesion after a 6-month course of penicillin.

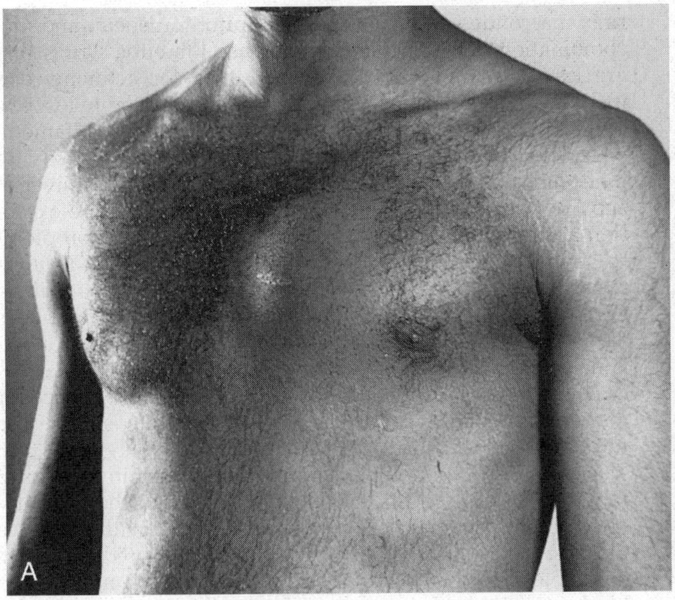

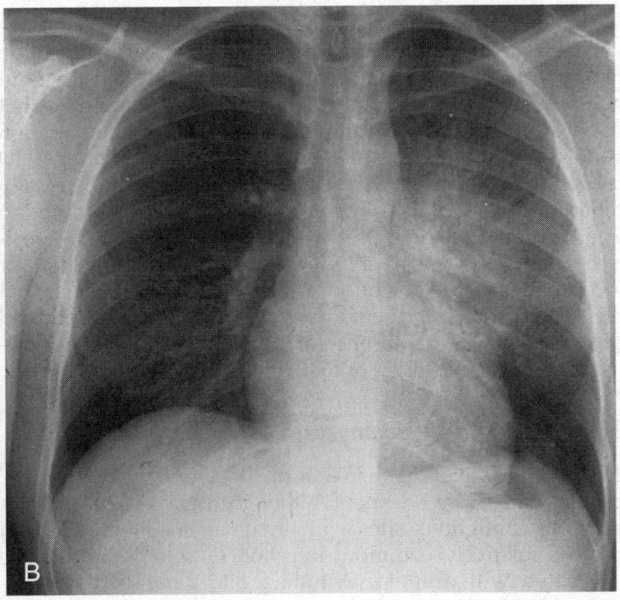

FIGURE 231–4 □ Thoracic actinomycosis. *A*, Initial presentation with a bulging mass lesion in the left chest wall with a central sinus tract. *B*, The chest radiograph with the associated pulmonary infiltrate.

wall, but there may be extension from the thorax or female genital tract or abdominal involvement after hematogenous dissemination. Most patients have had previous abdominal surgery, penetrating abdominal trauma, or a foreign body in the gastrointestinal tract. When there is antecedent surgery or trauma, the latent period may be several years.

The most common presentation, accounting for about two thirds of cases of abdominal actinomycosis, is appendicitis, usually with a periappendiceal mass. Less common sites of involvement include the colon, stomach, liver, gallbladder, pancreas, small bowel, anorectal area, pelvis, and abdominal wall.[18] No predisposing factors are noted in up to 50% of cases.[17, 18, 64] Hepatic involvement accounts for 5% to 15% of abdominal actinomycosis cases.[20] Some patients present with an intramural gastric lesion that simulates gastric carcinoma.[67] Liver function test results in these cases are often normal, neoplasm is often suspected, and there are often multiple small liver abscesses.[71–73] Retroperitoneal involvement may result from hematogenous dissemination or direct extension; presentations include pyelonephritis, renal abscess, perinephric abscess, and a mass simulating a bladder tumor.[74, 75] The diagnosis could conceivably be made with recovery of the agents of actinomycosis in urine culture, but it is not customary to process these specimens anaerobically.[76] Obstruction of the ureters with hydronephrosis is sometimes noted with mass lesions of the abdomen or pelvis.

Characteristic features of abdominal actinomycosis are similar to those noted before. Most patients have a slowly evolving inflammatory mass with microabscesses, abscesses, draining sinuses, or fistulous tracks. An extremely indurated or woody mass or actinomycetoma is often suggestive of a neoplasm.[77] Characteristic clinical features include fever, weight loss, palpable indurated masses, draining sinuses through the abdominal wall, and computed tomographic evidence of a multicystic contrast-enhancing mass.[18, 64, 65] In many cases, the diagnosis is established with an unnecessary laparotomy and histopathologic examination or recognition of characteristic features intraoperatively.[65] Needle aspiration with cytologic examination is an alternative method for establishing this diagnosis.[64] For patients who undergo surgery, an intraoperative frozen section will distinguish an inflammatory mass from carcinoma.[77, 78]

Pelvic Actinomycosis

The majority of cases in this category are found in association with IUDs. This association was originally noted in 1973 and subsequently popularized by Gupta and colleagues[78–84] with use of Papanicolaou smears for detection of the agents of actinomycosis. The Papanicolaou smear proved to be a relatively easy, inexpensive, and rapid method for detection of the agents of actinomycosis, but the major controversy concerns the implication of this observation in terms of management decisions. Two methods have been used: (1) the fast smears for detection of Gupta bodies consisting of amorphous material with radiating filaments[80] and (2) the fluorescent antibody conjugate stain for detection of specific agents of actinomycosis.[81–83] A survey of Papanicolaou smears from 69,925 women screened for *A. israelii* by use of the fluorescent antibody stain showed that this organism was not found in the absence of IUD use; the reported prevalence of *A. israelii* among IUD users is 1.6% to 5.3%.[85] In one report, 2 of 112 women with evidence of *A. israelii* had significant clinical infections, and the authors concluded that the majority with this organism had only superficial infections. In a comprehensive review in 1978, Gupta and coworkers[83] reported identification of agents of actinomycosis in 540 vaginal-pancervical (fast) smears from 520 women. Of these, 517 women used IUDs; the other 3 women had infections associated with other foreign bodies. Fluorescent antibody stains in 266 specimens showing cytologic evidence of actinomycosis indicated that *A. israelii* accounted for 250.[83] Most patients had IUD use of more than 2 years. These and other investigators have shown that culture is far less sensitive for detection, a not unexpected finding on the basis of the experience with microbial detection by culture at other anatomic sites.[86–88]

Pelvic actinomycosis associated with IUDs is highly variable and sometimes controversial. The range of clinical conditions includes vaginal discharge, pelvic inflammatory disease, tuboovarian abscess, and endometritis. In its most advanced and characteristic form, the consequences can be devastating: a frozen pelvis; urinary obstruction; and fistulae that extend to contiguous sites including gut, bladder, skin, or even a distant anatomic site.[65] In many cases, the nature of the infection simulates an advanced neoplasm.

The data summarized here have led to a somewhat controversial issue regarding management strategies. The detection of *Actinomyces* on smears seems to be relatively sensitive but not particularly specific for actinomycosis. It appears that IUDs are almost always implicated, although other foreign bodies account for a small portion of cases. Among IUD users, the prevalence of *Actinomyces* is relatively high, usually reported at 1% to 10%, but pelvic actinomycosis is rare.[79–89] The unknown factor in this association is whether the positive results by smear simply represent early infection or inconsequential colonization. Many authorities believe that this observation represents a contraindication to continued IUD use even in the absence of any symptoms. The alternative option is counseling of the patient and careful follow-up.

Musculoskeletal Actinomycosis

This is a relatively unusual form of actinomycosis as the primary site of involvement, although direct extension from multiple contiguous sites with involvement of muscle and bone is relatively common. Infection of soft tissue may be associated with trauma, including bite wounds.[90] Involvement of soft tissue including muscle may also result from hematogenous dissemination. The usual presentation is an indolent infection with induration and draining sinuses and typical granules. With involvement of feet, this is considered a mycetoma but should be called actinomycetoma. Osteomyelitis usually results when a bone is in the direction of contiguous spread. The most common bones are the mandible and vertebrae. With vertebral involvement, there is destruction of the vertebrae and adjacent ribs, but unlike tuberculosis, there is usually sparing of the disk space and no vertebral collapse.[47] Joint involvement is unusual, although agents of actinomycosis have been implicated in prosthetic joint infections.[91]

Central Nervous System Actinomycosis

These cases account for less than 5% of all cases of actinomycosis. Most represent hematogenous extension. In a review of 70 reported cases of central nervous system actinomycosis, brain abscess accounted for 67%, meningitis or meningoencephalitis accounted for 13%, actinomycetomas accounted for 7%, subdural empyemas accounted for 6%, and epidural abscesses accounted for 6%. The primary site of infection in these cases was usually the lung, oral cavity, abdomen, or pelvis, and this includes cases associated with IUD use.[92] As noted, brain abscess is the most frequent presentation; the usual clinical features are headache and focal neurologic findings with or without fever, and the computed tomographic scan generally shows a ring-enhancing lesion that may easily be mistaken for a neoplasm or pyogenic brain abscess. An actinomycetoma presents as a solid mass.[93] Cases classified as chronic meningitis often represent a parameningeal focus. Analysis of the cerebrospinal fluid usually shows an elevated protein level, lymphocytic cells, normal or low glucose level, and negative Gram stain and culture. The agents of actinomycosis are rarely grown from cerebrospinal fluid.[94] The diagnosis is usually made by neurosurgery; draining sinuses, sulfur granules, and other characteristic features of actinomycosis at alternative anatomic sites are not seen with central nervous system disease.

Treatment

Antibiotics have revolutionized the outcome of actinomycosis. Antimicrobial agents active in vitro include penicillin, ampicillin, antipseudomonad penicillins, most cephalosporins, macrolides, tetracyclines, rifampin, imipenem, and any combination of a β-lactam–β-lactamase inhibitor. Drugs that are less active and should not be used for actinomycosis include metronidazole, aminoglycosides, antistaphylococcal penicillins, cephalexin, ceftazidime, trimethoprim-sulfamethoxazole, and fluoroquinolones.[95–98] The lack of activity of metronidazole is curious in view of the nearly universal activity of this agent against obligate anaerobes. The exception appears to be the agents of actinomycosis and propionibacteria including *Propionibacterium acnes* as well as *P. propionicum*. On the basis of these observations, it is difficult to go wrong in terms of antibiotic selection. The main problems are dose, duration, the necessity of treating companion organisms, and the role of surgery.

The standard treatment based on decades of experience for most cases of actinomycosis at any anatomic site is high-dose intravenous penicillin (10 to 20 million units/d) for 2 to 6 weeks followed by oral penicillin V or amoxicillin for 6 to 12 months.[1, 7] The need for high doses is based on the difficulty of achieving therapeutic levels in dense tissue with extensive fibrosis. Consequently, early infections associated with less extensive lesions in terms of size and induration may probably be treated with less aggressive antibiotic treatment. For patients who cannot receive penicillin, the alternative drugs that have had most extensive use are clindamycin and tetracycline. The necessity of treating companion organisms is arbitrary, and most studies indicate that penicillin alone is adequate. There is one impressive reported response to imipenem in a complicated case of abdominal actinomycosis after failure to respond to surgery and high-dose penicillin.[99] It is obviously unclear whether this is related to superior activity against agents of actinomycosis or reflects activity against companion organisms.

The role of surgery is often controversial. Procedures sometimes advocated include incision and drainage of abscesses; debulking of large, inflammatory masses; and excision of sinus tracts. Some have reported impressive results with antibiotic treatment alone in patients with extensive disease.[100, 101] Percutaneous drainage of abscesses is another option.[102] In many instances, the most appropriate approach is aggressive antibiotic treatment, with surgery reserved for patients who fail to respond and who have the type of lesion or anatomic site of infection that suggests a successful surgical outcome.

References

1. Russo TA: Agents of actinomycosis. *In* Mandell GL, Bennett JE, Dolin R (eds): Principles and Practice of Infectious Diseases, ed 4. New York, Churchill Livingstone, 1995, pp 2280–2288.
2. Molto JE: Differential diagnosis of rib lesions: A case study from Middle Woodland Southern Ontario circa 230 A.D. Am J Phys Anthropol 83:439, 1990.
3. Bollinger O: Über eine neue Pilzkrankheit beim Rinde. Zentralbl Med Wiss 15:481, 1877.
4. Harz C: *Actinomyces bovis*, ein neuer Schimmel in den Geweben des Rinder. *In* Jahresbuch des Königlich Zentral-Thierarzneischule zu München 1877–1878. 5:125, 1879.
5. Israel J: Neue Beobachtungen auf dem Gebiete der Mykosen des Menschen. Arch Pathol Anat Physiol 74:15, 1879.
6. Erikson D: Pathogenic anaerobic organisms of the *Actinomyces* group. Br Med Res Council Spec Rep Ser 240:1, 1940.
7. Lerner PI: *Actinomyces* and *Arachnia*. *In* Gorbach S, Bartlett JG, Blacklow NR (ed): Infectious Diseases. Philadelphia, WB Saunders, 1992, pp 1626–1632.
8. Wolff M, Israel J: Über Reincultur des *Actinomyces* und seine Übertragbarkeit auf Thiere. Virchows Arch Pathol Anat 126:11, 1891.
9. Wright JH: The biology of the micro-organism of actinomycosis. J Med Res 13:349, 1905.
10. Kolouch F, Peltier LF: Actinomycosis. Surgery 20:401, 1946.

11. Pulverer G: Problems of human actinomycosis. Postepy Hig Med Dosw 28:253, 1974.
12. Bennhoff D: Actinomycosis: Diagnostic and therapeutic considerations and a review of 32 cases. Laryngoscope 94:1198, 1984.
13. Harvey JC, Cantrell JR, Fisher AM: Actinomycosis; its recognition and treatment. Ann Intern Med 46:868, 1957.
14. Eastridge C, Prather J, Hughes F, et al: Actinomycosis: A 24 year experience. South Med J 65:839, 1972.
15. Davis MIJ: Analysis of forty-six cases of actinomycosis with special reference to its etiology. Am J Surg 52:447, 1941.
16. Putman HC, Dockerty MB, Waugh JM: Abdominal actinomycosis; an analysis of 122 cases. Surgery 28:781, 1950.
17. Weese WC, Smith IM: A study of 57 cases of actinomycosis over a 36-year period. A diagnostic 'failure' with good prognosis after treatment. Arch Intern Med 135:1562, 1975.
18. Berardi RS: Abdominal actinomycosis. Surg Gynecol Obstet 149:257, 1979.
19. Drake DP, Holt RJ: Childhood actinomycosis; report of three recent cases. Arch Dis Child 51:979, 1976.
20. Coleman RM, Georg LK, Rozzell AR: *Actinomyces naeslundii* as an agent in human actinomycosis. Appl Microbiol 18:420, 1969.
21. Morris J, Kilbourn P: Systemic actinomycosis caused by *Actinomyces odontolyticus*. Ann Intern Med 81:700, 1974.
22. Eng R, Corrado M, Cleri D, et al: Infections caused by *Actinomyces viscosus*. Am J Clin Pathol 75:113, 1981.
23. Pordy R: Lumpy jaw due to *Actinomyces meyerii*: Report of the first case and review of the literature. Mt Sinai J Med 55:190, 1988.
24. Brock D, Georg L, Brown JM, et al: Actinomycosis caused by *Arachnia propionica*: Report of 11 cases. Am J Clin Pathol 59:66, 1973.
25. Gahrn-Hansen B, Frederiksen W: Human infections with *Actinomyces pyogenes (Corynebacterium pyogenes)*. Diagn Microbiol Infect Dis 15:349, 1992.
26. Georg LK: The agents of human actinomycosis. *In* Balows A (ed): Anaerobic Bacteria: Role in Disease. Springfield, IL, Charles C Thomas, 1974, pp 237–256.
27. Lewis R, McKenzie D, Bagg J, Dickie A: Experience with a novel selective medium for isolation of *Actinomyces* spp. from medical and dental specimens. J Clin Microbiol 33:1613, 1995.
28. Kramer J: Instant Replay. The Green Bay Diary of Jerry Kramer. The World Publishing Company, 1968, pp 48–50.
29. Holm P: Studies on aetiology of human actinomycosis. I. The other microbes of actinomycosis and their importance. Acta Pathol Microbiol Scand 27:736, 1950.
30. Holm P: Studies on aetiology of human actinomycosis. II. Do the other microbes of actinomycosis possess virulence? Acta Pathol Microbiol Scand 28:391, 1951.
31. Figures K, Douglas C: Actinomycosis associated with a root-treated tooth: Report of a case. Int Endodont J 24:326, 1991.
32. Harvey J, Cantrell J, Fisher A: Actinomycosis: Its recognition and treatment. Ann Intern Med 46:868, 1957.
33. Silbermann M, Chiminello F, Doku H, et al: Mandibular actinomycosis: Report of a case. J Am Dent Assoc 90:162, 1975.
34. Klapholz A, Talavera W, Rorat E, et al: Pulmonary actinomycosis in a patient with HIV infection. Mt Sinai J Med 56:300, 1989.
35. Yeager B, Hoxie J, Weisman R, et al: Actinomycosis in the acquired immunodeficiency syndrome–related complex. Arch Otolaryngol Head Neck Surg 112:1293, 1986.
36. Waksman SA, Henrici AT: The nomenclature and classification of the actinomycetes. J Bacteriol 46:337, 1943.
37. Brown J: Human actinomycosis. A study of 181 subjects. Hum Pathol 4:319, 1973.
38. Hillier S, Moncla B: Anaerobic gram-positive nonsporeforming bacilli and cocci. *In* Balows A (ed): Manual of Clinical Microbiology. Washington, DC, American Society for Microbiology, 1991, pp 522–533.
39. Happonen RP, Viander M: Comparison of fluorescent antibody technique and conventional staining methods in diagnosis of cervicofacial actinomycosis. J Oral Pathol 11:417, 1982.
40. Holmberg K: Diagnostic methods for human actinomycosis. Microbiol Sci 4:72, 1987.
41. Slack J: The source of infection in actinomycosis. J Bacteriol 43:193, 1942.
42. Pine L, Overman JR: Determination of the structure and composition of the sulphur granules of *Actinomyces bovis*. J Gen Microbiol 32:209, 1963.
43. Spilsbury B, Johnstone F: The clinical course of actinomycotic infections: A report of 14 cases. Can J Surg 5:33, 1962.
44. Weir J, Buck W: Periapical actinomycosis. Report of a case and review of the literature. Oral Surg 54:336, 1982.
45. Benhoff DF: Actinomycosis: Diagnostic and therapeutic considerations and a review of 32 cases. Laryngoscope 94:1198, 1984.
46. Lewis RP, Sutter VL, Finegold SM: Bone infections involving anaerobic bacteria. Medicine (Baltimore) 57:279, 1978.
47. Smith R, Henderson P: Actinomycotic canaliculitis. Aust J Ophthalmol 8:75, 1980.
48. Roussel T, Olson R, Rice T, et al: Chronic postoperative endophthalmitis associated with *Actinomyces* species. Arch Ophthalmol 109:60, 1991.
49. Har-el G, Prager D, De Soto F, et al: Actinomycotic granuloma masquerading as an infraorbital nerve neoplasm. Head Neck 12:261, 1990.
50. Chuong R, Goldberg M: CPC, case 60: Preauricular mass. J Oral Maxillofac Surg 44:214, 1986.
51. Arfeen S, Boast M, Large D: Unilateral thyroid swelling due to actinomycosis. Postgrad Med J 62:847, 1986.
52. Shelton C, Brackmann D: Actinomycosis otitis media. Arch Otolaryngol Head Neck Surg 114:88, 1988.
53. Kinnear W, MacFarlane J: A survey of thoracic actinomycosis. Respir Med 84:57, 1990.
54. Bates M, Cruickshank G: Thoracic actinomycosis. Thorax 12:99, 1957.
55. Heffner J: Pleuropulmonary manifestations of actinomycosis and nocardiosis. Semin Respir Infect 3:352, 1988.
56. Prather J, Eastridge C, Hughes FA, et al: Actinomycosis of the thorax. Ann Thorac Surg 9:307, 1970.
57. Morgan D, Nath H, Sanders C, et al: Mediastinal actinomycosis. AJR 155:735, 1990.
58. Fife T, Finegold S, Grennan T: Pericardial actinomycosis: Case report and review. Rev Infect Dis 13:120, 1991.
59. McQuarrie D, Hall W: Actinomycosis of the lung and chest wall. Surgery 64:905, 1968.
60. Flynn M, Felson B: The roentgen manifestations of thoracic actinomycosis. AJR 110:707, 1970.
61. Kwong J, Muller N, Godwin J, et al: Thoracic actinomycosis: CT findings in eight patients. Radiology 183:189, 1992.
62. Cole FH, Jarrett CL: Primary actinomycosis of the pericardium. South Med J 75:1028, 1982.
63. Lazzari G, Vineis C, Cugini A: Cytologic diagnosis of primary pulmonary actinomycosis: Report of two cases. Acta Cytol 25:299, 1981.
64. Cintron JR, Del Pino A, Duarte B, Wood D: Abdominal actinomycosis. Dis Colon Rectum 39:105, 1996.
65. Kaya E, Yilmazlar T, Emiroglu Z, et al: Colonic actinomycosis: Report of a case and review of the literature. Surg Today 25:923, 1995.
66. Brown JR: Human actinomycosis. A study of 181 subjects. Hum Pathol 4:319, 1973.
67. Skoutelis A, Panagopoulos C, Kalfarentzos F, Bassaris H: Intramural gastric actinomycosis. South Med J 88:647, 1995.
68. Putman H, Dockerty M, Waugh J: Abdominal actinomycosis. An analysis of 122 cases. Surgery 28:781, 1950.
69. Stringer M, Cameron A: Abdominal actinomycosis: A forgotten disease? Br J Hosp Med 38:125, 1987.
70. Deshmukh N, Heaney S: Actinomycosis at multiple colonic sites. Am J Gastroenterol 81:1212, 1986.
71. Cedermark B, Sundblad R, Willems JS: Suspected neoplasm of the liver with pulmonary metastases cured by surgery and penicillin. Disseminated actinomycosis revisited. Am J Surg 141:384, 1981.
72. Mongiardo M, DeRienzo B, Zanchetta G, et al: Primary hepatic actinomycosis. J Infect 12:65, 1986.
73. Smithers B, Wall D, Weedon D: Actinomycosis of the gallbladder. Aust N Z J Surg 53:587, 1983.
74. Ellis L, Kenny G, Nellans R: Urogenital aspects of actinomycosis. J Urol 122:132, 1979.
75. Ozyurt C, Yurtseven O, Kocak I, et al: Actinomycosis simulating bladder tumour. Br J Urol 76:263, 1995.
76. Piper J, Stoner B, Mitra SK, et al: Ileo-vesical fistula associated with pelvic actinomycosis. Br J Clin Pract 23:341, 1969.
77. Hinnie J, Jaques BC, Bell E, et al: Actinomycosis presenting as carcinoma. Postgrad Med J 71:749, 1995.

78. Muller-Holzner E, Ruth NR, Abfalter E, et al: IUD-associated pelvic actinomycosis: A report of five cases. Int J Gynecol Pathol 14:70, 1995.
79. Henderson S: Pelvic actinomycosis associated with an intrauterine device. Obstet Gynecol 41:726, 1973.
80. Gupta PK, Hollander DH, Frost JK: Actinomycetes in cervico-vaginal smears: An association with IUD usage. Acta Cytol 20:295, 1976.
81. Bhagavan BS, Gupta PK: Genital actinomycosis and intrauterine contraceptive devices. Cytopathologic diagnosis and clinical significance. Hum Pathol 9:567, 1978.
82. Spence MR, Gupta PK, Frost JK, King TM: Cytologic detection and clinical significance of *Actinomyces israelii* in women using intrauterine contraceptive devices. Am J Obstet Gynecol 131:295, 1978.
83. Gupta PK, Erozan YS, Frost JK: Actinomycetes and the IUD: An update. Acta Cytol 22:281, 1978.
84. Fiorino AS: Intrauterine contraceptive device–associated actinomycotic abscess and *Actinomyces* detection on cervical smear. Obstet Gynecol 87:142, 1996.
85. Valicenti JF, Pappas AA, Graber CD, et al: Detection and prevalence of IUD-associated *Actinomyces* colonization and related morbidity. JAMA 247:1149, 1982.
86. Mali B, Joshi J, Wagle U, et al: *Actinomyces* in cervical smears of women using intrauterine contraceptive devices. Acta Cytol 30:367, 1986.
87. Leslie D, Garland S: Comparison of immunofluorescence and culture for the detection of *Actinomyces israelii* in wearers of intra-uterine contraceptive devices. J Med Microbiol 35:224, 1991.
88. Jarvis D: Isolation and identification of actinomycetes from women using intrauterine contraceptive devices. J Infect 10:121, 1985.
89. Persson E: Genital actinomycosis and *Actinomyces israelii* in the female genital tract. Adv Contracept 3:115, 1987.
90. Reiner SL, Harrelson JM, Miller SE, et al: Primary actinomycosis of an extremity: A case report and review. Rev Infect Dis 9:581, 1987.
91. Cohen O, Keiser J, Pollner J, et al: Prosthetic joint infection with *Actinomyces viscosus*. Infect Dis Clin Pract 2:349, 1993.
92. Smego RA Jr: Actinomycosis of the central nervous system. Rev Infect Dis 9:855, 1987.
93. Sharma B, Banerjee A, Sobti M, et al: Actinomycotic brain abscess. Clin Neurol Neurosurg 92:373, 1990.
94. Bolton C, Ashenhurst E: Actinomycosis of the brain. Can Med Assoc J 90:922, 1964.
95. Lerner PI: Susceptibility of pathogenic actinomycetes to antimicrobial compounds. Antimicrob Agents Chemother 5:302, 1974.
96. Holmberg K, Nord C, Dornbusch K: Antimicrobial in vitro susceptibility of *Actinomyces israelii* and *Arachnia propionica*. Scand J Infect Dis 9:40, 1977.
97. Lerner P: Susceptibility of pathogenic *Actinomycetes* to antimicrobial compounds. Antimicrob Agents Chemother 5:302, 1974.
98. Martin M: Antibiotic treatment of cervicofacial actinomycosis for patients allergic to penicillin: A clinical and in vitro study. Br J Oral Maxillofac Surg 23:428, 1985.
99. Edelmann M, Cullmann W, Nowak KH, Kozuschek W: Treatment of abdominothoracic actinomycosis with imipenem. Eur J Clin Microbiol 6:194, 1987.
100. Schleck W, Gelfand M, Alper B, et al: Medical management of visceral actinomycosis. South Med J 76:921, 1983.
101. Wohlgemuth S, Gaddy M: Surgical implications of actinomycosis. South Med J 79:1574, 1986.
102. Goldwag S, Abbitt P, Watts B: Case report: Percutaneous drainage of periappendiceal actinomycosis. Clin Radiol 44:422, 1991.

232

Chlamydia

Julius Schachter

History

Chlamydia trachomatis was first visualized in 1907 by Halberstaedter and Prowazek in stained conjunctival scrapings taken from orangutans that had been inoculated with human trachomatous material.[1] Shortly thereafter, similar inclusions were identified in conjunctival scrapings from patients with trachoma and then from infants with inclusion blennorrhea. Inclusions were subsequently found in cervical cells of mothers of affected infants and in urethral cells of the fathers. In the first decade of this century, the presence of these inclusions was associated with nongonococcal urethritis.

C. trachomatis was first isolated from patients with lymphogranuloma venereum (LGV). In the 1930s, the growth cycle of the LGV organism (as seen after intracerebral inoculation in mice and then in eggs) was noted to be similar to that of *Chlamydia psittaci* that had been isolated during the psittacosis pandemic of 1929 to 1930. The trachoma agent proved more difficult to recover, not being infective for mice. It was isolated by inoculation of embryonated hens' eggs yolk sacs by T'ang and colleagues[2] in the 1950s. The first isolate of *Chlamydia* (other than LGV agents) from the genital tract was made in 1959 from the cervix of the mother of an infant with ophthalmia neonatorum.[3] In 1964, *Chlamydia* organisms were isolated from the urethras of men epidemiologically associated with conjunctivitis cases.[4, 5] In 1965, the introduction of a tissue culture isolation procedure for *C. trachomatis* made it possible to screen large numbers of specimens and to obtain the result of an isolation attempt in 48 to 72 hours.[6] This made the diagnosis clinically useful and led directly to identification of a broader clinical spectrum.

Disease associated with *C. psittaci* was first recognized in the latter part of the 19th century.[1] Sporadic outbreaks were associated with exposure to psittacine birds. Psittacosis attracted considerable attention as a result of a pandemic in 1929 to 1930. The causative agent was seen in impression smears from infected birds and human autopsy material and was isolated. In the preantibiotic era the case-fatality rate approached 20%. In the 1950s, it was recognized that there was a major reservoir in poultry. Psittacosis is now recognized as an occupational hazard to those exposed to infected turkeys in poultry processing plants. *C. psittaci* is also an important pathogen in domestic mammals, causing a number of diseases, such as abortion and arthritis, that have considerable economic impact.

Chlamydia pneumoniae was initially isolated from conjunctival specimens collected during trachoma surveys in Iran and Taiwan.[7] It has been shown to be widely distributed throughout the world. Seroepidemiologic studies indicated that 35% to 45% of adults in many countries have been exposed to the organism.[8] Infections begin relatively early in childhood. The organism has been associated with a wide variety of respiratory diseases including atypical pneumonia in young adults and mild epidemics of respiratory disease in military personnel.[9, 10] Severe and fatal cases have been observed in adults with underlying disease and in children

TABLE 232–1 ■ Characteristics of *Chlamydia* Species

SPECIES	ELEMENTARY BODY	SULFA SENSITIVITY	IODINE STAIN
C. trachomatis	Coccoid	+	+
C. psittaci	Coccoid	–	–
C. pneumoniae	Pear shaped	–	–
C. pecorum	Coccoid	–	–

in developing countries.[11, 12] This organism has also been implicated as a possible cause of coronary artery disease.[13]

A fourth species, *Chlamydia pecorum*, is a pathogen of mammals and is not considered an important cause of human disease.

Characteristics of the Pathogen

Taxonomy

The genus *Chlamydia* comprises four species, *C. trachomatis*, *C. psittaci*, *C. pneumoniae*, and *C. pecorum*(Table 232–1). They are obligate intracellular bacteria that have been placed in their own order and family (Chlamydiales, Chlamydiaceae).[14] These organisms are differentiated from other bacteria by a unique developmental cycle involving two morphologic forms—one adapted to extracellular survival and the other to intracellular multiplication. Because *Chlamydia* organisms are small and multiply only within susceptible cells, they were long thought to be viruses. However, their cellular organization, mechanisms of macromolecular synthesis and cell division, and antibiotic susceptibility are typically bacterial. *Chlamydia* organisms can be seen with the light microscope.

Many different strains of *Chlamydia* have been isolated from birds, humans, and other mammals. There is strong DNA homology within each species but surprisingly little among the four. Within species, biotypes and serotypes may be distinguished on the basis of host range, disease pattern, and antigenic composition.

C. trachomatis can be divided into three biotypes (Table 232–2). Two are associated with human diseases and can be differentiated serologically and by invasive properties. The LGV biotype can infect cultured cells efficiently, whereas the trachoma biotype requires mechanical assistance, such as centrifugation of the inoculum. In naturally occurring disease, the LGV biotype appears to infect endothelial and lymphoid cells and the trachoma biotype infects squamocolumnar cells. The murine biotype is represented by the mouse pneumonitis agent.

C. psittaci is virtually ubiquitous among avian species and is a common pathogen of mammals. It is known to infect humans only as zoonoses. It has been less well studied, and a systematic schema for differentiating its many biotypes and serotypes has not been developed. No animal reservoir has been identified for *C. pneumoniae*, although similar organisms have been isolated from a horse and a koala. It appears to be primarily a respiratory pathogen of humans.[15]

Developmental Cycle

The developmental cycle of *Chlamydia* species sets them apart from all other bacteria. There are some differences in inclusion morphology, but the species appear to have essentially identical developmental cycles. The cycle may be divided into several steps: (1) initial attachment of the elementary body (EB) to the host cell, (2) entry into the cell, (3) morphologic change to the reticulate body (RB) with intracellular growth and replication, (4) morphologic change of RBs to EBs, and finally (5) release of infectious particles.

ATTACHMENT

The attachment of *C. psittaci* and the LGV biotype of *C. trachomatis* to cells is highly efficient, as is penetration.[16] In contrast, the trachoma biotype attaches inefficiently. Attachment appears to be mediated by heparan sulfate–like molecules that act as a bridge between a specific receptor on the chlamydial particle and another on the susceptible host cell.[17] It is likely that this attachment process initiates a receptor-mediated endocytosis. Attachment may be partially charge dependent. Diethylaminoethyldextran pretreatment of cells leads to marked enhancement of attachment and entry of the trachoma biotype but not for most *C. psittaci* or the LGV biotype. Treatment with negatively charged molecules such as heparin can inhibit chlamydial infectivity and elute EBs from the surface of host cells. The attachment of *Chlamydia* to host cells and inhibition of phagolysosomal fusion are inhibited by specific antibody, mild heat treatment (56°C for 30 minutes), or trypsinization.[18, 19]

CELL ENTRY

Once attached, the EB is rapidly internalized by the host cell. If a mixture of EBs and *Escherichia coli* or yeast is presented to susceptible host cells, the *Chlamydia* organisms are preferentially ingested.[20] Many of the cells that *Chlamydia* species infect are not considered phagocytes. Moulder[21] has stressed the differentiation of host cells into professional and nonprofessional phagocytes and that *Chlamydia* induces phagocytosis by the nonprofessional phagocytes. The mechanism of chlamydial uptake is controversial. Ultrastructural studies suggest that *Chlamydia* organisms enter through clathrin-coated pits, via a pathway similar to that for receptor-mediated endocytosis.[22]

MORPHOLOGIC CHANGE AND REPLICATION

The infectious EB is relatively resistant to the extracellular environment. It is not metabolically active. EBs are 350 nm

TABLE 232–2 ■ Natural Host Ranges of *Chlamydia* Species and Human Diseases

SPECIES	NAURAL HOSTS	HUMAN DISEASES
C. psittaci	Birds, lower mammals	Psittacosis
C. pneumoniae	Humans	Respiratory
C. trachomatis		
Trachoma biotype	Humans	Trachoma, conjunctivitis, genital diseases, infant pneumonia
LGV biotype	Humans	LGV
Murine biotype	Mice	None known

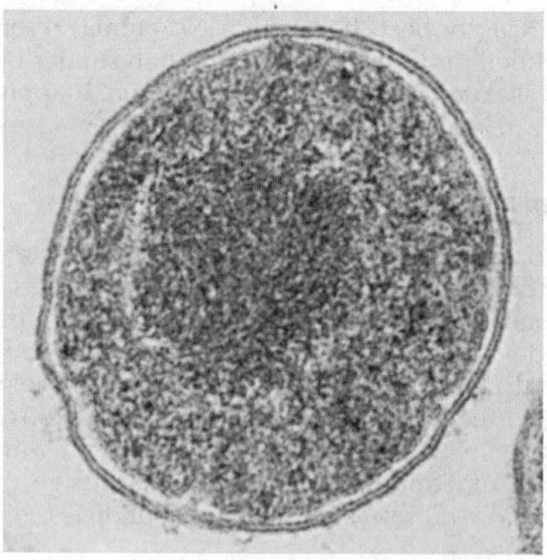

FIGURE 232–1 ▫ Electron micrograph of chlamydial elementary body showing inner and outer membranes and lack of peptidoglycan layer. Electron-dense centers also noted. (× 118,000.) (From Caldwell HD, Kromhout J, Schachter J: Purification and partial characterization of the major outer membrane protein of *Chlamydia trachomatis*. Infect Immun 31:1161–1176, 1981.)

in diameter and have an electron-dense center (Fig. 232–1). The EB changes to the metabolically active and dividing form, the RB, within the first 6 to 8 hours after entering the host cell. RBs are 1 μm in diameter and are not electron dense. Using the host cell pool of precursors, the RBs synthesize RNA, DNA, and protein.[23] The RBs divide by binary fission from 8 hours after entry into the cell to 18 to 24 hours. This is the stage of greatest metabolic activity, when the organisms are most sensitive to inhibitors of cell wall synthesis and inhibitors of bacterial metabolic activity. At 18 to 24 hours, some of the RBs reorganize into EBs (Fig. 232–2). This entire cycle takes place within the phagosome, which obviously undergoes a large increase in size. At some time between 48 and 72 hours the cell ruptures, releasing the infectious EBs.

Phagolysosomal fusion does not occur until the death of the cell is imminent. This inhibition has been attributed to a chlamydial surface antigen because antibody-treated EBs do not inhibit phagolysosomal fusion. Inhibition is specific to the chlamydial phagosome, as fusion can take place in other phagosomes in the same cell.[24]

The RBs are not stable outside the host cell. Thus, as part of their unique growth cycle, the *Chlamydia* strains have evolved two morphologic entities—the compact stable EB successfully persists in the extracellular environment and is responsible for cell-to-cell and host-to-host transmission, and the highly labile, noninfective RB is a metabolically active and vegetative form that does not survive outside the host cell.

Structure

The EB is a spherical particle with projections of the envelope (of unknown function) on one hemisphere[25] (Fig. 232–3). Electron microscopy reveals an outer membrane and an inner membrane. There is no peptidoglycan layer with muramic acid, but the presence of penicillin binding proteins suggests a related cross-linked structure.[26] The EB envelope is rigid and is relatively impermeable to macromolecules. The outer membrane contains lipopolysaccharide (LPS) and has a major outer membrane protein (MOMP) of 39,000 to 45,000 daltons. The MOMP is 60% of the weight of the outer membrane.[27] The structural rigidity of the EB appears to depend on disulfide cross-linking of MOMP molecules with each other and with other cysteine-rich proteins.[28] Soon after the EB enters the phagosome its envelope loses its rigidity and the subunit layer is disrupted and disappears. This reorganization to the more flexible and fragile structure of the RB probably involves reduction of the cross-linked disulfide bonds. The RB cell envelope is highly permeable.

Antigens

Chlamydia organisms contain a heat-stable LPS that is serologically the same in all members of the genus.[29] It is quite

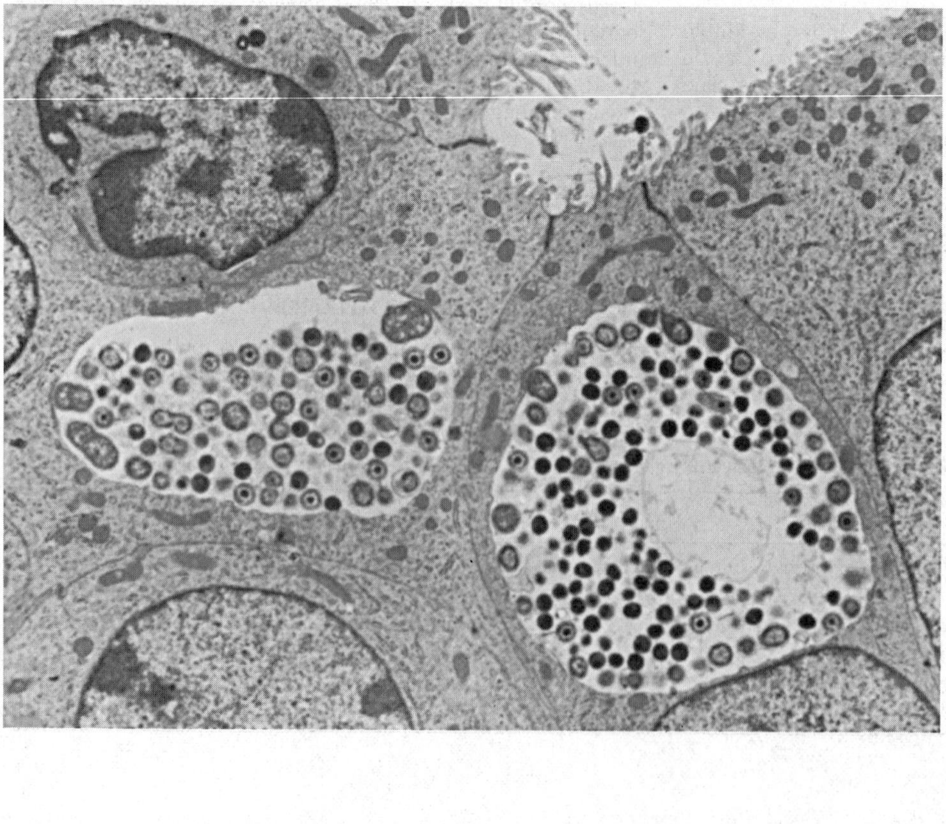

FIGURE 232–2 ▫ Chlamydial inclusions produced by the mouse pneumonitis agent in nonciliated cells in the murine oviduct. (× 7000.) (From Phillips DM, Swenson CE, Schachter J: Ultrastructure of *Chlamydia trachomatis* infection of the mouse oviduct. J Ultrastruct Res 88:244–256, 1984.)

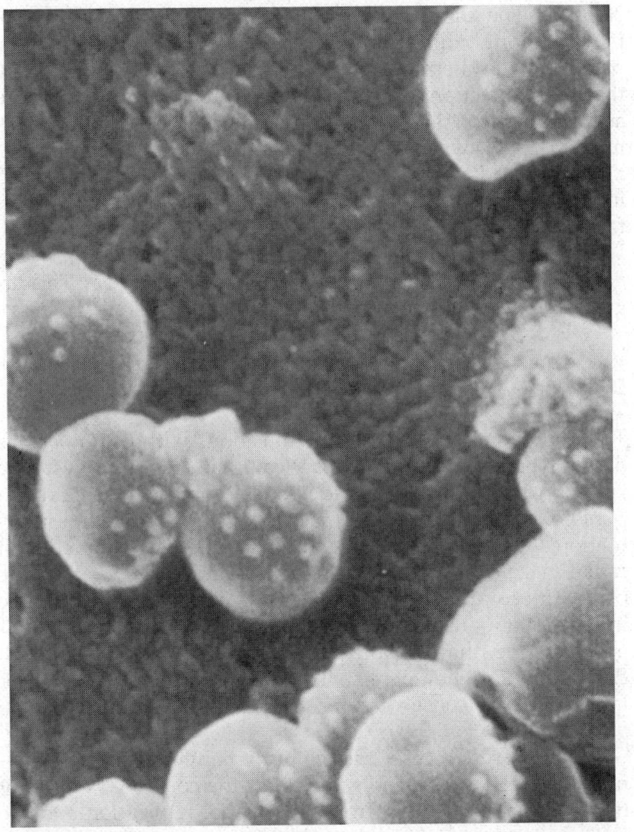

FIGURE 232–3 □ Electron micrograph of chlamydial particles showing hemispheric projections. (From Gregory WW, Gardner M, Byrne GI, Moulder JW: Arrays of hemispheric surface projections on *Chlamydia psittaci* and *Chlamydia trachomatis* observed by scanning electron microscopy. J Bacteriol 138:241–244, 1979.)

similar in structure to the LPS of such gram-negative bacteria as *Acinetobacter calcoaceticus* and Re mutants of *Salmonella typhimurium*. Heat-labile genus-specific antigens also exist. There are also species- and serotype-specific antigens. The human *C. trachomatis* pathogens can be divided into at least 15 serotypes by a microimmunofluorescent test.[30] The A, B, Ba, and C serotypes are associated with hyperendemic blinding trachoma, and the D to K serotypes are commonly associated with sexually transmitted disease. The L1, L2, and L3 serotypes represent the LGV biotype.[31] Antigens of species, serogroup (closely related serotypes), and serotype specificity can be found on the MOMP molecule.[32]

Only one serotype has been identified among *C. pneumoniae* isolates. There are many different serotypes among *C. psittaci*, but they have not been well characterized.

Metabolic Properties and Nucleic Acids

Chlamydia strains have been termed energy parasites because they do not generate their own adenosine triphosphate. In a sense, the endosome containing them functions as a reverse mitochondrion, taking in host cell–produced adenosine triphosphate and releasing adenosine diphosphate.[33] Typically, *Chlamydia* organisms require well-nourished host cells for their replication. They use the pool of host cell metabolites for their own synthesis.

The DNAs of *C. trachomatis* strains have a guanine plus cytosine content of approximately 44% to 45%.[34] At 6×10^5 to 8.5×10^5 base pairs, *Chlamydia* strains have one of the smallest bacterial genomes (one half the size of neisserial or rickettsial DNA).[35]

All *C. trachomatis* serotypes contain a 4.4-MDa plasmid.[36] It is present as a multimeric form. Restriction endonuclease cleavage patterns of the plasmid differed for the single LGV strain compared with the other *C. trachomatis* strains tested. Functions of the plasmid genes are not known, although some of the gene products are expressed during infection.

The sequence of the 16S RNA genes of *C. psittaci* and *C. trachomatis* has been determined, and there is only a 5% difference between the two species.[37] The sequence is similar to that of other eubacteria.

Chlamydial LPS has been successfully cloned into *E. coli* and is expressed in the outer membrane.[38] Because of its important structural and antigenic role, the genes responsible for MOMP have been of particular interest. The amino acid sequence of MOMP is now known for all serotypes. There are five conserved and four variable domains within the genes.[39] The most variable segments are approximately 11 amino acids long and occur one each in the N-terminal half and in the C-terminal half of the MOMP. These sites are responsible for the antigenic reactivity.[40]

Presence of a plasmid in *C. psittaci* strains appears to be variable. Morphologic evidence suggests that *Chlamydia* organisms may have bacteriophages.[41]

Epidemiology

Sexually Transmitted Chlamydial Infection

There appear to be two major modes of transmission of *C. trachomatis*. In industrialized Western society, virtually all *C. trachomatis* infections are sexually transmitted. *C. trachomatis* is now considered to be the most common sexually transmitted bacterial pathogen.[42] In the United States, it is estimated that more than 4 million new infections occur each year. These infections are just as important in the developing countries. Men who acquire the infection usually develop nongonococcal urethritis 1 to 3 weeks after infection.[43] Because cervical infection is often asymptomatic, it is difficult to assess incubation periods for women. Inapparent infections are common. If untreated, the infections can persist for years.

The highest rates of chlamydial infections are found in sexually active teenagers. Many studies have found approximately 1 in 6 female adolescents and 1 in 10 male adolescents to be infected.[44, 45] Risk factors for chlamydial infection include age, low socioeconomic status, recent change of partner, and use of oral contraceptives. Use of barrier methods of contraception is protective.[46, 47]

Ascending genital infections are common. The risk of men developing epididymitis is not known but is probably about 1%. Approximately 10% of young women with lower genital tract chlamydial infection have an episode of pelvic inflammatory disease.[48] Even more are likely to develop subclinical salpingitis.

Infants exposed to *Chlamydia* by passage through the infected birth canal may also acquire the infection and can develop a number of diseases, including conjunctivitis and pneumonia.[49] At least 60% to 70% of exposed infants acquire chlamydial infection. In adults, if infective genital tract discharges are inoculated into the eye either during sexual activity or by hand-to-eye contact, inclusion conjunctivitis may develop.[1]

Endemic Trachoma

In trachoma endemic areas, *C. trachomatis* is usually spread from child to child.[1] In many developing countries, trachoma is endemic and in some areas it is hyper- or holoendemic. Several hundred million people are known to be afflicted with trachoma and millions have been blinded. In holoendemic areas, children acquire the infection early. In some communities, all are infected by 2 years of age.[50] Poor hygiene and unsanitary conditions contribute to the spread of the organism. Flies act as mechanical vectors in spreading infective ocular discharges.[51] The disease begins as an acute mucopurulent conjunctivitis (often complicated by secondary bacterial infections [Fig. 232–4]) that becomes a chronic follicular keratoconjunctivitis, sometimes accompanied by a significant pannus (corneal neovascularization) formation. Active disease usually wanes when the children are 6 to 10 years old. Most of the children are left with minor sequelae when the disease becomes inactive, and there is no effect on vision. Some children with moderate to severe trachoma develop badly scarred conjunctivae. This scarring of the upper conjunctiva may, with time, result in distortion of the upper eyelid. The inturned upper lid margin causes the eyelashes to abrade and ultimately break down the corneal epithelium. It may take 25 or 30 years for this process to evolve fully, as the scars contract with age. The blindness seen in adults older than 40 years reflects early childhood trachoma. In a hyperendemic area, age-specific blindness rates at age 60 years may be 20% or more. Once common throughout the world, trachoma is now a major problem only in certain developing countries. Still, trachoma is the world's leading preventable cause of blindness.[52]

Psittacosis (Ornithosis)

Human psittacosis is a disease contracted from exposure to avian species infected with *C. psittaci*.[1] The term ornithosis is also used because the infection is not restricted to psittacines. The organism is ubiquitous among avian species, usually infecting the intestinal tract. It is also common in domestic mammals but they are seldom a source of human infection. This zoonosis is relatively uncommon, with only a few hundred cases occurring each year in the United States.

Chlamydia pneumoniae *Infection*

C. pneumoniae infections appear to occur relatively early in childhood.[8, 15] Serologic studies indicate an annual incidence of infection of at least 1% to 2%. Seroprevalence peaks at approximately 35% to 45% in most populations at about age 30 years. The clinical expression of these infections is uncertain. Although infection has been associated with severe pneumonia and epidemics of mild pneumonia,[9, 10] it is likely that most infections cause mild respiratory symptoms or are asymptomatic. Asymptomatic infections have been documented by recovery of the organism from healthy individuals. In Finland, epidemics of mild pneumonias have occurred in military trainees, and 6% to 8% of the soldiers were affected.[53]

Much evidence has been obtained indicating that *C. pneumoniae* may contribute to coronary artery disease.[54] The organism may be found within atheromatous lesions.[55]

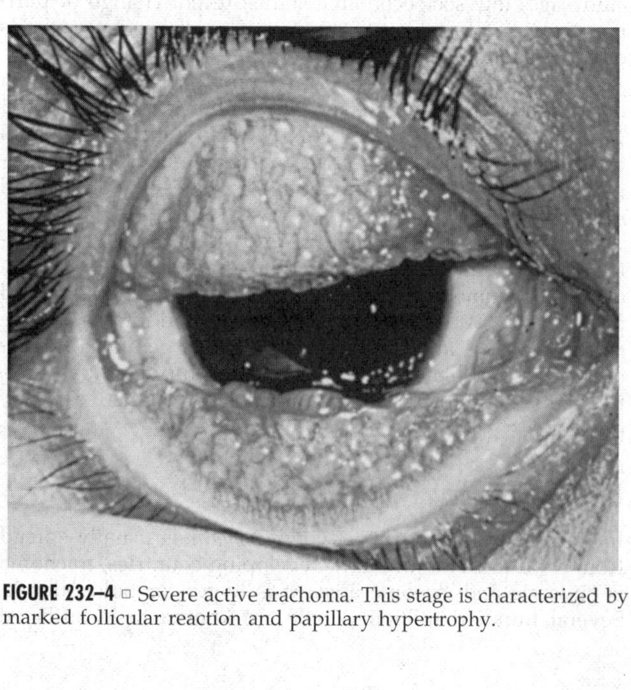

FIGURE 232–4 □ Severe active trachoma. This stage is characterized by marked follicular reaction and papillary hypertrophy.

Pathogenesis

The pathogenesis of any of the infections with *C. trachomatis* has not been elucidated. It is clear that LGV is a systemic infection involving lymphoid tissues. The organisms are capable of replicating within macrophages.[56] To date, all information suggests that the trachoma biotype has a limited host range in vivo. It appears to be almost exclusively a parasite of squamocolumnar epithelial cells. Because they are obligate intracellular parasites and kill host cells at the end of their growth cycle, these chlamydial strains must cause some cell damage where they persist. There is no in vivo evidence for latency in the sense of persistence of nonreplicating *Chlamydia*.

The disease process and clinical manifestations of chlamydial infections probably represent the combined effects of tissue damage resulting from chlamydial replication and the inflammatory responses caused by the presence of *Chlamydia* and necrotic material from the destroyed host cells. There is an abundant immune response to chlamydial infection (in terms of humoral or cell-mediated responses). There is now evidence that chlamydial diseases result in part from hypersensitivity or are diseases of immunopathology.[31, 57]

LGV is a truly lymphoproliferative disease. The trachoma biotype appears to cause a more localized lymphoproliferative response in the sense that it can induce follicle formation in the mucous membranes. Although such a response is best known for the conjunctiva (trachoma and inclusion conjunctivitis), follicular cervicitis, proctitis, and probably follicular urethritis are recognized. Follicles induced by *C. trachomatis* are true lymphoid follicles with germinal centers.

Trachoma has long been considered a disease in which reinfection is important.[31] In nonhuman primates, repeated (weekly) conjunctival instillation of *C. trachomatis* results in a disease with many of the manifestations of trachoma, including conjunctival scarring.[58] Similarly severe experimental salpingitis in nonhuman primates was also in part dependent on previous exposure to *Chlamydia*.[59] A common pathologic end point of chlamydial infection is scarring of mucous membranes. This is what ultimately leads to the blindness in trachoma and to infertility and ectopic pregnancy after acute salpingitis.

In a guinea pig model for *C. psittaci* infection a Triton (*t*-octylphenoxypolyethoxyethanol)–soluble extract of EBs induced an ocular hypersensitivity reaction if dropped onto the conjunctiva of previously infected, but not naive, animals.[60] The reactive material appears to be genus specific, as it induced conjunctivitis in nonhuman primates that had been infected with the trachoma agent.[57] The specific allergen for this ocular hypersensitivity reaction is probably a heat shock protein antigen of 57 kDa.[61] Current theory suggests that it is hypersensitivity to this heat shock protein (heat shock protein 60) that is specifically responsible for much of the chlamydial disease. It is known that this antigen is broadly cross-reactive, secreted by infected cells, and antibodies to it are found in high levels in women suffering from tubal factor infertility and ectopic pregnancy.[62, 63] Thus, the serologic tests may provide some support for a clinical diagnosis or have prognostic implications.

Immunology

Chlamydia species are highly complex organisms with antigens of genus, species, subspecies, and serotype specificity.[32] The most easily detected antigen is the genus-specific LPS antigen. It is responsible for the complement-fixing reactions commonly used to diagnose psittacosis or LGV.[64] Chlamydial LPS has two antigen sites. One is identical to that of other bacteria, and the other is *Chlamydia* specific.[65] *Acinetobacter* LPS can be used as the complement fixation antigen for antichlamydial antibodies, but not all serum samples positive against the chlamydial antigen react to the *Acinetobacter* LPS.[66]

The antigen responsible for delayed hypersensitivity (Frei test), which was used in diagnosing LGV, has not been studied with modern techniques. It is probably the LPS. The skin test antigen is heat stable and periodate sensitive. *C. psittaci* strains have been used to prepare Frei antigens.

Species-specific antigens are shared by all members of a chlamydial species. Subspecies- or serotype-specific antigens are common only to selected strains within chlamydial species. These antigens have been the basis for a variety of serologic tests used for the classification of *C. trachomatis*.[31] The responsible antigens appear to be on the MOMP molecule.

These serotypes fall into two broad complexes (B and C) by microimmunofluorescence.[30] Each complex shows extensive cross-reaction within the complex but little reaction with the other complex. Serotype-specific monoclonal antibodies are now available for typing purposes. It is likely that immunity to infection, although relatively weak, is serotype specific.

The MOMP molecule is cross-linked to 15- and 60-kDa proteins.[67] The 60-kDa proteins are important immunogens and are often found as a doublet.[68] Although MOMP appears to be the immundominant antigen, there may be a more selective response to 60- to 62-kDa proteins. The 60-kDa cystine-rich protein is surface exposed and has species-specific antigens. The 15-kDa proteins are not on the EB surface. They contain antigens of species and biotype specificity.[69] Monoclonal antibodies directed against MOMP have been shown capable of neutralizing infectivity in cell culture and prevent ocular infection in subhuman primates.[70]

Control of Chlamydial Infection by the Host

In the majority of chlamydial infections only a small proportion of cells at affected sites are infected. Because each inclusion releases hundreds of viable EBs and relatively few nearby cells are infected, there must be control mechanisms that limit infectivity. The mechanisms are not clear. Lymphokines have been shown to have an inhibitory effect on *Chlamydia*.[71] *C. trachomatis* is sensitive to interferon-α, -β, and -γ.[72] The latter appears to be most active. The lymphokine that inhibits *Chlamydia* in human macrophages and in mice has been identified as interferon-γ.[73, 74] It appears to delay the developmental cycle at the RB stage.[75] This may result in persistent inapparent infection and may also play a role in immunopathogenesis. The mode of action appears to be, as in other systems, depletion of tryptophan, making it unavailable to the *Chlamydia* organisms.[76]

Description

Chlamydia trachomatis *Infection*

TRACHOMA

Although onset can be insidious, the disease begins as a mucopurulent conjunctivitis, developing into a follicular keratoconjunctivitis.[1] Over time, some of the follicles necrose, resulting in scarring of the conjunctivae. The scars may slowly contract, distorting the eyelid and causing an inturning of the eyelashes so that they abrade the cornea (Fig. 232–5). This complex represents the blinding lesions of trachoma, called trichiasis and entropion. Trachoma often occurs in areas of the world where seasonal outbreaks of bacterial conjunctivitis make the disease worse. Severe lid deformity may not develop until 30 or 40 years after active disease has waned.

GENITAL TRACT INFECTION

In men, *C. trachomatis* causes 35% to 50% of cases of nongonococcal urethritis.[43] There is usually a mucopurulent discharge and dysuria. Ascending infections can occur. *C. trachomatis* is now recognized as the leading cause of epididymitis in sexually active young men.[77] Chlamydial proctitis is relatively common among homosexual men.[78]

In women, the most commonly affected site is the cervix, where the organism can cause a mucopurulent endocervicitis.[43] This condition is characterized by a mucopurulent endocervical discharge. Urethral infections occur and can cause a "sterile" pyuria in young women. Ascending genital infection is common.[48] *C. trachomatis* is found in the endometrium or fallopian tubes of approximately 25% of cases of acute salpingitis in the United States. *Chlamydia* strains are also an important cause of infertility and ectopic pregnancy as a result of tubal damage.[79] Unfortunately, the preceding chlamydial salpingitis can be clinically mild or even inapparent and thus may not be treated.

NEONATAL INFECTION

Approximately 60% to 70% of infants born through a *Chlamydia*-infected birth canal show serologic evidence of infection.[49, 80] About one in three of the exposed infants develops inclusion conjunctivitis of the newborn. It is a mucopurulent conjunctivitis with an incubation period of 5 to 21 days and usually resolves in a few months without treatment. Approximately one in six exposed infants develops a charac-

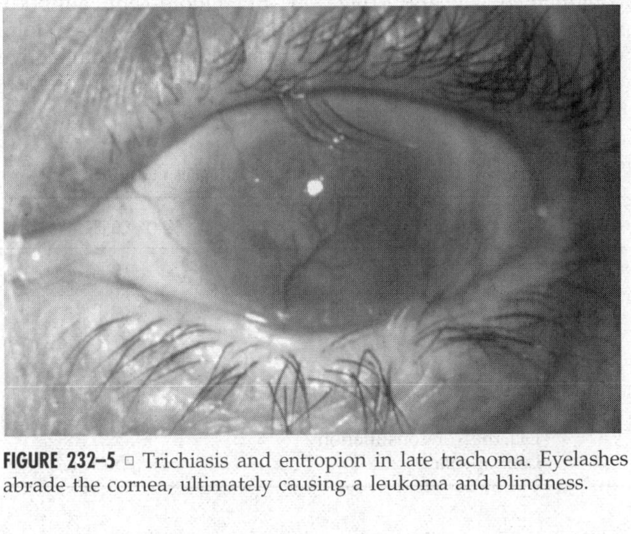

FIGURE 232–5 □ Trichiasis and entropion in late trachoma. Eyelashes abrade the cornea, ultimately causing a leukoma and blindness.

teristic pneumonia syndrome. The age at onset is usually between 2 and 12 weeks. The infants often have a prodrome of rhinitis, and many have conjunctivitis. Affected infants are usually afebrile, are markedly tachypneic and occasionally apneic, and have a staccato cough. Vaginal and gastrointestinal tract infections also occur but have no known clinical consequences.

Human Infection with Chlamydia psittaci

Psittacosis usually occurs in a respiratory or a typhoidal form.[1] Respiratory disease can be a mild influenzal disease or it can develop into a severe and fatal (if untreated) pneumonia. The incubation period is typically 1 to 3 weeks. Fever, chills, and severe headache usually occur (Table 232–3). Radiographs may show more extensive lung involvement than is expected from the respiratory difficulty. The typhoidal form of the disease involves a general toxic febrile state without respiratory findings. Person-to-person transmission is uncommon but has occurred.

Most human infections with *C. psittaci* from domestic mammals appear to be subclinical. They have been detected by serologic surveys. *C. psittaci* causing abortions in lower mammals may also cause abortions in humans.[81]

Chlamydia pneumoniae *Infection*

C. pneumoniae has been associated with relatively mild pneumonias in young adults. The clinical picture is similar to that seen with mycoplasmal pneumonia.[9] More severe disease is recognized but appears to be a function of underlying disease.[12]

Fatal infections have also been described in young Filipino children.[11] This is clearly an emerging area in infectious diseases and the clinical spectrum of *C. pneumoniae* infection is not clear. The spectrum is likely to range from inapparent infection to pharyngitis, bronchiolitis, and pneumonia. This organism's possible role in coronary artery disease is currently an active area of research.[13]

Diagnosis

Chlamydia trachomatis *Infection*

TRACHOMA

Trachoma diagnosis is based mainly on clinical findings: identification of follicular reaction, papillary hypertrophy, and scars within the conjunctiva.[82] Laboratory diagnosis is often based on demonstration of chlamydial inclusions in conjunctival smears[83] (Fig. 232–6). Fluorescent antibody methods are more sensitive than the classic Giemsa stain. *Chlamydia* organisms may be readily isolated from active cases in cell culture systems (Fig. 232–7). Detection of chlamydial genes by polymerase chain reaction is the most sensitive laboratory test. Serologic tests are not useful for diagnosing individual cases. In hyperendemic areas, the great majority of individuals have serum antibodies to *C. trachomatis*. Antibodies in tears correlate with intensity of the disease.[84]

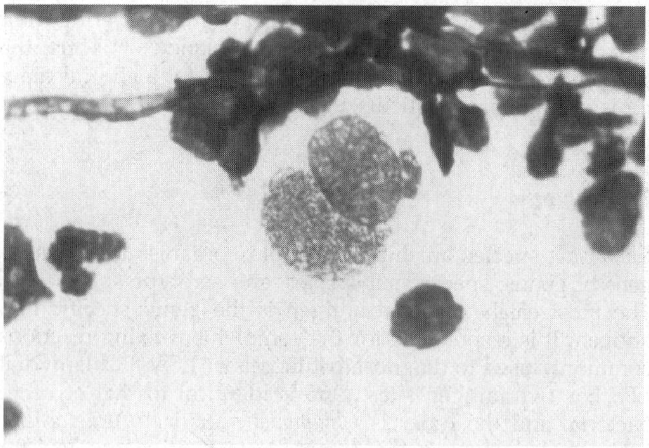

FIGURE 232–6 □ *C. trachomatis* inclusion in a conjunctival smear from a patient with trachoma. Giemsa stain. (Approximately × 1000.)

GENITAL TRACT INFECTION

Definitive diagnosis is made by isolation of the agent in cell culture systems.[85] Antigen detection, based on use of fluorescein-conjugated monoclonal antibodies or enzyme immunoassay, is simpler and less expensive but is also less sensitive than cell culture.[86, 87] Detection of chlamydial genes by DNA amplification tests (polymerase chain reaction, ligase chain reaction) is much more sensitive.[88, 89] These are likely to be the tests of choice in the future.

Serology does not play a role in diagnosing lower genital tract infections. The higher antibody levels seen by microimmunofluorescence in complications (e.g., epididymitis, salpingitis) may provide some support for a clinical diagnosis.

Some chlamydial diseases can be treated on a presumptive basis. Urethritis in men can be easily managed without a specific diagnosis, on the basis of a Gram stain (exclusion of gonorrhea by failure to demonstrate gram-negative diplococci in polymorphonuclear leukocytes). Women with mucopurulent endocervicitis or salpingitis should be automatically

TABLE 232–3 ■ Clinical Findings in Confirmed Human Psittacosis

SIGN OR SYMPTOM	% OF CASES
Fever	>95
Headache	>95
Chills	>95
Myalgias	>90
Sweats	50
Conjunctivitis or photophobia	50
Cough	50
Diarrhea or constipation	35
Leukopenia	25

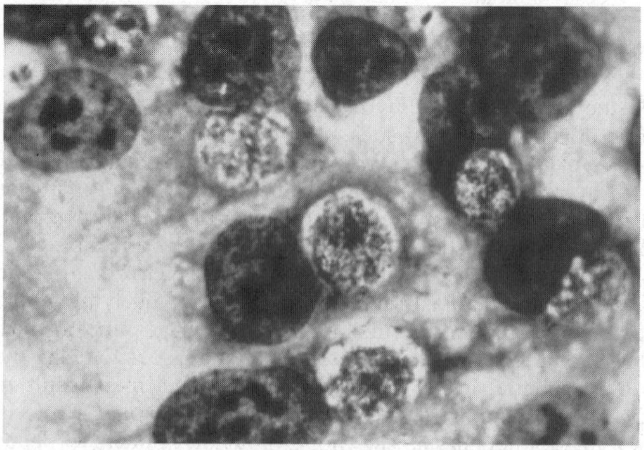

FIGURE 232–7 □ Giemsa stain of *C. trachomatis* inclusions in HeLa cells inoculated with a genital tract specimen. (Approximately × 1000.)

treated for chlamydial infection. Treatment of sexual partners is always indicated.

NEONATAL INFECTION

Conjunctivitis may be diagnosed readily by any of the cytologic tests. Giemsa stain is adequate in diagnosing severe cases, and the fluorescent antibody techniques are quite sensitive. The agent may be readily isolated.

A specific diagnosis for pneumonia may be more difficult because of sampling problems, but the organism can usually be isolated from the nasopharynx or tracheobronchial aspirates. Infants with chlamydial pneumonia almost always develop high immunoglobulin M antibody levels, and because of their defined exposure (at birth) the diagnosis may be readily established on the basis of a single-point determination of specific antichlamydial immunoglobulin M antibodies greater than 1:32 by microimmunofluorescence.[90]

Psittacosis

Clinical signs are not pathognomonic. The clinician's index of suspicion (asking questions about potential exposure to birds) is usually crucial to arriving at a diagnosis. Serodiagnosis is generally considered to be the method of choice, because isolation of the agent is seldom achieved. Rising antibody levels can be demonstrated by complement fixation or microimmunofluorescence. Other causes of atypical pneumonia must be considered when *C. psittaci* or *C. pneumoniae* infections are possibilities.

Chlamydia pneumoniae *Infection*

Specific serologic tests are available using modification of the microimmunofluorescent test with a *C. pneumoniae* antigen.[9] Seroconversion can also be demonstrated by the complement fixation test in approximately half the cases. A presumptive diagnosis may be made if the initial serum specimen has a *C. pneumoniae*–specific immunoglobulin M titer greater than 1:32 or immunoglobulin G titer greater than 1:512. Seroconversion can be delayed, taking more than 4 weeks.[9, 15] The organism can be isolated, with some difficulty, from respiratory tract specimens. Use of HL or HEp-2 cells provides a more sensitive culture system for *C. pneumoniae* than do cells such as McCoy or HeLa that are commonly used for culture of *C. trachomatis*.[91]

Treatment

Azithromycin given in a single 1-g dose is now considered the treatment of choice for uncomplicated lower genital tract infection with *C. trachomatis*.[92] This regimen is as effective as a 1-week course of doxycycline.[93] In general, tetracyclines are considered the drugs of choice for all other chlamydial infections, except when they are contraindicated or not tolerated. In those cases the alternative is erythromycin. Ofloxacin is also effective. Aminoglycosides are not active against *Chlamydia,* and this has led to their widespread use in controlling bacterial contamination in clinical specimens being tested for the presence of *Chlamydia*. Common antifungal drugs such as amphotericin B and nystatin are also inactive against *Chlamydia,* as are the nitroimidazoles used to treat *Trichomonas* infections. Cephalosporins are not active.

Although there are documented treatment failures in which *Chlamydia* organisms have been isolated from patients after treatment, the recovered agents have been found to be wholly susceptible to the antibiotics. There is a suggestion that relative resistance to erythromycin has been developing, but no data suggest that this has reached clinically relevant levels.[94] Rifampin, which is highly active in vitro, has not been widely used to treat human chlamydial infections. Rifampin resistance can be easily developed by passage in the laboratory.[95]

Chlamydia trachomatis *Infection*

TRACHOMA

To treat trachoma, 1% tetracycline ointment is usually applied on an intermittent basis. The goal of this therapy is to reduce the infectious load and reduce development of the blinding complications. This treatment is not an effective cure. Oral azithromycin is as effective as long-term topical tetracycline treatment, but this drug is too expensive for use in trachoma endemic areas.[96] Its value in controlling trachoma is currently under investigation.

GENITAL TRACT INFECTION

Treatment of uncomplicated genital tract infection is relatively easy, with 2 g of tetracycline per day for 7 days or doxycycline at 100 mg twice a day for 7 days, resulting in cure rates in excess of 95%.[92] Oral azithromycin in a 1-g single dose is the treatment of choice for uncomplicated genital tract infection; this results in cure rates greater than 95%. It is a coequal treatment of choice with a 7-day course of oral doxycycline (100 mg twice daily). However, it is currently too expensive for use in public clinics.

Erythromycin at 500 mg four times daily for 7 days is generally considered the treatment of choice for pregnant women and for those who are tetracycline intolerant. Ofloxacin is also effective. Upper genital tract infections call for longer courses of therapy.

NEONATAL INFECTION

Chlamydial infection in the infant calls for systemic therapy with erythromycin (50 mg/kg in divided doses each day), 7 to 14 days for conjunctivitis and 14 to 21 days for pneumonia. Topical therapy is not recommended because of relatively high failure rates and the need to eradicate extraocular infection and prevent subsequent development of pneumonia.

Psittacosis and Chlamydia pneumoniae *Infection*

Psittacosis is usually treated with tetracycline, 2 g daily for at least 10 to 14 days. Erythromycin is the alternative. Relapses are common if the duration of treatment is inadequate. Regimens for *C. pneumoniae* are likely to be similar, but sufficient experience is not yet available.

Prevention

Chlamydia trachomatis *Infection*

TRACHOMA

Experimental vaccines have induced a short-lived immune response, but some vaccinees developed more severe disease, suggesting hypersensitivity to the organism.[1, 31] Trachoma control is currently based on mass treatment of all affected individuals within a village setting with topical tetracycline ointment and on surgical intervention to correct lid deformities. These efforts are aimed at preventing blindness, not at curing trachoma. Improved living conditions provide the most effective control.

GENITAL TRACT INFECTION

No program for prevention of sexually transmitted chlamydial infection is in effect.[42] Guidelines for such a program have been developed, but economic considerations have prevented their implementation. Use of barrier contraceptives reduces transmission.

Psittacosis

Psittacosis is an occupational hazard for those in the poultry or pet bird industries. Chemoprophylaxis for exotic birds is available, and clean premises can be maintained by avoiding introduction of untreated birds.

Immunity

Immunity induced by chlamydial infection is not well understood. It is clear that single infections do not result in solid immunity to reinfection. Repeated infections are common. Some immunity probably develops after initial or serial infection. In screening studies, younger women are found to have higher cervical infection rates than older women, who often have higher antibody levels. This speculation is also consistent with the observation that many isolate-negative individuals attending sexually transmitted disease clinics have immunoglobulin M antibody to the organism.[97] This antibody could result from recent exposure and rapid resolution of the infection by an immune response.

The only human chlamydial infection that has been subjected to extensive vaccine studies is trachoma.[1, 31] Unfortunately, these studies were performed without a sophisticated knowledge of the chlamydial immune response. The results from field studies, vaccine trials, and infection of volunteers and subhuman primates indicate that there is a short-lived relative immunity to reinfection with homotypic challenge. Efforts to develop an effective vaccine are in the forefront of current chlamydial research.

NEONATAL INFECTION

Pregnant women can be screened for chlamydial infection; erythromycin treatment of those found to be infected prevents perinatal transmission.[98] Because attack rates for infant diseases have been fairly consistent in most studies, the prevalence of chlamydial infection in pregnant women determines the cost-benefit relationship of this stratagem.

References

1. Schachter J, Dawson CR (eds): Human Chlamydial Infections. Littleton, MA, PSG Publishing, 1978.
2. T'ang F-F, Chang H-L, Huang Y-T, et al: Trachoma virus in chick embryo. Natl Med J China 43:81, 1957.
3. Jones BR, Collier LH, Smith CH: Isolation of virus from inclusion blennorrhoea. Lancet 1:902, 1959.
4. Jones BR: Ocular syndromes of TRIC virus infection and their possible genital significance. Br J Vener Dis 40:3, 1964.
5. Rose L, Schachter J: Genitourinary aspects of inclusion conjunctivitis. Invest Ophthalmol 3:680, 1964.
6. Gordon FB, Quan AL: Isolation of the trachoma agent in cell culture. Proc Soc Exp Biol Med 118:354, 1965.
7. Grayston JT, Kuo C-C, Campbell LA: *Chlamydia pneumoniae* sp. nov. for *Chlamydia* strain TWAR. J Syst Bacteriol 39:88, 1989.
8. Forsey T, Darougar S, Treharne JD: Prevalence in human beings of antibodies to *Chlamydia* IOL-207, an atypical strain of *Chlamydia*. J Infect 12:145, 1986.
9. Grayston JT, Kuo C-C, Wang S-P, et al: A new *Chlamydia psittaci* strain, TWAR, isolated in acute respiratory tract infections. N Engl J Med 315:161, 1986.
10. Saikku P, Wang S-P, Kleemola M, et al: An epidemic of mild pneumonia due to an unusual strain of *Chlamydia psittaci*. J Infect Dis 151:832, 1985.
11. Saikku P, Ruutu P, Leinonen M, et al: Acute lower respiratory tract infection associated with *Chlamydia* TWAR antibody in Filipino children. J Infect Dis 158:1095, 1988.
12. Marrie TJ, Grayston JT, Wang S-P, et al: Pneumonia associated with the TWAR strain of *Chlamydia*. Ann Intern Med 106:507, 1987.
13. Saikku P, Leinonen M, Matilla K, et al: Serological evidence of an association of a novel *Chlamydia*, TWAR, chronic coronary heart disease and acute myocardial infarction. Lancet 2:983, 1988.
14. Moulder JW, Hatch TP, Kuo CC, et al: Order II. Chlamydiales Storz and Page 1971, 334. *In* Krieg NR, Holt JG (eds): Bergey's Manual of Systematic Bacteriology, Vol 1. Baltimore, Williams & Wilkins, 1984, pp 729–739.
15. Grayston JT, Aldous MB, Easton A, et al: Evidence that *Chlamydia pneumoniae* causes pneumonia and bronchitis. J Infect Dis 168:1231, 1993.
16. Kuo C-C, Wang SP, Grayston JT: Effect of polycations, polyanions and neuraminidase on the infectivity of trachoma-inclusion conjunctivitis and lymphogranuloma venereum organisms in HeLa cells: Sialic acid residues as possible receptors for trachoma-inclusion conjunctivitis. Infect Immun 8:74, 1973.
17. Zhang JP, Stephens RS: Mechanism of *C. trachomatis* attachment to eukaryotic host cells. Cell 89:861, 1992.
18. Byrne GI, Moulder JW: Parasite-specified phagocytosis of *Chlamydia psittaci* and *Chlamydia trachomatis* by L and HeLa cells. Infect Immun 19:598, 1978.
19. Byrne GI: Requirements of ingestion of *Chlamydia psittaci* by mouse fibroblasts (L cells). Infect Immun 14:645, 1976.
20. Brownridge EA, Wyrick PB: Interaction of *Chlamydia psittaci* reticulate bodies with mouse peritoneal macrophages. Infect Immun 24:697, 1979.
21. Moulder JW: Comparative biology of intracellular parasitism. Microbiol Rev 49:298, 1985.
22. Hodinka RL, Wyrick PB: Ultrastructural study of mode of entry of *Chlamydia psittaci* into L-929 cells. Infect Immun 54:855, 1986.
23. Moulder JW: The relation of the psittacosis group (chlamydiae) to bacteria and viruses. Annu Rev Microbiol 20:107, 1966.
24. Eissenberg LG, Wyrick PB: Inhibition of phagolysosome fusion is localized to *Chlamydia psittaci*–laden vacuoles. Infect Immun 32:889, 1981.
25. Gregory WM, Gardner M, Byrne G, et al: Arrays of hemispheric surface projections on *Chlamydia psittaci* and *Chlamydia trachomatis* observed by scanning electron microscopy. J Bacteriol 138:241, 1979.
26. Barbour AG, Amano K-I, Hackstadt T, et al: *Chlamydia trachomatis* has penicillin-binding proteins but not detectable muramic acid. J Bacteriol 151:420, 1982.
27. Caldwell HD, Kromhout J, Schachter J: Purification and partial characterization of the major outer membrane protein of *Chlamydia trachomatis*. Infect Immun 31:1161, 1981.
28. Newhall WJ: Biosynthesis and disulfide cross-linking of outer membrane components during the growth cycle of *Chlamydia trachomatis*. Infect Immun 55:162, 1987.
29. Brade L, Nurminen M, Makela PH, et al: Antigenic properties of *Chlamydia trachomatis* lipopolysaccharides. Infect Immun 48:569, 1985.
30. Wang S-P, Grayston JT: Immunologic relationship between genital TRIC, lymphogranuloma venereum and related organisms in a new microtiter indirect immunofluorescence test. Am J Ophthalmol 70:367, 1970.
31. Grayston JT, Wang S-P: New knowledge of chlamydiae and the diseases they cause. J Infect Dis 132:87, 1975.
32. Caldwell HD, Schachter J: Antigenic analysis of the major outer membrane protein of *Chlamydia* spp. Infect Immun 35:1024, 1982.
33. Hatch TP, Al-Hossainy E, Silverman JA: Adenine nucleotide and lysine transport in *Chlamydia psittaci*. J Bacteriol 150:662, 1982.
34. Kingsbury DT, Weiss E: Lack of deoxyribonucleic acid homology between species of the genus *Chlamydia*. J Bacteriol 96:1421, 1968.
35. Kingsbury DT: Estimate of the genome size of various microorganisms. J Bacteriol 98:1400, 1979.
36. Palmer L, Falkow S: A common plasmid of *Chlamydia trachomatis*. Plasmid 16:52, 1986.
37. Weisburg WG, Hatch TP, Woese CR: Eubacterial origin of chlamydiae. J Bacteriol 167:570, 1986.

38. Nano FE, Caldwell HD: Expression of chlamydial genus-specific lipopolysaccharide epitope in *Escherichia coli*. Science 228:742, 1985.
39. Stephens RS, Sanchez-Pescador R, Wagar EA, et al: Diversity of *Chlamydia trachomatis* major outer membrane protein genes. J Bacteriol 169:3879, 1987.
40. Stephens RS, Wagar EA, Schoolnik GK: High-resolution mapping of serovar-specific and common antigenic determinants of the major outer membrane protein of *Chlamydia trachomatis*. J Exp Med 167:817, 1988.
41. Richmond SJ, Stirling P, Ashley CR: Virus infecting the reticulate bodies of an avian strain of *Chlamydia*. FEMS Microbiol Lett 14:31, 1982.
42. Centers for Disease Control and Prevention: Recommendations for the prevention and management of *Chlamydia trachomatis* infections, 1993. MMWR Morbid Mortal Wkly Rep 42(RR-12):1, 1993.
43. Stamm WE, Holmes KK: *Chlamydia trachomatis* infections of the adult. *In* Holmes KK, Mardh P-A, Sparling PF, et al (eds): Sexually Transmitted Diseases. San Francisco, McGraw-Hill, 1990, pp 181–193.
44. Shafer MA, Blain B, Beck A, et al: *Chlamydia trachomatis*: Important relationships to race, contraception, lower genital tract infection, and Papanicolaou smears. J Pediatr 104:141, 1984.
45. Shafer MA, Prager V, Shalwitz J: Prevalence of urethral *Chlamydia trachomatis* and *Neisseria gonorrhoeae* among asymptomatic, sexually active adolescent boys. J Infect Dis 156:223, 1987.
46. Schachter J, Stoner E, Moncada J: Screening for chlamydial infections in women attending family planning clinics: Evaluations of presumptive indicators for therapy. West J Med 138:375, 1983.
47. Handsfield HH, Jasman LL, Roberts PL: Criteria for selective screening for *Chlamydia trachomatis* infection in women attending family planning clinics. JAMA 255:1730, 1986.
48. Westrom LV, Mardh P-A: Acute pelvic inflammatory disease (PID). *In* Holmes KK, Mardh P-A, Sparling PF, et al (eds): Sexually Transmitted Diseases. San Francisco, McGraw-Hill, 1990, pp 593–613.
49. Alexander ER, Harrison HR: Role of *Chlamydia trachomatis* in perinatal infection. Rev Infect Dis 5:713, 1983.
50. Dawson CR, Daghfous T, Messadi M, et al: Severe endemic trachoma in Tunisia. Br J Ophthalmol 60:245, 1976.
51. Forsey T, Darougar S: Transmission of chlamydiae by the housefly. Br J Ophthalmol 65:147, 1981.
52. Jones BR: Prevention of blindness from trachoma. Trans Ophthalmol Soc UK 95:16, 1975.
53. Kleemola M, Saikku P, Visakorpi R, et al: Epidemics of pneumonia caused by TWAR, a new *Chlamydia* organism, in military trainees in Finland. J Infect Dis 157:230, 1988.
54. Saikku P, Leinonen M, Tenkanen L, et al: Chronic *Chlamydia pneumoniae* infection as a risk factor for coronary heart disease in the Helsinki heart study. Ann Intern Med 116:273, 1992.
55. Kuo CC, Shor A, Campbell LA, et al: Demonstration of *Chlamydia pneumoniae* in atherosclerotic lesions of coronary arteries. J Infect Dis 167:841, 1993.
56. Kuo CC: Cultures of *Chlamydia trachomatis* in mouse peritoneal macrophages: Factors affecting organism growth. Infect Immun 20:439, 1978.
57. Taylor HR, Johnson SL, Schachter J, et al: Pathogenesis of trachoma: The stimulus for inflammation. J Immunol 138:3023, 1987.
58. Taylor HR, Johnson SL, Prendergast RA, et al: An animal model of trachoma. II. The importance of repeated reinfection. Invest Ophthalmol Vis Sci 23:507, 1982.
59. Patton DL, Kuo C-C, Wang S-P, et al: Distal tube obstruction induced by repeated *Chlamydia trachomatis* salpingeal infections in pig-tailed macaques. J Infect Dis 155:1292, 1987.
60. Watkins NG, Hadlow WJ, Moos AB, et al: Ocular delayed hypersensitivity: A pathogenic mechanism of chlamydial conjunctivitis in guinea pigs. Proc Natl Acad Sci USA 83:7480, 1986.
61. Morrison RP, Belland RJ, Lyng K, Caldwell HD: Chlamydial disease pathogenesis. The 57-kD chlamydial hypersensitivity antigen is a stress response protein. J Exp Med 170:1271, 1989.
62. Wagar EA, Schachter J, Bavoil P, Stephens RS: Differential human serologic response to two 60,000 molecular weight *Chlamydia trachomatis* antigens. J Infect Dis 162:922, 1990.
63. Toye B, Laferriere C, Claman P, et al: Association between antibody to the chlamydial heat-shock protein and tubal infertility. J Infect Dis 168:1236, 1993.
64. Schachter J: Chlamydiae. *In* Rose NR, Conway de Macario E, Fahey JL, et al (eds): Manual of Clinical Laboratory Immunology, ed 4. Washington, DC, American Society for Microbiology, 1992, pp 661–666.
65. Brade L, Nurminen M, Makela PH, et al: Antigenic properties of *Chlamydia trachomatis* lipopolysaccharides. Infect Immun 48:569, 1985.
66. Nurminen M, Wahlstrom E, Kleemola M, et al: Immunologically related ketodeoxyoctonate-containing structures in *Chlamydia trachomatis*, Re mutants of *Salmonella* species, and *Acinetobacter calcoaceticus* var. *antitratus*. Infect Immun 44:609, 1984.
67. Hatch TP, Miceli M, Sublett JE: Synthesis of disulfide-bonded outer membrane proteins during the developmental cycle of *Chlamydia psittaci* and *Chlamydia trachomatis*. J Bacteriol 165:379, 1986.
68. Newhall WJ, Batteiger B, Jones RB: Analysis of the human serological response to protein of *Chlamydia trachomatis*. Infect Immun 38:1181, 1982.
69. Zhang X-Y, Watkins NG, Stewart S, Caldwell HD: The low-molecular-mass, cystein-rich outer membrane protein of *Chlamydia trachomatis* possesses both biovar- and species-specific epitopes. Infect Immun 55:2570, 1987.
70. Zhang X-Y, Stewart S, Joseph T, et al: Protective monoclonal antibodies recognize epitopes located on the outer membrane protein of *Chlamydia trachomatis*. J Immunol 138:575, 1987.
71. Byrne GI, Faubion CL: Lymphokine-mediated microblastic mechanisms restrict *Chlamydia psittaci* growth in macrophages. J Immunol 128:469, 1982.
72. Czarniecki CW, Peterson EM, de la Maza LM: Interferon-induced inhibition of *Chlamydia trachomatis*: Dissociation from other biological activities of interferons. *In* Friedman RM, Merigan T, Sreevaksan T (eds): Interferons as Cell Growth Inhibitors and Antitumor Factors. New York, Alan R Liss, 1986, pp 467–480.
73. Rothermel CD, Rubin BY, Murray HW: Gamma interferon is the factor in lymphokine that activates human macrophages to inhibit intracellular *Chlamydia psittaci* replication. J Immunol 131:2542, 1983.
74. Byrne GI, Kreuger DA: Lymphokine-mediated inhibition of *Chlamydia* replication in mouse fibroblasts is neutralized by anti–gamma interferon immunoglobulin. Infect Immun 42:1152, 1983.
75. Shemer Y, Sarov I: Inhibition of growth of *Chlamydia trachomatis* by human gamma interferon. Infect Immun 48:592, 1985.
76. Byrne GI, Lehmann LK, Landry GJ: Introduction of tryptophan catabolism is the mechanism for gamma-interferon–mediated inhibition of intracellular *Chlamydia psittaci* replication. Infect Immun 53:347, 1986.
77. Berger RE, Alexander ER, Monda GE, et al: *Chlamydia trachomatis* as a cause of acute "idiopathic" epididymitis. N Engl J Med 298:301, 1978.
78. Quinn TC, Goodell SE, Mkrtichian E, et al: *Chlamydia trachomatis* proctitis. N Engl J Med 305:195, 1981.
79. Westrom L, Joesoef R, Reynolds G, et al: Pelvic inflammatory disease and fertility. A cohort study of 1,844 women with laparoscopically verified diseases and 657 control women with normal laparoscopic results. Sex Transm Dis 19:185, 1992.
80. Schachter J, Grossman M, Sweet RL, et al: Prospective study of perinatal transmission of *Chlamydia trachomatis*. JAMA 255:3374, 1986.
81. Johnson FWA, Matheson BA, Williams H, et al: Abortion due to infection with *Chlamydia psittaci* in a sheep farmer's wife. Br Med J 290:592, 1985.
82. Dawson CR, Jones BR, Garizzo ML: Guide to Trachoma Control. Geneva, World Health Organization, 1981.
83. Schachter J: Chlamydiae. *In* Balows A, Hausler WJ Jr, Hermann KL, et al (eds): Manual of Clinical Microbiology, ed 5. Washington, DC, American Society for Microbiology, 1991, pp 1045–1053.
84. Treharne JD, Dwyer R, Darougar S, et al: Antichlamydial antibody in tears and sera, and serotypes of *Chlamydia trachomatis* isolated from school children in southern Tunisia. Br J Ophthalmol 62:509, 1978.
85. Schachter J: Immunodiagnosis of sexually transmitted disease. Yale J Biol Med 58:443, 1985.
86. Tam MR, Stamm WE, Handsfield HH, et al: Culture-independent diagnosis of *Chlamydia trachomatis* using monoclonal antibodies. N Engl J Med 310:1146, 1984.
87. Howard LV, Coleman PF, England BJ, et al: Evaluation of chla-

mydiazyme for the detection of genital infections caused by *Chlamydia trachomatis*. J Clin Microbiol 23:329, 1986.
88. Bobo L, Coutlee F, Yolken RH, et al: Diagnosis of *Chlamydia trachomatis* cervical infection by amplified DNA with an enzyme immunoassay. J Clin Microbiol 28:1968, 1990.
89. Schachter J, Stamm WE, Quinn TC, et al: Ligase chain reaction to detect *Chlamydia trachomatis* infection of the cervix. J Clin Microbiol 32:2540, 1994.
90. Schachter J, Grossman M, Azimi PH: Serology of *Chlamydia trachomatis* in infants. J Infect Dis 146:530, 1982.
91. Cles LD, Stamm WE: Use of HL cells for improved isolation and passage of *Chlamydia pneumoniae*. J Clin Microbiol 28:938, 1990.
92. Centers for Disease Control and Prevention: 1993 sexually transmitted diseases treatment guidelines. MMWR Morbid Mortal Wkly Rep 42(RR-14):1, 1993.
93. Martin D, Mroczkowski T, Dalu AZ, et al: A controlled trial of a single dose of azithromycin for the treatment of chlamydial urethritis and cervicitis. N Engl J Med 327:921, 1992.
94. Mourad A, Sweet RL, Sugg N, Schachter J: Relative resistance to erythromycin in *Chlamydia trachomatis*. Antimicrob Agents Chemother 18:696, 1980.
95. Schachter J: Rifampin in *Chlamydia* infections. Rev Infect Dis 5:S562, 1983.
96. Bailey RL, Arullendran P, Whittle HC, Mabey DC: Randomised controlled trial of single-dose azithromycin intreatment of trachoma. Lancet 342:453, 1993.
97. Philip RN, Casper EA, Gordon FB, Quan AL: Fluorescent antibody responses to chlamydial infection in patients with lymphogranuloma venereum and urethritis. J Immunol 112:2126, 1974.
98. Schachter J, Sweet RL, Grossman M, et al: Experience with the routine use of erythromycin for chlamydial infections in pregnancy. N Engl J Med 314:276, 1986.

233

Mycoplasmas and Ureaplasmas

Marinella Cardello Cummings
William M. McCormack

History

Mycoplasmal species were first encountered in diseases of animals. By the end of the 19th century, the first known member of the group had been identified as the etiologic agent of contagious bovine pleuropneumonia, an important disease of cattle. This agent, now called *Mycoplasma mycoides*, was cultivated by Nocard and Roux in 1898 on serum-enriched, cell-free medium.[1] Similar organisms subsequently isolated from various species were called pleuropneumonia-like organisms, or PPLO. In 1937, Dienes and Edsall were first to report the isolation from a human of a mycoplasma (most likely *Mycoplasma hominis*), in a Bartholin gland abscess.[2]

Twelve mycoplasmal species—*Mycoplasma buccale, Mycoplasma faucium, Mycoplasma fermentans, Mycoplasma genitalium, Mycoplasma hominis, Mycoplasma lipophilum, Mycoplasma pneumoniae, Mycoplasma orale, Mycoplasma salivarium, Ureaplasma urealyticum, Mycoplasma primatum,* and *Acholeplasma laidlawii*—have been isolated from human sources, mainly from the mucous membranes of the urogenital and upper respiratory tracts. Four of the human mycoplasmal species, *M. pneumoniae, M. hominis, M. genitalium,* and *U. urealyticum,* have been shown to be pathogenic and will be dealt with in detail. Three mycoplasmal species have been recovered from patients with human immunodeficiency virus (HIV) infection, although their role in the pathogenesis of HIV and HIV-associated conditions is speculative. *M. fermentans* has been isolated from the blood[3] and urine[4] of HIV-infected persons and has been identified in renal tissue of patients who have acquired immunodeficiency syndrome–associated nephropathy.[5] Antibodies to *Mycoplasma penetrans* were found in about one third of homosexual men who had HIV infection and in almost 60% of HIV-infected homosexual men who had Kaposi's sarcoma.[6] Table 233–1 lists the human mycoplasmas, indicates their usual habitats, and lists prominent features of each species.[1,7]

Characteristics of the Pathogen

Mycoplasmas are small pleomorphic organisms, 0.3 to 0.8 μm in diameter, that lack a cell wall. They are bounded only by a plasma membrane. They belong to the class Mollicutes, order Mycoplasmatales, family Mycoplasmataceae. *Mycoplasma* and *Ureaplasma* species of the family Mycoplasmataceae infect only animals. Mycoplasmataceae require sterols for growth and differ widely in their metabolic activities. Some degrade glucose by the glycolytic pathway; some convert arginine to citrulline or ornithine by the arginine dihydrolase pathway. The ability of the genus *Ureaplasma* to hydrolyze urea sets it apart from the genus *Mycoplasma*.[7]

Mycoplasmas differ from viruses in that they contain both RNA and DNA. They resemble chlamydiae, rickettsiae, and viruses in filterability through a 45-μm filter, but they differ in being able to grow on cell-free media. Although cell wall–deficient bacterial variants (L forms, spheroplasts, protoplasts) form colonies that resemble those of mycoplasmas and although they share some other properties with the mycoplasmas, the two are unrelated. The filterability of mycoplasmas is the result not only of their small size but also of the flexibility of their plasma membrane.[1]

On solid medium, most mycoplasmas form small colonies, 50 to 600 μm in diameter, which can be seen only with a hand lens or under low power of a microscope. The classic fried egg appearance of the usual colony is due to an opaque granular central zone of growth down into the agar and a flat translucent peripheral zone of growth on the surface. Not all mycoplasmas produce fried egg colonies, and variations in colonial morphology are frequently dependent on the constituents of the medium as well as on atmosphere and inoculum size.[7] Ureaplasmas were originally called tiny, or T, strains because they form small (15 to 30 μm) colonies that lack a peripheral area of surface growth.[1]

By reason of their limited biosynthetic abilities, these organisms are highly fastidious and require complex enriched culture media for growth. Media ordinarily contain a peptone, a cholesterol, or a related sterol supplied by animal serum; preformed nucleic acid precursors supplied by yeast extract; and a metabolite, such as glucose, arginine, or urea.[8] The optimal temperature for growth of all mycoplasmal and ureaplasmal species is 37°C. Most mycoplasmas are facultatively anaerobic, but the growth of some is enhanced by incubation in air with 5% carbon dioxide.[2]

Mycoplasmataceae are the simplest and smallest self-replicating prokaryotes. The 500 MDa (700 kilobase pairs) genome characterizing *Mycoplasma* and *Ureaplasma* and its extremely low guanine plus cytosine content impose considerable restrictions on coding capacity, explaining the small number of cell proteins produced, the scarcity of metabolic pathways,

TABLE 233–1 ■ Properties of Human Mycoplasmas and Ureaplasmas

	SUBSTRATES METABOLIZED				
SPECIES	Glucose	Arginine	Urea	USUAL HABITAT	DISEASE ASSOCIATION
Ureaplasma urealyticum	−	−	+	Genital tract	Nongonococcal urethritis Infertility and reproductive failure
Mycoplasma hominis	−	+	−	Genital tract	Pelvic inflammatory disease Postpartum fever
Mycoplasma genitalium	+	−	−	Genital tract	Nongonococcal urethritis
Mycoplasma fermentans	+	+	−	Genital tract	None
Mycoplasma pneumoniae	+	−	−	Respiratory tract	Upper respiratory and lower respiratory infections
Mycoplasma salivarium	−	+	−	Oropharynx	None
Mycoplasma orale	−	+	−	Oropharynx	None
Mycoplasma buccale	−	+	−	Oropharynx	None
Mycoplasma faucium	−	+	−	Oropharynx	None
Mycoplasma lipophilum	−	+	−	Oropharynx	None
Mycoplasma primatum	−	+	−	Genital tract (rare)	None
Acholeplasma laidlawii	+	−	−	Respiratory tract (rare)	None
Mycoplasma pirum	+	+	−	Unknown	Possibly human immunodeficiency virus (HIV) associated
Mycoplasma penetrans	+	+	−	Unknown	Possibly HIV associated

Adapted from Chanock RM, Tully JG: Mycoplasmas. *In* Davis BD, et al (eds): Microbiology, ed 3. New York, Harper & Row, 1980, pp 785–795; and Velleca WM, Bird BR: Laboratory Diagnosis of Mycoplasma Infections. Course 8226-C. Washington, DC, US Department of Health and Human Services, Public Health Science Center for Disease Control, October 1980.

and the complex nutritional requirements.[7] Like other prokaryotes, these organisms divide by binary fission, but cytoplasmic division and genomic replication are not precisely synchronized and are easily dissociated.[7]

Mycoplasmas and ureaplasmas have a circular genome of double-stranded DNA, one fifth to one half as large as that of most bacteria. They generally grow more slowly than bacteria, with a mean generation time of 1 to 3 hours.[1]

Classification of mycoplasmas is based primarily on serologic reactions. Tests that detect membrane antigens, such as growth inhibition, metabolism inhibition, and immunofluorescence, are specific enough to detect serologic differences within species.[10] In the growth inhibition test, growth of the organism on agar is inhibited in a zone around a filter paper disk impregnated with specific antiserum. The metabolism inhibition test is unique to mycoplasmas and is based on the premise that inhibition of the growth of the organism by specific antibody is reflected by the failure of the organism to produce normal metabolic end products.[1] The advantage of this test is that only a few organisms are required. However, the organisms must be living, and the end points change over time. The test apparently detects all immunoglobulin classes, but most of the activity is usually in the immunoglobulin fraction. The direct identification of mycoplasmal colonies on agar by immunofluorescence is rapid and specific and has the further advantage of detecting a mixture of mycoplasmas of different serotypes in the same culture.

Immunoassays have been used to detect antigens of various mycoplasmal species.[11] Diagnosis is relatively inexpensive, and results are obtained quickly. These tests, however, are not sensitive enough to replace culture; like the use of DNA/RNA probes, which hold promise, they are not commercially available.

Epidemiology

An unusual feature of infection with *M. pneumoniae* is its peak incidence in children 5 to 15 years of age. The organism accounts for 15% to 50% of all pneumonias in this age group. Infections occur throughout the year, with a predilection for late summer and early fall. Intensive exposure to infected persons appears to be required for transmission of *M. pneumoniae.* The organism is usually introduced into a household by a school-age child. Spread of the organism from person to person is quite slow and generally not achieved through casual contact. The incubation period is 2 to 3 weeks.[1]

The genital mycoplasmas, *M. hominis* and *U. urealyticum,* are common inhabitants of the genitourinary mucous membranes of humans. Infants presumably become colonized with genital mycoplasmas during passage through the birth canal. Infants delivered by cesarean section are colonized less often than those delivered vaginally.[12] Ureaplasmas have been isolated from the genitalia of up to one third of infant girls and *M. hominis* from a smaller proportion.[12] Mycoplasmas are recovered less frequently from infant boys.[13] Mycoplasmas, mainly ureaplasmas, have been isolated from the nose and throat of about 15% of infants of both sexes.[12]

Neonatal colonization tends not to persist. These organisms are seldom recovered from prepubertal boys. Five percent to 22% of prepubertal girls are colonized with *U. urealyticum* and 8% to 17% with *M. hominis.*[14] After puberty, colonization is closely associated with sexual experience.[15] With increasing sexual experience, colonization increases more rapidly in women than in men, suggesting that it is easier to transmit the organisms from men to women than from women to men. Colonization rates with both *M. hominis* and *U. urealyticum* are higher among clinic populations than among the patients of private obstetricians and gynecologists. In Boston, *M. hominis* was isolated from 53.6% and ureaplasmas from 76.3% of clinic patients at a municipal hospital, compared with 21.3% and 52.9%, respectively, of patients visiting private obstetricians and gynecologists in the same area.[16] Women who use barrier methods of contraception are less likely to be colonized than are women who use other methods or no method of contraception.[17]

Thus, these organisms can be isolated from a significant proportion of heterosexually active men and women. It is against this background that the role of *M. hominis* and *U. urealyticum* in human disease must be viewed.

Pathogenesis

Mycoplasmas are surface parasites that adhere to and colonize the mucous membranes of the host.[18] They only rarely invade tissue or the blood stream. Efficient adherence mechanisms are therefore a prerequisite for their survival and pathogenicity. Adherence must be firm enough to prevent detachment by mucous secretions or by the urinary stream. The absence of a cell wall makes possible close contact of the plasma membrane with the host cell membrane. This provides an opportunity for mycoplasmal cells to rearrange their membrane surface in response to outside stimuli and perhaps also to adapt their cell shape to the configuration of the host cell membrane. The acquisition of host cell antigens by mycoplasmas, as suggested by Wise and coworkers,[19] may help them avoid or alter the host immunologic response. On the other hand, the acquisition of mycoplasmal antigens by the host membrane may trigger autoimmune reactions, which are common in some mycoplasmal infections.[20]

M. pneumoniae can attach to the surface of the respiratory epithelium, binding to neuraminic acid receptors. The organism does not enter host cells, nor does it penetrate beneath the epithelial surface. In tracheal organ cultures its attachment leads to direct damage to the epithelium, with loss of cilia and finally cell death. This cell damage may be produced by hydrogen peroxide released by the organism. Children 2 to 5 years of age often possess mycoplasmacidal antibodies, and although the disease appears most often at age 5 to 15 years, it has been suggested that the pathogenic effects of *M. pneumoniae* may include an immunopathologic reaction in a host sensitized by prior subclinical infection.[1]

Clinical Manifestations

In humans, *M. pneumoniae* causes mild upper respiratory disease more often than it does pneumonia. The organism can cause bronchitis, laryngitis, pharyngitis, or otitis media. The onset of pneumonia is generally gradual, and the symptoms may be mild or moderately severe. Involvement is usually interstitial or bronchopneumonic, often limited to one of the lower lobes. The course of the pneumonia is variable, with remittent fever, cough, and headache lasting for several weeks. Convalescence may extend for 4 to 6 weeks even in the absence of complications.[1]

M. hominis and *U. urealyticum* are both commonly isolated from women who have bacterial vaginosis; these organisms appear to be part of the abnormal polymicrobial flora of this condition.[21] *M. hominis* and, less often, *U. urealyticum* have been isolated from upper genital tract specimens from some patients with pelvic inflammatory disease and are probably important pathogens in some women who have this condition. It is clear, however, that most cases of pelvic inflammatory disease are caused by *Chlamydia trachomatis* and *Neisseria gonorrhoeae*.[22]

M. hominis has been shown to cause fever after abortion and postpartum endometritis.[23] *M. hominis* may act as an opportunist, causing infections outside the genitourinary tract such as wound, joint, and central nervous system infections.[24] *U. urealyticum* has been shown to cause some cases of nongonococcal urethritis[25] and has been associated with chorioamnionitis[26] and low birth weight.[27] Waites and coworkers[28] studied meningitis in 100 predominantly preterm infants. They found that *M. hominis* and *U. urealyticum* were the most common microorganisms isolated from the cerebrospinal fluid of these neonates. Valencia and colleagues[29] recovered *M. hominis* from 9 and *U. urealyticum* from 1 of 69 infants who were evaluated for suspected sepsis. In this study, nasopharyngeal colonization with mycoplasmas was associated with the development of chronic pulmonary disease. In contrast, Heggie and colleagues[30] recovered ureaplasmas from two and *M. hominis* from none of the cerebrospinal fluid samples from 920 infants. These workers did not find any relation between the isolation of mycoplasmas from tracheal aspirates and the subsequent development of respiratory disease.

M. genitalium probably plays a role in human genital tract infections.[31] Hooton and associates[32] used a DNA probe to determine the prevalence of urethral infection with *M. genitalium*. It was found most frequently (27%) in men with persistent or recurrent nongonococcal urethritis, suggesting that it may account for some of these infections. The organism was isolated more frequently from homosexual and bisexual men than from heterosexual men. Taylor-Robinson and colleagues,[33] with the use of polymerase chain reaction, detected *M. genitalium* in the urethra of about 20% of men who had either acute or chronic nongonococcal urethritis. Further studies are necessary to fully establish the role that *M. genitalium* plays in human urethritis.

M. genitalium has also been implicated in pelvic inflammatory disease. Thirty-eight percent of women with pelvic inflammatory disease had no antibody to *M. hominis* or *C. trachomatis* but had a fourfold or greater increase in *M. genitalium* antibody titer.[34]

Both *M. hominis* and *U. urealyticum* have been shown to have multiple serotypes.[35] Although the data are scanty, none of the work to date has suggested that any particular serotype is associated with any particular disease process.[36]

Diagnosis

Tracheal aspirates, nasopharyngeal swabs, throat swabs, or a sputum specimen should be obtained for *M. pneumoniae* culture.[7] *M. hominis* and *U. urealyticum* organisms should be sought in urethral cultures from men.[11] In women, vaginal specimens are more likely to contain *M. hominis* and *U. urealyticum* than are specimens from the endocervical canal, posterior fornix, or urethra.[38] Urine culture is useful for large epidemiologic studies but is an indirect means of sampling and yields fewer isolates than do cultures obtained directly from the genital mucosa.[39]

Swabs are immersed in 2 mL of cold sterile transport medium immediately after collection. Trypticase soy broth (BBL, Cockeysville, Maryland) with 0.5% Bovalbumin (Gibco, Grand Island, New York) is the transport medium used for *M. pneumoniae*. Sputum samples are collected in the morning and diluted 1:10 and 1:100 in transport medium.

Transport medium used for *M. hominis* and *U. urealyticum* is prepared by combining 70 mL of PPLO broth without crystal violet, with 20 mL of horse serum, 10 mL of yeast extract, 1.0 mL of penicillin (50,000 units/mL), 1.0 mL of polymyxin B (5000 mg/mL), 0.1 mL of amphotericin (5000 μg/mL), and 0.5 mL of phenol red (0.4%). The pH is adjusted to 6.0 to 6.2 with 1 N HCl. Urine specimens are centrifuged, and the sediment is used for culture. Specimens should be kept on wet ice or at 4°C and transported to the laboratory as soon as possible. Specimens that cannot be delivered to the laboratory and inoculated within 24 hours of collection should be frozen at −70°C.

Methylene blue glucose diphasic medium and glucose agar medium are used to cultivate *M. pneumoniae*. The diphasic medium is prepared by using a mycoplasma broth base and a mycoplasma agar base, both of which are supplemented with 20% horse serum, 10% fresh yeast extract, 50% glucose, 0.4% phenol red, 1% methylene blue, 100,000 units/mL penicillin, and 10% thallium acetate. The pH of the medium is adjusted to 7.8 with sterile 1 N NaOH. Once the agar has solidified in 1-mL aliquots in 13 × 100 mm screw cap test tubes or 1 dram screw cap vials, it is overlaid with the broth.[7] Glucose agar medium is prepared by combining mycoplasma agar base with 20% horse serum, 10% fresh yeast extract, 50% glucose, 100,000 units/mL penicillin, and 10% thallium acetate. The pH is adjusted to 7.8 with sterile 1 N NaOH.[7]

A 0.3-mL aliquot of each specimen is inoculated into the diphasic medium, which is incubated at 36°C and examined daily for color change from blue to yellow. The color change usually begins along the interface of the agar and broth. A color change during the first week of incubation is usually due to a bacterial contaminant, but thereafter it is almost always caused by growth of *M. pneumoniae.* The diphasic medium must be subcultured to glucose agar as soon as the color begins to change because the organism will lose viability as the medium becomes more acidic. A 0.1-mL aliquot of the diphasic medium is inoculated onto two of more glucose agar plates.[7]

Presumptive identification of colonies of *M. pneumoniae* on agar can be accomplished using hemadsorption or beta hemolysis. *M. pneumoniae* colonies adsorb guinea pig erythrocytes, whereas other mycoplasmas do not. The red blood cells can be seen adhering to the colonies under the microscope at × 100. *M. pneumoniae* produces a β-hemolysin (peroxide) that causes complete lysis of guinea pig and sheep erythrocytes. No other mycoplasma will cause complete hemolysis of red blood cells from these species.[7]

Complement fixation is the most widely available serologic test. Serum samples obtained from patients early in their illness and 1 to 3 weeks later usually show a fourfold or greater rise in titer. The glycolipid antigen used in this test cross-reacts with a variety of microorganisms and body tissues. A more specific serologic technique is enzyme immunoassay, which allows detection of immunoglobulins G and M and uses a protein surface antigen purified from *M. pneumoniae.*[40]

Cold agglutinins are immunoglobulin M autoantibodies that agglutinate human red blood cells at 4°C. Serum cold agglutinins are positive, in titers greater than 1:32, in 33% to 76% of patients with *M. pneumoniae* pneumonia. Cold agglutinins usually appear at the end of the first week of illness and disappear in 2 to 3 months. The height of the cold agglutinin response is usually directly proportional to the severity of pulmonary involvement. Cold agglutinins may also be present in measles and other infections, but titers are unlikely to be higher than 1:32.[40]

Differences in metabolic activity provide a useful means of identification of genital mycoplasmas. The specific metabolites, arginine and urea, along with a phenol red indicator, are added to separate tubes of liquid mycoplasmal media, which are then inoculated with the organisms or clinical material to be studied. *M. hominis* organisms convert arginine to ornithine, whereas ureaplasmas utilize urea. Both these reactions are associated with a rise in pH. From tubes showing a change in color of the pH indicator, an aliquot is subcultured onto agar for definitive identification.[7]

M. hominis and *U. urealyticum* are grown in mycoplasma broth or agar supplemented with 20% horse serum, 10% fresh yeast extract, and phenol red. Penicillin, polymyxin B, and amphotericin B are added to inhibit other organisms.[41]

Ureaplasmal medium contains lincomycin, to inhibit *M. hominis,* and 0.1% urea. The pH is adjusted to 6.0. *U. urealyticum* agar is prepared with the same supplements as the broth plus manganous sulfate, cysteine HCl, and putrescine. Medium used to isolate *M. hominis* contains erythromycin, to inhibit ureaplasmas, and arginine. The pH is adjusted to 7.0.

An aliquot of the original specimen is inoculated into 1.0 mL of each specific broth. After inoculation, pH is recorded. Tubes are incubated and read for 8 days; they are discarded as negative if there is no significant pH change. Once a rise in pH is noted, an aliquot is plated onto the appropriate agar.

After the inoculum has dried, a disk containing 15 μg of erythromycin is placed on the ureaplasma agar. Similarly, a disk impregnated with specific antiserum is placed on *M. hominis* agar. Plates are incubated for a minimum of 48 hours in an anaerobic jar in an atmosphere containing 10% carbon dioxide and 90% nitrogen.

Plates are read with a microscope under low power (× 10). Colonies of *M. hominis* usually have a classic fried egg appearance. When crowded, the colonies appear smaller and have less peripheral growth. There is a zone of inhibition around the disk impregnated with specific antiserum. There are two colony types of *U. urealyticum:* small, even colonies looking like bits of dust; and large, uneven, textured colonies with dark black centers and little peripheral growth. The addition of manganous sulfate to ureaplasma agar causes the colonies to appear quite dark, golden brown to chestnut, with a well-defined periphery.[42]

M. hominis will produce nonhemolytic pinpoint colonies on blood agar, but the organisms cannot be visualized in Gram-stained smears of these colonies. *M. hominis* will also grow in some routine blood culture media.[43] *Ureaplasma* and *M. genitalium* will not grow in ordinary microbiologic media.

M. genitalium has been isolated in SP4 medium.[44] *M. genitalium* is a glucose fermenter. It is more fastidious than either *M. hominis* or *U. urealyticum* and will not grow in conventional mycoplasmal media. These organisms require other supplements, such as CMRL 1066 tissue culture supplement with glutamine, yeastolate, and fetal bovine serum. Modification of SP4 media with polymyxin B and amphotericin prevents contamination. SP4 media can also be used for *M. hominis.* Commercially available culture media for the genital mycoplasmas are available. Broitman and coworkers[45] found Mycotrim GU broth with either A7 or A8 agar to be more sensitive and cost-effective than the Mycotrim Triphasic flask system. The bio Merieux Mycoplasme-Lyo system has been evaluated and found to be suitable for detecting *M. hominis* and *U. urealyticum.*[46]

Treatment and Prevention

Mycoplasmas are not sensitive to inhibitors of cell wall synthesis. The organisms are not susceptible to sulfonamides and trimethoprim because they do not synthesize folic acid. Protein synthesis in mycoplasmas is prokaryotic; antibiotics that inhibit protein synthesis may be effective.[47, 48] Mycoplasmas are usually sensitive to tetracyclines, aminoglycosides, and macrolides, but individual strains and species vary. Tetracyclines and erythromycins are effective in the treatment of infections caused by *M. pneumoniae.* Clinical improvement occurs even though the organisms persist.

M. hominis organisms are susceptible to clindamycin, moderately susceptible to chloramphenicol, and resistant to erythromycin, rifampin, and azithromycin.[49] Aminoglyclosides have limited activity.[50] Tetracycline is the antibiotic that is most frequently used to treat infections caused by *M. homonis;* however, with the emergence of tetracycline-resistant *M. hominis* strains,[50, 51] other agents, such as clindamycin, should be considered.

It appears that *C. trachomatis, U. urealyticum,* and possibly *M. genitalium* are causes of nongonococcal urethritis; treatment with tetracycline or doxycycline is usually effective.

However, 10% of *U. urealyticum* strains are resistant to tetracycline.[51–53] Of the quinolones, ofloxacin shows the most activity against *U. urealyticum*.[54] Patients who have nongonococcal urethritis and show no response to tetracycline should be tested, if possible, for *U. urealyticum* and treated with erythromycin or a quinolone.[55]

There are no immunizing preparations available for the genital mycoplasmas. Use of barrier methods of contraception retards colonization with mycoplasmas,[17] but because the organisms are so widespread, a significant number of sexually experienced adults will eventually become colonized.

References

1. Chanock RM, Tully JG: Mycoplasmas. *In* Davis BD, et al (eds): Microbiology, ed 3. New York, Harper & Row, 1980, pp 785–795.
2. Dienes L, Edsall G: Observations on the L-organism of Klieneberger. Proc Soc Exp Biol Med 36:740, 1937.
3. Montagnier L, Blanchard A: Mycoplasmas as cofactors in infection due to the human immunodeficiency virus [Review]. Clin Infect Dis 17(Suppl 1):S309, 1993.
4. Chirgwin KD, Cummings MC, DeMeo LR, et al: Identification of mycoplasmas in urine from persons infected with human immunodeficiency virus. Clin Infect Dis 17(Suppl 1):S264, 1993.
5. Bauer FA, Wear DJ, Angritt P, Lo SC: *Mycoplasma fermentans* (incognitus strain) infection in the kidneys of patients with acquired immunodeficiency syndrome and associated nephropathy: A light microscopic, immunohistochemical, and ultrastructural study. Hum Pathol 22:63, 1991.
6. Wang RY-H, Shih JW-K, Weiss SH, et al: *Mycoplasma penetrans* infection in male homosexuals with AIDS: High seroprevalence and association with Kaposi's sarcoma. Clin Infect Dis 17:724, 1993.
7. Valleca WM, Bird BR: Laboratory Diagnosis of Mycoplasma Infections. Course 8226-C Washington, DC, US Department of Health and Human Services, Public Health Service Center for Disease Control, October 1980.
8. Kenny GE: Mycoplasmas. *In* Lennette EH, Balows A, Hausler WJ, Shadomy HJ (eds): Manual of Clinical Microbiology, ed 4. Washington DC, American Society for Microbiology, 1985, pp 407–411.
9. Razin S: Molecular biology and genetics of mycoplasmas (molecules). Microbiol Rev 49:419, 1985.
10. Miettinen A: *Mycoplasma hominis* infections in the female genital tract. Ser A, Vol 222. Tampere, Finland, University of Tampere, 1987.
11. Kotani H, Huang K-J, McGarrity GJ: New method of identification and serodiagnosis for genital mycoplasmas by immunobinding assays. Pediatr Infect Dis 5 (Suppl):S349, 1986.
12. Klein JO, Buckland D, Finland M: Colonization of newborn infants by mycoplasmas. N Engl J Med 280:1025, 1969.
13. Foy HM, Kenny GE, Levinsohn EM, Grayston JT: Acquisition of mycoplasmata and T-strains during infancy. J Infect Dis 121:579, 1970.
14. Hammerschlag MR, Alpert S, Rosner I, et al: Microbiology of the vagina in children: Normal and potentially pathogenic organisms. Pediatrics 62:57, 1978.
15. McCormack WM, Almeida PC, Bailey PE, et al: Sexual activity and vaginal colonization with genital mycoplasmas. JAMA 221:1375, 1972.
16. McCormack WM, Rosner B, Lee Y: Colonization with genital mycoplasmas in women. Am J Epidemiol 97:240, 1973.
17. McCormack WM, Rosner B, Alpert S, et al: Vaginal colonization with *Mycoplasma hominis* and *Ureaplasma urealyticum*. Sex Transm Dis 13:67, 1986.
18. Razin S: Mycoplasma adherence. *In* Razin S, Barile MF (eds): The Mycoplasmas, Vol IV. New York, Academic Press, 1985, pp 161–202.
19. Wise KS, Cassell GH, Acton RT: Selective association of murine T lymphoblastoid cell surface alloantigens with Mycoplasma hyorhinis. Proc Natl Acad Sci USA 75:4479, 1978.
20. Fernald GW: Immunologic interactions between host cells and mycoplasmas: An introduction. Rev Infect Dis 4(Suppl):201, 1982.
21. Gravett MG, Eschenbach DA: Possible role of *Ureaplasma urealyticum* in preterm premature rupture of the fetal membrane. Pediatr Infect Dis 5(Suppl):S253, 1986.
22. Moller BR: The role of mycoplasmas in the upper genital tract of women. Sex Transm Dis 10(Suppl):281, 1983.
23. Plummer DC, Garland SM, Gilbert GL: Bacteremia and pelvic infection in women due to *Ureaplasma urealyticum* and *Mycoplasma hominis*. Med J Aust 146:135, 1987.
24. Madoff S, Hooper DC: Nongenitourinary infections caused by *Mycoplasma hominis* in adults. Rev Infect Dis 10:602, 1988.
25. Brunner H, Wolfgang W, Hans-Gerd S: Quantitative studies on the role of *Ureaplasma urealyticum* in non-gonococcal urethritis and chronic prostatitis. Yale J Med Biol 56:545, 1983.
26. Hillier SL, Krohn MJ, Kiviat N, et al: The association of *Ureaplasma urealyticum* with preterm birth, chorioamnionitis, post partum fever, intrapartum fever and bacterial vaginosis. Pediatr Infect Dis 5 (Suppl):S349, 1986.
27. Braun P, Lee YH, Klein JO, et al: Birth weight and genital mycoplasmas in pregnancy. N Engl J Med 284:167, 1971.
28. Waites KB, Crouse DT, Nelson KG, et al: Chronic *Ureaplasma urealyticum* and *Mycoplasma hominis* infections of central nervous system in preterm infants. Lancet 1:17, 1988.
29. Valencia GB, Banzon F, Cummings M, et al: *Mycoplasma hominis* and *Ureaplasma urealyticum* in neonates with suspected infection. Pediatr Infect Dis J 12:571, 1993.
30. Heggie AD, Jacobs MR, Butler VT, et al: Frequency and significance of isolation of *Ureaplasma urealyticum* and *Mycoplasma hominis* from cerebrospinal fluid and tracheal aspirate specimens from low birth weight infants. J Pediatr 124:956, 1994.
31. Tully JG, Taylor-Robinson D, Rose DL, et al: Urogenital challenge of primate species with *M. genitalium* and characteristic of infection induced in chimpanzees. J Infect Dis 153:1046, 1986.
32. Hooton TM, Roberts PL, Stamm WE, et al: Prevalence of *Mycoplasma genitalium* determined by DNA probe in men with urethritis. Lancet 1:266, 1988.
33. Taylor-Robinson D, Gilroy CB, Hay PE: Occurrence of *Mycoplasma hominis* in different populations and its clinical significance. Clin Infect Dis 17(Suppl 1):S66, 1993.
34. Moller BR, Taylor-Robinson D, Furr PM: Serological evidence implicating *Mycoplasma genitalium* in PID. Lancet 1:1102, 1984.
35. Lin J-S, Kass EH: Serological reactions of *Mycoplasma hominis:* Differences among mycoplasmacidal, metabolic inhibition, and growth agglutination tests. Infect Immun 10:535, 1974.
36. Lin JS: Human mycoplasmal infections: Serologic observations. Rev Infect Dis 7:216, 1985.
37. Tarr PI, Lee Y-H, Alpert S, et al: Comparison of methods for the isolation of genital mycoplasmas from men. J Infect Dis 133:419, 1976.
38. McCormack WM, Rankin JS, Lee YH: Localization of genital mycoplasmas in women. Am J Obstet Gynecol 112:920, 1972.
39. Taylor-Robinson D, McCormack WM: Mycoplasmas in human genitourinary infections. *In* Tully JG, Whitcomb RF (eds): The Mycoplasmas, Vol 2. New York, Academic Press, 1979, pp 307–366.
40. Broughton RA: Infections due to *Mycoplasma pneumoniae* in childhood. Pediatr Infect Dis 5:71, 1986.
41. Freundt EA: Culture media for classical mycoplasmas. *In* Tully JG, Razin S (eds): Methods in Mycoplasmology, Section C7, Vol 1. New York, Academic Press, 1983.
42. Razin S: Urea hydrolysis. *In* Tully JG, Razin S (eds). Methods in Mycoplasmology, Section E4, Vol 1. New York, Academic Press, 1983.
43. Wallace RJ, Alpert S, Browne K, et al: Isolation of *Mycoplasma hominis* from blood cultures in patients with post partum fever. Obstet Gynecol 51:181, 1978.
44. Tully JG, Cole RM, Taylor-Robinson D, Rose DL: A newly discovered mycoplasma in the human urogenital tract. Lancet 1:1288, 1981.
45. Broitman NL, Floyd CM, Johnson CA, et al: Comparison of commercially available media for detection and isolation of *Ureaplasma urealyticum* and *Mycoplasma hominis*. J Clin Microbiol 30:1335, 1992.
46. Sillis M: Genital mycoplasmas revisited—An evaluation of a new culture medium. Br J Biomed Sci 50:89, 1993.
47. Stanbridge EJ, Reff ME: The molecular biology of mycoplasmas. *In* Barile MF, Razin S (eds): The Mycoplasmas, Vol 1, Cell Biology. New York, Academic Press, 1979, pp 157–185.
48. McCormack WM: Susceptibility of mycoplasmas to antimicrobial

agents: Clinical implications. Clin Infect Dis 17(Suppl 1):S200, 1993.
49. Rumpianesi F, Morandotti G, Sperning R, et al: In vitro activity of azithromycin against *Chlamydia trachomatis, Ureaplasma urealyticum* and *Mycoplasma hominis* in comparison with erythromycin, roxithromycin and minocycline. J Chemother 5:155, 1993.
50. Koutsky LA, Stamm WE, Brunham RC, et al: Persistence of *Mycoplasma hominis* after therapy: Importance of tetracycline resistance and co-existing vaginal flora. Sex Transm Dis 10:374, 1983.
51. Cummings MC, McCormack WM: Increase in resistance of *Mycoplasma hominis* to tetracyclines. Antimicrob Agents Chemother 34:2297, 1990.
52. Evans RT, Taylor-Robinson D: The incidence of tetracycline resistant strains of *Ureaplasma urealyticum.* J Antimicrob Chemother 4:57, 1978.
53. Taylor-Robinson D, Furr PM: Clinical antibiotic resistance of *Ureaplasma urealyticum.* Pediatr Infect Dis 5(Suppl): S335, 1986.
54. Aznar J, Caballero MC, Lozano MC, et al: Activities of new quinolone derivatives against genital pathogens. Antimicrob Agents Chemother 27:76, 1985.
55. Glatt AE, McCormack WM, Taylor-Robinson D: Genital mycoplasmas. *In* Holmes KK, Mardh P-A, Sparling PF, Wiesner PJ (eds): Sexually Transmitted Diseases. New York, McGraw-Hill, 1990, pp 279–293.

RICKETTSIA

234

Rickettsia rickettsii (Rocky Mountain Spotted Fever)

J. Stephen Dumler

History

The pioneering work of Howard Taylor Ricketts in his study of the "spotted fever" in the Bitterroot Valley of Montana in the early 1900s still stands as a model for scientific investigation of infectious diseases.[1] The illness apparently existed for many years before Ricketts arrived to investigate the problem that was impeding agricultural development in that region. The causative agent was identified by Ricketts, who further showed that the disease could be transmitted by the wood tick, *Dermacentor andersoni.* S. Burt Wolbach, the renowned Harvard pathologist, described the pathologic findings in great detail and provided the initial explanations of the pathophysiologic disturbances that lead to clinical rickettsial illness. Named for the geographic region in which it was first identified, Rocky Mountain spotted fever (RMSF) was shown to occur in much higher frequency in the southern and eastern parts of the United States by the 1930s. Retrospective studies now clearly show that RMSF existed and caused severe and fatal illness in the eastern United States at the same time the disease was characterized in the Rocky Mountain regions.[2] Because of Ricketts' remarkable contributions to the study of these obligate intracellular vasculotropic bacteria, and in tribute to his death while studying epidemic typhus in Mexico City, the genus and species that cause RMSF now bear his name.

Characteristics of the Pathogen

Classification

Rickettsia rickettsii is an obligate intracellular bacterium that has a life cycle partly within mammalian cells and partly within tick cells. Often considered to be less than bacteria but more than viruses, rickettsiae in fact are true bacteria that have evolved for millennia within the cytoplasmic confines of host cells such that the ability to survive in extracellular niches has been lost. Phylogenetic classification of rickettsiae that is based on nucleic acid sequence divergence in the 16S ribosomal RNA genes of *R. rickettsii* and other species previously designated as members of the *Rickettsia* genus shows that they have a phylogenetic position within the alpha subdivision of eubacterial genera.[3, 4] Other genera that are genetically close to the genus *Rickettsia* include those previously classified within the Rickettsiaceae family, such as *Bartonella* (including the former genus *Rochalimaea*). *Coxiella burnetii,* which causes Q fever, occupies a distant phylogenetic position in the gamma subdivision. Also, species known previously as veterinary pathogens, including *Ehrlichia, Cowdria, Anaplasma,* and *Neorickettsia,* are clearly close genetic relatives of members of the genus *Rickettsia.* The agent of scrub typhus, previously designated *Rickettsia tsutsugamushi,* although a close genetic relative of the genus *Rickettsia,* is divergent enough to warrant a new genus designation, *Orientia.*[5]

Structure and Function of Rickettsia rickettsii

R. rickettsii contains DNA, RNA, and ribosomes and divides by binary fission. Ultrastructural studies reveal that this species has a gram-negative–type cell wall. The organisms are small, approximately 0.3 × 1.5 μm, and stain poorly with the Gram stain and well with Giemsa and Gimenez stains. Like other gram-negative bacteria, *R. rickettsii* has an inner cell membrane separated from the inner cell wall leaflet by a periplasmic space. Attached to the outer leaflet of the cell wall are a "microcapsular layer" that may contain the spotted fever group lipopolysaccharides and an electron-lucent "slime layer" that may appear denser when it is stabilized with specific anti–*R. rickettsii* antibodies.[6]

Because of the association with the intracellular environment of a host cell, *R. rickettsii* has evolved mechanisms to obtain host cell nutrients, including an adenosine triphosphate/adenosine diphosphate translocase that shuttles host cell energy-rich phosphate molecules into the bacterium.[7] Otherwise, rickettsiae contain typical metabolic machinery that includes an intact tricarboxylic acid cycle and the appropriate enzymes to mediate the processes. Like Enterobacteriaceae, *R. rickettsii* contains a gene with an open reading frame analogous to the *firA*-ORF17-*lpxA* region of *Escherichia coli,* encoding the enzymatic machinery that mediates lipid A biosynthesis.[8]

The *Rickettsia* genus appears to have sufficient genetic similarity that at least some antigens continue to be shared by members of both the spotted fever and typhus serologic groups.[9] These genus-shared antigens appear to reside at least partly on proteins in the outer membrane of the cell wall.[10] The lipopolysaccharide antigens of the spotted fever group appear to be broadly conserved, and these antigens are the predominant basis for the serologic differentiation of the *Rickettsia* genus into the spotted fever and typhus groups.[11, 12] All spotted fever group rickettsiae contain these cross-reactive antigens that are generally identified by the indirect immunofluorescent antibody serologic test, so that differentiation among the species within this serologic group can be difficult or impossible by routine serologic testing.[12] Each species, including *R. rickettsii*, contains species-specific epitopes that can be identified by monoclonal antibodies.[10, 13]

R. rickettsii also contains several immunodominant outer membrane proteins (rOmp), including a 190-kDa rOmpA, a 120-kDa rOmpB, and a 17-kDa lipoprotein that appears to be conserved throughout the genus.[13–17] The rOmpA has a predicted molecular structure that is consistent with a surface-exposed ligand because the gene that encodes the protein has several tandem repeats,[16] a motif recognized frequently in cell-cell adherence. Monoclonal antibodies reactive with the rOmpA of the related spotted fever group *Rickettsia conorii* inhibit binding of spotted fever group rickettsiae to host cells, further supporting the role of this protein as the major rickettsial ligand for adherence to host cells.[18] Recombinant rOmpA was tested as an immunogen in mice and in guinea pigs and showed promise as a potential vaccine.[19, 20] The function of rOmpB is still not certain, but it is the major component of a paracrystalline surface array, or S layer, that may play an important role in maintenance of rickettsial structure.[21] All rickettsiae possess an rOmpB that appears to result from proteolysis of a larger precursor and yields an accessory 32-kDa β-fragment that may serve as a membrane anchor domain. However, an *R. rickettsii* rOmpB mutant appears to have diminished in vitro ability to form plaques; thus, a contribution of rOmpB toward host cell lysis is speculated.[22] Monoclonal antibodies reactive with rOmpB protect mice from lethal rickettsial challenge.[23] Data suggest that the rickettsial rOmpA and rOmpB are differentially expressed when the promoters from the encoding genes are cloned into *E. coli*. This results in 28-fold higher transcription and expression from *ompB* promoters, partly explaining the 9:1 predominance of rOmpB to rOmpA in *R. rickettsii*.[24]

Whether *R. rickettsii* contains a phospholipase has been an important question for several years. Experimental data seem to implicate the rickettsia itself as a source of phospholipase-mediated host cell membrane lysis, because phospholipase A_2 and phospholipase C antigens and activity have been localized within *R. rickettsii*.[25, 26]

Genes for many of these protein antigens and metabolic enzymes have been identified, sequenced, and cloned. Several appear to be useful markers with sufficiently unique sequences to serve as targets for molecular diagnostic methods.[27–29] Genetic manipulation by plasmid transformation, transposon mutagenesis, or other methods has not yet been successful for the genus *Rickettsia*; thus, there is limited knowledge of the molecular pathogenesis of rickettsial infection.

Pathogenesis of Spotted Fever Group Rickettsioses

Pathogenetic mechanisms in mammalian host cells directly attributable to the rickettsiae are difficult to elucidate given the intimate nature of the relationship between the infectious agent and its obligatory host cell. Like other bacteria that may be intracellular pathogens, *R. rickettsii* attaches to the surface of a eukaryotic cell and is internalized to occupy a niche within the cytoplasmic compartment.[18] The predominant host cell in vivo is the endothelial cell, although vascular smooth muscle and macrophages may on occasion be infected. In vitro, infection is easily established in a variety of cell types including endothelial cells, macrophages, and fibroblasts.

It has been proposed that after attachment of *R. rickettsii* to the surface of the endothelial cell, rickettsial phospholipases focally damage the host cell membrane.[25, 26, 30, 31] The focal injury results in endocytic internalization of the damaged host cell membrane (induced phagocytosis), taking with it the attached rickettsiae.[32] Continued phospholipase activity further degrades the endocytic vacuole to allow the rickettsiae free access to the cytoplasmic compartment of the host cell. Rickettsiae are freely mobile in the cytoplasm of the host cell by virtue of directional actin polymerization.[33] This mobility often leads to entry into the nucleus for *R. rickettsii* but not for other *Rickettsia* species, and extrusion of the agent from the infected cell into adjacent uninfected cells furthers the local infection without exposing the rickettsiae to the external milieu. Within the cytoplasm of the infected host cell, *R. rickettsii* divides by binary fission with a generation time of approximately 9 hours under optimal circumstances.

The rickettsiae greatly affect the host cell by free radical–mediated peroxidation of lipids in host cell membranes,[34] continued phospholipase activity,[25, 31] and protease activity.[31] The net result of these pathologic cellular insults is that the infected cell undergoes morphologic changes seen by light microscopy that include cell swelling, necrosis, karyorrhexis, and lysis. Ultrastructural evaluation indicates that these findings correspond to swelling of the endoplasmic reticulum, loss of the Golgi apparatus, and dissolution of cell membranes, probably leading to loss of cellular osmoregulation and cell lysis[35] (Fig. 234–1). The infectious agent may exit the cell before this or may be released as the cell finally lyses. Occasional endothelial cells in vivo may develop an appearance characteristic of apoptosis, suggesting the contribution of the host cell or host factors in the pathogenetic process. In vitro, infected endothelial cells have an up-regulated expression of (1) interleukin-1α,[36] (2) surface procoagulant activity including tissue factor[37] and release of large von Willebrand factor multimers,[38] and (3) E-selectin,[39] which may partly contribute to the recruitment of inflammatory cells leading to the pathologic lesion characteristic of the vasculotropic rickettsioses and RMSF vasculitis. These endothelial responses are apparently not related to rickettsial lipopolysaccharide or endotoxin, because the lipopolysaccharide of *R. rickettsii* has few or no endotoxic effects in vivo.[40] The occurrence of fulminant (less than 5 days) RMSF in glucose-6-phosphate dehydrogenase–deficient individuals in the absence of host inflammatory or immune responses indicates that *R. rickettsii* alone is sufficient to cause RMSF.[41]

Other host responses clearly influence the course of RMSF. Immune suppression, particularly lack of interferon-γ, results in more severe or lethal infection.[42] Animal models of spotted fever group rickettsiosis indicate that the proinflammatory cytokines interleukin-1 and tumor necrosis factor and interferon-γ and interleukin-6 appear within 5 days of intravenous inoculation and diminish as the infection becomes lethal.[43, 44] The antirickettsial protective effects of interferon-γ and tumor necrosis factor-α are synergistic and are mediated by induction of nitric oxide synthase and the resultant increases in nitric oxide in murine endothelial cells and by a process involving tryptophan limitation and hydrogen peroxide production in human endothelial cells.[43–45]

Ecology of *Rickettsia rickettsii*

The human is an accidental and dead-end host for *R. rickettsii*. In nature, *R. rickettsii* occupies at least part of its life cycle

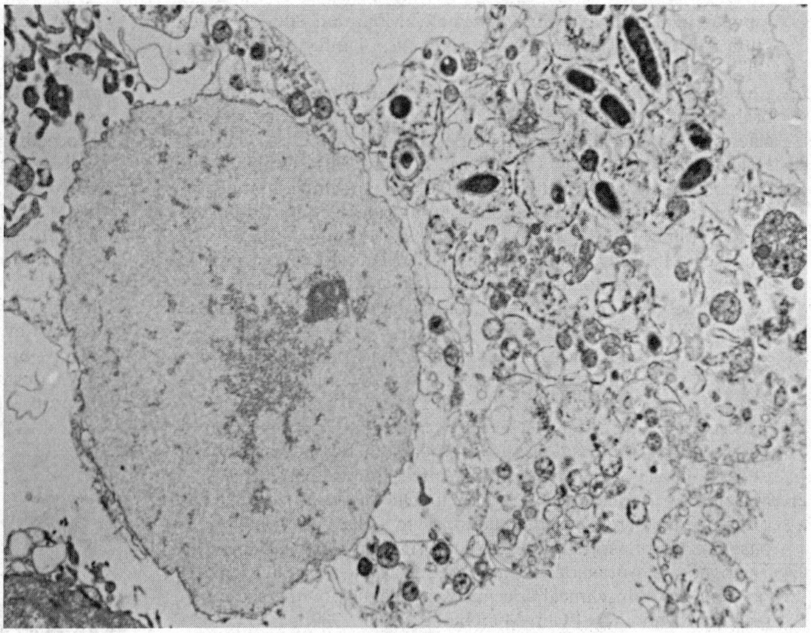

FIGURE 234–1 □ *Rickettsia rickettsii*–infected human umbilical vein endothelial cell with advanced cytopathologic changes. The rickettsiae appear in the cytoplasm as dark bacilli surrounded by a clear halo. The infected cell has lost osmoregulatory control and is near lysis. The rickettsiae may be freed from infected cells by lysis when the cell is severely injured or by propulsion with actin filament polymerization when the cell is less completely infected and damaged. Other characteristics here include nuclear condensation, which is a terminal effect of cell death. (From Silverman DJ: *Rickettsia rickettsii*–induced cellular injury of human vascular endothelium in vitro. Infect Immun 44:545–553, 1984.)

within a tick vector and part within the tissues and blood of small mammal hosts. Uninfected ticks acquire the infectious agent when a blood meal is taken from a rickettsemic animal, usually an infected small mammal.[46, 47] The rickettsiae attach to and infect the gut epithelial cells of the feeding tick and disseminate to infect most tick tissues, including salivary gland, while the tick is molting into its next life stage. Infected ticks may pass *R. rickettsii* from generation to generation (transovarial or vertical transmission) because of ovarian infection in adult female ticks; however, the infectious agent has a slightly deleterious effect by reducing the number of progeny that emerge in the next generation.[47] Thus, part of the natural maintenance of *R. rickettsii* depends on a degree of tick-mammal-tick transmission. Infected ticks transmit the rickettsiae to an uninfected mammalian host by regurgitation of salivary contents during feeding.

Because the rickettsiae require a short interval of reactivation by exposure to blood or increased temperature associated with the blood meal,[48] and a short interval is required before regurgitation of infected tick saliva, there is a "grace period" of approximately 48 hours or more during which there is a low likelihood of *R. rickettsii* transmission. After inoculation of the mammal by the bite of an infected tick, the animal may develop a period of rickettsemia, with or without overt clinical illness, that may last as long as several weeks before immunologic control of the infectious agent supervenes. During this interval, uninfected ticks feeding on the recently infected mammal may acquire the rickettsiae to renew the cycle. Transmission may occur by the bite of a tick at any life stage; however, it is predominantly the adult *Dermacentor* ticks in the United States that bite large mammals and are responsible for the occasional inadvertent transmission to humans.

References

1. Harden VA: Koch's postulates and the etiology of rickettsial diseases. J Hist Med Allied Sci 42:277, 1987.
2. Dumler JS: Fatal Rocky Mountain spotted fever in Maryland—1901. JAMA 265:718, 1991.
3. Weisburg WG, Dobson ME, Samuel JE, et al: Phylogenetic diversity of the rickettsiae. J Bacteriol 171:4202, 1989.
4. Stothard DR, Clark JB, Fuerst PA: Ancestral divergence of *Rickettsia bellii* from the spotted fever and typhus groups of *Rickettsia* and antiquity of the genus *Rickettsia*. Int J Syst Bacteriol 44:798, 1994.
5. Tamura A, Ohashi N, Urakami H, Miyamura S: Classification of *Rickettsia tsutsugamushi* in a new genus, *Orientia* gen. nov., as *Orientia tsutsugamushi* comb. nov. Int J Syst Bacteriol 45:589, 1995.
6. Silverman DJ, Wisseman CL Jr: Comparative ultrastructural study on the cell envelopes of *Rickettsia prowazekii*, *Rickettsia rickettsii*, and *Rickettsia tsutsugamushi*. Infect Immun 21:1020, 1978.
7. Winkler HH: Rickettsial permeability. An ADP-ATP transport system. J Biol Chem 251:389, 1976.
8. Shaw EI, Wood DO: Characterization of a *Rickettsia rickettsii* DNA fragment analogous to the *firA*-ORF17-*lpxA* region of *Escherichia coli*. Gene 140:109, 1994.
9. Ormsbee R, Peacock M, Philip R, et al: Antigenic relationships between the typhus and spotted fever groups of rickettsiae. Am J Epidemiol 108:53, 1978.
10. Anacker RL, Mann RE, Gonzales C: Reactivity of monoclonal antibodies to *Rickettsia rickettsii* with spotted fever and typhus group rickettsiae. J Clin Microbiol 25:167, 1987.
11. Walker DH, Gile JC, Feng H-M, et al: Diagnosis of spotted fever group rickettsioses by immunohistology with a group specific anti-lipopolysaccharide monoclonal antibody. Mod Pathol 7:128A, 1994.
12. Philip RN, Casper EA, Ormsbee RA, et al: Microimmunofluorescence test for the serological study of Rocky Mountain spotted fever and typhus. J Clin Microbiol 3:51, 1976.
13. Li H, Lenz B, Walker DH: Protective monoclonal antibodies recognize heat-labile epitopes on surface proteins of spotted fever group rickettsiae. Infect Immun 56:2587, 1988.
14. Gilmore RD Jr, Joste N, McDonald GA: Cloning, expression and sequence analysis of the gene encoding the 120 kD surface-exposed protein of *Rickettsia rickettsii*. Mol Microbiol 3:1579, 1989.
15. Gilmore RD Jr: Comparison of the *rompA* gene repeat regions of rickettsiae reveals species-specific arrangements of individual repeating units. Gene 125:97, 1993.
16. Anderson BE, McDonald GA, Jones DC, Regnery RL: A protective protein antigen of *Rickettsia rickettsii* has tandemly repeated, near-identical sequences. Infect Immun 58:2760, 1990.
17. Anderson BE, Tzianabos T: Comparative sequence analysis of a genus-common rickettsial antigen gene. J Bacteriol 171:5199, 1989.
18. Li H, Walker DH: Characterization of rickettsial attachment to host cells by flow cytometry. Infect Immun 60:2030, 1992.
19. McDonald GA, Anacker RL, Garjian K: Cloned gene of *Rickettsia rickettsii* surface antigen: Candidate vaccine for Rocky Mountain spotted fever. Science 235:83, 1987.
20. McDonald GA, Anacker RL, Mann RE, Milch LF: Protection of

guinea pigs from experimental Rocky Mountain spotted fever with a cloned antigen of *Rickettsia rickettsii*. J Infect Dis 158:228, 1988.
21. Ching W-M, Dasch GA, Carl M, Dobson ME: Structural analyses of the 120-kDa serotype protein antigens of typhus group rickettsiae. Ann N Y Acad Sci 590:334, 1990.
22. Hackstadt T, Messer R, Cieplak W, Peacock MG: Evidence for proteolytic cleavage of the 120-kilodalton outer membrane protein of rickettsiae: Identification of an avirulent mutant deficient in processing. Infect Immun 60:159, 1992.
23. Anacker RL, McDonald GA, List RH, Mann RE: Neutralizing activity of monoclonal antibodies to heat-sensitive and heat-resistant epitopes of *Rickettsia rickettsii* surface proteins. Infect Immun 55:825, 1987.
24. Policastro PF, Hackstadt T: Differential activity of *Rickettsia rickettsii ompA* and *ompB* promoter regions in a heterologous reporter gene system. Microbiology 140:2941, 1994.
25. Silverman DJ, Santucci L, Meyers N, Sekeyova Z: Penetration of host cells by *Rickettsia rickettsii* appears to be mediated by a phospholipase of rickettsial origin. Infect Immun 60:2733, 1992.
26. Manor E, Carbonetti NH, Silverman DJ: *Rickettsia rickettsii* has proteins with cross-reacting epitopes to eukaryotic phospholipase A_2 and phospholipase C. Microb Pathog 17:99, 1994.
27. Tzianabos T, Anderson BE, McDade JE: Detection of *Rickettsia rickettsii* DNA in clinical specimens by using polymerase chain reaction technology. J Clin Microbiol 27:2866, 1989.
28. Sexton DJ, Kanj SS, Wilson K, et al: The use of a polymerase chain reaction as a diagnostic test for Rocky Mountain spotted fever. Am J Trop Med Hyg 50:59, 1994.
29. Yan U, Uchiyama T, Uchida T: Nucleotide sequence of polymerase chain reaction product amplified from *Rickettsia japonica* DNA using *Rickettsia rickettsii* 190-kilodalton antigen gene primers. Microbiol Immunol 38:865, 1994.
30. Winkler HH, Miller ET: Phospholipase A and the interaction of *Rickettsia prowazekii* and mouse fibroblasts (L-929 cells). Infect Immun 38:109, 1982.
31. Walker DH, Firth WT, Ballard JG, Hegarty BC: Role of phospholipase-associated penetration mechanism in cell injury by *Rickettsia rickettsii*. Infect Immun 40:840, 1983.
32. Walker TS, Winkler HH: Penetration of cultured mouse fibroblasts (L cells) by *Rickettsia prowazekii*. Infect Immun 22:200, 1978.
33. Heinzen RA, Hayes SF, Peacock MG, Hackstadt T: Directional actin polymerization associated with spotted fever group rickettsia infection of Vero cells. Infect Immun 61:1926, 1993.
34. Silverman DJ, Santucci L: Potential for free radical–induced lipid peroxidation as a cause of endothelial cell injury in Rocky Mountain spotted fever. Infect Immun 56:3110, 1988.
35. Silverman DJ: *Rickettsia rickettsii*–induced cellular injury of human vascular endothelium in vitro. Infect Immun 44:545, 1984.
36. Sporn LA, Marder VJ: Interleukin-1α production during *Rickettsia rickettsii* infection of cultured endothelial cells: Potential role in autocrine cell stimulation. Infect Immun 64:1609, 1996.
37. Sporn LA, Haidaris PJ, Rui-Jin S, et al: *Rickettsia rickettsii* infection of cultured human endothelial cells induces tissue factor expression. Blood 83:1527, 1994.
38. Sporn LA, Rui-Jin S, Lawrence SO, et al: *Rickettsia rickettsii* infection of cultured endothelial cells induces release of large von Willebrand factor multimers from Weibel-Palade bodies. Blood 78:2595, 1991.
39. Sporn LA, Lawrence SO, Silverman DJ, Marder VJ: E-selectin–dependent neutrophil adhesion to *Rickettsia rickettsii*–infected endothelial cells. Blood 81:2406, 1993.
40. Kaplowitz LG, Lange JV, Fischer JJ, Walker DH: Correlation of rickettsial titers, circulating endotoxin, and clinical features in Rocky Mountain spotted fever. Arch Intern Med 143:1149, 1983.
41. Walker DH, Hawkins HK, Hudson P: Fulminant Rocky Mountain spotted fever. Its pathologic characteristics associated with glucose-6-phosphate dehydrogenase deficiency. Arch Pathol Lab Med 107:121, 1983.
42. Li H, Jerrells TR, Spitalny GL, Walker DH: Gamma interferon as a crucial host defense against *Rickettsia conorii* in vivo. Infect Immun 55:1252, 1987.
43. Feng H-M, Wen J, Walker DH: *Rickettsia australis* infection: A murine model of a highly invasive vasculopathic rickettsiosis. Am J Pathol 142:1471, 1993.
44. Feng H-M, Walker DH: Interferon-γ and tumor necrosis factor-α exert their antirickettsial effect via induction of synthesis of nitric oxide. Am J Pathol 143:1016, 1993.
45. Walker DH, Popov VL, Welsh JR, Feng H-M: Mechanisms of rickettsial killing within cytokine-stimulated endothelial cells. *In* Kazár J, Toman R (eds): Rickettsiae and Rickettsial Diseases, Proceedings of the Vth International Symposium. Bratislava, Slovak Republic, Slovak Academy of Sciences, Institute of Virology, 1996, pp 51–56.
46. Gage KL, Burgdorfer W, Hopla CE: Hispid cotton rats *(Sigmodon hispidus)* as a source for infecting immature *Dermacentor variabilis* (Acari: Ixodidae) with *Rickettsia rickettsii*. J Med Entomol 27:615, 1990.
47. McDade JE, Newhouse VF: Natural history of *Rickettsia rickettsii*. Annu Rev Microbiol 40:287, 1986.
48. Hayes SF, Burgdorfer W: Reactivation of *Rickettsia rickettsii* in *Dermacentor andersoni* ticks: An ultrastructural analysis. Infect Immun 37:779, 1982.

235

Rickettsia typhi and *Rickettsia prowazekii*

Joseph E. McDade
James G. Olson

Properties of *Rickettsia* Organisms

Rickettsia species are gram-negative, obligate intracellular bacteria. All species are associated with a mammalian host at some stage of their natural life cycles and are transmitted by arthropod vectors. For some species of *Rickettsia*, arthropods are both reservoirs and vectors. With the exception of epidemic typhus rickettsiae *(Rickettsia prowazekii)*, humans are not normal hosts in the life cycle of these organisms.

Rickettsiae are rod-shaped or coccobacillary microorganisms, ranging from 0.3 to 0.5 μm in diameter and from 0.8 to 2.0 μm in length. They do not possess flagella or pili (Fig. 235–1). Ultrastructurally, the outer envelope of a *Rickettsia* organism is typical of gram-negative bacteria.[1] The outer membrane contains 2-keto-3-deoxyoctonate, a marker of bacterial lipopolysaccharide.[2] Rickettsiae also contain a peptidoglycan layer that is presumed to be located between the outer leaflet of the cytoplasmic membrane and the inner leaflet of the cell wall.[1] The peptidoglycan is insoluble in sodium dodecyl sulfate, is sensitive to lysozyme, and contains glutamic acid, alanine, and diaminopimelic acid in a molar ratio of 1.0:2.3:1.0, which is characteristic of gram-negative bacteria. The peptidoglycan also contains lysine, which could provide a linkage site for lipoproteins.[3] Rickettsiae are surrounded by a polysaccharide slime layer that can be visualized by special stains.[4] The cytosol of rickettsiae contains nuclear structures, ribosomes, and other subcellular organelles typical of most bacteria. Multiplication occurs by binary fission.

Rickettsiae are capable of some independent metabolic activity, both energy producing and synthetic.[5] In addition,

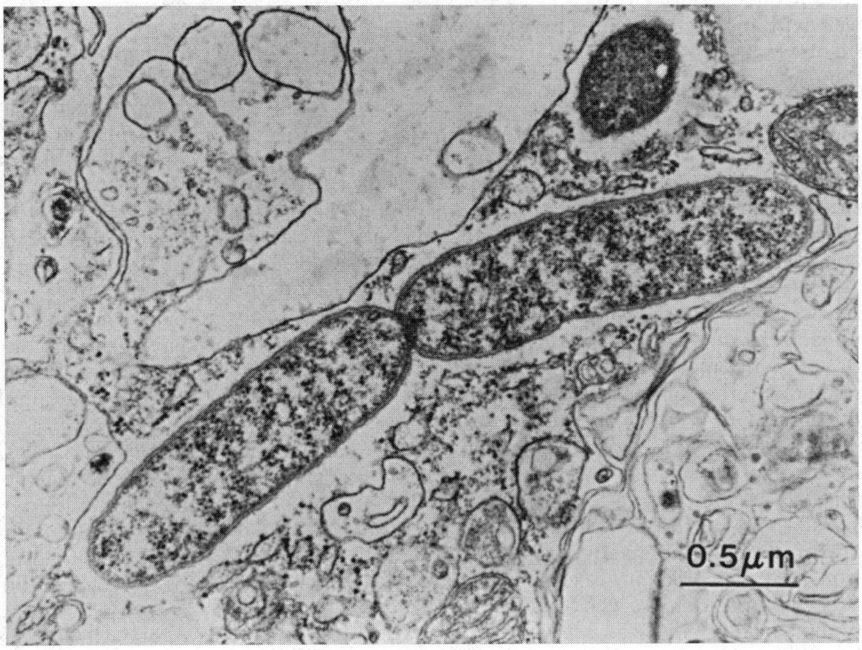

FIGURE 235–1 □ Electron photomicrograph of *Rickettsia prowazekii* cultivated on chick embryo cells. (Courtesy of Dr. David Silverman, University of Maryland School of Medicine, Baltimore, MD.)

rickettsiae possess numerous transport systems, which allow them to use metabolites present in host cells.[6] Perhaps most notable is the adenosine triphosphate/adenosine diphosphate translocase system that incorporates high-energy phosphate molecules. Rickettsiae are quite unstable outside their hosts, however, and are incapable of independent replication on synthetic or semisynthetic media.

R. prowazekii and *Rickettsia typhi* (formerly *Rickettsia mooseri*) are closely related phylogenetically and have common phenotypic characteristics.[7–10] The guanine plus cytosine content of their DNAs has been estimated at 29% to 30%[7]; interspecies DNA-to-DNA hybridization studies indicate 70% to 77% genetic relatedness.[8] The two species are virtually identical when compared by sequence analysis of DNA coding for 16S ribosomal RNA.[9] The size of the genomes of *R. typhi* and *R. prowazekii* has been estimated by pulsed-field gel electrophoresis as approximately 1100 kb.[11] Historically, *R. prowazekii* and *R. typhi* have been distinguished by their association with vectors and pathogenicity for certain experimental animals.[10] Human body lice are the vector for *R. prowazekii*, whereas fleas typically transmit *R. typhi*. Laboratory mice are susceptible to infection with *R. typhi* but generally are refractory to *R. prowazekii*. Both species share common antigens but they can be distinguished by monoclonal antibodies.[12] *R. typhi* and *R. prowazekii* also contain specific protein antigens that facilitate identification of the respective microorganisms. Purified specific antigens have also been used in the research laboratory for serodiagnosis of patients with epidemic or murine typhus, but they are not available commercially.[13, 14] Comparative properties of *R. prowazekii* and *R. typhi* are summarized in Table 235–1.

Rickettsiae can be cultivated in virtually any type of cell culture system; most species also grow extremely well in embryonated hens' eggs.[10] These organisms enter cells by induced phagocytosis and multiply within the cytosol unbounded by a phagosome.[15] As few as two microorganisms constitute a 50% infectious dose for *R. typhi* or *R. prowazekii*.[16] After a short lag phase, growth is exponential: the doubling time is approximately 9 hours.[17] Reasons for the slow growth rate are not known. *R. typhi* apparently moves freely from cell to cell in infected fleas,[18] whereas *R. prowazekii* accumulates within a single cell until it bursts.[17] Movement of rickett-

TABLE 235–1 ■ Selected Properties of Typhus *Rickettsia* Species

SPECIES	*RICKETTSIA PROWAZEKII*	*RICKETTSIA TYPHI*
Diseases	Louse-borne typhus, recrudescent typhus (Brill-Zinsser disease), flying squirrel–associated typhus fever	Murine typhus
Geographic distribution	Louse-borne typhus occurs in areas of Africa and of Central and South America where louse infestation is common. Recrudescent typhus occurs worldwide; follows the distribution of former typhus patients. Flying squirrel–associated typhus reported only in the United States, principally east of the Mississippi	Worldwide; usually follows the distribution of *Rattus* rats
Reservoirs	Humans primary; significance of flying squirrels as reservoirs not entirely clear	*Rattus* primarily; other rodents secondarily; fleas (*Xenopsylla cheopis*) also a possible reservoir
Vector	For epidemic typhus, body lice; method of transmission of flying squirrel–associated typhus fever uncertain	Asian rat flea (*Xenopsylla cheopis*) principal vector; cat flea (*Ctenocephalides felis*) also a vector
Strain variation	Strains remarkably similar, but flying squirrel isolates distinguishable from classic typhus strains by molecular techniques	No significant differences among strains

siae within host cells appears to be directed by actin filaments.[19]

Natural History of *Rickettsia typhi*

Commensal rats (*Rattus rattus* and *Rattus norvegicus*) are considered the primary reservoir of *R. typhi*, although numerous other rodents, including bandicoot rats (*Bandicota bengalensis* and *Bandicota indica*), the house mouse (*Mus musculus*), the African giant pouched rat (*Cricetomys gambianus*), and the house shrew (*Suncus murinus*), have been reported as reservoirs. Isolation of *R. typhi* has also been reported from domestic and peridomestic animals, such as cats and opossums, and numerous other animals have been infected experimentally. Infection with *R. typhi* apparently does not adversely affect mammalian reservoirs, although rodents remain rickettsemic for days to weeks and provide a source of typhus rickettsiae for ectoparasites during feeding.[18, 20]

The Asian rat flea (*Xenopsylla cheopis*) is the primary vector among *Rattus*; humans are accidental hosts in the transmission cycle (Fig. 235–2). Except as noted in the following, *X. cheopis* is considered a vector and not a reservoir of murine typhus rickettsiae. Fleas acquire *R. typhi* when feeding on infected rodent hosts. The rickettsiae multiply primarily within epithelial cells lining the midgut region of the fleas. Results of experimental infection studies indicate that *R. typhi* multiplies exponentially in *X. cheopis* during the first and second weeks after infectious feeding. Murine typhus rickettsiae are then released from infected midgut cells and accumulate in the gut lumen and in flea feces. High titers of *R. typhi* accumulate (10^5 to 10^7 plaque-forming units per flea) and persist indefinitely.[21] The growth rate in fleas is temperature dependent[22]: titers at 24°C and 30°C are two to three times higher than in fleas held at 18°C. Infection apparently is not harmful to fleas. They presumably remain infective for life (up to 1 year). Infection of humans and rodent hosts occurs by contamination of the bite site; in addition, irritation of the bite site induces scratching, allowing infection to occur via abraded skin. *X. cheopis* feeds rapidly and intermittently on hosts, facilitating transfer of *R. typhi*.[18]

During the third week after infectious feeding, *R. typhi* is also found in foregut tissue of *X. cheopis*, suggesting that *R. typhi* can be transmitted directly by flea bite. Under experimental conditions, transmission of infection occurs by bite at a rate of 20%, probably as a result of regurgitation of rickettsiae in the foregut but not via salivary secretions.[23] How frequently infection occurs by bite under natural conditions has not been determined.

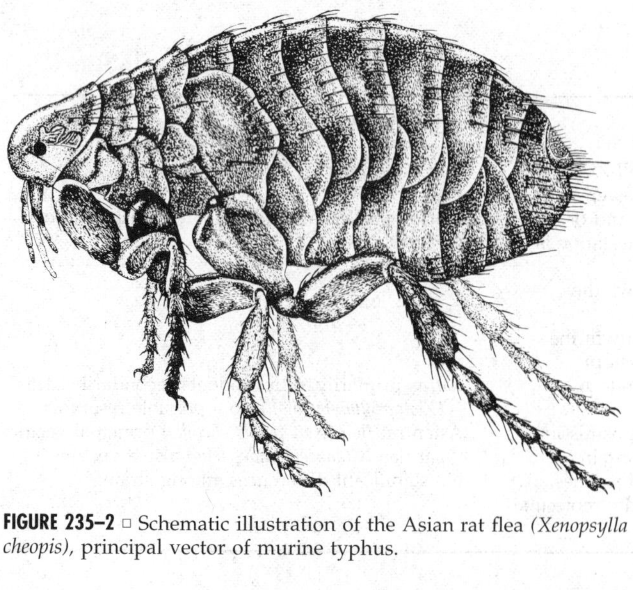

FIGURE 235–2 □ Schematic illustration of the Asian rat flea (*Xenopsylla cheopis*), principal vector of murine typhus.

Experimental infectivity studies indicate that transovarial transmission of *R. typhi* occurs at a low rate in *X. cheopis* and that fleas in the first filial generation are capable of transmitting *R. typhi* to other rodents.[24] Thus, fleas may be a secondary reservoir of *R. typhi* but with limited capability for maintaining this microorganism in nature.

Ten species of flea, three species of lice, and three species of mites have been implicated as actual or potential vectors of murine typhus.[18, 20] However, most of these ectoparasites have been discounted as vectors of murine typhus on epidemiologic grounds because they are unlikely to feed on humans. For example, comparative infectivity studies indicate that *R. typhi* accumulates to high titers in the mouse flea (*Leptopsylla segnis*)[21] and the cat flea (*Ctenocephalides felis*).[25] However, the mouse flea is presumed to be only a vector between mice as it is sessile and relatively host specific. In contrast, the high infectivity of *R. typhi* for *C. felis*, together with the broad host range of this flea, indicates that it may be a vector to humans. Cases of murine typhus have been reported in Los Angeles in association with seropositive domestic cats and peridomestic opossums, some of which were shown to be infested with cat fleas.[26, 27]

Natural History of *Rickettsia prowazekii*

R. prowazekii is the etiologic agent of epidemic typhus. It is unique among the rickettsiae in that humans are the principal reservoir. *R. prowazekii* is transmitted from person to person by infected body lice (*Pediculus humanus corporis*). Lice acquire the organism when they imbibe a blood meal from an infected person. Typhus rickettsiae infect cells lining the louse midgut, proliferate there, and progressively destroy the host cells in the process. *R. prowazekii* is then shed in louse feces. Humans become infected when contaminated feces come into contact with abraded skin.

Patients with epidemic typhus develop a nonsterile immunity after infection with *R. prowazekii*. Recrudescence of disease can occur from months to years after the primary infection, and if the ill person and contacts are infested with lice, another cycle of transmission can occur.[28] Exactly how *R. prowazekii* remains sequestered in humans is not known, although it has reportedly been isolated from the lymph nodes of former typhus patients during the course of elective surgery that was performed 20 years after their primary infection.[29] The digestive processes of lice may facilitate transmission of this organism from former typhus patients. Experimental data indicate that, in the course of digesting a blood meal, enzymes in the louse midgut modify or destroy antibody molecules and presumably render them incapable of neutralizing rickettsiae.[30] The transmission cycle of *R. prowazekii* in humans is shown in Figure 179–2.

Although humans are considered the primary reservoir, *R. prowazekii* has also been isolated from eastern flying squirrels (*Glaucomys volans volans*) captured in Florida and Virginia.[31] Numerous types of ectoparasites are known to infest flying squirrels, but lice (*Neohaematopinus sciuropteri*) and fleas (*Orchopeas howardii*) are the most likely vectors of *R. prowazekii* between animals. It has been isolated repeatedly from these ectoparasites but not from others. However, only squirrel lice become persistently infected with *R. prowazekii* under experimental conditions and transmit infection among flying squirrels.[32] Presumably, the sylvan cycle of typhus infection is maintained by lice in a manner analogous to epidemic typhus infection in humans. Serologic studies of flying squirrels indicate that most seroconversions to *R. prowazekii* occur in the autumn and early winter, when these animals are infested with the maximal number of ectoparasites. Apparently, infection persists for an indefinite period in a given focus; new infections occur each year among young, nonimmune animals.[33]

When the biologic and biochemical properties of flying squirrel isolates of *R. prowazekii* are compared with strains obtained from persons with louse-borne typhus, no significant differences are noted. Strains are 100% identical when compared by DNA-to-DNA hybridization studies.[8] In addition, the ability of different strains to form plaques on chicken embryo cell monolayers, to grow in embryonated hens' eggs, or to use glutamate as a substrate is the same. Susceptibility to erythromycin and electrophoretic properties of solubilized proteins of different isolates are also similar.[34, 35] However, isolates of *R. prowazekii* from humans and from flying squirrels can be distinguished by restriction endonuclease digestion of their respective DNAs.[36]

Human infections have been documented in the United States after known or suspected exposure to flying squirrels.[37, 38] Because patients did not report exposure to fleas, lice, or other vectors, the precise mode of transmission is uncertain. Infection is presumed to have occurred by inhalation of aerosolized feces from infected squirrel lice or fleas. The relative importance of flying squirrels in maintaining *R. prowazekii* in nature is uncertain.

References

1. Silverman DJ, Wisseman CL Jr: Comparative ultrastructural study on the cell envelopes of *Rickettsia prowazekii, Rickettsia rickettsii*, and *Rickettsia tsutsugamushi*. Infect Immun 21:1020, 1978.
2. Smith DK, Winkler HH: Separation of inner and outer membranes of *Rickettsia prowazekii* and characterization of their polypeptide composition. J Bacteriol 137:963, 1979.
3. Pang H, Winkler HH: Analysis of the peptidoglycan of *Rickettsia prowazekii*. J Bacteriol 176:923, 1994.
4. Silverman DJ, Wisseman CL Jr, Waddell AD, et al: External layers of *Rickettsia prowazekii* and *Rickettsia rickettsii*: Occurrence of a slime layer. Infect Immun 22:233, 1978.
5. Wisseman CL Jr: Some biologic properties of rickettsiae pathogenic for man. Zentralbl Bakteriol Parasitenkd Infektionskr Hyg 206:299, 1968.
6. Winkler HH: *Rickettsia* species (as organisms). Annu Rev Microbiol 44:131, 1990.
7. Tyeryar FJ Jr, Weiss E, Miller DB, et al: DNA base composition of rickettsiae. Science 180:415, 1973.
8. Myers WF, Wisseman CL Jr: Genetic relatedness among the typhus group of rickettsiae. Int J Syst Bacteriol 30:143, 1980.
9. Weisburg WG, Dobson ME, Samuel JE, et al: Phylogenetic diversity of the rickettsiae. J Bacteriol 171:4202, 1989.
10. Weiss E, Moulder JW: Order I. Rickettsiales Grieszczkiewicz 1939, 25. *In* Krieg NR, Holt JG (eds): Bergey's Manual of Systematic Bacteriology, Vol 1. Baltimore, Williams & Wilkins, 1984, pp 687-704.
11. Eremeeva ME, Roux V, Raoult D: Determination of the genome size and restriction pattern polymorphism of *Rickettsia prowazekii* and *Rickettsia typhi* by pulsed field gel electrophoresis. FEMS Microbiol Lett 112:105, 1993.
12. Black C, Tzianabos T, Roumillat LF, et al: Detection and characterization of mouse monoclonal antibodies to epidemic typhus rickettsiae. J Clin Microbiol 18:561, 1983.
13. Dasch GA: Isolation of species-specific protein antigens of *Rickettsia typhi* and *Rickettsia prowazekii* for immunodiagnosis and immunoprophylaxis. J Clin Microbiol 14:333, 1981.
14. Halle S, Dasch GA, Weiss E: Sensitive enzyme-linked immunosorbent assay for detection of antibodies against typhus rickettsiae, *Rickettsia prowazekii* and *Rickettsia typhi*. J Clin Microbiol 6:101, 1977.
15. Walker TS, Winkler HH: Penetration of cultured mouse fibroblasts (L cells) by *Rickettsia prowazekii*. Infect Immun 22:200, 1978.
16. Ormsbee R, Peacock M, Gerloff R, et al: Limits of rickettsial infectivity. Infect Immun 19:239, 1978.
17. Wisseman CL Jr, Waddell AD: In vitro studies on *Rickettsia*–host cell interactions: Intracellular growth cycle of virulent and attenuated *Rickettsia prowazekii* in chicken embryo cells in slide chamber cultures. Infect Immun 11:1391, 1975.
18. Azad AF: Epidemiology of murine typhus. Annu Rev Entomol 35:553, 1990.
19. Teysseire N, Chiche-Portiche C, Raoult D: Intracellular movements of *Rickettsia conorii* and *R. typhi* based on actin polymerization. Res Microbiol 143:821, 1992.
20. Traub R, Wisseman CL Jr, Farhang-Azad A: The ecology of murine typhus—A critical review. Trop Dis Bull 75:237, 1978.
21. Farhand-Azad A, Traub R, Wisseman CL Jr: *Rickettsia mooseri* infection in the fleas *Leptopsylla segnis* and *Xenopsylla cheopis*. Am J Trop Med Hyg 32:1392, 1983.
22. Farhang Azad A, Traub R: Transmission of murine typhus rickettsiae by *Xenopsylla cheopis*, with notes on experimental infection and effects of temperature. Am J Trop Med Hyg 34:555, 1985.
23. Azad AF, Traub R: Experimental transmission of murine typhus by *Xenopsylla cheopis* flea bites. Med Vet Entomol 3:429, 1989.
24. Farhang-Azad A, Traub R, Baqar S: Transovarial transmission of murine typhus rickettsiae in *Xenopsylla cheopis* fleas. Science 227:543, 1985.
25. Farhang-Azad A, Traub R, Sofi M, et al: Experimental murine typhus infection in the cat flea *Ctenocephalides felis* (Siphonaptera: Pulicidae). J Med Entomol 21:675, 1984.
26. Adams WH, Emmons RW, Brooks JE: The changing ecology of murine (endemic) typhus in southern California. Am J Trop Med Hyg 19:311, 1970.
27. Sorvillo FJ, Gondo B, Emmons R, et al: A suburban focus of endemic typhus in Los Angeles County: Association with seropositive domestic cats and opossums. Am J Trop Med Hyg 48:269, 1993.
28. Murray ES, Snyder JC: Brill's disease: Etiology. Am J Hyg 53:22, 1951.
29. Price WH: Studies on interepidemic survival of louse-borne epidemic typhus fever. J Bacteriol 69:106, 1955.
30. Wisseman CL Jr, Boese JL, Waddell AD, Silverman DJ: Modification of antityphus antibodies on passage through the gut of the human body louse with discussion of some epidemiologic and evolutionary implications. Ann N Y Acad Sci 266:6, 1975.
31. Bozeman FM, Masiello SA, Williams MS, et al: Epidemic typhus rickettsiae isolated from flying squirrels. Nature 255:545, 1975.
32. Bozeman FM, Sonenshine DE, Williams MS, et al: Experimental infection of ectoparasitic arthropods with *Rickettsia prowazekii* (GVF-16 strain) and transmission to flying squirrels. Am J Trop Med Hyg 30:253, 1981.
33. Sonenshine DE, Bozeman FM, Williams MS, et al: Epizootiology of epidemic typhus (*Rickettsia prowazekii*) in flying squirrels. Am J Trop Med Hyg 27:339, 1978.
34. Woodman DR, Weiss E, Dasch GA, et al: Biological properties of *Rickettsia prowazekii* strains isolated from flying squirrels. Infect Immun 16:853, 1977.
35. Dasch GA, Samms JR, Weiss E: Biochemical characteristics of typhus group rickettsiae with special attention to the *Rickettsia prowazekii* strains isolated from flying squirrels. Infect Immun 19:676, 1978.
36. Regnery RL, Zhang YF, Spruill CL: Flying squirrel–associated *Rickettsia prowazekii* (epidemic typhus rickettsiae) characterized by a specific DNA fragment produced by restriction endonuclease digestion. J Clin Microbiol 23:189, 1986.
37. Duma RJ, Sonenshine DE, Bozeman FM, et al: Epidemic typhus in the United States associated with flying squirrels. JAMA 245:2318, 1981.
38. McDade JE, Shepard CC, Redus MA, et al: Evidence of *Rickettsia prowazekii* infections in the United States. Am J Trop Med Hyg 29:277, 1980.

236

Rickettsia tsutsugamushi and Rickettsia akari

James G. Olson
Joseph E. McDade

Rickettsia tsutsugamushi

History of the Microorganism

Scrub typhus (chigger-borne rickettsiosis) can be traced to the third century AD, when the Chinese physician Keh-Hung provided the earliest known description of the disease.[1] Westerners became aware of scrub typhus in the mid-19th century, after Commodore Perry's visit to Japan opened the door to scientific and social interchange. Scrub typhus gained prominence in World War II when tens of thousands of soldiers in the Asiatic-Pacific theaters contracted the disease, with case-fatality rates ranging as high as 35%. Thousands of cases still occur each year in the endemic areas (see Fig. 179–3).

Characteristics of the Pathogen

R. tsutsugamushi is a small (0.5 to 1.2 μm), gram-negative, obligate intracellular bacterium. Like other rickettsiae, it has an arthropod vector (trombiculid mites) as part of its life cycle. Mice are the preferred laboratory hosts, although *R. tsutsugamushi* can also be cultivated in cell culture and in the yolk sac of embryonated eggs. Optimal growth is obtained at 32°C. In contrast to other rickettsiae, which grow optimally in vitro when the air is enriched (5%) for carbon dioxide, *R. tsutsugamushi* does not require carbon dioxide enrichment.[2] *R. tsutsugamushi* is best visualized when it is stained by a modification of the Gimenez technique.[3]

Evidence suggests that *R. tsutsugamushi* may be sufficiently different from other members of the genus *Rickettsia* to be assigned to a new genus.[4] Genetic analyses of 16S ribosomal RNA sequences show that *R. tsutsugamushi* is between 90.2% and 90.6% similar to *Rickettsia rickettsii, Rickettsia sibirica, Rickettsia prowazekii,* and *Rickettsia typhi.* The last four species share 98.1% similarity.[5] *R. tsutsugamushi* also differs morphologically from other members of the genus. The outer leaflet of its cell wall is much thicker than the inner leaflet; the opposite is true for the rest of the genus.[6] *R. tsutsugamushi* lacks peptidoglycan and lipopolysaccharide, substances found in all other members of the genus.[7] *R. tsutsugamushi* is soft and fragile, which also reflects its lack of peptidoglycan.[8, 9] Finally, *R. tsutsugamushi* is more resistant to penicillin than are other members of the genus.[10]

R. tsutsugamushi penetrates the plasma membrane of the host cell by active phagocytosis,[11] escapes from the phagosome, and then grows free within the cytoplasm. Organisms then move to the cell periphery and occasionally bud from the surface enclosed in host cell membrane[12, 13] (Fig. 236–1). Most observers have concluded that *R. tsutsugamushi,* like other rickettsiae, multiplies by transverse binary fission. Different isolates of *R. tsutsugamushi*, even strains collected in a limited geographic area, exhibit considerable antigenic diversity.[14] Group-specific antigens can be extracted from scrub typhus rickettsiae with ether, leaving the strain-specific antigens associated with the extracted organisms.[15, 16] Serologic and biochemical analyses of three prototype strains of *R. tsutsugamushi* (Karp, Gilliam, and Kato) have identified several quantitatively dominant antigenic proteins ranging in size from 50 to 63 kDa.[17] Analysis of one polypeptide with monoclonal antibodies showed that it contained both strain- and species-specific epitopes.[17] Both inbred and outbred strains of mice differ in their susceptibility to a given strain of *R. tsutsugamushi* inoculated intraperitoneally; of 15 strains of inbred mice, 9 strains were susceptible and 6 strains were resistant.[18] Subsequent genetic analyses of the inbred mice revealed that resistance was correlated with an autosomal dominant gene located on mouse chromosome 5.[19]

Natural History, Reservoirs, and Vectors

Leptotrombidium mites are both reservoirs and vectors of *R. tsutsugamushi*; infection is transmitted transovarially by females to their progeny. Although several species of rodents become infected with *R. tsutsugamushi* and maintain rickettsemia for several months,[20–22] there is no evidence that uninfected chiggers acquire *R. tsutsugamushi* from infected mammals.[23] The lack of horizontal transmission of *R. tsutsugamushi* is based on experimental investigations in which three species of *Leptotrombidium* failed to become infected while feeding on infected mammals.[23] Only larval mites (chiggers) feed on hosts; humans become infected when they intrude on areas that contain infected chiggers.

Field studies have shown a close correlation between the incidence of scrub typhus cases in humans and the population density of *Leptotrombidium deliense* collected from *Suncus murinus* and *Rattus* species.[24] In some geographic areas, there is an association between the species of mite and the serotype of *R. tsutsugamushi* they transmit. *Leptotrombidium scutellare* from Mount Fuji, Japan, was responsible for transmitting the Kawasaki serotype; *Leptotrombidium pallidum* transmitted the Karp serotype.[25]

Rickettsia akari

History of the Microorganism, Natural History, Reservoirs, and Vectors

R. akari is the etiologic agent of rickettsialpox. It was first isolated in 1946 in association with an outbreak of rickettsialpox at a housing development in New York City. *R. akari* was isolated from the blood of two patients, from a house mouse *(Mus musculus)* trapped on the premises, and from two pools of rodent mites *(Liponyssoides sanguineus)* that were collected at the same site. The investigation also revealed a strong association between mite exposure and rickettsialpox, further incriminating mites as vectors of the disease.[26–29] The relative contribution of mice and mites for maintaining *R. akari* in nature is not clear. *R. akari* has also been isolated from voles and may exist in other ecosystems.[30]

Characteristics of the Pathogen

R. akari is a small (0.6 × 1.0 μm), gram-negative, obligate intracellular bacterium. Mice are the preferred laboratory hosts, but guinea pigs are also susceptible. Outbred strains of mice are all susceptible to *R. akari*; inbred strains differ significantly in susceptibility.[31] Susceptibility or resistance in inbred mice has been correlated with the ability of their

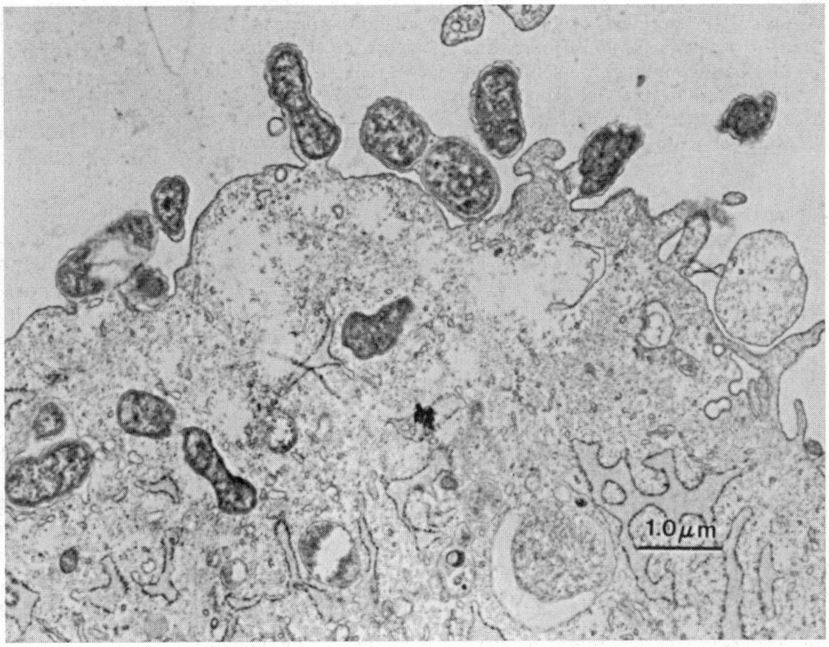

FIGURE 236–1 □ Electron micrograph of chick embryo cells infected with *Rickettsia tsutsugamushi,* the etiologic agent of scrub typhus. Note that the rickettsiae appear to bud from the chick cells enclosed in host cell membranes. (Courtesy Dr. David Silverman, University of Maryland School of Medicine, Baltimore.)

macrophages to phagocytose and kill *R. akari*.[32, 33] *R. akari* also grows well in tissue culture and the yolk sac of embryonated eggs.

R. akari grows primarily within the cytoplasm of the host cell, although it has also been observed within the nucleus. It can be visualized in infected tissue stained by the Gimenez, Giemsa, or Macchiavello methods.[3] *R. akari* is a member of the spotted fever group of rickettsiae. The guanine plus cytosine content of *R. akari* DNA, like other spotted fever group rickettsiae, is approximately 32% to 33%.[34] In DNA-to-DNA hybridization studies, 46% relatedness was observed between *R. akari* and *R. rickettsii*, the etiologic agent of Rocky Mountain spotted fever; other spotted fever rickettsiae are more closely related.[35] Antigenic analyses of *R. akari*, performed with convalescent human and guinea pig serum samples, have shown that *R. akari* possesses determinants that are common to all spotted fever group rickettsiae.[36] However, tests with polyvalent mouse antisera[37] and monoclonal antibodies[38] indicate that *R. akari* also contains species-specific antigens.

References

1. Farner DS, Katsampes CP: Tsutsugamushi disease. US Naval Med Bull 43:800, 1944.
2. Kopmans-Gargantiel AI, Wisseman CL Jr: Differential requirements for enriched atmospheric carbon dioxide content for intracellular growth in cell culture among selected members of the genus *Rickettsia*. Infect Immun 31:1277, 1981.
3. Elisberg BL, Bozeman FM: The rickettsiae. *In* Lennette EH, Schmidt NJ (eds): Diagnostic Procedures for Viral, Rickettsial and Chlamydial Infections. Washington, DC, American Public Health Association, 1979, pp 1061–1108.
4. Tamura A, Ohashi N, Urakami H, Miyamura S: Classification of *Rickettsia tsutsugamushi* in a new genus, *Orientia* gen. nov., as *Orientia tsutsugamushi* comb. nov. Int J Syst Bacteriol 45:589, 1995.
5. Ohashi N, Fukuhara M, Shimada M, Tamura A: Phylogenetic position of *Rickettsia tsutsugamushi* and relationship among its antigenic variants by analyses of 16S rRNA gene sequences. FEMS Microbiol Lett 125:299, 1995.
6. Silverman DJ, Wisseman CL Jr: Comparative ultrastructural study on the cell envelopes of *Rickettsia prowazekii, Rickettsia rickettsii*, and *Rickettsia tsutsugamushi*. Infect Immun 21:1020, 1978.
7. Amano K, Tamura A, Ohashi N, et al: Deficiency of peptidoglycan and lipopolysaccharide components in *Rickettsia tsutsugamushi*. Infect Immun 55:2290, 1987.
8. Takahashi M, Urakami H, Tamura A: Purification of cell envelopes of *Rickettsia tsutsugamushi*. Microbiol Immunol 29:475, 1985.
9. Tamura A, Urakami H, Tsuruhara T: Purification of *Rickettsia tsutsugamushi* by Percoll density gradient centrifugation. Microbiol Immunol 26:321, 1982.
10. Raoult D, Drancourt M: Antimicrobial therapy of rickettsial diseases. Antimicrob Agents Chemother 35:2457, 1991.
11. Cohn ZA, Bozeman FM, Campbell JH, et al: Study of growth of rickettsiae. V. Penetration of *Rickettsia tsutsugamushi* into mammalian cells in vitro. J Exp Med 109:271, 1959.
12. Ewing EP Jr, Takeuchi A, Shirai A, et al: Experimental infection of mouse peritoneal mesothelium with scrub typhus rickettsiae: An ultrastructural study. Infect Immun 19:1068, 1978.
13. Rikihisa Y, Ito S: Intracellular localization of *Rickettsia tsutsugamushi* in polymorphonuclear leukocytes. J Exp Med 150:703, 1979.
14. Traub R, Wisseman CL Jr: The ecology of chigger-borne rickettsiosis (scrub typhus). J Med Entomol 11:237, 1974.
15. Kobayashi Y, Nagai K, Tachibana N: Purification of complement fixing antigens of *Rickettsia orientalis* by ether extraction. Am J Trop Med Hyg 18:942, 1969.
16. Shishido A, Hikita M, Sat T, et al: Particulate and soluble antigens of *Rickettsia tsutsugamushi* in the complement fixation test. J Immunol 113:480, 1969.
17. Hanson B: Identification and partial characterization of *Rickettsia tsutsugamushi* major protein immunogens. Infect Immun 50:603, 1985.
18. Groves MG, Osterman JV: Host defenses in experimental scrub typhus: Genetics of natural resistance to infection. Infect Immun 19:583, 1978.
19. Groves MG, Rosenstreich DL, Taylor BA, Osterman JV: Host defenses in experimental scrub typhus: Mapping the gene that controls natural resistance in mice. J Immunol 125:1395, 1980.
20. Traub R, Wisseman CL Jr, Jones MR, O'Keefe JJ: The acquisition of *Rickettsia tsutsugamushi* by chiggers (trombiculid mites) during the feeding process. Ann N Y Acad Sci 266:91, 1975.
21. Strickman D, Smith CD, Corcoran KD, et al: Pathology of *Rickettsia tsutsugamushi* in *Bandicota savilei*, a natural host in Thailand. Am J Trop Med Hyg 51:416, 1994.
22. Van Peenen PFD, Ho CM, Bourgeois AL: Indirect immunofluorescence antibodies in natural and acquired *Rickettsia tsutsugamushi* infections of Philippine rodents. Infect Immun 15:813, 1977.
23. Walker JS, Chan CT, Manikumaran C, et al: Attempts to infect and demonstrate transovarial transmission of *R. tsutsugamushi* in three species of *Leptotrombidium* mites. Ann N Y Acad Sci 266:80, 1975.

24. Olson JG, Bourgeois AL, Fang RCY: Population indices of chiggers *(Leptotrombidium deliense)* and incidence of scrub typhus in Chinese military personnel, Pescadores Islands of Taiwan, 1976–1977. Trans R Soc Trop Med Hyg 76:85, 1982.
25. Kawamori F, Akiyama M, Sugeida M, et al: Epidemiology of tsutsugamushi disease in relation to the serotypes of *Rickettsia tsutsugamushi* isolated from patients, field mice, and unfed chiggers on the eastern slope of Mount Fuji, Shizuoka Prefecture, Japan. J Clin Microbiol 30:2842, 1992.
26. Huebner RJ, Jellison WL, Armstrong C: Rickettsialpox—A newly recognized rickettsial disease. V. Recovery of *Rickettsia akari* from a house mouse *(Mus musculus)*. Public Health Rep 62:777, 1947.
27. Huebner RJ, Jellison WL, Pomerantz C: Rickettsialpox—A newly recognized rickettsial disease. IV. Isolation of a rickettsia apparently identical with the causative agent of rickettsialpox from *Allodermanyssus sanguineus*, a rodent mite. Public Health Rep 61:1677, 1946.
28. Huebner RJ, Stamps P, Armstrong C: Rickettsialpox—A newly recognized rickettsial disease. I. Isolation of the etiologic agent. Public Health Rep 61:1605, 1946.
29. Greenberg M, Pellitteri OJ, Jellison WL: Rickettsialpox—A newly recognized rickettsial disease. III. Epidemiology. Am J Public Health 37:860, 1947.
30. Jackson EB, Danauskas JX, Coale MC, Smadel JE: Recovery of *R. akari* from the Korean vole *Microtus fortis pelliceus*. Am J Hyg 66:301, 1957.
31. Anderson GW Jr, Osterman JV: Host defenses in experimental rickettsialpox: Genetics of natural resistance to infection. Infect Immun 28:132, 1980.
32. Nacy CA, Meltzer MS: Macrophages in resistance to rickettsial infection: Strains of mice susceptible to the lethal effects of *Rickettsia akari* show defective macrophage rickettsiocidal activity in vitro. Infect Immun 36:1096, 1982.
33. Kokorin IN, Kabanova EA, Kyet CD, et al: Differences in the susceptibility of mouse cell lines to the rickettsia pox agent. Acta Virol 22:497, 1978.
34. Tyeryar FJJ, Weiss E, Millar DB, et al: DNA base composition of rickettsiae. Science 180:415, 1973.
35. Myers WF, Wisseman CL Jr: Genetic relationships within the spotted fever biotype of the genus *Rickettsia* (Abstr). Third National Meeting, American Society for Rickettsiology and Rickettsial Diseases; March 12–14, 1982; Atlanta, GA.
36. Bell EJ, Stoenner HG: Immunologic relationships among the spotted fever group of rickettsias determined by toxin neutralization tests in mice with convalescent animal serums. J Immunol 84:171, 1960.
37. Pickens EG, Bell EJ, Lackmen DB, et al: Use of mouse serum in identification and serologic classification of *Rickettsia akari* and *Rickettsia australis*. J Immunol 94:883, 1965.
38. McDade JE, Black CM, Roumillat LF, et al: Addition of monoclonal antibodies specific for *Rickettsia akari* to the rickettsial diagnostic panel. J Clin Microbiol 26:2221, 1988.

237

Coxiella burnetii (Q Fever)

Paul D. Holtom
John M. Leedom

History

Q fever is an infection caused by the organism *Coxiella burnetii*. Humans are usually infected by inhalation of aerosols from infected domestic animals. Q fever can present as an acute infection with an influenza-like illness, fever, and pulmonary and hepatic involvement or can develop into a chronic form with endocarditis and chronic hepatitis. Q fever (for *query*, to indicate the uncertain cause of the disease at the time of its description) was first described in 1936 by Derrick in Australia.[1] He reported detailed clinical data on nine abattoir workers who presented with febrile illnesses, and he successfully isolated the causal agent from human blood and urine by passage into guinea pigs. Burnet and Freeman[2] identified the organism as a rickettsia. Davis and Cox[3] independently isolated the same organism from ticks collected near Nine Mile Creek in Montana. In 1940, Cox proved that infection with this agent occurred in humans in the western United States. Subsequently, *C. burnetii* has been shown to have a worldwide distribution.

Characteristics of the Pathogen

C. burnetii has been classified as a member of the tribe Rickettsieae, family Rickettsiaceae, because it is a short (0.3 to 0.7 μm long), pleomorphic gram-negative rod that is an obligate intracellular parasite. However, studies have shown that *C. burnetii* is closest to *Legionella* phylogenetically and far removed from the Rickettsieae.[4,5] It can be isolated by intraperitoneal injection into guinea pigs, inoculation into the yolk sacs of embryonated chicken eggs, or tissue culture.

C. burnetii differs from the other rickettsiae in staining properties, DNA composition, energy production, antigen solubility, heat stability, antibiotic susceptibility, and mode of transmission.[6] Unlike the other rickettsiae, *C. burnetii* grows in the acidic environment of the phagolysosome of the cell rather than the cytoplasm or the nucleus.[7] It is resistant to inactivation and can survive for long periods in the environment.[8] The reason for this resistance may be the formation of an endospore-like cell variant.[9]

In passage through cell cultures or embryonated eggs, the lipopolysaccharide of *C. burnetii* undergoes an antigenic shift that is called phase variation.[10] Phase I is found in fresh isolates and is highly infectious. Conversion to phase II occurs after repeated passage through embryonated chicken eggs, although there is reversion to phase I with passage through laboratory animals. Although there is no morphologic difference between the two phases, there are differences in antigenic components, sugar composition of their lipopolysaccharides,[11] buoyant density, agglutinability, staining properties, and resistance to phagocytosis. A major difference is the presence of glucuronic acid on the surface antigen of the phase I organisms but not on those of phase II.[12] Plasmids have been identified in both phase I and phase II organisms, and some investigators have suggested a correlation between plasmid profile and clinical manifestations (acute or chronic infection), but this theory has not been confirmed by subsequent investigation.[13–15]

Epidemiology

C. burnetii is an extremely infectious organism. In fact, a single inhaled organism is sufficient to initiate infection.[16] It is endemic worldwide, with the exception of New Zealand.[17] *C. burnetii* infects many species of animals, and in animals the infection usually results in long-lasting parasitism. Mammals (both wild and domestic), birds, fish, and arthropods have been found to be infected with the organism.[18] Although many species of ticks have been found to be infected and there may be tick-borne transmission among animals, ticks apparently are not a source of infection in humans.

Q fever in humans is usually caused by the inhalation of aerosolized particles, which can be airborne even over long distances, although it it is often said to result from the ingestion of contaminated raw milk. A 1992 report[19] involved patients and staff of a psychiatric institution living in rural France. Some of the patients had direct contacts with goats. Others living 5 km away ingested raw milk products from the goats. Serologic evidence of *C. burnetii* infection or a history of compatible illness was significantly more common in persons who had tended goats, tended goats and ingested raw milk products, or only ingested raw milk products, compared with persons at the institution who were in none of these risk groups. Most reports associating Q fever with ingestion of raw dairy products are similar.[19, 20] That is, the infection occurs in rural settings where the possibility of inhalation of *C. burnetii,* dust-borne from the vicinity, cannot reasonably be excluded. It is of interest that direct studies of individuals ingesting contaminated milk in environments away from rural areas either show seroconversions without disease[21, 22] or are totally negative for evidence of *C. burnetii* infection.[23] Large numbers of *C. burnetii* organisms can be present in the parturient fluids of sheep, cattle, and cats and can also be shed in the urine, feces, and milk. Q fever is mainly an occupational or geographic disease associated with contact with farm animals such as cattle, sheep, and goats, although contacts with infected cats have been sources of urban outbreaks.[24, 25] There have been outbreaks among laboratory workers and workers in buildings where *C. burnetii* has been cultured.[26–28] Transmission of infection by blood transfusion[29] and during an autopsy[30] has been documented, but there have been no reports of transmission to health care providers caring for infected persons. Person-to-person transmission of Q fever is unusual but does occur.[31, 32] Although isolation and quarantine of patients with Q fever are not recommended, it should be remembered that such transmission has been documented.

Clinical Manifestations

Infection with *C. burnetii* can cause a wide spectrum of clinical findings, dependent at least in part on different host factors.[33] Many people who are infected with *C. burnetii* are asymptomatic; in a series from Switzerland, 54% of serologically diagnosed "cases" with a known exposure were asymptomatic.[34] In patients who have clinical illness, the most common presentations are an acute febrile systemic illness, pneumonia, hepatitis, or meningoencephalitis. Patients can develop a chronic illness characterized by endocarditis and a granulomatous hepatitis.

The incubation period for Q fever can be as short as 4 to 5 days,[35] but it typically ranges from 9 to 39 days. Fever is the most common symptom, occurring in 90%[36] to 100%[37] of patients, and the temperature often spikes to 40.0°C to 40.5°C (104°F to 105°F). Other signs and symptoms include chills, headache (often severe), retrobulbar pain, myalgias and arthralgias, neck pain and stiffness, pleuritic chest pain, cough, nausea and vomiting, diarrhea, jaundice, hepatomegaly, and splenomegaly. Unlike the other rickettsial diseases, Q fever does not usually present with a rash, although a transient erythematous macular rash has been noted in about 4% of patients. The manifestations of Q fever usually resolve within 2 to 4 weeks, although in some patients the fever has lasted as long as 9 weeks.[37] Case-fatality rates from acute Q fever are quite low (0% in most series), but in a French series of 323 hospitalized patients the case-fatality rate was 2.4%.[38]

The incidence of pulmonary involvement in patients with Q fever varies between 0% and 90%.[39] The reason for this wide variation is not known; possible explanations include geographic strain variation or the source, route, or dose of the infectious agent. In patients with pulmonary involvement, the chest radiograph can have patchy infiltrates resembling *Mycoplasma pneumoniae* infection or may show actual lobar consolidation.

Hepatic involvement in acute Q fever may range from minimal elevations of the hepatic transaminase values to a presentation indistinguishable from that of acute viral hepatitis. The incidence of hepatomegaly ranges from 11% to 65% in patients with acute Q fever; the reason for this reported variability is not known. Actual jaundice is uncommon and occurs in 4% to 5% of cases. Liver biopsy examinations in patients with Q fever hepatitis show a wide range of lesions, ranging from focal necrosis to severe, widespread liver cell necrosis with noncaseating granulomata. A characteristic granuloma has been described that consists of a clear central space surrounded by inflammatory cells and a fibrin ring.[40, 41]

In addition to the common manifestations of fever, pulmonary involvement, and hepatic involvement, there are many less common complications of Q fever. These include meningitis, encephalitis,[42, 43] optic neuritis,[44] Guillain-Barré syndrome,[45] myelopathy,[46] hemolytic anemia,[47] bone marrow necrosis,[48] arthritis, polyserositis, acute pleuropericarditis, myocarditis, thrombophlebitis, inflammatory pseudotumor of the lung, nephritis, orchitis, and epididymitis.

Chronic Q fever is usually manifested by endocarditis, although other manifestations have been described such as chronic hepatitis, infections of vascular prostheses, and aneurysms,[49] osteomyelitis, and interstitial pulmonary fibrosis.[50] Q fever endocarditis is usually accompanied by liver involvement and is a rare, severe, and often fatal complication of *C. burnetii* infection. The incidence of Q fever endocarditis appears to be increasing, but this may be due to improved diagnosis rather than a true change in epidemiology. In most of the cases, there is a history of preexisting valvular heart disease, and patients often have a prosthetic valve. The aortic valve is the most common site of infection.[51] The illness evolves slowly, presenting any time from 1 to 20 years after the acute infection, and presents clinically as a culture-negative endocarditis, although fever is often absent in Q fever endocarditis. Other findings include hepatomegaly, abnormal liver function tests, splenomegaly, anemia, microscopic hematuria, hyperglobulinemia, and thrombocytopenia. Chronic liver involvement in the absence of endocarditis has been reported but is uncommon.

Diagnosis

The clinical presentation of Q fever can resemble that of nearly any infectious disease. The diagnosis can be made only by the isolation of *C. burnetii* from a clinical sample or by serologic demonstration of infection. The other laboratory findings in acute and chronic Q fever are nonspecific. Although isolation of the organism is possible, it is seldom done because of the high risk of infection to laboratory personnel, and serologic tests are usually used to confirm the diagnosis.

Several tests are available to detect antibodies specific for *C. burnetii* in patients' serum samples. Complement fixation and indirect fluorescent antibody are the procedures most commonly used. The enzyme-linked immunosorbent assay has also been proposed as a method of diagnosing Q fever.[52] All three methods are highly specific. In acute *C. burnetii* infection in humans, antibodies to *C. burnetii* phase II antigen are produced, which generally become detectable 8 to 14 days after the onset of illness and peak around week 4 to 8 for indirect fluorescent antibody titers or week 12 to 13 for complement fixation titers. Although a phase II complement fixation titer of 1:8 is considered significant, confirmation of the diagnosis rests on demonstrating a fourfold or greater rise in complement fixation titer in paired serum specimens. Indirect fluorescent antibody titers for immunoglobulin G of 1:200 or greater and immunoglobulin M of 1:50 or greater are predictive of evolving acute or chronic infection.[53]

In chronic Q fever, the phase I antibody level becomes elevated. A phase I complement fixation antibody titer greater than 1:200 is considered diagnostic for chronic Q fever,[54] although some patients with endocarditis may have lower titers.

Treatment

Most acute Q fever infections resolve spontaneously, and symptoms respond to nonspecific therapy such as antipyretics and hydration. However, because of the concern for the development of chronic Q fever, and because some studies suggest that therapy shortens the duration of fever, specific antimicrobial therapy for acute Q fever is advisable. Tetracycline and its analogs are the mainstay of therapy. Tetracycline for 2 weeks at 25 mg/kg per day in four divided doses, or doxycycline, 100 mg twice a day for 15 to 21 days, is the recommended therapy for adults.

The treatment of chronic Q fever has never been the subject of controlled studies. No antibiotics have been found to be bactericidal for *C. burnetii,* although several (including tetracycline, doxycycline, trimethoprim-sulfamethoxazole, rifampin, and ciprofloxacin) have been shown to be bacteriostatic. The combination of rifampin with either doxycycline or trimethoprim-sulfamethoxazole has been recommended in the treatment of Q fever endocarditis. The optimal duration of therapy is also unknown; recommended treatment periods range from 12 months to an indefinite term.[55] Valve replacement surgery in Q fever endocarditis is indicated only for significant hemodynamic problems.

Prevention

Because *C. burnetii* organisms are widespread in the environment and relatively resistant to inactivation, control of the major reservoirs of the organism is impractical. There is a commercial vaccine available in Australia and in some European countries that is a formalin-inactivated whole-cell vaccine. The vaccine is made from phase I organisms and is highly effective.[56] At this time no vaccine is commercially available in the United States.

References

1. Derrick EH: "Q" fever, a new fever entity: Clinical features, diagnosis and laboratory investigation. Med J Aust 2:281, 1937.
2. Burnet FM, Freeman M: Experimental studies on the virus of Q fever. Med J Aust 2:299, 1937.
3. Davis GE, Cox HR: A filter-passing infectious agent isolated from ticks: I. Isolation from *Dermacentor andersoni,* reactions in animals, and filtration experiments. Public Health Rep 53:2259, 1938.
4. Stein A, Saunders NA, Taylor AG, Raoult D: Phylogenic homogeneity of *Coxiella burnetii* strains as determinated by 16S ribosomal RNA sequencing. FEMS Microbiol Lett 113:339, 1993.
5. Raoult D, Marrie T: Q fever. Clin Infect Dis 20:489, 1995.
6. Ormsbee RA: Rickettsiae (as organisms). Annu Rev Microbiol 23:275, 1969.
7. Baca OG, Li YP, Kumar H: Survival of the Q fever agent *Coxiella burnetii* in the phagolysosome. Trends Microbiol 2:476, 1994.
8. Sawyer LA, Fishbein DB, McDade JE: Q fever: Current concepts. Rev Infect Dis 9:935, 1987.
9. McCaul TF, Williams JC: Developmental cycle of *Coxiella burnetii:* Structure and morphogenesis of vegetative and sporogenic differentiations. J Bacteriol 147:1063, 1981.
10. Leedom JM: Q fever: An update. Curr Clin Top Infect Dis 1:304, 1980.
11. Schramek S, Mayer H: Different sugar compositions of lipopolysaccharides isolated from phase I and pure phase II cells of *Coxiella burnetii.* Infect Immun 38:53, 1982.
12. Jerrels JR, Hinricks DJ, Mallavia LP: Cell envelope analysis of *Coxiella burnetii* phase I and phase II. Can J Microbiol 20:1465, 1974.
13. Frazier ME, Mallavia LP, Samuel JE, Baca OG: DNA probes for the identification of *Coxiella burnetii* strains. Ann N Y Acad Sci 590:445, 1990.
14. Stein A: Lack of pathotype specific gene in human *Coxiella burnetii.* Microb Pathog 15:177, 1993.
15. Thiele D, Willems H: Is plasmid based differentiation of *Coxiella burnetii* in "acute" and "chronic" isolates still valid? Eur J Epidemiol 10:427, 1994.
16. Tigertt WD, Benenson AS, Bochenour WS: Airborne Q fever. Bacteriol Rev 25:285, 1961.
17. Hilbink F, Penrose M, Kovacova E, Kazar J: Q fever is absent from New Zealand. Int J Epidemiol 22:945, 1993.
18. Baca OG, Paretsky D. Q fever and *Coxiella burnetii:* A model for host-parasite interaction. Microbiol Rev 47:127, 1983.
19. Fishbein DB, Raoult D: A cluster of *Coxiella burnetii* infections associated with exposure to vaccinated goats and their unpasteurized dairy products. Am J Trop Med Hyg 47:35, 1992.
20. Brown GL, Colwell DC, Hooper WL: An outbreak of Q fever in Staffordshire. J Hyg 66:649, 1968.
21. Benson WW, Brock DW, Mather J: Serologic analysis of a penitentiary group using raw milk from a Q fever-infected herd. Public Health Rep 78:707, 1963.
22. Experimental Q fever in man (Editorial). Br Med J 1:1000, 1950.
23. Krumbiegel EF, Wisniewski HJ: Q fever in Milwaukee II. Consumption of raw milk by human volunteers. Arch Environ Health 21:63, 1970.
24. Langley JM, Marrie TJ, Covert A, et al: Poker players' pneumonia. N Engl J Med 319:354, 1988.
25. Marrie TJ, Durant H, Williams JC, et al: Exposure to parturient cats is a rick factor for acquisition of Q fever in Maritime Canada. J Infect Dis 158:101, 1988.
26. Meiklejohn G, Reimer LG, Graves PS, et al: Cryptic epidemic of Q fever in a medical school. J Infect Dis 144:107, 1981.
27. Bernard KW, Parham GL, Winkler WG, et al: Q fever control measures: Recommendations for research facilities using sheep. Infect Control 3:461, 1982.
28. Ruppanner R, Brooks D, Morrish D, et al: Q fever hazards from sheep and goats used in research. Arch Environ Health 37:103, 1982.
29. Heard SR, Ronalds CJ, Hearth RB: *Coxiella burnetii* infection in immunocompromised hosts. J Infect 11:15, 1985.
30. Harman JB: Q fever in Great Britain: Clinical account of eight cases. Lancet 2:1028, 1949.
31. Leedom JM: Q fever. *In* Spittle JA Jr (ed): Practice of Medicine, Vol 2. Hagerstown, MD, Harper & Row, 1981, pp 1–15.
32. Mann JS, Douglas JG, Inglis JN, et al: Q fever: Person to person transmission within a family. Thorax 41:974, 1985.
33. Raoult D: Host factors in the severity of Q fever. Ann N Y Acad Sci 590:33, 1990.
34. Dupuis G, Petite J, Peter O, Vouilloz M: An important outbreak of human Q fever in a Swiss Alpine valley. Int J Epidemiol 16:282, 1987.
35. Young FW: Q fever in Artesia, California. Calif Med 69:89, 1948.
36. Tselentis Y, Gikas A, Kofteridis D, et al: Q fever in the Greek island of Crete: Epidemiologic, clinical and therapeutic data from 98 cases. Clin Infect Dis 20:1311, 1995.
37. Clark WH, Lennette EH, Railsback OC, Romer MS: Q fever in California VII. Clinical features in 180 cases. Arch Intern Med 88:155, 1951.
38. Dupont HT, Raoult D, Brouqui P, et al: Epidemiologic features and clinical presentation of acute Q fever in hospitalized patients: 323 French cases. Am J Med 93:427, 1992.
39. Murray HW, Tuazon C: Atypical pneumonias. Med Clin North Am 64:507, 1980.
40. Hoffman CE, Heaton JW: Q fever hepatitis. Gastroenterology 83:474, 1982.

41. Travis LB, Travis WB, Li C-Y, et al: Q fever: A clinicopathologic study of five cases. Arch Pathol Lab Med 110:1017, 1986.
42. Ferrante MA, Dolan MJ: Q fever meningoencephalitis in a soldier returning from the Persian Gulf War. Clin Infect Dis 16:489, 1993.
43. Sempere AP, Elizaga J, Duarte J, et al: Q fever mimicking herpetic encephalitis. Neurology 43:2713, 1993.
44. Schuil J, Richardus JH, Baarsma GS, et al: Q fever as a possible cause of bilateral optic neuritis. Br J Ophthalmol 69:580, 1985.
45. Bernard E, Carles M, Laffant C, et al: Guillain-Barré syndrome associated with acute Q fever. Eur J Clin Microbiol Infect Dis 13:658, 1994.
46. Hwang YM, Lee MC, Suh DC, Lee WY: *Coxiella* (Q fever)–associated myelopathy. Neurology 43:338, 1993.
47. Cardellach F, Font J, Agusti AGN, et al: Q fever and hemolytic anemia. J Infect Dis 148:769, 1983.
48. Branda M, Bellingham AJ. Bone marrow necrosis and Q fever. Br Med J 210:148, 1980.
49. Piquet P, Raoult D, Tranier P, Mercier C: *Coxiella burnetii* infection of pseudoaneurysm of an aortic bypass graft with contiguous vertebral osteomyelitis. J Vasc Surg 19:165, 1994.
50. Brouqui P, Dupont HT, Drancourt M, et al: Chronic Q fever. Ninety-two cases from France, including 27 cases without endocarditis. Arch Intern Med 153:642, 1993.
51. Sawyer LA, Fishbein DB, McDade JE: Q fever: Current concepts. Rev Infect Dis 9:935, 1987.
52. Peter O, Dupuis G, Peacock MG, et al: Comparison of enzyme-linked immunosorbent assay and complement fixation and indirect fluorescent antibody tests for detection of *Coxiella burnetii* antibody. J Clin Microbiol 25:1063, 1987.
53. Tissot-Dupont H, Thirion X, Raoult D: Q fever serology: Cutoff determination for microimmunofluorescence. Clin Diagn Lab Immunol 1:189, 1994.
54. Turck WP, Howitt G, Turnberg LA, et al: Chronic Q fever. Q J Med 45:193, 1976.
55. Tobin MJ, Cahill N, Gearty G, et al: Q fever endocarditis. Am J Med 72:396, 1982.
56. Ackland JR, Worswick DA, Marmion BP: Vaccine prophylaxis of Q fever: A follow-up study of the efficacy of Qvac (CSL) 1985–1990. Med J Aust 160:704, 1994.

PART VIII VIRUSES

238

Virus Classification

Neil R. Blacklow

Viruses are not independently living microorganisms; they require host cells for their replication. This is because unlike all other forms of microorganisms—bacteria, fungi, protozoa, mycoplasmas, rickettsiae, and chlamydiae—viruses do not contain both DNA and RNA. Instead, they possess either DNA or RNA, and this feature represents the starting point for classification. Human virology in this textbook is therefore divided into the two categories of DNA and RNA viruses.

The presentation of human virology in an infectious diseases textbook should not only take into account principles of virus classification but also maintain a clinical orientation of epidemiology and pathogenesis. Thus, our coverage of human viruses follows virus classification where possible but deviates in a few areas in which characteristic diseases occur. In this chapter, I first cover basic information on the classification of human viruses relevant to readers who are working in or interested in the field of infectious diseases; then I explain how and why the book deviates in a few instances from this classification in its virology section.

Specifics of Virus Classification

After being divided into DNA and RNA categories, viruses are divided into families, which are designated by terms with the suffix -viridae. There are 20 families of viruses that contain human pathogens. Six families contain DNA and the remainder RNA (Table 238–1). A few viruses remain unclassified owing to insufficient information about their morphologic characteristics or nucleic acid.

Viruses are classified on the basis of shared biologic characteristics. Classification is based principally on (1) morphologic features and (2) genome (nucleic acid) structure and strategy of its replication. Morphologic features are determined predominantly by electron microscopy—virion size, shape, nucleocapsid symmetry, and presence or absence of an envelope (Fig. 238–1). Genome characteristics include predominantly molecular weight, "strandedness," polarity, and structure. The important properties of virions belonging to families of DNA viruses are outlined in Table 238–2 and those of RNA viruses in Table 238–3.

The highest taxonomic group for virus classification is the family, as just outlined. Further subdivisions into subfamilies, genera, and species are less clear-cut and agreed on, although schema exist. These subdivisions are based predominantly on antigenic differences between viruses. Interested readers are directed to other virology references for more details on viral taxonomy and nomenclature.[1–3] It should be noted that it is still customary and accepted virologic practice to use vernacular terms for virus species (e.g., mumps virus).

Epidemiologic Classification

In a less formal way, many viruses can be grouped clinically into four categories based on their modes of transmission.

1. *Enteric viruses.* Enteric viruses are normally acquired by ingestion (fecal-oral route) and localize to the intestinal tract. Examples are in the families Adenoviridae, Picornaviridae, Reoviridae, Astroviridae, and Caliciviridae.
2. *Respiratory viruses.* Respiratory viruses are usually acquired by inhalation (respiratory) or by fomites (hand to nose or mouth or eye) and typically localize to the respiratory

TABLE 238–1 ■ Families of Human Viruses, with Important Examples

FAMILY	EXAMPLES
DNA Viruses	
Adenoviridae	Adenovirus
Herpesviridae	Herpes simplex, Epstein-Barr, varicella-zoster viruses, cytomegalovirus
Poxviridae	Vaccinia, variola (smallpox), molluscum contagiosum viruses
Parvoviridae	Parvovirus B19
Papovaviridae	Papillomavirus, polyomavirus (JC, BK)
Hepadnaviridae	Hepatitis B virus
RNA Viruses	
Orthomyxoviridae	Influenza virus
Paramyxoviridae	Mumps, measles, parainfluenza, respiratory syncytial viruses
Coronaviridae	Coronavirus
Picornaviridae	Poliovirus, coxsackievirus, echovirus, other enteroviruses, hepatitis A virus, rhinovirus
Reoviridae	Rotavirus, reovirus, Colorado tick fever virus
Retroviridae	Human immunodeficiency virus (HIV) type 1, HIV-2, human T-cell lymphotrophic virus (HTLV) type I, HTLV-II
Togaviridae	Rubella virus; arthropod-borne viruses: eastern equine encephalitis, western equine encephalitis, Venezuelan equine encephalitis, chikungunya viruses
Flaviviridae	Arthropod-borne viruses: yellow fever, dengue, St. Louis encephalitis, Japanese encephalitis, Murray Valley encephalitis, tick-borne encephalitis, hepatitis C viruses
Bunyaviridae	Hantaan virus; arthropod-borne viruses: California encephalitis, sandfly fever, Rift Valley fever, Crimean-Congo hemorrhagic fever viruses
Arenaviridae	Rodent-borne viruses: lymphocytic choriomeningitis, Lassa fever, Machupo, Junin viruses
Filoviridae	Marburg, Ebola viruses
Rhabdoviridae	Rabies virus
Caliciviridae	Norwalk virus, hepatitis E virus
Astroviridae	Astrovirus
Unclassified Viruses	
Agent causing Creutzfeldt-Jakob disease, kuru agents—spongiform encephalopathies, prions	
Hepatitis D (delta) virus (a defective RNA-containing satellite of hepatitis B)	

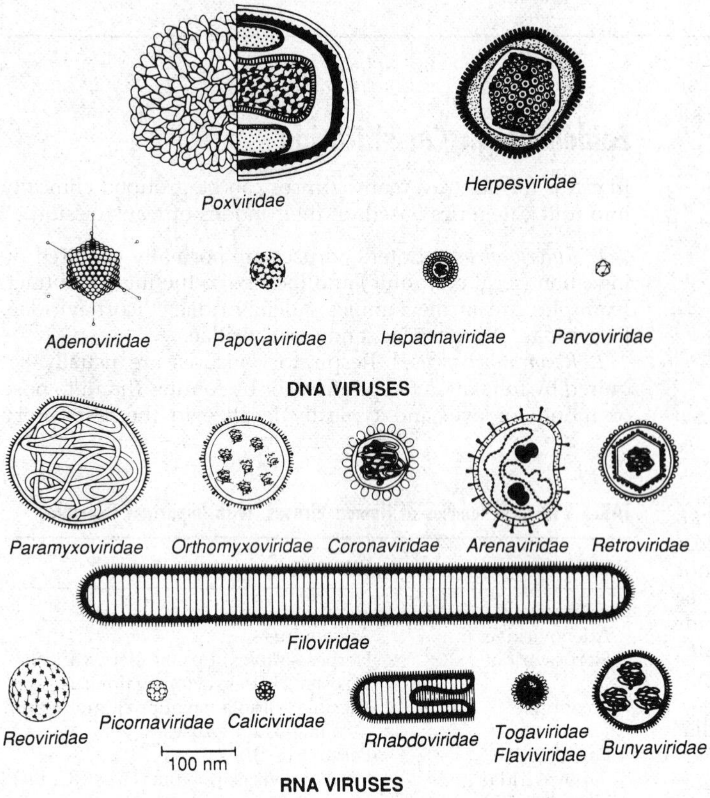

FIGURE 238–1 □ Shapes and sizes of viruses of families that include human pathogens. The virions are drawn to scale, but artistic license has been used in representing their structure. In some, the cross-sectional structure of capsid and envelope is shown, with a representation of the genome; with the extremely small virions, only size and symmetry are depicted. (From White DO, Fenner FJ: Classification and nomenclature of viruses. *In* White DO, Fenner FJ [eds]: Medical Virology, ed 4. San Diego, CA, Academic Press, 1994, pp 16–29.)

tract. Examples are in the families Adenoviridae, Orthomyxoviridae, Paramyxoviridae, Coronaviridae, and Picornaviridae.

3. *Arboviruses* (arthropod-borne viruses). Arboviruses replicate in arthropods that feed on the blood of humans. Examples are in the families Reoviridae, Togaviridae, Flaviviridae, and Bunyaviridae.

4. *Oncogenic viruses*. Oncogenic viruses are acquired by close contact or injection and typically become persistent and may progress to malignancy. Viruses that show these characteristics in experimental animals or humans are in the families Adenoviridae, Herpesviridae, Papovaviridae, Hepadnaviridae, and Retroviridae.

Important Virus Features Distinct from Formal Classification

Although viruses are classified into families, it is important to recognize that the epidemiologic or pathogenic characteristics of some virus infections are so distinctive that these viruses are best discussed either separately or in relation to viruses from a different family. Furthermore, viruses from one family can produce diverse clinical manifestations. The features of viruses that are distinct from their formal classification are covered in three categories:

Viruses in a Family Can Produce Diverse Diseases. Good

TABLE 238–2 ■ Properties of Virions of Families of DNA Viruses Infecting Humans

	VIRION					GENOME	
			Nucleocapsid				
FAMILY	Diameter (mm)	Envelope	*Symmetry*	*Capsomers*	Transcriptase	*Nature**	*Size† (kb, kbp)*
Parvoviridae	20	–	Icosahedral	32	–	ss, –, linear	5
Papovaviridae	45, 55‡	–	Icosahedral	72	–	ds, circular	5, 8‡
Adenoviridae	70	–	Icosahedral	252	–	ds, linear	36–38
Herpesviridae	150	+	Icosahedral	162	–	ds, linear	125–229
Poxviridae	250 × 200 × 200§	+‖	Complex	—	+	ds, linear	130–250
Hepadnaviridae	42	–	Icosahedral	?	+¶	ds, circular**	3.2

*All DNA virus genomes comprise a single molecule. ds, Double stranded; ss, single stranded; + or – indicates sense of single-stranded nucleic acid.
†For species that cause human infections.
‡Lower figure, *Polyomavirus;* higher figure, *Papillomavirus.*
§*Orthopoxvirus,* brick shaped; *Parapoxvirus,* ovoid, 260 × 160 nm.
‖Not essential for infectivity.
¶Reverse transcriptase.
**Circular molecule is double stranded for most of its length but contains a single-stranded region.
From White DO, Fenner FJ: Classification and nomenclature of viruses. *In* White DO, Fenner FJ (eds): Medical Virology, ed 4. San Diego, CA, Academic Press, 1994, pp 16–29.

TABLE 238–3 ■ Properties of Virions of Families of RNA Viruses Infecting Humans

	VIRION					GENOME	
			Nucleocapsid				
FAMILY	Diameter (nm)*	Envelope	*Symmetry*	*Capsomers*	Transcriptase	*Nature*†	*Size (kb, kbp)*
Picornaviridae	25–30	−	Icosahedral	60	−	ss, +	7.5–8.5
Caliciviridae	35–40	−	Icosahedral	32	−	ss, +	8.0
Astroviridae	28–30	−	Icosahedral	?	−	ss, +	7.5
Togaviridae	60–70	+‡	Icosahedral	60	−	ss, +	12
Flaviviridae	40–50	+‡	Icosahedral	?	−	ss, +	10
Coronaviridae	75–160	+‡	Helical	?	−	ss, +	27–33
Paramyxoviridae	150–300	+	Helical	?	+	ss, −	15–16
Rhabdoviridae	180 × 75	+	Helical	?	+	ss, −	13–16
Filoviridae	790–970 × 80	+	Helical	?	+	ss, −	12.7
Orthomyxoviridae	80–120	+	Helical	?	+	ss, 7–8, −	13.6
Arenaviridae	110–130	+‡	Helical	?	+	ss, 2, −	10–14
Bunyaviridae	90–120	+‡	Helical	?	+	ss, 3, −	13.5–21
Reoviridae	60–80	−	Icosahedral	32, 92§	+	ds, 10–12‖	18–27
Retroviridae	80–100	+‡	Icosahedral	?	+¶	ss, +	7–10**
Deltavirus††	32	−	Icosahedral	?	−	ss, −, circular	1.7

*Some enveloped viruses are quite pleomorphic and sometimes filamentous.
†All genomes except that of deltavirus are linear; ss, single stranded; ds, double stranded; 2–12, number of segments in segmented genomes; + or −, indicates sense of single-stranded nucleic acid.
‡No matrix protein.
§The 32 indicates the inner capsid of *Orbivirus, Rotavirus,* and *Orthoreovirus*; 92, outer capsid of *Orthoreovirus.*
‖*Orthoreovirus* and *Orbivirus,* 10; *Rotavirus,* 11; *Coltivirus,* 12.
¶Reverse transcriptase.
**Genome is diploid, two identical molecules being held together by hydrogen bonds at their 5′ ends.
††Currently unclassified as a family but does contain RNA and is a satellite of hepatitis B.
From White DO, Fenner FJ: Classification and nomenclature of viruses. *In* White DO, Fenner FJ (eds): Medical Virology, ed 4. San Diego, CA, Academic Press, 1994, pp 16–29.

examples of this can be found in the families Picornaviridae, Reoviridae, and Togaviridae (see Table 238–1). Clearly, in the Picornaviridae, rhinovirus produces an epidemiologic and pathogenic form of infection that is different from that of poliovirus or hepatitis A virus. In the Reoviridae, rotavirus infection differs markedly from that produced by the virus of Colorado tick fever. In the Togaviridae, rubella is quite distinct clinically from the other members, which are arthropod-borne viruses.

Epidemiology and Pathogenesis of Disease Syndromes Can Be Indistinguishable Between Viruses Belonging to Different Families. Two examples of this are exemplified by encephalitis viruses and hemorrhagic fever viruses. As Table 238–1 shows, viruses that produce clinically similar types of encephalitis by an arthropod-borne route belong to the Togaviridae, Flaviviridae, and Bunyaviridae families. Viruses that typically produce hemorrhagic fever belong to the Flaviviridae (dengue), Arenaviridae, and Filoviridae families.

Some Individual Viruses Produce Medically Distinctive Disease Syndromes. Some viruses produce a distinct clinical syndrome that is normally quite different from those produced by other members of their taxonomic family. Examples of this are yellow fever virus, rubella virus, poliovirus, and mumps virus (see Table 238–1). These are typical examples of viruses that retain the use of vernacular terms for species identification.

As a result of these important virus features that are distinct from formal classification, our coverage in the virology section of this book does not follow strictly the formal classification of viruses into families. The virology chapters are arranged in the order of the families as outlined in Table 238–1; however, some viruses from one family have individual chapters because of their medical importance (e.g., herpes simplex, Epstein-Barr, and varicella-zoster viruses and cytomegalovirus), other viruses are gathered together from different families because of their common clinical features (e.g., encephalitis viruses, hemorrhagic fever viruses), and still others are handled separately because of their distinctive clinical features (e.g., poliovirus, yellow fever virus). Our overriding goal is to present human virology in an organized but clinically relevant way for readers interested in the field of infectious diseases.

References

1. Murphy FA, Fauquet CM, Bishop DHL, et al: Virus Taxonomy: Sixth Report of the International Committee on Taxonomy of Viruses. Vienna, Springer-Verlag, 1995.
2. Murphy FA: Virus taxonomy and nomenclature. *In* Lennette EH, Halonen P, Murphy FA (eds): Laboratory Diagnosis of Infectious Diseases, Principles and Practice, Vol II. New York, Springer-Verlag, 1988, pp 153–176.
3. White DO, Fenner FJ: Classification and nomenclature of viruses. *In* White DO, Fenner FJ (eds): Medical Virology, ed 4. San Diego, CA, Academic Press, 1994, pp 16–29.

DNA VIRUSES

239

Adenoviruses

Marshall S. Horwitz

Adenoviruses are responsible for a variety of infections in the respiratory tract, conjunctiva, urinary tract, intestine, and occasionally other sites. Genetically altered adenoviruses are currently being studied intensively as vectors to deliver foreign genes, both for gene therapy and for immunization against other pathogens.[1, 2] In addition to the importance of adenoviruses as infectious agents, some members of this large family of viruses were the first human viruses shown to be oncogenic in rodents,[3, 4] in which they have served as excellent models for understanding viral transformation, oncogenes, and antioncogenes (reviewed in Shenk[5]); however, there is no evidence that adenoviruses are oncogenic in humans.[6] With the increasing numbers of patients with immunodeficiency caused by disease or by iatrogenic manipulations of the immune system, newer manifestations of adenovirus infections, such as a serious form of hepatitis, have been recognized.[7, 8]

History

Adenoviruses were discovered serendipitously in 1953 when an endogenous transmissable cytopathic agent emerged during attempts to establish tissue cultures of tonsils and adenoids from children undergoing surgical removal of these tissues.[9] The same agents were found in respiratory secretions obtained from febrile military recruits.[10, 11] With the availability of a culture system for adenoviruses, it was appreciated rapidly that a large number of acute respiratory diseases, including pneumonia,[12, 13] were caused by this family of viruses, which now includes 49 recognized distinct serotypes.[14] The association of some adenoviruses with keratoconjunctivitis helped explain previously reported epidemics of this clinical disease. Among shipyard workers whose occupational exposure frequently traumatized their eyes and required medical evaluation, ocular instruments contaminated with adenoviruses spread this disease iatrogenically.[15]

Characteristics of the Pathogen

Structure

All human adenoviruses share similar structural features: an icosahedron with fiber-like projections from each of the 12 vertices[16] (Fig. 239–1). The enteric adenoviruses have two fibers projecting from each vertex.[17] The length of the fiber, a trimer of identical subunits, varies among subgroups (see later) and depends on the number of repeating subunits in the shaft.[18–20] The fiber has a knoblike structure at its tip, which is the attachment site during infection,[21, 22] and the cell receptor for adenoviruses types 2 and 5 has been elucidated.[22a] The fiber is attached noncovalently to the icosahedron by a pentomeric polypeptide, named penton base, at each of the vertices. The major surface capsomere of the icosahedron is the trimeric polypeptide, the hexon, so named because it has six neighboring capsomeres on the face of the virus. There are other proteins (IIIa, VI, VIII, and IX; see Fig. 239–1*A*) necessary to hold the capsid together and to attach it to the linear genomic double-stranded DNA protected by both the capsid and two additional core basic proteins (V and VII; see Fig. 239–1*A*). The viral DNA is approximately 35 kb in length for most serotypes and has a terminal protein (TP) covalently linked to each 5′ end.[23] Major type-specific neutralizing epitopes appear on both the fiber and the hexon with minor sites on the penton base (reviewed in Pirofski and Horwitz[24]). However, all of these large surface proteins also have epitopes shared within the entire adenovirus family.[25] For example, the hexon has group-specific antigenic sites that are helpful in diagnostic virology. Thus, a single reference serum is capable of recognizing most of the human and animal adenoviruses in the *Mastadenovirus* genus but fails to recognize the chicken embryonic lethal virus (CELO) hexon of the *Aviadenovirus* genus (see later). This group-specific antigen was classically measured by complementation fixation tests, which have been supplemented by other serologic tests.[26] Many of the adenoviruses hemagglutinate rat and rhesus red blood cells and those of other species.[27] The hemagglutination test has led to a classification scheme of subgroups from A to E with the more recent addition of the enteric pathogenic types in subgroup F[28] (Table 239–1). The hemagglutinin is a property of the fiber protein, and there is usually a good correlation between the neutralization and hemagglutination inhibition (HI) tests. However, there are an increasing number of field isolates, especially in subgroups B and D,[29, 30] for which the neutralization and HI tests are divergent, probably because of recombination among different adenovirus isolates within subgroups. More distantly related adenoviruses seem to recombine infrequently.[31]

Biology

After adenovirus fibers attach to a cellular receptor, named CAR,[22a] the virus-cell interaction is augmented by the binding of penton base to cellular integrins.[32] The virus is internalized in endosomes where it undergoes initial uncoating during acidification of this structure.[33] Subsequent uncoating occurs in a stepwise fashion during transit of the particle to the nucleus,[34] where synthesis of early messenger RNA (mRNA) occurs. The early proteins synthesized before viral DNA replication begins include (1) a family of transforming proteins from the E1A and E1B regions at the left end of the genome (Fig. 239–2) (reviewed in Shenk[5] and Tooze[35]); (2) three proteins from the E2A and E2B regions, needed for replication of the viral genome: a 140-kDa DNA polymerase (pol), an 87-kDa precursor to the terminal protein (p-TP), and a DNA binding protein (DBP)[36]; (3) a group of proteins synthesized from early region three (E3) that controls the host immune and cytokine response to infection[37, 38] (see the later section on pathogenesis); and (4) a family of proteins from early region 4 (E4), one of which (E4, 34 kDa) binds to the E1B 55-kDa protein, which inhibits cellular mRNA accumulation in the cytoplasm but facilitates viral mRNA transcription.[39] The transforming proteins are responsible for some adenovirus serotypes' being oncogenic in rodents.[40]

An adenovirus E1A protein binds to the antioncogene retinoblastoma protein,[41, 42] freeing the transcription factor E2F

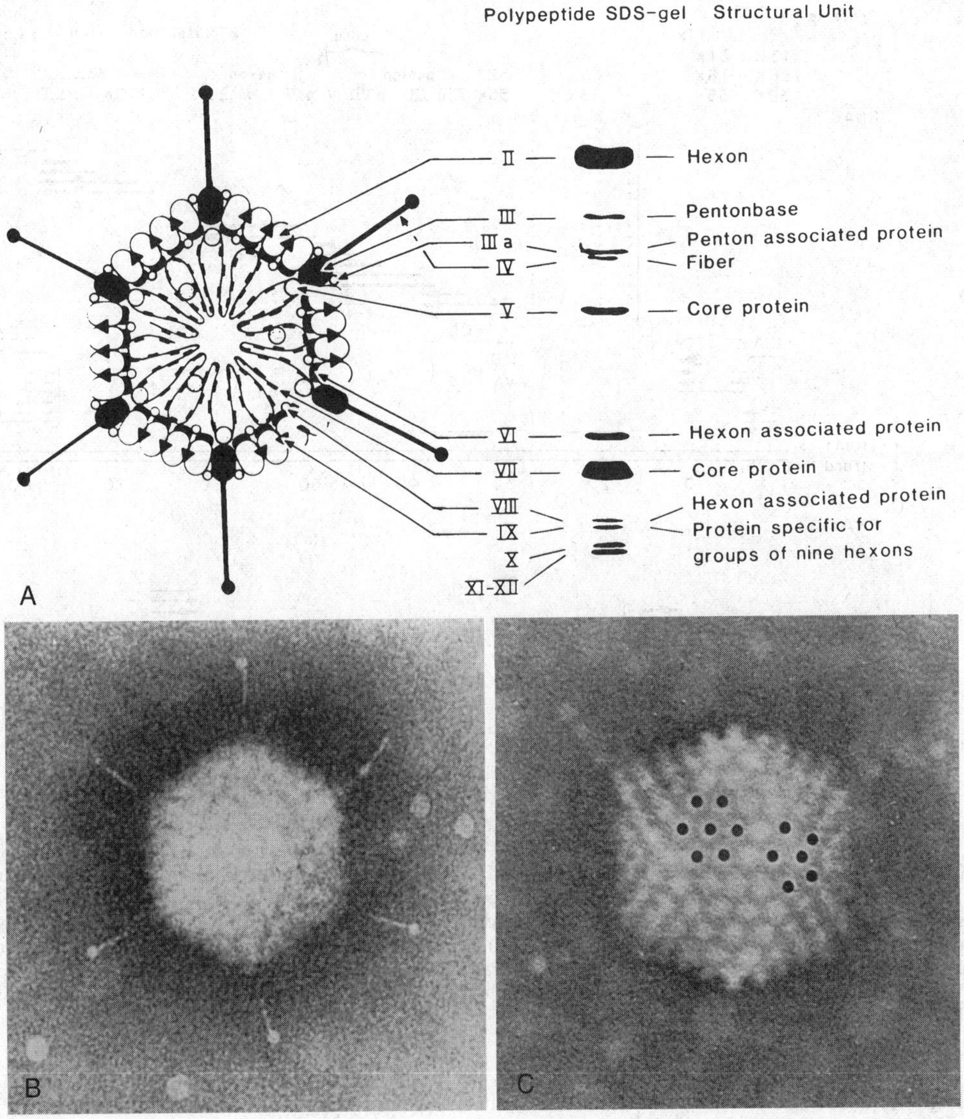

FIGURE 239–1 □ Adenovirus morphology and polypeptide composition. *A,* Schematic representation of the virion is shown together with a denaturing polyacrylamide gel stained with Coomassie blue to display the mobility and amount of each of the viral proteins (polypeptide I was an aggregate of some of the others and is not shown).[20] Polypeptides II, III, IIIA, IV, VI, VIII, and IX are components of the capsid, and core proteins are V and VII. The terminal proteins covalently linked to each 5′ end of the DNA are not shown. *B,* An electron micrograph of an adenovirus type 5, in which 6 of the 12 vertices (penton base plus fiber) are shown. *C,* The sixfold symmetry around each hexon and the fivefold capsomere configuration around each penton base are highlighted. (*A* from Persson H, Philipson L: Regulation of adenovirus. Curr Top Microbiol Immunol 97:157–203, 1982; *B* and *C* from Valentine RC, Periera HG: Antigens and structure of the adenovirus. J Mol Biol 13:13–20, 1965; Horwitz MS: Adenoviridae and their replication. *In* Fields BN, Knipe DM [eds]: Fields Virology, ed 2. New York, Raven Press, 1990, pp 1679–1721.)

TABLE 239–1 ■ Classification of Human Adenoviruses (*Mastadenovirus* h)

SUBGROUP	SEROTYPES	ONCOGENICITY IN RODENTS	HEMAGGLUTINATION Subgroup	HEMAGGLUTINATION Species*	GUANINE + CYTOSINE (%) OF DNA
A	12, 18, 31	High	3B†	R‡	48–49
B	3, 7, 11, 16, 34, 35	Weak	1A	My	50–52
	14, 21	Weak	1B§	My	
C	1, 2, 5, 6	Negative	3A	R‡	57–59
D‖	8, 9, 37	Negative	2A	R, Mo, H, Gp, D	57–61
	10, 19, 26, 27, 36, 38, 39	Negative	2B	R, Mo, H	
	13, 43	Negative	2C	R, Mo, H, My	
	15, 22, 23, 30, 44, 45, 46, 47	Negative	2D	R, Mo, My	
	17, 24, 32, 33, 42	Negative	2E	R, Mo	
	20, 25, 28, 29	Negative	2F§	R, My	
E	4	Negative	3A	R‡	57–59
F	40, 41	Negative	3A§	R‡	

*R, Rat; My, monkey, Mo, mouse; H, human; GP, guinea pig; D, dog.
†Very low titers.
‡Designates incomplete or atypical reaction.
§Moderate-range titers.
‖Two new serotypes, 48 and 49, are not included.[14]
Adapted from Horwitz MS: Adenoviridae and their replication. *In* Fields BN, Knipe DM (eds): Fields Virology, ed 2. New York, Raven Press, 1990, pp 1679–1721; and Hierholzer JC: Adenoviruses. *In* Balows A, Hausler WJ Jr, Herrmann KL, et al (eds): Manual of Clinical Microbiology, ed 5. Washington, DC, American Society for Microbiology, 1990, pp 896–903.

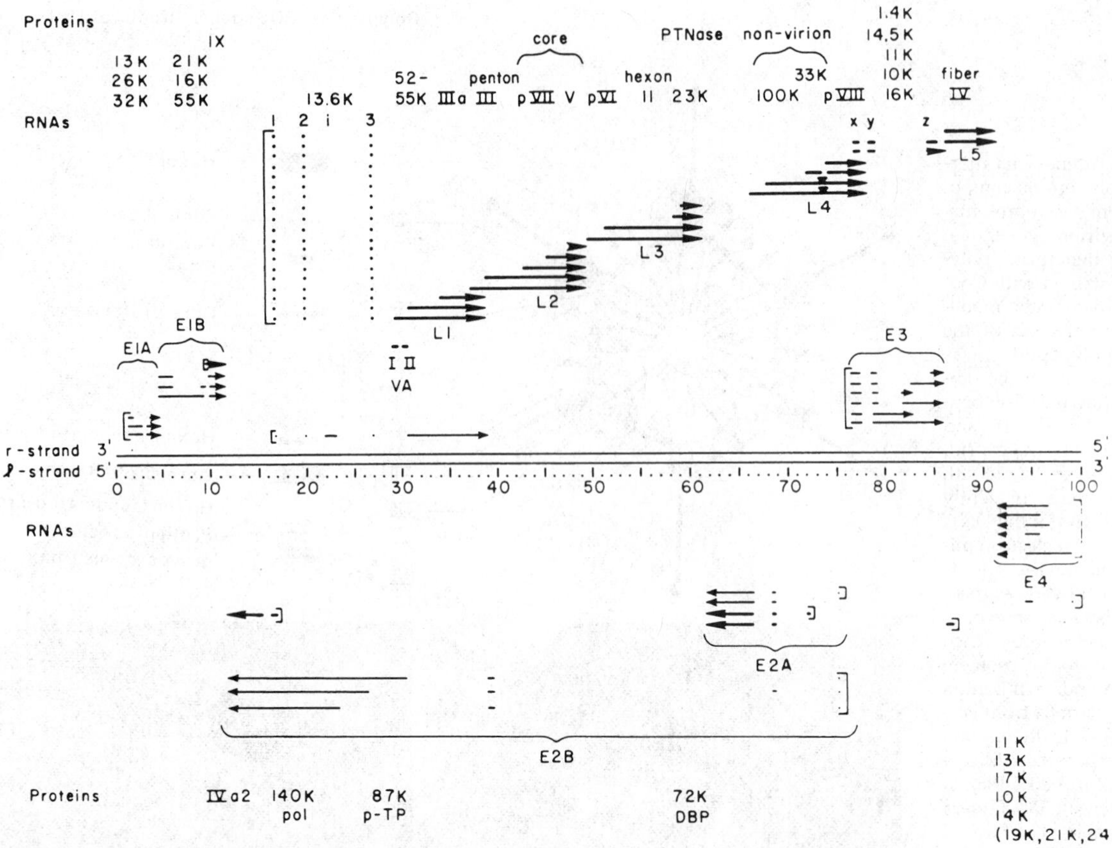

FIGURE 239–2 □ Transcription and translation map of early and late messenger RNA (mRNA) and protein products of adenovirus serotype 2. The thin lines represent early (E), and the thick lines, late (L) transcripts, with the arrowheads pointing in the 5′ to 3′ direction. L transcripts start at 16.3 map units and use the tripartite leader (1, 2, 3); for E transcripts also synthesized late, the arrow is also thick. Structural polypeptides are designated by roman numerals that correspond to polypeptides in Figure 239–1*A*; proteins synthesized as precursors that are later cleaved are designated by p. Nonstructural proteins are listed by size in kilodaltons (K). (Reprinted with permission from Broker TR: Animal virus RNA processing. *In* Apirion D [ed]: Processing of RNA. Boca Raton, FL, CRC Press, 1984, pp 181–212. Copyright CRC Press, Boca Raton, Florida.)

from its association with this protein and allowing E2F to transactivate other early viral genes such as E2. During the transformation cycle in rodent cells, this process alters transcription of mRNAs for proteins required for control of the cell cycle.[43] The function of E1A is augmented by proteins from the E1B region whose major function is to interact with the p53 antioncogene and prevent apoptosis.[44, 45] Inhibition of apoptosis early in infection could contribute to the survival of the cell until viral progeny are produced during the lytic cycle. During the transformation process in rodents, E1B could promote the immortalization of cells whose cell cycle control had been dysregulated by the E1A functions. The adenovirus structural proteins are synthesized primarily after viral DNA replication has been initiated. Viral DNA enters preformed empty capsids, assembled in the nucleus, to produce new progeny virus. Most of the structural proteins are synthesized from "late" mRNAs that originate at the strong major late promoter at 16.3 map units (see Fig. 239–2) and undergo multiple splices before functional mRNA is formed (reviewed in Philipson[46]). In fact, splicing of eukaryotic mRNAs was discovered in the adenovirus system.[47, 48]

Classification

Human adenoviruses are classified into subgroups by the hemagglutination pattern of red blood cells, the ability to cause tumors in rodents, or percentage of guanine plus cytosine content of their DNA (see Table 239–1). These viruses are included in the genus *Mastadenovirus,* which contains other viruses that infect simian, bovine, canine, and other mammals.[49] Aviadenoviruses contain additional members that naturally infect birds. Adenoviruses remain species specific in their natural patterns of infection and induction of disease; however, human serum samples have been shown to have antibodies to simian, canine, and bovine adenoviruses (reviewed in Taylor[50]). The guanine plus cytosine content of DNA is also reflected in sequence homology, which should be greater than 50% by hybridization of the entire viral genome for adenoviruses to be classified in the same subgroup.[51] There is some clinical significance to the classification scheme in that the manifestations of adenovirus diseases often correlate with the subgroup (Table 239–2). For example, when adenoviruses cause upper respiratory tract infections in children, they are usually group C agents, type 1, 2, 5, or 6. Adenoviruses related to lower respiratory tract infection and pneumonia are often group B, types 3, 7, and 21, or group E, type 4. Epidemic keratoconjunctivitis is most often associated with group D adenoviruses, type 8, 19, or 37. Hemorrhagic cystitis in normal children is often caused by a subgroup B adenovirus, type 11 or 21, whereas, persistent adenoviruses in the urinary tract in immunosuppressed patients are also commonly group B, serotypes 34 and 35. Although adenoviruses of a variety of subgroups can be isolated from fecal samples, only subgroup F, types 40 and 41, appear to cause diarrhea. Subgroup A is also commonly isolated from stool specimens but is not often associated with any disease syndrome other than an occasional case of meningoencephalitis in humans; however, it is highly oncogenic after experimental infection of hamsters. These patterns are not absolute, and exceptions to these serotype patterns do occur. Approximately two thirds of all adenovirus serotypes are uncommonly isolated, and their relationship with diseases is poorly defined. Human adenoviruses show a strong preference for growth in human tissue culture as described in the later section on viral diagnosis.

Pathogenesis

Manifestations of adenovirus diseases are probably the results of the cytolytic properties of the virus as well as the immunologic and cytokine responses of the host. In tissue-cultured cells, adenoviruses can lyse cells by inhibiting both host macromolecular synthesis[52] and transport of cellular mRNA to the cytoplasm.[53] The initial immune response probably is natural killer cell and monocyte recognition of infected cells, which evokes a cytokine response of interleukins-1 and -6 and tumor necrosis factor-α, as demonstrated in animal models.[54, 55] This phase is followed by the induction of cytotoxic T cells and the appearance of a variety of neutralizing and nonneutralizing antibodies to viral components such as hexon, fiber, and penton base (reviewed in Pirofski and Horwitz[24]). Elevated levels of interleukins-6 and -8 and tumor necrosis factor-α in serum during adenovirus infection correlate with more severe adenovirus infections in humans.[56] Adenoviruses also elaborate excess amounts of their penton base protein, which causes cells to round up and detach from tissue culture monolayers.[57] Such effects may be cytotoxic in vivo, and penton base protein has been demonstrated in the blood obtained from a few patients with fatal adenovirus pneumonia,[58] but the significance of this mechanism in most adenovirus-infected patients has not been further clarified.

Adenoviruses contain genes whose products can affect the immune response (reviewed in references 37, 59). The virus-associated RNA can inhibit the action of interferons (reviewed in Kitajewski and colleagues[60] and Mathews and Shenk[61]), and the E1B proteins inhibit apoptosis,[45] which otherwise might abort the production of adenoviruses in infected cells. An adenovirus E3 gene codes for a 19-kDa glycoprotein that retains the class I major histocompatibility complex in the endoplasmic reticulum and reduces the amount of this complex on the plasma membrane. This mechanism inhibits the presentation of viral peptides that are the signals for cytotoxic T-cell lysis.[59] Because various herpesviruses have been demonstrated to have comparable mechanisms for reducing cytotoxic T-cell lysis by inhibiting the cellular transporters of peptides to the class I major histocompatibility complex,[62] this general process to prevent immune cytolysis may be important in viral pathogenesis. Other E3 proteins inhibit tumor necrosis factor-α–mediated cytolysis and might also be directed at preventing destruction of infected cells before the full amount of adenovirus is produced.[63] Although the structural differences between these E3 genes from various adenovirus serotypes have not yet been correlated with differences in pathogenesis,[64] the concept that adenoviruses may control the manifestations of disease by altering the immune response is being actively pursued in animal models.[54, 55, 65, 66] Some of the histologic findings in adenoviral disease may be due to immunopathologic changes.[55] The effectiveness of the adenovirus E3 genes as antiinflammatory immunomodulators even when removed from the context of the virus has been shown in a number of animal models, including one in which functional E3 genes, placed into pancreatic islets, permitted the allogeneic transplantation of these immunologically altered donor cells.[38] Although adenoviruses do not cause transformation or tumors during infections of humans, they can remain latent or persistent within the human host.[66a] In addition to the intermittent shedding of adenoviruses for several years after a primary infection, even in the presence of a neutralizing antibody response,[67] adenovirus sequences have been found in human lymphocytes[68] and tonsils.[69] The prevalence of these sequences increases from childhood to adulthood, further suggesting that they are acquired during infection. In addition, there has been a report of adenovirus sequences found in lung tissue from patients with chronic obstructive pulmonary disease.[70]

Clinical Features

Respiratory Diseases

CHILDREN

Approximately 5% of all upper respiratory infections in children younger than 5 years[71] and 10% of pneumonias of childhood[72] are caused by adenoviruses. Coryza, cough, and a follicular distribution of exudate on the tonsils may be confused with other respiratory viruses (parainfluenza, influenza, and respiratory syncytial viruses) or group A streptococcal infection.[73, 74] Systemic manifestations such as fever,

TABLE 239–2 ■ Illnesses Associated with Adenovirus Infections

DISEASE	INDIVIDUALS MOST AT RISK	PRINCIPAL SEROTYPES
Acute febrile pharyngitis	Infants, young children	1–3, 5–7
Pharyngoconjunctival fever	School-age children	3, 7, 14
Acute respiratory disease	Military recruits	3, 4, 7, 14, 21
Pneumonia	Infants, young children	1–3, 7
Pneumonia	Military recruits	4, 7
Epidemic keratoconjunctivitis	Any age group	8, 11, 19, 37
Pertussis-like syndrome	Infants, young children	5
Acute hemorrhagic cystitis	Young children	11, 21
Gastroenteritis	Infants, young children	40, 41
Meningoencephalitis	Children and immunocompromised hosts	7, 12, 32
Hepatitis	Infants and children with liver transplants	1, 2, 5
Persistence of virus in urinary tract	Bone marrow transplant recipients, patients with acquired or other immunodeficiency syndrome or other immunosuppression	34, 35

Modified from Kasel JA: Adenoviruses. *In* Lennette EH, Schmidt NJ (eds): Diagnostic Procedures for Viral, Rickettsial and Chlamydial Infections, ed 5. Washington, DC, American Public Health Association, 1979, pp 229–256. Copyright 1979 by the American Public Health Association. Reprinted with permission; and Horwitz MS: Adenoviruses. *In* Fields BN, Knipe DM (eds): Fields Virology, ed 2. New York, Raven Press, 1990, pp 1723–1740.

malaise, myalgia, and headache may accompany these infections, which are commonly due to serotype 1, 2, 5, or 6 (subgroup C) or occasionally serotype 3 (subgroup B). When pneumonia occurs with these agents, it is usually mild to moderate in severity with subsequent recovery in most patients. However, there have been severe cases of adenovirus type 7 or type 21 pneumonias with residual pulmonary damage such as bronchiectasis or fatalities.[75, 76] The relationship between adenovirus infection and the whooping cough syndrome has received considerable attention. Although adenovirus infection can occasionally be accompanied by a severe cough and lymphocytosis,[77] whooping cough is caused by *Bordetella pertussis* and does not require adenoviruses as obligate coinfecting organisms.[78] However, it has been noted that during *B. pertussis* infections, adenoviruses are isolated more frequently than from control subjects.[79] Whether the extensive cough or putative cytokine release during *Bordetella* infection facilitates the isolation of adenoviruses has not been resolved.

ADULTS

Adults can develop similar respiratory symptoms with manifestations limited to the upper respiratory tract or extension to the lungs in the form of pneumonia.[80] The serotypes involved are usually 4, 7, and occasionally 3. The change in serotypes reflects the immunity that most people develop to types 1, 2, 5, and 6 during childhood. Adenovirus disease, especially early after induction into the military services with the accompanying crowding, fatigue, and new exposure to infectious diseases, was called ARD (acute respiratory disease).[81] ARD often affected many of the new recruits, causing tracheobronchitis and pneumonia requiring hospitalization. Although complete recovery was usual after 3 to 5 days of illness from adenovirus-induced ARD, the disruption of military maneuvers prompted the development of vaccines against types 4 and 7 (see later).

Pharyngoconjunctival Fever

Although adenoviral pharyngoconjunctival fever can occur sporadically, it usually appears as small outbreaks in children, especially in summer camps.[82] A granular palpebral and bulbar conjunctivitis, which may sequentially affect both eyes, is often accompanied by a febrile pharyngitis, cervical adenitis, and rhinitis.[83, 84] The incubation period is 6 to 9 days but was shorter in experimentally infected volunteers.[85, 86] Symptoms lasted 3 to 5 days, and there were usually no sequelae. Adenovirus serotypes most commonly involved, especially when a common source such as a pool or lake was incriminated in swimming pool conjunctivitis, were types 3 and 7[87]; however, many other serotypes from subgroups B, C, D, and E have been implicated in this disease. Although the epidemiologic association with a common source has been strong and adenoviruses are isolated from conjunctival swabs from infected patients, the virus has not been isolated from water samples from the implicated source.

Epidemic Keratoconjunctivitis

Epidemic keratoconjunctivitis is a more serious adenovirus infection of the eye that is highly contagious. It is caused by type 8, 19, or 37 and begins after an 8- to 10-day incubation period.[88–90] A follicular conjunctivitis accompanied by lid edema, photophobia, lacrimation, and pain is commonly followed by corneal infiltration of the subepithelial layer. Preauricular adenopathy is a common finding, and the initially unilateral disease often spreads to the other eye. If the disease progresses to a hemorrhagic conjunctivitis, it may be difficult to distinguish from that caused by enterovirus type 70. Although the inflammatory phase may last several weeks before resolution, corneal opacities may require months or even years to completely resolve. In adults, constitutional symptoms are not common, but children may have generalized adenopathy and fever.

Acute Hemorrhagic Cystitis

Hemorrhagic cystitis in the immunocompetent host is usually a self-limited infection with serotype 11 or 21 and is more common in males.[91, 92] The gross hematuria must be distinguished from more serious renal diseases and bacterial infections of the urinary tract. Children between the ages of 6 and 15 years are more commonly affected. They usually are afebrile and do not have any renal functional abnormalities. This disease also occurs in immunosuppressed patients such as renal transplant recipients in whom the infectious adenoviruses, including types 34 and 35, may have been latent in the transplanted kidney.[93, 94] Cytotoxic immunosupressive drugs in the latter setting may also cause red blood cells to appear in the urine, and some patients have hematuria from both of these processes.[95]

Gastrointestinal Disease

Although many adenovirus serotypes can be isolated from the intestine during respiratory adenovirus infections or even from asymptomatic children, only types 40 and 41 (subgroup F) appear to be associated with diarrhea.[96–98] Nosocomial infections have been reported from pediatric wards in patients younger than 4 years, and respiratory symptoms often accompany the gastrointestinal disease.[98] The incidence of diarrhea caused by adenoviruses varies greatly in the various reports; however, rotaviruses usually are the more common etiologic agents in most of these studies.[99] During outbreaks of adenovirus diarrhea in daycare settings, many unaffected children will also be found to have the agent in their stool samples.[100] By the age of 4 years, 50% of children have antibodies to the enteric adenoviruses.[101, 102] Intussusception has also been linked to adenovirus infection but not to the enteric types.[103, 104]

Adenovirus serotypes 1, 2, 5, and 6 (subgroup C) have been isolated from children with intussusception both from intestinal lymph nodes removed during surgery for bowel resection and from stool samples. Whether the enlarged mesenteric lymph nodes that might accompany an adenovirus infection could serve as a lead point for the intussusception or whether the hypermotility of irritated bowel is more likely to cause telescoping of the intestine has not been clarified.[105] Because most patients with intussusception do not have evidence of adenovirus infection, the role of virus infection in this syndrome has not been elucidated further.

Because there is some structural homology between the adenovirus type 12 E1B protein and A-gliadin, which is a component of wheat proteins known to activate celiac disease, a role of virus infection in inducing or aggravating this malabsorption syndrome has been proposed. Molecular mimicry can result in cross-reacting antibodies between A-gliadin and the adenovirus E1B protein.[106] Although adenovirus type 12 can persist in the intestine for long periods, its relationship with gluten-induced enteropathy has not been resolved.[107, 108]

Meningoencephalitis

Adenoviruses have been isolated from brain and cerebrospinal fluid obtained from patients with meningoencephalitis but are not a common cause of this disease.[109, 110] Meningoencephalitis has accompanied outbreaks of type 7 pneumonia, but in most of these cases the virus was isolated from extraneural sites.[111] There are no pathognomonic findings to distinguish adenovirus infections of the central nervous system from those caused by other etiologic agents.

Adenovirus Infections in Immunocompromised Hosts

Adenovirus infections of various organs and by different serotypes are usually more severe in immunocompromised patients,[112–114] even those with isolated hypogammaglobulinemia.[115] However, several situations deserve further elaboration. Hepatitis due to common group C serotypes (1, 2, and 5) is a problem after pediatric liver transplantation.[8, 116] It is not clear whether the infection is acute or results from reactivation of latent virus in the transplant or the tissues of the host. Of 484 pediatric hepatic transplantation patients, 49 had adenoviruses isolated from at least one sampled site, 20 had invasive disease, and 9 died.[8] Discontinuation of immunosuppressive therapy at the time of severe adenovirus infection has not always been successful in reversing the effects of the virus infection. Adenovirus hepatitis has also ended fatally in patients with the severe combined immunodeficiency syndrome, acquired immunodeficiency syndrome (AIDS), and bone marrow transplantation.

In AIDS patients, subgroup B adenoviruses were found in 12% of urine samples,[29] and subgroup D adenoviruses of multiple serotypes have been isolated from numerous stool samples. In 21% of bone marrow transplant recipients, subgroup B adenoviruses (primarily types 34 and 35) were isolated and significant disease occurred in 6.5%[117]; however, full evaluation of these latter agents revealed that some of them had hemagglutinins of other group B serotypes, indicating that there had been intrasubgroup recombination. The presence of adenoviruses in stool samples and at the site of colonic damage in AIDS patients has suggested that these agents might be responsible for some of their cases of chronic diarrhea.[118] However, most of the gastrointestinal problems in AIDS patients are probably due to other causes.

Epidemiology

Adenoviruses are ubiquitous agents that cause both sporadic and epidemic diseases. Each mammalian species has distinct adenovirus serotypes that share structural and some antigenic cross-reactivity with human adenoviruses[49]; however, there is no significant crossover of infectivity from animals to humans (reviewed in Taylor[50]). From longitudinal epidemologic observations[71, 119] and "virus watch" studies performed in New York and Seattle,[67, 120] a number of seminal observations have been made: (1) many adenovirus infections documented by virus isolation or serology were asymptomatic; (2) there is a high degree of intermittent adenovirus shedding, especially in stool specimens; (3) 7% of febrile illnesses in children are due to adenovirus infection. Group C serotypes 1, 2, and 5 are most common during childhood, and 40% to 60% of older children have antibodies to these types[71, 121, 122]; infection with types 3, 4, and 7 are uncommon in childhood, and thus these serotypes are more common as causes of respiratory disease in adults. Group B serotypes 11, 21, 34, and 35 have a predilection for the urinary tract[91, 92, 123] but can also cause pneumonias.[114] Group F serotypes 40 and 41 cause diarrhea in young children,[96–98] but group D serotypes are often isolated from stool samples of adult AIDS patients.[118] Group D adenoviruses of three serotypes (8, 19, and 37) are responsible for most cases of epidemic keratoconjunctivitis.[88–90] Epidemic keratoconjunctivitis formerly followed infections that could be traced to contaminated ophthalmologic equipment, when tonometers that contacted the corneas were used. However, as a highly transmissable infection, direct person-to-person spread and spread from contaminated objects such as shared towels are currently more common.

The biochemical basis of relative serotype specificity for each of these disease syndromes or sites of adenovirus replication have not been elucidated (see the section on pathogenesis). The unique occurence during World War II of ARD in new military recruits and the failure of ARD to spread to their civilian contacts was contrasted with influenza outbreaks in which there was no such separation of involved persons.[11, 124, 125] This is even more surprising because controlled studies showed, that during type 4 or 7 experimental infections, the infection was airborne.[126] Most other adenovirus transmissions are contact infections (either person to person, water-borne for adenoviral pharyngoconjunctival fever, or from contaminated instruments for some cases of epidemic keratoconjunctivitis). Additional information about the epidemiology appears in the sections describing each of the adenovirus syndromes.

Diagnosis

Except for keratoconjunctivitis, adenovirus syndromes are difficult to diagnose by clinical criteria without the help of the laboratory. Laboratory diagnosis may be required for epidemiologic characterization of outbreaks, including hospital-acquired adenovirus gastroenteritis, serious cases of pneumonia that can occur even in immunocompetent hosts, and the hepatitis that complicates therapy of immunosuppressed patients, including liver transplant recipients. Tissue biopsies or exfoliated cells may show intranuclear inclusions (characteristically without giant cell formation) or cell degeneration, described as smudge cell formation, particularly in pulmonary tissue (Fig. 239–3). Virus isolation is more reliable than histologic study and begins with inoculation of patient samples into tissue culture cells of human origin. Primary human embryonic kidney is optimal but expensive and is often replaced by a human continuous lung line, A549.[127] The 293 cell, which was derived by transformation of human embryonic kidney with the adenovirus E1 genes,[128] is often used when isolation of enteric adenoviruses is attempted.[129, 130] The E1B 55-kDa gene appears to facilitate the isolation of enteric adenoviruses.[131] Although a variety of antigen detection techniques are available for examining exfoliated cells[132, 133] and latex agglutination tests have been developed for stool sample diagnosis of enteric adenovirus infections,[134] both appear to be inferior to the sensitivity and specificity of polymerase chain reaction–based techniques.[135–137] Polymerase chain reaction, however, remains available only in research laboratories, and questions about specificity have been raised.[138] Once an adenovirus suspected because of typical tissue culture cytopathologic findings has been isolated, it is usually confirmed by group-specific reference sera.[50, 139] Subsequently, serotype can be determined by first grouping the isolate by hemagglutination pattern with rat and rhesus red blood cells and then by HI.[27, 140] Further characterization by neutralization of growth with type-specific sera prepared in various animals can be done.[27] When there is a discrepancy between serum neutralization and HI typing, the isolate is classified by numbers corresponding to serum neutralization and HI, which usually indicates recombination of adenoviruses within a subgroup.[30, 123, 141] This can be further clarified by looking at the entire viral genome using restriction endonuclease digestion to indicate the pattern of sequence-specific sites of cleavage. If *Sma*I digestion is supplemented by the use of several other restriction endonucleases, differences between serotypes and the presence of recombinants usually

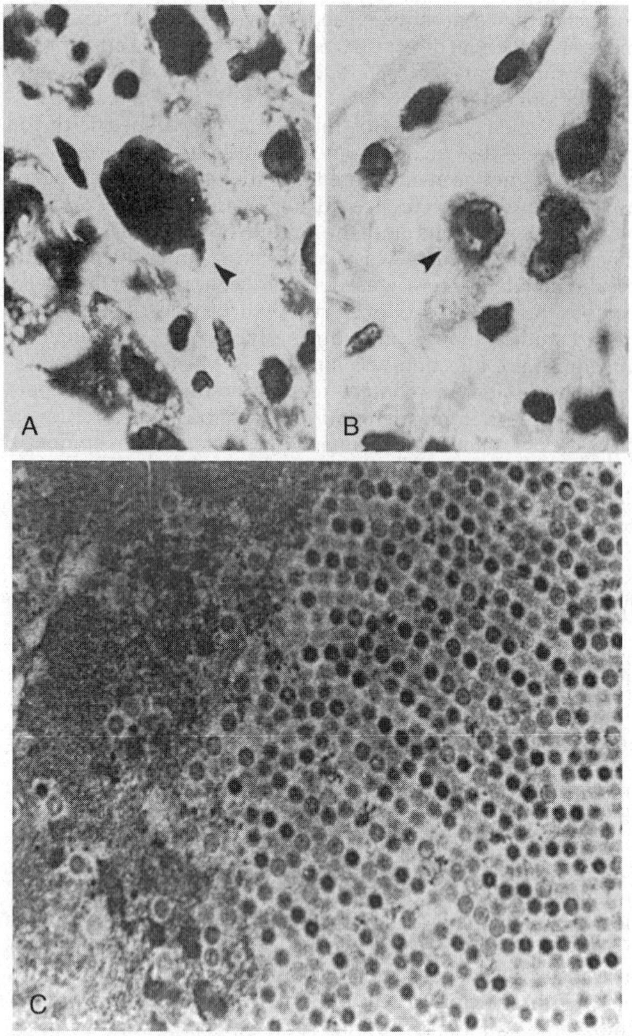

FIGURE 239–3 □ Adenovirus cytopathologic findings in human tissue. A "smudge cell" *(A)* designated by an arrow is shown in lung tissue from a fatal case of adenovirus pneumonia; a basophilic inclusion fills the nucleus and obliterates the nuclear membrane of a desquamated alveolar cell. A smaller intranuclear inclusion *(B)* contains many virions *(C)*, as illustrated by electron microscopy. (*A* to *C* from Myerowitz RL, Stalder H, Oxman MN, et al: Fatal disseminated adenovirus infection in a renal transplant recipient. Am J Med 59:591–598, 1975. Adapted with permission from American Journal of Medicine.)

can be detected.[123, 142, 143] Serologic diagnosis on paired serum samples to search for rising antibody titers between the acute and convalescence phase of an illness can also be done by a variety of techniques that have included complement fixation, HI,[144] serum neutralization,[145] and enzyme-linked immunoabsorbent assay[146] (reviewed in Hierholzer[26]).

Therapy

There are no effective antiviral agents, either for systemic use or for topical administration to the eyes, that have been proved to benefit patients with any of the adenovirus syndromes; however, many antiviral compounds inhibit adenovirus replication in tissue culture.[147–150] One of these agents [(*S*)-1-(3-hydroxy-2-phosphonylmethoxypropyl)cytosine] has been tried with some limited success as a topical agent in a rabbit ocular model of infection with adenovirus type 5.[151] Ribavirin has been used to treat hemorrhagic cystitis in several human bone marrow transplant patients, but no controlled trials are available to judge its efficacy.[95] Treatment of adenovirus infections is thus symptomatic and supportive, with recovery in most cases except for immunosuppressed patients with hepatitis and some cases of pneumonia. There are fatalities reported from adenovirus type 7 pneumonia even in immunocompetent patients, and a particularly virulent form (adenovirus type 7h) circulating in South America was reported in 1993.[152]

Prevention

Oral enteric-coated adenovirus serotypes 4 and 7 live vaccines exist for prevention of ARD in military recruits and have been effective.[153, 154] These serotypes have been attenuated only by physically coating the infectious agent to bypass the oropharynx and be displayed first in the intestine. They are not available for civilian populations, because the diseases they prevent are not as dramatic as ARD epidemics and most are self-limited. In addition, there has been some reluctance to use adenovirus vaccines in the general population, because these viruses have transforming genes[3, 5]; however, after several decades of use on young adults in the military, there is no evidence that these vaccine viruses are harmful in humans (reviewed in Horwitz[155]). Early batches of these adenovirus vaccines were contaminated by recombinant adenovirus–simian virus 40 hybrid strains,[156, 157] and simian virus 40 is oncogenic in rodents. However, this problem of simian virus 40 contamination introduced by using monkey kidney tissue culture has been completely eliminated by newer tissue culture and detection techniques.

Adenoviruses as Vectors for Delivery of Therapeutic Genes

Adenoviruses are currently being explored intensively as tools for the delivery of foreign DNAs.[1, 158] The goal of introducing DNA in such vectors is either to overexpress epitopes for immunization against a great variety of other infectious agents,[159] or to correct a genetic defect in the recipient cell, animal[160–162] or human.[163–166] Some of the advantages of adenovirus vectors (in contrast to retrovirus vectors) are that they can express genes in nonreplicating cells. Adenoviruses can be grown to high titers and are thus available in large quantities for subsequent use. Most of the foreign DNA inserted into adenoviruses used to deliver immunogenic proteins has involved substitutions in place of the E3 region, which is not essential for virus growth in tissue culture. Proteins such as the hepatitis B surface[159] or core antigen, the glycoprotein of rabies virus,[167] various human immunodeficiency virus type 1 proteins,[168] and numerous others have been expressed as immunogens in the E3 region of adenoviruses.

In contrast, adenoviruses used as vectors usually have both the E3 and E1 regions deleted to make the vectors' replication incompetent in the recipient host and to accommodate large inserts, up to 8.3 kb of foreign DNA, within the capsid. These defective adenoviruses can be grown in human embryonic kidney 293 cells, which were described earlier. Numerous genes have been inserted into the adenovirus E1 region. The *CFTR* gene, which is defective in cystic fibrosis, has been inserted into adenovirus vectors and has undergone limited safety trials in patients with cystic fibrosis.[169, 170] One of the problems with the use of adenovirus delivery systems is the type-specific immune response to the vector itself. It appears that both humoral and T-cell–based immunity decrease the longevity of foreign gene expression from adenovirus vectors.[171] Although recloning an immunogenic foreign protein into multiple distinct adenovirus serotypes might overcome the problem of repeated administration of such a protein to elicit an immune response,[172] such an approach would appear impractical when considering lifelong administration of a gene product to correct a genetic defect. Adenoviruses can also facilitate the entry of aggregates of foreign DNA complexed with polylysine external to the virion.[173–175] Although this last technique is useful for introducing DNA into tissue-cultured cells and may be helpful in local introduction of genes into animals, it is not effective for systemic instillation and expression of genes.

The reinsertion of the E3 region, which might abrogate some class I cytotoxic T-cell– and tumor necrosis factor-α–mediated responses (see section on pathogenesis), is under active investigation to decrease the immunogenicity of the vector. We have been successful in engineering an E3-containing adenovirus vector that elicited only low levels of virus-specific cytotoxic T cells and virtually no antibody response in a rat model. Because of this "immunologic ignorance," we were able to readminister the viral vector to achieve long-term expression of a therapeutic gene in such an animal model.[176] Thus, in addition to the role of adenoviruses as disease-causing agents described in this chapter, adenoviruses and their immunoregulatory genes might eventually be useful as therapeutic agents in a variety of clinical situations.

References

1. Grunhaus A, Horwitz MS: Adenoviruses as cloning vectors. *In* Rice C (ed): Seminars in Virology. London, WB Saunders, 1992, pp 237–252.
2. Bett AJ, Haddara W, Prevec L, et al: An efficient and flexible system for construction of adenovirus vectors with insertions or deletions in early regions 1 and 3. Proc Natl Acad Sci USA 91:8802–8806, 1994.
3. Trentin JJ, Yabe Y, Taylor G: The quest for human cancer viruses. Science 137:835–849, 1962.
4. Huebner RJ, Casey MJ, Chanock RM, et al: Tumors induced in hamsters by a strain of adenovirus type 3. Sharing of tumor antigens and "neoantigens" with those produced by adenovirus type 7 tumors. Proc Natl Acad Sci USA 54:381–388, 1965.
5. Shenk T: Adenoviridae: The viruses and their replication. *In* Fields BN, Knipe DM, Howley PM (eds): Fields Virology, ed 3. Philadelphia, Lippincott-Raven, 1996, pp 2111–2148.
6. Wold WSM, Mackey JK, Rigden P, et al: Analysis of human cancer DNAs for DNA sequences of human adenovirus serotypes 3, 7, 11, 14, 16, and 21 in group B. Cancer Res 39:3479–3484, 1979.
7. Krilov LR, Rubin LG, Frogel M, et al: Disseminated adenovirus infection with hepatic necrosis in patients with human immunodeficiency virus infection and other immunodeficiency states. Rev Infect Dis 12:303–307, 1990.
8. Michaels MG, Green M, Wald ER, et al: Adenovirus infection in pediatric liver transplant recipients. J Infect Dis 165:170–174, 1992.
9. Rowe WP, Huebner RJ, Gillmore LK, et al: Isolation of a cytopathogenic agent from human adenoids undergoing spontaneous degeneration in tissue culture. Proc Soc Exp Biol Med 84:570–573, 1953.
10. Hilleman MR, Werner JH: Recovery of new agents from patients with acute respiratory illness. Proc Soc Exp Biol Med 85:183–188, 1954.
11. Hilleman MR: Epidemiology of adenovirus respiratory infections in military recruit populations. Ann N Y Acad Sci 67:262–272, 1957.
12. Dingle J, Langmuir AD: Epidemiology of acute respiratory disease in military recruits. Am Rev Respir Dis 97:1–65, 1968.
13. Commission on Acute Respiratory Disease: Experimental transmission of minor respiratory illness to human volunteers by filter-passing agents. Demonstration of two illnesses characterized by long and short incubation periods and different clinical features. J Clin Invest 26:957–973, 1947.
14. Schnurr D, Dondero ME: Two new candidate adenovirus serotypes. Intervirology 36:79–83, 1993.
15. Jawetz E: The story of shipyard eye. Br Med J 1:873–878, 1959.
16. Stewart PL, Fuller SD, Burnett RM: Difference imaging of adenovirus: bridging the resolution gap between X-ray crystallography and electron microscopy. EMBO J 12:2589–2599, 1993.
17. Kidd AH, Chroboczek J, Cusack S, et al: Adenovirus type 40 virions contain two distinct fibers. Virology 192:73–84, 1993.
18. Green NM, Wrigley NG, Russell WC, et al: Evidence for a repeating cross-β sheet structure in the adenovirus fibre. EMBO J 2:1357–1365, 1983.
19. Maizel JV Jr, White DO, Scharff MD: The polypeptides of adenovirus. II. Soluble proteins, cores, top components and structure of the virion. Virology 36:126–136, 1968.
20. Maizel JV Jr, White DO, Scharff MD: The polypeptides of adenoviruses. I. Evidence for multiple protein components in the virion and a comparison of types 2, 7, 12. Virology 36:115–125, 1968.
21. Devaux C, Caillet-Boudin ML, Jacrot B, et al: Crystallization, enzymatic cleavage, and the polarity of the adenovirus type 2 fiber. Virology 161:121–128, 1987.
22. Belin M-T, Boulanger P: Involvement of cellular adhesion sequences in the attachment of adenovirus to the HeLa cell surface. J Gen Virol 74:1485–1497, 1993.

22a. Bergelson JM, Cunningham JA, Kurt-Jones E, et al: Isolation of a common receptor for coxsackie B viruses and adenoviruses 2 and 5. Science (in press).

23. Friefeld BR, Lichy JH, Field J, et al: The in vitro replication of adenovirus DNA. Curr Top Microbiol Immunol 110:221–255, 1984.
24. Pirofski L, Horwitz MS: Adenovirus, infection and immunity. *In* Roitt IV, Delves PS (eds): Encyclopedia of Immunology. London, Academic Press, 1992, pp 19–22.
25. Norrby E, Van der Veen J, Espmark A: A new serological technique for identification of adenovirus infections. Proc Soc Exp Biol Med 134:889–895, 1970.
26. Hierholzer JC: Adenoviruses. *In* Balows A, Hausler WJ Jr, Herrmann KL, et al (eds): Manual of Clinical Microbiology, ed 5. Washington, DC, American Society for Microbiology, 1991, pp 896–903.
27. Hierholzer JC: Further subgrouping of the human adenoviruses by differential hemagglutination. J Infect Dis 128:541–550, 1973.
28. Horwitz MS: Adenoviridae and their replication. *In* Fields BN, Knipe DM, Chanock RM, et al (eds): Virology, ed 2. New York, Raven Press, 1990, pp 1679–1721.
29. Horwitz MS, Valderrama G, Hatcher V, et al: Characterization of adenovirus isolates from AIDS patients. Ann N Y Acad Sci 437:161–174, 1985.
30. Hierholzer JC, Wigand R, Anderson LJ, et al: Adenovirus from patients with AIDS: A plethora of serotypes and a description of five new serotypes of subgenus D (types 43–47). J Infect Dis 158:804–813, 1988.
31. Gruber WC, Russell DJ, Tibbetts C: Fiber gene and genomic origin of human adenovirus type 4. Virology 196:603–611, 1993.
32. Wickham TJ, Mathias P, Cheresch DA, et al: Integrins of alpha v beta 3 and alpha v beta 5 promote adenovirus internalization but not virus attachment. Cell 73:309–319, 1993.
33. Pastan I, Seth P, FitzGerald D, et al: Adenovirus entry into cells: Some new observations on an old problem. *In* Notkins AL, Oldstone MBA (eds): Concepts in Viral Pathogenesis II. New York, Springer-Verlag, 1986, pp 141–146.
34. Greber UF, Willetts M, Webster P, et al: Stepwise dismantling of adenovirus 2 during entry into cells. Cell 75:477–486, 1993.
35. Tooze J: DNA Tumor Viruses, ed 2. Cold Spring Harbor, NY, Cold Spring Harbor Laboratory, 1981, pp 943–1054.
36. Chen M, Mermod N, Horwitz MS: Protein-protein interactions between adenovirus DNA polymerase and nuclear factor I mediate formation of the DNA replication preinitiation complexes. J Biol Chem 265:18634–18642, 1990.
37. Wold WSM, Tollefson AE, Hermiston TW: The E3 transcription unit of adenovirus. Curr Top Microbiol Immunol 199:237–274, 1995.
38. Efrat S, Fejer G, Brownlee M, et al: Prolonged survival of pan-

creatic islet allografts mediated by adenovirus immunoregulatory transgenes. Proc Natl Acad Sci USA 92:6947–6951, 1995.
39. Babiss LE, Ginsberg HS, Darnell JE Jr: Adenovirus E1B proteins are required for accumulation of late viral mRNA and for effects on cellular mRNA translation and transport. Mol Cell Biol 5:2552–2558, 1985.
40. Gallimore PH: Tumour production in immunosuppressed rats with cells transformed in vitro by adenovirus type 2. J Gen Virol 16:99–102, 1972.
41. Whyte P, Buchkovich KJ, Horowitz JM, et al: Association between an oncogene and an anti-oncogene: The adenovirus E1A proteins bind to the retinoblastoma gene product. Nature 334:124–129, 1988.
42. Howe JA, Bayley ST: Effects of Ad5 E1A mutant viruses on the cell cycle in relation to the binding of cellular proteins including the retinoblastoma protein and cyclin A. Virology 186:15–24, 1992.
43. Faha B, Harlow E, Lees E: The adenovirus E1A-associated kinase consists of cyclin E-p33cdk2 and cyclin A-p33cdk2. J Virol 67:2456–2465, 1993.
44. White E, Sabbatini P, Debbas M, et al: The 19-kilodalton adenovirus E1B transforming protein inhibits programmed cell death and prevents cytolysis by tumor necrosis factor α. Mol Cell Biol 12:2570–2580, 1992.
45. Rao L, Debbas M, Sabbatini P, et al: The adenovirus E1A proteins induce apoptosis, which is inhibited by the E1B 19-kDa and Bcl-2 proteins. Proc Natl Acad Sci USA 89:7742–7746, 1992.
46. Philipson L: Adenovirus assembly. *In* Ginsberg H (ed): The Adenoviruses. New York, Plenum Publishing, 1984, pp 309–337.
47. Berget SM, Moore C, Sharp PA: Spliced segments at the 5′ terminus of adenovirus 2 late mRNA. Proc Natl Acad Sci USA 74:3171–3175, 1977.
48. Chow LT, Roberts JM, Lewis JB, et al: A map of cytoplasmic RNA transcripts from lytic adenovirus type 2, determined by electron microscopy of RNA: DNA hybrids. Cell 11:819–836, 1977.
49. Ishibashi M, Yasue H: Adenoviruses of animals. *In* Ginsberg HS (ed): The Adenoviruses. New York, Plenum Publishing, 1984, pp 497–562.
50. Taylor PE: Adenoviruses: Diagnosis of infections. *In* Kurstak E, Kurstak C (eds): Comparative Diagnosis of Viral Disease. New York, Academic Press, 1977, pp 86–170.
51. Pina M, Green M: Biochemical studies on adenovirus multiplication. IX. Chemical and base composition analysis of 28 human adenoviruses. Proc Natl Acad Sci USA 54:547–551, 1965.
52. Horwitz MS: Intermediates in the synthesis of type 2 adenovirus deoxyribonucleic acid. J Virol 8:675–683, 1971.
53. Pilder S, More M, Logan J, et al: The adenovirus E1B-55K transforming polypeptide modulates transport or cytoplasmic stabilization of viral and host cell mRNAs. Mol Cell Biol 6:470–476, 1986.
54. Ginsberg HS, Moldawer LL, Sehgal PB, et al: A mouse model for investigating the molecular pathogenesis of adenovirus pneumonia. Proc Natl Acad Sci USA 88:1651–1655, 1991.
55. Prince GA, Porter DD, Jenson AB, et al: Pathogenesis of adenovirus type 5 pneumonia in cotton rats *(Sigmodon hispidus)*. J Virol 67:101–111, 1993.
56. Mistchenko AS, Diez RA, Mariani AL, et al: Cytokines in adenoviral disease in children: Association of interleukin-6, interleukin-8, and tumor necrosis factor alpha levels with clinical outcome. J Pediatr 124:714–719, 1994.
57. Bai M, Harfe B, Freimuth P: Mutations that alter an Arg-Gly-Asp (RGD) sequence in the adenovirus type 2 penton base protein abolish its cell-rounding activity and delay virus reproduction in flat cells. J Virol 67:5198–5205, 1993.
58. Ladisch S, Lovejoy FH, Hierholzer JC, et al: Extrapulmonary manifestations of adenovirus type 7 pneumonia simulating Reye syndrome and the possible role of adenovirus toxin. J Pediatr 95:348–355, 1979.
59. Wold WSM, Hermiston TW, Tollefson AE: Adenovirus proteins that subvert host defenses. Trends Microbiol 2:437–443, 1994.
60. Kitajewski J, Schneider RJ, Safer B, et al: Adenovirus VAI RNA antagonizes the antiviral action of interferon by preventing activation of the interferon-induced eIF-2 alpha kinase. Cell 45:195–200, 1986.
61. Mathews MB, Shenk T: Adenovirus virus-associated RNA and translation control (Review). J Virol 65:5657–5662, 1991.
62. Hill A, Jugovic P, York I, et al: Herpes simplex virus turns off the TAP to evade host immunity. Nature 375:411–415, 1995.
63. Wold WSM: Adenovirus genes that modulate the sensitivity of virus-infected cells to lysis by TNF. J Cell Biochem 53:329–335, 1993.
64. Flomenberg PR, Chen M, Horwitz MS: Characterization of a major histocompatibility complex class I antigen-binding glycoprotein from adenovirus type 35, a type associated with immunocompromised hosts. J Virol 61:3665–3671, 1987.
65. Tufariello J, Cho S, Horwitz MS: The adenovirus E3 14.7-kilodalton protein which inhibits cytolysis by tumor necrosis factor increases the virulence of vaccinia virus in a murine pneumonia model. J Virol 68:453–462, 1994.
66. Fejer G, Gyory I, Tufariello J, et al: Characterization of transgenic mice containing the adenovirus early region 3 genomic DNA. J Virol 68:5871–5881, 1994.
66a. Lukashok S, Horwitz MS: Adenovirus persistence. *In* Ahmed R, Chen I (eds): Persistent Viral Infections. London, John Wiley & Sons (in press).
67. Fox JP, Brandt CD, Wassermann FE, et al: The Virus Watch Program: A continuing surveillance of viral infections in metropolitan New York families. VI. Observations of adenovirus infections: Virus excretion patterns, antibody response, efficiency of surveillance, patterns of infection and relation to illness. Am J Epidemiol 89:25–50, 1969.
68. Horvath J, Palkonyay L, Weber J: Group C adenovirus DNA sequences in human lymphoid cell. J Virol 59:189–192, 1986.
69. Neumann R, Genersch E, Eggers HJ: Detection of adenovirus nucleic acid sequences in human tonsils in the absence of infectious virus. Virus Res 7:93–97, 1987.
70. Matsuse T, Hayashi S, Kuwano K, et al: Latent adenoviral infection in the pathogenesis of chronic airways obstruction. Am Rev Respir Dis 146:177–184, 1992.
71. Brandt CD, Kim HW, Vargosdo AJ: Infections in 18,000 infants and children in a controlled study of respiratory tract disease. I. Adenovirus pathogenicity in relation to serologic type and illness syndrome. Am J Epidemiol 90:484–500, 1969.
72. Mallet R, Riberre M, Bonnenfant F, et al: Les pneumopathies graves à adéno-virus. Arch Fr Pediatr 23:1057–1073, 1966.
73. Ginsberg HS, Gold E, Jordan WS Jr, et al: Relation of the new respiratory agents to acute respiratory diseases. Am J Public Health 45:915–922, 1955.
74. Harris DJ, Wulff R, Ray CG, et al: Viruses and disease. III. An outbreak of adenovirus type 7A in a children's home. Am J Epidemiol 93:399–402, 1971.
75. Lang WR, Howden CW, Laws J, et al: Bronchopneumonia with serious sequelae in children with evidence of adenovirus type 21 infection. Br Med J 1:73–79, 1969.
76. Simila S, Ylikorkala O, Wasz-Hockert O: Type 7 adenovirus pneumonia. J Pediatr 79:605–611, 1971.
77. Collier AM, Connor JD, Irving WR Jr: Generalized type 5 adenovirus infection associated with pertussis syndrome. J Pediatr 69:1073–1078, 1966.
78. Sturdy PM, Court SDM, Gardner PS: Viruses and whooping cough. Lancet 2:978–979, 1971.
79. Nelson KE, Gavitt F, Batt MD, et al: The role of adenoviruses in the pertussis syndrome. J Pediatr 86:335–341, 1975.
80. Mogabgab WJ: Mycoplasma pneumonia and adenovirus respiratory illnesses in military and university personnel, 1959–1966. Am Rev Respir Dis 97:345–358, 1968.
81. Miller LF, Rytel M, Pierce WE, et al: Epidemiology of nonbacterial pneumonia among naval recruits. JAMA 185:92–99, 1963.
82. Bell JA, Rowe WP, Engler JI, et al: Pharyngoconjunctival fever. Epidemiological studies of a recently recognized disease entity. JAMA 175:1083–1092, 1955.
83. Bennett FM, Law BB, Hamilton W, et al: Adenovirus eye infections in Aberdeen. Lancet 2:670–673, 1957.
84. Murray ES, Chang RS, Bell SD Jr, et al: Agents recovered from acute conjunctivitis cases in Saudia Arabia. Am J Ophthalmol 43:32–35, 1957.
85. Kaji M, Kimura M, Kamiya S, et al: An epidemic of pharyngoconjunctival fever among school children in an elementary school in Fukuoka Prefecture. Kyushu J Med Sci 12:1–8, 1961.
86. Bell JA, Ward TG, Huebner RJ, et al: Studies of adenoviruses (APC) in volunteers. Am J Public Health 46:1130–1146, 1956.

87. Foy HM, Cooney MK, Hatlen JG: Adenovirus type 3 epidemic associated with intermittent chlorination of a swimming pool. Arch Environ Health 17:795–802, 1968.
88. Dawson CR, O'Day D, Vastine D: Adenovirus 19, a cause of epidemic keratoconjunctivitis, not acute hemorrhagic conjunctivitis. N Engl J Med 293:45–46, 1975.
89. Dawson CR, Hanna L, Wood TR, et al: Adenovirus type 8 keratoconjunctivitis in the United States. Am J Ophthalmol 69:473–480, 1970.
90. Kemp MC, Hierholzer JC, Cabradilla CP, et al: The changing etiology of epidemic keratoconjunctivitis: Antigenic and restriction enzyme analysis of adenovirus types 19 and 37 isolated over a 10 year period. J Infect Dis 148:29–33, 1983.
91. Numazaki Y, Kumasaka T, Yano N, et al: Further study of acute hemorrhagic cystitis due to adenovirus type 11. N Engl J Med 289:344–347, 1973.
92. Mufson MA, Belshe RB, Horrigan TJ, et al: Cause of acute hemorrhagic cystitis in children. Am J Dis Child 126:605–609, 1973.
93. Harnett GB, Buckens MR, Clay SJ, et al: Acute hemorrhagic cystitis caused by adenovirus type 11 in a recipient of a transplanted kidney. Med J Aust 1:565–567, 1982.
94. Koga S, Shindo K, Matsuya F, et al: Acute hemorrhagic cystitis caused by adenovirus following renal transplantation: Review of the literature. J Urol 149:838–839, 1993.
95. Murphy GF, Wood DJ Jr, McRoberts JW, et al: Adenovirus-associated hemorrhagic cystitis treated with intravenous ribavirin. J Urol 149:565–566, 1993.
96. Wigand R, Baumeister HG, Maass G, et al: Isolation and identification of enteric adenoviruses. J Med Virol 11:233–240, 1983.
97. Wood DJ: Adenovirus gastroenteritis. Br Med J 296:229–230, 1988.
98. Yolken RH, Lawrence F, Leister F, et al: Gastroenteritis associated with enteric type adenovirus in hospitalized infants. J Pediatr 101:21–26, 1982.
99. Reina J, Hervas J, Ros MJ: Differential clinical characteristics among pediatric patients with gastroenteritis caused by rotavirus and adenovirus [in Spanish]. Enferm Infecc Microbiol Clin 12:378–384, 1994.
100. Van R, Wun CC, O'Ryan ML, et al: Outbreaks of human enteric adenovirus types 40 and 41 in Houston day care centers. J Pediatr 120:516–521, 1992.
101. Shinozaki T, Araki K, Ushijima H, et al: Antibody response to enteric adenovirus types 40 and 41 in sera from people in various age groups. J Clin Microbiol 25:1679–1682, 1987.
102. Lew JF, Moe CL, Monroe SS, et al: Astrovirus and adenovirus associated with diarrhea in children in day care settings. J Infect Dis 164:673–678, 1991.
103. Bhisitkul DM, Todd KM, Listernick R: Adenovirus infection and childhood intussusception. Am J Dis Child 146:1331–1333, 1992.
104. Yunis EJ, Atchison RW, Michaels RH, et al: Adenovirus and iliocecal intussusception. Lab Invest 33:347–351, 1975.
105. Yunis EJ, Hashida Y: Electron microscopic demonstration of adenovirus in appendix vermiformis in a case of ileocecal intussusception. Pediatrics 51:566–570, 1973.
106. Kagnoff MF, Paterson VJ, Kumar PJ, et al: Evidence for the role of a human intestinal adenovirus in the pathogenesis of coeliac disease. Gut 28:995–1001, 1987.
107. Mahon J, Blair GE, Wood GM, et al: Is persistent adenovirus 12 infection involved in coeliac disease? A search for viral DNA using the polymerase chain reaction. Gut 32:1114–1116, 1991.
108. Vesy CJ, Greenson JK, Papp AC, et al: Evaluation of celiac disease biopsies for adenovirus 12 DNA using a multiplex polymerase chain reaction. Mod Pathol 6:61–64, 1993.
109. Chou SM, Roo R, Burrell R, et al: Subacute focal adenovirus encephalitis. J Neuropathol Exp Neurol 32:34–50, 1973.
110. Kelsey DS: Adenovirus meningoencephalitis. Pediatrics 61:291–293, 1978.
111. Simila S, Jouppila R, Salmi A, et al: Encephalomeningitis in children associated with an adenovirus type 7 epidemic. Acta Pediatr Scand 59:310–316, 1970.
112. Zahradnik JM, Spencer MJ, Parker DD: Adenovirus infection in the immunocompromised patient. Am J Med 68:725–732, 1980.
113. Wigger HJ, Blanc WA: Fatal hepatic and bronchial necrosis in adenovirus infection with thymic alymphoplasia. N Engl J Med 275:870–874, 1966.
114. Myerowitz R, Stalder H, Oxman M, et al: Fatal disseminated adenovirus infection in a renal transplant recipient. Am J Med 59:591–598, 1975.
115. Siegal FP, Dikman SH, Arayata RB, et al: Fatal disseminated adenovirus 11 pneumonia in an agammaglobulinemic patient. Am J Med 71:1062–1067, 1981.
116. Cames B, Rahier J, Burtomboy G, et al: Acute adenovirus hepatitis in liver transplant recipients. J Pediatr 120:33–37, 1992.
117. Flomenberg P, Babbitt J, Drobyski WR, et al: Increasing incidence of adenovirus disease in bone marrow transplant recipients. J Infect Dis 169:775–781, 1994.
118. Janoff EN, Orenstein JM, Manischewitz JF, et al: Adenovirus colitis in the acquired immunodeficiency syndrome. Gastroenterology 100:976–979, 1991.
119. Vihma L: Surveillance of acute viral respiratory disease in children. Acta Paediatr Scand 92:8–52, 1969.
120. Fox JP, Hall CE, Cooney MK: The Seattle virus watch. VII. Observations of adenovirus infections. Am J Epidemiol 105:362–396, 1977.
121. Huebner RJ, Rowe WP, Ward TG, et al: Adenoidal-pharyngoconjunctival agents. N Engl J Med 251:1077–1086, 1954.
122. Jordan WS Jr, Badger GF, Curtiss C, et al: A study of illness in a group of Cleveland families. X. The occurrence of adenovirus infections. Am J Hyg 64:336–348, 1956.
123. Flomenberg PR, Chen P, Munk G, et al: The molecular epidemiology of adenovirus type 35 isolates from immunocompromised hosts. J Infect Dis 155:1127–1134, 1987.
124. Hilleman MR, Werner JH, Dascomb HE, et al: Epidemiology of RI (RI-67) group respiratory virus infections in recruit populations. Am J Hyg 62:29–43, 1955.
125. Rowe WP, Hartley JW, Huebner RJ: Additional serotypes of the APC virus group. Proc Soc Exp Biol Med 91:260–262, 1956.
126. Couch RB, Cate TR, Douglas RG Jr, et al: Effect of route of inoculation of experimental volunteers and evidence for airborne transmission. Bacteriol Rev 30:517–529, 1966.
127. Krisher KK, Menegus MA: Evaluation of three types of cell culture for recovery of adenovirus from clinical specimens. J Clin Microbiol 25:1323–1324, 1987.
128. Graham FL, Smiley J, Russell WC, et al: Characteristics of a human cell line transformed by DNA from human adenovirus type 5. J Gen Virol 36:59–72, 1977.
129. Takiff HE, Strauss SE, Garon CF: Propagation and in vitro studies of previously non-cultivable enteral adenoviruses in 293 cells. Lancet 2:832–834, 1981.
130. Shinozaki T, Araki K, Ushijima H, et al: Use of Graham 293 cells in suspension for isolating enteric adenoviruses from the stools of patients with acute gastroenteritis. J Infect Dis 156:246, 1987.
131. Mautner V, MacKay N, Steinthorsdottir V: Complementation of enteric adenovirus type 40 for lytic growth in tissue culture by E1B 55K function of adenovirus types 5 and 12. Virology 171:619–622, 1989.
132. Gardner PS, McQuillin J: Adenoviruses. *In* Gardner PS (ed): Rapid Virus Diagnosis: Application of Immunofluorescence. London, Butterworth, 1974, pp 181–193.
133. Grandien M, Pettersson CA, Gardner PS, et al: Rapid viral diagnosis of acute respiratory infections: Comparison of enzyme-linked immunosorbent assay and the immunofluorescence technique for detection of viral antigens in nasopharyngeal secretions. J Clin Microbiol 22:757–760, 1985.
134. Grandien M, Pettersson CA, Svensson L, et al: Latex agglutination test for adenovirus diagnosis in diarrheal disease. J Med Virol 23:311–316, 1987.
135. Wu TC, Kanayama MD, Hruban RH, et al: Virus-associated RNAs (VA-I and VA-II). An efficient target for the detection of adenovirus infections by in situ hybridization. Am J Pathol 140:991–998, 1992.
136. Turner PC, Bailey AS, Cooper RJ, et al: The polymerase chain reaction for detecting adenovirus DNA in formalin-fixed, paraffin-embedded tissue obtained post mortem. J Infect 27:43–46, 1993.
137. Hierholzer JC, Halonen PE, Dahlen PO, et al: Detection of adenovirus in clinical specimens by polymerase chain reaction and liquid-phase hybridization quantitated by time-resolved fluorometry. J Clin Microbiol 31:1886–1891, 1993.
138. Allard A, Albinsson B, Wadell G: Detection of adenoviruses in

stools from healthy persons and patients with diarrhea by two-step polymerase chain reaction. J Med Virol 37:149–157, 1992.
139. Kasel JA: Adenoviruses. *In* Lennette EH, Schmidt NJ (eds): Diagnostic Procedures for Viral, Rickettsial and Chlamydial Infections, ed 5. Washington, DC, American Public Health Association, 1979, pp 229–256.
140. Rosen I, Hovis JF, Bell JA: Further observation of typing adenoviruses and a description of two possible additional serotypes. Proc Soc Exp Biol Med 110:710–713, 1962.
141. Hierholzer JC, Torrence AC, Wright PR: Generalized viral illness caused by an intermediate strain of adenovirus (21/H21 + 35). J Infect Dis 14:281–288, 1980.
142. DeJong PJ, Valderrama G, Spigland I, et al: Adenovirus isolates from the urines of patients with the acquired immunodeficiency syndrome. Lancet 1:1293–1296, 1983.
143. Wadell G, Hammarskjold ML, Winberg G, et al: Genetic variability of adenoviruses. Ann N Y Acad Sci 354:16–42, 1980.
144. Mei YF, Wadell G: Hemagglutination properties and nucleotide sequence analysis of the fiber gene of adenovirus genome types 11p and 11a. Virology 194:453–462, 1993.
145. Toogood CI, Crompton J, Hay RT: Antipeptide antisera define neutralizing epitopes on the adenovirus hexon. J Gen Virol 73:1429–1435, 1992.
146. Herrmann JE, Perron-Henry DM, Blacklow NR: Antigen detection with monoclonal antibodies for the diagnosis of adenovirus gastroenteritis. J Infect Dis 155:1167–1171, 1987.
147. Dudgeon J, Bhargara SK, Ross CA: Treatment of adenovirus infection of the eye with 5'-iodo-2'-deoxyuridine. A double blind trial. Br J Ophthalmol 53:530–533, 1969.
148. Waring GO, Laibson PR, Satz JE, et al: Use of vidarabine in epidemic keratoconjunctivitis due to adenovirus types 3, 7, 8 and 19. Am J Ophthalmol 82:781–785, 1976.
149. Baba M, Mori S, Shigeta S, De Clercq E: Selective inhibitory effect of (*S*)-9-(3-hydroxy-2-phosphonylmethoxypropyl)adenine and 2'-nor-cyclic GMP on adenovirus replication in vitro. Antimicrob Agents Chemother 31:337–339, 1987.
150. Gordon YJ, Romanowski E, Araullo-Cruz T, et al: Inhibitory effect of (*S*)-HPMPC, (*S*)-HPMPA, and 2'-nor-cyclic GMP on clinical ocular adenoviral isolates is serotype-dependent in vitro. Antiviral Res 16:11–16, 1991.
151. Gordon YJ, Romanowski E, Araullo-Cruz T, et al: Pretreatment with topical 0.1% (*S*)-1-(3-hydroxy-2-phosphonylmethoxypropyl)cytosine inhibits adenovirus type 5 replication in the New Zealand rabbit ocular model. Cornea 11:529–533, 1992.
152. Murtagh P, Cerqueiro C, Halac A, et al: Adenovirus type 7h respiratory infections: A report of 29 cases of acute lower respiratory disease. Acta Paediatr 82:557–561, 1993.
153. Top FH Jr: Control of adenovirus acute respiratory disease in U.S. army trainees. Yale J Biol Med 48:185–195, 1975.
154. Top FH Jr, Buescher EL, Bancroft WH, et al: Immunization with live types 7 and 4 adenovirus vaccines. II. Antibody response and protective effect against acute respiratory disease due to adenovirus type 7. J Infect Dis 124:155–160, 1971.
155. Horwitz MS: Adenoviruses. *In* Fields BN, Knipe DM, Howley PM (eds): Fields Virology, ed 3. Philadelphia, Lippincott-Raven, 1996, pp 2149–2171.
156. Heubner RJ, Chanock RM, Rubin BA, et al: Induction by adenovirus type 7 of tumor in hamster having the antigenic characteristics of SV40 virus. Proc Natl Acad Sci USA 52:1333–1349, 1964.
157. Rowe WP, Baum SG: Studies of adenovirus SV40 hybrid viruses. II. Defectiveness of the hybrid particles. J Exp Med 122:955–966, 1965.
158. Yang Y, Nunes FA, Berencsi K, et al: Inactivation of E2a in recombinant adenoviruses improves the prospect for gene therapy in cystic fibrosis. Nat Genet 7:362–369, 1994.
159. Morin JE, Lubeck MD, Barton JE, et al: Recombinant adenovirus induces antibody response to hepatitis B virus surface antigen in hamsters. Proc Natl Acad Sci USA 84:4626–4630, 1987.
160. Jaffe HA, Danel C, Longenecker G, et al: Adenovirus-mediated in vivo gene transfer and expression in normal rat liver. Nat Genet 1:372–378, 1992.
161. Rosenfeld MA, Siegfried W, Yoshimura K, et al: Adenovirus-mediated transfer of a recombinant α-1–antitrypsin gene to the lung epithelium in vivo. Science 252:431–434, 1991.
162. Lemarchand P, Jones M, Yamada I, et al: In vivo gene transfer and expression in normal uninjured blood vessels using replication-deficient recombinant adenovirus vectors. Circ Res 72:1132–1138, 1993.
163. Zabner J, Couture LA, Gregory RJ, et al: Adenovirus-mediated gene transfer transiently corrects the chloride transport defect in nasal epithelia of patients with cystic fibrosis. Cell 75:207–216, 1993.
164. Rosenfeld MA, Yoshimura K, Trapnell BC, et al: In vivo transfer of the human cystic fibrosis transmembrane conductance regulator gene to the airway epithelium. Cell 68:143–155, 1992.
165. Bajocchi G, Feldman SH, Crystal RG, et al: Direct in vivo gene transfer to ependymal cells in the central nervous system using recombinant adenovirus vectors. Nat Genet 3:229–234, 1993.
166. Crystal RG, McElvaney NG, Rosenfeld MA, et al: Administration of an adenovirus containing the human CFTR cDNA to the respiratory tract of individuals with cystic fibrosis. Nat Genet 8:42–50, 1994.
167. Prevec L, Campbell JB, Christie BS, et al: A recombinant human adenovirus vaccine against rabies. J Infect Dis 161:27–30, 1989.
168. Dewar RL, Natarajan V, Vasudevachari MB, et al: Synthesis and processing of human immunodeficiency virus type 1 envelope proteins encoded by a recombinant human adenovirus. J Virol 63:129–136, 1989.
169. Rosenfeld MA, Yoshimura K, Trapnell BC, et al: In vivo transfer of the human cystic fibrosis transmembrane conductance regulator gene to the airway epithelium. Cell 68:143–155, 1992.
170. Crystal RG, McElvaney NG, Rosenfeld MA, et al: Administration of an adenovirus containing the human CFTR cDNA to the respiratory tract of individuals with cystic fibrosis. Nat Genet 8:42–50, 1994.
171. Yang Y, Li Q, Ertl HC, et al: Cellular and humoral immune responses to viral antigens create barriers to lung-directed gene therapy with recombinant adenoviruses. J Virol 69:2004–2015, 1995.
172. Hse KHL, Lubeck MD, Davis AR, et al: Immunogenicity and protective efficacy of adenovirus vectored respiratory syncytial virus vaccine. *In* Chanock RM, Ginsberg HS, Brown F, et al (eds): Vaccines 91: Modern Approaches to New Vaccines Including Prevention of AIDS. Plainview, NY, Cold Spring Harbor Laboratory Press, 1991, pp 293–297.
173. Yoshimura K, Rosenfeld MA, Seth P, et al: Adenovirus-mediated augmentation of cell transfection with unmodified plasmid vectors. J Biol Chem 268:2300–2303, 1993.
174. Cotten M, Wagner E, Zatloukal K, et al: Chicken adenovirus (CELO virus) particles augment receptor-mediated DNA delivery to mammalian cells and yield exceptional levels of stable transformants. J Virol 67:3777–3785, 1993.
175. Curiel DT, Agarwal S, Wagner E, et al: Adenovirus enhancement of transferrin-polylysine–mediated gene delivery. Proc Natl Acad Sci USA 88:8850–8854, 1991.
176. Ilan Y, Droguett G, RoyChowdhury N, et al: Insertion of the adenoviral E3 region into a recombinant viral vector prevents antiviral humoral and cellular immune responses and permits long term gene expression. Proc Natl Acad Sci USA (in press).

240

Herpes Simplex Viruses

Michael N. Oxman

Herpes simplex viruses (HSVs) are ubiquitous, remarkably host-adapted human pathogens. Initial (primary) HSV infection is usually asymptomatic or mild and self-limited, but instead of disappearing from the body during convalescence, the virus establishes a latent infection that persists for life. This latent infection is subject to intermittent reactivation that results in recurrent disease or asymptomatic virus shedding, transforming each affected person into a lifelong reservoir of HSV infection. As a consequence, HSV is endemic in virtually every human population. There are two HSVs, type 1 (HSV-1) and type 2 (HSV-2), which are closely related but differ in their epidemiology. HSV-1 is transmitted chiefly by contact with infected saliva, whereas HSV-2 is transmitted sexually or from a mother's genital tract infection to her newborn. This difference in transmission results in differences in the age-specific prevalence of infection and in the anatomic sites involved. HSV-1 infections occur frequently in children and most often involve the mouth, lips, pharynx, eyes, and skin sites above the waist. HSV-2 infections occur after the onset of sexual activity and involve predominantly the genitalia and skin sites below the waist. Severe disease is rare in otherwise healthy persons, but HSV infections are frequently life threatening to newborns and immunocompromised persons. Our current understanding of HSV, although incomplete, provides a rational basis for the development of effective methods for the diagnosis, treatment, and prevention of HSV infections.

History

The term *herpes* (from the Greek ερπειν, "to creep") has been used to describe a variety of cutaneous eruptions since the time of Hippocrates, but the first clear description of herpes labialis (herpes febrilis, fever blister, cold sore) as the herpetic eruption that appears about the mouth at the crisis of simple fevers is attributed to Herodotus, a Roman physician of the first century AD.[1–4] The often embarrassing lesions of herpes labialis were well recognized in 16th century England; in Shakespeare's *Romeo and Juliet*, Romeo's friend Mercutio describes their pathogenesis in women of romantic inclination: "O'er ladies' lips, who straight on kisses dream, Which oft the angry Mab with blisters plagues, Because their breaths with sweetmeats tainted are."[4, 5] Genital herpes (herpes genitalis, herpes progenitalis) was not well described until the 18th century, when Astruc, physician to the King of France, published a vivid description of the disease in men and women.[6, 7] By the end of the 19th century, human-to-human transmission of HSV had been documented, and the histopathologic appearance of herpetic lesions, particularly the characteristic multinucleated giant cells, had been described.[3, 4, 6, 8]

In the first part of this century, Grüter, Löwenstein, Doerr, Lipschütz, and other European investigators established the infectious nature of herpes labialis, genital herpes, and herpetic keratitis by transmitting infection from lesions in humans to experimental animals.[3, 4, 9–13] They also differentiated these HSV infections from herpes zoster, which could not be similarly transmitted, and demonstrated biologic and antigenic differences between the viruses responsible for herpes labialis and genital herpes.[13] Studies in rabbits demonstrated the neurotropism of HSV, its ability to spread along axonal pathways, its predilection for sensory ganglia, and its capacity to establish latent infections and to reactivate, either spontaneously or in response to external stimuli.[9, 14–19]

The involvement of sensory ganglia in recurrent herpes was recognized at the beginning of the century. Cushing[20] observed that section of the dorsal (sensory) root of the trigeminal ganglion was regularly followed by herpes labialis in the newly denervated area, provided that the peripheral sensory nerve remained intact, and Howard[21, 22] observed characteristic histopathologic changes in sensory ganglia innervating cutaneous sites of recurrent herpes. These observations and the work of Goodpasture and colleagues[15, 18] set the stage for elegant studies in the early 1970s, reviewed by Baringer[23] and Stevens,[24] that established the sensory neuron as the site of HSV latency and led to the recovery of latent HSV from human trigeminal and sacral ganglia. The first studies of the immune response to HSV demonstrated that herpes labialis occurred exclusively in persons who had preexisting neutralizing antibody,[25] a paradoxic finding in view of the classical dictum that immunity to infectious agents is associated with protection from disease. These observations supported the hypothesis that herpes labialis results from reactivation of a latent HSV infection in the trigeminal ganglion that had been initiated by an earlier primary infection of the oral mucosa.[18, 20, 23, 24] The typical clinical manifestations of that primary infection were not recognized until 1938, when HSV was shown to be the cause of acute gingivostomatitis, and it was further demonstrated that the disease occurred only in infants and young children who had no preexisting antibodies to HSV.[26–28] In 1946, Slavin and Gavett[29] described the conjugal transmission of genital herpes and demonstrated that the resulting "herpetic vulvovaginitis" was a manifestation of primary HSV infection. However, the preponderance of recurrent (endogenous) genital herpes obscured the contagious nature of the disease, and genital herpes was still not widely accepted as a sexually transmitted disease (STD) until rediscovery of the two HSV serotypes in the late 1960s made it possible to delineate the epidemiology of HSV-2 infection.[2, 30–32]

The past three decades have seen enormous advances in our understanding of HSV and its complex interactions with its human hosts. The organization and nucleotide sequence of the HSV-1 and HSV-2 genomes have been determined, and the structure and function of a number of viral gene products elucidated.[33, 34] Much has been learned about HSV replication, the regulation of viral gene expression, and the interactions of the virus with the infected cell.[34–37] Our understanding of HSV latency, although still incomplete, has been greatly expanded, and we are beginning to decipher the host immune responses to HSV infection.[24, 37–43] These advances have led to a number of new developments with far-reaching clinical implications. These include type-specific serologic assays that have provided a clear picture of the epidemiology of HSV-1 and HSV-2 infections and revealed the biologic effects of heterotypic immunity; new tools for molecular diagnosis and for the analysis of HSV infection and latency that have greatly expanded our understanding of the natural history and pathogenesis of HSV infections; and selective antiviral agents that are effective for the treatment and suppression of HSV infections. These advances have also led to the development of a variety of candidate HSV vaccines that are now undergoing clinical evaluation and to the construction of HSV vectors for gene therapy.

Characteristics of the Pathogen

Classification

HSV-1 (officially designated human herpesvirus [HHV] type 1) and HSV-2 (officially designated HHV-2) are classified as members of the family Herpesviridae (the herpesvirus family) on the basis of virion architecture and genome structure.[44, 45] The other human herpesviruses discovered to date are varicella-zoster virus (HHV-3), Epstein-Barr virus (HHV-4), human cytomegalovirus (HHV-5), HHV-6 (the cause of roseola infantum), HHV-7, and HHV-8 (which is etiologically linked to Kaposi's sarcoma). Nearly 100 different members of this remarkably successful family of viruses have already been identified in a wide variety of species ranging from fungi to humans, and new herpesviruses are still being discovered.

Members of the herpesvirus family are classified into three

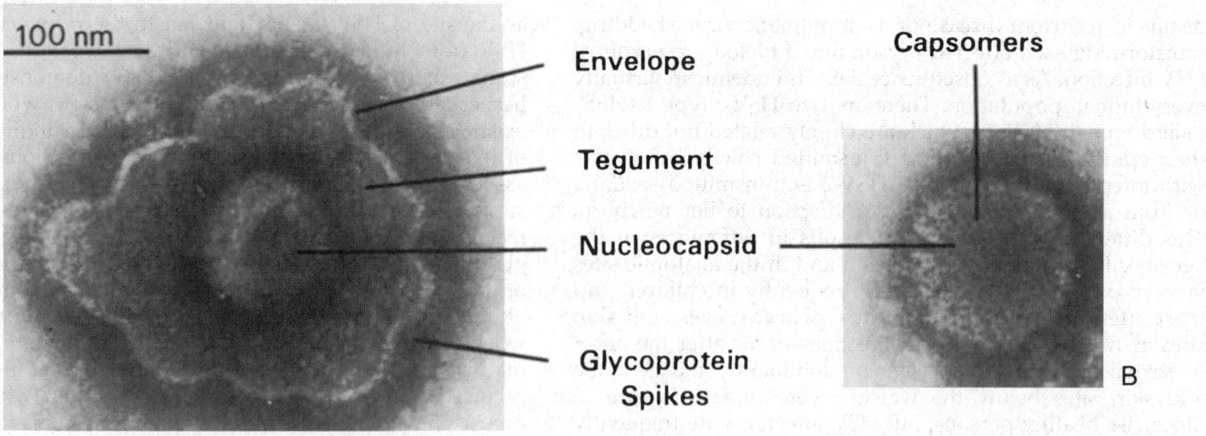

FIGURE 240–1 □ Atypical herpesvirus negatively stained with phosphotungstic acid. *A*, The complete virion. *B*, The nucleocapsid. (Magnification, × 40,000.) (From Straus SE, Ostrove JM, Inchauspe G, et al: Varicella zoster virus infections: Biology, natural history, treatment, and prevention. Ann Intern Med 108:221–237, 1988.)

subfamilies—Alphaherpesvirinae, Betaherpesvirinae, and Gammaherpesvirinae—on the basis of their biologic properties.[44, 45] HSV-1 and HSV-2 are classified as alphaherpesviruses because of their broad host range, relatively short replication cycle, rapid spread in cell culture, efficient lysis of productively infected cells, and capacity to establish latent infections primarily (although not exclusively) in sensory ganglia.[34, 44, 45]

Structure

The virions of HSV-1 and HSV-2, like those of all members of the herpesvirus family,[44, 45] consist of a central core that contains the viral genome, a linear molecule of double-stranded DNA, together with several viral proteins.[34, 46] The core is enclosed within an icosahedral shell or capsid approximately 100 nm in diameter that is composed of 162 identical protein subunits or capsomers. The resulting structure, the nucleocapsid (Fig. 240–1), is surrounded by an amorphous layer of viral protein of variable thickness (the tegument) and, finally, by a lipoprotein envelope derived from the nuclear membrane of the infected host cell (see Fig. 240–1). The complete virion is roughly spherical, with a diameter of 150 to 200 nm. Embedded in the lipid bilayer of the virus envelope and visible in electron micrographs as radially oriented spikes (see Fig. 240–1) are viral glycoproteins that interact with the surface of susceptible host cells to mediate virus attachment and enable the nucleocapsid to penetrate into the cell cytoplasm.[34, 47–49] Because of the essential role of these envelope glycoproteins, only intact enveloped virions are fully infectious, and this accounts for the lability of herpesviruses; infectivity is rapidly destroyed by organic solvents, detergents, proteolytic enzymes, heat, drying, and extremes of pH. HSV virions also contain large amounts of the polyamines spermine and spermidine, which may facilitate packaging of the viral genome by neutralizing the charge of DNA phosphate groups.[34, 50]

The genomes of HSV-1 and HSV-2 share about half their nucleotide sequences and are colinear.[9, 33, 34, 51–53] Each HSV-1 gene appears to have a functionally interchangeable HSV-2 homolog with which it shares at least some nucleotide sequences, and homologous genes occupy identical positions in each genome so that a single map suffices for both.[33, 52–59] Genetic recombination occurs readily between HSV-1 and HSV-2, and intertypic recombinants are viable.[58, 59] Nevertheless, many homologous coding and noncoding regions differ in length because of type-specific insertions and deletions of genetic information. This results in type-specific differences in restriction endonuclease cleavage sites and in the sizes of viral proteins, which form the basis of useful laboratory techniques to differentiate HSV-1 from HSV-2.[53, 58–63]

Strains belonging to a single HSV serotype also exhibit genetic variation, but the differences observed are much smaller than those that distinguish HSV-1 from HSV-2. This results in restriction endonuclease polymorphisms that are easily detected among epidemiologically unrelated strains of HSV-1 and HSV-2 and serve as useful markers for epidemiologic investigations.[60, 64–69]

The HSV genome is a linear, double-stranded molecule of DNA of approximately 150 kb (molecular weight about 100 $\times 10^6$) with a guanine plus cytosine content of 68% (HSV-1) or 69% (HSV-2). It consists of two covalently linked components designated L (long) and S (short). Each component consists of a stretch of unique sequences (U_L and U_S) bracketed by inverted repeats.[33, 34, 70, 71] The terminal and internal repeats bracketing U_L are designated TR_L (or *ab*) and IR_L (or *b′a′*); those bracketing the U_S are designated IR_S (or *a′c′*) and TR_S (or *ca*) (Fig. 240–2). The number of *a* sequence repeats at the L-S junction and at the L terminal is variable.[34] The L

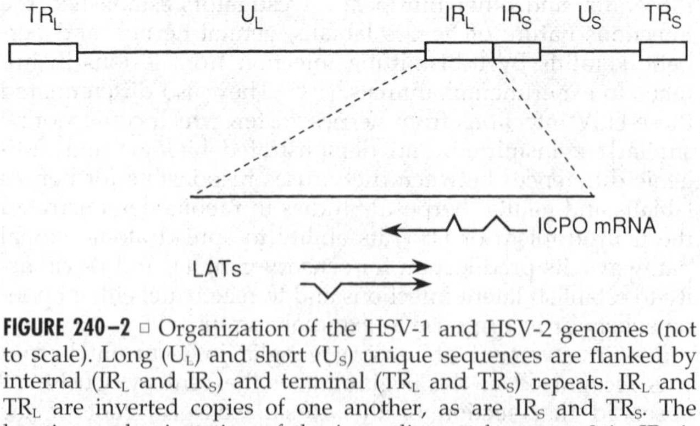

FIGURE 240–2 □ Organization of the HSV-1 and HSV-2 genomes (not to scale). Long (U_L) and short (U_S) unique sequences are flanked by internal (IR_L and IR_S) and terminal (TR_L and TR_S) repeats. IR_L and TR_L are inverted copies of one another, as are IR_S and TR_S. The location and orientation of the immediate early gene α0 in IR_L is indicated by the location and orientation of its messenger RNA (mRNA), which encodes infected cell protein 0 (ICP0). The location and orientation of the latency-associated transcripts (LATs) are also indicated. The sequences encoding ICP0 and LATs are repeated in the opposite orientation in TR_L. (Modified from Croen KD, Ostrove JM, Dragovic L, Straus SE: Characterization of herpes simplex type 2 latency-associated transcription in human sacral ganglia and in cell culture. J Infect Dis 163:23–28, 1991. © by the University of Chicago.)

and S components of HSV can invert relative to each other, yielding four linear isomers, and DNA extracted from clinical (wild-type) isolates of HSV-1 and HSV-2 contains equimolar quantities of all four.[72, 73] Curiously, however, the capacity to form these isomers is not essential for growth in cell culture. Mutants lacking most of the internal repeats, and thus "frozen" in one isomeric form, have been constructed in each of the four arrangements of L and S, and all are viable in cell culture.[34, 74] The HSV-1 and HSV-2 genomes each encode more than 80 different polypeptides.[33, 34, 37, 62, 63, 75–78] In addition to structural proteins, these include a large array of enzymes involved in nucleic acid synthesis (e.g., thymidine kinase, ribonucleotide reductase, deoxyuridine triphosphatase), DNA synthesis (e.g., DNA polymerase, helicase), and protein processing (e.g., protein kinase) and other proteins involved in DNA replication (e.g., DNA binding proteins).[34]

HSV virions contain at least 33 distinct virus-encoded proteins, including several core proteins associated with the viral DNA; seven or more capsid proteins; and a number of tegument proteins, including the α trans-inducing factor (VP16, Vmw65), which activates transcription of the HSV immediate early genes, and the virus host shutoff protein (VHS, U_L41) responsible for the early shutoff of host cell macromolecular synthesis.[34] There are also 11 envelope glycoproteins—gB, gC, gD, gE, gG, gH, gI, gJ, gK, gL, and gM—some of which have been shown to be components of the envelope spikes.[34, 75–77] The specific functions of most of the virion proteins remain to be determined. Only four of the envelope glycoproteins, gB, gD, gH, and gL, are required for virus replication in cultures of nonpolarized epithelial cells.[34, 77–82]

Biologic Properties

The most significant biologic property of HSV, which it shares with other members of the herpesvirus family, is its ability to establish lifelong persistent infections that ensure its perpetuation in the human population.[83] Primary infection, which occurs relatively early in life, is usually asymptomatic and rarely causes severe disease; however, despite the development of humoral and cell-mediated immunity, virus persists in the form of an asymptomatic latent infection in sensory neurons innervating the initially infected peripheral site. A variety of provocative factors, such as fever, trauma, emotional stress, sunlight, or menstruation, can reactivate the latent virus and produce a brief, self-limited episode of recurrent infection with peripheral shedding of HSV. When symptomatic, these episodes of reactivation present as herpes labialis, recurrent genital herpes, and the like (Table 240–1), but they are more often asymptomatic and detectable only by the presence of HSV in the saliva, genital secretions, or skin. Neither the persistence of HSV nor its periodic reactivation

TABLE 240–1 ■ Differences Between Herpes Simplex Virus Types 1 and 2

CHARACTERISTICS	HSV-1	HSV-2
Clinical		
Manifestations of primary infection		
Acute herpetic gingivostomatitis	+*	−†
Acute herpetic pharyngotonsillitis	+	−‡
Acute herpetic keratoconjunctivitis	+	−
Neonatal herpes simplex infections	±§	+
Manifestations of recurrent infection		
Herpes labialis	+	−
Herpes keratitis	+	−
Manifestations of primary or recurrent infection		
Cutaneous herpes		
Skin above the waist	+	−
Skin below the waist	−	+
Hands or arms	+	+
Herpetic whitlow	+	+
Eczema herpeticum	+	−
Herpes genitalis	±‖	+
Herpes simplex encephalitis	+	−
Herpes simplex meningitis	±¶	+
Disseminated HSV infection in immunocompromised patients	+	+
Epidemiologic		
Transmission	Nonsexual	Sexual
Epidemiologic association with carcinoma of the cervix	−	+
Latency		
In trigeminal and cervical sensory ganglia	+	−
In sacral sensory ganglia	−	+
Frequency of recurrence when latent in trigeminal and cervical sensory ganglia	+	−
Frequency of recurrence when latent in sacral sensory ganglia	−	+
Biochemical		
DNA guanine + cytosine	68%	69%
Homology between viral DNAs	Approximately 50%	
Stability of virus-specific thymidine kinase at 40°C	+	−
Biology		
Neurotropism in mice on peripheral inoculation	Less neurotropic	More neurotropic
Pock size on chick chorioallantoic membrane	Small	Large
Plaque formation in chick embryo cell monolayer culture	−	+
Temperature sensitivity of replication (40°C)	−	+
Inhibition of replication by heparin, neomycin, polylysine	+	−
Inhibition of replication by thymidine	−	+

HSV-1 and HSV-2 can be differentiated unequivocally by serologic techniques, by DNA-to-DNA hybridization, by restriction endonuclease fingerprinting of viral DNA, and by electrophoretic analysis of virus-specified proteins.

*+, Frequent or predominant cause, or significantly greater than the other serotype.
†−, Infrequent cause (except under special epidemiologic circumstances), or significantly less or lower than the other serotype.
‡HSV-2 is frequently isolated when pharyngotonsillitis is associated with orogenital sexual contact.
§HSV-1 is isolated from approximately 30% of cases, reflecting the increasing frequency with which HSV-1 causes genital herpes (in the mother) as well as some cases of infection acquired postnatally from individuals shedding HSV-1.
‖HSV-1 is now being isolated from 10% to 40% of patients with primary genital herpes, reflecting the growing proportion of the population that is reaching the age of sexual activity without having experienced orolabial HSV-1 infection and the prevalence of orogenital sexual contact. Herpetic vulvovaginitis in infants is generally caused by HSV-1, acquired from adults or by autoinoculation of infected saliva.
¶Some cases reported, but insufficient data to estimate frequency.
Modified from Oxman MN: Herpes stomatitis. *In* Braude AI (ed): Infectious Diseases and Medical Microbiology, ed 2. Philadelphia, WB Saunders, 1986.

significantly impairs the long-term survival or reproductive capacity of its host, and thus most infected persons remain in the community as lifelong carriers of HSV. The periodic reactivation of latent HSV infection provides ample opportunity for the virus to be transmitted to new susceptible persons before the adult carriers succumb to old age or other diseases (Fig. 240–3). In this regard, it is probably no accident that herpes labialis is frequently brought on by the fever associated with life-threatening bacterial infections; the deathbed kiss provides one last opportunity for HSV to be transmitted to the next generation. The remarkable adaptation of HSV to its natural host is underlined by its more destructive behavior in other species. For example, in rabbits and mice, HSV infections are often severe and not infrequently fatal. Similarly, *Herpesvirus simiae* causes severe, often fatal encephalomyelitis in humans, whereas it causes a mild or asymptomatic infection in its natural simian host followed by lifelong latency that is analogous to HSV in humans.[84] It seems likely that the many HSV genes that are dispensable for virus replication in cell culture[34] are involved in the establishment and maintenance of this remarkable virus-host interaction, the central feature of which is virus latency.

HSV-1 and HSV-2 cause a variety of clinical syndromes (see Table 240–1), depending on the virus type, the anatomic site involved, and the age and immune status of the host.[32, 51, 83, 85, 86] The outcome of HSV infection is also influenced by a number of more subtle and less well characterized properties of the virus and host.[32, 51, 83, 85, 86] There is growing evidence that HSV-1 and HSV-2 are adapted, respectively, to oral-facial-ocular and to genital tissues. For example, the monthly recurrence rate is substantially higher when genital herpes is caused by HSV-2 than by HSV-1 (0.34 and 0.08, respectively), whereas the recurrence rate of orofacial herpes is substantially higher when it is caused by HSV-1 than by HSV-2 (0.12 and 0.001, respectively).[87–91] Gentry and colleagues[92] have hypothesized, on the basis of comparative sequence analysis of herpesvirus enzymes, that HSV-1 and HSV-2 evolved from a common ancestral human herpesvirus that initially depended, as does *H. simiae*, on both oral and genital transmission. Their divergence and separate evolution, estimated to have begun 8 to 10 million years ago, are thought to have followed the adoption by our earliest human ancestors of bipedal stance and face-to-face mating posture, which provided the required microbiologic separation of oral and genital sites of infection.

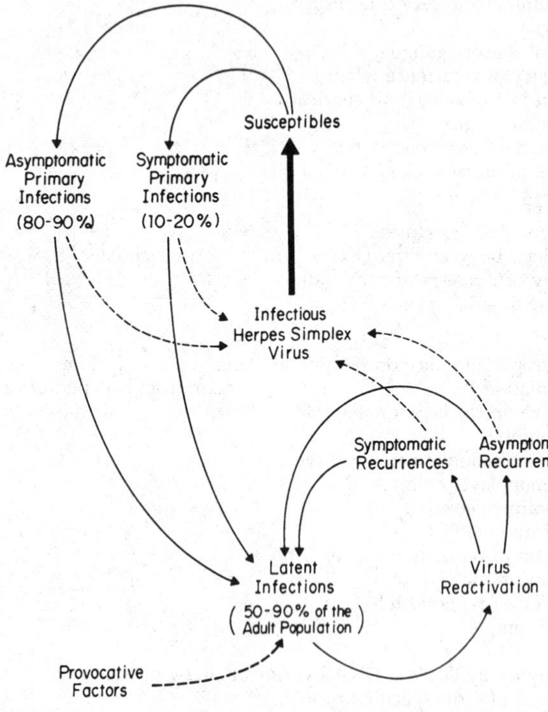

FIGURE 240–3 □ The ecology of HSV. The 50% to 90% of adults with latent infections are the reservoir of HSV. New susceptible individuals (usually children in the case of HSV-1) are infected when children or adults with latent infections shed virus during recurrences (for example, episodes of herpes labialis). During their primary infection, which is usually asymptomatic, the newly infected individuals develop latent infection and join the pool of lifelong virus carriers. (From Oxman MN: Herpes stomatitis. *In* Braude AI, Davis CE, Fierer J [eds]: Infectious Diseases and Medical Microbiology, ed 2. Philadelphia, WB Saunders, 1986, pp 752–772.)

HSV differs from all of the other human herpesviruses in having a broad host range. HSV-1 and HSV-2 can infect many experimental animals, including rats, mice, hamsters, guinea pigs, rabbits, nonhuman primates, and chick embryos, as well as a wide variety of cell cultures derived from human and animal tissues. HSV is also characterized by a rapid replication cycle that results in the death of the productively infected cell.[34]

Replication

Infection of susceptible cells is initiated when HSV envelope glycoproteins bind to components of the host cell surface in a series of interactions that culminate in penetration of the viral nucleocapsid and surrounding tegument into the cell cytoplasm.[34, 47–49, 77, 93, 94] Initial adsorption of the virion to nonpolarized cells in culture appears to be mediated by the binding of two viral glycoproteins, gB and gC, to heparan sulfate, a ubiquitous component of cell surface proteoglycans.[34, 47–49, 77, 78, 95–100] This is followed by binding of a third envelope glycoprotein, gD, to a different, less numerous but still ubiquitous receptor molecule that appears to be protease sensitive.[47–49, 80, 81, 101–105] Binding of gD to the plasma membrane is followed by penetration of the HSV nucleocapsid and tegument into the cell cytoplasm, a process that requires the participation of gB and gH and involves pH-independent fusion of the virion envelope with the plasma membrane of the cell.[47–49, 77–81, 102–107] Only three envelope glycoproteins, gB, gD, and gH, are required for this phase of infection in cultures of nonpolarized cells, although additional glycoproteins (e.g., gC) participate and under certain circumstances may even substitute for the required ones.[34, 47–49, 77–80, 97, 105–109]

In vivo, HSV must be able to infect epithelial cells and neurons, highly polarized cells that sort membrane and secreted proteins to one surface or another: in epithelial cells, to apical and basal surfaces; in neurons, to axons and dendrites.[34, 110] It appears that in vivo different receptors, recognized by different HSV glycoproteins, are expressed on the apical and basal surfaces of epithelial cells and the axons of sensory neurons, whereas nonpolarized cells in culture express more than one receptor on the same surface. Thus, gC is required for attachment of HSV to the apical surface of polarized epithelial cells, but not for attachment to the basal surface of the same cells or for attachment to nonpolarized epithelial cells.[34, 110] The complement receptor CRI (CD35) has been identified as the receptor for gC-dependent attachment of HSV-1 to the apical surface of polarized epithelial cells.[34] Glycoproteins gG, gE, and gI are also required for postattachment entry at the apical surface of polarized epithelial cells, and gE and gI are required for basolateral transmission of HSV infection.[34] Glycoprotein gL forms a complex with gH and is required for the transport of both proteins to the plasma membrane. Thus, gL is required for the incorporation of gH into the virion envelope, and HSV mutants unable to express gL lack gH. They attach to cells but are unable to enter.[34, 82, 111–113] Some of the envelope glycoproteins that are dispensable for HSV replication in cell culture appear to protect virions and HSV-infected cells from host defense mechanisms that operate in the whole animal (see later).

After entering the cytoplasm, HSV nucleocapsids are transported to nuclear pores and the viral DNA is released into the nucleus, a process that requires the activity of at least one virion protein.[114] The viral genes are transcribed by cell RNA polymerase II in a coordinately regulated and sequentially ordered cascade controlled by viral regulatory proteins.[34, 37, 115] HSV genes can be divided into three major classes on the basis of the temporal sequence of their transcription.[34, 37] First to be expressed are five immediate early or α genes, α0, α4, α22, α27, and α47, which are transcribed in the absence of viral protein synthesis. The α genes share a common cis-acting regulatory element upstream of their messenger RNA cap site that contains the octomer-related TAATGARAT motif and is responsive to a transactivating viral protein (α trans-inducing factor, VP16, or Vmw65), which is located in the tegument and thus introduced into the infected cell with the nucleocapsid.[34, 37, 116–120] VP16 does not bind directly to these cis-acting elements but forms a multicomponent DNA binding complex that incorporates two or more cellular factors, one of which is the ubiquitous octamer binding protein Oct-1.[34, 37, 121–129] HSV mutants lacking functional VP16 are deficient in α gene expression and do not replicate, although the defect can be overcome by infecting cells at high multiplicity.[130] Four of the α genes (α0, α4, α22, and α27) encode regulatory proteins, one of which (infected cell protein 4 [ICP4], encoded by the α4 gene) is required for transcription of early or β genes.[34, 37] ICP4 is also required for the expression of late genes.[34, 37] ICP0, the product of the α0 gene, transactivates a wide range of viral promoters and enhances the function of ICP4. Although not essential for HSV replication in cell culture, defects in ICP0 delay expression of β and γ genes and impair virus replication, especially at low multiplicities of infection.[34, 37] ICP0 may also be important for reactivation of latent HSV in the absence of α trans-inducing factor.[131, 132] ICP27, the product of the α27 gene, is an essential gene product that appears to have a number of different activities.[34, 37] It acts in concert with ICP4 and ICP0 to regulate the expression of a broad range of HSV genes and is required for the transition from early to late HSV gene expression and for efficient viral DNA replication.[133–137] ICP27 also inhibits the nuclear localization of ICP4 and ICP0, perhaps by altering the posttranslational modification of these regulatory proteins.[138–140] In addition, ICP27 inhibits RNA splicing, which may provide a selective advantage to HSVs whose messenger RNAs are predominantly unspliced.[34, 37, 141]

One α gene (α47) encodes a protein (ICP47) that blocks the presentation of antigenic HSV peptides by class I major histocompatibility complex (MHC) molecules and thus prevents the recognition and lysis of HSV-infected cells by $CD8^+$ cytotoxic T lymphocytes.[142–145] ICP47 binds to the transporter for antigen procession (TAP), preventing it from binding and transporting the antigenic HSV peptides into the endoplasmic reticulum–cis Golgi apparatus where they would ordinarily form a trimolecular complex with the MHC class I heavy chain and β_2-microglobulin that is transported to the cell surface and recognized by $CD8^+$ T lymphocytes.[144, 145] The β genes encode enzymes (e.g., DNA polymerase, thymidine kinase, ribonucleotide reductase) and other proteins (e.g., the major single-stranded DNA binding protein ICP8) involved in HSV DNA replication.[34, 37, 146] The late or γ genes, which are transcribed only after α and β gene expression, encode most of the virion proteins and glycoproteins.[34, 37, 147, 148] They have been subdivided into two groups. The γ_1 (delayed early or βγ) genes, which include the genes encoding envelope glycoproteins gB and gD, are expressed early in infection without the need for prior viral DNA replication; γ_2 (true late) genes, exemplified by the gene encoding gC, are expressed late in infection and only after viral DNA replication has commenced.[34, 37, 147, 148]

After synthesis in the cytoplasm, most of the viral proteins are extensively processed (by cleavage, phosphorylation, sulfation, glycosylation, myristylation, adenosine diphosphate–ribosylation, and nucleotidylylation) and are transported to the nucleus, where they serve as regulatory factors, enzymes involved in DNA replication, or structural components of progeny virions. The biosynthesis of HSV glycoproteins appears to parallel that of host cell glycoproteins and to involve cellular rather than viral enzymes.[34, 47] After processing in the Golgi apparatus, the HSV glycoproteins are transported to the plasma membrane and can be found in all cell membranes except mitochondrial membranes.[34, 47, 77] The HSV envelope glycoproteins associate with each other to form both homooligomers and heterooligomers detectable in the virion envelope and in the plasma membrane of the infected cell.[111–113]

In the nucleus, viral DNA appears to be replicated by a rolling circle mechanism that yields long head-to-tail concatemers.[34, 149, 150] These concatemers are then cleaved into monomers that are packaged into empty capsids previously assembled in the nucleus under the control of assembly proteins.[34] The assembly proteins include a viral protease and an abundant scaffolding protein (ICP35) that is required for the nuclear transport of the major capsid protein (VP5), for capsid assembly, and for DNA packaging.[34, 151–158] HSV DNA cleavage and encapsidation are tightly coupled processes that require the activity of a number of viral genes and lead to the formation of stable nucleocapsids that contain the complete HSV genome.[34, 151–159] HSV nucleocapsids with a full complement of viral DNA are able to undergo further maturation to infectious virus.[34, 159, 160] Newly assembled nucleocapsids acquire their tegument and envelope by budding through patches of the inner lamella of the nuclear membrane modified by the incorporation of viral glycoproteins and by the aggregation of tegument proteins on their inner surface (Fig. 240–4). Mature virions in the perinuclear space appear to exit the cell by way of the Golgi apparatus and transport vesicles, using the same pathway as secreted soluble proteins.[34, 77, 160, 161] Prior incorporation of glycoprotein gD (a γ_1 gene product) into all of the involved cellular membranes prevents progeny virions from penetrating into the cytoplasm from cytoplasmic vesicles or the cell surface and thus from being deenveloped.[47, 77, 101, 162–164] Electron microscopic evidence suggests that many HSV virions that are enveloped at the inner lamella of the nuclear membrane are subsequently deenveloped and then reenveloped at cytoplasmic membranes.[34] However, many of the nucleocapsids associated with cytoplasmid membranes appear to be partially degraded, and it is possible that this pathway is taken by the large fraction of progeny virions that lack a full complement of HSV DNA and are noninfectious.[34]

More than 80 HSV-encoded proteins are synthesized in infected cells from messenger RNA that is capped and polyadenylated but generally unspliced.[34, 37] More than half of these viral proteins are dispensable for virus replication in nonpolarized cells in culture.[34] However, even a virus as large as HSV is unlikely to carry superfluous genetic information, and thus the many viral genes that are dispensable for replication in cell culture are almost certain to have a role in the pathogenesis of infection in vivo and in the remarkable adaptation of HSV to its human host. For example, HSV thymidine kinase is dispensable for virus replication in cell culture and in epithelial cells in vivo, but thymidine kinase–negative mutants generally exhibit reduced pathogenicity in animal models, impaired replication in neurons (which do

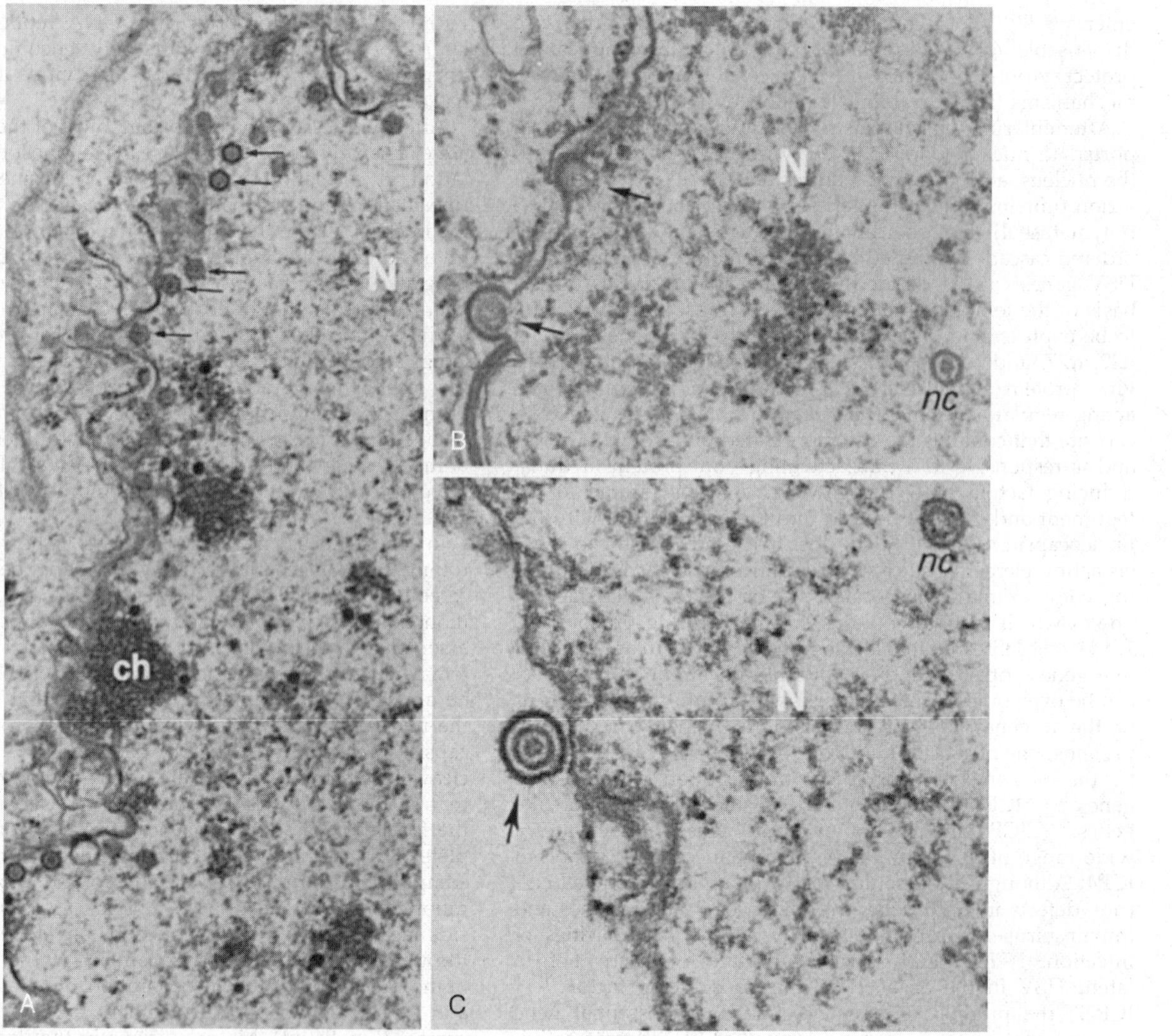

FIGURE 240–4 □ Assembly and maturation of HSV. *A*, An infected neuron from the brain of a patient with herpes simplex encephalitis shows the nucleus (N) with many HSV nucleocapsids adjacent to the inner surface of the nuclear membrane *(arrows)*. Also seen along the inner surface of the nuclear membrane are collections of condensed marginated chromatin (ch). (Magnification, × 30,000.) *B*, Higher magnification (× 50,000) showing HSV nucleocapsids in the process of budding through the inner lamella of the nuclear membrane in areas thickened by the incorporation of HSV glycoproteins and the aggregation of tegument proteins on the inner surface *(arrows)*; nc, nucleocapsids within the nucleus. C, The process of budding completed, a mature enveloped HSV virion *(arrow)* is seen in the perinuclear space adjacent to the nuclear membrane. (Magnification × 75,000.) (*A* to *C* from Oxman MN: Herpes simplex encephalitis and meningitis. *In* Braude AI, Davis CE, Fierer J [eds]: Infectious Diseases and Medical Microbiology, ed 2. Philadelphia, WB Saunders, 1986, pp 1114–1132.)

not multiply in vivo and have low levels of thymidine kinase and other enzymes involved in DNA synthesis), and reduced capacity to reactivate from latency.[34, 165–170] Similar results have also been reported for another β gene product, ribonucleotide reductase.[34, 171–173] Several of the dispensable envelope glycoproteins enable HSV to infect polarized epithelial cells and neurons and to spread efficiently from cell to cell; the products of other dispensable viral genes enable HSV to evade immunologic and other host defenses.[34] The low density of essential genetic information in the HSV genome permits the insertion and deletion of genetic material without loss of viability, facilitating the preparation of genetically engineered viruses for use as live attenuated HSV vaccines and vectors for the delivery of heterologous genetic material into cells for gene therapy.[34, 36, 174, 175]

Cytopathic Effects

HSV infection results in the rapid shutoff of host cell macromolecular synthesis, and cells in which virus replicates do not survive.[34] The process begins with virus entry; a tegument protein (the product of a γ_1 gene called VHS, for virion host shutoff protein) introduced into the cell with the nucleocapsid causes destabilization and degradation of messenger RNA.[34, 37, 176–181] The product of one of the α genes (ICP27 encoded by α27) inhibits RNA splicing, markedly reducing the production of cellular messenger RNA with little effect on the production of HSV messenger RNA, which is predominantly unspliced.[34, 37] HSV infection of human cells also activates a cellular protein kinase that phosphorylates a cellular translation factor (eukaryotic initiation factor 2α), shutting off all protein synthesis.[182] This results in rapid cell death and premature termination of HSV replication. However, the product of an HSV gene (γ_1 34.5), dispensable for HSV replication in nonhuman cells, prevents activation of the protein kinase and ensures that the infected cell survives long enough to produce progeny virus.[34, 182] Interestingly, deletion of the γ_1 34.5 gene markedly reduces the virulence of HSV in rodent models of HSV infection.[183] Further inhibition of host cell synthetic functions occurs at the time of β gene expression, although the responsible viral proteins remain to be identified.[34, 37, 181] The onset of HSV DNA replication is associated with a restructuring of the nucleus. Initially distributed diffusely, ICP4 and ICP8 (the major single-stranded DNA binding protein) condense with ICP0, ICP27, and HSV DNA into discrete foci or "replication compartments" that are the site of HSV DNA replication and γ gene transcription.[37] Cessation of host cell synthetic functions and the accumulation of viral gene products in the infected cells cause profound changes in cell morphology (cytopathic effects), which can be observed in vivo as well as in cell culture. These consist of "ballooning degeneration," the production of Cowdry type A intranuclear inclusion bodies, and the formation of multinucleated giant cells. Individual infected cells become greatly enlarged, with pale vacuolated cytoplasm and swollen nuclei (ballooning degeneration). The nuclei exhibit nucleolar fragmentation and margination of their chromatin (see Fig. 240–4), and they develop inclusion bodies. These are initially homogeneous and slightly basophilic, and they often fill the nucleus. However, they rapidly condense and evolve into sharply demarcated acidophilic inclusion bodies that are separated from the deeply basophilic ring of marginated chromatin at the nuclear membrane by a clear zone or halo (Fig. 240–5). The appearance of viral glycoproteins in the plasma membrane of infected cells causes them to fuse with adjacent cells, forming multinucleated giant cells (Fig. 240–6). Fusion of infected cells with adjacent uninfected cells provides an efficient method for the cell-to-cell spread of HSV infection, even in the presence of antibodies capable of neutralizing extracellular virions. The formation of multinucleated giant cells containing eosinophilic Cowdry type A intranuclear inclusion bodies is the hallmark of HSV infection and provides a means for rapid diagnosis.

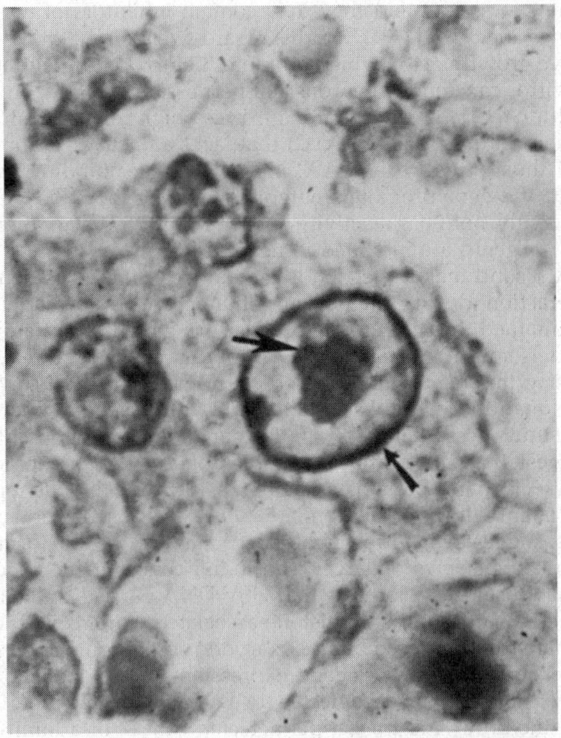

FIGURE 240–5 □ HSV cytopathic effects: intranuclear inclusion body. Section of liver from a malnourished child who died with disseminated HSV infection. A parenchymal cell shows ballooning degeneration with an enlarged nucleus containing a typical eosinophilic Cowdry type A intranuclear inclusion body (*large arrow*), which is separated from the basophilic ring of marginated chromatin at the nuclear membrane (*small arrow*) by a clear zone or halo. (H&E, × 2000.) (From Oxman MN: Herpes stomatitis. *In* Braude AI, Davis CE, Fierer J [eds]: Infectious Diseases and Medical Microbiology, ed 2. Philadelphia, WB Saunders, 1986, pp 752–772.)

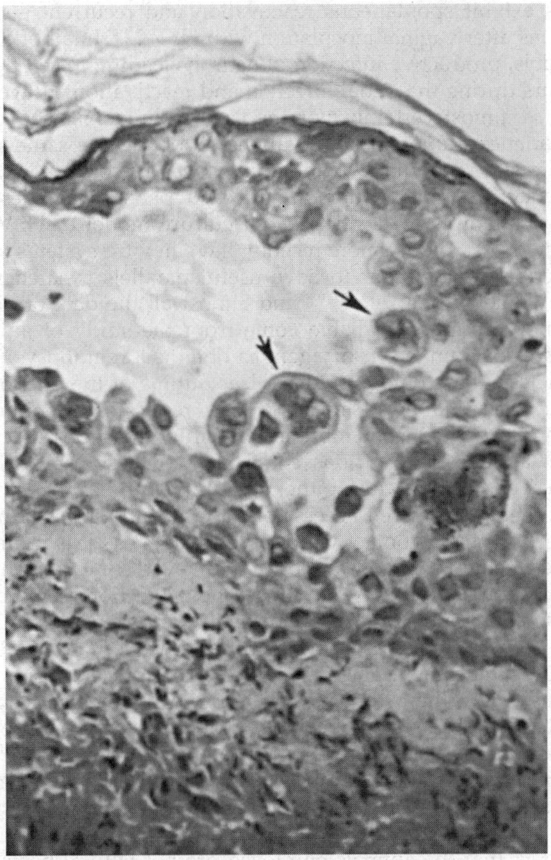

FIGURE 240–6 □ HSV cytopathic effects: multinucleated giant cells. Section of an intraepidermal vesicle produced by HSV infection of the skin. Infected epithelial cells show ballooning degeneration with the formation of multinucleated giant cells (*arrows*). Edema fluid has elevated the overlying stratum corneum. The underlying dermis shows edema and mononuclear cell infiltration. (H&E, × 200.) (Courtesy of Dr. R.J. Barr. From Oxman MN: Herpes stomatitis. *In* Braude AI, Davis CE, Fierer J [eds]: Infectious Diseases and Medical Microbiology, ed 2. Philadelphia, WB Saunders, 1986, pp 752–772.)

Herpes Simplex Virus Latency

The capacity of HSV to persist for life in its natural (human) host, as well as its long-term persistence in human populations, depends on its capacity to establish and maintain latent infections and to periodically reactivate. This remarkable adaptation, in which initial infection, latency, and reactivation are largely asymptomatic and unrecognized and almost never compromise the host's longevity or reproductive capacity, ensures the survival of HSV in nature (see Fig. 240–3). Because this benign virus-host interaction is the result of millions of years of coevolution, it seems unlikely that any animal model of HSV latency will exactly reproduce the situation in humans. Nevertheless, a number of animal models have been developed and intensively studied.[24, 34, 38, 39, 184–189] HSV latency is readily established in the mouse after corneal, skin, or footpad inoculation, but spontaneous reactivation is extremely rare.[184] HSV latency in the rabbit, established by corneal inoculation, resembles HSV latency in humans; reactivation occurs spontaneously and can be induced by iontophoresis of epinephrine into the cornea.[185–187] Guinea pigs exhibit spontaneous reactivation and recurrent genital lesions after vaginal inoculation with HSV-2.[188] In all of these models, productive infection of neurons leading to cell death occurs during the initial infection and reactivation. However, this is almost certainly not the case in humans, who may experience numerous reactivations involving the same anatomic site without developing any local sensory deficit.[38, 83] Latency and reactivation are in vivo phenomena; despite many attempts to develop a cell culture model of HSV latency,[34, 38, 190, 191] only more recently have in vitro systems been described that appear to have useful parallels to latency in the whole animal,[34, 38, 192–198] and almost all the data on HSV latency presently available come from the study of animal models or human sensory ganglia obtained at autopsy. Nevertheless, these data provide a clear outline of the phenomenon.* On initiation of infection, HSV replicates in epithelial cells of the mucous membranes or skin at the site of inoculation, and progeny virions come into contact with sensory nerve endings in the epithelium. Initial replication at the periphery is not even necessary if a large amount of virus is placed in direct contact with nerve endings, as it is in many experiments in animal models.[173] However, some peripheral replication is probably required when infection is initiated by small amounts of virus deposited on mucous membranes, as is generally the case during natural infection.

After attachment and penetration, HSV nucleocapsids are released into the cytoplasm of the nerve endings and transported by rapid retrograde axonal flow to the neuronal soma, where the viral DNA is released into the nucleus.[15, 199–201] In animal models, there is a brief period of virus replication in the sensory ganglia (which is probably an experimental artifact caused by the inoculation of large amounts of virus or the fact that the animals employed are not natural hosts for HSV), but there is no evidence that this occurs during natural infection in humans. Even in these animal models, all evidence of virus replication disappears within 2 to 4 weeks after infection. Periodically thereafter, latent virus reactivates, either spontaneously or in response to certain stimuli,[18–24, 184–186, 202–204] and is transported within the axons of sensory neurons back to the periphery, where it may again infect epithelial cells and produce the lesions of recurrent herpes or be shed into the environment in small amounts without producing signs or symptoms of disease. If the latently infected sensory ganglia are removed between these episodes of reactivation, no infectious virus can be recovered and no signs of virus replication can be detected. However, if the ganglia are explanted in culture, either whole or as dissociated viable ganglionic cells, infectious HSV emerges, usually within a week or so.[23, 24, 205–208] Thus, whereas latently infected ganglia are free of infectious virus, they contain cells, unequivocally shown to be neurons,[23, 24, 209–212] that retain the capacity to produce it.

Several important questions with implications for the prevention and treatment of HSV infections remain to be answered. The first is the mechanism by which HSV latency is established in sensory neurons. Studies with a variety of "replication-negative" HSV mutants, as well as the use of antiviral agents that block HSV DNA synthesis, have shown that latency can be established in the absence of detectable HSV replication, although without virus replication at the periphery, the number of latently infected neurons and the amount of HSV DNA per latently infected ganglion are reduced.[165–170, 173, 213–221] Of particular interest is the observation that an HSV mutant defective in VP16 and thus unable to transactivate its α genes and replicate nevertheless established latent infections in sensory neurons in vivo after peripheral inoculation.[221] Furthermore, this VP16-negative mutant exhibited no deficit in its capacity to persist in latent form or to reactivate.[221] Thus, whereas VP16 plays an essential role in the lytic pathway of HSV gene expression, it is not required for the establishment, maintenance, or reactivation of HSV latency. Studies with other replication-negative HSV mutants, including α4 (ICP4) deletion mutants, have demonstrated that latency can be established in sensory neurons in the absence of significant α gene expression.[37–39, 218–222] Thus, the establishment of HSV latency appears to be a passive process governed by neuronal factors rather than by any viral gene products.

These observations leave unanswered the questions of how sensory neurons infected in vivo with replication-competent wild-type HSV are able to avoid productive lytic infection and survive, given the fact that neurons and most other cells infected in culture undergo productive infection and are destroyed. One key to this crucial difference may be VP16, the tegument protein required to transactivate α gene expression (see earlier). During natural infection in vivo, virions produced in epithelial cells at the periphery infect the termini of sensory nerves, which are several centimeters from the nucleus of the neuron, a distance more than 1000 times greater than that separating the cell surface and nucleus in the epithelial cells and in most cells in culture. Nucleocapsids are efficiently transported to the neuronal nucleus by rapid retrograde axonal flow,[15, 199–201] but the amount of VP16 that reaches the nucleus may be insufficient to transactivate α gene expression and initiate productive HSV infection. In addition to this deficiency in VP16, sensory neurons in vivo may lack one or more of the cellular transcription factors required for VP16 transactivation or even for basal level α gene expression, and they may contain inhibitors of α gene expression.[121–128, 129, 223–225] In this regard, we already know that nerve growth factor, which promotes neuronal differentiation in vitro, can render neurons nonpermissive for HSV in cell culture[194, 195] and that neurons express high levels of an octamer binding protein (Oct-2) that lacks an activator domain and thus binds to the TAATGARAT octamer binding motif in HSV α gene promoters without activating them.[224, 225] Consequently, both basal activity and VP16-induced activation of HSV α genes are inhibited in neurons.[224, 225]

A second major question is the nature of the virus-neuron interaction during latency and the means by which it is maintained. In latently infected sensory ganglia from animal models and humans, HSV DNA appears to persist in a form lacking the free terminals observed in linear virion DNA.[214–216] The quantity of viral DNA detected and the fact that neurons constitute less than 10% of the ganglionic cell population suggest that the number of copies of the HSV genome is relatively high, perhaps as many as 10 to 20 HSV genomes per latently infected neuron.[34, 38, 39, 214–216] The absence of terminals suggests that this viral DNA may be in the form of circular episomes or large head-to-tail concatemers. Studies in a mouse model indicate that HSV DNA persists in latently infected neurons as a histone-associated supercoiled episomal structure resembling eukaryotic chromatin.[226] There is little evidence of viral gene expression during latency. No HSV proteins can be detected in latently infected neurons, and the only viral transcripts detected consist of a family of two or three overlapping RNAs transcribed from a diploid gene within the long inverted repeat sequences IR_L and TR_L (see Fig. 240–2). These transcripts, called latency-associated transcripts (LATs), have some unusual properties and may be present at as many as 20,000 to 50,000 copies per latently infected neuron.[34, 37, 40, 210–212, 227–236] They overlap the α0 gene, which encodes the immediate early protein ICP0, but they are transcribed from the DNA strand opposite that from which ICP0 messenger RNA is transcribed, and in the oppo-

*References 9, 18, 23, 24, 34, 37–41, 83, 167, 184, 189.

site direction (see Fig. 240–2). They are unusually stable introns, 2.0 and 1.5 kb in size, that are derived from an 8.5-kb primary transcript. The 2.0- and 1.5-kb LATs are not capped or polyadenylated and, unlike functional messenger RNA, are retained in the nucleus (Fig. 240–7). Moreover, no LAT-encoded protein has yet been identified in latently infected neurons. Evidence suggests that the 2.0- and 1.5-kb LATs may owe their stability, at least in part, to a stable lariat structure.[237] Because they are, in part, complementary to the 3′-terminal portion of ICP0 messenger RNA, it has been suggested that LATs might function as antisense RNA, to prevent the expression of the α0 gene.[210] Because ICP0 appears capable of trans-activating other α and β genes, including α4, in the absence of VP16,[34, 37, 40, 193, 217] its suppression by LATs might be expected to prevent productive HSV infection and thus play an important role in the establishment and maintenance of neuronal latency. Consistent with such a role in maintaining neuronal latency is the observation that the LAT promoter is more active in cells of neuronal origin than in nonneuronal cells.[34, 37, 40, 238–241] However, deletion mutants unable to express LATs show no defect in their capacity to establish and maintain neuronal latency in animal models, although they often exhibit a reduction in their efficiency of reactivation.[242–251] Thus, the role of LATs remains to be determined.

The absence of detectable HSV gene expression in latently infected neurons and the ability of replication-negative HSV mutants to establish and maintain latency in animal models indicate that HSV DNA replication, at least that catalyzed by HSV-encoded DNA polymerase, is not required to maintain the HSV genome in latently infected neurons. Consistent with this conclusion is the clinical observation that prolonged suppression of recurrent genital herpes with acyclovir, which blocks HSV DNA synthesis catalyzed by the viral DNA polymerase, fails to abolish latent HSV infection in the sacral ganglia.[252–254]

Although no HSV gene has yet been identified that is required for the establishment or maintenance of neuronal latency, two HSV genes have been implicated in reactivation. One, α0, encodes the immediate early protein ICP0. The other encodes the LATs. ICP0 is capable of trans-activating α and β gene expression in the absence of VP16, but it is dispensable for HSV replication in cell culture and in epithelial cells in vivo.[34, 37, 40, 131, 132, 193, 217] Despite their normal ability to establish and maintain latency in neurons, ICP0⁻ HSV mutants appear to be deficient in their capacity to reactivate in some (but not all) animal and cell culture models of HSV latency.[132, 193, 217, 255] In addition, the use of an adenovirus vector to introduce individual HSV genes into latently infected cells in culture has demonstrated that ICP0 is able to reactivate latent HSV, whereas ICP4, the critical α gene for HSV replication, is not.[131, 255, 256] Taken together, these data suggest that replication of HSV in permissive cells infected with HSV virions and reactivation of latent HSV in neurons involve different pathways. The initial event in the exogenous HSV infection of permissive cells is the VP16-stimulated expression of the α4 gene, whereas the initial event in the reactivation of latent HSV in neurons appears to be the expression of the α0 gene under the control of host cell factors.

LAT⁻ HSV mutants have also proved to be deficient in their capacity to reactivate in some but not all animal model systems,[242–251] suggesting that at least in some circumstances, both ICP0 and LATs are required for reactivation of latent

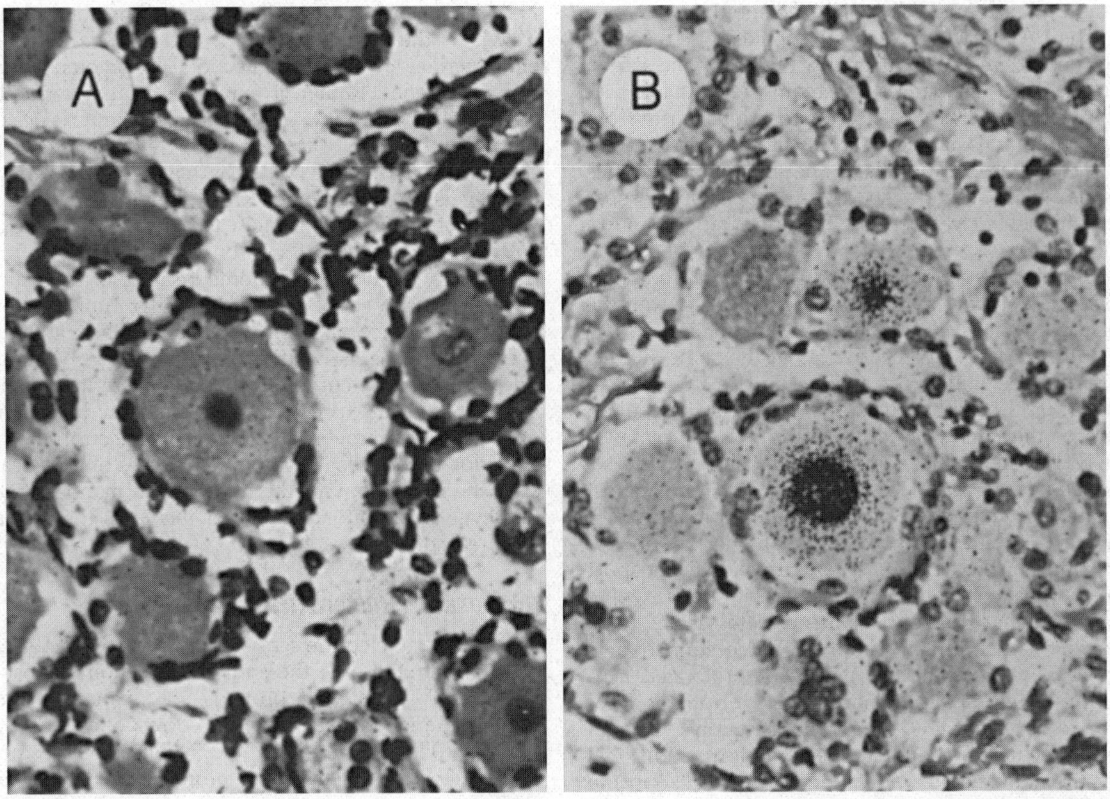

FIGURE 240–7 □ Detection of HSV LATs in human sensory ganglia by in situ hybridization. (Magnification, × 200.) *A*, Absence of ICP0 messenger RNA. Hybridization with sulfur S 35–labeled RNA complementary to ICP0 messenger RNA reveals no hybridization signal. *B*, Presence of LATs in the nuclei of two sensory neurons. Hybridization with ^{35}S-labeled RNA complementary to LATs reveals a dense accumulation of silver grains over two neuronal nuclei. (*A* and *B* from Croen KD, Ostrove JM, Dragovic L, Straus SE: Characterization of herpes simplex type 2 latency-associated transcription in human sacral ganglia and in cell culture. J Infect Dis 163:23–28, 1991.)

HSV. In one study, latency and reactivation by LAT⁻ ICP0⁺ and LAT⁺ ICP0⁺ HSV mutants were compared in the rabbit cornea model of HSV latency.[249] Although there was no difference in the number of latently infected neurons or in the amount of HSV DNA in trigeminal ganglia from LAT⁺ and LAT⁻ infected rabbits, both spontaneous and epinephrine iontophoresis–induced reactivation were reduced by 80% to 90% in the rabbits latently infected with LAT⁻ virus. Epinephrine iontophoresis induced low levels of productive-cycle transcription (i.e., transcription of α, β, and γ HSV genes) in only 1% to 10% of the latently infected neurons, and this was transient. Moreover, whereas infectious virus appeared in the periphery, no viral DNA replication and no infectious virus could be detected in the ganglia at any time after inductions, and there was no net increase in the amount of HSV DNA.[249] These observations indicate that LATs, although not absolutely required, play a major role in facilitating spontaneous and epinephrine-induced reactivation of latent HSV. They also suggest that only a small proportion of stimulated neurons go on to replicate viral genomes and that if any infectious virus is produced in the ganglion, it is transported rapidly to the periphery and reinitiates infection there efficiently. Moreover, the failure of productive-phase transcription to persist suggests that neurons induced to express productive-phase transcripts quickly reestablish their latent-phase transcription pattern. Furthermore, the absence of detectable differences in viral gene expression or in the recovery of viral DNA from ganglia latently infected with LAT⁻ and LAT⁺ viruses suggests that LAT exerts its effect in a critical subpopulation of sensory neurons or in peripheral tissues in which reactivated virus first replicates.[249] A similar study of LAT⁺ and LAT⁻ mutants of HSV-2 in a guinea pig model of genital herpes yielded similar results.[257] Expression of HSV-2 LATs had no effect on the establishment or maintenance of latency, but it markedly enhanced spontaneous reactivation.[257] The LAT function affecting spontaneous reactivation is reported to reside in the first 1.5 kb of the 8.5-kb primary transcript in sequences upstream of the stable 2.0- and 1.5-kb LATs.[258, 259] The absence of infectious virus from the ganglia in animals shedding HSV at the periphery is consistent with the observation that in neurons, noninfectious nucleocapsids are axonally transported to the periphery separately from HSV glycoproteins and enveloped at the neuroepithelial junction.[260]

The important question of the fate of the neuron after reactivation of latent HSV remains unresolved. However, the absence of sensory loss in the affected skin in individuals who have suffered repeated recurrences at the same site for many years and the failure of the specific site involved to gradually shift (as would be expected if reactivation resulted in the death of the latently infected neuron) argue in favor of the survival of neurons after reactivation in vivo.[38, 83, 184] Survival of the neuron after HSV reactivation would suggest that reactivation in vivo may not involve the normal cycle of HSV replication. It might involve only an increase in the number of copies of the HSV genome, with axonal transport of some to epithelial cells at the periphery; or it might involve formation and axonal transport of incomplete virions (e.g., nucleocapsids)[260]; or it might simply involve limited and short-lived HSV replication. The failure of prolonged acyclovir therapy to eliminate asymptomatic peripheral HSV shedding or to abolish latent ganglionic infection[252–254] from patients with recurrent genital herpes provides additional support for the notion that reactivation of latent HSV in the neuron involves a different pathway from that involved in HSV replication. The resistance of asymptomatic HSV shedding to acyclovir suggests that this pathway may involve little or no production of HSV-encoded thymidine kinase and use cellular rather than HSV-encoded DNA polymerase to replicate the HSV DNA. The presence of a host-dependent origin of DNA replication within the HSV genome is consistent with the possibility that cellular machinery in the neuron amplifies the HSV genome during latency and reactivation.[34]

It is clear that the phenomenon of HSV latency is heavily dependent on the unique properties of the sensory neuron. Selective pressures during the millennia have led HSV to develop the ability to establish and maintain latent infections in sensory neurons while at the same time retaining its capacity to induce productive lytic infections in epithelial cells. In view of the importance of latency for the survival of HSV in nature, it would seem logical that HSV genes should play a major role in the establishment and maintenance of latency. Some of the HSV genes that are dispensable for virus replication in epithelial cells would be good candidates. However, no HSV gene required for the establishment or maintenance of neuronal latency has yet been identified. This might imply that neuronal latency simply reflects the inability of HSV to initiate α gene expression in the absence of VP16 and the failure of this tegument protein to reach the nucleus of the infected neuron. However, the subsequent occurrence of spontaneous and induced HSV reactivation demonstrates that the latent HSV genome is capable of reactivation even in the absence of VP16. The application of extremely sensitive in situ polymerase chain reaction (PCR) techniques has revealed that at least in mouse models of HSV latency, HSV genomes can be detected in the majority of ganglionic neurons—many more than express abundant LATs detectable by conventional in situ hybridization.[261, 262] Most or all of these neurons appear to be producing low levels of LATs detectable by in situ PCR.[262] Moreover, the use of PCR techniques has also revealed low levels of transcription of α (ICPU4) and β (thymidine kinase) genes in latently infected ganglia.[263] These results suggest that reactivation of latent HSV in sensory neurons is not an all-or-none phenomenon in which the cascade of α, β, and γ gene expression that characterizes productive infection is triggered by transcription of α genes. Rather, it may be a multistep uphill process in which progression from one step to the next occurs at low frequency because of the inhospitable environment provided by the neurons. Thus, whereas many neurons may express low levels of α messenger RNA, these may not be sufficient to produce enough α protein to activate β gene expression, and so on. Clearly, the neuron plays a key role in limiting the activity of the HSV genome because of both the absence of adequate levels of required cellular transcription factors and the presence of neuron-specific inhibitors of HSV gene expression.* The association of the latent HSV genome with nucleosomes in a chromatin-like structure may also serve to limit HSV gene expression during latency by making much of the viral genome unavailable for transcription.[226] Presumably, dorsal root section and other causes of HSV reactivation alter the physiology of the neuron in a manner that reduces the level of inhibitory factors or increases the availability of required cofactors.

Antigenic Characteristics

Because the nucleotide sequences shared by HSV-1 and HSV-2 are distributed over the entire HSV genome, most if not all of the HSV-1–encoded proteins are related in amino acid sequence and structure to the corresponding proteins encoded by HSV-2.[9, 33, 34, 47, 51–57, 270–272] Consequently, most of the structural and nonstructural proteins of HSV-1 and HSV-2 elicit cross-reactive immune responses.[2, 30, 31, 41, 42, 47, 51, 270–274] This provides some degree of heterotypic immunity when persons infected with one HSV serotype are subsequently

*References 34, 37, 128, 129, 219, 223–225, 238–241, 264–269.

exposed to the other (see later), but it has complicated serodiagnosis and seroepidemiologic investigations.[47, 51, 275–281] Fortunately, two of the HSV envelope glycoproteins, gC and gG, elicit mainly type-specific immune responses, and this has permitted the development of type-specific immunoassays for identification of HSV isolates, serologic diagnosis of infection, and seroepidemiologic investigations.[47, 85, 272–274, 282–306]

Epidemiology

HSVs are worldwide in distribution. Despite the susceptibility of a variety of animals to experimental infection, humans are the only natural reservoir, and no vectors are involved in transmission. The capacity of HSVs to establish lifelong latent infections with periodic reactivation and virus shedding (see Fig. 240–3) ensures their survival in populations too small and isolated to support the continuous circulation of viruses that cause epidemic diseases like measles and influenza. Consequently, HSV is endemic in virtually every human society throughout the world, from large urban populations to remote geographically isolated native tribes.[276, 307, 308]

Geographic variations in the pattern of diseases caused by HSV (e.g., the occurrence of fatal disseminated HSV in African children or of HSV pharyngotonsillitis in American university students) reflect differences in the conditions of the host population and in the age at acquisition of infection, not variations in the parasite. Whereas the genomic DNA of isolates of HSV-1 and HSV-2 from different geographic locations (and even of epidemiologically unrelated isolates from the same location) have distinct restriction endonuclease "fingerprints," no consistent biologic differences have been documented.[34, 60, 64–69, 83, 85, 276, 309, 310] There is no evidence of differing racial or sexual susceptibility to HSV or of significant seasonal or sexual variation in the incidence of overt disease. However, genital herpes is transmitted more efficiently from men to women than from women to men.[277, 318–320]

The principal mode of transmission of HSV is close personal contact, which mediates the direct transfer of virus by infected secretions or from an infected mucocutaneous surface to the recipient's mucous membranes or skin. Because the intact stratum corneum is resistant to HSV infection, transmission to cutaneous sites generally requires some disruption of this barrier, either by trauma or by disease. HSV is labile. Consequently, despite experimental evidence that it can survive for hours on a variety of contaminated surfaces, there is no documented transmission from inanimate objects (such as toilet seats) or from swimming pools or hot tubs, and there is no evidence of natural transmission by aerosols.[32, 85, 276, 311–315] Epidemiologic studies have been complicated by two characteristics of HSV: the prevalence of occult infections and the nature of the immune response.

More than two thirds of initial HSV-1 and HSV-2 infections are asymptomatic or unrecognized, and reactivation of latent HSV infection far more often results in asymptomatic virus shedding than in overt disease.* Consequently, at any point in time, persons shedding HSV asymptomatically (many of whom are totally unaware of ever having been infected with HSV) far outnumber those with clinical disease. Thus, clinical surveys greatly underestimate the incidence and prevalence of HSV infection.[32, 83, 275–277, 291–306, 313–317] Furthermore, although the amount of virus in the lesions of overt disease is greater than that shed asymptomatically, most new HSV-1 and HSV-2 infections result from contact with persons who are shedding HSV in the absence of recognized symptoms or lesions.[32, 83, 275–277, 297, 298, 313–357]

The immune response to HSV is largely to type-common antigenic determinants, making it difficult to identify antibodies to one HSV serotype in persons previously infected with the other.* This problem has been solved by the development of serologic assays employing as antigens the gG envelope glycoproteins of HSV-1 and HSV-2, which elicit primarily type-specific immune responses.[282–306]

The prevalence of HSV-1 and HSV-2 infections is best assessed by serologic surveys that identify previously infected persons, most or all of whom shed HSV intermittently and thus constitute the source of virus responsible for new infections. The only infected persons not detected by such surveys are newly infected ones who are tested before their antibody response has exceeded the threshold of the assay and the occasional person who fails to mount a detectable immune response to the particular HSV antigen or antigens employed. Clinical surveys fail to detect the majority of primary infections, which are subclinical, but when they are prospective and combined with virologic and serologic studies, they provide the most reliable data on the incidence of both symptomatic and asymptomatic infections and can identify unexpected clinical presentations of primary infection, such as pharyngotonsillitis and a mononucleosis-like syndrome in HSV-infected adults.[330, 359, 360]

The different epidemiologic patterns of HSV-1 and HSV-2 infections reflect differences in the mode of transmission. Because HSV-1 is transmitted principally by contact with infected oral secretions or lesions, the incidence and prevalence of infection are influenced by factors that affect the degree of exposure to these sources of infection, such as crowding, poor hygiene, and age. Thus, the rate of acquisition of HSV-1 infection is inversely related to socioeconomic status.[3, 28, 276, 296, 314, 315, 322, 331] This was shown by early serologic studies, which revealed that the age-specific prevalence of antibodies to HSV-1 was lower in upper-income groups (e.g., medical students) than in lower-income groups (e.g., ward patients).[28, 361] A number of later seroepidemiologic studies† have demonstrated that in children of low-income families in developing countries, seroconversion (i.e., primary HSV-1 infection) occurs early in life: the majority acquire antibodies to HSV-1 by 5 years of age, and 95% are seropositive by age 15 years. Similar results were obtained in low-income families in the United States and Western Europe during the 1950s, although the rate of acquisition of antibodies was somewhat lower: about 30% of 5-year-olds and more than 80% of 15-year-olds were seropositive. Predictably, the age-specific prevalence of antibodies to HSV-1 has been decreasing during the past 40 years in Western industrialized countries, especially in middle-class populations, as the standard of living has improved.‡ Studies indicate that the prevalence of antibodies to HSV-1 in white adults in the United States is now 50% to 60%, but it is only 25% in white 14-year-olds and 25% to 30% in white college students; the figures are much higher in blacks (70% in 14-year-olds and 50% to 60% in college students), undoubtedly reflecting lower socioeconomic status and crowding during childhood.§ In a study of college students, only 30% of whom were initially seropositive for HSV-1, primary infections occurred in nearly 10% of the susceptible students per year.[330] Thus, whereas primary HSV-1 infections are largely confined to early childhood in developing countries, and even in poor urban populations in the United States, the majority of middle- and upper-income children in Western societies escape HSV-1 infections during

*References 32, 42, 43, 51, 83, 85, 89–91, 275–277, 291–306, 313–357.

*References 2, 30, 31, 42, 47, 51, 85, 276, 277, 281, 313–315, 358.

†References 276, 292, 294–296, 299, 301, 302, 304, 306, 314, 315.

‡References 276, 292, 294–296, 299, 301, 302, 304, 306, 314, 315, 362–364.

§References 85, 276, 292, 294–296, 299, 301, 302, 304, 306, 314, 315, 330, 362–364.

childhood and experience a second peak of infections in adolescence and early adult life.[276, 296, 314] Because the clinical manifestations of primary oropharyngeal HSV infection differ in young children (gingivostomatitis) and adults (pharyngotonsillitis and a mononucleosis-like syndrome), this epidemiologic change has resulted in the appearance of a previously unrecognized disease in young adults: acute herpetic pharyngotonsillitis. Moreover, the increasing proportion of the population now reaching puberty without having been infected with HSV-1, which induces partial immunity to subsequent HSV-2 infection, is an important factor in the current epidemic of genital herpes (see later).

Clinical surveys indicate that 15% to 45% of adults in Western countries suffer herpes labialis, the majority experiencing no more than one episode per year, but approximately one third have two to six episodes per year, and about 5% have recurrences as often as once per month.[314, 331, 335, 365–374] The frequency and severity of episodes tend to decrease with age, perhaps reflecting decreased temporal proximity to the initial infection.[314, 316, 331, 371–373] Persons with a history of herpes labialis compose only 30% to 70% of those infected with HSV-1 (i.e., those with antibodies to HSV-1). Seropositive children and adults, including those with no history of symptomatic primary or recurrent infections, periodically shed HSV asymptomatically in their saliva and are the major source of virus that causes new HSV-1 infections. The proportion shedding virus at any given point in time appears to range from 1% to 10%, but it may be greater in children during the first year or two after primary infection and is markedly increased in immunosuppressed patients.[26, 83, 85, 276, 325–335, 373, 374] Current data on seroprevalence indicate that approximately 130 million U.S. citizens of all ages (50%) are infected with HSV-1.

HSV-2, the predominant cause of genital herpes, is transmitted sexually by contact with infected genital secretions or mucocutaneous surfaces. Thus, HSV-2 infection is rare before puberty, and its acquisition thereafter is related to sexual activity. The highest rates of infection occur between ages 15 and 35 years, and more than 80% of all primary HSV-2 infections occur in this age group. The prevalence of antibodies to HSV-2 varies from essentially zero in children younger than 14 years and celibate adults to more than 80% in prostitutes.* Once an uncommon disease among members of the white middle class in Western industrialized countries, symptomatic genital herpes has increased dramatically in prevalence since the mid-1960s.† In white middle-class communities in the United States, physician visits for initial episodes of symptomatic genital herpes now exceed 1 per 1000 persons per year,‡ and symptomatic genital herpes accounts for 1% to 8% of visits to STD clinics, 0.1% to 1% of visits to general gynecology clinics, and 0.6% to 4% of visits to university health services.[85, 276, 277, 296, 313–315, 381–385] Factors that contribute to this increasing prevalence of symptomatic genital herpes in white middle-class populations include the increasing sexual activity of adolescents,[386] the decreased use of barrier contraceptives, and the reduced proportion of white middle-class adolescents who have partial immunity to HSV induced by childhood HSV-1 infection.§ Because only a minority of HSV-2 infections are symptomatic, the incidence of seroconversion and the prevalence of antibodies to HSV-2 provide the most reliable estimates of the true incidence and prevalence of HSV-2 infection. Studies employing type-specific serologic assays indicated that the incidence of primary HSV-2 infection is about 1% to 2% per year in college students, 2% per year in middle-class women of childbearing age, 5% to 10% per year in multipartnered heterosexual STD clinic patients, and 5% per year in sexually active homosexual men.* These assays revealed HSV-2 antibody prevalence rates of less than 1% in a group of South Carolina college freshmen, 20% to 22% in pregnant women in California and women attending family planning clinics in western Pennsylvania, more than 30% in pregnant women in Seattle and middle-class women receiving care in an Atlanta health maintenance organization, and 16% in a representative cross-section of 15- to 74-year-old men and women in the United States sampled between 1976 and 1980.† Antibody prevalence is substantially higher in men and women attending STD clinics and in sexually active homosexuals.[276, 277, 296, 314, 315, 375, 381] Risk factors for HSV-2 infection include multiple sexual partners, early age at first intercourse, years of sexual activity, history of other STDs, low family income, and race; the age-specific prevalence of antibodies to HSV-2 is more than three times higher in blacks than in whites.‡ As in the case of HSV-1, latency and asymptomatic virus shedding play a critical role in maintaining HSV-2 in human populations, and the majority of new HSV-2 infections are acquired from a sexual partner shedding virus in the absence of recognized signs or symptoms of disease.[276, 277, 318–320, 356, 357] All seropositive persons have latent infection and probably experience reactivation at least occasionally. In otherwise healthy men and women with antibody to HSV-2, the prevalence of asymptomatic virus shedding from the genital tract is generally 1% to 2% on any given day, but it is substantially higher (e.g., 6% or more) in the first few months after initial HSV-2 infection, in the days immediately before and after a symptomatic recurrence, and in persons with frequent symptomatic recurrences.§ HSV DNA can be detected by PCR at a rate approximately eight times higher than that reported for infectious virus,[388, 389] but the biologic significance of low levels of HSV DNA in the absence of infectious virus remains to be determined.

The data outlined indicate that there are now 40 to 60 million people in the United States (16% to 22%) infected with HSV-2 and that more than 1 million new infections occur each year. Although HSV-1 and HSV-2 appear to be adapted to different anatomic sites (see Table 240–1), the decreasing prevalence of HSV-1 infections before puberty in affluent populations and the increasing popularity of orogenital sexual practices are changing the epidemiology of HSV-1 and HSV-2 infections. HSV-1 is now causing disease in territory formally inhabited exclusively by HSV-2 and vice versa. In the United States and Western Europe, 10% to 40% or more of initial episodes of genital herpes are now caused by HSV-1.‖ Although comparable in severity to genital herpes caused by HSV-2, genital infections with HSV-1 recur much less frequently.[51, 87–91] Genital herpes is discussed in more detail in Chapter 113.

Neonatal HSV infections, two thirds of which are caused by HSV-2, are usually acquired during passage through the infected birth canal of a mother with asymptomatic genital herpes.¶ Infection may also be acquired postnatally from the mother or another adult with nongenital HSV infection or by

*References 2, 32, 51, 85, 276, 290–306, 313–315, 321–323, 352, 375, 376.

†References 32, 51, 85, 276, 277, 296, 313–323, 354, 375, 377–383.

‡References 276, 277, 296, 315, 377, 379, 381–383.

§References 276, 277, 292–306, 314, 315, 375, 381.

*References 85, 276, 277, 291–306, 321–324, 354, 375.

†References 51, 85, 276, 277, 291–306, 313–315, 321–324, 354, 375, 381–383.

‡References 85, 276, 277, 291–306, 314, 315, 375, 381–386.

§References 32, 51, 85, 89–91, 276, 277, 296, 313, 315, 317, 323, 336–357, 375, 381–383, 387.

‖References 51, 89, 91, 276, 277, 296, 317, 323, 347, 375–381, 384–386, 390, 391.

¶References 32, 43, 51, 85, 276, 296, 315, 321–323, 354, 375, 392.

nosocomial transmission in the nursery. The risk for infection is much greater for infants born to mothers with primary than with recurrent genital HSV infections. The incidence of neonatal HSV infection in the United States is estimated to be between 1 in 3000 and 1 in 5000 live births, and it may be increasing in some populations because of the increasing incidence of genital herpes and the decreasing prevalence of prior HSV-1 infection, which may reduce the risk for transmission from mother to infant.*

Certain HSV infections are a particular hazard for special groups.[276] Herpetic whitlow caused by HSV-1 is an occupational hazard for medical, dental, and nursing personnel whose hands are exposed to infected oropharyngeal secretions.[332, 393, 394] HSV-1 skin infections (herpes gladiatorum) are common in high-school and college wrestlers.[395–397] Nosocomial outbreaks of HSV-1 infection in patients and personnel have occurred in neonatal nurseries and intensive care units as well as in dental practices.[66, 398–402] HSV-1 may also spread rapidly through closed, susceptible populations of young children, such as hospital wards, orphanage nurseries, and daycare centers.[325–328, 403, 404] Prostitutes are at high risk for genital herpes caused predominantly by HSV-2,[376] and anal and perianal HSV-2 infections are common among sexually active homosexual men.[405, 406]

Pathogenesis

HSV infection is usually cytolytic, and the resulting pathologic process is a consequence of necrosis of infected cells plus local inflammatory responses. Exogenous HSV infection is initiated when virus comes into contact with a mucosal surface (e.g., oropharynx, conjunctivae, cervix) or penetrates the stratum corneum of the skin at a site where this barrier has been disrupted by small cracks, minor trauma, or disease. HSV replicates locally in cells of the stratum spinosum, which undergo ballooning degeneration and loss of intercellular bridges and are soon separated by intercellular edema. At this stage, the lesions are papular and contain a few small multinucleated giant cells, the result of the fusion of HSV-infected cells with their infected and uninfected neighbors. Typical eosinophilic intranuclear inclusion bodies are already present. In the skin, the papular lesions evolve rapidly into intraepidermal vesicles as a result of the infection and degeneration of more epithelial cells and the influx of edema fluid, which elevates the stratum corneum to form a delicate, clear vesicle (see Fig. 240–6). The vesicle fluid contains fibrin, degenerating epithelial cells, multinucleated giant cells, and a large amount of cell-free virus. Capillary dilatation and infiltration by inflammatory cells are pronounced in the underlying dermis, but necrosis is absent. Inflammatory cells soon invade the vesicle, turning the fluid cloudy and transforming it into a pustule. The fluid is then absorbed, leaving a flat, adherent crust that is subsequently detached when subjacent epithelial cells grow back. The lesions heal without scars. Lesions in mucous membranes develop in the same way, but the thin roof of the vesicle quickly breaks down, leaving a shallow ulcer.

In most infected persons, even those who have a primary infection (i.e., the initial HSV infection of a host with no immunity to HSV-1 or HSV-2), virus replication and cell destruction are rapidly terminated at the site of inoculation, and the infection remains asymptomatic or unrecognized. In some cases, however, virus replication and cell destruction are more extensive, resulting in clinically manifest disease at the portal of entry, spread of virus to regional lymph nodes, and some degree of viremia.[407–411] In the normal host, nonspecific and specific defense mechanisms combine to localize infection, terminate virus replication, and eventually eliminate infectious virus from tissues at the portal of entry and at any sites of viremic spread. The incubation period for symptomatic infections is usually 3 to 7 days (range, 1 day to more than 2 weeks).

Early in the course of both symptomatic and asymptomatic infections, virus invades local sensory or autonomic nerve endings and is transported within axons to regional sensory or autonomic ganglia,[206, 207, 412–415] where lifelong latent infections are established in neurons (see earlier). Thereafter, despite the host's immunity, this latent virus is periodically reactivated, either spontaneously or by various stimuli, including trauma to the ganglion or nerve root, fever, menstruation, ultraviolet light, sexual intercourse, and emotional stress.* The reactivated virus then travels within axons back to the periphery and reinfects epithelial cells in the skin or mucous membranes at the original portal of entry. There, virus replication and cell-to-cell spread may produce intraepidermal vesicles like those produced during primary infection. When reactivation of latent HSV results in clinically manifest disease, it is called a recurrence or an episode of recurrent HSV infection. In the normal host, immune mechanisms rapidly limit local virus replication and spread so that recurrent HSV infections are generally less severe, less extensive, and of shorter duration than primary infections. In fact, in the majority of instances, the local infection is so circumscribed that no recognizable lesions are produced and reactivation results only in asymptomatic virus shedding. The lesions produced by HSV-1 and HSV-2 are identical to and indistinguishable pathologically from those caused by varicella-zoster virus.

Immune Responses and Other Host Defenses

The manifestations of HSV infection are determined to a large extent by an array of interacting and overlapping local and systemic host defense mechanisms that limit HSV replication and spread, destroy HSV-infected cells, and eventually eliminate infectious virus.[42] These host defenses fall into two categories, nonspecific and specific, which are most clearly differentiated during primary HSV infections. Only nonspecific defenses are operative during the first several days of primary infection (i.e., until specific immune responses develop).

The normal cornified epithelium is an important nonspecific barrier to the initiation and spread of HSV infection. In patients with defects in this host defense (e.g., those who have atopic eczema, Darier disease, pemphigus, and burns) HSV infections are frequently severe, widespread, and occasionally disseminated.[420–425]

Once primary HSV infection is initiated in the skin or mucous membranes, a number of nonspecific defense mechanisms are mobilized, producing a local inflammatory response. Complement is activated at the surface of infected epithelial cells and virions, and there is local production of interferon-α and other lymphokines. Macrophages are activated and neutrophils migrate into the infected epithelium, followed by monocytes and lymphocytes, including a subset of lymphocytes called natural killer (NK) cells, which are activated by interferon-α. Monocytes and macrophages (and probably also neutrophils) ingest and destroy cell-free virus, and virus-infected epithelial cells are destroyed by NK cells and probably also by monocytes and macrophages.[42, 426–433] In addition to activating NK cells, monocytes, and macrophages, locally produced interferon-α inhibits virus multiplication in epithelial cells directly. Together, these nonspecific

*References 43, 51, 85, 276, 277, 315, 321–323, 354, 375, 392.

*References 3, 20, 23, 24, 202–204, 331, 365–367, 369–374, 416–419.

host defense mechanisms slow HSV replication and limit its spread.

Antibodies to HSV are first detected several days after the onset of infection; they are elicited by epitopes on most of the HSV-encoded proteins, but those that are protective are primarily to epitopes on the envelope glycoproteins.[42, 47, 285, 433–441] Protective antibodies include complement-dependent and complement-independent neutralizing antibodies; antibodies that mediate the complement-dependent lysis of HSV-infected cells; and antibodies that mediate antibody-dependent cellular cytotoxicity (ADCC): lysis of HSV-infected cells by Fc receptor–bearing effector cells, principally NK cells but also subpopulations of monocytes, macrophages, and neutrophils.[42, 440] These specific immune responses, especially ADCC, further inhibit virus replication at the portal of entry and at any sites of viremic spread, and they prevent further virus dissemination.[42, 440] Somewhat later, during the second week of infection, HSV-immune T lymphocytes can be detected. These include lymphocytes that proliferate and produce interferon-γ and other lymphokines in response to HSV antigens and lymphocytes that are cytolytic for HLA-matched HSV-infected cells.[42, 430–433, 436, 442] In addition to recognizing and lysing syngeneic target cells expressing HSV glycoproteins,[442–450] the HSV-reactive cytotoxic T lymphocytes lyse target cells that express the HSV immediate early proteins ICP4 and ICP27.[451, 452] Consequently, they are able to destroy HSV-infected cells early in the virus replication cycle, before any progeny virus is produced.

Because of the multiplicity of overlapping and redundant host defenses, it has been difficult to determine the exact role and relative importance of each. Nevertheless, observations in humans with various deficiencies in host defenses and experiments in animal models appear to identify several critically important host defense mechanisms. The natural resistance of the normal epithelium and the virucidal and cytolytic capacities of macrophages and NK cells play a crucial role in localizing infection at the portal of entry and slowing virus replication during the first few days, before specific immune responses have developed. When these defenses are deficient, as they are in patients with eczema or extensive burns and in newborns, there is risk for early virus dissemination and overwhelming systemic infection.[42, 420–425, 433, 440] ADCC, the appearance of which coincides with resolution of the systemic symptoms of primary HSV infections, also plays a crucial role in limiting virus replication at the portal of entry and preventing visceral dissemination. For example, the presence of antibodies mediating ADCC is predictive of better outcome in neonatal HSV infections; the capacity of ADCC to protect against high-dose virus challenge has been demonstrated in a number of animal experiments; and deficiencies in ADCC, due primarily to numeric or functional deficiencies in effector cells, are associated with a markedly increased risk for severe disseminated HSV infection in humans.[42, 323, 438–440, 453–456] Finally, HSV-reactive T lymphocytes appear to be required to eradicate infectious virus from mucocutaneous sites of infection.[42, 383, 436, 442, 443] Experimentally infected nude mice, which lack T lymphocytes but have supernormal macrophage and NK cell activity, do not suffer the early disseminated disease observed in human neonates but die late in infection, when specific T-lymphocyte–mediated responses normally develop; and patients with deficient T-lymphocyte function (e.g., patients with acquired immunodeficiency syndrome [AIDS]) develop severe, persistent, locally progressive herpetic lesions but rarely have hematogenous dissemination.[42, 405, 429, 432, 442, 443] The T-cell response to HSV infection is predominantly a Th1 response.[42, 443, 446–449, 457–460] $CD4^+$ T cells are the predominant inflammatory cells infiltrating early recurrent herpetic lesions, and interferon-γ, produced at lesion sites, is associated with induction of MHC class II antigens.[446–449, 457–461] The predominant HSV-specific cytotoxic T cells are $CD4^+$,[448, 449, 459–461] presumably because of the inhibition of MHC class I antigen presentation by ICP47.[142–145, 449, 462, 463] Although patients with deficient cell-mediated immunity are subject to more frequent and more severe HSV recurrences, as well as a much greater frequency of asymptomatic shedding, no specific defect has been consistently identified in otherwise healthy persons who suffer frequent episodes of recurrent genital or labial herpes.[42, 85, 276, 331, 375, 429, 443] However, peripheral blood mononuclear cells from healthy persons infected with HSV-1 who have infrequent episodes of herpes labialis produce higher levels of interferon-γ and interleukin-2 when stimulated with HSV antigen than do peripheral blood mononuclear cells from persons who experience frequent episodes of herpes labialis.[331, 449, 461]

In addition to mediating virus attachment and entry into susceptible host cells, HSV envelope glycoproteins interact with host defense mechanisms.[464] At least three, gC, gE, and gI, appear to protect virions and virus-infected cells from destruction by host immune defenses. Glycoprotein gC functions as a receptor for complement component C3b and interferes with the lytic function of both the classical and the alternative complement pathways.[465] Consequently, it protects cell-free virus from complement-mediated neutralization and HSV-infected cells from complement-mediated immune lysis.[466–468] Envelope glycoproteins gE and gI form a complex that functions as a receptor for the Fc domain of immunoglobulin G, and gE alone serves as a receptor for immunoglobulin G aggregates.[469, 470] In the presence of nonimmune immunoglobulin G and immunoglobulin G aggregates, these receptors protect cell-free HSV from neutralization and HSV-infected cells from antibody-plus-complement–mediated cytolysis and destruction by sensitized lymphocytes.[469–471] In addition, by binding the Fc portion of immune immunoglobulin G already bound to an antigenic site by its Fab end, these receptors may protect HSV-infected cells from ADCC-mediated cytolysis.[472] Similarly, the immediate early gene product ICP47, which is also dispensable for growth in cell culture, protects HSV-infected cells from immune lysis by blocking HSV antigen presentation by MHC class I molecules (see earlier). These "dispensable" glycoproteins and the gene for ICP47 are invariably present on clinical isolates of HSV, despite that they are all dispensable for virus replication in cell culture and that mutants lacking them are readily obtained. Thus, the involved host defense mechanisms are likely to be important in vivo.

Because of the nature of the immunity induced by HSV and the prevalence of asymptomatic infection, the characterization of HSV infections as either primary (i.e., the initial HSV infection of a host with no immunity to either HSV-1 or HSV-2) or recurrent (i.e., symptomatic HSV infection caused by the reactivation of latent [endogenous] HSV) does not reflect the true complexity of the situation. Immunity to HSV is incomplete, as evidenced by the frequent recurrence of disease (e.g., herpes labialis, recurrent genital herpes) in the presence of homologous humoral and cellular immunity and by the ability to induce symptomatic infection in sero-positive persons by inoculating their skin with homologous virus.[473] Nevertheless, the clinical efficacy of homologous immunity is considerable, as indicated by the reduced extent and severity of recurrent compared with primary infections and by the presence of substantial, although incomplete, resistance to exogenous reinfection by the same HSV serotype. For example, restriction endonuclease analysis of HSV isolates from sequential episodes of recurrent genital herpes has shown that most recurrences are caused by reactivation of endogenous virus latent in sacral sensory ganglia.[474] Exogenous reinfection with a different strain of the same HSV serotype does occur, but it is rare, presumably because of the host's resistance to exogenous reinfection.[67, 474] Furthermore, because of the extensive antigenic cross-reactivity of HSV-1 and HSV-2 (see earlier), both HSV serotypes induce heterologous humoral and cellular immunity. Consequently, infection with one HSV serotype reduces susceptibility to infection by the other and moderates the severity of those infections that do occur. For example, serologic studies in a large population of women revealed that the prevalence of antibodies to HSV-2 was lower in women with antibodies to HSV-1 than in women without HSV-1 antibodies, indicating that HSV-1 infection, presumably acquired in childhood, provided partial protection from subsequent HSV-2 infection.[294, 318–320] These same studies also showed that women with antibodies only to HSV-2 were more likely to have a history of symptomatic genital herpes than were women with antibodies to both viruses, indicating that preexisting immunity to HSV-1 reduces the severity of those HSV-2 infections that do occur, so that a higher proportion are subclinical. The effect of heterologous immunity was also demonstrated in prospective clinical studies of the transmission and natural history of genital herpes. In couples in which one partner had genital herpes and the other was seronegative for HSV-2, the annual rate of transmission of HSV-2 infection to the susceptible partner was much higher when the potential recipients were HSV-seronegative than when they had preexisting antibodies to HSV-1.[318–320] Initial episodes of genital herpes caused by HSV-2 were observed to be less severe in patients with serologic evidence of prior HSV-1 infection (i.e., in persons with nonprimary first-episode HSV-2 infections) than in those with no preexisting antibodies to HSV-1 or HSV-2 (i.e., those with true primary HSV-2 infections).[32, 85, 347, 375] In addition, HSV-1 was isolated from a much larger proportion of patients with primary genital herpes than with nonprimary first episodes, indicating that previous, presumably oropharyngeal, HSV-1 infection protects against genital herpes caused by the same HSV serotype. Finally, because most primary and nonprimary first-episode infections are asymptomatic but still result in the establishment of latent infections that are subject to periodic reactivation, many people experiencing their first recognized episode of symptomatic infection are not, as they believe, experiencing an initial episode of exogenous infection. Instead, they are suffering their first symptomatic recurrence due to reactivation of a latent infection established in the course of an earlier asymptomatic primary infection.[32, 85, 347, 375]

Clinical Manifestations

The clinical manifestations of HSV infection are determined by the portal of entry of the virus; the prior experience of the host with HSV (i.e., whether the infection is primary, nonprimary first episode, or recurrent); the serotype and amount of virus initiating infection; and such host factors as age, immunocompetence, nutritional status, and presence or absence of conditions like eczema or burns that compromise the normal resistance of the skin. The major clinical syndromes caused by HSV are listed in Table 240–1, together with an estimate of the proportion of each caused by HSV-1 and HSV-2. Whereas the proportion of cases caused by each HSV serotype varies widely, depending on the syndrome, there is generally no discernible difference between the clinical presentation and course when a given syndrome is caused by HSV-1 or by HSV-2. One exception appears to be the frequency of recurrences of oropharyngeal and genital HSV infections caused by the two viruses.[87–91] When 39 adults with concurrent primary HSV infections of the oropharynx and genitalia caused by the same virus in each person (HSV-1 in 12 and HSV-2 in 27) were observed, the pattern of subsequent recurrences was found to differ according to virus type and anatomic site. The mean monthly rate of recurrence was 0.34 for genital herpes caused by HSV-2, 0.08 for genital herpes caused by HSV-1, 0.12 for orolabial herpes caused by HSV-1, and 0.001 for orolabial herpes caused by HSV-2.[87–91] Because transmission of HSV and thus its survival in human populations depend chiefly on recurrent infections, the greater recurrence rate of HSV-1 than HSV-2 in orolabial infections and of HSV-2 than HSV-1 in genital infections may reflect the adaptation of the two serotypes to their respective anatomic niches (see earlier). These differences help to explain why HSV-1 is isolated from lesions of recurrent infection so much less frequently than from lesions of primary genital herpes and why HSV-2 is almost never isolated from lesions of herpes labialis.

Oropharyngeal Infections

ACUTE HERPETIC GINGIVOSTOMATITIS*

Acute herpetic gingivostomatitis, a manifestation of primary oropharyngeal HSV-1 infection, most often affects children between 6 months and 5 years of age, but it is being reported with increasing frequency in older children and adults. The source of infection is usually an adult with herpes labialis or an asymptomatic recurrence who is shedding HSV-1 in saliva, but it may also be another infected child, especially in a household or institutional outbreak. The incubation period is usually 3 to 6 days (range, 2 days to 2 weeks). Onset is abrupt, with temperature to 102°F to 104°F (38.9°C to 40.6°C), anorexia, and listlessness. The mouth becomes sore before oral lesions appear, and the infant is restless, irritable, and unwilling to eat or drink. Gingivitis is the most constant and striking manifestation of the disease. The gums are first hyperemic and then become markedly swollen (sometimes almost covering the teeth), reddened, friable, and exquisitely tender. They bleed easily, sometimes spontaneously, and there is a bright red line along the dental margin (Fig. 240–8). In most patients, vesicular lesions develop on the oral mucous membranes; they begin as tiny vesicles surrounded by narrow zones of erythema but quickly rupture, leaving tender, round, 1- to 3-mm, shallow, yellowish gray, indurated ulcers or plaques. These often coalesce and are surrounded by a thin, red halo. They may occur anywhere on the mucous membrane of the mouth or pharynx but are most common on the tongue, the inner surface of the lips, and the buccal and sublingual mucosa (Fig. 240–9). Lesions occur less fre-

*References 26–28, 83, 325, 326, 328, 329, 475, 476.

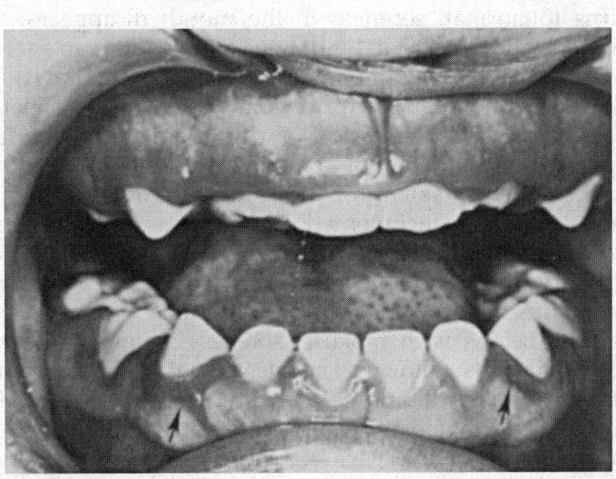

FIGURE 240–8 □ Acute herpetic gingivostomatitis: gingivitis. In this child with acute herpetic gingivostomatitis, the gums are tender, swollen, and hyperemic, and there is a bright red line *(arrows)* along the dental margin. (From Oxman MN: Herpes stomatitis. *In* Braude AI, Davis CE, Fierer J [eds]: Infectious Diseases and Medical Microbiology, ed 2. Philadelphia, WB Saunders, 1986, pp 752–772.)

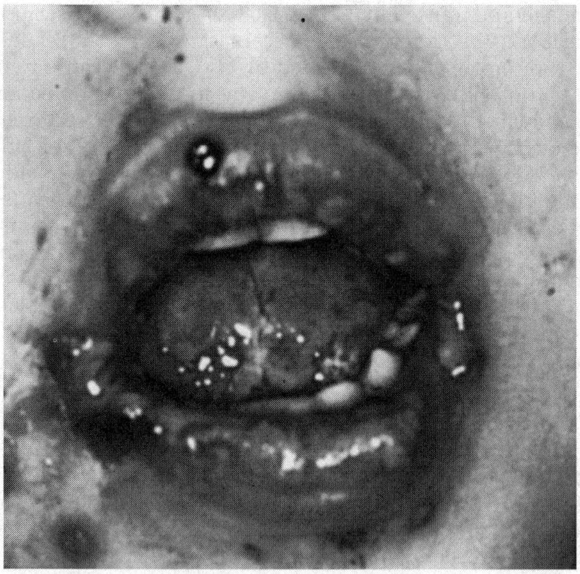

FIGURE 240–9 □ Acute herpetic gingivostomatitis. In addition to having vesicles on the oral mucosa, palate, and tongue, this child with acute herpetic gingivostomatitis has herpetic vesicles on the lips and perioral skin. (From Oxman MN: Herpes stomatitis. *In* Braude AI, Davis CE, Fierer J [eds]: Infectious Diseases and Medical Microbiology, ed 2. Philadelphia, WB Saunders, 1986, pp 752–772.)

quently on the soft palate and on the gums themselves, occasionally in the pharynx, and rarely in the larynx. The submandibular and anterior cervical lymph nodes are enlarged and tender. Salivation and drooling are marked, and the breath is fetid owing to overgrowth of anaerobic oral bacteria. Herpetic lesions also develop often in areas of skin contaminated with infected saliva, which contains large quantities of HSV. Thus, many children develop herpetic vesicles in the perioral skin (see Fig. 240–9), and herpetic paronychia is seen in finger suckers. Autoinoculation may also result in herpetic vulvovaginitis and HSV infections of the eye. The disease is self-limited and without sequelae in normal children, but it varies considerably in severity and duration. On occasion, infants are extremely ill with high fever, systemic toxicity, and severe and extensive mucosal lesions that prevent adequate oral intake of fluids. The acute phase generally lasts 5 to 7 days, after which the temperature returns to normal, soreness in the mouth disappears, and oral lesions begin to heal. Symptoms subside after an average of 12 to 14 days, but gingivitis may resolve more slowly, and adenopathy often persists for several weeks. HSV-1 is readily isolated from saliva and stool during the acute illness, and despite the development of neutralizing antibodies, it continues to be shed in saliva for weeks after recovery. Although viremia is rarely documented, it probably occurs in many cases of uncomplicated herpetic gingivostomatitis.

Primary infection with HSV-1 causes acute herpetic gingivostomatitis in adults as well as in children.[477–479] The disease in adults begins with malaise; soreness in the mouth and throat; pain on swallowing; swollen, tender, bleeding gums; and anterior cervical and submandibular lymphadenopathy. Pharyngitis is much more prominent than in children, occurring in nearly every case. One to 3 days after onset, vesicular lesions appear on the oral and pharyngeal mucosa, the tongue, the inner surface of the lips, and the palate. They are identical in appearance and evolution to the lesions of children, but the disease is generally less severe. Drooling is not a problem, perioral skin lesions are uncommon, and lesions produced by autoinoculation are rare.

ACUTE HERPETIC PHARYNGOTONSILLITIS[330, 359, 360]

In adults, primary oropharyngeal HSV-1 infection causes pharyngitis and tonsillitis much more frequently than gingivostomatitis. The illness begins with fever, malaise, headache, and sore throat. Tiny vesicles appear on the tonsils and posterior pharynx, but they quickly break down to form shallow ulcers that run together. A grayish yellow exudate forms on the tonsils and posterior pharynx in more than half the patients, but lesions in the anterior mouth or lips are seen in less than 10%. The disease is usually indistinguishable clinically from pharyngotonsillitis caused by the group A β-hemolytic streptococcus, and it may also be confused with infectious mononucleosis caused by Epstein-Barr virus. In college and university students, more than 70% of whom are seronegative for HSV-1 and HSV-2, HSV is a major cause of pharyngitis and tonsillitis. Although most cases appear to be caused by HSV-1, HSV-2 is being isolated with increasing frequency, especially when pharyngotonsillitis is associated with orogenital contact or occurs in the course of symptomatic genital herpes (see Chapter 113). Persons seropositive for HSV as a result of previous herpetic pharyngotonsillitis are latently infected and may subsequently develop herpes labialis and asymptomatic shedding of HSV in saliva. However, the incidence of recurrent HSV pharyngotonsillitis remains to be determined.

HERPES LABIALIS*

Herpes labialis (cold sore, fever blister) is the most common manifestation of recurrent HSV-1 infection. Most patients (50% to 80%) have a prodrome of pain, burning, tingling, or itching at the site of the subsequent eruption, which usually precedes its onset by 6 hours or less but occasionally lasts 24 to 48 hours. This is followed by the appearance of a small cluster of erythematous papules that rapidly develop into tiny, thin-walled, intraepidermal vesicles (Fig. 240–10). These generally become pustular and then either burst, leaving shallow ulcers, or dry and form a scab. Left undisturbed, the

*References 83, 204, 331, 333–335, 365–373, 478–482.

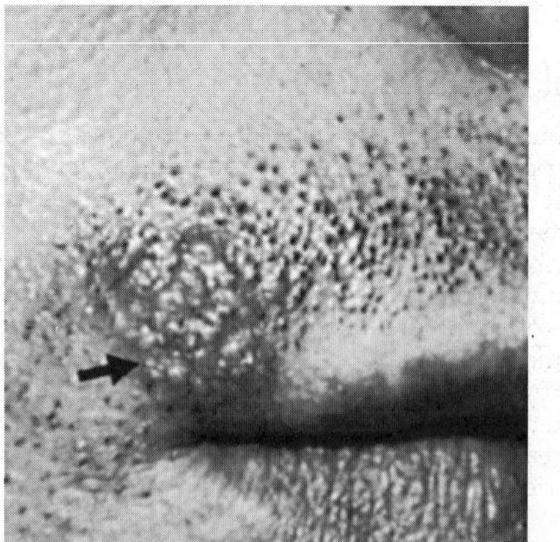

FIGURE 240–10 □ Herpes labialis. After a 12-hour prodrome of localized itching and burning, this medical student developed a small group of erythematous papules that quickly evolved into a typical cluster of vesicles *(arrow)* on an erythematous base. (From Oxman MN: Herpes stomatitis. *In* Braude AI, Davis CE, Fierer J [eds]: Infectious Diseases and Medical Microbiology, ed 2. Philadelphia, WB Saunders, 1986, pp 752–772.)

scab is displaced by the regrowth of epithelium. The evolution of the lesions is generally rapid, the papular stage lasting only a few hours and the vesicles crusting within 2 days. Lesion area (usually less than 100 mm^2) and pain are maximal during the vesicular stage and decline rapidly thereafter. Healing is completed, with loss of scabs and without scarring, in 6 to 10 days. Patients sometimes have local lymphadenopathy but no constitutional symptoms.

The most common site of herpes labialis is the vermilion border of the lip (95%), usually the outer third and more often the lower lip than the upper. Other sites include the nose, the chin, the cheek, and rarely the oral mucosa. Although HSV occasionally causes recurrent lesions of the oral mucosa, it is not the cause of recurrent aphthous ulcers, which afflict many persons with no history of HSV infection and no antibodies to HSV.[365–367, 483, 484] Most people subject to herpes labialis suffer fewer than two episodes per year, but a small minority have recurrences at intervals of a month or less. In a given person, the lesions generally recur at the same site, and the provoking factor (e.g., exposure to sunlight, menses, fever, stress) may also be stereotyped.

The quantity of HSV present is highest (more than 10^5 infectious doses per milliliter of vesicle fluid) during the first 24 hours, when the lesions are vesicular, and it decreases steadily thereafter; rarely is virus recovered after 5 days. HSV is usually present in the saliva during episodes of herpes labialis, and it can also be recovered from 1% to 5% of saliva samples obtained when persons are free of disease, although the concentration of virus is considerably lower. Intraoral lesions are rarely present, and HSV is not recovered from parotid gland secretions. Thus, the source of virus in the saliva remains a mystery.

Ocular Infections[485–497]

Primary HSV infections of the eye occur most commonly in children, often as a result of autoinoculation during acute herpetic gingivostomatitis or asymptomatic oropharyngeal HSV infection. The conjunctiva may also be the portal of entry of HSV and infection of the eye the sole manifestation of primary HSV infection. Most infections are asymptomatic or unrecognized, but even when ocular disease is obvious, the causal role of HSV is often unappreciated. Except in newborns, HSV infection of the eye is almost always caused by HSV-1.

When symptomatic, primary HSV infection is usually manifested as unilateral follicular conjunctivitis, often accompanied by blepharitis and preauricular lymphadenopathy. There may be herpetic vesicles on the lid margins and periorbital skin. Symptoms typically include photophobia, excessive lacrimation, chemosis, and edema of the eyelids, and many patients also have fever and constitutional symptoms. In the majority of cases, there is no obvious corneal involvement and the infection resolves spontaneously and completely in 2 to 3 weeks. Some primary infections do involve the cornea, producing acute herpetic keratoconjunctivitis. Minute vesicles develop near the corneal margin and may progress to form characteristic branching "dendritic" lesions or larger "ameboid" or "geographic" ulcers. Keratoconjunctivitis is usually accompanied by pain and a foreign body sensation. Deeper tissues are generally not involved during primary infection, except in newborns and in patients inadvertently treated with corticosteroids, and the process tends to resolve spontaneously without obvious sequelae. When infection does involve the underlying stroma, it may result in corneal edema, infection of other intraocular tissues, extensive scarring, and corneal perforation. Even when asymptomatic, primary infection results in the establishment of HSV latency in the trigeminal ganglion and periodic reactivation thereafter. Most reactivations are asymptomatic, with shedding of HSV in tears, but some result in symptomatic recurrences.

Ocular HSV infection may recur in the form of keratitis, blepharitis, or keratoconjunctivitis. Recurrences develop in at least 25% of patients who have symptomatic primary infection and in many persons who are seropositive with no history of disease. More than 40% of persons who have two or more episodes suffer another within 2 years. Recurrent infections tend to involve the underlying stroma; with repeated recurrences, there may be progressive corneal scarring and neovascularization, with eventual loss of vision. HSV is the leading infectious cause of blindness in the United States. Damage appears to be caused both by direct infection and cytolysis and by an immunopathologic inflammatory response to viral antigens. Corneal transplantation is frequently performed for end-stage corneal scarring caused by HSV. Unfortunately, some recipients develop recurrent HSV infection of the graft, which is easily confused with allograft rejection. Acute retinal necrosis is a rare, rapidly progressive HSV retinitis that occurs in immunocompetent as well as in immunocompromised persons.

In newborns, HSV infections of the eye are caused by HSV-2 more often than by HSV-1, reflecting the maternal genital source of most infections. Keratoconjunctivitis may progress by direct extension to chorioretinitis, but retinal involvement is usually a consequence of viremia, which occurs, generally in the absence of corneal involvement, in neonates and in immunosuppressed children and adults with disseminated HSV infections. HSV may also reach the retina by direct extension from the brain in patients with HSV encephalitis.

Infections of the Skin

Because of the resistance of the intact cornified epithelium, isolated exogenous HSV infections of the skin are uncommon in normal adults. When they do occur, they are usually associated with cutaneous trauma. Most primary cutaneous HSV infections occur in the course of acute herpetic gingivostomatitis or primary genital herpes. The skin lesions usually result from autoinoculation or zosteriform spread from an infected mucosal site in the same dermatome.[3, 83, 397, 439, 498–501] Vesicles tend to be discrete, rather than grouped, and heal without scarring in 7 to 14 days. A normal person with acute herpetic gingivostomatitis or primary genital herpes occasionally develops widespread cutaneous dissemination, resulting in a varicella-like rash. This is accompanied by malaise and fever, but rarely is there serious visceral infection. These skin lesions, the result of viremia, also resolve without scarring in 7 to 14 days.

Regardless of their location or pathogenesis, cutaneous HSV infections result in the establishment of latency in corresponding sensory ganglia, and the patient is subject to recurrences. Because the virus responsible for recurrent infections originates in sensory ganglia and is transported to the skin by sensory nerves, the lesions of recurrent cutaneous herpes may assume a segmental or dermatomal distribution that resembles that of herpes zoster, and they generally appear as grouped vesicles (see Fig. 240–10) rather than the individual vesicles seen in primary infections. A prodrome of pain, burning, itching, or tingling usually heralds the herpetic eruption, preceding it by 2 or 3 hours to 2 or 3 days. Lesions begin as grouped, erythematous papules that progress to vesicles, pustules, and crusts and then heal without scarring in 6 to 10 days. There is often regional lymphadenopathy, but constitutional symptoms are rare. Recurrent cutaneous herpes is sometimes associated with severe local neuralgia, and recurrences on the extremities may be accompanied by local edema and lymphangitis.[3, 32, 83, 332, 502–505]

In contrast to herpes zoster, recurrent HSV infections tend to recur repeatedly in the same dermatome.

TRAUMATIC HERPES[3, 32, 395, 396, 506, 507]

Primary cutaneous HSV infections occasionally appear in normal persons in the absence of oropharyngeal or genital herpes. Such lesions generally result from direct exogenous infection of skin rendered susceptible by trauma. They may occur when an adult shedding HSV in saliva "kisses away" the pain of a child's abrasion or tends an infant with diaper rash. Primary cutaneous herpes is also seen in wrestlers and rugby players (herpes gladiatorum, scrumpox); presumably, traumatized skin is infected by contact with an adversary's cutaneous lesions or virus-bearing saliva. In addition to local vesicular lesions, which are generally confined to the area of traumatized skin, there is usually regional lymphadenopathy, and constitutional symptoms are often present. Recurrences are common, often heralded by a prodrome of pain, burning, tingling, or itching. They are frequently accompanied by regional lymphadenopathy but almost never by symptoms of systemic illness.

INFECTIONS OF ABNORMAL SKIN[420–425, 508–511]

Cutaneous HSV is often severe and life threatening when it occurs in patients with disorders of the skin, such as eczema, Darier disease, pemphigus, or burns, which permit more extensive local virus replication and spread and facilitate visceral dissemination. Infection may be acquired nosocomially or by autoinoculation from symptomatic oropharyngeal or genital lesions or asymptomatic virus shedding. The lesions are often ulcerative and nonspecific in appearance, although careful examination may reveal vesicles, especially in adjacent normal skin. Thus, diagnosis requires a high index of suspicion, with prompt biopsy and culture for virus. Patients are febrile and toxic and without specific therapy may die with widespread visceral dissemination. Enormous amounts of virus are present in the lesions, and such patients are often a source of nosocomial infections. Recurrences are common, but although they may be extensive, they are usually less severe than the primary infection.

HERPETIC WHITLOW[3, 332, 393, 512–515]

Herpetic whitlow (or herpetic paronychia) is a painful HSV infection of a terminal phalanx. The thumb or index finger is most often involved, and the portal of entry is usually a damaged cuticle. Involvement of more than one finger is uncommon. In children, it is usually caused by HSV-1 and occurs in the course of primary oropharyngeal infection as a result of finger sucking. The source of infection may also be an adult who kisses away the pain of an injured finger. In adults, it is a preventable (by using gloves) occupational disease of medical and dental personnel exposed to oropharyngeal secretions containing HSV-1. However, the majority of adult cases are caused by HSV-2, acquired by autoinoculation during concurrent genital herpes.[515] Although it can occur in persons with antibodies to HSV-1 or HSV-2, most initial episodes of herpetic whitlow are primary exogenous infections.

The whitlow begins 2 to 7 days after exposure, with intense itching, pain, and erythema in the infected finger. Within a day, a deep vesicle appears, soon followed by others (Fig. 240–11), which then tend to coalesce. The process continues, destroying considerable tissue. In many cases, there appears to be pus under the cuticle, but incision discloses only a little clear fluid or, at a later stage, thick, yellow, necrotic debris. Intense local pain is always present. Systemic symptoms and epitrochlear or axillary lymphadenopathy are common, and lymphangitis and neuralgia may occur. The lesions tend to progress for about 10 days, during which time pain persists unabated. There is then abrupt improvement, and the lesions begin to dry. Resolution is usually complete in 18 to 20 days. If the lesion is incised, the period of disability is prolonged and there is risk for secondary bacterial infection. Recurrences at the same site are common.

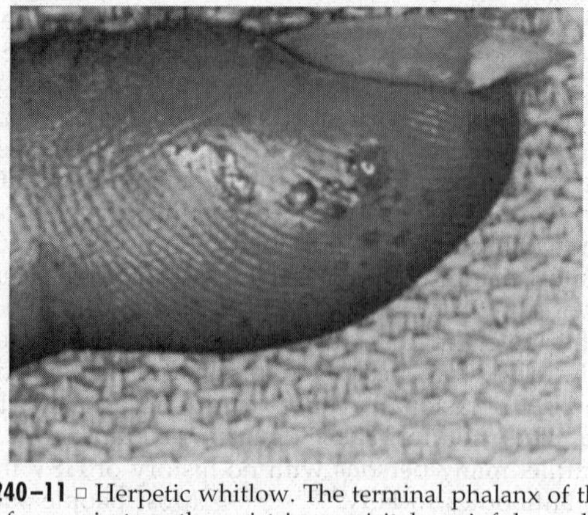

FIGURE 240–11 □ Herpetic whitlow. The terminal phalanx of the index finger of a respiratory therapist is exquisitely painful, swollen, and erythematous, with multiple deep and superficial vesicles. HSV-1 was isolated from vesicle fluid. (From Oxman MN: Herpes stomatitis. *In* Braude AI, Davis CE, Fierer J [eds]: Infectious Diseases and Medical Microbiology, ed 2. Philadelphia, WB Saunders, 1986, pp 752–772.)

Recurrent herpetic whitlows are often as painful as the primary infection, but they tend to be somewhat shorter in duration and are rarely accompanied by constitutional symptoms. The recurrent whitlow is frequently heralded and accompanied by severe neuralgic pain in the hand and arm, and it is often associated with swelling and edema of the hand, lymphangitis, and regional lymphadenopathy.

Central Nervous System Infections

In children and adults, central nervous system infections with HSV are relatively uncommon complications of primary or recurrent infections at peripheral sites. In contrast, central nervous system infection is a major component of neonatal HSV infection, occurring in at least 50% of affected newborns. Neonatal HSV infections are discussed in reference 323 and in Chapter 113.

HERPES SIMPLEX ENCEPHALITIS[43, 85, 86, 516–530]

Herpes simplex encephalitis is an acute necrotizing viral encephalitis that, beyond the neonatal period, is nearly always caused by HSV-1. It has a higher mortality rate than most other forms of viral encephalitis (greater than 70% in the absence of specific therapy). Although rare, it is the most common cause of sporadic acute necrotizing encephalitis in the United States; there are probably more than 1000 cases each year. Serologic data indicate that herpes simplex encephalitis occurs as a primary infection in about 50% of patients and as a recurrent infection in the remainder, but there is no obvious difference between the two groups in presentation, clinical course, or outcome.

The mode of presentation, clinical manifestations, and sequelae are determined largely by the nature and distribution of the pathologic process—acute asymmetric necrotizing encephalitis that involves primarily the orbitofrontal and temporal cortex and the limbic system. Although the manifestations and rate of progression are variable, most patients present with two recognizable groups of findings: (1) nonspecific changes seen in most forms of encephalitis, which include fever, headache, signs of meningeal irritation, nausea, vomiting, global confusion, generalized seizures, and alteration of consciousness; and (2) changes referable to focal necrosis of the orbitofrontal and temporal cortex and the limbic system, which include anosmia, memory loss, peculiar behavior, defects of speech (especially expressive aphasia), hallucinations (particularly olfactory and gustatory hallucinations), and focal seizures. There is rapid progression in some cases, with the appearance of reflex asymmetry, focal paralysis, hemiparesis, and coma. Cerebral edema contributes to these manifestations and plays an important role in the outcome of the disease. Other patients have a more protracted course, with several days of mild, nonspecific illness punctuated by intermittent periods of bizarre behavior alternating with lethargy or sleep. These patients may present a picture of acute psychosis or delirium tremens and be admitted to hospital for psychiatric care until the appearance of localizing neurologic signs, seizures, and coma alerts their physicians to the severe organic nature of their disease. Cerebrospinal fluid examination usually reveals a moderate pleocytosis with mononuclear cells and polymorphonuclear leukocytes, mildly elevated protein concentration, normal glucose concentration, and often a moderate number of erythrocytes. HSV is rarely isolated from the cerebrospinal fluid. Magnetic resonance imaging appears to be the most sensitive imaging procedure. Detection of HSV DNA in cerebrospinal fluid after PCR amplification provides a rapid and definitive diagnosis. Sensitivity and specificity of this technique approach 100%, and it has replaced brain biopsy as the primary means of establishing the diagnosis of herpes simplex encephalitis.[43, 85, 521, 523] Mortality and morbidity can be reduced by early initiation of antiviral therapy, but 5% or more of patients suffer a clinical relapse after antiviral therapy has been discontinued.

HERPES SIMPLEX MENINGITIS[86, 347, 531–539]

Herpes simplex meningitis is an acute, generally benign lymphocytic meningitis that occurs in otherwise normal adults, often in association with primary genital herpes. Most documented cases have been caused by HSV-2, which can frequently be isolated from the cerebrospinal fluid. Symptoms, which include headache, fever, photophobia, nausea and vomiting, myalgia, and nuchal rigidity, usually resolve in about a week, but 15% to 25% of patients experience one or more recurrences, sometimes in association with an episode of recurrent genital herpes. Except for its association with genital herpes, HSV meningitis resembles benign recurrent lymphocytic (Mollaret) meningitis. The detection of HSV-2 DNA in the cerebrospinal fluid after PCR amplification in 10 of 13 patients with benign recurrent lymphocytic (Mollaret) meningitis suggests that HSV-2 may be the principal cause of this heretofore idiopathic syndrome.[538, 539] Herpes simplex meningitis has also been observed in children, from whose cerebrospinal fluid HSV-1 has been isolated. Herpes simplex meningitis is discussed further in Chapter 113.

GANGLIONITIS AND MYELITIS ASSOCIATED WITH HERPES SIMPLEX VIRUS INFECTIONS[32, 86, 503, 505, 535, 540–546]

Genital and anorectal HSV infections may be complicated by lumbosacral ganglionitis, radiculitis, and ascending myelitis. Clinical manifestations include urinary retention, obstipation, abdominal and lower extremity muscle weakness, paresthesia and anesthesia over sacral dermatomes, and severe sacral neuralgia. These symptoms usually resolve spontaneously after a week or two, but some, especially sacral neuralgia, recur in association with episodes of recurrent genital or anorectal herpes. These complications are discussed in Chapter 113.

Genital Infections

ACUTE HERPETIC VULVOVAGINITIS IN INFANTS AND CHILDREN

In young infants and children, acute herpetic vulvovaginitis may result from autoinoculation during symptomatic or asymptomatic primary oropharyngeal HSV-1 infection or from contact with an adult shedding HSV (e.g., when diapers are changed). Because it may also occur as a result of sexual abuse (in which case it may be caused by HSV-2), its occurrence warrants a thorough and sensitive appraisal of the child's social situation and possible contacts. Every attempt should be made to isolate and type the responsible virus, which should then be saved for possible restriction endonuclease fingerprinting and comparison with isolates from suspected contacts. Symptoms include fever and malaise, and the perineal area is red, edematous, and studded with tiny vesicles that rapidly evolve into shallow, yellowish white ulcers 2 to 4 mm in diameter. The lesions are extremely painful and often coalesce to form larger ulcers. HSV urethritis is also generally present, and dysuria may lead to urinary retention. The inguinal lymph nodes are enlarged and tender. Fever and constitutional symptoms subside in a week, and healing is complete without scarring in 12 to 18 days.

PRIMARY, INITIAL NONPRIMARY, AND RECURRENT GENITAL HERPES AND ANORECTAL HERPES SIMPLEX VIRUS INFECTIONS

All are discussed in Chapter 113.

Neonatal Infections[32, 43, 85, 321–323, 354, 375]

Because newborn infants are unable to limit the replication and spread of HSV, neonatal infection is virtually always symptomatic and almost never trivial. In the absence of specific antiviral therapy, the mortality rate exceeds 5%, and most survivors have serious sequelae. This is in contrast to most other HSV infections, which are usually asymptomatic and rarely life threatening. The majority of neonatal infections are acquired during passage through the infected birth canal of a mother with asymptomatic genital herpes. Most of the remainder are acquired post partum, by nosocomial transmission within the nursery or from an adult who has a nongenital HSV infection such as herpes labialis or who is shedding HSV asymptomatically in saliva. Rarely, infection is acquired in utero, as a result of maternal viremia or ascending infection from the cervix. Approximately two thirds of neonatal HSV infections are caused by HSV-2. The interval between birth and onset of symptoms is variable, but most infants present during the second week of life. In about one third of patients, the disease resembles neonatal sepsis, whereas signs and symptoms of encephalitis predominate in many others. Diagnosis is hampered by the absence of skin lesions in 30% or more of infected infants. The oropharynx is probably an important portal of entry, but infected infants rarely have gingivostomatitis. Other portals of entry include the skin, respiratory tract, gastrointestinal tract, and conjunctivae. Neonatal HSV infections are discussed further in Chapter 113.

Herpes Simplex Virus Infections at Other Sites

Transient viremia is probably common during primary HSV infections in normal persons, but nonspecific and immune host defense mechanisms generally limit virus replication so that foci of hematogenous infection in the skin ɩal organs remain subclinical. These host defenses .t the direct extension of HSV infection from the .ynx to the trachea and esophagus. Nevertheless, al- ı it is much more common in immunocompromised ɴts, clinically manifest disease due to hematogenous emination or direct extension of HSV infection does occur normal hosts.

DISSEMINATED HERPES SIMPLEX VIRUS INFECTIONS*

Primary oropharyngeal and genital HSV infections in apparently normal children and adults are occasionally complicated by clinically significant viremia, with cutaneous or visceral dissemination. This may even occur during otherwise asymptomatic primary infections, in the absence of signs or symptoms of disease at the portal of entry. In most cases, clinically significant dissemination is confined to the skin, producing an illness that is virtually indistinguishable from varicella (except when oropharyngeal or genital lesions are present). The illness is self-limited and resolves in 7 to 14 days. Rarely, however, there is severe, often fatal visceral dissemination, which may or may not be accompanied by vesicular lesions in the skin. Multiple organs are involved, but fulminant HSV hepatitis is usually clinically predominant, and it is generally accompanied by leukopenia, thrombocytopenia, and disseminated intravascular coagulation. This syndrome, which is fatal in the majority of cases, occurs with greatest frequency in pregnant women, usually during the third trimester. Disseminated HSV-1 and HSV-2 infections in apparently normal children and adults have also been associated with herpetic esophagitis, adrenal necrosis, interstitial HSV pneumonitis, HSV cystitis, monarticular HSV arthritis, HSV meningitis, and rarely HSV encephalitis.

RESPIRATORY TRACT AND GASTROINTESTINAL TRACT INFECTIONS CAUSED BY HERPES SIMPLEX VIRUS[3, 32, 43, 83, 85, 375, 552, 569–584]

Apparently normal persons may develop herpetic tracheobronchitis due to aspiration of oropharyngeal secretions containing HSV-1. This occurs most often in the elderly and in association with endotracheal intubation. Clinical manifestations range from asymptomatic infection to severe tracheobronchitis with widespread mucosal ulceration. Focal or multifocal HSV pneumonitis may result from further aspiration or contiguous spread of infection, and these patients often have concurrent HSV esophagitis. Viremic infection of the lungs, which is common in immunosuppressed patients and results in bilateral interstitial pneumonitis, is rare in immunocompetent persons.

HSV esophagitis, a common manifestation of HSV infection in immunocompromised patients, can also occur in otherwise normal children and adults, especially in the presence of a nasogastric tube. It may present with fever, odynophagia, dysphagia, substernal pain, and rarely hematemesis, but it is often asymptomatic. Endoscopy reveals typical shallow herpetic ulcers of the esophageal mucosa. Herpetic esophagitis usually results from direct extension of symptomatic oropharyngeal infection or from infection of traumatized esophageal mucosa by HSV shed in saliva. It can, however, be a recurrent infection resulting from reactivation of virus latent in the vagus ganglion.[413, 585] Symptoms usually resolve spontaneously within a day or two after removal of the nasogastric tube.

*References 3, 32, 43, 83, 85, 354, 375, 411, 547–568.

Herpes Simplex Virus Infections in Immunocompromised Hosts

Patients whose host defenses are compromised by congenital immunodeficiencies, malnutrition, immunosuppressive diseases (including hematologic and lymphoreticular malignant neoplasms and AIDS), iatrogenic immunosuppression, and certain diseases of the skin are at increased risk for severe and even fatal HSV infections. Severe, frequently fatal HSV infections are common in malnourished children, especially in association with measles, and in children with primary immunodeficiency diseases that seriously impair their cellular immunity.[3, 407, 409, 586] The disease begins with acute herpetic gingivostomatitis, which is followed by sustained viremia with dissemination of infection to the liver, adrenal glands, lungs, and other viscera. Cutaneous dissemination is common, and there is also extensive infection of the esophagus and intestinal mucosa, which is due either to viremia or to large amounts of swallowed virus. These events are the result of primary HSV infection, and a similar syndrome has been observed after primary oropharyngeal or genital HSV infections in other immunocompromised children and adults.[3, 32, 83, 85, 586–600] The rare dissemination of primary HSV infections in pregnant women (see earlier) may be related to the depression of cellular immunity observed during the third trimester.[601]

The frequency and severity of HSV infections are markedly increased in patients with hematologic and lymphoreticular malignant neoplasms, in patients with AIDS, and in organ and bone marrow allograft recipients, particularly during the first 4 to 6 weeks after transplantation when immunosuppression is greatest.[83, 85, 405, 587–600, 602–613] These infections occur mainly in patients with preexisting antibodies to HSV, and this generally reflects reactivation of endogenous latent infection. Most seropositive transplant recipients shed HSV, most often from the oropharynx. Whereas these HSV infections are sometimes asymptomatic, they are usually associated with symptomatic mucocutaneous disease (e.g., herpes labialis, recurrent genital herpes). These recurrent infections often behave normally and resolve without complications. Sometimes, however, the local lesions do not resolve but slowly enlarge, ulcerate, become necrotic, and extend to deeper tissues. Satellite lesions develop, and mucous membrane involvement is often extensive, with ulcerative, sometimes nodular, lesions on the lips, buccal mucosa, tongue, and palate. Pain and chronicity are hallmarks of the disease; lesions may persist for 10 weeks or more, during which time the saliva and involved tissues contain large amounts of virus. These chronic atypical mucocutaneous HSV infections, which involve the perioral or anogenital region, are a major cause of morbidity in profoundly immunosuppressed patients. They are a frequent occurrence in patients with AIDS.[405, 599] Latent HSV is also reactivated during postchemotherapy mucositis; the majority of patients who develop stomatitis after cancer chemotherapy shed HSV in saliva, and it is generally difficult to assess the relative contribution of chemotherapy and HSV to the mucosal disease.[612] HSV dissemination is rarely associated with any of these chronic mucocutaneous HSV infections in seropositive patients, but local extension to the esophagus and trachea can be a major problem.

Virus can spread from the oropharynx to the esophagus and trachea, where infection is facilitated by mucosal damage caused by radiation, chemotherapy, or intubation. Herpetic esophagitis is a common but often unrecognized complication of oropharyngeal HSV infection in immunocompromised and debilitated patients, especially in the presence of a nasogastric tube.[552, 579, 614] There are typical herpetic ulcers of the esophageal mucosa that may become confluent in the lower third. Herpetic esophagitis can lead to viremia with infection of the liver and other organs, and the mucosal lesions are often superinfected with *Candida* species, which further obscures the diagnosis.

The lungs may also be infected by HSV, either by direct extension of infection from the oropharynx or as a consequence of viremia.[569–574, 613] Direct extension is facilitated by injury to the respiratory epithelium (e.g., by endotracheal intubation, chemotherapy, radiation, or burn injury). This probably explains the high incidence of herpetic tracheobronchitis in hospitalized burn victims and the frequency of local HSV infection in patients intubated for adult respiratory distress syndrome.[423, 425, 574] In these settings, most patients have focal or multifocal pneumonia, and concurrent HSV esophagitis is common.[569–574, 613] There is usually evidence of active oropharyngeal infection long before the onset of pneumonia. Diffuse bilateral interstitial pneumonia, a consequence of hematogenous HSV dissemination, is rare except in profoundly immunosuppressed patients and is much more likely to occur in the course of a primary rather than a recurrent HSV infection.

Herpes Simplex Virus Infection as a Cause of Erythema Multiforme

Recurrent HSV infections may be associated with allergic cutaneous and mucocutaneous disorders, especially erythema multiforme.[615–621] Fifteen percent or more of cases of erythema multiforme are regularly preceded by a symptomatic attack of recurrent herpes simplex, and the disease has been induced by the intradermal inoculation of inactivated HSV antigens in patients who suffer erythema multiforme but not in persons who have a history of uncomplicated recurrent herpes simplex.[615, 616] The erythema multiforme usually begins 3 to 10 days after the appearance of the herpetic lesions. It can range in severity from mild disease with typical target (iris) lesions on the extremities (erythema multiforme minor) to severe and extensive disease with lesions over the entire body, including the palms and soles (Fig. 240–12), and painful bullous-erosive lesions on the mucous membranes of the eyes, nose, oropharynx, genitalia, and anus (erythema multiforme major or Stevens-Johnson syndrome). Although the mucosal lesions may be confused with lesions caused directly by HSV infection, their histopathologic appearance is different.[622] The lesions of erythema multiforme result from vasculitis, and vesicles, when present, are subepidermal. Their formation represents an allergic response, presumably to circulating HSV antigens or antigen-antibody complexes, and these have been detected in the serum and in the skin lesions.[618, 620] The lesions do not result from virus replication in the skin, and thus they do not contain inclusion bodies or multinucleated giant cells, and they almost never yield HSV on culture. In many patients, the frequency of attacks has been reduced by suppressing HSV recurrences with long-term acyclovir prophylaxis.

Herpes Simplex Virus and Idiopathic Neurologic Syndrome

The intimate association of HSV with neurons has aroused suspicion that it may be involved in the pathogenesis of a variety of neurologic syndromes of unknown cause, including trigeminal neuralgia, atypical pain syndromes, idiopathic facial paralysis (Bell palsy), temporal lobe epilepsy, recurrent psychosis, and multiple sclerosis.[3, 83, 86, 623–638] However, the ubiquity of HSV, its lifelong latent residence in seropositive persons, and its frequent reactivation by a variety of stimuli minimize the etiologic significance of any temporal association between the occurrence or recurrence of HSV infection and the onset of another disease. The association of HSV with atypical pain syndromes, including trigeminal neuralgia, enjoys a measure of clinical and serologic support. Recurrent cutaneous HSV infections are sometimes associated with a prodrome of severe neuralgic pain,[83, 502–505] and repeated attacks for a period of years have occasionally resulted in the development of chronic pain and permanent sensory loss.[3, 504, 625, 626] The association of recurrent HSV with trigeminal neuralgia, which, like herpes labialis, almost always involves the second and third divisions of the trigeminal nerve, is supported by serologic data[3] and by the association of some cases with recurrent cutaneous herpes in the same area.[416, 504] These associations do not prove causality, however, and the absence of antibodies to HSV in some patients with trigeminal neuralgia indicates that even if HSV does cause the syndrome, it is not the only cause. The association of HSV with idiopathic facial palsy (Bell palsy), previously based primarily on serologic data,[628–632, 635] has been greatly strengthened by the detection of HSV DNA after PCR amplification in endoneurial fluid from 11 of 14 patients with acute Bell palsy but from none of 8 "control" patients with Ramsay Hunt syndrome. Varicella-zoster virus DNA was detected in all eight of the Ramsay Hunt patients but in none of the Bell palsy patients.[634, 637]

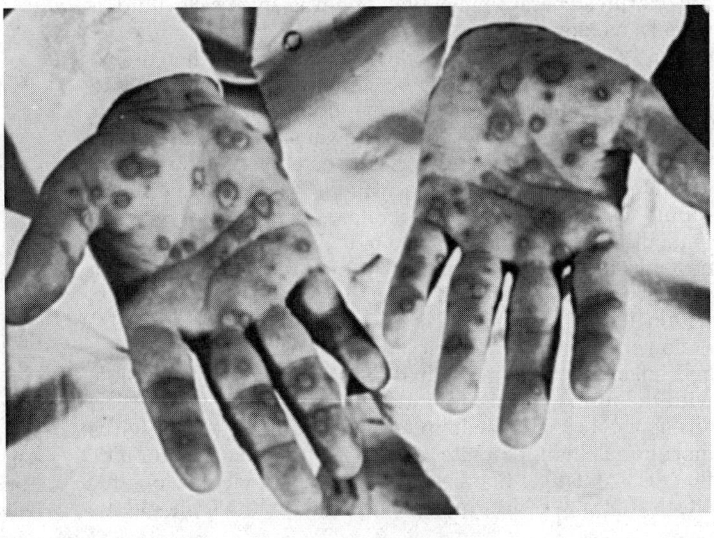

FIGURE 240–12 □ Recurrent erythema multiforme associated with recurrent herpes simplex. A young man with recurrent herpes simplex involving a small area of skin over his left scapula (herpes gladiatorum) regularly develops erythema multiforme 3 to 5 days after the onset of each herpetic recurrence. The rash consists of characteristic target (iris) lesions and involves primarily the skin of the trunk and extremities, including the palms and soles. HSV-1 is regularly isolated from the herpetic lesions over the scapula but not from the target lesions, and no multinucleated giant cells or intranuclear inclusion bodies have been detected in biopsy specimens of the erythema multiforme lesions. (From Oxman MN: Herpes stomatitis. *In* Braude AI, Davis CE, Fierer J [eds]: Infectious Diseases and Medical Microbiology, ed 2. Philadelphia, WB Saunders, 1986, pp 752–772.)

Herpes Simplex Virus Infection and Cancer

The capacity of HSV to induce cell transformation in vitro and the observation made in many (but not all) seroepidemiologic studies that the prevalence of antibodies to HSV-2 is higher in women with carcinoma of the cervix than in matched control subjects led to the suggestion that HSV-2 might play a causal role in cervical carcinoma.[314, 639] The epidemiologic studies indicated only that HSV-2 infection and cervical carcinoma are covariable: both are linked to sexual promiscuity and early age at first coitus.[639–641] Convincing evidence of any more direct linkage is lacking. Compelling data have been obtained implicating human papillomaviruses in the causation of cervical carcinoma (see Chapter 246).

Diagnosis

Although a presumptive diagnosis can often be made on clinical grounds (e.g., in patients with herpes labialis), many HSV infections are easily confused with other diseases. Thus, laboratory diagnosis is frequently necessary, and it is always desirable. The availability of specific antiviral therapy now places a high premium on early and reliable diagnosis.

Virus Isolation

Virus isolation remains the "gold standard" for the diagnosis of most HSV infections. It offers good sensitivity and unsurpassed specificity, and it yields virus for subsequent studies (e.g., sensitivity to specific antiviral drugs, restriction endonuclease fingerprinting). Experimental animals and embryonated eggs, although sensitive, have been replaced in most laboratories by cell culture techniques. HSV-1 and HSV-2 can be propagated in a wide variety of human and animal cells, but the most sensitive for direct isolation of HSV from clinical specimens include primary human embryonic kidney, primary human amnion, primary guinea pig embryo, and primary rabbit kidney cells as well as diploid human embryonic lung and foreskin fibroblasts.[275, 278, 279, 642] Tissue for virus isolation should be finely minced or dispersed with collagenase or trypsin, washed with tissue culture medium, and inoculated into cell cultures. Inoculation of viable cells, rather than a clarified suspension of homogenized tissue, increases the likelihood of isolating HSV from specimens containing small quantities of virus, especially if antibodies are present or antiviral therapy has already been instituted. Fluid should be aspirated from fresh vesicles and inoculated directly into cell cultures. Because the titer of virus in vesicle fluid is usually maximal during the first 24 to 48 hours,[643] fluid for culture should be taken as early as possible. Other tissues and body fluids should also be cultured when they are suspect, including blood, cerebrospinal fluid, urine, stool, saliva, throat washings or swabs, urethral swabs, rectal swabs, seminal fluid, and vaginal and cervical secretions. Many require special preparation before inoculation.[275, 278, 279] All specimens should be carried to the laboratory *on ice* and processed immediately. They may be held at 0°C for several hours (but never in the freezer compartment of a refrigerator or in an ordinary −20°C freezer). If cell cultures cannot be inoculated within 12 to 24 hours, specimens should be stored at −70°C or lower. Typical cytopathic effects, consisting of rounding and enlargement of individual cells followed by cell fusion, with the formation of multinucleated giant cells (see earlier) are usually apparent within 24 to 48 hours when the virus inoculum is high. Low-titer specimens or specimens in fluids that also contain antibodies to HSV may not yield cytopathic effects for a week or more, and thus cultures should be observed for at least 2 weeks before being considered negative. Virus isolates should be confirmed as HSV (and may be typed as HSV-1 or HSV-2) by any of a variety of serologic techniques (e.g., virus neutralization, immunofluorescent staining of viral antigens) using specific antisera or type-specific monoclonal antibodies or by nucleic acid hybridization.[83, 275, 278, 279, 644–646] The application of rapid antigen or nucleic acid detection techniques (see later) to cell cultures within 24 to 48 hours after specimen inoculation can detect and identify replicating virus even before the appearance of characteristic cytopathic effects. This often speeds diagnosis but may reduce sensitivity, especially with low-titer specimens. Thus, a duplicate culture should continue to be observed if the rapid method yields negative results.

Rapid Diagnosis of Herpes Simplex Virus Infection

Many therapeutic decisions require diagnostic information in minutes to hours rather than days, and several methods for rapid diagnosis are available. The histologic appearance of the lesions caused by HSV provides a rapid and practical means of diagnosis. Multinucleated giant cells and epithelial cells containing eosinophilic intranuclear inclusion bodies distinguish the lesions of HSV from those produced by almost all other pathogens. Other than HSV, only measles and varicella-zoster virus produce multinucleated giant cells and eosinophilic intranuclear inclusion bodies. The rash of measles normally is not vesicular, the disease does not resemble HSV infection clinically or epidemiologically, and the skin lesions of measles are histologically distinct from those of HSV. The characteristic cytologic changes induced by HSV (and varicella-zoster virus) can be easily demonstrated in Tzanck smears prepared at the bedside (Fig. 240–13). Cells are scraped from the base of an early vesicle, spread gently on a glass microscope slide, and stained with hematoxylin-eosin, Giemsa, Papanicolaou, or Paragon multiple stain.[83, 275, 278, 279, 647] Punch biopsy provides more reliable material for histologic examination, especially when lesions are secondarily infected with bacteria or fungi. Biopsy also facilitates diagnosis in the prevesicular stage. Biopsy specimens should

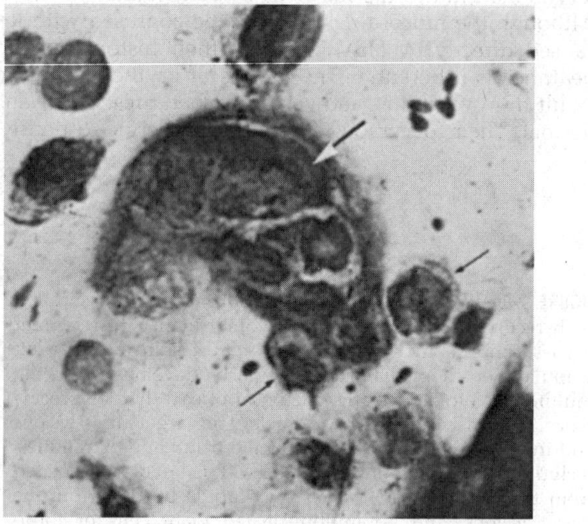

FIGURE 240–13 □ Tzanck smear showing a multinucleated giant cell. Cells scraped from the base of a herpetic vesicle were smeared on a glass slide and stained with Giemsa. The multinucleated giant cell contains a dense clump of nuclei *(large arrow)*. Two adherent cells *(small arrows)* are probably in the process of fusing with the giant cell. (From Oxman MN: Herpes stomatitis. *In* Braude AI, Davis CE, Fierer J [eds]: Infectious Diseases and Medical Microbiology, ed 2. Philadelphia, WB Saunders, 1986, pp 752–772.)

be obtained from the edges of lesions and should be fixed in Bouin fluid or another acid fixative to best demonstrate intranuclear inclusion bodies. Scrapings, vesicle fluid, and biopsy specimens can also be examined for virus particles by electron microscopy. However, neither electron microscopy nor histopathologic examination can distinguish HSV from varicella-zoster virus infection. This can be done only by virus isolation or by the direct detection and identification of HSV antigens or nucleic acids in tissue or vesicle fluid.

Rapid direct detection and identification of HSV antigens or nucleic acids in clinical specimens is now a reality. These techniques are specific and sensitive when they are applied to the evaluation of herpetic lesions, and they can even detect viral proteins and nucleic acids late in the course of disease when infectious virus may not be recovered; however, they often lack the sensitivity required to detect the small quantities of virus shed during asymptomatic recurrences, which, for example, are responsible for about 50% of neonatal HSV infections.[278, 279, 323, 645, 646, 648, 649] Because of its extraordinary sensitivity, the PCR technique is revolutionizing the diagnosis of HSV infections. In herpes simplex encephalitis, it provides a noninvasive diagnostic technique that is at least as sensitive as brain biopsy. As noted before, it has identified HSV-2 as the principal cause of benign recurrent lymphocytic (Mollaret) meningitis and established a strong association between HSV-1 infection and Bell palsy.[538, 539] It has also proved to be approximately eight times more sensitive than virus culture in detecting asymptomatic virus shedding by women with recurrent genital herpes.[388, 389, 650] However, in that situation, the epidemiologic significance of small amounts of HSV DNA in the absence of infectious virus remains to be determined.

Serologic Tests

The utility of serologic assays for the diagnosis of HSV infections has been limited by the need to obtain a sample of convalescent-phase serum to demonstrate sero-conversion; by the fact that recurrent infections, which account for much of the morbidity caused by HSV, generally do not stimulate a significant increase in antibody titers; and by the antigenic cross-reactivity of HSV-1 and HSV-2.[51, 83, 85, 275–281, 646, 651, 652] Nevertheless, serologic assays have been valuable for epidemiologic surveys and can give a retrospective diagnosis of primary HSV infection. Their utility for both purposes has been greatly enhanced by the development of serotype-specific assays.[278, 279, 282–306]

Prevention and Treatment

When we consider prevention and treatment, it is useful to outline potential goals. This requires that we recognize the differences between primary and recurrent HSV infections, distinguish between infection and disease, and take into account a number of unique characteristics of the HSV-host interaction:

- Most primary and recurrent HSV infections are asymptomatic.
- In primary infection of the normal host, HSV replication occurs during the incubation period, peaks soon after the onset of symptoms, and declines spontaneously thereafter as a consequence of the action of normal host defense mechanisms.
- Both symptomatic and asymptomatic HSV infections result in lifelong HSV latency.
- HSV latency is established early in the incubation period.
- Persons shed infectious HSV during both symptomatic and asymptomatic primary and recurrent HSV infections.
- Most primary HSV infections are acquired by contact with someone who is shedding HSV asymptomatically.
- Symptomatic and asymptomatic recurrent HSV infections occur despite the presence of normal humoral and cell-mediated immunity.
- There are two HSV serotypes, HSV-1 and HSV-2.

With respect to primary HSV infection, reasonable goals for prevention and treatment include the following:

1. Prevent primary HSV infection in persons exposed to HSV.
2. Failing that, prevent the development of disease in infected persons.
3. Failing that, reduce the duration and severity of disease in infected persons.
4. Prevent the establishment of HSV latency.
5. Failing that, reduce the frequency and severity of subsequent recurrences in latently infected persons.
6. Reduce transmission of HSV infection.

With respect to recurrent HSV infections, reasonable goals for prevention and treatment include the following:

1. Eradicate latent HSV infection.
2. Failing that, prevent the development of symptomatic and asymptomatic recurrences.
3. Failing that, prevent the development of symptomatic recurrences.
4. Failing that, reduce the frequency of recurrent infections and the duration and severity of recurrences that do occur.
5. Failing that, reduce the duration and severity of recurrent disease.
6. Reduce transmission of HSV infection.

Prevention of Herpes Simplex Virus Infection

Potential approaches to prevention of primary HSV infection include (1) avoidance of exposure to HSV; (2) preexposure prophylaxis by active or passive immunization or with antiviral agents; and (3) postexposure prophylaxis by active or passive immunization or with antiviral agents.

PREVENTION OF EXPOSURE

Avoidance of exposure is, at present, the only proven means of preventing HSV infection. However, the high incidence of asymptomatic virus shedding, usually by persons who have no history of symptomatic infection to alert them to their potential infectiousness, makes avoiding exposure impractical except in special circumstances. For example, medical and dental personnel should wear gloves to prevent contact with potentially infectious oropharyngeal and respiratory secretions. Practices and procedures in the newborn nursery should be designed to protect infants from nosocomial HSV infection (see Chapter 113). Health care workers who have herpetic whitlows should not engage in direct care of patients. Hospitalized patients with extensive HSV infections, such as eczema herpeticum, should be isolated. Persons with herpes labialis and recurrent genital herpes should avoid sexual contact when active lesions are present, and all sexually active persons should be aware that infection can be acquired during episodes of asymptomatic virus shedding. Use of barrier contraceptives and spermicides containing surfactants should be considered to decrease transmission during episodes of asymptomatic virus shedding (see Chapter 113). Pregnant women who have active genital herpes at term should be delivered by cesarean section before membranes rupture to reduce the risk for neonatal HSV infection. Susceptible pregnant women with seropositive sexual partners should practice abstinence during the 6 weeks before delivery to avoid acquiring primary infection near term.

PREEXPOSURE PROPHYLAXIS

No means of prophylaxis has yet been proved to be effective in humans. In addition, the high proportion of HSV infections that follow unrecognized exposures suggests that even if they were effective, short-lived forms of prophylaxis, such as the administration of acyclovir or preparations containing high titers of antibodies to HSV, would have little practical application. On the other hand, active preexposure immunization, if effective, would provide an ideal means of prophylaxis. The problem in the case of HSV is complicated by the phenomenon of latency and by the incomplete immunity provided by natural infection. Nevertheless, there are reasons for optimism. These include the reduction in the incidence and severity of HSV-2 infections in persons previously infected with HSV-1, the rarity of superinfection with a different strain of the same HSV serotype in immunocompetent persons, and the antigenic stability of HSV-1 and HSV-2. Moreover, a number of studies in animal models have demonstrated significant protection from exogenous HSV infection by immunizations with inactivated, attenuated, and replication-incompetent whole-virus vaccines; purified and recombinant envelope glycoprotein vaccines; and viral DNA vaccines.[653–667] Several experimental vaccines have entered clinical trials, and preliminary data suggest that with appropriate adjuvants, recombinant glycoprotein vaccines induce good levels of humoral and cell-mediated immunity in seronegative individuals. Placebo-controlled efficacy studies of the capacity of these vaccines to prevent primary genital herpes are currently under way.

Therapeutic immunization to reduce the frequency of recurrent HSV infections has a long and colorful history.[668] A placebo-controlled trial employing a recombinant HSV-2 glycoprotein D vaccine showed a small reduction in recurrences.[669] Further studies employing this approach are likely to follow.

Taken together, currently available clinical and experimental data suggest that whereas vaccination against HSV is unlikely to result in the sort of solid immunity seen with vaccines against measles, mumps, rubella, and poliomyelitis, it will probably reduce the risk for infection in seronegative persons significantly, especially when they are exposed to the small amounts of virus shed during asymptomatic recurrences. Immunization may also reduce the frequency and severity of disease in persons who are already infected, thus increasing the proportion who are asymptomatic. By reducing the duration and intensity of virus shedding by infected persons, immunization might also reduce transmission of HSV, but the expected increase in the proportion of infected persons who are asymptomatic but still shedding virus could have the opposite effect.

POSTEXPOSURE PROPHYLAXIS

The short incubation period of symptomatic HSV infection, the early establishment of latency, and the ability of replication-negative HSV mutants to establish latency all suggest that postexposure prophylaxis will be ineffective in preventing HSV infection or the establishment of latency. However, the efficacy of passive immunization in animal models[437–440, 670] and of antiviral chemotherapy in humans (see later) suggests that postexposure prophylaxis with antibodies to HSV, with antiviral agents, or with combinations of the two may reduce the incidence and severity of disease. This approach is being evaluated in clinical trials of acyclovir prophylaxis in newborns exposed to HSV at delivery, in the hope of improving the results achieved with antiviral therapy initiated after the onset of the symptoms and signs of neonatal HSV infection.[323, 671–674]

Treatment of Primary and Initial Nonprimary Herpes Simplex Virus Infections

A number of nucleoside derivatives that interfere with HSV DNA synthesis have been evaluated as potential antiviral agents, and additional compounds are under development. Four—idoxuridine, trifluorothymidine, vidarabine, and acyclovir—have been proved effective and are licensed for use in the United States. Idoxuridine and trifluorothymidine are effective for topical treatment of HSV keratitis, but they are too toxic for systemic use. Vidarabine and acyclovir are licensed for both topical and systemic use. Antiviral therapy is discussed in more detail in Chapter 32.

Vidarabine has been shown in double-blind, placebo-controlled studies to reduce the mortality and morbidity of neonatal HSV infections and of herpes simplex encephalitis (only about half of which are primary infections).[672, 675] Topical vidarabine is more effective than topical idoxuridine in treating HSV keratitis.[676]

Acyclovir, the first truly selective inhibitor of HSV replication to be evaluated clinically, is actively phosphorylated by HSV-encoded thymidine kinase but is a poor substrate for cellular thymidine kinases. Consequently, the concentration of acyclovir monophosphate is 30 to 100 times greater in HSV-infected cells than in uninfected cells.[677] Cellular enzymes then convert the acyclovir monophosphate to acyclovir triphosphate, which is a selective inhibitor of HSV-encoded DNA polymerase.[677] Acyclovir is more soluble and less toxic than vidarabine and is available in topical, intravenous, and oral formulations. It has been compared with vidarabine in two studies of patients with HSV encephalitis.[678, 679] In both, morbidity and mortality rates were significantly lower in patients treated with acyclovir than in patients treated with vidarabine. Thus, intravenous acyclovir, 10 mg/kg every 8 hours for 10 days, is now the treatment of choice for herpes simplex encephalitis. Because some patients have a relapse after therapy is completed, longer durations of treatment are currently being evaluated. A similar comparison in infants with neonatal HSV infections showed no significant difference in outcome between those treated with acyclovir and vidarabine.[673] Because of its lower toxicity and greater ease of administration, intravenous acyclovir, 10 mg/kg every 8 hours for 10 days, is currently the preferred treatment of neonatal HSV infections. Despite therapy, mortality and morbidity rates are still considerable in both diseases, and attempts to develop better therapeutic regimens continue. However, because no antiviral drug can restore life to neurons destroyed by HSV infection, further improvement in outcome will also require the development and application of techniques that permit earlier diagnosis and, thus, earlier initiation of therapy.

Acyclovir has proved to be effective treatment of primary and nonprimary first episodes of genital herpes.[680–691] Oral and intravenous therapy substantially shortened the duration of local symptoms and virus shedding; accelerated healing; and decreased new lesion formation, dysuria, vaginal discharge, and extragenital manifestations of infection. Topical acyclovir had a less marked effect on local lesions and did not decrease new lesion formation or extragenital signs and symptoms. Unfortunately, no form of therapy reduced the frequency or severity of subsequent recurrences, despite the observation that recurrences in untreated patients are more frequent in those who develop high titers of neutralizing antibodies,[87] presumably reflecting greater virus replication and HSV antigen production during primary infection. It may be that the events involved in the establishment of latent infection were completed before the initiation of treatment with acyclovir or placebo, so that subsequent inhibition of HSV replication by acyclovir had no effect. For most initial infections, oral therapy, 200 mg five times per day for 10 days, is recommended; 400 mg three times daily appears to be equally effective and is more convenient. Intravenous therapy, 5 mg/kg every 8 hours for 7 days, is reserved for disease severe enough to require hospitalization, especially if there are such extragenital manifestations as HSV meningitis. Topical acyclovir would appear to have no role in the therapy for initial genital HSV infections. The management of genital herpes is discussed in Chapter 113.

On the basis of anecdotal experience and analogy to initial genital herpes, it seems appropriate to administer oral or intravenous acyclovir to immunocompetent persons who have severe herpetic gingivostomatitis or pharyngotonsillitis, initial episodes of herpetic whitlow, and primary herpetic infections of the skin such as herpes gladiatorum.

Treatment of Recurrent Herpes Simplex Virus Infections

In immunocompetent hosts, recurrent HSV infections are generally limited in duration and extent and resolve spontaneously without complications.* Nevertheless, they cause sufficient physical and psychologic distress to cause most afflicted persons to seek some form of relief. Oral acyclovir, even begun during the prodrome, has a modest effect on the course of herpes labialis and recurrent genital herpes, and it does not appear to alter the frequency or severity of subsequent recurrences.[331, 482, 688–691, 693, 694] However, oral acyclovir, 200 mg five times daily for 5 days or 400 mg three times daily for 5 days beginning as early as possible, preferably during the prodrome, does provide meaningful relief to the minority of patients who have more prolonged episodes of recurrent genital herpes or herpes labialis. A study of recurrent HSV-2 infections of the hand (presumably herpetic whitlow), which tend to be more severe and prolonged than herpes labialis or recurrent genital herpes, demonstrated that oral acyclovir, at a dose of 2 g/d for 10 days, markedly shortened the clinical and virologic course of the disease.[695] Topical acyclovir is generally ineffective for recurrent HSV infections in normal hosts.

Prophylaxis (Suppression) of Frequently Recurring Herpes Simplex Virus Infections

Long-term prophylaxis with oral acyclovir has been shown to markedly reduce the incidence and severity of recurrent genital herpes in persons who suffer frequent recurrences. However, it does not prevent asymptomatic HSV shedding or abolish latency, even when it is continued for more than 5 years; recurrences resume when suppressive therapy is stopped.[252, 253, 277, 693–701] Whereas suppression with acyclovir does not eliminate asymptomatic shedding, it markedly reduces it.[387, 389] Thus, it may reduce the risk for transmission. Effective dosing schedules included 200 mg three times per day, 400 mg twice daily, 800 mg twice daily, and 800 mg once daily (see Chapter 113). Suppression with prophylactic oral acyclovir also appears to be beneficial for patients whose recurrences are associated with severe complications such as recurrent meningitis, erythema multiforme, and severe neuralgia, although controlled studies of such patients are lacking.

Two placebo-controlled studies of natural sunlight–induced and experimental ultraviolet light–induced herpes labialis demonstrated that prophylaxis with oral acyclovir reduced the incidence of lesion formation and the severity of the lesions that did occur.[702, 703] Interestingly, the occurrence of lesions was biphasic; 20% to 30% occurred within 48 hours of induction and the remaining 70% to 80% after 2 to 7 days. Acyclovir prophylaxis, even when it was begun a week before induction, did not prevent the development of the early lesions.[331, 702, 703] Two recently licensed prodrugs, famciclovir and valacyclovir, have much greater oral bioavailability than acyclovir does.[704–706] This permits less frequent dosing and results in blood levels of antiviral activity heretofore achievable only with intravenous acyclovir. Administered twice daily for episodic treatment of recurrent genital herpes, both prodrugs achieved results that were comparable to those achieved with acyclovir administered at a dose of 200 mg five times daily.[707, 708] However, treatment with 400 mg of acyclovir three times daily, which is only slightly less convenient, is likely to be less expensive.

*References 32, 43, 83, 85, 277, 373, 375, 480, 481, 692.

Treatment and Prophylaxis of Recurrent Herpes Simplex Virus Infections in Immunocompromised Patients

Recurrent HSV infections are a major cause of illness in patients undergoing organ or bone marrow transplantation or remission-induction chemotherapy for acute leukemia; 60% to 90% of seropositive patients develop mucocutaneous HSV infections during the early posttransplant period, when immunosuppression is greatest (see earlier). A number of placebo-controlled studies have shown that acyclovir, 250 mg/m^2 or 5 mg/kg intravenously every 8 to 12 hours or 200 to 400 mg per os three to five times per day, provides effective prophylaxis, reducing the frequency of recurrences by 90% or more.[709–713] At comparable doses, oral acyclovir and intravenous acyclovir have also been shown to provide effective treatment for mucocutaneous HSV infections in these patients,[609, 714, 715] and topical therapy with acyclovir cream provides a reasonable alternative when lesions are accessible.[611]

Development of Resistance to Antiviral Drugs

The increasing use of acyclovir has predictably led to the emergence of acyclovir-resistant HSV mutants. Because the selective antiviral activity of acyclovir involves two HSV-encoded enzymes, thymidine kinase and DNA polymerase, mutations altering either one can lead to resistance. Resistant mutants, most of which are thymidine kinase deficient, are readily selected in the laboratory. Acyclovir-resistant strains of HSV have also been isolated sporadically from patients receiving acyclovir, often before the initiation of treatment. In the past, these resistant isolates have almost all been thymidine kinase–deficient mutants with reduced pathogenicity in animal models, and generally there has been no correlation between acyclovir resistance and clinical response to treatment.[716–719] However, the development of clinical resistance in profoundly immunosuppressed patients receiving acyclovir therapy for persistent mucocutaneous HSV infections has been accompanied by the appearance of acyclovir-resistant HSV mutants.[720–723] Most of these have been thymidine kinase deficient and responsive to treatment with foscarnet or vidarabine, which do not require HSV-encoded thymidine kinase for activity, but they have not lost their pathogenicity in animal models and obviously produce disease in their human hosts. Even more disturbing has been the emergence of DNA polymerase mutants, which are still pathogenic and are resistant to foscarnet as well as to acyclovir.[724–726] In addition to complicating the care of the patients involved, the emergence and potential spread of such drug-resistant mutants places at risk our recently acquired capacity to treat HSV infections. The subject of drug-resistant mutants of HSV is discussed in references 727 to 733 and in Chapter 32.

References

1. Beswick TSL: The origin and the use of the word herpes. Med Hist 6:214, 1962.
2. Nahmias AJ, Dowdle WR: Antigenic and biologic differences in herpesvirus hominis. Prog Med Virol 10:110, 1968.
3. Juel-Jensen BE, MacCallum FO: Herpes Simplex, Varicella and Zoster. Philadelphia, JB Lippincott, 1972.
4. Wildy P: Herpes: History and classification. *In* Kaplan AS (ed): The Herpesviruses. New York, Academic Press, 1973, pp 1–25.
5. Shakespeare W: Romeo and Juliet. Act I; scene 4; lines 74–76.
6. Hutfield DC: History of herpes genitalis. Br J Vener Dis 42:263, 1966.
7. Astruc J: De Morbis Venereis, Libri Sex. Paris, Cavelier, 1736, pp 254–255.
8. Unna PG: The Histopathology of the Diseases of the Skin. Edinburgh, Clay, 1896, p 145.
9. Wildy P: Herpesviruses. *In* Fenner F, Gibbs A (eds): Portraits of Viruses: A History of Virology. Basel, S Karger, 1988, pp 230–253.
10. Grüter W: Experimentelle und klinische Untersuchungen über den sogenannten Herpes Comea. Berl Dtsch Ophthalmol Ges 42:162, 1920.
11. Löwenstein A: Aetiologische Untersuchungen über den fieberhaften Herpes. Munch Med Wochenschr 66:769, 1919.
12. Doerr R: Sitzungsberichte der Gesellschaft der schweizerischen Augenartzte. Diskussion. Klin Monatsblt Augenheilkd 65:104, 1920.
13. Lipschütz B: Untersuchungen über die Atiologie der Krankheiten der Herpesgruppe (herpes zoster, herpes genitalis and herpes febrilis). Arch Dermatol Res 136:428, 1921.
14. Friedenwald JS: Studies on the virus of herpes simplex. Arch Ophthalmol N Y 52:105, 1923.
15. Goodpasture EW, Teague O: Transmission of the virus of herpes fibrilis along nerves in experimentally infected rabbits. J Med Res 44:139, 1923.
16. Marinesco G, Draganesco S: Recherches experimentales sur le neurotropisme du virus herpetique. Ann Inst Pasteur 37:753, 1923.
17. Perdrau JR: Persistence of the virus of herpes in rabbits immunized with living virus. J Pathol 47:447, 1938.
18. Goodpasture EW: Herpetic infections with special reference to involvement of the nervous system. Medicine (Baltimore) 8:223, 1929.
19. Good RA, Campbell B: The precipitation of latent herpes simplex encephalitis by anaphylactic shock. Proc Soc Exp Biol Med 68:82, 1948.
20. Cushing H: The surgical aspects of major neuralgia of the trigeminal nerve. A report of 20 cases of operation upon the gasserian ganglion with anatomic and physiologic notes on the consequence of its removal. JAMA 44:773, 860, 920, 1002, 1088, 1905.
21. Howard WT: The pathology of labial and nasal herpes and of herpes of the body occurring in acute croupous pneumonia and their relation to so-called herpes zoster. Am J Med Sci 125:256, 1903.
22. Howard WT: Further observations on the relation of lesions of the gasserian and posterior root ganglia to herpes occurring in pneumonia and cerebrospinal meningitis. Am J Med Sci 130:1012, 1905.
23. Baringer JR: Herpes simplex virus infection of nervous tissue in animals and man. Prog Med Virol 20:1, 1975.
24. Stevens JG: Latent herpes simplex virus and the nervous system. Curr Top Microbiol Immunol 70:31, 1975.
25. Andrews CH, Carmichael EA: A note on the presence of antibodies to herpesvirus in postencephalitic and other human sera. Lancet 1:857, 1930.
26. Dodd K, Johnston LM, Buddingh GJ: Herpetic stomatitis. J Pediatr 12:95, 1938.
27. Black WC: Acute infectious gingivostomatitis ("Vincent's stomatitis"). Am J Dis Child 56:126, 1938.
28. Burnet FM, Williams SW: Herpes simplex: A new point of view. Med J Aust 1:637, 1939.
29. Slavin HB, Gavett E: Primary herpetic vulvovaginitis. Proc Soc Exp Biol Med 63:343, 1946.
30. Schneweis KE: Serologische Untersuchungen zur Typendifferenzierung des Herpesvirus hominis. Z Immunitätsforsch Exp Ther 124:24, 1962.
31. Plummer G: Serological comparison of the herpesvirus. Br J Exp Pathol 45:135, 1964.
32. Oxman MN: Genital herpes. *In* Braude AI, Davis CE, Fierer J (eds): Infectious Diseases and Medical Microbiology, ed 2. Philadelphia, WB Saunders, 1986, pp 1041–1054.
33. McGeoch DJ: The genomes of the human herpesvirus: Contents, relationships, and evolution. Annu Rev Microbiol 43:235, 1989.
34. Roizman B, Sears AE: Herpes simplex viruses and their replication. *In* Fields BN, Knipe DM, Howley PM (eds): Fields Virology, ed 3. Philadelphia, Lippincott-Raven, 1996, pp 2231–2295.
35. Hay J, Ruyechan WT: Regulation of herpes simplex virus type 1 gene expression. Curr Top Microbiol Immunol 179:1, 1992.
36. Ward PL, Roizman B: Herpes simplex genes: The blueprint of a successful human pathogen. Trends Genet 10:267, 1994.
37. Wagner EK, Guzowski JF, Singh J: Transcription of the herpes simplex virus genome during productive and latent infection. Prog Nucleic Acid Res Mol Biol 51:123, 1995.
38. Stevens JG: Human herpesviruses: A consideration of the latent state. Microbiol Rev 53:318, 1989.
39. Stevens JG: Overview of herpesvirus latency. Semin Virol 5:191, 1994.
40. Fraser NW, Block TM, Spivack JG: The latency-associated transcripts of herpes simplex virus: RNA in search of function. Virology 191:1, 1992.
41. Simmons A, Tscharke D, Speck P: The role of immune mechanisms in control of herpes simplex virus infection of the peripheral nervous system. Curr Top Microbiol Immunol 179:31, 1992.
42. Lopez C, Arvin AM, Ashley R: Immunity to herpesvirus infections in humans. *In* Roizman B, Whitley RJ, Lopez C (eds): The Human Herpesviruses. New York, Raven Press, 1993, p 397.
43. Whitley RJ, Roizman B: Herpes simplex viruses. *In* Richman DD, Whitley RJ, Hayden FG (eds): Clinical Virology. New York, Churchill Livingstone, 1997, pp 375–410.
44. Roizman B: Herpesviridae. *In* Fields BN, Knipe DM, Howley PM (eds): Fields Virology, ed 3. Philadelphia, Lippincott-Raven, 1996, pp 2221–2230.
45. Roizman B, Destrosiers RC, Fleckenstein B, et al: The family Herpesviridae: An update. Arch Virol 123:425, 1992.
46. Furlong D, Swift H, Roizman B: Arrangement of herpesvirus deoxyribonucleic acid in the core. J Virol 10:1071, 1972.
47. Spear PG: Glycoproteins specified by herpes simplex viruses. *In* Roizman B (ed): The Herpesviruses, Vol 3. New York, Plenum Publishing, 1985, pp 315–356.
48. Spear PG: Entry of alphaherpesviruses into cells. Semin Virol 4:167, 1993.
49. Spear PG: Membrane fusion induced by herpes simplex virus. *In* Bentz (ed): Viral Fusion Mechanisms. Boca Raton, FL, CRC Press, 1993, pp 201–232.
50. Gibson W, Roizman B: Compartmentalization of spermine and spermidine in the herpes simplex virion. Proc Natl Acad Sci USA 68:2818, 1971.
51. Corey L, Spear PG: Infections with herpes simplex viruses. N Engl J Med 314:686, 749, 1986.
52. Kieff ED, Bachenheimer SL, Roizman B: Size, composition and structure of the DNA of subtypes 1 and 2 herpes simplex virus. J Virol 8:125, 1971.
53. Honess RW, Watson DH: Unity and diversity in the herpesviruses. J Gen Virol 37:15, 1977.
54. McGeoch DJ, Dolan A, Donald S, Rixon FJ: Sequence determination and genetic content of the short unique region in the genome of herpes simplex virus type 1. J Mol Biol 181:1, 1985.
55. McGeoch DJ, Dolan A, Donald S, Brauer DHK: Complete DNA sequence of the short repeat region in the genome of herpes simplex virus type 1. Nucleic Acids Res 14:1727, 1986.
56. McGeoch DJ, Dalrymple MA, Davison AJ, et al: The complete DNA sequence of the long unique region in the genome of herpes simplex virus type 1. J Gen Virol 69:1531, 1988.
57. McGeoch DJ: DNA sequence and genetic content of the *Hind* III 1 region in the short unique component of the herpes simplex virus type 2 genome: Identification of the gene encoding glycoprotein G, and evolutionary comparisons. J Gen Virol 68:19, 1987.
58. Morse LS, Pereira L, Roizman B, Schaffer PA: Anatomy of HSV DNA. XI. Mapping of viral genes by analysis of polypeptides

and functions specified by HSV-1 × HSV-2 recombinants. J Virol 26:389, 1978.
59. Preston VG, Davison AJ, Marsden HS, et al: Recombinants between herpes simplex virus types 1 and 2: Analyses of genome structures and expression of immediate-early polypeptides. J Virol 28:499, 1978.
60. Hayward GS, Frenkel N, Roizman B: The anatomy of herpes simplex virus DNA: Strain differences and heterogeneity in the locations of restriction endonuclease cleavage sites. Proc Natl Acad Sci USA 72:1768, 1975.
61. Lonsdale DM: A rapid technique for distinguishing herpes simplex virus type 1 from type 2 by restriction enzyme technology. Lancet 1:849, 1979.
62. Cassai EN, Sarmiento M, Spear PG: Comparison of the virion proteins specified by herpes simplex virus types 1 and 2. J Virol 16:1327, 1975.
63. Marsden HS, Stow ND, Preston VG, et al: Physical mapping of herpes simplex virus induced polypeptides. J Virol 28:624, 1978.
64. Buchman TG, Simpson T, Nosal C, et al: The structure of herpes simplex virus DNA and its application to molecular epidemiology. Ann N Y Acad Sci 354:279, 1980.
65. Roizman B, Tognon M: Restriction endonuclease patterns of herpes simplex virus DNA: Application to diagnosis and molecular epidemiology. Curr Top Microbiol Immunol 104:275, 1983.
66. Buchman TG, Roizman B, Adams G, Stover BH: Restriction endonuclease fingerprinting of herpes simplex virus DNA: A novel epidemiologic tool applied to a nosocomial outbreak. J Infect Dis 138:488, 1978.
67. Buchman TG, Roizman B, Nahmias AJ: Demonstration of exogenous reinfection with herpes simplex virus type-2 by restriction endonuclease fingerprinting of viral DNA. J Infect Dis 140:295, 1979.
68. Lakeman FD, Nahmias AJ, Whitley RJ: Analysis of DNA from recurrent genital herpes simplex virus isolates by restriction endonuclease digestion. J Sex Transm Dis 13:61, 1986.
69. Schmidt OW, Fife KH, Corey L: Reinfection is an uncommon occurrence in patients with symptomatic recurrent genital herpes. J Infect Dis 149:645, 1984.
70. Sheldrick P, Berthelot N: Inverted repetitions in the chromosome of herpes simplex virus. Cold Spring Harb Symp Quant Biol 39:667, 1975.
71. Wadsworth S, Jacob RJ, Roizman B: Anatomy of herpes simplex virus DNA. II. Size, composition and arrangement of inverted terminal repetitions. J Virol 15:1487, 1975.
72. Hayward GS, Jacob RJ, Wadsworth SC, Roizman B: Anatomy of herpes simplex virus DNA: Evidence for four populations of molecules that differ in the relative orientations of their long and short segments. Proc Natl Acad Sci USA 72:4243, 1975.
73. Delius H, Clements JB: A partial denaturation map of herpes simplex virus type 1 DNA: Evidence for inversions of the unique DNA regions. J Gen Virol 33:125, 1976.
74. Jenkins FJ, Roizman B: Herpes simplex virus recombinants with noninverting genomes frozen in different isomeric arrangements are capable of independent replication. J Virol 59:494, 1986.
75. Honess RW, Roizman B: Proteins specified by herpes simplex virus XI. Identification and relative molar rates of synthesis of structural and non-structural herpesvirus polypeptides in infected cells. J Virol 12:1346, 1973.
76. Stannard LM, Fuller AO, Spear PG: Herpes simplex virus glycoproteins associated with different morphological entities projecting from the virion envelope. J Gen Virol 68:715, 1987.
77. Spear PG: Biology of the herpesviruses. *In* Holmes KK (ed): Sexually Transmitted Diseases, ed 2. New York, McGraw-Hill, 1990, pp 379–389.
78. Cai W, Gu B, Person S: Role of glycoprotein B of herpes simplex virus type 1 in viral entry and cell fusion. J Virol 62:2596, 1988.
79. Desai PJ, Schaffer PA, Minson AC: Excretion of non-infectious virus particles lacking glycoprotein H by a temperature-sensitive mutant of herpes simplex virus type 1: Evidence that gH is essential for virion infectivity. J Gen Virol 69:1147, 1988.
80. Ligas MW, Johnson DC: A herpes simplex virus mutant in which glycoprotein D sequences are replaced by β-galactosidase sequences binds to but is unable to penetrate into cells. J Virol 62:1486, 1988.
81. Fuller AO, Lee WC: Herpes simplex virus type 1 entry through a cascade of virus-cell interactions requires different roles of gD and gH in penetration. J Virol 66:5002, 1992.
82. Roop C, Hutchinson L, Johnson DC: A mutant herpes simplex virus type 1 unable to express glycoprotein L cannot enter cells, and its particles lack glycoprotein H. J Virol 67:2285, 1993.
83. Oxman MN: Herpes stomatitis. *In* Braude AI (ed): Infectious Diseases and Medical Microbiology, ed 2. Philadelphia, WB Saunders, 1986, pp 752–772.
84. Whitley RJ: Cercopithecine herpes virus 1 (B virus). *In* Fields BN, Knipe DM, Howley PM (eds): Fields Virology, ed 3. Philadelphia, Lippincott-Raven, 1996, pp 2623–2635.
85. Whitley RJ: Herpes simplex viruses. *In* Fields BN, Knipe DM, Howley PM (eds): Fields Virology, ed 3. Philadelphia, Lippincott-Raven, 1996, pp 2297–2342.
86. Oxman MN: Herpes simplex encephalitis and meningitis. *In* Braude AI, Davis CE, Fierer J (eds): Infectious Diseases and Medical Microbiology, ed 2. Philadelphia, WB Saunders, 1986, pp 1114–1132.
87. Reeves WC, Corey L, Adams HG, et al: Risk of recurrence after first episodes of genital herpes: Relation to HSV type and antibody response. N Engl J Med 305:315, 1981.
88. Lafferty WE, Coombs RW, Benedetti J, et al: Recurrences after oral and genital herpes simplex virus infection. Influence of site of infection and viral type. N Engl J Med 316:1444, 1987.
89. Koelle DM, Benedetti J, Langenberg A, et al: Asymptomatic reactivation of herpes simplex virus in women after the first episode of genital herpes. Ann Intern Med 116:433, 1992.
90. Benedetti JK, Corey L, Ashley R: Recurrence rates in genital herpes after symptomatic first-episode infection. Ann Intern Med 121:847, 1994.
91. Wald A, Zeh J, Selke S, et al: Virologic characteristics of subclinical and symptomatic genital herpes infections. N Engl J Med 333:770, 1995.
92. Gentry GA, Lowe M, Alford G, Nevins R: Sequence analysis of herpesviral enzymes suggests an ancient origin for human sexual behavior. Proc Soc Natl Acad Sci USA 85:2658, 1988.
93. Morgan C, Rose HM, Mednis B: Electron microscopy of herpes simplex virus. I. Entry. J Virol 2:507, 1968.
94. Fuller AO, Spear PG: Anti-gD antibodies that permit adsorption but block infection by herpes simplex virus prevent virion-cell fusion at the cell surface. Proc Natl Acad Sci USA 84:5454, 1987.
95. Wudunn D, Spear PG: Initial interaction of herpes simplex virus with cells in binding to heparin sulfate. J Virol 63:52, 1989.
96. Kuhn JE, Kramer MD, Willenbacher W, et al: Identification of herpes simplex virus type 1 glycoproteins interacting with the cell surface. J Virol 64:2491, 1990.
97. Herold BC, Wudunn D, Soltys N, Spear PG: Glycoprotein C of herpes simplex virus type 1 plays a principal role in the adsorption of virus to cells and in infectivity. J Virol 65:1090, 1991.
98. Spear PG, Shieh M-T, Herold BC, et al: Heparan sulfate glycosaminoglycans as primary cell surface receptors for herpes simplex virus. *In* Lane DA, Bjork I, Lindahl U (eds): Heparin and Related Polysaccharides. New York, Plenum Publishing, 1992, pp 341–353.
99. Tal-Singer R, Peng C, Ponce de Leon M, et al: Interaction of herpes simplex virus glycoprotein gC with mammalian cell surface molecules. J Virol 69:4471, 1995.
100. Williams RK, Straus SE: Specificity and affinity of binding of herpes simplex virus type 2 glycoprotein B to glycosaminoglycans. J Virol 71:1375, 1997.
101. Huang T, Campadelli-Fiume G: Anti-idiotypic antibodies mimicking glycoprotein D of herpes simplex virus identify a cellular protein required for virus spread from cell to cell and virus-induced polykaryocytosis. Proc Natl Acad Sci USA 93:1836, 1996.
102. Campadelli-Fiume G, Avitabile E, Fini S, et al: Herpes simplex virus glycoprotein D is sufficient to induce spontaneous pH-independent fusion in a cell line that constitutively expresses the glycoprotein. Virology 166:598, 1988.
103. Johnson DC, Burke RL, Gregory T: Soluble forms of herpes simplex virus glycoprotein D bind to a limited number of cell surface receptors and inhibit virus entry into cells. J Virol 64:2569, 1990.
104. Long D, Cohen GH, Muggeridge MI, Eisenberg RJ: Cysteine mutants of herpes simplex virus type 1 glycoprotein D exhibit temperature-sensitive properties in structure and function. J Virol 64:5542, 1990.

105. Highlander SL, Sutherland SL, Gage PJ, et al: Neutralizing monoclonal antibodies specific for herpes simplex virus glycoprotein D inhibit virus penetration. J Virol 61:3356, 1987.
106. Highlander SL, Cai WH, Persons S, et al: Monoclonal antibodies define a domain on herpes simplex virus glycoprotein B involved in virus penetration. J Virol 62:1881, 1988.
107. Fuller AO, Santos RS, Spear PG: Neutralizing antibodies specific for glycoprotein H of herpes simplex virus permit viral attachment to cells but prevent penetration. J Virol 63:3435, 1989.
108. Weber PC, Levine M, Glorioso JC: Rapid identification of nonessential genes of herpes simplex virus type 1 by Tn*5* mutagenesis. Science 236:576, 1987.
109. Campadelli-Fiume G, Stirpe D, Boscano A, et al: Glycoprotein C–dependent attachment of herpes simplex virus to susceptible cells leading to productive infection. Virology 178:213, 1990.
110. Sears AE, McGwire BS, Roizman B: Infection of polarized MDCK cells with herpes simplex virus 1: Two asymmetrically distributed cell receptors interact with different viral proteins. Proc Natl Aca Sci USA 88:5087, 1991.
111. Handler CG, Cohen GH, Eisenberg RJ: Cross-linking of glycoprotein oligomers during herpes simplex virus type 1 entry. J Virology 70:6076, 1996.
112. Handler CG, Eisenberg RJ, Cohen GH: Oligomeric structure of glycoproteins in herpes simplex virus type 1. J Virol 70:6067, 1996.
113. Hutchinson L, Browne H, Wargent V, et al: A novel herpes simplex virus glycoprotein, gL, forms a complex with glycoprotein H (gH) and affects normal folding and surface expression of gH. J Virol 66:2240, 1992.
114. Batterson W, Furlong D, Roizman B: Molecular genetics of herpes simplex virus. VII. Further characterization of a *ts* mutant defective in release of viral DNA and in other stages of viral reproductive cycle. J Virol 45:397, 1983.
115. Honess RW, Roizman B: Regulation of herpesvirus macromolecular synthesis. I. Cascade regulation of the synthesis of three groups of viral proteins. J Virol 14:8, 1974.
116. Mackem S, Roizman B: Structural features of the α gene 4, 0, and 27 promoter-regulatory sequences which confer α regulation on chimeric thymidine kinase genes. J Virol 44:939, 1982.
117. Batterson W, Roizman B: Characterization of the herpes simplex virion–associated factor responsible for the induction of α genes. J Virol 46:371, 1983.
118. Campbell MEM, Palfreyman JW, Preston CM: Identification of herpes simplex virus DNA sequences which encode a transacting polypeptide responsible for stimulation of immediate early transcription. J Mol Biol 180:1, 1984.
119. Kristie TM, Roizman B: Separation of sequences defining basal expression from those conferring α gene recognition within the regulatory domains of herpes simplex virus 1 α genes. Proc Natl Acad Sci USA 81:4065, 1984.
120. Pellett PE, McKnight JLC, Jenkins FJ, Roizman B: Nucleotide sequence and predicted amino acid sequence of a protein encoded in a small herpes simplex virus DNA fragment capable of *trans*-inducing α genes. Proc Natl Acad Sci USA 82:5870, 1985.
121. McKnight JLC, Kristie TM, Roizman B: Binding of the virion protein mediating α gene induction in herpes simplex virus 1–infected cells to its cis site requires cellular proteins. Proc Natl Acad Sci USA 84:7061, 1987.
122. O'Hare P, Goding CR, Haigh A: Direct combinatorial interaction between a herpes simplex virus regulatory protein and a cellular octamer-binding factor mediates specific induction of virus immediate-early gene expression. EMBO J 7:4231, 1988.
123. Triezenberg SJ, Lamarco KL, McKnight SL: Evidence of DNA:protein interactions that mediate HSV-1 immediate early gene activation by VP16. Genes Dev 85:6347, 1988.
124. Gerster T, Roeder RG: A herpesvirus transactivating protein interacts with transcription factor OTF-1 and other cellular proteins. Proc Natl Acad Sci USA 85:6347, 1988.
125. Goding CR, O'Hare P: Herpes simplex virus Vmw65–octamer-binding protein interaction: A paradigm for combinatorial control of transcription. Virology 173:363, 1989.
126. Kristie TM, Lebowitz JH, Sharp PA: The octamer-binding proteins form multiprotein-DNA complexes with the HSV αTIF regulatory protein. EMBO J 8:4229, 1989.
127. Xiao P, Capone JP: A cellular factor binds to the herpes simplex virus type 1 transactivator Vmw65 and is required for Vmw65-dependent protein-DNA complex assembly with Oct-1. Mol Cell Biol 10:4974, 1990.
128. Hayes S, O'Hare P: Mapping of a major surface-exposed site in herpes simplex virus protein Vmw65 to a region of direct interaction in a transcription complex assembly. J Virol 67:852, 1993.
129. Wilson AC, LaMarco K, Peterson MG, et al: The VP16 accessory protein HCF is a family of polypeptides processed from a large precursor protein. Cell 74:115, 1993.
130. Ace CI, McKee TA, Ryan JM, et al: Construction and characterization of a herpes simplex virus type 1 mutant unable to transinduce immediate-early gene expression. J Virol 63:2260, 1989.
131. Zhu XX, Chen J, Young CSH, Silverstein S: Reactivation of latent herpes simplex virus by adenovirus recombinants encoding mutants IE-0 gene products. J Virol 64:4489, 1990.
132. Cai W, Astor LM, Liptak C, et al: The herpes simplex virus type 1 regulatory protein ICP0 enhances virus replication during acute infection and reactivation from latency. J Virol 67:7501, 1993.
133. Sacks WR, Greene CC, Aschman DP, et al: Herpes simplex virus type 1 ICP27 is an essential regulatory protein. J Virol 55:796, 1985.
134. McCarthy AM, McMahan L, Schaffer PA: Herpes simplex virus type 1 ICP27 deletion mutants exhibit altered patterns of transcription and are DNA deficient. J Virol 63:18, 1989.
135. Smith IL, Hardwicke MA, Sandri-Goldin RM: Evidence that the herpes simplex virus immediate early protein ICP27 acts post-transcriptionally during infection to regulate gene expression. Virology 186:74, 1992.
136. Rice SA, Lam V: Amino acid substitution mutations in the herpes simplex virus ICP27 protein define an essential gene regulation function. J Virol 68:823, 1994.
137. Samaniego LA, Webb AL, DeLuca NA: Functional interactions between herpes simplex virus immediate-early proteins during infection: Gene expression as a consequence of ICP27 and different domains of ICP4. J Virol 69:5705, 1995.
138. Zhu Z, Cai W, Schaffer PA: Cooperativity among herpes simplex virus type 1 immediate-early regulatory proteins: ICP4 and ICP27 affect the intracellular localizations of ICP0. J Virol 68:3027, 1994.
139. Zhu Z, Schaffer PA: Intracellular localization of the herpes simplex virus type 1 major transcriptional regulatory protein, ICP4, is affected by ICP27. J Virol 69:49, 1995.
140. Panagiotidis CA, Lium EK, Silverstein SJ: Physical and functional interactions between herpes simplex virus immediate-early proteins ICP4 and ICP27. J Virol 71:1547, 1997.
141. Hardy WR, Sandri-Goldin RM: Herpes simplex virus inhibits host cell splicing, and regulatory protein ICP27 is required for this effect. J Virol 68:7790, 1994.
142. Koelle DM, Tigges MA, Burke RL, et al: Herpes simplex virus infection of human fibroblasts and keratinocytes inhibits recognition by cloned $CD8^+$ cytotoxic T lymphocytes. J Clin Invest 91:961, 1993.
143. York IA, Roop C, Andrews DW, et al: A cytosolic herpes simplex virus protein inhibits antigen presentation to $CD8^+$ T lymphocytes. Cell 77:525, 1994.
144. Ahn K, Meyer TH, Uebel S, et al: Molecular mechanism and species specificity of TAP inhibition by herpes simplex virus ICP47. EMBO J 15:3247, 1996.
145. Tomazin R, Hill AB, Jugovic P, et al: Stable binding of the herpes simplex virus ICP47 protein to the peptide binding site of TAP. EMBO J 15:3256, 1996.
146. Honess RW, Roizman B: Regulation of herpesvirus macro-molecular synthesis: Sequential transition of polypeptide synthesis requires functional viral polypeptides. Proc Natl Acad Sci USA 72:1276, 1975.
147. O'Hare P, Hayward GS: Evidence for a direct role for both the 175,000 and 110,000 molecular weight immediate-early proteins of herpes simplex virus in the transactivation of delayed-early promoters. J Virol 53:751, 1984.
148. Holland LE, Anderson KP, Shipman C, Wagner EK: Viral DNA synthesis is required for the efficient expression of specific herpes virus type 1 mRNA species. Virology 101:10, 1980.
149. Jacob RJ, Roizman B: Anatomy of herpes simplex virus DNA. VIII. Properties of the replicating DNA. J Virol 23:394, 1977.

150. Jacob RJ, Morse LS, Roizman B: Anatomy of herpes simplex virus DNA. XIII. Accumulation of head-to-tail concatemers in nuclei of infected cells and their role in the generation of the four isomeric arrangements of viral DNA. J Virol 29:448, 1979.
151. Tengelsen LA, Pederson NE, Shaver PR, et al: Herpes simplex virus type 1 DNA cleavage and encapsidation require the product of the UL28 gene: Isolation and characterization of two UL28 deletion mutants. J Virol 67:3470, 1993.
152. Newcomb WW, Brown JC: Structure of the herpes simplex virus capsid: Effects of extraction with guanidine hydrochloride and partial reconstitution of extracted capsids. J Virol 65:613, 1991.
153. Newcomb WW, Trus BL, Booy AC, et al: Structure of the herpes simplex virus capsid: Molecular composition of the pentons and the triplexes. J Mol Biol 232:499, 1993.
154. Nicholson P, Addison C, Cross AM, et al: Localization of the herpes simplex virus type 1 major capsid protein VP5 to the cell nucleus requires the abundant scaffolding protein VP22a. J Gen Virol 75:1091, 1994.
155. Matusick-Kumer L, Hurlburt W, Weinheimer SP, et al: Phenotype of the herpes simplex virus type 1 protease substrate ICP35 mutant virus. J Virol 68:5384, 1994.
156. Matusick-Kumar L, Newcomb WW, Brown JC, et al: The C-terminal 25 amino acids of the protease and its substrate ICP35 of herpes simplex virus type 1 are involved in the formation of sealed capsids. J Virol 69:4347, 1995.
157. Desai P, Deluca NA, Glorioso JC, et al: Mutations of herpes simplex type 1 genes encoding VP5 and VP23 abrogate capsid formation and cleavage of replicated DNA. J Virol 67:1357, 1993.
158. Newcomb WW, Homa FL, Thomsen DR, et al: Assembly of the herpes simplex virus capsid: Identification of intermediates in cell-free capsid formation. J Mol Biol 263:432, 1996.
159. Vlazny DA, Kwong A, Frenkel N: Site specific cleavage packaging of herpes simplex virus DNA and the selective maturation of nucleocapsids containing full length viral DNA. Proc Natl Acad Sci USA 79:1423, 1982.
160. Baines JD, Roizman B: The U_L11 gene of herpes simplex virus 1 encodes a function that facilitates nucleocapsid envelopment and egress from cells. J Virol 66:5168, 1992.
161. Johnson DC, Spear PG: Monensin inhibits the processing of herpes simplex virus glycoproteins, their transport to the cell surface, and the egress of virions from infected cells. J Virol 43:1102, 1982.
162. Tognon M, Furlong D, Conley AJ, Roizman B: Molecular genetics of herpes simplex virus. V. Characterization of a mutant defective in ability to form plaques at low temperatures and in a viral function which prevents accumulation of coreless capsids at nuclear pores late in infection. J Virol 40:870, 1981.
163. Johnson RM, Spear PG: Herpes simplex virus glycoprotein D mediates interference with herpes simplex virus infection. J Virol 63:819, 1989.
164. Campadelli-Fiume G, Qi S, Avitabile E, et al: Glycoprotein D of herpes simplex virus encodes a domain which precludes penetration of cells expressing the glycoprotein by superinfecting herpes simplex virus. J Virol 64:6070, 1990.
165. Field HJ, Wildy P: The pathogenicity of thymidine kinase–deficient mutants of herpes simplex virus in mice. J Hyg 81:267, 1978.
166. Price RW, Kahn A: Resistance of peripheral autonomic neurons to in vivo productive infection by herpes simplex virus mutants deficient in thymidine kinase activity. Infect Immun 43:571, 1981.
167. Wildy P, Field HJ, Nash AA: Classical herpes latency revisited. *In* Mahy BWJ, Minson AC, Darby GK (eds): Virus Persistence. Cambridge, MA, Cambridge University Press, 1982, pp 133–167.
168. Coen DM, Kosz-Vnenchak M, Jacobson JG, et al: Thymidine kinase–negative herpes simplex virus mutants establish latency in mouse trigeminal ganglia but do not reactivate. Proc Natl Acad Sci USA 86:4736, 1989.
169. Leist TP, Sandri-Goldin RM, Stevens JG: Latent infections in spinal ganglia with thymidine kinase–deficient herpes simplex virus. J Virol 63:4976, 1989.
170. Tenser RB, Hay KA, Edris WA: Latency-associated transcript but not reactivatable virus is present in sensory ganglion neurons after inoculation of thymidine kinase–negative mutants of herpes simplex virus type 1. J Virol 63:2861, 1989.
171. Goldstein DJ, Weller SK: Herpes simplex virus type 1–induced ribonucleotide reductase activity is dispensable for virus growth and DNA synthesis: Isolation and characterization of an ICP6 *lacZ* insertion mutant. J Virol 62:196, 1988.
172. Cameron JM, McDougall I, Marsden HS, et al: Ribonucleotide reductase encoded by herpes simplex virus is a determinant of the pathogenicity of the virus in mice and a valid antiviral target. J Gen Virol 69:2607, 1988.
173. Katz JP, Bodin ET, Coen DM: Quantitative polymerase chain reaction analysis of herpes simplex virus DNA in ganglia of mice infected with replication-incompetent mutants. J Virol 64:4288, 1990.
174. Roizman B, Jenkins FJ: Genetic engineering of novel genomes of large DNA viruses. Science 129:1208, 1985.
175. Glorioso JC, DeLuca NA, Fink DJ: Development and application of herpes simplex virus vectors for human gene therapy. Annu Rev Microbiol 49:675, 1995.
176. Fenwick ML, Walker MJ: Suppression of the synthesis of cellular macromolecules by herpes simplex virus. J Gen Virol 41:37, 1978.
177. Kwong AD, Frenkel N: Herpes simplex virus–infected cells contain a function(s) that destabilizes both host and viral mRNAs. Proc Natl Acad Sci USA 84:1926, 1987.
178. Kwong AD, Kruper JA, Frenkel N: Herpes simplex virus virion host shutoff function. J Virol 62:912, 1988.
179. Oroskar AA, Read GS: Control of mRNA stability by the virion host shutoff function of herpes simplex virus. J Virol 63:1897, 1989.
180. Read GS, Karr BM, Knight K: Isolation of a herpes simplex virus type 1 mutant with deletion in the virion host shutoff gene and identification of multiple forms of the *vhs* (U_L41) polypetide. J Virol 67:7149, 1993.
181. Silverstein S, Engelhardt EL: Alterations in the protein synthetic apparatus of cells infected with herpes simplex virus. Virology 95:324, 1979.
182. Chou J, Chen J-J, Gross M, et al: Association of a M_r 90,000 phosphoprotein with protein kinase PKR in cells exhibiting enhanced phosphorylation of translation initiation factor eIF-2 alpha and premature shutoff of protein synthesis after infection with gamma 1 34.5 – mutants of herpes simplex virus 1. Proc Natl Acad Sci USA 92:10516, 1995.
183. Whitley RJ, Kern ER, Chatterjee S, et al: Replication, establishment of latency, and induced reactivation of herpes simplex virus γ_1 34.5 deletion mutants in rodent models. J Clin Invest 91:2837, 1993.
184. Hill TJ: Herpes simplex virus latency. *In* Roizman B (ed): The Herpesviruses, Vol 3. New York, Plenum Publishing, 1985, pp 175–240.
185. Nesburn AB, Elliot JM, Leibowitz HM: Spontaneous reactivation of experimental herpes simplex keratitis in rabbits. Arch Ophthalmol 78:523, 1967.
186. Laibson PR, Kibrick S: Recurrence of herpes simplex virus in rabbit eyes: Results of a three-year study. Invest Ophthalmol 8:346, 1969.
187. Hill JM, Rayfield MA, Haruta Y: Strain specificity of spontaneous and adrenergically induced HSV-1 ocular reactivation in latently infected rabbits. Curr Eye Res 6:91, 1987.
188. Stanberry LR, Kern ER, Richards JT, et al: Genital herpes in guinea pigs: Pathogenesis of the primary infection and description of recurrent disease. J Infect Dis 146:397, 1982.
189. Stanberry LR: Pathogenesis of herpes simplex virus infections and animal models for its study. Curr Top Microbiol Immunol 179:15, 1992.
190. Wigdahl BL, Scheck AC, DeClerq E, Rapp F: High-efficiency latency and reactivation of herpes simplex virus in human cells. Science 217:1145, 1982.
191. Wigdahl BL, Scheck AC, Ziegler RJ, et al: Analysis of the herpes simplex virus genome during in vitro latency in human diploid fibroblasts and rat sensory neurons. J Virol 49:205, 1984.
192. Russell J, Preston CM: An in vitro latency system for herpes simplex virus type 2. J Gen Virol 67:397, 1986.
193. Russell J, Stow ND, Stow EC, Preston CM: Herpes simplex virus genes involved in latency in vitro. J Gen Virol 68:3009, 1987.
194. Wilcox CL, Johnson EM Jr: Nerve growth factor deprivation results in the reactivation of latent herpes simplex virus in vitro. J Virol 61:2311, 1987.
195. Wilcox CL, Johnson EM Jr: Characterization of nerve growth

factor–dependent herpes simplex virus latency in neurons in vitro. J Virol 62:393, 1988.
196. Doerig C, Pizer LI, Wilcox CL: Detection of the latency associated transcript in neuronal cultures during the latent infection with herpes simplex virus type 1. Virology 183:423, 1991.
197. Jamieson DR, Robinson LH, Daksis JI, et al: Quiescent viral genomes in human fibroblasts after infection with herpes simplex virus type 1 Vmw65 mutants. J Gen Virol 76:1417, 1995.
198. Syrjanen S, Mikola H, Nykanen M, Hukkanen V: In vitro establishment of lytic and nonproductive infection by herpes simplex virus type 1 in three-dimensional keratinocyte culture. J Virology 70:6524, 1996.
199. Cook ML, Stevens JG: Pathogenesis of herpetic neuritis and ganglionitis in mice: Evidence of intraaxonal transport of infection. Infect Immun 7:272, 1973.
200. Lycke E, Kristensson K, Svennerholm B, et al: Uptake and transport of herpes simplex virus in neurites of rat dorsal root ganglia cells in culture. J Gen Virol 65:55, 1984.
201. Kristensson K, Lycke E, Roytta M, et al: Neuritic transport of herpes simplex virus in rat sensory neurons in vitro. Effects of substances interacting with microtubular function and axonal flow [nocodazole, taxol and erythro-9-3-(2-hydroxynonyl)adenine]. J Gen Virol 67:2023, 1986.
202. Warren SL, Carpenter CM, Boak RA: Symptomatic herpes, a sequela of artificially 'induced' fever: Incidence and clinical aspects; recovery of virus from herpetic vesicles and comparison with a known strain of herpes virus. J Exp Med 71:155, 1940.
203. Ellison SA, Carlton CA, Rose HM: Studies of recurrent herpes simplex infections following section of the trigeminal nerve. J Infect Dis 105:161, 1959.
204. Pazin GJ, Ho M, Jannetta PJ: Herpes simplex reactivation after trigeminal nerve root decompression. J Infect Dis 138:405, 1978.
205. Stevens JG, Cook ML: Latent herpes simplex virus in spinal ganglia of mice. Science 173:843, 1971.
206. Bastian FO, Rabson AS, Yee CL, Tralka TS: Herpesvirus hominis: Isolation from human trigeminal ganglion. Science 178:306, 1972.
207. Baringer JR, Swoveland P: Recovery of herpes simplex virus from human trigeminal ganglia. N Engl J Med 288:648, 1973.
208. Baringer JR, Swoveland P: Persistent herpes simplex virus infection in rabbit trigeminal ganglia. Lab Invest 30:230, 1974.
209. McLennan JL, Darby G: Herpes simplex virus latency: The cellular location of virus in dorsal root ganglia and the fate of the infected cell following virus activation. J Gen Virol 51:233, 1980.
210. Stevens JG, Wagner EK, Devi-Rao GB, et al: RNA complementary to a herpesvirus alpha gene mRNA is prominent in latently infected neurons. Science 253:1056, 1987.
211. Croen KL, Ostrove JD, Dragovic LJ, et al: Latent herpes simplex virus in human trigeminal ganglia: Detection of an immediate early gene "anti-sense" transcript by in situ hybridization. N Engl J Med 317:1427, 1987.
212. Croen KD, Ostrove JM, Dragovic L, Straus SE: Characterization of herpes simplex type 2 latency-associated transcription in human sacral ganglia and in cell culture. J Infect Dis 163:23, 1991.
213. Efstathiou S, Kemp S, Darby G, Minson AC: The role of herpes simplex virus type 1 thymidine kinase in pathogenesis. J Gen Virol 70:869, 1989.
214. Rock DL, Fraser NW: Latent herpes simplex virus type 1 DNA contains two copies of the virion DNA joint region. J Virol 55:849, 1985.
215. Efstathiou S, Minson AC, Field HJ, et al: Detection of herpes simplex virus–specific DNA sequences in latently infected mice and in humans. J Virol 57:446, 1986.
216. Mellerick DM, Fraser NW: Physical state of the latent herpes simplex virus genome in a mouse model system: Evidence suggesting an episomal state. Virology 158:265, 1987.
217. Leib DA, Coen DM, Bogard CL, et al: Immediate-early regulatory gene mutants define different stages in the establishment and reactivation of herpes simplex virus latency. J Virol 63:759, 1989.
218. Kosz-Vnenchak M, Coen DM, Knipe DM: Restricted expression of herpes simplex virus lytic genes during establishment of latent infection by thymidine kinase–negative mutant viruses. J Virol 64:5396, 1990.
219. Margolis TP, Sedarati F, Dobsone AT, et al: Pathways of viral gene expression during acute neuronal infection with HSV-1. Virology 189:150, 1992.
220. Sedarati F, Margolis TP, Stevens JG: Latent infection can be established with drastically restricted transcription and replication of the HSV-1 genome. Virology 192:687, 1993.
221. Steiner I, Spivack JG, Deshmane SL, et al: A herpes simplex virus type 1 mutant containing a nontransducing Vmw65 protein establishes latent infection in vivo in the absence of viral replication and reactivates efficiently from explanted trigeminal ganglia. J Virol 64:1630, 1990.
222. Roizman B, Sears AE: An inquiry into the mechanism of herpes simplex virus latency. Annu Rev Microbiol 41:543, 1987.
223. Knipe DM: The role of viral and cellular nuclear proteins in herpes simplex virus replication. Adv Virus Res 37:85, 1990.
224. Kemp LM, Dent CL, Latchman DS: Octamer motif mediates transcriptional repression of HSV immediate-early genes and octamer-containing cellular promoters in neuronal cells. Neuron 4:215, 1990.
225. Lillycrop KA, Estridge JK, Latchman DS: The octamer binding protein Oct-2 inhibits transactivation of the herpes simplex virus immediate-early genes by the virion protein Vmw65. Virology 196:888, 1993.
226. Deshmane SL, Fraser NW: During latency, herpes simplex virus type 1 DNA is associated with nucleosomes in a chromatin structure. J Verol 63:943, 1989.
227. Deatley A, Spivack JG, Lavi E, Fraser NW: RNA from an immediate early region of the HSV-1 genome is present in the trigeminal ganglia of latently infected mice. Proc Natl Acad Sci USA 84:3204, 1987.
228. Rock DL, Nesburn AB, Ghiasi H, et al: Detection of latency-related viral RNAs in trigeminal ganglia of rabbits latently infected with herpes simplex virus type 1. J Virol 62:3820, 1987.
229. Puga A, Notkins AL: Continued expression of a poly(A) transcript of herpes simplex virus type 1 in trigeminal ganglia of latently infected mice. J Virol 61:1700, 1987.
230. Krause PR, Croen KD, Straus SE, Ostrove JM: Detection and preliminary characterization of herpes simplex virus type 1 transcripts in latently infected human trigeminal ganglia. J Virol 62:4819, 1988.
231. Stevens JG, Haarr L, Porter DP, et al: Prominence of the herpes simplex virus latency-associated transcript in trigeminal ganglia from seropositive humans. J Infect Dis 158:117, 1988.
232. Wagner EK, Devi-Rao G, Feldman LT, et al: Physical characterization of the herpes simplex virus latent-associated transcript in neurons. J Virol 62:1194, 1988.
233. Wagner EK, Flanagan M, Devi-Rao G, et al: The herpes simplex virus latency-associated transcript is spliced during the latent phase of infection. J Virol 62:4577, 1988.
234. Gordon YJ, Johnson B, Romanowski E, Araullo-Cruz T: RNA complementary to herpes simplex virus type 1 ICP0 gene demonstrated in neurons of human trigeminal ganglia. J Virol 62:1832, 1988.
235. Krause PR, Croen KD, Ostrove JM, Straus SE: Structural and kinetic analysis of herpes simplex type 1 latency-associated transcripts in human trigeminal ganglia and cell culture. J Clin Invest 86:235, 1990.
236. Mitchell WJ, Deshmane SL, Dolan A, et al: Characterization of herpes simplex virus type 2 transcription during latent infection of mouse trigeminal ganglia. J Virol 64:5342, 1990.
237. Wu TT, Su YH, Block TM, Taylor JM: Evidence that two latency-associated transcripts of herpes simplex virus type 1 are nonlinear. J Virol 70:5962, 1996.
238. Zwaagstra JC, Ghiasi H, Nesburn AB, et al: In vitro promoter activity associated with the latency-associated transcript gene of herpes simplex virus type 1. J Gen Virol 70:2163, 1989.
239. Batchelor AH, Ohare P: Regulation and cell type–specific activity of a promoter located upstream of the latency-associated transcript of herpes simplex virus type 1. J Virol 64:3269, 1990.
240. Zwaagstra JC, Ghiasi H, Nesburn AB, et al: Identification of a major regulatory sequence in the latency associated transcript (LAT) promoter of herpes simplex virus type 1 (HSV-1). Virology 182:287, 1991.
241. Kenny JJ, Krebs FC, Hartle HT, et al: Identification of a second ATF/CREB-like element in the herpes simplex virus type 1 (HSV-1) latency-associated transcript (LAT) promoter. Virology 200:220, 1994.

242. Javier RT, Stevens JG, Dissette VB, Wagner EK: A herpes simplex virus transcript abundant in latently infected neurons is dispensable for establishment of the latent state. Virology 166:254, 1988.
243. Steiner I, Spivack JG, Lirrete RP, et al: Herpes simplex virus type 1 latency-associated transcripts are evidently not essential for latent infection. EMBO J 8:505, 1989.
244. Leib DA, Bogard CI, Kosz-Vnenchak M, et al: A deletion mutant of the latency-associated transcript of herpes simplex virus type 1 reactivates from the latent state with reduced frequency. J Virol 63:2893, 1989.
245. Sedarati F, Izumi KM, Wagner EK, Stevens JG: Herpes simplex type 1 latency associated transcription plays no role in establishment or maintenance of a latent infection in murine sensory neurons. J Virol 63:4455, 1989.
246. Hill JM, Sedarati F, Javier RT, et al: Herpes simplex virus latent phase transcription facilitates in vivo reactivation. Virology 174:117, 1990.
247. Izumi KM, McKelvey AM, Devi-Rao G, et al: Molecular and biological characterization of a type 1 herpes simplex virus (HSV-1) specifically deleted for expression of the latency-associated transcript (LAT). Microb Pathog 7:121, 1989.
248. Devi-Rao GB, Bloom DC, Stevens JG, Wagner EK: Herpes simplex virus type 1 DNA replication and gene expression during explant-induced reactivation of latently infected murine sensory ganglia. J Virol 68:1271, 1994.
249. Bloom DC, Devi-Rao GB, Hill JM, et al: Molecular analysis of herpes simplex virus type 1 during epinephrine-induced reactivation of latently infected rabbits in vivo. J Virol 68:1283, 1994.
250. Bourne N, Stanberry LR, Connelly B, et al: Quantity of latency-associated transcript produced by herpes simplex virus is not predictive of the frequency of experimental recurrent genital herpes. J Infect Dis 169:1084, 1994.
251. Trousdale MD, Steiner I, Spivack JG, et al: In vivo and in vitro reactivation impairment of a herpes simplex virus type 1 latency-associated transcript variant in a rabbit eye model. J Virol 65:6989, 1991.
252. Straus SE, Seidlin M, Takiff HE, et al: Effect of oral acyclovir treatment on symptomatic and asymptomatic virus shedding in recurrent genital herpes. Sex Transm Dis 16:107, 1989.
253. Goldberg LH, Kaufman R, Kurtz TO, et al: Long-term suppression of recurrent genital herpes with acyclovir. A 5-year benchmark. Acyclovir study group. Arch Dermatol 129:582, 1993.
254. Fife KH, Crumpacker CS, Mertz GJ, et al: Recurrence and resistance patterns of herpes simplex virus following cessation of ≥6 years of chronic suppression with acyclovir. J Infect Dis 169:1338, 1994.
255. Clements GB, Stow ND: A herpes simplex virus type 1 mutant containing a deletion within immediate early gene 1 is latency-competent in mice. J Gen Virol 70:2501, 1989.
256. Harris RA, Everett RD, Zhu X, et al: Herpes simplex virus type 1 immediate-early protein Vmw110 reactivates latent herpes virus type 2 in an in vitro latency system. J Virol 63:3513, 1989.
257. Krause PR, Stanberry LR, Bourne N, et al: Expression of the herpes simplex virus type 2 latency-associated transcript enhances spontaneous reactivation of genital herpes in latently infected guinea pigs. J Exp Med 181:297, 1995.
258. Perng G, Ghiasi H, Stanina S, et al: The spontaneous reactivation function of the herpes simplex virus type 1 LAT gene resides completely within the first 1.5 kilobases of the 8.3-kilobase primary transcript. J Virol 70:976, 1996.
259. Farrell MJ, Hill JM, Margolis TP, et al: The herpes simplex virus type 1 reactivation function lies outside the latency-associated transcript open reading frame. J Virol 67:3653, 1993.
260. Penfold ME, Armati P, Cunningham AL: Axonal transport of herpes simplex virions to epidermal cells: Evidence for a specialized mode of virus transport and assembly. Proc Natl Acad Sci USA 91:6529, 1994.
261. Ramakrishnan R, Fink DJ, Jiang G, et al: Competitive quantitative PCR analysis of herpes simplex virus type 1 DNA and latency-associated transcript RNA in latently infected cells of the rat brain. J Virol 68:1864, 1994.
262. Ramakrishnan R, Poliani PL, Levine M, et al: Detection of herpes simplex virus type 1 latency-associated transcript expression in trigeminal ganglia by in situ reverse transcriptase PCR. J Virol 70:6519, 1996.
263. Kramer MF, Coen DM: Quantification of transcripts from the ICP4 and thymidine kinase genes in mouse ganglia latently infected with herpes simplex virus. J Virol 69:1389, 1995.
264. Valy-Nagy T, Deshmane SL, Spivack JG, et al: Investigation of herpes simplex virus type 1 (HSV-1) gene expression and DNA synthesis during the establishment of latent infection by an HSV-1 mutant, in1814, that does not replicate in mouse trigeminal ganglia. J Gen Virol 72:641, 1991.
265. Smith RL, Pizer LI, Johnson EM, Wilcox CL: Activation of second-messenger pathways reactivates latent herpes simplex virus in neuronal cultures. Virology 188:311, 1992.
266. Gu B, DeLuca N: Requirements for activation of the herpes simplex virus glycoprotein C promoter in vitro by the viral regulatory protein ICP4. J Virol 68:7953, 1994.
267. Smith CA, Bates P, Rivera-Gonzalez R, et al: ICP4, the major transcriptional regulatory protein of herpes simplex virus type 1, forms a tripartite complex with TATA-binding protein and TFIIB. J Virol 67:4676, 1993.
268. Zwaagstra JC, Ghiasi H, Slanina SM, et al: Activity of herpes simplex virus type 1 latency-associated transcript (LAT) promoter in neuron-derived cells: Evidence for neuron specificity and for a large LAT transcript. J Virol 64:5019, 1990.
269. Guzowski JF, Singh J, Wagner EK: Transcriptional activation of the herpes simplex virus type 1 U_L38 promoter conferred by the cis-acting downstream activation sequence is mediated by a cellular transcription factor. J Virol 68:7774, 1994.
270. Bzik DJ, Debroy C, Fox BA, et al: The nucleotide sequence of the gB glycoprotein gene of HSV-2 and comparison with the corresponding gene of HSV-1. Virology 155:322, 1986.
271. Watson RJ: DNA sequence of the herpes simplex virus type 2 glycoprotein D gene. Gene 26:307, 1983.
272. Swain MA, Peet RW, Galloway DA: Characterization of the gene encoding herpes simplex virus type 2 glycoprotein C and comparison with the type 1 counterpart. J Virol 53:561, 1985.
273. Pereira L, Dondero DV, Gallo D, et al: Serological analysis of herpes simplex virus types 1 and 2 with monoclonal antibodies. Infect Immun 35:363, 1982.
274. Kimmel KA, Dolter KE, Toth GM, et al: Serologic type conversion of a herpes simplex virus type 1 (HSV-1) to an HSV-2 epitope caused by a single amino acid substitution in glycoprotein C. J Virol 64:4033, 1990.
275. Rawls WE: Herpes simplex virus types 1 and 2 and *Herpesvirus simiae*. *In* Lennette EH, Schmidt NJ (eds): Diagnostic Procedures for Viral, Rickettsial and Chlamydial Infections. Washington, DC, American Public Health Association, 1979, p 309.
276. Nahmias AJ, Keyserling H, Lee FK: Herpes simplex viruses 1 and 2. *In* Evans AS (ed): Viral Infections of Humans: Epidemiology and Control. New York, Plenum Publishing, 1989, pp 393–417.
277. Mertz GJ: Epidemiology of genital herpes infections. Infect Dis Clin North Am 7:825, 1993.
278. Ashley R: Laboratory techniques in the diagnosis of herpes simplex infection. Genitourin Med 69:174, 1993.
279. Ashley R: Current concepts in laboratory diagnosis of herpes simplex infection. *In* Sacks SL, Straus SE, Whitley RJ, Griffiths PD (eds): Clinical Management of Herpes Viruses. New York, IOS Press, 1995, pp 137–174.
280. Ashley R, Cent A, Maggs V, et al: Inability of enzyme immunoassays to discriminate between infections with herpes simplex virus types 1 and 2. Ann Intern Med 115:520, 1991.
281. Field PR, Ho DW, Irving WL, et al: The reliability of serological tests for the diagnosis of genital herpes: A critique. Pathology 25:175, 1993.
282. Arvin AM, Koropchak CM, Yeager AS, Pereira L: The detection of type specific antibody to herpes simplex virus type 1 by radioimmunoassay using HSV-1 glycoprotein C purified with monoclonal antibody. Infect Immun 40:184, 1983.
283. Lee FK, Coleman RM, Pereira L, et al: Detection of herpes simplex virus type-2 specific antibody with glycoprotein G. J Clin Microbiol 22:641, 1985.
284. Ashley RL, Militoni J, Lee F, et al: Comparison of Western blot (immunoblot) and glycoprotein G–specific immunodot enzyme assay for detecting antibodies to herpes simplex virus types 1 and 2 in human sera. J Clin Microbiol 26:662, 1988.
285. Bernstein DI, Bryson YJ, Lovette MA: Antibody response to type-common and type-unique epitopes of herpes simplex virus polypeptides. J Med Virol 15:251, 1985.

286. Bernstein DI, Garratty E, Lovett MA, et al: Comparison of Western blot analysis to microneutralization for the detection of type-specific herpes simplex virus antibodies. J Med Virol 15:223, 1985.
287. Ho DW, Field PR, Irving WL, et al: Detection of immunoglobulin M antibodies to glycoprotein G-2 by Western blot (immunoblot) for diagnosis of initial herpes simplex virus type 2 genital infections. J Clin Microbiol 31:3157, 1993.
288. Levi M, Ruden U, Wahren B: Peptide sequences of glycoprotein G-2 discriminate between herpes simplex virus type 2 (HSV-2) and HSV-1 antibodies. Clin Diagn Lab Immunol 3:265, 1996.
289. Safrin S, Arvin A, Mills J, Ashley R: Comparison of the Western immunoblot assay and a glycoprotein G enzyme immunoassay for detection of serum antibodies to herpes simplex virus type 2 in patients with AIDS. J Clin Microbiol 30:1312, 1992.
290. Sanchez-Martinez D, Schmid DS, Whittington W, et al: Evaluation of a test based on baculovirus-expressed glycoprotein G for detection of herpes simplex virus type-specific antibodies. J Infect Dis 164:1196, 1991.
291. Sullender WM, Yasukawa LL, Schwartz M, et al: Type-specific antibodies to herpes simplex virus type 2 (HSV-2) glycoprotein G in pregnant women, infants exposed to maternal HSV-2 infection at delivery, and infants with neonatal herpes. J Infect Dis 157:164, 1988.
292. Ashley RL, Militoni J, Lee F, et al: Comparison of Western blot (immunoblot) and glycoprotein G–specific immunodot enzyme assay for detecting antibodies to herpes simplex virus types 1 and 2 in human sera. J Clin Microbiol 26:662, 1988.
293. Johnson RE, Nahmias AJ, Magder LS, et al: A seroepidemiologic survey of the prevalence of herpes simplex virus type 2 infection in the United States. N Engl J Med 321:7, 1989.
294. Breinig MK, Kingsley LA, Armstrong JA, et al: Epidemiology of genital herpes in Pittsburgh: Serologic, sexual, and racial correlates of apparent and inapparent herpes simplex infections. J Infect Dis 162:299, 1990.
295. Gibson JJ, Hornung CA, Alexander GR, et al: A cross-sectional study of herpes simplex virus types 1 and 2 in college students: Occurrence and determinants of infection. J Infect Dis 162:306, 1990.
296. Nahmias AJ, Lee FK, Bechman-Nahmias S: Sero-epidemiological and -sociological patterns of herpes simplex virus infection in the world. Scand J Infect Dis 69:19, 1990.
297. Koutsky LA, Ashley RL, Holmes KK, et al: The frequency of unrecognized type 2 herpes simplex virus infection among women. Implications for the control of genital herpes. Sex Transm Dis 17:90, 1990.
298. Kulhanjian JA, Soroush V, Au DS, et al: Identification of women at unsuspected risk of primary infection with herpes simplex virus type 2 during pregnancy. N Engl J Med 326:916, 1992.
299. Siegel D, Golden E, Washington AE, et al: Prevalence and correlates of herpes simplex infections. The population-based AIDS in multiethnic neighborhoods study. JAMA 268:1702, 1992.
300. Boucher FD, Yasukawa LI, Bronzan RN, et al: A prospective evaluation of primary genital herpes simplex virus type 2 infections acquired during pregnancy. Pediatr Infect Dis J 9:499, 1990.
301. Christenson B, Bottiger M, Svensson A, Jeansson S: A 15-year surveillance study of antibodies to herpes simplex virus types 1 and 2 in a cohort of young girls. J Infect 25:147, 1992.
302. Cunningham AL, Lee FK, Ho DWT, et al: Herpes simplex virus type 2 antibody in patients attending antenatal or STD clinics. Med J Aust 158:525, 1993.
303. Brown ZA, Benedetti JK, Watts DH, et al: Diagnosis of genital herpes complicating pregnancy. Am J Obstet Gynecol 172:1299, 1995.
304. Garland SM, Lee TN, Ashley RL, et al: Automated microneutralization: Method and comparison with Western blot for type-specific detection of herpes simplex antibodies in two pregnant populations. J Virol Methods 55:285, 1995.
305. Oberle MW, Rosero-Bixby L, Lee FK, et al: Herpes simplex virus type 2 antibodies: High prevalence in monogamous women in Costa Rica. Am J Trop Med Hyg 41:224, 1989.
306. Oliver L, Wald A, Kim M, et al: Seroprevalence of herpes simplex virus infections in a family medicine clinic. Arch Fam Med 4:228, 1995.
307. Black FL, Hierholzer WJ, Pinheiro F, et al: Evidence for persistence of infectious agents in isolated human populations. Am J Epidemiol 100:230, 1974.
308. Black FL: Infectious diseases in primitive societies. Science 187:515, 1975.
309. Hammer SM, Buchman TG, D'Angelo LJ, et al: Temporal cluster of herpes simplex encephalitis: Investigation by restriction endonuclease cleavage of viral DNA. J Infect Dis 141:436, 1980.
310. Whitley RJ, Lakeman AD, Nahmias AJ, Roizman B: DNA restriction enzyme analysis of herpes simplex virus isolates obtained from patients with encephalitis. N Engl J Med 307:1060, 1982.
311. Nerurkar LS, West F, May M, et al: Survival of herpes simplex virus in water specimens collected from hot tubs in spa facilities and on plastic surfaces. JAMA 250:3081, 1983.
312. Douglas JM, Corey L: Fomites and herpes simplex viruses: A case for nonveneral transmission? JAMA 250:3093, 1983.
313. Guinan ME, Wolinsky SM, Reichman RC: Epidemiology of genital herpes simplex virus infection. Epidemiol Rev 7:127, 1985.
314. Rawls WE, Campione-Piccardo J: Epidemiology of herpes simplex virus type 1 and 2. *In* Nahmais A, Dowdle W, Schinazi R (eds): The Human Herpesviruses: An Interdisciplinary Perspective. Amsterdam, Elsevier North Holland, 1981, pp 137–152.
315. Whitley RJ, Gnann JW: The epidemiology and clinical manifestations of herpes simplex virus infections. *In* Roizman B, Whitley RJ, Lopez C (eds): The Human Herpesviruses. New York, Raven Press, 1993, p 69.
316. Cowan FM, Johnson AM, Ashley R, et al: Relationship between antibodies to herpes simplex virus (HSV) and symptoms of HSV infection. J Infect Dis 174:470, 1996.
317. Koutsky LA, Stevens CE, Holmes KK, et al: Underdiagnosis of genital herpes by current clinical and viral-isolation procedures. N Engl J Med 326:1533, 1992.
318. Mertz GJ, Coombs RW, Ashley R, et al: Transmission of genital herpes in couples with one symptomatic and one asymptomatic partner: A prospective study. J Infect Dis 157:1169, 1988.
319. Mertz GJ, Benedetti J, Ashley R, et al: Risk factors for the sexual transmission of genital herpes. Ann Intern Med 116:197, 1992.
320. Bryson YJ, Dillon M, Bernstein DI, et al: Risk of acquisition of genital herpes simplex virus type 2 in sex partners of persons with genital herpes: A prospective couple study. J Infect Dis 167:942, 1993.
321. Prober CG, Corey L, Brown ZA, et al: The management of pregnancies complicated by genital infections with herpes simplex virus. Clin Infect Dis 15:1031, 1992.
322. Prober CG: Herpes simplex infections in pregnancy: Preventing neonatal herpes infections. *In* Sacks SL, Straus SE, Whitley RJ, Griffiths PD (eds): Clinical Management of Herpes Viruses. New York, IOS Press, 1995, pp 87–100.
323. Whitley RJ, Arvin A: Herpes simplex virus infection. *In* Remington J, Klein J (eds): Infectious Diseases of the Fetus and Newborn Infant, ed 4. Philadelphia, WB Saunders, 1995, pp 354–376.
324. Brown ZA, Benedetti J, Ashley R, et al: Neonatal herpes simplex virus infection in relation to asymptomatic maternal infection at the time of labor. N Engl J Med 324:1247, 1991.
325. Scott TF, Steigman AJ, Convey JH: Acute infectious gingivostomatitis: Etiology, epidemiology, and clinical pictures of a common disorder caused by the virus of herpes simplex. JAMA 117:999, 1941.
326. Buddingh GJ, Schrum DI, Lanier JC, Guidy DJ: Studies of the natural history of herpes simplex infections. Pediatrics 11:595, 1953.
327. Scott TF: Epidemiology of herpetic infections. Am J Ophthalmol 43:134, 1957.
328. Juretic M: Natural history of herpetic infection. Helv Paediatr Acta 21:356, 1966.
329. Cesario TC, Poland JD, Wulff H, et al: Six years' experiences with herpes simplex virus in a children's home. Am J Epidemiol 90:416, 1969.
330. Glezen WP, Fernald GW, Lohr JA: Acute respiratory disease of university students with special reference to the etiologic role of herpesvirus hominis. Am J Epidemiol 101:111, 1975.
331. Spruance SL: Herpes simplex labialis. *In* Sacks SL, Straus SE, Whitley RJ, Griffiths PD (eds): Clinical Management of Herpes Viruses. New York, IOS Press, 1995, pp 3–42.
332. Stern H, Elek SD, Miller DM, Anderson HF: Herpetic whitlow, a form of cross-infection in hospitals. Lancet 2:871, 1959.
333. Douglas RG Jr, Couch RB: A prospective study of chronic herpes simplex virus infection and recurrent herpes labialis in humans. J Immunol 104:289, 1970.

334. Lindgren KM, Douglas RG Jr, Couch RB: Significance of herpesvirus hominis in respiratory secretions of man. N Engl J Med 276:517, 1968.
335. Hatherley LI, Hayes K, Jack I: Herpesvirus in an obstetric hospital. Asymptomatic virus excretion in staff members. Med J Aust 2:273, 1980.
336. Ng ABP, Reagin JW, Yen SS: Herpes genitalis—Clinical and cytopathologic experience with 256 patients. Obstet Gynecol 36:645, 1970.
337. Adam E, Kaufman RH, Mirkovic RR, Melnick JL: Persistence of virus shedding in asymptomatic women after recovery from herpes genitalis. Obstet Gynecol 54:171, 1979.
338. Rattray MC, Corey L, Reeves WC, et al: Recurrent genital herpes among women: Symptomatic versus asymptomatic viral shedding. Br J Vener Dis 54:252, 1978.
339. Ekwo E, Wong YW, Myers M: Asymptomatic cervicovaginal shedding of herpes simplex virus. Am J Obstet Gynecol 134:102, 1979.
340. Tejani N, Klein SW, Kaplan M: Subclinical herpes simplex genitalis infections in the perinatal period. Am J Obstet Gynecol 135:547, 1979.
341. Boehm FH, Estes W, Wright PE, Growdon JF Jr: Management of genital herpes simplex virus infection occuring during pregnancy. Am J Obstet Gynecol 141:735, 1980.
342. Adam E, Dreesman GE, Kaufman RH, Melnick JL: Asymptomatic virus shedding after herpes genitalis. Am J Obstet Gynecol 137:827, 1980.
343. Whitley RJ, Nahmias AJ, Visintine AM, et al: The natural history of herpes simplex virus infection of mother and newborn. Pediatrics 66:489, 1980.
344. Scher J, Bottone E, Desmond E, Simons W: The incidence and outcome of asymptomatic herpes simplex genitalis in an obstetric population. Am J Obstet Gynecol 144:906, 1982.
345. Vontver LA, Hickok DE, Brown Z, et al: Recurrent herpes simplex virus infection in pregnancy: Infant outcome and frequency of asymptomatic recurrences. Am J Obstet Gynecol 142:75, 1982.
346. Mayer AR, Duff P: Longitudinal screening for herpes simplex virus in obstetric patients. Mil Med 147:492, 1982.
347. Corey L, Adams HG, Brown ZA, Holmes KK: Genital herpes simplex virus infections: Clinical manifestations, course, and complications. Ann Intern Med 98:958, 1983.
348. Harger JH, Pazin GJ, Armstrong JA, et al: Characteristics and management of pregnancy in women with genital herpes simplex virus infection. Am J Obstet Gynecol 145:784, 1983.
349. Hankins GDV, Cunningham FG, Luby JP, et al: Asymptomatic genital excretion of herpes simplex virus during early labor. Am J Obstet Gynecol 150:100, 1984.
350. Wittek AE, Yeager AS, Au DS, Hensleigh PA: Asymptomatic shedding of herpes simplex virus from the cervix and lesion site during pregnancy. Am J Dis Child 138:439, 1984.
351. Arvin AM, Hensleigh PA, Prober CG, et al: Failure of antepartum maternal cultures to predict the infant's risk of exposure to herpes simplex virus at delivery. N Engl J Med 315:796, 1986.
352. Prober CG, Hensleigh PA, Boucher FD, et al: Use of routine viral cultures at delivery to identify neonates exposed to herpes simplex virus. N Engl J Med 318:887, 1988.
353. Simkovich JW, Soper DE: Asymptomatic shedding of herpesvirus during labor. Am J Obstet Gynecol 158:588, 1988.
354. Prober CG, Arvin AM: Genital herpes and the pregnant woman. Curr Clin Top Infect Dis 10:1, 1989.
355. Yeager AS, Arvin AM: Reasons for the absence of a history of recurrent genital herpes infections in mothers of neonates infected with herpes simplex virus. Pediatrics 73:188, 1984.
356. Mertz GJ, Schmidt O, Jourden JL, et al: Frequency of acquisition of first-episode genital infection with herpes simplex virus from symptomatic and asymptomatic source contacts. Sex Transm Dis 12:33, 1985.
357. Rooney JF, Felser JM, Ostrove JM, Straus SE: Acquisition of genital herpes from an asymptomatic sexual partner. N Engl J Med 314:1561, 1986.
358. McClung H, Seth P, Rawls WE: Relative concentrations in human sera of antibodies to cross-reacting and specific antigens of herpes simplex virus types 1 and 2. Am J Epidemiol 104:192, 1976.
359. Evans AS, Dick EC: Acute pharyngitis and tonsillitis in University of Wisconsin students. JAMA 190:699, 1964.
360. McMillan JA, Weiner LB, Higgins AM, Lamparella VJ: Pharyngitis associated with herpes simplex virus in college students. Pediatr Infect Dis 12:280, 1993.
361. Andrewes CH, Carmichael EA: A note on the presence of antibodies to herpes virus in postencephalitic and other human sera. Lancet 1:857, 1930.
362. Smith IW, Peutherer JF, MacCallum FO: The incidence of *Herpesvirus hominis* antibody in the population. J Hyg (Camb) 65:395, 1967.
363. Wentworth BB, Alexander ER: Seroepidemiology of infections due to members of the herpesvirus group. Am J Epidemiol 94:496, 1971.
364. Hatherley LI, Hayes K, Jack I: Herpesvirus in an obstetric hospital. Prevalence of antibodies in patients and staff. Med J Aust 2:325, 1980.
365. Ship II, Morris AL, Durocher RT, Burket LW: Recurrent aphthous ulcerations and recurrent herpes labialis in a professional school student population. I. Experience. Oral Surg Oral Med Oral Pathol 13:1191, 1960.
366. Ship II, Morris AL, Durocher RT, Burket LW: Recurrent aphthous ulcerations in a professional school student population. IV. Twelve-month study of natural disease patterns. Oral Surg Oral Med Oral Pathol 14:30, 1961.
367. Ship II, Brightman VJ, Laster LL: The patient with recurrent aphthous ulcers and the patient with recurrent herpes labialis: A study of two population samples. J Am Dent Assoc 75:645, 1967.
368. Embil JA, Stephens RG, Manuel FR: Prevalence of recurrent herpes labialis and aphthous ulcers among young adults on six continents. Can Med Assoc J 113:627, 1975.
369. Young SK, Rowe NH, Buchanan RA: A clinical study for the control of facial mucocutaneous herpes virus infections. I. Characterization of natural history in a professional school population. Oral Surg Oral Med Oral Pathol 41:498, 1976.
370. Friedman E, Katcher AH, Brightman VJ: Incidence of recurrent herpes labialis and upper respiratory infection: A prospective study of the influence of biologic, social, and psychologic predictors. Oral Surg Oral Med Oral Pathol 43:873, 1977.
371. Ship II, Miller MF, Ram C: A retrospective study of recurrent herpes labialis (RHL) in a professional population, 1958–1971. Oral Surg Oral Med Oral Pathol 44:723, 1977.
372. Grout P, Barber VE: Cold sores—An epidemiological survey. J R Coll Gen Pract 26:428, 1976.
373. Overall JC Jr: Dermatologic viral diseases. *In* Gallasso GJ, Mirigan TC, Buchanen RA (eds): Antiviral Agents and Viral Diseases of Man, ed 2. New York, Raven Press, 1984, pp 247–312.
374. Greenberg MS, Brightman VJ, Ship II: Clinical and laboratory differentiation of recurrent intraoral herpes simplex virus infections following fever. J Dent Res 48:385, 1969.
375. Corey L: Genital herpes. *In* Holmes KK (ed): Sexually Transmitted Diseases, ed 2. New York, McGraw-Hill, 1990, pp 391–413.
376. Duenas A, Adam E, Melnick JL, Rawls WE: Herpesvirus type-2 in a prostitute population. Am J Epidemiol 95:483, 1972.
377. Chuang T-Y, Su WP, Perry HO, et al: Incidence and trend of herpes progenitalis. A 15-year population study. Mayo Clin Proc 58:436, 1983.
378. Becker TM, Blount JH, Guinan ME: Trends in genital herpes infections in private practice in the United States, 1966–1981. JAMA 253:1601, 1985.
379. Genital herpes infections—United States, 1966–1984. MMWR Morbid Mortal Wkly Rep 35:402, 1986.
380. Catterall RD: Biological effects of sexual freedom. Lancet 1:315, 1981.
381. Corey L: The current trend in genital herpes. Progress in prevention. Sex Transm Dis 21(Suppl 2):S38, 1994.
382. Catalano PM, Meritt AO, Mead PB: Incidence of genital herpes simplex virus at the time of delivery in women with known risk factors. Am J Obstet Gynecol 164:1303, 1991.
383. Corey L, Wald A: New developments in the biology of genital herpes. *In* Sacks SL, Straus SE, Whitley RJ, Griffiths PD (eds): Clinical Management of Herpes Viruses. New York, IOS Press, 1995, pp 43–54.
384. Sumaya CV, Marx J, Ullis K: Genital infections with herpes simplex virus in a university student population. Sex Transm Dis 7:16, 1980.
385. Kalinyak JE, Fleagle G, Docherty JJ: Incidence and distribution of herpes simplex virus types 1 and 2 from genital lesions in college women. J Med Virol 1:173, 1977.

386. Premarital sexual experience among adolescent women—United States, 1970–1988. MMWR Morbid Mortal Wkly Rep 39:929, 1991.
387. Wald A, Zeh J, Barnum G, et al: Suppression of subclinical shedding of herpes simplex virus type 2 with acyclovir. Ann Intern Med 124:8, 1996.
388. Cone RW, Hobson AC, Brown Z, et al: Frequent detection of genital herpes simplex virus DNA by polymerase chain reaction among pregnant women. JAMA 272:792, 1994.
389. Wald A, Corey L, Cone R, et al: Frequent genital herpes simplex virus 2 shedding in immunocompetent women: Effect of acyclovir treatment. J Clin Invest (in press).
390. Ross JD, Smith IW, Elton RA: The epidemiology of herpes simplex types 1 and 2 infection of the genital tract in Edinburgh 1978–1991. Genitourin Med 69:381, 1993.
391. Scoular A, Leask BGS, Carrington D: Changing trends in genital herpes due to herpes simplex virus type 1 in Glasgow. Genitourin Med 66:226, 1990.
392. Stanberry LR: Genital and neonatal herpes simplex virus infections: Epidemiology, pathogenesis and prospects for control. Rev Med Virol 3:37, 1993.
393. Rosato FE, Rosato EF, Plotkin SA: Herpetic paronychia: An occupational hazard of medical personnel. N Engl J Med 283:804, 1970.
394. Gill MJ, Arlette J, Buchan K: Herpes simplex virus infection of the hand. Am J Med 84:89, 1988.
395. Selling B, Kibrick S: An outbreak of herpes simplex among wrestlers (herpes gladiatorium). N Engl J Med 270:979, 1964.
396. Herpes gladiatorum at a high school wrestling camp—Minnesota. MMWR Morbid Mortal Wkly Rep 39:69, 1990.
397. Cockerell C: Diagnosis and treatment of cutaneous herpes simplex virus infections. West J Med 164:518, 1996.
398. Linnemann CC Jr, Buchman TG, Light IJ, et al: Transmission of herpes simplex virus type-1 in a nursery for the newborn: Identification of viral species isolated by DNA fingerprinting. Lancet 1:964, 1978.
399. Light IJ: Postnatal acquisition of herpes simplex virus by the newborn infant: A review of the literature. Pediatrics 63:480, 1979.
400. Manzella JP, McConville JH, Valente E, et al: An outbreak of herpes simplex virus type 1 gingivostomatitis in a dental hygiene practice. JAMA 252:2019, 1984.
401. Francis DP, Herrmann KL, MacMahon JR, et al: Nosocomial and maternally acquired herpesvirus hominis infections: A report of four fatal cases in neonates. Am J Dis Child 129:889, 1975.
402. Perl TM, Haugen TH, Pfaller MA, et al: Transmission of herpes simplex virus type 1 infection in an intensive care unit. Ann Intern Med 117:584, 1992.
403. Hale BD, Rendtorff RC, Walker LC, Roberts AN: Epidemic herpetic stomatitis in an orphanage nursery. JAMA 183:1068, 1963.
404. Schmitt DL, Johnson DW, Henderson FW: Herpes simplex type 1 infections in group day care. Pediatr Infect Dis J 10:729, 1991.
405. Siegal FP, Lopez C, Hammer GS, et al: Severe acquired immunodeficiency in male homosexuals, manifested by chronic perianal ulcerative herpes simplex lesions. N Engl J Med 305:1039, 1981.
406. Goodell SE, Quinn RC, Mkrtichian E, et al: Herpes simplex virus proctitis in homosexual men. Clinical, sigmoidoscopic, and histopathological features. N Engl J Med 308:868, 1983.
407. Kipping R, Downie A: Generalized infection with herpes simplex. Br Med J 10:247, 1948.
408. Ruchman J, Dodd K: Recovery of herpes simplex virus from the blood of a patient with herpetic rhinitis. J Lab Clin Med 35:434, 1950.
409. Becker WB, Kipps A, McKenzie D: Disseminated herpes simplex virus infection: Its pathogenesis based on virological and pathological studies in 33 cases. Am J Dis Child 115:1, 1968.
410. Craig CP, Nahmias AJ: Different patterns of neurologic involvement with herpes simplex virus types 1 and 2: Isolation of herpes simplex virus type 2 from the buffy coat of two adults with meningitis. J Infect Dis 127:365, 1973.
411. Stanberry LR, Floyd-Reising SA, Connelly BL, et al: Herpes simplex viremia: Report of eight pediatric cases and review of the literature. Clin Infect Dis 18:401, 1994.
412. Baringer JR: Recovery of herpes simplex virus from human sacral ganglions. N Engl J Med 291:828, 1974.
413. Warren KG, Brown SM, Wrobelwska Z, et al: Isolation of latent herpes simplex virus from the superior cervical and vagus ganglions of human beings. N Engl J Med 298:1068, 1978.
414. Takasu T, Furuta Y, Sato KC, et al: Detection of latent herpes simplex virus DNA and RNA in human geniculate ganglia by the polymerase chain reaction. Acta Otolaryngol (Stockh) 112:1004, 1992.
415. Furuta Y, Takasu T, Sato KC, et al: Latent herpes simplex virus type 1 in human geniculate ganglia. Acta Neuropathol (Berl) 84:39, 1992.
416. Carton CA, Kilbourne ED: Activation of latent herpes by trigeminal sensory-root section. N Engl J Med 246:172, 1952.
417. Segal AL, Katcher AH, Brightman VG, Miller MF: Recurrent herpes labialis, recurrent aphthous ulcers and the menstrual cycles. J Dent Res 53:797, 1974.
418. Kriesel JD, Pisani PL, McKeough MB: Correlation between detection of herpes simplex virus in oral secretions by PCR and susceptibility to experimental UV radiation–induced herpes labialis. J Infect Dis 170:1046, 1994.
419. Spruance SL, Freeman DJ, Stewart JCB, et al: The natural history of ultraviolet radiation–induced herpes simplex labialis and response to therapy with peroral and topical formulations of acyclovir. J Infect Dis 163:728, 1991.
420. Wenner HA: Complications of infantile eczema caused by the virus of herpes simplex: Description of the clinical characteristics of an unusual eruption and identification of an associated filterable virus. Am J Dis Child 67:247, 1944.
421. Ruchman I, Welsh AL, Dodd K: Kaposi's varicelliform eruption: Isolation of the virus of herpes simplex from cutaneous lesions of three adults and one infant. Arch Dermatol Syphilol 56:846, 1947.
422. Wheeler CE Jr, Abele DC: Eczema herpeticum, primary and recurrent. Arch Dermatol 93:162, 1966.
423. Foley FD, Greenwald KA, Nash G, Pruitt BA: Herpesvirus infection in burned patients. N Engl J Med 282:652, 1970.
424. Goodyear HM, McLeish P, Randall S, et al: Immunological studies of herpes simplex virus infection in children with atopic eczema. Br J Dermatol 134:85, 1996.
425. Hayden FG, Himel HN, Heggers JP: Herpesvirus infections in burn patients. Chest 106:15S, 1994.
426. Hirsch MS, Zisman B, Allison AC: Macrophages and age-dependent resistance to herpes simplex virus in mice. J Immunol 104:1160, 1970.
427. Sit MF, Tenney DJ, Rothstein JL, et al: Effect of macrophage activation on resistance of mouse peritoneal macrophages to infection with herpes simplex virus types 1 and 2. J Gen Virol 69:1999, 1988.
428. Lopez C: Resistance to herpes simplex virus–type 1 (HSV-1). Curr Top Microbiol Immunol 92:15, 1981.
429. Wilson CB: Developmental immunology and role of host defenses in neonatal susceptibility. *In* Remington JS, Klein JO (eds): Infectious Diseases of the Fetus and Newborn Infant, ed 3. Philadelphia, WB Saunders, 1990, pp 17–67.
430. Kirchner H: Immunobiology of infection with herpes simplex virus. Monogr Virol 13:1, 1982.
431. Fitzgerald-Bocarsly T, Howell DM, Pettera L, et al: Immediate early gene expression is sufficient for induction of natural killer cell indicated lysis of herpes simplex virus type 1 infection fibroblasts. J Virol 65:2666, 1991.
432. Hirsch MS: Herpes group virus infections in the compromised host. *In* Rubin RH, Young LS (eds): Clinical Approach to Infection in the Immunocompromised Host, ed 2. New York, Plenum Publishing, 1988, p 347.
433. Kohl S: Herpes simplex virus immunology: Problems, progress and promises. J Infect Dis 152:435, 1985.
434. Kohl S, Adam E, Matson DO, et al: Kinetics of human antibody responses to primary genital herpes simplex virus infection. Intervirology 18:164, 1982.
435. Oh SH, Douglas JM, Corey L, Kohl S: Kinetics of humoral immune response measured by antibody-dependent cell-mediated cytotoxicity and neutralization assays in genital herpes virus infections. J Infect Dis 159:328, 1989.
436. Blacklaws BA, Nash AA: Immunologic memory to herpes simplex virus type 1 glycoproteins B and D in mice. J Gen Virol 7:863, 1990.
437. Balachandran N, Bacchetti S, Rawls WE: Protection against lethal challenge of BALB/c mice by passive transfer of mono-

clonal antibodies to five glycoproteins of herpes simplex virus type 2. Infect Immun 37:1132, 1982.
438. Kohl S, Strynadka NCJ, Hodges RS, Periera LA: Analysis of the role of antibody-dependent cellular cytotoxic antibody activity in murine neonatal herpes simplex virus with antibodies to synthetic peptides of glycoprotein D and monoclonal antibodies to glycoprotein B. J Clin Invest 86:273, 1990.
439. Mester JC, Glorioso JC, Rouse BT: Protection against zosteriform spread of herpes simplex virus by monoclonal antibodies. J Infect Dis 263:263, 1991.
440. Kohl S: Role of antibody-dependent cellular cytotoxicity in defense against herpes simplex virus infections. Rev Infect Dis 13:108, 1991.
441. Kurtz JB: Specific IgG and IgM antibody responses in herpes simplex virus infections. J Med Microbiol 7:333, 1974.
442. Nash AA, Leung KN, Wildy P: The T-cell–mediated immune response of mice to herpes simplex virus. *In* Roizman B, Lopez C (eds): The Herpesviruses, Vol 4. New York, Plenum Publishing, 1985, pp 87–102.
443. Schmid DS, Rouse BT: The role of T-cell immunity in control of herpes simplex virus. Curr Top Microbiol Immunol 179:961, 1992.
444. Glorioso JC, Kees U, Kumel G, et al: Identification of herpes simplex virus type 1 (HSV-1) glycoprotein gC as the immunodominant antigen for HSV-1 specific memory cytotoxic T lymphocytes. J Immunol 135:575, 1985.
445. Martin S, Cantin E, Rouse BT: Evaluation of antiviral immunity using vaccinia virus recombinants expressing cloned genes for herpes simplex virus type 1 glycoproteins. J Gen Virol 70:1359, 1989.
446. Tigges MA, Koelle D, Hartog K, et al: Human CD8$^+$ herpes simplex virus–specific cytotoxic T-lymphocyte clones recognize diverse virion protein antigens. J Virol 66:1622, 1992.
447. Mikloska Z, Kesson AM, Penfold MET, et al: Herpes simplex virus protein targets for CD4 and CD8 lymphocyte cytotoxicity in cultured epidermal keratinocytes treated with interferon-γ. J Infect Dis 173:7, 1996.
448. Spruance SL, Evans TG, McKeough MB, et al: Th1/Th2-like immunity and resistance to herpes simplex labialis. Antiviral Res 28:39, 1995.
449. Carmack MA, Yasukawa LL, Chang SY, et al: T-cell recognition and cytokine production elicited by common and type-specific glycoproteins of herpes simplex virus type 1 and type 2. J Infect Dis 174:899, 1996.
450. Witmer LA, Rosenthal KL, Graham FL, et al: Cytotoxic T lymphocytes specific for herpes simplex virus (HSV) studied using adenovirus vectors expressing HSV glycoproteins. J Gen Virol 71:387, 1990.
451. Martin S, Zhu X, Silverstein SJ, et al: Murine cytotoxic T lymphocytes specific for herpes simplex virus type 1 recognize the immediate early protein ICP4 but not ICP0. J Gen Virol 71:2391, 1990.
452. Banks TA, Aleen EM, Dasgupta S, et al: Herpes simplex virus type 1 specific cytotoxic T lymphocytes recognize immediate-early protein ICP27. J Virol 65:3185, 1991.
453. Kohl S, West MS, Prober CG, et al: Neonatal antibody-dependent cellular cytotoxicity antibody levels are associated with the clinical presentation of neonatal herpes simplex virus infection. J Infect Dis 160:770, 1989.
454. Kohl S: Protection against murine neonatal herpes simplex infections by lymphokine-treated human leukocytes. J Immunol 144:307, 1990.
455. Prober CG, Sullender WM, Yasukawa LL, et al: Low risk of herpes simplex virus infections in neonates exposed to the virus at the time of vaginal delivery to mothers with recurrent genital herpes simplex virus infections. N Engl J Med 316:240, 1987.
456. Ashley RL, Dalessio J, Burchett S, et al: Herpes simplex virus-2 (HSV-2) type-specific antibody correlates of protection in infants exposed to HSV-2 at birth. J Clin Invest 90:511, 1992.
457. Burchett SK, Corey L, Mohan KM, et al: Diminished interferon-γ and lymphocyte proliferation in neonatal and postpartum primary herpes simplex virus infection. J Infect Dis 165:813, 1992.
458. Cunningham AL, Turner RR, Miller AC, et al: Evolution of recurrent herpes simplex lesions: An immunohistologic study. J Clin Invest 75:226, 1985.
459. Koelle DM, Abbo H, Peck A, et al: Direct recovery of herpes simplex virus (HSV)–specific T lymphocyte clones from recurrent genital HSV-2 lesions. J Infect Dis 169:956, 1994.
460. Koelle DM, Corey L, Burke RL, et al: Antigenic specificities of human CD4$^+$ T-cell clones recovered from recurrent genital herpes simplex virus type 2 lesions. J Virol 68:2803, 1994.
461. Torseth JW, Merigan TC: Significance of local γ-interferon in recurrent herpes simplex infection. J Infect Dis 153:979, 1986.
462. Früh K, Ahn K, Djaballah H, et al: A viral inhibitor of peptide transporters for antigen presentation. Nature 375:415, 1995.
463. Hill A, Jugovic P, York I, et al: Herpes simplex virus turns off the TAP to evade host immunity. Nature 375:411, 1995.
464. Banks TA, Rouse BT: Herpesvirus—Immune escape artists? Clin Infect Dis 14:933, 1992.
465. Fries LF, Friedman HM, Cohen GH, et al: Glycoprotein C of herpes simplex virus type 1 is an inhibitor of the complement cascade. J Immunol 137:1636, 1986.
466. McNearney TA, Odell C, Holers VM, et al: Herpes simplex virus glycoproteins gC-1 and gC-2 bind to the third component of complement and provide protection against complement-mediated neutralization of viral infectivity. J Exp Med 166:1525, 1987.
467. Harris SL, Frank I, Yee A, et al: Glycoprotein C of herpes simplex virus type 1 prevents complement-mediated cell lysis and virus neutralization. J Infect Dis 162:331, 1990.
468. Friedman HM, Wang L, Fishman NO, et al: Immune evasion properties of herpes simplex virus type 1 glycoprotein gC. J Virol 70:4253, 1996.
469. Dowler KW, Veltri RW: In vitro neutralization of HSV-2: Inhibition by binding of normal IgG and purified Fc to virion Fc receptors (FcR). J Med Virol 13:251, 1984.
470. Dubin G, Frank I, Friedman HM: Herpes simplex virus type 1 encodes two Fc receptors which have different binding characteristics for monomeric immunoglobulin G (IgG) and IgG complexes. J Virol 64:2725, 1990.
471. Adler R, Glorioso JC, Cossman J, Levin M: Possible role of Fc receptors on cells infected and transformed by herpesvirus: Escape from immune cytolysis. Infect Immun 21:442, 1978.
472. Frank I, Friedman HM: A novel function of the herpes simplex virus type 1 Fc receptor: Participation in bipolar bridging of antiviral immunoglobulin G. J Virol 63:4479, 1989.
473. Lazar MP: Vaccination for recurrent herpes simplex infection: Initiation of a new disease site following use of unmodified material containing the live virus. Arch Dermatol 73:70, 1956.
474. Schmidt OW, Fife KH, Corey L: Reinfection is an uncommon occurrence in patients with symptomatic recurrent genital herpes. J Infect Dis 149:645, 1984.
475. Kloene W, Bang FB, Chakroborty SM, et al: A two-year respiratory virus survey in four villages in West Bengal, India. Am J Epidemiol 92:307, 1970.
476. Connelly BL, Stanberry LR: Herpes simplex virus infections in children. Curr Opin Pediatr 7:19, 1995.
477. Rogers AM, Coriell LL, Blank H, Scott TFM: Acute herpetic gingivostomatitis in adults. N Engl J Med 241:330, 1949.
478. Farmer ED: Diseases of the mouth caused by herpes simplex virus. Proc R Soc Med 49:640, 1956.
479. Sheridan PJ, Herrmann EC: Intraoral lesions of adults associated with herpes simplex virus. Oral Surg Oral Pathol 32:390, 1971.
480. Spruance SL, Overall JC Jr, Kern ER, et al: The natural history of recurrent herpes simplex labialis. Implications for antiviral therapy. N Engl J Med 297:69, 1977.
481. Bader C, Crumpacker CS, Schnipper LE, et al: The natural history of recurrent facial-oral infection with herpes simplex virus. J Infect Dis 138:897, 1978.
482. Spruance SL, Stewart JCB, Rowe NH, et al: Treatment of recurrent herpes simplex labialis with oral acyclovir. J Infect Dis 161:185, 1990.
483. Blank H, Burgoon CF, Coriell LL, Scott TFM: Recurrent aphthous ulcers. JAMA 142:125, 1950.
484. Weather DR, Griffin JW: Intraoral ulcerations of recurrent herpes simplex and recurrent aphthae: Two distinct clinical entities. J Am Dent Assoc 81:81, 1970.
485. Binder PA: Herpes simplex keratitis. Surv Ophthalmol 21:313, 1977.
486. Darougar S, Wishart MS, Viswalingam ND: Epidemiological and clinical features of primary herpes simplex virus ocular infection. Br J Ophthalmol 69:2, 1985.

487. Poirier RH: Herpetic ocular infections of childhood. Arch Ophthalmol 98:704, 1980.
488. Kaufman HE: Viral keratoconjunctivitis. *In* Braude AI (ed): Infectious Diseases and Medical Microbiology, ed 2. Philadelphia, WB Saunders, 1986, pp 1453–1457.
489. Wilhelmus KR, Coster DJ, Donovan HC, et al: Prognostic indicators of herpetic keratitis. Analysis of a five-year observation period after corneal ulceration. Arch Ophthalmol 99:1578, 1981.
490. Shuster JJ, Kaufman HE, Nesburn AB: Statistical analysis of the rate of recurrence of herpes virus ocular epithelial disease. Am J Ophthalmol 91:328, 1981.
491. Nahmias AJ, Visintine AM, Caldwell DR, et al: Eye infections with herpes simplex viruses in neonates. Surv Ophthalmol 21:100, 1976.
492. Uninsky E, Jampol LM, Kaufman S, et al: Disseminated herpes simplex with retinitis in a renal allograft recipient. Ophthalmology 90:175, 1983.
493. Bloom JN, Katz JI, Kaufman HE: Herpes simplex retinitis and encephalitis in an adult. Arch Ophthalmol 95:1798, 1964.
494. Minckler DS, McLean ED, Shaw CH, Hendrickson A: *Herpesvirus hominis* encephalitis and retinitis. Arch Ophthalmol 94:89, 1976.
495. Johnson BL, Wisotzkey HM: Neuroretinitis associated with herpes simplex encephalitis in an adult. Am J Ophthalmol 83:481, 1977.
496. Dawson C: Management of herpes simplex eye diseases. *In* Sacks SL, Straus SE, Whitley RJ, Griffiths PD (eds): Clinical Management of Herpes Viruses. New York, IOS Press, 1995, pp 127–136.
497. Cunningham ET Jr, Short GA, Irvine AR, et al: Acquired immunodeficiency syndrome–associated herpes simplex virus retinitis. Clinical description and use of a polymerase chain reaction–based assay as a diagnostic tool. Arch Ophthalmol 114:834, 1996.
498. Stanberry LR, Kern ER, Richard JT, et al: Genital herpes in guinea pigs: Pathogenesis of the primary infection and description of recurrent disease. J Infect Dis 146:397, 1982.
499. Blyth WA, Harbour DA, Hill JT: Pathogenesis of zosteriform spread of herpes simplex virus in the mouse. J Gen Virol 65:1477, 1984.
500. Kalman CM, Laskin OL: Herpes zoster and zosteriform herpes simplex virus infections in immunocompetent adults. Am J Med 81:775, 1986.
501. Benedetti JK, Zeh J, Selke S, Corey L: Frequency and reactivation of nongenital lesions among patients with genital herpes simplex virus. Am J Med 98:237, 1995.
502. Nicolau S, Poincloux P: Etude clinique et experimentale d'un cas d'herpès récividant du doigt. Ann Inst Pasteur 38:977, 1924.
503. Slavin HB, Ferguson JJ: Zosterlike eruptions caused by the virus herpes simplex. Am J Med 8:456, 1950.
504. Behrman S, Knight G: Herpes simplex associated with trigeminal neuralgia. Neurology 4:525, 1954.
505. Layzer RB, Conant MA: Neuralgia in recurrent herpes simplex. Arch Neurol 31:233, 1974.
506. Shute P, Jeffries DJ, Maddocks AC: Scrumpox caused by herpes simplex virus. Br Med J 2:1629, 1979.
507. White WB, Grant-Kels JM: Transmission of herpes simplex virus type 1 infection in rugby players. JAMA 252:533, 1984.
508. Pugh RCB, Dudgeon JA, Bodia M: Kaposi's varicelliform eruption (eczema herpeticum) with typical visceral necrosis. J Pathol Bacteriol 69:67, 1955.
509. Terezhalmy GT, Tyler MT, Ross GR: Eczema herpeticum: Atopic dermatitis complicated by primary herpetic gingivostomatitis. Oral Surg Oral Med Oral Pathol 48:513, 1979.
510. Hazen PG, Eppes RB: Eczema herpeticum caused by herpes virus type 2, a case in a patient with Darier's disease. Arch Dermatol 113:1085, 1977.
511. Orenstein JM, Castadot MJ, Wilens ST: Fatal herpes hepatitis associated with pemphigus vulgaris and steroids in an adult. Hum Pathol 5:489, 1974.
512. Greaves WL, Kaiser AB, Alford RH, Schaffner W: The problem of herpetic whitlow among hospital personnel. Infect Control 1:381, 1980.
513. Fedler HM, Long SS: Herpetic whitlow: Epidemiology, clinical characteristics, diagnosis and treatment. Am J Dis Child 137:861, 1983.
514. Gill MJ, Arlette J, Buchan K: Herpes simplex virus infection of the hand. Am J Med 84:89, 1988.
515. Glogau R, Hanna L, Jawetz E: Herpetic whitlow as part of genital virus infection. J Infect Dis 136:689, 1977.
516. Drachman DA, Adams RD: Herpes simplex and inclusion-body encephalitis. Arch Neurol 7:61, 1962.
517. Whitley RJ, Soong SJ, Dolin R, et al: The NIAID Collaborative Antiviral Study Group. Adenine arabinoside therapy of biopsy-proven herpes simplex encephalitis. N Engl J Med 297:289, 1977.
518. Whitley RJ, Soong SJ, Hirsch MS, et al: The NIAID Collaborative Antiviral Study Group. Herpes simplex encephalitis: Vidarabine therapy and diagnostic problems. N Engl J Med 304:313, 1981.
519. Whitley RJ, Soong SJ, Linneman C, et al: The NIAID Collaborative Antiviral Study Group. Herpes simplex encephalitis. Clinical assessment. JAMA 247:317, 1982.
520. Nahmias AJ, Whitley RJ, Visintine AN, et al: Herpes simplex virus encephalitis: Laboratory evaluations and their diagnostic significance. J Infect Dis 145:829, 1982.
521. Whitley RJ, Lakeman F: Herpes simplex virus infections of the central nervous system: Therapeutic and diagnostic considerations. Clin Infect Dis 20:414, 1995.
522. Barnett EM, Jacobsen G, Evans G, et al: Herpes simplex encephalitis in the temporal cortex and limbic system after trigeminal nerve inoculation. J Infect Dis 169:782, 1994.
523. Lakeman FD, Whitley RJ: Diagnosis of herpes simplex encephalitis: Application of polymerase chain reaction to cerebrospinal fluid from brain-biopsied patients and correlation with disease. J Infect Dis 171:857, 1995.
524. Marton R, Gotlieb-Steimatsky T, Klein C, Arlazoroff A: Acute herpes simplex encephalitis: Clinical assessment and prognostic data. Acta Neurol Scand 93:149, 1996.
525. Aurelius E, Johansson B, Sköldenberg B, et al: Rapid diagnosis of herpes simplex encephalitis by nested polymerase chain reaction assay of cerebrospinal fluid. Lancet 337:189, 1991.
526. Sköldenberg B: Herpes simplex encephalitis. Scand J Infect 78:40, 1991.
527. Rose JW, Stroop WG, Matsuo F, Henkel J: Atypical herpes simplex encephalitis: Clinical, virologic, and neuropathologic evaluation. Neurology 42:1809, 1992.
528. Whitley R, Arvin A, Prober C, et al: Predictors of morbidity and mortality in neonates with herpes simplex virus infections. N Engl J Med 324:450, 1991.
529. Burke JW, Mathews VP, Elster AD, et al: Contrast-enhanced magnetization transfer saturation imaging improves MR detection of herpes simplex encephalitis. Am J Neuroradiol 17:773, 1996.
530. Demaerel PH, Wilms G, Robberecht W, et al: MRI of herpes simplex encephalitis. Neuroradiology 34:490, 1992.
531. Terni M, Caccialanza P, Cassai E, Kieff E: Aseptic meningitis in association with herpes progenitalis. N Engl J Med 285:503, 1971.
532. Craig CP, Nahmias AJ: Different patterns of neurologic involvement with herpes simplex virus type 1 and 2: Isolation of herpes simplex virus 2 from the buffy coat of two adults with meningitis. J Infect Dis 127:365, 1973.
533. Stalder H, Oxman MN, Dawson DM, Levin MJ: Herpes simplex meningitis: Isolation of herpes simplex virus type 2 from cerebrospinal fluid. N Engl J Med 289:1296, 1973.
534. Sköldenberg B, Jeansson S, Wolontis S: Herpes simplex virus type 2 and acute aseptic meningitis: Atypical features of cases with isolation of herpes simplex virus from cerebrospinal fluids. Scand J Infect Dis 7:227, 1975.
535. Bergström T, Vahlne A, Alestig K, et al: Primary and recurrent herpes simplex virus type 2–induced meningitis. J Infect Dis 162:322, 1990.
536. Sawanobori S, Onishi S, Matsuyama S, Irie H: HSV-1 and acute aseptic meningitis. Lancet 1:756, 1974.
537. Harford CG, Wellinghoff W, Weinstein RA: Isolation of herpes simplex virus from the cerebrospinal fluid in viral meningitis. Neurology 25:198, 1975.
538. Tedder DG, Ashley R, Tyler KL, Levin MJ: Herpes simplex virus infection as a cause of benign recurrent lymphocytic meningitis. Ann Intern Med 121:334, 1994.
539. Yamato LJ, Tedder DG, Ashley R, Levin MJ: Herpes simplex virus type 1 DNA in cerebrospinal fluid of a patient with Mollaret's meningitis. N Engl J Med 325:1082, 1991.
540. Caplan LR, Kleeman FJ, Berg S: Urinary retention probably secondary to herpes genitalis. N Engl J Med 297:918, 1977.

541. Oates JK, Greenhouse PRDH: Retention of urine in anogenital herpetic infection. Lancet 1:691, 1979.
542. Chang T-W: Transient neurogenic bladder in genital herpes. J Infect 1:375, 1979.
543. Hunt BP, Comer EO'B: Herpetic meningoencephalitis accompanying cutaneous herpes simplex. Am J Med 19:814, 1955.
544. Klastersky J, Cappel R, Snoeck JM, et al: Ascending myelitis in association with herpes-simplex virus. N Engl J Med 287:182, 1972.
545. Hinthorn DR, Baker LH, Romig DA, Liu C: Recurrent conjugal neuralgia caused by herpesvirus hominis type 2. JAMA 236: 587, 1976.
546. Gerber SI, Cromie WJ: Herpes simplex virus type 2 infection associated with urinary retention in the absence of genital lesions. J Pediatr 128:250, 1996.
547. Young EJ, Chafizadeh E, Oliveira VL, Genta RM: Disseminated herpesvirus infection during pregnancy. Clin Infect Dis 22:51, 1996.
548. Auch Moedy JL, Lerman SJ, White RJ: Fatal disseminated herpes simplex virus infection in a healthy child. Am J Dis Child 135:45, 1981.
549. Connor RW, Lorts G, Gilbert DN: Lethal herpes simplex virus type 1 hepatitis in a normal adult. Gastroenterology 76:590, 1979.
550. Flewett TH, Parker RGF, Philip WM: Acute hepatitis due to herpes simplex virus in an adult. J Clin Pathol 22:60, 1969.
551. Schneider V, Behm FG, Mumaw VR: Ascending herpetic endometritis. Obstet Gynecol 59:259, 1982.
552. Buss DH, Scharyj M: Herpesvirus infection of the esophagus and other visceral organs in adults. Incidence and clinical significance. Am J Med 66:457, 1979.
553. Eron L, Kosinski K, Hirsch MS: Hepatitis in an adult caused by herpes simplex virus type 1. Gastroenterology 71:500, 1976.
554. Joseph TJ, Vogt PJ: Disseminated herpes with hepatoadrenal necrosis in an adult. Am J Med 56:735, 1974.
555. Whorton CM, Thomas DM, Denham SW: Fatal systemic herpes simplex virus type 2 infection in a healthy young woman. South Med J 76:81, 1983.
556. Long JC, Wheeler CE, Briggaman RA: Varicella-like infection due to herpes simplex. Arch Dermatol 114:406, 1978.
557. Francis TJ, Osuntokum BO, Kemp GE: Fulminant hepatitis due to herpes hominis in an adult human. Am J Gastroenterol 57:329, 1972.
558. Goyette RE, Donowho EM, Hieger LR, Plunkett G: Fulminant herpesvirus hominis hepatitis during pregnancy. Obstet Gynecol 43:191, 1974.
559. Young EJ, Killam AP, Greene JF: Disseminated herpesvirus infection associated with primary genital herpes in pregnancy. JAMA 235:2731, 1976.
560. Hensleigh PA, Glover DB, Cannon M: Systemic herpesvirus hominis in pregnancy. J Reprod Med 22:171, 1979.
561. Kobbermann T, Clark L, Griffin WT: Maternal death secondary to disseminated herpesvirus hominis. Am J Obstet Gynecol 6:742, 1980.
562. Peacock JE Jr, Sarubbi FA: Disseminated herpes simplex virus infection during pregnancy. Obstet Gynecol 61:13S, 1983.
563. Chase RA, Pottage JC Jr, Haber MH, et al: Herpes simplex virus hepatitis in adults: Two case reports and review of the literature. Rev Infect Dis 9:329, 1987.
564. Lagrew DC, Furlow TG, Hager D, Yarrish YL: Disseminated herpes simplex virus infection in pregnancy. Successful treatment with acyclovir. JAMA 252:2058, 1984.
565. Gelven PL, Gruber KK, Swiger FK, et al: Fatal disseminated herpes simplex in pregnancy with maternal and neonatal death. South Med J 89:732, 1996.
566. Naraqi W, Jackson GG, Jonasson OM: Viremia with herpes simplex type 1 in adults: Four nonfatal cases, one with features of chickenpox. Ann Intern Med 85:165, 1976.
567. Remafedi G, Muldoon RL: Acute monarticular arthritis caused by herpes simplex virus type 1. Pediatrics 72:882, 1983.
568. Whittaker JA, Hardson MD: Severe thrombocytopenia after generalized HSV-2 infection. South Med J 72:864, 1978.
569. Schuller D, Spessert C, Fraser VJ, Goodenberger DM: Herpes simplex virus from respiratory tract secretions: Epidemiology, clinical characteristics, and outcome in immunocompromised and nonimmunocompromised hosts. Am J Med 94:29, 1993.
570. Nash G, Major MC, Foley FD: Herpetic infection of the middle and lower respiratory tract. Am J Clin Pathol 54:857, 1970.
571. Ramsey PG, Fife KH, Hackman RC, et al: Herpes simplex virus pneumonia: Clinical, virologic and pathologic features in 20 patients. Ann Intern Med 97:813, 1982.
572. Graham BS, Snell JD Jr: Herpes simplex virus infection of the adult lower respiratory tract. Medicine (Baltimore) 62:384, 1983.
573. Herout F, Vortel V, Vondrackova A: Herpes simplex involvement of the lower respiratory tract. Am J Clin Pathol 46:411, 1966.
574. Tuxen DV, Cade JF, McDonald MI, et al: Herpes simplex virus from the lower respiratory tract in adult respiratory distress syndrome. Am Rev Respir Dis 126:416, 1982.
575. Bastian JF, Kaufman IA: Herpes simplex esophagitis in a healthy 10-year-old boy. J Pediatr 100:426, 1982.
576. Deprew WT, Prentice RSA, Beck IT, et al: Herpes simplex ulcerative esophagitis in a healthy subject. Am J Gastroenterol 68:381, 1977.
577. Pazin GJ: Herpes simplex esophagitis after trigeminal nerve surgery. Gastroenterology 74:741, 1978.
578. Owensby LC, Stammer JL: Esophagitis associated with herpes simplex infection in an immunocompetent host. Gastroenterology 74:1305, 1978.
579. Nash G, Ross JS: Herpetic esophagitis. A common cause of esophageal ulceration. Hum Pathol 5:339, 1974.
580. Camazine B, Antkowiak JG, Nava MER, et al: Herpes simplex viral pneumonia in the postthoracotomy patient. Chest 108: 876, 1995.
581. Greenberg SB: Respiratory herpesvirus infections: An overview. Chest 106:1S, 1994.
582. Klainer AS, Oud L, Randazzo J, et al: Herpes simplex virus involvement of the lower respiratory tract following surgery. Chest 106:8S, 1994.
583. Prellner T, Flamholc L, Haidl S, et al: Herpes simplex virus—The most frequently isolated pathogen in the lungs of patients with severe respiratory distress. Scand J Infect Dis 24:283, 1992.
584. Sofer S, Pagtakha RD, Hoogstratten J: Fatal lower respiratory tract infection due to herpes simplex virus in a previously healthy child. Clin Pediatr 23:406, 1984.
585. Flowers RH, Kernodle DS: Vagal mononeuritis caused by herpes simplex virus: Association with unilateral vocal cord paralysis. Am J Med 88:686, 1990.
586. Kohl S: Postnatal herpes simplex virus infections. *In* Feigin RD, Cherry JD (eds): Textbook of Pediatric Infectious Diseases, ed 2. Philadelphia, WB Saunders, 1987, pp 1577–1601.
587. Taylor RJ, Saul SH, Dowling JN, et al: Primary disseminated herpes simplex infection with fulminant hepatitis following renal transplantation. Arch Intern Med 141:1519, 1981.
588. Keane JR, Malkinson FD, Bryant J, Levin S: Herpesvirus hominis hepatitis and disseminated intravascular coagulation. Arch Intern Med 136:1312, 1976.
589. Anuras S, Summers R: Fulminant herpes simplex hepatitis in an adult: Report of a case in a renal transplant recipient. Gastroenterology 70:425, 1976.
590. Muller SA, Hermann EC, Winkilmann RK: Herpes simplex infections in hematologic malignancies. Am J Med 52:102, 1972.
591. Montgomerie JZ, Becroft DMO, Croxson MC, et al: Herpessimplex virus infection after renal transplantation. Lancet 2:867, 1969.
592. Korsager B, Spencer ES, Mordhorst C-H, Andersen HK: Herpesvirus hominis infections in renal transplant patients. Scand J Infect Dis 7:11, 1975.
593. Lopyan L, Young AW, Menegus M: Generalized acute mucocutaneous herpes simplex type 2 with fatal outcome. Arch Dermatol 113:816, 1977.
594. Elliott WC, Houghton DC, Bryant RE, et al: Herpes simplex type 1 hepatitis in renal transplantation. Arch Intern Med 140:1656, 1980.
595. Walker DP, Longson M, Lawler W, et al: Disseminated herpes simplex virus infection with hepatitis in an adult renal transplant recipient. J Clin Pathol 34:1044, 1981.
596. Meyers JD, Flournoy N, Thomas ED: Infection with herpes simplex virus and cell-mediated immunity after marrow transplant. J Infect Dis 142:338, 1980.
597. Rand KH, Rasmussen LE, Pollard RB, et al: Cellular immunity and herpesvirus infections in cardiac-transplant patients. N Engl J Med 296:1372, 1977.

598. Pollard RB, Arvin AM, Gamberg P, et al: Specific cell-mediated immunity and infections with herpes viruses in cardiac transplant recipients. Am J Med 73:679, 1982.
599. Stewart JA, Reef SE, Pellett PE, et al: Herpesvirus infections in persons infected with human immunodeficiency virus. Clin Infect Dis 21(Suppl 1):S114, 1995.
600. Kusne S, Schwartz M, Breinig MK, et al: Herpes simplex virus hepatitis after solid organ transplantation in adults. J Infect Dis 163:1001, 1991.
601. Kumar A, Madden DL, Nankervis Ga: Humoral and cell-mediated immune responses to herpesvirus antigens during pregnancy—A longitudinal study. J Clin Immunol 4:12, 1984.
602. Pass RF, Whitley RJ, Whelchel JD, et al: Identification of patients with increased risk of infection with herpes simplex virus after renal transplantation. J Infect Dis 140:487, 1979.
603. Naraqi W, Jackson GG, Jonasson O, Yamashiroya HM: Prospective study of prevalence, incidence and source of herpes-virus infection in patients with renal allografts. J Infect Dis 136:531, 1977.
604. Arvin AM, Pollard RB, Rasmussen LE, Merigan TC: Cellular and humoral immunity in the pathogenesis of recurrent herpes viral infections in patients with lymphoma. J Clin Invest 65:869, 1980.
605. Wade JC, Day LM, Crowley JJ, Meyers JD: Recurrent infection with herpes simplex virus after marrow transplantation: Role of the specific immune response and acyclovir treatment. J Infect Dis 149:750, 1984.
606. Logan WS, Tindall JP, Elson MI: Chronic cutaneous herpes simplex. Arch Dermatol 103:606, 1971.
607. Schneidman DW, Barr RJ, Graham JH: Chronic cutaneous herpes simplex. JAMA 241:592, 1979.
608. Lam TM, Pazin GJ, Armstrong JA, Ho M: Herpes simplex infection in acute myelogenous leukemia and other hematologic malignancies: A prospective study. Cancer 48:2168, 1981.
609. Wade JC, Newton B, McLaren C, et al: Intravenous acyclovir to treat mucocutaneous herpes simplex virus infection after marrow transplantation. Ann Intern Med 96:265, 1982.
610. Whitley R, Barton N, Collins E, et al: Mucocutaneous herpes simplex virus infections in immunocompromised patients. A model for evaluation of topical antiviral agents. Am J Med 73:236, 1982.
611. Whitley RJ, Levin M, Barton N, et al: Infections caused by herpes simplex virus in the immunocompromised host. Natural history and topical acyclovir therapy. J Infect Dis 150:323, 1984.
612. Rand KH, Kramer B, Johnson AC: Cancer chemotherapy associated symptomatic stomatitis. Role of herpes simplex virus (HSV). Cancer 50:1262, 1982.
613. Neiman PE, Reeves W, Ray G, et al: A prospective analysis of interstitial pneumonia and opportunistic viral infection among recipients of allogeneic bone marrow grafts. J Infect Dis 136:754, 1977.
614. Cirillo NW, Lyon DT, Schuller AM: Tracheoesophageal fistula complicating herpes esophagitis in AIDS. Am J Gastroenterol 88:587, 1992.
615. Nasemann T: Über das postherpetische Erythema exsudativum multiforme. Hautarzt 15:346, 1964.
616. Shelly WB: Herpes simplex virus as a cause of erythema multiforme. JAMA 201:153, 1967.
617. Britz M, Sibulkin D: Recurrent erythema multiforme and herpes genitalis (type 2). JAMA 233:812, 1975.
618. Kazmierowski JA, Peizner DS, Wuepper KR: Herpes simplex antigen in immune complexes of patients with erythema multiforme: Presence following recurrent herpes simplex infection. JAMA 247:2547, 1982.
619. Fiumara NJ, Solomon J: Recurrent herpes simplex virus infections and erythema multiforme: A report of three patients. Sex Transm Dis 10:144, 1983.
620. Orton PW, Huff JC, Tonnesen MG, et al: Detection of a herpes simplex viral antigen in skin lesions of erythema multiforme. Ann Intern Med 101:48, 1984.
621. Weston WL, Brice SL, Jester JD, et al: Herpes simplex virus in childhood erythema multiforme. Pediatrics 89:32, 1992.
622. Lever WF: Histopathology of the Skin, ed 5. Philadelphia, JB Lippincott, 1975.
623. Constantine VS, Francis RD, Montes LF: Association of herpes simplex with neuralgia. JAMA 205:131, 1968.
624. Nahmias AJ, Roizman B: Infection with herpes simplex virus 1 and 2. N Engl J Med 289:677, 1973.
625. Finelli PF: Herpes simplex virus and the human nervous system. Current concepts and review. Mil Med 140:765, 1975.
626. Krohel GB, Richardson JR, Farelli DF: Herpes simplex neuropathy. Neurology 26:596, 1976.
627. Ellison GW: Multiple sclerosis: A fever blister of the brain. Lancet 2:664, 1974.
628. McCormick DP: Herpes simplex virus as a cause of Bell's palsy. Lancet 1:937, 1972.
629. Adour KK, Bell DN, Hilsinger RL Jr: Herpes simplex virus in idiopathic facial paralysis (Bell palsy). JAMA 233:527, 1975.
630. Adour KK, Hilsinger RL Jr, Byl FM: Herpes simplex polyganglionitis. Otolaryngol Head Neck Surg 88:270, 1980.
631. Vahlne A, Edström S, Arstila P, et al: Bell's palsy and herpes simplex virus. Arch Otolaryngol 107:79, 1981.
632. Mertens T, Thomas JP, Zippel C, Eggers HJ: Peripheral facial palsy and viral infections—Findings and problems. Med Microbiol Immunol 171:77, 1982.
633. Shearer ML, Finch SM: Periodic organic psychosis associated with recurrent herpes simplex. N Engl J Med 271:494, 1964.
634. Murakami S, Mizobuchi M, Nakashior Y, et al: Bell palsy and herpes simplex virus: Identification of viral DNA in endoneurial fluid and muscle. Ann Intern Med 124:27, 1996.
635. Spruance SL: Bell palsy and herpes simplex virus. Ann Intern Med 120:1045, 1994.
636. Adour KK, Ruboyianes JM, Von Doersten PG: Bell's palsy treatment with acyclovir and prednisone compared with prednisone alone: A double-blind, randomized, controlled trial. Ann Otol Rhinol Laryngol 105:371, 1996.
637. Baringer JR: Herpes simplex virus and Bell palsy. Ann Intern Med 124:63, 1996.
638. Devriese PP: Bell palsy and herpes simplex virus. Ann Intern Med 125:698, 1996.
639. Melnick JL, Rawls WE, Adam E: Cervical Cancer. *In* Evans AS (ed): Viral Infections of Humans: Epidemiology and Control. New York, Plenum Publishing, 1989, pp 687–711.
640. Paavonen J, Koutsky LA, Kiviat N: Cervical neoplasia and other STD-related genital and anal neoplasias. *In* Holmes KK (ed): Sexually Transmitted Diseases, ed 2. New York, McGraw-Hill, 1990, pp 561–591.
641. Shah KV: Biology of human genital tract papillomaviruses. *In* Holmes KK (ed): Sexually Transmitted Diseases, ed 2. New York, McGraw-Hill, 1990, pp 425–431.
642. Landry, ML, Mayo DR, Hsiung GD: Comparison of guinea pig embryo cells, rabbit kidney cells, and human embryonic lung fibroblast cell stains for isolation of herpes simplex virus. J Clin Microbiol 15:842, 1982.
643. Spruance SL, Overall JC, Kern ER, et al: The natural history of recurrent herpes simplex labialis: Implications for antiviral therapy. N Engl J Med 297:69, 1977.
644. Goldstein LC, Corey L, McDougall JK, et al: Monoclonal antibodies to herpes simplex viruses: Use in antigenic typing and rapid diagnosis. J Infect Dis 147:829, 1983.
645. Richman DD, Cleveland PH, Redfield DC, et al: Rapid viral diagnosis. J Infect Dis 149:298, 1984.
646. Fife KH, Corey L: Herpes simplex virus. *In* Holmes KK (ed): Sexually Transmitted Diseases, ed 2. New York, McGraw-Hill, 1990, pp 941–952.
647. Barr RJ, Herten RJ, Graham JH: Rapid method for Tzanck preparations. JAMA 237:1119, 1977.
648. Verano L, Michalski FJ: Herpes simplex virus antigen direct detection in standard transport medium by DuPont Herpchek enzyme-linked immunosorbent assay. J Clin Microbiol 28:2555, 1990.
649. Kudesia G, Van Hegan A, Wake S, et al: Comparison of cell culture with an amplified enzyme immunoassay for diagnosing genital herpes simplex infection. J Clin Pathol 44:778, 1991.
650. Hardy DA, Arvin AM, Yasukawa LL, et al: Use of polymerase chain reaction for successful identification of asymptomatic genital infections with herpes simplex virus in pregnant women at delivery. J Infect Dis 162:1031, 1990.
651. Corey L, Holmes KK: Genital herpes simplex virus infections: Current concepts in diagnosis, therapy and prevention. Ann Intern Med 98:973, 1983.
652. Simmons A, Nash AA: Role of antibody in primary and recurrent herpes simplex virus infection. J Virol 53:944, 1985.

653. Hall MJ, Katrak K: The quest for a herpes simplex virus vaccine: Background and recent development. Vaccine 4:138, 1986.
654. Stanberry LR, Bernstein DI, Burke RL, et al: Vaccination with recombinant herpes simplex virus glycoproteins: Protection against initial and recurrent genital herpes. J Infect Dis 155: 914, 1987.
655. Rooney JF, Wohlenberg C, Cremer KJ, et al: Immunization with a vaccinia virus recombinant expressing herpes simplex virus type I glycoprotein D: Long-term protection and effect of revaccination. J Virol 62:1530, 1988.
656. Meignier B, Jourdier TM, Norrild B, et al: Immunization of experimental animals with reconstituted glycoprotein mixtures of herpes simplex virus 1 and 2: Protection against challenge with virulent virus. J Infect Dis 155:921, 1987.
657. Meignier B, Longnecker R, Mavromara-Nazos P, et al: Virulence of and establishment of latency by genetically engineered deletion mutants of herpes simplex virus 1. Virology 162:251, 1988.
658. Meignier B, Martin B, Whitley RJ, Roizman B: In vivo behavior of genetically engineered herpes simplex viruses R7017 and R7020. II. Studies in immunocompetent and immunosuppressed owl monkeys (*Aotus trivirgatus*). J Infect Dis 162:313, 1990.
659. Burke RL: Development of a herpes simplex virus subunit glycoprotein vaccine for prophylactic and therapeutic use. Rev Infect Dis 13:S906, 1991.
660. Whitley RJ, Meignier B: Herpes simplex vaccines. *In* Ellis RW (ed): Vaccines: New Approaches to Immunological Problems. Boston, Butterworth, 1991, p 223.
661. Burke RL: Current status of HSV vaccine development. *In* Roizman B, Whitley RJ, Lopez C (eds): The Human Herpesviruses. New York, Raven Press, 1993, p 367.
662. Stanberry LR: Herpes simplex virus vaccines as immunotherapeutic agents. Trends Microbiol 3:244, 1995.
663. Morrison LLA, Knipe DM: Immunization with replication-defective mutants of herpes simplex virus type 1: Sites of immune intervention in pathogenesis of challenge virus infection. J Virol 68:689, 1994.
664. Morrison LA, Knipe DM: Mechanisms of immunization with a replication-defective mutant of herpes simplex virus 1. Virology 220:402, 1996.
665. Langenberg AG, Burke RL, Adair SF, et al: A recombinant glycoprotein vaccine for herpes simplex virus type 2: Safety and immunogenicity [corrected] [published erratum in Ann Intern Med 123:395, 1995]. Ann Intern Med 122:889, 1995.
666. Bourne N, Stanberry LR, Bernstein DI, et al: DNA immunization against experimental genital herpes simplex virus infection. J Infect Dis 173:800, 1996.
667. Boursnell MEG, Entwiste C, Blakeley D, et al: A genetically inactivated herpes simplex virus type 2 (HSV2) vaccine provides effective protection against primary and recurrent HSV2 disease. J Infect Dis 175:16, 1997.
668. McKenzie R, Straus SE: Therapeutic immunization for recurrent herpes simplex virus infections. Adv Exp Med Biol 394:67, 1996.
669. Straus SE, Corey L, Burke, RL, et al: Placebo-controlled trial of vaccination with recombinant glycoprotein D of herpes simplex virus type 2 for immunotherapy of genital herpes [see comments]. Lancet 343:1460, 1994.
670. Shimeld C, Hill TJ, Blyth WA, Easty DL: Passive immunization protects the mouse eye from damage after herpes simplex virus infection by limiting spread of virus in the nervous system. J Gen Virol 71:681, 1990.
671. Kimberlin D, Powell D, Gruber W, et al: Administration of oral acyclovir suppressive therapy after neonatal herpes simplex virus disease limited to the skin, eyes and mouth: Results of a phase I/II trial. Pediatr Infect Dis J 15:247, 1996.
672. Whitley RJ, Nahmias AJ, Soong S-J, et al: Vidarabine therapy of neonatal herpes simplex virus infection. Pediatrics 60:495, 1980.
673. Whitley R, Arvin A Prober C, et al: A, controlled trial comparing vidarabine with acyclovir in neonatal herpes simplex virus infection. N Engl J Med 324:444, 1991.
674. Whitley R, Arvin A, Prober C, et al: Predictors of morbidity and mortality in neonates with herpes simplex virus infections. N Engl J Med 324:450, 1991.
675. Whitley RJ, Soong S-J, Dolin R, et al: Adenine arabinoside therapy of biopsy-proven herpes simplex encephalitis. N Engl J Med 297:289, 1977.
676. Pavan-Langston D, Buchanan RA: Vidarabine therapy of simple and IUD-complicated herpes keratitis. Trans Am Acad Ophthalmol Otolaryngol 81:813, 1976.
677. Elion GB: Mechanism of action and selectivity of acyclovir. Am J Med 73:7, 1982.
678. Sköldenberg B, Forsgren M, Alestig K, et al: Acyclovir versus vidarabine in herpes simplex encephalitis. Randomised multicentre study in consecutive Swedish patients. Lancet 2:707, 1984.
679. Whitley RJ, Alford CA, Hirsch MS, et al: Vidarabine versus acyclovir therapy in herpes simplex encephalitis. N Engl J Med 314:144, 1986.
680. Mindel A, Adler MW, Sutherland S, Fiddian AP: Intravenous acyclovir treatment for primary genital herpes. Lancet 1:697, 1982.
681. Corey L, Fife KH, Benedetti JK, et al: Intravenous acyclovir for the treatment of primary genital herpes. Ann Intern Med 98:914, 1983.
682. Peacock JE Jr, Kaplowitz LG, Sparling PF, et al: Intravenous acyclovir therapy of first episodes of genital herpes: A multicenter double-blind, placebo-controlled trial. Am J Med 85:301, 1988.
683. Nilsen AE, Aasen T, Halsos AM, et al: Efficacy of oral acyclovir in the treatment of initial and recurrent genital herpes. Lancet 2:571, 1982.
684. Bryson YJ, Dillon M, Lovett M, et al: Treatment of first episodes of genital herpes simplex virus infection with oral acyclovir: A randomized double-blind controlled trial in normal subjects. N Engl J Med 308:916, 1983.
685. Mertz GJ, Critchlow CW, Benedetti J, et al: Double-blind placebo-controlled trial of oral acyclovir in first-episode genital herpes simplex virus infection. JAMA 252:1147, 1984.
686. Corey L, Nahmias AJ, Guinan ME, et al: A trial of topical acyclovir in genital herpes simplex virus infections. N Engl J Med 306:1313, 1982.
687. Reichman RC, Badger GJ, Guinan ME, et al: Topically administered acyclovir in the treatment of recurrent herpes simplex genitalis: A controlled trial. J Infect Dis 147:336, 1983.
688. Guinan ME: Oral acyclovir for treatment and suppression of genital herpes simplex virus infection: A review. JAMA 255:1747, 1986.
689. Stone KM, Whittington WL: Treatment of genital herpes. Rev Infect Dis 12(Suppl 6):610, 1990.
690. Whitley RJ, Gnann JW Jr: Acyclovir: A decade later. N Engl J Med 327:782, 1992.
691. Mertz GJ: Management of genital herpes. Adv Exp Med Biol 394:1, 1996.
692. Guinan ME, MacCalman J, Kern ER: The course of untreated recurrent genital herpes simplex infection in 27 women. N Engl J Med 304:759, 1981.
693. Reichman RC, Badger GJ, Mertz GJ, et al: Treatment of recurrent genital herpes simplex infections with oral acyclovir: A controlled trial. JAMA 251:2103, 1984.
694. Raborn GW, McGaw WT, Grace M, et al: Oral acyclovir and herpes labialis: A randomized, double-blind, placebo-controlled study. J Am Dent Assoc 115:38, 1987.
695. Gill JM, Bryant HE: Oral acyclovir therapy of recurrent herpes simplex virus type 2 infection of the hand. Antimicrob Agents Chemother 35:382, 1991.
696. Straus SE, Takiff HE, Seidlin M, et al: Suppression of frequently recurring genital herpes: A placebo-controlled double-blind trial of oral acyclovir. N Engl J Med 310:1545, 1984.
697. Douglas JM, Critchlow C, Benedetti J, et al: A double-blind study of oral acyclovir for suppression of recurrences of genital herpes simplex virus infection. N Engl J Med 310:1551, 1984.
698. Straus SE, Croen KD, Sawyer MH, et al: Acyclovir suppression of frequently recurring genital herpes: Efficacy and diminishing need during successive years of treatment. JAMA 260:2227, 1988.
699. Mertz GJ, Jones CC, Mills J, et al: Acyclovir Study Group. Long-term acyclovir suppression of frequently recurring genital herpes simplex virus infection: A multicenter double-blind trial. JAMA 260:201, 1988.
700. Gold D, Corey L: Acyclovir prophylaxis for herpes simplex virus infection. Antimicrob Agents Chemother 31:361, 1987.
701. Mattison HR, Reichman RC, Benedetti J, et al: Double-blind placebo-controlled trial comparing long-term suppressive with short-term oral acyclovir therapy for management of recurrent genital herpes. Am J Med 85(2A):20, 1988.

702. Spruance SL, Hammil MS, Hoge WS, et al: Acyclovir prevents reactivation of herpes labialis in skiers. JAMA 260:1597, 1988.
703. Spruance SL, Freeman DJ, Stewart JCB, et al: The natural history of ultraviolet radiation–induced herpes simplex labialis and response to therapy with peroral and topical formulations of acyclovir. J Infect Dis 163:728, 1991.
704. Perry CM, Wagstaff AJ: Famciclovir. A review of its pharmacological properties and therapeutic efficacy in herpesvirus infections. Drugs 50:396, 1995.
705. Sacks SL: Use of penciclovir and famciclovir in the management of genital herpes. Curr Probl Dermatol 24:219, 1996.
706. Weller S, Blum MR, Doucette M, et al: Pharmacokinetics of the acyclovir pro-drug valaciclovir after escalating single- and multiple-dose administration to normal volunteers. Clin Pharmacol Ther 54:595, 1993.
707. Sacks SL, Aoki FY, Diaz-Mitoma F, et al: Patient-initiated, twice-daily oral famciclovir for early recurrent genital herpes: A randomized, double-blind multicenter trial. JAMA 276:44, 1996.
708. Spruance SL, Tyring SK, DeGregorio B, et al: A large-scale, placebo-controlled, dose-ranging trial of peroral valaciclovir for episodic treatment of recurrent herpes genitalis. Arch Intern Med 156:1729, 1996.
709. Saral R, Ambinder RF, Burns WH: Acyclovir prophylaxis against herpes simplex virus infection in patients with leukemia. A randomized double-blind placebo-controlled study. Ann Intern Med 99:773, 1983.
710. Saral R, Burns WH, Laskin OL, et al: Acyclovir prophylaxis of herpes-simplex virus infections: A randomized double-blind controlled trial in bone marrow transplant recipients. N Engl J Med 305:63, 1981.
711. Hann IM, Prentice HF, Blacklock HA, et al: Acyclovir prophylaxis against herpes virus infections in severely immunocompromised patients: Randomised double blind trial. Br Med J 287:384, 1983.
712. Gluckman E, Devergie A, Melo R, et al: Prophylaxis of herpes infections after bone marrow transplantation by oral acyclovir. Lancet 2:706, 1983.
713. Saral R: Management of mucocutaneous herpes simplex virus infections in immunocompromised patients. Am J Med 85:57, 1988.
714. Meyers JD, Wade JC, Mitchell CD, et al: Multicenter collaborative trial of intravenous acyclovir for treatment of mucocutaneous herpes simplex virus infection in the immunocompromised host. Am J Med 73(1A):229, 1982.
715. Shepp DH, Newton BA, Dandliker PS, et al: Oral acyclovir therapy for mucocutaneous herpes simplex virus infections in immunocompromised marrow transplant recipients. Ann Intern Med 102:783, 1985.
716. Collins P: Viral sensitivity following the introduction of acyclovir. Am J Med 85(2A):129, 1988.
717. Burns WH, Saral R, Santos GW, et al: Isolation and characterisation of resistant herpes simplex virus after acyclovir therapy. Lancet 1:421, 1982.
718. Lehrman SN, Douglas JM, Corey L, Barry DW: Recurrent genital herpes and suppressive oral acyclovir therapy: Relation between clinical outcome and in-vitro drug sensitivity. Ann Intern Med 104:786, 1986.
719. Straus SE, Croen KD, Sawyer MH, et al: Acyclovir suppression of frequently recurring genital herpes: Efficacy and diminishing need during successive years of treatment. JAMA 260:2227, 1988.
720. Hirsch MS, Schooley RT: Resistance to antiviral drugs: The end of innocence. N Engl J Med 320:313, 1989.
721. Chatis PA, Miller CH, Schrager LE, Crumpacker CS: Successful treatment with foscarnet of an acyclovir-resistant mucocutaneous infection with herpes simplex virus in a patient with acquired immunodeficiency syndrome. N Engl J Med 320:297, 1989.
722. Erlich KS, Mills J, Chatis P, et al: Acyclovir-resistant herpes simplex virus infections in patients with the acquired immunodeficiency syndrome. N Engl J Med 320:293, 1989.
723. Gately A, Gander RM, Johnson PC, et al: Herpes simplex virus type 2 meningoencephalitis resistant to acyclovir in a patient with AIDS. J Infect Dis 161:711, 1990.
724. Birch CJ, Tachedjian G, Doherty RR, et al: Altered sensitivity to antiviral drugs of herpes simplex virus isolated from a patient with acquired immunodeficiency syndrome. J Infect Dis 162:731, 1990.
725. Collins P, Larder BA, Oliver NM, et al: Characterization of a DNA polymerase mutant of herpes simplex virus from a severely immunocompromised patient receiving acyclovir. J Gen Virol 70:375, 1989.
726. Sacks SL, Wanklin RJ, Reece DE, et al: Progressive esophagitis from acyclovir-resistant herpes simplex. Clinical roles for DNA polymerase mutants and viral heterogeneity? Ann Intern Med 111:893, 1989.
727. Balfour HH, Benson C, Braun J, et al: Management of acyclovir-resistant herpes simplex and varicella-zoster virus infections. J Acquir Immune Defic Syndr 7:254, 1994.
728. Chatis PA, Crumpacker CS: Resistance of herpesviruses to antiviral drugs. Antimicrob Agents Chemother 36:1589, 1992.
729. Coen DM: Acyclovir-resistant, pathogenic herpesviruses. Trends Microbiol 2:481, 1994.
730. Coen DM: Antiviral drug resistance in herpes simplex virus. Adv Exp Med Biol 394:49, 1996.
731. Laufer DS, Starr SE: Resistance to antivirals. Pediatr Clin North Am 42:583, 1995.
732. Pottage JC, Kessler HA: Herpes simplex virus resistance to acyclovir: Clinical relevance. Infect Agents Dis 4:115, 1995.
733. Safrin S: Treatment of acyclovir-resistant herpes simplex and varicella zoster virus infections. Adv Exp Med Biol 394:59, 1996.

241

Human Herpesvirus 6 and Other Newly Recognized Human Herpesviruses

Kathleen M. Neuzil
Donald H. Rubin

Advances in molecular biology have linked specific microbiologic agents to the pathogenesis of clinical syndromes ranging from childhood exanthems to cancer and peptic ulcer disease. No group of organisms better exemplifies these advances than the human herpesvirus group. In the past decade, three new members, human herpesvirus 6 types A and B (HHV-6), human herpesvirus 7 (HHV-7), and human herpesvirus 8 (HHV-8) (or Kaposi's sarcoma–associated herpesvirus), have been added to the family previously composed of herpes simplex virus types 1 and 2, cytomegalovirus, Epstein-Barr virus, and varicella-zoster virus. Although the diverse manifestations of these organisms continue to be defined, epidemiologic, clinical, and virologic studies indicate that these viruses have roles in some human disease and are implicated as causal agents in others.

Human Herpesvirus 6

History

A virus morphologically and genetically similar to human herpesviruses was originally isolated in 1986 from the peripheral blood leukocytes of patients with human immunodeficiency virus (HIV) infection and lymphoproliferative malignancies and was designated human B-lymphotropic virus.[1,2] Subsequently, the virus was shown to have a marked tropism for T lymphocytes bearing the CD4 antigen, and it was renamed HHV-6. In 1988, Yamanishi and colleagues[3] isolated HHV-6 from the peripheral blood lymphocytes of patients with exanthem subitum (roseola infantum, sixth disease). Since that time, epidemiologic and clinical studies have linked this virus to common febrile illnesses in children, including exanthem subitum, as well as less common maladies in children and adults (Table 241–1).

Characteristics of the Pathogen

HHV-6 has been classified as a member of the β-herpesvirus subgroup based on its morphologic, genomic, and lymphotropic characteristics. By serology, there are two variants of HHV-6, designated A and B. It is a large virus with a total diameter of 160 to 200 nm, and a 20- to 40-nm-thick envelope that is acquired from the nuclear and cytoplasmic membranes of the host cell.[1] The characteristic icosahedral symmetry of the viral nucleocapsid, approximately 90 to 100 nm in diameter, can be seen in the nucleus and cytoplasm of infected cells. Mature virions are released by exocytosis. The double-stranded 160- to 170-kb DNA genome has a guanine plus cytosine content of 43% to 44%, which is lower than that of other human herpesviruses.[2] HHV-6 is most closely related to cytomegalovirus, based on its hybridization to a fragment of the cytomegalovirus genome.[4]

Primary human lymphocytes from peripheral or cord blood readily support the growth of HHV-6, as does the human diploid lung fibroblast cell line MRC-5. $CD4^+$ T cells are the most readily affected cells in tissue culture.[5] Growth in primary lymphocytes requires stimulation by phytohemagglutinin and interleukin-2. Tissue culture–adapted HHV-6 grows in diverse cell lines of hematologic, epithelial, and neurologic origin. $CD4^+$ T cells are also the primary target in acute HHV-6 infection in vivo, although other hematopoietic cells, liver cells, kidney cells, salivary and bronchial gland cells, and brain cells may be infected.[6,7] In primary cell cultures, infection with HHV-6 produces large refractile cells with intranuclear or intracytoplasmic inclusion bodies, resulting in virus production and cell death.[1]

Similar to the other human herpesviruses, HHV-6 establishes lifelong latent infection in the host. Peripheral blood mononuclear cells, cerebrospinal fluid, and saliva are all potential reservoirs for latent virus.[8,9] HHV-6 possesses the ability to transform human epidermal cells and lymphocytes[10–12] and affect gene transcription of other human viruses, including papillomaviruses and human immunodeficiency virus.[13,14]

TABLE 241–1 ■ Clinical Manifestations of Human Herpesvirus 6 Infection

CHILDREN	ADULTS	IMMUNOCOMPROMISED PERSONS*
Fever and rash†	Fever, lymphadenopathy	Fever†
Fever and otitis†	Mononucleosis-like syndrome	Fever and rash†
Febrile seizures†	Hepatitis	Meningoencephalitis
Hepatitis	Meningoencephalitis	Pneumonitis (?)
Meningoencephalitis		Bone marrow suppression (?)
Intussusception		
Idiopathic thrombocytopenic purpura		

*(?), Causation not established.
†Common manifestation.

Epidemiology

Primary infection with HHV-6 is almost universal. Seroprevalence studies indicate that 95% to 100% of cord blood samples have antibody to HHV-6.[15] This maternally derived antibody declines in the ensuing months, with the lowest antibody levels detected in infants between 4 and 7 months of age. Seroconversion occurs between 6 months and 2 years of age in most children.[16–18] Eighty percent to 100% of healthy adults younger than 40 years have antibodies to HHV-6, with declining titers thereafter.[15,19,20] Antibody is acquired at an earlier age and is more prevalent in the Far East compared with Western countries.[15,20,21]

The widespread occurrence of HHV-6 in childhood suggests a facile and efficient means of transmission. Oral virus shedding may be the predominant mode of spread, as HHV-6 can be detected in the saliva of more than 85% of adults.[7,9,20,22,23] In addition, isolates from the saliva of mothers and the peripheral blood of their infants were genetically related, as determined by restriction enzyme analysis of purified DNA.[24] There is a high prevalence of HHV-6 DNA in peripheral blood mononuclear cells of healthy adults.[9,25,26] The relevance of this finding to blood product safety is uncertain.[27] Perinatal transmission occurs, and viral DNA detected by polymerase chain reaction (PCR) in the vaginal secretions of healthy women suggests the possibility for sexual transmission as well.[18] The virus has not been detected in human breast milk.[28] HHV-6 can infect renal and hepatic tissues and has caused primary infection in seronegative kidney and liver transplant recipients.[29,30]

HHV-6 type B is the predominant type in infants with primary HHV-6 infection, as well as healthy adult blood donors.[31,32] In contrast, either type or both types have been isolated from adult bone marrow transplant recipients.[33–35] The reasons for these epidemiologic differences are unclear; type A infection may occur later in life, may be clinically inapparent, or may have a higher propensity for reactivation.

Our understanding of the relationship of HHV-6 to malignancy is evolving. Seroepidemiologic surveys report a greater HHV-6 seropositivity among patients with Hodgkin's lymphoma compared with control subjects.[36–39] Furthermore, PCR detects HHV-6 DNA in the peripheral blood and lymph nodes of patients with Hodgkin's disease at rates greater than those found in the healthy population, but less than is seen in populations with reactive lymphadenopathies.[32,37,40] Further studies are needed to determine if HHV-6 has a role in the pathogenesis of Hodgkin's disease or if the immune status of Hodgkin's disease patients allows for the reactivation of latent virus. There is no evidence for an etiologic role of HHV-6 in the development of other lymphoproliferative malignancies.[40] As HHV-6 can activate transcription of human papillomavirus-transforming genes, it may be a cofactor in the development of cervical cancer.[41] In one study, four of six patients with HPV-6–related cervical neoplasias also had HHV-6 in cervical tissue detected by PCR. None of the 30 normal cervical specimens had HHV-6 DNA.[13] Patients with oral cancers have a higher seroprevalence to HHV-6 compared with healthy control persons; the significance of these findings remains to be determined.[36,42]

Pathogenesis

In acute infection with HHV-6, the virus replicates in peripheral blood mononuclear cells, salivary glands, and neuronal tissue, from which it is readily isolated.[18,43] In vitro, only activated, mature T lymphocytes support virus replication.[44,45] The clinical consequences of acute infection are presumed secondary to direct cytotoxicity, although some manifestations, such as idiopathic thrombocytopenic purpura, may be immune mediated. After primary infection, the virus establishes latency in several organs, including the lymph nodes, kidneys, liver, salivary glands, and peripheral blood mononuclear cells.[23, 30, 46] Viral DNA can be detected by PCR techniques in the peripheral blood of healthy subjects during clinical latency.[18, 25] The virus reactivates in recipients of bone marrow and solid organ transplants and in children in the early convalescent stage of measles infection, suggesting a role for T lymphocytes in the suppression of endogenous replication in healthy persons.[47, 48]

HHV-6 infection induces antibodies to a number of structural and nonstructural viral proteins that persist for many years.[49–52] Although neutralizing antibody is present in cord blood in high titer, the duration and degree of protection conferred from passive antibody is uncertain, as primary HHV-6 infection is not rare in the first 6 months of life.[15, 18] Serum from patients in the convalescent stage of exanthem subitum acquires neutralizing antibody, and the neutralizing antibody titer remains high throughout life.[15, 53] Second episodes of exanthema subitum are rare, supporting the correlation of antibody production with immunity and further suggesting that HHV-6 is the predominant virus producing this syndrome.

Clinical Manifestations

CHILDREN

Primary HHV-6 infection in children is almost universal by age 3, being most common between 6 and 12 months of age.[16, 18, 54, 55] The illness does not have a seasonal predilection.[18, 54] Children with primary HHV-6 infection generally have a febrile illness with or without rash; primary illness without fever and asymptomatic seroconversions have been reported.[55–57] Otitis and irritability are common components of the febrile illness. Fever lasts an average of 4 days. Children younger than 6 months have more diarrhea than older children and are more likely to require hospitalization.[18, 54] Although exanthem subitum is a common manifestation of primary HHV-6 infection in Japan, it accounts for a minority of symptomatic infections in the United States.[18, 54]

Seizures are the most common complication of primary HHV-6 infection in children, occurring in up to 25% of cases.[8, 58, 59] In patients with exanthem subitum, all seizures occur before the development of the rash.[58, 60] Status epilepticus has been reported.[60] Up to one third of all febrile seizures in children younger than 2 years are associated with primary HHV-6 infection. Meningoencephalitis has also been reported as a manifestation of primary infection.[58, 61] HHV-6 viral DNA in the cerebrospinal fluid can be detected by PCR in the majority of children with neurologic symptoms. HHV-6 has been implicated in the etiology of recurrent seizures in children, based on the persistence of viral genome in the cerebrospinal fluid.[8, 62] Other complications of primary HHV-6 infection in childhood include intussusception, thought to be secondary to enlarged mesenteric lymph nodes, and idiopathic thrombocytopenic purpura.[63–66]

ADULTS

Information regarding the clinical manifestations of primary HHV-6 infection in immunocompetent adults is limited but parallels that seen with primary cytomegalovirus or Epstein-Barr infection in adulthood. A nonspecific illness with lymphadenopathy, a mononucleosis-type syndrome, and hepatitis have been reported.[67–73] A feature of the mononucleosis-like syndrome in a subset of these patients is the presence of a generalized erythematous rash. A skin biopsy from such a patient showed lymphocytes infected with HHV-6 by immunohistochemistry and in situ hybridization.[67]

IMMUNOCOMPROMISED HOSTS

Recipients of bone marrow and kidney transplants may reactivate HHV-6 in the early posttransplant period, usually between weeks 2 and 4.[30, 48, 74, 75] Most patients develop fever. In bone marrow transplant recipients, an erythematous papular rash, similar to the rash seen with graft-versus-host disease, may accompany the fever.[48, 76, 77] HHV-6 DNA has been detected in the skin biopsy specimens of these patients by use of the PCR technique.[76, 77] Fatal encephalitis with invasion of brain tissue by the virus has been reported in a bone marrow transplant recipient.[35] HHV-6 DNA has been detected in the lungs of all seropositive bone marrow transplant patients with idiopathic pneumonitis at higher levels than are found in healthy control persons; causality has not been established.[9] Likewise, HHV-6 DNA levels in the peripheral blood of bone marrow transplant recipients correlate with the development of graft-versus-host disease and bone marrow suppression.[34, 78, 79] Whether HHV-6 causes the immune system abnormalities or is reactivated secondary to them has not been determined.

The relationship between HIV and HHV-6 infection is equally enigmatic. HHV-6 has been proposed as a cofactor for progression of HIV infection based on the viruses' common tropism for $CD4^+$ T lymphocytes, their synergistic cytopathic effects, and the ability of HHV-6 to transactivate HIV regulatory genes.[14, 80] Moreover, infection of peripheral blood mononuclear cells by HHV-6 in vitro results in immunosuppression characterized by reduced interleukin-2 synthesis and diminished $CD4^+$ and $CD8^+$ T-lymphocyte proliferation.[81] However, clinical data to support this hypothesis are limited. HHV-6 is widely disseminated at autopsy in patients with end-stage acquired immunodeficiency syndrome, affecting lung, lymph node, spleen, liver, kidney, and brain tissue.[82, 83] Lymphocytes and lymphatic tissue are disproportionately affected.[82, 84] It has been postulated that HHV-6 may contribute to disease in these patients based on its presence in tissue and the pathogenicity of other herpesviruses in HIV-infected persons. Prospective studies of large numbers of HIV-infected patients are needed to determine the relationship of disease to HHV-6 infection.

Diagnosis

Primary infection with HHV-6 can be diagnosed by isolation of the virus from blood or by serology. Serologic diagnosis of primary HHV-6 infection is based on the presence of immunoglobulin M antibody, which appears about 5 days after onset of disease and persists for approximately 1 month, or a fourfold rise in HHV-6–specific immunoglobulin G antibody. Newer enzyme-linked immunosorbent assays correlate well with the results of traditional immunofluorescent assays.[85, 86] The HHV-6 anticomplement immunofluorescent assay and enzyme-linked immunosorbent assay are specific, demonstrating no cross-reactivity to other herpesviruses, including cytomegalovirus.[87] Virus isolation from peripheral blood mononuclear cells, although cumbersome, is a useful confirmatory test for primary infection or reactivation. PCR methods are available for the detection of HHV-6 DNA, but these do not distinguish between active and latent infections.[9, 25]

Therapy

There have been no clinical trials of antiviral therapy for HHV-6 infection. HHV-6 replication is readily inhibited by foscarnet and ganciclovir in vitro.[49, 88, 89] Reports on the susceptibility of HHV-6 to acyclovir are discrepant and may reflect differences in virus strains or lack of assay standards.

However, HHV-6 appears similar to cytomegalovirus in its susceptibility to acyclovir, requiring high doses in most studies to inhibit replication.[88–93]

High-dose (>10 units/mL) recombinant interleukin-2 eliminates the cytopathic effect and the presence of extracellular virions in peripheral blood mononuclear cells infected with HHV-6.[44] Likewise, exogenous interferon-α suppresses HHV-6 replication in peripheral blood mononuclear cells in vitro.[94] Although interleukin-2 has been shown to increase the number of CD4+ cells in HIV-infected hosts, interferon alfa therapy has been disappointing.[95] Whether either of these immunoregulators used in HIV infection affects concomitant HHV-6 infection has not been determined. Therefore, whether early intervention to decrease HHV-6 replication in the setting of concomitant HIV infection would affect HIV progression remains unknown.

Human Herpesvirus 7

HHV-7 is a prevalent human herpesvirus that infects during childhood but at a later age than that documented for HHV-6. Like HHV-6, the prevalence of HHV-7 antibody is high at birth and declines in the first 6 months of life. There is an increased prevalence of antibody by the end of the first year, consistent with seroconversion. The seroprevalence to HHV-7 plateaus between the ages of 4 and 10 years.[96, 97] HHV-7 seroconversion may occur in the presence of high titers of HHV-6 antibody, suggesting lack of protection of HHV-6 against HHV-7.[98]

HHV-7 is a T-lymphotropic virus that infects CD4+ and CD8+ lymphocytes.[99, 100] It is frequently shed in the saliva of healthy adults, providing a potential mode of transmission.[101–104] HHV-7 is another causal agent of exanthem subitum; other clinical manifestations of this virus remain to be defined.[105, 106]

Human Herpesvirus 8, or Kaposi's Sarcoma–Associated Virus

A third new member of the human herpesvirus group has been identified by PCR in Kaposi's sarcoma lesions of patients with and without HIV infection, and in acquired immunodeficiency syndrome–related body cavity–based lymphomas.[107–109] A definitive causal relationship to Kaposi's sarcoma or these body cavity lymphomas has not been proved. Sequence analysis of PCR products demonstrates that the genome has similarities to, but is distinct from, Epstein-Barr virus, a member of the gammaherpesvirinae subfamily.[108] The number of virus copies per cell may be exceedingly low in disease states in which the virus may be associated. This may suggest that virus replication is preexistent in these cells and may not be necessary for disease; disease prevention in this setting would require effective immunization to prevent virus acquisition. Further characterization of the virus, including its mode of transmission and etiologic role in the development of disease, requires additional study.

References

1. Salahuddin S, Ablashi D, Markham P: Isolation of a new virus, HBLV, in patients with lymphoproliferative disorders. Science 234:596–598, 1986.
2. Josephs S, Salahuddin S, Ablashi D, et al: Genomic analysis of the human B-lymphotropic virus (HBLV). Science 234:601–603, 1986.
3. Yamanishi K, Okuno T, Shiraki K, et al: Identification of human herpesvirus-6 as a causal agent for exanthem subitum. Lancet 1:1065–1067, 1988.
4. Lawrence G, Chee M, Craxton M, et al: Human herpesvirus 6 is closely related to human cytomegalovirus. J Virol 64:287–299, 1990.
5. Takahashi K, Sonoda S, Higashi K, et al: Predominant CD4 T-lymphocyte tropism of human herpesvirus 6–related virus. J Virol 63:3161–3163, 1989.
6. Asano Y, Yoshikawa T, Suga S, et al: Human herpesvirus 6 harbouring in kidney (Letter). Lancet 2:1391, 1989.
7. Jarrett R, Clark D, Josephs S, et al: Detection of human herpesvirus-6 DNA in peripheral blood and saliva. J Med Virol 32:73–76, 1990.
8. Caserta M, Hall C, Schnabel K, et al: Neuroinvasion and persistence of human herpesvirus 6 in children. J Infect Dis 170:1586–1589, 1994.
9. Cone R, Huang M, Ashley R, et al: Human herpesvirus 6 DNA in peripheral blood cells and saliva from immunocompetent individuals. J Clin Microbiol 31:1262–1267, 1993.
10. Razzaque A: Oncogenic potential of human herpesvirus-6 DNA. Oncogene 5:1365–1370, 1990.
11. Razzaque A, Williams O, Wang J, et al: Neoplastic transformation of immortalized human epidermal keratinocytes by two HHV-6 DNA clones. Virology 195:113–120, 1993.
12. Puri R, Leland P, Razzaque A: Antigen(s)-specific tumour-infiltrating from tumour induced by human herpes virus-6 (HHV-6) DNA transfected NIH 3T3 transformants. Clin Exp Immunol 83:96–101, 1991.
13. Chen M, Wang H, Woodworth C, et al: Detection of human herpesvirus 6 and human papillomavirus 16 in cervical carcinoma. Am J Pathol 145:1509–1516, 1994.
14. Horvat R, Wood C, Balachandran N: Transactivation of human immunodeficiency virus promoter by human herpesvirus 6. J Virol 63:970–973, 1989.
15. Yoshikawa T, Suga S, Asano Y, et al: Neutralizing antibodies to human herpesvirus-6 in healthy individuals. Pediatr Infect Dis J 9:589–590, 1990.
16. Yanagi K, Harada S, Ban F, et al: High prevalence of antibody to human herpesvirus-6 and decrease in titer with age in Japan. J Infect Dis 161:153–154, 1990.
17. Asano Y, Yoshikawa T, Suga S, et al: Fatal fulminant hepatitis in an infant with human herpesvirus-6 infection. Lancet 335: 862–863, 1990.
18. Hall C, Long C, Schnable K, et al: Human herpes virus-6 infection in children. A prospective study of complications and reactivation. N Engl J Med 331:432–438, 1994.
19. Brown N, Sumaya C, Liu C, et al: Fall in human herpesvirus 6 seropositivity with age (Letter). Lancet 2:396, 1988.
20. Levy J, Ferro F, Greenspan D, et al: Frequent isolation of HHV-6 from saliva and high seroprevalence of the virus in the population. Lancet 335:1047–1050, 1990.
21. Kangro H, Osman H, Lau Y, et al: Seroprevalence of antibodies to human herpesviruses in England and Hong Kong. J Med Virol 43:91–96, 1994.
22. Harnett G, Farr T, Pietroboni G, et al: Frequent shedding of human herpesvirus 6 in saliva. J Med Virol 30:128–130, 1990.
23. Fox J, Briggs M, Ward P, et al: Human herpesvirus 6 in salivary glands. Lancet 336:590–593, 1990.
24. Mukai T, Yamamoto T, Kondo T, et al: Molecular epidemiological studies of human herpesvirus 6 in families. J Med Virol 42:224–227, 1994.
25. Cuende J, Ruiz J, Civeira M, et al: High prevalence of HHV-6 DNA in peripheral blood mononuclear cells of healthy individuals detected by nested-PCR. J Med Virol 43:115–118, 1994.
26. Luppi M, Barozzi P, Marasca R, et al: Human herpesvirus-6 (HHV-6) in blood donors. Br J Haematol 89:943–945, 1995.
27. Sayers M: Transfusion-transmitted viral infections other than hepatitis and human immunodeficiency virus infection. Cytomegalovirus, Epstein-Barr virus, human herpesvirus 6, and human parvovirus B19. Arch Pathol Lab Med 118:346–349, 1994.
28. Dunne W Jr, Jevon M: Examination of human breast milk for evidence of human herpesvirus 6 by polymerase chain reaction (Letter). J Infect Dis 168:250, 1993.
29. Ward K, Gray JJ, Efstathiou S: Brief report: Primary human herpesvirus 6 infection in a patient following liver transplantation from a seropositive donor. J Med Virol 28:69–72, 1989.

30. Okuno T, Higashi K, Shiraki K, et al: Human herpesvirus-6 infection in renal transplantation. Transplantation 49:519–522, 1990.
31. Dewhurst S, McIntyre K, Schnable K, et al: Human herpes 6 (HHV-6) variant B accounts for the majority of symptomatic primary HHV-6 infections in a population of U.S. infants. J Clin Microbiol 31:416–418, 1993.
32. DiLuca D, Dolcetti R, Mirandola P, et al: Human herpesvirus 6: A survey of presence and variant distribution in normal peripheral lymphocytes and lymphoproliferative disorders. J Infect Dis 170:211–215, 1994.
33. Drobski W, Eberle M, Majewski D, et al: Prevalence of human herpesvirus 6 variant A and B infections in bone marrow transplant recipients as determined by polymerase chain reaction and sequence-specific oligonucleotide probe hybridization. J Clin Microbiol 31:1515–1520, 1993.
34. Drobyski W, Dunne W, Burd E, et al: Human herpesvirus 6 (HHV-6) infection in allogeneic bone marrow transplant recipients: Evidence of a marrow suppressive role for HHV-6 in vivo. J Infect Dis 167:735–739, 1993.
35. Drobyski WR, Knox K, Majewski D, et al: Brief report: Fatal encephalitis due to variant B human herpesvirus-6 infection in a bone marrow transplant–recipient. N Engl J Med 330:1356–1360, 1994.
36. Shanavas K, Kala V, Vasudevan D, et al: Anti-HHV-6 antibodies in normal population and in cancer patients in India. J Exp Pathol 61:95–105, 1992.
37. Torelli G, Marasca R, Montorsi M, et al: Human herpesvirus 6 in non-AIDS related Hodgkin's and non-Hodgkin's lymphomas. Leukemia 6(Suppl 3):46S–48S, 1992.
38. Clark D, Alexander F, McKinney P, et al: The seroepidemiology of human herpesvirus-6 from a case-control of leukaemia and lymphoma. Int J Cancer 45:829–833, 1990.
39. Levine P, Ebbesen P, Ablashi D, et al: Antibodies to human herpes virus-6 and clinical course in patients with Hodgkin's disease. Int J Cancer 51:53–57, 1992.
40. Sumiyoshi Y, Kikuchi M, Ohshima K, et al: Analysis of human herpes virus-6 genomes in lymphoid malignancy in Japan. J Clin Pathol 46:1137–1138, 1993.
41. DiPaolo J, Popescu N, Ablashi D, et al: Multistage carcinogenesis utilizing human genital cells and human papillomaviruses. Toxicol Lett 72:7–11, 1994.
42. Yadav M, Chandrashekran A, Vasudevan D, et al: Frequent detection of human herpesvirus 6 in oral carcinoma. J Natl Cancer Inst 86:1792–1794, 1994.
43. Luppi M, Barozzi P, Maiorana A, et al: Human herpesvirus 6 infection in normal human brain tissue (Letter). J Infect Dis 169:943–944, 1994.
44. Roffman E, Frenkel N: Interleukin-2 inhibits the replication of human herpesvirus-6 in mature thymocytes. Virology 175:591–594, 1990.
45. Frenkel N, Schirmer E, Katsafanas G, et al: T-cell activation is required for efficient replication of human herpesvirus 6. J Virol 64:598–602, 1990.
46. Yoshikawa T, Suga S, Asano Y, et al: A prospective study of human herpesvirus-6 infection in renal transplantation. Transplantation 54:879–883, 1992.
47. Suga S, Yoshikawa T, Asano Y, et al: Activation of human herpesvirus-6 in children with acute measles. J Med Virol 38: 278–282, 1992.
48. Yoshikawa T, Suga S, Asano Y, et al: Human herpesvirus-6 infection in bone marrow transplantation. Blood 78:1381–1384, 1991.
49. Shiraki K, Okuno T, Yamanishi K, et al: Virion and nonstructural polypeptides of human herpesvirus-6. Virus Res 13:173–178, 1989.
50. Balachandran N, Amelse R, Zhou W, et al: Identification of proteins specific for human herpesvirus 6-infected human T cells. J Virol 63:2835–2840, 1989.
51. Littler E, Lawrence G, Liu M, et al: Identification, cloning, and expression of the major capsid protein gene of human herpesvirus 6. J Virol 64:714–722, 1990.
52. Yamamoto M, Black J, Stewart J, et al: Identification of a nucleocapsid protein as a specific serological marker of human herpesvirus 6 infection. J Clin Microbiol 28:1957–1962, 1990.
53. Asada H, Yalcin S, Balachandra K, et al: Establishment of titration system for human herpesvirus 6 and evaluation of neutralizing antibody response to the virus. J Clin Microbiol 27:2204–2207, 1989.
54. Asano Y, Yoshikawa T, Suga S, et al: Clinical features of infants with primary human herpesvirus 6 infection (exanthem subitum, roseola infantum). Pediatrics 93:104–108, 1994.
55. Pruksananonda P, Hall C, Insel R, et al: Primary human herpesvirus-6 infection in young children. N Engl J Med 326:1445–1450, 1992.
56. Suga S, Yoshikawa T, Asano Y, et al: Human herpesvirus-6 infection (exanthem subitum) without rash. Pediatrics 83:1003–1006, 1989.
57. Yoshiyama H, Suzuki E, Yoshida T, et al: Role of human herpesvirus 6 infection in infants with exanthema subitum. Pediatr Infect Dis J 9:71–74, 1990.
58. Suga S, Yoshikawa T, Asano Y, et al: Clinical and virological analyses of 21 infants with exanthem subitum (roseola infantum) and central nervous system complications. Ann Neurol 33:597–603, 1993.
59. Ward KN, Gray JJ: Primary human herpesvirus-6 infection is frequently overlooked as a cause of febrile fits in young children. J Med Virol 42:119–123, 1994.
60. Jones C, Dunn H, Thomas E, et al: Acute encephalopathy and status epilepticus associated with human herpes virus 6 infection. Dev Med Child Neurol 36:646–650, 1994.
61. Ishiguro N, Yamada S, Takahashi T, et al: Meningo-encephalitis associated with HHV-6 related exanthem subitum. Acta Paediatr Scand 79:987–989, 1990.
62. Kondo K, Hayakawa Y, Mori H, et al: Detection by polymerase chain reaction amplification of human herpesvirus 6 DNA in peripheral blood of patients with exanthem subitum. J Clin Microbiol 28:970–974, 1990.
63. Komura E, Hashida T, Otsuka T, et al: Human herpesvirus 6 and intussusception (Letter). Pediatr Infect Dis J 12:788–789, 1993.
64. Kitamura K, Ohta H, Ihara T, et al: Idiopathic thrombocytopenic purpura after human herpesvirus 6 infection (Letter). Lancet 344:830, 1994.
65. Asano Y, Yoshikawa T, Suga S, et al: Simultaneous occurrence of human herpesvirus 6 infection and intussusception in three infants. Pediatr Infect Dis J 10:335–357, 1991.
66. Yoshikawa T, Asano Y, Kobayashi I, et al: Exacerbation of idiopathic thrombocytopenic purpura by primary human herpesvirus 6 infection. Pediatr Infect Dis J 12:409–410, 1993.
67. Sumiyoshi Y, Askashi K, Kikuchi M: Detection of human herpes virus 6 in the skin of a patient with primary HHV 6 infection and erythroderma. J Clin Pathol 47:762–763, 1994.
68. Akashi K, Eizuru Y, Sumiyoshi Y, et al: Brief report: Severe infectious mononucleosis–like syndrome and primary human herpes virus 6 infection in an adult. N Engl J Med 329:168–171, 1993.
69. Sobue R, Miyazaki H, Okamoto M, et al: Fulminant hepatitis in primary human herpesvirus-6 infection (Letter). N Engl J Med 324:1290, 1991.
70. Read R, Larson E, Harvey J, et al: Clinical and laboratory findings in the Paul-Bunnell negative glandular fever–fatigue syndrome. J Clin Microbiol 21:157–165, 1990.
71. Goedhard J, Galama J, Wagenvoort J: Active human herpesvirus 6 in an adolescent male. Clin Infect Dis 20:1070–1071, 1995.
72. Niederman J, Liu C, Kaplan M, et al: Clinical and serological features of human herpesvirus-6 infection in three adults. Lancet 2:817–819, 1988.
73. Steeper T, Horwitz C, Ablashi D, et al: The spectrum of clinical and laboratory findings resulting from human herpesvirus-6 (HHV-6) in patients with mononucleosis-like illnesses not resulting from Epstein-Barr virus or cytomegalovirus. Am J Clin Pathol 93:776–783, 1990.
74. Yoshikawa T, Asano Y, Kojima S: Human herpesvirus-6 infection in bone marrow transplantation (Review). Leuk Lymphoma 8:65–73, 1992.
75. Asano Y, Yoshikawa T, Suga S, et al: Reactivation of herpesvirus type 6 in children receiving bone marrow transplants for leukemia (Letter). N Engl J Med 324:634–635, 1991.
76. Appleton A, Peiris J, Taylor C, et al: Human herpesvirus 6 DNA in skin biopsy tissue from marrow graft recipients with severe combined immunodeficiency. Lancet 344:1361–1362, 1994.
77. Michel D, Muller S, Worz S, et al: Human herpesvirus 6 DNA

in exanthematous skin in BMT patient (Letter). Lancet 344:686, 1994.
78. Carrigan D, Knox K: Human herpesvirus 6 isolation from bone marrow: HHV-6-associated bone marrow suppression in bone marrow transplant patients. Blood 84:3307–3310, 1994.
79. Wilborn F, Brinkmann V, Schmidt C, et al: Herpesvirus type 6 in patients undergoing bone marrow transplantation: Serologic features and detection by polymerase chain reaction. Blood 83:3052–3058, 1994.
80. Levy J, Landay A, Lennette E: Human herpesvirus 6 inhibits human immunodeficiency virus type 1 replication in cell culture. J Clin Microbiol 28:2362–2364, 1990.
81. Flamand L, Gosselin J, Stefanescu I, et al: Immunosuppressive effect of human herpesvirus 6 on T-cell functions: Suppression of interleukin-2 synthesis and cell proliferation. Blood 85:1263–1271, 1995.
82. Knox K, Carrigan D: Disseminated active HHV-6 infections in patients with AIDS. Lancet 343:577–578, 1994.
83. Corbellino M, Lusso P, Gallo RC, et al: Disseminated human herpesvirus 6 infection in AIDS (Letter). Lancet 342:1242, 1993.
84. Dolcetti R, Di Luca D, Mirandola P, et al: Frequent detection of human herpesvirus 6 DNA in HIV-associated lymphadenopathy (Letter). Lancet 344:543, 1994.
85. Robert C, Agut H, Aubin J, et al: Detection of antibodies to human herpesvirus-6 using immunofluorescence assay. Res Virol 141:545–555, 1990.
86. Cermelli C, Morori A, Montorsi M, et al: Comparison between immunofluorescence and enzyme-linked-immunosorbent assay in the determination of serum HHV-6 IgG. Microbiologica 17:69–73, 1994.
87. Asano Y, Yoshikawa T, Suga S, et al: Enzyme-linked immunosorbent assay for detection of IgG antibody to human herpesvirus 6. J Med Virol 32:119–123, 1990.
88. Agut H, Collandre H, Aubin J, et al: In vitro sensitivity of human herpesvirus-6 to antiviral drugs. Res Virol 140:219–228, 1989.
89. Agut H, Huraux JM, Collandre H, Montagnier L: Susceptibility of human herpesvirus 6 to acyclovir and ganciclovir (Letter). Lancet 2:626, 1989.
90. Burns W, Sandford G: Susceptibility of human herpesvirus 6 to antivirals in vitro. J Infect Dis 162:634–637, 1990.
91. Russler SK, Tapper MA, Carrigan DR: Susceptibility of human herpesvirus 6 to acyclovir and ganciclovir (Letter). Lancet 2:382, 1989.
92. DiLuca D, Katsafanas G, Schirmer E, et al: The replication of viral and cellular DNA in human herpesvirus 6-infected cells. Virology 175:199–210, 1990.
93. Kikuta H, Lu H, Matsumoto S: Susceptibility of human herpesvirus 6 to acyclovir. Lancet 2:861, 1989.
94. Kikuta H, Nakane A, Lu H, et al: Interferon induction by human herpesvirus 6 in human mononuclear cells. J Infect Dis 162:35–38, 1990.
95. Kovacs JA, Basder M, Dewar RJ, et al: Increases in CD4 T lymphocytes with intermittent courses of interleukin-2 in patients with human immunodeficiency virus infection. N Engl J Med 332:567–575, 1995.
96. Clark D, Freeland M, Mackie L, et al: Prevalence of antibody to human herpesvirus 7 by age (Letter). J Infect Dis 168:251–252, 1993.
97. Yoshikawa T, Asano Y, Kobayashi I, et al: Seroepidemiology of human herpesvirus 7 in healthy children and adults in Japan. J Med Virol 41:319–323, 1993.
98. Wyatt L, Rodriquez W, Balachandran N, et al: Human herpesvirus 7: Antigenic properties and prevalence in children and adults. J Virol 65:6260–6265, 1991.
99. Frenkel N, Schirmer E, Wyatt L, et al: Isolation of a new herpesvirus from human CD4+ T cells. Proc Natl Acad Sci USA 87:748–752, 1990.
100. Berneman Z, Ablashi D, Li G, et al: Human herpesvirus 7 is a T-lymphotropic virus and is related to, but significantly different from human herpesvirus 6 and human cytomegalovirus. Proc Natl Acad Sci USA 89:10552–10556, 1992.
101. Wyatt L, Frenkel N: Human herpesvirus 7 is a constitutive inhabitant of adult human saliva. J Virol 66:3206–3209, 1992.
102. Ueda K, Kusuhara K, Okada K, et al: Primary human herpesvirus 7 infection and exanthema subitum (Letter). Pediatr Infect Dis J 13:167–168, 1994.
103. Hidaka Y, Liu Y, Yamamoto M, et al: Frequent isolation of human herpesvirus 7 from saliva samples. J Med Virol 40:343–346, 1993.
104. DiLuca D, Mirandola P, Ravaioli T, et al: Human herpesviruses 6 and 7 in salivary glands and shedding in saliva of healthy and human immunodeficiency virus positive individuals. J Med Virol 45:462–468, 1995.
105. Tanaka K, Kondo T, Toriogoe S, et al: Human herpesvirus 7: Another causal agent for roseola (exanthem subitum). J Pediatr 125:1–5, 1994.
106. Asano Y, Suga S, Yoshikawa T, et al: Clinical features and viral excretion in an infant with primary human herpesvirus 7 infection. Pediatrics 95:187–190, 1995.
107. Cesarman E, Chang Y, Moore PS, et al: Kaposi's sarcoma–associated herpesvirus-like DNA sequences in AIDS-related body-cavity–based lymphomas. N Engl J Med 332:1186–1191, 1995.
108. Moore PS, Chang Y: Detection of herpesvirus-like DNA sequences in Kaposi's sarcoma patients with and without HIV infection. N Engl J Med 332:1181–1185, 1995.
109. Chang Y, Cesarman E, Pessin M, et al: Identification of herpesvirus-like DNA sequences in AIDS-associated Kaposi's sarcoma. Science 266:1865–1869, 1994.

242

Epstein-Barr Virus

Kenneth M. Kaye
Elliott Kieff

Classification

Epstein-Barr virus (EBV) specifically infects lymphocytes and is therefore classified as a gammaherpesvirus.[1] In another nomenclature, EBV was renamed human herpesvirus 4, although the term EBV is most widely used. Humans serve as the only natural host for EBV.

Virus Structure

The structure of EBV virions is similar to that of other herpesviruses. EBV has a protein core surrounded with DNA and a nucleocapsid surrounded by a protein tegument. This structure is surrounded by an envelope, which is surrounded by an outer envelope that has glycoprotein spikes. Unlike most herpesviruses, EBV has one predominant glycoprotein in the outer envelope.[1–9] The most abundant EBV envelope and tegument proteins (350/220 and 152 kDa, respectively) differ in size from major envelope and tegument proteins of herpes simplex virus type 1 (HSV-1).[2, 3, 10–16] However, similar to HSV-1, the sizes of the major EBV capsid proteins are 160, 47, and 28 kDa.[2, 3]

Genome

The 172-kb EBV genome is rich in guanine and cytosine, which compose 60% of the genome.[17–26] The EBV genome contains 0.5-kb terminal direct repeats[21, 27, 28] and four internal repeat elements.[19, 20, 29–31] The internal repeat elements divide the genome into unique sequence domains termed U1 to U5

(Fig. 242–1). The terminal repeats fuse the genome into a circular episome in latently infected cells. The terminal repeats are often used to study EBV clonality because an EBV strain tends to maintain a constant number of terminal repeat elements in latently infected cells,[32–35] and different isolates of EBV often differ in their number of terminal repeat elements. The number of repeat elements is easily tested by Southern blot analysis, which tests the size of the DNA fragment containing the terminal repeat elements after restriction endonuclease digestion of sites flanking the fused terminal repeats in EBV from latently infected cells. The presence of more than one size of restriction fragment indicates the presence of more than one isolate. However, the presence of only one restriction fragment indicates that the infected cells are likely to be clonal in nature, arising from one infected cell.[36, 37] Burkitt lymphoma and nasopharyngeal tumors are often monoclonal in nature.[32, 35]

EBV was the first herpesvirus to be cloned and sequenced.[18] Because the *Bam*HI restriction enzyme was used to generate the initial library that was sequenced, EBV open reading frames are frequently referred to by their *Bam*HI fragments.[17, 38] Thus, the EBV DNA polymerase gene is frequently referred to as *BALF3* (*Bam*HI A fragment, leftward open reading frame number 3). The DNA of the initially cloned strain (termed B95-8) contains a deletion when it is compared with other wild-type EBV sequences.[39] Several EBV clone libraries are now available.[39–44] When other herpesviruses were later sequenced, regions of homology with EBV were noted despite large differences in base composition (43% guanine plus cytosine for varicella-zoster virus; 71% guanine plus cytosine for HSV.[17, 45–55] These regions encode genes involved in lytic replication. However, despite some similarity, there are significant differences between homologous domains of the herpesviruses. For instance, EBV DNA fails to cross-hybridize to homologous HSV, varicella-zoster virus, or cytomegalovirus DNA. Also, antigenic cross-reactivity is extremely limited between EBV and other human herpesvirus proteins.

In contrast to most genes expressed in lytic infection, EBV latent genes have no homology to other herpesvirus genes but instead in some cases are related to cellular genes, from which they may have arisen. This evidence is strongest for EBV nuclear antigen-1 (EBNA-1). Monoclonal antibodies directed against the glycine-alanine repeat element in EBNA-1 cross-react with cell protein,[56] and there are two known cellular proteins that specifically bind the same DNA sequence that EBNA-1 binds.[57] Some lytic infection genes are also related to cellular genes. For instance, the EBV immediate early gene *BZLF1* is related to the *jun-fos* transcriptional activators.[58] Also, the early lytic gene *BHRF1* is homologous to the *bcl*-2 protooncogene, which inhibits cellular apoptosis.[59, 60] The late lytic gene *BCRF1* is homologous to human *IL10*.[61, 62]

There are two EBV types, termed type 1 and type 2, that differ significantly only in nuclear genes that are expressed in latent infection.[23, 24, 33, 34, 63–76] Specifically, differences are found in EBNA–leader protein (LP), EBNA-2, EBNA-3A, EBNA-3B, and EBNA-3C. The type 1 and 2 genes for EBNA-2, EBNA-3A, EBNA-3B, and EBNA-3C differ in amino acid sequence by 47%, 16%, 20%, and 28%, respectively.[63, 64, 69]

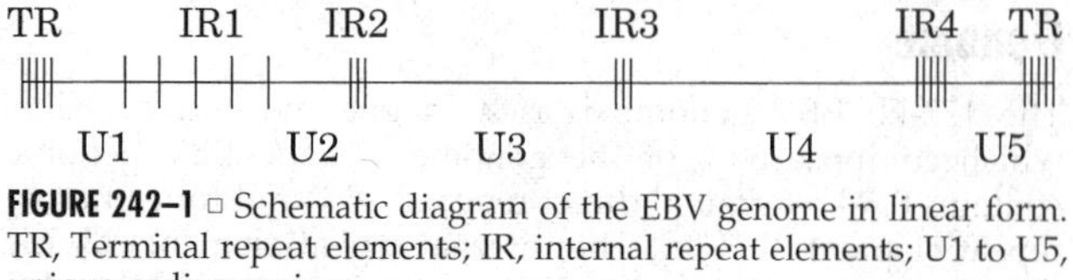

FIGURE 242–1 ▫ Schematic diagram of the EBV genome in linear form. TR, Terminal repeat elements; IR, internal repeat elements; U1 to U5, unique coding regions.

EBNA-LP differs by even less.[64, 77] In contrast, the integral membrane proteins expressed in latent infection, latent infection membrane protein (LMP)–1 or LMP-2, differ little between types 1 and 2.[36, 78, 79] Overall, the differences between EBV types 1 and 2 are significantly less than the differences between HSV types 1 and 2.[18, 24, 25, 33, 34, 39, 42, 74, 80–82] EBV type 1 appears to be more common in the Western world, whereas both types 1 and 2 are prevalent in Africa.[68, 72–74] In fact, almost half of African patients with Burkitt lymphoma are latently infected with EBV type 2. In the Western world, EBV type 2 DNA is frequently detected in oropharyngeal secretions; type 1 EBV is usually recovered from peripheral blood lymphocytes.[70, 72–74, 83]

Virus Infection

Adsorption, Penetration, Uncoating, and Early Intracellular Events in Infection

The B-cell receptor for EBV is the type 2 complement receptor (CR2), which is usually referred to as CD21.[1, 14, 84–87] The EBV envelope glycoprotein, gp350/220, binds to CD21 with an affinity of 1.2×10^{-8} M.[88–91] Of note, the gp350/220 amino acid sequence EDPGFFNVEI is similar to the sequence EDPGKQLYNVEA through which the C3d component of complement binds to CD21.[89, 90, 92] The messenger RNA for gp220 is a spliced variant of gp350.[93–95] CD21 may also be the EBV receptor on epithelial cells. CD21 is expressed at low levels in an epithelial cell line[96] and has been detected in nasopharyngeal carcinoma cells.[97] However, CD21 has not yet been demonstrated to serve as the EBV receptor on normal epithelial cells.

After adsorbing to the B cell by CD21, EBV causes CD21 and surface immunoglobulin to aggregate in the plasma membrane. This is followed by internalization of virus into cytoplasmic vesicles,[90, 98, 99] which then fuse with the virus envelope, releasing EBV nucleocapsid and tegument into the cytoplasm. B cells can similarly process gp350/220 coated beads into the cytoplasm. Although it is possible that gp350/220 is involved in the fusion of the virus envelope with the vesicle,[90, 93] it is more likely that gp85 directs fusion of the EBV envelope with the vesicle. Gp85 is homologous to the HSV-1 gH gene, which is important in HSV-1 envelope and cell membrane fusion,[100–102] and monoclonal antibodies to gp85 inhibit fusion of the EBV envelope and cell membranes.[103]

Compared with the better studied herpesviruses, much remains to be discovered regarding EBV capsid dissolution or DNA transport to the nucleus. By 16 hours after infection in B lymphocytes, the EBV genome circularizes.[104, 105] Cellular factors may then determine whether latent or lytic infection follows. Although transfection of HSV, varicella-zoster virus, or cytomegalovirus DNA into cells results in lytic replication, similar experiments with EBV DNA have not produced either lytic or latent infection.[106–109]

Lytic Epstein-Barr Virus Infection

EBV infection of B cells usually results in latent infection. Therefore, lytic EBV infection is primarily studied under artificial conditions with inducers of lytic virus replication.[110–116] Phorbol esters (such as 12-*O*-tetradecanoylphorbol-13-acetate) are often used to induce lytic infection and probably induce replication through protein kinase C activation of *jun-fos* transactivation through AP-1 sites upstream of immediate early EBV genes such as BZLF1 and BRLF1.[38, 117–122] A latently infected B lymphoma cell line termed Akata can be induced for lytic EBV replication in 20% to 50% of cells by cross-linking surface immunoglobulin.[123–126] Surface immunoglobulin cross-linking induces activation of phospholipase C, which produces inositol 1,4,5-trisphosphate and diacylglycerol, leading to mobilization of free calcium that activates protein kinase C.[127–129] As for other herpesviruses, viral DNA is synthesized in the nucleus where nucleocapsids assemble and virus becomes enveloped by budding through the inner nuclear membrane while host cell protein synthesis is inhibited.[130] As in other herpesviruses, lytic genes are classified by the order of their expression.[38, 126] Immediate early genes are expressed earliest, and expression is independent of new protein synthesis. Early genes are expressed next, and expression is not altered by inhibition of viral DNA synthesis. Late genes are expressed last, and expression is markedly reduced if viral DNA synthesis is inhibited.

IMMEDIATE EARLY GENES

Because lytic EBV infection can be studied only by induction of replication in cells already latently infected with EBV, the definition of immediate early genes must be slightly altered from that for other herpesviruses because it is not possible to rule out effects due to EBV latent genes already being expressed. Induction of lytic replication in latently infected Akata cells in the presence of cycloheximide (which inhibits protein synthesis) results in expression of BZLF1 and BRLF1, which are therefore defined as immediate early genes.[126] Another immediate early gene is BI′LF4, which has host cell–restricted transactivating effects.[131] BZLF1, BRLF1, and BI′LF4 each transactivate early EBV genes. Furthermore, transfection of BZLF1 under the control of a constitutively active promoter activates lytic EBV infection.[77, 132–135]

BRLF1 has been extensively studied. Its messenger RNA consists of three exons, each of which encodes a functional domain.[136, 137] The first exon (amino acids 1 to 167) encodes a transactivating domain.[138–140] The second exon (amino acids 168 to 202) encodes a basic domain homologous to a domain in the *fos-jun* transcription factor family[120] conferring the ability of BRLF1 to interact with AP-1 DNA sites[137, 141, 142] and also targets BRLF1 to the nucleus.[143] The third exon (amino acids 203 to 245) encodes a coiled coil leucine or isoleucine repeat capable of dimer formation.[120, 121, 137, 140, 141, 144–146] BRLF1 is phosphorylated on serine 336, possibly regulating its DNA binding activity.[127, 147] BRLF1 may also associate with the cellular protein p53 and possibly inhibits p53-mediated apoptosis in cells infected with EBV.[148] BRLF1 binds specifically to DNA and has distant homology to the cellular c-*myb* gene.[149, 150] Amino acids 520 to 605 contain a potent acidic transactivating domain.

EARLY GENES

EBV early genes are differentiated from late genes by persistent synthesis despite the presence of DNA synthesis inhibitors. At least 30 EBV early genes and almost 30 EBV late genes have been described throughout the EBV genome.[17, 38, 94, 119, 151–158] The functions of these genes have largely been postulated on the basis of homology to other herpesvirus genes that have previously been described. In many instances, these postulated functions have been confirmed experimentally. The BALF2 protein[159] is homologous to the HSV DNA binding protein ICP8 and is important in DNA replication.[160] BHRF1, another EBV early gene,[60] is homologous to the cellular protooncogene *bcl*-2, which inhibits cell apoptotic death. The role of BHRF1 is probably to prevent apoptotic cell death during lytic infection, thus allowing production of infectious virions. Other EBV early genes include several linked to DNA replication, including BALF5, the DNA polymerase; BALF2, the major DNA binding protein; BORF2 and BARF1, ribonucleotide reductase; BXLF1, thymidine kinase; and BGLF5, alkaline exonuclease.

LATE GENES

EBV late genes serve as structural proteins or are involved in virus envelopment or budding from the cell. Late genes encoding nonglycoproteins include BCLF1, probably the major nucleocapsid protein that is homologous to the major HSV capsid protein[50]; BNRF1, the major virion external nonglycoprotein and probably a tegument protein[161]; and BXRF1, a basic core protein that is homologous to the varicella-zoster virus basic virion core protein.[46, 47, 162]

Late genes encoding glycoproteins include BLLF1 (gp350/220), BALF4 (gp110), BXLF2 (gp85), ILF2 (gp55/80), and BDLF3 (gp42).[93, 101, 107, 163–167] BALF4 is homologous to HSV-1 gB, a major virus glycoprotein.[55, 163, 168] BLLF1 and BXLF2 are found on virus and in the plasma membrane of lytically infected cells.[2, 3, 16, 93, 101, 163, 164, 166, 169–173]

The EBV late gene BCRF1 is homologous to the cellular IL10 gene.[174, 175] Although IL10 can stimulate B-cell growth,[62] BCRF1 has no obvious effect on the ability of EBV to transform B lymphocytes because EBV mutants null for BCRF1 expression can fully transform B lymphocytes in vitro.[176] Instead, BCRF1 may function during lytic EBV infection in vivo as a negative regulator of cytotoxic T lymphocytes.[62] BCRF1 may blunt release of interferon-γ; the initiation of B-cell growth transformation is sensitive to interferon.[176, 177]

Latent Infection

EBV infection of B lymphocytes usually results in latent infection. At least 11 EBV genes are expressed in latent infection, which work in concert to growth transform B lymphocytes into immortalized lymphoblastoid cell lines in vitro. These genes include two small, non-polyadenylated RNAs (EBER-1 and EBER-2), six nuclear proteins (EBNA-1, EBNA-2, EBNA-3A, EBNA-3B, EBNA-3C, and EBNA-LP), and three integral membrane proteins (LMP-1, LMP-2A, and LMP-2B). Some authors use different nomenclatures for EBNA-3A, EBNA-3B, and EBNA-3C and for LMP-2A and LMP-2B, referring to EBNA-3B and EBNA-3C as EBNA-4, EBNA-5, or EBNA-6 (depending on the author) and LMP-2A and LMP-2B as TP-1 and TP-2.[178, 179]

EBNA-LP is encoded within the leader sequence of EBNA messenger RNAs. The IR1 EBV repeat (see Fig. 242–1) consists of alternating W1 and W2 sequences and encodes EBNA-LP exons. Because the number of IR1 repeat elements differs between EBV isolates, the size of EBNA-LP varies among isolates.[136, 180, 181] EBNA-LP is expressed throughout the cell nucleus but is also concentrated in small nuclear granules.[181, 182] Genetic analysis of EBNA-LP in recombinant EBV has demonstrated that deletion of the last two exons results in reduction in transformed cell outgrowth after plating in soft agarose.[183] Other experiments with similar mutated EBNA-LP recombinants have required fibroblast feeder layers to support the outgrowth of transformed B lymphoblastoid cell lines.[184] In experiments, expression of EBNA-LP and EBNA-2 in B cells costimulated with gp350 induced G_0 to G_1 cell cycle transition.[185] It has been reported that there is an association of EBNA-LP with the Rb and p53 cell genes.[186, 187] Expression of EBNA-LP in transgenic mice caused animals to die of heart failure through an unclear mechanism.[188]

The EBNA-2 gene is essential for EBV-induced growth transformation of B lymphocytes. Experiments demonstrating this finding took advantage of an EBV mutant termed P3HR-1,[123] which is not competent for transformation but is carried in continuous cell culture in a latently infected

B lymphoma cell line.[189, 190] P3HR-1 is deleted for EBNA-2 and the last two exons of EBNA-LP.[65, 180, 181, 191–193] When wild-type EBV DNA that spans the deletion is transfected into P3HR-1 cells and lytic infection is induced, 1 in 10^5 progeny virus is restored for the deleted DNA by homologous recombination, and these progeny are then competent to growth transform primary B lymphocytes.[183, 194]

EBNA-2 localizes to the cell nucleus within large nuclear granules[182, 193] and serves to transactivate cell and viral genes. EBNA-2 induces expression of CD23,[195] CD21,[196] *c-fgr*,[197] LMP-1,[198–203] and LMP-2[204, 205] (Fig. 242–2). Recombinant molecular genetic analyses of EBNA-2 demonstrate that three regions are required for B-cell transformation and that at least two of these regions are critical for transactivation activity. Of the 484 EBNA-2 amino acids, essential regions include amino acids 95 to 110, 280 to 337, and 425 to 462. Amino acids 425 to 462 have acidic transactivating characteristics, and amino acids 280 to 337 interact with DNA sequence-specific binding proteins that bring EBNA-2 in proximity to its response elements. However, the role of amino acids 95 to 110 is unclear. The EBNA-2 acidic transactivating domain (amino acids 425 to 462) is similar to the prototype HSV VP16 acidic domain.[206–208] Both the EBNA-2 and VP16 acidic domains have affinity for transcription factors TFIIB, TAF40, TFIIH, and RPA70[209] and probably recruit TFIIB, TAF40, and TFIIH to responsive promoters.

EBNA-2 associates with DNA by binding to the J kappa (Jκ) recombination signal sequence binding protein,[210–212] which binds to the consensus GTGGGAA Jκ recognition site in DNA. Jκ probably serves as an adapter protein in cells to recruit regulatory proteins. However, Jκ interaction with EBNA-2 accounts for only part of EBNA-2 transactivation of LMP-1 because mutation of EBNA-2 amino acids W319W320 that interact with Jκ reduces EBNA-2 responsiveness only 50%. PU.1 is another cellular DNA binding protein important for EBNA-2 transactivation of the LMP-1 promoter because mutation of the PU.1 DNA binding site reduces EBNA-2 function even more than mutating the Jκ binding site. Therefore, EBNA-2 is probably recruited to responsive promoters by Jκ or PU.1 and then recruits the basal transcription factors TFIIB, TAF40, and TFIIH, resulting in transcriptional activation.[213]

The EBNA-3A, EBNA-3B, and EBNA-3C genes encode proteins of 944, 938, and 992 amino acids, respectively, and are located consecutively in the EBV genome.[69, 214–222] Each gene consists of two exons and a short intron and has repeat

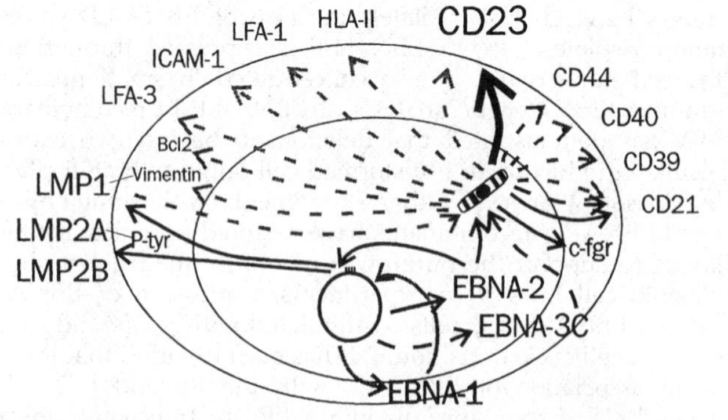

FIGURE 242–2 □ Induction of cellular and viral genes by EBV latent gene products. EBNA-2 induces expression of CD21, CD23, *c-fgr*, and LMP. EBNA-3C induces expression of CD21. LMP-1 induces expression of the cytoskeletal protein vimentin, ICAM-1, LFA-1, LFA-3, *bcl*-2, HLA-II, CD21, CD23, CD39, CD40, and CD44. (From Kieff E: Epstein-Barr virus and its replication. *In* Fields BN, Knipe DM, Howley PM [eds]: Fields Virology, ed 3. Philadelphia, Lippincott-Raven, 1996, pp 2343–2396.)

elements near the C-terminal.[214–217, 219–227] All the EBNA-3 genes encode hydrophilic proteins containing approximately 20% charged amino acids. Immunofluorescent microscopy demonstrates that the EBNA-3A, and EBNA-3B, and EBNA-3C proteins accumulate in B-cell nuclei, localizing to large clumps, but spare the nucleolus.[182, 214, 219, 220]

Analysis of the EBNA-3 genes in recombinant EBV has demonstrated that EBNA-3A and EBNA-3C are essential for EBV-mediated transformation of primary B lymphocytes but that EBNA-3B is dispensable for transformation. EBV recombinants that are null for EBNA-3A or EBNA-3C are not competent to transform primary B lymphocytes unless wild-type EBNA-3 gene is provided to the infected cell by means of a helper virus. In contrast, EBV recombinants that are null for EBNA-3B are fully competent to transform B lymphocytes in vitro.[228, 229] EBNA-3C induces expression of cellular CD21 (see Fig. 242–2). EBNA-3C competes with EBNA-2 for binding to the Jκ protein and modulates the ability of the Jκ–EBNA-2 complex to transactivate the LMP-1 promoter. Furthermore, when EBNA-3C binds to Jκ, it inhibits the ability of Jκ to bind to its consensus DNA binding sequence. Therefore, EBNA-3C probably plays an important role in down-modulating EBNA-2 transactivation in EBV-transformed B lymphocytes. EBNA-3A and EBNA-3B also bind to Jκ and inhibit its binding to DNA and are also likely to be involved in regulation of EBNA-2 transactivation.[230, 230a]

The EBNA-1 gene encodes 641 amino acids and binds specifically to a DNA partial palindrome.[210, 231–233] The EBNA-1 binding sequences are located at three different sites in EBV.[231, 232, 234] The site with highest EBNA-1 binding affinity is located at the left end of the EBV genome and contains 20 tandem direct 30 base pair repeats. The binding site with the next highest affinity contains two binding sequences in dyad symmetry and two in tandem and is located approximately 1 kb to the right of the first binding site within the EBV genome. The third binding site is located about 10 kb downstream of the EBNA-2 gene.[232] The first two EBNA-1 binding sites enable covalently closed circular DNA molecules to replicate as episomes in cells expressing EBNA-1 and are important for EBV maintenance in an episomal state in latently infected cells. For this reason, the DNA encoding these regions is referred to as *oriP* (plasmid DNA replication origin).[235–242]

LMP-1 is a dominant transforming gene expressed in latent EBV infection. LMP-1 is a 386–amino acid protein that consists of an N-terminal 25–amino acid cytoplasmic domain, six hydrophobic 20–amino acid transmembrane segments separated by five reverse turns, and a 200–amino acid cytoplasmic C-terminal. LMP-1 has no homology to known proteins.[243–245] When expressed in cells, LMP-1 constitutively forms patches that coalesce into caps in the plasma membrane, similar to activated growth factor receptors.[245, 246] LMP-1 has transforming effects when it is expressed in many different cell lines including rodent fibroblast cells.[247–250] In rodent fibroblast cell lines, LMP-1 causes cells to have altered morphologic features, allows cells to grow in medium with low serum, and causes cells to lose contact inhibition so that they heap up on one another.[250] LMP-1 also induces loss of anchorage dependence so that cells are able to grow as colonies in soft agar.[247, 249, 250] In addition, LMP-1 causes Rat-1 fibroblast cells to be tumorigenic in nude mice.[250] Expression of LMP-1 in EBV-negative B lymphoma cells[251–259] induces many of the changes seen when EBV transforms primary B lymphocytes. These include cell clumping, increased villous projections, and increased cell surface expression of B-cell activation markers and adhesion molecules such as CD23, CD39, CD40, CD44, human leukocyte antigen (HLA) class II, lymphocyte function–associated antigen (LFA)–1, intercellular adhesion molecule (ICAM)–1, and LFA-3 (see Fig. 242–2).

LMP-1 also protects B cells from apoptosis[256, 260, 261] through induction of expression of the cellular *bcl*-2 protooncogene.[256, 261, 262] LMP-1 induces the zinc finger protein A20, which protects cells from tumor necrosis factor-α toxicity.[263] LMP-1 also induces nuclear factor-κB to translocate to the nucleus.[263, 264] When expressed in epithelial cells, LMP-1 causes cells to have altered morphologic features and blocks terminal differentiation in a cell line that can be induced to differentiate.[265–269] Mice transgenic for LMP-1 have epidermal hyperplasia and altered expression of keratin.[268]

Analysis of LMP-1 in recombinant EBV has demonstrated that LMP-1 is essential for EBV-mediated primary B lymphocyte growth transformation.[270–272] Further genetic analysis in recombinant virus has demonstrated that the short cytoplasmic N-terminal is not essential for transformation and probably serves to anchor the first LMP-1 transmembrane domain.[270] In contrast, the C-terminal cytoplasmic domain is essential for LMP-1 function because EBV recombinants lacking this domain are not competent to transform primary B lymphocytes. Further analysis of the C-terminal domain demonstrated that deletion of all but the first 44 amino acids of the C-terminal results in the ability to transform primary B lymphocytes, but with a diminished capacity.[272] Thus, there appear to be at least two functional components within the C-terminal, one located within the first 44 amino acids of the C-terminal and one within the rest of the C-terminal. The first 44 amino acids of the LMP-1 cytoplasmic C-terminal interact with cellular factors termed TRAFs (tumor necrosis factor receptor–associated factors).[273, 273a, 273b] TRAFs also interact with the cellular receptor CD40, which, when stimulated, causes B-cell activating effects, many of which are similar to the ones that LMP-1 causes.[274–276] It is possible that LMP-1 mimics a constitutively stimulated CD40 receptor[277] (Fig. 242–3).

Except for their first exons, LMP-2A and LMP-2B are identical. The first exon of LMP-2A encodes a 119-residue N-terminal cytoplasmic domain in contrast to the first exon of LMP-2B, which is much shorter.[278, 279] Otherwise, LMP-2A and LMP-2B both have 12 hydrophobic integral membrane sequences separated by short reverse turns and a short 27-residue cytoplasmic C-terminal domain. In cells, LMP-2 colocalizes with LMP-1 in plasma membrane patches.[280, 281] LMP-2A and LMP-2B are dispensable for EBV-mediated B-cell transformation because recombinant EBV null for these genes is fully competent to transform primary B cells in vitro.[281–284]

LMP-2A is a substrate for Src family tyrosine kinases and associates with Src family kinases including Syk, Fyn, and Lyn.[280, 285] LMP-2 blocks the calcium flux normally seen after cross-linking surface immunoglobulin M or class II major histocompatibility complex antigens in B cells.[286] It is possible that LMP-2 interaction with Src family kinases inhibits the ability of these kinases to participate in signal transduction pathways that normally result in calcium mobilization. This LMP-2 effect may have important consequences in vivo because blocking calcium flux results in blocking a switch from latent to lytic EBV infection.[286–288] Prevention of a switch to lytic infection in cells that have their B-cell receptors activated would prevent antibody neutralization of infectious virions as well as a cytotoxic T-cell response to newly infected cells.

EBER-1 and EBER-2 are small non-polyadenylated RNAs that are abundantly expressed in EBV latent infection.[289–292] EBERs localize to the B-cell nucleus and form complexes with cellular La protein.[291, 293] Many patients with systemic lupus erythematosus have autoantibodies directed against the La protein. EBER-1 and EBER-2 have homology to the adenovirus VA1 and VA2 genes and also to cell U6 small RNAs.[294, 295] EBER-1 and EBER-2 are dispensable for EBV-mediated B-lymphocyte transformation because EBV recombinants deleted for the EBER genes are fully competent to growth transform primary B cells.[296] However, it is possible that the EBERs play an important role in EBV infection in vivo. Owing to their high abundance in the nuclei of latently infected cells, EBERs have served as useful markers in hybridization assays looking for evidence of EBV infection in tumors.

Epstein-Barr Virus Recombinant Genetics

EBV recombinant genetics has lagged behind recombinant genetics of other herpesviruses because of the limitation of

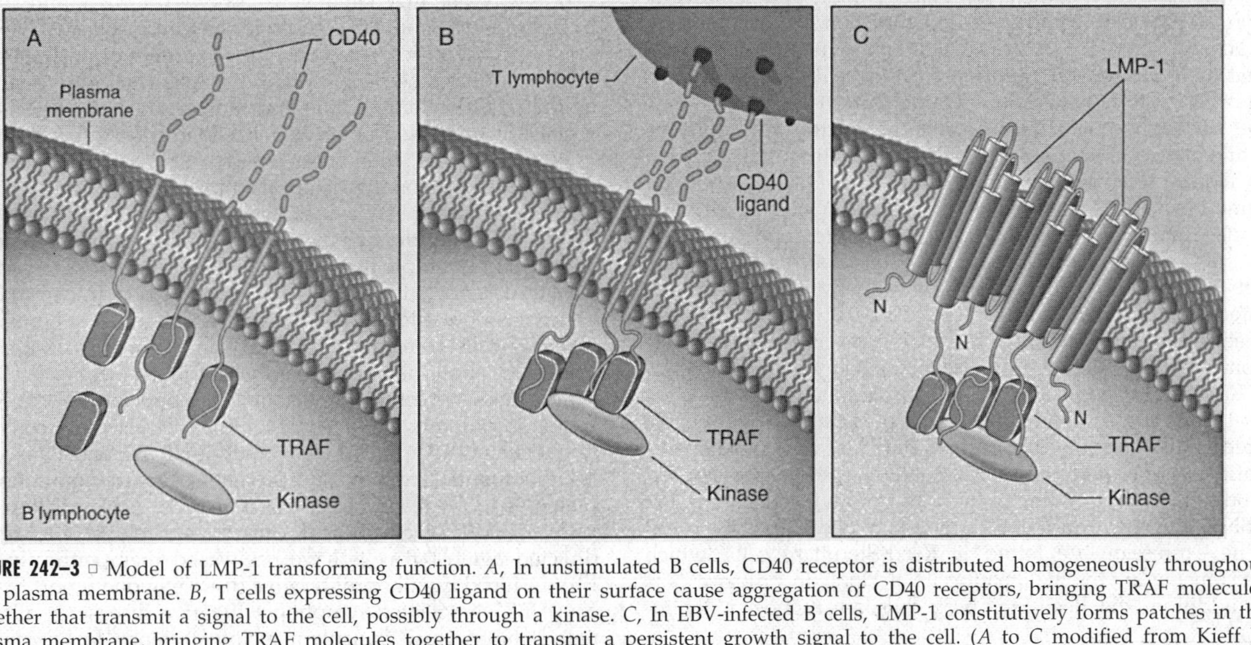

FIGURE 242–3 □ Model of LMP-1 transforming function. *A*, In unstimulated B cells, CD40 receptor is distributed homogeneously throughout the plasma membrane. *B*, T cells expressing CD40 ligand on their surface cause aggregation of CD40 receptors, bringing TRAF molecules together that transmit a signal to the cell, possibly through a kinase. *C*, In EBV-infected B cells, LMP-1 constitutively forms patches in the plasma membrane, bringing TRAF molecules together to transmit a persistent growth signal to the cell. (*A* to *C* modified from Kieff E: Epstein-Barr virus—Increasing evidence of a link to carcinoma. N Engl J Med 333:724–726, 1995. Reprinted by permission of The New England Journal of Medicine. Copyright 1995, Massachusetts Medical Society.)

in vitro EBV infection to human B lymphocytes and the nonpermissivity of these cells for EBV replication. However, in the past several years, an experimental system has bypassed these difficulties, allowing generation of recombinant EBV. This system uses a B lymphoma cell line that is latently infected with a strain of EBV termed P3HR-1, which is competent for lytic replication but incompetent for primary B-cell transformation because of deletion of DNA encoding the EBV latent genes EBNA-LP and EBNA-2. If wild-type EBNA-LP and EBNA-2 DNA is transfected into these cells and lytic virus replication is induced, some virus progeny will incorporate the wild-type DNA by homologous recombination and will be competent to transform primary B lymphocytes. If EBV DNA containing a specifically mutated gene is cotransfected with the wild-type EBNA-LP and EBNA-2 DNA and lytic replication is induced, some progeny virions will undergo two homologous recombination events, incorporating the wild-type EBNA-LP and EBNA-2 DNA and also the mutated EBV gene. This system therefore allows mutation of any EBV gene. Primary B lymphocytes are then infected with progeny virus to test recombinant virus for the ability to transform cells into continuous lymphoblastoid cell lines. Because primary B lymphocytes are dependent on EBV infection for immortalization in culture, mutations in essential transforming genes abolish the ability of EBV to immortalize B cells. Such virus will transform B cells only when the mutated gene is complemented by the wild-type gene provided by helper virus. This helper virus is the parental P3HR-1 that lacks EBNA-2 and EBNA-LP and therefore is incompetent to transform B lymphocytes by itself.*

Epstein-Barr Virus–Associated Malignant Neoplasms

EBV infection is associated with numerous human malignant neoplasms, which include endemic African Burkitt lymphoma, Hodgkin's disease, lymphoproliferative disease in immunocompromised hosts, and anaplastic nasopharyngeal carcinomas[307, 308, 308a] (Table 242–1). The associations of EBV and malignant neoplasms are based on high titers of anti-EBV antibodies in patients with these tumors and demonstration of EBV DNA and expressed EBV genes in tumor cells. Study of different EBV-associated tumors has demonstrated that there are several patterns of EBV latent gene expression in different tumor types. In endemic Burkitt lymphoma, only the EBNA-1 gene, which is responsible for EBV episome maintenance, is expressed.[309, 310] The Burkitt tumors appear to require a second event in addition to EBV infection for tumorigenicity because they also have a characteristic chromosomal translocation involving the c-*myc* protooncogene.[311, 312] A study of African children demonstrated an association between children with higher EBV antibody titers after initial infection and later development of Burkitt lymphoma, suggesting that increased EBV replication during primary infection may be a risk factor for tumor development.[313, 314]

EBV is also associated with approximately 50% of cases of Hodgkin's disease, most commonly in nonlymphocyte predominant forms, in younger patients, and in Hispanic patients. The pattern of EBV latent gene expression in Hodgkin's disease differs from Burkitt lymphoma in that EBNA-1, LMP-1, and LMP-2 are expressed. EBV DNA and gene expression are found in Reed-Sternberg cells, which presumably are the malignant cells of Hodgkin's disease.[315, 316] In addition, the Reed-Sternberg cells are monoclonally infected with EBV, indicating that EBV infection occurred before the onset of tumor formation.[315, 317, 318]

*References 176, 183, 184, 194, 208, 228, 229, 270–272, 281, 283, 284, 296–306.

TABLE 242–1 ■ Epstein-Barr Virus–Associated Malignancies

MALIGNANT NEOPLASM	EPSTEIN-BARR VIRUS ASSOCIATED (%)	EPSTEIN-BARR VIRUS LATENT ANTIGENS EXPRESSED*
African (endemic) Burkitt lymphoma	100	EBNA-1
Hodgkin's disease	50	EBNA-1, LMP-1, LMP-2
Lymphoproliferative disease (immunocompromised hosts)	100	EBNA-1, EBNA-2, EBNA-3A, EBNA-3B, EBNA-3C, EBNA-LP, LMP-1, LMP-2
Nasopharyngeal carcinoma	100	EBNA-1, LMP-1 +/−, LMP-2

*EBNA, Epstein-Barr virus nuclear antigen; LP, leader protein; LMP, latent infection membrane protein.

Adapted from Rickinson AB, Kieff E: Epstein-Barr virus. *In* Fields B, Knipe D, Howley P (eds): Fields Virology, ed 3. Philadelphia, Lippincott-Raven, 1996, pp 2397–2446.

The most common EBV-associated malignant neoplasm is anaplastic nasopharyngeal carcinoma, which is among the most common malignant neoplasms in southern China and in Aleuts.[319–322] It is likely that host genetic factors play a role in development of nasopharyngeal carcinoma. Initial evidence for the association of EBV and nasopharyngeal carcinoma was provided by the demonstration that patients with nasopharyngeal carcinoma had higher titers of EBV antibodies than did control subjects.[323, 324] More recently, immunoglobulin A antibodies to EBV replication proteins have been used to screen high-risk populations for nasopharyngeal carcinoma development and also to monitor responses to therapy for nasopharyngeal carcinoma.[325–327] In addition to an association between EBV antibodies and nasopharyngeal carcinoma, EBV latent infection of tumor cells has been demonstrated by the presence of EBV DNA and EBV latent gene expression. The EBV latent genes EBNA-1, LMP-1, and LMP-2 are most commonly expressed in the tumor cells.[328–331] LMP-1 may play a critical role in the development of nasopharyngeal carcinoma because LMP-1 has been shown to affect epithelial cell differentiation and morphologic characteristics when it is expressed in epithelial cells in culture.[331a, 331b, 331c]

When patients with either solid organ or bone marrow transplants develop lymphoproliferative disease, the tumors are almost always EBV associated and contain EBV DNA.[332–335] EBV is probably the driving tumorigenic force in these cells, and the full complement of EBV latent genes expressed in EBV-transformed B cells in vitro is expressed in the malignant cells. The tumor cells also have phenotypes similar to those of cells transformed by EBV in vitro, expressing the same activation markers and adhesion molecules.[336–338] These tumors may be either oligoclonal or monoclonal.[339, 340] EBV lymphoproliferative disease tends to be refractory to conventional chemotherapy and also to acyclovir. The most successful therapeutic strategy in recipients of solid organ transplants is to decrease immunosuppressive therapy, allowing recovery of host cytotoxic T cells.[341] Monoclonal antibodies directed against B cells have been used therapeutically for EBV-induced lymphoproliferative disease in one report.[342] Because EBV-associated lymphoproliferative disease in allogeneic bone marrow transplant recipients tends to be caused by the donor's B cells, strategies have included infusing donor white blood cells into affected patients. The donor leukocytes include T cells that are sensitized to EBV and therefore attack tumor cells that express EBV antigens.[343]

Individuals with acquired immunodeficiency syndrome tend to develop non-Hodgkin's lymphoma in late stages of disease when there is significant immunosuppression.[344] The most common of these lymphomas is histologically classified as immunoblastic, and 80% of these are EBV associated.[345, 346] EBV-associated lymphomas involving the central nervous system are common and are often immunoblastic.[347, 348] The immunoblastic lymphomas commonly express the full complement of EBV latent genes, similar to lymphoproliferative disease in transplant recipients.[346] A second pattern of latent gene expression seen in immunoblastic lymphomas consists of expression of LMP-1, LMP-2, and EBNA-1.

References

1. Kieff E: Epstein-Barr virus and its replication. *In* Fields BN, Knipe DM, Howley PM (eds): Fields Virology, ed 3. Philadelphia, Lippincott-Raven, 1996, pp 2343–2396.
2. Dolyniuk M, Pritchett R, Kieff E: Proteins of Epstein-Barr virus. I. Analysis of the polypeptides of purified enveloped Epstein-Barr virus. J Virol 17:935–949, 1976.
3. Dolyniuk M, Wolff E, Kieff E: Proteins of Epstein-Barr virus. II. Electrophoretic analysis of the polypeptides of the nucleocapsid and the glucosamine- and polysaccharide-containing components of enveloped virus. J Virol 18:289–297, 1976.
4. Epstein M, Achong B, Barr Y: Morphological and biological studies on a virus in cultured lymphoblasts from Burkitt's lymphoma. J Exp Med 121:761–770, 1965.
5. Epstein M, Achong B, Barr Y: Virus particles in cultured lymphoblasts from Burkitt's lymphoma. Lancet 1:702–703, 1964.
6. Pope JH, Achong BG, Epstein MA: Cultivation and fine structure of virus-bearing lymphoblasts from a second New Guinea Burkitt lymphoma: Establishment of sublines with unusual cultural properties. Int J Cancer 3:171–182, 1968.
7. Epstein MA, Achong BG: Discovery and general biology of the virus. *In* Epstein M, Achong B (eds): The Epstein-Barr Virus. Berlin, Springer-Verlag, 1979, pp 1–22.
8. Epstein M, Achong B: The Epstein-Barr Virus: Recent Advances. London, William Heinemann, 1986.
9. Epstein M, Achong B: The Epstein Barr virus. Annu Rev Microbiol 27:413–436, 1973.
10. Mueller-Lantzsch N, Georg B, Yamamoto N, zur Hausen H: Epstein-Barr virus–induced proteins. II. Analysis of surface polypeptides from EBV-producing and -superinfected cells by immunoprecipitation. Virology 102:401–411, 1980.
11. Qualtiere LF, Pearson GR: Epstein-Barr virus–induced membrane antigens: Immunochemical characterization of Triton X-100 solubilized viral membrane antigens from EBV-superinfected Raji cells. Int J Cancer 23:808–817, 1979.
12. Qualtiere LF, Pearson GR: Radioimmune precipitation study comparing the Epstein-Barr virus membrane antigens expressed on P3HR-1 virus–superinfected Raji cells to those expressed on cells in a B-95 virus–transformed producer culture activated with tumor-promoting agent (TPA). Virology 102:360–369, 1980.
13. Taylor N, Countryman J, Rooney C, et al: Expression of the *BZLF1* latency-disrupting gene differs in standard and defective Epstein-Barr viruses. J Virol 63:1721–1728, 1989.
14. Tedder TF, Weis JJ, Clement LT, et al: The role of receptors for complement in the induction of polyclonal B-cell proliferation and differentiation. J Clin Immunol 6:65–73, 1986.
15. Thorley-Lawson DA: Characterization of cross-reacting antigens on the Epstein-Barr virus envelope and plasma membranes of producer cells. Cell 16:33–42, 1979.
16. Thorley-Lawson DA, Edson CM: Polypeptides of the Epstein-Barr virus membrane antigen complex. J Virol 32:458–467, 1979.
17. Baer R, Bankier AT, Biggin MD, et al: DNA sequence and expression of the B95-8 Epstein-Barr virus genome. Nature 310:207–211, 1984.
18. Dambaugh T, Beisel C, Hummel M, et al: Epstein-Barr virus (B95-8) DNA VII: Molecular cloning and detailed mapping. Proc Natl Acad Sci USA 77:2999–3003, 1980.
19. Given D, Kieff E: DNA of Epstein-Barr virus. VI. Mapping of the internal tandem reiteration. J Virol 31:315–324, 1979.
20. Given D, Kieff E: DNA of Epstein-Barr virus. IV. Linkage map of restriction enzyme fragments of the B95-8 and W91 strains of Epstein-Barr virus. J Virol 28:524–542, 1978.
21. Given D, Yee D, Griem K, Kieff E: DNA of Epstein-Barr virus. V. Direct repeats of the ends of Epstein-Barr virus DNA. J Virol 30:852–862, 1979.
22. Jehn U, Lindahl T, Klein C: Fate of virus DNA in the abortive infection of human lymphoid cell lines by Epstein-Barr virus. J Gen Virol 16:409–412, 1972.
23. Kawai Y, Nonoyama M, Pagano JS: Reassociation kinetics for Epstein-Barr virus DNA: Nonhomology to mammalian DNA and homology of viral DNA in various diseases. J Virol 12:1006–1012, 1973.
24. Pritchett R, Pendersen M, Kieff E: Complexity of EBV homologous DNA in continuous lymphoblastoid cell lines. Virology 74:227–231, 1976.
25. Pritchett RF, Hayward SD, Kieff ED: DNA of Epstein-Barr virus. I. Comparative studies of the DNA of Epstein-Barr virus from HR-1 and B95-8 cells: Size, structure, and relatedness. J Virol 15:556–559, 1975.
26. Wagner EK, Roizman B, Savage T, et al: Characterization of the DNA of herpesviruses associated with Lucke adenocarcinoma of the frog and Burkitt lymphoma of man. Virology 42:257–261, 1970.
27. Hayward SD, Kieff E: DNA of Epstein-Barr virus. II. Comparison of the molecular weights of restriction endonuclease fragments of the DNA of Epstein-Barr virus strains and identification of end fragments of the B95-8 strain. J Virol 23:421–429, 1977.
28. Kintner C, Sugden B: Identification of antigenic determinants unique to the surfaces of cells transformed by Epstein-Barr virus. Nature 294:458–460, 1981.
29. Cheung A, Kieff E: Epstein-Barr virus DNA. X. Direct repeat within the internal direct repeat of Epstein-Barr virus DNA. J Virol 40:501–507, 1981.
30. Cheung A, Kieff E: Long internal direct repeat in Epstein-Barr virus DNA. J Virol 44:286–294, 1982.
31. Hayward SD, Nogee L, Hayward GS: Organization of repeated regions within the Epstein-Barr virus DNA molecule. J Virol 33:507–521, 1980.
32. Brown NA, Liu C, Garcia CR, et al: Clonal origins of lymphoproliferative disease induced by Epstein-Barr virus. J Virol 58:975–978, 1986.
33. Dambaugh T, Raab-Traub N, Heller M, et al: Variations among isolates of Epstein-Barr virus. Ann N Y Acad Sci 354:309–325, 1980.
34. Heller M, Dambaugh T, Kieff E: Epstein-Barr virus DNA. IX. Variation among viral DNAs from producer and nonproducer infected cells. J Virol 38:632–648, 1981.
35. Raab-Traub N, Flynn K: The structure of the termini of the Epstein-Barr virus as a marker of clonal cellular proliferation. Cell 47:883–889, 1986.
36. Busson P, Zhang Q, Guillon JM, et al: Elevated expression of ICAM1 (CD54) and minimal expression of LFA3 (CD58) in Epstein-Barr-virus–positive nasopharyngeal carcinoma cells. Int J Cancer 50:863–867, 1992.
37. Spaete RR, Mocarski ES: The alpha sequence of the cytomegalovirus genome functions as a cleavage/packaging signal for herpes simplex virus defective genomes. J Virol 54:817–824, 1985.
38. Farrell PJ: Epstein-Barr virus. *In* O'Brien SJ (ed): Genetic Maps. Cold Spring Harbor, NY, Cold Spring Harbor Press, 1992, pp 120–133.
39. Raab-Traub N, Dambaugh T, Kieff E: DNA of Epstein-Barr virus VIII: B95-8, the previous prototype, is an unusual deletion derivative. Cell 22(pt 1):257–267, 1980.
40. Arrand JR, Rymo L, Walsh JE, et al: Molecular cloning of the complete Epstein-Barr virus genome as a set of overlapping restriction endonuclease fragments. Nucleic Acids Res 9:2999–3014, 1981.
41. Buell GN, Reisman D, Kintner C, et al: Cloning overlapping DNA fragments from the B95-8 strain of Epstein-Barr virus reveals a site of homology to the internal repetition. J Virol 40:977–982, 1981.
42. Fischer DK, Miller G, Gradoville L, et al: Genome of a mononu-

cleosis Epstein-Barr virus contains DNA fragments previously regarded to be unique to Burkitt's lymphoma isolates. Cell 24:543–553, 1981.
43. Polack A, Hartl G, Zimber U, et al: A complete set of overlapping cosmid clones of M-ABA virus derived from nasopharyngeal carcinoma and its similarity to other Epstein-Barr virus isolates. Gene 27:279–288, 1984.
44. Skare J, Strominger JL: Cloning and mapping of *Bam*HI endonuclease fragments of DNA from the transforming B95-8 strain of Epstein-Barr virus. Proc Natl Acad Sci USA 77:3860–3864, 1980.
45. Cho MS, Bornkamm GW, zur Hausen H: Structure of defective DNA molecules in Epstein-Barr virus preparations from P3HR-1 cells. J Virol 51:199–207, 1984.
46. Davison AJ, Scott JE: The complete DNA sequence of varicella-zoster virus. J Gen Virol 67(pt 9):1759–1816, 1986.
47. Davison AJ, Taylor P: Genetic relations between varicella-zoster virus and Epstein-Barr virus. J Gen Virol 68(pt 4):1067–1079, 1987.
48. Davison AJ, Wilkie NM: Nucleotide sequences of the joint between the L and S segments of herpes simplex virus types 1 and 2. J Gen Virol 55(pt 2):315–331, 1981.
49. Kouzarides T, Bankier AT, Satchwell SC, et al: Large-scale rearrangement of homologous regions in the genomes of HCMV and EBV. Virology 157:397–413, 1987.
50. McGeoch DJ, Dalrymple MA, Davison AJ, et al: The complete DNA sequence of the long unique region in the genome of herpes simplex virus type 1. J Gen Virol 69(pt 7):1531–1574, 1988.
51. Nicholas J, Cameron KR, Honess RW: *Herpesvirus saimiri* encodes homologues of G protein–coupled receptors and cyclins. Nature 355:362–365, 1992.
52. Nicholas J, Cameron KR, Coleman H, et al: Analysis of nucleotide sequence of the rightmost 43 kbp of *Herpesvirus saimiri* (HVS) L-DNA: General conservation of genetic organization between HVS and Epstein-Barr virus. Virology 188:296–310, 1992.
53. Cameron KR, Stamminger T, Craxton M, et al: The 160,000-M_r virion protein encoded at the right end of the *Herpesvirus saimiri* genome is homologous to the 140,000-M_r membrane antigen encoded at the left end of the Epstein-Barr virus genome. J Virol 61:2063–2070, 1987.
54. Costa RH, Draper KG, Kelly TJ, Wagner EK: An unusual spliced herpes simplex virus type 1 transcript with sequence homology to Epstein-Barr virus DNA. J Virol 54:317–328, 1985.
55. Pellett PE, Biggin MD, Barrell B, Roizman B: Epstein-Barr virus genome may encode a protein showing significant amino acid and predicted secondary structure homology with glycoprotein B of herpes simplex virus 1. J Virol 56:807–813, 1985.
56. Luka J, Kreofsky T, Pearson GR, et al: Partial purification and characterization of a cellular protein crossreacting with the 72K EBNA. J Virol 52:833–838, 1984.
57. Wen LT, Lai PK, Bradley G, et al: Interaction of Epstein-Barr viral (EBV) origin of replication *(oriP)* with EBNA-1 and cellular anti–EBNA-1 proteins. Virology 178:293–296, 1990.
58. Packham G, Economou A, Rooney CM, et al: Structure and function of the Epstein-Barr virus BZLF1 protein. J Virol 64:2110–2116, 1990.
59. Cleary ML, Smith SD, Sklar J: Cloning and structural analysis of cDNAs for *bcl*-2 and a hybrid *bcl*-2/immunoglobulin transcript resulting from the t(14;18) translocation. Cell 47:19–28, 1986.
60. Pearson GR, Luka J, Petti L, et al: Identification of an Epstein-Barr virus early gene encoding a second component of the restricted early antigen complex. Virology 160:151–161, 1987.
61. Moore KW, O'Garra A, de Waal Malefyt R, et al: Interleukin-10. Annu Rev Immunol 11:165–190, 1993.
62. Moore KW, Vieira P, Fiorentino DF, et al: Homology of cytokine synthesis inhibitory factor (IL-10) to the Epstein-Barr virus gene *BCRFI* [published erratum in Science 250:494, 1990]. Science 248:1230–1234, 1990.
63. Adldinger HK, Delius H, Freese UK, et al: A putative transforming gene of Jijoye virus differs from that of Epstein-Barr virus prototypes. Virology 141:221–234, 1985.
64. Apolloni A, Sculley TB: Detection of A-type and B-type Epstein-Barr virus in throat washings and lymphocytes. Virology 202:978–981, 1994.
65. Dambaugh T, Hennessy K, Chamnankit L, Kieff E: U2 region of Epstein-Barr virus DNA may encode Epstein-Barr nuclear antigen 2. Proc Natl Acad Sci USA 81:7632–7636, 1984.
66. Gerber P, Nkrumah FK, Pritchett R, Kieff E: Comparative studies of Epstein-Barr virus strains from Ghana and the United States. Int J Cancer 17:71–81, 1976.
67. King W, Dambaugh T, Heller M, et al: Epstein-Barr virus DNA XII. A variable region of the Epstein-Barr virus genome is included in the P3HR-1 deletion. J Virol 43:979–986, 1982.
68. Rowe M, Young LS, Cadwallader K, et al: Distinction between Epstein-Barr virus type A (EBNA 2A) and type B (EBNA 2B) isolates extends to the EBNA 3 family of nuclear proteins. J Virol 63:1031–1039, 1989.
69. Sample J, Young L, Martin B, et al: Epstein-Barr virus types 1 and 2 differ in their EBNA-3A, EBNA-3B, and EBNA-3C genes. J Virol 64:4084–4092, 1990.
70. Sculley TB, Sculley DG, Pope JH, et al: Epstein-Barr virus nuclear antigens 1 and 2 in Burkitt lymphoma cell lines containing either 'A'- or 'B'-type virus. Intervirology 29:77–85, 1988.
71. Seibl R, Motz M, Wolf H: Strain-specific transcription and translation of the *Bam*HI Z area of Epstein-Barr virus. J Virol 60:902–909, 1986.
72. Sixbey JW, Shirley P, Chesney PJ, et al: Detection of a second widespread strain of Epstein-Barr virus. Lancet 2:761–765, 1989.
73. Young LS, Yao QY, Rooney CM, et al: New type B isolates of Epstein-Barr virus from Burkitt's lymphoma and from normal individuals in endemic areas. J Gen Virol 68(pt 11):2853–2862, 1987.
74. Zimber U, Adldinger HK, Lenoir GM, et al: Geographical prevalence of two types of Epstein-Barr virus. Virology 154:56–66, 1986.
75. Levy JA, Levy SB, Hirshaut Y, et al: Presence of EBV antibodies in sera from wild chimpanzees. Nature 233:559–560, 1971.
76. Nonoyama M, Pagano JS: Homology between Epstein-Barr virus DNA and viral DNA from Burkitt's lymphoma and nasopharyngeal carcinoma determined by DNA-DNA reassociation kinetics. Nature 242:44–47, 1973.
77. Jenson HB, Farrell PJ, Miller G: Sequences of the Epstein-Barr virus (EBV) large internal repeat form the center of a 16-kilobase-pair palindrome of EBV (P3HR-1) heterogeneous DNA [published erratum appears in J Virol 61:2950, 1987]. J Virol 61:1495–1506, 1987.
78. Hu LF, Zabarovsky ER, Chen F, et al: Isolation and sequencing of the Epstein-Barr virus BNLF-1 gene (LMP1) from a Chinese nasopharyngeal carcinoma. J Gen Virol 72(pt 10):2399–2409, 1991.
79. Sample J, Kieff EF, Kieff ED: Epstein-Barr virus types 1 and 2 have nearly identical LMP-1 transforming genes. J Gen Virol 75 (pt 10):2741–2746, 1994.
80. Dambaugh T, Hennessy K, Chamasukit L, Kieff E: The Epstein-Barr virus genome and its expression in latent infection. *In* Epstein M, Achong B (eds): The Epstein-Barr Virus: Recent Advances. London, William Heinemann, 1986, pp 13–45.
81. Rymo L, Lindahl T, Adams A: Sites of sequence variability in Epstein-Barr virus DNA from different sources. Proc Natl Acad Sci USA 76:2794–2798, 1979.
82. Rymo L, Lindahl T, Povey S, Klein G: Analysis of restriction endonuclease fragments of intracellular Epstein-Barr virus DNA and isoenzymes indicate a common origin of the Raji, NC-37, and F-265 human lymphoid cell lines. Virology 115:115–124, 1981.
83. Bornkamm GW, von Knebel-Doeberitz M, Lenoir GM: No evidence for differences in the Epstein-Barr virus genome carried in Burkitt lymphoma cells and nonmalignant lymphoblastoid cells from the same patients. Proc Natl Acad Sci USA 81:4930–4934, 1984.
84. Fingeroth JD, Weis JJ, Tedder TF, et al: Epstein-Barr virus receptor of human B lymphocytes is the C3d receptor CR2. Proc Natl Acad Sci USA 81:4510–4514, 1984.
85. Frade R, Barel M, Ehlin-Henriksson B, Klein G: gp140, the C3d receptor of human B lymphocytes, is also the Epstein-Barr virus receptor. Proc Natl Acad Sci USA 82:1490–1493, 1985.
86. Nemerow GR, Wolfert R, McNaughton ME, Cooper NR: Identification and characterization of the Epstein-Barr virus receptor on human B lymphocytes and its relationship to the C3d complement receptor (CR2). J Virol 55:347–351, 1985.
87. Weis JJ, Tedder TF, Fearon DT: Identification of a 145,000 M_r

membrane protein as the C3d receptor (CR2) of human B lymphocytes. Proc Natl Acad Sci USA 81:881–885, 1984.
88. Nemerow GR, Houghten RA, Moore MD, Cooper NR: Identification of an epitope in the major envelope protein of Epstein-Barr virus that mediates viral binding to the B lymphocyte EBV receptor (CR2). Cell 56:369–377, 1989.
89. Nemerow GR, Mold C, Schwend VK, et al: Identification of gp350 as the viral glycoprotein mediating attachment of Epstein-Barr virus (EBV) to the EBV/C3d receptor of B cells: Sequence homology of gp350 and C3 complement fragment C3d. J Virol 61:1416–1420, 1987.
90. Tanner J, Weis J, Fearon D, et al: Epstein-Barr virus gp350/220 binding to the B lymphocyte C3d receptor mediates adsorption, capping, and endocytosis. Cell 50:203–213, 1987.
91. Wells A, Koide N, Klein G: Two large virion envelope glycoproteins mediate Epstein-Barr virus binding to receptor-positive cells. J Virol 41:286–297, 1982.
92. Lambris JD, Ganu VS, Hirani S, Muller-Eberhard HJ: Mapping of the C3d receptor (CR2)–binding site and a neoantigenic site in the C3d domain of the third component of complement. Proc Natl Acad Sci USA 82:4235–4239, 1985.
93. Beisel C, Tanner J, Matsuo T, et al: Two major outer envelope glycoproteins of Epstein-Barr virus are encoded by the same gene. J Virol 54:665–674, 1985.
94. Biggin M, Farrell PJ, Barrell BG: Transcription and DNA sequence of the *Bam*HI L fragment of B95-8 Epstein-Barr virus. EMBO J 3:1083–1090, 1984.
95. Whang Y, Silberklang M, Morgan A, et al: Expression of the Epstein-Barr virus gp350/220 gene in rodent and primate cells. J Virol 61:1796–1807, 1987.
96. Birkenbach M, Tong X, Bradbury LE, et al: Characterization of an Epstein-Barr virus receptor on human epithelial cells. J Exp Med 176:1405–1414, 1992.
97. Martin DR, Yuryev A, Kalli KR, et al: Determination of the structural basis for selective binding of Epstein-Barr virus to human complement receptor type 2. J Exp Med 174:1299–1311, 1991.
98. Carel JC, Myones BL, Frazier B, Holers VM: Structural requirements for C3d,g/Epstein-Barr virus receptor (CR2/CD21) ligand binding, internalization, and viral infection. J Biol Chem 265:12293–12299, 1990.
99. Nemerow GR, Cooper NR: Early events in the infection of human B lymphocytes by Epstein-Barr virus: The internalization process. Virology 132:186–198, 1984.
100. Gompels U, Minson A: The properties and sequence of glycoprotein H of herpes simplex virus type 1. Virology 153:230–247, 1986.
101. Heineman T, Gong M, Sample J, Kieff E: Identification of the Epstein-Barr virus gp85 gene. J Virol 62:1101–1107, 1988.
102. Oba DE, Hutt-Fletcher LM: Induction of antibodies to the Epstein-Barr virus glycoprotein gp85 with a synthetic peptide corresponding to a sequence in the *BXLF2* open reading frame. J Virol 62:1108–1114, 1988.
103. Miller N, Hutt-Fletcher LM: A monoclonal antibody to glycoprotein gp85 inhibits fusion but not attachment of Epstein-Barr virus. J Virol 62:2366–2372, 1988.
104. Alfieri C, Birkenbach M, Kieff E: Early events in Epstein-Barr virus infection of human B lymphocytes [published erratum in Virology 185:946, 1991]. Virology 181:595–608, 1991.
105. Hurley EA, Thorley-Lawson DA: B cell activation and the establishment of Epstein-Barr virus latency. J Exp Med 168:2059–2075, 1988.
106. Graessmann A, Wolf H, Bornkamm GW: Expression of Epstein-Barr virus genes in different cell types after microinjection of viral DNA. Proc Natl Acad Sci USA 77:433–436, 1980.
107. Grogan E, Miller G, Henle W, et al: Expression of Epstein-Barr viral early antigen in monolayer tissue cultures after transfection with viral DNA and DNA fragments. J Virol 40:861–869, 1981.
108. Volsky DJ, Gross T, Sinangil F, et al: Expression of Epstein-Barr virus (EBV) DNA and cloned DNA fragments in human lymphocytes following Sendai virus envelope–mediated gene transfer. Proc Natl Acad Sci USA 81:5926–5930, 1984.
109. Volsky DJ, Shapiro IM, Klein G: Transfer of Epstein-Barr virus receptors to receptor-negative cells permits virus penetration and antigen expression. Proc Natl Acad Sci USA 77:5453–5437, 1980.
110. Ben-Sasson SA, Klein G: Activation of the Epstein-Barr virus genome by 5-aza-cytidine in latently infected human lymphoid lines. Int J Cancer 28:131–135, 1981.
111. Hudewentz J, Bornkamm GW, zur Hausen H: Effect of the diterpene ester TPA on Epstein-Barr virus antigen and DNA synthesis in producer and nonproducer cell lines. Virology 100:175–178, 1980.
112. Luka J, Kallin B, Klein G: Induction of the Epstein-Barr virus (EBV) cycle in latently infected cells by *n*-butyrate. Virology 94:228–231, 1979.
113. Ragona G, Ernberg I, Klein G: Induction and biological characterization of the Epstein-Barr virus (EBV) carried by the Jijoye lymphoma line. Virology 101:553–557, 1980.
114. Saemundsen AK, Kallin B, Klein G: Effect of *n*-butyrate on cellular and viral DNA synthesis in cells latently infected with Epstein-Barr virus. Virology 107:557–561, 1980.
115. zur Hausen H, Bornkamm GW, Schmidt R, Hecker E: Tumor initiators and promoters in the induction of Epstein-Barr virus. Proc Natl Acad Sci USA 76:782–785, 1979.
116. zur Hausen H, O'Neill F, Freese U, Hecher E: Persisting oncogenic herpesvirus induced by tumor promoter TPA. Nature 272:373–375, 1978.
117. Angel P, Imagawa M, Chiu R, et al: Phorbol ester–inducible genes contain a common cis element recognized by a TPA-modulated trans-acting factor. Cell 49:729–739, 1987.
118. Lee W, Mitchell P, Tjian R: Purified transcription factor AP-1 interacts with TPA-inducible enhancer elements. Cell 49:741–752, 1987.
119. Farrell P, Rowe D, Rooney C, Kouzarides T: Latent and lytic cycle promoters of the Epstein-Barr virus. EMBO J 2:1331–1338, 1983.
120. Farrell PJ, Rowe DT, Rooney CM, Kouzarides T: Epstein-Barr virus *BZLF1* trans-activator specifically binds to a consensus AP-1 site and is related to c-*fos*. EMBO J 8:127–132, 1989.
121. Flemington E, Speck SH: Identification of phorbol ester response elements in the promoter of Epstein-Barr virus putative lytic switch gene *BZLF1*. J Virol 64:1217–1226, 1990.
122. Laux G, Freese UK, Fischer R, et al: TPA-inducible Epstein-Barr virus genes in Raji cells and their regulation. Virology 162:503–507, 1988.
123. Hinuma Y, Konn M, Yamaguchi J, et al: Immunofluorescence and herpes-type virus particles in the P3HR-1 Burkitt lymphoma cell line. J Virol 1:1045–1051, 1967.
124. Miller G, Shope T, Lisco H, et al: Epstein-Barr virus: Transformation, cytopathic changes, and viral antigens in squirrel monkey and marmoset leukocytes. Proc Natl Acad Sci USA 69:383–387, 1972.
125. Takada K: Cross-linking of cell surface immunoglobulins induces Epstein-Barr virus in Burkitt lymphoma lines. Int J Cancer 33:27–32, 1984.
126. Takada K, Ono Y: Synchronous and sequential activation of latently infected Epstein-Barr virus genomes. J Virol 63:445–449, 1989.
127. Daibata M, Humphreys RE, Sairenji T: Phosphorylation of the Epstein-Barr virus *BZLF1* immediate-early gene product ZEBRA. Virology 188:916–920, 1992.
128. Daibata M, Humphreys RE, Takada K, Sairenji T: Activation of latent EBV via anti–IgG-triggered, second messenger pathways in the Burkitt's lymphoma cell line Akata. J Immunol 144:4788–4793, 1990.
129. Matsuo T, Heller M, Petti L, et al: Persistence of the entire Epstein-Barr virus genome integrated into human lymphocyte DNA. Science 226:1322–1325, 1984.
130. Gergely L, Klein G, Ernberg I: Host cell macromolecular synthesis in cells containing EBV-induced early antigens, studied by combined immunofluorescence and radioautography. Virology 45:22–29, 1971.
131. Marschall M, Schwarzmann F, Leser U, et al: The BI'LF4 trans-activator of Epstein-Barr virus is modulated by type and differentiation of the host cell. Virology 181:172–179, 1991.
132. Grogan E, Jenson H, Countryman J, et al: Transfection of a rearranged viral DNA fragment, WZhet, stably converts latent Epstein-Barr viral infection to productive infection in lymphoid cells. Proc Natl Acad Sci USA 84:1332–1336, 1987.
133. Jenson HB, Miller G: Polymorphisms of the region of the Epstein-Barr virus genome which disrupts latency. Virology 165:549–564, 1988.

134. Jenson HB, Rabson MS, Miller G: Palindromic structure and polypeptide expression of 36 kilobase pairs of heterogeneous Epstein-Barr virus (P3HR-1) DNA. J Virol 58:475–486, 1986.
135. Miller G, Rabson M, Heston L: Epstein-Barr virus with heterogeneous DNA disrupts latency. J Virol 50:174–182, 1984.
136. Finke J, Rowe M, Kallin B, et al: Monoclonal and polyclonal antibodies against Epstein-Barr virus nuclear antigen 5 (EBNA-5) detect multiple protein species in Burkitt's lymphoma and lymphoblastoid cell lines. J Virol 61:3870–3878, 1987.
137. Lieberman PM, Berk AJ: In vitro transcriptional activation, dimerization, and DNA-binding specificity of the Epstein-Barr virus Zta protein. J Virol 64:2560–2568, 1990.
138. Chi T, Carey M: The ZEBRA activation domain: Modular organization and mechanism of action. Mol Cell Biol 13:7045–7055, 1993.
139. Flemington EK, Borras AM, Lytle JP, Speck SH: Characterization of the Epstein-Barr virus BZLF1 protein transactivation domain. J Virol 66:922–929, 1992.
140. Lieberman PM, Berk AJ: The Zta trans-activator protein stabilizes TFIID association with promoter DNA by direct protein-protein interaction. Genes Dev 5:2441–2454, 1991.
141. Chang YN, Dong DL, Hayward GS, Hayward SD: The Epstein-Barr virus Zta transactivator: A member of the bZIP family with unique DNA-binding specificity and a dimerization domain that lacks the characteristic heptad leucine zipper motif. J Virol 64:3358–3369, 1990.
142. Flemington EK, Lytle JP, Cayrol C, et al: DNA-binding–defective mutants of the Epstein-Barr virus lytic switch activator Zta transactivate with altered specificities. Mol Cell Biol 14:3041–3052, 1994.
143. Mikaelian I, Drouet E, Marechal V, et al: The DNA-binding domain of two bZIP transcription factors, the Epstein-Barr virus switch gene product EB1 and Jun, is a bipartite nuclear targeting sequence. J Virol 67:734–742, 1993.
144. Kouzarides T, Packham G, Cook A, Farrell PJ: The BZLF1 protein of EBV has a coiled coil dimerisation domain without a heptad leucine repeat but with homology to the C/EBP leucine zipper. Oncogene 6:195–204, 1991.
145. Flemington E, Speck SH: Evidence for coiled-coil dimer formation by an Epstein-Barr virus transactivator that lacks a heptad repeat of leucine residues. Proc Natl Acad Sci USA 87:9459–9463, 1990.
146. Lieberman PM, Hardwick JM, Sample J, et al: The zta transactivator involved in induction of lytic cycle gene expression in Epstein-Barr virus–infected lymphocytes binds to both AP-1 and ZRE sites in target promoter and enhancer regions. J Virol 64:1143–1155, 1990.
147. Kolman JL, Taylor N, Marshak DR, Miller G: Serine-173 of the Epstein-Barr virus ZEBRA protein is required for DNA binding and is a target for casein kinase II phosphorylation. Proc Natl Acad Sci USA 90:10115–10119, 1993.
148. Zhang Q, Gutsch D, Kenney S: Functional and physical interaction between p53 and BZLF1: Implications for Epstein-Barr virus latency. Mol Cell Biol 14:1929–1938, 1994.
149. Gruffat H, Sergeant A: Characterization of the DNA-binding site repertoire for the Epstein-Barr virus transcription factor R. Nucleic Acids Res 22:1172–1178, 1994.
150. Gutsch DE, Holley-Guthrie EA, Zhang Q, et al: The bZIP transactivator of Epstein-Barr virus, BZLF1, functionally and physically interacts with the p65 subunit of NF-kappa B. Mol Cell Biol 14:1939–1948, 1994.
151. Bankier AT, Deininger PL, Satchwell SC, et al: DNA sequence analysis of the *Eco*RI Dhet fragment of B95-8 Epstein-Barr virus containing the terminal repeat sequences. Mol Biol Med 1:425–445, 1983.
152. Biggin M, Bodescot M, Perricaudet M, Farrell P: Epstein-Barr virus gene expression in P3HR1-superinfected Raji cells. J Virol 61:3120–3132, 1987.
153. Gibson T, Stockwell P, Ginsburg M, Barrell B: Homology between two EBV early genes and HSV ribonucleotide reductase and 38K genes. Nucleic Acids Res 12:5087–5099, 1984.
154. Gibson TJ, Barrell BG, Farrell PJ: Coding content and expression of the EBV B95-8 genome in the region from base 62,248 to base 82,920. Virology 152:136–148, 1986.
155. Hatfull G, Bankier AT, Barrell BG, Farrell PJ: Sequence analysis of Raji Epstein-Barr virus DNA. Virology 164:334–340, 1988.
156. Hudson GS, Bankier AT, Satchwell SC, Barrell BG: The short unique region of the B95-8 Epstein-Barr virus genome. Virology 147:81–98, 1985.
157. Hudson GS, Gibson TJ, Barrell BG: The *Bam*HI F region of the B95-8 Epstein-Barr virus genome. Virology 147:99–109, 1985.
158. Hudson GS, Farrell PJ, Barrell BG: Two related but differentially expressed potential membrane proteins encoded by the *Eco*RI Dhet region of Epstein-Barr virus B95-8. J Virol 53:528–535, 1985.
159. Hummel MA: Mapping of RNAs and proteins specified by Epstein-Barr virus in productively infected cells. Diss Abstr Int (Sci) 43:633-B, 1982.
160. Fixman ED, Hayward GS, Hayward SD: Trans-acting requirements for replication of Epstein-Barr virus ori-Lyt. J Virol 66:5030–5039, 1992.
161. Hummel M, Kieff E: Mapping of polypeptides encoded by the Epstein-Barr virus genome in productive infection. Proc Natl Acad Sci USA 79:5698–5702, 1982.
162. Freese UK, Laux G, Hudewentz J, et al: Two distant clusters of partially homologous small repeats of Epstein-Barr virus are transcribed upon induction of an abortive or lytic cycle of the virus. J Virol 48:731–743, 1983.
163. Gong M, Ooka T, Matsuo T, Kieff E: Epstein-Barr virus glycoprotein homologous to herpes simplex virus gB. J Virol 61:499–508, 1987.
164. Heineman T: Glycoproteins of Epstein-Barr Virus. Chicago, The University of Chicago; 1988. PhD dissertation.
165. Hummel M, Thorley-Lawson D, Kieff E: An Epstein-Barr virus DNA fragment encodes messages for the two major envelope glycoproteins (gp350/300 and gp220/200). J Virol 49:413–417, 1984.
166. Mackett M, Conway MJ, Arrand JR, et al: Characterization and expression of a glycoprotein encoded by the Epstein-Barr virus *Bam*HI I fragment. J Virol 64:2545–2552, 1990.
167. Nuebling CM, Mueller-Lantzsch N: Identification of the gene product encoded by the PstI repeats (IR4) of the Epstein-Barr virus genome. Virology 185:519–523, 1991.
168. Emini EA, Luka J, Armstrong ME, et al: Identification of an Epstein-Barr virus glycoprotein which is antigenically homologous to the varicella-zoster virus glycoprotein II and the herpes simplex virus glycoprotein B. Virology 157:552–555, 1987.
169. Gong M, Kieff E: Intracellular trafficking of two major Epstein-Barr virus glycoproteins, gp350/220 and gp110. J Virol 64:1507–1516, 1990.
170. Hoffman GJ, Lazarowitz SG, Hayward SD: Monoclonal antibody against a 250,000-dalton glycoprotein of Epstein-Barr virus identifies a membrane antigen and a neutralizing antigen. Proc Natl Acad Sci USA 77:2979–2983, 1980.
171. Strnad BC, Neubauer RH, Rabin H, Mazur RA: Correlation between Epstein-Barr virus membrane antigen and three large cell surface glycoproteins. J Virol 32:885–894, 1979.
172. Thorley-Lawson DA, Geilinger K: Monoclonal antibodies against the major glycoprotein (gp350/220) of Epstein-Barr virus neutralize infectivity. Proc Natl Acad Sci USA 77:5307–5311, 1980.
173. Thorley-Lawson DA, Poodry CA: Identification and isolation of the main component (gp350-gp220) of Epstein-Barr virus responsible for generating neutralizing antibodies in vivo. J Virol 43:730–736, 1982.
174. Hsu DH, de Waal Malefyt R, Fiorentino DF, et al: Expression of interleukin-10 activity by Epstein-Barr virus protein BCRF1. Science 250:830–832, 1990.
175. Vieira P, de Waal Malefyt R, Dang MN, et al: Isolation and expression of human cytokine synthesis inhibitory factor cDNA clones: Homology to Epstein-Barr virus open reading frame BCRFI. Proc Natl Acad Sci USA 88:1172–1176, 1991.
176. Swaminathan S, Hesselton R, Sullivan J, Kieff E: Epstein-Barr virus recombinants with specifically mutated *BCRF1* genes. J Virol 67:7406–7413, 1993.
177. Garner JG, Hirsch MS, Schooley RT: Prevention of Epstein-Barr virus–induced B-cell outgrowth by interferon alpha. Infect Immun 43:920–924, 1984.
178. Klein G: Advances in Viral Oncology. New York, Raven Press, 1987.
179. Miller G: The Epstein-Barr virus. *In* Fields BN, Knipe DM (eds): Fields Virology, ed 2. New York, Raven Press, 1990, pp 1921–1958.

180. Dillner J, Kallin B, Alexander H, et al: An Epstein-Barr virus (EBV)–determined nuclear antigen (EBNA5) partly encoded by the transformation-associated *Bam* WYH region of EBV DNA: Preferential expression in lymphoblastoid cell lines. Proc Natl Acad Sci USA 83:6641–6645, 1986.
181. Wang F, Petti L, Braun D, et al: A bicistronic Epstein-Barr virus mRNA encodes two nuclear proteins in latently infected, growth-transformed lymphocytes. J Virol 61:945–954, 1987.
182. Petti L, Sample C, Kieff E: Subnuclear localization and phosphorylation of Epstein-Barr virus latent infection nuclear proteins. Virology 176:563–574, 1990.
183. Hammerschmidt W, Sugden B: Genetic analysis of immortalizing functions of Epstein-Barr virus in human B lymphocytes. Nature 340:393–397, 1989.
184. Mannick JB, Cohen JI, Birkenbach M, et al: The Epstein-Barr virus nuclear protein encoded by the leader of the EBNA RNAs is important in B-lymphocyte transformation. J Virol 65:6826–6837, 1991.
185. Sinclair AJ, Palmero I, Peters G, Farrell PJ: EBNA-2 and EBNA-LP cooperate to cause G_0 to G_1 transition during immortalization of resting human B lymphocytes by Epstein-Barr virus. EMBO J 13:3321–3328, 1994.
186. Jiang WQ, Szekely L, Wendel-Hansen V, et al: Co-localization of the retinoblastoma protein and the Epstein-Barr virus–encoded nuclear antigen EBNA-5. Exp Cell Res 197:314–318, 1991.
187. Szekely L, Selivanova G, Magnusson KP, et al: EBNA-5, an Epstein-Barr virus–encoded nuclear antigen, binds to the retinoblastoma and p53 proteins. Proc Natl Acad Sci USA 90:5455–5459, 1993.
188. Huen DS, Fox A, Kumar P, Searle PF: Dilated heart failure in transgenic mice expressing the Epstein-Barr virus nuclear antigen-leader protein. J Gen Virol 74(pt 7):1381–1391, 1993.
189. Menezes J, Leibold W, Klein G: Biological differences between Epstein-Barr virus (EBV) strains with regard to lymphocyte transforming ability, superinfection and antigen induction. Exp Cell Res 92:478–484, 1975.
190. Miller G, Robinson J, Heston L, Lipman M: Differences between laboratory strains of Epstein-Barr virus based on immortalization, abortive infection, and interference. Proc Natl Acad Sci USA 71:4006–4010, 1974.
191. Dillner J, Kallin B, Klein G, et al: Antibodies against synthetic peptides react with the second Epstein-Barr virus–associated nuclear antigen. EMBO J 4:1813–1818, 1985.
192. Dillner J, Sternas L, Kallin B, et al: Antibodies against a synthetic peptide identify the Epstein-Barr virus–determined nuclear antigen. Proc Natl Acad Sci USA 81:4652–4656, 1984.
193. Hennessy K, Kieff E: A second nuclear protein is encoded by Epstein-Barr virus in latent infection. Science 227:1238–1240, 1985.
194. Cohen JI, Wang F, Mannick J, Kieff E: Epstein-Barr virus nuclear protein 2 is a key determinant of lymphocyte transformation. Proc Natl Acad Sci USA 86:9558–9562, 1989.
195. Wang F, Gregory CD, Rowe M, et al: Epstein-Barr virus nuclear antigen 2 specifically induces expression of the B-cell activation antigen CD23. Proc Natl Acad Sci USA 84:3452–3456, 1987.
196. Wang F, Gregory C, Sample CE, et al: Epstein-Barr virus nuclear protein 2 and latent membrane protein (LMP1) are effectors of phenotypic changes in human B lymphoma cells; EBNA-2 and LMP1 cooperatively induce CD23 (Abstr). FASEB J 4:A1880, 1990.
197. Knutson JC: The level of c-*fgr* RNA is increased by EBNA-2, an Epstein-Barr virus gene required for B-cell immortalization. J Virol 64:2530–2536, 1990.
198. Abbot SD, Rowe M, Cadwallader K, et al: Epstein-Barr virus nuclear antigen 2 induces expression of the virus-encoded latent membrane protein. J Virol 64:2126–2134, 1990.
199. Fahraeus R, Jansson A, Ricksten A, et al: Epstein-Barr virus–encoded nuclear antigen 2 activates the viral latent membrane protein promoter by modulating the activity of a negative regulatory element. Proc Natl Acad Sci USA 87:7390–7394, 1990.
200. Fahraeus R, Jansson A, Sjoblom A, et al: Cell phenotype-dependent control of Epstein-Barr virus latent membrane protein 1 gene regulatory sequences. Virology 195:71–80, 1993.
201. Ghosh D, Kieff E: cis-acting regulatory elements near the Epstein-Barr virus latent-infection membrane protein transcriptional start site. J Virol 64:1855–1858, 1990.
202. Tsang SF, Wang F, Izumi KM, Kieff E: Delineation of the cis-acting element mediating EBNA-2 transactivation of latent infection membrane protein expression. J Virol 65:6765–6771, 1991.
203. Wang F, Tsang SF, Kurilla MG, et al: Epstein-Barr virus nuclear antigen 2 transactivates latent membrane protein LMP1. J Virol 64:3407–3416, 1990.
204. Zimber-Strobl U, Kremmer E, Grasser F, et al: The Epstein-Barr virus nuclear antigen 2 interacts with an EBNA2 responsive cis-element of the terminal protein 1 gene promoter. EMBO J 12:167–175, 1993.
205. Zimber-Strobl U, Suentzenich KO, Laux G, et al: Epstein-Barr virus nuclear antigen 2 activates transcription of the terminal protein gene. J Virol 65:415–423, 1991.
206. Cohen JI: A region of herpes simplex virus VP16 can substitute for a transforming domain of Epstein-Barr virus nuclear protein 2. Proc Natl Acad Sci USA 89:8030–8034, 1992.
207. Cohen JI, Kieff E: An Epstein-Barr virus nuclear protein 2 domain essential for transformation is a direct transcriptional activator. J Virol 65:5880–5885, 1991.
208. Cohen JI, Wang F, Kieff E: Epstein-Barr virus nuclear protein 2 mutations define essential domains for transformation and transactivation. J Virol 65:2545–2554, 1991.
209. Tong X, Wang F, Thut CJ, Kieff E: The Epstein-Barr virus nuclear protein 2 acidic domain can interact with TFIIB, TAF40, and RPA70 but not with TATA-binding protein. J Virol 69:585–588, 1995.
210. Ambinder RF, Shah WA, Rawlins DR, et al: Definition of the sequence requirements for binding of the EBNA-1 protein to its palindromic target sites in Epstein-Barr virus DNA. J Virol 64:2369–2379, 1990.
211. Grossman SR, Johannsen E, Tong X, et al: The Epstein-Barr virus nuclear antigen 2 transactivator is directed to response elements by the J κ recombination signal binding protein. Proc Natl Acad Sci USA 91:7568–7572, 1994.
212. Henkel T, Ling PD, Hayward SD, Peterson MG: Mediation of Epstein-Barr virus EBNA2 transactivation by recombination signal-binding protein J κ. Science 265:92–95, 1994.
213. Johannsen E, Koh E, Mosialos G, et al: Epstein-Barr virus nuclear protein 2 transactivation of the latent membrane protein 1 promoter is mediated by J κ and PU.1. J Virol 69:253–262, 1995.
214. Hennessy K, Fennewald S, Kieff E: A third viral nuclear protein in lymphoblasts immortalized by Epstein-Barr virus. Proc Natl Acad Sci USA 82:5944–5948, 1985.
215. Hennessy K, Wang F, Bushman EW, Kieff E: Definitive identification of a member of the Epstein-Barr virus nuclear protein 3 family. Proc Natl Acad Sci USA 83:5693–5697, 1986.
216. Joab I, Rowe DT, Bodescot M, et al: Mapping of the gene coding for Epstein-Barr virus–determined nuclear antigen EBNA3 and its transient overexpression in a human cell line by using an adenovirus expression vector. J Virol 61:3340–3344, 1987.
217. Kallin B, Dillner J, Ernberg I, et al: Four virally determined nuclear antigens are expressed in Epstein-Barr virus–transformed cells. Proc Natl Acad Sci USA 83:1499–1503, 1986.
218. Kerdiles B, Walls D, Triki H, et al: cDNA cloning and transient expression of the Epstein-Barr virus–determined nuclear antigen EBNA3B in human cells and identification of novel transcripts from its coding region. J Virol 64:1812–1816, 1990.
219. Petti L, Kieff E: A sixth Epstein-Barr virus nuclear protein (EBNA3B) is expressed in latently infected growth-transformed lymphocytes. J Virol 62:2173–2178, 1988.
220. Petti L, Sample J, Wang F, Kieff E: A fifth Epstein-Barr virus nuclear protein (EBNA3C) is expressed in latently infected growth-transformed lymphocytes. J Virol 62:1330–1338, 1988.
221. Ricksten A, Kallin B, Alexander H, et al: BamHI E region of the Epstein-Barr virus genome encodes three transformation-associated nuclear proteins. Proc Natl Acad Sci USA 85:995–999, 1988.
222. Sixbey JW, Shirley P, Sloas M, et al: A transformation-incompetent, nuclear antigen 2–deleted Epstein-Barr virus associated with replicative infection. J Infect Dis 163:1008–1015, 1991.
223. Bodescot M, Brison O, Perricaudet M: An Epstein-Barr virus transcription unit is at least 84 kilobases long. Nucleic Acids Res 14:2611–2620, 1986.
224. Bodescot M, Chambraud B, Farrell P, Perricaudet M: Spliced RNA from the IR1-U2 region of Epstein-Barr virus: Presence of an open reading frame for a repetitive polypeptide. EMBO J 3:1913–1917, 1984.

225. Bodescot M, Perricaudet M: Epstein-Barr virus mRNAs produced by alternative splicing. Nucleic Acids Res 14:7103–7114, 1986.
226. Bodescot M, Perricaudet M, Farrell PJ: A promoter for the highly spliced EBNA family of RNAs of Epstein-Barr virus. J Virol 61:3424–3430, 1987.
227. Sculley TB, Walker PJ, Moss DJ, Pope JH: Identification of multiple Epstein-Barr virus–induced nuclear antigens with sera from patients with rheumatoid arthritis. J Virol 52:88–93, 1984.
228. Tomkinson B, Kieff E: Use of second-site homologous recombination to demonstrate that Epstein-Barr virus nuclear protein 3B is not important for lymphocyte infection or growth transformation in vitro. J Virol 66:2893–2903, 1992.
229. Tomkinson B, Robertson E, Kieff E: Epstein-Barr virus nuclear proteins EBNA-3A and EBNA-3C are essential for B-lymphocyte growth transformation. J Virol 67:2014–2025, 1993.
230. Robertson ES, Grossman S, Johannsen E, et al: Epstein-Barr virus nuclear protein 3C modulates transcription through interaction with the sequence-specific DNA-binding protein J kappa. J Virol 69:3108–3116, 1995.
230a. Robertson ES, Lin J, Kieff E: The amino-terminal domains of Epstein-Barr virus nuclear proteins 3A, 3B and 3C interact with RBPJκ. J Virol 70:3068–3074, 1996.
231. Jones CH, Hayward SD, Rawlins DR: Interaction of the lymphocyte-derived Epstein-Barr virus nuclear antigen EBNA-1 with its DNA-binding sites. J Virol 63:101–110, 1989.
232. Kimball AS, Milman G, Tullius TD: High-resolution footprints of the DNA-binding domain of Epstein-Barr virus nuclear antigen 1. Mol Cell Biol 9:2738–2742, 1989.
233. Rawlins DR, Milman G, Hayward SD, Hayward GS: Sequence-specific DNA binding of the Epstein-Barr virus nuclear antigen (EBNA-1) to clustered sites in the plasmid maintenance region. Cell 42:859–868, 1985.
234. Su W, Middleton T, Sugden B, Echols H: DNA looping between the origin of replication of Epstein-Barr virus and its enhancer site: Stabilization of an origin complex with Epstein-Barr nuclear antigen 1. Proc Natl Acad Sci USA 88:10870–10874, 1991.
235. Chittenden T, Lupton S, Levine AJ: Functional limits of *oriP*, the Epstein-Barr virus plasmid origin of replication. J Virol 63:3016–3025, 1989.
236. Middleton T, Sugden B: Retention of plasmid DNA in mammalian cells is enhanced by binding of the Epstein-Barr virus replication protein EBNA1. J Virol 68:4067–4071, 1994.
237. Reisman D, Yates J, Sugden B: A putative origin of replication of plasmids derived from Epstein-Barr virus is composed of two cis-acting components. Mol Cell Biol 5:1822–1832, 1985.
238. Sugden B, Marsh K, Yates J: A vector that replicates as a plasmid and can be efficiently selected in B-lymphoblasts transformed by Epstein-Barr virus. Mol Cell Biol 5:410–413, 1985.
239. Yates J, Warren N, Reisman D, Sugden B: A cis-acting element from the Epstein-Barr viral genome that permits stable replication of recombinant plasmids in latently infected cells. Proc Natl Acad Sci USA 81:3806–3810, 1984.
240. Yates JL, Camiolo SM: Dissection of DNA replication and enhancer activation functions of Epstein-Barr virus nuclear antigen 1. Cancer Cells 6:197–205, 1988.
241. Yates JL, Guan N: Epstein-Barr virus–derived plasmids replicate only once per cell cycle and are not amplified after entry into cells. J Virol 65:483–488, 1991.
242. Yates JL, Warren N, Sugden B: Stable replication of plasmids derived from Epstein-Barr virus in various mammalian cells. Nature 313:812–815, 1985.
243. Fennewald S, van Santen V, Kieff E: Nucleotide sequence of an mRNA transcribed in latent growth-transforming virus infection indicates that it may encode a membrane protein. J Virol 51:411–419, 1984.
244. Liebowitz D, Kopan R, Fuchs E, et al: An Epstein-Barr virus transforming protein associates with vimentin in lymphocytes. Mol Cell Biol 7:2299–2308, 1987.
245. Liebowitz D, Wang D, Kieff E: Orientation and patching of the latent infection membrane protein encoded by Epstein-Barr virus. J Virol 58:233–237, 1986.
246. Hennessy K, Fennewald S, Hummel M, et al: A membrane protein encoded by Epstein-Barr virus in latent growth-transforming infection. Proc Natl Acad Sci USA 81:7207–7211, 1984.
247. Baichwal VR, Sugden B: Transformation of Balb 3T3 cells by the *BNLF-1* gene of Epstein-Barr virus. Oncogene 2:461–467, 1988.
248. Moorthy RK, Thorley-Lawson DA: All three domains of the Epstein-Barr virus–encoded latent membrane protein LMP-1 are required for transformation of rat-1 fibroblasts. J Virol 67:1638–1646, 1993.
249. Wang D, Liebowitz D, Kieff E: The truncated form of the Epstein-Barr virus latent-infection membrane protein expressed in virus replication does not transform rodent fibroblasts. J Virol 62:2337–2346, 1988.
250. Wang D, Liebowitz D, Kieff E: An EBV membrane protein expressed in immortalized lymphocytes transforms established rodent cells. Cell 43(pt 2):831–840, 1985.
251. Birkenbach M, Liebowitz D, Wang F, et al: Epstein-Barr virus latent infection membrane protein increases vimentin expression in human B-cell lines. J Virol 63:4079–4084, 1989.
252. Liebowitz D, Kieff E: Epstein-Barr virus latent membrane protein: Induction of B-cell activation antigens and membrane patch formation does not require vimentin. J Virol 63:4051–4054, 1989.
253. Liebowitz D, Mannick J, Takada K, Kieff E: Phenotypes of Epstein-Barr virus LMP1 deletion mutants indicate transmembrane and amino-terminal cytoplasmic domains necessary for effects in B-lymphoma cells. J Virol 66:4612–4616, 1992.
254. Moorthy R, Thorley-Lawson DA: Processing of the Epstein-Barr virus–encoded latent membrane protein p63/LMP. J Virol 64:829–837, 1990.
255. Peng M, Lundgren E: Transient expression of the Epstein-Barr virus LMP1 gene in human primary B cells induces cellular activation and DNA synthesis. Oncogene 7:1775–1782, 1992.
256. Rowe M, Peng-Pilon M, Huen DS, et al: Upregulation of *bcl*-2 by the Epstein-Barr virus latent membrane protein LMP1: A B-cell–specific response that is delayed relative to NF-kappa B activation and to induction of cell surface markers. J Virol 68:5602–5612, 1994.
257. Wang D, Liebowitz D, Wang F, et al: Epstein-Barr virus latent infection membrane protein alters the human B-lymphocyte phenotype: Deletion of the amino terminus abolishes activity. J Virol 62:4173–4184, 1988.
258. Wang F, Gregory C, Sample C, et al: Epstein-Barr virus latent membrane protein (LMP1) and nuclear proteins 2 and 3C are effectors of phenotypic changes in B lymphocytes: EBNA-2 and LMP1 cooperatively induce CD23. J Virol 64:2309–2318, 1990.
259. Zhang Q, Brooks L, Busson P, et al: Epstein-Barr virus (EBV) latent membrane protein 1 increases HLA class II expression in an EBV-negative B cell line. Eur J Immunol 24:1467–1470, 1994.
260. Gregory CD, Dive C, Henderson S, et al: Activation of Epstein-Barr virus latent genes protects human B cells from death by apoptosis. Nature 349:612–614, 1991.
261. Henderson S, Rowe M, Gregory C, et al: Induction of *bcl*-2 expression by Epstein-Barr virus latent membrane protein 1 protects infected B cells from programmed cell death. Cell 65:1107–1115, 1991.
262. Martin JM, Veis D, Korsmeyer SJ, Sugden B: Latent membrane protein of Epstein-Barr virus induces cellular phenotypes independently of expression of Bcl-2. J Virol 67:5269–5278, 1993.
263. Laherty CD, Hu HM, Opipari AW, et al: The Epstein-Barr virus LMP1 gene product induces A20 zinc finger protein expression by activating nuclear factor κ B. J Biol Chem 267:24157–24160, 1992.
264. Hammarskjold ML, Simurda MC: Epstein-Barr virus latent membrane protein transactivates the human immunodeficiency virus type 1 long terminal repeat through induction of NF-kappa B activity. J Virol 66:6496–6501, 1992.
265. Dawson CW, Rickinson AB, Young LS: Epstein-Barr virus latent membrane protein inhibits human epithelial cell differentiation. Nature 344:777–780, 1990.
266. Fahraeus R, Rymo L, Rhim JS, Klein G: Morphological transformation of human keratinocytes expressing the LMP gene of Epstein-Barr virus. Nature 345:447–449, 1990.
267. Fairbairn LJ, Stewart JP, Hampson IN, et al: Expression of Epstein-Barr virus latent membrane protein influences self-renewal and differentiation in a multipotential murine haemopoietic 'stem cell' line. J Gen Virol 74(pt 2):247–254, 1993.
268. Wilson JB, Weinberg W, Johnson R, et al: Expression of the *BNLF-1* oncogene of Epstein-Barr virus in the skin of transgenic mice induces hyperplasia and aberrant expression of keratin 6. Cell 61:1315–1327, 1990.

269. Hu LF, Chen F, Zheng X, et al: Clonability and tumorigenicity of human epithelial cells expressing the EBV encoded membrane protein LMP1. Oncogene 8:1575–1583, 1993.
270. Izumi KM, Kaye KM, Kieff ED: Epstein-Barr virus recombinant molecular genetic analysis of the LMP1 amino-terminal cytoplasmic domain reveals a probable structural role, with no component essential for primary B-lymphocyte growth transformation. J Virol 68:4369–4376, 1994.
271. Kaye KM, Izumi KM, Kieff E: Epstein-Barr virus latent membrane protein 1 is essential for B-lymphocyte growth transformation. Proc Natl Acad Sci USA 90:9150–9154, 1993.
272. Kaye KM, Izumi KM, Mosialos G, Kieff E: The Epstein-Barr virus LMP1 cytoplasmic carboxy terminus is essential for B-lymphocyte transformation; fibroblast cocultivation complements a critical function within the terminal 155 residues. J Virol 69:675–683, 1995.
273. Mosialos G, Hanissian SH, Jawahar S, et al: A Ca^{2+}/calmodulin-dependent protein kinase, CaM kinase-Gr, expressed after transformation of primary human B lymphocytes by Epstein-Barr virus (EBV) is induced by the EBV oncogene *LMP1*. J Virol 68:1697–1705, 1994.
273a. Kaye KM, Devergne O, Harada JN, et al: Tumor necrosis factor receptor associated factor 2 is a mediator of NF-κB activation by latent infection membrane protein 1, the Epstein-Barr virus transforming protein. Proc Natl Acad Sci USA 93:11085–11090, 1996.
273b. Devergne O, Hatzivassiliou E, Izumi KM, et al: Association of TRAF1, TRAF2, and TRAF3 with an Epstein-Barr virus LMP1 domain important for B-lymphocyte transformation: Role in NF-κB activation. Mol Cell Biol 16:7098–7108, 1996.
274. Hu H, O'Rourke K, Boguski M, et al: A novel RING finger protein interacts with the cytoplasmic domain of CD40. J Biol Chem 269:20069–20072, 1994.
275. Sato T, Irie S, Reed J: A novel member of the TRAF family of putative signal transducing proteins binds to the cytosolic domain of CD40. FEBS Lett 358:113–118, 1995.
276. Cheng G, Cleary A, Ye Z, et al: Involvement of CRAF1, a relative of TRAF, in CD40 signaling. Science 267:1494–1498, 1995.
276a. Rothe M, Sarma V, Dixit M, Goeddel DV: TRAF2-mediated activation of NF-κB by TNF receptor 2 and CD40. Science 269:1424–1427, 1995.
276b. Cheng G, Baltimore D: TANK, a co-inducer with TRAF2 of TNF- and CD40L-mediated NF-κB activation. Genes Dev 10:963–973, 1996.
277. Kieff E: Epstein-Barr virus—Increasing evidence of a link to carcinoma. N Engl J Med 333:724–726, 1995.
278. Laux G, Perricaudet M, Farrell PJ: A spliced Epstein-Barr virus gene expressed in immortalized lymphocytes is created by circularization of the linear viral genome. EMBO J 7:769–774, 1988.
279. Sample J, Liebowitz D, Kieff E: Two related Epstein-Barr virus membrane proteins are encoded by separate genes. J Virol 63:933–937, 1989.
280. Longnecker R, Druker B, Roberts TM, Kieff E: An Epstein-Barr virus protein associated with cell growth transformation interacts with a tyrosine kinase. J Virol 65:3681–3692, 1991.
281. Longnecker R, Miller CL, Miao XQ, et al: The only domain which distinguishes Epstein-Barr virus latent membrane protein 2A (LMP2A) from LMP2B is dispensable for lymphocyte infection and growth transformation in vitro; LMP2A is therefore nonessential. J Virol 66:6461–6469, 1992.
282. Kim OJ, Yates JL: Mutants of Epstein-Barr virus with a selective marker disrupting the TP gene transform B cells and replicate normally in culture. J Virol 67:7634–7640, 1993.
283. Longnecker R, Miller CL, Miao XQ, et al: The last seven transmembrane and carboxy-terminal cytoplasmic domains of Epstein-Barr virus latent membrane protein 2 (LMP2) are dispensable for lymphocyte infection and growth transformation in vitro. J Virol 67:2006–2013, 1993.
284. Longnecker R, Miller CL, Tomkinson B, et al: Deletion of DNA encoding the first five transmembrane domains of Epstein-Barr virus latent membrane proteins 2A and 2B. J Virol 67:5068–5074, 1993.
285. Burkhardt AL, Bolen JB, Kieff E, Longnecker R: An Epstein-Barr virus transformation-associated membrane protein interacts with src family tyrosine kinases. J Virol 66:5161–5167, 1992.
286. Miller CL, Longnecker R, Kieff E: Epstein-Barr virus latent membrane protein 2A blocks calcium mobilization in B lymphocytes. J Virol 67:3087–3094, 1993.
287. Miller CL, Lee JH, Kieff E, Longnecker R: An integral membrane protein (LMP2) blocks reactivation of Epstein-Barr virus from latency following surface immunoglobulin crosslinking. Proc Natl Acad Sci USA 91:772–776, 1994.
288. Miller CL, Burkhardt AL, Lee JH, et al: Integral membrane protein 2 of Epstein-Barr virus regulates reactivation from latency through dominant negative effects on protein-tyrosine kinases. Immunity 2:155–166, 1995.
289. Arrand JR, Rymo L: Characterization of the major Epstein-Barr virus–specific RNA in Burkitt lymphoma–derived cells. J Virol 41:376–389, 1982.
290. Howe JG, Shu MD: Epstein-Barr virus small RNA (EBER) genes: Unique transcription units that combine RNA polymerase II and III promoter elements. Cell 57:825–834, 1989.
291. Howe JG, Steitz JA: Localization of Epstein-Barr virus–encoded small RNAs by in situ hybridization. Proc Natl Acad Sci USA 83:9006–9010, 1986.
292. Tugwood JD, Lau WH, O SK, et al: Epstein-Barr virus–specific transcription in normal and malignant nasopharyngeal biopsies and in lymphocytes from healthy donors and infectious mononucleosis patients. J Gen Virol 68(pt 4):1081–1091, 1987.
293. Lerner MR, Andrews NC, Miller G, Steitz JA: Two small RNAs encoded by Epstein-Barr virus and complexed with protein are precipitated by antibodies from patients with systemic lupus erythematosus. Proc Natl Acad Sci USA 78:805–809, 1981.
294. Glickman JN, Howe JG, Steitz JA: Structural analyses of EBER1 and EBER2 ribonucleoprotein particles present in Epstein-Barr virus–infected cells. J Virol 62:902–911, 1988.
295. Rosa MD, Gottlieb E, Lerner MR, Steitz JA: Striking similarities are exhibited by two small Epstein-Barr virus–encoded ribonucleic acids and the adenovirus-associated ribonucleic acids Vai and Vaii. Mol Cell Biol 1:785–796, 1981.
296. Swaminathan S, Tomkinson B, Kieff E: Recombinant Epstein-Barr virus with small RNA (EBER) genes deleted transforms lymphocytes and replicates in vitro. Proc Natl Acad Sci USA 88:1546–1550, 1991.
297. Lee MA, Kim OJ, Yates JL: Targeted gene disruption in Epstein-Barr virus. Virology 189:253–265, 1992.
298. Lee MA, Yates JL: *BHRF1* of Epstein-Barr virus, which is homologous to human proto-oncogene *bcl*2, is not essential for transformation of B cells or for virus replication in vitro. J Virol 66:1899–1906, 1992.
299. Marchini A, Cohen JI, Wang F, Kieff E: A selectable marker allows investigation of a nontransforming Epstein-Barr virus mutant. J Virol 66:3214–3219, 1992.
300. Marchini A, Kieff E, Longnecker R: Marker rescue of a transformation-negative Epstein-Barr virus recombinant from an infected Burkitt lymphoma cell line: A method useful for analysis of genes essential for transformation. J Virol 67:606–609, 1993.
301. Marchini A, Longnecker R, Kieff E: Epstein-Barr virus (EBV)–negative B-lymphoma cell lines for clonal isolation and replication of EBV recombinants. J Virol 66:4972–4981, 1992.
302. Marchini A, Tomkinson B, Cohen JI, Kieff E: *BHRF1*, the Epstein-Barr virus gene with homology to Bc12, is dispensable for B-lymphocyte transformation and virus replication. J Virol 65:5991–6000, 1991.
303. Robertson ES, Tomkinson B, Kieff E: An Epstein-Barr virus with a 58-kilobase-pair deletion that includes *BARF0* transforms B lymphocytes in vitro. J Virol 68:1449–1458, 1994.
304. Tomkinson B, Kieff E: Second-site homologous recombination in Epstein-Barr virus: Insertion of type 1 EBNA 3 genes in place of type 2 has no effect on in vitro infection. J Virol 66:780–789, 1992.
305. Tomkinson B, Robertson E, Yalamanchili R, et al: Epstein-Barr virus recombinants from overlapping cosmid fragments. J Virol 67:7298–7306, 1993.
306. Wang F, Marchini A, Kieff E: Epstein-Barr virus (EBV) recombinants: Use of positive selection markers to rescue mutants in EBV-negative B-lymphoma cells. J Virol 65:1701–1709, 1991.
307. Rickinson AB, Kieff E: Epstein-Barr virus. *In* Fields B, Knipe D, Howley P (eds): Fields Virology, ed 3. Philadelphia, Lippincott-Raven, 1996, pp 2397–2446.
308. Kieff E: Tumor viruses. *In* Abeloff M, Armitage J, Lichter A, et

al (eds): Clinical Oncology. New York, Churchill Livingstone, 1995, pp 135–150.

308a. Klein G: Epstein-Barr virus strategy in normal and neoplastic B cells. Cell 77:791–793, 1994.

309. Rowe M, Rowe DT, Gregory CD, et al: Differences in B cell growth phenotype reflect novel patterns of Epstein-Barr virus latent gene expression in Burkitt's lymphoma cells. EMBO J 6:2743–2751, 1987.

310. Lenoir GM, Philip T, Sohier R: Burkitt-type lymphoma: EBV association and cytogenetic markers in cases from various geographic locations. Prog Cancer Res Ther 27:283–295, 1984.

311. Magrath I, Jain V, Bhatia K: Epstein-Barr virus and Burkitt's lymphoma. Semin Cancer Biol 3:285–295, 1992.

312. Magrath I: The pathogenesis of Burkitt's lymphoma. Adv Cancer Res 55:133–270, 1990.

313. Fahraeus R, Chen W, Trivedi P, et al: Decreased expression of E-cadherin and increased invasive capacity in EBV-LMP–transfected human epithelial and murine adenocarcinoma cells. Int J Cancer 52:834–838, 1992.

314. Henle W, Henle G: Seroepidemiology of the virus. *In* Epstein M, Achong B (eds): The Epstein-Barr Virus. Berlin, Springer-Verlag, 1979, pp 61–78.

315. Herbst H, Dallenbach F, Hummel M, et al: Epstein-Barr virus latent membrane protein expression in Hodgkin and Reed-Sternberg cells. Proc Natl Acad Sci USA 88:4766–4770, 1991.

316. Pallesen G, Hamilton-Dutoit SJ, Rowe M, et al: Expression of Epstein-Barr virus replicative proteins in AIDS-related non-Hodgkin's lymphoma cells. J Pathol 165:289–299, 1991.

317. Jarrett RF, Gallagher A, Jones DB, et al: Detection of Epstein-Barr virus genomes in Hodgkin's disease: Relation to age [see comments]. J Clin Pathol 44:844–848, 1991.

318. Pallesen G, Hamilton-Dutoit SJ, Rowe M, Young LS: Expression of Epstein-Barr virus latent gene products in tumour cells of Hodgkin's disease [see comments]. Lancet 337:320–322, 1991.

319. Levine P, Connelly R: Epidemiology of nasopharyngeal cancer. *In* Wittes R (ed): Head and Neck Cancer. New York, John Wiley & Sons, 1985, pp 13–34.

320. Muir C, Waterhouse J, Mack T, et al: Cancer Incidence in Five Continents, Vol 5. Lyon, France, International Agency for Research in Cancer, 1987. IARC publication 88.

321. Wolf H, zur Hausen H, Becker V: EB viral genome in epithelial nasopharyngeal carcinoma cells. Nature New Biol 244:245–247, 1973.

322. Zur Hausen H, Schulte-Holthauzen H, Klein G, et al: EBV DNA in biopsies of Burkitt tumours and anaplastic carcinomas of the nasopharynx. Nature 228:1956–1958, 1970.

323. Henle W, Henle G, Ho HC, et al: Antibodies to Epstein-Barr virus in nasopharyngeal carcinoma, other head and neck neoplasms, and control groups. J Natl Cancer Inst 44:225–231, 1970.

324. Old L, Clifford P, Boyse E, et al: Precipitating antibody in human serum to an antigen present in cultured Burkitt's lymphoma cells. Proc Natl Acad Sci USA 56:1699–1704, 1966.

325. de The G, Zeng Y: Population screening for EBV markers: Toward improvement of nasopharyngeal carcinoma control. *In* Epstein M, Achong B (eds): The Epstein-Barr Virus: Recent Advances. London, William Heinemann, 1986, pp 237–249.

326. Henle G, Henle W: Epstein-Barr virus–specific IgA serum antibodies as an outstanding feature of nasopharyngeal carcinoma. Int J Cancer 17:1–7, 1976.

327. Zeng Y: Seroepidemiological studies on nasopharyngeal carcinoma in China. Adv Cancer Res 44:121–138, 1985.

328. Brooks L, Yao QY, Rickinson AB, Young LS: Epstein-Barr virus latent gene transcription in nasopharyngeal carcinoma cells: Coexpression of EBNA1, LMP1, and LMP2 transcripts. J Virol 66:2689–2697, 1992.

329. Busson P, McCoy R, Sadler R, et al: Consistent transcription of the Epstein-Barr virus LMP2 gene in nasopharyngeal carcinoma. J Virol 66:3257–3262, 1992.

330. Fahraeus R, Fu HL, Ernberg I, et al: Expression of Epstein-Barr virus–encoded proteins in nasopharyngeal carcinoma. Int J Cancer 42:329–338, 1988.

331. Young LS, Dawson CW, Clark D, et al: Epstein-Barr virus gene expression in nasopharyngeal carcinoma. J Gen Virol 69(pt 5):1051–1065, 1988.

331a. Wilson JB, Weinberg W, Johnson R, et al: Expression of the BNLF-1 oncogene of Epstein-Barr virus in the skin of transgenic mice induces hyperplasia and aberrant expression of keratin 6. Cell 61:1315–1327, 1990.

331b. Fåhraeus R, Rymo L, Rhim JS, Klein G: Morphological transformation of human keratinocytes expressing the LMP gene of Epstein-Barr virus. Nature 345:447–449, 1990.

331c. Dawson CW, Rickinson AB, Young LS: Epstein-Barr virus latent membrane protein inhibits human epithelial cell differentiation. Nature 344:777–780, 1990.

332. Locker J, Nalesnik M: Molecular genetic analysis of lymphoid tumours arising after organ transplantation. Am J Pathol 135:977–987, 1989.

333. Shapiro RS, McClain K, Frizzera G, et al: Epstein-Barr virus associated B cell lymphoproliferative disorders following bone marrow transplantation. Blood 71:1234–1243, 1988.

334. Weiss LM, Movahed LA: In situ demonstration of Epstein-Barr viral genomes in viral-associated B cell lymphoproliferations. Am J Pathol 134:651–659, 1989.

335. Zutter MM, Martin PJ, Sale GE, et al: Epstein-Barr virus lymphoproliferation after bone marrow transplantation. Blood 72:520–529, 1988.

336. Gratama JW, Zutter MM, Minarovits J, et al: Expression of Epstein-Barr virus–encoded growth-transformation–associated proteins in lymphoproliferations of bone-marrow transplant recipients. Int J Cancer 47:188–192, 1991.

337. Thomas JA, Hotchin NA, Allday MJ, et al: Immunohistology of Epstein-Barr virus–associated antigens in B cell disorders from immunocompromised individuals. Transplantation 49:944–953, 1990.

338. Young L, Alfieri C, Hennessy K, et al: Expression of Epstein-Barr virus transformation-associated genes in tissues of patients with EBV lymphoproliferative disease. N Engl J Med 321:1080–1085, 1989.

339. Cohen JI: Epstein-Barr virus lymphoproliferative disease associated with acquired immunodeficiency. Medicine (Baltimore) 70:137–160, 1991.

340. Purtilo D, DeFlorio DJ, Huff L, et al: Variable phenotypic expression of an X-linked lymphoproliferative syndrome. N Engl J Med 297:1077–1081, 1977.

341. Starzl T, Nalesnik M, Porter K, et al: Reversibility of lymphomas and lymphoproliferative lesions developing under cyclosporin A–steroid therapy. Lancet 1:583–587, 1984.

342. Fischer A, Blanche S, Le Bidois J, et al: Anti–B-cell monoclonal antibodies in the treatment of severe B-cell lymphoproliferative syndrome following bone marrow and organ transplantation. N Engl J Med 324:1451–1456, 1991.

343. Papadopoulos EB, Ladanyi M, Emanuel D, et al: Infusions of donor leukocytes to treat Epstein-Barr virus–associated lymphoproliferative disorders after allogeneic bone marrow transplantation [see comments]. N Engl J Med 330:1185–1191, 1994.

344. Pedersen C, Gerstoft J, Lundgren JD, et al: HIV-associated lymphoma: Histopathology and association with Epstein-Barr virus genome related to clinical, immunological and prognostic features. Eur J Cancer 27:1416–1423, 1991.

345. Epstein-Barr virus and AIDS-associated lymphomas. Lancet 338:979–981, 1991.

346. Hamilton-Dutoit SJ, Rea D, Raphael M, et al: Epstein-Barr virus–latent gene expression and tumor cell phenotype in acquired immunodeficiency syndrome–related non-Hodgkin's lymphoma. Correlation of lymphoma phenotype with three distinct patterns of viral latency. Am J Pathol 143:1072–1085, 1993.

347. Hamilton-Dutoit SJ, Raphael M, Audouin J, et al: In situ demonstration of Epstein-Barr virus small RNAs (EBER 1) in acquired immunodeficiency syndrome–related lymphomas: Correlation with tumor morphology and primary site. Blood 82:619–624, 1993.

348. MacMahon EM, Glass JD, Hayward SD, et al: Epstein-Barr virus in AIDS-related primary central nervous system lymphoma. Lancet 338:969–973, 1991.

243

Varicella-Zoster Virus

Charles Grose
John A. Zaia

Structure of the Virus and Its Genome

Varicella-zoster virus (VZV) is one of the seven human herpesviruses; the other six are herpes simplex virus (HSV) types 1 and 2, human cytomegalovirus, Epstein-Barr virus, and human herpesvirus types 6, 7, and 8. Like the other members of the herpesvirus family, VZV is an enveloped virus that contains double-stranded DNA within its protein core. The viral particle is an icosahedron. The complete enveloped virion measures between 150 and 200 nm in diameter; the naked particle is about 95 nm in diameter (Fig. 243–1).

The linear duplex VZV DNA has a buoyant density of 1.705 g/cm^3 in cesium chloride.[1, 2] The relative molecular mass of the VZV genome has been calculated from its rate of sedimentation in neutral sucrose to be approximately 92 to 110 × 10^6 daltons.[2, 3] When measured by electron microscopy and compared with a known standard, the relative mass was found to be 80 × 10^6 daltons,[4, 5] and this has been confirmed by electrophoretic analyses.[5] This viral DNA exists predominantly as two isomers.[5–7] In the conventional arrangement established for the DNA of the prototype HSV, VZV DNA can be divided into two segments, long (L) and short (S), separated by a joint region. The long segment is composed almost entirely of a unique sequence (UL). In contrast, the short segment contains a central unique sequence (US) flanked by internal and terminal inverted repeated sequences (IRs and TRs). Because of the presence of these repeated sequences, the short segment can be found in either of two equimolar orientations relative to the long segment of the VZV genome. These two arrangements are the basis for the two isomers of VZV DNA, in contrast to HSV, which, because both UL and US can invert relative to each other, exists as four isomers.[8]

The entire sequence of the VZV genome has been determined by M13-dideoxynucleotide technology.[9] The sequence includes 124,884 base pairs. The sequence data imply that the VZV genome contains 71 open reading frames, among which are six that encode VZV glycoproteins. These glycoprotein genes have been designated *gB, gC, gE, gH, gI,* and *gL*.[10] Among the human herpesviruses, VZV appears to code for the fewest glycoproteins. A comprehensive review of the VZV glycoproteins has been published.[11]

Replication of the Virus in Tissue Culture

Before the development of adequate virologic methods for isolation of VZV in tissue culture, clinical observation suggested that the causative agents of chickenpox and herpes zoster were similar.[12] Varicella was observed to occur not only after exposure to zoster but also after inoculation of susceptible children with vesicle fluid from persons with acute herpes zoster. The major significant advance in understanding the nature of these agents, however, was contributed by Weller and coworkers, who demonstrated the method for isolation and serial propagation of VZV.[13, 14] To study virus replication, growth kinetic experiments have been carried out in cell culture.[15] One of the peculiar properties of VZV is its propensity to remain cell associated (i.e., the viral particle remains attached to the outer cell membrane and is not released into the cell culture medium). Therefore, cell-free virus is difficult to prepare and viral infectivity titers are invariably low. The preferred method of obtaining cell-free virus is sonic disruption of VZV-infected cells that have first been dislodged from the culture flask with a rubber policeman.[16] Generally, titers of cell-free virus range from 1000 to 10,000 plaque-forming units per milliliter. As an alternative to cell-free virus, single-cell suspensions can be obtained by trypsin dispersion of VZV-infected monolayers and then used as a cell-associated virus inoculum.

The spread of virus from cell to cell has also been documented by fluorescent antibody staining.[15] Viral antigens are first detected in the nucleus of the newly infected cell within 4 hours of infection. Subsequently, the pattern of virus-specific fluorescence spreads to the cytoplasm by 14 hours and to neighboring cells by 18 hours after infection. Thus, a single

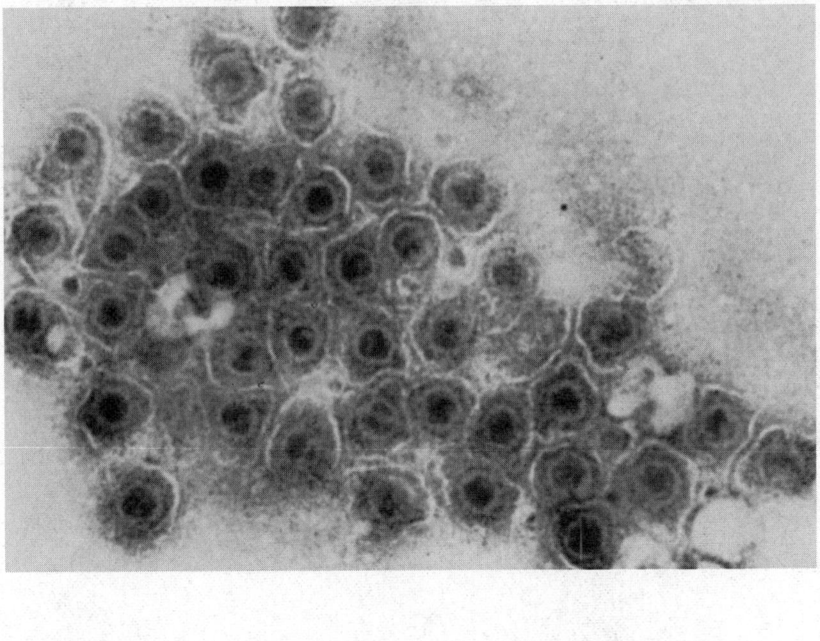

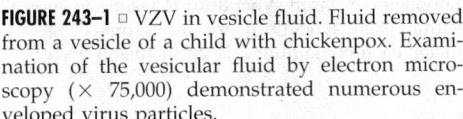

FIGURE 243–1 □ VZV in vesicle fluid. Fluid removed from a vesicle of a child with chickenpox. Examination of the vesicular fluid by electron microscopy (× 75,000) demonstrated numerous enveloped virus particles.

VZV replication cycle is estimated to last approximately 18 hours. To obtain maximal titers of infectivity in an infected monolayer, the virus appears to pass through two or three replication cycles.

The regulatory mechanisms affecting VZV replication have not been well delineated, but they probably resemble those already described for HSV replication.[17] Based on an operational definition, this regulatory cycle is divided into a minimum of three phases, which have been designated immediate early, early, and late. The synthesis of proteins in each phase is said to be coordinately regulated and sequentially ordered in a cascade pattern; otherwise stated, groups of viral peptides appear in an infected cell in a predictable pattern and the synthesis of the later-appearing proteins is dependent on the prior synthesis of earlier proteins. The last viral proteins to be synthesized during the late phase are the structural components of the virion.

The cytopathic effect of VZV infection is shown in Figure 243–2. In tissue culture, the virus spreads through the cell monolayer at a slower rate than HSV, presumably because of the relatively small amount of extracellular virus. The resultant cell-to-cell spread of virus produces a linear focality of cytopathic effect in vitro. Infected cells contain an intranuclear inclusion body indistinguishable from the Cowdry type A inclusions first described in HSV infection. In clinical disease a similar inclusion body is observed in infected tissue; this cytopathologic finding is identical for both chickenpox and herpes zoster.[14, 18]

Electron micrographic analysis of vesicle fluid from children with chickenpox demonstrates cell-free enveloped virions (see Fig. 243–1). The mechanism by which the VZV particle becomes enveloped and exits from an infected cell is not known. Based on the presence of enveloped virions within cytoplasmic vesicles, it is presumed that VZV does not acquire its envelope by budding through the outer cell membrane as do RNA viruses.[19] Instead, the nucleocapsid is formed in the nucleus and surrounds the newly synthesized viral DNA; it acquires an envelope after it exits the nucleus and buds into a cytoplasmic vacuole. These cytoplasmic vacuoles, which are thought to be derived from the Golgi apparatus, carry the enveloped virions to the outer cell membrane, where exocytosis occurs.[19]

Host Immune Response to Infection

Our understanding of the host immune response to VZV infection has changed with the technology available for immune analyses. For example, the antibody response to VZV has been measured by several methods with various degrees of sensitivity. In the 1950s and 1960s, the usual procedure was the complement fixation (CF) test. When serum samples from persons with chickenpox were assayed for CF antibody, it was observed that almost all children developed VZV antibody by the second week of illness. Within 1 year after chickenpox, VZV antibody was no longer detectable in 75% of the subjects. Thus, the VZV CF test is a poor assay for determining humoral immune status in the general population.

This deficiency was overcome in the 1970s by the development of an indirect fluorescent method, which used live VZV-infected cells as a substrate.[20, 21] In this assay, serum is incubated with an infected cell suspension or cell monolayer, after which a fluorescein-tagged antihuman globulin is added to the mixture. If the patient's serum sample contains VZV antibodies, they adhere to the viral antigens in the membranes of the infected cell and can then be detected by fluorescein-conjugated second antibody. This test has been called by the acronym FAMA (fluorescent antibody to membrane antigen). Because the FAMA test is more sensitive than the CF test, it can detect low levels of VZV-specific antibody in the serum of persons who had chickenpox long ago. With this test, it is possible to determine the humoral immune status in populations at high risk, such as children with leukemia or adult health care providers exposed to chickenpox.[22]

The nature of the fluorescent test was further defined by a comparison between the FAMA test and a VZV-specific neutralization assay.[23] The results showed a high degree of concordance between the two tests (i.e., nearly all persons

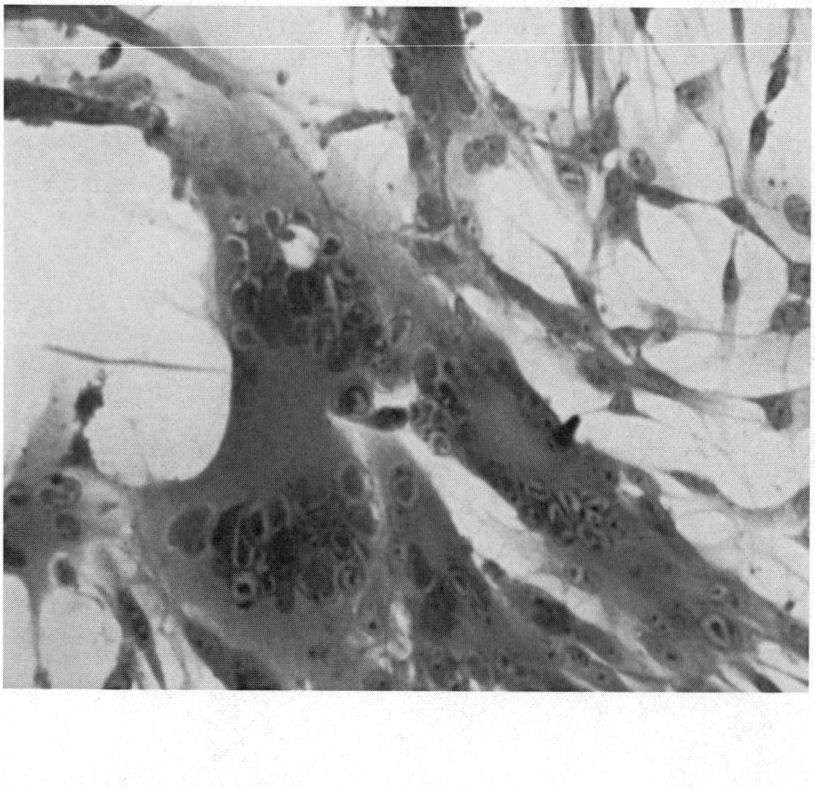

FIGURE 243–2 ▫ Cytopathic effect induced by VZV infection in human melanoma cell tissue culture monolayer. A large syncytium is visible in center. Within each syncytium are numerous clustered nuclei, each containing a large inclusion body.

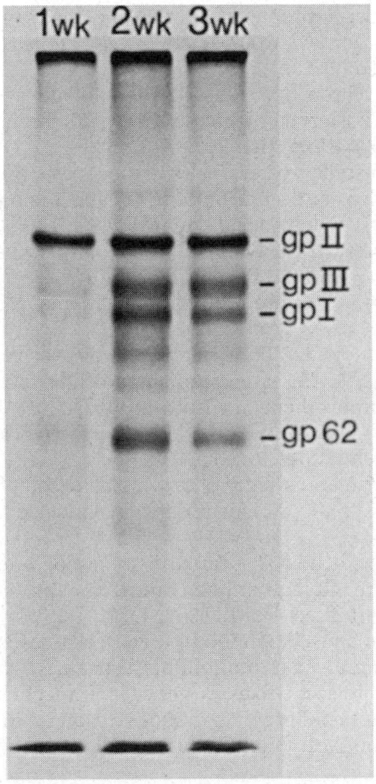

FIGURE 243–3 □ The immunoglobulin G response to the VZV glycoproteins during chickenpox. Serum from a healthy child with chickenpox was collected weekly, and all three samples were analyzed for immunoglobulin G antibodies to VZV glycoproteins by radioimmunoprecipitation methods. The autoradiographic profiles indicated the presence of antibody to VZV gpII during the first week (wk) of chickenpox (lane 1), whereas antibodies to gpI and gpIII appeared during the second week of illness (lanes 2 and 3). The new nomenclature for the VZV glycoproteins is as follows: gpI is now gE; gpII, gB; gpIII, gH; and gp62, gI. (From Grose C, Litwin V: Immunology of the varicella-zoster viral glycoproteins. J Infect Dis 157:877–881, 1988.)

with a positive FAMA titer also had demonstrable anti-VZV neutralizing antibody). This study suggested that the two assays were measuring a similar set of antibodies and, furthermore, that the neutralization determinants were present on the outer membrane of the infected cells.

These neutralization epitopes are harbored in the VZV glycoproteins, which are present on the cell surface.[11, 23] The humoral immune response to the individual VZV glycoprotein antigens can be assessed by immunoprecipitation reactions between crude radiolabeled VZV antigens and human serum samples (Fig. 243–3). By this method, antibody to at least one of the major VZV glycoproteins is easily demonstrable within 1 week after onset of chickenpox. By 2 weeks, antibodies to two more viral glycoproteins are present. The amount of glycoprotein antibody reaches a peak by 4 to 8 weeks, before a gradual decline occurs over the years after the episode of chickenpox.

As measured by lymphocyte proliferation assays, susceptible persons have no proliferative response in vitro to VZV antigens, and those with chickenpox also develop a cell-mediated immune response to the individual VZV glycoproteins.[24] These immunologic analyses suggest that viral glycoproteins are important for induction of a protective immune response to VZV.

Laboratory Diagnosis

Several methods are available for diagnosing VZV infection. Diagnosis can reliably be made on clinical grounds alone when there is a history of close exposure to chickenpox or herpes zoster in the past 10 to 21 days and a vesicular eruption consistent with chickenpox. In many situations, particularly those involving immunocompromised persons, often there are no clear historical data to support the diagnosis. In this situation, because treatment is of paramount importance, laboratory diagnosis is necessary. The earliest method for diagnosis was light microscopic examination of the vesicle contents stained with Wright-Giemsa stain to demonstrate multinucleated giant cells (Tzanck test). The presence of these giant cells strongly suggests a hepersvirus infection but not specifically VZV; for example, HSV infection causes similar cytopathology. Electron microscopic visualization of vesicular fluid also demonstrates VZV particles (see Fig. 243–1). Again, VZV particles cannot be differentiated from other herpesviruses by this diagnostic procedure.

In most virology laboratories, VZV infection is diagnosed by virus isolation in cell culture. Vesicular fluid is usually collected in sterile capillary tubes or tuberculin syringes, which are subsequently evacuated into culture medium. The medium is then layered over cultured cells, and in 3 to 5 days the cytopathic effect is visible in the monolayer. In human fibroblast cells, the result is multiple foci of swollen, rounded, refractile cells. In human melanoma cells, another excellent substrate for VZV isolation, the virus induces characteristic large syncytial foci whose nuclei are filled with inclusions (see Fig. 243–2). The extension of the cytopathic effect follows the longitudinal axis of the cell monolayer, a useful way of distinguishing this cytopathic effect from that of HSV. A definitive diagnosis of VZV infection is made by immunohistologic staining of the infected monolayer with a VZV-specific monoclonal antibody. VZV can also be isolated from the blood of viremic patients by inoculating buffy coat specimens onto cell monolayers.

A newer method for rapid diagnosis of VZV infection uses a fluorescein-conjugated VZV monoclonal antibody.[24] Samples of cells are obtained from the base of the vesicle lesion and dried onto a glass slide. The cells are then probed with the conjugated VZV-specific monoclonal antibody. In-

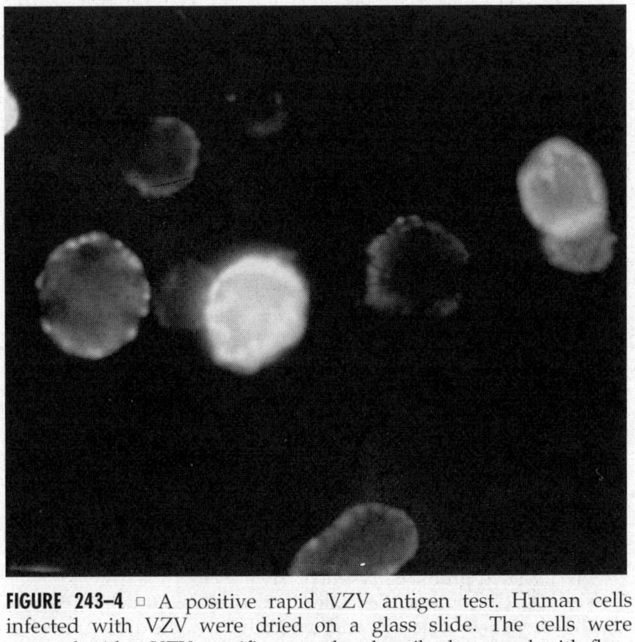

FIGURE 243–4 □ A positive rapid VZV antigen test. Human cells infected with VZV were dried on a glass slide. The cells were covered with a VZV-specific monoclonal antibody tagged with fluorescein. Bright surface staining is easily seen on several cells. Because the VZV rapid antigen test is more sensitive and specific, it should replace the Tzanck test.

fected cells that contain VZV antigens fluoresce brightly and are easily detectable. Rapid diagnosis by antigen detection can also be performed on punch biopsy specimens of vesicular lesions. The test requires only 1 or 2 hours and can quickly differentiate between vesicular rashes caused by VZV and HSV infection. Rapid diagnostic kits are available from commercial sources. Most kits use antibody to VZV gpI (now called VZV gE), because gE is the major cell surface antigen specified by VZV in infected cells (Fig. 243–4).

Serologic methods can be used to confirm the diagnosis, but because this requires acute- and convalescent-phase serum specimens, it is clearly not a method for rapid diagnosis.[22] Serum samples are obtained during the acute illness and then 14 to 28 days later. Titration of the level of VZV antibodies by either the CF test or the FAMA test shows a fourfold or greater rise in titer. The FAMA test can also be adapted to detect only VZV-specific immunoglobulin M antibody, a single positive result being diagnostic of acute VZV infection. Advances in serologic techniques to measure VZV antibody include the development of enzyme-linked immunosorbent assay, and commercially available assays are an acceptable alternative to FAMA for measurement of VZV antibody.[24]

Because they are so sensitive, the FAMA or enzyme-linked immunosorbent assays are reliable methods for demonstrating prior infection with VZV. For this reason, these tests are widely used as presumptive evidence of immunity after exposure to chickenpox. It should be noted that these assays are not reliable in persons who have received blood products and who might have acquired passive antibody. As mentioned earlier, the CF test, because it is insensitive for antibody, should not be used for determination of prior infection.

Acknowledgment

Research by the authors is supported by grants from the National Institutes of Health.

References

1. Ludwig H, Haines HG, Biswal N, Benyesh-Melnick M: The characterization of varicella-zoster virus DNA. J Gen Virol 14:111, 1972.
2. Iltis JP, Oakes JE, Hyman RW, Rapp F: Comparison of the DNAs of varicella-zoster viruses isolated from clinical cases of varicella and herpes zoster. Virology 82:345, 1977.
3. Rapp F, Iltis JP, Oakes JE, Hyman RW: A novel approach to study the DNA of herpes zoster virus. Intervirology 8:272, 1977.
4. Dumas AM, Geelen JLMC, Maris W, van der Noordaa J: Infectivity and molecular weight of varicella-zoster virus DNA. J Gen Virol 47:233, 1980.
5. Straus SE, Aulakh HS, Ruyechan WT, et al: Structure of varicella-zoster virus DNA. J Virol 40:516, 1981.
6. Ecker JR, Hyman RW: Varicella zoster virus DNA exists as two isomers. Proc Natl Acad Sci USA 79:156, 1982.
7. Hyman RW: The molecular genetics of varicella-zoster virus. *In* Hyman RW (ed): Natural History of Varicella-Zoster Virus. Boca Raton, FL, CRC Press, 1987, pp 131–162.
8. Roizman B: The structure and isomerization of herpes simplex virus genomes. Cell 16:481, 1979.
9. Davison AJ, Scott JE: The complete DNA sequence of varicella-zoster virus. J Gen Virol 67:1759, 1986.
10. Davison AJ, Edson CM, Ellis RW, et al: New common nomenclature for glycoprotein genes of varicella-zoster virus and their glycosylated products. J Virol 57:1195, 1986.
11. Grose C: Glycoproteins encoded by varicella-zoster virus: Biosynthesis, phosphorylation, and intracellular trafficking. Annu Rev Microbiol 44:59, 1990.
12. Zaia JA: Clinical spectrum of varicella-zoster virus infection. *In* Nahmias AJ, et al (eds): The Human Herpesviruses. Amsterdam, Elsevier North Holland, 1981.
13. Weller TH: Serial propagation in vitro of agents producing inclusion bodies derived from varicella and herpes zoster. Proc Soc Exp Biol Med 83:340, 1953.
14. Weller TH, Witton HM, Bell EJ: The etiologic agents of varicella and herpes zoster: serologic studies with the viruses as propagated in vitro. J Exp Med 108:843, 1958.
15. Grose C: Varicella zoster virus: Pathogenesis of the human diseases, the virus and viral replication, and the major viral glycoproteins and proteins. *In* Hyman RW (ed): Natural History of Varicella-Zoster Virus. Boca Raton, FL, CRC Press, 1987, pp 1–65.
16. Grose C, Perrotta DM, Brunell PA, Smith GC: Cell-free varicella-zoster virus in cultured human melanoma cells. J Gen Virol 43:15, 1979.
17. Honess RW, Roizman B: Regulation of herpesvirus macromolecular synthesis. I. Cascade regulation of the synthesis of three groups of viral proteins. J Virol 14:8, 1974.
18. Cowdry EV: The problem of intranuclear inclusions in virus diseases. Arch Pathol 18:527, 1934.
19. Harson R, Grose C: Egress of varicella-zoster virus from the melanoma cell: A tropism for the melanocyte. J Virol 69:4994, 1995.
20. Williams V, Gershon A, Brunell PA: Serologic response to varicella-zoster membrane antigens measured by indirect immunofluorescence. J Infect Dis 130:669, 1971.
21. Zaia JA, Oxman MN: Antibody to varicella-zoster virus–induced membrane antigen: Immunofluorescence assay using monodisperse glutaraldehyde-fixed target cells. J Infect Dis 136:519, 1977.
22. Gershon AA, Steinberg SP: Antibody response to varicella-zoster virus and the role of antibody in host defense. Am J Med Sci 282:12, 1981.
23. Grose C, Litwin V: Immunology of the varicella-zoster viral glycoproteins. J Infect Dis 157:877, 1988.
24. Grose C: Varicella-zoster virus infections—Chickenpox, shingles and varicella vaccine. *In* Glaser R (ed): Herpesvirus Infections. New York, Marcel Dekker, 1994, pp 117–186.

244

Cytomegalovirus

Sarah H. Cheeseman

History

Cytomegalovirus (CMV), originally called human salivary gland virus, was isolated independently in 1956 by Rowe and colleagues,[1] from adenoids of normal children undergoing tonsillectomy and adenoidectomy; by Smith,[2] from salivary glands of a child with disseminated disease and another dying of an unrelated tumor; and by Weller and colleagues,[3] from a liver biopsy specimen from a child with a congenital infection syndrome.

Characteristics of the Pathogen

Classification and Structure

CMV belongs to the family Herpesviridae, with whose other members it shares the characteristics of high frequency and lifelong persistence of infection and capability of reactivation. It is classified in the subfamily Betaherpesvirinae, along with human herpesviruses 6 and 7, on the basis of a number of properties, including restricted host range and long replication cycle. The viral particle is approximately 102 nm in diameter and (working from the outside in) consists of a lipid envelope studded with glycoproteins, surrounding a tegument (matrix) of phosphoproteins, an icosahedral nucleocapsid, and a DNA genome with a molecular mass of 155 kDa.

The CMV genome consists of linear double-stranded DNA arranged in long and short unique regions, each framed by repeating segments with mirror symmetry, called inverted terminal repeats. There is some homology between human DNA and the CMV long terminal repeats, so that molecular probes for hybridization must always take care to exclude this region. The entire genome has been sequenced, but the products and purpose of most of the 208 genes identified have not been defined.[4]

Viral components previously identified by their location, structure, and molecular weight are being renamed based on the segment (UL for unique long and US for unique short) of the genome where they are found and the map unit at which the open reading frame begins.[5] Thus, the lower matrix phosphoprotein, pp65, is designated ppUL83. This protein is the predominant CMV antigen in leukocytes of actively infected patients, the major component of the CMV complement fixation antigen, and a major target of $CD8^+$ lymphocyte cytotoxicity.[5, 6] A 150-kDa basic phosphoprotein, formerly pp150 and now known as ppUL32, is also a highly immunogenic component of the virus matrix.

Several human cellular proteins are found regularly in association with viral particles[7, 8] (Giugni TD, personal communication, March 15, 1995), but we do not know whether they are analogs encoded by the viral genome or are of cellular origin and incorporated in the process of virus assembly and release.

Replication

CMV initially attaches to heparan sulfate proteoglycans on the surface of cells via one or more of its envelope glycoprotein complexes.[9–13] The initial reversible attachment quickly becomes high-affinity binding, through either conformational change or the involvement of other molecules.[13] Interaction between CMV gpUL75 (glycoprotein gH, gp86) and a 92.5-kDa cellular protein appears to be responsible for fusion and viral penetration of the cell.[11] Several additional cell surface proteins involved in CMV binding and infection have been identified, including a 30- to 34-kDa protein that also binds viral glycoproteins[14–16] and a 130- to 150-kDa protein identical to human aminopeptidase N, which can render murine cells susceptible to human CMV.[8]

After fusion, CMV is transported to the nucleus, where viral tegument protein (ppUL83) may be detected.[5] The first new viral transcripts are the immediate early proteins; these appear to be transcribed directly from the inoculating viral sequence because they are expressed in the presence of a DNA polymerase inhibitor.[17] Thus, the expression of the major immediate early protein p72 in the nucleus may be the only evidence of infection in cells in which the virus does not complete its replicative cycle.[18] Among the activities of immediate early protein is binding to host cell as well as viral DNA,[19] but whether this is the mechanism for the stimulation of host cell macromolecular synthesis that follows CMV infection is unclear.

CMV immediate early and early proteins are produced within 1 to 2 hours and 2 to 24 hours, respectively, but late or structural proteins are not produced until 24 hours or more after infection, along with new copies of viral DNA.[20] Newly produced viral genomes along with tegument proteins are packaged and exported from the nucleus to the cytoplasm. The virus acquires its envelope in the course of passage through the Golgi apparatus or the plasma membrane.[20] The envelope glycoproteins undergo extensive post-translational processing to disulfide-linked complexes whose molecular weight designations vary maddeningly, but which the new nomenclature greatly simplifies. The predominant target of neutralizing antibody, glycoprotein B (gB),[21–27] is gpUL55 rather than gp55/116/130/150 or glycoprotein complex I. Glycoprotein H, the viral component that appears to fuse with the cell surface, is gpUL75 (previous designations were gp86 and glycoprotein complex III).[5]

After release from the cell, virus in the urine, and probably in other body fluids, adsorbs β_2-microglobulin, the light chain of class I human leukocyte antigen molecules.[28] This substance masks virus antigenic sites and prevents neutralization by antibody,[29] as well as augmenting infectivity, at least in some in vitro systems.[30, 31]

Biologic Properties

Host Range

Human CMV had been thought not to replicate in the cells of any other species, although a laboratory-attenuated strain (Towne) has been grown in primary chimpanzee skin fibroblasts.[32] Of common laboratory cells, only human fibroblasts support the replication of CMV, although they do not seem to be a target of the virus in vivo. Human endothelial cells can be infected by primary isolates but not by laboratory strains of the virus passaged in fibroblasts.[33] The virus displays a preference for differentiated cells.[34, 35]

Persistence

The capability of blood transfusions and organ transplants donated by seropositive persons to transmit CMV has long been established. Although CMV can be isolated from, and antigen can be detected in, circulating polymorphonuclear and mononuclear blood cells from actively infected immunocompromised patients, there has been only one report of isolation of infectious CMV from normal blood donors, despite efforts to repeat that observation by testing more than 1500 specimens.[36] The difficulty in getting peripheral blood or bone marrow cells to support the full cycle of CMV replication in vitro, despite evidence of infection by the production of immediate early antigen in vitro and in vivo,[37–42] focused attention on the likelihood that CMV exists in a latent state in these cells in healthy seropositive donors. The virus could then be reactivated after transfusion or transplantation, as allogeneic stimulation reactivates latent CMV in a murine model.[43] In fact, expression of CMV immediate early antigen does accompany in vitro differentiation to macrophages of monocytes from healthy CMV-seropositive donors.[35]

Polymerase chain reaction has made it possible to detect extremely low copy numbers of DNA or RNA transcripts within cells and thus to search directly for the site of viral persistence. By using this technique, CMV DNA has now been detected within the monocyte population of normal healthy persons seronegative and seropositive for CMV.[44] Quantitation of CMV DNA in peripheral blood leukocytes demonstrated low but comparable copy numbers in normal human immunodeficiency virus–negative, CMV-seronegative, and CMV-seropositive persons, as well as in asymptomatic human immunodeficiency virus–seropositive persons with $CD4^+$ cell counts greater than $100/mm^3$.[45] RNA transcripts for a late gene product of CMV have been detected with equal frequency (43% or 44%) in CMV-seropositive and -seronegative blood donor units.[46] Because selection of CMV-negative donors for blood transfusion and organ transplantation has been shown to prevent CMV infection in seronegative recipients, it is difficult to accept these results as evidence of either the site of viral latency or the lack of validity of conventional serology.

Vascular endothelial cells also support CMV replication and have the wide distribution required to explain transmission from all types of organ donation. The finding of circulating cytomegalic cells of endothelial origin in immunocompromised patients with active CMV infection shows that endothelial cells can be infected in vivo.[47] In an in vitro model, CMV can be transmitted from infected endothelial cell monolayers to monocytes and back to new endothelial cell monolayers.[48]

A possible alternative site of persistence is the lung. Human alveolar macrophages, highly differentiated cells of monocytic lineage, are fully permissive for the replication in vitro of CMV strain AD169.[49] In an autopsy study of 69 adults, CMV was isolated from the lungs of 8.[50] Four of these patients had not received exogenous immunosuppression, although some degree of immunosuppression, secondary to the debilitation of their terminal conditions, might be expected. A monoclonal antibody specific for an immediate early protein of CMV stained a wide number of cell types in various organs of six of nine seropositive individuals who died of trauma or other acute medical conditions not known to be immunosuppressive; kidney and lung were the most frequently positive organs, and endothelial cells stained positive in all tissues.[51]

Oncogenesis

Although CMV can be transforming in certain systems in vitro, there is little evidence to support a role in human carcinogenesis. Serologic associations and reports of detection of CMV nucleic acid in tumor cells formed the basis for debate about a causal relationship with Kaposi's sarcoma,[52–54] but it now appears that a distinct herpesvirus, more closely related to Epstein-Barr virus than CMV, is likely to be responsible for this entity.[55–57] Possible links to prostatic carcinoma[58] and to adenocarcinoma of the colon[59, 60] have also been proposed.

Antigenic Characteristics

Antigenic differences defined by avidity of reaction of various human serum samples to the laboratory prototype strains of CMV have been described, but these strain variations do not appear to have clinical import. Restriction endonuclease analysis of genomes from low-passage clinical isolates has been a more important tool for learning about the epidemiology of CMV infection, in particular for differentiating reactivation from reinfection.

Epidemiology

CMV can be transmitted from mother to child in utero (presumably via the transplacental route), during the birth process (from cervical and vaginal secretions), or in the early postnatal period, when breast milk is the most important vehicle.[61] Transmission of CMV among young children in daycare, their caretakers, and their parents is common, and isolates from different persons in this setting have been shown to be identical by DNA fingerprinting.[62]

After early childhood, the next major peak of CMV acquisition occurs in the late second and the third decade of life, when exchange of secretions with persons outside the family of origin again becomes common. Strong evidence points to venereal transmission of CMV: high rates of infection in patients attending clinics for sexually transmitted diseases[63] and in homosexual men,[64, 65] recovery of virus from genital secretions,[66, 67] and genomically identical virus isolated from sexual partners.[68] Nonvenereal transmission also continues to occur: the overall rate of acquisition in the adult population in the United States is 1% to 2% per year.

In general, CMV infection is acquired later in life than Epstein-Barr virus.[69] Throughout the world, the rate of congenital CMV infection is about 0.5% to 2.5%,[70] and differences in seroprevalence predominantly reflect the rate of acquisition in early childhood. In developing nations, in low socioeconomic conditions, as well as in highly developed nations with a pattern of group care for young children, this rate is quite high.[71] In the United States, in the early 1970s when the major studies of seroprevalence were performed, it was rather low: 13% in Rochester, New York,[72] and 30% in Washington, DC.[1] Nonetheless, by the age of 25 to 30 years, 35% to 40% of the U.S. population has antibody, and by age 60 years, 80% to 100%.[1, 63, 72] Surveys of volunteer blood donors cite seroprevalence rates for this young to middle-aged healthy population of 40% to 60%.[36, 46, 73]

Transmission of CMV may occur via blood transfusion and organ transplantation. White blood cells, platelets, and red blood cells have been implicated in transfusion-related infections. Lyophilized products of pooled plasma, such as factor VIII concentrates, do not appear to transmit the virus.[74] It is assumed that cellular blood products and organs used in transplantation contain, either in themselves or as a contaminant, cells with the capability of actively transmitting CMV. The effectiveness of methods that deplete contaminating leukocytes from transfused blood units in preventing CMV infection supports this assumption.[75]

Among patients with serologic evidence of prior infection with CMV, those who receive immunosuppressive drugs shed virus much more frequently (about 35% of urine samples) than do healthy persons.[76, 77] Nearly all organ transplant recipients who were seropositive before transplantation develop evidence of CMV activity after the transplantation—virus shedding and a significant increase in antibody titer, sometimes including an immunoglobulin M response. These observations led to the conclusion that in such patients, their own prior, persistent CMV infection was reactivated. Such reactivation is, indeed, the only current explanation for infection in seropositive patients whose blood and organ donors are all seronegative.

Reinfection does occur, however, as demonstrated by recovery of identical strains of CMV from the two seropositive recipients of kidneys from a single seropositive donor[78] and by isolation of CMV with different DNA restriction endonuclease patterns from the same individual, either simultaneously or sequentially.[79–82] In one case, the authors suspected a genotypic change without reinfection,[83] but in most of these instances, multiple exposures were likely. Prior natural infection reduces the likelihood of reinfection[84] and the severity of clinical manifestations (see Chapter 186), but deliberate reinfection of seropositive persons can produce symptomatic illness, viral excretion, and an immune response.[85]

Pathogenesis and Immune Response

The portals of entry for naturally occurring CMV infection imputed from its epidemiology are upper respiratory tract, gastrointestinal tract (through breast-feeding), and genital mucosal surfaces. Congenital infection is a natural example of the parenteral route of infection operative in transplantation and transfusion. The site of initial virus replication is unknown. In all likelihood, the route of spread throughout the body is viremia, which can be demonstrated in the acute phase of most cases of CMV mononucleosis[86] and is closely associated with symptomatic disease in transplant recipients.[87, 88]

CMV infection induces immunosuppression, with low CD4+ cell (helper cell) numbers and an inverted ratio of CD4+ cells to CD8+ cells in both experimental[85] and natural[89] CMV infection and after transplantation.[90] In vitro studies have identified alterations in cell processing of viral immediate early antigen[91] and down-regulation of cell surface human leukocyte antigen class I molecules as potential means of avoiding cytotoxic attack.[92] Absence of human leukocyte antigen class II antigens on CMV-infected alveolar epithelial cells suggests that similar phenomena occur in vivo as well.[93] The ability of lymphocytes to proliferate in response to stimulation with other herpesvirus antigens disappears for up to 2 months after the onset of symptoms of CMV mononucleosis,[94] apparently owing to suppressor cell activity.[95] Lymphoproliferative responsiveness returns during convalescence and includes a response to CMV antigen that persists for life.[6, 94, 96, 97]

Perhaps the most important protective response, at least in transplant recipients, is CMV-specific cytotoxicity. This response occurs early in the course of CMV infection, about 2 weeks after virus challenge.[85] Renal transplant recipients who fail to generate specific cytotoxicity have more severe disease and more prolonged viremia than do those whose lymphocytes kill CMV-infected targets.[98] In the absence of CMV-specific cytotoxicity, bone marrow recipients are much more likely to die of their infection than if they are able to make this response.[99, 100] Immune cytotoxic T cells can recognize the presence of the matrix proteins pp65 and pp150 early after cellular uptake of virus and lyse newly infected cells before the onset of viral protein synthesis.[101]

It is not clear that all immune responses are beneficial to the host. An excess of natural killer cells (morphologically defined as large granular lymphocytes) in bronchoalveolar lavage fluid has been associated with a poor outcome in CMV pneumonitis.[102]

Clinical Manifestations

Most CMV infections in normal hosts are subclinical at any age. The defined clinical syndromes are discussed in Chapter 186. Hypotheses that certain chronic diseases arise as a result of a silent but common viral infection often posit CMV as the agent. Speculations concerning diabetes,[103, 104] atherosclerosis,[105] and immunoglobulin A nephropathy[106–108] have been published but not confirmed.[109]

Diagnosis

Virus Isolation

The traditional means of cultivating CMV has been inoculation into human diploid fibroblasts, such as human embryonic lung, human foreskin fibroblasts, MRC-5, or WI-38 cells. Virus recovery is best when subconfluent monolayers are used, and it may be augmented by blind passage (trypsinization, division, and reseeding of the cells). In this system, cytopathic effect consists of foci of enlarged, refractile, oval to round cells, often with a dirty pigmentary deposit, that progressively enlarge and seem to pull a hole in the monolayer in their midst. Most isolates are recognized in the second week of incubation, but the cytopathic effect may appear overnight in some specimens, as in urine from congenitally infected infants or lung from patients with severe interstitial pneumonitis; it may also be delayed as long as 5 to 6 weeks. The slow yield of conventional culture has been overcome by a shell-vial technique[110] that uses centrifugation to enhance infectivity through a mechanism not yet understood[111] and immunofluorescent staining for the major immediate early nuclear antigen. Cultures processed by this technique yield results within 24 hours, with nearly complete concordance with the conventional method for urine specimens handled in parallel. Additional approaches to detecting the virus and their clinical utility are discussed in Chapter 186.

Serologic Methods

The vast majority of CMV antibody assays use the AD169 strain as an antigen, although it may fail to detect a few infected persons who are seropositive to other laboratory prototype strains.[112] The level of complement-fixing antibody has long been known to rise and fall in sequential blood samples from normal healthy persons[113]; to avoid misclassification of seropositivity as seronegativity, glycine-extracted antigen and extremely low dilutions of serum must be used. Alternative assays are now widely available, including enzyme-linked immunosorbent methods, indirect hemagglutination, and a latex agglutination test.[114–119]

More problematic is the detection of CMV-specific immunoglobulin M antibody. Because CMV induces Fc receptors on infected cells, assays that use an antigen derived from infected cells carry the risk of binding immunoglobulin heavy chains nonspecifically and, in particular, binding rheumatoid factor. Even assays that control stringently for rheumatoid factor detect immunoglobulin M in some subjects who previously had CMV infection.[120–122] Preliminary studies using recombinant antigens suggest that reactivity with nonstructural proteins, particularly p52, is more characteristic of acute primary CMV infection, whereas individuals with long-term seropositivity have antibody to the basic matrix phosphoprotein p150.[20]

Treatment

Two antiviral compounds that have useful activity against CMV are ganciclovir and foscarnet. Ganciclovir is a nucleoside analog that is phosphorylated to the triphosphate within the cell and functions as a DNA chain terminator. Its major clinical toxicity is bone marrow suppression, which may force dose reduction or interruption of treatment, but it also causes aspermatogenesis in animals and is carcinogenic in several animal model systems. Foscarnet is a pyrophosphate analog that functions as a relatively selective inhibitor of viral DNA polymerase. It is nephrotoxic but not myelotoxic. Resistance to both drugs has developed in isolates of CMV obtained from patients on therapy. Use of these agents is discussed in greater detail in Chapter 186.

Prevention

Prevention of CMV infection by avoidance of exposure is not generally practical: there is rarely a choice among suitable organ donors; women of childbearing age are unlikely to avoid young children, who seem to be among the most infectious shedders of virus; and those who will be at risk for CMV disease due to immunocompromise have often been infected earlier in life. An exception is the case of transfusion, where donor selection or filtration of blood to remove contaminating leukocytes is highly effective.[75, 123]

Passive antibody (CMV immunoglobulin) and prophylactic antiviral agents are the major approaches in current use (see

Chapter 186), while efforts to develop a protective vaccine continue. The Towne strain of CMV has been investigated as a live attenuated vaccine. About 50% of recipients experience a local reaction, with soreness and induration in the arm; humoral and cellular immune responses develop, including cytotoxic and lymphoproliferative reactions.[85, 124] Challenge of healthy vaccinees 1 year after immunization failed to produce serologic or clinical evidence of infection with 10 plaque-forming units of wild-type virus, but vaccine seemed less protective than natural immunity against challenge with 100 plaque-forming units.[125] In seronegative patients who received vaccine or placebo while awaiting renal transplantation, there was no difference in rate of CMV infection or development of disease.[126] In the group at highest risk of serious CMV disease—seronegative (prevaccine) recipients of kidneys from seropositive donors—severe disease appeared to be more frequent among placebo recipients. The major excess related to renal dysfunction and superinfection with other opportunistic pathogens, resulting in a lower graft survival rate for cadaver kidneys but not for those from living related donors. A study in CMV-seronegative mothers of CMV-shedding children in daycare showed no protection against primary infection in those who received Towne strain vaccine compared with placebo recipients.[84]

Because of concerns about oncogenicity and the use of any live virus in potentially pregnant or immunocompromised hosts, a viral subunit vaccine may be more desirable. The envelope glycoprotein complex, gB (gpUL55), is being studied as a possible candidate for a subunit vaccine.[127] A vaccine cannot reasonably be expected to provide better protection than previous natural infection, which seems adequate to prevent the devastating form of congenital infection but can only modify transplant-related syndromes and is abrogated in patients who have the acquired immunodeficiency syndrome. In these cases, restoration of T-cell immunity may be critical. Early results from a trial of infusing bone marrow transplant recipients with an expanded population of their donors' CMV-specific cytotoxic T lymphocytes give hope that this approach may prevent viremia and severe disease.[128, 129]

Acknowledgment

I am grateful to Terence D. Giugni, PhD, for helpful discussion on issues of virus attachment to and entry into cells.

References

1. Rowe WP, Hartley JW, Waterman S, et al: Cytopathogenic agent resembling human salivary gland virus recovered from tissue cultures of human adenoids. Proc Soc Exp Biol Med 92:418, 1956.
2. Smith MG: Propagation in tissue cultures of a cytopathogenic virus from human salivary gland virus (SGV) disease. Proc Soc Exp Biol Med 92:424, 1956.
3. Weller TH, Macauley IC, Craig JM, Wirth P: Isolation of intranuclear inclusion producing agents from infants with illnesses resembling cytomegalic inclusion disease. Proc Soc Exp Biol Med 94:4, 1957.
4. Bankier AT, Beck S, Bohni R, et al: The DNA sequence of the human cytomegalovirus genome. J DNA Sequencing Mapp 2:1, 1991.
5. Spaete RR, Gehrz RC, Landini MP: Human cytomegalovirus structural proteins. J Gen Virol 75:3287, 1994.
6. Forman SJ, Zaia JA, Clark BR, et al: A 64,000 dalton matrix protein of human cytomegalovirus induces in vitro immune responses similar to those of whole viral antigen. J Immunol 134:3391, 1985.
7. Michelson S, Tardy-Panit M, Colimon R, Landini MP: A human cytomegalovirus-neutralizing monoclonal antibody recognizes a normal cell protein. J Gen Virol 70:673, 1989.
8. Soderberg C, Giugni TD, Zaia JA, et al: CD13 (human aminopeptidase N) mediates human cytomegalovirus infection. J Virol 67:6576, 1993.
9. Keay S, Merigan TC, Rasmussen L: Identification of cell surface receptors for the 86-kilodalton glycoprotein of human cytomegalovirus. Proc Natl Acad Sci USA 86:10100, 1989.
10. Kari B, Gehrz R: A human cytomegalovirus glycoprotein complex designated gC-II is a major heparin-binding component of the envelope. J Virol 66:1761, 1992.
11. Keay S, Baldwin B: Anti-idiotype antibodies that mimic gp86 of human cytomegalovirus inhibit viral fusion but not attachment. J Virol 65:5124, 1991.
12. Kari B, Gehrz R: Structure, composition and heparin binding properties of a HCMV glycoprotein complex designated gC-II. J Gen Virol 74:255, 1993.
13. Compton T, Nowlin DM, Cooper NR: Initiation of human cytomegalovirus infection requires initial interaction with cell surface heparan sulfate. Virology 193:834, 1993.
14. Nowlin DM, Cooper NR, Compton T: Expression of a human cytomegalovirus receptor correlates with infectibility of cells. J Virol 65:3114, 1991.
15. Adlish JD, Lahijani RS, St. Jeor SC: Identification of a putative cell receptor for human cytomegalovirus. Virology 176:337, 1990.
16. Taylor HP, Cooper NR: The human cytomegalovirus receptor on fibroblasts is a 30-kilodalton membrane protein. J Virol 64:2484, 1990.
17. Iwayama S, Yamamoto T, Furuya T, et al: Intracellular localization and DNA-binding activity of a class of viral early phosphoproteins in human fibroblasts infected with human cytomegalovirus (Towne strain). J Gen Virol 75:3309, 1994.
18. Mocarski ES, Stinski MF: Persistence of the cytomegalovirus genome in human cells. J Virol 31:761, 1979.
19. Landini MP, Michelson S: Human cytomegalovirus proteins. Prog Med Virol 35:152, 1988.
20. Landini MP, La Placa M: Humoral immune response to human cytomegalovirus proteins: A brief review. Comp Immun Microbiol Infect Dis 14:97, 1991.
21. Britt WJ: Neutralizing antibodies detect a disulfide-linked glycoprotein complex within the envelope of human cytomegalovirus. Virology 135:369, 1984.
22. Pereira L, Hoffman M, Tatsuno M, Dondero D: Polymorphism of human cytomegalovirus glycoproteins characterized by monoclonal antibodies. Virology 139:73, 1984.
23. Rasmussen L, Mullenax J, Nelson M, Merigan TC: Human cytomegalovirus polypeptides stimulate neutralizing antibody in vivo. Virology 145:186, 1985.
24. Mach M, Utz U: Mapping of the major glycoprotein gene of human cytomegalovirus. J Gen Virol 67:1461, 1986.
25. Gonczol E, Hudecz F, Ianacone J, et al: Immune responses to isolated human cytomegalovirus envelope proteins. J Virol 58:661, 1986.
26. Masuho Y, Matsumoto YI, Sugano T, et al: Human monoclonal antibodies neutralizing human cytomegalovirus. J Gen Virol 68:1457, 1987.
27. Britt WJ, Vugler L, Stephens EB: Induction of complement-dependent and -independent neutralizing antibodies by recombinant-derived human cytomegalovirus pg55-116 (gB). J Virol 62:3309, 1988.
28. Grundy JE, McKeating JA, Griffiths PD: Cytomegalovirus strain AD169 binds β_2-microglobulin in vitro after release from cells. J Gen Virol 68:777, 1987.
29. McKeating JA, Griffiths PD, Grundy JE: Cytomegalovirus in urine specimens has host β_2-microglobulin bound to the viral envelope: A mechanism of evading the host immune response? J Gen Virol 68:785, 1987.
30. Grundy JE, McKeating JA, Ward PJ, et al: β_2-Microglobulin enhances the infectivity of cytomegalovirus and when bound to the virus enables class I HLA molecules to be used as a virus receptor. J Gen Virol 68:793, 1987.
31. Beersma MFC, Wertheim-van Dillon PME, Geelen JLMC, Feltkamp TEW: Expression of HLA class I heavy chains and β_2-microglobulin does not affect human cytomegalovirus infectivity. J Gen Virol 72:2757, 1991.
32. Perot K, Walker CM: Primary chimpanzee skin fibroblast cells are fully permissive for human cytomegalovirus replication. J Gen Virol 72:3281, 1992.

33. Waldman WJ, Roberts WH, Davis DH, Williams MV, et al: Preservation of natural endothelial cytopathogenicity of cytomegalovirus by propagation in endothelial cells. Arch Virol 117:143, 1991.
34. Poland SD, Bambrick LL, Dekaban GA, Rice GPA: The extent of human cytomegalovirus replication in primary neurons is dependent on host cell differentiation. J Infect Dis 170:1267, 1994.
35. Taylor-Wiedeman J, Sissons P, Sinclair J: Induction of endogenous human cytomegalovirus gene expression after differentiation of monocytes from health carriers. J Virol 68:1597, 1994.
36. Adler SP: Transfusion-associated cytomegalovirus infections. Rev Infect Dis 5:977, 1983.
37. Rice GPA, Schrier RD, Oldstone MBA: Cytomegalovirus infects human lymphocytes and monocytes: Virus expression is restricted to immediate-early gene products. Proc Natl Acad Sci USA 81:6134, 1984.
38. Einhorn L, Ost A: Cytomegalovirus infection of human blood cells. J Infect Dis 149:207, 1984.
39. Reiser H, Kuhn J, Doerr HW, et al: Human cytomegalovirus replicates in primary human bone marrow cells. J Gen Virol 67:2595, 1986.
40. Schrier RD, Nelson JA, Oldstone MBA: Detection of human cytomegalovirus in peripheral blood lymphocytes in a natural infection. Science 230:1048, 1985.
41. Maciejewski JP, Bruening EE, Donahue RE, et al: Infection of hematopoietic progenitor cells by human cytomegalovirus. Blood 80:170, 1992.
42. Soderberg C, Larsson S, Bergstedt-Lindqvist S, Moller E: Definition of a subset of human peripheral blood mononuclear cells that are permissive to human cytomegalovirus infection. J Virol 67:3166, 1993.
43. Olding LB, Jensen FC, Oldstone MBA: Pathogenesis of cytomegalovirus infection. I. Activation of virus from bone marrow-derived lymphocytes by in vitro allogeneic reaction. J Exp Med 141:561, 1975.
44. Taylor-Wiedeman J, Sissons JGP, Borysiewicz LK, Sinclair JH: Monocytes are a major site of persistence of human cytomegalovirus in peripheral blood mononuclear cells. J Gen Virol 72:2059, 1991.
45. Rasmussen L, Morris S, Zipeto D, et al: Quantitation of human cytomegalovirus DNA from peripheral blood cells of human immunodeficiency virus–infected patients could predict cytomegalovirus retinitis. J Infect Dis 171:177, 1995.
46. Zhang LJ, Hanff P, Rutherford C, et al: Detection of human cytomegalovirus DNA, RNA, and antibody in normal donor blood. J Infect Dis 171:1002, 1995.
47. Grefte A, vander Giessen M, van Son W, The TH: Circulating cytomegalovirus (CMV)-infected endothelial cells in patients with an active CMV infection. J Infect Dis 167:270, 1993.
48. Waldman WJ, Knight DA, Huang EH, Sedmak DD: Bidirectional transmission of infectious cytomegalovirus between monocytes and vascular endothelial cells: An in vitro model. J Infect Dis 171:263, 1995.
49. Drew WL, Mintz L, Hoo R, Finley TN: Growth of herpes simplex and cytomegalovirus in cultured human alveolar macrophages. Am Rev Respir Dis 119:287, 1979.
50. Craighead JE: Pulmonary cytomegalovirus infection in the adult. Am J Pathol 63:487, 1971.
51. Toorkey CB, Carrigan DR: Immunohistochemical detection of an immediate early antigen of human cytomegalovirus in normal tissues. J Infect Dis 160:741, 1989.
52. Giraldo G, Beth E, Kourilsky FM, et al: Antibody patterns to herpes-viruses in Kaposi's sarcoma: Serological association of European Kaposi's sarcoma with cytomegalovirus. Int J Cancer 15:839, 1975.
53. Ambinder RF, Newman C, Hayward GS, et al: Lack of association of cytomegalovirus with endemic African Kaposi's sarcoma. J Infect Dis 156:193, 1987.
54. Hashimoto H, Muller H, Muller F, et al: In situ hybridization analysis of cytomegalovirus lytic infection in Kaposi's sarcoma associated with AIDS. Virchows Arch 411:441, 1987.
55. Moore PS, Chang Y: Detection of herpesvirus-like DNA sequences in Kaposi's sarcoma in patients with and without HIV infection. N Engl J Med 332:1181, 1995.
56. Huang YQ, Kaplan MH, Poiesz B, et al: Human herpesvirus-like nucleic acid in various forms of Kaposi's sarcoma. Lancet 345:759, 1995.
57. Dupin N, Grandadam M, Calvez V, et al: Herpesvirus-like DNA sequences in patient with Mediterranean Kaposi's sarcoma. Lancet 345:761, 1995.
58. Geder L, Rapp F: Herpesviruses and prostate carcinogenesis. Arch Androl 4:71, 1980.
59. Huang ES, Roche JK: Cytomegalovirus DNA and adenocarcinoma of the colon: Evidence for latent viral infection. Lancet 1:957, 1978.
60. Hashiro GM, Horikami S, Loh PC: Cytomegalovirus isolations from cell cultures of human adenocarcinomas of the colon. Intervirology 12:84, 1979.
61. Dworsky M, Yow M, Stagno S, et al: Cytomegalovirus infection of breast milk and transmission in infancy. Pediatrics 73:295, 1983.
62. Adler SP: Molecular epidemiology of cytomegalovirus: Viral transmission among children attending a day care center, their parents, and caregivers. J Pediatr 112:366, 1988.
63. Davis LE, Stewart JA, Garvin S: Cytomegalovirus infection: A seroepidemiologic comparison of nuns and women from a venereal disease clinic. J Epidemiol 102:327, 1975.
64. Lange M, Klein EB, Kornfield H, et al: Cytomegalovirus isolation from healthy homosexual men. JAMA 252:1908, 1984.
65. Drew WL, Mills J, Levy J, et al: Cytomegalovirus infection and abnormal T-lymphocyte subset ratios in homosexual men. Ann Intern Med 103:61, 1985.
66. Lang DJ, Kummer JF: Cytomegalovirus in semen: Observations in selected populations. J Infect Dis 132:422, 1975.
67. Montgomery R, Youngblood L, Medearis DN Jr: Recovery of cytomegalovirus from the cervix in pregnancy. Pediatrics 49:524, 1972.
68. Handsfield HH, Chandler SH, Caine VA, et al: Cytomegalovirus infection in sex partners: Evidence for sexual transmission. J Infect Dis 151:344, 1985.
69. Horwitz CA, Henle W, Henle G, et al: Clinical and laboratory evaluation of cytomegalovirus-induced mononucleosis in previously healthy individuals: Report of 82 cases. Medicine (Baltimore) 65:124, 1986.
70. Hanshaw JB, Dudgeon JA, Marshall WC: Viral Diseases of the Fetus and Newborn, ed 2. Philadelphia, WB Saunders, 1985, pp 92–131.
71. Weller TH: The cytomegaloviruses: Ubiquitous agents with protean clinical manifestations. II. N Engl J Med 285:267, 1971.
72. Deibel R, Smith R, Clarke LM, et al: Cytomegalovirus infections in New York State: Laboratory studies of patients and healthy individuals. N Y State J Med 74:785, 1974.
73. Bayer WL, Tegtmeier GE: The blood donor: Detection and magnitude of cytomegalovirus carrier states and the prevalence of cytomegalovirus antibody. Yale J Biol Med 49:5, 1976.
74. Cheeseman SH, Sullivan JL, Brettler DB, Levine PH: Analysis of cytomegalovirus and Epstein-Barr virus antibody responses in treated hemophiliacs: Implications for the study of acquired immune deficiency syndrome. JAMA 252:83, 1984.
75. Hillyer CD, Emmens RK, Zago-Novaretti M, Berkman EM: Methods for the reduction of transfusion-transmitted cytomegalovirus infection filtration versus the use of seronegative donor units. Transfusion 34:929, 1994.
76. Duvall CP, Casazza AR, Grimley PM, et al: Recovery of cytomegalovirus from adults with neoplastic disease. Ann Intern Med 64:531, 1966.
77. Henson D, Siegel SE, Fuccillo DA, et al: Cytomegalovirus infections during acute childhood leukemia. J Infect Dis 126:469, 1972.
78. Chou S. Acquisition of donor strains of cytomegalovirus by renal transplant recipients. N Engl J Med 314:1418, 1986.
79. Chandler SH, Handsfield HH, McDougall JK: Isolation of multiple strains of cytomegalovirus from women attending a clinic for sexually transmitted diseases. J Infect Dis 155:655, 1987.
80. Collier AC, Chandler SH, Handsfield HH, et al: Identification of multiple strains of cytomegalovirus in homosexual men. J Infect Dis 159:123, 1989.
81. Spector SA, Hirata KK, Neuman TR: Identification of multiple cytomegalovirus strains in homosexual men with acquired immunodeficiency syndrome. J Infect Dis 150:953, 1984.
82. Drew WL, Sweet ES, Miner RC, Moarski ES: Multiple infections

by cytomegalovirus in patients with acquired immunodeficiency syndrome. Documentation by Southern blot hybridization. J Infect Dis 150:952, 1984.
83. Shen CY, Chang SF, Chao MF, et al: Identification of a serial change in recurrent cytomegalovirus strains in a healthy child by polymerase chain reaction. J Infect Dis 168:252, 1993.
84. Adler SP, Starr SE, Plotkin SA, et al: Immunity induced by primary human cytomegalovirus infection protects against secondary infection among women of childbearing age. J Infect Dis 171:26, 1995.
85. Quinnan GV, Delery M, Rook AH, et al: Comparative virulence and immunogenicity of the Towne strain and a nonattenuated strain of cytomegalovirus. Ann Intern Med 101:478, 1984.
86. Rinaldo CR, Jr., Black PH, Hirsch MS: Interaction of cytomegalovirus with leukocytes from patients with mononucleosis due to cytomegalovirus. J Infect Dis 136:667, 1977.
87. Cheeseman SH, Rubin RH, Stewart JA, et al: Controlled clinical trial of prophylactic human-leukocyte interferon in renal transplantation: Effects on cytomegalovirus and herpes simplex virus infection. N Engl J Med 300:1345, 1979.
88. Meyers JD, Ljungman P, Fisher LD: Cytomegalovirus excretion as a predictor of cytomegalovirus disease after marrow transplantation: Importance of cytomegalovirus viremia. J Infect Dis 162:373, 1990.
89. Carney WP, Rubin RH, Hoffmann RA, et al: Analysis of T-lymphocyte subsets in cytomegalovirus mononucleosis. J Immunol 126:2114, 1981.
90. Schooley RT, Hirsch MS, Colvin RB, et al: Association of herpesvirus infections with T-lymphocyte subset alterations, glomerulopathy, and opportunistic infections after renal transplantation. N Engl J Med 308:307, 1983.
91. Gilbert MJ, Riddell SR, Cheng-Rong LI, Greenberg PD: Selective interference with class I major histocompatibility complex presentation of the major immediate-early protein following infection with human cytomegalovirus. J Virol 67:3461, 1993.
92. Yamashita Y, Shimokata K, Mizuno S, et al: Down regulation of the surface expression of class I MHC antigens by human cytomegalovirus. Virology 193:727, 1993.
93. Ng-Bautista CL, Sedmak DD: Cytomegalovirus infection is associated with absence of alveolar epithelial cell HLA class II antigen expression. J Infect Dis 171:39, 1995.
94. Levin MJ, Rinaldo CR, Leary PL, et al: Immune response to herpesvirus antigens in adults with acute cytomegaloviral mononucleosis. J Infect Dis 140:851, 1979.
95. Rinaldo CR, Carney WP, Richter BS, et al: Mechanisms of immunosuppression in cytomegaloviral mononucleosis. J Infect Dis 141:488, 1980.
96. Moller-Larsen A, Andersen HK, Heron I, Sarvo I: In vitro stimulation of human lymphocytes by purified cytomegalovirus. Intervirology 249:249, 1976.
97. Pollard RB, Rand KH, Arvin AM, Merigan TC: Cell-mediated immunity to cytomegalovirus infection in normal subjects and cardiac transplant recipients. J Infect Dis 137:541, 1978.
98. Rook AH, Quinnan GV, Frederick WJ Jr, et al: Importance of cytotoxic lymphocytes during cytomegalovirus infection in renal transplant recipients. Am J Med 76:385, 1984.
99. Quinnan GV, Burns WH, Kirmani N, et al: HLA-restricted cytotoxic T lymphocytes are an early immune response and important defense mechanism in cytomegalovirus infections. Rev Infect Dis 6:156, 1984.
100. Riddell RP, Meyers JD, Greenberg PD: Cytotoxic T-lymphocyte response to cytomegalovirus after human allogeneic bone marrow transplantation: Pattern of recovery and correlation with cytomegalovirus infection and disease. Blood 78:1373, 1991.
101. Riddell SR, Rabin M, Geballe A, et al: Class I MHC-restricted cytotoxic T lymphocyte recognition of cells infected with human cytomegalovirus does not require endogeneous viral gene expression. J Immunol 146:2795, 1991.
102. Escudier E, Fleury J, Cordonnier C, et al: Large granular lymphocytes in bronchoalveolar lavage fluids from immunocompromised patients with cytomegalovirus pneumonitis. J Clin Pathol 86:641, 1986.
103. Pak CY, McArthur RG, Eun HM, Yoon JW: Association of cytomegalovirus infection with autoimmune type 1 diabetes. Lancet 2:1, 1988.
104. Banatvala JE, Bryant J, Schernthaner G, et al: Coxsackie B, mumps, rubella, and cytomegalovirus specific IgM responses in patients with juvenile-onset, insulin-dependent diabetes mellitus in Britain, Austria, and Australia. Lancet 1:1409, 1985.
105. Adam E, Melnick JL, Probtsfield JL, et al: High levels of cytomegalovirus antibody in patients requiring vascular surgery for atherosclerosis. Lancet 2:291, 1987.
106. Gregory MC, Hammond ME, Brewer ED: Renal deposition of cytomegalovirus antigen in immunoglobulin-A nephropathy. Lancet 2:11, 1988.
107. Waldo FB, Tomana M, Britt WJ, et al: Nonspecific mesangial staining with antibodies against cytomegalovirus in immunoglobulin A nephropathy. Lancet 1:129, 1989.
108. Dueymes M, Mignon-Conte M, Dueymes JM, et al: Mesangial staining with cytomegalovirus antibodies in IgA nephropathy. Lancet 1:619, 1989.
109. Park JS, Song JH, Yang WS, et al: Cytomegalovirus is not specifically associated with immunoglobulin A nephropathy. J Am Soc Nephrol 4:1623, 1994.
110. Gleaves CA, Smith TF, Shuster EA, Pearson GR: Rapid detection of cytomegalovirus in MRC-5 cells inoculated with urine specimens by using low-speed centrifugation and monoclonal antibody to an early antigen. J Clin Microbiol 19:917, 1984.
111. Hudson JB: Further studies on the mechanism of centrifugal enhancement of cytomegalovirus infectivity. J Virol Methods 19:97, 1988.
112. Faix RG: Cytomegalovirus antigenic heterogeneity can cause false negative results in indirect hemagglutination and complement-fixation antibody assay. J Clin Microbiol 22:768, 1985.
113. Waner J, Weller TH, Kevy SV: Patterns of cytomegaloviral complement-fixing antibody activity: A longitudinal study of blood donors. J Infect Dis 127:538, 1973.
114. Yeager AS: Improved indirect hemagglutination test for cytomegalovirus using human O erythrocytes in lysine. J Clin Microbiol 10:64, 1979.
115. Kettering JD, Schmidt NJ, Galls D, et al: Anti-complement immunofluorescence test for antibodies to human cytomegalovirus. J Clin Microbiol 6:627, 1977.
116. Beckwith DG, Halstead DC, Alpaugh K, et al: Comparison of a latex agglutination test with five other methods for determining the presence of antibody against cytomegalovirus. J Clin Microbiol 21:328, 1985.
117. McHugh TM, Casavant CH, Wilber JC, Stites DP: Comparison of six methods for the detection of antibody to cytomegalovirus. J Clin Microbiol 22:1014, 1985.
118. Sererat MN, Schifano JV, Lau P, et al: Evaluation of cytomegalovirus (CMV) antibody screening tests for blood donors. Am J Clin Pathol 86:523, 1986.
119. Leland DS, Barth KA, Cunningham EB, et al: Evaluation of four methods for cytomegalovirus antibody detection for use by a bone marrow transplantation service. J Clin Microbiol 27:176, 1989.
120. Rasmussen L, Kelsall D, Nelson R, et al: Virus-specific IgG and IgM antibodies in normal and immunocompromised subjects infected with cytomegalovirus. J Infect Dis 145:191, 1982.
121. Stagno S, Tinker MK, Elrod C, et al: Immunoglobulin M antibodies detected by enzyme-linked immunosorbent assay and radioimmunoassay in the diagnosis of cytomegalovirus infections in pregnant women and newborn infants. J Clin Microbiol 21:930, 1985.
122. Chou S, Kim DY, Scott KM, Sewell D: Immunoglobulin M to cytomegalovirus in primary and reactivation infections in renal transplant recipients. J Clin Microbiol 25:52, 1987.
123. Sayers MH, Anderson KC, Goodnough LT, et al: Reducing the risk for transfusion-transmitted cytomegalovirus infection. Ann Intern Med 116:55, 1992.
124. Gehrz RC, Christianson WR, Linner KM, et al: Cytomegalovirus vaccine. Specific humoral and cellular immune responses in human volunteers. Arch Intern Med 140:936, 1980.
125. Plotkin SA, Starr SE, Friedman HM, et al: Protective effects of Towne cytomegalovirus vaccine against low-passage cytomegalovirus administered as a challenge. J Infect Dis 159:860, 1989.
126. Brayman KL, Dafoe DC, Smythe WR, et al: Prophylaxis of serious cytomegalovirus infection in renal transplant candidates using live human cytomegalovirus vaccine: Interim results of a randomized controlled trial. Arch Surg 123:1502, 1988.
127. Britt W, Fay J, Seals J, Kensil C: Formulation of an immunogenic

human cytomegalovirus vaccine: Responses in mice. J Infect Dis 171:18, 1995.
128. Riddell SR, Watanabe KS, Goodrich JM, et al: Restoration of viral immunity in immunodeficient humans by the adoptive transfer of T cell clones. Science 257:238, 1992.
129. Riddell SR, Gilbert MJ, Greenberg PD: CD8+ cytotoxic therapy of cytomegalovirus and HIV infection. Curr Opin Immunol 5:484, 1993.

245

Human Parvovirus

Neal S. Young

History[1-4]

Although parvoviruses commonly cause disease in animals, it was only in 1975 that the first human pathogen of this family was discovered by Cossart and colleagues[5] in screening normal blood bank donors' sera for hepatitis antigen (one of the donor's serum samples was coded B19). Epidemiologic surveys established that serum from approximately half of the adult population contained immunoglobulin G (IgG) antibodies to this virus,[6-8] suggesting acquisition of immunity during childhood. Evidence of recent infection (viral antigen or immunoglobulin M [IgM] antibody to virus) was first found in the blood of Jamaican children residing in London, all of whom had presented with transient aplastic crisis of sickle cell disease,[9] and the close association of parvovirus and aplastic crisis was confirmed in a large retrospective study of serum from sickle cell disease patients with this complication.[10] Later, B19 parvovirus was shown to be the etiologic agent of fifth disease in hematologically normal persons,[11] and, when infection of the mother occurred during pregnancy, of some cases of nonimmune hydrops fetalis.[12] B19 parvovirus infection can persist and cause chronic bone marrow failure.[13] B19 parvovirus also has been implicated in rheumatic syndromes and in vasculitis.

Characteristics of the Pathogen

Classification and Structure

A typical member of the Parvoviridae family has about 5000 nucleotides of single-stranded DNA encapsidated in a small (about 20 nm in diameter) icosahedrally symmetric and unenveloped structure[14-18] (Fig. 245–1). The subfamily Parvovirinae contains the autonomous animal parvoviruses (genus *Parvovirus*), viruses that require a helper virus for replication (genus *Dependovirus*), and B19 and its simian relatives (genus *Erythrovirus*).[19] B19 shares basic morphologic[5] and DNA structural features[20, 21] with other members of the Parvoviridae. Although minor variations among isolates of B19 parvovirus are detected by restriction enzyme mapping,[22, 23] parallel epidemic curves[24] and the illness produced in normal volunteers[25] strongly suggest that a single parvovirus species is responsible for all clinical manifestations of B19 parvovirus infection.

Although B19 is the only known human pathogenic parvovirus, there are other human parvoviruses. The adeno-associated viruses were discovered in tissue culture, but the prevalence of antibodies to them in humans indicates the occurrence of natural infection.[16-18] They have also been isolated from throat and anal swab specimens from healthy children. More closely related to B19 is simian parvovirus, which can cause fatal anemia in cynomolgus monkeys.[26]

Genomic Organization

B19 parvovirus has been cloned[27] and sequenced[28] and its pattern of transcription mapped[29] (Fig. 245–2). The two structural proteins of the capsid are encoded in overlapping transcriptional frames on the right side of the genome, and a single nonstructural protein is encoded on the left side.[29, 30] The smaller structural protein (58 kDa, vP2) is the major constituent of the capsid, and the larger protein (83 kDa, VP1), which differs by only 227 amino acids from VP2; is the minor.[31] The structural proteins can self-assemble into capsids, into which the DNA is inserted.[32] In contrast, expression of the nonstructural protein is lethal in cells in which the gene has been transfected.[33] The functions of the B19 nonstructural protein are unknown, although the nonstructural proteins of other parvoviruses have been shown to act as replication competence factors and enhancer elements and to bind DNA. Selective expression of the B19 nonstructural protein can lead to cell death in the absence of viral replication. In addition to nonstructural protein, small proteins of unknown function, encoded on the left side of the genome, are expressed during infection.[34]

Although the genomic organization of B19 is similar to that of other Parvoviridae organisms, it is much more complex and differs in significant features, including the presence of a single strong promoter at the left side, failure of all transcripts to coterminate at the right side, and extensive splicing of all but the nonstructural protein RNA.[29] RNA expression occurs in early and late stages: first, nonstructural protein transcription, followed by capsid protein RNA expression.[35] B19 parvovirus' genomic organization and the identical sequence of the left- and right-hand terminal repeats

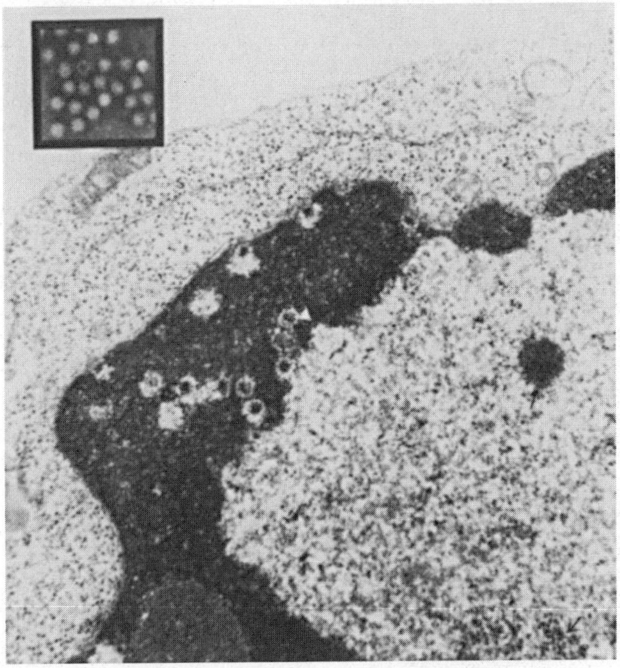

FIGURE 245–1 □ Electron micrographs of B19 parvovirus in a human erythroid progenitor cell infected in vitro and in serum *(inset)*.

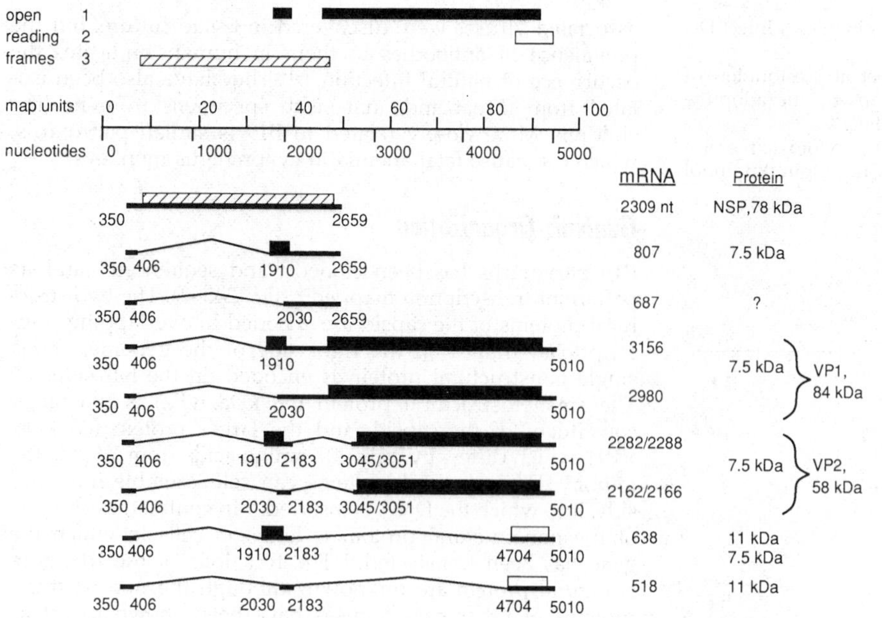

FIGURE 245–2 □ B19 parvovirus genomic organization. The 5400 nucleotides are divided into 100 map units for convenience. The molecular mass of the RNA transcripts is indicated on the left. The major capsid protein (VP2), minor capsid protein (VP1), and the nonstructural protein (NSP) and their molecular masses are indicated on the right. The coding sequences are shown by the open boxes with reading frames indicated by the numeral. All transcription begins at a single promoter on the far left-hand side of the genome. (Adapted from Luo W, Astell CR: A novel protein encoded by small RNAs of parvovirus B19. Virology 195:448–455, 1993.)

place it close to human adeno-associated virus, and the extreme tissue specificity of B19 parvovirus may be analagous to the defective nature of the dependoviruses.

Replication

The limited size of their genome makes parvoviruses dependent on actively cycling populations of cells for their own replication. Adeno-associated viruses need helper functions provided by other viruses, in particular adenovirus and herpesvirus[16–18, 36]; the relatedness of host cell and second virus help is suggested by the ability of adeno-associated virus to replicate in cells in which the cell cycle has been chemically manipulated.[37] Nuclear helper functions are also important in tissue tropism: minute virus of mice variants enter nonpermissive cells but are unable to complete their replicative cycle[38] (this difference is encoded, surprisingly, within the capsid genes[39]). Natural infections of parvoviruses usually occur in mitotically active tissues: this predilection results in infection of fetuses and young growing animals and in "embryonic" tissues of the lymphoid and hematopoietic systems.[40, 41] Three examples are worth citing: outbreaks of spontaneous abortions of pig litters caused by porcine parvovirus,[42] fatal myocarditis in puppies caused by canine parvovirus,[43] and infection of lymphocytes and bone marrow cells caused by feline parvovirus.[44]

Like that of other parvoviruses,[45–47] the replication strategy of B19 is based on the inverted terminal repeat structures.[27, 28] Replication of the single-stranded DNA of the Parvoviridae is initiated from these brief regions of double-strandedness, with formation of higher molecular weight intermediates visible on Southern blot analysis.[47] Thus, in clinical samples not only the presence of virus but also active viral replication can be detected.[48–50]

Pathogenesis (Figs. 245–3 and 245–4)

Host Cell

The bone marrow is a mitotically active tissue, and the only known natural host cell of B19 is the human erythroid progenitor cell. The virus also replicates in tissue culture of fetal liver[51] and peripheral blood cells.[52] B19 parvovirus can be propagated in some human megakaryocytoblastoid cell lines grown in the presence of erythropoietin.[53, 54] B19 inhibits erythroid, but not myeloid, colony formation,[55–57] and virus inoculation depletes suspension cultures of bone marrow of erythroid precursor cells.[58] B19 is cytotoxic to both early and late erythroid progenitors,[55, 57] inducing in vitro characteristic morphologic changes observed by light and electron microscopy[58, 59] similar to the appearance of bone marrow from patients with parvovirus infection.

Cellular Receptor and Tissue Specificity

Tissue specificity is largely determined by the nature of the cellular receptor, identified as erythrocyte P antigen or globoside, a glycolipid tetrohexoseceramide.[60] Virus binds with high affinity to P antigen, and infectivity in vitro can be blocked by either an excess of soluble globoside or monoclonal antibody to P antigen. Remarkably, rare individuals who lack globoside on the red blood cell surface (p phenotype) cannot be infected with B19.[61] Globoside is abundant

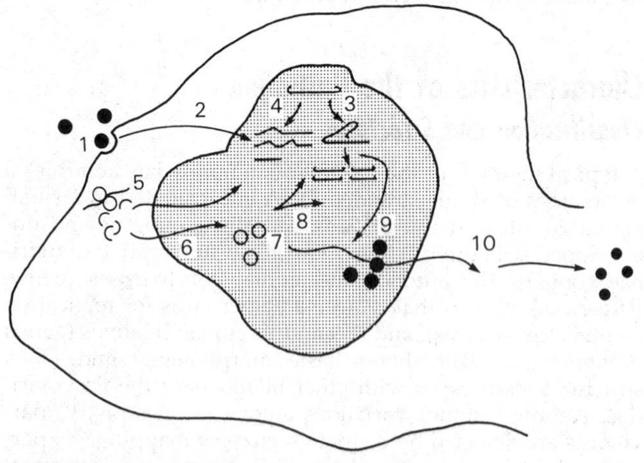

FIGURE 245–3 □ Life cycle of the B19 parvovirus: (1) binding to P antigen, the cellular receptor; (2) translocation to nucleus and encoding; (3) DNA replication; (4) RNA transcription; (5) protein translation; (6) protein trafficking to nucleus; (7) empty capsid assembly; (8) nonstructural protein effects; (9) DNA insertion; and (10) cell lysis and virus release.

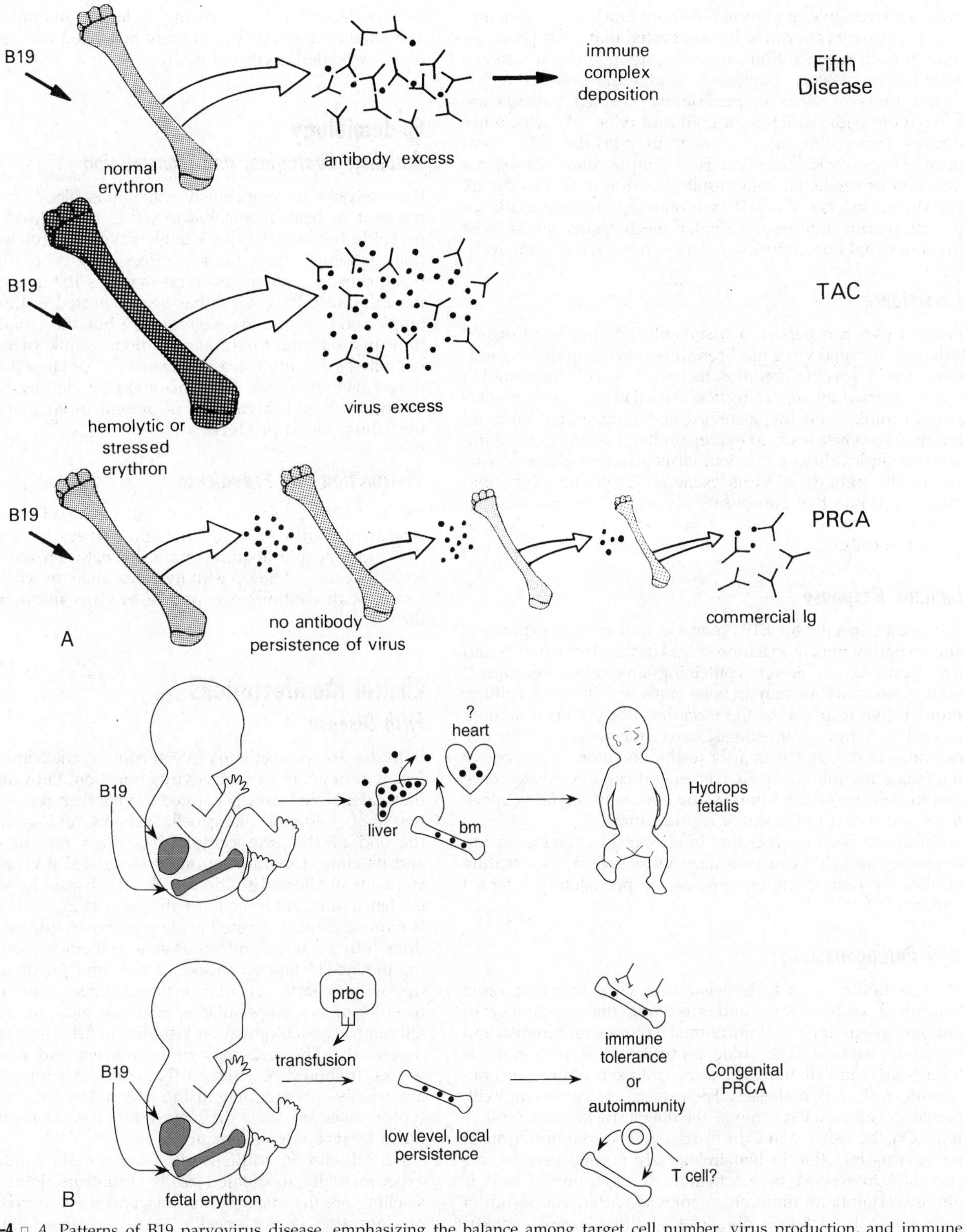

FIGURE 245–4 □ *A*, Patterns of B19 parvovirus disease, emphasizing the balance among target cell number, virus production, and immune response. TAC, Transient aplastic crisis; PRCA, pure red (blood) cell aplasia. *B*, Patterns of B19 parvovirus infection of the fetus, resulting in either death in utero or at birth or, when treated by transfusion of packed red blood cells (prbc), in PRCA. bm, Bone marrow.

on the red blood cell surface but is also found on megakaryocytes, endothelial cells, some placental cells, and fetal liver and heart.[62]

In addition to the P receptor, permissivity requires intracellular factors. The pattern of transcription of B19 parvovirus RNA differs between marrow cells and nonpermissive cell lines, suggestive of a transcription factor that enables capsid gene RNA expression.[63]

Cytotoxicity

Productive parvovirus infection is cytotoxic. The renewable nature of the erythroid progenitor target cell population is an important variable in clinical infection. Study of persistently infected patients over time has suggested that virus propagation and cell regeneration may alternate in cycles to achieve equilibrium between target cells and virus production.[49, 50] Lower titers of virus in persistently infected patients are compatible with depletion of erythroid cells.[64] As with other viruses, irreversible organ damage may be the only "footprint" of parvovirus infection. For example, feline parvovirus infection of cerebellar cells results in atrophy of this organ, and the persistence of ataxia in developing kittens is evidence of intrauterine infection.[65] Similar mechanisms might exist for congenital bone marrow failure syndromes in humans.[13]

Persistence

Parvoviruses can persist in tissue culture[66] and in animals.[41] Adeno-associated virus has been shown to integrate as concatemers at a specific chromosomal site[67] in cell lines, and it can be rescued by superinfection. Aleutian disease virus persists in minks, and the sustained and exaggerated humoral immune response leads to hypergammaglobulinemia and immune complex disease.[68] Latent virus infection is also apparent in the pattern of virus excretion in young pigs[42] and kittens.[69] While B19 parvovirus persists in patients, neither persistence nor integration of this virus has been demonstrated in cells.

Immune Response

Antibodies specific for B19 are made after natural exposure[70] and experimental inoculation,[25] IgM rising from day 5 and IgG from day 7. Serum containing antibodies neutralizes viral cytotoxicity for human bone marrow cells.[55, 71] A cellular proliferative response to the virus has not yet been demonstrated in vitro.[71] Immediately after infection, the immune response is directed primarily to the common sequences of the major and minor capsid species, but late in convalescence and in random serum samples, the dominant antibody specificity is directed to the minor capsid protein.[71]

Failure to produce IgG that binds capsid proteins on immunoblot and that can neutralize virus activity is a feature of the aberrant immune response of persistently infected patients.[49, 50, 64, 71]

B19 Pathogenesis

Marrow failure is an early event after virus infection, often coincident with viremia and preceding the appearance of antiparvovirus IgG[4, 24, 70]; in normal volunteers, viremia and the disappearance of reticulocytes from the circulation occur 5 days after inoculation, when the only symptoms are nonspecific rash and malaise.[24] These data are consistent with hematopoietic cells' serving as the major site of virus replication. On the other hand, fifth disease, the manifestation of parvovirus infection in hematologically normal persons, occurs late in respect to inoculation or exposure[24, 70] and is almost certainly an immune complex disorder. The serum of children with a clinical diagnosis of fifth disease contains IgM antibody to B19 parvovirus but rarely virus.[11, 72, 73] In normal volunteers, both the cutaneous and the rheumatic symptoms and signs of fifth disease occur 17 to 18 days after inoculation, when there are rising titers of specific antiviral immunoglobulins in the blood. Fifth disease can also be produced by infusion of immunoglobulins into chronically viremic patients.[50] Although patients with fifth disease are rarely viremic and probably not contagious, low concentrations of virus may be detectable for months after infection by polymerase chain reaction amplification.[64] A rash illness, even when anticipated, is rare enough after aplastic crisis to be reportable,[74] perhaps owing to larger quantities of virus and smaller amounts of antibody produced during infection of an expanded erythroid marrow.

Epidemiology

Stability, Contagion, and Transmission

Parvoviruses are notoriously contagious. They are relatively resistant to heat and stable to 60° C for at least 16 hours, probably because they lack labile envelope protein. In addition, extremely high titers of virus may be present in the blood during acute infection (as many as 10^{16} genomic copies per milliliter). Parvovirus has been detected in throat swabbings[70] and respiratory secretions,[25] but the usual route of transmission under natural conditions is unknown. Parvovirus may be acquired as a nosocomial[75–77] or laboratory[78] infection. Parvovirus may be transmitted by clotting factor concentrate,[79, 80] and, because it is present in circulating cells,[36] by cellular blood products.

Distribution and Prevalence

IgG to B19 is present in about half of the adult population worldwide, and seroepidemiologic surveys have suggested that most people acquire immunity between the ages of 5 and 19 years.[2, 6–8] Seropositivity rates increase with age, consistent with continuing exposure to virus throughout adult life.

Clinical Manifestations

Fifth Disease

Fifth disease, or erythema infectiosum, is the common manifestation of acute B19 parvovirus infection. Fifth disease was first categorized and separated from other related rash illnesses of childhood like rubella, rubeola, and scarlet fever at the end of the 19th century. The high rate of contagion and its clinical features strongly suggested a virus. Because virtually all affected children with fifth disease have serologic evidence of recent infection with parvovirus,[11, 72, 73] the illness is more accurately termed acute parvovirus infection. In children, fifth disease manifests as an exanthem, typically involving the face ("slapped cheek"), trunk, and proximal extremities with a lacy, reticular, erythematous eruption.[81–86] The macular or maculopapular appearance may mimic measles, although a vesiculopustular eruption in fifth disease has been described.[87] The rash may be evanescent and recurrent for weeks. It should be stressed that children with fifth disease are usually not extremely ill and may not be febrile. Although typical cases are easily diagnosed, fifth disease is often recognized by its epidemic character.

Fifth disease in adults is often a rheumatic syndrome.[81] In experimentally inoculated adult volunteers, joint pain and swelling are the major symptoms, and the pattern of cutaneous eruption is not specific.[24] The manifestations of fifth disease in adults have been described in patients newly diagnosed with arthritis, about 15% of whom have evidence of recent parvovirus infection.[88, 89] Polyarthralgia and frank arthritis may be acute, or the syndrome may persist for months and resemble rheumatoid arthritis in the pattern of joint involvement. Some patients have rheumatoid factor in the blood,[90] and B19 antigen has been detected in the synovial fluid.[91] However, B19 parvovirus does not have a general role in the etiology of rheumatoid arithritis.[92, 93]

Other rheumatic illnesses associated with B19 parvovirus infection include fibromyalgia[94] and a systemic lupus erythematosus–like syndrome.[95, 96] Infection has also been associated with some cases of vasculitis, including Wegener granulomatosis[97] and Kawasaki disease.[98]

Transient Aplastic Crisis

Transient aplastic crisis is a unique event in the life of persons with hemolytic disease, characterized by abrupt cessation of bone marrow erythropoiesis, reticulocytopenia, and severe but temporary anemia.[4, 10, 70, 98] Aplastic crisis occurs in virtually every hemolytic state, including sickle cell disease, hereditary spherocytosis, erythrocyte enzyme deficiencies, autoimmune hemolysis, paroxysmal nocturnal hemoglobinuria, and the thalassemias.[4] Although readily treated by red blood cell transfusions, anemia may precipitate fatal heart failure.[99] Virtually all cases of typical transient aplastic crisis are caused by B19 parvovirus infection,[4, 10] but erythroid marrow failure in these patients can also accompany serious systemic bacterial or mycobacterial infections.[99] Occasionally, parvovirus infection in a patient with underlying hemolysis is not followed by transient aplasia.[100]

The bone marrow of transient aplastic crisis shows an absence of erythroid precursor cells and the presence of striking giant pronormoblasts; rarely, necrosis of marrow may occur.[101] Reticulocytopenia and a fall in hemoglobin level are the sequelae of inoculation of parvovirus into hematologically normal volunteers,[24] associated with temporary cessation of marrow erythropoiesis.[102] Because of the 120-day average life span of a red blood cell in the circulation, this regular effect of B19 infection has hematologic consequences only for persons who have a heightened demand for red blood cells, usually owing to hemolysis. In cases of compensated hemolysis, in which a normal hemoglobin level is maintained by increased marrow activity, transient aplastic crisis can unmask the underlying hematologic disease.[103–105] Aplastic crisis caused by B19 infection can occur in persons with erythropoietic stress due to blood loss[106] or iron deficiency. Neutrophil and platelet numbers commonly fall during transient aplastic crisis,[99, 106–108] and parvovirus infection has been cited in cases of isolated thrombocytopenia[109] as well as transient[106–108] and permanent[110] pancytopenia. B19 parvovirus is a cause of hemophagocytic syndrome, in which variable pancytopenia occurs with characteristic bone marrow morphologic features.[111] However, idiopathic aplastic anemia and transient erythroblastopenia of childhood have not been associated by serologic studies with recent parvovirus infection.[112]

Chronic Bone Marrow Failure

B19 parvovirus can persist in immunosuppressed patients and cause chronic transfusion-dependent anemia, sometimes with severe neutropenia.[49, 50, 64, 113, 114] Anemia is commonly the only evidence of persistent B19 infection, and patients usually lack fever and fifth disease symptoms and signs. About 15% of cases of "idiopathic" pure red blood cell aplasia probably represent persistent parvovirus infection.[115] Persistent infection has been documented in congenital immunodeficiency syndromes,[49, 64] in acquired immunodeficiency syndrome caused by human immunodeficiency virus type 1 infection,[116] and in children with acute lymphocytic leukemia in remission who are receiving chemotherapy.[50, 113, 114] The congenital immunodeficiency state that predisposes to persistent infection has not been well characterized, although there are usually defects in both T- and B-cell function (Nezelof syndrome); anemia due to B19 may be the major clinical manifestation of the immunodeficiency state. Anemia may remit during periods in which virus is not present in the circulation.[49, 50, 64]

Hydrops Fetalis and Congenital Infection[2, 12, 117]

B19 infection is a cause of nonimmune hydrops fetalis, in which death of the term fetus is due to severe anemia and congestive heart failure.[118–126] Parvovirus has been demonstrated in fetal tissue by in situ hybridization, electron microscopy, and immunoblotting for proteins.[122–126] Similar to children and adults, the erythron appears to be the major target of virus infection, with characteristic morphologic changes and virus most consistently present in the liver, the major blood-producing organ of the fetus. Most women have been infected in the second trimester, so infection in the fetus is also presumably chronic. The role of B19 infection in early pregnancy in producing spontaneous abortions is unknown.[2, 127] Maternal fifth disease is not usually followed by a poor fetal outcome, and the risk of hydrops, although real, is probably not greater than 3% with documented exposure.[2, 127, 128]

Occasionally, parvovirus infection acquired during pregnancy can persist in the infant.[129] Hydropic infants treated in utero or at birth by red blood cell transfusions may remain anemic. The marrow may show red blood cell aplasia or dysplastic changes. Virus does not circulate and can be detected only by gene amplification of marrow. In contrast to persistent infection in later life, congenital infection does not respond to immunoglobulin therapy. There is little evidence to suggest that parvovirus is otherwise teratogenic in humans,[130] although virus has been detected in myocardial cells[131] which bear P antigen (and the puppy heart is a site of attack of canine parvovirus).

Diagnosis

Both capture radioimmunoassays[6, 132] and enzyme-linked immunoassays[7] have been employed to measure anti-B19 IgG and IgM in serum. Antibody quantities are usually reported in arbitrary units. The presence of high IgM levels to B19 in serum is evidence of recent infection; the quantity of IgG in exposed persons varies widely, and rising titers probably cannot be used to infer recent exposure. As described earlier, patients with persistent B19 parvovirus infection may not have serum antibodies to virus,[50] or antibodies that react by immunoassay but not on immunoblot to capsid proteins,[49, 71] or a pattern of antibody typical of early convalescence (IgM, and IgG directed mainly to the 58-kDa capsid protein).[64, 71]

The diagnosis of persistent B19 parvovirus infection depends on detecting virus itself rather than virus-specific antibody.[49, 50] Virus alone will also be present in serum from patients with transient aplastic crisis obtained at the onset of illness. DNA hybridization methods allow quantitation of virus as genome copy number.[132–136] In acute infection, the period of viremia is brief but often intense; there may be as many as 10^{16} genome copies per milliliter of serum. In persistent infection, 10^5 to 10^8 genome copies are more usual. Amplification of viral DNA by polymerase chain reaction is far more sensitive than direct hybridization methods, and viremia is more prolonged, even in acute infection, than was previously suspected.[137] The results of polymerase chain reaction studies should be interpreted cautiously—the sensitivity of the technique makes it susceptible to contamination and false-positive results. Replicating virus can be detected by Southern blot hybridization after restriction enzyme digestion. Parvovirus has been detected by blot and in situ hybridization and by immunofluorescence studies of bone marrow, spleen, and a variety of fetal organs.

Treatment

In normal children, fifth disease is a mild illness and no treatment is required. The polyarthralgia-arthritis syndrome in adults is usually a brief episode; more chronic rheumatic symptoms are treated with antiinflammatory drugs. The severity of anemia in transient aplastic crisis usually requires erythrocyte transfusion, but hospitalization is not mandatory. Hydrops fetalis can be diagnosed noninvasively in utero, and it may be possible to salvage the fetus with intrauterine transfusions.[136]

As described earlier, the defect in persistent parvovirus infection is humoral. Commercial immunoglobulin preparations contain anti-B19 parvovirus IgG.[70] Anemia due to persistent infection responds to infusions of commercial immunoglobulin,[64] and this treatment is recommended for immunodeficient anemic patients with evidence of B19 DNA in the blood. Fifth disease symptoms may result from formation of immune complexes between circulating virus and the administered immunoglobulin.

Prevention

Viremia accompanies transient aplastic crisis, and patients in crisis as well as persistently infected patients should be considered infectious, and, if hospitalized, separated from susceptible persons likely to suffer complications of parvovirus infection: patients who are immunosuppressed or have underlying hemolysis, and pregnant staff. Susceptibility can be predicted by the presence or absence of IgG antibody to virus in serum. The risk of contagion in typical fifth disease in the community is highest during the early phases of infection, when symptoms are least specific and the disease is most difficult to diagnose; the viremic patient can also be entirely asymptomatic, making control of spread of infection problematic. There is little rationale for excluding children with fifth disease exanthem from school.[2]

Animal parvovirus infections can be prevented by active immunization.[40, 41] Capsid proteins expressed in animal cells[31] or in a baculovirus system[138] self-assemble into empty capsids. These capsids are immunogenic in animals,[139] especially if enriched for VP1, the minor capsid protein that contains most of the linear neutralizing epitopes.[140] Recombinant capsids have entered phase I testing in human volunteers, and they should provide a safe and effective vaccine reagent.

References

1. Young NS: Parvoviruses. *In* Fields BM, Knipe DM, Howley PM (eds): Fields Virology, ed 3. Philadelphia, Lippincott-Raven, 1996, pp 2199–2220.
2. Centers for Disease Control: Risks associated with human parvovirus B19 infection. MMWR Morbid Mortal Wkly Rep 38:81, 1989.
3. Anderson LJ: Role of parvovirus B19 in human disease. Pediatr Infect Dis J 6:711, 1987.
4. Young NS: Hematologic and hematopoietic consequences of B19 parvovirus infection. Semin Hematol 25:159, 1988.
5. Cossart YE, Field AM, Cant B, et al: Parvovirus-like particles in human sera. Lancet 1:72, 1975.
6. Cohen BJ, Mortimer PP, Pereira MS: Diagnostic assays with monoclonal antibodies for the human serum parvovirus-like virus (SPLV). J Hyg 91:113, 1983.
7. Anderson LJ, Tsou C, Parker RA, et al: Detection of antibodies and antigens of human parvovirus B19 by enzyme-linked immunoabsorbent assays. J Clin Microbiol 24:533, 1986.
8. Cohen BJ, Buckley MM: The prevalence of antibody to human parvovirus B19 in England and Wales. J Med Microbiol 25:151, 1988.
9. Pattison JR, Jones SE, Hodgson J, et al: Parvovirus infections and hypoplastic crisis in sick-cell anaemia (Letter) Lancet 1:664, 1981.
10. Serjeant GR, Topley JM, Mason K, et al: Outbreak of aplastic crises in sickle cell anaemia associated with parvovirus-like agent. Lancet 2:595, 1981.
11. Anderson MJ, Lewis E, Kidd IM, et al: An outbreak of erythema infectiosum associated with human parvovirus infection. J Hyg 93:85, 1984.
12. Anderson LJ, Hurwitz ES: Human parvovirus B19 and pregnancy. Clin Perinatol 15:273, 1988.
13. Frickhofen N, Young NS: Persistent human parvovirus infection. Microb Pathogen 7:319, 1989.
14. Tattersall P, Cotmore SF: The nature of parvoviruses. *In* Pattison JR (ed): Parvoviruses and Human Diseases. Boca Raton, FL, CRC Press, 1988, pp 5–41.
15. Cotmore S, Tattersall P: The autonomously replicating parvoviruses of vertebrates. Adv Virus Res 33:91, 1987.
16. Blacklow NR: Adeno-associated viruses of humans. *In* Pattison JR (ed): Parvoviruses and Human Diseases. Boca Raton, FL, CRC Press, 1988, pp 165–174.
17. Berns KI, Bohenzky RA: Adeno-associated viruses: An update. Adv Virus Res 32:243, 1987.
18. Cukor G, Blacklow NR, Hoggan MD, et al: Biology of adeno-associated virus. *In* Berns KI (ed): The Parvoviruses. New York, Plenum Publishing, 1984, pp 33–66.
19. Pringle CR: Virus taxonomy update. Taxonomic decisions ratified at the plenary meeting of the ICTV at the 9th International Congress of Virology held in Glasgow on the 10th of August 1993. Arch Virol 133:491, 1993.
20. Summers J, Jones SE, Anderson MJ: Characterization of the genome of the agent of erythrocyte aplasia permits its classification as a human parvovirus. J Gen Virol 64:2527, 1983.
21. Clewley JP: Biochemical characterization of a human parvovirus. J Gen Virol 65:241, 1984.
22. Morinet F, Tratschin J-D, Perol Y, et al: Comparison of 17 isolates of the human parvovirus B19 by restriction enzyme analysis. Arch Virol 90:165, 1986.
23. Mori J, Beattie P, Melton DW, et al: Structure and mapping of the DNA of human parvovirus B19. J Gen Virol 68:2797, 1987.
24. Chorba TL, Coccia P, Holman RC, et al: The role of parvovirus B19 in aplastic crisis and erythema infectiosum (fifth disease). J Infect Dis 154:383, 1986.
25. Anderson MJ, Higgins PG, Davis LR, et al: Experimental parvoviral infection in humans. J Infect Dis 152:257, 1985.
26. O'Sullivan MG, Anderson DC, Fikes, JD et al: Identification of a novel simian parvovirus in cynomolgus monkeys with severe anemia: A paradigm of human B19 parvovirus infection. J Clin Invest 93:1571, 1993.
27. Cotmore SF, Tattersall P: Characterization and molecular cloning of a human parvovirus genome. Science 226:1161, 1984.
28. Shade RO, Blundell MC, Cotmore SF, et al: Nucleotide sequence and genome organization of human parvovirus B19 isolated from the serum of a child during aplastic crisis. J Virol 58:921, 1986.
29. Ozawa K, Ayub J, Hao Y-S, et al: Novel transcription map for the B19 (human) pathogenic parvovirus. J Virol 61:2395, 1987.
30. Cotmore SF, McKie VC, Anderson LJ, et al: Identification of the major structural and nonstructural proteins encoded by human parvovirus B19 and mapping of their genes by procaryotic expression of isolated genomic fragments. J Virol 60:548, 1986.
31. Ozawa K, Young NS: Characterization of capsid and noncapsid proteins of B19 parvovirus propagated in human erythroid bone marrow cell cultures. J Virol 61:2627, 1987.
32. Kajigaya S, Shimada T, Fujita S, et al: A genetically engineered cell line that produces empty capsids of B19 (human) parvovirus. Proc Natl Acad Sci USA 86:7601, 1989.
33. Ozawa K, Ayub J, Kajigaya S, et al: The gene encoding the nonstructural protein of B19 (human) parvovirus may be lethal in transfected cells. J Virol 62:2884, 1988.
34. Luo W, Astell CR: A novel protein encoded by small RNAs of parvovirus B19. Virology 195:448, 1993.
35. Shimomura S, Wong S, Komatsu N, et al: Early and late gene expression in UT-7 cells infected with B19 parvovirus. Virology 194:149, 1993.
36. Carter BJ, Laughlin CA: Adeno-associated virus defectiveness and the nature of the adenovirus helper function. *In* Berns KI (ed): The Parvoviruses. New York, Plenum Publishing, 1984, pp 67–128.
37. Yakobson B, Koch T, Winocour E: Replication of adeno-associ-

ated virus in synchronized cells without the addition of a helper virus. J Virol 61:972, 1987.
38. Spalholz BA, Tattersall P: Interaction of minute virus of mice with differentiated cells: Strain-dependent target cell specificity is mediated by intracellular factors. J Virol 46:937, 1983.
39. Antonietti JP, Sahli R, Beard P, et al: Characterization of the cell type–specific determinant in the genome of minute virus of mice. J Virol 62:552, 1988.
40. Siegl G: Biology of pathogenicity of autonomous parvoviruses. *In* Berns KI (ed): The Parvoviruses. New York, Plenum Publishing, 1984, pp 297–362.
41. Siegl G: Patterns of parvovirus disease in animals. *In* Pattison JR (ed): Parvoviruses and Human Diseases. Boca Raton, FL, CRC Press, 1988, pp 43–67.
42. Johnson RH, Collings DF: Transplacental infection of piglets with a porcine parvovirus. Res Vet Sci 12:570, 1971.
43. Siegl G: Canine parvovirus: Origin and significance of a "new" pathogen. *In* Berns KI (ed): The Parvoviruses. New York, Plenum Publishing, 1984, pp 363–388.
44. Kurtzman GJ, Platanias L, Lustig L, et al: Feline parvovirus propagates in cat bone marrow cultures and inhibits hematopoietic colony formation. Blood 74:71, 1989.
45. Ozawa K, Kurtzman G, Young N: Replication of the B19 parvovirus in human bone marrow cell cultures. Science 233:883, 1986.
46. Hauswirth WW: Autonomous parvovirus DNA structure and replication. *In* Berns KI (ed): The Parvoviruses. New York, Plenum Publishing, 1984, pp 129–152.
47. Berns KI, Hauswirth WW: Adeno-associated virus DNA structure and replication. *In* Berns KI (ed): The Parvoviruses. New York, Plenum Publishing, 1984, pp 1–31.
48. Kurtzman GJ, Gascon P, Caras M, et al: B19 Parvovirus replicates in circulating cells of acutely infected patients. Blood 71:1448, 1988.
49. Kurtzman GJ, Ozawa K, Hanson GR, et al: Chronic bone marrow failure due to persistent B19 parvovirus infection. N Engl J Med 317:287, 1987.
50. Kurtzman GJ, Cohen B, Meyers P, et al: Persistent B19 parvovirus infection as a cause of severe chronic anaemia in children with acute lymphocytic leukaemia. Lancet 2:1159, 1988.
51. Yaegashi N, Shiraishi H, Takeshita T, et al: Propagation of human parvovirus B19 in primary culture of erythroid lineage cells derived from fetal liver. J Virol 63:2422, 1989.
52. Schwarz TF, Serke S, Hottentrager B, et al: Replication of parvovirus B19 in hematopoietic progenitor cells generated in vitro from normal human peripheral blood. J Gen Virol 66:1273, 1992.
53. Shimomura S, Komatsu N, Frickhofen N, et al: First continuous propagation of B19 parvovirus in a cell line. Blood 79:18, 1992.
54. Munshi NC, Zhou S, Woody MJ, et al: Successful replication of parvovirus B19 in the human megakaryocytic cell line MB-02. J Virol 67:562, 1993.
55. Mortimer PP, Humphries RK, Moore JG, et al: A human parvovirus-like virus inhibits hematopoietic colony formation in vitro. Nature 302:426, 1983.
56. Takahashi T, Ozawa K, Takahashi K, et al: Susceptibility of human erythropoietic cells to B19 parvovirus in vitro increases with differentiation. Blood 75:603, 1990.
57. Srivastava A, Lu L: Replication of B19 parvovirus in highly enriched hematopoietic progenitor cells from normal human bone marrow. J Virol 62:3059, 1988.
58. Ozawa K, Kurtzman G, Young NS: Productive infection by B19 parvovirus of human erythroid bone marrow cells in vitro. Blood 70:384, 1987.
59. Young NS, Harrison M, Moore JG, et al: Direct demonstration of the human parvovirus in erythroid progenitor cells infected in vitro. J Clin Invest 74:2024, 1984.
60. Brown KE, Anderson SM, Young NS: Erythrocyte P antigen: Cellular receptor for B19 parvovirus. Science 262:114, 1993.
61. Brown KE, Hibbs JR, Gallinella G, et al: Resistance to parvovirus B19 due to lack of virus receptor (erythrocyte P antigen). N Engl J Med 330:1192, 1994.
62. Marcus DM, Kundu SK, Suzuki A: The P blood group system: Recent progress in immunochemistry and genetics. Semin Hematol 18:63, 1981.
63. Liu J, Green S, Shimada T, Young NS: A block in full-length transcript maturation in cells nonpermissive for B19 parvovirus. J Virol 66:4686, 1992.
64. Kurtzman GJ, Frickhofen N, Kimball J, et al: Pure red cell aplasia of ten years' duration due to B19 parvovirus infection and its cure with immunoglobulin therapy. N Engl J Med 321:519, 1989.
65. Kilham L, Margolis G: Viral etiology of spontaneous ataxia of cats. Am J Pathol 48:991, 1966.
66. Cheung AKM, Hoggan MD, Hauswirth WW, Berns KI: Integration of the adeno-associated virus genome into cellular DNA in latently infected human Detroit 6 cells. J Virol 33:739, 1980.
67. Kotin RM, Siniscalco M, Samulski RJ, et al: Site-specific interaction by adeno-associated virus. Proc Natl Acad Sci USA 87:2211, 1990.
68. Porter DD: Aleutian disease: A persistent parvovirus infection of mink with maximal but ineffective host humoral immune response. Prog Med Virol 33:42, 1986.
69. Csiza CK, Scott FW, de Lahunta A, Gillespie JH: Immune carrier state of feline panleukopenia virus–infected cats. Am J Vet Sci 32:419, 1971.
70. Saarinen UM, Chorba TL, Tattersall P, et al: Human parvovirus B19-induced epidemic red cell aplasia in patients with hereditary hemolytic anemia. Blood 67:1411, 1986.
71. Kurtzman GJ, Blaese M, Oseas R, et al: Immune response to B19 parvovirus infection. J Clin Invest 84:1114, 1989.
72. Plummer FA, Hammond GW, Forward K, et al: An erythema infectiosum-like illness caused by human parvovirus infection. N Engl J Med 313:74, 1985.
73. Okabe N, Kobayashi S, Tatsuzawa O, et al: Detection of antibodies to human parvovirus in erythema infectiosum (fifth disease). Arch Dis Child 59:1016, 1984.
74. Nunoue T, Koike T, Koike R, et al: Infection with human parvovirus (B19), aplasia of the bone marrow and a rash in hereditary spherocytosis. J Infect 14:67, 1987.
75. Evans JPM, Rossiter MA, Kumaran TO, et al: Human parvovirus aplasia: Case due to cross infection in a ward. Br Med J 288:681, 1984.
76. Pell LM, Naides SJ, Stollmon P, et al: Human parvovirus B19 infection among hospital staff members after contact with infected patients. N Engl J Med 321:485, 1989.
77. Seng C, Watkins P, Morse D, et al: Parvovirus B19 outbreak on an adult ward. Epidemiol Infect 113:345, 1994.
78. Cohen BJ, Courouce AM, Schwartz TF, et al: Laboratory infection with parvovirus B19 (Letter). J Clin Pathol 41:1027, 1988.
79. Mortimer PP, Luban NLC, Kelleher JF, et al: Transmission of serum parvovirus-like by clotting factor concentrates. Lancet 2:482, 1983.
80. Bartolomei Corsi O, Assi A, Morfini M, et al: Human parvovirus infection in haemophiliacs first infused with treated clotting factor concentrates. J Med Virol 25:165, 1988.
81. Ager EA, Chin TKY, Poland JP: Epidemic erythema infectiosum. N Engl J Med 275:1326, 1966.
82. Anderson MJ: Rash illness due to B19 virus. *In* Pattison JR (ed): Parvoviruses and Human Diseases. Boca Raton, FL, CRC Press, 1988, p 93–137.
83. Balfour HH Jr: Erythema infectiosum (fifth disease): Clinical review and description of 91 cases seen in an epidemic. Clin Pediatr 8:721, 1969.
84. Brass C, Elliott L, Stevens DA: Academy rash. A probable epidemic of erythema infectiosum ("fifth disease"). JAMA 248:568, 1982.
85. Cramp HE, Armstrong BDJ: Erythema infectiosum: An outbreak of "slapped cheek" disease in north Devon. Br Med J 1:885, 1976.
86. Lauer BA, MacCormack JN, Wilfert C: Erythema infectiosum. An elementary school outbreak. Am J Dis Child 130:252, 1976.
87. Naides SJ, Piette W, Veach LA, et al: Human parvovirus B19–induced vesiculopustular skin eruption. Am J Med 84:968, 1988.
88. Reid DM, Reid TMS, Brown T, et al: Human parvovirus-associated arthropathy. Lancet 1:419, 1985.
89. White DG, Woolf AD, Mortimer PP, et al: Human parvovirus arthropathy. Lancet 1:422, 1984.
90. Cohen BJ, Buckley MM, Clewley JP, et al: Human parvovirus infection in early rheumatoid and inflammatory arthritis. Ann Rheum Dis 45:832, 1986.
91. Stierle G, Brown KA, Rainsford SG, et al: Parvovirus associated antigen in the synovial membrane of patients with rheumatoid arthritis. Ann Rheum Dis 46:219, 1987.

92. Mimori A, Misaki Y, Hachiya T, et al: Prevalence of antihuman parvovirus B19 IgG antibodies in patients with refractory rheumatoid arthritis and polyarticular juvenile rheumatoid arthritis. Rheumatol Int 14:87, 1994.
93. Nikkari S, Luukkainen R, Möttönen T, et al: Does parvovirus B19 have a role in rheumatoid arthritis? Ann Rheum Dis 53:106, 1994.
94. Leventhal LJ, Naides SJ, Freundlich B: Fibromyalgia and parvovirus infection. Arthritis Rheum 34:1319, 1991.
95. Cope AP, Jones A, Brozovic M, et al: Possible induction of systemic lupus erythematosus by human parvovirus. Ann Rheum Dis 51:803, 1992.
96. Kalish RA, Knopf AN, Gary GW, Canoso JJ: Lupus-like presentation of human parvovirus B19 infection. J Rheumatol 19:169, 1992.
97. Finkel TH, Török TJ, Ferguson PJ, et al: Chronic parvovirus B19 infection and systemic necrotising vasculitis: Opportunistic infection or aetiological agent? Lancet 343:1255, 1994.
98. Nigro G, Zerbini M, Krzysztofiak A, et al: Active or recent parvovirus B19 infection in children with Kawasaki disease. Lancet 343:1260, 1994.
99. Serjeant GR, Goldstein AR: B19 virus infection and the aplastic crisis. *In* Pattison JR (ed): Parvoviruses and Human Diseases. Boca Raton, FL, CRC Press, 1988, pp 85–92.
100. Anderson MJ, Davis LR, Hodgson J, et al: Occurrence of infection with a parvovirus-like agent in children with sickle cell anaemia during a two-year period. J Clin Pathol 35:744, 1982.
101. Conrad ME, Studdard H, Anderson LJ: Case Report: Aplastic crisis in sickle cell disorders: Bone marrow necrosis and human parvovirus infection. Am J Med Sci 295:212, 1988.
102. Potter CG, Potter AC, Hatton CSR, et al: Variation of erythroid and myeloid precursors in the marrow and peripheral blood of volunteer subjects infected with human parvovirus (B19). J Clin Invest 79:1486, 1987.
103. Lefrere JJ, Courouce A-M, Girot R, et al: Six cases of hereditary spherocytosis revealed by human parvovirus infection. Br J Haematol 62:653, 1986.
104. McLellan NJ, Rutter N: Hereditary spherocytosis in sisters unmasked by parvovirus infection. Postgrad Med J 63:49, 1987.
105. Bertrand Y, Lefrere JJ, Leverger G, et al: Autoimmune hemolytic anaemia revealed by human parvovirus linked erythroblastopenia. Lancet 2:382, 1985.
106. Frickhofen N, Raghavachar A, Heit W, et al: Human parvovirus infection (Letter). N Engl J Med 314:646, 1986.
107. Saunders PWG, Reid MM, Cohen BJ: Human parvovirus induced cytopenias: A report of five cases (Letter). Br J Haematol 63:407, 1986.
108. Hanada T, Koike K, Takaya T, et al: Human parvovirus B19–induced transient pancytopenia in a child with hereditary spherocytosis. Br J Haematol 70:113, 1988.
109. Lefrere JJ, Got D: Peripheral thrombocytopenia in human parvovirus infection (Letter). J Clin Pathol 40:469, 1987.
110. Hamon MD, Newland AC, Anderson MJ: Severe aplastic anemia after parvovirus infection in the absence of underlying hemolytic anemia (Letter). J Clin Pathol 41:1242, 1988.
111. Shirono K, Tsuda H: Parvovirus B19–associated haemophagocytic syndrome in healthy adults. Br J Haematol 89:923, 1995.
112. Young NS, Mortimer PP, Moore JG, Humphries RK: Characterization of a virus that causes transient aplastic crisis. J Clin Invest 73:224, 1984.
113. Van Horn DK, Mortimer PP, Young N, et al: Human parvovirus associated red cell aplasia in the absence of underlying hemolytic anemia. Am J Pediatr Hematol Oncol 8:235, 1986.
114. Smith MA, Shah NR, Lobel JS, et al: Severe anemia caused by human parvovirus in a leukemia patient on maintenance chemotherapy. Clin Pediatr 27:383, 1988.
115. Frickhofen N, Chen ZJ, Young NS, et al: Parvovirus B19 as a cause of acquired chronic pure red cell aplasia. Br J Haematol 87:818, 1994.
116. Frickhofen N, Abkowitz JL, Safford M, et al: Persistent B19 parvovirus infection in patients infected with human immunodeficiency virus-1: A treatable cause of anemia in AIDS. Ann Intern Med 113:926, 1990.
117. Rodis JF, Hovick TJ Jr, Quinn DL, et al: Human parvovirus infection in pregnancy. Obstet Gynecol 72:733, 1988.
118. Brown T, Anand A, Ritchie LD, et al: Intrauterine parvovirus infection associated with hydrops fetalis. Lancet 2:1033, 1984.
119. Knott PD, Welply GAC, Anderson MJ: Serologically proved intrauterine infection with parvovirus. Br Med J 289:1660, 1984.
120. Anand A, Gray ES, Brown T, et al: Human parvovirus infection in pregnancy and hydrops fetalis. N Engl J Med 316:183, 1987.
121. Franciosi RA, Tattersall P: Fetal infection with human parvovirus B19. Hum Pathol 19:489, 1988.
122. Maeda H, Shimokawa H, Satoh S, et al: Nonimmunologic hydrops fetalis resulting from intrauterine human parvovirus B19 infection: Report of two cases. Obstet Gynecol 72:482, 1988.
123. Clewley JP, Cohen BJ, Field AM: Detection of parvovirus B19 DNA, antigen, and particles in the human fetus. J Med Virol 23:367, 1987.
124. Porter HJ, Khong TY, Evans MF, et al: Parvovirus as a cause of hydrops fetalis: Detection by in situ DNA hybridization. J Clin Pathol 41:381, 1988.
125. Knisely AS, O'Shea PA, McMillan P, et al: Electron microscopic identification of parvovirus virions in erythroid-line cells in fatal hydrops fetalis. Pediatr Pathol 8:163, 1988.
126. Caul EO, Usher MJ, Burton PA: Intrauterine infection with human parvovirus B19: A light and electron microscopy study. J Med Virol 24:55, 1988.
127. Kinney JS, Anderson LJ, Farrar J, et al: Risk of adverse outcomes of pregnancy after human parvovirus B19 infection. J Infect Dis 157:663, 1988.
128. Woernle CH, Anderson LJ, Tattersall P, et al: Human parvovirus B19 infection during pregnancy. J Infect Dis 156:17, 1987.
129. Brown KE, Green SW, Antunez de Mayolo J, et al: Congenital anaemia following transplacental B19 parvovirus infection. Lancet 343:895, 1994.
130. Weiland HT, Vermey-Keers C, Salimans MM, et al: Parvovirus B19 associated with fetal abnormality (Letter). Lancet 1:682, 1987.
131. Porter HJ, Quantrill AM, Fleming KA: B19 Parvovirus infection of myocardial cells (Letter). Lancet 1:535, 1988.
132. Cohen BJ: Laboratory tests for the diagnosis of infection with B19 virus. *In* Pattison JR (ed): Parvoviruses and Human Diseases. Boca Raton, FL, CRC Press, 1988, pp 69–83.
133. Anderson MJ, Jones SE, Minson AC: Diagnosis of human parvovirus infection by dot-blot analysis using cloned viral DNA. J Med Virol 15:163, 1985.
134. Clewley JP: Detection of human parvovirus using a molecularly cloned probe. J Med Virol 15:173, 1985.
135. Cunningham DA, Pattison JR, Craig RK: Detection of parvovirus DNA in human serum using biotinylated RNA hybridisation probes. J Virol Methods 19:279, 1988.
136. Schwarz TF, Roggendorf M, Hottentrager B, et al: Human parvovirus B19 infection in pregnancy (Letter). Lancet 2:566, 1988.
137. Clewley JP: Polymerase chain reaction assay of parvovirus B19 DNA in clinical specimens. J Clin Microbiol 27:2647, 1989.
138. Kajigaya S, Fujii H, Field A, et al: Self-assembled parvovirus capsids, produced in a baculovirus system, are antigenically and immunogenically similar to virions. Proc Natl Acad Sci USA 88:4646, 1991.
139. Bansal GP, Hatfield JA, Dunn FE, et al: Candidate recombinant vaccine for human B19 parvovirus. J Infect Dis 167:1034, 1993.
140. Saikawa T, Momoeda M, Anderson S, et al: Neutralizing linear epitopes of B19 parvovirus cluster in the VP1 unique and VP1-VP2 junction region. J Virol 67:3004, 1993.

246

Human Papillomaviruses (Including Wart Viruses)

Keerti V. Shah

History

The viral cause of human skin warts was established early in this century by experimental transmission of disease to susceptible persons with cell-free filtrate of wart extract.[1] In the 1930s, the studies of the cottontail rabbit papillomavirus provided the first example of a mammalian tumor virus,[2] but further progress in the characterization of papillomaviruses was hampered because they could not be propagated in tissue culture or transmitted to laboratory animals. This difficulty was bypassed to some extent by the advent of molecular cloning in the 1970s, when viral genomes in affected tissues were cloned directly in plasmid vectors. More than 70 individually distinct human papillomaviruses (HPVs) have been described to date.

HPVs infect the squamous epithelia of the skin and the mucous membranes.[3] Genital tract infections with HPVs are highly prevalent; they contribute to the occurrence of lower genital tract cancers and are linked etiologically to cancer of the cervix. Intrapartum transmission of HPVs from an infected mother to the offspring sometimes results in the production of respiratory papilloma in the exposed children. Cutaneous HPVs largely produce benign, self-limited warts; however, progression of warty lesions to squamous cell carcinomas may occur in the rare dermatologic disorder epidermodysplasia verruciformis.

Characteristics of the Pathogen

Papillomaviruses and polyomaviruses constitute two subfamilies of the family Papovaviridae. Papovaviruses are small, nonenveloped viruses with icosahedral symmetry, 72 capsomers, double-stranded circular DNA genome, and nucleus as the site of viral multiplication. The two subfamilies differ from each other with respect to virion size, genome size, and genetic organization and show no evidence of genetic or immunologic interrelatedness (Table 246–1). The viral genome is divided into an early region (about 4.5 kb), which is necessary for transformation; a late region (about 2.5 kb), which codes for the capsid proteins; and a regulatory region (about 1 kb), which contains the origin of replication and many of the control elements for transformation and replication (Fig. 246–1). There are eight open reading frames (ORFs E1 to E8) in the early region and two in the late region (ORFs L1 and L2), all of which are located on the same strand. Their functions are indicated in Table 246–2.

Papillomaviruses are classified on the basis of species of origin (e.g., human, bovine, rabbit) and the extent of genetic relatedness with other papillomaviruses from the same species. New types are defined on the basis of sequence variation from the known types in specific regions of the genome.[4] The papillomavirus virion contains a major capsid protein of 57 kDa and a minor capsid protein of 70 kDa. Species-specific and subfamily-specific determinants are located on the major capsid protein.

Papillomaviruses have not yet been propagated in tissue culture to yield virus particles, probably because full cellular differentiation required for virus production is not achieved in cultured cells. Infectious virus is produced when fragments of susceptible tissue are exposed to a condyloma extract that contains HPV-11 and transplanted beneath the renal capsule of athymic nude mice[5] or when HPV-infected keratinocytes are allowed to differentiate fully in the organotypic "raft" system.[6]

TABLE 246–1 ■ Differences Between Papillomavirus and Polyomavirus Subfamilies

MEASURE	PAPILLOMAVIRUS	POLYOMAVIRUS
Virion size (nm)	55	45
Genome size (base pairs)	8000	5000
Location of open reading frames	All on one strand	Distributed on both strands
Genetic and immunologic relatedness		
Between viruses of the same subfamily	Yes	Yes
Between viruses of different subfamilies	No	No
Association with naturally occurring tumors	Yes	No

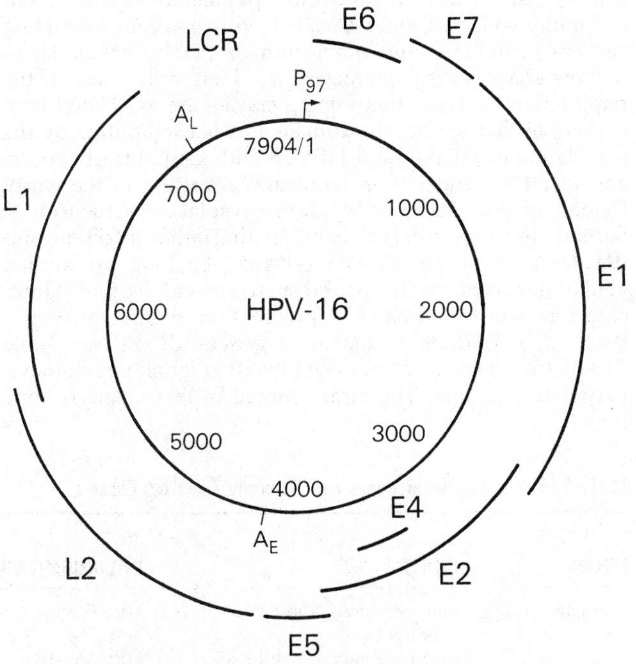

FIGURE 246–1 □ Genomic map of HPV-16 determined from the DNA sequence. The genome is a double-stranded circular DNA molecule of 7904 base pairs. Transcription occurs in a clockwise manner; the only transcriptional promoter mapped yet for HPV-16 is designated P97. The open reading frames deduced from the DNA sequence are designated E1 to E7, L1, and L2 and are indicated outside the circular genome. A_E and A_L represent the early and late polyadenylation sites. The viral long control region (LCR) contains transcriptional and replication regulatory elements. (From Shah KV, Howley PM: Papillomaviruses. *In* Fields BN, Knipe DM, Howley PM [eds]: Fields Virology, ed 3. Philadelphia, Lippincott-Raven, 1996, pp 2077–2109.)

TABLE 246–2 ■ Functions of Papillomavirus Open Reading Frames

OPEN READING FRAME	FUNCTION
E1	Plasmid replication
E2	Regulation of transcription; plasmid replication
E3, E8	Not known
E4	Coding for late cytoplasmic protein
E5, E6	Transformation (bovine papillomavirus)
E6, E7	Transformation (human papillomavirus)
L1	Coding for major capsid protein
L2	Coding for minor capsid protein

Papillomaviruses are highly species specific and also display a marked degree of cellular tropism. Mucosal HPVs are rarely detected on the skin (except in the genital area), and cutaneous HPVs are rarely detected at mucosal sites. All HPVs are strictly epitheliotropic, but a subset of animal papillomaviruses induce both dermal and epithelial proliferation to produce fibropapillomas.[7] Warts are thought to be of monoclonal origin, arising from the proliferation of a single infected basal cell.[8] Basal cells are presumably exposed to infectious virus after minor trauma to the epithelium, as would occur during sexual intercourse or after minor skin abrasions. All cells of a wart contain the viral genome, but the expression of viral genes is tightly linked to the state of cellular differentiation. Only the upper layers of the epithelium (which contain the differentiating and keratinizing cells) permit late gene expression and synthesis of viral particles. Virus multiplication is confined to the nucleus. Koilocytosis (cytoplasmic vacuolization) with an abnormal nucleus is a characteristic feature of productive papillomavirus infection.

Papillomaviruses are associated with naturally occurring cancers in humans and other animals (Table 246–3). These cancers share several characteristics. First, only some of the papillomavirus types that infect a species are associated with cancers in that species. In humans this is exemplified by the association of HPV-16 and HPV-18 with genital tract cancers and of HPV-5 and HPV-8 with cancers arising in the warty lesions of patients with epidermodysplasia verruciformis. Second, the time interval between the initial infection and development of invasive cancer may be long. In human genital tract cancers, this period spans several decades. Third, cofactors are required for progression to malignancy—sunlight, x-irradiation, diet, or a genetic defect (see Table 246–3). Cofactors have not been identified for all papillomavirus-related cancers. The viral genome in these cancers may be present in an integrated state (as in most human genital tract cancers) or in an extrachromosomal state (as in rabbit carcinomas), or it may be lost altogether with progression (as in bovine papillomavirus type 4–associated alimentary carcinomas of cattle).

Animal papillomaviruses that induce fibropapillomas in nature (e.g., bovine papillomavirus types 1 and 2) readily transform rodent cells in culture.[9] The transformed cells are tumorigenic in syngeneic animals. In contrast, HPVs can transform rodent cells only in cooperation with an activated *ras* oncogene.[10] The transforming activity of HPV types in vitro is correlated with their role in naturally occurring cancers. HPV-16 and HPV-18, which are associated with genital tract cancers, display greater transforming activity than HPV-6 and HPV-11, which are seldom found in genital tract cancers. Human keratinocytes transfected with HPV-16 and HPV-18 become immortal and carry the viral genome in an integrated state.[11] These cells are not tumorigenic in nude mice. In the collagen raft system, which permits epithelial cell differentiation, HPV-16– and HPV-18–transfected human keratinocytes stratify and show the morphologic features of intraepithelial neoplasia.[12] In quantitative assays of keratinocyte transformation by HPV DNAs, both oncogenic and nononcogenic HPVs induce transient cellular proliferation, but only the oncogenic HPVs give rise to immortalized cell lines.[13] The transforming activity of bovine papillomavirus type 1 is localized to the E5 and E6 ORFs, whereas that of HPVs is localized to the E6 and E7 ORFs.

Immune Response

Clinical observations have shown that conditions in which T-cell response is depressed (e.g., immunosuppressive therapy, organ transplantation, acquired immunodeficiency syndrome) are associated with a high prevalence and exacerbation of warts. Also, regressing flat skin warts show histologic evidence of a cell-mediated immune response. Infection appears to produce a low-titered antibody response to capsid proteins as measured by enzyme-linked immunosorbent assay with virus-like particles synthesized in recombinant baculovirus or vaccinia virus systems.[14, 15] Antibodies to the transforming proteins E6 and E7 are markers of HPV-associated invasive cervical cancer.[16]

Epidemiology and Clinical Features

The HPVs fall naturally into two groups, cutaneous HPVs and mucosal HPVs. The major clinical associations of HPV

TABLE 246–3 ■ Papillomaviruses and Naturally Occurring Cancers*

SPECIES	CANCER	PREDOMINANT VIRAL TYPES	STATE OF VIRAL GENOME IN CANCERS	COFACTORS
Humans	Skin carcinomas in EV patients	HPV-5, -8	Extrachromosomal	Sunlight; genetic defect
	Cervical, vulvar, penile carcinomas	HPV-16, -18	Integrated or extrachromosomal	Not known
	Malignant progression of respiratory papillomas	HPV-6, -11	Extrachromosomal	X-irradiation or not known
Cattle	Alimentary tract carcinoma	BPV-4	Absent	Bracken fern
	Eye and skin carcinoma	Not characterized	Not known	Sunlight
Sheep	Skin carcinoma	Not characterized	Not known	Sunlight
Cottontail rabbit	Skin carcinoma	CRPV	Extrachromosomal	Not known

*EV, Epidermodysplasia verruciformis; HPV, human papillomavirus; BPV, bovine papillomavirus; CRPV, cottontail rabbit papillomavirus.

TABLE 246–4 ■ Clinical Associations of Human Papillomavirus Types*

CLINICAL CONDITION	HUMAN PAPILLOMAVIRUS TYPE
Skin	
Plantar warts	1
Common warts	2, 4
Mosaic warts (superficial spreading wart)	2
Flat warts	3, 10, 28, 41
Macular plaques of epidermodysplasia verruciformis	5, 8, 9, 12, 14, 15, 17, 19, 20, 21, 22, 23, 24, 25, 36, 47, 50
Butchers' warts	7
Genital Warts	
Exophytic condyloma (any site)	6, 11
Flat condyloma (especially cervix)	6, 11, 16, 18, 31, others
Bowenoid papulosis	16
Giant condyloma (Buschke-Löwenstein tumor)	6, 11
Cervical cancer	
Strong association	16, 18
Moderate association	31, 33, 35, 45, 51, 52, 56
Weak association or none	6, 11, 42, 43, 44
Vulvar cancer	16
Respiratory papillomas	6, 11
Conjunctival papillomas	6, 11
Oral cavity	
Focal epithelial hyperplasia	13, 32
Mucosal warty lesions	6, 11, 16
Warts on lips	2

*HPV types for which information is limited are not listed.

infections are shown in Table 246–4. About 20 cutaneous HPVs have been recovered, almost exclusively from patients with epidermodysplasia verruciformis. Most of the mucosal HPVs reside in the genital tract, but two HPVs, HPV-13 and HPV-32, appear to infect the oral cavity exclusively. Genital tract HPVs also infect other mucosal sites, such as the respiratory tract, the oral cavity, and the conjunctiva. Infection is acquired through minor skin abrasions (cutaneous warts), by sexual intercourse (genital warts), or by transmission at birth from the genital tract of an infected mother to the offspring (respiratory papillomas).

Cutaneous Human Papillomavirus Infections

Skin warts are acquired by direct contact with an infected person or by contact with contaminated objects. Recreational activities (e.g., swimming), in which wet, bare skin is exposed in communally used facilities, increases the risk of acquiring plantar warts. Meat handlers, butchers, and abattoir personnel have a high prevalence of warts on their hands. These warts are caused by HPV infections and not by transmission of animal papillomaviruses. Skin warts are most common in older children and young adults and are rare before age 5 years. A majority of warts regress spontaneously within 2 years. There is a strong correlation between site and morphology of the wart and infecting HPV type (see Table 246–4).

Epidermodyplasia verruciformis is a rare dermatologic disorder of worldwide distribution in which a wart virus infection does not resolve.[17] The disease has a genetic basis; it is often familial, and patients frequently give a history of parental consanguinity. The lesions are either flat warts or reddish-brown macular plaques. In about a third of the cases, multiple foci of malignant transformation arise in the reddish brown plaques, most often in lesions that are exposed to sunlight and are caused by HPV-5 and HPV-8. The viral genome is present as multiple copies of unintegrated DNA.

Mucosal Human Papillomavirus Infections

Genital tract infections with HPVs are highly prevalent. It has been estimated that 10% to 20% of men and women in the age group 15 to 49 years (12 to 24 million persons) in the United States have prevalent HPV infection.[18] A large majority of these infections are clinically inapparent and show no cytologic or colposcopic abnormalities. The genital tract is frequently infected at multiple sites. Apparently normal epithelium adjacent to clinical lesions contains the viral genome.[19]

The most clearly recognized clinical manifestations of HPV infection are genital warts (condylomata). The incidence of genital warts has increased more than fivefold between 1966 and 1986.[20] Exophytic condylomata are largely the result of infections with HPV-6 and HPV-11. Flat condylomata are etiologically more heterogeneous and are associated with infections with many HPV types, including HPV types 6, 11, 16, 18, 31, 33, and 35. The predominant HPV lesions on the cervix are flat condylomata.[21]

Relationship to Cancers in the Genital Tract

SQUAMOUS CELL CARCINOMA OF THE CERVIX

Worldwide, about one-half million cases of cancer of the cervix are diagnosed annually. Cervical cancer accounts for about a quarter of all cancers in women in the developing world and for about 7% of cancers in women in the industrialized nations. The lifetime risk of developing cancer of the cervix varies as much as 10-fold in different geographic areas of the world. Squamous cell carcinoma of the cervix (about 85% of all cervical cancers) is associated with multiple sexual partners and has the characteristics of a sexually transmitted disease. Invasive cancer is preceded by a progressive series of abnormalities of the cervical epithelium that are classified as cervical intraepithelial neoplasia, grades 1, 2, or 3. The interval between mild cervical abnormalities grade 1 and invasive cancer may be several decades.

The evidence linking HPV infections and cervical cancer has been reviewed extensively[22, 23] and is summarized in Table 246–5. The epidemiologic evidence is strongly reinforced by laboratory studies, and together they make a compelling case for HPV as the cause of invasive cervical cancer.[23]

HPV infections by themselves are not sufficient to lead to cancer of the cervix. It is thought that HPVs increase the life span of the affected cells and that other cellular events (e.g., oncogene activation, inactivation of tumor suppressors, mutations) are necessary for progression to malignancy.[32] Epidemiologic studies have suggested that smoking and oral contraceptive use may be independent risk factors for cervical cancer.

OTHER CANCERS

Adenocarcinoma of the cervix, which constitutes about 10% to 15% of cervical cancers, is also associated with HPVs, especially HPV-18.[34] Some cancers of the penis, the vulva, the vagina, the anus, and the perineum are also HPV associated, but these cancers are much less common than cancer of the cervix. The lower incidence of malignancy at extracervical sites is ascribed to the absence at these sites of an area as susceptible to oncogenic transformation as the transformation zone at the squamocolumnar junction of the cervix.

TABLE 246–5 ■ Evidence Linking Human Papillomavirus Infections with Cervical Cancer*

HPVs are recovered from a large proportion of invasive cervical cancers as well as from CIN-1, -2, and -3, the precursor lesions of cancer.[22–26]
HPV-16 and HPV-18 (and some other HPV types) are preferentially associated with cancers. Between 50% and 60% of invasive cancers yield HPV-16 or HPV-18. Many other types (e.g., HPV-6 and HPV-11) are frequently found in mild cervical lesions and in inapparent infections but are virtually absent from invasive cancer. The viral genome in HPV-associated cancers is present in the cancer cells themselves in the primary tumor (as shown by hybridization studies in situ) as well as in metastatic tumors.[27, 28] The viruses found in cancer tissues are the ones that have transforming activity in studies in vitro.
The viral genome not only is present but also is transcriptionally active. ORFs E6 and E7 are consistently expressed in cancer tissues. Studies in vitro show that these ORFs code for the transforming proteins of HPVs.
In many invasive cancers, the viral genome is integrated into the cellular chromosomes. The integration appears to facilitate expression of E6 and E7. The circular viral genome breaks most often in the E1/E2 region for integration.[29, 30] This leaves intact the E6 and E7 ORFs and also removes the repressive effect, which E2 probably exercises on the promoter for E6 and E7.
Most of the cell lines derived from invasive cervical cancers contain HPV-16 or HPV-18.[30, 31] The viral genome is integrated in most HPV-associated cell lines and expresses E6 and E7 ORFs.
The viral transforming proteins E6 and E7 dysregulate the cell cycle by complexing, respectively, with cellular tumor suppressor proteins p53 and Rb. This leads to genetic instability and additional chromosmal changes, which underlie the development of invasive cancer.

*CIN, Cervical intraepithelial neoplasia; ORFs, open reading frames.

Human Papillomaviruses in the Respiratory Tract, Oral Cavity, and Conjunctiva

Adult-onset as well as juvenile-onset respiratory papillomas are caused by genital tract HPV-6 and HPV-11. It is likely that intrapartum transmission of HPV from infected mother to offspring is responsible for most of the cases of juvenile-onset respiratory papillomas. It has been estimated that only one of many children born to infected mothers develops respiratory papillomas.[35] The manner in which adult-onset respiratory HPV infection is acquired is not known. Most of the conjunctival papillomas are also caused by HPV-6 or HPV-11.

The oral cavity mucosa may be infected with HPVs that are peculiar to the oral cavity (HPV-13 and HPV-32) and by genital tract HPVs (HPV-6, -11, and -16). HPV-13 and HPV-32 are associated with a clinical condition called focal epithelial hyperplasia, which is common in indigenous populations of Central and South America and of Alaska and Greenland but is rare in whites.[37] HPV-2, the virus associated with common hand warts, is frequently identified in lesions on the lip vermilion.[38]

HPV-6 and HPV-11 are associated with the rare cases of severe dysplasia and malignant progression that occur in respiratory papillomas.[39] Although HPVs have been identified frequently in the common epithelial cancers of the respiratory tract and the oral cavity[40, 41] and in conjunctival carcinoma,[42] it is not clear whether their presence is of etiologic significance. Tonsillar carcinomas appear to be linked to HPV infections.[43]

Diagnosis

Diagnosis of HPVs requires nucleic acid hybridization studies. HPV sequences are detected by methods based on gene amplification by polymerase chain reaction or by direct hybridization of the genomes in the specimens, without prior amplification. The most commonly used polymerase chain reaction tests utilize consensus primers, which are capable of amplifying a large number of HPVs, and type-specific probes to identify the sequences in the polymerase chain reaction products.[44, 45] These tests have a high degree of analytic specificity and sensitivity. A U.S. Food and Drug Administration–approved, commercially available assay that screens for 14 genital HPV types by direct hybridization is also available.[46] HPV diagnosis may be useful, as an adjunct to the Papanicolaou smear, in identifying women with low-grade cervical cytologic abnormalities who harbor high-risk HPVs and may therefore be at risk for disease progression.

Treatment

Interferons administered into the lesions or given parenterally have been used successfully in treating refractory genital warts[47] but have been only marginally useful in the treatment of respiratory papillomas.[48] Traditional therapies include application of caustic agents (e.g., podophyllin, trichloroacetic acid), application of a DNA inhibitor (5-fluorouracil), cryotherapy, and surgical therapy. Cure rates of more than 90% are achieved in the treatment of cervical intraepithelial neoplasia lesions by any one of several treatment modalities, but the viruses may persist in a latent state.

Prevention

The development of HPV-based vaccines to prevent cervical cancer is an area of intensive investigation.[49, 50] In experimental studies, cattle, rabbits, and dogs can be protected against papilloma formation by immunization with virus-like particles that contain capsid proteins of the respective animal papillomaviruses. Therapeutic immunization with HPV-transforming proteins E6 and E7 may prove to have some value in the treatment of cervical cancer.

References

1. Ciuffo G: Innesto positivo con filtrato di verruca vulgare. G Ital Mal Venereol 48:12, 1907.
2. Shope R: Infectious papillomatosis of rabbits. J Exp Med 58:607, 1933.
3. Shah KV, Howley PM: Papillomaviruses. *In* Fields BN, Knipe DM, Howley PM (eds): Fields Virology, ed 3. Philadelphia, Lippincott-Raven, 1996, pp 2077–2109.
4. Delius H, Hofmann B: Primer-directed sequencing of human papillomavirus types. *In* Zur Hausen H (ed): Human Pathogenic Papillomaviruses. Heidelberg, Germany, Springer-Verlag, 1994, pp 13–31.
5. Kreider JW, Howett MK, Wolfe SA, et al: Morphological transformation in vivo of human uterine cervix with papillomavirus from condylomata acuminata. Nature 317:639, 1985.
6. Meyers C, Frattini GM, Hudson JB, et al: Biosynthesis of human papillomavirus from a continuous cell line upon epithelial differentiation. Science 257:971, 1992.
7. Lancaster W, Olson C: Animal papillomaviruses. Microbiol Rev 46:191, 1982.
8. Murray R, Hobbs J, Payne B: Possible clonal origin of common warts (verruca vulgaris). Nature 232:51, 1971.
9. Howley PM, Schlegel R: Papillomavirus transformation. *In* Salzman NP, Howley PM (eds): The Papovaviridae, Vol 2, The Papillomaviruses. New York, Plenum Publishing, 1987, pp 141–166.
10. Matlashewski G, Schneider J, Banks L, et al: Human papillomavirus type 16 DNA cooperates with activated *ras* in transforming primary cells. EMBO J 6:1741, 1987.

11. Durst M, Dzarlieva-Pertrusevzka P, Boukamp P, et al: Molecular and cytogenetic analysis of immortalized human primary keratinocytes obtained after transfection with human papilloma virus type 16 DNA. Oncogene 1:251, 1987.
12. McCance DJ, Kopan R, Fuchs E, et al: Human papillomavirus type 16 alters human epithelial cell differentiation in vitro. Proc Natl Acad Sci USA 85:7169, 1988.
13. Schlegel R, Phelps WC, Zhang Y-L, et al: Quantitative keratinocyte assay detects two biological activities of human papillomavirus DNA and identifies viral types associated with cervical carcinoma. EMBO J 7:3181, 1988.
14. Kirnbauer R, Hubbert NL, Wheeler CM, et al: A virus-like particle enzyme-linked immunosorbent assay detects serum antibodies in a majority of women infected with human papillomavirus type 16. J Natl Cancer Inst 86:494, 1994.
15. Hagensea ME, Yaegashi N, Galloway D: Self-assembly of human papillomavirus type 1 capsids by expression of the L1 protein alone or by co-expression of the L1 and L2 capsid proteins. J Virol 67:315, 1993.
16. Sun Y, Eluf-Neto J, Bosch FX, et al: Human papillomavirus (HPV)-related serologic markers of invasive cervical carcinoma in Brazil. Cancer Epidemiol Biomarkers Prev 3:341, 1994.
17. Orth G: Epidermodysplasia verruciformis. *In* Salzman NP, Howley PM (eds): The Papovaviridae, Vol 2, The Papillomaviruses. New York, Plenum Publishing, 1987, pp 199–243.
18. Koutsky LA, Galloway DA, Holmes KK: Epidemiology of genital human papillomavirus infection. Epidemiol Rev 10:122, 1988.
19. Ferenczy A, Mitao M, Nagai N, et al: Latent papillomavirus and recurring genital warts. N Engl J Med 313:784, 1985.
20. Becker TM, Stone KM, Alexander ER: Genital human papillomavirus infection: A growing concern. Obstet Gynecol Clin North Am 14:389, 1987.
21. Meisels A, Fortin R, Roy M: Condylomatous lesions of the cervix. II. Cytologic, colposcopic and histopathologic study. Acta Cytol 21:379, 1977.
22. Muñoz N, Bosch FX, Shah KV, Meheus A (eds): The Epidemiology of Human Papillomavirus and Cervical Cancer. IARC Publication 119. Lyon, France, International Agency for Research on Cancer, 1992.
23. IARC Monographs Working Group on the Evaluation of Carcinogenic Risks to Humans, Vol 64, Human Papillomaviruses. Lyon, France, International Agency for Research on Cancer, 1995.
24. Bosch FX, Manos MM, Muñoz N, et al: Prevalence of human papillomavirus in cervical cancer: A worldwide perspective. J Natl Cancer Inst 87:796, 1995.
25. Schiffman MH, Bauer HM, Hoover RN, et al: Epidemiologic evidence showing that HPV infection causes most cervical intraepithelial neoplasia. J Natl Cancer Inst 85:958, 1993.
26. Eluf-Neto J, Booth M, Muñoz N, et al: Human papillomavirus and invasive cervical cancer in Brazil. Br J Cancer 69:114, 1994.
27. Lancaster WD, Castellano C, Santos C, et al: Human papillomavirus deoxyribonucleic acid in cervical carcinoma from primary and metastatic sites. Am J Obstet Gynecol 154:115, 1986.
28. Fuchs PG, Girardi F, Pfister H: Human papillomavirus 16 DNA in cervical cancers and in lymph nodes of cervical cancer patients: A diagnostic marker for early metastases? Int J Cancer 43:41, 1989.
29. Baker CC, Phelps WC, Lindgren V, et al: Structural and transcriptional analysis of human papillomavirus type 16 sequences in cervical carcinoma cell lines. J Virol 61:962, 1987.
30. Schwarz E, Freese UK, Gissmann L, et al: Structure and transcription of human papillomavirus sequences in cervical carcinoma cells. Nature 314:111, 1985.
31. Yee C, Krishnan-Hewlett I, Baker CC, et al: Presence and expression of human papillomavirus sequences in human cervical carcinoma cell lines. Am J Pathol 119:361, 1985.
32. Howley PM: Papillomavirinae: The viruses and their replication. *In* Fields BN, Knipe DM, Howley PM (eds): Fields Virology, ed 3. Philadelphia, Lippincott-Raven, 1996, pp 2045–2076.
33. Zur Hausen H: Molecular pathogenesis of cancer of the cervix and its causation by specific human papillomavirus types. *In* Zur Hausen H (ed): Human Pathogenic Papillomaviruses. Heidelberg, Germany, Springer-Verlag, 1994, pp 131–156.
34. Tase T, Okagaki T, Clark BA, et al: Human papillomavirus types and localization in adenocarcinoma and adenosquamous carcinoma of the uterine cervix: A study by in situ DNA hybridization. Cancer Res 48:993, 1988.
35. Shah K, Kashima H, Polk BF, et al: Rarity of cesarean delivery in cases of juvenile-onset respiratory papillomatosis. Obstet Gynecol 68:795, 1986.
36. McDonnell PI, McDonnell JM, Kessis T, et al: Detection of human papillomavirus type 6/11 DNA in conjunctival papillomas by in situ hybridization with radioactive probes. Hum Pathol 18:1115, 1987.
37. Syrjanen SM: Human papillomavirus infections in the oral cavity. *In* Syrjanen K, Gissmann L, Koss LG (eds): Papillomaviruses and Human Disease. New York, Springer-Verlag, 1987, pp 104–137.
38. Eversole LR, Laipis PJ, Green TL: Human papillomavirus type 2 DNA in oral and labial verruca vulgaris. J Cutan Pathol 14:319, 1988.
39. Byrne JC, Tsao M-S, Fraser RS, et al: Human papillomavirus-11 DNA in a patient with chronic laryngotracheo-bronchial papillomatosis and metastatic squamous cell carcinoma of the lung. N Engl J Med 317:873, 1987.
40. Kiyabu M, Shibata D, Arnheim N, et al: Detection of human papillomavirus in formalin-fixed, invasive squamous carcinomas using the polymerase chain reaction. Am J Surg Pathol 13:221, 1989.
41. Maitland NJ, Cox MF, Lynas C, et al: Detection of human papillomavirus DNA in biopsies of human oral tissue. Br J Cancer 56:246, 1987.
42. McDonnell IM, Mayr AJ, Martin WJ: DNA of human papillomavirus type 16 in dysplastic and malignant lesions of the conjunctiva and cornea. N Engl J Med 320:1442, 1989.
43. Snijders PFJ, van den Brule AJC, Meijer DJLM, et al: Papillomaviruses and cancer of the upper digestive and respiratory tracts. *In* Zur Hausen H (ed): Human Pathogenic Papillomaviruses. Heidelberg, Germany, Springer-Verlag, 1994, pp 177–198.
44. Hildesheim A, Schiffman MH, Gravitt P, et al: Persistence of type-specific human papillomavirus infection among cytologically normal women in Portland, Oregon. J Infect Dis 169:235, 1994.
45. Jacobs MV, de Roda Husman AM, van den Brule AJC, et al: Group-specific differentiation between high- and low-risk human papillomavirus genotypes by general primer-mediated PCR and two cocktails of oligonucleotide probes. J Clin Microbiol 33:901, 1995.
46. Cox JT, Lorincz AT, Schiffman MH, et al: Human papillomavirus testing by hybrid capture appears to be useful in triaging women with a cytologic diagnosis of atypical squamous cells of undetermined significance. Am J Obstet Gynecol 172:946, 1995.
47. Eron LJ, Judson F, Tucker S, et al: Interferon therapy for condylomata acuminata. N Engl J Med 315:1059, 1986.
48. Kashima H, Leventhal B, Clark K, et al: Interferon α-N1 (Wellferon) in juvenile-onset recurrent respiratory papillomatosis: Results of a randomized study in twelve collaborative institutions. Laryngoscope 98:334, 1988.
49. Crawford L: Prospects for cervical cancer vaccines. Cancer Surveys 16:215, 1993.
50. Munoz N, Crawford L, Coursaget P: HPV vaccines and their potential use in the prevention and treatment of cervical neoplasia. Papillomavirus Rep 6:54, 1995.

247

Human Polyomavirus (Including the Agent Causing Progressive Multifocal Leukoencephalopathy)

Keerti V. Shah

Polyomavirus infections of humans were not recognized until 1971, when two polyomaviruses, BK virus (BKV) and JC virus (JCV), were isolated from immunosuppressed patients.[1, 2] JCV is the etiologic agent of progressive multifocal leukoencephalopathy (PML), a degenerative disease of the central nervous system.[3] BKV infection is associated with some urinary tract illnesses.[4] Millions of U.S. residents were inadvertently exposed to simian virus 40, an oncogenic polyomavirus of Asian macaques, because this virus was a frequent and unrecognized contaminant of inactivated poliovirus vaccines that were administered between 1955 and 1961. There is no firm evidence that simian virus 40 produced any ill effects in the exposed population.[5] Polyomaviruses are widely distributed in nature and cause a variety of illnesses in their natural hosts, affecting kidney, brain, lung, and other organs (Table 247–1). The viruses are species specific and infect only one or a few closely related species.

Characteristics of the Pathogen

The viral particle is small (diameter 45 nm), is nonenveloped, and has an icosahedral capsid with 72 capsomers. The structure and functions of polyomavirus genomes are known in great detail.[6, 7] The viral genome is a small, double-stranded, circular DNA molecule of about 5000 base pairs. It is functionally divided into an early region (2.3 kb) that codes for large and small T proteins, a late region (2.3 kb) that codes for viral capsid proteins, and a noncoding regulatory region (0.4 kb) that contains the origin of DNA replication and transcription control sequences. Viral DNA replication occurs bidirectionally starting from the origin of replication. The early and late regions are transcribed from different strands of the DNA molecule. The proteins coded by the viral genome are listed in Table 247–2. The large T antigen is a multifunctional, regulatory early protein. It binds to specific sites in the regulatory region of the viral genome and initiates viral DNA replication, activates cellular genes that mediate cellular DNA synthesis, and modulates early and late viral transcription. The major viral polypeptide VP1, a late protein, is the main component of the viral capsid, is involved in viral attachment to cellular receptors, and contains type-specific and type-common epitopes.

Polyomaviruses and papillomaviruses are classified as two subfamilies of the family Papovaviridae (see Chapter 246). Within each subfamily, the viruses show evidence of genetic relatedness (conserved nucleotide and amino acid sequences), but such evidence is lacking between viruses of the two subfamilies. BKV and JCV are closely related and their DNAs have an overall nucleotide sequence homology of 75%. The amino acid sequence homology between BKV and JCV proteins ranges from a high of 83% for large T protein to a low of 59% for the agnoprotein.

BKV and JCV are propagated in cell cultures of human origin. Primary human embryonic kidney cells and human diploid fibroblasts are suitable for primary isolation of BKV, whereas primary glial cells derived from fetal brains are suitable for primary isolation of JCV. Even in susceptible cells, the growth of BKV and JCV is inefficient and inconsistent.

BKV and JCV transform cells from a variety of rodent species. Ultraviolet-irradiated noninfectious BKV can transform human embryonic kidney cells. The BKV genome remains episomal in BKV-transformed human cells but is integrated in BKV-transformed rodent cells. Both viruses are oncogenic for newborn hamsters and produce cerebral tumors of many histologic types in intracerebrally inoculated animals.[8, 9] After intracerebral inoculation, BKV produces largely tumors of ventricular surfaces (e.g., ependymoma, choroid plexus papilloma) and JCV produces tumors of neural origin. Intravenous inoculation of BKV into hamsters produces insulinomas, osteosarcomas, and ependymomas. Intracerebral inoculation of JCV into owl and squirrel monkeys results in cerebral tumors, the only known example of a virus-induced central nervous system tumor in primates.[10]

TABLE 247–1 ■ Natural Hosts and Principal Characteristics of Polyomaviruses

NATURAL HOST	VIRUSES	TROPISM	ASSOCIATED ILLNESS
Humans	BK virus	Kidney epithelium	Hemorrhagic cystitis, ureteral stenosis
	JV virus	Kidney epithelium and brain oligodenodrocytes	Progressive multifocal leukoencephalopathy (PML)
Monkeys	Simian virus 40 of Asian macaques	Kidney epithelium	PML-like illness in some colonies
	Simian agent 12 of baboons	Kidney epithelium	None recognized
	Lymphotropic polyomavirus of African green monkeys	B lymphocytes	None recognized
Cattle	Bovine polyomavirus	Not known	None recognized
Rabbit	Rabbit kidney vacuolating virus	Kidney epithelium	None recognized
Mouse	Mouse polyoma virus	Kidney epithelium	Tumors in athymic mice
	K virus	Lung endothelium	Respiratory illness
Hamster	Hamster papovavirus	Not known	Cutaneous tumors
Athymic rat	Rat polyomavirus	Not known	Parotid gland abnormalities
Parakeet	Budgerigar fledgling disease virus	Many organs	Fatal illness in fledgling birds

TABLE 247–2 ■ Functions of Virus-Coded Polyomavirus Proteins

PROTEIN	NUMBER OF AMINO ACIDS*	FUNCTIONS
Early region		
Large T	708	Initiation of viral DNA replication, stimulation of host DNA synthesis, regulation of early and late transcription, establishment and maintenance of transformation
Middle T†	421‡	Cell transformation
Small T	174	Efficient viral DNA replication
Late region		
VP1	362	Major capsid protein, attaches to cellular receptors, mediates hemagglutination, has type-specific and type-common epitopes
VP2	352	Minor capsid protein
VP3	234	Minor capsid protein, subset of VP2
Agnoprotein	62	Not known

*For simian virus 40, except for middle T, as deduced from nucleotide sequence data.

†Middle T is found in mouse and hamster polyomaviruses but not in BKV, JCV, and simian virus 40.

‡For mouse polyomavirus.

Pathogenesis

The respiratory tract may be the site of entry of BKV and JCV. Mild respiratory illness may accompany primary BKV infection.[11] It is likely that the viruses multiply at the site of entry and are transported to the kidney in the blood stream. After primary infection, the virus may remain latent in the kidney of the immunocompetent host for an indefinite time and produce no ill effects. Viral genomic sequences have been detected in cadaver kidneys, B lymphocytes,[12, 13] and normal human brain.[14] Immunologic impairment, especially conditions that affect T-cell functions, bring about virus reactivation and viruria.

The viruses multiply exclusively in the nucleus of the infected cell. Productive infection in permissive cells is associated with a variety of nuclear changes (increase in size, occurrence of basophilic inclusions, and others) and results in cell death. The pathologic consequences of polyomavirus infections can be attributed to virus-induced destruction of infected cells. For example, infection and destruction of oligodendrocytes by JCV, and the resulting demyelination, account for the pathologic and clinical features of PML. Immunopathologic factors have not been implicated in diseases caused by polyomaviruses.

BKV and JCV differ in their biologic behavior and disease potential. Only JCV infects the central nervous system and produces PML.[3, 7] In bone marrow transplant recipients, BKV reactivation is far more common than JCV reactivation.[15]

Epidemiology and Clinical Features

Infections with BKV and JCV occur in childhood.[16] Serologic studies have shown that 50% of children in the United States are infected with BKV by age 3 or 4 years and with JCV by age 10 to 14 years. Although BKV and JCV have been recovered most often from urine, the rapid acquisition of antibodies in childhood is more consistent with an infection disseminated from the respiratory tract than from the urinary tract. With rare exceptions, illnesses caused by BKV and JCV are confined to immunocompromised persons.

Progressive Multifocal Leukoencephalopathy

PML is a rare, subacute, fatal demyelinating disease of the central nervous system of worldwide distribution. It occurs on a background of illnesses known to depress T-cell functions, for example, in patients with lymphoproliferative and chronic diseases, organ transplant recipients taking immunosuppressive therapy, and persons who have primary immunodeficiency diseases or acquired immunodeficiency syndrome. PML in patients with acquired immunodeficiency syndrome is reported to occur in nearly 4% of those with neurologic abnormalities,[17] and it accounts for the majority of PML cases in the United States.[18] The age distribution of PML cases has changed from that in the past. A few years ago it was predominantly a disease of the fifth and sixth decades of life, but it is now found increasingly in younger persons, including children.[7]

The onset of the disease is insidious. Early signs and symptoms suggest multifocal and asymmetric lesions in the brain. Impaired speech and vision and mental deterioration are common. As the disease progresses, paralysis of limbs, cortical blindness, and sensory abnormalities occur. Death usually takes place between 3 and 6 months after onset. Throughout the illness, the patient remains afebrile, with normal cerebrospinal fluid and without signs of increased intracranial pressure. Electroencephalograms show nonspecific changes. Until a few years ago, the diagnosis of PML could be established only by pathologic examination of a brain biopsy sample; however, more recently, noninvasive techniques such as computed tomography and magnetic resonance imaging have been effective in the diagnosis of PML.

The pathognomonic lesions of PML are the foci of demyelination surrounded by affected oligodendrocytes, which have inclusion-bearing, enlarged nuclei. In addition, many foci of demyelination contain within them abnormal astrocytes of greatly increased size and with bizarre nuclear changes. The demyelinating lesions are most frequent in the subcortical white matter, and the cerebrum is almost always affected. An inflammatory response is absent or mild.

Both viral particles and viral DNA are found in large quantities in PML brains. JCV is often detected in the cerebrospinal fluid of patients with acquired immunodeficiency syndrome.[19] The nuclei of affected oligodendrocytes contain abundant amounts of viral particles, often seen as dense crystalline arrays. Affected astrocytes only rarely contain viral particles but display JCV T antigen when they are cultured from PML patients' brains. It has been suggested that the oligodendrocytes and the astrocytes represent, respectively, productive infection and transformation by JCV. Patients who die with PML are found to have small amounts of virus at extraneural sites (kidney, liver, lung). The multifocal distribution of the discrete demyelinating foci in the brain suggests that the virus is seeded into the brain through the blood.[10]

Urinary Tract Illnesses

Virus reactivation and viruria occur frequently in pregnant women, in recipients of kidney and bone marrow allografts, and in others whose immunity is depressed.[4, 20] Reactivation in pregnancy has not been associated with any ill effect or with transmission of the infection to the newborn. About one fourth to one half of renal transplant recipients have BKV or JCV viruria. In some instances, the recipient is infected by the kidney from a seropositive donor. There is no firm evidence that BKV and JCV infections in renal transplant recipients are associated with loss of renal function or risk of dying, but these infections do contribute to the occurrence of ureteral stenosis, an infrequent and late complication of renal transplantation.[20] BKV viruria is associated with hemorrhagic cystitis in bone marrow transplant recipients,[15, 21] as well as with occasional cases of cystitis in otherwise healthy, immunocompetent children.[7] A case has been described in which atypical primary BKV infection in an immunologically defenseless child led to tubulointerstitial nephritis and irreversible renal damage.[22]

BK Virus and Simian Virus 40 in Human Tumors

Because of their oncogenic properties for laboratory animals and their ability to transform human cells, a variety of human tumors have been screened for BKV and JCV genomic sequences. In 1983, a variant extrachromosomal BKV genome was recovered from a pancreatic β-islet adenoma.[23] In some studies of brain tumors, extrachromosomal[24] or integrated[25] BKV sequences have been detected, but other investigations have had negative results.[26] Reports of the presence of simian virus 40 in brain tumors of children[27] and in adult mesotheliomas[28] remain to be confirmed.

Diagnosis

Serologic tests for BKV and JCV antibodies are not helpful for clinical diagnosis. Cytomorphology of urinary epithelial cells may be useful as an indicator of polyomavirus excretion in urine. The presence of virus in the urine or the brain can be demonstrated by a variety of techniques, including electron microscopy, isolation in tissue culture, enzyme-linked immunosorbent assay for viral antigens, nucleic acid hybridization assays for viral genomes, and gene amplification by polymerase chain reaction.[29]

Treatment

Treatment of PML by administration of nucleic acid analogs in an attempt to inhibit virus multiplication has been generally unsuccessful, although occasional remissions have been reported.[3] It is thought that reduction or elimination of iatrogenic immunosuppression in PML patients who have relatively intact immune functions (e.g., renal transplant recipients) may be beneficial.

Prevention

No efforts have been made to develop preventive measures against BKV and JCV infections.

Acknowledgment

This work was partially supported by Public Health Service grant P01 AI15969.

References

1. Gardner S, Field A, Coleman D, et al: New human papovavirus (B.K.) isolated from urine after renal transplantation. Lancet 1:1253, 1971.
2. Padgett BL, Walker DL, ZuRhein GM, et al: Cultivation of papova-like virus from human brain with progressive multifocal leucoencephalopathy. Lancet 1:1257, 1971.
3. Walker D, Padgett B: Progressive multifocal leukoencephalopathy. *In* Fraenkel-Conrat H, Wagner RR (eds): Comprehensive Virology, Vol 18. New York, Plenum Publishing, 1983, pp 161–193.
4. Arthur RR, Shah KV: The occurrence and significance of papovaviruses BK and JC in the urine. Prog Med Virol 36:42, 1989.
5. Shah K, Nathanson N: Human exposure to SV40: Review and comment. Am J Epidemiol 103:1, 1976.
6. Cole C. Polyomavirinae: The viruses and their replication. *In* Fields BN, Knipe DM, Howley PM (eds): Fields Virology, ed 3. Philadelphia, Lippincott-Raven, 1996, pp 1997–2026.
7. Frisque RJ, White FA: The molecular biology of JC virus, causative agent of progressive multifocal leukoencephalopathy. *In* Roos RP (ed): Molecular Neurovirology. Totowa, NJ: Humana Press, 1992, pp 25–58.
8. Zu Rhein GM: Studies of JC virus-induced nervous system tumors in the Syrian hamster: A review. *In* Sever JL, Madden DL (eds): Polyomaviruses and Human Neurological Diseases. New York, Alan R Liss, 1983, pp 205–221.
9. Corallini A, Altavilla G, Cecchetti MG, et al: Ependymomas, malignant tumors of pancreatic islets, and osteosarcomas induced in hamsters by BK virus, a human papovavirus. J Natl Cancer Inst 61:875, 1978.
10. Houff S, London W, Zu Rhein G, et al: New world primates as a model of viral-induced astrocytomas. *In* Sever JL, Madden DL (eds): Polyomaviruses and Human Neurological Diseases. New York, Alan R Liss, 1983, pp 223–226.
11. Sundsfjord A, Spein AR, Lucht E, et al: Detection of human polyomavirus BK DNA in nasopharyngeal aspirates from children with respiratory infections but not in saliva from immunodeficient and immunocompetent patients. J Clin Microbiol 32:1390, 1994.
12. Dorries K, Vogel E, Gunther S, et al: Infection of human polyomaviruses JC and BK in peripheral blood leukocytes from immunocompetent individuals. Virology 198:59, 1994.
13. Tornatore C, Berger JR, Houff SA, et al: Detection of JC virus DNA in peripheral lymphocytes from patients with and without progressive multifocal leukoencephalopathy. Ann Neurol 31:454, 1992.
14. White FA III, Ishaq M, Stoner GL, et al: JC virus DNA is present in many human brain samples from patients without progressive multifocal leukoencephalopathy. J Virol 66:5726, 1992.
15. Arthur RR, Shah KV, Baust SJ, et al: Association of BK viruria with hemorrhagic cystitis in recipients of bone marrow transplants. N Engl J Med 315:230, 1986.
16. Shah KV: Polyomaviruses. *In* Fields BN, Knipe DM, Howley PM (eds). Fields Virology, ed 3. Philadelphia, Lippincott-Raven, 1996.
17. Berger JR, Levy RM: The neurologic complications of human immunodeficiency virus infections. Med Clin North Am 77:1, 1993.
18. Holman RC, Janssen RS, Buehler JW, et al: Epidemiology of progressive multifocal leukoencephalopathy in the United States: Analysis of national mortality and AIDS surveillance data. Neurology 41:1733, 1991.
19. Gibson PI, Knowles WA, Hand JF, et al: Detection of JC virus DNA in the cerebrospinal fluid of patients with progressive multifocal leukoencephalopathy. J Med Virol 39:278, 1993.
20. Hogan TF, Padgett BL, Walker DL: Human polyomaviruses. *In* Belshe RB (ed): Textbook of Human Virology. Littleton, MA, PSG Publishing, 1984, pp 969–995.
21. Gluck TA, Knowles WA, Johnson MA, et al: BK virus-associated hemorrhagic cystitis in an HIV-infected man (Letter). AIDS 8:391, 1994.
22. Rosen S, Harmon W, Krensky A, et al: Tubulointerstitial nephritis associated with polyomavirus (BK type) infection. N Engl J Med 308:1192, 1983.
23. Caputo A, Corallini A, Grossi M, et al: Episomal DNA of a BK virus variant in a human insulinoma. J Med Virol 12:37, 1983.
24. Corallini A, Pagnani M, Viadana P, et al: Association of BK virus with human brain tumors and tumors of pancreatic islets. Int J Cancer 39:60, 1987.
25. Dorries K, Loeber G, Meixensberger J: Association of polyomaviruses JC, SV40, and BK with human brain tumors. Virology 160:268, 1987.
26. Arthur RR, Grossman SA, Ronnett BM, et al: Lack of association of human polyomaviruses with human brain tumors. J Neurooncol 20:55, 1994.

27. Bergsagel DJ, Finegold MJ, Butel JS, et al: DNA sequences similar to those of simian virus 40 in ependymomas and choroid plexus tumors of childhood. N Engl J Med 326:988, 1992.
28. Carbone M, Pass HI, Rizzo P, et al: Simian virus 40–like DNA sequences in human pleural mesothelioma. Oncogene 9:1781, 1994.
29. Arthur RR, Dagostin S, Shah KV: Detection of BKV and JCV in urine and brain tissue by the polymerase chain reaction. J Clin Microbiol 27:1174, 1989.

248

Hepatitis B Virus and Hepatitis D Virus

Raymond S. Koff

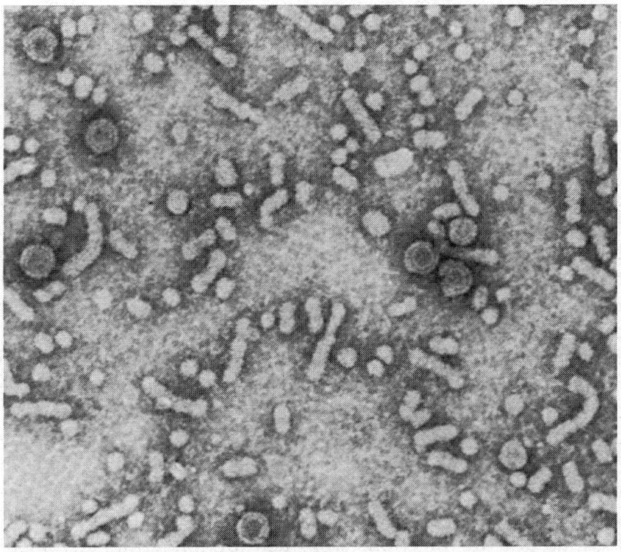

FIGURE 248–1 ▫ Electron micrograph of serum sample showing the 42-nm HBV particle and the smaller 22-nm spheres and tubules containing HBsAg envelope proteins and lipid.

Hepatitis B Virus

On a global basis, human hepatitis B virus (HBV) is the most common cause of persistent viremia and the most important cause of chronic liver disease and hepatocellular carcinoma. Clinically apparent HBV infections may have been extant for several millennia, but characterization of the responsible agent was achieved only in the past three decades.[1] HBV belongs to a family of genetically related but distinct hepatotropic DNA-containing animal viruses, now termed hepadnaviruses. The host range of these agents appears to be restricted to mammalian and avian species. The terms orthohepadnavirus and avihepadnavirus have been applied to the mammalian and avian genera, respectively; the family name Hepadnaviridae is also widely used.

Phylogenetic Relationships and Host Range

Human HBV and the other members of the Hepadnaviridae have morphologic and antigenic similarities, and some but not all are capable of inducing hepatocellular carcinoma. The viruses are double shelled, with a diameter of about 42 nm (Fig. 248–1). Each virus contains a small, partially double-stranded, partially single-stranded circular DNA with long, minus strands of nearly equal nucleotide length (Table 248–1). HBV is one of the smallest human viruses identified; it has a genome size of about 3.2 kb.

Because HBV and the other hepadnaviruses use reverse transcription during genome replication and may share some nucleotide sequences with the retroviruses, the possibility of an evolutionary relationship with the retroviruses has been suggested.[2] However, the replication cycle of the hepadnaviruses is distinct, and the relationship to the retroviruses remains speculative. An evolutionary relationship among the avian and mammalian hepadnaviruses has also been postulated on the basis of examination of specific genomic sequences, a limited number of which are shared. Human HBV, currently classified as hepadnavirus type 1, was the first recognized member of the orthohepadnavirus family. In addition to HBV, orthohepadnaviruses have been described in the Eastern woodchuck, the Beechey ground squirrel, and the tree squirrel. Avihepadnaviruses have been identified in the gray heron and in the domestic Pekin duck. Responsible agents are the woodchuck hepatitis virus, the ground squirrel hepatitis virus, the tree squirrel hepatitis virus, the gray heron hepatitis virus, and the duck hepatitis B virus. The tree squirrel and gray heron hepatitis viruses are less well characterized than the other agents. Chronic infections with human HBV, with woodchuck hepatitis virus and with ground squirrel hepatitis virus have been linked to the development of hepatocellular carcinoma. Although hepatocellular carcinoma has not been identified in duck hepatitis B virus–infected ducks in the United States, an association of duck hepatitis B virus with hepatocellular carcinoma in Qidong ducks in China has been suggested.[3] It is possible that "new" hepadnaviruses affecting different hosts and producing a broad spectrum of hepatic injury may be identified in future studies.

The host range of the known hepadnaviruses has been extended to other species (e.g., geese and chipmunks), but human beings probably cannot be infected by the nonhuman hepadnaviruses. The HBV host range appears to be limited to human beings and some nonhuman primate species. Experimental transmission of HBV to chimpanzees has served as a model for the study of infection; although rhesus and other monkeys may also be susceptible, infection in these animals has been inconsistent, and they have not proved useful for laboratory investigation.

Hepatitis B Virus Variants

As indicated before, and discussed later, HBV uses a reverse transcription step in genomic replication. As a consequence of the poor proofreading ability of the HBV DNA polymerase

TABLE 248–1 ■ **Genome Length of Representative Members of the Hepadnaviridae Family**

AGENT	MINUS STRAND NUCLEOTIDE LENGTH
Human hepatitis B virus	3188
Woodchuck hepatitis virus	3320
Ground squirrel hepatitis virus	3311
Duck hepatitis B virus	3021

protein, mutations are common and lead to a number of HBV genetic variants (HBV mutants).[4] At least some of these variants may arise by escaping from the host immunologic response (e.g., the so-called vaccine-induced HBV escape mutant). Nucleotide sequence studies of HBV DNA clones have revealed that deletions and point mutations may occur in each of the open reading frames. Multiple mutations have been reported in patients with chronic HBV infection. Statistical analysis indicates an increasing frequency of mutations from gene S (the lowest) to gene C, to gene P, to region X, to the precore (pre-C) region, and finally to the pre-S2/pre-S1 regions.[5] A number of these variants appear to differ in their biologic behavior compared with wild-type HBV; however, their role in the biology and natural history of HBV infection remains incompletely understood.[4] Some of the variants have been associated with increased pathogenicity (e.g., the precore mutant), whereas others may have lower pathogenicity (e.g., the X deletion mutants). Some may be associated with reduced replication; a number of variants have been described in hepatitis B surface antigen (HBsAg)–negative infections and in infections in which all conventionally measured markers of HBV infection are absent.[6] In one striking example, in which none of the usual markers of HBV infection was present, sequencing of amplified serum HBV DNA revealed a T to C mutation of DR2 and an 8-nucleotide deletion of the 3′ terminal end of the X gene.[7] These alterations result in the generation of a C-terminally truncated X protein and damage to the enhancer II–core promoter complex. Because DR2 has been implicated in the initiation of HBV DNA replication and because the X gene product is believed to transactivate the HBV enhancer and core promoter that regulates transcription of surface, core, and precore genes, it is not surprising that HBV replication is suppressed and expression of HBV gene products is reduced. In Table 248–2, some of the more commonly detected variants are listed.

Structure

HBV is a double-shelled, spherical particle, 42 nm in diameter, composed of a 27-nm-diameter, spherical, icosahedral nucleocapsid core and a surrounding envelope 7 nm in width.[8] HBV is associated with three particles that are readily visualized by electron microscopy of the serum of HBV-infected persons (see Fig. 248–1). These include the complete 42-nm HBV particle, smaller spherical particles about 22 nm (range of 15 to 25 nm) in diameter, and tubular particles with an average width of about 22 nm and a variable length of up to 200 nm. The small spherical and tubular particles are present in quantities far in excess of the 42-nm HBV particles. The 22-nm spherical and tubular particles are composed of the proteins, carbohydrate, and lipid of the envelope (surface or coat) of HBV but lack DNA or RNA transcripts and DNA polymerase activity. HBV infectivity can be destroyed by heating up to 98°C and by exposure to chemical agents such as glutaraldehyde. Even low-level quaternary ammonium germicides may be effective.[9]

TABLE 248–2 ■ Hepatitis B Virus Variants

Precore mutation at codon 28
Core deletion
Core point mutation at codons 48–60, 84–101, 147–155
Core promoter mutation
Encapsidation mutant
S point mutation at codons 145, 126, 131, 132
S deletion
Pre-S1/2 junction deletion
Pre-S1 deletion
Pre-S2/S promoter deletion
X deletion
Truncated X
Polymerase region mutation

TABLE 248–3 ■ Hepatitis B Virus Open Reading Frames, Gene Products, and Amino Acid Residues of Identified Proteins

OPEN READING FRAME	GENE PRODUCT	AMINO ACID RESIDUES OF IDENTIFIED PROTEIN
Pre-S1, pre-S2, S	Large HBsAg protein	400
Pre-S2, S	Middle HBsAg protein	281
S	Major HBsAg protein	226
Pre-C, C	HBeAg	189
C	HBcAg	212
P	DNA polymerase	844
X	HBxAg	154

ENVELOPE

The principal protein and antigenic material of the HBV envelope is the major protein of HBsAg, encoded by the S open reading frame of HBV DNA. The major HBsAg protein is composed of 226 amino acids. A group-specific determinant, labeled a, and a set of subtype determinants, labeled d and y and w and r, are also encoded by the S open reading frame and are present on the major HBsAg protein. The a determinant has been found in all HBV isolates and elicits protective immunity against infection by all HBV serotypes except in the rare case of the vaccine-induced escape mutant.[10] In addition to the major HBsAg protein, two other proteins, namely, the middle protein, encoded by the pre-S2 region and S open reading frame, and the large protein, encoded by pre-S1, pre-S2, and S, are expressed on the envelope of the HBV particle (Table 248–3). The large protein is present on the 22-nm spherical and tubular particles in a much smaller proportion than on the HBV particle. The major, middle, and large HBsAg proteins are present in both glycosylated and nonglycosylated forms. Interactions among the three HBsAg proteins appear to affect the biosynthesis, processing, and transport of the proteins. In addition to the glycosylated proteins, other carbohydrate components of the envelope may be present. Approximately one third of the content of the 22-nm particles appears to be host-derived lipid.

NUCLEOCAPSID (CORE)

The nucleocapsid consists of about 180 repeating subunits of its core protein, which contains C-terminal packaging signals and nuclear localization signals. Nucleocapsid particles can be released from intact HBV particles by treatment with nonionic detergents, which strip away the envelope, exposing free core particles and their associated antigens. The HBV nucleocapsid contains the circular DNA, a covalently attached primer protein, HBV DNA polymerase and reverse transcriptase activity, and protein kinase activity. The last serves to phosphorylate the core-associated proteins. The core protein expresses a major antigenic reactivity, the hepatitis B core antigen (HBcAg). HBcAg has been localized either to the surface or to internal locations of the core particle.[11] A related antigenic reactivity known as the hepatitis B e antigen (HBeAg) has also been characterized. It is a nonparticulate, soluble antigen derived from HBcAg by proteolytic self-cleavage and released into the circulation from infected hepatocytes. Whereas the presence of HBeAg in blood is generally correlated with active HBV replication, certain mutations in the precore and core region result in a replicating HBV variant in which HBeAg is not expressed.[12] The function of HBeAg in the life cycle of HBV remains incompletely understood. It may be an important target in the immune clearance of the virus and may also play a role in the in utero induction of T-lymphocyte tolerance.[13]

Genomic Structure of Hepatitis B Virus

OPEN READING FRAMES

The long, minus DNA strand of HBV is organized into four open reading frames: S, C, X, and P (Fig. 248–2). Two of these, S and C, have associated upstream regions termed pre-S and pre-C, respectively. The open reading frames, their gene products, and the amino acid residues of the products are listed in Table 248–3. The S open reading frame codes for the major HBsAg protein, containing 226 amino acids. The upstream pre-S2 region and the S open reading frame encode the middle-sized HBsAg protein; the pre-S1, pre-S2, and S encode the large HBsAg protein.

The pre-C region (containing a signal sequence) and the C open reading frame serve to specify the HBeAg; the C open reading frame encodes the HBcAg protein. Derived from a precursor protein (the precore protein) that harbors sequences essential for its secretion,[14] HBeAg contains an additional 10 amino acid residues at its N-terminal end but is truncated by about 35 amino acids at its C-terminal end. Mutations in the pre-C region abort translation of the HBeAg precursor, and mutations in the core promoter affect transcription of the HBeAg coding region. In both cases, HBV infections occur without detectable HBeAg.[12]

The longest open reading frame of the HBV genome is the P (pol or polymerase) open reading frame, which overlaps the others. P specifies the polypeptide with HBV DNA polymerase, reverse transcriptase, and ribonuclease H (RNase H) activities and at its N-terminal end contains the protein required for replication and packaging. Current information suggests that the reverse transcriptase activity is primed by a tyrosine residue within the N-terminal domain of the polypeptide.[15]

The X open reading frame encodes the X proteins (a full-length and shorter forms), which serve as transcriptional transactivators, enhancing the transcription and replication of HBV and other viruses. The mechanism by which the X proteins activate transcription is not understood. Limited available evidence suggests that the X protein is not necessary for the posttranscriptional phases of the processing of HBV DNA or HBV assembly into particles.

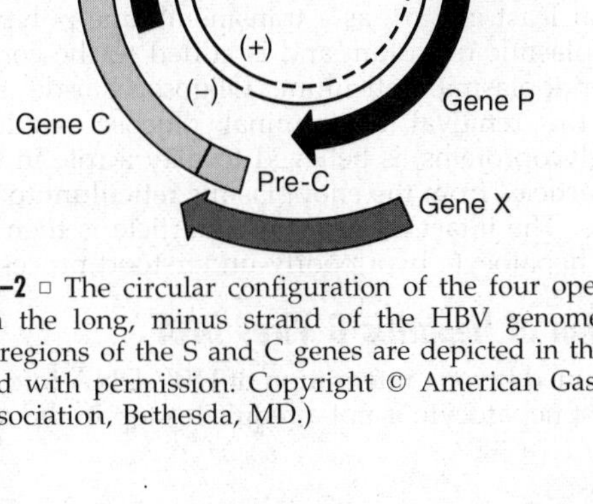

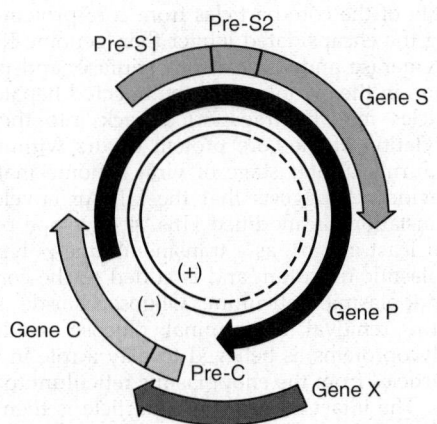

FIGURE 248–2 ▫ The circular configuration of the four open reading frames on the long, minus strand of the HBV genome and the upstream regions of the S and C genes are depicted in this illustration. (Used with permission. Copyright © American Gastroenterological Association, Bethesda, MD.)

PROMOTERS AND ENHANCERS

At least five promoters and two enhancer elements have been recognized on the DNA strand of the HBV genome.[16] Two separate promoters, the pre-S1 promoter and the S promoter, are used to code for the three HBsAg proteins. The pre-S1 produces a single transcript that codes for the large HBsAg, whereas the S promoter produces a number of transcripts that code for the middle and major HBsAg proteins. The third promoter, the core promoter, is associated with the open reading frame of HBcAg and codes for the 3.5-kb transcript that yields the core protein, serves as the template for translation of the polymerase protein, and serves as the pregenomic RNA from which HBV DNA is reverse transcribed. The fourth and fifth promoters are associated with the X open reading frame and give rise to transcripts that code for the full-length and shorter X proteins.[17] Binding sites for a number of transcription factors have been identified within the HBV promoters.[18] Two enhancer elements, enhancer I and enhancer II, which stimulate the transcriptional activity of the promoters, have also been identified. The enhancer I element is governed by cooperative interactions between enhancer binding proteins (e.g., nuclear receptors and liver-specific factors) and can up-regulate each of the promoters. The enhancer II element is also capable of binding with cellular factors. In addition, a glucocorticosteroid response element has been identified in the S open reading frame; it may increase expression of HBsAg in the presence of glucocorticoids. Other presently unidentified elements may also regulate the activity of HBV enhancers and promoters.

Replication in Vitro

Initial attempts to grow HBV in cell culture failed or yielded equivocal results. The hepatotropism displayed by HBV suggested that hepatocytes might prove more susceptible to in vitro infection than nonhepatic cells or tissue cultures derived from other cells. The demonstration that duck hepatitis B virus could be propagated in primary cultures of duck hepatocytes spurred further study of HBV replication in vitro. Several laboratories demonstrated that cloned, tandemly repeated multimers of HBV DNA could be used to transfect human hepatocellular carcinoma or hepatoblastoma cell lines. These transfected cell lines secreted HBsAg, HBeAg, HBV DNA polymerase activity, and HBV DNA associated with virus-like particles with the physical characteristics of HBV. The tandem nature of the DNA inserts permits the production of the 2.2-kb and 3.5-kb RNA replicative intermediates of HBV. The HBV produced by transfected cell lines has been shown to be capable of causing acute HBV infection in chimpanzees. Primary adult and fetal human hepatocytes have also been shown to support HBV infection and replication, but only a proportion of these cells are susceptible and they gradually lose their susceptibility over time.[19]

The tropism of HBV is not strictly restricted to the hepatocyte (see later) because infection in vivo has been demonstrated in extrahepatic sites. Suspension cultures of human bone marrow cells have been infected by HBV; both progenitor and stromal cells support HBV replication.[20] Unfortunately, none of the hepatocyte, hepatocyte-derived, or bone marrow cell tissue culture systems studied to date has permitted consistently high levels of HBV replication. In addition to mammalian cells, the HBV genome has been cloned in a variety of vectors, including bacterial and yeast cells.

Replication in Vivo

TARGETING TO HEPATOCYTES

The initiating events of HBV infection are poorly understood. HBV attachment to a specific receptor on the hepatocyte membrane has been postulated to involve binding affinity sites on the pre-S1 and pre-S2 proteins of the HBV envelope, but the nature of the receptor remains speculative. A number of proteins have been suggested as hepatocyte receptor candidates, but none has been identified as the responsible receptor. The demonstration of HBsAg binding by apolipoprotein H, a component of circulating lipoproteins, suggested a possible interaction between lipoprotein particles, HBsAg, and hepatocyte uptake of HBV.[21] However, apolipoprotein H appears to bind to the lipid rather than protein components of HBsAg[22]; its role in HBV uptake remains intriguing but uncertain. Regardless of the exact mechanism of attachment, after adsorption or penetration of the hepatocyte membrane, HBV DNA is transferred to the cell nucleus in an open, relaxed, circular form. Under conditions that have yet to be established, further processing of HBV DNA may be inhibited, and the infection remains latent. In such latent infections, extrachromosomal full-length, double-stranded, relaxed circular HBV DNA has been identified in hepatocyte nuclei without evidence of virus replication or the production of viral gene products. Most infections are not latent, however, and lead to HBV replication. Although integration of subgenomic fragments of HBV DNA or the intact HBV genome into the host genome of some hepatocytes may occur during HBV infection, integration of HBV DNA is not a required step in the replicative cycle of HBV (see the later section on HBV DNA integration).

SITE OF REPLICATION

The liver appears to be the major target organ of HBV infection and the principal but not the only site of HBV replication. Other hepadnaviruses have been shown to be capable of replication in extrahepatic tissues. Replication of duck hepatitis B virus in duckling liver in vivo is followed by replication in the pancreas, kidneys, and spleen. Peripheral blood lymphocytes of woodchuck hepatitis virus–infected woodchucks contain woodchuck hepatitis virus DNA in an episomal, nonreplicative state, which on appropriate stimulation can initiate woodchuck hepatitis virus replication. This suggests that extrahepatic tissues may serve as a reservoir of latent hepadnavirus infection and as a site for viral reactivation and amplification.

The presence of HBV DNA, HBV RNA, HBV replicative intermediates, and HBV proteins has now been described in a large number of extrahepatic organs and in a variety of cell types of individuals with chronic HBV infection[23] (Table 248–4). It is noteworthy that active replication of HBV and gene expression in these cells are not associated with injury or inflammation.[23] The precise importance of extrahepatic replication of HBV remains uncertain. Although it seems likely that these sites contribute in a limited manner to the large viral burden of infected individuals, they may play a role in some of the extrahepatic syndromes associated with HBV infection, in HBV reactivation, and in HBV recurrence after liver transplantation for chronic hepatitis B.

TABLE 248–4 ■ Hepatitis B Virus Replication-Competent Tissues and Cell Types

TISSUES	CELL TYPES
Liver	Hepatocytes, Kupffer cells, endothelial cells
Blood	Mononuclear cells/monocytes/lymphocytes
Spleen	Macrophage/monocyte, endothelial cells
Lymph node	Macrophage/monocyte, endothelial cells
Periadrenal ganglion	Neuronal cells, sustentacular cells
Skin	Basal keratinocytes, dermal stromal fibroblasts
Intestine	Mucosal endothelial cells, stromal fibroblasts, endothelial cells
Pancreas	Acinar cells, endothelial cells
Kidney	Endothelial cells
Bone marrow	Progenitor cells, stromal cells
Testes	Intertubular stromal fibroblasts

Adapted from Mason A, Wick M, White H, et al: Hepatitis B virus replication in diverse cell types during chronic hepatitis B virus infection. Hepatology 18:781–789, 1993.

MECHANISM

In the hepatocyte nucleus, the relaxed, circular HBV DNA is converted to a covalently closed circular DNA by repair of the positive DNA strand. This fully double-stranded DNA serves as a template for the synthesis of a series of RNA transcripts that include a longer than genome RNA and smaller RNA transcripts.[24] The longer than genome RNA (often termed pregenomic RNA), with about 3500 nucleotides, will serve as a template for reverse transcription, leading to production of full-length (about 3200 nucleotides), minus DNA strands of HBV.[25] The longer than genome RNA transcript and the HBV DNA polymerase and reverse transcriptase are encapsidated in core particles; it is within these particles within the cytoplasm of the cell that the minus DNA strand is produced by reverse transcription. Simultaneously, the RNA template is degraded. The structural and nonstructural viral proteins are translated from the smaller RNA transcripts, which vary in size from 700 to 2400 nucleotides. In contrast to reverse transcription of the long strand, the short positive-sense strands, which vary between 1700 and 2800 nucleotides in length, are believed to be generated from templates of negative-stranded DNA.

In addition to HBV DNA and HBV-specific RNA, superhelical, closed circular duplex DNA and incomplete HBV DNA forms comprising protein-linked minus strands, with or without plus strands, may be detected in infected hepatocytes. Incomplete HBV DNA forms and similarly identified HBV RNA-DNA hybrids are also considered intermediates in the biosynthesis of the HBV.

Assembly of the core particles from core protein subunits, containing the encapsidated longer than genome RNA, HBV DNA polymerase and reverse transcriptase, and protein kinase, occurs in the cytoplasm of the infected hepatocyte, but core particles may be transported back into the nucleus. Phosphorylation of the core protein occurs within the core particles during a later stage of viral genome maturation.[26] Current evidence suggests that the HBsAg envelope, with its posttranslationally modified HBsAg envelope proteins, is formed, at least in part, as a transmembrane polypeptide of the endoplasmic reticulum and is added to the core particle in the endoplasmic reticulum. Oligosaccharide trimming, namely, the removal of terminal glucose residues from HBsAg glycoproteins, is believed to play a role in the transport of particles from the endoplasmic reticulum to the Golgi apparatus. The intact nascent HBV particle is then exported from the hepatocyte by a poorly understood process.

Integration of Hepatitis B Virus DNA

As mentioned before, integration of HBV DNA into the DNA of the host hepatocyte is not a requisite step in the replicative cycle. Nonetheless, integration may occur randomly throughout the early phases of HBV infection. HBV DNA integrations are usually subgenomic. Hepatocytes with integrated HBV genomic fragments may express the gene products of the integrated genomic material but do not support genomic replication. The mechanisms subserving and controlling HBV DNA integration and the proportion of affected hepatocytes have yet to be established. Presumably, nearly all hepatocytes in which integration occurs are destroyed during the immune attack on infected cells. Those hepatocytes that survive may undergo clonal expansion, and some may be transformed into the malignant cells of hepatocellular carcinoma. The mechanisms by which HBV DNA integration leads to tumor development remain a subject of great interest. A direct transforming effect has been postulated that attributes transformation to the presence of chromosome abnormalities (deletions, duplications, and translocations) at the sites of HBV DNA integration. HBV DNA sequences, isolated from individual hepatocellular carcinomas, have been localized to a number of different chromosomes and translocation sites. A transforming effect has also been attributed to insertional mutagenesis as a consequence of HBV genomic integration into the cyclin A gene, the epidermal growth factor genes, the retinoic acid receptor gene, and the mevalonate kinase gene.[27] Activation of cellular oncogenes by adjacent HBV fragments has been implicated, but available evidence for this mechanism is limited. Finally, there is support for the notion that the production of the X protein by integrated genomic fractions containing the X open reading frame may play a key role in hepatocarcinogenesis.[27, 28]

Hepatitis D Virus

History

The existence of the hepatitis D (delta) virus (HDV) as an agent of viral hepatitis has been recognized only since 1977.[29] A link between HDV and HBV infections was apparent from the outset: the HDV antigen was initially detected in the liver of patients with chronic HBV infection. HDV is a defective, transmissible, RNA-containing satellite virus of HBV. It requires the helper or rescue function of HBV or other hepadnaviruses for its expression, assembly, and pathogenicity. Nonetheless, HDV replication may occur in the absence of hepadnavirus infection.[30] HDV appears to interfere with the synthesis of the helper HBV in most if not all dual HDV-HBV infections. HDV is not thought to be directly cytopathic.

Interaction of Hepatitis D and B Viruses

HDV infection is limited to persons who are infected by HBV: either HBV carriers superinfected with HDV or those who simultaneously contract primary infections with HBV and HDV, a circumstance termed coinfection. In the former case, the HBV of the persistently infected host serves the helper functions required by HDV. In coinfections, the helper functions are assumed by the infecting HBV accompanying HDV. Superimposition of HDV on chronic HBV infection often leads to chronic HDV infection. In contrast, because HDV infection cannot outlive infection with HBV, and because more than 95% of acute HBV infections in adults resolve, HDV infection and expression tend to be self-limited during coinfection with HBV.

Replicative Interactions

HDV invariably acquires by transcapsidation the HBsAg subtype of its host in superinfections or the HBsAg subtype of its accompanying HBV in coinfections. The HBsAg and pre-S proteins serve to encapsidate the newly synthesized HDV. Coincident with this process, the synthesis of preexisting HBV gene products (HBsAg and HBeAg) is diminished, and HBV replication may be transiently inhibited in most patients with HDV superinfections.[31, 32] In a few instances, HBsAg may be permanently lost; however, in some patients, presumably a minority, replication of HBV and HDV occurs concurrently without mutual inhibition.[32]

Morphology and Characteristics

HDV particles are 35 to 37 nm in diameter (Fig. 248–3) and are coated with HBsAg and small amounts of the pre-S proteins. The HBsAg and pre-S components of the coat material of HDV appear to be similar in composition to the small 22-nm HBsAg particles found in the circulation of HBV-infected persons, but the "large protein" is present in lower concentrations in HDV coat material. It has been suggested that HDV carries the pre-S HBV receptor in its coat material to attach to or exit from the plasma membrane of the hepatocyte. Electron microscopic examination of purified stable ribonucleoprotein complexes consisting of HDV antigen and HDV RNA has suggested the presence of a corelike structure with a diameter of about 19 nm.[33] Whether HDV has an internal core remains to be established.

The virus contains RNA and an antigenic nuclear phosphoprotein (HDV antigen) that binds RNA and exists in two isoforms, a 195–amino acid and a 214–amino acid protein.[34, 35] The open reading frame for the HDV antigen resides in antigenomic RNA (Fig. 248–4), but the editing necessary for the formation of the isoforms appears to occur posttranscriptionally in the genomic HDV RNA. The smaller HDV antigen transports RNA into the nucleus and is essential for HDV replication. The larger antigen is isoprenylated, a posttranslational change that enhances its inhibition of HDV RNA replication. The larger antigen also participates in the assembly of HDV particles. Both isoforms self-associate into multimers that are probably necessary for HDV assembly. Synthetic peptides that interfere with multimer formation have been described.[36]

RNA Genome

The RNA genome is single stranded, covalently closed, and circular, with slightly less than 1680 nucleotides.[34] It has structural and replicative similarities to certain infectious RNAs found in plants (see later), but its RNA is not homologous to the DNA of HBV. Genetic heterogeneity among HDV

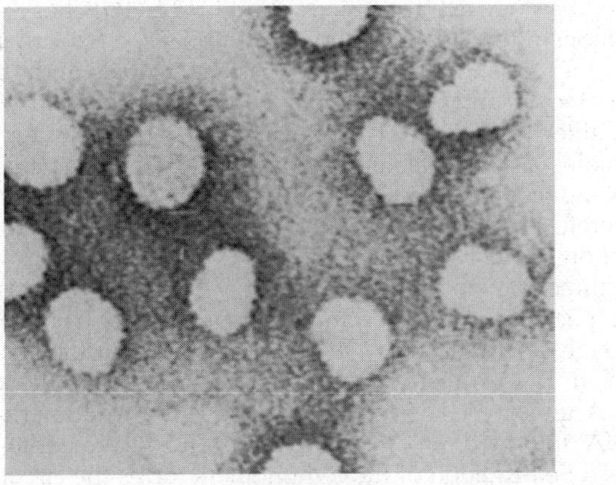

FIGURE 248–3 □ Electron micrograph of 35- to 37-nm HDV particles in serum.

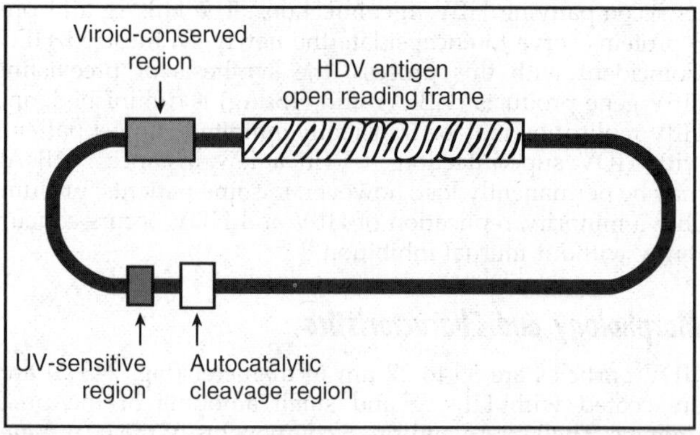

FIGURE 248–4 ▫ Schematic illustration of the HDV antigenome and identified regions. UV, Ultraviolet light. (Used with permission. Copyright © American Gastroenterological Association, Bethesda, MD.)

isolates is well known; at least three genotypes have been identified, but their relationship to disease persistence, severity, or outcome remains ill-defined. Despite its circular conformation, the RNA of HDV can form an unbranched rodlike structure by folding on itself through intramolecular base pairing, affecting 70% of the bases. A catalytic domain present on the genome is thought to represent a ribozyme that has a pseudoknot secondary structure[37] and that may also serve to stabilize downstream transcripts after polyadenylation.[38] The HDV antigenome (see Fig. 248–4) is a genome-complementary, circular RNA present in the infected hepatocyte and, to a lesser extent, in purified HDV particles. It contains, in addition to the open reading frame for HDV antigen, an autocatalytic cleavage region, a viroid-conserved region, and an ultraviolet light–sensitive region.

Classification

HDV is a highly unusual hepatitis agent with the smallest known and only circular RNA genome found in the animal viruses. HDV RNA has multiple features resembling those of viroid RNA (simple infectious RNAs), virusoids, and the RNAs of the circular plant satellite viruses. Hence, although it is still unclassified, the similarities to the plant satellite viruses are striking. Attempts to develop classification schemes that may encompass HDV within the known families of subviral satellite agents may eventually prove fruitful.

Mechanisms of Replication

HDV replication is presumed to occur in the hepatocyte only, because extrahepatic replication of HDV has yet to be demonstrated. HDV is thought to replicate efficiently in vivo, producing as many as 300,000 genomic copies in the average hepatocyte and as many as 2×10^{12} HDV particles per milliliter of serum. The precise mechanism of replication remains to be established; however, it is clear that HDV RNA does not encode an RNA-dependent RNA polymerase. Therefore, genomic replication is thought to involve the redirection of host RNA polymerase II. Although HBsAg is not required for the replication of HDV RNA, it is necessary for the packaging, release, and pathogenicity of HDV. HDV is thought to replicate by a "rolling circle" mechanism,[34, 35] in which RNA-directed RNA transcription from the circular RNA genome leads to the formation of a multimeric length RNA intermediate, which is then self-cleaved into monomers. Self-ligation of these monomers forms the circular antigenome, which through another cycle of the rolling circle mechanism produces nascent, progeny genomic RNA.

Variations in the folding of HDV RNA influence the rate of self-cleavage and may have important effects on the replication cycle.[39] The assembly of HDV particles appears to require interactions between HDV RNA and the HDV proteins and protein-protein interactions between HDV and HBsAg proteins.

Propagation

A variety of cell lines (primary chimpanzee or woodchuck hepatocytes, human hepatocellular carcinoma and fibrosarcoma cells) have been transfected with HDV complementary DNA constructs and express HDV RNA and HDV antigens. Expression of HDV complementary DNAs in transgenic mice does not appear to elicit a cytopathic effect.[40] Replication in vitro is not affected by treatment with interferon. HDV has been transmitted experimentally to chimpanzees infected with HBV[41]; more recently, HDV has been transmitted to the laboratory mouse, and evidence of replication has been reported in this model.[42]

References

1. Purcell RH: The discovery of the hepatitis viruses. Gastroenterology 104:955–963, 1993.
2. Miller RH, Robinson WS: Common evolutionary origin of hepatitis B virus and retroviruses. Proc Natl Acad Sci USA 83:2531–2535, 1986.
3. Duflot A, Mehrotra R, Yu S-Z, et al: Spectrum of liver disease and duck hepatitis B virus infection in a large series of Chinese ducks with hepatocellular carcinoma. Hepatology 21:1483–1491, 1995.
4. Feitelson MA: Biology of disease. Biology of hepatitis B virus variants. Lab Invest 71:324–349, 1994.
5. Lauder IJ, Lin H-J, Lau JYN, et al: The variability of the hepatitis B virus genome: Statistical analysis and biological implications. Mol Biol Evol 10:457–470, 1993.
6. Hou J, Karayiannis, Waters J, et al: A unique insertion in the S gene of surface antigen–negative hepatitis B virus Chinese carriers. Hepatology 21:273–278, 1995.
7. Uchida T, Shimojima M, Gotoh K, et al: "Silent" hepatitis B virus mutants are responsible for non-A, non-B, non-C, non-D, non-E hepatitis. Microbiol Immunol 38:281–285, 1994.
8. Tiollais P, Pourcel C, Dejean A: The hepatitis B virus. Nature 317:489–495, 1985.
9. Prince DL, Prince HN, Thraenhart O, et al: Methodological approaches to disinfection of human hepatitis B virus. J Clin Microbiol 31:3296–3304, 1993.
10. Carman WF, Zanetti AR, Karayiannis P, et al: Vaccine induced escape mutant of hepatitis B virus. Lancet 326:325–329, 1990.
11. Pushko P, Sallberg M, Borisova G, et al: Identification of hepatitis B virus core protein regions exposed or internalized at the surface of HBcAg particles by scanning with monoclonal antibodies. Virology 202:912–920, 1994.
12. Sato S, Suzuki K, Akahane Y, et al: Hepatitis B virus strains with mutations in the core promoter in patients with fulminant hepatitis. Ann Intern Med 122:241–248, 1995.
13. Milich DR, Jones JE, Hughes JL, et al: Is a function of the secreted hepatitis B e antigen to induce immunological tolerance in utero? Proc Natl Acad Sci USA 87:6599–6603, 1990.
14. Carlier D, Jean-Jean O, Fouillot N, et al: Importance of the C terminus of the hepatitis B virus precore protein in secretion of HBe antigen. J Gen Virol 76:1041–1045, 1995.
15. Zoulim F, Seeger C: Reverse transcription in hepatitis B virus is primed by a tyrosine residue of the polymerase. J Virol 68:6–13, 1994.
16. Yen TSB: Regulation of hepatitis B virus gene expression. Semin Virol 4:33–42, 1993.
17. Zheng Y-W, Riegler J, Wu J, et al: Novel short transcripts of hepatitis B virus X gene derived from intragenic promoter. J Biol Chem 269:22593–22598, 1994.
18. Raney AK, McLachlan A: Characterization of the hepatitis B

virus large surface antigen promoter Sp1 binding site. Virology 208:399–404, 1995.
19. Galle PR, Hagelstein J, Kommerell B, et al: In vitro experimental infection of primary human hepatocytes with hepatitis B virus. Gastroenterology 106:664–673, 1994.
20. Chai T, Prior S, Cooksley WGE, et al: Infection of human bone marrow stromal cells by hepatitis B virus: Implications for viral persistence and the suppression of hematopoiesis. J Infect Dis 169:871–874, 1994.
21. Mehdi H, Kaplan MJ, Anlar FY, et al: Hepatitis B virus surface antigen binds to apolipoprotein H. J Virol 68:2415–2424, 1994.
22. Neurath AR, Strick N: The putative cell receptors for hepatitis B virus (HBV), annexin V, and apolipoprotein H, bind to lipid components of HBV. Virology 204:475–477, 1994.
23. Mason A, Wick M, White H, et al: Hepatitis B virus replication in diverse cell types during chronic hepatitis B virus infection. Hepatology 18:781–789, 1993.
24. Ganem D, Varmus HE: The molecular biology of the hepatitis B virus. Annu Rev Biochem 56:651–693, 1987.
25. Lau JYN, Wright TL: Molecular virology and pathogenesis of hepatitis B. Lancet 342:1335–1340, 1993.
26. Kann M, Gerlich WH: Effect of core protein phosphorylation by protein kinase C on encapsidation of RNA within core particles of hepatitis B virus. J Virology 68:7993–8000, 1994.
27. Paterlini P, Poussin K, Kew M, et al: Selective accumulation of the X transcript of hepatitis B virus in patients negative for hepatitis B surface antigen with hepatocellular carcinoma. Hepatology 21:313–321, 1995.
28. Kim CM, Koike K, Saito I, et al: HBx gene of hepatitis B virus induces liver cancer in transgenic mice. Nature 351:317–320, 1991.
29. Rizzetto M, Canese MG, Arico S, et al: Immunofluorescence detection of new antigen-antibody system (delta/anti-delta) associated to hepatitis B virus in liver and serum of HBsAg carriers. Gut 18:997–1003, 1977.
30. Taylor J, Mason W, Summers J, et al: Replication of human hepatitis delta virus in primary cultures of woodchuck hepatocytes. J Virol 61:2891–2895, 1987.
31. Krogsgaard K, Aldershvile J, Kryger P, et al: Hepatitis B virus DNA, HBeAg and delta infection during the course from acute to chronic hepatitis B virus infection. Hepatology 5:778–782, 1985.
32. Bas C, Bartolome J, La Banda F, et al: Assessment of hepatitis B virus DNA levels in chronic HBsAg carriers with or without hepatitis delta virus superinfection. J Hepatol 6:208–213, 1988.
33. Ryu W-S, Netter HJ, Bayer M, Taylor J: Ribonucleoprotein complexes of hepatitis delta virus. J Virol 67:3281–3287, 1993.
34. Taylor JM: Genetic organization and replication strategy of hepatitis delta virus. Semin Virol 4:313–317, 1993.
35. Polish LB, Gallagher M, Fields HA, Hadler SC: Delta hepatitis: Molecular biology and clinical and epidemiological features. Clin Microbiol Rev 6:211–229, 1993.
36. Rozzelle JE Jr, Wang J-G, Wagner DS, et al: Self-association of a synthetic peptide from the N terminus of the hepatitis delta virus protein into an immunoreactive alpha-helical multimer. Proc Natl Acad Sci USA 92:382–386, 1995.
37. Kumar PKR, Taira K, Nishikawa S: Chemical probing studies of variants of the genomic hepatitis delta virus ribozyme by primer extension analysis. Biochemistry 33:583–592, 1994.
38. Tanner NK, Schaff S, Thill G, et al: A three-dimensional model of hepatitis delta virus ribozyme based on biochemical and mutational analyses. Curr Biol 4:488–498, 1994.
39. Gottlieb PA, Prasad Y, Smith JB, et al: Evidence that alternate foldings of the hepatitis delta RNA confer varying rates of self-cleavage. Biochemistry 33:2802–2808, 1994.
40. Guilhot S, Huang S-N, Xia YP, et al: Expression of the hepatitis delta virus large and small antigens in transgenic mice. J Virol 68:1052–1058, 1994.
41. Rizzetto M, Canese MG, Gerin JL, et al: Transmission of the hepatitis B virus–associated delta antigen to chimpanzees. J Infect Dis 141:590–602, 1980.
42. Netter HJ, Kajino K, Taylor JM: Experimental transmission of human hepatitis delta virus to the laboratory mouse. J Virol 67:3357–3362, 1993.

249

Poxviruses

Bernard Moss

The poxviruses constitute a large family of complex DNA viruses.[1, 2] Nine different poxviruses are associated with human disease, but only variola virus and molluscum contagiosum virus (MCV) are specific for humans (Table 249–1); the other infections are zoonoses.[3] The devastating effects of smallpox, caused by variola virus, and its successful eradication by immunization with vaccinia virus are recorded in detail.[4] Because variola virus appears to be absent from nature, the virus will be extinct when the planned destruction of laboratory stocks is implemented. Although vaccinia virus is no longer needed for routine smallpox vaccination, immunization of laboratory personnel working with large quantities of orthopoxviruses, including vaccinia virus itself, has been recommended.[5] In addition, vaccinia virus and avipoxviruses expressing genes of other pathogenic microorganisms are being tested as live recombinant vaccines.[6, 7]

Characteristics of Poxviruses

Classification

The infectious forms of poxviruses are large, complex, enveloped virions containing enzymes concerned with messenger RNA synthesis and a linear double-stranded DNA genome of 130 to 300 kilobase pairs.[1] Unlike other DNA viruses, poxviruses use the cytoplasmic compartment of the cell for transcription, replication, and assembly. The vertebrate poxviruses have been placed into eight genera: *Avipoxvirus*, *Capripoxvirus*, *Leporipoxvirus*, *Molluscipoxvirus*, *Orthopoxvirus*, *Parapoxvirus*, *Suipoxvirus*, and *Yatapoxvirus*.[2] Members of the same genus are antigenically related and have similar morphologies and host ranges. The genomes of vaccinia virus and variola virus are more than 90% identical.[8, 9]

TABLE 249–1 ■ Poxviruses That Cause Human Disease

GENUS	DISEASE	COMMON NAMES AND CHARACTERISTICS OF DISEASES
Orthopoxvirus	Variola	Smallpox; systemic; general rash; extinct
	Monkeypox	Systemic; general rash; rare zoonosis
	Vaccinia	Smallpox vaccine; local skin lesion
	Cowpox	Local skin lesion; rare zoonosis
Parapoxvirus	Orf	Local skin lesion; rare zoonosis
	Paravaccinia	Milker's nodules; rare zoonosis
Yatapoxvirus	Tanapox	Local skin lesion; rare zoonosis
	Yabapox	Local skin lesion; rare accidental infection
Molluscipoxvirus	Molluscum contagiosum	Multiple skin lesions; human transmission

Structure of the Virion

The infectious virus particles appear in electron microscopic images as oval or brick-shaped bodies between 200 and 400 nm long with a complex internal structure.[10–13] Vertebrate poxviruses have a characteristic biconcave core flanked by lateral bodies[14] (Fig. 249–1), although the latter appearance may be partly due to the method of sample preparation.[15] Intracellular mature virions (IMVs) have two closely opposed membranes now thought to be derived from cellular membranes of the intermediate compartment between the endoplasmic reticulum and the Golgi.[16] The extruded extracellular virions (EEVs) contain an additional membrane derived from the Golgi network.[17, 18] Both IMVs and EEVs are infectious.

Biochemical Components of the Virion

DNA is packaged within the virus core and consists of a linear duplex molecule with hairpin loops at each end.[19, 20] The nearly 200,000 base pair vaccinia virus genome is largely composed of unique sequences,[21] although there is a 10,000 base pair inverted terminal repetition[22, 23] within which are blocks of short tandem repeats as well as several genes.[24, 25] Most of the DNA is composed of closely spaced protein-coding regions separated by transcriptional regulatory sequences. The essential genes map within the conserved central region of the genome, whereas many that are dispensable for replication in tissue culture are nearer the ends.[26]

Proteins constitute 90% of the dry weight of vaccinia virions, and more than 100 polypeptides have been resolved by two-dimensional polyacrylamide gel electrophoresis.[27] In addition to structural proteins, more than a dozen enzymes are packaged in the virions.[28] Many of these, including a DNA-dependent RNA polymerase, capping and methylating enzymes, and poly(A) polymerase, are involved in messenger RNA synthesis. Nine polypeptides have been localized near the exterior of IMV particles and five associated with the membrane of EEVs.[1]

Lipids, mostly cholesterol and phospholipids, account for about 3% of the dry weight of vaccinia virus.[16, 29, 30] Other poxviruses, such as fowlpox virus, have much higher amounts of lipid including squalene and cholesterol esters.[31]

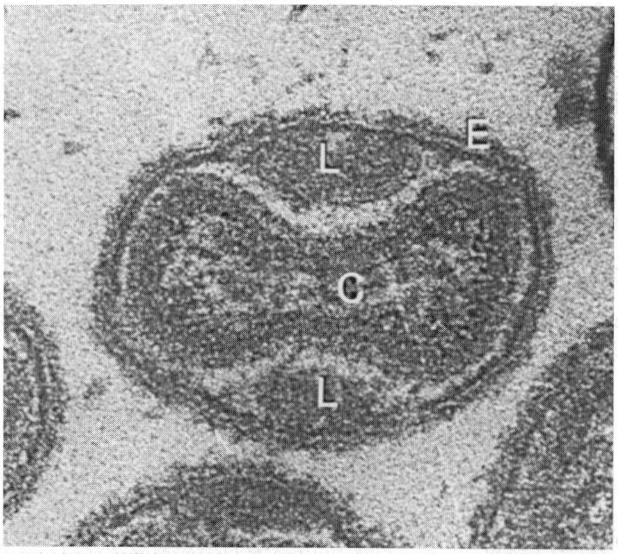

FIGURE 249–1 □ Electron micrograph of a thin-sectioned intracellular vaccinia virus particle. C, Core; L, lateral body; E, outer membrane. (From Pogo BGT, Dales S: Two deoxyribonuclease activities within purified vaccinia virus. Proc Natl Acad Sci USA 63:820–827, 1969.)

Virus Replication

Most of the detailed information regarding replication has been obtained with orthopoxviruses, especially vaccinia virus. Nevertheless, the main features are likely to be conserved among all members of the family.

Virus Entry

Both the IMVs and EEVs are infectious and enter cells primarily by pH-independent fusion with the cell membrane.[32–34] EEVs fuse with the plasma membrane at twice the rate of the IMVs[34] and penetrate cells more quickly.[35] The fusion process may be complex as EEVs have multiple membranes. Antibodies to several IMV proteins are neutralizing, suggesting that the latter are involved in cell attachment or penetration.[36–39] A proteolytic cleavage step may also be involved in penetration.[40] Another set of proteins may mediate the binding and fusion of the EEVs because an antibody that neutralized IMVs did not inhibit these steps.[34] The wide host range of vaccinia virus suggests that there is one common cellular receptor or multiple ones. A proposal that the epidermal growth factor receptor is an attachment site for vaccinia virus[41, 42] has been disputed.[43, 44]

Uncoating

The fusion of vaccinia virus with the plasma membrane and release of the core into the cytoplasm constitute the first stage of uncoating.[45] This step requires neither RNA nor protein synthesis. The second stage of uncoating, defined by the susceptibility of the genome to DNase, begins within 2 hours after infection and, unlike the first, is dependent on RNA and protein synthesis.[46]

Prereplicative Gene Expression

Expression of the poxvirus genome is regulated by a cascade mechanism that is divided into early, intermediate, and late phases[47] (Fig. 249–2). Regulation occurs primarily at the transcriptional level and early-, intermediate-, and late-stage genes have distinctive promoter sequences. Transcription of the early genes occurs on virus entry, coincident with the first stage of uncoating.[48, 49] RNA is synthesized, capped, and polyadenylylated by enzymes present in the virus core[50–52] and then translated on the cellular ribosomes. The DNA-dependent RNA polymerase is virus encoded[28, 53] but resembles its eukaryotic counterpart with regard to the large number and relative size of subunits. Sequence similarities indicate that the two largest subunits of poxvirus and eukaryotic RNA polymerases are homologous.[54, 55] An additional RNA polymerase–associated polypeptide, RAP94,[56] and a heterodimeric protein known as vaccinia virus early transcription factor[57–59] provide specificity for transcription of genes regulated by early promoters. This transcription factor binds to vaccinia virus early promoters, which are approximately 30 base pairs in length.[60] The sequence UUUUUNU, in which N can be any nucleotide, in the nascent RNA signals termination about 50 nucleotides downstream.[61, 62] The enzymes that cap,[63] methylate,[63, 64] and polyadenylylate[65] viral messenger RNAs are also virus encoded.[66–69] Some enzymes have multiple functions. For example, the capping enzyme also methylates the guanosine cap[63] and is a transcription termination factor.[70] A second RNA methyltransferase is also a subunit of the poly(A) polymerase.[69] The steps in initiation, elongation, and termination are under investigation.[71–73]

Postreplicative Gene Expression

Intermediate and late gene expressions occur after viral DNA replication. The intermediate and late messenger RNAs can

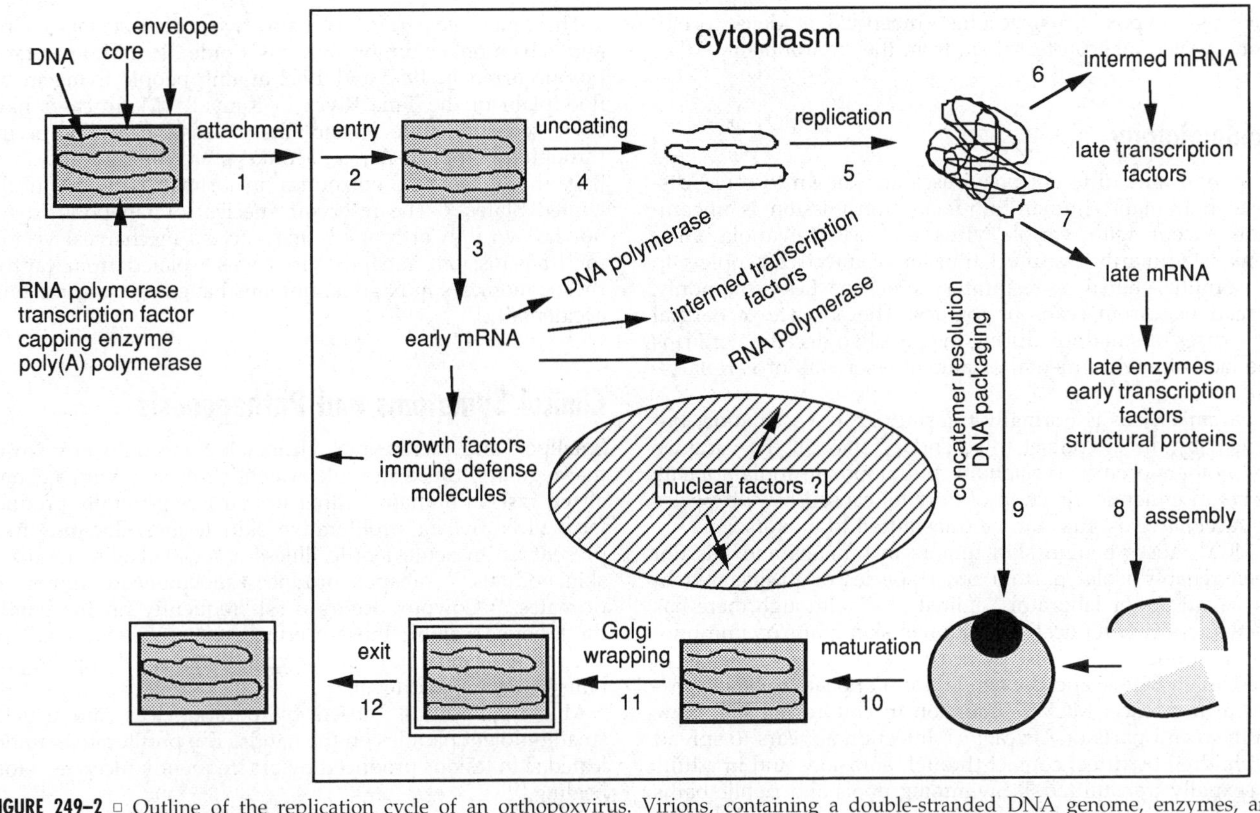

FIGURE 249–2 □ Outline of the replication cycle of an orthopoxvirus. Virions, containing a double-stranded DNA genome, enzymes, and transcription factors, attach to cells (1) and fuse with the cell membrane, releasing cores into the cytoplasm (2). The cores synthesize early messenger RNAs that are translated into a variety of proteins including growth factors, immune defense molecules, enzymes, and factors for DNA replication and intermediate transcription (3). Uncoating occurs (4), and the DNA is replicated to form concatemeric molecules (5). Intermediate genes in the progeny DNA are transcribed and the messenger RNAs are translated to form late transcription factors (6). The late genes are transcribed and the messenger RNAs are translated to form virion structural proteins, enzymes, and early transcription factors (7). Assembly begins with the formation of discrete membrane structures (8). The concatemeric DNA intermediates are resolved into unit genomes and packaged in immature virions (9). Maturation proceeds to the formation of infectious intracellular mature virions (10). The virions are wrapped by modified Golgi membranes and transported to the periphery of the cell (11). Fusion of the wrapped virions with the plasma membrane results in release of extracellular enveloped virus (12). Although replication occurs entirely in the cytoplasm, nuclear factors may be involved in transcription and assembly. (From Moss B: Poxviridae: The viruses and their replication. *In* Fields BN, Knipe DM, Howley PM [eds]: Fields Virology, ed 3. Philadelphia, Lippincott-Raven, 1996, pp 2637–2671.)

be distinguished from the majority of early messenger RNAs by their heterogeneous length and presence of a 5′ capped poly(A) leader of unknown function.[74–77] The enzymes and factors needed for intermediate transcription are synthesized early after infection.[78,79] At least three virus-encoded proteins, namely, RNA polymerase, capping enzyme, and an intermediate transcription factor,[80–83] are required for transcription of intermediate genes. The promoters recognized by the intermediate factors are similar in length but differ in sequence from early promoters.[84,85]

Three intermediate genes encode transcriptional transactivators of late genes.[79] At least two of these intermediate-stage proteins and one additional protein present in cells early in infection are required for transcription in vitro.[86–89] Late promoters differ in sequence from both early and intermediate promoters.[90] However, both intermediate and late promoters have an AAA at the transcriptional start site, which accounts for the generation of a novel 5′ poly(A) leader by slippage of the RNA polymerase.[91] The AAA sequence is occasionally found at the initiation site of early genes and then also leads to formation of a poly(A) leader.[92,93] The early transcription termination signal is not recognized during transcription of either intermediate or late genes, resulting in transcripts of heterogeneous length. However, the ends of some late transcripts are formed by cleavage.[94]

DNA Replication

Poxvirus DNA is replicated in the cytoplasm by a virus-encoded polymerase.[95,96] Concatemeric DNA structures are formed[97,98] and resolved into unit-size genomes by a site-specific mechanism[99,100] that requires one or more late viral proteins.[101,102]

Virus Assembly

Electron microscopic images suggest a sequence of developmental events (see Fig. 249–2) that begins in circumscribed granular regions of the cytoplasm with the formation of spicule-covered convex membranes within which a dense nucleoprotein mass forms and undergoes internal differentiation.[16,103,104] The resulting IMVs, although infectious, can be efficiently released only by cell lysis. As the IMVs move out of the assembly areas, some appear to be enveloped by Golgi membranes[17,18] and transported via actin filaments to the cell periphery, where budding through the plasma membrane may occur.[105–107] Many of the EEVs remain associated with the cell membrane and have been called cell-associated virions.[108] Cell-associated virions mediate cell-to-cell spread, whereas the released EEVs may be important for longer range virus spread within the host.[109] The virions of certain poxviruses, such as cowpox virus, become embedded in dense occlusions, which may protect them from the environment.[110, 111]

Epidemiology

Although nine different poxviruses are known to cause disease in humans, human-to-human transmission is uncommon except with variola virus and MCV. Variola virus spreads primarily by direct transfer of infective droplets to the oropharyngeal or respiratory mucosa.[4] Less commonly, spread was from scabs or fomites. The absence of natural new cases of smallpox during the past two decades confirms the lack of environmental or animal reservoirs of variola virus.

Vaccinia virus is normally transmitted by vaccination, but spread by direct contact to secondary sites on the vaccinee or to others occurs occasionally. Buffalopox in India appears to be an endemic infection of buffalo, caused by subspecies of vaccinia virus, that can be transmitted to milkers.[112]

MCV causes benign skin tumors in humans and has not been reliably isolated from other species or propagated in tissue culture or laboratory animals,[113, 114] although there has been a report of replication in human skin grafts on immunodeficient mice.[115] The disease occurs worldwide, including in the United States, and the genital form appears to be increasing in incidence. MCV is common in children of Fiji, New Guinea, and parts of Africa.[116, 117] Infection appears to spread in children by direct contact through abrasions and in adults is sexually transmitted.[118] Swimming pools and public baths have been implicated in Western countries. Analysis of the DNA by restriction endonuclease analysis indicated two major and at least one minor clinically indistinguishable variants.[119–124] Type I is more common than type II in the United Kingdom, Germany, Australia, Hong Kong, and Japan, although the ratios vary. MVC infections are common in patients with acquired immunodeficiency syndrome, and type II MCV infection may be proportionately higher than in the general population.[125] A molluscum contagiosum–like disease has been described in horses but has not been well characterized.[126, 127]

During the smallpox eradication campaign, a disease resembling smallpox was discovered in tropical rainforest areas of central and western Africa.[128] Between 1970 and 1986, 404 human cases were reported from seven countries. The disease is caused by monkeypox virus, which has been isolated from chimpanzees and several species of monkeys and squirrels. Squirrels are considered the most important reservoir. Human infections occur sporadically and affect mainly children in small remote villages whose population has frequent wild animal contacts. Usually, single cases occur but the virus can be transmitted with low frequency from human to human. Because smallpox vaccination provided protection against monkeypox, the incidence and duration of this disease could now increase. Offsetting this, however, are changes in dietary habits and customs that may lessen contacts with wild animals. DNA analyses suggest that there are geographically separated variants of monkeypox.[129, 130]

Although the traditional mode of human cowpox infection was milking of cows, bovine cowpox is uncommon. Cowpox virus has been isolated from cats and zoo animals, but rodents are thought to be the principal reservoir in Europe and Asia.[131, 132] Domestic cats are frequently implicated in human transmission.[133, 134]

Parapoxviruses infect domesticated animals including sheep, goats, cattle, and camels; humans are infected through skin abrasions. The disease acquired from sheep or goats is called orf and that from cows is called milker's nodules, paravaccinia, or pseudocowpox.[135–137]

The genus *Yatapoxvirus* contains two species: tanapox virus and Yaba monkey tumor poxvirus. Epidemics of human tanapox occurred in 1957 and 1962 among people living in the floodplain of the Tana River in Kenya.[138] Many cases have been seen in Zaire,[139] and the disease probably occurs throughout tropical Africa. Monkeys are infected and there have been tanapox epizootics in primate centers in the United States.[140] The reservoir species for tanapox virus is not known, but arthropods may act as mechanical vectors for transmission. Yabapox virus was isolated from captive rhesus monkeys in Nigeria; humans have been infected only accidentally.[141]

Clinical Symptoms and Pathogenesis

Smallpox and monkeypox viruses are the only poxviruses that regularly cause an acute systemic infection with a generalized rash in humans.[4] Other poxviruses generally produce local ulcerative or proliferative skin lesions. Tanapox may present as an acute febrile illness associated with localized skin nodules.[139] Yabapox produces subcutaneous tumors in primates.[142] Cowpox occurs most frequently on the hands; the lesions resemble those produced by a primary smallpox vaccination and may be accompanied by lymphangitis, lymphadenitis, and fever.[143]

Milker's nodules, caused by parapoxvirus, are usually small indolent papules on the hands. The proliferative umbilicated skin lesions produced by orf frequently ulcerate before healing.[144]

In molluscum contagiosum, firm, raised, flesh-colored nodules about 2 to 5 mm in diameter may occur singly or in clusters.[145] The lesions may occur anywhere on the body, but infrequently on the hands or soles, and may persist for months and years with little inflammatory reaction. The virus grows only in the epidermis, and no systemic spread occurs even when there is an immunodeficiency.

Poxviruses encode many proteins that influence virus pathogenicity.[146–151] These include growth factors and immune defense molecules including inhibitors of complement, interferons, interleukin-1, and tumor necrosis factor. The importance of cell-mediated immunity in the control of orthopoxvirus infection in humans was demonstrated by the progressive spread of vaccinia virus in infants and children who suffered from such deficiencies.[152, 153] By contrast, children with specific defects in antibody production usually reacted normally to vaccination.

Diagnosis

Poxvirus infection is usually suggested by the characteristic proliferative or ulcerative skin lesions and clinical history. Confirmation can be obtained by biopsy, electron microscopy of negatively stained material from scabs or vesicular fluid, detection of viral antigen, or virus isolation except in the case of MCV. Differentiation between poxviruses is made on the basis of biologic properties, specific serologic tests, or DNA analysis.[154–159]

Prevention and Treatment

Variola virus was eradicated by active immunization with live vaccinia virus.[4] Laboratory studies indicated that inactivated virus failed to elicit antibodies that neutralized enveloped virions, did not induce cytotoxic T cells, and gave lower levels of protection.[160, 161] Inactivated vaccines were not used for prevention of smallpox. Vaccinia immune globulin, however, provided protection when given during the incubation period and was beneficial for the treatment of vaccine complications. Methisazone (*N*-methylisatin β-thiosemicarbazone) was not effective in treating smallpox but probably had a beneficial effect when given prophylactically.[4]

References

1. Moss B: Poxviridae: The viruses and their replication. *In* Fields BN, Knipe DM, Howley PM (eds): Fields Virology, ed 3. Philadelphia, Lippincott-Raven, 1996, pp 2637–2671.
2. Murphy FA, Fauquet CM, Bishop DHL, et al: Virus taxonomy. Classification and nomenclature of viruses. Arch Virol Suppl 10:1, 1995.
3. Fenner F: Poxviruses. *In* Fields BN, Knipe DM, Howley PM (eds): Fields Virology, ed 3. Philadelphia, Lippincott-Raven, 1996, pp 2673–2702.
4. Fenner F, Henderson DA, Arita I, et al (eds): Smallpox and Its Eradication. Geneva, World Health Organization, 1988.
5. Richardson JH, Barkley WE (eds): Biosafety in Microbiological and Biomedical Laboratories. Washington, DC, US Department of Health and Human Services, 1984.
6. Moss B: Vaccinia virus: A tool for research and vaccine development. Science 252:1662, 1991.
7. Cox WI, Tartaglia J, Paoletti E: Poxvirus recombinants as live vaccines. *In* Binns MM, Smith GL (eds): Recombinant Poxviruses. Boca Raton, FL, CRC Press, 1992, pp 123–162.
8. Shchelkunov SN, Resenchuk SM, Totmenin AV, et al: Comparison of the genetic maps of variola and vaccinia viruses. FEBS Lett 327:321, 1993.
9. Massung RF, Liu L-I, Qi J, et al: Analysis of the complete genome of smallpox variola major virus strain Bangladesh-1975. Virology 201:215, 1994.
10. Peters D: Morphology of resting vaccinia virus. Nature 178:1453, 1956.
11. Nagington J, Horne RW: Morphological studies of orf and vaccinia viruses. Virology 16:248, 1962.
12. Westwood JCN, Harris WJ, Zwartouw HT, et al: Studies on the structure of vaccinia virus. J Gen Microbiol 34:67, 1964.
13. Easterbrook KB: Controlled degradation of vaccinia virions in vitro: An electron microscopic study. J Ultrastruct Res 14:484, 1966.
14. Pogo BGT, Dales S: Two deoxyribonuclease activities within purified vaccinia virus. Proc Natl Acad Sci USA 63:820, 1969.
15. Dubochet J, Adrian M, Richter K, et al: Structure of intracellular mature vaccine virus observed by cryoelectron microscopy. J Virol 68:1935, 1994.
16. Sodeik B, Doms RW, Ericsson M, et al: Assembly of vaccinia virus: Role of the intermediate compartment between the endoplasmic reticulum and the Golgi stacks. J Cell Biol 121:521, 1993.
17. Hiller G, Weber K: Golgi-derived membranes that contain an acylated viral polypeptide are used for vaccinia virus envelopment. J Virol 55:651, 1985.
18. Schmelz M, Sodeik B, Ericsson M, et al: Assembly of vaccinia virus: The second wrapping cisterna is derived from the trans Golgi network. J Virol 68:130, 1994.
19. Geshelin P, Berns KI: Characterization and localization of the naturally occurring cross-links in vaccinia virus DNA. J Mol Biol 88:785, 1974.
20. Baroudy BM, Venkatesan S, Moss B: Incompletely base-paired flip-flop terminal loops link the two DNA strands of the vaccinia virus genome into one uninterrupted polynucleotide chain. Cell 28:315, 1982.
21. Goebel SJ, Johnson GP, Perkus ME, et al: The complete DNA sequence of vaccinia virus. Virology 179:247, 1990.
22. Garon CF, Barbosa E, Moss B: Visualization of an inverted terminal repetition in vaccinia virus DNA. Proc Natl Acad Sci USA 75:4863, 1978.
23. Wittek R, Menna A, Muller K, et al: Inverted terminal repeats in rabbit poxvirus and vaccinia virus DNA. J Virol 28:171, 1978.
24. Wittek R, Moss B: Tandem repeats within the inverted terminal repetition of vaccinia virus DNA. Cell 21:277, 1980.
25. Wittek R, Cooper J, Barbosa E, et al: Expression of the vaccinia virus genome—Analysis and mapping of mRNAs encoded within the inverted terminal repetition. Cell 21:487, 1980.
26. Johnson GP, Goebel SJ, Paoletti E: An update on the vaccinia virus genome. Virology 196:381, 1993.
27. Essani K, Dales S: Biogenesis of vaccinia: Evidence for more than 100 polypeptides in the virion. Virology 95:385, 1979.
28. Moss B, Ahn B-Y, Amegadzie B, et al: Cytoplasmic transcription system encoded by vaccinia virus. J Biol Chem 266:1355, 1991.
29. Stern W, Dales S: Biogenesis of vaccinia: Concerning the origin of the envelope phospholipids. Virology 62:293, 1974.
30. Hiller G, Eibl H, Weber K: Acyl bis(monoacylglycero)phosphate, assumed to be a marker for lysosomes, is a major phospholipid of vaccinia virions. Virology 113:761, 1981.
31. Lyles DS, Randall CC, Gafford LG, et al: Cellular fatty acids during fowlpox virus infection of three different host systems. Virology 70:227, 1976.
32. Chang A, Metz DH: Further investigations on the mode of entry of vaccinia virus into cells. J Gen Virol 32:275, 1976.
33. Janeczko RA, Rodriguez JF, Esteban M: Studies on the mechanism of entry of vaccinia virus into animal cells. Arch Virol 92:135, 1987.
34. Doms RW, Blumenthal R, Moss B: Fusion of intra- and extracellular forms of vaccinia virus with the cell membrane. J Virol 64:4884, 1990.
35. Payne LG, Norrby E: Adsorption and penetration of enveloped and naked vaccinia virus particles. J Virol 27:19, 1978.
36. Gordon J, Mohandas A, Wilton S, et al: A prominent antigenic surface polypeptide involved in the biogenesis and function of the vaccinia virus envelope. Virology 181:671, 1991.
37. Rodriguez JF, Esteban M: Mapping and nucleotide sequence of the vaccinia virus gene that encodes a 14-kilodalton fusion protein. J Virol 61:3550, 1987.
38. Ichihashi Y, Takahashi T, Oie M: Identification of a vaccinia virus penetration protein. Virology 202:834, 1994.
39. Wolffe EJ, Vijaya S, Moss B: A myristylated, membrane protein encoded by the vaccinia virus L1R open reading frame is the target of potent neutralizing monoclonal antibodies. Virology 211:53, 1995.
40. Ichihashi Y, Oie M: Proteolytic activation of vaccinia virus for the penetration phase of infection. Virology 116:297, 1982.
41. Eppstein DA, Marsh YV, Schreiber AB, et al: Epidermal growth factor receptor occupancy inhibits vaccinia virus infection. Nature 266:550, 1985.
42. Marsh YV, Eppstein DA: Vaccinia virus and the EGF receptor: A portal of entry for infectivity? J Cell Biochem 34:239, 1987.
43. Buller RML, Smith GL, Cremer K, et al: Decreased virulence of recombinant vaccinia virus expression vectors is associated with a thymidine kinase–negative phenotype. Nature 317:813, 1985.
44. Hugin AW, Hauser C: The epidermal growth factor receptor is not a receptor for vaccinia virus. J Virol 68:8409, 1994.
45. Joklik WK: The intracellular uncoating of poxvirus DNA. I. The fate of radioactively-labeled rabbitpox virus. J Mol Biol 8:263, 1964.
46. Joklik WK: The intracellular uncoating of poxvirus DNA. II. The molecular basis of the uncoating process. J Mol Biol 8:277, 1964.
47. Moss B: Vaccinia virus transcription. *In* Conaway R, Conaway J (eds): Transcription Mechanisms and Regulation. New York, Raven, 1993, pp 185–205.
48. Munyon WH, Kit S: Induction of cytoplasmic ribonucleic acid synthesis in vaccinia-infected LM cells during inhibition of protein synthesis. Virology 29:303, 1966.
49. Kates JR, McAuslan B: Messenger RNA synthesis by a "coated" viral genome. Proc Natl Acad Sci USA 57:314, 1967.
50. Kates JR, McAuslan BR: Poxvirus DNA–dependent RNA polymerase. Proc Natl Acad Sci USA 58:134, 1967.
51. Munyon WE, Paoletti E, Grace JT Jr: RNA polymerase activity in purified infectious vaccinia virus. Proc Natl Acad Sci USA 58:2280, 1967.
52. Wei CM, Moss B: Methylated nucleotides block 5′-terminus of vaccinia virus mRNA. Proc Natl Acad Sci USA 72:318, 1975.
53. Jones EV, Puckett C, Moss B: DNA-dependent RNA polymerase subunits encoded within the vaccinia virus genome. J Virol 61:1765, 1987.
54. Broyles SS, Moss B: Homology between RNA polymerases of poxviruses, prokaryotes, and eukaryotes: Nucleotide sequence and transcriptional analysis of vaccinia virus genes encoding 147-kDa and 22-kDa subunits. Proc Natl Acad Sci USA 83:3141, 1986.

55. Patel DD, Pickup DJ: The second-largest subunit of the poxvirus RNA polymerase is similar to the corresponding subunits of procaryotic and eucaryotic RNA polymerases. J Virol 63:1076, 1989.
56. Ahn B-Y, Moss B: RNA polymerase–associated transcription specificity factor encoded by vaccinia virus. Proc Natl Acad Sci USA 89:3536, 1992.
57. Broyles SS, Yuen L, Shuman S, et al: Purification of a factor required for transcription of vaccinia virus early genes. J Biol Chem 263:10754, 1988.
58. Broyles SS, Fesler BS: Vaccinia virus gene encoding a component of the viral early transcription factor. J Virol 64:1523, 1990.
59. Gershon PD, Moss B: Early transcription factor subunits are encoded by vaccinia virus late genes. Proc Natl Acad Sci USA 87:4401, 1990.
60. Davison AJ, Moss B: The structure of vaccinia virus early promoters. J Mol Biol 210:749, 1989.
61. Yuen L, Moss B: Oligonucleotide sequence signaling transcriptional termination of vaccinia virus early genes. Proc Natl Acad Sci USA 84:6417, 1987.
62. Shuman S, Moss B: Bromouridine triphosphate inhibits transcription termination and mRNA release by vaccinia virions. J Biol Chem 264:21356, 1989.
63. Martin SA, Paoletti E, Moss B: Purification of mRNA guanylyltransferase and mRNA (guanine 7-)methyltransferase from vaccinia virus. J Biol Chem 250:9322, 1975.
64. Barbosa E, Moss B: mRNA (nucleoside-2′-)-methyltransferase from vaccinia virus. Purification and physical properties. J Biol Chem 253:7692, 1978.
65. Moss B, Rosenblum EN, Paoletti E: Polyadenylate polymerase from vaccinia virions. Nat New Biol 245:59, 1973.
66. Morgan JR, Cohen LK, Roberts BE: Identification of the DNA sequences encoding the large subunit of the mRNA capping enzyme of vaccinia virus. J Virol 52:206, 1984.
67. Niles EG, Lee-Chen G-J, Shuman S, et al: Vaccinia virus gene *D12L* encodes the small subunit of the viral mRNA capping enzyme. Virology 172:513, 1989.
68. Gershon PD, Ahn BY, Garfield M, et al: Poly(A) polymerase and a dissociable polyadenylation stimulatory factor encoded by vaccinia virus. Cell 66:1269, 1991.
69. Schnierle BS, Gershon PD, Moss B: Cap-specific mRNA (nucleoside-$O^{2\prime}$-)-methyltransferase and poly(A) polymerase stimulatory activities of vaccinia virus are mediated by a single protein. Proc Natl Acad Sci USA 89:2897, 1992.
70. Shuman S, Broyles SS, Moss B: Purification and characterization of a transcription termination factor from vaccinia virions. J Biol Chem 262:12372, 1987.
71. Baldick CJ, Cassetti MC, Harris N, et al: Ordered assembly of a functional preinitiation transcription complex, containing vaccinia virus early transcription factor and RNA polymerase, on an immobilized template. J Virol 68:6052, 1994.
72. Hagler J, Shuman S: A freeze-frame view of eukaryotic transcription during elongation and capping of nascent mRNA. Science 255:983, 1992.
73. Li J, Broyles SS: The DNA-dependent ATPase activity of vaccinia virus early gene transcription factor is essential for its transcription activation function. J Biol Chem 268:20016, 1993.
74. Schwer B, Visca P, Vos JC, et al: Discontinuous transcription or RNA processing of vaccinia virus late messengers results in a 5′ poly(A) leader. Cell 50:163, 1987.
75. Bertholet C, Van Meir E, ten Heggeler-Bordier B, et al: Vaccinia virus produces late mRNAs by discontinuous synthesis. Cell 50:153, 1987.
76. Ahn B-Y, Moss B: Capped poly(A) leader of variable lengths at the 5′ ends of vaccinia virus late mRNAs. J Virol 63:226, 1989.
77. Baldick CJ Jr, Moss B: Characterization and temporal regulation of mRNAs encoded by vaccinia virus intermediate stage genes. J Virol 67:3515, 1993.
78. Vos JC, Stunnenberg HG: Derepression of a novel class of vaccinia virus genes upon DNA replication. EMBO J 7:3487, 1988.
79. Keck JG, Baldick CJ, Moss B: Role of DNA replication in vaccinia virus gene expression: A naked template is required for transcription of three late transactivator genes. Cell 61:801, 1990.
80. Vos JC, Sasker M, Stunnenberg HG: Promoter melting by a stage-specific vaccinia virus transcription factor is independent of the presence of RNA polymerase. Cell 65:105, 1991.
81. Vos JC, Sasker M, Stunnenberg HG: Vaccinia virus capping enzyme is a transcription initiation factor. EMBO J 10:2553, 1991.
82. Rosales R, Harris N, Ahn B-Y, et al: Purification and identification of a vaccinia virus–encoded intermediate stage promoter–specific transcription factor that has homology to eukaryotic transcription factor SII (TFIIS) and an additional role as a viral RNA polymerase subunit. J Biol Chem 269:14260, 1994.
83. Harris N, Rosales R, Moss B: Transcription initiation factor activity of vaccinia virus capping enzyme is independent of mRNA guanylylation. Proc Natl Acad Sci USA 90:2860, 1993.
84. Hirschmann P, Vos JC, Stunnenberg HG: Mutational analysis of a vaccinia virus intermediate promoter in vivo and in vitro. J Virol 64:6063, 1990.
85. Baldick CJ, Keck JG, Moss B: Mutational analysis of the core, spacer and initiator regions of vaccinia virus intermediate class promoters. J Virol 66:4710, 1992.
86. Wright CF, Keck JG, Moss B: A transcription factor for expression of vaccinia virus late genes is encoded by an intermediate gene. J Virol 65:3715, 1991.
87. Keck JG, Kovacs GR, Moss B: Overexpression, purification and late transcription factor activity of the 17-kDa protein encoded by the vaccinia virus *A1L* gene. J Virol 67:5740, 1993.
88. Kovacs GR, Rosales R, Keck JG, et al: Modulation of the cascade model for regulation of vaccinia virus gene expression: Purification of a prereplicative, late-stage-specific transcription factor. J Virol 68:3443, 1994.
89. Wright CF, Coroneos AM: Purification of the late transcription system of vaccinia virus: Identification of a novel transcription factor. J Virol 67:7264, 1993.
90. Davison AJ, Moss B: The structure of vaccinia virus late promoters. J Mol Biol 210:771, 1989.
91. Stunnenberg HG, de Magistris L, Schwer B: The generation of poly(A) heads on vaccinia late mRNA: A proposal of a slippage mechanism. *In* Cech TR (ed): Molecular Biology of RNA. New York, Alan R Liss, 1989, pp 199–208.
92. Ink BS, Pickup DJ: Vaccinia virus directs the synthesis of early mRNAs containing 5′ poly(A) sequences. Proc Natl Acad Sci USA 87:1536, 1990.
93. Ahn B-Y, Jones EV, Moss B: Identification of the vaccinia virus gene encoding an 18-kilodalton subunit of RNA polymerase and demonstration of a 5′ poly(A) leader on its early transcript. J Virol 64:3019, 1990.
94. Antczak JB, Patel DD, Ray CA, et al: Site-specific RNA cleavage generates the 3′ end of a poxvirus late mRNA. Proc Natl Acad Sci USA 89:12033, 1992.
95. Earl PL, Jones EV, Moss B: Homology between DNA polymerases of poxviruses, herpesviruses, and adenoviruses: Nucleotide sequence of the vaccinia virus DNA polymerase gene. Proc Natl Acad Sci USA 83:3659, 1986.
96. Traktman P: Molecular genetic and biochemical analysis of poxvirus DNA replication. Semin Virol 2:291, 1991.
97. Moyer RW, Graves RL: The mechanism of cytoplasmic orthopoxvirus DNA replication. Cell 27:391, 1981.
98. Merchlinsky M, Garon C, Moss B: Molecular cloning and sequence of the concatemer junction from vaccinia virus replicative DNA: Viral nuclease cleavage sites in cruciform structures. J Mol Biol 199:399, 1988.
99. Merchlinsky M, Moss B: Resolution of linear minichromosomes with hairpin ends from circular plasmids contining vaccinia virus concatemer junctions. Cell 45:879, 1986.
100. DeLange AM, McFadden G: Efficient resolution of replicated poxvirus telomeres to native hairpin structures requires two inverted symmetrical copies of a core target DNA sequence. J Virol 61:1957, 1987.
101. Merchlinsky M, Moss B: Resolution of vaccinia virus DNA concatemer junctions requires late gene expresssion. J Virol 63:1595, 1989.
102. DeLange AM: Identification of temperature-sensitive mutants of vaccinia virus that are defective in conversion of concatemeric replicative intermediates to the mature linear DNA genome. J Virol 63:2437, 1989.
103. Dales S, Pogo BGT (eds): Biology of Poxviruses. New York, Springer-Verlag, 1981.
104. Morgan C: Vaccinia virus reexamined: Development and release. Virology 73:43, 1976.
105. Hiller G, Weber K, Schneider L, et al: Interaction of assembled

progeny pox viruses with the cellular cytoskeleton. Virology 98:142, 1979.
106. Stokes GV: High-voltage electron microscope study of the release of vaccinia virus from whole cells. J Virol 18:636, 1976.
107. Cudmore S, Cossart P, Griffiths G, et al: Actin-based motility of vaccinia virus. Nature 378:636, 1995.
108. Blasco R, Moss B: Role of cell-associated enveloped vaccinia virus in cell-to-cell spread. J Virol 66:4170, 1992.
109. Boulter EA, Appleyard G: Differences between extracellular and intracellular forms of poxvirus and their implications. Prog Med Virol 16:86, 1973.
110. Ichihashi Y, Matsumoto S, Dales S: Biogenesis of poxviruses: Role of A-type inclusions and host cell membranes in virus dissemination. Virology 46:507, 1971.
111. Funahashi S, Sato T, Shida H: Cloning and characterization of the gene encoding the major protein of the A-type inclusion body of cowpox virus. J Gen Virol 69:35, 1988.
112. Dumbell K, Richardson M: Virological investigations of specimens from buffaloes affected by buffalopox in Maharashtra State, India between 1985 and 1987. Arch Virol 128:257, 1993.
113. Epstein WL: Molluscum contagiosum. Semin Dermatol 11:184, 1992.
114. Porter CD, Blake NW, Cream JJ, et al: Molluscum contagiosum virus. Mol Cell Biol Hum Dis 1:233, 1992.
115. Buller RML, Burnett J, Chen W, et al: Replication of molluscum contagiosum virus. Virology 213:655, 1995.
116. Postlethwaite R, Watt JA, Hawley TG, et al: Features of molluscum contagiosum virus in the northeast of Scotland and in Fijian village settlements. J Hyg (Lond) 65:281, 1967.
117. Sturt RJ, Muller HK, Francis GD: Molluscum contagiosum in villages of the West Sepik district of New Guinea. Med J Aust 2:751, 1971.
118. Brown ST, Nalley JF, Kraus SJ: Molluscum contagiosum. Sex Transm Dis 8:527, 1981.
119. Darai G, Reisner H, Scholz J, et al: Analysis of the genome of molluscum contagiosum virus by restriction endonuclease analysis and molecular cloning. J Med Virol 18:29, 1986.
120. Scholz J, Rosen-Wolff A, Bugert J, et al: Epidemiology of molluscum contagiosum using genetic analysis of the viral DNA. J Med Virol 27:87, 1989.
121. Porter CD, Muhlemann MF, Cream JJ, et al: Molluscum contagiosum: Characterization of viral DNA and clinical features. Epidemiol Infect 99:563, 1987.
122. Porter CD, Archard LC: Characterisation by restriction mapping of three subtypes of molluscum-contagiosum virus. J Med Virol 38:1, 1992.
123. Thompson CH, De Zwart-Steffe RT, Biggs IM: Molecular epidemiology of Australian isolates of molluscum contagiosum. J Med Virol 32:1, 1990.
124. Nakamura J, Arao Y, Yoshida M, et al: Molecular epidemiological study of molluscum contagiosum virus in two urban areas of western Japan by the in-gel endonuclease digestion method. Arch Virol 125:339, 1992.
125. Thompson CH, de Zwart-Steffe RT, Donovan B: Clinical and molecular aspects of molluscum contagiosum infection in HIV-1 positive patients. Int J STD AIDS 3:101, 1992.
126. Van Rensburg IB, Collett MG, Ronen N, et al: Molluscum contagiosum in a horse. J S Afr Vet Assoc 62:72, 1991.
127. Lange L, Marett S, Maree C, et al: Molluscum contagiosum in three horses. J S Afr Vet Assoc 62:68, 1991.
128. Jezek Z, Fenner F: Human monkeypox. Monogr Virol 17:1, 1988.
129. Richardson M, Dumbell K: Comparisons of monkeypox viruses from animal and human infections in Zaire. Trop Geogr Med 46:327, 1994.
130. Douglass NJ, Richardson M, Dumbell KR: Evidence for recent genetic variation in monkeypox viruses. J Gen Virol 75:1303, 1994.
131. Marennikova SS, Ladnyj ID, Ogorodnikova SI, et al: Identification and study of a poxvirus isolated from wild rodents in Turkmenia. Arch Virol 56:7, 1978.
132. Bennett M, Gaskell CJ, Baxby D, et al: Feline cowpox virus infection. A review. J Small Anim Pract 14:167, 1990.
133. Baxby D, Bennett M, Getty B: Human cowpox 1969–1993: A review based on 54 cases. Br J Dermatol 131:598, 1994.
134. Zhukova OA, Tsanava SA, Marennikova SS: Experimental infection of domestic cats by cowpox virus. Acta Virol 36:329, 1992.
135. Mayr A, Büttner M: Ecthyma (orf) virus. *In* Dinter Z, Morein B (eds): Virus Infections of Ruminants. Amsterdam, Elsevier, 1990, pp 33–42.
136. Mayr A, Büttner M: Milker's node virus. *In* Dinter Z, Morein B (eds): Virus Infections of Ruminants. Amsterdam, Elsevier, 1990, pp 29–32.
137. Mayr A, Büttner M: Bovine papular stomatitis virus. *In* Dinter Z, Morein B (eds): Virus Infections of Ruminants. Amsterdam, Elsevier, 1990, pp 23–28.
138. Downie AW, Taylor-Robinson CH, Caunt AE, et al: Tanapox: A new disease caused by a poxvirus. Br Med J 1:363, 1971.
139. Jezek Z, Arita I, Szczeniowski M, et al: Human tanapox in Zaire: Clinical and epidemiological observations on cases confirmed by laboratory studies. Bull World Health Organ 63:1027, 1985.
140. Downie AW, España C: Comparison of Tanapox virus and Yaba-like viruses causing epidemic disease in monkeys. J Hyg (Lond) 70:23, 1972.
141. Grace JT, Mirand EA: Human susceptibility to a simian tumor virus. Ann N Y Acad Sci 108:1123, 1963.
142. Niven JSF, Armstrong JA, Andrewes CH, et al: Subcutaneous "growths" in monkeys produced by a poxvirus. J Pathol Bacteriol 81:1, 1961.
143. Downie AW: A study of the lesions produced experimentally by cowpox virus. J Pathol Bacteriol 48:361, 1939.
144. Johannessen JV, Krogh H-K, Solberg I, et al: Human orf. J Cutan Pathol 2:265, 1975.
145. Gottlieb SL, Myskowski PL: Molluscum contagiosum. Int J Dermatol 33:453, 1994.
146. Buller RML, Chakrabarti S, Cooper JA, et al: Deletion of the vaccinia virus growth factor gene reduces virus virulence. J Virol 62:866, 1988.
147. Buller RML, Palumbo GJ: Poxvirus pathogenesis. Microbiol Rev 55:80, 1991.
148. Isaacs SN, Kotwal GJ, Moss B: Vaccinia virus complement-control protein prevents antibody-dependent complement-enhanced neutralization of infectivity and contributes to virulence. Proc Natl Acad Sci USA 89:628, 1992.
149. Ray CA, Black RA, Kronheim SR, et al: Viral inhibition of inflammation: Cowpox virus encodes an inhibitor of the interleukin-1β converting enzyme. Cell 69:597, 1992.
150. McFadden G, Graham K: Modulation of cytokine networks by poxviruses: The myxoma virus model. Semin Virol 5:421, 1994.
151. Alcamí A, Smith GL: Cytokine receptors encoded by poxviruses: A lesson in cytokine biology. Immunol Today 16:474, 1995.
152. Freed ER, Duma RJ, Escobar MR: Vaccinia necrosum and its relationship to impaired immunologic responsiveness. Am J Med 52:411, 1972.
153. Fulginiti VA, Kempe CH, Hathaway EE, et al: Progressive vaccinia in immunologically deficient individuals. Birth Defects 4:129, 1968.
154. Fenner F, Nakanao JH: Poxviridae: The poxviruses. *In* Lennette EH, Halonen P, Murphy FA (eds): The Laboratory Diagnosis of Infectious Diseases: Principles and Practice. New York, Springer-Verlag, 1988, pp 177–210.
155. Ropp SL, Jin Q, Knight JC, et al: PCR strategy for identification and differentiation of small pox and other orthopoxviruses. J Clin Microbiol 33:2069, 1995.
156. Esposito JJ, Obijeski JF, Nakano JH: Orthopoxvirus DNA: Strain differentiation by electrophoresis of restriction endonuclease fragmented virion DNA. Virology 89:53, 1978.
157. Pfeffer M, Meyer H, Wiedmann M: A ligase chain reaction targeting two adjacent nucleotides allows the differentiation of cowpox virus from other *Orthopoxvirus* species. J Virol Methods 49:353, 1994.
158. Meyer H, Pfeffer M, Rziha H-J: Sequence alterations within and downstream of the A-type inclusion protein gene allow differentiation of *Orthopoxvirus* species by polymerase chain reaction. J Gen Virol 75:1975, 1994.
159. Meyer H, Osterrieder N, Pfeffer M: Differentiation of species of the genus *Orthopoxvirus* in a dot blot assay using digoxigenin-labeled DNA-probes. Vet Microbiol 34:333, 1993.
160. Appleyard G, Hapel AJ, Boulter EA: An antigenic difference between intracellular and extracellular rabbitpox virus. J Gen Virol 13:9, 1971.
161. Boulter EA, Zwartouw HT, Titmuss DHJ, et al: The nature of the immune state produced by inactivated vaccinia virus in rabbits. Am J Epidemiol 94:612, 1971.

RNA VIRUSES

250

Influenza Viruses

Charles B. Smith

History

Epidemic influenza remains the last great uncontrolled plague of mankind.

F. M. DAVENPORT[1]

The clinical syndrome of acute fever, cough, headache, myalgias, and malaise that characterizes influenza, combined with the typical pattern of occurrence in epidemics with associated increased mortality, suggests that influenza virus has been an important pathogen for many centuries.[2] Although the virus was not identified until 1933, studies of influenza antibodies in serum of persons born before and after 1918 clearly identified type A influenza virus as the cause of the great pandemic of 1918, which resulted in more than 20 million fatalities worldwide and greatly overshadowed World War I as a cause of death and suffering.[3]

Since it was first isolated from humans in 1933,[4] this virus has probably been studied more intensively than any other human virus. Its structure has been well-defined; segments of the genome have been sequenced; and the best efforts of modern science have been directed at developing vaccines and antiviral drugs. Despite these scientific advances, influenza virus infections continue to cost several billion dollars each year in the United States,[5] and they remain a major cause of morbidity and mortality throughout the world.

Characteristics of the Pathogen

Influenza viruses are members of the Orthomyxoviridae family and are structurally characterized by a ribonucleoprotein core arranged as a helical nucleocapsid and surrounded by a pleomorphic, lipid-containing envelope that has two distinct glycoproteins extending from the surface (Fig. 250–1). The viral genome is single stranded and of negative polarity, so that early in the replication process, an RNA transcriptase contained in the virus assists in the synthesis of a positive strand of RNA, which serves as messenger RNA for synthesis of new viral proteins and also as the template for synthesis of new viral RNA. The orthomyxoviruses differ from the paramyxoviruses (rubeola) primarily in that they have a genome that is divided into eight separate segments. This relatively unusual characteristic allows them to undergo genetic reassortment and thus enjoy a remarkable degree of genetic variability.[6]

The hemagglutinin (HA) glycoprotein extending out from the lipid envelope (see Fig. 250–1) is involved with attachment of the virus to neuraminic acid–containing mucopolysaccharide receptors on the cell surface membrane and also in the penetration of the virus into the cell.[7] The function of the neuraminidase (NA) glycoprotein on the surface of the virion is not as well understood, but it probably is involved in cleaving the HA–neuraminic acid receptor bond during the early stages of penetration of the virus, and possibly during the late stages of virus release from the infected cell. The matrix protein (M), which is found inside the lipid envelope, is involved in assembly and budding of the virion from the cell. The nucleocapsid contains at least three distinct proteins that have polymerase activity and another structural nucleoprotein.

The influenza viruses are classified principally according to the antigenicity of the components. The three major types of influenza viruses (A, B, and C) are distinguished by the antigenicity of the internal nucleoproteins. The genes that code for these antigens are relatively stable, possibly because antibodies do not have access to the antigens and there is no selective advantage for mutants. Types A and B influenza are most important clinically, and in this chapter I focus on them.

Because the HA and NA glycoproteins are situated on the surface of the virion and are involved in the critical initial steps of attachment to and penetration of host cells, they are most important in determining immunity to influenza. Antibodies to these surface glycoproteins can prevent infection in cell cultures as well as in animals, and it is not surprising that the influenza viruses have evolved several mechanisms for changing their antigenic coats so as to evade the important antibody arm of host defenses. Influenza type A viruses have evolved at least 13 subtypes of the HA (H1, H2, and so on) and at least nine subtypes of the NA (N1, N2, . . .). Many of the subtypes are found principally in animals, and during the past 50 years, the majority of human infections have been associated with three subtypes of HA and two subtypes of NA. Because the genes for the HA and NA are separate and subject to reassortment, a variety of combinations of the two antigens have been seen (e.g., H3N2, H1N1). The current custom of identifying type A influenza viruses recognizes the prototype isolate by type, place and year of isolation, and the subtypes of the HA and NA. Thus, the prototype virus for a subtype that circulated in 1987 was influenza virus A/Sichuan/2/87 (H3N2).

Epidemiology

The epidemiology of type A influenza virus infections is unique for respiratory viruses and is sufficiently characteristic to be helpful in identifying influenza outbreaks (Table 250–1). The unusual pattern of yearly occurrence of endemic influenza, with focal epidemics every 2 or 3 years and major

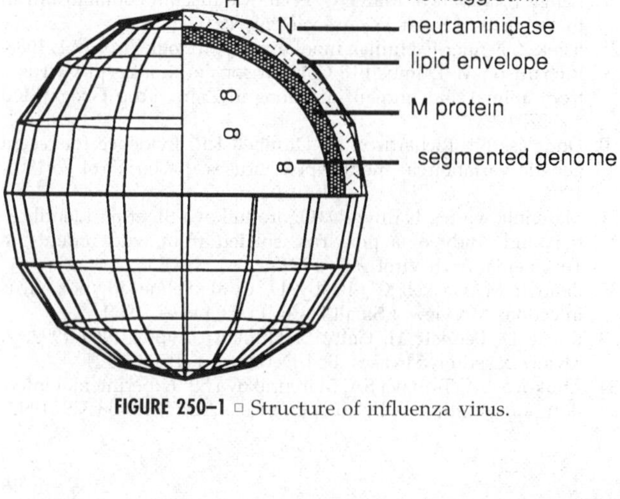

FIGURE 250–1 □ Structure of influenza virus.

TABLE 250–1 ■ Epidemiologic Characteristics of Influenza

Pandemics	Worldwide influenza, due to antigenic shift (reassortment)
Epidemics	Local outbreaks, due to antigenic drift (mutation)
Endemic	Sporadic cases each year
Seasonal	Winter months in northern latitudes—school related; abrupt onset and cessation of epidemics
Age factors	Infection rate: chidren > adults Morbidity and mortality: elders > children
Community clues	Increased absenteeism in schools, increased hospitalizations and mortality from pneumonia

worldwide pandemics every 10 or 20 years, can best be explained by understanding the mechanisms used by the type A influenza viruses to alter their antigenicity and thus escape host immune defenses.[8] Pandemic influenza has generally been associated with the appearance of new subtypes of HA or NA antigens of the virus, or both (antigenic shift), which spread rapidly because most of the population lack antibody. Studies of the genomes of these new strains indicate that genetic reassortment of the genes for different subtypes of the virus is involved in antigenic shift.[9] For example, the new influenza virus A/Hong Kong/68 (H3N2) differed from strains of the H2N2 virus that had circulated in previous years only in the replacement of the H2 genome with the H3 genome.[10] Evidence that animals may serve as the reservoir for introduction of new subtypes of HA genomes includes amino acid sequence homology between the HA of influenza type A strains found in domestic animals and human strains and demonstration that reassortment can occur between human and animal strains.[7, 11]

The genes that code for the HA and NA surface antigens of type A influenza viruses are relatively unstable, and they appear to continuously undergo mutations that alter antigenicity (antigenic drift) and thus provide a selective advantage for the mutant.[12] Antigenic variants may still be classified in the same subtype when tested by gel diffusion with polyclonal antisera, but people with antibody to the parent of the mutant may no longer be protected from infection and illness and antigenic variants can cause focal epidemics.[8] Regular antigenic drift of type A influenza viruses is the reason that recent isolates of the virus are used to prepare new influenza vaccine each year.

Host and environmental factors also influence the epidemiology of influenza. Although antibody levels slowly decline after infections, and older persons are usually reinfected by strains that show antigenic drift, older persons generally retain some immunologic resistance, and the prevalence of influenza is highest among children who are exposed for the first time to a particular virus subtype.[13] Children are important vectors in the spread of influenza, and the timing of local epidemics often relates to crowding of children into schoolrooms, where aerosol spread is most efficient.[14] Influenza outbreaks typically are confined to the midwinter months in the northern climates, and the tendency for the virus to survive best in aerosol droplet nuclei in an environment of low temperature and low humidity may be responsible for this seasonal pattern.[15]

The epidemiology of influenza is also characterized by a remarkable association of influenza epidemics with an increase in morbidity and mortality in the community.[16] Significant increases in absenteeism from schools and industries often coincides with an influenza outbreak, and physicians' knowledge of this can increase their accuracy in diagnosing influenza in individual patients. Although infection rates may be lower for older persons during an influenza epidemic, the infection is much more severe in elders and chronically ill persons, and this is often manifested by an easily documentable increase in mortality from pneumonias and influenza-like illnesses.[17] The Centers for Disease Control and Prevention and state health departments maintain continuous surveillance of these mortality figures. Like the absenteeism signal, significant increases in pneumonia and influenza mortality rates above those predicted signal the need for prophylaxis and therapy of type A influenza virus infections.

Pathogenesis

Initial infection with influenza viruses can occur in either the upper or the lower respiratory tract, although the lower tract appears to be more susceptible.[18] Virus multiplication is detectable within 24 hours and peaks around 72 hours, by which time clinical illness is usually evident. Virus excretion in respiratory secretions continues during the 3- to 5-day period of clinical illness, and usually disappears by 7 days, as the patient recovers.

The lower respiratory tract is the site of greatest pathologic changes: there is gross evidence of hyperemia and edema of bronchial surfaces and microscopic evidence of loss of ciliated and other bronchial epithelial cells.[19] In cases of primary influenza viral pneumonia, damage extends to the level of the alveolar cells.[20] Secondary bacterial infection is the principal complication of influenza, and several mechanisms have been postulated. In addition to direct physical damage to bronchial epithelium, normal ciliary activity is impaired by influenza virus infection and may impair physical clearance of bacteria from the lung.[21, 22] *Staphylococcus aureus* adheres more efficiently to influenza virus–infected cells.[23] Both polymorphonuclear[24] and alveolar macrophage[25] phagocytic functions are depressed during acute influenza virus infection.

The immune response to infection with influenza viruses is broad and includes the full spectrum of systemic and secretory immunoglobulins as well as generation of cytotoxic and natural killer lymphocytes.[26, 27] Recovery from acute influenza occurs before new antibody is detectable in serum or secretions and appears to correlate with the production of interferon,[28] and most important, with the generation of cytotoxic lymphocytes.[29, 30] Immunity of these cytotoxic cells to influenza viruses is cross-reactive for different subtypes of type A influenza viruses, recognizing common nucleoprotein antigens and epitopes of the HA molecule, which are conserved between subtypes.[31] This cross-reactivity is particularly interesting because it suggests that a vaccine might be developed that utilizes antigens that are stable and common to all subtypes of type A influenza virus.

Immunity to reinfection with influenza viruses is mediated principally by antibodies in serum and respiratory tract secretions.[32] Although antibodies are generated against both the internal and the external antigens of the virus, the greatest degree of protection is given by antibodies directed against the specific subtype antigens of the HA and NA. The degree of immunity varies with the level and specificity of these antibodies. When measured by the hemagglutination inhibition assay against the infecting virus, persons who have no detectable antibody have a high incidence of infection and illness, those with low levels of antibody may develop asymptomatic infections, and those with high levels of antibody are protected against infection and illness.[27] The general tendency for older persons to be less susceptible to infection with new antigenic variants or new subtypes of type A influenza viruses may be due to the limited degree of cross-reactivity with HA antigens that develops with repeated infection, or it may be a reflection of humoral or cytotoxic lymphocyte immunity to nucleoprotein or other antigens common to the type A viruses.

Clinical Manifestations

In otherwise healthy adults, the clinical picture (Fig. 250–2) of acute onset of fever, cough, and constitutional symptoms of headache, myalgias, and malaise that are severe enough to cause the patient to go to bed differentiates influenza virus infection from those of other respiratory viruses, particularly when influenza virus is known to be circulating in the community.[33] Coryza, nasal obstruction, and sore throat commonly accompany the illness, but they are less prominent than cough in the symptom complex of influenza when it is differentiated from "colds" caused by other respiratory viruses. The temperature is typically 38°C or higher and lasts for 3 to 4 days, as do the constitutional symptoms. The cough generally remains nonproductive and may persist for more than a week in uncomplicated cases. Malaise and fatigue usually disappear with defervescence, although in patients prone to depression, it may last for many weeks.[34] Nausea and vomiting occur in less than 25% of cases during the onset, and diarrhea and other abdominal complaints are uncommon in adults. Children are more likely to have diarrhea and other abdominal complaints, particularly with type B influenza virus infection.[35] Influenza in young children is more difficult to differentiate from other respiratory viral infections and may present as croup, bronchiolitis, or pneumonia.

The most distinctive disease process associated with influenza virus infection occurs in the lower respiratory tract, and the most common complications involve the lung: abnormalities in bronchial reactivity and in small airways function may persist for several weeks.[36] These effects vary in severity from transient, exercise-induced asthma to exacerbations of asthma that require hospitalization and to acute bronchitis in patients with chronic obstructive pulmonary disease.[37, 38] Secondary bacterial pneumonia is a common complication of influenza virus infection, particularly in elders and persons who have underlying chronic heart or lung disease.[39] This illness typically occurs 5 to 7 days after the onset of clinical influenza, at a time when the patient appears to have recovered. The common respiratory bacterial pathogens (pneumococci, *Haemophilus influenzae*, staphylococci) typically cause the secondary bacterial pneumonia, and the clinical picture does not differ from that of pneumonia due to these bacteria in other settings, except that the illness may be more severe.[40] Less common but more often fatal is primary influenza virus pneumonia.[41] This illness is also more likely to occur in patients with underlying illness; those at increased risk include patients with mitral stenosis and women in the third trimester of pregnancy, possibly because these conditions are associated with increased pulmonary capillary hypertension.[42] Primary influenza pneumonia has an onset within the first few days of the influenza illness and is typically rapidly progressive with diffuse bilateral involvement, hypoxemia, and a clinical picture of the adult respiratory distress syndrome with associated high mortality rate. Combined influenza viral and secondary bacterial pneumonias also occur, and they are often fatal.[41] Toxic shock syndrome has been described as a complication of acute influenza infection: toxin-producing *S. aureus* organisms are recovered from respiratory secretions.[43]

Influenza viruses may invade the blood stream[44] and damage other organs and tissues. The myalgias experienced by most patients with influenza may progress to frank myositis, rhabdomyolysis, and myoglobinuria.[45] Myocarditis and pericarditis with tamponade are recognized complications of influenza.[46] A variety of neurologic complications have been described, ranging from encephalopathy and myelitis to peripheral radiculopathy of the Guillain-Barré type.[47] Because the onset of neurologic complications varies from a few days to several weeks after onset of influenza, the relative importance of direct viral invasion and secondary immune pathogenesis has not been clarified. The fact that some influenza vaccines were associated with the Guillain-Barré syndrome supports an immune mechanism.[48] A role has been postulated for influenza virus in the pathogenesis of postencephalitic[49] and idiopathic[50] Parkinson disease.

Influenza viruses, particularly type B, are an important cause of Reye's syndrome,[51] which typically affects children recovering from an acute viral illness and is characterized by rapid onset of encephalopathy and associated hepatic dysfunction (see Chapter 165). The blood ammonia, hepatic enzyme, and creatine kinase values are elevated and the blood glucose level may be low. The syndrome is thought to be related to a generalized injury to mitochondria, and an important role for aspirin as a risk factor is well established.[52] Therapy is supportive, and prevention is best achieved by immunizing against influenza and avoiding salicylates for acute viral respiratory illnesses during the influenza season.

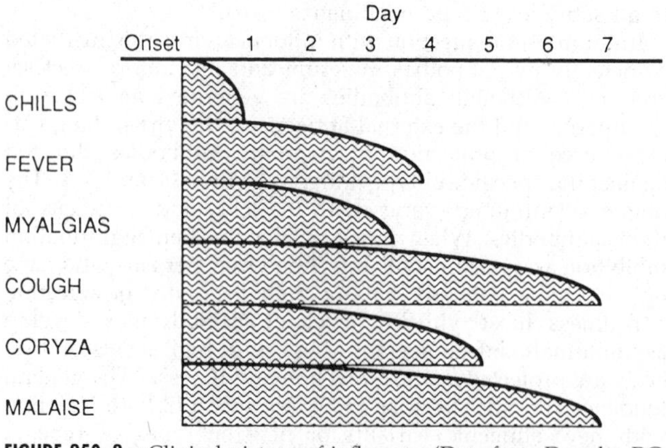

FIGURE 250–2 □ Clinical picture of influenza. (Data from Douglas RG: Influenza in man. *In* Kilbourne ED [ed]: The Influenza Viruses and Influenza. New York, Academic Press, 1975, pp 419–443; and Stuart-Harris CH: Clinical picture of influenza. *In* Stuart-Harris CH [ed]: Influenza and Other Virus Infections of the Respiratory Tract. London, E Arnold, 1965, pp 8–21.)

Diagnosis

A large number of infectious diseases can first present with an influenza-like illness characterized by acute onset of chills, fever, myalgias, headache, and malaise. The inclusion of prominent cough in the syndrome helps separate influenza from systemic infections that do not involve the respiratory tract primarily. Other respiratory pathogens that need to be considered in the differential diagnosis of influenza in adults include adenoviruses, *Chlamydia psittaci, Mycoplasma pneumoniae, Francisella tularensi, Legionella,* and occasionally pneumococci and other bacterial pathogens. The unique epidemiology of influenza is particularly helpful in identifying influenza infections during a documented outbreak.

Propagating the pathogen in culture is the most rapid and reliable method for laboratory diagnosis of influenza virus infections.[53] Secretions obtained by swab or wash from the upper respiratory tract, and sputum, when available, should be transported rapidly to the laboratory in virus transport medium at a cold temperature for immediate inoculation onto tissue culture cells. The classic cell culture method for identifying influenza virus usually requires 3 to 5 days and is most sensitive. More helpful to the clinician are newer rapid diagnostic techniques that utilize fluorescent-labeled

TABLE 250–2 ■ Indications for Use of Amantadine or Rimantadine

Prophylaxis
- *Control of influenza A outbreaks* in institutions housing persons at high risk, such as nursing homes. All patients and staff, regardless of vaccination status, should receive amantadine or rimantadine for duration of influenza activity in the community.
- *Adjunct to late vaccination* of persons at high risk for 2-wk period before vaccine takes effect.
- *To reduce the spread of infection* and to maintain care for persons at high risk in the home, home caregivers should be protected.
- *For immunodeficient persons,* such as those with acquired immunodeficiency syndrome, who have a poor antibody response to influenza vaccine.
- *For persons for whom influenza vaccine is contraindicated.*

Therapy (to be effective, therapy must begin within 24–48 h of onset of illness)
- *For influenza-like illness* in patients at high risk of developing complications of influenza type A.
- *Healthy adults* who want to reduce the severity of influenza illness.*
- *Persons hospitalized* with serious influenza illness.*

*Indications suggested by author.
Adapted from Centers for Disease Control and Prevention: Prevention and control of influenza Part II, Antiviral agents. MMWR Morbid Mortal Wkly Rep 43(RR-15):1, 1994.

murine monoclonal antibodies to identify viral antigen in shell vial cell cultures 24 hours after inoculation.[54] Attempts to identify viral antigen by enzyme-linked immunosorbent assay or viral genome by nucleic acid hybridization on smears of respiratory tract secretions have so far been too insensitive to be of clinical value.[55] Detection of influenza virus RNA in respiratory secretions by the polymerase chain reaction amplification technique holds promise for being more sensitive and rapid than virus culture in diagnosis.[56]

Antibodies to influenza viruses can be detected by a wide variety of techniques. Most often, the complement fixation test is used, and comparison of serum samples collected at the onset and 2 weeks later usually shows a diagnostic fourfold rise in antibody titer.[53] Most state health department laboratories are eager to receive specimens for diagnosis of influenza so that the presence of the virus in the community can be documented.

Treatment

Amantadine and its derivative rimantadine are antiviral agents currently approved for prophylaxis and therapy of type A influenza virus infections in adults (Table 250–2). Because rimantadine has been less thoroughly studied, it is not approved for therapy in children. In studies of naturally occurring type A influenza virus infections in both adults and children, amantadine or rimantadine therapy begun within 48 hours of onset of illness was associated with significant reductions in days of fever and severity of illness scores.[57, 58] Reduction of virus secretion is seen during therapy, indicating a direct antiviral effect; however, treated patients may have increased levels of the virus after cessation of therapy and resistance of posttherapy isolates of the virus to both agents has been detected.[58] The current recommendation is to use amantadine or rimantadine for therapy of acute influenza in patients who are at high risk of developing complications of the infection, such as the elderly and those with underlying heart and lung disease.[59] Some infectious disease clinicians use amantadine or rimantadine for therapy of patients hospitalized with serious influenza. Amantadine causes nervousness and insomnia in 7% to 10% of recipients, and high blood levels have been associated with more serious side effects of delirium and seizures. Because amantadine is primarily excreted by the kidney, dosage should be reduced in patients with decreased renal function and in the elderly.[59] Rimantadine is less dependent on renal excretion for clearance, approximately 40% being cleared by the liver, and it is associated with fewer side effects, particularly in the elderly. See Chapter 32 on antiviral agents for dosage recommendations.

Ribavirin is an antiviral drug that has been approved for aerosol therapy of severe lower respiratory tract infection with respiratory syncytial virus (see Chapter 32). The drug is active against both types A and B influenza viruses in vitro, and there are conflicting reports of the efficacy of oral and aerosol therapy for clinical influenza.[61, 62] It is not currently approved for use in influenza.

Prevention

The antiviral drugs amantadine and rimantadine have been 70% effective when used for prophylaxis against type A influenza virus infection.[59, 63] Antiviral prophylaxis is indicated for adults at high risk of developing complications of influenza infection who are unprotected by recent vaccination and are caught in the midst of a type A influenza outbreak[59, 60] (see Table 250–2). The indications for prophylaxis of families with index cases of influenza are unclear because of the appearance and transmission of resistant mutants in influenza A virus to family members.[64]

Inactivated influenza virus vaccines are the most important preventive measure against influenza.[60] In those years when the virus subtypes used in the vaccine reasonably matched the epidemic virus strains, vaccine use was associated with 70% or greater protection against influenza virus infection or influenza illness.[65, 66] A well-controlled trial indicated that the vaccine was highly effective in protecting against infection and illness with influenza virus in subjects aged 60 years or older.[67] The Immunization Practices Advisory Committee of the Centers for Disease Control and Prevention has recommended the use of vaccine for persons at high risk of being infected with influenza (such as health care workers) or at high risk of developing complications of the infection[60] (Table 250–3).

Because the current inactivated vaccines are made from virus grown in embryonated hens' eggs, patients with known egg allergy should not receive them. Compared with older preparations of the vaccine, current vaccines are highly purified and thus less likely to be associated with fevers and local reactions. Tenderness at the vaccination site is usually mild and occurs in less than 20% of recipients; systemic reactions of fever and myalgias occur in less than 5% of elderly adults.[60] The influenza vaccine prepared in 1976 was associated with the Guillain-Barré syndrome,[48] but subsequent preparations have not been implicated.[60]

Annual immunization is recommended because immunity

TABLE 250–3 ■ Indications for Use of Inactivated Influenza Vaccine

- *Persons at high risk* >6 mo of age, including elders, nursing home residents, and persons with chronic heart or lung disease, diabetes, renal dysfunction, and immunosuppression
- *Children and teenagers receiving long-term aspirin therapy* who are at risk for Reye's syndrome
- *Adults and children* who want to reduce their chances of developing influenza
- *Medical care workers* and household contacts of persons at high risk

from the vaccine generally does not last more than 1 year and the virus subtypes used in the vaccine are changed each year to most closely match the prevailing strains. Children younger than 12 years should receive two doses 1 month apart when receiving the vaccine for the first time. A single intramuscular dose is adequate for all others.

References

1. Davenport FM: Influenza viruses. *In* Evans AS (ed): Viral Infections of Humans. New York, Plenum Publishing, 1977, pp 273–296.
2. Hope-Simpson RE: The method of transmission of epidemic influenza: Further evidence from archival mortality data. J Hyg (Lond) 96:353, 1986.
3. Kilbourne ED: History of influenza. *In* Kilbourne ED (ed): Influenza. New York, Plenum Publishing, 1987, pp 1–22.
4. Smith W, Andrewes CH, Laidlaw PP: A virus obtained from influenza patients. Lancet 2:66, 1933.
5. Schoenbaum SC: Economic impact of influenza. Am J Med 82 (Suppl 6A):26, 1987.
6. Kingsbury DW: Orthomyxo- and paramyxoviruses and their replication. *In* Fields BN (ed): Virology. New York, Raven Press, 1985, pp 1157–1178.
7. Murphy BR, Webster RG: Influenza viruses. *In* Fields BN (ed): Virology. New York, Raven Press, 1985, pp 1179–1239.
8. Kendal AP: Epidemiologic implications of changes in the influenza virus genome. Am J Med 82(Suppl 6A):4, 1987.
9. Palese P, Young JF: Variation of influenza A, B and C viruses. Science 215:1468, 1982.
10. Nakajima K, Nakajima S, Sugiura A: The possible origin of H3N2 influenza virus. Virology 120:504, 1982.
11. Webster RG, Campbell CH, Granoff A: The in vivo production of new influenza A viruses. Virology 44:317, 1971.
12. Webster RG, Laver WG: Determination of the number of non overlapping antigenic areas on Hong Kong (H3N2) influenza virus hemagglutinin with monoclonal antibodies and the selection of variants with potential epidemiological significance. Virology 104:139, 1980.
13. Cate TR: Clinical manifestations and consequences of influenza. Am J Med 82(Suppl 6A):75, 1987.
14. Glezen WP: Consideration of the risk of influenza in children and indications for prophylaxis. Rev Infect Dis 2:408, 1980.
15. Hemmes JH, Winkler KC, Kool SM: Virus survival as a seasonal factor in influenza and poliomyelitis. Nature 188:430, 1960.
16. Glezen WP: Serious morbidity and mortality associated with influenza epidemics. Epidemiol Rev 2:26, 1982.
17. Baron RC, Dicker RC, Bussell KE, et al: Assessing trends in mortality in 121 US cities, 1970–79, from all causes and from pneumonia and influenza. Public Health Rep 103:120, 1988.
18. Douglas RG: Influenza in man. *In* Kilbourne ED (ed): The Influenza Viruses and Influenza. New York, Academic Press, 1975, pp 419–443.
19. Hers JF, Mulder J: Broad aspects of the pathology and pathogenesis of human influenza. Am Rev Respir Dis 83(Suppl):84, 1961.
20. Martin CM, Kunin LM, Gottlieb LS, et al: Asian influenza A in Boston, 1957–1958. Arch Intern Med 103:516, 1959.
21. Westerberg SC, Smith CB, Wiley BB: Pathogenesis of influenza virus infection in mouse tracheal organ cultures. Proc Soc Exp Biol Med 140:846, 1972.
22. Wilson R, Alton E, Rutman A: Upper respiratory tract viral infection and mucociliary clearance. Eur J Respir Dis 70:272, 1987.
23. Sanford BA, Davison VE, Ramsay MA: *Staphylococcus aureus* adherence to influenza A virus-infected and control cell cultures: Evidence for multiple adhesions. Proc Soc Exp Biol Med 181:104, 1986.
24. Hartshorn KL, Tauber AI: The influenza virus–infected phagocyte. A model of deactivation. Hematol Oncol Clin North Am 2:301, 1988.
25. Astry CL, Jakob GJ: Influenza virus–induced immune complexes suppress alveolar macrophage phagocytosis. J Virol 50:287, 1984.
26. Welliver RC, Ogra PL: Immunology of respiratory viral infections. Annu Rev Med 39:147, 1988.
27. Kilbourne ED: Influenza in man. *In* Kilbourne ED (ed): Influenza. New York, Plenum Publishing, 1987, pp 184–195.
28. Iwasaki T, Nozima T: Defense mechanisms against primary influenza infection in mice. I. The roles of interferon and neutralizing antibodies and thymus dependence of interferon and antibody production. J Immunol 118:256, 1977.
29. McMichael AJ, Gotch FM, Noble GR: Cytotoxic T-cell immunity to influenza. N Engl J Med 309:13, 1983.
30. Wells MA, Ennis FA, Albrecht P: Recovery from vital respiratory infection II. Passive transfer of immune spleen cells to mice with influenza pneumonia. J Immunol 126:1042, 1981.
31. Kuwano K, Scott M, Young JF, et al: HA2 subunit of influenza AH1 and H2 subtype viruses induces a protective cross-reactive cytotoxic T-lymphocyte response. J Immunol 140:1264, 1988.
32. Clements ML, Betts RF, Tierney EL, et al: Serum and nasal wash antibodies associated with resistance to experimental challenge with influenza A wild-type virus. J Clin Microbiol 24:157, 1986.
33. Stuart-Harris CH: Clinical picture of influenza. *In* Stuart-Harris CH (ed): Influenza and Other Virus Infections of the Respiratory Tract. London, E Arnold, 1965, pp 8–21.
34. Imboden JB, Canter A, Cluff LE: Convalescence from influenza: A study of psychological and clinical determinants. Arch Intern Med 108:115, 1961.
35. Glezen WP, Paredes A, Taber LH: Influenza in children: Relationship to other respiratory agents. JAMA 243:1345, 1980.
36. Little JW, Hall WJ, Douglas RG Jr, et al: Airway hyperactivity and peripheral airway dysfunctions in influenza A infection. Am Rev Respir Dis 118:295, 1978.
37. Minor TE, Dick AN, Baker JJ: Rhinovirus and influenza A infections as precipitants of asthma. Am Rev Respir Dis 113:149, 1976.
38. Smith CB, Golden CA, Kanner RE, et al: Association of viral and *M. pneumoniae* infections with acute respiratory illness in patients with chronic obstructive pulmonary disease. Am Rev Respir Dis 121:225, 1980.
39. Louria DB, Blumenfield HL, Ellis JT, et al: Studies in influenza in the pandemic of 1957–1958. 11. Pulmonary complications of influenza. J Clin Invest 38:213, 1959.
40. Barker WH: Excess pneumonia- and influenza-associated hospitalization during influenza A epidemics in the US, 1970–1978. *In* Kendal AP, Patriarca PA (eds): Options for the Control of Influenza. UCLA Symposia on Molecular and Cellular Biology New Series, Vol 36. New York, Alan R Liss, 1986, pp 75–87.
41. Ruben FL, Cate TR: Influenza pneumonia. Semin Respir Infect 2:122, 1987.
42. Stevens KM: Cardiac stroke volume as a determinant of influenza fatality. N Engl J Med 295:1363, 1976.
43. MacDonald KL, Osterholm MT, Hedberg CW, et al: Toxic shock syndrome. A newly recognized complication of influenza and influenza-like illness. JAMA 257:1053, 1987.
44. Naficy K: Human influenza infection with proved viremia. N Engl J Med 269:264, 1963.
45. Minow RA, Gorbach S, Johnson BL, et al: Myoglobinuria associated with influenza A infection. Ann Intern Med 80:359, 1974.
46. Proby CM, Hackett D, Gupta S, et al: Acute myopericarditis in influenza A infection. Q J Med 60:887, 1986.
47. Wells CEC: Neurologic complications of so-called "influenza." A winter study in southeast Wales. Br Med J 1:369, 1971.
48. Marks JS, Halpin TJ: Gullain-Barré syndrome in recipients of A/New Jersey influenza vaccine. JAMA 243:2490, 1980.
49. Gamboa ET, Wolf A, Yahr MD, et al: Influenza virus antigen in postencephalitic parkinsonism brain. Arch Neurol 31:228, 1974.
50. Mattock C, Marmot M, Stern G: Could Parkinson's disease follow intrauterine influenza? A speculative hypothesis. J Neurol Neurosurg Psychiatry 51:753, 1988.
51. LaMontagne JR: Summary of a workshop on disease mechanisms and prospects for prevention of Reye's syndrome. J Infect Dis 148:943, 1983.
52. Forsyth BW, Horwitz RI, Acampora D, et al: New epidemiologic evidence confirming that bias does not explain the aspirin–Reye's syndrome association. JAMA 261:2517, 1989.
53. Jackson GG, Muldoon RL: Viruses causing common respiratory infections in man. V. Influenza A (Asian). J Infect Dis 131:308, 1975.
54. Stokes CE, Bernstein JM, Kyger SA, et al: Rapid diagnosis of influenza A and B by 24-hour fluorescent focus assays. J Clin Microbiol 26:1263, 1988.
55. Coonrod JD, Karathenasis P, Betts RF, et al: Enzyme-linked immunosorbent assay of core antigens for clinical diagnosis of influenza. J Med Virol 25:399, 1988.

56. Cherian T, Bobo L, Steinhoff MC, et al: Use of PCR–enzyme immunoassay for identification of influenza A virus matrix RNA in clinical samples negative for cultivable virus. J Clin Microbiol 32:623, 1994.
57. VanVoris LP, Betts RF, Hayden FG, et al: Successful treatment of naturally occurring influenza A/USSR/77 HN. JAMA 245:1128, 1981.
58. Hall CB, Dolin R, Gale CL: Children with influenza infection: Treatment with rimantadine. Pediatrics 80:275, 1987.
59. Center for Disease Control and Prevention: Prevention and control of influenza. Part II, Antiviral agents. MMWR Morbid Mortal Wkly Rep 43(RR-15):1, 1994.
60. Margolis KL, Nichol KL, Poland GA, Pluhar RE: Frequency of adverse reactions to influenza vaccine in the elderly. JAMA 264:1139, 1990.
61. Stein DS, Creticos CM, Jackson GG, et al: Oral ribavirin treatment of influenza A and B. Antimicrob Agents Chemother 31:1285, 1987.
62. Bernstein DI, Revman PD, Sherman JR: Ribavirin small-particle aerosol treatment of influenza B virus infection. Antimicrob Agents Chemother 32:761, 1988.
63. Dolin R, Reichman RC, Mynard R: A controlled trial of amantadine and rimantadine in the prophylaxis of influenza A infection. N Engl J Med 307:580, 1982.
64. Hayden FG, Belshe RB, Clover RD, et al: Emergence and apparent transmission of rimantadine-resistant influenza A virus in families. N Engl J Med 321:1696, 1989.
65. Barker WT, Mullooly JP: Influenza vaccination of elderly persons. Reduction of pneumonia and influenza hospitalization and deaths. JAMA 244:2547, 1980.
66. Patriarca PA, Weber JA, Parker RA, et al: Efficacy of influenza vaccine in nursing homes. Reduction of illness and complications during an influenza A (H3N2) epidemic. JAMA 253:1136, 1985.
67. Govaert TM, Thijs CT, Masurel N, et al: The efficacy of influenza vaccination in elderly individuals. A randomized double-blind placebo-controlled trial. JAMA 272:1661, 1994.

251

Parainfluenza Viruses

Brian R. Murphy

History and Classification

The parainfluenza viruses, medium-sized, enveloped viruses having a single-stranded, nonsegmented, negative-sense RNA genome, are important respiratory tract pathogens in infants and children.[1] Between 1956 and 1960, the four human parainfluenza viruses were first recovered and were quickly shown to be major causes of severe lower respiratory tract disease, including croup, bronchiolitis, and pneumonia.[2–7]

Two of the five human parainfluenza viruses, that is, parainfluenza virus (PIV) type 1 and PIV-3, belong to the genus *Paramyxovirus* in the Paramyxoviridae family (Table 251–1); the *Rubulavirus* genus contains the remaining three human parainfluenza viruses, namely PIV-2, PIV-4, and mumps virus. These five viruses have a common structure and genome organization and are antigenically related[1, 8]; in addition, they share an attachment protein with both hemagglutination and neuraminidase activities. In contrast, viruses of the *Morbillivirus* genus have an attachment protein that has hemagglutination but not neuraminidase activity. The attachment glycoprotein of the pneumoviruses lacks both hemagglutination and neuraminidase activity. Paramyxoviruses in various mammalian and avian species are antigenically related to human strains[9–13] (see Table 251–1).

Characteristics of the Pathogen

Morphology

Parainfluenza viruses are pleomorphic and range in average diameter from 150 to 200 nm.[1] Virions contain spikes projecting from the lipid bilayer (Fig. 251–1) consisting of a hemagglutinin-neuraminidase (HN) glycoprotein or a fusion (F) glycoprotein embedded in the lipid bilayer by a hydrophobic anchor sequence and also contain a "tail" that extends into the virion. Underlying the lipid bilayer is a layer of matrix (M) protein that interacts with the surface glycoproteins, the lipid bilayer, and the nucleocapsid. The nucleocapsid consists of RNA, the nucleoprotein (NP), and the L and P proteins, which constitute the polymerase complex. The L and P proteins colocalize in clusters in nucleocapsids isolated from infected cells.[14, 15] Nucleocapsids also contain some M protein.

Virions bud from the plasma membrane of infected cells. It is thought that HN, F, and M proteins colocalize on the plasma membrane through an interaction of the M protein with the transmembrane or tail region of the surface glycoproteins. Nucleocapsids next interact with the M protein, and budding is initiated.

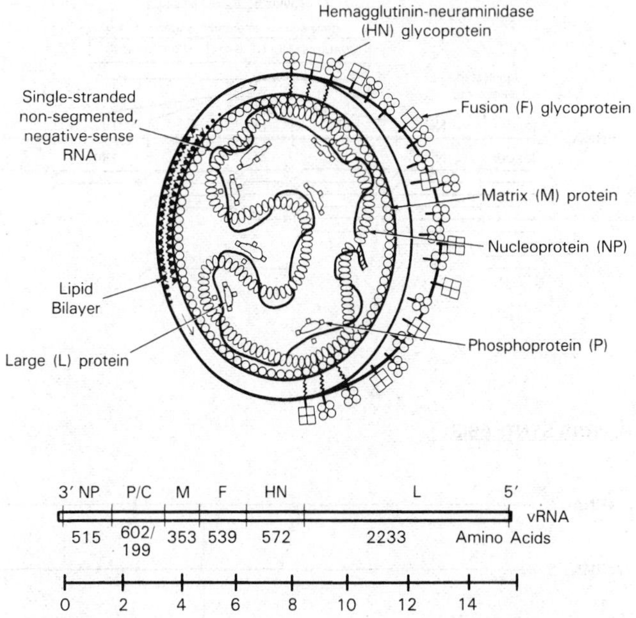

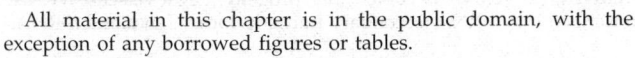

FIGURE 251–1 □ Parainfluenza virus virion. Viral glycoproteins are homotetramers (hemagglutinin-neuraminidase [HN] glycoprotein) or homotrimers (fusion [F] glycoprotein) that are inserted into the lipid bilayer by a hydrophobic anchor domain. Under the lipid bilayer is the M protein, which interacts with the nucleocapsid containing nucleoprotein (NP), P protein, and L protein and RNA. The RNA has terminal complementarity that can arrange into a panhandle. The NP protein protects the RNA from digestion with ribonuclease. The L and P proteins constitute the virion-associated polymerase.

TABLE 251–1 ■ Classification of the Viruses Within the Paramyxoviridae Family

	ACTIVITY OF ATTACHMENT GLYCOPROTEIN			RELATED ANIMAL VIRUSES	
GENUS	Hemagglutinin	Neuraminidase	HUMAN VIRUSES*	Name of Prototype Animal Virus	Species
Paramyxovirus	+	+	PIV-1	Sendai virus	Murine
	+	+	PIV-3	Shipping fever virus	Bovine
Rubulavirus	+	+	PIV-2	Simian virus 5	Canine
	+	+	PIV-4A, −4B	—	—
	+	+	Mumps virus	—	—
	+	+	—	Newcastle disease virus (seven serotypes)	Avian
Morbillivirus	+	0	Measles virus	Distemper virus	Canine
				Rinderpest virus	Bovine
Pneumovirus	0	0	RSV (subgroups A and B)	Bovine RSV	Bovine
				Pneumonia virus of mice	Murine
				Rhinotracheitis virus	Avian

*PIV, Parainfluenza virus; RSV, respiratory syncytial virus.

Organization of the Genome

The genome of human PIV-3 has been completely characterized and forms the basis for discussion here.[16–25] The linear genome is single stranded, negative sense, and 15,461 nucleotides in length and is transcribed into six messenger RNAs (mRNAs) that encode seven proteins (Fig. 251–2; see Fig. 251–1). One mRNA encodes two proteins (P and C) that are translated in different reading frames. The C protein is present in infected cells but not in virions. Although the other parainfluenza viruses have gene products and gene maps that are similar to those of PIV-3, they employ several different strategies for encoding their nonstructural proteins, which are described in detail elsewhere.[1, 26–31] Also, it was shown that several paramyxoviruses synthesize two forms of the P mRNA, one that is an exact copy of the genomic RNA and a second that contains the insertion of one or two nontemplated nucleotides. The insertion changes the reading

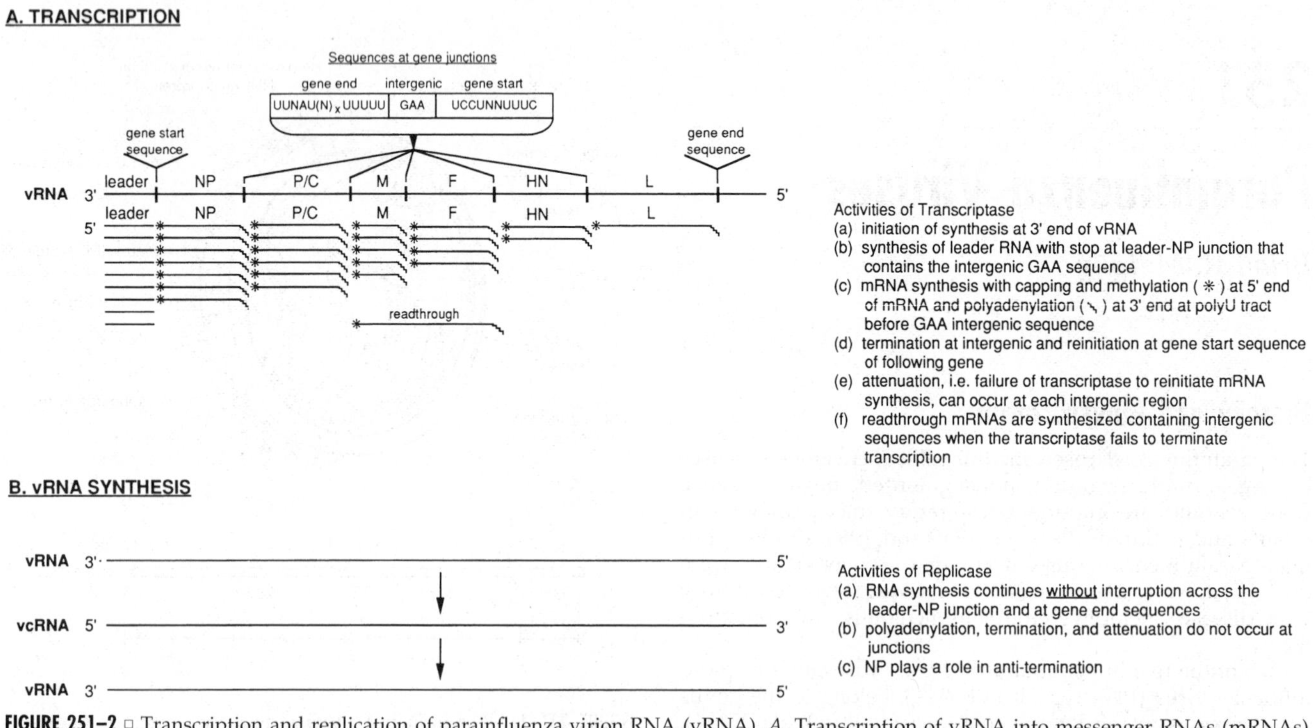
A. TRANSCRIPTION
Sequences at gene junctions
gene end
intergenic
gene start
UUNAU(N)x UUUUU
GAA
UCCUNNUUUC
gene start sequence
gene end sequence
vRNA 3'
leader
NP
P/C
M
F
HN
L
5'
readthrough
Activities of Transcriptase
(a) initiation of synthesis at 3' end of vRNA
(b) synthesis of leader RNA with stop at leader-NP junction that contains the intergenic GAA sequence
(c) mRNA synthesis with capping and methylation (✻) at 5' end of mRNA and polyadenylation at 3' end at polyU tract before GAA intergenic sequence
(d) termination at intergenic and reinitiation at gene start sequence of following gene
(e) attenuation, i.e. failure of transcriptase to reinitiate mRNA synthesis, can occur at each intergenic region
(f) readthrough mRNAs are synthesized containing intergenic sequences when the transcriptase fails to terminate transcription
B. vRNA SYNTHESIS
vRNA 3'
5'
vcRNA 5'
3'
vRNA 3'
5'
Activities of Replicase
(a) RNA synthesis continues without interruption across the leader-NP junction and at gene end sequences
(b) polyadenylation, termination, and attenuation do not occur at junctions
(c) NP plays a role in anti-termination

FIGURE 251–2 □ Transcription and replication of parainfluenza virion RNA (vRNA). *A,* Transcription of vRNA into messenger RNAs (mRNAs) is mediated by the L and P proteins. Transcription is initiated at a single promoter at the 3′ end and proceeds sequentially along the entire genome. The junctional sequences (i.e., gene end, intergenic, and gene start) indicated are those for human PIV-3. This drawing is a composite that incorporates information derived from other parainfluenza viruses, such as Sendai virus and Newcastle disease virus.[97, 98] Conserved intergenic sequences are a feature of PIV-3 and Sendai viruses, but mumps virus, simian virus 5, and Newcastle disease virus have intergenic sequences that vary in length. The decrease in the mRNA abundance as transcription proceeds from the 3′ to the 5′ end of vRNA is thought to be a consequence of polymerase falloff at intergenic regions during sequential transcription. *B,* RNA replication has two steps: (1) negative-sense vRNA is copied into positive-sense, virion-complementary RNA (vcRNA); (2) vcRNA is copied into progeny, negative-sense vRNA. The newly synthesized vRNA can be either incorporated into virions or transcribed into mRNA (secondary transcription). (Genes and mRNAs are not drawn to scale.)

frame, and the two different mRNAs encode P proteins that have the same N-terminals but that have different C-terminals.[26, 30] In addition, translational initiation can occur at internal AUG codons in both the P and C open reading frames, resulting in the synthesis of truncated forms of these proteins. Finally, mumps virus and simian virus 5 encode an additional protein, a small hydrophobic (SH) protein, from a separate mRNA located between the F and HN genes.[31, 32] The functions of the nonstructural and SH proteins are not known.

The 5′ and 3′ ends of the virion RNA are highly complementary in nucleotide sequence and presumably can form a panhandle, a structure thought to be important in replication.[20] Conserved nucleotide sequences are present at the end of genes, between genes (i.e., intergenic region), and at the start of genes that play a role in regulating transcription (see Fig. 251–2). The genome contains cis-acting promoter sequences at the 3′ end of virion RNA and virion-complementary RNA (see Fig. 251–2*B*). Parainfluenza viruses do not undergo genetic recombination, but complementation is efficient.[33]

Proteins

HN Glycoprotein. The HN protein is responsible for attachment of virus to neuraminic acid–containing glycolipid or glycoprotein cellular receptors and for release of virus from infected cells.[34, 35] The attachment function of the HN protein is responsible for agglutination of red blood cells (which have neuraminic acid–containing receptors on their surface) and for hemadsorption, in which red blood cells bind to HN proteins displayed on the plasma membrane of infected cells. The HN protein has enzymatic activity that cleaves neuraminic acid from cell receptors and from itself, which permits release of virus from infected cells and prevents self-aggregation of virions.

The PIV-3 HN glycoprotein, which contains 572 amino acids, forms a tetramer that is anchored to the virion membrane by a hydrophobic domain located near the N-terminal of the protein.[36] The globular ectodomain contains six antigenic sites, three of which are recognized by neutralizing antibodies.[37–39] An immune response to the HN protein is protective.[25, 40]

Fusion Glycoprotein. The F glycoprotein, which is a homotrimer,[41] is responsible for viral penetration by promoting fusion of the viral envelope with the plasma membrane of the cell. Like the HN protein, the F glycoprotein is displayed on the surface of infected cells. A cell that expresses F protein can fuse with a contiguous cell, leading to the formation of a syncytium, the characteristic cytopathic behavior of these viruses in tissue culture. Coexpression of the HN glycoprotein with the F glycoprotein is required for efficient fusion of contiguous cells.[42]

The PIV-3 F glycoprotein, which, like the HN glycoprotein, contains asparagine-linked carbohydrate, is 539 amino acids in length and contains an N-terminal hydrophobic signal sequence, an internal hydrophobic domain (the fusion domain) that is highly conserved among paramyxoviruses, and a hydrophobic anchor domain near its C-terminal.[23] Cleavage of the F protein ($F_0 \rightarrow F_1 + F_2$) into disulfide-linked subunits by host cell proteases is required for viral infectivity. As a result of this cleavage, the fusion domain of the F_0 becomes located at the new N-terminal of F_1 and is responsible for initiating the fusion of the viral and cellular membranes.[43] The relative cleavability of the F_0 glycoprotein is associated with the level of virulence of a virus and its ability to cause systemic disease.[44–46] The F glycoprotein of PIV-3 contains eight antigenic sites, four of which are recognized by antibodies with neutralizing or fusion-inhibiting activities.[47] Immunity to the F glycoprotein is protective.[25, 40]

M Protein. The PIV-3 M protein, 353 amino acids long, is a virion structural protein that is thought to play an important role in viral maturation and assembly via interactions with viral glycoproteins or the NP protein of the nucleocapsid.[19, 24, 48, 49]

NP Protein. The PIV-3 NP protein (515 amino acids long) is the most abundant virion protein (1600 to 2000 copies per virion).[17] The NP protein interacts with itself, with viral RNA, and with P protein in nucleocapsid assembly[50, 51] and is the major contributor to the helical symmetry of the ribonucleoprotein. In addition to its structural role, the NP protein is thought to play a role in the switch from transcription of virion RNA to replication of virion-complementary RNA[52] (see Fig. 251–2). Antibodies to the NP protein inhibit transcription of virion RNA in an in vitro reaction.[53]

P and L Proteins. The P and L proteins are responsible for transcriptase and replicase activities; in addition, the P protein functions in the assembly of nucleocapsids.[54] The relative contribution of each protein to nucleocapsid assembly and to the enzymatic activities is incompletely defined.[55] There are about 30 copies of L and 300 copies of P per virion.[50] The L and P proteins are 2233 and 602 amino acids long, respectively.[16, 20] Also, by the synthesis of a second form of the P mRNA containing nontemplated nucleotides as described earlier, parainfluenza viruses encode a second P-related protein that contains a different C-terminal domain containing a highly conserved cysteine-rich region that might have important biologic functions.[26, 30] A diagram of transcription and replication mediated by the L and P proteins is presented in Figure 251–2.

Epidemiology and Clinical Illness

PIV-1, -2, -3, and -4 have a worldwide distribution and are transmitted from person to person by aerosol or by contact with infected secretions. There is no known animal reservoir for the human parainfluenza viruses.

PIV-1, -2, -3, and -4 are unrelated by neutralization assays using postinfection animal serum[56] but share common antigens as revealed by complement fixation or radioimmunoprecipitation test.[57] The NP protein is antigenically related among the parainfluenza viruses and probably accounts for some of the elevation in heterotypic antibody titer that is common after infection with this group of viruses.[57–59] PIV-3 is a monotypic virus with highly conserved HN and F glycoproteins as revealed by antigenic analysis using monoclonal antibodies and sequence analysis of the HN and F genes of geographically diverse clinical isolates.[37, 60] PIV-1 and PIV-2 are also monotypic, like PIV-3, but PIV-4A and PIV-4B are distinct in cross-neutralization tests.[56, 61] Progressive accumulation of antigenic changes such as the antigenic drift of influenza A virus is not seen with the parainfluenza viruses.[59]

Parainfluenza viruses cause disease in infants, children, and adults, but serious disease generally occurs during the first 5 years of life.[7, 62–76] Usually the parainfluenza viruses cause febrile illness, consisting of rhinitis, pharyngitis, and bronchitis,[7, 64] but they can also cause a more serious lower respiratory tract disease that requires hospitalization of the patient (Table 251–2). PIV-3 is an important agent of bronchiolitis and pneumonia, being second only to respiratory syncytial virus (RSV) as a leading cause of lower respiratory tract disease in the pediatric age group. PIV-1, PIV-2, and PIV-3 are important causes of croup. PIV-4A and PIV-4B infrequently cause serious lower respiratory tract disease, but they are associated with mild upper tract disease.[59, 65, 77, 78]

TABLE 251–2 ■ Pediatric Respiratory Infections* in Inpatients† Caused by Parainfluenza Virus (PIV), Influenza Virus, or Respiratory Syncytial Virus (RSV)

		PATIENTS WITH EVIDENCE OF INFECTION (%)							
ILLNESS	NUMBER TESTED	RSV	PIV-3	PIV-1	PIV-2	Any PIV‡	Flu A H2N2‡	Flu A H3N2§	Flu B
Pneumonia	1162–1742	25.0	11.2	3.5	1.6	14.4	3.5	5.4	1.0
Bronchiolitis	873–1186	43.1	8.4	2.4	1.1	10.9	0.9	2.5	0.4
Croup	593–776	9.8	17.3	20.3	12.2	41.4	7.7	24.1	1.9
Pharyngitis-bronchitis	895–1337	10.6	11.0	3.7	2.0	14.7	2.0	4.6	0.9
Total respiratory	3523–5104	23.3	11.5	6.0	3.2	17.9	3.2	7.1	1.0
Inpatient control	1237–2155	5.4	5.0	1.9	1.2	7.5	0.5	0.9	0.5

*Infection documented by virus isolation or serum complement fixation antibody response.
†Studies performed at Children's Hospital National Medical Center from 1957 to 1976. Data from Kim et al (1973)[99] for RSV; Kim et al (1979)[100] for influenza; and Murphy et al[101] for PIV.
‡Tested from 1957 to 1968. Flu, influenza.
§Tested from 1968 to 1976.
Reprinted from Virus Res, volume 11, issue 1, Murphy BR, Prince GA, Collins PL, et al: Current approaches to the development of vaccines effective against parainfluenza and respiratory syncytial viruses, pages 1–15, with kind permission of Elsevier Science-NL, Sara Burgerhartstraat 25, 1055 KV Amsterdam, The Netherlands.

The upper and lower respiratory tract illnesses caused by RSV and the parainfluenza viruses are not clinically distinct, and identification of the agent requires virologic or immunologic techniques.

The most serious illness caused by PIV-3 occurs within the first 6 months of life, and in this way PIV-3 resembles RSV. In contrast, PIV-1 and PIV-2 generally cause serious illness after 6 months of life but before 5 years of age.[5, 65, 79] A large majority of children are infected by PIV-3 by age 2 years and by PIV-1 or PIV-2 by 5 years. First infections with these viruses are usually associated with febrile or respiratory illness, but usually less than 1% are severe enough to require hospitalization. Reinfections of decreasing severity are a hallmark of the parainfluenza viruses, particularly of PIV-3.[65, 67] Nosocomial infection occurs.[80] A comparison of the features of infection with RSV and the parainfluenza viruses is given in Table 251–3. In general, RSV and PIV-3 share the following characteristics: First, they undergo multiple-cycle replication in heteroploid cells in culture without exogenous trypsin (e.g., type 2 human epithelial [HEp-2] and Lewis lung carcinoma–monkey kidney [LLC-MK2] cells).[81] Second, they cause disease in the distal parts of the lung—the bronchioles and alveoli. Third, serious disease is caused within the first 4 months of life. Finally, severe disease with dissemination occurs in immunodeficient infants, children, and adults.[82, 83] It is possible that the differences between RSV and PIV-3, on the one hand, and PIV-1, on the other, are due to a greater cleavability of F glycoproteins of PIV-3 and RSV in heteroploid cells than of PIV-1, but this remains to be formally demonstrated in vivo. PIV-2 has the same cleavability as PIV-3 in heteroploid cells but is less virulent.

PIV-1 and PIV-2 cause discrete epidemics in the fall or winter, and PIV-3 causes endemic disease with periods of heightened activity, although significant variability in these epidemic patterns has been observed over time and in different locations.[5, 65, 67, 79, 84]

Pathogenesis and Immunity

The pathogenesis of PIV-1 infection in adults is depicted in Figure 251–3. In general, the incubation period for the parainfluenza viruses is between 2 and 6 days.[85, 86] Virus is generally cleared within 10 days of infection, but shedding of PIV-3 can be prolonged.[86, 87] Spread of the parainfluenza viruses outside the respiratory tract is rare,[87, 88] whereas for mumps and measles virus it is the rule. The mechanisms underlying the gradient in severity of disease caused by PIV-3 (bronchiolitis, pneumonia), PIV-1 and PIV-2 (croup), and PIV-4 (colds) are undefined. Interferon is seen in respiratory secretions after infection, and the parainfluenza viruses are interferon sensitive.[89]

Immunity to reinfection is conferred by prior infection with homologous virus but not by heterotypic virus.[11, 67] However, the homologous immunity induced is only partial, as indicated by frequent reinfection with homologous virus throughout the first 5 years of life. Evidence of immunity induced by prior infection is seen in the decrease in the frequency and severity of illness in persons undergoing reinfection with PIV-3.[65, 67] Several lines of evidence indicate that immunity to parainfluenza virus is mediated in part by antibody. First, there is sparing of PIV-1 and PIV-2 infections in the first 6 months of life when maternal antibody is present. Second, infants who possess a high level of maternal antibody to PIV-3 are less likely to develop illness caused by this virus within the first 5 months of life.[67] Third, a high level of neutralizing nasal wash immunoglobulin A antibody is associated with resistance to infection or illness caused by

TABLE 251–3 ■ Comparison of Human Paramyxoviruses That Cause Serious Lower Respiratory Tract Disease

VIRUSES	TRYPSIN REQUIRED FOR MULTISTEP REPLICATION IN HETEROPLOID CELLS	NUMBER OF BASIC AMINO ACIDS AT CLEAVAGE SITE*	CAUSE OF SEVERE PNEUMONIA OR BRONCHIOLITIS	CAUSE OF CROUP	SEVERE DISEASE IN IMMUNOCOMPROMISED HOST	AGE BY WHICH SEVERE LRT† DISEASE OCCURS (mo)
RSV	0	5	+ + + +	0	+ + +	≤4
PIV-3	0	3	+ + +	+ + +	+ + +	≤4
PIV-2	0	3	0	+ +	+	≥5
PIV-1	+	1	+	+ + + +	0	≥5

*The number of basic amino acids in the five C-terminal amino acids of F_1. The references for this are RSV,[102] PIV-3,[25] PIV-2,[103] and PIV-1.[104]
†LRT, Lower respiratory tract.

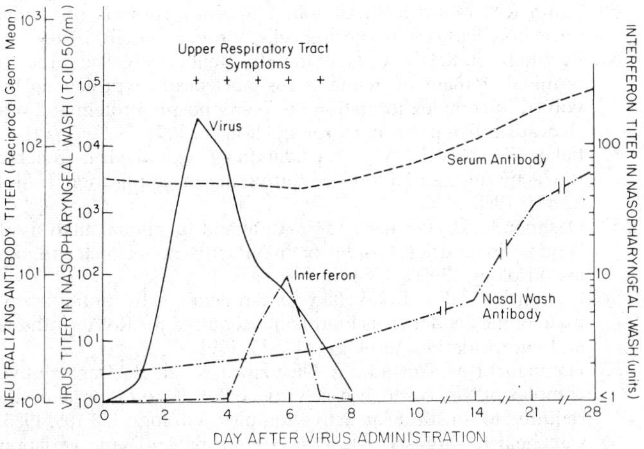

FIGURE 251–3 ▫ The response of adult volunteers to the intranasal administration of a median tissue culture infective dose of $10^{7.0}$ human PIV-1. (From Chanock RM, McIntosh K: Parainfluenza viruses. *In* Fields B [ed]: Fields Virology. New York, Raven Press, 1985, pp 1255–1284.)

PIV-1.[90] Fourth, passively transferred antibodies to the HN and F glycoproteins can protect experimental animals against infection or illness.[91] The role of cellular immune mechanisms in recovery from or resistance to human parainfluenza virus infection has not been defined. In experimental infection in mice, resolution of primary infection can be mediated by immune mechanisms dependent on functional $CD4^+$ T cells (and the antibody they provide help for) or $CD8^+$ T cells, indicating that the immune system is functionally redundant for clearance of primary infection.[92] Immunity to the HN and F glycoproteins is the major mediator of resistance to reinfection by paramyxoviruses.[25, 40, 91]

Diagnosis and Prevention

The respiratory tract illness caused by parainfluenza virus cannot be distinguished from those caused by other viral agents (e.g., rhinovirus, RSV, adenoviruses, orthomyxoviruses, or coronaviruses), by mycoplasmas, or by pathogenic bacteria. Specific laboratory diagnosis requires virus isolation with identification of the isolates using specific antisera (polyclonal or monoclonal) or identification of viral antigen (using specific monoclonal antibody) in secretions obtained from the respiratory tract.[69, 93] The parainfluenza viruses can be isolated in primary monkey kidney tissue or in a continuous line of LLC-MK2 cells with exogenous trypsin added.[81] Because heterotypic increases in antibody titers to members of the parainfluenza viruses occur in humans after infection, identification of the infecting virus by serologic techniques can be misleading. There are no specific antiviral therapies or vaccines for PIV-1, -2, -3, and -4. Inactivated vaccines against two other members of the Paramyxoviridae potentiated disease after natural infection with wild-type virus, which indicates that inactivated vaccine or subunit vaccines against the human parainfluenza viruses must be developed with considerable caution.[94, 95] New approaches to vaccine development have been reviewed.[96]

References

1. Kingsbury DW (ed): The Paramyxoviruses. New York, Plenum Publishing, 1991.
2. Beale AJ, McLeod DL, Stackiw W, Rhodes AJ: Isolation of cytopathogenic agents from the respiratory tract in acute laryngotracheobronchitis. Br Med J 1:303, 1958.
3. Chanock RM: Association of a new type of cytopathogenic myxovirus with infantile croup. J Exp Med 104:555, 1956.
4. Chanock RM, Parrott RH, Cook K, et al: Newly recognized myxoviruses from children with respiratory disease. N Engl J Med 258:207, 1958.
5. Glezen WP, Denny FW: Epidemiology of acute lower respiratory disease in children. N Engl J Med 288:498, 1973.
6. Johnson KM, Chanock RM, Cook MK, Huebner RJ: Studies of a new human hemadsorption virus. I. Isolation, properties and characterization. Am J Hyg 71:81, 1960.
7. Parrott RH, Vargosko A, Luckey A, et al: Clinical features of infection with hemadsorption viruses. N Engl J Med 260:731, 1959.
8. Pringle CR: The order Mononegavirales. Arch Virol 117:137, 1991.
9. Abinanti FR, Chanock RM, Cook MK, et al: Relationship of human and bovine strains of myxovirus para-influenza 3. Proc Soc Exp Biol Med 106:466, 1961.
10. Alexander DJ: Avian paramyxoviruses. Vet Bull 50:737, 1980.
11. Cook MK, Chanock RM: In vivo antigenic studies of parainfluenza viruses. Am J Hyg 77:150, 1963.
12. Chanock RM, Johnson KM, Cook MK, et al: The hemadsorption technique, with special reference to the problem of naturally occurring simian parainfluenza virus. Am Rev Respir Dis 83:125, 1961.
13. Goswami KKA, Russell WC: A comparison of paramyxoviruses by immunoprecipitation. J Gen Virol 60:177, 1982.
14. Portner A, Murti KG: Localization of P, NP, and M proteins on Sendai virus nucleocapsid using immunogold labeling. Virology 150:469, 1986.
15. Portner A, Murti KG, Morgan EM, Kingsbury DW: Antibodies against Sendai virus L protein: Distribution of the protein in nucleocapsids revealed by immunoelectron microscopy. Virology 163:236, 1988.
16. Galinski MS, Mink MA, Lambert DM, et al: Molecular cloning and sequence analysis of the human parainfluenza 3 virus mRNA encoding the P and C proteins. Virology 155:46, 1986.
17. Galinski MS, Mink MA, Lambert DM, et al: Molecular cloning and sequence analysis of the human parainfluenza 3 virus RNA encoding the nucleocapsid protein. Virology 149:139, 1986.
18. Galinski MS, Mink MA, Pons MW: Molecular cloning and sequence analysis of the human parainfluenza 3 virus genes encoding the surface glycoproteins, F and HN. Virus Res 8:205, 1987.
19. Galinski MS, Mink MA, Lambert DM, et al: Molecular cloning and sequence analysis of the human parainfluenza 3 virus gene encoding the matrix protein. Virology 157:24, 1987.
20. Galinski MS, Mink MA, Pons MW: Molecular cloning and sequence analysis of the human parainfluenza 3 virus gene encoding the L protein. Virology 165:499, 1988.
21. Spriggs MK, Collins PL: Human parainfluenza virus type 3: Messenger RNAs, polypeptide coding assignments, intergenic sequences, and genetic map. J Virol 59:646, 1986.
22. Spriggs MK, Collins PL: Sequence analysis of the P and C protein genes of human parainfluenza virus type 3: Patterns of amino acid sequence homology among paramyxovirus proteins. J Gen Virol 67:2705, 1986.
23. Spriggs MK, Olmsted RA, Venkatesan S, et al: Fusion glycoprotein of human parainfluenza virus type 3: Nucleotide sequence of the gene, direct identification of the cleavage-activation site, and comparison with other paramyxoviruses. Virology 152:241, 1986.
24. Spriggs MK, Johnson PR, Collins PL: Sequence analysis of the matrix protein gene of human parainfluenza virus type 3: Extensive sequence homology among paramyxoviruses. J Gen Virol 68:1491, 1987.
25. Spriggs MK, Murphy BR, Prince GA, et al: Expression of the F and HN glycoproteins of human parainfluenza virus type 3 recombinant vaccinia viruses: Contributions of the individual proteins to host immunity. J Virol 61:3416, 1987.
26. Thomas SM, Lamb RA, Paterson RG: Two mRNAs that differ by two nontemplated nucleotides encode the amino co-terminal proteins P and V of the paramyxovirus SV5. Cell 54:891, 1988.
27. Takeuchi K, Hishiyama M, Yamada A, Sugiura A: Molecular

cloning and sequence analysis of the mumps virus gene encoding the P protein: Mumps virus P gene is monocistronic. J Gen Virol 69:2043, 1988.
28. Curran J, Kolakofsky D: Ribosomal initiation from an ACG codon in the Sendai virus P/C mRNA. EMBO J 7:245, 1988.
29. Collins PL, Huang YT, Wertz GW: Identification of a tenth mRNA of respiratory syncytial virus and assignment of polypeptides to the ten viral genes. J Virol 49:572, 1984.
30. Cattaneo R, Kaelin K, Baczko K, Billeter MA: Measles virus editing provides an additional cysteine-rich protein. Cell 56:759, 1989.
31. Hiebert SW, Richardson CD, Lamb RA: Cell surface expression and orientation in membranes of the 44 amino acid SH protein of simian virus 5. J Virol 62:2347, 1988.
32. Elango N, Varsanyi TM, Kovamees J, Norrby E: Molecular cloning and characterization of six genes, determination of gene order and intergenic sequences and leader sequence of mumps virus. J Gen Virol 69:2893, 1988.
33. Bratt MA, Hightower LE: Genetics and paragenetic phenomena of paramyxoviruses. *In* Fraenkel-Conrat H, Wagner RR (eds): Comprehensive Virology. Regulation and Genetics. Genetics of Animal Viruses, Vol 9. New York, Plenum Publishing, 1977, pp 457–533.
34. Suzuki Y, Suzuki T, Matsumoto M: Isolation and characterization of receptor sialoglycoprotein for hemagglutinating virus of Japan (Sendai virus) from bovine erythrocyte membrane. J Biochem (Tokyo) 93:1621, 1983.
35. Umeda M, Nojima S, Inoue K: Activity of human erythrocyte gangliosides as a receptor to HVJ. Virology 133:172, 1984.
36. Elango N, Coligan JE, Jambou RC, Venkatesan S: Human parainfluenza type 3 hemagglutinin-neuraminidase glycoprotein: Nucleotide sequence of mRNA and limited amino acid sequence of the purified protein. J Virol 57:481, 1986.
37. van Wyke Coelingh KL, Winter CC, Murphy BR: Antigenic variation in the hemagglutinin-neuraminidase protein of human parainfluenza type 3 virus. Virology 143:569, 1985.
38. van Wyke Coelingh KL, Winter CC, Jorgensen ED, Murphy BR: Antigenic and structural properties of the hemagglutinin-neuraminidase glycoprotein of human parainfluenza virus type 3: Sequence analysis of variants selected with monoclonal antibodies which inhibit infectivity, hemagglutination, and neuraminidase activities. J Virol 61:1473, 1987.
39. Portner A, Scroggs RA, Metzer DW: Distinct functions of antigenic sites of the HN glycoprotein of Sendai virus. Virology 158:61, 1987.
40. Paterson RG, Lamb RA, Moss B, Murphy BR: Comparison of the relative roles of the F and HN surface glycoproteins of the paramyxovirus simian virus 5 in inducing protective immunity. J Virol 61:1972, 1987.
41. Russell R, Paterson RG, Lamb RA: Studies with cross-linking reagents on the oligomeric form of the paramyxovirus fusion protein. Virology 199:160, 1994.
42. Sergel T, McGinnes LW, Morrison TG: The fusion promotion activity of the NDV HN protein does not correlate with neuraminidase activity. Virology 196:831, 1993.
43. Lamb RA: Paramyxovirus fusion: A hypothesis for changes. Virology 197:1, 1993.
44. Glickman RL, Syddall RJ, Iorio RM, et al: Quantitative basic residue requirements in the cleavage-activation site of the fusion glycoprotein as a determinant of virulence for Newcastle disease virus. J Virol 62:354, 1988.
45. Toyoda T, Sakaguchi JT, Imai K, et al: Structural comparison of the cleavage-activation site of the fusion glycoprotein between virulent and avirulent strains of Newcastle disease virus. Virology 158:242, 1987.
46. Tashiro M, Pritzer E, Khoshnan MA, et al: Characterization of a pantropic variant of Sendai virus derived from a host range mutant. Virology 165:577, 1988.
47. van Wyke Coelingh K, Tierney EL: Human parainfluenza type 3 fusion glycoprotein: Antigenic and functional organization. J Virol 63:375, 1989.
48. Sanderson CM, Wu H-H, Nayak DP: Sendai virus M protein binds independently to either the F or the HN glycoprotein in vivo. J Virol 68:69, 1994.
49. Peeples ME: Paramyxovirus M proteins: Pulling it all together and taking it on the road. *In* Kingsbury DW (ed): The Paramyxoviruses. New York, Plenum Publishing, 1991, pp 427–456.
50. Lamb RA, Mahy BWJ, Chopin PW: The synthesis of Sendai virus polypeptides in infected cells. Virology 69:116, 1976.
51. Buchholz CJ, Retzler C, Homann HE, Neubert WJ: The carboxy-terminal domain of Sendai virus nucleocapsid protein is involved in complex formation between phosphoprotein and nucleocapsid-like particles. Virology 204:770, 1994.
52. Baker SC, Moyer SA: Encapsidation of Sendai virus genome RNAs by purified NP protein during in vitro replication. J Virol 62:834, 1988.
53. Deshpande KL, Portner A: Structural and functional analysis of Sendai virus nucleocapsid protein NP with monoclonal antibodies. Virology 139:32, 1984.
54. Curran J, Pelet T, Kolakofsky D: An acidic activation-like domain of the Sendai virus P protein is required for RNA synthesis and encapsidation. Virology 202:875, 1994.
55. Hamaguchi M, Yoshida T, Nishikawa K, et al: Transcriptive complex of Newcastle disease virus. I. Both L and P proteins are required to constitute an active complex. Virology 128:105, 1983.
56. Canchola J, Vargosko AJ, Kim HW, et al: Antigenic variation among newly isolated strains of parainfluenza type 4 virus. Am J Hyg 79:357, 1964.
57. Ito Y, Tsurudome M, Hishiyama M, Yamada A: Immunological interrelationships among human and nonhuman paramyxoviruses revealed by immunoprecipitation. J Gen Virol 68:1289, 1987.
58. Chanock RM, Wong DC, Huebner RJ, Bell JA: Serologic response of individuals infected with parainfluenza viruses. Am J Public Health 50:1858, 1960.
59. Killgore GE, Dowdle WR: Antigenic characterization of parainfluenza 4A and 4B by the hemagglutination-inhibition test and distribution of HI antibody in human sera. Am J Epidemiol 91:308, 1970.
60. van Wyke Coelingh KL, Winter C, Murphy BR: Nucleotide and deduced amino acid sequence of hemagglutinin-neuraminidase genes of human type 3 parainfluenza viruses isolated from 1957 to 1983. Virology 162:137, 1988.
61. Komada H, Kusagawa S, Orvell C, et al: Antigenic diversity of human parainfluenza virus type 1 isolates and their immunological relationship with Sendai virus revealed by using monoclonal antibodies. J Gen Virol 73:875, 1992.
62. Denny FW, Murphy TF, Clyde WA Jr, et al: An 11 year study in a pediatric practice. Pediatrics 71:871, 1983.
63. Welliver RC, Wong DT, Sun M, McCarthy N: Parainfluenza virus bronchiolitis: Epidemiology and pathology. Am J Dis Child 140:34, 1986.
64. Parrott RH, Vargosko AJ, Kim HW, et al: Myxoviruses: Parainfluenza. Am J Public Health 52:907, 1962.
65. Chanock RM, Parrott RH, Johnson KM, et al: Myxoviruses: Parainfluenza. Am Rev Respir Dis 88:152, 1963.
66. Glezen WP, Loda FA, Denny FW: Parainfluenza viruses. *In* Evans AS (ed): Viral Infections of Humans: Epidemiology and Control. New York, Plenum Publishing, 1982, pp 441–454.
67. Glezen WP, Frank AL, Taber LH, Kasel JA: Parainfluenza virus type 3: Seasonality and risk of infection and reinfection in young children. J Infect Dis 150:851, 1984.
68. Clarke SKR: Parainfluenza virus infections. Postgrad Med J 49:792, 1973.
69. Gardner PS, McQuillin J, McGuckin R, Ditchburn RK: Observations on clinical and immunofluorescent diagnosis of parainfluenza virus infections. Br Med J 2:7, 1971.
70. Fox JP, Hall CE: Infections with other respiratory pathogens: Influenza, parainfluenza, mumps, and respiratory syncytial viruses; *Mycoplasma pneumoniae*. *In* Fox JP, Hall CE (eds): Viruses in Families. Littleton, MA, PSG Publishing, 1980, pp 335–381.
71. Evans AS, Dick EC: Acute pharyngitis and tonsillitis in University of Wisconsin students. JAMA 190:699, 1964.
72. Bloom HH, Johnson KM, Jacobsen R, Chanock RM: Recovery of parainfluenza viruses from adults with upper respiratory illness. Am J Hyg 74:50, 1961.
73. Mufson MA, Webb PA, Kennedy H, et al: Etiology of upper respiratory tract illnesses among civilian adults. JAMA 195:91, 1965.
74. Hall CB, Geiman JM, Breese BB, Douglas RG Jr: Parainfluenza viral infections in children: Correlation of shedding with clinical manifestations. J Pediatr 91:194, 1977.
75. Monto AS: The Tecumseh study of respiratory illness. V. Pat-

terns of infection with the parainfluenza viruses. Am J Epidemiol 97:338, 1973.
76. Downham MAPS, McQuillin J, Gardner PS: Diagnosis and clinical significance of parainfluenza virus infections in children. Arch Dis Child 49:8, 1974.
77. Gardner SD: The isolation of parainfluenza 4 subtypes A and B in England and serological studies of their prevalence. J Hyg (Lond) 67:545, 1969.
78. Rubin EE, Quennec P, McDonald JC: Infections due to parainfluenza virus type 4 in children. Clin Infect Dis 17:998, 1993.
79. Chanock RM, Parrott RH: Acute respiratory disease in infancy and childhood: Present understanding and prospects for prevention. Pediatrics 36:21, 1965.
80. Mufson MA, Mocega HE, Krause HE: Acquisition of parainfluenza 3 virus infection by hospitalized children. I. Frequencies, rates, and temporal data. J Infect Dis 128:141, 1973.
81. Frank AL, Couch RB, Griffis CA, Baxter BD: Comparison of different tissue cultures for isolation and quantitation of influenza and parainfluenza viruses. J Clin Microbiol 10:32, 1979.
82. Fishaut M, Tubergen D, McIntosh K: Cellular response to respiratory viruses with particular reference to children with disorders of cell-mediated immunity. J Pediatr 96:179, 1980.
83. Whimbey E, Bodey GP: Viral pneumonia in the immunocompromised adult with neoplastic disease: The role of common community respiratory viruses. Semin Respir Infect 7:122, 1992.
84. Knott AM, Long CE, Hall CB: Parainfluenza viral infections in pediatric outpatients: Seasonal patterns and clinical characteristics. Pediatr Infect Dis J 13:269, 1994.
85. Murphy BR, Richman DD, Chalhub EG, et al: Failure of attenuated temperature-sensitive influenza A (H3N2) virus to induce heterologous interference in humans to parainfluenza type 1 virus. Infect Immun 12:62, 1975.
86. Frank AL, Taber LH, Wells CR, et al: Patterns of shedding of myxoviruses and paramixoviruses in children. J Infect Dis 144:433, 1981.
87. Gross PA, Green RH, Curnen MGM: Persistent infection with parainfluenza type 3 virus in man. Am Rev Respir Dis 108:894, 1973.
88. Wong VK, Steinberg E, Warford A: Parainfluenza virus type 3 meningitis in an 11 month old infant. Pediatr Infect Dis J 7:300, 1988.
89. Hall CB, Douglas RG, Simons RL, Geiman JM: Interferon production in children with respiratory syncytial, influenza, and parainfluenza virus infections. J Pediatr 93:28, 1978.
90. Smith CB, Purcell RH, Bellanti JA, Chanock RM: Protective effect of antibody to parainfluenza type 1 virus. N Engl J Med 275:1145, 1966.
91. Örvell C, Grandien M: The effects of monoclonal antibodies on biologic activities of structural proteins of Sendai virus. J Immunol 129:2779, 1982.
92. Hou S, Doherty PC, Zijlstra M, et al: Delayed clearance of Sendai virus in mice lacking class I MHC–restricted $CD8^+$ T cells. J Immunol 149:1319, 1992.
93. Chanock RM: Parainfluenza viruses. *In* Lennette EH, Schmidt NJ (eds): Diagnostic Procedures for Viral, Rickettsial and Chlamydial Infections. Washington, DC, American Public Health Association, 1979, pp 611–632.
94. Fulginiti VA, Eller JJ, Downie AW, Kempe CH: Altered reactivity to measles virus. Atypical measles in children previously immunized with inactivated measles virus vaccines. JAMA 202:1075, 1967.
95. Kim HW, Canchola JG, Brandt CD, et al: Respiratory syncytial virus disease in infants despite prior administration of antigenic inactivated vaccine. Am J Epidemiol 89:422, 1969.
96. Murphy BR, Hall SL, Kulkarni AB, et al: An update on approaches to the development of respiratory syncytial virus (RSV) and parainfluenza virus type 3 (PIV3) vaccines. Virus Res 32:13, 1994.
97. Chambers P, Millar NS, Bingham RW, Emmerson PT: Molecular cloning of complementary DNA to Newcastle disease virus, and nucleotide sequence analysis of the junction between the genes encoding the haemagglutinin-neuraminidase and the large protein. J Gen Virol 67:475, 1986.
98. Hiebert SW, Paterson RG, Lamb RA: Identification and predicted sequence of a previously unrecognized small hydrophobic protein, SH, of the paramyxovirus simian virus 5. J Virol 55:744, 1985.
99. Kim HW, Arrobio JO, Brandt CD, et al: Epidemiology of respiratory syncytial virus infection in Washington, D.C. I. Importance of the virus in different respiratory tract disease syndromes and temporal distribution of infection. Am J Epidemiol 98:216, 1973.
100. Kim HW, Brandt CD, Arrobio JO, et al: Influenza A and B virus infection in infants and young children during the years 1957–1976. Am J Epidemiol 109:469, 1979.
101. Murphy BR, Prince GA, Collins PL, et al: Current approaches to the development of vaccines effective against parainfluenza and respiratory syncytial viruses. Virus Res 11:1, 1988.
102. Collins PL, Huang YT, Wertz GW: Nucleotide sequence of the gene encoding the fusion (F) glycoprotein of human respiratory syncytial virus. Proc Natl Acad Sci USA 81:7683, 1984.
103. Hu X, Compans RW, Matsuoka Y, Ray R: Molecular cloning and sequence analysis of the fusion glycoprotein gene of human parainfluenza virus type 2. Virology 179:915, 1990.
104. Merson JR, Hull RA, Estes MK, Kasel JA: Molecular cloning and sequence determination of the fusion protein gene of human parainfluenza virus type 1. Virology 167:97, 1988.

252

Mumps Virus

Hillel K. Janai
Adriano Arguedas
Melvin I. Marks

History and Epidemiology

Mumps, derived from the English dialectal *mump,* meaning "grimace," obtained its name from the most frequently associated physical finding—painful parotid swelling. Until the current era of virologic and serologic diagnostic capabilities, mumps was called epidemic parotitis. Although the mumps virus is the most common pathogen causing parotitis, other viruses have been identified as a cause of parotid swelling.[1]

A virus was first described as a cause of epidemic parotitis in 1934.[2] The authors of this elegant study showed that when saliva from patients with epidemic parotitis was inoculated into the parotid glands of monkeys, the monkeys developed parotitis. The parotid tissues were then excised, filtered, and inoculated into parotid glands of other monkeys. Identical parotid inflammation occurred.

As techniques of viral culture improved, the mumps virus was cultivated in embryonated chicken eggs. By using this technique to isolate the antigen, serologic and skin tests for delayed hypersensitivity to mumps virus were developed.[3] Virus inactivation with formalin and vaccine production proved to be effective in disease prevention; however, the protective period was short and this preparation was never widely used as a vaccine.[4] A live, attenuated mumps vaccine was developed by virus attenuation through passage in tissue culture and was licensed in 1967.[5]

Mumps is a contagious disease, and 90% of infections occur in the pediatric age group. Infectivity rates are difficult to evaluate because 30% to 40% of infections are subclinical. It is endemic throughout the year, with epidemics occurring among unvaccinated children and young adults, usually congregated in a kindergarten, school, or military camp.

Clinical Manifestations and Complications

Clinical manifestations of mumps in early childhood are mild, the most common being fever and painful parotid swelling. In older children and young adults, complications of mumps occur more often. These commonly include meningitis or meningoencephalitis, and orchitis. Other uncommon complications include pancreatitis, arthritis, labyrinthitis, myocarditis, and thyroiditis.[6] (For details, see Chapter 150.)

Virus Structure

Mumps virus belongs to the Paramyxoviridae family. Other viruses in this family include human pathogens, parainfluenza and measles viruses, as well as animal pathogens, such as Newcastle disease virus and simian viruses. Viruses from this family are usually spherical and measure 150 to 200 nm in diameter. Pleomorphism may exist with variant viral dimensions ranging between 100 and 700 nm[7] (Figs. 252–1 and 252–2).

The genetic material of mumps virus is encoded in a single-stranded RNA. After infecting a cell, messenger RNA is transcribed from the viral RNA by polymerase enzymes of viral origin. The core of the viral particle is helical and contains RNA incorporated with capsid proteins. This core is surrounded by an envelope composed of lipid and glycoprotein projections. The glycoproteins have two distinct properties. One has both hemagglutinin and neuraminidase activity, and the other, fusion and hemolysin properties.[8]

Mumps virus produces inclusion bodies in the cytoplasm of infected human cells in vivo but, unlike other paramyxoviruses, the mumps virus also produces intranuclear inclusions in infected tissue culture cells. These inclusions are called nucleocapsid antigen or soluble antigen. Antibodies directed against this soluble antigen persist for only a short period, and their detection may represent a recent infection. Cross-reactions may occur due to the presence of similar binding sites to other paramyxoviruses (simian virus 5, parainfluenza virus, Newcastle disease virus).

Infected cells can be identified by the appearance of two surface glycoproteins on their cell membrane, the hemagglutinin and the hemolysin-fusion antigens. The hemagglutinin is responsible for the hemadsorption phenomenon (adherence of erythrocytes to mumps-infected cells) and is used in the hemagglutination inhibition test, which quantitates specific mumps antibodies. The hemolysin-fusion glycoprotein causes fusion of cell membranes and the creation of multinucleated giant cells both in vivo and in vitro. The hemolysin-fusion glycoprotein also has an important pathogenic role in central nervous system manifestations of mumps. Monoclonal antibodies against this particular antigen prevent mumps-induced encephalitis and brain necrosis in animal models injected with the mumps virus intracerebrally.[9]

Immune Response

Mumps virus induces host immune responses primarily by humoral antibody formation and secondary cellular T-lymphocyte activation. The immune response does not differ between natural mumps infection and vaccine-induced immunity. Immunoglobulin (Ig) G is the major quantitative isotope followed by IgM, IgA, and IgE. IgG2 and IgG4 play almost no role in human immune response to mumps virus.[10]

The dynamics of immunoglobulin production in the cerebrospinal fluid of children with mumps meningitis are of interest. In children with meningoencephalitis, specific mumps immunoglobulin levels are detected earlier and remain higher than in children with meningitis alone. There is no shift from IgM to IgG as observed in the humoral response.[11] After infection, neutralizing antibodies maintain low but protective concentrations. Most persons have clinically apparent mumps only once in a lifetime. It is possible that subclinical mumps infections may occur after protective levels of neutralizing antibodies decline, thereby boosting immune response and protecting patients from clinical illness.[12]

Although a striking feature of mumps is parotid gland swelling, clinical infection with mumps can occur in its absence. Moreover, even with the lack of meningeal findings, cerebrospinal pleocytosis may frequently be found.[13]

Like other viruses, mumps virus activates lymphocytes. Studies in mice have shown that mumps virus induces pro-

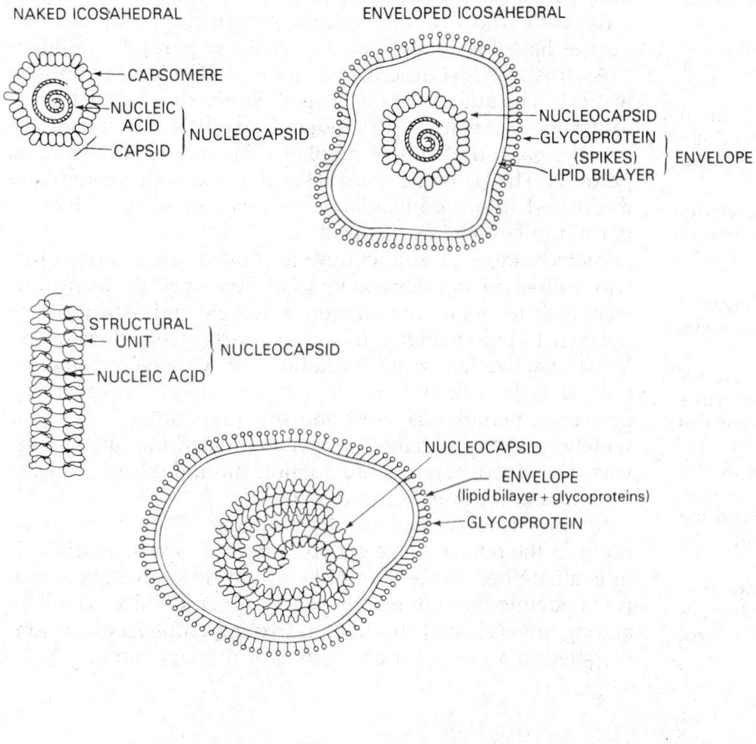

FIGURE 252–1 □ Schematic representation of mumps virus. (From Rippon JW: Medical mycology: The pathogenic fungi and the pathogenic actinomycetes. *In* Freeman BA [ed]: Burrows Textbook of Microbiology. Philadelphia, WB Saunders, 1979, pp 717–784.)

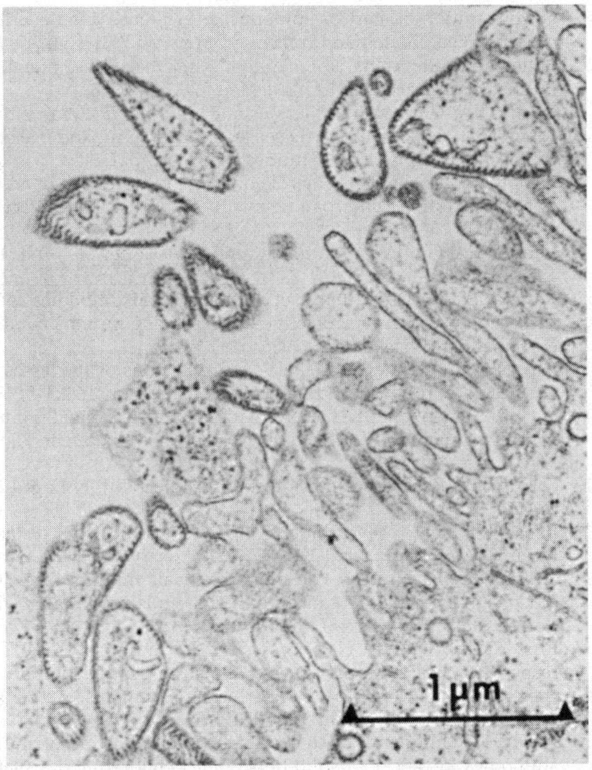

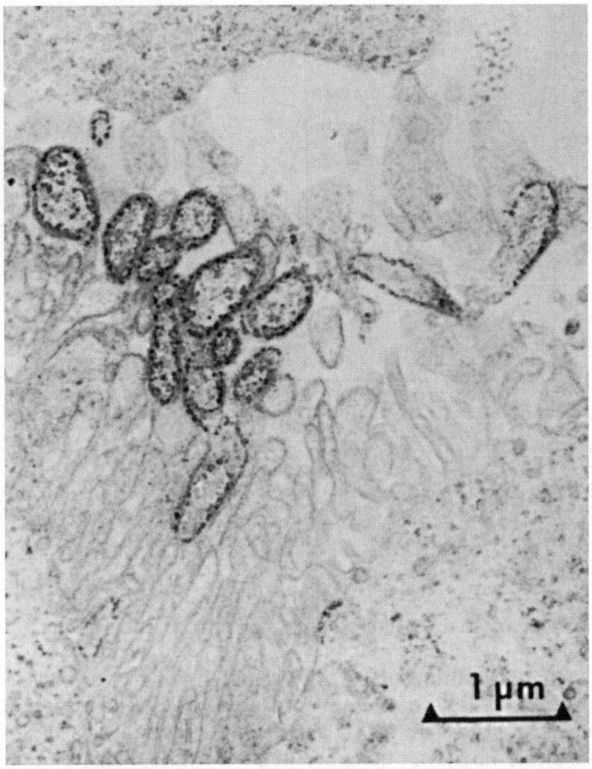

FIGURE 252–2 ▫ Mumps virions budding from epithelial cells of a hamster during experimental infection. (From Wolinsky JS, Servér AC: Mumps virus. *In* Fields BN [ed]: Virology. New York, Raven Press, 1985, pp 1255–1284.)

duction of helper T cells and killer cells, some of which have tumoricidal activity. Human studies in Japan have used mumps virus as immunotherapy in some types of advanced gynecologic cancers.[14] Patients were sensitized subcutaneously with mumps virus and later injected locally or systemically with the virus. Clinical improvement and tumor regression were observed in the majority of patients. The T-cell response to mumps virus is regulated by human leukocyte antigen restriction elements. (For a more detailed review of this phenomenon, see Bruserud and colleagues.[15])

The fact that mumps infection may induce islet cell antibodies has led to hypotheses linking mumps virus to the cause of type I diabetes mellitus.[16] Despite this, however, Schulz and colleagues[17] did not find any relationship between mumps infection and type I diabetes mellitus in a well-designed prospective study.

Diagnosis

The diagnosis of mumps is usually made on clinical grounds. A child with the typical appearance of swollen parotid glands and fever and a negative history of mumps immunization does not usually require serodiagnosis. If required, however, additional diagnostic methods are available (Table 252–1).

Mumps virus can be isolated from clinical specimens of patients with mumps, with or without parotitis. Saliva, urine, and cerebrospinal fluid specimens can be cultivated on a variety of cell line cultures. Syncytium formation can be pathognomonic, but hemadsorption and indirect immunofluorescence are both more sensitive.[18] Serologic tests for mumps virus have employed different methodologies with variable sensitivity and specificity, mainly because of cross-reactivity with other paramyxovirus antigens. For example, complement fixation of V and S antigens may cross-react with parainfluenza and other viral antigens. The hemagglutination inhibition test has the same cross-reactivity problems. The viral neutralization test, although specific, is complex and time-consuming.

Current laboratory methods for determining infection with mumps virus include measurement of the serum IgG component using an enzyme-linked immunoabsorbent assay in both acute and convalescent serum samples. Techniques have become available that allow measurement of IgM by a variation of the enzyme-linked immunosorbent assay known as antibody capture. By using this method, the assay can be performed in 6 hours, yielding results that are both highly sensitive and highly specific.[19,20] Also, polymerase chain reaction is available as a rapid method for detecting mumps virus within 48 hours.[21]

Prevention

No effective anti–mumps virus therapy exists, and passive immunization attempts have failed. Primary prevention with live, attenuated mumps virus has proved to be effective. Although antibody levels are 8- to 10-fold lower in postvacci-

TABLE 252–1 ■ Diagnostic Tests for Mumps Virus

Virus isolation
Viral culture (urine, saliva, cerebrospinal fluid)
Direct fluorescent antibody test (urine, saliva)
Serologic methods
Complement fixation for soluble antigen
Indirect fluorescent antibody test
Enzyme-linked immunosorbent assay
Antibody capture enzyme immunoassay

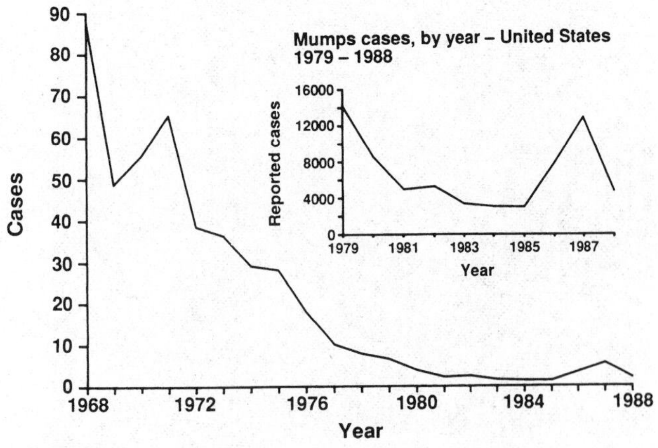

*Provisional data.

FIGURE 252–3 □ Mumps: reported cases per 100,000 population, by year, in the United States, 1968 to 1988. (From MMWR Morbid Mortal Wkly Rep 38:226, 1989.)

nation serum than in convalescent serum, neutralization of the clinical infection rate is high.[22]

As current immunization provides high, long-term protection, complications of mumps are now rarely encountered. However, a study from England, using 8716 samples of serum collected by five public health laboratories, revealed that 80% of children between 1 and 2 years of age lacked antibodies to mumps.[23] In the 3- to 4-year-old group, 55% were susceptible to mumps. In the United States between 1968 and 1985, reported cases of mumps decreased by 98.1%; however, in 1986, the reported cases of mumps more than doubled.[24] Furthermore, two large mumps outbreaks were reported to occur in 1987[24, 25] (Fig. 252–3). Questions about long-term efficacy of the vaccine have been raised. Cochi and colleagues[26] reviewed the data available on mumps vaccine since its introduction. Their survey pointed out that, after licensure, a decade elapsed before mumps vaccine was accepted as a routine immunization. Therefore, children born between 1967 and 1977 were not fully immunized, resulting in outbreaks within this high-risk group, especially in states that did not enforce vaccine administration before children entered school. Without enforcement of vaccine requirements, such epidemics may occur and may also affect part of the previously immunized population (in which vaccine efficacy ranges from 40% to 100%).[27–29]

Measles-mumps-rubella vaccine is commercially available, is safe and highly immunogenic, and provides protection. There are some fears of side effects because these vaccines contain animal and avian proteins with potential for allergic reactions. A new vaccine prepared with only human tissue provides similar antibody response and safety and is now commercially available.[28–30] (For more information, see Chapter 150.)

References

1. Tolpin MD, Schauf V: Mumps virus. *In* Belshe R (ed): Textbook of Human Virology. Littleton, MA, PSG Publishing, 1985, pp 311–331.
2. Johnson CD, Goodpasture EW: An investigation of the etiology of mumps. J Exp Med 59:1, 1934.
3. Enders JF: Mumps: Techniques of laboratory diagnosis, tests for susceptibility, and experiments on specific prophylaxis. J Pediatr 29:129, 1946.
4. Habel K: Vaccination of human beings against mumps: Vaccine administration at start of epidemic. I. Incidence and severity of mumps in vaccinated and control groups. Am J Hyg 54:295, 1951.
5. Hilleman MR, Buynak EB, Weibel RE, et al: Live, attenuated mumps-virus vaccine. N Engl J Med 278:227, 1968.
6. Young NA: Chickenpox, measles and mumps. *In* Remington JS, Klein JO (eds): Infectious Diseases of the Fetus and Newborn Infant. Philadelphia, WB Saunders, 1976, pp 521–586.
7. Choppin PW, Scheid A: The role of viral glycoproteins in adsorption, penetration, and pathogenicity of virus. Rev Infect Dis 2:40, 1980.
8. Lerner AM: Guide to immunization against mumps. J Infect Dis 122:116, 1970.
9. Love A, Rydbeck R, Utter G, et al: Monoclonal antibodies against the fusion protein are protective in necrotizing mumps meningoencephalitis. J Virol 58:220, 1986.
10. Sarnesto A, Julkunen I, Makela O: Proportions of Ig classes and subclasses in mumps antibodies. Scand J Immunol 22:345, 1985.
11. Statz A, Felgenhauer K: Differentiation of cerebrospinal immunoglobulins in mumps meningoencephalitis. Monatsschr Kinderheilkd 135:265, 1987.
12. Chang TW: Recurrent viral infection (reinfection). N Engl J Med 284:765, 1971.
13. Bank HO, Bang J: Involvement of the central nervous system in mumps. Acta Med Scand 113:487, 1943.
14. Shimizu Y, Hasumi K, Okudaira Y, et al: Immunotherapy of advanced gynecologic cancer patients utilizing mumps virus. Cancer Detect Prev 12:487, 1988.
15. Bruserud O, Paulsen G, Thorsby E: The mumps-specific T-cell response in healthy individuals and insulin-dependent diabetics: Preferential restriction by DR4-associated elements. Acta Pathol Microbiol Immunol Scand 95:173, 1987.
16. Hyoty H, Hiltunen M, Reunanen A, et al: Decline of mumps antibodies in type 1 (insulin-dependent) children and a plateau in the rising incidence of type 1 diabetes after introduction of the mumps-measles-rubella vaccine in Finland. Diabetologia 12:1303, 1993.
17. Schulz B, Michaelis D, Hildmann W, et al: Islet cell surface antibodies (ICSA) in subjects with a previous mumps injection—A prospective study over a 4 year period. Exp Clin Endocrinol 90:62, 1987.
18. Due-Nguyer H: Hemadsorption of mumps virus examined by light and electron microscopy. J Virol 2:494, 1968.
19. Sakata H, Tsurudome M, Hishiyama M, et al: Enzyme-linked immunosorbent assay for mumps IgM antibody: Comparison of IgM capture and indirect IgM assay. J Virol Methods 12:303, 1985.
20. Glikmann G, Pedersen M, Mordhorst CH: Detection of specific immunoglobulin M to mumps virus in serum and cerebrospinal fluid samples from patients with acute mumps infection, using an antibody-capture enzyme immunoassay. Acta Pathol Microbiol Immunol Scand 94:145, 1986.
21. Boriskin Y, Booth JC, Yamada A: Rapid detection of mumps virus by the polymerase chain reaction. J Virol Methods 42:23, 1993.
22. Fedova D, Bruckova M, Plesnik V, et al: Detection of post vaccination mumps virus antibody by neutralization test, enzyme-linked immunosorbent assay and sensitive hemagglutination inhibition test. J Hyg Epidemiol Microbiol Immunol 31:409, 1987.
23. Morgan-Capner P, Wright J, Miller CL, Miller E: Surveillance of antibody to measles, mumps, and rubella by age. BMJ 297:770, 1988.
24. Wharton M, Cochi SL, Hutcheson RH, et al: A large outbreak of mumps in the postvaccine era. J Infect Dis 158:1253, 1988.
25. Kaplan KM, Marder DC, Cochi SL, et al: Mumps in the workplace. Further evidence of the changing epidemiology of a childhood vaccine-preventable disease. JAMA 260:1434, 1988.
26. Cochi SL, Preblud SR, Orenstein WA: Perspectives on the relative resurgence of mumps in the United States. Am J Dis Child 142:499, 1988.
27. Fahlgren K: Two doses of MMR vaccine—Sufficient to eradicate measles, mumps and rubella? Scand J Soc Med 16:129, 1988.
28. Forsey T: Mumps vaccines—Current status (Editorial). J Med Microbiol 4:1, 1994.
29. Hersh BS, Fine PEM, Kent WK, et al: Mumps outbreak in a highly vaccinated population. J Pediatr 119:187, 1991.
30. Just M, Berger R, Gluck R, et al: Evaluation of combined vaccine against measles-mumps-rubella produced on human diploid cells. Dev Biol Stand 65:25, 1986.

253

Rubeola (Measles) and Subacute Sclerosing Panencephalitis Virus

David I. Bernstein
Peter D. Reuman
Gilbert M. Schiff

Rubeola

Measles virus causes a relatively distinct exanthematous disease characterized by a prodrome of fever, cough, coryza, and conjunctivitis followed by an erythematous, maculopapular, confluent rash and a pathognomonic enanthema (Koplik spots). Because of this and its highly contagious nature and high morbidity, measles (rubeola) was recognized in early civilizations, although it was frequently confused with smallpox and other exanthematous diseases.[1] Thanks to the introduction of effective vaccines, serious complications involving the respiratory tract and central nervous system (CNS) now occur only rarely in developed countries, but they were common earlier and remain a major cause of mortality and morbidity in underdeveloped countries.

History

The first description of measles as an entity distinct from smallpox was credited to Rhazes, a 10th century Persian physician, although he quoted other authors as far back as the 7th century.[2] Even during the Middle Ages, smallpox and measles continued to be confused, and it was not until the early 17th century that the distinction between the two diseases was relatively clear.[3] John Hall was the first to describe measles in America, reporting on a 1657 epidemic in Boston.[4] The pathognomonic enanthema of measles was first reported by Koplik[5] in 1896, although Koplik spots were recognized about a century earlier by John Quier and Richard Hazeltine.[4, 6] The extraordinary work and report of Panum[7] on an epidemic in the Faroe Islands defined the 14-day incubation period and lifetime immunity.

Measles was first transmitted to monkeys by Josias in 1898; Anderson and Goldberger (in 1911) and Blake and Trask (in 1921) demonstrated that monkeys could be infected with blood and nasopharyngeal secretions obtained from measles patients.[8] Plotz in 1938 and Rake and Shaffer in 1942 reported the adaptation of measles virus to chick embryos, although reliable tissue culture methods did not become available until a decade later.[3] In 1954, Enders and Peebles[9] reported isolating measles virus in human and rhesus monkey kidney tissue culture and the neutralization of the cytopathic effect by measles convalescent-phase serum. During the 1960s, the relationship between acute measles and the rare development of a late progressive encephalitis (subacute sclerosing panencephalitis [SSPE]) was uncovered.[10]

The further adaptation of measles virus to grow in chicken embryo tissue culture[11] led the way for the development of measles vaccines. Extensive trials of killed and attenuated (live) measles vaccines were conducted from 1958 to 1962. In 1963, both became available for general use, followed by the development and widespread use after 1965 of live, further attenuated measles vaccines. Since the Childhood Immunization Initiative and the Measles Elimination Program, which began in 1978, the incidence of measles in the United States has fallen dramatically. However, continued outbreaks of measles in the United States[12, 13] demonstrate that elimination of measles remains a difficult goal despite predictions that it would be eliminated by 1982.[14] The current Expanded Programme on Immunizations of the World Health Organization has a global target of reducing measles incidence by 90% and mortality by 95% from preprogram levels by 1995.[15]

Characteristics of the Pathogen

CLASSIFICATION

Measles virus is a member of the genus *Morbillivirus* in the family Paramyxoviridae. Included in this genus are canine distemper and rinderpest viruses, which share close immunologic relationships to measles.[16–18] More recently, morbilliviruses have been recognized in disease outbreaks in aquatic mammals.[19] Morbilliviruses differ from other paramyxoviruses in that they lack detectable neuraminidase activity and interact with cellular receptors that are insensitive to neuraminidase treatment.[16] Measles virus is a relatively large enveloped RNA virus with a spherical but pleomorphic shape. The diameter of the particle varies between 100 and 250 nm (mean, about 150 nm).

STRUCTURE

The measles virus is composed of an outer lipoprotein envelope surrounding a helical nucleocapsid.[16] The lipid in the virus envelope is derived from the host cell as it buds from the cell membrane. Six viral structural proteins and one nonstructural protein have been identified[18, 20] (Fig. 253–1). The nucleocapsid is a coiled rod that contains the viral genome RNA. About 5% of the nucleocapsid is RNA (molecular mass approximately 4.8 MDa). The outer envelope is 10 to 22 nm thick and contains the H (hemagglutinin) and F (fusion) factors, which are inserted into the lipid envelope as short surface projections or spikes, as well as the M (matrix) protein. The H and F proteins are glycosylated. The H protein is responsible for hemagglutination and mediates the adsorption of virus to the host cell. The H peplomers are formed by more than one and possibly three H molecules. The H and F proteins appear to function together for cell fusion of virus and host cell.[21] The F protein is synthesized as a 55- to 60-kDa glycoprotein; the fusion activity is generated by cleavage into a nonglycosylated F_1 part and a glycosylated F_2 part. The M protein is nonglycosylated and is associated with the inner lipid bilayer of the envelope. It appears to play a role in assembly of the virus.

The virus genome is linear, negative-sense RNA that is complexed with three viral proteins. Thus, the genome RNA must first be transcribed into message sense before production of virus-coded proteins. Sequence data are available for much of the genome. The linear order of genes is 3′-N-P/C-M-F-H-L-5′, the same as for Sendai virus.[18] The NP (nucleoprotein) is the major internal protein. It is phosphorylated and protects the viral RNA. The other internal virion components are the L, large protein, and the P, polymerase (phospho) protein. Both are believed to be part of the transcription complex. In addition to these six structural proteins, there is a nonstructural protein, C protein. Measles virions also contain an internal RNA-dependent RNA polymerase like other negative-sense RNA viruses.[22]

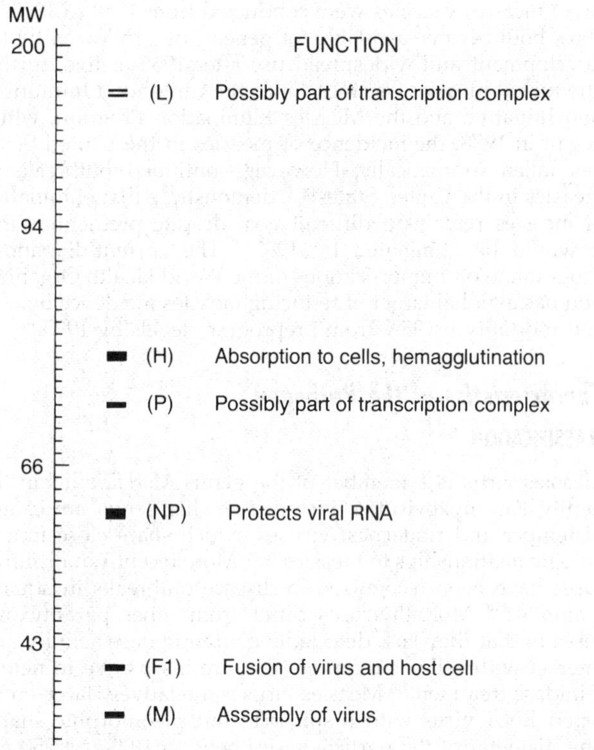

FIGURE 253–1 ▫ Schematic representation of sodium dodecyl sulfate–polyacrylamide gel electrophoresis pattern of measles virus proteins and their corresponding function. On the left are molecular weight standards ($\times 10^{-3}$).

BIOLOGIC AND BIOCHEMICAL PROPERTIES

Only a small fraction of virions produced in culture are infectious[16] because many noninfective particles are synthesized and infectious particles are rapidly inactivated. Infectious virions are rapidly inactivated by heat, ultraviolet light, lipid solvents, and extremes of acidity and alkalinity (pH below 5 or above 10).[23] Their lability at room temperature is of major importance in the handling of vaccines. Measles virus suspensions that have been stabilized with protein can be stored at −70°C for years without significant loss of infectivity.

REPLICATION

Measles virus can infect a broad range of nucleated cells, although it is not easily isolated from infected patients.[24] The human CD46 molecule or membrane cofactor protein has been identified as a major measles virus receptor.[25] Recovery of virus from infected persons occurs best with primary human and monkey kidney culture.[26] Isolation of virus from patients with SSPE requires cocultivation of explant cultures of brain tissue with cells susceptible to measles virus, although the viruses recovered by this method are often defective replicating viruses.

Two distinct types of cytopathic effects are seen in tissue culture.[16] Syncytium formation, or giant cells, form when boundaries of adjoining cells are lost and nuclei aggregate to the center. Ten to 50 nuclei containing intranuclear inclusion bodies may be present. The second form of cytopathic effect is characterized by a change of individual polygonal-looking cells into a spindle or stellate form that is often refractile. The proportion of the various changes depends on the virus strain, passage conditions, and host cells. Replication in tissue culture proceeds through an attachment phase followed by the adsorption of virus and an eclipse phase of 6 to 12 hours. Measles antigen can first be detected at about 12 hours. Most virus remains cell associated. Persistent infection can also develop readily in cells that are usually lysed by infection.[16] Giant cell formation can also occur during measles infection. Giant cells in lymphoid tissue are called Warthin-Finkeldey cells. Giant cells can also be formed by fusion of epithelial cells in the upper and lower respiratory tract, causing syncytium formation. These may be found in the nasal secretions.

Humans are the only natural host for measles virus, although primates can easily be infected by contact with measles patients. Infection of primates is usually subclinical, with the exception of the marmoset, which may develop severe symptoms. Laboratory strains of measles virus have been adapted for experimental studies in calves, lambs, dogs, ferrets, and rats but have been studied most extensively in hamsters and mice.

ANTIGENIC CHARACTERISTICS

Although the measles virus is considered a monotypic, antigenically stable virus, nucleotide sequence analysis of the genes of the measles virus has identified distinct differences in the N, H, P, and M genes of the wild-type measles virus, allowing the characterization of distinct lineages.[27] In contrast, the sequence of vaccine virus differed by less than 0.6%. Antigenic variations in the H and F proteins have also been demonstrated by use of monoclonal antibodies.[16] Cross-reactivity has been demonstrated with the three members of the *Morbillivirus* genus but not with other members of the Paramyxoviridae family.[17] The F component of measles and canine distemper virus are highly conserved, whereas the M and NP, and possibly the P, components show moderate antigenic relationships. The H protein of measles appears to be more closely related to rinderpest than to canine distemper virus.

Epidemiology

Measles is highly communicable and is found worldwide.[3, 28] It spreads from the infected person by the respiratory route through aerosolized droplets of respiratory secretions. It appears that infection is spread predominantly by persons ill with measles, although a role in the spread of measles for patients with mild, modified, or asymptomatic infections may exist, especially in populations in which many people are immunized. During epidemics in densely vaccinated populations, mild cases of measles may be missed because they do not meet typical clinical criteria.[29, 30] Direct contact accounts for the majority of infections, although indirect contact in a house or hospital ward is also possible. Infected persons are most contagious during the catarrhal stage of illness, which is marked by extensive virus excretion in respiratory secretions. Patients should be considered contagious from 1 to 2 days before the onset of symptoms (3 to 5 days before the rash) to at least 7 days after the onset of symptoms or 4 days after the appearance of the rash. Patients with SSPE are not infectious.

The prevalence of measles is affected by population density and, in more recent years, by the availability of measles vaccine. In the temperate zones among unimmunized populations, measles usually occurs in winter-spring epidemics in 2- or 5-year cycles that last 3 or 4 months. In rural settings or among isolated communities, populations can reach adult life without having been exposed. When measles virus is introduced into these communities, the results can be devastating. A classic description of such an outbreak in 1846 in the Faroe Islands was reported by Panum.[7]

In the prevaccine era, measles was a disease of children, the highest rate being among those 5 to 10 years of age. For example, between 1960 and 1964, about half of all measles patients were in this age group. In developing countries, measles generally occurs before age 5 years. Because of protection from maternal antibody, infection before the age of 6 months is, however, rare. In many developing countries, measles is the most important cause of death from age 1 through 5 years and accounts for between 1 and 2 million deaths per year worldwide. The frequency of measles is the same in males and females, although the complication rate may be higher among males (including the frequency of SSPE).[3] Measles susceptibility does not differ by race.

The introduction of measles vaccine has markedly altered the age incidence of measles. The prevaccine incidence of measles in those older than 10 years of age was less than 10%. In 1985, however, more than 60% of measles cases occurred in persons older than 10 years, and approximately half occurred in adolescents and young adults.[3] More recently, outbreaks on college campuses account for a significant proportion of all reported cases.[12, 31] Two main patterns of outbreaks in the United States have been seen. Outbreaks have been detected in highly immunized populations who had received one dose of vaccine; other outbreaks occurred in unvaccinated children of ethnic or racial minorities.[32–34]

Pathogenesis

Infection occurs as a result of contact by nasopharyngeal or possibly conjunctival epithelial surfaces with measles-contaminated respiratory droplets.[3, 16] The virus initially spreads to regional lymphatics; this is followed by a presumed primary viremia. This leads to viral replication in the reticuloendothelial system, including regional and distant sites, as well as in respiratory epithelium at the site of initial infection. A secondary viremia occurs on the fifth to seventh day after inoculation, which produces a more extensive and prolonged infection that seeds virus to lymphatic cells throughout the body.

The characteristic feature of virus multiplication in lymphoid tissues is the formation of multinucleated giant cells similar to those seen in tissue culture.[3, 28] Warthin-Finkeldey giant cells are seen in reticuloendothelial cells, including the adenoids, tonsils, Peyer patches, appendix, lymph nodes, spleen, and thymus. Giant cells are also readily detected on respiratory and other epithelial surfaces (including Koplik spots).

The viral content of the blood and respiratory tract is greatest between the 11th and 14th days after inoculation. By the time prodromal symptoms appear, virus is widely disseminated in epithelial membranes, small blood vessels, lymphocytes, and in many cases the CNS. Pleocytosis in the cerebrospinal fluid (CSF) is seen in approximately 10% of all cases[35]; changes on the electroencephalogram have been detected by Gibbs and associates[36] in 51% of 680 measles patients. Clinical encephalitis occurs in only 0.5 to 1 in 1000 measles cases. Studies support a direct role for virus in the pathogenic process,[37] although immune mechanisms are probably involved.[38]

A distinct clinical syndrome of measles (atypical measles) has been observed in some persons who were previously immunized with inactivated measles vaccine (see Chapter 146). Although the pathogenic mechanisms responsible for this syndrome are still unclear, patients with atypical measles lack antibody to the F protein (probably because the antigenic properties of this protein were destroyed by formalin inactivity) and have exaggerated or altered cellular responses to measles antigens with a predominance of Th1-type response.[3, 27, 39] Thus, the infecting virus replicated and spread, initiating pathologic immune reactions of the Arthus type.

Immune Response

Measles virus infection induces both antibody and cell-mediated immunity and provides lifelong immunity. Primary infection initially induces a humoral immunoglobulin M response that is short-lived, and then an immunoglobulin G response that persists for life. A local immunoglobulin A response also occurs in nasal secretions. Neutralizing antibody and hemagglutination inhibitory antibody appear in serum about the 14th day and peak 4 to 6 weeks after either natural infection or immunization. Complement-fixing antibody appears slightly later than hemagglutination inhibitory antibody.

Cell-mediated immune responses appear to be especially important in limiting the initial infection. Thus, persons with defects in cell-mediated immunity seem susceptible to fatal disseminated infections,[40] whereas agammaglobulinemic patients can recover from their infections.[40] Although substantial knowledge of the role of antibody, particularly to the H and F proteins, in host defense against measles has been obtained, the specificities of cellular immune responses are poorly understood. After infection, a lymphoproliferative response to measles can be demonstrated.[41, 42] T-cell clones of both $CD4^+$ class II–restricted helper cytotoxic T cells and $CD8^+$ class I–restricted cytotoxic T cells have also been established from healthy seropositive adults,[42] although cytotoxic T cells appear to be primarily restricted to class II.[43] Clones specific for the H, F, M, and NP proteins have been demonstrated.[42, 43] Increased levels of interferon-γ are seen during the rash of measles, but as the rash subsides, interleukin-4 levels increase and remain elevated for weeks, indicating a predominant Th2-type response.[39, 40] It has been suggested that measles infection initially produces a $CD8^+$ T-cell response that decreases virus replication,[44] followed by a Th2-type $CD4^+$ T-cell response that is required for optimal antibody production.[39]

Measles infection also induces a number of immune dysfunctions. Leukopenia is readily observed after infection and can also be seen after vaccination. Numbers of both neutrophils and lymphocytes are reduced, including T, B, and null cells, although the ratio between helper and suppressor cytotoxic T cells appears to be unchanged. Delayed hypersensitivity responses are also suppressed after both natural infection and measles vaccination. This includes skin test reactivity to common antigens and measured blastogenic responses to mitogens and specific antigens in vitro. Further natural killer cell activity and immunoglobulin synthesis of B cells are also impaired. It is still unclear, however, what the basic mechanisms of inhibition are. Monocytes are also affected during measles, and levels of tumor necrosis factor-α are decreased.[39] Deficiencies of tumor necrosis factor-α could contribute to a decrease in lymphoproliferative or other cell-related responses. Similarly, increased levels of interleukin-4 found in measles-infected patients could down-regulate macrophage-activated lymphoproliferative and delayed-type hypersensitivity responses.[39]

Clinical Manifestations

After an incubation period of 10 to 14 days and a prodromal stage characterized by cough, coryza, conjunctivitis, and fever, the typical rash appears.[3, 8] The pathognomonic Koplik spots can be seen before the rash as 1- to 3-mm pale bluish white spots on an erythematous background on the lateral buccal mucosa. The characteristic macular or maculopapular rash first appears on the forehead and behind the ears and then spreads over the face, neck, trunk, and limbs within 24 to 48 hours.

Respiratory tract involvement is common after measles infection. Manifestations include laryngitis, tracheobronchitis, bronchiolitis, and pneumonia. Secondary bacterial pneumonia and otitis media caused by typical respiratory pathogens are also not uncommon. Other complications, including cardiac and acute neurologic involvement, may be seen.

The diagnosis of measles in an epidemic setting can usually be made by history and physical findings, although as the number of physicians trained who have not regularly seen measles increases and the number of epidemics decreases, laboratory confirmation becomes more important. Although virus isolation and identification of measles antigens in nasopharyngeal secretions are possible, laboratory confirmation is usually accomplished by serologic determination of an elevation of measles antibody titer. (See Chapter 152 for a detailed discussion of viral exanthems.)

Subacute Sclerosing Panencephalitis

SSPE is a rare degenerative neurologic disease of children and adolescents produced by persistent measles virus infection of the CNS. Dawson,[45] in 1933, first noted viral inclusions in the neurons of patients who were dying of this disease. Measles viral antigen was found in brain tissue[46] in 1967, and several groups of investigators in 1969 succeeded in cultivating a measles-like virus from a patient's brain tissue.[47, 48]

Pathogenesis and Pathology

The seeding of the CNS with measles virus probably occurs during natural infection. Half to one third of children who acquire measles infection naturally have CSF pleocytosis and transient electroencephalographic changes,[49] and disease is more severe in younger children. Neither infectious virus nor viral particles are detectable within the CNS, but viral nucleoprotein structures are seen as inclusion bodies by electron microscopy. This is accompanied by a strong inflammatory response. When SSPE first appears, measles virus ribonucleocapsids have begun to spread to the entire CNS without formation of viral particles despite humoral and cellular immune responses.

The inability of SSPE virus (measles virus that is recovered from SSPE patients) to produce infectious virus was initially attributed to the absence of the M protein. Subsequent studies have shown transcriptional and translational changes that affect the expression, stability, and formation of the H, F, and especially M genes. Other studies have shown that several measles genes are affected by mutation.[27, 50–52] The M gene is most affected, but deletion in the cytoplasmic domain of the F protein may also be important in the altered growth properties of the virus. It is still unclear how SSPE virus can spread throughout the CNS without formation of infectious viral particles in the presence of a strong immune response. It is also unclear whether the pathologic changes are due to virus-mediated cell destruction or to immune or autoimmune responses.

In the assessment of the SSPE pathophysiologic process, it is important to recognize the dynamic nature of this disease; inflammation leads to necrosis and destruction, then to reparative or gliotic changes, and these dynamic processes move in a rostrocaudad direction.[53] Intranuclear and intracytoplasmic eosinophilic inclusions, best seen in oligodendroglia, vary in size from 2 to 10 μm, are more readily demonstrated in patients who have a shorter course of clinical disease, and are difficult to find in brain biopsy material. The characteristic gross histopathologic features—subacute inflammatory vascular changes, subacute demyelination, extensive gliosis, and neuronal and glial cell inclusions—can also be found in other diseases.[54]

Epidemiology

The incidence of SSPE is estimated to be between 0.6 and 2.2 cases for every 100,000 cases of measles. The risk of SSPE is greater for children who acquire the disease at an early age; half of SSPE patients have a history for measles infection before age 2 years and three fourths before age 4 years. Males outnumber females by 2 to 1, and cases more commonly come from rural areas, especially the southeastern United States and the Ohio River Valley. The lack of any consistent association with human leukocyte antigens suggests that variability in disease occurrence by ethnic group probably does not reflect genetic predisposition to the disease. Use of measles vaccine has resulted in a marked decline in SSPE cases.

Clinical Symptoms

The initial clinical manifestations of SSPE typically appear 6 to 8 years after measles infection. The onset of disease (stage 1) is insidious, the first symptoms being progressive behavioral and intellectual deterioration that can include psychologic difficulties, personality changes, declining school performance, impaired memory, altered judgment, and motor incoordination. Stage 2 disease appears with the onset of myoclonic spasms that are characteristically repetitive with rapid onset and a delayed relaxation phase. Once they have developed, seizures of this type often repeat at intervals of 10 to 60 seconds. Ocular abnormalities, ataxia, dyskinesia, focal neurologic deficits, and visual and speech impairment are also noted during this stage. Progression leads to stage 3 disease, with stupor, dementia, mutism, coma, and decerebrate rigidity. Patients with stage 4 disease show diminished muscle tone, central blindness, and decorticate rigidity and have difficulty feeding, chewing, and swallowing. At this advanced stage, unexplained episodes of hyperthermia and profuse diaphoresis are seen and myoclonus may disappear. Deterioration continues, and the majority of patients die in 1 to 3 years.[49]

Laboratory Diagnosis

The diagnosis of SSPE is based on a combination of clinical and laboratory factors, including the electroencephalogram and measles antibody titers. An electroencephalogram with typical burst-suppression pattern–paroxysmal complexes of 2 to 3 per second synchronous spike wave discharges with interim suppression of electrical activity occurring at 5- to 8-second intervals is diagnostic of SSPE. This pattern is characteristic of stage 2 disease before the onset of dementia,[45] and it deteriorates in later stages. Serum complement fixation titers to measles antibodies are greater than those in acute measles infection (accepted minimal serum titer 1:128).[54] There are increased antibody levels to the N and P proteins, with less increase to F and H and little or no antibodies to M in serum and CSF.[52] The CSF commonly shows no abnormalities of pressure, cell count, total protein, or glucose level but does contain abnormal oligoclonal immunoglobulin G bands.[55] This oligoclonal immunoglobulin G is antibody directed against measles antigen[56] and is present in CSF/serum ratios that indicate intrathecal measles antibody synthesis usually not found in acute infection (accepted minimal diagnostic CSF measles complement fixation titer is 1:8).[38] Computed tomography and magnetic resonance imaging can be used to confirm the clinical picture, but findings may be normal early in the disease.[57] As the disease progresses, the computed tomographic scan is more predictive, showing enlarging ventricles and widened sulci with multifocal low-density lesions probably indicating cerebral atrophy with areas of demyelination and encephalitis.[57, 58]

Treatment

No treatment is of proven benefit.[59] The rarity of the disease makes it difficult to perform randomized prospective controlled studies. Transfer factor, thymectomy, 5-bromodeoxyuridine and pyran copolymer, levodopa, carbodopa, nialamide, rifampin, ether, corticosteroids, 5-iodo-2′-deoxyuridine, and other agents have been tested, with little success.[59] Although amantadine and inosine pranobex (isoprinosine) have been tried, the experience is inconclusive.[53] Palliative treatments of importance include anticonvulsants, nutritional supplements, antibiotics when needed, physical therapy, and mental and behavioral control therapies.[48] Most recently, the combination of oral inosine pranobex and intraventricular interferon alpha was reported to have some effect[60]; intrathecal ribavirin was effective in a hamster model.[61]

References

1. Babbott FL Jr, Gordon JE: Modern measles. Am J Med Sci 228:334, 1954.
2. Black FL: Measles. *In* Evans AS (ed): Viral Infections of Humans; Epidemiology and Control. New York, Plenum Publishing, 1976, pp 297–316.
3. Cherry JD: Measles. *In* Feigin RD, Cherry JR (eds): Textbook of Pediatric Infectious Diseases. Philadelphia, WB Saunders, 1987, pp 1607–1628.
4. Caulfield E: Early measles epidemics in America. Yale J Biol Med 15:531, 1943.
5. Koplik H: The diagnosis of the invasion of measles from a study of the exanthema as it appears in the buccal mucous membrane. Arch Pediatr 13:918, 1896.
6. Brem J: Koplik spots for the record. An illustrated historical note. Clin Pediatr 11:161, 1972.
7. Panum PL: Observations made during the epidemic of measles on the Faroe Islands in the year 1846. Med Classics 3:829, 1939.
8. Measles (rubeola). *In* Krugman S, Katz SL, Gershon AA, et al (eds): Infectious Diseases of Children. St. Louis, CV Mosby, 1985, pp 152–166.
9. Enders JF, Peebles TC: Propagation in tissue cultures of cytopathogenic agents from patients with measles. Proc Soc Exp Biol Med 86:277, 1954.
10. Sever JL, Zenman W (eds): Proceedings of Symposium on Measles Virus and Subacute Sclerosing Panencephalitis. Neurology 18:1, 1968.
11. Katz SL, Milovanovic MV, Enders JF: Propagation of measles virus in cultures of chick embryo cells. Proc Soc Exp Biol Med 97:23, 1958.
12. Markowitz LE, Preblud SR, Orenstein WA, et al: Patterns of transmission in measles outbreaks in the United States 1985–1986. N Engl J Med 320:75, 1989.
13. Centers for Disease Control: Measles—Los Angeles County, California, 1989. MMWR Morbid Mortal Wkly Rep 38:49, 1989.
14. Centers for Disease Control: Goal to eliminate measles from the United States. MMWR 27:391, 1978.
15. Cutts FT, Markowitz LE: Successes and failures in measles control. J Infect Dis 170(Suppl):S32, 1994.
16. Norrby E: Measles Virus. *In* Fields BN, Knipe DM (eds): Fields Virology, ed 2. New York, Raven Press, 1990, pp 1013–1044.
17. Sheshberadaran H, Norrby E, McCullough KC, et al: The antigenic relationship between measles, canine distemper and rinderpest viruses studied with monoclonal antibodies. J Gen Virol 67:1381, 1986.
18. Barrett T: The molecular biology of the morbillivirus (measles) group. Biochem Soc Symp 53:25, 1987.
19. Osterhaus ADME, de Vries P, van Binnendijk RS: Measles vaccines: Novel generations and new strategies. J Infect Dis 170(Suppl):S42, 1994.
20. Tyrrell DLJ, Norrby E: Structural polypeptides of measles virus. J Gen Virol 39:219, 1978.
21. Wild TF, Malvoisin E, Buckland R: Measles virus: Both the haemagglutinin and fusion glycoproteins are required for fusion. J Gen Virol 72:439, 1991.
22. Seifried AS, Albrecht P, Milstien JB: Characterization of an RNA dependent RNA polymerase activity associated with measles virus. J Virol 25:781, 1978.
23. Musser SJ, Underwood GE: Studies on measles virus. II. Physical properties and inactivation studies of measles virus. J Immunol 85:292, 1960.
24. Naniche D, Varior-Krishnan G, Cervoni F, et al: Human membrane cofactor protein (CD46) acts as a cellular receptor for measles virus. J Virol 67:6025, 1993.
25. Dorig RE, Marcil A, Chopra A, Richardson CD: The human CD46 molecule is a receptor for measles virus (Edmonston strain). Cell 75:295, 1993.
26. Fuccillo DA, Sever JL: Measles virus. *In* Schmidt NJ, Emmons RW (eds): Diagnostic Procedures for Viral, Rickettsial and Chlamydial Infections, ed 6. Washington, DC, American Public Health Association, 1989, pp 713–730.
27. Bellini WJ, Rota JS, Rota PA: Virology of measles virus. J Infect Dis 170(Suppl):S15, 1994.
28. Preblud SR, Katz SL: Measles vaccine. *In* Plotkin SA, Mortimer EA Jr (eds): Vaccines. Philadelphia, WB Saunders, 1988, pp 182–202.
29. Wintermeyer L, Myers MG: Measles in a partially immunized community. Am J Public Health 69:923, 1979.
30. Edmondson MB, Addiss DG, Berg JL: Mild measles during a sustained outbreak in a highly vaccinated population. Pediatr Res 25:99A, 1989.
31. Centers for Disease Control: Measles on college campuses—United States, 1985. MMWR 34:445, 1985.
32. Gustafson TL, Brunell PA, Lievens AW, et al: Measles outbreak in a "fully immunized" secondary school population. N Engl J Med 316:771, 1987.
33. Hersh BS, Markowitz LE, Maes EF, et al: The geographic distribution of measles in the United States, 1980 through 1989. JAMA 267:1936, 1992.
34. Centers for Disease Control and Prevention: Retrospective assessment of vaccination coverage among school-aged children—Selected US cities, 1991. MMWR Morbid Mortal Wkly Rep 41:103, 1992.
35. Ojala A: On changes in the cerebrospinal fluid during measles. Ann Med Fenn 36:321, 1947.
36. Gibbs FA, Gibbs EL, Carpenter PR, et al: Electroencephalographic abnormality in "uncomplicated" childhood diseases. JAMA 171:1050, 1959.
37. Meulen VT, Kackell Y, Muller D, et al: Isolation of infectious measles virus in measles encephalitis. Lancet 2:1172, 1972.
38. Johnson RT, Griffin DE, Hirsch RL, et al: Measles encephalomyelitis—clinical and immunologic studies. N Engl J Med 310:137, 1984.
39. Griffin DE, Ward BJ, Esolen LM: Pathogenesis of measles virus infection: An hypothesis for altered immune responses. J Infect Dis 170:S24, 1994.
40. Griffin DE: Immune responses during measles virus infection. Curr Top Microbiol Immunol 191:117, 1995.
41. Greenstein JI, McFarland HF: Response of human lymphocytes to measles virus after natural infection. Infect Immun 40:198, 1983.
42. van Binnendijk RS, Poelen MCM, deVries P: Measles virus specific human T cell clones. J Immunol 142:2847, 1989.
43. Jacobson S, Sekaly RP, Jacobson CL, et al: HLA class II restricted presentation of cytoplasmic measles virus antigen to cytotoxic T cells. J Virol 63:1756, 1989.
44. Van Binnendijk RS, Poelen MCM, Kuijpers KC, et al: The predominance of $CD8^+$ T cells after infection with measles virus suggests a role for $CD8^+$ class I MHC-restricted cytotoxic T lymphocytes (CTL) in recovery from measles. Clonal analyses of human $CD8^+$ class I MHC-restricted CTL. J Immunol 144:2394, 1990.
45. Dawson JR Jr: Cellular inclusions in cerebral lesions of lethargic encephalitis. Am J Pathol 9:7, 1933.

46. Connolly JH, Allen IV, Hurwitz LJ, et al: Measles virus antibody and antigen in subacute sclerosing panencephalitis. Lancet 1:542, 1967.
47. Chen TT, Watanabe I, Zemon W, et al: Subacute sclerosing panencephalitis propagation of measles virus from brain biopsy in tissue culture. Science 163:1193, 1969.
48. Payne FE, Baublis JV, Itabashi HH: Isolation of measles virus from cell cultures of brain from a patient with subacute sclerosing panencephalitis. N Engl J Med 281:585, 1969.
49. Groves MC: Subacute sclerosing panencephalitis. Neurol Clin 2:267, 1984.
50. Hirano A, Ayata M, Wang AH, Wong TC: Functional analysis of matrix proteins expressed from cloned genes of measles virus variants that cause subacute sclerosing panencephalitis reveals a common defect in nucleocapsid binding. J Virol 67:1848, 1993.
51. Schmid A, Spielhofer P, Cattaneo R, et al: Subacute sclerosing panencephalitis is typically characterized by alterations in the fusion protein cytoplasmic domain of the persisting measles virus. Virology 188:910, 1992.
52. Billeter MA, Cattaneo R, Spielhofer P, et al: Generation and properties of measles virus mutations typically associated with subacute sclerosing panencephalitis. Ann N Y Acad Sci 724:367, 1994.
53. Dyken PR: Subacute sclerosing panencephalitis. Neurol Clin 3:179, 1985.
54. Anderson JR: Viral encephalitis and its pathology. Curr Top Pathol 76:23, 1988.
55. Meulen TV, Carter MT: Measles virus persistency and disease. Prog Med Virol 30:44, 1984.
56. Mehta PD, Patrick BA, Thormar H: Identification of virus-specific oligoclonal bands in subacute sclerosing panencephalitis by immunofixation after isoelectric focusing and peroxidase staining. J Clin Microbiol 16:985, 1982.
57. Duda EE, Huttenlocher PR, Patronas NJ: CT of subacute sclerosing panencephalitis. Am J Neuroradiol 1:35, 1980.
58. Bohlega S, al-Kawi MZ: Subacute sclerosing panencephalitis. Imaging and clinical correlation. J Neuroimaging 4:71, 1994.
59. Taylor WJ, DuPont RH, Dyken PR: Treatment of subacute sclerosing panencephalitis. Drug Intell Clin Pharmacol 18:375, 1984.
60. Gascon G, Yamini S, Crowell J, et al: Combined oral isoprinosine–intraventricular alpha-interferon therapy for subacute sclerosing panencephalitis. Brain Dev 15:346, 1993.
61. Honda Y, Hosoya M, Ishii T, et al: Effect of ribavirin on subacute sclerosing panencephalitis virus infections in hamsters. Antimicrob Agents Chemother 38:653, 1994.

254

Hantaviruses

Frederick T. Koster
Steven A. Jenison

Human hantavirus infections cause two distinct syndromes. Acute infection with the Eurasian hantaviruses causes the hemorrhagic fever renal syndrome (HFRS),[1–3] and acute infection with the North American hantaviruses causes the hantavirus pulmonary syndrome (HPS).[4–7] Although multiple North American hantaviruses may cause HPS (Table 254–1), the predominant HPS agent has been called Four Corners virus, Muerto Canyon virus, Sin Nombre virus (SNV), and Convict Creek virus. Because the nomenclature has not yet been formalized, we refer to the hantavirus that is endemic among deer mice *(Peromyscus maniculatus)* in western North America and that causes HPS in humans as SNV.

HPS was recognized first in a cluster of cases that occurred in the Four Corners region of the southwestern United States in the spring and summer of 1993.[8–12] The Four Corners is a region that surrounds the common borders of New Mexico, Arizona, Utah, and Colorado. Most of the initial cases occurred in young adults who had previously been healthy, and many were Navajo who lived in remote rural areas of northwestern New Mexico and northeastern Arizona. Prominent disease characteristics included rapidly progressive respiratory insufficiency, diffuse noncardiogenic pulmonary edema, vascular volume contraction, and depressed cardiac output,[4, 13] features indicating a massive pulmonary capillary leak syndrome. Soon after the outbreak began, serum samples of patients with HPS were found to contain immunoglobulin M antibodies that reacted with the Hantaan, Seoul, and Puumala hantaviruses in enzyme immunoassays.[8] By use of hantavirus consensus oligonucleotide primers in the reverse transcription–polymerase chain reaction (RT-PCR), genetic sequences of a previously uncharacterized hantavirus were amplified from human lung tissue.[5] Animal trappings in the Four Corners region demonstrated a high prevalence of infections with this hantavirus among deer mice *(P. maniculatus)*, common rodents of western North America.[14] The HPS agent was subsequently isolated in cell culture.[15, 16]

Characteristics of the Pathogen

Hantavirus is a genus of enveloped RNA viruses in the family Bunyaviridae.[17–19] The *Hantavirus* genus includes Hantaan virus (HTN), Seoul virus (SEO), Puumala virus (PUU), Prospect Hill virus (PHV), and SNV. Hantavirus virions consist of an RNA genome encased within a nucleocapsid shell and coated by an outer lipid envelope.[20–23] The RNA genome includes three segments called long, medium, and short. The shell is composed of a single nucleocapsid protein (N) encoded by the short segment.[22] The lipid envelope contains two glycoproteins (G1 and G2) encoded by the medium segment.[23] The long segment encodes the viral RNA-dependent RNA replicase.

Hantaviruses normally infect rodents, and human infections result from incidental rodent-to-human transmission. Each *Hantavirus* species normally infects a single rodent species. The prototypic hantavirus, HTN, infects the Asian striped field mouse *(Apodemus agrarius)* and is the etiologic agent of Korean hemorrhagic fever in humans.[24, 25] SEO infects the urban rat *(Rattus norvegicus)* and causes a human disease that is similar to Korean hemorrhagic fever.[26–29] SEO, like its rodent host, is cosmopolitan and infects rats in coastal cities of the United States.[26] PUU, which is enzootic among bank voles *(Clethrionomys glareolus)* in northern Europe, causes a relatively mild form of hemorrhagic fever called nephropathia epidemica.[30–36] The diseases caused by HTN, SEO, and PUU share many features and are known collectively as HFRS.

Before the recognition of HPS and the identification of SNV, PHV was the only known indigenous New World hantavirus. PHV is a North American hantavirus that infects a microtine rodent, the meadow vole *(Microtus pennsylvanicus)*; PHV is not known to cause human disease.[37–39] Subsequent to the discovery of SNV, several other North American hantaviruses have been identified and characterized. Hantaviruses that are genetically similar to PHV infect other microtine rodent species, including the California meadow mouse *Microtus californicus* (Isla Vista virus) and the prairie vole *Microtus ochrogaster* (Bloodland Lake virus) (Song W, et al, unpublished data). These common rodents are widely distributed in North America. It is unknown whether the han-

TABLE 254–1 ■ The Hantaviruses

HANTAVIRUS STRAIN	HOST RODENT (SPECIES)	GEOGRAPHIC RANGE	SYNDROME IN HUMANS*	MORTALITY RATE
Hantaan	Striped field mouse (*Apodemus agrarius*)	Eastern Asia	HFRS	5%
Seoul	Common rat (*Rattus norvegicus*)	Urban worldwide	HFRS	1%–2%
Puumala	Bank vole (*Clethrionomys glareolus*)	Northern Europe	Nephropathia epidemica	0.1%–1.0%
Dobrava	Yellow-necked field mouse (*Apodemus falvicollis*)	Balkans	HFRS	15%
Sim Nombre	Deer mouse (*Peromyscus maniculatus*)	Western North America	HPS	52%
New York	White-footed mouse (*Peromyscus leucopus*)	Eastern North America	HPS	1 fatal case
Black Creek Canal	Cotton rat (*Sigmodon hispidus*)	Florida	HPS with hemorrhage	1 case
Bayou	Not known	Louisiana	HPS with hemorrhage	1 fatal case
Prospect Hill	Meadow vole (*Microtus pennsylvanicus*)	Eastern North America	None known	—
El Moro Canyon	Western harvest mouse (*Reithrodontomys megalotis*)	Western states and central Mexico	None known	—
Isla Vista	California meadow mouse (*Microtus californicus*)	California, Oregon, Baja	None known	—
Tula	Common vole (*Microtus arvalis*)	Asia, Russia	None known	—

*HFRS, Hemorrhagic fever renal syndrome; HPS, hantavirus pulmonary syndrome.

taviruses that infect these microtine rodents can also infect humans.

SNV, the first identified HPS agent, infects the deer mouse (*P. maniculatus*).[5, 14, 40, 41] *P. maniculatus*, which is distributed throughout the western two thirds of North America, is a species within the rodent subfamily Sigmodontinae, family Muridae. To date, SNV has been implicated in the majority of HPS cases in North America. At least two HPS cases acquired in the eastern United States were caused by unique hantaviruses of other sigmodontine rodent species, including the white-footed mouse *Peromyscus leucopus* (New York virus)[42–45] and the cotton rat *Sigmodon hispidus* (Black Creek Canal virus).[43, 46] A fatal HPS case that occurred in Louisiana was caused by a unique hantavirus (Bayou virus) for which the rodent host is unknown.[47] SNV, New York virus, Black Creek Canal virus, and Bayou virus constitute a monophyletic genetic lineage that includes all of the known North American HPS agents. The North American HPS agents are most closely related to one another, are closely related to PHV and PUU, and are more distantly related to SEO and HTN.

Two additional hantaviruses of the phylogenetic grouping that includes the North American HPS agents have been identified in New World sigmodontine rodents of the genus *Reithrodontomys*. El Moro Canyon virus infects the western harvest mouse (*Reithrodontomys megalotis*),[48] which is distributed throughout the western United States and Mexico. Rio Segundo virus is known only from the prototype genome amplified from a *Reithrodontomys mexicanus* specimen obtained in Costa Rica.[49] Human infections with *Reithrodontomys* hantaviruses have not been reported.

The HPS outbreak in the Four Corners did not result from the sudden emergence of a new pathogen. Rather, the close clustering of cases in 1993 drew attention to a virus that was enzootic among deer mice and that rarely caused human infections. Nucleotide sequence analysis of SNV complementary DNAs showed that SNV was a unique hantavirus more closely related to PUU and PHV and more distantly related to SEO and HTN.[40, 41] Each of the three SNV genomic segments was similarly diverged from the homologous genomic segments of other hantaviruses. Genetic analysis of SNV complementary DNA clones from throughout the western United States and Canada indicated that although nucleotide sequence variations existed regionally, SNV amino acid sequences were highly conserved.[5, 50] The phylogenetic relatedness of different hantaviruses parallels the phylogenetic relatedness of their rodent hosts, suggesting that the hantaviruses are coevolving with their hosts[51, 52]; this holds true for SNV and its rodent host *P. maniculatus*. Therefore, there is no evidence that the 1993 HPS outbreak in Four Corners resulted from the sudden emergence of a new human pathogen through mutation or gene segment reassortment. Indeed, SNV infections among *P. maniculatus* and HPS cases in humans that occurred more than a decade before the 1993 HPS outbreak have been documented.[53–55]

Epidemiology of Hemorrhagic Fever Renal Syndrome and Hantavirus Pulmonary Syndrome

Wild rodents are the primary hosts of hantaviruses.[25–28, 37, 38] Rodents develop chronic hantavirus infections that do not appear to result in tissue damage or disease. Most human hantavirus infections appear to result from exposure to wild rodents or their habitats. Rodent urine and feces contain infectious virus, and humans may acquire infection through inhaling airborne particles of rodent excreta that contain viable virus. No arthropod vector has been implicated in the transmission of hantaviruses, but this possibility deserves further investigation. Human hantavirus infections that resulted from laboratory accidents have been reported, both as a result of rodent bites and through the inoculation of rodent blood.[56–58] HFRS has also resulted from even brief exposure to infected laboratory rats,[59, 60] and more than 100 laboratory-acquired cases have been documented in Japan alone.[57]

HTN infects more than 100,000 people in China each year, with a mortality rate of approximately 5%. The frequency of

HTN infection is highest among workers in certain agricultural occupations,[61, 62] who are more likely to disturb the habitats of the striped field mouse. HPS is distinctly less common, with approximately 110 cases having been documented between 1993 and 1995. Similar to HTN infections, human SNV infections occur more commonly in rural settings.[63, 64] HPS patients have often reported having entered or disturbed a dwelling, agricultural building, or automobile that was infested with mice.[64] There is no evidence that hantavirus infections have been transmitted from humans to other humans, and infected humans are not thought to represent a risk to health care workers. HPS patients have ranged in age from 11 to 69 years, with a mean of 35 years.[4] There is a slight excess of males and a relative overrepresentation (approximately one third of cases) of Native Americans among HPS case patients.

Clinical Features

Hemorrhagic Fever Renal Syndrome

Whereas the clinical features of infection by HTN, Dobrava, SEO, and PUU viruses clearly define HFRS,[3] morbidity and mortality vary considerably among the different viral strains[65–75] (see Table 254–1). The incubation period ranges from 12 to 21 days, with incubation as long as 6 weeks noted.[65] The ratio of mild and subclinical infection to severe infection is reported to be as high as 5:1, but prospective studies have not carefully defined this ratio. The syndrome is divided into five phases: febrile, shock, oliguria, diuresis, and convalescence (Fig. 254–1). In the febrile phase, common nonspecific symptoms include high temperature, chills, dizziness, headache, myalgias, abdominal pain, back pain, nausea, and vomiting (Table 254–2). A dry cough and shortness of breath precede the onset of mild pulmonary edema in 10% to 20% of the cases. The physical examination is notable for conjunctival effusion without erythema and an erythematous flush over the face, neck, chest, and nail beds. Petechiae may appear before the shock phase on the palate, face, chest, hips, thighs, and skinfolds. Flank tenderness may be prominent in severe cases.

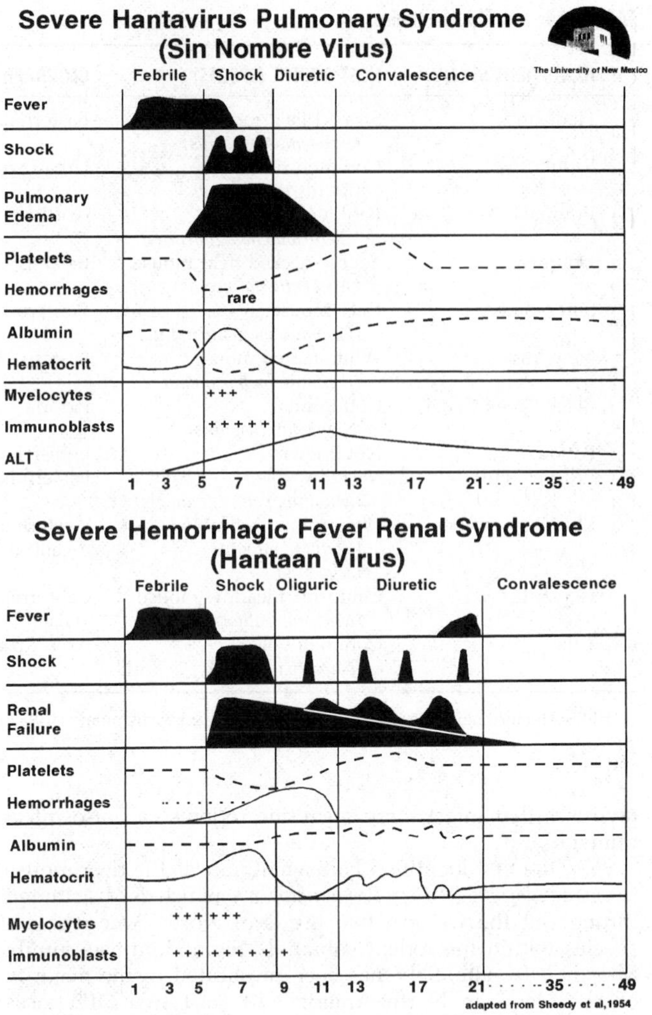

FIGURE 254–1 □ Evolution of hantavirus pulmonary syndrome (HPS) and hemorrhagic fever renal syndrome (HFRS), comparing organ-specific and laboratory abnormalities for each phase of illness. ALT, Alanine aminotransferase. (Adapted and reprinted by permission of the publisher from Sheedy JA, Froeb HF, Batson HA, et al: The clinical course of epidemic hemorrhagic fever. Am J Med 16:619, 1954. Copyright 1954 by Excerpta Medica Inc.)

TABLE 254–2 ■ Comparison of the Clinical Features of Known Pathogenic Hantaviruses Worldwide

	% POSITIVE			
CLINICAL FEATURE	**Sin Nombre**	**Hantaan**	**Seoul**	**Puumala**
Fever	100	100	100	100
Myalgias	100	69–78	52	20
Chills	80	92	70	60
Nausea and vomiting	71	72–82	61	78
Backache	29	95	90	82
Abdominal pain	24	23–25	65	67
Diarrhea	59	11–37	24	12
Dizziness, vertigo	41	41–100	7	12
Headache	71	83–86	43	90
Conjunctival suffusion	18	23–64	79	18
Cough	71	40	20	10
Dyspnea	95	<10	<10	<10
Lymphadenopathy	0	3–38	15	15
Petechiae	0	32–56	31	12
Hemorrhage	0	31–72	26	10
Platelets <100,000/mm³	100	54–78	70	80
White cell count >1000/mm³	88	92	41	57
Hypotension (pressure <90/60 mm Hg)	40	42–80	22	40
Pulmonary edema	100	20	10	10
Ventilator dependent	71	5	Rare	2
Oliguria <500 mL/24 h	41	59–67	37	54
Creatinine >2.0 mg/dL	17	94–100	50	70
Proteinuria >1+	17	96	94	100

After the petechiae appear, the hematocrit rises, and plasma volume falls as plasma fluid is leaking through the injured capillaries into tissue spaces. Death from primary shock accounts for one third of the fatalities. Proteinuria becomes massive, and oliguria progresses from irregularly present to well established to mark the oliguric phase.[76] Renal failure persists for 1 to 6 days, and dialysis may be required until diuresis begins. Recovery is impaired primarily by subcortical hemorrhage.[77] The hematocrit falls as extravascular edema fluid is reabsorbed into the circulation. Spontaneous diuresis of 4 to 8 L/d leads to a rapid decrease in azotemia but may be complicated by electrolyte disorders requiring careful monitoring.[78]

The clinical course extends for 2 to 4 weeks, with slow recovery in the majority. There is evidence of only slight residual tubule injury after recovery from acute renal failure in Korean hemorrhagic fever and nephropathia epidemica.[79, 80] Fatal hemorrhage, particularly in the central nervous system, remains rare, usually occurring in the shock and oliguric phases. Hematologic changes include elevated leukocyte count with marked left shift to the myeloid precursors, severe thrombocytopenia, and circulating atypical lymphocytes. Evidence for a consumptive coagulopathy includes prolonged bleeding time, prolonged prothrombin and activated partial thromboplastin times, circulating D-dimer, and decreased fibrinogen levels.[81–83]

Hantavirus Pulmonary Syndrome

The clinical course of HPS bears both similarities and striking differences compared with HFRS. The incubation period of HPS has been calculated to be 8 to 21 days in the few cases in which exposure was clearly defined. Subclinical infections appear to be uncommon, and no children younger than 11 years have been diagnosed with HPS. HPS is divided into four phases: febrile, shock, diuresis, and convalescence (see Fig. 254–1). HPS begins with an acute influenza-like phase, lasting 1 to 12 days,[4] characterized by the abrupt onset of fever, myalgias, malaise, nausea and vomiting, headache, and dizziness (see Table 254–2). Because the early symptoms of HPS mimic a host of other viral and bacterial infections, the clinician is faced with a difficult task in the early recognition of HPS before the onset of pulmonary edema. Abdominal pain, diarrhea, nausea, and vomiting may mimic acute appendicitis. The physical examination reveals an acutely ill person with tachypnea and tachycardia, but additional features such as pulmonary rales, abdominal tenderness, and conjunctival effusion are seen only in the minority of patients. After 1 to 5 days of high temperature, the appearance of dry cough and shortness of breath heralds the onset of pulmonary edema.

The second phase, or shock phase, is characterized by the abrupt onset of shortness of breath and hypoxemia due to pulmonary edema, progressing during a 6- to 12-hour period to severe hypoxemia requiring mechanical ventilation in 75% of cases. Early pulmonary edema is characterized by bronchiolar cuffing and Kerley B lines, with rapid progression to bilateral interstitial edema and alveolar flooding 6 to 12 hours later.[84] In spite of its severity, pulmonary edema persists only 2 to 4 days and is followed by a spontaneous diuresis lasting 3 to 4 days in patients who survive the shock phase. Hypotension with hemoconcentration may vary from profound to absent, and a cardiac index of less than 2.0 L/min per m^2 and a plasma lactate value of greater than 4.0 mmol/L are grave prognostic signs.[85] Shock in HPS is characterized by a low cardiac index and normal to elevated systemic vascular resistance,[85] in contrast to typical septic shock in which the cardiac index is elevated and systemic vascular resistance is diminished. In contrast to HFRS, HPS rarely has significant proteinuria, and elevations of creatinine values reflect volume depletion and prerenal azotemia only. Consistently abnormal laboratory findings include elevated serum lactate dehydrogenase and aspartate aminotransferase values and decreased serum bicarbonate and albumin levels.[4] The convalescent phase may last several months with weakness and postexertional fatigue. Limited follow-up studies in patients 6 months to 1 year after HPS have failed to demonstrate any persistent abnormalities in lung, cardiac, liver, or hematologic function.

The platelet count begins to decrease during the prodrome phase and is the earliest laboratory abnormality that would distinguish HPS from the host of other influenza-like syndromes. Hematologic changes are distinguished by a leukocytosis with marked left shift and by the appearance of circulating immunoblasts (atypical lymphocytes) coincident with the development of pulmonary edema.[4, 86] The triad of thrombocytopenia, circulating myelocytes, and circulating immunoblasts is highly specific and sensitive for the presumptive diagnosis of HPS (Foucar K, unpublished data). This triad of hematologic findings is not always present during the febrile phase, and serologic diagnosis is always required at any stage of the disease. A mild coagulopathy is demonstrable in all cases of HPS,[4, 86] yet petechiae, ecchymoses, and frank hemorrhage in the pulmonary tree have not yet been documented. Significant hemorrhage, in less than 5% of HPS cases, occurs as minor gastrointestinal hemorrhage and bleeding from venipuncture sites.

Pathogenesis

The clinical features of both HPS and HFRS are largely the result of a capillary leak syndrome and the coagulopathy, but the disease in the target organs is strikingly different for each syndrome. In both HPS and HFRS, inhalation of virus into the lungs appears to initiate the infection. A viremia is detected in HPS.[87] Viral nucleocapsid antigen is identified in capillary endothelial cells in many organs by immunohistochemistry. The kidneys from patients dying in the acute phase of Korean hemorrhagic fever contain dense precipitates, typical inclusion bodies, and Hantaan virion–like structures.[88] The lungs from patients dying of acute HPS contain typical inclusion bodies, but hantavirus-like virions are uncommon.[86, 89]

The evidence for altered vascular permeability in HFRS is widespread capillary engorgement, focal hemorrhage, and interstitial edema in many organs.[90] Retroperitoneal edema is massive in some cases, with histologic evidence for renal medullary congestion, pituitary necrosis, and adrenal hemorrhage and necrosis in many fatal cases. In HPS, the most striking finding at autopsy is edematous lungs with pleural effusions as large as 8 L.[86] The heart, kidneys, brain, and adrenals are grossly and histologically normal. The liver may be slightly enlarged and has microscopic evidence of triaditis. The pulmonary alveoli are filled with acellular proteinaceous fluid with hyaline-like membranes. The modestly thickened septa contain primarily large mononuclear cells, including immunoblasts, monocytes, and plasma cells but few polymorphonuclear leukocytes, and the alveolar epithelial cells are intact. This is in marked contrast to adult respiratory distress syndrome, characterized by thickened septa, hyaline membranes, and neutrophilic inflammatory infiltrate in the septa and alveoli.

Cellular immune responses appear to play a role in the pathogenesis of both HFRS and HPS. In HFRS, the presence of activated T cells, soluble interleukin-2 receptors, and interferon-γ–producing cells in peripheral blood is evidence of highly activated T cells.[91] The immunoblasts populating the lung, pleural effusion, liver, spleen, lymph nodes, and blood stream are a striking feature of HPS. Immunoperoxidase studies document activated T cells in lung parenchyma.[86] Flow cytometry studies identified the large blastlike cells in blood and pleural fluid as predominantly activated $CD8^+$ T cells, and elevated plasma levels of interleukin-2, interleukin-2 receptors, interferon-γ, interleukin-6, and soluble receptors for tumor necrosis factor suggest marked cytokine activation (unpublished data). Activated immunoblastic cells are not found infiltrating the kidney, heart, and most other tissues.[89] In HFRS, circulating immune complexes are detected,[92] and the classical complement pathway is activated.[93] Moreover, the kidney in the acute phase of nephropathia epidemica contains deposits of immunoglobulin and complement beneath the basement membrane,[94] suggesting that immune complexes may have a role in the immunopathogenesis of the renal lesion in HFRS. In contrast, in HPS, circulating immune complexes are not detected, and serum levels of activated complement components are normal.

These observations suggest that immunopathologic mechanisms may mediate the capillary leak syndrome in both HFRS and HPS. In this hypothesis, hantavirus-infected endothelial cells may be the target of attack by virus-specific cytolytic T cells, which appear in the circulation several days after virus-specific immunoglobulin M and immunoglobulin G antibody, both of which are present at onset of symptoms. Local secretion of cytokines may control viral replication but also injures the endothelial cell, creating temporary paracellular gaps that permit the escape of plasma fluid but not cells out of the capillary into the interstitium and alveolus, a scenario suggested by in vitro models.[95]

Diagnosis of Hantavirus Infections

Acute hantavirus infections are diagnosed by detecting immunoglobulin G and immunoglobulin M antibodies in serum that react with hantavirus antigens.[96–102] In acute SNV infections, SNV RNA can be detected in peripheral blood mononuclear cells by the RT-PCR.[87] The propagation of hantaviruses in cell culture or in laboratory animals is not currently a practical diagnostic modality.[15, 16, 25, 28, 103]

Hantavirus nucleocapsid proteins are highly antigenic, and high titers of immunoglobulin M and immunoglobulin G N antibodies are detected in serum at the onset of symptoms in HFRS and in HPS.[96–98, 100] N immunoglobulin G antibodies reach high titers and can be detectable for decades.[54, 97, 100, 104, 105] N polyclonal responses include antibodies that cross-react with the N proteins of related hantaviruses, and the strength of the cross-reactivity varies with the closeness of the evolutionary relatedness of the viruses.[52, 106–108] In both human and *P. maniculatus* SNV infections, an immunodominant region has been localized within the N-terminal 59 amino acids of SNV N.[98, 109] Antibodies that react within this region cross-react strongly with PUU N and PHV N and cross-react weakly with SEO N and HTN N. Therefore, the detection of hantavirus N antibody responses is a sensitive indicator of current or past hantavirus infection but generally cannot differentiate between infections caused by different hantavirus species.

In contrast, envelope glycoprotein (G1 and G2) responses tend to be more virus type specific and include neutralizing antibodies that block virus infectivity in vitro and in laboratory animals.[38, 98, 107, 110–119] The observation that G1 and G2 antibodies neutralize virus infectivity in vitro forms the basis for the plaque reduction neutralization test, a complicated assay for detecting hantavirus type–specific antibody reactivities.[21, 38, 107, 120] In SNV infections, SNV virus type–specific antibody reactivities to SNV G1 recombinant antigens have been described. The detection of these SNV G1 reactivities permits the virus type–specific diagnosis of SNV infections.[98] SNV G1 immunoglobulin G antibodies are detected at onset of disease symptoms, but immunoglobulin M antibodies are sometimes present at low or undetectable levels. A dominant linear epitope recognized by human SNV G1 antibodies has been mapped to an N-proximal portion of G1 (between amino acids 58 and 88).[98]

In nephropathia epidemica, PUU G1 antibodies are detected in acute and early convalescent serum samples, lagging somewhat behind PUU N antibody responses.[97, 100–102] PUU G2 antibody reactivities are not detected within the first 5 weeks after infection but rise gradually to high titers in subsequent weeks. N, G1, and G2 antibodies are detected at high titers 2 years after acute infection.[97, 100]

The detection of SNV N and SNV G1 antibodies in serum is the basis for virus type–specific diagnosis of human SNV infections. Hantavirus recombinant proteins have commonly been used as antigen targets in serodiagnostic assays because of the difficulty in obtaining adequate amounts of native viral proteins.[96, 98, 99, 101, 102] In the SNV Western blot assay, serum samples are tested for the presence of immunoglobulin G and immunoglobulin M antibodies that react with recombinant SNV N and G1 proteins.[98] Immunoglobulin G and immunoglobulin M antibodies to SNV N, and immunoglobulin G antibodies to SNV G1, are present in acute HPS. Immunoglobulin M antibodies to SNV G1 are often but not invariably detected (Fig. 254–2). The presence of immunoglobulin G and immunoglobulin M antibodies to SNV N indicates that the patient is infected with a hantavirus. The presence of SNV G1 antibodies indicates that the patient is infected with SNV or a closely related hantavirus. The SNV N and G1 recombinant proteins, and synthetic peptides derived from epitope mapping studies, are being adapted to a strip immunoblot assay format similar to that used in commercial tests for hepatitis C virus antibodies.

SNV RNA can be detected in the peripheral blood of patients with acute HPS by RT-PCR.[87] Various different hantavirus RNAs can be amplified in the RT-PCR by use of oligonucleotide primers derived from hantavirus consensus sequences. SNV RNA is most readily detected in peripheral blood mononuclear cell preparations, but it is also detected in plasma in some patients. SNV is detected during acute HPS and is not detected after convalescence. In cases in which the identity of the infecting hantavirus is in doubt, owing to either confusing epidemiologic factors or ambiguous serologic results, RT-PCR and nucleotide sequencing can provide a definitive identification.[43, 44, 46, 47, 87]

In fatal cases of hantavirus infections in which serum and fresh tissue samples are not available for study, hantavirus antigens can be detected by immunohistochemical staining

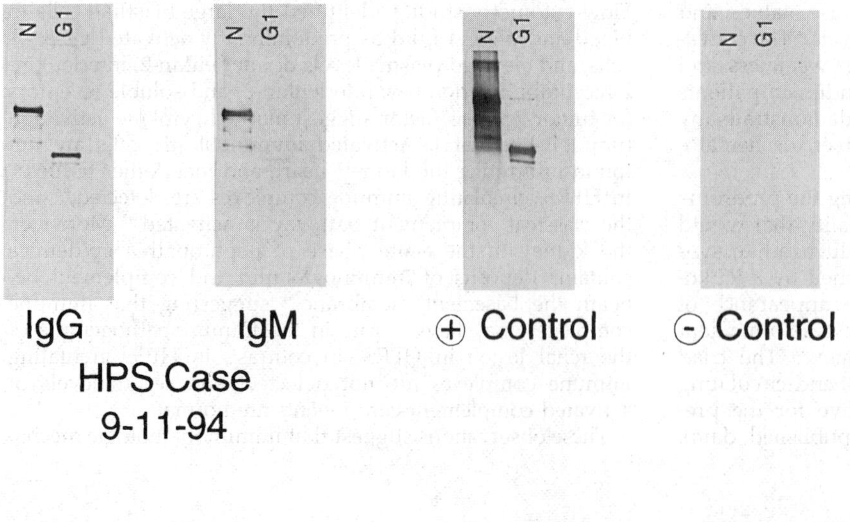

FIGURE 254–2 □ SNV recombinant Western blot assay. Each panel is a replicate Western blot that contains SNV N (N) and SNV G1 (G1) proteins in separate lanes.[98] Samples were reacted with serum from a patient with a clinical syndrome consistent with HPS. Separate blots were used to detect immunoglobulin G (IgG) antibodies and immunoglobulin M (IgM) antibodies. The serum sample was found to contain strong immunoglobulin G and immunoglobulin M reactivities to SNV N, a strong immunoglobulin G reactivity to SNV G1, and a weak immunoglobulin M reactivity to SNV G1. This pattern is typically seen in patients presenting with acute HPS. Positive and negative control serum samples, respectively, were tested with blots shown.

of paraffin-embedded tissue sections.[89] High densities of hantavirus antigens are observed in renal endothelial cells in fatal cases of HFRS and in pulmonary endothelial cells in fatal HPS cases. In most instances, the antibodies used for immunohistochemical staining have been mouse polyclonal antisera or monoclonal antibodies that react with hantavirus nucleocapsid proteins.[89, 115] Therefore, these antibodies can detect hantavirus antigens in tissues but cannot identify which hantavirus is present. Specific diagnosis by immunohistochemical staining will require the availability of hantavirus type–specific monoclonal antibodies.

Management

The management of HFRS focuses on restoring fluid balance, correcting electrolyte disorders, and treating hypotension with judicious fluid replacement.[78] Peritoneal dialysis or hemodialysis is essential for acute renal failure. Corticosteroids may predispose the patient to nosocomial pneumonia and are not recommended. Intravenous ribavirin has been shown in a placebo-controlled, randomized trial to reduce morbidity and mortality of HFRS in China for patients receiving at least 5 days of therapy.[121]

The management of HPS must focus on the prompt recognition of the syndrome and transfer of the patient to an intensive care unit.[13, 85] In the hypotensive patient, placement of a pulmonary artery catheter to measure pulmonary wedge pressures will help avoid excessive fluid replacement and exacerbation of alveolar flooding. The use of diuretics may exacerbate the volume depletion and shock, without alleviating the pulmonary edema. Pressors for inotropic support, such as dobutamine, should be used to restore blood pressure, urine output, and peripheral circulation. For patients with severe gas exchange abnormalities with a partial pressure of arterial oxygen/fraction of inspired oxygen (PaO_2/FIO_2) of less than 100, mechanical ventilation with high levels of positive end-expiratory pressure and conventional volume-controlled ventilation are necessary. Complete paralysis with vecuronium bromide, and the experimental reversed ratio ventilation, may be necessary in selected patients. Indicators of a high risk for mortality include admission serum lactate level above 4.0 μg/dL and a cardiac index less than 2.1 L/min per m^2.[85] Experience with two critically ill HPS patients treated with extracorporeal membrane oxygenation suggests that this experimental modality should be considered when it is available for patients with a high risk for mortality. Until HPS is diagnosed by serology, presumptive antibiotic therapy for common causes of sepsis must be instituted in every patient. Available uncontrolled data on ribavirin in HPS do not permit conclusions on efficacy (Chapman LE, Mertz G, unpublished data) until a nationwide placebo-controlled trial is completed.

Prevention

The Centers for Disease Control and Prevention has issued interim guidelines for reducing the risk for transmission of hantavirus infections.[122] These guidelines emphasize practical recommendations for preventing rodent infestations, for cleaning up rodent-infested sites, and for trapping and disposing of rodents.

Recombinant protein vaccines have been developed for HTN.[116] Studies indicate that immunization with hantavirus glycoproteins (G1 and G2) induces neutralizing antibody responses.[116, 117] It is conceivable that recombinant SNV glycoprotein vaccines could be useful when the risk for SNV transmission is high. The identification of a dominant G1 epitope that is recognized by human antibodies during acute SNV infections may be useful in the design of recombinant SNV vaccines.[98]

References

1. Earle DP: Symposium on epidemic hemorrhagic fever. Am J Med 16:617, 1954.
2. Lee HW, Lee PW, Lahdevirta J, Brummer-Korventkontio M: Aetiological relation between Korean haemorrhagic fever and nephropathia epidemica. Lancet 1:186, 1979.
3. World Health Organization: Hemorrhagic fever with renal syndrome—Memorandum from a WHO meeting. Bull World Health Organ 61:269, 1983.
4. Duchin JS, Koster FT, Peters CJ, et al: Hantavirus pulmonary syndrome: A clinical description of 17 patients with a newly recognized disease. N Engl J Med 330:949, 1994.
5. Nichol ST, Spiropoulou CF, Morzunov S, et al: Genetic identification of a novel hantavirus associated with an outbreak of acute respiratory illness in the southwestern United States. Science 262:914, 1993.
6. Hjelle B, Jenison SA, Goade DE, et al: Hantaviruses: Clinical, microbiologic and epidemiologic aspects. Crit Rev Clin Lab Sci 32:469, 1995.
7. Jenison S, Hjelle B, Simpson S, et al: Hantavirus pulmonary syndrome: Clinical, diagnostic, and virologic aspects. Semin Respir Infect 10:259, 1995.
8. Centers for Disease Control and Prevention: Outbreak of acute illness—Southwestern United States, 1993. MMWR Morbid Mortal Wkly Rep 42:421, 1993.
9. Centers for Disease Control and Prevention: Update: Outbreak of hantavirus infection—Southwestern United States, 1993. MMWR Morbid Mortal Wkly Rep 42:441, 1993.
10. Centers for Disease Control and Prevention: Update: Outbreak of hantavirus infection—Southwestern United States, 1993. MMWR Morbid Mortal Wkly Rep 42:477, 1993.
11. Centers for Disease Control and Prevention: Update: Outbreak of hantavirus infection—Southwestern United States, 1993. MMWR Morbid Mortal Wkly Rep 42:495, 1993.
12. Centers for Disease Control and Prevention: Update: Outbreak of hantavirus infection—United States, 1993. MMWR Morbid Mortal Wkly Rep 42:612, 1993.
13. Levy H, Simpson SQ: Hantavirus pulmonary syndrome. Am J Respir Crit Care Med 149:1710, 1994.
14. Childs JE, Ksiazek TG, Spiropoulou CF, et al: Serologic and genetic identification of *Peromyscus maniculatus* as the primary rodent reservoir for a new hantavirus in the southwestern United States. J Infect Dis 169:1271, 1994.
15. Elliott LH, Ksiazek TG, Rollin PE, et al: Isolation of the causative agent of hantavirus pulmonary syndrome. Am J Trop Med Hyg 51:102, 1994.
16. Schmaljohn AL, Li D, Negley DL, et al: Isolation and initial characterization of a newfound hantavirus from California. Virology 206:963, 1995.
17. McCormick JB, Palner EL, Sasso DR, et al: Morphological identification of the agent of Korean hemorrhagic fever (Hantaan virus) as a member of the Bunyaviridae. Lancet 1:765, 1982.
18. Schmaljohn CS, Dalrymple JM: Analysis of Hantaan virus RNA: Evidence for a new genus of Bunyaviridae. Virology 131:482, 1983.
19. Sugiyama K, Morikawa S, Matsuura Y, et al: Four serotypes of haemorrhagic fever with renal syndrome viruses identified by polyclonal and monoclonal antibodies. J Gen Virol 68:979, 1987.
20. Elliott LH, Kiley MP, McCormick JB: Hantaan virus: Identification of virion proteins. J Gen Virol 65:1285, 1984.
21. Schmaljohn CS, Hasty SE, Dalrymple JM, et al: Antigenic and genetic properties of viruses linked to hemorrhagic fever with renal syndrome. Science 227:1041, 1985.
22. Schmaljohn CS, Jennings JB, Hay J, et al: Coding strategy of the S genome segment of Hantaan virus. Virology 155:633, 1986.
23. Schmaljohn CS, Schmaljohn AL, Dalrymple JM: Hantaan virus M RNA: Coding strategy, nucleotide sequence, and gene order. Virology 157:31, 1987.
24. French GR, Foulke RS, Brand OA, et al: Korean hemorrhagic

fever: Propagation of the etiologic agent in a cell line of human origin. Science 211:1046, 1981.
25. Lee HW, Lee PW, Johnson KM: Isolation of the etiologic agent of Korean hemorrhagic fever. J Infect Dis 137:298, 1978.
26. Childs JE, Korch GW, Glass GE, et al: Epizootiology of hantavirus infections in Baltimore: Isolation of a virus from Norway rats, and characteristics of infected rat populations. Am J Epidemiol 126:55, 1987.
27. LeDuc JW, Smith GA, Johnson KM: Hantaan-like viruses from domestic rats captured in the United States. Am J Trop Med Hyg 33:992, 1984.
28. Lee HW, Baek LJ, Johnson KM: Isolation of Hantaan virus, the etiologic agent of Korean hemorrhagic fever from wild urban rats. J Infect Dis 146:638, 1983.
29. Song G, Hang CS, Liao HX, et al: Antigenic difference between viral strains causing classical and mild types of epidemic hemorrhagic fever with renal syndrome in China. J Infect Dis 150:889, 1984.
30. Brummer-Korvenkontio M, Vaheri A, von Bonsdorff C-H, et al: Nephropathia epidemica: Detection of antigen in bank voles and serologic diagnosis of human infection. J Infect Dis 141:131, 1980.
31. Mustonen J, Brummer-Korvenkontio M, Hedman K, et al: Nephropathia epidemica in Finland: A retrospective study of 126 cases. Scand J Infect Dis 26:7, 1994.
32. Niklasson B, LeDuc JW: Epidemiology of nephropathia epidemica in Sweden. J Infect Dis 155:269, 1987.
33. Plyusnin A, Vapalahti O, Ulfves K, et al: Sequences of wild Puumala virus genes show a correlation of genetic variation with geographic origin of the strains. J Gen Virol 75:405, 1994.
34. Settergren B: Nephropathia epidemica (hemorrhagic fever with renal syndrome) in Scandinavia. Rev Infect Dis 13:736, 1991.
35. Vapalahti O, Kallio-Kokko H, Salonen EM, et al: Cloning and sequencing of Puumala virus Sotkamo strain S and M segments: Evidence for strain variation in hantaviruses and expression of the nucleocapsid protein. J Gen Virol 73:829, 1992.
36. Yanagihara R, Amyx HL, Gajdusek DC: Experimental infection with Puumala virus, the etiologic agent of nephropathia epidemica, in bank voles *(Clethrionomys glareolus)*. J Virol 55:34, 1985.
37. Lee PW, Yanagihara R, Franko MC, et al: Preliminary evidence that Hantaan or a closely related virus is enzootic in domestic rodents. N Engl J Med 307:624, 1982.
38. Lee PW, Gibbs CJ Jr, Gajdusek DC, et al: Serotypic classification of hantaviruses by indirect immunofluorescent antibody and plaque reduction neutralization tests. J Clin Microbiol 22:940, 1985.
39. Yanagihara R: Hantavirus infection in the United States: Epizootiology and epidemiology. Rev Infect Dis 12:449, 1990.
40. Hjelle B, Jenison S, Torrez-Martinez N, et al: A novel hantavirus associated with an outbreak of fatal respiratory disease in the southwestern United States: Evolutionary relationships to known hantaviruses. J Virol 68:592, 1994.
41. Spiropoulou CF, Morzunov S, Feldmann H, et al: Genome structure and variability of a virus causing hantavirus pulmonary syndrome. Virology 200:715, 1994.
42. Brackett LE, Rotenberg J, Sherman CB: Hantavirus pulmonary syndrome in New England and Europe. N Engl J Med 331:545, 1994.
43. Centers for Disease Control and Prevention: Hantavirus pulmonary syndrome—Northeastern United States. MMWR Morbid Mortal Wkly Rep 43:549, 1994.
44. Hjelle B, Krolikowski J, Torrez-Martinez N, et al: Phylogenetically distinct hantavirus implicated in a case of hantavirus pulmonary syndrome in the northeastern United States. J Med Virol 46:21, 1995.
45. Song J-W, Baek L-J, Gajdusek DC, et al: Isolation of pathogenic hantavirus from white footed mouse *(Peromyscus leucopus)*. Lancet 344:1637, 1994.
46. Centers for Disease Control and Prevention: Newly identified hantavirus—Florida. MMWR Morbid Mortal Wkly Rep 43:99, 1994.
47. Morzunov SP, Feldmann H, Spiropoulou CF, et al: A newly recognized virus associated with a fatal case of hantavirus pulmonary syndrome in Louisiana. J Virol 69:1980, 1995.
48. Hjelle B, Chavez-Giles F, Torrez-Martinez N, et al: Genetic identification of a novel hantavirus of the harvest mouse *Reithrodontomys megalotis*. J Virol 68:6751, 1994.
49. Hjelle B, Anderson B, Torrez-Martinez N, et al: Prevalence and geographic genetic variation of hantaviruses of New World harvest mice *(Reithrodontomys)*: Identification of a divergent genotype from a Costa Rican *Reithrodontomys mexicanus*. Virology 207:452, 1995.
50. Hjelle B, Chavez-Giles F, Torrez-Martinez N, et al: Dominant glycoprotein epitope of Four Corners hantavirus is conserved across a wide geographical area. J Gen Virol 75:2881, 1994.
51. Puthavathana P, Dobbs M, Baek LJ, et al: Comparison of nucleotide sequences among hantaviruses belonging to the same serotype: An analysis of amplified DNA by thermal cycle sequencing. Virus Res 30:161, 1993.
52. Xiao S-Y, LeDuc JW, Chu Y-K, et al: Phylogenetic analysis of virus isolates of the genus *Hantavirus*, family Bunyaviridae. Virology 198:205, 1994.
53. Nerurkar VR, Song K-J, Song J-W, et al: Genetic evidence for a hantavirus enzootic in deer mice *(Peromyscus maniculatus)* a decade before the recognition of hantavirus pulmonary syndrome. Virology 204:563, 1994.
54. Wilson C, Hjelle B, Jenison S: A probable case of hantavirus pulmonary syndrome that occurred in New Mexico in 1975. Ann Intern Med 120:813, 1994.
55. Zaki SR, Albers RC, Greer PW, et al: Retrospective diagnosis of a 1983 case of fatal hantavirus pulmonary syndrome. Lancet 343:1037, 1994.
56. Dournon E, Moriniere B, Matheron S, et al: HFRS after a wild rodent bite in the Haute-Savoie and risk of exposure to Hantaan-like virus in a Paris laboratory. Lancet 1:676, 1984.
57. Kawamata J, Yamanouchi T, Dohmae K, et al: Control of laboratory acquired hemorrhagic fever with renal syndrome. Lab Anim Sci 37:431, 1987.
58. Tsai TF: Hemorrhagic fever with renal syndrome: Mode of transmission to humans. Lab Anim Sci 37:428, 1987.
59. Lee HW, Johnson KM: Laboratory-acquired infections with Hantaan virus, the etiologic agent of Korean hemorrhagic fever. J Infect Dis 146:645, 1982.
60. Umenai T, Lee HW, Lee PW, et al: Korean haemorrhagic fever in staff in an animal laboratory. Lancet 1:1314, 1979.
61. Ruo SL, Li YL, Tong Z, et al: Retrospective and prospective studies of hemorrhagic fever with renal syndrome in rural China. J Infect Dis 70:527, 1994.
62. Xu Z-Y, Guo C-S, Wu Y-L, et al: Epidemiological studies of hemorrhagic fever with renal syndrome: Analysis of risk factors and mode of transmission. J Infect Dis 152:137, 1985.
63. Flood J, Mintz L, Jay M, et al: Hantavirus infection following wilderness camping in Washington State and northeastern California. West J Med 163:162, 1995.
64. Zeitz PS, Butler JC, Cheek JE, et al: A case-control study of hantavirus pulmonary syndrome during an outbreak in the southwestern United States. J Infect Dis 171:864, 1995.
65. Counts EF, Seltzer R: The early diagnosis of endemic hemorrhagic fever. Ann Intern Med 38:67, 1953.
66. Sheedy JA, Froeb HF, Batson HA, et al: The clinical course of epidemic hemorrhagic fever. Am J Med 16:619, 1954.
67. Powell GM: Hemorrhagic fever: A study of 300 cases. Medicine (Baltimore) 33:97, 1954.
68. Lee HW, van der Groen G: Hemorrhagic fever with renal syndrome. Prog Med Virol 36:62, 1989.
69. Giles RB, Sheedy JA, Ekman CN, et al: The sequelae of epidemic hemorrhagic fever: With a note on causes of death. Am J Med 16:629, 1954.
70. Lee JS, Lee MC, Choi SJ, et al: Clinical features of serologically proven Korean hemorrhagic fever patients. Seoul J Med 21: 163, 1980.
71. Cohen MS, Casals J, Hsiung GD, et al: Epidemic hemorrhagic fever in Hubei Province, the People's Republic of China: A clinical and serological study. Yale J Biol Med 54:41, 1981.
72. Morimoto Y, Kishimoto S, Yamanouchi T, et al: Clinical features of hemorrhagic fever with renal syndrome in Japan: A clinical and laboratory study on 27 cases in Osaka in the 1960s and the 1980s. Jpn J Infect Dis 59:439, 1985.
73. Byun KS, Seo JB, Lee MS, et al: A clinical study of hemorrhagic fever with renal syndrome caused by Seoul viral infection. Korean J Infect Dis 18:11, 1986.

74. Lahdevirta J: Nephropathia epidemica in Finland: A clinical, serological and epidemiological study. Ann Clin Res 3(Suppl 8):1, 1971.
75. Antoniadis A, LeDuc JW, Acritidis N, et al: Hemorrhagic fever with renal syndrome in Greece: Clinical and laboratory characteristics. Rev Infect Dis 11(Suppl 4):S891, 1989.
76. Froeb HF, McDowell ME: Renal function in epidemic hemorrhagic fever. Am J Med 16:629, 1954.
77. Oliver J, MacDowell M: The renal lesion in epidemic hemorrhagic fever. J Clin Invest 36:99, 1957.
78. Earle DP: Analysis of sequential physiologic derangements in epidemic hemorrhagic fever. Am J Med 16:690, 1954.
79. Rubini ME, Jablon S, McDowell ME: Renal residuals of acute epidemic hemorrhagic fever. Arch Intern Med 128:378, 1960.
80. Lahdevirta J, Collan Y, Jokinen EJ, Hiltunen R: Renal sequelae to nephropathia epidemica. Acta Pathol Microbiol Scand A 86:265, 1978.
81. Settergren B, Juto P, Trollifors B: Hemorrhagic complications and other clinical findings in nephropathia epidemica in Sweden. A study of 355 serologically verified cases. J Infect Dis 157:380, 1988.
82. Lee HW: Hemorrhagic fever with renal syndrome in Korea. Rev Infect Dis 11(Suppl 4):S864, 1989.
83. Guang MY, Liu GZ, Cosgriff TM: Hemorrhage in hemorrhagic fever with renal syndrome in China. Rev Infect Dis 11(Suppl 4):S884, 1989.
84. Ketai LH, Williamson MR, Telepak RJ, et al: Hantavirus pulmonary syndrome (HPS): Radiographic findings in 16 patients. Radiology 191:665, 1994.
85. Hallin GW, Simpson SQ, Crowell RE, et al: Hantavirus pulmonary syndrome: Experience at the University of New Mexico Hospital. Crit Care Med 24:252, 1996.
86. Nolte KB, Feddersen RM, Foucar K, et al: Hantavirus pulmonary syndrome in the United States: Pathologic description of a disease caused by a new agent. Hum Pathol 26:110, 1995.
87. Hjelle B, Spiropoulou CF, Torrez-Martinez N, et al: Detection of Muerto Canyon virus RNA in peripheral blood mononuclear cells from patients with hantavirus pulmonary syndrome. J Infect Dis 170:1013, 1994.
88. Tao H, Jing-Yi Z, Yun-Ming T, et al: Identification of Hantaan virus–related structures in kidneys of cadavers with haemorrhagic fever with renal syndrome. Arch Virol 122:187, 1992.
89. Zaki SR, Greer PW, Coffield LM, et al: Hantavirus pulmonary syndrome—Pathogenesis of an emerging infectious disease. Am J Pathol 146:552, 1995.
90. Lukes RJ: The pathology of thirty-nine fatal cases of epidemic hemorrhagic fever. Am J Med 16:639, 1954.
91. Huang C, Jin B, Wang M, et al: Hemorrhagic fever with renal syndrome: Relationship between pathogenesis and cellular immunity. J Infect Dis 169:868, 1994.
92. Luo DD, Wang XH, Jin WE, Fan JZ: Detection and analysis of specific circulating immune complexes in epidemic hemorrhagic fever. Chin J Infect Dis 3:86, 1985.
93. Yan D, Gu X, Wang D, Yang S: Studies on immunopathogenesis in epidemic hemorrhagic fever: Sequential observations on activation of the first complement component in sera from patients with epidemic hemorrhagic fever. J Immunol 127:1064, 1981.
94. Jokinen EJ, Lahdevirta J, Collan Y: Nephropathia epidemica: Immunohistochemical study of pathogenesis. Clin Nephrol 9:1, 1978.
95. Goldblum SE, Hennig B, Jay M, et al: Tumor necrosis factor–induced pulmonary vascular endothelial injury. Infect Immun 57:1218, 1989.
96. Feldmann H, Sanchez A, Morzunov S, et al: Utilization of autopsy RNA for the synthesis of the nucleocapsid antigen of a newly recognized virus associated with hantavirus pulmonary syndrome. Virus Res 30:351, 1993.
97. Groen J, Dalrymple J, Fisher-Hoch S, et al: Serum antibodies to structural proteins of hantavirus arise at different times after infection. J Med Virol 37:283, 1992.
98. Jenison S, Yamada T, Morris C, et al: Characterization of human antibody responses to Four Corners hantavirus infections among patients with hantavirus pulmonary syndrome. J Virol 68:3000, 1994.
99. Kallio-Kokko H, Vapalahti O, Hedman K, et al: Puumala virus antibody and immunoglobulin G avidity assays based on a recombinant nucleocapsid antigen. J Clin Microbiol 31:677, 1993.
100. Lundkvist ÅA, Hörling J, Niklasson B: The humoral response to Puumala virus infection (nephropathia epidemica) investigated by viral protein specific immunoassays. Arch Virol 130:121, 1993.
101. Zöller LG, Yang S, Gött P, et al: A novel μ-capture enzyme-linked immunosorbent assay based on recombinant proteins for sensitive and specific diagnosis of hemorrhagic fever with renal syndrome. J Clin Microbiol 31:1194, 1993.
102. Zöller LG, Yang S, Gött P, et al: Use of recombinant nucleocapsid proteins of the Hantaan and nephropathia epidemica serotypes of hantaviruses as immunodiagnostic antigens. J Med Virol 39:200, 1993.
103. Lee PW, Amyx HL, Yanagihara R, et al: Partial characterization of Prospect Hill virus isolated from meadow voles in the United States. J Infect Dis 152:826, 1985.
104. Nuti M, Agostini M, Albini E, et al: Hantaan antibody in Italian ex-soldiers who served in the Balkans. Lancet 338:1277, 1991.
105. Settergren B, Ahlm C, Juto P, et al: Specific Puumala IgG virus half a century after haemorrhagic fever with renal syndrome. Lancet 338:66, 1991.
106. Asada H, Tamura M, Kondo K, et al: Cross-reactive immunity among different serotypes of virus causing hemorrhagic fever with renal syndrome. J Gen Virol 70:819, 1989.
107. Chu YK, Lee HW, LeDuc JW, et al: Serological relationships among viruses in the *Hantavirus* genus, family Bunyaviridae. Virology 198:196, 1994.
108. Xiao S-Y, Chu Y-K, Knauert FK, et al: Comparison of hantavirus isolates using a genus-reactive primer pair polymerase chain reaction. J Gen Virol 73:567, 1992.
109. Yamada T, Hjelle B, Lanzi R, et al: Antibody responses to Four Corners hantavirus infections in the deer mouse *(Peromyscus maniculatus):* Identification of an immunodominant region of the viral nucleocapsid protein. J Virol 69:1939, 1995.
110. Arikawa J, Schmaljohn AL, Dalrymple JM, et al: Characterization of Hantaan virus envelope glycoprotein antigenic determinants defined by monoclonal antibodies. J Gen Virol 70:615, 1989.
111. Arikawa J, Yao J-S, Yoshimatsu K, et al: Protective role of antigenic sites on the envelope protein of Hantaan virus defined by monoclonal antibodies. Arch Virol 126:271, 1992.
112. Dantas JR Jr, Okuno Y, Asada H, et al: Characterization of glycoproteins of viruses causing hemorrhagic fever with renal syndrome (HFRS) using monoclonal antibodies. Virology 151:379, 1986.
113. Lundkvist ÅA, Niklasson B: Bank vole monoclonal antibodies against Puumala virus envelope glycoproteins: Identification of epitopes involved in neutralization. Arch Virol 126:93, 1992.
114. Pensiero MN, Jennings GB, Schmaljohn CS, et al: Expression of the Hantaan virus M genome segment by using a vaccinia virus recombinant. J Virol 62:692, 1988.
115. Ruo SL, Sanchez A, Elliott LH, et al: Monoclonal antibodies to three strains of hantaviruses: Hantaan, R22, and Puumala. Arch Virol 119:1, 1991.
116. Schmaljohn CS, Chu YK, Schmaljohn AL, et al: Antigenic subunits of Hantaan virus expressed by baculovirus and vaccinia virus recombinants. J Virol 64:3162, 1990.
117. Wang M, Pennock DG, Spik KW, et al: Epitope mapping studies with neutralizing and non-neutralizing monoclonal antibodies to the G1 and G2 envelope glycoproteins of Hantaan virus. Virology 197:757, 1993.
118. Xu X, Ruo SL, McCormick JB, et al: Immunity to hantavirus challenge in *Meriones unguiculatus* induced by vaccinia-vectored viral proteins. Am J Trop Med Hyg 47:397, 1992.
119. Yoshimatsu K, Yoo Y-C, Yoshida R, et al: Protective immunity of Hantaan virus nucleocapsid and envelope protein studies using baculovirus-expressed proteins. Arch Virol 130:365, 1993.
120. Chu YK, Jennings G, Schmaljohn A, et al: Cross-neutralization of hantaviruses with immune sera from experimentally infected animals and from HFRS or HPS patients. J Infect Dis 172:1581, 1995.
121. Huggins JW, Hsiang CM, Cosgriff TM, et al: Prospective, double-blind, concurrent, placebo-controlled clinical trial of intravenous ribavirin therapy for hemorrhagic fever with renal syndrome. J Infect Dis 164:119, 1991.
122. Centers for Disease Control and Prevention: Hantavirus infection in the southwestern United States: Interim recommendations for risk reduction. MMWR Morbid Mortal Wkly Rep 42(RR-11):1, 1993.

255

Respiratory Syncytial Virus

Robert C. Welliver
Pearay L. Ogra

Respiratory syncytial virus (RSV) is the single most common cause of severe lower respiratory tract infections in infancy. Its worldwide distribution and unique seasonal occurrence in temperate climates, its potential for causing life-threatening or fatal respiratory illness, the possible role of the immune system in the pathogenesis of pulmonary disease, and its ability to cause reinfection in the presence of preexisting immunity have stimulated considerable investigative interest. Available modes of specific and nonspecific treatment do not yield impressive therapeutic outcomes, making the development of effective means of prevention a high priority.

Characteristics of the Pathogen

Classification

RSV is a member of the paramyxovirus family and has been assigned to the genus *Pneumovirus* because of certain differences from other paramyxoviruses, principally the lack of a hemagglutinin.[1] The virus contains a single, unsegmented strand of RNA of negative polarity.

Structure

RSV is an enveloped virus with a diameter of 300 to 350 nm, exhibiting spherical and filamentous forms.[2] It is currently believed that the genome of RSV codes for the synthesis of at least 10 viral proteins[3] shown in Table 255–1. Two nonglycosylated proteins are associated with the inner virion membrane, but, much more important, two glycoproteins are also found extending from the surface of the virion.[4, 5] One of these glycoproteins has a molecular mass of 68 kDa and functions as the fusion protein after proteolytic cleavage into subunits with molecular masses of 48 kDa (F_1) and 20 kDa (F_2).[6] The larger G glycoprotein has a molecular mass of approximately 90 kDa and has been identified as the attachment protein of RSV.[7] Within the envelope is a helical nucleocapsid.

TABLE 255–1 ■ Major Proteins Associated with Respiratory Syncytial Virus

Envelope (host cell membrane derived)
Matrix (M), 28 kDa
Large glycoprotein (G), 90 kDa
Fusion protein (F), 70 kDa
F_1 subunit, 50 kDa
F_2 subunit, 20 kDa
Other, 22 kDa
Internal viral nucleocapsid (RNA)
Nucleoprotein (NP), 42 kDa
Phosphoprotein (P), 34 kDa
Large protein (L), 200 kDa
Other proteins
Virion associated (1A), 9.5 kDa
Nonstructural
1B, 11 kDa
1C, 14 kDa

Replication

Replication of viral nucleic acid appears to proceed in a manner similar to that of other paramyxoviruses and is inhibited by 6-azauridine, an inhibitor of RNA replication,[8] but not by actinomycin D.[9]

Antigenic Characteristics

In the past it was believed that only one serotype of RSV existed; with animal serum, neutralizing titers vary somewhat against various strains of RSV. However, human convalescent serum seems to manifest essentially equivalent neutralizing antibody titers against all strains tested.[10] Panels of monoclonal antibodies have been developed against multiple epitopes on various viral proteins. Analysis of RSV strains using these antibodies in enzyme-linked immunosorbent assay (ELISA) and immunofluorescence assays has demonstrated that there is considerable homology among RSV proteins produced by most strains of the virus but that some variability in the antigenic structure of the G protein is evident among different strains.[11] On the basis of this type of analysis, two distinct subtypes of human RSV have been identified—subtype A and subtype B.[12] It has also been demonstrated that the degree of antigenic relatedness between the G proteins of the two subgroups is only about 5% whereas the relatedness between the fusion (F) proteins of the two subgroups is nearly 50%.[13] A further analysis of strains within each subgroup was carried out by determining the antigenic characteristics and size of structural proteins of 20 subgroup A and 43 subgroup B strains. Subgroup A strains are relatively uniform, whereas subgroup B strains vary to a much greater extent and have tentatively been divided into B1 and B2 variants on the basis of differences residing principally in the G and P proteins.[14]

Epidemiology

Distribution

Serologic surveys from essentially all areas of the world indicate that infection with RSV occurs commonly in all geographic and climatic areas.[15] In the United States and other countries in the temperate zones, sharp annual outbreaks of RSV occur during the colder months, in both the Northern and the Southern hemispheres.[16–18] It is apparent that both subtype A and subtype B strains may be present simultaneously or follow each other by several weeks in one epidemic season.[19–21] In the tropics and subtropical areas, outbreaks of RSV may be spread over several months and have less obvious peaks of activity. Interestingly, outbreaks in these areas occur during the hotter rainy seasons.[22] This peculiar epidemiologic pattern may be related to an increased amount of time spent indoors and to greater crowding during cold or rainy seasons. Other attempts to explain the onset and termination of RSV outbreaks on the basis of climatic conditions, such as temperature and hours of sunlight, have been generally unsuccessful.[23]

Prevalence

Most estimates of the prevalence of RSV infection have used hospitalization rates for bronchiolitis caused by RSV as the principal indicator of disease activity. This is because RSV infections in older persons are generally, but certainly not always, mild enough that they do not require medical attention. The risk of hospitalization for RSV bronchiolitis in infancy has been estimated to be between 1 and 7 per thousand.[15, 24, 25] Increased rates of hospitalization are observed in younger infants and those from lower socioeconomic circumstances. In one study, the rate of hospitalization for RSV infection of infants 1 to 3 months old in industrialized areas was 24.5 per thousand.[26] Estimates of the frequency with which RSV infects older persons are not easily obtained.

Among children in daycare centers, 75% were reinfected during their second exposure to virus in the classroom, and 65% were infected during the third exposure.[27] Adults are readily infected when RSV is introduced into a household[28] or during occupational exposure to infants with RSV.[29] Serologic evidence of past RSV infection is almost uniform among older children and adults,[30, 31] suggesting that reinfection occurs with sufficient frequency to maintain serum antibody titers at high levels.

Transmission

RSV is spread by self-inoculation after contact with virus, in secretions or on fomites, and possibly by large-droplet inoculation. In one study, five of seven persons who had direct physical contact with infected infants for 2 to 4 hours became infected, whereas none of 14 persons who sat at a distance of 6 feet or more from an infant's bed for 3 hours became infected. Ten other volunteers entered a patient's room only after the infant had been removed and then touched the bed and other objects that had been contaminated with secretions. Four of them became infected after touching the mucous membranes of their nose or eyes upon leaving the room.[29] Despite its reputation as an extraordinarily labile virus, RSV is capable of surviving on hands and inanimate objects as long as several hours after inoculation[32] (Table 255–2).

TABLE 255–2 ■ Survival of Respiratory Syncytial Virus in Patients' Secretions on Fomites

OBJECT INOCULATED	TIME UNTIL NO VIRUS RECOVERABLE (h)
Skin	0.5
Cloth	1
Paper tissue	1
Gloves	2
Countertop	7

Data from Hall CB, Douglas RG Jr, Geiman JM: Possible transmission by fomites of respiratory syncytial virus. J Infect Dis 141:98–102, 1980.

Pathogenesis

Antibody-Mediated Immunity

Antibody responses in the immunoglobulin (Ig) G, IgM, and IgA isotypes develop in serum and secretions after primary RSV infection.[33, 34] In some studies,[35] the appearance of secretory IgA antibody to RSV in the nasopharynx was associated with termination of virus shedding, and in another study[34] antibody was present in the respiratory tract at a time when virus shedding would be expected to be ongoing. Therefore, the role of secretory antibody in termination of RSV infection remains controversial.

Repeated infections with RSV result in progressively milder forms of clinical illness,[27] suggesting that some component of the immune system may provide partial protection against reinfection. Secretory antibody responses have been shown to be enhanced after secondary RSV infection.[34] Because virus shedding decreases with repeated infection, it may be true that enhanced secretory antibody responses with repeated infection account for partial immunity seen in older individuals. In addition, there is a correlation between the quantity of serum antibody acquired transplacentally and protection against illness caused by RSV infection in the first few months of life.[25] Nevertheless, infection occurs readily in the presence of reasonably large quantities of antibody acquired transplacentally or from a previous infection.[25, 30, 31] The method by which RSV escapes neutralization by preexisting antibody is unclear. Subtype differences in RSV do not completely account for this phenomenon, because consecutive infections with virus strains of the same subtype have also been observed.[36]

The development of RSV-specific IgE antibody has been demonstrated in both the nasopharyngeal secretions and the serum of infants with acute RSV infection. Titers of this antibody were significantly higher in patients with wheezing than in patients who had RSV infection without wheezing,[37, 38] and the titer seemed to correlate with the severity of illness.[37] Airway obstruction may be related to the IgE-directed release of chemical mediators that cause bronchoconstriction or excessive mucus secretion, such as histamine[37] or leukotriene C_4.[39]

Cell-Mediated Immunity

Cell-mediated immune mechanisms presumably play a role in limiting RSV infection, because it has been shown that RSV infections are particularly prolonged or severe in persons who have defects of cell-mediated immunity.[40, 41] In contrast, cell-mediated immune hypersensitivity, whether a result of previous immunization with inactivated vaccines[42] or natural infection,[43] has been associated with more severe forms of illness. RSV-specific cytotoxic T lymphocytes have been demonstrated, and their role in termination or enhancement of infection remains to be determined.[44, 45] These RSV-specific cells seem to recognize different viral proteins, including nucleoprotein, and may therefore be able to respond equally to infection with different viral subtypes.[46]

Other Defense Mechanisms

Cells infected with RSV have been shown to activate the complement cascade as well as neutrophil-mediated cytotoxicity mechanisms.[47, 48] The role of these mechanisms in limiting infection or in disease pathogenesis is unknown at present. Finally, RSV is a relatively poor inducer of interferon, and, even though RSV may be particularly susceptible to self-induced interferon, the course of illness appears to be unrelated to the quantity of interferon produced during natural infection.[35]

Clinical Manifestations

The major clinical manifestations associated with RSV infection are shown in Table 255–3.

Bronchiolitis

The most common form of severe illness caused by RSV infection is bronchiolitis. This illness most frequently affects infants from 2 to 6 months old, infrequently younger ones, and is progressively less frequent after 6 months of age.

TABLE 255-3 ■ Major Clinical Syndromes Associated with Respiratory Syncytial Virus Infection

Bronchiolitis in infancy
Asthma in children and adults
Pneumonia
Croup
Otitis media
Apnea in early infancy
Sudden infant death syndrome

Illness generally begins with symptoms of mild upper respiratory tract infection, with progression of cough and the development of wheezing. Fever is usually of low grade, but dyspnea and respiratory distress may be quite prominent. Auscultation of the chest reveals coarse inspiratory rales with rhonchi and wheezing on expiration. Significant hypoxemia may be present. Clinical improvement usually occurs in 3 to 4 days despite continued virus shedding and continued hypoxemia. Fatalities are extremely uncommon in the absence of underlying cardiac or pulmonary disease,[49] in which fatality rates may approach 5%. Recurrent episodes of wheezing (resulting from repeated RSV infection and other causes) occur commonly throughout infancy and early childhood, and evidence of pulmonary dysfunction has frequently been demonstrated on long-term follow-up of patients who had bronchiolitis in infancy.[50, 51] Whether these long-term abnormalities are the result of damage to the airway at a critical time in development or a manifestation of an inborn tendency toward small-airway dysfunction that is first signaled by the development of RSV bronchiolitis remains uncertain.

Pneumonia

RSV has been implicated as a frequent cause of pneumonia in infants and young children, particularly in those admitted to the hospital. Curves reflecting the incidence of pneumonia in infants and young children parallel the seasonal incidence of bronchiolitis as well as the frequency of isolation of RSV from inpatients. In fact, pneumonia and bronchiolitis are often diagnosed concurrently and are difficult to separate clinically in RSV-infected infants.[52]

Although RSV pneumonia is a rare event in immunocompetent older children and adults, it is becoming recognized as an important problem in recipients of organ transplantation.[53] Prolonged shedding of the virus is the rule, and some deaths appear to have been caused by RSV pneumonia in this population.

Croup

RSV can be recovered from approximately 10% of children with croup, especially during the first few years of life.[54] Croup caused by RSV may be milder in nature but otherwise indistinguishable from croup caused by the parainfluenza viruses, which are the most common causes of this illness.

Otitis Media

Viral agents are rarely recovered from the middle-ear cavities of children with acute otitis media, although this may be because viruses are responsible only for obstruction of the eustachian tube without direct invasion of the middle-ear cavity. In children who have acute otitis media during the RSV season, evidence of concurrent RSV infection has been found in up to 40% of cases.[55]

Apnea

Infants younger than 6 months old who have RSV infection may present with apnea early in the course of illness. It has been demonstrated that apnea caused by RSV may be followed by mild upper respiratory tract infection alone, or patients may later develop lower respiratory tract disease.[56] In the authors' experience, RSV may be recovered from the respiratory tract of infants who present with idiopathic apnea in the total absence of any symptoms of respiratory infection.

Sudden Infant Death Syndrome

RSV and other viral agents may be identified in the lung of as many as 30% of infants with sudden infant death syndrome. It is unclear how fairly minor infections with these agents may contribute to the development of sudden infant death.[57]

Clinical Course

As noted earlier, most RSV infections resolve spontaneously or with supportive therapy during a period of several days. Infections that are more severe or more persistent may occur in immunocompromised children[41] and adults[58] or in infants with bronchopulmonary dysplasia[59] or cyanotic congenital heart disease.[60] Even in otherwise healthy adults, RSV infection may result in pneumonia,[61] primary episodes of obstructive airway disease,[61] and abnormalities on pulmonary function tests that may last for up to 8 weeks after infection.[62]

Laboratory Findings

The results of routine laboratory investigations are so nonspecific in RSV infection as to be useless in identifying a specific agent. The usual findings at chest radiography include diffusely increased interstitial markings, areas of consolidation, which may vary considerably in size, and, most consistently, hyperinflation.[63, 64]

Diagnosis

The specific diagnosis of RSV infection is best made by isolation of the virus in tissue culture, identification of viral antigen, or specific serologic procedures.

Cell Culture

RSV can be recognized in cell culture by the formation of characteristic syncytia. These may be evident as early as a few days after inoculation of cell culture if conditions are optimal.[65] Maximal sensitivity is achieved by using low-passage human epithelial (HEp-2) cell lines. RSV is recovered much more frequently if clinical specimens are obtained by nasal washing or aspiration than if throat swabs or nasopharyngeal swabs are used.[66]

Shell vial procedures have replaced standard cell culture techniques in many diagnostic laboratories. Samples of respiratory secretions are centrifuged (700 × *g*) onto monolayers of culture cells in tubes, fresh medium is added, and the cell sheet is examined at various intervals for a cytopathic effect. The cell sheet can also be stained using immunofluorescence techniques for RSV antigen.[67, 68] In general, shell vial assays have proved to be as accurate as cell culture, with results available in 1 to 2 days, compared with an average of 4 to 5 days for cell culture. Cell culture using a variety of cell

TABLE 255–4 ■ Features of Various Diagnostic Tests for Respiratory Syncytial Virus Infection

TECHNIQUE	TIME UNTIL DEFINITIVE RESULT	COMMENT
Antigen detection using enzyme immunoassay or immunofluorescence	Several hours	Fastest and most sensitive assays False-positive results must be excluded Live virus not required
Polymerase chain reaction	4–12 h	Approximately as sensitive as cell culture Live virus not required
Shell vial assays	16–40 h	As accurate as cell culture, with earlier availability of results False-negative results later in illness Specimens must be handled carefully and promptly to avoid loss of infectivity
Cell culture	4–5 d on average	Highest specificity Identifies the presence of viruses other than RSV Specimens must be handled carefully and promptly to avoid loss of infectivity

lines may identify the presence of other viral agents more frequently (Table 255–4).

Rapid Diagnostic Tests

ANTIGEN DETECTION TECHNIQUES

The diagnosis of RSV infection has been greatly facilitated by the development of rapid diagnostic tests for identification of viral antigen in nasopharyngeal secretions, in bronchoalveolar lavage specimens, or in tissues obtained by biopsy or at autopsy. The accuracy of several commercially available kits that use indirect immunofluorescence, ELISA, or enzyme immunoassay procedures, is shown in Table 255–5. When compared with cell culture, there are probably no major differences in the sensitivity and specificity of each of these kits for diagnosis of RSV infection. There is considerable evidence that the rapid diagnostic assays are, in fact, far more sensitive for the detection of RSV infection than cell culture or shell vial assays.[65, 69–71] This is because as much as 40% of infectivity of a specimen may be lost even during storage in transport media at 4°C[72] and because antigen detection assays can still identify viral antigen in secretions or on the surface of exfoliated epithelial cells obtained several days into the course of illness, at a time when virus is no longer being shed. In the vast majority of instances when antigen detection assays yield positive results and the virus isolation assay is negative, appropriate blocking experiments have confirmed that positive results in antigen detection techniques represent true positive findings.[69–71] It should be noted that specimens obtained by nasopharyngeal aspiration also yield positive results by antigen detection techniques more commonly than specimens obtained by swabbing.[72]

TABLE 255–5 ■ Accuracy of Commercial Rapid Diagnostic Kits for Identification of Respiratory Syncytial Virus Infection

TECHNIQUE*	MANUFACTURER	% SENSITIVITY†	% SPECIFICITY†	REFERENCE
IFA	Burroughs-Wellcome	92‡	94	65
IFA	Burroughs-Wellcome	61	89	72
ELISA	Ortho	88§	94	71
ELISA	Ortho	69	100	72
EIA	Abbott	96§	96	70
EIA	Abbott	88	95	69

*IFA, Indirect immunofluorescence assay; ELISA, enzyme-linked immunosorbent assay; EIA, enzyme immunoassay.

†Versus tissue culture.

‡Immunofluorescence performed on tissue culture to confirm IFA-positive, culture-negative tests as true-positive results.

§Blocking assays used to confirm ELISA or EIA-positive, culture-negative result.

Commercially available kits often employ monoclonal antibodies as the detector antibody, because the background reactivity is quite low using monoclonal, versus polyclonal, antibodies. Some concern has arisen that highly specific monoclonal antibodies might not have broad enough reactivity to identify antigenically variant strains of RSV; however, antigen detection kits that utilize pools of monoclonal antibodies to RSV-containing antibodies to the fusion (F) protein and nucleoprotein react quite well with strains from either nucleoprotein subtype A or B.[11]

POLYMERASE CHAIN REACTION TECHNOLOGY

The polymerase chain reaction technique has also been adapted for the diagnosis of RSV infection.[73] A reverse transcription method proved to be approximately as sensitive and specific as conventional cell culture. Results were available with polymerase chain reaction in 8 to 24 hours, versus several days for cell culture. The polymerase chain reaction assay amplified a 243–base pair segment of the genome that codes for the F_1 subunit of the fusion protein, which is identical in subtype A and B strains. The lower limit of detection was 10 median tissue culture infectious doses.

Serologic Diagnosis

A variety of serologic techniques have been used in attempts to diagnose RSV infection. Of these, complement fixation techniques have been shown to be insensitive to RSV infection in infants, the age group in which the most severe form of illness occurs.[74] Immunofluorescence can be adapted to demonstrate RSV-specific responses in the IgG, IgM, and IgA isotypes, and increased sensitivity of the immunofluorescent technique in comparison with complement fixation techniques has been demonstrated in the diagnosis of RSV infection in infancy.[75] ELISAs have also been used to determine isotype-specific antibody responses to RSV. Although extensive evaluations have not been carried out, the sensitivity of ELISAs in infancy appears to be greater than that of complement fixation assays and approximately equal to that of immunofluorescent assays.[74] Neutralization assays using standard techniques have approximately the same sensitivity as ELISA or immunofluorescent assays.[74, 75] Complement-enhanced neutralization assays[75] are probably the most sensitive method for detection of RSV antibody in general use, but all neutralization assays have the disadvantage of being tedious and do not provide information on isotype-specific responses.

Each of the foregoing assay systems yields evidence of seroconversion to RSV only inconsistently in patients in the age group at which serious RSV infections occur most commonly, that is, 1 to 3 months. Each is probably equally useful in diagnosis of RSV infection in older children and adults. Only complement fixation and neutralization assays have been standardized, and these are the usual methods utilized for serologic detection of RSV infection.

Differential Diagnosis

Illness caused by RSV does not seem to be clinically distinguishable from that related to infections caused by other viruses,[76, 77] with the possible exception that the most severe forms of bronchiolitis are almost always associated with RSV infection. Parainfluenza and influenza virus bronchiolitis most closely mimics the severity of RSV-related disease. It is nearly impossible to distinguish RSV bronchiolitis from the first episode of true infantile asthma. In fact, RSV infection may provoke the first asthmatic episode in many children.

Treatment

Specific Antiviral Therapy

Ribavirin is a synthetic nucleoside that possesses in vitro antiviral properties against a variety of RNA and DNA viruses. When given by aerosol to infants with RSV infection, ribavirin has been associated with more rapid improvement in clinical illness scores and in oxygenation when compared with those of patients inhaling water as a control.[78, 79] Although there was initially some concern that ribavirin, because of its tendency to precipitate in the circuits of mechanical ventilators, could not be used to treat infants who needed mechanically assisted ventilation, the drug can nevertheless be administered safely to such patients provided that filters are placed and changed appropriately in the ventilatory circuits.[80]

The adequacy of the experimental design and methods of data evaluation in studies of the efficacy of ribavirin have been challenged.[81] The greatest benefit of ribavirin therapy was reported in a study of infants and young children who required mechanically assisted ventilation because of RSV infection.[82] In this study, in which water was used as the placebo, the time of ventilation and the duration of oxygen therapy were reduced by about one half in ribavirin recipients. Nevertheless, inhalation of water may cause bronchospasm or changes in diffusion capacity. A second study, using saline as a placebo, showed only slight differences favoring ribavirin use, which were not statistically significant.[83] Given the limited benefits and high costs of ribavirin, it should be used for only the most seriously ill infants with respiratory failure, if it is to be used at all. The effectiveness of ribavirin in transplant recipients who have RSV pneumonia has not been studied adequately.

Nonspecific Therapy

Most patients hospitalized for mild to moderate forms of RSV infection recover within a few days with supportive therapy alone. This includes administration of supplemental oxygen and replacement of fluid deficits. Unfortunately, there is not much to offer those with more severe forms of RSV infection. Despite continuing controversy, there is little convincing evidence that aerosolized bronchodilators,[84–86] theophylline,[87] or corticosteroids[88] are beneficial to the majority of patients with bronchiolitis. A small percentage of infants with bronchiolitis may respond favorably to aerosol therapy with β-adrenergic agents, but it appears impossible to identify them in advance.

Prevention

Nosocomial Infection

Hospital-acquired RSV infections are common on pediatric wards. Although these infections are usually not severe, they often prolong hospital stays unnecessarily. Occasionally, however, severe or fatal illness does occur.[89, 90] Hospital staff play a significant role in the spread of these infections, and the use of protective coverings such as gowns, masks, and goggles has been advocated to assist in reducing the rate of infection of health care workers.[91, 92] Although use of such articles is effective (either by protecting the worker or by reducing the number of visits to patients by such workers), their cost can be considerable. It may also be true that equally acceptable results can be attained by ensuring that medical personnel comply with simple hand-washing procedures,[93] which would be effective in removing RSV from the hands of health care providers.[94]

Immunization

ACTIVE

There is a clear need for effective immunoprophylaxis of RSV infection both in the United States and throughout the world. Because the major impact of the virus is expressed during the first half-year of life, programs for immunization against RSV face the considerable challenges of developing a vaccine that can be given in a single dose and is safe for this quite young, relatively unstable population. Prevention of spread of infection to infants might seem achievable by vaccination of adults and older children, but reinfection is common in these age groups, even in the presence of preexisting immunity. In all likelihood, secondary spread to infants could not be prevented.

A highly antigenic, formalin-inactivated RSV vaccine used in the 1960s did not provide protection against infection, and enhanced disease was observed in many vaccine recipients.[95] The focus of RSV vaccine development therefore switched to the development of live, attenuated vaccines. Temperature-sensitive mutant strains of RSV were produced, with the expectation that virus could grow at the relatively lower temperature of the nasopharynx but not in the lungs. Infection of seronegative children with these candidate vaccines resulted in shedding of virus strains that had reverted back to to the virulent (wild-type) strains.[96] Otitis media occurred in some recipients of the live vaccine. An inactivated vaccine consisting of purified preparations of the RSV F protein or attachment protein has been developed. Immunization of cotton rats with either of these vaccines results in the development in serum of antibody with neutralizing activity against RSV. This antibody was capable of protecting the lungs from virus replication on subsequent challenge, although replication did occur in the nasopharynx.[97]

An F protein vaccine is currently under investigation in humans. Adequate responses developed in seropositive children 18 to 36 months of age but not in younger infants.[98] Further trials of the F protein on a more potent adjuvant are in progress. In addition, trials of live, further attenuated RSV vaccines are being conducted.

Concern has arisen about whether immunization against one subtype of RSV provides adequate protection against the other subtype. Infants and children undergoing natural infection with one RSV subtype have been shown to develop fourfold or greater increases in neutralizing activity against each subtype with approximately equal frequency, although titers were significantly higher against the homologous infecting strain.[99] This would suggest that infection with a strain of one subtype would provide at least partial protection against subsequent infection with either subtype. However, neutralizing antibody (and antibody against either the F or attachment glycoprotein) does not provide complete protection against infection.[100] Further information about the exact mechanism of resistance to RSV infection may be required before an effective vaccine can be developed.

PASSIVE

An interesting development is the use of a hyperimmune human globulin in the prevention of RSV infection in infants and children with underlying cardiac or pulmonary disease.[101] These children are at high risk for severe illness at the time of RSV infection. A double-blind study indicated that monthly infusions of the hyperimmune globulin throughout the RSV season reduced the rate of hospitalization for RSV and the number of days in intensive care substantially. Side effects such as volume overload occurred with a negligible frequency. Children with these underlying illnesses whose health is particularly tenuous may benefit from preventive therapy with a similar compound when it is approved. The use of standard intravenous immune globulin preparations would not be expected to be of benefit, because the RSV neutralizing antibody content is much less than in the hyperimmune globulin.

References

1. Kingsbury DW, Bratt MA, Choppin PW, et al: Paramyxoviridae. Intervirology 10:137, 1978.
2. Berthiaume L, Joncas J, Pavilanis V: Comparative structure, morphogenesis and biological characteristics of the respiratory syncytial virus and the pneumonia virus of mice (PVM). Arch Gesamte Virusforsch 45:39, 1974.
3. Huang YT, Collins PL, Wertz GW: Characterization of the 10 proteins of human respiratory syncytial virus: Identification of a fourth envelope-associated protein. Virus Res 2:157, 1985.
4. Routledge EG, Willcocks MM, Morgan L, et al: Expression of the respiratory syncytial virus 22K protein on the surface of infected HeLa cells. J Gen Virol 68:1217, 1987.
5. Ueba O: Respiratory syncytial virus. II. Isolation and morphology of the glycoproteins. Acta Med Okayama 34:245, 1980.
6. Gruber C, Levine S: Respiratory syncytial virus polypeptides. III. The envelope-associated proteins. J Gen Virol 64:825, 1983.
7. Levine S, Klaiber-Franco R, Paradiso PR: Demonstration that glycoprotein G is the attachment protein of respiratory syncytial virus. J Gen Virol 68:2521, 1987.
8. Levine S, Peeples M, Hamilton R: Effective respiratory syncytial virus infection of HeLa cells macro-molecular synthesis. J Gen Virol 37:53, 1977.
9. Lambert DM, Pons MW, Mbuy GN, et al: Nucleic acids of respiratory syncytial virus. J Virol 36:837, 1980.
10. Coates HV, Alling DW, Channock RM: An antigenic analysis of respiratory syncytial virus isolates by a plaque reduction neutralization test. Am J Epidemiol 83:299, 1966.
11. Anderson LJ, Hierholzer JC, Tsou C, et al: Antigenic characterization of respiratory syncytial virus strains with monoclonal antibodies. J Infect Dis 151:626, 1985.
12. Mufson MA, Orvell C, Rafnar B, et al: Two distinct subtypes of human respiratory syncytial virus. J Gen Virol 66:2111, 1985.
13. Johnson PR Jr, Olmsted RA, Prince GA, et al: Antigenic relatedness between the glycoproteins of human respiratory syncytial virus subgroups A and B: Evaluation of the contributions of F and G glycoproteins to immunity. J Virol 61:3163, 1987.
14. Akerlind B, Norrby E, Orvell C, et al: Respiratory syncytial virus: Heterogeneity of subgroup B strains. J Gen Virol 69:2145, 1988.
15. Channock RM, Kim HW, Brandt CD, et al: Respiratory syncytial virus. *In* Evans AS (ed): Viral Infections of Humans, Epidemiology and Control, ed 2. New York, Plenum Publishing, 1983, pp 471–490.
16. Kim HW, Arrobio JA, Brandt CD, et al: Epidemiology of respiratory syncytial virus infection in Washington, DC. Am J Epidemiol 98:216, 1973.
17. Florman AL, McLaren LC: The effect of altitude and weather on the occurrence of outbreaks of respiratory syncytial virus infections. J Infect Dis 158:1401, 1988.
18. DeSilva LM, Hanlon MG: Respiratory syncytial virus: A report of a 5 year study at a children's hospital. J Med Virol 19:299, 1986.
19. Mufson MA, Belshe RB, Orvell C, et al: Respiratory syncytial virus epidemics: Variable dominance of subgroups A and B strains among children, 1981–1986. J Infect Dis 157:143, 1988.
20. Akerlind B, Norrby E: Occurrence of respiratory syncytial virus subtypes A and B strains in Sweden. J Med Virol 19:241, 1986.
21. Hendry RM, Talis AL, Godfrey E, et al: Concurrent circulation of antigenically distinct strains of respiratory syncytial virus during community outbreaks. J Infect Dis 153:291, 1986.
22. Spence L, Barratt N: Respiratory syncytial virus associated with acute respiratory infections in Trinidadian patients. Am J Epidemiol 88:256, 1968.
23. Sung RYT, Murray HGS, Chan RCK, et al: Seasonal patterns of respiratory syncytial virus infection in Hong Kong: A preliminary report. J Infect Dis 156:527, 1987.
24. Glezen WP: Pathogenesis of bronchiolitis—Epidemiologic considerations. Pediatr Res 11:239, 1977.
25. Glezen WP, Paredes A, Allison JE, et al: Risk of respiratory syncytial virus infection for infants from low-income families in relationship to age, sex, ethnic group, and maternal antibody level. J Pediatr 98:708, 1981.
26. Respiratory syncytial virus infection: Admissions to hospital in industrial, urban, and rural areas. Report to the Medical Research Council Subcommittee on Respiratory Syncytial Virus Vaccines. Br Med J 2:796, 1978.
27. Henderson FW, Collier AM, Clyde WA Jr, et al: Respiratory syncytial virus infections, reinfections and immunity. N Engl J Med 300:530, 1979.
28. Hall CB, Geiman JM, Biggar R, et al: Respiratory syncytial virus infections within families. N Engl J Med 294:414, 1976.
29. Hall CB, Douglas RG Jr: Modes of transmission of respiratory syncytial virus. J Pediatr 99:100, 1981.
30. Beem M, Egerer R, Anderson J: Respiratory syncytial virus neutralizing antibodies in persons residing in Chicago, Illinois. Pediatrics 34:761, 1964.
31. Johnson KM, Bloom HH, Mufson MA, et al: Natural reinfection of adults by respiratory syncytial virus. N Engl J Med 267:68, 1962.
32. Hall CB, Douglas RG Jr, Geiman JM: Possible transmission by fomites of respiratory syncytial virus. J Infect Dis 141:98, 1980.
33. Welliver RC, Kaul TN, Putnam TI, et al: The antibody response to primary and secondary infection with respiratory syncytial virus: Kinetics of class-specific responses. J Pediatr 96:808, 1980.
34. Kaul TN, Welliver RC, Wong DT, et al: Secretory antibody response to respiratory syncytial virus infection. Am J Dis Child 135:1013, 1981.
35. McIntosh K: Interferon in nasal secretions from infants with viral respiratory tract infections. J Pediatr 93:33, 1978.
36. Mufson MA, Belshe RB, Orvell C, et al: Subgroup characteristics of respiratory syncytial virus strains recovered from children with two consecutive infections. J Clin Microbiol 25:1535, 1987.
37. Welliver RC, Wong DT, Sun M, et al: The development of respiratory syncytial virus–specific IgE and the release of histamine in nasopharyngeal secretions after infection. N Engl J Med 305:841, 1981.
38. Bui RHD, Monilaro GA, Kettering JD, et al: Virus-specific IgE and IgG4 antibodies in serum of children infected with respiratory syncytial virus. J Pediatr 110:87, 1987.
39. Volovitz B, Welliver RC, DeCastro G, et al: The release of leukotrienes in the respiratory tract during infection with respiratory syncytial virus: Role in obstructive airway disease. Pediatr Res 24:504, 1988.

40. Fishaut M, Tubergen D, McIntosh K: Cellular response to respiratory viruses with particular reference to children with disorders of cell-mediated immunity. J Pediatr 96:179, 1980.
41. Hall CB, Powell KR, MacDonald NE, et al: Respiratory syncytial viral infection in children with compromised immune function. N Engl J Med 315:77, 1986.
42. Kim HW, Leikin SL, Arrobio J, et al: Cell-mediated immunity to respiratory syncytial virus induced by inactivated vaccine or by infection. Pediatr Res 10:75, 1976.
43. Welliver RC, Kaul A, Ogra PL: Cell-mediated immune response to respiratory syncytial virus infection: Relationship to the development of reactive airway disease. J Pediatr 94:370, 1979.
44. Bangham CRM, McMichael AJ: Specific human cytotoxic T cells recognize B-cell lines persistently infected with respiratory syncytial virus. Proc Natl Acad Sci USA 83:9183, 1986.
45. Isaacs D, Bangham CRM, McMichael AJ: Cell-mediated cytotoxic response to respiratory syncytial virus in infants with bronchiolitis. Lancet 2:769, 1987.
46. Bangham CRM, Openshaw PJM, Ball LA, et al: Human and murine cytotoxic T cells specific to respiratory syncytial virus recognize the viral nucleoprotein (N), but not the major glycoprotein (G), expressed by vaccinia virus recombinants. J Immunol 137:3973, 1986.
47. Kaul TN, Faden H, Baker R, et al: Virus-induced complement activation and neutrophil-mediated cytotoxicity against respiratory syncytial virus (RSV). Clin Exp Immunol 56:501, 1984.
48. Smith TH, McIntosh K, Fishaut M, et al: Activation of complement by cells infected with respiratory syncytial virus. Infect Immun 33:43, 1981.
49. Wohl MEB, Chernick V: Bronchiolitis. Am Rev Respir Dis 118:759, 1978.
50. Gurwitz D, Mindorff C, Levison H: Increased incidence of bronchio-reactivity in children with a history of bronchiolitis. J Pediatr 98:551, 1981.
51. Kattan M, Keenes TG, Lapierre JG, et al: Pulmonary function abnormalities in symptom-free children after bronchiolitis. Pediatrics 59:683, 1977.
52. Murphy TF, Henderson FW, Clyde WA Jr, et al: Pneumonia: An 11 year study in a pediatric practice. Am J Epidemiol 113:12, 1981.
53. Whimbey E, Champlin RE, Couch RB, et al: Community respiratory virus infections among hospitalized adult bone marrow transplant recipients. Clin Infect Dis 22:778, 1996.
54. Denny FW, Murphy TF, Clyde WA Jr, et al: Croup: An 11 year study in a pediatric practice. Pediatrics 71:871, 1983.
55. Berglund B, Salmivalli A, Toivanen P, et al: Isolation of respiratory syncytial virus from middle ear exudates of infants. Arch Dis Child 41:554, 1966.
56. Bruhn FW, Mokrohisky ST, McIntosh K: Apnea associated with respiratory syncytial virus infection in young infants. J Pediatr 90:382, 1977.
57. Uren EC, Williams AL, Jack I, et al: Association of respiratory virus infection with sudden infant death syndrome. Med J Aust 1:417, 1980.
58. Englund JA, Sullivan CJ, Jordan MC, et al: Respiratory syncytial virus infection in immunocompromised adults. Ann Intern Med 109:203,1988.
59. Groothuis JR, Gutierrez KM, Lauer BA: Respiratory syncytial virus infection in children with bronchopulmonary dysplasia. Pediatrics 82:199, 1988.
60. MacDonald NE, Hall CB, Suffin SC, et al: Respiratory syncytial viral infection in infants with congenital heart disease. N Engl J Med 307:397, 1982.
61. Vikerfors T, Grandien M, Olcen P: Respiratory syncytial virus infections in adults. Am Rev Respir Dis 136:561, 1987.
62. Hall WJ, Hall CB, Speers DM: Respiratory syncytial virus infection in adults: Clinical, virologic and serial pulmonary function studies. Ann Intern Med 88:203, 1978.
63. Simpson W, Hacking PM, Court SDM, et al: The radiologic findings in respiratory syncytial virus infection in children. II. The correlation of radiological categories with clinical and virological findings. Pediatr Radiol 2:155, 1974.
64. Rice RP, Loda F: A roentgenographic analysis of respiratory syncytial virus pneumonia in infants. Radiology 87:1021, 1966.
65. Kaul A, Scott R, Gallagher M, et al: Respiratory syncytial virus infection: Rapid diagnosis in children by use of indirect immunofluorescence. Am J Dis Child 132:1088, 1978.
66. Treuhaft MW, Soukup JM, Sullivan BJ: Practical recommendations for the detection of pediatric respiratory virus infections. J Clin Microbiol 22:270, 1985.
67. Smith MC, Creutz C, Huang YT: Detection of respiratory syncytial virus in nasopharyngeal secretions by shell vial technique. J Clin Microbiol 29:463, 1991.
68. Pedneault L, Robillard L, Turgeon JP: Validation of respiratory syncytial virus enzyme immunoassay and shell vial assay results. J Clin Microbiol 32:2861, 1994.
69. Swenson PD, Kaplan MH: Rapid detection of respiratory syncytial virus in nasopharyngeal aspirates by a commercial enzyme immunoassay. J Clin Microbiol 23:485, 1986.
70. Bromberg K, Tannis G, Daidone B, et al: Comparison of HEp-2 cell culture and Abbot respiratory syncytial virus enzyme immunoassay. J Clin Microbiol 24:434, 1987.
71. Lauer BA, Masters HA, Wren CG, et al: Rapid detection of respiratory syncytial virus in nasopharyngeal secretions by enzyme-linked immunosorbent assay. J Clin Microbiol 22:782, 1985.
72. Ahluwalia G, Embree J, McNicol P, et al: Comparison of nasopharyngeal aspirate and nasopharyngeal swab specimens for respiratory syncytial virus diagnosis by cell culture, indirect immunofluorescence assay, and enzyme-linked immunosorbent assay. J Clin Microbiol 25:763, 1987.
73. Paton AW, Paton JC, Lawrence AJ, et al: Rapid detection of respiratory syncytial virus in nasopharyngeal aspirates by reverse transcription and polymerase chain reaction amplification. J Clin Microbiol 30:901, 1992.
74. Richardson LS, Yolken RH, Belshe RB, et al: Enzyme-linked immunosorbent assay for measurement of serologic response to respiratory syncytial virus infection. Infect Immun 20:660, 1978.
75. Kaul TN, Welliver RC, Ogra PL: Comparison of fluorescent antibody, neutralizing antibody, and complement-enhanced neutralizing antibody assays for detection of serum antibody to respiratory syncytial virus. J Clin Microbiol 13:957, 1981.
76. Valenti WM, Clarke TA, Hall CB, et al: Concurrent outbreaks of rhinovirus and respiratory syncytial virus in an intensive care nursery: Epidemiology and associated risk factors. J Pediatr 100:722, 1982.
77. Caul EO, Waller DK, Clarke SKR: A comparison of influenza and respiratory syncytial virus infections among infants admitted to hospital with acute respiratory infections. J Hyg (Lond) 77:383, 1976.
78. Hall CB, McBride JT, Walsh EE, et al: Aerosolized ribavirin treatment of infants with respiratory syncytial viral infection. N Engl J Med 308:1443, 1983.
79. Rodriguez WJ, Kim HW, Brandt CD, et al: Aerosolized ribavirin in the treatment of patients with respiratory syncytial virus disease. Pediatr Infect Dis J 6:159, 1987.
80. Outwater KM, Meissner C, Peterson MB: Ribavirin administration to infants receiving mechanical ventilation. Am J Dis Child 142:512, 1988.
81. Wald ER, Dashefsky B, Green M: In re ribavirin: A case of premature adjudication? J Pediatr 112:154, 1988.
82. Smith DW, Frankel LR, Mathers LH, et al: A controlled trial of aerosolized ribavirin in infants receiving mechanical ventilation for severe respiratory syncytial virus infection. N Engl J Med 325:24, 1991.
83. Meert KL, Sarnaik AP, Gelmini MJ, et al: Aerosolized ribavirin in mechanically ventilated children with respiratory syncytial virus lower respiratory tract disease: A prospective, double-blind, randomized trial. Crit Care Med 22:566, 1994.
84. Rutter N, Milner AD, Hiller EJ: Effect of bronchodilators on respiratory resistance in infants and young children with bronchiolitis and wheezy bronchitis. Arch Dis Child 50:719, 1975.
85. Lenney W, Milner AD: Alpha and beta adrenergic stimulants in bronchiolitis and wheezy bronchitis in children under 18 months of age. Arch Dis Child 53:707, 1978.
86. Hughes DM, Lesouef PN, Landau LI: Effect of salbutamol on respiratory mechanics in bronchiolitis. Pediatr Res 22:83, 1987.
87. Brooks LJ, Cropp GJA: Theophylline therapy in bronchiolitis: A retrospective study. Am J Dis Child 135:934, 1981.
88. American Academy of Pediatrics Committee on Drugs: Should steroids be used in treating bronchiolitis? Pediatrics 46:640, 1970.
89. Simms DG, Downham MA, Webb JK, et al: Hospital cross-

infection on children's wards with respiratory syncytial virus and the role of adult carriage. Acta Paediatr Scand 64:541, 1975.
90. Hall CB, Douglas RG Jr, Geiman JM, et al: Nosocomial respiratory syncytial virus infection. N Engl J Med 293:1343, 1975.
91. Murphy D, Todd JK, Chao RK, et al: The use of gowns and masks to control respiratory illness in pediatric hospital personnel. J Pediatr 99:746, 1981.
92. Agah R, Cherry JD, Garakian AJ, et al: Respiratory syncytial virus (RSV) infection rate in personnel caring for children with RSV infections. Am J Dis Child 141:695, 1987.
93. Leclair JM, Freeman J, Sullivan BF, et al: Prevention of nosocomial respiratory syncytial virus infections through compliance with glove and gown isolation precautions. N Engl J Med 317:329, 1987.
94. Albert RK, Condie F: Hand washing patterns in medical intensive care units. N Engl J Med 304:1465, 1981.
95. Kapikian AZ, Mitchell RH, Chanock RM, et al: An epidemiologic study of altered clinical reactivity to respiratory syncytial (RS) virus infection in children previously vaccinated with an inactivated RS virus vaccine. Am J Epidemiol 89:405, 1969.
96. Hodes DS, Kim HW, Parrott RH, et al: Genetic alteration in a temperature sensitive mutant of respiratory syncytial virus after replication in vivo. Proc Soc Exp Biol Med 145:1158, 1974.
97. Walsh EE, Hall CB, Briselli M, et al: Immunization with glycoprotein subunits of respiratory syncytial virus to protect cotton rats against viral infection. J Infect Dis 155:1198, 1987.
98. Tristram DA, Welliver RC, Mohar CK, et al: Immunogenicity and safety of respiratory syncytial virus subunit vaccine in seropositive children 18–36 months old. J Infect Dis 167:191, 1993.
99. Hendry RM, Burns JC, Walsh EE, et al: Strain-specific serum antibody responses in infants undergoing primary infection with respiratory syncytial virus. J Infect Dis 157:640, 1988.
100. Levine S, Dajani A, Klaiber-Franco R: The response of infants with bronchiolitis to the proteins of respiratory syncytial virus. J Gen Virol 69:1229, 1988.
101. Groothuis JR, Simoes EAF, Levin MJ, et al: Prophylactic administration of respiratory syncytial virus immune globulin to high-risk infants and young children. N Engl J Med 329:1524, 1993.

256

Coronavirus

Ella M. Swierkosz
C. George Ray

History

Diseases caused by animal coronaviruses have been recognized since the 1930s. The first human coronaviruses (HCVs) were reported in 1965, when respiratory specimens from patients with common colds that had been inoculated into organ cultures (OCs) of human fetal tracheal or nasal epithelium yielded cytopathic agents that were designated OC43 and OC38.[1] The 229E virus was subsequently isolated during studies of medical students with acute upper respiratory tract illnesses.[2] The designation of these agents as coronaviruses was proposed in 1968, because their fringe of petal-shaped spikes resembled a "crown like the corona spinarum in religious art."[3] Coronavirus-like particles in human feces were described later[4] and subsequently have been associated with diarrheal diseases. The nature of these agents is still somewhat obscure; it is considered separately at the end of this chapter.

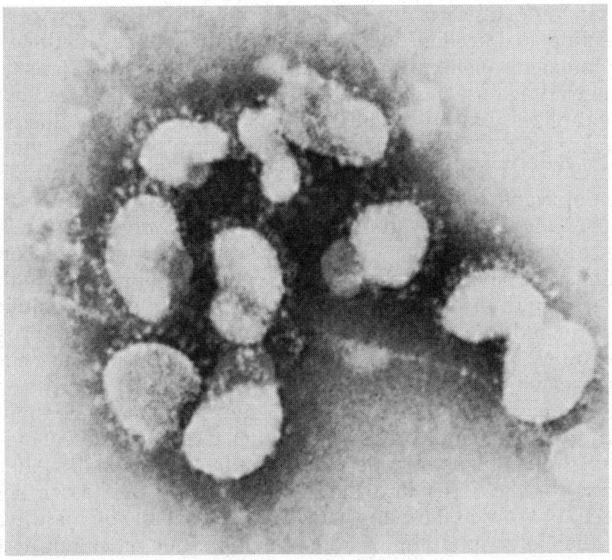

FIGURE 256–1 □ Electron micrograph of HCV 229E demonstrates the petal-shaped peplomers projecting from the envelope surfaces. (Courtesy of Dr. Claire M. Payne, University of Arizona College of Medicine, Tucson, AZ.)

Characteristics of the Pathogen

The family Coronaviridae has been divided into two genera: coronaviruses and toroviruses.[5,6] The genus *Coronavirus* consists of enveloped, generally spherical virions with helical nucleocapsids, ranging from 80 to 160 nm in diameter. They are distinguished by prominent petal-shaped spikes (peplomers) up to 20 nm in length that cover the entire envelope surface and give them the coronal appearance (Fig. 256–1). The single positive-polarity RNA genome functions as a messenger for the translation of protein. There are three or four major structural proteins: the S or spike glycoprotein (formerly E2) composes the peplomers on the virion envelope; the matrix glycoprotein, designated M (formerly E1); the hemagglutinin-esterase (HE) glycoprotein (formerly E3), which is found in the envelope of some antigenic group 2 viruses (including HCV OC43) and in turkey coronavirus (Table 256–1); and the nucleocapsid phosphoprotein, N, which binds to virion RNA, providing the structural basis for the helical nucleocapsid.[7]

The S glycoprotein mediates attachment to sialic acid–

TABLE 256–1 ■ Antigenic Groups of Coronaviridae

GROUP	REPRESENTATIVE STRAINS	HOST
1	HCV 229E	Human
	Canine coronavirus	Dog
	Feline enteric coronavirus	Cat
	Feline infectious peritonitis virus	Cat
	Porcine transmissible gastroenteritis virus	Pig
2	HCV OC43	Human
	Mouse hepatitis virus	Mouse
	Bovine coronavirus	Cattle
	Rabbit coronavirus	Rabbit
	Sialodacryadenitis virus	Rat
3	Avian bronchitis virus	Chicken
4	Bluecomb disease virus	Turkey

Adapted from Holmes KV: Coronaviridae and their replication. *In* Fields BN, Knipe DM (eds): Fields Virology, ed 2. New York, Raven Press, 1990, pp 841–856.

containing residues in the plasma membrane of host cells leading to infection and induces cell fusion[8]; cell-mediated cytotoxicity against mouse hepatitis virus–infected cells is directed against S glycoprotein.[9] Antibody to S glycoprotein neutralizes viral infectivity and inhibits the fusion-inducing ability of the virus.[10] The M glycoprotein forms the viral envelope and determines virion budding from the rough endoplasmic reticulum and Golgi membranes.[7] Antibodies to the M glycoprotein can neutralize the virus only in the presence of complement.[10] The HE glycoprotein, found only on some coronaviruses, shares some sequence homology with hemagglutinin of influenza C virus. It exhibits hemagglutinating and esterase activities, which permits elution of virus adsorbed to erythrocytes.[7] Antibody to HE glycoprotein neutralizes viral infectivity.[11]

Coronaviruses bind to cells via S glycoprotein and possibly HE glycoprotein, if present. A cellular receptor for coronavirus 229E, human aminopeptidase, has been described.[12] After entry of the virus into the cell, replication and assembly occur entirely in the cytoplasm. Virions assemble by budding at the Golgi apparatus or rough endoplasmic reticulum and are released by cell lysis or via cellular secretory mechanisms.[7]

Coronaviruses have been divided into four antigenic groups based on serologic comparisons.[7] There is a wide diversity of agents that affect birds and mammals, many of which are important in veterinary medicine and agriculture (see Table 256–1). The two recognized prototypic human strains, 229E and OC43, are in groups 1 and 2, respectively, along with other mammalian strains. Nearly all other HCVs that have been described are antigenically related to either 229E or OC43. Groups 3 and 4 include avian strains. Extensive genetic variation within strains is well recognized for the mammalian agents; this also occurs with those among humans, but the extent and significance are not yet well defined. There is no evidence for cross-species transmission in nature.

Epidemiology

Respiratory transmission from person to person is apparently common. Serologic surveys from different areas of the world have shown antibody prevalences among adults of 87% to 100% for HCV OC43, and 86% to 94% for HCV 229E.

Infections with HCV have been reported to account for a significant proportion of respiratory infections in adults and children.[13, 14] Their overall importance and possible sequelae, however, are not well understood, principally owing to the lack of reliable cell culture and other systems that can be conveniently used for their detection. Thus, most information about diseases produced by HCV has been derived from retrospective serologic determinations and infection of volunteer subjects.

Coronaviruses have been determined to be responsible for about 15% of upper respiratory tract infections in adults[15]: as many as 35% of adults show seroconversion to one strain or another during an epidemic. It has also been shown that seroconversion rates are highest among young children; they then drop during the second decade and adult years.[16]

One study used an enzyme immunoassay with polyclonal antibodies to detect HCV antigens in nasal secretions of infants and children 6 months to 6 years of age.[17] Antigens were detected in 30% of 108 acute respiratory episodes experienced by 30 children with a history of recurrent respiratory infections, and in 29% of 51 acute respiratory illnesses among their siblings. Most infections were due to HCV 229E; incidences peaked in the late fall or early winter and early summer. In contrast, other studies have shown that the highest frequency of antibody rises to both agents occurred during the winter months. Children were affected three times more often than adults, and serologic evidence suggesting reinfection was frequently observed during a 3-year period.[18]

Pathogenesis

Studies in HCV-infected human embryonic tracheal organ cultures[1, 15] and exfoliated cells from the nasopharynx of experimentally inoculated volunteers[19] indicate that a cytolytic effect on ciliated epithelial cells occurs and that this likely results in an inflammatory host response. In contrast, strain 229E can establish a persistent infection of cell cultures,[20] but the role of viral persistence in natural infection is not known. Immunologic injury mediates feline infectious peritonitis,[21] an animal coronavirus infection, and mouse hepatitis virus induces autoimmune-mediated demyelination in rodents,[22] but the importance of immune factors in the pathogenesis of HCV remains unknown.

Neurotropism of murine strains of coronaviruses is well recognized, and there is a close analogy between rodent demyelinating disease and multiple sclerosis.[23] Numerous studies have reported an association of HCV with multiple sclerosis,[24–26] and coronavirus antigen and RNA sequences have been detected in brain tissue of patients with multiple sclerosis.[27] Although these data do not establish coronavirus as the cause of multiple sclerosis, further work is warranted.

A high frequency of mutation and recombination has been observed among animal coronaviruses and may contribute to the large number of serotypes.[7] The number of serotypes of HCV has not been determined primarily because of the difficulty in culture-adapting these viruses, but strain differences have been observed among HCVs.[28] Because immunity is serotype specific, antigenic heterogeneity presumably allows for multiple symptomatic reinfections to occur.

Clinical Manifestations

The incubation period of HCV infections ranges from 2 to 5 days, and the usual illness lasts 3 to 18 days (mean, 7 days). In adults for whom data have been gathered by observation of natural illness and inoculation of volunteers, HCV usually produces an illness resembling that associated with rhinovirus infections. Symptoms of nasal discharge and malaise seem to be more prominent in coronavirus infections and cough more common in rhinovirus infections.[15]

The exact role of HCV in lower respiratory tract infections is less clear. It appears that HCV OC43 infections can produce cough as well as nasal symptoms in adults,[29, 30] and HCV infection has been associated with pneumonia and pleural reaction in military recruits.[31] In children, sore throat, cough, coryza, and fever are common, and pulmonary crackles have been noted in 5% of patients.[29] Acute attacks of wheezing can also occur, particularly among those known to be asthmatic or disposed to recurrent lower respiratory tract infections.[17, 33] Exacerbations of symptoms among persons with chronic obstructive pulmonary disease have also been reported.[34] Fatalities directly attributable to HCV appear to be exceedingly rare.

Diagnosis

Primary isolation of HCV is difficult. HCV 229E can be cultivated in several human diploid fibroblast cell strains or lines, but organ cultures remain the system of choice for HCV OC43. Both viruses can be adapted to replicate in a variety of diploid and heteroploid cell lines, and OC43 strains have been adapted in vivo in suckling mouse brains. Because of these difficulties, diagnoses have usually been made serologically, using complement fixation or more sensitive tests, such as enzyme immunoassay, indirect immunofluorescence, or hemagglutination inhibition (OC43 only).[13, 14, 18, 29–34] An indirect enzyme immunoassay for the detection of OC43 antibody has been found to be considerably more sensitive than hemagglutination inhibition, with high specificity.[35]

Antigen detection methods that use immunofluorescence of respiratory cells or enzyme immunoassay of respiratory secretions have been reported.[17, 19] Nucleic acid hybridization and reverse transcription–polymerase chain reaction have also been applied to the detection of HCV 229E RNA sequences.[36, 37]

The differential diagnosis of HCV infections encompasses the spectrum of agents that can affect the respiratory tract. These include rhinoviruses, myxoviruses, paramyxoviruses, adenoviruses, respiratory syncytial virus, Epstein-Barr virus, herpes simplex virus, some enteroviruses, and *Streptococcus pyogenes*. The severe coryza and occasional wheezing sometimes encountered can also mimic acute allergic rhinitis or asthma.

Treatment and Prevention

Symptomatic supportive care is all that is available. No specific preventive measures other than good hygiene are known. It is unlikely that any vaccine will be developed in the near future, and specific antiviral agents have not been tested for clinical efficacy in the prophylaxis or treatment of HCV infections.

Enteric Coronavirus-Like Particles

Coronavirus-like particles have been observed by direct electron microscopy of stool samples from patients with epidemic sprue, neonatal necrotizing enterocolitis, and gastroenteritis, particularly among premature infants and young children.[4, 38–40] A particularly high frequency of occurrence of these particles in diarrheal stool specimens submitted for electron microscopic examination has been noted in southern Arizona[41]; however, high rates of asymptomatic virus shedding have also been noted in some areas of the world.[42]

It is not yet clear whether this agent (or agents) belongs to the family Coronaviridae.[43] Isolation in cell cultures has been reported but not confirmed, but some strains have been reported to be propagated with difficulty in human fetal intestinal organ cultures.[39] Antigenic relatedness to HCV OC43 has been reported for some strains[44]; however, studies of other strains have not demonstrated such a relationship.[39, 40] Considerably more epidemiologic and biologic data will be needed before the role of these particles in human disease can be clearly ascertained.

References

1. Tyrrell DAJ, Bynoe ML: Cultivation of a novel type of common-cold virus in organ cultures. Br Med J 1:1467, 1965.
2. Hamre D, Procknow JJ: A new virus isolated from the human respiratory tract. Proc Soc Exp Biol Med 121:190, 1966.
3. Tyrrell DAJ, Almeida JD, Berry DM, et al: Coronaviruses. Nature 220:650, 1968.
4. Mathan M, Mathan VI, Swaminathan SP, et al: Pleomorphic virus-like particles in human faeces. Lancet 1:1068, 1975.
5. Cavanagh D, Brian DA, Brinton MA, et al: The Coronaviridae now comprises two genera, *Coronavirus* and *Torovirus*: Report of the Coronaviridae Study Group. Adv Exp Med Biol 342:255, 1993.
6. Snijder EJ, Horzinek MC, Spaan WJM: The Coronavirus-like superfamily. Adv Exp Med Biol 342:235, 1993.
7. Holmes KV: Coronaviridae and their replication. *In* Fields BN, Knipe DM (eds): Fields Virology, ed 2. New York, Raven Press, 1990, pp 841–856.
8. Vlasak R, Luytjes W, Spaan W, et al: Human and bovine coronaviruses recognize sialic acid–containing receptors similar to those of influenza C viruses. Proc Natl Acad Sci USA 85:4526, 1988.
9. Holmes KV, Welsh RM, Haspel MV: Natural cytotoxicity against mouse hepatitis virus-infected target cells. I. Correlation of cytotoxicity with virus binding to leukocytes. J Immunol 136:1446, 1986.
10. Collins AR, Knobler RL, Powell H, et al: Monoclonal antibodies to murine hepatitis virus-4 (strain JHM) define the viral glycoprotein responsible for attachment and cell-cell fusion. Virology 119:358, 1982.
11. Deregt D, Babiuk LA: Monoclonal antibodies to bovine coronavirus: Characteristics and topographical mapping of neutralizing epitopes on the E2 and E3 glycoproteins. Virology 161:410, 1987.
12. Yeager CL, Ashmun RA, Williams RK, et al: Human aminopeptidase N is a receptor for human coronavirus 229E. Nature 357:420, 1992.
13. Hamre D, Beem M: Virologic studies of acute respiratory disease in young adults. V. Coronavirus 229E infections during six years of surveillance. Am J Epidemiol 96:94, 1972.
14. Monto AS, Lim SK: The Tecumseh study of respiratory illness. VIII. Acute infection in chronic respiratory disease and comparison groups. Am Rev Respir Dis 111:27, 1985.
15. Bradburne AF, Bynoe ML, Tyrrell DAJ: Effects of the "new" human respiratory virus in volunteers. Br Med J 3:767, 1967.
16. Monto AS, Lim SK: The Tecumseh study of respiratory illness. VI. Frequency of and relationship between outbreaks of coronavirus infections. J Infect Dis 129:271, 1974.
17. Isaacs D, Flowers D, Clarke JR, et al: Epidemiology of coronavirus respiratory infections. Arch Dis Child 59:500, 1983.
18. Schmidt OW, Allan ID, Cooney MK, et al: Rises in titers of antibody to human coronaviruses OC43 and 229E in Seattle families during 1975–1979. Am J Epidemiol 123:862, 1986.
19. McIntosh K, McQuillin J, Reed SE, et al: Diagnosis of human coronavirus infection by immunofluorescence: Method and application to respiratory disease in hospitalized children. J Med Virol 2:341, 1978.
20. Chaloner-Larsson G, Johnson-Lussenberg CM. Establishment and maintenance of a persistent infection of L132 cells by human coronavirus strain 229E. Arch Virol 69:117, 1981.
21. Jacobse-Geels H, Daha MR, Horinek M: Isolation and characterization of feline C3 and evidence for the immune complex pathogenesis of feline infectious peritonitis. J Immunol 125:1606, 1980.
22. Watanabe R, Wege H, ter Meulen V: Adoptive transfer of EAE-like lesions from rats with coronavirus-induced demyelinating encephalomyelitis. Nature 305:150, 1983.
23. ter Meulen V, Masa PT, Dörries R: Coronaviruses. *In* McKendall RR (ed): Handbook of Clinical Neurology, Vol 12, Viral Disease. New York, Elsevier, 1989, pp 439–451.
24. Tanaka R, Iwaskai Y, Koprowski H: Intracisternal virus-like particles in brain of multiple sclerosis patient. J Neurol Sci 28:121, 1976.
25. Burks JS, DeVald BL, Jankovsky LD, et al: Two coronaviruses isolated from central nervous system tissue of two multiple sclerosis patients. Science 209:933, 1980.
26. Fleming JO, El Zaatari FAK, Gilmore W, et al: Antigenic assessment of coronaviruses isolated from patients with multiple sclerosis. Arch Neurol 45:629, 1988.
27. Murray RS, Brown B, Brian D, et al: Detection of coronavirus RNA and antigen in multiple sclerosis brain. Ann Neurol 31:525, 1992.
28. Reed SE: The behavior of recent isolates of human respiratory coronaviruses in vitro and in volunteers: Evidence of heterogeneity among 229E-related strains. J Med Virol 13:179, 1984.
29. Kaye HS, Marsh HB, Dowdle WR: Seroepidemiologic survey of coronarvirus (strain OC43)-related infection in a children's population. Am J Epidemiol 94:43, 1971.
30. Hendley JO, Fishburne HB, Gwaltney JM Jr.: Coronavirus infec-

tions in working adults: Eight year study with 229E and OC43. Am Rev Respir Dis 105:805, 1972.
31. Wenzel RP, Hendley JO, Davies JA, et al: Coronavirus infections in military recruits. Am Rev Respir Dis 109:621, 1974.
32. Kaye HS, Dowdle WR: Seroepidemiologic survey of coronavirus (strain 229E) infections in a population of children. Am J Epidemiol 101:238, 1975.
33. McIntosh K, Ellis EF, Hoffman LS, et al: The association of viral and bacterial respiratory infections with exacerbations of wheezing in young asthmatic children. J Pediatr 82:578, 1973.
34. Smith CB, Golden CA, Kanner RE, et al: Association of viral and *Mycoplasma pneumoniae* infections with acute respiratory illness in patients with chronic obstructive pulmonary diseases. Am Rev Respir Dis 121:225, 1980.
35. Gill EP, Dominguez EA, Greenberg SB, et al: Development and application of an enzyme immunoassay for coronavirus OC43 antibody in acute respiratory illness. J Clin Microbiol 32:2372, 1994.
36. Myint S, Harmsen D, Raabe T, et al: Characterization of nucleic acid probe for the diagnosis of human coronavirus 229E infections. J Med Virol 31:165, 1990.
37. Talbot PJ, Ekande S, Cashman NR, et al: Neurotropism of human coronavirus 229E. Adv Exp Med Biol 342:339, 1993.
38. Vaucher YE, Ray CG, Minnich LL, et al: Pleomorphic, enveloped, virus-like particles associated with gastrointestinal illness in neonates. J Infect Dis 145:27, 1982.
39. Resta S, Luby JP, Rosenfield CR, et al: Isolation and propagation of a human enteric coronavirus. Science 229:978, 1985.
40. Mortensen ML, Ray CG, Payne CM, et al: Coronavirus-like particles in human gastrointestinal disease. Am J Dis Child 139:928, 1985.
41. Payne CM, Ray CG, Borduin V, et al: An eight year study of the viral agents of acute gastroenteritis in humans: Ultrastructural observations and seasonal distribution with a major emphasis on coronavirus-like particles. Diagn Microbiol Infect Dis 5:39, 1986.
42. Sitborn M: Human enteric coronavirus-like particles (CVLP) with different epidemiological characteristics. J Med Virol 16:67, 1985.
43. Beards GM, Brown DWG, Green J, et al: Preliminary characterisation of torovirus-like particles of humans: Comparison with Berne virus of horses and Breda virus of calves. J Med Virol 20:67, 1986.
44. Battaglia M, Passarani N, DiMatteo A, et al: Human enteric coronaviruses: Further characterization and immunoblotting of viral proteins. J Infect Dis 155:140, 1987.

257

Poliovirus

Mark A. Pallansch
Larry J. Anderson
Olen M. Kew

History

Poliomyelitis is a disease of great antiquity. Perhaps the earliest description is evident in an Egyptian stele from around 1350 BC depicting a young man with typical asymmetric flaccid paralysis and atrophy of the leg. Several scattered reports of the disease also appear in the literature from the 17th and 18th centuries. By the mid-19th century, the industrial revolution had brought increased urbanization to Europe and North America and with it significant changes and improvements in living conditions. Coincident with these massive changes was the advent of larger and more frequent outbreaks of poliomyelitis. From the late 1800s, outbreaks were occurring in several European countries and in the United States, and they remained a dominant public health problem in the developed world for the first half of the 20th century.[1]

A major landmark in the study of poliomyelitis was the successful passage of the virus to nonhuman primates by Landsteiner and Popper in 1909.[2] The availability of animal models provided the first opportunity to study the disease outside of human patients and produced important information on the process of infection and the pathophysiology of the disease. Further studies on the infectious agent awaited the crucial development by Enders and colleagues[3] in 1949 of tissue culture systems for in vitro propagation of the virus. This advance and the recognition of three distinct serotypes[4] opened the way for all subsequent work on vaccines and study of the biochemical and biophysical properties of the polioviruses.

By the 1950s, two different approaches to the prevention of poliomyelitis by vaccination were developed. The first successful polio vaccine was produced by Salk and Younger in 1954 by chemical inactivation of tissue culture–propagated virus using formaldehyde.[5] This vaccine was completely noninfectious, yet after injection it elicited an immune response that was protective against paralytic disease. During the same period, many laboratories sought to produce live, attenuated polio vaccines. The oral polio vaccine (OPV) strains of Sabin were licensed in 1961, and mass immunization campaigns in the United States began in 1963.[6] Both the inactivated polio vaccine (IPV) and OPV contain three components, one for each immunologically distinct serotype of poliovirus.

Widespread immunization with IPV, and since 1963 with OPV, has virtually eliminated poliomyelitis in most developed countries.[7] An example of this progress can be seen in the data from the United States, where the annual number of cases of paralytic disease has fallen from the peak of more than 20,000 cases in 1952 to an average of less than 10 per year since 1980[8–10] (Fig. 257–1). None of the cases in the United States since 1980 have been caused by endemic wild

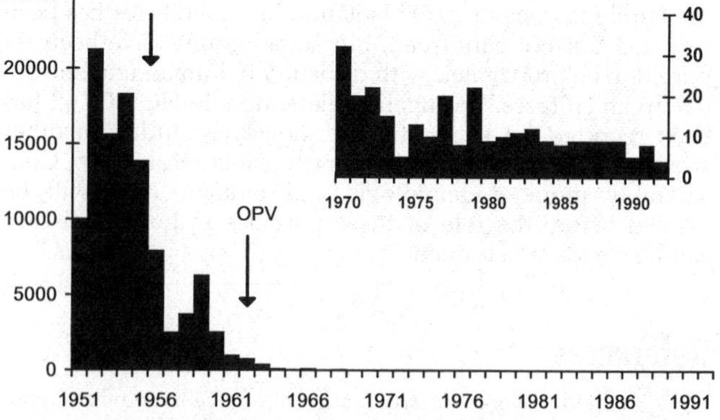

FIGURE 257–1 □ Incidence of paralytic poliomyelitis in the United States from 1951 to 1992. Number of cases reported during the period immediately before and after the introduction of both inactivated (IPV) and oral (OPV) polio vaccines in large-scale campaigns. No case since 1980 has been due to endemic wild poliovirus. Note the change in scale for the inset. (Data from references 8 to 10 and unpublished data.)

All material in this chapter is in the public domain, with the exception of any borrowed figures or tables.

poliovirus; however, poliomyelitis remains a major health problem in many other parts of the world. The World Health Organization estimates that nearly 100,000 cases occurred worldwide in 1993, primarily in children younger than 2 years.[11] Great strides have been made to increase vaccine coverage, and the World Health Assembly has declared a goal of worldwide poliomyelitis eradication by the year 2000. This goal is attainable because humans are the only known reservoir for poliovirus. The thrust of the effort is to achieve high vaccine coverage in all regions of the world coupled with supplemental immunization campaigns and aggressive investigation of all suspect cases of acute flaccid paralysis to identify wild virus circulation.[12]

Characteristics of the Pathogen

The polioviruses belong to the genus *Enterovirus* in the family Picornaviridae.[13] All are small, round 30-nm particles with icosahedral symmetry, and they contain no essential lipid. Polioviruses share most of their biochemical and biophysical characteristics with the other enteroviruses[14] and are different from some of the other picornaviruses (Table 257–1). The viral particles have a buoyant density of 1.34 g/cm^3 in cesium chloride and a sedimentation coefficient of approximately 156S. The infectious particles are relatively heat resistant (when stabilized by magnesium cations), resistant to acid pH (pH 3 to 5 for 1 to 3 hours), and also resistant to many common detergents and disinfectants, including common soap, nonionic detergents, ether, chloroform, and other lipid solvents.[15, 16] The virus is stable for weeks at 4°C and for days at room temperature. Drying, ultraviolet light, high heat (in the absence of magnesium cation), formaldehyde, and free chlorine, however, readily inactivate the virus.

Polioviruses and the enteroviruses are distinguished from the other picornaviruses on the basis of physical properties such as buoyant density in cesium chloride and stability in weak acid. The three poliovirus serotypes are distinguished from the other enteroviruses by neutralization with serotype-specific antiserum and the propensity to cause paralytic illness. The Mahoney strain of type 1 poliovirus is the prototype for the polioviruses, the genus *Enterovirus,* and the family Picornaviridae. It is among the most studied and best characterized agents of human disease.

The poliovirion consists of 60 copies each of four polypeptide chains that form a highly structured shell. Located inside this shell, the viral genome consists of a single molecule of RNA, which is about 7500 nucleotides long. The four capsid polypeptides are produced by the proteolytic cleavage of a single polyprotein precursor. These four virion polypeptides are designated VP1 through VP4 and in poliovirus type 1 (Mahoney strain) have molecular masses of 33.5, 30.1, 26.4, and 7.4 kDa, respectively. In addition, one small protein, VPg, is covalently attached to the 5′ end of the virion RNA. A major advance in studies on the structure of polioviruses occurred with the solution of the crystal structure to a resolution of 0.29 nm.[17] From the three-dimensional structure of the poliovirion, VP1 contributes the majority of the amino acid residues on the virion surface, VP2 and VP3 are partially exposed on the surface, and VP4 is completely internal.

The information concerning the surface of the virion also has been particularly useful in understanding the neutralization of poliovirus by antibodies. These efforts have culminated with the three-dimensional description of three neutralizing antigenic sites on type 1 poliovirus.[18] These antigenic sites consist of four principal epitopes, three of which are discontinuous, and two span different polypeptide chains. The observed structure of the antigenic sites explains why antigenicity of the virus is destroyed by disruption of the virion structure. In addition, other antigenic sites that elicit an immune response are not neutralizing.

The poliovirus-neutralizing antibody response is serotype specific, with the exception of some minor cross-reaction between poliovirus types 1 and 2. Heat-disrupted virions, particularly those heated in the presence of detergent, induce antibodies that react with many enteroviruses.[19, 20] These broadly reacting antibodies are generally not neutralizing. Antisera raised in animals to each of the viruses are largely type specific and are used for the determination of serotype in a neutralization assay. The virus also contains more than one T-cell epitope,[21] although the role of cell-mediated immunity in controlling infection is not determined.

Polioviruses are among the simplest viruses in terms of genetic complexity and size. The RNA genomes from all three serotypes of poliovirus have been cloned and sequenced.[22] The genomic RNA is infectious and serves as messenger RNA for viral protein synthesis. The RNA is translated in a single open reading frame into one large polyprotein, which is then processed through proteolytic cleavage by two distinct virus-encoded proteases into the functional viral proteins.[23]

Despite much research and the simple nature of the virus, the details of RNA replication have been elusive. The process begins when virion RNA is transcribed by the viral polymerase beginning at the 3′ end of the infecting viral RNA to generate a complementary RNA. In the next step, which is dependent on a "host factor," the progeny viral RNA is synthesized from the complementary RNA. The newly synthesized viral RNA is covalently linked to the VPg protein at the 5′ end of the RNA and then only the positive-sense strand of RNA is encapsidated in the viral structural proteins to form infectious viral particles.[24] The extensive studies of virus replication and assembly have resulted in the remarkable accomplishment of complete cell-free replication of poliovirus beginning with only the viral RNA.[25]

TABLE 257–1 ■ Comparative Physical and Biochemical Properties of Picornaviruses

PROPERTY	POLIO-VIRUS	NONPOLIO ENTEROVIRUS	RHINO-VIRUS	HEPATITIS A VIRUS
Acid stability*	+	+	–	+
Buoyant density†	1.34	1.34	1.40	1.34
Stable at 50°C‡	–	–	+	+
Stable at 65°C	–	–	–	+
Serotypes	3	62	100	1

*Incubation at pH 3.0 for 1 h.

†Cesium chloride equilibrium density expressed as grams per cubic centimeter.

‡Infectivity stable for 1 h in the absence of magnesium cations.

Data from Melnick JL: Portraits of viruses: The picornaviruses. Intervirology 20:61–100, 1983; and Melnick JL, Wenner HA, Phillips CA: Enteroviruses. *In* Lennette EH, Schmidt NJ (eds): Viral, Rickettsial and Chlamydial Infections, ed 5. Washington, DC, American Public Health Association, 1979, pp 471–534.

Epidemiology

There are several routes of poliovirus transmission.[26] In most developing countries the most important route is probably the fecal-oral route. The virus replicates efficiently in the intestinal tract and is shed in the stool for 2 to 4 weeks, and sometimes for several weeks longer. Shedding may be intermittent and is affected by the immune status of the individual. Past natural infection with wild poliovirus and vaccination with OPV serve to significantly reduce the extent and duration of poliovirus shedding. Enhanced IPV and competing enteric infections may also reduce the extent and duration of virus shedding in stool to a lesser degree.[27, 28]

Because virus also replicates in the upper respiratory tract, polioviruses are spread through upper respiratory tract secretions as well. Virus can be recovered from throat swabs and washings during the early acute phases of infection. Factors that affect transmission of the virus include extent of crowding, levels of hygiene, water quality, and sewage handling facilities. In areas with poor sanitary conditions and contaminated surface water or water supplies, the most important route of transmission is probably the fecal-oral route. In areas with good sanitary conditions and uncontaminated drinking water, other routes of transmission are probably more important. Studies with nonpolio enteroviruses suggest that respiratory tract secretions are infectious and may provide a source of virus for close contact spread through direct person-to-person contact, large-particle aerosols, or fomites. For example, during an outbreak of poliomyelitis in Finland in 1984[29, 30] person-to-person spread was probably the principal mode of transmission. During this outbreak an estimated 100,000 people were infected with type 3 poliovirus during a 1-month period in winter. This occurred despite little opportunity for widespread fecal-oral transmission through exposure to contaminated drinking or surface water.

Poliovirus can be effectively controlled with either IPV or OPV. This has been conclusively demonstrated by the elimination of endemic poliovirus from developed and developing countries in the Americas, Europe, most of east Asia, and Australia. Most of the cases reported since the 1970s in the United States are associated with exposure to OPV, either directly as vaccine recipient (usually first dose) or indirectly through contact with vaccine recipients.[31] The incidence of disease associated with use of OPV is 1 case in 1.4 million doses among first-dose recipients and 1 case in 6.4 million doses among contacts for all doses.[10] Occasionally, paralytic illness clinically indistinguishable from poliomyelitis has occurred after infection with other enteroviruses, particularly enterovirus 71. Such cases are infrequent and are discussed further in Chapter 258.

In many developing countries, poliomyelitis from wild polioviruses continues to be a major public health problem (Fig. 257–2). Large areas of Africa, the Middle East, and South Asia have extensive circulation of wild poliovirus, and children in these areas can be exposed to more than one serotype of wild virus before 1 year of age. To combat this problem, in 1988 the World Health Organization, through the Expanded Programme on Immunization, established the goal to eradicate poliomyelitis worldwide by the year 2000. Progress in this program has been significant: poliovaccine coverage in developing countries has increased to above 80%.[11] As another indication of the tremendous progress, the Pan American Health Organization effort to eliminate poliomyelitis resulted in the declaration of the Americas as the first region to be free of endemic poliovirus transmission.[32]

An extremely powerful tool for tracking the circulation of wild poliovirus strains is the molecular characterization of the virus genomes from clinical isolates. By comparing the changes that are observed between virus strains, the geographic and temporal origin of a virus can be determined.[33, 34] Building upon a nucleic acid sequence database of poliovirus

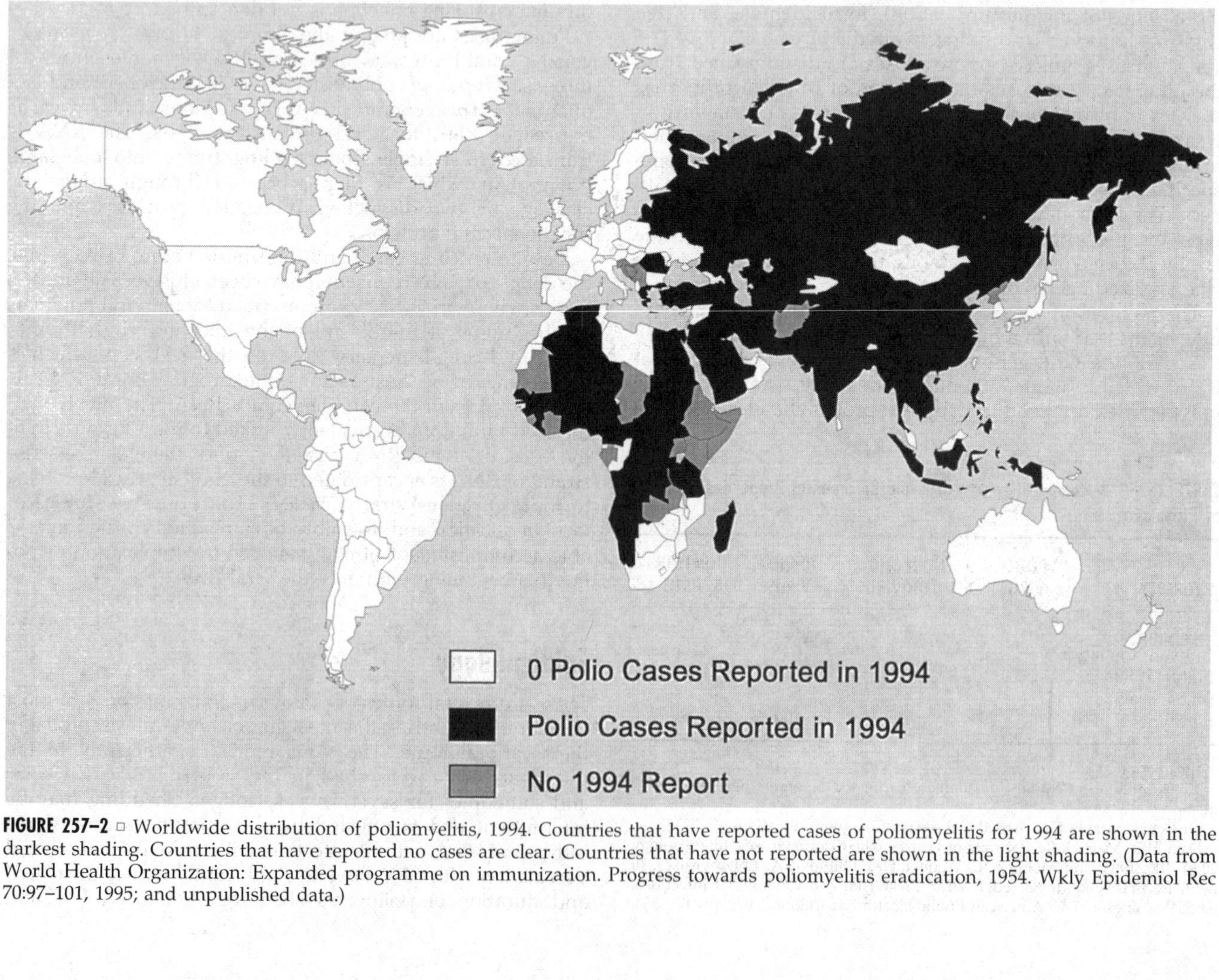

FIGURE 257–2 ▫ Worldwide distribution of poliomyelitis, 1994. Countries that have reported cases of poliomyelitis for 1994 are shown in the darkest shading. Countries that have reported no cases are clear. Countries that have not reported are shown in the light shading. (Data from World Health Organization: Expanded programme on immunization. Progress towards poliomyelitis eradication, 1954. Wkly Epidemiol Rec 70:97–101, 1995; and unpublished data.)

strains worldwide, it has been possible to develop rapid approaches to tracking wild poliovirus strains.

Any area with endemic wild polioviruses can serve as a reservoir for reintroduction of poliovirus to areas that have no endemic circulation of wild poliovirus.[35] For example, a type 1 poliovirus from the Middle East was responsible for a series of cases of poliomyelitis in the Netherlands, Canada, and the United States in 1979.[36] A type 3 virus from the Mediterranean region introduced into Finland resulted in many cases of paralytic disease and extensive spread within the country in 1984.[37] A type 3 poliovirus from South Asia caused another outbreak in the Netherlands in 1993, and although the virus was found in western Canada, no paralytic disease resulted.[38, 39] Similar smaller introductions into countries that are free of endemic virus occur nearly every year. The frequency and ease of international travel probably result in continuous introduction of wild poliovirus in all regions of the world, and a large proportion of the population must be vaccinated if poliomyelitis epidemics are to be prevented.

Pathogenesis

Disease associated with poliovirus infection results from tissue-specific cell destruction. Polioviruses are cytolytic both in vivo and in tissue culture. On entering a cell by way of specific receptors, the virus rapidly takes over cellular protein synthesis and inhibits cellular RNA transcription and DNA replication. Consequently, the cells degenerate and lyse, releasing the progeny virus. In culture, several thousand infectious progeny viruses are released for every infected cell. Because the process typically takes about 6 hours, a small inoculum can be amplified rapidly and can spread quickly through the host.

The site of virus replication is dependent on the presence of virus-specific receptors. By using mouse-human hybrid cell lines, it has been possible to localize the gene that encodes for a cellular receptor for poliovirus to human chromosome 19.[40] The gene for a poliovirus receptor has been sequenced and shown to belong to the immunoglobulin (Ig) superfamily.[41] Identification and characterization of the specific receptor have resulted in the construction of transgenic mice that express the human poliovirus receptor. Studies with these mice have provided insights into the pathogenesis of poliomyelitis.[42, 43]

In humans, the primary sites of infection are epithelial cells in the intestinal and respiratory tract. After primary infection, more extensive virus replication occurs in lymphoid tissue in tonsillar tissue and Peyer patches, and from there the virus enters the blood and infects other tissues, occasionally including motor neurons. The paralytic illness follows directly from the lytic infection of motor neurons: in the anterior horn for spinal poliomyelitis, or in the medulla for bulbar poliomyelitis.[44] Sensory neurons are spared. Several factors are associated with an increased risk of paralytic disease, including strenuous exercise, injections, tonsillectomy, and pregnancy, presumably by increasing the chance of the virus' infecting and lysing motor neurons.[45, 46]

A fundamental question about the pathogenesis of poliomyelitis is the identity of viral factors responsible for neurovirulence, which most other enteroviruses and poliovaccine viruses lack. Comparisons by molecular biologic techniques of the attenuated Sabin oral vaccine viruses and their virulent parents or natural virulent revertants have identified several potential sites that confer attenuation on the virus. Studies of natural vaccine virus revertants and artificially generated recombinant viruses have identified changes in the 5′ noncoding region and two sites within the capsid proteins that contribute to attenuation.[47, 48] Such studies are likely to improve our understanding of the pathogenesis of poliomyelitis and the virus functions modified in the attenuated vaccine strains.

Primary infection induces a strong humoral immune response. Typically this includes the production of an IgM response within 7 to 10 days of infection, followed by an IgG response beginning about 14 days after infection. Since the first symptoms occur from 3 to 14 days after infection, serum specimens taken early in the clinical illness often already have poliovirus antibody. Within a few months of initial infection the titer of IgM antibody begins to fall; however, the neutralizing IgG antibodies persist, providing long-term protection from viremia and disease. Infection with one serotype of poliovirus does not protect against infection and disease with other poliovirus serotypes, and patients have had additional episodes of paralytic disease from other serotypes. Therefore, immunization of patients with acute poliomyelitis is appropriate, because disease indicates susceptibility to poliovirus because of the absence of or ineffective prior immunization. It is important that specimens be obtained to confirm the diagnosis before vaccination.

Clinical Manifestations

The sequence of clinical symptoms parallels the sequence of sites of virus replication.[26, 44] The primary site of infection in epithelial and lymphoid tissue of the pharynx and gut may be associated with no specific symptoms or with mild systemic symptoms such as fever, headache, malaise, and occasionally mild gastrointestinal symptoms. If the virus secondarily infects the central nervous system, a second phase of illness (aseptic meningitis, paralysis, or both) occurs 3 to 10 days after the first phase of mild systemic symptoms. The clinical course of poliovirus aseptic meningitis is identical to that associated with the other enteroviruses and is described in Chapter 159. The tendency of poliovirus to infect motor neurons distinguishes its clinical picture from that of other enteroviruses.

Paralysis is usually associated with fever, stiff neck, muscle aches, and headaches; it develops rapidly and is typically asymmetric. It is a flaccid paralysis that most often affects the lower extremities and is associated with reduced or absent deep tendon reflexes and no sensory defects. During the period immediately after the primary illness, some recovery of function can be noted and complete functional recovery can occur. The permanent loss of motor neurons results in denervation atrophy of the affected muscles.

Poliomyelitis should be considered in all cases of pure motor paralysis and is usually associated with a normal or slightly elevated value for cerebrospinal fluid (CSF) protein, a normal CSF glucose value, and moderate mononuclear pleocytosis in CSF. Early in the illness, polymorphonuclear cells may predominate in the CSF, followed by a shift to mononuclear cells. Defects in the ventral horns of the spinal cord can be observed by magnetic resonance imaging. The lesion seen by magnetic resonance imaging corresponds to the innervation pattern of the affected extremity. Electromyography and nerve conduction velocities generally fail to show evidence of a conduction block.

The differential diagnosis includes spinal cord compression, stroke, neuropathy, and Guillain-Barré syndrome. Spinal cord compression is unlikely in the absence of central involvement in neural imaging. Lack of sensory involvement would exclude neuropathies. For stroke in the setting of meningoencephalitis, flaccid paralysis sometimes occurs, but the classic spasticity of upper motor lesions should follow. In Guillain-Barré syndrome, protein concentration is markedly elevated in the CSF and pleocytosis is mild or absent. Fever is usually absent, and paralysis is usually symmetric and ascending with evidence of conduction block by nerve conduction velocities (Table 257–2).

Delayed progression of neuromuscular symptoms may occur 20 years or longer after the initial paralysis due to poliovirus.[49] This postpolio syndrome is characterized by new muscle weakness associated with dysfunction of surviving motor neurons. The illness is usually associated with deterioration of those nerves involved in reinnervation during recovery from the original poliovirus infection. Inflammation is sometimes present in association with degenerating neurons.[50] It is believed that the life span of these nerves has been shortened by the process of reinnervation. This syndrome is not a form of amyotrophic lateral sclerosis. It does not appear that reactivation or replication of poliovirus is involved, but current data are not conclusive.[51, 52]

Diagnosis

The key to laboratory confirmation of poliovirus infection is the collection of appropriate clinical specimens.[14, 53] Good specimens are important for confirmation of the diagnosis of suspected poliomyelitis. Isolation of the virus also makes it possible to determine whether the virus is wild or vaccine related. In areas considered to be free of wild poliovirus this information may be important to public health officials, who must decide whether control programs are needed to prevent further cases of poliomyelitis. Laboratory studies can also be used to support the diagnosis of poliovirus infection when the patient has no knowledge of any exposure to the virus or has an atypical disease presentation.

Poliovirus infection can be demonstrated either by isolation of the virus or by serologic evidence of recent viral infection.[14] Virus is most frequently detected from stool specimens or rectal swabs, and less frequently in throat swabs, throat washings, or CSF. Fecal specimens for virus isolation should always be obtained from suspected cases, because the virus is shed the longest and in highest titer from the intestinal tract. Early in the acute phase of the illness, virus is frequently isolated from the throat. Isolation of virus from CSF provides the most direct link to disease but is usually less successful. The earlier in the course of illness that CSF specimens are collected, the more likely will virus be isolated. Nucleic acid probes can be used to determine whether the isolate is vaccine derived or wild poliovirus. For wild polioviruses, probes can identify the specific strain and therefore its probable geographic origin. Methods have been developed using the polymerase chain reaction assay for rapid detection and characterization of polioviruses.[54] Further development is necessary to achieve better sensitivity than by virus isolation from all types of specimens.

TABLE 257–2 ■ Differential Diagnosis of Poliomyelitis and Guillain-Barré Syndrome

SYMPTOM	POLIOMYELITIS	GUILLAIN-BARRÉ SYNDROME
Paralysis	Asymmetric	Symmetric, ascending
Fever	Present	Absent
Protein in cerebrospinal fluid	Normal	Elevated
Pleocytosis	Yes	Mild or absent
NCV*	No block	Block

*Electromyography nerve conduction velocities.

Poliovirus infection can also be confirmed by demonstrating a rise in titers of neutralizing antibody to one of the polioviruses. Other antibody assays such as complement fixation or enzyme immunoassays for poliovirus IgM antibodies have been described.[14, 55] These assays have not been sufficiently evaluated to determine their sensitivity and specificity in comparison to other reference techniques. The most common infectious agents that can mimic poliovirus disease are other enteroviruses, which are discussed further in Chapter 258.

Treatment

Treatment of acute poliomyelitis consists principally of supportive therapy and reduced physical activity. Mechanical ventilation is sometimes required in severe cases.

Specific antiviral treatment for poliovirus has been pursued for many years. Several classes of compounds have been identified that exhibit antiviral activity against poliovirus in tissue culture and experimental animals.[56–58] These newer drugs have not completed clinical trials, and no treatment has been shown to alter the clinical course of poliomyelitis.

Prevention

Immunization is the primary means of poliomyelitis prevention. Two highly effective vaccines are available, and immunization with one or the other is part of routine childhood immunization schedules in most of the world. Recommended vaccination schedules vary among countries. In the United States, the Immunization Practices Advisory Committee recommends three primary doses of OPV to be given at 2, 4, and 6 months of age.[59]

The World Health Organization recommends for developing countries that three routine doses be given at 6, 10, and 14 weeks of age and an additional dose at birth in endemic regions where exposure of very young infants to wild virus can be expected.[60] Supplementary pulse immunization through national immunization days have proved to be the most effective means of breaking the chain of wild virus transmission in endemic areas.[12]

Several European countries use enhanced IPV as the sole vaccine for routine childhood immunization.[5] These vaccines are administered with diphtheria-pertussis-tetanus vaccine or as a combined formulation, usually at 2, 4, and 15 months of age.[61] An additional booster dose is recommended at 5 years of age or before entering school. If polio immunization is indicated, enhanced IPV is the recommended vaccine for persons with congenital immunodeficiency disease, acquired immunodeficiency syndrome, or other altered immune status resulting from disease or immunosuppressive therapy. For unvaccinated adults at increased risk of exposure to poliovirus, a primary series of enhanced IPV is recommended.

Discussion continues on the relative merits of the two vaccines.[62–64] The advantages of OPV are low cost per dose; easy vaccine delivery; possible immunizing or booster effect for contacts of immunized persons; and less shedding of virus by immunized persons who are subsequently infected with wild poliovirus, resulting in reduced risk of spread within a community. The advantages of IPV include no vaccine-associated paralytic disease; greater stability for easier transport; and high efficacy after two doses. The major disadvantage of OPV is its reversion to neurovirulence and the rare associated cases of paralytic disease among vaccinees and their contacts. The major disadvantages of IPV are greater cost, requirement for injection, and its inability to increase vaccine coverage indirectly. Investigations of several outbreaks in developing countries have also noted lower than expected rates of seroconversion and inferred protection despite adequate vaccination programs for both OPV and IPV.[65, 66] The basis for decreased efficacy of OPV in some settings is under investigation.[67]

The relative importance of the advantages and disadvantages of OPV and IPV in different populations is the subject of ongoing debate. Although both vaccines have been effective in eliminating disease due to wild poliovirus in many countries, neither is yet able to meet all the requirements for highly effective vaccination programs in developing countries. Some authorities have advocated using combined IPV and OPV immunization schedules to take advantage of the strengths of both vaccines,[68] and the adoption of this approach in the United States seems likely.

The presence of a patient hospitalized with poliomyelitis has elicited concerns from hospital personnel who are unfamiliar with the risks associated with poliovirus infection. High rates of vaccine coverage and the rarity of wild poliovirus infections have essentially eliminated the risk of nosocomial poliomyelitis in the developed world. Because paralytic disease can also be caused by other infectious agents, such as enterovirus 71 and rabies virus, infection control practices should be appropriate for all potential agents until clinical, epidemiologic, or laboratory data have identified the likely agent. All immunocompetent patients with suspected or confirmed poliomyelitis should be placed in contact isolation, and in a private room if hygiene is poor, during the first 7 days of their illness. Staff should wear gowns and gloves if contact with infectious material (primarily feces) is likely.[69] Staff should also be aware of the risk of transmitting virus to other patients who may not be immunized or are at increased risk of paralytic disease because of immune system deficiency. The immunization status of staff should also be reviewed, and staff with a history of inadequate vaccination should be excluded from caring for patients with poliomyelitis and given the appropriate doses of vaccine. Public health officials should be notified immediately, so they can determine whether wild poliovirus may be involved, and community prevention programs are warranted.

References

1. Paul JR: A History of Poliomyelitis. New Haven, CT, Yale University Press, 1971.
2. Landsteiner K, Popper E: Uebertragung der Poliomyelitis acuta auf Affen. Ztschr Immunitatsforsch Exp Ther Jena 2:377, 1909.
3. Enders JF, Weller TH, Robbins FC: Cultivation of the Lansing strain of poliomyelitis virus in cultures of various human embryonic tissues. Science 109:85, 1949.
4. Bodian D, Morgan IM, Howe HA: Differentiation of three types of poliomyelitis viruses. III. The grouping of fourteen strains into three immunological types. Am J Hyg 49:234, 1949.
5. Salk J, Salk D: Control of poliomyelitis and influenza with killed virus vaccines. Science 195:834, 1977.
6. Sabin AB: Oral poliovirus vaccine: History of its development and use, and current challenge to eliminate poliomyelitis from the world. J Infect Dis 151:420, 1985.
7. Henderson RH, Keja J, Hayden GA, et al: Immunizing the children of the world: Progress and prospects. Bull World Health Organ 66:535, 1988.
8. Centers for Disease Control: Poliomyelitis Surveillance Summary 1979. Atlanta, US Department of Health and Human Services, 1981.
9. Nkowane BM, Wassilak SGF, Orenstein WA, et al: Vaccine-associated paralytic poliomyelitis. United States: 1973–1984. JAMA 257:1335, 1987.
10. Strebel PM, Sutter RW, Cochi SL, et al: Epidemiology of poliomyelitis in the United States one decade after the last reported case of indigenous wild virus-associated disease. Clin Infect Dis 14:568, 1992.
11. World Health Organization: Expanded programme on immunization—Progress towards poliomyelitis eradication, 1994. Wkly Epidemiol Rec 70:97, 1995.
12. Hull HF, Ward NA, Hull BP, et al: Paralytic poliomyelitis: Seasoned strategies, disappearing disease. Lancet 343:1331, 1994.
13. Melnick JL: Portraits of viruses: The picornaviruses. Intervirology 20:61, 1983.
14. Melnick JL, Wenner HA, Phillips CA: Enteroviruses. *In* Lennette EH, Schmidt NJ (eds): Viral, Rickettsial and Chlamydial Infections, ed 5. Washington, DC, American Public Health Association, 1979, pp 471–534.
15. Schürmann W, Eggers HJ: An experimental study on the epidemiology of enteroviruses: Water-and-soap washing of poliovirus 1-contaminated hands, its effectiveness and kinetics. Med Microbiol Immunol 174:221, 1985.
16. Mbithi JN, Springthorpe VS, Sattar SA: Comparative in vivo efficiencies of hand-washing agents against hepatitis A virus (HM-175) and poliovirus type 1 (Sabin). Appl Environ Microbiol 59:3463, 1993.
17. Hogle JM, Chow M, Filman DJ: Three-dimensional structure of poliovirus at 2.9 Å resolution. Science 229:1358, 1985.
18. Page GS, Mosser AG, Hogle JM, et al: Three-dimensional structure of poliovirus serotype 1-neutralizing determinants. J Virol 62:1781, 1988.
19. Mertens T, Pika U, Eggers HJ: Cross-antigenicity among enteroviruses as revealed by immunoblot technique. Virology 129:431, 1983.
20. Emini EA, Schleif WA, Colonno RJ, et al: Antigenic conservation and divergence between the viral-specific proteins of poliovirus type 1 and various picornaviruses. Virology 140:13, 1985.
21. Graham S, Wang EC, Jenkins O, et al: Analysis of the human T-cell response to picornaviruses: Identification of T-cell epitopes close to B-cell epitopes in poliovirus. J Virol 67:1627, 1993.
22. Toyoda H, Kohara M, Kataoka Y, et al: Complete nucleotide sequences of all three poliovirus serotype genomes. Implication for genetic relationship, gene function and antigenic determinants. J Mol Biol 174:561, 1984.
23. Pallansch MA, Kew OM, Semler BL, et al: Protein-processing map of poliovirus. J Virol 49:873, 1984.
24. Novak JE, Kirkegaard K: Improved method for detecting poliovirus negative strands used to demonstrate specificity of positive-strand encapsidation and the ratio of positive to negative strands in infected cells. J Virol 65:3384, 1991.
25. Molla A, Paul AV, Wimmer E: Cell-free, de novo synthesis of poliovirus. Science 254:1647, 1991.
26. Melnick JL: Enteroviruses. *In* Evans AS (ed): Viral Infections of Humans: Epidemiology and Control. New York, Plenum Publishing, 1982, pp 187–251.
27. Chin TDY: Immunity induced by inactivated poliovirus vaccine and excretion of virus. Rev Infect Dis 6(Suppl 2):S369, 1984.
28. Dömök I, Balayan MS, Fayinka OA, et al: Factors affecting the efficacy of live poliovirus vaccine in warm climates. Bull World Health Organ 51:333, 1974.
29. Kinnunen E, Hovi T, Stenvik M: Outbreak of poliomyelitis in Finland in 1984–5. Description of the nine paralytic cases. Scand J Infect Dis 18:15, 1986.
30. Poyry T, Stenvik M, Hovi T: Viruses in sewage waters during and after a poliomyelitis outbreak and subsequent nationwide oral poliovaccination campaign in Finland. Appl Environ Microbiol 54:371, 1988.
31. Sutter RW, Brink EW, Cochi SL, et al: A new epidemiologic and laboratory classification system for paralytic poliomyelitis cases. Am J Public Health 79:495, 1989.
32. The certification of wild poliovirus eradication from the Western Hemisphere. Epidemiol Bull 15:1, 1994.
33. Crainic R, Kew O: Evolution and polymorphism of poliovirus genomes. Biologicals 21:379, 1993.
34. Kinnunen L, Poyry T, Hovi T: Genetic diversity and rapid evolution of poliovirus in human hosts. Curr Top Microbiol Immunol 176:49, 1992.
35. Kubli D, Steffen R, Schär M: Importation of poliomyelitis to industrialized nations between 1975 and 1984: Evaluation and conclusions for vaccination recommendations. Br Med J 295:169, 1987.
36. Nottay BK, Kew OM, Hatch MH, et al: Molecular variation of type 1 vaccine-related and wild polioviruses during replication in humans. Virology 108:405, 1981.

37. Kew OM, Nottay BK, Rico-Hesse RR, et al: Molecular epidemiology of wild poliovirus transmission. *In* Kurstak E, Marusyk RG, Murphy FA, van Regenmortel MHV (eds): Applied Virology Research, Vol 2. New York, Plenum Publishing, 1990, pp 199–221.
38. Oostvogel PM, van der Avoort HG, Mulders MN, et al: Virological and serological aspects of the Dutch polio epidemic in 1992. Ned Tijdsch Geneeskd 137:1404, 1993.
39. Expanded programme on immunization. Wild poliovirus isolated in Alberta, 1993. Wkly Epidemiol Rec 68:235, 1993.
40. Bernhardt G, Bibb JA, Bradley J, et al: Molecular characterization of the cellular receptor for poliovirus. Virology 199:105, 1994.
41. Mendelsohn CL, Wimmer E, Racaniello VR: Cellular receptor for poliovirus: Molecular cloning, nucleotide sequence, and expression of a new member of the immunoglobulin superfamily. Cell 56:855, 1989.
42. Horie H, Koike S, Kurata T, et al: Transgenic mice carrying the human poliovirus receptor: new animal models for study of poliovirus neurovirulence. J Virol 68:681, 1994.
43. Racaniello VR, Ren R, Bouchard M: Poliovirus attenuation and pathogenesis in a transgenic mouse model for poliomyelitis. Dev Biol Stand 78:109, 1993.
44. Sabin AB: Paralytic poliomyelitis: Old dogmas and new perspectives. Rev Infect Dis 3:543, 1981.
45. Russell WR: The pre-paralytic stage and the effect of physical activity on the severity of paralysis. Br Med J 2:1023, 1947.
46. Wyatt HV: Provocation of poliomyelitis by multiple injections. Trans R Soc Trop Med Hyg 79:355, 1985.
47. Mento SJ, Weeks-Levy C, Tatem JM, et al: Significance of a newly identified attenuating mutation in Sabin 3 oral poliovirus vaccine. Dev Biol Stand 78:93, 1993.
48. Ren RB, Moss EG, Racaniello VR: Identification of two determinants that attenuate vaccine-related type 2 poliovirus. J Virol 65:1377, 1991.
49. Wiechers DO: Late effects of polio: Historical perspectives. Birth Defects 24:1, 1987.
50. Dalakas MC: New neuromuscular symptoms after old polio ("the post-polio syndrome"): Clinical studies and pathogenetic mechanisms. Birth Defects 24:241, 1987.
51. Melchers W, de Visser M, Jongen P, et al: The postpolio syndrome: No evidence for poliovirus persistence. Ann Neurol 32:728, 1992.
52. Sharief MK: Poliovirus persistence in the postpolio syndrome. Ann Neurol 34:415, 1993.
53. Kapenberg JG: Picornaviridae: The enteroviruses (polioviruses, coxsackieviruses, echoviruses). *In* Lennette EH, Halonen P, Murphy FA (eds): Laboratory Diagnosis of Infectious Diseases: Principles and Practices. Vol 2, Viral, Rickettsial, and Chlamydial Diseases. New York, Springer-Verlag, 1988, pp 692–722.
54. Yang CF, De L, Yang SJ, et al: Genotype-specific in vitro amplification of sequences of the wild type 3 polioviruses from Mexico and Guatemala. Virus Res 24:277, 1992.
55. Roivainen M, Agboatwalla M, Stenvik M, et al: Intrathecal immune response and virus-specific immunoglobulin M antibodies in laboratory diagnosis of acute poliomyelitis. J Clin Microbiol 31:2427, 1993.
56. Garozzo A, Pinizzotto MR, Guerrera F, et al: Antipoliovirus activity of isothiazole derivatives: mode of action of 5,5′-diphenyl-3,3′-diisothiazole disulfide (DID). Arch Virol 135:1, 1994.
57. Rombaut B, Andries K, Boeye A. A comparison of WIN 51711 and R 78206 as stabilizers of poliovirus virions and procapsids. J Gen Virol 72:2153, 1991.
58. De Meyer N, Haemers A, Mishra L, et al: 4′-Hydroxy-3-methoxyflavones with potent antipicornavirus activity. J Med Chem 34:736, 1991.
59. Immunization Practices Advisory Committee: General recommendations on immunization. MMWR Morbid Mortal Wkly Rep 38:205, 1989.
60. World Health Organization: Immunization Policy. Geneva, World Health Organization, 1986.
61. Immunization Practices Advisory Committee: Poliomyelitis prevention: Enhanced-potency inactivated poliomyelitis vaccine—Supplementary statement. MMWR Morbid Mortal Wkly Rep 36:795, 1987.
62. Amren DP, Mayer TR: National immunization policymaking: A controversial endeavor. Postgrad Med 77:93, 1985.
63. Sabin AB: Commentary: Is there a need for a change in poliomyelitis immunization policy? Pediatr Infect Dis J 6:887, 1987.
64. Salk J: Commentary: Poliomyelitis vaccination—Choosing a wise policy. Pediatr Infect Dis J 6:889, 1987.
65. Patriarca P, Laender F, Palmeira G, et al: Randomised trial of alternative formulations of oral poliovaccine in Brazil. Lancet 1:429, 1988.
66. Centers for Disease Control: Paralytic poliomyelitis—Senegal, 1986–1987: Update on the N-IPV efficacy study. MMWR Morbid Mortal Wkly Rep 37:257, 1988.
67. Patriarca PA, Wright PF, John TJ. Factors affecting the immunogenicity of oral poliovirus vaccine in developing countries: Review. Rev Infect Dis 13:926, 1991.
68. McBean AM, Modlin JF: Rationale for the sequential use of inactivated poliovirus vaccine and live attenuated poliovirus vaccine for routine poliomyelitis immunization in the United States. Pediatr Infect Dis J 6:881, 1987.
69. Garner JS, Simmons BP: CDC guideline for isolation precautions in hospitals. *In* Guidelines for Protecting the Safety and Health of Health Care Workers. US Department of Health and Human Services. Washington, DC, US Government Printing Office, 1988, pp A8-1–84.

258

Coxsackievirus, Echovirus, and Other Enteroviruses

Mark A. Pallansch
Larry J. Anderson

History

The discovery of the enteroviruses was closely associated with the extensive effort to control poliomyelitis.[1] The development of better systems for growing poliovirus resulted in the detection of numerous agents that are pathogenic for laboratory animals or cytopathic for tissue culture cells. Many of these agents are presently classified as nonpoliovirus enteroviruses and are associated with a variety of clinical illnesses.

In searching for suitable animals to replace monkeys for poliomyelitis studies, Dalldorf and Sickles (1948) inoculated suckling mice with fecal suspensions from two suspected cases of poliomyelitis. The mice became paralyzed, not with poliovirus, but with the first isolate of a new virus group that subsequently was named for the patient's home town, Coxsackie, New York. Further isolation studies with mice identified several additional members of this group. With some isolates, however, the mice developed a spastic rather than the typical flaccid paralysis. This difference in pathogenicity in mice led to classification of isolates as either group A viruses (flaccid paralysis) or group B (spastic paralysis). The flaccid paralysis associated with group A viruses results from a generalized myositis, whereas the spastic paralysis of group B virus infection results from generalized degeneration of brain and other organs with only focal lesions of striated muscle. The discovery of these agents led to the realization that some cases of "nonparalytic poliomyelitis" or aseptic meningitis were due to these agents and not necessarily to poliovirus. Many other illnesses were soon recognized as being related to infection with the coxsackieviruses, including herpangina, rash, pleurodynia, and myocarditis.

Tissue culture studies led to the isolation of other enteroviruses from the stools of persons with aseptic meningitis and from asymptomatic persons. The viruses caused cytopathic effects in tissue culture but did not kill suckling mice. Because they were isolated from stool specimens, cytopathic for tissue culture, and not initially linked to disease, they were called enteric cytopathic human orphan viruses, which eventually evolved to the designation echoviruses. The fundamental similarities among the coxsackieviruses, echoviruses, and polioviruses caused them to be grouped in the genus *Enterovirus,* in the family Picornaviridae.

During the next 20 years, more than 60 antigenically distinct virus isolates were described. The isolates were numbered sequentially as they were described within the three groups, coxsackievirus A, coxsackievirus B, or echovirus (e.g., echovirus 11). It was eventually discovered that serotypically related virus isolates could have different degrees of pathogenicity in mice. With use of this classification scheme, some isolates of the same serotype would be classified as coxsackievirus and other isolates as echovirus. Consequently, no new enterovirus serotype isolated since 1967 has been classified as echovirus or coxsackievirus; all were assigned to the enterovirus group and numbered sequentially, beginning with 68. In addition, with the exception of poliovirus, the classification scheme is based on pathogenicity in suckling mice, not humans.

Just as the discovery of this large group of viruses followed from isolation studies of polioviruses, much of our understanding of the structure, mode of transmission, and biology of these viruses is based on studies of poliovirus. The reader is referred to Chapter 257 for a review of this information.

Characterization of the Pathogen

The genus *Enterovirus* in the family Picornaviridae consists of 66 recognized viruses,[2, 3] including the three serotypes of poliovirus described in Chapter 257. A summary of the classification scheme for enteroviruses is shown in Table 258–1 with the numbers of serotypes in each group. The great diversity of serotypes of nonpoliovirus enteroviruses presents considerable problems for laboratory diagnosis and epidemiologic investigations, but the serotype usually has minimal relevance to the diagnosis and management of an individual patient.

The structure and physical properties of enteroviruses are nearly identical to those of poliovirus. Although detailed structural and antigenic analyses are only beginning, many parallels between structural components of poliovirus and the other enteroviruses are evident from biochemical studies. Antisera to each of the viruses raised in animals are usually type specific and provide reference reagents for the serotype determination of the enterovirus isolates.[4] These antigenic differences are the primary means of distinguishing different enterovirus isolates. Infection with one serotype provides long-term protection from infection by that serotype but little protection, if any, from infection by other serotypes. Antigenic differences among isolates in the same serotype can be complex. For example, studies with monoclonal antibodies have shown a large number of antigenic variants among coxsackievirus B4 isolates,[5] including differences in neutralizing epitopes.[6] Variation at one or several epitopes, however, does not change the serotype as determined by polyclonal antibodies.

The RNA genomes from several enteroviruses have been cloned, sequenced, and found to have genetic organization similar to that of poliovirus.[7–10] Continued characterization of echoviruses 22 and 23 has demonstrated that these two viruses are genetically distinct from the other enteroviruses.[11] In addition, the clinical and epidemiologic features of these two viruses may also be atypical for enteroviruses.[12] Further study is needed to more completely describe the genetic relationships between serotypes. This information may also help us understand the genetic basis for pathogenic differences between isolates.

TABLE 258–1 ■ Classification of Enteroviruses

VIRUS	SEROTYPES	MOUSE PATHOGENICITY	TISSUE CULTURE GROWTH
Poliovirus	1–3	−*	+
Coxsackievirus A	1–22, 24	+	±†
Coxsackievirus B	1–6	+	+
Echovirus	1–7, 9, 11–27, 29–33	−	+
Enterovirus	68–71	−	+

*Some strains of poliovirus have been adapted to grow in mice, but poliovirus is not normally pathogenic for mice.

†Although originally only a few coxsackieviruses A could be grown in tissue culture, use of additional cell lines has enabled nearly all of this group to grow in tissue culture.

Epidemiology

The patterns of virus shedding and routes of transmission for enteroviruses are the same as those for poliovirus. The virus is isolated in the highest titer and for the longest time in stool specimens but can also be isolated from respiratory secretions. Therefore, both fecal-oral transmission and spread by contact with respiratory secretions (person to person, fomites, and possibly large-particle aerosol) are considered the most important modes of transmission for these viruses. The relative importance of the different modes probably varies with the virus and the environmental setting. In addition, enteroviruses that cause a vesicular exanthem can, presumably, be spread by direct or indirect contact with vesicular fluid that contains infectious virus.[13] Exceptions to the usual mode of enterovirus transmission are the agents of acute hemorrhagic conjunctivitis, enterovirus 70 and coxsackievirus A24 variant. These two viruses are seldom isolated from respiratory tract or stool specimens and are probably spread primarily by direct or indirect contact with eye secretions.[14]

An important concept in understanding the epidemiology of the enteroviruses is variation: by serotype, by time, by geographic location, and by disease. This concept is illustrated in surveillance studies of nonpoliovirus enterovirus infections.[15] For example, Figure 258–1 summarizes the data for the 28 years from 1961 to 1988 for the coxsackievirus B isolates in the United States collected and analyzed by the Centers for Disease Control and Prevention.[16–23] These data illustrate two patterns of enterovirus prevalence—endemic and epidemic. The epidemic pattern, as typified by coxsackievirus B5, is characterized by sharp peaks in numbers of isolations followed by periods with few isolations. During the study period, there were four major epidemics of coxsackievirus B5 in the United States: 1961, 1967, 1972, and 1983. By contrast, endemic viruses such as coxsackieviruses B2 and B4 were isolated nearly every year and in about the same numbers each year. Even with endemic viruses, larger outbreaks do occasionally occur, as with coxsackievirus B3 in

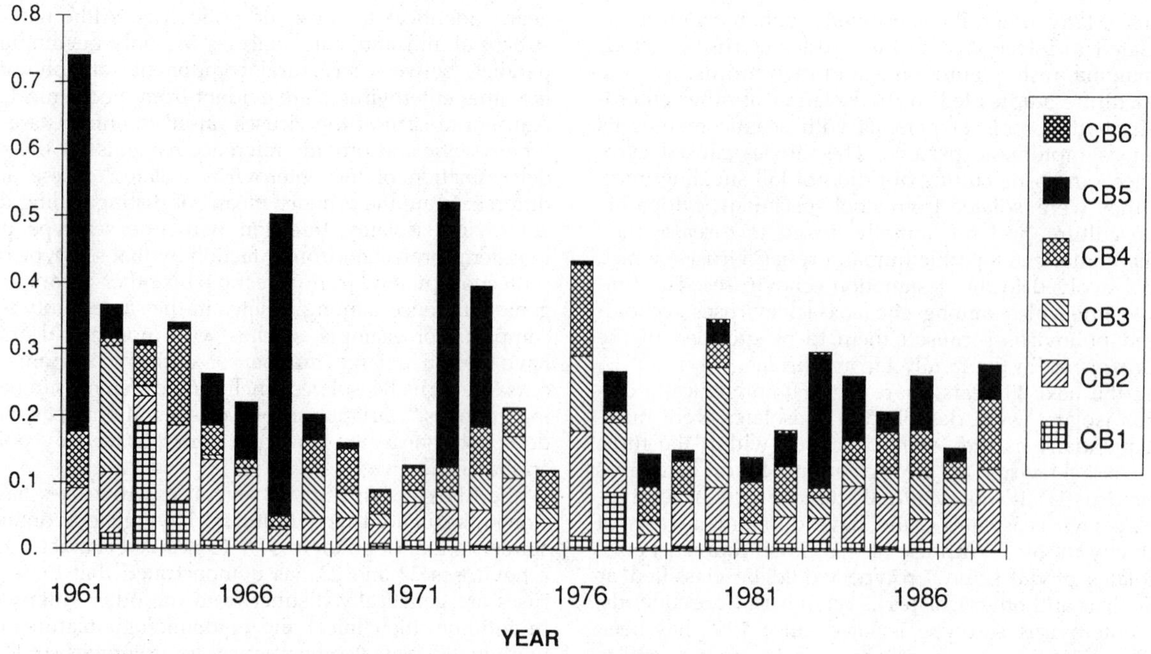

FIGURE 258–1 □ Temporal prevalence of coxsackievirus B isolates in the United States from 1961 to 1988. The graph shows the fraction of all nonpoliovirus enteroviruses that each of the serotypes of the coxsackievirus B group represents in each year. The key identifies the corresponding serotype. The fraction of all isolates is used rather than the number of isolates to compensate for variation in the number of reporting laboratories over time.

1980. Similar endemic and epidemic patterns are seen for the echoviruses and coxsackieviruses A.

Variation by location is also a major characteristic of enteroviruses. Outbreaks can be restricted to small groups such as schools and daycare centers or to selected communities, or they may become widespread at the regional, national, or even international level. Outbreaks in small groups can sometimes be linked epidemiologically to a breakdown in hygiene practices. Even during national outbreaks of a specific serotype, the location of virus activity may not be uniform. An example of regional variability in enterovirus activity is given in Figure 258–2, which illustrates echovirus 11 isolates in 1985 and 1986, when this virus was the enterovirus isolated most frequently in the United States. This activity was concentrated in the South and the West Coast in 1985 and in the East and Mountain States in 1986. By contrast, the epidemics of coxsackievirus B5 in 1961 and 1972 were nationwide: almost every state was affected.

Variation of enterovirus isolates can also be demonstrated by phenotypic markers in vitro. Attempts to understand this variation have often focused on studies of pathogenic potential in mice[24–26] and cell growth characteristics.[27–29] These studies have so far failed to identify any antigenic or other viral marker that correlates with human disease. To further confound studies of viral markers that predict disease, isolates from one patient consist of a collection of distinct variants that have different biologic properties.[30, 31] Thus, the diversity of variants within an isolate makes it difficult to identify what variants, and therefore which viral markers, might be responsible for the disease.

Many studies have examined the prevalence of antibodies to the enteroviruses in specific populations.[32–39] Several important conclusions can be drawn from these serosurveys. First, the number of persons who have neutralizing antibody to any given enterovirus is large, indicating a high rate of past infection. A high rate of recent infection is also suggested by immunoglobulin M surveys, which typically show 4% to 6% positivity. Second, infections with one serotype of enterovirus can boost the antibody titers to other enterovirus serotypes as measured by either immunoglobulin M or neutralization. The pattern of the heterotypic response varies by serotype and among individuals. Third, the pattern of antibody prevalence by serotype varies by geographic location, by time, and by age. Thus, prevalence data from different years and locations are not directly comparable. These three points must be considered when interpreting the findings of serologic studies of associations between enterovirus infection and disease.

Pathogenesis

Enteroviruses are cytopathic, and much of the associated disease presumably results from tissue-specific cell destruction. Some disease also results from the immune response to the infection. For example, enteroviral exanthems and myocarditis[2, 3, 40] are thought to result from the host response to the infection. The actual mechanisms of virus-induced disease, however, have not been well characterized. Some insight into human myocarditis has been gained from studies using animal model systems.[41, 42] Typically, the primary site of infection is the epithelial cells of the respiratory or gastrointestinal tract, followed by a viremia that may lead to a secondary site of tissue infection. Secondary infection of the central nervous system results in aseptic meningitis or, rarely, encephalitis or paralysis. Other tissue-specific infection can result in pleurodynia or myocarditis. Disseminated infection can lead to exanthems, nonspecific myalgias, or severe multiorgan disease in neonates.

Virus infection is dependent on the presence of specific receptors. Two distinct receptors for enteroviruses have been identified from human cells, an integrin and a decay-accelerating factor.[43, 44] Studies of the virus-receptor interactions should improve our understanding of the pathogenesis of enteroviral disease and, possibly, help develop prevention or treatment strategies.

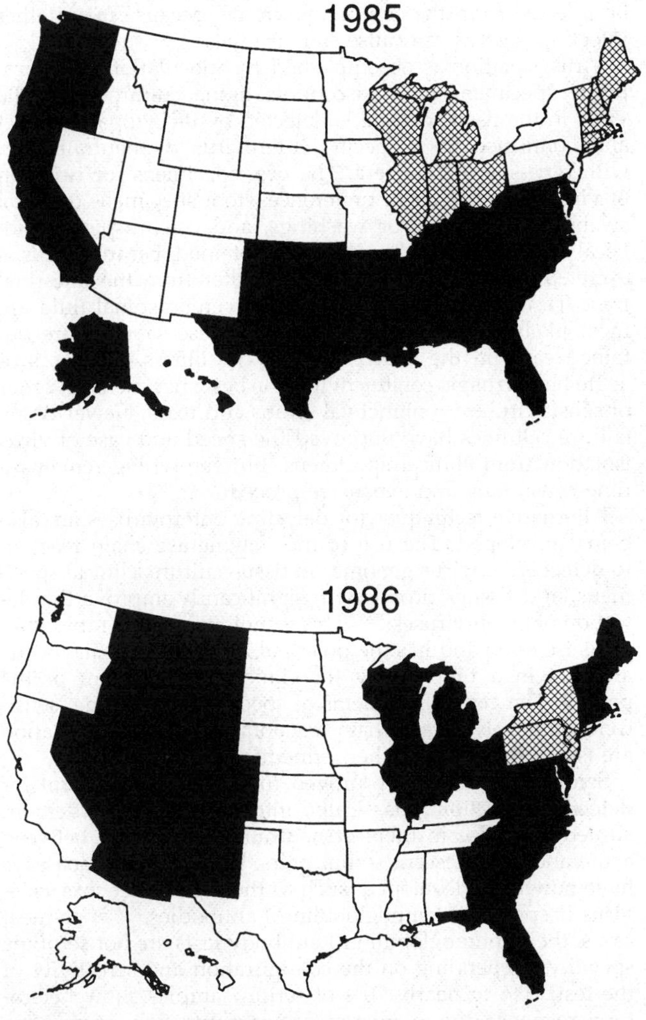

FIGURE 258–2 □ Geographic distribution of echovirus 11 isolates in the United States for 1985 and 1986. By using previously defined regions,[23] the relative ranking of echovirus 11 among all nonpoliovirus enteroviruses for each year in each region is represented by the degree of shading. Black areas indicate that the virus was the most common enterovirus in that region for that year. Moderate shading indicates that the virus was the second most common, and no shading indicates that echovirus 11 was not one of the three most common for that year. In both years, echovirus 11 was the most common enterovirus isolated in the United States.

Infection with enteroviruses elicits a strong humoral immune response. Often this response is heterotypic, that is, infection with one serotype induces an immune response to several other serotypes.[45, 46] Young children develop a more homotypic response, whereas older children and adults develop a more heterotypic response. This age difference in the specificity of the antibody response to an enterovirus infection probably reflects exposure to a greater number of serotypes with advancing age. The basis of this heterotypic response is not known, but it may be shared epitopes present in multiple serotypes. The subclass of the immunoglobulin G response has also been studied and is most often from the immunoglobulin G1 and G3 subclass of antibody.[47]

Clinical Manifestations

Enterovirus infections can result in a wide variety of disease syndromes. A summary of these syndromes in given in Table 258–2, and details of viral meningitis, encephalitis, pericarditis, myocarditis, and conjunctivitis can be found in other chapters. The most common result of enterovirus infection is either no symptoms or mild upper respiratory tract symptoms.[2, 3, 13, 15] Other mild enteroviral illness, consisting of fever, headache, malaise, and occasionally mild gastrointestinal symptoms, may also occur. Much less frequently, serious illness brings the patient to the attention of a physician.

The link between an enterovirus infection and a disease syndrome should be made with caution. Inapparent infections and prolonged excretion of virus, especially in stools, are common. A link cannot be made between infection and disease on the basis of isolating virus from the stool of an individual patient. A link can be inferred if the virus is isolated from a site that corresponds to the clinical symptoms and if that site is otherwise sterile. The association between infection and disease has most often been made from studies of outbreaks in which a large number of persons with the same clinical signs and symptoms have evidence of infection with the same serotype. Such studies have clearly demonstrated that enterovirus infection can cause aseptic meningitis, pericarditis, pleurodynia, myocarditis, and encephalitis. When an individual patient has a disease syndrome shown clearly to be associated with enterovirus infection and there is no evidence for involvement by another agent, infection probably implies causation.

The most commonly recognized serious manifestation of enterovirus infection is central nervous system disease, usually aseptic meningitis but sometimes encephalitis or paralysis. Enterovirus-associated central nervous system disease is reviewed elsewhere,[2, 3, 13, 15] and the clinical descriptions are found in the corresponding chapters of this book. Acute myocarditis and pericarditis are also discussed elsewhere in this book, and enterovirus involvement is reviewed elsewhere.[40, 48] Although the association between myocarditis and pericarditis and enterovirus infection is clearly established, it is not yet clear how often enterovirus infections are responsible for the disease syndromes. One study has shown that coxsackievirus B immunoglobulin M in a group of patients with acute myocarditis is significantly higher than in control subjects.[49] Enterovirus RNA has also been detected in myocardial biopsy specimens from patients with myocarditis.[50, 51] These and other studies suggest, but do not clearly show, that coxsackievirus B infection may be associated with a large fraction of cases of acute myocarditis. By contrast, different studies have failed to show conclusive evidence for the

TABLE 258–2 ■ Clinical Syndromes Associated with Enterovirus Infection

Central nervous system	
	Aseptic meningitis
	Encephalitis
	Flaccid paralysis
Respiratory	
	Mild upper respiratory tract symptoms
	Lymphonodular pharyngitis
Exanthems	
	Hand-foot-and-mouth disease
	Herpangina
Cardiac	
	Myocarditis
	Pericarditis
Other	
	Pleurodynia
	Acute hemorrhagic conjunctivitis
	Neonatal disseminated disease
	Chronic infection of agammaglobulinemic patients

Data from references 2, 3, 13, 15.

involvement of enterovirus infection in idiopathic dilated cardiomyopathies.[52–56]

A number of enterovirus serotypes have been associated with severe illness in neonates, including sepsis and generalized disseminated infection. The most systematic study of such illness, reported by Kaplan and coworkers,[57] covered records for a 10-year period in Nassau County, New York. Among hospitalized neonates were 77 patients with coxsackievirus B infection documented by isolation, and 6 died. The investigators estimated that 1 of every 2000 infants was hospitalized during the first 3 months of life in that area. This probably underestimates the true rate, because virus isolation studies miss some infections and other enteroviruses can also cause this syndrome. The contribution of echoviruses to neonatal illness has also been reviewed.[58]

Two enterovirus serotypes, enterovirus 70 and coxsackievirus A24 variant, are associated with acute hemorrhagic conjunctivitis. This disease is different from other enteroviral illness, having occurred in global pandemics since its introduction around 1969. The incubation period for these agents is shorter than that for other enteroviruses (24 to 72 hours), systemic illness is much less common, and conjunctival replication is the rule. The disease is characterized by acute onset of lacrimation, severe pain, chemosis and periorbital edema, photophobia, conjunctival hyperemia, and mild to severe subconjunctival hemorrhages. The disease is usually bilateral.

Association between enterovirus infection and other disease syndromes is less clearly defined. Of considerable interest is the possible association with several chronic diseases—diabetes mellitus, chronic heart disease, and arthritis. The most significant potential association is with juvenile-onset insulin-dependent diabetes mellitus. This potential association has been reviewed elsewhere.[59, 60] Several case-control studies and individual case reports suggest that enteroviruses can cause insulin-dependent diabetes mellitus, but it is not yet known whether they are a common or uncommon cause.[61–66]

Although there are few studies that examine the relationship between enterovirus infection and adverse effects on the fetus, one study found serologic evidence of central nervous system infection with coxsackievirus B in ventricular fluid from 4 of 28 newborns with congenital neural tube defects.[67] The infants had neutralizing antibody to only one coxsackievirus B serotype in the ventricular fluid but to several in serum. The unique distribution of antibodies in the ventricular fluid compared with that in serum supports the purported association. The mothers had antibodies to the same serotype as well as some other coxsackievirus B serotypes. No virus was isolated from infants or mothers. Two other studies have documented an association between enterovirus infection and miscarriages and stillbirths.[68, 69] Further studies are needed to assess the possibility of enterovirus infection of the fetus.

The chronic fatigue syndrome, also called epidemic neuromyasthenia or epidemic myalgic encephalomyelitis, has been linked to coxsackievirus B infection in some studies. In this poorly defined syndrome, the patient experiences excessive muscle fatigue with exercise accompanied by myalgia, and dysphasia, unexplained by other possible causes. Although there have been multiple studies showing either a serologic or a virologic association with enteroviruses, other studies contradict these findings.[70–74]

Diagnosis

The key to laboratory confirmation of enterovirus infection is the collection of appropriate clinical specimens for virus isolation or serologic studies.[4] Enterovirus infection cannot be inferred from the clinical syndrome, because many other infectious agents can cause similar illness.

Virus isolation is accomplished by inoculation of appropriate specimens onto susceptible tissue culture cells. The virus in the tissue culture is detected by its cytopathic effect and confirmed as a specific enterovirus by neutralization with type-specific antisera. The best specimens for isolation of virus are, in order of preference, stool specimens or rectal swabs, throat swabs or washings, and cerebrospinal fluid. Fecal specimens should always be obtained, because virus is excreted longest and in the highest titer from the intestinal tract. Throat swabs or washings and cerebrospinal fluid are most likely to yield virus isolates if these samples are obtained early in the acute phase of the illness. For cases of acute hemorrhagic conjunctivitis, the best specimens, in order of sensitivity, are conjunctival swabs and tears. Newer tissue culture cell lines have improved the speed and ease of virus isolation from clinical specimens, but serotyping remains a time-consuming and expensive procedure.[4, 75–77]

Alternative techniques for detecting enteroviruses are also being developed. The use of the polymerase chain reaction to detect enterovirus genomes in tissue culture, clinical specimens, and tissues promises to significantly improve the detection of enteroviruses.[78–80] This technique is more rapid than virus isolation and has the potential for providing diagnostic answers in a timely way for clinical management of the patient. The general problems of specimen processing, sensitivity, and polymerase chain reaction product contamination are issues that need further refinement.

Serologic studies have proved to be extremely useful for detecting infection. Classically, infection has been demonstrated by a rise in titers of neutralizing antibody between acute and convalescent serum pairs. Enzyme immunoassays have now been developed, such as those to detect coxsackievirus B–specific immunoglobulin M antibodies.[45, 81–83] In most cases, the immunoglobulin M antibody tests are not serotype specific.[46] Depending on the configuration and sensitivity of the test, 10% to nearly 70% of serum samples show heterotypic response due to other enterovirus infections. A positive result with either of these methods indicates recent viral infection, although with immunoglobulin M assays, the infecting serotype may not be the same one determined by the assay.

Treatment

Because no antiviral therapy is presently available for enterovirus infections, treatment is directed toward alleviating symptoms. Drugs have been identified that exhibit antiviral activity against several enteroviruses including poliovirus in tissue culture and experimental animals.[84, 85] These drugs, however, have not completed clinical trials. Interferon has been proposed for treatment of acute hemorrhagic conjunctivitis, but this awaits further evaluation.

In patients with agammaglobulinemia, chronic enterovirus infections have been treated with immune globulin, and this has controlled the infection in some cases.[86] Use of immune globulin in other clinical illness has not been systematically evaluated.

Prevention

There are no vaccines available for nonpoliovirus enteroviruses. General preventive measures include enteric precautions and good personal hygiene. Enteroviruses can be a cause of nosocomial infection. Serious infection is most common in newborns, although persons with compromised immune systems are also at high risk. Hospital staff can inadvertently carry the virus between patients or become infected themselves and spread the virus. Patients with suspected enterovirus infection should be managed with enteric precautions.[87] Patients and staff can be cohorted during outbreaks; during several newborn outbreaks, neonatal nurseries were closed to new admissions.

References

1. Melnick JL: Portraits of viruses: The picornaviruses. Intervirology 20:61, 1983.
2. Melnick JL: Enteroviruses: Polioviruses, coxsackieviruses, echoviruses, and newer enteroviruses. *In* Fields BN, Knipe DM (eds): Fields Virology, ed 2. New York, Raven Press, 1990, pp 549–606.
3. Modlin JF: Coxsackieviruses, echoviruses, and newer enteroviruses. *In* Mandell GL, Douglas RG Jr, Bennett JE (eds): Principles and Practice of Infectious Diseases, ed 3. New York, John Wiley & Sons, 1990, pp 1367–1383.
4. Grandien M, Forsgren M, Ehrnst A: Enteroviruses and reoviruses. *In* Schmidt NJ, Emmons RW (eds): Diagnostic Procedures for Viral, Rickettsial and Chlamydial Infections. Washington, DC, American Public Health Association, 1989, pp 513–569.
5. Prabhakar BS, Haspel MV, McClintock PR, et al: High frequency of antigenic variants among naturally occurring human coxsackie B4 virus isolates identified by monoclonal antibodies. Nature 300:374, 1982.
6. Prabhakar BS, Menegus MA, Notkins AL: Detection of conserved and nonconserved epitopes on coxsackievirus B4: Frequency of antigenic change. Virology 146:302, 1985.
7. Iizuka N, Kuge S, Nomoto A: Complete nucleotide sequence of the genome of coxsackievirus B1. Virology 156:64, 1987.
8. Lindberg AM, Stalhandske PO, Pettersson U: Genome of coxsackievirus B3. Virology 156:50, 1987.
9. Jenkins O, Booth JD, Minor PD, et al: The complete nucleotide sequence of coxsackievirus B4 and its comparison to other members of the Picornaviridae. J Gen Virol 68:1835, 1987.
10. Zhang G, Wilsden G, Knowles NJ, McCauley JW: Complete nucleotide sequence of a coxsackie B5 virus and its relationship to swine vesicular disease virus. J Gen Virol 74:845, 1993.
11. Stanway G, Kalkkinen N, Roivainen M, et al: Molecular and biological characteristics of echovirus 22, a representative of a new picornavirus group. J Virol 68:8232, 1994.
12. Ehrnst A, Eriksson M: Epidemiological features of type 22 echovirus infection. Scand J Infect Dis 25:275, 1993.
13. Melnick JL: Enteroviruses. *In* Evans AS (ed): Viral Infections of Humans: Epidemiology and Control. New York, Plenum Publishing, 1982, pp 187–251.
14. Hierholzer JC, Hatch MH: Acute hemorrhagic conjunctivitis. *In* Darrell RW (ed): Viral Diseases of the Eye. Philadelphia, Lea & Febiger, 1985, pp 165–196.
15. Morens DM, Pallansch MA, Moore M: Polioviruses and other enteroviruses. *In* Belshe RB (ed): Textbook of Human Virology. St. Louis, Mosby–Year Book, 1991, pp 427–497.
16. Centers for Disease Control: Neurotropic Viral Diseases Surveillance, Enterovirus Infections, Annual Summary, 1969. Atlanta, Centers for Disease Control, 1970.
17. Centers for Disease Control: Neurotropic Viral Diseases Surveillance, Enterovirus Infections, January-September, 1970. Atlanta, Centers for Disease Control, 1970.
18. Centers for Disease Control: Neurotropic Diseases Surveillance, Enterovirus Infections, Annual Summary, 1970. Atlanta, Centers for Disease Control, 1971.
19. Center for Disease Control: Enteric and Neurotropic Diseases Surveillance, Enterovirus Surveillance, 1971–1975. Atlanta, Centers for Disease Control, 1977.
20. Centers for Disease Control: Enterovirus Surveillance, Summary 1970–1979. Atlanta, Centers for Disease Control, 1981.
21. Morens DM, Zweighaft RM, Bryan JM: Non-polio enterovirus disease in the United States, 1971–1975. Int J Epidemiol 8:49, 1979.
22. Moore M: Enteroviral disease in the United States, 1970–1979. J Infect Dis 146:103, 1982.
23. Strikas RA, Anderson LJ, Parker RA: Temporal and geographic patterns of isolates of nonpolio enterovirus in the United States, 1970–1983. J Infect Dis 153:346, 1986.
24. Cao Y, Schnurr DP, Schmidt NJ: Monoclonal antibodies for study of antigenic variation in coxsackievirus type B4—Association of antigenic determinants with myocarditic properties of the virus. J Gen Virol 65:925, 1984.
25. Cao Y, Schnurr DP, Schmidt NJ: Differing cardiotropic and myocarditic properties of group B type 4 coxsackievirus strains. Arch Virol 80:119, 1984.
26. Jordan GW, Bolton V, Schmidt NJ: Diabetogenic potential of coxsackie B viruses in nature. Arch Virol 86:213, 1985.
27. Jimes S, Jamison RM: Coxsackievirus B4: In vitro genetic markers and virulence. Arch Virol 77:1, 1983.
28. Jimes S, Jamison RM, Grafton WD: Coxsackievirus B4: In vitro genetic markers and cardiovirulence. Arch Virol 81:345, 1984.
29. Jordan GW, Bolton V: Interferon-sensitive coxsackievirus variants in nature. J Interferon Res 5:289, 1985.
30. Hartig PC, Webb SR: Heterogeneity of a human isolate of coxsackie B4: Biological differences. J Infect 6:43, 1983.
31. Hartig PC, Madge GE, Webb SR: Diversity within a human isolate of coxsackie B4: Relationship to viral-induced diabetes. J Med Virol 11:23, 1983.
32. Bell EJ, McCartney RA: A study of coxsackie B virus infections, 1972–1983. J Hyg (Lond) 93:197, 1984.
33. Danes L, Jaresova I: Neutralization microtest with human coxsackievirus and echovirus serotypes. J Hyg Epidemiol Microbiol Immunol 29:399, 1985.
34. Manjunath N, Balaya S, Seth P: Serologic survey for neutralizing antibodies against group B coxsackieviruses in normal population in Delhi area. Indian J Med Res 76:656, 1982.
35. Mukundan P, John TJ: Prevalence and titres of neutralizing antibodies to group B coxsackieviruses. Indian J Med Res 77:577, 1983.
36. Santhanam S, Choudhury DS: Antibodies against coxsackie B2 virus in infants and children in Delhi. J Commun Dis 16:304, 1984.
37. Morag A, Margalith M, Shuval HI, et al: Acquisition of antibodies to various coxsackie and echo viruses and hepatitis A virus in agricultural communal settlements in Israel. J Med Virol 14:39, 1984.
38. Margalith M, Fattal B, Shuval HI, et al: Prevalence of antibodies to enteroviruses and varicella-zoster virus among residents and overseas volunteers at agricultural settlements in Israel. J Med Virol 20:189, 1986.
39. Lau RC: Coxsackie B virus infections in New Zealand patients with cardiac and noncardiac diseases. J Med Virol 11:131, 1983.
40. Woodruff JF: Viral myocarditis: A review. Am J Pathol 101:427, 1980.
41. Kandolf R, Klingel K, Zell R, et al: Molecular mechanisms in the pathogenesis of enteroviral heart disease: Acute and persistent infections. Clin Immunol Immunopathol 68:153, 1993.
42. Gauntt C, Higdon A, Bowers D, et al: What lessons can be learned from animal model studies in viral heart disease? Scand J Infect Dis Suppl 88:49, 1993.
43. Bergelson JM, Shepley MP, Chan BM, et al: Identification of the integrin VLA-2 as a receptor for echovirus 1. Science 255:1718, 1992.
44. Bergelson JM, Chan M, Solomon KR, et al: Decay-accelerating factor (CD55), a glycosylphosphatidylinositol-anchored complement regulatory protein, is a receptor for several echoviruses. Proc Natl Acad Sci USA 91:6245, 1994.
45. Dörries R, Ter Meulen V: Specificity of IgM antibodies in acute human coxsackievirus B infections, analysed by indirect solid phase enzyme immunoassay and immunoblot technique. J Gen Virol 64:159, 1983.
46. Pattison JR: Tests for coxsackie B virus–specific IgM. J Hyg (Lond) 90:327, 1983.
47. Torfason EG, Pallansch M, Reimer CB, et al: Immunoglobulin class and subclass-specific monoclonal antibody sandwich ELISA for the detection of antibodies against coxsackieviruses B, types 1–5. J Virol Methods 37:289, 1992.
48. Reyes MP, Lerner AM: Coxsackievirus myocarditis—With special reference to acute and chronic effects. Prog Cardiovasc Dis 27:373, 1985.
49. Frisk G, Torfason EG, Diderholm H: Reverse radioimmunoassays of IgM and IgG antibodies to coxsackie B viruses in patients with acute myopericarditis. J Med Virol 14:191, 1984.

50. Khan M, Why H, Richardson P, Archard L: Nucleotide sequencing of PCR products shows the presence of coxsackie-B3 virus in endomyocardial biopsies from patients with myocarditis or dilated cardiomyopathy. Biochem Soc Trans 22:176S, 1994.
51. Why HJ, Meany BT, Richardson PJ, et al: Clinical and prognostic significance of detection of enteroviral RNA in the myocardium of patients with myocarditis or dilated cardiomyopathy. Circulation 89:2582, 1994.
52. Satoh M, Tamura G, Segawa I, et al: Enteroviral RNA in dilated cardiomyopathy. Eur Heart J 15:934, 1994.
53. Giacca M, Severini GM, Mestroni L, et al: Low frequency of detection by nested polymerase chain reaction of enterovirus ribonucleic acid in endomyocardial tissue of patients with idiopathic dilated cardiomyopathy. J Am Coll Cardiol 24:1033, 1994.
54. Weiss LM, Liu XF, Chang KL, Billingham ME: Detection of enteroviral RNA in idiopathic dilated cardiomyopathy and other human cardiac tissues. J Clin Invest 90:156, 1992.
55. Keeling PJ, Jeffery S, Caforio AL, et al: Similar prevalence of enteroviral genome within the myocardium from patients with idiopathic dilated cardiomyopathy and controls by the polymerase chain reaction. Br Heart J 68:554, 1992.
56. Keeling PJ, Lukaszyk A, Poloniecki J, et al: A prospective case-control study of antibodies to coxsackie B virus in idiopathic dilated cardiomyopathy. J Am Coll Cardiol 23:593, 1994.
57. Kaplan MH, Klein SW, McPhee J, et al: Group B coxsackievirus infections in infants younger than three months of age: A serious childhood illness. Rev Infect Dis 5:1019, 1983.
58. Modlin JF: Perinatal echovirus infection: Insights from a literature review of 61 cases of serious infection and 16 outbreaks in nurseries. Rev Infect Dis 8:918, 1986.
59. Barrett-Conner E: Is insulin-dependent diabetes mellitus caused by coxsackievirus B infection? A review of the epidemiologic evidence. Rev Infect Dis 7:207, 1985.
60. Fohlman J, Friman G: Is juvenile diabetes a viral disease? Ann Med 25:569, 1993.
61. Frisk G, Fohlman J, Kobbah M, et al: High frequency of coxsackie-B-virus-specific IgM in children developing type I diabetes during a period of high diabetes morbidity. J Med Virol 17:219, 1985.
62. Banatvala JE, Bryant J, Schernthaner G, et al: Coxsackie B, mumps, rubella, and cytomegalovirus specific IgM responses in patients with juvenile-onset insulin-dependent diabetes mellitus in Britain, Austria, and Australia. Lancet 1:1409, 1985.
63. Schernthaner G, Banatvala JE, Scherbaum W, et al: Coxsackie-B-virus-specific IgM responses, complement-fixing islet-cell antibodies, HLA DR antigens, and C-peptide secretion in insulin-dependent diabetes mellitus. Lancet 2:630, 1985.
64. Frisk G, Nilsson E, Tuvemo T, et al: The possible role of coxsackie A and echo viruses in the pathogenesis of type I diabetes mellitus studied by IgM analysis. J Infect 24:13, 1992.
65. D'Alessio DJ: A case-control study of group B coxsackievirus immunoglobulin M antibody prevalence and HLA-DR antigens in newly diagnosed cases of of insulin-dependent diabetes mellitus. Am J Epidemiol 135:1331, 1992.
66. Frisk G, Friman G, Tuvemo T, et al: Coxsackie B virus IgM in children at onset of type 1 (insulin-dependent) diabetes mellitus: Evidence for IgM induction by a recent or current infection. Diabetologia 35:249, 1992.
67. Gauntt CJ, Gudvangen RJ, Brans YW, et al: Coxsackievirus group B antibodies in the ventricular fluid of infants with severe anatomic defects in the central nervous system. Pediatrics 76:64, 1985.
68. Frisk G, Diderholm H: Increased frequency of coxsackie B virus IgM in women with spontaneous abortion. J Infect 24:141, 1992.
69. Axelsson C, Bondestam K, Frisk G, et al: Coxsackie B virus infections in women with miscarriage. J Med Virol 39:282, 1993.
70. Yousef GE, Bell EJ, Mann GF, et al: Chronic enterovirus infection in patients with postviral fatigue syndrome. Lancet 1:146, 1988.
71. Bowles NE, Bayston TA, Zhang HY, et al: Persistence of enterovirus RNA in muscle biopsy samples suggests that some cases of chronic fatigue syndrome result from a previous, inflammatory viral myopathy. J Med 24:145, 1993.
72. Gow JW, Behan WM, Simpson K, et al: Studies on enterovirus in patients with chronic fatigue syndrome. Clin Infect Dis 18(Suppl 1):S126, 1994.
73. Swanink CM, Melchers WJ, van der Meer JW, et al: Enteroviruses and the chronic fatigue syndrome. Clin Infect Dis 19:860, 1994.
74. Miller NA, Carmichael HA, Calder BD, et al: Antibody to coxsackie B virus in diagnosing postviral fatigue syndrome. BMJ 302:140, 1991.
75. Patel JR, Daniel J, Mathan M, Mathan VI: Isolation and identification of enteroviruses from faecal samples in a differentiated epithelial cell line (HRT-18) derived from human rectal carcinoma. J Med Virol 14:255, 1984.
76. Patel JR, Daniel J, Mathan VI: A comparison of the susceptibility of three human gut tumour-derived differentiated epithelial cell lines, primary monkey kidney cells and human rhabdomyosarcoma cell line to 66-prototype strains of human enteroviruses. J Virol Methods 12:209, 1985.
77. Dagan R, Menegus MA: A combination of four cell types for rapid detection of enteroviruses in clinical specimens. J Med Virol 19:219, 1986.
78. Zoll GJ, Melchers WJ, Kopecka H, et al: General primer-mediated polymerase chain reaction for detection of enteroviruses: Application for diagnostic routine and persistent infections. J Clin Microbiol 30:160, 1992.
79. Glimaker M, Johansson B, Olcen P, et al: Detection of enteroviral RNA by polymerase chain reaction in cerebrospinal fluid from patients with aseptic meningitis. Scand J Infect Dis 25:547, 1993.
80. Nicholson F, Meetoo G, Aiyar S, et al: Detection of enterovirus RNA in clinical samples by nested polymerase chain reaction for rapid diagnosis of enterovirus infection. J Virol Methods 48:155, 1994.
81. Chan D, Hammond GW: Comparison of serodiagnosis of group B coxsackie virus infections by an immunoglobulin M capture enzyme immunoassay versus microneutralization. J Clin Microbiol 21:830, 1985.
82. Boman J, Nilsson B, Juto P: Serum IgA, IgG, and IgM responses to different enteroviruses as measured by a coxsackie B5–based indirect ELISA. J Med Virol 38:32, 1992.
83. McCartney RA, Banatvala JE, Bell EJ: Routine use of μ-antibody–capture ELISA for the serological diagnosis of coxsackie B virus infections. J Med Virol 19:205, 1986.
84. See DM, Tilles JG: Treatment of coxsackievirus A9 myocarditis in mice with WIN 54954. Antimicrob Agents Chemother 36:425, 1992.
85. Andries K, Dewindt B, Snoeks J, et al: In vitro activity of pirodavir (R 77975), a substituted phenoxy-pyridazinamine with broad-spectrum antipicornaviral activity. Antimicrob Agents Chemother 36:100, 1992.
86. O'Neil KM, Pallansch MA, Winkelstein JA, et al: Chronic group A coxsackievirus infection in agammaglobulinemia: Demonstration of genomic variation of serotypically identical isolates persistently excreted by the same patient. J Infect Dis 157:183, 1988.
87. Garner JS, Simmons BP: CDC guideline for isolation precautions in hospitals. *In* Guidelines for Protecting the Safety and Health of Health Care Workers. US Department of Health and Human Services. Washington, DC, US Government Printing Office, 1988, pp A8–1–84.

259

Rhinoviruses

Roland A. Levandowski

The rhinoviruses are picornaviruses that infect the respiratory tract of humans to produce the syndrome known as the common cold. Since the first strains were isolated in tissue cultures in the 1950s, more than 100 individual serotypes have been identified and numbered on the basis of a panel of specific neutralizing antibodies.[1–5] The numbering system roughly reflects the chronology of isolation of the prototypic strains of each serotype: the lowest numbered strains were isolated and submitted for typing earliest. Strategies for the rapid identification and control of rhinovirus infections are being developed as information on the physical composition of rhinoviruses and the mechanisms of cellular parasitism accumulates. Although the diversity of serotypes has been viewed as an obstacle to the production and implementation of a vaccine,[6] properties common to rhinoviruses such as receptor binding domains and the host's inflammatory responses are being explored for potentially broad applications to prevent and treat rhinovirus infections.

Characteristics of the Pathogen

The rhinovirus, like other picornaviruses, consists of a single-stranded RNA genome (in positive, or messenger, sense in the intact virion) surrounded by a non–lipid-enveloped protein capsid.[7] The virion has a total molecular mass of approximately 8 MDa and a diameter of 30 nm. The capsid is composed of 60 identical subunits arranged as 12 pentamers in an icosahedron[8] (Fig. 259–1). Each subunit includes one strand of each of the four structural proteins (VP1 to VP4). VP1, VP2, and VP3 have exterior projections that interact with neutralizing antibodies and correspond to the portions of the viral genome that demonstrate the greatest variability.[9–12] The defined receptor binding site of the virion resides in a depression in the surface of the capsid around the fivefold axis and consists of residues that are well conserved.[9–13] Associated with the receptor binding site is a more internally located hydrophobic pocket that may have a function in maintaining the structural integrity of the viral capsid and in facilitating the conformational changes needed for uncoating of viral RNA.[14, 15] This pocket is also identified as the site of binding of antiviral agents that stabilize the capsid and prevent uncoating of viral RNA.[15] The antigenic sites for the attachment of neutralizing antibodies (corresponding to surface loop projections from VP1, VP2, and VP3) border the receptor binding site.[10, 16] Antibodies binding nearer the receptor site neutralize viruses more efficiently and may interact directly with amino acid residues within the receptor site.[16a, 16b] The epitopes recognized by neutralizing antibodies include both linear and conformational amino acid sequences.[16–18] Permissible variation in the surface loop projections is potentially great, because antigens foreign to the rhinovirus capsid can be incorporated in the loop structures by site-directed mutagenesis.[19] VP4, which is exclusively internal, and VP2 result from a precursor (VP0) cleaved autocatalytically during encapsidation of the RNA[20, 21] (Fig. 259–2). Cleavage of VP0 to VP4 and VP2 appears to be a necessary step in the replication cycle, because mutation at the cleavage site results in a defective virus incapable of establishing infection even though it binds to receptors and undergoes conformational alterations similar to those of wild-type rhinoviruses.[22] The nonstructural proteins include two proteases with specific viral cleavage sites, an RNA-dependent RNA polymerase, and a small protein, VPg, that is covalently bound to the 5′ end of the viral RNA.[23–30] The P2A protease appears to function not only in viral protein processing but also in inactivating the complex required for binding of the host cell RNAs to ribosomes.[31] Translation of the genome is monocistronic, requires no cap, and is internally initiated at a site within the 550 to 600 nontranslated nucleotides at the 5′ end of the RNA.[32–35] Binding of ribosomes in the 5′-nontranslated region is restricted and specified by the secondary structure of the RNA.[36]

Thirty percent of the molecular weight of the virion is contributed by the viral RNA, which is composed of approximately 7200 nucleotides.[27–30] Although the nontranslated nucleotides are well conserved, hypervariable regions located in the domain of the structural proteins correspond to the antigenic sites where neutralizing antibodies attach to the rhinovirus capsid proteins.[10, 15, 34] VPg permits binding of the viral RNA to membranes for transcription and is found on both positive- and negative-stranded intermediates.[26] The 3′ end of the genome is polyadenylated.

The rhinovirus particle is variably susceptible to physical

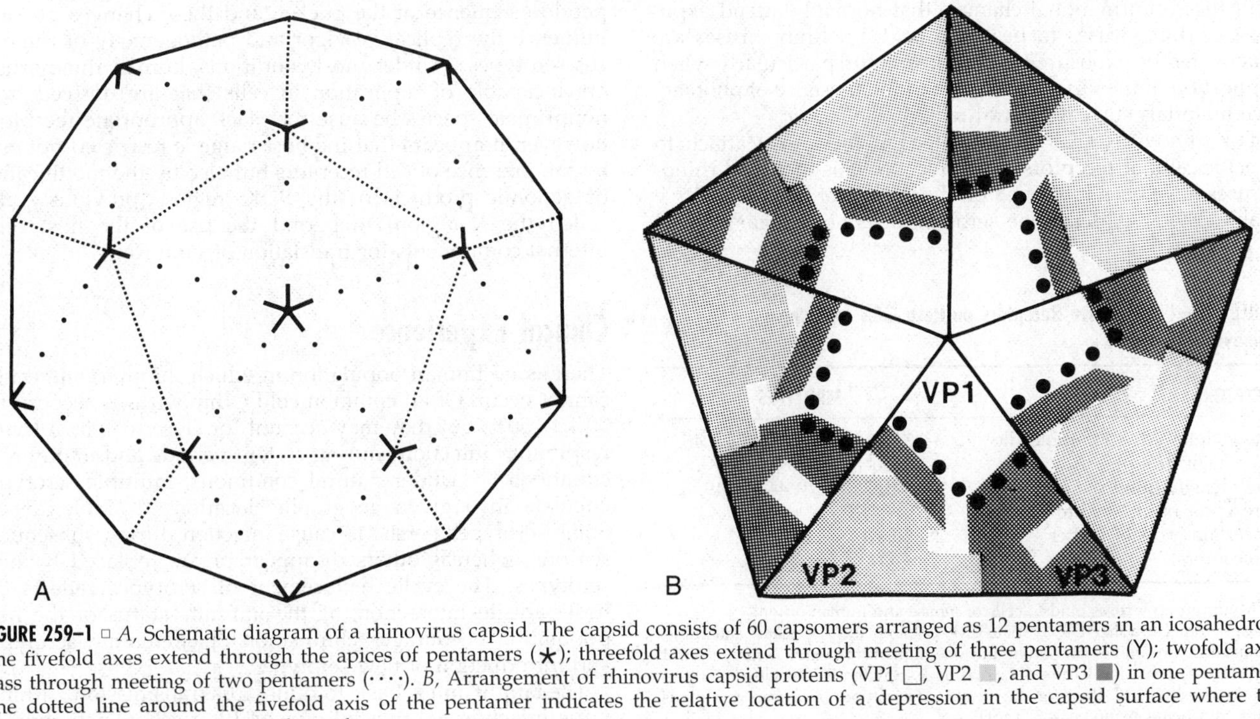

FIGURE 259–1 □ *A*, Schematic diagram of a rhinovirus capsid. The capsid consists of 60 capsomers arranged as 12 pentamers in an icosahedron. The fivefold axes extend through the apices of pentamers (★); threefold axes extend through meeting of three pentamers (Y); twofold axes pass through meeting of two pentamers (····). *B*, Arrangement of rhinovirus capsid proteins (VP1 □, VP2 ▒, and VP3 ■) in one pentamer. The dotted line around the fivefold axis of the pentamer indicates the relative location of a depression in the capsid surface where the putative receptor binding site is located.

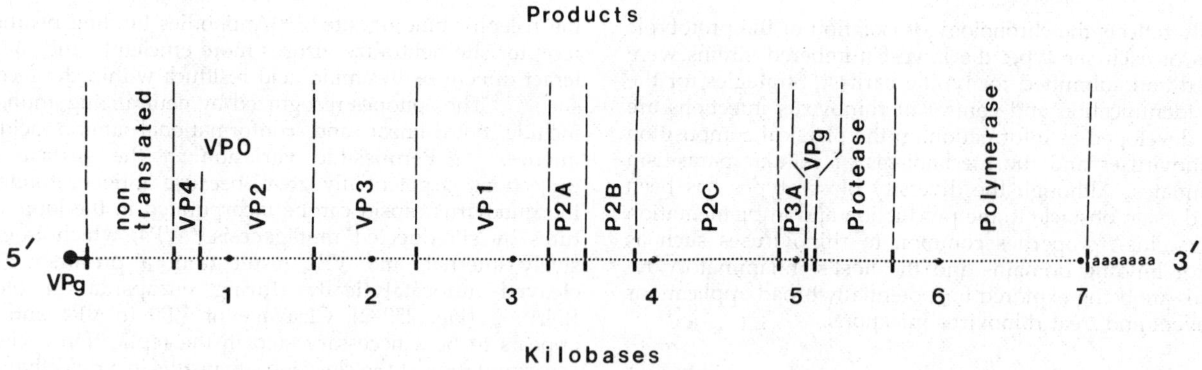

FIGURE 259–2 □ Sequence and sizes of genes from a representative rhinovirus. Products are labeled according to convention, as given by Rueckert and Wimmer.[21]

agents. The virion is not inactivated by organic solvents such as ether and chloroform because the capsid is not enveloped by a lipid membrane.[1] Rhinoviruses are also resistant to trichlorofluoroethane, ethanol, and weak phenol.[37] Although acid-resistant rhinoviruses have been selected from wild-type virus populations by repeated passage after exposure to low pH, the capsids of extracellular rhinoviruses normally undergo an irreversible conformational change and are inactivated when the pH is less than 5.[38, 39] However, the change in conformation of the capsid under acidic conditions is a critical part of the process of uncoating of intracellular virions.[40] Other human picornaviruses (poliovirus, coxsackievirus, and echovirus) are not inactivated by exposure to acidic conditions and therefore can be easily differentiated from the rhinoviruses.[41] Rhinoviruses also undergo conformational changes at increased temperature. The infectivity of rhinoviruses is indefinitely stable at −70°C. At 37°C the half-life of inactivation is on the order of hours to a day, and at 56°C it is minutes to a few hours. In some circumstances the virion may be temperature stabilized by divalent cations, although the effect is variable for different serotypes.[42] The antiviral agents that bind to the hydrophobic pocket near the receptor binding site also stabilize the viral capsid and prevent the conformational changes that normally attend exposure of rhinoviruses to heat and acid.[14, 15] Rhinoviruses are inactivated by exposure to ultraviolet light, particularly when replication of the virus takes place in the presence of photoactive materials such as neutral red.

For rhinoviruses to initiate infection they must attach to specific cellular receptors. Two glycoproteins that bind rhinoviruses have been identified on the surface of human cells[43, 44] (Table 259–1). At least one serotype does not appear to bind to either of the identified glycoproteins, and data from other studies suggest that other cellular receptors may exist.[14, 45–47] More than 80% of serotypes tested bind to a receptor that has been identified as a leukocyte attachment protein known as intercellular adhesion molecule 1 (ICAM-1).[48–51] ICAM-1 has been detected on most cells of human origin including HeLa cells, fibroblasts, and cells in the respiratory epithelium. A minority of serotypes bind to a second receptor on human cells identified as the low-density lipoprotein receptor.[45] Unlike the serotypes in the larger group (referred to as the major group), rhinoviruses binding to the low-density lipoprotein receptor also bind to a receptor on cells of murine origin.[52]

Penetration and uncoating of the virion after receptor attachment result in the release of viral RNA into the cytoplasm of the host cell, where the assembly of new virions occurs from replicative products. The uncoating process requires a compartment, possibly an endosome, in which acidification occurs, and a conformational change in the capsid frees the RNA.[53] The viral capsid may be stabilized and the conformational change prevented by insertion of certain molecules into the pocket-like depression of the receptor binding site.[54–56] The relative antiviral activity of the stabilizing agents against rhinoviruses is affected by changes in the peptide sequence of the pocket, and these changes possibly influence the replicative vigor and pathogenicity of rhinovirus serotypes.[57] Under most conditions, human rhinoviruses are incapable of replication in cells that are derived from nonprimate species because they lack appropriate receptors; however, it appears that the host range is restricted not only by the presence of cell receptors but also by the modification of genomic products of the P2BC region (previously also called the X region) to permit the use of the host cell's internal components for translation of viral RNA.[58, 59]

TABLE 259–1 ■ Putative Receptors on HeLa Cells for Human Rhinovirus Serotypes

RECEPTOR	SEROTYPES
Intercellular adhesion molecule 1 (major group)	3–22, 24, 26–28, 32–43, 45, 46, 48, 50–86, 88, 89
Low-density lipoprotein receptor (minor group*)	1A, 1B, 2, 29–31, 44, 47, 49, 62
Uncertain (possibly other receptors)	23, 25, 87

*Minor group viruses bind to cells of mouse and human origin.

Data from Uncapher DR, DeWitt CM, Colonno RJ: The major and minor group receptor families contain all but one human rhinovirus serotype. Virology 180:814, 1991; and Crump CE, Arruda E, Hayden FG: In vitro inhibitory activity of soluble ICAM-1 for the numbered serotypes of human rhinovirus. Antiviral Chem Chemother 4:323, 1993.

Clinical Experience

There is no human population in which rhinovirus infection cannot occur. Of all common colds, rhinoviruses account for 30% to 50%, but they may account for close to 100% of viral respiratory infections during certain periods and in outbreak situations.[60–65] Under natural conditions, multiple serotypes circulate in a given geographic location[66–70] (Table 259–2). Some serotypes persist to cause infection during subsequent seasons, whereas others disappear or are replaced by new serotypes. The cyclic replacement of serotypes reflects the host-parasite interaction, as the immune status of the host population encourages elimination of circulating serotypes and introduction of new serotypes.

The family unit is basic to rhinovirus transmission.[61] Rhinovirus infection is often introduced by a school-age child or

TABLE 259–2 ■ Rhinovirus Serotypes Isolated in More Than 1 Year from Adult Medical Center Students and Personnel with Naturally Acquired Common Colds in Chicago*

	YEAR									
SEROTYPE†	1968	1969	1970	1971	1972	1973	1974	1975	1976	1977
7	+			+						
8				+	+					
9	+	+								
19			+		+	+				
21		+	+	+		+				+
25	+			+	+					
40			+			+				
41				+				+		
51			+							+
62									+	+
Total serotypes	11	9	9	11	6	4	ND‡	3	5	5

*Some serotypes appear in consecutive years. Other serotypes appear only sporadically. Serotypes isolated in only 1 year are included in the total number of serotypes for each year.

†All nontypeable strains counted as one serotype for each year. Typing done with specific antisera for serotypes 1A and 1B through 89.

‡ND, No data available.

Courtesy of G. G. Jackson, M. Rubenis, and R. A. Levandowski, University of Illinois, Chicago, IL.

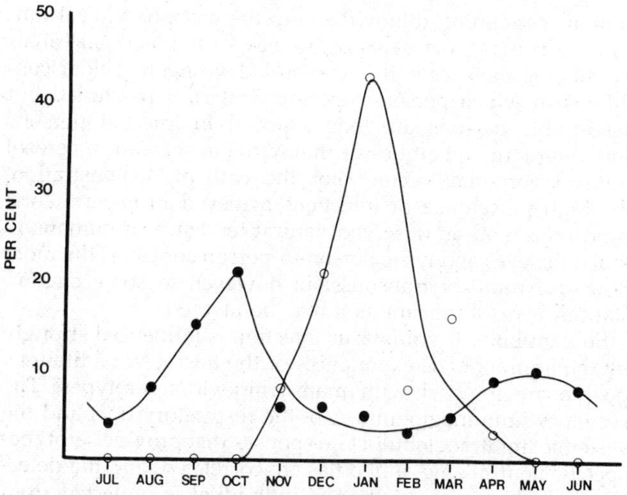

FIGURE 259–3 ▫ Monthly isolation of rhinoviruses as a percentage of all rhinovirus infections (●) and influenza virus isolates as a percentage of all influenza virus infections (○) during 20 years among adult medical center students and personnel in Chicago. The nadir of rhinovirus isolation in winter months between the fall and spring peaks coincides with the peak of influenza activity. Although influenza virus infection is absent between May and October, rhinovirus infections are observed throughout the year. (Courtesy of G. G. Jackson, M. Rubenis, and R. A. Levandowski, University of Illinois, Chicago, IL.)

one in daycare to other siblings and parents at home. Mothers are more often infected than fathers, presumably because of the increased intensity of personal contact with greater exposure and opportunity for transmission. Although susceptibility to rhinovirus infections decreases in adults because of multiple exposures over the years, the protection afforded by neutralizing antibody is incomplete, and infection on more than one occasion with the same serotype is possible if the infecting inoculum is adequately large.[71]

Fall and spring peaks have been documented for the occurrence of rhinovirus infection in temperate climates[61, 72, 73] (Fig. 259–3). The fall peak may be related partly to social events, as return to school means many more opportunities for transmission of rhinoviruses among larger groups of children. During the winter months of most years, the occurrence of rhinovirus infections in industrial countries is reduced (although not absent). It is possible that the reduced occurrence of rhinovirus infection reflects either direct interference by influenza virus and other more efficiently spread viruses or the induction of natural interferons, because interferon is induced by influenza and other respiratory viruses.[74] However, the lower relative humidity during cold months may contribute to the inactivation of rhinoviruses.[75]

The nasal secretions contain the greatest quantity of rhinovirus during infection.[76, 77] The quantity of virus present in secretions varies from person to person and from day to day in one infected person. Generally, the peak of shedding of a rhinovirus is on the second to fourth day after inoculation and parallels the severity of clinical symptoms (Fig. 259–4). Virus is usually shed for 7 to 10 days, but instances of shedding for several weeks are documented.[61, 76] Although the secretions of the nasopharynx traverse the posterior oropharynx, little infectious rhinovirus is found in oral secretions. The paucity of virus in oral secretions at least partly explains the inefficiency of oral secretions in transmitting infection.[77, 78] In families, the interval between the initial infection and subsequent ones is related to the quantity and duration of the shedding of virus and ranges up to 10 days with an average of 3 days.[77–80]

The transmission of rhinoviruses has been observed in experimental conditions during person-to-person contact, by exposure to fomites, and by aerosols. Which is the predominant natural mode of transmission has not been definitively demonstrated. Although rhinoviruses may persist for several hours after application to inanimate surfaces, transfer by contact with contaminated objects often does not occur.[75, 78, 81, 82] Transfer of rhinovirus from an infected person to a susceptible one can occur through hand touching of only a few seconds' duration.[83] In this setting, infection of the respiratory tract is achieved by direct self-inoculation of se-

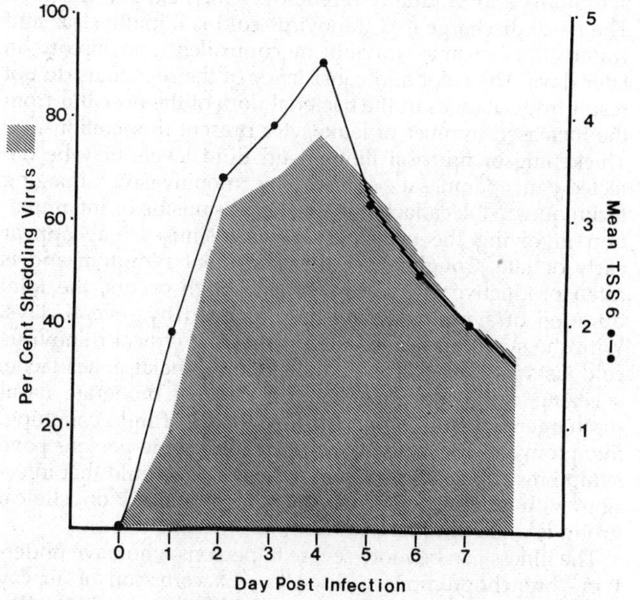

FIGURE 259–4 ▫ Percentage of volunteers shedding virus in nasal secretions and daily mean total symptom scores for six symptoms (TSS6) during the 7 days after experimental infection with rhinovirus serotype 25. The six symptoms are nasal obstruction, nasal discharge, sneezing, sore throat, cough, and headache graded to reflect the severity above the baseline day (day 0).

..retions containing rhinovirus onto the nasopharyngeal mucosa by rubbing the nares or by way of the lacrimal canals by rubbing the eyes with secretion-laden fingers. Under conditions in which person-to-person contact is precluded but susceptible persons are long exposed to infected persons shedding large quantities of rhinovirus in secretions, aerosol transmission may occur.[81] For the ease of demonstration, the high percentage of infections achieved in experimental conditions, and an observed natural tendency of humans to touch the eyes and nose, person-to-person contact is the more powerful route of transmission; however, in some circumstances, aerosol transmission may be favored.[65, 81]

Susceptibility to rhinovirus infection is influenced strongly by the immunologic experiences of the host. Over a lifetime, people are infected with many rhinovirus serotypes. The secretory immunoglobulin A of the respiratory tract and the systemic immunoglobulin G responses that provide serotype-specific neutralizing antibodies are correlated, and the detection of either suggests that an individual is protected from infection.[61] The protection afforded is relative, because the neutralizing capacity of antibodies can be overwhelmed by a large inoculum of rhinovirus.[71] Antibody is a relatively poor measure of exposure to rhinoviruses because serotype-specific lymphocyte proliferative responses may be detected even in the absence of neutralizing antibodies.[84, 85]

Women may have increased susceptibility to respiratory virus infection at the midpoint of the menstrual cycle.[86] Contrary to popular myth, susceptibility to rhinovirus infection is not increased by exposure to cold, as demonstrated in volunteers and in polar settlements.[65, 87, 88] The production of interferon in nasal secretions after a rhinovirus cold provides a natural resistance to infection that persists only long enough for specific neutralizing antibody to develop in 2 to 6 weeks.[89, 90]

The illness associated with rhinovirus infection appears after a 24- to 72-hour incubation period that follows the deposition of virus in the nasopharynx.[91] Sore throat and sneezing often herald the onset of a rhinovirus cold. Nasal discharge and nasal obstruction, the symptoms most typical of a cold, reach their peak within a day or two of onset of symptoms and gradually recede over the next several days. The nasal discharge in a rhinovirus cold is initially clear and watery but becomes variably mucopurulent and viscous in later days. The color and consistency of the secretions do not result from changes in the bacterial flora of the nose but from the increased number of leukocytes present in secretions.[91–93] Thickening of mucosal linings and fluid levels may be detected in paranasal sinuses by noninvasive imaging techniques.[94, 95] Headache as a result of sinusitis or inflammation involving the ostia of paranasal sinuses may appear early or late. Cough is a rather persistent symptom and is often productive of sputum. When cough occurs, the total duration of symptoms may be prolonged by several days. With the symptoms taken all together the typical rhinovirus cold lasts 5 to 7 days: 1 or 2 days of mild malaise, headache, sneezing, and sore throat; 3 to 6 days of moderate nasal discharge and obstruction; and 2 to 4 days of mild coughing. Symptom severity is highly variable, and some persons have symptoms suggestive of allergic rhinitis or so mild that infection with a rhinovirus may not be suspected on clinical grounds.

The illness can be more severe in persons who have underlying bronchopulmonary disorders. Exacerbation of airway obstruction in patients with asthma and chronic obstructive lung disease has been documented.[96–99] Changes in airways function may also be found in adults with special pulmonary function maneuvers, even in the absence of overt lung disease.[100, 101] The relation of these changes to direct involvement by replication of rhinovirus in the lower respiratory tract or to reflexive responses to upper airway infection is unclear. Although clearance of material from the nasopharynx and lung may be disordered by rhinovirus infection, ciliary function in the airways is not appreciably affected in otherwise healthy adults.[102–104]

The replication of rhinoviruses occurs predominantly in the upper airways, partly because the replication of rhinoviruses is maximal at nasal temperature, 33°C to 34°C.[105] Infected nasopharyngeal epithelial cells can be identified by a number of methods including immunologic staining methods and in situ hybridization, even though it is often difficult to demonstrate morphologic or functional abnormalities of the tissues involved.[92, 104, 106–108] Rhinoviruses have been isolated from the middle ear during otitis media[109] and from paranasal sinuses during acute sinusitis.[110] Rhinoviruses have been recovered from the bronchial secretions of infected volunteers, although it is not clear that the finding represents active replication of rhinovirus in the lower respiratory tract rather than the introduction of upper airway materials during the collection of secretions.[111] Rhinovirus has been recovered from heart blood at necropsy, but rhinoviremia has never been noted ante mortem.[112] Although large volumes of the nasal secretions enter the gastrointestinal tract, rhinoviruses have rarely been recovered from the stool. However, the absence of rhinovirus from the gut is not related simply to gastric acidity, because gastric aspirates inconsistently inactivate rhinoviruses.[113]

A multitude of interacting factors including cytokines and inflammatory mediators are implicated in the production of the nasopharyngeal symptoms during rhinovirus infection. Reflex mechanisms may account for some of the nasal discharge, as anticholinergic compounds reduce the quantity of nasal secretions.[114, 115] Kinins have been identified in the nasal secretions during acute rhinovirus infection and correlate with measures of vascular permeability and symptoms.[116] Exogenous kinins applied to the nasopharynx produce sore throat and stimulate nasal obstruction and discharge. The origin of the interferon found in nasal secretions during rhinovirus infection is presumably the cells of the nasopharyngeal tissues and may include the lymphocytes of the submucosa, because rhinoviruses potently induce interferon when cultured with mononuclear leukocytes in vitro.[117–119] Although interferon may limit the extent of viral replication, it may also modify the local inflammatory response and recruit lymphocytes from the blood pool for interactions in the respiratory mucosal environment.[120] The spectrum of other cytokines produced by mononuclear leukocytes in response to rhinovirus infections is not fully determined, but several such as interleukin-1, interleukin-6, interleukin-8, tumor necrosis factor-α, and interferon-γ have been detected by using sensitive assays, and their contributions to symptoms and airway reactivity are being investigated.[120a–120d]

During the first few days of rhinovirus infection, the number of polymorphonuclear leukocytes rises, while lymphocyte populations, particularly the T lymphocytes, are transiently reduced in the peripheral blood.[117, 121, 122] The destination of the lymphocytes after leaving the peripheral blood is uncertain, but lymphocytes and other mononuclear leukocytes can be found in submucosal sites in the respiratory tract.[123] Although the vast majority of leukocytes migrating into mucopurulent secretions are polymorphonuclear leukocytes, lymphocytes and other mononuclear leukocytes are also shed in increased numbers.[93, 122] The recruitment of large numbers of polymorphonuclear leukocytes to produce a mucopurulent nasal secretion is possibly specific, because cells infected with a rhinovirus produce a soluble chemoattractant.[124] Although the severity of symptoms in rhinovirus infections can be correlated with the magnitude of change in numbers of leukocytes, the role of specific leukocytes in the pathophysiology of rhinovirus infection is not established. It has been suggested that polymorphonuclear leukocytes may be responsible for release of factors that promote cell damage and increase inflammation.[125] The ability of rhinoviruses to activate mononuclear leukocytes including B cells, T cells, and natural killer cells and the association of cytokines with symptoms during rhinovirus infection suggest a role for mononuclear leukocytes also in local inflammation.[119, 120a–120d, 125a] As natural killer cell function is augmented by exposure to rhinovirus in vitro, it is of interest that virus replication and cell injury can be limited by natural killer cells in models of picornavirus infection.[119, 126, 127]

Laboratory Aspects

Although newer methods such as polymerase chain reaction are gaining acceptance and wider use, tissue cultures inoculated with secretions still provide the most direct and practical way for most clinical laboratories to identify rhinoviruses as agents of common colds. The yield is improved when nasal secretions are collected directly or are washed from the mucosal surface with a physiologic salt solution.[77] Oral secretions contain fewer infectious virions, and nasal swabs sample a smaller portion of the secretions than nasal washing. Collecting several samples daily and early from an infected person improves recovery, because the maximal titer of shed virus and the greatest proportion of shedders are found during the first days of infection[78] (see Fig. 259–4).

Rhinoviruses replicate in many tissue types, including human diploid fibroblasts (WI-38, MRC-5, foreskin), HeLa, KB, HEp-2, WISH, monkey kidney, human fetal tonsil, and nasal polyp explants.[4, 38, 61, 119, 128–134] Permissive HeLa strains provide high titers of rhinovirus, and diploid fibroblasts provide a system that facilitates identification of virus replication.[4, 38, 132, 133] Agitation and incubation at 33°C (the optimal temperature that mimics nasal conditions) encourage replication.[105] The cytopathologic appearance of the infected monolayer of tissue culture by itself is strongly suggestive of rhinovirus infection and is confirmed by acid lability and ether resistance of the isolate. Intersecting pools of sera may facilitate serotyping efforts, although cross-reactivity among serotypes is noted.[135, 136] The most widely used method for detecting antibodies to a specific rhinovirus is neutralization of virus using a standardized input of the median tissue culture infectious dose ($TCID_{50}$). The assay is maximally sensitive with a low viral inoculum of 10 to 100 $TCID_{50}$.[137] Acute- and convalescent-phase serum samples collected 2 to 6 weeks apart are used to determine whether antibody titer has risen significantly. Neither of the foregoing methods for identifying rhinovirus infection is optimal for implementation of therapeutic intervention with antiviral agents, because isolation of a rhinovirus from clinical samples may require up to 2 weeks and serodiagnosis of rhinovirus infection by specific neutralizing antibody is impractical, considering the multitude of serotypes.

Potential means of rapid rhinovirus detection include methods employed for other agents, such as immunoassay or probing with labeled DNA complementary to the viral genome.[138, 139] If the antigen concentration is low, an amplification step of replication in tissue cultures might be necessary. Detection of viral nucleic acid by amplification in polymerase chain reaction may also be possible and might be universal, as there are portions of the genome that are relatively well conserved among the serotypes examined.[140] The potential sensitivity (theoretically a single genome copy) and specificity of the polymerase chain reaction technique make the test a desirable addition to other methods. Furthermore, the identification process can be made at the serotype level in some instances by means of restriction enzymes that cleave the DNA produced by polymerase chain reaction to produce a pattern of fragments specific for a given serotype.[141] The detection of specific rhinovirus enzymes is also conceivable if appropriate substrates can be devised.[142]

Treatment and Prevention

Inactivated rhinoviruses produce immunity in volunteers after parenteral or intranasal inoculation[143–145]; however, the rhinovirus vaccines tested have conferred homotypic, but not heterotypic, protection. Animal studies with synthetic rhinovirus peptides suggest that a heterotypic antibody response may be induced, but it is not known whether the response is protective.[146, 147] Use of a multivalent rhinovirus vaccine in humans suggests that a variable response to the contained antigens occurs and that heterotypic immunity is not sufficiently increased.[148] Although serum antibody titers decline after natural infection, the durability of antibody after immunization is not defined. At present there is no useful vaccine to prevent infections caused by rhinoviruses.

The interruption of transmission of rhinoviruses from person to person begins with hand washing. In the laboratory and in field trials, the use of paper handkerchiefs permeated with chemical agents such as citric acid and iodine that inactivate rhinoviruses has reduced transmission and might be considered for circumstances of high transmission or severe consequences of infection.[149–151]

The evaluation of treatments designed to prevent attachment to specific cellular receptors is progressing. One approach has been to apply a monoclonal antibody directed against the ICAM-1 receptor on the cells of the nasal epithelium. However, data from an initial clinical trial suggest no prevention of infection and modest symptomatic benefit that may be insufficient to warrant clinical use.[152] A soluble form of ICAM-1 has been produced as a purified protein and has been shown to be capable of preventing infection of tissue cultures by most rhinovirus serotypes that bind to ICAM-1.[153, 154] A curious finding is that some serotypes (e.g., serotypes 23 and 25) are not well inhibited by the soluble ICAM-1, even though these serotypes had previously been identified as being in the ICAM-1 receptor group by blocking the receptor on HeLa cells with specific monoclonal antibodies. However, other studies indicate that serotypes 23 and 25 may use an alternative receptor and that strains of specific serotypes may develop a reduced affinity for ICAM-1.[47] Further clinical trials will determine the value of receptor blockade for the prevention and treatment of rhinovirus infections.

Many antiviral agents that are active against rhinoviruses are being identified and some have undergone clinical trials.[55, 155–164] Some are unacceptable because of toxicity. Others studied in clinical trials have had limited antiviral effects. Although some drugs have shown prophylactic effects in preventing rhinovirus infections, none has been shown to be beneficial after infection is established. In general, it appears that the strategy for drug delivery must be direct delivery via intranasal administration of powdered or dissolved drug. A limiting feature in some instances appears to be maintenance of adequate concentrations of drug at the target nasopharyngeal tissues, which are protected by complex clearance mechanisms. As an example, pirodavir when given as a nasal spray six times per day reduced infection rates by approximately half as compared with placebo but had no effect when given three times per day.[163] As another example, enviroxime, which is one of the most potent chemical inhibitors of rhinoviruses in tissue culture, had inconsistent effects in volunteer challenge studies, possibly because of the poor water solubility of the compound.[165–167] However, alternative formulations designed to bypass solubility barriers and to improve retention of the drug at the intranasal site may help to improve effectiveness.[168]

Many studies have shown the efficacy of interferon alpha or interferon inducers applied locally in the nasopharynx in preventing rhinovirus infection.[118, 169–174] Strategies for use are based on the observed seasonality and family clustering of infections with rhinoviruses. Administration of interferon alpha on a long-term basis results in infiltration of the nasal mucosa with increased numbers of lymphocytes and causes nasal bleeding (usually not sufficient to result in epistaxis) in 5% to 10% of recipients.[175, 176] Limiting the duration of use of interferon to a week or two after introduction of a respiratory virus into a family reduces some of the undesirable aspects of administration; however, when this approach is used rhinovirus infections are fewer but other common cold viruses such as parainfluenza virus are relatively unaffected.[171] The paucity of symptoms in many infected persons suggests that subclinical infections could also reduce the efficacy of interferon alpha used in this manner.[80] Preparations of interferon beta and interferon gamma have been less well studied. Although some reduction in symptoms caused by rhinovirus infection has been demonstrated, interferon beta does not appear to prevent acquisition of the infection either experimentally or naturally.[177, 178] Human interferon gamma not only fails to prevent rhinovirus infection but also may augment the symptomatic response.[179] No study with interferon has shown a therapeutic effect once infection has been established and symptoms have begun.

Ascorbic acid and zinc have received much popular attention as potential remedies for the common cold.[180–187] However, neither ascorbic acid nor zinc has been shown to prevent rhinovirus infection in volunteer challenge studies.[180, 184, 185] Although symptomatic benefits of administration of ascorbic acid or zinc have been described in studies of naturally occurring respiratory infections, the results have shown no consistent, reproducible pattern for the type of symptoms affected, the degree of relief, or the duration of symptoms. These inconsistencies may be attributed in some instances to the failure of "blinding" (because both ascorbic acid and zinc can be readily discerned by taste). In other instances, positive outcomes may reflect a statistical artifact.[181, 184, 185] The current data, however, indicate a modest effect at best and are insufficient to prompt a strong recommendation in favor of ascorbic acid except as supplementation in the case of dietary deficiency. Nevertheless, interest in ascorbic acid has continued because it seems to offer a simple, benign treatment for an infectious disease lacking a well-defined, specific remedy.[187]

In the absence of specific antiviral therapy, several simple measures may be readily undertaken in alleviating symptoms. Maintenance of hydration to keep secretions loose and the judicious use of nasal decongestant medications offer the most convenient combination for treatment. The nasal wash maneuver with room temperature physiologic salt solution is surprisingly pleasant and provides temporary opening of nasal passages by removing tenacious secretions and causing detumescence of the mucosa. Aspirin and other nonsteroidal antiinflammatory agents may improve systemic symptoms such as malaise but are of no clear benefit to local inflammatory symptoms.[188] Aspirin should be used cautiously and should not be given to children. Acetaminophen is preferred as the antiinflammatory agent for children, because many respiratory viruses can cause the common cold, the etiology of respiratory infection may not be determined easily, and aspirin administration has been implicated in the development of Reye's syndrome related to respiratory virus infection.[189] Antihistamines appear to be relatively ineffective, but pseudoephedrine has shown a benefit in relieving nasal congestion and anticholinergic agents have demonstrated some effect in reducing nasal secretions.[114, 115, 190, 191] A combination of several of these modalities has been suggested as a potential therapeutic approach. In a study of volunteers infected with a rhinovirus 1 day before beginning treatment, the combination of interferon alpha to reduce virus replication, naproxen as an antiinflammatory agent to reduce systemic symptoms, and ipratropium as an anticholinergic medication to reduce nasal secretions was effective in reducing symptoms without impairing immune responses to the infecting strain.[192] The promising results suggest that further investigation of similar rationalized regimens is warranted and may lead to relief from (if not a cure for) rhinovirus infection and the common cold.

References

1. Rhinoviruses: A numbering system. Nature 213:761, 1967.
2. A collaborative report: Rhinoviruses—Extension of the numbering system. Virology 43:524, 1971.
3. A collaborative report: Rhinoviruses—Extension of the numbering system from 89 to 100. Virology 159:191, 1987.
4. Conant RM, Hamparian VV: Rhinoviruses: Basis for a numbering system. I. HeLa cells for propagation and serologic procedures. J Immunol 100:107, 1968.
5. Conant RM, Hamparian VV: Rhinoviruses: Basis for a numbering system. II. Serologic characterization of prototype strains. J Immunol 100:114, 1968.
6. Fox JP: Is a rhinovirus vaccine possible? Am J Epidemiol 103:345, 1976.
7. Rueckert RR: On the structure and morphogenesis of picornaviruses. *In* Fraenkel-Conrat H, Wagner RR (eds): Comprehensive Virology, Vol 6. New York, Plenum Publishing, 1976, pp 131–213.
8. Luo M, Rossmann MG, Palmenberg AC: Prediction of three-dimensional models for foot-and-mouth disease virus and hepatitis A virus. Virology 166:503, 1988.
9. Rossman MG, Arnold E, Erickson JW, et al: Structure of a human common cold virus and functional relationship to other picornaviruses. Nature 317:146, 1985.
10. Sherry B, Mosser AG, Colonno RJ, et al: Use of monoclonal antibodies to identify four neutralization immunogens on a common cold picornavirus, human rhinovirus 14. J Virol 57:246, 1986.
11. Smith TJ, Olson NH, Cheng RH, et al: Structure of a human rhinovirus-bivalently bound antibody complex: Implications for viral neutralization and antibody flexibility. Proc Natl Acad Sci USA 90:7015, 1993.
12. Barnett PV, Rowlands DJ, Parry NR: Characterization of monoclonal antibodies raised against a synthetic peptide capable of inducing a neutralizing response to human rhinovirus type 2. J Gen Virol 74:1295, 1993.
13. Rossmann MG, Palmenberg AC: Conservation of the putative receptor attachment site in picornaviruses. Virology 164:373, 1988.
14. Rossmann MG: Viral cell recognition and entry. Protein Sci 3:1712, 1994.
15. Bibler-Muckelbauer JK, Kremer MJ, Rossmann MG, et al: Human rhinovirus 14 complexed with fragments of active antiviral compounds. Virology 202:360, 1994.
16. Appleyard G, Russell SM, Clarke BE, et al: Neutralization epitopes of human rhinovirus type 2. J Gen Virol 71:1275, 1990.

16a. Hewat EA, Blaas D: Structure of a neutralizing antibody bound bivalently to human rhinovirus 2. EMBO 15:1515, 1996.

16b. Smith TJ, Chase ES, Schmidt TJ, et al: Neutralizing antibody to human rhinovirus 14 penetrates the receptor-binding canyon. Nature 383:350, 1996.

17. Tormo J, Blaas D, Parry NR, et al: Crystal structure of a human rhinovirus neutralizing antibody complexed with a peptide derived from viral capsid protein VP2. EMBO J 13:2247, 1994.
18. Speller SA, Sangar DV, Clarke BE, et al: The nature and spatial distribution of amino acid substitutions conferring resistance to neutralizing monoclonal antibodies in human rhinovirus type 2. J Gen Virol 74:193, 1993.

19. Resnick DA, Smith AD, Geisler SC, et al: Chimera from a human rhinovirus 14–human immunodeficiency virus type 1 (HIV-1) V3 loop seroprevalence library induce neutralizing responses against HIV-1. J Virol 69:2406, 1995.
20. Arnold E, Luo M, Vriend G, et al: Implications of the picornavirus capsid structure for polyprotein processing. Proc Natl Acad Sci USA 84:21, 1987.
21. Rueckert RR, Wimmer E: Systematic nomenclature of picornavirus proteins. J Virol 50:957, 1984.
22. Lee WM, Monroe SS, Rueckert RR: Role of maturation cleavage in infectivity of picornaviruses: Activation of an infectosome. J Virol 67:2110, 1993.
23. Ivanoff L, Towatari T, Ray J, et al: Expression and site-specific mutagenesis of the poliovirus 3C protease in *E. coli.* Proc Natl Acad Sci USA 83:5392, 1986.
24. Sommergruber W, Zorn M, Blaas D, et al: Polypeptide 2A of human rhinovirus type 2: Identification as a protease and characterization by mutational analysis. Virology 169:68, 1989.
25. Korant BD, Lonberg-Holm K, LaColla P: Picornaviruses and togaviruses: Targets for design of antivirals. *In* De Clerq E, Walker RT (eds): Targets for the Design of Antiviral Agents. New York, Plenum Publishing, 1984, pp 61–98.
26. Semler BL, Anderson CL, Hanecak R, et al: A membrane-associated precursor to poliovirus VPg identified by immunoprecipitation with antibodies directed against a synthetic heptapeptide. Cell 28:405, 1982.
27. Stanway G, Hughes PJ, Mountford RC, et al: The complete nucleotide sequence of a common cold virus: Human rhinovirus 14. Nucleic Acids Res 12:7859, 1984.
28. Skern T, Sommergruber W, Blaas D, et al: Human rhinovirus 2: Complete nucleotide sequence and proteolytic processing signals in the capsid protein region. Nucleic Acids Res 13:2111, 1985.
29. Duechler M, Skern T, Sommergruber W, et al: Evolutionary relationships within the human rhinovirus genus: Comparison of serotypes 89, 2, and 14. Proc Natl Acad Sci USA 84:2605, 1987.
30. Hughes PJ, North C, Jellis CH, et al: The nucleotide sequence of human rhinovirus 1B: Molecular relationships within the rhinovirus genus. J Gen Virol 69:49, 1988.
31. Krausslich HG, Nicklin MJ, Toyoda H, et al: Poliovirus proteinase 2A induces cleavage of eucaryotic initiation factor 4F polypeptide p220. J Virol 61:2711, 1987.
32. Trono D, Andino R, Baltimore D: An RNA sequence of hundreds of nucleotides at the 5′ end of poliovirus RNA is involved in allowing viral protein synthesis. J Virol 62:2291, 1988.
33. Jackson RJ: RNA translation: Picornaviruses break the rules. Nature 334:292, 1988.
34. Rivera VM, Welsh JD, Maizel JV Jr: Comparative sequence analysis of the 5′ noncoding region of the enteroviruses and rhinoviruses. Virology 165:42, 1988.
35. Pilipenko EV, Blinov VM, Romanova LI, et al: Conserved structural domains in the 5′ untranslated region of picornaviral genomes: An analysis of the segment controlling translation and neurovirulence. Virology 168:201, 1989.
36. Rohll JB, Percy N, Ley R, et al: The 5′-untranslated regions of picornavirus RNAs contain independent functional domains essential for RNA replication and translation. J Virol 68:4384, 1994.
37. Hamparian VV, Ketler A, Hilleman MR: Recovery of new viruses (coryzavirus) from cases of common cold in human adults. Proc Soc Exp Biol Med 108:444, 1961.
38. Korant BD, Lonberg-Holm K, Noble J, et al: Naturally occurring and artificially produced components of three rhinoviruses. Virology 48:71, 1972.
39. Skern T, Torgersen H, Auer H, et al: Human rhinovirus mutants resistant to low pH. Virology 183:757, 1991.
40. Prchla E, Kuechler E, Blaas D, et al: Uncoating of human rhinovirus serotype 2 from late endosomes. J Virol 68:3713, 1994.
41. Tyrrell DAJ, Chanock RM: Rhinoviruses: A description. Science 141:152, 1963.
42. Dimmock NJ, Tyrrell DAJ: Some physicochemical properties of rhinoviruses. Br J Exp Pathol 45:271, 1964.
43. Tomassini JE, Colonno RJ: Isolation of a receptor protein involved in attachment of human rhinoviruses. J Virol 58:290, 1986.
44. Mischak H, Neubauer C, Kuechler E, et al: Characteristics of the minor group receptor of human rhinoviruses. Virology 163:19, 1988.
45. Hofer F, Gruenberger M, Kowalski H, et al: Members of the low density lipoprotein receptor family mediate cell entry of a minor-group common cold virus. Proc Natl Acad Sci USA 91:1839, 1994.
46. Uncapher CR, DeWitt CM, Colonno RJ: The major and minor group receptor families contain all but one human rhinovirus serotype. Virology 180:814, 1991.
47. Crump CE, Arruda E, Hayden FG: In vitro inhibitory activity of soluble ICAM-1 for the numbered serotypes of human rhinovirus. Antiviral Chem Chemother 4:323, 1993.
48. Colonno RJ, Callahan PL, Long WJ: Isolation of a monoclonal antibody that blocks attachment of the major group of human rhinoviruses. J Virol 57:7, 1986.
49. Greve JM, Davis G, Meyer AM, et al: The major human rhinovirus receptor is ICAM-1. Cell 56:839, 1989.
50. Staunton DE, Merluzzi VJ, Rothlein R, et al: A cell adhesion molecule, ICAM-1, is the major surface receptor for rhinoviruses. Cell 56:849, 1989.
51. Lineberger DW, Uncapher CR, Graham DJ, et al: Domains 1 and 2 of ICAM-1 are sufficient to bind human rhinoviruses. Virus Res 24:173, 1992.
52. Yin FH, Lomax NB: Host range mutants of human rhinovirus in which nonstructural proteins are altered. J Virol 48:410, 1983.
53. Neubauer C, Frasel L, Kuechler E, et al: Mechanism of entry of human rhinovirus 2 into HeLa cells. Virology 158:255, 1987.
54. Smith TJ, Kremer MJ, Luo M, et al: The site of attachment in human rhinovirus 14 for antiviral agents that inhibit uncoating. Science 233:1286, 1986.
55. Badger J, Minor I, Kremer MJ, et al: Structural analysis of a series of antiviral agents complexed with human rhinovirus 14. Proc Natl Acad Sci USA 85:3304, 1988.
56. Ismail-Cassim N, Chezzi C, Newman JFE: Inhibition of the uncoating of bovine enterovirus by short chain fatty acids. J Gen Virol 71:2283, 1990.
57. Andries K, Dewindt B, Snoeks J, et al: Two groups of rhinoviruses revealed by a panel of antiviral compounds present sequence divergence and differential pathogenicity. J Virol 64:1117, 1990.
58. Yin FH, Lomax NB: Establishment of a mouse model for human rhinovirus infection. J Gen Virol 67:2335, 1986.
59. Lomax NB, Yin FH: Evidence for the role of the P2 protein of human rhinovirus in its host range change. J Virol 63:2396, 1989.
60. Cooney MK, Hall CE, Fox JP: The Seattle virus watch. III. Evaluation of isolation methods and summary of infections detected by virus isolations. Am J Epidemiol 96:286, 1972.
61. Fox JP, Cooney MK, Hall CE: The Seattle virus watch. V. Epidemiologic observations of rhinovirus infections, 1965–1969, in families with young children. Am J Epidemiol 101:122, 1975.
62. Wulff H, Noble GR, Maynard JE, et al: An outbreak of respiratory infection in children with rhinovirus serotypes 16 and 29. Am J Epidemiol 90:304, 1969.
63. Phillips CA, Melnick JL, Grim CA: Rhinovirus infections in a student population: Isolation of five new serotypes. Am J Epidemiol 87:447, 1968.
64. Hamre D, Connelly AP Jr, Procknow JJ: Virologic studies of acute respiratory disease in young adults. III. Some biologic and serologic characteristics of seventeen rhinovirus serotypes isolated October, 1960 to June, 1961. J Lab Clin Med 64:450, 1964.
65. Warshauer DM, Dick EC, Mandel AD, et al: Rhinovirus infections in an isolated Antarctic station. Transmission of the viruses and susceptibility of the population. Am J Epidemiol 129:319, 1989.
66. Gwaltney JM Jr, Hendley JO, Simon G, et al: Rhinovirus infections in an industrial population. III. Number and prevalence of serotypes. Am J Epidemiol 87:158, 1968.
67. Calhoun AM, Jordan WS Jr, Gwaltney JM Jr: Rhinovirus infections in an industrial population. V. Change in distribution of serotypes. Am J Epidemiol 99:58, 1974.
68. Monto AS, Cavallaro JJ: The Tecumseh study of respiratory illness. IV. Prevalence of rhinovirus serotypes, 1966–1969. Am J Epidemiol 96:352, 1972.
69. Monto AS, Bryan ER, Ohmit S: Rhinovirus infections in Tecumseh, Michigan: Frequency of illness and number of serotypes. J Infect Dis 156:43, 1987.

70. Thwing CJ, Arruda E, Vieira Filho JPB, et al: Rhinovirus antibodies in an isolated Amazon Indian tribe. Am J Trop Med Hyg 48:771, 1993.
71. Hendley JO, Edmondson WP Jr, Gwaltney JM Jr: Relation between naturally acquired immunity and infectivity of two rhinoviruses in volunteers. J Infect Dis 125:243, 1972.
72. Monto AS, Sullivan KM: Acute respiratory illness in the community. Frequency of illness and the agents involved. Epidemiol Infect 110:145, 1993.
73. Aymard M, Chomel JJ, Allard JP, et al: Epidemiology of viral infections and evaluation of the potential benefit of OM-85 BV on the virologic status of children attending day-care centers. Respiration 61(Suppl 1):24, 1994.
74. Holmes MJ, Reed SE, Stott EJ, et al: Studies of experimental rhinovirus type 2 infections in polar isolation and in England. J Hyg (Lond) 76:379, 1976.
75. Reed SE: An investigation of the possible transmission of rhinovirus colds through indirect contact. J Hyg (Lond) 75:249, 1975.
76. Douglas RG Jr, Cate TR, Gerone PJ, et al: Quantitative rhinovirus shedding patterns in volunteers. Am Rev Respir Dis 94:159, 1966.
77. D'Alessio DJ, Peterson JA, Dick CR, et al: Transmission of experimental rhinovirus colds in volunteer married couples. J Infect Dis 233:28, 1976.
78. Hendley JO, Wenzel RP, Gwaltney JM Jr: Transmission of rhinovirus colds by self-inoculation. N Engl J Med 288:1361, 1973.
79. Gwaltney JM Jr, Hendley JO: Rhinovirus transmission: One if by air, and two if by hand. Am J Epidemiol 107:357, 1978.
80. Foy HM, Cooney MK, Hall C, et al: Case-to-case intervals of rhinovirus and influenza virus infections in households. J Infect Dis 157:180, 1988.
81. Dick EC, Jennings LC, Mink KA, et al: Aerosol transmission of rhinovirus colds. J Infect Dis 156:442, 1987.
82. Jennings LC, Dick EC, Mink KA, et al: Near disappearance of rhinovirus along a fomite transmission chain. J Infect Dis 158:888, 1988.
83. Gwaltney JM Jr, Moskalski PB, Hendley JO: Hand-to-hand transmission of rhinovirus colds. Ann Intern Med 88:463, 1978.
84. Levandowski RA, Pachucki CT, Rubenis M: Specific mononuclear cell response to rhinovirus. J Infect Dis 148:1125, 1983.
85. Hastings GZ, Francis MJ, Rowlands DJ, et al: Antigen processing and presentation of human rhinovirus to CD4 T cells is facilitated by binding to cellular receptors for virus. Eur J Immunol 23:1340, 1993.
86. Dowling HF, Jackson GG, Inouye T: Transmission of the experimental common cold in volunteers. II. The effect of certain host factors upon susceptibility. J Lab Clin Med 50:516, 1957.
87. Dowling HF, Jackson GG, Spiesman IG, et al: Transmission of the common cold to volunteers under controlled conditions. III. The effect of chilling of the subjects upon susceptibility. Am J Hyg 68:59, 1958.
88. Douglas RG Jr, Lindgren KM, Couch RB: Exposure to cold environment and rhinovirus common cold. Failure to demonstrate effect. N Engl J Med 279:742, 1968.
89. Fleet WF, Couch RB, Cate TR, et al: Homologous and heterologous resistance to rhinovirus common cold. Am J Epidemiol 82:185, 1965.
90. Cate TR, Rossen RD, Douglas RG Jr, et al: The role of nasal secretion and serum antibody in the rhinovirus common cold. Am J Epidemiol 84:352, 1966.
91. Jackson GG, Dowling HF, Spiesman IG, et al: Transmission of the common cold to volunteers under controlled conditions. I. The common cold as a clinical entity. Arch Intern Med 101:267, 1958.
92. Turner RB, Hendley JO, Gwaltney JM Jr: Shedding of infected ciliated epithelial cells in rhinovirus colds. J Infect Dis 145:849, 1982.
93. Levandowski RA, Weaver CW, Jackson GG: Nasal secretion leukocyte populations determined by flow cytometry during acute rhinovirus infection. J Med Virol 25:423, 1988.
94. Turner BW, Cail WS, Hendley JO, et al: Physiologic abnormalities in the paranasal sinuses during experimental rhinovirus colds. J Allergy Clin Immunol 90:474, 1992.
95. Gwaltney JM Jr, Phillips CD, Miller RD, et al: Computed tomographic study of the common cold. N Engl J Med 330:25, 1994.
96. Minor TE, Dick EC, Baker JW, et al: Rhinovirus and influenza A infections as precipitants of asthma. Am Rev Respir Dis 113:149, 1976.
97. Lemanske RF Jr, Dick EC, Swenson CA, et al: Rhinovirus upper respiratory infection increases airway hyperreactivity and late asthmatic reactions. J Clin Invest 83:1, 1989.
98. Stenhouse AC: Rhinovirus infection in acute exacerbations of chronic bronchitis: A controlled prospective study. Br Med J 3:461, 1967.
99. Calhoun WJ, Dick EC, Schwartz LB, et al: A common cold virus, rhinovirus 16, potentiates airway inflammation after segmental antigen bronchoprovocation in allergic subjects. J Clin Invest 94:2200, 1994.
100. Fridy WW Jr, Ingram RH Jr, Hierholzer JC, et al: Airways function during mild viral respiratory illnesses: The effect of rhinoviruses on cigarette smokers. Ann Intern Med 80:150, 1974.
101. Blair HT, Greenberg SB, Stevens PM, et al: Effects of rhinovirus infection on pulmonary function of healthy human volunteers. Am Rev Respir Dis 114:95, 1976.
102. Lourenço RV, Stanley ED, Gatmaitan B, et al: Abnormal deposition and clearance of inhaled particles during upper respiratory viral infections. J Clin Invest 50:62a, 1971.
103. Garrard CS, Levandowski RA, Gerrity TR, et al: The effects of acute respiratory virus infection upon tracheal mucus transport. Arch Environ Health 40:322, 1985.
104. Wilson R, Alton E, Rutman A, et al: Upper respiratory tract viral infection and mucociliary clearance. Eur J Respir Dis 70:272, 1987.
105. Tyrrell DAJ: Common cold viruses. Int Rev Exp Pathol 1:209, 1962.
106. Hamory BH, Hendley JO, Gwaltney JM Jr: Rhinovirus growth in nasal polyp organ culture. Proc Soc Exp Biol Med 155:577, 1977.
107. Bruce C, Chadwick P, Al-Nakib W: Detection of rhinovirus RNA in nasal epithelial cells by in situ hybridization. J Virol Methods 30:115, 1990.
108. Arruda E, Mifflin TE, Gwaltney JM Jr, et al: Localization of rhinovirus replication in vitro with in situ hybridization. J Med Virol 34:38, 1991.
109. Arola M, Ziegler T, Ruuskanen O, et al: Rhinovirus in acute otitis media. J Pediatr 113:693, 1988.
110. Hamory BH, Sande MA, Sydnor A Jr, et al: Etiology and antimicrobial therapy of acute maxillary sinusitis. J Infect Dis 139:197, 1979.
111. Halperin SA, Eggleston PA, Hendley JO, et al: Pathogenesis of lower respiratory tract symptoms in experimental rhinovirus infection. Am Rev Respir Dis 128:806, 1983.
112. Urquhart GED, Stott EJ: Rhinoviraemia. Br Med J 2:28, 1970.
113. Cate TR, Douglas RG Jr, Johnson KM, et al: Studies on the inability of rhinovirus to survive and replicate in the intestinal tract of volunteers. Proc Soc Exp Biol Med 124:1290, 1967.
114. Borum P, Olsen L, Winther B, et al: Ipratropium nasal spray: A new treatment for rhinorrhea in the common cold. Am Rev Respir Dis 123:418, 1981.
115. Gaffey MJ, Gwaltney JM Jr, Dressler WE, et al: Intranasally administered atropine methonitrate treatment of experimental rhinovirus colds. Am Rev Respir Dis 135:241, 1987.
116. Naclerio RM, Proud D, Lichentenstein LM, et al: Kinins are generated during experimental rhinovirus colds. J Infect Dis 157:133, 1988.
117. Cate TR, Couch RB, Johnson KM: Studies with rhinoviruses in volunteers, production of illness, effect of naturally acquired antibody, and demonstration of a protective effect not associated with serum antibody. J Clin Invest 43:56, 1964.
118. Panusarn C, Stanley ED, Dirda V, et al: Prevention of illness from rhinovirus infection by a topical interferon inducer. N Engl J Med 291:57, 1974.
119. Levandowski RA, Horohov DW: Rhinovirus induces natural killer-like cytotoxic cells and interferon alpha in mononuclear leukocytes. J Med Virol 35:116, 1991.
120. Hayden FG, Winther B, Donowitz GR, et al: Human nasal mucosal responses to topically applied recombinant leukocyte A interferon. J Infect Dis 156:64, 1987.
120a. Proud D, Gwaltney J Jr, Hendley JO, et al: Increased levels of interleukin-1 are detected in nasal secretions of volunteers during experimental rhinovirus colds. J Infect Dis 169:1007, 1994.
120b. Zhu Z, Tang W, Ray A, et al: Rhinovirus stimulation of interleukin-6 in vivo and in vitro: Evidence for nuclear factor

κB–dependent transcriptional activation. J Clin Invest 97:421, 1996.
120c. Gern JE, Dick EC, Lee WM, et al: Rhinovirus enters but does not replicate inside monocytes and airway macrophages. J Immunol 156:621, 1996.
120d. Johnston SL, Papi A, Monick MM, et al: Rhinoviruses induce interleukin-8 mRNA and protein production in human monocytes. J Infect Dis 175:323, 1997.
121. Douglas RG Jr, Alford RH, Cate TR, et al: The leukocyte response during viral respiratory illness in man. Ann Intern Med 64:521, 1966.
122. Levandowski RA, Ou DW, Jackson GG: Acute-phase decrease of T-lymphocyte subsets in rhinovirus infection. J Infect Dis 153:743, 1986.
123. Thomas LH, Fraenkel DJ, Bardin PG, et al: Leukocyte responses to experimental infection with human rhinovirus. J Allergy Clin Immunol 94:1255, 1994.
124. Turner RB: Rhinovirus infection of human embryonic lung fibroblasts induces the production of a chemoattractant for polymorphonuclear leukocytes. J Infect Dis 157:346, 1988.
125. Turner RB: The role of neutrophils in the pathogenesis of rhinovirus infections. Pediatr Infect Dis J 9:832, 1990.
125a. Gern JE, Vrtis R, Kelly EAB, et al: Rhinovirus produces nonspecific activation of lymphocytes through a monocyte-dependent mechanism. J Immunol 157:1605, 1996.
126. Gauntt CJ, Arizpe HM, Kung JT, et al: Antimyocarditic activity of the guanine derivative BIOLF-70 in a coxsackievirus B3 murine model. Antimicrob Agents Chemother 27:184, 1985.
127. Godeny EK, Gauntt CJ: Involvement of natural killer cells in coxsackievirus B3–induced murine myocarditis. J Immunol 137:1695, 1986.
128. Price WH: The isolation of a new virus associated with respiratory clinical disease in humans. Proc Natl Acad Sci USA 42:546, 1956.
129. Pelon W, Mogabgab WJ, Phillips IA, et al: A cytopathogenic agent isolated from naval recruits with mild respiratory illness. Proc Soc Exp Biol Med 94:262, 1957.
130. Mogabgab WJ, Pelon W: Problems in characterizing and identifying an apparently new virus found in association with mild respiratory disease in recruits. Ann N Y Acad Sci 67:403, 1957.
131. Haff RF, Wohlsen B, Force EE, et al: Growth characteristics of two rhinovirus strains in WI-26 and monkey kidney cells. J Bacteriol 91:2339, 1966.
132. Stott EJ, Tyrrell DAJ: Some improved techniques for the study of rhinoviruses using HeLa cells. Arch Gesamte Virusforsch 23:236, 1968.
133. Lewis FA, Kennet ML: Comparison of rhinovirus-sensitive HeLa cells and human embryo fibroblasts for isolation of rhinoviruses from patients with respiratory disease. J Clin Microbiol 3:528, 1976.
134. Hamory BH, Hendley JO, Gwaltney JM Jr: Rhinovirus growth in nasal polyp organ culture. Proc Soc Exp Biol Med 155:577, 1977.
135. Kenney GE, Cooney MK, Thompson DJ: Analysis of serum pooling schemes for identification of large numbers of viruses. Am J Epidemiol 91:439, 1970.
136. Cooney MK, Wise JA, Kenney GE, et al: Broad antigenic relationships among rhinovirus serotypes revealed by cross-immunization of rabbits with different serotypes. J Immunol 114:635, 1975.
137. Douglas RG Jr, Fleet WF, Cater TR, et al: Antibody to rhinovirus in human sera. I. Standardization of a neutralization test. Proc Soc Exp Biol Med 127:497, 1968.
138. Dearden CJ, Al-Nakib W: Direct detection of rhinoviruses by an enzyme-linked immunosorbent assay. J Med Virol 23:179, 1987.
139. Bruce CB, Al-Nakib W, Tyrrell DAJ, et al: Synthetic oligonucleotides as diagnostic probes for rhinoviruses. Lancet 2:53, 1988.
140. Gama RE, Hughes PJ, Bruce CB, et al: Polymerase chain reaction amplification of rhinovirus nucleic acids from clinical material. Nucleic Acids Res 16:9346, 1988.
141. Mori J, Clewley JP: Polymerase chain reaction and sequencing for typing rhinovirus RNA. J Med Virol 44:323, 1994.
142. Korant BD: Viral proteases—An emerging therapeutic target. Crit Rev Biotechnol 8:149, 1988.
143. Price WH: Vaccine for the prevention in humans of coldlike symptoms associated with the JH virus. Proc Natl Acad Sci USA 43:790, 1957.
144. Andrewes CH, Tyrrell DAJ, Stones PB, et al: Prevention of colds by vaccination against a rhinovirus. Br Med J 1:1344, 1965.
145. Perkins JC, Tucker DN, Knopf HLS, et al: Evidence of protective effect of an inactivated rhinovirus vaccine administered by the nasal route. Am J Epidemiol 90:319, 1969.
146. McCray J, Werner G: Different rhinovirus serotypes neutralized by antipeptide antibodies. Nature 329:736, 1987.
147. Francis MJ, Hastings GZ, Sangar DV, et al: A synthetic peptide which elicits neutralizing antibody against rhinovirus type 2. J Gen Virol 68:2687, 1987.
148. Hamory BH, Hamparian VV, Conant RM, et al: Human responses to two decavalent rhinovirus vaccines. J Infect Dis 132:623, 1975.
149. Gwaltney JM Jr, Moskalski PB, Hendley JO: Interruption of experimental rhinovirus transmission. J Infect Dis 142:811, 1980.
150. Dick EC, Hossain SU, Mink KA, et al: Interruption of transmission of rhinovirus colds among human volunteers using virucidal paper handkerchiefs. J Infect Dis 153:352, 1986.
151. Longhini IM Jr, Monto AS: Efficacy of virucidal nasal tissues in interrupting familial transmission of respiratory agents. A field trial in Tecumseh, Michigan. Am J Epidemiol 128:639, 1988.
152. Hayden FG, Gwaltney JM Jr, Colonno RJ: Modification of experimental rhinovirus colds by receptor blockade. Antiviral Res 9:233, 1988.
153. Ohlin A, Hoover-Litty H, Sanderson G, et al: Spectrum of activity of soluble intercellular adhesion molecule-1 against rhinovirus reference strains and field isolates. Antimicrob Agents Chemother 38:1413, 1994.
154. Crump CE, Arruda E, Hayden FG: Comparative antirhinoviral activities of soluble intercellular adhesion molecule-1 (sICAM-1) and chimeric ICAM-1/immunoglobulin A molecule. Antimicrob Agents Chemother 38:1425, 1994.
155. DeLong DC, Reed SE: Inhibition of rhinovirus replication in organ cultures by a potential antiviral drug. J Infect Dis 141:87, 1980.
156. Zerial A, Werner GH, Phillpotts RJ, et al: Studies on 44 081 R.P., a new antirhinovirus compound, in cell cultures and in volunteers. Antimicrob Agents Chemother 27:846, 1985.
157. Diana GD, Oglesby RC, Akullian V, et al: Structure-activity studies of 5-[[4-(4,5-dihydro-2-oxazolyl)phenoxy]alkyl]-3-methylisoxazoles: Inhibitors of picornavirus uncoating. J Med Chem 30:383, 1987.
158. Al-Nakib W, Willman J, Higgins PG, et al: Failure of intranasally administered 4′,6-dichloroflavan to protect against rhinovirus infection in man. Arch Virol 92:255, 1987.
159. Kenny MT, Torney HL, Dulworth JK: Mechanism of action of the antiviral compound MDL 20,610. Antiviral Res 9:249, 1988.
160. Al-Nakib W, Higgins PG, Barrow I, et al: Intranasal chalcone, Ro 09-0410, as prophylaxis against rhinovirus infection in human volunteers. J Antimicrob Chemother 20:887, 1987.
161. Fox MP, Otto MJ, McKinlay MA: The prevention of rhinovirus and poliovirus uncoating by WIN 51711: A new antiviral drug. Antimicrob Agents Chemother 30:110, 1986.
162. Al-Nakib W, Higgins PG, Barrow GI, et al: Suppression of colds in human volunteers challenged with rhinovirus by a new synthetic drug (R61837). Antimicrob Agents Chemother 33:522, 1989.
163. Hayden FG, Andries K, Janssen PAJ: Safety and efficacy of intranasal pirodavir (R77975) in experimental rhinovirus infection. Antimicrob Agents Chemother 36:727, 1992.
164. Denyer C, Jackson P, Loakes DM, et al: Isolation of antirhinoviral sesquiterpenes from ginger *(Zingiber officinale).* J Nat Prod 57:658, 1994.
165. Phillpotts RJ, DeLong DC, Wallace J, et al: The activity of enviroxime against rhinovirus infection in man. Lancet 1:1342, 1981.
166. Hayden FG, Gwaltney JM Jr: Prophylactic activity of intranasal enviroxime against experimentally induced rhinovirus type 39 infection. Antimicrob Agents Chemother 21:892, 1982.
167. Levandowski RA, Pachucki CT, Rubenis M, et al: Topical enviroxime against rhinovirus infection. Antimicrob Agents Chemother 22:1004, 1982.
168. Wyde PR, Six HR, Wilson SZ, et al: Activity against rhinoviruses, toxicity, and delivery in aerosol of enviroxime in liposomes. Antimicrob Agents Chemother 32:890, 1988.
169. Stanley ED, Jackson GG, Dirda V, et al: Effect of a topical

interferon inducer on rhinovirus infections in volunteers. J Infect Dis 133(Suppl): A121, 1976.
170. Scott GM, Wallace J, Greiner J, et al: Prevention of rhinovirus colds by human interferon-α_2 from *Escherichia coli.* Lancet 2:186, 1982.
171. Monto AS, Shope TC, Schwartz SA, et al: Intranasal interferon-α_{2b} for seasonal prophylaxis of respiratory infection. J Infect Dis 154:128, 1986.
172. Douglas RM, Moore BW, Miles HB, et al: Prophylactic efficacy of intranasal α_2-interferon against rhinovirus infections in the family setting. N Engl J Med 314:65, 1986.
173. Hayden FG, Albrecht JK, Kaiser DL, et al: Prevention of natural colds by contact prophylaxis with intranasal α_2-interferon. N Engl J Med 314:71, 1986.
174. Foy HM, Fox JP, Cooney MK: Efficacy of α_2-interferon against the common cold. N Engl J Med 315:513, 1986.
175. Douglas RM, Albrecht JK, Miles HB, et al: Intranasal interferon-α_2 prophylaxis of natural respiratory virus infection. J Infect Dis 151:731, 1985.
176. Hayden FG, Mills SE, Johns ME: Human tolerance and histopathologic effects of long-term administration of intranasal interferon-α_2. J Infect Dis 148:914, 1983.
177. Sperber SJ, Levine PA, Innes DJ, et al: Tolerance and efficacy of intranasal administration of recombinant β-serine interferon in healthy adults. J Infect Dis 158:166, 1988.
178. Sperber SJ, Levine PA, Sorrentino JV, et al: Ineffectiveness of recombinant interferon-beta serine nasal drops for prophylaxis of natural colds. J Infect Dis 160:700, 1989.
179. Higgins PG, Al-Nakib W, Barrow GI, et al: Recombinant human interferon-γ as prophylaxis against rhinovirus colds in volunteers. J Interferon Res 8:591, 1988.
180. Schwartz AR, Togo Y, Hornick RB, et al: Evaluation of the efficacy of ascorbic acid in prophylaxis of induced rhinovirus 44 infection in man. J Infect Dis 128:500, 1973.
181. Coulehan JL: Ascorbic acid and the common cold: Reviewing the evidence. Postgrad Med 66:153, 1979.
182. Eby GA, Davis DR, Halcomb WW: Reduction in duration of common colds by zinc gluconate lozenges in a double-blind study. Antimicrob Agents Chemother 25:20, 1984.
183. Douglas RM, Miles HB, Moore BW, et al: Failure of effervescent zinc acetate lozenges to alter the course of upper respiratory tract infections in Australian adults. Antimicrob Agents Chemother 31:1263, 1987.
184. Al-Nakib W, Higgins PG, Barrow I, et al: Prophylaxis and treatment of rhinovirus colds with zinc gluconate lozenges. J Antimicrob Chemother 20:893, 1987.
185. Farr BM, Conner EM, Betts RF, et al: Two randomized controlled trials of zinc gluconate lozenge therapy of experimentally induced rhinovirus colds. Antimicrob Agents Chemother 31:1183, 1987.
186. Mink KA, Dick EC, Jennings LC, et al: Amelioration of rhinovirus colds by vitamin C (ascorbic acid) supplementation. Med Virol 7:356, 1988.
187. Hemilä H: Does vitamin C alleviate the symptoms of the common cold?—A review of current evidence. Scand J Infect Dis 26:1, 1994.
188. Stanley ED, Jackson GG, Panusarn C, et al: Increased virus shedding with aspirin treatment of rhinovirus infection. JAMA 231:1248, 1975.
189. Fulginiti VA, Committee on Infectious Diseases: Special report: Aspirin and Reye's syndrome. Pediatrics 69:810, 1982.
190. Gaffey MJ, Gwaltney JM Jr, Sastre A, et al: Intranasally and orally administered antihistamine treatment of experimental rhinovirus colds. Am Rev Respir Dis 136:556, 1987.
191. Sperber SJ, Gwaltney JM Jr, Sorrentino JV, et al: Pseudoephedrine alone or combined with ibuprofen as treatment for experimental rhinovirus colds. *In* Program and Abstracts of the 27th Interscience Conference on Antimicrobial Agents and Chemotherapy. Washington, DC, American Society for Microbiology, 1987, p 184.
192. Gwaltney JM Jr: Combined antiviral and antimediator treatment of rhinovirus colds. J Infect Dis 166:776, 1992.

260

Hepatitis A Virus

Stanley M. Lemon

History

Although records dating as far back as Hippocrates describe epidemic jaundice, it was not until the early 20th century that "catarrhal jaundice" was suggested by Cockayne[1] to result from an infection of the liver. He proposed the term infective hepatitis for what we now know as type A viral hepatitis. The infectious, nonbacterial nature of the responsible agent was firmly established by the transmission of disease to human volunteers during World War II.[2] At that time, two forms of viral hepatitis, designated infectious hepatitis and homologous serum hepatitis, were differentiated on the basis of their epidemiology, incubation periods, and lack of protection in cross-challenge studies. The terms hepatitis A and hepatitis B were proposed shortly thereafter and are still used today. The virus itself was identified in 1973 by Feinstone and colleagues,[3] who applied immunoelectron microscopy to the examination of fecal suspensions collected from human volunteers (Fig. 260–1). Definitive propagation of hepatitis A virus (HAV) in cell culture followed about 6 years later.[4] In the interim, however, much had been learned about the biology of this virus and the pathogenesis of type A hepatitis by experimental inoculation of chimpanzees and several other species of higher primates.[5–8] These animals remain the only available animal models for the disease.

Characteristics of the Pathogen

The HAV virion is a small, nonenveloped, icosahedral particle approximately 27 nm in diameter that contains a single-

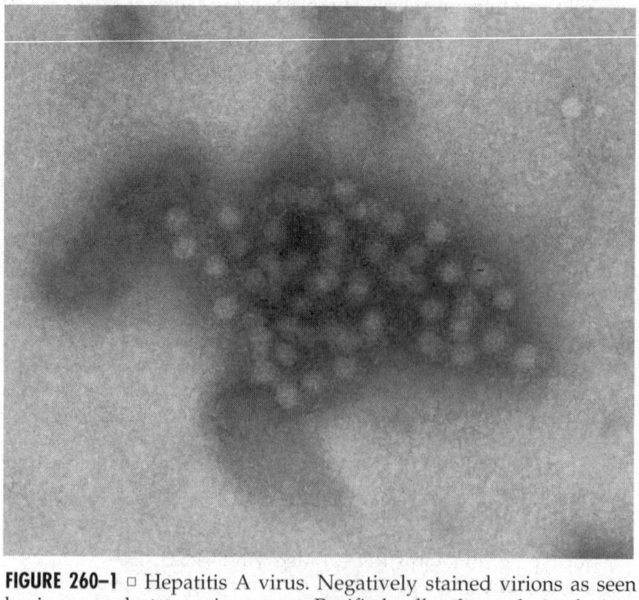

FIGURE 260–1 □ Hepatitis A virus. Negatively stained virions as seen by immunoelectron microscopy. Purified cell culture–derived virus has been aggregated by specific antibody. (× 100,000.) (Courtesy of Dr. S. M. Feinstone, Center for Biologics Evaluation and Research, Bethesda, MD.)

stranded RNA genome that is 7.5 kb in length. The general structure and genomic organization of the virus are similar in many respects to those of other mammalian picornaviruses. However, as detailed in the following, HAV has several unique features. Although the virus was formally classified as enterovirus type 72, these distinctive features of HAV, coupled with the fact that HAV shares little nucleotide sequence homology with other enteroviruses,[9] have led to its reclassification within a unique genus, *Hepatovirus*, of the Picornaviridae.[10] Several detailed reviews of the biology of HAV have been published.[11–14]

Physical Characteristics

The majority of infectious HAV particles sediment at 156S and band at a density of 1.325 g/cm^3 in cesium chloride.[15] However, infectious dense particles banding at 1.40 to 1.44 g/cm^3 in cesium constitute a small percentage of all virions and presumably represent virions with capsids that are permeable to cesium cations. Virus particles that band at much lower densities and are resistant to antibody-mediated neutralization probably represent virions that are complexed with lipid-containing cellular materials.[16, 17]

Like the enteroviruses, HAV is stable at low pH (less than pH 3.0).[18] However, the thermal stability of HAV is considerably greater than that of other picornaviruses, placing the virus among the most stable of all human viral pathogens.[19–21] Incubation of the virus for 4 weeks at room temperature results in only a 100-fold decrease in infectivity (thus, an inoculum of 10^8 infectious particles may be reduced to 10^6). When the virus is held at high temperatures for short periods (10 minutes), significant loss of infectivity does not occur until 60°C.[20] The virus capsid is significantly stabilized in the presence of 1 M Mg^{2+}, resulting in only a 100-fold decrease in infectivity on heating to 80°C for 10 minutes.[19] However, infectivity is destroyed almost instantaneously by heating above 90°C. HAV is highly resistant to drying, and infectious virus has been recovered from acetone-fixed cell sheets. It is also highly resistant to detergents, surviving a 1% concentration of sodium dodecyl sulfate. Significantly, the infectivity of HAV is not reduced by solvent-detergent inactivation procedures applied to blood products, explaining in part the occurrence of HAV transmission after administration of HAV-contaminated clotting factor concentrates in Europe.[22]

Capsid Composition

The highly stable capsid of HAV is composed of 60 copies each of three major structural proteins, VP1, VP2, and VP3, that are 300, 222, and 246 amino acids in length, respectively.[9] A fourth structural protein, VP4, with a predicted length of 23 amino acids is suggested by the genomic RNA sequence (see later) but has not been demonstrated in polyacrylamide gels.[13] The presence of a consensus myristylation signal within the putative VP4 coding region suggests that this protein may be only 17 amino acids in length, but data suggest that this site is not utilized.[23, 24] In this respect, HAV differs significantly from other picornaviruses, which have considerably larger and universally myristylated VP4 structural proteins.[25]

There is only one serotype of HAV. The virus is antigenically distinct from all other picornaviruses.[26, 27] The amino acid sequences of the HAV capsid proteins have been deduced from nucleotide sequences of several cloned human HAV strains.[9, 28, 29] These protein sequences demonstrate little relatedness to the capsid protein sequences of poliovirus or other human picornaviruses. However, among different strains of HAV recovered from humans there is approximately 97% amino acid conservation in the sequences of VP1, VP2, and VP3. Few strains of HAV have been well studied for antigenic variation. Classic polyclonal antibody cross-neutralization studies of human HAV (HM175 strain) and an owl monkey–derived (PA21) viral isolate have suggested no significant differences in the neutralization antigen(s) of these two disparate strains.[26] Although human strains of the virus may be distinguished antigenically from several strains that have been isolated from naturally infected nonhuman primates (cynomolgus and African green monkeys),[30, 31] all simian and human strains of HAV demonstrate significant antigenic cross-reactivity and probably stimulate cross-protective antibodies. Thus, there is good evidence for high-level antigenic conservation among HAV strains.

The analysis of mutant HAVs, selected in cell culture for resistance to neutralization by murine monoclonal antibodies to the virus, suggests that there is an array of closely spaced epitopes constituting an immunodominant neutralization site on the capsid surface.[32, 33] Several pieces of evidence indicate that these epitopes are assembled (that is, conformationally derived) rather than sequential (defined by linear amino acid sequence) structures. First, neutralizing murine monoclonal antibodies do not recognize denatured capsid proteins separated by sodium dodecyl sulfate–polyacrylamide gel electrophoresis. Second, antibody elicited to purified HAV capsid polypeptides only weakly recognizes native capsids and has limited neutralization activity.[34] Third, HAV proteins expressed from recombinant DNA as fusion proteins in *Escherichia coli* are capable of eliciting antibodies reactive with denatured capsid polypeptides, but these antibodies do not react with or neutralize native virus. These facts have made difficult the development of a vaccine based on recombinant DNA technology, which is unfortunate because growth of HAV in cell culture is relatively inefficient and not conducive to economical vaccine production (see later).

Virion RNA

The HAV genome is a single-stranded 35S RNA of positive polarity, 7478 bases in length and containing a 3′ terminal poly(A) tract[9, 13] (Fig. 260–2). As with other positive-strand viruses, isolated viral RNA is itself infectious and regenerates virus after transfection of permissive cells.[35] As with other picornaviruses, a small peptide, VPg, is covalently linked to the 5′ end of virion RNA.[36] Complementary DNA from several strains of virus has been molecularly cloned and the complete nucleotide sequences of these different HAVs are known.[9, 28, 35] The genome is organized in a fashion similar to that of poliovirus: it contains a long 5′-nontranslated region (5′ NTR) 734 bases in length and a shorter 3′ NTR. Both NTRs have substantial secondary RNA structure.[37] The 5′ NTR contains a 0.6-kb RNA segment termed an internal ribosomal entry site (IRES), which directs the binding of 40S ribosomal subunits to the viral RNA, thereby initiating viral translation in a 5′ cap-independent fashion.[38] The IRES of HAV is many times less active than the IRESs of other picornaviruses, resulting in inefficient translation of the viral message and contributing to the slow growth of the virus. IRES-directed translation utilizes one or more cell-specific translation initiation factors, and the affinity of the 5′ NTR for these factors probably plays a role in defining cellular tropisms of the virus.[39]

The noncoding regions flank a single large open reading frame that encodes a polyprotein that is processed into both structural (P1 region) and nonstructural (P2 and P3 genomic regions) viral proteins (see Fig. 260–2). Significantly, HAV differs from poliovirus and many other human picornaviruses in that the 2A protein lacks protease activity and remains attached to some fully formed virions.[12, 40, 41] In poliovirus-infected cells, this protein plays an important role in the

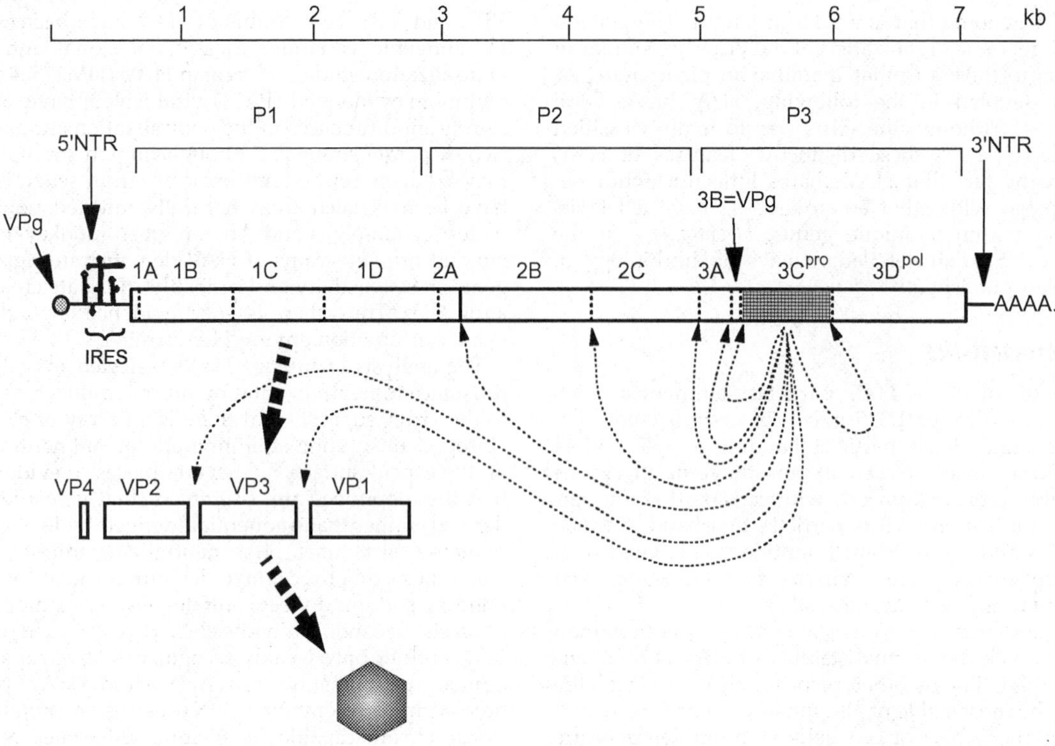

FIGURE 260–2 □ Organization of the HAV genome. The virion RNA is 7.5 kb in length, positive in sense, and thus able to function directly as messenger. It contains three major regions: the 5′- and 3′-nontranslated regions (5′NTR and 3′NTR) and a single large open reading frame encoding the viral polyprotein (shown as the large rectangular box). The 5′ terminal nucleotide of the 5′NTR is covalently attached to a small viral protein (3B, otherwise known as VPg). The 3′NTR has a 3′ terminal poly(A) tract. The 5′NTR contains substantial RNA secondary structure that forms the viral internal ribosomal entry site (IRES) that directs the cap-independent translation of the viral polyprotein. This polyprotein can be divided into three domains (P1, P2, and P3); each of these domains is proteolytically processed to yield smaller viral proteins (e.g., 1A, 1B, 1C). The capsid proteins, VP1 (1D), VP2 (1B), VP3 (1C) (and possibly VP4, 1A), are encoded by the P1 region, and nonstructural proteins involved in replication are encoded by the P2 and P3 regions. These include a nucleoside triphosphatase (2C) with possible helicase activity; VPg (3A), which may play a role in priming for new RNA synthesis; a virus-specific protease ($3C^{pro}$, shaded region); and an RNA-dependent RNA polymerase ($3D^{pol}$). Proteolytic processing of the polyprotein is directed entirely by $3C^{pro}$. Dotted lines indicate the cleavage activities of this protease, which also has RNA-binding activity and plays a role in RNA replication. Primary cleavage occurs between the 1D (VP1) and 2A proteins. Replication of viral RNA proceeds asymmetrically, as with poliovirus, resulting in production of a large excess of positive-sense over negative-sense RNAs. Only positive-sense RNA molecules are packaged in progeny virions.

shutdown of host cell macromolecular synthesis, a phenomenon not seen with HAV. Other proteins encoded by the P2 region (2B, 2C) are believed to have a role in RNA replication and probably contribute to host range specificity.[42, 43] The P3 nonstructural proteins include an RNA-dependent RNA polymerase ($3D^{pol}$) and a protease ($3C^{pro}$) that appears to be solely responsible for posttranslational processing of the viral polyprotein[44] (see Fig. 260–2).

Extensive analysis of partial genomic nucleotide sequences from a large number of human HAV strains has shown that circulating human strains of HAV are relatively closely related genetically, especially when compared with the genetic diversity evident among other picornaviruses such as poliovirus.[45, 46] These studies have documented the existence of two major human HAV genotypes (genotypes I and III), the sequences of which differ from each other at more than 15% of the bases studied (Fig. 260–3). At least two other human HAV isolates belong to other, much less common genotypes (II and VII). This genetic classification is of epidemiologic and evolutionary interest but is not of clinical significance with respect to severity of symptoms or other manifestations of hepatitis A. Strains of virus recovered from naturally infected nonhuman primates represent three additional genotypes (IV, V, VI) and, unlike the human genotypes, demonstrate subtle antigenic differences as described earlier.

The simian viruses are considered to have low pathogenicity for humans.[30, 31] Evidence suggests that they constititute a biologically distinct group of viruses that are capable of causing liver disease in infected cynomolgus and African green monkeys but not chimpanzees, which (like New World owl monkeys and certain tamarin species) develop acute hepatitis after challenge with human strains of HAV.[47] In contrast, human strains of HAV generally do not cause disease in the former primate species. These differences in virus host range may be due, at least in part, to differences in the cellular receptors utilized by these viruses.[27, 48] Strain-specific differences in virulence have not been described among human HAV strains.

Propagation in Cultured Cells

Investigators have known since the 1940s that both serum and fecal specimens could transmit HAV to humans, but attempts to grow the virus in a variety of primary cell cultures and continuous cell lines were unsuccessful for many years. These efforts probably failed because the virus grows slowly in cultured cells and usually does not induce a cytopathic effect. With the advent of serologic tests for viral antigen (see later) and the availability of specific antibodies, it became possible to monitor the replication of virus in cell cultures. HAV was first isolated in marmoset liver explant cultures and was subsequently propagated in continuous

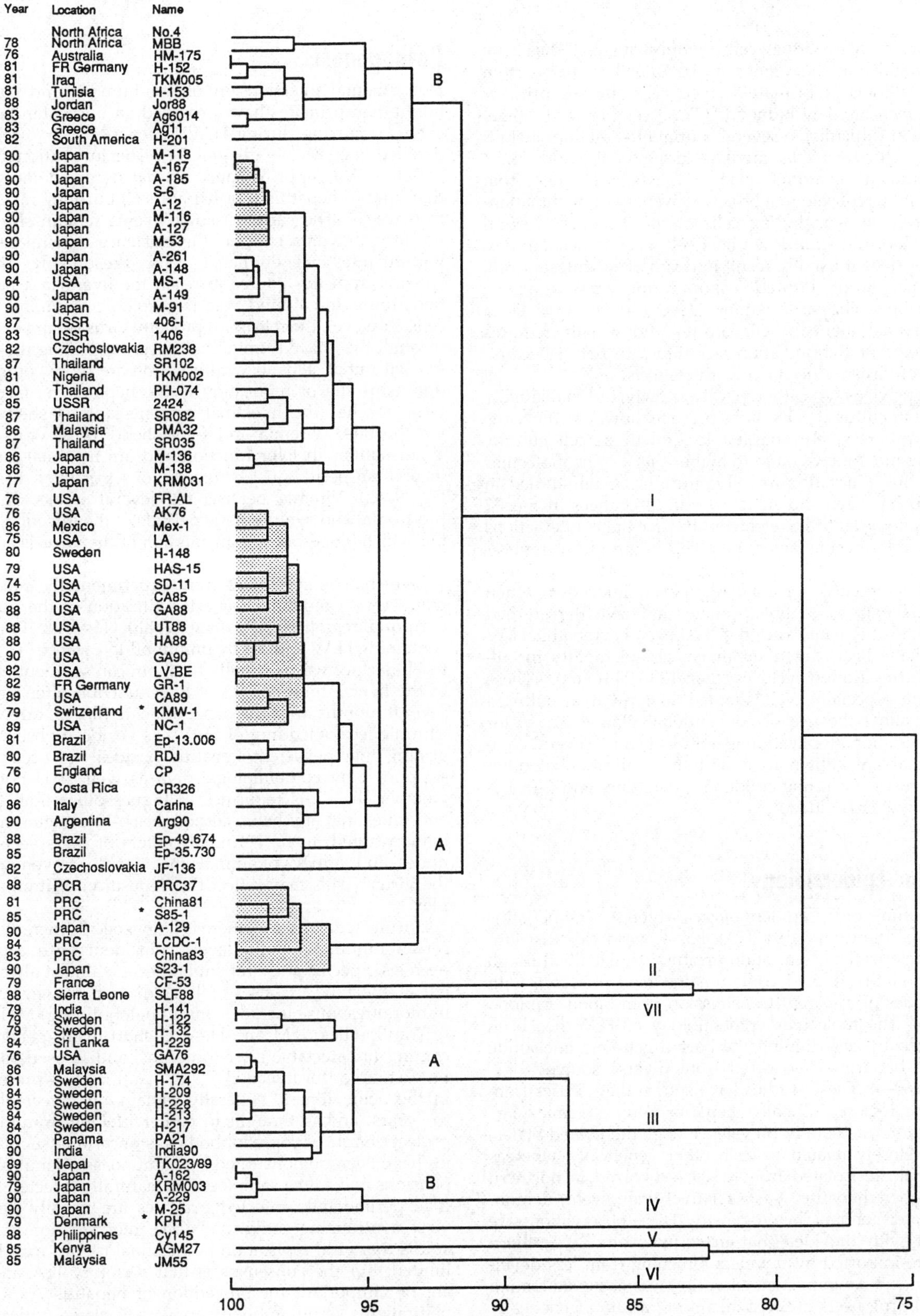

FIGURE 260–3 □ Genetic relatedness in 93 individual strains of HAV determined by a pairwise comparison of genomic RNA sequences within a 168-nucleotide segment of the polyprotein coding region corresponding to the 1D-2A junction. The year and geographic origin of each virus are indicated in the left-hand columns; the location of the most rightward node connecting any two viruses, on the scale at the bottom, indicates the approximate percentage nucleotide identity between those two viruses. Major genotypes (85% sequence identity) are designated by Roman numerals I through VII; subgenotypes (92.5% identity) are indicated by letters (e.g., IA and IB). Viruses that are the sole members of genotypes IV, V, and VI were each recovered from infected Old World monkeys. (From Robertson BH, Jansen RW, Khanna B, et al: Genetic relatedness of hepatitis A virus strains recovered from different geographic regions. J Gen Virol 73:1365–1377, 1992.)

fetal rhesus monkey kidney cells.[4, 49] Subsequent studies have demonstrated that the virus may be directly isolated from clinical materials in primate-derived cells such as primary African green monkey kidney (AGMK) cells or, with somewhat greater difficulty, in several continuous cell lines including BS-C-1 (*Cercopithecus* monkey kidney cells) and PLC/PRF/5 (human hepatoma cells).[50–52] There is evidence that the virus may replicate in a broader diversity of mammalian-derived cell types including cells of murine origin.[53] Viral infection does not shut down host cell macromolecular synthesis, nor does it usually result in death of the infected cell. Rather, infection of cultured cells uniformly leads to persistent infections. The virus requires several days to weeks to reach maximal titers in cell cultures and usually requires immunologic or hybridization techniques to detect because of a lack of virus-induced cytopathic effects.

Wild-type virus typically replicates slowly and to relatively low titers in cultured cells. With passage, however, the virus becomes progressively adapted to growth in cell culture, replicating more rapidly and to higher titers.[54] The molecular basis for this adaptation to cell culture has been studied in detail and has been shown to be due to changes in the P2 proteins and viral IRES element that facilitate interactions with host cell–specific factors involved in viral RNA replication and translation.[39, 42, 43] Highly cell culture adapted viruses are often attenuated (or no longer even infectious) when used to challenge susceptible primates and have been studied as candidate attenuated vaccines.[55, 56] Several cytopathic HAV variants have been described that replicate rapidly in cultured cells (replication cycle less than 18 to 24 hours).[20] These viruses are especially well adapted to growth in cultured cells and allow the use of conventional plaque assays for viral quantitation. Replication is not blocked by several compounds that are known to inhibit the replication of other picornaviruses, including arildone, guanidine, and 2-(α-hydroxybenzyl)benzimidazole.

Molecular Epidemiology

Classic features of the epidemiology of type A viral hepatitis are described in Chapter 91. HAV has a worldwide distribution characterized by fecal-oral transmission, usually through close personal contact or contaminated food or water, with rare episodes of apparent transmission from blood or blood products.[11] The molecular epidemiology of HAV has been investigated by determining the partial genomic nucleotide sequences of viruses recovered from diverse sources[45, 46, 57] (see Fig. 260–3). These studies have shown that viruses from geographic regions in which hepatitis A is endemic (e.g., China) or intermediate in prevalence (e.g., the United States) are often closely related to each other genetically, whereas viruses that are isolated from cases recognized in northern Europe (where hepatitis A is a relatively rare event) demonstrate greater genomic heterogeneity. These observations are consistent with the idea that most infections in northern Europe are imported by travelers returning from less developed regions.[45] An important exception was observed among parenteral drug users in Sweden, among whom a genetically distinct virus strain was observed to circulate during a number of years. This suggests that there may be small "pockets" of virus circulation among certain high-risk groups. In these Swedish individuals, it is likely that virus was transmitted by contaminated needles as with other agents of viral hepatitis. Partial genomic sequencing of virus strains has also been useful in identifying the source of virus in other epidemiologic studies, including one that demonstrated the transmission of HAV to hemophilic patients via high-purity, solvent-detergent–inactivated factor VIII preparations.[58]

Pathogenesis

Experimental infections involving humans and susceptible nonhuman primates have provided an understanding of the events occurring during HAV infection[5–8, 48, 59, 60] (for a more detailed review, see Chapter 91). The incubation period of hepatitis A is approximately 28 days (considerably shorter than that of hepatitis B or hepatitis C) but may range from 2 to 6 weeks. The early virologic events remain shrouded in mystery, but data support the existence of viral replication within intestinal epithelial cells. Presumably, the virus spreads from this source to reach the liver via a hematogenous route. In cultured polarized colonic carcinoma (Caco-2) cells, however, the release of progeny virus occurs exclusively through the apical (luminal) surface, suggesting the possibility that initial steps in viral invasion are more complex. The dominant site of replication is the hepatocyte, from which virus reaches the intestinal contents and is shed in feces via the bile.[5] Viremia and fecal shedding of virus precede abnormalities in liver function and are maximal late in the incubation period, just before the onset of liver disease (see Fig. 91–2). Viremia persists for several weeks during the prodromal and symptomatic periods of the infection,[48, 60] during which blood-borne transmission of the virus is a possibility.

Liver biopsy specimens from experimentally infected primates reveal mononuclear cell infiltration of the portal and periportal regions and swollen hepatocytes with 10% or more containing HAV antigen by immunofluorescence.[59, 61–65] Hepatocellular necrosis is usually focal but can span entire lobules of the liver. Abnormalities of liver function often persist for several months after the onset of acute illness, rarely longer. Chronic fecal shedding of HAV has not been observed, suggesting that persistent hepatitis A does not occur. This is supported by epidemiologic data as well. It is not known whether the virus replicates in tissues other than the liver and intestinal epithelia, although HAV antigen has been demonstrated in the germinal centers of the spleen, lymph nodes, and kidneys of animals inoculated intravenously with the virus.[59] This may reflect the deposition of immune complexes.

During acute disease, there is a nonspecific increase in total serum immunoglobulin levels coincident with acute liver necrosis. Specific antiviral antibodies are almost always present at the time of onset of liver disease, however.[66–68] The humoral response includes immunoglobulin (Ig) M, IgG, and IgA antibodies. IgM anti-HAV is short-lived, generally becoming undetectable after 6 months, and is used as a diagnostic marker for infection.[67, 69] IgG anti-HAV is present early in the acute illness, generally remains at detectable levels for years, and is thought to confer lifelong immunity. The protective role of coproantibodies is uncertain: such antibodies have been demonstrated by immunoassays, but fecal suspensions and saliva samples from naturally infected humans or experimentally infected primates are usually devoid of virus-neutralizing activity.[70, 71] One interpretation of this result is that viral replication in intestinal tissues may be quite limited, but the consensus is that secretory IgA antibodies are not important for prevention of hepatitis A. Although neutralizing serum antibody appears to play a critical role in protection against reinfection,[68, 72] other immune mechanisms such as natural killer cells, human leukocyte antigen–restricted T-cell–mediated cytotoxicity, and induction of interferons are likely to be important in clearing acute HAV infection.[73–75]

Clinical Manifestations

The clinical manifestations of HAV infection are reviewed in detail in Chapter 91. In the individual patient, clinical features of hepatitis A are indistinguishable from those of other types of viral hepatitis. In young children (younger than 2 years) most infections are anicteric and not recognized as caused by a hepatitis virus; in contrast, the majority of infected adults develop overt hepatitis.[11, 76] The severity of disease increases with age, but overall mortality is quite low.[77–79] HAV does not cause chronic viral hepatitis.

Diagnosis

Marked elevations of serum aspartate aminotransferase and alanine aminotransferase activities in the presence of a typical clinical illness should suggest the possibility of viral hepatitis caused by any of the classic hepatitis viruses (A, B, C, D, or E). The diagnosis of hepatitis A rests on the specific demonstration of serum IgM anti-HAV.[67, 69] The method of choice for detection of this antibody is a solid-phase IgM capture immunoassay (Fig. 260–4*C*). This method is quite sensitive, often detecting IgM anti-HAV at serum dilutions exceeding 1:10^6. Serum is thus diluted extensively before testing to improve the specificity of the procedure for recent infection. Under such conditions, IgM is usually no longer detectable after 6 months, although in occasional cases it may persist for up to a year. Rheumatoid factor (IgM anti-IgG) may interfere with such assays and is often present during acute hepatitis.[67] This is usually not a problem if serum samples are diluted before testing.

The other commonly used serum test is a competitive inhibition immunoassay that is not specific for any single immunoglobulin isotype[66, 80] (Fig. 260–4*B*). This test is useful in determining prior infection (and hence immunity) but is not specific for acute infection. In general, these tests are not extremely sensitive (detection threshold approximately 100 mIU/mL in comparison with a World Health Organization reference reagent) and usually fail to detect protective levels of antibody conferred by passive immunization with pooled immune globulins (IGs).[72] Without modifications, these tests also may not detect protective levels of antibody conferred by active immunization with a single dose of inactivated HAV vaccine (see Chapter 91). Although solid-phase immunoassays for HAV antigen have been developed (Fig. 260–4*A*), they are of little diagnostic value because most HAV shedding occurs before acute liver injury. Similarly, tissue culture isolation of the virus as described earlier is not achieved easily and its use is restricted to research laboratories. Reverse transcription of viral RNA to yield complementary DNA, followed by polymerase chain reaction amplification of the complementary DNA (reverse transcription–polymerase chain reaction assay), permits detection of HAV in feces and serum and may also provide information concerning the virus genotype.[45, 57] Although potentially useful in epidemiologic studies, this is likely to remain a research procedure.

Prevention

Inasmuch as HAV is generally transmitted via the fecal-oral route, one of the most effective methods of control is the maintenance of high standards of hygiene. This includes public sanitation measures to protect drinking water supplies and proper collection, treatment, and disposal of sewage. However, two forms of specific immunoprophylaxis are available for prevention of hepatitis A (see Chapter 91). Passive immunization with pooled IG provides a high level of protection when administered even as late as 2 weeks after exposure.[81] In addition, formalin-inactivated HAV vaccines have been shown to be extraordinarily effective in preventing symptomatic hepatitis A in immunized children, and two such vaccines are now licensed in the United States.[82, 83] However, both IG and vaccine immunoprophylaxis have significant shortcomings. The use of IG results in only short-term protection against disease and requires recognition of recent exposure. Moreover, supplies of IG for intramuscular use have been severely limited in the United States because

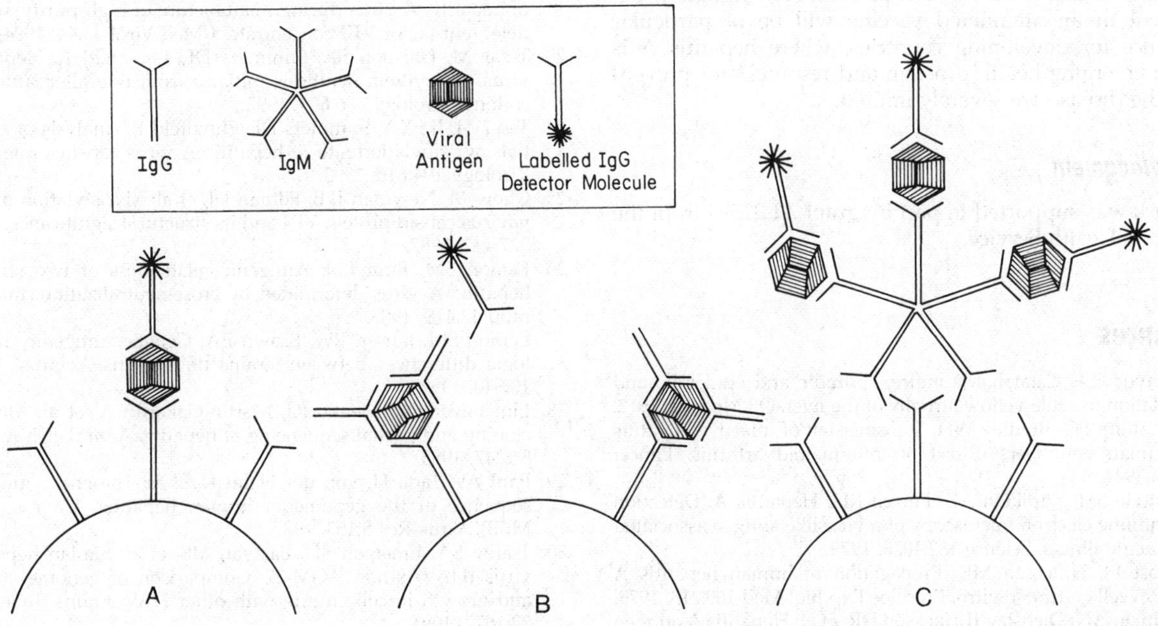

FIGURE 260–4 ▫ Solid-phase immunoassays for detection of HAV antigen and anti-HAV antibodies. *A*, Detection of HAV antigen: virus is captured by anti-HAV bound to a solid-phase support and subsequently detected by labeled anti-HAV IgG. *B*, Non–isotype-specific detection of anti-HAV: antibody of any isotype is detected by its ability to compete with labeled anti-HAV IgG for binding to captured virus. *C*, Isotype-specific detection of anti-HAV IgM: IgM antibody is captured with anti-human IgM antibody bound to the solid phase and is then probed sequentially with HAV antigen and labeled anti-HAV IgG. Detector IgG labels may be iodine 125 or enzymes such as alkaline phosphatase.

of extensive military purchases of IG during the Persian Gulf War or removal of lots of IG from distribution because of fears about the presence of contaminating hepatitis C virus RNA (despite the absence of evidence for hepatitis C transmission after administration of intramuscular IG). On the other hand, although the inactivated vaccine is both safe and effective, it is quite expensive and its high cost is likely to limit its use severely.[84] Thus, interest persists in the development of an attenuated vaccine that might be less expensive to manufacture and deliver and thus might allow more universal vaccine-induced protection against disease.

Attempts to produce an attenuated HAV strain for use as a live virus vaccine have been based on successive passage of virus in cell culture.[85] These efforts have resulted in cell culture–adapted strains that demonstrate an attenuation phenotype in nonhuman primates as well as human volunteers.[55, 56, 86, 87] Attenuation is likely to be due to mutations in the P2 proteins and possibly also the 5′ NTR of the viral genome that occurred during adaptation and passage of the virus in cell culture.[42, 88] However, these virus variants appear to have significantly reduced infectivity for humans and generally induce only low levels of protective antibodies. They are not infectious by the oral route. Although an attenuated vaccine has been used extensively in China,[89] no vaccine candidate has been clearly demonstrated to be acceptable in terms of both attenuation and immunogenicity. Development of attenuated vaccines has been made difficult by the absence of reliable markers for attenuation and the possibility of reversion of a vaccine strain to a pathogenic phenotype with spread to contacts. However, developments in understanding the molecular biology of HAV and the genetic basis for attenuation of the virus have suggested alternative strategies for development of live, attenuated viruses. Genetic modifications made to existing attenuated vaccine candidates might possibly improve their attenuation or immunogenicity phenotypes. Alternatively, viable mutant viruses have been constructed that have large deletions within the 5′ NTR and have striking temperature-sensitive replication phenotypes.[90] These viruses are being studied to determine whether they might have a useful attenuation phenotype. Ultimately, development of an attenuated vaccine will be of particular importance for developing countries, where hepatitis A is often an emerging health problem and resources for prevention of the disease are severely limited.

Acknowledgment

This work was supported in part by grant AI-32599 from the U.S. Public Health Service.

References

1. Cockayne EA: Catarrhal jaundice, sporadic and epidemic, and its relation to acute yellow atrophy of the liver. Q J Med 6:1, 1912.
2. MacCallum FO, Bradley WH: Transmission of infective hepatitis to human volunteers: Effect on rheumatoid arthritis. Lancet 2:228, 1944.
3. Feinstone SM, Kapikian AZ, Purcell RH: Hepatitis A: Detection by immune electron microscopy of a viruslike antigen associated with acute illness. Science 182:1026, 1973.
4. Provost PJ, Hilleman MR: Propagation of human hepatitis A virus in cell culture in vitro. Proc Soc Exp Biol Med 160:213, 1979.
5. Schulman AN, Dienstag JL, Jackson DR, et al: Hepatitis A antigen particles in liver, bile, and stool of chimpanzees. J Infect Dis 134:80, 1976.
6. Dienstag JL, Feinstone SM, Purcell RH, et al: Experimental infection of chimpanzees with hepatitis A virus. J Infect Dis 132:532, 1975.
7. Holmes AW, Deinhardt F, Wolfe L, et al: Specific neutralization of human hepatitis type A in marmoset monkeys. Nature 243:419, 1973.
8. Provost PJ, Villarejos VM, Hilleman MR: Suitability of the rufiventer marmoset as a host animal for human hepatitis A virus. Proc Soc Exp Biol Med 155:283, 1977.
9. Cohen JI, Ticehurst JR, Purcell RH, et al: Complete nucleotide sequence of wild-type hepatitis A virus: Comparison with different strains of hepatitis A virus and other picornaviruses. J Virol 61:50, 1987.
10. Francki RIB, Fauquet CM, Knudson DL, Brown F: Classification and Nomenclature of Viruses. New York, Springer-Verlag, 1991.
11. Lemon SM: Type A viral hepatitis: New developments in an old disease. N Engl J Med 313:1059, 1985.
12. Ticehurst JR, Cohen JI, Feinstone SM, et al: Replication of hepatitis A virus: New ideas from studies with cloned cDNA. *In* Ehrenfeld E, Semler BL (eds): Molecular Aspects of Picornavirus Infection and Detection. Washington, DC, ASM Press, 1989, p 27.
13. Lemon SM, Robertson BH: Current perspectives in the virology and molecular biology of hepatitis A virus. Semin Virol 4:285, 1993.
14. Lemon SM: Hepatitis A virus: Current concepts of the molecular virology, immunobiology, and approaches to vaccine development. Rev Med Virol 2:73, 1992.
15. Lemon SM, Jansen RW, Newbold JE: Infectious hepatitis A virus particles produced in cell culture consist of three distinct types with different buoyant densities in CsCl. J Virol 54:78, 1985.
16. Lemon SM, Binn LN: Incomplete neutralization of hepatitis A virus in vitro due to lipid-associated virions. J Gen Virol 66:2501, 1985.
17. Provost PJ, Wolanski BS, Miller WJ, et al: Biophysical and biochemical properties of CR326 human hepatitis A virus. Am J Med Sci 270:87, 1975.
18. Scholz E, Heinricy U, Flehmig B: Acid stability of hepatitis A virus. J Gen Virol 70:2481, 1989.
19. Siegl G, Weitz M, Kronauer G: Stability of hepatitis A virus. Intervirology 22:218, 1984.
20. Lemon SM, Murphy PC, Shields PA, et al: Antigenic and genetic variation in cytopathic hepatitis A virus variants arising during persistent infection: Evidence for genetic recombination. J Virol 65:2056, 1991.
21. Murphy P, Nowak T, Lemon SM, Hilfenhaus J: Inactivation of hepatitis A virus by heat treatment in aqueous solution. J Med Virol 41:61, 1993.
22. Lemon SM, Murphy PC, Smith A, et al: Removal/neutralization of hepatitis A virus during manufacture of high purity, solvent/detergent factor VIII concentrate. J Med Virol 43:44, 1994.
23. Tesar M, Harmon SA, Summers DF, Ehrenfeld E: Hepatitis A virus polyprotein synthesis initiates from two alternative AUG codons. Virology 186:609, 1992.
24. Tesar M, Jia X-Y, Summers DF, Ehrenfeld E: Analysis of a potential myristoylation site in hepatitis A virus capsid protein VP4. Virology 194:616, 1993.
25. Chow M, Newman JFE, Filman DJ, et al: Myristylation of picornavirus capsid protein VP4 and its structural significance. Nature 327:482, 1987.
26. Lemon SM, Binn LN: Antigenic relatedness of two strains of hepatitis A virus determined by cross-neutralization. Infect Immun 42:418, 1983.
27. Lemon SM, Jansen RW, Brown EA: Genetic, antigenic, and biologic differences between strains of hepatitis A virus. Vaccine 10:S40, 1992.
28. Linemeyer DL, Menke JG, Martin-Gallardo A, et al: Molecular cloning and partial sequencing of hepatitis A viral cDNA. J Virol 54:247, 1985.
29. Paul AV, Tada H, von der Helm K, et al: The entire nucleotide sequence of the genome of human hepatitis A virus (isolate MBB). Virus Res 8:153, 1987.
30. Tsarev SA, Emerson SU, Balayan MS, et al: Simian hepatitis A virus (HAV) strain AGM-27: Comparison of genome structure and growth in cell culture with other HAV strains. J Gen Virol 72:1677, 1991.
31. Nainan OV, Margolis HS, Robertson BH, et al: Sequence analysis of a new hepatitis A virus naturally infecting cynomolgus macaques *(Macaca fascicularis)*. J Gen Virol 72:1685, 1991.
32. Ping L-H, Jansen RW, Stapleton JT, et al: Identification of an immunodominant antigenic site involving the capsid protein VP3 of hepatitis A virus. Proc Natl Acad Sci USA 85:8281, 1988.

33. Ping L-H, Lemon SM: Antigenic structure of human hepatitis A virus defined by analysis of escape mutants selected against murine monoclonal antibodies. J Virol 66:2208, 1992.
34. Hughes JV, Bennett C, Stanton LW, et al: Hepatitis-A virus structural proteins: Sequencing and ability to induce virus-neutralizing antibody responses. *In* Lerner RA, Chanock RM, Brown F (eds): Vaccines 85: Molecular and Chemical Basis of Resistance to Parasitic, Bacterial and Viral Diseases. Cold Spring Harbor, NY, Cold Spring Harbor Laboratory, 1985, p 255.
35. Cohen JI, Ticehurst JR, Feinstone SM, et al: Hepatitis A virus cDNA and its RNA transcripts are infectious in cell culture. J Virol 61:3035, 1987.
36. Weitz M, Baroudy BM, Maloy WL, et al: Detection of a genome-linked protein (VPg) of hepatitis A virus and its comparison with other picornaviral VPgs. J Virol 60:124, 1986.
37. Brown EA, Day SP, Jansen RW, Lemon SM: The 5′ nontranslated region of hepatitis A virus: Secondary structure and elements required for translation in vitro. J Virol 65:5828, 1991.
38. Brown EA, Zajac AJ, Lemon SM: In vitro characterization of an internal ribosomal entry site (IRES) present within the 5′ nontranslated region of hepatitis A virus RNA: Comparison with the IRES of encephalomyocarditis virus. J Virol 68:1066, 1994.
39. Day SP, Murphy P, Brown EA, Lemon SM: Mutations within the 5′ nontranslated region of hepatitis A virus RNA which enhance replication in BS-C-1 cells. J Virol 66:6533, 1992.
40. Anderson DA, Ross BC: Morphogenesis of hepatitis A virus: Isolation and characterization of subviral particles. J Virol 64:5284, 1990.
41. Martin A, Escriou N, Chao S-F, et al: Identification and site-directed mutagenesis of the primary (2A/2B) cleavage site of the hepatitis A virus polyprotein: Functional impact on the infectivity of HAV RNA transcripts. Virology 213:213, 1995.
42. Emerson SU, Huang YK, McRill C, et al: Mutations in both the 2B and 2C genes of hepatitis A virus are involved in adaptation to growth in cell culture. J Virol 66:650, 1992.
43. Emerson SU, Huang YK, Purcell RH: 2B and 2C mutations are essential but mutations throughout the genome of HAV contribute to adaptation to cell culture. Virology 194:475, 1993.
44. Schultheiss T, Sommergruber W, Kusov Y, Gauss-Müller V: Cleavage specificity of purified recombinant hepatitis A virus 3C proteinase on natural substrates. J Virol 69:1727, 1995.
45. Jansen RW, Siegl G, Lemon SM: Molecular epidemiology of human hepatitis A virus defined by an antigen-capture polymerase chain reaction method. Proc Natl Acad Sci USA 87:2867, 1990.
46. Robertson BH, Jansen RW, Khanna B, et al: Genetic relatedness of hepatitis A virus strains recovered from different geographic regions. J Gen Virol 73:1365, 1992.
47. Purcell RH: Approaches to immunization against hepatitis A virus. *In* Hollinger FB, Lemon SM, Margolis HS (eds): Viral Hepatitis and Liver Disease. Baltimore, Williams & Wilkins, 1991, p 41.
48. Lemon SM, Binn LN, Marchwicki R, et al: In vivo replication and reversion to wild-type of a neutralization-resistant variant of hepatitis A virus. J Infect Dis 161:7, 1990.
49. Deinhardt F, Scheid R, Gauss-Muller V, et al: Propagation of human hepatitis A virus in cell lines of primary human hepatocellular carcinomas. Prog Med Virol 27:109, 1981.
50. Daemer RJ, Feinstone SM, Gust ID, Purcell RH: Propagation of human hepatitis A virus in African green monkey kidney cell culture: Primary isolation and serial passage. Infect Immun 32:388, 1981.
51. Binn LN, Lemon SM, Marchwicki RH, et al: Primary isolation and serial passage of hepatitis A virus strains in primate cell cultures. J Clin Microbiol 20:28, 1984.
52. Flehmig B, Vallbracht A, Wurster G: Hepatitis A virus in cell culture: III. Propagation of hepatitis A virus in human embryo kidney cells and human embryo fibroblast strains. Med Microbiol Immunol (Berl) 170:83, 1981.
53. Dotzauer A, Feinstone SM, Kaplan G: Susceptibility of nonprimate cell lines to hepatitis A virus infection. J Virol 68:6064, 1994.
54. Jansen RW, Newbold JE, Lemon SM: Complete nucleotide sequence of a cell culture–adapted variant of hepatitis A virus: Comparison with wild-type virus with restricted capacity for in vitro replication. Virology 163:299, 1988.
55. Midthun K, Ellerbeck E, Gershman K, et al: Safety and immunogenicity of a live attenuated hepatitis A virus vaccine in seronegative volunteers. J Infect Dis 163:735, 1991.
56. Sjogren MH, Purcell RH, McKee K, et al: Clinical and laboratory observations following oral or intramuscular administration of a live, attenuated hepatitis A vaccine candidate. Vaccine 10(Suppl 1):S135, 1992.
57. Robertson BH, Khanna B, Nainan OV, Margolis HS: Epidemiologic patterns of wild-type hepatitis A virus determined by genetic variation. J Infect Dis 163:286, 1991.
58. Mannucci PM, Gdovin S, Gringeri A, et al: Transmission of hepatitis A to patients with hemophilia by factor VIII concentrates treated with organic solvent and detergent to inactivate viruses. Ann Intern Med 120:1, 1994.
59. Mathiesen LR, Drucker J, Lorenz D, et al: Localization of hepatitis A antigen in marmoset organs during acute infection with hepatitis A virus. J Infect Dis 138:369, 1978.
60. Cohen JI, Feinstone S, Purcell RH: Hepatitis A virus infection in a chimpanzee: Duration of viremia and detection of virus in saliva and throat swabs. J Infect Dis 160:887, 1989.
61. Dienstag JL, Popper H, Purcell RH: The pathology of viral hepatitis types A and B in chimpanzees. Am J Pathol 85:131, 1976.
62. Shimizu YK, Shikata T, Beninger PR, et al: Detection of hepatitis A antigen in human liver. Infect Immun 36:320, 1982.
63. Murphy BL, Maynard JE, Bradley DW, et al: Immunofluorescence of hepatitis A virus antigen in chimpanzees. Infect Immun 21:663, 1978.
64. Teixera MR Jr, Weller IVD, Murray A, et al: The pathology of hepatitis A in man. Liver 2:53, 1982.
65. Keenan CM, Lemon SM, LeDuc JW, et al: Pathology of hepatitis A infection in the owl monkey *(Aotus trivirgatus).* Am J Pathol 115:1, 1984.
66. Mathiesen LR, Feinstone SM, Wong DC, et al: Enzyme-linked immunosorbent assay for detection of hepatitis A antigen in stool and antibody to hepatitis A antigen in sera: Comparison with solid-phase radioimmunoassay, immune electron microscopy, and immune adherence hemagglutination assay. J Clin Microbiol 7:184, 1978.
67. Lemon SM, Brown CD, Brooks DS, et al: Specific immunoglobulin M response to hepatitis A virus determined by solid-phase radioimmunoassay. Infect Immun 28:927, 1980.
68. Lemon SM, Binn LN: Serum neutralizing antibody response to hepatitis A virus. J Infect Dis 148:1033, 1983.
69. Decker RH, Kosakowski SM, Vanderbilt AS, et al: Diagnosis of acute hepatitis A by HAVAB-M, a direct radioimmunoassay for IgM anti-HAV. Am J Clin Pathol 76:140, 1981.
70. Coulepis AG, Locarnini SA, Lehmann NI, Gust ID: Detection of hepatitis A virus in the feces of patients with naturally acquired infections. J Infect Dis 141:151, 1980.
71. Stapleton JT, Lange DK, LeDuc JW, et al: The role of secretory immunity in hepatitis A virus infection. J Infect Dis 163:7, 1991.
72. Stapleton JT, Jansen RW, Lemon SM: Neutralizing antibody to hepatitis A virus in immune serum globulin and in the sera of human recipients of immune serum globulin. Gastroenterology 89:637, 1985.
73. Vallbracht A, Gabriel P, Maier K, et al: Cell-mediated cytotoxicity in hepatitis A virus infection. Hepatology 6:1308, 1986.
74. Maier K, Gabriel P, Koscielniak E, et al: Human gamma interferon production by cytotoxic T lymphocytes sensitized during hepatitis A virus infection. J Virol 62:3756, 1988.
75. Vallbracht A, Maier K, Stierhof Y-D, et al: Liver-derived cytotoxic T cells in hepatitis A virus infection. J Infect Dis 160:209, 1989.
76. Hadler SC, Webster HM, Erben JJ, et al: Hepatitis A in day-care centers: A community-wide assessment. N Engl J Med 302:1222, 1980.
77. Rakela J, Redeker AG, Edwards VM, et al: Hepatitis A virus infection in fulminant hepatitis and chronic active hepatitis. Gastroenterology 74:879, 1978.
78. Forbes A, Williams R: Changing epidemiology and clinical aspects of hepatitis A. Br Med Bull 46:303, 1990.
79. Hadler SC: Global impact of hepatitis A virus infection: Changing patterns. *In* Hollinger FB, Lemon SM, Margolis HS (eds): Viral Hepatitis and Liver Disease. Baltimore, Williams & Wilkins, 1991, p 14.
80. Purcell RH, Wong DC, Moritsugu Y, et al: A microtiter solid-phase radioimmunoassay for hepatitis A antigen and antibody. J Immunol 116:349, 1976.
81. Winokur PL, Stapleton JT: Immunoglobulin prophylaxis for hepatitis A. Clin Infect Dis 14:580, 1992.

82. Werzberger A, Mensch B, Kuter B, et al: A controlled trial of a formalin-inactivated hepatitis A vaccine in healthy children. N Engl J Med 327:453, 1992.
83. Innis BL, Snitbhan R, Kunasol P, et al: Protection against hepatitis A by an inactivated vaccine. JAMA 271:1328, 1994.
84. Lemon SM, Shapiro CN: The value of immunization against hepatitis A. Infect Agents Dis 3:38, 1994.
85. Siegl G, Lemon SM: Recent advances in hepatitis A vaccine development. Virus Res 17:75, 1990.
86. Provost PJ, Bishop RP, Gerety RJ, et al: New findings in live, attenuated hepatitis A vaccine development. J Med Virol 20:165, 1986.
87. Karron RA, Daemer RJ, Ticehurst JR, et al: Studies of prototype live hepatitis A virus vaccine in primate models. J Infect Dis 157:338, 1988.
88. Cohen JI, Rosenblum B, Feinstone SM, et al: Attenuation and cell culture adaptation of hepatitis A virus (HAV): A genetic analysis with HAV cDNA. J Virol 63:5364, 1989.
89. Mao JS, Dong DX, Zhang HY, et al: Primary study of attenuated live hepatitis A vaccine (H2 strain) in humans. J Infect Dis 159:621, 1989.
90. Shaffer DR, Brown EA, Lemon SM: Large deletion mutations involving the first pyrimidine-rich tract of the 5′ nontranslated RNA of hepatitis A virus define two adjacent domains associated with distinct replication phenotypes. J Virol 68:5568, 1994.

261

Hepatitis C Virus

Raymond S. Koff

History

The development of serologic tests for the diagnosis of hepatitis A and hepatitis B virus infections, achieved in the mid-1970s, resulted in awareness of the existence of other etiologic forms of viral hepatitis that were termed non-A, non-B hepatitis. Molecular cloning of the hepatitis C virus (HCV), the major responsible blood-borne pathogen of non-A, non-B hepatitis, a brilliant achievement but one that proved a painstakingly slow process, was first reported in 1989.[1] This extraordinary work resulted in an explosion of information about this important member of the Flaviviridae family and increased understanding of the importance of HCV as a major cause of chronic liver disease. Nonetheless, the complex biologic characteristics of the agent and the pathogenesis of its uncanny ability to evade the host immune system, thereby leading to persistent infections, remain ill-defined. Although HCV is now recognized to have been the predominant agent responsible for percutaneously transmitted non-A, non-B hepatitis during the past two decades, the existence of other, epidemiologically minor blood-borne hepatitis viruses continues to be an unresolved question. Whether such agents are related to HCV or to other Flaviviridae is also uncertain. Studies in which flavivirus-like genomes have been identified in the inoculum containing a non-C agent, known as the GB hepatitis agent, are intriguing, but information is fragmentary.[2] Analysis of the importance of non-C blood-borne agents is also complicated by the fact that homologous immunity to HCV infection has not been established in experimentally transmitted infection in chimpanzees[3] and that second infections (reinfections) with different HCV isolates have been reported in polytransfused individuals.[4]

Morphology and Characteristics of the Agent

HCV is a lipoprotein-enveloped, chloroform-sensitive, RNA-containing virus with a buoyant density in sucrose estimated to be 1.08 g/dL and a nucleocapsid buoyant density estimated to be 1.25 g/cm^3. Classic filtration studies suggested a diameter of between 38 and 60 nm for the HCV particle. Although considerable size heterogeneity of putative HCV particles has been observed, supporting the possible coexistence of small defective interfering particles, electron microscopy of an enriched plasma sample revealed the presence of spherical, enveloped 55-nm virus-like particles,[5] which are probably the actual virions. Treatment with detergent liberated 33-nm icosahedral particles presumed to be associated with the HCV nucleocapsid. Similar 55- to 65-nm particles with an inner core estimated to be 30 to 35 nm in diameter have been identified.[6] Envelope projections observed on the virus-like particles have included spikes, knobs, or neither. The lipid-rich envelope of HCV contains at least two glycoproteins containing antigenic domains that may elicit antibodies.

Hepatitis C Virus

HCV contains a positive-sense, single-stranded RNA molecule. The genome has a length of about 9400 nucleotides and contains a 5′-nontranslated region of about 332 to 342 nucleotides, which is well conserved in the different strains that have been studied, and a single, large open reading frame that encodes a large polyprotein of about 3000 amino acids. The putative structure of the HCV genome is shown in Figure 261–1, and the probable function and gene products of the genomic regions are shown in Table 261–1. The 5′-nontranslated region appears to play an important role in the regulation of HCV translation; an unusual folding region may encompass an internal ribosomal entry site.[7, 8] The 5′-nontranslated region contains multiple stem loops, a pseudoknot, three to six AUG codons, and a six-nucleotide motif that may be involved in modulating viral transcription.[9] After the large open reading frame, a short but variable (27 to 45 nucleotides in length) 3′-nontranslated region contains poly(U) or poly(A) sequences.

The large polyprotein encoded by the HCV open reading frame is subjected to posttranslational cleavage through the action of a cellular signalase (signal peptidase) and two or more virus-specific proteinases.[10] About one third of the polyprotein, after the 5′-nontranslated region, comprises a number of structural proteins. These are recognized to include an internal viral structural protein called the nucleocapsid or core (C) protein and two glycosylated envelope proteins, termed E1 and E2/NS1, which are present in the lipid-containing envelope of the virus and may generate neutralizing antibodies. The envelope glycoproteins and the core protein are cleaved from the polyprotein by the action of the cellular signalase. The HCV core protein is processed in vivo by cleavage of its C-terminal hydrophobic segment to generate the mature core protein (a phosphoprotein) that can bind RNA, is membrane associated, and may function as a transcriptional transactivator. Sequencing of the core gene has revealed the presence of two nuclear localization signals, a DNA-binding motif, a phosphorylation site, and hydrophilic domains containing immunogenic epitopes.[11] An HCV-encoded cleavage product, p7, is located between the E2 and NS2 proteins. It is preceded by a hydrophobic sequence in

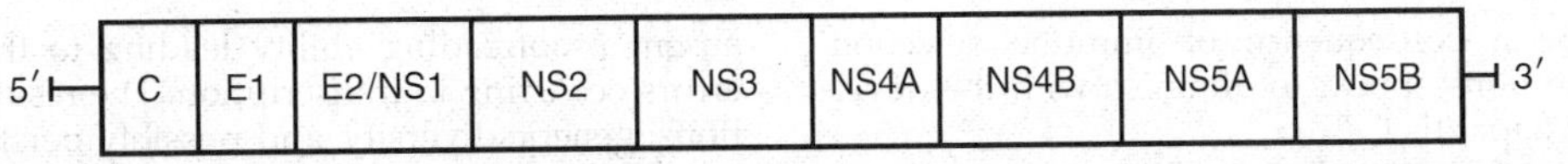

FIGURE 261–1 □ Genomic map of HCV RNA depicting the regions encoding the structural and nonstructural proteins. The 5′-nontranslated region and the shorter 3′-nontranslated region containing poly(U) or poly(A) sequences are indicated by the horizontal lines preceding the C region (on the left side) and following the NS5B region (on the right side).

E2 that may direct translocation into the endoplasmic reticulum.[12]

The remaining two thirds of the polyprotein is also cleaved into distinct proteins (termed NS2, NS3, NS4A, NS4B, NS5A, and NS5B) that are nonstructural and are likely to be involved in the replication of HCV. These proteins appear to have metalloproteinase, protease, helicase, and RNA polymerase activities (see Table 261–1). Processing of the nonstructural polyprotein involves at least two virus-encoded proteinases: one at NS2/3 and one at NS3. The NS2/3 enzyme is a zinc-dependent metalloproteinase; the NS3 enzyme is a chymotrypsin-like serine proteinase[13] that appears to function in both cis and trans cleavage modes.[14] NS4A sequences appear to be important in the polyprotein processing, particularly for the NS4B/5A cleavage site.[15] The functions of NS4B and NS5A are unknown. The RNA polymerase is encoded by the NS5B region.

Classification

Because of similarities in stretches of deduced amino acid sequences within their open reading frames, including motifs predictive of serine proteinases and other enzymatic activities, and similarities in the hydropathy profile of their proteins, HCV is currently classified as a separate third genus in the Flaviviridae, which includes both the *Flavivirus* genus and the *Pestivirus* genus. Although its genomic length is considerably shorter than that of typical pestiviruses and closer to that of the flaviviruses, other features (e.g., the presence of a long 5′-nontranslated region, the absence of vector transmission, and the frequency of persistent infections) suggest a closer relationship to the pestiviruses.

TABLE 261–1 ■ Hepatitis C Virus Genomic Regions: Functional Role and Gene Products

GENOMIC REGIONS	FUNCTIONAL ROLE AND GENE PRODUCTS
5′ Nontranslated	Internal ribosomal entry site
	? Modulation of virus transcription
C (core)	Nuclear localization signals
	DNA-binding motif
	Phosphorylation site
	Hydrophilic domains containing immunogenic epitopes
	Nucleocapsid phosphoprotein binds RNA, membrane associated, ? transcriptional transactivator
E1	Envelope glycoprotein (epitope)
E2/NS1	Envelope glycoprotein (epitope)
	Translocation signal to endoplasmic reticulum
NS2/3	Zinc-dependent metalloproteinase
NS3	Chymotrypsin-like serine proteinase
	Helicase
NS4A	Involved in polyprotein processing, at NS4B/5A cleavage site
NS4B	Unknown
NS5A	Unknown
NS5B	RNA-dependent RNA polymerase

Genetic Variation

HCV persistence may be a consequence of mutability of the RNA, leading to changes in the virus that permit escape from the immune mechanisms that would limit continuing replication. The basis for this theory is the identification of differences in HCV RNA from one strain to another. The complete nucleotide sequence of a number of HCV isolates has been published during the past few years. Comparison among distinct isolates has revealed marked differences among the sequenced nucleotides. This genomic heterogeneity led to the realization that distinct genotypes of HCV exist. Genotyping may be undertaken by sequence homology studies, restriction fragment length polymorphisms of amplified polymerase chain reaction products, polymerase chain reaction amplification with subtype-specific primers, or line probe hybridization assays.[16]

By general agreement, HCV genotypes have nucleotide divergence of more than 20%; within genotypes, nucleotide divergence does not exceed 10%. Initial attempts to classify these genotypes resulted in a number of confusing systems that have now been replaced, more or less, by a nomenclature that recognizes six distinct genotypes and at least an equal number of subtypes.[17] Subsequent preliminary observations suggest the existence of 10 genotypes and as many as 80 subtypes. In lieu of complete genome analysis involving all 9400 nucleotides, HCV genotypes can be identified by sequence analysis comparisons in subgenomic fragments of RNA. These include the HCV core, E1, NS5, and 5′-nontranslated regions.[18]

Early studies indicated that the worldwide distribution of these genotypes is variable.[19] HCV genotypes 1, 2, and subtype 3a appear to be the most prevalent in North America, Europe, and Japan. Type 4 may be prevalent in Africa. Among American patients with chronic hepatitis C, nearly 75% had HCV genotype 1; half of these were 1a and half were 1b.[20] Maps of the distribution of HCV genotypes remain incomplete at this time, but it is likely that the global picture will be filled in during the next few years.

In addition to geographic heterogeneity in HCV isolates and heterogeneity among isolates from different individuals in the same region, HCV isolates from the same individual may vary. Such isolates are called HCV quasi species. Changes in the HCV genome have been studied by serial nucleotide analysis both in an HCV-infected human being and in an experimentally infected chimpanzee. Mutation rates of approximately 1.44 to 1.92×10^{-3} base substitutions per site per year were identified. Amino acid substitutions in the 5′-terminal end of the E2/NS1 region (the hypervariable region) of HCV are frequent and have been recognized during acute HCV infection[21]; these may permit the virus to escape immune recognition by preexisting antibodies because this region appears to contain two B-cell epitopes. Neutralizing antibodies to HCV have been identified and appear to inhibit the replicative cycle of HCV. These antibodies have been shown to be isolate specific and appear to change over time as a consequence of the emergence of neutralization escape HCV mutants.[22] Genetic drift elsewhere in the viral RNA may also allow HCV to escape from cytotoxic T lymphocytes, thereby favoring persistent infection. This genetic variability may be a consequence of immune selection. Amino acid substitutions appear to diminish with the development of chronic hepatitis C.[21]

Propagation

Experimental transmission and serial passage of HCV in chimpanzees have been established unequivocally with inocula of either serum or plasma obtained from blood donors implicated in transfusion-associated hepatitis C or from patients with chronic hepatitis C. The importance of the chimpanzee in the study of HCV infection is also highlighted by the fact that the virus was originally cloned from nucleic acid extracted from large quantities of the plasma of an infected chimpanzee. Attempts to transmit HCV experimentally to cynomolgus monkeys, green monkeys, rhesus monkeys, Japanese monkeys, doguera baboons, and woodchucks have been unsuccessful.[23] Hence, the host range of HCV appears to be restricted.

Attempts to propagate HCV in cell culture systems using human lymphocytic cell lines have been reported.[24] In the initial studies, genomic replication of HCV was identified, but it was not entirely clear whether HCV infection of these cells is abortive or productive of infectious HCV particles. Subsequent studies correlating HCV infectivity in vivo with in vitro infectivity[25] indicated that infectious HCV could be produced in cell culture and that viral replication could be inhibited by interferon-α and interferon-β.[26] Primary chimpanzee hepatocyte cultures and primary human fetal liver cells may also support replication of HCV. Chimpanzee hepatocyte cultures inoculated with HCV were found to have both positive- and negative-stranded HCV RNA detected as early as 4 days after inoculation[27]; intracellular HCV RNA-negative strands became detectable 12 to 24 days after human fetal liver cells were exposed to HCV.[28] In addition to these studies of HCV propagation, it has been possible to establish cell lines (e.g., Chinese hamster ovary cells) in which specific HCV genes are expressed, and the expressed proteins may be isolated and further studied.[29] Although not yet widely used, these models may prove useful in the study of HCV biology and infectivity, in understanding the humoral response to infection, and in the screening of antiviral drugs.

Replication

HCV replication is thought to occur through the action of RNA-dependent RNA polymerase. Nonetheless, the precise replicative mechanisms remain poorly understood. In serum, HCV virions may be associated with circulating low-density lipoproteins; on the hepatocyte, HCV uptake may occur at the site of the low-density lipoprotein receptor. Presumably after the HCV envelope is uncoated, the positive-stranded RNA genome is transcribed into a negative strand, which then serves as a template for the transcription of a nascent positive RNA strand. The positive strand is subsequently encapsidated within a nucleocapsid containing the core protein. Although preliminary data have suggested that HCV RNA may be self-priming,[30] confirmation of this observation is not yet available. The HCV genome is translated by a mechanism involving an internal ribosomal entry site on the 5′-nontranslated region. HCV persistence may be a consequence of the extreme mutability of the RNA genome, leading to changes in the virus that permit escape from the immune mechanisms that would limit continuing replication. This theory is supported by the identification of differences in HCV RNA from one strain to another. HCV RNA replication rates are believed to be high and coupled with poor or absent proofreading ability leading to the failure to detect errors occurring in transcription. The result is multiple mutations, genetic diversity, and possibly persistent infection.

Site of Replication

The tissue sites at which HCV RNA replication occurs have yet to be fully determined. HCV replication occurs in liver and possibly in lymphocytes and bone marrow cells because negative-stranded HCV RNA was detected in these cells.[31, 32] However, because negative-stranded HCV RNA has also been detected in serum, in a lipid membrane structure linked with the E1 envelope protein,[33] contamination of tissues with blood may lead to detection of the negative strand even in the absence of extrahepatic replication. Although HCV RNA has been detected in some secretions and excretions (e.g., saliva, urine, seminal fluid, and ascites),[34, 35] evidence of replication in the tissue source is not available and contamination remains a possible explanation for its detection.

References

1. Choo Q-L, Kuo G, Weiner AJ, et al: Isolation of a cDNA clone derived from a blood-borne non-A, non-B viral hepatitis genome. Science 244:359–362, 1989.
2. Simons JN, Pilot-Matias TJ, Leary TP, et al: Identification of two flavivirus-like genomes in the GB hepatitis agent. Proc Natl Acad Sci USA 92:3401–3405, 1995.
3. Farci P, Alter HJ, Govindarajan S, et al: Lack of protective immunity against reinfection with hepatitis C virus. Science 258:135–140, 1992.
4. Lai ME, Mazzoleni AP, Argiolu F, et al: Hepatitis C virus in multiple episodes of acute hepatitis in polytransfused thalassaemic children. Lancet 343:388–390, 1994.
5. Takahashi K, Kishimoti S, Yoshizawa H, et al: p26 protein and 33-nm particle associated with nucleocapsid of hepatitis C virus recovered from the circulation of infected hosts. Virology 191:431–434, 1992.
6. Kaito M, Watanabe S, Tsukiyama-Kohara K, et al: Hepatitis C virus particle detected by immunoelectron microscopic study. J Gen Virol 75:1755–1760, 1994.
7. Le S-Y, Sonenberg N, Maizel JV Jr: Unusual folding regions and ribosome landing pad within hepatitis C virus and pestivirus RNAs. Gene 154:137–143, 1995.
8. Tsukiyama-Kohara K, Iizuka N, Kohara M, et al: Internal ribosome entry site within hepatitis C virus RNA. J Virol 66:1476–1483, 1992.
9. Vizmanos JL, Jauregui JI, Gullon A, et al: The GCGGAA gene-regulatory motif of herpes simplex virus type-1 is also found in hepatitis C virus. Gene 154:131–132, 1995.
10. Grakoui A, McCourt DW, Wychowski C, et al: Characterization of the hepatitis C virus–encoded serine proteinase: Determination of proteinase-dependent polyprotein cleavage site. J Virol 67:2832–2843, 1993.
11. Bukh J, Purcell RH, Miller RH: Sequence analysis of the core gene of 14 hepatitis C virus genotypes. Proc Natl Acad Sci USA 91:8239–8243, 1994.
12. Lin C, Lindenbach BD, Pragai BM, et al: Processing in the hepatitis C virus E2-NS2 region: Identification of p7 and two distinct E2-specific products with different C termini. J Virol 68:5063–5073, 1994.
13. Hahm B, Han DS, Back SH, et al: NS3-4A of hepatitis C virus is a chymotrypsin-like protease. J Virol 69:2534–2539, 1995.
14. Bartenschlager R, Ahlborn-Laake L, Yasargil K, et al: Substrate determinants for cleavage in cis and in trans by the hepatitis C virus NS3 proteinase. J Virol 69:198–205, 1995.
15. Bartenschlager R, Ahlborn-Laake L, Mous J, Jacobsen H: Kinetic and structural analyses of hepatitis C virus polyprotein processing. J Virol 68:5045–5055, 1994.
16. Andonov A, Chaudhary RK: Subtyping of hepatitis C virus isolates by a line probe assay using hybridization. J Clin Microbiol 33:254–256, 1995.
17. Simmonds P, Holmes EC, Cha T-A, et al: Classification of hepati-

tis C virus into six major genotypes and a series of subtypes by phylogenetic analysis of the NS-5 region. J Gen Virol 74:2391–2399, 1993.
18. Simmonds P, Smith DB, McOmish F, et al: Identification of genotypes of hepatitis C virus by sequence comparisons in the core, E1 and NS-5 regions. J Gen Virol 75:1053–1061, 1994.
19. Takada N, Takase S, Takada A, et al: Differences in the hepatitis C virus genotypes in different countries. J Hepatol 17:277–283, 1993.
20. Mahaney K, Tedeschi V, Maertens G, et al: Genotypic analysis of hepatitis C virus in American patients. Hepatology 20:1405–1411, 1994.
21. Yamaguchi K, Tanaka E, Higashi K, et al: Adaption of hepatitis C virus for persistent infection in patients with acute hepatitis. Gastroenterology 106:1344–1348, 1994.
22. Shimizu YK, Hijikata M, Iwamoto A, et al: Neutralizing antibodies against hepatitis C virus and the emergence of neutralization escape mutant viruses. J Virol 68:1494–1500, 1994.
23. Abe K, Kurata T, Teramoto Y, et al: Lack of susceptibility of various primates and woodchucks to hepatitis C virus. J Med Primatol 22:433–434, 1993.
24. Shimizu YK, Iwamoto A, Hijikata M, et al: Evidence for in vitro replication of hepatitis C virus genome in a human T-cell line. Proc Natl Acad Sci USA 89:5477–5481, 1992.
25. Shimizu YK, Purcell RH, Yoshikura H: Correlation between the infectivity of hepatitis C virus in vivo and its infectivity in vitro. Proc Natl Acad Sci USA 90:6037–6041, 1993.
26. Shimizu YK, Yoshikura H: Multicycle infection of hepatitis C virus in cell culture and inhibition by alpha and beta interferons. J Virol 68:8406–8408, 1994.
27. Lanford RE, Sureau C, Jacob JR, et al: Demonstration of in vitro infection of chimpanzee hepatocytes with hepatitis C virus using strand-specific RT/PCR. Virology 202:606–614, 1994.
28. Iacovacci S, Sargiacomo M, Parolini I, et al: Replication and multiplication of hepatitis C virus genome in human foetal liver cells. Res Virol 144:275–279, 1993.
29. Harada S, Suzuki R, Ando A, et al: Establishment of a cell line constitutively expressing E2 glycoprotein of hepatitis C virus and humoral response of hepatitis C patients to the expressed protein. J Gen Virol 76:1223–1231, 1995.
30. Kawano S, Ueno T, Fujiyama S, et al: Self-priming of hepatitis C virus RNA. Int Hepatol Commun 2:139–146, 1994.
31. Muller HM, Pfaff E, Goeser T, et al: Peripheral blood leukocytes serve as a possible extrahepatic site for hepatitis C virus replication. J Gen Virol 74:669–676, 1993.
32. Gabrielli A, Manzin A, Candela M, et al: Active hepatitis C virus infection in bone marrow and peripheral blood mononuclear cells from patients with mixed cryoglobulinemia. Clin Exp Immunol 97:87–93, 1994.
33. Shindo M, Di Bisceglie AM, Akatsuka T, et al: The physical state of the negative strand of hepatitis C virus RNA in serum of patients with chronic hepatitis C. Proc Natl Acad Sci USA 91:8719–8723, 1994.
34. Liou T-C, Chang T-T, Young K-C, et al: Detection of HCV RNA in saliva, urine, seminal fluid, and ascites. J Med Virol 37:197–202, 1992.
35. Young K-C, Chang T-T, Liou T-C, et al: Detection of hepatitis C virus RNA in peripheral blood mononuclear cells and in saliva. J Med Virol 41:55–60, 1993.

262

Hepatitis E Virus

Raymond S. Koff

An enterically transmitted form of virus causing hepatitis, resembling but not identical to hepatitis A virus in its epidemiologic behavior and serologically distinct from all other known hepatitis viruses, has been recognized to be responsible for outbreaks of predominantly water-borne hepatitis in the Indian subcontinent; central and Southeast Asia, including the central Asian republics of the former Soviet Union; the Middle East; northern Africa; and, in the Americas, Mexico.[1] The responsible agent, designated hepatitis E virus (HEV), has been partially characterized. It is a spherical, nonenveloped agent with a polyadenylated, positive-sense, single-stranded RNA molecule.[2] It may be a nonenveloped member of the alpha-like RNA virus supergroup. However, firm classification is not yet available. Serologically documented epidemics of hepatitis E have been extant at least since the mid-1950s.[3, 4] It is likely that this infection has a considerably longer history. It is now thought to be the major agent of sporadic hepatitis among young individuals in developing countries.

Another agent, serologically distinct from HEV, may also be responsible for water-borne hepatitis in India,[5] but information about this agent is exceedingly scarce. If this postulate is correct, this agent may be the sixth human hepatitis virus and the third to be spread enterically.

Morphology and Characteristics of the Agent

Spherical virus-like particles, 27 to 34 nm in diameter (Fig. 262–1), have been visualized by electron microscopy or immunoelectron microscopy of stool samples of naturally infected patients and experimentally infected human volunteers and nonhuman primates.[1] Isolates of these HEV particles, recovered from stool samples, have induced hepatitis in inoculated marmosets, cynomolgus and owl monkeys, and chimpanzees. The physicochemical properties of HEV are incompletely understood. HEV appears to be labile and can be inactivated by cycles of freeze-thawing or heating to 100°C. A sedimentation coefficient of 183S and a buoyant density of 1.29 g/cm^3 in a potassium tartrate–glycerol gradient have been reported. A poorly defined and characterized HEV antigen may be present on the surface of HEV particles; it has been identified in the cytoplasm of hepatocytes of experimentally infected cynomolgus macaques, chimpanzees, and *Aotus* monkeys.[6] Its importance remains ill-defined.

Hepatitis E Virus Genome

Molecular cloning of HEV has revealed its RNA genome to be about 7.5 kb in length.[3] Short untranslated regions have been identified at the 5′ and 3′ ends. Three separate, partially overlapping open reading frames (Table 262–1) encoding nonstructural proteins, at the 5′ end, and structural proteins, at the 3′ end, have been identified.[7] The first open reading frame, the longest, encodes a 1690–amino acid protein that is

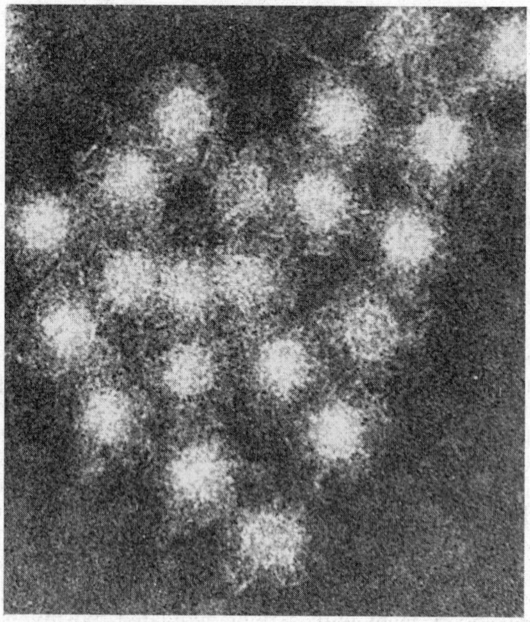

FIGURE 262–1 □ HEV particles, approximately 32 nm in diameter, isolated from stool and aggregated by anti-HEV in acute-phase serum (× 222,566). (Courtesy of Daniel Bradley.)

cleaved into nonstructural replicative proteins, including a methyltransferase, an RNA-dependent RNA polymerase (RNA replicase), a helicase, and a cysteine protease. The second open reading frame, encoding a protein of 660 amino acids, is believed to be the structural, capsid protein gene of HEV. Immunodominant epitopes have been identified in the structural protein encoded by the second open reading frame.[8] The function of the smallest open reading frame, which can encode a protein of 123 amino acids and contains epitopes recognized by antibodies in the sera of infected patients, remains uncertain.

Classification

A relationship of HEV to the caliciviruses was suggested on the basis of studies of its physicochemical properties, the genomic organization, and the electron microscopic observation of spikes and indentations on the surface of the HEV particle. Subsequent analysis of the nonstructural polyprotein domains of HEV has linked HEV to the alpha-like supergroup of positive-stranded RNA viruses.[9]

Genetic Variation

Whereas atypical strains that differ somewhat from the prototype strain in resistance to inactivation and immunoreactivity may exist,[10] it is generally believed that only one serotype of HEV has been identified to date. Nonetheless, few data indicate the existence of genetic variation in isolates from different regions. Nucleotide and amino acid sequence comparisons of a large number of HEV isolates have shown that most isolates within a given geographic region are genetically related.[11] However, isolates recovered from geographically more distant areas tend to show greater diversity. The RNA polymerase region appears to be more highly conserved than other genomic regions. HEV appears not to undergo rapid mutations[12]; strain differences may have emerged in the distant past and are restricted in their circulation. Homologous immunity is suggested by the observation that second attacks of HEV infection have yet to be described.

TABLE 262–1 ■ Hepatitis E Virus Open Reading Frames

OPEN READING FRAME NUMBER	ENCODED AMINO ACIDS	FUNCTION
1	1690	RNA-dependent RNA polymerase (RNA replicase) Helicase Cysteine protease Methyltransferase
2	660	Capsid protein with immunodominant epitopes
3	123	Epitopes (? function)

Propagation

Although propagation of HEV in human embryo lung diploid cells has been claimed,[13] confirmation is not available. In fact, growth of HEV in tissue culture has been unsuccessful in a variety of cell lines, and cytopathic effects have not been observed after direct inoculation of HEV. These studies have included primary African green monkey kidney, primary rhesus monkey kidney, continuous fetal rhesus kidney, continuous human embryonic kidney, and buffalo green monkey cell lines.

Replication

Replication of HEV may be limited to the hepatocyte. Direct studies of HEV replication in infected human beings are not yet available. Although the precise mechanism of replication remains ill-defined, it has been postulated that after HEV enters the hepatocyte, the positive-sense HEV RNA is translated to produce the nonstructural proteins needed for the generation of negative-stranded RNA (antigenomic RNA).[14] HEV antigenomic negative-stranded RNA replicative intermediates have been identified in the liver of experimentally infected rhesus monkeys.[15] Antigenomic RNA may then serve as a template for synthesis of positive-sense RNA and subgenomic RNAs, which produce the structural proteins that encapsidate the positive-sense RNA to form new viral particles. Extensive investigation of the morphogenesis and packaging of HEV in the hepatocyte remains to be undertaken.

References

1. Krawczynski K: Hepatitis E. Hepatology 17:932–941, 1993.
2. Reyes GR, Purdy MA, Kim JP, et al: Isolation of a cDNA from the virus responsible for enterically transmitted non-A, non-B hepatitis. Science 247:1335–1339, 1990.
3. Wong DC, Purcell RH, Sreenivasan MA, et al: Epidemic and endemic hepatitis in India: Evidence for a non-A, non-B hepatitis virus aetiology. Lancet 2:876–878, 1980.
4. Khuroo MS: Study of an epidemic of non-A, non-B hepatitis: Possibility of another human hepatitis virus distinct from post-transfusion non-A, non-B type. Am J Med 68:818–824, 1980.
5. Arankalle VA, Chadha MS, Tsarev SA, et al: Seroepidemiology of water-borne hepatitis in India and evidence for a third enterically-transmitted hepatitis agent. Proc Natl Acad Sci USA 91:3428–3432, 1994.
6. Krawczynski K, Bradley DW: Enterically transmitted non-A, non-B hepatitis: Identification of virus-associated antigen in experimentally infected cynomolgus macaques. J Infect Dis 159:1042–1049, 1989.
7. Tam AW, Smith MM, Guerra ME, et al: Hepatitis E virus (HEV):

Molecular cloning and sequencing of the full-length viral genome. Virology 185:120–131, 1991.
8. Khudyakov YE, Favorov MO, Jue DL, et al: Immunodominant antigenic regions in a structural protein of the hepatitis E virus. Virology 198:390–393, 1994.
9. Purdy MA, Tam AW, Huang C-C, et al: Hepatitis E virus: A nonenveloped member of the 'alpha-like' RNA virus supergroup. Semin Virol 4:319–326, 1993.
10. Chauhan A, Diliwari JB, Kaur U, et al: Atypical strain of hepatitis E virus (HEV) from north India. J Med Virol 44:22–29, 1994.
11. Yin S, Purcell RH, Emerson SU: A new Chinese isolate of hepatitis E virus: Comparison with strains recovered from different geographical regions. Virus Genes 9:23–32, 1994.
12. Yin S, Tsarev SA, Purcell RH, Emerson SU: Partial sequence comparison of eight new Chinese strains of hepatitis E virus suggests the genome sequence is relatively stable. J Med Virol 41:230–241, 1993.
13. Huang RT, Li R, Wei J, et al: Isolation and identification of hepatitis E virus in Xinjiang, China. J Gen Virol 73:1143–1148, 1992.
14. Reyes GR, Huang C-C, Tam AW, Purdy MA: Molecular organization and replication of hepatitis E virus (HEV). Arch Virol Suppl 7:15–25, 1993.
15. Nanda SK, Panda SK, Durgapal H, Jameel S: Detection of the negative strand of hepatitis E virus RNA in the livers of experimentally infected rhesus monkeys: Evidence for viral replication. J Med Virol 42:237–240, 1994.

263

Rotaviruses and Other Reoviridae

John E. Herrmann

The family Reoviridae consists of four genera that infect vertebrate animals: *Orthoreovirus, Coltivirus, Orbivirus,* and *Rotavirus.* Additional genera of viruses infect insects and plants, but these genera are not discussed. The reoviruses (respiratory enteric orphan viruses) were the first to be described. They are the type genus of the family and are the prototype viruses of the genus *Orthoreovirus.* All four of the Reoviridae genera share similar physiochemical characteristics in that they have nonenveloped virions approximately 70 to 80 nm in diameter with inner and outer capsids, and they are unique among viruses in containing double-stranded RNA. The diseases caused by each genus, however, are markedly different. The most important agents of human disease are the rotaviruses, which are the major cause of gastroenteritis in infants and young children. The reoviruses, although they were the first to be recognized and are widespread among animal species and humans, have not been clearly implicated as etiologic agents for any specific disease. The orbiviruses are more important as veterinary pathogens but cause febrile illnesses and possibly other illnesses in humans. Colorado tick fever virus is the important pathogen in the *Coltivirus* genus.

Rotavirus

Worldwide, acute diarrheal diseases are the greatest single cause of infectious disease morbidity and mortality. In Asia, Africa, and Latin America, an estimated 5 million deaths annually are attributed to infectious diarrhea, with the highest mortality occurring in infants and young children. In developed countries, infectious diarrhea is also important, and gastroenteritis due to rotavirus alone causes up to 50% of all pediatric hospitalizations during the winter months.

Although other viruses have been associated with diarrheal disease, the traditional (group A) rotaviruses are considered to be the major viral agents of gastroenteritis of infants and young children. Non–group A rotaviruses have been detected far less frequently. Group B rotaviruses have been associated with epidemics of gastroenteritis in China, primarily in older children and adults.[1] Group C rotaviruses have been implicated in occasional cases of diarrhea in many countries,[2] including the United States.[3]

Characteristics of the Pathogen

Rotaviruses contain double-stranded RNA enclosed in a double capsid (complete or double-shelled particles) and are approximately 70 nm in diameter. Incomplete (or single-shelled) particles of approximately 55 nm in diameter are also found. The intact particles as seen by negative-stain electron microscopy (Fig. 263–1) have a characteristic wheel (Latin *rota*) shape. Double-shelled particles have a density of 1.36 g/cm^3 in cesium chloride.[4, 5]

Electrophoretic analysis has shown the viral genome to be composed of 11 segments of double-stranded RNA. The segments have an estimated total mass of 1.1×10^7 daltons in cesium chloride, and single-shelled particles have a density of 1.38 g/cm^3 in cesium chloride.[4, 5]

Group A rotaviruses contain a group-specific common antigen designated VP6, a protein on the surface of the inner capsid protein. The more recently recognized non–group A rotaviruses, which currently include groups B to G and possi-

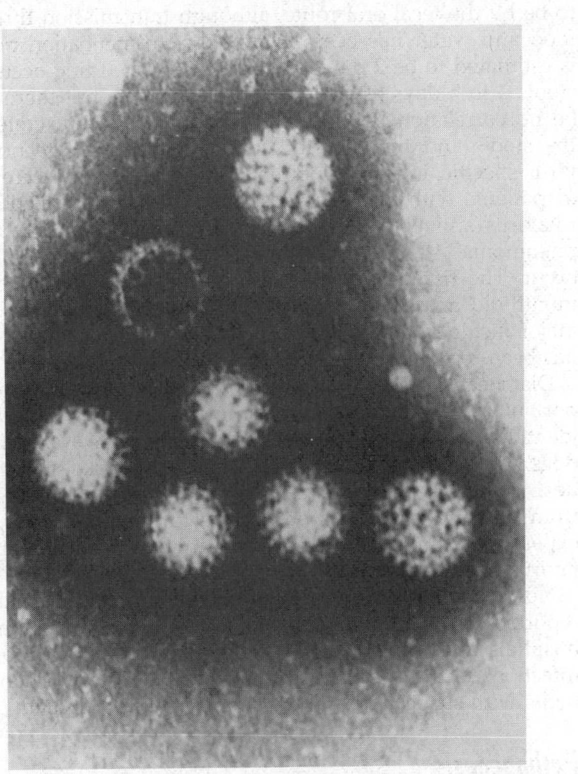

FIGURE 263–1 ▫ Rotavirus particles observed by negative-stain electron microscopy in a stool suspension of a child with diarrhea. (Courtesy of Dr. W. D. Cubitt, Institute of Child Health, London.)

bly others, are morphologically the same as group A rotaviruses but lack the group A common antigen. Group B through G rotaviruses have also been referred to in past studies as non–group A rotaviruses, atypical rotaviruses, or pararotaviruses. These rotaviruses have been detected in pigs,[6, 7] calves, lambs,[8] and chickens[9] as well as in humans.[10]

Serotypes of group A rotaviruses are based on differences in two viral proteins that elicit neutralizing antibodies, VP4 and VP7. Serotypes based on VP7 are designated G types (for glycoprotein), and serotypes based on VP4 are designated P types (for protease-sensitive protein).[5, 11, 12] Because of cross-reactivities seen with antibodies to VP4, P types have also been distinguished on the basis of gene sequences (genotypes). There are currently 14 G serotypes, 9 P serotypes, and 19 P genotypes. Human rotavirus isolates are most commonly in G serotypes 1 to 4 but are also found in G serotypes 6, 8 to 10, and 12. Eight human P serotypes have been described: 1A, 1B, 2, 3A, 3B, 4, 5, and 8. There are also two subgroups, based on antigenic differences in VP6, and numerous electropherotypes based on migration patterns of rotaviral RNA segments in gels.

Rotavirus strains have been shown to retain infectivity at pH 3.5 or pH 10.0 and after treatment with ether, chloroform, fluorocarbons, or proteases.[13] The most effective disinfectants for rotaviruses are 95% ethanol, formalin, and Lysol.[14, 15] Sodium hypochlorite may[16] or may not[15] be effective, and rotaviruses have been shown to survive chlorine treatment in community water supplies.[17]

Epidemiology

Group A rotavirus gastroenteritis occurs primarily in infants and young children. Outbreaks in adults have been reported[18, 19] but do not appear to be common. In temperate climates, rotavirus infections increase sharply during the winter months, whereas in tropical climates, infections usually occur year-round. Transmission of the virus is thought to be by the fecal-oral route, although transmission through food and water has been suggested. The incubation period is estimated to be 2 days. Maximal virus shedding occurs in stools 2 to 5 days after the onset of diarrhea, but there may be no correlation between the amount of virus excreted in the stools and the severity of the diarrhea.[20] Detection of virus-specific immunoglobulin A in pharyngeal secretions of patients with rotavirus gastroenteritis[20] and detection of rotavirus antigen in respiratory secretions of children with pneumonia[21] suggest that transmission by virus aerosols may occur. The frequency of disease is highest in the 6- to 24-month-old age group, and rotavirus is not thought to be a major factor in infant mortality in developing countries but has been reported.[22]

Diarrheal diseases due to rotavirus infections are also important in young farm animals, and rotaviruses have been identified in a number of species including monkeys, apes,[23–25] dogs,[26, 27] cats,[28] rabbits,[29] mice,[30] chickens, turkeys,[31, 32] and deer.[33] There is no evidence that natural virus transmission from humans to animals or animals to humans occurs, but experimental infection of newborn animals with human rotavirus strains may result in symptomatic infection.[34]

Nosocomial infections are not uncommon, and it has been reported that approximately 20% of rotavirus infections in hospitals were considered nosocomial.[35, 36] Thus, appropriate infection control measures should be undertaken when patients with suspected viral gastroenteritis are admitted.

Pathogenesis

Rotavirus-induced diarrhea appears to be due to decreased absorption of salt and water related to selective infection of the absorptive intestinal villus cells, which results in net fluid secretion. Depressed levels of disaccharidases[37] and impaired D-xylose absorption have been observed.[38] Pale, fatty stools have been associated with rotaviral diarrhea, suggesting that rotavirus infection may interfere with digestion of fats and pigmentation of feces.[39] Villus shortening, reticular cell enlargement, mitochondrial swelling, lymphocyte infiltration of the villous lamina propria, and irregular microvilli have been observed in histopathologic studies. The pathogenesis of non–group A rotavirus diarrhea appears to be similar, although the occurrence of syncytia on the surface of villi has been detected in a number of animal species and may be a pathognomonic lesion for non–group A rotavirus infections.[40]

Clinical Manifestations

Common clinical findings usually include vomiting, abdominal distress, diarrhea, and mild dehydration. Fever and vomiting frequently precede diarrhea. In one study of children with confirmed rotavirus gastroenteritis, temperature of 37.9°C to 39°C was found in 46% and greater than 39°C in 31% of these patients.[41] Other findings may include irritability and pharyngeal or tympanic membrane erythema. Stools are typically watery and usually do not contain blood or leukocytes. Dehydration and associated electrolyte imbalance may occur in severe cases, requiring hospitalization. Fatalities are rare in developed nations but are common in developing nations, where rotavirus produces more severe dehydration than bacterial diarrheas do. The course of rotavirus disease is generally 3 to 9 days, and the mean time of hospitalization when required is 4 days.[42]

Rotavirus infections have been associated with a variety of conditions such as intussusception, Reye's syndrome, hemolytic-uremic syndrome, and Kawasaki syndrome, but disease association with rotavirus is strongest for some cases of neonatal necrotizing enterocolitis.[43] Chronic symptomatic infections occur in patients with primary immunodeficiency diseases, and severe disease may occur in those who are immunosuppressed for bone marrow transplantation.

Asymptomatic rotavirus infections are common, especially in newborn children, and the association of illness with rotavirus infection increases with the age of the child up to the age of 2 years. Virus shedding was associated with diarrhea in 29% of neonates, in 50% of children age 1 to 6 months, and in 74% of children 7 to 24 months old.[44] Infection in adults is usually asymptomatic, but severe illness has been reported both in elderly patients[18] and in apparently normal young adults.[19] Severe gastroenteritis in adults due to non–group A rotaviruses has been reported in China.[1] In a comparison of rotavirus illness in children and adults in families, the infection rate was 32% in children compared with 17% for adults, and 70% of infected children were symptomatic, whereas only 40% of the infected adults were symptomatic.[45] The strains that infect newborns asymptomatically may not be different from the strains causing illness in older infants.[46]

Diagnosis

Before virus cultivation techniques and immunoassays were developed for rotavirus detection, electron microscopy was the major technique used. For isolation of rotavirus from clinical materials, the use of primary African green monkey kidney or cynomolgus monkey kidney cells appears to be more effective than MA104 cells,[47–49] but isolation of human strains is still considered to be inefficient, and the methods are time-consuming.

Several tests have been developed for diagnosis of rotavirus infection, but antigen detection by enzyme-linked immunosorbent assay (ELISA) is now the preferred method, and tests are available from a number of manufacturers. Commercially produced tests that use polyclonal serum may give false-positive results, especially in stool samples from neonates.[50–52] The use of monoclonal antibody to the rotaviral group antigen in ELISA has been found to give higher sensitivity than polyclonal antibodies, and it eliminates the problems of nonspecificity.[53, 54] An ELISA that uses sensitized latex particles on membrane filters is more rapid than standard ELISAs are, but the test has been found unreliable for use with frozen stool samples.[55] An ELISA for non–group A rotaviruses has been described[56] but is not widely available. Whether routine testing for the non–group A rotaviruses will become necessary depends on the results of future epidemiologic studies. Latex agglutination tests for detection of rotavirus antigen in stool samples are also available from several commercial sources. To date, all use polystyrene particles sensitized with polyclonal antibody, although monoclonal antibody–based tests have been reported.[57] The tests are convenient to use and can usually be done more rapidly than ELISA but may be far less sensitive than ELISA.[58–60]

The preferred specimen for viral antigen detection is a freshly collected undiluted stool sample, although other specimens such as anal swabs can be used. Samples to be assayed for rotavirus may be shipped on wet ice, and stored for a few days at 4°C, but the preferred method for handling virus samples is to send them on dry ice, with subsequent storage at −70°C.

Additional tests may be necessary for confirmation if a definitive diagnosis cannot be obtained with commercially produced or other rotavirus assays. The best method is gel electrophoresis; electron microscopy or immunoelectron microscopy can also be used, if available.

The availability of monoclonal antibodies to subgroup antigens[61, 62] and to specific G and P serotypes[63, 64] permits diagnosis of rotaviruses as to specific subgroup and serotype, but this is not routinely done or required because the disease produced by different subgroups or serogroups is indistinguishable. Use of these antibodies does, however, facilitate classification of rotavirus isolates in epidemiologic studies. The use of polymerase chain reaction may not result in increased sensitivity over other methods, but it does permit serotype identification.[65]

Treatment

There is presently no specific antiviral therapy for rotavirus infections. Ribavirin has been shown to inhibit animal rotaviruses in vitro, but it was not effective against murine rotavirus infection in vivo.[66] Treatment with rotavirus-specific neutralizing antibodies given orally to infants with acute gastroenteritis was not effective,[67] but it was effective in resolving chronic rotavirus diarrhea in immunodeficient children.[68] Treatment, therefore, is usually directed at prevention of severe dehydration and electrolyte imbalance. Use of oral rehydration salt solutions containing glucose or sucrose has been shown to be as effective as intravenous fluid therapy for mild to moderately severe dehydrating rotavirus gastroenteritis.[69] The standard World Health Organization formula consists, per liter of water, of glucose 20 g, sodium chloride 3.5 g, sodium bicarbonate 2.5 g, and potassium chloride 1.5 g. Oral rehydration solutions are also commercially available. Intravenous therapy must be administered if oral rehydration is not successful in replacing fluids and electrolytes or if the patient is in shock or is severely dehydrated.

Prevention

It is thought that diarrhea in developing countries is not likely to be reduced by improved sanitation and water supplies; thus, control measures will require effective vaccines.[70] The principal approach taken in more recent years has been active immunization with live, attenuated rotavirus. The first series of studies were done with orally administered animal strains of rotavirus, and three vaccines have been used the most in field trials. One uses the Nebraska calf diarrhea virus strain of bovine rotavirus, another the WC3 bovine rotavirus strain, and the third a rhesus rotavirus strain.

Field trials in Finland with the Nebraska calf diarrhea virus vaccine, designated RIT 4237, indicated that a high level of protection was obtained in infants vaccinated at age 6 to 12 months. Infants vaccinated at age 7 days were also found to be protected in two of three studies.[71] Seroconversion occurred in approximately 50% of the vaccine recipients. The RIT 4237 vaccine was also found efficacious in protecting children in Lima, Peru.[72] Studies in Butare, Rwanda, with the same vaccine, however, did not show any protective effect.[73] Further, there was no significant difference in the rates of seroconversion between the 122 vaccine and 123 placebo recipients. Lack of protection was also found in a study of Gambian children, which involved 170 vaccine and 83 placebo recipients.[74] There were no clear reasons for the failure of the vaccine in either study, although interference by other enteric viruses might be a factor.[75, 76] Because of these vaccine failures, the manufacturer withdrew RIT 4237 from further studies. It has also been suggested that breast-feeding could interfere with vaccines owing to antirotavirus antibody and nonspecific rotavirus inhibitors.[75–78] To avoid these potential problems, vaccination of neonates was investigated by Vesikari and colleagues,[79] who administered RIT 4237 vaccine to 119 newborn infants and placebo to 120 others in Finland. The vaccine gave no protection against rotavirus infection but did appear to lessen the severity of diarrhea. In naturally occurring outbreaks in neonates, protection against gastroenteritis seemed to be serotype specific and to be related to levels of neutralizing antibody against the homotypic virus.[80] This suggests that a rotavirus vaccine may need to contain all four of the known medically important serotypes to produce sufficient protection.

The rhesus rotavirus vaccine has been found to be more immunogenic than vaccines based on bovine rotavirus strain.[81] In clinical trials with the rhesus rotavirus vaccine, a study involving 41 vaccines and 32 control children in the United States found no significant differences in the frequency of rotavirus diarrhea among vaccine or placebo recipients.[82] Other studies have shown protection to vary from year to year.[83, 84] The vaccine has also been evaluated in Venezuela,[85] where it was found during a 1-year surveillance period that there were 5 episodes of rotavirus diarrhea in the 123 vaccinated infants, compared with 16 episodes in the 124 infants who had received placebo. It may be that this vaccine is more effective in inducing protection against its close human serotype 3 relative, rather than against the other human serotypes. These two animal virus vaccines have not been directly compared for efficacy in preventing rotavirus diarrhea, but the rhesus rotavirus vaccine has been tested in Finland in a setting comparable to the one used for the RIT 4237 vaccine trials.[86] Of 100 children receiving vaccine, there were two episodes of rotavirus diarrhea compared with six in the 100 receiving placebo, leading the authors to conclude that the degree of protection was similar to that obtained with the RIT 4237 vaccine. The WC3 bovine rotavirus vaccine has also shown variable rates of protection[87, 88] and was particularly ineffective in developing countries.[89]

Efforts to improve efficacy of the animal vaccines are being undertaken by production of viral gene reassortants with human virus strains to produce vaccines that express human G proteins but retain the attenuated characteristics of the animal strains.[90–94] Both rhesus rotavirus and bovine WC3 rotavirus reassortant vaccines containing gene segments coding for neutralization proteins for human G serotypes have been prepared and tested for safety, immunogenicity, and efficacy in humans. The vaccines have given protection rates of 63% to 77% in studies to date.[93–95] Further details on various reassortant vaccines under development have been reviewed.[94]

Rotavirus strains of human origin have also been evaluated for use as vaccines. A naturally attenuated nursery strain vaccine that cross-reacts with G serotypes 1 through 4 has been tested but did not provide protection against rotavirus disease.[96] Cold-adapted human rotaviruses were found to give irregular neutralizing antibody responses of low titer.[94]

Methods for passive immunization have been investigated as well. Human breast milk contains rotavirus-specific immunoglobulin, and this immunoglobulin A can be transferred to neonates and detected in the neonates' feces.[97] This may account, in part, for the protective, antiinfective properties of breast milk.[98] Passive immunization by artificial means has been successfully demonstrated to prevent rotavirus illness in animals, as has oral administration of rotavirus-specific antibodies to neonates[99] or children.[100] Current interest in prevention, however, has concentrated on vaccine development. Because the current vaccines do not provide complete protection, new approaches to immunization will continue to be needed.

New approaches that have shown promise in animal models of rotavirus infection include the use of virus-like particles prepared from recombinant proteins[101] and plasmid DNA vaccines encoding specific rotavirus proteins.[102]

Reovirus

Serologic surveys indicate that reovirus infections in humans are common and widespread, but most of these infections appear either to be inapparent or to result in mild symptoms. At one time, these viruses were included among the echoviruses (enteric cytopathic human orphan viruses) before more complete characterization. When they were reclassified as reoviruses,[103] the orphan label was retained to indicate the lack of association with specific diseases. A more extensive review of these viruses is available.[104]

Characteristics of the Pathogen

Reoviruses (which are also called orthoreoviruses to avoid confusion with the family Reoviridae) are nonenveloped viruses of approximately 75 nm in diameter. Complete particles have a double capsid, and the virions contain double-stranded RNA that has 10 segments. Reoviruses can be inactivated by treatment with 70% ethanol for 1 hour at room temperature, but they may not be inactivated by other commonly used disinfectants.[105, 106] There are three distinct serotypes of human reoviruses, but all three share a common group antigen as detected by complement fixation or immunodiffusion.[103, 107]

Epidemiology

Reoviruses have frequently been isolated from the stool samples of infants and children, and seroepidemiologic studies indicate that more than 70% of children acquire antibodies to reovirus before the age of 5 years.[108] Thus, it appears that reovirus infections occur primarily in younger children, although no definitive association with disease has been established. The mode of transmission has also not been established, but the ability to isolate these viruses from stools and respiratory secretions along with their relatively stable nature suggests that reoviruses are transmitted by a fecal-oral route, and possibly by a respiratory route, in a manner similar to that proposed for enteroviruses and rotaviruses.

Reovirus infections have also been reported in a variety of animal species, including farm animals, cats, dogs, and nonhuman primates.[107] There are avian strains that do not share mammalian reovirus group antigens. There is no evidence of transmission of reoviruses between humans and animals.

Clinical Manifestations

Reovirus infections in avian and mammalian animal species are clearly associated with respiratory illnesses,[109, 110] but no specific clinical manifestations are well documented for human infections. However, there has been some correlation of minor respiratory symptoms both in children and in adult volunteers.[111, 112] An association of reovirus type 3 with biliary atresia in infants has been reported,[113, 114] and reoviruses have also been associated with neurologic and exanthemal illnesses,[109, 114] but the significance of these findings remains to be established.

Diagnosis

Detection of either reovirus antigen or antibody can be used to diagnose reovirus infections. Isolation of virus in primary *Macaca* kidney cell cultures or in mouse L cells is usually from fecal samples or from throat and nasal swabs. Direct detection of antigen in fixed tissues by immunofluorescent or immunoperoxidase staining can also be done. Paired acute- and convalescent-phase serum samples can be used to detect seroconversion by hemagglutination inhibition, complement fixation, or virus neutralization. Details of methods for detection of reovirus and antibodies are available elsewhere.[104, 115]

Treatment and Prevention

No specific treatment or prevention measures have been recommended for reovirus infections in humans because of the lack of definitive association with disease. Vaccine preparations are available for veterinary use.[109]

Orbivirus

Orbiviruses are arthropod-borne viruses classified as a genus of the family Reoviridae; the genus contains viruses that cause infections in animals and in humans. The most important diseases in animals are bluetongue in sheep and other ruminants and African horse sickness. The importance and epidemiology of orbiviruses in humans are not well defined, but several have been associated with disease. Tick-borne viruses of the Kemerovo serogroup have caused severe febrile illness in eastern Europe and in the western United States.[116] Other orbiviruses that have been implicated in febrile illnesses include Changuinola virus (Panama), Lebombo virus, and Orungo virus (Africa).

Characteristics of the Pathogen

All of the orbiviruses have nonenveloped virions of approximately 80 nm in diameter with a double capsid. The inner capsid contains circular capsomers, hence the genus name (Latin *orbis,* meaning "orbit" or "circle"). The double-stranded RNA contains 10 segments. There are more than

100 subtypes as distinguished by virus neutralization tests, but orbiviruses do not share a group antigen.

Coltivirus

There are two recognized serotypes (Eyach and Colorado tick fever viruses) and nine probable serotypes in this genus.[116] Colorado tick fever virus was originally classified as an orbivirus, but because it has 12 rather than 10 genome segments, it is now classified in the *Coltivirus* genus.[116] Colorado tick fever is the only well-defined disease caused by coltiviruses and is the only one discussed here.

Epidemiology

The geographic distribution of colorado tick fever virus is similar to that of its tick vector, *Dermacentor andersoni,* and includes the western United States and parts of Alberta and British Columbia in Canada. The virus is transmitted to humans by infected ticks; the major occurrence is in spring and early summer. Other tick species may be infected but have not been shown to be a vector for human disease. Rodents, especially ground squirrels and chipmunks, are important reservoirs for the virus. Infections of humans are associated with occupational or recreational exposure to infected ticks in epidemic areas. There are approximately 100 to 200 cases reported per year, although the true incidence is thought to be several times higher.[117] Infection of *D. andersoni* ticks may be as high as 20% in some areas.[118]

Pathogenesis and Clinical Manifestations

Colorado tick fever virus infects erythrocyte precursors in bone marrow and may persist in erythrocytes for up to 20 weeks[119] without apparent lysis or damage of the cells. Pathogenesis in humans is not well characterized, but infection may cause pathologic changes, especially in the myocardium and liver.[120, 121]

After an incubation period of 3 to 6 days, illness may include high fever, chills, lethargy, nausea, myalgia, and ocular pain. Fever is biphasic in about 50% of cases. A macular rash may or may not be present. Neurologic symptoms may also occur. The disease is rarely fatal, and recovery is usually complete after 7 to 10 days, although convalescence may be prolonged.[122] A rapid drop in the peripheral leukocyte count to 2000 to 3000/mm^3 is the major laboratory finding.

Diagnosis

Viral antigen can be detected directly by immunofluorescent staining of blood smears[123] or by immunofluorescent staining of blood smears after inoculation of suckling mice with patients' blood. Colorado tick fever virus can be cultivated in cell culture, but the technique is not considered sensitive enough for primary virus isolation. If paired acute- and convalescent-phase serum samples are available, an indirect immunofluorescent test with cell culture infected with high-titer virus stocks can be used to demonstrate seroconversion to Colorado tick fever virus.[124] ELISA procedures for detection of immunoglobulin G and immunoglobulin M antibodies to Colorado tick fever virus have also been described.[125]

Treatment and Prevention

Specific antiviral therapy is not available, and treatment for the disease is symptomatic (antipyretic, analgesic). There are no vaccines available for general use, although experimental vaccines have been reported,[126] so prevention is accomplished by avoidance of tick-infested areas, use of tick repellents, and rapid removal of ticks before they become attached. To prevent possible Colorado tick fever virus transmission by transfusion, patients should not donate blood for 6 months after recovery.

References

1. Hung T, Chen G, Wang C, et al: Waterborne outbreak of rotavirus diarrhoea in adults in China caused by a novel rotavirus. Lancet 1:1139, 1984.
2. Penaranda M, Cubitt WD, Sinarachatanant P, et al: Group C rotavirus infection in patients with diarrhea in Thailand, Nepal and England. J Infect Dis 160:392, 1989.
3. Jiang B, Dennehy PH, Spangenberger S, et al: First detection of group C rotavirus in fecal specimens of children with diarrhea in the United States. J Infect Dis 172:45, 1995.
4. Kapikian AZ, Kalica AR, Shih JW, et al: Buoyant density in cesium chloride of the human reovirus-like agent of infantile gastroenteritis by ultracentrifugation, electron microscopy, and complement fixation. Virology 70:564, 1976.
5. Estes MK, Cohen J: Rotavirus gene structure and function. Microbiol Rev 53:410, 1989.
6. Bohl EH, Saif LJ, Theil KW, et al: Porcine pararotavirus: Detection, differentiation from rotavirus, and pathogenesis in gnotobiotic piglets. J Clin Microbiol 15:312, 1982.
7. Bridger JC, Clarke IN, McCrae MA: Characterization of an antigenically distinct porcine rotavirus. Infect Immun 35:1058, 1982.
8. Snodgrass DR, Herring AJ, Campbell JM, et al: Comparison of atypical rotaviruses from calves, piglets, lambs and man. J Gen Virol 65:909, 1984.
9. McNulty MS, Allan GM, Todd D, et al: Isolation from chickens of a rotavirus lacking the group antigen. J Gen Virol 55:405, 1981.
10. Espejo RT, Puerto F, Soler C, et al: Characterization of human pararotavirus. Infect Immun 44:112, 1984.
11. Gorziglia M, Larralde G, Kapikian AZ, Chanock RM: Antigenic relationships among human rotaviruses as determined by outer capsid protein VP4. Proc Natl Acad Sci USA 87:7155, 1990.
12. Larralde G, Gorziglia M: Distribution of conserved and specific epitopes on the VP8 subunit of rotavirus VP4. J Virol 66:7438, 1992.
13. Estes MK, Palmer EL, Obijeski JF: Rotaviruses: A review. Curr Top Microbiol Immunol 105:123, 1985.
14. Tan JA, Schnagl RD: Inactivation of a rotavirus by disinfectants. Med J Aust 1:19, 1981.
15. Snodgrass DR, Herring JA: The activity of disinfectant on lamb rotavirus. Vet Rec 101:81, 1977.
16. Tan JA, Schnagl RD: Rotavirus inactivated by a hypochlorite-based disinfectant: A reappraisal. Med J Aust 1:550, 1983.
17. Smith EM, Gerba CP: Development of a method for detection of human rotavirus in water and sewage. Appl Environ Microbiol 43:1440, 1982.
18. Marrie TJ, Lee SHS, Faulkner RS, et al: Rotavirus infection in a geriatric population. Arch Intern Med 142:313, 1982.
19. Echeverria P, Blacklow NR, Cukor G, et al: Rotavirus as a cause of severe gastroenteritis in adults. J Clin Microbiol 18:663, 1983.
20. Stals F, Walther FJ, Bruggeman CA: Faecal and pharyngeal shedding of rotavirus and rotavirus IgA in children with diarrhoea. J Med Virol 14:333, 1984.
21. Santocham M, Yolken RH, Quiroz E, et al: Detection of rotavirus in respiratory secretions of children with pneumonia. J Pediatr 103:583, 1983.
22. Carlson JAK, Middleton PJ, Szymanski M, et al: Fatal rotavirus gastroenteritis: An analysis of 21 cases. Am J Dis Child 132:477, 1978.
23. Malherbe HH, Strickland-Cholmley M: Simian virus SA-11 and the related "O" agent. Arch Ges Virusforsch 22:235, 1967.
24. Stuker G, Oshiro LS, Schmidt NJ, et al: Virus detection in monkeys with diarrhea: The association of adenoviruses with diarrhea and the possible role of rotaviruses. Lab Anim Sci 29:610, 1979.
25. Ashley CR, Caul EO, Clark SKR, et al: Rotavirus infections of apes. Lancet 2:477, 1978.

26. Roseto A, Lema F, Sitbon M, et al: Detection of rotavirus in dogs. Soc Occup Med 7:478, 1979.
27. England JJ, Poston RP: Electron microscopic identification and subsequent isolation of a rotavirus from a dog with fatal neonatal diarrhea. Am J Vet Res 41:782, 1980.
28. Snodgrass DR, Angus KW, Gray EW: A rotavirus from kittens. Vet Rec 104:222, 1979.
29. Bryden AS, Thouless ME, Flewett TH: A rabbit rotavirus. Vet Rec 99:323, 1976.
30. Much D, Zajac I: Purification and characterization of epizootic diarrhea of infant mice virus. Infect Immun 6:1019, 1972.
31. Jones RC, Hughes CS, Henry RR: Rotavirus infection in commercial laying hens. Vet Rec 104:22, 1979.
32. McNulty MS, Allan GM, Todd D, et al: Isolation and cell culture propagation of rotaviruses from turkeys and chickens. Arch Virol 61:13, 1979.
33. Tzipori S, Caple TW, Butler R: Isolation of a rotavirus from deer. Vet Rec 99:398, 1976.
34. Wyatt RG, Mebus CA, Yolken RH, et al: Rotaviral immunity in gnotobiotic calves: Heterologous resistance to human virus induced by bovine virus. Science 203:548, 1979.
35. Ryder RW, McGowan JE, Hatch MH, et al: Reovirus-like agent as a cause of nosocomial diarrhea in infants. J Pediatr 90:698, 1977.
36. Black RE, Merson MH, Rahman ASMM, et al: A two-year study of bacterial, viral and parasitic agents associated with diarrhea in rural Bangladesh. J Infect Dis 142:660, 1980.
37. Bishop RF, Davidson GP, Holmes IH, et al: Virus particles in epithelial cells of duodenal mucosa from children with viral gastroenteritis. Lancet 2:1281, 1973.
38. Mavromichalis J, Evans N, McNeish AS, et al: Intestinal damage in rotavirus and adenovirus gastroenteritis assessed by D-xylose malabsorption. Arch Dis Child 52:589, 1977.
39. Thomas MEM, Luton P, Matimer JY: Virus diarrhoea associated with pale fatty faeces. J Hyg (Lond) 87:313, 1981.
40. Hall GA: Comparative pathology of infection by novel diarrhoea viruses. Ciba Found Symp 128:218, 1987.
41. Rodriguez WJ, Kim HW, Arrobio JO, et al: Clinical features of acute gastroenteritis associated with human reovirus-like agent in infants and young children. J Pediatr 91:188, 1977.
42. Middleton PJ, Szymanski MT, Petric M: Viruses associated with acute gastroenteritis in young children. Am J Dis Child 131:733, 1977.
43. Rotbart HA, Nelson WL, Glode MP, et al: Neonatal rotavirus associated necrotizing enterocolitis: Case control study and prospective surveillance during an outbreak. J Pediatr 112:87, 1988.
44. Champsaur H, Questiaux E, Prevot J, et al: Rotavirus carriage, asymptomatic infection and disease in the first years of life. I. Virus shedding. J Infect Dis 149:667, 1984.
45. Wenman WM, Hinde D, Feltham S, et al: Rotavirus infection in adults: Result of a prospective family study. N Engl J Med 301:303, 1979.
46. Vial PA, Kotloff KL, Losonsky GA: Molecular epidemiology of rotavirus infection in a room for convalescing newborns. J Infect Dis 157:668, 1988.
47. Hasegaws A, Matsuno S, Inouye S, et al: Isolation of human rotavirus in primary cultures of monkey kidney cells. J Clin Microbiol 16:387, 1982.
48. Ward RL, Knowlton DR, Pierce MJ: Efficiency of human rotavirus propagation in cell culture. J Clin Microbiol 19:748, 1984.
49. Naguib T, Wyatt RG, Mohieldin MS, et al: Cultivation and subgroup determination of human rotaviruses from Egyptian infants and young children. J Clin Microbiol 19:210, 1984.
50. Krause PJ, Hyams JS, Middleton PJ, et al: Unreliability of Rotazyme ELISA test in neonates. J Pediatr 103:259, 1983.
51. Chrystie IL, Totterdell BM, Banatvala JE: False positive Rotazyme tests on faecal samples from babies. Lancet 2:1028, 1983.
52. Rotbart HA, Yolken RH, Nelson WL, et al: Confirmatory testing of Rotazyme results in neonates. J Pediatr 107:289, 1985.
53. Herrmann JE, Blacklow NR, Perron DM, et al: Monoclonal antibody enzyme immunoassays for the detection of rotavirus in stool specimens. J Infect Dis 152:830, 1985.
54. Dennehy PH, Gauntlet DR, Tente WE: Comparison of nine commercial immunoassays for the detection of rotavirus in fecal specimens. J Clin Microbiol 26:1630, 1988.
55. Brooks RG, Brown L, Franklin RB: Comparison of a new rapid test (Test Pack Rotavirus) with standard enzyme immunoassay and electron microscopy for the detection of rotavirus in symptomatic hospitalized children. J Clin Microbiol 27:775, 1989.
56. Brown DWG, Beards GM, Guang-Mu C, et al: Prevalence of antibody to group B (atypical) rotavirus in humans and animals. J Clin Microbiol 25:316, 1987.
57. Pothier P, Limone F, Kohli E, et al: Development and preliminary evaluation of a latex agglutination test using a monoclonal antibody for rotavirus detection in stool specimens. Ann Inst Pasteur 138:523, 1987.
58. Morinet F, Ferchal F, Colimon R, et al: Comparison of six methods for detecting human rotavirus in stools. Eur J Clin Microbiol 3:136, 1984.
59. Knisley CV, Bednarz-Prashad AJ, Pickering LK: Detection of rotavirus in stool specimens and monoclonal and polyclonal antibody-based assay system. J Clin Microbiol 23:897, 1986.
60. Doern GV, Herrmann JE, Henderson P, et al: Detection of rotavirus with a new polyclonal antibody enzyme immunoassay (Rotazyme II) and a commercial latex agglutination test (Rotalex): Comparison with a monoclonal antibody enzyme immunoassay. J Clin Microbiol 23:226, 1986.
61. Lambert KP, Marbehant P, Marissens D, et al: Monoclonal antibodies directed against different antigenic determinants of rotavirus. J Virol 51:47, 1984.
62. Taniguchi K, Urasawa T, Urasawa S, et al: Production of subgroup-specific monoclonal antibodies against human rotavirus and their application to an enzyme-linked immunosorbent assay for subgroup determination. J Med Virol 14:115, 1984.
63. Coulson BS, Unicomb LE, Pitson GA, et al: Simple and specific enzyme immunoassay using monoclonal antibodies for serotyping human rotaviruses. J Clin Microbiol 25:509, 1987.
64. Taniguchi K, Urasawa T, Morita Y, et al: Direct serotyping of human rotaviruses in stools by an enzyme-linked immunosorbent assay using serotype 1-, 2-, 3- and 4-specific monoclonal antibodies to VP7. J Infect Dis 155:1159, 1987.
65. Gouveau V, Glass P, Woods K, et al: Polymerase chain reaction amplification and typing of rotavirus nucleic acids from stool specimens. J Clin Microbiol 28:276, 1990.
66. Schoub BD, Prozesky DW: Antiviral activity of ribavirin in rotavirus gastroenteritis in mice. Antimicrob Agents Chemother 12:543, 1977.
67. Hilpert H, Brussow H, Mieten C, et al: Use of bovine milk concentrate containing antibody to rotavirus to treat rotavirus gastroenteritis in infants. J Infect Dis 156:158, 1987.
68. Guarino A, Guandalini S, Albano F, et al: Enteral immunoglobulins for treatment of protracted rotaviral diarrhea. Pediatr Infect Dis 10:612, 1991.
69. Santosham M, Daun RS, Dillman L, et al: Oral rehydration therapy of infantile diarrhea. A controlled study of well-nourished children hospitalized in the United States and Panama. N Engl J Med 306:159, 1985.
70. Bishop RF: Development of candidate rotavirus vaccines. Vaccine 11:247, 1993.
71. Vesikari T: Clinical trials of live oral rotavirus vaccines: The Finnish experience. Vaccine 2:255, 1993.
72. Lanata CF, Black RE, del Aguila R, et al: Protection of Peruvian children against rotavirus diarrhea of specific serotypes by one, two, or three doses of the RIT 4237 attenuated bovine rotavirus vaccine. J Infect Dis 159:453, 1989.
73. DeMol P, Zissis G, Butzler JP, et al: Failure of live, attenuated oral rotavirus vaccine. Lancet 2:108, 1986.
74. Hanlon P, Marsh V, Shenton F, et al: Trial of an attenuated bovine rotavirus vaccine (RIT 4237) in Gambian infants. Lancet 1:1342, 1986.
75. Edelman R: Perspective on the development and deployment of rotavirus vaccine. Pediatr Infect Dis J 6:704, 1987.
76. Albert MG: Failure of live, oral vaccine in developing countries. J Infect Dis 155:1350, 1987.
77. McLean BS, Holmes IH: Effects of antibodies, trypsin and trypsin inhibitors on susceptibility of neonates to rotavirus infection. J Clin Microbiol 13:33, 1981.
78. Berger R, Hadziselimovic F, Just M, Reigel F: Influence of breast milk on nosocomial rotavirus infection in infants. Infection 12:171, 1984.
79. Vesikari T, Isolauri E, Delem A, et al: Clinical efficacy of the RIT 4237 live attenuated bovine rotavirus vaccine in infants vaccinated before a rotavirus epidemic. J Pediatr 107:189, 1985.

80. Chiba S, Yokoyama T, Nakata S, et al: Protective effect of naturally acquired homotypic and heterotypic rotavirus antibodies. Lancet 2:417, 1986.
81. Vesikari T, Kapikian AZ, Delem A, et al: A comparative trial of rhesus monkey (RRV-1) and bovine (RIT 4237) oral rotavirus vaccines in young child. J Infect Dis 153:832, 1986.
82. Wright PF, Tajima T, Thompson J, et al: Candidate rotavirus vaccine (rhesus rotavirus strain) in children: An evaluation. Pediatrics 80:473, 1987.
83. Christy C, Madore HP, Pichichero ME, et al: Field trial of rhesus rotavirus vaccines in infants. Pediatr Infect Dis J 7:647, 1988.
84. Madore HP, Christy C, Pichichero M, et al: Field trial of rhesus rotavirus or human-rhesus rotavirus reassortant vaccine of vp7 serotype 3 or 1 specificity in infants. J Infect Dis 166:235, 1992.
85. Flores J, Perez-Schael I, Gonzalez M, et al: Protection against severe rotavirus diarrhoea by rhesus rotavirus vaccine in Venezuelan infants. Lancet 1:822, 1987.
86. Vesikari T, Isoauri E, Ruuska T, et al: Clinical trials of rotavirus vaccines. Ciba Found Symp 128:218, 1987.
87. Clark HF, Borian FE, Bell LM, et al: Protective effect of WC3 vaccine against rotavirus diarrhea in infants during a predominantly serotype 1 rotavirus season. J Infect Dis 158:570, 1988.
88. Bernstein DI, Smith VE, Sander DS, et al: Evaluation of WC3 rotavirus vaccine and correlates of protection in healthy infants. J Infect Dis 162:1055, 1990.
89. Georges-Courbot MC, Monges J, Siopathis MR, et al: Evaluation of the efficacy of a low passage bovine rotavirus vaccine (strain WC3) in children in Central Africa. Res Virol 142:405, 1991.
90. Midthun K, Greenberg B, Hoshino Y, et al: Reassortant rotaviruses as potential live rotavirus vaccine candidates. J Virol 53:949, 1985.
91. Hoshino Y, Saif LJ, Sereno NM, et al: Infection immunity of piglets to either VP3 or VP7 outer capsid protein confers resistance to challenge with a virulent rotavirus bearing the corresponding antigen. J Virol 62:744, 1988.
92. Halsey NA, Anderson EL, Sears SD, et al: Human-rhesus reassortant vaccines: Safety and immunogenicity in adults, infants, and children. J Infect Dis 158:1261, 1988.
93. Vesikari T, Ruuska T, Green K, et al: Protective efficacy against serotype 1 rotavirus diarrhea by live oral-rhesus reassortant rotavirus vaccines with human rotavirus vp7 serotype 1 or 2 specificity. Pediatr Infect Dis J 11:535, 1992.
94. Offitt PA, Clark HF: Vaccines for enteric viral pathogens. *In* Blaser MJ (ed): Infections of the Gastrointestinal Tract. New York, Raven Press, 1995, pp 1471–1478.
95. Bernstein DI, Glass RI, Rodgers G, et al: Evaluation of rhesus rotavirus monovalent and tetravalent reassortant vaccines in US children. US Rotavirus Vaccine Efficacy Group. JAMA 273: 1191, 1995.
96. Vesikari T, Ruuska T, Koivu H-P, et al: Evaluation of the M37 human rotavirus vaccine in 2- to 6-month-old infants. Pediatr Infect Dis J 10:912, 1991.
97. Rahmen MM, Yamauchi M, Hanada N, et al: Local production of rotavirus-specific IgA in breast tissue and transfer to neonates. Arch Dis Child 62:401, 1987.
98. Welsh JK, May TT: Anti-infective properties of breast milk. J Pediatr 94:1, 1979.
99. Barnes GL, Doyle IW, Hewson PH, et al: A randomised trial of oral gammaglobulin in low-birth-weight infants infected with rotavirus. Lancet 1:1371, 1983.
100. Ebina T, Sato A, Umezu K, et al: Prevention of rotavirus infection by cow colostrum containing antibody against human rotavirus. Lancet 2:1029, 1983.
101. Conner ME, Crawford SE, Barone C, et al: Rotavirus subunit vaccines. Arch Virol Suppl 12:199, 1996.
102. Herrmann JE, Chen SC, Fynan EF, et al: DNA vaccines against rotavirus infections. Arch Virol Suppl 12:207, 1996.
103. Sabin AB: Reoviruses, a new group of respiratory and enteric viruses formerly classified as ECHO type 10 is described. Science 103:1387, 1959.
104. Tyler KL, Fields BN: Reoviridae: The reoviruses. *In* Lennette EH, Halonen P, Murphy FA (eds): Laboratory Diagnosis of Infectious Diseases, Principles and Practice, Vol II. New York, Springer-Verlag, 1988, pp 353–374.
105. Stanley NF, Dorman DC, PonsFord J: Studies on the pathogenesis of a hitherto undescribed virus (hepatoencephalomyelitis) producing unusual symptoms in suckling mice. Aust J Exp Biol 31:147, 1953.
106. Stanley NF, Dorman DC, PonsFord J: Studies on the hepatoencephalomyelitis virus. Aust J Exp Biol 32:543, 1954.
107. Leers WD, Rozee KR, Wardlow HC: Immunodiffusion and immunoelectrophoretic studies of reovirus antigens. Can J Microbiol 14:161, 1968.
108. Lerner AM, Cherry JD, Klein JO, et al: Infections with reoviruses. N Engl J Med 267:947, 1962.
109. Thein P, Scheid R: Reoviral infections. *In* Steele (ed): CRC Handbook Series in Zoonoses, Section B, Viral Zoonoses, Vol II. Boca Raton, FL, CRC Press, 1981, pp 191–216.
110. Stanley NF: Diagnosis of reovirus infections: Comparative aspects. *In* Kurstak E, Kurstak K (eds): Comparative Diagnosis of Viral Diseases. New York, Academic Press, 1977, pp 385–421.
111. Rosen L, Hovis JF, Mastrota FM, et al: An outbreak of infection with a type 1 reovirus among children in an institution. Am J Hyg 71:266, 1960.
112. Rosen L, Evans HE, Spickard A: Reovirus infections in human volunteers. Am J Hyg 77:29, 1963.
113. Morecki R, Glaser JH, Cho S, et al: Biliary atresia and reovirus type 3 infection. N Engl J Med 307:481, 1982.
114. Glaser JH, Balistreri WF, Morecki R: Role of reovirus type 3 in persistent infantile cholestasis. J Pediatr 105:912, 1984.
115. Rosen L: Reoviruses. *In* Lennette EH, Schmidt NJ (eds): Diagnostic Procedures for Viral, Rickettsial, and Chlamydial Infections, ed 5. Washington, DC, American Public Health Association, 1979, pp 577–584.
116. Calisher CH: Medically important arboviruses of the United States and Canada. Clin Microbiol Rev 7:89, 1994.
117. Emmons RW: Reoviridae: The orbiviruses (Colorado tick fever). *In* Lennette EH, Halonen P, Murphy FA (eds): Laboratory Diagnosis of Infectious Diseases, Principles and Practice, Vol II. New York, Springer-Verlag, 1988, pp 375–383.
118. Monath TP: Orbivirus (Colorado tick fever). *In* Mandell GL, Douglas RG, Bennett JE (eds): Principles and Practice of Infectious Diseases, ed 2. New York, John Wiley & Sons, 1985, pp 931–932.
119. Philip RN, Casper EA, Cory J, et al: The potential for transmission of arboviruses by blood transfusion with particular references to Colorado tick fever. *In* Greenwalt TJ, Jamieson GA (eds): Transmissible Disease and Blood Transfusion. New York, Grune & Stratton, 1975, pp 175–195.
120. Emmons RW, Schade HI: Colorado tick fever simulating acute myocardial infarction. JAMA 222:87, 1972.
121. Loge RV: Acute hepatitis associated with Colorado tick fever. West J Med 142:91, 1985.
122. Goodpasture HC, Poland JD, Francy DB, et al: Colorado tick fever: Clinical, epidemiologic, and laboratory aspects of 228 cases in Colorado in 1973–1974. Ann Intern Med 88:303, 1978.
123. Emmons RW, Lennette EH: Immunofluorescent staining in the laboratory diagnosis of Colorado tick fever. J Lab Clin Med 68:923, 1966.
124. Emmons RW, Dondero DV, Devlin V, et al: Serologic diagnosis of Colorado tick fever. A comparison of complement-fixation, immunofluorescence, and plaque-reduction methods. Am J Trop Med Hyg 18:796, 1969.
125. Calisher CH, Poland JD, Calisher SB, et al: Diagnosis of Colorado tick fever virus infection by enzyme immunoassays for immunoglobulin M and G antibodies. J Clin Microbiol 22:84, 1985.
126. Thomas LA, Philip RN, Patzer E, et al: Long duration of neutralizing-antibody response after immunization of man with a formalinized Colorado tick fever vaccine. Am J Trop Med Hyg 16:60, 1967.

264

Human Immunodeficiency Virus and Other Retroviruses

Zene Matsuda
James A. Hellinger
Max Essex

Historical Background

Viruses that cause leukemia in chickens—subsequently known as RNA tumor viruses or retroviruses—have been recognized for more than 80 years.[1] Mammalian retroviruses were first identified by Ludwig Gross almost half a century later, in the early 1950s, through careful selection of inbred strains of mice prone to leukemia.[2] By the mid-1960s, it was widely recognized that mammalian and avian retroviruses often had a high degree of genetic relatedness to normal cellular genes. This recognition was due to both the presence of retrovirus-transduced oncogenes and the existence of a vast family of endogenous xenotropic murine retroviruses that apparently are not pathogenic.

The recognition that such inherited retroviruses did not cause disease, combined with a failure to find human retroviruses by electron microscopy, led to a deemphasis on such research for a time. Concurrently, however, it was found that retroviruses do cause leukemia in at least one species, domestic cats.[3] Soon after, it was further recognized that such feline retroviruses often caused lethal immune suppression.[4]

The first human retrovirus—human T-cell lymphotropic virus type I, or HTLV-I—was described in 1980 by Gallo and colleagues[5] (Table 264–1). This agent was associated with a characteristic type of hematopoietic disease called adult T-cell leukemia (ATL), a syndrome described a few years earlier by Takatsuki and colleagues.[6] In 1981, the same virus was independently described by Hinuma and colleagues[7] as the ATL virus. It soon became apparent that HTLV-I was regularly associated with ATL, a disease that was more common in areas such as southwestern Japan. Cloning, sequencing, and functional analysis of this virus revealed that it contained at least two important regulatory genes that were not present in earlier analyzed retroviruses of cats or mice.[8–10] The second human retrovirus, HTLV-II, was identified in a patient who had hairy cell leukemia.[11] It was immediately recognized as related to but distinct from HTLV-I.

Attempts to find the cause of acquired immunodeficiency syndrome (AIDS) revealed a third human retrovirus, human immunodeficiency virus type 1 (HIV-1). Although AIDS was recognized as a new disease,[12] most early hypotheses suggested that it was caused by drugs or alloantigenic stimulation.[13] When cases of AIDS were observed in blood transfusion recipients and hemophiliacs, hypotheses of an infectious agent emerged. Only those familiar with T-lymphotropic human leukemia viruses or the retroviruses that cause immunosuppression in cats, however, had much enthusiasm for the idea of a retrovirus as the cause of human AIDS. The first identification by Barre-Sinoussi and colleagues[14] of a retrovirus in a homosexual patient with lymphadenopathy—initially designated lymphadenopathy-associated virus (LAV)—combined with other reports,[15, 16] focused attention on retroviruses. Extensive analysis by Gallo and colleagues[17, 18] later provided conclusive evidence that this virus was the cause of AIDS. Initially referred to as LAV,[14] HTLV-III,[18] AIDS-related virus,[19] and HTLV-III/LAV, this virus is now generally designated HIV-1.

Human immunodeficiency virus type 2 (HIV-2) was identified in West Africa as a virus related to but distinct from HIV-1.[20] Initially designated HTLV-IV,[21] it is much more closely related to a simian immunodeficiency virus (SIV) of monkeys[22] than to HIV-1. Largely restricted to West Africa,[23] HIV-2, although biologically similar to HIV-1, has reduced pathogenicity compared with HIV-1[24] (Table 264–2).

Human Retrovirology

Retroviruses

Retroviruses utilize two identical RNA molecules as their genome in the virion.[25] As with other retrotransposons, the genome of all replication-competent retroviruses contains direct repeats (R) at both ends[26] and two unique sequences, one immediately after the direct repeat in the 5′ end, U5, and the other immediately preceding the direct repeat in the 3′ end, U3. The retrovirus genome contains three essential structural genes *gag* (group-specific antigen), *pol* (polymerase), and *env* (envelope), which are arranged in this order from the 5′ to 3′ direction (Fig. 264–1). The structural proteins are first synthesized as precursor polyproteins and processed into mature products by proteolytic cleavage. Proteolytic processing of Gag and Pol is catalyzed by a virally encoded protease, and processing of Env is catalyzed by cellular proteases.

Products of the *gag* gene constitute the viral core and include the matrix protein (MA), the capsid protein (CA), and the nucleocapsid protein (NC). The *pol* gene encodes multiple enzymes required for the virus life cycle such as reverse transcriptase, ribonuclease H, integrase, and protease.

TABLE 264–1 ■ Properties of Human Retroviruses

PROPERTIES	HTLV-I	HTLV-II	HIV-1	HIV-2
Morphology	Oncovirus	Oncovirus	Lentivirus	Lentivirus
Macrophage tropism	?	?	+	+
CD4+ lymphocyte tropism	+	+	+	+
Primary cell receptor	?	?	CD4	CD4
Cytopathic (c) or transforming (t) in vitro	t	t	c	c
Additional genes (regulatory genes)	2	2	6+	6+
Transactivation	+	+	+	+
Chronic infection	+	+	+	+

TABLE 264–2 ■ Pathogenic Human Retroviruses

CHARACTERISTICS	HIV-1	HIV-2	HTLV-I	HTLV-II
Geography	Worldwide, but especially sub-Saharan Africa and Southeast Asia	West Africa primarily	Worldwide with high prevalence in southern Japan, Asia, and the Caribbean	Distribution not known; highest seroprevalence in injection drug users
Transmission				
Sexual	Heterosexual and homosexual	Similar to HIV-1	Male-to-female transmission more efficient	Unknown, but presumed to be same as for HTLV-I
Parenteral	Cellular and cell-free blood products	Similar to HIV-1	Cellular blood products (not cell free)	Cellular blood products (not cell free)
Perinatal	Occurs in approximately 25%–35%	Infrequent	Occurs in about 25%, mainly related to breast-feeding	Unknown, but presumed to be same as for HTLV-I
Clinical illness				
Induction period	7–10 y median duration before AIDS; more rapid progression in infants and elders	Clearly linked to AIDS; but less frequent progression and/or more prolonged incubation period than with HIV-1	Adult T-cell leukemia/lymphoma in 1%–5% after > 20 y latency TSP/HAM develops 1–4 y after HTLV-I–contaminated blood transfusion	Isolated from atypical T-cell variant hairy cell leukemias
Type disease	Prominent immune defects and neurologic manifestations	Clinical AIDS similar to HIV-1	Clinical illness infrequent, involves immune defects, neurologic disease; atypical lymphocytosis, skin involvement may precede adult T-cell leukemia/lymphoma	Association with disease not yet established
Associated cancers	Lymphoma, Kaposi's sarcoma	Similar to HIV-1	Adult T-cell leukemia/lymphoma, B-cell chronic lymphocytic leukemia	Atypical variant hairy cell leukemia

Both Gag and Pol polyproteins are translated from full-length messenger RNA (mRNA), which also serves as the genomic RNA. Because *pol* of human retroviruses does not have an initiation codon and it is encoded in a different frame than that of *gag*, the *pol* product is translated as a *gag-pol* fusion protein by frameshifting. The frameshift signal is located near the beginning of *pol*.[27–29] This frameshift regulates the ratio of *gag* and *pol* products. The *env* gene encodes an external surface protein (SU) and a transmembrane protein (TM). The surface protein is a major determinant of retrovirus tropism because it binds to specific host cell receptors. The transmembrane protein anchors the surface protein into a

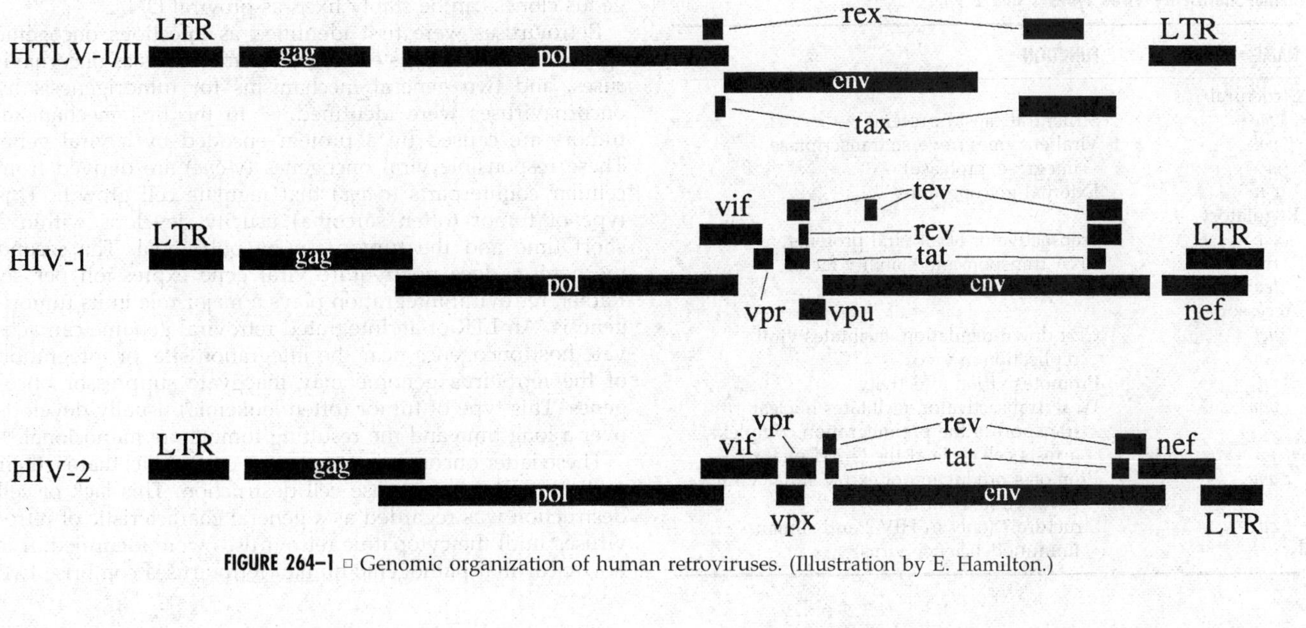

FIGURE 264–1 □ Genomic organization of human retroviruses. (Illustration by E. Hamilton.)

TABLE 264–3 ■ Efficiency of Human Retrovirus–Specific Proteins for Serum Detection of Antibodies in Infected People*

HIV GENE†	HIV ANTIGEN‡	EFFICIENCY§ OF HIV-1 PROTEINS FOR Ab DETECTION IN		EFFICIENCY§ OF HIV-2 PROTEINS FOR Ab DETECTION IN	HTLV GENE	HTLV ANTIGEN‡	EFFICIENCY§ OF HTLV-I PROTEINS FOR Ab DETECTION IN	
		Healthy	AIDS	Healthy			Healthy	ATL
gag	p55/24/17	H	M	H	*gag*	p55/24/19	H	H
pol	p64/53/34	H	H	H	*pol*	Not known		
env	gp120/41	H	H	H	*env*	gp61–68/46/21	H	H
tat	p14	L	L	NT	*tax*	p42	M	M-H
rev	p19	L	M-H‖	NT	*rex*	p27	NT	L
vif	p23	M	L	NT				
nef	p27	M	L	M				
vpr	p10	M-H¶	M	L-M				
vpu	p16	H¶	M	NA				
vpx	p12	NA	NA	L				

*Ab, Antibody; NT, not tested; ATL, adult T-cell leukemia; NA, not applicable.
†HIV-1 does not contain *vpx* and HIV-2 does not contain *vpu*.
‡p, Protein; gp, glycoprotein; size of protein, kilodaltons.
§H, High; M, moderate; L, low efficiency in detection of serum antibodies.
‖Highest in Walter Reed stage 5 or early AIDS.
¶Highest at seroconversion.

viral lipid membrane and is important for fusion between viral and cellular lipid membranes in the initial steps of infection. Although simple animal retroviruses are composed only of these three structural genes, human retroviruses have a more complex genomic organization and contain several additional genes[30] (Tables 264–3 and 264–4).

As with other viruses, the retrovirus life cycle starts when a virion binds to a specific receptor expressed on the target cell. Although studies have revealed the presence of partially reverse-transcribed DNA in retrovirus virions,[31, 32] complete conversion of the RNA genome into a DNA form (reverse transcription) occurs once the retrovirus infects the target cell. This DNA form of the retrovirus is called the provirus.[33] Reverse transcription generates a long terminal repeat (LTR) at both ends of the provirus.[34] LTRs contain several transcriptional and posttranscriptional control elements. These include enhancers, a promoter, and a polyadenylation signal. HTLV-I contains a cis regulatory element called *rex*-responsive element in the 3′ LTR.[35–37]

TABLE 264–4 ■ Functions of Genes and Their Products for Human Immunodeficiency Virus Types 1 and 2

NAME	FUNCTION
Structural	
gag	Structural capsid proteins
pol	Viral enzymes (reverse transcriptase, integrase, protease)
env	External glycoproteins
Regulatory	
tat	Transactivator of all viral proteins
rev	RNA transport and stability factor
tev	? (*tat* + *rev* function)
Accessory	
nef	CD4 down-regulation, facilitates viral replication in vivo
vif	Promotes virion infectivity
vpr	Weak transactivator, facilitates nuclear transport of the preintegration complex, arrests cell cycle at the G_2/M phase
vpu	Promotes production of extracellular viral particles (only in HIV-1)
vpx	Structural? (only in HIV-2 and simian immunodeficiency virus)

The provirus is transported into the nucleus of the cell, where it is spliced at the end of its LTR into the host genome (integration). Thereafter, it becomes a part of the host genome. Reverse transcription and integration at the end of the LTR are two unique characteristics of retroviruses. These processes are catalyzed by reverse transcriptase and integrase, respectively. Viral mRNAs are transcribed from the integrated provirus by host transcription machinery. Human retroviruses carry a specific transcription activator on their own LTR.[38–41] After posttranscriptional processing, transcribed mRNAs are transported to the cytoplasm and translated to produce viral proteins. Human retroviruses have specific gene products for posttranscriptional regulation of mRNA species.[42–45] Viral proteins are transported to assembly sites, where they bud out to produce a virion. Further proteolytic processing of Gag and Gag-Pol proteins takes place and the virus becomes a mature infectious virion. The details of virus assembly and maturation of retroviruses are still not well understood. Having both RNA and DNA forms in their life cycles, retroviruses have characteristics of both RNA and DNA viruses. Like RNA viruses, retroviruses can generate diverse genotypes after each replication, yet some advantageous clones can be stably fixed as proviral DNA.

Retroviruses were first identified as infectious oncogenic agents in animals. This established retroviruses as oncornaviruses, and two general mechanisms for tumorigenesis by oncornaviruses were identified.[3, 25] In the first mechanism, tumors are caused by a protein encoded by a viral gene. These responsible viral oncogenes (v-*onc*) are derived from cellular counterparts (c-*onc*) that regulate cell growth. This type of tumor (often sarcoma) usually develops within a short time and the tumor can be polyclonal. The second mechanism does not require viral gene expression per se. Rather, retroviral integration plays a major role in its tumorigenesis. An LTR of an integrated retroviral genome can activate host oncogenes near the integration site, or integration of the retrovirus genome may inactivate suppressor oncogenes. This type of tumor (often leukemia) usually develops over a long time and the resulting tumors are monoclonal.[46]

These latter oncornaviruses are not cytopathic; that is, their replication does not cause cell destruction. This lack of cell destruction was regarded as a general characteristic of retroviruses until the cytopathic retroviruses were identified. It is now clear that pathogenic human retroviruses comprise two distinct families—one is oncogenic (HTLV-I) and the other is cytopathic (HIV-1 and -2).

Human Retroviruses and Diseases

HTLV-I AND ATL

HTLV-I is etiologically linked with an aggressive type of T-cell leukemia, ATL, which was first described in Japan.[6] Different from animal oncoviruses, it contains two unique genes, *tax* and *rex*, in addition to the three essential structural genes, *gag*, *pol*, and *env*. The *tax* gene is located between *env* and the 3′ LTR in the HTLV-I genome.[9] This is where the oncogene v-*src* is observed in Rous sarcoma virus. However, unlike v-*src*, *tax* does not have a cellular counterpart.[9] Tax activates transcription from its own LTR and is essential to the viral life cycle.[38, 39] Tax is also known for its transcriptional activation of several cellular genes via interaction with bZIP proteins.[47] These characteristics of Tax suggest that Tax plays a critical role in leukemogenesis by HTLV-I. Retention of this region of the HTLV-I genome in a majority of leukemic cells in ATL patients further supports this hypothesis.[48] However, transgenic mice expressing *tax* do not develop leukemia; rather, they develop neurofibromas.[49] Moreover, few successful transformations of primary human lymphocytes by transduction of a *tax* expression vector have been reported.[50] This suggests that *tax* alone may not be sufficient for leukemogenesis or that the system used was not appropriate. For example, it is possible that rodent cells lack specific factors important for Tax function.

To reconcile these experimental data, autocrine immortalization accompanied by secondary events has been proposed for leukemogenesis by HTLV-I. Under this hypothesis, Tax transactivates cellular genes such as those for interleukin-2 (IL-2) and IL-2 receptor in the target T cell. Indeed, tumor cells derived from ATL patients show high levels of IL-2 receptor expression. With autocrine stimulation of IL-2 receptor by IL-2, HTLV-I–infected T cells enter immortal cell growth.[51] During this unregulated cell growth, secondary events are postulated to occur that trigger transformation of T cells. However, no clear candidate for these secondary events has been identified. It has been postulated that these secondary events are rare; therefore, only a fraction of people infected by HTLV-I develop ATL.[52, 53]

It is noteworthy that ATL develops only after a long time from the initial infection.[54, 55] This long interval is reminiscent of tumorigenesis by retroviral integration at specific sites. However, early studies of ATL cells by Southern blot analysis revealed that HTLV-I does not integrate at a specific loci.[56] Therefore, it seems unlikely that ATL is caused by specific insertional activation or inactivation of a particular gene. ATL does not have to be caused by activation or inactivation of a single particular gene. Its etiology can be multiple.[57] During the incubation period, many virus-infected cells are presumably destroyed by the host immune system and eliminated. Only the viruses that acquire mutations to escape from the immune system may be responsible for ATL. In agreement with this hypothesis, many HTLV-I genomes in tumor cells are defective.[48]

HTLV-I research has lagged behind that of HIV-1 despite its earlier identification. This is mainly due to its ineffectiveness at cell-free infection[58, 59] and the lack of an infectious molecular clone. The characterization of an infectious molecular clone[60] should help answer many questions in this area of research. It is now possible to determine the role of each gene experimentally in the virus life cycle and in the process of leukemogenesis.

CYTOPATHIC RETROVIRUSES AND AIDS

An important conceptual change in retrovirology came from the study of feline leukemia virus.[4, 61] Despite its classification as an oncornavirus, the major cause of death in infected cats is primarily due to immunodeficiency, not to cancer. It is clear that retrovirus-induced pathogenesis is not limited to tumorigenesis. Indeed, the second major category of pathogenic human retroviruses consists of cytopathic retroviruses. This group includes HIV-1 and HIV-2.[14, 18–20] HIV-1 was first noticed among U.S. homosexual men[12] and was identified as the causative agent of AIDS. HIV-1 is the cause of the current worldwide epidemic of AIDS. HIV-2, although it can cause AIDS, is much less pathogenic than HIV-1.[24] Both HIV-1 and HIV-2 have similar genomic organizations (see Table 264–4). The only difference in the gene components is the presence of one of two accessory genes. HIV-1 has *vpu* but not *vpx*[62–64] and HIV-2 has *vpx* but not *vpu*.[65, 66] However, it seems that this simple difference alone may not be able to account for their differences in pathogenesis. HIV-1 has several apparent similarities to HTLV-I. It is $CD4^+$ T-cell tropic in part and its essential regulatory genes *tat* and *rev* correspond to *tax* and *rex*, respectively. However, HIV-1 belongs to a different family of retroviruses, lentiviruses, and its life cycle and pathogenesis are quite different from those of oncornaviruses. The natural course of HIV infection progresses for several years. HIVs maintain persistent infection and are cytopathic to their major target cells, $CD4^+$ T cells. The number of $CD4^+$ cells of infected individuals decreases gradually during a period of several years. Parallel with this decrease of $CD4^+$ cells, the immune system of the infected individual slowly deteriorates, as $CD4^+$ T cells are the major modulator of the immune system. Once $CD4^+$ T cells decrease below a threshold level, the patient starts to suffer from opportunistic infections. These opportunistic infections are often fatal because of immune system collapse.

Human Immunodeficiency Virus Types 1 and 2

Biology

VIRAL STRUCTURE AND LIFE CYCLE

The HIVs are spherical viruses of about 100 nm in diameter. The core or nucleocapsid is condensed into a cylindrical, trapezoidal, or triangular shape instead of the spherical shape seen with the HTLVs. When the HIV core is sectioned on end, it may appear as a small sphere, usually not centered in the particle (Figs. 264–2 and 264–3).

HIV-1 and HIV-2 may be slightly distinguishable from each other by the degree of condensation of the nucleocapsid, particularly as it separates from the envelope.[67] HIV-2 appears to retain more peplomer proteins at the outer surface than does HIV-1, which confers a fuzzy appearance.

The HIVs have a sophisticated replication cycle, involving at least nine functional genes with identified products. The replication cycle may vary in regulatory mechanisms for different cell types. While providing numerous opportunities for targeting antiviral drugs, it also provides many loopholes for virus survival.

Apart from the existence of sophisticated regulatory genes, the general replication cycle for the HIVs is the same as for other retroviruses (see Fig. 264–2). Reverse transcription follows attachment to CD4 and penetration, and the resulting DNA is transported to the nucleus, where it integrates into the host genome. Transcription and splicing of the various messages occur in the nucleus, using the integrated chromosomal provirus as template. Both genomic and nongenomic forms of RNA are transported to the cytoplasm, where trans-

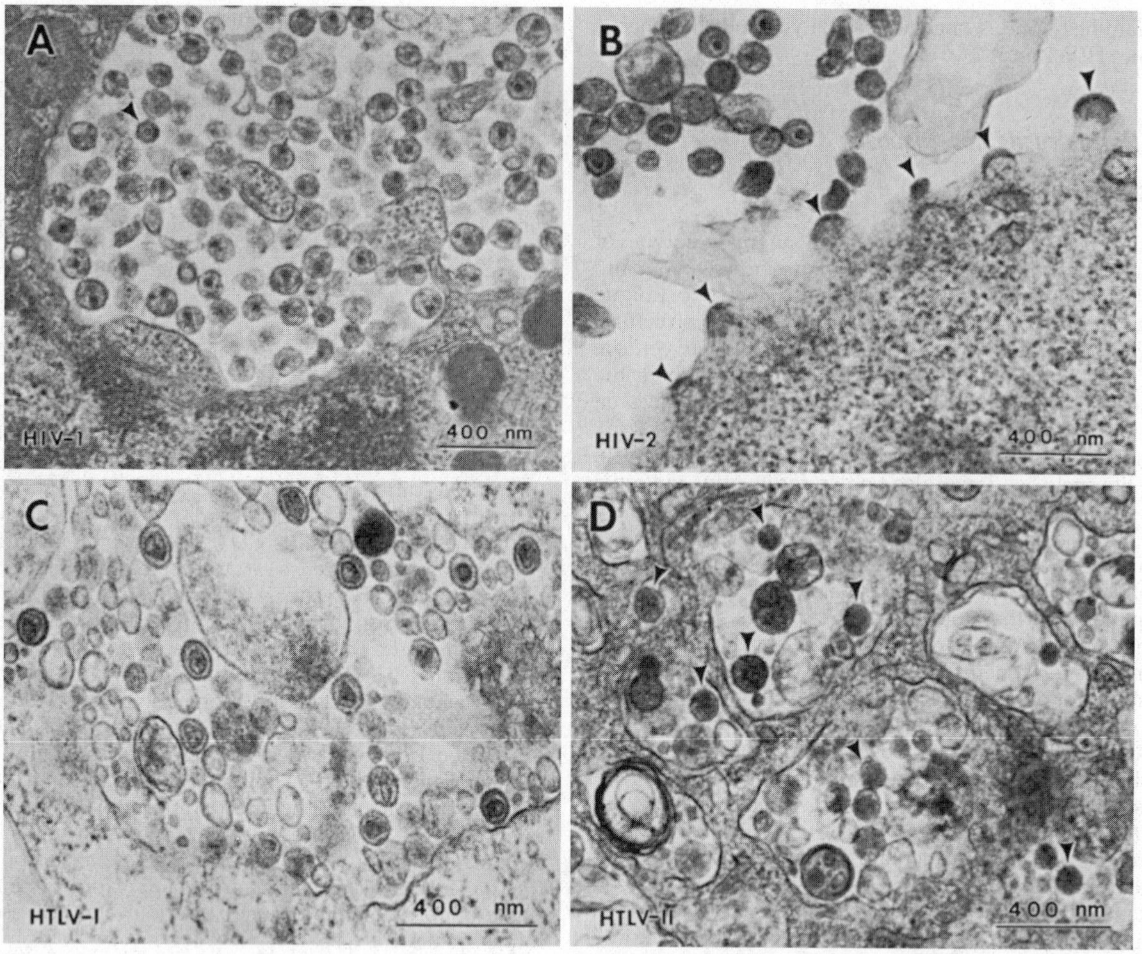

FIGURE 264–2 □ Electron micrographs showing the typical appearance of HIV-1 particles in intracellular vacuole *(A);* HIV-2 budding from cell surface in Sup T lymphocytes *(B);* HTLV-I *(C);* and HTLV-II particles within a promonocyte *(D).* (Courtesy of Q. C. Yu, MD, PhD, Harvard School of Public Health, Boston, MA.)

lation occurs. Viral genomes and newly produced structural proteins are transported to assembly sites at the cytoplasmic membrane, where morphogenesis and budding of progeny virus occur. Both HIV-1 and HIV-2 bud from cytoplasmic membranes and perhaps from vacuolar membranes as well. Whereas the budding of most retroviruses has no deleterious effects on the infected cells, the production of large amounts of HIV can cause the lysis of lymphocytes.[68] In vitro, HIV may cause cell lysis or multinuclear cell (syncytium) formation (Fig. 264–4).

GENES OF HUMAN IMMUNODEFICIENCY VIRUSES (see Tables 264–3 and 264–4)

In the initial phase of HIV-1 and HIV-2 or SIV research, relatively few isolates were studied, usually using virus from established T-cell tumor cell lines. During this period, most of the gene products were identified and classified into three categories. The first are three structural genes, *gag*, *pol*, and *env.* The second are the essential regulatory genes *tat*[40, 41] (transactivator of transcription) and *rev*[42, 43] (regulator of viral gene expression). Other genes were called accessory genes because mutations of these genes did not abolish the capacity of virus replication in established cell lines.[69, 70] These accessory genes are *vif* (virus infectivity factor),[71–73] *nef* (negative regulatory factor),[64, 74] *vpr* (virus protein R),[75–77] *vpu* (virus protein U),[62–64] and *vpx* (viral protein X).[65, 66] It seems that some of these accessory genes were actually not dispensable in the natural life cycle of HIV-1 and HIV-2 or SIV in the host. The majority of the information on the function of each gene is derived from study of HIV-1, except for *vpx*, which is unique to HIV-2 and SIV. Given the similarity of their genomic organization as well as homology in primary structures, it is generally assumed that the functions of the corresponding accessory genes in the HIV-1 and HIV-2–SIV groups are similar to each other. However, it remains to be determined experimentally whether the particular function described for an HIV-1 gene is completely applicable for that of HIV-2 or SIV and vice versa. In the following section, the description is generally for HIV-1 gene products unless otherwise described.

Structural Genes

The HIV-1 *gag* gene encodes a polyprotein of about 55 kDa that is made from a full-genomic-length form of mRNA. Pol precursor of 160 kDa is also made from the same mRNA by frameshifting. Both polyproteins are myristylated at their N-terminals and are cleaved by the viral protease to form the final products. The myristylation seems important for proper targeting of the Gag precursor. The Gag precursor is processed into mature products: matrix MA (p17), CA (p24), NC (p9), and p6. The myristylated residues remain associated with the N-terminal cleavage product, p17, the majority of which become situated at the inner surface of the virus envelope. Some fractions of p17 are phosphorylated and as-

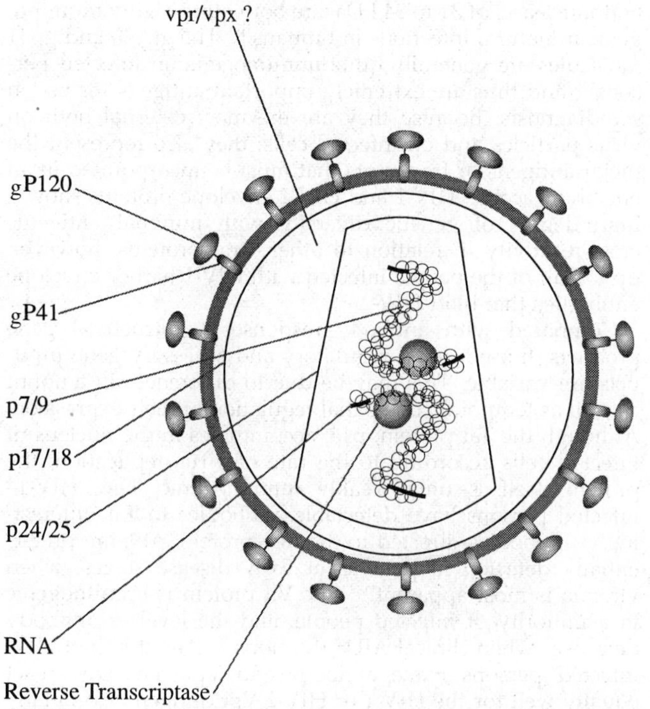

FIGURE 264–3 □ Virion structure of HIV. (Illustration by E. Hamilton.)

sociated with the core structure.[78] MA is important not only for incorporation of the envelope protein into mature virions but also to assist with transport of the preintegration complex of HIV-1 into nucleus.[79–81] The nuclear localization signal of the matrix protein MA of HIV-1 allows the establishment of infection in macrophages and quiescent T lymphocytes.[82] Because of its affinity for the inner glycoprotein envelope, p17 plays an important role in positioning viral cores at

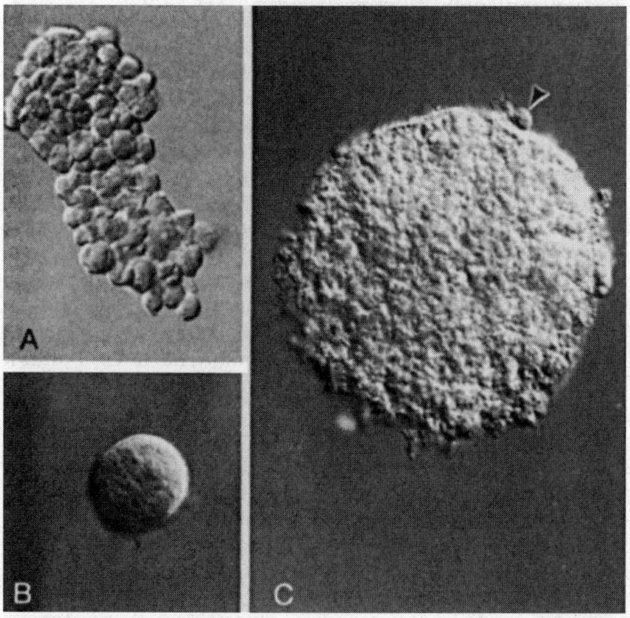

FIGURE 264–4 □ HIV infection of CD4$^+$ T lymphocytes inducing cell aggregation *(A);* multinuclear cell (syncytium) formation, which is accompanied by depletion of cell numbers in vitro *(B);* and a single lymphocyte *(arrowhead)* (C). (*A* to *C* courtesy of Q. C. Yu, MD, PhD, Harvard School of Public Health, Boston, MA.)

budding sites in the cell. Another cleavage product of the Gag polyprotein is p24, the major structural capsid protein that constitutes the virus core. Interaction between HIV-1 p24 and cyclophilin A seems essential for virus infectivity.[83, 84] The smaller core protein products of the *gag* polyprotein, p9 and p6, are rapidly cleaved from an intermediate p15. These proteins are situated at the C-terminal of the translation product and at the innermost region of the virus core. As in other retroviruses, p9 is the nucleocapsid protein that binds directly to the viral RNA. The most C-terminal *gag* protein p6 seems important for efficient viral release from the HIV-1–infected cells.[85] Three-dimensional structures of both p17 and p9 have been determined by nuclear magnetic resonance.[86, 87]

The *pol* gene products provide various essential enzyme functions. In addition to protease, which is at the N-terminal, the *pol* gene encodes reverse transcriptase, ribonuclease H, and integrase. Reverse transcriptase and associated ribonuclease H activity make the first proviral DNA strand. After the DNA provirus is made, the integrase or endonuclease integrates this provirus into the chromosomal DNA of the cell. Integration itself seems necessary for virus replication in T lymphocytes, but it is not clear whether other cells, such as macrophages, have the same requirement. As all *pol* products are enzymes that can be targeted for therapeutic intervention, the structure of all *pol* products has been determined and structure-oriented drug design has been attempted.[88–91]

The *env* gene also encodes a polyprotein, gp160, which is subsequently cleaved to form the external glycoprotein, gp120, and the transmembrane protein, gp41.[92–94] The gp120 binds strongly to the CD4 molecule.[95] The primary region for gp120 binding to the CD4 molecule has been mapped to the C-terminal,[96, 97] but it appears that an additional portion of the binding site is present at the N-terminal of the molecule.[98] Other antibody-neutralizing sites have been mapped within gp120,[99] and sites for syncytium formation have been mapped to the N-terminal of gp41.[100]

The gp120 molecule is highly glycosylated, with a mean of 24 different sites harboring residues of either mannose or other complex sugars.[101] As a result, more than half of the mass of the molecule is carbohydrate.

Regulatory and Accessory Genes

Along with the manufacture and assembly of the virus and its components, a major activity of HIV-type viruses is the regulation of replication. There are two essential regulatory genes in primate lentiviruses, *tat* and *rev.*

The *tat* gene is an efficient transactivator of transcription.[40, 41] HIVs that lack *tat* gene function cannot replicate.[102] One proposed mechanism of transactivation by Tat is facilitation of elongation of the transcript. Tat functions as an antiterminator via binding to the TAR region, which is present in all viral transcripts.[103–106] Tat binds to TAR together with cellular proteins.[107, 108]

The *rev* gene is another essential regulator of posttranscriptional events.[42, 43, 109] Rev is required for the expression of virus structural proteins. Rev alleviates the negative effects of a cis-acting repression sequence via binding to *rev*-responsive elements.[110, 111] It has been shown to interact with a cellular protein that has similarity to nuclear pore proteins.[112–114] The cis-acting repression sequence is present in at least the *gag* and *env* regions.[115, 116] The *rev*-responsive element is located within the *env* gene.[117]

A third major category of HIV genes is the accessory gene, which is regularly present in HIV-1 and HIV-2 but is apparently not absolutely necessary for virus replication in established T-cell lines. It is possible, indeed likely on the basis of current observations, that accessory genes perform important functions at the host level, perhaps preferentially in cells other than T lymphocytes.

HIV-1 and HIV-2 or SIV have three common accessory genes *vif*,[71–73] *vpr*,[75–77] and *nef*.[74] In addition to these, HIV-1 uniquely contains *vpu*[62–64] and HIV-2 and SIV uniquely contain *vpx*.[65, 66] The functions of most of the accessory genes are still not clearly understood at a molecular level. Some of the functions are inferred from the phenotypes of the mutants.

The *vif* gene of HIV-1 encodes a 23-kDa protein.[71–73] Mutations in *vif* affect the ability of viruses to infect in a cell-free manner but cell-to-cell transmission of viruses does not seem to be effected.[118, 119] Interestingly, this defect is partially compensated in some T-cell lines, suggesting that some cellular factors modify *vif* function.[120]

The *vpr* gene encodes a protein of about 12 kDa that is present in virus particles as well as in infected cells.[75, 77] It is conserved between HIV-1 and HIV-2–SIV. Although it apparently is not essential for replication in T-cell lines, the replication of *vpr* mutant viruses is affected in macrophages. The *vpr* gene facilitates the transport of a preintegration complex to the nucleus together with MA in HIV-1.[81, 82] HIV-1 *vpr* manifests pleiotropic effects such as transactivation of several promoters and arrest of the cell cycle at the G_2/M phase.[76, 121] The physiologic importance of this effect of *vpr* is still not clear. In the SIV model, *vpr* seems important to maintain virus replication in vivo,[122] but it is not necessary to induce simian AIDS in young animals with immature immune systems.[123]

The p27 *nef* product[74] is a myristylated protein. Nef was originally described as a putative negative regulator of transcription,[124] as *nef* mutants replicate better than wild-type virus.[125] However its function as a negative regulator is now controversial. SIV_{mac} with a mutated *nef* gene shows attenuated replication in vivo, suggesting a positive effect of *nef* in the viral life cycle.[126] It is known that *nef* down-modulates surface expression of CD4 in infected cells.[127, 128] However, it is not clear whether this function is responsible for the apparent positive effect of *nef* SIV_{mac} in monkeys. HIV-1 *nef* seems to bind cellular proteins via its PxxP motif.[129]

The *vpu* gene makes a 16-kDa product. It is an integral membrane phosphoprotein and forms multimers.[130] With mutated *vpu*, virions manifest abnormal morphologic characteristics and are inefficiently released from infected cells.[131] It may play a role in degrading CD4 intracellularly.[132] The *vpu* gene is uniquely observed in HIV-1 and is missing from HIV-2 and SIV.

In contrast to *vpu*, the *vpx* gene is present in HIV-2 and in related SIVs but not in HIV-1. The *vpx* gene is thought to be derived from *vpr* by gene duplication and its gene product, Vpx, is a virion-associated protein, as is Vpr.[133] Mutations of *vpx* attenuate the replication capacity of viruses in peripheral blood mononuclear cells, especially in macrophages.[134] Why *vpu* and *vpx* are uniquely distributed in distinct primate lentiviruses and their effects on pathogenesis remain to be elucidated.

Antibody Responses to HIV Proteins (see Table 264–3)

Perhaps partly because of their abundance in virions, HIV structural proteins induce a prominent antibody response in infected individuals. Among Gag proteins, the matrix protein p17 quite regularly induces antibodies in infected persons. As p24 is both present in large amounts in virus particles and quite regularly antigenic in infected persons, it is a useful diagnostic antigen. It is well known that in the late stage of AIDS the anti-p24 titer drops because of high antigenemia. Antibodies to p9 and p6 can be detected in some infected persons if the proper assay systems are used. The polymerase, which can occur in forms of 64 and 53 kDa, and the endonuclease, of 31 to 34 kDa, are both quite highly immunogenic in natural infections in humans.[135] The gp120 and gp41 molecules are generally quite immunogenic in infected persons[136] and thus are extremely important antigens for use in serodiagnosis. Because they are the most external both on virus particles and on infected cells, they also represent the major antigens or fragments that must be incorporated in an effective vaccine. HIV-1 and HIV-2 envelope proteins show a high degree of genetic diversity with minimal antigenic cross-reactivity in relation to other viral proteins; however, up to half of the people infected with HIV-1 harbor envelope antibodies that bind HIV-2.[137]

Compared with antibody responses to structural gene products, those against regulatory and accessory gene products are variable. This may be due to differences in amount as well as temporal and spatial regulation of their expression. Although the Tat protein, p14, accumulates in the nucleus of infected cells according to the rate of virus replication, the protein itself is only weakly immunogenic. Few HIV-1–infected persons have detectable antibodies to Tat. Interestingly, antibodies directed to the Rev protein, p19, are preferentially detected in patients at early disease stages, when viremia is most apparent.[138] The Vif protein is immunogenic in a minority of infected people, and the level of antibody decreases when clinical AIDS develops.[139] About half of HIV-infected persons make antibodies to Vpr that cross-react equally well for the HIV-1 or HIV-2 Vpr antigen.[140] As many as half of HIV-1–infected people make antibodies to the Nef protein, but the detectability of such antibodies drops as clinical AIDS progresses.[139] Some HIV-1–infected persons make antibodies to Vpu preferentially at early stages of infection or at the final stages of clinical AIDS.[62] The presence of antibodies to Vpu is definitive proof of HIV-1 infection, as it is not present in HIV-2. Similarly, the Vpx protein, p14, which is weakly immunogenic, serves as an antigen to confirm that the infecting agent is HIV-2 rather than HIV-I.[65]

TROPISM OF HUMAN IMMUNODEFICIENCY VIRUSES AND THE ENVELOPE PROTEIN

The major cellular preference or tropism of HIVs is determined by the interaction between viral surface protein and cellular receptors. The CD4 molecule—the principal receptor for attachment of gp120—has greater specific binding affinity for gp120 than it has for its natural binding ligand, the class II major histocompatibility complex.[141–143] Cells that express the CD4 molecule, lymphocytes and monocytes, constitute the major targets of HIV infection. Experimental evidence for CD4 as the major specific receptor for HIV-1 includes the following observations: (1) monoclonal antibodies to fragments of the CD4 molecule block HIV infection in most cell types,[141–143] (2) insertion and expression of CD4 gene in a nonsusceptible cell type render it susceptible to HIV infection,[144] (3) segments (epitopes) of CD4 are critical to viral binding,[145] and (4) synthetic peptide fragments of CD4 inhibit HIV infection.[146] Therapeutic approaches, such as use of recombinant soluble CD4, take advantage of viral CD4 binding.

Other mechanisms for viral entry into cells may contribute to HIV-1 and HIV-2 infection of cells that may have few or no CD4 receptors. Cells of monocyte/macrophage lineage are infected through their CD4 receptors and by phagocytic uptake. In vitro, HIV-specific antibody at low levels binds virus and, once complexed, is targeted for macrophage uptake by the Fc receptor of the antibody. Like the antibody-dependent enhancement of infection reported in dengue hemorrhagic fever, this mechanism may selectively target macrophages for antibody-mediated viral uptake, and it may have significant implications for the design of a safe vaccine. The clinical significance of this mechanism in HIV infection has not been established.[147–150] Sequence analysis of the envelope region suggests that changes in the relatively limited region of envelope can affect macrophage and T-cell tropism.[151]

Other cell types are susceptible to HIV-1, although the mechanism is unknown. These are endothelial, cervical, and colorectal cells, transformed B cells, and a number of cells of monocyte/macrophage lineage—pulmonary macrophages and Langerhans, follicular dendritic, and glial cells.[152–160] The affinity of gp120 to carbohydrate molecules (galactosylceramides) expressed on glial cells has been shown, which may explain one mechanism of infection of non-CD4$^+$ cells by HIV-1.[161] Although *env* is a major determinant of tropism, other genes may play a role. For example, *rev* does not function well in rodent cells.[162] Coreceptors of the fusin and chemokine receptor families have been identified on some susceptible cells.

VIRUS REPLICATION AND GENERATION OF HETEROGENEITY

The presence of multiple regulatory and accessory genes clearly separates HIVs from typical animal oncornaviruses. Indeed, HIVs are quite different from typical oncornaviruses with regard to replication. HIVs can infect nondividing cells such as macrophages. The MA of the *gag* gene and Vpr of HIV-1 seem important for this function.[82] Second, the virus' ability to replicate in the presence of host immune responses is amazingly robust. Its envelope, for example, is heavily glycosylated to evade the host immune response, reminiscent of trypanosome coat protein.[101] Furthermore, the reverse transcriptase of HIV-1 is more error prone than that of other oncornaviruses. With its robust replication, error-prone reverse transcriptase rapidly creates a quasi species of viruses within each host.[163] The generation of quasi species is a hallmark of HIV-1 infection. It is also an effective way for virus to survive under the many negative selection forces such as the host immune responses and the administration of drugs. HTLV-I is presumably also replicating, yet its magnitude may be much smaller and the mutation frequency is much lower. Indeed, most HTLV-I isolates are highly conserved even when isolated from different geographic regions. The closely related lentivirus HIV-2 seems to have less variation than HIV-1. Given the relatively similar error rates of HIV-1 and HIV-2 reverse transcriptases,[164] this might suggest that HIV-1 replicates much faster than HIV-2. In any event, the high mutation rate, presumably related to high replication of HIV-1, poses a major challenge to any therapeutic or preventive intervention.

A variety of related HIV quasi species may be present in the cells and free in the plasma of HIV-infected persons at any given time. Viral variability may reflect differences in viral target cell specificity and clinical manifestations.

Human Immunodeficiency Virus Pathogenesis and Establishment of Infection

PROGRESSION OF INFECTION

Viral Quasi Species

After HIV-1 is introduced into a host, virus presumably replicates in local lymphoid organs. During the early period of infection, which is sometimes accompanied by influenza-like symptoms, virus is believed to spread within the host body. It is now clear that during the subsequent asymptomatic phase, which may span several years, virus replication and the host immune response are under a dynamic equilibrium, which slightly favors the virus. During this period, virus isolation is often difficult and viral load, as monitored in peripheral blood mononuclear cells, is deceivingly low. However, studies have shown that virus is actively replicating in lymph nodes, and presumably in other lymphoid organs, during this period.[165, 166] The immune system then gradually erodes, as manifested by the destruction of lymph node organization, and eventually disease begins. Data from clinical trials of antiviral drugs with careful monitoring of viral load and species genotype suggest that the half-life of virus is only a few days and it is accompanied by massive death and regeneration or redistribution of CD4$^+$ cells.[167, 168] This leads to high rates of virus replication in a short period, resulting in an enormous range of virus quasi species.

Some investigators have correlated the varied clinical features of HIV infection with biologic differences among isolates. There are some discernible differences in HIV strains isolated from patients whose clinical status is different (asymptomatic, HIV-related neurologic manifestations, full-blown AIDS) or isolates from different sites in the same patient (blood, cerebrospinal fluid [CSF]). The most extensive studies are based on sequence analyses of the *env* gene. Some of the sequence differences correlate with the different biologic properties of viruses such as CD4$^+$ cell killing as tested in vitro.[169] One example is the conversion to syncytium-inducing ability of HIV-1 and disease progression. About 50% of HIV-1–infected individuals who develop AIDS switch from non–syncytium-inducing to syncytium-inducing phenotypes. A sequence change in V3 as well as in the V1-V2 region of *env* is correlated with this change.[170] However, it has not been possible to establish a conclusive correlation between particular changes in the primary sequence of a gene and changes in disease status. An accumulation of HIV-1 mutations that result in more positively charged amino acids in the V3 loop of gp120 seems to be most regularly correlated with virus syncytium-inducing ability and cytotoxic effects. However, because the viruses analyzed came only from blood rather than from lymph nodes, one cannot assume that this genotype is responsible for the observed systemic deterioration. Disparate findings may be related to methodologic differences such as the use of specific cell lines, culture-adapted virus isolates, mitogens, and cytokines such as IL-2 used to amplify viral and T-cell replication in vitro.[171–176]

HOST IMMUNE RESPONSE TO HUMAN IMMUNODEFICIENCY VIRUS

HIV infection induces both humoral and cell-mediated immune responses that are present throughout progression to disease and ultimately fail to control the persistent viremia. Within a few weeks of infection a high peak viremia occurs and declines, presumably because of an immune response that is temporarily effective. After a few years, the viremia gradually returns to above a minimal threshold level and continues to rise as the patient's clinical status declines. During all periods, virus replication in lymphoid tissue is much higher than that in blood.

Insight into a protective immune response and methods of viral immune evasion and persistence have a critical bearing on prevention strategies. Humoral immunity to HIV infection involves the production of antibodies to viral antigens, including cytolytic antibodies that activate the complement cascade to kill free virus or infected cells, and neutralizing antibodies. HIV-specific antibodies that are able to mediate neutralization and antibody-dependent cellular cytotoxicity (ADCC) have been found in the peripheral blood and CSF of infected persons.[177] Neutralizing antibodies are present in most HIV-infected persons, including those with progressive disease, but they have not been clearly correlated with prognosis. In vitro, neutralization-resistant variants of HIV-1 generated by growth in the presence of neutralizing serum have specific point mutations in the envelope gene. Nevertheless, neutralizing antibodies are useful tools for identifying critical viral epitopes as potential components of effective immunity.[178, 179] Neutralizing antibodies are directed against the outer viral envelope glycoproteins (gp120 and gp41). Epitope mapping studies have identified conserved areas of gp120 that induce group-specific neutralizing antibody responses in systems in vitro and in experimental animals able to neutralize diverse viral isolates. In contrast, type-specific antibodies inhibit only a narrow spectrum of single viral isolates. The principal neutralizing determinant of HIV-1 has been mapped to a 24–amino acid sequence of the envelope protein gp120.[180, 181] A smaller eight–amino acid fragment of this sequence contains a central Gly-Pro-Gly sequence conserved between isolates that is flanked by variable regions that differ with isolates. Vaccine mixtures of peptides to these regions have the potential to elicit neutralizing antibodies that are group specific.[182]

High titers of the antibodies that mediate ADCC in conjunction with natural killer cells are present in most HIV-infected persons. These antibodies are reported to decline with progression to AIDS, as does the antiviral activity of these antibody-armed natural killer cells.[183–188] Clinical correlation of ADCC with neutralizing antibodies and other markers of clinical stage may better establish the precise mechanisms of protective immunity.[189]

Cytotoxic reactivity to HIV-infected cells occurs through the non–human leukocyte antigen–restricted CD16$^+$ natural killer cells and through the major histocompatibility complex–restricted cytotoxic T lymphocytes (CTLs). Natural killer cell activity is reported to diminish in later stages of HIV infection and may be enhanced in vitro by either IL-2 or interferon-α.[183, 190] CTLs may be reactive to several antigens including those of Env, Pol, Gag, and the regulatory Nef protein. These cells are usually CD8$^+$ in vivo and are reported to decline with progression to AIDS.[191–196] A similar population of CD8$^+$ cells is reported to hinder viral culture attempts in vitro.[197] Current research efforts are directed at discovering epitopes of viral antigens that induce broadly protective ADCC and CTLs, analogous to the group-specific reactivity of the principal neutralizing determinant.

The immune responses to HIV-1 and HIV-2 appear similar, but HIV-2 has not been studied as extensively. HIV-2–infected persons have antibodies to many viral proteins, neutralizing antibodies, and evidence of ADCC.[189, 198] Neutralizing antibodies and ADCC to HIV-2 frequently have broad, group-specific reactivity.[199] Future research must distinguish protective immune responses from other mechanisms exploited by HIV for viral persistence, replication, and dissemination.

IMMUNOPATHOGENESIS AND IMMUNE DEFECTS

HIV preferentially infects the immune system, leading to depletion of helper T cells and the unique clinical manifestations of HIV infection, AIDS.[12, 200–204] Exposure to HIV leads to a lifelong infection characterized by HIV DNA provirus integration into the host cell genome. It is presumed that the HIV genome must integrate into cellular DNA to replicate and express viral proteins and that integration leads to chronic infection. Cell death associated with virus production is thought to be the means for eliminating infected cells.

HIV-Induced Immune Defects

HIV-1 infection of two critical components of the immune system, lymphocytes and macrophages, results in a cascade of predictable quantitative and qualitative defects in cellular and humoral immunity. Through CD4$^+$ cell depletion and dysfunction, HIV infection disrupts the normal function of the CD4$^+$ cell, which activates macrophages, secretes IL-2 and other cytokines for lymphoid and hematopoietic growth and differentiation, and induces cytotoxic and suppressor T cells and B cells. In addition, HIV probably disrupts many of the essential activities of the macrophage, including phagocytosis and destruction of foreign antigens, presentation of antigens to lymphocytes, and secretion of cytokines.[205–208] Current data suggest that monocyte chemotaxis is frequently impaired and that many of the functional defects seen in HIV-infected monocytes are the result of failure of CD4$^+$ cells to signal cytokine induction. For example, in vitro, addition of one of these deficient cytokines, interferon-γ, only partially reconstitutes the defective monocyte respiratory burst that is important in eliminating foreign organisms.[206–208]

Characteristic immunologic abnormalities of HIV infection include lymphopenia with depletion of CD4$^+$ helper T cells, impaired delayed-type hypersensitivity reactions, polyclonal B-cell activation and increased immunoglobulin production, decreased humoral responses to immunization, decreased T- and B-cell proliferative responses, altered production of specific cytokines, decreased interferon-γ, decreased IL-2, increased tumor necrosis factor-α (TNF-α), increased levels of acid-labile interferon, and diminished cell-mediated cytotoxicity.[209–212] The consequences of a defective humoral response are particularly severe in persons who were not previously exposed to a bacterial pathogen and who therefore depend on the primary immunoglobulin M response for immune protection.[213, 214] Selective immune defects make HIV-infected persons susceptible to immunologic abnormalities and a wide range of opportunistic infections and tumors that differ depending on the individual's route of HIV infection and endemic geographic exposures to other infections.[215–217] Patients who have HIV-2–associated AIDS appear to have similar forms of immune compromise.[218, 219]

Theories of Immunopathogenesis

Mechanisms of immunopathogenesis, although their exact nature is speculative, must account for the chronicity of HIV infection, the cellular and tissue distribution of virus, and the estimates of less than 1 in 100 HIV-infected peripheral blood mononuclear cells in AIDS patients. Although there is evidence of higher rates of HIV infection of lymphoid tissues, theories of immunopathogenesis must explain the inability of the T-cell pool to compensate for cell destruction by producing mature cells. Current theories of cytopathicity include (1) high-level virus budding with increases in cell permeability; (2) shortened life of infected cells caused by HIV-induced terminal differentiation; (3) syncytium formation by fusion of infected cells with many uninfected cells; (4) toxic effects resulting from accumulation of viral proteins or circular proviral DNA[220]; (5) a critical cofactor of virulent HIV infection such as *Mycoplasma*, a second viral infection, or a toxic agent[221–225]; and (6) HIV-induced autoimmune cell destruction. Theories of HIV-induced autoimmune processes speculate on the immune clearance of uninfected cells with free HIV envelope proteins bound to their CD4 protein and the development of cytotoxic cells that target CD4$^+$ cells or major histocompatibility complex class II antigen–containing cells.[226, 227]

In vitro, both HIV-1 and HIV-2 are cytopathic for some T-cell lines but infect cells of monocyte/macrophage lineage without cytopathic effects. The lack of cytopathicity may be related to the propensity of HIV in these cells to bud into and accumulate in intracytoplasmic vacuoles, where HIV remains immunologically sequestered.[228] In the human host, noncytopathic, latent infection of monocyte/macrophage lineage cells (including bone marrow precursors) and microglial cells in the nervous system may thus provide a reservoir where HIV can persist and be reactivated.[226, 227]

In vitro, silently infected cells can be activated to produce virus by a variety of agents, including specific antigens and mitogens, ultraviolet light, coinfecting viruses (herpesviruses, hepatitis B virus, HTLV-I), and cytokines (granulocyte-macrophage colony-stimulating factor [GM-CSF] and TNF-α).[209] Enhanced HIV expression (by cytokines and other agents) may involve the effect of a DNA binding protein on the HIV promoter region.[229] Future research must clarify mechanisms of viral persistence and activation and how they interact with the host immune response.

NEUROPATHOGENESIS OF HUMAN IMMUNODEFICIENCY VIRUS

Besides immunodeficiency, HIV-1 infection may present as neurologic disorders. Neurologic and neuropsychologic signs and symptoms occur in a significant number of AIDS patients. These symptoms may be directly derived from HIV-1 infection of the nervous system or may be due to associated opportunistic infections or cancers. Neurologic manifestations range from acute aseptic meningitis and inflammatory neuropathies, which are seen early in HIV infection, to AIDS dementia complex, chronic meningitis, mononeuritis, myelopathies, and sensory neuropathies, which are seen in patients with AIDS-related complex and AIDS.[230, 231] Pediatric HIV infection of the nervous system results in AIDS encephalopathy, neurodevelopmental delays, seizures, spastic paraparesis, and dementia. Neuropathologic findings in children are similar to those in adults but more frequently involve calcification, especially in the basal ganglia.[232–235]

Forty percent to 60% of AIDS patients develop AIDS dementia complex, which may be the presenting feature of both HIV-1 and HIV-2 infections.[231, 236] This syndrome, also known as AIDS encephalopathy or subacute encephalitis, refers to the typical neurologic deficits and neuropathology seen in AIDS patients. Direct evidence that HIV-1 causes AIDS dementia complex is based on (1) detection of HIV-1 RNA and DNA in brain tissue by hybridization methods,[233] (2) intrathecal production of HIV-specific immunoglobulin,[237] and (3) viral detection by electron microscopy and isolation from CSF and brain tissue of patients.[230, 232] (Evidence of intrathecal immunoglobulin production is based on comparison of titers in CSF and blood.)

The subtle, early clinical features of AIDS dementia complex—diminished memory and poor concentration—may become more evident during intercurrent illness or opportunistic infections; in later stages it progresses to psychomotor retardation and apathy. Cranial computed tomography may reveal evidence of cerebral atrophy, which on T2-weighted magnetic resonance images shows as diffuse white matter abnormalities.[235, 238–240]

The CSF findings may be completely normal in 20% of HIV-infected persons, but more often they show mildly elevated protein concentration and mononuclear pleocytosis.[241, 242] CSF abnormalities, including intrathecal HIV immunoglobulin G synthesis, are not specific for AIDS dementia complex and can be seen in HIV-infected persons who have no overt neurologic symptoms.[236, 243] The fact that results of CSF viral culture are more often positive for persons with both abnormal CSF and positive plasma viral culture suggests that these persons have higher titers of HIV. Isolated replication of HIV-1 exclusively from the CSF is rare.[244] Reports of high levels of unintegrated viral DNA identified by polymerase chain reaction (PCR) in patients with AIDS dementia may indicate increased viral expression, as it does in cats infected with the feline leukemia virus.[220, 245, 246] Data indicate that treatment with zidovudine (previously azidothymidine, or AZT) has caused the incidence of AIDS dementia complex among AIDS patients to decline and that it inhibits virus replication in the central nervous system.[247]

Autopsy studies indicate that HIV infection of the nervous system is evident in approximately 90% of HIV-infected persons and may involve the brain, spinal cord, or peripheral nerves. These studies often uncover evidence of disease that was not clinically evident.[231, 248–251] Neuropathologic evaluation reveals multinucleated giant cells (syncytia), white matter gliosis and demyelination, microglial nodules, focal necrosis of neurons, and perivascular inflammation.[248, 252, 253]

Pathogenesis of Nervous System Infection

Current data obtained by immunochemical staining and hybridization methods for HIV-1 antigen and nucleic acids in brain tissue indicate that most HIV in the nervous system of infected patients is present in monocyte/macrophages and in related cells—microglial cells and multinucleated giant cells of monocyte origin.[254–256] Neurons and vascular endothelial cells rarely contain HIV, although they may have relatively few CD4 receptors.[257]

Mechanisms proposed to account for HIV-related neurologic disease must account for the disproportionate severity of brain disease and the paucity of infected neurons and other cells. These theories focus on cytotoxic inflammatory products and cytokines released by the HIV-infected macrophage, the combined effects of the virus and viral envelope on cells in the central nervous system, altered permeability of the blood-brain barrier, the role of coinfection by other neurotropic viruses, and toxicity related to autoimmune mechanisms.

It has been proposed that HIV-infected macrophages may play a central but indirect role in the pathogenesis of HIV-related neurologic disease.[258] In vitro data indicate that macrophages express a low density of CD4 on their cell surface and are susceptible to infection but are refractory to syncytium formation and cell killing.[259, 260] Resistance to direct HIV cytopathicity has led investigators to propose that infected monocytes and macrophages serve as a reservoir of persistent infection. As with the visna lentivirus infection of sheep, human monocytes infected in the periphery may serve as a "Trojan horse" to transport virus silently across the blood-brain barrier into the central nervous system. Terminal differentiation of monocytes into tissue macrophages may stimulate HIV replication, release of mediators of inflammation including cytokines, and subsequent central nervous system disease.[261, 262]

It has been proposed that HIV-infected monocyte/macrophages initiate central nervous system damage by releasing cytokines or proteolytic enzymes toxic to adjacent neural cells (the "innocent bystanders"), including endothelial cells, astrocytes, and neurons. Disruption of the blood-brain barrier by injury to endothelial cells (or by direct infection of these cells) may allow toxic agents to enter from the blood stream, which cause further damage. A number of research groups are studying TNF-α (also called cachectin), a cytokine involved in immune and inflammatory reactions that is released by activated macrophages. In vitro, TNF is cytotoxic to glioma-derived cell lines and damages myelin and oligodendrocytes of the spinal cord.[263, 264] HIV-1 stimulates TNF-α and TNF-β production from both peripheral blood mononuclear cells and T lymphocytes. In addition, exogenous addition of specific cytokines such as TNF-α (or TNF-β or interferon-γ) strongly enhances HIV syncytium formation in both cell types.[265] TNF appears to induce HIV-1 transcription by acting on a κB-like enhancer element of the LTR via a nuclear factor-κB–like protein factor.[266]

In the nervous system, HIV infection of neurons and glial cells may result in cell killing by the virus itself and by CTL recognition and killing of infected cells.[267] In vitro support for this hypothesis includes direct infection of neurons and glial cell lines,[159, 173, 268] evidence of HIV-1 and HIV-2 isolates from CSF or brain with monocyte/macrophage tropism, and correlation of biologic features with viral virulence in the host.[260, 269] However, the small fraction of HIV-1–infected cells in the nervous system of AIDS patients suggests that these mechanisms of cell killing are not primary in neuropathogenesis but may be adjunctive.

It has been proposed that neurotoxic effects of viral products such as gp120 have a role in neuropathogenesis by causing innocent bystander destruction of adjacent cells, which induces release of mediators of inflammation and neurotoxic cytokines such as TNF and IL-1. Few experimental data indicate that viral envelope proteins have direct neurotoxic effects on mouse hippocampal neurons and rat retinal ganglion neurons that may be blocked by calcium channel antagonists.[270, 271] The glycoprotein gp120 shares partial sequence homology with neuroleukin, a putative neurotropic factor, subsequently identified as the essential cellular glycolytic enzyme glucophosphoisomerase.[272, 273] There is also a report of the presence of antigenic similarity between the V3 region of the HIV-1 envelope and cellular proteins, which may serve as target for the immune system.[274] The nature of the cellular protein is unknown. Data based on envelope sequence analysis of brain-derived HIV-1 suggest that there might be an association between a particular envelope sequence and AIDS dementia complex.[275] However, a more detailed analysis of other regions of the viral genome may be needed to clarify further the significance of this association. The relative contributions of these mechanisms of neuropathogenesis of HIV await further study.

Epidemiology

GEOGRAPHIC DISTRIBUTION

HIV-1 is distributed worldwide, the greatest seroprevalence being in persons with multiple sexual contacts and in injection drug users (IDUs) in urban centers of North America, South America, the Caribbean, Western Europe, sub-Saharan Africa, Thailand, and India (see Table 264–2). Elevated incidence rates in regions of lower prevalence indicate further international spread. HIV-2 appears to be largely limited in distribution to West Africa, although low rates of infection have been reported in the United States, Portugal, India, Mozambique, Angola, and elsewhere[276] (see Chapter 131).

NATURAL HISTORY

After infection with HIV-1, many infected persons remain asymptomatic, but some develop a mild to severe mononucleosis-like syndrome of fever, myalgia, headache, sore throat, and rash after an incubation period that lasts a few days to 3 months.[277, 278] Median time from infection to seroconversion is estimated as 2.1 months, 95% being detected by 5.8 months.[279] Silent HIV infection—a prolonged seronegative state in which virus can be cultured and viral nucleotides can be detected by PCR methods—is unusual.[280–283] Once an adult person is infected with HIV, the virus is virtually always detectable; in a few rare cases of reversion from HIV-seropositive status to -seronegative status, PCR techniques have demonstrated continued evidence of HIV genome.[282] A few studies of African commercial sex workers with regular frequent exposure to HIV-1 suggest that a few people may become infected locally and develop a Th1 cellular immune response without developing antibodies or systemic infection.[284] Whether such individuals were actually either transiently or persistently infected in a local site awaits further evidence.

Clinical progression of HIV infection to symptomatic illness, regardless of route of transmission, involves a prolonged but variable incubation period with a median of 7 to 10 years in persons older than 12 years. The incubation period is substantially shorter in mother-to-infant cases.[285–288] A small fraction of infected individuals, perhaps 1% to 4%, become long-term nonprogressors, showing no reductions in $CD4^+$ cell count or immune functions until at least 10 years after infection.[289, 290] Although HIV-2 infection is clearly linked to AIDS in some persons, increasing seroprevalence of this infection with age suggests either a longer incubation period than for HIV-1 in most carriers or a benign clinical course in a significant fraction of infected persons.[24] Current theories on causes of individual differences in rates of progression to AIDS include host genetics,[205] virulence of viral strains, nutritional factors,[291] and immune stress related to coinfections with other microorganisms such as mycoplasma, HTLV-I, or herpesviruses (herpes simplex virus, cytomegalovirus, human herpesvirus type 6).[292]

MODES OF TRANSMISSION

The natural history of HIV infection is quite varied and may reflect differences in host immune response, virus dose, viral virulence, and route of infection, all of which may influence susceptibility to infection, rate of progression to AIDS, and transmissibility of the virus to others.[138] For example, the immune system of a person infected by an HIV-contaminated blood transfusion must respond immediately to a greater antigenic load of cell-associated and cell-free virus than that of someone infected by exposure because of a limited dilution of virus by vaginal intercourse. In parenteral infections, HIV is likely to disseminate via the blood stream, promptly invade other sites such as lymph nodes, and secondarily induce a mucosal immune response. In contrast, infections transmitted by sexual or mucosal contact may elicit a more vigorous, primary local immunity, which may have a role in immune containment and degree of infectivity.[293] HIV-exposed cells at mucosal surfaces may act to contain local infection, transmit infection, and prevent superinfection. Whereas direct infection in the blood is likely to begin in monocytes and/or T lymphocytes, infection via vaginal intercourse is more likely to begin in Langerhans cells.[294, 295] Insights into these issues may prove useful in the development of HIV vaccine candidates that are able to initiate immunity protective against sexual, parenteral, and perinatal transmission.

Sexual Transmission

Sexual transmission is the dominant mode of HIV spread in the developing world. About 50% of all AIDS cases in the United States were acquired by homosexual contact and less than 10% by vaginal sex. Heterosexual HIV transmission is becoming increasingly common in the United States. In sub-Saharan Africa and Thailand, sexual transmission accounts for about 90% of reported cases of AIDS.[296] Although sexual contact is clearly the most important determinant of HIV transmission, biologic factors of both host and virus may significantly alter transmission efficiency and play a substantial role in the dynamics of the HIV epidemic.[138, 297, 298]

The most reliable data on heterosexual HIV transmission efficiency involve spouses of hemophiliacs and transfusion recipients.[299–303] In these groups, the rate of male-to-female HIV transmission is estimated to be less than 0.2% per contact in the West, although substantially higher rates are observed in Africa and Asia.[304, 305] Sexual transmission of HIV among homosexual men is thought to be substantially less efficient than that of hepatitis B virus. Several reports indicate lower sexual transmission efficiency from a female infected index case than from a male, a characteristic seen with several sexually transmitted diseases.[138, 306, 307]

Cofactors of Transmission and Host Infectivity. Sexually transmitted diseases may act to enhance host infectiousness or to increase susceptibility to HIV by genital tract inflammation, which disrupts epithelial integrity and brings more susceptible cells in contact with infective secretions. Breaks in the integrity of the mucosal barrier (vaginal, oral, rectal) or of penile squamous epithelium facilitate HIV transmission to exposed persons. Increased risk of HIV transmission results from contact with more virus, either free virus or cell-associated virus in infective secretions. Specific risk factors that may involve this mechanism include the physical trauma of receptive anal intercourse, the presence of diseases that cause genital ulceration, and the presence of other sexually transmitted diseases.[308]

Data for heterosexual male patients with chancroid or syphilis and homosexual males in San Francisco who have herpes simplex clearly document a greater risk of HIV seroconversion associated with prior or coexisting causes of genital ulceration.[304, 309, 310] Nevertheless, the link between HIV and sexually transmitted diseases must be evaluated cautiously, as association may be confounded by shared risk factors such as sexual activity and socioeconomic status.[138, 306, 309, 311]

Currently, host infectiousness is best understood in terms of viral titers in blood, both free in plasma and within mononuclear cells. HIV can be cultured from nearly all infected persons at any stage of infection, and viral titers may increase 10- to 100-fold in symptomatic patients. Viral titers in other tissues and fluids probably increase with progression of HIV infection.[312–314]

Persons with symptomatic HIV infection or low $CD4^+$ cell counts are more likely to transmit infection, probably because they have higher titers of virus in infective body fluid.[315, 316] Failure to transmit HIV to long-standing sexual partners suggests that some hosts may be minimally infectious or that their partners may be resistant to infection. One study of female sexual partners of hemophiliacs reported that seroconversion occurred early and was not related to clinical or immune status of the index case.[317] Case clusters include one study that found an elevated number of $CD8^+$ cells (often seen early in HIV infection) with a normal $CD4^+$ cell level in efficient homosexual male transmitters.[318, 319] Maternal antibodies to gp120 may be protective in limiting perinatal transmission; antibodies to gp120 should be evaluated for their protective role in other modes of transmission as well.[320]

HIV in Semen and the Reproductive Tract. Although results of comparable quantitative viral studies have not been reported, correlation between plasma viral titers and stages of infection may also apply to other body compartments and fluids. In addition, differences in viral titer and location (free or cell-associated virus) may underlie differences in infectivity of semen and vaginal secretions. Virus and HIV antibodies are present in vaginal secretions, semen, and saliva of HIV-infected persons.[152, 313, 314, 321–325] At present, studies in vitro are technically difficult owing to the immunomodulatory effects of seminal plasma[326] and reproductive tract secretions on lymphocytes and macrophages. Semen from American homosexual males who test positive for HIV has elevated numbers of white blood cells, but virus cultures are positive more often with seminal plasma than with the cellular fraction of semen. Local inflammation increases the numbers of all types of white blood cells in semen and may activate lymphocytes and macrophages to produce HIV.[327, 328] Although spermatozoa have few to no CD4 receptors, several reports offer contradictory evidence about whether HIV attaches to or enters them.[329–331] The roles of mucosal immune defense against HIV, antibodies (mucosal immunoglobulin A, immunoglobulin G), and cellular immunity in preventing or facilitating transmission have not been adequately evaluated.

Parenteral Transmission

HIV is transmitted by both cell-free and cell-associated blood products. Before the institution of routine blood screening for HIV in the spring of 1985, substantial numbers of transfusion recipients and hemophiliacs were infected by HIV-contaminated blood products. Nearly 100% of transfusion recipients of HIV-contaminated blood exhibit seroconversion.[332, 333] Needle sharing among HIV-infected IDUs is a particularly risky and efficient route of spread.[334]

Perinatal Transmission

Perinatal HIV infection is common in areas with significant seroprevalence of HIV-1 among women of childbearing age. Perinatal transmission causes almost all of the pediatric HIV infections in the world. HIV-1–seropositive women, particularly if they are symptomatic or have less than 400 $CD4^+$ cells per mm^3, transmit infection to their infants at rates of 13% to 50%,[335–337] but diagnosis is usually delayed because antibodies found in newborns do not distinguish between active infection and passively acquired maternal antibodies until after 12 to 15 months.[337, 338] Enzyme-linked immunosorbent assay (ELISA) p24 antigen testing, viral culture, and especially PCR analysis are useful for earlier detection in infants.[339] A positive PCR result at 3 to 4 months of age should be a reliable indicator of infection of the infant. At earlier periods, small numbers of positive cells in a PCR assay might represent infected maternal cells that can be carried over to the infant. Infected infants reveal no clinical correlates of infection at the time of birth. Although controversy exists over whether HIV-infected infants suffer from prematurity or low birth weight, clearly many die of AIDS within their first 2 years.[340–342] Although few data are available, perinatal transmission of HIV-2 appears to be rare.[343–347]

At present, the time and predominant route of perinatal HIV transmission remain to be clarified. It is increasingly clear that the largest fraction of neonatal infections occur at the time of passage through the birth canal. This fraction is also the most sensitive to prevention by the administration of antiviral drugs to the mother. Placental transfer in utero and transmission during birth have been documented by virus isolation and antigen detection from aborted fetuses, although maternal blood contamination of fetal tissues cannot be excluded.[348] Either way, transplacental transmission would account for only a minority of infant infections. Evidence for some postnatal infection via infected breast milk has also emerged.[349, 350] The current lack of either early diagnostic methods for infants or a clear understanding of the role of breast milk in HIV immunity and transmission has created confusion over recommendations about breast-feeding practices.[335, 351] At present, it should not be recommended that infected mothers breast-feed when sterile equipment with breast milk substitutes is readily available. In developing countries where sterile equipment for breast milk substitutes may not be readily available, breast-feeding is still recommended. Several studies suggest that maternal transmission may be associated with some antibodies to gp120 epitopes.[320, 352, 353] It was demonstrated that the administration of zidovudine to HIV-infected mothers for several months before delivery can reduce the rate of infection in infants by 67%.[354] This has major ramifications and indicates that HIV antibody screening of pregnant women may be important. The value of this regimen in developing countries is unclear, because of the expense involved.[353] Several trials are about to begin to determine whether shorter periods of zidovudine administration just before birth would also decrease maternal transmission rates.

Diagnosis and Prognosis of Infection with Human Immunodeficiency Virus Types 1 and 2

DIAGNOSTIC TECHNIQUES

Techniques for diagnosing HIV range from direct isolation of replication-competent viruses to detection of viral antigens, detection of viral transcripts (mRNA), detection of unintegrated or integrated proviral DNA, and detection of host immune responses to viral antigens. Because of ease, sensitivity, and specificity, serologic methods are used for the routine diagnosis of HIV-1 infection. Serologic methods such as ELISA, particle agglutination, Western blot, immunofluorescence, and radioimmunoprecipitation are described in Chapter 126. According to transfusion studies, HIV seroconversion occurs during a 2- to 6-week period. The earliest detectable antibodies are produced to gp120, followed by antibodies to p24 and *pol* gene products (reverse transcriptase, endonuclease—p64, p53, p34); antibodies to gp41 may not be detectable for up to 6 weeks[355] (see Table 264–3). In contrast to the HIV-1 structural gene products, none of the HIV-1 regulatory gene products is highly immunogenic. Antibody response to these or other gene products, however, may prove useful for diagnosis or prognosis. The most commonly used screening and confirmatory tests, such as the ELISA and Western blot technique, use extracellular virus or synthetic peptides as antigen sources to detect circulating antibodies to HIV.

Current ELISA format tests have greater than 98% to 99% sensitivity and specificity for HIV infection. Positive predictive value is greater than 99% for strongly reactive samples from persons at high risk but is quite dependent on the pretest probability of test positivity. False-positive results occur at higher frequency with samples from people with alcoholic hepatitis, neoplasms, immune abnormalities, multiple transfusions, multiparity, leprosy, and malaria.[356–358] HIV-2–seropositive persons have 59% to 91% cross-reactivity in HIV-1 ELISA tests and can be identified directly by using HIV-2–specific ELISA tests, which are now available in the United States. A combined HIV-1–HIV-2 screening assay may be useful in geographic areas where both viruses exist.[359] The N-terminal region of HIV-2 gp35 is highly immunogenic and allows specific confirmation of HIV-2 infection by Western blotting.[360, 361]

Samples that are repeatedly reactive by ELISA may be confirmed by Western blotting or by less available techniques such as immunofluorescence or radioimmunoprecipitation. The Western blot technique identifies bands of HIV antibodies to discrete viral antigens that are electrophoretically separated and transferred to nitrocellulose paper. This method is more specific than ELISA for detecting HIV infection but varies in test performance characteristics, depending on reagents and methods used. Criteria for a positive result include the presence of bands from at least two gene products: *env*, gp120 or gp41; *gag*, p24 or p19; and *pol*, p64/53 or p34.[362] Negative samples have no bands. Reasons for indeterminate patterns that do not meet the criteria for positive results are not well understood, but these patterns may indicate an early stage of seroconversion, loss of p24 antibodies in progression to AIDS, or HIV-2 infection. Isolated faint reactivity to p24 is often nonspecific. Patterns with reactivity to *pol* antigens usually indicate HIV exposure.[363]

PCR, a method of DNA or RNA amplification, uses whole blood cells or plasma to detect as few as one or several copies of viral genome. This method is highly sensitive and useful for confirming HIV in indeterminate or antibody-negative samples or perinatal infection and detecting HIV in tissue samples. PCR quantification may prove useful in monitoring response to therapy and disease progression.[364, 365] Quantitative competitive PCR is designed to quantitate viral load in an infected individual by measuring viral RNA in plasma samples.[366] Combinations of PCR, especially long-distance PCR, and DNA sequencing can offer precise information about the viral genome over long distances.[367] For rapid classification, for example, to different clades, methods such as the single-strand conformational polymorphism technique can be used after PCR. In situ PCR methods can also be used to provide anatomic or morphologic information such as the type of cells infected and distribution of infected cells in tissues.

Virus isolation, the most specific HIV diagnostic method, remains the "gold standard." Technical improvements allow virus isolation from blood in nearly 100% of HIV-infected persons at stages of infection after the first few months. Virus isolation is done by cocultivation of body fluids with uninfected, mitogen-stimulated peripheral blood mononuclear cells. Isolation takes several weeks and is based on elevation of p24 antigen or reverse transcriptase in the supernatant or on immunofluorescence of infected cells. Virus is commonly isolated, cell free or cell associated, from peripheral blood, bone marrow, genital secretions, brain, and CSF.[313, 325] Isolation from saliva or urine is much less frequent.[368]

MARKERS OF AIDS PROGRESSION

To date, the most useful clinical predictors of progression to AIDS are a decrease in the $CD4^+$ lymphocyte count and a decrease in the ratio of $CD4^+$ to $CD8^+$ cells (which is not dependent on leukocyte count and therefore varies less than the total $CD4^+$ cell count). Using a nonspecific indicator of immune stimulation—elevation in either β_2-microglobulin or neopterin—in conjunction with either of these markers further improves prediction of prognosis. Serum levels of immunoglobulin A, IL-2 receptor, and p24 antigen provide only scant additional information.[369, 370]

Although doing so is technically difficult, HIV-1 can be isolated from both cell-free plasma and peripheral blood mononuclear cells from most infected persons. Several studies indicate that patients in Centers for Disease Control and Prevention stage 4 disease or who have AIDS have 10 to 100 times greater levels of both plasma viremia (free virus) and cell-associated virus than do healthy HIV-seropositive persons. Viral titers in vivo are not closely linked to either p24 antibody or p24 antigen, both of which may be difficult to measure in circulating immune complexes.[313, 314, 371] The titer of antibodies to p24 appears to follow a pattern reciprocal to that of p24 antigen. Levels of p24 antigen correlate with virus replication in vitro and in primary infection. Antibodies to p24 increase and remain high during latency, often in association with a drop in measurable free p24 antigen, and may fall as HIV symptoms develop and p24 antigenemia increases. Viral heterogeneity, circulating immune complexes, or other factors may underlie problems with use of currently available ELISAs as potential prognostic markers. Plasma HIV RNA is a useful clinical marker that indicates both long-term prognosis and response to effective antiretroviral therapies.

HIV-2–associated AIDS appears to have an immune profile comparable to that of HIV-1 AIDS—skin test anergy, diminished $CD4^+$ cell count, and elevated β_2-microglobulin and neopterin levels. Although the natural history has not been fully characterized, in persons followed prospectively,[372, 373] HIV-2 infection appears to induce progressive decreases in $CD4^+$ lymphocytes, although less rapidly than does HIV-1.[24]

Biomedical Prevention and Control Strategies and Prospects

APPROACHES TO RETROVIRAL THERAPY

Current HIV therapies aim to prevent HIV-related disease by attacking actively replicating virus and enhancing the host immune system. These strategies identify or target HIV-infected cells that express viral gene products within the cell or on its surface. Besides these approaches against already infected cells, strategies to protect uninfected cells from being infected by HIVs are also important. Characteristics of the ideal antiretroviral agent include high viral inhibitory activity with low toxicity during prolonged use and excellent penetration into lymphocytes, macrophages, the nervous system, and other immunologically privileged cells or tissues that may harbor virus. Future therapies will most likely employ both antiviral agents and immunomodulators for long-term control of HIV infection. Optimal combinations of drugs and strategies with different mechanisms of action and synergistic anti-HIV effects are required not only to minimize toxicity but also to prevent the emergence of drug resistance.[374] At present, no single antiviral agent has been demonstrated to prevent progression to AIDS except for brief periods. The major cause of the failure is the presence of viral mutant quasi species, which results in the growth of the clone that is resistant to that particular drug. Most recently, combination chemotherapy that includes a protease inhibitor has shown great promise in HIV reduction and prolongation of life.

ANTIRETROVIRAL THERAPIES

Antiretroviral agents can be classified into two major categories on the basis of their molecular weight. Agents with a low molecular weight include several enzyme inhibitors, peptides, or other compounds. These agents are usually administered as drugs and do not need a special delivery system. Another group of agents are molecules with higher molecular weight. These include recombinant proteins and nucleic acid derivatives. These agents may be administered as they are or delivered via special transfer techniques.

Enzyme Inhibitors. Inhibitors of enzymes that are required for HIV replication potentially control HIV infection by interfering at critical steps in the viral life cycle (Fig. 264–5). Currently these represent a major group of antiviral drugs. Potential target enzymes are reverse transcriptase, protease, and integrase. Nucleoside analogs, including zidovudine, which are phosphorylated by cellular kinases, act to competitively inhibit viral reverse transcriptase and terminate DNA chain synthesis. Several nucleoside analogs are reviewed in detail in Chapter 127.

HIV protease is another major target of enzyme inhibitors. The structure of protease has been determined and this information has been used to guide development of inhibitors.[88] The development of inhibitors of integrase is still in an early stage.

Therapeutic Macromolecules. This group contains a broad range of molecules aimed at various steps of virus replication. Advances in knowledge of the HIV-1 life cycle and the introduction of the concept of intracellular immunization guided this approach.[375] Candidate therapeutic molecules range from proteins to nucleic acids. The initial step of viral infection, the binding of virus to a CD4 receptor, can theoretically be inhibited by recombinant proteins such as soluble CD4 (recombinant soluble CD4) and immunoadhesin (CD4-Fc antibody chimera).[376] The infected cells that express viral envelope gp120 may be selectively eliminated by CD4 linked to ricin or other toxins. An approach of gene therapy can be utilized to transduce therapeutic trans-dominant negative mutants of viral genes, ribozymes, and antisense oligonucleotides into infected as well as uninfected target cells.[377] Depending on the kind of molecules and the genes targeted, a

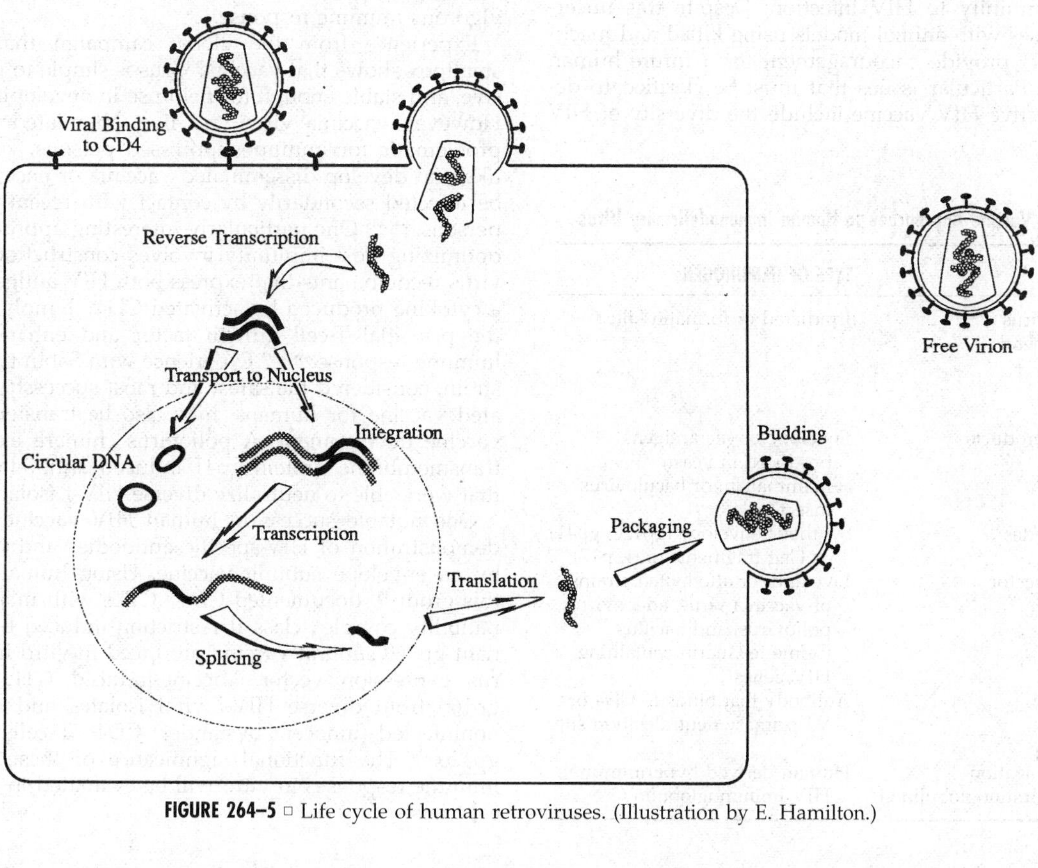

FIGURE 264–5 □ Life cycle of human retroviruses. (Illustration by E. Hamilton.)

variety of steps of virus replication can be attacked. Although some of the agents are quite effective in vitro, a major problem is the low efficiency of delivery and the difficulty of specific targeting to appropriate cell populations.

PROGRESS IN HUMAN IMMUNODEFICIENCY VIRUS VACCINE DEVELOPMENT

A wide range of antigens and delivery vehicles are in development as potential vaccine candidates for HIV (Table 264–5). Vaccine candidates are selected for further testing on the basis of evidence that they elicit HIV-specific immune responses in animals. Human testing ordinarily follows extensive testing of safety, toxicity, and immunogenicity in animals, including primates.

A major difficulty in the development of HIV vaccines is the lack of an appropriate animal model for testing antigen preparations. Two primate models are relevant for testing HIV products. One, the chimpanzee, is extremely expensive, limited in numbers, and representative only for limiting infection rather than disease because chimpanzees usually do not become ill with HIV. The second is the rhesus group of monkeys, which can be similarly infected, without disease development, using simian-human recombinant viruses called simian-human immunodeficiency viruses.[378] Made with envelope genes of HIV-1 and other genes of SIV, these recombinants can be used to challenge after immunization with HIV-1 envelope preparations.

The ideal HIV vaccine should be easy to administer, stable, and inexpensive; have minimal adverse effects; and induce a durable and protective immune response against diverse HIV-1 isolates. In areas of West Africa where the incidence of both viruses is significant, an HIV vaccine should ideally protect against both HIV-1 and HIV-2 infection.

Current approaches to HIV vaccination to prevent infection and immunotherapy to prevent progression to AIDS are limited by a lack of understanding of the critical components of protective immunity to HIV infection. Despite this uncertainty, successes with animal models using killed and inactivated SIV[379, 380] provide encouragement for a future human HIV vaccine. Particular issues that must be clarified to develop an effective HIV vaccine include the diversity of HIV isolates, the high mutation rate of envelope glycoproteins, and the nature of protective immunity.[381–383]

TABLE 264–5 ■ Vaccine Approaches to Human Immunodeficiency Virus

VACCINE	TYPE OF IMMUNOGEN
Killed whole virus blood peripheral lymphocytes + γ-irradiation Formalin	Irradiated or formalin killed
Recombinant products	Envelope or *gag* antigens produced in yeast, mammalian, or baculovirus insect cells
Synthetic peptides	Synthetic envelope (gp120, gp41) or Gag fragments (p24, p17)
Recombinant vector	Live and/or attenuated strains of vaccinia virus, adenovirus, poliovirus, and bacillus Calmette-Guérin containing HIV genes
Antiidiotype Anti-CD4 Anti–V3 loop	Antibody that binds to CD4 or V3 primary neutralization site
Passive immunization Anti–HIV immunoglobulin G	Human-derived hyperimmune HIV immunoglobulin G

SUBUNIT VACCINES, ADJUVANTS, AND LIVE REPLICATION VECTORS

Although current vaccine approaches are quite varied, the earliest and greatest efforts have involved production of subunit vaccines composed of synthetic or recombinant viral envelope proteins (gp41, gp120, and gp160). These approaches generally focus on envelope proteins because they are targets for neutralizing antibodies and cell-mediated immune responses, and they induce protective immunity to feline leukemia virus in cats.[384]

Recombinant methods allow efficient production of large quantities of purified viral antigens and pose no risk of transmitting infectious live virus. Limitations of this approach include the potential for direct toxicity of the viral products, the induction of narrow immunity to the specific antigens used, and the cost, which may be particularly high if glycoproteins must be produced in animal cells.[385] Recombinant viral proteins expressed in prokaryotic cells *(Escherichia coli)* or eukaryotic cells (mammalian cells, yeast, and insect cells containing baculovirus) have different conformation and glycosylation patterns that influence their immunogenicity as vaccines.

Methods for enhancing immunogenicity of these proteins include delivering the proteins with adjuvants that can stimulate T-cell and B-cell activation and using live viral or bacterial recombinants as delivery vectors. New adjuvants, such as saponins[386] and polyphosphazines,[387] may greatly enhance the immune response.[388] Expression of recombinant viral genes in the human host by a replicating viral vector, such as vaccinia virus, adenovirus, and poliovirus, or Ty, the yeast transposon, is a promising approach that has several distinct advantages.[389–393] This method, by using a replicating attenuated vector (containing HIV-1 envelope genes) that produces viral proteins, may more closely simulate natural infection, resulting in greater antigen exposure and a broader, more vigorous immune response.

Experience from the global campaign that eliminated smallpox shows that vaccinia virus is simple to use, inexpensive, and stable enough for field use in developing countries. However, vaccinia virus and live, attenuated vaccines are problematic for immunosuppressed persons, who are more likely to develop disseminated vaccinia or encephalitis or to be infected secondarily by contact with recently vaccinated persons.[394, 395] One particularly interesting approach aimed at optimizing host immunity involves construction of vaccinia virus recombinants that express both HIV antigens and IL-2, a cytokine produced by activated $CD4^+$ lymphocytes that is the principal T-cell growth factor and enhances the host immune response.[396, 397] Experience with Sabin type 1 vaccine strain, considered the safest and most successful live attenuated vaccine for humans, may also be transferable to HIV vaccine development. A poliovirus chimera expressing the transmembrane protein gp41 induced antibodies in rabbits that were able to neutralize diverse HIV-1 isolates.[398]

One notable success in human HIV vaccine trials is the demonstration of HIV-specific antibodies and CTLs elicited by an envelope subunit vaccine. Using human volunteers, this group[385] documented $CD4^+$ CTLs with major histocompatibility complex class II restriction induced by a recombinant gp160 subunit vaccine produced in vitro in a baculovirus expression vector. Vaccine-induced CTLs recognized gp160 from diverse HIV-I viral isolates and did not lyse noninfected (innocent bystander) $CD4^+$ T cells coated with gp120.[385] The functional significance of these HIV-specific immune responses in vitro will be evaluated in further clinical trials.

OTHER APPROACHES

Killed virus vaccines have proved successful as retroviral vaccines in animal models, but the possibility of inadequate inactivation of a lethal virus makes use of killed HIV vaccine in uninfected humans a greater concern. Virus inactivation by irradiation, heat, or chemicals (formalin, psoralen, or propionolactone) destroys infectivity by disrupting viral RNA but preserves viral antigenicity. In one trial, formalin-inactivated whole SIV potentiated with alum, muramyl dipeptide, or both conferred protection to challenge doses of live SIV in eight of nine rhesus macaques.[379, 399] Postexposure immunization in humans using irradiated or inactivated HIV-1 has been reported, but its efficacy is unclear.[400, 401] Immunization with defective genetically engineered nonpathogenic viral strains that are able to express viral antigens but unable to replicate has also been proposed.[124]

Different approaches using HIV-specific antibody immunization include passive immunotherapy and antiidiotype vaccination. To date, one study has shown that HIV hyperimmune globulin extracted from infected persons does not confer protection to virus challenge when injected into chimpanzees.[402] Hyperimmunization, which has been useful in preventing perinatal transmission of hepatitis B virus, has also been proposed to prevent perinatal transmission of HIV. The antiidiotype approach involves the production of antibody with CD4-like conformation that has high binding affinity for gp120. In theory, this antibody binds envelope gp120 without exposing the vaccinee to the potential risks of the viral antigens, but it may itself impair the immune system by preventing normal interaction of CD4 receptors with major histocompatibility complex antigens.[403, 404]

HUMAN IMMUNODEFICIENCY VIRUS VACCINE TRIALS: THE BROADER CONTEXT

The rapid spread and worldwide distribution of HIV infection require that many and different potential vaccines be expedited through animal testing for prompt evaluation in human subjects. Despite the urgent need for a vaccine, human trials must be carefully planned and follow rigorous ethical guidelines tailored to the cultural sensitivities of the participants.[405] Human phase I and II vaccine trials evaluating safety, immunogenicity, and dosing schedules are done in healthy adults at low risk of infection to minimize the possibility that an HIV-specific immune response is due to occult or intercurrent HIV infection or is influenced by another infection or a disease cofactor present in a high-risk group.[406] Patterns of HIV transmission and host immune response may differ because of sexual habits, genetic differences, or endemic infectious exposures that may be related to geographic origin.[216, 217] Trials should maintain strict confidentiality of study participants to avoid possible economic and social discrimination that may result from association with an HIV vaccine trial. Vaccine recipients must anticipate vaccine-induced HIV seroconversion and possible restrictions on foreign travel, blood donation, insurance, and job eligibility.

Currently, the HIV-1 that is spreading most rapidly in developing countries in Asia and Africa is different in envelope subtype specificity (e.g., HIV-1 A, C, D, E) from the HIV-1 that is endemic in the United States and Western Europe. Although the vaccine trials would be most efficient in sites such as Thailand or sub-Saharan Africa, Western commercial companies have little incentive to make a vaccine with those strains or subtypes because they are not currently present in the West. This dilemma has diminished the pace of HIV vaccine development.[407]

Human T-Cell Lymphotropic Virus Types I and II

Biology

VIRAL STRUCTURE

The HTLVs are spherical, enveloped type C oncoviruses of approximately 100 nm (see Fig. 264–2). They emerge from infected cells by budding from the cytoplasmic membrane or at vacuolar membranes. A proviral genome of HTLV-I and HTLV-II is presented in Figure 264–1. The genotypes of different isolates of HTLV-I are closely related to each other, 95% to 99% related at the sequence level. HTLV-II is about 60% related to HTLV-I at the sequence level. The closest relatives of the HTLV-type viruses are bovine leukemia virus and simian T-cell leukemia virus of Old World monkeys and apes. Whereas bovine leukemia virus has minimal sequence homology with the HTLVs, the simian T-leukemia virus is quite closely related to HTLV-I.[408]

Structural Genes

As described earlier, the overall organization of the HTLV-I genome is similar to that of other retroviruses. The *gag* gene encodes a polyprotein of approximately 55 kDa that is processed into 19-, 24-, and 15-kDa proteins. The 19-kDa protein is a matrix protein. It is perhaps the most type specific for distinguishing between HTLV-I and HTLV-II. It is myristylated, phosphorylated, and situated at the inner surface of the outer viral envelope. The p24 capsid protein makes up the major capsid structure and is usually highly immunogenic. Most HTLV-infected persons make antibodies to both p24 and p19. The viral protein at the C-terminal, p15, is found internally at the nucleocapsid. Infected cells often contain breakdown products of a polyprotein encoded by portions of p24 and p19. The *pol* gene encodes protease, reverse transcriptase, and integrase. The protease catalyzes cleavage of the Gag and Pol polyproteins. Frequent genetic changes in the protease gene may be one reason for the general lack of infectious molecular clones. The Gag and Pol products can be translated from a single message by ribosomal frameshifting.[29, 409] Other polymerase products include a reverse transcriptase molecule and a nuclease-integrase molecule. These protein products have not yet been characterized for the HTLVs. The HTLVs differ from most conventional leukemia viruses in that reverse transcriptase utilizes Mg^{2+} as its divalent cation, rather than Mn^{2+}. The *env* gene encodes a polyprotein of approximately 61 kDa (gp61). It is glycosylated but not as heavily as the analogous, much larger proteins of HIV. The envelope polyprotein undergoes cleavage to form the outer spike peplomer protein (gp46) and the 21-kDa transmembrane protein, both of which are highly immunogenic. For some strains of HTLV-I, Tax-Env fusion proteins may be seen at various sizes from 60 to 70 kDa. There is also slight size polymorphism for different isolates of HTLV-I and HTLV-II, so that the polyprotein may be as large as 67 kDa and the N-terminal cleavage product may be as large as 52 kDa.

REGULATORY GENES

As with HIVs, HTLVs make mRNA for two key regulatory nuclear proteins, Tax and Rex, from doubly spliced RNA. The *tax* genes of HTLV-I and HTLV-II encode proteins of about 40 kDa that function as efficient transactivators for transcription from the virus 5′ LTR[38, 39, 410] (see Fig. 264–1). Tax can also activate other heterologous promoters via its interaction with other transcriptional factors.[47] As described earlier, this indirect mechanism of transactivation function for Tax may be responsible for immortalization or transformation. One candidate is target gene IL-2 and/or its receptor.[51]

The *rex* gene encodes at least two proteins of approximately 21 and 27 kDa.[44, 45] The *rex* gene, like the *tax* gene, is essential for virus replication. p27 Rex apparently functions at a posttranscriptional level to regulate mRNA splicing.[411] p27 facilitates the expression of viral structural genes *(gag, pol, env)* and reduces proportionally the expression of *tax* and *rex* (the regulatory genes). The function of p21 Rex is still not understood. As with Rev of HIVs, Rex functions through the cis-acting sequences located in the 3′ LTR called *rex*-responsive element.[35–37] Rex can complement Rev function but not vice versa.[412] The pX region also encodes several small proteins.[413, 414]

LIFE CYCLE

It is assumed that HTLVs have a replication cycle similar to that of other retroviruses. The HTLV-I life cycle is, however, much less well understood than the life cycles of the HIVs. This is in part because an infectious molecular clone of HTLVs has not been available until lately and infection of cells with intact virus HTLVs is inefficient. Although the exact receptor to which the HTLVs bind has not been identified, it is clearly highly represented on T lymphocytes and perhaps on other cells, including selected cultured cells of myeloid,[415] fibroblast, and epithelial origin.[416, 417] Because circulating T cells of certain lower species can also be infected,[418] this receptor is presumably conserved. In humans the gene for the receptor is located on chromosome 17.[419] As HTLV is usually present in low titer and is defective in cell-free form, infection of other cells is usually more efficient by cocultivation with infected cells. As infectious molecular clones of the virus have been extremely difficult to obtain, it is possible that extracellular virus is usually replication defective.

Immune Response and Immune Defects Associated with Human T-Cell Lymphotropic Virus Infection

Studies of recipients of HTLV-I–contaminated transfused blood demonstrate detectable antibodies by standard serologic tests within 3 to 6 weeks after infection. Titers of immunoglobulin M antibodies detected early fall as immunoglobulin G levels rise during the first several months of infection.[420] The major structural gene products of *gag* (p19, p24, p15), envelope (gp46), and transmembrane protein (gp21) and to a lesser extent the regulatory *tax* gene product are immunogenic in infected individuals. Given the low variability of the HTLV-I genome, HTLV-I–specific antibodies, especially antibody to the gp46 viral envelope, probably modify the course of HTLV infection. An important question remains about the possibility of delayed antibody expression and a prolonged seronegative state for months or years, particularly after neonatal exposure. A study that screened for prolonged incubation of HTLV-I infection in relatives of patients with tropical spastic paraparesis, an HTLV-I–associated myelopathy (TSP/HAM), found no evidence among seronegative first-degree relatives for latent viral genomes using PCR techniques.[421] Current data suggest that anti-Tax antibody is a marker for increased HTLV-I infectivity in perinatal transmission and for increased sexual transmission.[422–424]

Cell-mediated immune control mechanisms described for HTLV-I include CTLs, natural killer cell activity, and ADCC.[425–428] The mapping of functional domains of the gp46 envelope glycoproteins of HTLV-I and HTLV-II, the primary targets of ADCC, may provide insights important for vaccine development.[429] The relative contributions of humoral and cellular immunity in controlling primary infection, viral persistence, and disease expression have not been clearly delineated.

HTLV-I–related dysfunction in cell-mediated immunity includes depressed delayed-type hypersensitivity skin testing responses in HTLV-I carriers, which is most apparent in patients at least 60 years of age.[430] Increased susceptibility to common infections and possibly to cancers appears to be related to HTLV-I seropositivity alone, as distinct from the immunocompromise associated with chronic and acute forms of ATL/lymphoma (ATLL). Indirect evidence also comes from elevated seroprevalence rates among persons with infectious diseases and among cancer patients in Japan.[431, 432]

Studies in vitro indicate that HTLV-I infection induces an immune deficit, including altered T-cell functions such as reduced T-cell memory responses to Epstein-Barr virus,[433] functional alterations of $CD4^+$ tumor cells in ATLL so that they behave more as suppressor cells,[434] and diminished cytotoxic activity.[435] Segments of transmembrane protein gp21 inhibit lymphoproliferation in mice and may participate in HTLV-I–related immunosuppression.[436] The progressive irreversible depletion of helper T cells and lymphocytes characteristic of HIV-I infection is not seen with HTLV-I infection.

Although HTLV-II also appears to alter T-cell function, it has been studied less than HTLV-I.[437] One report of immunologic evaluation of 11 IDUs in New Orleans who were infected with HTLV-I, HTLV-II, or both described abnormal T-cell–dependent B-cell proliferative response as assessed by the pokeweed mitogen response.[438]

Epidemiology

GEOGRAPHIC DISTRIBUTION

There is a unique clustered geographic distribution of HTLV-I in the world. Greatly elevated rates of infection occur in southwestern Japan, on the islands of Kyushu, Shikoku, and Okinawa.[439] Within this region, there also exists local clustering of HTLV-I infection. The highest rates occur in coastal towns such as Kagoshima in Kyushu, where more than a quarter of the adults may be infected with HTLV-I. Areas in the middle region of Japan, such as the Tokyo area, have low rates of HTLV-I infection. Relatively few comprehensive studies have been done elsewhere in Asia, but it is clear that the virus is present in other regions, such as Taiwan.[440]

The second major region of the world where elevated rates of HTLV-I were described early is the Caribbean basin.[441] In all instances, rates of infection increased with advancing age. Elevated rates of HTLV-I also occur in South America,[442] Central America, and sub-Saharan Africa.[443, 444] The wide distribution of HTLV-I suggests that this virus has been in the human population considerably longer than HIV-1 or HIV-2.

Because many of the studies of geographic distribution of HTLV have relied on serologic evaluations that are extensively cross-reactive between HTLV-I and HTLV-II, less is known about the distribution of HTLV-II. For many infections reported primarily on the basis of antibody prevalence the pathogen could have been either virus. More extensive analysis suggests that, at least in the southwestern regions of Japan, the agent is primarily or exclusively HTLV-I. In the United States, however, HTLV-II seems at least as common as HTLV-I.[445] In Europe, the rates of infection with both HTLV-I and HTLV-II appear to be low, except in certain populations of migrants or IDUs.[446] One possible interpretation of the elevated rates for HTLV-II among IDUs is that this virus is transmitted more efficiently than HTLV-I by the parenteral route.

MODES OF TRANSMISSION

HTLV-I is highly cell associated and is efficiently transmitted by exposure to blood containing HTLV-I–infected cells. A number of studies demonstrate that seroconversion occurs in 48% to 82% of recipients of HTLV-I–contaminated cellular products, but no risk is associated with factor concentrates or noncellular blood products.[420, 447] The fact that virus can be identified from nearly 100% of HTLV-I–seropositive healthy donors indicates that all asymptomatic carriers are potentially infectious.[448] Routine blood screening for HTLV-I should substantially reduce the risk of HTLV-I infection for leukemia patients and others who receive multiple transfusions.[449, 450]

Parenteral Transmission

Blood exposure through needle sharing appears to be an efficient means of HTLV transmission. Serologic evidence of HTLV-II infection is reported in IDUs in New York City, New Orleans, and Great Britain. In one study, 19 of 169 IDUs in New York City had evidence of HTLV-II by PCR assay and high rates of dual or triple infection with HTLV-I and HIV-1.[445, 451–453]

Sexual Transmission

Elevated rates of HTLV-I seropositivity among sexual partners of patients with ATLL, female sex workers, homosexual men, and persons with sexually transmitted diseases indicate that HTLV-I is transmitted sexually and more efficiently from male to female than from female to male. HTLV-I has been detected in 1% of lymphocytes in semen of a carrier, but viral genomes have not been quantified or correlated systematically with the stage of infection.[454] In Japan, both prospective and cross-sectional studies of spouses show more efficient male-to-female sexual transmission.[423, 455, 456] More efficient sexual spread from male to female may be related to prolonged retention of infective semen in the female reproductive tract. Higher rates of HTLV-I infection were associated with increasing age, multiple sexual partners, and genital ulcerations, including lesions of syphilis. In these aspects, HTLV-I sexual transmission may be similar to that of HIV-1, which is also enhanced by genital ulcerations and is transmitted more efficiently from male to female.[304] These factors may alter the dose and likelihood of exposure, host susceptibility, and transmissibility of HTLV-I infection.[457, 458] A prospective study of HTLV-I in couples from Japan provided evidence that antibody to p40 Tax protein may serve as a marker of relative infectivity in HTLV-I–seropositive men.[422, 423]

Perinatal Transmission

Although breast-feeding is thought to be the primary factor in perinatal transmission of HTLV-I, only 25% of breast-fed children of HTLV-I carrier mothers were infected.[459] Numerous reports, both cross-sectional surveys and prospective evaluations, established a high risk of postnatal transmission to infants of seropositive mothers and a lower risk for bottle-fed infants.[460] Bottle feeding is an effective measure to control the endemic cycle of HTLV-I transmission and should significantly reduce the incidence of carriers and future ATLL cases. Further study is required to establish optimal recommendations for seropositive mothers in developing countries, as breast-feeding is a simple and effective measure to reduce infant mortality in those areas.[455, 461]

Several cross-sectional studies suggest that antibody to p40 Tax protein is a marker for infectivity, as hepatitis e antigen is in hepatitis B infections. These studies found significantly higher rates of HTLV-I in mothers with antibody to p42 Tax protein. Clarification of the role of this antibody may require prospective evaluation controlling for breast-feeding practices.[422, 424, 462]

Adult T-Cell Leukemia/Lymphoma

INCIDENCE

The typical presentation of ATLL is in adults with a mean age of approximately 50 years.[54, 55] Infection of an immature immune system early in life may be critical to ATLL development, which typically occurs more than 20 years after infection. Lifetime risk of ATLL among HTLV-I carriers is estimated as 1% to 5%.[52, 53] The best population level data are available from Japan, where there are approximately 1.2 million carriers, primarily from endemic areas in the southern and western prefectures, and 700 new cases of ATLL each year. Familial case clustering may be related to greater risk associated with perinatal transmission or to shared environmental or genetic susceptibility.[463] In the United States, ATLL has been reported most frequently from endemic areas in the southeast, especially in black persons and in migrants from HTLV-I endemic areas.[464, 465] The American Adult T-Cell Leukemia/Lymphoma Registry, established in 1987 at the National Cancer Institute, may facilitate epidemiologic studies and expedite identification of HTLV-I infection in endemic areas in the United States.

CLINICAL FEATURES

HTLV-I–Associated Hematologic Abnormalities

HTLV-I–associated hematologic abnormalities span a clinical spectrum that may involve progression from asymptomatic carrier to a preleukemic state (pre-ATL), chronic and smoldering ATL, and acute ATL and lymphoma. At each stage there is evidence of monoclonal or oligoclonal provirus integration into the host cellular genome. Asymptomatic carriers may be identified when blood screening is performed for other purposes.

Pre-ATL is often found unexpectedly in asymptomatic carriers who show leukocytosis or morphologically abnormal lymphocytes associated with monoclonal or oligoclonal proviral integration. About half of these persons experience spontaneous resolution of the leukocytosis; in the remainder, leukocytosis persists or evolves to acute ATLL. Approximately 30% of patients have a smoldering or chronic phase that involves skin lesions, without visceral involvement, and absent (smoldering) or mild (chronic) elevation of total white cell count. Superficial dermatophytosis is common in these patients. Progression from pre-ATL, chronic, and smoldering states may occur during a period of months to years.[54, 466–469]

Clinical Manifestations

ATLL[6] is an aggressive neoplasm characterized by proliferation of T cells with one or several HTLV-I proviruses integrated into the cellular genome. Progression to ATLL involves transformation and growth of a dominant clonal population of lymphocytes. As with other infectious agents, a major reason to assume that HTLV-I causes ATLL is the observation that the virus is regularly present in the tumor cells. The monoclonal integration sites observed for the provirus in all primary tumors indicate that all cells in a given tumor (even when they are dispersed in leukemia) originate from the one cell initially infected by virus.[470]

In the past, the differential diagnosis of HTLV-I–associated hematologic abnormalities and ATLL has been hindered by a lack of HTLV-I diagnostic methods. ATLL should be distinguished from other T-cell malignancies, including non-Hodgkin's lymphoma, T-cell chronic lymphocytic leukemia, and two other conditions with prominent skin manifestations, mycosis fungoides and Sézary syndrome.

Presenting clinical features include lymphadenopathy that

does not involve the mediastinum, hepatomegaly and splenomegaly, skin lesions, hypercalcemia, and opportunistic infections. In acute T-cell leukemia, peripheral blood smears reveal a raised white cell count and abnormal T lymphocytes with lobulated or indented nuclei.[471] Up to a third of cases are of the lymphomatous type, however, and have no circulating tumor cells. Leukemic cell infiltration may result in skin lesions, interstitial pneumonitis, and ascites.[472]

Granulocytosis and eosinophilia are common and may result from increased production of GM-CSF. In vitro, HTLV-I and HTLV-II *tax* gene transactivates the GM-CSF promoter, leading to constitutive GM-CSF production.[473] Elevations in serum calcium, lactate dehydrogenase, and bilirubin values are common. Hypercalcemia often occurs in association with lytic bone lesions and may result from the activity of tumor cells to convert vitamin D precursor to the highly active 1,25-dihydroxyvitamin D_3.[474]

ATLL leads to immune compromise and may present opportunistic infections identical to those seen in AIDS, such as *Pneumocystis carinii* pneumonia and superficial or disseminated fungal infections, including cryptococcal meningitis, *Candida* esophagitis, and cytomegalovirus pneumonia. Recurrent *Strongyloides stercoralis* infection has been reported in association with both smoldering and acute ATLL.[475, 476]

Immunophenotyping of tumor cells in blood and tissue demonstrates diffuse pleomorphic large-cell non-Hodgkin's lymphoma, with characteristics of a mature activated helper T cell: Tac antigen$^+$/IL-2 receptor$^+$, terminal deoxytransferase–negative (TdT$^-$), and E rosette–positive. The cells are usually CD4$^+$ but occasionally CD4$^-$/CD8$^+$. ATLL cells frequently show different karyotypic abnormalities but no particular chromosomal abnormality that occurs regularly.[477, 478]

Markers that are reported to correlate with poor prognosis include the presence of ascites, marked white blood cell increase, pronounced hypercalcemia, and serum levels of soluble IL-2 receptor.[479–482] The level and significance of antibody to p42 Tax protein in patients with ATLL have varied in reports.[424, 483]

THERAPY

At present, there is no effective treatment for ATLL. Acute, full-blown ATLL is highly aggressive and usually resistant to standard combination chemotherapies designed for the treatment of acute lymphoblastic leukemia and non-Hodgkin's lymphoma.[484–486] Despite promising initial findings, the therapeutic efficacy of deoxycoformycin has not been clearly demonstrated. Interferon-β and interferon-γ have also been used to treat ATLL.

Unlike resting T cells, HTLV-I–infected T cells in ATLL and TSP/HAM express Tac peptide and high levels of IL-2 receptor. Therefore, therapies may be targeted to exploit altered cell surface proteins of HTLV-I–infected cells. Targeted approaches such as administration of anti-Tac antibody and IL-2–linked diphtheria toxin may afford selective killing of HTLV-I–transformed T cells of ATLL.[487] It may be possible to screen potential therapeutic agents using a rabbit model in which newborn animals injected with HTLV-I develop ascites with leukemic infiltrates comparable to that seen in ATLL.[488]

Human T-Cell Lymphotropic Virus and Neurologic Disease

TSP/HAM

HTLV-I is also linked with another disease entity—TSP/HAM. Since the first report from the Caribbean, TSP/HAM has been reported from HTLV-I endemic areas of Japan, Latin America, the Caribbean, and other parts of the world.[489–493] TSP/HAM is discussed in detail in Chapter 130.

OTHER NEUROLOGIC CONDITIONS

Reports of a possible association between HTLV-I and inflammatory neural diseases such as multiple sclerosis have been difficult to verify, and at present there is no convincing evidence to support an association.[494, 495] Results of studies using highly sensitive techniques such as PCR conflict and do not support a role for HTLV-I in multiple sclerosis.[496, 497]

COMPARISON OF PATHOGENESIS OF ATLL AND TSP/HAM

Case reports of TSP/HAM patients developing ATLL and patients with ATLL before TSP/HAM suggest that different, but to date incompletely understood, pathogenic mechanisms underlie these conditions. Since the first cases of TSP/HAM were identified by their clinical similarities and response to steroids, investigators have speculated about a possible immune pathogenesis of this condition. It is difficult at present to separate the complex interaction of viral factors and host immune response in the pathogenesis of TSP/HAM. Several studies have documented a higher load of HTLV-I viral genome in patients with TSP/HAM than in asymptomatic persons who are seropositive.[498–500] To date, no drastic differences have been identified by sequence analysis between HTLV-I isolates from persons with TSP/HAM and isolates from patients with ATLL.[501, 502] However, it is possible some subtle changes in HTLV-I genes such as *tax* may be associated with the different pathologic outcome.[503]

Other Illnesses Possibly Associated with Human T-Cell Lymphotropic Virus Type I

HTLV-I may also be involved in B-cell chronic lymphocytic leukemia. Evidence for this association includes the increased seroprevalence of HTLV-I in Caribbean and African patients with chronic lymphocytic leukemia[504] and the fact that hybridoma cell lines derived from two patients with this disorder produced HTLV-I–specific antibodies.[505] The HTLV-I *tax* gene product may be associated with the development of chronic B-cell leukemia in humans.[505, 506] Nevertheless, B-cell chronic lymphocytic leukemia is not common in Japan, and in two cases studied, tumor cells did not have integrated HTLV-I provirus.[507] Case reports also suggest association of HTLV-I seropositivity with idiopathic adult polymyositis and leprosy.[508–510]

Interaction Between Human T-Cell Lymphotropic Virus and Human Immunodeficiency Virus

HTLV-I shares cell tropism for CD4$^+$ cells with HIV-1 and may interact to promote HIV expression.[511, 512] HIV replication is enhanced and sustained in HTLV-I– and HTLV-II–infected cell lines.[513] The envelope of HTLV-I or HTLV-II can independently activate T cells, leading to HIV expression.[514] Although the viral transactivating proteins—Tax of HTLV-I and HTLV-II and Tat of HIV-1—do not cross-activate the heterologous promoters, HTLV-I and HTLV-II *rex* regulatory gene product can function interchangeably with *rev* in HIV-1 (but not vice versa).[412, 515, 516]

These data suggest that clinically significant interactions may occur in persons coinfected with HTLV and HIV. To date, most reports of viral cofactors have examined the role of HTLV as a cofactor in altering disease progression to AIDS in persons infected with HIV. A number of reports of persons infected with both HTLV-I and HIV-1 identified shared risk factors, such as injection drug use, blood product exposure, and multiple sexual partners.[451, 517, 518] Preliminary clinical reports of accelerated progression to AIDS in coinfected patients in Trinidad have not been confirmed, however,[519, 520] and the effect has not been found in some other populations.[521, 522] A prospective study of IDUs in Miami documented a threefold greater risk of AIDS among persons with seroprevalent infections of both HTLV-I and -II and HIV-1 infections than among those infected only with HIV-1. The implications of the results are limited, however, in the absence of knowledge of duration of HIV seropositivity; dual infection may indicate more prolonged HIV infection.[523] Interesting case reports include ATL in a 19-year-old woman from West Africa[524] who was seropositive for HTLV-I, HIV-2, and human herpesvirus 6. Prospective studies of larger groups are needed to clarify the role of both viruses and cofactors in disease progression. Further study of viral interactions is important, as those who have dual infection may warrant more frequent observation in asymptomatic stages, earlier intervention, and more aggressive therapy to prevent disease progression.

Associations Between Human T-Cell Lymphotropic Virus Type II and Disease

The clinical spectrum of HTLV-II–associated disease is not known and may be somewhat confounded by the serologic cross-reactivity with HTLV-I. Although no convincing clinical association with HTLV-II has been established, the virus has been isolated on a number of occasions from patients with a T-cell variant of hairy cell leukemia.[11, 525, 526] The leukemic cells are predominantly T cells, may appear atypical in the circulation, show hairy cell morphology, and may stain positive for tartrate-resistant acid phosphatase. One patient with evidence of a double lymphoproliferative disease involving clonal expansion of $CD8^+$ T cells with integrated HTLV-II provirus also had evidence of an aggressive B-cell hairy cell leukemia. Tumor cells from the more common B-cell hairy cell leukemia do not harbor HTLV-II genome.[527, 528] Individual case reports described virus isolation or serologic evidence of HTLV-II in patients with T-cell chronic lymphocytic leukemia with neutropenia, T-cell prolymphocytic leukemia, hemophilia A with pancytopenia, AIDS, and exfoliative erythrodermatitis.[453, 526, 529, 530]

Diagnosis of Infection with Human T-Cell Lymphotropic Virus Types I and II

Although only a small percentage of HTLV-I–infected persons develop disease and the fraction who develop HTLV-II disease may be even smaller, both viruses are transmitted efficiently with whole blood or blood cells.[420] When appropriate assay systems are used, antibodies to the Env and Gag antigens can be detected readily. Almost all infected persons have antibodies to the Env external glycoprotein gp45, the transmembrane protein p21, and the Env polyprotein gp61.[531, 532] Most also have antibodies to the virus core proteins p24 and p19 as well as the Gag precursor p55. The majority of infected persons also have antibodies to the Tax protein p42,[39, 410] but the possibility remains that a small fraction of latently infected persons may make antibodies to the Tax protein in the absence of antibodies to the virus structural proteins. Only a small fraction of HTLV-infected people have detectable antibodies to the Rex proteins (see Table 264–3).

The currently available commercial tests contain either whole disrupted virus antigens or recombinant expressed virus structural proteins in an ELISA format or an agglutination format. Although at least half of the HTLV-infected persons in the United States are infected with HTLV-II rather than HTLV-I,[445] all of the current tests contain only HTLV-I antigen. As a result, 10% to 20% of HTLV-II infections may be scored (false) negative.

Tests that are made with whole disrupted virus may also miss some people who have antibodies directed primarily at the envelope proteins. As the outer envelope glycoprotein is fragile and HTLV is expensive to produce, most "whole virus" antigen preparations contain only borderline amounts of these important antigens. In addition, the existing agglutination tests may give false-negative reactions with high-titer antibodies owing to a prozone effect.[533]

Antibodies to the Tax protein are more prevalent in persons who became infected from their mothers,[424] and the presence of these antibodies in men indicates an increased risk for sexual transmission of HTLV-I to the spouse.[423] These observations suggest that the presence of Tax antibodies may indicate elevated levels of replicating virus.

For confirmatory tests, Western blotting is most often used, but radioimmunoprecipitation and immunofluorescence may also be used.[534] The criterion for confirming infection is the presence of antibodies to the products of two of the following three genes: for *gag* p19 or p24, for *tax* p42, and for *env* gp45 or gp61.

Some regions of the external glycoprotein are more immunogenic than others,[535, 536] and some domains are relatively type specific for HTLV-I or HTLV-II. When used appropriately, this allows one to identify the type of infection.[536] PCR can also be used to confirm infection with HTLV-I or HTLV-II when whole blood is available for DNA. With the use of appropriate primers and probes, PCR tests can detect both HTLV-I and HTLV-II or distinguish between them.[445]

Treatment and Vaccine Prospects

THERAPY

Currently, there is no indication for treating asymptomatic persons with evidence of HTLV-I or HTLV-II exposure. In vitro, zidovudine inhibits infectivity of HTLV-I, but efficacy and toxicity have not been evaluated directly in HTLV-I–seropositive persons.[537] Chemotherapies identified for their anti–HIV-1 activity should be evaluated for activity against HTLV-I. Basic similarities in structure and function of essential retroviral genes such as *pol* (reverse transcriptase, protease, integrase) may indicate shared drug sensitivity.

PREVENTION AND CONTROL STRATEGIES

Since 1986, Japan has instituted prevention programs for HTLV-I infection, including blood screening and vigorous injunctions against breast-feeding by seropositive mothers. Blood screening alone is expected to eliminate 16% of new HTLV-I infections in Japan. Avoidance of breast-feeding may substantially reduce the risk of perinatal transmission, although changes in prevalence of HTLV-I infection and HTLV-I complications in endemic areas may not be evident on a population level for years.[538]

Although the geographic distribution and risk groups for HTLV-I and HTLV-II infection in the United States are less clearly established than in Japan, blood screening for HTLV-I infection will limit transmission. However, the precise impact of this intervention in the United States may be difficult to estimate. Owing to the similarities in HTLV and HIV transmission and epidemiologic risks, current methods of blood donor screening substantially reduce risk of HTLV-I infection by blood products.

VACCINE APPROACHES

In the AIDS era, vaccine prevention of HTLV-I has not received high priority because HTLV-I carriers develop disease relatively infrequently. Current research priorities emphasize

HIV-1 vaccine development, which may provide important directions for work on HTLV-I. Documentation of effective humoral immune responses to vaccine candidates and passive immunization in animal models are important steps toward the development of a vaccine for HTLV-I.[539]

References

1. Ellerman V, Bang O: Zentrabl Bakteriol Parasitenkd Infectionskr Hyg 46:596, 1908.
2. Gross L: "Spontaneous" leukemia developing in C3H mice following inoculation in infancy with AK-leukemic extracts or AK embryos. Proc Soc Exp Biol Med 78:27, 1953.
3. Jarrett B, Crawford E, Martin WB, et al: Leukemias in the cat: A virus-like particle associated with leukemia (lymphosarcoma). Nature 202:567, 1964.
4. Essex M: Horizontally and vertically transmitted oncornavirus of cats. Adv Cancer Res 21:175–248, 1975.
5. Poiesz BJ, Ruscetti FW, Gazdar AF, et al: Detection and isolation of type C retrovirus particles from fresh and cultured lymphocytes of a patient with cutaneous T-cell lymphoma. Proc Natl Acad Sci USA 77:7415–7419, 1980.
6. Takatsuki K, Uchiyama T, Sagawa K, et al: Adult T-cell leukemia in Japan. Excerpta Med Int Congr Ser 415:73, 1977.
7. Hinuma Y, Nagata K, Hanaoka M, et al: Adult T-cell leukemia: Antigen in an ATL cell line and detection of antibodies to the antigen in human sera. Proc Natl Acad Sci USA 78:6476–6480, 1981.
8. Wong-Staal F, Hahn B, Manzari V, et al: A survey of human leukaemias for sequences of a human retrovirus. Nature 302:626–628, 1983.
9. Seiki M, Hattori S, Hirayama Y, et al: Human adult T-cell leukemia virus: Complete nucleotide sequence of the provirus genome integrated in leukemia cell DNA. Proc Natl Acad Sci USA 80:3618–3622, 1983.
10. Haseltine WA, Sodroski J, Patarca R, et al: Structure of 3′ terminal region of type II human T lymphotropic virus: Evidence for new coding region. Science 225:419–421, 1984.
11. Kalyanaraman VS, Sarngadharan MG, Robert-Guroff M, et al: A new subtype of human T-cell leukemia virus (HTLV-II) associated with a T-cell variant of hairy cell leukemia. Science 218:571–573, 1982.
12. Gottlieb MS, Schroff R, Schanker HM, et al: *Pneumocystis carinii* pneumonia and mucosal candidiasis in previously healthy homosexual men: Evidence of a new acquired cellular immunodeficiency. N Engl J Med 305:1425–1431, 1981.
13. Francis DP, Curran JW, Essex M: Epidemic acquired immune deficiency syndrome: Epidemiologic evidence for a transmissible agent. J Natl Cancer Inst 71:1–4, 1983.
14. Barre-Sinoussi F, Chermann JC, Rey F, et al: Isolation of a T-lymphotropic retrovirus from a patient at risk for acquired immune deficiency syndrome (AIDS). Science 220:868–871, 1983.
15. Essex M, McLane MF, Lee TH, et al: Antibodies to cell membrane antigens associated with human T-cell leukemia virus in patients with AIDS. Science 220:859–862, 1983.
16. Gelmann EP, Popovic M, Blayney D, et al: Proviral DNA of a retrovirus, human T-cell leukemia virus, in two patients with AIDS. Science 220:862–865, 1983.
17. Popovic M, Sarngadharan MG, Read E, et al: Detection, isolation, and continuous production of cytopathic retroviruses (HTLV-III) from patients with AIDS and pre-AIDS. Science 224:497–500, 1984.
18. Gallo RC, Salahuddin SZ, Popovic M, et al: Frequent detection and isolation of cytopathic retroviruses (HTLV-III) from patients with AIDS and at risk for AIDS. Science 224:500–503, 1984.
19. Levy JA, Hoffman AD, Kramer SM, et al: Isolation of lymphocytopathic retroviruses from San Francisco patients with AIDS. Science 225:840–842, 1984.
20. Barin F, M'Boup S, Denis F, et al: Serological evidence for virus related to simian T-lymphotropic retrovirus III in residents of West Africa. Lancet 2:1387–1389, 1985.
21. Kanki PJ, Barin F, M'Boup S, et al: New human T-lymphotropic retrovirus related to simian T-lymphotropic virus type III (STLV-IIIAGM). Science 232:238–243, 1986.
22. Kanki PJ, McLane MF, King NW Jr, et al: Serologic identification and characterization of a macaque T-lymphotropic retrovirus closely related to HTLV-III. Science 228:1199–1201, 1985.
23. Romieu I, Marlink R, Kanki P, et al: HIV-2 link to AIDS in West Africa. J Acquir Immune Defic Syndr 3:220–230, 1990.
24. Marlink R, Kanki P, Thior I, et al: Reduced rate of disease development after HIV-2 infection as compared to HIV-1. Science 265:1587–1590, 1994.
25. Weiss RA, Teich N, Varmus H, et al: RNA Tumor Viruses. Cold Spring Harbor, NY, Cold Spring Harbor Laboratory Press, 1984.
26. Doolittle RF, Feng DF, McClure MA, et al: Retrovirus phylogeny and evolution. Curr Top Microbiol Immunol 157:1–18, 1990.
27. Wilson W, Braddock M, Adams SE, et al: HIV expression strategies: Ribosomal frameshifting is directed by a short sequence in both mammalian and yeast systems. Cell 55:1159–1169, 1988.
28. Mador N, Panet A, Honigman A: Translation of *gag*, *pro*, and *pol* gene products of human T-cell leukemia virus type 2. J Virol 63:2400–2404, 1989.
29. Hatfield D, Oroszlan S: The where, what and how of ribosomal frameshifting in retroviral protein synthesis. Trends Biochem Sci 15:186–190, 1990.
30. Gallo R, Wong-Staal F, Montagnier L, et al: HIV/HTLV gene nomenclature. Nature 333:504, 1988.
31. Zhang H, Zhang Y, Spicer TP, et al: Reverse transcription takes place within extracellular HIV-1 virions: Potential biological significance. AIDS Res Hum Retroviruses 9:1287–1296, 1993.
32. Trono D: Partial reverse transcripts in virions from human immunodeficiency and murine leukemia viruses. J Virol 66:4893–4900, 1992.
33. Temin H: Nature of the provirus Rous sarcoma. Natl Cancer Inst Monogr 17:557–570, 1964.
34. Gilboa E, Mitra SW, Goff S, et al: A detailed model of reverse transcription and tests of crucial aspects. Cell 18:93–100, 1979.
35. Toyoshima H, Itoh M, Inoue J, et al: Secondary structure of the human T-cell leukemia virus type 1 *rex*-responsive element is essential for *rex* regulation of RNA processing and transport of unspliced RNAs. J Virol 64:2825–2832, 1990.
36. Grassmann R, Berchtold S, Aepinus C, et al: In vitro binding of human T-cell leukemia virus rex proteins to the rex-response element of viral transcripts. J Virol 65:3721–3727, 1991.
37. Unge T, Solomin L, Mellini M, et al: The Rex regulatory protein of human T-cell lymphotropic virus type I binds specifically to its target site within the viral RNA. Proc Natl Acad Sci USA 88:7145–7149, 1991.
38. Sodroski JG, Rosen CA, Haseltine WA: Trans-acting transcriptional activation of the long terminal repeat of human T lymphotropic viruses in infected cells. Science 225:381–385, 1984.
39. Slamon DJ, Shimotohno K, Cline MJ, et al: Identification of the putative transforming protein of the human T-cell leukemia viruses HTLV-I and HTLV-II. Science 226:61–65, 1984.
40. Sodroski J, Rosen C, Wong-Staal F, et al: Trans-acting transcriptional regulation of human T-cell leukemia virus type III long terminal repeat. Science 227:171–173, 1985.
41. Arya SK, Guo C, Josephs SF, et al: Trans-activator gene of human T-lymphotropic virus type III (HTLV-III). Science 229:69–73, 1985.
42. Feinberg MB, Jarrett RF, Aldovini A, et al: HTLV-III expression and production involve complex regulation at the levels of splicing and translation of viral RNA. Cell 46:807–817, 1986.
43. Sodroski J, Goh WC, Rosen C, et al: A second post-transcriptional trans-activator gene required for HTLV-III replication. Nature 321:412–417, 1986.
44. Orita S, Takagi S, Saiga A, et al: Human T cell leukaemia virus type 1 p21X mRNA: Constitutive expression in peripheral blood mononuclear cells of patients with adult T cell leukaemia. J Gen Virol 73:2283–2289, 1992.
45. Nagashima K, Yoshida M, Seiki M: A single species of pX mRNA of human T-cell leukemia virus type I encodes trans-activator p40x and two other phosphoproteins. J Virol 60:394–399, 1986.
46. Hayward WS, Neel BG, Astrin SM: Activation of a cellular *onc* gene by promoter insertion in ALV-induced lymphoid leukosis. Nature 290:475–480, 1981.
47. Wagner S, Green MR: HTLV-I Tax protein stimulation of DNA binding of bZIP proteins by enhancing dimerization. Science 262:395–399, 1993.

48. Korber B, Okayama A, Donnelly R, et al: Polymerase chain reaction analysis of defective human T-cell leukemia virus type I proviral genomes in leukemic cells of patients with adult T-cell leukemia. J Virol 65:5471–5476, 1991.
49. Nerenberg M, Hinrichs SH, Reynolds RK, et al: The *tat* gene of human T-lymphotropic virus type 1 induces mesenchymal tumors in transgenic mice. Science 237:1324–1329, 1987.
50. Grassmann R, Dengler C, Muller-Fleckenstein I, et al: Transformation to continuous growth of primary human T lymphocytes by human T-cell leukemia virus type I X-region genes transduced by a *Herpesvirus saimiri* vector. Proc Natl Acad Sci USA 86:3351–3355, 1989.
51. Maruyama M, Shibuya H, Harada H, et al: Evidence for aberrant activation of the interleukin-2 autocrine loop by HTLV-1–encoded p40x and T3/Ti complex triggering. Cell 48:343–350, 1987.
52. Murphy EL, Hanchard B, Figueroa JP, et al: Modelling the risk of adult T-cell leukemia/lymphoma in persons infected with human T-lymphotropic virus type I. Int J Cancer 43:250–253, 1989.
53. Kondo T, Kono H, Nonaka H, et al: Risk of adult T-cell leukaemia/lymphoma in HTLV-I carriers. Lancet 2:159, 1987.
54. Kawano F, Yamaguchi K, Nishimura H, et al: Variation in the clinical courses of adult T-cell leukemia. Cancer 55:851–856, 1985.
55. Bunn PA Jr, Schechter GP, Jaffe E, et al: Clinical course of retrovirus-associated adult T-cell lymphoma in the United States. N Engl J Med 309:257–264, 1983.
56. Seiki M, Eddy R, Shows TB, et al: Nonspecific integration of the HTLV provirus genome into adult T-cell leukaemia cells. Nature 309:640–642, 1984.
57. Shimoyama M, Kagami Y, Shimotohno K, et al: Adult T-cell leukemia/lymphoma not associated with human T-cell leukemia virus type I. Proc Natl Acad Sci USA 83:4524–4528, 1986.
58. Miyoshi I, Kubonishi I, Yoshimoto S, et al: Type C virus particles in a cord T-cell line derived by co-cultivating normal human cord leukocytes and human leukaemic T cells. Nature 294:770–771, 1981.
59. De Rossi A, Aldovini A, Franchini G, et al: Clonal selection of T lymphocytes infected by cell-free human T-cell leukemia/lymphoma virus type I: Parameters of virus integration and expression. Virology 143:640–645, 1985.
60. Zhao TM, Robinson MA, Bowers FS, et al: Characterization of an infectious molecular clone of human T-cell leukemia virus type I. J Virol 69:2024–2030, 1995.
61. Essex M, Hardy WD Jr, Cotter SM, et al: Naturally occurring persistent feline oncornavirus infections in the absence of disease. Infect Immun 11:470–475, 1975.
62. Matsuda Z, Chou MJ, Matsuda M, et al: Human immunodeficiency virus type 1 has an additional coding sequence in the central region of the genome. Proc Natl Acad Sci USA 85:6968–6972, 1988.
63. Strebel K, Klimkait T, Martin MA: A novel gene of HIV-1, *vpu*, and its 16-kilodalton product. Science 241:1221–1223, 1988.
64. Cohen EA, Terwilliger EF, Sodroski JG, et al: Identification of a protein encoded by the *vpu* gene of HIV-1. Nature 334:532–534, 1988.
65. Yu XF, Ito S, Essex M, et al: A naturally immunogenic virion-associated protein specific for HIV-2 and SIV. Nature 335:262–265, 1988.
66. Henderson LE, Sowder RC, Copeland TD, et al: Isolation and characterization of a novel protein (X-ORF product) from SIV and HIV-2. Science 241:199–201, 1988.
67. Yu QC, Matsuda Z, Yu X, et al: An electron-lucent region within the virion distinguishes HIV-1 from HIV-2 and simian immunodeficiency virus. AIDS Res Hum Retroviruses 10:757–761, 1994.
68. Leonard R, Zagury D, Desportes I, et al: Cytopathic effect of human immunodeficiency virus in T4 cells is linked to the last stage of virus infection. Proc Natl Acad Sci USA 85:3570–3574, 1988.
69. Subbramanian RA, Cohen EA: Molecular biology of the human immunodeficiency virus accessory proteins. J Virol 68:6831–6835, 1994.
70. Trono D: HIV accessory proteins: Leading roles for the supporting cast. Cell 82:189–192, 1995.
71. Lee TH, Coligan JE, Allan JS, et al: A new HTLV-III/LAV protein encoded by a gene found in cytopathic retroviruses. Science 231:1546–1549, 1986.
72. Sodroski J, Goh WC, Rosen C, et al: Replicative and cytopathic potential of HTLV-III/LAV with *sor* gene deletions. Science 231:1549–1553, 1986.
73. Kan NC, Franchini G, Wong-Staal F, et al: Identification of HTLV-III/LAV *sor* gene product and detection of antibodies in human sera. Science 231:1553–1555, 1986.
74. Allan JS, Coligan JE, Lee TH, et al: A new HTLV-III/LAV encoded antigen detected by antibodies from AIDS patients. Science 230:810–813, 1985.
75. Yuan X, Matsuda Z, Matsuda M, et al: Human immunodeficiency virus *vpr* gene encodes a virion-associated protein. AIDS Res Hum Retroviruses 6:1265–1271, 1990.
76. Cohen EA, Terwilliger EF, Jalinoos Y, et al: Identification of HIV-1 *vpr* product and function. J Acquir Immune Defic Syndr 1990;3:11–18, 1990.
77. Cohen EA, Dehni G, Sodroski JG, Haseltine WA: Human immunodeficiency virus *vpr* product is a virion-associated regulatory protein. J Virol 64:3097–3099, 1990.
78. Gallay P, Swingler S, Aiken C, et al: HIV-1 infection of nondividing cells: C-terminal tyrosine phosphorylation of the viral matrix protein is a key regulator. Cell 80:379–388, 1995.
79. Yu X, Yuan X, Matsuda Z, et al: The matrix protein of human immunodeficiency virus type 1 is required for incorporation of viral envelope protein into mature virions. J Virol 66:4966–4971, 1992.
80. Dorfman T, Mammano F, Haseltine WA, et al: Role of the matrix protein in the virion association of the human immunodeficiency virus type 1 envelope glycoprotein. J Virol 68:1689–1696, 1994.
81. von Schwedler U, Kornbluth RS, Trono D: The nuclear localization signal of the matrix protein of human immunodeficiency virus type 1 allows the establishment of infection in macrophages and quiescent T lymphocytes. Proc Natl Acad Sci USA 91:6992–6996, 1994.
82. Bukrinsky MI, Haggerty S, Dempsey MP, et al: A nuclear localization signal within HIV-1 matrix protein that governs infection of non-dividing cells. Nature 365:666–669, 1993.
83. Franke EK, Yuan HE, Luban J: Specific incorporation of cyclophilin A into HIV-1 virions. Nature 372:359–362, 1994.
84. Thali M, Bukovsky A, Kondo E, et al: Functional association of cyclophilin A with HIV-1 virions. Nature 372:363–365, 1994.
85. Gottlinger HG, Dorfman T, Sodroski JG, Haseltine WA: Effect of mutations affecting the p6 gag protein on human immunodeficiency virus particle release. Proc Natl Acad Sci USA 88:3195–3199, 1991.
86. Matthews S, Barlow P, Boyd J, et al: Structural similarity between the p17 matrix protein of HIV-1 and interferon-gamma. Nature 370:666–668, 1994.
87. Summers MF, Henderson LE, Chance MR, et al: Nucleocapsid zinc fingers detected in retroviruses: EXAFS studies of intact viruses and the solution-state structure of the nucleocapsid protein from HIV-1. Protein Sci 1:563–574, 1992.
88. Erickson J, Kempf D: Structure-based design of symmetric inhibitors of HIV-1 protease. Arch Virol Suppl 9:19–29, 1994.
89. Davies JF, Hostomska Z, Hostomsky Z, et al: Crystal structure of the ribonuclease H domain of HIV-1 reverse transcriptase. Science 252:88–95, 1991.
90. Kohlstaedt LA, Wang J, Friedman JM, et al: Crystal structure at 3.5 Å resolution of HIV-1 reverse transcriptase complexed with an inhibitor. Science 256:1783–1790, 1992.
91. Dyda F, Hickman AB, Jenkins TM, et al: Crystal structure of the catalytic domain of HIV-1 integrase: Similarity to other polynucleotidyl transferases. Science 266:1981–1986, 1994.
92. Allan JS, Coligan JE, Barin F, et al: Major glycoprotein antigens that induce antibodies in AIDS patients are encoded by HTLV-III. Science 228:1091–1094, 1985.
93. Barin F, McLane MF, Allan JS, et al: Virus envelope protein of HTLV-III represents major target antigen for antibodies in AIDS patients. Science 228:1094–1096, 1985.
94. McCune JM, Rabin LB, Feinberg MB, et al: Endoproteolytic cleavage of gp160 is required for the activation of human immunodeficiency virus. Cell 53:55–67, 1988.
95. Lasky LA, Nakamura G, Smith DH, et al: Delineation of a region of the human immunodeficiency virus type 1 gp120

glycoprotein critical for interaction with the CD4 receptor. Cell 50:975–985, 1987.
96. Clayton LK, Hussey RE, Steinbrich R, et al: Substitution of murine for human CD4 residues identifies amino acids critical for HIV-gp120 binding. Nature 335:363–366, 1988.
97. Jameson BA, Rao PE, Kong LI, et al: Location and chemical synthesis of a binding site for HIV-1 on the CD4 protein. Science 240:1335–1339, 1988.
98. Syu WJ, Huang JH, Essex M, et al: The N-terminal region of the human immunodeficiency virus envelope glycoprotein gp120 contains potential binding sites for CD4. Proc Natl Acad Sci USA 87:3695–3699, 1990.
99. Hwang SS, Boyle TJ, Lyerly HK, et al: Identification of envelope V3 loop as the major determinant of CD4 neutralization sensitivity of HIV-1. Science 257:535–537, 1992.
100. Kowalski M, Potz J, Basiripour L, et al: Functional regions of the envelope glycoprotein of human immunodeficiency virus type 1. Science 237:1351–1355, 1987.
101. Robey WG, Safai B, Oroszlan S, et al: Characterization of envelope and core structural gene products of HTLV-III with sera from AIDS patients. Science 228:593–595, 1985.
102. Dayton AI, Sodroski JG, Rosen CA, et al: The trans-activator gene of the human T cell lymphotropic virus type III is required for replication. Cell 44:941–947, 1986.
103. Berkhout B, Silverman RH, Jeang KT: Tat trans-activates the human immunodeficiency virus through a nascent RNA target. Cell 59:273–282, 1989.
104. Selby MJ, Peterlin BM: Trans-activation by HIV-1 Tat via a heterologous RNA binding protein. Cell 62:769–776, 1990.
105. Marciniak RA, Calnan BJ, Frankel AD, et al: HIV-1 Tat protein trans-activates transcription in vitro. Cell 63:791–802, 1990.
106. Kato H, Sumimoto H, Pognonec P, et al: HIV-1 Tat acts as a processivity factor in vitro in conjunction with cellular elongation factors. Genes Dev 6:655–666, 1992.
107. Cordingley MG, LaFemina RL, Callahan PL, et al: Sequence-specific interaction of Tat protein and Tat peptides with the transactivation-responsive sequence element of human immunodeficiency virus type 1 in vitro. Proc Natl Acad Sci USA 87:8985–8989, 1990.
108. Weeks KM, Ampe C, Schultz SC, et al: Fragments of the HIV-1 Tat protein specifically bind TAR RNA. Science 249:1281–1285, 1990.
109. Terwilliger E, Burghoff R, Sia R, et al: The *art* gene product of human immunodeficiency virus is required for replication. J Virol 62:655–658, 1988.
110. Dayton ET, Powell DM, Dayton AI: Functional analysis of CAR, the target sequence for the Rev protein of HIV-1. Science 246:1625–1629, 1989.
111. Malim MH, Hauber J, Le SY, et al: The HIV-1 *rev* trans-activator acts through a structured target sequence to activate nuclear export of unspliced viral mRNA. Nature 338:254–257, 1989.
112. Fritz CC, Zapp ML, Green MR: A human nucleoporin-like protein that specifically interacts with HIV Rev. Nature 376:530–533, 1995.
113. Bogerd HP, Fridell RA, Madore S, et al: Identification of a novel cellular cofactor for the Rev/Rex class of retroviral regulatory proteins. Cell 82:485–494, 1995.
114. Stutz F, Neville M, Rosbash M: Identification of a novel nuclear pore–associated protein as a functional target of the HIV-1 Rev protein in yeast. Cell 82:495–506, 1995.
115. Schwartz S, Campbell M, Nasioulas G, et al: Mutational inactivation of an inhibitory sequence in human immunodeficiency virus type 1 results in Rev-independent *gag* expression. J Virol 66:7176–7182, 1992.
116. Olsen HS, Cochrane AW, Rosen C: Interaction of cellular factors with intragenic cis-acting repressive sequences within the HIV genome. Virology 191:709–715, 1992.
117. Rosen CA, Terwilliger E, Dayton A, et al: Intragenic cis-acting *art* gene–responsive sequences of the human immunodeficiency virus. Proc Natl Acad Sci USA 85:2071–2075, 1988.
118. Strebel K, Daugherty D, Clouse K, et al: The HIV 'A' *(sor)* gene product is essential for virus infectivity. Nature 328:728–730, 1987.
119. Fisher AG, Ensoli B, Ivanoff L, et al: The *sor* gene of HIV-1 is required for efficient virus transmission in vitro. Science 237:888–893, 1987.
120. Gabuzda DH, Lawrence K, Langhoff E, et al: Role of *vif* in replication of human immunodeficiency virus type 1 in CD4+ T lymphocytes. J Virol 66:6489–6495, 1992.
121. Rogel ME, Wu LI, Emerman M: The human immunodeficiency virus type 1 *vpr* gene prevents cell proliferation during chronic infection. J Virol 69:882–888, 1995.
122. Lang SM, Weeger M, Stahl-Hennig C, et al: Importance of *vpr* for infection of rhesus monkeys with simian immunodeficiency virus. J Virol 67:902–912, 1993.
123. Baba TW, Jeong YS, Penninck D, et al: Pathogenicity of live, attenuated SIV after mucosal infection of neonatal macaques. Science 267:1820–1825, 1995.
124. Fisher AG, Ratner L, Mitsuya H, et al: Infectious mutants of HTLV-III with changes in the 3′ region and markedly reduced cytopathic effects. Science 233:655–659, 1986.
125. Luciw PA, Cheng-Mayer C, Levy JA: Mutational analysis of the human immunodeficiency virus: The orf-B region down-regulates virus replication. Proc Natl Acad Sci USA 84:1434–1438, 1987.
126. Kestler HW III, Ringler DJ, Mori K, et al: Importance of the *nef* gene for maintenance of high virus loads and for development of AIDS. Cell 65:651–662, 1991.
127. Aiken C, Konner J, Landau NR, et al: Nef induces CD4 endocytosis: Requirement for a critical dileucine motif in the membrane-proximal CD4 cytoplasmic domain. Cell 76:853–864, 1994.
128. Garcia JV, Miller AD: Serine phosphorylation–independent downregulation of cell-surface CD4 by *nef*. Nature 350:508–511, 1991.
129. Saksela K, Cheng GH, Baltimore D: Proline-rich (PxxP) motifs in HIV-1 Nef bind to SH3 domains of a subset of Src kinases and are required for the enhanced growth of Nef+ viruses but not for down-regulation of CD4. EMBO J 14:484–491, 1995.
130. Schubert U, Henklein P, Boldyreff B, et al: The human immunodeficiency virus type 1 encoded Vpu protein is phosphorylated by casein kinase-2 (CK-2) at positions Ser52 and Ser56 within a predicted alpha-helix-turn-alpha-helix-motif. J Mol Biol 236:16–25, 1994.
131. Klimkait T, Strebel K, Hoggan MD, et al: The human immunodeficiency virus type 1–specific protein vpu is required for efficient virus maturation and release. J Virol 64:621–629, 1990.
132. Bour S, Schubert U, Strebel K: The human immunodeficiency virus type 1 Vpu protein specifically binds to the cytoplasmic domain of CD4: Implications for the mechanism of degradation. J Virol 69:1510–1520, 1995.
133. Tristem M, Marshall C, Karpas A, Hill F: Evolution of the primate lentiviruses: Evidence from *vpx* and *vpr*. EMBO J 11:3405–3412, 1992.
134. Kappes JC, Conway JA, Lee SW, et al: Human immunodeficiency virus type 2 *vpx* protein augments viral infectivity. Virology 184:197–209, 1991.
135. Allan JS, Coligan JE, Lee TH, et al: Immunogenic nature of a Pol gene product of HTLV-III/LAV. Blood 69:331–333, 1987.
136. Kitchen LW, Barin F, Sullivan JL, et al: Aetiology of AIDS—Antibodies to human T-cell leukaemia virus (type III) in haemophiliacs. Nature 312:367–369, 1984.
137. Syu WJ, Du B, Essex M, et al: Association between cross-reactive HIV-2 gp120 antibody and disease progression in HIV-1 infection. *In* Brown F, Chanock RM, Ginsberg HS, et al (eds): Vaccines 1990. Cold Spring Harbor, NY, Cold Spring Harbor Laboratory Press, 1990, pp 373–377.
138. Holmberg SD, Horsburgh CR Jr, Ward JW, et al: Biologic factors in the sexual transmission of human immunodeficiency virus. J Infect Dis 160:116–125, 1989.
139. Lee TH, Chou MJ, Huang JH, et al: Association between antibody to envelope glycoprotein gp120 and the outcome of human immunodeficiency virus infection. *In* Ginsberg H, Lerner R (eds): Vaccines 1988. Cold Spring Harbor, NY, Cold Spring Harbor Laboratory Press, 1988, pp 373–377.
140. Yu XF, Matsuda M, Essex M, et al: Open reading frame *vpr* of simian immunodeficiency virus encodes a virion-associated protein. J Virol 64:5688–5693, 1990.
141. Dalgleish AG, Beverley PC, Clapham PR, et al: The CD4 (T4) antigen is an essential component of the receptor for the AIDS retrovirus. Nature 312:763–767, 1984.
142. Klatzmann D, Champagne E, Chamaret S, et al: T-lymphocyte T4 molecule behaves as the receptor for human retrovirus LAV. Nature 312:767–768, 1984.

143. McDougal JS, Kennedy MS, Sligh JM, et al: Binding of HTLV-III/LAV to T4+ T cells by a complex of the 110K viral protein and the T4 molecule. Science 231:382–385, 1986.
144. Maddon PJ, Dalgleish AG, McDougal JS, et al: The T4 gene encodes the AIDS virus receptor and is expressed in the immune system and the brain. Cell 47:333–348, 1986.
145. Sattentau QJ, Dalgleish AG, Weiss RA, et al: Epitopes of the CD4 antigen and HIV infection. Science 234:1120–1123, 1986.
146. Lifson JD, Hwang KM, Nara PL, et al: Synthetic CD4 peptide derivatives that inhibit HIV infection and cytopathicity. Science 241:712–716, 1988.
147. Halstead SB, O'Rourke EJ: Dengue viruses and mononuclear phagocytes. I. Infection enhancement by non-neutralizing antibody. J Exp Med 146:201–217, 1977.
148. Robinson WE Jr, Montefiori DC, Mitchell WM: Antibody-dependent enhancement of human immunodeficiency virus type 1 infection. Lancet 1:790–794, 1988.
149. McKeating JA, Griffiths PD, Weiss RA: HIV susceptibility conferred to human fibroblasts by cytomegalovirus-induced Fc receptor. Nature 343:659–661, 1990.
150. Homsy J, Meyer M, Tateno M, et al: The Fc and not CD4 receptor mediates antibody enhancement of HIV infection in human cells. Science 244:1357–1360, 1989.
151. Hwang SS, Boyle TJ, Lyerly HK, et al: Identification of the envelope V3 loop as the primary determinant of cell tropism in HIV-1. Science 253:71–74, 1991.
152. Pomerantz RJ, de la Monte SM, Donegan SP, et al: Human immunodeficiency virus (HIV) infection of the uterine cervix. Ann Intern Med 108:321–327, 1988.
153. Salahuddin SZ, Rose RM, Groopman JE, et al: Human T lymphotropic virus type III infection of human alveolar macrophages. Blood 68:281–284, 1986.
154. Tschachler E, Groh V, Popovic M, et al: Epidermal Langerhans cells—A target for HTLV-III/LAV infection. J Invest Dermatol 88:233–237, 1987.
155. Adachi A, Koenig S, Gendelman HE, et al: Productive, persistent infection of human colorectal cell lines with human immunodeficiency virus. J Virol 61:209–213, 1987.
156. Dewhurst S, Sakai K, Bresser J, et al: Persistent productive infection of human glial cells by human immunodeficiency virus (HIV) and by infectious molecular clones of HIV. J Virol 61:3774–3782, 1987.
157. Nelson JA, Wiley CA, Reynolds-Kohler C, et al: Human immunodeficiency virus detected in bowel epithelium from patients with gastrointestinal symptoms. Lancet 1:259–262, 1988.
158. Pomerantz RJ, Kuritzkes DR, de la Monte SM, et al: Infection of the retina by human immunodeficiency virus type I. N Engl J Med 317:1643–1647, 1987.
159. Cheng-Mayer C, Rutka JT, Rosenblum ML, et al: Human immunodeficiency virus can productively infect cultured human glial cells. Proc Natl Acad Sci USA 84:3526–3530, 1987.
160. Montagnier L, Gruest J, Chamaret S, et al: Adaptation of lymphadenopathy associated virus (LAV) to replication in EBV-transformed B lymphoblastoid cell lines. Science 225:63–66, 1984.
161. Yahi N, Baghdiguian S, Moreau H, et al: Galactosyl ceramide (or a closely related molecule) is the receptor for human immunodeficiency virus type 1 on human colon epithelial HT29 cells. J Virol 66:4848–4854, 1992.
162. Winslow BJ, Trono D: The blocks to human immunodeficiency virus type 1 Tat and Rev functions in mouse cell lines are independent. J Virol 67:2349–2354, 1993.
163. Coffin JM: HIV population dynamics in vivo: Implications for genetic variation, pathogenesis, and therapy. Science 267:483–489, 1995.
164. Bakhanashvili M, Hizi A: Fidelity of the reverse transcriptase of human immunodeficiency virus type 2. FEBS Lett 306:151–156, 1992.
165. Pantaleo G, Graziosi C, Demarest JF, et al: HIV infection is active and progressive in lymphoid tissue during the clinically latent stage of disease. Nature 362:355–358, 1993.
166. Embretson J, Zupancic M, Ribas JL, et al: Massive covert infection of helper T-lymphocytes and macrophages by HIV during the incubation period of AIDS. Nature 362:359–362, 1993.
167. Wei X, Ghosh SK, Taylor ME, et al: Viral dynamics in human immunodeficiency virus type 1 infection. Nature 373:117–122, 1995.
168. Ho DD, Neumann AU, Perelson AS, et al: Rapid turnover of plasma virions and CD4 lymphocytes in HIV-1 infection. Nature 373:123–126, 1995.
169. Yu X, McLane MF, Ratner L, et al: Killing of primary CD4+ cells by non–syncytium-inducing macrophage-tropic human immunodeficiency virus type 1. Proc Natl Acad Sci USA 91:10237–10241, 1994.
170. Groenink M, Fouchier RA, Broerson S, et al: Relation of phenotype evolution of HIV-1 to envelope V2 configuration. Science 260:1513–1516, 1993.
171. Anand R, Siegal F, Reed C, et al: Non-cytocidal natural variants of human immunodeficiency virus isolated from AIDS patients with neurological disorders. Lancet 2:234–238, 1987.
172. Kotler DP, Gaetz HP, Lange M, et al: Enteropathy associated with the acquired immunodeficiency syndrome. Ann Intern Med 101:421–428, 1984.
173. Koyanagi Y, Miles S, Mitsuyasu RT, et al: Dual infection of the central nervous system by AIDS viruses with distinct cellular tropisms. Science 236:819–822, 1987.
174. Asjo B, Morfeldt-Manson L, Albert J, et al: Replicative capacity of human immunodeficiency virus from patients with varying severity of HIV infection. Lancet 2:660–662, 1986.
175. Evans LA, McHugh TM, Stites DP, et al: Differential ability of human immunodeficiency virus isolates to productively infect human cells. J Immunol 138:3415–3418, 1987.
176. Hoxie JA, Haggarty BS, Rackowski JL, et al: Persistent noncytopathic infection of normal human T lymphocytes with AIDS-associated retrovirus. Science 229:1400–1402, 1985.
177. Ljunggren K, Chiodi F, Broliden PA, et al: HIV-1–specific antibodies in cerebrospinal fluid mediate cellular cytotoxicity and neutralization. AIDS Res Hum Retroviruses 5:629–638, 1989.
178. Robert-Guroff M, Brown M, Gallo RC: HTLV-III–neutralizing antibodies in patients with AIDS and AIDS-related complex. Nature 316:72–74, 1985.
179. Weiss RA, Clapham PR, Cheingsong-Popov R, et al: Neutralization of human T-lymphotropic virus type III by sera of AIDS and AIDS-risk patients. Nature 316:69–72, 1985.
180. Rusche JR, Javaherian K, McDanal C, et al: Antibodies that inhibit fusion of human immunodeficiency virus–infected cells bind a 24-amino acid sequence of the viral envelope, gp120. Proc Natl Acad Sci USA 85:3198–3202, 1988.
181. Ho DD, Kaplan JC, Rackauskas IE, et al: Second conserved domain of gp120 is important for HIV infectivity and antibody neutralization. Science 239:1021–1023, 1988.
182. Javaherian K, Langlois AJ, McDanal C, et al: Principal neutralizing domain of the human immunodeficiency virus type 1 envelope protein. Proc Natl Acad Sci USA 86:6768–6772, 1989.
183. Weinhold KJ, Lyerly HK, Matthews TJ, et al: Cellular anti-GP120 cytolytic reactivities in HIV-1 seropositive individuals. Lancet 1:902–905, 1988.
184. Blumberg RS, Paradis T, Hartshorn KL, et al: Antibody-dependent cell-mediated cytotoxicity against cells infected with the human immunodeficiency virus. J Infect Dis 156:878–884, 1987.
185. Ljunggren K, Chiodi F, Biberfeld G, et al: Lack of cross-reaction in antibody-dependent cellular cytotoxicity between human immunodeficiency virus (HIV) and HIV-related West African strains. J Immunol 140:602–605, 1988.
186. Lyerly HK, Matthews TJ, Bolognesi DP, et al: Human T-cell lymphotropic virus IIIB glycoprotein (gp120) bound to CD4 determinants on normal lymphocytes and expressed by infected cells serves as target for immune attack. Proc Natl Acad Sci USA 84:4601–4605, 1987.
187. Rook AH, Lane HC, Folks T, et al: Sera from HTLV-III/LAV antibody–positive individuals mediate antibody-dependent cellular cytotoxicity against HTLV-III/LAV–infected T cells. J Immunol 138:1064–1067, 1987.
188. Tyler DS, Lyerly HK, Weinhold KJ: Anti–HIV-1 ADCC. AIDS Res Hum Retroviruses 5:557–563, 1989.
189. Ljunggren K, Moschese V, Broliden PA, et al: Antibodies mediating cellular cytotoxicity and neutralization correlate with a better clinical stage in children born to human immunodeficiency virus–infected mothers. J Infect Dis 161:198–202, 1990.
190. Cai Q, Huang XL, Rappocciolo G, et al: Natural killer cell responses in homosexual men with early HIV infection. J Acquir Immune Defic Syndr 3:669–676, 1990.
191. Culmann B, Gomard E, Kieny MP, et al: An antigenic peptide

of the HIV-1 NEF protein recognized by cytotoxic T lymphocytes of seropositive individuals in association with different HLA-B molecules. Eur J Immunol 19:2383–2386, 1989.
192. Walker BD, Flexner C, Birch-Limberger K, et al: Long-term culture and fine specificity of human cytotoxic T-lymphocyte clones reactive with human immunodeficiency virus type 1. Proc Natl Acad Sci USA 86:9514–9518, 1989.
193. Walker BD, Chakrabarti S, Moss B, et al: HIV-specific cytotoxic T lymphocytes in seropositive individuals. Nature 328:345–348, 1987.
194. Walker BD, Flexner C, Paradis TJ, et al: HIV-1 reverse transcriptase is a target for cytotoxic T lymphocytes in infected individuals. Science 240:64–66, 1988.
195. Plata F, Autran B, Martins LP, et al: AIDS virus-specific cytotoxic T lymphocytes in lung disorders. Nature 328:348–351, 1987.
196. Walker BD, Plata F: Cytotoxic T lymphocytes against HIV. AIDS 4:177–184, 1990.
197. Walker CM, Moody DJ, Stites DP, et al: $CD8^+$ lymphocytes can control HIV infection in vitro by suppressing virus replication. Science 234:1563–1566, 1986.
198. Ljunggren K, Biberfeld G, Jondal M, et al: Antibody-dependent cellular cytotoxicity detects type- and strain-specific antigens among human immunodeficiency virus types 1 and 2 and simian immunodeficiency virus SIVmac isolates. J Virol 63:3376–3381, 1989.
199. Bottiger B, Karlsson A, Andreasson PA, et al: Cross-neutralizing antibodies against HIV-1 (HTLV-IIIB and HTLV-IIIRF) and HIV-2 (SBL-6669 and a new isolate SBL-K135). AIDS Res Hum Retroviruses 5:525–533, 1989.
200. Masur H, Michelis MA, Greene JB, et al: An outbreak of community-acquired *Pneumocystis carinii* pneumonia: Initial manifestation of cellular immune dysfunction. N Engl J Med 305:1431–1438, 1981.
201. Poon MC, Landay A, Prasthofer EF, et al: Acquired immunodeficiency syndrome with *Pneumocystis carinii* pneumonia and *Mycobacterium avium-intracellulare* infection in a previously healthy patient with classic hemophilia. Clinical, immunologic, and virologic findings. Ann Intern Med 98:287–290, 1983.
202. Siegal FP, Lopez C, Hammer GS, et al: Severe acquired immunodeficiency in male homosexuals, manifested by chronic perianal ulcerative herpes simplex lesions. N Engl J Med 305:1439–1444, 1985.
203. Fauci AS, Masur H, Gelmann EP, et al: NIH conference. The acquired immunodeficiency syndrome: An update. Ann Intern Med 102:800–813, 1985.
204. Hymes KB, Cheung T, Greene JB, et al: Kaposi's sarcoma in homosexual men—A report of eight cases. Lancet 2:598–600, 1981.
205. Spear GT, Kessler HA, Rothberg L, et al: Decreased oxidative burst activity of monocytes from asymptomatic HIV-infected individuals. Clin Immunol Immunopathol 54:184–191, 1990.
206. Smith PD, Ohura K, Masur H, et al: Monocyte function in the acquired immune deficiency syndrome. Defective chemotaxis. J Clin Invest 74:2121–2128, 1984.
207. Poli G, Bottazzi B, Acero R, et al: Monocyte function in intravenous drug abusers with lymphadenopathy syndrome and in patients with acquired immunodeficiency syndrome: Selective impairment of chemotaxis. Clin Exp Immunol 62:136–142, 1985.
208. Pennington JE, Groopman JE, Small GJ, et al: Effect of intravenous recombinant gamma-interferon on the respiratory burst of blood monocytes from patients with AIDS. J Infect Dis 153:609–612, 1986.
209. Hirsch MS, Curran J: Human immunodeficiency viruses. *In* Fields BN, Knipe DN (eds): Fields Virology, ed 2. New York, Raven Press, 1990, pp 1545–1570.
210. Lane HC, Masur H, Edgar LC, et al: Abnormalities of B-cell activation and immunoregulation in patients with the acquired immunodeficiency syndrome. N Engl J Med 309:453–458, 1983.
211. Pahwa SG, Quilop MT, Lange M, et al: Defective B-lymphocyte function in homosexual men in relation to the acquired immunodeficiency syndrome. Ann Intern Med 101:757–763, 1984.
212. Redfield RR, Wright DC, Tramont EC: The Walter Reed staging classification for HTLV-III/LAV infection. N Engl J Med 314:131–132, 1986.
213. Ammann AJ, Schiffman G, Abrams D, et al: B-cell immunodeficiency in acquired immune deficiency syndrome. JAMA 251:1447–1449, 1984.
214. Polsky B, Gold JW, Whimbey E, et al: Bacterial pneumonia in patients with the acquired immunodeficiency syndrome. Ann Intern Med 104:38–41, 1986.
215. Piot P, Plummer FA, Mhalu FS, et al: AIDS: An international perspective. Science 239:573–579, 1988.
216. Quinn TC, Piot P, McCormick JB, et al: Serologic and immunologic studies in patients with AIDS in North America and Africa. The potential role of infectious agents as cofactors in human immunodeficiency virus infection. JAMA 257:2617–2621, 1987.
217. Marlink RG, Essex M: Africa and the biology of human immunodeficiency virus. JAMA 257:2632–2633, 1987.
218. Clavel F, Mansinho K, Chamaret S, et al: Human immunodeficiency virus type 2 infection associated with AIDS in West Africa. N Engl J Med 316:1180–1185, 1987.
219. Naucler A, Andreasson PA, Costa CM, et al: HIV-2–associated AIDS and HIV-2 seroprevalence in Bissau, Guinea-Bissau. J Acquir Immune Defic Syndr 2:88–93, 1989.
220. Pang S, Koyanagi Y, Miles S, et al: High levels of unintegrated HIV-1 DNA in brain tissue of AIDS dementia patients. Nature 343:85–89, 1990.
221. Fauci AS: The human immunodeficiency virus: Infectivity and mechanisms of pathogenesis. Science 239:617–622, 1988.
222. Ho DD, Kaplan JC: Pathogenesis of human immunodeficiency virus infection and prospects for control. Yale J Biol Med 60:589–600, 1987.
223. Levy JA: Mysteries of HIV: Challenges for therapy and prevention. Nature 333:519–522, 1988.
224. Seligmann M, Pinching AJ, Rosen FS, et al: Immunology of human immunodeficiency virus infection and the acquired immunodeficiency syndrome. An update. Ann Intern Med 107:234–242, 1987.
225. Lemaitre M, Guetard D, Henin Y, et al: Protective activity of tetracycline analogs against the cytopathic effect of the human immunodeficiency viruses in CEM cells. Res Virol 141:5–16, 1990.
226. Klatzmann D, Barre-Sinoussi F, Nugeyre MT, et al: Selective tropism of lymphadenopathy associated virus (LAV) for helper-inducer T lymphocytes. Science 225:59–63, 1984.
227. Folks TM, Kessler SW, Orenstein JM, et al: Infection and replication of HIV-1 in purified progenitor cells of normal human bone marrow. Science 242:919–922, 1988.
228. Gendelman HE, Orenstein JM, Martin MA, et al: Efficient isolation and propagation of human immunodeficiency virus on recombinant colony-stimulating factor 1–treated monocytes. J Exp Med 167:1428–1441, 1988.
229. Nelbock P, Dillon PJ, Perkins A, et al: A cDNA for a protein that interacts with the human immunodeficiency virus Tat transactivator. Science 248:1650–1653, 1990.
230. Ho DD, Rota TR, Schooley RT, et al: Isolation of HTLV-III from cerebrospinal fluid and neural tissues of patients with neurologic syndromes related to the acquired immunodeficiency syndrome. N Engl J Med 313:1493–1497, 1985.
231. Navia BA, Cho ES, Petito CK, et al: The AIDS dementia complex: II. Neuropathology. Ann Neurol 19:525–535, 1986.
232. Belman AL, Lantos G, Horoupian D, et al: AIDS: Calcification of the basal ganglia in infants and children. Neurology 36:1192–1199, 1986.
233. Shaw GM, Harper ME, Hahn BH, et al: HTLV-III infection in brains of children and adults with AIDS encephalopathy. Science 227:177–182, 1985.
234. Sharer LR, Epstein LG, Cho ES, et al: Pathologic features of AIDS encephalopathy in children: Evidence for LAV/HTLV-III infection of brain. Hum Pathol 17:271–284, 1986.
235. Pizzo PA: Pediatric AIDS: Problems within problems. J Infect Dis 161:316–325, 1990.
236. Klemm E, Schneweis KE, Horn R, et al: HIV-II infection with initial neurological manifestation. J Neurol 235:304–307, 1988.
237. Resnick L, diMarzo-Veronese F, Schupbach J, et al: Intra-blood-brain-barrier synthesis of HTLV-III–specific IgG in patients with neurologic symptoms associated with AIDS or AIDS-related complex. N Engl J Med 313:1498–1504, 1985.
238. Ho DD, Bredesen DE, Vinters HV, et al: The acquired immunodeficiency syndrome (AIDS) dementia complex. Ann Intern Med 111:400–410, 1989.

239. Snider WD, Simpson DM, Nielsen S, et al: Neurological complications of acquired immune deficiency syndrome: Analysis of 50 patients. Ann Neurol 14:403–418, 1983.
240. Navia BA, Jordan BD, Price RW: The AIDS dementia complex: I. Clinical features. Ann Neurol 19:517–524, 1986.
241. Levy RM, Bredesen DE, Rosenblum ML, et al: Central nervous system disorders in AIDS. *In* Levy JA (ed): AIDS: Pathogenesis and Treatment. New York, Marcel Dekker, 1989, pp 371–401.
242. Levy RM, Bredesen DE, Rosenblum ML: Neurological manifestations of the acquired immunodeficiency syndrome (AIDS): Experience at UCSF and review of the literature. J Neurosurg 62:475–495, 1985.
243. Sonnerborg AB, von Sydow MA, Forsgren M, et al: Association between intrathecal anti–HIV-1 immunoglobulin G synthesis and occurrence of HIV-1 in cerebrospinal fluid. AIDS 3:701–705, 1989.
244. Sonnerborg A, Ehrnst A, Strannegard O: Relationship between the occurrence of virus in plasma and cerebrospinal fluid of HIV-1 infected individuals. J Med Virol 27:258–263, 1989.
245. Hoover EA, Mullins JI, Quackenbush SL, et al: Experimental transmission and pathogenesis of immunodeficiency syndrome in cats. Blood 70:1880–1892, 1987.
246. Mullins JI, Chen CS, Hoover EA: Disease-specific and tissue-specific production of unintegrated feline leukaemia virus variant DNA in feline AIDS. Nature 319:333–336, 1986.
247. Portegies P, de Gans J, Lange JM, et al: Declining incidence of AIDS dementia complex after introduction of zidovudine treatment. BMJ 299:819–821, 1989.
248. Petito CK, Cho ES, Lemann W, et al: Neuropathology of acquired immunodeficiency syndrome (AIDS): An autopsy review. J Neuropathol Exp Neurol 45:635–646, 1986.
249. Parry GJ: Peripheral neuropathies associated with human immunodeficiency virus infection. Ann Neurol 23(Suppl):S49–S53, 1988.
250. Dalakas MC, Pezeshkpour GH: Neuromuscular diseases associated with human immunodeficiency virus infection. Ann Neurol 23(Suppl):S38–S48, 1988.
251. Wilkes MS, Fortin AH, Felix JC, et al: Value of necropsy in acquired immunodeficiency syndrome. Lancet 2:85–88, 1988.
252. Lantos PL, McLaughlin JE, Schoitz CL, et al: Neuropathology of the brain in HIV infection. Lancet 1:309–311, 1989.
253. Anders KH, Guerra WF, Tomiyasu U, et al: The neuropathology of AIDS. UCLA experience and review. Am J Pathol 124:537–558, 1986.
254. Gabuzda DH, Ho DD, de la Monte SM, et al: Immunohistochemical identification of HTLV-III antigen in brains of patients with AIDS. Ann Neurol 20:289–295, 1986.
255. Koenig S, Gendelman HE, Orenstein JM, et al: Detection of AIDS virus in macrophages in brain tissue from AIDS patients with encephalopathy. Science 233:1089–1093, 1986.
256. Nuovo GJ, Gallery F, MacConnell P, et al: In situ detection of polymerase chain reaction–amplified HIV-1 nucleic acids and tumor necrosis factor-alpha RNA in the central nervous system. Am J Pathol 144:659–666, 1994.
257. Wiley CA, Schrier RD, Nelson JA, et al: Cellular localization of human immunodeficiency virus infection within the brains of acquired immune deficiency syndrome patients. Proc Natl Acad Sci USA 83:7089–7093, 1986.
258. Epstein LG, Gendelman HE: Human immunodeficiency virus type 1 infection of the nervous system: Pathogenetic mechanisms. Ann Neurol 33:429–436, 1993.
259. Ho DD, Rota TR, Hirsch MS: Infection of monocyte/macrophages by human T lymphotropic virus type III. J Clin Invest 77:1712–1715, 1986.
260. Gartner S, Markovits P, Markovitz DM, et al: The role of mononuclear phagocytes in HTLV-III/LAV infection. Science 233:215–219, 1986.
261. Haase AT: Pathogenesis of lentivirus infections. Nature 322:130–136, 1986.
262. Gendelman HE, Narayan O, Kennedy-Stoskopf S, et al: Tropism of sheep lentiviruses for monocytes: Susceptibility to infection and virus gene expression increase during maturation of monocytes to macrophages. J Virol 58:67–74, 1986.
263. Rutka JT, Giblin JR, Berens ME, et al: The effects of human recombinant tumor necrosis factor on glioma-derived cell lines: Cellular proliferation, cytotoxicity, morphological and radioreceptor studies. Int J Cancer 41:573–582, 1988.
264. Selmaj KW, Raine CS: Tumor necrosis factor mediates myelin and oligodendrocyte damage in vitro. Ann Neurol 23:339–346, 1988.
265. Vyakarnam A, McKeating J, Meager A, et al: Tumour necrosis factors (alpha, beta) induced by HIV-1 in peripheral blood mononuclear cells potentiate virus replication. AIDS 4:21–27, 1990.
266. Israel N, Hazan U, Alcami J, et al: Tumor necrosis factor stimulates transcription of HIV-1 in human T lymphocytes, independently and synergistically with mitogens. J Immunol 143:3956–3960, 1989.
267. Sethi KK, Naher H, Stroehmann I: Phenotypic heterogeneity of cerebrospinal fluid–derived HIV-specific and HLA-restricted cytotoxic T-cell clones. Nature 335:178–181, 1988.
268. Chiodi F, Fuerstenberg S, Gidlund M, et al: Infection of brain-derived cells with the human immunodeficiency virus. J Virol 61:1244–1247, 1987.
269. Cheng-Mayer C, Seto D, Tateno M, et al: Biologic features of HIV-1 that correlate with virulence in the host. Science 240:80–82, 1988.
270. Brenneman DE, Westbrook GL, Fitzgerald SP, et al: Neuronal cell killing by the envelope protein of HIV and its prevention by vasoactive intestinal peptide. Nature 335:639–642, 1988.
271. Dreyer EB, Kaiser PK, Offermann JT, et al: HIV-1 coat protein neurotoxicity prevented by calcium channel antagonists. Science 248:364–367, 1990.
272. Lee MR, Ho DD, Gurney ME: Functional interaction and partial homology between human immunodeficiency virus and neuroleukin. Science 237:1047–1051, 1987.
273. Chaput M, Claes V, Portetelle D, et al: The neurotrophic factor neuroleukin is 90% homologous with phosphohexose isomerase. Nature 332:454–455, 1988.
274. Trujillo JR, McLane MF, Lee T-H, et al: Molecular mimicry between human immunodeficiency virus type 1 gp120 V3 loop and human brain proteins. J Virol 67:7711–7715, 1993.
275. Power C, McArthur JC, Johnson RT, et al: Demented and nondemented patients with AIDS differ in brain-derived human immunodeficiency virus type 1 envelope sequences. J Virol 68:4643–4649, 1994.
276. Essex M, Kanki P: Human immunodeficiency virus type 2 (HIV-2). *In* Broder S, Merigan T (eds): Textbook of AIDS Medicine. Baltimore, Williams & Wilkins, 1994, pp 873–886.
277. Ho DD, Sarngadharan MG, Resnick L, et al: Primary human T-lymphotropic virus type III infection. Ann Intern Med 103:880–883, 1985.
278. Cooper DA, Gold J, Maclean P, et al: Acute AIDS retrovirus infection. Definition of a clinical illness associated with seroconversion. Lancet 1:537–540, 1985.
279. Horsburgh CR Jr, Ou CY, Jason J, et al: Duration of human immunodeficiency virus infection before detection of antibody. Lancet 2:637–640, 1989.
280. Ranki A, Valle SL, Krohn M, et al: Long latency precedes overt seroconversion in sexually transmitted human-immunodeficiency-virus infection. Lancet 2:589–593, 1987.
281. Loche M, Mach B: Identification of HIV-infected seronegative individuals by a direct diagnostic test based on hybridisation to amplified viral DNA. Lancet 2:418–421, 1988.
282. Farzadegan H, Polis MA, Wolinsky SM, et al: Loss of human immunodeficiency virus type 1 (HIV-1) antibodies with evidence of viral infection in asymptomatic homosexual men. A report from the Multicenter AIDS Cohort Study. Ann Intern Med 108:785–790, 1988.
283. Imagawa DT, Lee MH, Wolinsky SM, et al: Human immunodeficiency virus type 1 infection in homosexual men who remain seronegative for prolonged periods. N Engl J Med 320:1458–1462, 1989.
284. Rowland-Jones S, Sutton J, Ariyoshi K, et al: HIV-specific cytotoxic T-cells in HIV-exposed but uninfected Gambian women. Nat Med 1:59–62, 1995.
285. Hessol NA, Lifson AR, O'Malley PM, et al: Prevalence, incidence, and progression of human immunodeficiency virus infection in homosexual and bisexual men in hepatitis B vaccine trials, 1978–1988. Am J Epidemiol 130:1167–1175, 1989.
286. Anderson RM, May RM: Epidemiological parameters of HIV transmission. Nature 333:514–519, 1988.
287. Curran JW, Jaffe HW, Hardy AM, et al: Epidemiology of HIV infection and AIDS in the United States. Science 239:610–616, 1988.

288. Rogers MF, Thomas PA, Starcher ET, et al: Acquired immunodeficiency syndrome in children: Report of the Centers for Disease Control National Surveillance, 1982 to 1985. Pediatrics 79:1008–1014, 1987.
289. Pantaleo G, Menzo S, Vaccarezza M, et al: Studies in subjects with long term nonprogressive human immunodeficiency virus infection. N Engl J Med 332:209–216, 1995.
290. Cao YZ, Qin LM, Zhang LQ, et al: Virologic and immunologic characterization of long-term survivors of human immunodeficiency virus type 1 infection. N Engl J Med 332:201–208, 1995.
291. Moseson M, Zeleniuch-Jacquotte A, Belsito DV, et al: The potential role of nutritional factors in the induction of immunologic abnormalities in HIV-positive homosexual men. J Acquir Immune Defic Syndr 2:235–247, 1989.
292. Gendelman HE, Phelps W, Feigenbaum L, et al: Trans-activation of the human immunodeficiency virus long terminal repeat sequence by DNA viruses. Proc Natl Acad Sci USA 83:9759–9763, 1986.
293. Haseltine WA: Silent HIV infections. N Engl J Med 320:1487–1489, 1989.
294. Braathen LR, Ramirez G, Kunze RO, Gelderblom H: Langerhans cells as primary target cells for HIV infection (Letter). Lancet 2:1094, 1987.
295. Delorme P, Dezutter-Dambuyant C, Ebersold A, et al: In vitro infection of epidermal Langerhans cells with human immunodeficiency virus type 1 (HTLV-IIIB isolate). Res Virol 144:53–58, 1993.
296. Piot P, Laga M: Epidemiology of AIDS in the developing world. *In* Broder S, Merigan TC Jr, Bolognesi D (eds): Textbook of AIDS Medicine. Baltimore, Williams & Wilkins, 1994, pp 109–132.
297. Rowley JT, Anderson RM, Ng TW: Reducing the spread of HIV infection in sub-Saharan Africa: Some demographic and economic implications. AIDS 4:47–56, 1990.
298. Soto-Ramirez LE, Renjifo B, McLane MF, et al: HIV-1 Langerhans' cell tropism associated with heterosexual transmission. Science 271:1291-1293, 1996.
299. Jason JM, McDougal JS, Dixon G, et al: HTLV-III/LAV antibody and immune status of household contacts and sexual partners of persons with hemophilia. JAMA 255:212–215, 1986.
300. Peterman TA, Stoneburner RL, Allen JR, et al: Risk of human immunodeficiency virus transmission from heterosexual adults with transfusion-associated infections. JAMA 259:55–58, 1988.
301. Kreiss JK, Kitchen LW, Prince HE, et al: Antibody to human T-lymphotropic virus type III in wives of hemophiliacs. Evidence for heterosexual transmission. Ann Intern Med 102:623–626, 1985.
302. Redfield RR, Markham PD, Salahuddin SZ, et al: Frequent transmission of HTLV-III among spouses of patients with AIDS-related complex and AIDS. JAMA 253:1571–1573, 1985.
303. Kingsley LA, Rinaldo CR Jr, Lyter DW, et al: Sexual transmission efficiency of hepatitis B virus and human immunodeficiency virus among homosexual men. JAMA 264:230–234, 1990.
304. Cameron DW, Simonsen JN, D'Costa LJ, et al: Female to male transmission of human immunodeficiency virus type 1: Risk factors for seroconversion in men. Lancet 2:403–407, 1989.
305. Piot P, Plummer FA, Rey MA, et al: Retrospective seroepidemiology of AIDS virus infection in Nairobi populations. J Infect Dis 155:1108–1112, 1987.
306. Johnson AM, Laga M: Heterosexual transmission of HIV. AIDS 2(Suppl 1):S49–S56, 1988.
307. Haverkos HW, Edelman R: The epidemiology of acquired immunodeficiency syndrome among heterosexuals. JAMA 260:1922–1929, 1988.
308. Kreiss JK, Koech D, Plummer FA, et al: AIDS virus infection in Nairobi prostitutes. Spread of the epidemic to East Africa. N Engl J Med 314:414–418, 1986.
309. Simonsen JN, Cameron DW, Gakinya MN, et al: Human immunodeficiency virus infection among men with sexually transmitted diseases. Experience from a center in Africa. N Engl J Med 319:274–278, 1988.
310. Holmberg SD, Stewart JA, Gerber AR, et al: Prior herpes simplex virus type 2 infection as a risk factor for HIV infection. JAMA 259:1048–1050, 1988.
311. Pepin J, Plummer FA, Brunham RC, et al: The interaction of HIV infection and other sexually transmitted diseases: An opportunity for intervention. AIDS 3:3–9, 1989.
312. Redfield RR, Markham PD, Salahuddin SZ, et al: Heterosexually acquired HTLV-III/LAV disease (AIDS-related complex and AIDS). Epidemiologic evidence for female-to-male transmission. JAMA 254:2094–2096, 1985.
313. Ho DD, Modgil T, Alam M: Quantitation of human immunodeficiency virus type 1 in the blood of infected persons. N Engl J Med 321:1621–1625, 1989.
314. Coombs RW, Collier AC, Allain JP, et al: Plasma viremia in human immunodeficiency virus infection. N Engl J Med 321:1626–1631, 1989.
315. Osmond D, Bacchetti P, Chaisson RE, et al: Time of exposure and risk of HIV infection in homosexual partners of men with AIDS. Am J Public Health 78:944–948, 1988.
316. Ward JW, Holmberg SD, Allen JR, et al: Transmission of human immunodeficiency virus (HIV) by blood transfusions screened as negative for HIV antibody. N Engl J Med 318:473–478, 1988.
317. Ragni MV, Kingsley LA, Nimorwicz P, et al: HIV heterosexual transmission in hemophilia couples: Lack of relation to T4 number, clinical diagnosis, or duration of HIV exposure. J Acquir Immune Defic Syndr 2:557–563, 1989.
318. Clumeck N, Taelman H, Hermans P, et al: A cluster of HIV infection among heterosexual people without apparent risk factors. N Engl J Med 321:1460–1462, 1989.
319. Seage GR, Horsburgh CR Jr, Hardy AM, et al: Increased suppressor T cells in probable transmitters of human immunodeficiency virus infection. Am J Public Health 79:1638–1642, 1989.
320. Goedert JJ, Mendez H, Drummond JE, et al: Mother-to-infant transmission of human immunodeficiency virus type 1: Association with prematurity or low anti-gp120. Lancet 2:1351–1354, 1989.
321. Belec L, Georges AJ, Steenman G, et al: Antibodies to human immunodeficiency virus in the semen of heterosexual men. J Infect Dis 159:324–327, 1989.
322. Belec L, Georges AJ, Steenman G, et al: Antibodies to human immunodeficiency virus in vaginal secretions of heterosexual women. J Infect Dis 160:385–391, 1989.
323. Vogt MW, Witt DJ, Craven DE, et al: Isolation of HTLV-III/LAV from cervical secretions of women at risk for AIDS. Lancet 1:525–527, 1986.
324. Wofsy CB, Cohen JB, Hauer LB, et al: Isolation of AIDS-associated retrovirus from genital secretions of women with antibodies to the virus. Lancet 1:527–529, 1986.
325. Levy JA: The transmission of AIDS: The case of the infected cell. JAMA 259:3037–3038, 1988.
326. Alexander NJ, Anderson DJ: Immunology of semen. Fertil Steril 47:192–205, 1987.
327. Wolff H, Anderson DJ: Male genital tract inflammation associated with increased numbers of potential human immunodeficiency virus host cells in semen. Andrologia 20:404–410, 1988.
328. Anderson DJ, Wolff H, Pudney J, et al: Presence of HIV in semen (Abstr). Presented at the VIth International Conference on AIDS; June 20–21, 1990; San Francisco, CA.
329. Borzy MS, Connell RS, Kiessling AA: Detection of human immunodeficiency virus in cell-free seminal fluid. J Acquir Immune Defic Syndr 1:419–424, 1988.
330. Bagasra O, Freund M, Weidmann J, et al: Interaction of human immunodeficiency virus with human sperm in vitro. J Acquir Immune Defic Syndr 1:431–435, 1988.
331. Anderson DJ, Wolff H, Pudney J, et al: Presence of HIV in semen. *In* Alexander NJ (ed): Heterosexual Transmission of AIDS. New York, Wiley-Liss, 1990, pp 167–180.
332. Anderson KC, Gorgone BC, Marlink RG, et al: Transfusion-acquired human immunodeficiency virus infection among immunocompromised persons. Ann Intern Med 105:519–527, 1986.
333. Ward JW, Deppe DA, Samson S, et al: Risk of human immunodeficiency virus infection from blood donors who later developed the acquired immunodeficiency syndrome. Ann Intern Med 106:61–62, 1987.
334. Chaisson RE, Moss AR, Onishi R, et al: Human immunodeficiency virus infection in heterosexual intravenous drug users in San Francisco. Am J Public Health 77:169–172, 1987.
335. Blanche S, Rouzioux C, Moscato ML, et al: A prospective study of infants born to women seropositive for human immunodeficiency virus type 1. HIV Infection in Newborns French Collaborative Study Group. N Engl J Med 320:1643–1648, 1989.
336. Ryder RW, Nsa W, Hassig SE, et al: Perinatal transmission

of the human immunodeficiency virus type 1 to infants of seropositive women in Zaire. N Engl J Med 320:1637–1642, 1989.
337. Hira SK, Kamanga J, Bhat GJ, et al: Perinatal transmission of HIV-I in Zambia. BMJ 299:1250–1252, 1989.
338. Pyun KH, Ochs HD, Dufford MT, et al: Perinatal infection with human immunodeficiency virus. Specific antibody responses by the neonate. N Engl J Med 317:611–614, 1987.
339. Marshall GS, Barbour SD, Plotkin SA: AIDS in a child without antibody to HIV. Lancet 1:446–447, 1987.
340. Lallemant M, Lallemant-Le-Coeur S, Cheynier D, et al: Mother-child transmission of HIV-1 and infant survival in Brazzaville, Congo. AIDS 3:643–646, 1989.
341. Scott GB, Hutto C, Makuch RW, et al: Survival in children with perinatally acquired human immunodeficiency virus type 1 infection. N Engl J Med 321:1791–1796, 1989.
342. The European Collaborative Study: Mother-to-child transmission of HIV infection. Lancet 2:1039–1043, 1988.
343. Poulsen AG, Kvinesdal B, Aaby P, et al: Prevalence of and mortality from human immunodeficiency virus type 2 in Bissau, West Africa. Lancet 1:827–831, 1989.
344. Andreasson P-A, Dias F, Goudiaby JMT, et al: HIV-2 infection in prenatal women and vertical transmission of HIV-2 in Guinea-Bissau (Abstr). Presented at the IVth International Conference on AIDS and Associated Cancers in Africa; October 1989; Marseilles, France.
345. Hojlyng N, Kvinesdal BB, Molbak K, et al: Vertical transmission of HIV-2: Does it occur? (Abstr). Presented at the IVth International Conference on AIDS and Associated Cancers in Africa; October 1989; Marseilles, France.
346. Gnaore E, Gayle H, Adjorlolo G, et al: HIV infection in 1008 children and their mothers in Abidjan, Côte d'Ivoire (Abstr). Presented at the IVth International Conference on AIDS and Associated Cancers in Africa; October 1989; Marseilles, France.
347. Kanki P, Ricard D, Mboup S, et al: Perinatal transmission of HIV-2 (Abstr). Presented at the IVth International Conference on AIDS; June 12–16, 1988; Stockholm, Sweden.
348. Maury W, Potts BJ, Rabson AB: HIV-1 infection of first-trimester and term human placental tissue: A possible mode of maternal-fetal transmission. J Infect Dis 160:583–588, 1989.
349. Ryder RW, Hassig SE: The epidemiology of perinatal transmission of HIV. AIDS 2(Suppl 1):S83–S89, 1988.
350. Thiry L, Sprecher-Goldberger S, Jonckheer T, et al: Isolation of AIDS virus from cell-free breast milk of three healthy virus carriers. Lancet 2:891–892, 1985.
351. Oxtoby MJ: Human immunodeficiency virus and other viruses in human milk: Placing the issues in broader perspective. Pediatr Infect Dis J 7:825–835, 1988.
352. Rossi P, Moschese V, Broliden PA, et al: Presence of maternal antibodies to human immunodeficiency virus 1 envelope glycoprotein gp120 epitopes correlates with the uninfected status of children born to seropositive mothers. Proc Natl Acad Sci USA 86:8055–8058, 1989.
353. Lallemant M, Le Coeur S, Tarantola D, et al: Antiretroviral prevention of HIV perinatal transmission. Lancet 343:1429–1430, 1994.
354. Connor EM, Sperling RS, Gelber R, et al: Reduction of maternal-infant transmission of human immunodeficiency virus type 1 with zidovudine treatment. Pediatric AIDS Clinical Trials Group Protocol 076 Study Group. N Engl J Med 331:1173–1180, 1994.
355. Chou MJ, Lee TH, Hatzakis A, et al: Antibody responses in early human immunodeficiency virus type 1 infection in hemophiliacs. J Infect Dis 157:805–811, 1988.
356. Steckelberg JM, Cockerill FR: Serologic testing for human immunodeficiency virus antibodies. Mayo Clin Proc 63:373–380, 1988.
357. Mendenhall CL, Roselle GA, Grossman CJ, et al: False positive tests for HTLV-III antibodies in alcoholic patients with hepatitis. N Engl J Med 314:921–922, 1986.
358. Kashala O, Marlink R, Ilunga M, et al: Infections with human immunodeficiency virus type 1 (HIV-I) and human T cell lymphotropic viruses among leprosy patients and contacts: Correlation between HIV-I cross-reactivity and antibodies to lipoarabinomannan. J Infect Dis 169:296–304, 1994.
359. Ayres L, Avillez F, Garcia-Benito A, et al: Multicenter evaluation of a new recombinant enzyme immunoassay for the combined detection of antibody to HIV-1 and HIV-2. AIDS 4:131–138, 1990.
360. De Cock KM, Brun-Vezinet F: Epidemiology of HIV-2 infection. AIDS 3(Suppl 1):S89–S95, 1989.
361. Zuber M, Samuel KP, Lautenberger JA, et al: Bacterially produced HIV-2 *env* polypeptides specific for distinguishing HIV-2 from HIV-1 infections. AIDS Res Hum Retroviruses 6:525–534, 1990.
362. The Consortium for Retrovirus Serology Standardization: Serological diagnosis of human immunodeficiency virus infection by Western blot testing. JAMA 260:674–679, 1988.
363. Essex M, Kanki PJ, Marlink R, et al: Antigenic characterization of the human immunodeficiency viruses. J Am Acad Dermatol 22:1206–1210, 1990.
364. Ou CY, Kwok S, Mitchell SW, et al: DNA amplification for direct detection of HIV-1 in DNA of peripheral blood mononuclear cells. Science 239:295–297, 1988.
365. Laure F, Courgnaud V, Rouzioux C, et al: Detection of HIV1 DNA in infants and children by means of the polymerase chain reaction. Lancet 2:538–541, 1988.
366. Piatak M Jr, Saag MS, Yang LC, et al: High levels of HIV-1 in plasma during all stages of infection determined by competitive PCR. Science 259:1749–1754, 1993.
367. Barnes WM: PCR amplification of up to 35-kb DNA with high fidelity and high yield from lambda bacteriophage templates. Proc Natl Acad Sci USA 91:2216–2220, 1994.
368. Groopman JE, Salahuddin SZ, Sarngadharan MG, et al: HTLV-III in saliva of people with AIDS-related complex and healthy homosexual men at risk for AIDS. Science 226:447–449, 1984.
369. Moss AR, Bacchetti P, Osmond D, et al: Seropositivity for HIV and the development of AIDS or AIDS related condition: Three year follow up of the San Francisco General Hospital cohort. Br Med J 296:745–750, 1988.
370. Fahey JL, Taylor JM, Detels R, et al: The prognostic value of cellular and serologic markers in infection with human immunodeficiency virus type 1. N Engl J Med 322:166–172, 1990.
371. Allain JP, Laurian Y, Paul DA, et al: Long-term evaluation of HIV antigen and antibodies to p24 and gp41 in patients with hemophilia. Potential clinical importance. N Engl J Med 317:1114–1121, 1987.
372. Kanki PJ, Marlink RG, Siby T, et al: Biology of HIV-2 infection in West Africa. *In* Papas TS (ed): Gene Regulation and AIDS. Houston, Portfolio Publishing Company of Texas, 1990, pp 255–272.
373. Siby T, Thior I, Marlink R, et al: Clinico-immunologic evaluation of HIV-2 infection in Senegal (Abstr). Presented at the Vth International Conference on AIDS in Africa; October 10–12, 1990; Kinshasa, Zaire.
374. Hirsch MS: Chemotherapy of human immunodeficiency virus infections: Current practice and future prospects. J Infect Dis 161:845–857, 1990.
375. Baltimore D: Gene therapy. Intracellular immunization. Nature 335:395–396, 1988.
376. Schooley RT, Merigan TC, Gaut P, et al: Recombinant soluble CD4 therapy in patients with the acquired immunodeficiency syndrome (AIDS) and AIDS-related complex. A phase I-II escalating dosage trial. Ann Intern Med 112:247–253, 1990.
377. Morgan RA, Anderson WF: Human gene therapy. Annu Rev Biochem 62:191–217, 1993.
378. Li J, Lord CI, Haseltine W, et al: Infection of cynomolgus monkeys with a chimeric HIV-I/SIVmac virus that expresses the HIV-I envelope glycoproteins. J Acquir Immune Defic Syndr 5:639–646, 1992.
379. Murphey-Corb M, Martin LN, Davison-Fairburn B, et al: A formalin-inactivated whole SIV vaccine confers protection in macaques. Science 246:1293–1297, 1989.
380. Gibbs CJ: HIV immunization and challenge of HIV-seropositive and -seronegative chimpanzees (Abstr). Presented at the Vth International Conference on AIDS; June 4–9, 1989; Montreal, Canada.
381. Fauci AS, Gallo RC, Koenig S, et al: NIH conference. Development and evaluation of a vaccine for human immunodeficiency virus (HIV) infection. Ann Intern Med 110:373–385, 1989.
382. Koff WC, Hoth DF: Development and testing of AIDS vaccines. Science 241:426–432, 1988.
383. Koff WC, Fauci AS: Human trials of AIDS vaccines: Current status and future directions. AIDS 3(Suppl 1):S125–S129, 1989.
384. Lewis MG, Mathes LE, Olsen RG: Protection against feline

leukemia by vaccination with a subunit vaccine. Infect Immun 34:888–894, 1981.
385. Orentas RJ, Hildreth JE, Obah E, et al: Induction of CD4+ human cytolytic T cells specific for HIV-infected cells by a gp160 subunit vaccine. Science 248:1234–1237, 1990.
386. Newman MJ, Wu JY, Gardner BH, et al: Saponin adjuvant induction of ovalbumin-specific CD8+ cytotoxic T lymphocyte responses. J Immunol 148:2357–2362, 1992.
387. Payne L, Jenkins SA, Andrianov A, et al: Water soluble phosphazene polymers for parenteral and mucosal vaccine delivery. *In* Powell MF, Neuman MJ (eds): Vaccine Design. New York, Plenum Publishing, 1995, pp 473–493.
388. Morein B: The iscom antigen-presenting system. Nature 332:287–288, 1988.
389. Brown F, Schild GC, Ada GL: Recombinant vaccinia viruses as vaccines. Nature 319:549–550, 1986.
390. Hu SL, Kosowski SG, Dalrymple JM: Expression of AIDS virus envelope gene in recombinant vaccinia viruses. Nature 320:537–540, 1986.
391. Chakrabarti S, Robert-Guroff M, Wong-Staal F, et al: Expression of the HTLV-III envelope gene by a recombinant vaccinia virus. Nature 320:535–537, 1986.
392. Moss B, Flexner C: Vaccinia virus expression vectors. Annu Rev Immunol 5:305–324, 1987.
393. Davis AR, Kostek B, Mason BB, et al: Expression of hepatitis B surface antigen with a recombinant adenovirus. Proc Natl Acad Sci USA 82:7560–7564, 1985.
394. Fenner F, Henderson DA, Arita I, et al: Developments in vaccination and control between 1900 and 1966. *In* Fenner F, Henderson DA, Arita I, et al (eds): Smallpox and Its Eradication. Geneva, World Health Organization, 1988, pp 277–314.
395. Redfield RR, Wright DC, James WD, et al: Disseminated vaccinia in a military recruit with human immunodeficiency virus (HIV) disease. N Engl J Med 316:673–676, 1987.
396. Flexner C, Hugin A, Moss B: Prevention of vaccinia virus infection in immunodeficient mice by vector-directed IL-2 expression. Nature 330:259–262, 1987.
397. Ramshaw IA, Andrew ME, Phillips SM, et al: Recovery of immunodeficient mice from a vaccinia virus/IL-2 recombinant infection. Nature 329:545–546, 1987.
398. Evans DJ, McKeating J, Meredith JM, et al: An engineered poliovirus chimaera elicits broadly reactive HIV-1 neutralizing antibodies. Nature 339:385–388, 1989.
399. Desrosiers RC, Wyand MS, Kodama T, et al: Vaccine protection against simian immunodeficiency virus infection. Proc Natl Acad Sci USA 86:6353–6357, 1989.
400. Salk J: Prospects for the control of AIDS by immunizing seropositive individuals. Nature 327:473–476. 1987.
401. Ezzell C: Another AIDS vaccine. Nature 330:509, 1987.
402. Prince AM, Horowitz B, Baker L, et al: Failure of a human immunodeficiency virus (HIV) immune globulin to protect chimpanzees against experimental challenge with HIV. Proc Natl Acad Sci USA 85:6944–6948, 1988.
403. Dalgleish AG, Thomson BJ, Chanh TC, et al: Neutralisation of HIV isolates by anti-idiotypic antibodies which mimic the T4 (CD4) epitope: A potential AIDS vaccine. Lancet 2:1047–1050, 1987.
404. Habeshaw JA, Dalgleish AG: The relevance of HIV *env*/CD4 interactions to the pathogenesis of acquired immune deficiency syndrome. J Acquir Immune Defic Syndr 2:457–468, 1989.
405. Barry M: Ethical considerations of human investigation in developing countries: The AIDS dilemma. N Engl J Med 319:1083–1086, 1988.
406. Nabel GJ, Rice SA, Knipe DM, et al: Alternative mechanisms for activation of human immunodeficiency virus enhancer in T cells. Science 239:1299–1302, 1988.
407. Essex M: Confronting the AIDS vaccine challenge. Technol Rev 97:23–29, 1994.
408. Watanabe T, Seiki M, Tsujimoto H, et al: Sequence homology of the simian retrovirus genome with human T-cell leukemia virus type I. Virology 144:59–65, 1985.
409. Varmus H: Retroviruses. Science 240:1427–1435, 1988.
410. Lee TH, Coligan JE, Sodroski JG, et al: Antigens encoded by the 3′-terminal region of human T-cell leukemia virus: Evidence for a functional gene. Science 226:57–61, 1984.
411. Hidaka M, Inoue J, Yoshida M, Seiki M: Post-transcriptional regulator *(rex)* of HTLV-1 initiates expression of viral structural proteins but suppresses expression of regulatory proteins. EMBO J 7:519–523, 1988.
412. Rimsky L, Hauber J, Dukovich M, et al: Functional replacement of the HIV-1 *rev* protein by the HTLV-1 rex protein. Nature 335:738–740, 1988.
413. Koralnik IJ, Gessain A, Klotman ME, et al: Protein isoforms encoded by the pX region of human T-cell leukemia/lymphotropic virus type I. Proc Natl Acad Sci USA 89:8813–8817, 1992.
414. Berneman ZN, Gartenhaus RB, Reitz MS Jr, et al: Expression of alternatively spliced human T-lymphotropic virus type I pX mRNA in infected cell lines and in primary uncultured cells from patients with adult T-cell leukemia/lymphoma and healthy carriers. Proc Natl Acad Sci USA 89:3005–3009, 1992.
415. Gomez-Lucia E, Chen YA, Yu QC, et al: Infection of a promonocytic cell line with HTLV-I and II. *In* Jolicoeur P, Linial M (eds): RNA Tumor Viruses. Cold Spring Harbor, NY, Cold Spring Harbor Press, 1990, p 270.
416. Yoshikura H, Nishida J, Yoshida M, et al: Isolation of HTLV derived from Japanese adult T-cell leukemia patients in human diploid fibroblast strain IMR90 and the biological characters of the infected cells. Int J Cancer 33:745–749, 1984.
417. Hoshino H, Shimoyama M, Miwa M, et al: Detection of lymphocytes producing a human retrovirus associated with adult T-cell leukemia by syncytia induction assay. Proc Natl Acad Sci USA 80:7337–7341, 1983.
418. Miyoshi I, Yoshimoto S, Taguchi H, et al: Transformation of rabbit lymphocytes with T-cell leukemia virus. Gann 74:1–4, 1983.
419. Sommerfelt MA, Williams BP, Clapham PR, et al: Human T cell leukemia viruses use a receptor determined by human chromosome 17. Science 242:1557–1559, 1988.
420. Okochi K, Sato H, Hinuma Y: A retrospective study on transmission of adult T cell leukemia virus by blood transfusion: Seroconversion in recipients. Vox Sang 46:245–253, 1984.
421. Cruickshank JK, Richardson JH, Morgan OS, et al: Screening for prolonged incubation of HTLV-I infection in British and Jamaican relatives of British patients with tropical spastic paraparesis. BMJ 300:300–304, 1990.
422. Kashiwagi S, Kajiyama W, Hayashi J, et al: Antibody to p40tax protein of human T cell leukemia virus 1 and infectivity. J Infect Dis 161:426–429, 1990.
423. Chen YM, Okayama A, Lee TH, et al: Sexual transmission of human T-cell leukemia virus type I associated with the presence of anti-Tax antibody. Proc Natl Acad Sci USA 88:1182–1186, 1991.
424. Okayama A, Chen YM, Tachibana N, et al: High incidence of antibodies to HTLV-I tax in blood relatives of adult T cell leukemia patients. J Infect Dis 163:47–52, 1991.
425. Miyakoshi H, Koide H, Aoki T: In vitro antibody-dependent cellular cytotoxicity against human T-cell leukemia/lymphoma virus (HTLV)–producing cells. Int J Cancer 33:287–291, 1984.
426. Kannagi M, Sugamura K, Sato H, et al: Establishment of human cytotoxic T cell lines specific for human adult T cell leukemia virus–bearing cells. J Immunol 130:2942–2946, 1983.
427. Ruscetti FW, Mikovits JA, Kalyanaraman VS, et al: Analysis of effector mechanisms against HTLV-I– and HTLV-III/LAV–infected lymphoid cells. J Immunol 136:3619–3624, 1986.
428. Tanaka Y, Tozawa H, Koyanagi Y, et al: Recognition of human T cell leukemia virus type I (HTLV-I) *gag* and *pX* gene products by MHC-restricted cytotoxic T lymphocytes induced in rats against syngeneic HTLV-I–infected cells. J Immunol 144:4202–4211, 1990.
429. Zhang XQ, Yang L, Ho DD, et al: Human T lymphotropic virus types I– and II–specific antibody-dependent cellular cytotoxicity: Strain specificity and epitope mapping. J Infect Dis 165:805–812, 1992.
430. Tachibana N, Okayama A, Ishizaki J, et al: Suppression of tuberculin skin reaction in healthy HTLV-I carriers from Japan. Int J Cancer 42:829–831, 1988.
431. Gibbs WN, Lofters WS, Campbell M, et al: Non-Hodgkin lymphoma in Jamaica and its relation to adult T-cell leukemia-lymphoma. Ann Intern Med 106:361–368, 1987.
432. Essex M, McLane MF, Tachibana N, et al: Seroepidemiology of human T-cell leukemia virus in relation to immunosuppression and the acquired immunodeficiency syndrome. *In* Gallo RC,

Essex M, Gross L (eds): Human T-Cell Leukemia/Lymphoma Viruses. Cold Spring Harbor, NY, Cold Spring Harbor Laboratory Press, 1984, pp 355–362.
433. Katsuki T, Katsuki K, Imai J, et al: Immune suppression in healthy carriers of adult T-cell leukemia retrovirus (HTLV-I): Impairment of T-cell control of Epstein-Barr virus-infected B-cells. Jpn J Cancer Res 78:639–642, 1987.
434. Yamada Y: Phenotypic and functional analysis of leukemic cells from 16 patients with adult T-cell leukemia/lymphoma. Blood 61:192–199, 1983.
435. Yssel H, de Waal Malefyt R, Duc Dodon MD, et al: Human T cell leukemia/lymphoma virus type I infection of a $CD4^+$ proliferative/cytotoxic T cell clone progresses in at least two distinct phases based on changes in function and phenotype of the infected cells. J Immunol 142:2279–2289, 1989.
436. Ruegg CL, Monell CR, Strand M: Identification, using synthetic peptides, of the minimum amino acid sequence from the retroviral transmembrane protein p15E required for inhibition of lymphoproliferation and its similarity to gp21 of human T-lymphotropic virus types I and II. J Virol 63:3250–3256, 1989.
437. Popovic M, Flomenberg N, Volkman DJ, et al: Alteration of T-cell functions by infection with HTLV-I or HTLV-II. Science 226:459–462, 1984.
438. deShazo RD, Chadha N, Morgan JE, et al: Immunologic assessment of a cluster of asymptomatic HTLV-I–infected individuals in New Orleans. Am J Med 86:65–70, 1989.
439. Hinuma Y, Komoda H, Chosa T, et al: Antibodies to adult T-cell leukemia-virus–associated antigen (ATLA) in sera from patients with ATL and controls in Japan: A nation-wide sero-epidemiologic study. Int J Cancer 29:631–635, 1982.
440. Wang CH, Chen CJ, Hu CY, et al: Seroepidemiology of human T-cell lymphotropic virus type I infection in Taiwan. Cancer Res 48:5042–5044, 1988.
441. Blattner WA, Kalyanaraman VS, Robert-Guroff M, et al: The human type-C retrovirus, HTLV, in blacks from the Caribbean region, and relationship to adult T-cell leukemia/lymphoma. Int J Cancer 30:257–264, 1982.
442. Merino F, Robert-Guroff M, Clark J, et al: Natural antibodies to human T-cell leukemia/lymphoma virus in healthy Venezuelan populations. Int J Cancer 34:501–506, 1984.
443. Saxinger W, Blattner WA, Levine PH, et al: Human T-cell leukemia virus (HTLV-I) antibodies in Africa. Science 225:1473–1476, 1984.
444. Biggar RJ, Saxinger C, Gardiner C, et al: Type-I HTLV antibody in urban and rural Ghana, West Africa. Int J Cancer 34:215–219, 1984.
445. Lee H, Swanson P, Shorty VS, et al: High rate of HTLV-II infection in seropositive i.v. drug abusers in New Orleans. Science 244:471–475, 1989.
446. Gradilone A, Zani M, Barillari G, et al: HTLV-I and HIV infection in drug addicts in Italy. Lancet 2:753–754, 1986.
447. Williams AE, Fang CT, Slamon DJ, et al: Seroprevalence and epidemiological correlates of HTLV-I infection in U.S. blood donors. Science 240:643–646, 1988.
448. Morishima Y, Ohya K, Ueda R, et al: Detection of adult T-cell leukemia virus (ATLV) bearing lymphocytes in concentrated red blood cells derived from ATL associated antibody (ATLA-Ab) positive donors. Vox Sang 50:212–215, 1986.
449. Larson CJ, Taswell HF: Human T-cell leukemia virus type I (HTLV-I) and blood transfusion. Mayo Clin Proc 63:869–875, 1988.
450. Minamoto GY, Gold JW, Scheinberg DA, et al: Infection with human T-cell leukemia virus type I in patients with leukemia. N Engl J Med 318:219–222, 1988.
451. Robert-Guroff M, Weiss SH, Giron JA, et al: Prevalence of antibodies to HTLV-I, -II, and -III in intravenous drug abusers from an AIDS endemic region. JAMA 255:3133–3137, 1986.
452. Tedder RS, Shanson DC, Jeffries DJ, et al: Low prevalence in the UK of HTLV-I and HTLV-II infection in subjects with AIDS, with extended lymphadenopathy, and at risk of AIDS. Lancet 2:125–128, 1984.
453. Ehrlich GD, Glaser JB, LaVigne K, et al: Prevalence of human T-cell leukemia/lymphoma virus (HTLV) type II infection among high-risk individuals: Type-specific identification of HTLVs by polymerase chain reaction. Blood 74:1658–1664, 1989.
454. Nakano S, Ando Y, Ichijo M, et al: Search for possible routes of vertical and horizontal transmission of adult T-cell leukemia virus. Gann 75:1044–1045, 1984.
455. Tajima K, Tominaga S, Suchi T, et al: Epidemiological analysis of the distribution of antibody to adult T-cell leukemia-virus–associated antigen: Possible horizontal transmission of adult T-cell leukemia virus. Gann 73:893–901, 1982.
456. Kajiyama W, Kashiwagi S, Ikematsu H, et al: Intrafamilial transmission of adult T cell leukemia virus. J Infect Dis 154:851–857, 1986.
457. Murphy EL, Figueroa JP, Gibbs WN, et al: Sexual transmission of human T-lymphotropic virus type I (HTLV-I). Ann Intern Med 111:555–560, 1989.
458. Riedel DA, Evans AS, Saxinger C, et al: A historical study of human T lymphotropic virus type I transmission in Barbados. J Infect Dis 159:603–609, 1989.
459. Nakano S, Ando Y, Saito K, et al: Primary infection of Japanese infants with adult T-cell leukaemia–associated retrovirus (ATLV): Evidence for viral transmission from mothers to children. J Infect 12:205–212, 1986.
460. Ando Y, Nakano S, Saito K, et al: Transmission of adult T-cell leukemia retrovirus (HTLV-I) from mother to child: Comparison of bottle- with breast-fed babies. Jpn J Cancer Res 78:322–324, 1987.
461. Hino S, Yamaguchi K, Katamine S, et al: Mother-to-child transmission of human T-cell leukemia virus type-I. Jpn J Cancer Res 76:474–480, 1985.
462. Kamihira S, Toriya K, Amagasaki T, et al: Antibodies against p40tax gene product of human T-lymphotropic virus type-I (HTLV-I) under various conditions of HTLV-I infection. Jpn J Cancer Res 80:1066–1071, 1989.
463. The third nation-wide study on adult T-cell leukemia/lymphoma (ATL) in Japan: Characteristic patterns of HLA antigen and HTLV-I infection in ATL patients and their relatives. The T- and B-Cell Malignancy Study Group. Int J Cancer 41:505–512, 1988.
464. Weinberg JB, Spiegel RA, Blazey DL, et al: Human T-cell lymphotropic virus I and adult T-cell leukemia: Report of a cluster in North Carolina. Am J Med 85:51–58, 1988.
465. Blayney DW, Blattner WA, Robert-Guroff M, et al: The human T-cell leukemia-lymphoma virus in the southeastern United States. JAMA 250:1048–1052, 1983.
466. Kinoshita K, Amagasaki T, Ikeda S, et al: Preleukemic state of adult T cell leukemia: Abnormal T lymphocytosis induced by human adult T cell leukemia-lymphoma virus. Blood 66:120–127, 1985.
467. Broder S, Bunn PA Jr, Jaffe ES, et al: NIH conference. T-cell lymphoproliferative syndrome associated with human T-cell leukemia/lymphoma virus. Ann Intern Med 100:543–557, 1984.
468. Ratner L, Griffith RC, Marselle L, et al: A lymphoproliferative disorder caused by human T-lymphotropic virus type I. Demonstration of a continuum between acute and chronic adult T-cell leukemia/lymphoma. Am J Med 83:953–958, 1987.
469. Kinoshita K, Hino S, Amagasaki T, et al: Development of adult T-cell leukemia-lymphoma (ATL) in two anti–ATL-associated antigen–positive healthy adults. Gann 73:684–685, 1982.
470. Yoshida M, Hattori S, Seiki M: Molecular biology of human T-cell leukemia virus associated with adult T-cell leukemia. Curr Top Microbiol Immunol 115:157–175, 1985.
471. Rosenblatt JD, Chen IS, Wachsman W: Infection with HTLV-I and HTLV-II: Evolving concepts. Semin Hematol 25:230–246, 1988.
472. Takatsuki K, Yamaguchi K, Kawano F, et al: Clinical diversity in adult T-cell leukemia-lymphoma. Cancer Res 45:4644s–4645s, 1985.
473. Nimer SD, Gasson JC, Hu K, et al: Activation of the GM-CSF promoter by HTLV-I and -II tax proteins. Oncogene 4:671–676, 1989.
474. Reichel H, Koeffler HP, Norman AW: 25-Hydroxyvitamin D_3 metabolism by human T-lymphotropic virus–transformed lymphocytes. J Clin Endocrinol Metab 65:519–526, 1987.
475. Nakada K, Kohakura M, Komoda H, et al: High incidence of HTLV antibody in carriers of *Strongyloides stercoralis*. Lancet 1:633, 1984.
476. O'Doherty MJ, Van de Pette JE, Nunan TO, et al: Recurrent *Strongyloides stercoralis* infection in a patient with T-cell lymphoma-leukaemia. Lancet 1:858, 1984.

477. Fukuhara S, Hinuma Y, Gotoh YI, et al: Chromosome aberrations in T lymphocytes carrying adult T-cell leukemia–associated antigens (ATLA) from healthy adults. Blood 61:205–207, 1983.
478. Miyamoto K, Tomita N, Ishii A, et al: Chromosome abnormalities of leukemia cells in adult patients with T-cell leukemia. J Natl Cancer Inst 73:353–362, 1984.
479. Takatsuki K, Yamaguchi K, Kawano F, et al: Clinical aspects of adult T-cell leukemia/lymphoma (ATL). Princess Takamatsu Symp 15:51–57, 1984.
480. Jaffe ES, Blattner WA, Blayney DW, et al: The pathologic spectrum of adult T-cell leukemia/lymphoma in the United States. Human T-cell leukemia/lymphoma virus–associated lymphoid malignancies. Am J Surg Pathol 8:263–275, 1984.
481. Yamaguchi K, Nishimura Y, Kiyokawa T, et al: Elevated serum levels of soluble interleukin-2 receptors in HTLV-I–associated myelopathy. J Lab Clin Med 114:407–410, 1989.
482. Blayney DW, Jaffe ES, Fisher RI, et al: The human T-cell leukemia/lymphoma virus, lymphoma, lytic bone lesions, and hypercalcemia. Ann Intern Med 98:144–151, 1983.
483. Yokota T, Cho MJ, Tachibana N, et al: The prevalence of antibody to p42 of HTLV-I among ATLL patients in comparison with healthy carriers in Japan. Int J Cancer 43:970–974, 1989.
484. Lofters W, Campbell M, Gibbs WN, et al: 2′-Deoxycoformycin therapy in adult T-cell leukemia/lymphoma. Cancer 60:2605–2608, 1987.
485. Shimoyama M, Ota K, Kikuchi M, et al: Chemotherapeutic results and prognostic factors of patients with advanced non-Hodgkin's lymphoma treated with VEPA or VEPA-M. J Clin Oncol 6:128–141, 1988.
486. Yamaguchi K, Yul LS, Oda T, et al: Clinical consequences of 2′-deoxycoformycin treatment in patients with refractory adult T-cell leukaemia. Leuk Res 10:989–993, 1986.
487. Waldmann TA: Anti–IL-2 receptor monoclonal antibody (anti-Tac) treatment of T-cell lymphoma. Important Adv Oncol 131-141, 1994.
488. Seto A, Kawanishi M, Matsuda S, et al: Adult T cell leukemia–like disease experimentally induced in rabbits. Jpn J Cancer Res 79:335–341, 1988.
489. Cruickshank EK: A neuropathic syndrome of uncertain origin—Review of 100 cases. West Indian Med J 5:147, 1956.
490. Montgomery RD, Cruickshank EK, Robertson WB, et al: Clincial and pathological observations on Jamaican neuropathy. A report on 206 cases. Brain 87:425, 1964.
491. Gessain A, Barin F, Vernant JC, et al: Antibodies to human T-lymphotropic virus type-I in patients with tropical spastic paraparesis. Lancet 2:407–410, 1985.
492. Osame M, Usuku K, Izumo S, et al: HTLV-I associated myelopathy, a new clinical entity. Lancet 1:1031–1032, 1986.
493. Osame M, Matsumoto M, Usuku K, et al: Chronic progressive myelopathy associated with elevated antibodies to human T-lymphotropic virus type I and adult T-cell leukemialike cells. Ann Neurol 21:117–122, 1987.
494. Lolli F, Fredrikson S, Kam-Hansen S, et al: Increased reactivity to HTLV-I in inflammatory nervous system diseases. Ann Neurol 22:67–71, 1987.
495. Mora CA, Garruto RM, Brown P, et al: Seroprevalence of antibodies to HTLV-I in patients with chronic neurological disorders other than tropical spastic paraparesis. Ann Neurol 23(Suppl):S192–S195, 1988.
496. Nishimura M, Adachi A, Maeda M, et al: Human T lymphotrophic virus type I may not be associated with multiple sclerosis in Japan. J Immunol 144:1684–1688, 1990.
497. Bangham CRM, Nightingale S, Cruickshank JK, et al: PCR analysis of DNA from multiple sclerosis patients for the presence of HTLV-I. Science 246:821–824, 1989.
498. Yoshida M, Osame M, Kawai H, et al: Increased replication of HTLV-I in HTLV-I–associated myelopathy. Ann Neurol 26:331–335, 1989.
499. Gessain A, Saal F, Gout O, et al: High human T-cell lymphotropic virus type I proviral DNA load with polyclonal integration in peripheral blood mononuclear cells of French West Indian, Guianese, and African patients with tropical spastic paraparesis. Blood 75:428–433, 1990.
500. Greenberg SJ, Jacobson S, Waldmann TA, et al: Molecular analysis of HTLV-I proviral integration and T cell receptor arrangement indicates that T cells in tropical spastic paraparesis are polyclonal. J Infect Dis 159:741–744, 1989.
501. Tsujimoto A, Teruuchi T, Imamura J, et al: Nucleotide sequence analysis of a provirus derived from HTLV-1–associated myelopathy (HAM). Mol Biol Med 5:29–42, 1988.
502. Daenke S, Nightingale S, Cruickshank JK, et al: Sequence variants of human T-cell lymphotropic virus type I from patients with tropical spastic paraparesis and adult T-cell leukemia do not distinguish neurological from leukemic isolates. J Virol 64:1278–1282, 1990.
503. Renjifo B, Essex M: *Tax* mutation associated with tropical spastic paraparesis/human T-cell leukemia virus type 1–associated myelopathy. J Virol 69:2611–2615, 1995.
504. Blattner WA, Gibbs WN, Saxinger C, et al: Human T-cell leukaemia/lymphoma virus–associated lymphoreticular neoplasia in Jamaica. Lancet 2:61–64, 1983.
505. Mann DL, DeSantis P, Mark G, et al: HTLV-I–associated B-cell CLL: Indirect role for retrovirus in leukemogenesis. Science 236:1103–1106, 1987.
506. Harper ME, Kaplan MH, Marselle LM, et al: Concomitant infection with HTLV-I and HTLV-III in a patient with T8 lymphoproliferative disease. N Engl J Med 315:1073–1078, 1986.
507. Clark JW, Hahn BH, Mann DL, et al: Molecular and immunologic analysis of a chronic lymphocytic leukemia case with antibodies against human T-cell leukemia virus. Cancer 56:495–499, 1985.
508. Verdier M, Denis F, Sangare A, et al: Antibodies to human T lymphotropic virus type 1 in patients with leprosy in tropical areas. J Infect Dis 161:1309–1310, 1990.
509. Morgan OS, Rodgers-Johnson P, Mora C, et al: HTLV-1 and polymyositis in Jamaica. Lancet 2:1184–1187, 1989.
510. Nerenberg MI, Wiley CA: Degeneration of oxidative muscle fibers in HTLV-1 *tax* transgenic mice. Am J Pathol 135:1025–1033, 1989.
511. De Rossi A, Franchini G, Aldovini A, et al: Differential response to the cytopathic effects of human T-cell lymphotropic virus type III (HTLV-III) superinfection in T4$^+$ (helper) and T8$^+$ (suppressor) T-cell clones transformed by HTLV-I. Proc Natl Acad Sci USA 83:4297–4301, 1986.
512. Zack JA, Cann AJ, Lugo JP, et al: HIV-1 production from infected peripheral blood T cells after HTLV-I induced mitogenic stimulation. Science 240:1026–1029, 1988.
513. Montefiori DC, Mitchell WM: Infection of the HTLV-II–bearing T-cell line C3 with HTLV-III/LAV is highly permissive and lytic. Virology 155:726–731, 1986.
514. Gallo RC: Mechanism of disease induction by HIV. J Acquir Immune Defic Syndr 3:380–389, 1990.
515. Lewis N, Williams J, Rekosh D, et al: Identification of a cis-acting element in human immunodeficiency virus type 2 (HIV-2) that is responsive to the HIV-1 *rev* and human T-cell leukemia virus types I and II *rex* proteins. J Virol 64:1690–1697, 1990.
516. Felber BK, Derse D, Athanassopoulos A, et al: Cross-activation of the Rex proteins of HTLV-I and BLV and of the Rev protein of HIV-1 and nonreciprocal interactions with their RNA responsive elements. New Biol 1:318–328, 1989.
517. Cortes E, Detels R, Aboulafia D, et al: HIV-1, HIV-2, and HTLV-I infection in high-risk groups in Brazil. N Engl J Med 320:953–958, 1989.
518. Murphy EL, Gibbs WN, Figueroa JP, et al: Human immunodeficiency virus and human T-lymphotropic virus type I infection among homosexual men in Kingston, Jamaica. J Acquir Immune Defic Syndr 1:143–149, 1988.
519. Bartholomew C, Blattner W, Cleghorn F: Progression to AIDS in homosexual men co-infected with HIV and HTLV-I in Trinidad. Lancet 2:1469, 1987.
520. Bartholomew C, Cleghorn F, Hull B, et al: Update on coinfection with HIV and HTLV-I in Trinidad (Abstr). Presented at the VIth International Conference on AIDS; June 20–21, 1990; San Francisco, CA.
521. Okubo S, Yasunaga K: Significance of viral co-infections by HIV, HTLV-1, Epstein-Barr virus and cytomegalovirus for immunological conditions in Japanese hemophiliacs. AIDS 2:318–319, 1988.
522. Hattori T, Koito A, Takatsuki K, et al: Frequent infection with human T-cell lymphotropic virus type I in patients with AIDS but not in carriers of human immunodeficiency virus type 1. J Acquir Immune Defic Syndr 2:272–276, 1989.

523. Page JB, Lai SH, Chitwood DD, et al: HTLV-I/II seropositivity and death from AIDS among HIV-1 seropositive intravenous drug users. Lancet 335:1439–1441, 1990.
524. Baurmann H, Miclea JM, Ferchal F, et al: Adult T-cell leukemia associated with HTLV-I and simultaneous infection by human immunodeficiency virus type 2 and human herpesvirus 6 in an African woman: A clinical, virologic, and familial serologic study. Am J Med 85:853–857, 1988.
525. Saxon A, Stevens RH, Golde DW: T-lymphocyte variant of hairy-cell leukemia. Ann Intern Med 88:323–326, 1978.
526. Rosenblatt JD, Golde DW, Wachsman W, et al: A second isolate of HTLV-II associated with atypical hairy-cell leukemia. N Engl J Med 315:372–377, 1986.
527. Rosenblatt JD, Giorgi JV, Golde DW, et al: Integrated human T-cell leukemia virus II genome in CD8+ T cells from a patient with "atypical" hairy cell leukemia: Evidence for distinct T and B cell lymphoproliferative disorders. Blood 71:363–369, 1988.
528. Lion T, Razvi N, Golomb HM, et al: B-lymphocytic hairy cells contain no HTLV-II DNA sequences. Blood 72:1428–1430, 1988.
529. Sohn CC, Blayney DW, Misset JL, et al: Leukopenic chronic T cell leukemia mimicking hairy cell leukemia: Association with human retroviruses. Blood 67:949–956, 1986.
530. Cervantes J, Hussain S, Jensen F, et al: T-prolymphocytic leukemia associated with human T-cell lymphotropic virus II (Abstr). Clin Res 34:454A, 1986.
531. Lee TH, Coligan JE, Homma T, et al: Human T-cell leukemia virus-associated membrane antigens: Identity of the major antigens recognized after virus infection. Proc Natl Acad Sci USA 81:3856–3860, 1984.
532. Lee TH, Coligan JE, McLane MF, et al: Serological cross-reactivity between envelope gene products of type I and type II human T-cell leukemia virus. Proc Natl Acad Sci USA 81:7579–7583, 1984.
533. Chen YM, Gomez-Lucia E, Okayama A, et al: Antibody profile of early HTLV-I infections. Lancet 336:1214–1216, 1990.
534. Weinhold KJ, Tyler DS, Lyerly HK: Measurement of direct and indirect forms of anti-HIV-1 ADCC: Implications for other retroviral disease. Dev Biol Stand 72:343–348, 1990.
535. Chen YM, Lee TH, Samuel KP, et al: Antibody reactivity to different regions of human T-cell leukemia virus type 1 gp61 in infected people. J Virol 63:4952–4957, 1989.
536. Chen YM, Lee TH, Wiktor SZ, et al: Type-specific antigens for serological discrimination of HTLV-I and HTLV-II infection. Lancet 336:1153–1155, 1990.
537. Matsushita S, Mitsuya H, Reitz MS, et al: Pharmacological inhibition of in vitro infectivity of human T lymphotropic virus type I. J Clin Invest 80:394–400, 1987.
538. Osame M, Janssen R, Kubota H, et al: Nationwide survey of HTLV-I–associated myelopathy in Japan: Association with blood transfusion. Ann Neurol 28:50–56, 1990.
539. Takehara N, Iwahara Y, Uemura Y, et al: Effect of immunization on HTLV-I infection in rabbits. Int J Cancer 44:332–336, 1989.

265

Rubella Virus

Alexander Rakowsky
John L. Sever

History

It appears that rubella was known to the early Arabian physicians under the name *al-hamikah*, but two German physicians, de Bergen in 1752 and Orlow in 1758, are generally credited with first recognizing rubella clinically and calling it *Rotheln*.[1] In all three cases, however, rubella was seen as a variant of measles or scarlet fever, and it was Manton[2] in 1815 who first described the illness as a separate clinical entity. During the period from the mid-18th to the mid-19th centuries, this illness was of great interest to German physicians, and thus the name German measles came about as the popular name for rubella.[1] The actual term rubella was coined in 1861 by Veale,[3] a Scottish physician who found the German name *Rotheln* too harsh and foreign in sound.

In 1881 at the International Congress of Medicine in London, rubella was officially recognized as a distinct illness, and a complete description of acquired rubella infection was known by the early 20th century.[1] However, it was thought to be a mild, self-limited illness that rarely produced complications. This view was changed in 1941 when Gregg,[4] an Australian ophthalmologist, published a paper in which he noted an association between maternal rubella infection and congenital defects. Although this association was initially doubted, by 1944 Gregg's observations were confirmed by fellow Australians Swan and colleagues and by investigators in the United States.[1] Verification of the viral agent did not occur until 1962, when two separate teams, Weller and Neva[5] at Harvard University and Parkman and coworkers[6] at Walter Reed Hospital, independently isolated the virus in cell culture.

The information contained in this chapter reflects the views of the authors only and not necessarily those of the Food and Drug Administration.

Characteristics of the Pathogen

Classification

Rubella virus belongs to the togavirus family and is the only member of the genus *Rubivirus*. Only one immunologically distinct type has been described, and no common serologic relationship exists between the rubella virus and other viruses, although the rubella virus is physiochemically similar to the other members of the Togaviridae family (*Alphavirus*, *Flavivirus*, and *Pestivirus*).[1] Humans are the only known host.

Structure

The rubella virus is essentially spherical,[7] measuring 60 to 70 nm in diameter, with an electron-dense central nucleoid measuring 30 nm. This central nucleoid is contained within a 10-nm-thick, single-layered envelope acquired during the process of viral budding into cytoplasmic vesicles or through the plasma membrane. The envelope is lipoprotein in nature and being nonrigid gives rise to pleomorphic viral particles. Also, virus-specified polypeptides are found on viral surface projections that are 5 to 6 nm long.

The nucleic acid of wild rubella virus is a single positive-sense strand of RNA with a molecular mass of 3.2 to 3.8 $\times 10^6$ daltons, which is associated with arginine-rich protein.[8] DNA has not been detected in wild virus preparation; however, after growth in baby hamster kidney cells, viral variants that are recombinants between rubella and a latent retrovirus have been detected. These variants contain DNA, reverse transcriptase, and DNA-directed DNA polymerase. If this phenomenon occurs naturally, it could explain the possible persistence of rubella virus in some humans.

Biologic and Biochemical Properties

The virus is heat labile and has a half-life of 1 hour at 37°C.[6] Infectivity is lost within 2 minutes at 100°C, but Kistler and Sapatino[9] have noted that even after heating at 70°C for 60 minutes, some infectivity persists. In regard to colder temperatures, infectivity is rapidly lost during storage at −10°C to −20°C. However, in the presence of 2% albumin, infectivity is maintained for a week or more at 4°C and indefinitely at −60°C. Heat inactivation can be prevented through stabilization by the addition of magnesium sulfate to the viral suspension; protein stabilization allows survival of rapid freeze-thaw cycles.[1]

Infectivity is also lost at pH levels below 6.8 or above 8.1 and in the presence of ultraviolet light, lipid-active solvents, or other chemicals such as formalin, ethylene oxide, deoxycholate, proteolytic enzymes (trypsin), and β-propiolactone. Thimerosal will not inactivate the virus.[1]

In cell culture, rubella virus infectivity is inhibited by amantadine, yet the drug has not shown clinical efficacy.[10] Attenuated virus strains show decreased infectivity in some laboratory animals owing to the failure of attenuated virus to multiply at 39°C, the body temperature of rabbits.

Antigenic Characteristics

The rubella virion contains three major structural polypeptides, E1, E2 and C, whose molecular masses are 58, 42 to 47, and 33 kDa, respectively.[11–14] E1 and E2 are envelope glycoproteins, and they form the projections located on the viral membrane. The E1 glycoprotein has been shown to possess hemagglutinating activity (demonstrated by use of monoclonal antibodies), and both E1 and E2 have demonstrated viral neutralizing activity. E1 appears to be the more exposed of the two glycoproteins, with E2 being buried topologically under E1 on the virion surface.[11–14] The exact function of E2 is not clear, but it appears to play a role in the cell surface expression of E1.[11–14] Structural protein C, which is not glycosylated, is associated with the genomic RNA, and together they form the nucleocapsid.

Two precipitating antigens have been identified, designated theta and iota, and these are associated with the viral envelope and core, respectively. Natural infection with rubella virus leads to the formation of antibody against both of these precipitating antigens. Earlier vaccines led to antibody formation against the theta component only; the presently used vaccine (the RA 27/3 vaccine) produces a strong response against the theta component and a weak response to the iota component.[12–14]

The antigenic sites responsible for complement fixation and platelet aggregation have not yet been identified, although there now appears to be two distinct rubella complement-fixing antigens.

Culture Techniques

Rubella virus grows in a wide variety of primary cell cultures (such as human, simian, bovine, rabbit, canine, and duck) but does not produce a cytopathic effect.[15] Instead, the rubella virus is detected by its ability to produce interference to superinfection by a wide variety of viruses, with this effect being due to interferon production. The African green monkey kidney cell culture is the best suited and is the one most frequently used in clinical laboratories for isolation of the rubella virus by the interference technique.

When grown in continuous cell lines (hamster, rabbit, simian, human), rubella virus can lead to a wide variety of cytopathic effects. The continuous cell lines RK-13 (rabbit kidney line) and Vero (vervet kidney line) produce a good cytopathic effect uncomplicated by adventitious simian agents, provided that conditions are well controlled.[16] Because of the inability of the continuous cell lines BHK-21 and Vero to produce interferon, high titers of rubella virus are produced, and this allows the use of these cell lines for antigen production (to be used in serologic testing). Viral plaquing, which is the basis for the neutralization assays, can be performed with RK-13, BHK-21, SIRC (rabbit cornea), or Vero cells.[17]

Immune Responses to Rubella Virus

Immune Response to Acquired Infection

HUMORAL IMMUNE RESPONSE

Multiple antibody measurement techniques have been developed for use in rubella virus infections. The earliest two described were the neutralizing antibody in 1964[18] and the hemagglutination inhibition (HAI) test in 1967.[19] Both techniques can detect immunoglobulin (Ig) G at 2 to 3 days after onset of rash (approximately 2 weeks after becoming infected), peak within a month, and persist, although with decreasing titers, for years and possibly lifelong.[18, 19] The distinguishing feature of these two antibody measurement techniques is that they measure the inhibition of the infectivity of the rubella virus.[20] The neutralizing antibody test has the best correlation with protective immunity of all the available antibody measurement techniques, but the HAI test also correlates well.[20]

Because the neutralizing antibody and HAI tests are time-consuming, expensive, and difficult to perform, other techniques were developed. These include latex agglutination, immunofluorescence, radioimmunoassay, dot immunoassay, and enzyme immunoassay (EIA).[21] By these techniques, IgG typically becomes detectable within 5 to 15 days after rash onset, peaks at 15 to 30 days, and then gradually declines to a persistent titer. In most cases, there is persistence for life. In addition, passive hemagglutination can be used to measure IgG antibody.[22] However, the passive hemagglutination antibody is first detectable 15 to 20 days after rash onset and peaks by 200 days.[22] This is followed by persistence of antibody. Overall, IgG1 appears to be the predominant IgG subclass involved.[1]

Of all these techniques, the most commonly used in clinical laboratories are the EIAs because of their ease and low expense. However, IgG titers detected by these methods, compared with the neutralizing antibody and HAI tests, do not necessarily equate with protective immunity. High titers of IgG (by EIA and similar techniques) appear to indicate true protection, but it is well recognized that reinfection can occur in subjects with even moderate IgG levels but no antibody titer by either the neutralizing antibody or HAI test.[20, 23]

Rubella-specific IgM antibody response can also be measured by HAI, radioimmunoassay, immunofluorescence, or EIA.[24] IgM antibodies are detectable 5 to 10 days after the onset of rash, peak at 20 days, and then disappear within 50 to 70 days. In some subjects, low levels of IgM can persist longer, with up to 4 years being documented.

Complement fixation antibodies and precipitins are also detectable.[25, 26] Of the precipitins, the theta titer rises promptly, persists, and is seen after both natural infection and administration of any of the approved rubella vaccines. The iota titer rises slowly and is induced only by the RA 27/3 vaccine. The complement fixation and iota titers become detectable 10 days after onset of rash and slowly rise to a peak between 30 and 90 days out. The iota precipitins are present for only a few months.

IgA mediates the local nasopharyngeal immune response and appears within 10 days after infection. With natural infection, the IgA antibody persists for up to 1 year and at times longer.[27] On the contrary, after rubella vaccination, a lack of local nasopharyngeal IgA is usually seen,[28] except in cases in which the vaccine is administered intranasally. This method of administration is not done, however, because of a weaker systemic response. IgD and IgE antibodies become detectable within 6 to 9 days after infection; IgE peaks earlier than IgD, remains elevated for approximately 2 months, and then declines by 6 months.

CELLULAR IMMUNE RESPONSE

Cell-mediated immunity usually precedes humoral immunity by a week. Peak activity of cell-mediated immunity is concurrent with peak antibody responses and may persist for life. Cellular immune response to rubella virus can be measured by lymphocyte transformation response, levels of interferon and macrophage inhibitory factor, response of delayed hypersensitivity to skin testing, and release of lymphokines by lymphocytes.[29]

Proper T-cell function is needed to clear rubella virus appropriately. The E1 polypeptide appears to be the major antigenic source for T-cell response.[12–14] Several studies appear to indicate that the development of chronic arthritis after natural infection is secondary to altered T-cell recognition of the appropriate rubella virus antigens.[30–32] If there was a poor recognition, then the virus can possibly persist and lead to joint complications in this manner. If the recognition triggered a hyperimmune response, then the joint complications would be caused by an immune mechanism.

CURRENT AND FUTURE ADVANCES

Several studies have examined the efficacy of using either saliva or oral fluid to measure an immune response to rubella. Both IgA and IgG can be measured in these fluids, and results indicate good correlation with the standard serum EIA to determine the immune status of a subject.[33, 34]

There has been considerable work done in mapping the various potential antigenic sites on the rubella virus. On the basis of these results, synthetic peptides can be developed that simulate the antigenic sites. These synthetic peptides may potentially be used to develop vaccines with lower complication rates than of the one presently used and could be used to create antigens for EIAs.[12–14]

In addition, polymerase chain reaction techniques have been studied in the diagnosis of congenital rubella infection in utero. By this method, viral RNA has been detected in specimens of chorionic villus specimens from infected infants as early as 15 weeks of gestation.[35]

Immune Response to Congenital Infection

HUMORAL IMMUNE RESPONSE

Transplacental maternal antibody transfer is poor during the first half of gestation, and the fetal humoral immune response is also minimal during this time. Thus, measurements of either IgG or IgM levels in fetal blood samples before 16 weeks of gestation are difficult to determine.[35] As the pregnancy progresses, IgG is transferred to the child and IgM is produced by the fetal immune system. At birth, presence of an IgM level in an infant indicates (with high probability, assuming minimal blood exchange at birth) an intrauterine rubella infection.[23]

There are several complications of the humoral immune system related to congenital rubella infection. Hypogammaglobulinemia can occur, with only IgA being affected typically. Also, there is a persistence of rubella-specific IgM, with the mechanism for this not being clear. The IgM levels remain elevated in 60% of infants during the first 4 months of life and in 40% of infected infants aged 8 to 12 months. When measured by sensitive serologic tests, such as radioimmunoassay and immunofluorescence, IgM levels may persist beyond 1 year of life.[36, 37] Last, there is a slow maturation of IgG1 avidity. After an acquired rubella infection, the IgG1 antibody initially has a low avidity or functional affinity.[37] However, this quickly changes to high-avidity rubella-specific IgG1 antibody production. After congenital infection, the avidity of the IgG1 antibodies remains low for a prolonged time; up to 40% of congenitally infected infants in one study still produced low-avidity IgG1 antibodies 3 years after birth. The investigators of this one study have proposed that low-avidity IgG1 antibody levels be used as a test for confirmation of a congenital rubella infection because of their persistence.[37, 38]

CELLULAR IMMUNE RESPONSE

The cellular immune response in congenitally infected children may also be impaired. Studies have shown selective tolerance to the E1 protein of the rubella virus, leading to inadequate T-cell response and persistence of live virus. This persistence of a low level of active infection leads to the development of the delayed manifestations seen in congenitally infected infants. The etiology of this selective tolerance is not clear.[12]

Conclusions

Patients with congenital rubella infection are an immunologic paradox. They have high levels of rubella-specific IgG and persistence of high levels of rubella-specific IgM and yet present with complications indicative of persistent active infection. The slow maturation of the avidity of the IgG1 subclass, the major IgG subclass in rubella infections, and the selective tolerance of T cells to the E1 antigen most likely explain this situation.

References

1. Cherry JD: Rubella. *In* Feigin RD, Cherry JD (eds): Textbook of Pediatric Infectious Diseases, ed 3. Philadelphia, WB Saunders, 1992, pp 1792–1817.
2. Manton WG: Some accounts of rash liable to be mistaken for scarlatina. Med Trans R Coll Physicians (Lond) 5:149, 1815.
3. Veale H: History of epidemic Rotheln, with observations on its pathology. Edinb Med J 12:404, 1866.
4. Gregg NM: Congenital cataracts following German measles in the mother. Trans Ophthalmol Soc Aust 3:35, 1941.
5. Weller TH, Neva FA: Propagation in tissue culture of cytopathic agents from patients with rubella-like illness. Proc Soc Exp Biol Med 111:225, 1962.
6. Parkman PD, Buescher EL, Artenstein MS, et al: Studies of rubella. I. Properties of the virus. J Immunol 93:595, 1964.
7. Oshiro JS, Schmidt MJ, Lennette EH: Electron microscopic studies of rubella virus. J Gen Virol 5:205, 1969.
8. Bardeletti G, Kessler N, Aymard-Henry M: Morphology, biochemical analysis and neuraminidase activity of rubella virus. Arch Virol 49:175, 1975.
9. Kistler GS, Sapatino V: Temperature- and UV-light resistance of rubella virus infectivity. Arch Ges Virusforsch 38:11, 1972.
10. Gershon A: Rubella virus (German measles). *In* Mandell G, Bennett J, Dolin R (eds): Principles and Practice of Infectious Diseases, ed 4. New York, Churchill Livingstone, 1995, pp 1242–1247.
11. Bowden DS, Westway EG: Rubella virus: Structural and nonstructural proteins. J Gen Virol 65:933, 1984.
12. Mauracher CA, Mitchell LA, Tingle AJ: Selective tolerance to the E1 protein of rubella virus in congenital rubella syndrome. J Immunol 151:2041, 1993.
13. Chaye H, Ou D, Chong P, et al: Human T- and B-cell epitopes of E1 glycoprotein of rubella virus. J Clin Immunol 13:93, 1993.
14. Ou D, Chong P, Tingle AJ: Mapping T-cell epitopes of rubella virus structural proteins E1, E2, and C recognized by T-cell lines

and clones derived from infected and immunized populations. J Med Virol 40:175, 1993.
15. Parkman PD, Buescher EL, Artenstein MS: Recovery of rubella virus from army recruits. Proc Soc Exp Biol Med 111:225, 1962.
16. McCarthy K, Taylor-Robinson CH: Rubella. Br Med Bull 23:185, 1967.
17. Hermann KL: Rubella virus. *In* Lennette EH, Schmidt NJ (eds): Diagnostic Procedures for Viral, Rickettsial and Chlamydial Infections. Washington, DC, American Public Health Association, 1979, p 725.
18. Parkman PD, Mundon FK, McCown JM, et al: Studies of rubella. II. Neutralization of the virus. J Immunol 93:608, 1964.
19. Stewart GL, Parkman PD, Hopps HE, et al: Rubella virus hemagglutination inhibition test. N Engl J Med 276:554, 1967.
20. Zrein M, Joncas JH, Pedneault L, et al: Comparison of a whole-virus enzyme immunoassay (EIA) with a peptide-based EIA for detecting rubella virus immunoglobulin G antibodies following rubella vaccination. J Clin Microbiol 31:1521, 1993.
21. Hermann KL: Available rubella serologic tests. Rev Infect Dis 7(Suppl 1):S108, 1985.
22. Hauknes G: Experience with an indirect (passive) hemagglutination test for the demonstration of rubella virus antibody. Acta Pathol Microbiol Scand 88:85, 1980.
23. The American College of Obstetricians and Gynecologists (ACOG): Rubella and pregnancy: ACOG technical bulletin number 171—August 1992. Int J Gynecol Obstet 42:60, 1993.
24. Cubie H, Edmond E: Comparison of five different methods of rubella IgM antibody testing. J Clin Pathol 38:203, 1985.
25. Sever JL, Huebner RJ, Castellano GA, et al: Rubella complement fixation test. Science 148:385, 1965.
26. Cappel R, Schluederberg A, Horstmann DM: Large-scale production of rubella precipitinogens and their use in the diagnostic laboratory. J Clin Microbiol 1:201, 1975.
27. Salonen EM, Hove T, Meurman O, et al: Kinetics of specific IgA, IgD, IgE, IgG, and IgM antibody responses in rubella. J Med Virol 16:1, 1985.
28. Saule H, Enders G, Zeller J, et al: Congenital rubella infection after previous immunity of the mother. Eur J Pediatr 147:195, 1988.
29. Buimovici-Klein E, Cooper LZ: Cell-mediated immune response to rubella infections. Rev Infect Dis 7(Suppl 1):S123, 1985.
30. Ueno Y: Rubella arthritis. An outbreak in Kyoto. J Rheumatol 21:874, 1994.
31. Mitchell LA, Decarie D, Shukin R, et al: Cellular hyperimmunoreactivity to rubella virus synthetic peptides in chronic rubella associated arthritis. Ann Rheum Dis 52:590, 1993.
32. Mitchell LA, Tingle AJ, Shukin R, et al: Chronic rubella vaccine–associated arthropathy. Arch Intern Med 153:2268, 1993.
33. Thieme T, Piacentini S, Davidson S, et al: Determination of measles, mumps, and rubella immunization status using oral fluid samples. JAMA 272:219, 1994.
34. Perry KR, Brown DWG, Parry JV, et al: Detection of measles, mumps, and rubella antibodies in saliva using antibody capture radioimmunoassay. J Med Virol 40:235, 1993.
35. Valente P, Sever JL: In utero diagnosis of congenital infections by direct fetal sampling. Israel J Med Sci 30:416, 1994.
36. Cooper LZ: Congenital rubella in the United States. *In* Krugman S, Gershon AA (eds): Infections of the Fetus and Newborn Infant: Progress in Clinical and Biological Research, Vol 3. New York, Alan R Liss, 1975, pp 1–22.
37. Thomas HIJ, Morgan-Capner P, Cradock-Watson JE, et al: Slow maturation of IgG1 avidity and persistence of specific IgM in congenital rubella: Implications for diagnosis and immunopathology. J Med Virol 41:196, 1993.
38. Williams LL, Shannon BT, Leguire LE, et al: Persistently altered T cell immunity in high school students with the congenital rubella syndrome and profound hearing loss. Pediatr Infect Dis J 12:831, 1993.

266

Yellow Fever Virus

Theodore F. Tsai

History

Yellow fever epidemics of major proportions plagued Europe and America in the 18th and 19th centuries. Outbreaks in the United States spread in a saltatory pattern from sailing ships originating in the West Indies to coastal and river port cities, reaching as far north as Boston and St. Louis. Frequently these epidemics were associated with attack rates of 33% and mortality rates of 10%. The last yellow fever outbreaks in the United States occurred in 1905 in the Mississippi delta. The mosquito-borne transmission of yellow fever, championed by Carlos Finlay, was proved in 1900 by a U.S. Army commission led by Walter Reed. This understanding made it possible to prevent the disease through the control of vector mosquitoes, although the viral origin of the disease was not proved until 1928.[1, 2]

Characteristics of the Pathogen

Yellow fever virus is the type species of RNA viruses in the family Flaviviridae. Hepatitis C virus, although classified in the Flaviviridae because of its similar genomic organization, is antigenically distinct from the arthropod-borne flaviviruses. Virions are enveloped and spherical, with a diameter of approximately 40 nm. The lipid bilayer envelope contains a matrix (M) protein and the envelope (E) protein, which is variably glycosylated. The genome, a single segment of positive-sense RNA, is bound into a nucleocapsid with a basic capsid (C) protein. Virions enter host cells by receptor-mediated endocytosis. Viral RNA synthesis occurs in the cytoplasm, and protein synthesis proceeds in an extensively proliferated endoplasmic reticulum. Virions mature within the endoplasmic reticulum and are released through the plasma membrane by exocytotic fusion.

The 11-kb viral genome has a single open reading frame of 10,233 nucleotides. The polyprotein product is cleaved during and after translation into the three structural proteins (C, M, and E) and several nonstructural proteins (NS1, NS2a, NS2b, NS3, NS4a, NS4b, and NS5). NS1, a glycosylated protein found on the cell surface is involved in viral assembly and release and induces protective antibodies. NS5 is believed to be the viral RNA polymerase. Other nonstructural proteins have cleavage (NS2b and NS3) and replicative functions such as protease, nucleotide triphosphatase, and helicase activity.[3, 4]

The E protein (53 to 54 kDa) has a major role in virion attachment to host cells, hemagglutination, and virus neutralization. Changes in the protein are associated with virulence and attenuation. Crystallographic studies have disclosed rodlike E homodimers lying horizontally on the viral surface. The third of three distinct domains on the protein is an immunoglobulin-like domain containing an RGD sequence motif recognized by integrins.[5] The consensus complete nucleotide sequence of yellow fever 17D vaccine strains differs from the wild-type Asibi virus in 48 nucleotides scattered throughout the genome, leading to substitutions of 22 amino acids.[6] Phenotypic attributes associated with these changes are now amenable to study in viruses generated with infectious complementary DNA.

Yellow fever virus is antigenically related to several African flaviviruses, including Uganda S, Bouboui, Wesselsbron, Banzi, and Zika viruses. Molecular taxonomic studies of the complete E protein gene sequence have differentiated yellow fever strains into three topotypes representing East and West Africa and the New World. Western Hemisphere and West African strains are closely related, suggesting that yellow fever virus may have been introduced to the New World by trading ships from Africa. Biologic differences among the three topotypes, such as immunity provided by existing vaccines, have not been shown.

Epidemiology

Yellow fever occurs in tropical America and in Africa in endemic zones bounded approximately by 15 degrees north latitude and 15 degrees south latitude (Fig. 266–1). Epidemic (urban) yellow fever is transmitted in an interhuman cycle by *Aedes aegypti* mosquitoes. After feeding on viremic humans, infected mosquitoes may transmit infections to other hosts for 1 to 2 weeks.

Only the sylvatic cycle of transmission, involving forest mosquitoes and monkeys, currently occurs in South America. Most cases are in men who work in forested areas. Sporadic cases and outbreaks occur principally during the late rainy season (January to May), when vector *Haemagogus* mosquitoes are most abundant. No urban *A. aegypti*–borne transmission of yellow fever has occurred in the Western Hemisphere since 1954. But the reentrenchment of *A. aegypti* in urban and rural locations, overlapping areas with sylvatic transmission, has increased the risk of epidemic urban transmission, especially in coastal cities with nonimmunized populations.[7]

Enzootic transmission occurs in the high forests of West and Central Africa with the occurrence of sporadic human cases. In the transition zone of forest to savanna and in the moist savanna, recurrent viral activity each rainy season leads to a high level of enzootic and endemic transmission among monkeys and humans, and periodically to outbreaks. Cases originating in these emergence areas may spread to the dry savanna and to urban areas where there is a risk for interhuman *A. aegypti*–borne epidemic transmission. The first such urban outbreak in Africa in 40 years was reported from western Nigeria in 1987. A yellow fever outbreak in Kenya in 1992 illustrates the emergence of the infection from a previously silent focus in East Africa.[8, 9]

Yellow fever is significantly underreported in both Africa and South America. In most instances only fatal cases are recognized, and officially reported cases may represent only 1% of true morbidity. Outbreaks in Nigeria in 1987 may have produced as many as 120,000 cases and 25,000 deaths.

Resistance to acquiring yellow fever may be associated with cross-immunity to dengue fever virus and other flaviviruses. This cross-reactive immunity may explain the absence of yellow fever in Asia. Genetic factors as well may be associated with host resistance.

Clinical Features

Classic yellow fever is a biphasic illness progressing through three stages—infection, remission, and intoxication. Infection

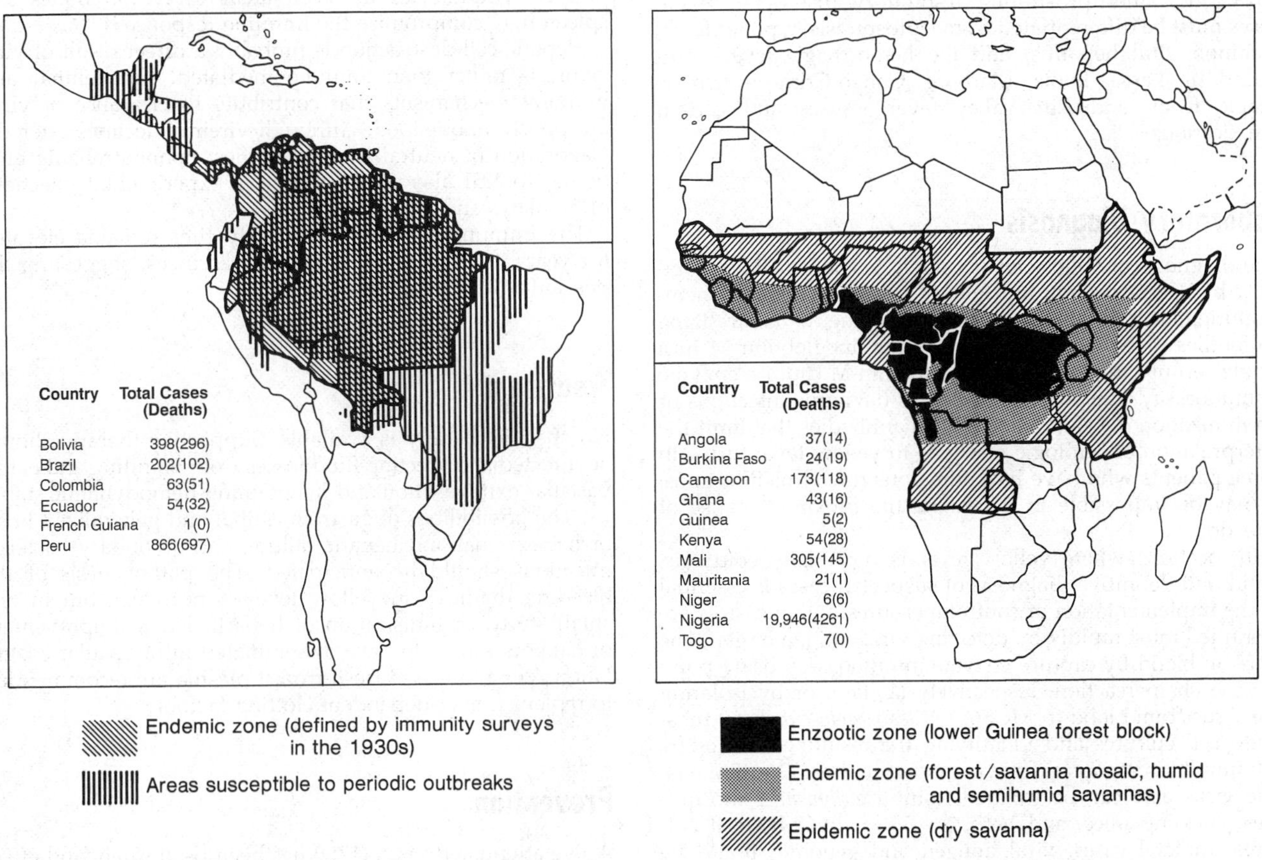

Country Total Cases (Deaths)
Bolivia 398(296)
Brazil 202(102)
Colombia 63(51)
Ecuador 54(32)
French Guiana 1(0)
Peru 866(697)
Country Total Cases (Deaths)
Angola 37(14)
Burkina Faso 24(19)
Cameroon 173(118)
Ghana 43(16)
Guinea 5(2)
Kenya 54(28)
Mali 305(145)
Mauritania 21(1)
Niger 6(6)
Nigeria 19,946(4261)
Togo 7(0)
Endemic zone (defined by immunity surveys in the 1930s)
Areas susceptible to periodic outbreaks
Enzootic zone (lower Guinea forest block)
Endemic zone (forest/savanna mosaic, humid and semihumid savannas)
Epidemic zone (dry savanna)

FIGURE 266–1 □ Geoecologic distribution of yellow fever, and reported cases, 1980 to 1990.

may result in subclinical infection, self-limited influenza, or fulminating illness that leads to death within days. After an incubation period of 3 to 6 days, abrupt onset of fever and chills is followed rapidly by headache, backache, generalized myalgias, nausea, and vomiting. Few physical signs are present other than flushing of the face and conjunctivae and Faget sign, a relative bradycardia. After 3 to 4 days, symptoms and fever remit for a period of hours to 1 or 2 days, only to recur and intensify during the period of intoxication. Jaundice, the clinical sign for which the disease is named, evidence of renal dysfunction, and a hemorrhagic diathesis develop in varying degrees. Mucosal bleeding and gastrointestinal hemorrhage, the black vomit mentioned in early descriptions of the disease, originate from reduced hepatic synthesis of clotting factors and disseminated intravascular coagulation. Oliguria and azotemia reflect fluid loss through vomiting, extravascular extravasation, and possibly primary glomerular and interstitial nephritis. Acute tubular necrosis may follow as a late event associated with hypotension. Myocarditis may lead to cardiac dysfunction and arrhythmias. Signs and symptoms of encephalopathy may be associated with hepatic and renal failure, and in rare cases with central nervous system infection. Secondary bacterial infections may complicate the course of illness. The overall case-fatality rate is 5% to 10%, but 20% to 50% of patients entering the stage of intoxication may die.

Clinical laboratory abnormalities include leukopenia, albuminuria, prolonged prothrombin time, and elevations in serum transaminase and indirect and direct bilirubin values. Early and marked transaminase and bilirubin elevations signal a poor outcome. Mild chemical disturbances in liver function may be present in anicteric cases. Thrombocytopenia and other signs of consumptive coagulopathy are present in some cases. Hepatic damage may lead to hypoglycemia.

The differential diagnosis includes malaria, dengue, influenza, and other prostrating respiratory disorders. Severe cases must be differentiated from leptospirosis, typhoid fever, common viral hepatitis, and the hemorrhagic fevers produced by Lassa, Ebola, Marburg, Congo-Crimean hemorrhagic fever, and Rift Valley fever viruses and certain intoxications.[10, 11]

Laboratory Diagnosis

The diagnosis of yellow fever usually is confirmed serologically by demonstrating fourfold or greater increases in hemagglutination inhibition, complement fixing, or neutralizing antibodies or by detecting specific immunoglobulin M in a single serum sample by immunoglobulin M capture enzyme immunoassay. Patients with previous flavivirus infections or immunization develop heterologous antibodies that limit the interpretation of serologic reactions to yellow fever virus. In some patients who have had numerous flavivirus infections, it may be impossible to determine the proximate cause of infection.

In locations where yellow fever is potentially epidemic, rapid and definitive diagnosis of suspected cases is essential to the implementation of control measures. Viremic cases are identified most rapidly by detecting viral antigen or genomic RNA in blood by capture enzyme immunoassay or by polymerase chain reaction, respectively (1 day), or by isolating the virus from blood in MOS61 *(Aedes pseudoscutellaris)* mosquito cell cultures and identifying the resulting isolates by immunofluorescence or enzyme immunoassay (3 to 5 days). The virus also can be isolated from *Toxorhynchites* mosquitoes, suckling mice, and Vero, C6/36, or $LLCMK_2$ cell cultures. In fatal cases, viral antigen and genome should be sought in liver tissue by immunohistochemical staining or in situ hybridization, respectively. Ordinary histopathologic examination of viscerotomy samples is a widely used approach to surveillance, but it is contraindicated for critically ill patients; moreover, other toxic and infectious agents, especially other hemorrhagic fever viruses, can produce similar pathologic patterns.[12, 13]

Pathology and Pathophysiology

The initial replicative sites probably are reticuloendothelial cells of local lymph nodes, bone marrow, spleen, and Kupffer cells. Virions disseminate hematogenously to multiple sites during the early period of infection. The principal pathologic finding is a patchy, primarily midzonal eosinophilic necrosis of hepatocytes with minimal inflammatory or proliferative responses. Hepatocytes surrounding the central vein and portal areas are spared to a greater degree and the reticular architecture is largely preserved. Hepatocytes undergo an acidophilic degeneration progressing from a cloudy appearance to progressive shrinkage of the cytoplasm and formation of Councilman bodies. Accumulation of ceroid pigment and microvesicular fat is prominent. Torres bodies, intranuclear inclusions, are found occasionally. Viral antigen is found in hepatocytes and within Councilman bodies. Only nonspecific changes of hepatitis are found after the acute stages of illness. Complete resolution is the rule, but chronic active hepatitis was reported in one case. The kidneys are enlarged and edematous. Glomeruli may show mesangial proliferation and capillary endothelial swelling. The interstitium is edematous; tubular epithelial cells are swollen and may contain viral antigen. Degeneration and necrosis of the myocardium and lesions in the conduction system may be present. Viral antigen can be detected in occasional myocardial fibers. Depletion of lymphocytes in B-cell areas of lymph nodes and spleen may compromise the immune response.[14, 15]

Hepatic cell destruction is probably a direct result of viral cytolysis rather than immune mediated. The cellular and humoral mechanisms that contribute to clearance of virus are poorly understood. Although viremia declines after the elaboration of neutralizing antibodies, nonneutralizing antibodies to NS1 also are protective in experimental infections of monkeys and mice.

The immunoglobulin M antibody titer remains elevated for years in some patients and in vaccinees, suggesting the possibility of viral persistence.

Treatment

No specific therapy is available. Supportive therapy should be directed at correcting fluid losses from vomiting and extravascular extravasation and maintaining hemodynamic stability. The possibilities of gastrointestinal and generalized hemorrhages, renal and hepatic failure, and secondary bacterial infections should be anticipated. The pathogenesis of the bleeding diathesis in yellow fever is not clear, but in one small study, administration of heparin led to improvement of patients shown to have disseminated intravascular coagulation. Vitamin K and fresh-frozen plasma are recommended to replenish liver-dependent clotting factors.[15]

Prevention

A live attenuated virus (17D) has been used safely and effectively as a vaccine for 50 years. The strain was derived from a human isolate (Asibi) and was attenuated by serial passages in mouse and chick embryo cells.[16, 17] Vaccine-related adverse events are generally mild and occur in less than 5% of vaccinees. A residual neurotropic potential is seen in an age-related encephalitis that occurs exclusively in children, especially infants younger than 4 months. Eighteen cases, one fatal, have been reported. The vaccine is contraindicated for infants younger than 4 months. Immunization of children aged 4 to 6 months is recommended only if they cannot avoid epidemic areas. After age 6 months, infants may be immunized if they reside in rural areas of endemic zones. Immunization should be deferred until age 9 to 12 months for residents of urban areas. Congenital infection without malformation was demonstrated in one case after inadvertent immunization during the first trimester of pregnancy. The protection afforded by immunization to mildly immunosuppressed persons, to asymptomatic human immunodeficiency virus–seropositive persons, and to pregnant women may outweigh the risks of the vaccine if the potential for exposure to yellow fever is judged to be high. Immunogenicity and safety of yellow fever vaccine were shown in human immunodeficiency virus–infected adults with $CD4^+$ cell counts greater than 200/mm^3. However, infants with human immunodeficiency virus infection without acquired immunodeficiency syndrome have responded poorly to the vaccine when it was given at 1 year of age. When important, antibody responses to vaccination should be determined in persons with human immunodeficiency virus infection or other immunosuppressive conditions.

A single 0.5-mL subcutaneous dose confers long-lasting immunity after 7 to 10 days. Measurable neutralizing antibody may persist for more than 40 years, but reimmunization at 10-year intervals is required for international travelers. Yellow fever vaccine can be given concurrently with immune serum globulin, chloroquine, and other vaccines such as hepatitis B vaccine and intramuscular typhoid polysaccharide vaccine. Coadministration of the last may have an adjuvant effect. Cholera vaccine may interfere with the immune response if it is given within 3 weeks of yellow fever immunization. The current chick embryo–derived vaccine may be allergenic to persons allergic to eggs. Diluted intradermal test doses have been immunogenic in some cases. Candidate vaccine virus generated from infectious complementary DNA has been tested for safety and immunogenicity with promising results.[18]

Protective measures against mosquito bites, such as application of repellents to skin and clothing and the use of bed netting, are well advised.

References

1. Duffy J: Yellow fever in the continental United States during the nineteenth century. Bull N Y Acad Med 44:687, 1968.
2. Smith HH, Downs WG: Historical perspectives on yellow fever vector research. Curr Top Vector Res 1:1, 1983.
3. Chambers TJ, Hahn CS, Galler R, Rice CM. Flavivirus genome organization, expression and replication. Annu Rev Microbiol 44:649, 1990.
4. Monath TP, Heinz FX: Flaviviruses. *In* Fields BN, Knipe DM, Howley PM (eds): Fields Virology, ed 3. Philadelphia, Lippincott-Raven, 1996, pp 961–1034.
5. Rey FA, Heinz FX, Mandl C, et al: The envelope glycoprotein from tick-borne encephalitis virus at 2 Å resolution. Nature 375:291, 1995.
6. dos Santos CN, Post PR, Carvalho R, et al: Complete nucleotide sequence of yellow fever virus vaccine strains 17DD and 17D-213. Virus Res 35:35, 1995.
7. Monath TP: Yellow fever and dengue—The interactions of virus, vector and host in the re-emergence of epidemic disease. Semin Virol 5:133, 1994.
8. Chang GJ, Cropp BC, Kinney RM, et al: Nucleotide sequence variation of the envelope protein gene identifies two distinct genotypes of yellow fever virus. J Virol 69:5773, 1995.
9. Nasidi A, Monath TP, DeCock K, et al: Urban yellow fever epidemic in western Nigeria, 1987. Trans Soc Trop Med Hyg 83:401, 1989.
10. Kerr JA: The clinical aspects and diagnosis of yellow fever. *In* Strode GK (ed): Yellow Fever. New York, McGraw-Hill, 1951, p 385.
11. Monath TP: Yellow fever: A medically neglected disease. Report on a seminar. Rev Infect Dis 9:165, 1987.
12. Bres PLJ: A century of progress in combating yellow fever. Bull WHO 64:775, 1986.
13. Monath TP: Yellow fever. *In* Monath TP (ed): Arboviruses: Epidemiology and Ecology. Boca Raton, FL, CRC Press, 1989, pp 139–231.
14. Francis TI, Moore DL, Edington GM, Smith JA: A clinicopathological study of human yellow fever. Bull WHO 46:659, 1972.
15. deBrito T, Sigueira SAC, Santos RTM, et al: Human fatal yellow fever—Immunohistochemical detection of viral antigens in the liver, kidney and heart. Pathol Res Pract 188:177, 1992.
16. 1990—Yellow fever vaccine. Recommendations of the Immunization Practices Advisory Committee (ACIP). MMWR Morbid Mortal Wkly Rep 39(RR-6): 1, 1990.
17. Freestone DS: Yellow fever vaccine. *In* Plotkin SA, Mortimer EA (eds): Vaccines, ed 2. Philadelphia, WB Saunders, 1994, pp 741–779.
18. Marchevsky RS, Mariano J, Ferreira VS, et al: Phenotypic analysis of yellow fever virus derived from complementary DNA. Am J Trop Med Hyg 52:75, 1995.

267

Dengue Viruses

Scott B. Halstead

History

The dengue syndrome is an acute febrile viral exanthem accompanied by headache, myalgia, anorexia, gastrointestinal disturbances, and prostration caused by viruses transmitted by mosquitoes. Outbreaks of febrile exanthems were reported widely before the agents were identified, and serologic tests were available during the period of European colonization. Classic dengue fever was first described by Benjamin Rush, who treated cases during the 1780 outbreak in Philadelphia. An earlier account of a dengue-like disease in Batavia (Jakarta, Indonesia) by David Bylon was probably caused by chikungunya, a togavirus also transmitted by the bite of *Aedes aegypti*.[1] Four serotypes are known: Dengue types 1 and 2 were isolated during World War II by Japanese and U.S. workers.[2] Types 3 and 4 were recovered in the Philippines in 1956.[3] Dengue syndromes caused by dengue viruses and those caused by chikungunya, o'nyong-nyong, and West Nile viruses, although often temporarily incapacitating, were generally known to have a good prognosis. This view changed in Manila in 1956, with the recognition of the dengue hemorrhagic fever–dengue shock syndrome (DHF-DSS). Since that time, more than 3 million children have been hospitalized and 57,000 have died with this syndrome, principally in tropical Asia, and more recently in Caribbean and South American countries.

Characteristics of the Pathogen

The four dengue viruses are single-stranded, enveloped positive-sense RNA viruses of the family of Flaviviridae (type species, yellow fever virus). The family is composed of 54 serologically related viruses.[4, 5] Flaviviruses are spherical, 35- to 45-nm virions consisting of a nucleocapsid core approximately 30 nm in diameter surrounded by a lipoprotein envelope. The envelope, studded with poorly resolved projections, is composed of many replicates of the E protein (54 kDa) embedded in a lipid bilayer. When assembled on the virion, the E protein bears epitopes that are specific to the virus serotype. Presumably these serve as sites for viral attachment to and transport through host cell plasma membranes. Other epitopes are shared between dengue viruses (dengue subgroup antigens) or nondengue flaviviruses (group antigens). Although the functional significance of these conformational sites is not known, neutralization can be achieved only when antibody attaches to several discontinuous segments of the E protein.[6]

Complete gene sequences are known for dengue virus types 1, 2, 3, and 4, and complete or partial sequences are known for several dengue virus 1 through 4 strains that have distinctive geographic or temporal origin or biologic properties.[7, 8] Flavivirus genomes are 11 kb long and contain a single, long open reading frame with short nontranslated portions at the 3′ and 5′ ends. The gene is translated as a single polyprotein with structural proteins at the 5′ end. Once in cytosol, like other RNA viruses, dengue virus uses cellular cytoplasmic ribosomes to produce proteins that, together with positive RNA copies, are assembled into complete virions in cytoplasmic vacuoles. Virions are exfoliated by reverse pinocytosis.

Dengue viruses have a narrow biologic range in vivo. Viremia follows subcutaneous inoculation only in primate species. Virus replication in primates appears to be restricted to cells of mononuclear phagocyte lineage.[9] In vitro, dengue viruses replicate in a wide range of cell culture types of vertebrate and invertebrate origin. In addition, dengue viruses of all four types can be selected for their ability to replicate in central nervous system tissue of laboratory animals, such as mice, rats, and hamsters. Passage in mice and in some tissue cultures (e.g., primary dog kidney) places selective pressure on dengue viruses that reduces their ability to produce viremia in monkeys or clinical disease in humans. Antibodies directed at any virion epitope, when present at subneutralizing concentrations and when incubated with dengue viruses in the presence of primate monocytes, result in enhanced infection,[10, 11] a phenomenon called antibody-dependent enhancement.

Antigenic subtypes of dengue types 3 and 4 virus have been discovered. Dengue type 3 viruses recovered in the Caribbean in 1963 and in Tahiti in 1969 differ from prototype dengue type 3 viruses and recent isolates from Southeast Asia. Antibody raised to the subtype poorly neutralizes Southeast Asian dengue type 3 virus strains.[12] A similar but reverse serologic relationship was observed with a dengue type 4 virus strain isolated in the Caribbean in 1981.[13] Nucleotide sequence data reveal geographic homologies (genotypes) among dengue viruses. Currently, two genotypes have been described for dengue virus strain 1, five for dengue 2, four for dengue 3, and two for dengue 4.[8, 14] Viruses recovered from a region at an interval of 20 years show greater homology than strains of the same serotype recovered concurrently from different regions.[8]

Epidemiology

Dengue viruses are transmitted by mosquitoes of the day-time-biting Stegomyia family, principally *A. aegypti.* In most tropical areas, *A. aegypti* is highly urbanized, breeding in water stored for drinking or bathing or in rainwater collected in manufactured or natural containers. In Southeast Asia, there is a jungle cycle with high rates of dengue virus transmission among several species of monkeys. In Malaysia, dengue virus may be maintained in a cycle involving *Aedes nivius,* which feed on both monkeys and humans.[15] In suburban and rural areas, limited transmission from person to person may be sustained by *Aedes albopictus.* Outbreaks attributed solely to *A. albopictus* occurred in Japan during World War II and more recently on the Seychelles.[16] In general, this species is not sufficiently anthropophilic to serve as an efficient epidemic vector, as evidenced by the absence of dengue transmission in areas where *A. albopictus* is widely distributed, including China, Japan, Korea, Taiwan, the Hawaiian islands, and 25 states of the United States.[17] Dengue viruses are introduced often in these areas by viremic tourists, who acquire infections on visits to tropical countries.

Currently, *A. aegypti* is almost universally distributed in the tropics between 30 degrees north and 20 degrees south latitude, an area in which nearly half of the world's population live.[18] Dengue viruses have spread throughout this range. Most transmission occurs at altitudes below 2000 feet and during the rainy season. Frosts or sustained cold weather destroys adult mosquitoes and interrupts transmission. *A. aegypti* has a short flight range, and the dispersal of dengue viruses is almost entirely due to the movement of viremic human beings.[19] Under epidemic conditions, dengue usually spreads along major transportation arteries. Typically, it exhibits the epidemiologic features of a respiratory tract disease. An infected index case introduces virus into a household infested with *A. aegypti* and, after the combined extrinsic (mosquito) and intrinsic (host) incubation periods, secondary cases occur. As a result, dengue transmission is intense in crowded, urban areas. In some countries, middle- and upper-income housing provides more mosquito-breeding sites than does that of the urban poor.

Nonimmune populations support outbreaks of classic dengue fever. In certain areas where multiple dengue types are endemic, outbreaks of DHF are common. Between 250,000 and 500,000 DHF-DSS cases occur throughout the world annually; the case-fatality rate is 1% to 5%. Countries principally involved are China (Hainan), the Philippines, Vietnam, Laos, Cambodia, Thailand, Malaysia, Indonesia, Myanmar, India, and Sri Lanka. In 1981, Cuba experienced a sharp DHF outbreak: 116,143 persons were hospitalized in a 3-month period, including 10,000 for shock.[20] After an absence of dengue virus transmission for 40 years, dengue 1 was introduced in 1977 and dengue 2 in 1981. There is some evidence to suggest that the responsible dengue 2 strain was imported from Southeast Asia.[8, 14, 21] Subsequent to the outbreak in Cuba, Venezuela, Colombia, and Brazil have experienced DHF-DSS outbreaks caused by the same sequence of dengue viruses. An important observation in the Cuban outbreak was that black children, although exposed to dengue virus 1 and 2 infections at the same or greater rates than whites, experienced DHF-DSS only one fifth to one tenth as often.[22] This implies that during secondary dengue virus infection severity of human disease is under host genetic control. Human dengue virus infections in Africa have been unusually mild.[23] Dengue viruses of multiple serotypes have circulated in Bangladesh, India, and Sri Lanka, where DHF-DSS occurred only sporadically until 1988.[24] Since then, sharp outbreaks of DHF-DSS in New Delhi and in Sri Lanka suggest that viral strain differences are responsible for clinically overt versus clinically silent areas.

Pathogenesis

Retrospective and prospective epidemiologic data show that DHF-DSS occurs in two immunologic settings: infections in infants born to dengue-immune mothers and second infections in children older than 1 year.[25] In the latter category, infection sequences most frequently associated with DHF-DSS are dengue virus types 1, 2; 3, 2; 4, 2, and some or all secondary infection sequences end with type 3.[26, 27] Secondary dengue 3 infections are known to be pathogenic. The severity of secondary dengue virus type 1 and 4 infections is not well studied. The circulation of infection-enhancing antibody, passively or actively acquired, is the pathogenetic mechanism common to seemingly unrelated immunologic settings.[28, 29] If the same serum contains antibody that neutralizes infecting virus even at low dilutions, DHF does not occur. Persons who have experienced two different dengue virus infections or more are not at risk for DHF-DSS during third or fourth infections, presumably because of down-modulation of infection by low-level cross-reactive neutralizing antibodies.

In monkeys, and from limited experimental and autopsy studies of human cases, it appears that dengue viruses replicate in dermal histiocytes at locations where virus has been injected.[30, 31] Virus spreads to macrophages in draining lymph nodes, then to macrophages in the spleen, Kupffer cells in the liver, bone marrow mononuclear cells, blood monocytes, and finally mononuclear phagocytes throughout the skin.[30] Antibody-dependent enhancement increases the number of infected cells and might drive virus into cells that are not normally involved. The late and sudden appearance of increased vascular permeability suggests that early interactions between elements of the immune response and dengue virus–infected mononuclear phagocytes result in activation of complement and release of monokines (Fig. 267–1). Although human cytotoxic and helper T lymphocytes exhibiting specificity for dengue viral antigens have been detected and lymphokines released using dengue virus–infected monocytes as targets,[32, 33] the cytokines that produce dengue shock remain to be identified; interferon-γ and interleukin-2 do appear to play a role in this process.

Host factors such as ethnicity, age, and sex influence the severity of dengue illness, but virus factors also contribute.[9, 34] For example, in the American tropics dengue 2 viruses associated with secondary infection DHF-DSS are always of recent Southeast Asian origin and not of the American genotype.[14] Infection-enhancing and -neutralizing antibodies modulate the severity of infection upward or downward. Antibody specificities are presumably determined by antigen presentation and are thus under control of the viral genome.[34] It is also possible that quantitative aspects of human antibody responses determine that in one individual enhancing antibodies (low responses) circulate, whereas in another protec-

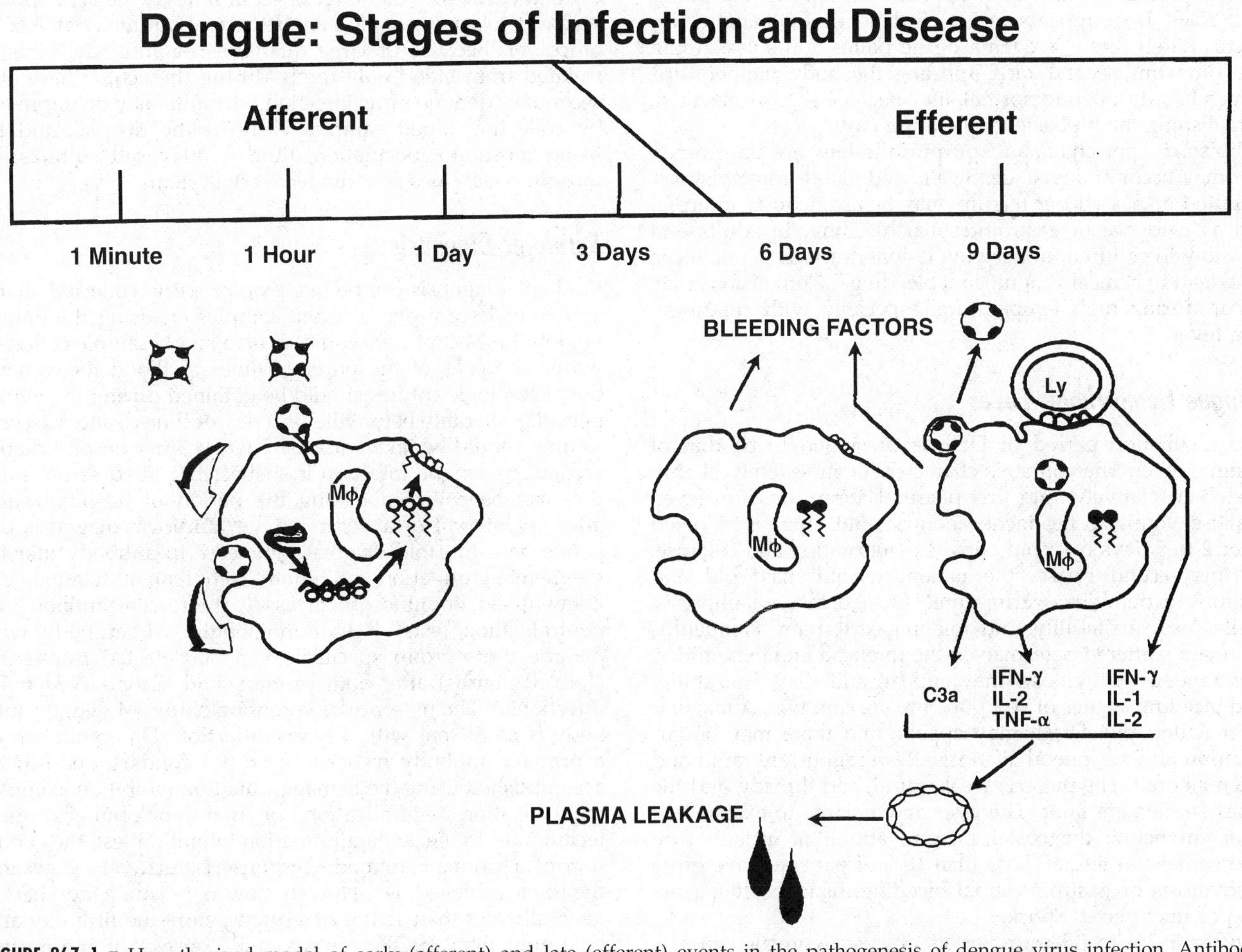

FIGURE 267–1 ▫ Hypothesized model of early (afferent) and late (efferent) events in the pathogenesis of dengue virus infection. Antibody-dependent enhancement of infection of mononuclear phagocytes is an afferent event that regulates the production of cytokines, which results in the signs and symptoms of dengue hemorrhagic fever–dengue shock syndrome.

tive antibodies (high responses) do. Finally, the ability of virus to replicate to high titer in human mononuclear phagocytes may be a critical pathogenic factor.

Clinical Manifestations

Dengue Fever

Manifestations vary with age and from patient to patient. In infants and young children, the disease may be undifferentiated or characterized by a 1- to 5-day fever, pharyngeal inflammation, rhinitis, and mild cough.[35] In outbreaks, a majority of infected older children and adults exhibit most of the findings described here.[36]

After an incubation period of 1 to 7 days, there is sudden onset of fever; the temperature rapidly rises to 39.4°C to 41.1°C (100°F to 106°F), usually accompanied by frontal or retroorbital headache. Occasionally, back pain antedates the fever. A transient, macular, generalized rash that blanches under pressure may appear. The pulse may be slow relative to the degree of fever. Myalgia or arthralgia occurs soon after the onset and increases in severity. Involvement of the joints may be particularly severe in patients with chikungunya or o'nyong-nyong infection. From the second to the sixth days of fever, nausea and vomiting are apt to occur, and generalized lymphadenopathy, cutaneous hyperesthesia or hyperalgesia, taste aberrations, and pronounced anorexia may develop.

One to two days after defervescence, a generalized, morbilliform, maculopapular rash appears that spares the palms and soles. It disappears in 1 to 5 days; desquamation may occur. Rarely, there is edema of the palms and soles. About the time this second rash appears, the body temperature, which had dropped to normal, may become slightly elevated, establishing the biphasic temperature curve.

Epistaxis, petechiae, and purpuric lesions are uncommon but may occur at any stage. Swallowed blood from epistaxis, vomited or passed per rectum, may be erroneously interpreted as evidence of gastrointestinal bleeding. In adults and possibly in children, underlying lesions, such as peptic ulcer, may lead to clinically significant bleeding.[37] Convulsions may occur during high temperature, especially with chikungunya fever.

Dengue Hemorrhagic Fever

The incubation period of DHF is presumed to be that of dengue fever. The course is characteristic in severely ill children.[38] A relatively mild first phase of abrupt onset of fever, malaise, vomiting, headache, anorexia, and cough is followed after 2 to 5 days by rapid clinical deterioration and collapse. In this second phase, the patient usually has cold and clammy extremities, warm trunk, flushed face, diaphoresis, restlessness, irritability, and midepigastric pain. Frequently, there are scattered petechiae on the forehead and extremities; spontaneous ecchymosis may appear, and easy bruisability and bleeding at sites of venipuncture are common. A macular or maculopapular rash may appear, and there may be circumoral and peripheral cyanosis. Respirations are rapid and often labored. The pulse is weak, rapid, and thready, and the heart sounds are faint. The liver may enlarge to extend to 4 to 6 cm below the costal margin, and it is usually firm and somewhat tender. Less than 10% of patients have gross ecchymosis or gastrointestinal bleeding, usually after a period of uncorrected shock.

After a 24- to 36-hour period of crisis, convalescence is fairly rapid for the children who recover. The temperature may return to normal before or during the stage of shock. Bradycardia and ventricular extrasystoles are common during convalescence. Infrequently, there is residual brain damage due to prolonged shock, or occasionally to intracranial hemorrhage.

Laboratory Findings

The most common hematologic abnormalities during clinical shock are a 20% or greater increase in hematocrit value over the recovery value,[38] thrombocytopenia, mild leukocytosis (the cell count values seldom exceeding 10,000/mm^3), prolonged bleeding time, and moderately decreased prothrombin level (seldom less than 40% of control values).[39] Fibrinogen levels may be subnormal, and fibrin split products elevated.[40]

Other abnormalities include hypocomplementemia, moderate elevations of the serum transaminase value, mild metabolic acidosis with hyponatremia, and, at times, hypochloremia, slight elevation of serum urea nitrogen, and hypoalbuminemia.[38, 41] Radiographs of the chest reveal pleural effusions in nearly all patients. Sonograms reveal pleural effusions, ascites, and edema of gallbladder.

Diagnosis

Virus Isolation

Blood should be obtained during the febrile period, preferably before the fifth day after onset of illness. The acute-phase serum or plasma sample may be frozen, optimally at −65°C or colder. Because of large quantities of antibody, virus is isolated from blood only rarely during the acute phase of a secondary dengue virus infection.[42] Results may be improved by collecting blood samples early in the disease, and by using mosquito inoculation, fluid overlay cell cultures, or mosquito cell lines as virus recovery systems.[43, 44]

Serologic Diagnosis

Etiologic diagnosis can be made on properly collected acute- and convalescent-phase serum samples or, using the immunoglobulin M capture technique, on a single sample collected within 6 weeks of the onset of illness.[45] Blood for conventional serologic studies should be obtained during the febrile period, preferably before the fifth day of illness, and a second sample should be taken at least 2 weeks after onset. When a secondary dengue infection is suspected, paired serum samples can be collected during the period of hospitalization after an interval of at least 1 day.[46] Serologic diagnosis depends on a fourfold or greater increase in antibody titer by the hemagglutination inhibition, complement fixation, enzyme-linked immunosorbent assay, fluorescent antibody, or neutralization test.[46, 47] Immunoglobulin M antibody with dengue virus group specificity can be detected transiently (1 to 3 months) after both primary and secondary dengue infections.[45] The presence of immunoglobulin M dengue antibody is consistent with a recent infection. Differentiation of a primary antibody response from a secondary one can be accomplished using the hemagglutination inhibition, complement fixation neutralization, or immunoglobulin capture techniques. In the hemagglutination inhibition test, the evolution of a primary antibody response is relatively slow and the titer achieved is relatively low.[45, 46] Thus, the titer is generally less than 1:20 if measured before the fifth day and not more than 1:1280 if measured 2 weeks or more after onset. In a secondary response, the hemagglutination inhibition titer is generally greater than 1:20 before the fifth day after onset and rises to 1:2560 or higher, often so rapidly that high fixed titers are observed. In the complement fixation and neutralization tests, primary infections result in relatively dengue type–specific responses in convalescent-phase serum, whereas a broadly reactive response, usually involving all four types, characterizes a secondary-type antibody response. In the immunoglobulin M/immunoglobulin G capture test the ratio of immunoglobulin M to immunoglobulin G is greater than 1:1 in the acute phase of primary infections and less than 1:1 in secondary infections.[45]

Differential Diagnosis

Dengue Fever. Clinical diagnosis derives from a high index of suspicion and a knowledge of the geographic distribution and environmental cycles of causal viruses. Travelers may be exposed to dengue in hotels and during daytime shopping trips in epidemic or endemic areas. The differential diagnosis includes a number of viral respiratory tract and influenza-like diseases plus the early stages of malaria, scrub typhus, hepatitis, and leptospirosis. Abortive forms of each of these diseases modified by therapy or vaccine may never evolve beyond a dengue-like stage.

Clinical dengue fever may be caused by chikungunya, o'nyong-nyong, or West Nile virus. Chikungunya, a togavirus, is distributed in Africa and throughout Southeast Asia. The period of fever lasts a mean of 3 days, and infection is usually accompanied by arthralgia.[47] O'nyong-nyong, also a togavirus, transmitted by *Anopheles* species, produced a sizable epidemic in Tanzania in 1952.[48] West Nile virus, a flavivirus distributed in western India and East Africa, produces a syndrome indistinguishable from that caused by dengue viruses.[49]

Four arboviral diseases have dengue-like courses but without rash: Colorado tick fever, sandfly fever, Rift Valley fever, and Ross River fever.[50] Colorado tick fever occurs sporadically among campers and hunters in the western United States; sandfly fever, in the Mediterranean region, the Middle East, southern Russia, and parts of the Indian subcontinent; Rift Valley fever, in North, East, Central, and South Africa; and Ross River fever is endemic in much of eastern Australia with epidemic extension to Fiji. In adults, Ross River fever often produces protracted and crippling arthralgia involving weight-bearing joints. Because clinical findings vary and there are many possible agents, the term dengue-like disease should be used until a specific diagnosis is established.

Dengue Hemorrhagic Fever. In endemic areas, hemorrhagic fever should be suspected in children who have a febrile illness and exhibit a positive response to the tourniquet test, hemoconcentration, thrombocytopenia, and hemorrhagic manifestations, with or without shock in confirmed dengue infections.[51] Pleural effusion or signs of shock are pathognomonic. Because many rickettsial diseases, meningococcemia, and other severe illnesses caused by a variety of agents may produce hemorrhagic phenomena, the term DHF-DSS should be used only when epidemiologic, virologic, or serologic evidence suggests the possibility of dengue infection. Hemorrhagic manifestations have been described in other diseases known or presumed to be viral, including the clinically distinguishable hemorrhagic fevers described in Chapter 269.

Treatment

Dengue Fever. Treatment is supportive. Bed rest is recommended during the febrile period. Antipyretic drugs or cold water sponging should be used to keep body temperature below 40°C (104°F). Analgesics or mild sedation may be required to control pain. Because of its effects on hemostasis, aspirin should not be given. Fluid and electrolyte replacement is required when there are deficits due to sweating, fasting, thirst, vomiting, or diarrhea.

Dengue Hemorrhagic Fever–Dengue Shock Syndrome. Management requires immediate evaluation of vital signs and of the degree of hemoconcentration, dehydration, and electrolyte imbalance.[46, 50] Close monitoring is essential for at least 48 hours, because shock may occur or recur precipitously early in the disease. Patients who are cyanotic or have labored breathing should be given oxygen. Rapid intravenous replacement of fluids and electrolytes can frequently sustain patients until spontaneous recovery occurs. When elevation of the hematocrit persists after replacement of fluids, plasma or plasma colloid preparations are indicated. Care must be taken to avoid overhydration, which may contribute to cardiac failure. Transfusions of fresh blood or of platelets suspended in plasma may be necessary to control bleeding; they should not be given during hemoconcentration but only after evaluation of hemoglobin or hematocrit values. Salicylates are contraindicated because of their effect on blood clotting.

Paraldehyde or chloral hydrate may be required for children who are markedly agitated. Use of pressor amines, β-adrenergic blocking agents, and aldosterone has not significantly reduced the mortality rate compared with simple supportive therapy. Steroids do not shorten the duration of disease or improve prognosis for children receiving conscientious supportive therapy.[52]

Hypervolemia during the fluid reabsorptive phase may be life threatening and is heralded by a drop in hematocrit with wide pulse pressure. Diuretics and digitalis therapy may be necessary.

Prevention

Attenuated vaccines for dengue virus types 1, 2, 3, and 4 are under development in Thailand.[53] A killed vaccine for chikungunya is efficacious but not generally available.[54] Prophylaxis consists of avoiding mosquito bites by use of insecticides, repellents, protective clothing, screening in houses, and destruction of *A. aegypti* breeding sites.[55] If water storage is mandatory, a tight-fitting lid or a thin layer of oil on all containers may prevent egg laying or hatching. A larvicide, such as temephos [Abate: *O,O'*-(thiodi-4,1-phenylene)phosphorothioic acid *O,O,O,O'*-tetramethyl ester], available as a 1% sand-granule formulation and effective at a concentration of one part per million, may be added safely to drinking water. Ultra–low-volume spray equipment effectively dispenses malathion from truck or airplane for rapid killing of adult mosquitoes during an epidemic. Only personal antimosquito measures are effective against mosquitoes in the field, forest, or jungle.

References

1. Carey SE: Chikungunya and dengue: A case of mistaken identity? J Hist Med Allied Sci 26:243, 1971.
2. Sabin AB: Research on dengue during World War II. Am J Trop Med 1:30, 1952.
3. Hammon W McD, Rudnick A, Sather GE: Viruses associated with hemorrhagic fevers of the Philippines and Thailand. Science 131:1102, 1960.
4. Westaway EG, Brinton MA, Gaidamovich SYA, et al: Flaviviridae. Intervirology 24:183, 1985.
5. Karabatsos N (ed): International Catalog of Arbovirus 1985. Ft. Collins, CO, American Society of Tropical Medicine and Hygiene, 1985.

6. Mason PW, Dalrymple JM, Gentry MK, et al: Molecular characterization of a neutralizing domain of the Japanese encephalitis virus structural glycoprotein. J Gen Virol 8:2037, 1989.
7. Hahn YS, Galler R, Hunkapiller T, et al: Nucleotide sequence of dengue 2 RNA and comparison of the encoded proteins with those of other flaviviruses. Virology 162:167, 1988.
8. Lewis JA, Chang G-J, Lanciotti RS, et al: Phylogenetic relationships of dengue-2 viruses. Virology 197:216, 1993.
9. Halstead SB: Pathogenesis of dengue: Challenges to molecular biology. Science 239:476, 1988.
10. Halstead SB, O'Rourke EJ: Dengue viruses and mononuclear phagocytes. I. Infection enhancement by nonneutralizing antibody. J Exp Med 146:201, 1977.
11. Halstead SB, O'Rourke EJ, Allison AC: Dengue viruses and mononuclear phagocytes. II. Identity of blood and tissue leukocytes supporting in vitro infection. J Exp Med 146:218, 1977.
12. Russell PK, McCown JM: Comparison of dengue 2 and dengue 3 virus strains by neutralization tests and identification of a subtype of dengue 3. Am J Trop Med Hyg 21:97, 1972.
13. Henchal EA, Repik PM, McCown JM, et al: Identification of an antigenic and genetic variant of dengue 4 virus from the Caribbean. Am J Trop Med Hyg 35:393, 1986.
14. Rico-Hesse R: Molecular evolution and distribution of dengue viruses type 1 and 2 in nature. Virology 174:479, 1990.
15. Rudnick A: Ecology of dengue virus. Asian J Infect Dis 2:156, 1977.
16. Metselaar D, Grainger CR, Oei KG, et al: An outbreak of type 2 dengue fever in the Seychelles, probably transmitted by *Aedes albopictus* (Skuse). Bull World Health Organ 58:937, 1980.
17. Centers for Disease Control: Update: *Aedes albopictus* infestation—United States, Mexico. MMWR Morbid Mortal Wkly Rep 38:440, 1989.
18. WHO Vector Biology and Control Division: Geographical Distribution of Arthropod-Borne Diseases and Their Principal Vectors. Geneva, World Health Organization, 1989.
19. Sheppard PM, MacDonald WW, Tonn RJ, et al: The dynamics of an adult population of *Aedes aegypti* in relation to dengue hemorrhagic fever in Bangkok. J Anim Ecol 38:661, 1969.
20. Kouri GP, Guzman MG, Bravo JR, Triana C: Dengue hemorrhagic fever/dengue shock syndrome: Lessons from the Cuban epidemic, 1981. Bull World Health Organ 67:375, 1989.
21. Deubel V, Nogueira RM, Drouet MT, et al: Direct sequencing of genomic cDNA fragments amplified by the polymerase chain reaction for molecular epidemiology of dengue-2 viruses. Arch Virol 129:197, 1993.
22. Guzman MG, Kouri GP, Bravo J, et al: Dengue hemorrhagic fever in Cuba, 1981. A retrospective seroepidemiologic study. Am J Trop Med Hyg 84:179, 1990.
23. Saluzzo JF, Cornet M, Castagnet P, et al: Isolation of dengue 2 and 4 viruses from patients in Senegal. Trans R Soc Trop Med Hyg 80:5, 1986.
24. Carey DE, Myers RM, Reuben R, et al: Studies on dengue in Vellore, South India. Am J Trop Med Hyg 15:580, 1966.
25. Halstead SB, Nimmannitya S, Cohen SN: Observations related to pathogenesis of dengue hemorrhagic fever. IV. Relation of disease severity to antibody response and virus recovered. Yale J Biol Med 42:311, 1970.
26. Sangkawibha N, Rojanasuphot S, Ahandvik S, et al: Risk factors in dengue shock syndrome. A prospective epidemiological study in Rayong, Thailand. I. The 1980 outbreak. Am J Epidemiol 120:653, 1984.
27. Burke DS, Nisalak A, Johnson DE, et al: A prospective study of dengue infections in Bangkok. Am J Trop Med Hyg 38:172, 1988.
28. Kliks S, Nimmannitya S, Nisalak A, et al: Evidence that maternal dengue antibodies are important in the development of dengue hemorrhagic fever in infants. Am J Trop Med Hyg 38:411, 1988.
29. Kliks S, Nisalak A, Brandt WE, et al: Antibody dependent enhancement in human monocytes as a risk factor for dengue hemorrhagic fever. Am J Trop Med Hyg 40:444, 1989.
30. Marchette NJ, Halstead SB, Falkler WA Jr, et al: Studies on the pathogenesis of dengue infection in monkeys. III. Sequential distribution of virus in primary and heterologous infections. J Infect Dis 128:23, 1973.
31. Boonpucknavig S, Boonpucknavig V, Bhamarapravati N, et al: Immunofluorescence study of skin rash in patients with dengue hemorrhagic fever. Arch Pathol Lab Med 103:463, 1979.
32. Kurane I, Meager A, Ennis FA: Dengue virus–specific human T-cell clones. Serotype cross-reactive proliferation, interferon γ production, and cytotoxic activity. J Exp Med 170:763, 1989.
33. Hober D, Poli L, Roblin B, et al: Serum levels of tumor necrosis factor-α (TNFα), interleukin-6 (IL-6) and interleukin-1β (IL-1β) in dengue-infected patients. Am J Trop Med Hyg 48:324, 1993.
34. Morens DM, Halstead SB: Disease severity–related antigenic differences in dengue 2 strains detected by dengue 4 monoclonal antibodies. J Med Virol 22:163, 1987.
35. Halstead SB, Nimmannitya S, Margiotta MR: Dengue and chikungunya infection in man in Thailand, 1962–1964. II. Observations on disease in outpatients. Am J Trop Med Hyg 18:972, 1969.
36. Simmons JS, St John HH, Reynolds FHK: Experimental studies of dengue. Philipp J Sci 44:1, 1931.
37. Tsai CJ, Kuo CH, Chen PC, et al: Upper gastrointestinal bleeding in dengue fever. Am J Gastroenterol 86:33, 1991.
38. Cohen SN, Halstead SB: Shock associated with dengue infection. I. The clinical and physiologic manifestations of dengue hemorrhagic fever in Thailand, 1964. J Pediatr 68:448, 1966.
39. Weiss HJ, Halstead SB: Studies of hemostasis in Thai hemorrhagic fever. J Pediatr 66:918, 1965.
40. Bokisch VA, Top FH Jr, Russell PK, et al: The potential pathogenic role of complement in dengue hemorrhagic shock syndrome. N Engl J Med 289:996, 1973.
41. Memoranda: Pathogenic mechanisms in dengue hemorrhagic fever. Report of an international collaborative study. Bull WHO 48:117, 1973.
42. Nisalak A, Halstead SB, Singharaj P, et al: Observations related to pathogenesis of dengue hemorrhagic fever. III, Virologic studies of fatal disease. Yale J Biol Med 42:293, 1970.
43. Rosen L, Gubler D: The use of mosquitoes to detect and propagate dengue viruses. Am J Trop Med Hyg 23:1153, 1974.
44. Igarashi A: Isolation of a Singh's *Aedes albopictus* cell clone sensitive to dengue and chikungunya viruses. J Gen Virol 40:531, 1978.
45. Innis BL, Nisalak A, Nimmannitya S, et al: An enzyme-linked immunosorbent assay to characterize dengue infections where dengue and Japanese encephalitis co-circulate. Am J Trop Med Hyg 40:418, 1989.
46. Dengue Hemorrhagic Fever: Diagnosis, Treatment and Control. Geneva, World Health Organization, 1995, pp 1–93.
47. Carey DE, Myers RM, DeRantiz KM, et al: The 1964 chikungunya epidemic at Vellore, South Africa, including observations on concurrent dengue. Trans R Soc Trop Med Hyg 63:434, 1969.
48. Robinson MC: An epidemic of virus disease in Southern Province Tanganyika Territory in 1952–1953. I. Clinical features. Trans R Soc Trop Med Hyg 49:28, 1955.
49. Carey DE, Rodrigues FM, Myers RM, et al: Arthropod-borne viral infections in children in Vellore, South India, with particular references to dengue and West Nile viruses. India Pediatr 5:285, 1968.
50. Feigin RD, Cherry JD (eds): Textbook of Pediatric Infectious Diseases, ed 4. Philadelphia, WB Saunders, 1997.
51. Nimmannitya S, Halstead SB, Cohen SV, et al: Dengue and chikungunya virus infection in man in Thailand, 1962–1964. I. Observations on hospitalized patients with hemorrhagic fever. Am J Trop Med Hyg 18:954, 1969.
52. Tassniyom S, Vasanawathana S, Chirawatkul A, et al: Failure of high-dose methylprednisolone in established dengue shock syndrome: A placebo-controlled, double-blind study. Pediatrics 92:111, 1993.
53. Bhamarapravati N, Yoksan S, Chayaniyayothin T, et al: Immunization with a live attenuated dengue-2-virus candidate vaccine (16681-PDK 53): Clinical, immunological and biological responses in adult volunteers. Bull World Health Organ 65:189, 1987.
54. Harrison VR, Binn LN, Randall R: Comparative immunogenicities of chikungunya vaccines prepared in avian and mammalian tissues. Am J Trop Med Hyg 16:786, 1967.
55. Halstead SB: Selective primary health care: Strategies for control of disease in the developing world. XI. Dengue. Rev Infect Dis 6:251, 1984.

268

Encephalitis Viruses Belonging to the Families Flaviviridae, Togaviridae, and Bunyaviridae

Charles H. Hoke, Jr.

History

Seven families of viruses contain human pathogens that cause encephalitis. Four of those families contain the bulk of these pathogens: the Flaviviridae, Togaviridae, Bunyaviridae, and Herpesviridae (Table 268–1). The first three of these families are discussed in this chapter. Encephalitides caused by viruses of the family Flaviridae are St. Louis encephalitis (SLE), Japanese encephalitis (JE), Murray Valley encephalitis (MVE), tick-borne encephalitis (including Central European and Russian spring-summer encephalitis), and Powassan encephalitis. Members of the genus *Alphavirus* of the family Togaviridae cause eastern equine encephalitis (EEE), western equine encephalitis (WEE), and Venezuelan equine encephalitis (VEE). Encephalitogenic members of the Bunyaviridae family are in the California serogroup and cause California, La Crosse, and Jamestown Canyon encephalitis.[1]

The first viral agent of encephalitis was demonstrated when SLE virus was isolated in 1933 from a patient who died in an outbreak in St. Louis and Kansas City, Missouri.[2] In relatively quick succession, most of the known agents of other types of viral encephalitis were discovered.[3–14] In 1986, infection by human immunodeficiency virus was demonstrated to be a cause of viral encephalitis.[15]

Additional causes of acute viral encephalitis may exist. For clinical and public health reasons, it is important to pursue the diagnosis of such cases, particularly fatal cases. Blood and cerebrospinal fluid rarely yield virus isolates. Brain tissue may be required. In fatal cases of viral encephalitis, postmortem tissue should be sought. The laboratory evaluation of viral encephalitis must be carefully planned in coordination with available microbiologic services. Because the capability to isolate etiologic agents is highly specialized, evaluations may require participation of state and national laboratories. A wide range of cells and animals may be required for virus isolation. Serologic confirmation of most etiologies can be made by virus-specific immunoglobulin M (IgM) capture assays and other types of serologic tests.

Characteristics of the Pathogen

Flaviviridae

JAPANESE ENCEPHALITIS VIRUS

History and Geographic Location. JE virus was isolated from a human in 1935[3] and from the vector mosquito, *Culex tritaeniorhynchus*, in 1938. Numerous summertime epidemics of encephalitis had occurred in Japan and Korea in the preceding decades. Once a virus was isolated, subsequent encephalitis epidemics were clearly associated with the JE virus. After World War II, intensive study of the ecology of the virus in Japan and Korea was undertaken and a great deal was learned about its transmission to the bird population and to semidomestic pigs. Crude vaccines were developed for U.S. soldiers during and after the war. A vaccine was developed in Japan in the early 1960s for use in Japanese children, and a purified version was introduced in 1966. Widespread use of the vaccine along with improved living standards was associated with a reduction in the annual incidence from several thousand cases to about 10. In 1988, the vaccine was proved efficacious under field conditions in Thailand.[16] The disease is important in many Asian countries. China probably has between 10,000 and 50,000 cases per year. As a consequence, China manufactures many millions of doses of vaccine for its children each year. Taiwan, Korea, Thailand, Sri Lanka, and India also have immunization programs. Morbidity and mortality among children are considerable in Nepal, Thailand, Sri Lanka, India, the Philippines, and Vietnam.

Classification. JE virus is a member of the family Flaviviridae, along with the agents of yellow fever, dengue fever, MVE, SLE, and West Nile encephalitis.

Structure. The Flaviviridae have a spherical nucleocapsid surrounded by a lipid-containing envelope with surface projections. The particles are 40 to 70 nm in diameter and contain a single molecule of single-stranded RNA, which is positive sense (the genome and the messenger RNA are the same). The entire genome contains about 10,000 base pairs. There are three structural polypeptides, the envelope, the matrix, and the capsid (abbreviated E, M, and C), which are glycosylated, and several nonstructural proteins.

Biologic and Biochemical Properties. JE virus replicates to high titer in a number of vertebrate and insect cell lines, causing a cytopathic effect (CPE).[17] It readily infects the brain of many animals, but only on direct injection into the brain or after intravenous injection with mechanical disruption of the blood-brain barrier.

The proteins of the virus, especially the envelope protein and the NS1 nonstructural protein, can be readily observed in antigenically reactive form on polyacrylamide gel electrophoresis. The complete genome has been cloned, sequenced, and expressed in a number of prokaryotic and eukaryotic expression systems.[18, 19] Infectious complementary DNA has been made, and mutants with reduced neurovirulence have been recovered.[20]

Replication. The virus replicates in inoculated mosquitos, in cell lines derived from them, and in vertebrates and their cells.[20a] The virus membrane fuses with the cell membrane and penetrates the cytoplasm, where replication of the positive-sense genome and synthesis of both structural and nonstructural proteins takes place. The structural proteins are assembled into virion particles, which then bud from the surface of infected cells.[21]

Antigenic Characteristics. JE virus was originally classified with yellow fever and dengue viruses as a group B arbovirus. This assignment was based on cross-reactions observed using the hemagglutination inhibition test.[22] This classification was, unfortunately, a confusing coincidence, because this B is unrelated to the B originally used in the now obsolete term Japanese B encephalitis. The B in this term was used to distinguish encephalitis caused by JE virus from von Economo encephalitis lethargica, which was called type A. Neutralization of the virus using specific monkey or mouse serum confirms its identity. Specific monoclonal antibodies have been developed that are now in wide use for unequivo-

TABLE 268–1 ■ Initial Isolations of Flaviviridae, Togaviridae, and Bunyaviridae Associated with Viral Encephalitis

	ANIMAL HOST		HUMANS		VECTOR		
VIRUS AND ENCEPHALITIS TYPE	**Animal**	**Year**	**Location**	**Year**	**Location**	**Species**	**Year**
Family Flaviviridae							
St. Louis	Birds	1955	St. Louis Kansas City, MO	1933	Yakima, WA	*Culex pipiens* *Culex tarsalis*	1941
Japanese	Horses	1937	Nagasaki, Japan Tokyo	1934 1938	Japan	*Culex tritaeniorhynchus*	1930
Tick-borne	Insectivores, rodents, birds	1939(?)	Far Eastern Russia Former Czechoslovakia	1937 1948	Far Eastern Russia	*Ixodes persulcatus*	1937
Murray Valley	Horses	1984	Australia	1951	Australia	*Culex annulirostris*	1960
West Nile	Horses	1968	West Nile Province, Uganda	1937	Egypt	*Culex* species	1952
Powassan	Squirrels	1968	Ontario, Canada	1958	Colorado	*Dermacentor andersoni*	1952
Rocio	Sparrows	1975	Rural São Paolo, Brazil	1975	Brazil	*Psorophora ferox*	1978
Family Togaviridae, genus *Alphavirus*							
Eastern equine	Horses	1933	Massachusetts	1938	Georgia	*Coquillettidia perturbans*	1949
Western equine	Horses	1930	California	1938	Washington State	*Aedes aegypti* *Culex tarsalis*	1941
Venezuelan equine	Horses	1936	Trinidad	1944	Trinidad	*Mansonia titillans*	1944
Members of the family Bunyaviridae, California serogroup							
California	Unknown		San Joaquin, CA	1945	California	*Aedes malanimon*	1943
La Crosse	Squirrels	1970	La Crosse, WI	1964	Wisconsin	*Aedes triseriatus*	1972
Jamestown Canyon	White-tailed deer	1973	Wisconsin	1965	Colorado	*Culiseta inornata*	1962

cal identification of JE virus. Nucleotide sequence amplification techniques have been used to determine the genetic relatedness of isolates.

Laboratory Demonstration of Infection. Occasionally the virus can be isolated from cerebrospinal fluid, particularly in fulminant disease when there is abundant virus replication. Post mortem, the virus can be isolated from virtually any site in the brain. Specimens from several areas are best cultivated. Minced material is placed in culture with an appropriate cell line. Cultures derived from hamster, porcine, chicken, monkey, and mosquito cells (AP61 or C6/36) are useful for isolating the virus. Once a CPE is observed, the virus' identity may be confirmed by use of an enzyme-linked immunosorbent assay (ELISA). Alternatively, it may be identified by demonstration of a reduction in the number of virus plaques after treatment with virus-specific antiserum. A technique of historical interest only is neutralization of the lethal effect of the virus on suckling mice by specific serum.

Diagnosis can be made unequivocally by demonstrating virus-specific antiviral IgM antibody in the cerebrospinal fluid or serum, which was present in the specimens of 80% of patients collected at the time of admission to a hospital in rural Thailand. One hundred percent of specimens collected 3 days later contained virus-specific IgM antibody.[23, 24]

ST. LOUIS ENCEPHALITIS VIRUS

History and Geographic Location. SLE virus was isolated from a human brain in 1933,[2] and proof of natural infection of *Culex tarsalis* mosquito vectors came during study of an outbreak in 1941.[25] Since 1933, both urban and rural outbreaks have occurred, some focal and some widespread. Urban outbreaks have occurred in many cities. Notable outbreaks have occurred in Missouri, Illinois, Kentucky, Texas, Arizona, Colorado, New Jersey, California, and Florida; significant ones occurred in 1932, 1937, 1954, 1962, 1972, 1980, 1984, and 1990.

Classification. SLE virus is a member of the family Flaviviridae. It is grouped in the JE complex.

Structure. SLE virus is structurally identical to other flaviviruses: they have a single strand of RNA of positive polarity about 11,000 base pairs long. The nucleotide sequence of the RNA is known, and the genes are arranged in the following order: capsid, pre-M, envelope, NS1, NS1a, NS2b, NS3, NS4a, NS4b, NS5. The virus particle is constructed only from the first three proteins. The NS, or nonstructural, proteins are involved in the replication of RNA or the transport and assembly of the virus but are not included in the final structure.

A single long open reading frame (contains no natural stopping codons) allows the protein to be transcribed as a single amino acid chain, which is later cleaved into individual proteins.[26] The RNA is complexed with a highly basic capsid protein. The nucleocapsid is surrounded by a lipid bilayer. Two proteins, the M protein and the E, or envelope, protein, surround the lipid bilayer.

Biologic and Biochemical Properties. The virus can be grown in a number of cell lines (BHK-21 [baby hamster kidney], Vero, LLC-MK_2, MA-104, and porcine kidney) in which a CPE occurs and, under proper conditions, plaques are formed.[27] Baby mice and hamsters are highly susceptible to intracerebral infection. The virus can be identified by its susceptibility to neutralization by specific monkey or human serum or in ELISAs using appropriate reagents.

Replication. After the virus enters the cell, the nucleocapsid is uncoated. Translation of the RNA into a long protein begins at a single site. Individual proteins are cut from the long polyprotein. The RNA is also transcribed into complementary (negative-sense) RNA strands, which in turn are transcribed into more full-length genomes, which can be either translated or assembled as genome into new viral particles. The RNA and the proteins are assembled into viral packages in a poorly understood process that aligns the membrane proteins together around the nucleocapsid and ultimately allows budding from the cell membrane.

Antigenic Characteristics. SLE virus is most closely related to the JE, MVE, and West Nile viruses, and these viruses have been grouped using mouse hyperimmune ascites fluid in the JE antigenic complex, along with several other viruses.[28] With monoclonal antibodies, some variation in SLE virus isolates has been detected.

Laboratory Demonstration of Infection. As with JE virus, isolation is most often successful with postmortem tissue. Virus antigen can be demonstrated by specific staining methods. IgM antibody capture ELISA can be used to establish the diagnosis. Other forms of antibody tests (complement fixation, hemagglutination inhibition, neutralization) have been used in the past.

CENTRAL EUROPEAN ENCEPHALITIS (TICK-BORNE AND RUSSIAN SPRING-SUMMER ENCEPHALITIS) VIRUS

History and Geographic Location. Tick-borne encephalitis was first recognized in 1932 in Far Eastern Russia. The virus was isolated from human brain in 1937 and that same year was shown to be transmissible by ticks.[29, 30] In 1948, the disease was described in the Strakonice District of Czechoslovakia. A virus isolated from a patient with the disease was shown to be similar to the one that had been isolated from the cases in Far Eastern Russia.[31] Most affected persons are exposed to ticks in woodland areas between May and October, although the disease may also be acquired by consuming raw milk.

Classification. Formerly, the names Russian spring-summer encephalitis and tick-borne encephalitis virus were widely used. Because no virus named tick-borne encephalitis virus has been entered in the *International Catalog of Arboviruses*, Calisher[32] proposed that the complex be referred to as Central European encephalitis virus.

Structure. The structure of viruses of this complex is the same as that of other flaviviruses.

Biologic and Biochemical Properties. Flaviviruses are generally stable between pH 7 and 9, but Central European encephalitis virus is stable at lower pH.[33] This property may account for its infectiousness when ingested orally.

The virus replicates in a large range of cells, including human, chicken (egg and cell culture), cow, pig, monkey, reptile, and amphibian.[34] It also replicates in ticks: *Ixodes persulcatus* and *Ixodes ricinus* have been shown experimentally to be competent vectors.[29, 35] Virus disseminates in the ticks after a meal of infected blood and is subsequently transmissible when the tick feeds.

Many small mammals, including shrews, moles, voles, hamsters, and mice, are highly susceptible to infection and are heavily infested by vector ticks in the wild. These mammals serve as maintenance hosts for the virus. Cows and mice become viremic after being bitten by infected ticks and subsequently shed virus in milk.[36] Animals may be infected for long periods. Intracerebral inoculation of sheep and monkeys causes encephalitis.[37]

The molecular structure of the virus has been studied in detail. The nucleotide sequence of the genome and the amino acid sequence of the proteins have been determined. The large degree of sequence homology with other flaviviruses confirms that the serologic system that classifies these viruses together has a good genetic foundation.[38]

The binding sites of monoclonal antibodies to component proteins and the location of disulfide cross-links in the envelope glycoprotein have been determined. The genetic changes responsible for developing resistance to some neutralizing monoclonal antibodies have been identified.[39] Analysis of the binding of monoclonal antibodies suggests that the virus antigens in strains isolated over a wide range in Austria have been stable during a 14-year period.[40]

Replication. Replication of Central European encephalitis virus is similar to that of other flaviviruses.

Antigenic Characteristics. The hemagglutination inhibition test shows Central European encephalitis virus to be antigenically related to the other members of the family Flaviviridae. Neutralization tests afford serologic identification of infecting flaviviruses.

Through studies of the antigen sites on the envelope glycoprotein, the binding of a number of monoclonal antibodies to a series of important epitopes has been mapped. Other studies using various molecular fragments or disrupted molecular structures have contributed to the development of a widely accepted two-dimensional diagram of this protein. Full crystallographic definition of the tertiary structure has been achieved.[41] Glycosylation appears to have no effect on the immunoreactive structures.[41a]

Laboratory Demonstration of Infection. Early in the illness, virus may be isolated from the blood. In fatal cases, it can be isolated from brain tissue in infant mice and a number of types of cell culture.[31] As for other flaviviruses, IgM capture ELISA has replaced older serologic tests.[42]

MURRAY VALLEY ENCEPHALITIS VIRUS

History and Geographic Location. Although outbreaks of MVE had been noted as early as 1917, the virus was not characterized until 1951.[10] Epidemics occurred in Australia in 1956, 1971, 1974, 1978, 1981, and 1984.[31] Cases have been confirmed in New Guinea.[43]

Classification. MVE virus is antigenically and genetically similar to JE virus. It is classified as a member of the JE virus complex.[28]

Structure. The structure is similar to that of the other flaviviruses.

Biologic and Biochemical Properties. MVE virus grows in a variety of cells[44] and in infant mice, hamsters, and chickens.

Replication. MVE virus replicates in a manner similar to that of other flaviviruses.

Antigenic Characteristics. The virus is antigenically similar to other flaviviruses. Consequently, antibody detected by hemagglutination inhibition may cross-react with those viruses.

Laboratory Demonstration of Infection. The virus can be isolated from the brain post mortem in cultures of chick embryo and infant mice cells. Hemagglutination inhibition, complement fixation, and neutralizing antibody tests can be used to confirm infection by demonstrating at least a fourfold increase in antibody titer from acute- to convalescent-phase specimens. Detection of virus-specific IgM is useful in diagnosis.[45]

Togaviridae

The Togaviridae that cause encephalitis—EEE, WEE, and VEE viruses—are all members of the genus *Alphavirus*. EEE virus readily causes serious brain infection. WEE virus tends to cause encephalitis in very young children. VEE virus generally causes only a debilitating febrile disease and rarely encephalitis.

Alphaviruses are 60 to 65 nm in diameter and spherical. The single-stranded RNA genome is contained in a nucleocapsid core. A lipid bilayer is surrounded by an outer glycoprotein shell[46] from which glycoprotein spikes protrude. The genome is about 11,700 bases long. The genome codes for four nonstructural proteins of unknown function. All members of the genus have a similarly organized genome. There are strong antigenic cross-reactions among the alphaviruses, and many serologic assays cross-react. Hemagglutination inhibition is somewhat more specific.[5] The alphaviruses replicate and produce CPE in a wide variety of vertebrate cells. Plaque assays sensitive to a single infectious particle can be performed readily on a variety of cells. CPE is much less notable in invertebrate cell lines. Animals may be readily infected. Horses develop encephalitis after inoculation with WEE, EEE, or VEE virus. Inoculated infant mice develop fatal encephalitis.[5]

EASTERN EQUINE ENCEPHALITIS VIRUS

History and Geographic Location. EEE virus was first isolated in 1933.[6] It is transmitted between birds and humans by the mosquito vector. It causes fatal encephalitis in humans along the East Coast of the United States and in some inland locations in New York, Michigan, and South Dakota.[5]

Classification. EEE is a member of the genus *Alphavirus* of the Togaviridae family.

Structure. The structure of EEE is that described earlier for members of the *Alphavirus* genus of Togaviridae.

Biologic and Biochemical Properties. EEE virus replicates well in BHK cells, Vero cells, and avian embryo cells. It causes a CPE and can be plaqued on these cells. The molecular basis of its invasiveness and virulence for children is not known.

Replication. The virus attaches to specific receptors on the surface of target cells and undergoes endocytosis.[47] RNA serves as the template for both new protein synthesis and RNA synthesis. Replication takes place in the cytoplasm.

Antigenic Characteristics. EEE shares antigenic determinants with other alphaviruses as determined by immunofluorescence, ELISA, and radioimmunoassays or complement fixation tests. It can be distinguished from other strains by neutralization or modified hemagglutination inhibition tests.[48]

Laboratory Demonstration of Infection. Virus may be isolated from serum collected early in infection[49] and from the brain of fatal cases. Serologic tests are used to demonstrate development of specific antibody during acute illness. An IgM capture ELISA can be used to confirm infection with a single specimen.[50]

WESTERN EQUINE ENCEPHALITIS VIRUS

History and Geographic Location. WEE virus was first isolated from the brain of a horse that became ill in a major epizootic outbreak in the San Joaquin Valley of California.[4] It was isolated in 1938 from the brain of a child who had died of encephalitis, and from mosquitos in 1941.[51] It is found in western North and South America.

Classification. WEE is a member of the genus *Alphavirus* in the family Togaviridae.

Structure. The structure of WEE is similar to that of EEE and other alphaviruses.

Biologic and Biochemical Properties. WEE is less neuroinvasive than EEE[51] but infects similar cells. It grows especially well in suckling mice and embryonated eggs. Analysis of the genomes of WEE, EEE, and Sindbis virus, an *Alphavirus* from the Old World, has led to the suggestion that WEE was derived from a recombination of genetic material from EEE and Sindbis virus.[52]

Replication. Replication is similar to that of EEE.

Antigenic Characteristics. WEE may be distinguished from other alphaviruses on the basis of the hemagglutination inhibition test or neutralization tests with specific antisera or monoclonal antibodies.

Laboratory Demonstration of Infection. Virus may be isolated post mortem from brain tissue. The antibody tests described for EEE may be used to demonstrate increased antibody titer or the presence of virus-specific IgM.[50] Occasionally, it can be isolated from throat swab samples or cerebrospinal fluid.[53]

VENEZUELAN EQUINE ENCEPHALITIS VIRUS

History and Geographic Location. VEE virus was isolated from the brain of a horse in an outbreak of fatal encephalomyelitis in Venezuela in 1936.[54] Having been distinguished from the already isolated EEE and WEE viruses, it was named for that country.[55] The first recognized human cases were reported in 1944 in Trinidad. Epizootic infections occurred between 1955 and 1972 with associated epidemics. In 1979, disease in humans and horses spread through northern Central America and into Texas.[56, 57]

Classification. VEE virus is a member of the genus *Alphavirus* of the family Togaviridae.

Structure. VEE virus is, like other alphaviruses, a spherical particle about 60 nm in diameter. A nucleocapsid core containing genomic RNA and nucleocapsid protein is contained within a lipid bilayer and an outer glycoprotein shell. Glycoprotein spikes on the surface are made up of trimers of the proteins E1 and E2. The genome of the virus is contained on a single strand of RNA.[46] The genome contains approximately 11,700 bases, which contain the genes for eight proteins: four nonstructural proteins, a capsid, a p62 (or E2) protein, 6K, and E1. The last four proteins, along with new RNA, are assembled into the final particle.[58]

Biologic and Biochemical Properties. VEE viruses grow well in newborn mice and in cultures of mammalian and insect cells.

Replication. Replication of VEE probably begins in lymph nodes draining the site of inoculation, and, when the central nervous system is invaded, in neural cells. The virus enters cells by a process called adsorptive endocytosis. Nucleocapsids are released, and viral RNA is uncoated for replication. Viral RNA serves as messenger RNA, and the resulting nonstructural proteins serve as catalysts for subsequent RNA transcription. The genomic RNA is also transcribed into a full length negative-sense RNA, which in turn is transcribed into a genomic positive-sense RNA. Viral structural proteins are produced by translation of a subgenomic piece of the RNA (called subgenomic RNA because it contains only the portion of the genome that codes for the structural proteins). The structural proteins are assembled into viral particles by a physical process that is driven by the nature of the proteins, their proximity to one another, and their insertion into internal cell membranes.[58]

Antigenic Characteristics. Isolates of VEE virus have been grouped into a complex containing several subtypes (I through VI) based on distinctions detectable in the hemagglutination inhibition test. Subtype I has been subdivided into variants A through F, and variants IA, IB, and IC are associated with epizootics and human cases.[5]

Laboratory Demonstration of Infection. Virus may be isolated by inoculating specimens from serum and throat swabs into suckling mice or Vero cells. Serologic diagnosis can be made using hemagglutination inhibition and neutralization tests or an IgM capture ELISA.[50, 59–61]

Bunyaviridae

The family Bunyaviridae (the name of which was derived from the name of the town in Uganda where the prototype virus, Bunyamwera virus, was isolated from mosquitos) contains more than 250 individual species in five genera. The encephalitis viruses, members of the California serogroup, cause California, Jamestown Canyon, and La Crosse encephalitis. Occasionally, a member of the phlebovirus genus, Rift Valley fever virus, has been associated with encephalitis.

History and Geographic Location. The California encephalitis virus was isolated during studies of arbovirus encephalitis in Kern County, California, in 1943. Serologic studies confirmed that it had caused three cases of viral encephalitis.[13, 62] Further cases of encephalitis caused by this virus have not been observed, but a serologically related virus, La Crosse virus, was first isolated from a fatal human case in Wisconsin in 1960,[14] and this virus has been associated with human disease across the midwestern United States.[63] Jamestown Canyon virus, discovered subsequently, has caused occasional cases of encephalitis.[64, 65]

Classification. Viruses of the Bunyaviridae family have been classified on the basis of complement fixation analysis. Cross-neutralization and hemagglutination inhibition tests have been used to develop the serogroups. Comparing different members, genomes are organized similarly and protein-coding mechanisms are similar. Molecular characteristics are used to define the genera.[66]

Structure. Bunyavirus lipid-enveloped particles contain two glycoproteins. Glycoprotein spikes, which bear type-specific antigenic determinants, protrude from a lipid membrane. Contained within the particles are three negative-sense (proteins are translated from complementary messenger RNA), single-stranded RNA molecules, each one contained in a viral nucleoprotein, and an enzyme with transcriptase activity. The virions are between 80 and 120 nm in diameter. The RNA genome has a small, a medium-sized, and a large segment. The M segment codes for the two structural glycoproteins, G1 and G2. The large, small, and medium-sized segments also code for nonstructural proteins.[66]

Biologic and Biochemical Properties. Most of these viruses are transmitted to animal hosts by arthropods.[67] They may be isolated in cell culture, in which a CPE is observed, or by suckling mouse brain inoculation. California encephalitis virus is found in the western United States and Canada and may be isolated from the principal mosquito vector, *Aedes melanimon*. The principal vertebrate hosts are rodents and rabbits. Isolation from humans is uncommon. Cultures may be propagated in mice or BHK-21 cells. La Crosse virus, which occurs in the central and eastern United States, is transmitted by *Aedes triseriatus*. The principal vertebrate hosts are chipmunks and squirrels. The virus may be isolated by inoculation of suckling mouse brains or cultivation in BHK-21 cells. Jamestown Canyon virus occurs in North America. The animal host is the white-tailed deer. Although many human infections have occurred, only a few cases of human encephalitis have been identified.[68]

Replication. Bunyaviruses attach to the surface of host cells by means of interactions between surface glycoproteins and host cells. After fusion of cell and virion membranes, the virus is uncoated. The genome RNA is transcribed into complementary messenger RNA using virion-associated polymerase. The large and small segments are translated by free ribosomes, and the medium-sized segment is translated by membrane-bound ribosomes. The genome is replicated using the previously synthesized complementary RNA. G1 and G2 proteins are glycosylated. As they accumulate in the Golgi apparatus, modified host membrane is acquired as particles bud into the Golgi cisternae. Finally, cytoplasmic vesicles fuse with the plasma membrane and virus particles are released from the cell. Virus replication slows cell protein synthesis and may or may not destroy the host cell.[66]

Antigenic Characteristics. Immune response is directed

principally against the G1 and G2 glycoproteins on the surface of the particles and the nucleoprotein capsid protein. Bunyaviruses share complement fixation antigens.[69] Blocking of viral hemagglutination by antibody forms the basis of the hemagglutination inhibition assay. Antibody that neutralizes the ability to form plaques is stimulated by infection. Monoclonal antibodies have proved useful for distinguishing isolates.[70]

Laboratory Demonstration of Infection. Rising antibody titers during the course of acute infection indicate infection by a suspected virus. Virus may be isolated post mortem from brain tissue by inoculating suckling mouse brain or by cultivating specimens in cell lines such as the BHK-21 cell line. Isolates are identified serologically.[71]

References

1. Westaway EG, Brinton MA, Gaidamovich SY, et al: Flaviviridae. Intervirology 24:183, 1985.
2. Webster LT, Fite GL: A virus encountered in the study from cases of encephalitis in the St. Louis and Kansas City epidemic of 1933. Science 78:463, 1933.
3. Mitamura T, Kitaoka M, Watanabe M, et al: Study on Japanese encephalitis virus. Animal experiments and mosquito transmission experiments. Kansai Iji 1:260, 1936.
4. Meyer KF, Harung CM, Howitt B: The etiology of epizootic encephalomyelitis of horses in the San Joaquin Valley, 1930. Science 74:227, 1931.
5. Peters CJ, Dalrymple JM: Alphaviruses. *In* Fields BN, Knipe DM (eds): Fields Virology, ed 2. New York, Raven Press, 1990, pp 713–761.
6. TenBroeck C, Merrell MH: A serological difference between eastern and western equine encephalomyelitis virus. Proc Soc Exp Biol Med 31:217, 1933.
7. Farber S, Hill A, Connerley ML, Dingle JH: Encephalitis in infants and children caused by the virus of eastern variety of equine encephalitis. JAMA 114:1725, 1940.
8. Randall R, Mills JW: Fatal encephalitis in man due to the Venezuelan virus of equine encephalomyelitis in Trinidad. Science 99:225, 1944.
9. Smorodintsev AA: Tick-borne spring-summer encephalitis. Prog Med Virol 1:210, 1958.
10. French EL: Murray Valley encephalitis: Isolation and characterization of the etiological agent. Med J Aust 1:100, 1952.
11. McLean CM, Donohue WL: Powassan virus: Isolation of virus from a fatal case of encephalitis. Can Med Assoc J 80:708, 1959.
12. Lopes O, Coimbra TLM, Sacchetta L de A, et al: Emergence of a new arbovirus disease in Brazil. I. Isolation and characterization of the etiologic agent, Rocio virus. Am J Epidemiol 107:444, 1978.
13. Reeves WC, Hammon WMcD: Epidemiology of the arthropod-borne viral encephalitides in Kern County, California, 1943–1952. Univ Calif Public Health 4:1, 1962.
14. Thompson WH, Kahlfayan B, Anslow RO: Isolation of California encephalitis group virus from a fatal human illness. Am J Epidemiol 81:245, 1965.
15. Bigger RJ, Johnson BK, Mrisoke SS, et al: Severe illness associated with appearance of antibody to human immunodeficiency virus in an African. Br Med J 293:1210, 1986.
16. Hoke CH, Nisalak A, Sangawhipa N, et al: Protection against Japanese encephalitis by formalin-inactivated vaccines. N Engl J Med 319:608, 1988.
17. Leake CJ, Burke DS, Nisalak A, Hoke CH: Isolation of Japanese encephalitis virus from clinical specimens using a continuous mosquito cell line. Am J Trop Med Hyg 35:1045, 1986.
18. McAda PC, Mason PW, Schmaljohn CS, et al: Partial nucleotide sequence of the Japanese encephalitis virus genome. Virology 158:348, 1987.
19. Sumiyoshi H, Mori C, Fuke I, et al: Complete nucleotide sequence of the Japanese encephalitis virus genome RNA. Virology 161:497, 1987.
20. Sumiyoshi H, Tignor GH, Shope RE: Characterization of a highly attenuated Japanese encephalitis virus generated from molecularly cloned cDNA. J Infect Dis 171:1144, 1995.

20a. Beatty BJ, Calisher CH, Shope RE: Arboviruses. *In* Schmidt NJ, Emmons RW (eds): Diagnostic Procedures for Viral, Rickettsial and Chlamydial Infections. Washington, DC, American Public Health Association, 1989, pp 797–856.

21. Hase T, Summers PL, Dubois DR: Ultrastructural changes of mouse brain neurons infected by Japanese encephalitis virus. Int J Exp Pathol 71:493, 1990.
22. Casals J, Brown LV. Hemagglutination with arthropod-borne viruses. J Exp Med 99:429, 1954.
23. Burke DS, Nisalak A, Ussery MA, et al: Kinetics of IgM and IgG responses to Japanese encephalitis virus in human serum and cerebrospinal fluid. J Infect Dis 151:1093, 1985.
24. Burke DS, Nisalak A, Hoke CH Jr: Field trial of a Japanese encephalitis diagnostic kit. J Med Virol 18:41, 1986.
25. Hammon W McD, Reeves, WC, Brookman B, Gjullin CM: Mosquitoes and encephalitis in the Yakima Valley, Washington. V. Summary of case against *Culex tarsalis* Coquillett as a vector of the St. Louis and western equine viruses. J Infect Dis 70:278, 1942.
26. Trent DW, Kinney RM, Johnson BJ, et al: Partial nucleotide sequence of St. Louis encephalitis virus RNA: Structural proteins, NS1, ns2a, and ns2b. Virology 156:293, 1987.
27. Karabatsos N: General characteristics and antigenic relationships. *In* Monath TP (ed): St. Louis Encephalitis. Washington, DC, American Public Health Association, 1980, pp 105–158.
28. Calisher CH, Karabatsos N, Dalrymple JM, et al: Antigenic relationships between flaviviruses as determined by cross-neutralization tests with polyclonal antisera. J Gen Virol 70:37, 1989.
29. Zilber LA, Soloviev VD: Far Eastern tick-borne spring-summer (spring) encephalitis. Annu Rev Sov Med Spec 5 (Suppl):1, 1946.
30. Smorodintsev AA: Tick-borne spring-summer encephalitis. Prog Med Virol 1:210, 1958.
31. Monath TP, Heinz FX: Flaviviruses. *In* Fields BN, Knipe DM, Howley PM, et al (eds): Fields Virology, ed 3. Philadelphia, Lippincott-Raven, 1996, pp 961–1034.
32. Calisher CH: Antigenic classification and taxonomy of flaviviruses (family Flaviviridae) emphasizing a universal system for the taxonomy. Acta Virol 32:469, 1988.
33. Pogodina VV: The resistance of tick-borne encephalitis virus to the effects of gastric juice. Vopr Virusol 3:295, 1958.
34. Pudney M, Varma MGR: The growth of some tick-borne arboviruses in cell cultures derived from tadpoles of the common frog, *Rana temporaria*. J Gen Virol 10:131, 1971.
35. Rampas J, Gallia F: The isolation of encephalitis virus from *Ixodes ricinus* ticks. Cas Lek Cesk 88:1179, 1949.
36. Pogodina VV: Experimental study of the pathogenesis of tick-borne encephalitis on alimentary infection. II. Study of pathways of excretion of virus from white mice. Probl Virol 5:304, 1960.
37. Zilber LA: Pathogenicity of Far Eastern and Western (European) tick-borne encephalitis viruses in sheep and monkeys. *In* Libikova H (ed): Biology of Viruses of the Tick-Borne Encephalitis Complex. New York, Academic Press, 1960, pp 260–265.
38. Mandl CW, Heinz FX, Kunz C: Sequence of the structural proteins of tick-borne encephalitis virus (western subtype) and comparative analysis with other flaviviruses. Virology 166:197, 1988.
39. Heinz FX, Kunz C: Molecular epidemiology of tick-borne encephalitis virus: Peptide mapping of large nonstructural proteins of European isolates and comparison with other flaviviruses. J Gen Virol 62:271, 1982.
40. Guirakhoo F, Radda AC, Heinz FX, Kunz C: Evidence for antigenic stability of tick-borne encephalitis virus by the analysis of natural isolates. J Gen Virol 68:859, 1987.
41. Rey FA, Heinz FX, Mand IC, et al: The envelope glycoprotein from tick-borne encephalitis virus at 2 Å resolution. Nature 375:291, 1995.

41a. Winkler G, Heinz FX, Kunz C: Studies on the glycosylation of flavivirus E proteins and the role of carbohydrate in antigenic structure. Virology 159:237, 1987.

42. Heinz FX, Roggendorf M, Hofmann H, Kunz C: Comparison of two different enzyme immunoassays for detection of immunoglobulin M antibodies against tick-borne encephalitis virus in serum and cerebrospinal fluid. J Clin Microbiol 14:141, 1981.
43. French EL, Anderson SG, Price AVG, et al: Murray Valley encephalitis in New Guinea. I. Isolation of Murray Valley encephalitis virus from the brain of a fatal case of encephalitis occurring in a Papuan native. Am J Trop Med Hyg 6:827, 1957.
44. Westaway EG: Assessment and application of a cell line from

pig kidney for plaque assay and neutralization tests with twelve group B arboviruses. Am J Epidemiol 84:439, 1966.
45. Marshall ID: Murray Valley and Kunjin encephalitis. *In* Monath TP (ed): The Arboviruses: Epidemiology and Ecology. Boca Raton, FL, CRC Press, 1988, pp 151–190.
46. Harrison SC: Alphavirus structure. *In* Schlesinger S, Schlesinger MJ (eds): The Togaviridae and Flaviviridae. New York, Plenum Publishing, 1986, pp 21–34.
47. Kielian M, Helenius A: Entry of alphavirus. *In* Schlesinger S, Schlesinger MJ (eds): The Togaviridae and Flaviviridae. New York, Plenum Publishing, 1986, pp 91–119.
48. Karabatsos N: Antigenic relationships of group A arboviruses by plaque reduction neutralization testing. Am J Trop Med Hyg 24:527, 1975.
49. Clarke DH: Two nonfatal human infections with the virus of eastern encephalitis. Am J Trop Med Hyg 10:67, 1961.
50. Calisher CH, El-Kafrawi AO, Al-Deen Mahmud MI, et al: Complex-specific immunoglobulin M antibody patterns in humans infected with alphaviruses. J Clin Microbiol 23:155, 1986.
51. Hayes RO: Eastern and western encephalitis. *In* Beran GW (ed): Handbook Series in Zoonoses, Section B, Viral Zoonoses, Vol 1. Boca Raton, FL, CRC Press, 1981, pp 29–57.
52. Hahn CS, Lustig S, Strauss EG, Strauss JH: Western equine encephalitis virus is a recombinant virus. Proc Natl Acad Sci USA 85:5997, 1988.
53. Rozdilsky B, Robertson HE, Chorney J: Western encephalitis: Report of eight fatal cases: Saskatchewan epidemic, 1965. Can Med Assoc J 98:79, 1968.
54. Kubes V, Rios FA: The causative agent of infectious equine encephalomyelitis in Venezuela. Science 90:20, 1939.
55. Beck CE, Wyckoff RWG: Venezuelan equine encephalitis. Science 88:530, 1938.
56. Venezuelan encephalitis. *In* Proceedings of the Workshop-Symposium on Venezuelan Encephalitis Virus. Washington, DC, Pan American Health Organization, 1972. Scientific publication 243.
57. Walton TE, Grayson MA: Venezuelan equine encephalomyelitis. *In* Monath TP (ed): The Arboviruses, Epidemiology and Ecology, Boca Raton, FL, CRC Press, 1988.
58. Schlesinger S, Schlesinger MJ: Replication of Togaviridae and Flaviviridae. *In* Fields BN, Knipe DM (eds): Fields Virology, ed 2. New York, Raven Press, 1990, pp 697–711.
59. Briceno Rossi AL: Rural epidemic encephalitis in Venezuela caused by a group A arbovirus (VEE). *In* Melnick JL (ed): Progress in Medical Virology, Vol 9. Basel, S Karger, 1967, pp 176–203.
60. Dietz WH Jr, Peralta PH, Johnson KM: Ten clinical cases of human infection with Venezuelan equine encephalomyelitis virus, subtype ID. Am J Trop Med Hyg 28:329, 1979.
61. Sanchez JL, Lednar WM, Macasaet FF, et al: Venezuelan equine encephalomyelitis: Report of an outbreak associated with jungle exposure. Mil Med 149:618, 1984.
62. Hammon W McD, Reeves WC: California encephalitis virus—A newly described agent. I. Evidence of natural infection in man and other animals. Calif Med 77:303, 1952.
63. Kappus KD, Monath TP, Kaminski RM, et al: Reported encephalitis associated with California serogroup virus infections in the United States, 1963–1981. *In* Calisher CH, Thompson WH (eds): California Serogroup Viruses. New York, Alan R Liss, 1983, pp 31–41.
64. Deibel R, Srihongse S, Grayson MA, et al: Jamestown Canyon virus: The etiologic agent of an emerging human disease? *In* Calisher CH, Thompson WH (eds): California Serogroup Viruses. New York, Alan R Liss, 1983, pp 313–328.
65. Srihongse S, Grayson MA, Deibel R: California serogroup viruses in New York State: The role of subtypes in human infections. Am J Trop Med Hyg 33:1218, 1984.
66. Schmaljohn C: Bunyaviridae: The viruses and their replication. *In* Fields BN, Knipe DM, Howley PM (eds): Fields Virology, ed 3. Philadelphia, Lippincott-Raven, 1996, pp 1447–1471.
67. Bishop DHL, Calisher C, Casals J, et al: Bunyaviridae. Intervirology 14:125, 1980.
68. Grimstad PR, Calisher CH, Haroff RN, et al: Jamestown Canyon virus (California serogroup) is the etiologic agent of widespread infection in Michigan humans. Am J Trop Med Hyg 35:376, 1984.
69. Shope RE, Causey OR: Further studies on the serological relationships of group C arthropod-borne viruses and the application of these relationships to rapid identification of types. Am J Trop Med Hyg 11:886, 1962.
70. Gonzalez-Scarano F, Shope RE, et al: Characterization of monoclonal antibodies against the G1 and N proteins of La Crosse and Tahyna, two California serogroup bunyaviruses. Virology 120:42, 1982.
71. Calisher CH, Monath TP, Karabatsos N, Trent DW: Arbovirus subtyping: Applications to epidemiologic studies, availability of reagents, and testing services. Am J Epidemiol 114:619, 1981.

269

Hemorrhagic Fever Viruses Belonging to the Families Arenaviridae, Filoviridae, and Bunyaviridae

Kelly T. McKee, Jr.

The viral hemorrhagic fevers are a group of geographically diverse diseases with generally similar clinical, pathologic, and epidemiologic features. All are caused by RNA viruses, and those covered in this chapter derive from three taxonomic families (Table 269–1). Hemorrhagic fevers caused by flaviviruses (e.g., yellow fever, dengue hemorrhagic fever, Omsk hemorrhagic fever, Kayasanur Forest disease) are considered in (Chapters 266 and 267).

As a group, hemorrhagic fever viruses cause severe, often fatal, infections in humans. They are zoonoses whose distribution is closely tied to the ecology and population biology of specific rodents or arthropod vectors. The fundamental lesion in the viral hemorrhagic fever syndrome is disruption of the vascular bed; clinical manifestations relate to consequences of microvascular damage and increased vascular permeability. Person-to-person spread has been described for most of these diseases, and clustering of cases or community outbreaks are common.

Arenavirus Disease

Lymphocytic choriomeningitis virus (LCMV), the first arenavirus to be identified, was isolated by Armstrong and Lillie in 1933.[1] Two years later it was isolated from mice, in which it was found to produce a persistent infection. Studies of the virus in animals have made fundamental contributions to immunology and viral pathogenesis. LCMV infection in humans has received little attention, however, perhaps because of its relative infrequency. The discovery of other arenaviruses highly pathogenic for humans led to more extensive clinical observations and studies of human disease caused by these agents.

At least 16 arenaviruses are currently recognized; 6 are

The views presented are those of the author and do not necessarily represent the views of the Department of Defense or its components.

TABLE 269–1 ■ Viral Hemorrhagic Fevers of Humans

FAMILY	DISEASE	GEOGRAPHY	NATURAL TRANSMISSION	MORTALITY	PERSON-TO-PERSON SPREAD
Arenaviridae	South American hemorrhagic fevers	Rural Argentina Rural Bolivia Rural Venezuela Rural (?) Brazil	Rodent→human via inhalation or contact with contaminated secreta or excreta	10%–30% (untreated)	Yes
	Lassa fever	Rural West Africa		1%–3% overall (?); 20% in hospitalized patients (untreated)	Yes
Bunyaviridae	Hemorrhagic fever with renal syndrome	Rural Asia, Far East Rural Balkans Rural Scandinavia and Western Europe Urban centers worldwide	Same as Arenaviridae	<1%–15% (strain and geography dependent)	No
	Hantavirus pulmonary syndrome	Rural Americas	Same as Arenaviridae	≈50%	No
	Crimean-Congo hemorrhagic fever	Rural Africa, west Asia, central Europe	Tick bite; inhalation or contact with blood of infected mammals	Highly variable; 15%–40% in recognized cases	Yes
Filoviridae	Ebola hemorrhagic fever, Marburg disease	Rural sub-Saharan Africa	Unknown	30%–90%	Yes

known to cause disease in humans after natural exposure: LCMV (lymphocytic choriomeningitis), Lassa fever virus (Lassa fever), Junin virus (Argentine hemorrhagic fever [AHF]), Machupo virus (Bolivian hemorrhagic fever [BHF]), Guanarito virus (Venezuelan hemorrhagic fever), and Sabia virus (no specific disease designation) (Table 269–2). Several others reportedly have caused illness in laboratory workers. When viewed under the electron microscope, all arenaviruses appear alike: pleomorphic particles averaging 110 to 130 nm in diameter, with a unit membrane and 10-nm club-shaped projections. Individual virions contain electron-dense particles thought to represent cellular ribosomes captured during the viral maturation process.[2] Two virus-specific and two ribosomal (host-derived) RNA species can be isolated from intact virions. The small (S) segment codes for the three major structural proteins of the virus: N (nucleoprotein) and (via a precursor protein [GPC]) the two membrane glycoproteins (G1 and G2). The large (L) segment codes for a protein believed to represent an RNA-dependent RNA polymerase.[3]

A novel coding strategy has been recognized for arenaviruses. Termed ambisense, the 3′ half of the S RNA codes for the N protein in the viral complementary sense, whereas the 5′ half codes for GPC in the viral sense.[4]

Epidemiology

All arenaviruses naturally pathogenic for humans are carried by rodents. Each virus is associated with a predominant host species, in which it establishes a chronic, persistent infection.[5] Chronically infected rodents shed large quantities of infectious virus in secreta and excreta (particularly saliva and urine). Arenaviruses are spread horizontally and vertically within susceptible reservoir populations. Infection of mature rodents is usually without evident effect, whereas decreased survivorship, growth, and reproduction may result from neonatal infections acquired vertically.[6, 7]

With the exception of *Mus musculus*, reservoir hosts for arenaviruses occupy rural or semirural habitats. Thus, most

TABLE 269–2 ■ Arenaviruses Pathogenic for Humans

VIRUS	DISEASE	GEOGRAPHY	PRINCIPAL RESERVOIR	CURRENT ANNUAL INCIDENCE	MORTALITY (UNTREATED)	SPECIFIC TREATMENT
Lymphocytic choriomeningitis (LCM)	LCM	Worldwide	*Mus musculus*	Unknown	<1%	None usually needed
Lassa fever	Lassa fever	West Africa	*Mastomys natalensis*	10^3–10^4	1%–3%; 20% in hospital	Ribavirin
Junin	Argentine hemorrhagic fever (HF)	Argentine pampas	*Calomys musculinus*	10^1–10^2	15%–20%	Immune plasma, ? ribavirin
Machupo	Bolivian HF	Beni Department, Bolivia	*Calomys callosus*	10^1	20%+	? Ribavirin
Guanarito	Venezuelan HF	Central plains of Venezuela	? *Sigmodon alstoni* ? *Zygodontomys brevicauda*	10^1–?10^2	20%–30%	? Ribavirin
Sabia	None designated	São Paulo State, Brazil	Unknown	Unknown	Unknown	? Ribavirin

naturally acquired arenavirus diseases occur in rural settings. Although mechanisms of transmission have not been precisely defined, evidence strongly suggests that humans become infected via percutaneous or mucous membrane inoculation with infectious virus, or inhalation of contaminated particles.

LYMPHOCYTIC CHORIOMENINGITIS

The majority of human LCMV infections have been reported from the Americas and Europe. The virus is more or less globally distributed, however, and the true extent of human illness worldwide is unknown. Early studies established the epidemiologic association of LCMV with feral rodents and subsequently house mice, particularly during the winter months.[8, 9] There has been a decline in reported human infections, thought to be due to some combination of changing virus-rodent dynamics, improvements in socioeconomic conditions, and underreporting of cases. Most cases of LCMV infection are currently identified through laboratory surveillance of neurotropic virus diseases, and through recognition of occasional outbreaks traceable to a specific source.

M. musculus is the natural reservoir for LCMV. Mice infected as newborns develop lifelong infections associated with virus shedding in secretions and excreta. Human infections are believed to occur subsequent to direct contact with infected excreta in aerosols or via inoculation of mucous membranes or abraded skin surfaces. In addition to sporadic commensal rodent-associated cases, mice and hamsters used as laboratory animals as well as pets have been repeatedly documented as sources of LCMV epidemics.[10–12] Even LCMV-infected tumors, passed in laboratory animals and subsequently infecting them, have provided a source for outbreaks.[11, 12] Person-to-person transmission of LCMV has not been documented.

LASSA FEVER

Lassa fever occurs exclusively in West Africa. Clinical disease has been documented in Sierra Leone, Liberia, and Nigeria; serologic evidence for infection has been reported from the Ivory Coast, Ghana, Senegal, Upper Volta, Mali, and Guinea. Lassa fever is an extremely common infection in endemic areas; estimates range from thousands to tens of thousands of cases annually, with no predilection for age or sex. In one study from Sierra Leone, antibody prevalence ranged from 8% to 52% and increased with age.[13] Illness/infection ratios of 9% to 26% have been suggested, but reinfection and seroreversion occur, complicating these estimates.[13] The multimammate rat *Mastomys natalensis* is the sole reservoir for Lassa virus. This common rodent is highly commensal with humans and regularly contaminates houses and peridomestic areas with infectious urine and respiratory secretions. Humans apparently become infected through contact with these infectious excreta as aerosols or fomites. Strongest associations occur for households with high rodent populations, indiscriminate food storage, and direct rodent contact.[14]

Lassa virus is transmitted from rodents to humans and from human to human, although the relative importance of each mode of spread remains poorly defined.[15, 16] Clustering of cases and seropositive subjects has been seen, but the presumed common source for exposure is usually unrecognized.[15] Person-to-person transmission of Lassa virus is well described. Infections have followed direct contact with febrile patients and via sexual transmission during incubation and convalescence. The virus has been recovered from breast milk, and transmission from nursing mothers to infants probably occurs. Nosocomial infections are well recognized, and explosive outbreaks, although uncommon, have occurred in Nigeria and Liberia.[17, 18] Experience in endemic areas indicates that application of barrier nursing and isolation practices can significantly reduce the risk of nosocomial spread.

Lassa fever is an important cause of morbidity and mortality among adults in parts of West Africa. In Sierra Leone, 10% to 16% of all adult medical hospitalizations, 39% to 47% of adult febrile admissions, and 30% of adult medical deaths were due to Lassa fever.[19] The case-fatality rate among hospitalized patients is 16% to 17%. The case-fatality rate among pregnant women is higher, reaching 30% or more during the third trimester.[20] In children, Lassa fever is similarly important. Studies suggest that more than 20% of febrile pediatric admissions in endemic areas are due to this disease; case-fatality rates in children younger than 15 years are estimated at 12% to 14%.[21]

SOUTH AMERICAN HEMORRHAGIC FEVERS

AHF is a seasonal disease endemic to the pampas of north-central Argentina. First described in 1955, the disease initially was limited to a 16,000 km^2 region of Buenos Aires Province. Since that time, however, the endemic area has expanded to the north and west, nearly eight times the area originally described; portions of three additional provinces are now involved.[22] During the 1980s, the annual incidence of AHF ranged from 200 to 500 cases, but numbers were higher in earlier decades.[23] The etiologic agent, Junin virus, is carried in nature by several field-dwelling rodent species, of which *Calomys musculinus* is the most important. Cases of AHF are diagnosed year-round, the vast majority occurring during a well-defined epidemic season lasting from February through July that coincides with autumn grain harvests and maximal rodent population densities. The male/female ratio is 4:1, with a preponderance of cases in 15 to 60-year-old males living or working in rural areas. Rodent-to-human transmission is the principal route of infection; cases are associated with inhalation of aerosols generated by mechanical grain harvesters, and exposure to linear habitats such as roadsides and fencerows inhabited by *C. musculinus*.[24, 25] Person-to-person transmission of Junin virus occurs uncommonly but is documented in sexual partners. Nosocomial transmission is rare. Infections occur in children, but relatively infrequently.

Machupo virus, the cause of BHF, exists in nature only in the Beni Department of northern Bolivia. From 1959 to 1962, nearly 500 cases of BHF were reported, with a 30% mortality rate[26]; then, between 1962 and 1964, a series of devastating epidemics in and around the community of San Joachin occurred after an influx of the principal virus reservoir, *Calomys callosus*, into the town.[27] Effective rodent surveillance and control programs subsequently eliminated epidemic BHF, and only sporadic cases have been recognized since. Although most BHF is thought to follow exposure to aerosolized urine from Machupo virus–infected rodents, case clusters in Cochabamba in 1971 and near the town of Magdalena in 1994, as well as anecdotal reports, provide strong evidence for person-to-person transmission of Machupo virus.[28, 29]

Venezuelan hemorrhagic fever was first recognized in 1989 and is known to occur only in the rural plains region of central Venezuela. From the time of its discovery until 1992, nearly 100 infections were reported; since then, few cases have been seen[30] (Tesh R, unpublished data). The epidemiologic aspects of the illness appear to be similar to those of sporadic AHF and BHF. The cotton rat *Sigmodon alstoni* was initially thought to be the natural reservoir for the etiologic agent, Guanarito virus.[31] However, more recent studies indicate that *S. alstoni* carries a virus serologically related to Guanarito (tentatively named Pirital virus), and that the cane rat *(Zygodontomys brevicauda)* is the legitimate host for Guanarito virus.[31a] Neither person-to-person nor laboratory-acquired infections with Guanarito virus have yet been reported, although there is no reason to suspect that they could not occur.

Naturally acquired Sabia virus infection has been documented only once, the virus having been recovered from a fatal human case of hemorrhagic fever in São Paulo State, Brazil.[32] The epidemiologic aspects remain undefined. Serious illness in laboratory workers exposed to aerosolized virus has validated its pathogenic potential, however.[33]

Pathogenesis

The principal target organs for arenaviruses appear to be macrophages and, to a lesser extent, vascular endothelium. Clinicopathologic manifestations stem from endogenous mediator release, extravasation of fluid into extravascular spaces, and activation of hematologic and immunologic cascades. Histopathologic findings are typically unimpressive, and, with the exception of LCMV, investigations into possible immunologic mechanisms of damage have yielded unconvincing results.

LYMPHOCYTIC CHORIOMENINGITIS

Neurologic disease in LCMV infection is believed to be immunologically mediated. Those patients with aseptic meningitis or other central nervous system lesions develop these manifestations during the second phase of a biphasic illness. Immunosuppressed patients inoculated with LCMV as experimental therapy for malignancy failed to develop neurologic disease despite high viremias and, in one case, high brain tissue titers.[34] Autopsy findings in otherwise normal patients have been remarkable for perivascular mononuclear cell infiltrates throughout the leptomeninges and brain substance.[35] Viral antigen is observed in the meninges and cortical cells by immunofluorescence (IF), consistent with virus replication in the central nervous system.

LASSA FEVER

Infection with Lassa virus results in widespread dissemination of virus, but damage is limited to focal hepatic necrosis without significant inflammatory response, some evidence of interstitial pneumonitis, and occasional focal adrenal cortical necrosis.[36] Liver damage is variable, with concomitant cellular injury, necrosis, and regeneration. Histopathologic changes are insufficient in themselves to account for death, however.

Outcome in Lassa fever correlates with the degree of virus replication[37] (Fig. 269–1). Increases of serum aspartate aminotransferase levels to greater than 150 IU/L, but not of other hepatic enzymes, are also associated with a poor prognosis[19, 37] (see Fig. 269–1). Cardiac involvement has been limited to hemorrhage and lymphocytic infiltrates in the pericardium, and occasional interstitial myocarditis. The severe retrosternal or epigastric pain present in many patients may be due to pleural or pericardial involvement.

Increased vascular permeability is significant. Important clinical events in fatal disease are a consequence of endothelial and platelet dysfunction (despite adequate numbers of circulating platelets).[38, 39] An inhibitor of platelet function has been identified in the serum of nonhuman primates and of patients with severe Lassa fever, specifically inhibiting platelet-dense granule and adenosine triphosphate release[40] and also suppressing superoxide generation in neutrophils.[41] Platelet and fibrinogen turnover is normal, and there is no increase in fibrinogen breakdown products[42]; therefore, disseminated intravascular coagulation is not significant.

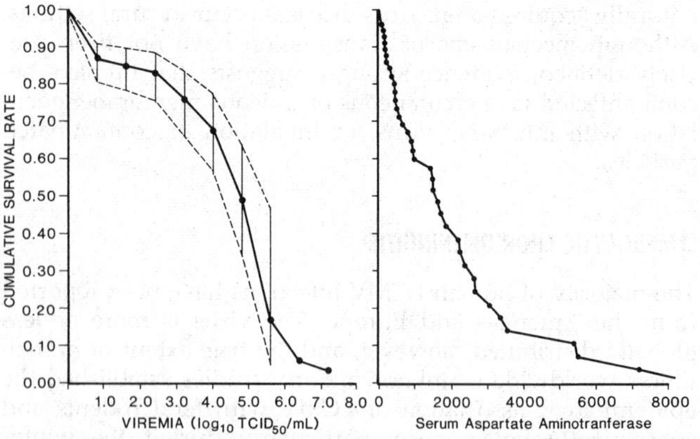

FIGURE 269–1 ▫ Relationship between viremia and aspartate aminotransferase (AST) levels in serum and outcome of Lassa fever by survival analysis. (Data from McCormick JB, King IJ, Webb PA, et al: A case-control study of the clinical diagnosis and course of Lassa fever. J Infect Dis 155:445–455, 1987; and Johnson KM, McCormick JB, Webb PA, et al: Clinical virology of Lassa fever in hospitalized patients. J Infect Dis 155:456–464, 1987.)

SOUTH AMERICAN HEMORRHAGIC FEVERS

Infection with Junin, Machupo, and Guanarito viruses produce similar lesions in humans. Multiple organs are involved, with changes most evident in the vascular, lymphoreticular, hematologic, and central nervous systems. Bleeding, rash, and extravasation of fluid into the soft tissues of the face implicate vascular damage complicated by thrombocytopenia as important elements in pathogenesis. Proteinuria is common, and renal tubular involvement is seen pathologically.[43] Macrophages and lymphocytes contain viral particles and antigen, although the mechanism of their destruction remains undefined.[44] Interferon-α levels in AHF are extremely high, ranging from 1000 to 16,000 IU/mL[45]; higher levels correlate with poor prognosis.[46] It is likely that the high and prolonged levels of circulating interferon are responsible for many of the clinical and pathologic changes observed, although a variety of other mediators (e.g., tumor necrosis factor-α) are likely candidates as well.[47] Involvement of the central nervous system is frequent; both neuroinvasion and neurovirulence have been demonstrated in animal models of these infections, and the occurrence of a late neurologic syndrome in AHF patients after treatment with immune plasma (see later) points to viral invasion of the brain in humans.[48]

Clinical Features

LYMPHOCYTIC CHORIOMENINGITIS

Lymphocytic choriomeningitis in humans follows an incubation period of 1 to 3 weeks.[8] In the largest existing study of human LCMV infections, 33 of 94 (35%) were asymptomatic, 47 (50%) were mild to moderate febrile illnesses without significant central nervous system manifestations, and 14 (15%) were typical lymphocytic choriomeningitis.[49] The typical disease begins with fever, malaise, weakness, anorexia, nausea, myalgia, and severe, often retroorbital, headache with photophobia. Fifty percent of patients may have sore throat, vomiting, or arthralgias; chest pain and pneumonitis occur less frequently. Alopecia, parotitis, orchitis, and transient arthritis of the hands have been reported. Physical examination shows pharyngeal inflammation, usually without exudate.

This phase lasts about 1 week, with a remission for a few days, which is then followed by a second and occasionally a third wave of fever. During these later febrile periods, neurologic involvement occurs. Most neurologic disease presents as aseptic meningitis, and about a third of these patients develop encephalopathy. Cerebrospinal fluid from patients with meningeal signs contains several hundred white cells per cubic millimeter, predominantly lymphocytes (>80%), with mildly increased protein and occasionally low glucose levels. Virus is often found in cerebrospinal fluid taken during the acute phase of disease.[50] Although rarely fatal, the disease can be severe, necessitating hospitalization, and a prolonged convalescence with persistent fatigue, somnolence, and dizziness. Neurologic sequelae are unusual but have been reported,[51] including a single reported case of permanent unilateral deafness similar to that associated with Lassa fever.[52] Infection with LCMV in pregnancy can result in fetal or early neonatal death, as well as microcephaly, hydrocephalus, chorioretinitis, and psychomotor retardation.[53, 54] A Lassa fever–like syndrome has been reported once.[55]

LASSA FEVER

The onset of Lassa fever is subtle. After an incubation period of 8 to 14 days (3 weeks at most), patients note the gradual onset of fever, malaise, and headache. During a period of several days, sore throat, myalgia, arthralgia, epigastric or retrosternal pain, severe frontal headache, and dry cough develop. By the end of the first week, patients are highly febrile and in a toxic condition. Conjunctivitis, lymphadenopathy, abdominal and muscle tenderness, hypotension, and relative bradycardia may be found at physical examination. A painful purulent pharyngitis is found in about 40% of cases and is sometimes associated with vesicles or ulcers. There is no characteristic rash, and neither cutaneous hemorrhages nor jaundice is seen early in the disease. With disease progression, edema of the face and neck and evidence of fluid buildup in the lungs occur. Hemorrhage is associated with fatal outcome but occurs in only 15% to 20% of patients; most often bleeding is from the gums and nose, less frequently from the gastrointestinal tract or vagina. About a fifth of patients have pleural or pericardial rubs.

Neurologic signs are infrequent; stupor, coma, and convulsions, as well as hemorrhage and severe hypotension, portend a poor prognosis. The duration of illness is typically about a month in survivors. Recovery is slow, and convalescence may be complicated by pericarditis, orchitis, uveitis, pleural effusion, or ascites. Acute-onset eighth cranial nerve deafness develops in up to 25% of patients and may be permanent.[56]

Lassa fever is particularly hazardous for pregnant women. The risk of death during the third trimester is nearly six times that during the first two.[20] Spontaneous or therapeutic abortion improves outcome, but fetal and perinatal wastage is high. Lassa fever in infants and extremely young children may present a "swollen baby" picture due to diffuse edema and abdominal distention.[57] In older children, cough and gastrointestinal symptoms may dominate the clinical picture.

Most clinical laboratory studies in Lassa fever are not diagnostically useful. Leukopenia may be present early, but normal or elevated white cell counts are more typical as the disease progresses. Platelet counts are normal or elevated, although platelets themselves are dysfunctional. Proteinuria is inconsistent. High serum viremia (>$10^{3.6}$ $TCID_{50}$ [median tissue culture infective doses] per mL) and aspartate aminotransferase values higher than 150 IU/L are associated with poor outcomes (50% and 73% mortality, respectively; 80% if both factors coexist).[37, 58]

Differentiating Lassa fever from arbovirus diseases, malaria, typhoid fever, and other febrile illnesses common to West Africa is difficult on clinical grounds. Triads of pharyngitis, retrosternal pain, and proteinuria, or pharyngitis, retrosternal pain, and vomiting, yielded the best combinations of sensitivity, specificity, and positive predictive value in a single published case-control study from Sierra Leone.[19]

SOUTH AMERICAN HEMORRHAGIC FEVERS

The clinical features of AHF, BHF, and Venezuelan hemorrhagic fever are remarkably similar.[24, 30, 59] Between 1 and 2 weeks after exposure to the virus, patients experience the gradual onset of fever, malaise, anorexia, and myalgia. Shortly afterward, headache, back pain, epigastric pain, dizziness, and gastrointestinal disturbances appear. Vascular phenomena such as flushing of the face and chest, conjunctival injection, and orthostatic hypotension become apparent. Cutaneous petechiae are seen in the majority of patients, most frequently involving the axillae and palate. Congestion and bleeding of the gums are common. The appearance of a hemorrhagic gingival margin at the point of dental insertion is a characteristic finding. Neurologic changes are almost universally present, with diminished deep tendon reflexes, tremors (particularly of the tongue), lethargy, and hyperesthesia being seen most often. Most patients improve after 7 to 10 days and go on to an uneventful recovery. However, in the more severely ill (about 30% of the total), the disease evolves along one of three fairly distinctive lines: (1) a pronounced hemorrhagic diathesis manifested by diffuse ecchymoses and bleeding from mucous membranes and puncture sites; (2) a neurologic syndrome characterized by delirium, obtundation, coma, and convulsions; or (3) a mixed hemorrhagic-neurologic syndrome with shock. If the disease is untreated, overall mortality may be as high as 20% to 30%.

Leukopenia (cell count of <4000/mm^3 with lymphocytes and neutrophils proportionally affected) and thrombocytopenia (cell count of <100,000/mm^3) are virtually invariable. Proteinuria is extremely common and may be accompanied by microscopic hematuria. Serum enzyme and renal function studies are not seriously abnormal, and routine clotting studies are within normal ranges except in severe cases. As in Lassa fever and lymphocytic choriomeningitis, convalescence is prolonged (3 to 6 weeks) and is characterized by weakness, weight loss, autonomic instability, and occassional alopecia.[60]

Diagnosis

Arenavirus infections are traditionally diagnosed by demonstration of a fourfold rise in virus-specific antibody titer, isolation of virus, or demonstration of high-titer immunoglobulin (Ig) G antibody and virus-specific IgM antibody in association with a compatible clinical illness.[61] Antigens may be prepared and inactivated so that serologic diagnosis can be performed without high-level safety precautions. Antibodies detectable by IF or enzyme immunoassay (EIA) appear earlier in illness in Lassa fever and lymphocytic choriomeningitis (within 1 to 2 weeks) than in South American hemorrhagic fevers (usually during the third week). Neutralizing antibodies are reliably detected in AHF and BHF after day 21 but are inconsistent and difficult to detect in Lassa fever and lymphocytic choriomeningitis.

Virus isolation is best performed by inoculation of body fluids or tissue samples onto Vero or other susceptible cell cultures and then staining of infected cells at periodic intervals using specific antisera for identification. Virus is readily recovered early in disease from serum in Lassa fever patients (and often from throat washing and urine) but is lower in titer and more difficult to detect in South American arenavirus infections. In patients with AHF, cocultivation of peripheral blood mononuclear cells with susceptible cell lines improves yields considerably.[62] Antigen detection by EIA has proved useful for Lassa fever and Machupo virus infections in humans.[28, 63] Application of newer technologies such as reverse transcription–polymerase chain reaction holds great promise for diagnosis of arenavirus infections in the future.[64]

Treatment

Fundamental to management of all arenavirus hemorrhagic fevers is careful attention to and correction of fluid, electrolyte, and osmotic disturbances that accompany these infections. Even vigorous support of these imbalances, however, may be insufficient in itself to prevent progression to death. Fortunately, advances in specific treatment for many arenavirus diseases have been made that have significantly improved outcome.

Administration of convalescent immune plasma has proved to be effective in treatment for AHF when given within the first 8 days of illness.[65] Therapeutic efficacy correlates with the amount of neutralizing antibody delivered[66, 67] (Table 269–3). Use of immune plasma has reduced mortality in AHF from 15% to 20% to less than 1% among patients treated within 8 days of disease onset. A curious side effect of immune plasma therapy has been the occurrence of a late neurologic syndrome of uncertain cause in about 10% of treated survivors.[65] This condition, characterized by fever, headache, ataxia, and intention tremors, begins 4 to 6 weeks after plasma treatment but is generally benign.

Ribavirin is effective in treating Lassa fever.[58] Although dosing by both oral and intravenous routes reduces mortality, parenterally administered drug is more effective. Optimal benefit is derived within the first 6 days of illness (Table 269–4). Preliminary studies of ribavirin in AHF have suggested benefit,[68] and the drug has been successfully used under compassionate protocol to treat patients with BHF[28] and Sabia virus infection.[33]

Prevention

On the basis of principles developed and implemented during BHF outbreaks of the 1960s,[69] surveillance and control of rodents in communities of the Bolivian Beni Department have effectively eliminated epidemic disease. The sylvatic nature of the reservoirs for Junin and Guanarito viruses make rodent population control to prevent AHF and VHF (and sporadic BHF) impractical, however. Similarly, control of rodents to prevent Lassa fever is not feasible.

A live attenuated vaccine against AHF has been developed and extensively tested in the United States and Argentina.[70] This vaccine, Candid No. 1, proved effective in preventing AHF under conditions of natural exposure in a double-blind, placebo-controlled field trial conducted in the AHF endemic area (McKee K, Maiztegui J, Enria D, et al, unpublished data). The vaccine has subsequently been administered to more than 100,000 persons in the endemic area without significant adverse effect.[71] Fewer than 10 cases of AHF have occurred to date among Candid No. 1 vaccines, and there has been a sharp drop in reported incidence of disease since implementation of widespread immunization (Enria D, unpublished data). Candid No. 1 also proved effective in prophylaxis against BHF in a rhesus macaque model of this infection (Jahrling PB, unpublished data), but its utility has not yet been assessed for disease prevention in Bolivia. Interestingly, the vaccine was of no benefit in animal model infection with Guanarito virus (Jahrling PB, unpublished data). A molecularly engineered Lassa fever virus vaccine has been developed and tested in animal models, but has not yet been evaluated in humans.[72]

In the event of significant exposure (e.g., needlestick or intimate personal contact) to Lassa virus (or any other pathogenic arenavirus), it has been recommended that oral ribavirin, 500 mg four times daily for 7 days, be administered.[73] The efficacy of this prophylactic regimen is unproved, however, and close monitoring of disease contacts for at least one normal incubation period, with initiation of therapy at the first sign of illness, represents an acceptable alternative.

TABLE 269–3 ■ Immune Plasma Therapy for Argentine Hemorrhagic Fever

EFFECT OF DAY OF THERAPY ON OUTCOME			
	<8 Days' Illness	>8 Days' Illness	
Fatality	1%	16%	
EFFECT OF DOSE*			
	1000–2000 TU	2000–3000 TU	>3000 TU
Fatality	8.3%	2.5%	0.8%

*Therapeutic units (TU): Σ (neutralizing antibody titer × plasma volume)/body weight (kg).

Data from Maiztegui JI, Fernandez NJ, de Damilano AJ: Efficacy of immune plasma in treatment of Argentine haemorrhagic fever and association between treatment and a late neurological syndrome. Lancet 2:1216–1217, 1979; and Enria D, France SG, Ambrosio A, et al: Current status of the treatment of Argentine hemorrhagic fever. Med Microbiol Immunol 175:173–176, 1986.

TABLE 269–4 ■ Ribavirin Therapy for Lassa Fever*

THERAPY	RISK FACTOR† Admission Viremia $10^{3.6}$ $TCID_{50}$/mL	Admission AST >150 IU/L
Treatment Within 6 Days of Onset of Illness		
None	15/20 (75%)	11/18 (61%)
Ribavirin PO	1/5 (20%)	1/5 (20%)
Ribavirin IV	1/11 (9%)	1/20 (5%)
Plasma	5/9 (56%)	6/16 (38%)
Treatment After 6 Days of Onset of Illness		
None	21/27 (78%)	22/44 (52%)
Ribavirin PO	2/5 (40%)	1/9 (11%)
Ribavirin IV	9/19 (47%)	11/43 (26%)
Plasma	7/12 (58%)	8/66 (66%)

*AST, Aspartate aminotransferase; $TCID_{50}$, median tissue culture infective dose; PO, by mouth; IV, intravenously.

†Number of deaths/total number of patients (% fatal).

Data from McCormick JB, King IJ, Webb PA, et al: Lassa fever. Effective therapy with ribavirin. N Engl J Med 314:20–26, 1986.

Hemorrhagic Fever with Renal Syndrome

Hemorrhagic fever with renal syndrome (HFRS) gained widespread attention as a serious and frequently fatal affliction of United Nations forces during the Korean War.[74] However, syndromes of fever, hematologic abnormality, and renal dysfunction had actually been recognized as distinct clinical entities throughout the Far East, Scandinavia, and central Europe for many years previously. In 1953, Gadjusek[75] noted clinical and epidemiologic similarities among these geographically diverse disorders and proposed a common cause. The causative agent of HFRS in Korea, Hantaan virus, was identified by Lee and Lee in 1976 through demonstration of antigen in the lungs of infected reservoir rodents, the striped field mouse *(Apodemus agrarius)*.[76, 77] Hantaan virus, together with similar but serologically distinct viruses recovered from humans and rodents worldwide, possesses the morphologic and biochemical characteristics of members of the Bunyaviridae family and represents a distinct genus within this large family.[78–80]

Hantaviruses are lipid-enveloped, negative-stranded RNA viruses with tripartite genomes.[80, 81] The medium-sized (M) RNA segment contains the gene encoding two envelope glycoproteins (G1 and G2); the L segment encodes the viral polymerase and the S segment encodes the nucleoprotein.[82, 83] Virus particles are typically spherical to oval, with diameters ranging from 80 to 115 nm.[78, 84] At least 11 hantaviruses are currently recognized, 8 of which have been linked definitively to human disease[85] (Table 269–5). All hantaviruses described to date are associated with a predominant rodent host in which they establish chronic inapparent infections.[86]

Epidemiology

The epidemiology of hantavirus infections is tightly linked to the ecology, population dynamics, and distribution of the various rodent reservoirs. Within endemic areas, circumscribed foci or microfoci of rodent infection and human disease are seen.[87] Chronically infected animals shed large amounts of virus in saliva, urine, and feces. It is thought that humans become infected through contact with these contaminated secreta and excreta via inhalation of small-particle aerosols or contact of mucous membrane or nonintact skin with infectious materials. Human HFRS cases number in the tens to thousands annually, depending on the infecting virus and the geographic setting.

With the exception of Seoul virus infections, HFRS is a rural disease. Hantaan virus circulates across eastern Russia, China, and the Korean peninsula, carried by the striped field mouse.[88] The bank vole *(Clethrionomys glareolus)* serves as principal reservoir for Puumala virus, the etiologic agent of HFRS in Scandinavia, northern Europe, and Russia west of the Ural Mountains.[88, 89] In the Balkans, HFRS has been associated with at least three viruses: Puumala, Hantaan, and Dobrava (also known as Belgrade), the last two being carried primarily by the yellow-necked field mouse *Apodemus flavicollis.*[90–92] *Rattus* species are hosts for Seoul-like viruses distributed worldwide; human infections are most frequently seen in eastern Asia. Inapparent infections of laboratory rats with Seoul-like viruses have resulted in outbreaks of severe and sometimes fatal HFRS among animal handlers, scientists, and others exposed to cages housing infected animals.[93]

In the United States, at least five hantaviruses are known to circulate: Seoul (or Seoul-like) virus, Prospect Hill virus, Sin Nombre virus, New York-1 virus, and Black Creek Canal virus. Seoul-like agents have been associated with human infections in several urban centers, but significant disease not been recognized.[94–96] Antibodies to Prospect Hill virus, associated with the meadow vole *Microtus pennsylvanicus,* have been found in selected groups (e.g., mammologists), but no association with human illness has been made.[97] In November 1993, a new hantavirus serotype, associated with a highly lethal disease now known as hantavirus pulmonary syndrome (HPS), was identified in deer mice *(Peromyscus maniculatus)* captured in the Four Corners area of the Southwest.[98–100] This virus, currently named Sin Nombre (formerly Four Corners, or Muerto Canyon, virus), has been shown to be well established in reservoir populations and is more closely related phylogenetically to Prospect Hill and Puumula viruses than to other hantaviruses.[98] Sin Nombre virus has been linked to more than 100 cases of HPS from at least 20 states, the vast majority of which lie within the recognized distribution of *P. maniculatus* (Fig. 269–2). Cases of HPS have also been identified outside the known range of *P. maniculatus,* leading to discovery and evidence of additional hantaviruses related to, but distinct from, Sin Nombre virus.[101–104] Clinical HPS is being increasingly recognized elsewhere in the Americas as well (e.g., Canada, Brazil, Argentina)[105] (Peters C, Enria D, personal communications, 1995).

HFRS is a seasonal disease, although individual cases are seen year-round.[89, 93] Far Eastern HFRS and Balkan HFRS occur primarily during the late fall and early winter, with smaller peaks in the spring and summer. Most European HFRS occurs between the late summer and early winter. Men 20 to 50 years of age occupationally or recreationally active in rural settings are most often affected, with agricultural workers, foresters, and soldiers in the field being at greatest risk for exposure. Infections due to Seoul (rat-borne) virus tend to occur more frequently during the warmer months and are more evenly distributed among the age and sex classes than are rural hantavirus infections, presumably because the reservoir predominates in peridomestic settings. In the United States, HPS has been seen primarily during the spring and early summer months.[104] Cases have been about equally distributed between the sexes, and the ages of those affected has ranged from 12 to 69 years (the majority being 20 to 40 years old).[103, 104]

Pathogenesis

The portal of viral entry is the respiratory tract (via inhalation) or mucous membranes and nonintact skin (via direct

TABLE 269–5 ■ Hantaviruses

VIRUS STRAIN	PRINCIPAL RESERVOIR	DISTRIBUTION	CLINICAL FORM
Hantaan	*Apodemus agrarius*	Northern Asia Far East	Severe hemorrhagic fever with renal syndrome (HFRS)
	Apodemus flavicollis	Balkans	
Seoul	*Rattus norvegicus, Rattus rattus*	Worldwide	Mild or moderate HFRS
Puumala	*Clethrionomys glareolus*	Scandinavia Northern Europe Balkans	Nephropathia epidemica (mild HFRS)
Dobrava/Belgrade	*A. flavicollis*	Balkans	Severe HFRS
Prospect Hill	*Microtus pennsylvanicus*	United States	None recognized
Sin Nombre*	*Peromyscus maniculatus*	United States	Hantavirus pulmonary syndrome (HPS)
New York-1	*Peromyscus leucopus*	United States	HPS
Black Creek Canal	*Sigmodon hispidus*	United States	HPS
Andes	Unknown	South America	HPS
Thottapalayam	*Suncus murinus*	India	None recognized
Thailand	*Bandicota indica*	Thailand	None recognized

*Also known as Muerto Canyon and Four Corners virus.

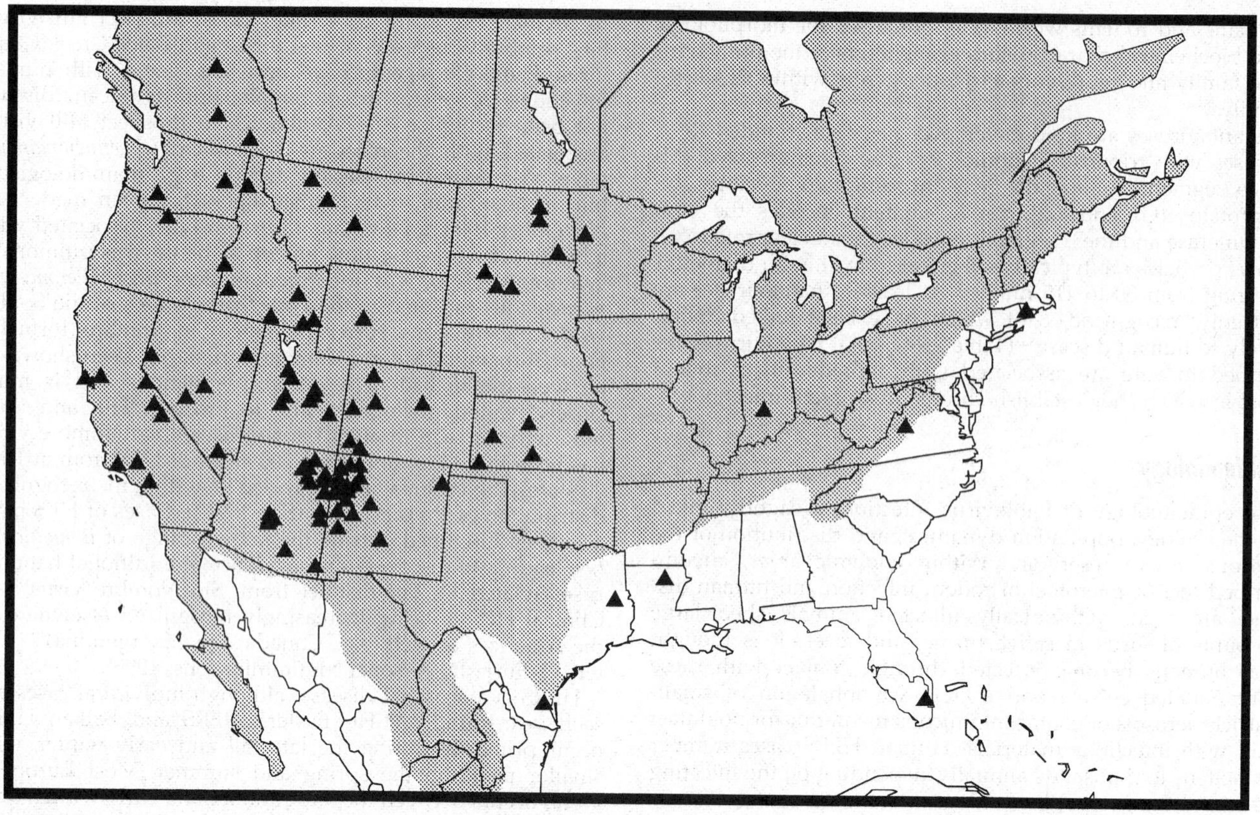

FIGURE 269–2 □ Geographic distribution of the deer mouse *Peromyscus maniculatus (shaded area)* and locations of confirmed human hantavirus pulmonary syndrome cases through February 1995. (Courtesy of Dr. Jim Mills and Ms. Judith Graber, Centers for Disease Control and Prevention, Atlanta, GA.)

contact or inoculation). Serum antibodies develop within 3 to 7 days of clinical presentation, and virus can be detected for 7 to 10 days after onset of illness from peripheral blood mononuclear cells (and possibly plasma).[106, 107] The renal, hematologic, and cardiovascular systems are most severely affected in HFRS caused by all but Sin Nombre virus. Pathologic changes in fatal cases of "classic" (non-HPS) HFRS involve multiple organ systems, but a triad of lesions consisting of hemorrhagic necrosis of the renal medulla, anterior pituitary, and cardiac right atrium is characteristic.[108] In HPS, few changes in the kidneys, brain, and heart have been observed; rather, the predominant findings at autopsy have involved the lungs. Pulmonary edema with large serous pleural effusions dominate the gross findings, with intraalveolar edema, interstitial mononuclear infiltrates, and focal hyaline membrane formation observed microscopically.[103, 109, 110] Interestingly, retroperitoneal effusions seen almost universally in classic HFRS are absent in HPS.

The underlying pathologic abnormality in human hantavirus infection is vascular endothelial damage. Although the cause of injury is unknown, both direct (cytopathic) and indirect (immune-mediated) mechanisms have been implicated. With endothelial compromise, capillaries and small blood vessels become grossly dilated; this leads to extravasation of fluid and, to a lesser extent, cellular elements, into surrounding tissues. Vascular dysregulation and release of soluble factors acting on hematologic and immunologic systems occur as well. The clinical features of classic HFRS, including flushing, facial edema, conjunctival effusion and injection, pulmonary edema, and petechiae, are manifestations of this generalized capillary and small vessel damage. The peculiar distribution of the triad lesions is poorly understood but probably reflects susceptibility of these organ sites to the volume shifts, pressure necrosis, and anoxia resulting from multisystem vascular insults. Selective damage to the pulmonary vascular bed observed in HPS is unexplained at present but suggests that cellular tropisms of Sin Nombre and related viruses differ from those of hantaviruses causing classic HFRS.

Clinical Features

HFRS is a complex, multiphasic disorder.[111–113] A spectrum of clinical severity, ranging from asymptomatic or mild disease to fulminant hemorrhagic fever or pulmonary failure and death, may be seen (Table 269–6). The incubation period ranges from 4 to 42 days, but most cases of HFRS (and presumably HPS) occur within 2 to 3 weeks after exposure. In classic HFRS caused by Hantaan virus, five phases of disease have been described: febrile, hypotensive, oliguric, diuretic, and convalescent. The phases often overlap or blend together, however. Prodromal symptoms are infrequent, and illness onset is typically abrupt. Presenting signs and symptoms include high temperature, chills, malaise, myalgias, headache, dizziness, and anorexia. Shortly afterward, severe back and abdominal pain appears, leading often to misdiagnosis as an acute abdomen. Erythematous facial flushing extending often to the neck, shoulders, and upper thorax is characteristic and is accompanied by periorbital swelling and conjunctival, palatal, and pharyngeal injection. Petechiae are frequently present on the soft palate and axillae. As the disease progresses, white cell counts gradually rise, platelet counts begin to drop, and protein becomes increasingly evident in the urine.

Within a week, a period of hypotension will ensue, beginning abruptly and coinciding with defervescence. The fall in

TABLE 269–6 ■ Clinical Features of Human Pathogenic Hantavirus Infections*

VIRUS	OVERALL SEVERITY	COMPLEXITY	SYSTEM AFFECTED: Renal	SYSTEM AFFECTED: Pulmonary	HEMORRHAGIC PHENOMENA	MORTALITY
Hantaan	2+–4+	Multiphasic	4+	1+–2+	1+–4+	1%–15%
Seoul	1+–3+	Multiphasic (blurred)	2+	0–1+	1+–2+	~1%
Puumala	1+–2+†	Biphasic	1+–2+	0–1+	0–1+	<1%
Dobrava/Belgrade	1+–4+‡	Multiphasic	4+‡	1+–2+‡	>10%‡	Unknown
Prospect Hill	0	NA	0	0	0	None observed
Sin Nombre	3+–4+	Biphasic	0–1+	4+	0–1+	~50%

*Scale 0–4+: assignments based on reported findings relative to other clinical types; NA, not available.
†Reports indicate that severe clinical forms of Puumala infection exist.
‡Association with human disease is not definitively established.

blood pressure may be acompanied in severe cases by typical signs of hypotensive shock: tachycardia, cold and clammy skin, and mental changes. By this stage, laboratory abnormalities are striking: leukocytosis with a marked shift to the left, profound thrombocytopenia, and massive proteinuria with hematuria. Although potentially serious, the hypotensive phase generally is brief: hours to a few days. Most patients then develop oliguria. The degree of oliguria varies from patient to patient, and output may decrease to the point of anuria in severely affected individuals. Pulmonary edema may suddenly appear. Serum urea nitrogen and creatinine levels may rise to extraordinary levels and are accompanied by metabolic changes typical of renal insufficiency. Dialysis at this point may be lifesaving. A more profound bleeding diathesis may supervene, resulting in potentially lethal pulmonary, gastrointestinal, or intracranial hemorrhages.

After 3 to 7 days, renal function is restored spontaneously, and patients enter a period of diuresis. Urine outputs typically exceed 5 to 6 L/d, and electrolyte disturbances consequent to massive diuresis may hazard recovery. Convalescence is prolonged, with complete clinical recovery often requiring several months. Anemia and hyposthenuria often persist for many months or years. Permanent sequelae of clinical significance are uncommon, but abnormalities in renal function have been described in a number of survivors years after infection, and evidence exists for an association with hypertensive renal disease.[114]

Severe HFRS occuring in the Balkan states is similar clinically to Hantaan virus disease. Seoul virus infections generally are somewhat milder than that just described, but fatalities have been reported. The syndrome associated with Puumala virus, nephropathia epidemica, is usually milder still and only rarely fatal; however, severe HFRS associated with Puumala-like strains has been reported from Germany and elsewhere.[115]

HPS, recognized in the United States since 1993, is a much more serious, life-threatening disorder with considerable morbidity and high mortality. In contrast to previously recognized hantavirus clinical syndromes, asymptomatic or mild infections appear to be infrequent.[103] The signs and symptoms of Sin Nombre and related virus infections are referable to the cardiopulmonary system; renal abnormalities are absent or insignificant in most cases. During the 3- to 6-day prodromal phase of HPS, fever and myalgia are almost universally present. Gastrointestinal distress, headache, and dizziness may be observed, but respiratory symptoms are generally absent early in the disease process. The prodrome is followed by a cardiopulmonary phase, heralded by progressive dyspnea and cough. Tachypnea and tachycardia accompany the preexisting fever, and hypotension occurs. Signs of generalized vascular dysregulation (flushing, injection, petechiae), so typical of classic HFRS, are conspicuously absent. Leukocytosis is common in HPS, and a left shift in the differential count (with or without leukocytosis) is frequent as well. Thrombocytopenia may also be seen but is not always present early. Atypical lymphocytes are visible in peripheral blood smears. Although mild proteinuria is frequent, frank renal insufficiency is rare.

Progressive hypoxemia and pulmonary edema requiring intubation and assisted ventilation have characterized the vast majority of HPS cases confirmed to date. The case-fatality rate in the first 17 cases described was greater than 75%; deaths were generally subsequent to cardiac dysrhythmias due to intractable hypotension 2 to 16 days after disease onset.[109] Mortality among more recently diagnosed cases is somewhat lower (45%), presumably because of increased disease awareness and consequent recognition of less severe cases.[104] Convalescence among survivors is characterized by an often rapid improvement in oxygenation and return to normal hemodynamic function. Long-term sequelae of HPS have not been described.

Diagnosis

A high index of suspicion is vital to early recognition of human hantavirus infection. The differential diagnosis of classic HFRS includes rickettsial, leptospiral, meningococcal, other viral, and poststreptococcal syndromes. Initial signs and symptoms mimic an acute intraabdominal process in some cases. The presentation of HPS may suggest pneumococcal pneumonia and sepsis, pneumonic plague, tularemia, legionellosis, histoplasmosis (or other fungal pulmonary infection), mycoplasmal pneumonia, psittacosis, or severe rickettsial disease. Laboratory diagnosis is made by demonstration of specific hantavirus IgM antibodies in acute serum by EIA, or a fourfold or greater rise in virus-specific IgG antibodies by EIA or IF.[100, 116] Purified recombinant hantavirus antigens have been produced for use in both EIA and Western blot assays, enhancing diagnostic specificity.[117–119] Neutralizing antibody tests are highly specific but are impractical for clinical use. Hantaviral antigens can be detected in tissues by immunohistochemical techniques,[110] and the availability of nucleic acid primers from several hantavirus strains has enabled amplification of nucleotide sequences from fresh or frozen tissues by reverse transcription–polymerase chain reaction.[98]

Isolation of hantaviruses from human specimens is difficult and technically demanding. Several cell lines are susceptible (e.g., Vero E-6, A549), and specific strains also grow in newborn mice, rats, and gerbils. Because of their aerosol infectivity, any attempts at isolation of hantaviruses should be made only under appropriately high levels of biocontainment (level 3 or 4).

Treatment

Close monitoring with emphasis on volume balance and electrolyte status is fundamental to successful treatment of HFRS. Early hospitalization, bed rest, and avoidance of trauma are necessary to minimize disruption of fragile vascular beds. Patients with severe classic HFRS and all cases of HPS should be managed in an intensive care environment. With classic HFRS, wide fluctuations in volume requirements often occur. Careful fluid restriction is necessary early in the disease; massive inputs to cover losses may be required later during diuretic periods. Severe renal failure with attendant fluid and metabolic complications should be anticipated in seriously ill patients; peritoneal dialysis or hemodialysis can be lifesaving.[102, 113]

In HPS, the goal of supportive therapy is maintenance of oxygenation and tissue perfusion. Hypoxemia should be managed through oxygen supplementation, with use of mechanical ventilation as necessary. Fluid input should be restricted expectantly. In light of capillary fragility, use of inotropic agents in lieu of fluids has been suggested to maintain tissue perfusion.[103]

Hantaviruses are susceptible in vitro to ribavirin. When given early in disease, intravenous ribavirin has been shown to reduce mortality and to reduce severity of renal dysfunction and hemorrhage in Chinese HFRS patients.[120] Although ribavirin has been used to treat patients with HPS through an open-label trial, confirmation of its effectiveness in this syndrome remains lacking.

Isolation of patients with HFRS (and presumably HPS, although experience is limited) is unnecessary, even under conditions of severe hemorrhage. Neither viremia nor virus shedding at the time of clinical presentation is easily demonstrated, and person-to-person transmission of hantaviruses has not been documented. Use of universal precautions in handling blood and body fluids is prudent, however. Physical barriers and respiratory protection should be employed when clinical procedures or specimen processing is likely to generate aerosols.

Prevention

The prevalence and ubiquity of reservoirs make rodent population control impractical in the field. However, measures to minimize infestations in peridomestic settings coupled with general guidelines for avoidance of rodents and their excreta should reduce exposure risk. Insecticides should be utilized simultaneously with rodent extermination techniques to control fleas, which may serve as vectors for other human pathogens (e.g., *Yersinia pestis*).

Candidate Hantaan virus vaccines have been developed using both classic and molecular techniques. Cell culture– and mouse brain–derived products have been tested widely in China and Korea, and a vaccinia-vectored recombinant immunogen (expressing M and S gene products from the prototype Hantaan strain) is under study in human volunteers in the United States (McClain D, personal communication). However, no vaccine has yet proved effective in preventing hantavirus infections in controlled clinical trials.

Marburg and Ebola Virus Diseases

Marburg and Ebola viruses constitute the Filoviridae, a family of RNA viruses capable of inducing severe and highly lethal hemorrhagic fevers in primates, including humans. These mysterious agents are maintained in nature through unknown mechanisms and have been responsible for sporadic disease and explosive outbreaks that have captured the attention of both the scientific and lay communities.[121] Marburg and Ebola viruses were initially believed to be exclusively African viruses; the discovery in 1989 of Ebola viruses in the United States and subsequently elsewhere among colonies of nonhuman primates originating in the Philippines prompted a reappraisal of this thinking.

The family Filoviridae presently consists of four viruses: Marburg virus and three Ebola viruses subtypes: Ebola-Sudan, Ebola-Zaire, and Ebola-Reston[122, 123] (Table 269–7). A probable fourth Ebola virus strain, yet unnamed, was recovered from a human infected in the Ivory Coast[124]; classification of this agent is incomplete at this time. A single, negative-sense RNA strand codes for seven polypeptides: a nucleoprotein, a glycoprotein, a polymerase, and four other proteins.[125–127] Morphology is unique, with particles assuming long (up to 14,000 nm), filamentous, often bizarre shapes (U, 6, or circular configurations) of constant 80-nm diameter.[128] Although biochemically similar in makeup, there is little serologic cross-reactivity between Marburg virus and the various Ebola virus strains, whereas all Ebola viruses recognized to date cross-react to varying degrees among themselves.[129–131]

Epidemiology

Marburg and Ebola viruses were unknown to science until 1967, when simultaneous outbreaks of hemorrhagic fever occurred in Marburg and Frankfurt, Germany, and Belgrade, Yugoslavia.[132] Thirty-one cases (25 primary and 6 secondary) of what came to be known as Marburg virus disease were recognized, 7 of which were fatal. Primary infections were linked to contact with African green monkeys shipped from a primate export facility in Uganda. The virus then disappeared from view until 1975, when a young Australian tourist who had traveled in Zimbabwe contracted Marburg virus infection and died in a Johannesburg, South Africa, hospital.[133] His female traveling companion became ill a week after onset in her partner, and a nurse in Johannesburg subsequently became infected, but both survived. Three additional cases make up the entire remaining experience with Marburg virus in humans[134, 135]: an expatriate engineer contracted the disease in northwestern Kenya in 1980 and died; the physician attending to the engineer became secondarily infected but survived; and in 1987, a Danish teenager contracted the disease in Kenya and died. Despite extensive investigation, no reservoir, vector, or naturally occurring source for any Marburg virus infection has ever been identified.

Two simultaneous, explosive, and apparently unrelated outbreaks of hemorrhagic fever in 1976 in northern Zaire and southern Sudan proved to be the sentinel cases of Ebola virus disease in humans.[136] These epidemics lasted for months and affected more than 500 persons. Mortality was quite high (nearly 90% in Zaire and 50% in Sudan), and secondary cases associated with exposure to blood or other body fluids (e.g., reuse of needles and syringes, sexual contacts) were common. Isolated Ebola virus cases in 1972 (1 putative nonfatal case retrospectively identified by serology, along with 1 probable fatal case),[137] 1976 (1 nonfatal laboratory infection)[138] and 1977 (a single fatal case in Tandala, Zaire),[139] together with a second outbreak in southern Sudan involving 34 persons (22 fatalities) in 1979,[140] round out the confirmed experience with these viruses in Africa before the 1990s. Although it is evident that close interpersonal contact or nosocomial transmission accounted for many of the Ebola cases recognized during the large Zaire and Sudan outbreaks, epidemiologic studies have failed to identify a reservoir, vector, or source for any of the naturally occurring human infections.

Like Marburg virus, Ebola virus seemed to disappear for a period. Then, in November 1989, an outbreak of hemorrhagic fever occurred among cynomolgus monkeys *(Macaca*

TABLE 269–7 ■ Currently Recognized Filoviruses

VIRUS STRAIN	ORIGIN	PATHOGENICITY FOR HUMANS	HOST OR RESERVOIR	REMARKS
Marburg	Central and southern Africa	High	Unknown	Caused lethal infections in African green monkeys; sporadic human cases
Ebola-Zaire	Zaire	High	Unknown	Caused community epidemics with high mortality, as well as sporadic human cases
Ebola-Sudan	Southern Sudan	High	Unknown	Caused community epidemics with high mortality
Ebola-Reston	Phillipines	? Low	Unknown	Caused lethal infections in cynomolgus macaques
Ebola-Ivory Coast*	Ivory Coast	? High	Unknown	Caused lethal infection in chimpanzees

*Single human case has been recognized; virus is not yet officially classified as distinct.

fascicularis) housed in a quarantine facility in Reston, Virginia.[141] While samples were processed for electron microscopy in animals from this suspected (and later confirmed) simian hemorrhagic fever epizootic, filovirus-like particles were spotted by an alert technician. Ebola virus was identified in culture fluids from several pathologic specimens, prompting investigations nationwide to assess the scope and significance of the problem.[142] Subsequently, Ebola virus was identified at facilities in Texas and Pennsylvania among colonies of sick and dying cynomolgus monkeys, most of which had been procured from a single source in the Philippines. Epidemiologic investigations in the Philippines confirmed the presence of widespread Ebola infections among captured and caged animals in the exporter's facilities but failed to clarify the source or extent of the infection in nature.[143] The virus either persisted or was later reintroduced into the Philippine export facility: infected macaques traced to this same source were detected in Italy in 1992.[144] Despite the high (>75%) case-fatality rates documented among these Asian macaques, however, no human illness has occurred among the several individuals shown virologically and serologically to have been infected with this virus strain.[145]

In November 1994, a Swiss ethnologist developed a hemorrhagic fever syndrome after dissecting one of several chimpanzees that had died of unknown causes in the Ivory Coast.[124] A strain of Ebola virus was recovered from her blood that proved to be distinct from previously recognized filoviruses. Although the ethnologist survived, her severe clinical illness was similar to that described for other African Ebola virus cases.

In early April 1995, a laboratory worker hospitalized in the village of Kikwit, Bandundu Province, Zaire, died after a febrile illness initially thought to be typhoid fever. Medical and surgical personnel caring for this patient became ill with fever, headache, myalgia, and hemorrhagic manifestations beginning about 4 days later. Ebola virus antigens and RNA were identified in samples sent from these and other patients shortly afterward; active surveillance indicated that several chains of infection had occurred up to 4 months previously.[146] Through June, nearly 300 people had been identified with hemorrhagic fever attributable to Ebola virus infection. The overall case-fatality rate was 79%. About a third of cases occurred among health care workers, in whom infections were associated with inadequate barrier nursing practices.[147] Sequence study of the virus glycoprotein gene indicated that the 1995 epidemic strain was closely related to the Zaire strain of Ebola virus isolated some 20 years previously.[146] In July 1996, yet another outbreak of Ebola virus began, this time in Gabon. By the time it was declared terminated in January 1997, 59 cases with 44 deaths had been recorded. A fatal nosocomial infection occurred in Johannesburg, South Africa, in conjunction with this outbreak. A nurse caring for a patient who had been unknowingly transported from Gabon was exposed to large volumes of blood in the course of her routine duties, became ill 4 days later, and subsequently died. The Ebola virus strain involved in this latest epidemic is uncharacterized at the time of this writing.

The natural history of filoviruses remains enigmatic. That these are zoonotic viruses is strongly suggested by the patterns of human infection, the biologic properties of the agents, and some intriguing epidemiologic associations (particularly with exposure to bats); despite extensive ecologic study, however, no natural source for any filovirus has been identified. Person-to-person transmission of both Ebola and Marburg viruses has been documented in association with parenteral or mucous membrane exposure to contaminated body fluids. The role of aerosol transmission is less clear, although experimental transmission of Marburg and Ebola viruses has been demonstrated,[130, 131] and droplet or aerosol spread of Ebola-Reston virus occurred among quarantined cynomolgus monkeys.[142]

Pathogenesis

Hematogenous spread of Ebola and Marburg viruses to multiple organs follows mucous membrane exposure or direct inoculation of virus. Extensive virus replication is associated with focal necrotic changes in liver, spleen, lymph nodes, kidney, lung, and gonads.[132, 136, 148] The most prominent pathologic changes are observed in the liver, where foci of parenchymal necrosis containing Councilman-like bodies are seen. The presence of virus is strongly correlated with visible necrosis. Few inflammatory cells accompany the hepatic lesions, however, and blood biochemical changes suggest that liver damage is not central to disease outcome.

The major manifestation of this usually severe disease is vascular failure. Pathologic features of fatal Marburg and Ebola virus infection typically include hemorrhages in skin, mucous membranes, alimentary luminal surfaces, and viscera.[132, 136, 148, 149] These abnormalities are temporally associated with increased vascular permeability. Extravasation of fluid into abdominal viscera, lungs, and kidneys precipitates organ dysfunction. Endothelial cell dysfunction and subsequent loss of vascular integrity appear to be due both to direct (cytopathology) and indirect (mediator induced) virus effects. Disseminated intravascular coagulation has been observed in primate models of Marburg virus infection, but its role in pathogenesis is less certain.

Humans and other primates fatally infected with filoviruses die with high viremias and little or no evidence of an effective humoral immune response. It has been postulated that cellular immunity is important in recovery (and probably protection) from infection, but evidence for this is circumstantial.[130]

Clinical Features

Clinical disease after infection with Marburg, Ebola-Zaire, and Ebola-Sudan viruses is severe, relentlessly progressive, and frequently fatal.[150, 151] As of this writing, there have been no reports of human illness after infection with filoviruses of Asian origin. However, experience with these latter agents is extremely limited, and they are closely related antigenically to African filoviruses[131]; thus, avirulence of these viruses for humans should not be generally assumed.

The incubation period for African filoviruses in humans typically ranges from 3 to 8 days but can be somewhat longer in secondary exposures. Onset of illness is sudden, with severe frontal headache, fever, chills, myalgias, extreme malaise, and anorexia. Nausea, vomiting, diarrhea, and abdominal pain are common early in disease. Conjunctivitis, pharyngitis, and oral ulcerations are frequently described as well. Patients appear prostrate and apathetic and may be disoriented. A maculopapular rash that ultimately desquamates in survivors appears on the trunk and back around the fifth day of illness. Gross bleeding is frequent and is most often seen from mucous membranes (including the gastrointestinal tract), nasopharynx, and vagina; petechiae and oozing from venipuncture sites are also commonly observed.

Thrombocytopenia and leukopenia with a left shift are present early in disease. After a few days, significant neutrophilia appears. Serum biochemical studies show elevated enzyme values (aspartate aminotransferase > alanine aminotransferase), with normal or only slightly elevated bilirubin values. Viremia is present during acute disease and can persist for weeks in visceral organs and other sites (e.g., semen, anterior chamber of the eye) after apparently normal recovery.[132, 133, 138]

Death due to intractable shock occurs on days 6 to 16 of illness. Infections in pregnancy produce many maternal deaths, and abortion or fetal demise is virtually universal. Convalescence is prolonged for survivors, requiring many weeks for recovery from the severe wasting that typically occurs.

Diagnosis

The method of choice for serologic diagnosis of recent filovirus infection historically has been the indirect IF assay, using virus-infected cells inactivated by γ-radiation and affixed to slides.[61, 152] Prompted by concerns over specificity of IF, particularly in epidemiologic studies,[130] enzyme EIAs for IgG and IgM antibodies[61, 131, 153] have been developed and tested. These assays have proved to be sensitive in diagnosis of documented African and Asian filovirus disease and have given negative results in suspect IF-positive serosurvey samples. It is thus important to confirm IF diagnoses of filovirus infections in single samples or serosurveys with another, more specific test. Other, more technically demanding, diagnostic tools such as Western blot and immunoprecipitation assays have been applied to serodiagnosis of filoviruses as well.[152, 154]

Infectious virus and viral antigen are present in blood and tissues of patients during acute disease and post mortem. However, isolation and other experimental manipulation of filoviruses in animals or cell culture systems are highly hazardous and should be undertaken only under maximal biologic safety (level 4) conditions. The E-6 clone of Vero cells has been most useful for initial propagation of African filoviruses from clinical specimens; MA-104 and SW-13 cells have proved sensitive for recovery of Ebola-Reston virus.[61] Some strains of filoviruses may be relatively fastidious, requiring passage in animals for recovery.

Viral antigen can be detected using antigen capture EIA.[155] The ability of this test to detect antigen in samples that have been inactived using γ-radiation or betapropiolactone provides an avenue for diagnosis in the absence of elaborate biologic containment facilities. Immunohistochemical techniques have been successfully applied to detection of antigen in tissues.[141]

The unique morphology of the Filoviridae makes electron microscopy potentially useful in examination of patients' specimens.[128, 131, 156] This tool has particular utility for assessment of infection retrospectively in tissues preserved by formalin fixation, where isolation is no longer possible.

A wide range of infectious diseases with similar presentations occur in those parts of sub-Saharan Africa where filovirus infections have occurred. Among these afflictions, malaria, typhoid, rickettsial diseases, and other viral hemorrhagic fevers represent particularly important and potentially treatable entitites that must be excluded.

Treatment

No specific treatment exists for hemorrhagic fevers caused by filoviruses. Supportive management of shock, organ failure, clotting disturbances, and volume shifts is most important. There is no effective antiviral therapy for these diseases. Human interferon, in conjunction with convalescent plasma, was used in a patient who survived,[138] although experimental studies have shown no in vitro sensitivity of filoviruses for interferon. Infusion of human convalescent plasma containing strain-specific antibodies would seem justified (assuming the infusate is free of other infectious agents), although this approach is without proven effect.

Prevention

No vaccine has been developed for Marburg or Ebola viruses. Poor understanding of mechanisms of protection and recovery from illness has complicated rational development of prophylactic measures. Experience in epidemic settings supports the central role of interruption of person-to-person transmission through early identification of cases and intervention in limiting spread of disease among close personal contacts.[73] Prevention of nosocomial spread can be accomplished through use of sterile equipment, adequate decontamination procedures, and application of barrier nursing practices. Absence of identified reservoirs or vectors precludes use of ecologic controls to limit acquisition of disease from natural sources. Recognition of risks to individuals involved in work with wild-caught monkeys or their tissues has resulted in institution of controls pertaining to importation and quarantine of animals.[157]

Crimean-Congo Hemorrhagic Fever

Crimean-Congo hemorrhagic fever (CCHF) is a tick-borne viral disease with a wide geographic distribution. Human infections have been recognized in Eastern Europe, the Middle East, across Asia as far east as China, and throughout Africa. The etiologic agent of what had been known since the 1930s as Crimean hemorrhagic fever was identified as a virus in 1947.[158] In 1969, however, a virus that had been recovered from a febrile patient in the Belgian Congo (now Zaire) in 1956 was found to be identical to the Crimean hemorrhagic fever agent, and the nomenclature was revised to reflect the linkage; hence the current name, CCHF.[159]

CCHF virus is a member of the *Nairovirus* genus in the Bunyaviridae family. All viruses of this genus are thought to be transmitted by ticks. As with other Bunyaviridae, virions are 90 to 120 nm in diameter, with 10-nm surface projections.

The tripartite negative-stranded RNA genome codes for two surface glycoproteins (via the M segment), a nucleoprotein (via the S segment), and a viral polymerase (via the L segment).

Epidemiology

The epidemiology of CCHF is tied to complex relationships that exist between the virus's arthropod vectors and their nonhuman vertebrate hosts.[160] The virus is a parasite of at least 24 species of ixodid (hard) ticks, particularly *Hyalomma* species. Transovarial and transstadial transmission of CCHF virus has been documented in several of these tick species, which presumably serve as both reservoir and vector of the agent. In addition, the ticks feed on (and infect) a wide variety of wild and domestic animals, including birds; the specific vertebrate host parasitized (and possibly infected) is both tick species and life cycle stage specific. Although quantitative studies are few, it is clear that vertebrate amplification of CCHF infection is a major contributor to sustainment and spread of the virus in nature. In general, wild hares and large herbivores represent the major vertebrate reservoirs. Human infections occur secondary to bites from infected ticks; exposure to viremic animal blood, tissues, and excreta; and nosocomially. The last route is particularly significant, inasmuch as several serious outbreaks of CCHF have occurred among hospital personnel after exposure to infectious materials from unsuspected cases.[161–163]

Seasonality of CCHF depends on local climatic conditions, and peaks correspond to periods of maximal tick infestation. CCHF is a rural disease, and many of the endemic areas are remote; information on incidence and prevalence is consequently variable in quality. A relatively high range of illness/infection ratios have been reported from some countries (from 20% to 50%), but human infections have not been recognized in some areas where infected ticks or seropositive animals and humans have been found (reviewed in Watts and colleagues[163] and Peters and LeDuc[164]). This variability is unexplained but may relate to geographic differences in virulence among CCHF virus strains, predominant mode of disease acquisition, or density of infection in reservoir or vector populations. Case-fatality rates among hospitalized patients in Eurasia have ranged from 13% to 50%; in southern Africa the mortality rate is approximately 30%, despite availability of relatively advanced medical care.[160, 165]

Pathogenesis

CCHF is a multisystem disease.[167] Generalized vascular damage, endothelial lesions, and scattered focal hemorrhages with edema are typically seen in multiple organs. IF studies have demonstrated the presence of viral antigen concentrated in the liver and spleen. Histologically, focal to massive necrosis of the liver is seen, but the degree of hepatic involvement is generally disproportionate to the amount of antigen present. It is unclear whether direct cytopathologic changes or circulating inflammatory mediators represent the major cause of damage. Disseminated intravascular coagulation is well documented as an early and prominent feature of CCHF, and the resultant microthrombus formation with subsequent infarction is undoubtedly critical in pathogenesis. In contrast to other viral hemorrhagic fevers, gross bleeding in CCHF is quite common, and the volume of blood loss may be significant. Anemia or circulatory collapse may contribute to death in fatal cases.

Clinical Features

The incubation period for CCHF is generally 2 to 7 days.[165, 166] Onset is abrupt, with high temperature, chills, severe headache, myalgias, weakness, epigastric pain, and nausea and vomiting. Conjunctival injection, flushing of the face and chest, pharyngeal hyperemia, and palatal petechiae are frequent. After 3 to 5 days, a brief remission of several hours' duration may be seen in one third to two thirds of patients, followed by a second, overtly hemorrhagic, phase of illness. During this latter period, bradycardia, pulmonary edema, and hypovolemic shock occur. Petechiae appear on most patients, distributed over the chest and abdomen. Epistaxes are common, and in more severe cases, uncontrolled bleeding at other mucosal surfaces, as well as venipuncture sites, may occur. In such cases, large pressure-associated ecchymoses frequently are seen (Fig. 269–3). This stage may last from 3 to 10 days and is associated with changes in mood and affect.

Leukopenia, thrombocytopenia, and elevated serum transaminase values are generally present at the time of initial clinical consultation. Studies of South African patients showed that leukocytosis (white cell count of ≥10,000/mm^3), severe thrombocytopenia (platelet count of ≤20,000/mm^3), or marked abnormalities of serum transaminase levels (aspartate aminotransferase ≥200 IU/L, alanine aminotransferase ≥150 IU/L) or coagulation (activated partial thromboplastin time ≥60 seconds or fibrinogen ≤110 mg/dL) were 90% predictive of a fatal outcome if seen during the first 5 days of illness.[166] Recovery in survivors is slow and prolonged.

Diagnosis

CCHF virus is readily recovered from blood after its inoculation into newborn mice or cell cultures. Viral antigen can be demonstrated in many organs of fatal cases by immunohistochemistry. In most patients, virus-specific IgM and IgG antibodies can be detected by indirect IF or EIA on days 7 to 9 of illness, with IgM falling to low or undetectable levels by

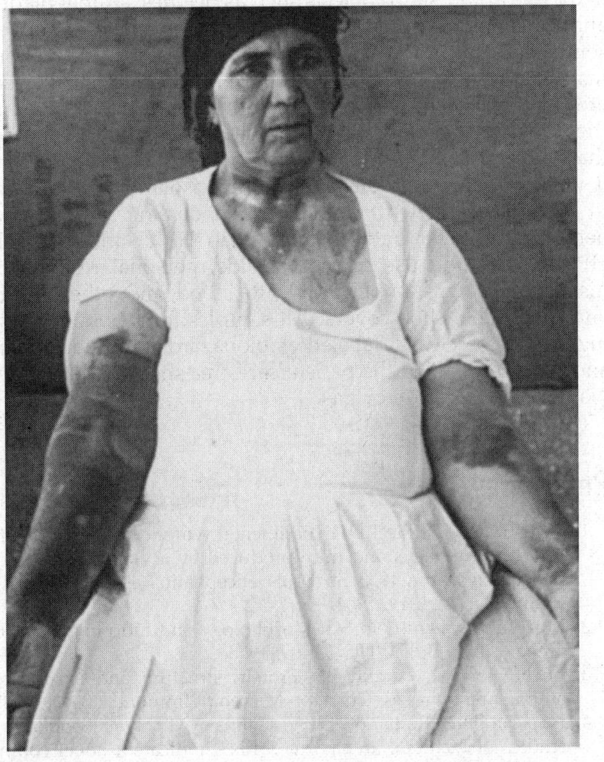

FIGURE 269–3 □ Patient with Crimean-Congo hemorrhagic fever virus infection illustrating extensive ecchymoses. (Courtesy of Dr. D. I. H. Simpson.)

3 to 5 months.[168] Neutralizing antibody appears toward the end of the first week of illness but reaches only modest titer (1:16 to 1:256) and persists only 4 to 5 months in survivors.[167]

Treatment

As with other viral hemorrhagic fevers, close attention to fluid, electrolyte, and volume status is critical to management. Treatment of CCHF with immune plasma has been generally unsuccessful.[168] The virus is sensitive in vitro to ribavirin,[168] and this drug has been reported to be useful in management of South African CCHF cases.

Prevention

Avoidance of tick bite is the most effective strategy for preventing infection. This is best done through use of personal protective measures such as repellents and sprays for impregnating clothing. Avoidance of mucous membrane or nonintact skin contact with human or animal blood in endemic areas, as well as avoidance of high-risk behaviors such as crushing ticks by hand, is prudent.

A formalin-inactivated mouse brain CCHF vaccine has been used in the former Soviet Union and Bulgaria, but no data on efficacy are available.

Isolation of Patients

With the exception of hantaviruses, the viral hemorrhagic fevers discussed in this chapter are renowned for their propensity for person-to-person spread in nosocomial and familial settings. Many of these transmissions can be traced to inoculation of infectious materials (e.g., shared needles) or exchange of body fluids (e.g., sexual transmission); however, not all case clusters or outbreaks are so readily explained. In general, application of universal precautions in handling of body fluids and sharp objects such as needles, scalpel blades, and broken glass implements by clinical and laboratory personnel will minimize the potential for spread of infectious materials in hospital settings. All hemorrhagic fever viruses are relatively stable as droplets and aerosols, however, and the potential for interpersonal spread under conditions other than direct inoculation or close contact thus exists. Therefore, it would appear prudent to maximize isolation precautions to the greatest extent possible when dealing with a viral hemorrhagic fever patient (other than HFRS and probably HPS), to include use of face shields, personal respirators, disposable gowns impermeable to blood and other fluids, and disposable shoe covers. All samples for laboratory testing should be clearly labeled as biohazards, and equipment and supplies leaving the patient care area should be sterilized via high temperature or gas.

References

1. Armstrong C, Lillie RD: Experimental lymphocytic choriomeningitis of monkeys and mice produced by a virus encountered in studies of the 1933 St. Louis encephalitis epidemic. Public Health Rep 49:1019, 1934.
2. Murphy FA, Whitfield SG: Morphology and morphogenesis of arenaviruses. Bull WHO 52:409, 1975.
3. Buchmeier MJ, Parekh BS: Protein structure and expression among arenaviruses. Curr Top Microbiol Immunol 133:41, 1987.
4. Auperin DD, Romanowski V, Galinski M, et al: Sequencing studies of Pichinde arenavirus S RNA indicate a novel coding strategy, an ambisense viral S RNA. J Virol 52:897, 1986.
5. Murphy FA, Walker DH: Arenaviruses: Persistent infection and viral survival in reservoir hosts. *In* Kurstak E, Maramorosch K (eds): Viruses and Environment. New York, Academic Press, 1978, pp 155–180.
6. Webb PA, Justines G, Johnson KM: Infection of wild and laboratory animals with Machupo and Latino viruses. Bull WHO 52:493, 1975.
7. Vitullo AD, Hodara VL, Merani MS: Effect of persistent infection with Junin virus on growth and reproduction of its natural reservoir, *Calomys musculinus.* Am J Trop Med Hyg 37:663, 1987.
8. Armstrong C, Sweet LK: Lymphocytic choriomeningitis. Public Health Rep 54:673, 1939.
9. Armstrong C: Studies on choriomeningitis and poliomyelitis. Bull N Y Acad Med 17:295, 1941.
10. Biggar RJ, Woodall JP, Walter PD, et al: Lymphocytic choriomeningitis outbreak associated with pet hamsters. Fifty-seven cases from New York State. JAMA 232:494, 1975.
11. Gregg MB: Recent outbreaks of lymphocytic choriomeningitis in the United States of America. Bull WHO 52:549, 1975.
12. Dykewicz CA, Data VM, Fisher-Hoch SP, et al: Lymphocytic choriomeningitis outbreak associated with nude mice in a research laboratory. JAMA 267:1349, 1992.
13. McCormick JB, Webb PA, Krebs JW, et al: A prospective study of the epidemiology and ecology of Lassa fever. J Infect Dis 155:437, 1987.
14. Monath TP, Newhouse VF, Kemp GE, et al: Lassa virus isolation from *Mastomys natalensis* rodents during an epidemic in Sierra Leone. Science 185:263, 1974.
15. Fraser DW, Campbell CC, Monath TP, et al: Lassa fever in the eastern province of Sierra Leone, 1970–1972. I. Epidemiologic studies. Am J Trop Med Hyg 23:1131, 1974.
16. Keenlyside RA, McCormick JB, Webb PA, et al: Case-control study of *Mastomys natalensis* and humans in Lassa virus–infected households in Sierra Leone. Am J Trop Med Hyg 32:829, 1983.
17. Carey DE, Kemp GE, White HA, et al: Lassa fever. Epidemiological aspects of the 1970 epidemic, Jos, Nigeria. Trans R Soc Trop Med Hyg 66:402, 1972.
18. Monath TP, Mertens PE, Patton R, et al: A hospital epidemic of Lassa fever in Zorzor, Liberia, March–April 1972. Am J Trop Med Hyg 22:773, 1973.
19. McCormick JB, King IJ, Webb PA, et al: A case-control study of the clinical diagnosis and course of Lassa fever. J Infect Dis 155:445, 1987.
20. Price ME, Fisher-Hoch SP, Craven RB, McCormick JB: A prospective study of maternal and fetal outcome in acute Lassa fever during pregnancy. BMJ 297:584, 1988.
21. Webb PA, McCormick JB, King IJ, et al: Lassa fever in children in Sierra Leone, West Africa. Trans R Soc Trop Med Hyg 80:577, 1986.
22. Maiztegui JI, Feuillade M, Briggiler A: Progressive extension of the endemic area and changing incidence of Argentine hemorrhagic fever. Med Microbiol Immunol 175:149, 1986.
23. Carballal G, Videla CM, Merani MS: Epidemiology of Argentine hemorrhagic fever. Eur J Epidemiol 4:259, 1988.
24. Maiztegui JI: Clinical and epidemiological patterns of Argentine haemorrhagic fever. Bull WHO 52:567, 1975.
25. Mills JN, Ellis BA, McKee KT Jr, et al: A longitudinal study of Junin virus activity in the rodent reservoir of Argentine hemorrhagic fever. Am J Trop Med Hyg 47:749, 1992.
26. Hemorrhagic Fever Commission of Bolivia: Hemorrhagic fever in Bolivia [in Spanish]. Bull Panam Health Organ 58:93, 1965.
27. MacKenzie RB: Epidemiology of Machupo virus infection. I. Pattern of human infection, San Joachin, Bolivia, 1962–1964. Am J Trop Med Hyg 14:808, 1965.
28. Centers for Disease Control: Bolivian hemorrhagic fever—El Beni Department, Bolivia, 1994. MMWR Morbid Mortal Wkly Rep 43:943, 1994.
29. Peters CJ, Kuehne RW, Mercado RR, et al: Hemorrhagic fever in Cochabamba, Bolivia, 1971. Am J Epidemiol 99:425, 1974.
30. Salas R, de Manzione N, Tesh RB, et al: Venezuelan haemorrhagic fever. Lancet 338:1033, 1991.
31. Tesh RB, Wilson ML, Salas R, et al: Field studies on the epidemiology of Venezuelan hemorrhagic fever. Am. J Trop Med Hyg 49:227, 1993.

31a. Fulhorst CF, Bowen MD, Salas R, et al: Isolation and characterization of Pirital virus, a newly discovered South American areuavirus. Am J Trop Med Hyg (in press).

32. Coimbra TLM, Nassar ES, Burattini MN, et al: New arenavirus isolated in Brazil. Lancet 343:391, 1994.
33. Barry M, Russi M, Armstrong L, et al: Brief Report: Treatment of a laboratory-acquired Sabia virus infection. N Engl J Med 333:294; 1995.
34. Horton J, Hotchin JE, Olson KB, et al: The effects of MP virus infection in lymphoma. Cancer Res 31:1066, 1971.
35. Warkel RL, Rinaldi CF, Bancroft WH, et al.: Fatal acute meningoencephalitis due to lymphocytic choriomeningitis virus. Neurology 23:198, 1973.
36. Walker DH, McCormick JB, Johnson KM, et al: Pathologic and virologic study of Lassa fever in man. Am J Pathol 107:349, 1982.
37. Johnson KM, McCormick JB, Webb PA, et al: Clinical virology of Lassa fever in hospitalized patients. J Infect Dis 155:546, 1987.
38. Fisher-Hoch SP, Mitchell SW, Sasso DR, et al: Physiologic and immunologic disturbances associated with shock in Lassa fever in a primate model. J Infect Dis 155:465, 1987.
39. Fisher-Hoch SP, McCormick JB, Sasso D, et al: Hematologic dysfunction in Lassa fever. J Med Virol 26:127, 1988.
40. Cummins D, Fisher-Hoch SP, Walshe KJ, et al: A plasma inhibitor of platelet aggregation in patients with Lassa fever. Br J Haematol 72:543, 1989.
41. Roberts PJ, Cummins D, Bainton AD, et al: Plasma from patients with severe Lassa fever profoundly modulates f-met-leu-phe induced superoxide generation in neutrophil. Br J Haematol 73:152, 1989.
42. Lange JV, Mitchell SW, McCormick JB, et al: Kinetic study of platelets and fibrinogen in Lassa virus–infected monkeys and early pathologic events in Mopeia virus–infected monkeys. Am J Trop Med Hyg 34:999, 1985.
43. Cossio P, Laguens R, Arana R, et al: Ultrastructural and immunochemical study of the human kidney in Argentine haemorrhagic fever. Virchows Arch 368:1, 1975.
44. Gonzales PH, Cossio PM, Arana R, et al: Lymphatic tissue in Argentine hemorrhagic fever. Arch Pathol Lab Med 104:250, 1980.
45. Levis SC, Saavedra MC, Ceccoli C, et al: Endogenous interferon in Argentine hemorrhagic fever. J Infect Dis 149:428, 1984.
46. Levis SC, Saavedra MC, Ceccoli C, et al: Correlation between endogenous interferon and the clinical evolution of patients with Argentine haemorrhagic fever. J Interferon Res 5:383, 1985.
47. Heller MV, Saavedra MC, Falcoff R, et al: Increased tumor necrosis factor-α levels in Argentine hemorrhagic fever. J Infect Dis 166:1203, 1992.
48. Peters CJ, Jahrling PB, Liu CT, et al: Experimental studies of arenaviral hemorrhagic fevers. Curr Top Microbiol Immunol 132:5, 1987.
49. Hinman AR, Fraser DW, Douglas RG, et al: Outbreak of lymphocytic choriomeningitis virus infections in medical center personnel. Am J Epidemiol 101:103, 1975.
50. Vanzee BE, Douglas RG Jr, Betts RF, et al: Lymphocytic choriomeningitis in university hospital personnel: Clinical features. Am J Med 58:803, 1975.
51. Meyer HM Jr, Johnson RT, Crawford IP, et al: Central nervous syndromes of "viral" etiology. Am J Med 29:334, 1960.
52. Ormay I, Kovacs P: Lymphocytic choriomeningitis causing unilateral deafness [in Hungarian]. Orv Hetil 130:789, 1989.
53. Sheinbergas MM: Antibody to lymphocytic choriomeningitis virus in children with congenital hydrocephalus. Acta Virol 19:165, 1975.
54. Barton LL, Budd SC, Morfitt WS, et al: Congenital lymphocytic choriomeningitis virus infection in twins. Pediatr Infect Dis J 12:942, 1993.
55. Smadel JE, Green RH, Pahtraul RM, et al: Lymphocytic choriomeningitis: Two human fatalities following an unusual febrile illness. Proc Soc Exp Biol Med 49:683, 1942.
56. Cummins D, McCormick JB, Bennet D, et al: Acute sensorineural deafness in Lassa fever. JAMA 264:2093, 1990.
57. Monson MH, Cole AK, Frame JD, et al: Pediatric Lassa fever: A review of 33 Liberian cases. Am J Trop Med Hyg 36:408, 1987.
58. McCormick JB, King IJ, Webb PA, et al: Lassa fever. Effective therapy with ribavirin. N Engl J Med 314:20, 1986.
59. Mackenzie RB, Beye HK, Valverde L, et al: Epidemic hemorrhagic fever in Bolivia. I. A preliminary report of the epidemiologic and clinical findings in a new epidemic area in South America. Am J Trop Med Hyg 13:620, 1964.
60. Weissenbacher MC, Laguens RP, Coto CE: Argentine hemorrhagic fever. Curr Top Microbiol Immunol 134:79, 1987.
61. Jahrling PB: Filoviruses and Arenaviruses. *In* Murray PR, Baron EJ, Pfaller MA, Tenover FC, Yolken RH (eds): Manual of Clinical Microbiology, ed 6. Washington, DC, ASM Press, 1995, pp 1068–1081.
62. Ambrosio AM, Enria DA, Maiztegui JI: Junin virus isolation from lymphomononuclear cells of patients with Argentine hemorrhagic fever. Intervirology 25:97, 1986.
63. Niklasson BS, Jahrling PB, Peters CJ: Detection of Lassa fever antigens and Lassa-specific immunoglobulin G and M by enzyme-linked immunosorbent assay. J Clin Microbiol 20:239, 1984.
64. Demby AH, Chamberlain J, Brown DWG, et al: Early diagnosis of Lassa fever by reverse transcription-PCR. J Clin Microbiol 32:2898, 1994.
65. Maiztegui JI, Fernandez NJ, de Damilano AJ: Efficacy of immune plasma in treatment of Argentine haemorrhagic fever and association between treatment and a late neurological syndrome. Lancet 2:1216, 1979.
66. Enria D, Briggiler AM, Fernandez NJ, et al: Importance of dose of neutralizing antibodies in treatment of Argentine haemorrhagic fever with immune plasma. Lancet 2:255, 1984.
67. Enria D, Franco SG, Ambrosio A, et al: Current status of the treatment of Argentine hemorrhagic fever. Med Microbiol Immunol 175:173, 1986.
68. Enria DA, Briggiler AM, Levis S., et al: Preliminary report. Tolerance and antiviral effect of ribavirin in patients with Argentine hemorrhagic fever. Antiviral Res 7:353, 1987.
69. Johnson KM, Webb PA, Justines G: Biology of Tacaribe-complex viruses. *In* Lehman-Grube F (ed): Lymphocytic Choriomeningitis Virus and Other Arenaviruses. Berlin, Springer-Verlag, 1973, pp 241–258.
70. Barrera Oro JG, McKee KT Jr: Toward a vaccine against Argentine hemorrhagic fever. Bull Pan Am Health Organ 25:118, 1991.
71. World Health Organization: Vaccination against Argentine haemorrhagic fever. Wkly Epidemiol Rec 68:233, 1993.
72. Fisher-Hoch SP, McCormick JB, Auperin D, et al: Protection of rhesus monkeys from fatal Lassa fever by vaccination with a recombinant vaccinia virus containing the Lassa virus glycoprotein gene. Proc Natl Acad Sci USA 85:1, 1988.
73. Centers for Disease Control: Management of patients with suspected viral hemorrhagic fever. MMWR Morbid Mortal Wkly Rep 37(Suppl 3):1, 1988.
74. Earle DP: Symposium on epidemic hemorrhagic fever. Am J Med 16:617, 1954.
75. Gajdusek DC: Acute infectious hemorrhagic fevers and mycotoxicoses in the Union of Soviet Socialist Republics. Washington, DC, Army Medical Service Graduate School, Walter Reed Army Medical Center, 1953. Medical Science publication 2.
76. Lee HW, Lee PW: Korean hemorrhagic fever. I. Demonstration of causative antigen and antibodies. Korean J Intern Med 19:371, 1976.
77. Lee HW, Lee PW, Johnson KM: Isolation of the etiologic agent of Korean hemorrhagic fever. J Infect Dis 137:298, 1978.
78. White JD, Shirey FG, French GR, et al: Hantaan virus, aetiological agent of Korean haemorrhagic fever, has Bunyaviridae-like morphology. Lancet 1:768, 1982.
79. McCormick JB, Sasso DR, Palmer EL, Kiley MP: Morphological identification of the agent of Korean haemorrhagic fever (Hantaan virus) as a member of the Bunyaviridae. Lancet 1:765, 1982.
80. Schmaljohn CS, Hasty SE, Dalrymple JM, et al: Antigenic and genetic properties of viruses linked to hemorrhagic fever with renal syndrome. Science 227:1041, 1985.
81. Schmaljohn CS, Hasty SE, Harrison SA, Dalrymple JM: Characterization of Hantaan virions, the prototype virus of hemorrhagic fever with renal syndrome. J Infect Dis 148:1005, 1983.
82. Schmaljohn CS, Dalrymple JM: Analysis of Hantaan virus RNA: Evidence for a new genus of Bunyaviridae. Virology 131:482, 1983.
83. Elliott RM, Schmaljohn CS, Collett MS: Bunyaviridae genome structure and gene expression. Curr Top Microbiol Immunol 169:91, 1991.
84. Hung T, Choi Z, Zhao T, et al: Morphology and morphogenesis of viruses of hemorrhagic fever with renal syndrome (HFRS). I. Some peculiar aspects of the morphogenesis of various strains of HFRS virus. Intervirology 23:97, 1985.

85. Xiao S-Y, LeDuc JW, Chu YK, et al: Phylogenetic analysis of virus isolates in the genus *Hantavirus*, family Bunyaviridae. Virology 198:205, 1994.
86. LeDuc JW: Epidemiology of Hantaan and related viruses. Lab Anim Sci 37:413, 1987.
87. Yanagihara R: Hantavirus infection in the United States: Epizootology and epidemiology. Rev Infect Dis 12:449, 1990.
88. Lee HW, Lee PW, Baek LJ, et al: Geographical distribution of hemorrhagic fever with renal syndrome and hantaviruses. Arch Virol 115(Suppl 1):5, 1990.
89. Settergren B: Nephropathia epidemica (hemorrhagic fever with renal syndrome) in Scandinavia. Rev Infect Dis 13:736, 1991.
90. Avsic-Zupanc T, Likar M, Novakovic S, et al: Evidence of the presence of two hantaviruses in Slovenia. Arch Virol 115(Suppl 1):87, 1990.
91. Avsic-Zupanc T, Xiao S-Y, Stojanovic R, et al: Characterization of Dobrava virus: A hantavirus from Slovenia. J Med Virol 38:132, 1992.
92. Gligic A, Dimkovic N, Xiao S-Y, et al: Belgrade virus: A new *Hantavirus* causing severe hemorrhagic fever with renal syndrome in Yugoslavia. J Infect Dis 166:113, 1992.
93. Lee HW: Epidemiology. *In* Lee HW, Dalrymple JM (eds): Manual of Hemorrhagic Fever with Renal Syndrome. Seoul, World Health Organization Collaborating Center for Virus Reference and Research Institute for Viral Diseases, Korea University, 1989, pp 39–48.
94. Childs JE, Glass GE, Korch GW, et al: Evidence of human infection with a rat-associated *Hantavirus* in Baltimore, Maryland. Am J Epidemiol 127:875, 1988.
95. Childs JE, Glass GE, Ksiazek TG, et al: Human-rodent contact and infection with lymphocytic choriomeningitis and Seoul viruses in an inner-city population. Am J Trop Med Hyg 44:117, 1991.
96. Yanagihara R, Chin CT, Weiss MB, et al: Serological evidence of *Hantavirus* infection in the United States. Am J Trop Med Hyg 34:396, 1985.
97. Yanagihara R, Gajdusek DC, Gibbs CJ Jr, et al: Prospect Hill virus: Serological evidence for infection in mammologists. N Engl J Med 310:1325, 1984.
98. Nichol ST, Spiropoulou CF, Morzunov S, et al: Genetic identification of a hantavirus associated with an outbreak of acute respiratory illness. Science 262:914, 1993.
99. Elliott LH, Ksiazek TG, Rollin PE, et al: Isolation of the causative agent of hantavirus pulmonary syndrome. Am J Trop Med Hyg 51:102, 1994.
100. Ksiazek TG, Peters CJ, Rollin PE, et al: Identification of a new North American hantavirus that causes acute pulmonary insufficiency. Am J Trop Med Hyg 52:117, 1995.
101. Rollin PE, Ksiazek TG, Elliott LH, et al: Isolation of Black Creek Canal virus, a new hantavirus from *Sigmodon hispidus* in Florida. J Med Virol 46:35, 1995.
102. Hantavirus pulmonary syndrome—Northeastern United States, 1994. MMWR Morbid Mortal Wkly Rep 43:99, 1994.
103. Butler JC, Peters CJ: Hantaviruses and hantavirus pulmonary syndrome. Clin Infect Dis 19:387, 1994.
104. Chapman LE, Khabbaz RF: Epidemiology and etiology of the Four Corners *hantavirus* outbreak. Infect Agents Dis 3:234, 1994.
105. Stephen C, Johnson M, Bell A: First reported cases of hantavirus pulmonary syndrome in Canada. Can Commun Dis Rep 20:121, 1994.
106. Hjelle B, Spiropoulou CF, Torrez-Martinez N, et al: Detection of Muerto Canyon virus RNA in peripheral blood mononuclear cells from patients with hantavirus pulmonary syndrome. J Infect Dis 170:1013, 1994.
107. Horling J, Lundkvist A, Persson K, et al: Detection and subsequent sequencing of Puumala virus from human specimens by PCR. J Clin Microbiol 33:277, 1995.
108. Hullinghorst RL, Steer A: Pathology of epidemic hemorrhagic fever. Ann Intern Med 38:77, 1953.
109. Duchin JS, Koster FT, Peters CJ, et al: Hantavirus pulmonary syndrome: A clinical description of 17 patients with a newly recognized disease. N Engl J Med 330:949, 1994.
110. Zaki SR, Greer PW, Coffield LM, et al: Hantavirus pulmonary syndrome: Pathogenesis of an emerging infectious disease. Am J Pathol 146:552, 1995.
111. Chun CH, Laehdevirta J, Lee HW: Clinical manifestations of HFRS. *In* Lee HW, Dalrymple JM (eds): Manual of Hemorrhagic Fever with Renal Syndrome. Seoul, World Health Organization Collaborating Center for Virus Reference and Research Institute for Viral Diseases, Korea University, 1989, pp 19–38.
112. McKee KT Jr, MacDonald C, LeDuc JW, et al: Hemorrhagic fever with renal syndrome—A clinical perspective. Mil Med 150:640, 1985.
113. Bruno P, Hassell LH, Brown J, et al: The protean manifestations of hemorrhagic fever with renal syndrome. A retrospective review of 26 cases from Korea. Ann Intern Med 113:385, 1990.
114. Glass GE, Watson AJ, LeDuc JW, et al: Infection with a ratborne *Hantavirus* in US residents is consistently associated with hypertensive renal disease. J Infect Dis 167:614, 1993.
115. Pilaski J, Feldmann H, Morzunov S, et al: Genetic identification of a new Puumala virus strain causing severe hemorrhagic fever with renal syndrome in Germany. J Infect Dis 170:1456, 1994.
116. Lee PW, Meegan JM, LeDuc JW, et al: Serologic techniques for detection of Hantaan virus infection, related antigens and antibodies. *In* Lee HW, Dalrymple JM (eds): Manual of Hemorrhagic Fever with Renal Syndrome. Seoul, World Health Organization Collaborating Center for Virus Reference and Research Institute for Viral Diseases, Korea University, 1989, pp 36–38.
117. Zoller L, Yang S, Gott P, et al: Use of recombinant nucleocapsid proteins of the Hantaan and nephropathia epidemica serotypes of hantaviruses as immunodiagnostic antigens. J Med Virol 39:200, 1993.
118. Feldmann H, Sanchez A, Morzunov S, et al: Utilization of autopsy RNA for the synthesis of the nucleocapsid antigen of a newly recognized virus associated with hantavirus pulmonary syndrome. Virus Res 30:351, 1993.
119. Jenison S, Yamada T, Morris C, et al: Characterization of human antibody responses to four corners hantavirus infections among patients with hantavirus pulmonary syndrome. J Virol 68:3000, 1994.
120. Huggins JW, Hsiang CM, Cosgriff TM, et al: Prospective, double-blind, concurrent, placebo-controlled clinical trial of intravenous ribavirin therapy of hemorrhagic fever with renal syndrome. J Infect Dis 164:1119, 1991.
121. Preston R. The Hot Zone. New York, Random House, 1994.
122. Kiley MP, Bowen ETW, Eddy GA, et al: Filoviridae: A taxonomic home for Marburg and Ebola viruses? Intervirology 18:24, 1982.
123. Feldmann H, Klenk H-D, Sanchez A: Molecular biology and evolution of filoviruses. Arch Virol 7(Suppl)1:81, 1993.
124. Le Guenno B, Formentry P, Wyers M, et al: Isolation and partial characterization of a new strain of Ebola virus. Lancet 345:1271, 1995.
125. Kiley MP, Cox NJ, Elliott LH, et al: Physiochemical properties of Marburg virus: Evidence for three distinct virus strains and their relationship to Ebola virus. J Gen Virol 69:1957, 1988.
126. Elliott LH, Kiley MP, McCormick JB: Descriptive analysis of Ebola virus proteins. Virology 147:169, 1985.
127. Sanchez A, Kiley MP, Holloway BP, et al: Sequence analysis of the Ebola virus genome: Organization, genetic elements, and comparison with the genome of Marburg virus. Virus Res 29:215, 1993.
128. Murphy FA, van der Groen G, Whitfield SG, et al: Ebola and Marburg virus morphology and taxonomy. *In* Pattyn SR: Ebola Virus Haemorrhagic Fever. Amsterdam, Elsevier North Holland, 1978, pp 61–84.
129. Bowen ETW, Platt GS, Lloyd G, et al: A comparative study of strains of Ebola virus isolated from southern Sudan and northern Zaire in 1976. J Med Virol 6:129, 1980.
130. Peters CJ, Sanchez A, Rollin PE, et al: Filoviridae: Marburg and Ebola viruses. *In* Fields BN, Knipe DM, Howley PM (eds): Fields Virology, ed 3. Philadelphia, Lippincott-Raven, 1996, pp 1161–1176.
131. Peters CJ, Sanchez A, Feldmann H, et al: Filoviruses as emerging pathogens. Semin Virol 5:147, 1994.
132. Martini GA, Siegert R (eds): Marburg Virus Disease. New York, Springer-Verlag, 1971.
133. Gear JSS, Cassel GA, Gear AJ, et al: Outbreak of Marburg virus disease in Johannesburg. Br Med J 4:489, 1975.
134. Smith DH, Johnson BK, Isaacson M, et al: Marburg-virus disease in Kenya. Lancet 1:816, 1982.
135. Johnson ED, Koimet E, Gitau LG, et al: Marburg virus disease: An environmental health threat in Kenya. *In* Kinoti SH, Waiyoki

PG, Were BO (eds): The Role of Man in Disease Control. Proceedings of the 11th Annual Medical Scientific Conference. African Medical and Research Foundation, 1990.
136. Pattyn SR (ed): Ebola Virus Haemorrhagic Fever. Amsterdam, Elsevier North Holland, 1978.
137. Johnson KM, Scribner CL, McCormick JB: Ecology of Ebola virus: A first clue? J Infect Dis 143:749, 1981.
138. Emond RTD, Evans B, Bowen ETW, et al: A case of Ebola virus infection. Br Med J 2:541, 1977.
139. Heymann DL, Weisfeld JS, Webb PA, et al: Ebola hemorrhagic fever: Tandala, Zaire, 1977–1978. J Infect Dis 142:372, 1980.
140. Baron RC, McCormick JB, Zubeir OA: Ebola hemorrhagic fever in southern Sudan: Hospital dissemination and intrafamiliar spread. Bull WHO 6:997, 1983.
141. Jahrling PB, Geisbert TW, Dalgard DW, et al: Preliminary report: Isolation of Ebola virus from monkeys imported to USA. Lancet 335:502, 1990.
142. Peters CJ, Johnson ED, Jahrling PB, et al: Filoviruses. *In* Morse S (ed): Emerging Viruses. New York, Oxford University Press, 1991, pp 159–175.
143. Hayes CG, Burans JP, Ksiazek TG, et al: Outbreak of fatal illness among captive macaques in the Philippines caused by an Ebola-related filovirus. Am J Trop Med Hyg 46:664, 1992.
144. World Health Organization: Viral haemorrhagic fever in imported monkeys. Wkly Epidemiol Rec 67:142, 1992.
145. Centers for Disease Control: Update: Filovirus infection among persons with occupational exposure to nonhuman primates. MMWR Morbid Mortal Wkly Rep 39:266, 1990.
146. World Health Organization: Ebola haemorrhagic fever. Wkly Epidemiol Rec 70:149; 1995.
147. American Health Consultants: Lack of barrier precautions linked to Ebola spread. Hosp Infect Control 22:101; 1995.
148. Murphy FA: Pathology of Ebola virus infection. *In* Pattyn SR (ed): Ebola Virus Haemorrhagic Fever. Amsterdam, Elsevier North Holland, 1978, pp 37–42.
149. Fisher-Hoch SP, Platt GS, Neild GH, et al: Pathophysiology of shock and hemorrhage in a fulminating viral infection (Ebola). J Infect Dis 152:887, 1985.
150. Gear JHS: Clinical aspects of African viral hemorrhagic fevers. Rev Infect Dis 11(Suppl 4):S777, 1989.
151. Surreau PH: Firsthand clinical observations of hemorrhagic manifestations in Ebola hemorrhagic fever in Zaire. Rev Infect Dis 11(Suppl 4):S790, 1989.
152. Elliott LH, Bauer SP, Perez-Oronoz G, et al: Improved specificity of testing methods for filovirus antibodies. J Virol Methods 43:85, 1993.
153. Ksiazek T: Laboratory diagnosis of filovirus infections in nonhuman primates. Lab Anim 20:34, 1991.
154. Richman DD, Cleveland PH, McCormick JB, et al: Antigenic analysis of strains of Ebola virus: Identification of two Ebola virus serotypes. J Infect Dis 147:268, 1983.
155. Ksiazek TG, Rollin PE, Jahrling PB, et al: Enzyme immunoassay for Ebola virus antigens in tissues of infected primates. J Clin Microbiol 30:947, 1992.
156. Geisbert TW, Jahrling PB: Use of immunoelectron microscopy to show Ebola virus during the 1989 United States epizootic. J Clin Pathol 43:813, 1990.
157. Centers for Disease Control: Update: Ebola-related filovirus infection in nonhuman primates and interim guidelines for handling nonhuman primates during transit and quarantine. MMWR Morbid Mortal Wkly Rep 39:22, 1990.
158. Chumakov MP: A new virus disease—Crimean hemorrhagic fever [in Russian]. Nov Med 4:9, 1947.
159. Casals J: Antigenic similarity between the virus causing Crimean hemorrhagic fever and Congo virus. Proc Soc Exp Biol Med 131:233, 1969.
160. Hoogstral H: The epidemiology of tick-borne Crimean-Congo hemorrhagic fever in Asia, Europe, and Africa. J Med Entomol 51:307, 1979.
161. Burney MI, Ghafoor A, Saleen M, et al: Nosocomial outbreak of viral hemorrhagic fever caused by Crimean hemorrhagic fever–Congo virus in Pakistan, January 1976. Am J Trop Med Hyg 29:941, 1980.
162. Simpson DIH, Knight EM, Courtois GH, et al: Congo virus: A hitherto undescribed virus occurring in Africa. I. Human isolations—Clinical notes. East Afr Med J 44:86, 1967.
163. Watts DM, Ksiazek TG, Linthicum KJ, et al: Crimean-Congo Hemorrhagic Fever. *In* Monath TP (ed): The Arboviruses: Epidemiology and Ecology, Vol 2. Boca Raton, FL, CRC Press, 1989, pp 177–222.
164. Peters CJ, LeDuc JW: Bunyaviridae: Bunyaviruses, Phleboviruses, and Related Viruses. *In* Belshe RB (ed): Textbook of Human Virology, ed 2. St. Louis, Mosby–Year Book, 1991, pp 571–614.
165. Swanepoel R, Shepherd AJ, Leman PA, et al: Epidemiologic and clinical features of Crimean-Congo hemorrhagic fever in Southern Africa. Am J Trop Med Hyg 36:120, 1987.
166. Swanepoel R, Gill DE, Shepherd AJ, et al: The clinical pathology of Crimean-Congo hemorrhagic fever. Rev Infect Dis 11(Suppl 4):S794, 1989.
167. Shepherd AJ, Swanepoel R, Leman PA: Antibody response in Crimean-Congo hemorrhagic fever. Rev Infect Dis 11(Suppl 4):S801, 1989.
168. Watts DM, Ussery MA, Nash D, et al: Inhibition of Crimean-Congo hemorrhagic fever viral infectivity in vitro by ribavirin. Am J Trop Med Hyg 41:581, 1989.

270

Rabies Virus

Charles E. Rupprecht
Makonnen Fekadu
James E. Childs

The acute, nearly invariably fatal encephalomyelitis that is one of the key defining hallmarks of the disease known as rabies is etiologically attributable to rabies virus and its neurotropic *Lyssavirus* relatives. All warm-blooded vertebrates are probably susceptible to experimental infection but in greatly varying degrees. In nature, mammals form the principal hosts, with distinct reservoirs among the Carnivora and Chiroptera. Owing to the insidious nature and near global distribution of this malady, the ultrastructural, biochemical, molecular, pathobiologic, and immunologic attributes of lyssaviruses are receiving increasing attention.[1–5]

Classification

Rabies has taxonomic affinity with the family Rhabdoviridae, which together with the Filoviridae and Paramyxoviridae form the order Mononegavirales. The Rhabdoviridae family consists of the genus *Vesiculovirus* (type species: vesicular stomatitis virus), the genus *Ephemerovirus* (type species: bovine ephemeral fever virus), the genus *Lyssavirus* (type species: rabies virus), and several uncharacterized rhabdoviruses isolated from a variety of plants, invertebrates, and vertebrates, primarily assigned on the basis of their distinctive rod- or bullet-shaped morphologic characteristics.[6] The genus *Lyssavirus* includes rabies virus and a group of antigenically and genetically related Old World viruses.[7] Previously, rabies and the rabies-related viruses were defined on the basis of morphology, serology, and the ability to cause encephalitis in

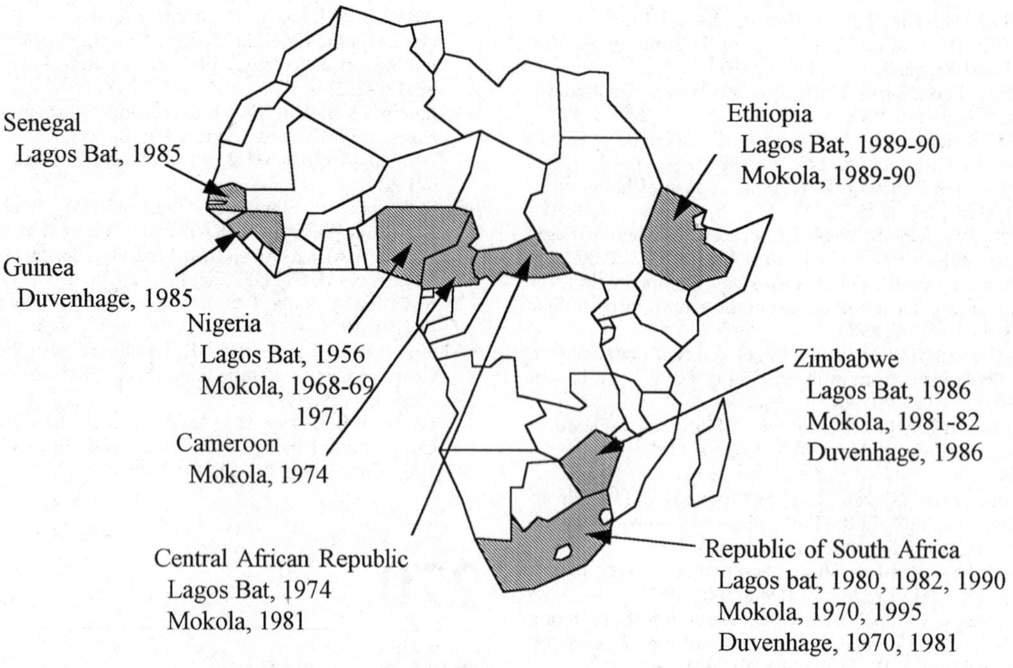

FIGURE 270–1 □ Isolations of lyssaviruses in Africa, 1956 to 1995.

laboratory animals[8]; two rhabdovirus species isolated from insects in Africa, Obodhiang and kotonkan, seemingly aligned with this group on the basis of serology, await further characterization. Tentatively, there are at least five distinct lyssaviruses related to rabies[9–12] but they are easily distinguished by their characteristic antigenic and genetic properties: (1) Lagos bat virus, first isolated from straw-colored fruit bats, *Eidolon helvum*, on Lagos Island, Nigeria, in 1956; (2) Mokola virus, first isolated from *Crocidura* shrews in Ibadan, Nigeria, during 1968; (3) Duvenhage virus, isolated from the brain of a man bitten on the lip by a bat during 1970, in Warmbaths, South Africa; and (4) two different European bat lyssaviruses, type 1 and type 2, isolated from insectivorous bats in western Europe commencing in 1968.

Originally, the nonrabies lyssaviruses were thought to be little more than biologic curiosities,[8] restricted in their geographic distribution to wildlife in regions of sub-Saharan Africa (Fig. 270–1). Although experimental vaccination of laboratory animals with traditional rabies virus vaccines did not provide good cross-reactive immunity to the nonrabies lyssaviruses, such as Mokola or Lagos bat virus, little concern was engendered initially because these viral species appeared limited in host range. Several observations have increased the level of concern of public health workers over the potential significance of the nonrabies lyssaviruses. Mokola and Lagos bat viruses have been isolated from vaccinated domestic animals, raising the possibility of more frequent bite transmission to humans in Africa.[10, 13, 14] Moreover, the finding of European bat lyssaviruses in 1981 from two bats in Western Germany, and later from *Eptesicus serotinus* and *Myotis* species bats throughout western Europe,[15] demonstrated that the distribution and incidence of infection were greater than previously believed (Fig. 270–2). Then, in 1985, a Finnish bat biologist died with type 2 European bat lyssavirus infection, presumably resulting from bat bite, although a definitive source of exposure was not identified. That same year, a child also died of a rabies-like illness in Russia, and the causative agent was later demonstrated to be type 1 European bat lyssavirus. Important questions remain to be answered about these rabies-related lyssaviruses. How widely distributed are these nonrabies lyssaviruses? What are their native reservoirs? How are these viruses transmitted among their reservoirs, and how are they transmitted to humans and domestic animals? What is the role of arthropods, if any, in the natural cycles of the African lyssaviruses, such as Mokola? Will it become necessary to develop new vaccines against these rabies-related viruses? What is the likelihood of translocation of lyssaviruses between the Old and New Worlds?

Besides their differentiation from the other lyssaviruses, isolates of rabies virus may be informally categorized as either fixed laboratory or vaccine strains (Table 270–1), adapted by passage in animals or cell culture, or street (wild-type) viruses. The use of monoclonal antibodies (MAbs) and genetic sequencing to differentiate street rabies viruses has been useful in identifying virus variants originating in major host reservoirs throughout the world[16–31] and has been essential in implicating the likely sources of human exposure when a definitive history of animal bite was unavailable. Great progress has been made since the late 1980s in the understanding of *Lyssavirus* epidemiology and phylogeny through

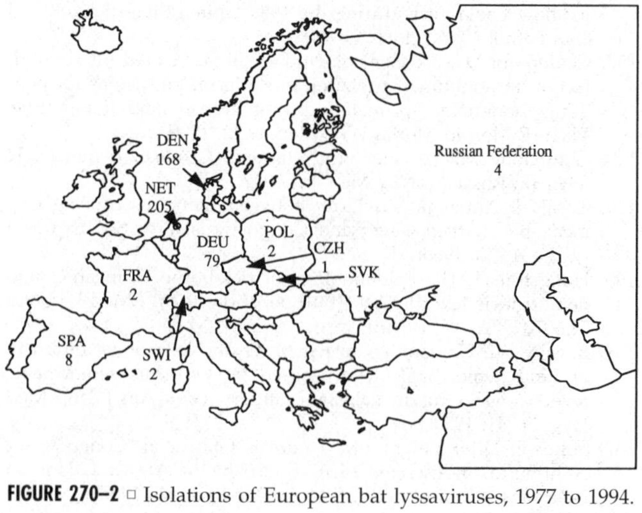

FIGURE 270–2 □ Isolations of European bat lyssaviruses, 1977 to 1994.

TABLE 270–1 ■ Tissue Culture Rabies Vaccines Used in Humans

VACCINE*	CELL SUBSTRATES FOR PRODUCTION	VIRUS STRAINS	CONCENTRATION OR PURIFICATION METHODS	INACTIVATION METHODS	ADJUVANT	LYOPHILIZED
HDCV	Human diploid MRC-5 fibroblasts	PM 1503	Ultrafiltration	Betapropiolactone	No	Yes
RVA	Fetal rhesus diploid lung cells	Kissling	Concentration via adsorption	Betapropiolactone	$AlPO_4$	No
PHKC	Primary hamster kidney cells	Vnukovo-32	Ultrafiltration and zonal centrifugation	Ultraviolet irradiation	No	Yes
PHKC	Primary hamster kidney cells	Beijing 31	Concentration	Inactivated by formalin	$Al(OH)_3$	No
PDKC	Primary dog kidney cells	PM 1503	Ultrafiltration	Betapropiolactone	$AlPO_4$	Yes
HDCV	Human diploid MRC-5 fibroblasts	SAD CL-60	Filtration and zonal centrifugation	Betapropiolactone	No	Yes
PCEC	Primary chick embryo fibroblasts	LEP	Filtration and zonal centrifugation	Betapropiolactone	No	Yes
PDEV	Primary duck embryo	PM 1503	Zonal centrifugation	Betapropiolactone	No	Yes
PVRV	Vero cell line	PM 1503	Density gradient centrifugation	Betapropiolactone	No	Yes

*HDCV, Human diploid cell vaccine; RVA, rabies vaccine, adsorbed; PCEC, purified chicken embryo cell; PVRV, purified Vero cell rabies vaccine.

the application of molecular techniques, particularly rabies virus nucleic acid detection by amplification of complementary DNA by the reverse transcription–polymerase chain reaction[32] with subsequent generation of viral nucleotide sequences. For example, such analyses have provided historical insights into the global dissemination of rabies virus variants by human colonization[25] and the significance of wildlife translocation in current disease distribution patterns.[33, 34] However, it is the extreme sensitivity of the reverse transcription–polymerase chain reaction technique that also greatly increases the probability of a false-positive diagnosis resulting from laboratory contamination. Moreover, because of *Lyssavirus* heterogeneity, false-negative results can occur if primer selection is inadequate to compensate for sequence heterogeneity; universal primers for all known global *Lyssavirus* variants have not been clearly identified or standardized. In view of these factors, the related costs, and the considerable expertise required for proper analysis and interpretation, such molecular techniques are not recommended for routine rabies diagnosis at present.[35]

Characteristics of the Pathogen

Lyssaviruses are single-stranded, negative-sense, unsegmented RNA viruses, with a molecular mass of some 4.6×10^6 daltons.[2] Although defective particles may be proportionately smaller, mature virions measure approximately 75 to 80 nm by 180 to 200 nm. The virion is composed of an internal ribonucleoprotein (RNP) core or nucleocapsid, containing the nucleic acid, and an outer envelope, a lipid-containing bilayer integument covered, except for a cavity at the blunt end, with transmembrane spikes of proteinaceous peplomers or homotrimers,[36] some projecting 6 to 10 nm long (Fig. 270–3).

Several nontranslated spacers or intergenic regions divide the 11.9-kb rabies viral genome (Fig. 270–4), which encodes five polypeptides. One region of the genome located between the end of the G (glycoprotein) protein coding sequence and the beginning of the L (large) protein coding sequence was previously suggested as representative of a remnant sixth *Lyssavirus* gene.[37] Additional data, however, indicate that this region of the genome encodes a G messenger RNA with a long 3′-noncoding region and does not possess evidence of a pseudogene.[38] The five expressed viral proteins are associated with either the symmetrically helical nucleocapsid complex or the viral envelope. The L (originally large or transcriptase protein), the N (nucleoprotein), and the NS (originally nonstructural transcriptase-associated, nominal phosphoprotein, or M1) proteins constitute, together with the linear viral RNA, the RNP complex. The M (matrix protein, or M2) and G proteins are associated with the envelope (7.5 to 10 nm) of neutral lipids, glycolipids, and phospholipids, derived within the host cell.

An understanding of the diverse functions of the five *Lyssavirus* proteins continues to evolve.[39] The relatively high molecular mass (but small copy number) L protein (approximately 185 to 244 kDa, 2142 amino acids) functions during transcription and replication, with associated RNA-dependent RNA polymerase, methylation, messenger RNA 5′-capping, 3′-poly(A), and protein kinase activities. The G protein (about 58 to 80 kDa, approximately 505 amino acids) forms protrusions that cover the outer surface of the virion envelope and may be N-glycosylated at several sites, as a prerequisite for efficient cell surface expression. The rabies G protein is responsible for reception at the host cell membrane,[40] induction of pH-mediated endocytosis, and serotype definition within the *Lyssavirus* genus. The G protein has received an enhanced degree of biomedical focus, because it is the only rabies protein known to induce virus-neutralizing antibody (VNA), in addition to its elicitation of cell-mediated immunity. As quasi species,[41] selection of rabies virus G protein point mutants has allowed definition of specific sites in the genome that may serve as prerequisites for virulence.[42] In contrast to the external G protein, the N protein (approximately 51 to 62 kDa, about 450 amino acids) is the major component of the nucleocapsid and determines the group specificity among lyssaviruses, owing to its considerable antigenic cross-reactivity.[43] It is associated with full-length negative- and positive-sense RNA. Although the precise role of the N protein is unclear, it is tightly bound to the viral RNA and may protect against cellular ribonucleases. In addition, the N protein can modulate transcription and appears to promote replication; phosphorylation of the N protein may involve a host cell protein kinase. The NS protein (approximately 33 to 40 kDa, about 297 amino acids) is necessary for transcription[44] and may prevent protein aggregation while assisting in the deposition of N protein onto RNA. Its phosphorylation probably involves the L viral protein kinase. The M protein (about 21 to 26 kDa, approximately 202 amino acids) is an integral structural component that appears to bind to the nucleocapsid and the cytoplasmic domain of

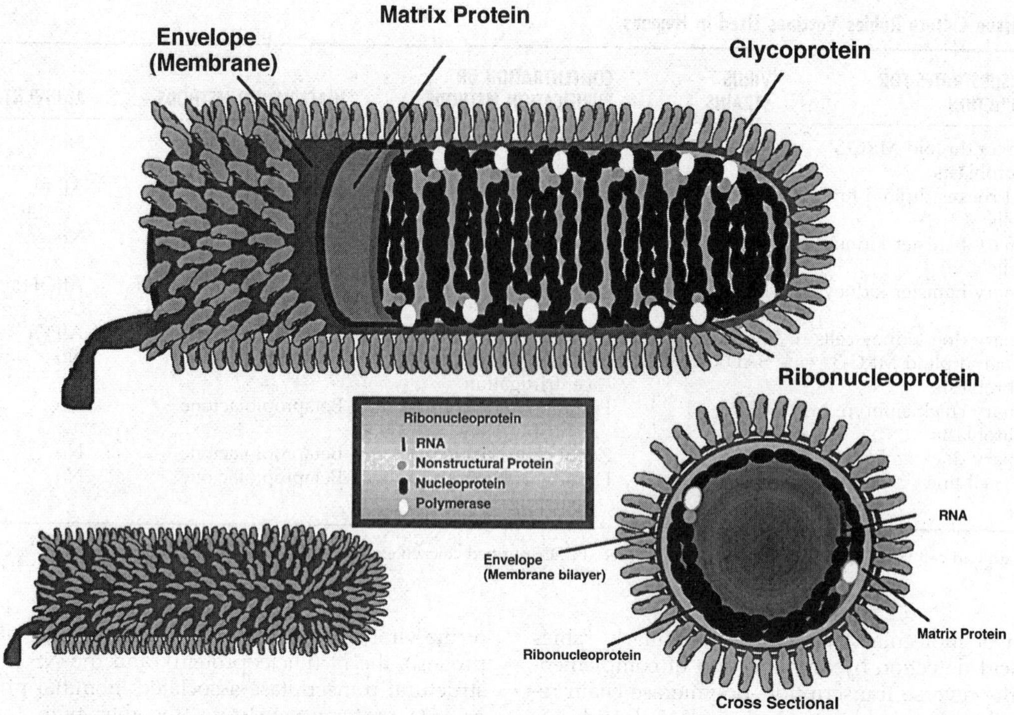

FIGURE 270–3 □ Rabies virions are bullet shaped and measure approximately 180 nm in length and 75 nm in diameter. The outer surface is covered by 10-nm spikelike glycoprotein peplomers inserted into the host cell membrane. The genome RNA encodes for five structural proteins: glycoprotein (G), nucleoprotein (N), nonstructural (NS), large polymerase (L), and matrix (M) proteins. The N, NS, and L proteins and the genomic RNA form the ribonucleoprotein (RNP) core. (Modified from Orciari LA: Genetic Analysis of Rabies Virus Isolates from Skunks in the United States. Athens, GA, University of Georgia, 1995. Master's dissertation.)

the G protein. The M protein, positioned beneath the lipid membrane bilayer, probably facilitates the viral assembly and budding process and may also assist in the regulation of RNA genome transcription.

Lyssaviruses do not persist in the environment. Their resistance to chemical and physical agents partly depends on the source and nature of the infectious material, such as brain tissue, a film of saliva, or purified virus. As an enveloped agent, the virus is sensitive to many lipid solvents.[45] It is rapidly destroyed by exposure to formalin, strong acids and bases, most detergents, and ultraviolet irradiation, including sunlight. Repeated freezing and thawing usually leads to a loss of viral infectivity. It may persist for minutes at 56°C, hours to days at 4°C, weeks to months at −20°C, and years in the proper diluent and sterile conditions at −70°C or colder.

Laboratory isolation of *Lyssavirus* can readily occur by either animal inoculation or cell culture.[46] Newborn, weanling, or young adult rodents (usually mice), inoculated intracranially with brain, saliva, or other material, are the typical hosts of choice for primary virus isolation. Animals are usually observed for a minimum of 4 weeks, although they may show clinical illness as early as 5 to 7 days after inoculation. A number of susceptible host cells, notably continuous lines of BHK-21 or murine neuroblastoma cells, have gradually replaced routine animal inoculation for virus isolation.

Virus Reproduction

Lyssavirus multiplication (Fig. 270–5) is believed to be similar to that of other negative-stranded RNA viruses that have been more intensively studied, such as vesicular stomatitis virus. The precise mechanism of entry of virus into the nerve is not clear. Some evidence supports the belief that rabies virus binds selectively at or near nicotinic acetylcholine receptors[47–55] via neuromuscular junctions. These sites are close to unsheathed nerves at synaptic clefts, where virus can gain ready access to the axoplasm. This intriguing hypothesis does not preclude alternative mechanisms or routes supportive of viral neurotropism, because other protein-based receptors

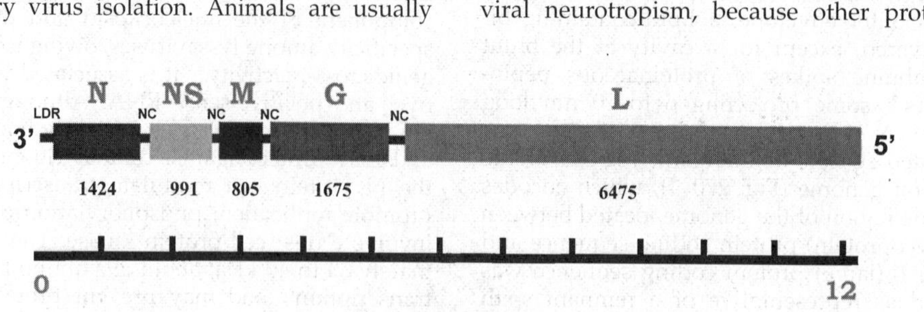

FIGURE 270–4 □ The rabies virus genome is single-stranded, antisense, nonsegmented RNA of approximately 12 kb. There is a leader of 50 nucleotides followed by N, NS, M, G, and L genes, which code for the five structural proteins. The intergenic noncoding regions are considered the most variable, especially the M-G and G-L genes. (Modified from Orciari LA: Genetic Analysis of Rabies Virus Isolates from Skunks in the United States. Athens, GA, University of Georgia, 1995. Master's dissertation.)

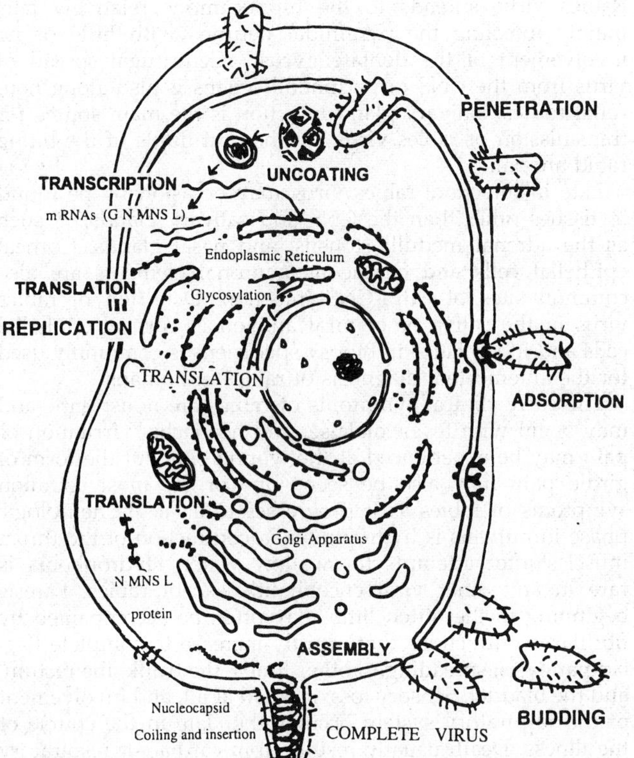

FIGURE 270–5 □ Generalized *Lyssavirus* cycle of infection and replication involves adsorption (virus peplomers–host cell receptor interaction); penetration (endocytosis or pinocytosis of the virus via clathrin-coated pits); uncoating (release of the RNP into the host cell cytoplasm); transcription (L + NS polymerase transcribe negative-sense RNA to form five capped, methylated, polyadenylated messenger RNAs (mRNAs) and 50-nt leader); translation (synthesis of N, NS, and M proteins on polyribosomes in the rough endoplasmic reticulum); processing (stepwise glycoprotein glycosylation, migration, and insertion into the cytoplasmic membrane); replication (production of plus strand genome template and complementary negative strand); assembly (binding of the N, NS, and L proteins, and RNA to form RNP, the formation of M-RNP complex, which binds to the cytoplasmic membrane containing glycoprotein inserts to form complete virus); and budding (release of completed virions). (Modified from Wagner RR, Thomas JR, McGowan JJ: Rhabdovirus cytopathopathology: Effects on cellular macromolecular synthesis. *In* Fraenkel-Courat H, Wagner RR [eds]: Comprehensive Virology, Vol 19. New York: Plenum Publishing, 1984, pp 223–295; and Dubois-Dalco M, Holmes KV, Rentier B: Assembly of Enveloped RNA Viruses. [Kingsbury DW, ed] New York, Springer-Verlag, 1984.)

can also bind rabies virus, and acetylcholine receptors are not exclusively found in some sites permissively supportive of rabies virus infection.[56, 57]

After eventual viral invasion at a host portal of entry (usually a bite wound), viral attachment to host cell membranes occurs via a conformational alteration in the G protein during receptor-mediated endocytosis or by planar fusion. After adsorption, viral particles may penetrate the cell cytoplasm within an endosome. Coated vesicles may fuse with lysosomes and are uncoated to RNP in a low-pH microenvironmental event, perhaps mediated by a putative fusion domain of the G protein.[58] In cellular locales rich in ribosomes, such as in the perikaryon or proximal dendrite, the RNP core initiates primary transcription of the five complementary monocistronic messenger RNAs by using the virion-associated RNA-dependent RNA polymerase. Each RNA is then translated into an individual viral protein. After viral proteins have been synthesized, replication of the genomic RNA continues with the synthesis of full-length, positive-stranded RNA, which acts as a template for the production of progeny negative-stranded RNA. Within the central nervous system (CNS), *Lyssavirus* replication has been associated almost exclusively with neurons,[1] and there is little evidence to suggest replication in astrocytes, glial cells, oligodendrocytes, or Schwann cells.

Whereas nucleocapsid production commences in the cytosol, the viral G protein appears to be synthesized and glycosylated on the rough endoplasmic reticulum as an approximately 524 amino acid precursor,[2] in which the N-terminal 19–amino acid leader or signal is cleaved, leaving a portion of about 505 amino acids. Primary structure of the G protein consists of a C-terminal cytoplasmic endodomain anchor, a transmembrane portion, and an antigenic ectodomain of some 439 amino acids; the removal of the approximately 44 amino acids of the endodomain and a portion of the transmembrane sequence results in a truncated soluble form of the G protein, which is ordinarily unable to induce protective immunity[59] without alteration.[60] Further G protein processing may occur via transport through the Golgi apparatus. A specific biochemical configuration appears to act in avoidance of nonspecific membrane fusion, until acquisition of its native state at the cell surface.[61] Viral assembly of nucleocapsid with membrane components and budding of the virion from the infected cell may occur by the inverse process of initial viral attachment and adsorption. In contrast, the process of envelope formation on cytoplasmic membranes is quite variable and may be exceedingly complex in its three-dimensional array.[1] A high proportion of amino acid substitutions in the G protein may be tolerated while molecular function is retained (provided that comparative charge and hydrophobicity or hydrophilicity is conserved), but even a single amino acid alteration at certain locations may be critical in the determination of relative virulence, in part because of influences on secondary structure, recognition at neural termini, restrictions in conformational epitopes, and subsequent viral clearance.[62–65] This last generation of viral escape mutants under neutralizing antibody pressure in vitro has proved useful in the delineation of operational antigenic sites, as well as in the development of apathogenic rabies virus vaccines.[66] Because a variety of hydrophobic membrane proteins have already been crystallized, future definition of the three-dimensional structure of the rabies G protein by x-ray crystallography may enable a better topographic localization of operationally defined viral epitopes by mapping of the amino acid substitutions of escape variants belonging to a particular antigenic group, so as to design novel antiviral agents.

Pathogenesis, Pathophysiology, Pathology, and Clinical Features

For more than a century, it has been appreciated that rabies is primarily caused by entry of an infectious agent into a wound, usually inflicted by a bite.[67] In 1804, the pathogenesis of rabies infection was described by Zinke, who experimentally transmitted rabies by swabbing the saliva of rabid dogs onto fresh wounds of rabbits and dogs and showed that saliva contained the infectious agent. He also indirectly confirmed the observations of Morgagni, who in 1769 described the "paresthesia" of early sensory and motor symptoms at the site of bite exposure as evidence that the infectious agent travels via the nervous system.

Centripetal spread of virus from the site of entry to the CNS occurs within motor and sensory axons of peripheral nerves. Sectioning of the sciatic nerve after ipsilateral footpad inoculation can prevent the development of rabies,[68] indicating that rabies virus spreads to the spinal cord via primary innervation pathways. Local application of microtubule-disrupting agents (active on tubulin-containing cytoskeletal structures) to the ischiatic nerve, thereby inhibiting axonal transport, succeeded in altering virus propagation, providing additional evidence for axonal transport of rabies virus.[69] This neurotropic ability of rabies virus provides utility as an efficient microanatomic tracer of neuronal networks in vivo[70]; after primary infection of hypoglossal motor neurons, retrograde transneuronal viral transfer occurred by 2 days after inoculation (unaccompanied by neuronal degeneration), with sequential involvement of second-order neurons and spread to higher order cortical and subcortical cell groups, but not to adjoining glial cells or uninfected fibers of passage.

The incubation period of rabies in humans and animals may vary from days to years.[23, 71] In nature, this usually slow course of productive infection in the proximate individual host may ensure rabies virus survival until new susceptible reservoir generations reach a density necessary for efficient virus transmission.[72] Long incubation periods may assist in the selection of a virus population that can reach and multiply in the salivary glands and be excreted in the saliva of a rabid individual. Yet, there is no great difference in the pathogenic behavior of the virus in foxes, skunks, and bats on the one hand and in cattle, horses, and humans on the other.[4] A primary difference in rabies infection between reservoir host species (i.e., species involved in virus transmission and perpetuation in nature, such as the mammalian carnivores and bats) and the "dead end" host or victim species (i.e., livestock and humans) may have more to do with different biting tendencies of each species when rabid than with the nature of the infection itself in the individual animal.

From experimental animal models, it has been shown that rabies virus may replicate in muscle cells during early stages of infection, before virus entry into the nerve endings, and that virus may remain at the site of entry for a prolonged time.[4, 73] Other experiments, however, demonstrated that virus replication in muscle cells before entry of the nerve endings is not necessarily a pathogenic requirement for the development of CNS infection.[74] Obviously, these somewhat conflicting observations do not adequately explain the precise location, the form of residual virus, or the mechanism by which virus can exist during this eclipse phase. A number of factors, alone or in combination, may be operative as potential explanations. Virus may be sequestered at the original site of entry, undergoing no, or only minimal, replication in muscle or associated tissue, until some unknown future stimulus or event brings it into proximity with a nerve ending. In contrast, the sequestration site may not necessarily be nonneural in origin but may be at the level of the dorsal root ganglia and involve RNP[75] with little replicative activity owing to some defect in the available biochemical milieu. If frank disease has an immunologic basis, the incubation period may equate with a dynamic stasis, perhaps related to a delayed immunologic surveillance via antigen-presenting cells.[76] In theory, inocula may also contain defective interfering particles that limit neuronal access until after a variable delay. Regardless, unusually long incubation periods, exceeding 4 to 6 weeks, tend to be the exception rather than the observed rule.

During the centripetal transport of rabies virus locally to the brain, insufficient viral antigen may be detected by the immune system to induce an immune response.[5] No reliable diagnostic method is currently available to qualitatively determine a case of rabies in humans or animals during the incubation period,[68] before the prodromal stage. Once the CNS neurons become infected, there is rapid dissemination of the virus along neuronal pathways. The infection spreads to the brain stem tegmentum and deep cerebellar nuclei, cerebellar Purkinje cells, and neurons in the cerebral cortex. Rabies virus spreads to the hippocampus relatively late, mainly infecting the pyramidal neurons with little or no involvement of the dentate gyrus.[77] Centrifugal spread of virus from the CNS to peripheral organs is also along neuronal routes. Salivary gland infection is the main source for transmission of rabies virus via the oral fluids of the biting rabid animal.

Late in infection, rabies virus may occasionally be found in tissues other than the CNS and salivary glands,[4, 78] such as the adrenal medulla, tonsils, and nasal glands. Corneal epithelial cells and cutaneous neuronal elements are also common sites of extra-CNS infection. Detection of rabies virus in the saliva or of viral antigen in corneal epithelial cells and in nuchal skin biopsy specimens is commonly used for the antemortem diagnosis of rabies in humans.[79]

The early clinical symptoms of rabies are nonspecific and may begin with fever, malaise, and headache.[80] Irritation or pain may be experienced at the wound site, but the form of girdle pain may also be seen. One of the most common symptoms of rabies as it progresses to an acute neurologic phase in humans is hydrophobia, a contraction of the throat muscles after attempts to swallow water. Hydrophobia is rare in any other viral encephalitis except rabies. Paresis beginning in the bitten limb may often be accompanied by fibrillary contractions that rapidly increase to complete flaccid paralysis, spreading to other limbs, the trunk, the rectum, and the bladder. Sensory loss, if noted at all, and involvement of the respiratory system occur rather late in the course of the illness. Death usually results from cardiac or respiratory failure. In rabies enzootic areas, any patient who develops an acute neurologic disease of viral cause should be suspected of having rabies. Definitive rabies diagnosis requires a careful evaluation of the epidemiology of animal rabies in the area where the patient may have been exposed, in addition to the clinical examination of the patient.

Rabies is usually considered to be invariably fatal. However, recovery from rabies, usually with severe neurologic sequelae, has been documented in a few naturally infected humans and animals.[81, 82] Similar observations have also been made in experimentally infected animals.[83–88]

Despite its acute onset, striking clinical manifestations, and overt lethality, and the often extensive neuronal involvement of the CNS, the pathologic findings associated with rabies are relatively mild, with little to no cell destruction or cytopathic changes. Typically, no gross pathologic changes are visible other than a variable degree of cerebral edema and meningeal congestion. Nonspecific inflammation of variable severity can be observed in the brain, spinal cord, and ganglia. Inflammatory infiltration, consisting primarily of mononuclear cells, may be detected in the leptomeninges. The severity of infection and to some extent the location of pathologic changes may be directly proportional to the duration of the morbidity period. Long morbidity periods can result in greater pathologic changes and a wider distribution of virus in the CNS and peripheral organs.[89] Microscopic changes, including perivascular cuffing, neuronophagia, and modest neuronal necrosis, tend to be sparse in relation to the overall extent of viral antigen detection by immunofluorescence.[90–92]

Light microscopic histopathologic study, focused on identification of the eosinophilic intracytoplasmic pathognomic inclusion body (Negri body) of rabies virus in infected neurons, underestimates the wide distribution of viral antigen in the brain. Negri bodies are haloed, ovoid cytoplasmic bodies; their development is usually related to the morbidity period of the victim.[93] These inclusions are typically detected by light microscopy in only 50% to 75% of specimens otherwise found positive by virus isolation, immunofluorescence, or ultrastructural microscopy.[79] Negri bodies are seen most frequently in the Purkinje cells in the cerebellum and the pyramidal cells in the hippocampus, and less often in the medulla, spinal cord, cerebral cortex, basal ganglia, and peripheral ganglia. Negri bodies consist of viral nucleocapsid protein, identical to the mass of matrices seen by electron microscopy[94]; these matrices correspond to the site of virus replication. Neurons containing viral matrices, accompanied by prolific numbers of viral particles budding from membranes of the rough endoplasmic reticulum and the plasma membrane, are usually seen by ultrastructural microscopy.[1] Less commonly appreciated as a pathologic manifestation of rabies, induced spongiform change of the gray matter, affecting the neuropil and neuronal cell bodies of the thalamus and cerebral cortex, has been documented in experimental and naturally occurring cases.[95, 96]

Rather than physical destruction of microscopic elements, select organic dysfunction, owing to pathophysiologic disruption in critical neuronal activities and neurotransmitter imbalance, may ultimately explain the underlying mechanisms of apparent viral virulence.[97] Recognition of the functional interaction that exists between the immune system and the CNS during health and disease is also clearly indicated. For example, during rabies virus encephalitis, brain receptors for interleukin-1 may decrease while local interleukin-1 concentrations are increasing.[98, 99] Moreover, copious amounts of nitric oxide may be produced locally in the brain in response to rabies infection.[100, 101] A combined, targeted immunopharmacologic rationale, following rapid, accurate diagnosis, may hold the future approach toward resolution of lethal rabies encephalomyelitis.[102]

Host Immune Mechanisms

Immunity to rabies potentially involves the induction of both nonspecific and specific immune responses in the host. Exposure to virus may or may not lead to productive infection, and either outcome may or may not result in detectable immune responses,[5, 103] depending on an interplay of viral and host factors. In the nontreated patient, rabies-specific VNA may be only rarely detected in serum at the onset of illness and usually does not occur, if at all, until later stages of disease. Antibody in high titer in the cerebrospinal fluid of infected individuals, in contrast to the vaccinee, is considered a reliable indication of CNS infection. The immune reaction can be appropriate and protective or may in some instances be detrimental and actually contribute to the pathogenesis of clinical disease.[104–106] Administration of humoral antibody alone immediately after exposure may actually prolong the incubation period of rabies infection, as demonstrated by passive immunization in experimental animals. Immunosuppression, either induced or genetic, may also prolong the incubation period; conversely, administration of rabies VNA may induce what has been termed the early death phenomenon, associated with inflammatory neuronal lesions. Primates inoculated with low-potency vaccines after rabies virus exposure died earlier than did nonimmunized rabies-infected control animals, suggesting that clinical rabies may involve immunopathologic mechanisms.

Cytokines such as interferon[107–110] can also be involved in the immunity or pathogenesis of rabies. Although rabid patients have relatively low levels of endogenous interferon in the terminal CNS, virus replication can be inhibited by interferon administration early after infection. Nevertheless, the experimental administration of interferon was not found to be therapeutic when administered either peripherally or intrathecally 1 to 2 weeks after the onset of disease.

Although rabies virus particles represent complex antigens consisting of five different structural proteins, the induction of protective antiviral immunity has focused primarily on the response to the surface G protein. Historically, rabies VNAs were believed to play the major role in immune protection against rabies.[111, 112] However, comparison of VNA titers and mortality in laboratory animals immunized with whole-virus vaccine or viral G protein does not always delineate a clear relationship between absolute titer level of VNA and vaccine-induced resistance to rabies.[113] Rather, some immunization experiments indicate that protective activity may correlate more with a vaccine's ability to induce immunologic memory. This lack of a firm correlation between absolute VNA titers and survivorship in immunized animals suggested that, in addition to the G protein and VNA alone, other antigens and immune effector mechanisms were likely to be involved in the protection against lethal rabies virus infection, in either pre- or postexposure situations.

Identification of the relative contribution of the individual *Lyssavirus* antigens in humoral versus cellular immunity has been slowly forthcoming. To this end, the relative role of different *Lyssavirus* antigens in helper T-cell activation has been approached experimentally by measuring antigen-mediated lymphokine release to various rabies structural proteins.[114] Intact virus usually induces the highest lymphokine secretion, with the greatest response to purified viral antigens being to the N, G, NS, and M proteins, respectively. In addition, several human T-lymphocyte clones from rabies vaccine recipients have been isolated and characterized.[115–118] Most of these rabies-reactive clones were of the helper/inducer class of T lymphocytes. These T-cell clones were tested in proliferation assays for their ability to recognize antigenic determinants in rabies virus and related lyssaviruses. Some of the T cells cross-reacted with classic fixed rabies viruses and also with Duvenhage and Mokola viruses. The majority of these cross-reactive helper T cells recognized determinants present in the viral RNP. In addition, rabies cytotoxic T-cell responses were evident against antigenic determinants of both the RNP and the G proteins. Those T-cell clones that exhibited different cross-reactivity patterns among several viruses were found to recognize closely situated epitopes, presented in the context of the same major histocompatibility complex molecule. Thus, lack of recognition of a particular *Lyssavirus* by a given T-cell clone may be attributable in some cases to amino acid variation in the antigen of question. Moreover, rabies virus T-cell responses in humans are apparently restricted by more than a single product of the human leukocyte antigen–gene complex. These data also suggest that besides the external G protein, internal proteins are a major target for rabies-specific helper T cells.

Certain internal *Lyssavirus* antigens may possess an inherent capacity to enhance immune responsiveness,[119] characterized by some as having the qualities of a superantigen.[120] In lieu of other antigens, rabies RNP is capable of inducing protection against a peripheral rabies virus challenge,[121, 122] in the absence of VNA. A single inoculation of RNP prepared from either rabies or Mokola virus resulted in 80% to 90% protection against a peripheral lethal rabies challenge. In addition, administration of Mokola or rabies virus RNP resulted in substantial protection of mice challenged with Duvenhage virus, indicating that immunization with RNP can confer cross-protective immunity against infection to heterologous lyssaviruses. One of the significant functions of these RNP-specific immune responses may be the promotion of viral RNP attachment via Fc receptors to phagocytic cells, which are then stimulated by virus to produce cytokines such as interferon, inhibiting virus replication.

The last century has exploited the small advances made in applied immunology in the development of a plethora of rabies vaccines.[123] Ideally, these biologicals should maximize potency, purity, safety, efficacy, and cost. Although a few live virus vaccines were effective in rabies prophylaxis, did not require adjuvant, and induced a long-lasting immune response that involved the full spectrum of immune effectors, these traditionally carried the risk of vaccine-induced disease,[124] especially in the immunocompromised host. Inactivated animal neural vaccines eliminated the potential for vaccine-associated rabies but were hampered by low potency and adverse reactions due to myelin basic proteins. The research focus in rabies vaccinology during the past 30 years[125] has been toward inactivated tissue culture rabies vaccines for domestic animal[126] and human use (see Table 270–1), which vary in the nature of the cell substrate, seed strain, method of concentration and inactivation, adjuvant type, and phase for storage. Modern methods of vaccine production are finally able to begin to reach those populations in the developing world most at risk for rabies.[127–135]

Human rabies postexposure treatment typically includes the simultaneous administration of vaccine and polyclonal antirabies immunoglobulin. This extremely effective treatment regimen (with relatively few exceptions[125, 136, 137]) still presents certain practical obstacles arising from availability, quality assurance, and cost. In addition, passively administered antibodies may interfere with the induction of immune effectors, such as helper T-cell and cytotoxic T-cell responses. Thus, novel biologicals, such as murine antirabies MAbs, may fill a niche in the postexposure treatment of humans against rabies.[138, 139] However, murine MAbs may induce an immune response in humans to mouse allotypes, which may later interfere with the use of other mouse MAbs (e.g., MAbs used for cancer treatment). Recombinant DNA techniques can minimize this problem by "humanizing" mouse MAb genes. Alternatively, hybridomas that secrete rabies virus antigen-specific human MAbs have been generated.[140–144] Protection experiments in rabies virus–infected animals revealed that MAbs may be effective in preventing lethal rabies virus infection even after the virus may have entered the CNS.[145] Such an MAb cocktail might offer several distinctive advantages over hyperimmune serum: the specific virus-neutralizing activity and protective activity would be higher than those of rabies immunoglobulin; only relatively small quantities of MAbs have to be utilized based on protein content; and use of MAbs may be superior for local wound treatment, when only small volumes can be inoculated at the actual bite site. If selective, cost-effective, panreactive antibodies can be developed, which efficaciously neutralize virus but do not interfere with active immunization from vaccine,[146] these might form the basis for the development of a more rational treatment protocol, perhaps involving MAbs and a next generation of recombinant-derived *Lyssavirus* biologicals.[147, 148]

Both G and N protein genes have now been effectively expressed in a number of prokaryotic and eukaryotic systems[34, 149–162] for parenteral and oral applications. The productive analysis of these and other *Lyssavirus* genes may eventually contribute to a better understanding of the precise role of individual proteins in the effective induction of protective immune mechanisms. Clearly, host defense against rabies infection is an extremely complex and still poorly understood phenomenon a century after Pasteur's death. Despite numerous and intensive studies of rabies pathogenesis and immunity, the appreciation of the virus-host interaction in this almost invariably fatal viral infection is far from complete.

References

1. Gosztonyi G: Reproduction of lyssaviruses: Ultrastructural composition of *Lyssavirus* and functional aspects of pathogenesis. Curr Top Microbiol Immunol 187:43, 1994.
2. Wunner WH: The chemical composition and molecular structure of rabies viruses. *In* Baer GM (ed): The Natural History of Rabies, ed 2. Boca Raton, FL, CRC Press, 1991, p 31.
3. Tordo N, Kouknetzoff A: The rabies virus genome: An overview. Onderstepoort J Vet Res 60:263, 1993.
4. Charlton KM: The pathogenesis of rabies and other lyssaviral infections: Recent studies. Curr Top Microbiol Immunol 187:95, 1994.
5. Lafon M: Immunobiology of lyssaviruses: The basis for immunoprotection. Curr Top Microbiol Immunol 187:145, 1994.
6. Wunner WH, Calisher CH, Dietzgen RG, et al: Rhabdoviridae. Arch Virol Suppl 10:275, 1995.
7. Bourhy H, Kissi B, Tordo N: Molecular diversity of the *Lyssavirus* genus. Virology 194:70, 1993.
8. Shope RE: Rabies-related viruses. Yale J Biol Med 55:271, 1982.
9. Rupprecht CE, Dietzschold B, Wunner WH, et al: Antigenic relationships of lyssaviruses. *In* Baer GM (ed): The Natural History of Rabies, ed 2. Boca Raton FL, CRC Press, 1991, pp 69–100.
10. Swanepoel R, Barnard BJH, Meredith CD, et al: Rabies in southern Africa. Onderstepoort J Vet Res 60:325, 1993.
11. Schneider LG, Cox JH: Bat lyssaviruses in Europe. Curr Top Microbiol Immunol 187:207, 1994.
12. King AA, Meredith CD, Thomson GR: The biology of southern African lyssavirus variants. Curr Top Microbiol Immunol 187:267, 1994.
13. Foggin CM: Mokola virus infection in cats and a dog in Zimbabwe. Vet Rec 113:115, 1983.
14. Wiktor TJ, Macfarlan RI, Foggin CM, et al: Antigenic analysis of rabies and Mokola virus from Zimbabwe using monoclonal antibodies. Dev Biol Stand 57:199, 1984.
15. Muller WW: Review of reported rabies case data in Europe to the WHO Collaborating Centre Tübingen from 1977 to 1994. Rabies Bull Eur 18:17, 1994.
16. Dietzschold B, Tollis M, Rupprecht CE, et al: Antigenic variation in rabies and rabies-related viruses: Cross-protection independent of glycoprotein-mediated virus-neutralizing antibody. J Infect Dis 156:815, 1987.
17. Dietzschold B, Rupprecht CE, Tollis M, et al: Antigenic diversity of the glycoprotein and nucleocapsid proteins of rabies and rabies-related viruses: Implications for epidemiology and control of rabies. Rev Infect Dis 10(Suppl 4):S785, 1988.
18. Bourhy H, Kissi B, Lafon M, et al: Antigenic and molecular characterization of bat rabies virus in Europe. J Clin Microbiol 30:2419, 1992.
19. Kissi B, Tordo N, Bourhy H: Genetic polymorphism in the rabies virus nucleoprotein gene. Virology 209:526, 1995.
20. Bourhy H, Kissi B, Tordo N: Taxonomy and evolutionary studies on lyssaviruses with special reference to Africa. Onderstepoort J Vet Res 60:277, 1993.
21. Smith JS: Rabies virus epitopic variation: Use in ecologic studies. Adv Virus Res 36:215, 1989.
22. Smith JS, Yager PA, Bigler WJ, et al: Surveillance and epidemiologic mapping of monoclonal antibody-defined rabies variants in Florida. J Wildl Dis 26:473, 1990.
23. Smith JS, Fishbein DB, Rupprecht CE, et al: Unexplained rabies in three immigrants in the United States. A virologic investigation. N Engl J Med 324:205, 1991.
24. Smith JS, Orciari LA, Yager PA, et al: Epidemiologic and historical relationships among 87 rabies virus isolates as determined by limited sequence analysis. J Infect Dis 166:296, 1992.
25. Smith JS, Seidel HD: Rabies: A new look at an old disease. Prog Med Virol 40:82, 1993.
26. Mccoll KA, Gould AR, Selleck PW, et al: Polymerase chain reaction and other laboratory techniques in the diagnosis of long incubation rabies in Australia. Aust Vet J 70:84, 1993.
27. Smith JS, Orciari LA, Yager PA: Molecular epidemiology of rabies in the United States. Semin Virol 6:387, 1995.
28. Sacramento D, Bourhy H, Tordo N: PCR technique as an alternative method for diagnosis and molecular epidemiology of rabies virus. Mol Cell Probes 5:229, 1991.
29. Orciari LA: Genetic Analysis of Rabies Virus Isolates from Skunks in the United States. Athens, GA, University of Georgia, 1995. Master's dissertation.
30. Nadin-Davis SA, Casey GA, Wandeler AI: A molecular epidemiological study of rabies virus in central Ontario and western Quebec. J Gen Virol 75:2575, 1994.
31. Mebatsion T, Cox JH, Conzelmann KK: Molecular analysis of rabies-related viruses from Ethiopia. Onderstepoort J Vet Res 60:289, 1993.

32. Ermine A, Larzul D, Ceccaldi PE, et al: Polymerase chain reaction amplification of rabies virus nucleic acids from total mouse brain RNA. Mol Cell Probes 4:189, 1990.
33. Centers for Disease Control and Prevention: Translocation of coyote rabies—Florida, 1994. MMWR Morbid Mortal Wkly Rep 44:580, 1995.
34. Rupprecht CE, Smith JS, Fekadu M, et al: The ascension of wildlife rabies: A cause for public health concern or intervention? Emerging Infect Dis 1:107, 1995.
35. World Health Organization: WHO Workshop on Genetic and Antigenic Molecular Epidemiology of Lyssaviruses. Geneva, World Health Organization, 1994.
36. Gaudin Y, Ruigrok RW, Tuffereau C, et al: Rabies virus glycoprotein is a trimer. Virology 187:627, 1992.
37. Tordo N, Poch O, Ermine A, et al: Walking along the rabies genome: Is the large G-L intergenic region a remnant gene? Proc Natl Acad Sci USA 83:3914, 1986.
38. Ravkov EV, Smith JS, Nichol ST: Rabies virus glycoprotein gene contains a long 3′ noncoding region which lacks pseudogene properties. Virology 206:718, 1995.
39. Kawai A, Morimoto K: Functional aspects of lyssavirus proteins. Curr Top Microbiol Immunol 187:27, 1994.
40. Gaudin Y, Ruigrok RW, Knossow M, et al: Low-pH conformational changes of rabies virus glycoprotein and their role in membrane fusion. J Virol 67:1365, 1993.
41. de la Torre JC, Holland JJ: RNA virus quasispecies populations can suppress vastly superior mutant progeny. J Virol 64:6278, 1990.
42. Coulon P, Lafay F, Tuffereau C, Flamand A: The molecular basis for altered pathogenicity of lyssavirus variants. Curr Top Microbiol Immunol 187:69, 1994.
43. Kissi B, Tordo N, Bourhy H: Genetic polymorphism in the rabies virus nucleoprotein gene. Virology 209:526, 1995.
44. Chenik M, Chebli K, Gaudin Y, et al: In vivo interaction of rabies virus phosphoprotein (P) and nucleoprotein (N): Existence of two N-binding sites on P protein. J Gen Virol 75:2889, 1994.
45. Kaplan MM: Safety precautions in handling rabies virus. *In* Meslin F-X, Kaplan MM, Koprowski H (eds): Laboratory Techniques in Rabies, ed 4. Geneva, World Health Organization, 1996, pp 3–8.
46. Sureau P, Ravisse P, Rollin PE: Rabies diagnosis by animal inoculation, identification of Negri bodies, or ELISA. *In* Baer GM (ed): The Natural History of Rabies, ed 2. Boca Raton, FL, CRC Press, 1991, pp 203–217.
47. Lentz TL, Burrage TG, Smith AL, et al: Is the acetylcholine receptor a rabies virus receptor? Science 215:182, 1982.
48. Lentz TL, Burrage TG, Smith AL, et al: The acetylcholine receptor as a cellular receptor for rabies virus. Yale J Biol Med 56:315, 1983.
49. Lentz TL, Wilson PT, Hawrot E, et al: Amino acid sequence similarity between rabies virus glycoprotein and snake venom curaremimetic neurotoxins. Science 226:847, 1984.
50. Lentz TL, Benson RJ, Klimowicz D, et al: Binding of rabies virus to purified *Torpedo* acetylcholine receptor. Brain Res 387:211, 1986.
51. Lentz TL, Hawrot E, Wilson PT: Synthetic peptides corresponding to sequences of snake venom neurotoxins and rabies virus glycoprotein bind to the nicotinic acetylcholine receptor. Proteins 2:298, 1987.
52. Lentz TL, Hawrot E, Donnelly-Roberts D, et al: Synthetic peptides in the study of the interaction of rabies virus and the acetylcholine receptor. Adv Biochem Psychopharmacol 44:57, 1988.
53. Lentz TL: Rabies virus binding to an acetylcholine receptor alpha-subunit peptide. J Mol Recognit 3:82, 1990.
54. Baer GM, Shaddock JH, Quirion R, et al: Rabies susceptibility and acetylcholine receptor (Letter). Lancet 335:664, 1990.
55. Lentz TL: Structure-function relationships of curaremimetic neurotoxin loop 2 and of a structurally similar segment of rabies virus glycoprotein in their interaction with the nicotinic acetylcholine receptor. Biochemistry 30:10949, 1991.
56. Reagan KJ, Wunner WH: Rabies virus interaction with various cell lines is independent of the acetylcholine receptor. Arch Virol 84:277, 1985.
57. Broughan JH, Wunner WH: Characterization of protein involvement in rabies virus binding to BHK-21 cells. Arch Virol 140:75, 1995.
58. Durrer P, Gaudin Y, Ruigrok RWH, et al: Photolabeling identifies a putative fusion domain in the envelope glycoprotein of rabies and vesicular stomatitis viruses. J Biol Chem 270:17575, 1995.
59. Dietzschold B, Wiktor TJ, Wunner WH, et al: Chemical and immunological analysis of the rabies soluble glycoprotein. Virology 124:330, 1983.
60. Wojczyk B, Shakin-Eshleman SH, Doms RW, et al: Stable secretion of a soluble, oligomeric form of rabies virus glycoprotein: Influence of N-glycan processing on secretion. Biochemistry 34:2599, 1995.
61. Gaudin Y, Tuffereau C, Durrer P, et al: Biological function of the low-pH, fusion-inactive conformation of rabies virus glycoprotein (G): G is transported in a fusion-inactive state-like conformation. J Virol 69:5528, 1995.
62. Dietzschold B, Wunner WH, Wiktor TJ, et al: Characterization of an antigenic determinant of the glycoprotein that correlates with pathogenicity of rabies virus. Proc Natl Acad Sci USA 80:70, 1983.
63. Dietzschold B, Wiktor TJ, Trojanowski JQ, et al: Differences in cell-to-cell spread of pathogenic and apathogenic rabies virus in vivo and in vitro. J Virol 56:12, 1985.
64. Dietzschold B, Tollis M, Lafon M, et al: Mechanisms of rabies virus neutralization by glycoprotein-specific monoclonal antibodies. Virology 161:29, 1987.
65. Flamand A, Coulon P, Gaudin Y, et al: Reversible conformational changes of the rabies glycoprotein that mask or expose epitopes involved in virulence. J Cell Biochem Suppl 19A:277, 1995.
66. Lafay F, Benejean J, Tuffereau C, et al: Vaccination against rabies: Construction and characterization of SAG2, a double avirulent derivative of SADBern. Vaccine 12:317, 1994.
67. Steele JH, Fernandez PJ: History of rabies and global aspects. *In* Baer GM (ed): The Natural History of Rabies, ed 2. Boca Raton, FL, CRC Press, 1991, p 1.
68. Baer GM, Cleary WF, Diaz AM, et al: Characteristics of 11 rabies virus isolates in mice: Titers and relative invasiveness of virus, incubation period of infection, and survival of mice with sequelae. J Infect Dis 136:336, 1977.
69. Tsiang H: Evidence for an intraaxonal transport of fixed and street rabies virus. J Neuropathol Exp Neurol 38:286, 1979.
70. Ugolini G: Specificity of rabies virus as a transneuronal tracer of motor networks: Transfer from hypoglossal motoneurons to connected second-order and higher order central nervous system cell groups. J Comp Neurol 356:457, 1995.
71. Para M: An outbreak of post-vaccinal rabies (rage de laboratoire) in Fortaleza, Brazil, in 1960. Residual fixed virus as the etiological agent. Bull WHO 33:177, 1965.
72. Wandeler AI, Nadin-Davis SA, Tinline RR, Rupprecht CE: Rabies epidemiology: Some ecological and evolutionary perspectives. Curr Top Microbiol Immunol 187:297, 1994.
73. Murphy FA, Bauer SP: Early street rabies virus infection in striated muscle and later progression to the central nervous system. Intervirology 3:256, 1974.
74. Shankar V, Dietzschold B, Koprowski H: Direct entry of rabies virus into the central nervous system without prior local replication. J Virol 65:2736, 1991.
75. Gosztonyi G, Dietzschold B, Kao M, et al: Rabies and borna disease. A comparative pathogenetic study of two neurovirulent agents. Lab Invest 68:285, 1993.
76. Ray NB, Ewalt LC, Lodmell DL: Rabies virus replication in human and murine macrophage-like cell lines: Implications for viral persistence. J Virol 69:764, 1995.
77. Jackson AC, Reimer DL: Pathogenesis of experimental rabies in mice: An immunohistochemical study. Acta Neuropathol (Berl) 78:159, 1989.
78. Balachandran A, Charlton KM: Experimental rabies infection of non-nervous tissues in skunks (*Mephitis mephitis*) and foxes (*Vulpes vulpes*). Vet Pathol 31:93, 1994.
79. Smith JS: Rabies Virus. *In* Murray PR, Baron EJ, Pfaller MA, et al (eds): Manual of Clinical Microbiology, ed 6. Washington, DC, ASM Press, 1995, pp 997–1003.
80. Hemachuda T: Rabies. *In* Vinken PJ, Bruyn GW, Klawans HL (eds): Handbook of Clinical Neurology. Amsterdam, Elsevier Science Publishers, 1989, pp 383–404.
81. Hattwick MA, Weis TT, Stechschulte CJ, et al: Recovery from rabies. A case report. Ann Intern Med 76:931, 1972.

82. Alvarez AL, Fajardo R, Lopez ME, et al: Partial recovery from rabies in a nine-year-old boy. Pediatr Infect Dis J 13:1154, 1994.
83. Miller A, Morse HC III, Winkelstein J, et al: The role of antibody in recovery from experimental rabies. I. Effect of depletion of B and T cells. J Immunol 121:321, 1978.
84. Fekadu M, Baer GM: Recovery from clinical rabies of 2 dogs inoculated with a rabies virus strain from Ethiopia. Am J Vet Res 41:1632, 1980.
85. Fekadu M, Shaddock JH, Baer GM: Intermittent excretion of rabies virus in the saliva of a dog two and six months after it had recovered from experimental rabies. Am J Trop Med Hyg 30:1113, 1981.
86. Prabhakar BS, Fischman HR, Nathanson N: Recovery from experimental rabies by adoptive transfer of immune cells. J Gen Virol 56:25, 1981.
87. Jackson AC, Reimer DL, Ludwin SK: Spontaneous recovery from the encephalomyelitis in mice caused by street rabies virus. Neuropathol Appl Neurobiol 15:459, 1989.
88. Fekadu M, Summer JW, Shaddock JH, et al: Sickness and recovery of dogs challenged with a street rabies virus after vaccination with a vaccinia virus recombinant expressing rabies virus N protein. J Virol 66:2601, 1992.
89. Dupont JR, Earle KM: Human rabies encephalitis. A study of forty-nine fatal cases with a review of the literature. Neurology 15:1023, 1965.
90. Trimarchi CV, Debbie J: The fluorescent antibody in rabies. *In* Baer GM (ed): The Natural History of Rabies, ed 2. Boca Raton, FL, CRC Press, 1991, pp 219–233.
91. Dean DJ, Abelseth MK: The fluorescent antibody test. *In* Kaplan MM, Koprowski H (eds): Laboratory Techniques in Rabies. Geneva, World Health Organization, 1973, pp 73–84.
92. Velleca WM, Forrester FT. Laboratory Methods for Detecting Rabies. Washington, DC, US Government Printing Office, 1981.
93. Murphy FA, Harrison AK, Winn WC, et al: Comparative pathogenesis of rabies and rabies-like viruses: Infection of the central nervous system and centrifugal spread of virus to peripheral tissues. Lab Invest 29:1, 1973.
94. Matsumoto S: Electron microscopy of nerve cells infected with street rabies virus. Virology 17:198, 1962.
95. Charlton KM: Rabies: spongiform lesions in the brain. Acta Neuropathol (Berl) 63:198, 1984.
96. Charlton KM, Casey GA, Webster WA, et al: Experimental rabies in skunks and foxes. Pathogenesis of the spongiform lesions. Lab Invest 57:634, 1987.
97. Tsiang H: Pathophysiology of rabies virus infection of the nervous system. Adv Virus Res 42:375, 1993.
98. Marquette C, Ceccaldi P-E, Weber P, et al: Brain interleukin-1 receptors during rabies virus infection. J Neuroimmunol 54:179, 1994.
99. Haour F, Marquette C, Ban E, et al: Receptors for interleukin-1 in the central nervous and neuroendocrine systems: Role in infection and stress. Ann Endocrinol (Paris) 56:173, 1995.
100. Koprowski H, Zheng YM, Heber-Katz E, et al: In vivo expression if inducible nitric oxide synthase in experimentally induced neurologic disease. Proc Natl Acad Sci USA 90:3024, 1993.
101. Koprowski H, Zheng YM, Fu ZF, et al: NOS expression in experimentally induced neurologic diseases. J Neurochem 64:S32, 1995.
102. Hemachudha T: Human rabies: Clinical aspects, pathogenesis, and potential therapy. Curr Top Microbiol Immunol 187:121, 1994.
103. Follmann EH, Ritter DG, Beller M: Survey of trappers in northern Alaska for rabies antibody. Epidemiol Infect 113:137, 1994.
104. Prabhakar BS, Nathanson N: Acute rabies death mediated by antibody. Nature 290:590, 1981.
105. Smith JS, McCelland CL, Reid FL, et al: Dual role of the immune response in street rabiesvirus infection of mice. Infect Immun 35:213, 1982.
106. Nathanson N, Gonzalez-Scarano F: Immune response to rabies virus. *In* Baer GM (ed): The Natural History of Rabies, ed 2. Boca Raton, FL, CRC Press, 1991, pp 145–161.
107. Baer GM, Shaddock JH, Moore SA, et al: Successful prophylaxis against rabies in mice and Rhesus monkeys: The interferon system and vaccine. J Infect Dis 136:286, 1977.
108. Baer GM, Moore SA, Shaddock JH, et al: An effective rabies treatment in exposed monkeys: a single dose of interferon inducer and vaccine. Bull WHO 57:807, 1979.
109. Merigan TC, Baer GM, Winkler WG, et al: Human leukocyte interferon administration to patients with symptomatic and suspected rabies. Ann Neurol 16:82, 1984.
110. Baer GM, Shaddock JH, Levy H, et al: Interferon in rabies postexposure prophylasis. *In* Thraenhart O, Koprowski H, Bogel K, et al (eds): Progress in Rabies Control. Kent, UK, Wells Medical 1989, pp 245–250.
111. Bunn TO: Canine and feline vaccines, past and present. *In* Baer GM (ed): The Natural History of Rabies, ed 2. Boca Raton, FL, CRC Press, 1991, pp 415–425.
112. Wunderli PS, Shaddock JH, Schmid DS, et al: The protective role of humoral neutralizing antibody in the NIH potency test for rabies vaccines. Vaccine 9:638, 1991.
113. Rupprecht CE, Dietzschold B: Perspectives on rabies virus pathogenesis. Lab Invest 57:603, 1987.
114. Ertl HC, Dietzschold B, Gore M, et al: Induction of rabies virus-specific T-helper cells by synthetic peptides that carry dominant T-helper cell epitopes of the viral ribonucleoprotein. J Virol 63:2885, 1989.
115. Celis E, Ou DW, Dietzschold B, et al: Recognition of rabies and rabies-related viruses by T cells derived from human vaccine recipients. J Virol 62:3128, 1988.
116. Celis E, Karr RW, Dietzschold B, et al: Genetic restriction and fine specificity of human T cell clones reactive with rabies virus. J Immunol 141:2721, 1988.
117. Celis E, Ou D, Dietzschold B, et al: Rabies virus–specific T cell hybridomas: Identification of class II MHC-restricted T-cell epitopes using synthetic peptides. Hybridoma 8:263, 1989.
118. Celis E, Miller RW, Wiktor TJ, et al: Isolation and characterization of human T cell lines and clones reactive to rabies virus: Antigen specificity and production of interferon-gamma. J Immunol 136:692, 1986.
119. Hooper DC, Pierard I, Modelska A, et al: Rabies ribonucleocapsid as an oral immunogen and immunological enhancer. Proc Natl Acad Sci USA 91:10908, 1994.
120. Lafon M, Scott-Algara D, Marche PN, et al: Neonatal deletion and selective expansion of mouse T cells by exposure to rabies virus nucleocapsid superantigen. J Exp Med 180:1207, 1994.
121. Dietzschold B, Wang HH, Rupprecht CE, et al: Induction of protective immunity against rabies by immunization with rabies virus ribonucleoprotein. Proc Natl Acad Sci USA 84:9165, 1987.
122. Tollis M, Dietzschold B, Volia CB, et al: Immunization of monkeys with rabies ribonucleoprotein (RNP) confers protective immunity against rabies. Vaccine 9:134, 1991.
123. Vodopija I, Clark HF: Human vaccination against rabies. *In* Baer GM (ed): The Natural History of Rabies, ed 2. Boca Raton, FL, CRC Press, 1991, pp 571–595.
124. Bingham J, Foggin CM, Gerber H, et al: Pathogenicity of SAD rabies vaccine given orally in chacma baboons *(Papio ursinus)*. Vet Rec 131:55, 1992.
125. Thraenhart O, Marcus I, Kreuzfelder E: Current and future immunoprophylaxis against human rabies: Reduction of treatment of failures and errors. Curr Top Microbiol Immunol 187:173, 1994.
126. Jenkins SR, Clark KA, Debbie JG, et al: Compendium of animal rabies control, 1995. National Association of State Public Health Veterinarians, Inc. MMWR Morbid Mortal Wkly Rep 44:1, 1995.
127. Lin FT: The protective effect of the large-scale use of PHKC rabies vaccine in humans in China. Bull World Health Organ 68:449, 1990.
128. Chutivongse S, Wilde H, Supich C, et al: Postexposure prophylaxis for rabies with antiserum and intradermal vaccination. Lancet 335:896, 1990.
129. Chutivongse S, Wilde H, Fishbein DB, et al: One-year study of the 2-1-1 intramuscular postexposure rabies vaccine regimen in 100 severely exposed Thai patients using rabies immune globulin and Vero cell rabies vaccine. Vaccine 9:573, 1991.
130. Fishbein DB, Miranda NJ, Merrill P, et al: Rabies control in the Republic of the Philippines: Benefits and costs of elimination. Vaccine 9:581, 1991.
131. Sehgal S, Bhattacharya D, Bhardwaj M: Clinical evaluation of purified vero-cell rabies vaccine in patients bitten by rabid animals in India. J Commun Dis 26:139, 1994.
132. Dutta JK, Warrell JJ, Dutta TK: Intradermal rabies immunization for pre- and post-exposure prophylaxis. Nat Med J India 7:119, 1994.

133. Meslin FX, Fishbein DB, Matter HC: Rationale and prospects for rabies elimination in developing countries. Curr Top Microbiol Immunol 187:1, 1994.
134. Khawplod P, Glueck R, Wilde H, et al: Immunogenicity of purified duck embryo rabies vaccine (Lyssavac-N) with use of the WHO-approved intradermal postexposure regimen. Clin Infect Dis 20:646, 1995.
135. Wilde H, Glueck R, Khawplod P, et al: Efficacy study of a new albumin-free human diploid cell rabies vaccine (Lyssavac-HDC, Berna) in 100 severely rabies-exposed Thai patients. Vaccine 13:593, 1995.
136. Wilde H, Choomkasien P, Hemachudha T, et al: Failure of rabies postexposure treatment in Thailand. Vaccine 7:49, 1989.
137. Tabbara KF, Al-Omar O: Eyelid laceration sustained in an attack by a rabid desert fox. Am J Ophthalmol 119:651, 1995.
138. Schumacher CL, Dietzschold B, Ertl HC, et al: Use of mouse anti-rabies monoclonal antibodies in postexposure treatment of rabies. J Clin Invest 84:971, 1989.
139. Montano-Hirose JA, Lafage M, Weber P, et al: Protective activity of a murine monoclonal antibody against European bat lyssavirus 1 (EBL1) infection in mice. Vaccine 11:1259, 1993.
140. Lafon M, Edelman L, Bouvet JP, et al: Human monoclonal antibodies specific for the rabies virus glycoprotein and N protein. J Gen Virol 71:1689, 1990.
141. Dietzschold B, Gore M, Casali P, et al: Biological characterization of human monoclonal antibodies to rabies virus. J Virol 64:3087, 1990.
142. Cheung SC, Dietzschold B, Koprowski H, et al: A recombinant human Fab expressed in *Escherichia coli* neutralizes rabies virus. J Virol 66:6714, 1992.
143. Dorfman N, Dietzschold B, Kajiyama W, et al: Development of human monoclonal antibodies to rabies. Hybridoma 13:397, 1994.
144. Rando RF, Notkins, AL: Production of human monoclonal antibodies against rabies virus. Curr Top Microbiol Immunol 187:195, 1994.
145. Dietzschold B, Kao M, Zheng YM, et al: Delineation of putative mechanisms involved in antibody-mediated clearance of rabies virus from the central nervous system. Proc Natl Acad Sci USA 89:7252, 1992.
146. Schumacher CL, Ertl HC, Koprowski H, et al: Inhibition of immune responses against rabies virus by monoclonal antibodies directed against rabies virus antigens. Vaccine 10:754, 1992.
147. Schnell MJ, Mebatsion T, Conzelmann K-K: Infectious rabies viruses from cloned cDNA. EMBO J 13:4195, 1994.
148. Xiang ZQ, Spitalnik S, Tran M, et al: Vaccination with a plasmid vector carrying the rabies virus glycoprotein gene induces protective immunity against rabies virus. Virology 199:132, 1994.
149. Wiktor TJ, Macfarlan RI, Reagan KJ, et al: Protection from rabies by a vaccinia virus recombinant containing the rabies virus glycoprotein gene. Proc Natl Acad Sci USA 81:7194, 1984.
150. Prehaud C, Takehara K, Flammand A, et al: Immunogenic and protective properties of rabies virus glycoprotein expressed by baculovirus vectors. Virology 173:390, 1989.
151. Fekadu M, Shaddock JH, Summer JW, et al: Oral vaccination of skunks with raccoon poxvirus recombinants expressing the rabies glycoprotein or the nucleoprotein. J Wildl Dis 27:681, 1991.
152. Fu ZF, Dietzschold B, Schumacher CL, et al: Rabies virus nucleoprotein expressed in and purified from insect cells is efficacious as a vaccine. Proc Natl Acad Sci USA 88:2001, 1991.
153. Sumner JW, Fekadu M, Shaddock JH, et al: Protection of mice with vaccinia virus recombinants that express the rabies nucleoprotein. Virology 183:703, 1991.
154. Fu ZF, Rupprecht CE, Dietzschold B, et al: Oral vaccination of raccoons (*Procyon lotor*) with baculovirus-expressed rabies virus glycoprotein. Vaccine 11:925, 1993.
155. Klepfer SR, Debouck C, Uffelman J, et al: Characterization of rabies glycoprotein expressed in yeast. Arch Virol 128:269, 1993.
156. Goto H, Minamoto N, Ito H, et al: Expression of the nucleoprotein of rabies virus in *Escherichia coli* and mapping of antigenic sites. Arch Virol 140:1061, 1995.
157. Brochier B, Costy F, Pastoret P-P: Elimination of fox rabies from Belgium using a recombinant vaccinia-rabies vaccine: An update. Vet Microbiol 46:269, 1995.
158. Aubert MFA, Masson E, Artois M, Barrat J: Oral wildlife rabies vaccination field trials in Europe, with recent emphasis on France. Curr Top Microbiol Immunol 187:219, 1994.
159. Campbell JB: Oral rabies immunization of wildlife and dogs: Challenges to the Americas. Curr Top Microbiol Immunol 187:245, 1994.
160. Lutze-Wallace C, Sapp T, Sidhu M, et al: In vitro assessments of the genetic stability of a live recombinant human adenovirus vaccine against rabies. Can J Vet Res 59:157, 1995.
161. Taylor J, Meignier B, Tartaglia J, et al: Biological and immunogenic properties of a canarypox-rabies recombinant, ALVAC-RG (vCP65) in non-avian species. Vaccine 13:539, 1995.
162. Rupprecht CE, Shankar V, Hanlon CA, et al: Beyond Pasteur to 2001: Future trends in lyssavirus research? Curr Top Microbiol Immunol 187:325, 1994.

271

Caliciviruses and Astroviruses

Neil R. Blacklow

Viral gastroenteritis is a common, medically important illness that occurs worldwide. Despite its frequency and importance, no pathogens were identified until the early 1970s with the discovery of Norwalk virus.[1, 2] In the past, electron microscopic (EM) and antigen detection techniques were the prerequisite for the detection in stools and study of Norwalk virus and most other small round gastroenteritis viruses. This is because, despite intensive efforts, the viruses (with the exception of the astroviruses) have remained refractory to cultivation in vitro in cell culture. The cloning of the Norwalk virus genome has now established conclusively that the virus is a calicivirus.[3, 4] The understanding of Norwalk virus molecular virology has clarified the nature of several other related small round gastroenteritis viruses that are also caliciviruses. Most of our knowledge of the caliciviruses is derived from the study of Norwalk virus, the prototype and most extensively studied calicivirus. This discussion of caliciviruses therefore concentrates on Norwalk virus. In more recent years, other small round gastroenteritis viruses that are unrelated to caliciviruses have been extensively characterized and form a second major family of diarrheal agents, the astroviruses.[5] Less medically relevant information is known about astroviruses than caliciviruses. The syndrome of viral gastroenteritis is also produced by two other virus families that are larger in size than the small round caliciviruses and astroviruses, namely, the rotaviruses and enteric adenoviruses (covered in Chapters 239 and 263).

Classification and Comparative Virology of Small Round Gastroenteritis Viruses

The small round viruses that are associated with gastroenteritis are 20 to 40 nm in diameter and can be categorized morphologically into three groups on the basis of careful EM studies of the agents in stool specimens.[5, 6] The caliciviruses such as Norwalk virus and related agents form a first category. Sometimes referred to as small round structured viruses (SRSVs), or Norwalk-like viruses, these agents usually possess an amorphous surface structure with a feathery, ragged outline that lacks geometric symmetry (Fig. 271–1*A*). On the basis of biochemical and molecular virologic studies (see caliciviruses later), the SRSVs are now known to belong to the family Caliciviridae.[4] These viruses share characteristics of density in cesium chloride (1.34 to 1.42 g/cm^3), size (27 to 40 nm in diameter), and their derivation from epidemics or family outbreaks of gastroenteritis. The individual calicivirus strains are named after the location of the outbreak from which they are derived (e.g., Norwalk, Ohio; Hawaii; Snow Mountain, Colorado; Montgomery County, Maryland; Taunton, England; Otofuke and Sapporo, Japan). At least three of these virus strains (Norwalk, Hawaii, Snow Mountain) are immunologically distinct on the basis of immunoelectron microscopy (IEM) studies that employ human serum from infected and uninfected persons in the assays. These three viruses have also induced disease in volunteers (they do not produce disease in animals, including primates), and this has provided the necessary human clinical material for development of immunoassays to detect each of them in stools and their antibodies in serum.[7–10] Unlike the SRSV strains, some other calicivirus strains, detected in young children, demonstrate a virion surface structure with cup-shaped indentations or hollows (Latin *calix*, "cup") that may form a six-pointed star (Star of David, Fig. 271–1*B*), which is the classic appearance of the virus family Caliciviridae.[11, 12] SRSV strains only occasionally show this appearance.

The second category of small round gastroenteritis viruses consists of the agents belonging to the family Astroviridae. The astroviruses have a definitive, classic surface structure on EM.[12] They are 27 to 32 nm in diameter and have a five- or six-pointed star on their surface that consists of a continuous, rounded structure (Fig. 271–1*C*). This morphologic feature contrasts with that of classic caliciviruses, whose surface is broken by hollows, and with that of SRSV-appearing caliciviruses, whose surface is feathery and ragged. Biochemical and molecular virologic studies (see the section on astroviruses) also indicate the distinctiveness of astroviruses from caliciviruses. Immunoassays that now detect and quantify astroviruses have revealed their medical importance in the same way that immunoassay earlier permitted recognition of Norwalk virus as an important pathogen.[13, 14]

The third category of small round viruses said to be associated with gastroenteritis is the smallest (20 to 26 nm diameter). Their surface structures lack discernible features and a sharply delineated outer edge, in contrast to those of Norwalk virus, which are clearly defined, albeit feathery and ragged. These smallest agents include Ditchling, W (Wollan), cockle, and Parramatta, which have been visualized in stool specimens.[6] It now appears unlikely that these agents are medically important causes of diarrhea, and it is unclear whether they even cause gastroenteritis at all, because serologic evidence of recent infection is usually lacking (unlike the situation with caliciviruses and astroviruses). It is possi-

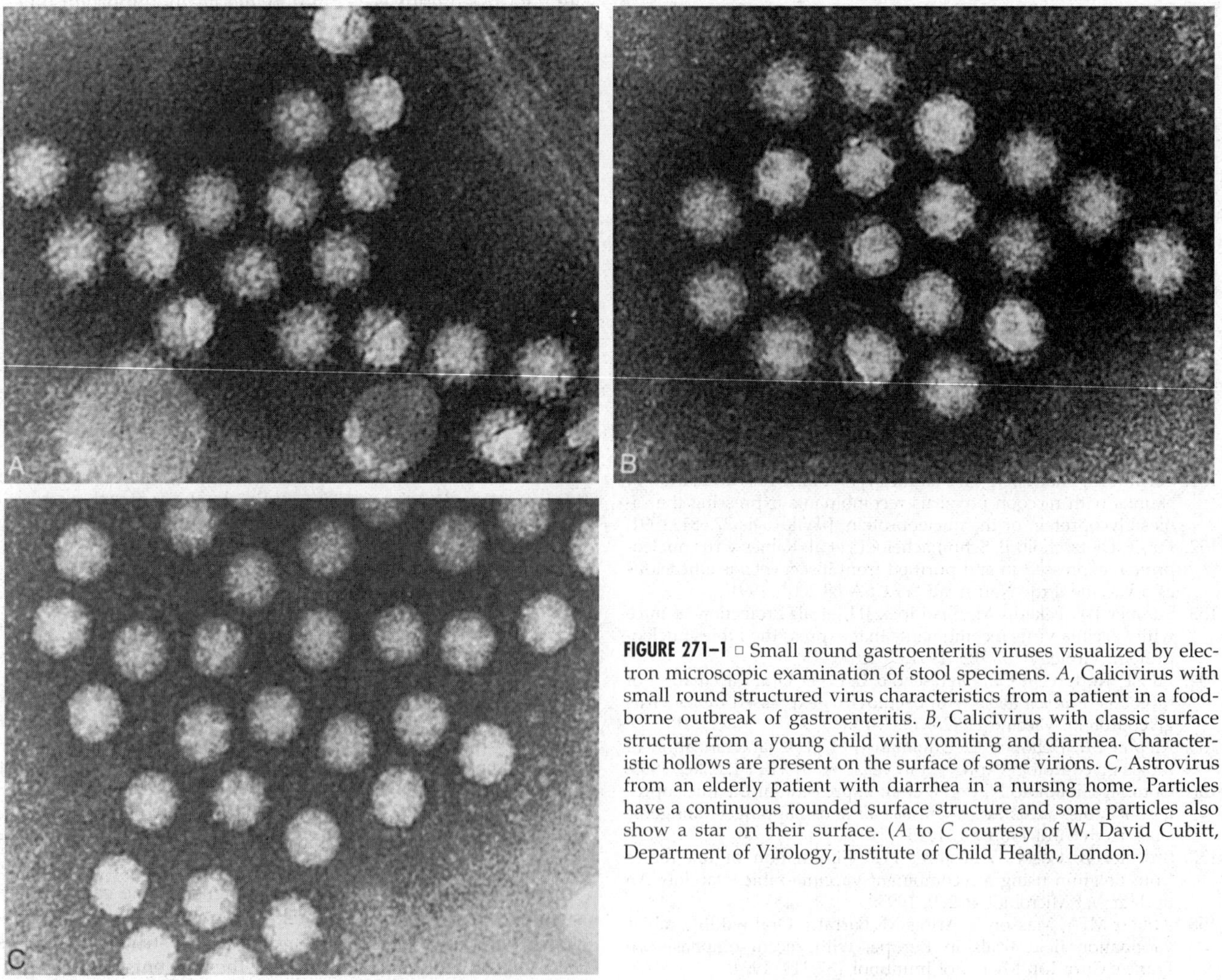

FIGURE 271–1 □ Small round gastroenteritis viruses visualized by electron microscopic examination of stool specimens. *A*, Calicivirus with small round structured virus characteristics from a patient in a foodborne outbreak of gastroenteritis. *B*, Calicivirus with classic surface structure from a young child with vomiting and diarrhea. Characteristic hollows are present on the surface of some virions. *C*, Astrovirus from an elderly patient with diarrhea in a nursing home. Particles have a continuous rounded surface structure and some particles also show a star on their surface. (*A* to *C* courtesy of W. David Cubitt, Department of Virology, Institute of Child Health, London.)

ble that these small agents represent passenger parvoviruses in feces that are unrelated to gastroenteritis,[6] and they are not discussed further here.

Caliciviruses

Characteristics of the Pathogen

Norwalk virus, the prototype calicivirus, is difficult to recognize in stools by direct EM owing to its small size and the fact that it is shed in relatively low titer in feces. It can be visualized by IEM reaction of feces with human convalescent-phase serum that contains Norwalk antibodies, which aggregate viral particles.[1] By IEM, the virions are round, nonenveloped, and 27 nm in average diameter; they have a ragged outline in which there is a suggestion of small indentations on the surface[15] (see Fig. 271–1*A* and *B*). New structural studies, based on recombinant Norwalk virus particles produced in insect cells by a baculovirus recombinant expressing the complementary DNA that encodes Norwalk capsid protein, now clearly demonstrate icosahedral particles with the cuplike depressions characteristic of caliciviruses.[16]

Norwalk virus and other caliciviruses have not been cultivated in vitro, nor do they produce disease in animal model systems. Biochemical studies of Norwalk virus, purified from human stool samples, indicate a single structural protein of about 60 kDa, which is characteristic of caliciviruses.[17] The viral genome has been molecularly cloned and characterized and contains single-stranded RNA of positive polarity, about 7.7 kb in size, permitting definitive classification in the family Caliciviridae.[4] The viral genome encodes three open reading frames, one of which codes for the 60-kDa structural protein of the viral capsid.

More than 50 SRSVs have had their genomic sequences analyzed, and it is clear that these agents are caliciviruses.[18–30] These caliciviruses can currently be categorized into three genogroups on the basis of their nucleotide–amino acid sequence homologies in the polymerase region and in the capsid region of their genomes. The genogroups include agents such as Norwalk, Southampton, and Desert Shield viruses in group I; Hawaii, Snow Mountain, Bristol, and Toronto ("minireovirus") viruses in group II; and Sapporo virus and classic EM-appearing strains of pediatric diarrhea in group III. These three genogroups are currently defined on the basis of arbitrary genetic criteria and do not necessarily relate to immunobiologic characteristics; for example, Hawaii and Snow Mountain viruses, both members of genogroup II, are distinct on the basis of IEM reactions with defined human serum.[31, 32] Medically relevant serotypic differences between the various calicivirus strains clearly await further delineation.

Epidemiology

Immunoassay techniques, using defined human clinical reagents, have been employed to determine the epidemiology of Norwalk virus as a medically important pathogen. Disease usually occurs in epidemic fashion, characterized by acute vomiting and diarrhea with a short incubation period (24 to 48 hours), and sweeps through communities. Forty-two percent of 74 acute nonbacterial gastroenteritis outbreaks studied in the United States were associated with Norwalk virus, and an additional 23% were provisionally associated (a minority of patients showed seroconversion) with the virus or a related calicivirus.[33] These outbreaks typically occur in certain settings (Table 271–1), such as contaminated drinking or swimming water, ingestion of raw or incompletely cooked shellfish, recreational camps, cruise ships, nursing homes, schools (elementary through college), and community or family locations. Outbreaks occur during all seasons, affecting older (school-age) children and adults and seemingly sparing infants and young children; however, there is the suggestion that more sensitive diagnostic assays could reveal outbreaks in very young populations.

TABLE 271–1 ■ Epidemiologic Settings for Gastroenteritis Outbreaks Caused by Norwalk Virus

Community or family locations
Schools (elementary through college)
Military troops
Recreational camps
Athletic teams
Cruise ships
Contaminated drinking or swimming water
Ingestion of incompletely cooked shellfish
Ingestion of fecally contaminated foods
Nursing homes

Classic EM-appearing calicivirus strains, unlike Norwalk virus and other SRSVs, typically cause gastroenteritis in infants and young children. Although less is known about their epidemiology than that of Norwalk virus, the illness resembles that produced by rotavirus and may cause 2% to 5% of pediatric diarrhea, including that found in daycare centers.[11, 34–36]

In the United States, antibody prevalence levels to Norwalk virus are low in childhood as determined by immunoassay using defined human clinical reagents. Antibody prevalence levels rapidly rise during adolescence and early adulthood, paralleling Norwalk disease expression, reaching about 60% of the population by middle age. In developing tropical nations, antibody prevalence increases at an earlier age, 2 to 6 years.[37, 38] Interestingly, a study of Finnish infants and young children provided evidence (seroconversions) for Norwalk virus infection when serum samples were tested in a more sensitive immunoassay containing baculovirus-expressed recombinant Norwalk virus capsid protein as antigen.[39] Whether the occurrence of Norwalk virus infection and disease in the very young is actually widespread and common remains to be determined.

Norwalk virus infection has been shown conclusively in volunteer studies to be spread by the fecal-oral route.[2] Some epidemiologic data suggest airborne transmission,[40] which is consistent with its reported presence in vomitus and also with the extremely rapid secondary spread of Norwalk virus infection that is often observed.

Pathogenesis

Volunteer studies performed with Norwalk and Hawaii viruses reveal that gastroenteritis occurs in about half of those administered the virus orally.[32] Illness is accompanied by a mucosal lesion of the proximal small intestine that is characterized by damage to villus absorptive cells, infiltration of the lamina propria by polymorphonuclear leukocytes and mononuclear cells, and villus shortening with crypt hypertrophy.[41, 42] These changes, associated with malabsorption of D-xylose, lactose, and fat, revert to normal within 2 weeks of the onset of illness. In contrast, the rectal mucosa and gastric mucosa are not altered during illness, although there is a marked delay in gastric motor function and emptying that is likely to be responsible for the nausea and vomiting.[43]

Norwalk virus illness commonly occurs in the presence of preexisting serum or intestinal antibodies to the virus.[8, 44–47] Uninfected volunteers are more likely to have absent or lower preexisting antibody titers than infected individuals. Volunteers who have been rechallenged with the virus approximately 2 to 4 years later develop illness again. Volunteers remain well if they did not become ill on the first challenge, and they usually lack or have low levels of serum or intestinal antibody. Thus, the rise in serum antibody titer seen after Norwalk virus illness appears to be a marker for infection in susceptible persons and can lack a protective role. The explanation for the confusing aspects of clinical immunity seen with Norwalk virus is not clear. Clarification may await more definitive, precise, and sensitive immunoassay methods. It is possible that the unusual pattern of clinical immunity is related to a genetic control of host susceptibility or the need for repeated exposures to the virus to generate illness and immune response. It does seem that immunity to Norwalk virus is not long lasting and that repeated bouts of illness throughout life are possible. After a sufficient number of repeated illnesses due to the virus, it is conceivable that clinical immunity could develop.

Clinical Manifestations

Norwalk virus illness is typically acute and explosive, characterized by rapid onset of vomiting, diarrhea, or both; it is accompanied by a varying spectrum of signs and symptoms, such as abdominal cramps, low-grade fever, nausea, headache, malaise, and myalgia.[2] Disease usually resolves spontaneously within 24 to 48 hours. Death is extremely rare; those who succumb are elderly or debilitated. A minority of patients may develop transient leukocytosis, and fecal leukocytes are nearly always absent.

Diagnosis

In an individual patient, a diagnosis of Norwalk virus gastroenteritis cannot be made on clinical grounds alone, because the entity can be consistent with other causes of acute noninflammatory infectious diarrhea. A presumptive diagnosis during a disease outbreak can be made if there is an absence of bacterial or parasitic pathogens, the presence of vomiting in a majority of cases, a duration of illness from 0.5 to 5 days, and an incubation period estimated at 1 to 2 days.[48]

A specific diagnosis of Norwalk virus gastroenteritis requires demonstration of the virus or its antigen in feces or a rise in specific serum antibody titer to the virus. (Norwalk virus and other caliciviruses are not normally found in the stool of asymptomatic persons.) Immunoassay techniques are developed for the specific diagnosis of Norwalk, Snow Mountain, and Hawaii gastroenteritis but are not commercially available because they are restricted to the few research laboratories that possess the human clinical diagnostic reagents necessary for performance of the tests.[7–10] Immunoglobulin M antibody responses to Norwalk virus can be detected and indicate recent infection, but the immunoglobulin M assays also require reagents derived from human volunteers.[49, 50] Use of IEM is impractical because it is too cumbersome for routine or rapid diagnosis. It is hoped that various diagnostic tests under development will lead to wider availability of specific laboratory diagnosis. These procedures still require considerable refinement and evaluation to establish their utility. They include tests such as an immunoassay that uses genetically assembled Norwalk virus capsid protein in place of relying on human clinical materials, a reverse transcription–polymerase chain reaction assay, and a monoclonal antibody–based immunoassay for Norwalk virus that also supplants human reagents.[30, 51–54]

Treatment and Prevention

Because no specific antiviral therapy is available for Norwalk virus gastroenteritis, therapy must be supportive—replacement of fluid and electrolytes, as for other infectious diarrheas. In one study, it was shown that oral administration of bismuth subsalicylate reduced the severity and duration of abdominal cramps in volunteers ill with Norwalk virus gastroenteritis and reduced the duration of gastrointestinal symptoms from 20 to 14 hours.[55] Secondary spread of infection, as in nosocomial settings, can be prevented by standard enteric precautions. The duration of virus shedding can be up to 7 days, which is considerably longer than the length of symptomatic illness, and volunteers exposed to the virus who remain asymptomatic may also shed it for up to a week.[47] These findings carry implications for infection control practices. It is unlikely that a useful vaccine will be easily developed for long-term prevention of Norwalk virus illness because the natural disease does not confer long-term immunity. It is possible that a vaccine could be developed for prevention of illness short term for travelers, for example, because volunteers who were previously ill remained well when challenged again 4 to 14 weeks later.[44]

Astroviruses

Characteristics of the Pathogen

Astrovirus can be visualized by direct EM examination of diarrheal stool samples from infants.[12] The virus is a 27- to 32-nm-diameter round particle that possesses a distinctive ultrastructure, exhibiting a five- or occasionally six-pointed starlike appearance on its surface and a continuous outer margin that forms a distinct rim (see Fig. 271–1C). The virus is named after the star shape that appears on the surface of some particles. The morphologic characteristics of the astroviruses clearly distinguish them from those of the caliciviruses.[12]

The virus can be cultivated in cell cultures treated with trypsin.[13, 55] This has facilitated viral characterization. The virus contains a positive-sense, single-stranded RNA genome of an approximate size of 7.2 kb.[56] Several astrovirus structural proteins are described, including an 87-kDa protein produced in infected cells that reacts with monoclonal antibody specific for viral capsids.[56] This protein may serve as a precursor to three to five smaller capsid proteins of approximately 30 kDa in size.[57] Sequence analysis of the viral genome, together with the size and number of structural proteins, as well as the replication strategy characteristics of the virus led to the official classification of astrovirus as a new family of RNA viruses, the Astroviridae.[58]

There are seven viral serotypes, defined by IEM.[13, 59] A monoclonal antibody has been prepared that reacts with a group-specific antigen shared by all viral serotypes.[13] When incorporated into an enzyme immunoassay format, the monoclonal antibody detects all astroviral serotypes in stool, thereby providing the framework for understanding the epidemiology and medical importance of the astroviruses.[60]

Epidemiology

Astrovirus gastroenteritis is most prominent in young children but also occurs in immunocompromised individuals and elderly institutionalized patients.[14, 61, 62] Peak occurrence is in the winter months in temperate regions and in the rainy season in tropical areas.[63, 64] Infection is spread person to person by the fecal-oral route and by contaminated food and water.[65]

The disease occurs in several clinical settings (Table 271–2). Most noteworthy is endemic childhood diarrhea, typically among children younger than 2 years, for which astrovirus appears to be responsible for about 3% to 9% of cases in

TABLE 271–2 ■ Clinical Settings for Astrovirus Infections

Endemic diarrhea of infants and young children
Daycare center diarrhea
Nosocomial diarrhea
Epidemic diarrhea of school-age children and adults
Nursing home diarrhea
Diarrhea in bone marrow transplant patients
Acute diarrhea in patients with acquired immunodeficiency syndrome

studies performed in Asia, Europe, Central America, and the United States.[14, 64, 66–70] Astrovirus is also an important pathogen in daycare settings, where it has caused 4% to 7% of cases of diarrhea.[71, 72] The virus seems to be a common cause of nosocomial outbreaks of infant diarrhea as well as of nonoutbreak nosocomial gastroenteritis.[73, 74] It appears to be an uncommon cause of epidemic diarrhea, unlike calicivirus, with only a few outbreaks reported.[75, 76] However, astrovirus infection does appear to produce significant clinical illness in elderly and immunocompromised patients in whom immunity may have waned.[61, 62, 77, 78] Several disease outbreaks have been diagnosed in residential facilities for the elderly and on geriatric wards.[62, 77, 78] In the most complete study reported to date of the role of enteric viruses in acute diarrhea of patients with acquired immunodeficiency syndrome (that employed a broad repertoire of assays to detect all known human diarrhea viruses), astrovirus was most commonly identified (12% of cases).[61] Indeed, it produced diarrhea more frequently than any pathogen, bacterial, parasitic, or viral. Last, in one study, astrovirus caused 4% of episodes of diarrhea occurring after bone marrow transplantation, equaling *Clostridium difficile* as the most common identifiable infectious agent.[79]

In the United Kingdom, antibody prevalence levels to astroviruses rise rapidly during early childhood, reaching more than 70% of the population by 3 to 4 years of age.[80] Most adults have serum antibodies. Antibodies to all viral serotypes are present in commercial preparations of human γ-globulin in the United States and Japan.[76, 81] Because most astrovirus disease occurs in the young, but disease outbreaks are found in the elderly, it may be that most young adults are protected by antibody levels that decline with age.

Pathogenesis

In the only reported histopathologic study to date, astrovirus has been visualized by EM in human intestinal epithelial cells obtained by small intestinal biopsy from two children who also shed the virus in diarrheal stool.[82] The only other pathogenesis data in humans are derived from limited volunteer studies. In two studies, a total of 36 adult volunteers were administered astrovirus orally, only 2 of whom developed unequivocal gastroenteritis.[62, 83] Virus-specific antibody rises (seroconversion) developed in the majority of volunteers, and fecal virus shedding in some. It therefore seems that astrovirus is of relatively low pathogenicity in immunocompetent, healthy young adults, in contrast to the effect of Norwalk virus in volunteers.

Clinical Manifestations

Astrovirus illness typically consists of watery diarrhea lasting 2 to 5 days in immunocompetent patients, with vomiting sometimes less common than that seen with calicivirus illness.[14, 62, 76] Accompanying findings include fever, anorexia, nausea, and abdominal pain. Dehydration in ill infants and young children occurs less commonly than with rotavirus disease.[14] Diarrhea may occasionally last 7 to 14 days with prolonged fecal virus shedding, and some patients can develop prolonged lactose intolerance.[84] Illness in immunocompromised patients can also be prolonged.[79, 84]

Diagnosis

The traditional "gold standard" for diagnosis has been examination of stool specimens by EM.[12] However, this technique is cumbersome, expensive, and restricted to highly experienced electron microscopists. A monoclonal antibody–based enzyme immunoassay test detects all astrovirus serotypes in stools with a high degree of sensitivity and specificity and has been the basis for many reported clinicoepidemiologic studies.[60] Although not currently commercially available, the enzyme immunoassay test makes the diagnosis of astrovirus infection much more practical and inexpensive than EM. Detection of astrovirus or its antigen in stool typically indicates symptomatic infection because the virus is not usually found in asymptomatic persons. A reverse transcription–polymerase chain reaction test to diagnose astrovirus infection in stools has also been developed, and its findings have closely correlated with and confirmed the enzyme immunoassay diagnostic test results.[61, 72, 79]

Treatment and Prevention

Therapy is supportive with replacement of fluid and electrolytes. Virus transmission is prevented by standard enteric precautions. Virus shedding in stool can continue for several days after resolution of diarrhea.[84] Further understanding of the economic importance of astrovirus diarrhea and of the mechanisms of immunity to the virus is necessary before vaccine development can be considered.

References

1. Kapikian AZ, Wyatt RG, Dolin R, et al: Visualization by immune electron microscopy of a 27 nm particle associated with acute infectious nonbacterial gastroenteritis. J Virol 10:1075, 1972.
2. Blacklow NR, Dolin R, Fedson DS, et al: Acute infectious nonbacterial gastroenteritis: Etiology and pathogenesis. Ann Intern Med 76:993, 1972.
3. Jiang X, Graham DY, Wang K, Estes MK: Norwalk virus genome cloning and characterization. Science 250:1580, 1990.
4. Jiang X, Wang M, Wang K, Estes MK: Sequence and genomic organization of Norwalk virus. Virology 195:51, 1993.
5. Caul EO, Appleton H: The electron microscopical and physical characteristics of small round human fecal viruses: An interim scheme for classification. J Med Virol 9:257, 1982.
6. Caul EO: Small round human fecal viruses. *In* Pattison JR (ed): Parvoviruses and Human Disease. Boca Raton, FL, CRC Press, 1988, pp 139–163.
7. Greenberg HB, Wyatt RG, Valdesuso J, et al: Solid-phase microtiter radioimmunoassay for detection of the Norwalk strain of acute nonbacterial epidemic gastroenteritis virus and its antibodies. J Med Virol 2:97, 1978.
8. Blacklow NR, Cukor G, Bedigian MK, et al: Immune response and prevalence of antibody to Norwalk enteritis virus as determined by radioimmunoassay. J Clin Microbiol 10:903, 1979.
9. Dolin R, Roessner KD, Treanor JJ, et al: Radioimmunoassay for detection of the Snow Mountain agent of viral gastroenteritis. J Med Virol 19:11, 1986.
10. Treanor JJ, Madore HP, Dolin R: Development of an enzyme immunoassay for the Hawaii agent of viral gastroenteritis. J Virol Methods 22:207, 1988.
11. Cubitt WD: The candidate caliciviruses. Ciba Found Symp 128:157, 1987.
12. Madeley CR: Comparison of the features of astroviruses and caliciviruses seen in samples of feces by electron microscopy. J Infect Dis 139:519, 1979.

13. Herrmann JE, Hudson RW, Perron-Henry DM, et al: Antigenic characterization of cell-cultivated astrovirus serotypes and development of astrovirus-specific monoclonal antibodies. J Infect Dis 158:182, 1988.
14. Herrmann JE, Taylor DN, Echeverria P, Blacklow NR: Astroviruses as a cause of gastroenteritis in children. N Engl J Med 324:1757, 1991.
15. Kapikian AZ, Chanock RM: Norwalk group of viruses. *In* Fields BN, Knipe DM (eds): Virology. New York, Raven Press, 1985, pp 1495–1517.
16. Prasad BVV, Rothnagel R, Jiang X, Estes MK: Three dimensional structure of baculovirus-expressed Norwalk virus capsids. J Virol 68:5117, 1994.
17. Greenberg HB, Valdesuso JR, Kalica AR, et al: Proteins of Norwalk virus. J Virol 37:994, 1981.
18. Green J, Norcott JP, Lewis D, et al: Norwalk-like viruses: Demonstration of genomic diversity by polymerase chain reaction. J Clin Microbiol 31:3007, 1991.
19. Lambden PR, Carl EO, Ashley CR, Clarke IN: Sequence and genome organization of a human small round-structured (Norwalk-like) virus. Science 259:516, 1993.
20. Moe CL, Gentsch J, Grohmann G, et al: Application of PCR to detect Norwalk virus in fecal specimens from outbreaks of gastroenteritis. J Clin Microbiol 32:642, 1994.
21. Lew JF, Petric M, Kapikian AZ, et al: Identification of "minireovirus" as a Norwalk-like virus in pediatric patients with gastroenteritis. J Virol 68:3391, 1994.
22. Lew JF, Kapikian AZ, Jiang X, et al: Molecular characterization and expression of the capsid protein of a Norwalk-like virus recovered from a Desert Shield troop with gastroenteritis. Virology 200:319, 1994.
23. Lew JF, Kapikian AZ, Valdesuso J, Green KY: Molecular characterization of Hawaii virus and other Norwalk-like viruses: Evidence for genetic polymorphism among human caliciviruses. J Infect Dis 170:535, 1994.
24. Wang J, Jiang X, Madore HP, et al: Sequence diversity of small round structured viruses. J Virol 68:5982, 1994.
25. Cubitt WD, Jiang XJ, Wang J, Estes MK: Sequence similarity of human caliciviruses and small round structured viruses. J Med Virol 43:252, 1994.
26. Green SM, Dingle KE, Lambden PR, et al: Human enteric caliciviridae: A new prevalent SRSV group defined by RNA-dependent RNA polymerase and capsid diversity. J Gen Virol 75:1883, 1994.
27. Matson DO, Zhong WM, Nakata S, et al: Molecular characterization of a human calicivirus with sequence relationships closer to animal caliciviruses than other known human caliciviruses. J Med Virol 45:215, 1995.
28. Ando T, Monroe SS, Gentsch JR, et al: Detection and differentiation of antigenically distinct small round-structured viruses (Norwalk-like viruses) by reverse transcription–PCR and Southern hybridization. J Clin Microbiol 33:64, 1995.
29. Liu BL, Clarke IN, Caul EO, Lambden PR: Human enteric caliciviruses have a unique genome structure and are distinct from the Norwalk-like viruses. Arch Virol 140:1345, 1995.
30. Jiang X, Wang J, Estes MK: Characterization of SRSVs using RT-PCR and a new antigen ELISA. Arch Virol 140:363, 1995.
31. Cubitt WD, Blacklow NR, Herrmann JE, et al: Antigenic relationships between human caliciviruses and Norwalk virus. J Infect Dis 156:806, 1987.
32. Blacklow NR, Greenberg HB: Viral gastroenteritis. N Engl J Med 325:252, 1991.
33. Kaplan JE, Gary GW, Baron RC, et al: Epidemiology of Norwalk gastroenteritis and the role of Norwalk virus in outbreaks of acute nonbacterial gastroenteritis. Ann Intern Med 96:756, 1982.
34. Cubitt WD, McSwiggan DA: Calicivirus gastroenteritis in North West London. Lancet 2:975, 1981.
35. Matson DO, Estes MK, Glass RI, et al: Human calicivirus-associated diarrhea in children attending day care centers. J Infect Dis 159:71, 1989.
36. Riepenhoff-Talty M, Saif LJ, Barrett HJ, et al: Potential spectrum of etiological agents of viral enteritis in hospitalized infants. J Clin Microbiol 17:352, 1983.
37. Greenberg HB, Valdesuso J, Kapikian AZ, et al: Prevalence of antibody to the Norwalk virus in various countries. Infect Immun 26:270, 1979.
38. Cukor G, Blacklow NR, Echeverria P, et al: Comparative study of the acquisition of antibody to Norwalk virus in pediatric populations. Infect Immun 29:822, 1980.
39. Lew JF, Valdesuso J, Vesikari T, et al: Detection of Norwalk virus or Norwalk-like virus infections in Finnish infants and young children. J Infect Dis 169:1364, 1994.
40. Sawyer LA, Murphy JJ, Kaplan JE, et al: 25- to 30 nm virus particle associated with a hospital outbreak of acute gastroenteritis with evidence for airborne transmission. Am J Epidemiol 127:1261, 1988.
41. Schreiber DS, Blacklow NR, Trier JS: The mucosal lesion of the proximal small intestine in acute infectious nonbacterial gastroenteritis. N Engl J Med 288:1318, 1973.
42. Schreiber DS, Blacklow NR, Trier JS: The small intestinal lesion induced by Hawaii agent acute infectious nonbacterial gastroenteritis. J Infect Dis 129:705, 1974.
43. Meeroff JC, Schreiber DS, Trier JS, Blacklow NR: Abnormal gastric motor function in viral gastroenteritis. Ann Intern Med 92:370, 1980.
44. Parrino TA, Schreiber DS, Trier JS, et al: Clinical immunity in acute gastroenteritis caused by Norwalk agent. N Engl J Med 297:86, 1977.
45. Greenberg HB, Wyatt RG, Kalica AR, et al: New insights in viral gastroenteritis. Perspect Virol 11:163, 1981.
46. Johnson PC, Mathewson JJ, DuPont HL, Greenberg HB: Multiple challenge study of host susceptibility to Norwalk gastroenteritis in U.S. adults. J Infect Dis 161:18, 1990.
47. Graham DY, Jiang X, Tanaka T, et al: Norwalk virus infection of volunteers: New insights based on improved assays. J Infect Dis 170:34, 1994.
48. Kaplan JE, Feldman R, Campbell DS, et al: The frequency of a Norwalk-like pattern of illness in outbreaks of acute gastroenteritis. Am J Public Health 72:1329, 1982.
49. Cukor G, Nowak NA, Blacklow NR: Immunoglobulin M responses to the Norwalk virus of gastroenteritis. Infect Immun 37:463, 1982.
50. Erdman DD, Gary GW, Anderson LJ: Development and evaluation of an IgM capture enzyme immunoassay for diagnosis of recent Norwalk virus infection. J Virol Methods 24:57, 1989.
51. Jiang X, Wang M, Graham DY, Estes MK: Expression, self-assembly, and antigenicity of the Norwalk virus capsid protein. J Virol 66:6527, 1992.
52. DeLeon R, Matsui SM, Baric RS, et al: Detection of Norwalk virus in stool specimens by reverse transcriptase–polymerase chain reaction and nonradioactive oligoprobes. J Clin Microbiol 30:3151, 1992.
53. Jiang X, Wang J, Graham DY, Estes MK: Detection of Norwalk virus in stool by polymerase chain reaction. J Clin Microbiol 30:2529, 1992.
54. Herrmann JE, Blacklow NR, Matsui SM, et al: Monoclonal antibodies for detection of Norwalk virus antigen in stools. J Clin Microbiol 33:2511, 1995.
55. Steinhoff MC, Douglas RG Jr, Greenberg HB, Callahan DR: Bismuth subsalicylate therapy of viral gastroenteritis. Gastroenterology 78:1495, 1980.
56. Lewis TL, Greenberg HB, Herrmann JE, et al: Analysis of astrovirus serotype 1 RNA, identification of the viral RNA-dependent RNA polymerase motif, and expression of a viral structural protein. J Virol 68:77, 1994.
57. Monroe SS, Stine SE, Goulkin L, et al: Temporal synthesis of proteins and RNAs during human astrovirus infection of cultured cells. J Virol 65:641, 1991.
58. Monroe SS, Jiang B, Stine SE, et al: Subgenomic RNA sequence of human astrovirus supports classification of Astroviridae as a new family of RNA viruses. J Virol 67:3611, 1993.
59. Lee TW, Kurtz JB: Prevalence of human astrovirus serotypes in the Oxford region 1976–92, with evidence for two new serotypes. Epidemiol Infect 112:187, 1994.
60. Herrmann JE, Nowak NA, Perron-Henry DM, et al: Diagnosis of astrovirus gastroenteritis by antigen detection with monoclonal antibodies. J Infect Dis 161:226, 1990.
61. Grohmann GS, Glass RI, Pereira HG, et al: Enteric viruses and diarrhea in HIV-infected patients. N Engl J Med 329:14, 1993.
62. Midthun K, Greenberg HB, Kurtz JB, et al: Characterization and seroepidemiology of a type 5 astrovirus associated with an outbreak of gastroenteritis in Marin County, California. J Clin Microbiol 31:955, 1993.

63. Bates PR, Bailey AS, Wood DJ, et al: Comparative epidemiology of rotavirus, subgenus F (types 40 and 41) adenovirus, and astrovirus gastroenteritis in children. J Med Virol 39:224, 1993.
64. Cruz JR, Bartlett AV, Herrmann JE, et al: Astrovirus-associated diarrhea among Guatemalan ambulatory rural children. J Clin Microbiol 30:1140, 1992.
65. Appleton H: Small round viruses: Classification and role in food-borne infections. Ciba Found Symp 128:108, 1987.
66. Kurtz JB, Lee TW, Pickering D: Astrovirus-associated gastroenteritis in a children's ward. J Clin Pathol 30:948, 1977.
67. Madeley CR, Cosgrove BP, Bell EJ, Fallon RJ: Stool viruses in babies in Glasgow. I. Hospital admission with diarrhea. J Hyg (Lond) 78:261, 1977.
68. Ashley CR, Caul EO, Paver WK: Astrovirus-associated gastroenteritis in children. J Clin Pathol 31:939, 1978.
69. Kotloff KL, Herrmann JE, Blacklow NR, et al: The frequency of astrovirus as a cause of diarrhea in Baltimore children. Pediatr Infect Dis 11:587, 1992.
70. Utagawa ET, Nishizawa S, Sekine S, et al: Astrovirus as a cause of gastroenteritis in Japan. J Clin Microbiol 32:1841, 1994.
71. Lew JF, Moe CL, Monroe SS, et al: Astrovirus and adenovirus associated with diarrhea in children in day care settings. J Infect Dis 164:673, 1991.
72. Mitchell DK, Van R, Morrow AL, et al: Outbreaks of astrovirus gastroenteritis in day care centers. J Pediatr 123:725, 1993.
73. Esahli H, Breback K, Bennet R, et al: Astroviruses as a cause of nosocomial outbreaks of infant diarrhea. Pediatr Infect Dis 10:511, 1991.
74. Ford-Jones EL, Mendorff CM, Langley JM, et al: Epidemiologic study of 4684 hospital-acquired infections in pediatric patients. Pediatr Infect Dis J 8:668, 1989.
75. Oishi I, Yamazaki K, Kimoto T, et al: A large outbreak of acute gastroenteritis associated with astrovirus among students and teachers in Osaka, Japan. J Infect Dis 170:439, 1994.
76. Konno T, Suzuki H, Ishida N, et al: Astrovirus-associated epidemic gastroenteritis in Japan. J Med Virol 9:11, 1982.
77. Gray JJ, Wreghitt TG, Cubitt WD, Elliot PR: An outbreak of gastroenteritis in a home for the elderly associated with astrovirus type 1 and human calicivirus. J Med Virol 23:377, 1987.
78. Lewis DC, Lightfoot NF, Cubitt WD, Wilson SA: Outbreaks of astrovirus type 1 and rotavirus gastroenteritis in a geriatric inpatient population. J Hosp Infect 14:9, 1989.
79. Cox GJ, Matsui SM, Lo RS, et al: Etiology and outcome of diarrhea after marrow transplantation: A prospective study. Gastroenterology 107:1398, 1994.
80. Kurtz J, Lee T: Astrovirus gastroenteritis age distribution of antibody. Microbiol Immunol 166:227, 1978.
81. LeBaron CW, Furutan NP, Lew JF, et al: Viral agents of gastroenteritis: Public health importance and outbreak management. MMWR Morbid Mortal Wkly Rep 39:1, 1990.
82. Phillips AD, Rice SJ, Walker-Smith JA: Astrovirus within human small intestinal mucosa. Gut 23:A923, 1982.
83. Kurtz JB, Lee TW, Craig JW, Reed SE: Astrovirus infection in volunteers. J Med Virol 3:221, 1979.
84. Kurtz JB, Lee TW: Astroviruses: Human and animal. Ciba Found Symp 128:92, 1987.

PART IX UNCONVENTIONAL AGENTS CAUSING SLOW INFECTIONS

272

Transmissible Spongiform Encephalopathies

David M. Asher

The transmissible spongiform encephalopathies (TSEs) comprise a group of slow infections of the nervous system (see Chapter 163) with unique agents whose nature remains controversial. At least four TSEs have been recognized in humans (Table 272–1): kuru,[1] Creutzfeldt-Jakob disease (CJD),[2] the Gerstmann-Sträussler syndrome (GSS),[3] and a newly described "variant" of CJD (V-CJD).[4] The syndrome of fatal familial insomnia (FFI)[5] may be associated with infection by a similar transmissible agent.

TSEs also affect a variety of animals: scrapie in sheep and goats,[6] transmissible mink encephalopathy (TME) in ranch mink,[7–9] and chronic wasting disease (CWD) in American elk and deer.[10, 11] In 1986, a bovine spongiform encephalopathy (BSE) was recognized among British cattle and other ungulates[12]; feline spongiform encephalopathy of domestic cats and felines in zoos may have originated from BSE.

The TSEs all share a generally similar clinical and histopathologic picture of progressive neurologic degeneration, differing in some features including the areas of central nervous system most affected, and all are associated with infectious agents similar in properties. The TSEs take their name from a striking neuropathologic change that occurs in each disease to a greater or lesser extent: neuronal vacuolation leading to spongy degeneration of the cerebral cortical gray matter (Fig. 272–1).

Etiologic Agents of Transmissible Spongiform Encephalopathies

Brain tissues (and other tissues less consistently) of humans and animals with TSEs harbor infectious agents demonstrable by experimental transmission of disease to susceptible animals[13] (Fig. 272–2). The infectious agents replicate in some cell cultures, but they do not achieve the high titers of infectivity found in brain tissues, nor do they cause recognizable cytopathic effects. (Although not replacing animals as an assay for infectivity, cell cultures have been useful for studying the synthesis and secretion of PrP—the protease-resistant protein associated with the agents—and the effects of drugs.[14–26]) Most studies characterizing the infectious agents and the pathogenesis of infection have employed the agent of sheep scrapie adapted to rodents.[27]

The pathogens transmitting TSEs were originally called viruses and still are by some authorities.[13] Titrations of infectivity by serial dilution of tissues taken from animals in successive passages clearly demonstrate that the agents replicate. The scrapie agent was retained by filters with average pore diameter of 50 nm or less,[28, 29] suggesting that it has the size of a small virus. However, the TSE agents are much more resistant to inactivation by a variety of chemical and physical treatments, including heat, ultraviolet light, and ionizing radiation, than are conventional viruses, stimulating hypotheses that they might be unique pathogens not containing nucleic acid.[30–32] The demonstration that infectivity of scrapie is substantially reduced by treatments that denature proteins[32, 33] indicated that the infectious moiety must either contain or be protected by a protein. Prusiner[32, 34] concluded that the pathogens causing TSEs are probably subviral in size, are devoid of nucleic acid, and contain protein, and he proposed that they be called prions.[32, 34] Proponents of a rival theory, that the agents are composed of a tiny unique nucleic acid protected by host components, suggested the term virino.[35, 36]

The prion or "all protein" hypothesis is widely but not universally accepted. The unusual resistance of TSE agents to heat and chemical exposures may repose in a tiny resistant fraction, the great bulk of infectivity being destroyed with kinetics of inactivation resembling those of known viruses.[37, 38] This resistant fraction may be protected from inactivation by host proteins and by aggregation into hydrophobic masses. These anomalies make it difficult to interpret inactivation studies as ruling out a nucleic acid component within the scrapie agent. Irradiation inactivation kinetic studies were reinterpreted as more consistent with the hypothesis that the scrapie agent might have a nucleic acid genome of small viral size.[39] Even proponents of the prion theory originally allowed for a possibility that the infectious particle might contain a small nucleic acid.[40–42]

Studies showed that transgenic mice overexpressing recombinant PrP genes became ill with a spongiform encepha-

TABLE 272–1 ■ Transmissible Spongiform Encephalopathies: Slow Infections of the Nervous System Caused by Unconventional Agents

DISEASE	NATURALLY INFECTED HOSTS	FAMILIAL OCCURRENCE
Kuru	Humans	No
Creutzfeldt-Jakob disease (CJD)	Humans	Sometimes
Variant Creutzfeldt-Jakob disease (V-CJD)*	Humans	No
Gerstmann-Sträussler syndrome (GSS)	Humans	Yes
Fatal familial insomnia (FFI)†	Humans	Yes
Scrapie	Sheep, goats	No
Transmissible mink encephalopathy (TME)	Mink	No
Chronic wasting disease (CWD)	Elk, deer	No
Bovine spongiform encephalopathy (BSE, "mad cow" disease)‡	Cattle, zoo ungulates	No
Feline spongiform encephalopathy (FSE)‡	House cats, zoo felines	No

*Not yet transmitted to animals.

†Transmitted to mice but not to primates. Histopathologically not spongiform.

‡Almost simultaneous outbreaks of BSE and FSE suggest that they are related.

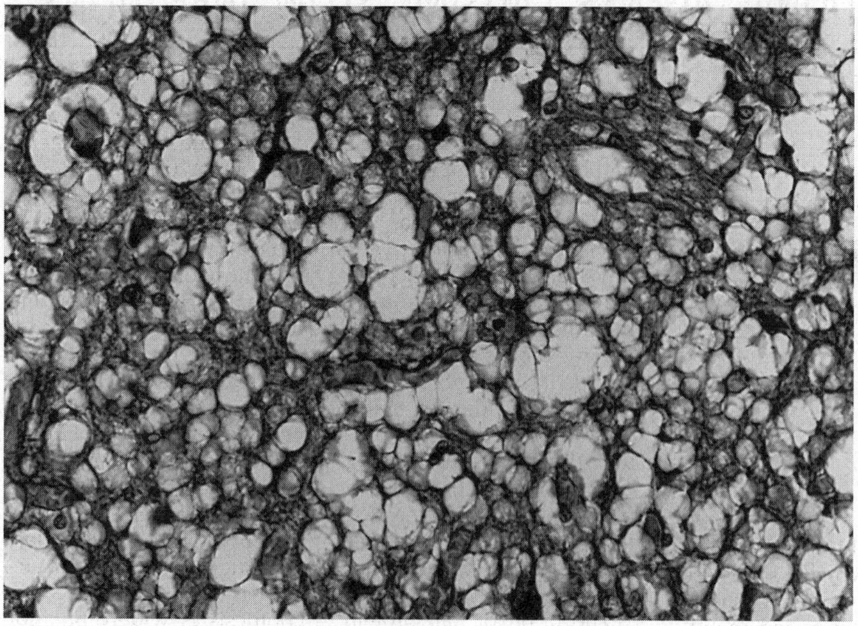

FIGURE 272–1 □ Status spongiosus: severe vacuolation in the cerebral cortex of a young man who died with familial CJD. (H&E.) (From Asher DM: Slow viral infections. *In* Scheld WM, Whitley RJ, Durack DT [eds]: Infections of the Central Nervous System, ed 2. Philadelphia, Lippincott-Raven, 1997, pp 199–221.)

lopathy,[43] and extracts of their brains (containing surprisingly little PrP) are claimed to have transmitted encephalopathy to hamsters and some transgenic mice, although not to ordinary mice,[44] in serial passage. If confirmed, those results strongly support the prion hypothesis.

Possible virus-like structures have been described in brain tissues from animals and humans with TSEs. Unique tubulovesicular particles have been regularly seen in thin sections of plastic-embedded infected tissue[45, 46] (Fig. 272–3), and tiny spherical particles were found in negatively stained extracts of tissue.[47, 48] Neither structure has been convincingly demonstrated either to contain nucleic acid or to be associated with infectivity. No nucleic acids unique to the TSEs have been

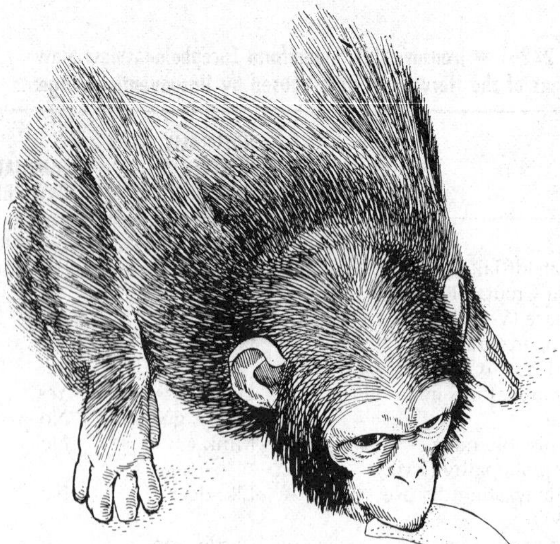

FIGURE 272–2 □ A chimpanzee in the intermediate stage of experimental kuru has lost normal prehension and eats directly from the floor. (From Asher DM, Gibbs CJ Jr, David E, et al: Experimental kuru in the chimpanzee. *In* Montagna W, McNulty WP [eds]: Symposia of the Fourth International Congress of Primatology. Beaverton, Oregon, Vol 4. Basel, S Karger, 1973, p 44. Reproduced with permission of S. Karger AG, Basel.)

identified,[49, 50] although those attempts should be repeated using more powerful molecular methodology now available.[51] Until their actual structure is determined unambiguously and the component encoding the self-replicating pathogenic information identified, it seems less contentious to call them simply TSE agents.

Merz and colleagues[52–54] observed scrapie-associated fibrils (Fig. 272–4), resembling but distinguishable from the amyloid fibrils that accumulate in brains of patients with Alzheimer disease, in extracts of tissues from patients and animals with TSEs. Prusiner and coworkers described a group of antigenically related, low-molecular-weight proteins, relatively resistant to protease digestion and ranging in mass from about 27 to 30 kDa (Fig. 272–5), in brains of animals with scrapie[55] and in patients with CJD[56, 57]; they postulated that the abnormal proteins might be the prions or a component of them, and they designated them the PrP or prion protein 27–30 (PrP27–30).[58] Scrapie-associated fibrils contain PrP27–30.[59–61] PrP27–30 is found consistently in brains of patients with TSEs[62] and in their amyloid plaques.[60] PrP generally copurifies with infectivity of scrapie,[34, 63] although several groups claimed to have separated infectivity from PrP[64, 65] or found differences between the physical behavior of the infectious entity and that of PrP.[66–68] So it remains controversial whether PrP constitutes the complete infectious agent or is a component or simply an important pathologic host protein not usually separated from the agent. The demonstration that PrP is encoded by a normal host gene[69, 70] with an amino acid sequence identical to that of the normal gene product[71] seemed to favor the last possibility, as did the recognition that there are distinct strains of scrapie agent.

There are substantial differences in several properties of disease transmitted by isolates of the same TSE to animals—differences in incubation periods[72, 73] and in histologic picture including presence and distribution of amyloid plaques in brain[72, 74] and distribution of vacuolation.[75] Those properties are determined by the agent and are usually not altered after serial passages in animals or even after passages through animals of another species expressing a different PrP.[76] Agent-specific properties occasionally change suddenly and then remain stable on subsequent passages in animals, a phenomenon resembling mutation.[73] It is not understood how agent-specific information can be transmitted and repli-

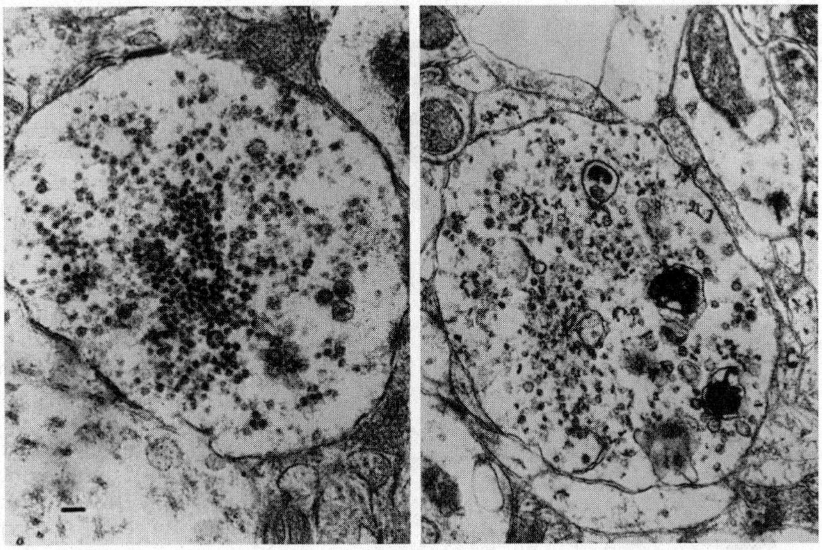

FIGURE 272–3 ▫ Tubulovesicular particles measuring about 23 nm across in the postsynaptic process of a mouse with scrapie *(left)* and a patient with CJD *(right)*. (Bar = 100 nm.) (Courtesy of Dr. Harash K. Narang, Public Health Laboratory, Newcastle upon Tyne, England.)

cated in the absence of some genetic material independent of the host. Ingenious hypotheses have been proposed to explain how a host-coded protein, the gene for which is present and expressed in all normal subjects, might replicate and transmit pathogenic information.[77–80] It was proposed that differences in protein conformation alone[13, 80–84] might serve to transmit self-replicating pathogenic information. One study found agent-associated differences in proteinase cleavage sites of PrP, suggesting that an altered folding might explain strain differences.[9, 85] Skeptics continue to suspect that the complete infectious agents more probably contain small unique nucleic acids as their information-bearing moieties.[86]

Whatever its relationship to the actual infectious particles, PrP clearly plays a central role in the pathogenesis of TSEs, and its expression in the cell is obligatory for replication of the infectious agent.[87] PrP27–30 is a glycoprotein[88] consisting of 55 amino acids[68] with attached carbohydrates, a neuraminic acid residue,[88] and an inositol[17] (Fig. 272–6). It has the physical properties of an amyloid protein[56]—staining with Congo red dye and birefringence in polarized light—presumably resulting from its high content of β-pleated-sheet structure. The PrPs of several species of animals are similar in amino acid sequence and antigenicity, although not identical.[89, 90] The primary structure of PrP is encoded by the host and is not influenced by the source of infectious agent provoking its formation,[91] although in chimeric animals expressing PrP genes from two rodent species, the PrP that accumulates is that of the species to which the infecting strain of agent was adapted.[92] PrP27–30 is cleaved from a larger precursor protein (designated PrP33–35, abbreviated as PrP[93]) consisting of about 250 amino acids.[94] It occurs in tissues of normal humans and animals as well as in those with TSE.[16]

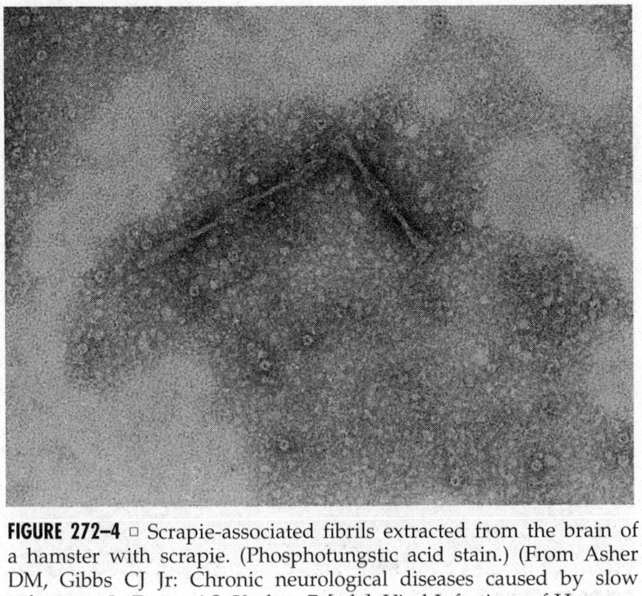

FIGURE 272–4 ▫ Scrapie-associated fibrils extracted from the brain of a hamster with scrapie. (Phosphotungstic acid stain.) (From Asher DM, Gibbs CJ Jr: Chronic neurological diseases caused by slow infections. *In* Evans AS, Kaslow R [eds]: Viral Infections of Humans, ed 2. New York, Plenum Publishing, 1997, pp 1027–1051.)

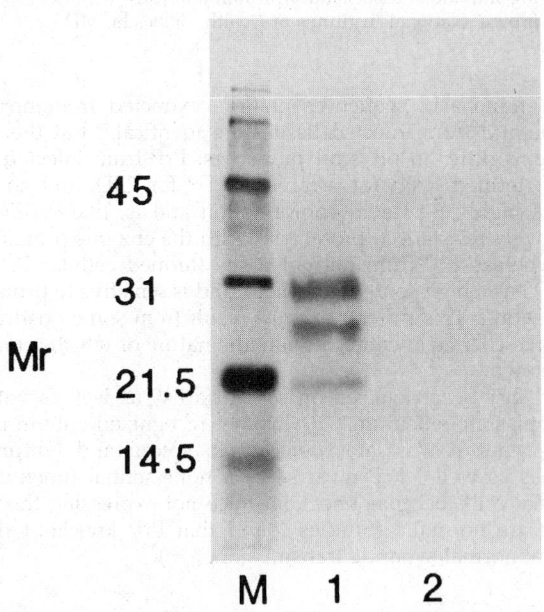

FIGURE 272–5 ▫ Imunoblot of brain extracts with antibodies to PrP27–30. Detergent–protease K extracts of brain tissues from a patient with GSS (1) and a patient without neurologic disease (2) were fractionated by polyacrylamide gel electrophoresis, transferred to a nitrocellulose membrane, incubated with rabbit antiserum to hamster PrP, and then stained by an indirect immunoperoxidase method. M, Molecular weight markers. (From Asher DM, Gibbs CJ Jr: Chronic neurological diseases caused by slow infections. *In* Evans AS, Kaslow R [eds]: Viral Infections of Humans, ed 2. New York, Plenum Publishing, 1997, pp 1027–1051.)

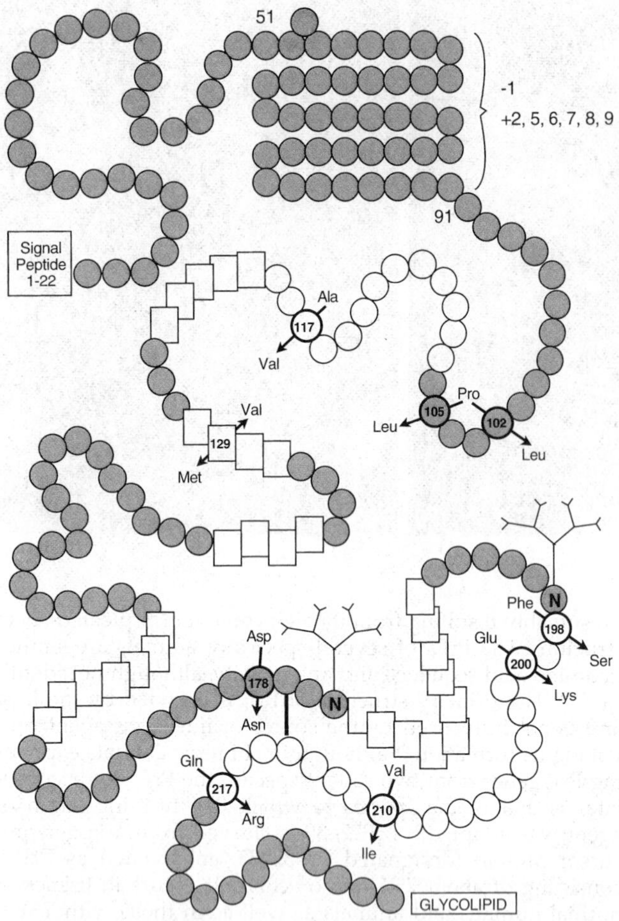

FIGURE 272–6 □ Schematic diagram of the amino acid structure of PrP showing mutations associated with familial TSEs. (Courtesy of Dr. Paul Brown, National Institutes of Health, Bethesda, MD.)

The amino acid sequences of PrPs extracted from normal tissue and from infected tissues are identical,[70] but the two proteins differ in physical properties: PrP from infected tissues (termed PrP^{Sc} for scrapie, PrP^{CJD} for CJD, and so on) has a highly β-pleated conformation and is, like PrP27–30, relatively resistant to proteolysis with the enzyme proteinase K, whereas PrP from normal tissue (termed cellular PrP or PrP^{C}) has a high content of α-helix and is sensitive to protease digestion.[95] This difference must result from some posttranslational change in conformation, the nature of which remains unknown.[83]

PrP has been detected on cell surfaces[17] as well as within endoplasmic reticulum.[96] It was first recognized only in neurons,[94] but it was later detected in spleen and lymphoid tissues as well.[97] PrP must serve a nonessential function in normal cells, because knockout mice not expressing the PrP gene are normal.[98] (Studies found that PrP knockout mice had abnormal synaptic transmission.[99, 100])

Pathology

Histopathologic changes in TSEs occur only in neural tissues. Typical changes are vacuolation and loss of neurons (Fig. 272–7) with hypertrophy and proliferation of astrocytes demonstrable by gold stain (Fig. 272–8) or by immunostaining of glial fibrillary acidic protein. Changes are more pronounced in the cerebral cortex in CJD and GSS and in the cerebellum in kuru and are typically most severe in gray matter. Patients with prominent white matter involvement have been described.[101, 102] Some loss of myelin is seen secondary to degeneration of neurons. There is no inflammation. Vacuoles vary in severity and distribution; they appear to arise by budding from cell membranes into the cytoplasm and later from the walls of existing vacuoles to form multiple vacuolations.[103]

Amyloid plaques (Fig. 272–9) are found in brains of all patients with GSS and V-CJD, in at least 70% of patients with kuru, and less commonly in typical sporadic CJD. Amyloid plaques are most common in the cerebellum but occur elsewhere in the brain as well. The plaques react with anti-PrP antibodies[74, 96, 104, 105] but not with antisera to the amyloid A protein in plaques of Alzheimer disease.[96, 106] In TSE brain specimens without typical plaques, PrP can usually be detected in the parenchyma by immunostaining,[107] which is enhanced by treatment of tissue sections with formic acid[74, 108] or autoclaving.[109, 110]

In eight patients who died with V-CJD, unusually prominent PrP plaques, often surrounded by halos of spongiform change, were noted throughout cerebellum and cerebrum, with smaller numbers in the basal ganglia, hypothalamus, and thalamus.[4] Such plaques have been seen rarely in sporadic CJD[111] and in scrapie and CWD.[10] The finding of similar plaques in brains of monkeys inoculated with suspensions of tissue from cows with BSE gives additional evidence suggesting a possible causal link between the two diseases.[112]

Pathogenesis

Little information is available about pathogenesis of human TSEs. The kuru agent probably entered the body through lesions in the skin or mouth[13] exposed to infected tissues during ritual cannibalism; incubation periods after exposure have been longer than 30 years.[113] In iatrogenic CJD, the agent is introduced into the body either directly into nervous system—brain or the eye—by surgery (with incubation periods of 15 months or more) or indirectly by subcutaneous injection of contaminated hormones (with incubation periods of several years). In GSS, familial CJD, and sporadic cases of CJD, the portal of entry (if any) of the infectious agent is not known. It remains to be determined whether exposure to BSE-contaminated beef transmitted V-CJD to humans and, if so, the vehicle and the portal of entry.

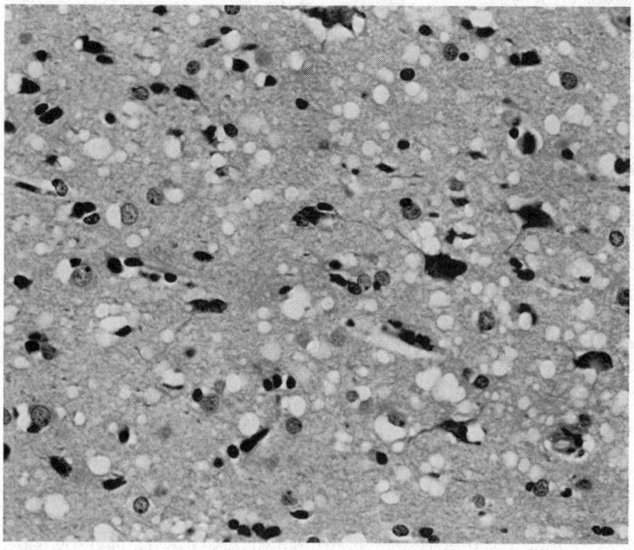

FIGURE 272–7 □ Vacuolation and loss of neurons in the cerebral cortex of a patient with GSS. (H&E.)

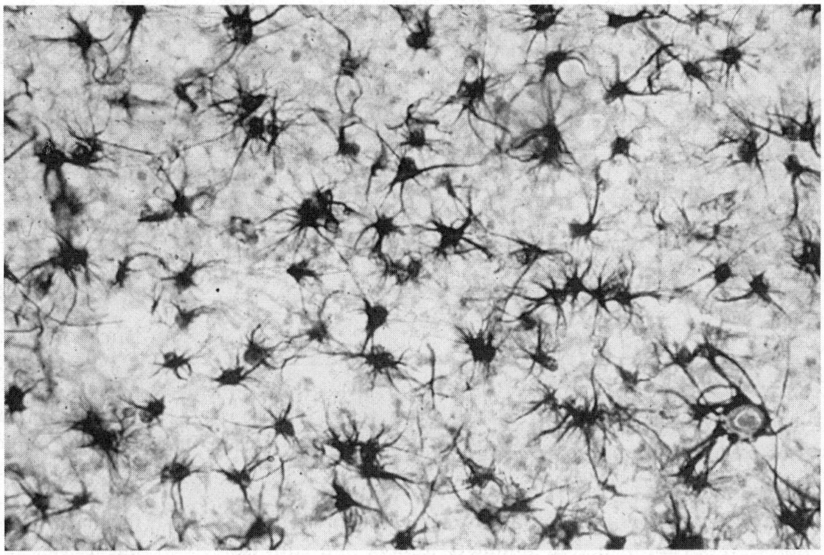

FIGURE 272–8 □ Proliferation and hypertrophy of astrocytes in the cerebral cortex of a chimpanzee with experimental kuru. (Cajal gold stain.) (Courtesy of Ms. Elisabeth Beck, Institutes of Psychiatry, London, UK.)

In sheep naturally exposed to scrapie, the infectious agent was first detected in intestines and mesenteric lymph nodes,[114] suggesting that the alimentary tract can be a portal of infection in that disease. Epidemiologic evidence suggests the same portal for BSE,[115] feline spongiform encephalopathy, and TME.[8] Nothing is known of sources of infection in CWD. Monkeys were experimentally infected with the agents of scrapie, kuru, and CJD by feeding them contaminated tissue.[116]

Spread of the TSE agents within the human body is also poorly understood. In animals inoculated intraperitoneally, subcutaneously, or orally, the first site of replication of the agents appears to be in tissues of the reticuloendothelial system.[114, 117] The agent has been detected in lymph nodes and spleens of occasional CJD patients at autopsy[118–120] (Table 272–2), suggesting that the same thing may be true in human disease.

It has not been determined with certainty whether the agent occurs in human blood during the incubation period or symptomatic illness with CJD. Transmissions of disease to

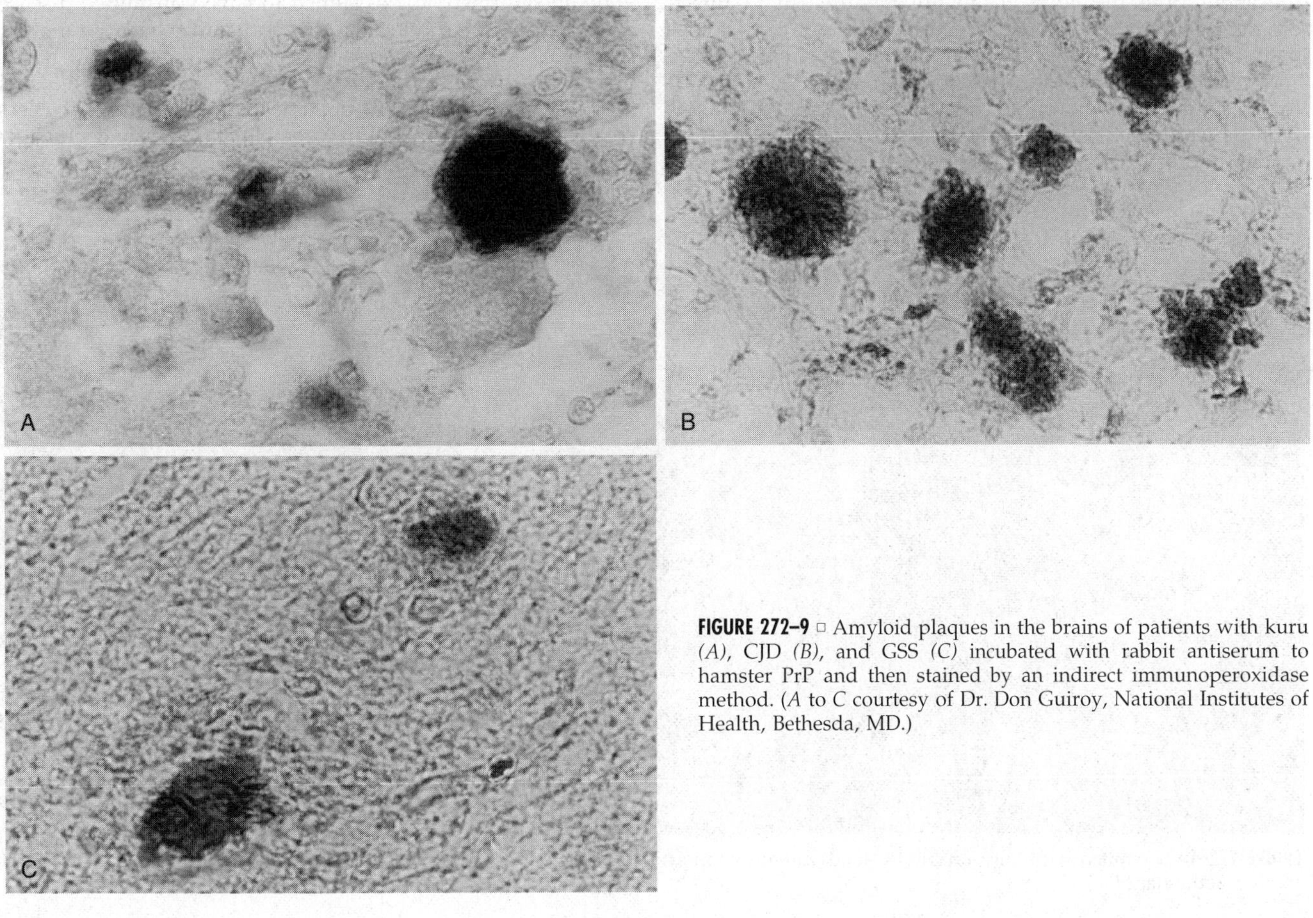

FIGURE 272–9 □ Amyloid plaques in the brains of patients with kuru *(A)*, CJD *(B)*, and GSS *(C)* incubated with rabbit antiserum to hamster PrP and then stained by an indirect immunoperoxidase method. (*A* to *C* courtesy of Dr. Don Guiroy, National Institutes of Health, Bethesda, MD.)

TABLE 272–2 ■ Infectivity of Tissues and Body Fluids from Patients with Creutzfeldt-Jakob Disease

CONSISTENTLY TRANSMIT INFECTIOUS AGENT (≥50% OF ATTEMPTS)	SOMETIMES TRANSMIT INFECTIOUS AGENT (40%–33% OF ATTEMPTS)	POSSIBLY TRANSMIT INFECTIOUS AGENT (OCCASIONAL REPORTS)
Brain	Kidney	Blood
Spinal cord	Liver	Urine
Eye	Lung	
	Lymph node	
	Spleen	
	CSF	

Modified from Asher DM: Slow viral infections of the central nervous system. *In* Scheld WM, Whitley RJ, Durack DT (eds): Infections of the Central Nervous System. New York, Raven Press, 1991, pp 145–166.

animals injected with human blood have been claimed,[121–124] although not confirmed in a limited number of attempts.[118, 120] Epidemiologic and clinical studies did not support the hypothesis that donors had transmitted CJD to recipients of blood or derivatives,[125, 126] although anecdotal reports raised that possibility.[127, 128] However, the agent of CJD was convincingly demonstrated in blood of experimentally infected rodents, associated with nucleated cells.[129, 130] In natural scrapie of sheep (in which no blood-borne agent has been detected), the agent first appears in the central nervous system rather late in disease, multiplying there to much higher levels than in lymphoid and other tissues infected earlier.[114] In experimental infections of mice, the scrapie agent appears to spread to the central nervous system by ascending peripheral nerves[117, 131] rather than through the blood stream.

In human kuru it is probable that the only portal of exit of the agent from the body, in quantities sufficient to infect others, was through infected tissues exposed during cannibalism[13]; in iatrogenically transmitted CJD the infected tissues of source patients provided a similar portal of exit.[132, 133] Brain, spinal cord, and eyes of patients with CJD are consistently infectious.[120] Several other human tissues and cerebrospinal fluid (CSF) sometimes contained the agent as well[118, 120] (see Table 272–2). A small number of studies failed to find infectious agent in secretions or excretions from patients with CJD,[120] although one report, never confirmed, claimed that urine transmitted disease to mice.[122]

No antibodies and no cell-mediated immunity to the infectious agents of the spongiform encephalopathies have been demonstrated in either patients or animals at any time during illness.[118] This apparent lack of immune response to infection remains unexplained.

Epidemiology and Mechanisms of Transmission

Kuru once affected many children 4 years old and older, adolescents, and adults, especially women, among the Fore people (Fig. 272–10) in a restricted area of Papua New Guinea. It is now found rarely (Fig. 272–11) and only in older adults.[13] Children born to and nursed by affected mothers have never developed kuru unless they also participated in cannibalism. No evidence indicates spread of kuru by any mechanism except by ritual cannibalism, which ended in the late 1950s.[113]

The epidemiology of CJD and its variants is more complicated than that of kuru. CJD has been recognized worldwide, at rates of 0.25 to 2 cases per million population per year,[134, 135] with foci of much higher incidence among Libyan Jews in Israel, in isolated villages of Slovakia, and in other limited areas.[13] Hypothetic mechanisms for the origin of sporadic CJD have been proposed, including exposure to a ubiquitous agent with a low transmission rate and appearance of spontaneous somatic mutations in the PrP yielding an infectious protein agent de novo.[136] Except for iatrogenic spread of CJD,[137] which accounts for a relatively small proportion of cases, and the cluster of V-CJD possibly linked to BSE,[4] none of the hypotheses has convincing support. Like kuru, CJD has not occurred in children born to affected mothers.[120, 133] One unconfirmed study claimed to have transmitted disease to mice inoculated with placenta and cord blood of a mother with CJD.[138]

Iatrogenic transmission of CJD from patients to uninfected subjects has been amply documented. More than 30 years ago, CJD was recognized in three patients who had previous neurosurgery performed in the same operating suite.[139, 140] CJD was accidentally transmitted by transplantation of a

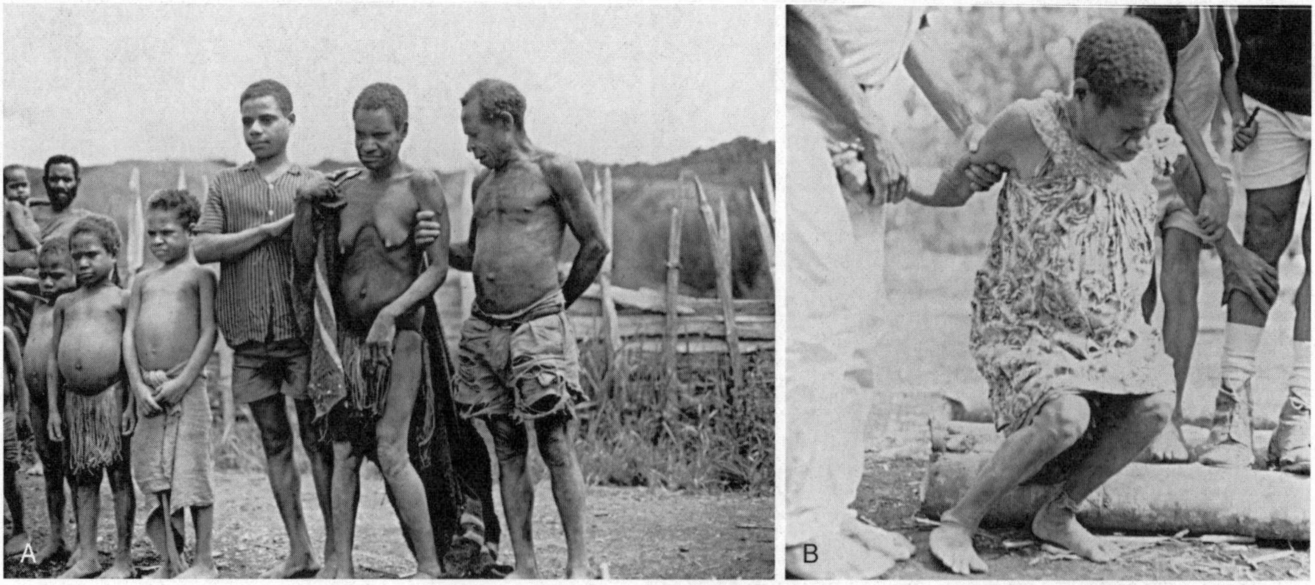

FIGURE 272–10 □ Women with kuru unable to stand without support. (*A* and *B* courtesy of Dr. D. Carleton Gajdusek, National Institutes of Health, Bethesda, MD.)

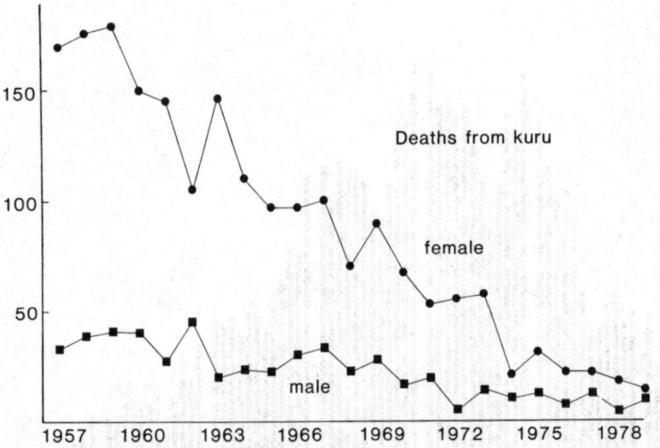

FIGURE 272–11 □ Deaths from kuru registered in Okapa, Papua New Guinea during the first 20 years of study. (Courtesy of Dr. D. Carleton Gajdusek, National Institutes of Health, Bethesda, MD.)

contaminated cornea[141] and by contaminated cortical electrodes used during epilepsy surgery.[142] CJD has affected more than 80 young people who received injections of human cadaveric pituitary growth hormone[137] involving at least five contaminated lots in three countries and several recipients of human pituitary gonadotropin,[143] with minimal incubation periods as long as 19 years. One sample of cadaveric growth hormone transmitted disease to a monkey.[132] Cases of CJD also occurred in patients who received grafts of lyophilized cadaveric dura mater.[144–152] However, for the great majority of sporadic cases of CJD no probable iatrogenic event can be identified.

Spouses and household contacts of patients are at low risk of acquiring CJD, although two conjugal cases have been reported,[153, 154] each more suggestive of common-source exposure than of case-to-case transmission. It was thought that medical personnel had no increased risk of CJD[135, 155]; reports of CJD in histopathology technicians,[156, 157] a neurosurgeon,[111] an orthopedist (who had collected dura),[158] a pathologist,[159] and at least 15 other health care workers[160] forced reconsideration of that issue.

The recognition in the United Kingdom of BSE among cattle (Fig. 272–12) and of similar TSEs affecting captive ungulates, domestic cats, and felines in zoos—apparently infected by eating contaminated feed[12, 115, 161, 162]—raised concern that the scrapie agent, never linked to human disease, had crossed a species barrier from sheep to cattle and acquired a broadened range of susceptible hosts, posing a potential danger for humans. Research findings suggesting that transgenic mice expressing the human PrP-encoding gene had no increased susceptibility to infection with the BSE agent[163] seemed initially reassuring. However, recognition of V-CJD, a new clinical-histopathologic variant of CJD affecting 10 relatively young people,[4] forced authorities in the United Kingdom to conclude that a "link with BSE . . . may be the most plausible explanation." After changes in feeding of cattle and in meat-cutting and -rendering procedures were introduced in the United Kingdom, intended to reduce opportunities for exposure of livestock to infection, cases of BSE have dropped markedly (Fig. 272–13), especially among younger cattle.[115] Those steps should also have reduced the likelihood of human exposure. BSE has never been recognized in the United States.

Scrapie has been recognized in Great Britain and on the European continent for more than 200 years; it was accidentally imported to the United States in 1947 and gradually spread, especially among sheep of the Suffolk breed.[6] Scrapie is transmitted laterally from infected sheep to uninfected sheep and goats exposed to them. Transmission from infected ewe to lamb appears to be especially important in maintaining scrapie in flocks. Postnatal infection clearly takes place, and some data suggest that transplacental transmission may also occur.[6] Although the mechanism for contact transmission of scrapie is not known, it has been proposed that parasites play some role. One report suggested hay mites as a possible vector.[164]

TME has occurred only in self-limited outbreaks in the United States. Both TME and BSE resemble kuru rather than scrapie in epidemiology; they appear to be strictly foodborne, and there is no evidence of contagion by contact or maternal transmission of infection in either disease.[8, 115] The epidemiology of CWD—its origin, spread through captive and wild herds, and possible relationship to other TSEs—is not yet understood.

Clinical Manifestations and Diagnosis

Kuru, the first human spongiform encephalopathy recognized to be a slow infection,[1, 165] is a progressive degenerative disease of the cerebellum and brain stem with less marked involvement of the cerebral cortex. The first sign of kuru is usually a cerebellar ataxia followed by progressive incoordination (see Fig. 272–10) and coarse shivering tremors. Variable abnormalities in cranial nerve function appear with frequent impairment in conjugate gaze and swallowing. Patients die of inanition and pneumonia, decubitus ulcers with septicemia, or accidental burns, usually less than a year after onset. Although changes in mentation are common, there is no frank dementia or progression to coma as in CJD. There are no signs of acute encephalitis—no fever (except during secondary infections), headaches, or convulsions.

CJD occurs throughout the world, affecting mainly middle-aged and older subjects (mean ages in most series from 60 to

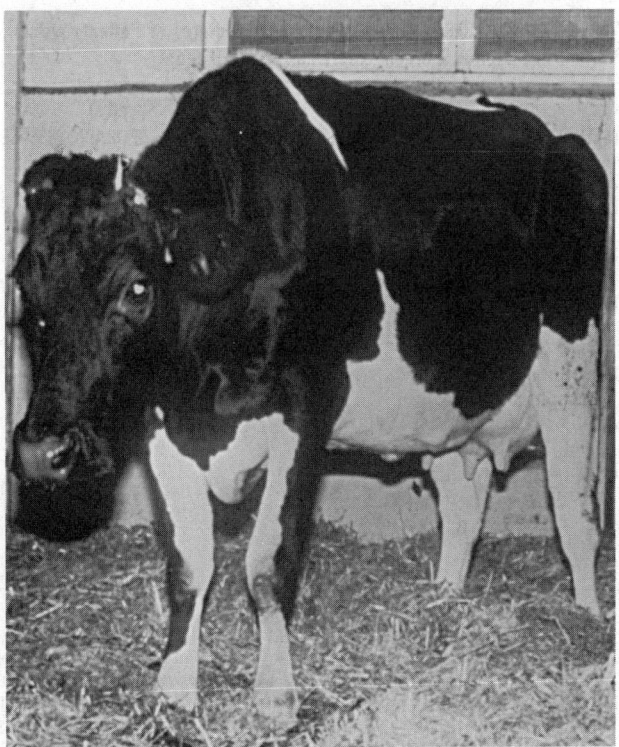

FIGURE 272–12 □ A British cow with BSE. (Courtesy of Dr. C. J. Gibbs, Jr., National Institutes of Health, Bethesda, MD.)

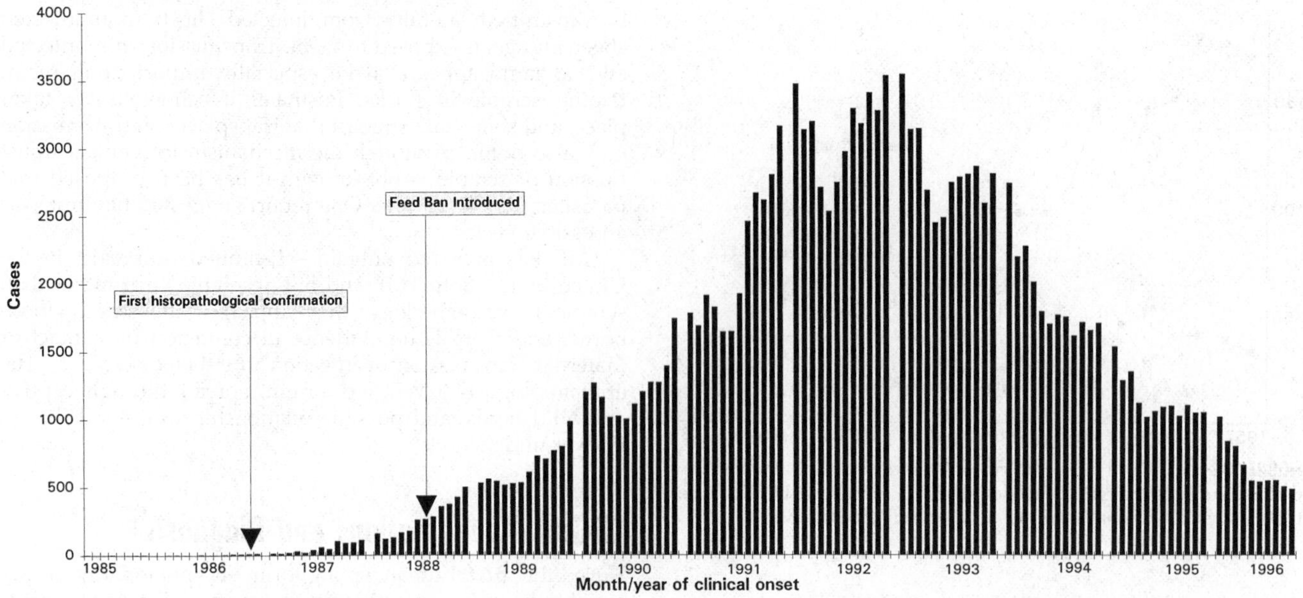

FIGURE 272–13 □ Confirmed cases of BSE registered by month and year of clinical onset. Data are valid to the end of October 1996; produced April 8, 1997. (Courtesy of the Ministry of Agriculture, Food and Fisheries, Hook Rise South, Tolworth, Surbiton, Surrey, UK.)

69 years[120]) and occurring rarely in older adolescents and young adults.[166–173] Patients initially have either sensory disturbances or confusion and inappropriate behavior, progressing in weeks or months to frank dementia and then coma. V-CJD, tentatively attributed to exposure to the BSE agent,[4] differs in several respects from typical sporadic CJD, most strikingly in younger age at onset, frequent early complaints of dyesthesias or pain in the extremities, and absence of periodic electroencephalographic changes (Table 272–3). Recipients of human pituitary hormones with iatrogenic CJD

TABLE 272–3 ■ Clinical and Histopathologic Features of Patients with Variant and Typical Sporadic Creutzfeldt-Jakob Disease

FEATURE	VARIANT DISEASE	TYPICAL SPORADIC DISEASE
Age* at death (y)	29 (range 19–41)	65
Duration* of illness (mo)	12 (range 8–23)	4
Presenting signs	Abnormal behavior Dysesthesia	Dementia
Later signs	Dementia Ataxia Myoclonus	Ataxia Myclonus
Periodic electroencephalography	None	Most
PRNP codon 129 Met/Met	100%	83%
Histopathologic changes	Vacuolation Neuronal loss Astrocytosis	Vacuolation Neuronal loss Astrocytosis
"Florid" PrP plaques†	100%	None

*Median age and duration for V-CJD, average for typical CJD.
†Dense plaques with pale periphery surrounded by a halo of spongiform change.
From Will RG, Ironside JW, Zeidler M, et al: A new variant of Creutzfeldt-Jakob disease in the UK. Lancet 347(9006):921–925, 1996. © by The Lancet Ltd. 1996. (Will et al. compared findings in 10 patients with V-CJD [February 1994–January 1996] and 185 with typical sporadic CJD [May 1990–January 1996].)

have typically presented with cerebellar ataxia and become demented only late in disease.[174] Most patients with CJD develop myoclonic jerking movements, frequently with generalized "startle" myoclonus. Mean survival of patients with CJD is less than a year from earliest signs of illness, although about 10% live for more than 2 years.[175] Reports of remission have never been confirmed.

GSS is a familial disease resembling CJD[3] but with more prominent cerebellar ataxia and later appearance of dementia and amyloid plaques at autopsy.

FFI, an inherited syndrome with an autosomal dominant pattern of occurrence, characterized by progressive severe insomnia and dysautonomia with selective atrophy of two thalamic nuclei, was described in several Italian kindreds.[5, 176–178] Patients with FFI have ataxia, myoclonus, and other signs resembling those of CJD and GSS. Only a few affected patients had spongiform changes in the cerebral cortex. Those findings suggested that FFI might be a new prion disease; indeed, protease-resistant PrP was detected in brains of patients with FFI, although it apparently differed somewhat from the PrP found in patients with CJD or GSS.[5] In a small number of attempts, FFI was not transmitted to primates[120]; transmission of encephalopathy from thalamic tissues of FFI patients to mice was claimed by two groups.[179, 180]

The TSEs of animals[6, 8, 11, 161] are all characterized by progressive incoordination and frequently by inappropriate behavior and inanition; tremors, abnormal movements, and convulsions are less common. Pruritus, not seen in the other TSEs, is often observed in sheep with scrapie[6] and polydipsia or polyuria in deer with CWD.[11]

Laboratory Findings

Most patients with sporadic, iatrogenic, and familial CJD have abnormal electroencephalographic findings at some time during the disease[120]; as the disease progresses, the background becomes slow and irregular with diminished amplitude. A variety of paroxysmal discharges (slow waves, sharp waves, spike and wave complexes) may also appear; these may sometimes be unilateral or focal as well as bilaterally synchronous. Paroxysmal discharges may be precipitated by loud noise. Many patients with CJD have typical periodic suppression-burst complexes of high-voltage slow activity on the electroencephalogram (Fig. 272–14) at some time during the illness.[181] Patients with V-CJD have thus far lacked typical electroencephalographic findings.[4]

Computed tomography may show cortical atrophy with large ventricles late in the course of CJD. There may also be some elevation of total CSF protein value. Abnormal liver function studies sometimes suggest hepatic parenchymal disease.[182] Results of other clinical laboratory tests are generally normal.

One additional laboratory test has been useful in establishing the diagnosis of CJD. Abnormal protein spots were detected in the CSF of most patients with CJD using two-dimensional gel electrophoresis–isoelectric focusing.[183] Two of these spots (originally designated 130 and 131) were found in fluids of patients with CJD (Fig. 272–15) and also in fluids of some patients with acute herpes simplex encephalitis but not in those of patients with Alzheimer disease. They were identified as 14-3-3 protein,[183a] a ubiquitous protein (possibly involved in signal transduction and the cell cycle[184]) present in the normal brain and other tissues but usually detected only in trace amounts in CSF.[185] Elevated levels of 14-3-3 in the CSF of a patient with appropriate clinical findings strongly suggest the diagnosis of CJD.[183a, 186, 187] (The 14-3-3 protein is not related antigenically to the PrP protein.)

Diagnosis and Differential Diagnosis

The demonstration of scrapie-associated fibrils[54] or PrP[188] in extracts of brain treated with detergent and proteinase K confirms the histopathologic diagnosis, although their absence does not absolutely rule it out. Transmission of disease to susceptible animals by inoculation of brain suspension is used in special cases. Chimpanzees and squirrel monkeys are consistently susceptible to the human TSEs with relatively shorter incubation periods than those of other primates[120, 189]; animals should be observed for at least 3 years before transmission attempts are considered to be tentatively negative. Transgenic mice expressing human PrP sequences are expected to replace monkeys as assay animals eventually. Unusual cases of CJD may be difficult to distinguish from Alzheimer disease; the finding of the 14-3-3 proteins in CSF (see Fig. 272–15) strongly suggests the former. The two diseases can sometimes be distinguished only at autopsy. The plaques of TSEs, where present, can be differentiated from those of Alzheimer disease by immunostaining with specific antisera[96, 106] (see Fig. 272–9).

Although brain biopsy is often diagnostic of TSE, this procedure can be recommended only if some other potentially treatable disease remains to be excluded or if rapid diagnosis is justified for reasons of public health.

Host Genetics and Transmissible Spongiform Encephalopathies

In most series of CJD, about 10% of cases have a family history of presenile dementia consistent with the disease,[190] the pattern of occurrence suggesting an autosomal dominant mode of inheritance. The clinical and histopathologic findings in patients with a family history of CJD (FCJD) resemble those in sporadic cases. GSS is defined as familial. The basis for the familial occurrence of TSEs lies in a series of mutations in the gene coding for PrP.

The gene coding for PrP is closely linked or identical to that controlling the incubation periods of scrapie in sheep[191] and both scrapie and CJD in mice,[191–193] and amino acid

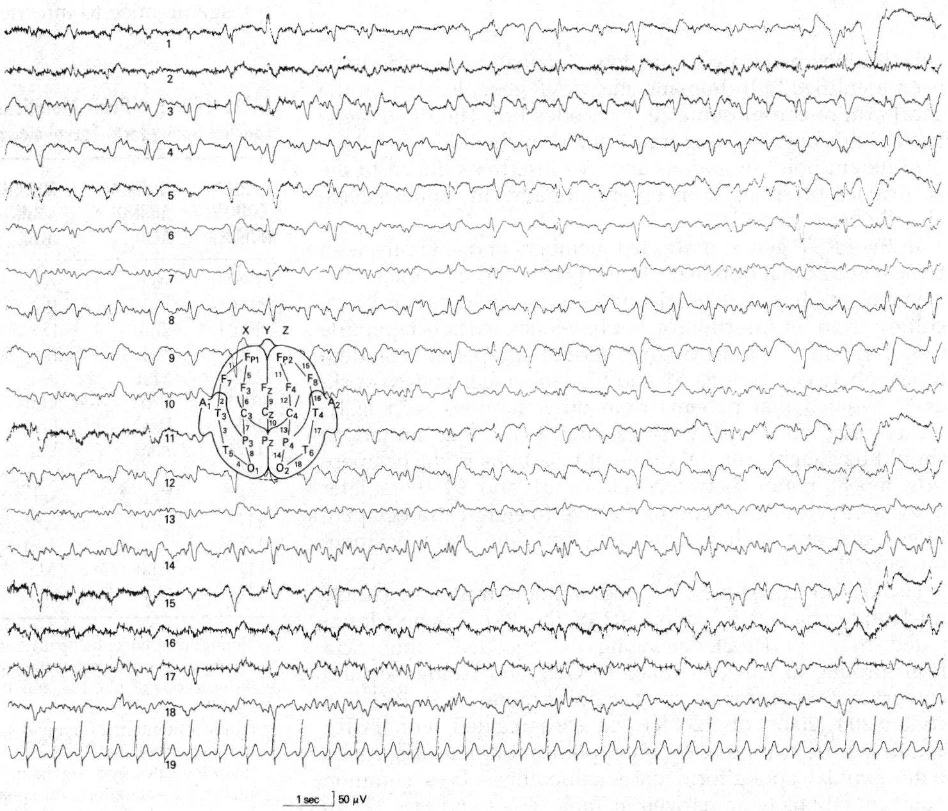

FIGURE 272–14 □ Electroencephalogram from a patient with CJD. Periodic high-voltage slow-wave complexes are present on a slow, poorly organized background. (Courtesy of Dr. Charles Henry, Department of Neurology, Medical College of Virginia, Richmond, VA.)

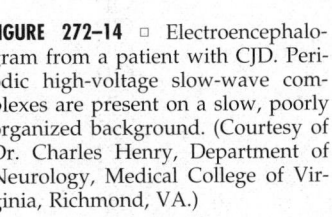

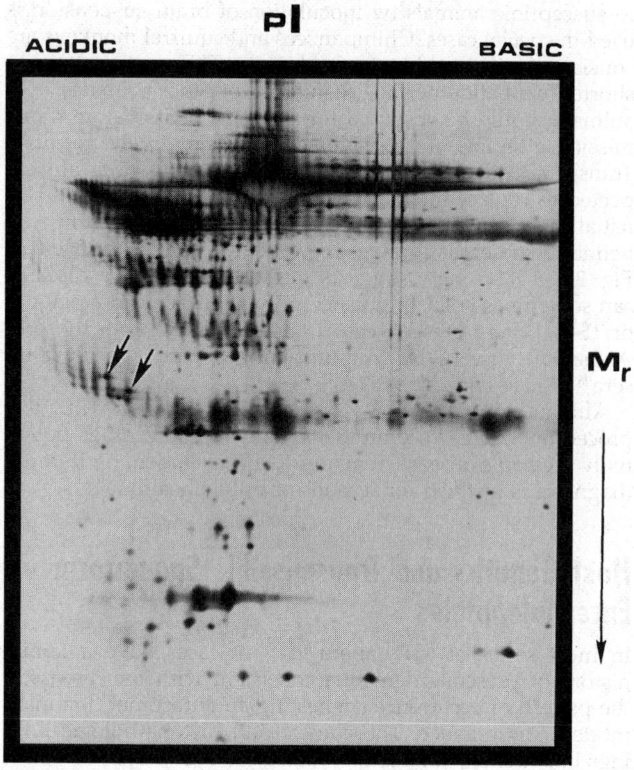

FIGURE 272–15 □ Polypeptides in CSF of a patient with CJD demonstrated by two-dimensional separation: electrophoresis–isolectric focusing and silver staining. Although not unique to CJD, the spots have not been seen in CSF of patients with Alzheimer disease or healthy older subjects. The image was digitized and computer enhanced. (Courtesy of Dr. Michael Harrington, California Institute of Technology, Pasadena, CA.)

substitutions associated with long incubation periods have been identified.[194] In humans, the *PRNP* gene, located on the short arm of chromosome 20,[195] encodes PrP. The *PRNP* gene has a single open reading frame of 750 nucleotides[90] in which 11 different point mutations and five insertions linked to the occurrence of spongiform encephalopathy in families have already been identified.

In the *PRNP* genes of affected members in one family with typical autosomal dominant FCJD, Owen and coworkers discovered an abnormal restriction endonuclease pattern[196] resulting from an insertion of 144 bases (six extra octapeptide repeats)[197] in a region of five normal octapeptide tandem repeats between codons 51 and 91. Goldgaber and coworkers[198] showed that patients from other families with FCJD lacked that abnormality, suggesting that other mutations should be sought. Several different insertions in the octapeptide repeat region between codons 51 and 91 were later associated with FCJD (coding for five to eight extra octapeptides) and one with GSS (coding for nine extra octapeptides).[199, 200]

Hsaio and colleagues[195] found a point mutation (single nucleotide change) in codon 102 of the *PRNP* gene (designated 102^{Leu} or P102L, changing the encoded amino acid from proline to leucine) linked to GSS, and Goldgaber and coworkers[201] soon found another point mutation in *PRNP* at codon 200 (200^{Lys} or E200K) that cosegregated with FCJD. Those are the two most common point mutations associated with familial spongiform encephalopathies. Less common point mutations (summarized in Table 272–4 and Fig. 272–6) were later demonstrated in other families with FCJD and GSS; in addition to the 200^{Lys} mutation, FCJD has been linked to each of four other point mutations (178^{Asn}, 180^{Ile}, 210^{Ile}, 232^{Met}) and GSS to point mutations at five other codons (105^{Leu}, 117^{Val}, 145^{Stop}, 198^{Ser}, 217^{Arg}) as well as to the more common 102^{Leu} mutation.[199] Patients with kuru had neither mutations nor insertions in their *PRNP* genes.[202] In patients with FFI a mutation was found in the *PRNP* gene at codon 178 (178^{Asn}), identical to that found in some kindreds with FCJD. However, the two groups of patients differed in *PRNP* sequences at codon 129 of the abnormal allele (a codon encoding methionine in about 60% of *PRNP* alleles of normal subjects and valine in the rest); FFI patients had 129^{Val} on the 178^{Asn} allele, whereas FCJD patients had 129^{Met}.[203, 204]

Homozygosity at the 129 locus is much more common in subjects with iatrogenic CJD[205] and sporadic CJD[206] than in general populations, suggesting that homozygosity at codon 129 may increase susceptibility to infection. In the cluster of V-CJD,[4] every patient tested has been homozygous for 129^{Met}, although that genotype is expected in less than half of the general population. (A similar association of scrapie with homozygosity of codon 171^{Gln} of the PrP gene in Suffolk sheep has been noted.[207])

In addition to the methionine-valine polymorphism at codon 129, there are other normal polymorphisms in the *PRNP* gene at codons 117 and 124 (silent polymorphisms with both variants encoding the same amino acid) and in the octapeptide repeat region between codons 51 and 91, where both deletions and short insertions of less than five extra repeats have been detected in healthy subjects.[13] It is not known whether these polymorphisms play any role in neurologic diseases.

Other genes may also influence susceptibility to spongiform encephalopathies; one study purported to show increased frequency of one allele of the apolipoprotein E gene in subjects with CJD compared with normal subjects from the same population,[208, 209] although that finding is disputed.[210, 211] Some factor other than PrP may also affect susceptibility of transgenic mice to infection with the CJD agents.[212]

TABLE 272–4 ■ Point Mutations in the *PRNP* Gene Associated with Familial Spongiform Encephalopathy

PRNP CODON NUMBER	NORMAL AMINO ACID	MUTANT AMINO ACID	ASSOCIATED POLYMORPHISM	SPONGIFORM ENCEPHALOPATHY
178*	Asp	Asn	129^{Val}	CJD
180	Val	Ile		CJD
200*†	Glu	Lys		CJD
210	Val	Ile		CJD
232	Met	Arg		CJD
102*†	Pro	Leu		GSS
105	Pro	Leu		GSS
117	Ala	Val		GSS
145	Tyr	Stop‡		GSS
198	Phe	Ser		GSS
217	Glu	Arg		GSS
178*§	Asp	Asn	129^{Met}	FFI
117	Ala	Ala		? None‖
124	Gly	Gly		? None

*Spongiform encephalopathy was transmitted to animals injected with suspensions of tissues from patients in these families (as well as from families with insertions of 120, 168, and 192 nucleotides in the region between codons 51 and 91).

†Largest numbers of familial spongiform encephalopathies were associated with these mutations.

‡Stop indicates stop codon/amber mutant.

§FFI, not a spongiform encephalopathy histopathologically, has been transmitted to mice but not to primates.

‖? None, ? normal polymorphism.

Not all subjects with mutations in the *PRNP* gene have expressed disease, even in affected families. Penetrance appears to be quite high for GSS patients with the 102^{Leu} mutation and for FCJD patients with the 178^{Asn} mutation; less than 60% of subjects with the 200^{Lys} mutation had CJD, at least by the usual expected age[199] (a life table analysis of 13 Libyan Jewish families with the 200^{Lys} mutation predicted that penetrance would be close to 100% in carriers surviving past the age of 80 years[213]). Several members of families with FFI have survived past the age of 60 years without showing signs of illness, although they bore the 178^{Asn} mutation. It is not known whether unaffected family members with such mutations in the *PRNP* gene have inapparent infections, perhaps because of exceptionally long incubation periods, or whether they escaped infection.

The mechanism by which the mutations act is also in dispute. Those favoring the prion hypothesis[34] postulate that mutations facilitate the folding of protein into an abnormal self-replicating β-sheet of amyloid, perhaps by nucleation,[13] whereas those who support the idea that the pathogen may contain a small nucleic acid attribute familial disease to a genetically controlled susceptibility, possibly involving increased affinity of PrP for the agent as a receptor protein on the host cell membrane or protecting the pathogen from inactivation, or both.

Therapy

Several substances—the polyanions HPA-23, carrageenan, and dextran sulfate,[214] as well as amphotericin B[215, 216] and a derivative compound[217]—interfered with experimental scrapie (prolonging the asymptomatic incubation period and reducing expression of PrP, although not infectivity) in rodents treated before or shortly after inoculation, but no treatment reversed an established infection of the central nervous system. The polyanion Congo red inhibited synthesis of PrP in scrapie-infected cells.[18, 218, 219] Remission of human CJD after treatment has never been confirmed.

Prevention of Infection and Disinfection of Contaminated Materials

Brain tissues of patients with all forms of TSEs—sporadic, iatrogenic, and familial—contain the infectious agents[3, 135] and pose a potential risk of accidental transmission to other patients and to medical personnel. Other tissues and CSF are less often infectious and probably contain smaller amounts of agent but must also be treated with respect. As noted earlier, although human blood has not been convincingly incriminated in transmission of spongiform encephalopathies, there has been concern about potential risk. Materials and surfaces contaminated with tissues or CSF from patients suspected of having CJD must be treated with care. Adherence to universal precautions for handling blood and body fluids[220] should reduce the chances of accidental exposure. Until proved otherwise, exposure to the BSE agent must also be considered a potential danger for humans.

Whenever possible, contaminated instruments should be discarded by careful packaging and transported to sites of incineration. Although no method of sterilization can be relied on to remove all infectivity from contaminated surfaces,[221] several methods reduce titers of infectivity markedly. Contaminated tissues and most biologic products can probably not be completely freed of infectivity without destroying structural integrity and biologic activity. (Organic solvent extraction was reported to free one class of biologics of scrapie infectivity.[222]) Medical and family histories of individual tissue donors should be carefully reviewed for dementia. Dural grafts should be obtained from selected donors, pooled grafts avoided, and graft materials of allogeneic human origin replaced with autologous or synthetic materials whenever possible. The preparation of hormones from pools of pituitary glands for use in humans has been discontinued in the United States.

Three treatments are currently recommended for disinfection of objects and surfaces contaminated by the infectious agents: heat, sodium hydroxide, and chlorine bleach.[223–225] Heating, by incineration of disposable items or by steam autoclaving under pressure for at least 2 hours (at 132°C or higher rather than 121°C), should be employed when possible. (One study found that some infectivity survived even harsher conditions of heating and actually appeared to be stabilized by treatment with formaldehyde before heating.[226]) Sodium hydroxide solutions (1 N or stronger) are effective in inactivating large amounts of both scrapie and CJD agents,[119] especially when combined with autoclaving; contaminated materials should be exposed for at least 1 hour. Sodium hypochlorite (5.25%) had considerable inactivating potency in several experimental studies and was more effective than 2 N sodium hydroxide in a comparison.[221] One study suggested that the same formic acid treatment used to enhance the immunostaining of amyloid in tissue sections reduced the infectivity of scrapie agent in the tissue markedly[226]; such treatment should be considered by pathology laboratories. One phenolic disinfectant was reported to be effective in eliminating infectivity.[223] Attempts to sterilize the spongiform encephalopathy agents with ethylene oxide gas and with a variety of commercial liquid disinfectants were ineffective.[227] Reliance on traditional methods to sterilize surgical instruments resulted in accidental iatrogenic transmissions of CJD.[133]

Other Degenerative Diseases of the Central Nervous System Caused by Unconventional Agents

It was claimed that other human diseases may be caused by infections with agents similar to those causing the spongiform encephalopathies: familial Alzheimer disease of adults[228] and Alpers disease (a convulsive disorder with hemiatrophy and status spongiosus of the cerebral gray matter) of young children.[229] These claims, as well as an assertion that the blood of many normal subjects contains a transmissible spongiform encephalopathy agent,[230] were not confirmed.[120, 231] A later claim that suspensions of brain tissues from subjects with Alzheimer disease transmitted a similar condition to marmosets[232] is also unsubstantiated.[233]

References

1. Gajdusek DC, Gibbs CJ Jr, Alpers M: Experimental transmission of a kuru-like syndrome in chimpanzees. Nature 209:794, 1966.
2. Gibbs CJ Jr, Gajdusek DC, Asher DM, et al: Creutzfeldt-Jakob disease (spongiform encephalopathy): Transmission to the chimpanzee. Science 161:388, 1968.
3. Masters CL, Gajdusek DC, Gibbs CJ Jr: Creutzfeldt-Jakob disease virus isolation from the Gerstmann-Sträussler syndrome, with an analysis of the various forms of amyloid deposition in the virus-induced spongiform encephalopathies. Brain 104:559, 1981.
4. Will RG, Ironside JW, Zeidler M, et al: A new variant of Creutzfeldt-Jakob disease in the UK. Lancet 347:921, 1996.
5. Medori R, Tritschler HJ, Leblanc A, et al: Fatal familial insomnia,

a prion disease with a mutation at codon-178 of the prion protein gene. N Engl J Med 326:444, 1992.
6. Detwiler LA: Scrapie. Rev Sci Tech 11:491, 1992.
7. Marsh RF, Burger D, Hanson RP: Transmissible mink encephalopathy: Behavior of the disease agent in mink. Am J Vet Res 30:1637, 1969.
8. Marsh RF, Hanson RP: On the origin of transmissible mink encephalopathy. *In* Prusiner SB, Hadlow WJ (eds): Slow Transmissible Diseases of the Nervous System, Vol 1. New York, Academic Press, 1979, pp 451–460.
9. Marsh RF, Bessen RA: Physicochemical and biological characterizations of distinct strains of the transmissible mink encephalopathy agent. Philos Trans R Soc Lond B Biol Sci 343:413, 1994.
10. Williams ES, Young S: Neuropathology of chronic wasting disease of mule deer *(Odocoileus hemionus)* and elk *(Cervus elaphus nelsoni).* Vet Pathol 30:36, 1993.
11. Williams ES, Young S: Chronic wasting disease of mule deer: A spongiform encephalopathy. J Wildl Dis 16:89, 1980.
12. Wilesmith JW: Epidemiology of bovine spongiform encephalopathy and related diseases. Arch Virol Suppl 7:245, 1993.
13. Gajdusek DC: Infectious amyloids. Subacute spongiform encephalopathies as transmissible cerebral amyloidoses. *In* Fields BN, Knipe DM, Howley PM (eds): Fields Virology, ed 3. Philadelphia, Lippincott-Raven, 1996, pp 2851–2900.
14. Butler DA, Scott MR, Bockman JM, et al: Scrapie-infected murine neuroblastoma cells produce protease-resistant prion proteins. J Virol 62:1558, 1988.
15. Caughey B, Race R, Vogel M, et al: In vitro expression of cloned PrP cDNA derived from scrapie-infected mouse brain: Lack of transmission of scrapie infectivity. Ciba Found Symp 135:197, 1988.
16. Caughey B, Race RE, Chesebro B: Detection of prion protein mRNA in normal and scrapie-infected tissues and cell lines. J Gen Virol 69:711, 1988.
17. Caughey B, Race RE, Ernst D, et al: Prion protein biosynthesis in scrapie-infected and uninfected neuroblastoma cells. J Virol 63:175, 1989.
18. Caughey B, Raymond GJ: Sulfated polyanion inhibition of scrapie-associated PrP accumulation in cultured cells. J Virol 67:643, 1993.
19. Oleszak EL, Murdoch G, Manuelidis L, et al: Growth factor production by Creutzfeldt-Jakob disease cell lines. J Virol 62:3103, 1988.
20. Priola SA, Caughey B, Race RE, et al: Heterologous PrP molecules interfere with accumulation of protease-resistant PrP in scrapie-infected murine neuroblastoma cells. J Virol 68:4873, 1994.
21. Race RE, Fadness LH, Chesebro B: Characterization of scrapie infection in mouse neuroblastoma cells. J Gen Virol 68:1391, 1987.
22. Priola SA, Caughey B, Raymond GJ, et al: Prion protein and the scrapie agent: In vitro studies in infected neuroblastoma cells. Infect Agents Dis 3:54, 1994.
23. Race RE, Caughey B, Graham K, et al: Analyses of frequency of infection, specific infectivity, and prion protein biosynthesis in scrapie-infected neuroblastoma cell clones. J Virol 62:2845, 1988.
24. Rubenstein R, Deng H, Race R, et al: Scrapie strain infection in vitro induces changes in neuronal cells. Mol Neurobiol 8:129, 1994.
25. Scott MR, Butler DA, Bredesen DE, et al: Prion protein gene expression in cultured cells. Protein Eng 2:69, 1988.
26. Asher DM, Yanagihara RT, Gajdusek DC, et al: Studies of spongiform encephalopathies in cell culture. *In* Prusiner S, Hadlow W (eds): Slow Transmissible Agents of the Nervous System, Vol 2. New York, Academic Press, 1979, pp 235–242.
27. Kimberlin RH, Walker CA: Pathogenesis of scrapie (strain 263K) in hamsters infected intracerebrally, intraperitoneally or intraocularly. J Gen Virol 67:255, 1986.
28. Gibbs C Jr: Search for infectious etiology in chronic and subacute degenerative diseases of the central nervous system. Curr Top Microbiol Immunol 40:44, 1967.
29. Gibbs C Jr, Gajdusek D, Latarjet R: Unusual resistance to ionizing radiation of the viruses of kuru, Creutzfeldt-Jakob disease and scrapie. Proc Natl Acad Sci USA 75:6268, 1978.
30. Gibbons RA, Hunter GD: Nature of the scrapie agent. Nature 215:1041, 1967.
31. Lewin P: Scrapie: An infective peptide? Lancet 1:748, 1972.
32. Prusiner SB: Novel proteinaceous infectious particles cause scrapie. Science 216:136, 1982.
33. Cho H: Requirement of a protein component for scrapie infectivity. Intervirology 14:213, 1980.
34. Prusiner S: Scrapie prions. Annu Rev Microbiol 43:345, 1989.
35. Kimberlin R: Scrapie agent: Prions or virinos. Nature 297:107, 1982.
36. Carp RI, Kascsak RJ, Rubenstein R, et al: The puzzle of PrP (Sc) and infectivity—Do the pieces fit? Trends Neurosci 17:148, 1994.
37. Rohwer RG: Virus-like sensitivity of scrapie agent to heat inactivation. Science 223:600, 1984.
38. Rohwer RG: Scrapie infectious agent is virus-like in size and susceptibility to inactivation. Nature 308:658, 1984.
39. Rohwer RG: Estimation of scrapie nucleic acid MW from standard curves for virus sensitivity to ionizing radiation. Nature 320:381, 1986.
40. Riesner D, Kellings K, Wiese U, et al: Prions and nucleic acids: Search for residual nucleic acids and screening for mutations in the PrP gene. Dev Biol Stand 80:173, 1993.
41. Kellings K, Prusiner SB, Riesner D: Nucleic acids in prion preparations—Unspecific background or essential component. Philos Trans R Soc Lond B Biol Sci 343:425, 1994.
42. Bellinger-Kawahara C, Cleaver JE, Diener TO, et al: Purified scrapie prions resist inactivation by UV irradiation. J Virol 61:159, 1987.
43. Hsiao KK, Scott M, Foster D, et al: Spontaneous neurodegeneration in transgenic mice with mutant prion protein. Science 91:1587, 1990.
44. Hsiao KK, Groth D, Scott M, et al: Serial transmission in rodents of neurodegeneration from transgenic mice expressing mutant prion protein. Proc Natl Acad Sci USA 91:9126, 1994.
45. David-Ferreira JF, David-Ferreira KL, Gibbs CJ Jr, et al: Scrapie in mice: Ultrastructural observations in the cerebral cortex. Proc Soc Exp Biol Med 28:313, 1968.
46. Narang HK, Asher DM, Pomeroy KL, et al: Abnormal tubulovesicular particles in brains of hamsters with scrapie. Proc Soc Exp Biol Med 184:504, 1987.
47. Özel M, Xi YG, Baldauf E, et al: Small virus-like structure in brains from cases of sporadic and familial Creutzfeldt-Jakob disease. Lancet 344:923, 1994.
48. Özel M, Diringer H: Small virus-like structure in fractions from scrapie hamster brain. Lancet 343:894, 1994.
49. Borras T, Gibbs CJ Jr: Molecular hybridization studies with scrapie brain nucleic acids. I. Search for specific DNA sequences. Arch Virol 88:67, 1986.
50. Duguid JR, Rohwer RG, Seed B: Isolation of cDNAs of scrapie-modulated RNAs by subtractive hybridization of a cDNA library. Proc Natl Acad Sci USA 85:5738, 1988.
51. Lisitsyn N, Lisitsyn N, Wigler M: Cloning the differences between two complex genomes. Science 259:946, 1993.
52. Merz PA, Somerville RA, Wisniewski HM, et al: Scrapie-associated fibrils in Creutzfeldt-Jakob disease. Nature 306:474, 1983.
53. Merz PA, Somerville RA, Wisniewski HM, et al: Abnormal fibrils from scrapie-infected brain. Acta Neuropathol (Berl) 54:63, 1981.
54. Merz PA, Rohwer RG, Kascsak R, et al: Infection-specific particles from the unconventional slow-virus diseases. Science 225:437, 1984.
55. Bolton DC, McKinley MP, Prusiner SB: Identification of a protein that purifies with the scrapie prion. Science 218:1309, 1982.
56. Bockman JM, Kingsbury DT, McKinley MP, et al: Creutzfeldt-Jakob disease prion proteins in human brains. N Engl J Med 312:73, 1985.
57. Bendheim PE, Bockman JM, McKinley MP, et al: Scrapie and Creutzfeldt-Jakob disease prion proteins share physical properties and antigenic determinants. Proc Natl Acad Sci USA 82:997, 1985.
58. McKinley MP, Bolton DC, Prusiner SB: A protease-resistant protein is a structural component of the scrapie prion. Cell 35:57, 1983.
59. Barry RA, McKinley MP, Bendheim PE, et al: Antibodies to the scrapie protein decorate prion rods. J Immunol 135:603, 1985.
60. DeArmond SJ, McKinley MP, Barry RA, et al: Identification of prion amyloid filaments in scrapie-infected brain. Cell 41:221, 1985.

61. Diringer H, Gelderblom H, Hilmert H, et al: Scrapie infectivity, fibrils and low molecular weight protein. Nature 306:476, 1983.
62. Brown P, Coker-Vann M, Pomeroy K, et al: Diagnosis of Creutzfeldt-Jakob disease by Western blot identification of marker protein in human brain tissue. N Engl J Med 314:547, 1986.
63. Ceroni M, Piccardo P, Safar J, et al: Scrapie infectivity and prion protein are distributed in the same pH range in agarose isoelectric focusing. Neurology 40:508, 1990.
64. Miyamoto T, Sakaguchi S, Katamine S, et al: The infectivity is dissociated from PrP accumulation in salivary gland of Creutzfeldt-Jakob disease agent–inoculated mice. Ann N Y Acad Sci 724:310, 1994.
65. Xi YG, Ingrosso L, Ladogana A, et al: Amphotericin-B treatment dissociates in vivo replication of the scrapie agent from PrP accumulation. Nature 356:598, 1992.
66. Manuelidis L, Sklaviadis T, Akowitz A, et al: Viral particles are required for infection in neurodegenerative Creutzfeldt-Jakob disease. Proc Natl Acad Sci USA 92:5124, 1995.
67. Manuelidis L, Manuelidis EE: Creutzfeldt-Jakob disease and dementias. Microb Pathog 7:157, 1989.
68. Multhaup G, Diringer H, Hilmert H, et al: The protein component of scrapie-associated fibrils is a glycosylated low molecular weight protein. EMBO J 4:1495, 1985.
69. Chesebro B, Race R, Wehrly K, et al: Identification of scrapie prion protein–specific mRNA in scrapie-infected and uninfected brain. Nature 315:331, 1985.
70. Basler K, Oesch B, Scott M, et al: Scrapie and cellular PrP isoforms are encoded by the same chromosomal gene. Cell 46:417, 1986.
71. Hope J, Morton LJ, Farquhar CF, et al: The major polypeptide of scrapie-associated fibrils (SAF) has the same size, charge distribution and N-terminal protein sequence as predicted for the normal brain protein (PrP). EMBO J 5:2591, 1986.
72. Bruce ME, Dickinson AG: Genetic control of amyloid plaque production and incubation period in scrapie-infected mice. J Neuropathol Exp Neurol 44:285, 1985.
73. Bruce ME, Dickinson AG: Biological evidence that scrapie agent has an independent genome. J Gen Virol 68:79, 1987.
74. McBride PA, Bruce ME, Fraser H: Immunostaining of scrapie cerebral amyloid plaques with antisera raised to scrapie-associated fibrils (SAF). Neuropathol Appl Neurobiol 14:325, 1988.
75. Bruce M, Chree A, McConnell I, et al: Transmission of bovine spongiform encephalopathy and scrapie to mice—Strain variation and the species barrier. Philos Trans R Soc Lond B Biol Sci 343:405, 1994.
76. Kimberlin RH, Walker CA, Fraser H: The genomic identity of different strains of mouse scrapie is expressed in hamsters and preserved on reisolation in mice. J Gen Virol 70:2017, 1989.
77. Weissmann C: A 'unified theory' of prion propagation. Nature 352:679, 1991.
78. Wills PR: Potential pseudoknots in the PrP-encoding messenger RNA. J Theor Biol 159:523, 1992.
79. Wills PR: Self-organization of genetic coding. J Theor Biol 162:267, 1993.
80. Prusiner SB: Human prion diseases and neurodegeneration. Curr Top Microbiol Immunol 207:1, 1996.
81. Prusiner SB: Biology and genetics of prion diseases. Annu Rev Microbiol 48:655, 1994.
82. Safar J, Roller PP, Gajdusek DC, et al: Thermal stability and conformational transitions of scrapie amyloid (prion) protein correlate with infectivity. Protein Sci 2:2206, 1993.
83. Safar J, Roller PP, Gajdusek DC, et al: Scrapie amyloid (prion) protein has the conformational characteristics of an aggregated molten globule folding intermediate. Biochemistry 33:8375, 1994.
84. Baldwin MA, Pan KM, Nguyen J, et al: Spectroscopic characterization of conformational differences between PrPc and PrPsc—An alpha-helix to beta-sheet transition. Philos Trans R Soc Lond B Biol Sci 343:435, 1994.
85. Bessen RA, Marsh RF: Distinct PrP properties suggest the molecular basis of strain variation in transmissible mink encephalopathy. J Virol 68:7859, 1994.
86. Chesebro B, Caughey B: Scrapie replication without the prion protein? Curr Biol 3:696, 1993.
87. Sailer A, Bueler H, Fischer M, et al: No propagation of prions in mice devoid of PrP. Cell 77:967, 1994.
88. Bolton DC, Meyer RK, Prusiner SB: Scrapie PrP 27–30 is a sialoglycoprotein. J Virol 53:596, 1985.
89. Bode L, Pocchiari M, Gelderblom H, et al: Characterization of antisera against scrapie-associated fibrils (SAF) from affected hamster and cross-reactivity with SAF from scrapie-affected mice and from patients with Creutzfeldt-Jakob disease. J Gen Virol 66:2471, 1985.
90. Kretzschmar HA, Stowring LE, Westaway D, et al: Molecular cloning of a human prion protein cDNA. DNA 5:315, 1986.
91. Bockman JM, Prusiner SB, Tateishi J, et al: Immunoblotting of Creutzfeldt-Jakob disease prion proteins: Host species–specific epitopes. Arch Neurol 21:589, 1987.
92. Prusiner SB, Scott M, Foster D, et al: Transgenetic studies implicate interactions between homologous PrP isoforms in scrapie prion replication. Cell 63:673, 1990.
93. Braig HR, Diringer H: Scrapie: Concept of a virus-induced amyloidosis of the brain. EMBO J 4:2309, 1985.
94. Kretzschmar HA, Prusiner SB, Stowring LE, et al: Scrapie prion proteins are synthesized in neurons. Am J Pathol 122:1, 1986.
95. Meyer RK, McKinley MP, Bowman KA, et al: Separation and properties of cellular and scrapie prion proteins. Proc Natl Acad Sci USA 83:2310, 1986.
96. Piccardo P, Safar J, Ceroni M, et al: Immunohistochemical localization of prion protein in spongiform encephalopathies and normal tissue. Neurology 40:518, 1990.
97. Doi S, Ito M, Shinagawa M, et al: Western blot detection of scrapie-associated fibril protein in tissues outside the central nervous system from preclinical scrapie-infected mice. J Gen Virol 69:955, 1988.
98. Büeler H, Aguzzi A, Sailer A, et al: Mice devoid of PrP are resistant to scrapie. Cell 73:1339, 1993.
99. Collinge J, Whittington MA, Sidle KCL, et al: Prion protein is necessary for normal synaptic function. Nature 370:295, 1994.
100. Whittington MA, Sidle KCL, Gowland I, et al: Rescue of neurophysiological phenotype seen in PrP null mice by transgene encoding human prion protein. Nat Genet 9:197, 1995.
101. Tateishi J, Ohta M, Koga M, et al: Transmission of chronic spongiform encephalopathy with kuru plaques from humans to small rodents. Ann Neurol 5:581, 1979.
102. Tateishi J, Sato Y, Koga H, et al: Experimental transmission of human spongiform encephalopathy to small rodents. 1. Clinical and histological observations. Acta Neuropathol (Berl) 51:127, 1980.
103. Beck E, Daniel PM, Davey AJ, et al: A note on membrane lamellation. Brain 108:153, 1985.
104. Baron H, Baron-van Evercooren A, Brucher JM: Antiserum to scrapie-associated fibril protein reacts with amyloid plaques in familial transmissible dementia. J Neuropathol Exp Neurol 47:158, 1988.
105. Kitamoto T, Tateishi J, Tashima T, et al: Amyloid plaques in Creutzfeldt-Jakob disease stain with prion protein antibodies. Ann Neurol 20:204, 1986.
106. Bobin SA, Currie JR, Merz PA, et al: The comparative immunoreactivities of brain amyloids in Alzheimer's disease and scrapie. Acta Neuropathol (Berl) 74:313, 1987.
107. Kitamoto T, Tateishi J: Immunohistochemical confirmation of Creutzfeldt-Jakob disease with a long clinical course with amyloid plaque core antibodies. Am J Pathol 131:435, 1988.
108. Kitamoto T, Ogomori K, Tateishi J, et al: Formic acid pretreatment enhances immunostaining of cerebral and systemic amyloids. Lab Invest 57:230, 1987.
109. Hayward PAR, Bell JE, Ironside JW: Prion protein immunocytochemistry: Reliable protocols for the investigation of Creutzfeldt-Jakob disease. Neuropathol Appl Neurobiol 20:375, 1994.
110. Haritani M, Spencer YI, Wells GAH: Hydrated autoclave pretreatment enhancement of prion protein immunoreactivity in formalin-fixed bovine spongiform encephalopathy–affected brain. Acta Neuropathol (Berl) 87:86, 1994.
111. Gajdusek DC, Gibbs CJ Jr, Earle K, et al: Transmission of subacute spongiform encephalopathy to the chimpanzee and squirrel monkey from a patient with papulosis maligna of Köhlmeyer-Degos. Excerpta Med Int Congr Ser 319:390, 1974.
112. Lasmezas CI, Deslys JP, Demalmay R, et al: BSE transmission to macaques. Nature 381:743, 1996.
113. Klitzman RL, Alpers MP, Gajdusek DC: The natural incubation period of kuru and the episodes of transmission in three clusters of patients. Neuroepidemiology 3:3, 1984.

114. Hadlow WJ, Kennedy RC, Race RE: Natural infection of Suffolk sheep with scrapie virus. J Infect Dis 146:657, 1982.
115. Wilesmith JW: An epidemiologist's view of bovine spongiform encephalopathy. Philos Trans R Soc Lond B Biol Sci 343:357, 1994.
116. Gibbs C Jr, Amyx H, Bacote A, et al: Oral transmission of kuru, Creutzfeldt-Jakob disease, and scrapie to nonhuman primates. J Infect Dis 142:205, 1980.
117. Kimberlin RH: Scrapie: How much do we really understand? Neuropathol Appl Neurobiol 12:131, 1986.
118. Asher DM, Gibbs CJ Jr, Gajdusek DC: Pathogenesis of spongiform encephalopathies. Ann Clin Lab Sci 6:84, 1976.
119. Asher DM: Slow viral infections. *In* Scheld WM, Whitley RJ, Durack DT (eds): Infections of the Central Nervous System, ed 2. Philadelphia, Lippincott-Raven, 1997, pp 199–221.
120. Brown P, Gibbs CJ Jr, Rodgers-Johnson P, et al: Human spongiform encephalopathy: The NIH series of 300 cases of experimentally transmitted disease. Ann Neurol 35:513, 1994.
121. Manuelidis EE, Kim JH, Mericangas JR, et al: Transmission to animals of Creutzfeldt-Jakob disease from human blood. Lancet 2:896, 1985.
122. Tateishi J: Transmission of Creutzfeldt-Jakob disease from human blood and urine into mice. Lancet 2:1074, 1985.
123. Tamai Y, Kojima H, Kitajima R, et al: Demonstration of the transmissible agent in tissue from a pregnant woman with Creutzfeldt-Jakob disease. N Engl J Med 327:649, 1992.
124. Deslys JP, Lasmezas C, Dormont D: Selection of specific strains in iatrogenic Creutzfeldt-Jakob disease. Lancet 343:848, 1994.
125. Esmonde TF, Will RG, Slattery JM, et al: Creutzfeldt-Jakob disease and blood transfusion. Lancet 341:205, 1993.
126. Heye N, Hensen S, Muller N: Creutzfeldt-Jakob disease and blood transfusion. Lancet 343:298, 1994.
127. Klein R, Dumble LJ: Transmission of Creutzfeldt-Jakob disease by blood transfusion. Lancet 341:768, 1993.
128. Créange A, Gray F, Cesaro P, et al: Creutzfeldt-Jakob disease after liver transplantation. Ann Neurol 38:269, 1995.
129. Kuroda Y, Gibbs CJ Jr, Amyx HL, Gajdusek DC: Creutzfeldt-Jakob disease in mice: Persistent viremia and preferential replication of virus in low-density lymphocytes. Infect Immun 41:154, 1983.
130. Manuelidis EE, Gorgacz EJ, Manuelidis L: Viremia in experimental Creutzfeldt-Jakob disease. Science 200:1069, 1978.
131. Kimberlin RH, Walker CA: Pathogenesis of experimental scrapie. Ciba Found Symp 135:37, 1988.
132. Gibbs CJ Jr, Asher DM, Brown PW, et al: Creutzfeldt-Jakob disease infectivity of growth hormone derived from human pituitary glands. N Engl J Med 328:358, 1993.
133. Gibbs CJ Jr, Asher DM, Kobrine A, et al: Transmission of Creutzfeldt-Jakob disease to a chimpanzee by electrodes contaminated during neurosurgery. J Neurol Neurosurg Psychiatry 57:757, 1994.
134. Holman RC, Khan AS, Kent J, et al: Epidemiology of Creutzfeldt-Jakob disease in the United States, 1979–1990: Analysis of national mortality data. Neuroepidemiology 14:174, 1995.
134a. Holman RC, Khan AS, Belay ED, Schonberger LB: Creutzfeldt-Jakob disease in the United States, 1979–1994: Using national mortality data to assess the possible occurrence of variant cases. Emerg Infect Dis 2:333, 1996.
135. Masters CL, Harris JO, Gajdusek DC, et al: Creutzfeldt-Jakob disease: Patterns of world wide occurrence and the significance of familial and sporadic clustering. Ann Neurol 5:177, 1979.
136. Prusiner SB: Genetic and infectious prion diseases. Arch Neurol 50:1129, 1993.
137. Brown P, Preece MA, Will RG: Friendly fire in medicine—Hormones, homografts, and Creutzfeldt-Jakob disease. Lancet 340:24, 1992.
138. Tamai Y, Kojima H, Kitajima R, et al: Demonstration of the transmissible agent in tissue from a pregnant woman with Creutzfeldt-Jakob disease. N Engl J Med 327:649, 1992.
139. Will RG, Matthews WB: Evidence for case-to-case transmission of Creutzfeldt-Jakob disease. J Neurol Neurosurg Psychiatry 45:235, 1982.
140. Nevin S, McMenemy WH, Behrman D, et al: Subacute spongiform encephalopathy: A subacute form of encephalopathy attributed to vascular dysfunction (spongiform cerebral atrophy). Brain 83:519, 1960.
141. Duffy P, Collins G, Devoe AG, et al: Possible person-to-person transmission of Creutzfeldt-Jakob disease. N Engl J Med 290:693, 1974.
142. Bernoulli C, Siegfried J, Baumgartner G, et al: Danger of accidental person-to-person transmission of Creutzfeldt-Jakob disease by surgery. Lancet 1:478, 1977.
143. Cochius JI, Hyman N, Esiri MM: Creutzfeldt-Jakob disease in a recipient of human pituitary–derived gonadotrophin—A second case. J Neurol Neurosurg Psychiatry 55:1094, 1992.
144. Martinez-Lage JF, Poza M, Sola J, et al: Accidental transmission of Creutzfeldt-Jakob disease by dural cadaveric grafts. J Neurol Neurosurg Psychiatry 57:1091, 1994.
145. Martinez-Lage JF, Poza M, Tortosa JG: Creutzfeldt-Jakob disease in patients who received a cadaveric dura mater graft—Spain, 1985–1992. MMWR Morbid Mortal Wkly Rep 42:560, 1993.
146. Centers for Disease Control: Rapidly progressive dementia in a patient who received a cadaveric dura mater graft. MMWR Morbid Mortal Wkly Rep 36:49, 1987.
147. Centers for Disease Control: Update: Creutzfeldt-Jakob disease in a second patient who received a cadaveric dura mater graft. MMWR Morbid Mortal Wkly Rep 38:37, 1989.
148. Diringer H, Braig HR: Infectivity of unconventional viruses in dura mater. Lancet 1:439, 1989.
149. Martinez-Lage JF, Sola J, Poza M, et al: Pediatric Creutzfeldt-Jakob disease—Probable transmission by a dural graft. Childs Nerv Syst 9:239, 1993.
150. Masullo C, Pocchiari M, Macche G, et al: Transmission of Creutzfeldt-Jakob disease by dural cadaveric graft. J Neurosurg 71:954, 1989.
151. Nisbet TJ, MacDonaldson I, Bishara SN: Creutzfeldt-Jakob disease in a second patient who received a cadaveric dura mater graft. JAMA 261:1118, 1989.
152. Thadani V, Penar PL, Partington J, et al: Creutzfeldt-Jakob disease probably acquired from a cadaveric dura mater graft. Case report. J Neurosurg 69:766, 1988.
153. Jellinger K, Seitelberger F, Heiss W-D, et al: Konjugale Form der subakuten spongiöse Enzephalopathie (Jakob-Creutzfeldt Erkrankung). Wien Klin Wochenschr 84:245, 1972.
154. Matthews WB: Epidemiology of Creutzfeldt-Jakob disease in England and Wales. J Neurol Neurosurg Psychiatry 38:210, 1975.
155. Gajdusek DC, Gibbs CJ Jr, Asher DM, et al: Precautions in medical care of and in handling materials from patients with transmissible virus dementia (Creutzfeldt-Jakob disease). N Engl J Med 297:1253, 1977.
156. Miller D: Creutzfeldt-Jakob disease in histopathology technicians. N Engl J Med 318:853, 1988.
157. Sitwell L, Lach B, Atack E, et al: Creutzfeldt-Jakob disease in histopathology technicians. N Engl J Med 318:854, 1988.
158. Weber T, Tumani H, Holdorff B, et al: Transmission of Creutzfeldt-Jakob disease by handling of dura mater. Lancet 341:123, 1993.
159. Gorman DG, Benson DF, Vogel DG, et al: Creutzfeldt-Jakob disease in a pathologist. Neurology 42:463, 1992.
160. Berger JR, David NJ: Creutzfeldt-Jakob disease in a physician—A review of the disorder in health care workers. Neurology 43:205, 1993.
161. Bradley R, Wilesmith JW: Epidemiology and control of bovine spongiform encephalopathy (BSE). Br Med Bull 49:932, 1993.
162. Kimberlin RH: Bovine spongiform encephalopathy: An appraisal of the current epidemic in the United Kingdom. Intervirology 35:208, 1993.
163. Collinge J, Palmer MS, Sidle KC, et al: Unaltered susceptibility to BSE in transgenic mice expressing human prion protein. Nature 378:779, 1995.
164. Wisniewski HM, Sigurdarson S, Rubenstein R, et al: Mites as vectors for scrapie. Lancet 347:1114, 1996.
165. Gajdusek DC, Zigas V: Degenerative disease of the central nervous system in New Guinea: Epidemic occurrence of "kuru" in the native population. N Engl J Med 257:974, 1957.
166. Lacey RW, Dealler SF: The transmission of prion disease. Vertical transfer of prion disease. Hum Reprod 9:1792, 1994.
167. Berman PH, Davidson GS, Becker LE: Progressive neurological deterioration in a 14-year-old girl. Pediatr Neurosci 14:42, 1988.
168. Brown P, Cathala F, Labauge R, et al: Epidemiologic implications of Creutzfeldt-Jakob disease in a 19 year-old girl. Eur J Epidemiol 1:42, 1985.

169. Brown P, Cervenakova L, Goldfarb LG, et al: Molecular genetic testing of a fetus at risk of Gerstmann-Sträussler-Scheinker syndrome. Lancet 343:181, 1994.
170. Brown P: Vertical transmission of prion disease. Hum Reprod 9:1796, 1994.
171. Monreal J, Collins GH, Masters CL, et al: Creutzfeldt-Jakob disease in an adolescent. J Neurol Sci 52:341, 1981.
172. Packer RJ, Cornblath DR, Gonatas NK, et al: Creutzfeldt-Jakob disease in a 20-year-old woman. Neurology 30:492, 1980.
173. Will RG, Wilesmith JW: Response to the article: 'Vertical transfer of prion disease' by Lacey and Dealler. Hum Reprod 9:1797, 1994.
174. Brown P, Cervenakova L, Goldfarb LG, et al: Iatrogenic Creutzfeldt-Jakob disease—An example of the interplay between ancient genes and modern medicine. Neurology 44:291, 1994.
175. Brown P, Rodgers-Johnson P, Cathala F, et al: Creutzfeldt-Jakob disease of long duration: Clinicopathological characteristics, transmissibility, and differential diagnosis. Ann Neurol 16:295, 1984.
176. Medori R, Montagna P, Tritschler HJ, et al: Fatal familial insomnia—A second kindred with mutation of prion protein gene at codon-178. Neurology 42:669, 1992.
177. Manetto V, Medori R, Cortelli P, et al: Fatal familial insomnia—Clinical and pathologic study of five new cases. Neurology 42:312, 1992.
178. Gambetti P, Petersen R, Monari L, et al: Fatal familial insomnia and the widening spectrum of prion diseases. Br Med Bull 49:980, 1993.
179. Collinge J, Palmer MS, Sidle KC, et al: Transmission of fatal familial insomnia to laboratory animals. Lancet 346:569, 1995.
180. Tateishi J, Brown P, Kitamoto T, et al: First experimental transmission of fatal familial insomnia. Nature 376:434, 1995.
181. Gloor P, Kalabay O, Giard N: The electroencephalogram in diffuse encephalopathies: Electroencephalographic correlates of grey and white matter lesions. Brain 91:779, 1968.
182. Roos R, Gajdusek DC, Gibbs CJ Jr: The clinical characteristics of transmissible Creutzfeldt-Jakob disease. Brain 96:1, 1973.
183. Harrington MG, Merril CR, Asher DM, et al: Abnormal proteins in the cerebrospinal fluid of patients with Creutzfeldt-Jakob disease. N Engl J Med 315:279, 1986.
183a. Hsich G, Kenney K, Gibbs CJ Jr, et al: 14-3-3 protein: A diagnostic cerebrospinal fluid marker for transmissible spongiform encephalopathies. N Engl J Med 335:924, 1996.
184. Burbelo PD, Hall A: Hot numbers in signal transduction. Curr Biol 5:95, 1995.
185. Boston PF, Jackson P, Thompson RJ: Human 14-3-3 protein: Radioimmunoassay, tissue distribution, and cerebrospinal fluid levels in patients with neurological disorders. J Neurochem 38:1475, 1982.
186. Blisard K, Davis L, Harrington M, et al: Pre-mortem diagnosis of Creutzfeldt-Jakob disease by detection of abnormal cerebrospinal fluid proteins. J Neurol Sci 99:75, 1990.
187. Yun M, Wu W, Hood L, et al: Human cerebrospinal fluid protein database—Edition 1992. Electrophoresis 13:1002, 1992.
188. Serban D, Taraboulos A, DeArmond SJ, et al: Rapid detection of Creutzfeldt-Jakob disease and scrapie prion proteins. Neurology 40:110, 1990.
189. Asher DM, Gibbs CJ Jr, Sulima MP, et al: Transmission of human spongiform encephalopathies to experimental animals—comparison of the chimpanzee and squirrel monkey. Dev Biol Stand 80:9, 1993.
190. Asher DM, Masters CL, Gajdusek DC, et al: Familial spongiform encephalopathies. *In* Kety SS, Rowland LP, Sidman RL, et al (eds): Genetics of Neurological and Psychiatric Disorders. New York, Raven Press, 1983, pp 273–291.
191. Hunter N, Foster JD, Dickinson AG, et al: Linkage of the gene for the scrapie-associated fibril protein (PrP) to the *Sip* gene in Cheviot sheep. Vet Rec 124:364, 1989.
192. Carlson GA, Kingsbury DT, Goodman PA, et al: Linkage of prion protein and scrapie incubation time genes. Cell 46:503, 1986.
193. Westaway D, Goodman PA, Mirenda CA, et al: Distinct prion proteins in short and long scrapie incubation period mice. Cell 51:651, 1987.
194. Westaway D, Carlson GA, Prusiner SB: Unraveling prion diseases through molecular genetics. Trends Neurosci 12:221, 1989.
195. Hsiao K, Baker HF, Crow TJ, et al: Linkage of a prion protein missense variant to Gerstmann-Sträussler syndrome. Nature 338:342, 1989.
196. Owen F, Poulter M, Lofthouse R, et al: A rare Msp1 polymorphism in the human prion gene in a family with a history of early onset dementia. Neurosci Lett Suppl 32:S53, 1988.
197. Owen F, Poulter M, Lofthouse R, et al: Insertion in prion protein gene in familial Creutzfeldt-Jakob disease. Lancet 1:51, 1989.
198. Goldgaber D, Teener JW, Goldfarb LG, et al: No Msp 1 polymorphism in the open reading frame of the PrP gene in patients with familial Creutzfeldt-Jakob disease. Alzheimer Dis Assoc Disord 2:311, 1988.
199. Goldfarb LG, Brown P: The transmissible spongiform encephalopathies. Annu Rev Med 46:57, 1995.
200. Goldfarb LG, Brown P, Gajdusek DC: The molecular genetics of human transmissible spongiform encephalopathy. *In* Prusiner SB, Collinge J, Powell J, et al (eds): Prion Diseases of Humans and Animals. New York, Ellis Horwood, 1992, pp 139–153.
201. Goldgaber D, Goldfarb LG, Brown P, et al: Mutations in familial Creutzfeldt-Jakob disease and Gerstmann-Sträussler-Scheinker's syndrome. Exp Neurol 106:204, 1989.
202. Goldfarb LG, Brown P, Goldgaber DG, et al: Creutzfeldt-Jakob disease and kuru patients lack a mutation consistently found in the Gerstmann-Sträussler-Scheinker syndrome. Exp Neurol 108:247, 1990.
203. Medori R, Tritschler HJ: Prion protein gene analysis in 3 kindreds with fatal familial insomnia (FFI)—Codon-178 mutation and codon-129 polymorphism. Am J Hum Genet 53:822, 1993.
204. Goldfarb LG, Petersen RB, Tabaton M, et al: Fatal familial insomnia and familial Creutzfeldt-Jakob disease: Disease phenotype determined by a DNA polymorphism. Science 258:806, 1992.
205. Collinge J, Palmer MS, Dryden AJ: Genetic predisposition to iatrogenic Creutzfeldt-Jakob disease. Lancet 337:1441, 1991.
206. Palmer MS, Dryden AJ, Hughes JT, et al: Homozygous prion protein genotype predisposes to sporadic Creutzfeldt-Jakob disease. Nature 352:340, 1991.
207. Westaway D, Zuliani V, Cooper CM, et al: Homozygosity for prion protein alleles encoding glutamine-171 renders sheep susceptible to natural scrapie. Genes Dev 8:959, 1994.
208. Amouyel P, Vidal O, Launay JM, et al: The apolipoprotein E alleles as major susceptibility factors for Creutzfeldt-Jakob disease. Lancet 344:1315, 1994.
209. Amouyel P, Alperovitch A, Delasnerie-Laupretre N, et al: Apolipoprotein E in Creutzfeldt-Jakob disease. Lancet 345:595, 1995.
210. Roses AD, Saunders AM, Strittmatter WJ, et al: Apolipoprotein E in Creutzfeldt-Jakob disease (Letter). Lancet 345:69, 1995.
211. Zerr I, Helmhold M, Armstrong VW, et al: Apolipoprotein E in Creutzfeldt-Jakob disease. Lancet 345:266, 1995.
212. Telling GC, Scott M, Mastrianni J, et al: Prion propagation in mice expressing human and chimeric PrP transgenes implicates the interaction of cellular PrP with another protein. Cell 83:79, 1995.
213. Spudich S, Mastrianni JA, Wrensch M, et al: Complete penetrance of Creutzfeldt-Jakob disease in Libyan Jews carrying the E200K mutation in the prion protein gene. Mol Med 1:607, 1995.
214. Kimberlin RH, Walker CA: Suppression of scrapie infection in mice by heteropolyanion 23, dextran sulfate, and some other polyanions. Antimicrob Agents Chemother 30:409, 1986.
215. Pocchiari M, Schmittinger S, Masullo C: Amphotericin B delays the incubation period of scrapie in intracerebrally inoculated hamsters. J Gen Virol 68:219, 1987.
216. Pocchiari M, Casaccia P, Ladogana A: Amphotericin B: A novel class of antiscrapie drugs. J Infect Dis 160:795, 1989.
217. Demaimay R, Adjou K, Lasmezas C, et al: Pharmacological studies of a new derivative of amphotericin B, MS-8209, in mouse and hamster scrapie. J Gen Virol 75:2499, 1994.
218. Caughey B: Scrapie associated PrP accumulation and its prevention—Insights from cell culture. Br Med Bull 49:860, 1993.
219. Caughey B, Brown K, Raymond GJ, et al: Binding of the protease-sensitive form of prion protein PrP to sulfated glycosaminoglycan and Congo red. J Virol 68:2135, 1994.
220. Occupational Safety and Health Administration, US Department of Labor: Occupational exposure to bloodborne pathogens; final rule (29 CFR Part 1910.1030). Fed Regist 56:64175, 1991.

221. Taylor DM, Fraser H, McConnell I, et al: Decontamination studies with the agents of bovine spongiform encephalopathy and scrapie. Arch Virol 139:313, 1994.
222. DiMartino A, Safar J, Ceroni M, et al: Purification of non-infectious ganglioside preparations from scrapie-infected brain tissue. Arch Virol 124:111, 1992.
223. Ernst DR, Race RE: Comparative analysis of scrapie agent inactivation methods. J Virol Methods 41:193, 1993.
224. Brown P, Rohwer RG, Gajdusek DC: Sodium hydroxide disinfection of Creutzfeldt-Jakob disease virus. N Engl J Med 310:727, 1984.
225. Taylor DM: Inactivation of SE agents. Br Med Bull 49:810, 1993.
226. Brown P, Liberski PP, Wolff A, et al: Resistance of scrapie infectivity to steam autoclaving after formaldehyde fixation and limited survival after ashing at 360°C: Practical and theoretical implications. J Infect Dis 161:467, 1990.
227. Asher DM, Gibbs CJ Jr, Gajdusek DC: Slow viral infections: Safe handling of the agents of the subacute spongiform encephalopathies. *In* Miller B, Gröschel D, Richardson J, et al (eds): Laboratory Safety: Principles and Practice. Washington, DC, American Society for Microbiology, 1986, pp 59–71.
228. Manuelidis EE, de Figueiredo JM, Kim JH, et al: Transmission studies from blood of Alzheimer disease patients and healthy relatives. Proc Natl Acad Sci USA 85:4898, 1988.
229. Manuelidis EE, Rorke LB: Transmission of Alpers' disease (chronic progressive encephalopathy) produces experimental Creutzfeldt-Jakob disease in hamsters. Neurology 39:615, 1989.
230. Manuelidis EE, Manuelidis L: A transmissible Creutzfeldt-Jakob disease–like agent is prevalent in the human population. Proc Natl Acad Sci USA 90:7724, 1993.
231. Godec MS, Asher DM, Kozachuk WE, et al: Blood buffy coat from Alzheimer's disease patients and their relatives does not transmit spongiform encephalopathy to hamsters. Neurology 44:1111, 1994.
232. Baker HF, Ridley RM, Duchen LW, et al: Induction of beta(A4)-amyloid in primates by injection of Alzheimer's disease brain homogenate. Comparison with transmission of spongiform encephalopathy. Mol Neurobiol 8:25, 1994.
233. Goudsmit J, Morrow CH, Asher DM, et al: Evidence for and against the transmissibility of Alzheimer's disease. Neurology 30:945, 1980.

PART X MYCOBACTERIA

273

Mycobacterium tuberculosis and Other Mycobacteria

Zahra Toossi
Jerrold J. Ellner

The genus *Mycobacterium* consists of slow-growing, rod-shaped, obligate aerobic organisms that, once stained, characteristically resist destaining by acid alcohol treatment and thus are referred to as acid-fast bacilli. They are ubiquitous and range from organisms that have no pathogenicity for humans to such highly virulent species as *Mycobacterium tuberculosis* and *Mycobacterium leprae*. Because of the lack of effective vaccines, infections with these two mycobacteria still plague humans.

Mycobacterium tuberculosis

Characteristics of the Pathogen

Of the four species of *M. tuberculosis* complex, only *M. tuberculosis* and *Mycobacterium bovis* are associated with substantial disease in humans. *Mycobacterium microti* is a pathogen of rodents, and *Mycobacterium africanum* is a rare cause of tuberculosis in Africa. Humans are the only reservoir for *M. tuberculosis*, despite its ability to infect other primates.

M. tuberculosis is a strictly aerobic, non–spore-forming, nonmotile rod that grows slowly (doubling time, 12 to 18 hours). On complex solid media (Löwenstein-Jensen or Middlebrook 7H10 agar) incubated at 37°C, buff-colored colonies are visible in 3 to 6 weeks. Growth is enhanced by 10% carbon dioxide. Virulent strains form strands or cords. A high lipid content (25%, in contrast to 0.5% for gram-positive bacteria and 3% for gram-negative bacteria) characterizes all mycobacteria. Mycolic acid is the principal component of the complex lipids of mycobacteria, which include mycosides, wax D, cord factor, and sulfolipids.[1] The contribution of each constituent to virulence remains obscure. For instance, wax D, a complex of peptides, polysaccharides, and mycolic acid, enhances cell-mediated immune responses against mycobacterial proteins. Cord factor is lethal to mice and inhibits polymorphonuclear leukocyte migration. Sulfolipids inhibit activation of macrophages and, thus, production of microbicidal molecules.[2] Theoretically, a permeability barrier consequent to the complexing of carbolfuchsin with mycolic acid residues in the cell wall of mycobacteria is the basis for the phenomenon of acid fastness, a property shared by some strains of *Nocardia*.

M. tuberculosis can be differentiated from other mycobacteria by its production of niacin, reduction of nitrates, production of a heat-labile catalase, and sensitivity to isoniazid (INH). Catalase is not produced by 25% of INH-resistant strains, and this phenotype is associated with lack or dysfunction of the *katG* gene. A second gene, *inhA*, is important in cell wall mycolic acid synthesis, and its lack is associated with resistance to INH and ethionamide. Most strains of *M. bovis* do not produce niacin (96%) or reduce nitrates (91%). A radiometric method using Middlebrook 7H12 culture medium with radiolabeled fatty acid (palmitate labeled with carbon 14) as substrate (BACTEC) has reduced the time required for isolation and identification of *M. tuberculosis* by half, from 4 weeks to 2 on average. Tubercle bacilli can be distinguished from nontuberculous mycobacteria by their sensitivity to *p*-nitro-*o*-acetylamino-3-hydroxypropiophenone, which is added to BACTEC vials once the growth index is significant. Identification of *M. tuberculosis* from the BACTEC system with use of the commercially available DNA probe (GenProbe) has become a powerful tool for the rapid diagnosis of tuberculosis.[3, 4] GenProbe identified *M. tuberculosis* in 21% of cultures within 1 week and in 66% of cultures within 2 weeks. The radiometric procedure has also been applied to drug susceptibility testing of *M. tuberculosis* and may be superior to conventional susceptibility testing using solid media because of its rapidity.[5] A promising approach for rapid drug susceptibility testing is the use of luciferase reporter mycobacteriophages to infect *M. tuberculosis*. In the presence of added substrate (luciferin), only metabolizing (live) organisms produce light, which can then be measured by a luminometer.[6] Phage typing has been employed in epidemiologic investigations to identify various strains of *M. tuberculosis*.[7] However, this method does not provide adequate specificity because many isolates fall into a few major types. DNA fingerprinting by restriction fragment length polymorphism has been successfully applied in several outbreaks of tuberculosis.[8] The most widely used system is based on restriction fragment length polymorphism with detection of the insertion element IS6110, which is present only in isolates of *M. tuberculosis* complex and in high copy numbers in *M. tuberculosis* isolates.[9]

Transmission and Epidemiology

The portal of entry for tubercle bacilli is the lung. Aerosolization of pulmonary secretions by patients with active pulmonary tuberculosis while coughing, sneezing, speaking, or singing leads to formation of droplet nuclei, which, if small enough (1 to 10 μm), remain floating in the air for some time. These droplet nuclei can reach terminal bronchioles and alveoli once they are inhaled, evading the mucociliary mechanisms of the lower respiratory tract. The efficiency of transmission of infection depends on the presence of lung cavitation, the expulsive force of the cough, and the liquidity of secretion. Thus, close contacts of a smear-positive patient are at maximal risk for being infected. Roughly 25% to 50% of those exposed become infected, and the attack rate may be as high as 80% if a sustained, heavy exposure occurs.[10, 11] The rate of infection for contacts of smear-negative, culture-positive patients (5%)[12] is no different from that in the community. Transmission by other means is rare. Infection can occur by dermal inoculation of bacilli, occasionally seen in hospital personnel handling infected tissues and cultures. In the developed countries, infection with *M. bovis* through milk from infected cows has been eliminated by pasteurization of milk. In some developing countries, however, this route of infection may still be operant.

Spread of tuberculosis can be rapid in certain situations of overcrowding. Case rates among prison inmates, likely to come from segments of society in which the prevalence of tuberculosis and human immunodeficiency virus (HIV) infection is high, are much higher than in the general population.[13] Nursing home residents also have higher case rates than those of age-matched control subjects who live at home, probably owing to cohabitation with infectious patients with tuberculosis and to waning of immunocompetence secondary to aging.[14] In such populations, tuberculin skin testing on entry and annually to detect new infection is crucial. Greater ease of transmission occurs in overcrowded and economically deprived segments of populations of urban cities, which accounts for the persistence of tuberculosis in countries where the overall prevalence is low. Only 5% to 10% of persons infected with *M. tuberculosis* develop clinical disease. Worldwide, 3 to 4 million new smear-positive cases—and an equal number of cases of smear-negative and extrapulmonary tuberculosis—occur each year. The annual death rate is 2 to 3 million.[15] Morbidity and mortality from tuberculosis are greater at the extremes of age and greater among males than females in all groups except young adults. The risk for developing tuberculosis is twice as great for single or widowed men and four times as great for divorced men than for married men, which implicates emotional stress and lack of social support in progression to disease.[16] Other factors associated with increased risk for tuberculosis are alcoholism, diabetes mellitus, gastrectomy, chronic renal insufficiency, cancer, silicosis, immunosuppressive therapy, and HIV infection.[17] The risk for developing disease after infection of an otherwise normal host with *M. tuberculosis* is about 3% to 5% during the first year and persists at a lower rate for life, declining to less than 0.1% per year in adults with normal findings at chest radiography. Positive tuberculin reactors with pulmonary scars, however, have 0.8% risk for developing disease sometime during their lifetime.[18] HIV infection constitutes the greatest risk factor (15%) for development of tuberculosis by persons who had a prior infection with *M. tuberculosis*.[19] At the present time, 95% of tuberculosis occurs in developing countries, with highest case rates in countries in sub-Saharan Africa. Further, of the 1.7 billion people infected with *M. tuberculosis* worldwide, the majority reside in developing countries and 75% are younger than 50 years, indicating continued transmission to each new generation. In high-frequency areas such as Africa, HIV infection will adversely affect tuberculosis control measures, because prior tuberculosis infection is common in the group of 20- to 50-year-olds. However the ultimate impact of HIV infection and acquired immunodeficiency syndrome (AIDS) on tuberculosis remains to be seen.

The prevalence of tuberculosis has been declining in many developed countries, a reflection mainly of improvement in standards of living. However, the rate of decline was clearly accelerated by the discovery and use of INH. In the United States, the decline in prevalence of tuberculosis was negatively affected in the late 1970s, probably secondary to arrival of Indochinese refugees. In 1986, the annual decline of 2.5% reversed (Fig. 273–1) coincident with the epidemic of HIV infection. In fact, the principal increase in the number of tuberculosis patients occurred in the 25- to 44-year-old age group, and the majority of cases have been reported from locations with high HIV prevalence such as New York City, Newark (New Jersey), and Florida. Seroprevalence studies in the tuberculosis clinics have shown a high prevalence of HIV coinfection among patients with tuberculosis. Matching of the tuberculosis and the AIDS registries revealed that 4.9% of AIDS patients suffered from tuberculosis. Although the fraction of tuberculosis patients with HIV infection may be large, the absolute number of such cases probably will be too low to affect the control of tuberculosis in developed countries. In the United States, there has been a substantial drop in the number of reported cases of tuberculosis during 1992 to 1995, reflecting to some extent decreased transmission of *M. tuberculosis* due to improved implementation of public health measures such as infection control guidelines and directly observed treatment of active cases.[20] Approximately 30% of tuberculosis in this country is in foreign-born subjects. The geographic distribution of tuberculosis is uneven in the United States; the majority of cases are in large cities in the East and Southeast of the country and in Native American reservations. Approximately 70% of tuberculosis in this country occurs in racial and ethnic minorities. Case rates have increased more rapidly in urban areas and among African-American, Hispanics, Asians, and Pacific Islanders (Fig. 273–2). Compared with a case rate of 4.2 per 100,000 in non-Hispanic whites, case rates are 10-fold higher among Asians, 8-fold higher among African-Americans, and 5-fold higher among Hispanics and Native Americans. Outbreaks of tuberculosis have occurred in a variety of settings, such as correctional facilities, residences for AIDS patients, nursing homes, and hospitals, raising the concern of spread of tuberculosis, especially to immunocompromised individuals. Nosocomial tuberculosis involving multidrug-resistant strains of *M. tuberculosis* with transmission to patients and health care professionals has been particularly alarming.[21] Also, shelters have

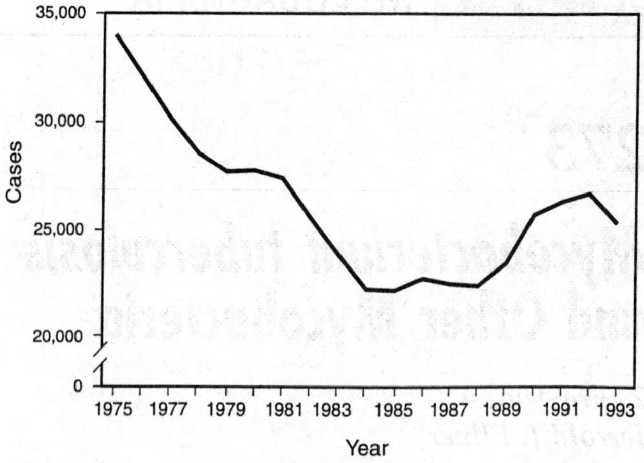

FIGURE 273–1 ▫ Reported cases of tuberculosis in the United States. (From Centers for Disease Control and Prevention: Expanded tuberculosis surveillance and tuberculosis morbidity—United States, 1993. MMWR Morbid Mortal Wkly Rep 43:361–366, 1994.)

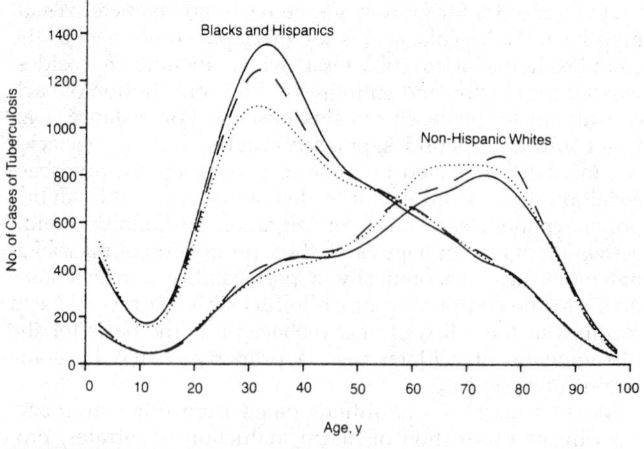

FIGURE 273–2 ▫ Frequency distribution of reported cases of tuberculosis by age among non-Hispanic whites and blacks and Hispanics combined for 1985 *(dotted line)*, 1986 *(dashed line)*, and 1987 *(solid line)*.

been identified as sources of tuberculosis outbreaks.[22] The prevalence of tuberculosis in homeless persons is substantially higher than in the general population; both primary and progressive primary tuberculosis are more common in the urban homeless.

Immunopathogenesis

The implantation of inhaled droplet nuclei containing a few (one to three) tubercle bacilli into terminal airspaces and subsequent ingestion of mycobacteria by macrophages lining the alveoli initiate the tuberculous focus of infection. Because of greater airflow to the lower and middle lung fields, bacilli tend to be deposited in these regions. *M. tuberculosis* grows slowly without elaboration of exotoxins. Within tissue macrophages, mycobacteria evade host microbicidal killing by virtue of virulence factors. Mycobacteria may block phagolysosomal fusion and so may not encounter cellular hydrolytic lysosomal enzymes. Also, the production of superoxide anion, a potent microbicidal molecule, is suppressed by mycobacterial sulfolipids.

Unimpeded growth in the lungs is associated with lymphohematogenous spread to the hilar nodes and extrapulmonary sites. Infected persons develop cell-mediated immunity in 4 to 6 weeks, and tuberculous foci are subsequently infiltrated by blood mononuclear cells. Proteins of low molecular weight (cytokines) are generated by activated T lymphocytes. Some, such as interferon-γ, may enable the tissue macrophages and the newly arrived blood monocytes to destroy mycobacteria. Other cytokines, such as interleukin-2, clonally expand *Mycobacterium*-specific T-cell populations, further amplifying the host immune response. A tubercle is formed with a caseous, necrotic center consisting of dead and live bacilli and cellular debris surrounded by granulation tissue containing lymphocytes and macrophages. Activated macrophages (epithelioid cells) may fuse into Langhans giant cells. Whether the lesion will progress or regress depends on the ability of activated macrophages to further ingest and destroy the pathogen. In 90% of patients, immune mechanisms halt tuberculous infection. Small caseous foci are dissolved and replaced by fibrous tissue. Larger foci (greater than 5 mm) develop fibrous capsules, which may calcify with time. These larger foci may be reactivated years later if the host's antimycobacterial immune response is compromised. Also, in approximately 2% to 8% of patients with primary infection, cell-mediated immunity is apparently inadequate and parenchymal disease progresses. In both reactivation tuberculosis and progressive primary infection, the mycobacterial load within the caseous center increases. Delayed-type hypersensitivity, incapable of containing the infection, contributes to tissue damage. Tumor necrosis factor, produced by both lymphocytes and macrophages, and procoagulant factors generated by macrophages lead to thrombosis of blood vessels, ischemia, and necrosis. Release of reactive oxygen metabolites by mononuclear phagocytes leads to further tissue damage. Release of macrophage proteinases and lipases, which hydrolyze and liquefy the caseum, is a key factor in lung damage. Extracellular bacillary growth is enhanced within this milieu. Finally, adjacent bronchioles become necrotic, and cavity formation occurs.

Tuberculin Skin Testing

Tuberculin skin testing is the standard method for identifying persons infected with *M. tuberculosis*. Intracutaneous administration of 5 tuberculin units (TU) of purified protein derivative (PPD) (Mantoux test) is superior to the multiple puncture method (tine test), although the latter is still used for screening large populations at low risk. Cross-reactions are due to infection with mycobacteria other than *M. tuberculosis* and vaccination with bacille Calmette-Guérin (BCG).[23] In general, the larger the induration, the greater the probability of infection with *M. tuberculosis*. The use of 250 TU of PPD results in an increased proportion of nonspecific reactions. The significance of the size of the reaction to 5TU depends primarily on the presence of mycobacteria other than *M. tuberculosis* in the environment. For instance, in Alaska, where there are no known cross-reacting mycobacteria, a 5-mm induration at 48 hours is indicative of tuberculous infection. In Georgia, nontuberculous mycobacteria, such as *Mycobacterium avium*, are common, and a 15-mm reaction is more suggestive of true infection with *M. tuberculosis*. In most geographic areas, using 15 mm of induration as the cutoff point will best identify infection with *M. tuberculosis*. A reaction larger than 5 mm should be considered positive, however, in persons who have recently had close contact with a patient with tuberculosis; in persons whose chest radiographs are consistent with tuberculosis; and in immunosuppressed persons who are likely to show blunted response to the organism, such as HIV-infected persons.

Waning of skin test reactivity can occur with advancing age, at a rate of 5% per year. Reactivity can be accentuated by repeated testing (booster effect) and can be confused with a true new skin test conversion. The booster effect is more common in the elderly and in areas where nontuberculous mycobacteria are common. Among older adults, the booster effect may become apparent after application of a third or fourth sequential PPD test. In situations in which repeated skin testing is expected (i.e., yearly testing of hospital employees), a second skin test should be done a week after a negative initial test result[24] to establish a new baseline. False-negative tuberculin reactions are associated with cellular immune hyporesponsiveness. Concurrent viral infections (HIV infection, measles, varicella), lymphoreticular malignant neoplasms, malnutrition, sarcoidosis, immunosuppressive drugs, chronic renal failure, and overwhelming illness of any kind fall in this category. Approximately 50% of patients with miliary disease and 25% of those with pulmonary tuberculosis have a negative skin test result.[25] Despite its limitations, tuberculin skin testing may be useful both to assist in the diagnosis of suspected cases of tuberculosis and to identify persons who may need preventive therapy. However, even in the presence of a reaction to control antigens such as mumps, a negative tuberculin skin test result does not exclude the diagnosis of tuberculosis.

Prevention

VACCINATION

The value of BCG vaccination as protection against tuberculosis remains unclear. Protection rates of 0% to 80% have been reported, and no good explanation for such variability in effectiveness has been forthcoming. Analysis of limited available data from human studies suggests that BCG strain differences are not a significant determinant of overall efficacy in the prevention of tuberculosis.[26] BCG vaccination may be beneficial in reducing miliary and meningeal disease in children. Adverse reactions due to BCG vaccination are uncommon and include regional adenitis and osteitis. BCG should not be administered to children or adults who have symptomatic HIV infection, because it may lead to disseminated BCG infection. However, the World Health Organization recommends BCG vaccination for asymptomatic HIV-infected children who are at increased risk for tuberculous infection. In developed countries, BCG vaccination renders useless the tuberculin reaction and, so, should not be employed. The use of BCG in health care workers at risk for development of tuberculosis is presently controversial.[27]

PREVENTIVE THERAPY

The main application of chemoprophylaxis is to prevent the development of clinical tuberculosis from latent infection. INH, 300 mg daily for 6 to 12 months, is now the established regimen of chemoprophylaxis. In controlled trials conducted by the U.S. Public Health Service, INH therapy has reduced the prevalence of disease by 54% to 88%.[28] The major determinant of efficacy in different studies has been the compliance rate. In fact, among compliant infected persons with abnormal findings on chest radiographs, the success rate was above 90%.[29] Also, in recently infected nursing home patients, the efficacy of INH preventive therapy was 98%. The major concern about INH chemotherapy remains its potential hepatotoxicity. Although about 10% of patients have abnormal results on liver function tests, only 1% develop clinical hepatitis. Hepatitis usually occurs 4 to 8 weeks after the start of therapy. The rate of occurrence of hepatitis increases with age and is nil for patients younger than 20 years, 0.03% at 20 to 34 years, 0.2% at 35 to 49 years, and 2.3% at 50 to 69 years. Daily use of alcohol is a risk factor for development of hepatitis.

Tuberculin-reactive persons at high risk (Table 273–1) should receive preventive therapy regardless of their age. Management of tuberculin reactors who have additional risk factors (so-called low-risk tuberculin reactors) is controversial. The current recommendation is to treat those younger than 35 years whose tuberculin skin test reaction is larger than 15 mm of induration at 48 hours. Treatment is also recommended for children younger than 5 years who are tuberculin-negative and have had recent contact with persons with active disease (primary prophylaxis). The skin test is repeated after 3 months, and treatment is continued only if the result is positive. When the possibility of INH resistance exists, preventive therapy with another agent, for example, rifampin, is logical, but it was associated in at least one instance with development of rifampin-resistant strains.[30] HIV-infected subjects living in areas where tuberculosis is prevalent may benefit from INH preventive therapy even if their PPD skin test result is negative.[31] INH prophylaxis is indicated in any HIV-infected patient who is exposed to a patient with tuberculosis. Also, a repeated course of preventive therapy is indicated in an HIV-positive subject who has received prior INH prophylaxis and has been reexposed to tuberculosis.

Environmental Control

To prevent transmission of tuberculosis, it is desirable to limit contact, especially of smear-positive patients, with uninfected persons. Usually, by the time the diagnosis is made, the patient's close contacts have been much exposed, and hospitalization does not reduce the number of secondary cases.[32] Patients should be advised to stay at home to limit further exposure to new contacts and urged to cover the nose and mouth while coughing or sneezing. Prompt institution of effective therapy for compliant patients remains the key to preventing spread of tuberculosis in the population. Once sputum smears become negative in response to treatment, the patient can be considered noninfectious. Hospitalized patients receiving treatment for newly diagnosed tuberculosis are usually considered noninfectious after 14 days' therapy, provided that the number of acid-fast bacilli on sputum smears declines. Use of high-efficiency particulate respirators instead of surgical masks by health care workers who care for patients with smear-positive tuberculosis has been recommended by both the Centers for Disease Control and Prevention and the Occupational Safety and Health Administration; it is, however, an extremely costly means of preventing tuberculosis.[33]

TABLE 273–1 ■ Tuberculin-Reactive High-Risk Groups to be Considered for Tuberculosis Prophylaxis

Close contacts of newly diagnosed patients with infectious tuberculosis
Recent tuberculin skin test converters
Persons with abnormal findings on chest radiographs compatible with inactive tuberculosis
Foreign-born persons (and their families) from high-prevalence areas who have entered the United States within the past 2 y
Persons with known or suspected human immunodeficiency virus infection
Persons with medical or iatrogenic conditions that increase the risk for tuberculosis—silicosis, gastrectomy, jejunoileal bypass, weight of 10% or more below ideal, chronic renal failure, diabetes mellitus, corticosteroid or other immunosuppressive therapy, hematopoietic malignant neoplasm, other malignant neoplasm, and other conditions in which immunosuppression results from the disease or its treatment

Mycobacteria Other Than *Mycobacterium tuberculosis*

Several features distinguish nontuberculous mycobacteria from *M. tuberculosis*. Nontuberculous mycobacteria are ubiquitous in nature, have a varied spectrum of pathogenicity for humans, colonize rather than invade the host to cause disease, and do not pose public health hazards because they are in general not transmitted from person to person. Also, in contrast to *M. tuberculosis*, these mycobacteria are usually drug resistant. With the greater frequency of disease due to some nontuberculous mycobacteria and occurrence in immunocompromised patients, recognition of these infections is important. Table 273–2 is a classification based on Runyon's more recent grouping and the biochemical and microbiologic properties of nontuberculous mycobacteria that may be recovered in the laboratory from human specimens.[34–36] High-performance liquid chromatography has been used in speciating mycobacteria on the basis of their mycolic acid pattern. This technique has been useful in the identification of rare and newly recognized species such as *Mycobacterium celatum* and *Mycobacterium genavense*.[37]

Mycobacterium avium-intracellulare

M. avium and *M. intracellulare*, previously differentiated by their virulence for chickens and rabbits, respectively, are similar biochemically and antigenically and today are referred to as *M. avium* complex (MAC). Growth is slow, during 6 to 8 weeks, and optimal at 37°C. Colonies are usually not pigmented and are either opaque and domed or transparent and flat. On the basis of seroreactivity with mycobacterial cell wall glycopeptidolipids, there are 28 serotypes of MAC. Thin-layer chromatography has been applied to differentiate serotypes. Environmental sources of MAC include water, soil, dust, air, and dried plants. Possible water-associated disease has been reported for MAC.[38] Interestingly, 50% of clinical isolates, 75% of aerosol isolates, 25% of water isolates, and 5% of soil isolates contained plasmids.[39] Enhanced virulence has been shown to be associated with plasmids.[40] Disease due to MAC, which has been recognized as a human pathogen only since 1943, has increased steadily in the last decade. This cannot be attributed solely to the epidemic of HIV infection, despite that as many as half of AIDS patients develop MAC infection.

In immunocompetent hosts, MAC is mildly pathogenic;

TABLE 273–2 ■ Some Characteristics of Medically Important Nontuberculous Mycobacteria*

SPECIES	OPTIMAL TEMPERATURE (°C)	GROWTH RATE (wk)	NIACIN PRODUCTION	NITRATE REDUCTION	TWEEN HYDROLYSIS	UREASE	ARYLSULFATASE (10 d)	CATALASE PRODUCTION	
								25°C–37°C	68°C
Photochromogens									
M. kansasii	37	2–3	−	+	+	+	+	Strong	+
M. marinum	32	1–2	−	−	+	+	+	Weak	+
M. simiae	37	1–2	+	−	−	+	+	Strong	+
Scotochromogens									
M. scrofulaceum	37	2–4	−	−	−	+	−	Strong	+
M. xenopi	42	2–4	−	−	−	−	+	Weak	+
M. szulgai	37*	2–4	−	+	±	+	±	Strong	+
M. gordonae†	37	2–4	−	−	−	−	±	Strong	+
M. flavescens†	37	1–2	−	+	+	+			
Nonchromogens									
M. avium complex	37‡	4–6	−	−	−	−	±	Weak	+
M. malmoense	22, 37	2–12	−	−	+	±	±	NA§	NA
M. haemophilum	<32	1–8	−	±	−	−	+	NA	NA
M. ulcerans	32	4–8	±	−	−	−	±	Weak	+
M. terrae-triviale‡	37	2–3	+	+	+	−	±	Strong	+
Rapid Growers									
M. fortuitum	37	1	+	+	±	+	+	Strong	+
M. chelonae	37	1	−	−	±	+	+	Strong	+
M. thermoresistible‡	37, 45	1	−	+	+	+	−	Strong	+

*Photochromogenic at 25°C.
†Saprophytic in humans; case reports of disease due to these mycobacteria exist.
‡Some strains produce yellow pigment that intensifies with age.
§NA, Not available.
Data from references 34 to 36.

rather than causing disease, it usually colonizes the tracheobronchial tree, preexisting areas of bronchiectasis, or old cavities. Thus, strict criteria for diagnosis of infection, such as the presence of cavities or infiltrates on chest radiographs, repeated isolation of MAC from sputum (even during the initial few weeks of treatment), associated clinical symptoms, and isolation from sterile sources, have been recommended. Pulmonary infection due to MAC usually occurs in association with preexisting lung disease—silicosis, chronic bronchitis, emphysema, healed tuberculosis, or bronchiectasis. The patient is often white, middle-aged, and male; however, an increasing number of MAC infections have been identified in patients who have no predisposing factors, 80% of whom are women, usually in the sixth decade of life.[41] These patients present with symptoms similar to those of persons with underlying lung disease; their chest radiographs show multiple nodules rather than cavities, and disease is often progressive without treatment. Disseminated MAC disease affects immunocompromised hosts, specifically AIDS patients.[42] Cervical lymphadenitis (especially in children), bone and joint infection, urinary tract involvement, and cutaneous infections including panniculitis have been reported.

Chemotherapy for MAC is difficult, because isolates usually demonstrate resistance to antituberculous agents. For asymptomatic immunocompetent patients with pulmonary infiltrates alone, bronchial toilet is recommended. When disease is symptomatic, treatment regimens with three to five agents should be given for 18 to 24 months. Extrapulmonary disease should be treated for 24 to 36 months. Modern treatment of MAC in AIDS patients involves the use of a macrolide antibiotic such as azithromycin or clarithromycin, ethambutol or rifabutin, and a third drug such as ciprofloxacin.[43] Addition of intravenous amikacin has not been shown to enhance efficacy. Clofazimine has been found to be particularly toxic in AIDS patients. Clinical response to antimycobacterial therapy is usually coincident with a reduction in growth of MAC by blood culture. Optimal duration of therapy in this population is unclear, however, and it is often continued for life. Preventive therapy with rifabutin against MAC has been advocated in patients with $CD4^+$ lymphocyte counts of less than $100/mm^3$.[44] The results of a retrospective study have indicated that in HIV-infected patients, a regimen of dapsone-pyrimethamine as prophylaxis against *Pneumocystis carinii* and *Toxoplasma* infection in comparison to aerosolized pentamidine was also effective in preventing mycobacterial infections including MAC and *M. genavense* and *M. tuberculosis*.[45]

Mycobacterium kansasii

Initially isolated in 1953, *M. kansasii* has occasionally been cultured from milk or water supplies; its natural reservoir is unknown. On smear examination, organisms appear long, thick, and crossbarred. Most strains are photochromogenic (development of 13-carotene crystals on exposure to light) and grow within 3 weeks on solid media. Unlike other photochromogens, they reduce nitrate. *M. kansasii* is antigenically close to *M. tuberculosis*, so cross-reaction with PPD-S is common. Countries of highest prevalence appear to be the United States, England, and Wales. In the United States, the prevalence of *M. kansasii* disease is greatest in the metropolitan areas of the Southeast and Midwest; the male/female ratio is 4:1. Eighty percent of patients are white; their median age is 50 years. Chronic obstructive lung disease and pneumoconiosis predispose to infection. Miners, welders, sandblasters, and painters are at highest risk for development of disease. Interestingly, guinea pigs exposed to *M. kansasii* developed progressive lung disease only if the inoculum contained dust aerosols.[46]

The most common form of disease due to *M. kansasii* is an indolent pneumonia, generally milder than tuberculosis. Multiple cavities that are often thin walled (33%), scarring (70%), and endobronchial spread (70%) are seen on chest radiographs.[47] Extensive unilateral upper lobe disease is more common than with MAC infection, but none of the radiographic features is specific for any of the mycobacterioses, including tuberculosis. Cervical lymphadenitis (especially in children), cutaneous abscesses or cellulitis mimicking pyogenic infection, and musculoskeletal involvement including arthritis, fasciitis, tenosynovitis, or osteomyelitis have been reported. Dissemination rarely occurs with far-advanced disease or in immunocompromised hosts such as AIDS patients.[48] In most forms of disease, caseating or noncaseating granulomata, with or without acid-fast bacilli, are seen on histologic examination. Skin lesions may show granulomata or collections of acute- and chronic-phase inflammatory cells. *M. kansasii* is sensitive to most antituberculous drugs. Sputum conversion can be achieved in 90% to 100% with two- or three-drug regimens,[49] although unless the regimen contains rifampin, the relapse rate is high (5% to 15%). Both sulfamethoxazole and quinolones are active against *M. kansasii* and hold promise as future therapeutic options. Surgery may rarely be necessary to manage disease but does not avoid the need for drug treatment because sputum conversion and relapse are not affected by surgery alone.

Mycobacterium marinum

The reservoirs for *M. marinum* are water and aquatic organisms. A photochromogen, *M. marinum* grows optimally at 32°C; colonies appear in 8 to 14 days. Cutaneous disease usually occurs as a result of trauma to skin in contaminated, nonchlorinated fresh, or salty water. Two to 3 weeks after inoculation, a single papulonodular lesion develops, which may later ulcerate. A sporotrichoid pattern, with abscess formation and secondary nodules along the lymphatics, can also occur. Dissemination in immunocompromised hosts, synovitis, and osteomyelitis have been reported. On pathologic examination, early lesions show collections of polymorphonuclear cells surrounded by histiocytes. Older lesions consist of lymphocytes, epithelioid cells, and occasionally, Langhans giant cells, usually without caseation. Most strains are resistant to INH and streptomycin and susceptible to rifampin and ethambutol. Despite the organism's sensitivity to trimethoprim-sulfamethoxazole treatment, treatment failures have been reported. The duration of treatment depends on the promptness of response and can range from 6 weeks to 18 months. Spontaneous resolution can also occur.

Mycobacterium simiae

Also known as *Mycobacterium habana*, *M. simiae* elaborates pigments only after prolonged exposure to light. It has been isolated from both wild and captured monkeys and in cultures of hospital water. Colonization or pulmonary disease mimicking tuberculosis can occur, and a few cases of disseminated infection have been reported. Owing to variable susceptibility and multiple drug resistance, treatment is usually unsuccessful.

Mycobacterium scrofulaceum

Initially isolated in 1956, *M. scrofulaceum* is a scotochromogen that grows at 25°C to 37°C in 4 to 6 weeks. Because of antigenic and drug susceptibility similarities with MAC, some authors have classified the two together, as MACS complex. The most common form of disease is cervical lymphadenitis in children 1 to 5 years of age, involving a single node or a cluster in the submandibular area. The portal of entry is believed to be the oral cavity. Infection may first be noticed when the node ruptures, but at times fibrosis and calcification occur. Involvement of lymph nodes of the head and extremities is infrequent. Differentiation from lymphadenitis due to *M. tuberculosis* and MAC is important. Surgical excision of the lymph node and overlying skin is the mainstay of therapy. Progressive pulmonary disease, bone and soft tissue disease, or disseminated disease occurs uncommonly. Susceptibility to antituberculous drugs is variable. Both erythromycin and sulfonamides demonstrate activity against *M. scrofulaceum*. Clinical outcome depends on the presence and nature of the underlying disease.

Mycobacterium ulcerans

M. ulcerans is endemic to Australia, Africa, and Mexico. In the United States, a few cases have been reported in Nigerian immigrants. Rough, nonpigmented colonies, often with cord formation, appear in 4 to 6 weeks of incubation at 33°C. Also known as Bairnsdale ulcer (in Australia) and Buruli ulcer (in Uganda), cutaneous disease due to *M. ulcerans* often involves the leg and is preceded by trauma. During many weeks, a single ulcer with necrosis develops, without systemic symptoms or adenopathy. Satellite ulcers may develop. Histologic examination reveals mononuclear cell infiltration, rare Langhans giant cells, and central necrosis containing acid-fast bacilli. Surgical excision, especially of early lesions, can be curative. More limited surgery, combined with a regimen of dapsone and streptomycin for 2 weeks, has been successful.

Mycobacterium haemophilum

Unique among mycobacteria in its absolute requirement for iron, *M. haemophilum* is a nonchromogen that grows at temperatures below 32°C. Growth may take 1 to 8 weeks and is stimulated by the presence of 10% carbon dioxide. Individuals with profound deficits in cell-mediated immune response, such as patients with HIV infection,[50] recipients of organ transplants undergoing immunosuppressive treatments, and patients with lymphoma, are at risk for development of infections with *M. haemophilum*.[51] Skin and soft tissue infection is the main form of *M. haemophilum* disease. Multiple painful nodules or ulcers, commonly on the extremities, may develop into abscesses with the drainage of purulent material. Pathologic examination shows an inflammatory infiltrate with occasional giant cells and a necrotic noncaseous center containing AFB. Osteomyelitis and arthritis have also been reported. Resistance to INH, streptomycin, and ethambutol and susceptibility to rifampin—and occasionally to tetracycline and sulfamethoxazole—are seen. Surgical débridement in combination with antibiotics is indicated, but the outcome depends on improvement of the immune status of the host.

Mycobacterium genavense

This new species of mycobacteria is a slowly growing fastidious organism that fails to grow on solid media; however, it does grow slowly (8 to 12 weeks) in BACTEC 13A vials.[52] Analysis (by sequencing) of ribosomal RNA genes after amplification in blood culture and tissue biopsy specimens may allow the detection of growth-deficient mycobacteria such as *M. genavense*.[53, 54] *M. genavense* infection has thus far been described only in AIDS patients, in whom it causes a syndrome indistinguishable from MAC and is estimated to be responsible for 10% of disseminated nontuberculous mycobacterial infections.[55] Fever, weight loss, diarrhea, hepatomegaly, splenomegaly, and anemia are common. Response to antimycobacterial therapy directed against MAC and survival in patients with *M. genavense* infection are similar to those with MAC infection and are dependent on absolute CD4+ cell levels.

Rapidly Growing Mycobacteria

Among the more than 20 species of the ubiquitous rapidly growing mycobacteria, two—*Mycobacterium fortuitum* and *Mycobacterium chelonae*—are human pathogens. Nonpigmented colonies grow at 25°C to 40°C in 7 days on both mycobacterial medium and routine bacteriologic medium. Because of resistance to staining, results of tests for acid fastness are at times negative, even when the organism is isolated in culture. Specimen decontamination with sodium hydroxide, commonly used in mycobacteriology laboratories, is toxic to these microorganisms.

Subspecies of *M. fortuitum* (*M. fortuitum* biovar *fortuitum*, *M. fortuitum* biovar *peregrinum*, and an unnamed biovariant complex) and of *M. chelonae* (*M. chelonae* subsp. *abscessus* and *M. chelonae* subsp. *chelonae*) have different susceptibility patterns to drugs. In general, these mycobacteria are resistant to antituberculous drugs except amikacin and are sensitive to cefoxitin, sulfamethoxazole, erythromycin, and imipenem. Skin and soft tissue infection, the most common clinical form of disease, is usually secondary to a puncture wound and occurs within 6 weeks to 6 months. Systemic symptoms are absent, and dissemination is extremely unusual. Outbreaks of wound infection in association with vaccination have been reported. Spontaneous resolution in 1 to 2 years occurs in as many as 20% of cases. Infection of indwelling peritoneal catheters or long-term intravenous catheters can occur. Breast infection after augmentation mammaplasty and sternal wound infection after cardiac bypass surgery have been reported. Disseminated disease is uncommon in severely immunocompromised persons and is associated with a high rate of mortality. Chronic pneumonia due to *M. fortuitum* and *M. chelonae* presents in a manner indistinct from disease caused by other mycobacteria.[56] The majority of patients are women—nonsmokers who have no preexisting lung disease. Predisposing conditions are achalasia, cystic fibrosis, lipoid pneumonia, and healed tuberculosis. On radiographic examination, a reticulonodular pattern is seen, usually bilateral, sparing the upper lobes, and rarely associated with cavities. Clinical exacerbations occur during a period of years, but there is no spontaneous resolution. A combination of parenteral antibiotics (amikacin-cefoxitin) followed by oral drugs for up to 6 months has been effective. Surgical resection for infection by drug-resistant species (*M. chlelonae* subsp. *abscessus*) and with unilateral localized disease may be considered.

Mycobacterium xenopi

This scotochromogen grows optimally at 42°C and only after prolonged incubation at 37°C. Colonies are smooth and on cornmeal agar have filamentous extension. Whereas birds are the natural reservoir, *M. xenopi* has been isolated from tap water, hot-water generators, and storage tanks of hospitals; it has been implicated in nosocomial pulmonary infections indistinguishable from those due to other mycobacteria.[57] Extrapulmonary and disseminated disease has been reported. Treatment of *M. xenopi* infection is unpredictable because of variable resistance to a number of antimicrobial agents.

Mycobacterium szulgai

These mycobacteria, discovered in 1972,[58] are scotochromogenic when grown at 37°C and photochromogenic at 25°C. Their natural reservoir is not known. Most patients infected with *M. szulgai* have chronic pulmonary disease that is clinically similar to disease due to other nontuberculous mycobacteria. Response to three-drug regimens is good.

Mycobacterium malmoense

Originally reported in 1977,[59] these organisms grow in 2 to 12 weeks as colorless, smooth colonies at temperatures ranging from 22°C to 37°C. Most cases have been reported from Sweden, England, and Wales. Patients typically present with a chronic pulmonary infection and have preexisting pneumoconiosis. The response to antimicrobial agents is unpredictable.

References

1. Besra GS, Chatterjee D: Lipids and carbohydrates of *Mycobacterium tuberculosis*. *In* Bloom BR (ed): Tuberculosis: Pathogenesis, Protection, and Control. Washington, DC, ASM Press, 1994, pp 285–306.
2. Pabst MJ, Gross IMS, Brozna JP, Goren MB: Inhibition of macrophage priming by sulfatids from *Mycobacterium tuberculosis*. J Immunol 140:634, 1988.
3. Heifets LB, Good RC: Current laboratory methods for the diagnosis of tuberculosis. *In* Bloom BR (ed). Tuberculosis: Pathogenesis, Protection, and Control. Washington, DC, ASM Press, 1994, pp 85–110.
4. Ellner PD, Kiehn TE, Cammarata R, et al: Rapid detection and identification of pathogenic mycobacteria by combining radiometric and nucleic acid probe methods. J Clin Microbiol 26:1349, 1988.
5. Heifets L: Qualitative and quantitative drug susceptibility tests in mycobacteriology. Am Rev Respir Dis 137:1217, 1988.
6. Jacobs WR, Barletta RG, Udani R, et al: Rapid assessment of drug susceptibilities of *Mycobacterium tuberculosis* by means of luciferase reporter phages. Science 260:819, 1993.
7. Snider DE Jr, Jones WD, Good RC: The usefulness of phage typing *Mycobacterium tuberculosis* isolates. Am Rev Respir Dis 130:1095, 1984.
8. Shoemaker SA, Fisher JH, Jones WD Jr, Scoggin CH: Restriction fragment analysis of chromosomal DNA defines different strains of *Mycobacterium tuberculosis*. Am Rev Respir Dis 134:210, 1986.
9. Small PM, Schafer RW, Hopewell PC, et al: Exogenous reinfection with multi-drug–resistant *Mycobacterium tuberculosis* in patients with advanced HIV infection. N Engl J Med 328:1137, 1993.
10. Stead WW: Tuberculosis among elderly persons: An outbreak in a nursing home. Ann Intern Med 94:606, 1981.
11. Honk VH, Kent DC, Baker JH: The Byrd study. In depth analysis of a micro-outbreak of tuberculosis in a closed environment. Arch Environ Health 16:4, 1968.
12. Stylbo K: Recent advances in epidemiological research in tuberculosis. Adv Tuberc Res 20:1, 1980.
13. Stead WW: Undetected tuberculosis in prison. Source of infection for community at large. JAMA 240:2544, 1978.
14. Stead WW, Lofgren JP, Warren E, Thomas C: Tuberculosis as an endemic and nosocomial infection among the elderly in nursing homes. N Engl J Med 312:1483, 1985.
15. Raviglione MC, Snider DE, Kochi A: Global epidemiology of tuberculosis. Morbidity and mortality of a worldwide epidemic. JAMA 273:220, 1995.
16. Horwitz O: Tuberculosis risk and marital status. Am Rev Respir Dis 104:22, 1971.
17. Reider HL, Canthen GM, Kelly DG, et al: Tuberculosis in the United States. JAMA 262:385, 1989.
18. American Thoracic Society: Preventive treatment of tuberculosis: Statement of the American Thoracic Society, National Tuberculosis and Respiratory Disease Association and the Centers for Disease Control. Am Rev Respir Dis 104:460, 1971.
19. Selwyn PA, Hartel D, Lewis VA, et al: A prospective study of the risk of tuberculosis among intravenous drug users with human immunodeficiency virus infection. N Engl J Med 320:545, 1989.
20. Centers for Disease Control and Prevention: Tuberculosis morbidity—United States, 1995. MMWR Morbid Mortal Wkly Rep 45:365, 1996.
21. Pearson ML, Jereb JA, Frieden TR, et al: Nosocomial transmission of multidrug-resistant *Mycobacterium tuberculosis* infections: Factors in transmission to staff and HIV-infected patients. Ann Intern Med 117:191, 1992.
22. Barnes PF, Hiyam E, Susan PM, et al: Transmission of tuberculosis among the urban homeless. JAMA 275:305, 1996.
23. Cauthen MG, Snider DE, Onorato IM: Boosting of tuberculin sensitivity among Southeast Asian refugees. Am J Respir Crit Care Med 149:1597, 1994.
24. Huebner RE, Schein MF, Bass JB Jr: The tuberculin skin test. Clin Infect Dis 17:968, 1993.
25. Nash DR, Douglass JE: Anergy in active pulmonary tuberculosis. Chest 77:32, 1980.
26. Brewer TF, Graham AC: Relationship between bacille Calmette-Guérin (BCG) strains and the efficacy of BCG in the prevention of tuberculosis. Clin Infect Dis 20:126, 1995.
27. Centers for Disease Control and Prevention: The role of BCG vaccine in the prevention and control of tuberculosis in the United States. MMWR Morbid Mortal Wkly Rep 45(RR-4):1, 1996.
28. American Thoracic Society: Treatment of tuberculosis infection in adults and children. Am J Respir Crit Care Med 149:1359, 1994.
29. International Union Against Tuberculosis: Efficacy of various duration of isoniazid preventive therapy for tuberculosis. Bull World Health Organ 50:555, 1982.
30. Livingood JR, Sigler TG, Foster LR, et al: INH-resistant tuberculosis: A community outbreak and report of a rifampin prophylaxis failure. JAMA 253:2847, 1985.
31. Pape JW, Jean SS, Ho JL, et al: Effect of isoniazid prophylaxis on incidence of active tuberculosis and progression of HIV infection. Lancet 342:268, 1993.
32. Gunnels N, Bates JH, Swindoll H: Infectivity of sputum positive tuberculosis patients on chemotherapy. Am Rev Respir Dis 109:323, 1974.
33. Nettleman MD, Fredrickson M, Good NL, et al: Tuberculosis control strategies: The cost of particulate respirators. Ann Intern Med 121:37, 1994.
34. Runyon EH: Anonymous mycobacteria in pulmonary disease. Med Clin North Am 43:273, 1959.
35. Wolinsky E: Nontuberculous mycobacteria and associated diseases. Am Rev Respir Dis 119:107, 1979.
36. Woods GL, Washington JA: Mycobacteria other than *M. tuberculosis*: Review of microbiological and clinical aspects. Rev Infect Dis 9:275, 1987.
37. Tortoli E, Bartoloni A, Burrini C, et al: Utility of high-performance liquid chromatography for identification of mycobacterial species rarely encountered in clinical laboratories. Eur J Clin Microbiol Infect Dis 14:240, 1995.
38. Moulin GC, Sherman IH, Hoaglin DC: *Mycobacterium avium* complex, an emerging pathogen in Massachusetts. J Clin Microbiol 22:9, 1985.
39. Meissner PS, Falkinham JO III: Plasmid DNA profiles as epidemiological markers for clinical and environmental isolates of *M. avium*, *M. intracellulare*, and *M. scrofulaceum*. J Infect Dis 153:325, 1986.
40. Crawford JT, Bates JH: Analysis of plasmids in *Mycobacterium avium-bintracellulare* isolates from persons with acquired immunodeficiency syndrome. Am Rev Respir Dis 134:659, 1986.
41. Brince DS, Peterson DD, Steiner RM: Infection with *Mycobacterium avium* complex in patients without predisposing conditions. N Engl J Med 321:863, 1989.
42. Greene JB, Sidhu GS, Lewin S, et al: *Mycobacterium avium-intracellulare*: A cause of disseminated lifethreatening infection in homosexuals and drug abusers. Ann Intern Med 97:539, 1982.
43. Chaisson RE, Benson CA, Dube MP, et al: Clarithromycin therapy for bacteremic *Mycobacterium avium* complex disease. A randomized double blind dose ranging study in patients with AIDS. Ann Intern Med 121:974, 1995.
44. Dubin DS, Rahal JJ: *Mycobacterium avium* complex. Infect Dis Clin North Am 8:413, 1994.
45. Opravil M, Pechere M, Lazzarin A, et al: Dapsone/pyrimethamine may prevent mycobacterial disease in immunosuppressed patients infected with the human immunodeficiency virus. Clin Infect Dis 20:244, 1995.
46. Geruez-Rienx C, Tacquet A, Devulder B: Experimental study of interactions of pneumoconiosis and mycobacterial infections. Ann N Y Acad Sci 200:106, 1972.

47. Christensen EE, Dietz GW, Ahn CH: Radiographic manifestations of pulmonary *Mycobacterium kansasii* infections. Am J Roentgenol 131:985, 1978.
48. Sherer R, Sable R, Sonnenberg M: Disseminated infection with *Mycobacterium kansasii* in AIDS. Ann Intern Med 105:710, 1986.
49. Ahn CH, Lowell IR, Ahn SS: Chemotherapy for disease due to *Mycobacterium kansasii:* Efficacies of some individual drugs. Rev Infect Dis 3:1028, 1981.
50. Rogers PL, Walker RE, Lane MC: Disseminated *Mycobacterium haemophilum* infection in two patients with AIDS. Am J Med 84:640, 1988.
51. Straus LW, Ostroff MS, Jernigan DB, et al: Clinical and epidemiologic characteristics of *Mycobacterium haemophilum*, an emerging pathogen in immunocompromised patients. Ann Intern Med 120:118, 1994.
52. Emler S, Bottger ED, Broers B, et al: Growth-deficient mycobacteria in patients with AIDS: Diagnosis by analysis of DNA amplified from blood or tissue. Clin Infect Dis 20:772, 1995.
53. Bottger EC, Teske A, Kirschner P, et al: Disseminated "*Mycobacterium genavense*" infection in patients with AIDS. Lancet 340:76, 1992.
54. Bessessen MT, Shlay J, Stone-Venohr B, et al: Disseminated *Mycobacterium genavense* infection: Clinical and microbiological features and response to therapy. AIDS 7:1357, 1993.
55. von-Overbeck J, Clark RA, Tortoli E, et al: Treatment of disseminated *Mycobacterium genavense* infection. Arch Intern Med 155: 400, 1995.
56. Griffith DE, Wallace RJ: Pulmonary disease due to rapidly growing mycobacteria. Semin Respir Med 9:505, 1988.
57. Costrini AM, Mahler DA, Gross WM, et al: Clinical and roentgenographic features of nosocomial infection due to *Mycobacterium xenopi*. Am Rev Respir Dis 123:104, 1981.
58. Marks J, Jenkins PA, Tsukamura M: *Mycobacterium szulgai*—A new pathogen. Tubercle 53:210, 1972.
59. Schroder KH, Juhlin I: *Mycobacterium malmoense* sp. Int Syst Bacteriol 27:241, 1977.

274

Mycobacterium leprae

Diana N. J. Lockwood
Keith P. W. J. McAdam

Microbial Agent

Leprosy is caused by *Mycobacterium leprae*, an acid-fast intracellular organism that is not cultivatable on artificial media.

The presence of acid-fast rods in the nodules of patients with lepromatous leprosy was first recorded in 1874 by Armauer Hansen,[1] who postulated that these bacilli caused leprosy. To his chagrin he was unable to fulfill the Koch postulates and thereby demonstrate that these organisms caused leprosy, and the postulates remain unproved today because of a continuing inability to grow *M. leprae* in vitro.

M. leprae is a straight rod-shaped organism with rounded ends, 1 to 8 μm long and 0.3 μm wide. Like other mycobacteria, it is gram-positive and remains acid-fast after staining with carbolfuchsin.[2] It is an obligate intracellular parasite with a special affinity for skin macrophages and peripheral nerve Schwann cells. Under circumstances permitting uncontrolled growth, organisms cluster into globi (Fig. 274–1). Uniform acid-fast staining is seen in only a small proportion of *M. leprae* organisms from biopsies. Irregularly stained bacteria are nonviable, because of partial loss of cell contents after death.

Assessing the Bacillary Load

The acid-fast bacillary load of a patient is determined by Ziehl-Neelsen staining of smears made from skin slits. Suspect lesions and sites commonly affected in lepromatous leprosy should be sampled (forehead, earlobes, chin, extensor surface of the forearm, buttocks, and trunk). The density of bacilli is expressed using a logarithmic scale extending from few acid-fast bacilli (AFB) to many per high-power field. The number of AFB per field is scored according to the scale in Table 274–1. A mean score, the bacterial index (BI), is derived by adding the scores from individual sites and dividing by the number of sites sampled.[3] In untreated lepromatous leprosy the BI is 5+ or 6+. The BI falls to zero in polar tuberculoid disease.[4] Slit skin smears detect only bacilli present at a concentration greater than 10^4 per gram of tissue and so cannot be used as a test of microbiologic cure.

Morphologic Index

The morphologic index is used as a guide to the numbers of viable *M. leprae* present. Only solid-staining organisms are viable, their numbers being expressed as a percentage of a representative count of organisms.[5] The morphologic index is a useful index of progress under treatment and changes more rapidly than the BI. A rising morphologic index indicates either a failure of taking or absorbing antileprotic drugs or the development of bacillary resistance.

In Vivo Cultivation of *Mycobacterium leprae*

In 1960, the first useful laboratory growth of *M. leprae* was achieved when Shepard[6] demonstrated bacillary multiplication in the mouse footpad of *M. leprae* derived from nasal washings of lepromatous patients. The growth of a typical inoculum of 10^3 AFB is slow and limited, with an initial lag phase followed by multiplication to 10^6 organisms during 6 months. *M. leprae* may also be grown in immunodeficient mice (thymectomized-irradiated and congenitally athymic) with yields of up to 10^9 organisms after a year, accompanied by hematogenous spread.[7]

The nine-banded armadillo is extremely unusual in being naturally susceptible to *M. leprae* infection,[8] which may be related to the animal's low core temperature. Infection is progressive and systemic with dissemination of AFB particularly to the skin, lymph nodes, liver, and spleen. Wild armadillos have been found in Louisiana with naturally occurring *M. leprae* infections.[9]

Experimental transmission to rhesus, mangabey, and African green monkeys has been achieved.[10] However, unlike the armadillo, these primates do not provide large amounts of

TABLE 274–1 ■ Bacterial Index

SCORE	BACILLI PER FIELD
6+	Many clumps (1000) in an average field
5+	100–1000 bacilli in an average field
4+	10–100 bacilli in an average field
3+	1–10 bacilli in an average field
2+	1–10 bacilli in 10 fields
1+	1–10 bacilli in 100 fields

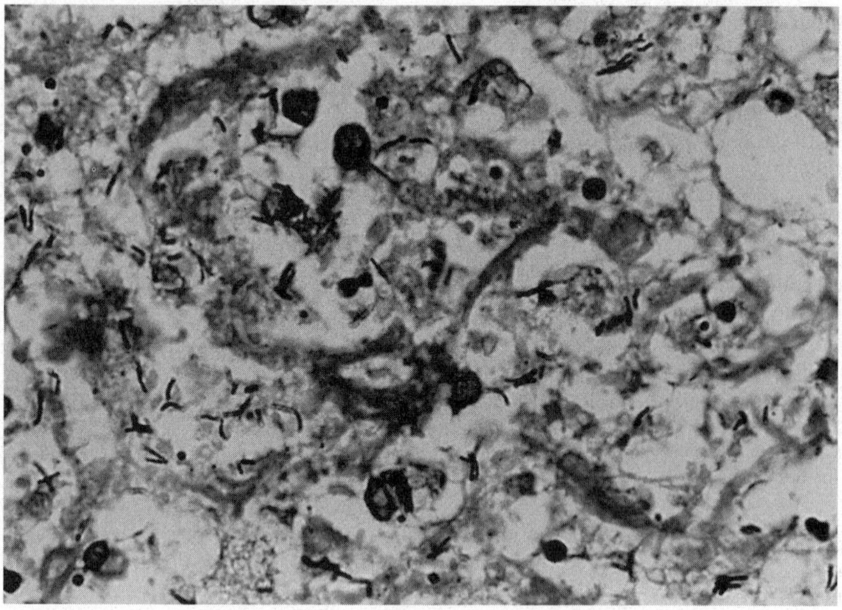

FIGURE 274–1 □ Skin biopsy specimen showing numerous intracellular acid-fast bacilli clumping into globi. (Wade-Fite stain, ×1000.)

antigen. The mouse and armadillo models of *M. leprae* infection have enabled the biologic characteristics of *M. leprae* to be elucidated and banks of purified antigen to be established.

Biologic Characteristics (Table 274–2)

M. leprae is a stable and remarkably hardy organism; AFB in nasal discharges collected from lepromatous patients may remain viable for up to 10 days after drying.[11] *M. leprae* has a doubling time of 12 days (compared with 20 minutes for *Escherichia coli*). The optimal growth temperature is 27°C to 30°C, which is consistent with the clinical observation of maximal *M. leprae* growth at cool superficial sites (skin, nasal mucosa, and peripheral nerves). The minimal infecting dose in the mouse footpad model is 3 to 40 solid-staining bacteria.[12] There is no change in pathogenicity with serial passage through mice and armadillos. *M. leprae* appears to be a single species with isolates having similar biologic characteristics and identical genotypes (using restriction fragment length polymorphism analysis) regardless of the type of leprosy and race or geographic origin of the patient.[13] The only strain differences demonstrable are isolate-stable differences in drug resistance, growth rates, and yields in infected animals.[14]

TABLE 274–2 ■ Biologic Characteristics of *Mycobacterium leprae*

Minimal countable numbers as acid-fast bacilli (AFB)	5×10^4
Routine infecting dose (total AFB)	5×10^3–10^4
Minimal infecting dose (solid-staining AFB)	3–40
Temperature for optimal growth	27°C–30°C
Doubling time (logarithmic phase)	12.5 d
Plateau yield	1×10^6
Resistance to 0.5 N sodium hydroxide	Exposure < 20 min
Retention of viability in tissues or homogenates at 4°C	7–10 d
Survival in dried nasal discharge at 26.7°C, 77.6% humidity	<14 d
Growth rate and pathogenicity after 26–42 serial mouse passages (in 16–24 y)	Unchanged

Adapted from Rees RJW: The contribution of Charles C. Shepard to leprosy research: From the mouse footpad model to new DNA technology. Lepr Rev 57(Suppl):1–14, 1986.

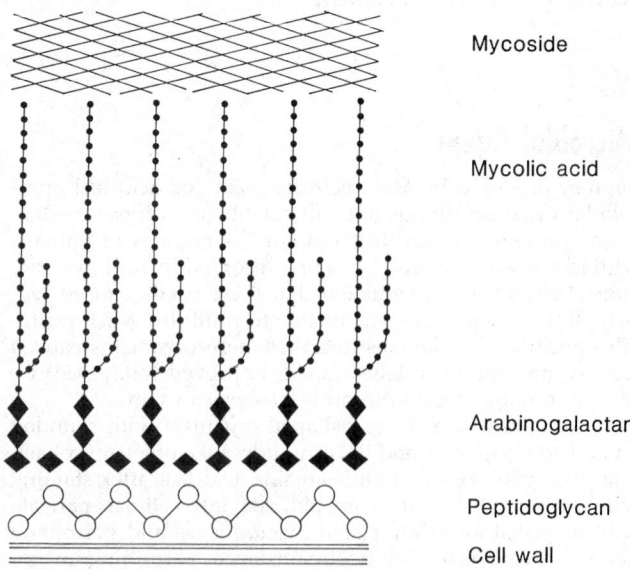

Mycobacterial Structure and Metabolism

M. leprae is characterized by a thick and unusually lipophilic mycobacterial cell wall that endows the organism with its characteristics of acid-fastness, aggregation of cells, and resistance to many bactericidal agents and may also retard the transport of nutrients into the cell. The cell wall is a complex lipid structure with a phospholipid envelope abutting a peptidoglycan backbone, which supports an arabinogalactan matrix[15] (Fig. 274–2). Within this matrix are numerous complex molecules, notably phenolic glycolipid (PGL), which is unique to *M. leprae*.

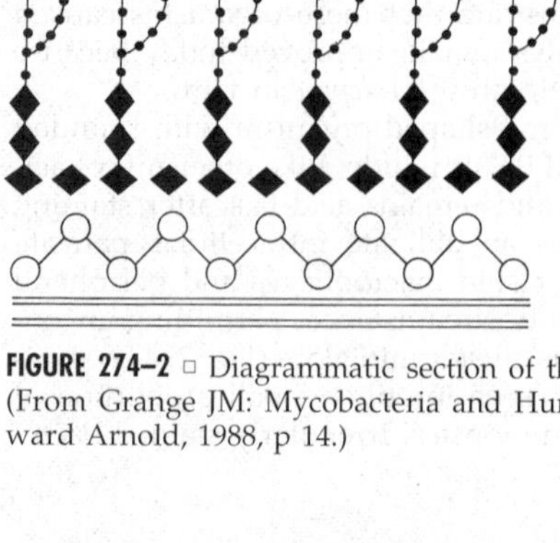

FIGURE 274–2 □ Diagrammatic section of the mycobacterial cell wall. (From Grange JM: Mycobacteria and Human Disease. London, Edward Arnold, 1988, p 14.)

Understanding the particular metabolism of an organism is crucial to the development of new agents directed against that organism. With *M. leprae* an important goal is to establish the quirk of metabolism that prevents growth of the organism in vitro. Inside host cells (e.g., human and armadillo), a complex array of host-derived nutrients is available to the mycobacterium, thus disguising which metabolites *M. leprae* may be incapable of producing. *M. leprae* has competent catabolic pathways for energy generation, is capable of producing its own adenosine triphosphate, and can take up amino acids and incorporate them into proteins.[16] However, it is unable to synthesize the purine ring and probably depends on host purines in the form of adenine nucleotides.[17] It also has two other unusual metabolic abilities: utilization of the carbon source 6-phosphogluconate, which is formed rapidly in activated macrophages, and the ability to oxidize dopa.[18]

The pathogenicity of a microorganism is partly determined by its ability to acquire iron from its host. Mycobacteria are unusual in synthesizing two sets of iron-chelating molecules, exochelins and mycobactins. Exochelins are low-molecular-weight extracellular peptides that solubilize and chelate iron from the environment. Iron is then transferred to the cellular mycobactins for transport across the cell wall and intracellular storage.[19] Both the biosynthesis and the function of the exochelins and mycobactins are potential targets for antimycobacterial drugs, although no success has been achieved to date.

The successful survival of *M. leprae* within macrophages is probably partly due to a lipoidal layer that forms outside the cell wall, containing PGL and other polar mycosides that bind and probably exclude macrophage-produced toxic oxygen metabolites and hydrolytic enzymes.[20] Another protective mechanism used by the leprosy bacillus within the macrophage is that of inhibition of phagosome-lysosome fusion, so enabling the bacillus to escape into the cytoplasm and avoid contact with harmful lysosome enzymes.[21] Two enzymes, superoxide dismutase and peroxidase, partially protect *M. leprae* from the toxic oxygen metabolites generated by the macrophage respiratory burst.[22] However, *M. leprae* lacks catalase and so is probably killed by hydrogen peroxide, which it is unable to reduce to a less toxic form.[23]

Mycobacterial Antigens

Identifying the antigens that determine recognition and handling of *M. leprae* is important both for analyzing the immune response to mycobacteria and as a basis for vaccine and diagnostic reagent development. The two major types of antigens in *M. leprae* are the carbohydrate-lipid group and the protein antigens. The dominant carbohydrate epitopes are contained within three classes, the PGLs, lipoarabinomannan (LAM), and the arabinogalactan-peptidoglycan complex.[24] *M. leprae* synthesizes a species-specific lipid, PGL, which has a unique disaccharide terminal residue.[25, 26] Substantial quantities of PGL have been found in tissues surrounding foci of infection.[27] Immunofluorescent studies using PGL monoclonal antibodies showed that PGL is a significant component of the bacterial surface capsule.[28] The importance of PGL as an antigen is borne out by several pieces of evidence: high titers of antibodies directed against PGL are found only in leprosy patients,[28] more than 90% of patients with lepromatous leprosy have PGL antibodies, and after antileprosy treatment is started both the PGL antibody titer and the PGL antigen levels fall.[29, 30] In contrast, less than 50% of tuberculoid patients have PGL antibodies,[31] which limits the usefulness of PGL antibody in the detection of early leprosy in population surveys. A fivefold rise in immunoglobulin M antibodies to synthetic PGL in patients with BI values between 0 and 1 has been demonstrated, suggesting that PGL antibodies may be a good indicator of early bacillary multiplication in close contacts of leprosy patients.[32]

The two other major carbohydrate antigens are LAM and the arabinogalactan-peptidoglycan complex. Serum from leprosy patients, including those with tuberculoid disease, has high-titer antibodies to LAM[33], but so also does serum from patients with other mycobacterial infections. Therefore, although LAM antibodies are a more sensitive indicator of mycobacterial infection than are PGL antibodies, their lack of specificity limits their use in early diagnosis. LAM has now been recognized to be highly immunogenic, both as a B-cell antigen[34] and in its effects on the cellular immune system. LAM isolated from *Mycobacterium tuberculosis* has been shown to suppress T-cell activation[35], inhibit interferon-γ activation of macrophages[36], induce the release of tumor necrosis factor,[37] and mediate a generalized inhibition of antigen presentation.[38] LAM also plays a pivotal role in the intracellular survival of mycobacteria within the macrophage, because it down-regulates macrophage effector function by scavenging potentially cytotoxic oxygen free radicals, inhibits protein kinase C activity, and may block transcription of inducible interferon-γ genes.[39, 40]

Polyacrylamide gel electrophoresis of disrupted *M. leprae* organisms separates at least 50 proteins ranging from 10 to 100 kDa.[41] The relative importance of these proteins has been assessed by using several different techniques. First, analysis of murine monoclonal antibodies produced from mice immunized with *M. leprae* lysates showed at least six *M. leprae* proteins important in the generation of an immune response[42]; second, a genomic library of *M. leprae* has been constructed and recombinant clones produced from this library have been screened with antibody and oligonucleotide probes[43, 44]; and third, T-cell responses of leprosy patients to recombinant protein antigens have been measured.[45]

By use of the murine monoclonal antibodies, six immunodominant *M. leprae* proteins (70, 65, 36, 30, 28, and 18 kDa) were identified.[46] The 70- and 65-kDa proteins stimulate strong cellular immune responses in patients and their contacts.[47–49] The 28-kDa protein is a superoxide dismutase enzyme with close homology to a human mitochondrial enzyme.[50] The 18-kDa protein is clearly a major immunogen, stimulating *M. leprae*–specific T-cell clones[51] and eliciting peripheral blood T-cell and antibody responses in leprosy patients.[45, 52, 53]

The responses of the contacts of leprosy patients are particularly interesting, for this group is most likely to have encountered *M. leprae* and thus to have developed protective immunity if not incubating disease. Potentially protective antigens should stimulate T cells to proliferate and secrete cytokines such as interferon-γ, which would activate macrophages to kill mycobacteria. So far no single antigen has been shown to be associated with protective immunity. It seems likely therefore that protective immunity is not determined by a single antigen but results from several antigens that initiate a complex balance of responses.

Cloning mycobacterial genes and expressing the gene product have been vital steps in permitting the analysis of the protein antigens of *M. leprae*. The most successful approach to cloning the *M. leprae* genes has been the cloning of small fragments of *M. leprae* DNA into an *E. coli* λgt11 phage expression vector with resultant expression of *M. leprae* proteins.[43] Genetic engineering techniques can then be applied to enable *E. coli* to produce large amounts of mycobacterial proteins. Another approach has been to transfer larger fragments of mycobacterial DNA in cosmids into *E. coli* and establish DNA libraries.[44] Expression of *M. leprae* proteins is detected immunologically by using monoclonal antibodies against *M. leprae;* the entire gene can then be sequenced and high-level protein expression obtained. An ordered library of cloned DNA fragments and a genetic map of *M. leprae* have now been constructed with complete coverage of the chromosome and location of many genetic loci (more than 70 as of 1995).[54]

M. leprae proteins may be classified according to their location: cell wall associated, membrane associated, cytoplasmic, or secreted. Cell wall fractions containing antigenic proteins have been used with some success to protect mice against footpad infection.[53, 55] Hunter and colleagues[56] isolated two major membrane proteins of 35 and 22 kDa. The 35-kDa protein contains *M. leprae*–specific epitopes[57] and T-cell epitopes.[58] Rivoire and coworkers[59] isolated the major *M. leprae* cytosolic protein of 10 kDa, sequenced and amplified the gene for this protein, and produced a promising 10-kDa skin test reagent. The 36- and 30/31-kDa proteins and antigen 85 complex are secreted antigens released by viable mycobacteria. A recombinant 30-kDa protein stimulated *M. leprae*–reactive T-cell clones and reacted with serum from patients with lepromatous leprosy.[60] These antigens have not been extensively studied but may prove to be important in the development of an early protective response, because they are encountered by the immune system at an early stage.

The *M. leprae* 10-, 70-, and 65-kDa protein antigens have been shown to be structural homologs of heat shock proteins that are synthesized by cells in response to hostile environmental conditions.[61] Heat shock proteins may provide some structural function that is necessary for cellular integrity, especially in response to environmental stresses, and so constitute an important adaptive survival mechanism. Both antibodies and T cells directed against the 65-kDa protein have been demonstrated in people with mycobacterial infections and people immunized with bacillus Calmette-Guérin (BCG) or heat-killed *M. leprae.*[62] The gene encoding the 65-kDa protein is highly conserved, with the amino acid sequences of this protein in *M. leprae, M. tuberculosis,* and *Mycobacterium bovis*-BCG displaying greater than 95% homology, even though the total genomes of these organisms show only 20% homology.[63] Monoclonal antibodies directed against the mycobacterial 65-kDa protein detect similar antigens in gram-negative and gram-positive bacteria, spirochetes, and rickettsiae. The widespread cross-species conservation of sequence and structure of this protein suggests that it is biologically important, perhaps a major immune target, and contributes to the immune protection conferred by BCG.

The application of molecular biology technology to the analysis of *M. leprae* has resulted in the development of several polymerase chain reaction probes (18, 36, and 65 kDa and ribosomal RNA sequences) for the detection of *M. leprae* DNA. *M. leprae* sequences have been detected in tissues from patients who have bacteriologically negative results on conventional Fite-Faraco staining. These techniques may help to resolve diagnostic problems in patients with tuberculoid disease in whom no *M. leprae* organisms can be found.

Detection of rifampin resistance takes between 6 to 12 months for *M. leprae,* using the currently available mouse footpad culture techniques. The molecular basis for rifampin resistance has now been elucidated in *M. leprae,* and the mutations responsible for resistance have been shown to lie within a region of 23 amino acids. It is now possible, using a polymerase chain reaction–single-strand polymorphism technique, to identify rifampin-resistant isolates within hours.[64]

Vaccines Against Leprosy

There is substantial cross-reactivity between BCG and *M. leprae,* and this has been exploited in attempts to develop a vaccine against leprosy. Trials of BCG as a vaccine against leprosy in Uganda, New Guinea, Myanmar (Burma), and South India showed it to confer statistically significant but variable protection, ranging from 80% in Uganda to 20% in Myanmar.[65] In northern Malawi, BCG gave 50% protection against leprosy but no significant protection against tuberculosis.[66] A case-control study in Venezuela showed that BCG vaccination gave 56% protection to the household contacts of leprosy patients.[67] The variability and unpredictability of BCG have led to various attempts to improve its protective efficacy. Combining BCG and killed *M. leprae* is one approach, but trials in Venezuela[68] and Malawi[69] have not shown an advantage for BCG plus *M. leprae* over BCG alone.[68] Results are currently awaited from a trial in South India where BCG has been combined with an atypical mycobacterium. One explanation for the variable protection induced by BCG is that early contact with environmental mycobacteria primes the immune system, and perhaps the immunity toward mycobacterial antigens shared between environmental species and *M. leprae* confers protective immunity against *M. leprae.* Vaccination with BCG after contact with environmental mycobacteria would then contribute little toward inducing improved immunity against *M. leprae.*[70]

Assessing a leprosy vaccine is a complex problem, because one is vaccinating against a disease of long incubation and low prevalence with different manifestations. It has been estimated that evaluating a vaccine requires 10 or more years with populations of 80,000 to 100,000 being vaccinated. There is also a fear that vaccination of people with subclinical infection or undiagnosed disease may potentiate T-cell–mediated responses against infected host cells, producing immunopathology and particularly nerve damage. Furthermore, the success of multidrug therapy has reduced the need for a vaccine against leprosy.

Manipulation of mycobacterial genes is opening up new approaches to studies of pathogenicity, diagnosis, and chemotherapy. Synthetic peptides based on known protein sequences can be developed for use in diagnosis, and mycobacterial enzymes that are potential targets for drugs can be produced by cloning and expressing the appropriate genes, thereby enabling in vitro drug screening of potential new antileprotic agents. Cloning and expressing *M. leprae* genes using a λgt11 phage vector in an *E. coli* expression system may result in important genes being missed, and products such as PGL may not be produced. Complex lipids may be missed because they are not single-gene products but instead are produced by biosynthetic pathways catalyzed by the products of several genes. Other cloning hosts such as *Mycobacterium smegmatis* and *M. bovis* BCG, which might provide a more appropriate environment for gene action, are therefore being sought. *Streptomyces lividans* is another potentially useful host because of its taxonomic closeness to the mycobacteria.[50]

The understanding of the structure and metabolism of *M. leprae* is still far from complete, and the steps involved in the development of both immune and pathologic responses to the organism remain unclear. The development of new drugs, new diagnostic tests, and ultimately a rational vaccine remains contingent on a better understanding of the organism and the human immune response to it.

References

1. Hansen GA: Undersolgelser angraaende spedalskhedens aasger. Nor Mag Laeg 4:1, 1874.
2. Rees RJW, Young DB: The microbiology of leprosy. *In* Hastings RC (ed): Leprosy. Edinburgh, Churchill Livingstone, 1994, pp 49–86.

3. Ridley DS: Therapeutic trials in leprosy using serial biopsies. Lepr Rev 29:45, 1958.
4. Ridley DS, Jopling WH: Classification of leprosy according to immunity. A five-group system Int J Lepr Other Mycobact Dis 34:255, 1966.
5. Waters MFR, Rees RJW: Changes in the morphology of *Mycobacterium leprae* in patients under treatment. Int J Lepr Other Mycobact Dis 34:255, 1962.
6. Shepard CC: Acid-fast bacilli in nasal excretions in leprosy and results of inoculation of mice. Am J Hyg 71:147, 1960.
7. Colston MJ, Hilson GRF: Growth of *Mycobacterium leprae* and *M. marinum* in congenitally athymic (nude) mice. Nature 262:399, 1976.
8. Kircheimer WF, Storrs EE: Attempts to establish the armadillo (*Dasypus novemcinctus* Linn) as a model for the study of leprosy. I. Report of lepromatoid leprosy in an experimentally infected armadillo. Int J Lepr Other Mycobact Dis 39:693, 1971.
9. Walsh GP, Meyers WM, Binford CH: Leprosy—A zoonosis. Lepr Rev 52(Suppl):77, 1981.
10. Wolf RN, Gormus BJ, Martin LN: Experimental transmission of *Mycobacterium leprae* to primates. Science 227:529, 1986.
11. Davey TF, Rees RJW: The nasal discharge in leprosy: Clinical and bacteriological aspects. Lepr Rev 45:121, 1974.
12. Rees RJW: The contribution of Charles C. Shepard to leprosy research: From mouse footpad model to new DNA technology. Lepr Rev 57(Suppl):10, 1986.
13. Williams DL, Gillis TP: A study of the relatedness of *Mycobacterium leprae* isolates using restriction fragment length polymorphism analysis. Acta Leprol 7(Suppl 1):226, 1989.
14. Shepard CC, McRae DH: Hereditary characteristic that varies amongst isolates of *Mycobacterium leprae*. Infect Immun 3:121, 1971.
15. Wheeler PR, Ratledge C: Metabolism in *Mycobacterium leprae, Mycobacterium tuberculosis*, and other pathogenic mycobacteria. Br Med Bull 44:547, 1988.
16. Khanolkar SR: Preliminary studies of the metabolic activity of purified suspensions of *Mycobacterium leprae*. J Gen Microbiol 128:423, 1982.
17. Wheeler PR: Biosynthesis and scavenging of purines by pathogenic mycobacteria including *Mycobacterium leprae*. J Gen Microbiol 133:2999, 1987.
18. Wheeler PR: Metabolism in *M. leprae*: Its relation to other research on *M. leprae* and to aspects of metabolism in other mycobacteria and intracellular parasites. Int J Lepr Other Mycobact Dis 52:208, 1984.
19. Hall RM, Ratledge C: Exochelin-mediated iron acquisition by the leprosy bacillus, *Mycobacterium leprae*. J Gen Microbiol 133:193, 1987.
20. Ryter A, Fretel C, Rastogi N, David N: Macrophage interaction with mycobacteria, including *M. leprae*. Acta Leprol 21:2116, 1984.
21. Sibley LD, Franzblau SG, Krahenbuhl JL: Intracellular fate of *Mycobacterium leprae* in normal and activated mouse macrophages. Infect Immun 55:680, 1987.
22. Wheeler PR, Gregory D: Superoxide dismutase, peroxidatic activity and catalase in *Mycobacterium leprae* purified from armadillo liver. J Gen Microbiol 121:457, 1980.
23. Sharp AK, Colston MJ, Banerjee DK: Susceptibility of *Mycobacterium leprae* to the bactericidal activity of mouse macrophages and to hydrogen peroxide. J Med Microbiol 19:77, 1985.
24. Gaylord H, Brennan PJ: Leprosy and the leprosy bacillus: Recent developments in characterization of antigens and immunology of the disease. Annu Rev Microbiol 41:645, 1987.
25. Hunter SW, Brennan PJ: A novel phenolic glycolipid from *Mycobacterium leprae* possibly involved in immunogenicity and pathogenicity. J Bacteriol 147:728, 1994.
26. Hunter SW, Fujiwara T, Brennan PJ: Structure and antigenicity of the major specific glycolipid antigen of *Mycobacterium leprae*. J Biol Chem 257:15072, 1982.
27. Young DB: Detection of mycobacterial lipids in skin biopsies from leprosy patients. Int J Lepr Other Mycobact Dis 49:198, 1981.
28. Young DB, Khanolkar SR, Barg LL: Generation and characterization of monoclonal antibodies to the phenolic glycolipid of *Mycobacterium leprae*. Infect Immun 43:183, 1984.
29. Cho S, Yanagihara DI, Hunter SW, et al: Serological specificity of phenolic glycolipid 1 from *Mycobacterium leprae* and use in serodiagnosis of leprosy. Infect Immun 41:1077, 1983.
30. Cho S, Hunter SW, Gelber RH, et al: Quantitation of the phenolic glycolipid of *Mycobacterium leprae* and relevance to glycolipid antigenemia in leprosy. J Infect Dis 153:560, 1986.
31. Young DB, Dissanayake S, Miller RA, et al: Humans respond predominantly with IgM immunoglobulin to the species specific glycolipid of *Mycobacterium leprae*. J Infect Dis 149:870, 1984.
32. Hussain R, Jamil S, Kifayet A: Quantitation of IgM antibodies to the *M. leprae* synthetic disaccharide can predict early bacterial multiplication in leprosy. Int J Lepr Other Mycobact Dis 58:491, 1990.
33. Brennan PJ: The carbohydrate-containing antigens of *M. leprae*. Lepr Rev 57:39, 1986.
34. Chatterjee D, Bozie CM, McNeill M, Brennan PJ: Structural features of the arabinan component of the lipoarabinomannan of *Mycobacterium tuberculosis*. J Biol Chem 266:9652, 1991.
35. Kaplan G, Ghandhi RR, Weinstein DE, et al: *Mycobacterium leprae* antigen induced suppression of T cell proliferation in vitro. J Immunol 138:3028, 1987.
36. Sibley LD, Hunter SW, Brennan PJ, Krahenbuhl JL: Mycobacterial lipoarabinomannan inhibits gamma interferon–mediated activation of macrophages. Infect Immun 56:1232, 1988.
37. Barnes PF, Fong S, Brennan PJ: Local production of tumour necrosis factor and IFN-γ in tuberculous pleuritis. J Immunol 145:149, 1990.
38. Moreno C, Mehlert A, Lamb J: The inhibitory effects of mycobacterial lipoarabinomannan and polysaccharide upon polyclonal and monoclonal human T cell proliferation. Clin Exp Immunol 74:206, 1988.
39. Chan J, Fujiwara T, Brennan PJ, et al: Microbial glycolipids: Possible virulence factors that scavenge oxygen radicals. Proc Natl Acad Sci USA 86:2453, 1989.
40. Chan J, Fan X, Hunter SW, et al: Lipoarabinomannan, a possible virulence factor involved in persistence of *Mycobacterium tuberculosis* within macrophages. Infect Immun 59:1755, 1991.
41. Chakrabarty AK, Maire MA, Lambert PH: SDS-PAGE analysis of *M. leprae* protein antigens reacting with antibodies from sera from lepromatous patients and infected armadillos. Clin Exp Immunol 49:523, 1982.
42. Kaufmann SHE, Young DB: Vaccination against tuberculosis and leprosy. Immunobiology 184:208, 1992.
43. Young RA, Mehra V, Sweetser D, et al: Genes for the major protein antigens of the leprosy parasite *Mycobacterium leprae*. Nature 316:450, 1985.
44. Clark-Curtiss JE, Jacobs WR, Docherty MA: Molecular analysis of DNA and construction of genomic libraries of *Mycobacterium leprae*. J Bacteriol 161:1093, 1985.
45. Dockrell HM, Stoker NG, Lee SP, et al: T-cell recognition of the 18-kilodalton antigen of *Mycobacterium leprae*. Infect Immun 57:1979, 1989.
46. Engers HD, Abe M, Bloom BR, et al: Results of a World Health Organisation–sponsored workshop on monoclonal antibodies to *Mycobacterium leprae*. Infect Immun 48:603, 1985.
47. Ottenhoff THM, Haanen JBAG, Geluk A, et al: Regulation of mycobacterial heat shock reactive T-cells by HLA class II molecules: Lessons from leprosy. Immunol Rev 121:171, 1991.
48. Adams E, Garsia RJ, Hellqvist L, et al: T cell reactivity to the purified mycobacterial antigens p65 and p70 in leprosy patients and their contacts. Clin Exp Immunol 80:206, 1990.
49. Britton WJ, Hellqvist L, Basten A, Inglis A: Immunoreactivity of a 70 kD protein purified from *Mycobacterium bovis* bacillus Calmette-Guérin by monoclonal antibody affinity chromatography. J Exp Med 164:695, 1986.
50. Thangaraj HS, Lamb FI, Davis EO, et al: Identification, sequencing and expression of *Mycobacterium leprae* superoxide dismutase, a major antigen. Infect Immun 58:1937, 1990.
51. Mustafa AS, Gill HK, Nerland A, et al: Human T-cell clones recognize a major *M. leprae* protein antigen expressed in *E. coli*. Nature 319:63, 1986.
52. Roche PW, Prestige RL, Watson JD, Britton WJ: Antibody responses to the 18kD protein of *Mycobacterium leprae* in leprosy and tuberculosis patients. Int J Lepr Other Mycobact Dis 60:201, 1992.
53. Doherty TM, Booth RJ, Love SG, et al: Characterisation of an antibody-binding epitope from the 18-kDa protein on *Mycobacterium leprae*. Infect Immun 142:1691, 1989.
54. Eiglmeier K, Honore N, Woods SA, et al: Use of an ordered

cosmid library to deduce the genomic organisation of *Mycobacterium leprae*. Mol Microbiol 7:197, 1993.
55. Roche PW, Neupane KD, Britton WJ: Cellular immune response to the cell walls of *Mycobacterium leprae* in leprosy patients and healthy subjects exposed to leprosy. Clin Exp Immunol 89:110, 1992.
56. Hunter SW, Rivoire S, Mehra V, et al: The major native proteins of the leprosy bacillus. J Biol Chem 265:14065, 1990.
57. Roche PW, Britton WJ, Failbus SS, et al: Operational value of serological measurements in multibacillary leprosy patients: Clinical and bacteriological correlates of antibody responses. Int J Lepr Other Mycobact Dis 58:480, 1990.
58. Mohagheghpour N, Munn MW, Gelber RH, Engeleman EG: Identification of an immunostimulatory protein from *Mycobacterium leprae*. Infect Immun 58:703, 1990.
59. Rivoire B, Pessolani MCV, Bozic CM, et al: Chemical definition, cloning and expression of the major protein of the leprosy bacillus. Infect Immun 62:2417, 1994.
60. Thole JER, Schoringh R, Janson AA, et al: Molecular and immunological analysis of a fibronectin-binding protein secreted by *Mycobacterium leprae*. Mol Microbiol 6:153, 1992.
61. Young DB, Lathigra R, Hendrix R, et al: Stress proteins are immune targets in leprosy and tuberculosis. Proc Natl Acad Sci USA 85:4267, 1988.
62. Shinnick TM, Vodkin MH, Williams JC: The *Mycobacterium tuberculosis* 65-kilodalton antigen is a heat shock protein which corresponds to common antigen and to the *Escherichia coli* GroEL protein. Infect Immun 56:446, 1988.
63. Shinnick TM, Sweetser D, Thole J, et al: The etiologic agents of leprosy and tuberculosis share an immunoreactive protein antigen with the vaccine strain *Mycobacterium bovis* BCG. Infect Immun 55:1932, 1987.
64. Honore N, Perrani E, Telenti A, et al: A simple and rapid technique for the detection of rifampin resistance in *Mycobacterium leprae*. Int J Lepr Other Mycobact Dis 61:600, 1993.
65. Fine PEM, Rodrigues LC: Modern vaccines: Mycobacterial diseases. Lancet 335:1016, 1990.
66. Ponnighaus JM, Fine PEM, Sterne JAC, et al: Efficacy of BCG vaccine against leprosy and tuberculosis in northern Malawi. Lancet 339:636, 1992.
67. Convit J, Smith PG, Zuniga M, et al: BCG vaccination protects against leprosy in Venezuela: A case control study. Int J Lepr Other Mycobact Dis 61:185, 1993.
68. Convit J, Sampson C, Zuniga M, et al: Immunoprophylactic trial with combined *Mycobacterium leprae*/BCG vaccine against leprosy: Preliminary results. Lancet 339:446, 1992.
69. Randomised controlled trial of single BCG, repeated BCG, or combined BCG and killed *Mycobacterium leprae* for prevention of leprosy and tuberculosis in Malawi. Karonga Prevention Trial Group. Lancet 348:17, 1996.
70. Bettering BCG (Editorial). Lancet 339:462, 1992.

275

Candida albicans and Related Species

Janine R. Maenza
William G. Merz

Candida species are the most common fungal pathogens affecting humans. These organisms cause a wide spectrum of opportunistic diseases, from noninvasive superficial skin infections to deep-seated infections of solid organs. The past few decades have seen increasing numbers of *Candida* infections, both community acquired and nosocomial, reflecting, among other factors, the use of broad-spectrum antibacterials, use of intravascular devices, and a growing population of immunosuppressed patients.

Characteristics of the Pathogen

There are nearly 200 *Candida* species, of which fewer than 20 are capable of causing disease in humans. Most species may be seen morphologically as budding yeast, hyphal, or pseudohyphal forms, but some, such as *Candida (Torulopsis) glabrata,* are found only as yeast or hyphae. The genus *Candida* is not a tight taxonomic group based on true phylogenetic relationships but rather a somewhat diverse group of asexual organisms with similar phenotypic characteristics. When the sexual form of a *Candida* species is identified, the organism is classified into the proper sexual species that does reflect phylogenetic relationship. Thus, for example, the sexual form of *Candida krusei* is *Issatchenkia orientalis*, that of *Candida lusitaniae* is *Clavispora lusitaniae*, that of *Candida guilliermondii* is *Yamadazyma guilliermondii*, and that of *Candida kefyr* is *Kluyveromyces marxianus*. This variety of sexual genera attests to the diversity of this group of microorganisms.

Candida albicans is the species most commonly found as both a colonizer and a pathogen. Other frequently encountered species include *C. guilliermondii*, *C. kefyr* (previously known as *Candida pseudotropicalis*), *C. krusei*, *C. lusitaniae*, *Candida parapsilosis*, and *Candida tropicalis*. Most authorities also now recognize the commonly encountered organism *Torulopsis glabrata* as a *Candida* species, thus leading to its renaming as *C. glabrata*. *Candida* species less frequently found as human colonizers or pathogens include *C. lipolytica*, *C. rugosa*, *C. viswanathii*, *C. haemulonii*, *C. norvegensis*, *C. catenulata*, *C. intermedia*, *C. lambica*, and *C. zeylanoides*. *Saccharomyces cerevisiae* and *Hansenula anomala*, although not *Candida* species, are mentioned here because they are yeasts that have similar phenotypic characteristics and can cause some infections that are indistinguishable from those caused by *Candida* species.

Anatomic areas colonized by *Candida* species include skin, mouth, rectum, and vagina, from which *C. albicans* is frequently isolated; other species are not as common and tend to colonize fewer anatomic sites. *C. glabrata* is known to colonize the mouth, rectum, and vagina; *C. parapsilosis* may be found in rectal and skin cultures; and *C. tropicalis* may be isolated from the mouth and skin.[1]

Pathogenesis

There are significant differences in virulence among different *Candida* species, as evidenced by clinical data and animal models. There is no single fungal factor, however, but multiple factors that contribute to their ability to cause infection[2] (Table 275–1). One notable factor associated with the virulence of *C. albicans* is the presence of surface molecules that permit the organism to adhere to epithelial cells, endothelial cells, extracellular matrix, and hardware. Production of surface molecules that mimic host substances and thereby allow avoidance of immune surveillance has been described. An additional factor that may be involved in host invasion is the production of hydrolytic enzymes (including acid proteases and phospholipases). The ability of *C. albicans* to convert rapidly to a hyphal form (with either true hyphae or pseudohyphae) may also contribute to pathogenicity.[3] Loss of a single factor does not appear to be sufficient to render an isolate avirulent, although it may restrict its ability to cause all types of infections. Evidence for this comes from mutants of *C. albicans* that produce no or lower levels of acid protease and grow more slowly than wild-type strains but are not completely avirulent.[4] In fact, the ability of this genus to cause disease depends as much, if not more, on host defects as on any particular virulence factor inherent to the organism. Structural host defects associated with *Candida* infection include breaks in the integrity of the skin or mucous membranes due to burns, trauma, or occlusion and maceration. Exogenous causes of host defects include the use of antimicrobials that change the normal colonizing flora and procedures resulting in the presence of prosthetic materials. Endogenous host factors include the extremes of age, diabetes, and immunologic abnormalities including specific lymphocyte deficiencies and granulocyte and complement abnormalities.

Epidemiology

Although *Candida* organisms can be isolated from environmental sources (soil, foods, water, plants), most infections are acquired from endogenous flora.[5, 6] The evidence for endoge-

TABLE 275–1 ■ Virulence Factors of *Candida albicans*

Adhesion
Ability to transform rapidly from yeast to hyphae
Production of hydrolytic enzymes
Acid proteinase secretion
Phospholipase secretion
Phenotypic switching and chromosomal instability
Antigenic variation
Host mimicry
Toxin production

Adapted from Bodey GP: Candidiasis. Pathogenesis, Diagnosis, and Treatment. New York, Raven Press, 1993; and Cutler JE: Putative virulence factors of *Candida albicans*. Annu Rev Microbiol 45:187–218, 1991. With permission from the Annual Review of Microbiology, Volume 45, © 1991, by Annual Reviews Inc.

nous sources of infection comes from molecular typing systems with use of DNA-based methods including restriction endonuclease fragment polymorphisms analyzed by electrophoresis (normal or pulsed field), electrophoretic karyotyping, and rapid arbitrarily primed polymerase chain reaction amplification.[7] Data support that most patients are colonized with a distinct strain of *Candida*; if a blood stream or other infection occurs, the infecting strain is frequently the same strain as the colonizer.[5, 6] An exception to this scenario may be *C. parapsilosis*, which is reported to cause infection from exogenous sources without prior colonization[8] and has been responsible for outbreaks related to intravenous infusions.[9] In addition, neonatal *Candida* infections usually occur by person-to-person transmission, and there are isolated reports of nosocomial transmission of a single *C. albicans* strain between patients in other settings.[8, 10]

Different types of *Candida* infections are associated with different host populations. Cutaneous *Candida* infections and *Candida* vaginitis may occur in immunologically intact hosts. Mucocutaneous candidiasis of the oropharynx is usually found in patients with defects of cell-mediated immunity, although it may also be seen in patients with diabetes mellitus and patients receiving broad-spectrum antibacterials. Blood stream and associated solid organ *Candida* infections are most commonly seen in burn patients, postsurgical patients, and immunocompromised patients. Specific risk factors associated with candidemia and deep tissue infections in these populations include the use of indwelling intravascular catheters, parenteral hyperalimentation, broad-spectrum antibacterials, and intensive chemotherapy regimens leading to prolonged neutropenia.[11, 12] In addition, among surgical patients, gastrointestinal procedures are associated with an increased rate of candidemia, probably related to disruption of bowel mucosa colonized with *Candida*. Neonatal candidemia is associated with prematurity and low birth weight.

Clinical Diseases

The many clinical syndromes associated with *Candida* species are most frequently caused by *C. albicans*. As these clinical entities are described, other species known to be responsible are noted as appropriate.

Cutaneous Candidiasis

Cutaneous candidiasis may be seen in normal as well as in immunocompromised hosts. In normal hosts, risk factors for the development of infection include moist or occluded areas, friction, burn sites, or skin areas that have been irradiated. Cutaneous candidiasis is more frequent in diabetic than in nondiabetic individuals.[13] The infection manifests as intense erythema of intertriginous areas. The erythematous areas may be papular, plaquelike, or confluent. Satellite lesions consisting of pustules or erythematous papules may surround these areas. Commonly involved sites include the axillae, inguinal regions, perineum, skin beneath the breasts, and digital web spaces. *Candida* folliculitis may also be seen, especially in moist or occluded areas.

Sterile lesions, which may be hyperkeratotic, papular, or eczematous, can occur in locations separate from the sites of *Candida* infection. These lesions represent allergic reactions, known as id reactions, and have been seen in patients with mucous membrane as well as cutaneous candidiasis.[1, 14] Resolution of the id reaction is seen with antifungal treatment of the initiating infection.

Candidiasis may also involve the nails and nail folds. Onychomycosis, with nail discoloration or destruction, may occur in previously damaged nails or with a concomitant paronychial infection. Unlike dermatophyte infections of the nails, *Candida* onychomycosis is often painful.[1] *Candida* paronychial infections present as erythematous lesions, often lacking the purulence seen in bacterial infections. Both onychomycosis and paronychial infections are usually found as occupational infections in people whose hands remain wet for long periods (e.g., dishwashers).

Diagnosis of these cutaneous disorders is often made on clinical grounds, although confirmation may be added by detection of the budding yeast and hyphal forms on direct microscopic examination (potassium hydroxide) of skin or nail scrapings. Cultures are not routinely done because they are unlikely to add to the results of the microscopic examination and may reflect only fungal colonization. Skin lesions may also be a manifestation of disseminated candidiasis. These secondary lesions arise from hematogenous spread and may include erythematous macronodular papules, subcutaneous nodules, lesions resembling ecthyma gangrenosum, and rarely purpuric lesions.[15–17] These lesions are more common with *C. tropicalis* and *C. krusei* than with *C. albicans*. A distinct syndrome of cutaneous candidiasis was described in European heroin users in the mid-1980s. Use of a new form of the drug known as brown heroin led to episodes of disseminated candidiasis with skin findings manifested as multiple nodules and extensive areas of folliculitis.[18–20]

Chronic Mucocutaneous Candidiasis

Chronic mucocutaneous candidiasis includes a group of somewhat heterogeneous syndromes in patients with T-cell abnormalities. The defect may be specifically related to *Candida* only or to other antigens also. Not all patients have the same deficits, but the immunologic abnormalities may include additional abnormalities of T-lymphocyte function as well as occasional dysfunction of B cells, granulocytes, or complement.[21]

The clinical manifestations grouped together as chronic mucocutaneous candidiasis are thus varied. Most patients present in infancy or early childhood. The first signs may be oral thrush or perineal candidiasis. Some patients may develop more widespread cutaneous candidiasis and onychomycosis, others may have only localized skin involvement, and others may have disease involving only the nails. Invasive infections are rare in all forms of this disease.[22]

In some instances, syndromes of chronic mucocutaneous candidiasis are associated with other disorders, such as multiple endocrine abnormalities[23] and recurrent viral and bacterial pulmonary or sinus infections.[24] In patients in whom the diagnosis of chronic mucocutaneous candidiasis is suspected, an initial evaluation should include phenotypic characterization of lymphocyte subsets and investigation of T-cell function (e.g., response to mitogens).

Oral and Esophageal Candidiasis

Systemic factors associated with the development of upper gastrointestinal candidiasis include the use of antibiotics, diabetes, hematologic malignant neoplasms, medication-induced immunosuppression, and human immunodeficiency virus (HIV) infection. Local structural or functional factors may also be associated with disease development; disorders of esophageal motility in particular are associated with *Candida* overgrowth. In the newborn, oral candidiasis may occur as a consequence of colonization or infection from the mother's vaginal flora or other exogenous sources. In immunosuppressed patients with mucositis, oral and esophageal candidiasis must be considered potential sources of disseminated candidiasis. The majority of cases of oral and esophageal candidiasis are caused by *C. albicans*, but *C. glabrata*, *C.*

krusei, C. tropicalis, C. parapsilosis, S. cerevisiae, and *H. anomala* are also reported to cause this disease.[25–28]

Oral candidiasis may present with different clinical manifestations. The most common is typical oral thrush, or the pseudomembranous form of oral candidiasis. In this form, white pseudomembranous plaques are seen on the surfaces of the oropharynx. Less commonly seen are erythematous candidiasis (red mucosal patches in the absence of pseudomembranes), hyperplastic candidiasis or *Candida* leukoplakia (rough plaques that cannot be removed by scraping), and angular cheilitis (in which the corners of the lips are involved with erythema and cracking). The diagnosis of oral candidiasis is usually made clinically by noting one of these typical appearances on physical examination. Confirmation can be obtained by direct microscopic examination. Culture is not generally helpful given the high colonization rate of the oropharynx with *Candida* species.

Esophageal candidiasis also has a range of clinical manifestations from superficial infection to deep invasive disease. This diversity is most commonly due to varying host defects, with superficial disease seen in patients with HIV infection and deep infection in neutropenic patients. It may present with or without concomitant oral infection. Symptoms are indistinguishable from those of other infectious and noninfectious causes of esophagitis and include dysphagia, odynophagia, and retrosternal chest pain. Patients may also be asymptomatic even with extensive disease. Complications of esophageal candidiasis include perforation; bleeding; a risk for dissemination; and, in chronic *Candida* esophagitis, esophageal stenosis. The diagnosis of esophageal candidiasis is frequently made on clinical grounds in high-risk populations. For example, a patient with HIV infection, oral thrush, and esophageal symptoms may be treated empirically for *Candida* esophagitis. In neutropenic patients with concomitant thrombocytopenia, the potential bleeding complications of endoscopy may preclude the use of this diagnostic procedure, and empirical treatment may again be used. In instances of esophageal symptoms when the diagnosis is less certain or in patients who do not respond to empirical treatment, a definitive diagnosis can be made by endoscopy and biopsy (Fig. 275–1). Endoscopy may also be useful for obtaining cultures for species identification and susceptibility testing in HIV-infected patients who are refractory to azole treatment.

Oral and esophageal candidiasis that is clinically refractory to ketoconazole, fluconazole, and itraconazole has been documented, most frequently in HIV-infected patients. Fluconazole resistance, in particular, has been well described[29–36] and is more likely to occur in HIV-infected patients with advanced immunosuppression (low $CD4^+$ lymphocyte counts), multiple prior episodes of thrush or esophagitis, and extensive previous exposure to systemic azoles.[28] Fluconazole-resistant candidiasis represents a significant clinical problem because many patients with this disease require treatment with parenteral amphotericin B.[28, 34] In patients with advanced HIV infection, the prevalence of fluconazole resistance may be substantial. In a cross-sectional study we performed[37] of patients with $CD4^+$ lymphocyte counts less than 200/mm^3, 46% of patients with positive fungal cultures had at least one organism that showed in vitro fluconazole resistance (as defined by a minimal inhibitory concentration of 8 μg/mL or greater). Importantly, 31% of the *C. albicans* isolates showed fluconazole resistance, and the presence of this organism correlated with clinical thrush.[37] Another study found a prevalence of in vitro fluconazole resistance of 32% in HIV-infected patients with recurrent oropharyngeal candidiasis.[38] Strategies to prevent the development of fluconazole resistance have not been clearly delineated but may include using topical agents as first-line therapy for oral thrush and reserving systemic azoles for patients who are refractory to topical treatment or have esophageal involvement.

Vulvovaginal Candidiasis

Vulvovaginal candidiasis is a common fungal infection both in normal women and in women with deficits of cell-mediated immunity. The infection causes vulvar itching and a thick vaginal discharge. Physical examination usually reveals vulvar erythema and an adherent white discharge. The use of antibacterial agents, which change the normal vaginal flora, is frequently associated with the development of this disease.[39, 40] Pregnancy[41] and diabetes[42] are also associated with *Candida* vaginitis, and some studies have suggested the use of oral contraceptives as a risk factor.[43, 44]

C. albicans is the cause of more than 80% of cases of vulvovaginal candidiasis,[45] but non-*albicans* species are also reported as pathogens.[46] *C. tropicalis* and *C. glabrata* are the most commonly identified non-*albicans* species, although *C. parapsilosis* and *S. cerevisiae* have also been described.[47]

Recurrent vulvovaginal candidiasis, usually defined as three or four episodes in a year,[1] may be more common in

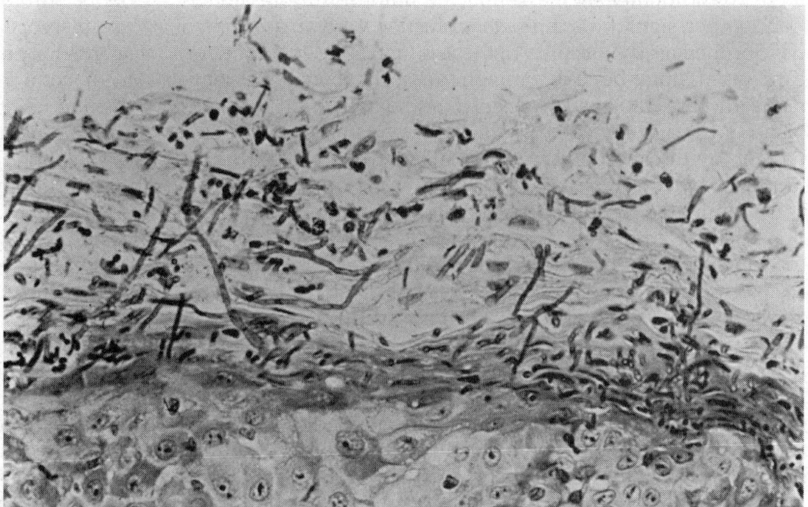

FIGURE 275–1 □ Histologic specimen demonstrating *Candida* esophagitis.

women with immune defects.[45, 48] A recurrent infection within 3 months is usually due to reinfection with the same *Candida* strain; after 3 months, reinfection with a different strain is more common.[49, 50] Some data suggest that persistence of vaginal organisms after treatment,[51] rather than a gastrointestinal reservoir[45, 49] or sexual transmission,[52–54] is responsible for recurrent episodes. Theories to explain the mechanism of recurrent disease include (1) deficiencies in normal bacterial flora, (2) a *Candida*-specific deficiency in T-lymphocyte activity, and (3) an acquired hypersensitivity reaction to *Candida*.[45] Management of recurrent disease may require long courses of antifungal therapy or chronic antifungal prophylaxis.[50]

Because *Candida* species may be found as normal vaginal flora in 40% of women,[55] the diagnosis of *Candida* vaginitis should not be made in the absence of symptoms. In addition, because the signs and symptoms may overlap those of bacterial vaginitis, history and physical examination alone cannot be relied on with diagnostic certainty. The diagnosis is usually made by consistent clinical findings combined with a microscopic examination of a saline wet preparation to ensure the absence of clue cells and *Trichomonas* organisms and a potassium hydroxide preparation to look for the presence of yeast or hyphal forms. Cultures may be necessary in unusual presentations, in recurrent episodes, or for assessing therapy in selected patients.

Candidemia

Candidemia is uncommon as a community-acquired infection, except in intravenous drug users, but is a frequent nosocomial complication. Inpatient populations most at risk for the development of candidemia include burn patients, postsurgical patients, oncology patients, and patients who are immunosuppressed after solid organ transplantation. The frequency of nosocomial *Candida* blood stream infections increased up to fourfold during the 1980s[56, 57] (Fig. 275–2). Factors related to the development of candidemia include the use of central venous catheters, parenteral alimentation, broad-spectrum antibacterials, and intensive chemotherapy and immunosuppressive regimens.[11, 12]

The greatest concern with the patient with candidemia is that the blood stream infection is a marker for disseminated disease with invasive solid organ infection as well. The attributable mortality of nosocomial candidemia has been shown to be as high as 38%.[58] The organs most frequently involved in disseminated infection are eye, kidney, and heart. It is also possible to see gastrointestinal, cutaneous, and joint involvement. Candidemia in the setting of immunosuppression is frequently a sign of disseminated infection with an associated risk for increased mortality. In the immunocompetent patient, candidemia may be less commonly associated with disseminated disease and may frequently be related to an infection of an intravascular catheter. In a study of nonneutropenic patients with candidemia, 72% of all episodes were thought to arise from vascular catheters.[59]

Disseminated candidiasis often occurs in the absence of documented candidemia. An autopsy study demonstrated that only 43% of cases of invasive candidiasis were diagnosed by antemortem blood cultures.[60] This presents a difficult situation in a disease with few specific findings in which a diagnosis of disseminated candidiasis must frequently be made on clinical grounds. Diagnostic clues may include skin lesions associated with disseminated candidiasis (see cutaneous candidiasis), endophthalmitis (in nonneutropenic patients), esophagitis, myalgias, and myositis. In any neutropenic patient with fever unresponsive to broad-spectrum antibacterial therapy, the diagnosis must be considered likely.

The difficulty of diagnosis of disseminated candidiasis in the absence of positive blood cultures has been a major impetus in the development of nonculture methods. These techniques (discussed later) lack the sensitivity to be uniformly recommended. Specificity of the tests is also variable, but a positive result should be regarded as an additional piece of evidence suggesting disseminated infection.

Fungal surveillance cultures of urine, stool, and respiratory secretions have also been studied as possible predictors of systemic fungal infections in oncology patients. Positive cultures for *C. tropicalis* have been shown to correlate with systemic disease, whereas cultures of *C. albicans* do not.[61] A benefit of surveillance cultures is that species identification may be predicted when deep tissue or blood cultures first become positive for yeast. Negative surveillance cultures are predictive of the absence of systemic disease.[61]

Although, in general, *C. albicans* remains the most common cause of candidemia, non-*albicans* species cause a substantial number of infections. At Johns Hopkins Hospital, we have observed a clear difference in the frequency of non-*albicans* infections in oncology patients compared with nononcology patients; during the years 1992 to 1995, 47% of candidemia episodes in nononcology patients were caused by non-*albicans* species, compared with 81% of the episodes in oncology patients.[62] This frequency of non-*albicans* infections is higher than has been described historically; a review found that 46% of the reported infections in oncology patients during the past 40 years were due to non-*albicans* species (predominantly *C. tropicalis, C. glabrata, C. parapsilosis,* and *C. krusei*).[63] Specific associations were also found between patients with leukemia and *C. tropicalis* infections and between bone marrow transplant recipients and *C. krusei* or *C. lusitaniae* infections. In addition, the prophylactic use of fluconazole in these patients has been associated with the emergence of *C. krusei* and *C. glabrata* infections.[64, 65]

Urinary Tract Infections

Candida species may colonize the lower urinary tract and cause either lower or upper urinary tract infections. In patients with lower tract infections, symptoms include the classic findings of cystitis: urgency, frequency, and dysuria, indistinguishable from bacterial infections. Upper tract infections may result either from a primary ascending (lower) urinary tract infection or from seeding of the kidney from a hematogenous infection. Multiple microabscesses, perinephric abscess, papillary necrosis, and fungus balls have been seen as manifestations of upper tract *Candida* infections.

Candida urinary infections are most commonly seen in patients with indwelling urinary catheters. Diabetes and the use of broad-spectrum antibacterials or immunosuppressive agents may also be risk factors for infection. *C. albicans* is the most common cause of *Candida* urinary infections, but *C. glabrata, C. guilliermondii, C. kefyr, C. lusitaniae, C. tropicalis,* and *S. cerevisiae* have all been reported to cause cystitis.[1]

The finding of candiduria may reflect anything from contamination to asymptomatic colonization to a localized lower or upper urinary tract infection to disseminated candidiasis with the kidney as a target organ. Thus, a urine culture showing *Candida* must be interpreted in light of the clinical picture including the patient's underlying risk factors, symptoms, physical examination findings, and history of urinary catheterization or instrumentation. Unlike the situation with bacteriuria, there is no specific breakpoint at which colony counts are considered significant; there is not necessarily a correlation between severity of disease and colony count in urine.[1] To assess for true infection, an indwelling catheter should be changed if one is present, and urinalysis and culture should be repeated. If there is no history of recent genitourinary instrumentation, patients should be evaluated both for the presence of a urinary obstruction or other struc-

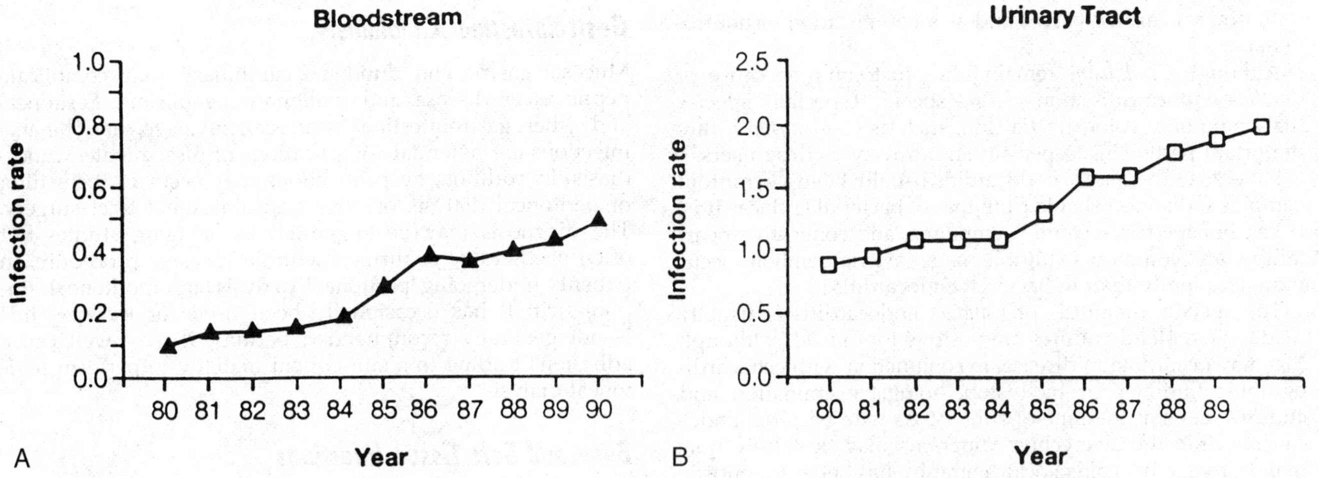

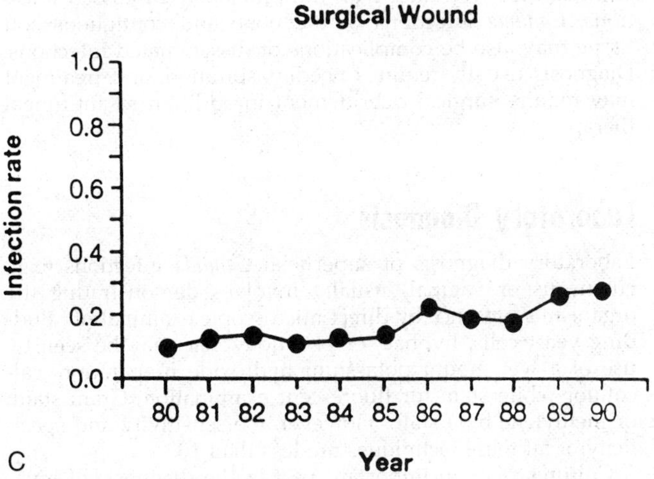

FIGURE 275–2 □ Data from the National Nosocomial Infections Surveillance System showing trends in the rates of nosocomial fungal infections (shown as rate per 1000 hospital discharges) from 1980 to 1990. *A*, Blood stream infections. *B*, Urinary tract infections. *C*, Surgical wound infections. (*A* to *C* from Jarvis WR: Epidemiology of nosocomial fungal infections, with emphasis on *Candida* species. Clin Infect Dis 20:1526–1530, 1995. Copyright by The University of Chicago.)

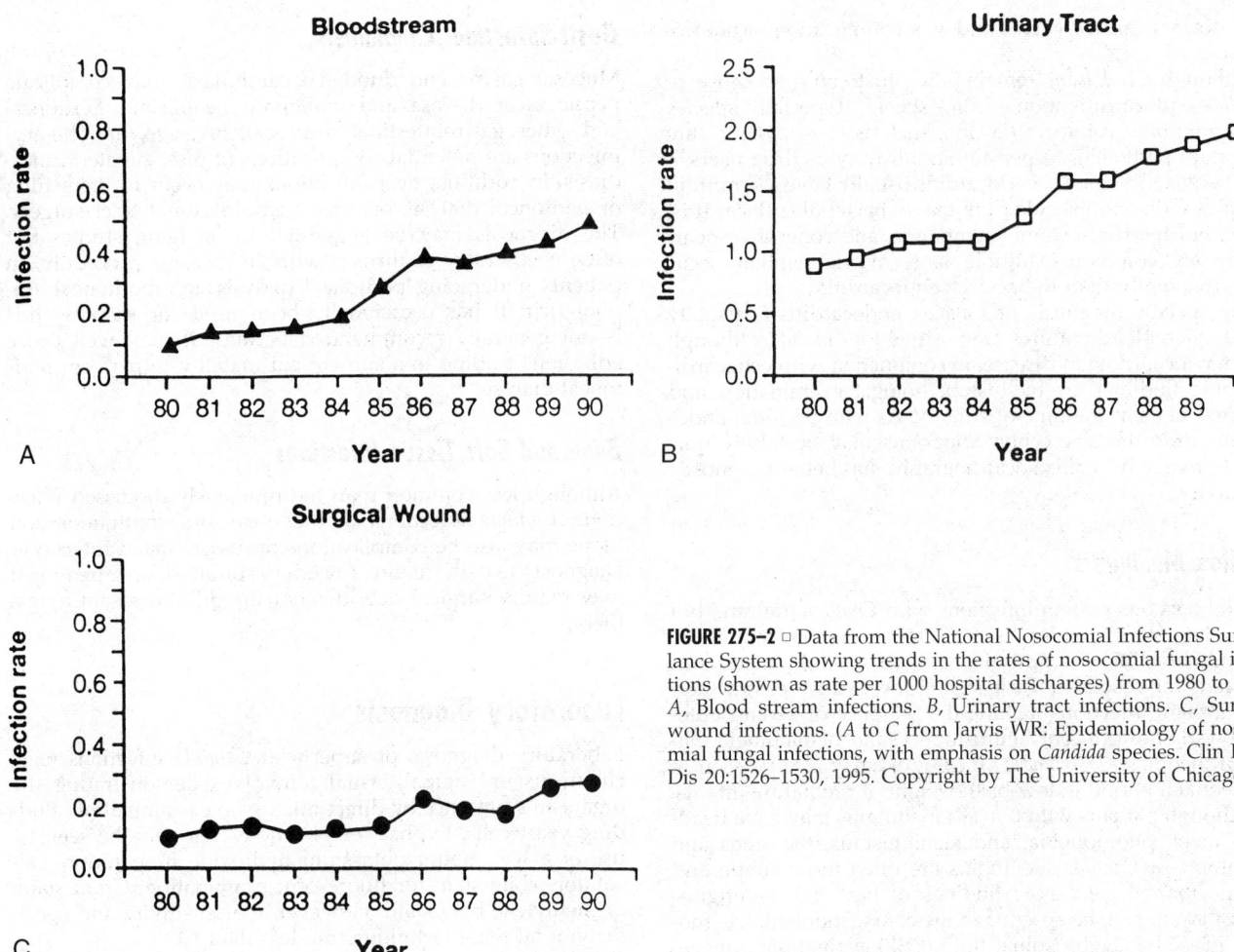

tural abnormality and for evidence of disseminated candidiasis.[66]

Ocular Infections

Although *Candida* species can cause infection of almost any area of the eye, the most common and serious ocular infection is *Candida* endophthalmitis. Most cases are due to *C. albicans*, but rare cases of *C. parapsilosis* and *C. krusei* infection are reported.[67–70] Endophthalmitis can occur either as a primary event, with direct infection of the eye in the setting of trauma or surgery, or as a secondary process in patients with candidemia. The latter is becoming increasingly frequent, and because the disease may be asymptomatic, all patients with candidemia should have an ophthalmoscopic examination to assess for its presence. Ophthalmoscopic examination to assess for the presence of *Candida* endophthalmitis is also useful as a method to detect deep tissue infection in the absence of positive blood cultures. Diagnosis of *Candida* endophthalmitis is usually made clinically by the typical appearance of the retina on ophthalmoscopic examination: a white lesion with indistinct margins. There may be extension into the vitreous or associated hemorrhage. In patients who do have symptoms, both ocular pain and visual disturbances have been reported. Ocular symptoms and the classic findings of *Candida* endophthalmitis are unusual in neutropenic patients.[2]

When the clinical picture is uncertain, a definitive diagnosis can be made by either a vitreous tap or a partial vitrectomy. Partial vitrectomy is also used as a therapeutic technique in some patients.[71] Early diagnosis is important to avoid disease progression that could require enucleation. Even with early institution of antifungal therapy, however, *Candida* endophthalmitis may lead to vitreal scarring with permanent visual impairment.

Candida keratitis, or keratoconjunctivitis, is an uncommon, exogenous, superficial *Candida* eye infection. The disease most often occurs after trauma or in patients receiving long-term steroid eyedrops. The diagnosis of fungal infection may be suggested by physical examination revealing ulcerative lesions with spidery borders or inflammation, but corneal scrapings for histopathologic examination and culture are necessary to establish the specific cause. A specific culture method is employed in which plates are streaked by the ophthalmologist immediately on obtaining cultures. The streaking is done in patterns, and fungal growth that is not in the area of streaking is not interpreted as a positive result.

Candida *Endocarditis*

Members of the genus *Candida* are the most common cause of fungal endocarditis. This infection is increasing in frequency in conjunction with the increased rates of the underlying risk factors for the disease. These risk factors include cardiac surgery, prosthetic heart valves, central venous catheters, and intravenous drug use. *Candida* endocarditis may also occur in the setting of a structurally abnormal native valve or as a secondary infection in patients with bacterial endocarditis. It is an extremely rare occurrence in patients with normal cardiac valves and as a complication of neutropenia.

Although *C. albicans* remains the most common cause of *Candida* endocarditis, non-*albicans* species, especially species that commonly colonize the skin, such as *C. parapsilosis*, are important pathogens, especially in intravenous drug users.[72]

Patients with *Candida* endocarditis usually have a symptom complex indistinguishable from that of bacterial endocarditis. Fever, nonspecific systemic symptoms, and congestive heart failure are common. Multiple large arterial emboli occur more frequently than in bacterial endocarditis.

The specific diagnosis of *Candida* endocarditis is usually made when blood cultures are positive for *Candida*, although this may occur late in disease, in conjunction with echocardiographic findings, or by histopathologic examination and cultures taken at the time of surgery. As with bacterial endocarditis, transthoracic echocardiograms may be falsely normal; transesophageal echocardiography has better diagnostic sensitivity.

Candida *Meningitis*

Central nervous system infections with *Candida* are rare, but when they occur, meningitis is the most common manifestation. Other clinical syndromes include mycotic aneurysms and cerebral abscesses. Risk factors for *Candida* central nervous system infections include the presence of a ventriculoperitoneal shunt, recent neurosurgery, and hematologic malignant neoplasms.[73] *Candida* meningitis may also be seen in the neonatal period in low-birth-weight or premature infants.

Although patients with *Candida* meningitis may have headache, fever, photophobia, and meningismus, the signs and symptoms of *Candida* meningitis are often more subtle and chronic than these classic findings of bacterial meningitis. Fever may, in fact, be absent and the course indolent. Diagnosis is made by cerebrospinal fluid (CSF) evaluation; nonspecific findings include a CSF pleocytosis (of either neutrophils or lymphocytes), increased protein concentration, and low glucose level. A CSF Gram stain may be positive, but the diagnosis is most often made by culture. It may, however, be necessary to perform repeated CSF analyses before documentation of a positive culture in patients with chronic *Candida* meningitis. In a review of 18 cases of chronic *Candida* meningitis, only 8 patients had a positive culture from the first CSF sample.[74] In contrast, cultures may be readily positive with postneurosurgical *Candida* meningitis or shunt infections. In addition to *C. albicans, C. tropicalis, C. parapsilosis, C. lusitaniae,* and *C. glabrata* have been identified as rare causes of postneurosurgical *Candida* meningitis or shunt infections.[75, 76]

Hepatosplenic Candidiasis

Hepatosplenic candidiasis is a syndrome of disseminated candidiasis found in patients being treated for acute leukemia or bone marrow transplant recipients who have had long periods of severe neutropenia. The disease is most often diagnosed when the neutrophil count is recovering. The patients have multifocal hepatic and splenic abscesses. At this point, patients may be noted to have fever once empirical antifungal therapy is stopped. Signs and symptoms, in addition to fever, usually include right upper quadrant abdominal pain, elevated liver function test results, and hepatosplenomegaly. Blood cultures are rarely positive, and the diagnosis is usually made by the characteristic appearance of multiple focal lesions in the liver and spleen as seen by computed tomography or ultrasonography. Computed tomography has been reported to have a higher sensitivity (93%) than ultrasonography (less than 50%).[77]

Gastrointestinal Candidiasis

Mucosal gastric and duodenal candidiasis may complicate peptic ulcer disease and malignant neoplasms. Peritoneal and other gastrointestinal (mucosal, invasive, and biliary) infections are potential complications of disseminated candidiasis. In addition, deep infections may occur in the setting of peritoneal dialysis or after gastrointestinal tract surgery. The diagnosis may be suggested by imaging studies but often needs to be confirmed with an invasive procedure. In patients undergoing peritoneal dialysis, intraperitoneal amphotericin B has occasionally been used for therapy; this is not generally recommended because it may well cause adhesions leading to a subsequent inability to perform peritoneal dialysis.

Bone and Soft Tissue Infections

Although less common than the previously discussed infections, *Candida* infections of the bone and contiguous soft tissue may also be complications of disseminated infections. Diagnosis usually requires needle aspiration, and treatment may require surgical débridement in addition to antifungal therapy.

Laboratory Diagnosis

Laboratory diagnosis of superficial *Candida* infections (e.g., cutaneous or vaginal) usually involves demonstrating the organism's presence by direct microscopic examination. Budding yeast cells, hyphae, or pseudohyphae may be seen by use of a wet mount potassium hydroxide preparation, calcofluor white stain for fluorescent examination, Gram stain, or methylene blue stain. However, the sensitivity and specificity of all these techniques are less than 100%.

Cultures play an important part in the diagnosis of invasive forms of candidiasis. However, a positive culture from the gastrointestinal or respiratory tract may represent colonization, and contamination of other specimens may occur; therefore, biopsy for histologic examination is necessary to prove invasion. Cultures from sterile sites, however, need to be interpreted as evidence of disease.

The techniques for culturing blood for *Candida* have improved in more recent years. There has been increased frequency and speed of recovery of yeast by the use of lysis-centrifugation techniques and automated continuously monitoring systems. Automated continuously monitoring systems detect the growth of organisms by means of a metabolic signal. Currently available automated systems include BACTEC 9240, BacT/Alert, ESP, and Vital. Although the total recovery of yeast and time to recovery are improved with use of these systems, there is some concern for false-negative results with candidemia because there may be instances in which organisms grow in the media but do not produce a metabolic signal.[78]

Once a culture is positive, species identification can be made by a number of different tests. *C. albicans* may be identified morphologically by means of the germ tube test (in which hyphae are produced from the yeast cells when the organism is incubated in serum at 37°C for 2 to 3 hours)[1] or by rapid commercially available enzymatic assays. Additional identification involves biochemical reactions done manually or with commercial automated systems. Reactions include urease activity, carbohydrate fermentation reactions, carbon assimilation patterns, and chromogenic enzymatic reactions. CHROMagar Candida is a new medium that allows presumptive identification of *Candida* species on the basis of reactions of species-specific enzymes with substrates in the medium that develop into different colors.[79] This medium is useful for detection of multiple yeast species in a specimen and for more rapid identification of these species. Finally, DNA-based assays have been shown to be feasible for the detection of *Candida* and are likely to play a larger role in the future for species identification.[80]

As noted previously, the lack of sensitivity of blood cultures for the diagnosis of disseminated candidiasis has been a major factor leading to the development of nonculture detection systems. Among studied techniques, enzyme-linked immunosorbent assay and latex agglutination tests have been shown to have low sensitivity in immunocompromised patients and low specificity in immunocompetent patients. Most antigen detection tests (including those for mannan and enolase) also lack the sensitivity and specificity to be clinically relied on.[81, 82] Detection of fungus-specific metabolites has the potential to be useful for diagnosis. One study has shown that elevated levels of D-arabinitol have a 74% sensitivity for the detection of fungemia and are present earlier than positive blood cultures; thus, D-arabinitol determination may be useful in addition to performing blood cultures.[83] DNA-based techniques, using polymerase chain reaction amplification methods, are also being developed as nonculture methods for detection of candidemia. A variety of DNA sequences, including those for 14-α-lanosterol demethylase, actin, and aspartic proteinase, have been studied as potential targets. Compared with cultures, these assays have a sensitivity ranging from 79% to 100%[80]; however, their sensitivity and specificity for the diagnosis of disseminated candidiasis, especially in patients with the absence of positive blood cultures, remain to be determined in large clinical trials.

In some situations, antifungal susceptibility testing should be performed to help guide therapeutic decisions. Susceptibility testing may be useful in the clinical setting of oral or esophageal candidiasis that is clinically refractory to systemic azole therapy, with breakthroughs of prophylaxis, for specific species (e.g., *C. lusitaniae,* which may develop resistance to amphotericin B),[84] and possibly for all positive blood cultures in patients for whom fluconazole therapy is contemplated. In vitro susceptibility testing has become more standardized in the past few years. Guidelines from the National Committee on Laboratory Standards recommend a system of broth macrodilution involving a series of tube dilutions. The minimal inhibitory concentration of an antifungal agent is the lowest concentration of that agent that inhibits the growth of the organism. These end points are clear with amphotericin B but tend to be less sharp with azoles. Therefore, because the amount of slight turbidity is usually the same for all concentrations above the minimal inhibitory concentration, an 80% inhibition standard is used to define the minimal inhibitory concentration for azoles. Although susceptibility testing has become more reproducible with use of these guidelines, breakpoints for susceptibility or resistance and development of easier methods, such as microtiter dilutions, need to be established. Further correlation of in vitro and in vivo results will be necessary to determine breakpoints.

Treatment

Treatment of *Candida* infections varies substantially on the basis of the anatomic location of disease, the patient's underlying risk factors for infection, the specific species responsible for infection, and in some cases the strain's susceptibility to drug. In general, the classes of agents used to treat candidiasis include allylamines (terbinafine), azoles (e.g., clotrimazole, ketoconazole, fluconazole, itraconazole), polyenes (e.g., nystatin, amphotericin B), and nucleoside analogs (flucytosine). Newer agents include lipid formulations of amphotericin B (amphotericin B lipid complex and liposomal amphotericin B). These medications were designed on the basis of the theory that toxicity could be decreased by providing site-specific delivery of amphotericin B by the use of phospholipid membranes or vesicles, thereby directly transferring the drug to the fungal membranes. Available data indicate that liposomal amphotericin B and amphotericin B lipid complex are less toxic than conventional amphotericin B, but there is also a substantial cost difference. There are currently insufficient data to determine how efficacious they are, and it is therefore not clear what the role of these alternative formulations will be. Newer agents that inhibit cell wall synthesis are in the early stages of clinical trials.[85]

Superficial, cutaneous infections may be treated with any of a number of topical agents, if the infection is localized and lacking nail involvement. Available topical agents include clotrimazole, ketoconazole, miconazole, nystatin, and terbinafine. With extensive cutaneous infection in immunocompromised patients, with folliculitis, or with nail involvement, treatment should usually include a systemic agent (most frequently an oral azole), with or without concomitant topical therapy.

Oral candidiasis may be treated with a topical agent (nystatin, clotrimazole, or amphotericin B oral suspension) or systemically with an oral azole or parenteral amphotericin B (in patients with azole resistance). *Candida* esophagitis requires systemic therapy, usually an oral azole, but parenteral amphotericin B may be similarly needed in patients who do not respond to azole therapy or in whom there is a concern for disseminated candidiasis.

Candida vaginitis is usually treated with a topical agent, but oral azoles have been shown to have clinical and microbiologic efficacy. The oral agents may also be useful in that they decrease gastrointestinal carriage of *Candida*, thought by some to be a reservoir that may lead to recurrent infections. Recurrent vulvovaginal infections do, in fact, often require chronic or prophylactic oral azole therapy for control.[50] There is no evidence from controlled trials to indicate that treatment of male sexual partners reduces recurrences in women[45]; however, such treatment is recommended by some clinicians.

Candidemia requires treatment in all populations of patients. Candidemia and disseminated candidiasis in neutropenic patients should be treated with parenteral amphotericin B (to a total dose of 0.5 to 1.0 g). *C. albicans* and *C. glabrata* infections may be treated with low to moderate doses of amphotericin B (0.5 to 0.6 mg/kg per day). Treatment with higher doses is often recommended for *C. krusei* and *C. tropicalis* infections (greater than 0.7 mg/kg per day, and often 1.0 mg/kg per day), whereas *C. parapsilosis* may show amphotericin B tolerance requiring moderate to high doses of amphotericin B often in combination with flucytosine. *C. lusitaniae* may be resistant to amphotericin B; susceptibility testing should be performed on this organism, and optimal therapy is likely to be a combination. Flucytosine should almost never be used alone because of the potential for the rapid development of resistance. When it is used in combination with amphotericin B or fluconazole, serum levels should be monitored (peak 70 to 80 μg/mL, trough 30 to 40 μg/mL) to prevent dose-related toxic effects. White blood cell growth factors, both granulocyte colony-stimulating factor and granulocyte-macrophage colony-stimulating factor, are often used to reduce the duration of neutropenia in these patients as an adjunctive measure in the treatment of infectious complications. There are no data on the specific role that these substances play in helping to prevent or treat *Candida* infections[81]; however, one study showed that bone marrow transplant patients with invasive candidiasis who received macrophage colony-stimulating factor had improved survival compared with historical control subjects.[86]

In nonneutropenic patients, fluconazole (400 mg/d for 14 days beyond the time of the last positive blood culture) can be used for the treatment of candidemia in relatively noncritically ill patients.[59] However, fluconazole should not be used in patients with infections due to *C. glabrata* or *C. krusei* given the lower susceptibility of these organisms to this agent. In addition to antifungal therapy, a crucial component of managing candidemia is the removal of intravenous catheters. When intravenous lines cannot be changed (e.g., because of severity of illness, thrombocytopenia, or a coagulopathy), aggressive therapy should be instituted with the realization that cultures remaining positive in this setting herald a poor prognosis.

Treatment of *Candida* urinary tract infections should involve changing the urinary catheter if one is present. Antifungal therapy should be with parenteral amphotericin B if there is a concern that candiduria is a manifestation of systemic infection; otherwise, oral azoles (e.g., fluconazole 100 mg/d) or amphotericin B bladder washings (50 mg of amphotericin B in 1 L of sterile water per day) may be used.[66]

Standard treatment of *Candida* endophthalmitis involves the use of parenteral amphotericin B with or without concomitant flucytosine. Intravitreal injection of antifungals is advocated by some. In some centers, partial vitrectomy is used as a therapeutic modality.[71] Although there are reports of successful use of systemic azole therapy,[87] none of these agents has been evaluated prospectively for use in endophthalmitis.

There are also case reports of successful medical therapy for *Candida* endocarditis,[88, 89] but in general, treatment of this disease requires a combined medical-surgical approach. Treatment with amphotericin B (0.6 to 0.8 mg/kg per day) should be initiated once the diagnosis is made. Valve replacement should then be performed and amphotericin B continued postoperatively. Recommendations are usually for a total duration of 6 to 10 weeks or a total dose of 1 to 2 g. Some authors recommend following amphotericin B therapy with fluconazole suppression.

Candida meningitis should be treated with amphotericin B (0.6 to 0.8 mg/kg per day), with or without flucytosine. Some patients are treated with intrathecal amphotericin B in addition to systemic therapy. Durations of therapy are not well defined but often extend to 6 weeks. Treatment of meningitis that occurs in the setting of a CSF shunt usually requires removal or replacement of the shunt.

Prophylaxis

Prophylaxis to prevent *Candida* infections has been used mainly in three groups of patients: those with HIV infection, patients who are neutropenic during cancer chemotherapy or after bone marrow transplantation, and solid organ transplant recipients.

In HIV-infected patients, a study comparing systemic fluconazole (200 mg/d) with topical clotrimazole in patients with $CD4^+$ cell counts less than 200/mm^3 showed that fluconazole prevented the development of esophageal candidiasis and other deep fungal infections but had no effect on mortality.[90] Nevertheless, because of concerns about cost, drug-drug interactions, and the potential development of azole resistance, fluconazole prophylaxis is still a matter of debate for this group of patients.

In neutropenic patients, prophylactic strategies have been considered in light of information that fungal colonization often precedes infection. Oral fluconazole (400 mg/d) has been shown to decrease fungal colonization, superficial and hematogenous infections, and mortality in bone marrow transplant patients and has been used in oncology centers for the purpose of preventing invasive candidiasis.[91–93] In patients with leukemia, however, a study comparing fluconazole with placebo during the period of neutropenia failed to show a difference in the rate of invasive fungal infections or mortality.[94] In addition, fluconazole has been shown in some studies to change the species responsible for colonization of these patients, with increases in *C. glabrata* and *C. krusei*.[64, 65]

Antifungal prophylaxis after solid organ transplantation, especially after liver transplantation, has often been recommended because of the high risk for fungal infections immediately after transplantation.[95–97] A randomized trial supported the use of fluconazole for this purpose. Compared with nystatin, fluconazole (100 mg/d) reduced both *Candida* colonization and infection after liver transplantation.[98]

Azole resistance is not commonly reported in *C. albicans* isolated from oncology or organ transplant patients. It is likely that the short courses of azole prophylaxis used in these populations lead to a lower risk for the development of resistance than is seen in HIV-infected patients who may receive extended azole therapy.

References

1. Odds FC: *Candida* and Candidiasis. A Review and Bibliography. Philadelphia, WB Saunders, 1988.
2. Bodey GP: Candidiasis. Pathogenesis, Diagnosis, and Treatment. New York, Raven Press, 1993.
3. Cutler JE: Putative virulence factors of *Candida albicans*. Annu Rev Microbiol 45:187, 1991.
4. Edison AM, Manning-Zweerink M: Comparison of the extracellular proteinase activity produced by a low-virulence mutant of *Candida albicans* and its wild-type parent. Infect Immun 56:1388, 1988.
5. Reagan DR, Pfaller MA, Hollis RJ, et al: Characterization of the sequence of colonization and nosocomial candidemia using DNA fingerprinting and a DNA probe. J Clin Microbiol 28:2733, 1990.
6. Voss A, Hollis RJ, Pfaller MA, et al: Investigation of the sequence of colonization and candidemia in nonneutropenic patients. J Clin Microbiol 32:975, 1994.
7. Pfaller MA: Epidemiology of fungal infections: The promise of molecular typing. Clin Infect Dis 20:1535, 1995.
8. Pfaller MA: Nosocomial candidiasis: Emerging species, reservoirs, and modes of transmission. Clin Infect Dis 22(Suppl 2):S89, 1996.
9. Plouffe JF, Brown DG, Silva J Jr, et al: Nosocomial outbreak of *Candida parapsilosis* fungemia related to intravenous infusions. Arch Intern Med 137:1686, 1977.
10. Bart-Delabesse E, Van Deventer H, Goessens W, et al: Contribution of molecular typing methods and antifungal susceptibility testing to the study of a candidemia cluster in a burn care unit. J Clin Microbiol 33:3278, 1995.
11. Fraser VJ, Jones M, Dunkel J, et al: Candidemia in a tertiary care hospital: Epidemiology, risk factors, and predictors of mortality. Clin Infect Dis 15:414, 1992.
12. Wey SB, Mori M, Pfaller MA, et al: Risk factors for hospital-acquired candidemia: A matched case-control study. Arch Intern Med 149:2349, 1989.
13. Vazquez JA, Sobel JD: Fungal infections in diabetes. Infect Dis Clin North Am 9:97, 1995.
14. Hosen H: Id reactions from focal fungus infections treated by immunological methods. Tex Med 69:83, 1973.
15. Bodey GP, Luna M: Skin lesions associated with disseminated candidiasis. JAMA 229:1466, 1974.
16. Jarowski CI, Fialk MA, Murray HW, et al: Fever, rash, and muscle tenderness: A distinctive clinical presentation of disseminated candidiasis. Arch Intern Med 138:544, 1978.
17. Marcus J, Grossman ME, Yunakov MJ, et al: Disseminated candidiasis, *Candida* arthritis, and unilateral skin lesions. J Am Acad Dermatol 26:295, 1992.

18. Calandra T, Francioli P, Glauser MP, et al: Disseminated candidiasis with extensive folliculitis in abusers of brown Iranian heroin. Eur J Clin Microbiol 4:340, 1985.
19. Darcis JM, Etienne M, Demonty J, et al: *Candida albicans* septicemia with folliculitis in heroin addicts. Am J Dermatopathol 8:501, 1986.
20. Dupont B, Drouhet E: Cutaneous, ocular, and osteoarticular candidiasis in heroin addicts: New clinical and therapeutic aspects in 38 patients. J Infect Dis 152:577, 1985.
21. Herrod HG: Chronic mucocutaneous candidiasis in childhood and complications of non-*Candida* infection: A report of the Pediatric Immunodeficiency Collaborative Study Group. J Pediatr 116:377, 1990.
22. Kauffman CA, Shea MJ, Frame PT: Invasive fungal infections in patients with chronic mucocutaneous candidiasis. Arch Intern Med 141:1076, 1981.
23. Edwards JE, Lehner RI, Stiehm ER, Fisher TJ: Severe candidal infections: Clinical perspective, immune defense mechanisms, and current concepts of therapy. Ann Intern Med 89:91, 1978.
24. Chipps BE, Saulsbury FT, Hsu SH, et al: Noncandidal infections in children with chronic mucocutaneous candidiasis. Johns Hopkins Med J 122:175, 1979.
25. Powderly WG: Mucosal candidiasis caused by non-*albicans* species of *Candida* in HIV-positive patients. AIDS 6:604, 1992.
26. Cameron ML, Schell WA, Bruch S, et al: Correlation of in vitro fluconazole resistance of *Candida* isolates in relation to therapy and symptoms of individuals seropositive for human immunodeficiency virus type 1. Antimicrob Agents Chemother 37:2449, 1993.
27. Chavanet P, Lopez J, Grappin M, et al: Cross-sectional study of the susceptibility of *Candida* isolates to antifungal drugs and in vitro–in vivo correlation in HIV-infected patients. AIDS 8:945, 1994.
28. Maenza JR, Keruly JC, Moore RD, et al: Risk factors for fluconazole-resistant candidiasis in human immunodeficiency virus–infected patients. J Infect Dis 173:219, 1996.
29. Vuffray A, Durussel C, Boerlin P, et al: Oropharyngeal candidiasis resistant to single-dose therapy with fluconazole in HIV-infected patients (Letter). AIDS 8:708, 1994.
30. Boken DJ, Swindells S, Rinaldi MG: Fluconazole-resistant *Candida albicans*. Clin Infect Dis 17:1018, 1993.
31. Redding S, Smith J, Farinacci G, et al: Resistance of *Candida albicans* to fluconazole during treatment of oropharyngeal candidiasis in a patient with AIDS: Documentation by in vitro susceptibility testing and DNA subtype analysis. Clin Infect Dis 18:240, 1994.
32. Newman SL, Flanigan TP, Fisher A, et al: Clinically significant mucosal candidiasis resistant to fluconazole treatment in patients with AIDS. Clin Infect Dis 19:684, 1994.
33. White A, Goetz MB: Azole-resistant *Candida albicans*: Report of two cases of resistance to fluconazole and review. Clin Infect Dis 19:687, 1994.
34. Bailey GG, Perry FM, Denning DW, Mandal BK: Fluconazole-resistant candidosis in an HIV cohort. AIDS 8:787, 1994.
35. Sangeorzan JA, Bradley SF, Xiaogang H, et al: Epidemiology of oral candidiasis in HIV-infected patients: Colonization, infection, treatment, and emergence of fluconazole resistance. Am J Med 97:339, 1994.
36. Sanguineti A, Carmichael K, Campbell K: Fluconazole-resistant *Candida albicans* after long-term suppressive therapy. Arch Intern Med 153:1122, 1993.
37. Maenza JR, Merz WG, Romagnoli MJ, et al: Infection due to fluconazole-resistant *Candida* in patients with AIDS: Prevalence and microbiology. Clin Infect Dis 24:28, 1997.
38. Revankar SG, Kirkpatrick WR, McAtee RK, et al: Detection and significance of fluconazole resistance in oropharyngeal candidiasis in human immunodeficiency virus–infected patients. J Infect Dis 174:821, 1996.
39. Caruso LJ: Vaginal moniliasis after tetracycline therapy: The effects of amphotericin B. Am J Obstet Gynecol 90:374, 1967.
40. Oriel JD, Waterworth PM: Effects of minocycline and tetracycline on the vaginal yeast flora. J Clin Pathol 28:403, 1975.
41. Morton RS, Rashid S: Candidal vaginitis: Natural history, predisposing factors, and prevention. Proc R Soc Med 70(Suppl 4):3, 1977.
42. Fleury FJ: Adult vaginitis. Clin Obstet Gynecol 24:407, 1981.
43. Catterall RD: Influence of estrogenic contraceptive pills on candidiasis. Br J Vener Dis 47:45, 1971.
44. Oriel JD, Partridge BM, Denny MJ, et al: Genital yeast infections. Br Med J 4:761, 1972.
45. Sobel JD: Pathophysiology of vulvovaginal candidiasis. J Reprod Med 34(Suppl 8):572, 1989.
46. Horowitz BJ, Giaquinta D, Ito S: Evolving pathogens in vulvovaginal candidiasis: Implications for patient care. J Clin Pharmacol 32:248, 1992.
47. Spinillo A, Michelone G, Cavanna C, et al: Clinical and microbiological characteristics of symptomatic vulvovaginal candidiasis in HIV-seropositive women. Genitourin Med 70:268, 1994.
48. Monif GRG: Classification and pathogenesis of vulvovaginal candidiasis. Am J Obstet Gynecol 152:935, 1985.
49. O'Connor MI, Sobel JD: Epidemiology of recurrent vulvovaginal candidiasis: Identification and strain differentiation of *Candida albicans*. J Infect Dis 154:358, 1986.
50. Sobel JD: Recurrent vulvovaginal candidiasis: A prospective study of the efficacy of maintenance ketoconazole therapy. N Engl J Med 315:1455, 1986.
51. Sobel JD: Epidemiology and pathogenesis of recurrent vulvovaginal candidiasis. Am J Obstet Gynecol 152:924, 1985.
52. Calderson-Marquez JJ: Itraconazole in the treatment of vaginal candidiasis and the effect of treatment of the sexual partner. Rev Infect Dis 9(Suppl 1):S143, 1987.
53. Buch A, Christensen ES: Treatment of vaginal candidiasis with natamycin and effect of treating the partner at the same time. Acta Obstet Gynecol Scand 61:393, 1982.
54. Bisschop MP, Merkus JM, Scheygrond H, van Cutsem J: Cotreatment of the male partner in vaginal candidiasis: A double-blind randomized control study. Br J Obstet Gynaecol 93:79, 1986.
55. Soll DR, Galask R, Schmid J, et al: Genetic dissimilarity of commensal strains of *Candida* spp. carried in different anatomical locations of the same healthy women. J Clin Microbiol 29:1702, 1991.
56. Banerjee SN, Emori TG, Culver DH, et al: Secular trends in nosocomial primary bloodstream infections in the United States, 1980–1989. Am J Med 91(Suppl 3B):86S, 1991.
57. Jarvis WR: Epidemiology of nosocomial fungal infections, with emphasis on *Candida* species. Clin Infect Dis 20:1526, 1995.
58. Wey SB, Mori M, Pfaller MA, et al: Hospital-acquired candidemia: The attributable mortality and excess length of stay. Arch Intern Med 148:2642, 1988.
59. Rex JH, Bennett JE, Sugar AM, et al: A randomized trial comparing fluconazole with amphotericin B for the treatment of candidemia in patients without neutropenia. N Engl J Med 331:1325, 1994.
60. Berenguer J, Buck M, Witebsky F, et al: Lysis-centrifugation blood cultures in the detection of tissue-proven invasive candidiasis. Diagn Microbiol Infect Dis 17:103, 1993.
61. Sanford GR, Merz WG, Wingard JR, et al: The value of fungal surveillance cultures as predictors of systemic fungal infections. J Infect Dis 142:503, 1980.
62. Maenza JR, Merz WG: Candidemia: Epidemiology and laboratory detection. Infect Dis Clin Pract 2:83, 1997.
63. Wingard JR: Importance of *Candida* species other than *C. albicans* as pathogens in oncology patients. Clin Infect Dis 20:115, 1995.
64. Wingard JR, Merz WG, Rinaldi MG, et al: Increase in *Candida krusei* infection among patients with bone marrow transplantation and neutropenia treated prophylactically with fluconazole. N Engl J Med 325:1274, 1991.
65. Wingard JR, Merz WG, Rinaldi MG, et al: Association of *Torulopsis glabrata* infections with fluconazole prophylaxis in neutropenic bone marrow transplant patients. Antimicrob Agents Chemother 37:1847, 1993.
66. Fisher JF, Newman CL, Sobel JD: Yeast in the urine: Solutions for a budding problem. Clin Infect Dis 20:183, 1995.
67. Weens JJ Jr: *Candida parapsilosis*: Epidemiology, pathogenicity, clinical manifestations, and antimicrobial susceptibility. Clin Infect Dis 14:756, 1992.
68. McQuillen DP, Zingman BS, Meunier F, Levitz SM: Invasive infections due to *Candida krusei*: Report of ten cases of fungemia that include three cases of endophthalmitis. Clin Infect Dis 14:472, 1992.
69. Joshi N, Hamory BH: Endophthalmitis caused by non-*albicans* species of *Candida*. Rev Infect Dis 13:281, 1991.

70. O'Day DM, Head WS, Robinson RD: An outbreak of *Candida parapsilosis* endophthalmitis: Analysis of strains by enzyme profile and antifungal susceptibility. Br J Ophthalmol 71:126, 1987.
71. Snip RC, Michels RG: Pars plana vitrectomy in the management of endogenous *Candida* endophthalmitis. Am J Ophthalmol 82:699, 1976.
72. Andriole VT: Endocarditis in the drug user. Conn Med 34:327, 1970.
73. Bayer AS, Edwards JE Jr, Seidel JS, Guze LB: *Candida* meningitis. Report of seven cases and review of the English literature. Medicine (Baltimore) 55:477, 1976.
74. Voice RA, Bradley SF, Sangeorzan JA, Kauffman CA: Chronic candidal meningitis: An uncommon manifestation of candidiasis. Clin Infect Dis 19:60, 1994.
75. Nguyen MH, Yu VL: Meningitis caused by *Candida* species: An emerging problem in neurosurgical patients. Clin Infect Dis 21:323, 1995.
76. Sánchez-Portocarrero J, Martín-Rabadán, Saldaña CJ: *Candida* cerebrospinal fluid shunt infection. Diagn Microbiol Infect Dis 20:33, 1994.
77. Anttila Veli-Jukka, Ruutu P, Bondestam S, et al: Hepatosplenic yeast infection in patients with acute leukemia: A diagnostic problem. Clin Infect Dis 18:979, 1994.
78. Wakefield T, Wagner D, Antik N, et al: Importance of >5 day incubation or terminal subculture of BacT/Alert and BACTEC 460 blood culture systems (Abstr C-72). *In* Abstracts of the General Meeting of the American Society for Microbiology; May 16–20, 1993; Atlanta; p 458.
79. Odds FC, Bernaerts R: CHROMagar Candida, a new differential isolation medium for presumptive identification of clinically important *Candida* species. J Clin Microbiol 32:1923, 1994.
80. Mitchell TG, Sandin RL, Bowman BH, et al: Molecular mycology: DNA probes and applications of PCR technology. J Med Vet Mycol 32(Suppl 1):351, 1994.
81. Swerdloff JN, Filler SG, Edwards JE Jr: Severe candidal infections in neutropenic patients. Clin Infect Dis 17(Suppl 2):S457, 1993.
82. Harley WB, Dummer JS: Diagnosis of disseminated candidiasis by detection of antigenemia: A critical review. Infect Dis Clin Pract 3:168, 1994.
83. Walsh TJ, Merz WG, Lee JW, et al: Diagnosis and therapeutic monitoring of invasive candidiasis by rapid enzymatic detection of serum D-arabinitol. Am J Med 99:164, 1995.
84. Edwards JE Jr, Filler SG: Current strategies for treating invasive candidiasis: Emphasis on infections in nonneutropenic patients. Clin Infect Dis 14(Suppl 1):S106, 1992.
85. Hector RF: Compounds active against cell walls of medically important fungi. Clin Microbiol Rev 6:1, 1993.
86. Nemunaitis J, Shannon-Dorcy K, Appelbaum FR, et al: Long-term follow-up of patients with invasive fungal disease who received adjunctive therapy with recombinant human macrophage colony-stimulating factor. Blood 82:1422, 1993.
87. Akler ME, Vellend H, McNeely DM, et al: Use of fluconazole in the treatment of candidal endophthalmitis. Clin Infect Dis 20:657, 1995.
88. Wells CJ, Leech GJ, Lever AML, Wansbrough-Jones MH: Treatment of native valve *Candida* endocarditis with fluconazole. J Infect 31:233, 1995.
89. Zahid MA, Klotz SA, Hinthorn DR: Medical treatment of recurrent candidemia in a patient with probable *Candida parapsilosis* prosthetic valve endocarditis. Chest 105:1597, 1994.
90. Powderly WG, Finkelstein DM, Feinberg J, et al: A randomized trial comparing fluconazole with clotrimazole troches for the prevention of fungal infections in patients with advanced human immunodeficiency virus infection. N Engl J Med 332:700, 1995.
91. Uzan O, Anaissie EJ: Antifungal prophylaxis in patients with hematologic malignancies: A reappraisal. Blood 86:2063, 1995.
92. Goodman JL, Winston DJ, Greenfield RA, et al: A controlled trial of fluconazole to prevent fungal infections in patients undergoing bone marrow transplantation. N Engl J Med 326:845, 1992.
93. Slavin MA, Osborne B, Adams R, et al: Efficacy and safety of fluconazole prophylaxis for fungal infections after marrow transplantation—A prospective, randomized, double-blind study. J Infect Dis 171:1545, 1995.
94. Winston DJ, Chandrasekar PH, Lazarus HM: Fluconazole prophylaxis of fungal infections in patients with acute leukemia. Ann Intern Med 188:495, 1993.
95. Paya CV: Fungal infections in solid-organ transplantation. Clin Infect Dis 16:677, 1993.
96. Warnock DW: Fungal complications of transplantation: Diagnosis, treatment and prevention. J Antimicrob Chemother 36(Suppl B):73, 1995.
97. Kung N, Fisher N, Gunson B, et al: Fluconazole prophylaxis for high-risk liver transplant recipients. Lancet 345:1234, 1995.
98. Lumbreras C, Cuervas-Mons V, Jara P, et al: Randomized trial of fluconazole versus nystatin for the prophylaxis of *Candida* infection following liver transplantation. J Infect Dis 174:583, 1996.

276

Cryptococcus neoformans

John R. Graybill

History

Cryptococcus neoformans, the agent of cryptococcosis, has been recognized as a pathogen in humans since 1894, but it was considered an uncommon cause of disease until recent years.

Characteristics of the Pathogen

C. neoformans is familiar to us as the only encapsulated fungus, a characteristic that is relevant not only to classification but also to pathogenicity. *C. neoformans* was formerly considered an asexually reproducing yeast, but Kwon-Chung[1] was able to identify mating types and convert the organism to its perfect mycelial form, *Filobasidiella neoformans.* When the basidiospores are plated onto routine culture media or inoculated into mice, they convert to typical encapsulated cryptococci within a few days.

When cultured either from the environment or from patients, the fungus appears as small, yeastlike cells with narrow-based budding daughter cells.[2] The capsule is composed of α-kinked D-mannopyranoside residues.[3, 4] The presence of a capsule is readily detected by the India ink or nigrosin test, in which a specimen is mixed with either India ink or nigrosin and examined under a microscope. A halo effect about the organism distinguishes the capsule. Capsular material can also be stained in tissues with mucicarmine. Indirectly, the capsular polysaccharide can be identified immunologically with specific antibodies raised against it. This is the basis of the diagnostic latex cryptococcal agglutination test (LCAT).[5] The LCAT has been modified as an enzyme-linked immunosorbent assay (cryptococcal antigen test). Finally, *C. neoformans* colonies can be identified in culture media containing caffeic acid.[6] *C. neoformans* can uniquely metabolize caffeic acid to a melanin-like pigment, making the brown cryptococcal colonies readily distinguishable from other fungal colonies.

Epidemiology

C. neoformans has been divided into *C. neoformans* var. *neoformans* (serotypes A and D) and *C. neoformans* var. *gattii* (serotypes B and C). *C. neoformans* var. *gattii* has caused cryptococcosis mainly in patients without acquired immunodeficiency syndrome (AIDS), largely in Australia, with a few cases along the southern California coast and in the tropical Americas. The ecologic niche of the mycelial form of *C. neoformans* var. *gattii* is *Eucalyptus camaldulensis*, the Australian red river gum tree. It is likely that the organism reached the Americas with importation of this tree. Such a natural plant reservoir for the globally distributed *C. neoformans* var. *neoformans* has not yet been appreciated. *C. neoformans* var. *neoformans* has been recovered from pigeon droppings, excreta of other birds, and a variety of fruits. All four serotypes are pathogenic to humans, but *C. neoformans* var. *neoformans* causes most human disease, and the most common serotype is A.[4]

Among the groups most commonly exposed to *C. neoformans* are pigeon fanciers. These people rarely become ill with cryptococcosis, but they develop delayed-type hypersensitivity to cryptococcal antigens, indicating prior infection. Most of those who become ill with cryptococcosis are immunosuppressed. In the past, this population included mostly patients who had depressed cell-mediated immunity[7–10] as a result of lymphocytic leukemia, lymphomas, steroid therapy, or another underlying disorder. These groups accounted for 300 to 500 cases per year in the United States. At present, by far the most commonly affected group is patients with AIDS; 5% to 7% of AIDS patients in the United States and up to 30% in Africa develop cryptococcosis.[11] The organism is thought to be transmitted only by the respiratory route and not directly from one human to another.

Pathogenesis

Much of our understanding of the pathogenesis and host defense mechanisms comes from studies of animal models, especially mice. Presumably, after being inhaled, *C. neoformans* is ingested by alveolar macrophages. The efficiency of phagocytosis in vivo is not clear and may depend in part on the antiphagocytic properties of the capsule.[12] Unencapsulated yeast cells are readily phagocytosed and killed, whereas encapsulated cells are more resistant. Both macrophages and polymorphonuclear leukocytes can ingest and kill cryptococci, and the process may depend in part on opsonization by complement and antibody directed at the capsule.[13–17] Monoclonal antibodies to capsular polysaccharide have been used successfully to passively immunize mice against *C. neoformans*.[16] Antibodies derived from humans immunized with cryptococcal capsular polysaccharide antigens are protective in mice.[18] Thus, humoral immune mechanisms are important in resistance to *C. neoformans*. Various cell-mediated mechanisms have also been demonstrated in the murine model. Among these, there is evidence that natural killer cells may participate in early killing of cryptococci and that antibody-dependent cell-mediated killing may be operative as well.[17, 19, 20] Within the first week after immunization of mice with cryptococcal antigens, helper T-lymphocyte activity can be demonstrated[21]; in the first week after infection, first-order suppressor T cells are also generated, which stimulate second-order suppressor cells, which suppress the helper T cells.[21] Yet a third order of suppressor T cells has been discovered.[22] The exact effect of suppressor cells in vivo is not clear. In a successful host response, there is an increase in helper T-cell activity, skin test conversion, and reduction of *C. neoformans* organisms in tissue counts.[12, 23] Therefore, it is clear in mice that T lymphocytes are critical to successful host defenses, and the clinical settings of cryptococcosis strongly support a similar role in humans.

C. neoformans may pass through the lungs clinically unsuspected, the later development of meningitis being the first indication of disease. Alternatively, if the infection is contained in the lungs, it may cause pneumonia, poorly defined mass lesions, pulmonary nodules, occasional hilar adenopathy, and rarely pleural effusion.[7, 8, 24] Patients with disease limited to the lungs often have no major defects of cell-mediated immunity, although immune defects are common to patients with disseminated disease.

When *C. neoformans* escapes from the lungs, the major secondary site of infection is the meninges. In AIDS patients, the infection is usually widely distributed and also commonly infects the prostate.[25] The prostate and central nervous system are major sources of relapse for AIDS patients if therapy is interrupted.

Either the enzyme phenoloxidase or its product melanin is the major virulence factor in the neurotropism of *C. neoformans*, but the exact mechanism is not worked out. In patients who do not have AIDS, a chronic lymphocytic inflammatory response is elicited in the cerebrospinal fluid (CSF). There are usually 10 to 100 lymphocytes per mm^3, reduced CSF glucose value, and elevated protein level. As many as two thirds of patients have positive LCAT results for antigen. The LCAT or cryptococcal antigen test result is positive in most patients.

The chronic inflammation may involve the aqueduct of Sylvius, producing obstructive hydrocephalus. There may also be vasculitis, with subsequent focal ischemic damage to the brain or cranial nerves. There may be diffuse inflammation of the meninges, which impairs reabsorption of CSF and causes communicating hydrocephalus. Extracerebral foci of infection may also include the skin, prostate, other soft tissues, and bones.

Clinical Course of Infection

Although the first encounter of humans with *C. neoformans* occurs in the lungs, it is surprising that cryptococcal pneumonia occurs in less than 15% of patients (Fig. 276–1). Pulmonary infection may be manifested by cough that produces mucoid sputum, by chest pain, and sometimes by fever. Cavitations and calcification are rare. One study of patients with cryptococcal infection confirmed that many of them were either only modestly symptomatic or asymptomatic during their pulmonary infection, but the patients with immune suppression tended to develop meningitis, whereas immunocompetent patients have disease confined to the lungs.[8]

The most dangerous form of disease, and that most frequently encountered, is meningitis. This takes the form of

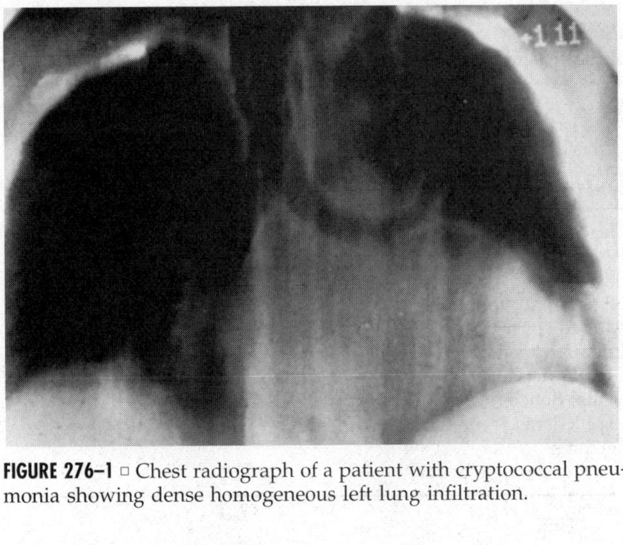

FIGURE 276–1 □ Chest radiograph of a patient with cryptococcal pneumonia showing dense homogeneous left lung infiltration.

chronic meningitis, with progressive headache, personality changes, dementia, and focal neurologic findings related to vascular or cranial nerve involvement (Table 276–1). Loss of vision may be associated with papilledema and high CSF pressure or may be due to direct involvement of the optic nerve by *C. neoformans*. More than half of the patients have no meningismus or fever. Cryptococcal meningitis may be completely asymptomatic early in the course.[26] Less commonly, there may be nodular or ulcerative skin lesions.[27] Focal osteomyelitis may also occur.

Intracerebral hypertension causes a potentially lethal syndrome of increased headache, papilledema, obtundation, and coma.[28] This occurs during the first week of treatment in up to 5% of patients. The mechanism for intracerebral hypertension is unclear but may relate to either the load of fungal organisms impeding CSF drainage or osmotic effects of high CSF capsular polysaccharide. Computed tomography does not usually show evidence of obstructive hydrocephalus, and the pressure may be relieved by serial lumbar punctures with drainage of large volumes of fluid. Rapid attention to this acute problem may be the major reason for the sharp reduction of early mortality to less than 10% in cryptococcal meningitis. This was seen in the most recent study of the Mycoses Study Group and AIDS Clinical Trials Group (Saag M, Graybill JR, unpublished observations).

Diagnosis

The diagnosis of cryptococcosis depends on demonstrating the organism or its capsular polysaccharide in tissues or body fluids.[5, 9] Because *C. neoformans* may be a commensal organism, its recovery from sputum cultures does not establish a diagnosis of invasive cryptococcosis; however, multiple cultures, when associated with pulmonary infiltrates or mass lesions, do support a diagnosis of pulmonary cryptococcal disease.[7, 24] Recovery of *C. neoformans* from tissue biopsy specimens, urine, blood, bone marrow, or CSF establishes the diagnosis of invasive cryptococcosis. In the case of tissue obtained without cultures, Gomori methenamine silver stain identifies yeast cells, but mucicarmine stain is necessary to confirm that the organism is *C. neoformans*. Unfortunately, some clinical isolates of *C. neoformans* have produced minimal polysaccharide, and the findings of mucicarmine stain examination may be equivocal (Rinaldi MG, Graybill JR, unpublished observations).

Demonstration of the pathogen on an India ink preparation is pathognomonic for *C. neoformans* infection, but the observer must distinguish yeast cells from talc granules (which come from the gloves used during lumbar puncture), erythrocytes, and leukocytes (Table 276–2). The India ink preparation finding is positive in more than half of non-AIDS patients with meningitis and in even more of those with AIDS.[29, 30]

TABLE 276–1 ■ Signs and Symptoms of Cryptococcal Meningoencephalitis at the Time of Hospitalization

SIGN OR SYMPTOM	NUMBER: Not Immunosuppressed	NUMBER: Acquired Immunodeficiency Syndrome
Headache	91	82
Fever	64	75
Stiff neck	75	33
Nausea and vomiting	55	46
Altered consciousness	50	24
Impaired mentation	41	16
Cranial nerve lesion	50	15
Visual deficits	27	10
Papilledema	27	8
Seizures	7	18
Focal neurologic deficits	11	5

TABLE 276–2 ■ Typical Cerebrospinal Fluid Findings in Cryptococcal Meningitis*

MEASURE	NON-AIDS	AIDS
Leukocytes per mm³	10–300	<5
Differential	>80% lymphocytes	>80% lymphocytes
Glucose value	<40 mg/dL	>40 mg/dL
Protein level	100–300 mg/dL	20–100 mg/dL
Positive finding on India ink preparation	60%–70%	>90%
Cerebrospinal fluid CRAG titer	1:1–1:512 Usually <1:1000	1:1–1:1,000,000 Frequently >1:1000
Serum CRAG test result positive	70%	>90%

*AIDS, Acquired immunodeficiency syndrome; CRAG, cryptococcal antigen. Data from references 5, 9, 12, 29, 30, 34.

A positive LCAT or cryptococcal antigen test result is significant for diagnosis in any titer. In the serum, false-positive results may be associated with antigen-antibody complexes and rarely with infection caused by *Trichosporon beigelii*, an organism with cell wall antigens similar to those of *C. neoformans*. One may either boil the serum or treat it with pronase to denature proteins; the capsular polysaccharide antigen is not affected by these treatments. The LCAT result is positive in the serum of about 70% of non-AIDS patients with cryptococcosis and in more than 90% of patients with AIDS and cryptococcosis. The significance of a positive serum LCAT result in non-AIDS patients is not clear. However, there is general agreement that a positive serum antigen test result in patients with AIDS, even with no recovery of organisms from any tissue, is an indication for treatment to prevent meningitis. The CSF LCAT is useful for both diagnosis and prognosis. Whereas there is no correlation of serum titer with outcome, a high initial CSF titer greater than 1:1024 in patients with AIDS is a predictor of a fatal outcome[25] (Table 276–3). Obtundation and CSF cell counts below 20/mm³ are also predictors of a poor outcome. During therapy for acute infection, an unchanged or rising CSF (but not serum) LCAT titer is predictive of treatment failure, and a rise of the titer during long-term suppressive therapy is predictive of relapse.[31]

The differential diagnosis of cryptococcosis, particularly meningitis, is broad. It includes chronic infectious meningitis, as from syphilis, brucellosis, tuberculosis, histoplasmosis, coccidioidomycosis, cysticercosis, or even epidural abscess; neoplastic processes, such as lymphoma or carcinomatous meningitis; autoimmune diseases, such as systemic lupus erythematosus; and a variety of miscellaneous diseases, including sarcoidosis.

Treatment

Treatment of cryptococcal meningitis has undergone dramatic changes, and these are continuing at present. Most investigations have been concentrated in patients infected with human immunodeficiency virus, who represent the majority of those with cryptococcosis. The traditional therapy for patients without AIDS has been 0.3 mg/kg of amphotericin B per day, given intravenously and up to 150 mg/kg per day of flucytosine, given orally, for as long as 6 weeks.[32] This

TABLE 276–3 ■ Value of Cryptococcal Antigen Measurement in Management of Acquired Immunodeficiency Syndrome–Associated Cryptococcal Meningitis

		INDICATED TITER CHANGE					
		Decrease		No change		Increase	
GROUP		*N*	%	*N*	%	*N*	%
INITIAL TREATMENT: Baseline cerebrospinal fluid titer ≥1:8							
Responders	(*N* = 21)	18	86	2	9	1	5
Failures	(*N* = 25)	11	44	12	48	2	8
$P < .01$ for responders versus failures							
LONG-TERM SUPPRESSION AFTER INITIAL TREATMENT							
Cerebrospinal Fluid Titer							
Success	(*N* = 126)	74	59	46	36	6	5
Relapse	(*N* = 14)	4	29	4	29	6	43
$P = .001$ for successful suppression versus relapse							
Serum Titer							
Success	(*N* = 157)	67	43	68	43	22	14
Relapse	(*N* = 13)	6	46	5	39	2	15
No correlation of serum titer with relapse							

Data from Powderly WG, Cloud GA, Dismukes WA, Saag MS: Measurement of cryptococcal antigen in serum and cerebrospinal fluid: Value in the management of AIDS-associated cryptococcal meningitis. Clin Infect Dis 18:789–792, 1992.

regimen is curative in up to 75% of non-AIDS patients. A shorter 4-week course in patients who have uncomplicated disease has been suggested but is not generally accepted.[33]

Much more is known about treatment response in patients with AIDS and cryptococcosis. Initial reports noted high treatment failure and relapse rates after amphotericin B and flucytosine administration was terminated.[29, 34] Two large randomized studies indicated that long-term fluconazole suppression therapy (2% to 3% relapse) was more effective in preventing relapse than placebo (37%) or weekly amphotericin B (18%) and better tolerated than amphotericin B.[25, 35] Thus, after initial treatment, there is widespread agreement that fluconazole should be continued indefinitely at 200 mg/d to prevent relapse. It is not known whether late relapses are caused by noncompliance with suppressive treatment or by emergence of fluconazole-resistant isolates[36, 37] (Table 276–4).

Although there is agreement on suppressive therapy, there is little concordance on initial regimens. Initial reports of fluconazole and itraconazole were encouraging for clinical responses. However, less than 50% of patients showed CSF culture result conversion to negative, and there were late microbiologic relapses noted for itraconazole recipients.[25, 36, 38] Further, in two comparative trials of fluconazole versus amphotericin B, responses to amphotericin B (conversion of CSF culture results to negative) occurred more frequently and also more rapidly than to fluconazole (Table 276–5). The median time of conversion was 42 days for amphotericin B versus 64 days for fluconazole.[25] In the most recent investigations, two directions were taken to increase the rate and rapidity of initial response. The Mycoses Study Group evaluated 2 weeks of amphotericin B with or without flucytosine followed by long-term triazole therapy or fluconazole (Mycoses Study Group 17, results unpublished). The other approach was taken by the California Cooperative Treatment Group, which evaluated an oral regimen of fluconazole (400 mg/d) plus flucytosine (150 mg/kg per day).[39] Preliminary findings suggest advantages in both approaches.

In the initial series by the California Cooperative Treatment Group, 67% of patients had culture result conversion of their CSF during the 8-week course of therapy evaluated. With use of the oral regimen, the toxic effect of flucytosine was still a problem in some patients at the high dose of 150 mg/kg per day; 28% of 20 patients stopped therapy because of intolerance to flucytosine.[40] However, responses were rapid, and this approach may reduce flucytosine toxicity and yet still allow rapid CSF culture result conversions, totaling 75% in 32 patients in 10 weeks. In continuing studies, not yet published, the California Cooperative Treatment Group had data suggesting that the addition of flucytosine to fluconazole and raising the starting dose of fluconazole to as high as 1600 mg/d both have therapeutic value. This less toxic oral regimen is favored by some on the grounds of efficacy and reduced toxicity.

The approach taken by the Mycoses Study Group and AIDS Clinical Trials Groups has been to treat with amphotericin B for 2 weeks and to follow this with antifungal triazole therapy for an additional 8 weeks for "induction" therapy.[41] The initial 2-week period included either amphotericin B at 0.7 mg/kg per day or amphotericin B plus flucytosine at 100 mg/kg per day orally. With careful observation of CSF pressure and repeated mechanical drainage of CSF for high pressures (few patients had obstructive hydrocephalus at computed tomography), the mortality during the first 2 weeks of treatment was less than 6%. Of 381 patients entered into the study, approximately 80% of either treatment group had clinically improved by 2 weeks of therapy. Those who received amphotericin B alone had 51% negative culture results versus 60% for those receiving combined amphotericin B and flucytosine ($P = .06$). Few people left the study because of flucytosine toxic effects, suggesting that flucytosine was well tolerated. In addition, flucytosine was administered without blood level measurement, and dose adjustment was based on renal function and peripheral blood cell counts. At a 1-year follow-up of patients who achieved negative CSF culture results during primary therapy, only 2 flucytosine recipients relapsed versus 13 of those who had not received

TABLE 276–4 ■ Percent Relapses with Long-Term Suppressive Therapy

	PLACEBO		AMPHOTERICIN B		FLUCONAZOLE		ITRACONAZOLE	
STUDY	*N*	%	*N*	%	*N*	%	*N*	%
Bozette et al[25]*	27	37			34	3		
Powderly et al[39]†			78	18	111	2		
Mycoses Study Group 025‡ (unpublished data)					51	4	57	23

*Fluconazole at 200 mg/d superior to placebo.
†Fluconazole at 200 mg/d superior to amphotericin B at 1 mg/kg/wk.
‡Fluconazole at 200 mg/d superior to itraconazole at 200 mg/d.

TABLE 276–5 ■ Results of Initial Treatment of Cryptococcal Meningitis in Patients with Acquired Immunodeficiency Syndrome*

STUDY	AMPHOTERICIN B ± FLUCYTOSINE		FLUCONAZOLE		ITRACONAZOLE		FLUCONAZOLE + FLUCYTOSINE	
	N	% Success	N	% Success	N	% Success	N	% Success
Larsen et al[36]	6	100	14	43				
Saag et al[18]	63	40	131	34				
Moskovitz et al[45]					29	38	37	41
Larsen et al[38]							32	75

*Successful treatment is defined as conversion of cerebrospinal fluid culture results to negative within 10 wk.

flucytosine. On the basis of these findings, 2 weeks of combined amphotericin B and flucytosine therapy is recommended. After completion of 2 weeks of therapy, fluconazole or itraconazole at 400 mg/d was given for an additional 8 weeks.[42] Clinical responses and negative CSF culture results were similar for both groups. Itraconazole was as effective as fluconazole at 400 mg/d from weeks 2 to 10. However, at 200 mg/d for long-term suppressive therapy, fluconazole was superior (2 of 51 patients microbiologically relapsed) to itraconazole (13 of 57 patients relapsed).[43] Thus, this study also supports fluconazole at 200 mg/d for long-term suppressive therapy.

As we look forward, new agents appearing on the horizon may further modify these recommendations. One is a reduction of amphotericin B toxicity by using lipid-associated forms of amphotericin B, such as liposomes (AmBisome [Nexstar, San Dimas, CA]), amphotericin B lipid complex (Liposome Company, Princeton, NJ), or amphotericin B colloidal dispersion (Amphocil [Zeneca, Macclesfield, UK, and Sequus, Menlo Park, CA]). All have some efficacy and reduced toxicity compared with amphotericin B. They are also costly, and it is unclear whether they will replace amphotericin B, given the modest indication of reduced toxicity.

Finally, there is renewed interest in using cytokines such as granulocyte stimulation factor, interferon-γ, and others in a combined cytokine–antifungal drug regimen.[44] There has also been an increased interest in treatment with monoclonal antibodies to *C. neoformans*.[18] Such antibodies prolong survival in infected mice and may help to eliminate capsular polysaccharide antigen from the CSF and thus prevent CSF hypertension. There are no published clinical studies, however. A vaccine in early stages of development has been produced to immunize against *C. neoformans* by generating high-titer protective antibodies in normal humans. It may be placed into comparative trial in the near future.[40, 45]

References

1. Kwon-Chung KJ: A new genus, *Filobasidiella*, the perfect state of *Cryptococcus neoformans*. Mycologia 67:1197, 1975.
2. Neilson JB, Fromtling RA, Bulmer GS: *Cryptococcus neoformans*: Size range of infectious particles from aerosolized soil. Infect Immun 17:634, 1977.
3. Bhattacharjee AK, Kwon-Chung KJ, Glaudemans CP: On the structure of the capsular polysaccharide from *Cryptococcus neoformans* serotype C. Immunochemistry 15:673, 1978.
4. Bhattacharjee AK, Bennett JE, Glaudemans CPJ: Capsular polysaccharide from *Cryptococcus neoformans*. Rev Infect Dis 6:619, 1984.
5. Kaufman CA, Bergman AG, Severance PJ, et al: Detection of cryptococcal antigen: Comparison of two latex agglutination tests. Am J Clin Pathol 81:106, 1980.
6. Wang HS, Zeimis RT, Roberts GD: Evaluation of a caffeic acidferric citrate test for rapid identification of *Cryptococcus neoformans*. J Clin Microbiol 6:445, 1977.
7. Hammerman KG, Powell KE, Christianson CS, et al: Cryptococcosis: Clinical forms and treatment. Am Rev Respir Dis 108:1116, 1973.
8. Kerkering TM, Duma RJ, Shadomy S: The evolution of pulmonary cryptococcosis. Ann Intern Med 94:611, 1981.
9. Diamond RD, Bennett JE: Prognostic factors in cryptococcal meningitis: A study of 111 cases. Ann Intern Med 80:175, 1974.
10. Kaplan MH, Rosen PP, Armstrong D: Cryptococcosis in a cancer hospital. Clinical and pathological correlates in forty-six patients. Cancer 39:2265, 1977.
11. Dismukes WE: Cryptococcal meningitis in patients with AIDS. J Infect Dis 157:624, 1988.
12. Fromtling RA, Shadomy HJ: Immunity in cryptococcosis: An overview. Mycopatholgia 77:183, 1982.
13. Diamond, RD, Root RK, Bennett JE: Factors influencing killing of *Cryptococcus neoformans* by human leukocytes in vitro. J Infect Dis 125:367, 1972.
14. Graybill JR, Ahrens J: Immunization and complement interaction in host defense against cryptococcosis. J Reticuloend Soc 30:347, 1981.
15. Macher AM, Bennett JE, Gadek JE, et al: Complement depletion in cryptococcal sepsis. J Immunol 120:1685, 1978.
16. Dromer F, Charrier J, Contrepois A, et al: Protection of mice against experimental cryptococcosis by anti--*Cryptococcus neoformans* monoclonal antibody. Infect Immun 55:749, 1987.
17. Miller GPG, Kohl S: Antibody-dependent leukocyte killing of *Cryptococcus neoformans*. J Immunol 131:1455.
18. Saag MS, Powderly WG, Cloud GA, et al: Comparison of amphotericin B with fluconazole in the treatment of acute AIDS-associated cryptococcal meningitis. N Engl J Med 326:83, 1992.
19. Hidore MR, Murphy JW: Correlation of natural killer cell activity and clearance of *Cryptococcus neoformans* from mice after adoptive transfer of splenic nylon wool-nonadherent cells. Infect Immun 51:547, 1986.
20. Nabavi N, Murphy JW: Antibody-dependent natural killer cell–mediated growth inhibition of *Cryptococcus neoformans*. Infect Immun 51:536, 1986.
21. Murphy JW: Effects of first-order *Cryptococcus*-specific T-suppressor cells on induction of cells responsible for delayed-type hypersensitivity. Infect Immun 48:439, 1985.
22. Khakpour FR, Murphy JW: Characterization of a third-order suppressor T cell (Ts3) induced by cryptococcal antibody. Infect Immun 51:556, 1986.
23. Graybill JR, Alford RH: Cell-mediated immunity in cryptococcosis. Cell Immunol 14:12, 1974.
24. Balmes JR, Hawkins JG: Pulmonary cryptococcosis. Semin Respir Med 9:180, 1987.
25. Bozette SA, Larsen RA, Chiu J, et al: A placebo-controlled trial of maintenance therapy with fluconazole after treatment of cryptococcal meningitis in the acquired immunodeficiency syndrome. N Engl J Med 324:580, 1991.
26. Liss HP, Rimland D: Asymptomatic cryptococcal meningitis. Am Rev Respir Dis 124:88, 1981.
27. Schupbach CW, Wheeler CF, Briggaman RA: Cutaneous manifestations of disseminated cryptococcosis. Arch Dermatol 112:1734, 1976.
28. Blasi E, Barluzzi R, Mazzolla R, et al: Biomolecular events involved in anticryptococcal resistance in the brain. Infect Immun 63:1218, 1995.
29. Kovacs JA, Kovacs AA, Polis M, et al: Cryptococcosis in the

acquired immunodeficiency syndrome. Ann Intern Med 103: 533, 1985.
30. Zugar A, Louie E, Holzman RS, et al: Cryptococcal disease in patients with the acquired immunodeficiency syndrome. Ann Intern Med 104:234, 1986.
31. Graybill JR, Craven PC, Michell L, Drutz DJ: Interaction of chemotherapy and immune defenses in experimental murine cryptococcosis. Antimicrob Agents Chemother 14:659, 1978.
32. Bennett JE, Dismukes WE, Duma RJ, et al: A comparison of amphotericin B alone and combined with flucytosine. N Engl J Med 301:126, 1979.
33. Dismukes WE, Cloud G, Gallis HA, et al: Treatment of cryptococcal meningitis with combination amphotericin B and flucytosine for four as compared with six weeks. N Engl J Med 317:334, 1987.
34. Eng RHK, Bishburg E, Smith SM, et al: Cryptococcal infections in patients with the acquired immunodeficiency syndrome. Am J Med 81:19, 1986.
35. Powderly WG, Cloud GA, Dismukes WA, Saag MS: Measurement of cryptococcal antigen in serum and cerebrospinal fluid: Value in the management of AIDS-associated cryptococcal meningitis. Clin Infect Dis 18:789, 1992.
36. Larsen RA, Leal MA, Chan LS: Fluconazole compared with amphotericin B plus flucytosine for cryptococcal meningitis in AIDS. Ann Intern Med 113:183, 1990.
37. Currie BP, Casadevall A: Estimation of the prevalence of cryptococcal infection among patients infected with the human immunodeficiency virus in New York City. Clin Infect Dis 19:1029, 1994.
38. Larsen RA, Bozette SA, Jones BE, et al: Fluconazole combined with flucytosine for treatment of cryptococcal meningitis in patients with AIDS. Clin Infect Dis 19:745, 1991.
39. Powderly WG, Saag MS, Cloud GA, et al: A controlled trial of fluconazole or amphotericin B to prevent relapse of cryptococcal meningitis in patients with the acquired immunodeficiency syndrome. N Engl J Med 326:83, 1992.
40. Denning DW, Armstrong RW, Lewis BH, et al: Elevated cerebrospinal fluid pressures in patients with cryptococcal meningitis and acquired immunodeficiency syndrome. Am J Med 91:267, 1991.
41. Van der Horst C, Saag M, Cloud G, et al: Part I. Randomized double blind comparison of amphotericin B plus flucytosine (AMB + FC) to AMB alone (step 1) followed by a comparison of fluconazole to itraconazole (step 2) in the treatment of acute cryptococcal meningitis in patients with AIDS (Abstr I216). Presented at the 35th Interscience Conference on Antimicrobial Agents and Chemotherapy; September 1995; San Francisco, CA.
42. Saag M, van der Horst C, Cloud G, et al: Part 2. Randomized double blind comparison of amphotericin B plus flucytosine (AMB + FC) to AMB alone (step 1) followed by a comparison of fluconazole to itraconazole (step 2) in the treatment of acute cryptococcal meningitis in patients with AIDS (Abstr I217). Presented at the 35th Interscience Conference on Antimicrobial Agents and Chemotherapy; September 1995; San Francisco, CA.
43. Saag MS, Cloud GC, Graybill JR, et al: Comparison of fluconazole (FLU) versus itraconazole (ITRA) as maintenance therapy of AIDS associated cryptococcal meningitis (CM) (Abstr I218). Presented at the 35th Interscience Conference on Antimicrobial Agents and Chemotherapy; September 1995; San Francisco, CA.
44. Rozenbaum R, Goncalves JR: Clinical epidemiology study of 171 cases of cryptococcosis. Clin Infect Dis 18:369, 1994.
45. Moskovitz BL, Wiesinger B: (Abstr 34). Presented at the First National Conference on Human Retroviruses and Infections; December 1993; Washington, DC.

277

Aspergillus Species

Richard D. Meyer

History

The term aspergillosis refers to a diverse set of conditions that range from intoxication through colonization or provocation of an allergic reaction to either localized or widespread invasive disease. *Aspergillus* species, of which more than 90 have been described, show mycelial morphology whether in a saprophytic state or in invasive disease.[1] Disease in humans has been related to at least 19 species, most commonly *Aspergillus fumigatus* and *Aspergillus flavus*, and to a lesser extent, *Aspergillus niger* and others.[2]

Aspergillus species were described in the 18th century, and first in avian and then in human disease in the mid-19th century. Subsequently, Virchow and Olser independently described cases of pulmonary infection. In 1890, Dieulafoy associated the pulmonary form with pigeon feeder's disease.[1, 3] By the turn of the century Renon described pulmonary disease in wig cleaners and concluded that moldy grain was the source of the conidia. Animal intoxications putatively caused by aflatoxins were reported, and soon thereafter the majority of veterinary forms of the disease were described.[1, 3] Various workers then described the saprophytic pulmonary, and more recently the allergic, forms of the disease; in the latter half of this century much emphasis has been placed on the well-known importance of the increased incidence of *Aspergillus* species as opportunistic pathogens in invasive infections.[1]

Characteristics of the Pathogen

Aspergillus species are members of the Eumycetes. They grow in nature in the same way that they do on appropriate culture media. They reproduce by enteroblastic development, wherein the inner wall of the fertile hypha helps to form the conidia (spore); the conidiogenous cell is phialidic.[1] *A. fumigatus*, for example, grows into gray-green colonies with a conidial mass and, on microscopic examination, displays septate hyphae branched at 45-degree angles with conidiophores up to 300 μm long and 5 to 8 μm in diameter; each in turn merges into a vesicle topped with phialides.[1] Aflatoxins and endotoxins produced by *Aspergillus* species play a role in intoxication; the aflatoxin from *A. flavus* is a potent carcinogen. *Aspergillus* species have antigenic moieties that elicit antibody responses in patients with allergic forms of the disease or with mycetoma.

Epidemiology

Aspergillus species are truly ubiquitous in nature; they are saprobic in soil and water, on various foodstuffs, and in decaying vegetation. They can be found in air sampled anywhere on earth.[1] The conidia, which under auspicious circumstances will form hyphae, are unevenly distributed, as has been noted in the occupational risks of disease.

Human disease may be community acquired (more common in noninvasive forms of aspergillosis) or nosocomial (more common in invasive disease because of the complex interaction of the amount of inoculum with host defenses). The principal route of transmission is airborne. The pathogen enters the respiratory tract, or sometimes an operative site. A secondary transmission route is contact, usually with skin or a wound.[4] Invasive aspergillosis is second in frequency to candidiasis among invasive mycoses in patients with leukemia and lymphoma.

Nosocomial point-source acquisition of invasive aspergillosis has been increasingly recognized as an important source of invasive disease. Walsh and Pizzo[4] classified most of those cases as directly hospital acquired by airborne transmission. Subclasses of sources include nonfiltered, nonventilated air as indirectly documented; contaminated intake ducts, exhaust ducts, or filters in ventilation systems (documented in several outbreaks); construction, either installation of contaminated fireproofing materials or inadequate barriers between construction, demolition, or renovation sites; areas for care of patients; and contaminated surfaces and ornamental plants.[4] These authors also summarized data on contact transmission from contaminated dressings for skin or bone or from inadvertent intraperitoneal administration of *Aspergillus* organisms.[4] Moreover, inadvertent infusion of *A. fumigatus* in a contaminated intravenous solution has led to one instance of transient illness and fungemia followed by recovery without specific therapy.[5] Use of marijuana contaminated with *A. fumigatus* has also led to disseminated disease.[6]

Several typing systems based on phenotypic or genomic features have been described to distinguish *A. fumigatus* strains. The latter include restriction endonuclease analysis of DNA, randomly amplified polymorphic DNA markers, and moderately repetitive sequences; analysis of moderately repetitive sequences has linked invasive isolates to the environment.[7]

Pathogenesis

Aspergillus organisms may colonize preexisting pulmonary cavities and grow saprobically but subsequently only rarely invade tissue. The greatest risk factor for invasive aspergillosis is granulocytopenia, particularly if it is protracted; patients with T-cell dysfunction are also at increased risk, but in the absence of granulocytopenia they account for a small minority of cases.[4, 8–12] Thus, patients with hematologic and other malignancies, organ allograft recipients, and those receiving immunosuppressive therapy, for example, for rheumatologic disorders, are all at increased risk. Corticosteroid therapy in renal allograft recipients and in neutropenic bone marrow transplant recipients enhances the risk of aspergillosis, as does use of T-cell–depleted human leukocyte antigen–mismatched donor marrow for transplantation.[12–14] In one study of orthotopic liver transplantation recipients, risk factors for invasive pulmonary aspergillosis were increased serum creatinine concentration and use of OKT-3.[15]

Patients with chronic granulomatous disease of childhood are also at increased risk.[16] Invasive aspergillosis has been reported in acquired immunodeficiency syndrome; it was included at first as an indicator disease but was removed in 1987 because of low frequency. The frequency of occurrence now appears to have risen. When it does occur, it is usually late in the course of disease, sometimes as a nosocomial complication. Almost all cases occur in patients with $CD4^+$ lymphocyte counts of less than 50/mm^3. A wide spectrum of pulmonary infection, as well as less common infection at other sites, including the paranasal sinuses, is noted.[17–19]

Many of these associations correlate with the primary importance of the granulocytes and alveolar macrophages in containment of *Aspergillus*. Nonetheless, invasive paranasal sinus, pulmonary, and disseminated aspergillosis in previously normal hosts or those with miscellaneous medical conditions has been described.[20] Some of these "normal" hosts have underlying alcoholic liver disease. Failure to contain *Aspergillus* organisms in the lung is followed by hematogenous dissemination. Invasive pulmonary aspergillosis rarely complicates viral influenza.

Correlates in experimental laboratory studies show that corticosteroids blunt the lysosomal response in forming phagocytic vacuoles in neutrophils of mice exposed to *Aspergillus* spores.[21] Alveolar, but not peritoneal, macrophages inhibit germination of and then kill spores by a mechanism independent of oxidative killing mechanisms or T-cell activation.[22] Normal monocytes can also damage them.[23] Granulocytes ingest but may not kill spores, and although they are unable to engulf hyphae of aspergilli because of the size discrepancy, they nonetheless cause damage to the hyphae.[24] Granulocytes, like monocytes, damage the hyphal form via an oxidative mechanism.[25]

Aspergilli colonizing the respiratory tract can lead to both specific (directed against aspergilli) and nonspecific increases in serum immunoglobulin (Ig) E levels.[26]

Clinical Manifestations

Classification of clinical syndromes of aspergillosis sometimes lacks precision because of the frequent overlap in findings. The following schema modified from Pennington[27] applies to pulmonary aspergillosis and demonstrates the wide spectrum of underlying host conditions.

Aspergillus *Hypersensitivity Lung Diseases*

EXTRINSIC ASTHMA

Inhalation of spores from the environment provokes IgE-mediated sensitized mast cell mechanisms in airways of allergic persons.[27]

EXTRINSIC ALLERGIC ALVEOLITIS

Aspergillus species spores—on moldy barley, oats, corn, or hay—are among the many precipitants of this syndrome, commonly also referred to as farmer's lung. Cough, dyspnea, and sometimes fever and chills follow inhalation of spores by a sensitized person. Diffuse pulmonary infiltrates and a restrictive pattern on pulmonary function testing result; eventually pulmonary fibrosis may ensue. Skin testing with *Aspergillus* antigen usually shows an Arthus reaction, *Aspergillus* serum precipitin levels are elevated, and corticosteroid therapy is usually salutary, perhaps because of a role of lymphocyte transformation in pathogenesis.[27, 28]

ALLERGIC BRONCHOPULMONARY ASPERGILLOSIS

Allergic bronchopulmonary aspergillosis (ABPA) principally occurs in previously allergic asthma patients, usually adults, and has been found in patients with cystic fibrosis. Exposure may be environmental or from colonization in the respiratory tract; the latter is associated with plugs of viscous material containing aspergilli.[26] Clinical features include worsening bronchospasm, and less commonly nonspecific complaints and low-grade fever; up to two thirds of patients have cough with brownish sputum, and sputum shows *Aspergillus* organisms.[26–29] Radiographic infiltrates may or may not be present but they commonly involve upper lobes (Fig. 277–1). Bronchi-

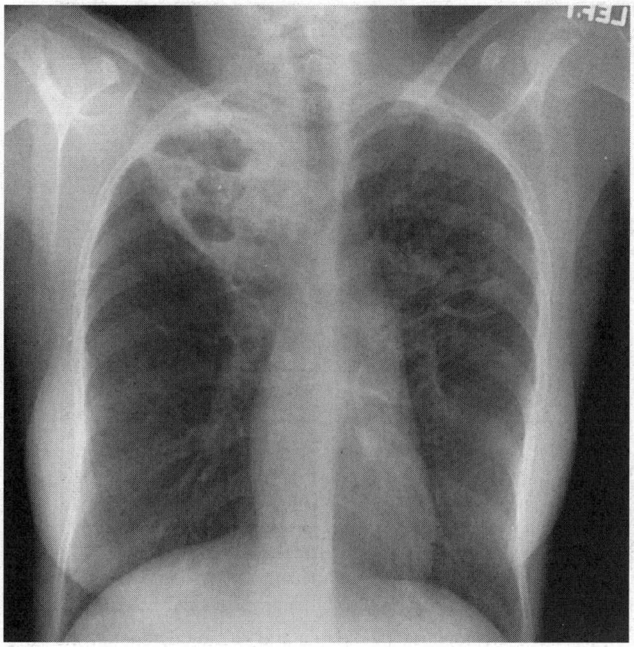

FIGURE 277–1 □ Posteroanterior chest radiograph from a 20-year-old woman marijuana smoker with *Aspergillus fumigatus* in sputum and recurrent wheezing and fever. Bilateral upper lobe infiltrates with prominence on right and cavitation are seen. Antibacterial and prednisone therapy given for allergic bronchopulmonary apergillosis led to resolution.

ectasis is a common result if ABPA is not treated promptly; pulmonary fibrosis is another sequela. IgE and IgG antibodies, as well as cellular immune mechanisms, are likely to be important in pathogenesis. Criteria for diagnosis include asthma, peripheral eosinophilia, immediate reaction to *Aspergillus* skin testing, serum precipitins against *Aspergillus*, an elevated serum IgE level, elevated levels of serum IgG and IgE against *Aspergillus*, pulmonary infiltrates, and central bronchiectasis.[28, 30] A useful guide for staging and therapy is available.[30] Early therapy with corticosteroids with tapering of doses after remission, if possible, is indicated.[29] Itraconazole has been promising in pilot studies in reduction of colonization in ABPA.[31] High-dose inhaled corticosteroids have also been anecdotally reported as a beneficial adjunct to oral corticosteroids in control of both symptoms and pulmonary infiltrates.[32] Although ABPA is typically not associated with invasion, *A. fumigatus* has been found in lung parenchyma after corticosteroid therapy, and rarely it has even disseminated.[33, 34] The ABPA syndrome is rarely associated with other fungal precipitants.

Bronchocentric granulomatosis associated with chronic asthma is associated with aspergilli in some cases and may resemble ABPA (overlap syndrome[35]). Allergic *Aspergillus* sinusitis affects allergic persons with nasal polyps and shares certain features of ABPA: aspergilli, mucoid impaction and inflammatory debris in paranasal sinuses, and serum antibodies to *A. fumigatus*.[28]

Mucoid Impaction Syndrome

Mucoid impaction of the bronchi is associated with asthma, ABPA, and eosinophilic pneumonia; the last condition has been ascribed to hypersensitivity to fungi, including aspergilli, and may overlap with ABPA.[35] Mucoid impaction of bronchi includes obstruction of proximal bronchi by plugs larger than those seen in ABPA, some of which contain aspergilli. Patients usually suffer from asthma or chronic bronchitis. Common presenting features are cough, fever, chest pain, hemoptysis, and expectoration of mucous plugs. By definition, hypersensitivity to aspergillus is not found. Mucolytic agents are used for therapy.[35]

Noninvasive Pulmonary Aspergillosis

MYCETOMATA

Aspergillus species are the pathogens of the vast majority of these fungus balls, which grow in preexisting cavities, usually from antecedent tuberculosis; fungus balls develop less commonly in other underlying pulmonary disorders, such as cystic cavities.[27, 28] Mats of hyphae grow saprobically with host material in the cavities, but limited local invasion into the cavity wall may also occur. Hemoptysis is the most common presenting complaint, although cough and weight loss have also been described.[27]

A chest radiograph of such a patient with hemoptysis (or, frequently, an asymptomatic patient) shows the fungus ball with a surrounding air-crescent shadow. A similar or even eidetic radiographic appearance may be seen with an entirely different pathogenesis in the evolution of necrotic lung parenchyma into an abscess or sequestrum-like mass (Fig. 277–2). A patient with an aspergilloma generally shows serum IgG precipitins to *Aspergillus* organisms, and sputum cultures usually propagate the organism.[27]

The natural history of an aspergilloma is variable, and a small number remain inactive or resolve spontaneously. Overlap syndrome with ABPA has been reported.[36] Opinions on management are controversial. Bronchoscopy may be indicated to localize a bleeding source. Systemic antifungal therapy is of benefit if there is overlap into invasion with the chronic necrotizing form of pulmonary aspergillosis (see later[28]). Supportive therapy suffices for the vast majority of patients, although those with life-threatening hemoptysis require surgical intervention.[27] Fatal hemoptysis still occurs and has been reported with an aspergilloma in the presence of human immunodeficiency virus infection.[37] Surgery may be difficult because of underlying disease and may be complicated by inadvertent spillage of fungi into the pleural cavity and subsequent empyema thoracis, dissemination, or both.[38] Direct intracavitary instillation of various antimycotic medicaments (amphotericin B, nystatin, miconazole, iodides) has not led to any consistent improvement, although certain patients may benefit.[39] Preliminary results with oral itraconazole therapy are encouraging.[40, 41]

Invasive Pulmonary Aspergillosis

The confounded nosology and possibility of overlap syndromes are exemplified by descriptions of a semiinvasive or slowly progressing chronic necrotizing form of aspergillosis.[42, 43] The presence of underlying systemic or lung disease or mild immunosuppressive therapy with radiation, chemotherapy, or corticosteroids preceded development of a smoldering (usually for 1 to 6 months) infection followed by cavity formation, which is often associated with an air-crescent sign.[42, 43]

The lung is the site most commonly involved in invasive disease and is a way station for disseminated disease in at least a quarter of patients with classic invasive pulmonary aspergillosis.[8, 9] In patients at risk (see earlier), this frequently occurs in the setting of relapse of the underlying condition or immunosuppressive therapy (especially with granulocytopenia), and prior antibacterial therapy without sustained response. Invasive paranasal sinus disease occurs in the same setting[44] and in patients with acquired immunodeficiency syndrome.[19] Endobronchial invasion may precede pulmonary

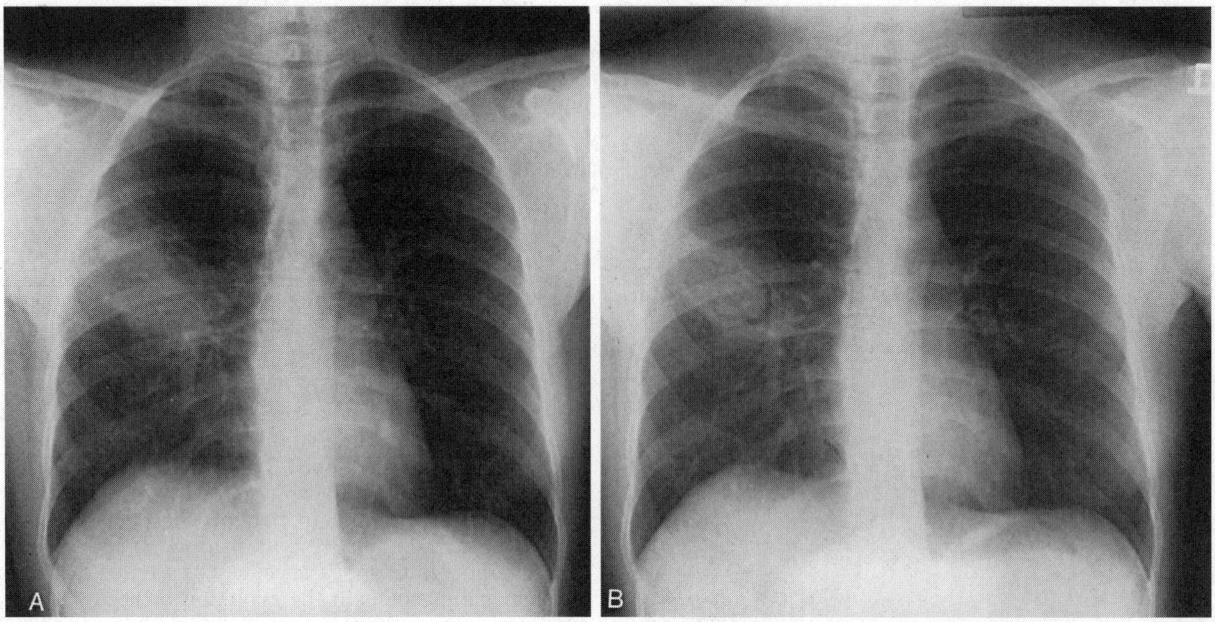

FIGURE 277–2 □ Posteroanterior chest radiographs from a 28-year-old woman with acute myelogenous leukemia and granulocytopenia showing wedge-shaped right upper lobe infiltrate *(A)* and air-crescent sign around sequestrum *(B)*. Surgical resection was curative with remission of leukemia. (*A* and *B* from Meyer RD, Young LS, Armstrong D, Yu B: Aspergillosis complicating neoplastic disease. Am J Med 54:6–15, 1973.)

parenchymal invasion at a stage before radiographic infiltrates are evident.[3] Necrotizing bronchitis with pseudomembrane formation has been described as a variant form in patients with acquired immunodeficiency syndrome[17] and had occurred in other types of patients. Unremitting fever and new pulmonary infiltrates are common features, as are dyspnea and nonproductive cough. Pleural pain and the findings of a pleural rub occur in a minority of patients and with other findings (hemoptysis, tachycardia) mimic the syndrome of pulmonary embolus with infarction; this results from hemorrhagic infarction secondary to blood vessel invasion by aspergilli.[8] Massive hemoptysis is uncommon. Physical examination may also disclose findings of dullness, rales, or pulmonary consolidation.

Radiographic changes are quite varied. They most often show patchy or bronchopneumonic infiltrates, wedge-shaped pleural-based infiltrates, or nodular densities (Fig. 277–3*A*; see Fig. 277–2*A*). Interstitial infiltrates or sequestrum formation (see Fig. 277–2*B*) is less common. Computed tomographic findings include multiple small masses, clusters of nodules, and a computed tomographic halo sign around a pulmonary mass. Generally 2 to 3 weeks elapses before cavitation ensues.[45] Other patients show a much more fulminant course, with rapidly progressive pulmonary infiltrates, fever, and death. Pneumothorax may develop from a cavity.

Other Forms of Invasive Aspergillosis

Disseminated disease almost always results from a primary pulmonary infection, but it can also occur from skin inoculation or when no likely entry source is identifiable. Virtually any site can be involved as a result of hematogenous dissemination, including the central nervous system, heart (abscesses or pericarditis), gastrointestinal tract, kidney, liver (resembling hepatosplenic candidiasis), thyroid, or spleen. Clinical findings related to abscesses and infarcts vary according to the involved site and range from dramatic to silent.[8, 9]

Central nervous system aspergillosis as part of disseminated disease is usually manifested by infarcts, which are frequently multiple and associated with vascular invasion and hemorrhage, and occasionally abscess formation.[8, 46–48] Onset of seizure activity, focal neurologic deficits, and depressed levels of consciousness are common clinical findings.[8] Chronic meningitis and ventriculitis are unusual findings in immunocompromised patients. Manifestations in intravenous drug abusers include necrotizing vasculitis, granulomata, meningitis, and ventriculitis.[49] Endophthalmitis may be secondary to trauma, endogenous (e.g., from intravenous narcotic abuse or as part of disseminated disease), or from direct extension.[2, 50–52] *Aspergillus* species, particularly *A. niger,* cause otomycosis, an almost always benign condition of the external ear canal and pinna. On the other hand, severe external otitis with invasion and necrosis from aspergillosis resembles that caused by *Pseudomonas aeruginosa* and requires an aggressive surgical approach and amphotericin B therapy.[53, 54]

Aspergillosis of the paranasal sinuses has been caused by *A. flavus* in the Sudan, and elsewhere by it and other species. It is classified as (1) a chronic noninvasive form characterized by a luminal mass that may cause inflammation but does not invade and that is treated by surgical removal of the mass or (2) invasive disease, which is either acute (as in granulocytopenic or immunosuppressed patients) or chronic and also requires systemic antifungal chemotherapy.[44] Chronic noninvasive disease and chronic invasive disease are distinguished with computed tomography or magnetic resonance imaging or at surgery.[55] Nasal and orbitonasal disease with black, necrotic eschars also occurs, and necrotizing epiglottitis has been described in an immunosuppressed patient.[56]

Endocarditis on a native or prosthetic valve or in a mural location is characterized by negative results of blood cultures and peripheral embolization.[57, 58] Diagnosis is usually made by examination of an embolus. Primary therapy is surgical, with amphotericin B as an adjunct. Mycotic aneurysm with embolization and vascular graft infections have also been reported.[59, 60]

Pleural aspergillosis, or empyema thoracis, usually follows surgery complicated by a bronchopleural or pleurocutaneous fistula, much less commonly follows another episode of aspergillosis, and has rarely been related to silk suture material acting as a nidus.[38, 61–63] Therapy consists of surgical management, removal of foreign bodies, and, on an individualized

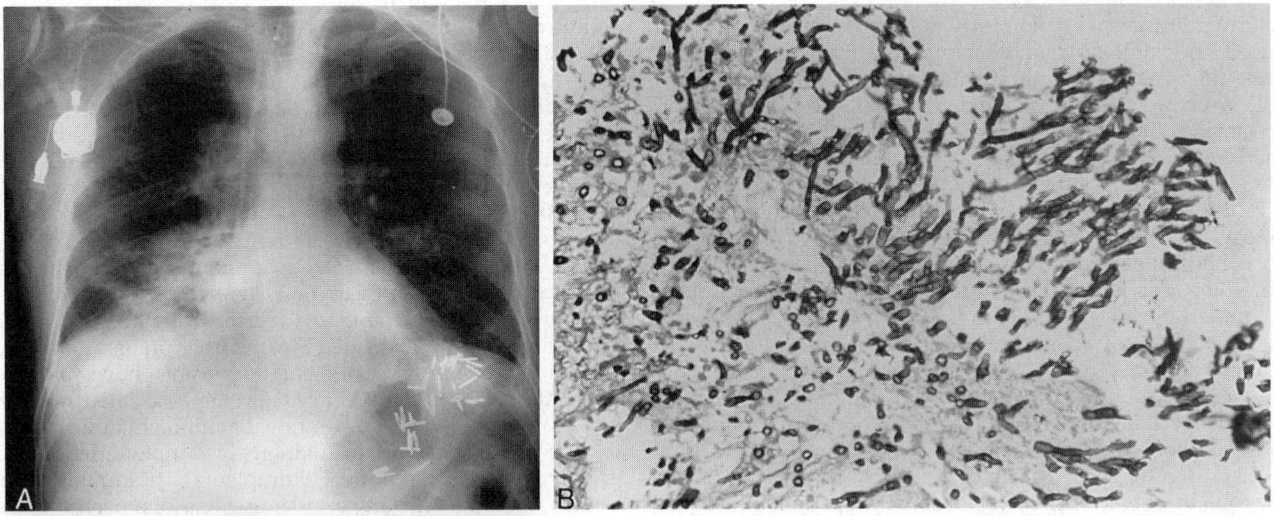

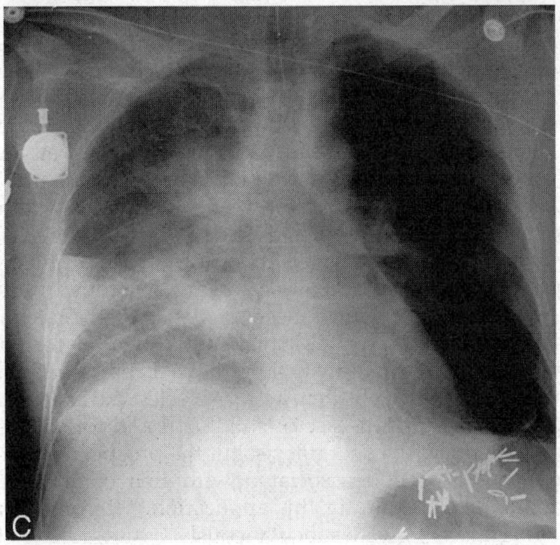

FIGURE 277–3 ▫ *A*, Posteroanterior chest radiograph from a 57-year-old man with lymphoma (undergoing methylprednisolone therapy) and granulocytopenia shows a hazy nodular right lower lobe and right upper lobe infiltrates that arose over 2 weeks. *B*, Histopathologic examination of a transbronchial biopsy specimen shows hyphae of aspergilli (cytologic preparation of bronchoalveolar lavage specimen also showed hyphae). *C*, Fatal progression of infiltrates followed despite amphotericin B therapy.

basis, intravenous amphotericin B, perhaps with itraconazole follow-up therapy. Local instillation of amphotericin B has been recommended, but its role is not clear.[62]

Osteomyelitis in children usually results from contiguous spread from pulmonary infection into rib or vertebra, usually in the setting of chronic granulomatous disease of childhood; a similar process rarely occurs in immunocompromised adults.[16, 64, 65] Sternal infection with *Aspergillus* may follow median sternotomy incisions.[66] In immunocompromised adults, hematogenous spread to, most commonly, the vertebrae, and both vertebral osteomyelitis and discitis in drug abusers have been reported separately.[64, 67, 68] Articular aspergillosis is rare and when it does occur is part of hematogenously disseminated disease, usually in immunosuppressed patients; birefringent crystals thought to be calcium oxalate may be found on fluid analysis.[69]

Cutaneous aspergillosis occurs as a result of hematogenous spread in a small number of cases of dissemination; multiple erythematous papules that form pustules secondary to microabscesses and large necrotic lesions resembling ecthyma gangrenosum have been noted.[70, 71] Similar erythematous to violaceous, edematous, indurated plaques that become eschars probably result from primary cutaneous inoculation, and some spread distantly.[72–74] Biopsy is required for diagnosis. Operative débridement, control of the underlying disorder, and intravenous amphotericin B are recommended therapy, even without documented dissemination. Cutaneous seeding and formation of a nodule have also followed transthoracic needle biopsy in a leukemic patient with pulmonary aspergillosis.[75] *Aspergillus* burn wound infection is treated with wide débridement or amputation.[76] Sources for listings of other miscellaneous anatomic sites involved are available.[2, 8, 9]

Diagnosis

General guidelines for therapy and reference sources for therapy of noninvasive aspergillosis have been listed.[3, 28, 30] The clinical constellation of fever unresponsive to optimal antibacterial therapy in the presence of granulocytopenia or immunosuppressive therapy, especially with new pulmonary infiltrates, should lead to immediate consideration of performance of diagnostic procedures and empirical use of amphotericin B therapy. The disappointingly low number (only 10% or slightly more) of cultures of respiratory tract material taken noninvasively that yield aspergilli in the face of invasive pulmonary or disseminated disease is well known.[2, 3, 8, 9] Moreover, aspergilli seen on direct examination or cultured from sputum specimens of patients at risk for invasive disease may represent only colonization.[8] Isolation of *A. fumigatus* or *A. flavus* alone from sputum cultures of patients at risk frequently is not due to contamination and cannot be ignored in patients who have acute leukemia, granulocytopenia or solid organ transplantation, or who have received antibiotic therapy or cytotoxic chemotherapy.[77, 78, 78a] Some investigators stress the utility of submitting multiple sputum specimens.[78a] Follow-up assessment is required. Ideally, examination of specimens obtained by bronchoalveolar lavage or transbronchial biopsy (or percutaneous transthoracic biopsy or open lung biopsy) should be used to confirm tissue invasion (Fig. 277–3*B*). In patients with acute leukemia, a transbronchial biopsy specimen is likely to add little to findings of examination of bronchoalveolar lavage and brushing specimens; open lung biopsy is likewise likely to have limited value, unless the underlying disease is controlled.[75, 79, 80] Other species, such as *Aspergillus terreus*, are much less likely to cause invasion but also do so; even they cannot be dismissed summarily.[47, 81] Isolation of aspergilli from nasal cultures of granulocytopenic patients receiving antibiotics has been reported as significant in a study of hyperendemic aspergillosis.[82]

Definitive diagnosis can be made only by finding tissue invasion by characteristic structures at histopathologic examination with appropriate stains (calcofluor white and others) *and* confirming the findings by culture. Even with use of fluorescent antibody directed against *Aspergillus*, morphologic criteria are not totally reliable for diagnosis owing to confusion with other fungi.[2] Eumycetes confused with aspergilli on histopathologic examination include *Pseudoallescheria boydii* (*Scedosporium apiospermum*, treated with imidazoles rather than amphotericin B), *Fusarium* species, and Mucoraceae. Biopsy of skin and of other involved sites should be performed whenever possible, together with histopathologic examination and culture of skin scrapings and biopsy specimens.

Blood cultures almost never yield aspergilli in the face of invasive disease. Examination of cerebrospinal fluid in central nervous system aspergillosis typically shows red blood cells and small numbers of mononuclear cells, but culture of cerebrospinal fluid only rarely yields the organism.[8] Persistent neutrophilia in cerebrospinal fluid is unusual.[47] Computed tomography shows infarcts or abscesses.

Serologic tests for antibody, despite their utility in diagnosis of allergic forms of the disease, have no established value in the diagnosis of invasive aspergillosis. Detection of circulating antigen in serum and cerebrospinal fluid of patients with invasive disease has been reported promising with both radioimmunoassay and enzyme-linked immunosorbent assay methods, but neither is widely available.[47, 83–85] Preliminary reports of polymerase chain reaction techniques applied to respiratory tract specimens indicate that they can retrospectively confirm some cases but are fraught with too many false-positive results to be useful.[86, 87]

Treatment

Surgical drainage, débridement, or resection should generally be carried out whenever feasible for invasive disease such as sinusitis, cutaneous aspergillosis, or empyema thoracis. Removal of the catheter is a cornerstone of therapy of aspergillosis complicating chronic peritoneal dialysis. Successful resection for sequestrum formation in invasive pulmonary aspergillosis has been carried out both without and with systemic antifungal treatment.[8, 88] Resection has also been useful in pulmonary aspergillosis in renal transplantation patients.[89]

Amphotericin B remains the mainstay of systemic therapy for invasive aspergillosis and in pulmonary or disseminated forms is given in daily doses of up to 0.75 mg/kg (occasionally up to 1.0 mg/kg), if tolerated, to a total dose of at least 30 mg/kg. The course of the underlying disorder greatly affects duration of therapy. Long-term survival rates for leukemia and lymphoma patients are at least 10% but are higher (~25%) for treated renal allograft recipients, including those who undergo pulmonary resection.[89] Either flucytosine or rifampin has been used empirically with amphotericin B in an attempt to enhance activity, but no clear-cut results support this practice.[2, 47, 90, 91] Flucytosine given alone likely plays no role in therapy.

Amphotericin B incorporated into multilamellar vesicles (liposomal amphotericin B) is remarkably nontoxic to host kidneys and has been used to treat paranasal pulmonary and cerebral aspergillosis cases that were refractory to varying amounts of standard amphotericin B. It is not yet commercially available in the United States. Other preparations, such as lipid complex and colloidal dispension, have just been introduced in the United States and are associated with less nephrotoxicity than is conventional amphotericin B.

Direct injection or instillation of amphotericin B by subconjunctival, intravitreal, intrapleural, or intraperitoneal routes or lavage of paranasal sinuses may be useful in specific patients.[50, 51, 93, 94]

Itraconazole, an imidazole antifungal agent, is approved for use in therapy of pulmonary and extrapulmonary aspergillosis, including disseminated disease, in patients who have failed to respond to or are intolerant of amphotericin B therapy.[41, 95–97] It may also be tried in patients with relatively less serious infections or greater immunocompetence. Long-term therapy is necessary, and therapy with "off-label" doses greater than 400 mg/d may be required. Suspension preparation leads to higher blood levels than does capsule preparation. Other experimental triazoles are being developed. Terbinafine, which has been introduced in the United States, is active in vitro but likely will not be investigated for this indication. Granulocyte transfusions have been used with continued amphotericin B therapy for selected patients with chronic granulomatous disease of childhood and for selected leukemia patients with aspergillosis, but the prospect of acute respiratory deterioration associated with this combination has tempered enthusiasm for this application.[99] Recombinant human interferon-γ given subcutaneously as an adjunct to antifungal chemotherapy is promising in selected chronic granulomatous disease patients.[100] The use of granulocyte-macrophage colony-stimulating factor, sargramostim, with amphotericin B deserves further investigation. The importance of in vitro susceptibility test results of aspergilli is uncertain, and usually testing versus amphotericin B is not recommended.[101]

Prevention

Environmental control measures to prevent conidia from reaching patients at risk are indicated, including during construction activities.[4, 102, 103] Additional measures such as whole-wall laminar air flow units with high-efficiency particulate air filters reduce the risk but are generally not used because of their expense and lack of tolerance by some patients, among other reasons.[4, 104] Ketoconazole or fluconazole is not effective in prophylaxis; other azoles are entering trials. A nasal spray of topical amphotericin B—an attempt to reduce paranasal sinus and respiratory colonization—looks promising in initial European studies.[102, 105]

References

1. Rippon JW: Medical Mycology: The Pathogenic Fungi and the Pathogenic Actinomycetes, ed 3. Philadelphia, WB Saunders, 1988.
2. Rinaldi M: Invasive aspergillosis. Rev Infect Dis 5:1061, 1983.

3. Dar MA, Ahman M, Weinstein AJ, et al: Thoracic aspergillosis. Cleve Clin Q 51:615, 1984.
4. Walsh TJ, Pizzo PA: Nosocomial fungal infections: A classification for hospital-acquired fungal infections and mycoses arising from endogenous flora or reactivation. Annu Rev Microbiol 42:517, 1988.
5. Daisy JA, Abrutyn EA, MacGregor RR: Inadvertent administration of intravenous fluids contaminated with fungus. Ann Intern Med 91:563, 1979.
6. Hamadeh R, Ardehali A, Locksley RM, York MK: Fatal aspergillosis associated with smoking contaminated marijuana, in a marrow transplant recipient. Chest 94:432, 1988.
7. Girardin H, Sarfati J, Traoré F, et al: Molecular epidemiology of nosocomial invasive aspergillosis. J Clin Microbiol 32:684, 1994.
8. Meyer RD, Young LS, Armstrong D, Yu B: Aspergillosis complicating neoplastic disease. Am J Med 54:6, 1973.
9. Young RC, Bennett JE, Vogel CL, et al: Aspergillosis: The spectrum of disease in 98 patients. Medicine (Baltimore) 49:147, 1970.
10. Gerson SL, Talbot GH, Hurwitz S, et al: Discriminant scorecard for diagnosis of invasive pulmonary aspergillosis in patients with acute leukemia. Am J Med 79:57, 1985.
11. Lake KB, Browne PM, Van Dyke JJ, Ayers L: Fatal disseminated aspergillosis in an asthmatic patient treated with corticosteroids. Chest 83:138, 1983.
12. Gustafson TL, Schaffner W, Lavely GB, et al: Invasive aspergillosis in renal transplant recipients: Correlation with corticosteroid therapy. J Infect Dis 148:230, 1983.
13. Wingard JR, Beals SU, Santos GW, et al: *Aspergillus* infections in bone marrow transplant recipients. Bone Marrow Transplant 2:175, 1987.
14. Pirsch JD, Maki DG: Infectious complications in adults with bone marrow transplantation and T-cell depletion of donor marrow. Ann Intern Med 104:619, 1986.
15. Kusne S, Torre-Cisneros J, Manez R, et al: Factors associated with invasive lung aspergillosis and the significance of positive aspergillus culture after liver transplantation. J Infect Dis 166:1379, 1992.
16. Cohen MS, Isturiz RE, Malech HL, et al: Fungal infection in chronic granulomatous disease. Am J Med 71:59, 1981.
17. Denning DW, Follansbee SE, Scolaro M, et al: Pulmonary aspergillosis in the acquired immunodeficiency syndrome. N Engl J Med 324:654, 1991.
18. Lortholary O, Meyohas M-C, Dupont B, et al: Invasive aspergillosis in patients with acquired immunodeficiency syndrome: Report of 33 cases. Am J Med 95:177, 1993.
19. Meyer RD, Gaultier CG, Yamashita JT, et al: Fungal sinusitis in patients with AIDS: Report of four cases and review of the literature. Medicine (Baltimore) 73:69, 1994.
20. Karam GH, Griffin FM Jr: Invasive pulmonary aspergillosis in nonimmunocompromised nonneutropenic hosts. Rev Infect Dis 8:357, 1986.
21. Merkow L, Pardo M, Epstein SM, et al: Lysosomal stability during phagocytosis of *Aspergillus flavus* spores by alveolar macrophages of cortisone-treated mice. Science 160:79, 1968.
22. Schaffner A, Douglas H, Braude AI, Davis CE: Killing of *Aspergillus* spores depends on the anatomical source of the macrophage. Infect Immun 42:1109, 1983.
23. Diamond RD, Huber E, Haudenschild CC: Mechanisms of destruction of *Aspergillus fumigatus* hyphae mediated by human monocytes. J Infect Dis 147:474, 1983.
24. Diamond RD, Krzesicki R, Epstein B, Jao W: Damage to hyphal forms of fungi by human leukocytes in vitro. Am J Pathol 91:313, 1978.
25. Rex JH, Bennett JE, Gallin JI, et al: Normal and deficient neutrophils can cooperate to damage *Aspergillus fumigatus* hyphae. J Infect Dis 162:523, 1990.
26. Patterson R, Rosenberg M, Roberts M: Evidence that *Aspergillus fumigatus* growing in the airway of man can be a potent stimulus of specific and nonspecific IgE formation. Am J Med 63:257, 1977.
27. Pennington JE: *Aspergillus* lung disease. Med Clin North Am 64:475, 1980.
28. Levitz SM: Aspergillosis. Infect Dis Clin North Am 3:1, 1989.
29. Fink JN: Allergic bronchopulmonary aspergillosis. Chest 87(Suppl): 81S, 1985.
30. Greenberger PA, Patterson R: Allergic bronchopulmonary aspergillosis: Model of bronchopulmonary disease with defined serologic, radiologic, pathologic and clinical findings from asthma to fatal destructive lung disease. Chest 91(Suppl):165S, 1987.
31. Bodey GP, Glann AS: Central nervous system aspergillosis following steroidal therapy for allergic bronchopulmonary aspergillosis. Chest 103:299, 1993.
32. Imbeault B, Cormien Y: Usefulness of inhaled high-dose corticosteroids in allergic bronchopulmonary aspergillosis. Chest 103:1614, 1993.
33. Riley DJ, MacKenzie JW, Uhlman WE, Edelman NH: Allergic bronchopulmonary aspergillosis: Evidence of limited tissue invasion. Am Rev Respir Dis 111:232, 1975.
34. Denning DW, Van Wye JE, Lewiston NJ, Stevens DA: Adjunctive therapy of allergic bronchopulmonary aspergillosis with itraconazole. Chest 100:813, 1991.
35. Katzenstein AL, Liebow AA, Friedman PJ: Bronchocentric granulomatosis, mucoid impaction, and hypersensitivity reactions to fungi. Am Rev Respir Dis 111:497, 1975.
36. Ein ME, Wallace RJ, Williams TW: Allergic bronchopulmonary aspergillosis-like syndrome consequent to aspergilloma. Am Rev Respir Dis 119:811, 1979.
37. Lombardo GT, Anandarao N, Lin CS, et al: Fatal hemoptysis in a patient with AIDS-related complex and pulmonary aspergilloma. N Y State J Med 87:306, 1987.
38. Rosenberg RS, Creviston SA, Schonfeld AJ: Invasive aspergillosis complicating resection of a pulmonary aspergilloma in a nonimmunocompromised host. Am Rev Respir Dis 126:1113, 1982.
39. Hargis JL, Bone RC, Stewart J, et al: Intracavitary amphotericin B in the treatment of symptomatic pulmonary aspergillomas. Am J Med 68:389, 1980.
40. Dupont B: Itraconazole therapy in aspergillosis: Study in 49 patients. J Am Acad Dermatol 23:607, 1990.
41. DeBeule K, DeDoncker P, Cauwenbergh G, et al: The treatment of aspergillosis and aspergilloma with itraconazole: Clinical results of an open international study (1982–1987). Mycoses 31:476, 1988.
42. Gefter WB, Weingrad TR, Epstein DM, et al: "Semi-invasive" pulmonary aspergillosis. Radiology 140:313, 1981.
43. Binder RE, Faling LJ, Pugatch RD, et al: Chronic necrotizing pulmonary aspergillosis: A discrete clinical entity. Medicine (Baltimore) 61:109, 1982.
44. Talbot GH, Huang A, Provencher M: Invasive aspergillus rhinosinusitis in patients with acute leukemia. Rev Infect Dis 13:219, 1991.
45. Kuhlman JE, Fishman EK, Burch PA, et al: CT of invasive pulmonary aspergillosis. AJR 150:1015, 1988.
46. Walsh TJ, Hier DB, Caplan LR: Aspergillosis of the central nervous system: Clinicopathological analysis of 17 patients. Ann Neurol 18:574, 1985.
47. Peacock JE Jr, McGinnis MR, Cohen MS: Persistent neutrophilic meningitis: Report of four cases and review of the literature. Medicine (Baltimore) 63:379, 1984.
48. Boon AP, Adams DH, Buckels U, McMaster P: Cerebral aspergillosis in liver transplantation. J Clin Pathol 43:114, 1990.
49. Morrow R, Wong B, Finkelstein WE, et al: Aspergillosis of the cerebral ventricles in a heroin abuser. Arch Intern Med 143:161, 1983.
50. Roney P, Barr CC, Chun CH, Raff MJ: Endogenous *Aspergillus* endophthalmitis. Rev Infect Dis 8:955, 1986.
51. Naidoff MA, Green WR: Endogenous *Aspergillus* endophthalmitis occurring after kidney transplant. Am J Ophthalmol 79:502, 1975.
52. Barr CC, Walsh A, Wainscott B, Finger R: *Aspergillus* endophthalmitis in intravenous-drug users—Kentucky. MMWR Morbid Mortal Wkly Rep 39:48, 1990.
53. Cunningham M, Yu VL, Turner J, Curtin H: Necrotizing otitis externa due to *Aspergillus* in an immunocompetent patient. Arch Otolaryngol Head Neck Surg 114:554, 1988.
54. Gordon G, Giddings NA: Invasive otitis externa due to *Aspergillus* species: Case report and review. Clin Infect Dis 19:866, 1994.
55. Washburn RG, Kennedy DW, Begley MG, et al: Chronic fungal sinusitis in apparently normal hosts. Medicine (Baltimore) 67:231, 1988.

56. Bolivar R, Gomez LG, Luna M, et al: *Aspergillus* epiglottitis. Cancer 51:367, 1983.
57. Woods GL, Wood RP, Shaw BW Jr: Aspergillus endocarditis in patients without prior cardiovascular surgery: Report of a case in a liver transplant recipient and review. Rev Infect Dis 11:263, 1989.
58. Lang DM, Leisen JCC, Elliott JP, et al: Echocardiographically silent *Aspergillus* mural endocarditis. West J Med 149:334, 1988.
59. Rose HD, Stuart JL: Mycotic aneurysm of the thoracic aorta caused by *Aspergillus fumigatus*. Chest 70:81, 1976.
60. Aguado JM, Valle R, Anjons R, et al: Aortic bypass graft infection due to *Aspergillus*: Report of a case and review. Clin Infect Dis 14:916, 1992.
61. Parry MF, Coughlin FR, Zambetti FX: *Aspergillus* empyema. Chest 81:768, 1982.
62. Stamatis G, Greschuchna D: Surgery for pulmonary aspergilloma and pleural aspergillosis. Thorac Cardiovasc Surg 36:356, 1988.
63. Hendrix WC, Arudo LK, Platts-Mills TAE, et al: *Aspergillus* epidural abscess and hand compression in a patient with aspergillosis and empyema. Survival and response to high dose amphotericin B therapy. Am Rev Respir Dis 145:1483, 1992.
64. Tack KJ, Rhame FS, Brown B, Rhompson RC Jr: *Aspergillus* osteomyelitis. Am J Med 73:295, 1982.
65. Caligiuri P, MacMahon H, Courtney J, Weiss L: Opportunistic pulmonary aspergillosis with chest wall invasion. Arch Intern Med 143:2323, 1983.
66. Barzaghi N, Emmi V, Mencherini S, et al: Sternal osteomyelitis due to *Aspergillus fumigatus* after cardiac surgery. Chest 105:1275, 1994.
67. Holmes PF, Osterman DW, Tullos HS: *Aspergillus* discitis. Clin Orthop 226:240, 1988.
68. Brown DL, Musher DM, Taffet GE: Hematogenously acquired *Aspergillus* vertebral osteomyelitis in seemingly immunocompetent drug addicts. West J Med 147:84, 1987.
69. Alvarez L, Calvo E, Abril C: Articular aspergillosis: Case report. Clin Infect Dis 20:457, 1995.
70. Vedder JS, Schorr WF: Primary disseminated pulmonary aspergillosis with metastatic skin nodules. JAMA 209:1191, 1969.
71. Keating MJ, Bodey GP, McCredie KB, et al: Disseminated aspergillosis during remission induction in a long-term survivor with acute promyelocytic leukemia. Med Grand Rounds 2:170, 1983.
72. Prystowsky SD, Vogelstein B, Ettinger DS, et al: Invasive aspergillosis. N Engl J Med 295:655, 1976.
73. McCarty JM, Flam MS, Pullen G, et al: Outbreak of primary cutaneous aspergillosis related to intravenous arm boards. J Pediatr 108:721, 1986.
74. Allo MD, Miller J, Townsend T, Tan C: Primary cutaneous aspergillosis associated with Hickman intravenous catheters. N Engl J Med 317:1105, 1987.
75. Jobin EH, Westenfeld F, Dietrich PA: Cutaneous infection due to *Aspergillus* species after transthoracic lung biopsy (Letter). Clin Infect Dis 17:955, 1993.
76. Bruck HM, Nash G, Foley FD, Pruitt BA: Opportunistic fungal infection of the burn wound with Phycomycetes and *Aspergillus*. Arch Surg 102:476, 1971.
77. Nalesnik MA, Myerowitz RL, Jenkins R, et al: Significance of *Aspergillus* species isolated from respiratory secretions in the diagnosis of invasive pulmonary aspergillosis. J Clin Microbiol 11:370, 1980.
78. Treger TR, Visscher DW, Bartlett MS, Smith JW: Diagnosis of pulmonary infection caused by *Aspergillus*: Usefulness of respiratory cultures. J Infect Dis 152:572, 1985.
78a. Horvath JD, Dummer S: The use of respiratory-tract cultures in the diagnosis of invasive pulmonary aspergillosis. Am J Med 100:171, 1996.
79. Albelda SM, Talbot GH, Gierson SL, et al: Role of fiberoptic bronchoscopy in the diagnosis of invasive pulmonary aspergillosis in patients with acute leukemia. Am J Med 76:1027, 1984.
80. McCabe RE, Brooks RG, Mark JBD, Remington JS: Open lung biopsy in patients with acute leukemia. Am J Med 78:609, 1985.
81. Trite DM, Woods GL: Fatal disseminated infection with *Aspergillus terreus* in immunocompromised hosts. Clin Infect Dis 16:118, 1993.
82. Aisner J, Murillo J, Schimpff SC, et al: Invasive aspergillosis in acute leukemia. Correlation with nose culture and antibiotic use. Ann Intern Med 90:4, 1979.
83. Burnie JP, Matthews R: Heat shock protein 88 and *Aspergillus* infection. J Clin Microbiol 29:2099, 1991.
84. Patterson TF, Miniter P, Patterson JE, et al: *Aspergillus* antigen detection in the diagnosis of invasive aspergillosis. J Infect Dis 171:1553, 1995.
85. Rogers TR, Haynes KA, Barnes RA: Value of antigen detection in predicting invasive pulmonary aspergillosis. Lancet 336: 1210, 1990.
86. Spreadburg C, Hoblen D, Aufauvre-Brown A, et al: Detection of *Aspergillus fumigatus* by polymerase chain reaction. J Clin Microbiol 31:615, 1993.
87. Bretagne S, Costa J-M, Marmorat-Khuong A, et al: Detection of *Aspergillus* species DNA in bronchoalveolar lavage samples by competitive PCR. J Clin Microbiol 33:1164, 1995.
88. Kibbler CC, Milkins SR, Bhamra A, et al: Apparent pulmonary mycetoma following invasive aspergillosis in neutropenic patients. Thorax 43:108, 1988.
89. Weiland D, Ferguson RM, Peterson PK, et al: Aspergillosis in 25 renal transplant patients: Epidemiology, clinical presentation, diagnosis, and management. Ann Surg 198:622, 1983.
90. Denning DW, Stevens DA: The treatment of invasive aspergillosis: Surgery and antifungal therapy of 2121 published cases. Rev Infect Dis 12:1147, 1990.
91. Meyer RD: Current role of therapy with amphotericin B. Clin Infect Dis 14(Suppl 1):S154, 1992.
92. Lopez-Berestein G, Bodey GP, Fainstein V, et al: Treatment of systemic fungal infections with liposomal amphotericin B. Arch Intern Med 149:2533, 1989.
93. Kravitz SP, Berry PL: Successful treatment of *Aspergillus* peritonitis in a child undergoing continuous cycling peritoneal dialysis. Arch Intern Med 146:2061, 1986.
94. Cochrane LJ, Morano JU, Norman JR, Manset JK: Use of intracavitary amphotericin B in a patient with aspergilloma and recurrent hemoptysis (Letter). Am J Med 90:654, 1991.
95. Denning DW, Tucker RM, Hanson LH, Stevens DA: Treatment of invasive aspergillosis with itraconazole. Am J Med 86:791, 1989.
96. Peters-Christodoulou MN, de Beer FC, Bots GTAM, et al: Treatment of postoperative *Aspergillus fumigatus* spondylodiscitis with itraconazole. Scand J Infect Dis 23:373, 1991.
97. Denning DW, Stepan DE, Blume KG, Stevens DA: Control of invasive pulmonary aspergillosis with oral itraconazole in a bone marrow transplant patient. J Infect 24:73, 1992.
98. Shadomy S, Espinel-Ingroff A, Gebhart RJ: In vitro studies with SF 86-327, a new orally active allylamine derivative. J Med Vet Mycol 23:125, 1985.
99. Wright DG, Robichaud KJ, Pizzo PA, Deisseroth AB: Lethal pulmonary reactions associated with the combined use of amphotericin B and leukocyte transfusions. N Engl J Med 304:1185, 1981.
100. Bernhisel-Broadbent J, Camargo EE, Jaffe HS, Lederman HM: Recombinant human interferon-γ as adjunct therapy for *Aspergillus* infection in a patient with chronic granulomatous disease. J Infect Dis 163:908, 1991.
101. Drutz DJ: In vitro antifungal susceptibility testing and measurement of levels of antifungal agents in body fluids. Rev Infect Dis 9:392, 1987.
102. Meunier F: Prevention of mycoses in immunocompromised patients. Rev Infect Dis 9:408, 1987.
103. Loo VG, Bertrand C, Dixon C, et al: Control of construction-associated nosocomial aspergillosis in an antiquated hematology unit. Infect Control Hosp Epidemiol 17:360, 1996.
104. Sherertz RJ, Belani A, Kramer BS, et al: Impact of air filtration of nosocomial *Aspergillus* infections: Unique risk of bone marrow transplant recipients. Am J Med 83:709, 1987.
105. Conneally E, Cafferkey MT, Daly PA, et al: Nebulized amphotericin B as prophylaxis against aspergillosis in granulocytopenic patients. Bone Marrow Transplant 5:403, 1990.

278

Histoplasma

Joe Wheat

History

Darling first described the disease in 1905 in autopsy material from a case seen in the Panama Canal Zone and identified the organism to be *Leishmania*. He named these structures *Histoplasma capsulatum* because they resembled plasmodium-like organisms within histocytes.[1] The apparent capsule proved to be a staining artifact caused by cytoplasmic shrinkage. In 1945, Christie and Peterson,[2] recognizing the frequency of pulmonary calcifications in children with negative tuberculin skin tests, suspected histoplasmosis to be a common but benign pulmonary infection. Edwards and colleagues,[3] in 1969, reported the geographic distribution of histoplasmosis in the United States. Emmons[4] isolated the organism from soil in 1949. Furcolow[4a] detected the organism in air samples in 1954, supporting earlier suspicions that the disease was acquired when conidia were inhaled. Zeidberg and coworkers,[5] in 1952, reported the importance of bird droppings for growth of *H. capsulatum* in soil.

Characteristics of the Pathogen

H. capsulatum var. *capsulatum* is an ascomycete of the family Arthrodermataceae.[6] Its telemorphic state is *Ajellomyces capsulatus*. *H. capsulatum* grows as a mold in the soil and is found primarily in microfoci containing large amounts of rotted guano where starlings have roosted or bats have inhabited. The mold consists of hyphae bearing large tuberculate macroconidia (8 to 14 μm in diameter), which are characteristic of *H. capsulatum*, and smaller (2 to 5 μm) microconidia, which are the infectious form of the organism (Fig. 278–1).

At temperatures above 35°C, *H. capsulatum* grows as a yeast measuring 2 to 3 by 3 to 4 μm in diameter (Fig. 278–2). The yeast form is typically found in infected tissues; however, hyphal elements have been seen in cardiac vegetations and other sites of intravascular infection.[7, 8]

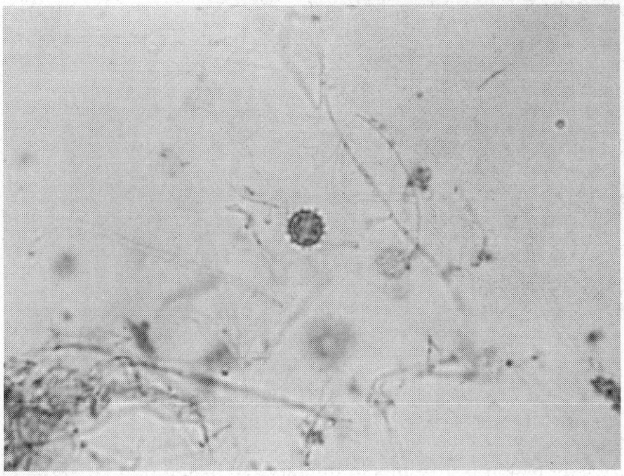

FIGURE 278–1 □ Mold phase of *Histoplasma capsulatum* showing tuberculate macroconidia and hyphae bearing microconidia.

Growth on fungal media at room temperature is relatively slow; incubation for 1 to 4 weeks is required. Definitive identification as *H. capsulatum* var. *capsulatum* requires conversion of the mold to the yeast, demonstration of specific reactivity with anti–*H. capsulatum* antisera (exoantigen tests), or reactivity with DNA probes specific for *Histoplasma* messenger RNA.[9]

Epidemiology

Although *H. capsulatum* is recognized as endemic in certain areas of North America and Latin America,[3] its distribution is much wider. Cases of histoplasmosis have been reported from Europe and Asia. In the United States, most cases have occurred within the Ohio and Mississippi River valleys (Fig. 278–3). Factors accounting for this distribution are not fully understood; however, humid environmental conditions[1, 10] and acidic, permeable soil characteristics[5] appear to be important. Bird and bat excrement enhances growth of the organism in soil by accelerating sporulation. These unique growth requirements, in part, explain the localization of *Histoplasma* into so-called microfoci (Table 278–1). Activities that disturb such sites are associated with exposure to *H. capsulatum* (see Table 278–1). Spores can be blown by the wind for miles, exposing individuals who had no direct contact with the contaminated site.[11] Also, sites not visibly contaminated with droppings may harbor the organism.

Attack rates and severity of clinical disease after exposure vary greatly. Exposure in enclosed areas usually causes more severe illnesses than exposure occurring out-of-doors.[12] Attack rates are higher when exposure occurs in schools or other areas involving children, as children are less likely than adults to have developed immunity as a result of previous infection.[13]

Pathogenesis

Infection with *H. capsulatum* develops when microconidia are inhaled into the lungs. These spores germinate into yeasts, which promote the influx of neutrophils, macrophages, and natural killer cells, serving to inhibit progression of the infection. *H. capsulatum* parasitizes macrophages, which may assist in dissemination throughout the reticuloendothelial system.

T-cell immunity plays the key role in determining the outcome of infection with *H. capsulatum*.[14] With development of specific cellular immunity, cytokines arm macrophages to kill the fungus and halt progression of the disease.[15] These defense mechanisms are generally sufficient to control the infection in immunocompetent individuals, explaining the subclinical or self-limited course characteristic of acute histoplasmosis. Individuals with underlying conditions that impair these defenses, such as acquired immunodeficiency syndrome (AIDS), are at risk for developing more severe, and often fatal, progressive forms of infection.

Reinfection and reactivation of clinically "quiescent" infection also occur in histoplasmosis. T-cell immunity may wane in the absence of occasional reexposure, or exposure to heavy inocula may overcome immune mechanisms, permitting reinfection to occur. Illnesses are thought to be milder after reinfection.[16]

Reactivation of latent histoplasmosis may occur in immunocompromised patients.[17, 18] Identification of a mitochondrial DNA pattern characteristic of that found in Panamanian strains in five Puerto Rican immigrants to New York City

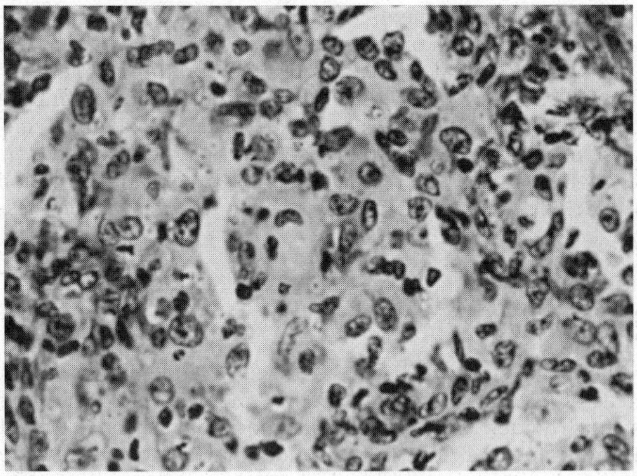

FIGURE 278–2 ▫ Hematoxylin-eosin stain of tissue showing typical yeast-phase organisms demonstrating capsule-like staining artifact surrounding the yeast.

TABLE 278–1 ■ Sources of Exposure to *Histoplasma capsulatum*

MICROFOCUS	ACTIVITIES
Caves	Spelunking
Chicken coops	Cleaning, demolition, use of bird droppings in garden
Bird roosts	Excavation, camping
Bamboo canebrakes	Cutting cane, recreation
Schoolyards	Routine activities, cleaning
Prison grounds	Routine activities, cleaning
Decayed woodpiles	Transporting or burning wood
Dead trees	Recreational, cutting wood
Contaminated chimneys	Cleaning, demolition
Old buildings	Demolition, remodeling, cleaning
Any of above	Epidemiologic studies at contaminated microfoci
Laboratories	Research

supports the hypothesis that reactivation accounts for some cases of disseminated histoplasmosis in patients with AIDS.[19]

Clinical Manifestations

After low-inoculum exposure, about 1 in 100 exposed individuals develops symptomatic histoplasmosis; the remainder experience clinically unrecognized infection (Table 278–2). Underlying host factors, including presence of immunodeficiency, specific immunity to *H. capsulatum*, pulmonary disease, and extent of exposure, interact to influence the outcome of infection.

Self-limited Syndromes

Most clinically recognized infections are self-limited in the absence of underlying immune deficiency or chronic pulmonary disease.[20, 21] The common self-limited presentations include acute pulmonary histoplasmosis, pericarditis,[22] and rheumatologic syndromes,[23] often resembling sarcoidosis.[24, 25]

Acute Pulmonary Histoplasmosis. Acute self-limited illnesses constitute the majority of symptomatic cases (see Table 278–2). About 80% present with influenza-like, acute pulmonary symptoms of fever, chills, headache, myalgia, anorexia, nonproductive cough, and retrosternal or pleuritic chest

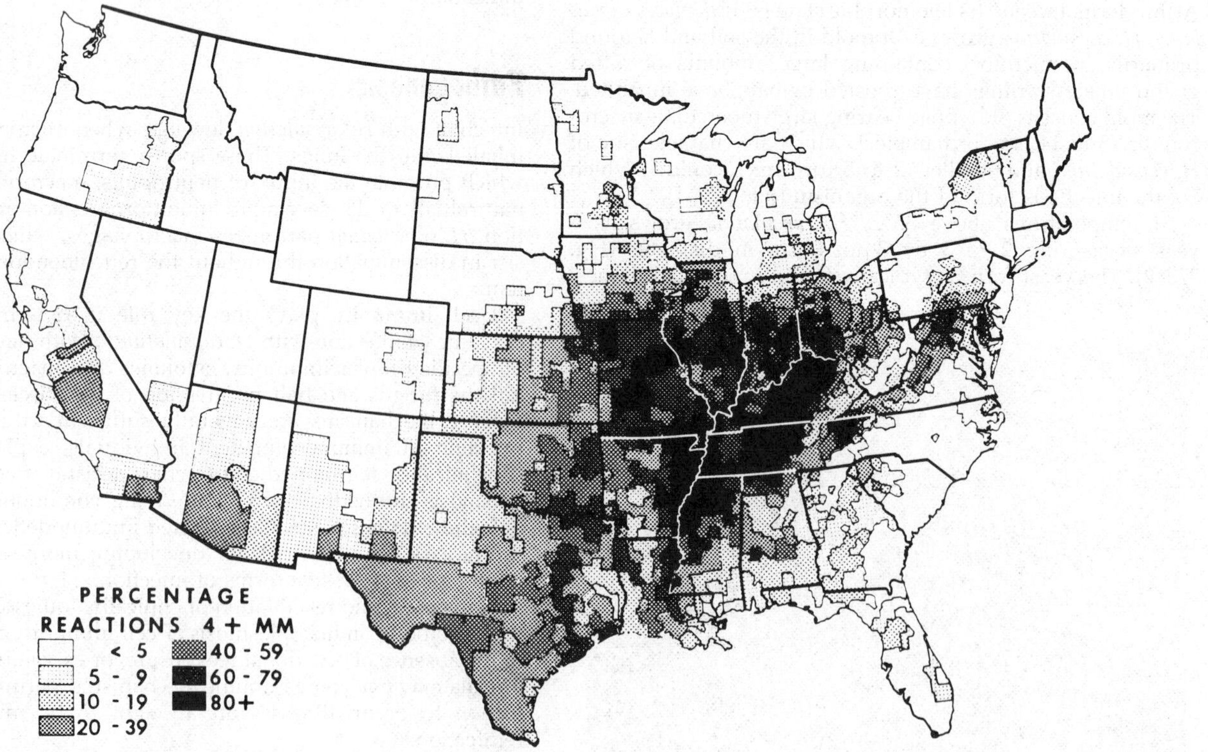

FIGURE 278–3 ▫ Endemic distribution of histoplasmosis in the United States based on skin test results in military recruits. (From Edwards LB, Acquaviva FA, Livesay VT, et al: An atlas of sensitivity to tuberculin, PPD-B and histoplasmin in the United States. Am Rev Respir Dis 99[Suppl]:1–18, 1969.)

TABLE 278–2 ■ Clinical Manifestations of Histoplasmosis

MANIFESTATIONS	HEAVY INOCULUM (%)	LIGHT INOCULUM (%)
Asymptomatic	10–50	99
Self-limited	50–90	1
Pulmonary (80% of symptomatic)		
Arthritis with erythema nodosum (5%–10%)		
Pericarditis (5%–10%)		
Mediastinal granuloma (unknown)		
Disseminated	Unknown	0.05
Chronic pulmonary	Unknown	0.05
Inflammatory or fibrotic	Unknown	0.02
Fibrosing mediastinitis		
Sarcoid-like		
Constrictive pericarditis		
Broncholithiasis		

pain.[26] Chest radiographs show enlarged hilar or mediastinal lymph nodes with patchy infiltrates.[26] Rarely, cavitation may occur in patients with acute pulmonary histoplasmosis.[27, 28] These patients improve within a few weeks[13] but may experience fatigue for months. After heavy exposure, most patients develop symptomatic infection and many present with diffuse pulmonary involvement causing respiratory insufficiency.[29] Concurrent dissemination probably occurs more commonly in such patients than in patients with more focal pulmonary histoplasmosis after low-inoculum exposure.

Mediastinal Granuloma. Patients may present with obstructive symptoms resulting from enlarged mediastinal lymph nodes.[30] These nodes may block the airways or pulmonary arteries in young children or may erode into adjacent structures.

Rheumatologic Syndromes. Five percent to 10% of symptomatic patients present with arthritis or severe arthralgia accompanied by erythema nodosum.[23, 31] These manifestations may linger for months and are best managed by treatment with antiinflammatory agents. Arthritis may rarely be a manifestation of disseminated infection.[32]

Pericarditis. Pericarditis is another inflammatory complication of acute self-limited histoplasmosis, also occurring in 5% to 10% of symptomatic cases.[22] Clinical findings resemble those of viral pericarditis, except that chest radiographs usually show mediastinal lymphadenopathy. Pericardial fluid is often bloody. These patients typically respond to antiinflammatory treatment but up to a quarter exhibit pericardial tamponade. Late constriction is rare.[33] Pericarditis may also be a complication of disseminated histoplasmosis.[34]

Chronic Pulmonary Histoplasmosis

Chronic pulmonary histoplasmosis is characterized by slowly progressive pulmonary disease producing fibrotic apical lung infiltrates with cavitation.[21, 35] Whereas most patients with chronic pulmonary histoplasmosis exhibited symptoms for months before diagnosis, cases have been described after acute exposure to contaminated microfoci.[36, 37] The dominant factor predisposing to chronic pulmonary histoplasmosis is underlying obstructive lung disease.

Symptoms include cough, dyspnea, chest pain, hemoptysis, weakness, fatigue, fever, sweats, and weight loss. Upper lobe infiltrates are present in nearly all cases and cavities occur in 65% to 87% (Fig. 278–4). Other radiographic findings include bullae, mediastinal or pulmonary calcifications, pleural thickening, and hilar retraction. Air-fluid levels may be seen within the cavities, often as a result of concurrent bacterial infection. Fungus balls may develop as a consequence of superinfection with *Aspergillus*.

Progression in chronic pulmonary histoplasmosis is manifested by formation of new cavities, spread to new areas of the lungs, and cavity enlargement in most cases.[38] Bronchopleural fistula is a rare complication.[38]

Disseminated Histoplasmosis

The definition of disseminated histoplasmosis includes a progressive clinical illness with extrapulmonary spread of infection.[20, 39] Progressive disseminated histoplasmosis occurs in about 1 in 2000 acute infections.[20] Underlying immunosuppressive conditions and extremes of age are risk factors for dissemination.[40] AIDS has been identified as a major risk factor,[18] and disseminated histoplasmosis has been reported in patients with idiopathic $CD4^+$ lymphocytopenia.[41] Other chronic debilitating diseases may also predispose to dissemination.

Clinical manifestations are more severe in patients with immune dysfunction. Patients may present shortly after the exposure or years later and may experience asymptomatic periods interrupted by symptomatic relapses.[39] Fever and weight loss are the most common symptoms. Examination reveals hepatomegaly or splenomegaly in about half of cases and lymphadenopathy in a third. Shock, respiratory distress, hepatic and renal failure, and coagulopathy may complicate severe cases.[18] Central nervous system involvement occurs in 10% to 20% of cases, presenting as chronic meningitis or focal brain lesions.[42] Rarely, *Histoplasma* may infect the spinal cord.[43, 44] Other frequent sites of dissemination include the oropharyngeal or gastrointestinal mucosa and skin. Gastrointestinal lesions include ulcerations or polypoid masses, leading to misdiagnosis as colitis or malignancy.[45–49] Lesions most often involve the ileal cecal area but may occur from the

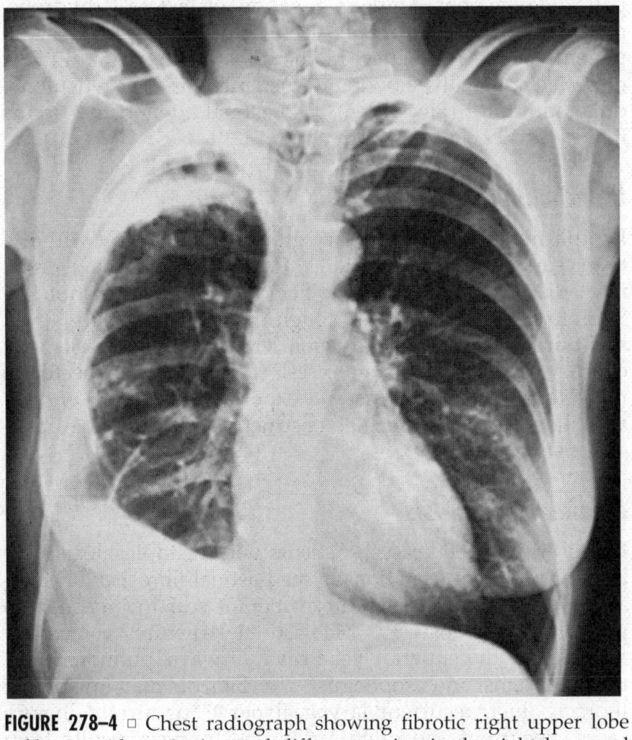

FIGURE 278–4 ▫ Chest radiograph showing fibrotic right upper lobe infiltrate with cavitation and diffuse scarring in the right lung and elevation of the right diaphragm in a patient with concurrent sarcoidosis.

TABLE 278–3 ■ Focal Manifestations of Disseminated Histoplasmosis

Central nervous system: meningitis, abscess, encephalitis, myelopathy
Chorioretinitis
Mouth ulcers or masses
Laryngeal ulcer or mass
Esophageal mass or ulcer
Cardiac: endocarditis, myocarditis, pericarditis
Gastrointestinal: mucosal mass or ulcer
Pancreatitis
Granulomatous hepatitis
Adrenal mass or Addison disease
Genitourinary: interstitial nephritis, epididymitis, penile or vaginal ulcer
Soft tissue: carpal tunnel syndrome, cutaneous ulcers, cellulitis
Bone: lytic lesion

mouth to the anus. Skin lesions may be erythematous maculopapular, pustulonecrotic, hyperpigmented, or crateriform in character.[50–52]

Adrenal involvement is found in 80% to 90% of autopsied cases but Addison disease is uncommon (<10% of cases).[39] Physicians should exclude histoplasmosis in patients with adrenal masses or Addison disease and should rule out adrenal insufficiency in patients with disseminated histoplasmosis who have hyperkalemia, hyponatremia, or hypotension.

Hypercalcemia, presumably caused by increased sensitivity to vitamin D, has rarely been described.[53, 54] Other rare manifestations of dissemination include chorioretinitis,[55] pleuritis,[56] pericarditis,[34] endocarditis,[57, 58] peritonitis,[59] pancreatitis,[20] cholecystitis,[60] prostatitis,[61] panniculitis,[62] mastitis,[63] epididymitis,[64] and involvement of the penis[65, 66] and vagina[65] (Table 278–3).

Laboratory findings of anemia, leukopenia, and thrombocytopenia suggest bone marrow involvement, and alkaline phosphatase elevation may be a clue to the presence of hepatic involvement. Marked elevation of lactate dehydrogenase has been an especially useful clue to the diagnosis in patients with AIDS. Chest radiographs are abnormal in 70% of patients, usually showing diffuse interstitial or reticulonodular infiltrates (Fig. 278–5); mediastinal adenopathy occurs in 20% and cavitation is rare.[18, 20, 67]

Broncholithiasis

Lymph nodes and pulmonary granulomata calcify within a few years of initial infection.[68] Calcified nodes may erode into adjacent bronchi, causing hemoptysis or obstruction.[69, 70] Symptoms include chronic cough, hemoptysis, chills, fever, and purulent sputum production.[70] Massive hemoptysis may complicate the more severe cases.[70] Patients may expectorate rocklike particles of tissue and experience recurrent and severe hemoptysis, bronchial obstruction, or tracheoesophageal fistula.

Mediastinal Fibrosis

Rarely (~1 in 5000 cases), patients with histoplasmosis may present with manifestations of mediastinal fibrosis.[30, 71] Mediastinal fibrosis represents an exuberant scarring reaction to prior histoplasmosis.[30, 71] Mediastinal structures commonly affected are the superior vena cava, airways, pulmonary arteries or veins, and esophagus.[30, 71, 72] Fibrosis may invade the thoracic duct, recurrent laryngeal nerve, or atrium in rare cases. Recurrent and often serious hemoptysis results from lung or airway damage and vascular compromise. Respiratory failure ensues in one third of cases.

Chest radiographs are often normal but may show subcarinal or superior mediastinal widening, and computed tomographic scans reveal fibrotic restriction and invasion of mediastinal structures and calcification of the lymph nodes.

Presumed Ocular Histoplasmosis

A choroiditis often involving the macula and causing visual loss has been attributed to histoplasmosis.[73, 74] However, there is no scientific basis establishing *H. capsulatum* as its cause. *H. capsulatum* has not been demonstrated convincingly in the eye tissues of patients with this syndrome. Instead, the association has been based on high rates of skin test reactivity. However, careful epidemiologic studies with control subjects selected from the same geographic area as the cases have not been performed.[75] To be distinguished from this syndrome, however, is involvement of the eye during disseminated histoplasmosis.[76]

Diagnosis

Diagnosis of histoplasmosis requires a high index of clinical suspicion and awareness of the uses and limitations of a battery of serologic and mycologic tests. Diagnostic modalities include cultures, special stains of tissue, and tests for antibodies and antigens (Table 278–4). The role of each test varies with the severity of the infection.[77]

Antigen Detection

A rapid diagnosis is important in patients with severe manifestations of histoplasmosis. Detection of *Histoplasma* antigen in the body fluids offers a valuable approach to diagnosis in such cases,[77, 78] providing results within 24 to 48 hours. Antigen is found in the blood, urine, and bronchoalveolar lavage fluid of most individuals with disseminated histoplasmosis and in up to 75% of those with diffuse lung involvement during acute pulmonary histoplasmosis. Antigen may be found in cerebrospinal fluid of 25% to 50% of patients with chronic meningitis caused by histoplasmosis.[79]

Positive results caused by cross-reacting antigens occur in patients with disseminated blastomycosis, paracoccidioidomycosis, coccidioidomycosis, and *Penicillium marneffei* infection. Distinction between histoplasmosis and other mycoses

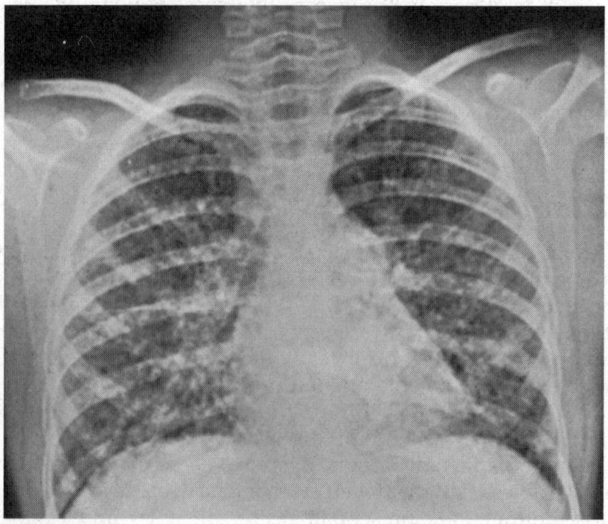

FIGURE 278–5 □ Chest radiograph of a patient with disseminated histoplasmosis showing diffuse interstitial alveolar infiltrates.

TABLE 278–4 ■ Summary of Diagnostic Test Results in Histoplasmosis

	POSITIVE (%)		
TEST	Self-limited	Cavitary	Disseminated
Antibody			
Immunodiffusion	75	100	63
Complement fixation	89	93	63
Either immunodiffusion or complement fixation	99	100	71
Antigen detection	40–75*	21	92
Culture	15	85	85

*Seventy-five percent with diffuse pulmonary infiltrates (Wheat J, unpublished, 1995).

From Williams B, Fojtasek M, Connolly-Stringfield P, Wheat J: Diagnosis of histoplasmosis by antigen detection during an outbreak in Indianapolis, Ind. Arch Pathol Lab Med 118:1205–1208, 1994.

that share cross-reacting antigens can usually be made on an epidemiologic, clinical, or laboratory basis, however.

Antigen levels decline during the first year after treatment or spontaneously in patients with self-limited histoplasmosis[80] and increase with relapse,[81] providing a tool for monitoring therapy.[81] Antigen testing is available at the Histoplasmosis Reference Laboratory, Indiana University School of Medicine, in Indianapolis.

Fungal Stain

Fungal staining of tissue sections or Wright stain of peripheral blood smears permits rapid diagnosis but with a lower sensitivity than culture or antigen detection. Fungal stains of tissues are positive in about half of disseminated cases.[20] The highest yield is from bone marrow.[18, 20] *H. capsulatum* may be seen in peripheral blood smears of patients with severe disease.[82, 83] The sensitivity may be lower if pathologists are inexperienced with recognition of *H. capsulatum* in tissues.

Organisms that may be misidentified as *H. capsulatum* include *Pneumocystis carinii*, *Candida glabrata*, and *Toxoplasma gondii*. Artifacts may also be mistaken for *H. capsulatum* in silver stains of tissues. Polymerase chain reaction may improve the accuracy of tests to identify *H. capsulatum* in tissues.

Fungal Cultures

Cultures provide the strongest proof for histoplasmosis but are limited by low sensitivity (10% to 15%) in self-limited infections and delayed growth (2 to 4 weeks)[77, 84] (see Table 278–4). In disseminated histoplasmosis, the highest yield is from bone marrow or blood, positive in more than 75% of cases.[18, 20] Cultures of urine and sputum are often (~50%) positive in patients with disseminated histoplasmosis.[85]

In cavitary histoplasmosis, organisms can be found in sputum of 60% to 85% of cases if multiple specimens are cultured.[77, 86] Cultures are usually negative in patients with mild acute pulmonary, pericardial, or rheumatologic manifestations and need not be performed.[77, 84]

Serologic Tests

High levels of antibodies develop within 4 to 6 weeks in most symptomatic infections and peak during the next few months. Serologic tests are positive in about 90% of patients with symptomatic histoplasmosis but in a lower percentage of patients who have asymptomatic infection[87] or who are immunosuppressed. Antibody levels decline after recovery from histoplasmosis and may increase with relapse, occasionally providing a useful method for monitoring response to treatment.

Commonly, physicians conjecture that serologic tests for antibodies are unreliable in patients from areas in which histoplasmosis is endemic, expecting that background seropositivity is high. Whereas the majority of adults residing within an endemic area have positive skin tests, only 5% are seropositive: less than 1% by immunodiffusion and 5% by complement fixation.[84] This disparity between high skin test positivity and low seropositivity can be explained by the weaker serologic response in asymptomatic cases and tendency for seropositivity to wane while skin test positivity persists after exposure to *H. capsulatum*.

Limitations of the serologic tests include a 4- to 6-week delay in diagnosis while antibodies are being produced after acute infection, false-negative results for immunocompromised patients, and false-positive results for patients with blastomycosis, coccidioidomycosis, and paracoccidioidomycosis.[88]

Also, high levels of antibodies persisting from past histoplasmosis may cause confusion in patients with other diseases such as malignancy or mycobacterial lung disease. A positive test for anti-*Histoplasma* antibodies may cause a misdiagnosis of histoplasmosis in such cases. Thus, serologic tests for antibodies must be interpreted with caution in individuals with diseases that are not highly suggestive of histoplasmosis. Attempts to establish a specific diagnosis on the basis of fungal stains or cultures or antigen detection are appropriate for such individuals.

Of the commercially available tests, the complement fixation test is the most sensitive.[84] Titers of at least 1:32 have the greatest significance but titers of 1:8 or 1:16 should not be disregarded. The immunodiffusion test is less sensitive and becomes positive later than the complement fixation test. The diagnostic yield is highest if both the immunodiffusion and complement fixation tests are performed.

Histoplasmin Skin Test

Skin tests are not useful diagnostically because of high background rates of skin test positivity (50% to 80%) in endemic areas, false-positive results for patients with other fungal diseases, and false-negative results for patients with disseminated disease.[3, 89] Furthermore, skin tests boost antibody levels, compromising interpretation of serologic tests.[90]

Summary of Diagnostic Approach

Self-limited Syndromes. Serologic tests for antibodies should be performed in all cases. Measurement of antigen in urine and bronchoalveolar lavage fluid and fungal stain, culture, and antibody tests should be considered for patients with respiratory compromise caused by diffuse pulmonary infiltrates, as a prompt diagnosis is needed if antifungal therapy is to be given in time to alter the course of the infection. Tests for antigen may also be useful in patients who present within the first month of suspected exposure when tests for antibodies may be negative.

Chronic Pulmonary Histoplasmosis. Serologic tests for antibodies and fungal cultures of sputum should be performed for patients with findings of chronic pulmonary histoplasmosis. Bronchoalveolar lavage and transbronchial lung biopsy should be considered if sputum cannot be obtained, sputum cultures are negative, or malignancy is suspected. If bronchoscopy is negative for other causes of infectious, inflammatory, or neoplastic lung disease, positive serologic tests for anti–*H. capsulatum* antibodies would provide an acceptable basis for diagnosis of histoplasmosis in patients with negative cultures for *H. capsulatum*.

Disseminated Histoplasmosis. Tests for antigen and fungal stains of lesions should be performed as they allow a rapid diagnosis. Fungal blood cultures and cultures of focal lesions should be obtained. Bone biopsy for stains and culture is appropriate for patients with negative tests for antigen especially if patients are anemic, leukopenic, or thrombocytopenic. Serologic tests for antibodies may provide a basis for performance of additional biopsies and assist in interpretation of positive tests for antigen in patients with negative cultures. Biopsy of other tissues may be appropriate in selected cases. Polymerase chain reaction applications may provide another useful method for rapid diagnosis of disseminated histoplasmosis.

***Histoplasma* Meningitis.** Diagnosis of meningitis is especially difficult.[42] Cultures of cerebrospinal fluid are positive in no more than half of patients. Such patients may have positive cultures from blood or other tissues involved in the generalized dissemination. In cases with isolated meningitis, however, diagnosis may be based on tests for antigen[79] or antibody[91] in the cerebrospinal fluid. In rare cases, meningeal or brain biopsy is needed to establish a diagnosis of meningeal or cerebral histoplasmosis.

Broncholithiasis. Although organisms may be demonstrated in fungal stains of calcified nodes in some patients, cultures are negative. Serologic tests may be positive but tests for antigens would be expected to be negative.

Fibrosing Mediastinitis. Although fungal stains of tissues are positive in more than half of cases, cultures are usually negative. Serologic tests are positive in two thirds of cases while tests for antigen are negative.

Treatment

Indications for Treatment

Acute Pulmonary Histoplasmosis. Patients with acute pulmonary histoplasmosis occasionally benefit from treatment. The clearest indication is for the patient with diffuse lung involvement after a heavy-inoculum exposure who presents with respiratory insufficiency[29] (Table 278–5). A brief course of amphotericin B and adjunctive corticosteroid therapy can be lifesaving in such patients. Patients with acute pulmonary histoplasmosis who are moderately symptomatic at the time of diagnosis or do not improve after a month of observation may benefit from therapy.

Mediastinal Granuloma. Patients typically recover without treatment.[92] Patients with severe or persistent obstructive symptoms or fistula may benefit from antifungal therapy.[93–95] Others have been treated successfully by surgical resection of obstructive masses.[69, 96–98]

TABLE 278–5 ■ Indications for Antifungal Therapy

INDICATED	NOT INDICATED
Acute pulmonary histoplasmosis with respiratory failure or prolonged symptoms	Acute self-limited pulmonary disease, rheumatologic pericarditis
Mediastinal granuloma with symptomatic obstruction	Fibrosing mediastinitis*
Disseminated histoplasmosis	Sarcoid-like disease
Chronic pulmonary histoplasmosis	Presumed ocular disease

*The benefit of therapy for patients with an elevated erythrocyte sedimentation rate and positive serologic test is controversial.

A trial of antifungal therapy with itraconazole or ketoconazole is reasonable to relieve symptoms, perhaps accompanied by adjunctive corticosteroid therapy in patients with symptomatic airway obstruction.[93]

Antifungal treatment or resection of enlarged mediastinal lymph nodes to prevent progression to fibrosing mediastinitis[99, 100] is not indicated, because progression of granulomatous mediastinitis to fibrosing mediastinitis has not been documented and must be rare.[30]

Rheumatologic Syndromes and Pericarditis. These are noninfectious inflammatory manifestations of acute histoplasmosis and respond to antiinflammatory therapy.[22, 23] Antifungal therapy is not indicated unless a bone, a joint, or the pericardium is a site of disseminated infection.

Chronic Pulmonary Histoplasmosis. The untreated course in patients with chronic pulmonary histoplasmosis is usually progressive. In the Centers for Disease Control Cooperative Mycosis Study of untreated patients, 21% died, 23% showed radiographic progression, and only 33% improved spontaneously.[101] Amphotericin B treatment improves survival, reduces symptoms, promotes radiographic healing, and eradicates *H. capsulatum* from the sputum.[102]

Disseminated Histoplasmosis. Treatment is indicated for all patients with disseminated disease. The mortality of patients with untreated disseminated histoplasmosis is 80%.[103] Mortality can be reduced to less than 25% with antifungal therapy.[20, 101, 104, 105]

Broncholithiasis. Antifungal therapy is not indicated. Surgical therapy is required for patients with significant hemoptysis or recurrent pneumonia and for repair of bronchoesophageal fistulae.[69]

Mediastinal Fibrosis. Antifungal treatment is not thought to improve the outcome of mediastinal fibrosis, but a few patients treated with ketoconazole have shown some improvement.[106] Antifungal therapy might be tried in patients with positive serologic tests and elevated erythrocyte sedimentation rates.[106] Although most authorities discourage surgical therapy, improvement after resection of the scar tissue has been reported.[107] Operative mortality is high (25%), however.

Presumed Ocular Histoplasmosis. Presumed ocular histoplasmosis, if indeed caused by *H. capsulatum*, does not represent an active infection and would not be expected to respond to antifungal therapy. Corticosteroids and laser therapy have been used for these patients.[74, 108, 109]

Selection of Antifungal Regimen

AMPHOTERICIN B

Amphotericin B is fungicidal and acts more rapidly than do other antifungal agents. Improvement of fever occurs within 1 week in more than 80% of patients with disseminated infection.[20] Amphotericin B is the treatment of choice for patients with moderately severe or severe clinical manifestations of histoplasmosis. Unfortunately, up to half of patients presenting with severe manifestations of disseminated histoplasmosis (shock or respiratory failure) die within the first week of treatment. Liposomal amphotericin B may permit more aggressive therapy of patients with life-threatening illnesses, improving the outcome of severe histoplasmosis.

Treatment could be changed to itraconazole or ketoconazole within 3 to 7 days in patients who respond rapidly and in 10 to 14 days in those with complications requiring longer hospitalization.

ITRACONAZOLE AND KETOCONAZOLE

Itraconazole and ketoconazole are effective for treatment of patients with mild or moderate manifestations of histoplasmosis. Itraconazole may be superior to ketoconazole. In noncomparative trials for treatment of disseminated histoplasmosis, itraconazole was successful in 85% to 100% of cases,[110, 111] compared with 56% to 70% for ketoconazole.[112, 113] Itraconazole was effective in 85% of cases of disseminated histoplasmosis in patients with AIDS, compared with 9% for ketoconazole.[110] Ketoconazole and itraconazole are also effective treatments for chronic pulmonary histoplasmosis, inducing responses in 75% to 85% of cases.[111, 113]

Both itraconazole and ketoconazole require an acidic environment for solubilization. They should be given with food or an acidic beverage such as cola. Medications that reduce gastric acidity (histamine H_2 antagonists or omeprazole) should be avoided. Histamine H_2 antagonists reduce blood concentrations of ketoconazole by up to 90%.[114] Sucralfate had a smaller impact on ketoconazole concentrations (30% reduction)[114] and might be used in place of histamine H_2 antagonists or omeprazole in patients who require treatment for gastritis or ulcer disease. Itraconazole blood levels were affected less by histamine H_2 antagonists, however (~20% reduction).[115]

Blood concentrations of itraconazole should be measured in all patients during the second week of therapy 2 to 4 hours after a dose. Absorption is highly variable, and treatment failure has occurred in patients with undetectable serum concentrations not attributable to use of interacting medications.[110] Dosage could be reduced to 200 mg once daily in patients with concentrations of at least 10 μg/mL as measured by bioassay.

Itraconazole and ketoconazole are eliminated exclusively by hepatic metabolism. Accordingly, hepatic enzyme inducers (e.g., rifampin, rifabutin, phenytoin, phenobarbital) reduce blood concentrations of these agents by up to 90%[116, 117] and should be avoided. Enzyme induction persists for several weeks after discontinuing the interacting medication, potentially delaying response to treatment or causing treatment failure.

Itraconazole and ketoconazole reduce metabolism of other drugs by inhibition of hepatic cytochrome P-450 enzymes. This interaction causes increase in blood concentrations of terfenadine (Seldane), astemizole (Hismanal), and cisapride (Propulsid), potentially causing serious ventricular arrhythmias and even death.[118] Such combinations should be strictly avoided. Interactions increasing the blood concentrations and toxicities of phenytoin, warfarin (Coumadin), oral hypoglycemics, digitalis, and cyclosporine must also be recognized so that these treatments can be monitored appropriately.[119]

FLUCONAZOLE

Fluconazole is less effective than itraconazole for treatment of histoplasmosis. Fluconazole at 200 to 400 mg induced responses in 40% and 75% of cases in chronic pulmonary and disseminated histoplasmosis, respectively (Pappas P, unpublished). Treatment with 800 mg/d induced remission in 74% of AIDS patients with mild to moderately severe manifestations of disseminated histoplasmosis, but one third had relapses during maintenance treatment with 400 mg/d (Wheat J, unpublished).

Fluconazole might be appropriate for patients with mild illnesses who require treatment with medications that contraindicate use of itraconazole or ketoconazole or who do not absorb itraconazole or ketoconazole. Fluconazole dosage for induction therapy should be 800 mg/d, and 400 mg/d may be adequate for maintenance therapy. Absorption is predictable, and drug interactions that reduce fluconazole concentrations are rare, precluding the need to measure blood concentrations. Fluconazole, like itraconazole and ketoconazole, slows the metabolism and clearance of other medications by inhibition of hepatic cytochrome P-450 enzymes.

Treatment of Meningitis

Sixty percent to 80% of patients with meningitis caused by *H. capsulatum* respond to treatment with amphotericin B, but half have relapses 6 to 24 months later.[42] The benefit of higher daily doses, higher total doses, or intraventricular administration of amphotericin B is unknown. Intraventricular therapy could be reserved for patients who have failed to respond to systemic amphotericin B followed by suppression with itraconazole or fluconazole. Fluconazole, although less active than itraconazole for histoplasmosis, may have an advantage in therapy of meningitis because it achieves good concentrations in the cerebrospinal fluid. Cerebrospinal fluid findings should be monitored for at least 1 year after therapy.

Duration of Therapy

The optimal duration of therapy for histoplasmosis has not been defined adequately. If amphotericin B is used exclusively, at least 30 mg/kg should be given for 2 to 4 months, usually at a dose of about 50 mg or 0.7 mg/kg per day. After 1 week of daily therapy, most patients have improved sufficiently to reduce the frequency of amphotericin B to alternate days, thus reducing toxicity.

If an azole is used as the mainstay of therapy, it should be given for at least 12 months for disseminated disease and often longer for chronic pulmonary histoplasmosis. Shorter courses (3 months) should suffice in patients with acute pulmonary histoplasmosis or granulomatous mediastinal lymphadenitis.

Chronic suppressive or so-called maintenance therapy is indicated in some patients. Relapse occurs in 80% of patients with AIDS if treatment is stopped [18] and in a lower percentage of other cases (<20%).[20] Suppressive treatment is indicated for all patients with AIDS and for others who have had relapses after adequate courses of amphotericin B or itraconazole. Weekly or biweekly amphotericin B (50 to 100 mg)[18, 120] and itraconazole (200 to 400 mg/d)[121] are more than 90% effective as maintenance therapy. Fluconazole at 400 mg/d is inferior to itraconazole and should be reserved for patients who cannot take itraconazole.

Prevention

Epidemiologists who are collecting soil samples at suspected sites and workers involved in cleanup of those sites should follow procedures described by the Centers for Disease Control and Prevention to avoid inhalation exposure. Individuals who are collecting samples should wear masks. Those who are cleaning up bird or bat droppings or debris at contaminated sites should wear respirators.[122] Sites growing *H. capsulatum* should be decontaminated with formalin before cleanup or excavation, when possible.[122, 123]

Laboratory employees who are working with *H. capsulatum* are at risk for exposure by inhalation of infectious conidia or accidental inoculation. Workers who are identifying cultures that might contain *H. capsulatum* must observe Centers for Disease Control and Prevention level II precautions; those who are propagating mold-phase cultures are at a higher risk for exposure and must observe level III precautions.[124]

References

1. Furcolow ML: Environmental aspects of histoplasmosis. Arch Environ Health 10:4–10, 1965.

2. Christie A, Peterson JC: Pulmonary calcification in negative reactors to tuberculin. Am J Public Health 35:1131–1147, 1945.
3. Edwards LB, Acquaviva FA, Livesay VT, et al: An atlas of sensitivity to tuberculin, PPD-B and histoplasmin in the United States. Am Rev Respir Dis 99(Suppl):1–18, 1969.
4. Emmons CW: Isolation of *Histoplasma capsulatum* from soil. Am J Public Health 64:892–896, 1949.
4a. Furcolow ML: Recent studies on the epidemiology of histoplasmosis. Ann N Y Acad Sci 72:127–164, 1958.
5. Zeidberg LD, Ajello L, Dillon A, Runyon LC: Isolation of *Histoplasma capsulatum* from soil. Am J Public Health 42:930–935, 1952.
6. Bowman BH, Taylor JW, White TJ: Molecular evolution of the fungi: Human pathogens. Mol Biol Evol 9:893–904, 1992.
7. Hutton JP, Durham JB, Miller DP, Everett ED: Hyphal forms of *Histoplasma capsulatum*: A common manifestation of intravascular infections. Arch Pathol Lab Med 109:330–332, 1985.
8. Svirbely JR, Ayers LW, Buesching WJ: Filamentous *Histoplasma capsulatum* endocarditis involving mitral and aortic valve porcine bioprostheses. Arch Pathol Lab Med 109:273–276, 1985.
9. Stockman L, Clark KA, Hunt JM, Roberts GD: Evaluation of commercially available acridinium ester–labeled chemiluminescent DNA probes for culture identification of *Blastomyces dermatitidis*, *Coccidioides immitis*, *Cryptococcus neoformans*, and *Histoplasma capsulatum*. J Clin Microbiol 31:845–850, 1993.
10. Goodman NL, Larsh HW: Environmental factors and growth of *Histoplasma capsulatum* in soil. Mycopathol Mycol Appl 32:145–156, 1967.
11. Tosh FE, Doto IL, D'Alessio DJ, et al: The second of two epidemics of histoplasmosis resulting from work on the same starling roost. Am Rev Respir Dis 94:406–413, 1966.
12. Waldman RJ, England AC, Tauxe R, et al: A winter outbreak of acute histoplasmosis in northern Michigan. Am J Epidemiol 117:68–75, 1983.
13. Brodsky AL, Gregg MB, Kaufman L, Mallison GF: Outbreak of histoplasmosis associated with the 1970 Earth Day activities. Am J Med 54:333–342, 1973.
14. Deepe GS Jr, Bullock WE: Histoplasmosis: A granulomatous inflammatory response. *In* Gallin JI, Goldstein IM, Snyderman R (eds): Inflammation: Basic Principles and Clinical Correlates. New York, Raven Press, 1988, pp 733–749.
15. Wu-Hsieh BA, Lee GS, Franco M, Hofman FM: Early activation of splenic macrophages by tumor necrosis factor alpha is important in determining the outcome of experimental histoplasmosis in mice. Infect Immun 60:4230–4238, 1992.
16. Goodwin RA Jr, des Prez RM: Histoplasmosis. Am Rev Respir Dis 117:929–956, 1978.
17. Davies SF, Khan M, Sarosi GA: Disseminated histoplasmosis in immunologically suppressed patients. Am J Med 64:94–100, 1978.
18. Wheat LJ, Connolly-Stringfield PA, Baker RL, et al: Disseminated histoplasmosis in the acquired immune deficiency syndrome: Clinical findings, diagnosis and treatment, and review of the literature. Medicine (Baltimore) 69:361–374, 1990.
19. Keath EJ, Kobayashi GS, Medoff G: Typing of *Histoplasma capsulatum* by restriction fragment length polymorphisms in a nuclear gene. J Clin Microbiol 30:2104–2107, 1992.
20. Sathapatayavongs B, Batteiger BE, Wheat LJ, et al: Clinical and laboratory features of disseminated histoplasmosis during two large urban outbreaks. Medicine (Baltimore) 62:263–270, 1983.
21. Wheat LJ, Wass J, Norton J, et al: Cavitary histoplasmosis occurring during two large urban outbreaks: Analysis of clinical, epidemiologic, roentgenographic, and laboratory features. Medicine (Baltimore) 63:201–209, 1984.
22. Wheat LJ, Stein L, Corya BC, et al: Pericarditis as a manifestation of histoplasmosis during two large urban outbreaks. Medicine (Baltimore) 62:110–119, 1983.
23. Rosenthal J, Brandt KD, Wheat LJ, Slama TG: Rheumatologic manifestations of histoplasmosis in the recent Indianapolis epidemic. Arthritis Rheum 26:1065–1070, 1983.
24. Thornberry DK, Wheat LJ, Brandt KD, Rosenthal J: Histoplasmosis presenting with joint pain and hilar adenopathy: Pseudosarcoidosis. Arthritis Rheum 25:1396–1402, 1982.
25. Wheat LJ, French MLV, Wass JL: Sarcoidlike manifestations of histoplasmosis. Arch Intern Med 149:2421–2426, 1989.
26. Wheat LJ, Slama TG, Eitzen HE, et al: A large urban outbreak of histoplasmosis: Clinical features. Ann Intern Med 94:331–337, 1981.
27. Chick EW, Dillon ML, Tahanasab A: Acute cavitary histoplasmosis. Chest 71:674–675, 1977.
28. Bennish M, Radkowski MA, Rippon JW: Cavitation in acute histoplasmosis. Chest 84:496–497, 1983.
29. Kataria YP, Campbell PB, Burlingham BT: Acute pulmonary histoplasmosis presenting as adult respiratory distress syndrome: Effect of therapy on clinical and laboratory features. South Med J 74:534–537, 1981.
30. Loyd JE, Tillman BF, Atkinson JB, des Prez RM: Mediastinal fibrosis complicating histoplasmosis. Medicine (Baltimore) 67:295–310, 1988.
31. Medeiros AA, Marty SD, Tosh FE, Chin TDY: Erythema nodosum and erythema multiforme as clinical manifestations of histoplasmosis in a community outbreak. N Engl J Med 274:415–420, 1966.
32. Gass M, Kobayashi GS: Histoplasmosis. Arch Dermatol 100:724–727, 1969.
33. Wooley CF, Hosier DM: Constrictive pericarditis due to *Histoplasma capsulatum*. N Engl J Med 264:1230–1232, 1961.
34. Young EJ, Vainrub B, Musher DM: Pericarditis due to histoplasmosis. JAMA 240:1750–1751, 1978.
35. Goodwin RA Jr, Owens FT, Snell JD, et al: Chronic pulmonary histoplasmosis. Medicine (Baltimore) 55:413–452, 1976.
36. Davies SF, Sarosi GA: Acute cavitary histoplasmosis. Chest 73:103–105, 1978.
37. Latham RH, Kaiser AB, Dupont WD, Dan BB: Chronic pulmonary histoplasmosis following the excavation of a bird roost. Am J Med 68:504–508, 1980.
38. Furcolow ML: Course and prognosis of untreated histoplasmosis. JAMA 177:292–296, 1961.
39. Goodwin RA Jr, Shapiro JL, Thurman GH, et al: Disseminated histoplasmosis: Clinical and pathologic correlations. Medicine (Baltimore) 59:1–33, 1980.
40. Wheat LJ, Slama TG, Norton JA, et al: Risk factors for disseminated or fatal histoplasmosis. Ann Intern Med 96:159–163, 1982.
41. Smith DK, Neal JJ, Holmberg SD, Centers for Disease Control Idiopathic $CD4^+$ T-Lymphocytopenia Task Force: Unexplained opportunistic infections and $CD4^+$ T-lymphocytopenia without HIV infection. N Engl J Med 328:374–379, 1993.
42. Wheat LJ, Batteiger BE, Sathapatayavongs B: *Histoplasma capsulatum* infections of the central nervous system: A clinical review. Medicine (Baltimore) 69:244–260, 1990.
43. Bazan C III, New PZ: Intramedullary spinal histoplasmosis efficacy of gadolinium enhancement. Neuroradiology 33:190, 1991.
44. Livas IC, Nechay PS, Nauseef WM: Clinical evidence of spinal and cerebral histoplasmosis twenty years after renal transplantation. Clin Infect Dis 20:692–695, 1995.
45. Schneider RP, Edwards W: Histoplasmosis presenting as an esophageal tumor. Gastrointest Endosc 23:158–159, 1977.
46. Cimponeriu D, LoPresti P, Lavelanet M, et al: Gastrointestinal histoplasmosis in HIV infection: Two cases of colonic pseudocancer and review of the literature. Am J Gastroenterol 89:129–131, 1994.
47. Lee KR, Lin F: The radiology corner: Gastrointestinal histoplasmosis, roentgenographic, clinical and pathological correlation. Am J Gastroenterol 63:255–265, 1975.
48. Lee SH, Barnes WG, Hodges GR, Dixon A: Perforated granulomatous colitis caused by *Histoplasma capsulatum*. Dis Colon Rectum 28:171–176, 1985.
49. Morrison YY, Rathbun RC, Huycke MM: Disseminated histoplasmosis mimicking Crohn's disease in a patient with the acquired immunodeficiency syndrome. Am J Gastroenterol 89:1255–1257, 1994.
50. Hazelhurst JA, Vismer HF: Histoplasmosis presenting with unusual skin lesions in acquired immunodeficiency syndrome (AIDS). Br Med J 113:345–348, 1985.
51. Barton EN, Roberts L, Ince WE, et al: Cutaneous histoplasmosis in the acquired immune deficiency syndrome: A report of three cases from Trinidad. Trop Geogr Med 40:153–157, 1988.
52. Cott GR, Smith TW, Hinthorn DR, Liu C: Primary cutaneous histoplasmosis in immunosuppressed patients. JAMA 242:456–457, 1979.
53. Walker JV, Baran D, Yakub N, Freeman RB: Histoplasmosis with

hypercalcemia, renal failure, and papillary necrosis: Confusion with sarcoidosis. JAMA 237:1350–1352, 1977.
54. Murray JJ, Heim CR: Hypercalcemia in disseminated histoplasmosis: Aggravation by vitamin D. Am J Med 78:881–884, 1985.
55. Macher A, Rodrigues MM, Kaplan W, et al: Disseminated bilateral chorioretinitis due to *Histoplasma capsulatum* in a patient with the acquired immunodeficiency syndrome. Ophthalmology 92:1159–1164, 1985.
56. Kilburn CD, McKinsey DS: Recurrent massive pleural effusion due to pleural, pericardial, and epicardial fibrosis in histoplasmosis. Chest 100:1715–1717, 1991.
57. Gaynes RP, Gardner P, Causey W: Prosthetic valve endocarditis caused by *Histoplasma capsulatum*. Arch Intern Med 141:1533–1537, 1981.
58. Rogers EW, Weyman AE, Noble RJ, Bruins SC: Left atrial myxoma infected with *Histoplasma capsulatum*. Am J Med 64:683–690, 1978.
59. Reddy PA, Brasher CA, Christianson C, Gorelick DF: Peritonitis due to histoplasmosis. Ann Intern Med 72:79–81, 1969.
60. Patrick CC, Flynn PM, Henwick S, Pui CH: Disseminated histoplasmosis presenting as a cystic duct obstruction. Pediatr Infect Dis J 11:593–594, 1992.
61. Zighelboim J, Goldfarb RA, Mody D, et al: Prostatic abscess due to *Histoplasma capsulatum* in a patient with the acquired immunodeficiency syndrome. J Urol 147:167–168, 1992.
62. Pottage JC Jr, Trenholme GM, Aronson IK, Harris AA: Panniculitis associated with histoplasmosis and alpha 1-antitrypsin deficiency. Am J Med 75:150–153, 1983.
63. Osborne BM: Granulomatous mastitis cause by *Histoplasma* and mimicking inflammatory breast carcinoma. Hum Pathol 20:47–52, 1989.
64. Kauffman CA, Slama TG, Wheat LJ: *Histoplasma capsulatum* epididymitis. J Urol 125:434–435, 1980.
65. Sills M, Schwartz A, Weg JG: Conjugal histoplasmosis: A consequence of progressive dissemination in the index case after steroid therapy. Ann Intern Med 79:221–224, 1973.
66. Jayalakshmi P, Goh KL, Soo-Hoo TS, Daud A: Disseminated histoplasmosis presenting as penile ulcer. Aust N Z J Med 20:175–176, 1990.
67. Conces DJ Jr, Stockberger SM, Tarver RD, Wheat LJ: Disseminated histoplasmosis in AIDS: Findings on chest radiographs. AJR 160:15–19, 1993.
68. Goodwin RA, Loyd JE, des Prez RM: Histoplasmosis in normal hosts. Medicine (Baltimore) 60:231–266, 1981.
69. Garrett HE Jr, Roper CL: Surgical intervention in histoplasmosis. Ann Thorac Surg 42:711–722, 1986.
70. Arrigoni MG, Bernatz PE, Donoghue FE: Broncholithiasis. J Thorac Cardiovasc Surg 62:231–237, 1971.
71. Goodwin RA, Nickell JA, des Prez RM: Mediastinal fibrosis complicating healed primary histoplasmosis and tuberculosis. Medicine (Baltimore) 51:227–246, 1972.
72. Schowengerdt CG, Suyemoto R, Beachley F: Granulomatous and fibrous mediastinitis. J Thorac Cardiovasc Surg 57:365–379, 1969.
73. Woods AC, Wahlen HE: The probable role of benign histoplasmosis in the etiology of granulomatous uveitis. Am Heart J 49:205–220, 1960.
74. Schwarz J: Histoplasmosis of the eye. *In* Histoplasmosis. New York, Praeger, 1981, pp 317–350.
75. Spaeth GL: Presumed *Histoplasma* uveitis: Continuing doubts as to its actual cause. *In* Ajello L, Chick E, Furcolow M (eds): Histoplasmosis, Proceedings of the Second National Conference. Springfield, IL, Charles C Thomas, 1971, pp 221–230.
76. Specht CS, Mitchell KT, Bauman AE, Gupta M: Ocular histoplasmosis with retinitis in a patient with acquired immune deficiency syndrome. Ophthalmology 98:1356–1359, 1991.
77. Williams B, Fojtasek M, Connolly-Stringfield P, Wheat J: Diagnosis of histoplasmosis by antigen detection during an outbreak in Indianapolis, Ind. Arch Pathol Lab Med 118:1205–1208, 1994.
78. Wheat LJ, Kohler RB, Tewari RP: Diagnosis of disseminated histoplasmosis by detection of *Histoplasma capsulatum* antigen in serum and urine specimens. N Engl J Med 314:83–88, 1986.
79. Wheat LJ, Kohler RB, Tewari RP, et al: Significance of *Histoplasma* antigen in the cerebrospinal fluid of patients with meningitis. Arch Intern Med 149:302–304, 1989.
80. Wheat LJ, Connolly-Stringfield P, Blair R, et al: Effect of successful treatment with amphotericin B on *Histoplasma capsulatum* variety *capsulatum* polysaccharide antigen levels in patients with AIDS and histoplasmosis. Am J Med 92:153–160, 1992.
81. Wheat LJ, Connolly-Stringfield P, Blair R, et al: Histoplasmosis relapse in patients with AIDS: Detection using *Histoplasma capsulatum* variety *capsulatum* antigen levels. Ann Intern Med 115:936–941, 1991.
82. Kurtin PJ, McKinsey DS, Gupta MR, Driks M: Histoplasmosis in patients with acquired immunodeficiency syndrome: Hematologic and bone marrow manifestations. Am J Clin Pathol 93:367–372, 1990.
83. Zarabi CM, Thomas R, Adesokan A: Diagnosis of systemic histoplasmosis in patients with AIDS. South Med J 85:1171–1175, 1992.
84. Wheat LJ, French MLV, Kohler RB, et al: The diagnostic laboratory tests for histoplasmosis: Analysis of experience in a large urban outbreak. Ann Intern Med 97:680–685, 1982.
85. Smith JW, Utz JP: Progressive disseminated histoplasmosis: A prospective study of 26 patients. Ann Intern Med 76:557–565, 1972.
86. Sutcliffe MC, Savage AM, Alford RH: Transferrin-dependent growth inhibition of yeast-phase *Histoplasma capsulatum* by human serum and lymph. J Infect Dis 142:209–219, 1980.
87. Wheat LJ: Histoplasmosis. Infect Dis Clin North Am 2:841–859, 1988.
88. Wheat LJ, French MLV, Kamel S, Tewari RP: Evaluation of cross-reactions in *Histoplasma capsulatum* serologic tests. J Clin Microbiol 23:493–499, 1986.
89. Zeidberg LD, Dillon A, Gass RS: Some factors in the epidemiology of histoplasmin sensitivity in Williamson County, Tennessee. Am J Public Health 41:80–89, 1951.
90. Kaufman L, Terry RT, Schubert JH, McLaughlin D: Effects of a single histoplasmin skin test on the serological diagnosis of histoplasmosis. J Bacteriol 94:798–803, 1967.
91. Wheat LJ, French MLV, Batteiger B, Kohler RB: Cerebrospinal fluid *Histoplasma* antibodies in central nervous system histoplasmosis. Arch Intern Med 145:1237–1240, 1985.
92. Alcorn GL: Clinical problems in cardidopulmonary disease: Histoplasmosis with symptomatic lymphadenopathy, clinical evaluation by R.A. Goodwin, M.D. Chest 77:213–215, 1980.
93. Greenwood MF, Holland P: Tracheal obstruction secondary to *Histoplasma* mediastinal granuloma. Chest 62:642–645, 1972.
94. Jenkins DW, Fisk DE, Byrd RB: Mediastinal histoplasmosis with esophageal abscess. Gastroenterology 70:109–111, 1976.
95. Coss KC, Wheat LJ, Conces DJ Jr, et al: Esophageal fistula complicating mediastinal histoplasmosis: Response to amphotericin B. Am J Med 83:343–346, 1987.
96. Gilliland MD, Scott LD, Walker WE: Esophageal obstruction caused by mediastinal histoplasmosis: Beneficial results of operation. Surgery 95:59–62, 1984.
97. Woods LP: Mediastinal *Histoplasma granuloma* causing tracheal compression in a 4-year-old child. Surgery 58:448–452, 1965.
98. Landay MJ, Rollins NK: Mediastinal histoplasmosis granuloma: Evaluation with CT. Radiology 172:657–659, 1989.
99. Dines DE, Payne WS, Bernatz PE, Pairolero PC: Mediastinal granuloma and fibrosing mediastinitis. Chest 75:320–324, 1979.
100. Sakulsky SB, Harrison EG, Dines DE, Payne WS: Mediastinal granuloma. J Thorac Cardiovasc Surg 54:280–290, 1967.
101. Furcolow ML: Comparison of treated and untreated severe histoplasmosis. JAMA 183:121–127, 1963.
102. Sutliff WD, Andrews CE, Jones E, Terry RT: Histoplasmosis cooperative study: Veterans Administration–Armed Forces Cooperative Study on histoplasmosis. Am Rev Respir Dis 89:641–650, 1964.
103. Rubin H, Furcolow ML, Yates JL, Brasher CA: The course and prognosis of histoplasmosis. Am J Med 27:278–288, 1959.
104. Reddy P, Gorelick DF, Brasher CA, Larsh H: Progressive disseminated histoplasmosis as seen in adults. Am J Med 48:629–636, 1970.
105. Sarosi GA, Voth DW, Dahl BA, et al: Disseminated histoplasmosis: Results of long-term follow-up. Ann Intern Med 75:511–516, 1971.
106. Urschel HC Jr, Razzuk MA, Netto GJ, et al: Sclerosing mediastinitis: Improved management with histoplasmosis titer and ketoconazole. Ann Thorac Surg 50:215–221, 1990.
107. Mathisen DJ, Grillo HC: Clinical manifestation of mediastinal

fibrosis and histoplasmosis. Ann Thorac Surg 54:1053–1058, 1992.
108. Fine SL, Wood WJ, Isernhagen RD, et al: Laser treatment for subfoveal neovascular membranes in ocular histoplasmosis syndrome: Results of a pilot randomized clinical trial. Arch Ophthalmol 111:19–20, 1993.
109. Macular Photocoagulation Study Group: Laser photocoagulation for neovascular lesions nasal to the fovea: Results from clinical trials for lesions secondary to ocular histoplasmosis or idiopathic causes. Arch Ophthalmol 113:56–61, 1995.
110. Wheat J, Hafner R, Korzun AH, et al: Itraconazole treatment of disseminated histoplasmosis in patients with the acquired immunodeficiency syndrome. Am J Med 98:336–342, 1995.
111. Dismukes WE, Bradsher RW Jr, Cloud GC, et al: Itraconazole therapy for blastomycosis and histoplasmosis. Am J Med 93:489–497, 1992.
112. Slama TG: Treatment of disseminated and progressive cavitary histoplasmosis with ketoconazole. Am J Med 74:70–73, 1983.
113. Dismukes WE, Cloud G, Bowles C, et al: Treatment of blastomycosis and histoplasmosis with ketoconazole: Results of a prospective randomized clinical trial. Ann Intern Med 103:861–872, 1985.
114. Piscitelli SC, Goss TF, Wilton JH, et al: Effects of ranitidine and sulcralfate on ketoconazole bioavailability. Antimicrob Agents Chemother 35:1765–1771, 1991.
115. Stein AG, Daneshmend TK, Warnock DW, et al: The effects of H_2-receptor antagonists on the pharmacokinetics of itraconazole, a new oral antifungal. Br J Clin Pharmacol 27:105P–106P, 1989.
116. Tucker RM, Denning DW, Hanson LH, et al: Interaction of azoles with rifampin, phenytoin, and carbamazepine: In vitro and clinical observations. Clin Infect Dis 14:165–174, 1992.
117. Drayton J, Dickinson G, Rinaldi MG: Coadministration of rifampin and itraconazole leads to undetectable levels of serum itraconazole. Clin Infect Dis 18:266–266, 1994.
118. Pohjola-Sintonen S, Viitasalo M, Toivonen L, Neuvonen P: Torsades de pointes after terfenadine-itraconazole interaction. Am J Clin Pharmacol 275:105–106, 1989.
119. Wheat J: Itraconazole. Med Lett 35:7–10, 1993.
120. McKinsey DS, Gupta MR, Driks M, et al: Histoplasmosis in patients with AIDS: Efficacy of maintenance amphotericin B therapy. Am J Med 92:225–227, 1992.
121. Wheat J, Hafner R, Wulfsohn M, et al: Prevention of relapse of histoplasmosis with itraconazole in patients with the acquired immunodeficiency syndrome. The National Institute of Allergy and Infectious Diseases Clinical Trials and Mycoses Study Group Collaborators. Ann Intern Med 118:610–616, 1993.
122. Tosh FE: Histoplasmosis Control: Decontamination of Bird Roosts, Chicken Houses, and Other Point Sources. US Department of Health, Education and Welfare (Public Health Service), CDC Publication 00-3021.
123. Tosh FE, Weeks RJ, Pfeiffer FR, et al: The use of formalin to kill *Histoplasma capsulatum* at an epidemic site. Am J Epidemiol 85:259–265, 1967.
124. Centers for Disease Control: Fungal agents. *In* Richmond JY, McKinney RW (eds): Biosafety in Microbiological and Biomedical Laboratories. Washington, DC: US Government Printing Office, 1993, pp 78–83.

279

Coccidioides immitis

Stanley C. Deresinski
Carol A. Kemper

History[1,2]

In 1892, Alejandro Posada[3] reported the case history of an Argentinean soldier named Domingo Escurra who was afflicted with skin lesions thought to be those of mycosis fungoides, and when Posada discovered rounded microorganisms in the lesions, he believed he had discovered the cause of this disease. Shortly thereafter, Emmet Rixford and T. C. Gilchrist[4,5] reported finding apparently identical organisms in the cutaneous lesions of Joas Furtado Silverra and Jose Teixara Periera, both immigrants to California from the Azores.

All three investigators believed that the organism they had observed was a protozoan (a mistake Samuel Taylor Darling was to make 10 years later in his description of *Histoplasma capsulatum*). Rixford and Gilchrist believed it to be a sporozoan, and because of its resemblance to the coccidia, they named it *Coccidioides*. The isolate from Silverra was named *immitis* ("not minor") to indicate its apparent virulence. In 1900, Ophüls and Moffitt examined the "white mouldy growth" (also observed by Rixford and Gilchrist but discarded as a contaminant) recovered from the pleura and spleen of another Azorean immigrant with the infection and rapidly confirmed that the organism was a fungus, described its life cycle, and satisfied Koch's postulates.[6–8] In 1932, the fungus was isolated from soil under a Delano, California, bunkhouse where four Filipino farm workers who had developed serious coccidioidal infections had lived.[9]

Infections caused by the organism seemed to be almost invariably fatal.[8] Later laboratory, clinical, and epidemiologic observations by Dickson and Gifford[10,11] determined, however, that valley fever, a usually self-limited disease seen with great frequency in the San Joaquin Valley of California, was also caused by *Coccidioides immitis* (CI) and that the respiratory tract was its portal of entry. Smith subsequently developed an effective reagent (coccidioidin) for skin and serologic tests for coccidioidomycosis and, by means of clinical observation and enormous skin test and serologic surveys, further defined the nature and geographic extent of the disease in the San Joaquin Valley. Smith and colleagues[12–14] described the predisposition of certain groups to severe disease, demonstrated that self-limited exposure to the fungus appeared to protect individuals from subsequent infection, and reported the prognostic value of skin test reactivity and the intensity of the complement-fixing antibody response.

Characteristics of the Pathogen

Classification, Replication, and Structure

CI is a dimorphic fungus that has been proposed as a member of the family Onygenaceae, order Onygenales, division Ascomycotina.[15,16] Its guanine plus cytosine content is 49.41% to 49.61%,[17] and it is variously reported to have three or four pairs of chromosomes.[18, 19] CI exhibits the mycelial form in the saprobic state, whereas it exists as an endosporulating spherule in the parasitic (tissue) phase. In contrast to most other pathogenic dimorphs, its morphologic state is not thermally determined. Instead, a key factor in the formation of endosporulating spherules in vitro is the maintenance of carbon dioxide tension in the range of 20 to 60 torr.[20] These values encompass those found in the human and animal host and thus may also be critical for morphologic conversion in vivo. Polymorphonuclear leukocytes may play a role in maintaining the organism in the spherule-endospore phase in vivo.[21, 22]

The mode of reproduction of CI is unique.[23–25] Although mating and meiosis have not been observed, molecular population genetic and phylogenetic analyses have found evidence of recombination, indicating cryptic sexual reproduction.[25] The saprobic phase is seen in soil as well as under standard methods of cultivation in the laboratory (Fig. 279–1). Within several days of inoculation, conidia first appear on side branches of thin hyphae. Septa, which contain pores, arise from the inner layer of cell wall behind the growing hyphae, which eventually branch to form a mycelium. Multiple septa form simultaneously in fertile hyphae, creating cells. These divide with the subsequent internal (enteroarthric) development of thick-walled multinucleated arthroconidia alternating with thin-walled cells, which undergo autolysis (Fig. 279–2). As a consequence, arthroconidia, the infectious units of CI, readily disarticulate from the colony (in a process called rhexolytic secession) and may become airborne. Inhalation of the arthroconidia by an animal or human may then lead to infection.

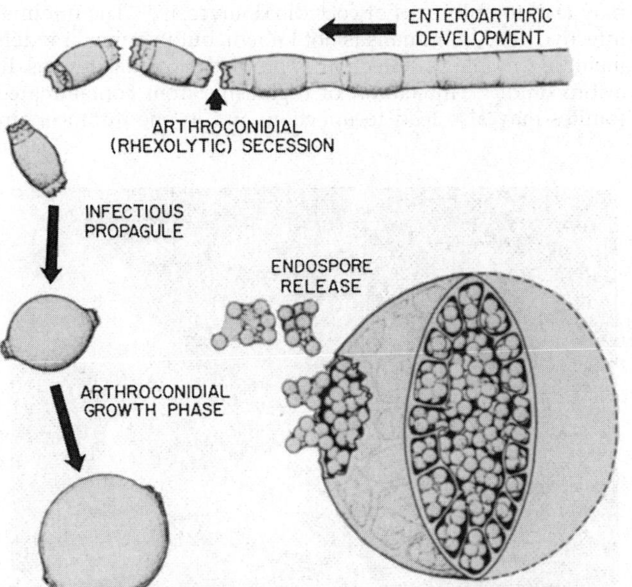

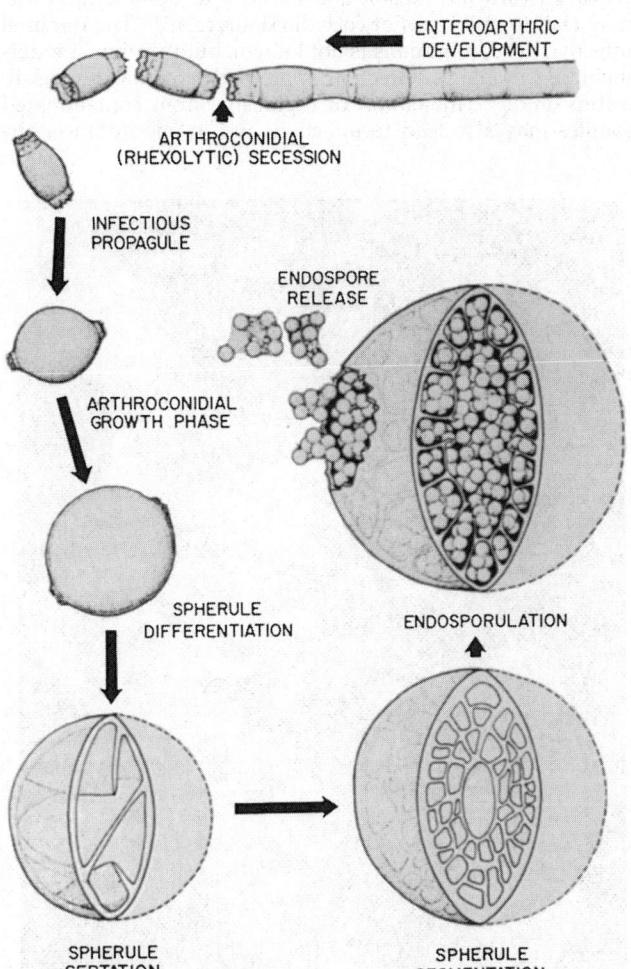

FIGURE 279–1 ▫ Life cycle of *Coccidioides immitis*. (From Cole GT, Sun SH: Arthroconidium-spherule-endospore transformation in *Coccidioides immitis*. *In* Szaniszlo PJ [ed]: Fungal Dimorphism: With Emphasis on Fungi Pathogenic for Humans. New York, Plenum Publishing, 1985, pp 281–336.)

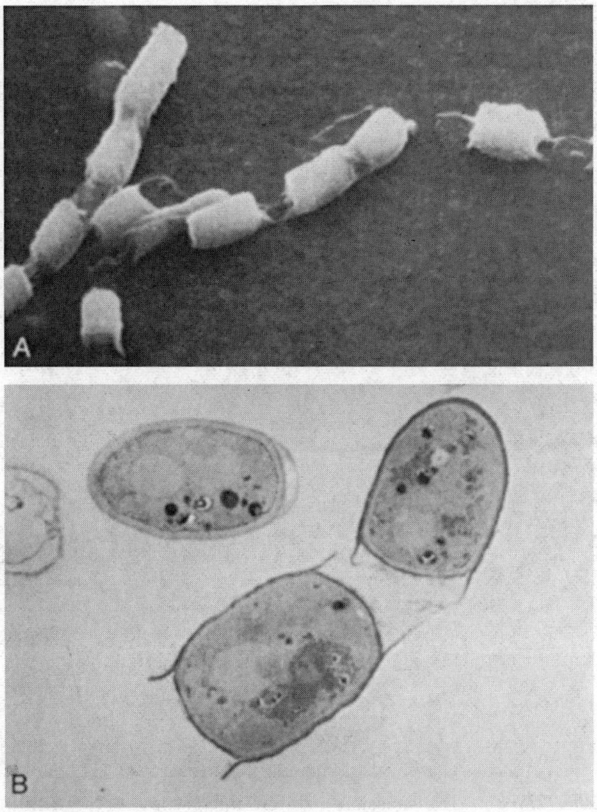

FIGURE 279–2 ▫ *A*, Scanning electron microscopy of mycelial fragment demonstrating arthroconidia alternating with "clear spaces." *B*, Transmission electron microscopy of arthroconidia undergoing rhexolytic secession with demonstration of retained hyphal outer wall. (*A* and *B* courtesy of Dr. S. H. Sun, Veterans Administration Medical Center, San Antonio, TX.)

Once in the host, the arthroconidia become uninucleated and, within 48 hours, convert to spherules, probably as a result of exposure to ambient concentrations of carbon dioxide[20] and, possibly, polymorphonuclear leukocytes.[22] The spherules enlarge, reaching a size of 20 to 150 μm in diameter, while their walls thicken. At the same time, the nucleus undergoes repeated synchronous divisions. After approximately 72 hours, and after cessation of mitosis, the spherule, by inward growth of cell wall matrix, undergoes septation that initially divides the internal contents into multinucleated masses of protoplasm. A β-glucosidase, which is identical to a known immunoglobulin M (IgM)–reactive 120-kDa antigen detected in the tube precipitin test, may be important in spherule morphogenesis.[26] Secondary cleavage further divides the coenocytic (multinucleated) protoplasm into uninucleated endospores (Fig. 279–3). The network of internal cleavage planes, called the segmentation apparatus, undergoes autolysis. This enzymatic breakdown does not affect the spherule or endospore walls and is therefore under both temporal and spatial control. A 36-kDa serine proteinase with broad substrate specificity appears to be at least partly responsible for this autolysis. This enzyme is present in the cell wall of the mycelial-phase as well as of the spherule-phase organism, but it reaches its highest concentration in

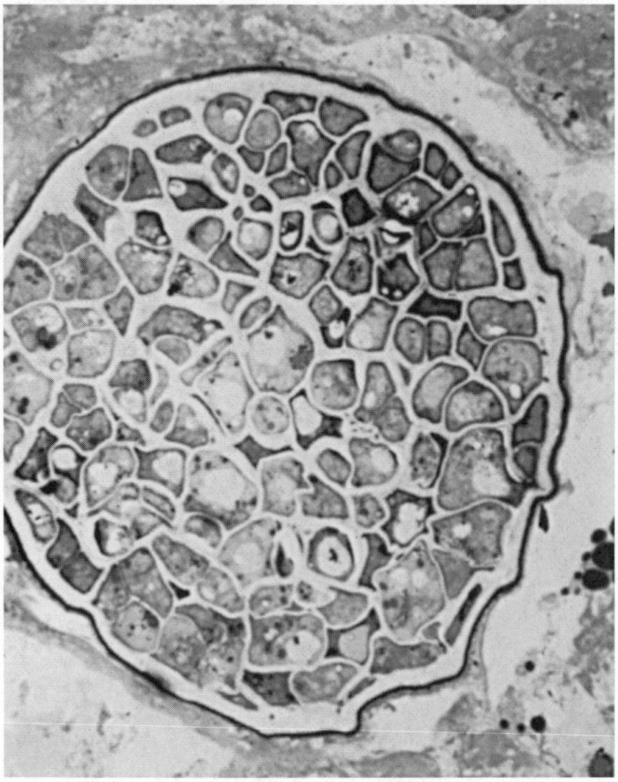

FIGURE 279–3 ▫ Transmission electron microscopy of segmenting spherule in vivo. (Courtesy of Dr. S. H. Sun, Veterans Administration Medical Center, San Antonio, TX.)

the wall of the segmentation apparatus just before segmentation and may be regulated, at least in part, by a low-molecular-weight proteinase inhibitor.[27, 28] The mature spherule may contain several hundred endospores, each 2 to 5 μm in diameter. Rupture of the spherule wall leads to release of the endospores in large "packets," with individual cells held together by fibrillar material from the inner spherule cell wall[29] (Fig. 279–4). The endospores then enlarge to become nascent spherules and repeat the parasitic-phase reproductive cycle.

Biologic and Biochemical Properties

Approximately half the mycelial cell wall is made up of protein and *N*-acetylglucosamine; the remainder is composed of other polysaccharides, particularly glucose and mannose.[30–33] The inner spherule wall consists of a matrix of chitin and β-(1→3)-glucan, whereas the outer part of the wall is primarily made up of the latter.[34] The chitin content of spherules is almost twice that of mycelia. Approximately 4% of the whole spherule wall is made up of lipid; 17% is peptide.[24]

CI is a strict aerobe and produces catalase.[35] Both morphologic forms of the fungus contain most or all of the enzymes of the Krebs, the pentose phosphate, and the Embden-Meyerhof pathways.[36] A wide variety of substrates can be used as carbon sources.[37, 38]

The rate of growth and release of endospores in vitro is stimulated, through binding to cytosol proteins, by testosterone, 17β-estradiol, and progesterone. In the case of the last two hormones, this is accomplished by concentrations that are physiologic during pregnancy,[39, 40] and they may thus contribute to the increased risk for dissemination during late gestation (see later).

Antigenic Characteristics

The antigenic characteristics of CI remain to be fully defined.[24, 41] "Antigen 2" is the sole antigen of alkali-soluble, water-soluble extracts of both mycelial and spherule cell walls and appears to be an important immunogen. It is reactive in the IgM tube precipitin antibody reaction.[42–44] This antigen is not unique to CI, however.[24] A spherule-derived β-glucosidase is reactive with IgM antibody in the tube precipitin test, and a 48-kDa chitinase is detected in the complement-fixing antibody test and in immunodiffusion.[26, 45]

Antigenic differences exist between arthrospores and spherules.[46] Coccidioidin, prepared from mycelia, contains at least 26 antigenic components, 16 of which are not found in the spherule-derived preparation, spherulin. Conversely, spherulin contains at least 16 antigens not present in coccidioidin.[47]

Epidemiology

Transmission

Infection is almost invariably the result of inhalation of airborne arthroconidia. Individuals who are routinely exposed to dust from infected soil, such as archaeologists, are at greatest risk. Natural phenomena, including earthquakes, which disturb the topsoil and allow it to become airborne, may lead to outbreaks of coccidioidomycosis.[47a] The minimal infective dose in humans is not known, but in animal models including monkeys, infection is produced with as few as 10 arthroconidia.[48] Inhalation of organisms from contaminated fomites may also lead to infection, and in one instance, air-

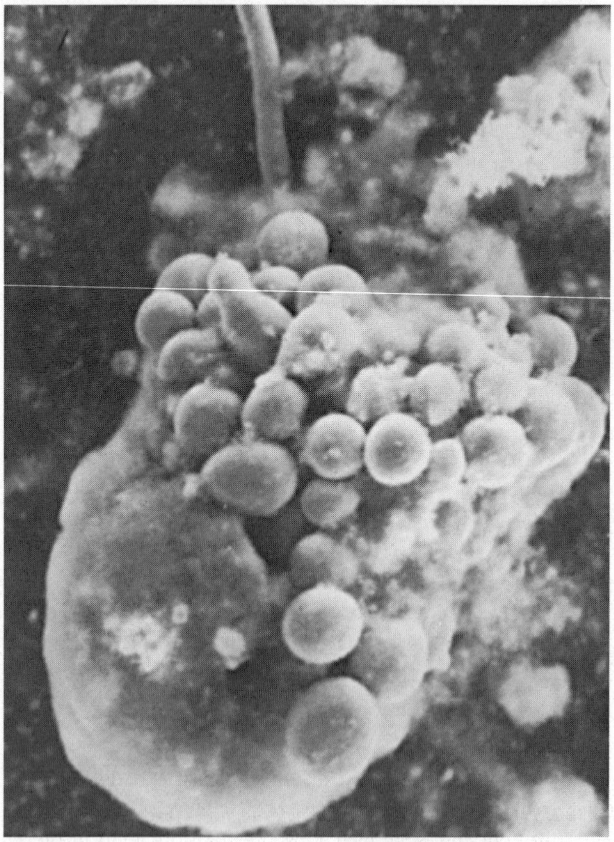

FIGURE 279–4 ▫ Scanning electron microscopy of spherule undergoing cell wall rupture with release of endospores. (Courtesy of Dr. S. H. Sun, Veterans Administration Medical Center, San Antonio, TX.)

borne transmission may have resulted from aerosol generated by use of a band saw used to cut through a patellar abscess during a postmortem examination.[49, 50] Infection may be the result, on rare occasion, of direct cutaneous inoculation, which occurs most commonly in laboratory workers but has also been reported in the embalmer of the body of an individual who had died with disseminated coccidioidomycosis.[51, 52] Infection in the neonate is reported, suggesting transmission from the mother.[53, 54]

Apparent sexual transmission has also been reported.[49] Transmission by fomite has been invoked to explain cases of primary coccidioidomycosis occurring outside the endemic area.[55–58] However, most presentations of primary coccidioidomycosis in nonendemic areas are the consequence of infection acquired within the endemic area that first becomes symptomatic after a traveler has returned home.[59]

Studies of transmission of CI infection have been limited by an inability to distinguish distinct phenotypes among isolates of CI. Molecular epidemiology holds more hope in this regard, although the available data are limited. Restriction fragment length polymorphism analysis of a small number of clinical isolates of CI revealed only two distinct groups, with 13 of 15 from California and 1 from Venezuela appearing identical.[60]

Distribution

The ecologic niche of CI is the soil of the Lower Sonoran Life Zone, a semiarid area with hot summers, infrequent winter freezes, and alkaline soil.[61] The areas of highest endemicity are in the southwestern United States and northern Mexico, although the soil in scattered areas of Central America (the Montagua Valley in Guatemala and the Comayagua Valley of Honduras) and South America (parts of Venezuela, Colombia, Paraguay, Bolivia, and Argentina) also harbors the fungus[62–65] (Fig. 279–5). Even within these areas, the distribution of the fungus, for poorly defined reasons, is spotty.

Infection may also occur outside the usual endemic area under unusual circumstances. Coccidioidomycosis occurred in epidemic form in a nonendemic area when a dust storm blew out of the Central Valley of California in 1977 and blanketed parts of the coastal region.[66]

Prevalence

Prevalence studies rely largely on skin test surveys. These indicate that with an annual rate of new infections of 3% to 5%, as many as 75% to 90% of long-term residents of highly endemic areas such as Tucson, Arizona, have been infected.[12, 66] Other studies, however, report a lower prevalence.[67] Skin test surveys may actually underestimate prevalence because some patients with proven coccidioidomycosis never develop dermal sensitivity to antigens of the etiologic agent and because of apparent waning of skin test reactivity with age.[66]

Data from skin test surveys have led to estimates that 25,000 to 100,000 new infections are acquired annually in the United States.[62] The average annual incidence of symptomatic coccidioidomycosis in students seen at the student health service of the University of Arizona in Tucson between 1979 and 1983 was 0.43%.[68] Attack rates of 60% to 93% have been reported in point exposures such as have occurred in archaeology students.[69–71]

The number of newly infected individuals reaches a peak in the dry period from summer to late fall in California; two seasonal peaks are seen in Arizona.[72, 73] Dust storms are associated with miniepidemics of infection.[66, 74] The annual number of cases reported in California, a number that remained relatively constant for more than a decade, has in-

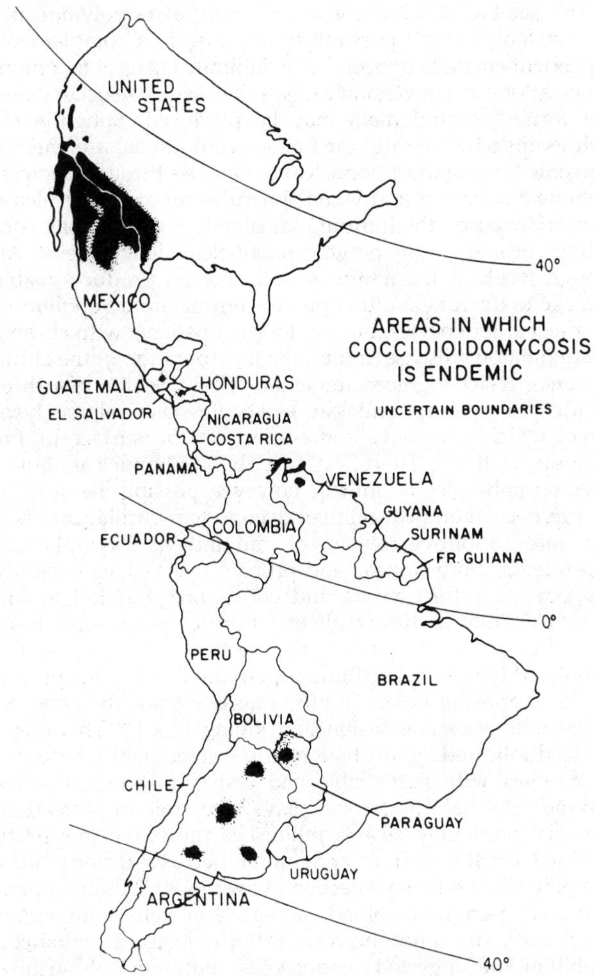

FIGURE 279–5 □ This map displays the regions in which coccidioidomycosis is most highly endemic. The stippled areas represent the uncertain boundaries. (From Pappagianis D. *In* Stevens DA [ed]: Coccidioidomycosis. New York, Plenum Publishing, 1980, p 64.)

creased almost 10-fold, to approximately 5000, in the last several years, most likely as the result of an unusual sequence of prolonged drought followed by heavy rains.[75]

Only approximately 40% of infected individuals develop symptomatic disease, whereas 5% to 10% may develop pulmonary residua such as nodules and cavities. Potentially life-threatening dissemination is seen in less than 1% of those infected, but this frequency varies widely depending on a number of demographic and clinical factors. Filipinos may have a risk for dissemination that is 10 to 175 times that of non-Hispanic whites. Black and Hispanic persons also have an increased risk for dissemination, although it is of lesser magnitude.[12, 73] Pregnancy abrogates the apparent relative protection of non-Hispanic white women from dissemination,[76, 77] possibly, in part, as a result of the trophic effects of estrogen and progesterone on CI.[39, 40] Immunosuppressive disease and therapies that affect cellular immune response also increase the risk for severe disease.[78, 79] Other demographic changes may also be important, including aging.[79a]

Pathogenesis and Immune Response

Inhaled arthroconidia reach the alveoli, where they convert to the spherule-endospore phase within 72 hours. The initial inflammatory response to the presence of the arthroconidia, which temporarily retain an antiphagocytic hyphal outer wall layer[80] (see Fig. 279–2*B*), consists of an influx of polymorphonuclear leukocytes,[81] possibly in response to a complement-dependent chemotaxinogen.[82] The infiltrate changes to a mononuclear one as conversion to the spherule phase occurs, and well-formed granulomata may be produced. Spherule (as well as mycelial) lysates, at low concentrations, are chemotaxigenic for polymorphonuclear leukocytes through complement activation,[82, 83] and when spherules rupture and release their endospores, the infiltrate transiently reverts to one consisting primarily of polymorphonuclear leukocytes.[6] Although weak in the ability to kill or even produce visible damage to the fungal ultrastructure, normal human polymorphonuclear leukocytes, but not those of patients with chronic granulomatous disease, inhibit the incorporation of the chitin precursor *N*-acetylglucosamine into cell wall chitin of arthroconidia.[84] Polymorphonuclear leukocytes also release lysozyme, which may have some effect on the surface of the spherule wall.[80, 85] The effect of polymorphonuclear leukocytes on spherules is limited, however, possibly because of the presence of an extracellular glycoprotein fibrillar matrix.[86]

In mice, adoptive transfer of immunity is T-lymphocyte dependent.[87] Both murine and primate macrophages readily phagocytose arthroconidia and endospores but fail to kill them, probably as the result of failure of phagosome-lysosome fusion.[88, 89] Activation, by incubation with spherule-stimulated lymphocyte culture supernatant, of murine peritoneal macrophages before in vitro infection leads to enhanced phagosome-lysosome fusion and killing of CI.[90] This effect can be duplicated by incubation with recombinant interferon-γ.[91] Studies with susceptible and resistant strains of mice also indicate that interferon-γ plays a key role in protection, whereas interleukin (IL)–4 diminishes protective immunity against CI.[92] IL-1α, IL-6, and tumor necrosis factor-α may also play a key role in protection in the mouse.[93] Pretreatment of human peripheral blood mononuclear cells with either interferon-γ or tumor necrosis factor-α leads to enhanced inhibition of ingested endospores but not of arthroconidia.[94, 95] Mature spherules are too large to be ingested by professional phagocytes, but they can induce murine peritoneal macrophages to produce tumor necrosis factor-α in vitro.[96]

These observations are consistent with studies involving experimental CI infection of congenitally athymic nude as well as experiments with beige mice (with dysfunctional polymorphonuclear leukocytes and natural killer cells), providing evidence that the primary effector cells in resistance to this fungus are polymorphonuclear leukocytes and macrophages.[97] The susceptibility of inbred strains of mice to infection with CI appears to be under the control of a single gene that is expressed by spleen cells and is associated with an acquired suppression of cell-mediated immunity.[98–100]

Lymphocytes from patients with coccidioidomycosis respond in vitro to soluble antigens of CI as well as to intact killed spherules, arthrospores, and endospores.[101, 102] The in vitro response of peripheral blood mononuclear cells from normal individuals with positive skin test responses to spherule-derived antigens includes enhanced production of IL-2 and interferon-γ, but the correlation of these responses with the intensity of the dermal hypersensitivity reaction to the same antigens is poor.[94] Human glass adherent peripheral blood mononuclear cells incubated with killed arthroconidia or spherules produce tumor necrosis factor-α, and these cells ingest killed endospores and can phagocytose arthroconidia and inhibit their growth.[103–105] Patients with disseminated disease often have impaired lymphocyte response to coccidioidal antigens, in parallel with defective cutaneous delayed hypersensitivity reactions.[13, 106, 107] In mice, loss of immunologic responsiveness appears to be due to the activation of a splenic suppressor cell population induced by circulating coccidioidal antigen.[108] In humans, suppression of lymphocyte response may be mediated by immunoglobulin G (IgG), either alone or in immune complexes.[109] This is consistent with the observation that serum antibody to CI is not protective. In fact, there is a generally direct relationship between the intensity of the complement-fixing antibody response and the extent of extrapulmonary dissemination of the fungus.[13, 14]

Although direct experimental evidence is as yet incomplete, the importance of the cellular immune response, together with the lack of protection afforded by antibody, suggests that the outcome of infection with CI depends on the development of a dominant Th1-type response.[110] The Th1 cytokine interferon-γ appears to play a key role in protective immunity, whereas the Th2 cytokine IL-4 impairs an effective immune response in a murine model.[92] IL-12 administration to mice significantly ameliorates systemic infection with CI, and this is associated with a shift from a Th2 to a Th1 cytokine pattern in pulmonary lymphocytes.[110a] Examination of cytokine production patterns of peripheral blood mononuclear cells obtained from patients with disseminated infection and from coccidioidal-immune control subjects also suggests that inadequate immunologic control of CI is associated with a diminished Th1 response.[110b] Furthermore, this hypothesis is also consistent with evidence of a correlation between elevated serum concentrations of immunoglobulin E and disease severity, because IL-4, a cytokine that is key to the Th2-dominant response, is responsible for B-cell switching to immunoglobulin E production.[111–113] Furthermore, IL-5, another cytokine associated with Th2 dominance, is the most potent regulator of eosinophilia, a laboratory finding that is sometimes associated with disseminated infection.[114] To the extent that Th1 dominance is important for recovery from infection with CI, cytokine therapy (e.g., IL-12, IL-2, interferon-γ) or anticytokine therapy (e.g., anti–IL-4) may prove effective therapeutically.

The characteristics of CI that account for its virulence are little understood. Endospores produce urease and respond to an acid environment by increased production of ammonium. Thus, endospores that have been ingested by phagocytic cells may increase the pH within the phagosome and thus avoid degradation by its acid proteases.[115]

An enzyme with elastase (and lesser collagenase) activity, possibly identical to or a subunit of the serine proteinase thought to be important in the dissolution of the segmentation apparatus during spherule-endospore reproduction, has been recovered from culture filtrates of the parasitic phase of CI. The activity of this enzyme peaks at the time of endospore release. This ability to enzymatically degrade connective tissue matrix macromolecules may have an important role in the pathogenesis of coccidioidomycosis. Breakdown of pulmonary connective tissue matrix at the time of endospore release may allow intrapulmonary and extrapulmonary spread of the organism and may contribute to progressive loss of pulmonary parenchyma.[116] In addition, the enzymatic breakdown products of elastin are chemotactic and may thus further contribute to the inflammatory response, which may also be destructive.[117]

Clinical Manifestations

Primary Infection

Infection results in clinically evident disease in only approximately 40% of individuals, and illness in most consists of a prolonged and sometimes severe but self-limited influenza-like illness, commonly with pneumonitis (Figs. 279–6 and 279–7). Approximately 5% are left with pulmonary residuals such as nodules and cavities, which may be variably symp-

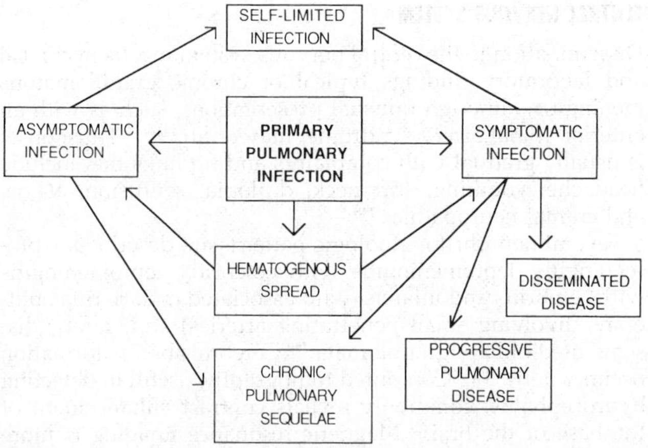

FIGURE 279–6 ▫ Suggested overall schema of infection with CI. The probable occurrence of asymptomatic dissemination is suggested by the frequent finding of chorioretinitis and by recovery of CI from the urine in patients without other clinical evidence of dissemination.

tomatic.[12] Less than 1% of patients develop clinically apparent extrapulmonary dissemination.

Complaints that occur in the majority of those who develop symptomatic infection are fatigue, cough, and chest pain. Approximately one half report fever, and one fifth complain of dyspnea. Arthralgia or myalgia and headache are each reported by one fifth.[118, 119] Patients with acute primary infection may develop a variety of presumably immune-mediated complications. Most prominent among these are a variety of exanthems, including nonspecific, often evanescent erythematous macular or confluent skin eruptions and erythrodermas, erythema multiforme, and erythema nodosum. Elements of more than one type of eruption may be present simultaneously. Erythema nodosum occurs most commonly in young, nongravid female patients and is reported to be an indicator of a good prognosis.[12]

Patients may also develop arthritis ("desert rheumatism") during this stage. This must be distinguished from joint infection due to hematogenous dissemination of CI.[118] Unusual examples of immune-mediated disease in CI infection include glomerulonephritis associated with mixed cryoglobulinemia and occult pulmonary coccidioidomycosis in which a cold-reacting protein contained IgG anticoccidioidin antibody.[120] Although transient eosinophilia is frequent, especially in patients with these immunologic manifestations, persistent eosinophilia may be an epiphenomenon of dissemination.[121] The total white cell count is usually normal.[119]

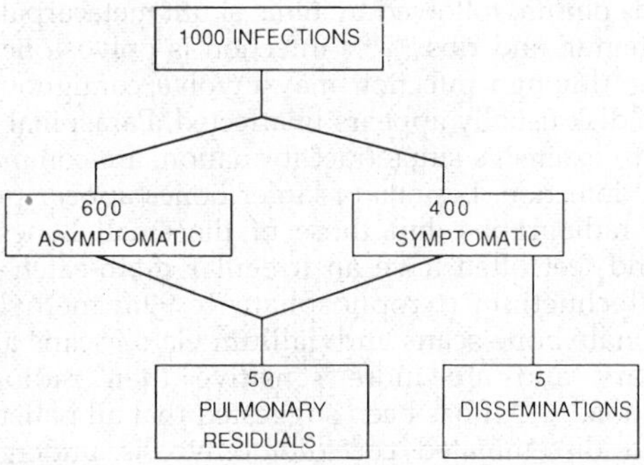

FIGURE 279–7 ▫ Outcome of infection. (Based on data from Smith CE, Beard RR, Whiting EG, Rosenberger HG: Varieties of coccidioidal infection in relation to the epidemiology and control of disease. Am J Public Health 36:1394, 1946.)

Pulmonary Disease

Pneumonia, usually self-limited, may be acutely progressive, leading to respiratory failure; a more chronic form of progressive pneumonitis is also recognized.[122–125] Abnormalities on the chest radiograph are evident in approximately half of patients with acute symptomatic infection[116] and consist most often of segmental or lobar consolidation or of nodular or patchy infiltrates. Hilar adenopathy, a finding that is thought to be associated with an increased risk for dissemination, is seen in approximately 20%, as are small pleural effusions.[126]

Acutely progressive pulmonary disease may be associated with a diffuse miliary or reticulonodular radiographic pattern, often together with mediastinal adenopathy. Exudative pleural and pericardial effusions may result from serosal involvement.[127–129] In one series, 48% of patients with pleural effusion had erythema nodosum or erythema multiforme.[130] Upper airway infection may present with hoarseness in patients with laryngeal involvement and may result, particularly in children, in upper airway obstruction.[131, 132] CI may cause endobronchial mass lesions. Cavitation (often thin walled) of lung parenchyma (Fig. 279–8) may regress, stabilize, or proceed progressively and inexorably; the subsequent clinical course may be benign or complicated by hemoptysis, mycetoma, rupture into the pleural space, and bacterial superinfection.[133–136] Residual asymptomatic pulmonary nodules, if first discovered at a time remote from the primary infection, may require distinction from malignant neoplasm. Other pulmonary residua include fibrosis, bronchiectasis, and calcifications.[126]

Disseminated Infection

At least two observations suggest that subclinical dissemination is probably common. Chorioretinal lesions can be found

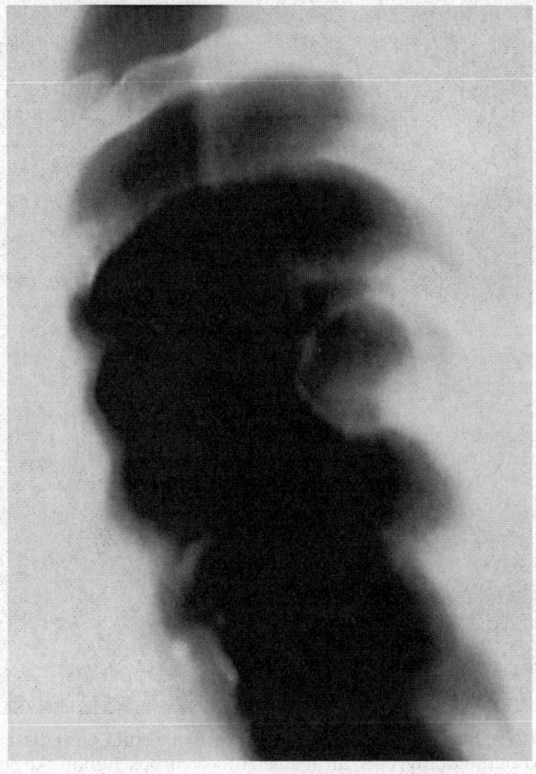

FIGURE 279–8 ▫ Thin-walled pulmonary cavity caused by CI. (Courtesy of Dr. David Stevens, Santa Clara Valley Medical Center, San Jose, California.)

in as many as 40% of patients without other clinical evidence of dissemination,[137, 138] and CI can frequently be recovered from urine of patients thought to have only pulmonary disease.[139, 140] Clinically evident dissemination, which is generally apparent within the first several months after primary infection, may be widespread, involving multiple sites. Often, however, the clinical disease resulting from dissemination may be apparently limited to just a few sites or even just one site. Sites of disseminated disease include skin and subcutaneous tissues, bones and joints, liver, lymph nodes, spleen, genitourinary tract, peritoneal cavity, eyes, thyroid,[141] and central nervous system. Infection of vascular graft material may occur as the result of dissemination.[142]

SKIN

Skin is the most commonly recognized site of dissemination. Manifestations of hematogenous skin infection include plaques, papules (which are often verrucous), pustules, granulomatous lesions, and subcutaneous abscesses[143] (Fig. 279–9). The prognosis for survival in patients with skin lesions depends on the extent of involvement of other organ systems; those with little or no disease apparent at other sites have an excellent outcome. The presence of an ulcerating subcutaneous lesion must lead to the consideration that it represents the egress site of a sinus tract. Such sinus tracts may be remarkably extensive and can be a reflection of distant disease, most commonly of bone. Direct inoculation of fungus into skin results in a primary chancriform lesion.

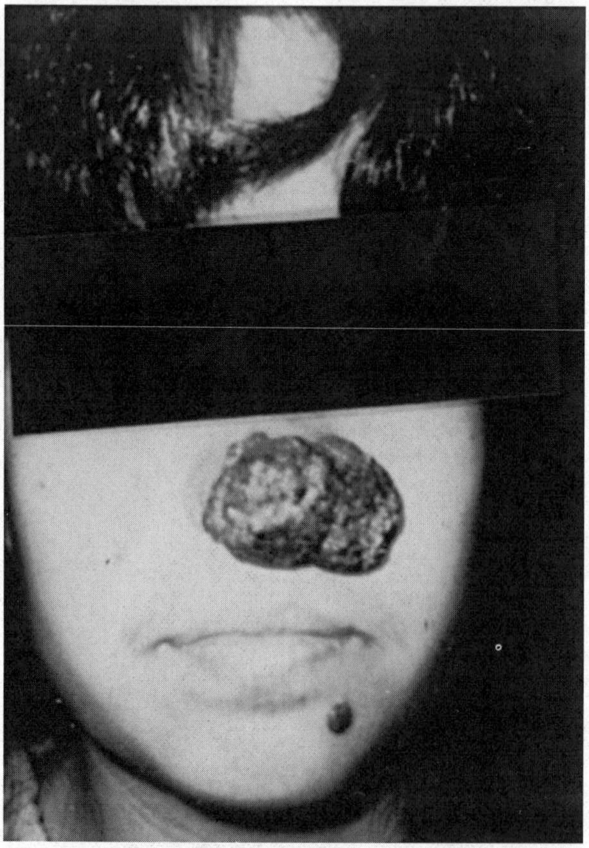

FIGURE 279–9 □ Two skin lesions on the face of a child with disseminated coccidioidomycosis: an exuberant verrucous tumor-like lesion of the nose and one of the chin that appears nodular and granulomatous. (Courtesy of Dr. Richard Tucker, Wenatchee Valley Clinic, Wenatchee, Washington.)

CENTRAL NERVOUS SYSTEM

Dissemination to the central nervous system results in clinical and laboratory findings typical of chronic granulomatous meningitis, although unusual presentations, such as with an anterior spinal artery syndrome, may occur.[144–147] Thus, onset is usually gradual with complaints and findings that include headache, vomiting, stiff neck, diplopia, confusion, ataxia, and cranial neuropathies.[148]

Several neurohistopathologic patterns are described: leptomeningitis, leptomeningitis with cerebritis, leptomeningitis with cerebritis and infarcts (with associated endarteritis obliterans involving small penetrating arteries) and, rarely, disseminated miliary granulomata.[149] Cerebral abscess formation occurs rarely.[150, 151] Computed tomography, useful in detecting hydrocephalus, commonly reveals contrast enhancement of the base of the brain. Magnetic resonance imaging is more sensitive and may detect intense contrast enhancement of the cervical subarachnoid space as well as of the basilar, sylvian, and interhemispheric cisterns. In addition, focal parenchymal signal abnormalities consistent with ischemia or infarction may be seen as may, on occasion, mass lesions that are usually hypodense and enhancing.[150–152]

Examination of cerebrospinal fluid (CSF) reveals a predominantly mononuclear pleocytosis (with the total white cell count generally in the range of 100 to 1500 cells per mm^3), high protein concentration, and, often, low glucose level. CSF eosinophilia is frequent; approximately one third of patients in one series had more than 10 eosinophils per mm^3 of CSF.[153] CSF protein concentration is, in the majority of cases, less than 300 mg/dL; a concentration approaching or exceeding 1000 mg/dL suggests the presence of obstruction to CSF flow. Tests performed on ventricular CSF may be misleading in that in the absence of ventriculitis (an infrequent complication), the abnormalities may be much more apparent in lumbar CSF. Because the organism is recovered from CSF in only a minority of cases, the etiologic diagnosis usually depends on the detection of IgG antibody to the fungus in the fluid. The development of hydrocephalus (most often communicating) is common and is probably the result of an ongoing inflammatory response with persisting pleocytosis and elevations of CSF concentrations of tumor necrosis factor-α and IL-1β.[154, 155] Ventricles may become isolated as the result of local areas of obstruction to CSF egress.[156] Large-vessel vasculitis, sometimes with the development of intracranial aneurysms, is associated with high mortality.[157, 158] Meningitis, which is uniformly fatal without treatment, remains a highly morbid and potentially lethal disease despite aggressive therapeutic management.

MUSCULOSKELETAL SYSTEM

The most common site of coccidioidal osteomyelitis is the vertebral column, followed by tibia, skull, metacarpals, metatarsals, femur, and ribs.[159–162a] Infection is polyostotic in 40% of cases. Although infection may involve contiguous vertebrae, the disk usually appears unaffected. Paraspinal masses, often with extensive sinus tract formation, are common with vertebral infection. Lesions of larger bones appear primarily lytic on radiographs, but those of the small bones of the hands and feet often have an irregular moth-eaten appearance.[163] Technetium pyrophosphate Tc 99m methylene diphosphonate bone scans and gallium Ga 67 scans are complementary and are more sensitive than radiographic examination.[164, 165] It has been suggested that all patients with suspected disseminated coccidioidomycosis undergo bone scanning.[164] Hypercalcemia has been reported in coccidioidomycosis, but not all affected patients have evident infection of bone, suggesting that an osteolytic substance is responsible.[166–168]

Patients with coccidioidal infection of joints[160–162, 168a] represent approximately 20% of those with disseminated disease. Conversely, dissemination is widespread in 25% of cases of coccidioidal arthritis at the time of presentation. Arthritis is monarticular in 90% of cases, with the large weight-bearing joints most commonly involved in adult patients. Thus, the knee is affected in approximately three fourths of cases and the ankle in 10%; the elbow, wrist, hip, and interphalangeal joints are less frequently involved. The small joints of the hands and feet appear to involved with greater frequency in children. Synovial effusions are exudative, with the protein concentration in excess of 3.0 g/dL and with total white cell counts ranging to as high as 50,000/mm^3 with a predominantly mononuclear cell pleocytosis. Culture of the fluid yields the organism approximately half the time; culture and histologic examination of synovial tissue may be more productive. Tenosynovitis without bone or joint infection is also reported.[169]

OTHER SITES

Sites of genitourinary tract infection include the kidneys, prostate, epididymis, and uterus.[170–173] CI may be recovered from urine in the absence of apparent urinary tract disease.[139, 140] Peritonitis with an exudative peritoneal effusion may occur and has been described in patients undergoing continuous ambulatory peritoneal dialysis[174, 175]; in this group, an eosinophilic effusion has been noted. Patients with intraabdominal infection may present with an omental mass.[176]

Ocular involvement may consist of asymptomatic chorioretinitis as well as necrotizing conjunctivitis and potentially sight-threatening iridocyclitis.[138, 139, 177, 178]

Infection in the Immunocompromised Host

Dissemination in the patient with impaired cellular immunity may occur as a result of recent infection or of reactivation of latent infection. In either case, the clinical presentation may be explosive, rapidly progressive, and often fatal.[179–181] Approximately 5% of cardiac allograft recipients in Arizona develop coccidioidomycosis, with reactivation of past infection being responsible in a number of these.[182] The risk for coccidioidomycosis in the first year after renal transplantation among patients in Arizona is, however, only 2% to 3% greater than that for subsequent years, suggesting that reactivation of latent infection accounts for only a small proportion of cases.[183] Whereas the risk for development of coccidioidal disease diminishes after the first posttransplant year, the potential for late reactivation remains significant and accounts for the likelihood that allograft recipients and other similarly immunocompromised patients will first present in a geographic location outside the endemic area.[102, 181, 183]

Because persisting antibody (but not skin test reactivity) appears to be a marker of increased risk for reactivation after immunosuppression, serum coccidioidal antibodies should be measured in any potential transplant recipient who has been in a coccidioidomycosis endemic area, even briefly or remotely in time. Those with serum antibody to CI before transplantation or with history of prior pulmonary coccidioidomycosis should be considered candidates to receive empirical antifungal therapy during the times of peak posttransplantation immunosuppression. Posttransplantation serologic surveillance may also be useful in these patients.[182, 183]

Coccidioidomycosis is reported with increasing frequency in patients infected with human immunodeficiency virus (HIV).[79] The estimated cumulative rate of active coccidioidomycosis among HIV-infected patients residing in an endemic area was 25% after 41 months of observation, with those with a diagnosis of acquired immunodeficiency syndrome (AIDS) or a CD4$^+$ lymphocyte count of less than 250/mm^3 being at greatest risk. Neither a positive skin test result nor a prior history of coccidioidomycosis contributed significantly to this risk.[183] As with organ transplant recipients, however, coccidioidal seropositivity may identify a group with increased risk for subsequent active coccidioidomycosis. In one study performed in an endemic area, seropositivity in the absence of contemporaneous active coccidioidomycosis was associated with an approximately 70% risk for active fungal infection at 36 months compared with a previously reported risk of approximately 25% during a similar period among HIV-infected patients who initially had no detectable antibody to coccidioidal antigens.[183, 184]

This problem is not limited to areas of CI endemicity; almost half of the HIV-infected patients reported to the Centers for Disease Control and Prevention with disseminated coccidioidomycosis resided in nonendemic counties in 35 states.[185] This observation, which is often most likely the consequence of late reactivation of dormant infection in the face of profound impairment of cellular immunity, demonstrates the importance of an accurate lifelong travel and residence history in HIV-infected patients.[185a] Whereas consideration has been given to prophylaxis with fluconazole in selected patients (e.g., those with low CD4$^+$ lymphocyte counts resident in or traveling to endemic areas and those with a positive serologic test result), no clinical trial data exist to validate this approach.[186, 187]

The presentation and course of CI infection in HIV-infected patients depend, to a large extent, on the level of immunocompromise as crudely reflected by the CD4$^+$ lymphocyte count. In patients with relatively intact cellular immunity, coccidioidomycosis most often resembles that observed in the general population. However, in patients with low CD4$^+$ lymphocyte counts, diffuse pulmonary disease, with radiographic evidence of diffuse bilateral reticulonodular infiltrates, and extrapulmonary dissemination appear to occur with increased frequency.[186] Those presenting with bilateral interstitial pulmonary infection have been reported to have a median survival of only 1 month, but those with only unilateral focal lung disease often have a relatively benign clinical course.[186]

The diagnosis of coccidioidomycosis in HIV-infected patients often requires a high index of suspicion. Not only may patients often first present outside endemic areas, but approximately 20%, mostly with only pulmonary infection, will have negative serologic test results.[186, 188] On the other hand, persisting seropositivity may be seen in HIV-infected patients without evidence of active coccidioidomycosis.[184] Furthermore, active coccidioidomycosis may coexist with other opportunistic infections. Of particular concern is its occasional presentation simultaneously with *Pneumocystis carinii* pneumonia. In that circumstance, coccidioidomycosis may become evident only as the result of clinical worsening in the face of adjunctive corticosteroid therapy given for *P. carinii* pneumonia.[189]

Pregnancy

Although largely based on historical data with possibly diminished contemporary relevance, the risk for dissemination is reported to be as much as 40 to 100 times greater than that of the general population when infection occurs during pregnancy.[190] It has been estimated that the rate of dissemination after infection in the first trimester is 23%; the risks in the second and third trimesters are, respectively, 59% and 68%.[190] Analysis of more recent data indicates an increased risk for coccidioidal meningitis in pregnant women relative to those not pregnant but fails to confirm an increased risk of dissemination after infection acquired in the third trimester relative to earlier trimesters.[191] Although neonatal coccidioidomycosis occurs, it does so only rarely, possibly because the placenta appears to be resistant to infection.[192] The normal placenta, however, produces cytokines, such as IL-4 and IL-10, that are associated with a Th2-like lymphocyte response and that may inhibit local Th1-like responses that could otherwise be injurious to the fetus.[193] Systemic spillover of this effect would be expected to lead to increased susceptibility to intracellular pathogens. The increasing risk for dissemination as pregnancy progresses is also consistent with both the trophic effects of estradiol and progesterone on CI as well as evidence of reduced cellular immunity to antigens of CI near term and in the postpartum period.[39, 40, 194]

Laboratory Diagnosis

Direct Examination

Direct examination of body tissues, exudates, and respiratory secretions may allow visualization of CI. In cases of widespread dissemination, bone marrow or liver biopsy specimens may prove useful.[195, 196] Pus and sputum may be examined by potassium hydroxide preparation with Parker superchrome ink or lactophenol cotton blue stain added to enhance visualization. A Papanicolaou stain of a cytologic preparation of sputum is superior to potassium hydroxide preparation, however.[197] Fungal stains, such as periodic acid–Schiff, are useful, as is calcofluor white.[198] Cytologic examination of bronchoalveolar lavage fluid obtained from patients with pulmonary coccidioidomycosis reveals the organism in approximately half of cases; culture and histologic examination of tissue obtained by transbronchial biopsy appear to be more sensitive.[199] Some pollen, especially that of the mulberry, cottonwood, and elm trees,[200] may resemble the spherules of CI. CI has also been visualized on Papanicolaou-stained cytologic preparations of anterior chamber fluid of patients with coccidioidal iridocyclitis.[178]

Specimens obtained from pulmonary lesions, including nodules, by fine-needle aspiration seldom yield evidence of granulomatous inflammation, but examination of cytologic preparations of these specimens commonly reveals the presence of endosporulating spherules.[201]

Histologic examination of biopsy specimens demonstrates the large endosporulating spherules, which are readily seen with routine staining with hematoxylin-eosin. The only fungus that produces a tissue phase that is morphologically similar is *Rhinosporidium seeberi*, which causes mucocutaneous infection of the nasal area. However, the sporangia of this organism are much larger (up to 350 μm in diameter) and, in contrast to CI, stain with mucicarmine. Small, immature, nonendosporulating spherules of CI may be confused with yeasts such as *Blastomyces dermatitidis* and *Cryptococcus neoformans*. The mycelial forms of CI are occasionally also visualized, especially in pulmonary cavities, where they have been reported to be present in up to 75% of specimens, and in approximately 30% of pulmonary granulomata.[202] Hyphal forms have also been recovered from coccidioidal pulmonary mycetomata and CSF obtained from a ventriculoperitoneal shunt in a patient with coccidioidal meningitis.[135, 203]

Culture

If coccidioidomycosis is suspected, the microbiology laboratory should be notified when it is sent samples for cultivation because of the significant biohazard involved.

CI may be isolated from a wide variety of clinical sources, including sputum, exudates, prostatic secretions, urine, tissue, bone marrow,[204] CSF, and blood. Potentially contaminated specimens, such as sputum, should be processed within 2 hours to minimize overgrowth of bacteria. CI will grow on most media, including those containing 0.4 mg/mL cycloheximide, which inhibits most morphologically similar nonpathogens. Growth is visible within 3 to 4 days of inoculation of Sabouraud dextrose agar and incubation at 25°C; the agar surface rapidly becomes covered. Colonies may initially appear smooth and moist but soon develop an abundant aerial mycelium. Colonies are initially white but, with continued incubation, darken to become tan or brown. As many as 20% of isolates may exhibit atypical morphologic features.[23]

CI can be recovered from the urine of 9% to 24% of patients with pulmonary coccidioidomycosis when large early morning urine volumes are processed. A minimum of 200 mL is centrifuged, and the sediment is inoculated onto appropriate media. Colony counts are only 0.03 to 17 per mL of urine. With prostatic involvement, expressed secretions may contain 15 to 120 colony-forming units per mL.[139, 140] CI has been recovered from blood, particularly in immunocompromised patients[205] after inoculation into trypticase soy broth (vented) and incubation for a median of 5 days. Inoculation of spherules into BACTEC 6B media yields visible growth within several days but fails to produce sufficient ^{14}C-labeled carbon dioxide in bottles containing trypticase soy broth incubated aerobically to exceed the bacterial radiometric growth index threshold.[206]

Microscopic examination of a culture tease preparation will demonstrate branched septate hyphae, approximately 2 μm wide, with alternating barrel-shaped arthroconidia and clear zones termed disjunctors. The arthroconidia are 3 to 4.5 μm wide and 3 to 12 μm long.[207] Although this morphologic appearance is strongly suggestive of CI, it is not pathognomonic. More than a dozen keratinophilic soil fungi produce arthroconidia and cannot be readily distinguished from CI morphologically when grown at 25°C.[208] These nonpathogenic mimes include *Trichosporon, Geotrichum, Arthroderma,* and *Auxarthron*.

Definitive morphologic identification of an isolate as CI requires demonstration of the endosporulating spherule. In the past, this required inoculation into animals with subsequent examination of infected tissue. Although more technically demanding, phase conversion can also be achieved in vitro at 37°C to 40°C in either liquid medium or agar slants under increased carbon dioxide tension.[209] The identification of antigens of CI in the concentrated supernatants of 3- to 6-day-old broth cultures by immunodiffusion obviates the need for phase conversion.[210, 211] A DNA probe that detects coccidioidal ribosomal RNA has also been used for rapid culture identification.[212]

Skin Test

The demonstration of a delayed dermal reaction to the administration of coccidioidal antigens is widely used to detect evidence of previous exposure to the fungus, because most infected persons develop delayed dermal hypersensitivity. Skin test reactivity may be detected as early as 3 days after onset of symptoms. Of those who develop a positive reaction, 83% do so in the first week, 93% by the end of the second week, and 99% by the end of the fourth week[213] (Fig. 279–10). Although reactivity may wane with time, it can persist for life, thus rendering the skin test useless as a diagnostic tool. Repeated skin testing may cause apparent conversion to a positive reaction because of a boosting phenomenon or by sensitization to noncoccidioidal antigens in the preparations[214]; as a result, even apparent skin test conversion may be suspect. Its utility, therefore, is largely as an epidemiologic and a prognostic tool. Patients who are anergic to coccidioidal skin test antigens (such anergy is often specific to anti-

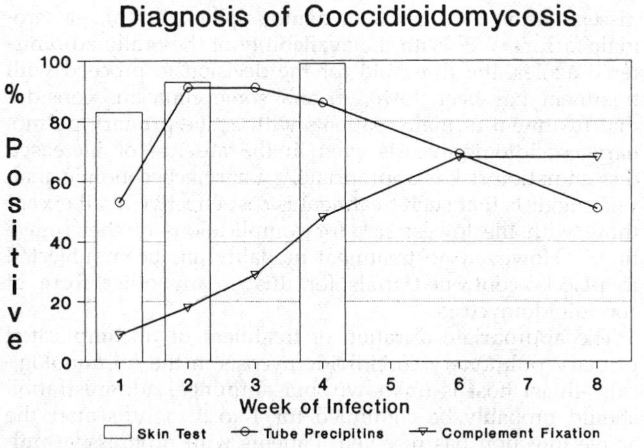

FIGURE 279–10 ▫ Skin test response to coccidioidin and tube precipitin and complement-fixing antibody responses in the first 8 weeks of symptomatic illness. (Provided by Dr. Richard Tucker and based on data in references 13, 14, 213.)

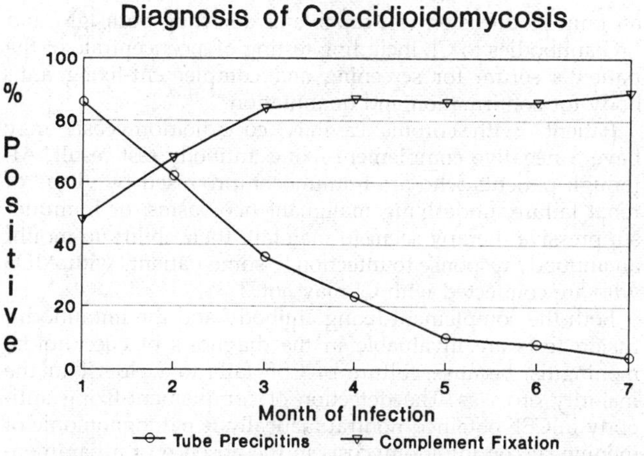

FIGURE 279–11 ▫ Tube precipitin and complement-fixing antibody test results from months 1 through 7 after the onset of symptomatic illness. (Provided by Dr. Richard Tucker and based on data in references 13, 14, 213.)

gens of this fungus) are more likely to suffer from disseminated infection[13] and to respond poorly to therapy. Restoration of skin test reactivity may occur with successful therapy.[106]

Two skin test reagents are available for detection of delayed dermal sensitivity to CI. Coccidioidin is a culture filtrate of the mycelial phase, whereas spherulin is a filtrate of the spherule-endospore phase of the organism. Both are mixtures of multiple, predominantly polysaccharide antigens and are standardized by bioequivalence testing. In each case, induration of at least 5 mm in diameter 24 to 72 hours after intradermal injection is considered a positive reaction. The majority of studies indicate that spherulin has a sensitivity equal to or greater than that of coccidioidin.[215–218] It may have less specificity, however. Because the number of false-positive reactions to either reagent appears to be greatest when the test is read at 24 hours, it has been suggested that later readings are preferable.[218] Neither coccidioidin nor spherulin skin testing elicits antibody responses to coccidioidal antigens.[219, 220] However, coccidioidin may elicit a serologic response to histoplasmin.[220]

Serology

Serologic tests are useful in the diagnosis and management of coccidioidomycosis[219] (Fig. 279–11; see also Fig. 279–10). The initial antibody response to infection with CI is, as expected, of the IgM class. This antibody has been demonstrated in 90% of patients within 1 to 3 weeks after the onset of symptoms of acute primary infection as a tube precipitin.[14] IgM antibody to the same tube precipitin antigen (factor 2 of coccidioidin)[41] can also be detected with somewhat greater sensitivity by immunodiffusion. The latex particle agglutination reaction, which also detects IgM antibody, may become positive before either the tube precipitin or the immunodiffusion assay for tube precipitin but has lesser specificity; all positive reactions should be confirmed by one of the last two methods. IgM antibodies are seldom detectable for more than 6 months after infection, and they have no prognostic value. These tests are not useful in the examination of CSF of patients suspected of having coccidioidomycosis.

IgG antibody to coccidioidin may be detected by sheep red blood cell complement fixation, immunodiffusion, or enzyme immunoassay. The immunodiffusion test detects an antibody that corresponds to the complement-fixing antibody detected by the sheep red blood cell method. Detection of complement-fixing antibody by the immunodiffusion assay has somewhat greater specificity than detection of complement-fixing antibody by the sheep red blood cell method.[221] A commercially available enzyme immunoassay correlates closely with results by complement fixation.[221a] IgG antibody is first detectable by either method several weeks after the onset of infection and after the responses to the tests that detect IgM have become positive. Seropositivity in the absence of active coccidioidomycosis is rare but has been reported to occur in HIV-infected patients and allograft recipients.[182, 184] In certain reference laboratories, the height of the complement-fixing antibody response by the sheep red blood cell method has a direct correlation with the extent of infection, with titers greater than 1:16 often signaling the presence of extrapulmonary dissemination[14] (Table 279–1). Patients with single-site dissemination (e.g., meninges, a solitary bone site) may have a lower titer. The immunodiffusion test with detection of complement-fixing antibody gives comparable qualitative results and may also be of value when it is used quantitatively.[222] An enzyme-linked immunosorbent assay capable of detecting IgM and IgG antibody to CI is also available; results obtained with this test appear to correlate with latex particle agglutination, immunodiffusion, and complement-fixing antibody results.[223] A practical strategy is to use

TABLE 279–1 ▪ Complement-Fixing Antibody Titer and Dissemination of Coccidioidomycosis

CLINICAL STATUS	PATIENTS (N)	COMPLEMENT-FIXING ANTIBODY TITER > 1:16 (%)
Not Disseminated		
Primary infection (no dissemination)	3154	5.3
Pulmonary residua (including cavities)	848	1.0
Disseminated		
All disseminated	709	61.0
Single site (not meningeal)	141	15.0
Meningitis	136	49.0
Extensive dissemination (not meningeal)	291	83.0

Adapted from Smith CE, Saito MT, Simmons SA: Pattern of 39,500 serologic tests in coccidioidomycosis. JAMA 160:546–552, 1956. Copyright 1956, American Medical Association.

an immunodiffusion test capable of detecting both IgM and IgG antibodies to CI, including testing of a concentrate of the patient's serum for screening and complement-fixing antibody for confirmation and quantitation.[65, 221]

Patients with chronic cavitary coccidioidomycosis may have a negative complement-fixing antibody test result. Although patients who are immunocompromised by virtue of renal failure, underlying malignant neoplasms, or immunosuppressive therapy seem to maintain their ability to mount an antibody response to infection,[179] some patients with AIDS who are coinfected with CI may not.[79, 224]

Both the complement-fixing antibody and the immunodiffusion tests are invaluable in the diagnosis of coccidioidal meningitis, because culture of CSF fails to yield CI in the majority of cases. The detection of complement-fixing antibody in CSF obtained nontraumatically is pathognomonic of meningeal coccidioidomycosis in the absence of a parameningeal focus of infection; however, the CSF of as many as 5% of cases will not have detectable antibody. Detection of antibodies to a 33-kDa spherule antigen by enzyme-linked immunosorbent assay may be even more sensitive. Effective therapy is reflected in a reduction of CSF complement-fixing antibody titer.[144, 145]

Whereas serologic tests for coccidioidomycosis are of enormous clinical value, caution must be exerted in their interpretation. Serologic cross-reactions with antigens of other fungi, including *H. capsulatum* and *B. dermatitidis,* have been reported. Sixteen percent of patients with acute histoplasmosis have complement-fixing antibody to CI.[225] Significant interlaboratory variation in the results of the complement fixation test, as well as variation in results obtained with different commercially available immunodiffusion kits, presents an important additional problem.[226]

One potential method of circumventing the vagaries of the host antibody response for diagnosis is to detect circulating fungal products. Antigens of CI have been detected in the serum of one half to three fourths of patients with active coccidioidomycosis. False-positive results may occur.[227–229]

Differential Diagnosis

The protean manifestations of coccidioidomycosis require consideration of a wide range of alternative diagnoses. When patients present with immunologic manifestations of acute primary infection, consideration must be given to diseases such as acute allergic reactions, serum sickness, rheumatoid arthritis, vasculitis, and many more. The differential diagnosis of acute pneumonia is broad. Patients with chronic cavitary disease or solitary pulmonary nodules must be evaluated for, among other things, the possibility of malignant neoplasm, other granulomatous infections such as tuberculosis, and histoplasmosis. Coccidioidomycosis has often been misdiagnosed as neoplastic disease.[3, 230, 231]

The differential diagnosis of chronic meningitis caused by CI encompasses many etiologic considerations.[232] These include tuberculosis, cryptococcosis, malignant neoplasm, and immunologic disease. Coccidioidal osteomyelitis or arthritis often resembles that due to *Mycobacterium tuberculosis.*[159–161]

Treatment[233]

Nonmeningeal Infection

Most cases of primary coccidioidomycosis are self-limited. For that reason, and because of the potential toxicity of amphotericin B, treatment has been reserved for instances in which the illness is unusually severe, the illness appears to be progressive, or the patient is in a high-risk category for dissemination as a result of demographic, clinical, or serologic factors.[234, 235] With the availability of the orally administered azoles, the threshold for the decision to proceed with treatment has been lowered, and some clinicians consider that treatment of many patients with active primary pulmonary coccidioidomycosis even in the absence of increased dissemination risk is appropriate.[236] Pharmacoeconomic analysis suggests that such treatment is cost-effective in all except those with the lowest risk for complications of their infection.[237] However, no treatment modality has been subjected to placebo-controlled trials for this or any other form of coccidioidomycosis.

The appropriate duration of treatment of uncomplicated primary pulmonary coccidioidomycosis in the immunologically intact host is unknown, but antifungal administration should probably be continued for 1 to 3 months after the active infection has resolved. Patients with progressive pulmonary or disseminated infection not involving the central nervous system should continue to receive chemotherapy for at least 6 months after the disease appears to have been rendered inactive. Treatment of those with ongoing severe immunocompromise should probably be of indefinite duration.[108]

Amphotericin B remains the treatment of choice for rapidly progressive or otherwise life-threatening infection. Patients are often given a total dose of at least 30 mg/kg. However, it may be reasonable in many instances in which the infection rapidly comes under control to change therapy to an orally administered azole before this somewhat arbitrarily chosen amount is reached.

Miconazole has been used in the treatment of coccidioidomycosis, but it is less effective than amphotericin B, with a high relapse rate, and has been supplanted by other azoles.[238, 239] Noncomparative trials using ketoconazole, which is available only for oral administration, indicate that it is efficacious in many instances, although the relapse rate is high; in the absence of randomized trial data, its efficacy relative to other agents, including amphotericin B, is unknown.[240–243]

Fluconazole, given orally in doses of 200 to 400 mg daily, appears to be reasonably effective in the treatment of chronic pulmonary and nonmeningeal disseminated coccidioidomycosis, although the relapse rate, even after prolonged therapy, is high.[244] Response rates similar to those obtained with fluconazole have been obtained with itraconazole, albeit in noncomparative trials.[245]

Immunomodulating therapy has been attempted with "transfer factor," an ill-defined heterogeneous product of antigen-stimulated peripheral blood mononuclear cells, but its efficacy remains untested.[246] The potential role of cytokines is under laboratory investigation. One of these, recombinant human IL-2, had no effect in a murine model of coccidioidomycosis.[247] Other potential candidates for investigation include IL-12, interferon-γ, and granulocyte-macrophage colony-stimulating factor.

Meningitis

The largest experience in the treatment of coccidioidal meningitis has been with amphotericin B, a drug that does not penetrate the CSF after intravenous administration and is ineffective when given by that route alone. Treatment of meningitis with this polyene antibiotic therefore requires its delivery directly into the intrathecal or intraventricular space. The drug may be administered into the lumbar space, into the cisterna magna, by lateral cervical puncture, or into a lateral ventricle after placement of an indwelling catheter with a subcutaneous reservoir. Because abnormalities of CSF flow patterns are common in these patients and, in fact, loculation of fluid may occur, it is important to define flow initially and at intervals thereafter, using radionuclide techniques.

When amphotericin B is administered into the lumbar space, it is probably best to use the so-called hyperbaric method in which the drug is mixed with 10% dextrose in water, given by barbotage, followed by immediate placement of the patient in a 30-degree head down position for approximately 45 minutes. This has two potential benefits: delivery of the drug to the site of maximal infection, the basal meninges; and rapid removal from the lumbar space, where the drug may cause arachnoiditis, radiculitis, myelitis, and spinal artery thrombosis. Whichever route is used, treatment is initiated with a dose of 0.01 to 0.05 mg given by barbotage. Each dose is administered in dextrose in water together with 25 mg of hydrocortisone. The dose is gradually increased, on a daily basis, until a dose of 0.5 to 1.0 mg is reached. At that point, it may be desirable to change the dosing interval to every other day. The dose and interval of administration may need to be altered at times because of toxic effect. As clinical and laboratory improvement occurs, the dosing interval may eventually be progressively prolonged. Whereas the desired total duration of therapy has not been well defined, one recommended approach is to discontinue treatment when the CSF has stably returned to normal or nearly normal and has remained so for at least 12 to 24 months, during which CSF should be examined and drug administered every 4 to 6 weeks. Periodic examination of CSF for at least a year after discontinuation of therapy is probably wise. However, relapse may occur many years later.[120, 248] As a result of the frequency of relapse, many patients receive oral azole therapy after initial therapy with intrathecally administered amphotericin B.

The role of concomitant systemic administration of amphotericin B in the absence of apparent disease outside the central nervous system is uncertain, but such therapy is often recommended, usually with a total dose of 1 g being given.

Miconazole has also been administered directly into CSF for the treatment of coccidioidal meningitis but is rarely indicated for this purpose.[249, 250] Administration of ketoconazole in high oral doses may decrease the total amount of intrathecal amphotericin B required for treatment.[251] Treatment with orally administered fluconazole, which penetrates the CSF well, alone in a dose of 400 mg once daily is reported to yield response rates comparable to those previously reported with intrathecally administered amphotericin B.[248, 252–254] The use of higher doses (e.g., 800 mg daily) may hasten the response to therapy but is associated with an increased risk of adverse reactions. Itraconazole therapy (300 to 400 mg daily) has also produced clinical and laboratory responses in patients with coccidioidal meningitis, despite the relative lack of penetration of this drug into CSF.[255] Treatment of coccidioidal meningitis with azoles may have to be given for the life of the patient because of the high risk for relapse when therapy is discontinued after apparent resolution of infection.[256]

Impairment of CSF flow resulting in hydrocephalus is a frequent complication of coccidioidal meningitis and is amenable to the placement of a CSF shunt.[257] Another cause for deterioration of the patient is bacterial superinfection of a CSF shunt or intra-CSF catheter, which may require removal of the foreign body for cure. Large-vessel vasculitis may also cause clinical worsening.[158]

Bone and Joint Infection

Coccidioidal infection of joints is difficult to eradicate. Intraarticular amphotericin B produces cartilage damage in experimental animals and thus probably carries some risk in humans. Radical synovectomy, although difficult to accomplish totally, may produce the best chance of cure in some cases of chronic disease. The patient with coccidioidal osteomyelitis often benefits from surgical débridement. Although topical irrigation of osteomyelitic lesions or of associated sinus tracts is commonly used, its role is uncertain.[159–161]

Pulmonary Cavity Infection

Cavitary lung lesions often respond poorly to chemotherapy.[258] Stable asymptomatic cavities may be best ignored, but rapidly expanding cavities, life-threatening hemoptysis, recurrent bacterial superinfection, and threatened rupture into the pleural space are indications for surgical resection.[259]

Ocular Infection

Ocular infection, such as chorioretinitis, granulomatous conjunctivitis, and iridocyclitis, should be treated with a systemically administered antifungal agent. Amphotericin B has been administered by intraocular injection.[178]

Special Underlying Conditions

PREGNANCY

The apparent high risk for dissemination of coccidioidomycosis during the second and third trimesters of pregnancy necessitates strong consideration of therapy in all patients whose infection presents during that period. Ketoconazole, miconazole, and itraconazole should not be considered safe for use in pregnancy because of their effects on hormonal metabolism. Inadequate data exist to affirm the safety of fluconazole in pregnancy; it causes fetal abnormalities when it is administered in high doses to pregnant rats, possibly as the result of its lowering of estrogen levels, an effect not seen in nonpregnant humans.[189, 260] Furthermore, several infants born to women who had received fluconazole during the first trimester of pregnancy have had anomalies similar to those described in animal studies.[260a] There is a reasonable record of safe use of amphotericin B in pregnancy, and thus this drug remains the systemic antifungal agent of choice for use in pregnancy.[190]

HUMAN IMMUNODEFICIENCY VIRUS INFECTION

Primary nonprogressive pulmonary coccidioidomycosis has resolved without treatment in some HIV-infected patients with relatively high $CD4^+$ lymphocyte counts. Nonetheless, we believe that all HIV-infected patients with active coccidioidomycosis should receive antifungal chemotherapy. Amphotericin B is the drug of choice in cases in which the fungal infection appears to be immediately life threatening. Those with disseminated infection or AIDS (including those so classified only on the basis of a $CD4^+$ lymphocyte count of 200/mm^3 or lower) should continue to receive antifungal therapy, usually with orally administered fluconazole, for the remainder of their lives.

The absorption of many drugs from the gastrointestinal tract may be reduced in patients with AIDS. This is especially true with drugs such as ketoconazole and itraconazole, which require low gastric pH for absorption, because hypochlorhydria is common in these patients.[261] An additional concern with regard to the use of the azoles is the potential for pharmacokinetic interactions with other drugs taken by AIDS patients, such as rifampin, rifabutin, and clarithromycin.[262]

Clinical studies are required to determine whether AIDS patients with positive serologic test responses for coccidioidomycosis in the absence of active fungal infection would benefit from preemptive therapy. Also to be determined is the potential benefit of prophylactic therapy in AIDS patients resident in or traveling to endemic areas.

Prevention

Immunization

A spherule-derived vaccine is immunogenic and protective in rodents and primates.[263] It is reasonably well tolerated in humans and can induce skin test conversion.[264] A trial of a spherule-derived vaccine in humans, however, failed to demonstrate efficacy.[265]

General Preventive Measures

Because no vaccine is available, prevention of infection entails avoidance of exposure to the fungus in either its natural setting or a laboratory setting. In addition, CI may be temporarily eliminated from small soil foci by the use of fungicides. In the health care setting, dressings should be changed daily, and material contaminated with infected body substances should be disposed of promptly. Disinfection of surfaces can be accomplished with iodophors, phenols, formaldehyde, and hypochlorite.[266, 267]

Acknowledgment

The authors would like to acknowledge the bibliographic assistance of Karen Moody, MLS, medical librarian, Sequoia Hospital, Redwood City, California.

References

1. Fiese MJ: Coccidioidomycosis. Springfield, IL, Charles C Thomas, 1958.
2. Deresinski SC: History of coccidioidomycosis: "Dust to dust." *In* Stevens DA (ed): Coccidioidomycosis: A Text. New York, Plenum Publishing, 1980, pp 1–20.
3. Posada A: Un nuevo caso de micosis fungoidea con psorospermias. An Circ Med Argent 15:585–597, 1892.
4. Rixford E: A case of protozoic dermatitis. Occident Med Times 8:704–707, 1894.
5. Rixford E, Gilchrist TC: Two cases of protozoan (coccidioidal) infection of the skin and other organs. Johns Hopkins Hosp Rep 1:209–268, 1896.
6. Ophüls W, Moffitt HC: A new pathogenic mould (formerly described as a protozoan *(Coccidioides immitis pyogenes)*: Preliminary report. Philadelphia Med J 5:1471–1472, 1900.
7. Ophüls W: Further observations on a pathogenic mould formerly described as a protozoan *(Coccidioides immitis, Coccidioides pyogenes)*. J Exp Med 6:443–486, 1905.
8. Ophüls W: Coccidioidal granuloma. JAMA 45:1201–1296, 1905.
9. Stewart RA, Meyer KF: Isolation of *Coccidioides immitis* from soil. Proc Soc Exp Biol Med 29:937–938, 1932.
10. Dickson EC: "Valley fever" of the San Joaquin Valley and fungus *Coccidioides*. Calif West Med 47:151–155, 1937.
11. Dickson EC, Gifford MA: *Coccidioides* infection (coccidioidomycosis). Arch Intern Med 62:853–871, 1938.
12. Smith CE, Beard RR, Whiting EG, Rosenberger HG: Varieties of coccidioidal infection in relation to the epidemiology and control of the disease. Am J Public Health 36:1394–1402, 1946.
13. Smith CE, Whiting EG, Baker EE, et al: The use of coccidioidin. Am Rev Tuberc 57:330–360, 1948.
14. Smith CE, Saito MT, Simmons SA: Pattern of 39,500 serologic tests in coccidioidomycosis. JAMA 160:546–552, 1956.
15. Currah RS: Taxonomy of the Onygenales: Arthrodermataceae, Gymnoascaceae, Myxotrichaceae and Onygenaceae. Mycotaxin 24:1–216, 1985.
16. Bowman BH, Taylor JW, White TJ: Molecular evolution of the fungi: Human pathogens. Mol Biol Evol 9:893–904, 1992.
17. Pappagianis D, Ornelas A, Hector R: Guanine plus cytosine content of the DNA of *Coccidioides immitis*. Sabouraudia 23:451–454, 1985.
18. Kwon-Chung KJ: *Coccidioides immitis*: Cytological study on the formation of the arthrospores. Can J Genet Cytol 11:43–53, 1969.
19. Sun SH, Huppert M: A cytological study of morphogenesis in *Coccidioides immitis*. Sabouraudia 14:185–198, 1976.
20. Klotz SA, Drutz DJ, Huppert M, et al: The critical role of CO_2 in the morphogenesis of *Coccidioides immitis* in cell-free subcutaneous chambers. J Infect Dis 150:127–134, 1984.
21. Baker O, Braude AI: A study of stimuli leading to the production of spherules in coccidioidomycosis. J Lab Clin Med 47:169–181, 1956.
22. Galgiani JN, Hayden R, Payne CM: Leukocyte effects on the dimorphism of *Coccidioides immitis*. J Infect Dis 146:56–63, 1982.
23. Huppert M, Sun SH: Overview of mycology and the mycology of *Coccidioides immitis*. *In* Stevens DA (ed): Coccidioidomycosis: A Text. New York, Plenum Publishing, 1980, pp 21–46.
24. Cole GT, Sun SH: Arthroconidium-spherule-endospore transformation in *Coccidioides immitis*. *In* Szaniszlo PJ (ed): Fungal Dimorphism: With Emphasis on Fungi Pathogenic for Humans. New York, Plenum Publishing, 1985, pp 281–336.
25. Burt A, Carter DA, Koenig GL, et al: Molecular markers reveal cryptic sex in the human pathogen *Coccidioides immitis*. Proc Natl Acad Sci USA 93:770–773, 1996.
26. Kruse D, Cole GT: A seroreactive 120-kilodalton beta-1,3-glucanase of *Coccidioides immitis* which may participate in spherule morphogenesis. Infect Immun 60:4350–4363, 1992.
27. Yuan L, Cole GT, Sun SH: Possible role of a proteinase in endosporulation of *Coccidioides immitis*. Infect Immun 56:1551–1559, 1988.
28. Yuan L, Cole GT: Characterization of a proteinase inhibitor isolated from the fungal pathogen *Coccidioides immitis*. Biochem J 257:729–736, 1989.
29. Huppert M, Sun SH, Harrison JL: Morphogenesis throughout sparobic and parasitic cycles of *Coccidiodes immitis*. Mycopathologia 78:107–122, 1982.
30. Wheat RW, Tritschler C, Conant NF, Lowe EP: Comparison of *Coccidioides immitis* arthrospore, mycelium and spherule cell walls, and influence of growth medium on mycelial cell wall composition. Infect Immun 17:91–97, 1977.
31. Wheat RW, Su Chung KS, Ornellas EP, Scheer ER: Extraction of skin test activity from *Coccidioides immitis* mycelia by water, perchloric acid and aqueous phenol extraction. Infect Immun 19:152–159, 1978.
32. Wheat RW, Su Chung KS: Antigenic fractions of *Coccidioides immitis*. *In* Ajello L (ed): Coccidioidomycosis: Current Clinical and Diagnostic Status. Miami, FL, Symposia Specialists, 1977, pp 453–460.
33. Wheat RW, Scheer E: Cell walls of *Coccidioides immitis*: Neutral sugars of aqueous alkaline extract polymers. Infect Immun 17:91–97, 1977.
34. Hector R, Pappagianis D: Enzymatic degradation of the walls of spherules of *Coccidioides immitis*. Exp Mycol 6:136–152, 1982.
35. Zimmer BL, Pappagianis D: Taxonomic and physiologic characteristics of *Coccidioides immitis*. *In* Leive L (ed): Microbiology. Washington, DC, American Society for Microbiology, 1986, pp 165–168.
36. Lones G: Studies of intermediary metabolism in *Coccidioides immitis*. *In* Ajello L (ed): Coccidioidomycosis: Proceedings of the 2nd Symposium on Coccidioidomycosis. Tucson, AZ, University of Arizona Press, 1965, pp 349–353.
37. Baker EE, Smith CE: Utilization of carbon and nitrogen compounds by *Coccidioides immitis* (Rixford and Gilchrist, 1896). J Infect Dis 70:51–53, 1942.
38. Sippel JE, Levine HB: Sugars and amino acids as carbon, nitrogen, or energy sources for *Coccidioides immitis* spherules and endospores. Appl Microbiol 18:522–524, 1969.
39. Powell BL, Drutz DJ, Huppert M, Sun SH: Relationship of progesterone- and estradiol-binding proteins in *Coccidioides immitis* to coccidioidal dissemination in pregnancy. Infect Immun 40:478–485, 1983.
40. Powell BL, Drutz DA: Identification of a high-affinity binder for estradiol and a low-affinity binder for testosterone in *Coccidioides immitis*. Infect Immun 45:784–786, 1984.
41. Reiss E: *Coccidioides immitis*. *In* Reiss E (ed): Molecular Immunology of Mycotic and Actinomycotic Infections. New York, Elsevier Science Publishing, 1986, pp 53–76.

42. Cox RA, Huppert M, Starr P, Britt LA: Reactivity of alkali-soluble, water-soluble cell wall antigen of *Coccidioides immitis* with anti-*Coccidioides* immunoglobulin M precipitin antibody. Infect Immun 43:502–507, 1984.
43. Ward ER, Cox RA, Schmitt JA, et al: Delayed-type hypersensitivity responses to cell wall fraction of the mycelial phase of *Coccidioides immitis*. Infect Immun 12:1093–1097, 1975.
44. Lecara G, Cox RA, Simpson RB: *Coccidioides immitis* vaccine: Potential of an alkali-soluble, water-soluble cell wall antigen. Infect Immun 39:437–475, 1983.
45. Johnson SM, Pappagianis D: The coccidioidal complement fixation and immunodiffusion–complement fixation antigen is a chitinase. Infect Immun 60:2588–2592, 1992.
46. Landay ME, Wheat RW, Conant NF, Lowe EP: Serological comparison of spherules and arthrospores of *Coccidioides immitis*. J Bacteriol 94:1400–1405, 1967.
47. Huppert M, Spratt NS, Vukovich KR, et al: Antigenic analysis of coccidioidin and spherulin determined by two dimensional immunoelectrophoresis. Infect Immun 20:541–551, 1978.
47a. Schneider E, Hajjeh RA, Spiegel RA, et al: A coccidioidomycosis outbreak following the Northridge, Calif, earthquake. JAMA 277:904–908, 1997.
48. Converse JL, Reed RE: Experimental epidemiology of coccidioidomycosis. Bacteriol Rev 30:678–695, 1966.
49. Perez JA, Abraham J: Coccidioidomycosis: A new sexually transmitted disease? Centennial Conference on Coccidioidomycosis (Abstr 28). 5th International Conference on Coccidioidomycosis; August 24–27, 1994; Stanford University, Stanford, CA.
50. Kohn GJ, Linne SR, Smith CM, Hoeprich PD: Acquisition of coccidioidomycosis at necropsy by inhalation of coccidioidal endospores. Diagn Microbiol Infect Dis 15:527–530, 1992.
51. Pappagianis D: Coccidioidomycosis. *In* Demis DJ (ed): Clinical Dermatology. Hagerstown, MD, Harper & Row, 1973, pp 1–11.
52. Wilson JW, Smith CE, Plunkett OA: Primary cutaneous coccidioidomycosis. Calif Med 79:233–239, 1953.
53. Bernstein DI, Tipton JR, Schoot SF, Cherry JD: Coccidioidomycosis in a neonate: Maternal-infant transmission. J Pediatr 99:752–754, 1981.
54. Spark RP: Does transplacental spread of coccidioidomycosis occur? Report of a neonatal fatality and review of the literature. Arch Pathol Lab Med 105:347–350, 1981.
55. Eckmann BH, Schaefer GL, Huppert MH: Bedside transmission of coccidioidomycosis via growth on fomites. Am Rev Respir Dis 89:1175–1185, 1964.
56. Gehlbach SH, Hamilton JD, Conant NF: Coccidioidomycosis. An occupational disease in cotton mill workers. Arch Intern Med 131:254–255, 1973.
57. Schwarz J, Kantman CA: Occupational hazards from deep mycoses. Arch Dermatol 113:1270–1275, 1977.
58. Velasco-Castrejón O, González-Ochoa A: Coccidioidomicosis adquirida en la ciudad de Mexico. Un caso atipico desde el punto de vista epidemiologico. Rev Invest Salus Publica 35:97–102, 1975.
59. Standaert SM, Schaffner W, Galgiani JN, et al: Coccidioidomycosis among visitors to a *Coccidioides immitis*–endemic area: An outbreak in a military reserve unit. J Infect Dis 171:1672–1675, 1995.
60. Zimmerman CR, Snedker CJ, Pappagianis D: Characterization of *Coccidioides immitis* isolates by restriction fragment length polymorphisms. J Clin Microbiol 32:3040–3042, 1994.
61. Maddy KT: The geographic distribution of *Coccidioides immitis* and possible ecologic implications. Ariz Med 15:178–188, 1958.
62. Pappagianis D: Epidemiology of coccidioidomycosis. *In* Stevens DA (ed): Coccidioidomycosis: A Text. New York, Plenum Publishing, 1980, pp 63–85.
63. Rippon JW: Medical Mycology. Philadelphia, WB Saunders, 1988, pp 435–439.
64. Pappagianis D: Epidemiology of coccidioidomycosis. Curr Top Med Mycol 2:199–238, 1988.
65. Hicks MJ, Hagaman RM, Barbee RA: The prevalence of cellular immunity to coccidioidomycosis in a highly endemic area. West J Med 144:425–428, 1986.
66. Pappagianis D, Einstein H: Tempest from Tehachapi takes toll. West J Med 129:527–530, 1978.
67. Dodge RR, Lebowitz MD, Barbee R, Burrows B: Estimates of *C. immitis* infection by skin test reactivity in an endemic area. Am J Public Health 75:863–865, 1985.
68. Kerrick SS, Lundergan LL, Galgiani JN: Coccidioidomycosis at a University Health Service. Am Rev Respir Dis 131:100–102, 1985.
69. Gilman DW, Wehrle PF, Cowper H: Coccidioidomycosis— Canoga Park, California. MMWR Morbid Mortal Wkly Rep 14:302–303, 1965.
70. Lacy GH, Swatek FE: *Coccidioides* in California. *In* Ajello L (ed): Coccidioidomycosis: Current Clinical and Diagnostic Status. Miami, FL, Symposia Specialists, 1977, pp 79–90.
71. Werner SB, Pappagianis D, Heindl I, Mickel A: An epidemic of coccidioidomycosis among archaeology students in northern California. N Engl J Med 286:507–512, 1972.
72. Smith CE, Beard RR, Rosenberger HG, Whiting EG: Effect of season and dust control on coccidioidomycosis. JAMA 132:833–838, 1946.
73. Hugenholtz P: Climate and coccidioidomycosis. *In* Ferguson MS (ed): Proceedings of the Symposium on Coccidioidomycosis. Atlanta, Communicable Disease Center, 1957, pp 136–143. US Public Health Service Publication 575.
74. Centers for Disease Control and Prevention: Coccidioidomycosis following the Northridge Earthquake—California, 1994. MMWR Morbid Mortal Wkly Rep 43:194–195, 1994.
75. Pappagianis D: Marked increase in cases of coccidioidomycosis in California: 1991, 1992, and 1993. J Infect Dis 19(Suppl 1):S14–S18, 1994.
76. Smale LE, Birsner JW: Maternal deaths from coccidioidomycosis. JAMA 140:1152–1154, 1949.
77. Wack EE, Ampel NM, Galgiani JN, Bronnimann DA: Coccidioidomycosis during pregnancy. An analysis of ten cases among 47,120 pregnancies. Chest 94:376–379, 1988.
78. Cohen IM, Galgiani JN, Potter D, Ogden DA: Coccidioidomycosis in renal replacement therapy. Arch Intern Med 142:489–494, 1982.
79. Bronnimann DA, Adam RD, Galgiani JN, et al: Coccidioidomycosis in the acquired immunodeficiency syndrome. Ann Intern Med 106:372–379, 1987.
79a. Coccidioidomycosis—Arizona, 1990–1995. MMWR Morbid Mortal Wkly Rep 45:1069–1073, 1996.
80. Drutz DJ, Huppert M: Coccidioidomycosis: Factors affecting the host-parasite interaction. J Infect Dis 147:372–390, 1983.
81. Savage DC, Madin SH: Cellular responses in lungs of immunized mice to intranasal infection with *Coccidioides immitis*. Sabouraudia 6:94–102, 1968.
82. Galgiani JN, Isenberg RA, Stevens DA: Chemotaxigenic activity of extracts from the mycelial and spherule phases of *Coccidioides immitis* for human polymorphonuclear leukocytes. Infect Immun 21:862–865, 1978.
83. Galgiani JN, Yam P, Petz LD, et al: Complement activation by *Coccidioides immitis*: In vitro and clinical studies. Infect Immun 28:944–949, 1980.
84. Galgiani JN, Payne CM, Jones JF: Human polymorphonuclear-leukocyte inhibition of chitin precursors into mycelia of *Coccidioides immitis*. J Infect Dis 149:404–411, 1984.
85. Collins MS, Pappagianis D: Effects of lysozyme and chitinase on the spherules of *Coccidioides immitis* and *Histoplasma capsulatum*. Contrib Microbiol Immunol 3:106–125, 1973.
86. Frey CL, Drutz DJ: Influence of fungal surface components on the interaction of *Coccidioides immitis* with polymorphonuclear neutrophils. J Infect Dis 153:933–943, 1986.
87. Beaman L, Pappagianis D, Benjamini E: Significance of T cells in resistance to experimental murine coccidioidomycosis. Infect Immun 17:580–585, 1977.
88. Beaman L, Benjamini E, Pappagianis D: Role of lymphocytes in macrophage-induced killing of *Coccidioides immitis* in vitro. Infect Immun 34:347–353, 1981.
89. Beaman L, Holmberg CA: In vitro response of alveolar macrophages to infection with *Coccidioides immitis*. Infect Immun 28:594–560, 1980.
90. Beaman L, Benjamini E, Pappagianis D: Activation of macrophages by lymphokines: Enhancement of phagosome-lysosome fusion and killing of *Coccidioides immitis*. Infect Immun 39:1201–1297, 1983.
91. Beaman L: Fungicidal activation of murine macrophages by recombinant gamma interferon. Infect Immun 55:2951–2955, 1987.
92. Magee DM, Cox RA: Roles of gamma interferon and interleu-

kin-4 in genetically determined resistance to *Coccidioides immitis*. Infect Immun 63:3514–3519, 1995.
93. Cox RA, Magee DM: Production of tumor necrosis factor alpha, interleukin-1 alpha, and interleukin-6 during murine coccidioidomycosis. Infect Immun 63:4178–4180, 1995.
94. Beaman L: Effects of recombinant gamma interferon and tumor necrosis factor on in vitro interactions of human mononuclear phagocytes with *Coccidioides immitis*. Infect Immun 59:4427-4429, 1991.
95. Ampel NM, Bejarano GC, Galgiani JN: Killing of *Coccidioides immitis* by human peripheral blood mononuclear cells. Infect Immun 60:4200–4204, 1992.
96. Slagle DC, Cox RA, Kuruganti U: Induction of tumor necrosis factor alpha by spherules of *Coccidioides immitis*. Infect Immun 57:1916–1921, 1989.
97. Clemons KV, Leathers CR, Lee KW: Systemic *Coccidioides immitis* infection in nude and beige mice. Infect Immun 47:814–821, 1985.
98. Kirkland TN, Fierer J: Inbred mouse strains differ in resistance to lethal *Coccidioides immitis* infection. Infect Immun 40:912–916, 1983.
99. Kirkland TN, Fierer J: Genetic control of resistance to *Coccidioides immitis*: A single gene that is expressed in spleen cells determines resistance. J Immunol 135:548–552, 1985.
100. Cox RA, Kennell W, Boncyk L, Murphy JW: Induction and expression of cell-mediated immune responses in inbred mice infected with *Coccidioides immitis*. Infect Immun 56:13–17, 1988.
101. Deresinski SC, Stevens DA, Applegate RJ, et al: Cellular immunity to *Coccidioides immitis*: In vitro lymphocyte response to spherules, arthrospores, and endospores. Cell Immunol 32:110–119, 1977.
102. Ampel NM, Bejarano GC, Salas SD, Galgiani JN: In vitro assessment of cellular immunity in human coccidioidomycosis: Relationship between dermal hypersensitiviy, lymphocyte transformation, and lymphokine production by peripheral blood mononuclear cells from healthy adults. J Infect Dis 165:710–715, 1992.
103. Ampel NM, Dols CL, Galgiani JN: Coccidioidomycosis during human immunodeficiency virus infection: Results of a prospective study in a coccidioidal endemic area. Am J Med 94:235–240, 1993.
104. Deresinski SC, Levine HB, Stevens DA: *Coccidioides immitis* endospores: Phagocytosis by human cells. Mycopathologia 3:179–181, 1978.
105. Ampel NM, Galgiani JN: Interaction of human peripheral blood mononuclear cells with *Coccidioides immitis* arthroconidia. Cell Immunol 133:253–262, 1991.
106. Cox RA, Vivas JR: Spectrum of in vivo and in vitro cell-mediated immune responses in coccidioidomycosis. Cell Immunol 31:130–141, 1977.
107. Cox RA, Vivas JR, Gross A, et al: In vivo and in vitro cell-mediated immune responses in coccidioidomycosis. I. Immunologic responses of persons with primary, asymptomatic infection. Am Rev Respir Dis 114:937–942, 1976.
108. Cox RA, Kennell W: Suppression of T-lymphocyte response by *Coccidioides immitis* antigen. Infect Immun 56:1424–1429, 1988.
109. Cox RA, Pope RM: Serum-mediated suppression of lymphocyte transformation responses in coccidioidomycosis. Infect Immun 55:1058–1062, 1987.
110. Deresinski SC: The immunology of coccidioidomycosis. *In* Friedman H, Chmel H, Bendinelli M (eds): Pulmonary Infections and Immunity. New York, Plenum Publishing, 1994, pp 29–49.
110a. Magee DM, Cox RA: Interleukin-12 regulation of host defenses against *Coccidioides immitis*. Infect Immun 64:3609–3613, 1996.
110b. Corry DB, Ampel NM, Christian L, et al: Cytokine production by peripheral blood mononuclear cells in human coccidioidomycosis. J Infect Dis 174:440–443, 1996.
111. Cox RA, Baker BS, Stevens DA: Specificity of immunoglobulin E in coccidioidomycosis and correlation with disease involvement. Infect Immun 37:609–616, 1982.
112. Shapira SK, Jabara HH, Thienes CP, et al: Deletional switch recombination occurs in interleukin-4–induced isotype switching to IgE expression by human B cells. Proc Natl Acad Sci USA 88:7528–7532, 1991.
113. Scott P: IL-12: Initiation cytokine for cell-mediated immunity. Science 260:496–497, 1993.
114. Sanderson CJ: Interleukin-5, eosinophils, and disease. Blood 79:3101–3109, 1992.
115. Cole GT: Ammonia production by *Coccidioides immitis* and its significance to the host-fungus interplay (Abstr L29). 5th Symposium on Topics in Mycology: Host-Fungus Interplay; June 27–30, 1995; Stanford University, Stanford, CA.
116. Resnick S, Pappagianis D, McKerrow JH: Proteinase production by the parasitic cycle of the pathogenic fungus *Coccidioides immitis*. Infect Immun 55:2807–2815, 1987.
117. Hunninghake GW, Davidson JM, Rennard S, et al: Elastin fragments attract macrophage precursors to diseased sites in pulmonary emphysema. Science 212:925–927, 1981.
118. Smith CE: Coccidioidomycosis. Med Clin North Am 27:790–807, 1943.
119. Yozwiak ML, Lundergan LL, Kerrick SS, Galgiani JN: Symptoms and routine laboratory abnormalities associated with coccidioidomycosis. West J Med 149:419–421, 1988.
120. Gamble CN, Ruggles SW: The immunopathogenesis of glomerulonephritis associated with mixed cryoglobulinemia. N Engl J Med 299:81–84, 1978.
121. Schermoly MJ, Hinthorn DR: Eosinophilia in coccidioidomycosis. Arch Intern Med 148:895–896, 1988.
122. Bayer AS: Fungal pneumonias: Pulmonary coccidioidal syndromes (part I). Primary and progressive primary coccidioidal pneumonias—Diagnostic, therapeutic, and prognostic considerations. Chest 79:575–583, 1981.
123. Bayer AS: Fungal pneumonias: Pulmonary coccidioidal syndromes (part 2). Miliary, nodular, and cavitary pulmonary coccidioidomycosis: Chemotherapeutic and surgical considerations. Chest 79:686–691, 1981.
124. Larsen RA, Jacobson JA, Morris AH, Benowitz BA: Acute respiratory failure caused by primary pulmonary coccidioidomycosis. Two case reports and a review of the literature. Am Rev Respir Dis 131:797–799, 1985.
125. Bayer AS, Yoshikawa TT, Guze LB: Chronic progressive coccidioidal pneumonitis. Report of six cases with clinical, roentgenographic, serologic and therapeutic features. Arch Intern Med 139:536–540, 1979.
126. Batra P: Pulmonary coccidioidomycosis. J Thorac Imaging 7:29–38, 1992.
127. Birsner JW: The roentgen aspects of five hundred cases of pulmonary coccidioidomycosis. Am J Roentgenol Radium Ther Nucl Med 72:4, 1954.
128. Schwartz EL, Waldmann EB, Payne RM, et al: Coccidioidal pericarditis. Chest 70:670–672, 1976.
129. Amundson DE: Perplexing pericarditis caused by coccidioidomycosis. South Med J 86:694–696, 1993.
130. Lonky SA, Catanzaro A, Moser KM, Einstein H: Acute coccidioidal pleural effusion. Am Rev Respir Dis 114:681–688, 1976.
131. Boyle JO, Coulthard SW, Mandel RM: Laryngeal involvement in disseminated coccidioidomycosis. Arch Otolaryngol Head Neck Surg 117:433–438, 1991.
132. Moskowitz PS, Sue JY, Gooding CA: Tracheal coccidioidomycosis causing upper airway obstruction in children. AJR 139:596–600, 1982.
133. Winn WA: A long term study of 300 patients with cavitary-abscess lesions of the lung of coccidioidal origin. An analytical study with special reference to treatment. Dis Chest 54(Suppl 1):12–16, 1968.
134. Putnam JS, Harper WK, Greene JF Jr, et al: *Coccidioides immitis*: A rare cause of pulmonary mycetoma. Am Rev Respir Dis 112:733–738, 1975.
135. Winn RE, Johnson R, Galgiani JN, et al: Cavitary coccidioidomycosis with fungus ball formation. Diagnosis by fiberoptic bronchoscopy with coexistence of hyphae and spherules. Chest 105:412–416, 1994.
136. Cunningham RT, Einstein H: Coccidioidal pulmonary cavities with rupture. J Thorac Cardiovasc Surg 84:172–177, 1982.
137. Blumenkranz MS, Stevens DA: Endogenous coccidioidal endophthalmitis. J Ophthalmol 87:974–984, 1980.
138. Rodenbiker HT, Ganley JP, Galgiani JN, Axline SG: Prevalence of chorioretinal scars associated with coccidioidomycosis. Arch Ophthalmol 99:71–75, 1981.
139. Petersen EA, Friedman BA, Crowder ED: Coccidioiduria: Clinical significance. Ann Intern Med 85:34–38, 1976.
140. DeFelice R, Wieden MA, Galgiani JN: The incidence and implications of coccidioiduria. Am Rev Respir Dis 125:49–52, 1982.

141. Loeb JM, Livermore BM, Wofsy D: Coccidioidomycosis of the thyroid. Ann Intern Med 91:409–412, 1979.
142. Schwartz DN, Fihn SD, Miller RA: Infection of an arterial prosthesis as the presenting manifestation of disseminated coccidioidomycosis: Control of disease with fluconazaole. Clin Infect Dis 16:486–488, 1993.
143. Jacobs PH: Cutaneous coccidioidomycosis. *In* Stevens DA (ed): Coccidioidomycosis: A Text. New York, Plenum Publishing, 1980, pp 213–224.
144. Kelly PC: Coccidioidal meningitis. *In* Stevens DA (ed): Coccidioidomycosis: A Text. New York, Plenum Publishing, 1980, pp 163–194.
145. Galgiani JN, Peng T, Lewis ML, et al: Cerebrospinal fluid antibodies detected by ELISA against a 33-kDa antigen from spherules of *Coccidioides immitis* in patients with coccidioidal meningitis. The National Institute of Allergy and Infectious Diseases Mycoses Study Group. J Infect Dis 173:499–502, 1996.
146. Bouza E, Dreyer JS, Hewitt WL, Meyer RD: Coccidioidal meningitis. An analysis of thirty-one cases and review of the literature. Medicine (Baltimore) 60:139–172, 1981.
147. Wrobel CJ, Rothrock J: Coccidioidomycosis meningitis presenting as anterior spinal artery syndrome. Neurology 42:1840, 1992.
148. Vincent T, Galgiani JN: The natural history of coccidioidomycosis: VA–Armed Forces Cooperative Studies, 1955–1958. Clin Infect Dis 16:247–254, 1993.
149. Sobel RA, Ellis WG, Nielsen SL, Davis RL: Central nervous system coccidioidomycosis: A clinicopathologic study of treatment with and without amphotericin B. Hum Pathol 15:980–995, 1984.
150. Mendel E, Milefchik EN, Ahmadi J, Gruen P: Coccidioidomycosis brain abscess. Case report. J Neurosurg 80:140–142, 1994.
151. Bañuelos AF, Williams PF, Johnson RH, et al: Central nervous system abscesses due to *Coccidioides* species. Clin Infect Dis 22:240–250, 1996.
152. Wrobel CJ, Meyer S, Johnson RH, Hesselink JR: MR findings in acute and chronic coccidioidomycosis meningitis. AJNR 13:1241–1245, 1992.
153. Ragland AS, Argura EL, Ismail Y, Johnson R: Eosinophilic pleocytosis in coccidioidal meningitis: Frequency and significance. Am J Med 95:254–257, 1993.
154. Shetter AG, Fischer DW, Flom RA: Computed tomography in cases of coccidioidal meningitis, with clinical correlation. West J Med 142:782–786, 1985.
155. Ampel NM, Ahmann DR, Delgado KL, et al, and the National Institute of Allergy and Infectious Diseases Mycoses Study Group: Tumor necrosis factor-alpha and interleukin-1 beta in cerebrospinal fluid of patients with coccidioidal meningitis during therapy with ketoconazole. J Infect Dis 171:1675–1678, 1995.
156. Harrison HR, Reynolds AF: Trapped fourth ventricle in coccidioidal meningitis. Surg Neurol 17:197–199, 1982.
157. Hadley MN, Martin NA, Spetzler RF, Johnson PC: Multiple intracranial aneurysms due to *Coccidioides immitis* infection. Case report. J Neurosurg 66:453–456, 1987.
158. Williams PL, Johnson R, Pappagianis D, et al: Vasculitic and encephalitic complications associated with *Coccidioides immitis* infection of the central nervous system in humans: Report of 10 cases and review. Clin Infect Dis 14:673–682, 1992.
159. Kemper CA, Deresinski SC: Fungal diseases of bones and joints. *In* Kibbler CC, Odds FC, MacKenzie DWR (eds): Principles and Practice of Mycology. Sussex, England, John Wiley & Sons, 1996, pp 49–68.
160. Deresinski SC: Coccidioidomycosis of bone and joints. *In* Stevens DA (ed): Coccidioidomycosis: A Text. New York, Plenum Publishing, 1980, pp 195–212.
161. Bried JM, Galgiani JN: *Coccidioides immitis* infections in bones and joints. Clin Orthop 211:235–243, 1986.
162. Kemper CA, Deresinski SC: Fungal arthritis. *In* Maddison PJ, Isenberg DA, Woo P, Glass DN (eds): The Oxford Texbook of Rheumatology. Oxford, Oxford University Press, 1993, pp 599–607.
162a. Kemper CA, Deresinski SC: Fungal diseases of bones and joints. *In* Kibbler CC, Odds FC, Mackenzie DWR (eds): Principles and Practice of Clinical Mycology. Sussex, UK, John Wiley & Sons, 1996, pp 49–68.
163. Dalinka MK, Dinnenberg S, Greendyke WH, Hopkins R: Roentgenographic features of osseous coccidioidomycosis. J Bone Joint Surg Am 53:1157–1164, 1971.
164. Boddicker JH, Fong D, Walsh TE, et al: Bone and gallium scanning in the evaluation of disseminated coccidioidomycosis. Am Rev Respir Dis 122:279–287, 1980.
165. Moreno AJ, Weisman I, Rodriguez AA, et al: Nuclear imaging in coccidioidal osteomyelitis. Clin Nucl Med 12:604–609, 1987.
166. Lee JC, Catanzaro A, Parthemore JG, et al: Hypercalcemia in disseminated coccidioidomycosis. N Engl J Med 297:431–433, 1977.
167. Walter RM Jr, Lawrence RM: Hypercalcemia in disseminated coccidioidomycosis. Am J Med Sci 281:97–99, 1981.
168. Parker MS, Dokoh S, Woolfenden JM, Buchsbaum HW: Hypercalcemia in coccidioidomycosis. Am J Med 76:341–344, 1984.
168a. Kemper CA, Deresinski SC: Fungal arthritis. *In* Gorbach S, Bartlett J, Blacklow N (eds): Oxford Textbook of Rheumatology. Oxford, UK, Oxford University Press (in press).
169. Reid GD, Klinkhoff A, Bozek C, Denegri JF: Coccidioidomycosis tenosynovitis: Case report and review of the literature. J Rheumatol 11:392–394, 1984.
170. Price MJ, Lewis EL, Carmalt JE: Coccidioidomycosis of prostate gland. Urology 19:653–655, 1982.
171. Chen KT: Coccidioidomycosis of the epididymis. J Urol 130:978–979, 1983.
172. Salgia K, Bhatia L, Rajashekaraiah KR, et al: Coccidioidomycosis of the uterus. South Med J 75:614–616, 1982.
173. Parker P, Adcock LL: Pelvic coccidioidomycosis. Obstet Gynecol Surv 36:225–229, 1981.
174. Chen KTK: Coccidioidal peritonitis. Am J Clin Pathol 80:514–516, 1983.
175. Ampel NM, White JD, Varanasi UR, et al: Coccidioidal peritonitis associated with continuous ambulatory peritoneal dialysis. Am J Kidney Dis 11:512–514, 1988.
176. Dooley DP, Reddy RK, Smith CE: Coccidioidomycosis presenting as an omental mass. Clin Infect Dis 19:802–803, 1994.
177. Maguire LJ, Campbell RJ, Edson RS: Coccidioidomycosis with necrotizing granulomatous conjunctivitis. Cornea 13:539–542, 1994.
178. Moorthys RS, Rao NA, Sidikaro Y, Foos RY: Coccidioidomycosis iridocyclitis. Ophthalmology 101:1923–1928, 1994.
179. Deresinski SC, Stevens DA: Coccidioidomycosis in compromised hosts. Experience at Stanford University Hospital. Medicine (Baltimore) 54:377–395, 1974.
180. Rutala PJ, Smith JW: Coccidioidomycosis in potentially compromised hosts: The effect of immunosuppressive therapy in dissemination. Am J Med Sci 275:283–295, 1982.
181. Seltzer J, Broaddus VC, Jacobs R, Golden JA: Reactivation of coccidioides infection. West J Med 145:96–98, 1986.
181a. Holt CD, Winston DJ, Kubak B, et al: Coccidioidomycosis in liver transplant patients. Clin Infect Dis 24:216–221, 1997.
182. Hall KA, Sethi GK, Rosado LJ, et al: Coccidioidomycosis and heart transplantation. J Heart Lung Transplant 12:525–526, 1993.
183. Hall KA, Copeland JG, Zukoski CF, et al: Markers of coccidioidomycosis before cardiac or renal transplantation and the risk of recurrent infection. Transplantation 55:1422–1424, 1993.
184. Arguinchona HL, Ampel NM, Dols CL, et al: Persistent coccidioidal seropositivity without clinical evidence of active coccidioidomycosis in patients infected with human immunodeficiency virus. J Infect Dis 20:1281–1285, 1995.
185. Jones JL, Fleming PL, Cieselski CA, et al: Coccidioidomycosis among persons with AIDS in the United States. J Infect Dis 171:961–966, 1995.
185a. Kemper CA, Linette A, Kane C, Deresinski SC: Travels with HIV: The effects of travel on the compliance and health of HIV infected adults. Int J STD AIDS 7:1–6, 1996.
186. Fish DG, Ampel NM, Galgiani JN, et al: Coccidioidomycosis during human immunodeficiency virus infection. A review of 77 patients. Medicine (Baltimore) 69:384–391, 1990.
187. McNeil MM, Ampel NM: Opportunistic coccidioidomycosis in patients infected with human immunodeficiency virus: Prevention issues and priorities. Clin Infect Dis 21(Suppl 1):S111–S113, 1995.
188. Antoniskis D, Larsen RA, Akil B, et al: Seronegative disseminated coccidioidomycosis in patients with HIV infection. AIDS 4:691–693, 1990.
189. Mahaffey KW, Hippenmeyer CL, Mandel R, Ampel NM: Unrec-

ognized coccidioidomycosis complicating *Pneumocystis carinii* pneumonia in patients infected with the human immunodeficiency virus and treated with corticosteroids. A report of two cases. Arch Intern Med 153:1496–1498, 1993.
190. Peterson CM, Schuppert K, Kelly PC, Pappagianis D: Coccidioidomycosis and pregnancy. Obstet Gynecol Surv 48:149–156, 1993.
191. Einstein H, Johnson R, Caldwell J, et al: Coccidioidomycosis and pregnancy: The Kern County experience (Abstr K202). Presented at the 35th Interscience Conference on Antimicrobial Agents and Chemotherapy; September 17–20, 1995; San Francisco, CA; p 324.
192. Park RO: Does transplacental spread of coccidioidomycosis occur? Report of a neonatal fatality and review of the literature. Arch Pathol Lab Med 105:347–350, 1981.
193. Wegmann TG, Lin H, Guilbert LJ, Mosmann TR: Bidirectional cytokine interactions in the maternal-fetal relationship. Is successful pregnancy a TH2 phenomenon? Immunol Today 14:353–356, 1993.
194. Barbee RA, Hicks MJ, Grosso D, Sandel C: The maternal immune response in coccidioidomycosis—Is pregnancy a risk factor for serious infection? Chest 100:709–715, 1991.
195. Howard PF, Smith JW: Diagnosis of disseminated coccidioidomycosis by liver biopsy. Arch Intern Med 143:1335–1338, 1983.
196. Wolfson D, Lee S: Coccidioidomycosis diagnosed from bone marrow smear. JAMA 266:707, 1991.
197. Warlick MA, Quan SF, Sobonya RE: Rapid diagnosis of pulmonary coccidioidomycosis. Cytologic v. potassium hydroxide preparations. Arch Intern Med 143:723–725, 1983.
198. Hageage GJ, Harrington BJ: Use of calcofluor white in clinical mycology. Lab Med 15:109–112, 1984.
199. DiTomasso JP, Ampel NM, Sobonya RE, Bloom JW: Bronchoscopic diagnosis of pulmonary coccidioidomycosis. Comparison of cytology, culture, and transbronchial biopsy. Diagn Microbiol Infect Dis 18:83–87, 1994.
200. Nunez D, Stanley C, Robertstad, Drow DL: Pseudoepidemic of coccidioidomycosis. Am J Infect Control 10:68–71, 1982.
201. Raab SS, Silverman JF, Zimmerman KG: Fine-needle aspiration biopsy of pulmonary coccidioidomycosis. Spectrum of cytologic findings in 73 patients. Am J Clin Pathol 99:582–587, 1993.
202. Puckett TF: Hyphae of *Coccidioides immitis* in tissues of the human host. Am Rev Tuberc 70:320–327, 1954.
203. Wages DS, Helfend L, Finkle H: *Coccidioides immitis* presenting as a hyphal form in a ventriculoperitoneal shunt. Arch Pathol Lab Med 119:91–93, 1995.
204. Fainstein V, Hopfer RL, Trier P, Bodey GP: Bone marrow cultures: Their value in diagnosing fungal and mycobacterial infection in patients with cancer. J Infect Dis 144:79, 1981.
205. Ampel NM, Ryan KJ, Carry PJ, et al: Fungemia due to *Coccidioides immitis*. An analysis of 16 episodes in 15 patients and a review of the literature. Medicine (Baltimore) 65:312–321, 1986.
206. Ampel NM, Wieden MA: Discrepancy between growth of *Coccidioides immitis* in bacterial blood culture media and a radiometric growth index. Diagn Microbiol Infect Dis 9:7–10, 1988.
207. Huppert M, Sun SH, Bailey JW: Natural variability in *Coccidioides immitis*. *In* Ajello L (ed): Coccidioidomycosis: Proceedings the 2nd Symposium on Coccidioidomycosis. Tucson, AZ, University of Arizona Press, 1965, pp 323–328.
208. Sigler L, Carmichaell JW: Taxonomy of *Malbranchea* and some other hyphomycetes with arthroconidia. Mycotaxon 4:349–488, 1976.
209. Brosbe EA: Use of refined agar for the in vitro propagation of spherule phase of *Coccidioides immitis*. J Bacteriol 93:497–498, 1967.
210. Standard PG, Kaufman L: Immunological procedure for the rapid and specific identification of *Coccidioides immitis* in cultures. J Clin Microbiol 5:149–153, 1977.
211. Kaufman L, Standard PG: Improved version of the exoantigen test for identification of *Coccidioides immitis* and *Histoplasma capsulatum*. J Clin Microbiol 8:42–45, 1978.
212. Beard JS, Benson PM, Skillman L: Rapid diagnosis of coccidioidomycosis with a DNA probe to ribosomal RNA. Arch Dermatol 129:1589–1593, 1993.
213. Smith CE: Diagnosis of pulmonary coccidioidomycosis. Calif Med 75:385, 1951.
214. Galgiani JN, and the Valley Fever Vaccine Study Group: Development of dermal hypersensitivity to coccidioidal antigens associated with repeated skin testing. Am Rev Respir Dis 191:1045–1047, 1986.
215. Levine HB, Gonzalez-Ochoa A, Ten Eyck DR: Dermal sensitivity to *Coccidioides immitis*. A comparison of responses elicited in man by spherulin and coccidioidin. Am Rev Respir Dis 107:379–385, 1973.
216. Stevens DA, Levine HB, Deresinski SC, Blaine LJ: Spherulin in clinical coccidioidomycosis. Chest 68:697–702, 1975.
217. Gifford J, Catanzaro A: A comparison of coccidioidin and spherulin skin testing in the diagnosis of coccidioidomycosis. Am Rev Respir Dis 124:440–444, 1981.
218. Woodruff WW III, Buckley CE III, Gallis HA, et al: Reactivity to spherule-derived coccidioidin in the southeastern United States. Infect Immun 43:860–869, 1984.
219. Pappagianis D, Smith CE, Campbell CC: Serologic status after positive coccidioidin skin reactions. Am Rev Respir Dis 96:520–523, 1967.
220. Deresinski SC, Levine HB, Kelly PC, et al: Spherulin skin testing and histoplasmal and coccidioidal serology: Lack of effect. Am Rev Respir Dis 116:1116–1118, 1977.
221. Pappagianis D, Zimmer BL: Serology of coccidioidomycosis. Clin Microbiol Rev 3:247–268, 1990.
221a. Zartarian M, Peterson EM, de la Maza LM: Detection of antibodies to *Coccidioides immitis* by enzyme immunoassay. Am J Clin Pathol 107:148–153, 1997.
222. Wieden MA, Galgiani JN, Pappagianis D: Comparison of immunodiffusion techniques with standard complement fixation assay for quantitation of coccidioidal antibodies. J Clin Microbiol 18:529–534, 1983.
223. Martins TB, Jaskowski TD, Mouritsen CL, Hill HR: Comparison of commercially available enzyme immunoassay with traditional serologic tests for detection of antibodies to *Coccidioides immitis*. J Clin Microbiol 33:940–943, 1995.
224. Roberts CJ: Coccidioidomycosis in acquired immune deficiency syndrome. Depressed humoral as well as cellular immunity. Am J Med 76:734–736, 1984.
225. Wheat J, French MLV, Kamel S, Tewari RP: Evaluation of cross-reactions in *Histoplasma capsulatum* serologic tests. J Clin Microbiol 23:493–499, 1986.
226. Johnson JE, Jeffery B, Huppert M: Evaluation of five commercially available immunodiffusion kits for detection of *Coccidioides immitis* and *Histoplasma capsulatum* antibodies. J Clin Microbiol 20:530–532, 1984.
227. Yoshinoya S, Cox RA, Pope RM: Circulating immune complexes in coccidioidomycosis. Detection and characterization. J Clin Invest 66:655–663, 1980.
228. Weiner MH: Antigenemia detected in human coccidioidomycosis. J Clin Microbiol 18:136–142, 1983.
229. Galgiani JN, Dugger KO, Ito JI, Wieden MA: Antigenemia in primary coccidioidomycosis. Am J Trop Med Hyg 33:645–649, 1984.
230. Oldfield EC III, Olson PE, Bone WD, et al: Coccidioidomycosis presenting as neoplasia: Another great imitator disease. Infect Dis Clin Pract 4:87–92, 1995.
231. Deresinski SC: Commentary: The masquerades of coccidioidomycosis. Infect Dis Clin Pract 4:93–94, 1995.
232. Wilhelm C, Ellner JJ: Chronic meningitis. Neurol Clin 4:115–141, 1986.
233. Deresinski SC: Coccidioidomycosis. *In* Schlossberg D (ed): Current Therapy of Infectious Disease. Philadelphia, Mosby–Year Book, 1996, pp 599–602.
234. Winn WA: Coccidioidomycosis and amphotericin B. Med Clin North Am 47:1131–1148, 1963.
235. Stevens DA: Coccidioidomycosis and the indications for chemotherapy. Drugs 26:334–336, 1983.
236. Caldwell J, Welch G, Johnson R, Einstein H: Evaluation of response to early azole treatment in primary coccidioidomycosis (Abstr 43). Centennial Conference on Coccidioidomycosis. 5th International Conference on Coccidioidomycosis; August 24–27, 1994; Stanford University, Stanford, CA.
237. Bauer R, Caldwell J, Johnson R: The pharmacoeconomics of early azoles in primary coccidioidomycosis (Abstr N5). Presented at the 35th Interscience Conference on Antimicrobial Agents and Chemotherapy; September 17–20, 1995; San Francisco, CA; p 346.

238. Stevens DA, Levine HB, Deresinski AC: Miconazole in coccidioidomycosis. II. Therapeutic and pharmacologic studies in man. Am J Med 60:191–202, 1976.
239. Hoeprich PD, Lawrence RM, Goldstein E: Treatment of coccidioidomycosis with miconazole. JAMA 243:1923–1926, 1980.
240. Galgiani JN, Stevens DA, Graybill JR, et al: Ketoconazole therapy of progressive coccidioidomycosis. Comparison of 400- and 800-mg doses and observations at higher doses. Am J Med 84:603–610, 1988.
241. Catanzaro A, Friedman PJ, Shillaci R, et al: Treatment of coccidioidomycosis with ketoconazole: An evaluation utilizing a new scoring system. Am J Med 74:58–63, 1983.
242. Stevens DA, Stiller RL, Williams PL, Sugar AM: Experience with ketoconazole in three major manifestations of progressive coccidioidomycosis. Am J Med 74:64–69, 1983.
243. Dismukes WE, Stamm AM, Graybill JR, et al: Treatment of systemic mycoses with ketoconazole: Emphasis on toxicity and clinical response in 52 patients. National Institute of Allergy and Infectious Diseases collaborative antifungal study. Ann Intern Med 98:13–20, 1983.
244. Catanzaro A, Galgiani JN, Levine BE, et al: Fluconazole in the treatment of chronic pulmonary and nonmeningeal disseminated coccidioidomycosis. Am J Med 98:249–256, 1995.
245. Graybill JR, Stevens DA, Galgiani JN, et al: Itraconazole treatment of coccidioidomycosis. NIAID Mycoses Study Group. Am J Med 89:282–290, 1990.
246. Catanzaro A, Spitler L, Moser KM: Immunotherapy of coccidioidomycosis. J Clin Invest 54:690–701, 1974.
247. Hoeprich PD, Merry JM: Effect of recombinant human interleukin 2 in experimental murine coccidioidomycosis. Diagn Microbiol Infect Dis 9:115–118, 1988.
248. Labadie EL, Hamilton RH: Survival improvement in coccidioidal meningitis by high-dose intrathecal amphotericin B. Arch Intern Med 146:2013–2018, 1986.
249. Deresinski SC, Lilly RB, Levine HB, et al: Treatment of fungal meningitis with miconazole. Arch Intern Med 137:1180–1185, 1977.
250. Shehab ZM, Britton H, Dunn JH: Imidazole therapy of coccidioidal meningitis in children. Pediatr Infect Dis J 7:40–44, 1988.
251. Craven PC, Graybill JR, Jorgensen JH, et al: High-dose ketoconazole for treatment of fungal infections of the central nervous system. Ann Intern Med 98:160–167, 1983.
252. Galgiani JN, Catanzaro A, Cloud GA, et al. Fluconazole therapy for coccidioidal meningitis. The NIAID Mycoses Study Group. Ann Intern Med 119:28–35, 1993.
253. Tucker RM, Galgiani JN, Denning DW, et al: Treatment of coccidioidal meningitis with fluconazole. Rev Infect Dis 12(Suppl 3):S380–S389, 1990.
254. Tucker RM, Williams PL, Arathoon EG, et al: Pharmacokinetics of fluconazole in cerebrospinal fluid and serum in human coccidioidal meningitis. Antimicrob Agents Chemother 32:369–373, 1988.
255. Tucker RM, Denning DW, Dupont B, Stevens DA: Itraconazole therapy for chronic coccidioidal meningitis. Ann Intern Med 112:108–112, 1990.
256. Dewsnup DH, Galgiani JN, Graybill JR, et al: Is it ever safe to stop azole therapy for *Coccidioides immitis* meningitis? Ann Intern Med 124:305–310, 1996.
257. Young RF, Gade G, Grinnell V: Surgical treatment for fungal infections in the central nervous system. J Neurosurg 63:371–381, 1985.
258. Catanzaro A, Drutz DJ: Pulmonary coccidioidomycosis. *In* Stevens DA (ed): Coccidioidomycosis: A Text. New York, Plenum Publishing, 1980, pp 147–161.
259. Salomon NW, Osborne R, Copeland JG: Surgical manifestations and results of treatment of pulmonary coccidioidomycosis. Ann Thorac Surg 30:433–438, 1980.
260. Washton H: Review of fluconazole: A new triazole antifungal agent. Diagn Microbiol Infect Dis 12:229S–233S, 1989.
260a. Pursley TJ, Blomquist IK, Abraham J, et al: Fluconazole-induced congenital anomalies in three infants. Clin Infect Dis 22:336–340, 1996.
261. Lake-Bakaar G, Tom W, Lake-Bakaar D, et al: Gastropathy and ketoconazole malabsorption in the acquired immunodeficiency syndrome (AIDS). Ann Intern Med 109:471–473, 1988.
262. Schafer-Korting M: Pharmacokinetic optimisation of oral antifungal therapy. Clin Pharmacokinet 25:329–341, 1993.
263. Segal E: Vaccines against fungal infections. Crit Rev Microbiol 14:229–271, 1987.
264. Williams PL, Sable DL, Sorgen SP, et al: Immunologic responsiveness and safety associated with the *Coccidioides immitis* spherule vaccine in volunteers of white, black, and Filipino ancestry. Am J Epidemiol 119:591–602, 1984.
265. Pappagianis D, and the Valley Fever Vaccine Study Group: Evaluation of the protective efficacy of the killed *Coccidioides immitis* vaccine in humans. Am Rev Respir Dis 148:656–670, 1993.
266. Kruse RH, Green TH, Chambers RC, Jones MW: Disinfection of aerosolized pathogenic fungi on laboratory surfaces. I. Tissue phase. Appl Microbiol 11:436–445, 1963.
267. Kruse RH, Green TH, Chambers RC, Jones MW: Disinfection of aerosolized pathogenic fungi on laboratory surfaces. II. Culture phase. Appl Microbiol 12:155–160, 1964.

280

Sporothrix schenckii

E. Nan Scott
Ronald A. Greenfield

History

Sporotrichosis is a chronic disease caused by a soil fungus, *Sporothrix schenckii*. Typically, the disease produces suppurating nodules along the lymphatics of the skin and subcutaneous tissues. Rarely, the process extends to other tissues, involving joints, bones, and tendons either directly or via the blood stream. Lesions occur in other organs even less frequently.

Characteristics of the Pathogen

S. schenckii is a dimorphic fungus capable of growing in yeast form at 37°C in culture and in infected hosts or as a mold at 25°C. At room temperature, rapidly growing, off-white mold colonies develop that become pigmented with age, turning yellow, brown, or black. Oval hyaline conidia (2 to 3 × 3 to 6 μm) are borne on conidiophores, which often form a cluster resembling a daisy or palm tree (Fig. 280–1). The flower-like cluster of conidia is characteristic of *S. schenckii* and is not produced by any other pathogenic fungus. In some isolates, conidia of a second type are seen that are thick walled, often triangular, and black and that arise laterally from the hyphae. Although in infected tissues they are usually present in small numbers, when found, *S. schenckii* cells appear as round, oval, or cigar-shaped yeasts that vary in size from 1 to 3 × 3 to 10 μm. The teleomorph (sexual) state of this organism remains unknown. It has been suggested that *S. schenckii* is a member of the *Ceratocystis* fungal complex.[1]

Epidemiology

S. schenckii organisms are widely distributed in nature, growing on plant debris in soils and on the bark of trees, on shrubs, and on garden plants. They have also been recovered from air, water, and a variety of other substrates. The organ-

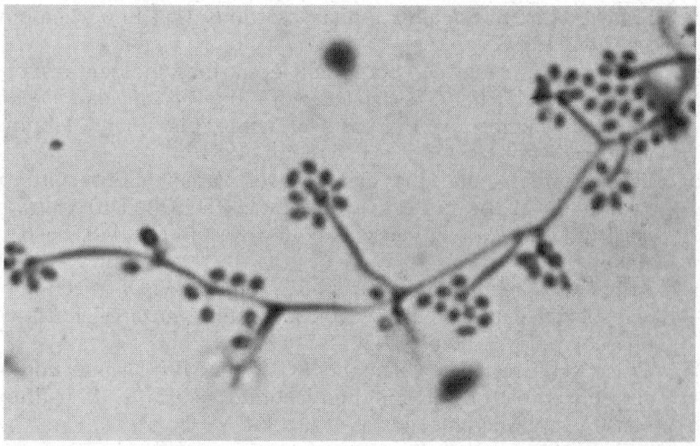

FIGURE 280–1 □ Daisy-like clusters of ovoid conidia are borne at the tips of slender conidiophores that arise at angles from a single hyphal filament. The photograph was made from a slide culture.

ism is widely, but not uniformly, distributed in the environment, and the conditions that determine its natural occurrence have not been delineated precisely. It has been suggested that the presence of other molds may promote or inhibit the growth of *S. schenckii*.[2] The fungus and the disease occur throughout much of the world, principally in temperate and tropical zones, but the abundance of the organism and the reported incidence of the disease show great geographic variation.

From its various environmental locations *S. schenckii* is readily available for traumatic inoculation into and beneath the skin of humans and other mammals. The agents of penetrating trauma, which introduces the conidia of the fungus, are most often splinters, thorns, or woody fragments of plants, but any activity involving contact with plant or plant products (e.g., sphagnum moss) and minor skin trauma may be adequate to initiate the infectious process.[3–5] These activities include occupational exposure such as basket weaving, adobe brick making, horticulture, and farming and outdoor activities such as hiking, camping, sports, and berry picking. The infecting trauma is often minor, and it is apparent from skin test studies that the majority of *S. schenckii* inoculations only promote immunity and do not produce clinical disease. In addition, transmission can occur from infected animals to animal handlers, particularly veterinarians.[6] These zoonotic sporotrichosis infections, although rare, are usually acquired from the handling of cats or horses with extensive skin lesions, resulting in transmission even without trauma. The use of gloves by anyone handling animals with cutaneous lesions should prevent most of these cases.

The prevalence of *S. schenckii* infection as determined by skin testing for delayed hypersensitivity was 26% in a few areas of Mexico[7] and 11% in 349 subjects tested in New Orleans.[8] A single seroepidemiologic study utilizing an enzyme immunoassay against a crude soluble *S. schenckii* antigen showed that 18% of 300 healthy residents of Oklahoma had measureable antibody.[9, 10] Serum from age group cohorts demonstrated that the acquisition of antibody to *S. schenckii* began as early as age 5 years. The low prevalence of clinical disease, compared with the frequency of cellular and humoral immunity demonstrated by these studies, suggests that there is strong natural resistance to this organism.

Lymphocutaneous sporotrichosis is the most common form of the disease, and patients who develop extracutaneous involvement are probably immunocompromised. Poverty and malnutrition appear to be immunocompromising factors, and alcoholism is noteworthy for its frequent association with extracutaneous sporotrichosis. It is not certain whether alcoholism incurs malnutrition, subjects the patient to more frequent and effective trauma, actually suppresses the immune responses, or poses a combination of these factors.

Patients with immunosuppression due to human immunodeficiency virus infection and the acquired immunodeficiency syndrome have been reported with disseminated cutaneous sporotrichosis and with disseminated sporotrichosis, including sporotrichal meningitis.[11–15] The incidence of sporotrichosis in acquired immunodeficiency syndrome is not precisely known; however, it would appear that disseminated sporotrichosis is more common in patients with human immunodeficiency virus infection than in the general population. Sporotrichosis is less common in human immunodeficiency virus infection than are other endemic mycoses and is not currently an acquired immunodeficiency syndrome–defining condition.

Pathogenesis

The initial reddish purple, necrotic, nodular sporotrichosis chancre appears 1 to 10 weeks or longer after the penetrating skin injury.[16] This lesion is a suppurating granuloma consisting of histiocytes and giant cells with neutrophils accumulating in the center, the whole surrounded by lymphocytes and plasma cells. Occasionally, an asteroid body may be seen in the center of the granuloma that consists of a basophilic yeast cell (3 to 5 μm) surrounded by eosinophilic material arranged in ray formation. This structure, described by Splendore,[17] was initially thought to be pathognomonic for sporotrichosis, but similar eosinophilic rays are seen in lesions of diseases such as actinomycosis, zygomycosis, and even around schistosome ova.[18]

From the initial lesion, the fungus spreads along local lymphatic channels, forming the chain of indolent nodular and ulcerating granulomata that typify lymphocutaneous sporotrichosis, and this form of the disease is by far the most common clinical presentation. Other tissues are involved by direct extension, and less often by hematogenous dissemination. Bones, joints, tendon sheaths, and bursae are the structures most frequently involved by the nonlymphocutaneous form. Pulmonary sporotrichosis is uncommon, and it is not clear whether it results from inhalation or from hematogenous spread of the fungus. Central nervous system sporotrichosis is rare.[10, 13, 14] This form of the disease results from hematogenous dissemination, and, because of the difficulty of establishing a definitive diagnosis, it is reasonable to believe that other, unrecognized cases occur.

Clinical Manifestations

Cutaneous Sporotrichosis

The primary lesion develops in the skin at the site of inoculation, typically the hand or fingers, but it can be located on any (exposed) part of the body, including the face. The initial small nodule slowly enlarges, turns red, becomes pustular, and ulcerates, releasing small amounts of purulent material from which the organism is readily cultured. In the lymphocutaneous form of the disease, extension along lymphatic channels of the skin is soon apparent, and a chain of nodules develops: the older, more distal lesions ulcerate and drain and the newer, more proximal lesions form subcutaneous nodules that attach to the skin as they age and begin to ulcerate (Fig. 280–2). The lesions usually are not painful, but extensive disease may cause functional impairment. Epitrochlear lymph nodes may be involved, but the axillary and inguinal nodes are usually spared. Some patients exhibit no lymphangitic spread, and the disease presents as an indolent,

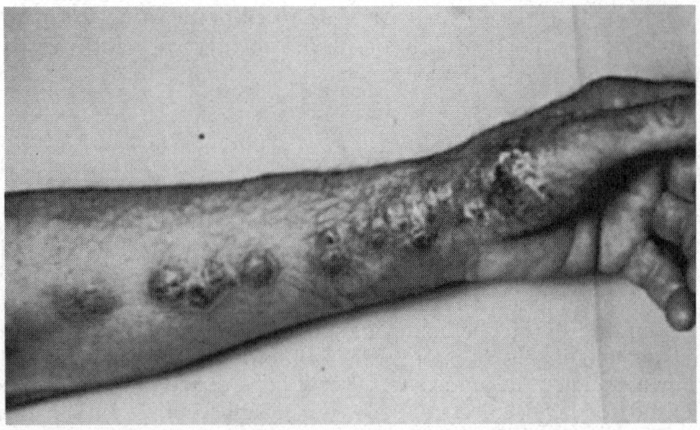

FIGURE 280–2 □ The chain of ulcerating, nodular skin lesions is typical of the cutaneous form of sporotrichosis. Characteristically, the older distal lesions show more ulceration and the younger proximal lesions have not yet broken down. The "bridges" of normal skin between lesions occur frequently, but a firm swollen lymphatic "cord" connecting the nodules can be felt under the skin.

ulcerating plaque that persists for years if it is not treated. This is called fixed cutaneous or plaque sporotrichosis. The frequency of this form of the disease varies from 10% in some series from the United States[19] to more than 50% in patients reported from other countries.[20] We speculate that immunity to the fungus established by prior contact plays a role in restricting the lesion to the area of a new traumatic reinoculation.

The thermal dimorphism of this fungus is also a factor in the restriction of lesions to skin and subcutaneous lymphatics, and many *S. schenckii* isolates from the fixed and lymphocutaneous lesions are unable to grow well at temperatures above 35°C.[21, 22]

Spontaneous healing of the cutaneous forms of sporotrichosis has been reported,[23, 24] but without treatment, as a rule, the lesions persist for years, progressing slowly with draining and scarring.

Extracutaneous Sporotrichosis

The fungus probably spreads to deeper tissues via hematogenous dissemination. Lesions may occur in almost any organ, but disease tends to localize in the joints, especially of the extremities, and in the adjacent long bones. The resulting arthritis is often confused with rheumatoid arthritis until bone destruction and draining fistulae suggest the need for cultures to establish the cause of the osteomyelitis. Lymphocutaneous lesions and lymphangitic spread are not prominent in these patients, although multiple joints may be involved successively.

The inflammatory response in sporotrichosis of bones, joints, and tendons is most often low grade and chronic, but the patient usually has pain and the involved areas may be warm and red. Functional impairment in joint sporotrichosis may be severe. Bone and joint destruction may require drainage and other procedures, including joint fusion, but these may fail owing to persistent osteomyelitis.

Pulmonary sporotrichosis typically presents as a chronic pneumonitis with cavitation, usually in the upper lobes, that is clinically indistinguishable from mycobacterial or other fungal infections.[25] Symptoms are productive cough and often minimal constitutional symptoms. Diagnosis requires culture of the organism from sputum or its histopathologic recognition in biopsy specimens.

Sporotrichosis lesions occasionally develop in a variety of other organs—eye, prostate, oral mucosa, larynx—and the clinical manifestations then depend on the organ involved. Involvement of the central nervous system and meninges is decidedly rare.[10, 13, 14] Because lesions in these organs all develop without contiguous skin lesions and without direct trauma to the infected site, they are presumed to result from hematogenous dissemination. Recovering the fungus from extracutaneous lesions may be difficult, particularly with central nervous system disease, perhaps because of the small number of organisms in the tissue. An elevated serum antibody titer, which is characteristic for these patients, should prompt repeated attempts at culture.

Other than serologic tests and cultures, most clinical laboratory studies are of little use in detecting sporotrichosis. The cerebrospinal fluid findings from patients with central nervous system sporotrichosis are those of chronic meningitis with elevated protein levels and a low-grade mononuclear pleocytosis. The glucose concentration may be normal or low.

Diagnosis

The characteristic chain of ulcerating skin nodules should stimulate a high degree of clinical suspicion, leading to appropriate cultures and serologic tests. Individual skin lesions have no diagnostic features, and laboratory assistance is required. The extracutaneous forms of the disease are even less distinctive, and again diagnosis depends on the laboratory findings. Recovery of the fungus on culture may be difficult in extracutaneous sporotrichosis, and repeated attempts may be necessary. A positive serologic test result provides strong support for the diagnosis and should stimulate repeated culturing.

Specific Laboratory Diagnosis

Demonstration of *S. schenckii* is necessary for definitive diagnosis of sporotrichosis, and this is best accomplished by recovery on culture and identification of the fungus. Infection caused by *S. schenckii* may be recognized by direct examination and culture of infected material or by serologic tests. The fungus can be identified in biopsied tissue by culture and direct immunofluorescence or immunoperoxidase staining techniques,[26] but such tests are not widely available. In the extracutaneous forms of *S. schenckii* infection (particularly central nervous system), tests for antibody are diagnostically important when clinical features are lacking and tissues, exudates, or fluids are more difficult to obtain for direct examination and culture. The tube and latex agglutination tests are reliable and sensitive,[27] and these antibody tests are based on the antibody response to the peptidorhamnomannan of the outer cell wall of the organism.[28] These tests are available both commercially and from reference laboratories. An enzyme-linked immunosorbent assay has been developed that is more sensitive and may prove to be valuable, particularly in cerebrospinal fluid, where the latex agglutination test result may be negative.[9, 10] Results with Western blot testing suggest that this technique may differentiate between cutaneous and extracutaneous disease,[29] but further data are needed.

Differential Diagnosis

The cutaneous forms of sporotrichosis are so characteristic that diagnosis rarely poses a problem, but it may have to be differentiated from syphilis, yaws, tuberculosis, tularemia, glanders, and involvement of the skin by other fungal pathogens. Extracutaneous sporotrichosis is not distinctive, and more thorough investigation may be necessary. Before draining fistulae develop, the bone and joint involvement may resemble that of rheumatoid arthritis. The cause of the osteomyelitis must be differentiated from bacterial and other fungal diseases as well as neoplasms. Recovery of *S. schenckii* on culture is conclusive, because it is not a laboratory contaminant.

Treatment

Agents used for treatment of sporotrichosis include saturated solution of potassium iodide, amphotericin B, ketoconazole, fluconazole, and itraconazole. Unfortunately, direct comparative analyses of treatment with various agents for various forms of sporotrichosis are not available.

High response rates (89% to 100%) have been demonstrated for treatment of cutaneous and lymphocutaneous sporotrichosis with itraconazole, 200 mg/d orally for 3 to 12 months.[30–32] This form of sporotrichosis often responds to treatment with saturated solution of potassium iodide. An initial dose of 10 drops diluted in liquid, preferably fruit juice, is given three times daily after meals, and increased dropwise to 120 drops per day or the maximum tolerated by the individual patient (usually less than 60 drops). This last dose is continued for 1 month or longer after the lesions appear to be fully healed. Although relatively inexpensive, this form of therapy is poorly accepted by many patients and often complicated by increased lacrimation, increased salivation, salivary gland swelling, gastrointestinal upset, and rash. The mechanism of action of potassium iodide is unknown; it is ineffective in vitro against *S. schenckii* and believed to facilitate killing by promoting the respiratory burst associated with superoxide formation in phagolysosomes.[33] Ketoconazole at 200 to 800 mg/d orally has been used for treatment of lymphocutaneous sporotrichosis and for treatment of deep-seated sporotrichosis,[34] but its use has largely been supplanted by itraconazole. Fluconazole at 200 to 800 mg/d orally appears less effective than oral itraconazole but may be useful in patients who cannot absorb itraconazole or who cannot tolerate itraconazole because of drug interactions or adverse effects (Mycosis Study Group, unpublished data, 1995). Local application of heat may be useful.[22, 35] Many *S. schenckii* isolates recovered from lymphocutaneous infection grow poorly at temperatures above 35°C.[21] Heat treatment may thus inhibit the growth of the fungus, increase blood flow thereby enhancing delivery of drug therapy, and enhance the phagocytic killing process (Mycosis Study Group, unpublished data, 1995).

Itraconazole at 200 mg orally twice daily is the preferred treatment for extracutaneous disease.[31] As in other bone and joint infections, drainage and débridement are often required in osteoarticular sporotrichosis.[36] Treatment with itraconazole should be continued for 12 to 18 months. Treatment with amphotericin B may be required for patients with disease unresponsive to itraconazole treatment or patients with meningitis. A total dose of 2.0 g of amphotericin B is usual, but relapses may occur even after such therapy. Both flucytosine and rifampin usually show in vitro synergism with amphotericin B.[37] The role of combination antifungal therapy for sporotrichosis is largely undefined, but these agents may be useful adjuncts in treatment of recalcitrant disease and in treatment of meningitis.

Prevention

Sporotrichosis can be prevented when environmental sources of *S. schenckii* are identified and avoided or eliminated. This has been accomplished in specific situations, such as those involving sphagnum moss[5] and mine timbers.[2] For the most part, however, the simple precautions needed to prevent infection in agricultural workers are difficult to achieve, because of the cost of the necessary protective clothing for hands, feet, arms, and legs.

References

1. Mariat F: Taxonomic problems related to the fungal complex *Sporothrix schenckii/Ceratocystis* spp. *In* Iwata K (ed): Recent Advances in Medical and Veterinary Mycology. Tokyo, University of Tokyo Press, 1977, pp 265–270.
2. Simson FW: The pathology of sporotrichosis in man and experimental animals. *In* Sporotrichosis Infection in Mines of the Witwatersrand. A Symposium. Proceedings of the Transvaal Mine and Medical Officers Association. Johannesburg, South Africa, The Transvaal Chamber of Mines, 1947, pp 34–58.
3. Centers for Disease Control: Multistate outbreak of sporotrichosis in seedling handlers, 1988. MMWR Morbid Mortal Wkly Rep 37:652, 1988.
4. D'Alessio DJ, Leavens LJ, Strumpf GB, et al: An outbreak of sporotrichosis in Vermont associated with sphagnum moss as the source of infection. N Engl J Med 272:1054, 1965.
5. Powell KE, Taylor A, Phillips BJ, et al: Cutaneous sporotrichosis in forestry workers. JAMA 240:232, 1978.
6. Reed KD, Moore FM, Geiger GE, et al: Zoonotic transmission of sporotrichosis: Case report and review. Clin Infect Dis 16:384, 1993.
7. Gonzales-Ochoa A, Ricoy E, Velasco O, et al: Valoracion comparatira de los antigenos polisacarido y cellular de *Sporothrix schenckii*. Rev Invest Salud Publica 30:303, 1970.
8. Schneidau JD, Lamar LM, Hairston MA: Cutaneous hypersensitivity to sporotrichin in Louisiana. JAMA 188:371, 1964.
9. Scott EN, Muchmore HG, Parkinson AJ: Enzyme and radioimmunoassays in human sporotrichosis. *In* Proceedings of the VIIIth Congress of the International Society of Human and Animal Mycology. Palmerston North, New Zealand, International Society of Human and Animal Mycology, 1982, pp 212–215.
10. Scott EN, Kaufman L, Brown AC, Muchmore HG: Serologic studies in the diagnosis and management of meningitis due to *Sporothrix schenckii*. N Engl J Med 317:935, 1987.
11. Heller HM, Fuhrer J: Disseminated sporotrichosis in patients with AIDS: Case report and review of the literature. AIDS 5:1243, 1991.
12. Keiser P, Whittle D: Sporotrichosis in human immunodeficiency virus-infected patients: Report of a case. Rev Infect Dis 13:1027, 1991.
13. Penn CC, Goldstein E, Bartholomew WR: *Sporothrix schenckii* meningitis in a patient with AIDS. Clin Infect Dis 15:741, 1992.
14. Donabedian H, O'Donnell E, Olszewski C, et al: Disseminated cutaneous and meningeal sporotrichosis in an AIDS patient. Diagn Microbiol Infect Dis 18:111, 1994.
15. Bolao F, Podzamczer D, Ventin M, et al: Efficacy of acute phase and maintenance therapy with itraconazole in an AIDS patient with sporotrichosis. Eur J Clin Microbiol Infect Dis 13:609, 1994.
16. Rippon JW: Sporotrichosis. *In* Rippon JW: Medical Mycology: The Pathogenic Fungi and the Pathogenic Actinomycetes, ed 3. Philadelphia, WB Saunders, 1988, pp 325–352.
17. Splendore A: Sobre acultura d'uma nova especie de cognumello pathogenico. Rev Soc Sci Sao Paulo 3:62, 1908.
18. Hoeppli R: Histologic observation in experimental schistosomiasis japonicum. Chin Med J 43:1179, 1932.
19. Dellatorre DL, Lattanand A, Buckley HR, Urbach F: Fixed cutaneous sporotrichosis of the face. Am Acad Dermatol 6:97, 1982.
20. Honbo S, Yamano T, Masaki J, Urabe H: Analytical studies on peculiar cases of sporotrichosis, the lesions of which contained numerous fungal elements. *In* Proceedings of the IXth Congress of the International Society of Human and Animal Mycology. Atlanta, International Society of Human and Animal Mycology, 1985, pp 11–12.
21. Kwon-Chung KJ: Comparison of isolates of *Sporothrix schenckii* obtained from fixed cutaneous lesions with isolates from other types of lesions. J Infect Dis 139:424, 1979.
22. MacKinnon JE, Conti-Diaz IA: The effect of temperature on sporotrichosis. Sabouraudia 2:56, 1962.
23. Iwatsu T, Nishmura K, Miyaji M: Spontaneous disappearance of cutaneous sporotrichosis. Int J Dermatol 24:524, 1985.
24. Pueringer RJ, Iber C, Deike MA, et al: Spontaneous remission of

extensive pulmonary sporotrichosis. Ann Intern Med 104:366, 1986.
25. Zvetina JR, Rippon JW, Daum V: Chronic pulmonary sporotrichosis. Mycopathologia 64:53, 1978.
26. Russell B, Beckett JH, Jacobs PH: Immunoperoxidase localization of *Sporothrix schenckii* and *Cryptococcus neoformans*. Arch Dermatol 115:433, 1979.
27. Kaufman L, Reiss E: Serodiagnosis of fungal diseases. *In* Rose NR, Friedman H, Fahey JL (eds): Manual of Clinical Laboratory Immunology, ed 3. Washington, DC, American Society for Microbiology, 1986, pp 446–466.
28. Travassos LR, Lloyd KO: *Sporothrix schenckii* and related species of *Ceratocystis*. Microbiol Rev 44:683, 1980.
29. Scott EN, Muchmore HG: Immunoblot analysis of antibody responses to *Sporothrix schenckii*. J Clin Microbiol 27:300, 1989.
30. Restrepo A, Robledo J, Gomez I, et al: Itraconazole therapy in lymphangitic and cutaneous sporotrichosis. Arch Dermatol 122:413, 1986.
31. Sharkey-Mathis PK, Kauffman CA, Graybill JR, et al: Treatment of sporotrichosis with itraconazole. NIAID Mycoses Study Group. Am J Med 95:279, 1993.
32. Kauffman CA: Newer developments in therapy for endemic mycoses. Clin Infect Dis 19S:S28, 1994.
33. Cunningham K, Bulmer G, Rhoades E: Phagocytosis and intracellular fate of *Sporothrix schenckii*. J Infect Dis 140:815, 1979.
34. Calhoun DL, Waskin H, White MP, et al: Treatment of systemic sporotrichosis with ketoconazole. Rev Infect Dis 13:47, 1991.
35. Hiruma M, Katoh T, Yamamoto I, Kagawa S: Local hyperthermia in the treatment of sporotrichosis. Mykosen 30:315, 1987.
36. Bayer AS, Scott VJ, Guze LB: Fungal arthritis. III. Sporotrichal arthritis. Semin Arthritis Rheum 9:66, 1979.
37. Winn RE: Sporotrichosis. Infect Dis Clin North Am 2:899, 1988.

281

Blastomyces and Paracoccidioides

George S. Deepe, Jr.

BLASTOMYCES

George S. Deepe, Jr.
Bruce S. Klein

History

In 1894, T. C. Gilchrist examined a skin biopsy specimen from the hand of a patient who had been diagnosed with scrofuloderma. He failed to detect tubercle bacilli but noted the presence of protozoan-like organisms that appeared budding and yeastlike.[1] Shortly thereafter, Gilchrist and Stokes[2, 3] identified a similar organism in the skin of a patient who was thought to have lupus vulgaris. They successfully cultured it on artificial medium and transferred the infection to a dog. Because the microbe resembled blastomycetes morphologically, the new pathogen was called *Blastomyces dermatitidis*.

Characteristics of the Pathogen

B. dermatitidis is a dimorphic fungus that exists as the mycelial form in nature and as the yeast form in tissues from infected humans and animals. In culture, the organism grows as a mycelium at room temperature and in the yeast phase at 37°C. In vitro the transition from the mycelial to the yeast phase can be divided into three stages. Stage 1 is characterized by uncoupling of oxidative phosphorylation and a decrement in cellular adenosine triphosphate levels. In stage 2, spontaneous respiration terminates. Subsequently, the cells enter stage 3, in which respiration recovers and the fungus transforms to the yeast phase. Cysteine is required during stage 2 for conversion to yeast cells.[4] Existence of this pathway in the dimorphic fungi, *Histoplasma capsulatum* and *Paracoccidioides brasiliensis*, suggests a common mechanism for survival in vivo.[4, 5]

On artificial media, such as Sabouraud, the mycelia grow as fluffy white colonies. Conidia range from 2 to 10 μm in diameter. Yeast colonies are wrinkled and folded. Yeast cells are multinucleate and form broad-based buds, and individual ones may vary from 8 to 30 μm in diameter.[6] *B. dermatitidis* possesses a sexual stage termed *Ajellomyces dermatitidis*. The organism is heterothallic, and both "positive" (pigmented colonies) and "negative" (white colonies) mating types have been identified.[7] Both mating types cause clinical disease, apparently in equal proportions, and both have been isolated from a single patient.[8, 9]

Two serotypes that differ in the expression of cell wall A antigen, and multiple genotypes, defined by restriction fragment length polymophisms, have been described.[10, 11]

Epidemiology

Infection with *B. dermatitidis* has been reported from North and South America, Europe, Africa, and Asia.[6] Precise delineation of the endemic regions, particularly in North America, has relied on case reports of human or animal infection because no widely available test exists to identify asymptomatic infection. In the United States, blastomycosis occurs in the Midwest and Southeast (except Florida), western Pennsylvania, and northern New York. Endemic zones are found in the Canadian provinces of Ontario, Quebec, and Alberta.

In the past, *B. dermatitidis* was rarely recovered from soil. Epidemiologic studies of outbreaks of blastomycosis in Wisconsin have uncovered a natural habitat: a high incidence of clinical illness was observed among persons exposed to soil along riverbanks. Cultures of soil and organic debris from these sites propagated *B. dermatitidis*. Hence, available evidence indicates that the environment along waterways represents an important reservoir for infection.[12, 13]

Clinical illness caused by *B. dermatitidis* develops nine times more frequently in males than in females,[14] a finding that has been attributed to sex differences in occupation and recreational activities. The vast majority of reported cases have occurred in manual laborers, hunters, and agricultural workers, and in the past these endeavors have been performed principally by males. In blastomycosis epidemics, documented infection is not more prevalent in males.

Exact information regarding incidence and prevalence of infection does not exist, because the illness is not reportable and a reliable diagnostic test is not widely available. Surveys of hospital discharges performed by the Centers for Disease Control and Prevention during 1970 and 1980 to 1982 indicate that the incidence of blastomycosis is 0.6 per million per year.[15] However, this figure underestimates the true occurrence of infection. Most cases are sporadic but several epidemics have been recognized.[12, 13, 16–18]

With the exception of rare cases of sexual transmission,[19, 20] blastomycosis is not transmitted from human to human. One report indicated that human blastomycosis resulted from the bite of an actively infected dog.[21] Several reports of inoculation blastomycosis in pathologists indicate the infection may be an occupational hazard.[22]

Pathogenesis

Presumably, infection with *B. dermatitidis* develops from accidental inhalation of hyphae and conidia from soil, although definitive proof is lacking.[23] The sequence of events in the early pathogenesis of disease has not been established. Most likely, the inhaled fungal elements settle into respiratory bronchioles or alveoli, where they transform within days into the yeast phase. The organisms then disseminate lymphohematogenously to regional lymph nodes and other organ systems.

Blastomyces organisms induce two distinct inflammatory responses. In visceral organ systems such as lung, liver, and genitourinary tract, the typical reaction, which is termed pyogranulomatous, is an admixture of suppuration and granulomatous inflammation with giant cells (Fig. 281–1). Although granulomata often surround areas of suppurative necrosis, tissue sections may contain fields composed either strictly of neutrophils and necrotic debris or of granulomata. Pyogranulomatous inflammation is also found in tissues of those infected with *Coccidioides immitis* and *P. brasiliensis*. The characteristic histopathologic picture of the skin and squamous mucosa (e.g., trachea, larynx) is that of pseudoepitheliomatous proliferation with intraepithelial microabscesses.[23] In visceral organs the evolution of the inflammatory response to *B. dermatitidis* yeasts has been ascertained from limited autopsy material and experimental models.[24–26] The earliest cellular infiltrate (within 24 hours) contains polymorphonuclear leukocytes. By 7 days, granulomata and suppurative necrosis can be detected.[25]

The incubation period for primary pulmonary blastomycosis is approximately 6 weeks and ranges from 21 to 106 days. It is shorter for occupational blastomycosis (median 14 days, range of 7 to 35 days).[22]

Blastomyces yeasts release a chemotactic factor that may induce influx of neutrophils and monocytes.[27] The pyogranulomatous reaction can be elicited by cell walls from virulent yeasts. Evidence suggests that phospholipid from this material may be responsible for producing the granulomatous response.[28, 29]

Immune Response and Host Defenses

Detection of antibody produced in response to infection by *B. dermatitidis* has been hampered by lack of a suitable antigen. The antigen blastomycin was not reliable; however, humoral responses to A antigen can be measured in many cases.[30] Unfortunately, A antigen contains carbohydrate epitopes that are shared with other dimorphic fungi, which causes the nonspecificity in commercial serologic assays for blastomycosis.[31] More recently, a 120-kDa antigen from the cell wall of *B. dermatitidis* yeasts appears to be a specific target of the humoral response of humans.[32] The antibodies are directed against a 25–amino acid repeat arrayed in tandem on this protein and also on A antigen.[31, 33] Specific antibody appears to have no role in host defenses.[34]

In vitro, human neutrophils and mononuclear phagocytes kill conidia, but these phagocytes, which are prominent in the inflammatory response, kill yeasts inefficiently.[35, 36] In cell-free systems, conidia and yeasts are susceptible to products of oxygen metabolism. Conidia are partially eliminated by hydrogen peroxide and are killed completely by hypochlorous acid or a combination of hydrogen peroxide, myeloperoxidase, and halide.[36, 37] Yeasts are much less susceptible to hydrogen peroxide. Killing by this substance can be augmented by addition of Fe^{2+} and halide.[38, 39]

Infection activates the cell-mediated immune system. The percentage of humans with blastomycosis who mount a skin test response to blastomycin has ranged from 0% to 50%.[40, 41] The high incidence of anergy is probably related to the poor antigenicity of blastomycin. In vitro, human monocyte-derived macrophages recognize the yeast through binding the 120-kDa cell wall protein with CR3 (CD11b/CD18) and CD14 receptors. Subsequent uptake of the yeast and processing of this and other antigens lead to outgrowth of $CD4^+$ T cells and is associated with development of acquired resistance.[42, 43] An alkali-soluble, water-soluble antigen from cell wall (B-ASWS)

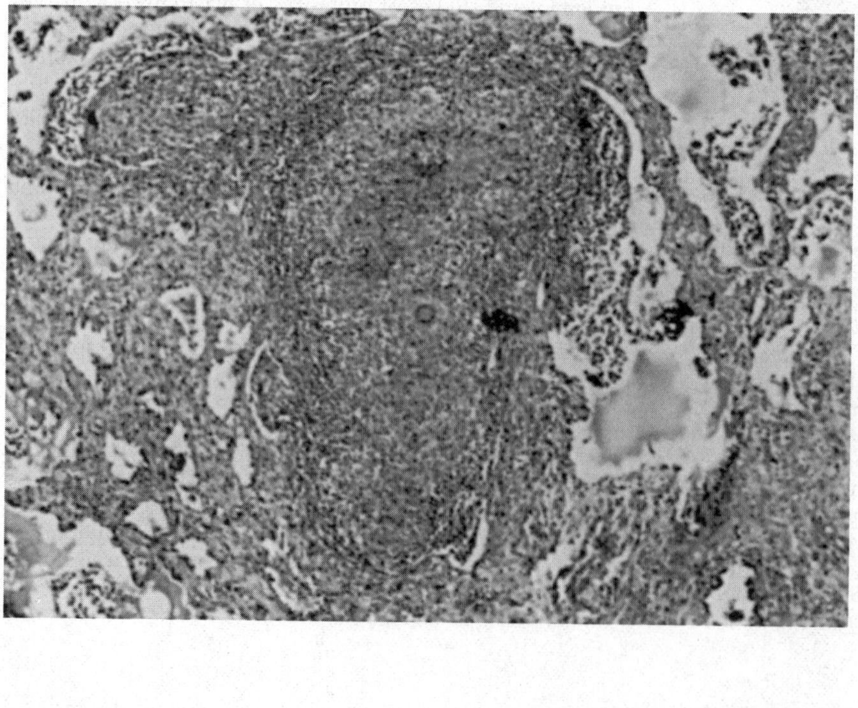

FIGURE 281–1 □ Pyogranulomatous response to *Blastomyces dermatitidis* in a lung specimen from a patient with pulmonary blastomycosis. A mantle of mononuclear cells surrounds the area of acute inflammation. A giant cell is seen in the middle of the field (× 165). (Courtesy of Judith Rhodes, PhD, University of Cincinnati College of Medicine, Cincinnati, OH.)

and the 120-kDa antigen share a determinant that induces antigen-specific proliferative responses by peripheral blood mononuclear cells of persons who have recovered from blastomycosis.[43, 44] The alkali-soluble, water-soluble antigen is useful for skin testing *B. dermatitidis*–infected animals but has not been studied in humans. Protective immunity is conferred by antigen-reactive T lymphocytes.[34] Interferon-γ enhances the anti-*Blastomyces* activity of neutrophils, monocytes, and macrophages.[45, 46]

Clinical Manifestations

Like other systemic mycoses, blastomycosis is a spectral disease. Most likely the majority of infections are asymptomatic. Clinical features of blastomycosis range from acute, self-limited pneumonia to a disseminated form (Table 281–1).

Pulmonary Disease

Acute pulmonary blastomycosis produces two distinct patterns of illness. One is a systemic, influenza-like illness characterized by fever, chills, myalgias, arthralgias, photophobia, and headache. A nonproductive cough can progress to a cough productive of mucopurulent sputum. The second type of illness consists of pleuritic chest pain of abrupt onset without constitutional symptoms. The pain usually lasts no longer than 48 hours. Occasionally, acute pulmonary infection fails to resolve and advances by bronchogenic spread from a localized pneumonia to widespread involvement of all lung fields.[47–49] Frequently, ulcerative bronchitis is present in pulmonary tissues of patients with this form of disease.[23] Chest radiographs of acute disease typically reveal segmental airspace disease, which varies from patchy, nodular opacities to extensive confluent densities (Fig. 281–2). Less common abnormalities include mass lesions, interstitial infiltrates, cavitation, and miliary pattern.[48, 50, 51]

Chronic pulmonary blastomycosis, defined by the presence of symptoms lasting longer than 3 weeks,[48] is clinically indistinguishable from pulmonary tuberculosis, histoplasmosis, or coccidioidomycosis. This illness may be the result of nonhealing acute pneumonia or reactivation of dormant disease foci. Fatigue, low-grade fever, malaise, and weight loss are often observed. Radiographic abnormalities, if present, are similar to those in acute pulmonary infection.

Extrapulmonary Blastomycosis

Evidence of dissemination is prevalent among patients with blastomycosis. Spread of the fungus beyond the lungs (Table 281–2) may result from progression of pulmonary infection or reactivated disease.[48, 52] The most common sites of involvement are skin, bone, genitourinary tract, and central nervous system.

TABLE 281–1 ■ Clinical Manifestations of Blastomycosis

Pulmonary blastomycosis
Acute (duration of symptoms ≤ 3 wk)
Asymptomatic
Influenza-like illness (fever, chills, cough, myalgias)
Pleuritic symptoms
Chronic (duration of symptoms > 3 wk)
Progression by bronchogenic spread from acute pulmonary disease
Endogenous reactivation
Extrapulmonary blastomycosis
Lymphohematogenous spread from advancing pneumonia
Endogenous reactivation

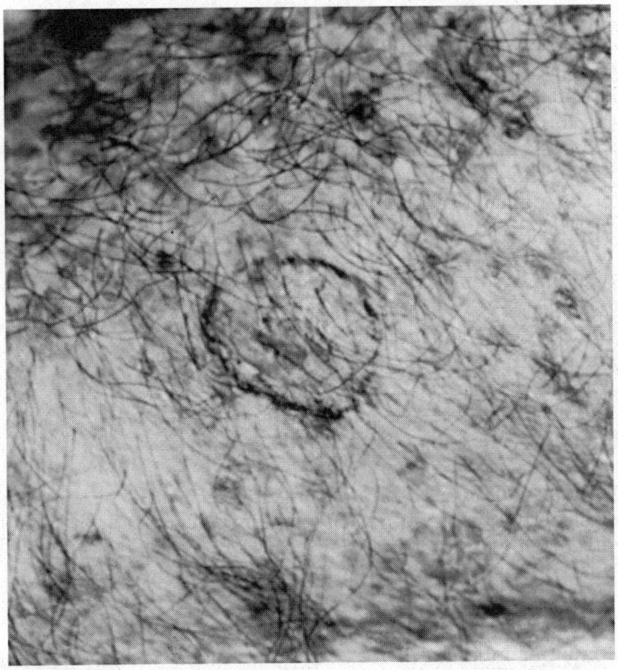

FIGURE 281–2 □ Early skin lesion of disseminated blastomycosis. A small papule is present on the forearm of a patient with systemic blastomycosis. (Courtesy of Corwin Dunn, MD, Christ Hospital, Cincinnati, OH.)

Cutaneous lesions begin as subcutaneous nodules or pustular papules, which can go unnoticed (Fig. 281–3). Untreated, they become ulcerated with verrucous borders. The center is crusted, and "black dots" (degenerated capillaries)[53] are present in the ulcer (Fig. 281–4). These lesions are usually distributed on exposed areas of skin but can also develop on mucocutaneous surfaces and may be misdiagnosed as carcinoma. A second type of skin manifestation is the papule that becomes ulcerated with a granulomatous base.

Bone is a frequent site of involvement in disseminated blastomycosis. Although any bone may be infected, ribs, vertebrae, long bones, skull, and facial bones are the most common. The lesions are painless and may be manifested only by a draining sinus or subcutaneous abscess. The characteristic radiographic feature of osseous disease is a lytic lesion.[54] The fungus can spread from bone to joints.[55]

Within the genitourinary tract, kidneys, prostate, epididymides, testes, seminal vesicles, and bladder can be infected by *B. dermatitidis*. In kidneys, *Blastomyces* yeasts and pyogran-

TABLE 281–2 ■ Prevalence of Extrapulmonary Blastomycosis by Site

SITE	PREVALENCE* (%)
Skin	68.8
Bone and joints	18.7
Genitourinary tract	14.5
Reticuloendothelial system (liver, spleen, lymph nodes, bone marrow)	9.4
Subcutaneous tissue	5.0
Mucosa†	4.3
Thyroid	2.2

*Percentages based on reviews of references 41, 48, 62, 66–70. Calculations include autopsy studies.

†Laryngeal, oropharyngeal, nasal.

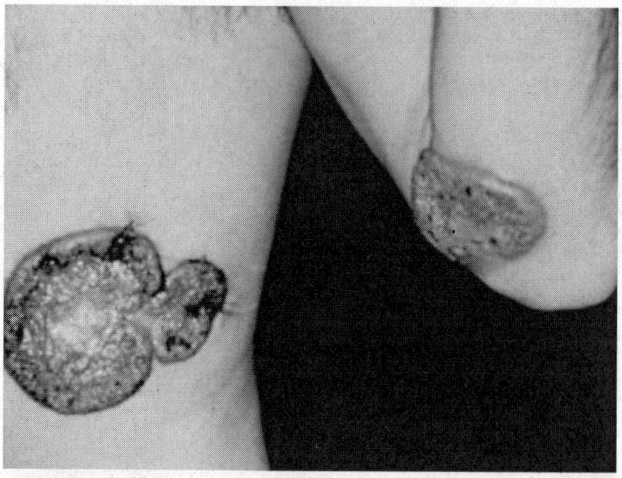

FIGURE 281–3 □ Advanced skin lesions of disseminated blastomycosis on the thorax and arm. The patient had an 18-month history of progressive skin disease. Note the verrucous borders and ulcerated center as well as the numerous black dots on the arm lesion.

ulomatous inflammation are more common in the cortex than in the medulla. Aggregates of yeast have been detected in glomeruli.[56] Involvement of the prostate may cause nonspecific prostatitis and symptoms of obstruction. Epididymitis can be recurrent. The last two diseases can be the presenting symptom of disseminated blastomycosis.[23, 41, 57]

Central nervous system infection has been reported in as many as 33% of autopsies, but clinically apparent disease is less frequent (see Table 281–2). The fungus elicits a granulomatous or suppurative mass lesion that may be mistaken for tumor. Chronic basilar meningitis is a late manifestation and is indistinguishable from other causes of this illness. Lymphocytic pleocytosis, hypoglycorrhachia, and elevated protein level are common laboratory findings in cerebrospinal fluid of persons with blastomycotic meningitis.[58]

Blastomyces organisms may spread to adrenals, larynx, thyroid, gastrointestinal tract, liver, and spleen. Hypoadrenalism is rare. Far fewer children than adults contract blastomycosis, but the spectrum of disease is similar in both.[59]

Blastomycosis is predominantly a disease of immunocompetent hosts, although infection does occur in patients who are immunosuppressed. Clinical manifestations of disseminated infection in immunocompromised persons are virtually the same as in those whose immune system is putatively intact, except that the disease progresses more rapidly.[49, 60]

Laboratory abnormalities can exist in all forms of blastomycosis, but they are nonspecific. Elevated erythrocyte sedimentation rates, leukocytosis with an increase in band forms of neutrophils, and anemia are often present.

Diagnosis

The yeasts can be visualized in specimens from body fluids or aspirated skin lesions. A wet mount preparation, with or without 10% potassium hydroxide, can be made and examined by light microscopy (Fig. 281–5). Cerebrospinal fluid, bronchoalveolar lavage fluid, urine, and pleural fluid specimens should be centrifuged to optimize the chance of detecting the organism. In such specimens, yeasts are characteristic. They are large and possess a broad-based bud and a refractile cell wall. These features help distinguish *B. dermatitidis* from *P. brasiliensis,* which has a narrow bud, and from *Cryptococcus neoformans,* which has a capsule. In skin aspirates, yeasts should not be confused with lipid droplets.

When blastomycosis is suspected or considered, histopathologic examination of tissue specimens should include staining with Gomori–methenamine silver because yeasts may not be seen with hematoxylin-eosin stain. The presence of pyogranulomatous inflammation should alert the physician to the possibility of blastomycosis. Periodic acid–Schiff stain colors the cell wall red and can be a useful adjunctive stain, because it allows evaluation of the inflammatory response and morphologic characteristics of the organism. If *Cryptococcus* is considered, mucicarmine, which stains the cell wall of *Cryptococcus* but not *Blastomyces*, may be used.

A portion of specimens should be submitted for culture. Material is plated on Sabouraud glucose agar and cultured at 30°C. Specimens contaminated with bacteria may be plated on agar containing penicillin and streptomycin or chloramphenicol. If the fungus is to be identified precisely, the yeast form must be grown, and this is accomplished by culturing on nutrient agar at 37°C.

Serologic tests are performed by immunodiffusion using the A antigen. Detectable precipitin antibodies are reported in up to 80% of cases.[29] An enzyme immunoassay using the A antigen is a more sensitive serologic test but has a higher frequency of false-positive results (20% to 25%). No reliable skin test reagent is available. Lymphocyte transformation studies in vitro with alkali-soluble, water-soluble antigen can identify a large proportion of infected patients, but the test is not feasible for most clinical laboratories.[12]

The differential diagnosis of acute pulmonary blastomycosis includes other fungal pneumonias acquired from nature, and bacterial pneumonias. Disseminated blastomycosis should be distinguished from disseminated coccidioidomycosis and paracoccidioidomycosis.

Treatment

Before the advent of effective antifungal therapy, the mortality rate of blastomycosis exceeded 60%. The introduction of 2-hydroxystilbamidine reduced mortality,[41, 61] but this drug is

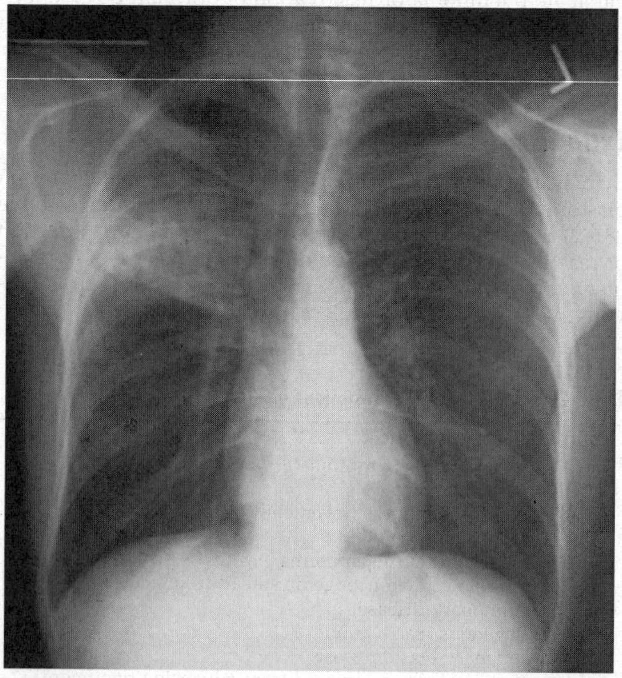

FIGURE 281–4 □ Pulmonary blastomycosis. Right upper lobe airspace disease is apparent.

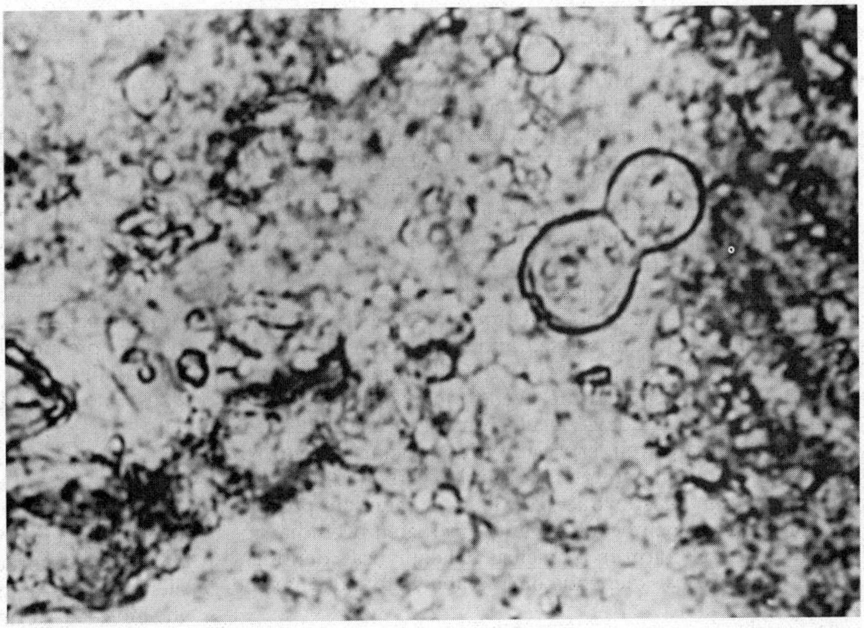

FIGURE 281–5 □ *Blastomyces* yeast in potassium hydroxide preparation from skin aspiration. Note the broad-based budding of this fungal form.

now largely of historical interest. Patients with acute blastomycosis may not require specific antifungal therapy if they have no significant underlying disease and if symptoms have been present less than 3 weeks, although this approach is controversial. No specific indices are available to aid the physician in determining who is at risk for progressive disease. Therefore, the patient should be observed for several months after the initial illness, to ensure that infection has not progressed.

Amphotericin B has been the mainstay of therapy for the past three decades. The exact amount of amphotericin B required to cure blastomycosis has not been determined, but previous studies have suggested that a total dose of less than 1.0 g is associated with a higher mortality and a total dose of less than 1.5 g with a higher rate of relapse. Therefore, recommendations for total dose usually range from 2.0 to 2.5 g of amphotericin B or 30 to 35 mg/kg. Even with this dose, approximately 10% to 20% of patients suffer a relapse 5 years after treatment is completed.[62] Many relapses respond to a second course of amphotericin B. Numerous schedules for amphotericin B administration have been published, but it is our practice to give 10 mg on the first day and increase the daily dose by 10 to 15 mg to a maximum of 50 mg. If the patient is seriously ill, amphotericin B is given daily until symptoms resolve, then three times a week. Patients who are less ill receive 50 mg three times a week.

Ketoconazole and itraconazole have emerged as important therapeutic options in the treatment of nonmeningeal blastomycosis in immunocompetent hosts. One clinical study has shown that a dose of ketoconazole of 400 mg/d for at least 6 months produced a cure rate of 79%, whereas 800 mg/d for the same period produced a 100% cure rate.[63] Similar cure rates have been reported in another study in which the 400 mg dose was employed.[64] It has been recommended that if ketoconazole is used for blastomycosis, the starting dose should be 400 mg/d because this dosage has a lower incidence of side effects. Should the patient not respond, a larger dose (600 or 800 mg/d) can be given. Treatment should continue for at least 6 months. Beyond that period of time, it can be discontinued when symptoms have dissipated or radiographic abnormalities have improved or stabilized. Although trials comparing the efficacy of amphotericin B and ketoconazole have not been conducted, the effectiveness of ketoconazole is similar to that reported for amphotericin in earlier studies.

A clinical trial showed that intraconazole therapy produced cure rates of 90% in nonmeningeal, non–life-threatening forms of blastomycosis and was less toxic than ketoconazole therapy. Many experts now prefer itraconazole to ketonazole because of its similar efficacy and lower toxicity. The recommended initial dose of itraconazole in adults is 200 mg/d. If disease persists or progresses, the dose should be increased in increments of 100 mg up to a maximum of 400 mg/d. Treatment should be continued for at least 6 months. There is little published clinical experience to recommend the use of itraconazole in children.[65]

Surgery has virtually no role in the treatment of blastomycosis, but it may be useful in establishing a diagnosis. As an adjunct to antimycotic therapy, surgery may be indicated for drainage of large quantities of empyema or pus from bone or subcutaneous tissues. As the sole treatment, surgical resection of infected tissues should not be considered curative.

PARACOCCIDIOIDES

Ana M. Gomez
George S. Deepe, Jr.

History

The first cases of paracoccidioidomycosis were described in Brazil by Adolfo Lutz in 1908.[71] He reported two patients with granulomatous disease of the nasopharynx and cervical lymphadenopathy. He identified in tissues the presence of a budding organism that resembled *C. immitis*. Material removed from the lymph nodes grew a filamentous organism that was indicative of a fungus. Lutz called the infectious process "hyphoblastomycosis." For many years, the illness was believed to be caused by *C. immitis* until Almeida provided evidence that hyphoblastomycosis was caused by a distinct pathogenic fungus.[72] Subsequently, the organism was named *P. brasiliensis*.

Characteristics of the Pathogen

The agent of paracoccidioidomycosis is the dimorphic fungus *P. brasiliensis*. In secretions from mucocutaneous lesions, in tissues, and in culture at 37°C, the fungus is found as a double-walled, oval to round yeast cell of 4 to 40 μm diameter. The yeast may exhibit single or multiple budding[73]; a yeast cell surrounded by numerous budding yeasts gives the appearance of a pilot wheel, which is characteristic of this pathogenic fungus (Fig. 281–6).

The fungus is usually grown on Sabouraud dextrose agar, although other media support its growth. At 37°C, the colonies are soft and cream colored and have a cerebriform, or wrinkled, appearance. At 19°C to 28°C the fungus grows as a mold; at room temperature, well-formed colonies do not appear until 20 to 30 days' incubation.[74] The mycelial phase does not sporulate well, especially if the organism is grown on media containing simple or complex carbohydrates, but when grown on yeast extract agar there is abundant production of conidia, arthroconidia, and arthroaleuroconidia approximately 2 to 5 μm in diameter.[74] Unequivocal identification of *P. brasiliensis* depends on the ability to cultivate the yeast phase.

The virulence of isolates of *P. brasiliensis* varies widely, which may account for marked differences in clinical manifestations of disease among individuals. Expression of virulence by *Paracoccidioides* has been correlated directly with α-glucan content in cell walls of yeasts.[75, 76]

Epidemiology

Paracoccidioidomycosis is limited geographically to Central and South America, from Mexico to Argentina. No endemic cases have been reported from Belize, Nicaragua, Surinam, Guyana, Chile, or the Caribbean islands.[77] Cases have been described in North America, Europe, and Asia, but in each instance, the victim had resided in endemic areas.[78, 79] Eighty percent of reported cases are from Brazil.[80]

Because the fungus has been isolated only rarely from nature its ecologic niche has been difficult to determine. Case reports and skin test results have been used to define endemic areas. Based on epidemiologic studies, the areas of highest prevalence are the rural and suburban regions of Brazil, Colombia, Venezuela, Ecuador, and Argentina.[77] It is thought that regions in these countries possess the climatic and ecologic conditions suitable for fungal growth in soil. This includes the combination of moderate temperatures, relatively high humidity, and rich vegetation.[81]

Clinically apparent disease is observed most commonly in men who are in close contact with nature. It is rare in women (male/female ratio is 15:1), adolescents, and children, but the prevalence of skin test reactivity in men and women is equal. In Colombia, Ecuador, and Argentina, the male/female ratio is approximately 150:1.[82] In the endemic regions, the estimated annual incidence is 1 to 3 clinical cases per 100,000 inhabitants, or 3000 to 10,000 new cases per year.[77] The infection is presumed to be acquired by inhalation of fungal propagules from the soil. Human-to-human transmission does not occur. Most patients work in agricultural activities.

Pathogenesis

Human infection with *P. brasiliensis* is acquired via accidental inhalation of airborne fungal propagules.[83] The small fungal elements settle into the small airways of the lungs. Once the mycelial forms have transformed into yeasts, an early neutrophilic response is followed by an influx of mononuclear cells. The yeasts spread from lung parenchyma lymphohematogenously to regional lymph nodes, forming a primary complex.[84] In addition, the organism can migrate to involve many visceral organs, especially those of the reticuloendothelial system. Healed lesions may calcify, but it seems to happen much less frequently than in tuberculosis or histoplasmosis. After spread to distant organs, the organism may become dormant or be completely eliminated from tissues.[84]

In visceral organs the typical inflammatory response to *P. brasiliensis* is characterized by an admixture of a necrotizing, suppurative process and granulomatous inflammation.[85] Most of what is known of the evolution of the inflammatory response is derived from animal studies,[86] which suggest that the earliest infiltrates (within 2 weeks) are composed of neutrophils that produce suppuration; granulomata are present from 2 weeks to a month after inoculation.

The increased frequency of disease in adult males suggests that hormonal factors may play a role in the pathogenesis of infection. Indeed, physiologic concentrations of estrogens, but not androgens, inhibit the transformation of mycelia to yeast.[87] Estrogens do not alter yeast growth or budding.[88]

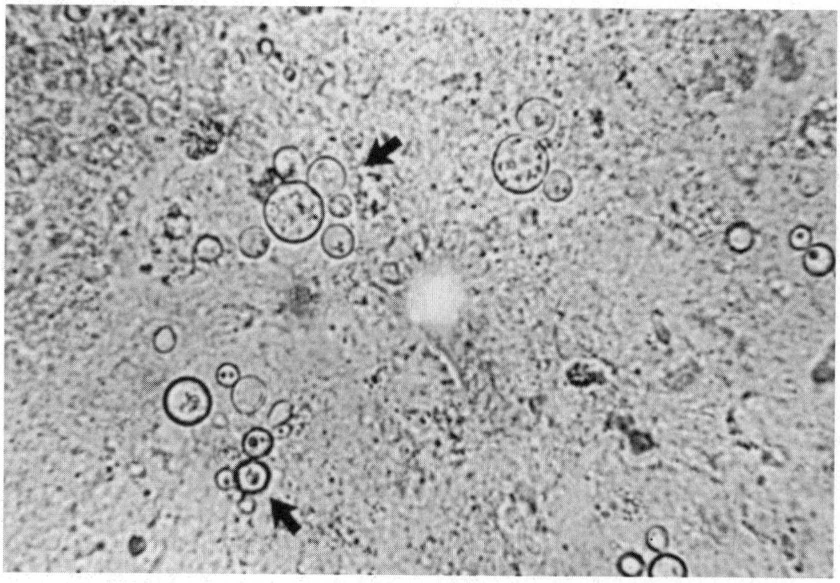

FIGURE 281–6 □ *Paracoccidioides brasiliensis* yeasts in potassium hydroxide–treated sputum sample. The arrows point to the pilot wheel appearance of the fungus. (Courtesy of Angela Restrepo, PhD, Mycology Unit, Corporacìon des Investigaciones Biológicas, Medellín, Colombia.)

Thus, the increased resistance of women to *P. brasiliensis* may be caused by circulating estrogens.

Immune Response and Host Defenses

Circulating specific antibody is detected in a large proportion of infected persons, and titers may escalate in progressive, disseminated forms of paracoccidioidomycosis.[89] Anti–*P. brasiliensis* antibody is an opsonin and enhances phagocytosis by macrophages.[90] Yeast cells trigger activation of the alternative pathway of complement, and constituents of the complement cascade can act as opsonins.[91]

Human neutrophils ingest yeast cells of *P. brasiliensis*, but it is not clear whether these phagocytes exert fungicidal activity.[92] In cell-free systems, large amounts of hydrogen peroxide kill yeasts, and adding a halide to this system reduces the concentration of hydrogen peroxide required to exert fungicidal activity.[93] Pulmonary macrophages from mice weakly kill isolates of *P. brasiliensis* yeasts. Exposure to interferon-γ can enhance the antifungal effects of these phagocytes.[94] Murine natural killer cells also can limit growth of yeast cells.[95]

The vast majority of patients with subclinical infection demonstrate cutaneous reactivity to paracoccidioidin, and their peripheral blood mononuclear cells mount a blastogenic response to this antigen in vitro.[96] In widely disseminated disease, generalized anergy is observed in a large proportion of patients, but cutaneous reactivity may be restored after therapy.[97] Likewise, mononuclear cells from these persons do not respond to mitogens or antigens in vitro.[98] The underlying causes of the anergic state are poorly understood; however, experimental evidence suggests that suppressor T cells, immune complexes, and a plasma inhibitory factor may be responsible, in part, for the observed depression of immune responses.[97, 99–101]

Clinical Manifestations

The clinicopathologic and immunologic manifestations of paracoccidioidomycosis, like those of histoplasmosis and tuberculosis, should be considered as occurring along a spectrum (Table 281–3). The clinical features of infection range from an acute pulmonary infection that is self-limited, to chronic pulmonary disease, to a progressive disseminated form with frequent involvement of mucocutaneous tissues, the reticuloendothelial system, and the adrenals.

Pulmonary Disease

In approximately 80% of adults infected with this fungus, pulmonary disease is evident by radiography, but the majority of infections are asymptomatic.[102, 103] A smaller proportion of patients exhibit persistent cough, purulent sputum, chest pain, weight loss, weakness, malaise, dyspnea, and fever.[104] Often, there are few auscultatory findings or none. The most common radiographic picture of the lungs in actively infected patients is diffuse interstitial and alveolar infiltrates (Fig. 281–7). The chest radiograph may also demonstrate nodules, cavitation, and hilar adenopathy. Rarely, a large cavitary mass, sometimes referred to as a paracoccidioidoma, is detected.[104]

Chronic pulmonary infections are generally associated with progressive fibrosis of the pulmonary parenchyma. As a consequence, deterioration of lung function and cor pulmonale may ensue.

The most frequent sites of dissemination are the mucosal tissues and skin: approximately 58% and 34% of patients, respectively, have such involvement.[104–106] These two sites are often infected concurrently. Oropharyngeal lesions begin as papules, which then progress to form ulcers (Fig. 281–8). The borders are heaped up, the base is infiltrated, and the lesions are typically dark purple. Small hemorrhagic spots can be seen in the base of the ulcer (Fig. 281–9). Skin lesions are often extensions of mucosal lesions, and their morphologic appearance is varied. Papules, ulcers, abscesses, and verrucous lesions may be observed.

Other sites of dissemination include lymph nodes, adrenals, liver, spleen, central nervous system, and bones. Enlarged cervical lymph nodes are associated with mucosal lesions, but other nodes can be affected. Involved nodes are firm and adherent to skin, and draining sinuses may arise from them. In autopsy series, *P. brasiliensis* is present in adrenal glands in as many as 95% of cases.[103] Decreased adrenal reserve is detected in as many as 48% of nonfatal cases.[107] The proportion of patients with overt Addison disease is smaller, but in one study was reported to be 14%.[108]

Children and young adults exhibit an acute or subacute form of the disease, with large numbers of yeasts in the reticuloendothelial system and fungemia. Cutaneous lesions are acneiform. The lung radiograph usually shows a miliary pattern.[104]

Diagnosis

Specimens such as sputum or pus should be examined directly on a slide with a drop of 10% potassium hydroxide. If

TABLE 281–3 ■ Clinicopathologic and Immunologic Manifestations of Paracoccidioidomycosis*

CLASSIFICATION	HYPERERGIC	INTERMEDIATE	ANERGIC
Clinical manifestations	Asymptomatic, paracoccidioidoma	Progressive pulmonary infection, with or without mucocutaneous involvement	Widespread involvement of reticuloendothelial system, lymphadenopathy, miliary lung disease
Immune reactions			
Positive skin test (%)	90–100	42–76	<30
Anti–*P. brasiliensis* antibodies (%)	<5	80–95	70–100
Blastogenic response to antigens and mitogens	+ + +	+ + / + + +	+ / −
Histopathology	Granuloma; rare yeast cells, if any	Granuloma and necrotizing suppuration; few yeast cells	Diffuse infiltration with polymorphonuclear leukocytes and macrophages; abundant yeasts

*+ + +, Stimulation index > 10; + +, stimulation index 5–10; +, stimulation index 3–5.
Data from references 85, 95, 96, 102.

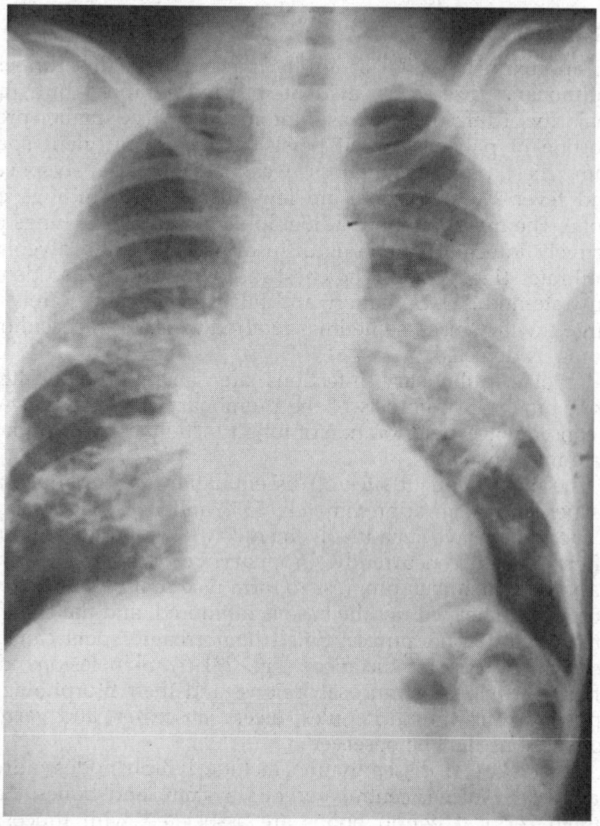

FIGURE 281–7 □ Pulmonary paracoccidioidomycosis. The chest radiograph reveals bilateral interstitial and alveolar infiltrates in the middle and lower lobes. The upper lobes are spared. (Courtesy of Angela Restrepo, PhD, Mycology Unit, Corporacìon des Investigaciones Biológicas, Medellín, Colombia.)

P. brasiliensis yeasts are present, they will appear as double-walled yeasts 4 to 40 μm in diameter. Identification of multiple budding yeasts with the pilot wheel appearance is indicative of *Paracoccidioides* infection. Repeated examinations should be performed if the initial examination is negative.

Tissue biopsy examination (excluding mucocutaneous tissue) reveals the typical admixture of necrotizing suppuration and granulomatous inflammation. Yeasts may be detected by hematoxylin-eosin staining (Fig. 281–10), but they are much more readily observed in specimens using silver stains such as Gomori–methenamine silver (Fig. 281–11). In contrast, histopathologic examination of the mucocutaneous lesions demonstrates pseudoepitheliomatous hyperplasia and intraepithelial microabscesses with yeast cells. In the visceral organs of children with disseminated paracoccidioidomycosis, yeast cells are abundant and tissues contain massive aggregates of macrophages.

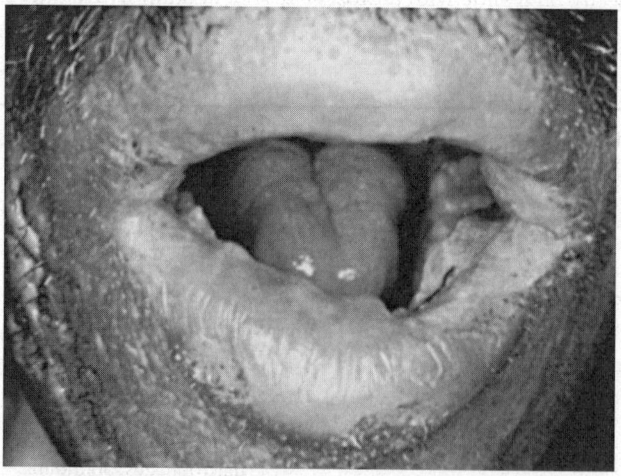

FIGURE 281–8 □ Angular cheilitis and lip lesions caused by *Paracoccidioides brasiliensis.* Hemorrhagic spots are evident at both angles of the lips. (Courtesy of Angela Restrepo, PhD, Mycology Unit, Corporacion des Investigaciones Biológicas, Medellín, Colombia.)

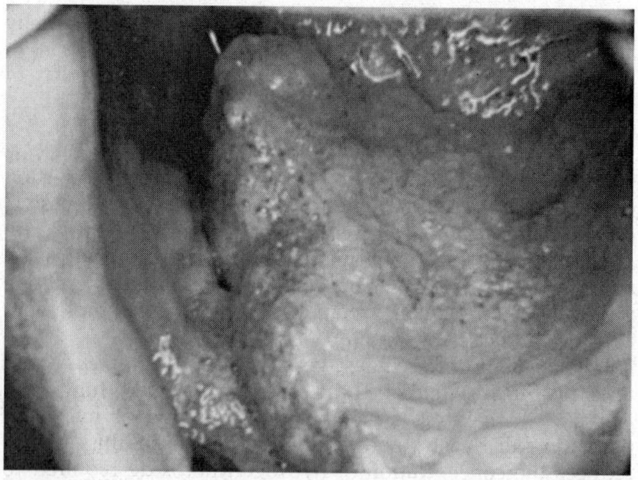

FIGURE 281–9 □ Large ulceration of the tongue caused by *Paracoccidioides.* Hemorrhagic spots are widely dispersed. (Courtesy of Angela Restrepo, PhD, Mycology Unit, Corporacìon des Investigaciones Biológicas, Medellín, Colombia.)

Unequivocal confirmation that the illness is caused by *P. brasiliensis* requires that cultures be performed. Material for culture is placed on Sabouraud dextrose agar or yeast extract agar containing antibiotics and cycloheximide and is incubated at room temperature. Mycelia are usually evident by 20 to 30 days. Because the organism does not produce characteristic conidia, the identity of the fungus must be established by conversion to the yeast phase at 37°C.

The common serologic assays used for diagnosis include immunodiffusion in agar gel and complement fixation. The former is a specific and sensitive assay, and detection of precipitation bands 1 and 2 is suggestive of either recent or remote infection.[109] As many as 95% of patients with active disease have antibodies detected by immunodiffusion.[74] The complement fixation test is positive in 80% to 95% of patients with active disease,[110] although there may be cross-reactivity with *Histoplasma* antigens. The quantitative nature of this test may provide a means to follow the response to therapy. Other serologic tests include immunoelectrophoresis, counterimmunoelectrophoresis, and enzyme-linked immunosorbent assay, but they are not widely used. A specific exoantigen has been detected in culture filtrates of *P. brasiliensis.* This 43-kDa antigen appears to be specific and has properties of a proteinase.[111–114] This antigen may provide a specific test for diagnosis of paracoccidioidomycosis.

Skin testing with paracoccidioidin is useful for epidemiologic studies but not for clinical diagnosis, because a large proportion of patients with active disease may have negative results on skin tests. Cross-reactivity with histoplasmin may be observed.

The principal differential diagnosis for paracoccidioidomycosis is tuberculosis. Concomitant infections with *P. brasiliensis* and *M. tuberculosis* may be present in as many as 25% of patients.[115] Other diseases that may mimic paracoccidioidomycosis include histoplasmosis, blastomycosis, leishma-

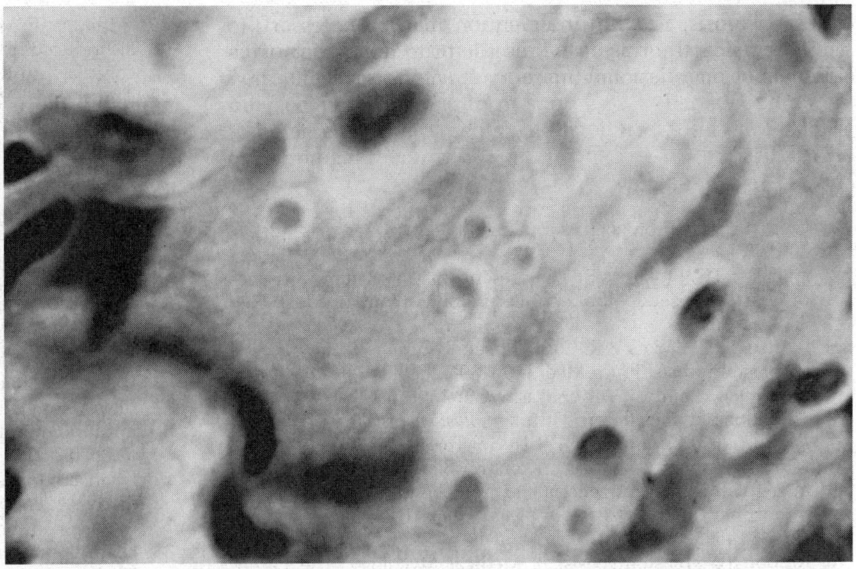

FIGURE 281–10 ▫ Photomicrograph of *Paracoccidioides* yeasts in tissue stained with hematoxylin-eosin. Multiple budding is present in addition to the "Mickey Mouse" configuration of budding yeasts. (Courtesy of Angela Restrepo, PhD, Mycology Unit, Corporacìon des Investigaciones Biológicas, Medellín, Colombia.)

niasis, and chromoblastomycosis. The extensive lymphadenopathy of patients with paracoccidioidomycosis may be misconstrued as lymphoma.

Treatment

Before the introduction of ketoconazole, sulfonamides were the primary treatment for paracoccidioidomycosis.[115] Sulfadiazine or sulfamerazine, 2 to 6 g/d, is administered daily for 4 weeks or until there is clinical or microbiologic evidence of improvement. Once this is attained, the dose is reduced to 2 to 3 g/d; treatment is continued for 3 to 5 years. Alternatively, long-acting sulfonamides such as sulfamethoxypyridazine may be given, 1 g/d for 1 week initially, followed by 500 mg/d for several years.[116] Treatment with sulfonamides is associated with a 15% relapse rate.

Amphotericin B is used for life-threatening infections or when sulfonamides are ineffective. The dose of amphotericin B ranges from 0.25 to 1.2 mg/kg, either every day if the patient is acutely ill, or every other day. Usually, a total dose of 1 to 3 g is sufficient. All patients who take a course of amphotericin B should be given ketoconazole for several months thereafter.

The oral azoles have become the mainstay of therapy for all forms of paracoccidioidomycosis because of their efficacy and ease of administration. Ketoconazole has been used extensively and is effective in more than 85% of cases. Relapse rates range from 0% to 11%. Therapy is initiated with 200 mg/d and continued for at least 6 months. If the response to this dose is poor or if disease is widely disseminated, the daily starting dose is 400 mg. Some physicians prescribe 400 mg/d routinely.[105, 106, 117, 118] Although ketoconazole produces excellent results, itraconazole appears to be superior. Its activity is higher, the duration of therapy can be reduced to 6 months, and a dosage of 100 mg/d is recommended. Relapses are less frequent (3% to 5%) with this drug. Thus, several experts in the field recommend itraconazole as the preferred drug for this disease.[119, 120]

There is little place for surgery in the treatment of paracoc-

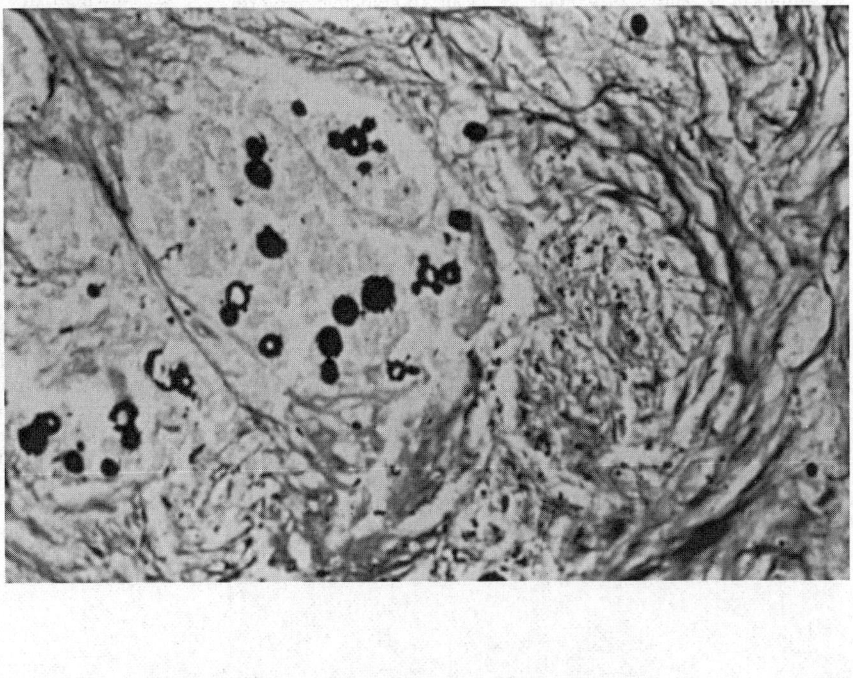

FIGURE 281–11 ▫ *Paracoccidioides* yeasts in tissue stained with Gomori–methenamine silver. Multiple budding yeasts are evident. (Courtesy of Judith Rhodes, PhD, University of Cincinnati College of Medicine, Cincinnati, OH.)

cidioidomycosis. Surgical intervention may be necessary to diagnose visceral forms of the disease or to remove paracoccidiomas or mass lesions caused by *P. brasiliensis*.

References

Blastomyces

1. Gilchrist TC: Protozoan dermatitis. J Cutan Gen Dis 12:496, 1894.
2. Gilchrist TC, Stokes WR: The presence of an oidium in tissues of a case of pseudo–lupus vulgaris. Johns Hopkins Hosp Rep 7:129, 1896.
3. Gilchrist TC, Stokes WR: Case of pseudo–lupus vulgaris caused by blastomycosis. J Exp Med 3:53, 1896.
4. Medoff G, Painter A, Kobayashi GS: Mycelial-to-yeast phase transitions of the dimorphic fungi *Blastomyces dermatitidis* and *Paracoccidioides brasiliensis*. J Bacteriol 169:4055, 1987.
5. Maresca B, Lambowitz AM, Kumar VB, et al: Role of cysteine in regulating morphogenesis and mitochondrial activity in the dimorphic fungus *Histoplasma capsulatum*. Proc Natl Acad Sci USA 78:4596, 1981.
6. Rippon JW: Blastomycosis. *In* Medical Mycology: The Pathogenic Fungi and the Pathogenic Actinomycetes, ed 2. Philadelphia, WB Saunders, 1982, pp 428–458.
7. McDonough ES, Lewis AL: *Blastomyces dermatitidis:* Production of a sexual stage. Science 156:528, 1967.
8. McDonough ES, McNamara WJ, Chan DM, et al: Geographic distribution of "+" and "−" isolates of *Blastomyces (Ajellomyces) dermatitidis* in North America. Am J Epidemiol 98:63, 1973.
9. McDonough ES, Chan DM, McNamara WJ: Dual infection by + and − mating types of *Ajellomyces (Blastomyces) dermatitidis*. Am J Epidemiol 106:67, 1977.
10. Kaufman L, Standard PG, Weeks RJ, et al: Detection of two *Blastomyces dermatitidis* serotypes by exoantigen analysis. J Clin Microbiol 18:110, 1983.
11. Fraser VJ, Keath EJ, Powderly WG: Two cases of blastomycosis from a common source: Use of DNA restriction analysis to identify strains. J Infect Dis 163:1378, 1991.
12. Klein BS, Vergeront JM, Weeks RJ, et al: Isolation of *Blastomyces dermatitidis* in soil associated with a large outbreak of blastomycosis in Wisconsin. N Engl J Med 314:529, 1986.
13. Klein BS, Vergeront JM, Disalvo AF, et al: Two outbreaks of blastomycosis along rivers in Wisconsin. Am Rev Respir Dis 136:1333, 1987.
14. Furculow ML, Chick EW, Busey JD, et al: Prevalence and incidence studies of human and canine blastomycosis. I. Cases in the United States, 1885–1968. Am Rev Respir Dis 102:60, 1970.
15. Reingold AL, Lu XD, Plikaytis BD, et al: Systemic mycoses in the United States, 1980–1982. J Med Vet Mycol 24:433, 1986.
16. Smith JR Jr., Harris JS, Conant NF, et al: An epidemic of North American blastomycosis. JAMA 158:641, 1970.
17. Tosh FE, Hammerman KJ, Weeks RJ, et al: A common source epidemic of North American blastomycosis. Am Rev Respir Dis 109:525, 1974.
18. Kitchen MS, Reiber CG, Eastin GB: An urban epidemic of North American blastomycosis. Am Rev Respir Dis 109:525, 1974.
19. Farber ER, Leahy MS, Meadows TR: Endometrial blastomycosis acquired by sexual contact. Obstet Gynecol 32:306, 1968.
20. Craig MW, Davey WN, Green RA: Conjugal blastomycosis. Am Rev Respir Dis 102:86, 1970.
21. Gnann JW Jr., Bressler GS, Bodet A III, et al: Human blastomycosis after a dog bite. Ann Intern Med 98:48, 1983.
22. Klein BS, Vergeront JM, Davis JP: Epidemiologic aspects of blastomycosis, the enigmatic systemic mycosis. Semin Respir Infect 1:29, 1986.
23. Schwarz J, Baum GL: Blastomycosis. Am J Clin Pathol 11:999, 1951.
24. Harvey RP, Schmid ES, Carrington CC, et al: Mouse model of pulmonary blastomycosis: Utility, simplicity, and quantitative parameters. Am Rev Respir Dis 117:695, 1978.
25. Deepe GS Jr., Taylor CL, Bullock WE: Evolution of the inflammatory response and cellular immune responses in a murine model of disseminated blastomycosis. Infect Immun 50:183, 1985.
26. Williams JE, Moser SA: Chronic murine pulmonary blastomycosis induced by intratracheally inoculated *Blastomyces dermatitidis* conidia. Am Rev Respir Dis 135:17, 1987.
27. Thurmond LM, Mitchell TG: *Blastomyces dermatitidis* chemotactic factor: Kinetics of production and biological characterization evaluated by a modified neutrophil chemotaxis assay. Infect Immun 46:87, 1984.
28. Cox RA, Mills LR, Best GK, et al: Histologic reaction to cell walls of an avirulent and virulent strain of *Blastomyces dermatitidis*. J Infect Dis 129:179, 1979.
29. Cox RA, Best GK: Cell wall composition of two strains of *Blastomyces dermatitidis* exhibiting differences in virulence for mice. Infect Immun 5:449, 1972.
30. Kaufman L, McLaughlin DW, Clark MJ, et al: Specific immunodiffusion test for blastomycosis. Appl Microbiol 26:244, 1973.
31. Klein BS, Jones JM: Purification and characterization of the major antigen WI-1 from *Blastomyces dermatitidis* yeasts and immunological comparison with A antigen. Infect Immun 62:3890, 1994.
32. Klein BS, Jones JM: Isolation, purification, and radiolabeling of a novel 120-kD surface protein on *Blastomyces dermatitidis* yeasts to detect antibody in infected patients. J Clin Invest 85:152, 1990.
33. Klein BS, Hogan LH, Jones JM: Immunological recognition of a 25 amino acid repeat arrayed in tandem on a major antigen of *Blastomyces dermatitidis*. J Clin Invest 92:330, 1993.
34. Brummer E, Morozumi PA, Vo PT, et al: Protection against pulmonary blastomycosis: Adoptive transfer with T lymphocytes, but not serum, from resistant mice. Cell Immunol 73:349, 1982.
35. Drutz DJ, Frey CL: Intracellular and extracellular defenses of human phagocytes against *Blastomyces dermatitidis* conidia and yeasts. J Lab Clin Invest 105:737, 1985.
36. Schaffner A, Davis CE, Schaffner T, et al: In vitro susceptibility of fungi to killing by neutrophil granulocytes discriminates between primary pathogenicity and opportunism. J Clin Invest 78:511, 1986.
37. Sugar AM, Picard M: Macrophage- and oxidant-mediated inhibition of the ability of live *Blastomyces dermatitidis* conidia to transform to the pathogenic yeast phase: Implications for the pathogenesis of dimorphic fungal infections. J Infect Dis 163:371, 1991.
38. Sugar AM, Chahal RS, Brummer E: Susceptibility of *Blastomyces dermatitidis* strains to products of oxidative metabolism. Infect Immun 41:908, 1983.
39. Sugar AM, Chahal RS, Brummer E: The iron-hydrogen peroxide system in fungicidal activity against the yeast phase of *Blastomyces dermatitidis*. J Leukoc Biol 36:545, 1984.
40. Smith DT: Immunologic types of blastomycosis: A report on 40 cases. Ann Intern Med 31:463, 1949.
41. Witorsch P, Utz JP: North American blastomycosis: A study of 40 patients. Medicine (Baltimore) 47:169, 1968.
42. Newman SL, Chatuverdi S, Klein BS: The WI-1 antigen of *Blastomyces dermatitidis* yeasts mediate binding to human macrophage CD11b/CD18 (CR3) and CD14. J Immunol 154:753, 1995.
43. Klein BS, Sondel PS, Jones JM: WI-1, a 120 kD surface protein on *Blastomyces dermatitidis* yeasts, is a target antigen of cell-mediated immunity in human blastomycosis. Infect Immun 60:4291, 1992.
44. Bradsher RW, Alford RH: *Blastomyces dermatitidis* antigen–induced lymphocyte reactivity in human blastomycosis. Infect Immun 33:485, 1981.
45. Brummer E, Morrison CJ, Stevens DA: Recombinant and natural γ-interferon activation of macrophages in vitro: Different dose requirements for induction of killing activity against phagocytizable and nonphagocytizable fungi. Infect Immun 49:787, 1984.
46. Morrison CJ, Brummer E, Isenberg RA, et al: Activation of murine polymorphonuclear neutrophils for fungicidal activity by recombinant γ interferon. J Leukoc Biol 41:434, 1987.
47. Sarosi GA, Hammerman KJ, Tosh FE, et al: Clinical features of acute pulmonary blastomycosis. N Engl J Med 290:540, 1974.
48. Sarosi GA, Davies SF: Blastomycosis. Am Rev Respir Dis 120:911, 1979.
49. Recht, LD, Philips JR, Eckman MR, et al: Self-limited blastomycosis: A report of thirteen cases. Am Rev Respir Dis 120:1109, 1979.

50. Cush R, Light RW, George RB: Clinical and roentgenographic manifestations of acute and chronic blastomycosis. Chest 69:345, 1976.
51. Halvorsen RA, Duncan JD, Merten DF: Pulmonary blastomycosis: Radiologic manifestations. Radiology 150:1, 1984.
52. Laskey W, Sarosi GA: Endogenous activation in blastomycosis. Ann Intern Med 88:50, 1978.
53. Leavell UW: Cutaneous North American blastomycosis and black dots. Arch Dermatol 92:155, 1965.
54. Gehweiler JA, Capp MP, Chick EW: Observations on the roentgen patterns in blastomycosis of bone. Am J Roentgenol Radium Ther Nucl Med 108:497, 1970.
55. Bayer AS, Scott VJ, Guze LB: Fungal arthritis. IV. Blastomycotic arthritis. Semin Arthritis Rheum 9:145, 1979.
56. Schwarz J, Salfelder K: Blastomycosis: A review of 152 cases. Curr Top Pathol 65:165, 1977.
57. Inoshita T, Youngberg GA, Boelen LJ, et al: Blastomycosis presenting with prostatic involvement: Report of two cases and review of the literature. J Urol 130:160, 1982.
58. Gonyea EF: The spectrum of primary pulmonary blastomycotic meningitis: A review of central nervous system blastomycosis. Ann Neurol 3:26, 1978.
59. Laskey WL, Sarosi GA: Blastomycosis in children. Pediatrics 65:111, 1980.
60. Recht LD, Davies SF, Eckman MR, et al: Blastomycosis in immunosuppressed patients. Am Rev Respir Dis 125:359, 1982.
61. Colsky J: Treatment of systemic blastomycosis with 2-hydroxystilbamidine. Arch Intern Med 93:796, 1954.
62. Parker JD, Doto IL, Tosh FE: A decade of experience with blastomycosis and its treatment with amphotericin B. Am Rev Respir Dis 99:895, 1969.
63. National Institute of Allergy and Infectious Diseases Study Group: Treatment of blastomycosis and histoplasmosis with ketoconazole. Results of a prospective randomized trial. Ann Intern Med 103:861, 1985.
64. Bradsher RW, Rice DC, Abernathy RS: Ketoconazole therapy for endemic blastomycosis. Ann Intern Med 103:872, 1985.
65. Dismukes WE, Bradsher RW, Cloud GC, et al: Itraconazole therapy for blastomycosis and histoplasmosis. Am J Med 93:489, 1992.
66. Cherniss EI, Waisbren BA: North American blastomycosis: A clinical study of 40 cases. Ann Intern Med 44:105, 1956.
67. Abernathy RS: Clinical manifestations of pulmonary blastomycosis. Ann Intern Med 51:707, 1959.
68. Lockwood WR, Allison F, Batson BE, et al: The treatment of North American blastomycosis: Ten years' experience. Am Rev Respir Dis 100:314, 1969.
69. Duttera MJ, Osterhout S: North American blastomycosis: A survey of 63 cases. South Med J 62:295, 1969.
70. Kepron MD, Schoemperlen B, Hershfield ES, et al: North American blastomycosis in central Canada. Can Med Assoc J 106:243, 1972.

Paracoccidioides

71. Lutz A: Una mycose pseudococcidioidica localizada no boca e observada no Brasil. Contribucao ao conhecimento dos hyphoblastomycoses americanas. Brasil Med 22:121, 1908.
72. Almeida F: Estudos comparativos do granuloma coccidioidica nos Estados Unidos e no Brasil. Novo genero para parasito brasilero. An Fac Med Univ Sao Paulo 5:3, 1930.
73. Padiha-Gonzalvez A: Paracoccidioidomycosis. Cutis 40:214, 1987.
74. Rippon JW (ed): Medical Mycology, ed 3. Philadelphia, WB Saunders, 1988, pp 506–531.
75. San Blas G, San Blas F, Serrano LE: Host-parasite relationship in the yeastlike form of *P. brasiliensis*. Infect Immun 15:343, 1977.
76. San Blas G, San Blas F: Variability in cell wall composition in *P. brasiliensis*. A study of two strains. Sabouraudia 20:31, 1982.
77. Restrepo A: The ecology of *Paracoccidioides brasiliensis:* A puzzle still unsolved. Sabouraudia 23:323, 1985.
78. Greer DL, Restrepo A: The epidemiology of paracoccidioidomycosis. *In* Al Doory Y (ed): The Epidemiology of Human Mycotic Diseases. Springfield, IL, Charles C Thomas, 1975, pp 117–130.
79. Bouzy E, Winston DJ, Rhodes JC, et al: Paracoccidoidomycosis (South American blastomycosis) in the United States. Chest 72:100, 1977.
80. Borelli D: Some ecological aspects of paracoccidioidomycosis. *In* Proceedings of the Pan American Symposium on Paracoccidioidomycosis. Washington, DC, Pan American Health Organization, 1972, pp 59–64.
81. Restrepo A: The ecology of *Paracoccidioides brasiliensis*: A puzzle still unresolved. J Med Vet Mycol 23:323, 1985.
82. Restrepo A: Immune response to *Paracoccidioides brasiliensis* in human and animal hosts. Curr Top Med Mycol 2:239, 1988.
83. Franco M: Host-parasite relationships in paracoccidioidomycosis. J Med Vet Mycol 25:5, 1986.
84. Franco M, Montenegro MR: Anatomia patologica. *In* Del Negro G, Lacaz CS, Fiorillo AM (eds): Paracoccidioidomycosis (Blastomicose Sul-Americana). São Paulo, Brazil, Sarvier Editores, 1982, pp 97–117.
85. Brummer E, Restrepo A, Stevens DA, et al: Murine model of paracoccidioidomycosis. Production of fatal acute pulmonary or chronic pulmonary and disseminated disease. Immunological and pathological observations. J Exp Pathol 1:241, 1984.
86. Restrepo A, Salazar ME, Cano LE, et al: Estrogens inhibit mycelial-to-yeast transformation in the fungus *P. brasiliensis*. Implications for resistance of females to paracoccidioidomycosis. Infect Immun 46:346, 1984.
87. Loose DS, Stover EP, Restrepo A, et al: Estradiol binds to a receptor-like cytosol-binding protein and initiates a biological response in *P. brasiliensis*. Proc Natl Acad Sci USA 80:7659, 1983.
88. Restrepo A, Moncada LH: Serologic procedures in the diagnosis of paracoccidioidomycosis. *In* Proceedings of the International Symposium on Mycoses. Washington, DC, Pan American Health Organization, 1977.
89. Restrepo A, Velez H: Efectos de la fagocitosis in vitro sobre *P. brasiliensis*. Sabouraudia 13:10, 1975.
90. Calich VLG, Kipnis TL, Mariano M, et al: The activation of the complement system by *P. brasiliensis* in vitro: Its opsonic effect and possible significance for an in vivo model of infection. Clin Immunol Immunopathol 12:20, 1979.
91. McEwen JG, Brummer E, Stevens DA, et al: Effect of murine polymorphonuclear leukocytes on the yeast form of *P. brasiliensis*. Am J Trop Med Hyg 36:603, 1987.
92. McEwen JG, Sugar AM, Brummer E, et al: Toxic effects of products of oxidative metabolism on the yeast phase form of *P. brasiliensis*. J Med Microbiol 18:423, 1984.
93. Brummer E, Hanson LH, Restrepo A, et al: In vivo and in vitro activation of pulmonary macrophages by IFN-γ for enhanced killing of *Paracoccidioides brasiliensis* or *Blastomyces dermatitidis*. J Immunol 140:2786, 1988.
94. Jimenez BE, Murphy JW: In vitro effects of natural killer cells against *Paracoccidioides brasiliensis* yeast phase. Infect Immun 46:552, 1984.
95. Mussatti CC, Rezkallah-Iwasso MT, Mendes E, et al: In vivo and in vitro evaluation of cell-mediated immunity in patients with paracoccidioidomycosis. Cell Immunol 24:365, 1978.
96. Costa PC, Pagnano PMG, Bechelli LM, et al: Lymphocyte transformation test in patients with paracoccidioidomycosis. Mycopathologia 84:55, 1983.
97. Mota NGS, Rezkallah-Iwasso MT, Peracoli MT, et al: Correlation between cell-mediated immunity and clinical forms of paracoccidioidomycosis. Trans R Soc Trop Med Hyg 79:765, 1985.
98. Arango M, Oropeza F, Anderson O, et al: Circulating immunocomplexes and in vitro cell reactivity in paracoccidioidomycosis. Mycopathologia 79:153, 1982.
99. Castaneda E, Brummer E, Pappagianis D, et al: Regulation of immune responses by T suppressor cells and by serum in paracoccidioidomycosis. Cell Immunol 117:1, 1988.
100. Jimenez-Finkel BE, Murphy JW: Induction of antigen-specific T suppressor cells by soluble *Paracoccidioides brasiliensis* antigen. Infect Immun 56:734, 1988.
101. Giraldo R, Restrepo A, Gutierrez F, et al: Pathogenesis of paracoccidioidomycosis: A model based on the study of 46 patients. Mycopathologia 58:63, 1976.
102. Pena CE: Deep mycotic infections in Colombia. A clinicopathological study of 102 cases. Am J Clin Pathol 47:505, 1967.
103. Restrepo A, Robledo M, Giraldo R, et al: The gamut of paracoccidioidomycosis. Am J Med 61:33, 1976.
104. Restrepo A, Gomez I, Cano LE, et al: Treatment of paracoccidioi-

domycosis with ketoconazole: A three year experience. Am J Med 74:48, 1983.
105. Vargas J, Recacoechea M: Ketoconazole in the treatment of paracoccidioidomycosis (South American blastomycosis). Experience in 30 cases in Bolivia. Mycoses 31:187, 1988.
106. Del Negro G, Melo EHL, Rodbard P, et al: Limited adrenal reserve in paracoccidioidomycosis: Cortisol and aldosterone response to 1-24 ACTH. Clin Endocrinol 13:553, 1980.
107. Abad A, Gomez I, Velez P, et al: Adrenal function in paracoccidioidomycosis: A prospective study in patients before and after ketoconazole therapy. Infection 14:22, 1986.
108. Restrepo A, Moncada LH: Characterization of the precipitin bands detected in the immunodiffusion test for paracoccidioidomycosis. Appl Microbiol 28:138, 1974.
109. Kauffman L: Evaluation of serological tests for paracoccidioidomycosis. Preliminary report. *In* Proceedings of the Pan American Symposium on Paracoccidioidomycosis. Washington DC, Pan American Health Organization, 1972, pp 221–224.
110. Puccia R, Schenkman PA, Travassos LR: Exocellular components of *Paracoccidioides brasiliensis*: Identification of a specific antigen. Infect Immun 53:199, 1986.
111. Mendes-Giannini MJS, Bueno JP, Shikanai-Yasuda MA, et al: Detection of the 43,000-molecular-weight glycoprotein in sera of patients with paracoccidioidomycosis. J Clin Microbiol 27:2842, 1989.
112. Puccia R, Travassos LR: The 43 kDa glycoprotein from the human pathogen *Paracoccidioides brasiliensis* and its deglycosylated form: Excretion and susceptibility to proteolysis. Arch Biochem Biophys 289:298, 1991.
113. Puccia R, Travassos LR: 43-Kilodalton glycoprotein from *Paracoccidioides brasiliensis:* Immunochemical reactions with sera from patients with paracoccidioidomycosis, histoplasmosis, or Jorge Lobo's disease. J Clin Microbiol 29:1610, 1991.
114. Salfelder K, Doehnert G: Paracoccidioidomycosis. Anatomic study with complete autopsies. Virchows Arch 348:51, 1969.
115. Negroni P: Prolonged therapy for paracoccidioidomycosis: Approaches, complications, and risks. *In* Proceedings of the Pan American Symposium on Paracoccidioidomycosis. Washington DC, Pan American Health Organization, 1977, pp 147–155. PAHO Scientific Publication 254.
116. Restrepo A, Gomez I, Cano LE, et al: Posttherapy status of paracoccidioidomycosis treated with ketoconazole. Am J Med 74:53, 1983.
117. Brummer E, Castaneda E, Restrepo A: Paracoccidioidomycosis: An update. Clin Microbiol Rev 6:89, 1993.
118. Munera MI, Naranjo MS, Gomez I, et al: Seguimiento postterapia de pacientes con paracoccidioidomicosis tratados con itraconazol. Medicina Univ Pontificia Bolivariana (Medellín) 8:33, 1989.
119. Naranjo MS, Trujillo M, Munera MI, et al: Treatment of paracoccidioidomycosis with itraconazole. J Med Vet Mycol 28:67, 1990.
120. Mok WY, Fava-Netto C: Paracoccidioidin and histoplasmin sensitivity in Coari (State of Amazonas), Brazil. Am J Trop Med Hyg 27:808, 1978.

282

Dematiaceous Fungi

Jill R. Rosenthal

The dematiaceous fungi are pigmented fungi that have brown or black cell walls in their conidia, mycelia, and sclerotic bodies and form brown to black colonies in culture. The pigment appears to be a form of melanin.[1] The taxonomy of this group has been controversial, and many of the organisms appear in the literature under multiple names. Identification is based on the morphologic features of conidia and conidiophores in culture; many species can form different types of conidia within a single culture, contributing to morphologic confusion.

Cutaneous diseases caused by this group of fungi include chromoblastomycosis, phaeohyphomycosis, and mycetoma. These diseases are characterized by their clinical appearance, the tissue form of the infecting organism, and the etiologic agent. The causative fungi are saprophytes and are usually found in soil or in association with decaying vegetable material. Disease is usually the result of traumatic implantation, such as by a wood splinter, and therefore usually involves an extremity. Both normal and immunocompromised hosts can be affected. Although most of the dematiaceous fungi tend to cause one type of disease, there are rare instances of fungi that usually cause chromoblastomycosis producing clinical presentations more suggestive of phaeohyphomycosis or mycetoma and vice versa.[2–5] This has led some authors to propose that the clinical syndrome produced may depend as much on the interaction between the organism and the host as on the identity of the infective agent.[4]

Chromoblastomycosis

Clinical Manifestations

The most common form of dematiaceous fungal infection is chromoblastomycosis (chromomycosis, verrucous dermatitis), a chronic, localized infection of the skin that follows traumatic inoculation of a causative organism. The most common infecting organisms are *Fonsecaea pedrosoi*, *Fonsecaea compacta*, *Phialophora verrucosa*, *Cladosporium carrionii*, and *Rhinocladiella aquaspersa*; *Exophiala jeanselmei* has also been reported as a cause.[6] In the United States, *P. verrucosa* is the most commonly isolated agent; worldwide, *F. pedrosoi* is most common.[7, 8] The disease occurs most commonly in tropical, rural areas but has been reported in Central America, South America, North America, Cuba, Jamaica, Martinique, India, South Africa, Madagascar, Australia, northern Europe, and Great Britain.[9(pp1205–1206)] The most commonly isolated fungi from woody materials, soil, and vegetable material are *F. pedrosoi*, *C. carrionii*, and *P. verrucosa*, their frequency in nature corresponding to the frequency with which these agents cause disease; woody plant materials are the most common sources of fungal isolates.[10]

Because the dematiaceous fungi are saprophytes found in soil, decomposing vegetation, and, in particular, decaying wood, and the disease is acquired by traumatic implantation, chromoblastomycosis is most commonly seen in adult male agricultural workers, who often work barefoot and may receive puncture wounds on the feet.[7, 9(pp1205–1206)] Lesions most commonly occur on exposed sites such as the feet and lower legs but have been reported on other sites, such as the hands, buttocks, face, neck, ears, or trunk. Infection is usually limited to the skin and subcutaneous tissue in the vicinity of the initial injury, which may be inconsequential and may pass unnoticed by the patient. There have been no cases of human-to-human transmission.[7]

Early descriptions of chromoblastomycosis describe five morphologic types of infection, including nodular, tumorous, verrucous, plaque, and cicatricial lesions.[11] Possibly these represent different stages of disease or vary with the site of involvement. Chromoblastomycosis begins as a small pink papule, usually on the exposed surface of the lower extremity, that gradually enlarges to form a superficial nodule. In time, the lesion forms a scaly and fissured pink, violaceous, or brownish plaque, which eventually becomes verrucous

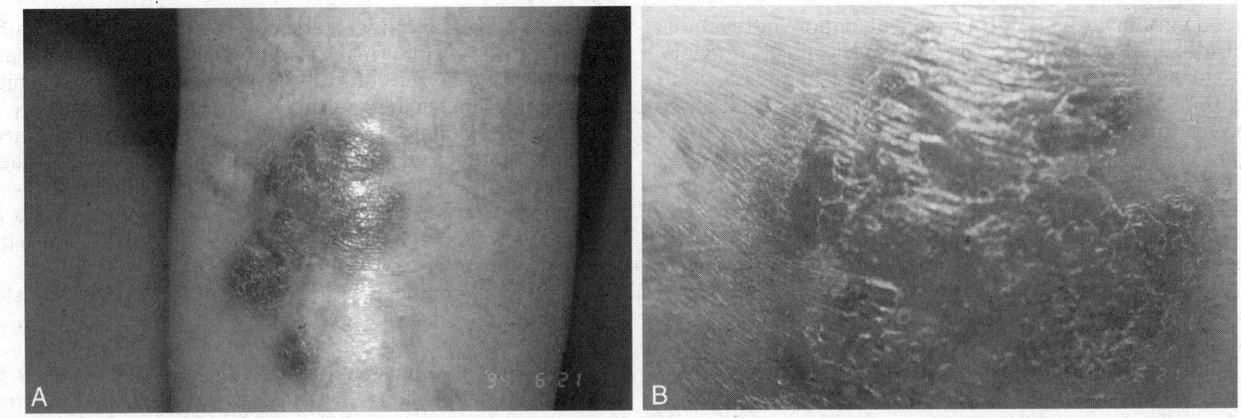

FIGURE 282–1 □ Chromoblastomycosis. *A*, Multiple plaques on the lower leg. *B*, Close-up of *A*. (See Color Plate 2.) (*A* and *B* courtesy of Nellie Konnikov, MD, New England Medical Center, Boston, MA.)

and may ulcerate with trauma (Fig. 282–1 [see Color Plate 2]). Small nodular lesions may develop into larger papillomatous or lobulated tumorous lesions with epidermal debris, crusting, and hyperkeratosis. Markedly verrucous lesions may occur on the sides of the feet (Fig. 282–2 [see Color Plate 2]). Ultimately, thick, crusted, tumorous hyperkeratotic masses may result, with ulceration due to trauma or secondary bacterial infection a frequent occurrence. Cicatricial lesions may result after peripheral enlargement with central healing, leading to atrophic scarring. Black dots may be visible on the surface of lesions and represent sites where blood and fungal cells (sclerotic bodies, "copper pennies") are expelled from the skin through transepidermal elimination; these may be sampled for skin scrapings or culture.[7] Chromoblastomycosis is usually asymptomatic in the absence of secondary infection. Satellite lesions may result from scratching or, more rarely, may occur via the lymphatic system.[12] Hematogenous spread is rare but has been reported to cause brain abscess.[9(pp1205–1206), 13] After many years, chronic and recurrent secondary infections may lead to elephantiasis due to lymphatic obstruction.[7, 9(pp1205–1206)]

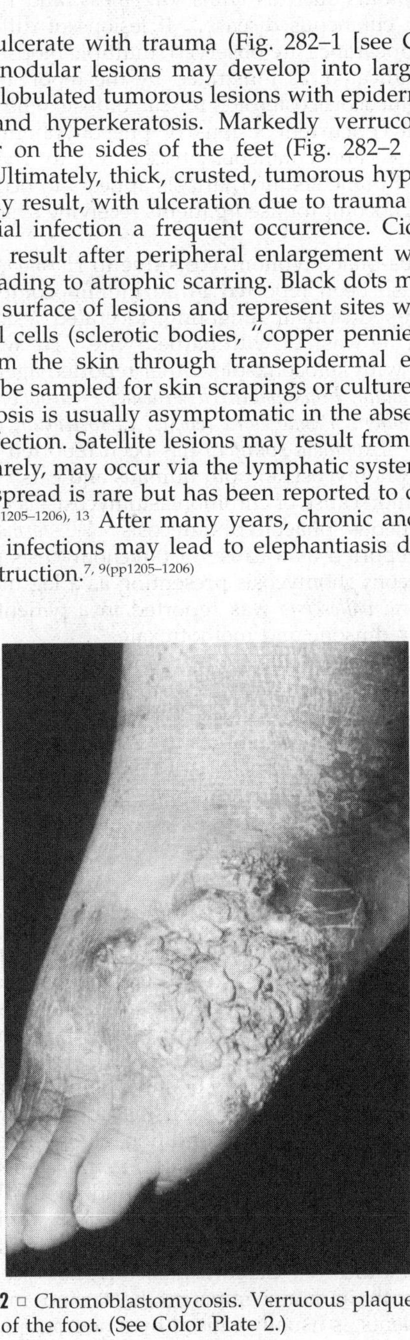

FIGURE 282–2 □ Chromoblastomycosis. Verrucous plaques on the lateral aspect of the foot. (See Color Plate 2.)

Differential Diagnosis

The differential diagnosis includes blastomycosis, cutaneous tuberculosis, leprosy, leishmaniasis, tertiary syphilis, yaws, and halogenoderma. Diagnosis is established by identification of pigmented thick-walled cells in clusters on microscopic examination of tissue scrapings in potassium hydroxide, fungal culture, or biopsy. Histopathologic examination reveals pseudoepitheliomatous hyperplasia with foreign body granulomata with focal abscess formation, chronic fibrosis, and the presence of brownish fungal cells within giant cells as well as in the stratum corneum, within abscesses, and free in tissue.[7, 9(pp1205–1206), 14] The brown, thick-walled, septate 5- to 12-μm cells are known variously as copper pennies, Medlar bodies, sclerotic bodies, and muriform cells, among other names, and represent the tissue form of the causative fungi.[7] The septa or cross-walls are seen in two planes; these bodies are seen only in chromoblastomycosis and are not seen in other dematiaceous fungal infections such as phaeohyphomycosis or mycetoma.[6, 7] Culture of crusts, exudate, pus, or biopsy specimens should be performed on plain Sabouraud glucose agar and Sabouraud glucose agar containing cycloheximide and chloramphenicol; verrucous lesions are said to have the highest yield for culture and for the visualization of sclerotic bodies.[15] Cultures should be kept at 25°C for at least 6 weeks, because the organisms that cause chromoblastomycosis grow slowly.[12] Unlike mycetoma, in which the morphologic appearance of the granules yields a clue to identity, the causative fungus in chromoblastomycosis cannot be identified by the appearance of the sclerotic bodies.[7] Identification of the causative agent is made by culture morphology and the microscopic appearance of the sporulation patterns. Serologic methods for the detection of complement-fixing and precipitating antibodies can also be used for diagnosis and for assessing response to treatment, although they are not routinely employed in the diagnosis of chromoblastomycosis.[7, 12, 14, 16, 17]

Treatment

Treatment of chromoblastomycosis is difficult, especially for infections caused by *F. pedrosoi*.[18] Therapy for small lesions, if possible, consists of wide and deep excision with skin grafting. With early lesions, excision may be curative. However, most patients present too late in the course to make this practical. Electrosurgical therapy is advocated by some authors and thought by others to produce a higher risk of recurrence. Cryosurgical destruction or local heat therapy may also be helpful.[19–21] Previously reported treatments have included various drugs singly or in combination: intravenous or intralesional amphotericin B, flucytosine, thiabendazole, and ketoconazole.[9(pp1205–1206), 18] Development of resistance to flucytosine may be a problem when this agent is used alone in the treatment of chromoblastomycosis, as it is with other fungal infections. Combination therapy with flucytosine and ketoconazole or amphotericin B appears to be synergistic.[7, 22, 23] Ketoconazole alone is slightly effective in mild disease, but its usefulness is limited by the risk of hepatotoxicity; fluconazole appears not to be useful in the treatment of chromoblastomycosis.[23, 24] Itraconazole at 200 mg daily for 6 to 24 months is effective in more than 60% of cases, even those due to *F. pedrosoi*.[18, 25, 26] Saperconazole, the newest triazole, not yet available in the United States, did well in a small series of patients at doses of 200 mg daily for 6 to 12 months and appears to be promising for the treatment of chromoblastomycosis, with response rates of about 75%.[18, 27] With additional studies, it may prove to be more effective than itraconazole, in briefer treatment courses. Rarely, amputation of the affected limb may be required as a last resort.

Phaeohyphomycosis

Phaeohyphomycosis refers to localized subcutaneous or deeper abscesses caused by *E. jeanselmei*, *Wangiella (Exophiala) dermatitidis*, and occasionally other agents. Infecting species include those from the genera *Exophiala*, *Exserohilum*, *Cladosporium*, *Bipolaris*, *Alternaria*, *Curvularia*, and *Wangiella*.[28] There are several different clinical syndromes ranging in severity. Infections may occur in both immunocompetent and immunocompromised patients and in animals as well as in humans. On histologic examination, pigmented yeastlike cells, hyphae, and pseudohyphae may be seen in infected tissue; sclerotic bodies, as seen in chromoblastomycosis, and grains, as seen in mycetoma, are absent. Both *E. jeanselmei* and *W. dermatitidis* have been recovered from soil, wood, and other plant materials.[14] The agents of phaeohyphomycosis have also been isolated from sewage, shower curtains, toilet bowls, bats, frogs, and wasp nests.[29]

Superficial, Cutaneous, and Subcutaneous Phaeohyphomycosis

Superficial phaeohyphomycosis includes tinea nigra and black piedra—superficial infections of the stratum corneum of the skin and of the hair, respectively (see Chapter 145). Examples of cutaneous phaeohyphomycosis include dermatomycoses produced by the nondermatophyte molds *Scytalidium* and *Hendersonula*, which produce chronic diseases of the skin and nails clinically similar to the dermatophytoses[6] (see Chapter 145). Colonization of fissured areas on the soles, skin ulcers, or dermatitic skin may also occur with dematiaceous fungi such as *Alternaria*, *Curvularia*, *Cladosporium*, and *Aureobasidium*.[29] Such colonization is not always pathogenic. These species may rarely cause skin or more invasive infection.

Like other dematiaceous fungal infections, subcutaneous phaeohyphomycosis begins after an abrasion or penetrating injury. Some patients are diabetic, but infections commonly occur in normal hosts as well.[29] Lesions of subcutaneous phaeohyphomycosis (phaeohyphomycotic cyst) begin with a firm nodule that may be tender and that may then develop into a large cyst or abscess up to several centimeters in diameter.[9(p1206)] A history of trauma may be obtained, and a wooden splinter is sometimes found in the tissue in association with the cyst.[30] Surgical excision is usually the treatment of choice. The most common cause of phaeohyphomycotic cyst is *E. jeanselmei*, although *W. dermatitidis* is more common in Japan.[29] Phaeohyphomycotic cysts have been mistaken for ganglion cysts, epidermal cysts, foreign body granulomata, and Baker cysts.[14] Lesions due to *W. dermatitidis* may exhibit more epidermal change, with a scaly or verrucous surface or pustules.[14] Diagnosis is established with potassium hydroxide preparation and culture of purulent aspirates, homogenized tissue from excision or biopsy specimens, or skin scrapings.[14] As for chromoblastomycosis, cultures should be inoculated onto Sabouraud glucose agar both with and without cycloheximide and chloramphenicol.

Unusual examples of traumatic inoculations causing phaeohyphomycosis include a mixed phaeohyphomycotic infection caused by *Exserohilum rostratum* and *Curvularia* in a cocaine user and phaeohyphomycosis due to *Curvularia lunata* after an explosion.[31, 32] *Curvularia geniculata* and *C. lunata* have also been reported to result from football injuries, eventuating in disseminated disease, and to cause fungal keratitis, mycetoma, and prosthetic valve endocarditis.[29] Systemic symptoms such as chills, dizziness, and nausea may accompany cutaneous disease.[33] If lesions of different morphologic appearance are observed, multiple biopsies and cultures are indicated, as illustrated by the report of a patient receiving glucocorticosteroids for sarcoidosis who developed distinct but concurrent lesions of phaeohyphomycosis due to *P. verrucosa* and cutaneous abscess due to *Mycobacterium fortuitum*.[34] Cutaneous alternariosis appears to occur primarily in immunocompromised patients receiving systemic corticosteroids.[35]

Cutaneous phaeohyphomycosis due to *Hormonema dematioides* has also been reported in an immunocompetent man who developed anular, fungating, ulcerated lesions on the hands after he was cut with barbed wire.[36] He was successfully cured with ketoconazole. Other reported agents include *Tetraploa aristata*, *Phialophora richardsiae*, *Pleurophoma* species, *Bipolaris spicifera*, *Phialophora repens*, *E. rostratum*, and many others.[33, 37–41] *Exophiala spinifera* has been reported as a cause of phaeohyphomycosis in both humans and cats.[42, 43] *P. verrucosa*, a common cause of chromoblastomycosis, is a rare cause of subcutaneous phaeohyphomycosis.[3] *W. dermatitidis* has also been reported as a cause of onychomycosis of the toenails.[44] Phaeohyphomycosis presenting as a leg ulcer caused by *Curvularia pallescens* was reported in a patient receiving low-dose prednisone and methotrexate.[45]

Fungal keratitis results from traumatic inoculation of dematiaceous fungi such as *W. dermatitidis*, which also causes cutaneous phaeohyphomycosis, and can occur after penetrating injury or ophthalmic surgery.[46] Other agents reported to cause fungal keratitis include *E. jeanselmei*, *Bipolaris hawaiiensis*, *Exserohilum longirostratum*, *E. rostratum*, *Fusarium*, *Curvularia*, and nondematiaceous agents such as *Aspergillus* and *Candida*.[47–51]

Systemic Phaeohyphomycosis

Systemic phaeohyphomycosis is usually an opportunistic infection.[29] However, agents causing cutaneous phaeohyphomycosis have also been described as causing aggressive sinus infections in immunocompetent hosts.[52–54] Dematiaceous fungi, including *Bipolaris*, *Exserohilum*, *Curvularia*, and *Alternaria* species, also appear to be more common causes than *Aspergillus* of allergic fungal sinusitis, an immunoglobulin E–mediated hypersensitivity condition, as opposed to a true invasive infection.[55–58] Disseminated *Fusarium* infections can occur in immunosuppressed patients and should be considered in patients with fever and neutropenia who present with myalgias and violaceous necrotic papules, vesicles, pustules, and nodules.[59, 60] Cerebral phaeohyphomycosis, which occurs in both immunocompetent hosts and immunosuppressed patients, is usually caused by a neurotropic dematiaceous fungus, *Xylohypha bantiana* (previously known as *Cladosporium bantianum* or *Cladosporium trichoides*).[61–64] Fatal cerebral phaeohyphomycosis has also been reported with *Chaetomium globosum* in a renal transplant patient and with *Ochroconis gallopavum* in a patient with large-cell lymphoma.[65, 66] Cerebral phaeohyphomycosis has also been caused by *F. pedrosoi*, which usually causes chromoblastomycosis, and by *W. dermatitidis*, which usually causes subcutaneous phaeohyphomycosis and has neurotropic tendencies with systemic infections.[67, 68] Cerebral phaeohyphomycosis due to *X. bantiana* usually presents only with cerebral lesions, without a known primary extra–central nervous system source, but cutaneous lesions may be seen in patients with disease due to *F. pedrosoi* or other agents that usually involve the skin.[63, 64, 69] The sinuses may be portals of entry for cerebral infection.[54] Inhalation of spores followed by hematogenous spread to the brain is another possibility.[63] Cerebral phaeohyphomycosis most commonly manifests as brain abscess, resulting in focal symptoms such as hemiparesis, but other symptoms such as headache, visual impairment, ataxia, incoordination, and seizures may be seen as well, and meningeal irritation or frank meningitis may be present.[69] The prognosis in cerebral phaeohyphomycosis is poor. Other systemic phaeohyphomycotic infections include pneumonia, tenosynovitis, septic arthritis, esophagitis, endophthalmitis, endocarditis, peritonitis, and osteomyelitis.[32, 54, 70]

Therapy for phaeohyphomycosis involves surgical débridement or excision and systemic antifungal therapy.[33, 70] Small cutaneous and subcutaneous lesions can be treated with surgery alone. Small cutaneous lesions have occasionally responded to topical imidazoles under occlusion, and localized heat application may also be considered.[39] Agents used include ketoconazole, itraconazole, flucytosine, fluconazole, and amphotericin B.[33, 68, 71, 72] In general, results are poor, except for small, localized lesions, but itraconazole may be helpful for some patients.[28] Keratitis is treated with systemic and topical antifungal agents. There appears to be no effective therapy yet for cerebral phaeohyphomycosis, and the prognosis for this disease is poor.[69]

Mycetoma

Mycetoma (Madura foot, maduromycosis), a localized chronic infection involving the skin, subcutaneous tissue, and sometimes bone, is characterized by swelling (tumefaction) and discharge of infected grains from draining sinuses (Fig. 282–3). The name mycetoma literally means fungal tumor. The process may be due to fungal infection (eumycotic mycetoma, or eumycetoma) or aerobic actinomycetes (actinomycotic mycetoma, or actinomycetoma). The various agents causing mycetoma are saprophytes found in soil and decaying vegetation. Infection occurs after traumatic inoculation, such as a puncture by a wooden splinter or a thorn. The condition is most common in tropical and subtropical regions, where people walk barefoot, and is most common in male agricultural workers between the ages of 20 and 50 years. Pathogenicity may be determined by many factors, including the thermal tolerance of the organisms. For example, most strains of *E. jeanselmei* isolated from soil are unable to grow at temperatures warmer than 30°C, in contrast to most specimens isolated from human infections, which grow readily at warmer temperatures.[73] The prevalence of the causative agents of eumycetoma and actinomycetoma varies by geographic location and soil type.[73] Mycetoma due to *Madurella grisea* has been reported in California. *Pseudallescheria boydii* has been isolated in sewage and has been reported as a cause of mycetoma in sewer workers in the United States.[73] The onset of disease may be many years, even several decades, after the initial injury.[9(pp1210–1213)]

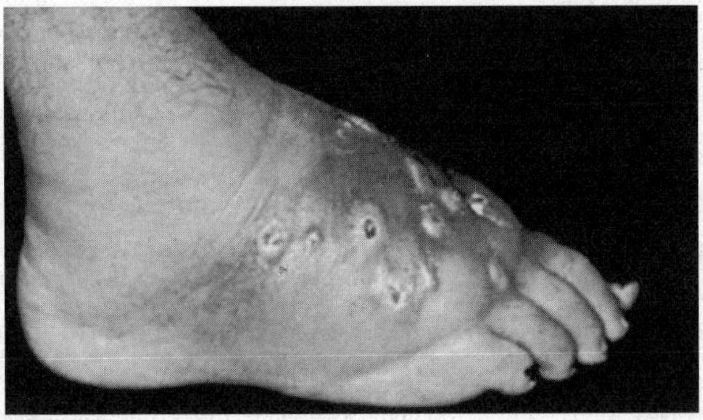

FIGURE 282–3 ◻ Mycetoma of the foot. (Courtesy of Victor Newcomer, MD, Santa Monica, CA.)

TABLE 282–1 ■ Appearance of Grains in Mycetoma

CAUSATIVE ORGANISM	GRAIN APPEARANCE
Actinomycetoma	
Nocardia asteroides	White, yellow to orange
Nocardia brasiliensis	Yellow-white
Actinomadura madurae	White to yellow or pink
Actinomadura pelletieri	Red
Streptomyces somaliensis	Yellow-white
Actinomyces israelii	White
Nocardia madurae	White; rarely pink
Mycotic Mycetoma	
Pseudallescheria boydii	White to yellow
Madurella grisea	Black
Madurella mycetomatis	Black
Exophiala jeanselmei	Black

Worldwide, actinomycotic mycetoma and eumycotic mycetoma occur with about equal frequency.[73] This may vary widely by area, however; for example, actinomycotic mycetoma accounts for 98% of cases in Mexico.[74] The agents most commonly responsible for causing actinomycotic mycetoma are *Nocardia brasiliensis, Actinomadura (Streptomyces) pelletieri, Streptomyces somaliensis,* and *Actinomadura madurae*; *Madurella mycetomatis* is the most common cause of eumycetoma.[9(pp1210–1213)] In the United States, however, *P. boydii* is the most common cause of eumycotic mycetoma.[8] *P. verrucosa*, which commonly causes chromoblastomycosis and rarely phaeohyphomycosis, has been reported as a cause of mycetoma.[3] *E. jeanselmei*, which usually causes phaeohyphomycosis, occasionally causes mycetoma. *Aspergillus, Fusarium*, and other agents have also rarely caused mycetoma.[73]

Mycetoma begins clinically with the development of firm, painless nodules that enlarge to produce a lumpy swelling. The lesions break down and discharge pus or a serous or serosanguineous drainage containing grains (tiny fungal or bacterial colonies that may have a crystalline matrix), the color and appearance of which may give a clue to the infecting organism (Table 282–1). Multiple sinus tracts may be present, and some may close and reopen or be replaced by new sinuses as the old ones heal with fibrosis. Raised borders or nodules around sinus tracts may be seen with *N. brasiliensis, A. madurae*, or *A. pelletieri*, giving a bumpy appearance; bone involvement is common with these organisms as well.[73] *S. somaliensis* tends to produce less bone involvement and is not characterized by raised sinus tract openings.[73] With time, infection may spread to deeper tissues, causing periostitis, osteomyelitis, and infectious arthritis.[9(pp1210–1213)] Although progression is slow, marked swelling and deformity may eventually result. Actinomycetoma tends to develop more rapidly than eumycetoma. Systemic spread is extremely unusual, although it may occur in actinomycetoma; spread on the skin may occur rapidly in actinomycetoma, especially when it is caused by *N. brasiliensis*.[73] Lesions are most commonly seen on the lower extremities, which are unprotected from trauma. It is thought that repeated punctures or lacerations result in inoculation of the causative organisms, perhaps accounting for the presence of multiple lesions. The back is a common site of infection in Mexico, where people may carry contaminated branches and other materials on their backs without protective clothing.[74] In Mexico and in Central and South America, *N. brasiliensis*, which causes the most aggressive form of actinomycetoma, accounts for almost 90% of cases of mycetoma.[74]

The differential diagnosis of mycetoma includes chronic osteomyelitis due to bacteria or mycobacteria; other deep fungal infections, such as blastomycosis, coccidioidomycosis, or sporotrichosis; botryomycosis; leishmaniasis; yaws; syphilis; and chromoblastomycosis. Botryomycosis is a bacterial infection in which abscesses also drain granules consisting of clusters of bacteria. It is usually caused by *Staphylococcus aureus* and occasionally by gram-negative bacteria such as *Pseudomonas aeruginosa*, *Escherichia coli*, or *Proteus* species; Gram stain, biopsy, and culture will distinguish it from actinomycotic mycetoma.

Diagnosis is made by microscopic examination with potassium hydroxide preparation, Gram stain, and acid-fast stains of smears of pus and granules and by culture of the grains. If possible, drug sensitivity testing should be performed. In some instances, serologic evaluation may be helpful. Early lesions may need incision and drainage for appropriate material to be obtained for diagnosis. If no sinuses are present, biopsy may be necessary for diagnosis. Histologic examination reveals granulation tissue with abscess formation and grains. The shape and color of the grains, along with their appearance in tissue on skin biopsy, may be helpful in identifying the causative agent.[74] Radiographs of bone should be performed to determine the presence and extent of bone involvement. Actinomycetoma is more likely to invade bone or other structures than is eumycetoma.[73]

Treatment of mycetoma is difficult, in part because the condition is usually far advanced by the time the diagnosis is made. Choice of therapy and response are determined by the causative organism, the site of involvement, and the degree of invasion. Specific identification of the etiologic agent is essential to guide therapy; the agents used for actinomycetoma and eumycetoma are different. Actinomycetoma should be treated with antibiotics such as trimethoprim-sulfamethoxazole plus streptomycin, dapsone plus streptomycin, penicillin, tetracycline, and rifampin, and surgical débridement.[9(pp1210–1213)] Trimethoprim-sulfamethoxazole with dapsone, sulfadoxine-pyrimethamine with either streptomycin or rifampin, sulfadiazine with tetracycline, and minocycline are regimens found useful by some authors.[73, 74] Prolonged treatment courses are necessary.

Wide excision may be curative of early, localized lesions of eumycetoma before bone involvement occurs, but relapse rates are high, and surgical therapy must be accompanied by appropriate antibiotic therapy guided by culture and in vitro susceptibility testing.[74] Eumycotic mycetoma is extremely resistant to medical therapy, in part because the organism is somewhat protected by its grain form in tissue in both eumycetoma and actinomycetoma.[75] Ketoconazole in high doses for prolonged courses appears effective in about 60% to 70% of patients with mycetoma caused by *M. mycetomatis*.[9(pp1210–1213), 76] However, eumycetoma due to *P. boydii* or *Acremonium* is refractory to therapy, although intravenous miconazole has been helpful in some patients with *P. boydii*.[18, 73, 77] Itraconazole appears less effective than ketoconazole in this condition but may be useful in mycetoma due to *Fusarium*.[18, 78, 79] Amphotericin appears not to be useful, except in occasional infections with *M. grisea* or *M. mycetomatis*.[73]

References

1. Dixon DM, Polak-Wyss A: The medically important dematiaceous fungi and their identification. Mycoses 34:1, 1991.
2. Sughayer M, DeGirolami PC, Khettry U, et al: Human infection caused by *Exophiala pisciphila*: Case report and review. Rev Infect Dis 13:379, 1991.
3. Turiansky GW, Benson PM, Sperling LC, et al: *Phialophora verrucosa*: A new cause of mycetoma. J Am Acad Dermatol 32:311, 1995.
4. Barba-Gómez JF, Mayorga J, McGinnis MR, et al: Chromoblastomycosis caused by *Exophiala spinifera*. J Am Acad Dermatol 26:367, 1992.
5. Zaharopoulos P, Schnadig VJ, Davie KD, et al: Multiseptate bodies in systemic phaeohyphomycosis diagnosed by fine needle aspiration cytology. Acta Cytol 32:885, 1988.
6. McGinnis MR, Hilger AE: Infections caused by black fungi. Arch Dermatol 123:1300, 1987.
7. Milam CP, Fenske NA: Chromoblastomycosis. Dermatol Clin 7:219, 1989.
8. Morris MI, Gurevitch A, Edwards JE Jr: Dematiaceae and agents of superficial mycoses. *In* Gorbach S, Bartlett JG, Blacklow NR (eds): Infectious Diseases. Philadelphia, WB Saunders, 1992, pp 1937–1941.
9. Hay RJ, Roberts SOB, MacKenzie DWR: Mycology. *In* Champion RH, Burton JL, Ebling FJG (eds): Rook/Wilkinson/Ebling Textbook of Dermatology, ed 5. Boston, Blackwell Scientific Publications, 1992, pp 1127–1216.
10. Okeke CN, Gugnani HC: Studies on pathogenic dematiaceous fungi. 1. Isolation from natural sources. Mycopathologia 94:19, 1986.
11. Carrion AL: Chromoblastomycosis. Ann N Y Acad Sci 50:1255, 1950.
12. Rippon JW: Chromoblastomycosis. *In* Rippon JW: Medical Mycology: The Pathogenic Fungi and the Pathogenic Actinomycetes, ed 3. Philadelphia, WB Saunders, 1988, pp 276–296.
13. Azulay RD, Serruya J: Hematogenous dissemination in chromomycosis. Arch Dermatol 95:57, 1967.
14. McGinnis MR: Chromoblastomycosis and phaeohyphomycosis: New concepts, diagnosis, and mycology. J Am Acad Dermatol 8:1, 1983.
15. Zaias N, Rebell G: A simple and accurate diagnostic method in chromoblastomycosis. Arch Dermatol 108:545, 1973.
16. Vollum DI: Chromomycosis: A review. Br J Dermatol 96:454, 1977.
17. Espinel-Ingroff A, Shadomy S, Dixon D, et al: Exoantigen test for *Cladosporium bantianum*, *Fonsecaea pedrosoi*, and *Phialophora verrucosa*. J Clin Microbiol 23:305, 1986.
18. Restrepo A: Treatment of tropical mycoses. J Am Acad Dermatol 31:S91, 1994.
19. Kinbara T, Fukushiro R, Eryu Y: Chromomycosis: Report of two cases successfully treated with local heat therapy. Mykosen 25:689, 1982.
20. Tagami H, Ginaza M, Imaizumi S, et al: Successful treatment of chromoblastomycosis with topical heat therapy. J Am Acad Dermatol 10:615, 1984.
21. Lubritz RR, Spence JE: Chromoblastomycosis: Cure by cryosurgery. Int J Dermatol 17:830, 1978.
22. Silber JG, Gombert ME, Green KM, Shalita AR: Treatment of chromomycosis with ketoconazole and 5-fluorocytosine. J Am Acad Dermatol 8:236, 1983.
23. Arenas R: Chromoblastomycosis. *In* Jacobs PH, Nall L (eds): Antifungal Drug Therapy: A Complete Guide for the Practitioner. New York, Marcel Dekker, 1990, pp 43–51.
24. Díaz M, Negroni R, Montero-Gei F, et al: A Pan American 5-year study of fluconazole therapy for deep mycoses in the immunocompetent host. Clin Infect Dis 14(Suppl 1):S68, 1992.

25. Tufanelli L, Milburn PB: Treatment of chromoblastomycosis. J Am Acad Dermatol 23:728, 1990.
26. Restrepo A, Gonzalez A, Gomez I, et al: Treatment of chromoblastomycosis with itraconazole. Ann N Y Acad Sci 544:504, 1988.
27. Franco L, Gomez I, Restrepo A: Saperconazole in the treatment of systemic and subcutaneous mycoses. Int J Dermatol 31:725, 1992.
28. Sharkey PK, Graybill JR, Rinaldi MG, et al: Itraconazole treatment of phaeohyphomycosis. J Am Acad Dermatol 23:577, 1990.
29. Rippon JW: Phaeohyphomycosis. *In* Rippon JW: Medical Mycology: The Pathogenic Fungi and the Pathogenic Actinomycetes, ed 3. Philadelphia, WB Saunders, 1988, pp 297–324.
30. Kawachi Y, Tateishi T, Shojima K, et al: Subcutaneous pheomycotic cyst of the finger caused by *Exophiala jeanselmei*: Association with a wooden splinter. Cutis 56:41, 1995.
31. Lavoie SR, Espinel-Ingroff A, Kerkering T: Mixed cutaneous phaeohyphomycosis in a cocaine user. Clin Infect Dis 17:114, 1993.
32. Grieshop TJ, Yarbrough D 3rd, Farrar WE: Case report: Phaeohyphomycosis due to *Curvularia lunata* involving the skin and subcutaneous tissue after an explosion at a chemical plant. Am J Med Sci 305:387, 1993.
33. Burges GE, Walls CT, Maize JC: Subcutaneous phaeohyphomycosis caused by *Exserohilum rostratum* in an immunocompetent host. Arch Dermatol 123:1346, 1987.
34. Faulk CT, Lesher JL: Phaeohyphomycosis and *Mycobacterium fortuitum* abscesses in a patient receiving corticosteroids for sarcoidosis. J Am Acad Dermatol 33:309, 1995.
35. Chaidemenos GC, Mourellou O, Karakatsanis G, et al: Cutaneous alternariosis in an immunocompromised patient. Cutis 56:145, 1995.
36. Coldiron BM, Wiley EL, Rinaldi MG: Cutaneous phaeohyphomycosis caused by a rare fungal pathogen, *Hormonema dematioides*: Successful treatment with ketoconazole. J Am Acad Dermatol 23:363, 1990.
37. Markham WD, Key RD, Padhye AA, et al: Phaeohyphomycotic cyst caused by *Tetraploa aristata*. J Med Vet Mycol 28:147, 1990.
38. Tam M, Freeman S: Phaeohyphomycosis due to *Phialophora richardsiae*. Australas J Dermatol 30:37, 1989.
39. Dooley DP, Beckius ML, Jeffery BS, et al: Phaeohyphomycotic cutaneous disease caused by *Pleurophoma* in a cardiac transplant patient. J Infect Dis 159:503, 1989.
40. Straka BF, Cooper PH, Body BA: Cutaneous *Bipolaris spicifera* infection. Arch Dermatol 125:1383, 1989.
41. Hironaga M, Nakano K, Yokoyama I, et al: *Phialophora repens*, an emerging agent of subcutaneous phaeohyphomycosis in humans. J Clin Microbiol 27:394, 1989.
42. Kotylo PK, Israel KS, Cohen JS, et al: Subcutaneous phaeohyphomycosis of the finger caused by *Exophiala spinifera*. Am J Clin Pathol 91:624, 1989.
43. Kettlewell P, McGinnis MR, Wilkinson GT: Phaeohyphomycosis caused by *Exophiala spinifera* in two cats. J Med Vet Mycol 27:257, 1989.
44. Matsumoto T, Matsuda T, Padhye AA, et al: Fungal melanonychia: Ungual phaeohyphomycosis caused by *Wangiella dermatitidis*. Clin Exp Dermatol 17:83, 1992.
45. Berg D, Garcia JA, Schell WA, et al: Cutaneous infection caused by *Curvularia pallescens*: A case report and review of the spectrum of disease. J Am Acad Dermatol 32:375, 1995.
46. Levenson JE, Duffin RM, Gardner SK, et al: Dematiaceous fungal keratitis following penetrating keratoplasty. Ophthalmic Surg 15:578, 1984.
47. Anandi V, Suryawanshi NB, Koshi G, et al: Corneal ulcer caused by *Bipolaris hawaiiensis*. J Med Vet Mycol 26:301, 1988.
48. Thomas PA: Mycotic keratitis—An underestimated mycosis. J Med Vet Mycol 32:235, 1994.
49. Bouchon CL, Greer DL, Genre CF: Corneal ulcer due to *Exserohilum longirostratum*. Am J Clin Pathol 101:452, 1994.
50. al-Hedaithy SS, al-Kaff AS: *Exophiala jeanselmei* keratitis. Mycoses 39:97, 1993.
51. Anandi V, George JA, Thomas R, et al: Phaeohyphomycosis of the eye caused by *Exserohilum rostratum* in India. Mycoses 34:489, 1991.
52. Aviv JE, Lawson W, Bottone EJ, et al: Multiple intracranial mucoceles associated with phaeohyphomycosis of the paranasal sinuses. Arch Otolaryngol Head Neck Surg 116:1210, 1990.
53. Rao A, Forgan-Smith R, Miller S, et al: Phaeohyphomycosis of the nasal sinuses caused by *Bipolaris* species. Pathology 21:280, 1989.
54. Lawson W, Blitzer A: Fungal infections of the nose and paranasal sinuses. Part II. Otolaryngol Clin North Am 26:1037, 1993.
55. Cody DT 2nd, Neel HB 3rd, Ferreiro JA, et al: Allergic fungal sinusitis: The Mayo Clinic experience. Laryngoscope 104:1074, 1994.
56. Manning SC, Schaefer SD, Close LG, et al: Culture-positive allergic fungal sinusitis. Arch Otolaryngol Head Neck Surg 117:174, 1991.
57. Manning SC, Mabry RL, Schaefer SD, et al: Evidence of IgE-mediated hypersensitivity in allergic fungal sinusitis. Laryngoscope 103:717, 1993.
58. Friedman GC, Hartwick RWJ, Ro JY, et al: Allergic fungal sinusitis: Report of three cases associated with dematiaceous fungi. Am J Clin Pathol 96:368, 1991.
59. Alvarez-Franco M, Reyes-Mugica M, Paller AS: Cutaneous *Fusarium* infection in an adolescent with acute leukemia. Pediatr Dermatol 9:62, 1992.
60. Bushelman SJ, Callen JP, Roth DN, et al: Disseminated *Fusarium solani* infection. J Am Acad Dermatol 32:346, 1995.
61. Sekhon AS, Galbraith J, Mielke BW, et al: Cerebral phaeohyphomycosis caused by *Xylohypha bantiana*, with a review of the literature. Eur J Epidemiol 8:387, 1992.
62. Borges MC Jr, Warren S, White W, et al: Pulmonary phaeohyphomycosis due to *Xylohypha bantiana*. Arch Pathol Lab Med 115:627, 1991.
63. Aldape KD, Fox HS, Roberts JP, et al: *Cladosporium trichoides* cerebral phaeohyphomycosis in a liver transplant recipient. Report of a case. Am J Clin Pathol 95:499, 1991.
64. Palaoglu S, Sav A, Basak T, et al: Cerebral phaeohyphomycosis. Neurosurgery 33:894, 1993.
65. Anandi V, John TJ, Walter A, et al: Cerebral phaeohyphomycosis caused by *Chaetomium globosum* in a renal transplant patient. J Clin Microbiol 27:2226, 1989.
66. Sides EH 3rd, Benson JD, Padhye AA: Phaeohyphomycotic brain abscess due to *Ochroconis gallopavum* in a patient with malignant lymphoma of a large cell type. J Med Vet Mycol 29:317, 1991.
67. al-Hedaithy SS, Jamjoom ZA, Saeed ES: Cerebral phaeohyphomycosis caused by *Fonsecaea pedrosoi* in Saudi Arabia. APMIS 3(Suppl):94, 1988.
68. Kenney RT, Kwon-Chung KJ, Waytes AT, et al: Successful treatment of systemic *Exophiala dermatitidis* infection in a patient with chronic granulomatous disease. Clin Infect Dis 14:235, 1992.
69. Salaki JS, Louria DB, Chmel H: Fungal and yeast infections of the central nervous system. A clinical review. Medicine (Baltimore) 63:108, 1984.
70. Gold WL, Vellend H, Salit IE, et al: Successful treatment of systemic and local infections due to *Exophiala* species. Clin Infect Dis 19:339, 1994.
71. Vukmir RB, Kusne S, Linden P, et al: Successful therapy for cerebral phaeohyphomycosis due to *Dactylaria gallopava* in a liver transplant recipient. Clin Infect Dis 19:714, 1994.
72. Noel SB, Greer DL, Abadie SM, et al: Primary cutaneous phaeohyphomycosis. Report of three cases. J Am Acad Dermatol 18:1023, 1988.
73. Rippon JW: Mycetoma. *In* Rippon JW: Medical Mycology: The Pathogenic Fungi and the Pathogenic Actinomycetes, ed 3. Philadelphia, WB Saunders, 1988, pp 80–118.
74. Magaña M, Magaña-García M: Mycetoma. Dermatol Clin 7:203, 1989.
75. Roberts SOB, MacKenzie DWR: Mycology. *In* Rook A, Ebling FJG, Wilkinson DS, et al (eds): Textbook of Dermatology, ed 4. Boston, Blackwell Scientific Publications, 1986, pp 980–982.
76. Mahgoub ES, Gumaa SA: Ketoconazole in the treatment of eumycetoma due to *Madurella mycetomii*. Trans R Soc Trop Med Hyg 78:376, 1984.
77. Hay RJ, MacKenzie DWR: Mycetoma (madura foot) in the United Kingdom: A survey of 44 cases. Clin Exp Dermatol 8:553, 1983.
78. Mahgoub ES: Mycetoma. *In* Tropical Mycoses. Beerse, Belgium, Janssen Research Council, 1990, pp 50–72.
79. Resnik BI, Burdick AE: Improvement of eumycetoma with itraconazole. J Am Acad Dermatol 33:917, 1995.

283

Phycomycetes

Burt R. Meyers
Alejandra C. Gurtman

The class Zygomycetes consists of two orders containing species pathogenic for humans, Mucorales and Entomophthorales. The order Mucorales is further divided into six genera, of which three, *Mucor, Rhizopus*, and *Absidia*, are the most important; infections with species of *Cunninghamella* and *Mortierella* have been described,[1–3] and, less commonly, infections with *Saksenaea, Syncephalastrum, Apophysomyces*, and *Thamnidium*[4–8] (Table 283–1). The order Mucorales is associated with mucormycosis and does not include infection with *Entomophthora* organisms. The two main pathogenic genera of Entomophthorales are *Conidiobolus* and *Basidiobolus*. Tropical subcutaneous phycomycosis and rhinoentomophthoromycosis are rather indolent infections associated with nodules and granuloma formation.[1, 9–11] Mucorales infections usually are rapidly progressive, invading blood vessels, leading to infarction of tissue involving vital organs such as the brain and lung,[12–17] and often associated with a fatal outcome.

Microbiology and Morphology of the Mucorales

Growth of these fungi on either food or agar is characterized by a white or gray woolly appearance (Fig. 283–1). This growth represents mycelia with multiple nuclei that are nonseptate. All the genera give rise to specialized mycelia known as conidiophores, which are sacs filled with asexual spores called sporangia. A rhizoid, filament-like mycelium that extends into the air is also seen. The genera can be further classified by differences in the origin of the rhizoids and sporangiophores for the genera *Rhizopus* and *Absidia* (Fig. 283–2); the genus *Mucor*, on the other hand, does not produce rhizoids and therefore appears less abundant in culture. The columella, the tip of sporangiophore appearing within the sporangium, differentiates *Cunninghamella* from the other genera, which do not possess this structure.

Colonies of Entomophthorales differ from those of Mucorales, being flat and covered with white fuzz. This order also produces septate hyphae, which differentiate it from the Mucorales, which are nonseptate. The genera can be further differentiated by the presence or absence of zygospores and other changes in conidiophores.

Epidemiology

Mucorales are ubiquitous saprophytes found throughout the world that usually thrive in any organic material. They can affect fruits (including strawberries) and sweet potatoes and account for the mold that grows on moist bread. *Aspergillus* species are often found in hospital environments, whereas Mucorales organisms are not. Mucormycosis involving the skin and subcutaneous tissue was reported in hospitals when contaminated elastic dressings were used.[18]

Cunninghamella

In 1988, 10 cases of infection secondary to *Cunninghamella* species were reported.[19] The fungus is a soil saprophyte that

TABLE 283–1 ■ Classification of Pathogenic Zygomycetes

PATHOGEN	COMMENTS
Order 1: Mucorales	
Family 1: Mucoraceae	Rhinocerebral, rhinoorbital/paranasal, cardiac involvement; pulmonary, gastrointestinal, skin and soft tissue involvement; disseminated disease; osteomyelitis; cerebral involvement; occurs in patients with chronic renal failure or hemodialysis taking deferoxamine
Genera: *Absidia, Apophysomyces, Mucor, Rhizomucor, Rhizopus*	
Pathogenic species: *Absidia corymbifera, Apophysomyces elegans, Mucor circinelloides, Mucor hiemalis, Mucor racemosus, Mucor ramosissimus, Rhizomucor miehei, Rhizomucor pusillus, Rhizopus arrhizus, Rhizopus microsporus, Rhizopus microsporus rhizopodiformis*	
Family 2: Mortierellaceae	Bovine abortion
Genus: *Mortierrella*	
Pathogenic species: *Mortierella wolfii*	
Family 3: Cunninghamellaceae	Disseminated disease, thrombocytopenia
Genus: *Cunninghamella*	
Pathogenic species: *Cunninghamella bertholletiae*	
Family 4: Sakenaeaceae	Subcutaneous infection, disseminated disease, osteomyelitis
Genus: *Saksenaea*	
Pathogenic species: *Saksenaea vasiformis*	
Family 5: Syncephalastraceae	
Genus: *Syncephalastrum*	
Pathogenic species: Not identified to species level	
Family 6: Thamnidiaceae	Chronic cystitis
Genus: *Cokeromyces*	
Pathogenic species: *Cokeromyces recurvatus*	
Order 2: Entomophthorales	
Family 1: Entomophthoraceae	Subcutaneous granuloma; rhinopharyngeal, sinus, and pulmonary involvement
Genus: *Conidiobolus*	
Pathogenic species: *Conidiobolus coronatus, Conidiobolus incongruus*	
Family 2: Basidiobolaceae	Subcutaneous granuloma, adenopathy
Genus: *Basidiobolus*	
Pathogenic species: *Basidiobolus ranarum*	

Adapted from Rinaldi MG: Zygomycosis. Infect Dis Clin North Am 3:19–41, 1989.

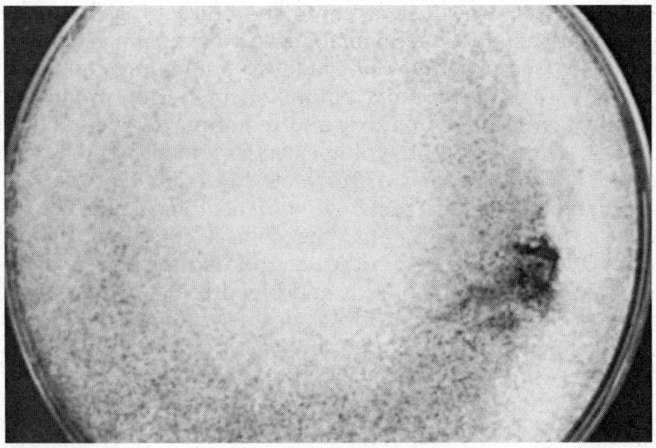

FIGURE 283–1 □ Moldlike growth of *Rhizopus* species covering the entire surface of a plate with Sabouraud agar after 48 hours' incubation at 37°C.

can cause disseminated disease; the only clinical presentation may be fever associated with thrombocytopenia.[20] There is only one report of disease without hematogenous spread, which presented as a chronic infection in the skin resembling an entomophthoromycosis infection. Sensitivity to amphotericin B varies.[21, 22]

Entomophthorales

Entomophthorales organisms are usually found in tropical climates and typically infect immunocompetent hosts. Infections with these organisms have not been described in the Western Hemisphere. Because the fungus grows poorly at 15°C, it has been suggested that in temperate climates it is disseminated only during warm months from its reservoir in reptiles that feed on insects. *Basidiobolus haptosporus* infection probably follows insect bites or minor trauma in children in this environment. Infection with *Conidiobolus coronatus* usually follows inhalation of spores and is observed in adult agricultural workers exposed to tropical rain forest vegetation.[23]

Although the organisms infect the nasal mucosa they usually do not cause tissue infarction, because blood vessels are not invaded. The affinity of these spores for the nasal mucosa has not been adequately described. Invasive disease caused by *Conidiobolus incongruus* has been reported in a granulocytopenic host.[74]

Mucormycosis has worldwide distribution and usually occurs in association with underlying conditions, including diabetes mellitus with or without ketoacidosis, lymphoid malignancy, burns, severe trauma, prolonged postoperative courses, multiple myeloma, hepatitis, cirrhosis, renal failure[25] steroid therapy, and immunodeficiency states (induced or acquired[26]), as well as use of contaminated Elastoplast bandages.[18] Uncontrolled diabetes with hyperglycemia and acidosis is often the setting for the development of serious infection with the Zygomycetes. High levels of glucose impair phagocytosis. Delayed or diminished neutrophil chemotaxis has been described in diabetic patients with ketoacidosis. Other studies in vitro have shown that *Rhizopus* favors an acid environment, a temperature of 39°C, and glucose-rich media.[27] A normal leukocyte complement is important in preventing mucormycosis, as demonstrated in animal infection,[28] because neutropenia reduces resistance to mucormycosis. Bronchoalveolar macrophages prevent spore germination and tissue invasion. In experimentally induced diabetic animal models or those treated with cortisone, phagocytosis is reduced and the macrophages allow spore germination and infection.[29] Other serum factors (i.e., antibodies) are probably necessary to inhibit spore germination.[30]

Infection is probably initiated by the inhalation of asexual sporangiospore spores through the nose and into the sinuses, from where the organism may extend into the cerebrum and retroorbital tissues; spores may enter the lower airways and settle in the alveoli or enter through denuded skin. When they cause infection, these fungi have a predilection for invading blood vessels, leading to venous and arterial thrombosis with subsequent ischemia and gangrene. Spores of Mucorales may also invade bronchi, stomach, and intestines of neutropenic patients.

The clinical states associated with mucormycosis include rhinocerebral-rhinoorbital-paranasal syndrome; pulmonary, gastrointestinal, cardiac, skin, and soft tissue involvement; a disseminated form; osteomyelitis; cerebritis; and chronic renal failure (in hemodialysis patients receiving deferoxamine).

With Entomophthorales infection, three clinical syndromes have been described: basidiobolomycosis, subcutaneous granuloma infiltrating muscle with lymph gland hyperplasia; rhinoentomophthoromycosis, granulomata of the inferior turbinate with superficial spread without ulceration to the nasopharynx or paranasal sinuses; and pulmonary infection by *C. incongruus*. In none of these cases does tissue destruction occur.

A common antigen is shared by *Absidia, Rhizopus,* and *Mucor* organisms. Although some specific antigens for each genus have been found by immunodiffusion, their role in the diagnosis of acute disease has not been elucidated. Fewer data are available for the Entomophthorales.

Clinical Syndromes

In patients who have a predisposing factor such as leukemia, malignancy, immunosuppression, or diabetes mellitus, infection may occur in the nasal turbinates, the paranasal sinuses, the palate, and the eye or retroorbital area with invasion into brain and cavernous sinus (Fig. 283–3). However, rarely, rhinocerebral infection may occur in a normal patient.[31] Symptoms depend on the areas involved. With the rhinocerebral form, fever, facial and orbital pain, headache, diplopia, loss of vision, and facial or orbital cellulitis may be noted. Facial anesthesia may be an early clinical sign. Cranial nerve involvement is not uncommon. Black nasal discharge in this setting is often mistaken for dried blood rather than evidence of tissue infarction. Careful physical examination of the pharynx, nasal turbinate, and palate for necrotic ulcerations is necessary. Physical signs may include proptosis, chemosis,

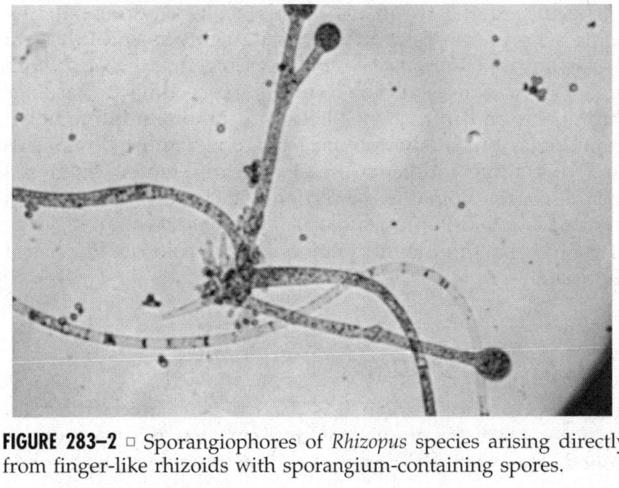

FIGURE 283–2 □ Sporangiophores of *Rhizopus* species arising directly from finger-like rhizoids with sporangium-containing spores.

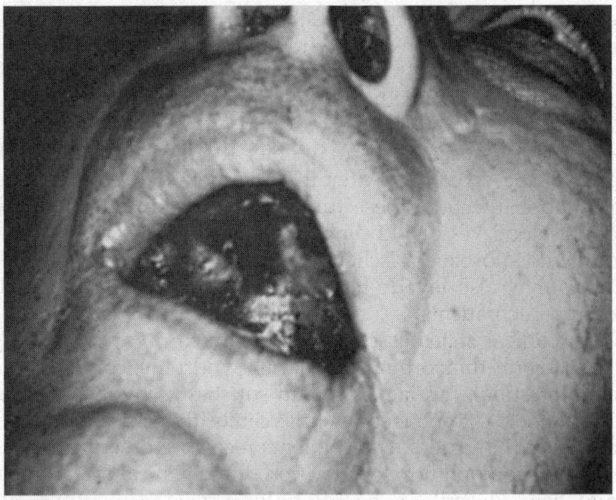

FIGURE 283–3 □ Necrosis of the hard palate secondary to invasion by *Rhizopus* species in a renal transplant patient taking corticosteroids.

and retinal infarction; thrombosis of the cavernous sinus or internal carotid artery may occur. Patients may develop seizures and epistaxis. Radiographic examination usually reveals evidence of destruction of the paranasal sinuses or of inflammation; computed tomography or magnetic resonance imaging best reveals involvement of the sinuses and orbital and retroorbital areas.

Diagnostic Procedures

The diagnosis is best established by direct examination and culture of infected tissue obtained by biopsy, because superficial culture of necrotic material may reveal only colonizing microorganisms; areas from which to obtain biopsy material include the buccal, nasal, and palatal mucosa or paranasal sinuses. Examination of a smear of tissue with direct light without staining may establish the diagnosis within minutes after the biopsy procedure. Morphologically, broad, nonseptate, nonpigmented hyphae 15 to 20 μm in diameter, up to 20 μm long, often with right-angled branching are noted. The hyphae of *Aspergillus* species are smaller and septate and branch at acute angles. Blood culture should be attempted, although the organism is rarely isolated. Spinal tap may reveal pleocytosis, usually with an elevated protein value; the glucose level may be normal. Culture of cerebrospinal fluid is necessary, but the organism has not been isolated from the central nervous system.

The differential diagnosis of this acute syndrome in patients who are at risk includes acute sinusitis secondary to *Aspergillus* or *Pseudomonas aeruginosa* infection, because both organisms can invade blood vessels, proceeding to vascular thrombosis and infarction. Malignant tumors, midline lethal granuloma, Burkitt lymphoma, and noma must be considered. For more indolent disease, the differential diagnosis includes granulomatous infections, including other fungi (i.e., blastomycosis), tuberculosis, syphilis, and leprosy, each of which can produce ulceration and invasion of the nasal turbinate.

Therapy and Outcome

Intravenous amphotericin B is the drug of choice; the total dose necessary for eradication and cure has not been determined. The empirical dose is 1 to 2 g; in some cases 4 g has been necessary to effect a cure. The efficacy of the azole compounds in the treatment of Zygomycetes infections is limited to one experimental model in guinea pigs and few human cases.[31a] Liposomal amphotericin B is a promising therapy, because it is nontoxic and requires a short period of infusion with low fluid volume, and premedication is not required. The liposomes disseminate in organs that are rich in reticuloendothelial cells.[32] If a patient has evidence of acidosis and hyperglycemia, the clinical condition should be reversed immediately; other supportive therapy may be necessary—intravenous fluids and blood pressure and ventilatory support. Synergy of flucytosine with rifampin and tetracycline has been reported. In some cases, local irrigation of infected sinuses with amphotericin B has been employed. The use of hyperbaric oxygen is suggested, although clinical trials have not determined its efficacy.[33, 34] In one study in which all patients had premortem diagnoses, patients with diabetes mellitus tended to survive, whereas those with acute leukemia and transplant recipients did not.[12] In another study, Parfrey[14] noted that survival before 1970 was 6% compared with 73% thereafter.[14] Another study reviewing survival in patients with paranasal sinus mucormycosis revealed that survival had increased to 70% in the years 1970 to 1979, compared with early estimates with lower survival data. It appears that the chance of survival is better for patients who have no underlying disease (75%) or diabetes (60%) than for those who have renal disease (25%); the overall survival rate, including cases before 1960, was 50% in the 179 cases surveyed. The authors noted that surgical débridement or radical resection and amphotericin B therapy significantly increased the chances of survival; 79% of diabetics who received the drug survived, versus 37% of those who did not receive the drug. With amphotericin B and surgery, 81% survived (and 89% of those who also had diabetes). Prognosis was poorer for patients with hemiplegia, facial necrosis, and nasal deformity. Survival was not related to age or sex, laterality of involvement, or x-ray findings.[13]

A review of 33 patients with mucormycosis revealed that patients with only rhinoorbital or paranasal involvement had a better prognosis than those with either cerebral or disseminated disease.[14] Invasive fungal sinusitis must be differentiated from chronic noninvasive disease, which has also been associated with fungal colonization. In the latter case, cure is usually associated with surgical removal of hyphal masses and draining of sinuses.[35] Itraconazole is generally not active against Zygomycetes.[36]

Specific Infections

Pulmonary Mucormycosis

Pulmonary mucormycosis is characterized by invasion of the pulmonary vessels, with lung infarction and pneumonia.[37, 38] Patients with underlying disease (diabetes, leukemia, lymphoma) and allograft recipients are at risk for infection. Spores of Mucorales enter through the nares into the nasal sinus, and subsequently to bronchi and lungs. The organism then invades blood vessels, causing pulmonary hemorrhage, infarction, and gangrene. Lymphatics may also be involved; the disease may run an indolent course and produce a solitary nodule on chest radiographs. On histologic section and examination, nonseptate hyphae surrounded by neutrophilic leukocytes are noted.

Clinically there is evidence of pulmonary infarction, pneumonia, lung abscess, or any combination of these. The presentation may be acute and fulminant or subacute. Patients with underlying disease who experience a new episode of chills, fever, and pulmonary infiltrates, especially if they are receiving antibiotics, should be suspected of having fungal infection. Sudden onset of pleuritic chest pain, bloody sputum, and pleural friction rub in this setting is highly suggestive; the x-ray appearance of an infarction with cavitation suggests either *Mucor* or *Aspergillus* species. Usually the patchy, heterogeneous infiltrate progresses, despite antibiotic therapy, into consolidation and cavity formation, often associated with a hemorrhagic pleural effusion. The condition may be complicated by massive hemoptysis and death, the pulmonary vessels being eroded by the fungus; endogenous spread to all organs has been described.[39] Severe bacterial superinfection by *Pseudomonas* or *Staphylococcus* has been reported.[16] The disease may be less fulminant in diabetic patients, producing a subacute pneumonitis, with or without cavitation.[40]

DIAGNOSIS

Pulmonary mucormycosis should be considered when immunocompromised patients have evidence of pulmonary infarction or acute pneumonitis that does not respond to antimicrobial agents. Because Mucorales organisms are rarely seen on Gram stain or isolated from sputum culture, further diagnostic studies may be necessary: bronchoalveolar lavage and broncoscopy with transbronchial biopsy of lung parenchyma for smear, culture, and histologic examination. Patients who are profoundly thrombocytopenic may require platelet transfusions before undergoing this procedure. On examination of the tissue, large, broad nonseptate hyphae with wide-angled branching suggest Mucorales. Isolates should be sent to the laboratory for plating on blood or Sabouraud agar at 37°C and kept for 10 to 14 days; growth usually occurs within 1 or 2 days. Direct plating of biopsy material on agar increases the yield.

The differential diagnosis includes other infectious agents (fungi, parasites) that produce pulmonary disease in immunocompromised hosts. *Nocardia asteroides* produces acute necrotizing pneumonia, often with cerebral involvement. Examination of sputum and tissue may reveal threadlike, beaded, branching, gram-positive filamentous rods that are also partially acid-fast. *Aspergillus* species can invade blood vessels and produce an identical clinical picture. Differentiation can be made only with tissue specimens or culture. Other organisms that cause pneumonia in immunocompromised hosts include *Pneumocystis carinii* and cytomegalovirus. In patients with these infections, pneumonia is diffuse, often associated with dyspnea and hypoxia; cavitation and hemoptysis do not usually occur. *Legionella* species may also produce pulmonary cavitation, but this is uncommon.

When *Mucor* infection is suspected, therapy should be instituted promptly with intravenous amphotericin B. In most cases treatment is empirical; patients receive between 1 and 2 g; the total dose necessary for cure is not known. Other imidazole agents are being studied. The role of neutrophil transfusions has not been studied. In some cases, surgical resection is necessary for cure, especially in nonimmunosuppressed patients.[41] Patients have survived even without the administration of amphotericin B.[42]

Gastrointestinal Zygomycosis

Patients with underlying conditions such as kwashiorkor, malnutrition, pellagra, amebic colitis, uremia, and typhoid fever are more susceptible to gastrointestinal zygomycosis[43]; the incidence is increased in South Africa compared with the rest of the world. Infection may occur in the neonatal period.[44] The route of infection is believed to be secondary to ingestion of fungi, which then may colonize or infect the gastrointestinal tract, especially in patients who had gastric ulcers; one third of patients are children. The stomach and large bowel are the organs most commonly involved; invasion of blood vessels causes ischemia, necrosis, and infarction. Symptoms include abdominal pain, diarrhea, hematemesis, and bloody stools. Erosive necrotic ulcers and gangrene, hemorrhages, peritonitis, and bowel infarction are associated. Diagnosis is made by biopsy and cultures; stool and gastric cultures should be obtained, although results are rarely positive. The cause of death is shock secondary to hemorrhagic infarction; most cases have been recognized at autopsy.

Cutaneous Zygomycosis

Cutaneous zygomycosis can be primary or secondary and has occurred in patients with burns,[45] diabetes mellitus,[45] postsurgical wound infections,[46] elastic (Elastoplast) bandages,[18] or as part of nodular lesions, secondary to hematogenous seeding. Primary cutaneous mucormycosis may follow trauma; outcome depends on the extension and location of the injury.[47, 48] Diagnosis is based on the demonstration of the fungus in culture or biopsy specimens. Parenteral amphotericin B or a solution containing 5 mg/mL applied with gauze or by atomization may be required.[49] When this therapy is not successful, patients may need aggressive surgical débridement, amputation, or both.

Disseminated Zygomycosis (Rare)

After primary infection in the lungs, the fungi can spread to the central nervous system, gastrointestinal tract, spleen, kidneys, and heart. The disseminated form of zygomycosis is more commonly seen in patients with lymphoid malignancies. It is uniformly fatal, and the diagnosis is usually made at necropsy.

Cardiac Mucormycosis

Endocarditis has been reported without prior cardiac involvement,[50] as well as in association with cardiac surgery and infection of prosthetic valves[51]; large vegetations with symptoms secondary to subsequent emboli may occur. Diffuse cardiac involvement may occur in patients with underlying diseases. Diagnosis is suggested by echocardiography, because blood cultures rarely propagate the pathogen. Surgical extirpation may be curative.

Septic Arthritis and Osteomyelitis

Osteomyelitis of the femur has been observed secondary to hematogenous spread[52]; cranial bone involvement in the absence of rhinocerebral involvement has been described. Recently after trauma, a patient with acquired immunodeficiency syndrome developed a cutaneoarticular form of *Cunninghamella* infection[53]; bone infection of the ankle secondary to a primary cutaneous infection has also been reported.[54]

Brain Abscess

After inadvertent direct intravenous injection of the fungus the most common presentation is brain abscess[55]; 22 cases have been reported in the literature, half of them in intravenous drug users.[56] The basal ganglia are most often affected; deep abscesses were noted.[57] The clinical presentation includes fever, headaches, and lethargy; hemiparesis and speech disturbances may be the initial presentation. Most patients died despite attempts at surgery and amphotericin B therapy.

Mucormycosis in Hemodialysis Patients

Mucormycosis has been seen with increased frequency in hemodialysis patients,[58] who received deferoxamine therapy for iron and aluminum overload.[19, 59] Iron is a growth factor for some bacteria and fungi. Patients who received iron have a greater incidence of infections such as tuberculosis, malaria, brucellosis, and amebiasis.[60] Deferoxamine might increase the availability of iron to the fungi, acting as a growth promoter. It is postulated that the microorganism may be unable to synthesize siderophores but has receptors for them; the organism might use deferoxamine as a siderophore as a source of iron. This may be the same mechanism that promotes *Yersinia* infection in these patients.[6]

Conclusion

Even though the treatment and prognosis of mucormycosis have improved, infection with these organisms still is associated with a high mortality rate. If prognosis and survival are to improve, early diagnosis must be achieved, as well as control of the underlying disorder, aggressive surgery when indicated, and systemic antifungal therapy.

References

1. Rinaldi MG: Zygomycosis. Infect Dis Clin North Am 3:19, 1989.
2. Rippon JW: Medical Mycology: The Pathogenic Fungi and the Pathogenic Actinomycetes, ed 2. Philadelphia, WB Saunders, 1988, pp 615–640.
3. Bottone EJ, Weitzman I, Hanna BA: *Rhizopus rhizopodiformis:* Emerging etiological agent of mucormycosis. J Clin Microbiol 9:530, 1979.
4. Pierce PF, Wood MB, Roberts GD, et al: *Saksenaea vasiformis* osteomyelitis. J Clin Microbiol 25:933, 1987.
5. Axelrod P, Kwon-Chung KJ, Frawley P, et al: Chronic cystitis due to *Cokeromyces recurvatus:* A case report. J Infect Dis 155:1062, 1987.
6. Padhye AA, Koshi G, Anandi V, et al: First case of subcutaneous zygomycosis caused by *Saksenaea vasiformis* in India. Diagn Microbiol Infect Dis 9:69, 1988.
7. Meis JPGM, Kullberg B-J, Pruszczynski M, Veth RPH: Severe osteomyelitis due to the zygomycete *Apophysomyces elegans*. J Clin Microbiol 32:3078, 1994.
8. Huffnagle KE, Southern PM Jr, Byrd LT, Gander RM: *Apophysomyces elegans* as an agent of zygomycosis in a patient following trauma. J Med Vet Mycol 30:83, 1992.
9. Braude AI: The zygomycetes. *In* Braude AI, Davis CE, Fierer J (eds): Infectious Diseases and Medical Microbiology, ed 2. Philadelphia, WB Saunders, 1986, pp 597–601.
10. Martinson FD: Phycomycosis (zgomycosis). *In* Braude AI, Davis CE, Fierer J (eds): Infectious Diseases and Medical Microbiology, ed 2. Philadelphia, WB Saunders, 1986, pp 743–748.
11. Burkitt DP, Wilson A, Jelliffe D: Subcutaneous phycomycosis: A review of 31 cases seen in Uganda. Br Med J 1:1669, 1964.
12. Meyers BR, Wormser G, Hirschman SZ, et al: Rhinocerebral mucormycosis. Diagnosis premortem and therapy. Arch Intern Med 139:557, 1979.
13. Blitzer A, Lawson W, Meyers BR, et al: Patient survival factors in paranasal sinus mucormycosis. Laryngoscope 90:635, 1980.
14. Parfrey NA: Improved diagnosis and prognosis of mucormycosis. Medicine (Baltimore) 65:113, 1986.
15. Lehrer R: Mucormycosis. Ann Intern Med 93:108, 1980.
16. Meyer RD, Rosen P, Armstrong D: Phycomycosis complicating leukemia and lymphoma. Ann Intern Med 77:871, 1972.
17. Marchevsky AM, Bottone EJ, Geller SA, et al: The changing spectrum of disease, etiology and diagnosis of mucormycosis. Hum Pathol 11:457, 1980.
18. Gartenberg G, Bottone E, Keusch G, et al: Hospital-acquired mucormycosis *(Rhizopus rhizopodiformis)* of skin and subcutaneous tissue: Epidemiology, mycology and treatment. N Engl J Med 299:1115, 1978.
19. Rex JM, Ginsberg AM, Fries LF, et al: *Cunninghamella bertholletiae* infection associated with deferoxamine therapy. Rev Infect Dis 10:1187, 1988.
20. McGinnis MR, Walker DM, Dominy IE, et al: Zygomycosis caused by *Cunninghamella bertholletiae.* Arch Pathol Lab Med 106:282, 1982.
21. Kolbeck PC, Makhoul RG, Randal Bollinger R, Sanfilippo F: Widely disseminated *Cunninghamella* mucormycosis in an adult renal transplant patient: Case report and review of the literature. Am J Clin Pathol 83:747, 1984.
22. McGinnis MR, Walker DH, Dominy IE, et al: Zygomycosis caused by *Cunninghamella bertholletiae.* Arch Pathol Lab Med 106:287, 1982.
23. Ng KH, Chin CS, Jalleh RD, et al: Nasofacial zygomycosis. Oral Surg Oral Med Oral Pathol 72:685, 1991.
24. Walsh TJ, Renshaw G, Andrews J, et al: Invasive zygomycosis due to *Conidiobolus incongruus.* Clin Infect Dis 19:423, 1994.
25. Hammer GS, Bottone EJ, Hirschman SZ: Mucormycosis in a transplant recipient. Am J Clin Pathol 64:389, 1975.
26. Cuadrado LM, Guerrero A, Lopez Garcia Asenjo GA, et al: Cerebral mucormycosis in two cases of acquired immunodeficiency syndrome. Arch Neurol 1:109, 1988.
27. Reinhardt FJ, Kaplan W, Ajello L: Experimental cerebral zygomycosis in alloxan-diabetic rabbits. I. Relationship of temperature tolerance of selected zygomycetes to pathogenicity. Infect Immun 2:404, 1970.
28. Artis WM, Fountain JA, Delcher HK, et al: A mechanism of susceptibility to mucormycosis in diabetic ketoacidosis: Transferrin and iron availability. Diabetes 31:1109, 1982.
29. Waldorf AR, Levitz SM, Diamond RD: In vivo bronchoalveolar macrophage defense against *Rhizopus oryzae* and *Aspergillus fumigatus.* J Infect Dis 150:752, 1984.
30. Waldorf AR, Halde C, Vedros NA: Murine model of pulmonary mucormycosis in cortisone-treated mice. Sabouraudia 20:217, 1982.
31. Radner AB, Witt MD, Edwards JE Jr: Acute invasive rhinocerebral zygomycosis in an otherwise healthy patient: Case report and review. Clin Infect Dis 20:163, 1995.

31a. Van Cutsem J, Van Gerven F, Fransen J, et al: Treatment of experimental zygomycosis in guinea pigs: Azoles and amphotericin B. Chemotherapy 35:267, 1989.

32. Lopez-Berestein G, Fainstein V, Hopfer R, et al: Liposomal amphotericin B for the treatment of systemic fungal infection in patients with cancer: A preliminary study. J Infect Dis 151:704, 1985.
33. Ferguson BJ, Mitchell TG, Moon R, et al: Adjunctive hyperbaric oxygen for treatment of rhinocerebral mucormycosis. Rev Infect Dis 10:551, 1988.
34. Couch L, Theilen F, Mader JT: Rhinocerebral mucormycosis with cerebral extension successfully treated with adjunctive hyperbaric oxygen therapy. Arch Otolaryngol Head Neck Surg 114: 791, 1988.
35. Washburn RG, Kennedy DW, Begley MG, et al: Chronic fungal sinusitis in apparently normal hosts. Medicine (Baltimore) 67: 231, 1988.
36. Grant SM, Clissold SP: Itraconazole—A review of its pharmacodynamic and pharmacokinetic properties, and therapeutic use in superficial and systemic mycoses. Drugs 37:310, 1989.
37. Meyers BR: Pulmonary mucormycosis. *In* Braude AI, Davis CE, Fierer J (eds): Infectious Diseases and Medical Microbiology, ed 2. Philadelphia, WB Saunders, 1986, pp 875–877.
38. Baker RD: Pulmonary mucormycosis. Am J Pathol 32:287, 1956.
39. Meyer R, Kaplan M, Ong M: Cutaneous lesions in disseminated mucormycosis. JAMA 225:737, 1973.
40. Murray HW: Pulmonary mucormycosis with massive fatal hemoptysis. Chest 68:65, 1975.
41. Temeck BK, Benzon DJ, Moskaluk CA, Pass HI: Thoracotomy for pulmonary mycoses in non–HIV-immunosuppressed patients. Ann Thorac Surg 58:333, 1994.
42. Gribetz AR, Chuang MT, Burrows L, et al: *Rhizopus* lung abscess in renal transplant patient successfully treated by lobectomy. Chest 77:102, 1980.
43. Calle S, Klatsky S: Interstitial phycomycosis (mucormycosis). Am J Clin Pathol 45:264, 1966.
44. Reimund E, Ramos A: Disseminated neonatal gastrointestinal mucormycosis: A case report and review of the literature. Pediatr Pathol 14:385, 1944.

45. Bruk HM, Nash G, Foley FD, et al: Opportunistic fungal infection of the burn wound with *Phycomycetes* and *Aspergillus*. Arch Surg 102:476, 1971.
46. Paparello SF, Parry RL, MacGillivray DC, et al: Hospital-acquired wound mucormycosis. Clin Infect Dis 14:350, 1992.
47. Johnson PC, Satter White RK, Monheit JE, et al: Primary cutaneous mucormycosis in trauma patients. J Trauma 27:437, 1987.
48. Vainrub B, Macarsno A, Mander S, et al: Wound zygomycosis (mucormycosis) in otherwise healthy adults. Am J Med 84:546, 1988.
49. Green JF, Dhaliwal AS: Cutaneous mucormycosis. Infect Med 4:423, 1987.
50. Virmani R, Connor DH, McAllister HA: Cardiac mucormycosis. Am J Clin Pathol 78:42, 1982.
51. Chaudhry R, Venugopal P, Chopra P: Prosthetic mitral valve mucormycosis caused by *Mucor* species. Int J Cardiol 17:333, 1987.
52. Echols RM, Selinger DS, Hallowell C, et al: *Rhizopus* osteomyelitis: A case report and review. Am J Med 66:141, 1979.
53. Mostaza JM, Barbado FJ, Fernandez-Martrin J, et al: Cutaneoarticular mucormycosis due to *Cunninghamella bertholletiae* in a patient with AIDS. Rev Infect Dis 77:316, 1989.
54. Maliwan N, Reyes CV, Rippon JW: Osteomyelitis secondary to cutaneous mucormycosis. Report of a case and a review of the literature. Am J Dermatol Pathol 6:479, 1984.
55. Pierce PF, Solomon SL, Kaufman L, et al: Zygomycetes brain abscesses in narcotic addicts with serological diagnosis. JAMA 248:2881, 1982.
56. Freeman Woods K, Hanna BJ: Brain stem mucormycosis in a narcotic addict with eventual recovery. Am J Med 80:126, 1986.
57. Stave GM, Heimberger T, Kerkering TM: Zygomycosis of the basal ganglia in intravenous drug users. Am J Med 86:115, 1989.
58. Boelaret JR, Fenves AZ, Coburn JW: Mucormycosis among patients on dialysis. N Engl J Med 321:190, 1989.
59. Boelaert JR, van Roost GF, Vergauwe PL, et al: The role of desferrioxamine in dialysis-associated mucormycosis: Report of three cases and review of the literature. Clin Nephrol 29:261, 1988.
60. Murray MJ, Murray AB: Adverse effect of iron repletion on infection (Abstr). Am J Clin Nutr 31:700, 1978.
61. Robins-Browne RM, Prpic JK: Effects of iron and desferrioxamine on infections with *Yersinia enterocolitica.* Infect Immun 47:774, 1985.

284

Miscellaneous Fungi

Alan M. Sugar

With each passing year, the list of fungi recovered from patients with a variety of infections increases. An ever-expanding array of fungi are identified as new pathogens and others, previously thought to be saprophytes, are implicated in serious invasive infections. The patients at greatest risk of developing such infections are those with the most seriously impaired immune systems. The importance of the neutrophil in protection against invasion from these organisms with low virulence is clear, and the role of high doses of corticosteroids in predisposing toward the development of these infections is appreciated. As the numbers of immunocompromised patients increases, the numbers of opportunistic fungal infections will also increase and will include infections with the more exotic organisms, some of which are reviewed here. An encyclopedic reference source is available for the interested reader and for the clinician confronted with a patient infected with one of the rarely recovered fungi.[1]

Fusarium Species

These molds are well-known plant pathogens, living in soil worldwide. Although now being encountered more frequently as agents of invasive infections, *Fusarium* species have been appreciated as rather common etiologic agents recovered from patients with fungal keratitis, mycetoma, and onychomycosis. The following species have been recovered from invasive infection:

Fusarium moniliforme
Fusarium proliferatum
Fusarium oxysporum
Fusarium solani
Fusarium napiforme

Given their widespread distribution in the environment, it is not surprising that the organism can be acquired through direct inoculation. This is the usual mode of transmission of infection in cases of corneal infection, endophthalmitis, continuous ambulatory peritoneal dialysis–associated peritonitis, localized skin disease, and nail infections.[2, 3] In the immunocompetent host, there is little risk of dissemination of the infection from the initial focus. However, in patients with neutropenia, and rarely in those receiving large doses of corticosteroids, disseminated disease has been increasingly recognized.[4–9]

Fusarium species grow in the environment and in tissue as molds. The characteristic microscopic appearance is that of narrow, septate hyphae, with acute angle branching. By histopathologic criteria, they are indistinguishable from several other fungi, especially *Aspergillus* species. The hyphae are most easily visualized in tissue after staining with periodic acid–Schiff or Gomori–methenamine silver.

In the laboratory, *Fusarium* grows rapidly on agar, but cycloheximide inhibits its growth. Mature colonies can produce a variety of pigments depending on the species. The genus derives from the characteristic morphology of the fusiform conidia.

Invasive fusariosis is primarily a disease of neutropenic patients. Thus, patients with leukemia and those undergoing bone marrow transplantation are at greatest risk for developing this mycosis during the neutropenic phase of their therapy. Most often beginning as fever during the neutropenic episode, clinically evident fusariosis is most commonly seen as a pulmonary illness, often with cutaneous manifestations. Blood culture results are frequently positive in patients with fusariosis, in contrast to the negative blood culture results in patients with aspergillosis. The chest film may demonstrate infiltrates or nodules, but the lesions are best seen by computed tomography of the lungs and are often evident as multiple nodular lesions. Because the organism is acquired through the respiratory tract, it is not surprising to see patients with sinusitis caused by *Fusarium*.

Many of the clinical and histopathologic manifestations of fusariosis overlap those of aspergillosis. Given the different antifungal susceptibility patterns of *Aspergillus* and *Fusarium* species, this distinction may be of great clinical utility. However, some features tend to favor one organism over the other. For example, positive blood culture results are distinctly uncommon in patients with aspergillosis but are common in patients with fusariosis (approximately 40%).[6] Skin lesions are also more commonly found in patients with fusarial infection, with up to 79% of such patients developing cutaneous manifestations of the infection.[8]

Mortality of patients with invasive fusariosis is high, the

causes likely being profound and continuing neutropenia combined with the relative lack of efficacy of amphotericin B.[10] However, clinical experience with other antifungal drugs is limited, and some authors still recommend amphotericin B as the drug of first choice in treating disseminated fusariosis.[8] Much of the mortality may be explained by the extremely immunocompromised nature of the patients with these infections and the lack of return of normal neutrophil counts. In such a setting, recovery would be exceptional and no antifungal drug can be expected to be efficacious. Liposomal amphotericin B has been reported to be active, perhaps because more amphotericin B can be administered to the patient.[11–13] Until more evidence is available, initial therapy should be with amphotericin B, either in the traditional formulation with deoxycholate or as one of the liposomal formulations. The role of azole therapy in disseminated fusarial infection remains undetermined.

Pseudallescheria/Scedosporium

Most recently known by the name *Pseudallescheria boydii*, this fungus is unique in medicine in that it is the sexual (perfect) stage which is most often recovered from human infections. The asexual (imperfect) stage is known as *Scedosporium apiospermum*. Other mycoses are typically caused by the asexual stages of the different fungi. To complicate matters further, the sexual stage of the fungus has been known by the now obsolete names of *Allescheria boydii* and *Petriellidium boydii* and the asexual stage was once called *Monosporium apiospermum*. An additional unique feature of these fungi is the innate resistance to amphotericin B and the need to treat disease with an azole derivative. Reports of various types of infection caused by *Pseudallescheria* and *Scedosporium* are found in the literature, often with no cross-reference to each other in the title of the paper[14–17] (Table 284–1).

The disease in immunocompetent patients is largely confined to localized infection, usually initiated as a result of penetrating trauma. Involvement of the eyes, bones, joints, brain, and subcutaneous tissue has been reported.[18–23] Several cases of endocarditis have been reported.[24, 25] Meningitis has also been reported.[18, 26, 27] Sinusitis and pneumonitis, both as invasive processes and as ones characterized by the formation of fungus balls, resembling in many ways aspergillosis, both occur.[28–30] Pulmonary infection typically occurs in patients with chronic obstructive pulmonary disease or other anatomic abnormalities of the lungs and their airways. The infection is marked by an extensive inflammatory response and tissue necrosis.

In immunocompromised patients, such as those with neutropenia and those who have been treated with high-dose corticosteroids, disseminated disease is the rule. The disease usually presents in these situations as fever, accompanied by pulmonary infiltrates, followed by extrapulmonary dissemination, usually to the brain or eye.[31, 32] As with *Aspergillus* species, vascular invasion occurs.

Infection caused by *Aspergillus* species or *Fusarium* species closely mimics the clinical presentations of infections caused by *Pseudallescheria*. Culture results of lesions are usually positive, but blood culture results are most often negative. The organism appears in tissue as septate hyphae, characterized by acute angle branching, much like *Aspergillus*. Growth in the laboratory occurs in several days, and colonies may progress from a whitish coloration to light or brownish gray. As for all molds, correct speciation is dependent on conidiation and evaluation of the morphology of those conidia and their associated structures.

Therapy for both forms of disease requires adequate surgical débridement whenever possible and the use of an antifungal drug. Because the experience with amphotericin B has been so poor, the azole derivatives have been used, including miconazole,[20, 33, 34] ketoconazole,[35, 36] fluconazole,[17] and itraconazole.[37–39] Given the positive anecdotal experience in treating these infections with itraconazole, many experts favor this drug over the more difficult to administer miconazole and the more toxic ketoconazole. The drug of choice, however, is not known. Consultation with a medical mycologist is desirable for patients not responding to therapy.

TABLE 284–1 ■ Pathogenic Species of *Pseudallescheria/Scedosporium**

Pseudallescheria boydii (Allescheria boydii, Petriellidium boydii)
Scedosporium inflatum (Scedosporium prolificans)
Scedosporium apiospermum (Monosporium apiospermum)

*Names in parentheses are obsolete.

Trichosporon

A member of the Cryptococcaceae family, *Trichosporon* species are being increasingly recognized as a cause of invasive infection in immunocompromised patients, especially those with chemotherapy-induced neutropenia.[40–43] Cases of endocarditis in immunocompetent patients[44, 45] and of invasive disease in patients with organ transplants, trauma, or acquired immunodeficiency syndrome have also been reported.[46–49] However, more commonly in the past, *Trichosporon* species have been recovered from superficial infections of the hair, known as white piedra. The principal species of *Trichosporon* recovered from patients with invasive disease is *Trichosporon beigelii*, formerly called *Trichosporon cutaneum*. Other members of the *Trichosporon* genus include *Trichosporon ovoides, Trichosporon inkin, Trichosporon asahii, Trichosporon asteroides*, and *Trichosporon mucoides*. For the most part, these other *Trichosporon* species are recovered from superficial infections of the skin and hair.

Invasive trichosporonosis is characterized by onset during periods of severe neutropenia (absolute neutrophil count $< 100/mm^3$) or other significant immunosuppression. Skin lesions are relatively common, as are positive blood culture results. An interesting and usually helpful finding is the cross-reactivity of the latex agglutination test for cryptococcosis.[50, 51] A positive latex agglutination test for cryptococcal antigen in a neutropenic patient almost always reflects infection with *Trichosporon* species and not with *Cryptococcus neoformans*.

Blastoschizomyces capitatus was once known as *Trichosporon capitatum* or *Geotrichum capitatum*. It can cause invasive disease in the immunocompromised patient, as well.[52] Pulmonary infiltrates are more commonly seen with this organism than with the other two closely related organisms. Patients are usually severely immunosuppressed and therefore have a high mortality rate. Therapy with amphotericin B may be successful if the underlying predispositions can be reversed.

Sucessful treatment of disseminated trichosporonosis depends in large part on the recovery of an adequate neutrophil count, if neutropenia was an important predisposing condition for the development of this infection. Reports on the utility of amphotericin B in treating invasive trichosporonosis have not been encouraging, and some evidence suggests that azoles, such as fluconazole, might be more effective.[53, 54] Selection of the most appropriate antifungal drug depends on the clinical situation and should be made, if possible, in consultation with a physician who has experience in treating these types of infections.

Malassezia

Malassezia furfur, also known as *Pityrosporum ovale*, is a lipophilic fungus, growing as a yeast. It is a normal inhabitant on human skin and is the etiologic agent of tinea versicolor. Folliculitis in cancer patients[55] and seborrheic dermatitis in patients with acquired immunodeficiency syndrome are more invasive manifestations of cutaneous disease.[56, 57] Invasive disease is most commonly manifested as intravenous catheter–associated sepsis, and most cases are in children, especially neonates,[58–61] but adults are not immune.[59, 62] Virtually all of the patients with this invasive form of infection are receiving parenteral lipids. *Malassezia pachydermatis* has also been associated with invasive infection.[63]

Because *M. furfur* requires lipids for its growth, special media containing fatty acids must be used in the laboratory for the fungus to be recovered from clinical specimens. The polymerase chain reaction technique has been reported to be useful in documenting spread of the organism within an intensive care unit.[64]

Treatment most often requires removal of the infected catheter and discontinuation of the lipid hyperalimentation. Antifungal drugs have not been demonstrated to be absolutely required in every case, and an attempt to eliminate the predisposing factors for the infection should be considered to be the most important therapeutic step. However, in the extremely ill patient with manifestations of sepsis, treatment with amphotericin B would be prudent.

Penicillium marneffei

This fungus is widely distributed in Southeast Asia, including Vietnam, Thailand, and southern China.[65–68] It is most prominently recognized as an important agent of invasive mycosis in human immunodeficiency virus–infected patients who have lived or traveled in that endemic area.[69–75] As the epidemic of acquired immunodeficiency syndrome progresses unabated, the importance of penicilliosis as a cause of significant morbidity and mortality should not be underestimated. In addition to the acquired immunodeficiency syndrome and other forms of immunocompromise, such as that induced by corticosteroid therapy, lymphoma predisposes to this infection.

The fungus is dimorphic, growing in the environment as a mold and in tissue as a yeastlike organism. In addition to humans, the bamboo rat and its surrounding underground living places have been found to harbor the fungus.[66, 76] In the yeastlike form, the fungus divides by fission, with the production of characteristic cross-walls, yielding a profile different from other more commonly seen fungi. In the laboratory, the fungus can be recognized by the production of a red pigment that surrounds the mold as it grows on agar.[77]

The presentation of penicilliosis is that of a chronic infection with the development of fever and weight loss. Skin lesions, cough, and generalized malaise are also often present. On physical examination, the patient is often found to have involvement of multiple organ systems, including lungs (pneumonia), bones (osteolytic lesions), hepatosplenomegaly, diffuse lymphadenopathy, skin (papular or ulcerated lesions), and subcutaneous abscesses. Laboratory evaluation may reveal evidence of anemia or thrombocytopenia. Thus, nothing is pathognomonic of the disease, and appropriate diagnostic tests must be guided by the clinical presentation and the presence of a travel history to the endemic regions.

Diagnosis is made by positive culture of material taken from appropriate lesions, histopathologic examination, and serology.[77–79] Preliminary criteria for interpretation of an indirect immunofluorescent antibody test have been proposed.[78]

The disease usually responds to therapy. Amphotericin B and itraconazole seem to be the most active agents.[80, 81] As with other infections in human immunodeficiency virus–infected persons, long-term suppressive therapy is thought to be necessary in patients who have had an initial response to antifungal therapy.[81, 82]

Dematiaceous Fungi

The fungi placed within this group contain melanin-like pigment in the cell walls of their hyphae or spores, or both. Classification of the organisms and the diseases they cause has generated considerable confusion, as is evident from the profusion of names by which clinical syndromes and the fungi are called. Ajello and colleagues[83] have proposed the term phaeohyphomycosis to cover all infections caused by hyphomycetes that grow in tissue as dark-walled hyphae. However, the definition has been extended over the years to include fungi in other classes. In addition, phaeohyphomycosis is a histopathologic designation and not one that is amenable to easy clinical description of a given disease. The suggestion made by Kwon-Chung and Bennett[84] that the clinical syndrome followed by the causative organism is a better way to communicate information about these diseases seems to be one that should be adapted. Many different dematiaceous fungi have been recovered from human disease and the list continues to grow (Table 284–2).

The dematiaceous molds typically give rise to infections of the skin and subcutaneous tissues, paranasal sinuses, and central nervous system. Manifestations of the former syndrome are of a single abscess, which can grow quite large. This usually appears at a site of trauma. Sinus involvement presents with a chronic course of nasal congestion and symptoms that may be confused with allergic sinusitis. The ethmoid sinus is most commonly involved. Facial pain develops, and examination of the sinuses is consistent with a mass filling the cavity. Systemic symptoms are absent. Evaluation with computed tomography or magnetic resonance imaging is useful in demonstrating the extent of the pathologic changes. Central nervous system involvement is usually manifested by the development of a brain abscess. Typical symptoms and signs reflect the anatomic location of the lesions.

For all types of phaeohyphomycosis, diagnosis depends on the visualization of the dark-walled hyphae in tissue and growth of the fungus from culture. The primary treatment has been surgical excision, but the supplemental use of itraconazole may be helpful.[85] The most appropriate drug, dose, and duration of medical therapy are unknown.

Rhinosporidium

Rhinosporidium seeberi causes a localized infection of the mucous membranes.[86] The infection is chronic, enlarging for months to years, forming a friable pedunculated polypoid lesion usually in the nose or conjunctiva. In tissue, the organism appears as a thick-walled cyst, from 10 to 200 μm in

TABLE 284–2 ■ Some Dematiaceous Fungal Species Associated with Human Disease

Alternaria	*Exophiala*
Aureobasidium	*Exserohilum*
Cladosporium	*Fonsecaea*
Curvularia	*Phialophora*
Dactylaria	*Sarcinomyces*

diameter. In the past, the organism had not been cultured, and confirmation of reports of successful in vitro propagation of the organism have not been forthcoming.[87, 88] However, in tissue culture, the life cycle of the organism can be maintained. The precise classification of this microorganism is in doubt, but it is thought to be a fungus, given the morphology observed in infected tissue. Although the disease is cosmopolitan, most patients have been from India and Sri Lanka. Therapy consists of surgical extirpation of the lesion.

Prototheca

The true classification of this organism is not clear, but it is thought to be an achloric alga. However, most discussions of this organism and of protothecosis, the resulting disease, are generally in the context of mycoses. *Prototheca wickerhamii* and *Prototheca zopfii* are the two species that have been recovered from humans with protothecosis. The organism lives in water and soil and causes a rare, noncontagious disease, primarily affecting adults. Involvement of skin and soft tissue has been reported,[89–92] as has olecranon bursitis.[93] The disease has been noted to occur in human immunodeficiency virus–infected patients.[94, 95] The typical skin lesions are papules or plaques, and ulcerations occur, but no systemic symptoms or signs of infection are noted. Diagnosis depends on visualizing the organism in tissue or isolating it in the microbiology laboratory. *Prototheca* species grow within 48 hours on Sabouraud agar and other agars not containing cycloheximide. Treatment is accomplished by surgical excision of the lesion, if possible. Amphotericin B and tetracycline, alone or in combination, have also been used successfully in some of the reported cases.

References

1. Kwon-Chung KJ, Bennett JE: Medical Mycology. Philadelphia: Lea & Febiger, 1992.
2. Nelson PE, Dignani MC, Anaissie EJ: Taxonomy, biology, and clinical aspects of *Fusarium* species. Clin Microbiol Rev 7:479–504, 1994.
3. Louie T, el Baba F, Shulman M, Jimenez-Lucho V: Endogenous endophthalmitis due to *Fusarium*: Case report and review. Clin Infect Dis 18:585–588, 1994.
4. Anaissie E, Kantarjian H, Ro J, et al: The emerging role of *Fusarium* infections in patients with cancer. Medicine (Baltimore) 67:77–83, 1988.
5. Robertson MJ, Socinski MA, Soiffer RJ, et al: Successful treatment of disseminated *Fusarium* infection after autologous bone marrow transplantation for acute myeloid leukemia. Bone Marrow Transplant 8:143–145, 1991.
6. Rabodonirina M, Piens MA, Monier MF, et al: *Fusarium* infections in immunocompromised patients: Case reports and literature review. Eur J Clin Microbiol Infect Dis 13:152–161, 1994.
7. Gais AS, Gudnason T, Giebink GS, Ramsay NKC: Disseminated infection with *Fusarium* in recipients of bone marrow transplants. Rev Infect Dis 13:1077–1088, 1991.
8. Martino P, Gastaldi R, Raccah R, Girmenia C: Clinical patterns of *Fusarium* infections in immunocompromised patients. J Infect 28(Suppl 1):7–15, 1994.
9. Guarro J, Gen J: Opportunistic fusarial infections in humans. Eur J Clin Microbiol Infect Dis 14:741–754, 1995.
10. Anaissie EJ, Hachem R, Legrand C, et al: Lack of activity of amphotericin B in systemic murine fusarial infection. J Infect Dis 165:1155–1157, 1992.
11. Viviani MA, Cofrancesco E, Boschetti C, et al: Eradication of *Fusarium* infection in a leukopenic patient treated with liposomal amphotericin B. Mycoses 34:255–256, 1991.
12. Wolff MA, Ramphal R: Use of amphotericin B lipid complex for treatment of disseminated cutaneous fusarium infection in a neutropenic patient. Clin Infect Dis 20:1568–1569, 1995.
13. Ellis ME, Clink H, Younge D, Hainau B: Successful combined surgical and medical treatment of *Fusarium* infection after bone marrow transplantation. Scand J Infect Dis 26:225–258, 1994.
14. Hofman P, Saintpaul MC, Garitoussaint M, et al: Disseminated infection due to *Scedosporium apiospermum* in liver transplantations—A differential diagnosis with invasive aspergillosis. Ann Pathol 13:332–335, 1993.
15. Hopwood V, Evans EGV, Matthews J, Denning DW: *Scedosporium prolificans*, a multi-resistant fungus, from a UK AIDS patient. J Infect 30:153–155, 1995.
16. Rabodonirina M, Paulus S, Thevenet F, et al: Disseminated *Scedosporium prolificans (S. inflatum)* infection after single-lung transplantation. Clin Infect Dis 19:138–142, 1994.
17. Tapia M, Richard C, Baro J, et al: *Scedosporium inflatum* infection in immunocompromised haematological patients. Br J Haematol 87:212–214, 1994.
18. Garcia JA, Ingram CW, Granger D: Persistent neutrophilic meningitis due to *Pseudallescheria boydii*. Rev Infect Dis 12:959–960, 1990.
19. Dellestable F, Kures L, Mainard D, et al: Fungal arthritis due to *Pseudallescheria boydii (Scedosporium apiospermum)*. J Rheumatol 21:766–768, 1994.
20. Dworzack DL, Clark RB, Borkowski WJ Jr, et al: *Pseudallescheria boydii* brain abscess: Association with near-drowning and efficacy of high-dose, prolonged miconazole therapy in patients with multiple abscesses. Medicine (Baltimore) 68:218–224, 1989.
21. Hung LH, Norwood LA: Osteomyelitis due to *Pseudallescheria boydii*. South Med J 86:231–234, 1993.
22. Bloom PA, Laidlaw DA, Easty DL, Warnock DW: Treatment failure in a case of fungal keratitis caused by *Pseudallescheria boydii*. Br J Ophthalmol 76:367–368, 1992.
23. Salitan ML, Lawson W, Som PM, et al: *Pseudallescheria* sinusitis with intracranial extension in a nonimmunocompromised host. Otolaryngol Head Neck Surg 102:745–750, 1990.
24. Welty FK, McLeod GX, Ezratty C, et al: *Pseudallescheria boydii* endocarditis of the pulmonic valve in a liver transplant recipient. Clin Infect Dis 15:858–860, 1992.
25. Raffanti SP, Fyfe B, Carreiro S, et al: Native valve endocarditis due to *Pseudallescheria boydii* in a patient with AIDS: Case report and review. Rev Infect Dis 12:993–996, 1990.
26. Peacock JE Jr: Persistent neutrophilic meningitis. Infect Dis Clin North Am 4:747–767, 1990.
27. Huang HJ, Zhu JY, Zhang YH: The first case of *Pseudallescheria boydii* meningitis in China—Electron microscopic study and antigenicity analysis of the agent. J Tongji Medical Univ 10:218–221, 1990.
28. Watters GW, Milford CA: Isolated sphenoid sinusitis due to *Pseudallescheria boydii*. J Laryngol Otol 107:344–346, 1993.
29. Hung CC, Chang SC, Yang PC, Hsieh WC: Invasive pulmonary pseudallescheriasis with direct invasion of the thoracic spine in an immunocompetent patient. Eur J Clin Microbiol Infect Dis 13:749–751, 1994.
30. Severo LC, Kaemmerer A, Camargo JJ, Porto NS: Actinomycotic intracavitary lung colonization. Mycopathologia 108:1–4, 1989.
31. Berenguer J, Diaz-Mediavilla J, Urra D, Munoz P: Central nervous system infection caused by *Pseudallescheria boydii*: Case report and review. Rev Infect Dis 11:890–896, 1989.
32. Caya JG, Farmer SG, Williams GA, et al: Bilateral *Pseudallescheria boydii* endophthalmitis in an immunocompromised patient. Wis Med J 87:11–14, 1988.
33. Collignon PJ, Macleod C, Packham DR. Miconazole therapy in *Pseudallescheria boydii* infection. Australas J Dermatol 26:129–132, 1985.
34. Grigg AP, Phillips P, Durham S, Shepherd JD: Recurrent *Pseudallescheria boydii* sinusitis in acute leukemia. Scand J Infect Dis 25:263–267, 1993.
35. Pluss JL, Opal SM: An additional case of pulmonary *Pseudallescheria boydii* improved with ketoconazole therapy. Chest 87:843, 1985.
36. Galgiani JN, Stevens DA, Graybill JR, et al: *Pseudallescheria boydii* infections treated with ketoconazole. Clinical evaluations of seven patients and in vitro susceptibility results. Chest 86:219–224, 1984.
37. Goldberg SL, Geha DJ, Marshall WF, et al: Successful treatment of simultaneous pulmonary *Pseudallescheria boydii* and *Aspergillus terreus* infection with oral itraconazole. Clin Infect Dis 16:803–805, 1993.

38. Walsh M, White L, Atkinson K, Enno A: Fungal *Pseudallescheria boydii* lung infiltrates unresponsive to amphotericin B in leukaemic patients. Aust N Z J Med 22:265–268, 1992.
39. Nomdedeu J, Brunet S, Martino R, et al: Successful treatment of pneumonia due to *Scedosporium apiospermem* with itraconazole: Case report. Clin Infect Dis 16:731–733, 1993.
40. Gueho E, Improvisi L, de Hoog GS, Dupont B: *Trichosporon* on humans: A practical account. Mycoses 37:3–10, 1994.
41. Naum S, Petursson SR, Weinbaum D, Rosenfeld CS: Long-term survival after allogenic bone marrow transplantation complicated by trichosporonosis. South Med J 87:286–287, 1994.
42. Grauer ME, Bokemeyer C, Bautsch W, et al: Successful treatment of a *Trichosporon beigelii* septicemia in a granulocytopenic patient with amphotericin B and granulocyte colony-stimulating factor. Infection 22:283–286, 1994.
43. Pierard GE, Read D, Pierard-Franchimont C, et al: Cutaneous manifestations in systemic trichosporonosis. Clin Exp Dermatol 17:79–82, 1992.
44. Sidarous MG, O'Reilly MV, Cherubin CE: A case of *Trichosporon beigelii* endocarditis 8 years after aortic valve replacement. Clin Cardiol 17:215–219, 1994.
45. Miralles A, Quiroga J, Farinola T, et al: Recurrent *Trichosporon beigelii* endocarditis after aortic valve replacement. Cardiovasc Surg 2:119–223, 1994.
46. Mirza SH: Disseminated *Trichosporon beigelii* infection causing skin lesions in a renal transplant patient. J Infect 27:67–70, 1993.
47. Ness MJ, Markin RS, Wood RP, et al: Disseminated *Trichosporon beigelii* infection after orthotopic liver transplantation. Am J Clin Pathol 92:119–123, 1989.
48. Miro O, Sacanella E, Nadal P, et al: *Trichosporon beigelii* fungemia and metastatic pneumonia in a trauma patient. Eur J Microbiol Infect Dis 13:604–606, 1994.
49. Nahass GT, Rosenberg SP, Leonardi CL, Penneys NS: Disseminated infection with *Trichosporon beigelii*. Report of a case and review of the cutaneous and histologic manifestations. Arch Dermatol 129:1020–1023, 1993.
50. McManus EJ, Jones JM: Detection of a *Trichosporon beigelii* antigen cross-reactive with *Cryptococcus neoformans* capsular polysaccharide in serum from a patient with disseminated *Trichosporon* infection. J Clin Microbiol 21:681–685, 1985.
51. Melcher GP, Reed KD, Rinaldi MG, et al: Demonstration of a cell wall antigen cross-reacting with cryptococcal polyssacharide in experimental disseminated trichosporonosis. J Clin Microbiol 29:192–196, 1991.
52. Martino P, Venditti M, Micozzi A, et al: *Blastoschizomyces captitus*: An emerging cause of invasive fungal disease in leukemia patients. Rev Infect Dis 12:570–582, 1990.
53. Walsh TJ, Melcher GP, Rinaldi MG, et al: *Trichosporon beigelii*, an emerging pathogen resistant to amphotericin B. J Clin Microbiol 28:1616–1622, 1990.
54. Anaissie E, Goaslan A, Hachem R, et al: Azole therapy for trichosporonosis: Clinical evaluation of eight patients, experimental therapy for murine infection, and review. Clin Infect Dis 45:781–787, 1992.
55. Sandin RL, Fang TT, Hiemenz JW, et al: *Malassezia furfur* folliculitis in cancer patients. The need for interaction of microbiologist, surgical pathologist, and clinician in facilitating identification by the clinical microbiology laboratory. Ann Clin Lab Sci 23:377–384, 1993.
56. Groisser D, Bottone EJ, Lebwohl M: Association of *Pityrosporum orbiculare (Malassezia furfur)* with seborrheic dermatitis in patients with acquired immunodeficiency syndrome (AIDS). J Am Acad Dermatol 20:770–773, 1989.
57. Ross S, Richardson MD, Graybill JR: Association between *Malassezia furfur* colonization and seborrhoeic dermatitis in AIDS patients. Mycoses 37:367–370, 1994.
58. Sizun J, Karangwa A, Giroux JD, et al: *Malassezia furfur*–related colonization and infection of central venous catheters. A prospective study in a pediatric intensive care unit. Intensive Care Med 20:496–499, 1994.
59. Barber GR, Brown AE, Kiehn TE, et al: Catheter-related *Malassezia furfur* fungemia in immunocompromised patients. Am J Med 95:365–370, 1993.
60. Marcon MJ, Powell DA: Human infections due to *Malassezia* spp. Clin Microbiol Rev 5:101–191, 1992.
61. Weiss SJ, Schoch PE, Cunha BA: *Malassezia furfur* fungemia associated with central venous catheter lipid emulsion infusion. Heart Lung 20:87–90, 1991.
62. Athar MA, Stafford L: *Malassezia furfur* fungemia: A case report. Can J Infect Control 8:63–64, 1993.
63. Welbel SF, McNeil MM, Pramanik A, et al: Nosocomial *Malassezia pachydermatis* bloodstream infections in a neonatal intensive care unit. Pediatr Infect Dis J 13:104–108, 1994.
64. van Belkum A, Boekhout T, Bosboom R: Monitoring spread of *Malassezia* infections in a neonatal intensive care unit by PCR-mediated genetic typing. J Clin Microbiol 32:2528–2532, 1994.
65. Deng Z, Ribas JL, Gibson DW, Connor DH: Infections caused by *Penicillium marneffei* in China and Southeast Asia: Review of eighteen published cases and report of four more Chinese cases. Rev Infect Dis 10:640–652, 1988.
66. Deng ZL, Yun M, Ajello L: Human penicilliosis marneffei and its relation to the bamboo rat *(Rhizomys pruinosus)*. J Med Vet Mycol 24:383–389, 1986.
67. Jayanetra P, Nitiyanant P, Ajello L, et al: Penicilliosis marneffei in Thailand: Report of five human cases. Am J Trop Med Hyg 33:637–644, 1984.
68. Imwidthaya P: Update of penicilliosis marneffei in Thailand. Review article. Mycopathologia 127:135–137, 1994.
69. Piehl MR, Kaplan RL, Haber MH: Disseminated penicilliosis in a patient with acquired immunodeficiency syndrome. Arch Pathol Lab Med 112:1262–1264, 1988.
70. Rokiah I, Ng KP, Soo-Hoo TS: *Penicillium marneffei* infection in an AIDS patient—A first case report from Malaysia. Med J Malaysia 50:101–104, 1995.
71. Wong KH, Lee SS, Lo YC, et al: Profile of opportunistic infections among HIV-1 infected people in Hong Kong. Chung Hua I Hsueh Tsa Chih 55:127–136, 1995.
72. Borradori L, Schmit JC, Stetzkowski M, et al: Penicilliosis marneffei infection in AIDS. J Am Acad Dermatol 31:843–836, 1994.
73. Sirisanthana V, Sirisanthana T: *Penicillium marneffei* infection in children infected with human immunodeficiency virus. Pediatr Infect Dis 12:1021–1025, 1993.
74. Hilmarsdottir I, Meynard JL, Rogeaux O, et al: Disseminated *Penicillium marneffei* infection associated with human immunodeficiency virus: A report of two cases and a review of 35 published cases. J Acquir Immune Defic Syndr 6:466–471, 1993.
75. Chiewchanvit S, Mahanupab P, Hirunsri P, Vanittanakom N: Cutaneous manifestations of disseminated *Penicillium marneffei* mycosis in five HIV-infected patients. Mycoses 34:245–249, 1991.
76. Li JC, Pan LQ, Wu SX: Mycologic investigation on *Rhizomys pruinous senex* in Guangxi as natural carrier with *Penicillium marneffei*. Chin Med J 102:477–485, 1989.
77. Deng ZL, Connor DH: Progressive disseminated penicilliosis caused by *Penicillium marneffei*. Report of eight cases and differentiation of the causative organism from *Histoplasma capsulatum*. Am J Clin Pathol 84:323–327, 1985.
78. Yuen KY, Wong SS, Tsang DN, Chau PY: Serodiagnosis of *Penicillium marneffei* infection. Lancet 344:444–445, 1994.
79. Supparatpinyo K, Sirisanthana T: Disseminated *Penicillium marneffei* infection diagnosed on examination of a peripheral blood smear of a patient with human immunodeficiency virus infection. Clin Infect Dis 18:246–247, 1994.
80. Supparatpinyo K, Khamwan C, Baosoung V, et al: Disseminated *Penicillium marneffei* infection in southeast Asia. Lancet 344:110–113, 1994.
81. Supparatpinyo K, Chiewchanvit S, Hirunsri P, et al: An efficacy study of itraconazole in the treatment of *Penicillium marneffei* infection. J Med Assoc Thail 75:688–691, 1992.
82. Supparatpinyo K, Nelson KE, Merz WG, et al: Response to antifungal therapy by human immunodeficiency virus–infected patients with disseminated *Penicillium marneffei* infections and in vitro susceptibilities of isolates from clinical specimens. Antimicrob Agents Chemother 37:2407–2411, 1993.
83. Ajello L, Georg LK, Steigbigel RT, Wang CJ: A case of phaeohyphomycosis caused by a new species of *Phialophora*. Mycologia 66:490–498, 1974.
84. Kwon-Chung KJ, Bennett JE: Medical Mycology. Philadelphia: Lea & Febiger, 1992, pp 620–677.
85. Sharkey PK, Graybill JR, Rinaldi MG, et al: Itraconazole treatment of phaeohyphomycosis. J Am Acad Dermatol 23:577–586, 1990.

86. Thianprasit M, Thagerngpol K: Rhinosporidiosis. Curr Top Med Mycol 3:64–85, 1989.
87. Levy MG, Meuten DJ, Breitschwerdt EB: Cultivation of *Rhinosporidium seeberi* in vitro: Interaction with epithelial cells. Science 234:474–476, 1986.
88. Krishnamoorthy S, Sreedharan VP, Koshy P, et al: K. Culture of *Rhinosporidium seeberi*: Preliminary report. J Laryngol Otol 103:178–180, 1989.
89. McAnally T, Parry EL: Cutaneous protothecosis presenting as recurrent chromomycosis. Arch Dermatol 121:1066–1069, 1985.
90. Goldstein GD, Bhatia P, Kalivas J: Herpetiform protothecosis. Int J Dermatol 25:54–55, 1986.
91. Nelson AM, Neafie RC, Connor DH: Cutaneous protothecosis and chlorellosis, extraordinary "aquatic-borne" algal infections. Clin Dermatol 5:76–87, 1987.
92. Modly CE, Burnett JW: Cutaneous algal infections: Protothecosis and chlorellosis. Cutis 44:23–24, 1989.
93. Demontclos M, Chatte G, Perrinfayolle M, Flandrois JP: Olecranon bursitis due to *Prototheca wickerhamii*, an algal opportunistic pathogen. Eur J Clin Microbiol Infect Dis 14:561–562, 1995.
94. Laeng RH, Egger C, Schaffner T, et al: Protothecosis in an HIV-positive patient. Am J Surg Pathol 18:1261–1264, 1994.
95. Woolrich A, Koestenblatt E, Don P, Szaniawski W: Cutaneous protothecosis and AIDS. J Am Acad Dermatol 31:920–924, 1994.

PROTOZOA

285

Entamoeba histolytica and Other Intestinal Amoebae

Sharon L. Reed

History

Dysentery was first well described by Hippocrates, but it was not until 1875 that Losch carefully characterized motile trophozoites from the stool of a Russian farmer. He fulfilled Koch's postulates by reproducing dysentery in a dog fed the infected stool and detecting similar parasites in submucosal ulcers at autopsy of the dog and the patient.[1] Koch first reported amebic liver abscesses in 1833. The name *Entamoeba histolytica* was coined by Dobell in his 1919 monograph entitled *The Amebae Living in Man.* One of the most dramatic outbreaks of amebiasis occurred in 1933 during the Chicago World's Fair, when 1400 people developed amebic dysentery after sewage and water pipes were connected in two hotels.[1] During the past 50 years, infection with *Entamoeba* has continued to be a public health problem in both developed and developing countries.

Characteristics of the Pathogen

Infection is acquired by the ingestion of environmentally resistant cysts, most often from infected food or water. Cysts of *E. histolytica* range in size from 10 to 20 μm and are characterized by four nuclei with a distinct, central karyosome. The chitinous cell wall of cysts contributes to their ability to remain viable for up to a month in moist conditions.[2] Motile trophozoites, which are released from the cysts after exposure to stomach acid, colonize the large intestine. In the majority of patients, infection is completely asymptomatic, and the trophozoites remain as harmless commensals in the bowel, phagocytosing erythrocytes and bacteria. At some stage during infection, unknown factors cause the trophozoites to encyst and complete the life cycle. In less than 10% of infected patients, trophozoites either invade the bowel locally, causing amebic dysentery, or enter the blood stream to cause distant abscesses, particularly of the liver. Although hematophagous trophozoites are often shed during active dysentery, they do not survive in the environment, and these patients rarely transmit infection.

Epidemiology

Up to 10% of the world's population is infected with *E. histolytica,* resulting in a morbidity second only to that of malaria and schistosomiasis.[3] In developed countries, the incidence of amebic infection is estimated at less than 5%,[4] but surveys in homosexuals have documented isolation of *E. histolytica* from up to 30% of stool specimens.[5] Infection is spread by fecal-oral transmission of infectious cysts. Although other primates can harbor *E. histolytica,* humans are the primary reservoir of infection, and asymptomatic carriers can excrete up to 15 million cysts per day.[2] Recent immigrants, institutionalized patients, and homosexuals are all at higher risk for amebiasis. Clinicians in developed countries should be aware of atypical mechanisms of transmission, including colonic irrigation[6] and use of imported water.[7]

E. histolytica infection can cause either asymptomatic infection or a wide spectrum of clinical disease. The relative roles of the host and parasite in determining the severity of infection have been a major area of debate. Despite anecdotal evidence for increased severity in pregnant women,[8] infants,[9] and patients treated with steroids,[10] epidemiologic and genetic studies now strongly support the hypothesis that intrinsic virulence properties of the infecting strain are the major determinant of infection. Brumpt[11] first hypothesized in 1925 that the epidemiology of amebic infection was best explained by the existence of two morphologically identical strains, *E. histolytica,* which was capable of invasion, and *Entamoeba dispar,* which was not. Landmark studies by Sargeaunt and colleagues[12, 13] of more than 6000 amebic isolates identified a series of distinct isoenzyme patterns (zymodemes) that differentiated between strains isolated from asymptomatic patients and those isolated from patients with colitis and liver abscess. When isoenzyme analysis was extended to isolates of *Entamoeba* cultured from homosexual men and patients with acquired immunodeficiency syndrome (AIDS), it was found that all harbored nonpathogenic zymodemes *(E. dispar)* and remained free of invasive amebiasis.[14–16] If untreated, these patients spontaneously cleared the parasite.[14, 16] Almost two thirds of symptomatic AIDS patients harbored other potential pathogens.[16] These data suggested that *E. dispar* does not cause detectable morbidity, even in AIDS patients. Thus, *Entamoeba* cysts detected in the stool of a symptomatic patient with AIDS cannot be assumed to be the cause of diarrhea. In longitudinal studies of asymptomatic carriers of pathogenic zymodemes *(E. histolytica),* only 10% developed invasive amebiasis within 1 year.[17]

Biologic and biochemical confirmation of Sargeaunt's data includes differences in surface antigens,[18, 19] ribosomal RNA sequences,[20, 21] and restriction fragment length polymorphisms of a number of genes between invasive and noninvasive *Entamoeba.*[22–24] These consistent differences support Brumpt's initial hypothesis that *Entamoeba* should be separated into two distinct species.[25, 26] Unfortunately, *E. dispar* and *E. histolytica* are morphologically identical, and their separation by routine diagnostic laboratories awaits the development of new diagnostic tests.

Pathogenesis

Successful invasion by *E. histolytica* trophozoites requires multiple steps, including attachment, degradation of the extracellular matrix to allow bowel invasion, killing of host cells, and evasion of local and systemic immunity. To initiate symptomatic infection, trophozoites within the bowel lumen must penetrate the mucous layer and adhere to the intestinal epithelium. A galactose-inhibitable lectin is critical for attachment to colonic mucins, bacteria, and host epithelial cells,[27–29] and immunization with the purified lectin has protected gerbils from the development of liver abscesses.[30] *E. dispar* produces a related lectin, but epitope differences revealed by monoclonal antibodies have served as the basis of a diagnostic test.[31]

The earliest pathologic changes of invasive amebiasis have been best characterized in rodent models in which epithelial cells undergo marked shortening of microvilli and apical separation before direct contact with trophozoites.[32, 33] Dissolution of the extracellular matrix is most likely mediated by extracellular cysteine proteinases, enzymes that degrade collagen, laminin, and extracellular matrix macromolecules.[34] Clinical isolates from patients with invasive amebiasis release significantly more cysteine proteinase activity, and patients with clinical amebiasis develop an antibody response to the amebic cysteine proteinase, demonstrating that it is released during the course of human infection.[35] Cysteine proteinases are encoded by at least six genes, one of which is present only in strains capable of invasion.[24, 35a] Pretreatment of trophozoites with cysteine proteinase inhibitors prevented, or significantly inhibited, amebic liver abscess formation in mice with severe combined immunodeficiency.[36]

After apical separation of epithelial cells, trophozoites can penetrate the interglandular epithelium, erode through the lamina propria, and extend laterally under epithelium that appears normal to produce the classic flask-shaped ulcer.[37] Trophozoites are usually detected by standard hematoxylin-eosin staining of tissues at the periphery of necrotic tissue. The bright pink staining with periodic acid–Schiff helps to differentiate trophozoites from phagocytic cells.[37] In amebic liver abscesses, the liver parenchyma is replaced by necrotic debris with few inflammatory cells. Trophozoites are usually detectable only near the capsule (Fig. 285–1).

Although well-established intestinal lesions and amebic liver abscesses are notable for the paucity of acute inflammatory cells, results of experimental animal infection suggest that an early neutrophil infiltrate occurs in both the intestine and the liver.[32, 38, 39] The initial signal to inflammatory cells may be derived from both a direct effect of *E. histolytica* products on leukocyte migration[40] and the local release of chemokines. Intestinal epithelial cells have significantly more complex functions than simple absorption of nutrients. A number of epithelial cell monolayers have been shown to express chemokines, including interleukin-8, interleukin-1β, interleukin-10, and tumor necrosis factor-α.[41] Coculture of trophozoites with human epithelial and stromal cell lines stimulates an array of potent chemoattractant and proinflammatory chemokines, including interleukin-8, growth-related oncogene-α, granulocyte-macrophage colony-stimulating factor, interleukin-1α, and interleukin-6.[42] The role of neutrophils in acute *E. histolytica* infection is unclear. Nonactivated neutrophils are lysed by virulent *E. histolytica* trophozoites in vitro,[43] but cytokine-activated neutrophils killed amoebae.[44] Thus, neutrophils may play a role in the first line of defense against acute *E. histolytica* infection.

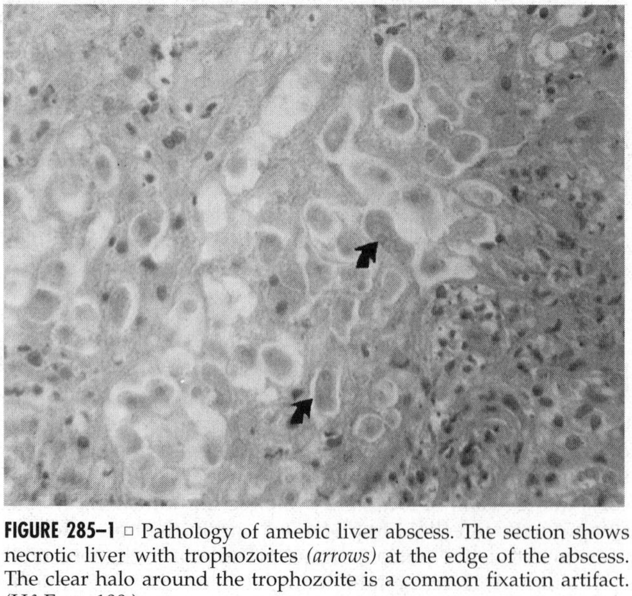

FIGURE 285–1 □ Pathology of amebic liver abscess. The section shows necrotic liver with trophozoites *(arrows)* at the edge of the abscess. The clear halo around the trophozoite is a common fixation artifact. (H&E, × 100.)

To kill epithelial cells, *E. histolytica* trophozoites must adhere to target cells by the galactose-inhibitable lectin.[45] Cell death can occur within seconds and is associated with increased intracellular calcium.[46] Cytotoxicity may be mediated by pore-forming peptides,[47] phospholipases,[48] or hemolysins.[49]

Once amoebae penetrate the mucosa of the bowel, they encounter components of the complement system. To cause a liver abscess, trophozoites must survive invasion through the blood stream. Indeed, studies of recent clinical isolates from patients with invasive disease revealed that they were resistant to complement-mediated lysis.[50] Resistance is mediated in part by the galactose-inhibitable lectin, which interferes with formation of the membrane attack complex.[51] In contrast, *E. dispar* trophozoites are rapidly lysed by fluid-phase activated components, limiting them to the bowel lumen.[50] *E. histolytica* trophozoites activate the alternative pathway of complement by a unique mechanism, specific cleavage of C3 by the extracellular cysteine proteinase.[52] Although hemolytically active C3b is generated, the remaining C3a portion of the molecule and C5a, which have anaphylatoxin and chemotactic activity, are rapidly degraded by the neutral cysteine proteinase.[53] Thus, *E. histolytica* trophozoites may circumvent normal host immunity by inactivating the proinflammatory factors C3a and C5a.[53]

The role of cell-mediated immunity in amebiasis is unclear. Activated macrophages kill trophozoites[54] and incubation of immune T cells with amebic antigen stimulates a cytotoxic T cell response[43] in vitro. However, the T cell–mediated response appears to be suppressed in patients with acute disease.[55] AIDS patients do not have an increased incidence of severe amebiasis, which suggests that cell-mediated immunity is not critical in controlling initial invasion.[56]

Serum antibodies are not protective; recurrent invasive amebiasis is rare but does occur. More than 95% of patients with acute amebiasis develop antibodies with titers that correlate best with the length of illness.[57] Studies of the mucosal immune response have revealed that antiamebic secretory immunoglobulin A can be detected in the saliva of patients with intestinal amebiasis.[58] Although specific secretory immunoglobulin A antibodies block attachment of trophozoites to epithelial cell monolayers,[58] whole parasites and lysates degrade humoral and secretory immunoglobulin A in vitro.[59] This degradation was inhibited by cysteine proteinase inhibitors. Thus, like mucosally invasive bacteria such as streptococci and *Neisseria meningitidis*,[60] *E. histolytica* may circumvent mucosal immunity by cleaving immunoglobulin A.

Clinical Manifestations

Intestinal Amebiasis

Asymptomatic Cyst Passers. Intestinal amebic infection is most commonly manifested as asymptomatic cyst shedding. Asymptomatic patients with no biopsy evidence of invasive disease spontaneously stop shedding within 5 months.[61] In developed countries, homosexual patients are the highest risk group, although the incidence has dropped from a high of 30% to less than 8%, possibly reflecting safer sexual practices.[62] Studies of 100 homosexual patients from London revealed that all patients were carriers of nonpathogenic zymodemes *(E. dispar)*, had negative amebic serologic results, and had no histologic evidence of disease.[14, 15] It is important to identify the rare asymptomatic patient who is harboring *E. histolytica*, however. A group of these patients were followed up for a year in Durban, South Africa, and 10% developed amebic colitis.[17] These patients represent a public health risk but can be identified by positive amebic serology.[17]

Amebic Colitis. Patients with amebic colitis typically present with a gradual onset of abdominal pain and frequent, watery stools containing blood and mucus. Symptoms of diarrhea, tenesmus, and back pain may be present for 1 to 2 weeks before patients seek medical attention. In contrast to the symptoms of bacterial dysentery, fever is uncommon. More than 80% of patients complain of localized abdominal tenderness.[63] Fulminant progression of amebic colitis, which is an unusual disease that occurs most often in children, is characterized by severe, bloody diarrhea and fever with rapid progression to acute abdominal tenderness.[64] More than 60% may have colonic and transmural necrosis on pathologic specimens.[65] Ameboma occurs in less than 1% of patients with invasive amebic intestinal disease.[63] Although the clinical presentation of a patient with an abdominal mass and radiographic studies with "apple core" lesions may mimic that of carcinoma,[66] the diagnosis of ameboma can be made by serology and biopsy.

Complications. The most common complication of intestinal amebiasis is peritonitis, which may develop gradually.[63] Hemorrhage and strictures of the anus or colon are less frequent.[63] Direct spread of infection can cause perianal cutaneous amebiasis with painful ulcers mimicking squamous cell carcinoma.[67]

Differential Diagnosis. Bacterial causes including *Shigella, Campylobacter, Salmonella, Vibrio,* and enteroinvasive *Escherichia coli* must be ruled out in any patient presenting with dysentery. Lack of fever and a paucity of fecal leukocytes are clues to amebiasis. Because amebic colitis may also mimic inflammatory bowel disease, it is particularly important to establish the correct diagnosis by serology or detection of the trophozoites in stools, as presumptive therapy with steroids may cause toxic megacolon.[68]

Extraintestinal Amebiasis

Amebic Liver Abscess. The most common complication of invasive amebiasis is amebic liver abscess.[69, 70] This condition can be challenging to diagnose as the symptoms may be nonspecific and develop months after the patient leaves an endemic area. The majority of patients present with less than 10 days of fever and right upper quadrant pain, often radiating to the shoulder.[57, 71] A tender, enlarged liver is detected in 80%.[71] Approximately 10% of patients have no abdominal findings and may present with fever of unknown origin.[71] All patients with extraintestinal amebiasis have preceding intestinal infection, but less than 30% have active diarrhea at the time of presentation.[71] The actual prevalence of asymptomatic colonization may be as high as 72% in these patients, however, when they are evaluated with amebic cultures.[72] A smaller subset of patients have a subacute course, presenting with hepatomegaly, weight loss, and anemia of more than 2 weeks' duration.

Pleuropulmonary Amebiasis. The most frequent complication of amebic liver abscess is pleuropulmonary involvement, which occurs in 10% to 20% of patients.[73] Half may have a small, serous pleural effusion. Localized, contiguous spread of an abscess into the pleural cavity usually responds to medical therapy alone. Hepatobronchial fistula is a rare but dramatic event sometimes accompanied by cough productive of large amounts of necrotic material, which may contain trophozoites. Unless aspiration occurs, medical therapy alone usually elicits a good response. The sudden development of pain and respiratory distress may herald the formation of an empyema that requires aggressive drainage.

Peritoneal Amebiasis. The second most common complication of amebic liver abscess is rupture into the peritoneum, which occurs in 2% to 5% of patients.[71] Because the contents of liver abscesses are sterile, the prognosis is much better than that for rupture of amebic colitis, and the complication can usually be treated with percutaneous catheter drainage.[74]

Pericardial Amebiasis. The most serious complication of amebic liver abscess is rupture into the pericardium, which has a mortality approaching 70%.[75] More than two thirds of these patients have abscesses of the left lobe of the liver. Patients usually have a preceding serous effusion but may rapidly deteriorate with cardiac tamponade, even when receiving medical therapy.[71] Open drainage may be required because of the development of loculations.

Cerebral Amebiasis. Cerebral amebiasis is usually diagnosed at autopsy in 1% to 2% of patients in large series.[71] Symptoms depend on the size and location of the lesion, but patients can die within 24 hours of cerebellar involvement. Because metronidazole penetrates well into the brain, the incidence of this unusual complication should decrease.

Genitourinary Amebiasis. Renal amebiasis can result from rupture of a hepatic abscess, hematogenous spread from lesions in the liver, or extension through the lymphatics. Patients usually respond well to aspiration and medical therapy.

Diagnosis

Microscopic Diagnosis

The identification of trophozoites or cysts of *E. histolytica* is critical to the early diagnosis of amebic colitis. Examination of a wet mount of a fresh stool sample or scrapings from the edge of a bowel ulcer for motile, hematophagous trophozoites results in the highest yield. Trophozoites are rapidly killed by drying, water, urine, barium, and several antibiotics. Because shedding of cysts may be intermittent, trichrome or iron-hematoxylin stains of the concentrates of at least three stool samples are recommended. Amebic cultures are much more sensitive than are standard stool examinations but are not available in most microbiology laboratories. Trophozoites are rarely detected in amebic liver aspirates unless part of the capsule is obtained. Cysts of invasive *E. histolytica* cannot be differentiated microscopically from those of noninvasive *E. dispar*.

Serologic Tests

Amebic serology is useful in the diagnosis of invasive amebiasis. The most commonly used tests, enzyme-linked immunosorbent assay, indirect hemagglutination, agar gel diffusion, and counterimmunoelectrophoresis, are positive in more than 90% of patients with invasive amebiasis, including asymptomatic carriers of invasive *E. histolytica*.[4, 17] Because the titer correlates with the duration of disease, up to 10% of patients presenting acutely with amebic liver abscess may have negative serologic results, but follow-up studies should show positive results within 2 weeks.[57] The diagnosis of acute amebiasis by indirect hemagglutination is problematic as titers can remain positive for years after successful treatment.[4] In contrast, enzyme-linked immunosorbent assay, counterim-

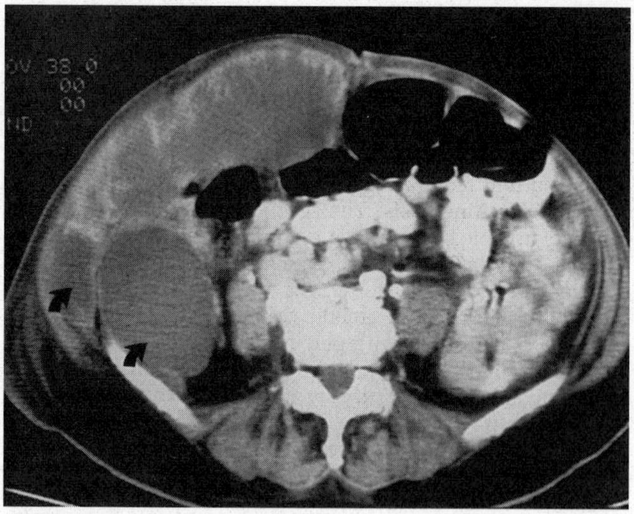

FIGURE 285–2 □ Computed tomographic scan of a patient with localized rupture of an amebic liver abscess *(arrows)*. (Courtesy of Department of Radiology, University of California at San Diego Medical Center, San Diego, CA.)

munoelectrophoresis, and agar gel diffusion results usually revert to negative within months, so a positive test is almost always indicative of acute disease.

Radiographic Studies

Noninvasive radiographic studies are critical to the early diagnosis of amebic liver abscess. Ultrasonography typically shows a round or oval hypoechoic area contiguous to the liver capsule with significant wall echoes.[76] Computed tomography (Fig. 285–2) and magnetic resonance imaging are sensitive procedures for detection of amebic liver abscesses. These studies are also useful guides to management of patients. More than 80% of patients with symptoms of more than 10 days' duration have a single abscess of the right lobe. In contrast, up to half of patients who present acutely have multiple lesions that may require diagnostic aspiration to rule out a bacterial cause. Imaging studies are useful for identifying abscesses of the left lobe of the liver, which increase the risk of rupture into the pericardium. Frequent radiographic studies may be confusing in patients responding well to medical management, as abscesses may actually increase in size during the first 2 weeks.[76] More than two thirds of patients have a normal ultrasound examination within 6 months, but abnormalities may persist longer than 1 year in 10%.[76]

Barium studies are relatively contraindicated in the diagnosis of acute amebic colitis because of the possibility of colon perforation.

Laboratory Tests

Routine laboratory tests are rarely helpful in the diagnosis of acute amebiasis. More than three fourths of patients with amebic liver abscesses have white cell counts greater than 10,000/mm^3.[57] Eosinophilia is not associated with amebiasis. The level of alkaline phosphatase is elevated in more than 75% of patients with amebic liver abscess. Transaminase values are elevated in less than 50% of patients with amebic liver abscesses, especially those with acute disease or complications.

Future Diagnostic Tests

Future diagnostic tests will focus on the early diagnosis of invasive amebiasis. Detection of specific immunoglobulin A in saliva correlated well with serum enzyme-linked immunosorbent assays.[77] The ability to differentiate *E. histolytica* from *E. dispar* directly in stool specimens will be especially useful. Monoclonal antibodies against pathogen-specific epitopes of the galactose-inhibitable lectin have been used in a stool enzyme-linked immunosorbent assay.[78] Conserved nucleotide sequences of ribosomal RNA that differentiate *E. histolytica* from *E. dispar* have been used as nucleotide probes[79] and for polymerase chain reaction amplification in stools.[80]

Treatment

The introduction of imidazoles has dramatically improved the therapy of invasive amebic disease. Metronidazole is well absorbed orally and can also be given intravenously. Standard therapy for amebic colitis or liver abscess is 750 mg (10 mg/kg) three times a day for 5 to 10 days (Table 285–1), although single-dose therapy of liver abscesses with 2 g of metronidazole, tinidazole, or ornidazole is effective in more than 80% of patients. The main side effects of metronidazole are nausea, vomiting, and a disulfiram-like effect with alcohol. There is little role for older treatment modalities. Emetine and dehydroemetine have potential cardiovascular and gastrointestinal side effects, and higher relapse rates are associated with chloroquine. With early diagnosis and effective treatment, mortality resulting from uncomplicated amebic liver abscesses has decreased to less than 1%.

TABLE 285–1 ■ **Treatment of Amebiasis**

SYNDROME	ADULT DOSAGE*	PEDIATRIC DOSAGE
Asymptomatic cyst passer, luminal agent		
Paromomycin (250-mg tablets)	500 mg tid × 7 d	30 mg/kg/d in three doses × 7 d
Iodoquinol (650-mg tablets)	650 mg tid × 20 d	20–40 mg/kg/d in three doses × 20 d
Diloxanide furoate† (500-mg tablets)	500 mg tid × 10 d	20 mg/kg/d in three doses × 10 d
Acute colitis		
Metronidazole (250- or 500-mg tablets)	750 mg tid × 5–10 d	30–50 mg/kg/d in three doses × 5–10 d
+ luminal agent (above)		
Amebic liver abscess		
Metronidazole	750 mg tid IV or PO × 5–10 d	30–50 mg/kg/d in three doses × 5–10 d
Tinidazole†	2 g PO	
Ornidazole†	2 g PO	
+ luminal agent (above)		

*tid, Three times daily; IV, intravenously; PO, orally.
†Not available in the United States.

Follow-up therapy with a luminal agent is important for all patients with invasive amebiasis. Only two luminal agents are available in the United States, iodoquinol and paromomycin, although diloxanide furoate is also quite effective (see Table 285–1). Iodoquinol is a halogenated hydroxyquinoline that must be given for a 20-day course. Paromomycin is a nonabsorbable aminoglycoside that is effective against both cysts and trophozoites.[81] Diloxanide furoate, a substituted acetanilide, has been extensively used outside the United States. All have efficacy rates of 85% to 95% for the eradication of cyst passage.[82] Treatment with a luminal agent is important because metronidazole is not effective against cysts. Although 50 patients with liver abscesses in a South African study rapidly responded to metronidazole, 55% still had cysts in their stool after treatment and 15% developed recurrent invasive disease.[72]

The majority of patients respond dramatically to therapy with metronidazole, with resolution of fever and abdominal pain within 72 hours.[83] Percutaneous drainage should be considered for patients who remain symptomatic. Aspiration should also be performed to rule out a pyogenic abscess, particularly if multiple abscesses are present, for imminent rupture with lesions larger than 12 cm, and to decrease the risk of rupture of an abscess of the left lobe of the liver into the pericardium.[84] Percutaneous drainage has proved so successful that open surgery is reserved for bowel perforation.

The two biggest dilemmas in the treatment of amebic infection involve the therapy of asymptomatic cyst passers and pregnant women. If a patient is asymptomatic and has negative serologic results, and the infecting strain can be identified as *E. dispar*, the patient can be safely followed up without therapy.[14] The treatment of pregnant women is problematic because there is anecdotal evidence that invasive amebic disease is more severe and the drug of choice, metronidazole, has potential teratogenic effects. One approach would be careful follow-up of asymptomatic pregnant women with negative serologic results or proven *E. dispar* infections without therapy, reserving treatment with metronidazole for those with invasive disease. Others would treat all pregnant women with mild to moderate intestinal disease with paromomycin.[82]

Prevention of Amebiasis

Transmission of amebiasis could be completely prevented with adequate sanitation, which requires both adequate disposal of human feces and sterilization of water. Cysts are resistant to levels of chlorination used in standard water purification, but filtration and precipitation are effective. Because infected food handlers are a major source of transmission, health education and early treatment of cyst passers and patients with invasive disease are critical. There is no effective chemoprophylaxis for the individual traveler. Risk of infection can be minimized by avoiding consumption of unpeeled fruits and vegetables and by using bottled water. Cysts are killed by boiling and by iodination.[85]

Other Intestinal Amoebae

E. histolytica is the only intestinal amoeba that causes human disease. The cysts must be differentiated from those of *Entamoeba coli*, which are larger (30 to 40 μm) and have up to eight nuclei with eccentric karyosomes. *Entamoeba hartmanni* is smaller (10 to 20 μm) and has a single nucleus. *Endolimax nana* contains a characteristic glycogen-containing vacuole. Infection by intestinal amoebae other than *E. histolytica* does not warrant treatment.

References

1. Kean BH: A history of amebiasis. *In* Ravdin JI (ed): Amebiasis. Human Infection by *Entamoeba histolytica*. New York, John Wiley & Sons, 1988, pp 1–10.
2. Walsh JA: Prevalence of *Entamoeba histolytica* infection. *In* Ravdin JI (ed): Amebiasis. Human Infection by *Entamoeba histolytica*. New York, John Wiley & Sons, 1988, pp 93–105.
3. Walsh JA: Problems in recognition and diagnosis of amebiasis: Estimation of the global magnitude of morbidity and mortality. Rev Infect Dis 8:228, 1986.
4. Healy GR: Immunologic tools in the diagnosis of amebiasis: Epidemiology in the United States. Rev Infect Dis 8:239, 1986.
5. William DC, Shookhoff HB, Felman YM, et al: High rates of enteric protozoal infections in selected homosexual men attending a veneral disease clinic. Sex Transm Dis 5:155, 1978.
6. Amebiasis associated with colonic irrigation. MMWR Morbid Mortal Wkly Rep 30:101, 1981.
7. Reed SL, Davis CE, Jinich H: Amebiasis from the "miraculous water of Tlacote." N Engl J Med 332:687, 1995.
8. Abioye AA: Fatal amoebic colitis in pregnancy and puerperium: A new clinico-pathological entity. J Trop Med Hyg 76:97, 1973.
9. Rode H, Davies MR, Cyives S: Amoebic liver abscesses in infancy and childhood. S Afr J Surg 16:131, 1978.
10. Stuvier PC, Goud TJ: Corticosteroids and liver amoebiasis. Br Med J 2:394, 1978.
11. Brumpt E: Étude sommaire de l'*Entamoeba dispar* n. sp. amibe akkystes quadrinuclées, parasite de l'homme. Bull Acad Natl Med (Paris) 94:942, 1925.
12. Sargeaunt PG, Williams JE, Greene JD: The differentiation of invasive and noninvasive *Entamoeba histolytica* by isoenzyme electrophoresis. Trans R Soc Trop Med Hyg 72:519, 1978.
13. Sargeaunt PG, Jackson TFHG, Simjee A: Biochemical heterogeneity of *Entamoeba histolytica* isolates, especially those from liver abscesses. Lancet 1:1386, 1982.
14. Allason-Jones E, Mindel A, Sargeaunt PG, Katz D: Outcome of untreated infection with *Entamoeba histolytica* in homosexual men with and without HIV antibody. BMJ 297:654, 1988.
15. Allason-Jones E, Mindel A, Sargeaunt PG, et al: *Entamoeba histolytica* as a commensal intestinal parasite in homosexual men. N Engl J Med 315:353, 1986.
16. Reed SL, Wessel DW, Davis CE: *Entamoeba histolytica* infection and AIDS. Am J Med 90:269, 1991.
17. Gathiram V, Jackson TFHG: A longitudinal study of asymptomatic carriers of pathogenic zymodemes of *Entamoeba histolytica*. S Afr Med J 72:669, 1987.
18. Reed SL, Flores BM, Batzer MA, et al: Molecular and cellular characterization of the 29-kDa peripheral membrane protein of *Entamoeba histolytica*: Differentiation between pathogenic and nonpathogenic isolates. Infect Immun 60:542, 1992.
19. Edman U, Meraz MA, Rausser S, et al: Characterization of an immuno-dominant variable surface antigen from pathogenic and nonpathogenic *Entamoeba histolytica*. J Exp Med 172:879, 1990.
20. Que X, Reed SL: Nucleotide sequence of a small subunit ribosomal RNA (16S-like rRNA) gene from *Entamoeba histolytica*: Differentiation of pathogenic from nonpathogenic isolates. Nucleic Acids Res 19:5438, 1991.
21. Clark CB, Diamond LS: Ribosomal RNA genes of 'pathogenic' and 'nonpathogenic' *Entamoeba histolytica* are distinct. Mol Biochem Parasitol 49:297, 1991.
22. Edman U, Meza I, Agabian N: Genomic and cDNA actin sequences from a virulent strain of *Entamoeba histolytica*. Proc Natl Acad Sci USA 84:3024, 1987.
23. Tannich E, Scholze H, Nickel R, et al: Homologous cysteine proteinases of pathogenic and nonpathogenic *Entamoeba histolytica*. J Biol Chem 266:4798, 1991.
24. Reed SL, Bouvier J, Pollack AS, et al: Cloning of a virulence factor of *Entamoeba histolytica:* Pathogenic strains possess a unique cysteine proteinase gene. J Clin Invest 91:1532, 1993.
25. Clark CG, Cunnick CC, Diamond LS: *Entamoeba histolytica*: Is conversion of "nonpathogenic" amebae to the "pathogenic" form a real phenomenon? Exp Parasitol 74:307, 1992.

26. Sargeaunt PG: '*Entamoeba histolytica*' is a complex of two species. Trans R Soc Trop Med Hyg 86:348, 1992.
27. Petri WA, Smith RD, Schlesinger PH, et al: Isolation of the galactose-binding lectin that mediates the in vitro adherence of *Entamoeba histolytica*. J Clin Invest 80:1238, 1987.
28. Petri WA, Chapman MD, Snodgrass T, et al: Subunit structure of the galactose and *N*-acetyl-D-galactosamine–inhibitable adherence lectin of *Entamoeba histolytica*. J Biol Chem 264:3007, 1989.
29. Chadee K, Petri WA, Innes DJ, et al: Rat and human colonic mucins bind to and inhibit adherence lectin of *Entamoeba histolytica*. J Clin Invest 80:1245, 1987.
30. Petri WA, Ravdin JI: Protection of gerbils from amebic liver abscess by immunization with the galactose-specific adherence lectin of *Entamoeba histolytica*. Infect Immun 59:97, 1991.
31. Petri WA, Jackson TFHG, Gathiram V, et al: Pathogenic and nonpathogenic strains of *Entamoeba histolytica* can be differentiated by monoclonal antibodies to the galactose-specific adherence lectin. Infect Immun 58:1802, 1990.
32. Chadee K, Meerovitch E: The pathology of experimentally induced cecal amebiasis in gerbils *(Meriones unguiculatus)*. Am J Pathol 119:485, 1985.
33. Takeuchi A, Phillips BP: Electron microscope studies of experimental *Entamoeba histolytica* infections in the guinea pig. I. Penetration of the intestinal epithelium by trophozoites. Am J Trop Med Hyg 24:34, 1975.
34. Keene WE, Pettit MG, Allen S, et al: The major neutral proteinase of *Entamoeba histolytica*. J Exp Med 163:536, 1986.
35. Reed SL, Keene WE, McKerrow JH: Thiol proteinase expression correlates with pathogenicity of *Entamoeba histolytica*. J Clin Microbiol 27:2772, 1989.
35a. Bruchhaus I, Jacobs T, Leippe M, Tannich E: *Entamoeba histolytica* and *Entamoeba dispar*: Differences in numbers and expression of cysteine proteinase genes. Mol Microbiol 22:255, 1996.
36. Stanley SL, Zhang T, Rubin D, et al: Role of the *Entamoeba histolytica* cysteine proteinase in amebic liver abscess formation in severe combined immunodeficient mice. Infect Immun 63:1587, 1995.
37. Joyce MP, Ravdin JI: Pathology of human amebiasis. *In* Ravdin JI (ed): Amebiasis. Human Infection by *Entamoeba histolytica*. New York, John Wiley & Sons, 1988, pp 129–165.
38. Brandt H, Perez-Tamayo R: Pathology of human amebiasis. Hum Pathol 1:351, 1970.
39. Chadee K, Meerovitch E: The pathogenesis of experimentally induced amebic liver abscess in the gerbil *(Meriones unguiculatus)*. Am J Pathol 117:71, 1984.
40. Chadee K, Moreau F, Meerovitch E: *Entamoeba histolytica:* Chemoattractant activity for gerbil neutrophils in vivo and in vitro. Exp Parasitol 64:12, 1987.
41. Eckmann L, Kagnoff MF, Fierer J: Epithelial cells secrete the chemokine interleukin-8 in response to bacterial entry. Infect Immun 61:4569, 1993.
42. Eckmann L, Reed SL, Smith JR, Kagnoff MF: *Entamoeba histolytica* trophozoites induce an inflammatory cytokine response by cultured human cells through the paracrine action of cytolytically released interleukin-1. J Clin Invest 96:1269, 1995.
43. Salata RA, Martinez-Palomo A, Murphy CF, et al: Patients treated for amebic liver abscesses develop a cell-mediated immune response effective in vitro against *Entamoeba histolytica*. J Immunol 136:2633, 1986.
44. Denis M, Chadee K: Human neutrophils activated by interferon-γ and tumour necrosis factor-α kill *Entamoeba histolytica* trophozoites in vitro. J Leukoc Biol 46:270, 1989.
45. McCoy JJ, Mann BJ, Petri WA: Adherence and cytotoxicity of *Entamoeba histolytica* or how lectins let parasites stick around. Infect Immun 62:3045, 1994.
46. Ravdin JI, Moreau F, Sullivan JA, et al: Relationship of free intracellular calcium to the cytolytic activity of *Entamoeba histolytica*. Infect Immun 56:1505, 1988.
47. Leippe M, Sebastian E, Schoenberger OL, et al: Pore-forming peptide of pathogenic *Entamoeba histolytica*. Proc Natl Acad Sci USA 88:7659, 1991.
48. Long-Krug SA, Fischer KJ, Hysmith RM, et al: Phospholipase A enzymes of *Entamoeba histolytica*: Description and subcellular localization. J Infect Dis 152:536, 1985.
49. Jansson A, Gillin F, Kagardt U, et al: Coding of hemolysins within the ribosomal RNA repeat on a plasmid in *Entamoeba histolytica*. Science 263:1440, 1994.
50. Reed SL, Gigli I: Lysis of complement-sensitive *Entamoeba histolytica* by activated terminal complement components. Initiation of complement activation by an extracellular neutral cysteine proteinase. J Clin Invest 86:1815, 1990.
51. Braga L, Ninomiya H, McCoy JJ, et al: Inhibition of the complement membrane attack complex by the galactose-specific adhesin of *Entamoeba histolytica*. J Clin Invest 90:1131, 1992.
52. Reed SL, Keene WE, McKerrow JH, et al: Cleavage of C3 by a neutral cysteine proteinase of *Entamoeba histolytica*. J Immunol 143:189, 1989.
53. Reed SL, Ember JA, Herdman DS, et al: The extracellular neutral cysteine proteinase of *Entamoeba histolytica* degrades anaphylatoxins C3a and C5a. J Immunol 155:266, 1995.
54. Salata RA, Pearson RD, Ravdin JI: Interaction of human leukocytes and *Entamoeba histolytica*. Killing of virulent amebae by the activated macrophage. J Clin Invest 76:491, 1985.
55. Salata RA, Martinez-Palomo A, Canales L, et al: Suppression of T-lymphocyte responses to *Entamoeba histolytica* antigen by immune sera. Infect Immun 58:2941, 1990.
56. Jessurun J, Barron-Rodriguez LP, Fernandez-Tinoco G, et al: The prevalence of invasive amebiasis is not increased in patients with AIDS. AIDS 6:307, 1992.
57. Katzenstein D, Rickerson V, Braude AI: New concepts of amebic liver abscess derived from hepatic imaging, serodiagnosis, and hepatic enzymes in 67 consecutive cases in San Diego. Medicine (Baltimore) 61:237, 1982.
58. Carrero JC, Diaz MY, Viveros M, et al: Human secretory immunoglobulin A anti–*Entamoeba histolytica* antibodies inhibit adherence of amebae to MDCK cells. Infect Immun 62:764, 1994.
59. Kelsall BL, Ravdin JI: Degradation of human immunoglobulin A by *Entamoeba histolytica*. J Infect Dis 168:1319, 1993.
60. Plaut AG: The IgA1 proteases of pathogenic bacteria. Annu Rev Microbiol 37:603, 1983.
61. Nanda R, Baveja U, Anand BS: *Entamoeba histolytica* cyst passers: Clinical features and outcome in untreated subjects. Lancet 2:301, 1984.
62. Sorvillo FJ, Lieb L, Mascola L, et al: Declining rates of amebiasis in Los Angeles County: A sentinel for decreasing acquired immunodeficiency syndrome (AIDS) incidence? Am J Public Health 79:1563, 1989.
63. Adams EB, MacLeod IN: Invasive amebiasis. I. Amebic dysentery and its complications. Medicine (Baltimore) 56:315, 1977.
64. Fuchs G, Ruiz-Palacios G, Pickering LK: Amebiasis in the pediatric population. *In* Ravdin JI (ed): Amebiasis. Human Infection by *Entamoeba histolytica*. New York, John Wiley & Sons, 1988, pp 594–613.
65. Aristizabal H, Acevedo J, Botero M: Fulminant amebic colitis. World J Surg 15:216, 1991.
66. Radke RA: Ameboma of the intestine: An analysis of the disease as presented in 78 collected and 41 previously unreported cases. Ann Intern Med 43:1048, 1955.
67. Mhlanga BR, Lanoie LO, Norris HJ, et al: Amebiasis complicating carcinomas: A diagnostic dilemma. Am J Trop Med Hyg 759: 764, 1992.
68. Patel AS, DeRidder PH: Amebic colitis masquerading as acute inflammatory bowel disease: The role of serology in its diagnosis. J Clin Gastroenterol 11:407, 1989.
69. Reed SL: Amebiasis: An update. Clin Infect Dis 14:385, 1992.
70. Bruckner DA: Amebiasis. Clin Microbiol Rev 5:356, 1992.
71. Adams EB, MacLeod IN: Invasive amebiasis. II. Amebic liver abscess and its complications. Medicine (Baltimore) 56:325, 1977.
72. Irusen EM, Jackson TFHG, Simjee AE: Asymptomatic intestinal colonization by pathogenic *Entamoeba histolytica* in amebic liver abscess: Prevalence, response to therapy, and pathogenic potential. Clin Infect Dis 14:889, 1992.
73. Ibarra-Perez C: Thoracic complications of amebic abscess of the liver. Report of 501 cases. Chest 79:672, 1981.
74. Ken JG, vanSonnenberg E, Casola G, et al: Perforated amebic liver abscesses: Successful percutaneous treatment. Radiology 170:195, 1989.
75. Ibarra-Perez C, Green L, Calvillo-Juarez M, et al: Diagnosis and treatment of rupture of amebic abscess of the liver into the pericardium. J Thorac Cardiovasc Surg 64:11, 1972.
76. Ralls PW, Quinn MF, Boswell WD, et al: Patterns of resolution in successfully treated hepatic amebic abscess: Sonographic evaluation. Radiology 149:541, 1983.

77. del Muro R, Acosta E, Merino E, et al: Diagnosis of intestinal amebiasis using salivary IgA antibody detection. J Infect Dis 162:1360, 1990.
78. Haque R, Kress K, Wood S, et al: Diagnosis of pathogenic *Entamoeba histolytica* infection using a stool ELISA based on monoclonal antibodies to the galactose-specific adhesin. J Infect Dis 167:247, 1993.
79. Garfinkel LI, Giladi M, Huber M, et al: DNA probes specific for *Entamoeba histolytica* possessing pathogenic and nonpathogenic zymodemes. Infect Immun 57:926, 1989.
80. Acuna Soto R, Samuelson J, De Girolami P, et al: Application of the polymerase chain reaction to the epidemiology of pathogenic and nonpathogenic *Entamoeba histolytica*. Am J Trop Med Hyg 48:58, 1993.
81. Sullam PM, Slutkin G, Gottlieb AB, et al: Paromomycin therapy of endemic amebiasis in homosexual men. Sex Transm Dis 13:151, 1986.
82. McAuley JB, Juranek DD: Luminal agents in the treatment of amebiasis. Clin Infect Dis 14:1161, 1992.
83. Thompson JE, Forlenza S, Verma R: Amebic liver abscess: A therapeutic approach. Rev Infect Dis 7:171, 1985.
84. vanSonnenberg E, Mueller PR, Schiffman HR, et al: Intrahepatic amebic abscesses: Indications for and results of percutaneous catheter drainage. Radiology 156:631, 1985.
85. Backer H: Field water disinfection. *In* Auerbach PS, Geehr EC (eds): Management of Wilderness and Environmental Emergencies. St. Louis, CV Mosby, 1989, pp 805–829.

286

Giardia lamblia

Michael J. G. Farthing

Giardiasis, the most common protozoal infection of the human intestinal tract, is found worldwide. Despite decades of debate as to whether the causative organism, *Giardia lamblia*, is a pathogen or a commensal organism, it is now clear that it is an important cause of diarrhea and intestinal malabsorption, particularly in young persons. *Giardia* organisms are widely disseminated in the environment, mainly in surface water and mammalian reservoirs. Although there is evidence to suggest that protective immunity eventually develops, this may not occur until several years after primary exposure, suggesting that, in highly endemic environments, multiple exposures are necessary to produce protective immunity. Developing new ways of controlling infection thus constitutes a major challenge for epidemiologists, clinicians, and scientists.

History

Giardia was probably first seen through a hand lens made by Anton van Leeuwenhoek in the late 17th century. At the time the Dutch microscopist was suffering from chronic diarrhea and saw the organism in his own feces.[1] He named it *pissabed*, which, in old Dutch, approximates "wood louse." Vilem Lambl formally rediscovered the parasite in 1859 and called it *Cercomonas intestinalis*. Some 20 years later, Kunstler identified a similar parasite in amphibians, which he called *Giardia agilis*, after his teacher and mentor, Alfred Giard. The binomial *G. lamblia* was introduced by Stiles in 1915, although the most widely accepted names are *Giardia intestinalis* (humans and some other mammals), *Giardia muris* (rodents), and *G. agilis* (amphibians). The first clear description of the pathogenicity of *Giardia* resulted when Fantham and Porter[2] experimentally infected young animals with cysts from humans and produced diarrhea, and in some instances weight loss. Knowledge of the parasite remained rudimentary until Meyer[3] successfully cultured the parasite axenically in 1976.

Characteristics of the Pathogen

Giardia is a flagellate protozoan (phylum Sarcomastigophora; class Zoomastigophorea; order Diplomonadida). The organism exists in two forms: the motile trophozoite, which is relatively fragile and cannot survive outside its host, and the cyst, which is the infective form of the parasite that can survive in the environment, particularly in moist, cool conditions.[4] The trophozoite has two nuclei and four pairs of flagella. The dorsal surface of the parasite is convex, whereas the ventral surface is occupied predominantly by the ventral disk, which is composed of contractile proteins generally considered to be involved in mechanical, and possibly hydrodynamic, mechanisms of attachment to the substratum.[5–7] One of these contractile proteins has been characterized and named giardin.[8] Another distinctive structure in the parasite is the median body. Morphologically, this differs among the three types of *Giardia*: hammer claw shaped in *G. intestinalis*, a pair of round bodies in *G. muris*, and teardrop shaped in *G. agilis* (Fig. 286–1). The function of the median body is not known. Studies suggest that two other morphologic variants exist: *Giardia psittaci*, which lacks the ventrolateral flange that in other types encircles the ventral disk,[9] and *Giardia ardeae*, an isolate from the great blue heron, which has a median body similar to those of *G. muris* and *G. intestinalis* but a ventral disk and single caudal flagellum more similar to *G. muris*.

The parasite surface membrane has not been well characterized, although there is antigenic diversity between isolates[10, 11] and *N*-acetyl-D-glucosamine is the major glycosyl residue.[12] Within the cytoplasm are rough endoplasmic reticulum, glycogen particles, and free ribosomes but no mito-

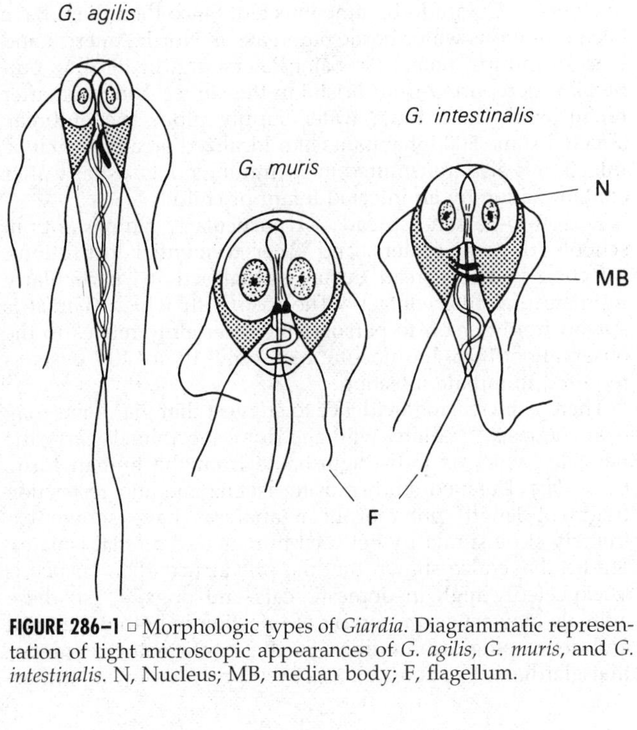

FIGURE 286–1 ▫ Morphologic types of *Giardia*. Diagrammatic representation of light microscopic appearances of *G. agilis*, *G. muris*, and *G. intestinalis*. N, Nucleus; MB, median body; F, flagellum.

chondria or Golgi bodies. *Giardia* is an aerotolerant anaerobe that uses an iron-sulfur protein and flavin electron transport system for respiration.[13] Glycolysis is the major pathway of carbohydrate metabolism, the necessary enzymes being located within the cytosol.[14, 15] The parasite is unable to synthesize phospholipids and sterols,[14] which it acquires by uptake from the intestinal lumen; bile must be a major source.[16] *Giardia* is unable to synthesize purines and pyrimidines but does have respective salvage pathways.[17, 18]

Although *Giardia* can be grown in culture in vitro, its growth requirements have not been clearly defined. The parasite is dependent on nutrients from the intestinal lumen, some of which, including bile salts and biliary lipids, have been shown to stimulate growth.[16, 19, 20] It is also likely that mucus acts as a nutrient for the parasite.

Although five morphologically distinct forms of the parasite have been identified, it is now well established that diversity exists among different isolates of *G. lamblia*. Phenotypic variation has been shown by analysis of surface antigens,[10, 11] isoenzyme analysis,[21, 22] and metabolic radiolabeling with [^{35}S]methionine.[23] In addition, genotypic variation has been shown by restriction fragment length polymorphism, chromosome analysis,[24, 25] and DNA fingerprinting.[26, 27] The relationship between these phenotypic and genotypic variations and the parasite's virulence and their effects on the host immune response have not been determined.

Epidemiology

G. lamblia organisms are found throughout the world, but their prevalence is greatest in developing countries, where peak prevalence rates in childhood can be 25% to 30%.[28, 29] In the industrialized world, prevalence rarely exceeds 7%,[30] although higher rates are reported from some areas of North America and Eastern Europe. Age-specific prevalence rates reported from Africa[31] and the Indian subcontinent[28] rise throughout childhood and begin to fall only during adolescence. Giardiasis is transmitted by water or contaminated food and also by direct person-to-person contact. The importance of water-borne spread of giardiasis became apparent in North America[32] during the mid-1960s, when a large number of skiers in Colorado became infected. Since then there have been numerous water-borne outbreaks in North America and Eastern Europe, notably in Saint Petersburg. In 1986, an outbreak was reported from Bristol in the United Kingdom after repair work on a town water supply pipe. The outbreak affected some 500 inhabitants of a localized area of the city.[33] Infection is also transmitted in swimming pools, usually after contamination by an infected infant or child.

Person-to-person spread is particularly important in schools, daycare centers, and other residential institutions. Infection is also spread during sexual activity, particularly intimate oral-anal contact.[34] The ease with which *Giardia* is spread from person to person almost certainly relates to the observation that an inoculum of only 10 to 100 cysts is required to initiate infection.

There is increasing evidence to suggest that giardiasis may be a zoonosis.[35–37] Many wild and domestic animals carry the parasite, which is indistinguishable from the human form, *G. lamblia*. Detailed studies using isoenzyme and restriction fragment length polymorphism analyses have shown extremely close similarity between human and animal isolates. Studies have also shown that the prevalence of *G. lamblia* is unexpectedly high in domestic cats and dogs,[38, 39] so these animals may act as a reservoir of infection in both developed and developing communities. Further confirmatory evidence that giardiasis is a zoonosis has been provided by an author-volunteer who successfully infected himself with an isolate obtained from a Gambian giant pouched rat.[40]

Pathogenesis

Colonization

Colonization may be considered a three-stage process: excystation, adherence, and multiplication. Excystation is thought to occur predominantly in the proximal small intestine, there being experimental evidence in vitro that it is triggered by exposure to gastric acid, and subsequently to pancreatic enzymes.[41, 42] Adherence to the epithelium is thought to play a major part in ensuring that the parasite remains within the gut and is not cleared distally by peristalsis. The ventral disk is traditionally considered the organelle of attachment, which is effected by a combination of hydrodynamic and mechanical forces.[5, 6] The disk contains contractile proteins that probably alter the shape of the disk (Figs. 286–2 and 286–3). Attachment to glass or plastic surfaces can be inhibited by agents that interfere with contractile protein function.[43]

More recently, a mannose-binding lectin has been identified in the surface membrane of *Giardia*, which, like bacterial colonization factors, may mediate attachment to the intestinal epithelium[44–46] (Fig. 286–4). This lectin appears to be involved in the attachment process to isolated enterocytes in vitro and is trypsin sensitive.[47] However, treatment of disrupted trophozoites with trypsin increases lectin activity, suggesting that the intracellular form of the molecule is a prolectin.[45] The lectin appears to be present over the entire parasite surface, having no predilection for the ventral disk. Lectin-mediated attachment may be the primary attachment mechanism before ventral disk–mediated mechanisms can operate.

The parasite multiplies by binary fission, which in vitro occurs every 6 to 10 hours. Bile stimulates parasite growth, principally because it contains phospholipid, uptake of which is facilitated by bile salts.[16, 19] Bile salts are also taken up

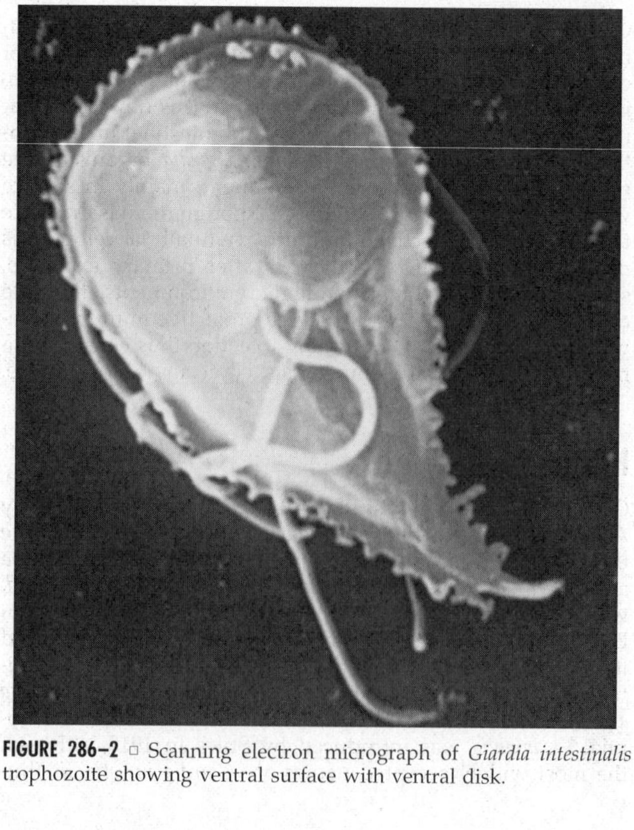

FIGURE 286–2 ▫ Scanning electron micrograph of *Giardia intestinalis* trophozoite showing ventral surface with ventral disk.

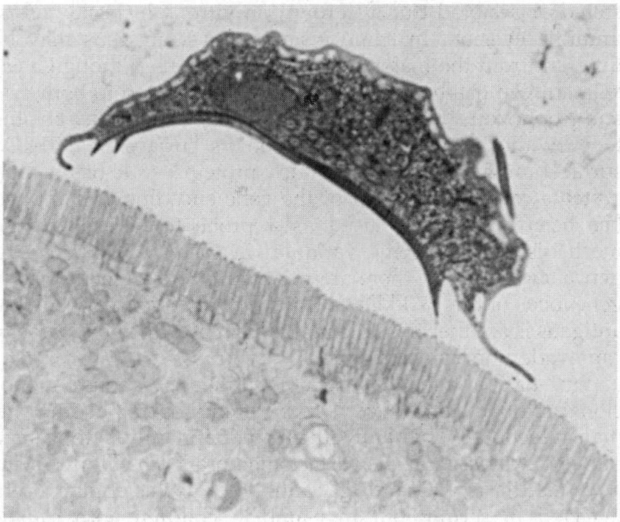

FIGURE 286–3 □ Transmission electron micrograph of *Giardia intestinalis* trophozoite in transverse section situated above the human jejunal microvillus membrane.

actively by the parasite by what appears to be an active transport process, possibly involving a carrier.[48] There is no evidence that the parasite metabolizes bile salts, and why it should take up substantial amounts of these substances remains unknown.[49] Interestingly, conjugated bile salts appear to be at least one of the promoting factors for encystation.[50]

Mechanisms of Diarrhea, Malabsorption, and Intestinal Damage

A unifying hypothesis that explains the diarrhea and malabsorption of giardiasis is not yet available. A variety of mechanisms have been proposed, some of which operate in the intestinal lumen and others in the intestinal mucosa.[51, 52]

LUMINAL FACTORS

The early belief that *Giardia* could prevent absorption by acting as a physical barrier to nutrients seems highly unlikely, largely because of the enormous functional reserve of the small intestine and the relatively small size of the parasite. There is no evidence that *Giardia* produces an enterotoxin by which it might induce water and electrolyte secretion, nor is there evidence that it causes direct epithelial damage by producing cytotoxin; however, bacterial overgrowth has been described in patients from India with giardiasis and also in overland travelers.[53, 54] It has been proposed that these bacteria deconjugate bile salts, which action leads to impaired lipid solubilization and fat malabsorption. Deconjugated bile salts were found in the luminal fluid of Indian patients with giardiasis,[53] although not in patients from the United Kingdom.[49] *Giardia* organisms do not themselves deconjugate bile salts, but they may reduce effective intraluminal concentrations by taking them up by active transport.[48] It is conceivable that during chronic infection this process might deplete the bile salt pool, particularly in infants and young children.

Duodenal concentrations of trypsin, chymotrypsin, and lipase have been shown to be reduced in symptomatic patients with giardiasis. This is not due to primary pancreatic insufficiency but to a direct effect of trophozoites on hydrolytic enzyme activity. The mechanism has not been established but may relate to an effect of one of *Giardia*'s own proteinases.[55, 56]

MUCOSAL INJURY

Some patients with giardiasis have morphologic abnormalities of the intestinal mucosa, namely reduction in villus height and increased numbers of lamina propria and intraepithelial lymphocytes.[57–59] Rarely, this can result in subtotal villus atrophy.[60] In others, there may be no obvious light microscopic abnormalities, although ultrastructural studies indicate that there can be damage to microvilli. There is a close relationship between the extent of the mucosal damage and the degree of impaired absorption of dietary substrates. The mechanism by which *Giardia* organisms damage the intestinal mucosa has not been determined. There is no evidence that it is a direct effect of the parasite, and invasion of the mucosa is seen only rarely.

Evidence is increasing that immune responses in the intestinal mucosa may be responsible for the abnormalities of villus architecture.[61] There is evidence from both animal and human studies that the increase in intraepithelial and lamina propria lymphocytes antedates the morphologic abnormalities in the villi. There is also a functional counterpart to this observation, because the intensity of the mucosal inflammatory response is related to the impairment of absorptive function. Furthermore, although T-cell–deficient, athymic (*nu/nu*) mice fail to clear the parasite, they sustain substantially less morphologic damage than do immunocompetent animals.[62] Finally, there is now clear evidence that T-cell activation in human fetal small intestine in vitro results in villus atrophy.[63] The possibility remains, therefore, that sensitization and subsequent activation of mucosal T cells by *Giardia* antigen(s) could account for the mucosal abnormalities, perhaps in the same way that intolerance to gluten and cow's milk protein produces similar effects in susceptible persons.

Whether *Giardia* lectin can act as a mitogen and directly activate mucosal T cells remains to be established.[44, 46]

Immune Responses

Immune responses are important in eradicating the parasite from the intestine during acute infection and also in the development of protective immunity.[64] Infection is more com-

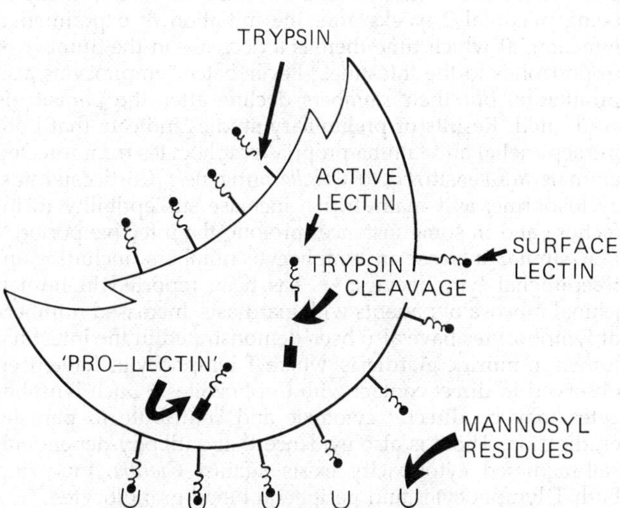

FIGURE 286–4 □ Some characteristics of the mannose-binding lectin of *Giardia intestinalis*.

mon in immunodeficiency states, particularly those associated with malnutrition, hypogammoglobulinemia, and human immunodeficiency virus infection.

ANTIBODY

Acute giardiasis is associated with serum immunoglobulin (Ig) M, IgA, and IgG responses. The specific anti-*Giardia* IgM response occurs early in infection and generally declines within 2 to 3 weeks.[65, 66] Current evidence suggests that an IgM response is present in the vast majority of patients with acute giardiasis, if not in all. Approximately 30% of patients also mount a serum IgA response, which, like IgM, is present in relatively low titer and is probably short-lived.[67] As with other acute infections, the IgG response occurs later and may persist for months or even years, particularly in highly endemic areas, where continued exposure to the parasite boosts the specific serum IgG response.[28, 65] Elevated IgG titers can be found in both infected and noninfected persons in endemic areas, whereas specific anti-*Giardia* IgM is generally found only during current infection, indicating that this antibody response may be helpful in diagnosis.

Occasionally, increased concentrations of total serum IgE have been reported in giardiasis, which in one case was not due to specific anti-*Giardia* IgE, but possibly to food antigens after increased intestinal permeability as a result of the infection.[68] Secretory IgA probably has a major role in parasite clearance and also in the development of protective immunity. Specific anti-*Giardia* surface IgA has been demonstrated in human jejunal fluid, human milk, and in experimental animals.[69, 70] During experimental infection, clearance of the parasite relates closely to rising concentrations of surface IgA and IgG in intestinal secretions,[71–73] and suckling mice can be protected from experimental *G. muris* infection by immune animals' milk.[74]

CELLULAR IMMUNE RESPONSE

The importance of cell-mediated immunity in clearing *Giardia* organisms has been clearly demonstrated in congenitally hypothymic, T-cell–deficient mice, which experience prolonged infections with *G. muris*.[75] In immunocompetent mice, lymphocyte numbers increase in the small intestinal epithelium, being maximal 2 weeks after the initiation of experimental infection, at which time there is a decrease in the number of trophozoites in the intestine.[76] Peyer patch lymphocytes also proliferate, but their numbers decline after the parasite is eradicated. Results of preliminary studies indicate that both intraepithelial and lamina propria lymphocytes from infected animals are sensitized to *Giardia* antigens.[76] Corticosteroids, cyclosporine, and malnutrition increase susceptibility to infection, and in some instances prolong the infective period.[64]

A similar increase in lymphocyte numbers, including intraepithelial lymphocytes,[59, 77] has been reported in human jejunal mucosa of patients with giardiasis. Increased numbers of lymphocytes have also been demonstrated in the intestinal lumen in murine giardiasis, where T lymphocytes have been observed in direct contact with trophozoites.[78] Such lymphocytes may be directly cytotoxic and contribute to parasite eradication. There is also evidence that antibody-dependent, cell-mediated cytotoxicity exists against *Giardia*, involving both T lymphocytes and peripheral blood granulocytes.[79]

***Giardia* Antigens.** A variety of surface antigens have been studied, including an 82- to 88-kDa protein that is an immunodominant antigen in human infections.[80–82] A 56-kDa antigen may also be important, as are other high-molecular-mass *Giardia* polypeptides and proteins of the cytoskeleton, such as the ventral disk protein giardin, which has a molecular mass of 31-kDa.[83–85] Some *Giardia* surface antigens are excreted or secreted during growth in vitro, which may assist immune evasion. In some instances, cyst antigens may be different from the major trophozoite antigens, although a 65-kDa antigen has been identified that is common to both cyst and trophozoite.[86, 87] Like other protozoa, *Giardia* may be able to vary the antigens expressed on its surface. A 170-kDa surface antigen may be one such protein.[88, 89] It has a high cysteine content, and part of the gene encoding this antigen has been cloned and used as a probe to investigate the mechanism of antigenic variation in *Giardia*.[90] Current evidence suggests that there are frequent rearrangements at the gene locus of this 170-kDa antigen. The ability to vary surface antigens is another possible mechanism by which the parasite can evade immune clearance.

A 57-kDa antigen has been identified by mouse monoclonal antibody and shown to be immunogenic during human infection.[91] This antigen in predominantly cytoplasmic but also expressed at the surface membrane. In children with *acute* giardiasis, IgG and IgA antibodies to this antigen were detected in serum, but in Gambian children with *chronic* giardiasis the IgA response was absent, suggestive that this antigen may be a determinant of immune clearance.[92, 93]

Clinical Manifestations

The vast majority of persons infected with *Giardia* have no symptoms, and there is little evidence that the parasite does them any harm. This situation is most common in highly endemic areas of the tropics and subtropics. It is probably this observation that led to the commonly held belief, during the first half of this century, that *Giardia* was a harmless commensal organism. There is no doubt, however, that *Giardia* is an important cause of acute diarrhea, particularly in travelers to endemic areas, in children, and in those involved in water-borne epidemics due to contaminated water. The symptom pattern has been particularly well documented in travelers[94, 95] (Table 286–1). Symptoms begin 1 to 3 weeks after cysts are ingested. Diarrhea may be watery initially, but it can resolve rapidly. Associated symptoms include nausea, anorexia, and abdominal bloating. Occasionally, allergic manifestations are reported, including arthralgia, myalgia, urticaria, and eosinophilia.[68] If their disease is not treated, 30% to 50% of these patients develop persistent diarrhea; half have biochemical evidence of malabsorption with steatorrhea and weight loss.[96–99] These symptoms may persist for many weeks, and in children, chronic giardiasis may be confused with celiac disease,[100] cow's milk protein enteropathy, and other noninfective causes of intestinal malabsorption.

TABLE 286–1 ■ Symptoms of Acute Giardiasis in Travelers

CLINICAL FEATURES	ASPEN, COLORADO (n = 324) (%)	FORMER SOVIET UNION (n = 56) (%)
Diarrhea	96	93
Weakness	72	80
Weight loss	62	73
Abdominal pain	61	77
Nausea	60	59
Steatorrhea	57	55
Flatulence	35	—
Vomiting	29	—
Fever	17	—

Data from Moore GT, Cross WM, McGuire D, et al: Epidemic giardiasis at a ski resort. N Engl J Med 281:402–407, 1969; and Brodsky RE, Spencer HC Jr, Schultz MG: Giardiasis in American travelers to the Soviet Union. J Infect Dis 130:319–323, 1974.

Since the 1920s, it has been alleged that *Giardia* infection can impair growth and development of children.[101] This has been confirmed by several hospital-based studies in which retarded growth and weight gain were demonstrated, predominately in preschool children.[101, 102] Results of community-based studies in The Gambia and Guatemala[29] also suggest that this parasite does have an independent inhibitory effect on growth, although the analyses required to show such an association were complex because all children had other intestinal, respiratory, and systemic infections at the same time.

Immunodeficiency states, particularly hypogammaglobulinemia and malnutrition, are apparently associated with increased susceptibility to giardiasis.[103] Although its prevalence is greater in homosexual males and patients with human immunodeficiency virus infection, unlike cryptosporidiosis it does not appear to be a major clinical problem for them. However, in hypogammaglobulinemic patients it may be extremely difficult, if not impossible, to eradicate the infection, despite multiple courses of appropriate antimicrobials, either single agents or combinations. Lymphoid nodular hyperplasia is a common finding in patients with giardiasis and hypogammaglobulinemia (Fig. 286–5).

Diagnosis

Clinical history may now be the most common approach to making a diagnosis of giardiasis, particularly in travelers who have moved from an area of low endemicity to one of high endemicity. Such persons often receive anti-*Giardia* chemotherapy before a precise microbiologic diagnosis is made and a good clinical response to therapy is often taken as confirmation. The "gold standard" for diagnosis is still the microscopic demonstration of the parasite (cysts, trophozoites, or both) in feces, duodenal fluid, or a jejunal mucosal biopsy specimen. A variety of immunodiagnostic approaches have also been used, and the application of DNA probes for diagnosis is still awaited (Table 286–2).

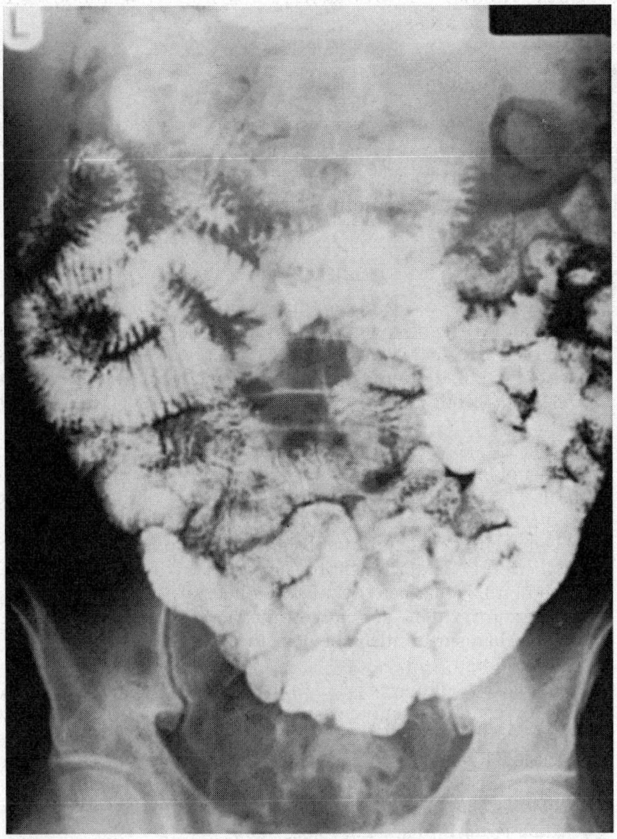

FIGURE 286–5 □ Barium follow-through examination in a man with chronic giardiasis and hypogammaglobulinemia, showing diffuse lymphoid nodular hyperplasia throughout the small intestine.

TABLE 286–2 ■ Diagnosis of Giardiasis

Clinical history (empirical treatment)
Microscopy: feces, duodenal juice, jejunal biopsy or smear
Immunodiagnosis*: serology (IgM, IgA), fecal antigen
DNA probes*: fecal *Giardia* DNA

*Research techniques.

Microscopy

Although our ability to detect *Giardia* forms in feces is enhanced by cyst concentration techniques, most studies indicate that even after examination of three consecutive specimens on different days, only about 80% of infections are detected.[104–106] This probably relates to the highly variable pattern of cyst excretion and the fact that the ability to detect cysts in feces is observer dependent. Although examination of duodenal fluid obtained either by aspiration or by the string test is often put forward as producing a higher diagnostic yield,[107] studies suggest that this may not be the case.[108] If repeated fecal specimens do not demonstrate the pathogen, and the clinical presentation strongly suggests giardiasis, this approach certainly complements fecal microscopy. Trophozoites can also be detected in jejunal mucosal biopsy specimens and impression smears taken from these specimens.

Immunodiagnosis

Serologic responses in giardiasis and the use of immunologic techniques to detect *Giardia* antigen in feces are potentially useful approaches for improving the speed and accuracy of diagnosis in giardiasis,[64] although these techniques are still largely restricted to research laboratories. The majority of patients with giardiasis have an increased specific anti-*Giardia* IgG antibody titer, but this comes relatively late in infection and can persist for many months, and possibly years.[28, 65] The IgG response in giardiasis is, therefore, not helpful in distinguishing past from present infection, and it accounts for the high prevalence of anti-*Giardia* IgG in noninfected persons in endemic areas. The anti-*Giardia* IgM response occurs relatively early in infection and is short-lived, probably lasting only a few weeks.[65, 66] The anti-*Giardia* IgM response does appear to distinguish current infections from past ones. Specific serum anti-*Giardia* IgA titers, like IgM titers, are lower than those of IgG and can be detected in only about 30% of patients.[67] Like the IgM response, however, it is relatively short-lived and so may be useful in identifying patients with current infection.

Several approaches have been used to detect specific *Giardia* antigens in feces by counterimmunoelectrophoresis or enzyme-linked immunosorbent assay.[109–111] Several groups have produced encouraging results with sensitivity better than 90%, and a simple, commercially available test is now available. A 65-kDa *Giardia* antigen has been identified in feces, and its detection has formed the basis of a diagnostic test based on counterimmunoelectrophoresis.[87] Whether this approach will survive in a routine diagnostic laboratory remains to be established. Specific *Giardia* DNA probes now being used in many research laboratories could theoretically

TABLE 286–3 ■ Drug Treatment of Giardiasis*

DRUG	DOSAGE	SIDE EFFECTS
Metronidazole	Adults: 1.2 g dose/d × 3 d, or 250 mg tid × 7 d	Metallic taste, peripheral neuropathy
	Children: 15 mg/kg/d (maximum, 750 mg) × 10 d	Disulfiram-like reaction with alcohol
Quinacrine	Adults: 100 mg tid daily × 7 d	Bitter taste, yellow discoloration of the skin and sclerae
	Children: 2 mg/kg tid × 7 d	Nausea, vomiting, toxic psychosis, exfoliative dermatitis, exacerbation of psoriasis
Furazolidone	Adults: 100 mg qid daily for 7–10 d	Nausea, vomiting, hemolysis in patients with glucose-6-phosphate dehydrogenase deficiency
	Children: 2 mg/kg tid × 10 d	

*tid, Three times daily; qid, four times daily.

be applied to the detection of *Giardia* DNA in feces.[112, 113] Release of DNA from cysts still appears to be a problem, making the technique relatively insensitive, although this should be possible to overcome using the polymerase chain reaction.

Treatment

The most widely used drugs to treat giardiasis are the nitroimidazole derivatives (metronidazole, tinidazole), the acridine dyes (mepacrine), and the nitrofurans (furazolidone). The regimens for adults and children are shown in Table 286–3. Unfortunately, none of these drugs is ideal, as they have a variety of unwanted adverse effects, and none is regarded as being safe in pregnancy. The drugs of choice are the nitroimidazole derivatives, because the high-dose, short-treatment regimen is usually acceptable to patients and generally ensures good compliance; however, in some countries they are not licensed for treatment of giardiasis. The search continues for new compounds, a variety of drugs having been shown to have anti-*Giardia* activity, including sodium fusidate, D-propranolol, tricyclic compounds, and mebendazole.[114–117] Studies suggest that albendazole has antigiardial activity in vitro, which is supported by clinical trial data in humans.

Treatment failures with nitroimidazole derivatives are common in giardiasis, and it is often necessary to give a second course of the drug. Failing this, a second-line drug such as mepacrine can be given alone or in combination with the nitroimidazole derivative. The reason for treatment failures has not been clearly established, although there is increasing evidence that *Giardia* may become relatively resistant to some anti-*Giardia* drugs.[118] The development of sensitivity assays in vitro should help plan further treatment when infection is difficult to eradicate.[119–121] It has been shown that the phenotype and genotype of *Giardia* isolates can change during the course of chronic infection, possibly owing to selection of relatively resistant strains after treatment with a nitroimidazole derivative.[26]

Prevention

Giardia organisms are widely distributed throughout the environment, in water and in human and animal reservoirs. It is unlikely that any single environmental intervention will eradicate the disease. Transmission, however, may be interrupted by ensuring high standards of water purification, it being particularly important not to rely on chlorination alone, because the effect on cyst viability is variable. Travelers to endemic areas should avoid consuming tap water and locally produced soft drinks and ice. Boiling water for 10 minutes destroys cysts, but the opportunity to do so is often not available to travelers.

Person-to-person spread can be controlled by ensuring high standards of personal hygiene and adequate supervision in nurseries and residential institutions. Avoidance of intimate oral-anal contact reduces the risk of transmission during sexual activity. Treating carriers in areas of low endemicity should help to control human reservoirs, although it is doubtful whether this would have any impact whatsoever in highly endemic areas.

Acknowledgments

I am grateful for the financial support of the Wellcome Trust and the Joint Research Board of St. Bartholomew's Hospital. Special thanks go to Ms. Nicola Herrera for her assistance in the preparation of this manuscript.

References

1. Dobell CA: The discovery of intestinal protozoa in man. Proc R Soc Med 13:1, 1920.
2. Fantham HB, Porter A: The pathogenicity of *Giardia lamblia intestinalis* from man to experimental animals. Br Med J 2:139, 1916.
3. Meyer EA: *Giardia lamblia*: Isolation and axenic cultivation. Exp Parasitol 39:101, 1976.
4. Feely DE, Erlandsen SL, Chase DG: Structure of the trophozoite and cyst. *In* Erlandsen SL, Meyer EA (eds): *Giardia* and Giardiasis. New York, Plenum Publishing, 1984, pp 3–31.
5. Holberton DV: Attachment of *Giardia*—A hydrodynamic model based on flagellar activity. J Exp Biol 60:207, 1974.
6. Holberton DV: Fine structure of the ventral disc apparatus and the mechanism of attachment in the flagellate *Giardia muris*. J Cell Sci 13:11, 1973.
7. Feely DE, Schollmeyer JV, Erlandsen SL: *Giardia* spp.: Distribution of contractile proteins in the attachment organelle. Exp Parasitol 53:145, 1982.
8. Crossley R, Holberton DV: Characterization of proteins from the cytoskeleton of *Giardia lamblia*. J Cell Sci 59:81, 1983.
9. Erlandsen SL, Bemrick WJ: SEM evidence for a new species, *Giardia psittaci*. J Parasitol 73:623, 1987.
10. Smith PD, Gillin FD, Kaushal NA, et al: Antigenic analysis of *Giardia lamblia* from Afghanistan, Puerto Rico, Ecuador and Oregon. Infect Immun 36:714, 1982.

11. Nash TE, Keister DB: Differences in excretory-secretory products and surface antigens among 19 isolates of *Giardia*. J Infect Dis 152:1166, 1985.
12. Ward HD, Alroy J, Lev BI, et al: Biology of *Giardia lamblia*. Detection of *N*-acetyl-D-glucosamine as the only surface saccharide moiety and identification of two distinct subsets of trophozoites by lectin binding. J Exp Med 167:73, 1988.
13. Weinbach EC, Claggett CE, Keister DB, et al: Respiratory metabolism of *Giardia lamblia*. J Parasitol 66:347, 1980.
14. Jarroll EL, Muller PJ, Meyer EA, et al: Lipid and carbohydrate metabolism of *Giardia lamblia*. Mol Biochem Parasitol 2:187, 1981.
15. Lindmark DG: Energy metabolism of the anaerobic protozoan *Giardia lamblia*. Mol Biochem Parasitol 1:1, 1980.
16. Farthing MJG, Keusch GT, Carey MC: Effect of bile and bile salts on growth and membrane lipid uptake by *Giardia lamblia*: Possible implications for pathogenesis of intestinal disease. J Clin Invest 76:1727, 1985.
17. Lindmark DG, Jarroll EL: Pyrimidine metabolism in *Giardia lamblia* trophozoites. Mol Biochem Parasitol 5:291, 1982.
18. Wang CC, Aldritt S: Purine salvage networks in *Giardia lamblia*. J Exp Med 158:1703, 1983.
19. Farthing MJG, Varon SR, Keusch GT: Mammalian bile promotes growth of *Giardia lamblia* in axenic culture. Trans R Soc Trop Med Hyg 77:467, 1983.
20. Keister DB: Axenic culture of *Giardia lamblia* in TYI-S-33 medium supplemented with bile. Trans R Soc Trop Med Hyg 77:487, 1983.
21. Bertram MA, Meyer EA, Lile JD, et al: A comparison of isoenzymes of five axenic *Giardia* isolates. J Parasitol 69:793, 1983.
22. Meloni BP, Lymbery AJ, Thompson RCA: Isoenzyme electrophoresis of 30 isolates of *Giardia* from humans and felines. Am J Trop Med Hyg 38:65, 1988.
23. Cevallos AM, Morrison AM, Archibald SC, et al: [^{35}S]-methionine biosynthetic radiolabelling of *Giardia lamblia*: Basis for a typing system? Gut 5:A748, 1989.
24. Nash TE, McCutchan T, Keister D, et al: Restriction-endonuclease analysis of DNA from 15 *Giardia* isolates from humans and animals. J Infect Dis 152:64, 1985.
25. Butcher PB, Clark C, Farthing MJG: *Giardia lamblia* cloned genomic DNA probes: Uses in faecal diagnosis and genetic analysis of clinical isolates. Gut 29:A722, 1988.
26. Butcher PD, Cevallos AM, Carnaby S, et al: Phenotypic and genotypic variation in *Giardia lamblia* isolates during chronic infection. Gut 35:51, 1993.
27. Carnaby S, Butcher PD, Summerbell CD, et al: Minisatellites corresponding to the human polycore probes 33.6 and 33.15 in the genome of the most "primitive" known eukaryote *Giardia lamblia*. Gene 166:167, 1995.
28. Gilman RH, Brown KH, Visvesvara GS, et al: Epidemiology and serology of *Giardia lamblia* in a developing country: Bangladesh. Trans R Soc Trop Med Hyg 79:469, 1985.
29. Farthing MJG, Mata L, Urrutia JJ, et al: Natural history of *Giardia* infection of infants and children in rural Guatemala and its impact on physical growth. Am J Clin Nutr 43:393, 1986.
30. Petersen H. Giardiasis (lambliasis). Scand J Gastroenterol 7:44, 1972.
31. Oyerinde JPO, Ogunbi O, Alonge AA: Age and sex distribution of infections with *Entamoeba histolytica* and *Giardia intestinalis* in the Lagos population. Int J Epidemiol 6:231, 1977.
32. Craun GF: Waterborne outbreaks of giardiasis. Current status. *In* Erlandsen SL, Meyer EA (eds): *Giardia* and Giardiasis. New York, Plenum Publishing, 1984, pp 243–261.
33. Jephcott AE, Begg NT, Baker IA: Outbreak of giardiasis associated with mains water in the United Kingdom. Lancet 1:730, 1986.
34. Owen RL: Direct fecal-oral transmission of giardiasis. *In* Erlandsen SL, Meyer EA (eds): *Giardia* and Giardiasis. New York, Plenum Publishing, 1984, pp 329–339.
35. Woo PK: Evidence for animal reservoirs and transmission of *Giardia* infection between animal species. *In* Erlandsen SL, Meyer EA (eds): *Giardia* and Giardiasis. New York, Plenum Publishing, 1984, pp 341–364.
36. Thompson RCA, Meloni BP, Lymbery AJ: Humans and cats have genetically identical forms of *Giardia*: Evidence of a zoonotic relationship (Letter). Med J Aust 148:207, 1988.
37. Bemrick WJ, Erlandsen SL: Giardiasis—Is it really a zoonosis? Parasitol Today 4:69, 1988.
38. Sykes TJ, Fox MT: Patterns of infection with *Giardia* in dogs in London. Trans R Soc Trop Med Hyg 83:239, 1989.
39. Winsland JKD, Nimmo S, Butcher PS, et al: Prevalence of *Giardia* in dogs and cats in the United Kingdom: Survey of an Essex veterinary clinic. Trans R Soc Trop Med Hyg 83:791, 1989.
40. Majewska AC: Successful experimental infections of a human volunteer and Mongolian gerbils with *Giardia* of animal origin. Trans R Soc Trop Med Hyg 88:360, 1994.
41. Bingham AK, Meyer EA: *Giardia* excystation can be induced in vitro in acidic solutions. Nature 277:301, 1979.
42. Rice EW, Schaefer FW: Improved in vitro excystation procedure for *Giardia lamblia* cysts. J Clin Microbiol 14:709, 1981.
43. Feely DE, Erlandsen SL: Effect of cytochalasin-B, low Ca^{++} concentration, iodoacetic acid and quinacrine-HC1 on the attachment of *Giardia* trophozoites in vitro. J Parasitol 68:869, 1982.
44. Farthing MJG, Perreira MEA, Keusch GT: Description and characterisation of a surface lectin from *Giardia lamblia*. Infect Immun 51:661, 1986.
45. Lev B, Ward H, Keusch GT, et al: Lectin activation in *Giardia lamblia* by host protease: A novel host-parasite interaction. Science 232:71, 1986.
46. Ward HD, Lev BI, Kane AV, et al: Identification and characterization of Taglin, a mannose-6-phosphate binding, trypsin-activated lectin from *Giardia lamblia*. Biochemistry 26:8669, 1987.
47. Inge PMG, Edson CM, Farthing MJG: Attachment of *Giardia lamblia* to mammalian intestinal cells. Gut 29:795, 1988.
48. Halliday CEW, Inge PM, Farthing MJ: Characterization of bile salt uptake by *Giardia lamblia*. Int J Parasitol 25:1089, 1995.
49. Halliday CEW, Inge PMG, Farthing MJG: *Giardia*–bile salt interactions. Trans R Soc Trop Med Hyg 82:428, 1988.
50. Gillin FD, Reiner DS, Boucher SE: Small intestinal factors promote encystation of *Giardia lamblia* in vitro. Infect Immun 56:705, 1988.
51. Katelaris, PH, Farthing MJG: Diarrhoea and malabsorption in giardiasis: A multifactorial process. Gut 33:295, 1992.
52. Farthing MJG: Pathogenesis of giardiasis. Trans R Soc Trop Med Hyg 87(Suppl 3):17, 1993.
53. Tandon BN, Tandon RK, Satpathy BK, et al: Mechanism of malabsorption in giardiasis: A study of bacterial flora and bile salt deconjugation in upper jejunum. Gut 18:176, 1977.
54. Tomkins AM, Drasar BS, Bradley AK, et al: Bacterial colonization of jejunal mucosa in giardiasis. Trans R Soc Trop Med Hyg 72:33, 1978.
55. Katelaris PH, Seow F, Ngu MC: The effect of *Giardia lamblia* trophozoites on lipolysis in vivo. Parasitology 103:35, 1991.
56. Seow F, Katelaris PH, Ngu MC: The effect of *Giardia lamblia* trophozoites on trypsin, chymotrypsin and amylase in vitro. Parasitology 106:233, 1993.
57. Yardley JH, Takano J, Hendrix TR: Epithelial and other mucosal lesions of the jejunum in giardiasis. Jejunal biopsy studies. Bull Johns Hopkins Hosp 115:389, 1964.
58. Hartong WA, Gourley WK, Arvanitakis C: Giardiasis: Clinical spectrum and functional-structural abnormalities of the small intestinal mucosa. Gastroenterology 77:61, 1979.
59. Wright SG, Tomkins AM: Quantification of the lymphocytic infiltrate in jejunal epithelium in giardiasis. Clin Exp Immunol 29:408, 1977.
60. Levinson JD, Nastro LJ: Giardiasis with total villous atrophy. Gastroenterology 74:271, 1978.
61. Farthing MJG: Host-parasite interactions in human giardiasis. Q J Med 70:191, 1989.
62. Roberts-Thomson IC, Mitchell GF: Giardiasis in mice. I. Prolonged infections in certain mouse strains and hypothymic (nude) mice. Gastroenterology 75:42, 1978.
63. MacDonald TT, Spencer J: Evidence that activated mucosal T cells play a role in the pathogenesis of enteropathy in human small intestine. J Exp Med 167:1341, 1988.
64. Farthing MJG, Goka AKJ: Immunology of giardiasis. Ballieres Clin Gastroenterol 1:589, 1987.
65. Goka AKJ, Rolston DDK, Mathan VI, et al: Diagnosis of giardiasis by specific IgM antibody enzyme-linked immunosorbent assay. Lancet 2:184, 1986.
66. Nash TE, Herrington DA, Losonsky GA, et al: Experimental human infections with *Giardia lamblia*. J Infect Dis 156:974, 1987.

67. Goka AKJ, Rolston DDK, Mathan VI, et al: Serum IgA response in human *Giardia lamblia* infection. Serodiagn Immunother 3:273, 1989.
68. Farthing MJG, Chong S, Walker-Smith JA: Acute allergic phenomena in giardiasis. Lancet 2:1428, 1984.
69. Briaud M, Morichau-Beauchant M, Matuchansky C, et al: Intestinal immune response in giardiasis. Lancet 2:358, 1981.
70. Miotti PG, Gilman RH, Pickering LK, et al: Prevalence of serum and milk antibodies to *Giardia lamblia* in different populations of lactating women. J Infect Dis 152:1025, 1985.
71. Snider DP, Gordon J, McDermott MR, et al: Chronic *Giardia muris* infection of anti-IgM–treated mice. I. Analysis of immunoglobulin- and parasite-specific antibody in normal and immunoglobulin-deficient animals. J Immunol 135:4153, 1985.
72. Snider DP, Underdown BJ: Quantitative and temporal analyses of murine antibody response in serum and gut secretions to infection with *Giardia muris*. Infect Immun 52:271, 1986.
73. Heyworth MF: Antibody response to *Giardia muris* trophozoites in mouse intestine. Infect Immun 52:568, 1986.
74. Andrews JS, Hewlett EL: Protection against infection with *Giardia muris* by milk containing antibody to *Giardia*. J Infect Dis 143:242, 1981.
75. Stevens DP, Frank DM, Mahmoud AAF: Thymus dependency of host resistance to *Giardia muris* infection: Studies in nude mice. J Immunol 120:680, 1978.
76. Kanwar SS, Ganguly NK, Walia BNS, et al: Enumeration of small intestinal lymphocyte population in *Giardia lamblia* infected mice. J Diarrhoeal Dis Res 2:243, 1984.
77. Ferguson A, McClure JP, Townley RRW: Intraepithelial lymphocyte counts in small intestinal biopsies from children with diarrhoea. Acta Paediatr Scand 65:541, 1976.
78. Heyworth MF, Owen RL, Seaman WE, et al: Harvesting of leukocytes from intestinal lumen in murine giardiasis and preliminary characterization of these cells. Dig Dis Sci 30:149, 1985.
79. Smith PD, Keister DB, Elson CO: Human host response to *Giardia lamblia* II. Antibody-dependent killing in vitro. Cell Immunol 82:308, 1983.
80. Edson CM, Farthing MJG, Thorley-Lawson DA, et al: An 88,000 M_r *Giardia lamblia* surface protein which is immunogenic in humans. Infect Immun 54:621, 1986.
81. Einfeld DA, Stibbs HH: Identification and characterization of a major antigen of *Giardia lamblia*. Infect Immun 46:377, 1984.
82. Kumkum, Khanna R, Khuller M, et al: Plasma membrane associated antigens of trophozoites of axenic *Giardia lamblia*. Trans R Soc Trop Med Hyg 82:439, 1988.
83. Torian BE, Barnes RC, Stephens RS, et al: Tubulin and high–molecular weight polypeptides as *Giardia lamblia* antigens. Infect Immun 46:152, 1984.
84. Clark JT, Holberton DV: Plasma membrane isolated from *Giardia lamblia*: Identification of membrane proteins. Eur J Cell Biol 42:200, 1986.
85. Taylor GD, Wenman WM: Human immune response to *Giardia lamblia* infection. J Infect Dis 155:137, 1987.
86. Gillin FD, Reiner DS, Gault MJ, et al: Encystation and expression of cyst antigens by *Giardia lamblia* in vitro. Science 235:1040, 1987.
87. Rosoff JD, Stibbs HH: Isolation and identification of a *Giardia lamblia*–specific stool antigen (GSA 65) useful in coprodiagnosis of giardiasis. J Clin Microbiol 23:905, 1986.
88. Aggarwal A, Nash TE: Antigenic variation of *Giardia lamblia* in vivo. Infect Immun 56:1420, 1988.
89. Adam RD, Aggarwal A, Lal AA, et al: Antigenic variation of a cysteine-rich protein in *Giardia lamblia*. J Exp Med 167:109, 1988.
90. Upcroft JA, Capon AG, Dharmkrong-At A, et al: *Giardia intestinalis* antigens expressed in *Escherichia coli*. Mol Exp Parasitol 26:267, 1987.
91. Char S, Shetty N, Elliott EJ, et al: Serum IgA response in children with *Giardia lamblia* infection and identification of an immunodominant 57-kDa antigen. Parasite Immunol 13:329, 1991.
92. Char S, Cevallos AM, Farthing MJG: An immunodominant antigen of *Giardia lamblia* is a heat shock protein. Biotechnol Ther 3:151, 1992.
93. Char S, Cevallos AM, Yamson P, et al: Impaired IgA response to *Giardia* heat shock antigen in children with persistent diarrhoea and giardiasis. Gut 34:38, 1992.
94. Moore GT, Cross WM, McGuire D, et al: Epidemic giardiasis at a ski resort. N Engl J Med 281:402, 1969.
95. Brodsky RE, Spencer HC, Schultz HG: Giardiasis in American travelers to the Soviet Union. J Infect Dis 130:319, 1974.
96. Cantor D, Biempica L, Toccalino H, et al: Small intestine studies in giardiasis. Am J Gastroenterol 47:134, 1967.
97. Tewari SG, Tandon BN: Functional and histological changes of small bowel in patients with *Giardia lamblia* infestation. Indian J Med Res 62:689, 1974.
98. Rabassa EB, Arbelo TF, Guillot CC, et al: Malabsorption por *Giardia lamblia*. Rev Cubana Pediatr 47:247, 1975.
99. Wright SG, Tomkins AM, Ridley DS: Giardiasis: Clinical and therapeutic aspects. Gut 18:343, 1977.
100. Cortner JA: Giardiasis: A cause of celiac syndrome. Am J Dis Child 98:311, 1959.
101. Farthing MJG: Giardiasis: Pathogenesis of chronic diarrhea and impact on child growth and development. *In* Lebenthal E (ed): Chronic Diarrhea in Children. New York, Raven Press, 1984, pp 253–267.
102. Kay R, Barnes GL, Townley RRW: *Giardia lamblia* infestation in 154 children. Aust Paediatr 13:98, 1977.
103. Webster ADB: Giardiasis and immunodeficiency diseases. Trans R Soc Trop Med Hyg 74:440, 1980.
104. Kamath KR, Murugasu R: A comparative study of four methods for detecting *Giardia lamblia* in children with diarrheal illness and malabsorption. Gastroenterology 66:16, 1974.
105. Madanagopalan N, Prabhakar Rao U, Somasundaram A, et al: A correlative study of duodenal aspirate and faeces examination in giardiasis before and after treatment with metronidazole. Curr Med Res Opin 3:99, 1975.
106. Thornton SA, West AH, Du Pont HL, et al: Comparison of methods for identification of *Giardia Lamblia*. Am J Clin Pathol 80:858, 1983.
107. Rosenthal P, Liebman WM: Comparative study of stool examinations: Duodenal aspiration and pediatric Entero-Test for giardiasis in children. J Pediatr 96:278, 1980.
108. Goka AKJ, Rolston DDK, Mathan VI, et al: The relative merits of faecal and duodenal juice microscopy in the diagnosis of giardiasis. Trans R Soc Trop Med Hyg 84:66, 1990.
109. Craft JC, Nelson JD: Diagnosis of giardiasis by counterimmunoelectrophoresis of feces. J Infect Dis 145:499, 1982.
110. Ungar BLP, Yolken PH, Nash TE, et al: Enzyme-linked immunosorbent assay for detection of *Giardia lamblia* in fecal specimens. J Infect Dis 149:90, 1984.
111. Green EL, Miles MA, Warhurst DC: Immunodiagnostic detection of *Giardia* antigen in faeces by a rapid visual enzyme-linked immunosorbent assay. Lancet 2:691, 1985.
112. Butcher PD, Farthing MJG: DNA probes for the faecal diagnosis of *Giardia lamblia* infections in man. Biochem Soc Trans 17:363, 1988.
113. Butcher PB, Clark C, Farthing MJG: *Giardia lamblia* cloned genomic DNA probes: Uses in faecal diagnosis and genetic analysis of clinical isolates. Gut 29:A722, 1988.
114. Farthing MJG, Inge PMG: Antigiardial activity of the bile salt-like antibiotic sodium fusidate. J Antimicrob Chemother 17:165, 1986.
115. Farthing MJG, Inge PMG, Pearson RM: Effect of D-propranolol on growth and motility of flagellate protozoa. J Antimicrob Chemother 20:519, 1987.
116. Hewlett EL, Pearson RD: Antiprotozoal activity of tricyclic compounds. Science 230:1063, 1985.
117. Al-Waili NS, Al-Waili BH, Saloom KY: Therapeutic use of mebendazole in giardial infections. Trans R Soc Trop Med Hyg 82:438, 1988.
118. Boreham PFL, Phillips RE, Shepherd RW: Heterogeneity in the responses of clones of *Giardia intestinalis* to antigiardial drugs. Trans R Soc Trop Med Hyg 81:406, 1987.
119. Jokipii L, Jokipii AMM: In vitro susceptibility of *Giardia lamblia* trophozoites to metronidazole and tinidazole. J Infect Dis 141:317, 1980.
120. Boreham PF, Phillips RE, Shepherd RW: The sensitivity of *Giardia intestinalis* to drugs in vitro. J Antimicrob Chemother 14:449, 1984.
121. Inge PMG, Farthing MJG: A radiometric assay for antigiardial drugs. Trans R Soc Trop Med Hyg 81:345, 1987.

287

Plasmodium and Babesia

David J. Wyler

Malaria

History

The history of malaria is a fascinating story of the human struggle with a debilitating and devastating illness that at one time afflicted more than two thirds of the world's population and helped shape the course of history.[1] Periodic fevers (malaria) were described more than 3000 years ago in early Chinese, Chaldean, and Hindu writings. By that time, certain herbal medications for malaria were probably already in use. One such traditional therapy (extracts from the plant *Artemesia annua*) that has been used for centuries in China has received substantial attention as a potential curative against multidrug-resistant strains of *Plasmodium falciparum*. The recognition by the Greeks in the fourth century BC of an association between exposure to swamps (mosquito breeding grounds) and periodic fevers led to drainage of swamps as a method to control malaria that is still in use today. By the 17th century, the bark of the quinaquina (cinchona) tree of South America was in widespread use for intermittent fever; quinine, the active alkaloid, was identified in the mid-19th century. The two discoveries that revolutionized the struggle with malaria came in the late 19th century, when Laveran first identified plasmodia as the pathogen and Ross demonstrated that mosquitos were the vector and delineated the parasite's life cycle (in avian malaria). Development in the 1940s of DDT, an efficacious residual insecticide, and synthesis of new antimalarial drugs (especially chloroquine) useful in treatment and chemoprophylaxis provided powerful new control modalities. As a result, the World Health Organization began a worldwide malaria eradication program in 1955. The program was officially declared a failure in 1976, when insecticide resistance in *Anopheles* vectors, drug resistance in strains of *P. falciparum*, and political and administrative disorganization in certain endemic regions severely undermined the initial successes of the program.[2] The development in the 1970s of methods for continuous cultivation in vitro of *P. falciparum*, for the production of monoclonal antibodies, and for genetic engineering for the first time permitted concerted efforts at developing a malaria vaccine.[3] A vaccine against the asexual blood stages of *P. falciparum* has proved partially effective in preventing malaria in field trials.[4, 5] Other vaccine candidates are in earlier stages of testing.[6] Clinical investigations are better at defining the pathogenesis of severe falciparum malaria and could provide novel approaches to clinical management.

Characteristics of the Pathogen

The genus *Plasmodium* is classified within the class Sporozoa (subphylum Apicomplexa), placing it in a class with *Toxoplasma gondii*, *Eimeria*, *Cryptosporidium*, and *Babesia*. Numerous *Plasmodium* species have been identified that naturally infect a variety of animals,[7] but only four species are important human pathogens: *P. falciparum*, *Plasmodium vivax*, *Plasmodium malariae*, and *Plasmodium ovale*. Each species has distinctive morphologic features that permit specific identification and biologic characteristics that are clinically important (Table 287–1).

Malaria is transmitted when infected female anopheline mosquitos inject sporozoites while taking a blood meal (or when infected erythrocytes are injected intravenously) (Fig. 287–1). Within minutes of entering the circulation, sporozoites invade hepatocytes, where they develop as hepatic exoerythrocytic forms. A distinctive protein that surrounds the sporozoite surface (the circumsporozoite protein) is believed to contain the ligand for association with the hepatocyte plasma membrane,[8] and it is the basis of a candidate antimalaria vaccine. When the parasite transforms and multiplies at this stage, it is referred to as a tissue schizont; after 1 to 2 weeks' intrahepatic development, merozoites emerge from the tissue schizonts, enter the circulation, and infect erythrocytes. It is estimated that each sporozoite can give rise to 10,000 to 30,000 merozoites, and the number of sporozoites injected influences the intensity of the subsequent asexual-stage infection (in falciparum malaria[9]). Latent exoerythrocytic schizonts (now called hypnozoites[10]) of *P. vivax* and *P. ovale* can persist for months or years and give rise to malaria

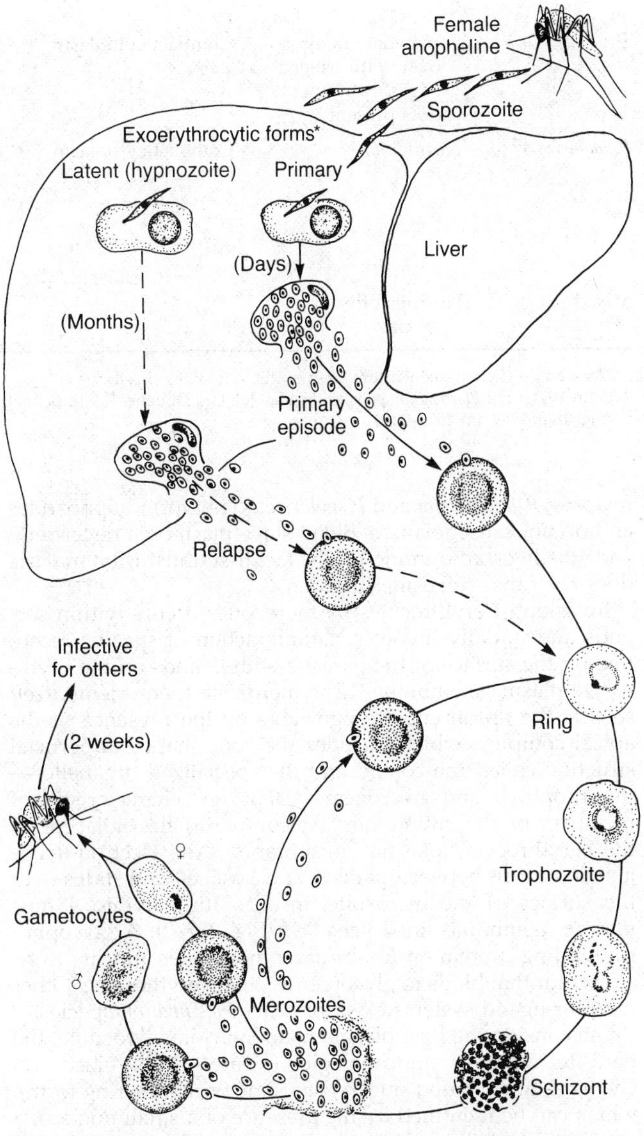

FIGURE 287–1 □ Life cycle of plasmodia in humans. *Exoerythrocytic forms are also called tissue schizonts.

TABLE 287–1 ■ Selected Diagnostic and Clinical Features of Human Malaria

PLASMODIUM SPECIES	MORPHOLOGIC CHARACTERISTICS USEFUL IN SPECIES DIAGNOSIS* Infected RBCs	Trophozoite	Schizont	Gametocyte	IMPORTANT CLINICAL FEATURES
P. falciparum	Normal size; multiply infected RBCs more frequent than in other species	Small rings with threadlike cytoplasm (blue) and double chromatin dots (red)	Seldom seen in peripheral blood smear	Diagnostic banana-shaped gametocyte	Can achieve intense parasitemia, causing death through complications (severe anemia, renal failure, cerebral dysfunction, pulmonary edema) *A medical emergency!* Failure to recognize *P. falciparum* and to treat appropriately can lead to death.
P. vivax	Enlarged; Schüffner dots (red) present	Ameboid cytoplasm	Visible on smear	Round	Infection limited to younger RBCs; danger of splenic rupture, relapse related to persistence of latent exoerythrocytic forms
P. ovale	Somewhat enlarged, oval, with fringed edges; Schüffner dots present	Compact cytoplasm	Visible on smear	Round	Same as *P. vivax*
P. malariae	Normal size	Compact cytoplasm	Merozoites arranged in rosette around central pigment clump	Round	Limited parasitemia; can be chronic in subclinical and subpatent forms; can cause nephritis in children
Mixed	Features of each species				

*As seen on Giemsa-stained thin smears. RBCs, Red blood cells.
From Wyler DJ: *Plasmodium* species. *In* Mandell GL, Douglas RG Jr, Bennett JE (eds): Principles and Practice of Infectious Diseases, ed 3. New York, Churchill Livingstone, 1989, pp 2056–2066.

relapses; *P. falciparum* and *P. malariae* do not form hypnozoites and do not cause relapses. Blood-stage plasmodia never reinvade the liver, accounting for the fact that transfusion malaria does not cause relapsing infection.

Invasion of erythrocytes by merozoites occurs within seconds and initially involves the interaction of specific receptors on the surface of the parasite with ligands on the erythrocyte plasma membrane.[11] The merozoite then orients itself so that the apical end (recognizable by the presence of the apical complex, which includes the cone-shaped superficial structure called the conoid and the specialized organelles—the rhoptries and micronemes—that are characteristic of members of the subphylum Apicomplexa) lies adjacent to the erythrocyte plasma membrane. An electron-dense junction forms between parasite and host cell and slides over the surface of the merozoite, incorporating it into a host plasma membrane–lined vacuole[12] (Fig. 287–2). A glycophorin binding protein on *P. falciparum* merozoites appears to be a receptor that binds to glycophorin on the erythrocyte. Other receptor-ligand systems exist for other *Plasmodium* species.

Once inside the host plasma membrane–lined vacuole, the parasite acquires morphologic features (recognized on Giemsa-stained blood smears) of a signet ring (the ring form), which can be identified by the presence of a small nucleus, a chromatin dot that stains purplish, from which emanates a fine ring of cytoplasm that stains blue (Fig. 287–3*A*). As the parasite matures, the cytoplasm progressively increases and acquires an ameboid configuration. This is the trophozoite stage (Fig. 287–3*B*). After the nucleus has divided for the first time, the stage is referred to as the schizont (Fig. 287–3*C*). Ultimately, 6 to 24 nuclei are discernible, the number depending on the species, which indicate the presence of the many merozoites that ultimately rupture out of the schizont. These merozoites rapidly invade uninfected erythrocytes and continue the asexual intraerythrocyte cycle. The process of intraerythrocytic development and replication, schizogony, requires 48 hours for *P. falciparum*, *P. vivax*, and *P. ovale* and 72 hours for *P. malariae*. Because fever[13] occurs in association with schizont rupture (Fig. 287–4), in cases in which all the asexual intraerythrocytic parasites are developing synchronously (as commonly occurs in semiimmune patients or in relapsing malaria), fever appears at either 48- or 72-hour intervals. In cases in which the parasite broods are developing asynchronously (as in nonimmune patients suffering a primary malaria attack), this periodicity is absent.

Innate host factors can influence invasion and intraerythrocyte parasite development.[14] For example, only young erythrocytes support the growth of *P. vivax* and *P. ovale*; it is believed that *P. malariae* develops only in more mature erythrocytes, whereas the intraerythrocyte development of *P. falciparum* is not restricted to a subpopulation of normal erythrocytes. The clinical implication is that only *P. falciparum* can

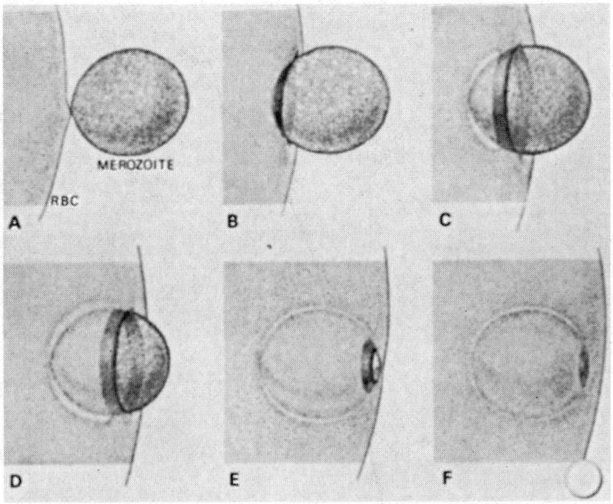

FIGURE 287–2 □ The sequence of events in merozoite entry into an erythrocyte. *A*, Initial attachment of merozoite at its apical pole. *B*, Formation of a circumferential junction between parasite and host cell. *C* to *E*, Movement of junction over merozoite surface with invagination of the erythrocyte plasma membrane. *F*, Resealing of erythrocyte membrane and creation of the host membrane–lined parasitophorous membrane. (*A* to *F* from Aikawa M, Miller LH, Johnson J, Rabbege J: Erythrocyte entry by malarial parasites. A moving junction between erythrocyte and parasite. J Cell Biol 77:72–82, 1978.)

proliferate to the high densities in circulation (parasitemia) that are associated with high mortality rates; the other species rarely cause lethal infections. On the other hand, erythrocytes that contain variant hemoglobin may fail to support the normal development of *P. falciparum* and prevent parasitemia from reaching potentially lethal levels. The clearest example is the protection imparted to patients with sickle hemoglobin (HbS).[15] This protection against lethal malaria accounts for the high frequency of the sickle allele in regions where *P. falciparum* malaria is or has been transmitted.[16] Because sickle cell anemia (SS hemoglobin) also carries a high mortality rate, the heterozygous state (AS hemoglobin) is maintained at a particularly high frequency in these regions (an example of the genetic principle of balanced polymorphism). The cellular basis of the protection apparently involves the leakage of potassium from infected cells that contain HbS when they are exposed to low oxygen tension.[17] Other erythrocyte variants, including those that contain HbF, those deficient in

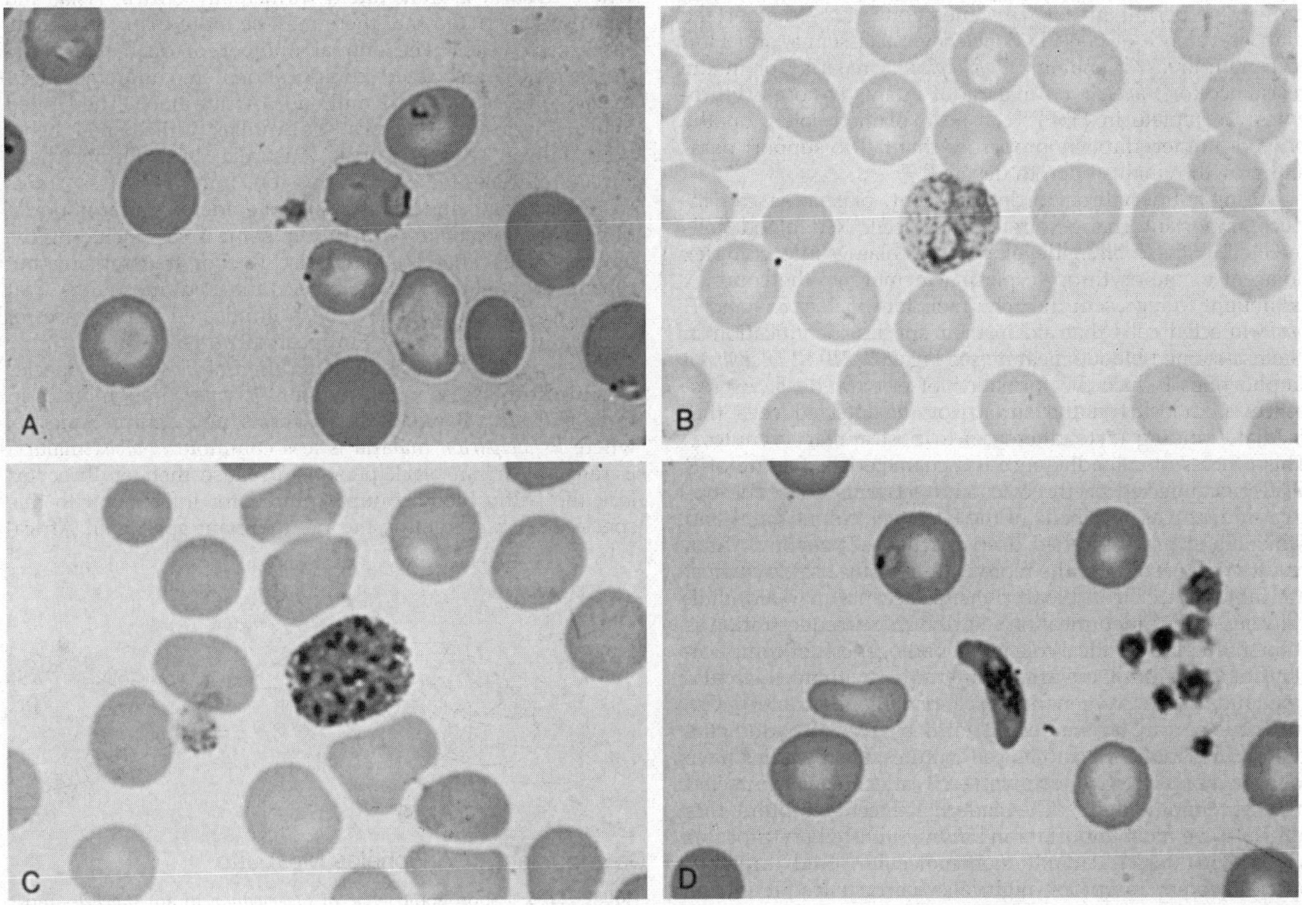

FIGURE 287–3 □ Representative stages in the life cycle of plasmodia that infect humans. *A*, Ring stage of *P. falciparum*. *B*, Trophozoite of *P. vivax* (note Schüffner dots and enlarged erythrocyte). *C*, Schizont of *P. vivax* (note multiple nuclei of merozoites). *D*, Macrogametocyte of *P. falciparum* (note crescentic shape).

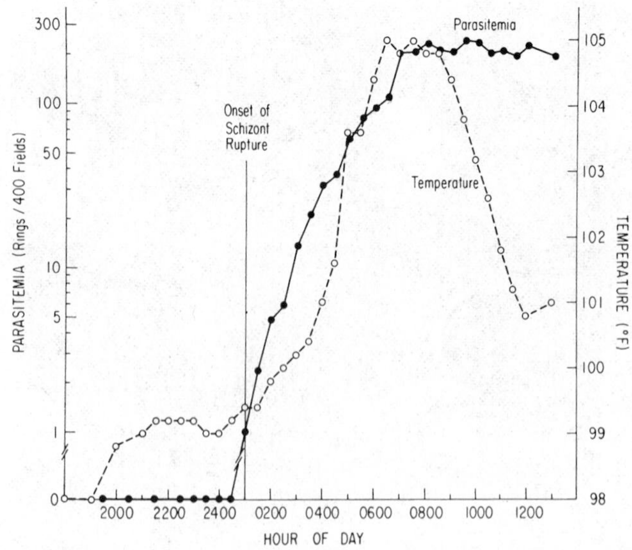

FIGURE 287–4 □ Relationship of fever to maturation of plasmodium (*P. vivax*) in malaria. Note temperature elevation at time of schizont rupture. Regular fever patterns are not an invariable feature of malaria and depend on the synchronized maturation of the intracellular asexual-stage parasites. (From Miller LH: Transfusion malaria. *In* Greenwalt TJ, Jamieson GA [eds]: Transmissible Disease and Blood Transfusion. New York, Grune & Stratton, 1975, pp 241–266.)

glucose-6-phosphate dehydrogenase (G-6-PD), and those with cytoskeletal defects, may fail to support *P. falciparum* growth or permit invasion by merozoites.[18-20] Whether the high prevalence of G-6-PD deficiency, thalassemia, and HbE in certain areas of endemic *P. falciparum* malaria[21] or innate resistance to *P. falciparum* malaria of infants (whose erythrocytes are replete in HbF)[18] can be explained solely on the basis of intraerythrocyte properties that fail to support parasite growth remains open to debate.[22, 23]

During intraerythrocyte development, plasmodia can induce important changes in the host cell. Red blood cells infected with *P. vivax* develop a caveolae-vesicle complex adjacent to the erythrocyte plasma membrane; the complex is thought to represent the Schüffner dots of *P. vivax*– and *P. ovale*–infected cells that aid in their species identification in Giemsa-stained blood smears[24] (see Fig. 287–3*B*). *P. falciparum* trophozoites induce the formation of electron-dense excrescences ("knobs") on the surface of the infected cells that mediate binding (cytoadherence) to postcapillary venules.[25] This process of cytoadherence is a characteristic feature of *P. falciparum*–infected erythrocytes and accounts for sequestration in deep vascular beds of the late-stage trophozoites and schizonts (a process called deep vascular schizogony). As a result of sequestration, the more mature forms of *P. falciparum* are rarely detected in blood films (a fact that may aid clinically in species identification). Furthermore, sequestration is thought to play a critical role in the pathogenesis of complications of *P. falciparum* malaria by interfering with microcirculation and tissue oxygenation (see pathogenesis later). Cytoadherence can be studied in vitro by use of endothelial cell or amelanotic melanoma cell cultures; such studies have identified putative ligands involved in attachment of infected cells to endothelium.[26] The endothelial cell receptors that appear to be most important in binding infected erythrocytes are CD36, intercellular adhesion molecule-1, and thrombospondin; other receptors might also participate.[27] It is currently believed that certain cytokines produced during falciparum malaria (such as tumor necrosis factor [TNF] and interleukin-1) up-regulate these endothelial receptors and augment cytoadherence in addition to mediating some features of the disease (such as fever). Sequestration of this type does not occur in malarias associated with the three other species.

The sexual cycle of plasmodial reproduction begins with development from a subpopulation of merozoites into gametocytes (see Fig. 287–3*D*). Distinctive morphologic appearance differentiates them from the asexual stages, distinguishes male and female forms, and may assist in species identification. For example, the macrogametocyte (female) of *P. falciparum* is uniquely falciform (crescentic) in shape. Within the gut of a female anopheline mosquito, gametes emerge from ingested gametocytes (Fig. 287–5). Here, spermlike microgametes fertilize the macrogametes, giving rise to the zygote; flagellated ookinetes develop from the zygotes and invade the gut epithelium. Oocysts are formed in the gut wall, and within these structures thousands of sporozoites develop. The sporozoites subsequently migrate to the salivary glands, whence they emerge during the mosquito's next blood meal. The sexual cycle of plasmodial development in the vector (sporogony) requires approximately 10 days. The sexual-stage development in the mosquito can be blocked if specific antibodies to gametes are present in the blood meal.[28] This observation has led to the development of experimental transmission-blocking vaccine.[29]

Epidemiology

Although reliable prevalence data are not available, it is estimated that hundreds of millions of people live in areas where malaria is transmitted (principally Africa, Asia, and Latin America) and that there may be more than 300 million cases each year.[30] The annual number of deaths resulting from malaria-associated complications in children is estimated to be as high as 1 million in Africa alone. The United States, Puerto Rico, Jamaica, the Antilles, Chile, Israel, Lebanon, Taiwan, North Korea, Australia, and Europe have successfully eliminated transmission. Imported cases, transfusion malaria,[31] and small localized epidemics after importation[32, 32a] still occur infrequently in some areas, including the United States, that are otherwise free of transmission but where anopheline vectors breed. Infected mosquitos that stow away on jetliners have been implicated in rare cases of malaria in residents near European airports.

The geographic distribution of different *Plasmodium* species is difficult to assess with precision. *P. vivax* predominates in India, Pakistan, Bangladesh, Sri Lanka, and Central America, where *P. falciparum* malaria is less common. *P. vivax* malaria is rare in African black persons, because their erythrocytes lack the Duffy blood group required for infection with this species.[33] *P. falciparum* is the predominant species in Africa,

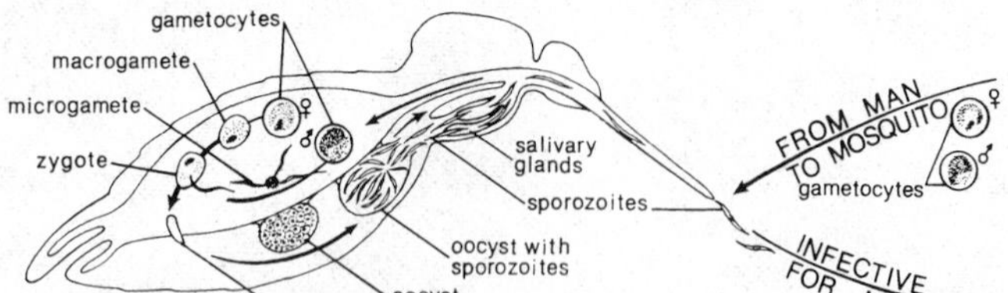

FIGURE 287–5 □ Sporogonic cycle of *Plasmodium* in an *Anopheles* mosquito (see text). (From Miller LH: Transfusion malaria. *In* Greenwalt TJ, Jamieson GA [eds]: Transmissible Disease and Blood Transfusion. New York, Grune & Stratton, 1975, pp 241–266.)

Haiti, and New Guinea. Both *P. vivax* malaria and *P. falciparum* malaria are prevalent in Southeast Asia, South America, and Oceania. *P. ovale*, the rarest species, is transmitted primarily in Africa; rarely, cases occur elsewhere. *P. malariae* is distributed widely and is frequently encountered in Africa. Imported malaria remains a problem in the United States, where approximately 1000 cases have been officially reported annually since the close of the Vietnam War era.[34] Thousands of cases of imported malaria occur annually in Europe.[35]

Fatal imported malaria has occurred in the United States and Europe because some physicians failed to make the correct diagnosis and institute appropriate therapy in a timely manner or failed to prescribe appropriate chemoprophylaxis and other preventive measures for travelers to malarious areas. On the other hand, transfusion malaria has decreased as a problem. The American Association of Blood Banks has published guidelines that reduce the risk for transmission by this route.[36] Because *P. malariae* can persist indetectably in circulation longer than 50 years without causing symptoms, the blood banking guidelines do not eliminate the risk for transfusion malaria due to this species. Congenital malaria in children born in the United States to mothers from malaria-endemic areas is reported occasionally.[37] Transmission in conjunction with transfusion of platelet[38] or leukocyte[39] concentrates or organ transplantation[40] has also been documented. In Saudi Arabia, *P. falciparum* was transmitted between patients when a single syringe was used sequentially to flush heparin locks.[40a]

Pathogenesis

Illness results exclusively during the asexual intraerythrocyte cycle; hepatic exoerythrocytic development causes no discernible disease, and patients with exclusively gametocyte parasitemia are asymptomatic. The pathogenesis of malaria remains poorly understood. Clinical illness arises from fever and its physiologic consequences, anemia, tissue hypoxia, and the initiation of certain immunopathologic events. Because of their lethal potential, the complications of *P. falciparum* malaria have received the closest scrutiny.

Fever is a consequence of pathophysiologic events triggered at the time of schizont rupture[13] (see Fig. 287–4). To explain this observation, it has been postulated that at the time of schizont rupture, substances are released that stimulate macrophages to produce pyrogenic cytokines such as interleukin-1 and TNF-α.[41] Vasodilation that results from the fever, as well as diaphoresis, vomiting, and decreased fluid intake, causes a decrease in effective plasma volume that can manifest as orthostatic hypotension. Secretion of antidiuretic hormone and aldosterone increases as a normal homeostatic response and can result in hyponatremia.[42] Inappropriate antidiuretic hormone secretion can also occur.[43]

Anemia in malaria results from hemolysis during schizont rupture and from other ill-defined mechanisms; the magnitude of the anemia is usually greater than can be accounted for on the basis of parasitemia alone.[44] Splenomegaly may result in erythrocyte sequestration,[45] and ineffective erythropoiesis with a delayed reticulocytosis response to the hemolytic anemia has been observed in cases of *P. falciparum* malaria, even after antimalarial treatment. Hemoglobinemia and hemoglobinuria occur mainly when hemolysis is massive, in blackwater fever. This condition is more common in nonimmune patients than in residents of areas where *P. falciparum* is endemic and is usually associated with high concentrations of *P. falciparum* organisms in blood. Less commonly, it occurs as an atypical (immune?) response during reinfection or in association with quinine administration or the ingestion of oxidant antimalarial agents by patients with G-6-PD deficiency. Thrombocytopenia frequently complicates malaria caused by all species and may be profound (cell count $<50,000/mm^3$), but this is rarely accompanied by serious spontaneous hemorrhage. Platelet sequestration (including in the spleen), not decreased production, is the mechanism of this complication.[46]

The potential complications of *P. falciparum* malaria include renal failure, pulmonary edema, cerebral dysfunction, and malabsorption.[47] Tissue hypoxia due to anemia and microvascular congestion is thought to be the cause of these disturbances, although the contribution of other factors (parasite toxins or host-derived cytokines) has been proposed.[48] Sequestration of *P. falciparum*–infected erythrocytes within microvascular beds of the affected organs (see earlier) is believed to result in sluggish blood flow, reduced oxygen delivery, and perhaps also loss of endothelial integrity, leading to leakage of fluid into the interstitium (e.g., pulmonary edema). Renal cortical ischemia and acute tubular necrosis have been documented histopathologically post mortem.[49] Microvascular congestion, interstitial edema, and hyaline membrane formation have been observed in specimens taken from patients who died with pulmonary edema. In fatal cases of cerebral malaria, microvascular congestion of the cerebral cortical gray matter, perivascular edema, hemorrhage (ring hemorrhage), and rarely glial reaction (malarial granuloma) have been observed. Studies, however, suggest that some of these changes may occur post mortem.[50] Malabsorption and enterocolitis, two rare complications, probably also occur as a result of the microcirculatory disorder and tissue hypoxia.[47] It is possible that gram-negative sepsis that sometimes complicates *P. falciparum* malaria[48] may be the result of invasion of bowel organisms through mucosa, the structural integrity of which has been compromised by this process.

Although the prothrombin and partial thromboplastin times are often prolonged in malaria patients and some patients may have reduced levels of factors V, VII, and X and fibrinogen, there is little evidence to suggest that disseminated intravascular coagulation is common in this disease. Clinically important bleeding probably affects no more than 5% of patients, even those with serious complications such as cerebral malaria.[48] Histologic evidence of disseminated intravascular coagulation is rarely detected in postmortem examinations of fatal cases.

Cerebral malaria, the most common serious complication of malaria, occurs only in *P. falciparum* infections.[51] Death occurs in 20% to 50% of cases.[48, 51] The pathogenesis of cerebral malaria is currently viewed in relation to the process of sequestration of parasitized erythrocytes in cerebral postcapillary venules. Precisely how sequestration and reduced microcirculation result in the variety of clinical expressions of cerebral dysfunction that are often reversible is less clear, however. There has been increased emphasis on the potential role of cytokines, particularly TNF-α, in the pathogenesis. One theory suggests that local production of TNF by cerebral endothelial cells triggers the generation of nitric oxide, which in turn leads to cerebrovascular dilatation, increased cerebrospinal fluid pressure, and possibly defective neurotransmission.[52] The most compelling evidence supporting the hypothesis is the observation that African children who have a genetic propensity to overexpress the TNF-α gene are at significantly greater risk for development of severe or life-threatening cerebral malaria.[53] Clinical studies have largely excluded the earlier perspectives by demonstrating that reduced total cerebral blood flow, cerebral edema, inflammation, and microthrombus formation are not features of this complication.[54] In some children, cerebral malaria may result in chronic neurologic deficits,[55] but sequelae are rare in adults. A transient neurologic syndrome with fine tremors, convulsions, or confusional states has been observed in a small percentage of adults and children in Southeast Asia during their recovery from severe falciparum malaria.[55a] A risk factor for developing the syndrome was receiving mefloquine after a course of parenteral antimalarial therapy. This observation strongly suggests that the syndrome represents a metabolic encephalopathy. Marked glucose use and lactate production by the sequestered parasites may also contribute to the encephalopathy.

Hypoglycemia and lactic acidosis have been identified as important potential complications of *P. falciparum* malaria. These metabolic derangements are frequently documented in infected pregnant women and in patients with severe disease (e.g., cerebral malaria[56]). Impaired hepatic glycogenolysis and gluconeogenesis in the face of increased anaerobic glycolysis by the parasite and the hypoxic tissues of the host may partially explain this condition. Because quinine is a potent secretagogue for insulin, its administration can aggravate hypoglycemia. Metabolic acidosis may contribute to respiratory distress in children with falciparum malaria.[56a]

The immune responses to malaria are rapid and profound, but those that confer some degree of protection (the ability to limit parasitemia) are most apparent in persons who have experienced numerous infections.[57] Malaria is accompanied by a brisk increase in immunoglobulins, many of which lack anti-*Plasmodium* specificity and may indeed be autoantibodies[58] or have specificities that provide for the biologic false-positive serologic reactions (such as in tests for syphilis or Epstein-Barr virus infection).[59, 60] The presence of a lymphocyte mitogen in plasmodia may account at least partially for this polyclonal B-cell hyperresponse.[61] Hyperplasia of the mononuclear phagocyte system (formerly called the reticuloendothelial system) is a similarly rapid and extensive response. Recruitment of blood monocytes to the spleen and liver probably results from the elaboration of chemotactic lymphokines produced in response to parasite products.[62] Splenomegaly can result and contributes to the clearance of infected erythrocytes, a process that apparently depends on the decreased deformability of these cells.[63] Sequestration of platelets and neutrophils in the spleen may explain the thrombocytopenia and neutropenia that frequently occur in malaria.

Despite the remarkable immunologic perturbations induced by malaria, there are relatively few chronic sequelae. Unmodified splenic enlargement can result in hyperreactive malarial splenomegaly (also known as tropical splenomegaly syndrome and big spleen disease) observed in a small subpopulation of patients living in Africa, New Guinea, and Indonesia.[64] A relatively small subpopulation of children chronically infected with *P. malariae* develop immune complex–mediated glomerulonephritis that is refractory to treatment with antimalarial and immunosuppressive agents.[65] The relatively high prevalence of Burkitt lymphoma in Africans living in malaria endemic regions is believed to result from an atypical response to Epstein-Barr virus infection.[66] Immunosuppression[67] and polyclonal B-cell stimulation induced by malaria infection might be cofactors in the oncogenesis.

In areas where *P. falciparum* malaria is endemic, older children and adults experience infection as a milder disease and with lower levels of parasitemia than do young children.[57] Pregnancy or prolonged residence outside an endemic area often results in the loss of this immunity. Because transfusion of γ-globulins from immune adults could impart limited protection to infected children,[68] there is reason to believe that antibody plays a role in defense to the blood-stage parasites. Neutralization of merozoite invasion may be one mechanism. Antibody-mediated clearance and opsonization are more likely to be instrumental in defense than are cytotoxic mechanisms. Antibody-independent, T-cell–mediated defense has been observed in certain rodent malaria models, but the underlying mechanism remains to be elucidated. Soluble products (such as toxic oxygen radicals) of macrophages activated by lymphokines are being considered by some as a potential molecular basis of defense.[69] Because splenectomy profoundly weakens a host's antimalarial defense, it seems likely that critical immune events take place in this organ.[70] Concepts of malarial defense that incorporate antigen-nonspecific mechanisms will have to reconcile the fact that immunity in malaria appears to be species and to some extent also strain specific.

Clinical Manifestations

The hallmark of malaria is the febrile paroxysm, during which patients typically experience high temperature (105°F), rigors, headache, abdominal pain, nausea, vomiting, and overwhelming malaise. The paroxysm is temporally associated with schizont rupture (see Fig. 287–4). When schizogony occurs in a synchronized manner—when all parasites are at approximately the same stage of development at any given time—the paroxysms occur at regular intervals of 48 (tertian malaria) or 72 hours (quartan malaria, due to *P. malariae*). When the paroxysm abates, diaphoresis, fatigue, and even euphoria dominate the clinical picture. The dramatic contrast of a deathly ill patient presented during a paroxysm and that of the same patient exhausted but relatively well a few hours later is rarely encountered in other infectious diseases. In patients in whom schizogony is asynchronous (typically those who have little antimalarial immunity, such as travelers to endemic areas), the periodicity of the fever and accompanying symptoms are usually irregular. Accordingly, there is no justification to exclude malaria from diagnostic consideration simply on the grounds of an irregular fever pattern.

For one or more days before the onset of the paroxysm, the patient may experience a prodrome of malaise, fatigue, and headache that mimics viral illness. Because some patients also experience localizing symptoms, such as chest, abdominal, or joint pain, physicians may be misled in their evaluation.[71] The ability of malaria to masquerade as a large number of other illnesses can contribute to a delay in establishing the correct diagnosis; in *P. falciparum* malaria, this delay can prove lethal. Fever in any patient with a history of possible exposure (travel, illicit intravenous drug use, transfusion, accidental inoculation with blood from an infected patient) should prompt an examination of blood smears. Because symptoms may appear before parasitized erythrocytes reach detectable levels in the blood, the search should be repeated on at least 3 consecutive days.

Physical examination of patients with malaria generally reveals tachycardia, and orthostatic hypotension is common. Splenomegaly and tender hepatomegaly are often present, but vigorous palpation for spenomegaly is inadvisable because the spleen can be ruptured. Lymphadenopathy is not a feature of malaria; this finding should prompt a search for another illness. A variety of other physical findings in patients with malaria have been reported: jaundice, urticaria, petechiae, conjunctival suffusion, scleral icterus, retinal vasospasm and hemorrhage, and herpes labialis. Scattered rales are occasionally heard when auscultation is carried out during a paroxysm. Flow murmurs resulting from fever and anemia are not uncommon. The abdomen may be tender. Despite musculoskeletal pain, signs of arthritis and myositis are absent. In uncomplicated cases, results of the neurologic examination are normal, except for minor behavioral changes attributable to high fever. Cerebral malaria occurs as a complication of *P. falciparum* infection; important neurologic dysfunction in the setting of malaria due to species other than *P. falciparum* should prompt a search for a disease other than malaria. The neurologic abnormalities associated with cerebral malaria include altered consciousness; acute organic brain syndrome (with altered intellectual function, behavioral changes, and hallucinations); major motor seizures; meningismus; and rarely focal abnormalities such as Babinski sign, hemiparesis, or movement disorders (tremors, myoclonus, choreiform movements). The results of lumbar puncture and analysis of cerebrospinal fluid are not diagnostic and serve principally to assist in identifying other causes of central nervous system dysfunction. An elevated opening pressure, increased cerebrospinal fluid protein and lactate concentrations, and low-grade pleocytosis are occasionally recorded, but hypoglycorrhachia does not occur. The presence of hypoglycemia may aggravate the neurologic abnormalities.[56] Febrile convulsions may be impossible to distinguish from cerebral malaria in infected children.

Malaria during pregnancy can increase the risk for low birth weight, prematurity, abortion, and stillbirth and may cause hypoglycemia. The choice of drugs for the treatment and prevention of malaria must consider potential adverse effects to the fetus.

Several abnormal results of laboratory tests have been encountered in acute malaria. Normocytic normochromic anemia, thrombocytopenia, and decreased neutrophil and lymphocyte counts are common.[72] Early infection may stimulate a leftward shift in the differential leukocyte count, however. Urinanalysis may disclose low-grade proteinuria, probably due to fever, but findings are otherwise normal if the patient is not suffering from malaria-induced acute tubular necrosis. Elevated blood urea nitrogen may reflect dehydration; elevation of the serum creatinine value suggests renal failure. Hyponatremia is often documented. Moderately elevated liver transaminase concentrations and mild bilirubinemia (mostly indirect) are not worrisome, whereas elevated alkaline phosphatase level or substantial transaminase elevation should suggest the presence of liver disease or centrilobular necrosis that occasionally complicates severe malaria. Hypoglycemia should be sought in patients who have *P. falciparum* malaria.

Diagnosis

The diagnosis of malaria is established by identifying parasitized erythrocytes on appropriately stained blood films. Serologic tests are available in the United States through the Centers for Disease Control and Prevention in Atlanta. These tests may not be reliable in establishing a diagnosis of malaria and are generally reserved for epidemiologic studies and to identify infected donors in cases of transfusion malaria.

Once a diagnosis of malaria is entertained on clinical grounds, several blood smears obtained in a period of 3 successive days should be carefully examined before excluding the diagnosis. In nonimmune patients, symptoms typically begin before parasites reach detectable levels in circulation. Because late trophozoites and schizonts of *P. falciparum* are sequestered out of the circulation, the period just after the end of the paroxysm is likely to reveal the greatest number of parasitized erythrocytes in *P. falciparum* malaria; however, the timing of obtaining blood smears is less important than that they be obtained and examined multiple times a day.

Careful preparation of the blood smears substantially enhances their utility. Ideally, smears should be prepared directly from a fresh finger or earlobe prick rather than from anticoagulated blood obtained by venipuncture (anticoagulants may distort the parasite's morphologic appearance, complicating species identification). Microscope slides should be thoroughly cleaned with alcohol and dried completely. Thick smears are prepared by spreading *one drop* of blood over an area the size of a dime (1.5 cm) with the pointed edge of a glass slide, a toothpick, or a wooden applicator stick. Thin smears are prepared in the same manner as ones used for hematologic examination. After thick smears have dried thoroughly (usually several hours), they are treated with distilled water to lyse erythrocytes and then stained with Giemsa or Wright-Giemsa. Thin smears can be fixed in alcohol minutes after they appear dry and then stained. A rapid method for preparing thick smears employs Field stain.[73]

Both thick and thin smears should be examined thoroughly. Species identification, carried out on thin smears, generally requires special experience of the examiner. When parasites are detected, some effort to quantify parasitemia is advisable, to provide a baseline value for monitoring response to therapy. With high parasite concentrations, the percentage of infected erythrocytes should be determined. With less severe parasitemia, determining the number of parasites per white blood cell permits estimation of the number per cubic millimeter (using the white cell count). In the absence of detectable parasites, the presence of granular brown pigment in monocytes can be a clue to the diagnosis.

The important decision that must be made once parasites are detected is whether the patient is infected with *P. falciparum*, because chloroquine-resistant strains of *P. falciparum* are now widely distributed geographically (Table 287–2). Chloroquine is the initial treatment for all the other species. Chloroquine-resistant strains of *P. vivax* occur in parts of Indonesia, Papua New Guinea, and Myanmar.[74] These strains respond to mefloquine treatment. The small size of the rings, the presence of double chromatin dots, the tendency for multiple rings to be present in individual erythrocytes, and the absence of trophozoite- and schizont-infected erythrocytes suggest *P. falciparum*. The pathognomonic banana-shaped (crescentic) gametocytes of this species are rarely detected early in acute infection. When 5% of the erythrocytes or more are infected, it is imperative to assume that the patient has *P. falciparum* malaria and to treat for hyperparasitemia (see section on treatment).

Treatment

P. falciparum malaria is a medical emergency because potentially lethal complications can develop rapidly. Institution of treatment should not be delayed. When a definitive species diagnosis cannot be made expeditiously or when simultaneous infection with more than one species is suspected, hospitalizing the patient and initiating chemotherapy directed at *P. falciparum* are appropriate. Monitoring the parasites' response to antimalarial drugs (examining blood smears two

TABLE 287–2 ■ Geographic Distribution of Chloroquine- and Fansidar-Resistant Strains

Chloroquine resistance reported from all regions with *P. falciparum* except
- Americas: Central America west of the Panama Canal, Haiti, Dominican Republic
- Asia: Middle East (most countries)

Fansidar resistance reported from
- Americas: Brazil, Panama
- Asia: Thailand,* Myanmar (formerly Burma),* Kampuchea,* Vietnam
- Africa: East Africa
- Oceania: Irian Jaya, Papua New Guinea, Vanuatu

*Because Fansidar resistance is widespread in these areas, therapy for *P. falciparum* malaria should include quinine and tetracycline. In other areas where Fansidar resistance is less common, initial treatment with quinine and antifolate metabolities is appropriate, but vigilance for recrudescene occurring within 90 days after treatment should be maintained.

or three times a day) is important, because this may permit early detection of treatment failure. Vigilant observation for clinical complications (such as repeated physical examination and blood gas and glucose determinations) is essential, even after treatment is instituted. Supportive care (fluid and electrolyte management, dialysis, blood transfusion, mechanically assisted ventilation) may be an important adjunct to antimicrobial chemotherapy in selected patients. In some cases (e.g., parasitemia of 5% or more infected erythrocytes, a condition referred to as hyperparasitemia), exchange blood transfusion may be lifesaving.[75] Corticosteroids are no longer recommended as adjunctive treatment for cerebral malaria because they are ineffective and may prove deleterious.[76]

The choice of antimalarial drugs in the treatment of *P. falciparum* malaria (Table 287–3) depends on where the infection was acquired (in view of the geographic distribution of multidrug-resistant strains [see Table 287–2]) and the clinical status of the patient. Because dissemination of drug-resistant strains can be expected to continue in the future, the view that any patient may be the index case for the appearance of a new drug-resistant strain in a particular geographic region is probably an appropriately cautious perspective. Thus, for example, resistance to antifolate metabolites such as Fansidar, which is characteristic of certain strains of *P. falciparum* encountered in parts of Southeast Asia, Brazil, and elsewhere (and dictates treatment with alternative drugs), is appearing

TABLE 287–3 ■ Treatment and Chemoprophylaxis of Malaria

		DOSE	
INDICATION	**DRUG AND ROUTE***	**Adult**	**Pediatric**
Uncomplicated infection with all species except chloroquine-resistant *P. falciparum*	Chloroquine phosphate PO	600 mg base (1 g) followed by 300 mg base (500 mg) in 6 h, then 300 mg base (500 mg)/d for 2 d	10 mg/kg (base) to maximum of 600 mg; followed by half of this dose in 6 h and then daily for 2 d
Patient unable to take oral medications	Chloroquine hydrochloride IM†	200 mg base (250 mL) q 6 h for maximum of 3 d	5 mg/kg (base) q 12 h for a maximum of 3 d
Severe (complicated) *P. falciparum* infection	Quinidine gluconate IV	Loading dose 10 mg of salt/kg body weight in 1–2 h, then 0.02 mg/kg/min continuous infusion‡	Same rate for adult
Uncomplicated infection due to chloroquine-resistant *P. falciparum*§	Combination of Quinine sulfate PO	650 mg q 8 h for 5–7 d	25 mg/kg/d in 3 doses for 5–7 d
	Pyrimethamine PO	25 mg bid for 3 d	<10 kg: 6.25 mg/d 10–20 kg: 12.5 mg/d 20–40 kg: 25 mg/d
	Sulfadiazine or sulfisoxazole PO	500 mg qid for 5 d	200 mg/kg/d in 4 doses (maximum 2 g d) for 5 d
Uncomplicated infection due to sulfonamide-pyrimethamine–resistant *P. falciparum*	Combination of Quinine sulfate PO	650 mg q 8 h for 5–7 d	25 mg/kg/d in 3 doses for 5–7 d
	Tetracycline PO *or*	250 mg PO qid for 7–10 d	6 mg/kg/PO qid for 7–10 d‖
	Clindamycin PO	900 mg tid × 3 d	20–40 mg/kg/d in 3 divided doses
Uncomplicated infection due to chloroquine- or sulfonamide-resistant *P. falciparum*: alternative regimen	Mefloquine PO	15 mg/kg (base) to 1000 mg maximum; single dose	Same rate as for adult
Prevention of relapses due to *P. vivax* and *P. ovale*	Primaquine phosphate PO	15 mg base (26.3 mg)/d for 14 d	0.3 mg base/kg/d for 14 d
Chemoprophylaxis of all species except chloroquine-resistant *P. falciparum*	Chloroquine phosphate PO	300 mg base (500 mg) once/wk; begin 2 wk before and continue for 4 wk after leaving area	<1 y: 37.5 mg base¶ 1–3 y: 75 mg base 4–6 y: 100 mg base 7–10 y: 150 mg base 11–16 y: 225 mg base
Chemoprophylaxis of chloroquine-resistant *P. falciparum*	Mefloquine PO	250 mg once/wk; begin 2 wk before and continue for 4 wk after leaving area	Mefloquine is not recommended for children
	or Doxycycline PO‖**	100 mg qd; begin 2 d before entering and continue for 4 wk after leaving area	Contraindicated in children <8 y

*IM, Intramuscularly; IV, intravenously; PO, orally; bid, twice daily; qd, every day; qid, four times daily; tid, three times daily.
†May cause potentially fatal side effects. See text.
‡Do not use loading dose if quinine, quinidine, or mefloquine has been administered in the prior 24 h.
§Infection in patients with sulfonamide-pyrimethamine–resistant strains (such as those acquired in Southeast Asia) may exhibit recrudescence after this treatment.
‖Tetracyclines should be avoided if possible in children younger than 8 years and in pregnant women.
¶Children may refuse to take chloroquine tablets because of their bitter taste; it may be necessary to disguise the taste by mixing ground tablets in food. Palatable liquid preparations for pediatric use are readily available in several countries where malaria transmission occurs.
**Tetracycline is recommended for travelers to areas of Southeast Asia with mefloquine-resistant strains of *P. falciparum* (see text).

in other areas of the world. Accordingly, the regimen summarized in Table 287–3 should be considered only as a general guideline; the most up-to-date information should be sought in treating a patient. If asexual-stage parasitemia does not begin to decline within 24 to 48 hours of instituting treatment or persists at a detectable level after 5 days, drug failure must be considered. In cases of low-grade drug resistance, recrudescence (resurgence of parasitemia due to replication of blood-borne parasites) can occur within 90 days or more after detectable parasitemia has cleared. It may be impossible to distinguish recrudescence from reinfection in patients residing where malaria transmission occurs.

Patients with parasitemias in excess of 5% or who are suffering from serious complications of *P. falciparum* infection should be admitted to an intensive care unit and treated with quinidine gluconate[75] by slow intravenous drip. This drug should never be given by intravenous push or by intramuscular injection; to do so could result in cardiovascular collapse. The electrocardiogram, vital signs, and blood glucose concentration should be monitored carefully. In addition, exchange transfusion can rapidly lower parasitemia and may be lifesaving.[75] The patient should be switched to oral medication as soon as this is feasible and when serious complications are controlled. A neurologic syndrome can develop when parenteral therapy is followed by oral mefloquine (see earlier[55a]). Choosing an appropriate alternative oral antimalarial drug seems advisable.

The safest and best studied regimen available for the treatment of uncomplicated chloroquine-resistant *P. falciparum* malaria is a combination of oral quinine, a sulfonamide, and pyrimethamine (see Table 287–3). Fansidar, a fixed-dose combination of sulfadoxine (500 mg per tablet), a long-acting sulfonamide, and pyrimethamine (25 mg per tablet) can be used (three tablets total for adults) in place of the individual antifolate metabolites. Patients with known hypersensitivity to sulfonamides should be treated with quinine and tetracycline, in the regimen recommended for antifolate-resistant strains of *P. falciparum* (see Table 287–3). Therapeutic and prophylactic use of Fansidar has been associated with severe and in some cases fatal reactions, including the Stevens-Johnson syndrome.[77] Infection with multidrug-resistant strains acquired in Southeast Asia and Brazil may respond initially to the quinine-antifolate regimen and then manifest delayed recrudescence. To minimize the risk of such recrudescence, *P. falciparum* malaria acquired in these areas should be treated with a combination of quinine and tetracycline or quinine and clindamycin (a therapeutic combination preferable for pregnant women and children younger than 8 years) (see Table 287–3). There is disturbing evidence that quinine resistance may be developing in some strains of *P. falciparum* in Southeast Asia.[78] Quinine administered orally can cause cinchonism, a condition characterized by tinnitus, headache, nausea, and altered vision. Quinine hypersensitivity is rare; its manifestations may include bronchospasm, hemolytic anemia, and thrombocytopenia. The daily dose of quinine should be reduced for patients with renal or hepatic failure; serum levels are not altered by peritoneal dialysis or hemodialysis.

Mefloquine and halofantrine have been introduced for the oral treatment of chloroquine-resistant *P. falciparum* malaria, although the latter drug is not currently (as of May 1997) marketed in the United States. Mefloquine resistance is a problem in strains of *P. falciparum* transmitted along the Thai borders with Cambodia and Myanmar, and drug failure has been reported sporadically from countries in South America, Asia, Africa, and the Middle East. Mefloquine therapy should not be used when chloroquine or sulfonamide-pyrimethamine combinations are effective primarily because of its potential toxicity and long elimination half-life. The formulation marketed in the United States contains 250 mg of mefloquine HCl and for the treatment of uncomplicated malaria is administered at a rate of 15 mg/kg of body weight, although higher doses (up to 25 mg/kg) have been used in some situations, but with greater intolerance (especially vomiting). If vomiting occurs within 1 hour of administration, the full dose should be repeated; this is unnecessary if vomiting occurs later. Tolerability can be improved by administering split doses at an interval of 6 to 24 hours. Vigilance for the development of bradycardia and sinus arrhythmias is appropriate. Because mefloquine can also prolong the QT_c interval, caution must be exercised in the coadministration of mefloquine with certain cardiotropic agents.

Because there is extensive cross-resistance between mefloquine and halofantrine, and because the latter has significant cardiotoxic potential (more than 13 halofantrine associated deaths have been reported), I believe that halofantrine should be reserved for exceptional circumstances when other alternatives are unacceptable.[79, 80]

To treat infections of all other species of *Plasmodium* and of sensitive strains of *P. falciparum*, chloroquine phosphate can be administered orally in the doses outlined in Table 287–3. (Apparent chloroquine-resistant strains of *P. vivax* can be treated with mefloquine.) Most patients experience some mild gastrointestinal irritation; other side effects, such as pruritus and exacerbation of psoriasis, headache, dizziness, blurred vision, and acute psychosis, are uncommon. Children should be observed for the first hour, because they may vomit the tablets. The drug can also be administered by nasogastric gavage. Intramuscular chloroquine hydrochloride administered to children has produced fatal reactions in isolated cases. Although this regimen was reported to be safe in a study conducted in West Africa,[81] it should be used with great caution.

Artemesinin is a sesquiterpene lactone compound derived from the wormwood plant *Artemisia annua*, extracts of which have been used for centuries in China in the empirical treatment of malarial fevers.[82] Artemesinin preparations are being used primarily in Asia and parts of Africa.

To prevent relapses of sporozoite-induced infections with *P. vivax* or *P. ovale*, patients should also receive a course of primaquine after completing a course of chloroquine, because chloroquine does not eradicate the hepatic exoerythrocytic forms (hypnozoites). Primaquine can induce hemolytic anemia in patients with G-6-PD deficiency; a laboratory test for this condition should be performed before the drug is administered. Patients with the Caucasian form of the deficiency should not receive primaquine. Those with the milder form may be given the drug, and their hematocrit should be carefully monitored. Hypnozoites of some strains of *P. vivax* are not eradicated by one course of primaquine[83]; a second course of longer duration or larger doses may be necessary. Because no hypnozoites form in blood-induced malaria, primaquine is not required.

Prevention

The mainstays of malaria prevention are reducing exposure to infected mosquitos and chemoprophylaxis. The former is accomplished by wearing appropriate clothing and using effective insect repellents (such as those with high DEET content) at night, employing window screens and bed netting (including permethrin-impregnated bed netting[84]) and spraying "knockdown" insecticides indoors at sundown. No chemoprophylactic regimen is sufficiently reliable to encourage a casual attitude about these preventive measures. Specific updated information on the risk for malaria by country and on chemoprophylaxis advice is available around-the-clock from the Centers for Disease Control and Prevention (telephone 404-639-1610) and in pamphlets such as "Health Information for International Travel" (Department of Health and Human Services publication available from the U.S. Government Printing Office).

Chemoprophylaxis of malaria[85] has been complicated by the dissemination of drug-resistant strains of *P. falciparum*. Hispaniola, Central America (north of Panama), and Egypt (Fayoum Governorate) are currently the only regions considered free of such resistant strains. Travelers to these regions and to countries where *P. falciparum* is not transmitted (Algeria, Morocco, Iraq, Syria, Turkey, Azerbaijan, and most of northern Iran and China with the exception of South China including Hainan Island) should receive chloroquine once per week (on the same day of the week) starting 2 weeks before entering a malarious area and continuing for 4 weeks after leaving the area. In doses used for malaria chemoprophylaxis, chloroquine does not cause retinal damage and is considered safe for use in pregnant women. Cases of vivax malaria that were incompletely responsive to chloroquine have been documented in Papua New Guinea, parts of Indonesia, and Myanmar, Mefloquine used as prophylaxis in these areas can be expected to prevent chloroqine-resistant *P. vivax* infection. On return from areas with high transmission levels of *P. vivax* or *P. ovale*, travelers who do not have G-6-PD deficiency are often given a course of primaquine to prevent relapsing malaria. In the United States, where primaquine supplies are limited from time to time, this recommendation depends on drug availability.

The chemoprophylaxis of chloroquine-resistant falciparum malaria is complicated; recommendations are subject to some controversy and change.[85] Because some patients have developed serious side effects from the prophylactic use of Fansidar, this regimen is now rarely employed. Travelers to most areas where chloroquine-resistant strains are transmitted should receive as chemoprophylaxis only mefloquine[86] (Lariam; for adults, the dose is one 250-mg tablet each week, beginning 2 weeks before entering the endemic area and continued for 4 weeks after leaving a malarious area).[85] Mefloquine is not recommended for individuals with known hypersensitivity to the drug, children weighing less than 15 kg (30 pounds), pregnant women, patients receiving β-blockers or certain other cardiotropic drugs, patients with a history of convulsive or certain psychiatric disorders, or individuals involved in essential tasks that involve fine motor coordination (such as airline pilots). For travelers who cannot take mefloquine, chloroquine can be recommended in the usual prophylactic regimen (see Table 287–3), and three Fansidar tablets can be provided for use as a lifesaving *temporary* measure if fever develops and immediate medical attention cannot be obtained (unless the patient has known hypersensitivity to sulfonamides). The traveler should then seek medical attention as soon as possible. For travelers with known sulfonamide allergy, an alternative self-treatment regimen (such as quinine and doxycycline) can be prescribed after consultation with a travel medicine specialist. Because of potentially severe side effects, mefloquine in therapeutic doses (1000 to 1200 mg) is not recommended as an alternative to Fansidar in these patients.

In some parts of the world, proguanil, an antifolate metabolite, is prescribed in combination with chloroquine to travelers entering areas with chloroquine-resistant strains of *P. falciparum*; proguanil is not sold in the United States, and the efficacy of this regimen is probably less than that of available alternatives.[87] Amodiaquine is no longer advised for malaria prophylaxis because it can cause fatal agranulocytosis. Doxycycline (100 mg) alone, one tablet taken daily, can be recommended during brief visits to forested areas of Thailand, Myanmar, and Kampuchea, where there may be a risk for acquiring multidrug-resistant malaria.[88, 89] This regimen should begin 1 to 2 days before entering the area and be continued for 4 weeks after leaving the area. It should not be administered to children younger than 8 years or to pregnant women. Tetracyclines can cause exaggerated sunburns and *Candida* vaginitis with prolonged use.

Pregnant women should not travel in tropical countries because of a variety of infectious disease risks. Chloroquine treatment and prophylaxis are generally safe for pregnant women and have not been considered to pose teratogenic risk. Although chloroquine is detectable in breast milk, breast-feeding is not a reliable means of providing chemoprophylaxis to infants. Teratogenic effects of folate antimetabolites have been noted in laboratory animals (but not in humans), suggesting that the prophylactic use of this category of drugs should be avoided in pregnant women. When it is decided that the use of pyrimethamine for 3 days (see Table 287–3) outweighs the risk for inadequately treatment of chloroquine-resistant *P. falciparum* malaria, it should be administered with folinic acid. For relapsing malaria, acute attacks should be prevented with chloroquine prophylaxis; after delivery, primaquine can be administered.

Patients who have undergone splenectomy or are functionally asplenic are theoretically at risk for more severe malaria infection because the spleen plays a critical role in antimalarial host defense.[90] It is difficult to emphatically discourage the travel of asplenic patients to malarious areas because suitable documentation on the course of malaria in such persons is lacking. Such patients should be informed of their potentially unique situation and given particularly detailed advice on malaria prevention and the need to seek immediate attention in the event of a febrile illness. Individuals with human immunodeficiency virus infection are not known to be at greater risk for complications from malaria.

In the last two decades, extraordinary efforts were applied to the development of a vaccine against malaria.[6] One strategy was to devise a means of preventing sporozoites from entering liver cells or developing into hepatic schizonts by inducing antibody against circumsporozoite protein. Unfortunately, results of clinical trials of an antisporozoite vaccine proved discouraging.[91] Results of field trials of a vaccine against asexual blood-stage parasite appear somewhat more hopeful.[4, 5]

Babesiosis

History

Babesiosis, a malaria-like illness transmitted by infected ticks, was in 1888 the first disease shown (in cattle) to be transmitted by an arthropod. The first well-documented human case (allegedly due to *Babesia bovis*) was reported in 1957, and a small number of cases due to *Babesia divergens* were subsequently reported from Europe. In the 1970s, cases of human babesiosis (due to *Babesia microti*), acquired on Nantucket Island and Martha's Vineyard in Massachusetts and on Shelter Island and eastern Long Island in New York, were reported from the United States.[92, 93] Additional cases have since been documented.[94, 95] Cases of transfusion-induced babesiosis have also been documented.[96] All told, more than 100 human cases of clinical and subclinical babesiosis have been reported.[97] Human cases of babesiosis due to a species related to *Babesia gibsoni* (a pathogen of dogs) have been reported from Washington and California.[98, 99]

Characteristics of the Pathogen

Babesia organisms are hematoprotozoa (class Piroplasmia) that undergo asexual reproduction by budding (generation time of *Babesia rodhaini*, 5 to 14 hours) within erythrocytes of mammalian hosts. The molecular basis for their attachment to and invasion of erythrocytes is unknown. Merozoites of *B. rodhaini*, a species that infects rodents, activate the alternative complement pathway and use the C3b receptor on erythrocytes to gain entry into host cells.[100] *B. microti* in erythrocytes can resemble ring stages of *P. falciparum*; the absence of parasite-associated pigment distinguishes *B. microti* and may be helpful diagnostically. Only merozoite and trophozoite stages have been observed in erythrocytes; no exoerythrocytic or sexual stage has yet been identified in mammalian hosts. In ticks, *Babesia* organisms divide by binary fission in the intestinal epithelium. The parasites subsequently spread to the tick salivary glands and are injected with saliva during a blood meal.

Epidemiology

Babesiosis (due to *B. bovis*, *Babesia bigemina*, *B. divergens*, and *Babesia major*) is an economically important disease of cattle in some parts of the world. Rodents can become infected with *B. microti* and *B. rodhaini*. The seven human cases of babesiosis reported from Europe (Yugoslavia, Ireland, Scotland, France, and the former Soviet Union) were probably caused by *B. divergens* or *B. bovis*; all involved splenectomized patients, most of whom died of the infection. In contrast, the cases acquired in the northeastern United States have been due to *B. microti* and occurred predominantly in patients with a spleen, most of whom survived. The results of seroepidemiologic surveys suggest that asymptomatic babesiosis exists in Mexico and Nigeria and is more common than symptomatic disease in regions of the northeastern United States where transmission occurs.[92]

Babesia of cattle can be transmitted by ixodid (hard) ticks, including *Dermacentor*, *Ixodes*, and *Rhipicephalus*. *B. microti* is transmitted by *Ixodes scapularis*, a species that feeds primarily on deer, mice, and voles. These rodents are the major identified reservoir of *B. microti* that is transmissible to humans in the United States. Humans encounter infected *I. scapularis* (usually the nymphs) principally in marsh, scrub, and heathland. Because this tick species also transmits Lyme borreliosis (see Chapter 224), simultaneous infection with *B. microti* and *Borellia burgdorferi* is not surprising.[101]

Pathogenesis

The limited knowledge available on the pathogenesis of babesiosis derives from observations of naturally infected cattle and experimentally infected rodents.[102] Anemia, a major complication of infection, results from hemolysis of infected erythrocytes; premature removal of uninfected erythrocytes may also occur. Erythrophagocytosis can be appreciated histologically. No convincing evidence has been presented of an autoimmune mechanism. Hemoglobinemia, production of immune complexes, and activation of the clotting and complement systems[103] might contribute to the pathogenesis of renal failure that can complicate severe infections. A role for macrophage-derived TNF-α has been postulated in host defense and pathogenesis.[104]

Clinical Manifestations

Human babesiosis due to *B. microti* infection can vary from inapparent to overwhelming. Younger patients are more likely to be asymptomatic than patients older than 50 years. Splenectomized patients, and perhaps those otherwise immunocompromised, generally experience more severe disease. In *B. microti* infection, symptoms may begin 1 to 2 weeks after the tick bite. Symptoms are similar to those of malaria and influenza: malaise, fatigue, fever, rigors, myalgia, and headache. Lassitude and depression may be striking and can dominate the clinical presentation. Symptoms may wax and wane for weeks, during which hepatomegaly and splenomegaly may be present. Infection is accompanied by normochromic, normocytic anemia that can be mild or moderately severe. Mild neutropenia may be present. Atypical lymphocytosis has been documented in several cases.[105] Mild elevations of transaminase, alkaline phosphatase, and bilirubin values have been observed. Most patients with a spleen recover spontaneously after a prolonged course of several months; splenectomized patients experience more intense parasitemia and more severe anemia but generally recover.[97] Acute respiratory failure due to noncardiogenic pulmonary edema can complicate infections, even during treatment.[106] In contrast, infection with *B. divergens* in splenectomized patients causes severe anemia, hemoglobinemia, hemoglobinuria, renal and hepatic failure, hypotension, and in most cases death.

Diagnosis

Examination of Giemsa-stained blood smears for the presence of intraerythrocytic parasites is the most rapid and specific test for establishing a diagnosis[107] (Fig. 287–6). Because symptoms are similar and *B. microti* organisms resemble ring stages of *P. falciparum*, it may be difficult to distinguish babesiosis from malaria. The travel history may be helpful. In addition, the presence in erythrocytes of four daughter cells (tetrads) held together by cytoplasmic bridges (resembling a Maltese cross) is particularly distinctive; the absence of parasite-associated pigment also distinguishes *Babesia* from *Plasmodium* infection. *B. divergens* can be round, oval, piriform, or ring shaped. Two rather than four daughter cells are observed after division. Examination of blood smears by an experienced parasitologist may be necessary to confirm the diagnosis. Injection of infected blood into hamsters or jirds (preferably splenectomized) can be expected to induce a patent parasitemia with *B. microti* in 2 to 4 weeks. Serologic tests for babesiosis are available from the Centers for Disease Control and Prevention.

Treatment and Prevention

The treatment of choice for *B. microti* infection is a combination of quinine, 650 mg orally, and clindamycin, 600 mg orally, both given every 8 hours for 7 days.[108] For overwhelm-

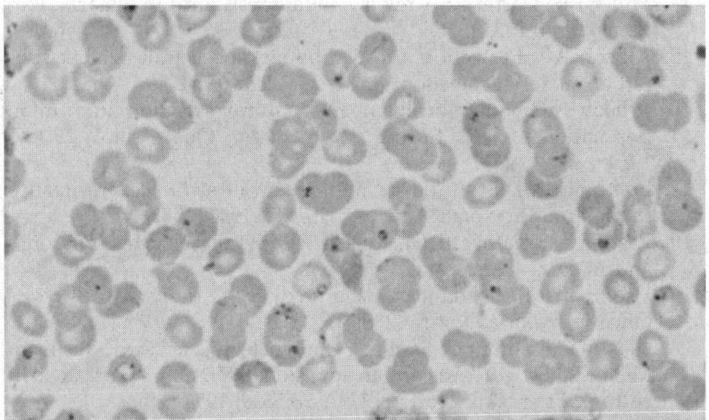

FIGURE 287–6 □ *Babesia microti*–infected erythrocytes from a case of transfusion-induced babesiosis. Note ring and one tetrad form.

ing infection (due to *B. microti* or *B. divergens*) in splenectomized patients, exchange transfusion may be lifesaving. Pentamidine isethionate reduces fever and parasitemia but is not curative and is toxic. Chloroquine is not efficacious.[109] Avoiding contact with ticks, using repellants, and inspecting for and removing ticks after exposure to tick-infested vegetation are the only modalities available for personal protection. People who lack a spleen or are functionally asplenic should be particularly cautious about avoiding contact with ticks. Environmental control of tick populations has been achieved in selected circumstances by malathion spraying. Deer and rodent control, although theoretically beneficial, has not been instituted on a large scale as a public health measure in areas of *B. microti* transmission.

References

1. Bruce-Chwatt LJ: History of malaria from prehistory to eradication. *In* Wernsdorfer WH, McGregor I (eds): Malaria: Principles and Practice of Malariology. New York, Churchill Livingstone, 1988, pp 1–59.
2. Farid MA: The malaria programme—From euphoria to anarchy. World Health Forum 1:8, 1980.
3. Wyler DJ: Malaria—Resurgence, resistance and research. N Engl J Med 308:875, 1983.
4. Alonso PL, Smith T, Armstrong JRM, et al: Randomised trial of efficacy of SPf66 vaccine against *Plasmodium falciparum* malaria in children in southern Tanzania. Lancet 344:1175, 1994.
5. Noya O, Gabaldon. BY, Alarcon de Noya B, et al: A population-based clinical trial with the SPf66 synthetic *Plasmodium falciparum* vaccine in Venezuela. J Infect Dis 170:396, 1994.
6. Jones TR, Hoffman SL: Malaria vaccine development. Clin Microbiol Rev 7:303, 1994.
7. Garnham PCC: Malaria Parasites and Other Hemosporidia. Oxford, Blackwell Scientific Publications, 1966.
8. Frevert U: Malaria sporozoite-hepatocyte interactions. Exp Parasitol 79:206, 1994.
9. McElroy PD, Beier JC, Oster CN, et al: Predicting outcome in malaria: Correlation between rate of exposure to infected mosquitoes and level of *Plasmodium falciparum* parasitemia. Am J Trop Med Hyg 51:523, 1994.
10. Krotoski WA, Collins WE, Bray RS, et al: Demonstration of hypnozoites in sporozoite-transmitted *Plasmodium vivax* infection. Am J Trop Med Hyg 31:1291, 1982.
11. Coppel R: Malaria—Revealing the tie that binds. Parasitol Today 8:393, 1992.
12. Aikawa M, Miller LH, Johnson J, Rabbege J: Erythrocyte entry by malarial parasites. A moving junction between erythrocyte and parasite. J Cell Biol 77:72, 1978.
13. Neva FA, Howard WA, Glew RH, et al: Relationship of serum complement levels to events of the malarial paroxysm. J Clin Invest 54:451, 1974.
14. Miller LH, Carter R: A review. Innate resistance in malaria. Exp Parasitol 40:132, 1976.
15. Allison AC: Protection afforded by sickle cell trait against subtertian malarial infection. Br Med J 1:290, 1954.
16. Allison AC: Polymorphism and natural selection in human populations. Cold Spring Harb Symp Quant Biol 29:137, 1964.
17. Friedman MJ: Erythrocytic mechanism of sickle cell resistance to malaria. Proc Natl Acad Sci USA 75:1994, 1978.
18. Pasvol G, Weatherall DJ, Wilson RJM, et al: Fetal haemoglobin and malaria. Lancet 1:1269, 1976.
19. Friedman MJ: Oxidant damage mediates variant red cell resistance to malaria. Nature 280:245, 1979.
20. Kidson C, Lamont G, Saul A, et al: Ovalocytic erythrocytes from Melanesians are resistant to invasion by malaria parasites in culture. Proc Natl Acad Sci USA 78:5829, 1981.
21. Luzzatto L: Genetics of red cells and susceptibility to malaria. Blood 54:961, 1979.
22. Gilles HM, Fletcher KA, Hendrickse RG, et al: Glucose-6-phosphate dehydrogenase deficiency, sickling and malaria in African children in South Western Nigeria. Lancet 1:138, 1979.
23. Martin SK, Miller LH, Alling D, et al: Severe malaria and glucose-6-phosphate dehydrogenase deficiency: Reappraisal of the malaria G-6-PD hypothesis. Lancet 1:524, 1979.
24. Aikawa M, Miller LH, Rabbege J: Caveola-vesicle complexes in the plasmalemma of erythrocytes infected with *Plasmodium vivax* and *P. cynomolgi*. Am J Pathol 79:285, 1975.
25. Udeinya IJ, Schmidt JA, Aikawa M, et al: Falciparum malaria infected erythrocytes specifically bind to cultured endothelial cells. Science 213:555, 1981.
26. Pasloske BL, Russell RJ: Malaria, the red cell, and the endothelium. Annu Rev Med 45:283, 1994.
27. Ockenhouse CF, Tegoshi T, Maeno Y, et al: Human vascular endothelial cell adhesion receptors for *Plasmodium falciparum*–infected erythrocytes: Roles for endothelial leukocyte adhesion molecule 1 and vascular cell adhesion molecule 1. J Exp Med 176:1183, 1992.
28. Rener J, Graves PM, Carter R, et al: Target antigens of transmission blocking immunity on gametes of *Plasmodium falciparum*. J Exp Med 158:976, 1983.
29. Meuwissen JHET: Current studies related to the development of transmission blocking malaria vaccines: A review. Trans R Soc Trop Med Hyg 83(Suppl):57, 1989.
30. Stürchler D: How much malaria is there worldwide? (Letter) Parasitol Today 5:39, 1989.
31. Guerrero IC, Weniger BC, Schultz MG: Transfusion malaria in the United States, 1972–1981. Ann Intern Med 99:221, 1983.
32. Maldonado YA, Nahlen BL, Roberts RR, et al: Transmission of *Plasmodium vivax* in San Diego County, California, 1986. Am J Trop Med Hyg 42:3, 1990.

32a. Zucker JR: Changing patterns of autochthonous malaria transmission in the United States: A review of recent outbreaks. Emerg Infect Dis 2:37, 1996.

33. Miller LH, Mason SJ, Clyde DF, et al: The resistance factor to *Plasmodium vivax* in blacks: The Duffy blood-group genotype, *Fy Fy*. N Engl J Med 295:302, 1976.
34. Centers for Disease Control and Prevention: Malaria Surveillance Annual Summary 1991; issued April 1994.
35. Phillips-Howard PA, Bradley DJ: Epidemiology of malaria in European travelers. *In* Steffen R, Lobel HO, Haworth J, Bradley DJ (eds): Travel Medicine. Berlin, Springer-Verlag, 1989, pp 90–101.
36. Standards for Blood Banks and Transfusion Services, ed 16. Arlington, VA, American Association of Blood Banks, 1994.
37. Hubert TV: Congenital malaria in the United States: Report of a case and review. Clin Infect Dis 14:922, 1992.
38. Garfield MD, Ershler WB, Maki DG: Malaria transmission by platelet concentrate transfusion. JAMA 240:2285, 1978.
39. Dover AS, Guinee VF: Malaria transmission by leukocyte component therapy. JAMA 217:1701, 1971.
40. Lefavour GS, Pierce JC, Frame JD: Renal transplant–associated malaria. JAMA 244:1820, 1980.

40a. Abulrahi HA, Bohlega EA, Fontaine RE, et al: *Plasmodium falciparum* malaria transmitted in hospital through heparin locks. Lancet 349:23, 1997.

41. White NJ, Ho M: The pathophysiology of malaria. Adv Parasitol 31:84, 1992.
42. Malloy JP, Brooks MH, Barry KG: Pathophysiology of acute falciparum malaria. II. Fluid compartmentalization. Ann Intern Med 43:745, 1967.
43. Holst FGE, Hemmer CJ, Kern P, et al: Inappropriate secretion of antidiuretic hormone and hyponatremia in severe falciparum malaria. Am J Trop Med Hyg 50:602, 1994.
44. Phillips RE, Pasvol G: Anemia of *Plasmodium falciparum* malaria. Baillieres Clin Haematol 5:315, 1992.
45. Looareesuwan S, Ho M, Wattanagoon Y, et al: Dynamic alternation in splenic function during acute *falciparum* malaria. N Engl J Med 317:675, 1987.
46. Kelton JG, Keystone J, Moore J, et al: Immune-mediated thrombocytopenia of malaria. J Clin Invest 71:832, 1983.
47. Olsson RA, Johnston EH: Histopathologic changes and small bowel absorption in falciparum malaria. Am J Trop Med Hyg 18:355, 1969.
48. World Health Organization Malaria Action Programme: Severe and complicated malaria. Trans R Soc Trop Med Hyg 80(Suppl): 1, 1986.
49. Trang TT, Phu NH, Vinh H, et al: Acute renal failure in patients with severe falciparum malaria. Clin Infect Dis 15:874, 1992.

50. MacPherson GG, Warrell MJ, White NJ, et al: Human cerebral malaria: A quantitative ultrastructure analysis of parasitized erythrocyte sequestration. Am J Pathol 19:385, 1985.
51. Hamer DH, Wyler DJ: Cerebral malaria. Semin Neurol 13:180, 1993.
52. Clark IA, Rockett KA, Cowden WB: Possible central role of nitric oxide in conditions clinically similar to cerebral malaria. Lancet 340:894, 1992.
53. McGuire W, Hill AV, Allsopp CE, et al: Variation in the TNF-alpha promoter region associated with susceptibility to cerebral malaria. Nature 371:508, 1994.
54. Wyler DJ: Steroids are out in the treatment of cerebral malaria: What's next? J Infect Dis 158:320, 1988.
55. Brewster DR, Kwaitkowski D, White NJ: Neurological sequelae of cerebral malaria in children. Lancet 336:1039, 1990.
55a. Nguyen TH, Day NP, Ly VC, et al: Post-malaria neurological syndrome. Lancet 348:917, 1996.
56. White NJ, Warrell DA, Chantavanich P, et al: Severe hypoglycemia and hyperinsulinemia in falciparum malaria. N Engl J Med 309:61, 1983.
56a. English M, Waruiru C, Amukoye E, et al: Deep breathing in children with severe malaria: Indicator of metabolic acidosis and poor outcome. Am J Trop Med Hyg 55:521, 1996.
57. McGregor IA, Gilles HM, Walters JH, et al: Effects of heavy and repeated malarial infections on Gambian infants and children: Effects of erythrocytic parasitization. Br Med J 2:686, 1956.
58. Voller A: Immunopathology of malaria. Bull World Health Organ 50:177, 1974.
59. Haghighi L, Doust JY, Boroomand K: Biological false positive VDRL test in malaria. Trop Geogr Med 22:482, 1970.
60. Reed RE: False-positive Monospot tests in malaria. Am J Clin Pathol 61:173, 1974.
61. Wyler DJ, Oppenheim JJ: Lymphocyte transformation in human *Plasmodium falciparum* malaria. J Immunol 113:449, 1974.
62. Wyler DJ, Gallin JI: Spleen-derived mononuclear chemotactic factor in malaria infections: A possible mechanism for splenic macrophage accumulation. J Immunol 118:478, 1977.
63. Wyler DJ, Quinn TC, Chen L-T: Relationship of alterations in splenic clearance function and microcirculation to host defense in acute rodent malaria. J Clin Invest 67:1400, 1981.
64. Greenwood BM, Fakunle VM: The tropical splenomegaly syndrome: A review of its pathogenesis. *In* The Role of the Spleen in the Immunology of Parasitic Diseases. Basel, Schwabe, 1979, p 229.
65. Hendrickse RG, Adeniyi A: Quartan malarial nephrotic syndrome in children. Kidney Int 16:64, 1979.
66. Morrow RH Jr: Epidemiological evidence for the role of falciparum malaria in the pathogenesis of Burkitt's lymphoma. IARC Sci Publ 60:177, 1985.
67. Wyler DJ: Cellular aspects of immunoregulation in malaria. Bull World Health Organ 57(Suppl):239, 1979.
68. Cohen S, McGregor IA, Carrington SP: Gamma-globulin and acquired immunity to human malaria. Nature 192:733, 1961.
69. Clark IA, Virelizier JL, Carswell EA, et al: Possible importance of macrophage-derived mediators in acute malaria. Infect Immun 32:1058, 1981.
70. Wyler DJ: The spleen and malaria. Ciba Found Symp 94:98–111, 1983.
71. Kean BH, Reilly PC: Malaria the mime: Recent lessons from a group of civilian travellers. Am J Med 61:159, 1976.
72. Perrin LH, Mackey LJ, Miescher PA: The hematology of malaria in man. Semin Hematol 19:70, 1982.
73. Russell PF, West LS, Manwell RD, et al: Practical Malariology, ed 2. New York, Oxford University Press, 1963.
74. Murphy GS, Basri H, Purnomo, et al: Vivax malaria resistant to treatment and prophylaxis with chloroquine. Lancet 341:96, 1993.
75. Miller KD, Greenberg AE, Campbell CC: Treatment of severe malaria in the United States with a continuous infusion of quinidine gluconate and exchange transfusion. N Engl J Med 321:65, 1989.
76. Warrell DA, Looareesuwan S, Warrell MJ, et al: Dexamethasone proves deleterious in cerebral malaria. A double-blind trial in 100 comatose patients. N Engl J Med 306:313, 1982.
77. Olsen VV, Loft S, Christensen K: Serious reaction during malaria prophylaxis with pyrimethamine-sulfadoxine (Letter). Lancet 2:994, 1982.
78. Pukrittaya S, Supanaranond W, Looareesuwan S, et al: Quinine in severe malaria: Evidence of declining efficacy in Thailand. Trans R Soc Trop Med Hyg 88:324, 1994.
79. Bryson HM, Goa KL: Halofantrine. A review of its antimalarial activity, pharmacokinetic properties and therapeutic potential. Drugs 43:236, 1992.
80. Weinke T, Loscher T, Fleischer K, et al: The efficacy of halofantrine in the treatment of acute malaria in nonimmune travelers. Am J Trop Med Hyg 47:1, 1992.
81. White NJ, Miller KD, Churchill FC, et al: Chloroquine treatment of severe malaria in children: Pharmacokinetics, toxicity and new dosage recommendations. N Engl J Med 319:1493, 1988.
82. White NJ: Artemesinin: Current status. Trans R Soc Trop Med Hyg 88(Suppl 1):S3, 1994.
83. Miller LH, Wyler DJ, Glew RH, et al: Sensitivity of four strains (Central American) of *Plasmodium vivax* to primaquine. Am J Trop Med Hyg 23:309, 1974.
84. Choi HW, Bremen JG, Teutsch SM, et al: The effectiveness of insecticide-impregnated bed nets in reducing cases of malaria infection: A meta-analysis of published results. Am J Trop Med Hyg 52:377, 1995.
85. Wyler DJ: Malaria chemoprophylaxis for the traveler. N Engl J Med 329:31, 1993.
86. World Health Organization: Development of mefloquine as an anti-malarial drug. Bull World Health Organ 61:169, 1983.
87. Lobel HD, Miani M, Eng T, et al: Long-term malaria prophylaxis with weekly mefloquine. Lancet 341:848, 1993.
88. Webster HK, Thaithong S, Pavanand K, et al: Cloning and characterization of mefloquine-resistant *Plasmodium falciparum* from Thailand. Am J Trop Med Hyg 34:1022, 1985.
89. Pang LW, Boudreau EF, Limsomwong N, et al: Doxycycline prophylaxis for *falciparum* malaria. Lancet 1:1161, 1987.
90. Looareesuwan S, Suntharasamai P, Webster HK, et al: Malaria in splenectonized patients. Clin Infect Dis 16:361, 1993.
91. Herrington DA, Clyde DF, Losonsky G, et al: Safety and immunogenicity in man of a synthetic peptide malaria vaccine against *Plasmodium falciparum* sporozoites. Nature 328:257, 1987.
92. Ruebush TR, Juranek DD, Chisholm ES, et al: Human babesiosis on Nantucket Island: Evidence for self-limited and subclinical infections. N Engl J Med 297:825, 1977.
93. Grunwaldt E: Babesiosis in Shelter Island. N Y State J Med 77:1320, 1977.
94. Meldrum SC, Birkhead GS, White DJ, et al: Human babesiosis in New York State: An epidemiological description of 136 cases. Clin Infect Dis 15:1019, 1992.
95. Krause PJ, Telford SR, Ryan R, et al: Geographical and temporal distribution of babesial infection in Connecticut. J Clin Microbiol 29:1, 1991.
96. Jacoby GA, Hunt JV, Kosinski KS, et al: Treatment of transfusion-transmitted babesiosis by exchange transfusion. N Engl J Med 303:1098, 1980.
97. Rosner F: Babesiosis in splenectomized adults: Review of 22 reported cases. Am J Med 76:696, 1984.
98. Quick RE, Herwaldt BL, Thomford JW, et al: Babesiosis in Washington State: A new species of *Babesia*? Ann Intern Med 119:284, 1993.
99. Pershing DH, Herwaldt BL, Glaser C, et al: Infection with babesia-like organism in northern California. N Engl J Med 332:298, 1995.
100. Jack RM, Ward PA: *Babesia rodhaini* interactions with complement: Relationship to parasite entry into red cells. J Immunol 124:1566, 1980.
101. Benach JL, Coleman JL, Habicht GS, et al: Serological evidence for simultaneous occurrences of Lyme disease and babesiosis. J Infect Dis 152:473, 1985.
102. Callow LL, Dalgliesch RJ: Immunity and immunopathology in babesiosis. *In* Cohen S, Warren KS (eds): Immunology of Parasitic Infections, ed 2. Boston, Blackwell Scientific Publications, 1982, pp 475–526.
103. Chapman WE, Ward PE: The complement profile in babesiosis. J Immunol 117:935, 1976.
104. Clark IA, Wills EJ, Richmond JE, et al: Suppression of babesiosis in BCG-infected mice and its correlation with tumour inhibition. Infect Immun 17:430, 1977.
105. Rosenbaum GS, Johnson DH, Cunha BA: Atypical lymphocytosis in babesiosis (Letter). Clin Infect Dis 20:203, 1995.

106. Boustani MR, Lepore TJ, Gelfand JA, et al: Acute respiratory failure in patients treated for babesiosis. Am J Respir Crit Care Med 149:1689, 1994.
107. Healy GR, Ruebush TK: Morphology of *Babesia microti* in human blood smears. Am J Clin Pathol 73:107, 1980.
108. Wittner M, Rowink S, Tanowitz HB, et al: Successful chemotherapy of transfusion babesiosis. Ann Intern Med 96:601, 1982.
109. Miller LH, Neva FA, Gill F: Failure of chloroquine in human babesiosis *(Babesia microti):* Case report and chemotherapeutic trials in hamsters. Ann Intern Med 88:200, 1978.

288

Leishmania

Philip D. Marsden
Warren D. Johnson, Jr.

Few infectious diseases are as complex as leishmaniasis. An endemic disease of the tropics and subtropics, human leishmaniasis assumes a bewildering variety of forms in the skin. Visceral leishmaniasis (kala-azar) has a more typical presentation.

It was in the liver of a British soldier returned from India that William Boog Leishman found leishmanial amastigotes. These amastigotes, or *Leishmania donovani* bodies, are the smallest major parasites of humans, measuring 2 μm and characterized by a nucleus and a rod-shaped kinetoplast (Fig. 288–1*A*). *Trypanosoma cruzi* amastigotes are indistinguishable, but the type of cells the parasites invade (muscle cells for *T. cruzi*) provides the distinction. Leishmanial amastigotes are found only in phagocytic cells such as skin and splenic macrophages and Kupffer cells of the liver. The amastigote form is found only in humans, but ingestion of this form by the phlebotomine sandfly vector results in the development of a flagellated promastigote form (Fig. 288–1*B*), which effects transmission when the female fly feeds again. Promastigote forms also grow when infected tissues are cultivated in blood agar medium at a temperature of 24°C to 26°C. Books and reviews are available for readers who wish to know more of the medical microbiology and epidemiology of this group of diseases.[1–3]

Geographic Distribution

The family Trypanosomatidae, defined by Doflein in 1901, has two genera, *Trypanosoma* and *Leishmania,* that cause disease in humans. Trypanosomal diseases are limited in their geographic distribution by vector presence. The glossinae (tsetse flies) are restricted to Africa, and the great majority of triatomine bugs exist in the New World. Leishmaniasis has no such vector restriction, although specific sandflies are involved in the transmission cycles. Early explorers such as the Portuguese probably spread leishmaniasis around the world from its original locality. Figure 288–2 shows the distribution of the major clinical types of leishmaniasis, namely visceral and cutaneous forms. Phlebotomines do not survive in cold climates; however, rapid air travel and the slow genesis of *Leishmania* infections mean that cases now can be seen anywhere in the world.

The clinical aspects of *Leishmania* infections may differ depending on where the infections are contracted. Visceral leishmaniasis affects mainly adults in India, but in the Mediterranean and Brazil it is a disease of childhood. Lymphadenopathy is relatively common in Sudanese visceral leishmaniasis. No animal reservoir has been documented in India, although in the Mediterranean, Brazil, and China dogs have epidemiologic importance. Although the parasites are morphologically indistinguishable, patients' responses to treatment are quite different in these locations.

Cutaneous leishmaniasis also has multiple geographic variants. The classic oriental sore of the Middle East is often a closed, nodular, chronic skin granuloma, although it ulcerates with time. The lesions of Ethiopian cutaneous leishmaniasis may remain closed but gradually increase in diameter. The most common form of cutaneous leishmaniasis in South America is a rapidly ulcerating lesion. In Brazil, Venezuela, Ethiopia, and the Dominican Republic, a curious disseminated form of cutaneous leishmaniasis associated with anergy rarely occurs. This clinical form is called diffuse cutaneous leishmaniasis.

Mucosal leishmaniasis is more restricted geographically, and most cases come from South America; occasional reports of autochthonous cases have appeared from Texas and Europe. The Sudan is a special case, as mucosal leishmaniasis is sufficiently common to generate a series of published reports.

Taxonomy

Because all leishmanias are morphologically identical, the different types of leishmaniasis were initially defined by their geographic distribution, epidemiology, sandfly vectors, animal reservoirs, and clinical presentation. Parasites are now grouped into species and subspecies according to a variety of biologic and biochemical criteria. The latter include DNA buoyant density, restriction enzyme analysis of kinetoplast DNA, radiorespirometry, isoenzymes, antigenic analysis using monoclonal antibodies, and molecular karyotyping. Despite these new techniques, the classification of leishmania remains cumbersome and controversial and the biochemical and genomic analyses often conflict.

L. donovani, the agent of visceral leishmaniasis, appears to be a relatively uniform organism and the subdivision into *Leishmania donovani donovani* (India), *L. d. chinensis* (China), *L. d. archibaldi* (East Africa), *L. d. infantum* (Mediterranean basin), and *L. d. chagasi* (South America) is probably not warranted. We discuss visceral leishmaniasis as a single entity and indicate important regional differences. Cutaneous leishmaniasis is divided into Old World and New World disease (Table 288–1). Mucosal leishmaniasis is predominantly caused by *Leishmania viannia braziliensis,* which is discussed separately.

The taxonomy of *Leishmania* organisms is rarely available at the time of consultation, because it takes weeks to isolate and characterize the organisms. It is important for clinicians who see patients with leishmaniasis to know what species of

TABLE 288–1 ■ Causative Organisms of Cutaneous Leishmaniasis*

Old World	New World
Leishmania tropica	*Leishmania mexicana mexicana*
Leishmania major	*Leishmania mexicana amazonensis*
Leishmania aethiopica	*Leishmania viannia braziliensis*
	Leishmania viannia panamensis
	Leishmania viannia guyanensis
	Leishmania viannia peruviana

*Rarely, *L. donovani* has been known to cause purely cutaneous disease.

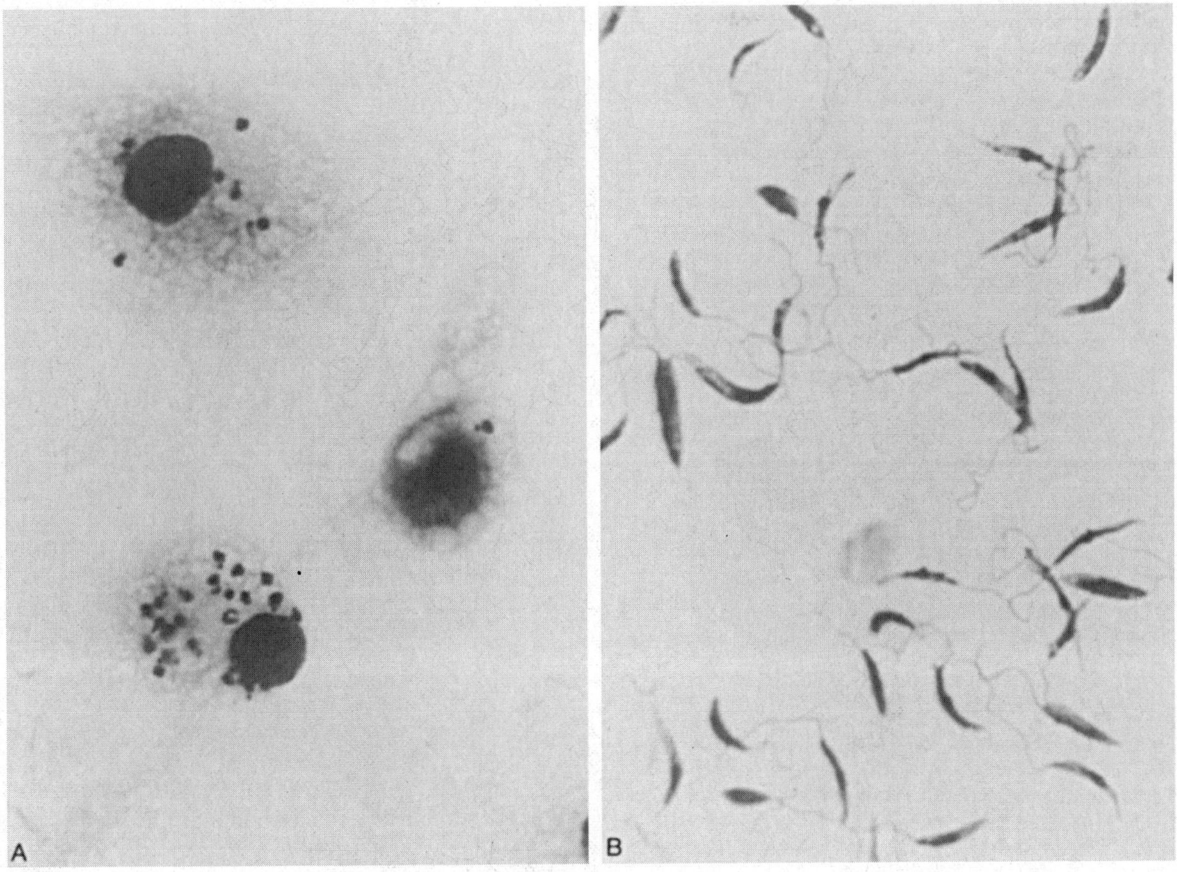

FIGURE 288–1 □ *A,* Leishmanial amastiogotes within host macrophages. *B,* Flagellated promastigote leishmanial forms found in the sandfly vector.

Leishmania are present in the area. For example, in northeastern Brazil the great majority of patients have *L. v. braziliensis* infection, which is important because it is more resistant to treatment and is the species most commonly associated with mucosal disease.

Visceral Leishmaniasis, or Kala-Azar

Kala-azar is a Hindi term meaning black fever or fatal fever. The *Leishmania* life cycle was discovered in India by the Kala-azar Commission, which was founded because so many people died of this disease in Bengal, India. The patient with visceral leishmaniasis presents with a history of recurrent fever, weakness, and weight loss. Sweating may occur at night. On examination, the patient is thin, which tends to emphasize the abdominal prominence caused by a marked enlargement of the liver and spleen. These organs are firm and nontender on palpation, although the patient may complain of discomfort resulting from the splenic enlargement. Anemia and thrombocytopenia are common, and bleeding phenomena result, particularly epistaxis. In India and in parts of China, visceral leishmaniasis affects mainly adults, but elsewhere, especially in Brazil and the Mediterranean, it is a disease of children. It has been suggested that malnutrition is an important determinant of the development of clinical visceral leishmaniasis; if so, persons in the first decade of life would be most vulnerable.[4]

Laboratory investigation confirms the presence of a normocytic, normochromic anemia, which is often severe. Pancytopenia is usual, with a low white cell count caused by a marked reduction in granulocytes, especially neutrophils. In occasional patients one or all of these three elements are relatively normal. The serum globulin level is often markedly elevated (4 to 8 g/dL), and electrophoresis shows a polyclonal increase of the immunoglobulin fractions. This finding provided the basis for the old tests for visceral leishmaniasis in which one drop of commercial formalin or antimonial drug would solidify the patient's serum (formol gel test).

With these findings, the clinician must then seek the organism. The safest procedure is bone marrow aspiration. Giemsa-stained smears are prepared from the aspirate and scrutinized for the characteristic amastigotes within macrophages. The bone marrow should also be cultured in Nicolle-Novy-MacNeal medium (10% defibrinated rabbit blood in agar) at 26°C and examined weekly for 4 weeks for the appearance of the flagellated *Leishmania* promastigote forms. A definitive diagnosis is established by this procedure in 90% of cases. If the clinical suspicion is strong but bone marrow findings are negative, splenic aspiration is indicated. A fine intramuscular needle attached to a syringe is inserted into the nonmobile spleen and negative pressure is applied. The needle is withdrawn immediately and the aspirated splenic pulp is used to prepare Giemsa-stained slides and to seed cultures. This procedure should not be performed if the platelet count is 80,000/mm^3 or less, the prothrombin activity is 60% or less of the control value,[5] the spleen is palpable less than 4 cm below the costal margin, or the physician is inexperienced with the technique. The potential risk is that of tearing the splenic capsule, but the value of the procedure, particularly in the evaluation of treatment, is undisputed.[6] A liver biopsy examination, a more familiar but less sensitive procedure, may also reveal amastigotes. Touch preparations of the biopsy on a clean slide and Giemsa staining make the amastigotes easier to identify.

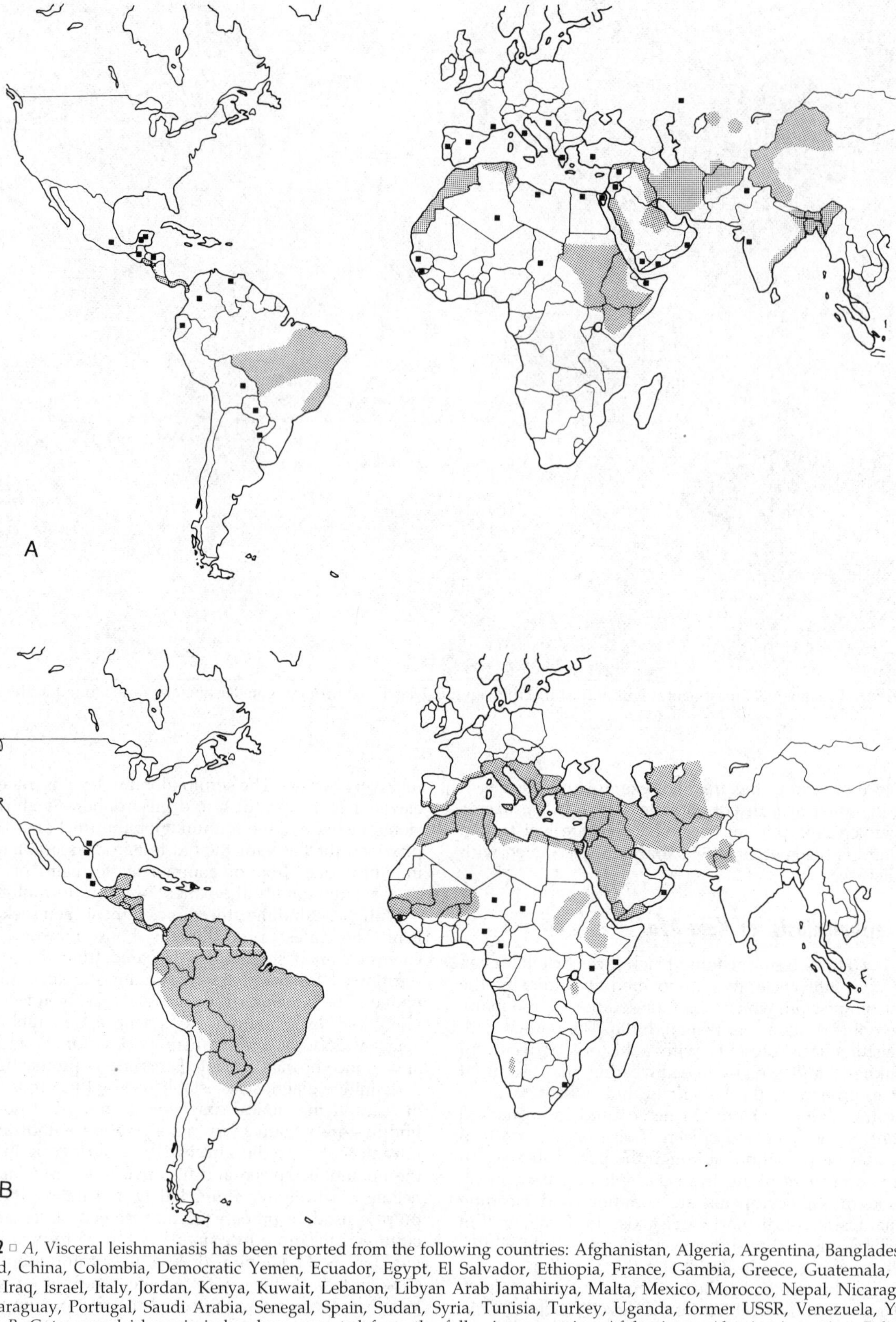

FIGURE 288–2 □ *A,* Visceral leishmaniasis has been reported from the following countries: Afghanistan, Algeria, Argentina, Bangladesh, Bolivia, Brazil, Chad, China, Colombia, Democratic Yemen, Ecuador, Egypt, El Salvador, Ethiopia, France, Gambia, Greece, Guatemala, Honduras, India, Iran, Iraq, Israel, Italy, Jordan, Kenya, Kuwait, Lebanon, Libyan Arab Jamahiriya, Malta, Mexico, Morocco, Nepal, Nicaragua, Oman, Pakistan, Paraguay, Portugal, Saudi Arabia, Senegal, Spain, Sudan, Syria, Tunisia, Turkey, Uganda, former USSR, Venezuela, Yemen, and Yugoslavia. *B,* Cutaneous leishmaniasis has been reported from the following countries: Afghanistan, Algeria, Argentina, Belize, Bolivia, Brazil, Burkina Faso, Cameroon, Chad, Colombia, Costa Rica, Democratic Yemen, Dominican Republic, Ecuador, Egypt, Ethiopia, French Guiana, Gambia, Greece, Guatemala, Guyana, Honduras, India, Iran, Iraq, Israel, Jordan, Kenya, Kuwait, Lebanon, Libyan Arab Jamahiriya, Mali, Mauritania, Mexico, Morocco, Nicaragua, Niger, Nigeria, Oman, Pakistan, Panama, Paraguay, Peru, Saudi Arabia, Senegal, Sudan, Suriname, Syria, Tunisia, Turkey, United States, Venezuela, former USSR, and Yemen. (*A* and *B* data from Guidelines for Leishmaniasis Control at Regional and Subregional Levels. Geneva, World Health Organization, 1988.)

A number of minor accessory signs occur in visceral leishmaniasis. Hair changes similar to those seen in kwashiorkor may be present, and the eyelashes may be long. Kala-azar is called black fever because of the increased pigmentation on the face and trunk, which seems to be more frequent in India. Lymphadenopathy may be present, especially in the East African and Mediterranean cases. *Leishmania* amastigotes have been recovered from affected lymphatic glands. Histologic examination of the liver shows normal hepatocytes but masses of parasites in the Kupffer cells. Slight increases in transaminase and alkaline phosphatase levels are common but jaundice is rare. The prothrombin time is usually normal. The spleen shows massive parasite involvement, with plasma cells and lymphocyte activity. Rare complications of established kala-azar are intralobular cirrhosis (Rogers cirrhosis), glomerulonephritis caused by immunoglobulin deposition in the basement membrane, and amyloidosis.

We now have a working knowledge of the basic immunology of leishmaniasis. The parasites reside and multiply exclusively in mononuclear phagocytes (monocytes and various populations of macrophages) in their mammalian hosts. Acute visceral leishmaniasis is accompanied by depressed cellular responses to leishmania antigen. Delayed hypersensitivity skin test responses are negative, and peripheral blood mononuclear cells do not proliferate or produce interferon-γ (IFN-γ) or interleukin (IL)–2 when cultured in vitro with leishmania antigen.[7, 8] These mononuclear cells produce IL-2 and IFN-γ when challenged with mitogens or unrelated antigens. Although leukopenia occurs in patients with acute disease, the fact that there is no significant decrease in total numbers of circulating lymphocytes would indicate that the observed suppression is not due merely to the lack of available lymphocytes. In fact, there are circulating T cells in patients with acute visceral leishmaniasis that are capable of suppressing antigen-driven lymphocyte proliferation.[6] During the recovery phase of the illness, the Th1 cytokines (IFN-γ, IL-2) are elaborated in response to leishmania antigens and the Th2 cytokines (IL-4, IL-5, IL-10) are reduced or absent.[8] Although anti-*Leishmania* antibodies are readily detectable during acute infection, there is no evidence that they are important in recovery from acute disease or in resistance to reinfection.

Anti-*Leishmania* drugs are often evaluated in patients with visceral leishmaniasis because of the multiplicity of signs, which disappear with successful treatment. Thus, the fever remits; anemia, leukopenia, and thrombocytopenia improve; and the liver and spleen diminish in size. The serum γ-globulin value takes longer to return to normal. Results of the *Leishmania* delayed hypersensitivity skin test become positive. In therapeutic studies, the presence of amastigotes in splenic aspirates is the best guide to treatment success, but it is likely that amastigotes persist silently and indefinitely in privileged sites, as in *Mycobacterium tuberculosis* infection.

Relapse in the skin is frequently documented in India and less frequently in East Africa and Brazil. This post–kala-azar dermal leishmaniasis was described in 5% of Indian visceral leishmaniasis patients after antimonial treatment. It is polymorphic and may present as hypopigmented or erythematous macules or as nodules resembling leprosy. The nodules are rich in parasites. In India, where there is no animal reservoir, such patients must be important in maintaining the cycle.

Untreated visceral leishmaniasis is often fatal, death being due to intercurrent respiratory or intestinal infection or to bleeding. For every classic case of visceral leishmaniasis in an endemic region there are many other persons who have been bitten by infected sandflies but have not developed disease.[9] The longest incubation period known to us is 9 years,[10] but it is usually measured in weeks or months. Visceral leishmaniasis is also being recognized with increasing frequency as an opportunistic infection in immunosuppressed patients, including persons with human immunodeficiency virus infection.

The differential diagnosis of visceral leishmaniasis must include the two other great tropical infections that cause hepatosplenomegaly, malaria and schistosomiasis. Hyperimmune malarial splenomegaly is characterized by high immunoglobulin M levels and hepatic sinusoidal lymphocytosis. Hepatosplenic schistosomiasis associated with *Salmonella* septicemia may closely resemble visceral leishmaniasis, but *Schistosoma mansoni* eggs are present in the stool. The hepatosplenomegaly of visceral leishmaniasis is often so marked that conditions with an equivalent degree of enlargement of these organs, namely leukemias, lymphomas, myelosclerosis, chronic brucellosis, and deposition disorders (Gaucher disease), are part of the differential diagnosis. In early visceral leishmaniasis with modest splenomegaly, typhoid fever and acute malaria must be excluded, as well as a host of fungal, bacterial, rickettsial, and viral infections.

Cutaneous Leishmaniasis

THE OLD WORLD

The increase in tourism has resulted in cases of cutaneous leishmaniasis appearing all over the world. The urban (dry) type of oriental sore caused by *Leishmania tropica* presents as a firm, erythematous papule that is usually no larger than 2 to 4 cm and occurs on an exposed part of the body where the female sandfly had an opportunity to bite. As the lesion enlarges, a serous crust forms and the reddish, inflamed border is elevated above the level of the surrounding skin (the so-called volcano sign). Clinical variants include a psoriasiform type with marked scaling and warty hyperkeratosis. The lesion remains static for 4 to 6 months, but fibrosis gradually effects healing, leaving a well-defined and characteristic scar. Immunity is usually lifelong. This type of leishmaniasis is frequently contracted in cities of the Middle East. For this reason, a number of epithets for oriental sore name cities (Aleppo or Bagdad boil, Biskra button).

The so-called wet type of Old World leishmaniasis is prone to earlier ulceration, is found principally in rural areas of the endemic zone, and is caused by *Leishmania major.* It must be stressed that these are general distinctions, and rapidly ulcerating lesions can be found that are due to *L. tropica* and vice versa. The ulcer of the wet type is a larger lesion with a granulomatous base and an active, firm, erythematous border. It is slow to heal, but most lesions close within the year.

Some 5% to 10% of both types of lesions follow an atypical course, with failure to heal and persistence of active foci in the form of nodules or papules at the extremity of the lesion for many years. The similarity to lupus vulgaris has given rise to the term lupoid leishmaniasis. Biopsy of cutaneous leishmaniasis lesions initially shows a poorly organized granulomatous inflammation with a massive infiltration of lymphocyte and plasma cells and epithelioid cell formation. In established cases such as lupoid leishmaniasis, well-defined tubercle formation with giant cells is seen, but parasites are scarce at this stage. Lesions that persist many years at the limits of the old scar of acute disease are referred to as leishmaniasis recidivans.

Ethiopian cutaneous leishmaniasis caused by *Leishmania aethiopica* also presents as a chronic skin granuloma, which may not ulcerate but may persist for many years and gradually extend. Ethiopia is one of the areas of the world where diffuse anergic cutaneous leishmaniasis has been well documented. These patients develop widespread cutaneous nodules that are rich in amastigotes and resemble those of lepromatous leprosy. The histologic examination shows an absence of lymphocytes and plasma cells and the result of the leishmanin skin test is negative. Patients respond poorly to treatment.

Biopsy for cutaneous leishmaniasis should always involve the active edge of the lesion to avoid histologic changes produced by necrosis or secondary infection. The granulomatous reaction is not diagnostic, because there are other types of skin granulomata, including tuberculosis, sarcoid, and foreign body granulomata. Skin malignancies may present as ulcers similar to those of leishmaniasis.

The definitive diagnosis requires demonstration of the parasite. Parasites may be seen in hematoxylin-eosin–stained sections of the biopsy specimen. Aspiration of the dermis at the active border of the lesion usually demonstrates parasites in Giemsa-stained smears or after culture in Nicolle-Novy-MacNeal medium. Immunologic tests such as the leishmanin skin test or detection of circulating antibodies by immunofluorescence or enzyme-linked immunosorbent assay aid in diagnosis. In general, the older the lesion, the more difficult it is to find parasites, with the notable exception of the rare diffuse anergic cutaneous leishmaniasis.

THE NEW WORLD

These causative *Leishmania* organisms are divided into the *Leishmania mexicana* and the *L. viannia* subgenera[3] (see Table 288–1).

Leishmania mexicana **Group.** Initial work in Mexico defined a limited type of cutaneous leishmaniasis that was particularly prevalent in the Yucatan peninsula and that closely resembled dry oriental sore *(L. mexicana mexicana),* although the ear pinna was involved more frequently and infections at this site tended to last a long time. This unusual localization probably reflects the vector phlebotomines' preferential feeding site. Later work in Belém, Brazil, defined a second *L. mexicana* subspecies, *L. m. amazonensis.* Human infections with this organism are relatively uncommon because the vector fly rarely bites humans but maintains a zoonotic cycle. An important clinical aspect of these parasitoses is that, to date, only *L. m. amazonensis* parasites have produced disseminated anergic cutaneous leishmaniasis in the New World. Cases have been reported from Venezuela, Brazil, and the Dominican Republic. In immunocompetent hosts, *L. m. amazonensis* infections produce relatively small lesions resembling Old World leishmaniasis, which may or may not ulcerate and frequently are self-healing within a year.

Leishmania viannia **Group.** The *L. braziliensis* subgenus was renamed to honor the physician who introduced antimonials for the treatment of leishmaniasis. The individual parasites merit brief separate consideration. *L. v. braziliensis* is the most destructive in terms of the rapidity of skin ulceration and evidence of metastatic lesions. The skin ulcers tend to be large, deep, and slow to heal. Histologic examination reveals the usual granulomatous process, but necrosis is marked. Lymphatic dissemination occurs but not as frequently as one would expect for the organism that is primarily responsible for mucosal metastasis. Sometimes active skin and mucosal lesions are seen together. Lesions are slow to resolve, but spontaneous healing without therapy does occur. Rarely, hyperkeratotic plaquelike lesions are seen, and leishmaniasis recidivans is documented. The geographic distribution of *L. v. braziliensis* is extensive in Latin America. It also occurs in countries east of the Andes and has been documented as far north as Belize. Isolation of *L. v. braziliensis* is difficult. Parasites are scant in the lesion and grow poorly in culture in vitro and in the hamster. With experience, parasites can be isolated from about half of patients. The leishmanin skin test and circulating antibodies assume increased diagnostic importance.

L. v. panamensis is said to be associated with mucosal metastasis. The skin ulcers are smaller than those caused by *L. v. braziliensis,* and the parasite seems to be less destructive in the skin. *L. v. guyanensis* was initially defined in French Guyana. This parasite has been reported in patients with mucosal disease. It causes small skin ulcers that are frequently multiple and ascend the lymphatics. These lesions must be differentiated from sporotrichosis. Cases have been reported only north of the Amazon River. *L. v. peruviana* has been reported only from the western slopes of the Andes and the Argentine highlands. There are usually single ulcers that are self-healing and no evidence of metastasis.

Mucosal leishmaniasis (espundia) is virtually restricted to South America because of the distribution of *L. v. braziliensis.*[11] It is especially common in central Brazil, where *L. v. braziliensis* is the dominant species. We estimate that less than 5% of patients who develop an *L. v. braziliensis* primary skin lesion develop mucosal disease.[12, 13] Initial symptoms are nasal blockage, epistaxis, and tissue coming from the nose. The granuloma frequently begins on the nasal septum, which usually perforates. Exuberant granulation tissue may block one or both nostrils. The process extends from the floor of the nose to the hard and soft palate. The pharynx and larynx may be involved, and a hoarse voice is a valuable sign. Tissue destruction may result in loss of the cartilaginous nose or lips. Aspiration pneumonia and laryngeal closure may result in a fatal outcome.

At the initial consultation, a careful history must be obtained and the *Leishmania* scar (usually on the limbs) located. Only 10% of patients do not have a scar. There is evidence that multiple skin lesions and previous inadequate therapy are more frequently associated with mucosal leishmaniasis. It is probable that amastigotes reach the mucosal vasculature relatively early after skin infection with *L. v. braziliensis.* We know little of the genesis of mucosal disease or the effect of factors such as temperature, trauma, and the immune response of cartilage. There is no evidence of a cellular immune defect in these patients. The intradermal skin test and lymphocyte proliferative responses are maintained. Lymphocytes from these patients produce IFN-γ, which inhibits intracellular replication of *Leishmania* organisms. It has been suggested that mucosal leishmaniasis may represent a hypersensitivity to *Leishmania.* Antibody titers of patients with mucosal disease are high. Indirect methods of diagnosis such as these are valuable in mucosal leishmaniasis, because the parasite is difficult to isolate. *L. v. braziliensis* is difficult to grow, and bacterial and fungal flora of the nose and mouth often contaminate the cultures. The best culture method is to take a biopsy of an active granuloma, triturate it, and inoculate it into the nose and the hind feet of a hamster. Subsequent aspiration and culture from these sites may yield *Leishmania* organisms but often only after a period of several months.

Systemic mycoses with skin manifestations are also important in the differential diagnosis, including lobomycosis and particularly paracoccidioidomycosis, which can affect the nasal mucosa in a similar manner. The differential diagnosis also includes tertiary treponematoses, cancer, leprosy, rhinoscleroma, and lethal midline granuloma.

Treatment

The treatment of all forms of leishmaniasis is most unsatisfactory. The first-line therapy remains the pentavalent antimonials (Sb^v), which were introduced more than 70 years ago. Pentostam (sodium stibogluconate) is marketed by Wellcome, and Specia (Rhodia) makes Glucantime (meglumine antimonate). Pentostam is in common use in English-speaking countries (available from the Centers for Disease Control and Prevention in Atlanta), and Glucantime is used in Francophone and Latin American countries. Pentavalent antimonials have been the subject of several reviews.[14–16] They are unstable compounds and should be stored at 4°C in the dark.

Visceral Leishmaniasis

Thakur and coworkers[6] reported that 20 mg of Sb^v per kg of body weight per day for 40 days was the most effective regimen for Indian visceral leishmaniasis. This regimen has also been used with success in East African visceral leishmaniasis. Visceral leishmaniasis is more difficult to treat successfully in India than in the Mediterranean, Africa, China, or South America. We still await satisfactory studies from some of these areas, but on the current evidence Sb^v, a dose of 20 mg/kg per day for 20 to 28 days, depending on the area, is recommended.[17] The combination of IFN-γ and pentavalent antimony is effective in a majority of patients with either refractory or relapsing visceral leishmaniasis.[18]

Evaluation of treatment is based on clinical criteria, such as absence of fever, regression of hepatosplenomegaly, normalization of hematopoietic parameters, and decrease in serum globulin levels. After therapy, a repeated bone marrow examination or splenic aspiration and a search for *Leishmania* organisms by using Giemsa-stained smears and culture may be indicated if the clinical response is incomplete. Follow-up for a 2-year period is desirable.

Cutaneous Leishmaniasis

Primary *L. tropica* infections could probably be treated with a single 20-day course of Sb^v, at 10 mg/kg per day.[17] Chronic infections such as lupoid leishmaniasis or leishmaniasis recidivans require Sb^v, 20 mg/kg per day, for longer periods. *L. aethiopica* skin infections are relatively resistant to treatment, so the higher dose would have to be used.

In Brazil, we use Sb^v, at 20 mg/kg per day for 20 days, for primary infections. This dose is probably adequate for the great majority of *L. v. guyanensis, L. v. panamensis,* and *L. v. peruviana* primary infections. *L. mexicana* primary infections respond to lower doses, with the notable exception of disseminated anergic cutaneous leishmaniasis. In both the Old World and the New World, this syndrome is notoriously difficult to treat, and the 20 mg/kg per day dose of Sb^v may be needed for months to revert the result of the leishmanin skin test and achieve healing of the skin lesions. The combination of IFN-γ and antimony may be efficacious in this form of leishmaniasis.

Mucosal Leishmaniasis

The current recommendation for treatment of mucosal leishmaniasis is Sb^v, at 20 mg/kg per day for 40 days. At that time the activity of the lesion is assessed clinically, histologically, and parasitologically. Signs of persistent activity by any of these parameters is an indication to continue treatment, which in our experience has been as long as 3 months.[19]

Pentavalent antimonials should be administered in a single slow intravenous or intramuscular injection. Antimonials have a bad reputation, largely because of the marked side effects of the obsolete trivalent antimonial compounds. The adverse reactions associated with pentavalent antimonials are much less serious, although still significant. They are dose related and include arthralgias, pancreatitis, abnormal liver function test results (transaminases, alkaline phosphatase), and prolongation of the ST interval or inversion of the T wave. The development of electrocardiographic abnormalities is an indication for stopping treatment.[20] Weekly electrocardiographic examinations are indicated after the first 2 weeks of therapy.

Second-line drugs include pentamidine and amphotericin B.[17] Pentamidine isethionate is given intramuscularly at 2 to 4 mg/kg per day for up to 15 doses. Serious side effects include hypotension and hypoglycemia. Amphotericin B is used in a dose of 0.25 to 1 mg/kg per day to a total of 30 mg/kg or a maximal total dose of 2.5 g.

The Future

Effective oral drug treatment is a priority in leishmaniasis research. Oriental sore is said to respond well to topical creams,[21] but they cannot be used for cutaneous leishmaniasis that has the potential for metastatic lesions. In oriental sore, in which spontaneous healing is the rule, the patient may opt for natural healing if the lesion is not in an exposed site.

Prophylaxis and Control

Personal prophylaxis in endemic areas should include restricting activity in crepuscular hours when phlebotomines are active. For example, in Amazonas, military troops take their bath in the afternoon to avoid nocturnal phlebotomines. Repellents and clothing cover are only partially effective, but an insecticide-impregnated mosquito net covering the bed is a good precaution.

Effective control measures depend to a certain extent on what is known of the transmission cycle.[22] The former Soviet Union has had success in controlling *L. major* transmission by attacking the giant gerbil (*Rhombomys opimus,* the main animal reservoir) and the vector *Phlebotomus papatasi.* In various countries, DDT residual spraying of houses for malaria control has reduced the prevalence of visceral leishmaniasis. This is the case in Brazil, where the only control measures adopted at the Ministry of Health level are for visceral leishmaniasis, namely domiciliary spraying and destruction of infected dogs. Sylvatic leishmaniasis is impossible to control at the present time.

The former Soviet Union, Israel, and Iran have used leishmanial vaccines containing live attenuated promastigotes. Between 1982 and 1986, 1.2 million people were vaccinated in Iran. Vaccination with killed promastigotes has been tried in Brazil, but the scientific effort and coordination in leishmania vaccine research have been haphazard to date, and no firm opinion can be given on the efficacy of these initiatives.[3]

Acknowledgments

We wish to acknowledge support from the National Institutes of Health for our research (AI 16282).

References

1. Chang K-P, Bray RS: Leishmaniasis. Amsterdam, Elsevier, 1985.
2. Peters W, Killick-Kendrick R (eds): The Leishmaniases in Biology and Medicine. London, Academic Press, 1987.
3. Grimaldi G Jr, McMahon-Pratt D: Leishmaniasis and its etiologic agents in the New World: An overview. Prog Clin Parasitol 2:73, 1991.
4. Cerf BJ, Jones TC, Badaro R, et al: Malnutrition as a risk factor for severe visceral leishmaniasis. J Infect Dis 156:1030, 1987.
5. Bryceson A: Splenic aspiration procedure. *In* Peters W, Killick-Kendrick R (eds): The Leishmaniases in Biology and Medicine, Vol 2. London, Academic Press, 1987, pp 728–729.
6. Thakur CP, Kumar M, Kumar P, et al: Rationalisation of regimens

of treatment of kala-azar with sodium stibogluconate in India: A randomised study. Br Med J 296:1557, 1988.
7. Carvalho EM, Bacellar O, Barral A, et al: Antigen-specific immunosuppression in visceral leishmaniasis is cell mediated. J Clin Invest 83:860, 1989.
8. Ho JL, Badaro R, Hatzigeorgiou D, et al: Cytokines in the treatment of leishmaniasis: From studies of immunopathology to patient therapy. Biotherapy 7:223, 1994.
9. Badaro R, Jones TC, Carvalho EM, et al: New perspectives on a subclinical form of visceral leishmaniasis. J Infect Dis 154:1003, 1986.
10. Wright MI: Kala azar of unusual duration associated with agammaglobulinaemia. Br Med J 1:1218, 1959.
11. Marsden PD: Mucosal leishmaniasis ("espundia" Escomel, 1911). Trans R Soc Trop Med Hyg 80:859, 1986.
12. Jones TC, Johnson WD Jr, Barretto AC, et al: Epidemiology of American cutaneous leishmaniasis due to *Leishmania braziliensis braziliensis.* J Infect Dis 156:73, 1987.
13. Netto EM, Marsden PD, Llanos-Cuentas EA, et al: Long-term follow-up of patients with *Leishmania (viannia) braziliensis* infection and treated with glucantime. Trans R Soc Trop Med Hyg 84:367, 1990.
14. Marsden PD: Pentavalent antimonials: Old drugs for new diseases. Rev Soc Bras Med Trop 18:187, 1985.
15. Bryceson A: Therapy in man. *In* Peters W, Killick-Kendrick R (eds): The Leishmaniases in Biology and Medicine, Vol 2. London, Academic Press, 1987, pp 847–907.
16. Berman JD: Chemotherapy for leishmaniasis. Biochemical mechanisms, clinical efficacy and future strategies. Rev Infect Dis 10:560, 1988.
17. Drugs for parasitic infection. Med Lett 35:111, 1993.
18. Badaro R, Falcoff E, Badaro FS, et al: Treatment of visceral leishmaniasis with pentavalent antimony and interferon-γ. N Engl J Med 322:16, 1990.
19. Marsden PD, Sampaio RNR, Carvalho EM, et al: High continuous antimony therapy in two patients with unresponsive mucosal leishmaniasis. Am J Trop Med Hyg 34:710, 1985.
20. Chulay JD, Spencer HC, Mugambi M: Electrocardiographic changes during treatment of leishmaniasis with pentavalent antimony (sodium stibogluconate). Am J Trop Med Hyg 34:702, 1985.
21. El-On J, Jacobs GP, Weinrausch L: Topical chemotherapy of cutaneous leishmaniasis. Parasitol Today 4:76, 1988.
22. Marsden PD: Selective primary health care: Strategies for control of disease in the developing world. XIV. Leishmaniasis. Rev Infect Dis 6:736, 1984.
23. Guidelines for Leishmaniasis Control at Regional and Subregional Levels. Geneva, World Health Organization, 1988.

289

Trypanosoma

James H. Maguire

Four flagellated protozoans of the genus *Trypanosoma* infect human beings.[1] In Africa, *Trypanosoma brucei rhodesiense* and *Trypanosoma brucei gambiense* produce sleeping sickness. *Trypanosoma cruzi,* the agent of Chagas disease, and the nonpathogenic *Trypanosoma rangeli* are endemic to the Americas. Like *Leishmania* and other members of the family Trypanosomatidae, trypanosomes pass through morphologically and physiologically distinct developmental stages in their insect vectors and mammalian hosts. Each stage contains a kinetoplast, a dark-staining structure that consists of tight coils of DNA lying within the terminal portion of the organism's single mitochondrion (Fig. 289–1).

African Trypanosomes

Characteristics of the Pathogen

The two subspecies of *T. brucei* that infect human beings are morphologically identical but produce epidemiologically and clinically distinct patterns of disease.[2–4] In West and Central Africa, *T. b. gambiense* causes Gambian sleeping sickness, and in East Africa, *T. b. rhodesiense* causes Rhodesian sleeping sickness. A closely related third subspecies, *Trypanosoma brucei,* is responsible for nagana, an infection of livestock that seriously limits cattle production in Africa.

Within the mammalian host, African trypanosomes assume the fusiform trypomastigote stage (see Fig. 289–1). This stage of the parasite, which measures 15 to 40 μm long, is propelled by a single anterior flagellum that extends from a lateral undulating membrane. Trypomastigotes circulate extracellularly in the blood, lymph, and interstitial fluids and replicate by longitudinal binary fission. Early generations of parasites are long and slender, whereas later generations that are infectious to the tsetse fly vector are short and stumpy. Trypomastigotes are covered by a thick glycoprotein surface coat that undergoes antigenic variation during infection, a process that allows the organism to evade lysis by specific antibodies.[5, 6]

The other phase of the parasite's life cycle takes place in the blood-sucking tsetse fly vector (genus *Glossina*). The fly ingests trypomastigotes with a blood meal from an infected mammal. The trypomastigotes transform into procyclic forms that multiply and then later penetrate the insect's midgut and migrate to the salivary glands, where they transform into epimastigotes, which also replicate. After about 3 weeks, infective metacyclic trypanosomes develop from the epimastigotes. Transmission to the mammalian host occurs when the tsetse fly inoculates saliva containing metacyclic forms during feeding. These forms transform into blood stream trypomastigotes, replicate locally, and then spread to the blood stream, lymphatics, and interstitial spaces.

Epidemiology

Transmission of African trypanosomiasis is limited to focal areas of sub-Saharan Africa between latitudes 14 degrees north and 29 degrees south.[2–4] Each year, about 25,000 cases are reported and an estimated 50 million persons live at risk of being infected.[4] Epidemics have claimed tens to hundreds of thousands of lives in the past and may occur in the future if political instability or economic constraints interfere with sleeping sickness control programs.

In West and Central Africa, the vectors of Gambian trypanosomiasis are species of tsetse flies such as *Glossina palpalis, Glossina tachinoides,* and *Glossina fuscipes,* which inhabit forested riverbanks and similar humid areas.[2] Human beings in nearby settlements are the major reservoir of infection, although pigs and other domestic animals may harbor the parasite.

T. b. rhodesiense is transmitted by *Glossina morsitans* and related species that live in the sparsely inhabited savannahs of East Africa. Wild animals, such as the bushbuck and hartebeest, are important reservoirs, and except under epidemic conditions, human beings become infected when they enter areas of natural transmission to hunt, fish, collect honey, or visit wild game parks.

Reported cases of African trypanosomiasis caused by congenital infection, blood transfusion, and laboratory accident

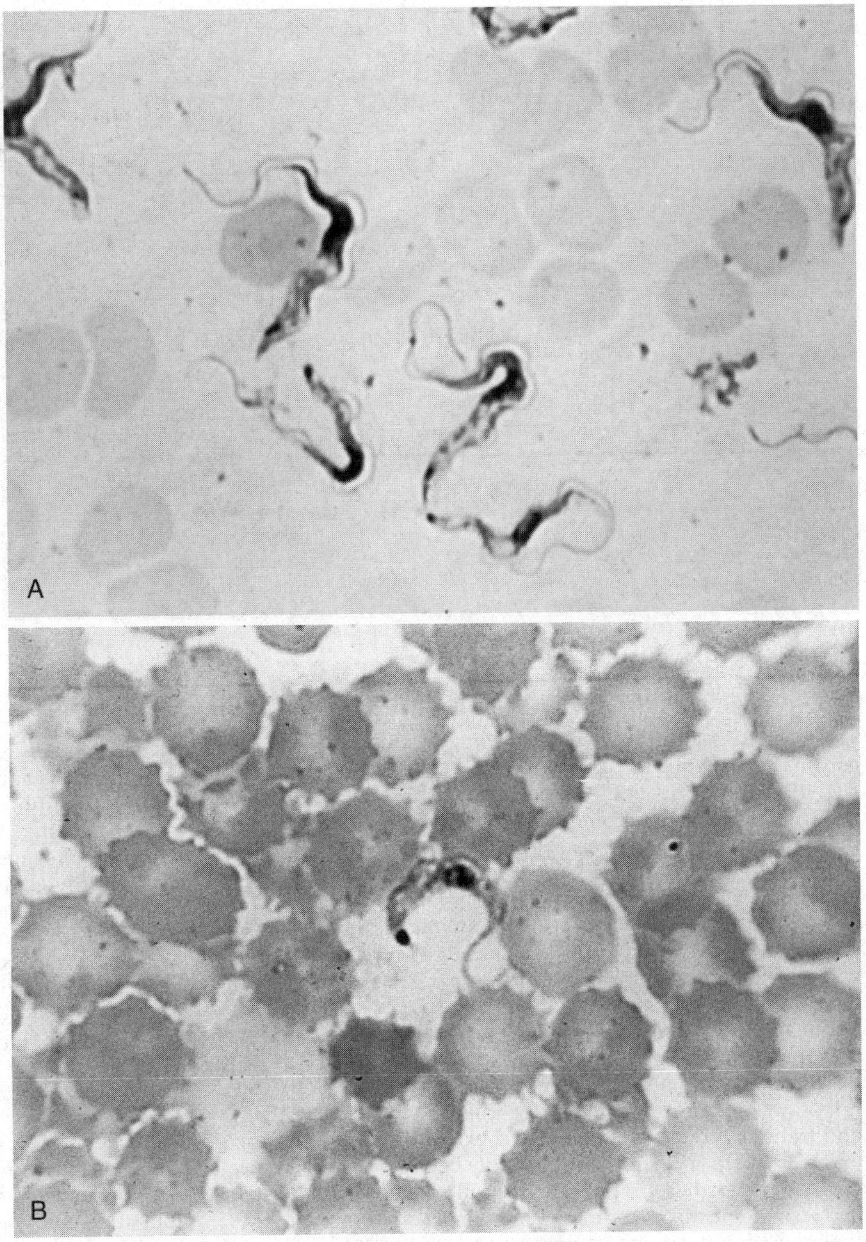

FIGURE 289–1 ▫ Blood stream trypomastigotes (slender forms) in the peripheral blood of a patient with Gambian sleeping sickness *(A)* and a patient with acute Chagas disease *(B)*. Note the free flagellum extending from the anterior end and the dotlike, posteriorly situated kinetoplast (approximately × 1200). (*A* and *B* from the teaching collection of the Department of Tropical Public Health, Harvard School of Public Health, Boston, MA.)

are rare.[7] In the United States, there were 17 cases of imported infections during a 20-year period, most of which were due to *T. b. rhodesiense* acquired in game parks.[8]

Pathogenesis

An inflamed nodule or trypanosomal chancre forms at the site of the bite, where the parasites are inoculated and multiply outside the cells in the subcutaneous tissue. The organism gradually spreads from the local site of infection to the lymphatics, blood stream, and interstitial spaces, where they continue extracellular replication. The parasitemia increases until specific antibodies produced by the host cause a sharp decline of parasite numbers.[5, 6] Parasites that have different surface antigen variants escape destruction and give rise to a new wave of parasitemia. Because each organism contains the genetic code for numerous variants, the waves of parasitemia continue to recur for months. After months to years of blood and lymph involvement, the organisms penetrate the central nervous system (CNS).

The mechanisms by which African trypanosomes produce disease are not well understood.[9, 10] Antigens from the recurrent waves of parasitemia activate lymphocytes and macrophages, resulting in enlargement of lymph nodes and the spleen and massive production of immunoglobulins, particularly immunoglobulin M (IgM), that are mostly nonspecific and nonprotective. Circulating immune complexes, lymphokines and kinins, and toxins produced by the parasite may all play a role in the pathogenesis of the illness. In the later stage of disease, lymphocytes and plasma cells infiltrate the pia and arachnoid of the brain and form cuffs around blood vessels, especially in the heart and CNS, where parasites are located (Fig. 289–2). Perivascular demyelinization, proliferation of astrocytes, and focal hemorrhages are seen in the brain. Pancarditis frequently occurs in Rhodesian disease. Generalized immunosuppression and associated secondary infections are common during the later phases of the disease.

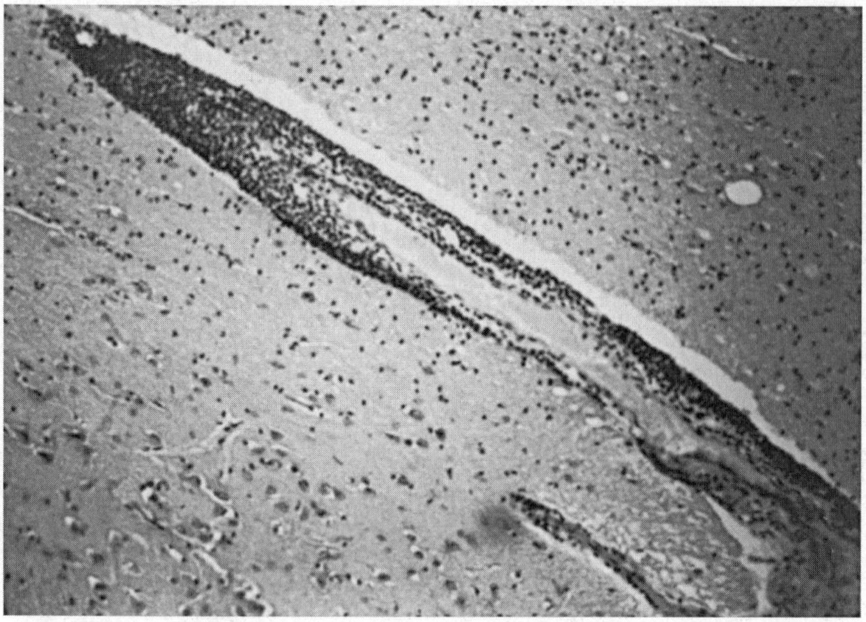

FIGURE 289–2 □ Section of human brain from a fatal case of Gambian sleeping sickness. An infiltrate of lymphocytes and plasma cells forms a cuff around the blood vessel. Parasites are rarely seen in tissue sections (approximately × 200). (From the teaching collection of the Department of Tropical Public Health, Harvard School of Public Health; and courtesy of Dr. S. C. Pan, Harvard School of Public Health, Boston, MA.)

Clinical Manifestations

The clinical features of African trypanosomiasis vary according to the stage of infection and the subspecies of parasite.[11–13] Without treatment, both infections are invariably fatal. The course of Rhodesian disease is more rapid and severe than that of Gambian disease.

First symptoms appear several days to 2 weeks after the tsetse bite. A tender, red nodule, the trypanosomal chancre, may develop in the subcutaneous tissue at the site of initial parasite replication, which heals after a few weeks. With systemic dissemination of the infection, patients experience headache, myalgia, malaise, and episodes of fever that recur with each wave of parasitemia. Lymphadenopathy is a more prominent feature of Gambian trypanosomiasis. The characteristic enlargement of posterior cervical nodes, the Winterbottom sign, may suggest the diagnosis. Splenomegaly and transient edema of the face and extremities are common, and a circinate erythematous rash may be observed in Caucasians. Amenorrhea, impotence, hypothyroidism, and other endocrinologic disorders may result from lesions of the hypothalamus, pituitary, and peripheral endocrine glands.[2, 14]

Anemia, monocytosis, and markedly elevated levels of IgM in the serum are characteristic of both forms of the disease.[11] In Rhodesian infections, the signs and symptoms of systemic disease appear within a week or two of inoculation, and the course is often complicated by congestive heart failure or arrhythmias related to myocarditis, by secondary infection, or by disseminated intravascular coagulation.[13] Death caused by *T. b. rhodesiense* occurs within weeks to months, frequently before the CNS is invaded. In contrast, the symptoms of the disseminated phase of Gambian trypanosomiasis are often mild or absent, and the infection may not be recognized for several years until CNS invasion occurs.

The CNS becomes involved within a few months of inoculation in persons with Rhodesian disease and after months to several years in persons with Gambian disease. CNS disease usually progresses gradually over several weeks to months, although occasionally coma and death can occur within a few days. Characteristic symptoms and signs include a persistent headache; inability to concentrate; personality changes; seizures; motor disturbances including tremors, choreoathetosis, and ataxia; and finally coma. Daytime somnolence (sleeping sickness) is due to disruption of normal circadian alternation of sleeping and waking rather than to hypersomnia.[14, 15] With CNS involvement, the cerebrospinal fluid (CSF) is under increased pressure and has elevated protein and IgM concentrations and a mononuclear pleocytosis consisting predominantly of lymphocytes and an occasional morula cell of Mott (plasma cell that contains aggregates of immunoglobulin). In time, patients lapse into coma and die with malnutrition and secondary infection or in status epilepticus.

Human immunodeficiency virus infection, which is highly prevalent in many parts of sub-Saharan Africa, does not appear to have a major impact on the incidence or severity of African trypanosomiasis.[16] Persons infected with both human immunodeficiency virus and *T. b. gambiense,* however, may be at higher risk of relapse after treatment with eflornithine.

Diagnosis

The diagnosis of African trypanosomiasis cannot be made solely on clinical grounds. Early disease may be confused with malaria, Epstein-Barr virus or cytomegalovirus infection, tuberculosis, or lymphoma; late-stage disease mimics psychiatric illness or meningoencephalitis of another infectious cause.

Definitive diagnosis of African trypanosomiasis is made by microscopic identification of trypanosomes in the blood, CSF, or fluid aspirated from a chancre or a lymph node.[17] Motile trypanosomes can be seen in fresh preparations, and the morphologic characteristics can be further studied in Giemsa- or Wright-stained smears. In the early stage of disease, *T. b. gambiense* is more readily detected in lymph node aspirates and *T. b. rhodesiense* in blood. The sensitivity of parasitologic diagnosis can be increased by examining thick blood films, buffy coat preparations from centrifuged microhematocrit tubes, or eluates of blood fractionated on diethylaminoethyl cellulose anion-exchange columns.[18] The quantitative buffy coat technique, which employs acridine orange to stain parasites that have been separated from blood components by centrifugation, is extremely sensitive and easily performed.[19] With all of these techniques, repeated examinations may be necessary because of fluctuating levels of parasitemia. Parasites can be isolated by inoculation of body fluids or tissue into culture media or, in the case of Rhodesian but not Gambian trypanosomiasis, laboratory rodents.

A variety of sensitive serologic tests detect specific antibodies within several weeks of infection but require parasitologic tests to confirm the diagnosis.[17, 20] The card agglutination test for trypanosomiasis is widely used for screening rural populations because it is easily performed under field conditions.[21] The sensitivity of antigen detection tests and polymerase chain reaction–based assays is under evaluation.[22, 23]

In all cases of African trypanosomiasis, the CSF should be examined for evidence of CNS involvement, even if neurologic examination findings are normal. Identification of parasites, increased numbers of mononuclear cells, or an increased protein level indicates CNS invasion. A double-centrifugation technique has been shown to enhance detection of trypanosomes in CSF.[24]

Treatment

Specific treatment of African trypanosomiasis is most effective in reducing mortality and preventing permanent neurologic damage if administered early in the course of infection, before involvement of the CNS.[2, 25, 26] The choice of antitrypanosomal drugs depends on the stage and the geographic origin of infection. Because the drugs are toxic and several different treatment regimens have been proposed, expert advice should be sought before therapy is administered. In the United States, such assistance, as well as several of the antitrypanosomal drugs listed in Table 289–1, can be obtained from the Parasitic Disease Drug Service, Centers for Disease Control and Prevention in Atlanta.

All four drugs listed in Table 289–1 are effective for treatment of *T. b. gambiense* infections. The drug of choice is eflornithine (difluoromethylornithine, Ornidyl) because of its low toxicity and excellent CNS penetration.[27] Although it is active in both early- and late-stage disease, in endemic countries its high cost and requirement for multiple intravenous doses limit its use to late-stage infections that are refractory to melarsoprol. About 50% of persons receiving standard doses of eflornithine develop a mild and reversible bone marrow depression. Seizures occur infrequently and are associated with high CNS levels of the drug.

TABLE 289–1 ■ Therapeutic Dosages for Treatment of African and American Trypanosomiasis

DISEASE AND DRUG	DOSE*
African Trypanosomiasis	
Pentamidine isethionate	Base: 4 mg/kg/d or every other day IM or IV × 10 doses
Suramin†	4 mg/kg (test dose) IV on day 1; 10 mg/kg IV on day 3; beginning on day 5, 20 mg/kg/d (maximum 1 g) IV q 6 d × five doses
Melarsoprol†	1.5 mg/kg IV on day 1; 2.0 mg/kg IV on day 2; 2.2 mg/kg IV on day 3; 2.5 mg/kg IV on day 10; 3.0 mg/kg IV on day 11; and 3.6 mg/kg IV on days 12, 20, 21, 22
Eflornithine	Adults: 100 mg/kg IV q 6 h × 2 wk; then 75 mg/kg PO q 6 h × 4 wk
	Children: 150 mg/kg IV q 6 h × 2 wk, then 75 mg/kg PO q 6 h × 4 wk
American Trypanosomiasis	
Nifurtimox†	Adults: 8–10 mg/kg/d in four doses PO × 90 d
	Youths 11–16 y: 12.5–15 mg/kg/d in four doses PO × 90 d
	Children <11 y: 15–20 mg/kg/d in four doses PO × 90 d
Benznidazole	5 mg/kg/d PO × 60 d

*IM, Intramuscularly; IV, intravenously; PO, orally.
†Available in the United States from the Parasitic Disease Drug Service, Centers for Disease Control and Prevention, Atlanta, Georgia.

Pentamidine (Pentam 300, Pentacarinat) and suramin (Bayer 205) are useful for the treatment of early- but not late-stage Gambian disease because they do not cross the blood-brain barrier. Pentamidine is preferred over suramin, which is more toxic and more expensive. Suramin may be used if pentamidine resistance is suspected, such as in areas where pentamidine has been used widely for prophylaxis. A regimen consisting of only six doses of pentamidine and two full (20 mg/kg) doses of suramin has little toxicity and appears more effective than therapy with either drug alone.[25]

Pentamidine can cause sterile abscesses when injected intramuscularly, but it can be given safely by slow intravenous infusion for 2 hours. Persons who receive pentamidine should be monitored closely for hypotension, hypoglycemia, bone marrow toxicity, nephrotoxicity, and hepatotoxicity. Therapy with suramin should begin with a small test dose to check for idiopathic hypersensitivity reactions to the drug or anaphylactoid reactions related to the action of the drug on *Onchocerca volvulus*, a filarial parasite endemic to parts of Africa. Renal insufficiency, fever, arthralgia, rash, and neuropathy may complicate suramin therapy. If evidence of nephrotoxicity develops, the drug should be withheld until renal function improves.

The trivalent arsenical derivative melarsoprol (mel B, Arsobal) is widely used for late-stage Gambian infection because of the unavailability of eflornithine. Two doses of pentamidine or a test dose and one full dose of suramin are administered first to clear the blood stream of trypanosomes. Melarsoprol induces a life-threatening encephalopathy in 2% to 10% of persons and may cause exfoliative dermatitis, diarrhea, or jaundice.[12, 28] Administration of corticosteroids reduces the incidence and mortality of reactive arsenical encephalopathy.

Because *T. b. brucei* infections respond poorly to eflornithine and pentamidine, suramin is used for early infections and melarsoprol is used for CNS infections. Patients who relapse after melarsoprol should be offered a second course of melarsoprol before receiving toxic alternatives such as nitrofurazone or nifurtimox.[25]

All persons treated for African trypanosomiasis should be followed up for a minimum of 2 years for evidence of relapse. The CSF should be examined at the end of treatment and 3, 6, 12, 18, and 24 months later for signs of CNS involvement.

Prevention

The only sure means of preventing infection is by avoiding areas infested by tsetse flies. Using heavy, protective, and light-colored clothing and insect repellents reduces the risk of infection. Pentamidine is no longer recommended as a prophylactic drug because the dose used is not curative, may mask infection until CNS invasion occurs, and promotes the emergence of drug-resistant strains of the parasite.

Current strategies for controlling sleeping sickness in West and Central Africa involve systematic surveillance of populations at risk and early detection and treatment of infected persons to reduce the human reservoir of disease.[2, 4] In these regions and in East Africa, vector control efforts are directed at reducing contact between humans and flies by using simple, inexpensive, and nonpolluting technologies such as tsetse traps and screens.[29]

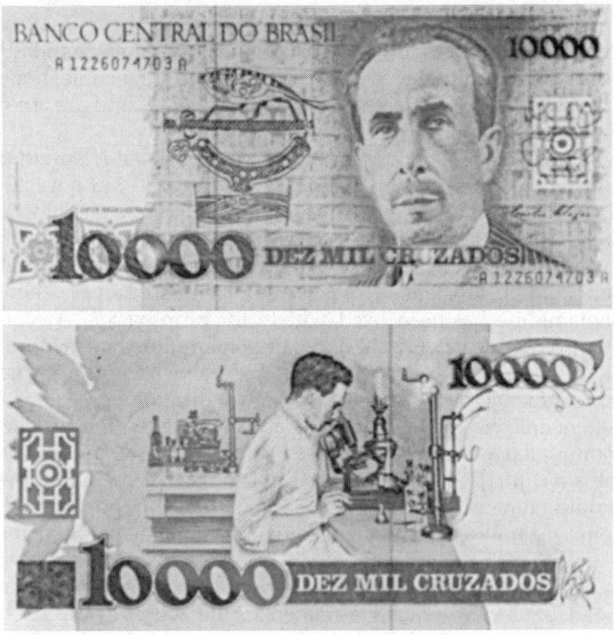

FIGURE 289–3 ▫ Carlos Chagas, the discoverer of *Trypanosoma cruzi*, honored on Brazilian currency. To the left of the portrait of Chagas in the top panel is a schematic diagram of the life cycle of the parasite in its insect and mammalian hosts.

Trypanosoma cruzi

In 1909, the Brazilian physician Carlos Chagas (Fig. 289–3) discovered *T. cruzi* and described the clinical features of American trypanosomiasis, or Chagas disease. *T. cruzi* is found only in the Western Hemisphere, where it is transmitted by reduviid bugs to more than 100 different species of wild and domestic animals as well as to human beings.[30–33] Chagas disease is a leading cause of cardiovascular death and gastrointestinal disease in South America.

In contrast to the African trypanosomes, the infective metacyclic trypomastigote stage of *T. cruzi* is discharged in the feces of the infected insect vector during or shortly after the taking of a blood meal. Metacyclic trypomastigotes enter the host through the bite wound or mucous membranes and invade host cells. Within the cell, the parasite loses its flagellum and transforms into a round amastigote 3 to 4 μm in diameter (Fig. 289–4), which replicates by binary fission. When the dividing amastigotes have about filled the host cell, they transform into flagellated, motile trypomastigotes, which are released into the interstitial spaces and the blood stream on host cell lysis. Trypomastigotes have the ability to invade other host cells and continue the intracellular multiplication cycle. Trypomastigotes of *T. cruzi* are distinguished from those of African trypanosomiasis by their inability to multiply, their larger kinetoplast, and their C- or S-shaped appearance (see Fig. 289–1).

Reduviid bugs become infected by ingesting trypomastigotes in the blood taken from a mammalian host. In the bug's midgut, trypomastigotes transform into epimastigotes, which replicate by binary fission and assume the infective metacyclic stage in the hindgut about 2 weeks later.

Infection with *T. cruzi* persists for the life of the host. The mechanisms by which the parasite escapes the host's immune defenses are not well understood.[34, 35] Trypomastigotes are able to escape from phagocytic vacuoles within the host cell. Extracellular trypomastigotes can be lysed by antibody in vitro but are not completely cleared from the blood of immune hosts. There is no evidence that *T. cruzi* organisms have the kind of surface antigenic variation that occurs in African trypanosomiasis.

Epidemiology

Reduviid bugs, also called kissing bugs or assassin bugs, and sylvatic mammals infected with *T. cruzi* are found throughout warmer regions of the Americas, including southern portions of the United States as far north as Maryland.[32, 33] Within this area an estimated 16 million to 18 million humans are infected, and an additional 90 million are at risk of infection. The geographic distribution of human infection and disease is focal: the greatest numbers of infected persons live in Brazil, Bolivia, Argentina, Chile, and Venezuela. Chagas disease is enzootic in the Caribbean. Trinidad and Tobago have reported a small number of human cases.[33]

The distribution of human infection is affected by the range and habits of the insect vector and by the degree of contact between humans and the vector. Rates of transmis-

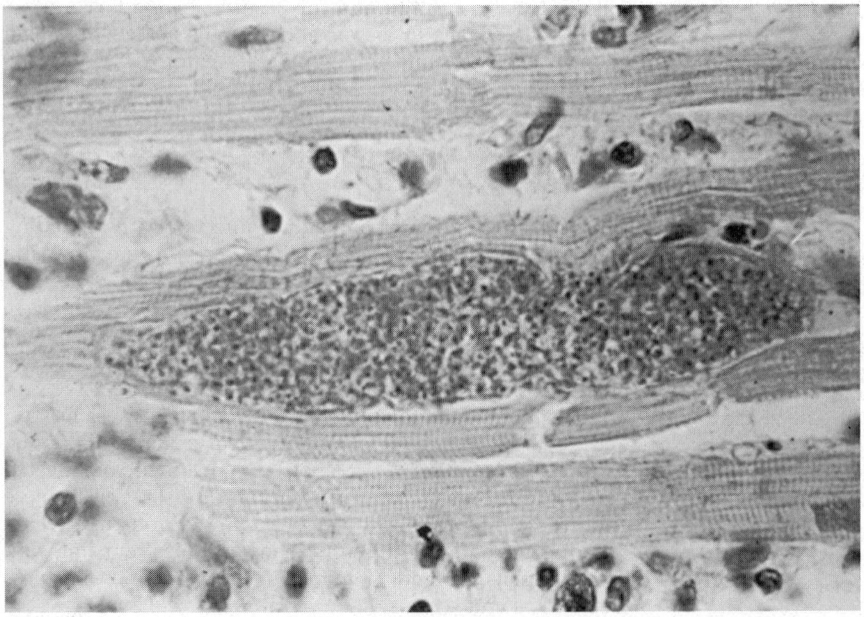

FIGURE 289–4 ▫ Heart tissue from a fatal case of acute Chagas disease. A nest of intracellular amastigotes fills the cardiac muscle cell, and mononuclear cell infiltrates and edema separate intact and degenerating fibers (approximately × 1000). (Courtesy of Dr. S. C. Pan, Harvard School of Public Health, Boston, MA.)

sion are highest in tropical areas where highly domesticated vectors such as *Triatoma infestans, Rhodnius prolixus,* and *Panstrongylus megistus* colonize human dwellings. The bugs hide in cracks in the walls and in the thatch of roofs during the day and emerge at night to take their blood meal from sleeping residents. Transmission occurs principally in the impoverished mud-stick houses of rural areas or the slums surrounding large cities. In the United States, only a few autochthonous cases of human infection have been reported.[36] The potential for transmission is low in the United States because the vector bugs prefer sylvatic habitats and do not infest houses. It is estimated, however, that 100,000 to 370,000 chronically infected immigrants from Latin America are living in the United States.[33, 37]

Vector control programs have markedly reduced the incidence of new cases in several countries, most notably Argentina, Brazil, Chile, Uruguay, and Venezuela.[33] The "southern cone" countries, which account for more than two thirds of infected people, are nearing their goal of eradicating the vector *T. intestans*.[38]

Transmission of *T. cruzi* via blood products from chronically infected donors is a frequent and serious occurrence, especially in large Latin American cities to which persons from rural areas have migrated in great numbers.[39] The risk of transmission of the parasite from a chronically infected donor may be as high as 10% to 15% per unit of blood. In many endemic areas, reliable serologic screening of blood is not uniformly available. Although only a few cases of transfusion-induced Chagas disease have been reported in the United States, the problem could intensify with the large numbers of immigrants from endemic areas of Latin America.[40] Currently, blood is not screened for *T. cruzi* in the United States.

T. cruzi can also be transmitted across the placenta, a phenomenon that occurs in 1% to 3% of pregnancies of chronically infected women.[41] Other, less frequent, routes of transmission include organ allografts and accidents among laboratory personnel who work with live parasites.[42]

Pathogenesis

Infection with *T. cruzi* has an initial acute stage that lasts for several weeks and a chronic phase that persists for the life of the host. After replicating at the site of entry, large numbers of parasites disseminate via the circulation and infect all types of nucleated cells but preferentially muscle cells, macrophages, and neurons and supporting cells of the central and peripheral nervous systems (see Fig. 289–4). Rupture of parasitized cells provokes an intense mononuclear cell inflammatory response and in severe cases causes acute myocarditis, destruction of autonomic ganglia in the heart and gastrointestinal tract, and meningoencephalitis.[43, 44] With development of humoral and cell-mediated immunity, the parasitemia falls to a subpatent level, and the number of parasites in the tissues declines dramatically, which signals an end to the acute phase.[34, 35]

Despite the appearance of the immune response, persons remain infected for life with both circulating and intracellular parasites. The majority of chronically infected individuals remain asymptomatic, and tissue damage is limited to small foci of inflammation and scars in various tissues and some loss of autonomic ganglia. About 10% to 30% of chronically infected persons sustain progressive damage to the heart or gastrointestinal tract that is sufficient to produce clinical disease.[43–46]

In chronic Chagas heart disease, there is a slowly progressive myocarditis that leads to flaccid dilatation of all four chambers and, in some cases, an apical aneurysm. On histologic examination, the heart has widespread destruction of myocardial cells, diffuse fibrosis, edema and mononuclear cell infiltration of the myocardium, and scarring of the conduction system with fibrous and adipose tissues.[45] The pathogenesis of chronic Chagas heart disease is poorly understood. An autoimmune process is suspected because the intensity of chronic inflammation appears to be out of proportion to the few parasites found in affected tissues.[35] Abnormalities in the coronary microvasculature and focal hypoperfusion may contribute to the myocardial damage.[47]

Chronic Chagas gastrointestinal disease is caused by destruction of autonomic ganglia.[46] Impaired motility and emptying of the esophagus and the colon lead to hypertrophy and dilatation of these organs, the so-called megasyndromes.

Clinical Manifestations

The acute stage of *T. cruzi* infection is usually asymptomatic or may present as influenza-like illness.[30] Symptoms first appear 1 to 2 weeks after exposure to infected reduviid bugs or as long as several months after transfusion of infected blood. There may be a characteristic unilateral edema of the eyelids (Romaña sign) or an indurated erythematous lesion of the skin (chagoma) at the site of inoculation. Acute infection may be accompanied by fever, malaise, generalized lymphadenopathy, and hepatosplenomegaly that lasts 4 to 8 weeks. The peripheral blood shows increased numbers of lymphocytes, atypical lymphocytes, and trypomastigotes, and parasites can be isolated from the CSF with ease.[48] About 10% of acute Chagas disease patients, most commonly young children, develop severe acute myocarditis or meningoencephalitis that may be fatal. Acute transfusion-induced infection may be fulminant and produce life-threatening involvement of the heart and CNS, especially in immunocompromised patients.[40, 49]

Survivors of the acute stage of infection, whether apparent or inapparent, enter an asymptomatic chronic "indeterminate" stage. The indeterminate stage may last for life, but about 10% to 30% of patients develop chronic myocarditis or gastrointestinal tract disease after several years or decades. An early sign of chronic Chagas myocarditis is an abnormal electrocardiogram with right bundle branch block, which may be present years before symptoms appear.[50, 51] Symptoms of heart disease appear most frequently in early adulthood or middle age. The most common presentation is biventricular congestive heart failure that is often complicated by systemic and pulmonary thromboembolism (Fig. 289–5*A*). Some patients complain of anginal or atypical chest pain even though coronary angiography shows no lesions.[52, 53] Complete atrioventricular block or ventricular arrhythmias may cause syncopal episodes or sudden cardiac death, even in persons with no prior cardiac symptoms. Less than one third of patients with symptomatic chronic Chagas heart disease survive longer than 2 years.

Denervation of the esophagus in Chagas disease leads to a clinical syndrome identical to idiopathic achalasia of the esophagus.[54] Failure of the lower esophageal sphincter to relax and disordered peristalsis cause dysphagia, regurgitation, recurrent episodes of aspiration pneumonia, and eventually permanent dilatation of the esophagus (megaesophagus). Chagas megacolon resembles Hirschsprung disease of the colon and is characterized by prolonged periods of obstipation and occasionally intestinal obstruction or volvulus. Barium contrast radiographs readily demonstrate megaesophagus, megacolon, and the associated motor disorders (Fig. 289–5*B*).

Chagas gastrointestinal disease is common south of the Amazon basin but seldom occurs in northern South America or Central America. Regional variation in the clinical features

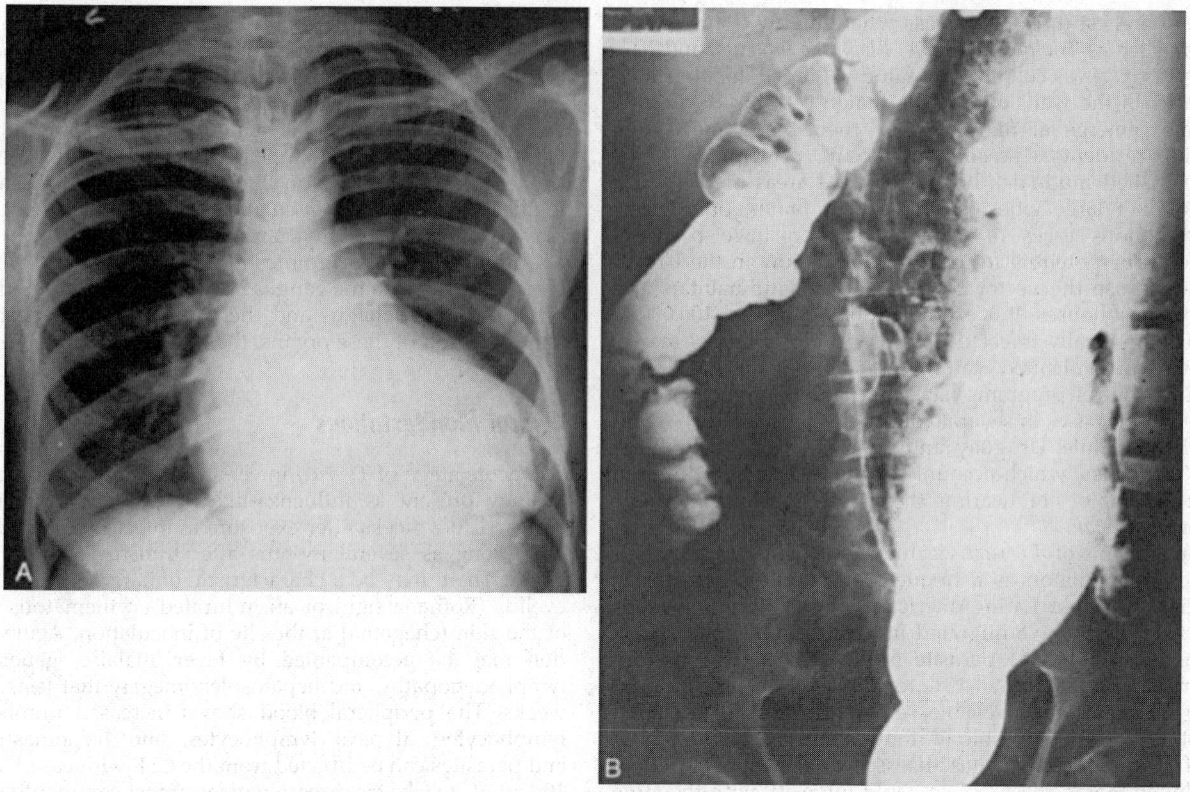

FIGURE 289–5 □ *A,* Chest radiograph from a 27-year-old woman with chronic Chagas cardiomyopathy. Global enlargement of the heart and clear lung fields are seen. *B,* Radiograph from a patient with Chagas megacolon (with barium contrast). Marked dilatation of the descending colon and retention of feces are present despite attempts to clear the bowel before the procedure. (*A* and *B* from the teaching collection of the Department of Tropical Public Health, Harvard School of Public Health, Boston, MA.)

of chronic Chagas disease may be due to infection with different strains of *T. cruzi.*[55]

Persons with acquired immunodeficiency syndrome or persons receiving immunosuppressive therapy may experience an exacerbation of chronic infection.[56, 57] Fever, myocarditis, and skin lesions are common among recipients of cardiac allografts, whereas patients with acquired immunodeficiency syndrome frequently have lesions of the CNS that resemble the lesions of cerebral toxoplasmosis or lymphoma at computed tomography or magnetic resonance imaging. Parasites are occasionally seen in blood smears and are readily detected in biopsy specimens of heart, skin, or brain.

Congenital infection with *T. cruzi* leads to abortion, stillbirth, or an acute disease that is apparent at birth or develops within weeks after delivery.[41] Congenital Chagas disease of the newborn is characterized by fever, jaundice, anemia, thrombocytopenia, hepatosplenomegaly, and skin lesions that contain parasites. Mortality in the congenital disease is usually due to myocarditis, pneumonitis, or encephalitis. Severe disease has been reported in children infected with both *T. cruzi* and human immunodeficiency syndrome at birth.[58]

Diagnosis

The diagnosis of acute Chagas disease and congenital Chagas disease is established by detection of trypomastigotes in the peripheral blood.[30, 59] Wet mounts of whole blood, buffy coat, or centrifuged serum should be examined microscopically for motile parasites, and smears should be stained with Giemsa or Wright stain. When parasites are not identified by direct observation during the acute stage, they can be isolated by cultivation of blood on Novy-MacNeal-Nicolle or another special medium, by animal inoculation, or by xenodiagnosis (allowing laboratory-reared, uninfected reduviid bugs to feed on the patient or the patient's blood and examining them for the presence of trypanosomes 3 to 4 weeks later).

Detection of parasites by culture, animal inoculation, or xenodiagnosis does not distinguish acute from chronic infection. In cases with negative smears, recently acquired infection can be demonstrated by the presence of specific IgM antibodies by the enzyme-linked immunosorbent assay or indirect fluorescent antibody test or by observing a fourfold rise of specific immunoglobulin G titers.

Because the parasitemia is subpatent during the chronic stage, the diagnosis usually relies on serologic tests for immunoglobulin G antibody to *T. cruzi.* Complement fixation (Machado-Guerreiro), indirect fluorescent antibody, enzyme-linked immunosorbent assay, and indirect hemagglutination antibody tests for *T. cruzi* infection are sensitive and specific. Use of purified glycoprotein antigens or recombinant antigens avoids the occasional false-positive reactions that occur in persons with mucocutaneous or visceral leishmaniasis or infection with the nonpathogenic *T. rangeli.*[60–62] In the United States, serologic testing is available at the Centers for Disease Control and Prevention, and enzyme-linked immunosorbent assay–based kits are available commercially for clinical testing. It is seldom necessary, for clinical purposes, to confirm a serologic diagnosis of chronic *T. cruzi* infection by culture or xenodiagnosis. Assays based on the polymerase chain reaction are more sensitive for detecting parasitemia in the chronic stage of infection than is xenodiagnosis or culture.[63]

Treatment

Antitrypanosomal therapy is indicated for acute or congenital Chagas disease and for reactivated infections in immunocompromised persons. It is not recommended for chronic infection because of the limited effectiveness and toxicity of available drugs.[30, 64] Both nifurtimox (Lampit) and benznidazole (Rochagan, see Table 289–1) clear the parasitemia and reduce the severity and duration of the acute illness. Except in parts of Argentina and Chile, where parasites may be more susceptible, these drugs rarely eradicate the infection. It is not known whether treatment during the acute phase prevents the complications of chronic Chagas disease. Cure of infection is difficult to document and should be regarded as certain only when serologic tests, xenodiagnosis, culture, and polymerase chain reaction–based assays fail to demonstrate parasites for several years. The addition of interferon-γ to either nifurtimox or benznidazole may shorten the acute phase of illness.[49]

The long course of treatment with either nifurtimox or benznidazole (see Table 289–1) requires meticulous monitoring because of the high incidence of adverse effects. Nifurtimox causes severe anorexia and weight loss, and both drugs may cause neuropathy, psychotic reactions, rashes, and gastrointestinal upset.

The toxic antitrypanosomal drugs are not indicated for chronic *T. cruzi* infection because of the low rate of "parasitologic cure" and the lack of effect on preventing progression of the chronic disease. Allopurinol is currently under evaluation for treatment of chronic infections because of its low toxicity, its activity against *T. cruzi* in mice, and its apparent ability to suppress parasitemia in chronically infected persons.[65] Management of patients with chronic asymptomatic infection entails close clinical monitoring for complications. Persons who develop symptomatic heart disease may require treatment with diuretics, vasodilators, antiarrhythmic agents, pacemakers, or, in selected cases, cardiac transplantation.[57] Mechanical dilatation of the esophagus affords temporary relief of megaesophagus, and both megaesophagus and megacolon can be effectively treated by surgery.

Prevention

No vaccine or chemoprophylactic agent prevents *T. cruzi* infection. Travelers should avoid sleeping in houses or outdoor areas that may be infested with reduviid bugs. Transfusion-induced Chagas disease can be prevented by careful serologic screening of blood donors or by treating donor blood with gentian violet for at least 24 hours before transfusion. Efforts to prevent transmission of *T. cruzi* by reduviid vectors in endemic areas have focused on improvement of housing to discourage colonization by reduviids and application of insecticides in houses by sprays, fumigant canisters, and impregnated paints.

References

1. Hoare CA: The Trypanosomes of Mammals: A Zoological Monograph. Oxford, Blackwell Scientific Publications, 1972.
2. World Health Organization: Epidemiology and control of African trypanosomiasis. Report of a WHO Expert Committee. World Health Organ Tech Rep Ser 739:1, 1986.
3. Apted FIC: Present status of chemotherapy and chemoprophylaxis of human trypanosomiasis in the eastern hemisphere. Pharmacol Ther 11:391, 1980.
4. Kuzoe FA: Current situation of African trypanosomiasis. Acta Trop 54:153, 1993.
5. Vickerman K: Antigenic variation in trypanosomes. Nature 273:613, 1978.
6. Borst P, Rudenko G: Antigenic variation in African trypanosomes. Science 264:1872, 1994.
7. Receveur MC, Le Bras M, Vincendeau P: Laboratory-acquired Gambian trypanosomiasis. N Engl J Med 329:209, 1993.
8. Bryan RT, Waskin HA, Richards RO, et al: African trypanosomiasis in American travelers: A 20 year review. *In* Steffen R (ed): International Travel Medicine. Berlin, Springer-Verlag, 1990, pp 121–123.
9. Greenwood BM, Whittle HC: The pathogenesis of sleeping sickness. Trans R Soc Trop Med Hyg 74:716, 1980.
10. Pentreath VW: Royal Society of Tropical Medicine and Hygiene Meeting at Manson House, London, 19 May 1994. Trypanosomiasis and the nervous system. Pathology and immunology. Trans R Soc Trop Med Hyg 89:9, 1995.
11. Wéry M, Mulumba PM, Lambert PH, Kazyumba L: Hematologic manifestations, diagnosis, and immunopathology of African trypanosomiasis. Semin Hematol 19:83, 1982.
12. Haller L, Adams H, Merouze F, et al: Clinical and pathological aspects of human African trypanosomiasis *(T. b. gambiense)* with particular reference to reactive arsenical encephalopathy. Am J Trop Med Hyg 35:94, 1986.
13. Gear JHS, Miller GB: The clinical manifestations of Rhodesian trypanosomiasis: An account of cases contracted in the Okavango swamps of Botswana. Am J Trop Med Hyg 35:1146, 1986.
14. Radomski MW, Buguet A, Montmayeur A, et al: Twenty-four-hour plasma cortisol and prolactin in human African trypanosomiasis patients and healthy African controls. Am J Trop Med Hyg 52:281, 1995.
15. Buguet A, Bert J, Tapie P, et al: Sleep-wake cycle in human African trypanosomiasis. J Clin Neurophysiol 10:190, 1993.
16. Pepin J, Ethier L, Kazadi C, et al: The impact of human immunodeficiency virus infection on the epidemiology and treatment of *Trypanosoma brucei gambiense* sleeping sickness in Nioki, Zaire. Am J Trop Med Hyg 47:133, 1992.
17. Van Meirvenne N: Diagnosis of human African trypanosomiasis. Ann Soc Belg Med Trop 72(Suppl 1):53, 1992.
18. Lanham SM, Godfrey DG: Isolation of salivarian trypanosomes from man and other animals using DEAE-cellulose. Exp Parasitol 28:521, 1970.
19. Bailey JW, Smith DH: The quantitative buffy coat for the diagnosis of trypanosomes. Trop Doct 24:54, 1994.
20. Noireau F, Lemesre JL, Nzoukoudi MY, et al: Serodiagnosis of sleeping sickness in the Republic of Congo: Comparison of indirect immunofluorescent antibody test and card agglutination test. Trans R Soc Trop Med Hyg 82:237, 1988.
21. Asonganyi T, Bedifeh BA, Ade SS, et al: An evaluation of the reactivity of the card agglutination test for trypanosomiasis (CATT) reagent in the Fontem sleeping sickness focus, Cameroon. Afr J Med Med Sci 23:39, 1994.
22. Nantulya VM, Doua F, Molisho S: Diagnosis of *Trypanosoma brucei gambiense* sleeping sickness using an antigen detection enzyme-linked immunosorbent assay. Trans R Soc Trop Med Hyg 86:42, 1992.
23. Bromidge T, Gibson W, Hudson K, et al: Identification of *Trypanosoma brucei gambiense* by PCR amplification of variant surface glycoprotein genes. Acta Trop 53:107, 1993.
24. Cattand P, Miezan BT, De Raadt P: Human African trypanosomiasis: Use of double centrifugation of cerebrospinal fluid to detect trypanosomes. Bull WHO 66:83, 1986.
25. Pepin J, Milord F: The treatment of human African trypanosomiasis. Adv Parasitol 33:1, 1994.
26. Van Nieuwenhove S: Advances in sleeping sickness therapy. Ann Soc Belg Med Trop 72(Suppl 1):39, 1992.
27. Milord F, Pepin J, Loko L, et al: Efficacy and toxicity of eflornithine for treatment of *Trypanosoma brucei gambiense* sleeping sickness. Lancet 340:652, 1992.
28. Pepin J, Milord F, Khonde AN, et al: Risk factors for encephalopathy and mortality during melarsoprol treatment of *Trypanosoma brucei gambiense* sleeping sickness. Trans R Soc Trop Med Hyg 89:92, 1995.
29. Rogers DJ, Hendrickx G, Slingenbergh JH: Tsetse flies and their control. Rev Sci Tech 13:1075, 1994.
30. Brener Z, Andrade Z (eds): *Trypanosoma cruzi* e Doença de Chagas. Rio de Janeiro, Guanabara Koogan, 1979.
31. Marsden PD: The transmission of *Trypanosoma cruzi* to man and its control. *In* Croll NA, Cross JH (eds): Human Ecology and Infectious Disease. New York, Academic Press, 1983, pp 253–289.
32. World Health Organization: Control of Chagas disease. Report of a WHO Expert Committee. World Health Organ Tech Rep Ser 811:1, 1991.

33. Schmunis GA: American trypanosomiasis as a public health problem. *In* Chagas' Disease and the Nervous System. Washington, DC, Pan American Health Organization, 1994, pp 3–29.
34. Hoff R, Boyer MH: Immunology of Chagas' disease. *In* Tizard I (ed): Immunology and Pathogenesis of Trypanosomiasis. Boca Raton, FL, CRC Press, 1985, pp 185–199.
35. Brener Z: The pathogenesis of Chagas' disease: An overview of current theories. *In* Chagas' Disease and the Nervous System. Washington, DC, Pan American Health Organization, 1994, pp 30–46.
36. Schiffler RJ, Mansur GP, Navin TR: Indigenous Chagas' disease (American trypanosomiasis) in California. JAMA 251:2983, 1984.
37. Kirchhoff LV: Current concepts: American trypanosomiasis (Chagas' disease)—A tropical disease now in the United States. N Engl J Med 329:639, 1993.
38. World Health Organization: Chagas disease. Interruption of transmission. Wkly Epidemiol Rec 70:13, 1995.
39. Schmunis GA: *Trypanosoma cruzi,* the etiologic agent of Chagas' disease: Status in the blood supply in endemic and nonendemic countries. Transfusion 31:547, 1991.
40. Cimo PL, Luper WE, Scouros MA: Transfusion-associated Chagas' disease in Texas: Report of a case. Tex Med 89:48, 1993.
41. Bittencourt AL: Congenital Chagas' disease, a review. Am J Dis Child 130:99, 1976.
42. Herwaldt BL, Juranek DD: Laboratory-acquired malaria, leishmaniasis, trypanosomiasis, and toxoplasmosis. Am J Trop Med Hyg 48:313, 1993.
43. Andrade ZA: Mechanisms of myocardial damage in *Trypanosoma cruzi* infection. Ciba Found Symp 99:214, 1983.
44. Santos-Buch CA, Acosta AM: Pathology of Chagas' disease. *In* Tizard I (ed): Immunology and Pathogenesis of Trypanosomiasis. Boca Raton, FL, CRC Press, 1985, pp 145–183.
45. Andrade ZA, Andrade SG, Oliveira GB, et al: Histopathology of the conducting tissue of the heart in Chagas' myocarditis. Am Heart J 95:316, 1978.
46. Koberle F: Chagas' disease and Chagas' syndromes: The pathology of American trypanosomiasis. Adv Parasitol 6:63, 1968.
47. Rossi MA, Bestetti RB: The challenge of chagasic cardiomyopathy. The pathologic roles of autonomic abnormalities, autoimmune mechanisms and microvascular changes, and therapeutic implications. Cardiology 86:1, 1995.
48. Hoff R, Teixeira RS, Carvalho JS, et al: *Trypanosoma cruzi* in the cerebrospinal fluid during the acute stage of Chagas' disease. N Engl J Med 298:604, 1978.
49. Grant IH, Gold JWM, Wittner M, et al: Transfusion-associated acute Chagas' disease acquired in the United States. Ann Intern Med 111:849, 1989.
50. Laranja FS, Dias E, Nobrega G, et al: Chagas' disease: Clinical, epidemiologic, and pathologic study. Circulation 14:1035, 1956.
51. Maguire JH, Hoff R, Sherlock I, et al: Cardiac morbidity and mortality due to Chagas' disease: Prospective electrocardiographic study of a Brazilian community. Circulation 75:1140, 1987.
52. Hagar JM, Rahimtoola SH: Chagas' heart disease in the United States. N Engl J Med 325:763, 1991.
53. Torres FW, Acquatella H, Condado JA, et al: Coronary vascular reactivity is abnormal in patients with Chagas' heart disease. Am Heart J 129:995, 1995.
54. Tanowitz HB, Simon D, Gumprecht JP, et al: Gastrointestinal manifestations of Chagas' disease. *In* Rustgi VK (ed): Gastrointestinal Infections in the Tropics. Basel, S Karger, 1990, pp 56–75.
55. Miles MA, Povoa MM, Prata A, et al: Do radically dissimilar *Trypanosoma cruzi* strains (zymodemes) cause Venezuelan and Brazilian forms of Chagas' disease? Lancet 1:1338, 1981.
56. Rocha A, de Meneses AC, da Silva AM, et al: Pathology of patients with Chagas' disease and acquired immunodeficiency syndrome. Am J Trop Med Hyg 50:261, 1994.
57. Bocchi EA, Bellotti G, Uip D, et al: Long-term follow-up after heart transplantation in Chagas' disease. Transplant Proc 25:1329, 1993.
58. Freilij H, Altcheh J, Muchinik G: Perinatal human immunodeficiency virus infection and congenital Chagas' disease. Pediatr Infect Dis J 14:161, 1995.
59. Frasch ACC, Reyes MB, Sánchez DO: Diagnosis of Chagas' disease: Present and future. *In* Chagas' Disease and the Nervous System. Washington, DC, Pan American Health Organization, 1994, pp 47–53.
60. Winkler MA, Brashear RJ, Hall HJ, et al: Detection of antibodies to *Trypanosoma cruzi* among blood donors in the southwestern and western United States. II. Evaluation of a supplemental enzyme immunoassay and radioimmunoprecipitation assay for confirmation of seroreactivity. Transfusion 35:219, 1995.
61. Pastini AC, Iglesias SR, Carricarte VC, et al: Immunoassay with recombinant *Trypanosoma cruzi* antigens potentially useful for screening donated blood and diagnosing Chagas disease. Clin Chem 40:1893, 1994.
62. D'Alessandro A: Biology of *Trypanosoma (Herpetosoma) rangeli* Tejera, 1920. *In* Lumsden WHR, Evans DA (eds): Biology of the Kinetoplastida, Vol 1. London, Academic Press, 1976, pp 327–403.
63. Britto C, Cardoso MA, Vanni CM, et al: Polymerase chain reaction detection of *Trypanosoma cruzi* in human blood samples as a tool for diagnosis and treatment evaluation. Parasitology 110:241, 1995.
64. de Castro SL: The challenge of Chagas' disease chemotherapy: An update of drugs assayed against *Trypanosoma cruzi.* Acta Trop 53:83, 1993.
65. Gallerano RH, Marr JJ, Sosa RR: Therapeutic efficacy of allopurinol in patients with chronic Chagas' disease. Am J Trop Med Hyg 43:159, 1990.

290

Toxoplasma gondii

Craig Roberts
Rima McLeod

Taxonomy

Toxoplasma gondii is in the phylum Apicomplexa and the class Sporozoea. Isolates of *T. gondii* have been called strains (e.g., the RH strain or the ME49 strain). There are three patterns of virulence of *T. gondii* tachyzoites for mice, measured as differences in survival. Restriction fragment length polymorphism patterns and isoenzyme zymodemes are characteristic for each of these three phenotypes of virulence (I, similar to the RH strain of *T. gondii*; II, similar to the ME49 strain of *T. gondii*; and III, similar to the C56 strain of *T. gondii*). Virulence varies (i.e., differences in lethality and for cyst numbers produced in mice); isolates proliferate at different rates in tissue culture and produce different neurologic manifestations (i.e., variable destruction and inflammatory responses). The RH strain, the most commonly used laboratory strain, does not undergo gametogenesis in cat intestine and proliferates rapidly.

Morphology and Composition

Tachyzoites (see Chapter 182, Fig. 182–1*A* to *C*) and bradyzoites (see Fig. 182–1*D* to *F*) are crescentic and measure approximately 6 × 2 μm. Tachyzoites have a nucleus, mitochondria, Golgi apparatus, and endoplasmic reticulum (Fig. 290–1; see also Fig. 182–1*A* to *C*). They have three unit membranes that compose their pellicle (see Fig. 182–1*A*). Their outer membrane is continuous; their two inner membranes are discontinuous, are closely apposed, and end at internal structures (located at either end of the tachyzoite) called polar rings. These inner membranes have holes called micro-

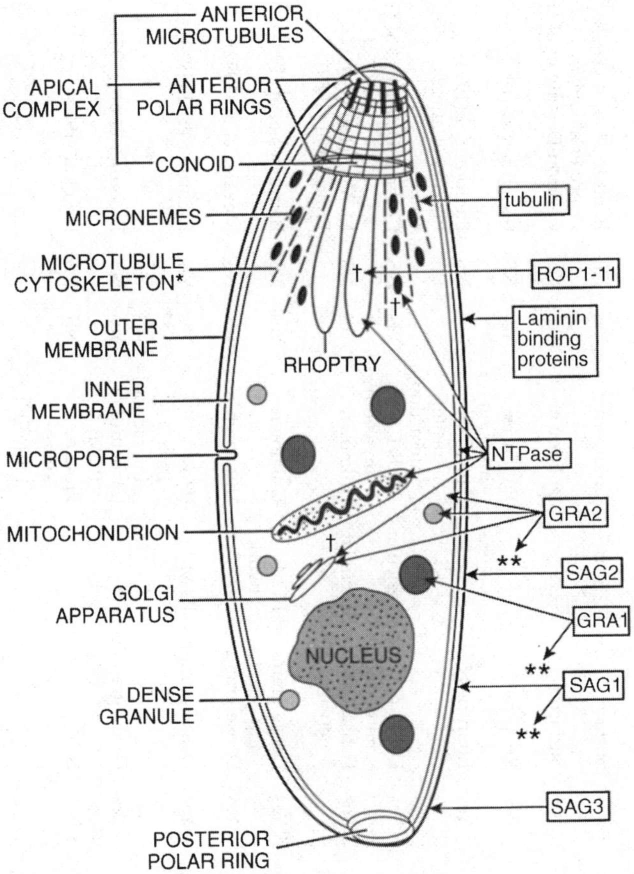

FIGURE 290–1 □ Diagrammatic representation of *Toxoplasma gondii* tachyzoite. Representative proteins and glycoproteins are indicated by a square outline that encloses them. Their locations are indicated by arrowheads. NTPase, Nucleoside triphosphate hydrolases. *The cytoskeleton of *T. gondii* is composed of 22 microtubules; these actually extend posteriorly but are indicated schematically in this figure only at the anterior end. **Parasitophorous vacuole. †Locations of adenosine triphosphatase activity, not necessarily the cloned 63-kDa protein. (Redrawn from McLeod R, Mack D, Brown C: *Toxoplasma gondii*—New advances in cellular and molecular biology. Exp Parasitol 72:109–121, 1991.)

pores. Under the pellicle, extending from the anterior polar ring almost the length of the tachyzoite, are 22 microtubules (the cytoskeleton). A hollow, truncated cone of fibers, probably microtubules, wound in a spiral (the conoid) is present at the anterior end of the parasite and protrudes as tachyzoites enter host cells. Rhoptries (club-shaped, dense, osmophilic structures with narrow ends that terminate in the conoid), micronemes (osmophilic vesicles between the few rhoptries), and a plastid (a multilamellar structure that contains unique extranuclear DNA, thought to be related to chloroplasts) are characteristic of Apicomplexa, and the first two organelles may be important during entry into host cells. Electron-dense granules contain proteins that are secreted. SAG1 is a unique tachyzoite antigen. Temperature-sensitive and drug-resistant mutant tachyzoites have been produced.

Bradyzoites (see Fig. 182–1*D* to *F*) are resistant to pepsin, induce oocyst formation in the week after they are ingested by cats, have unique antigens not present in tachyzoites, have electron-dense rhoptries, and have unique cytoplasmic granules (perhaps stored carbohydrates). Cysts contain bradyzoites (a few to 10,000). The cyst wall is argyrophilic and stains weakly with periodic acid–Schiff stain. Bradyzoites stain well with the periodic acid–Schiff stain. High or low pH, nitric oxide, and other "stresses" lead to tachyzoite to bradyzoite interconversion. A 5-hydroxynaphthoquinone–resistant mutant organism expresses bradyzoite antigens.

Oocysts (see Fig. 182–1*H*) form after five stages of schizogony (detectable by light microscopy). By the third stage, gametes are either male (microgamete with increased DNA content, a flagellum, and cytoplasm with a nucleus and a mitochondrion) or female (macrogamete, large, spherical cell with two types of peripheral cytoplasmic granules). These granules contribute to the outer and inner layers of the rigid, impervious oocyst wall. Sporulation, which requires aeration for 1 to 3 days at room temperature, produces eight sporozoites (in two sporocysts) in an oocyst wall. Sporozoites and the inside of the oocyst wall have stage-specific antigens. Drug-resistant mutants incapable of forming oocysts have been identified.

Deoxyribonucleic Acid

The sporozoite contains approximately 0.1 pg of DNA and approximately 8×10^7 base pairs per cell (haploid DNA content). Mitochondrial DNA is approximately 3% of the total DNA. The plastid also contains DNA. Nucleotide sequences for a number of proteins are known (Table 290–1), and complementary DNA and genomic libraries have been produced. Some of the *T. gondii* genes identified have introns. Information about translation as well as transcription has been reviewed (McLeod et al, 1991). Data concerning sequences of complementary DNAs from tachyzoite and bradyzoite complementary DNA libraries should greatly facilitate understanding of the biology of this parasite.

Ribonucleic Acid

T. gondii ribosomal RNA has a typical large and small molecule. Its messenger RNA has a 3′-polyadenylated tail. This has been translated in heterologous systems producing *T. gondii* proteins. *T. gondii* has an RNase P that cleaves transfer RNA.

Antigens

The tachyzoite contains at least 1000 proteins. Many of the antigens and proteins of *T. gondii* have now been named. They are designated with three letters and a number, according to the life cycle stage from which they were isolated, their location within the organism, or their function. The surface antigens of tachyzoites are designated SAG; proteins found within the micronemes, MIC; those in the rhoptries, ROP; and those in the dense granules, GRA. Antigens found in the bradyzoite stage, but not in the tachyzoite stage, are designated BAG; those secreted by bradyzoites to form the cyst matrix are called MAG. Some of these, their localization, and characteristics of the genes that encode them are shown in Figure 290–1 and Table 290–1. Major surface proteins of 14, 22, 30, 46, and 66 kDa have been identified. Antibody to a 6-kDa carbohydrate antigen is present early during infection. The most abundant surface protein is the 30-kDa antigen (molecular mass, 30 to 35 kDa under reducing conditions and 27 to 28 kDa under nonreducing conditions) called SAG1 or P30. Antibodies to SAG1 have been identified in sera from acutely and chronically infected adults and congenitally infected persons. It is detected only in tachyzoites (not bradyzoites or sporozoites) and is approximately 5% of the total tachyzoite protein. It is homogeneously distributed on the tachyzoite surface, within the tachyzoite, and within the vesicular network of the parasitophorous vacuole. It is hydrophobic with a slightly acidic isoelectric point and is prob-

TABLE 290–1 ■ Cloned Genes and the Proteins They Encode*

PRODUCT	COPY NUMBER	INTRONS	TOTAL GENE SEQUENCE	mRNA SIZE	POST-TRANSLATIONAL MODIFICATION	PRODUCT SIZE (PREDICTED)	GPI ANCHOR	ESA	LOCATION	FUNCTION (POSTULATED)	PRESENT IN T†	PRESENT IN B†	AUTHORS (DATE OF PUBLICATION)
SAG1 (P30) (gp30)	1	No	Yes	1500 nt	Yes	30–35 kDa	Yes	Yes	Surface; vacuolar network	Unknown	Yes	No	Burg et al (1988)
SAG2 (gp22)	1	No	Yes	1600 nt	Yes	22 kDa	Yes	NS	Surface	Unknown	Yes	No	Boothroyd et al (1987) Prince et al (1990)
SAG3 (P43)	1	NS	Yes	2000 nt	NS	43 kDa	Yes	NS	Surface	Unknown	Yes	Yes	Cesbron-Delauw et al (1994)
ROP1	1	No	Yes	2100 nt	Probably	60 kDa	NS	NS	Rhoptries	Enhances invasion	Yes	NS	Ossorio et al (1992)
ROP2 (P54)	NS	No	Yes	2234 nt	Yes	66 kDa	NS	Yes	Rhoptries	(Host-parasite interaction)	Yes	NS	Herion et al (1993) Beckers et al (1994)
GRA1 (P23)	1	No	Yes	1400 nt	Yes	24 kDa	Yes	Yes	Dense granules; vesicular network; PV	Binds Ca^{2+} (invasion)	Yes	NS	Cesbron-Delauw et al (1989)
GRA2 (gp28.5) (gp28)	1	Yes	Yes	1100 nt	Yes	28–28.5 kDa	Yes	Yes	Dense granules; vacuolar network; PV	Unknown	Yes	NS	Mercier et al (1993) Prince et al (1989)
GRA3	1	No	Yes	NS	Probably	30 kDa	No	Yes	Dense granules; PVM; intravacuolar network	Unknown	Yes	NS	Bermudes et al (1994a)
GRA4 (P40)	1	No	Yes	1900 nt	Yes	40 kDa	No	Yes	Dense granules	Unknown	Yes	NS	Mevelec et al (1992)
GRA5 (P21)	1	No	Yes	850 nt	Probably	21 kDa	NS	Yes	Dense granules; PVM	(Host-parasite interaction)	Yes	Yes	Lecordier et al (1993)
GRA6	NS	No	Yes	NS	Potentially *N*-glycosylated	32 kDa	NS	Yes	Dense granules; PV	(Structure of PVM)	Yes	NS	Lecordier et al (1995)
TOX PK1	NS	Yes	No	NS	NS	NS	NS	NS	NS	Protein kinase [enzyme]	NS	NS	Ng et al (1995)

TOX PK2	NS	Yes	No	NS	NS	NS	NS	NS	NS	Protein kinase [enzyme]	NS	NS	Ng et al (1995)
NTPase (P63)	5	No	No	2800 nt	Unknown	50 kDa	NS	NS	Submembrane; mitochondria	(Purine salvage) [enzyme]	Yes	NS	Johnson et al (1989)
NTPase 1 (NTPase I)	NS	NS	Yes	NS	NS	66–67 kDa	NS	Yes	Vesicular structures; PVM; vacuolar space	Host-parasite interaction NTPase [enzyme]	Yes	NS	Bermudes et al (1994b) Asai et al (1995)
NTPase 2	NS	NS	Yes	NS	NS	NS	NS	Yes			NS	NS	
NTPase 3 (NTPase II)	NS	NS	Yes	NS	NS	66–67 kDa		Yes			Yes	NS	
DHFR-TS	1	Yes	Yes	NS	NS	(69 kDa)	NS	NS	NS	DHFR-TS [enzymes]	Yes	NS	Roos (1993)
α-Tubulin (P54)	1	Yes	No	1347 nt	Yes	54 kDa	NS	NS	Subpellicular; microtubules	Motility (invasion)	Yes	NS	Boothroyd et al (1987)
β-Tubulin (P54)	1	Yes	No	1362 nt	Yes	54 kDa	NS	NS	Subpellicular; microtubules	Motility (invasion)	Yes	NS	Schwartzman et al (1983) Nagel and Boothroyd (1988)
Gene B1	50	Yes	Yes	1600 nt	Yes	NS	NS	NS	NS	Unknown	Yes	NS	Burg et al (1988)
HGPRT	NS	NS	Yes	NS	NS	(25 kDa)	NS	NS	NS	HGPRT [enzyme]	NS	NS	Vasanthakumar et al (1994)
LDH	NS	NS	Yes	NS	NS	(35 kDa)	NS	NS	NS	LDH [enzyme]	No	Yes	Yang and Parmley (1995)
BAG5 (BAG1) (HSP30)	NS	NS	NS	NS	NS	28–30 kDa	NS	NS	Cytosol	HSP (stage conversion)	No	Yes	Parmley et al (1995) Bohne et al (1995)
MAG1 (P65)	1	Yes	Yes	NS	NS	65 kDa	NS	Yes	Cyst matrix; cyst wall	(Cyst matrix structure)	No	Yes	Parmley et al (1994)

*B, Bradyzoites; DHFR-TS, dihydrofolate reductase–thymidylate synthase; ESA, excretory secretory antigen; GPI, glycosyl phosphatidylinositol; HGPRT, hypoxanthine-guanine phosphoribosyltransferase; HSP, heat shock protein; LDH, lactate dehydrogenase; mRNA, messenger RNA; NS, not stated in original paper; nt, nucleotides; NTPase, nucleoside triphosphate hydrolase; PV, parasitophorous vacuole; PVM, parasitophorous vacuole membrane; T, tachyzoites.

†A yes or no indicates the presence or absence of either complementary DNA or protein in this life cycle stage.

ably glycosylated. Several closely related forms of this protein are resolved by two-dimensional gel electrophoresis. The gene encoding SAG1 has been cloned and sequenced, has a single open reading frame, is a single copy, and contains no introns. The primary translation product has a C-terminal hydrophobic tail, which predicts posttranslational cleavage and modification with a glycolipid anchor. The SAG1 messenger RNA transcript is 1500 nucleotides in length and polyadenylated. Antibodies to SAG1 reduce but do not completely prevent host cell invasion. They are shed as a result of a tight moving junction at the interface of parasite and host cell membrane. Antibody to SAG1 and complement lyse tachyzoites. Paradoxically, passive protection studies using monoclonal antibodies to SAG1 have reported either partial protection or increased mortality.

Some genes encoding proteins present in either the rhoptries or the dense granules of tachyzoites have been cloned. Many of these products are released during or after cell invasion. ROP1 appears to enhance invasion, whereas ROP2 is found on the parasitophorous vacoule membrane, suggesting that it is involved in the host-parasite interaction. The genes encoding six GRA proteins have been cloned. Their protein products have been immunolocalized to the parasitophorous vacuole including its membrane. These proteins may be important to the structure of the parasitophorous vacuole and allow parasite exploitation of the host cell environment. Vaccination with GRA2 can protect mice from infection (i.e., increase their survival rate).

A gene that encodes a bradyzoite-specific cytosolic protein has been cloned and designated by different investigators as *BAG1* and *BAG5*; it encodes a molecule of 28 to 30 kDa, which has homology with the small heat shock proteins of plants. It is induced when tachyzoites are stressed (by high pH) in tissue culture and may play a role in the interconversion of tachyzoites and bradyzoites. A gene encoding MAG1, a protein expressed by bradyzoites and rapidly secreted to become associated with the cyst matrix, has also been cloned. MAG1 is recognized by immune serum from many hosts including humans.

T. gondii is not capable of de novo purine synthesis. *T. gondii* cannot use preformed folates, and thus its dihydrofolate reductase has been a major target for antimicrobial agents. *T. gondii* dihydrofolate reductase has both dihydrofolate reductase and thymidylate synthase activity.

Three nucleoside triphosphate hydrolases have been cloned from a virulent strain of *T. gondii*, two of which are expressed and secreted into the parasitophorous vacuole. These enzymes become associated with the parasitophorous vacuole membrane and may use host adenosine triphosphate as a substrate to supply the parasite with energy. In contrast to virulent strains, all avirulent strains of *T. gondii* examined to date express one of these nucleoside triphosphate hydrolases. Both expressed isoenzymes have markedly enhanced hydrolytic activity in the presence of dithiothreitol. They differ in their ability to hydrolyze triphosphate and diphosphate substrates.

A lactate dehydrogenase gene expressed in the bradyzoite stage but not in the tachyzoite stage has been cloned. The tachyzoite stage appears to express a different isoform of this enzyme, which may account for the greater functional activity of lactate dehydrogenase observed in this life cycle stage compared with the bradyzoite stage.

Invasion of Host Cells by Tachyzoites and Replication

During invasion, the *T. gondii* rhoptry and plasma membrane fuse; within 15 seconds, *T. gondii* is within a parasitophorous vacuole in the cell cytoplasm. There is some evidence to suggest that secretion by *T. gondii* and a phenomenon reminiscent of attachment and shedding of the host cell membrane may be involved in entry. The parasitophorous vacuole becomes surrounded by mitochondria and does not fuse with lysosomes or thus become acidified. *T. gondii* organisms then multiply by a type of binary fission called endodyogeny within the parasitophorous vacuole. During division, the nuclear membrane of *T. gondii* remains intact and chromosomes do not condense at metaphase (in contrast to mitosis in higher eukaryotes). Without appreciably disrupting the host cell's function, the tachyzoite divides until the vacuolar membrane and host cell lyse, releasing many tachyzoites. Mutant parasites, mutant host cells, and inhibitors of cellular processes have been used to study biochemical interactions between *T. gondii* and host cells. *T. gondii* needs host cell purines to replicate. *T. gondii*'s hypoxanthine-guanine phosphoribosyltransferase can provide sufficient purine salvage. None of the following host cell processes is needed for replication: synthesis of nucleic acids, proteins, oxidative phosphorylation, and adenosine triphosphate synthesis by mitochondria. The role of host cell lipid synthesis is not known.

Life Cycle (see also Chapter 182)

T. gondii is an obligate intracellular protozoan parasite that can infect a wide variety of birds and mammals. It can enter all host cells. There appears to be a special propensity for cyst formation and recrudescence with tissue destruction in the central nervous system.

In the acute infection, the tachyzoite (formerly called trophozoite and sometimes endozoite) proliferates within cells in many tissues. In persons who have a competent immune system, cyst formation begins about 8 days after infection, and cysts persist for the remainder of the host's life. The cysts form in many tissues but especially in muscle and brain. The wall of these cysts is derived partly from the host cell. The cysts contain hundreds of the slowly replicating form of the parasite, bradyzoites, which are more resistant than tachyzoites to acid and pepsin. If tissues that contain cysts are ingested by a carnivore, bradyzoites are released from the cyst in the intestine and again disseminate from the intestine to cause acute, and then chronic, infection. Cats, which develop acute infection with tachyzoites and then form cysts as described before for all other hosts, are also the definitive host for the sexual phase of the life cycle. After a cat ingests cysts, bradyzoites invade their intestinal cells. After several stages of schizogony, they yield male and female gametes, which fuse and form a zygote. The zygote synthesizes a protective wall and is excreted by the cat as a single-celled, unsporulated oocyst. At 37°C, the excreted oocyst sporulates, dividing three times, which yields eight infectious sporozoites that are still contained within the oocyst wall. The oocyst can remain viable for more than a year in warm, moist soil. When oocysts are ingested by a mammal or bird, sporozoites are released and again infect intestinal epithelial cells, becoming tachyzoites and finally, again, encysted bradyzoites.

Propagation and Isolation

Isolation of the organism is discussed in Chapter 182. Tachyzoites and bradyzoites can be isolated by use of animal inoculation or tissue culture. Tachyzoites can be maintained in culture, and addition of interferon-γ to the media or change in pH or nitric oxide concentration leads to cyst formation in vitro. Velocity and equilibrium sucrose gradient centrifugation is used to purify unsporulated oocysts. The oocyst stage has not been propagated in vitro.

Immune Responses to *Toxoplasma gondii*

Humoral immunity and cell-mediated immunity contribute to protection against *T. gondii*. Natural killer cells and macrophage interactions are the first line of defense, with macrophage-produced interleukin-12 and tumor necrosis factor-α inducing natural killer cells to produce interferon-γ. Interferon-γ and tumor necrosis factor-α activate macropages to kill intracellular organisms by oxygen-dependent and oxygen-independent mechanisms. Interleukin-12 produced by macrophages facilitates the expansion of helper/inducer T cells, which prevent dissemination of *T. gondii* by secreting interferon-γ and interleukin-2. Cytotoxic T cells, which have been shown to lyse *T. gondii*–infected cells in vitro, are present in infected hosts. Interleukin-4, interleukin-10, and transforming growth factor-β can diminish resistance to infection. Secretory immunoglobulin A specific for *T. gondii* is secreted intestinally and in the milk of infected mothers. Numbers of cysts that form after peroral infection are determined by class I and class II immune response (i.e., major histocompatibility complex) genes of the host. A number of genes including the immune response genes influence survival in experimental models of disease.

Related Organism

An encysted organism *(Neospora caninum)* that appears similar to *T. gondii* in preparations examined with light microscopy (with electron-dense rhoptries) has been described in tissues from a number of animals, such as dogs and cats, but not in humans. This organism is serologically distinct from *T. gondii*, however, and no association with disease in humans has been recognized.

Antimicrobial Susceptibility Testing

Studies in vitro and in vivo (in mice) have demonstrated inhibition of replication of *T. gondii* tachyzoites by pyrimethamine, sulfadiazine (and sulfamerazine and sulfamethazine), and spiramycin. Pyrimethamine and these sulfonamides act synergistically. Studies in vitro (with longer incubation times) and in vivo have demonstrated efficacy for clindamycin. The relevance of these data to antimicrobial levels needed for treatment of toxoplasmosis in humans remains to be determined.

Surface Decontamination

Tachyzoites are easily destroyed by desiccation, heat, and pepsin. Cysts are destroyed by cooling below −20°C and heating above 60°C. Bradyzoites are resistant to pepsin. The oocyst wall is not disrupted by 0.5% ammonium sulfate, sodium hydroxide, or sodium hypochlorite. Disinfection of a cat litter box can be accomplished by burning feces or flushing them in the toilet and then soaking the tray in boiling water for 5 minutes or strong (7%) ammonia for 3 hours. Disposal by drying, surface burial, freezing, chlorine bleach, dilute ammonia, quaternary ammonium compounds, or any general disinfectant cannot be relied on to destroy oocysts.

Bibliography

- Asai T, Miura S, Sibley D, et al: Biochemical and molecular characterization of nucleoside triphosphate hydrolase isozymes from the parasitic protozoan *Toxoplasma gondii*. J Biol Chem 270:11391, 1995.
- Beckers CJM, Dubremetz J-F, Mercereau-Puijalon O, Joiner KA: The *Toxoplasma gondii* rhoptry protein ROP2 is inserted into the parasitophorous vacuole membrane, surrounding the intracellular parasite, and is exposed to the host cell cytoplasm. J Cell Biol 127:947, 1994.
- Bermudes D, Dubremetz J-F, Achbarou A, Joiner KA: Cloning of a cDNA encoding the dense granule protein GRA3 from *Toxoplasma gondii*. Mol Biochem Parasitol 68:247, 1994a.
- Bermudes D, Peck KR, Afifi MA, et al: Tandemly repeated genes encode nucleoside triphosphate hydrolase isoforms secreted into the parasitophorous vacuole of *Toxoplasma gondii*. J Biol Chem 269:29252, 1994b.
- Bohne W, Heesemann J, Gross U: Reduced replication of *Toxoplasma gondii* is necessary for induction of bradyzoite-specific antigens—A possible role for nitric oxide in triggering stage conversion. Infect Immun 62:1761, 1994.
- Bohne W, Gross U, Ferguson DJ, Heesemann J: Cloning and characterization of a bradyzoite-specifically expressed gene (hsp30/bag1) of *Toxoplasma gondii*, related to genes encoding small heat-shock proteins of plants. Mol Microbiol 16:1221, 1995.
- Boothroyd JC, Burg JL, Nagel SD, et al: Antigen and tubulin genes of *Toxoplasma gondii*. *In* Agabian N, Goodman H, Nogueira N (eds): Molecular Strategies of Parasitic Invasion. New York, Alan R Liss, 1987, pp 237–250.
- Brown CR, McLeod R: Class I MHC genes and CD8+ T cells determine cyst number in *Toxoplasma gondii* infection. J Immunol 145:3438, 1990.
- Burg JL, Perelman D, Kasper L, et al: Molecular analysis of the gene encoding the major surface antigen of *Toxoplasma gondii*. J Immunol 141:3584, 1988.
- Burg JL, Grover M, Pouletty P, Boothroyd JC: Direct and sensitive detection of a pathogenic protozoan, *Toxoplasma gondii*, by polymerase chain reaction. J Clin Microbiol 27:1787, 1989.
- Cesbron-Delauw MF, Guy B, Torpier G, et al: Molecular characterization of a 23-kilodalton major antigen secreted by *Toxoplasma gondii*. Proc Natl Acad Sci USA 86:7537, 1989.
- Cesbron-Delauw M-F, Tomavo S, Beauchamp P, et al: Similarities between the primary structures of two distinct major surface proteins of *Toxoplasma gondii*. J Biol Chem 269:16217, 1994.
- Darde ML, Bouteille B, Pestre-Alexandre M: Isoenzymic characterization of seven strains of *Toxoplasma gondii* by isoelectrofocusing in polyacrylamide gels. Am J Trop Med Hyg 39:551, 1988.
- Deroin F, Thulliez P, Candolfi, et al: Early prenatal diagnosis of congenital toxoplasmosis using amniotic fluid samples and tissue culture. Eur J Clin Microbiol 7:423, 1988.
- Donald RGK, Roos DS: Stable molecular transformation of *Toxoplasma gondii*: A selectable dihydrofolate reductase-thymidylate synthase marker based on drug-resistance mutations in malaria. Proc Natl Acad Sci USA 90:11703, 1993.
- Dubey JP, Swan GV, Frenkel JK: A simplified method for isolation of *Toxoplasma gondii* from the feces of cats. J Parasitol 58:1005, 1972.
- Gazzinelli RT, Wysocka M, Hayashi S, et al: Parasite-induced IL-12 stimulates early INF-gamma synthesis and resistance during acute infection with *Toxoplasma gondii*. J Immunol 153:2533, 1994.
- Grover CM, Thulliez P, Remington JS, Boothroyd JC: Rapid prenatal diagnosis of congenital *Toxoplasma* infection by using polymerase chain reaction and amniotic fluid. J Clin Microbiol 28:2297, 1990.
- Herion P, Hernandez-Pando R, Dubremetz J-F, Saavedra R: Subcellular localization of the 54-kDa antigen of *Toxoplasma gondii*. J Parasitol 79:216, 1993.
- Johnson AM, Illana S, McDonald PJ, Asai T: Cloning, expression and nucleotide sequence of the gene fragment encoding an antigenic portion of the nucleoside triphosphate hydrolase of *Toxoplasma gondii*. Gene 85:215, 1989.
- Joiner KA, Dubremetz JF: *Toxoplasma gondii*: A protozoan for the nineties. Infect Immun 61:1169, 1993.
- Kasper LH, Crabb JH, Pfefferkorn ER: Isolation and characterization of a monoclonal antibody–resistant antigenic mutant of *Toxoplasma gondii*. J Immunol 129:1694, 1982.
- Kim K, Soldati D, Boothroyd JC: Gene replacement in *Toxoplasma*

gondii with chloramphenicol acetyltransferase as selectable marker. Science 262:911, 1993.
- Lecordier L, Mercier C, Torpier G, et al: Molecular structure of a *Toxoplasma gondii* dense granule antigen (GRA-5) associated with the parasitophorous vacuole membrane. Mol Biochem Parasitol 59:143, 1993.
- Lecordier L, Moleon-Borodowski I, Dubremetz J-F, et al: Characterization of a dense granule antigen of *Toxoplasma gondii* (GRA6) associated to the network of the parasitophorous vacuole. Mol Biochem Parasitol 70:85, 1995.
- Mack D, McLeod R: A new micromethod to study effects of antimicrobial agents on *Toxoplasma gondii*: Comparison of sulfadoxine and sulfadiazine and study of clindamycin, metronidazole, and cyclosporine A. Antimicrob Agents Chemother 26:26, 1984.
- McLeod R, Mack D, Brown C: *Toxoplasma gondii*—New advances in cellular and molecular biology. Exp Parasitol 72:109, 1991.
- Mercier C, Lecordier L, Darcy F, et al: Molecular characterization of a dense granule antigen (Gra2) associated with the network of the parasitophorous vacuole in *Toxoplasma gondii*. Mol Biochem Parasitol 58:71, 1993.
- Mevelec M-N, Chardes T, Mercereau-Puljalon O, et al: Molecular cloning of GRA4, a *Toxoplasma gondii* dense granule protein, recognized by mucosal IgA antibodies. Mol Biochem Parasitol 56:227, 1992.
- Nagel SD, Boothroyd JC: The alpha- and beta-tubulins of *Toxoplasma gondii* are encoded by single copy genes containing multiple introns. Mol Biochem Parasitol 29:261, 1988.
- Ng HC, Singh M, Jeyaseelan K: Identification of two protein serine/threonine kinase genes and molecular cloning of a *SNF1* type protein kinase gene from *Toxoplasma gondii*. Biochem Mol Biol Int 35:155, 1995.
- Ossorio PN, Schwartzman JD, Boothroyd JC: A *Toxoplasma gondii* rhoptry protein associated with host cell penetration has unusual charge asymmetry. Mol Biochem Parasitol 50:1, 1992.
- Parmley S, Weiss LM, Yang S: Cloning of a bradyzoite-specific gene of *Toxoplasma gondii* encoding a cytoplasmic antigen. Mol Biochem Parasitol 73:253, 1995.
- Parmley S, Yang S, Harth G, et al: Molecular characterization of a 65-kilodalton *Toxoplasma gondii* antigen expressed abundantly in the matrix of tissue cysts. Mol Biochem Parasitol 66:283, 1994.
- Pfefferkorn ER: Cellular biology of *Toxoplasma gondii*. *In* Wyler D (ed): Modern Parasite Biology: Cellular, Immunological, and Molecular Aspects. New York, WH Freeman, 1990, pp 26–50.
- Prince JB, Araujo F, Remington J, et al: Cloning of cDNAs encoding a 28 kilodalton antigen of *Toxoplasma gondii*. Mol Biochem Parasitol 34:3, 1989.
- Prince JB, Auer KL, Huskinson SF, et al: Cloning, expression, and cDNA sequence of surface antigen P22 from *T. gondii*. Mol Biochem Parasitol 43:97, 1990.
- Roos D: Primary structure of the dihydrofolate reductase–thymidylate synthase gene from *Toxoplasma gondii*. J Biol Chem 268:6269, 1993.
- Schwartzman JD, Pfefferkorn ER: Immunofluorescent localization of myosin at the anterior pole of the coccidian *Toxoplasma gondii*. J Protozool 30:657, 1983.
- Sharma SD: Immunology of *Toxoplasma gondii* infection. *In* Wyler D (ed): Modern Parasite Biology: Cellular, Immunological, and Molecular Aspects. New York, WH Freeman, 1990, pp 184–199.
- Sharma SD, Araujo FG, Remington JS: *Toxoplasma* antigen isolated by affinity chromatography with monoclonal antibody protects mice against lethal infection with *Toxoplasma gondii*. J Immunol 133:2818, 1984.
- Sibley LD, Sharma SD: Ultrastructural localization of an intracellular *Toxoplasma* protein that induces protection in mice. Infect Immun 55:2137, 1987.
- Sibley LD, Pfefferkorn ER, Boothroyd JC: Development of genetic systems for *Toxoplasma gondii*. Parasitol Today 9:392, 1993.
- Sibley LD, Weidner E, Krahenbuhl JL: Phagosome acidification blocked by intracellular *Toxoplasma gondii*. Nature 315:416, 1985.
- Sibley LD, Adams LD, Fukutomi Y, Krahenbuhl JL: Tumor necrosis factor-α triggers antitoxoplasmal activity of IFN-γ primed macrophages. J Immunol 147:2340, 1991.
- Vasanthakumar G, van Ginkel S, Parish G: Isolation and sequencing of a cDNA encoding the hypoxanthine-guanine phosphoribosyltransferase from *Toxoplasma gondii*. Gene 147:153, 1994.
- Weiss L, LaPlace D: Development of bradyzoites of *Toxoplasma gondii* in vitro. J Eukaryot Microbiol 41:18S, 1994.
- Yang S, Parmley SF: A bradyzoite stage–specifically expressed gene of *Toxoplasma gondii* encodes a polypeptide homologous to lactate dehydrogenase. Mol Biochem Parasitol 73:291, 1995.

291

Pneumocystis carinii

Walter T. Hughes

Pneumocystis carinii is a unique microbe that is found almost exclusively in the lungs of immunocompromised mammalian hosts. It has not been found outside the animal reservoir, and the only known mode of transmission is from animal to animal by the respiratory route. Most humans are believed to have contracted asymptomatic infection with *P. carinii* in infancy and childhood and to maintain a latent, indetectable infection throughout life. If the host's immunity is compromised, life-threatening *P. carinii* pneumonitis may develop.

Morphology

Three structural forms of *P. carinii* are the cyst, sporozoite, and trophozoite. The cyst, the largest of the three forms, often measures 5 to 6 μm in diameter. The fully developed cyst has a thick cell wall, providing a sturdy round, oval, or cup-shaped structure while it is intact. The cyst wall is generally about 0.1 to 0.3 μm thick in most areas, but some sites may be twice that. The sporozoite is an intracystic cell about 1 to 2 μm in diameter. As many as eight sporozoites may be found in the intact cyst. These cells appear fragile and pleomorphic with punctate, eccentric nuclei. The trophozoite (2 to 5 or 6 μm in diameter) is believed to be the excysted sporozoite. The cell wall is thinner than that of the cyst.

The method used for staining preparations of *P. carinii* determines the visibility of the three forms. Polychrome stains such as Giemsa or Wright stain the trophozoites and sporozoites but not the cyst (Fig. 291–1). The Gomori-Grocott methenamine–silver nitrate and toluidine blue O stains color the cysts but do not permit visualization of the sporozoites and trophozoites (Fig. 291–2).

Classification

Early investigators such as Chagas, Carini, and the Delanoes considered the organism a protozoan without question. More recently, Yoneda and coworkers[1, 2] supported the protozoan classification by demonstrating evidence of membrane fusion. Vossen and colleagues[3] also argued that the organism was a protozoan because of the presence of a microtubular system similar to that of the Sporozoa. Gradus and associates[4] found that the DNA content per cell of *P. carinii* more nearly matches that of protozoa than that of fungi, yet the guanine plus cytosine proportion of *P. carinii* DNA is 33 mol/L, a value not sufficiently distinct. Jackson and coworkers[5] were unable to detect characteristic fungal protein elongation factor-3 in *P. carinii*. *P. carinii* is susceptible to the antiprotozoan drugs pentamidine (*Trypanosoma, Leishmania* species),

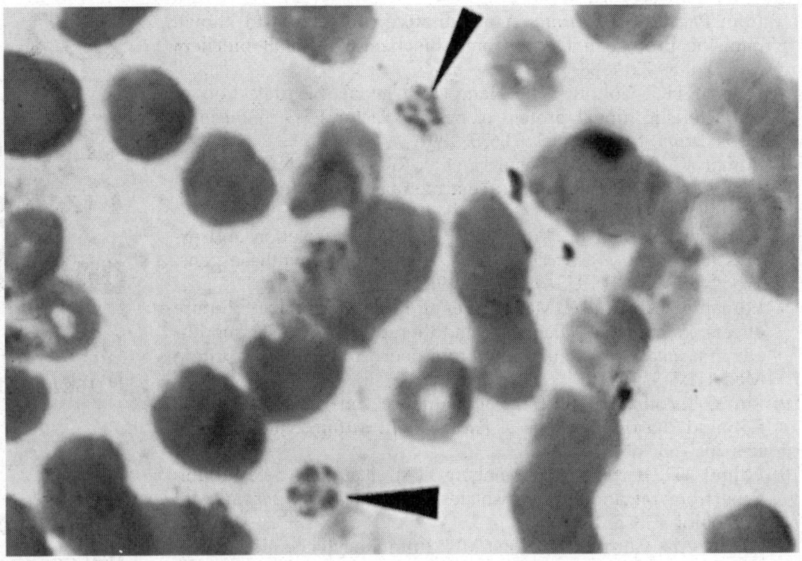

FIGURE 291–1 ▫ Imprint of lung biopsy specimen stained with Giemsa method. Clusters of *Pneumocystis carinii* sporozoites *(arrowheads)* are located within the cyst. The cyst wall does not stain, but an area of rarefaction is usually discernible.

trimethoprim-sulfamethoxazole *(Isospora)*, pyrimethamine-sulfonamide (*Toxoplasma, Plasmodium* species), and dapsone (*Plasmodium* species). Antifungal drugs in clinical use tested to date (amphotericin B, ketoconazole, gentian violet, nystatin) are ineffective.

Edman and colleagues found the ribosomal RNA sequences,[6] thymidylate synthase,[7] and dihydrofolate reductase[8] of *P. carinii* to be more similar to those of the ascomycetes than to those of protozoa. Liu and coworkers[9] compared 26S ribosomal RNA genes in *P. carinii, Saccharomyces cerevisiae*, and *Trypanosoma pyriformis* and found greater resemblance to the yeast than to the protozoan. Analysis of amino acid sequences of β-tubulin showed close matches with certain fungi.[10] The cyst form of *P. carinii* has chitin in the cell wall, in common with the fungi.[11] Pixley and coworkers[12] concluded that the mitochondrial DNA of *P. carinii* is more like that of fungi than of protozoa. Eriksson[13] reviewed available taxonomic features of *P. carinii* and proposed placement in a new family, Pneumocystidaceae, and a new order, Pneumocystidales (Ascomycota). The isolation and culture of *P. carinii* in pure form will allow conclusive taxonomic placement.

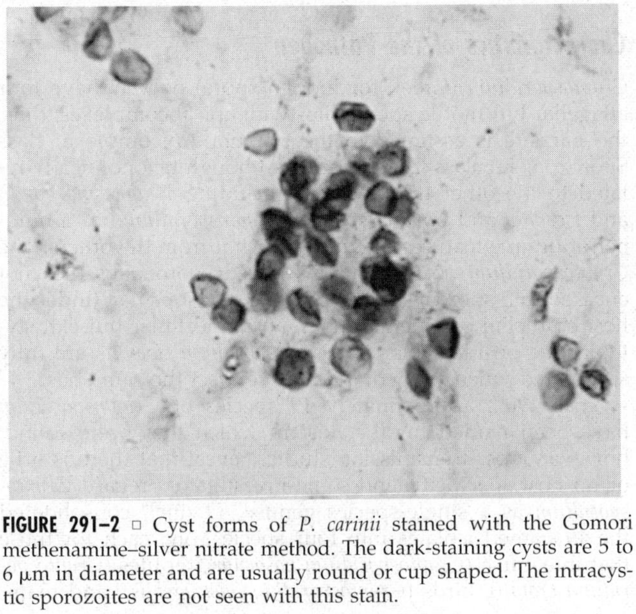

FIGURE 291–2 ▫ Cyst forms of *P. carinii* stained with the Gomori methenamine–silver nitrate method. The dark-staining cysts are 5 to 6 μm in diameter and are usually round or cup shaped. The intracystic sporozoites are not seen with this stain.

Life Cycle

The complete life cycle of *P. carinii* has not been firmly established; however, microscopic observations from infections in vivo and propagation of *P. carinii* in vitro provide information on the replicative cycle.[14, 15] The most mature form is the thick-walled cyst containing up to eight sporozoites. Through breaks in the cyst wall, the small sporozoites excyst, after which they are referred to as trophozoites. The mechanism by which the trophozoite proceeds through a replicative system is not known. Replication by sexual, asexual, and combined sexual-asexual pathways has been proposed.

Antigenic Structure

Some understanding of the antigenic features of *P. carinii* has come from studies using monoclonal antibodies that recognize specific epitopes on *P. carinii* from various animal species, including rats, rabbits, ferrets, and humans.[16, 17] Antigens ranging from 25 to 120 kDa have been described for *P. carinii*. There is evidence that organisms derived from humans are different from those of lower animals. Passive administration of a monoclonal antibody to a purified surface glycoprotein has been shown to reduce the severity of *P. carinii* infection in ferrets, suggesting biologic activity of the monoclonal antibody in vivo.[18]

References

1. Yoneda K, Walzer PD, Rickey CS, Birk MG: *Pneumocystis carinii*: Freeze-fracture study of stages of the organism. Exp Parasitol 53:68, 1982.
2. Yoneda K, Walzer PD: Attachment of *Pneumocystis carinii* to type 1 alveolar cells studied by freeze-fracture electron microscopy. Infect Immun 40:812, 1983.
3. Vossen MEMH, Beckers PJA, Meuwissen JHETh, Stadhowders AM: Microtubules in *Pneumocystis carinii*. Z Parasitenkd 49:291, 1976.
4. Gradus MS, Gilmore M, Lerner M: An isolation method of DNA

from *Pneumocystis carinii*: A quantitative comparison to known parasitic protozoan DNA. Comp Biochem Physiol B Biochem Mol Biol 89:75, 1988.
5. Jackson HC, Colthurst D, Hancock V, et al: No detection of characteristic fungal protein elongation factor EF-3 in *Pneumocystis carinii*. J Infect Dis 163:675, 1991.
6. Edman JC, Kovacs JA, Masur H, et al: Ribosomal RNA sequence shows *Pneumocystis carinii* to be a member of the fungi. Nature 334:519, 1988.
7. Edman U, Edman JC, Lundgren B, Santi DV: Isolation and expression of the *Pneumocystis carinii* thymidylate synthase gene. Proc Natl Acad Sci USA 86:6503, 1989.
8. Edman JC, Kovacs JA, Masur H, et al: Molecular biology: Future effects on taxonomy, diagnosis, and therapy. *In* Masur H, moderator: *Pneumocystic* pneumonia: From bench to clinic. Ann Intern Med 111:813, 1989.
9. Liu Y, Rocourt M, Pan S, et al: Sequence and variability of the 5.8S and 26S rRNA genes of *Pneumocystis carinii*. Nucleic Acids Res 20:3763, 1992.
10. Edlind TD, Bartlett MS, Weinberg GA, et al: The beta-tubulin gene from rat and human isolates of *Pneumocystis carinii*. Mol Microbiol 6:3365, 1992.
11. Walker AN, Garner RD, Horst MN: Immunocytochemical detection of chitin in *Pneumocystis carinii*. Infect Immun 58:412, 1990.
12. Pixley FJ, Wakefield AE, Banergfi S, Hopkin JM: Mitochondrial gene sequences show fungal homology for *Pneumocystis carinii*. Mol Microbiol 5:1347, 1991.
13. Eriksson OE: *Pneumocystis carinii*, a parasite in lungs of mammals, referred to a new family and order (Pneumocystidaceae, Pneumocystidales, Ascomycota). Syst Ascomycetym 13:165, 1994.
14. Cushion MT, Ruffolo JJ, Walzer PD: Analysis of the developmental stages of *Pneumocystis carinii* in vitro. Lab Invest 58:324, 1988.
15. Barton EG Jr, Campbell G: *Pneumocystis carinii* in lungs of rats treated with cortisone acetate. Ultrastructural observation relating to the life cycle. Am J Pathol 54:209, 1969.
16. Gigliotti F, Stokes DC, Cheatham AB, et al: Development of monoclonal antibodies to *Pneumocystis carinii*. J Infect Dis 154:315, 1986.
17. Kovacs JA, Helpern JL, Lundgren B, et al: Monoclonal antibodies to *Pneumocystis carinii*: Identification of specific antigens and characterization of antigenic difference between rat and human isolates. J Infect Dis 159:60, 1989.
18. Gigliotti F, Hughes WT: Passive immunoprophylaxis with specific monoclonal antibody confers partial protection against *Pneumocystis carinii* pneumonitis in animal models. J Clin Invest 81:1666, 1988.

292

Cryptosporidium, Isospora, Cyclospora, Microsporidia, and Dientamoeba

Lawrence J. Davis
Rosemary Soave

Cryptosporidium

History

Only since the early 1980s has the coccidian protozoan *Cryptosporidium* become well recognized as a significant pathogen of humans. First recognized by Tyzzer[1] in 1907 in the gastric glands of asymptomatic laboratory mice, the protozoan was considered a benign commensal organism for nearly 50 years. In 1955, *Cryptosporidium* was first implicated as the cause of disease in animals when it was found in fowl with fatal enteritis.[2] Since the 1970s, *Cryptosporidium* has been identified in the gastrointestinal or respiratory tract of most species of animals, including mammals, reptiles, birds, and fish. The parasite is also responsible for major agricultural losses each year.[3–5]

Although human cryptosporidiosis was first reported in 1976,[6] appreciation of its pathogenic potential for humans came in the early 1980s, when *Cryptosporidium* was detected in acquired immunodeficiency syndrome (AIDS) patients with severe enteritis.[7, 8] Subsequent reports of cryptosporidial disease outbreaks in animal handlers and travelers[9, 10] demonstrated that it could parasitize the immunocompetent population as well.[7, 9–11] As familiarity with diagnostic techniques has improved, the number of reported cases has continued to increase, and *Cryptosporidium* has become recognized as a common cause of enteritis for both immunocompetent and immunocompromised hosts worldwide.[12–16]

Characteristics of the Pathogen

Cryptosporidium (Greek for hidden spore) oocysts have four aflagellar but motile sporozoites with apical complexes; thus, the parasite is assigned to the phylum Apicomplexa, class Sporozoa, subclass Coccidiasina. Although taxonomically related to the other true coccidia, including *Toxoplasma gondii* and *Isospora* and *Eimeria* species, *Cryptosporidium* has a number of unique features that distinguish it from the others. The *Cryptosporidium* oocyst contains naked sporozoites (i.e., not encased in a sporocyst). The parasite develops just under the host epithelial cell membrane in an intracellular but extracytoplasmic position. Finally, *Cryptosporidium* oocysts are fully sporulated when formed and may reinfect the same host.[12–16]

Since 1907, approximately 19 species of *Cryptosporidium* have been named for the host in which they were found; however, cross-transmission studies reveal that there is little or no host specificity, and some investigators regard *Cryptosporidium* as a single-species genus.[17] Levine[18] consolidated the 19 named isolates into four species, one each for those that infect fish *(Cryptosporidium nasorum)*, reptiles *(Cryptosporidium crotali)*, birds *(Cryptosporidium meleagridis)*, and mammals *(Cryptosporidium muris)*, but at least one has been found to be invalid.[19] The exact number of distinct *Cryptosporidium* species and the nature of differences among various isolates have not been determined. Upton and Current[20] have proposed two species of *Cryptosporidium* that infect mammals: *Cryptosporidium parvum* (4- to 6-μm-diameter oocyst), which causes disease in humans and cattle; and *C. muris* (5- to 8-μm-diameter oocyst), which infects the stomach of cattle.

The *Cryptosporidium* life cycle, like that of other coccidia, can be divided into five stages: excystation (release of infective sporozoites from the oocyst), merogony (asexual replication), gametogony (formation of microgametes and macrogametes), fertilization, and oocyst formation.[21] Infection is initiated by ingestion, or perhaps inhalation, of oocysts.[21] The acid-fast oocyst is 4 to 6 μm in diameter and, when mature (sporulated), contains four thin, flat, motile sporozoites (Fig. 292–1). On dissolution of a single suture on the oocyst wall, the sporozoites excyst and move freely by gliding. They implant in the host epithelium, where they subsequently develop into trophozoites. Asexual multiplication (merogony) results in the formation of type 1 and type 2 meronts (schizonts) that contain eight and four merozoites, respectively. The merozoites closely resemble sporozoites and may reinvade the host and reinitiate merogony, or they may differentiate into microgametocytes (male) or macrogametocytes (female), which then initiate fertilization. Fertilized macrogametes develop into oocysts that can either reinfect the host or exit the body in search of a new host. Two types of oocysts have been identified: thin-walled oocysts, which are more likely to reinfect; and thick-walled oocysts, which are more likely to be expelled into the environment.[19]

Epidemiology

The major modes of *Cryptosporidium* transmission appear to be human to human or through contaminated water.[12–16, 19, 22, 23] Transmission by the animal-to-human, human-to-animal, and food-borne routes also occurs.[7, 23] A small oral inoculum of oocysts is sufficient to cause human illness.[24]

Water-borne outbreaks account for the greatest number of cryptosporidiosis cases identified to date. Contaminated municipal drinking water was responsible for a diarrhea outbreak involving approximately 400,000 cases in Milwaukee, Wisconsin, in 1993 and has been implicated in five other major outbreaks in the United States.[23, 25–27] Filtration of municipal water can reduce oocyst contamination, but protection is not absolute; the municipal water systems that were implicated in outbreaks included filtration treatment, and small numbers of oocysts have been detected in filtered municipal water in 27% to 54% of municipalities tested.[23, 28, 29] Endemic transmission of *Cryptosporidium* through drinking water has not been demonstrated but is under investigation. Swimming in fresh surface water (i.e., lakes or rivers) or in swimming pools has also been associated with the acquisition of cryptosporidial infection.[30–32] *Cryptosporidium* oocysts have been demonstrated in 65% to 97% of surface water bodies tested.[29, 30, 33–35]

A 1993 diarrhea outbreak in Maine traced to consumption of contaminated apple cider was the first documentation of food-borne transmission.[36] Human-to-human spread is responsible for infection in daycare center attendees, household contacts of index cases, hospitalized patients, and health care workers.[37–41] Transmission related to animal contact has been well documented in handlers of calves[42, 43] and other mammals, particularly neonates.[23] Travelers are at increased risk for cryptosporidiosis, probably because of ingestion of contaminated water or possibly food.[9, 10, 44] Spread of the parasite by aerosolization and fomites has been suggested but not confirmed.

Cryptosporidiosis has been described in more than 50 countries worldwide.[12–16, 22] Its true prevalence is currently not known. Surveys of selected populations have revealed rates of infection from 0.6% to 20% in developed countries and 4% to 32% in underdeveloped countries. Higher infection rates appear to be associated with younger age and a warm, humid climate.[12–16, 22, 45, 46] Both sexes are affected equally. Breast-feeding may confer protection, although this remains controversial.[22, 47] Various serologic surveys have revealed greater than expected rates of seropositivity, suggesting that active or recent infection is common in the general population.[48, 49]

As of 1986, the Centers for Disease Control and Prevention estimated that 3% to 4% of all AIDS patients had cryptosporidiosis as their AIDS-defining opportunistic infection.[50] In later studies, the parasite was identified in 15% of patients with AIDS and diarrhea at the National Institutes of Health[51] and in 16% of those at the Johns Hopkins Hospital.[52] In Haiti and Africa, up to 50% of AIDS patients are infected.[53]

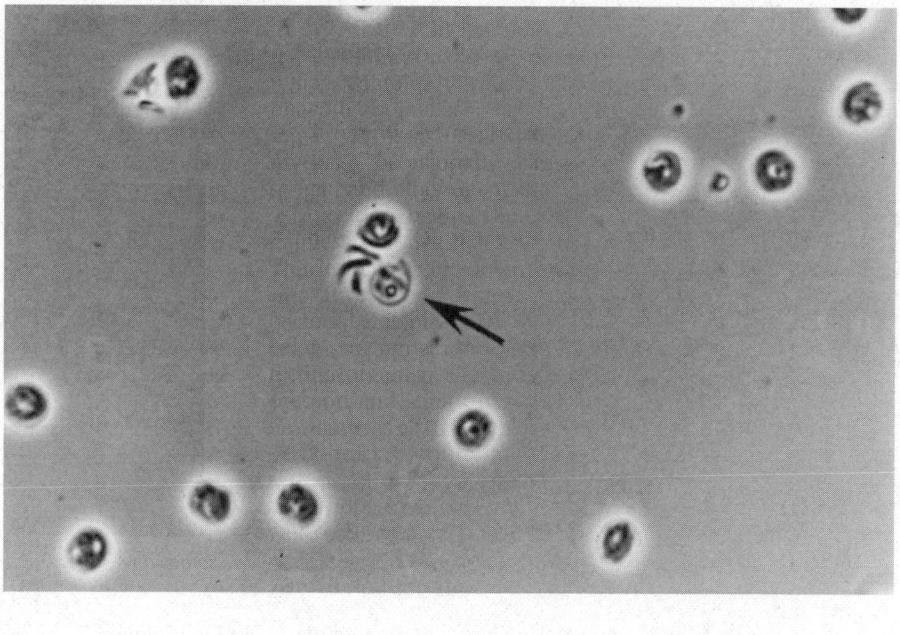

FIGURE 292–1 □ Human stool–derived *Cryptosporidium* oocysts. Excysting oocyst *(arrow)* is releasing three of its four sporozoites. (Phase-contrast microscopy × 630.)

Although an asymptomatic carrier state has been described for *Cryptosporidium,* its frequency is not known.[54] Whether cryptosporidiosis in an immunocompromised host represents reactivation of previous infection or infection de novo also remains to be determined.[55]

Pathology and Pathogenesis

Evaluation of tissue biopsy specimens obtained primarily from immunocompromised patients provides the basis for most of our understanding of the histopathologic process of cryptosporidiosis.[8, 56, 57] Cryptosporidia are most often seen along the apical surfaces of epithelial cells of the small intestine (Fig. 292–2); however, the parasite has also been detected throughout the alimentary tract, including the esophagus, stomach, small and large intestine[8, 12–16, 56, 57]; gallbladder and bile and pancreatic ducts[58–60]; within colonic submucosal vessels[61]; and in the respiratory tract.[62–64] Histologic changes are nonspecific and mild despite the presence of numerous organisms. They include blunting or complete loss of villi, elongation of crypts, and infiltration of the lamina propria with polymorphonuclear leukocytes, lymphocytes, and plasma cells.[65] Histologic changes do not correlate with the degree of clinical symptoms. Ultrastructural studies of infected intestine reveal the parasite ensconced between microvilli and enclosed within a parasitophorous vacuole just under the host cell membrane yet outside the host cytoplasm, a unique "intracellular yet extracytoplasmic" position.[12–16, 56, 57]

The pathogenic mechanisms in intestinal cryptosporidiosis remain to be fully elucidated. Diminished small intestinal glucose, electrolyte, and water absorption has been demonstrated in conjunction with characteristic histopathologic features of cryptosporidiosis in an animal model.[66] Enterotoxic or humoral factors may play a role[67]; in vitro findings suggest that increased local prostanoid production contributes to impaired enterocyte sodium-coupled glucose transport.[68]

Cryptosporidial cholecystitis or cholangitis is a fairly frequent finding in immunocompromised patients with cryptosporidial enteritis. Such patients have marked histopathologic changes in the biliary tract and gallbladder, ranging from acute inflammation to gangrenous necrosis. Cryptosporidia are found adherent to the biliary epithelium and in the bile.[56, 58–60] A number of patients with cryptosporidial cholecystitis were also found to have concurrent cytomegalovirus infection of the biliary tract.[58] Pancreatitis has been reported in association with cryptosporidiosis in both immunocompetent and immunocompromised patients.[69, 70]

Although cryptosporidia have been isolated from sputum, tracheal aspirates, bronchoalveolar lavage fluid, and lung tissue, whether they are pathogens, colonizers, or contaminants from the gastrointestinal tract has not been determined.[62–64] Cryptosporidial involvement of the biliary and pulmonary tracts has not been described for immunocompetent patients with cryptosporidial infection.

Clinical Manifestations

The hallmark of human cryptosporidiosis in both immunocompetent and immunocompromised hosts is voluminous watery diarrhea.[8, 12–16, 71, 72] It is usually accompanied by crampy abdominal pain (often after eating), weight loss, flatulence, and malaise. Nausea, vomiting, myalgias, and fever are less common. Fecal examination reveals *Cryptosporidium* oocysts and mucus but rarely blood or leukocytes. Peripheral blood leukocytosis and eosinophilia are also uncommon. Fat, carbohydrate, and vitamin B_{12} malabsorption is well documented and contributes significantly to the wasting syndrome that is seen in patients with AIDS. Radiographic findings are nonspecific and include mucosal thickening and disordered small bowel motility.

The incubation period for cryptosporidiosis is typically 2 to 14 days. The severity and duration of the illness are determined by the immune status of the host.[8, 11, 12–16] For the immunocompetent host, symptoms may have an explosive onset and last 10 to 14 days.[11, 12–16] Clearance of the oocysts (and the potential for contagion) may lag behind clinical improvement by 1 to 2 weeks.[73]

In immunocompromised persons, including those with AIDS, the disease often develops insidiously; however, as immune competence wanes, clinical symptoms frequently worsen. Patients may experience voluminous (1 to 25 L daily) watery diarrhea, profound weight loss, electrolyte imbalance, and severe dehydration, requiring hospitalization for months, often until they die.[8, 12–16, 72, 74]

Patients with biliary cryptosporidiosis often have classic signs of cholangitis: right upper quadrant pain, nausea, vomiting, and enteritis.[58–60] The serum alkaline phosphatase and

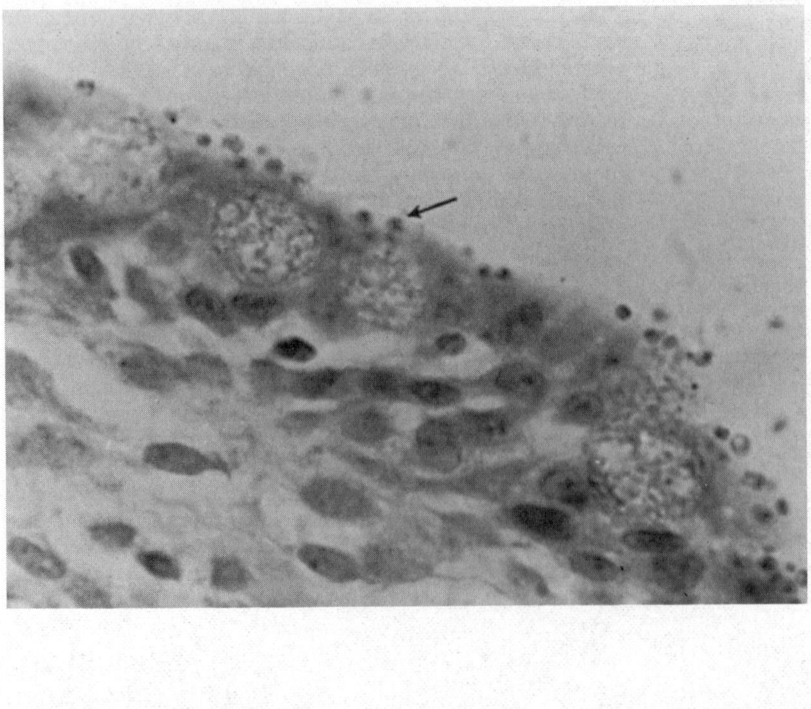

FIGURE 292–2 □ Cryptosporidia *(arrow)* studding the small bowel epithelial surface of a patient with AIDS. (Giemsa stain, × 450.)

γ-glutamyl transpeptidase levels are usually elevated, whereas bilirubin and transaminase values remain normal. On radiographic examination, the gallbladder may be dilated, with thickened walls and luminal irregularities suggestive of sclerosing cholangitis. Patients who underwent cholecystectomy or endoscopic retrograde cholangiopancreatography have been found to have cryptosporidia studding the gallbladder epithelial surface and in the bile. The patients' symptoms improved transiently after either cholecystectomy or endoscopic papillotomy. Pancreatitis complicating cryptosporidial infection has also been described.[69, 70]

Diagnosis

The diagnosis of cryptosporidial enteritis is made by detection of oocysts in fecal or intestinal biopsy specimens. Since 1981, many staining techniques for detecting the parasite in stool specimens have been popularized.[75, 76] Most widely accepted have been modified acid-fast stains, which readily distinguish the acid-fast *Cryptosporidium* oocysts from yeasts, which although similar in shape and size are not acid-fast. However, data indicate that acid-fast staining lacks sensitivity, especially when stool is formed. Concentration by centrifugation may improve sensitivity.

A direct immunofluorescent antibody stain using monoclonal murine immunoglobulin M to the oocyst wall (Meridian) and enzyme-linked immunosorbent assays for detection of cryptosporidial antigen in stool specimens are now commercially available and in use in some clinical laboratories. Studies to determine the sensitivity, specificity, and predictive value of these techniques are ongoing. Although these newer technologies may enhance detection of *Cryptosporidium*,[77] for the present, *Isospora* and *Cyclospora* can be detected only by microscopic examination, enhanced by acid-fast staining.

Immunofluorescence and enzyme-linked immunosorbent assays have been developed to detect anticryptosporidial immunoglobulins in serum and various secretions.[48, 78, 79] Both immunocompetent and immunocompromised patients generate immunoglobulin G in response to infection with *Cryptosporidium*. Whereas patients with AIDS seldom generate anticryptosporidial immunoglobulin M, immunocompetent patients usually exhibit an increase in immunoglobulin M antibody early in the course of cryptosporidial infection. Current work at the Centers for Disease Control and Prevention is aimed at identifying *Cryptosporidium* epitopes responsible for the early antibody response that might be useful diagnostically.[80]

Treatment

No consistently effective therapy for human cryptosporidiosis is currently known. Research has been hindered by difficulty in cultivating the organism and by the absence of a suitable in vitro model for screening drugs. Symptomatic small-animal models are being developed but have not been widely accepted.[71] A wide variety of antimicrobial and immunomodulating agents as well as special diets have been tested in an unprecedented fashion on a compassionate basis for AIDS patients with cryptosporidiosis; although most have been unsuccessful, a few have shown limited promise.[12, 19, 71, 72, 81, 82]

Interest in macrolide antibiotics for cryptosporidiosis began with anecdotal reports of responses to spiramycin in the mid-1980s.[83] In the first placebo-controlled trial for AIDS-related cryptosporidiosis, oral spiramycin was found to be no more efficacious than placebo, probably owing to poor absorption in the target population.[81] Results of a single-blind placebo-controlled trial of intravenous spiramycin suggest that despite modest anticryptosporidial activity, use of this form of the agent is limited by toxic effects. Controlled trials of oral spiramycin in immunocompetent children have provided both positive[84] and negative[85] results, possibly related to inadequate dosing.

The newer macrolide azithromycin may be more promising. Preliminary results of a randomized, double-blind, placebo-controlled crossover trial in 80 AIDS patients suggest that a lactose-free form of oral azithromycin, 900 mg once daily, conferred modest, statistically insignificant, clinical and parasitologic improvement.[86] Preliminary regression analysis of the data suggests a statistically significant decrease in stool oocyst counts in patients who achieved higher serum azithromycin levels.[86] Anecdotal reports of improved liver function after treatment with intravenous azithromycin have prompted further study of this route.[87] Pilot clinical trials of the macrolides roxithromycin and clarithromycin for AIDS-related cryptosporidiosis are in progress.[81]

Diclazuril and letrazuril, benzeneacetonitrile derivatives active against coccidian infection in poultry, were found to lack efficacy in placebo-controlled trials in AIDS patients.[81, 88]

Paromomycin is a nonabsorbable aminoglycoside that concentrates in the colon. Data are conflicting on the efficacy of paromomycin for AIDS-related cryptosporidiosis. In one double-blind, placebo-controlled trial, 1.5 to 2 g/d for 14 days was associated with partial symptomatic and parasitologic responses, consistent with other anecdotal observations.[89–92] However, in an AIDS Clinical Trials Group–sponsored multicenter, double-blind, placebo-controlled trial, paromomycin at 2 g/d for 21 days was associated with no significant benefit relative to placebo.[93] Clinical use of paromomycin has been disappointing because clinical response may not correlate with reduction in parasite shedding, response may be transient, and eradication appears unusual.

Nitazoxanide (NTZ) is a nitrothiazole benzamide compound with a broad spectrum of antimicrobial activity. In an open-label trial of nitazoxanide at 0.5 to 2 g/d orally for 4 weeks, 43% of patients with AIDS-related cryptosporidiosis had a 50% or greater reduction in diarrheal frequency and/or a significant reduction in oocyst shedding in stool; some patients experienced additional benefit with extended therapy.[94] An AIDS Clinical Trials Group–sponsored, multicenter, placebo-controlled trial of nitazoxanide is in progress.

Given the limitations of antimicrobial chemotherapy for cryptosporidiosis, strategies for immunotherapy are of great interest. Novel therapies, including hyperimmune bovine colostrum, bovine colostral immunoglobulins, and cow's milk globulin, have resulted in both success and failure in humans and animals when they were administered orally.[72, 95–98] The use of bovine transfer factor also appeared promising, but more investigation is required, including identification of the active component.[99] Clinical investigation of various novel immunomodulatory agents including a hyperimmune egg yolk preparation containing high titers of anticryptosporidial antibody is under way.

Anecdotal reports of AIDS patients experiencing improvement in cryptosporidial enteritis while receiving zidovudine therapy[72, 100, 101] may be explained by improved immune function rather than specific anticryptosporidial activity.

Cryptosporidiosis in immunocompetent hosts is self-limited, although the enteritis can be severe. In the absence of defined specific therapy, management is generally limited to supportive measures. Cryptosporidiosis in patients with weakened immunity due to exogenous factors such as chemotherapy may resolve if immunoreductive therapy is lessened or interrupted. Cryptosporidiosis in AIDS is commonly chronic and unremitting; supportive measures are often vital, and an attempt at specific anticryptosporidial therapy is usually justified.

Fluid and electrolyte management, with oral or intravenous repletion as needed, is crucial for supportive therapy. AIDS patients with chronic cryptosporidiosis may benefit from parenteral nutrition. Nonspecific antidiarrheal agents such as kaolin plus pectin (Kaopectate), loperamide (Imodium), diphenoxylate (Lomotil), bismuth subsalicylate (Pepto-Bismol), or opiates may provide symptomatic relief, but safety has not been investigated in cryptosporidiosis. The long-acting parenteral somatostatin analog octreotide has provided symptomatic relief in some patients with AIDS and cryptosporidiosis,[102] although no consistent benefit was observed in a prospective, multicenter clinical trial.[103]

Prevention

The *Cryptosporidium* oocyst is hardy and resistant to many disinfectants used in hospitals and laboratories, including 3% hypochlorite solution, iodophor, cresylic acid, benzalkonium chloride, and 5% formaldehyde.[12, 19] Oocyst infectivity appears to be eliminated by exposure to temperatures above 73°C for 1 minute[104] and reduced by prolonged exposure to undiluted bleach or 5% ammonia. Whether freezing reduces or eliminates infectivity is under study.

Persons who are immunocompromised should be advised that certain activities are risks for cryptosporidiosis and should be avoided. These include unprotected physical contact with infected persons or animals, swimming in pools, and consumption of or swimming in freshwater. Data on the risk associated with the consumption of municipal water are insufficient to recommend preventive measures, but immunocompromised individuals who wish to do so can eliminate the risk for transmission from tap water by boiling it for at least 1 minute, by drinking bottled water from safe sources (such as steam-distilled water), or by the correct use of certain types of water filtration units.[23, 29]

Isospora belli

History

Human infection with *I. belli* was first described in 1915.[105] Although it has been recognized as a pathogen for many years, much remains to be learned about infection with this parasite.

Characteristics of the Pathogen

I. belli, like *Cryptosporidium* and *Cyclospora*, is a true coccidian. Its oocysts are elliptical and substantially larger (22 to 33 μm by 10 to 15 μm), and each contains two sporocysts. Inside each sporocyst are four sporozoites. Clinical disease is acquired through ingestion of the mature (sporulated) oocyst. The parasite invades host intestinal epithelium and, once in the enterocyte cytoplasm, passes through the asexual (merogony) and sexual (gametogony) phases of its life cycle. Unsporulated oocysts are shed in the feces and must mature outside the host to become infective.

Epidemiology

The prevalence of *I. belli* in humans is not known. It is distributed throughout the world but is more common in tropical and subtropical climates. Endemic areas include Latin America, the Caribbean, Africa, Australia, and Southeast Asia.[106–109] In the United States, *I. belli* has been implicated in several institutional outbreaks of diarrhea, as the cause of enteritis in World War II veterans returning from the Pacific, and as a cause of traveler's diarrhea.[106–108, 110] Isosporiasis has been documented in 0.2% to 1.0% of all AIDS patients in the United States and in 5% to 19% of AIDS patients in Haiti and Africa.[108, 111–113] The relative infrequency of clinical *I. belli* infection among AIDS patients in the United States may be due to the use of trimethoprim-sulfamethoxazole (TMP-SMX) for *Pneumocystis carinii* prophylaxis. The mode of transmission is not well worked out; acquisition from infected animals and humans, and through contaminated water, is suspected but not confirmed.

Pathology and Pathogenesis

Histopathologic evaluation of small bowel biopsy specimens from infected patients reveals atrophic mucosa, shortened villi, hypertrophic crypts, and infiltration of the lamina propria with inflammatory cells, particularly eosinophils.[106, 114, 115] Electron microscopic examination has demonstrated parasites within cytoplasmic vacuoles of enterocytes. Extraintestinal isosporiasis is well documented in cats[116] but rarely described in humans. *I. belli* has been identified in the lymph nodes of one patient with AIDS and in the gallbladder lumen of an AIDS patient with acalculous cholecystitis.[117, 118]

Clinical Manifestations

Signs and symptoms of isosporiasis include watery diarrhea without blood or inflammatory cells, cramping abdominal pain, anorexia, and weight loss. Low-grade fever may be present. Fat malabsorption is common; peripheral eosinophilia has been documented in some cases. Immunocompetent adults usually have a self-limited diarrheal illness, but there have been case reports of prolonged illness.[110] AIDS patients and immunocompetent infants and children often have a chronic or relapsing form of the disease.[107, 112, 119–121]

Diagnosis

Diagnosis is established by finding *Isospora* oocysts in fecal specimens (Fig. 292–3). Like *Cryptosporidium* and *Cyclospora*, they are acid-fast but are easily distinguished by their larger size and ellipsoid shape. *Isospora* organisms may also be identified with a fluorescent auramine stain. Other methods of identifying *Cryptosporidium*, including serologic tests, have not been extended to *Isospora*. *Isospora* oocysts may be shed only intermittently, suggesting that specimen concentration or obtaining multiple specimens may be useful in diagnosis.[110]

Treatment

Unlike cryptosporidiosis, isosporiasis promptly responds to therapy. One week of oral double-strength TMP-SMX, 160 mg of TMP and 800 mg of SMX four times a day, usually effects a clinical and parasitologic cure, with response evident, on average, within 3 days.[121, 122] AIDS patients have a high rate of relapse but respond well to retreatment with TMP-SMX. To prevent relapse, AIDS patients can be maintained with long-term suppressive therapy; double-strength TMP-SMX three times weekly or pyrimethamine, 25 mg, plus sulfadiazine, 500 mg (Fansidar), once weekly appears effective.[122] There have been scattered anecdotal reports of response to pyrimethamine alone[123] and to the experimental agents roxithromycin[124] and diclazuril.[125] Results of treatment with metronidazole, quinacrine, and nitrofurantoin have been mixed.[106, 114, 122, 126] Controlled studies are needed to establish the precise dose and duration of induction and maintenance therapy. Better alternative therapy is needed.

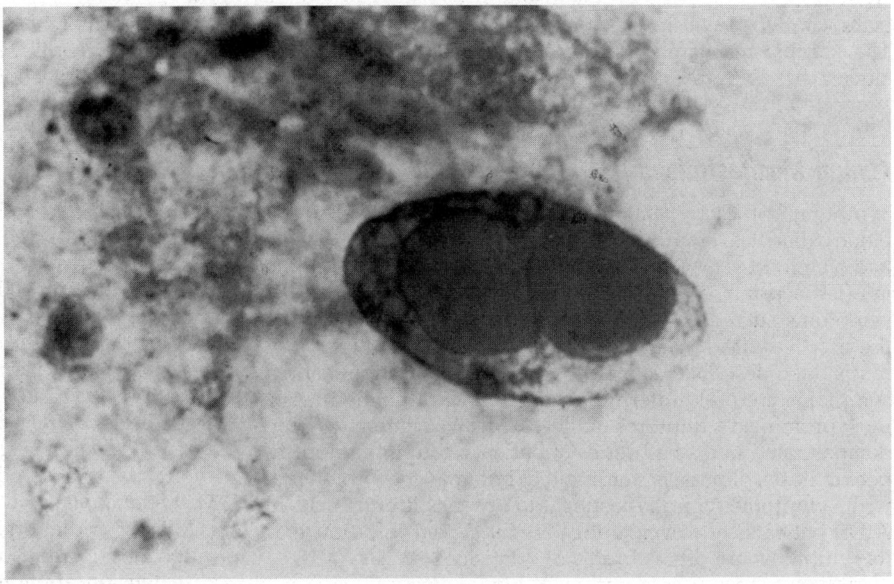

FIGURE 292–3 □ Acid-fast *Isospora belli* oocyst in the stained smear of a fecal specimen from a patient with AIDS and diarrhea. (× 450.) (Courtesy of Madeleine Boncy, Haitian Study Group on Kaposi's Sarcoma and Opportunistic Infection [GHESKIO], Port-au-Prince, Haiti.)

Cyclospora

History

Cyclospora is the newest coccidian to be discovered in humans. Since 1986, and possibly as early as 1979, a unique acid-fast organism resembling a "large *Cryptosporidium*" has been characterized in humans with diarrheal illness.[127, 128] Although variously termed a coccidian-like body, a cyanobacterium (blue-green algae), and a cyanobacterium-like body, similarities between these reports suggest that they describe the same parasite.[129–135] Sporulation, excystation, and ultrastructural analyses support the classification of this pathogen as *Cyclospora*.[131, 133]

Characteristics of the Pathogen

Cyclospora is an intracellular enteric parasite. The genus is in the phylum Apicomplexa, class Sporozoa, subclass Coccidiasina, suborder Eimeriorina. The species name *Cyclospora cayetanensis* has been proposed for the human pathogen,[133] although the degree of relatedness between *Cyclospora* identified in diverse human cohorts remains under study. *Cyclospora* species reported in several animal hosts appear to be distinct from *Cyclospora* species in humans.[131, 134]

The round *Cyclospora* oocysts contain two sporocysts, each of which envelops two sporozoites. *Cyclospora* oocysts identified in human fecal specimens are typically 8 to 10 μm in diameter, distinct from oocysts of *Cryptosporidium* (also round, but 4 to 6 μm) and *Isospora* (elliptical, 28 × 13 μm). Although the complete life cycle of *Cyclospora* and the nonhuman vectors remain unknown, human infection appears to begin with oral ingestion.[129, 130]

Epidemiology

Human *Cyclospora* appears to be globally distributed, with reports matching its description in residents and travelers from North America, Central America, South America, the Caribbean islands, Eastern Europe, India, Nepal, Bangladesh, and Southeast Asia.[135–137] Incidence is seasonal, with most cases reported from Nepal and Peru occurring during the warm, rainy months, and from the United States between May and July.[129–131, 134] Symptomatic infection occurs in all ages and in immunocompetent and immunocompromised hosts alike. Persons native to endemic areas appear less susceptible to clinical infection, suggesting that past infection may confer some degree of immunity.[130] Prevalence data are limited. In endemic areas, investigators identified *Cyclospora* in 6% to 18% of children aged 1 to 24 months in Lima, Peru, shantytowns, and in 12% of Nepalese children with diarrhea aged 18 to 60 months, but in no Nepalese or Haitian children with diarrhea younger than 18 months.[131, 138, 139] Among Haitian adults with chronic diarrhea, *Cyclospora* was detected in 11% of human immunodeficiency virus (HIV)–seropositive, but none of the HIV-seronegative, patients tested.[138] In the United States and England, which have not been considered endemic areas, *Cyclospora* was identified in 0.1% to 0.5% of stool specimens received in three clinical laboratories.[134, 135, 139a, 139b]

There was a surge in non–travel-related cases in the New York City and Palm Beach, Florida, metropolitan areas in May to June 1995, and nearly 1450 sporadic and cluster-related cases were reported in 20 states, Washington, DC, and two Canadian provinces in May to June 1996.[134, 135, 139c, 139d] The risk factors involved have not been identified, although preliminary epidemiologic investigation has suggested an association with eating fresh fruits (particularly raspberries). Whether growing awareness and more aggressive testing for *Cyclospora* have played a role in this apparent rising incidence is not known.

Although the range of exposure risks for *Cyclospora* infection remains to be defined, humans appear to have contracted *Cyclospora* from contaminated water in outbreaks in Nepal and Chicago.[129, 140] One case of infection after ingestion of lettuce contaminated with cyanobacterium-like bodies has also been reported.[130] Direct transmission from animals or from person to person has not been documented.

Pathology and Pathogenesis

Diarrhea associated with *Cyclospora* infection is typically watery and negative for occult blood or leukocytes, consistent with a noninvasive process.[130] Small bowel injury is prominent. Endoscopy reveals duodenal erythema in some patients[141]; histologic features on duodenal[141] and jejunal[142] biopsy include villous atrophy, crypt hyperplasia, and epithelial disarray, with acute and chronic inflammation.

Electron microscopic analysis of jejunal biopsy specimens has demonstrated intracytoplasmic parasites within enterocytes, contained within vacuoles toward the luminal poles.[142] The specific mechanism of intestinal injury remains to be elucidated. Extraintestinal infection (cholangitis) has been suggested in two patients with AIDS.[142a]

Clinical Manifestations

Symptoms of *Cyclospora* infection commonly include nonbloody diarrhea, cramping abdominal pain, nausea, anorexia, and weight loss.[142a–146] In contrast to cryptosporidiosis, fatigue is often a principal complaint, and fever and influenza-like symptoms such as myalgias are common, especially during the first few days. Diarrhea may not be consistently watery but is often described as urgent or explosive. Gastrointestinal symptoms are often intermittent and may not be the first or most prominent symptoms of illness. Malabsorption has been demonstrated in a small series of patients.[141] In immunocompetent hosts, illness is self-limited but may be prolonged, with symptoms typically lasting 2 to 6 weeks if untreated. In AIDS patients, however, untreated *Cyclospora* infection and its symptoms are often chronic or relapsing.[138, 147]

Diagnosis

Diagnosis of *Cyclospora* infection is established by identifying the oocysts in stool. *Cyclospora* oocysts are round and 8 to 10 μm in diameter; on unstained wet preparations, they are nonrefractile and contain globular inclusions.[131] Although morphologically similar, *Cryptosporidium* oocysts are smaller (4 to 6 μm); careful measurement allows differentiation. Modified acid-fast staining greatly facilitates detection of *Cyclospora* and should be requested; the intensity of oocysts staining within a smear is often highly variable,[133] in contrast to *Cryptosporidium*, which stains more homogeneously. In addition, *Cyclospora* oocysts characteristically autofluoresce blue-green under ultraviolet epifluorescence microscopy. Direct immunofluorescent stains specific for *Cryptosporidium* do not appear to react with *Cyclospora*.[131]

Cyclospora oocysts have also been identified in duodenal aspirates and in small bowel biopsy specimens examined by electron microscopy.[142]

Treatment

The illness associated with human *Cyclospora* infection responds promptly to oral TMP-SMX, much like isosporiasis but in contrast to cryptosporidiosis. For adults, TMP at 160 mg and SMX at 800 mg twice daily for 7 days in immunocompetent patients,[143, 145] and four times daily for 10 days in patients with AIDS,[138] has been associated with resolution of symptoms and eradication of *Cyclospora* from stool. Relapse subsequent to therapy is common in AIDS patients but responds to retreatment; long-term suppressive therapy with TMP at 160 mg and SMX at 800 mg three times a week appears to greatly reduce recurrence.[138] Further study is needed to define (1) appropriate children's dosages, (2) alternative therapy for TMP-SMX–intolerant patients, and (3) whether a smaller TMP-SMX dose than that suggested for adults with AIDS would be as effective.

Microsporidia

History

Microsporidial organisms are obligate intracellular spore-forming protozoan parasites long recognized as pathogens in mammals, fish, crustaceans, and insects.[148, 149] Until the AIDS epidemic, association of human disease with microsporidial infection was rare; first reported in 1959,[150] only eight cases were known until 1985. Subsequently, however, human microsporidial infection associated with varied clinical syndromes, predominantly among HIV-infected persons, has been described with increasing frequency.[151–154]

Characteristics of the Pathogen

Microsporidia is the term used to refer to members of the phylum Microspora, order Microsporida. The phylum contains more than 1000 species within approximately 100 genera.[148, 149] Six genera have been described in human infection (Table 292–1): *Encephalitozoon* (including *Encephalitozoon intestinalis*, formerly *Septata intestinalis*[155]), *Enterocytozoon, Pleistophora, Nosema*, and the more recently designated *Vittaforma* (one species, *Vittaforma corneae*, formerly *Nosema corneum*[155a]) and *Trachipleistophora*.[156] Microsporidia that are not well enough characterized to assign to a genus have been named *Microsporidium* sp.

Microsporidial organisms are primitive eukaryotes lacking mitochondria and Golgi. Spores contain a coiled polar tubule, an extension apparatus, and sporoplasm, which consists of cytoplasm and one or two nuclei. In the appropriate environment, spores extrude their tubule, which then penetrates a host cell and provides a conduit for the transfer of the sporoplasm into the host cytoplasm. Merogony and sporogony follow. The resultant new spores are released when the host cell ruptures, remaining within the host or passing into the environment.[148, 154, 157]

Spores are typically ovoid or piriform. Dimensions vary by species and range from 1 to 20 μm in diameter. Microsporidial spores found in humans are relatively small at 1 to 2

TABLE 292–1 ■ Clinical Manifestations of Microsporidia Infection, by Species and Host

	HOST	
SPECIES	HIV Infected	Non-HIV Infected
Encephalitozoon cuniculi	Disseminated infection	Seizures[a]
Encephalitozoon hellem	Keratoconjunctivitis, disseminated infection	—
Encephalitozoon intestinalis[b]	Enteritis, disseminated infection	—
Enterocytozoon bieneusi	Enteritis, cholangitis, respiratory infection	Enteritis[c]
Pleistophora species	Myositis	Myositis[d]
Trachipleistophora hominis	Myositis	—
Nosema connori	—	Disseminated infection[e]
Nosema ocularum		Keratitis[f]
Vittaforma corneae[g]	—	Keratitis[h]
Microsporidium africanum	—	Corneal ulcer[i]
Microsporidium ceylonensis	—	Corneal ulcer[j]

[a]Two cases, one with decreased CD4/CD8.[150, 171]
[b]Formerly *Septata intestinalis.*
[c]Two cases, one an organ recipient receiving immunosuppressive therapy.[154, 221]
[d]One case, cellular immunity impaired.[196]
[e]One case, thymic aplasia.[222]
[f]One case, immunocompetent.[185, 200]
[g]Formerly *Nosema corneum.*
[h]One case, immunocompetent.[155a]
[i]One case, immunocompetent.[148, 200]
[j]One case, immunocompetent.[148, 199]

μm. Shape, position of nuclei, and number of nuclei and coils of the polar tubule also vary. Classification of microsporidian species into various genera is determined by morphologic features and the mode of replication within the host cell.[148, 157]

Epidemiology

The majority of microsporidiosis cases have been reported in AIDS patients, including nearly all cases of *Enterocytozoon bieneusi* and all cases of *Encephalitozoon hellem* and *E. intestinalis*.[158] Only 10 non–HIV-related cases of microsporidiosis have been documented; four of these were in immunocompromised individuals[150, 154] (see Table 292–1).

Human microsporidiosis has a worldwide distribution, with cases in HIV-infected patients reported from North and South America, Europe, Africa, Asia, and Australia.[148, 151, 158] The actual prevalence of microsporidial infection in humans is unknown, because diagnostic techniques are limited, and studies have been few. Microsporidia have been identified in 7.5% to 50% of AIDS patients with previously unexplained diarrhea.[159–164] Most[165] but not all[166] studies reveal a strong correlation between intestinal microsporidiosis and clinical enteritis, suggesting that microsporidia, particularly *E. bieneusi*, are an important cause of AIDS-related diarrhea. However, asymptomatic enteric carriage may be common in HIV infection.[166–168]

The modes by which humans become infected with microsporidia are unknown. Spores may be shed in feces, urine, or respiratory secretions of infected humans.[158, 169] Fecal-oral and sexual modes of transmission from human to human have been proposed[151] but not documented. Microsporidial spores have been identified in surface water,[170] but only of species not known to infect humans. Microsporidia species are found in numerous animal hosts representing most phyla and including fish and crustacean species consumed by humans.[148, 149] However, other than several mammalian hosts in which *Encephalitozoon cuniculi* has been identified, the animal reservoirs of microsporidia species pathogenic to humans remain unknown, and zoonotic transmission to humans has yet to be demonstrated.

Pathology and Pathogenesis

Tissue distribution, histopathologic features, and propensity to disseminate vary widely among species of microsporidia recognized in human disease.[151, 154] Pathophysiologic mechanisms and the full range of organ involvement remain to be elucidated for these organisms. Impaired cellular immunity is a factor in host susceptibility; nearly all cases of human microsporidiosis have been in HIV-infected individuals.[152, 154]

Human infection with *E. bieneusi* is virtually always limited to intestinal and biliary tissue.[171, 172] Organisms have been observed from duodenum to colon, in biliary and gallbladder epithelia, and in the pancreatic duct.[173] Whereas the greatest density is typically in the duodenum or proximal jejunum,[172] predominantly biliary infestation has been reported.[163, 174, 175] Infection is nearly always limited to the epithelial cell layer, with organisms evident within apical cytoplasm. Histopathologic features range from minimal injury to marked epithelial cell dystrophy, vesiculation, and sloughing.[175] Intraepithelial and lamina propria mononuclear cell infiltrates are variable. Damage to small intestinal villous architecture may be minimal or extreme with atrophy and crypt elongation and often correlates with the degree of infestation.[167, 176] Infection of biliary epithelia has been linked to sclerosing cholangitis, acalculous cholecystitis, and papillary stenosis,[175, 177] although histopathologic changes are often minimal.[154] There have been rare reports of *E. bieneusi* in nasal and tracheobronchial tissue.[178]

Human infection with *Encephalitozoon* species is frequently disseminated. *E. intestinalis* is, like *E. bieneusi*, associated with gastroenteritis.[179] Small bowel villous atrophy, enterocyte sloughing, and acute inflammatory infiltrates are variably present.[179, 180] However, in contrast to *E. bieneusi*, *E. intestinalis* organisms are commonly demonstrable in apical and basal enterocyte cytoplasm as well as within macrophages from lamina propria to submucosa.[179, 181] In addition, disseminated *E. intestinalis* infection, with hepatobiliary, bronchial, and renal involvement, has been reported.[181, 182] *E. intestinalis* has been identified in the urine or respiratory secretions of several patients with enteritis,[183, 184] suggesting that disseminated infection is underrecognized.

E. hellem has been identified in superficial corneal and conjunctival epithelia.[185–189] Inflammatory changes are variable. Subclinical, systemic infection may accompany ocular disease, with spores demonstrable in respiratory secretions and urine.[190] Superficial respiratory epithelial cell infection has been demonstrated in symptomatic tracheitis, bronchiolitis, and sinusitis.[186, 191, 192] *E. hellem* was demonstrated in the bronchi, kidneys, ureters, bladder, and corneas of a patient with advanced AIDS who died of renal and respiratory failure.[192]

E. cuniculi has been identified in hepatocytes and in omental tissue of two AIDS patients with granulomatous hepatitis[193] and peritonitis,[194] respectively.

Myositis has been reported associated with *Pleistophora* infection (one AIDS patient[195] and one HIV-seronegative individual with impaired cellular immunity[196]) and with *Trachipleistophora* infection (one AIDS patient[155a]). Organisms were demonstrated among atrophic muscle fibers.[155a, 195, 196]

Clinical Manifestations

Clinical features of microsporidiosis include chronic diarrhea, keratoconjunctivitis, myositis, nephritis, hepatitis, sinusitis, and pneumonia.[153, 154]

Enteritis due to *E. bieneusi* or *E. intestinalis* is the most common clinical manifestation of microsporidiosis in patients with AIDS.[159, 162] Diarrhea is typically chronic and intermittent, loose to watery, and nonbloody.[153, 154, 159, 162] Fecal leukocytes are usually absent. Anorexia, weight loss, and dehydration are common, and findings on D-xylose testing are often abnormal, consistent with malabsorption.[162, 173] Abdominal cramping, nausea, and vomiting may occur. Density of *E. bieneusi* infestation and associated histopathologic appearance may not correlate with severity of enteritis, and chronic asymptomatic carriage has been documented.[168] Concomitant infection with other opportunistic gastrointestinal pathogens, such as *Cryptosporidium* or cytomegalovirus, is often present.[164, 197]

E. bieneusi and *E. intestinalis* have been implicated in biliary disease, including cholangitis and acalculous cholecystitis.[171, 175, 181] Patients may present with right upper quadrant pain or intractable nausea. The alkaline phosphatase level is often elevated, whereas bilirubin and transaminase levels are typically normal. Radiologic imaging may reveal dilatation or luminal irregularities of biliary ducts and gallbladder distention or thickening.[175]

Although *E. intestinalis* infection has been recognized chiefly in association with intestinal and biliary disease,[179] dissemination is underrecognized and extragastrointestinal manifestations remain poorly characterized.

Infection with *E. hellem* in patients with AIDS is most commonly associated with keratoconjunctivitis.[187, 188] Ocular pain or pruritus, foreign body sensation, lacrimosis, and blurred vision may be present. Infection may be bilateral, and bacterial superinfection has been reported. Isolated cases of bronchitis, nephritis, and cystourethritis associated with *E.*

hellem infection have been reported.[188] However, asymptomatic or cryptic disseminated infection may be underrecognized.

E. cuniculi has been identified in single cases of hepatitis,[193] peritonitis[194] and generalized infection,[154] all HIV-infected patients. *E. cuniculi* has also been reported in two children with seizure disorders,[150, 198] one of whom had a decreased CD4/CD8 ratio.

Pleistophora species have been identified on skeletal muscle biopsy specimens in two patients presenting with generalized muscle weakness: a patient with AIDS[195] and an HIV-negative individual with decreased cell-mediated immunity.[196] Creatine kinase and aldolase values were elevated in the former but not the latter case, and electromyography was consistent with inflammatory myopathy in both.

Vittaforma corneae, Nosema ocularum, and *Microsporidium* species not belonging to recognized genera have been identified in rare cases of keratitis with or without iritis in immunocompetent hosts[148, 155a, 199, 200] (see Table 292–1).

Diagnosis

Diagnosis of microsporidiosis requires demonstration of organisms in tissue, stool, or body fluids. Electron microscopic examination of tissue specimens remains the "gold standard" for species identification, but improvements in the sensitivity of various staining techniques that employ light microscopy have made testing for microsporidia easier and more accessible.[154, 161, 175] With use of chromotrope-based stains (trichrome blue stain, Weber chromotrope stain),[189, 201, 202] spores appear pink and refractile, and some have a darker staining band along the shorter axis, making them distinct from other stained elements. With chemofluorescence (Uvitex 2B, calcofluor white 2MR), spore walls can be identified under fluorescence microscopy.[203, 204] Because nonmicrosporidial elements may be stained and the morphologic appearance is not distinctive, the specificity of chemofluorescence is suboptimal. Giemsa stains[158] are more useful for body fluid specimens than for stool. Immunofluorescent stains for *Encephalitozoon* species are under development.[205, 206] The relative sensitivity, specificity, and predictive value of the different diagnostic methods have not yet been determined, and the number of negative specimens needed to confirm a true negative result is unknown. Concentration of body fluid specimens may improve yield but has not been consistently helpful for stool specimens.[165, 202]

Studies suggest that stool examination is as sensitive as endoscopic biopsy for detection of microsporidia.[154, 165] Still, when microsporidiosis is suspected despite negative findings on stool examination, small bowel biopsy is advisable. Although microsporidial infestation is frequently densest in jejunum,[164, 173] biopsy of duodenum often provides the diagnosis.[162] Colonic biopsy is insensitive for microsporidiosis, although infection may be detected in the terminal ileum.[207]

Light microscopic examination of histologic specimens for microsporidia is complicated by the small size of these organisms and the sometimes near-normal appearance of infected tissue.[159, 162] Hematoxylin-eosin and Giemsa stains are commonly used,[158, 208] although tissue Gram stains (e.g., Brown-Brenn)[165] or chromotrope stains[209] may provide increased contrast of microsporidia spores against surrounding tissue. Microsporidia have also been visualized on touch preparations of small intestinal biopsy specimens with Giemsa staining.[210]

Encephalitozoon keratoconjunctival infection may be diagnosed by chromotrope or Giemsa staining of scrapings or smears from swabs of cornea or conjunctiva.[190, 206, 211] Examination of urine or sputum for microsporidia may assist in diagnosis, even in the absence of urinary or respiratory symptoms.

Speciation of human microsporidia is useful clinically, because disease manifestations and responsiveness to therapy vary from species to species. However, speciation by light microscopy is difficult owing to the small size and similar shapes of these organisms. Whereas *Encephalitozoon* and *Nosema* species have been successfully cultured,[186, 192, 211–213] the process is not useful for routine diagnosis. Serologic assays[198, 214] and polymerase chain reaction method[213] are under development.

Treatment

Therapeutic options for human microsporidiosis are few, and their effectiveness appears to vary among species. Controlled studies are lacking, and most of the available information is based on anecdotal data.

To date, albendazole (at doses of 400 mg orally twice daily for a minimum of 4 weeks) has been the most successful agent used in the treatment of AIDS-related microsporidiosis, but whereas *E. intestinalis* and *E. cuniculi* appear susceptible, *E. bieneusi* seems much less responsive.[169, 213, 215, 216] Even in responders, microsporidia may not be eradicated, and chronic maintenance therapy may be required.[215] A placebo-controlled, multicenter trial of albendazole for intestinal microsporidiosis is under way. Metronidazole was associated with clinical improvement of *E. bieneusi* enteritis in one study, but parasite infestation was not affected, and subsequent investigations found no benefit.[159, 216, 217] Atovaquone in patients with *E. bieneusi* infection was associated with improvement in diarrhea but limited reduction in parasite burden in one small series.[218] Supportive measures to address chronic diarrhea, fluid and electrolyte loss, and malabsorption remain the principal component of management in most cases of intestinal microsporidiosis.

Improvement in *E. hellem* keratoconjunctivitis has been reported with topical fumagillin[219] and oral itraconazole[220] therapy, but controlled trials have not been performed.

Dientamoeba fragilis

History

D. fragilis was described by Weynon[223] in 1915 and reported as a new species by Jepps and Dobell[224] in 1918. Although it is ubiquitous, *D. fragilis* is often overlooked by standard parasitologic techniques, and it remains poorly understood.

Characteristics of the Pathogen

D. fragilis appears to exist only in the trophozoite form. The lack of a cyst stage may account for the difficulty in identifying it on standard ova and parasite preparations. Although initially assigned to the phylum Sarcodina,[224] it is now considered to be more closely related to the flagellate genera *Histomonas* and *Trichomonas*.[225, 226] The organism has an ameboid shape and measures 5 to 12 μm in diameter. It is binucleate, with central nuclear granules and cytoplasmic vacuoles.

Epidemiology

D. fragilis has a worldwide distribution, but its true prevalence is not known.[226] It has been variously reported to be common and rare. Its frequency appears to be higher in studies that employ preserved stool specimens, permanently stained fecal smears, and multiple stool examinations. In various surveys in the United States, the prevalence of the parasite has ranged from 1.4% to 18.6%.[225]

The mode of transmission of *D. fragilis* is not known. Dientamoebiasis rarely occurs in conjunction with the other parasitic enteritides that are typically transmitted by fecally contaminated food and water. Some researchers have suggested that *D. fragilis* may be transmitted by the ova of the human pinworm *Enterobius vermicularis*.[226]

Pathology and Pathogenesis

D. fragilis may colonize the cecum and proximal large intestine but does not cause invasive disease. Local irritation has been suggested as the mechanism whereby it produces gastrointestinal symptoms.[226]

Clinical Manifestations

Clinical disease occurs in 50% of infected adults and almost all infected children.[226] Dientamoebiasis is not known to be more severe or more common in immunocompromised hosts. Symptoms are nonspecific and typically include intermittent diarrhea, cramping, and bloating. Biliary involvement may occur. Peripheral eosinophilia has been documented principally in children.[227]

Diagnosis

Diagnosis requires demonstration of the *D. fragilis* trophozoite in stool; it is not detectable by biopsy. Specimens are optimal if they are submitted fresh for immediate processing or preserved in polyvinyl alcohol, sodium acetate–acetic acid–formalin, or Schaudinn fixative; other preservatives, such as formalin alone, may substantially lower yield.[228] Hematoxylin-Kinyoun or trichrome staining of stool smears facilitates detection.[229] Multiple specimens obtained on different days may enhance the chances of finding this organism.

Treatment

As yet, no therapy for dientamoebiasis has been approved by the U.S. Food and Drug Administration; however, some benefit has been obtained from treatment with iodoquinol, 650 mg three times daily for 20 days[230]; tetracycline, 500 mg four times daily for 10 days[225]; or paromomycin, 25 to 30 mg/kg per day in three doses for 7 days.[231]

References

Cryptosporidium

1. Tyzzer EE: A sporozoan found in the peptic glands of the common mouse. Proc Soc Exp Biol Med 5:12, 1907–1908.
2. Slavin D: *Cryptosporidium meleagridis* (sp. nov.). J Comp Pathol Ther 65:262, 1955.
3. Panciera RJ, Thomassen RW, Garner FM: Cryptosporidial infection in a calf. Vet Pathol 8:479, 1971.
4. Angus KW: Cryptosporidiosis in man, domestic animals and birds: A review. J R Soc Med 76:62, 1983.
5. Tzipori S: Cryptosporidiosis in animals and humans. Microbiol Rev 47:84, 1983.
6. Nime FA, Burek JD, Page DL, et al: Acute enterocolitis in a human being infected with the protozoan *Cryptosporidium*. Gastroenterology 70:592, 1976.
7. Current WL, Reese NC, Ernst JV, et al: Human cryptosporidiosis in immunocompetent and immunodeficient persons: Studies of an outbreak and experimental transmission. N Engl J Med 308:1252, 1983.
8. Soave R, Danner RL, Honig CL, et al: Cryptosporidiosis in homosexual men. Ann Intern Med 110:504, 1984.
9. Jokipii L, Pohjola S, Valle SL, Jokipii AM: Cryptosporidiosis associated with traveling and giardiasis. Gastroenterology 4:838, 1985.
10. Soave R, Ma P: Cryptosporidiosis: Traveler's diarrhea in two families. Arch Intern Med 145:70, 1985.
11. Wolfson JS, Richter JM, Waldron MA, et al: Cryptosporidiosis in immunocompetent patients. N Engl J Med 312:1278, 1985.
12. Fayer R, Ungar BLP: *Cryptosporidium* spp. and cryptosporidiosis. Microbiol Rev 50:458, 1986.
13. Soave R, Armstrong D: *Cryptosporidium* and cryptosporidiosis. Rev Infect Dis 8:1012, 1986.
14. Janoff EN, Barth Reller L: *Cryptosporidium* species, a protean protozoan. J Clin Microbiol 25:967, 1987.
15. Tzipori S: Cryptosporidiosis in perspective. Adv Parasitol 27:63, 1988.
16. Crawford FG, Vermund SH: Human cryptosporidiosis. Crit Rev Microbiol 16:113, 1988.
17. Tzipori S, Angus KW, Campbell I, Gray EW: *Cryptosporidium*: Evidence for a single-species genus. Infect Immun 30:884, 1980.
18. Levine ND: Taxonomy and review of the coccidian genus *Cryptosporidium* (protozoa, apicomplexa). J Protozool 31:94, 1984.
19. Current WL: *Cryptosporidium*: Its biology and potential for environmental transmission. Crit Rev Environ Control 17:21, 1985.
20. Upton SJ, Current WL: The species of *Cryptosporidium* (Apicomplexa: cryptosporididae) infecting mammals. J Parasitol 71:625, 1985.
21. Hojlyng N, Holten-Andersen W, Jepsen S: Cryptosporidiosis: A case of airborne transmission. Lancet 2:271, 1987.
22. Navin TR: Cryptosporidiosis in humans: Review of recent epidemiologic studies. Eur J Epidemiol 1:77, 1985.
23. Juranek DD: Cryptosporidiosis: Sources of infection and guidelines for prevention. Clin Infect Dis 21:S57, 1995.
24. Dupont HL, Chappell CL, Sterling C, et al: The infectivity of *Cryptosporidium parvum* in healthy volunteers. N Engl J Med 332:855, 1995.
25. D'Antonio RG, Winn RE, Taylor JP, et al: A waterborne outbreak of cryptosporidiosis in normal hosts. Ann Intern Med 103:886, 1985.
26. MacKenzie WR, Hoxie NJ, Proctor ME, et al: A massive outbreak in Milwaukee of *Cryptosporidium* infection transmitted through the public water supply. N Engl J Med 331:161, 1994.
27. Hayes EB, Matte TD, O'Brien TR, et al: Contamination of a conventionally treated filtered public water supply by *Cryptosporidium* associated with a large community outbreak of cryptosporidiosis. N Engl J Med 320:1372, 1989.
28. LeChevallier MW, Moser RH: Occurrence of *Giardia* and *Cryptosporidium* in raw and finished drinking water. J Am Water Works Assoc 87:54, 1995.
29. Centers for Disease Control and Prevention: Assessing the public health threat associated with waterborne cryptosporidiosis: Report of a workshop. MMWR Morbid Mortal Wkly Rep 44(RR-6):1, 1995.
30. Gallaher MM, Herndon JL, Nimo LJ, et al: Cryptosporidiosis and surface water. Am J Public Health 79:39, 1988.
31. Centers for Disease Control and Prevention: *Cryptosporidium* infections associated with swimming pools—Dane County, Wisconsin, 1993. MMWR Morbid Mortal Wkly Rep 43:561, 1994.
32. Joce RF, Brace J, Kiely D, et al: An outbreak of cryptosporidiosis associated with a swimming pool. Epidemiol Infect 107:497, 1991.
33. Madore MS, Rose JB, Gerba CP, et al: Occurrence of *Cryptosporidium* oocysts in sewage effluents and select surface waters. J Parasitol 73:702, 1987.
34. LeChevallier MW, Norton WD, Lee RG: Occurrence of *Giardia* and *Cryptosporidium* in surface water supplies. Appl Environ Microbiol 57:2617, 1991.
35. Rose JB, Gerba CP, Jakubowski W: Survey of potable water supplies for *Cryptosporidium* and *Giardia*. Environ Sci Technol 25:1393, 1991.
36. Millard PS, Gensheimer KF, Addiss DG, et al: An outbreak of cryptosporidiosis from fresh-pressed apple cider. JAMA 272:1592, 1994.
37. Heijbel H, Slaine K, Seigel B, et al: Outbreak of diarrhea in a day care center with spread to household members: The role of *Cryptosporidium*. Pediatr Infect Dis J 6:532, 1987.
38. Dryjanski J, Gold JW, Ritchie MT, et al: Cryptosporidiosis. Case report in a health team worker. Am J Med 80:751, 1986.
39. Koch KL, Phillips DJ, Aber RC, Current WL: Cryptosporidiosis in hospital personnel. Evidence for person-to-person transmission. Ann Intern Med 102:593, 1985.

40. Martino P, Gentile G, Caprioli A, et al: Hospital acquired cryptosporidiosis in a bone marrow transplantation unit. J Infect Dis 158:647, 1988.
41. Cordell RL, Addiss DG: Cryptosporidiosis in child care settings: A review of the literature and recommendations for prevention and control. Pediatr Infect Dis J 13:310, 1994.
42. Lengerich FJ, Addiss DG, Marx JJ, et al: Increased exposure to cryptosporidia among dairy farmers in Wisconsin. J Infect Dis 167:1252, 1993.
43. Miron D, Kenes J, Dagan R: Calves as a source of an outbreak of cryptosporidiosis among young children in an agricultural closed community. Pediatr Infect Dis J 10:483, 1991.
44. Ma P, Kaufman DL, Helmick CG, et al: Cryptosporidiosis in tourists returning from the Caribbean. N Engl J Med 312:647, 1985.
45. Caprioli A, Gentile G, Baldassarri L, et al: *Cryptosporidium* as a common cause of childhood diarrhea in Italy. Epidemiol Infect 102:537, 1989.
46. Casemore DP, Jackson B: Sporadic cryptosporidiosis in children. Lancet 2:679, 1983.
47. Mata L, Bolanos H, Pizarro D, Vives M: Cryptosporidiosis in children from some highland Costa Rican rural and urban areas. Am J Trop Med Hyg 33:24, 1984.
48. Ungar BLP, Soave R, Fayer R, Nash TE: Enzyme immunoassay detection of immunoglobulin M and G antibodies to *Cryptosporidium* in immunocompetent and immunocompromised patients. J Infect Dis 153:570, 1986.
49. Ungar BLP, Mulligan M, Nutman TB: Serologic evidence of *Cryptosporidium* infection in US volunteers before and during Peace Corps Service in Africa. Arch Intern Med 149:894, 1989.
50. Navin TR, Harden AM: Cryptosporidiosis in patients with AIDS. J Infect Dis 155:150, 1987.
51. Smith PD, Lane HC, Gill VJ, et al: Intestinal infections in patients with the acquired immunodeficiency syndrome (AIDS). Ann Intern Med 108:328, 1988.
52. Laughon BE, Druckman DA, Vernon A, et al: Prevalence of enteric pathogens in homosexual men with and without acquired immunodeficiency syndrome. Gastroenterology 94:984, 1988.
53. Quinn TC, Mann JM, Curran JW, Piot P: AIDS in Africa: An epidemiologic paradigm. Science 234:955, 1986.
54. Roberts WG, Green PHR, Ma J, et al: Prevalence of cryptosporidiosis in patients undergoing endoscopy: Evidence for an asymptomatic carrier state. Am J Med 87:537, 1989.
55. Holley HP, Thiers BH: Cryptosporidiosis in a patient receiving immunosuppressive therapy. Possible activation of latent infection. Dig Dis Sci 31:1004, 1986.
56. Guarda LA, Stein SA, Cleary KA, Ordonez NG: Human cryptosporidiosis in the acquired immune deficiency syndrome. Arch Pathol Lab Med 107:562, 1983.
57. Lefkowitch JH, Krumholz S, Feng-Chen K-C: Cryptosporidiosis of the human small intestine: A light and electron microscopic study. Hum Pathol 15:746, 1984.
58. Blumberg RS, Kelsey P, Perrone T, et al: Cytomegalovirus- and cryptosporidium-associated acalculous gangrenous cholecystis. Am J Med 76:118, 1984.
59. Margulis SJ, Honig CL, Soave R, et al: Biliary tract obstruction in the acquired immunodeficiency syndrome. Ann Intern Med 105:207, 1986.
60. Schneiderman DJ, Cello JP, Laing FC: Papillary stenosis and sclerosing cholangitis in the acquired immunodeficiency syndrome. Ann Intern Med 106:546, 1987.
61. Gentile G, Baldassarri L, Caprioli A, et al: Colonic vascular invasion as a possible route of extra-intestinal cryptosporidiosis. Am J Med 82:574, 1987.
62. Forgacs P, Tarshis A, Ma P, et al: Intestinal and bronchial cryptosporidiosis in an immunodeficient homosexual man. Ann Intern Med 99:793, 1983.
63. Kocoshis SA, Cibull ML, Davis TE, et al: Intestinal and pulmonary cryptosporidiosis in an infant with severe combined immune deficiency. J Pediatr Gastroenterol Nutr 3:49, 1984.
64. Miller RA, Wasserheit JN, Kirihara J, Coyle MB: Detection of *Cryptosporidium* oocysts in sputum during screening for *Mycobacterium*. J Clin Microbiol 20:1992, 1984.
65. Current WL, Garcia LS: Cryptosporidiosis. Clin Microbiol Rev 4:325, 1991.
66. Argenzio RA, Liacos JA, Levy ML, et al: Villous atrophy, crypt hyperplasia, cellular infiltration, and impaired glucose-Na absorption in enteric cryptosporidiosis of pigs. Gastroenterology 98:1129, 1990.
67. Guarino A, Canani RB, Pozio E, et al: Enterotoxic effect of stool supernatant of *Cryptosporidium*-infected calves on human jejunum. Gastroenterology 106:28, 1994.
68. Argenzio RA, Lecce J, Powell DW: Prostanoids inhibit intestinal NaCl absorption in experimental porcine cryptosporidiosis. Gastroenterology 104:440, 1993.
69. Gross TL, Wheat J, Bartlett M, et al: AIDS and multiple system involvement with *Cryptosporidium*. Am J Gastroenterol 81:456, 1986.
70. Hawkins SP, Thomas RP, Tesdate C: Acute pancreatitis: A new finding in *Cryptosporidium* enteritis. Br Med J 294:483, 1987.
71. Peterson C: Cryptosporidiosis in patients with the human immunodeficiency virus. Clin Infect Dis 15:903, 1992.
72. Mannheimer SB, Soave R: Protozoal infections in patients with AIDS: Cryptosporidiosis, isosporiasis, cyclosporiasis and microsporidiosis. Infect Dis Clin North Am 8:483, 1994.
73. Jokipii L, Jokipii AMM: Timing of symptoms and oocyst excretion in human cryptosporidiosis. N Engl J Med 315:1643, 1986.
74. Soave R, Johnson WD: AIDS commentary: Cryptosporidiosis and *Isospora belli* infections. J Infect Dis 157:225, 1988.
75. Garcia LS, Bruckner DA, Brewer TC, Shimizu RY: Techniques for the recovery and identification of *Cryptosporidium* oocysts from stool specimens. J Clin Microbiol 18:185, 1983.
76. Ma P, Soave R: Three step stool examination for cryptosporidiosis in ten homosexual men with protracted watery diarrhea. J Infect Dis 147:824, 1983.
77. Sterling CR, Arrowood MJ: Detection of *Cryptosporidium* and cryptosporidiosis. Rev Infect Dis 8:1012, 1986.
78. Campbell PM, Current WL: Demonstration of serum antibodies to *Cryptosporidium* sp. in normal and immunodeficient humans with confirmed infections. J Clin Microbiol 18:165, 1983.
79. Tzipori S, Campbell I: Prevalence of *Cryptosporidium* antibodies in 10 animal species. J Clin Microbiol 14:455, 1981.
80. Moss DM, Bennett SN, Arrowood MJ, et al: Kinetic and isotypic analysis of specific immunoglobulins from crew members with cryptosporidiosis on a U.S. Coast Guard Cutter. J Eukaryot Microbiol 41:52S, 1994.
81. Blagburn BL, Soave R: Prophylaxis and chemotherapy: Human and animal. *In* Fayer R (ed): *Cryptosporidium* and Cryptosporidiosis. Boca Raton, FL, CRC Press, 1997, pp 111–128.
82. Ritchie DJ, Becker ES: Update on the management of intestinal cryptosporidiosis in AIDS. Ann Pharmacol 28:767, 1994.
83. Moskovitz BL, Stanton TL, Kusmierek JJE: Spiramycin therapy for cryptosporidial diarrhea in immunocompromised patients. J Antimicrob Chemother 22(Suppl B):189, 1988.
84. Saez-Llorens X, Odio CM, Umana MA, et al: Spiramycin vs. placebo for treatment of acute diarrhea caused by *Cryptosporidium*. Pediatr Infect Dis 8:136, 1989.
85. Wittenberg DF, Miller NM, van den Ende J: Spiramycin is not effective in treating *Cryptosporidium* diarrhea in infants: Results of a double-blind randomized trial. J Infect Dis 159:131, 1989.
86. Soave R, Havlir D, Lancaster D, et al: Azithromycin (AZ) therapy of AIDS-related cryptosporidial diarrhea (CD): A multicenter, placebo-controlled, double-blind study (Abstr 405). *In* Programs and Abstracts of the 33rd Interscience Conference on Antimicrobial Agents and Chemotherapy; October 1993; New Orleans, LA; p 193.
87. Friedman CR, Soave R: Intravenous azithromycin for cryptosporidiosis in AIDS (Abstr 190). *In* Programs and Abstracts of the 31st Annual Meeting of the Infectious Disease Society of America; October 16–18, 1993; New Orleans, LA; p 33-A.
88. Soave R, Dieterich D, Kotler D, et al: Oral diclazuril for cryptosporidiosis (Abstr Th.B.520). *In* Programs of the Sixth International Conference on AIDS; June 1990; San Francisco, CA; p 252.
89. Scaglia M, Atzori C, Marchetti G, et al: Effectiveness of aminosidine (paromomycin) sulfate in chronic *Cryptosporidium* diarrhea in AIDS patients: An open, uncontrolled, prospective clinical trial. J Infect Dis 170:1349, 1994.
90. White AC, Chappell CL, Hayat CS, et al: Paromomycin for cryptosporidiosis in AIDS: A prospective, double blind trial. J Infect Dis 170:419, 1994.
91. Clezy K, Gold J, Blaze J, et al: Paromomycin for the treatment of cryptosporidial diarrhoea in AIDS patients. AIDS 5:1146, 1991.

92. Fitchenbaum CJ, Ritchie DJ, Powderly WG: Use of paromomycin for treatment of cryptosporidiosis in patients with AIDS. Clin Infect Dis 16:298, 1993.
93. Hewitt RG, Yiannoutsos CT, Carey J, et al: A double-blind, placebo-controlled trial of paromomycin for the treatment of cryptosporidiosis in patients with advanced HIV disease and CD_4 counts under 150 (ACTG 192) (Abstr). Abstracts of the Fourth Conference on Retroviruses and Opportunistic Infections; January 22–26, 1997; Washington DC; p 65.
94. Davis LJ, Soave R, Dudley RE, et al: Nitazoxanide for AIDS-related cryptosporidial diarrhea: An open-label safety, efficacy and pharmacokinetic study (Abstr LM50). Presented at the Interscience Conference on Antimicrobial Agents and Chemotherapy; September 15–18, 1996; New Orleans, LA; p 289.
95. Saxon A, Weinstein W: Oral administration of bovine colostrum anticryptosporidia antibody fails to alter the course of human cryptosporidiosis. J Parasitol 73:413, 1987.
96. Tzipori S, Roberton D, Chapman C: Remission of diarrhoea due to cryptosporidiosis in an immunodeficient child treated with hyperimmune bovine colostrum. Br Med J 293:1276, 1986.
97. Tzipori S, Robertson D, Cooper DA, White L: Chronic cryptosporidial diarrhoea and hyperimmune cow colostrum. Lancet 2:344, 1987.
98. Ungar BLP, Ward DJ, Fayer R, Quinn CA: Cessation of *Cryptosporidium*-associated diarrhea in an acquired immunodeficiency syndrome patient after treatment with hyperimmune bovine colostrum. Gastroenterology 98:486, 1990.
99. McMeeking M, Borkowsky W, Klesius PH, et al: A controlled trial of bovine dialyzable leukocyte extract for cryptosporidiosis in patients with AIDS. J Infect Dis 161:108, 1990.
100. Flanigan T, Whalen C, Turner J, et al: *Cryptosporidium* infection and CD4 counts. Ann Intern Med 116:840, 1992.
101. Greenberg RE, Mir R, Bank S, et al: Resolution of intestinal cryptosporidiosis after treatment of AIDS with AZT. Gastroenterology 97:1327, 1989.
102. Cook DJ, Kelton JG, Stanisz AM, Collins SM: Somatostatin treatment for cryptosporidial diarrhea in a patient with the acquired immunodeficiency syndrome. Ann Intern Med 108: 708, 1988.
103. Romeau J, Miro JM, Siera G, et al: Efficacy of octreotide in the management of chronic diarrhoea in AIDS. AIDS 5:1495, 1991.
104. Fayer R: Effect of high temperature on infectivity of *Cryptosporidium parvum* oocysts in water. Appl Environ Microbiol 60:2732, 1994.

Isospora belli

105. Woodcock HM: Notes on the protozoan parasites in the excreta. Br Med J 2:709, 1915.
106. Brandborg LL, Goldberg SB, Briedenbach WC: Human coccidiosis—A possible cause of malabsorption. The life cycle in small bowel mucosal biopsies as a diagnostic feature. N Engl J Med 283:1306, 1970.
107. Lindsay DS, Dubey JP, Blagburn BL: Biology of *Isospora* spp. from humans, nonhuman primates, and domestic animals. Clin Microbiol Rev 10:19, 1997.
108. Sorvillo FJ, Lieb LE, Seidel J, et al: Epidemiology of isosporiasis among persons with acquired immunodeficiency syndrome in Los Angeles County. Am J Trop Med Hyg 53:656, 1995.
109. Prociv P, Luke R, Quayle P: Isosporiasis in the aboriginal population of Queensland. Med J Aust 156:115, 1992.
110. Shaffer N, Moore L: Chronic traveler's diarrhea in a normal host due to *Isospora belli*. J Infect Dis 159:596, 1989.
111. Smith PD, Quinn TC, Strober W, et al: Gastrointestinal infections in AIDS. Ann Intern Med 116:63, 1992.
112. DeHovitz JA, Pape JW, Boncy M, Johnson WD Jr: Clinical manifestations and therapy of *Isospora belli* infection in patients with acquired immunodeficiency syndrome. N Engl J Med 315:87, 1986.
113. Tarimo DS, Killewo JZJ, Minjas JN, et al: Prevalence of intestinal parasites in adult patients with enteropathic AIDS in north-eastern Tanzania. E Afr Med J 73:397, 1996.
114. Trier JS, Moxey PC, Schimmel EM, Robles E: Chronic intestinal coccidiosis in man: Intestinal morphology and response to treatment. Gastroenterology 6:923, 1974.
115. Webster BH: Human isosporiasis: A report of three cases with necropsy findings in one case. Am J Trop Med 6:86, 1957.
116. Dubey JP, Frenkel JK: Extraintestinal stages of *Isospora felis I. rivolta* (protozoa: Eimeridiae) in cats. J Protozool 19:89, 1972.
117. Restrepo C, Macher AM, Radany EH: Disseminated extraintestinal isosporiasis in a patient with acquired immunodeficiency syndrome. Am J Clin Pathol 87:536, 1987.
118. Benator DA, French AL, Beaudet LM, et al: *Isospora belli* infection associated with acalculous cholecystitis in a patient with AIDS. Ann Intern Med 121:663, 1994.
119. Liebman WM, Thaler MM, DeLorimier A, et al: Intractable diarrhea of infancy due to intestinal coccidiosis. Gastroenterology 78:579, 1980.
120. Forthal DN, Guest SS: *Isospora belli* enteritis in three homosexual men. Am J Trop Med Hyg 33:1060, 1984.
121. Pape JW, Johnson WD: *Isospora belli* infections. Prog Clin Parasitol 2:119, 1991.
122. Pape JW, Verdier R, Johnson WD, et al: Treatment and prophylaxis of *Isospora belli* infection. N Engl J Med 320:1044, 1989.
123. Weiss LM, Perlman DC, Sherman J, et al: *Isospora belli* infection: Treatment with pyrimethamine. Ann Intern Med 109:474, 1988.
124. Musey KL, Chidiac C, Beaucaire G, et al: Effectiveness of roxithromycin for treating *Isospora belli* infection. J Infect Dis 158:646, 1988.
125. Kayembe K, Desmet P, Henry MC, et al: Diclazuril for *Isospora belli* infection in AIDS. Lancet 1:1397, 1989.
126. Ma P, Kaufman D, Montana J: *Isospora belli* diarrheal infection in homosexual men. AIDS Res 1:327, 1984.

Cyclospora

127. Soave R, Dubey JP, Ramos LJ, et al: A new intestinal pathogen? Clin Res 34:533A, 1986.
128. Ashford RW: Occurrence of an undescribed coccidian in man in Papua New Guinea. Ann Trop Med Parasitol 73:497, 1979.
129. Centers for Disease Control and Prevention: Outbreaks of diarrheal illness associated with cyanobacteria (blue-green algae)–like bodies—Chicago and Nepal, 1989 and 1990. MMWR Morbid Mortal Wkly Rep 40:325, 1991.
130. Hoge CW, Shlim DR, Rajah R, et al: Epidemiology of diarrhoeal illness associated with a coccidian-like organism among travelers and foreign residents in Nepal. Lancet 341:1175, 1993.
131. Ortega YR, Sterling CR, Gilman RH, et al: *Cyclospora* species—A new protozoan pathogen of humans. N Engl J Med 328:1308, 1993.
132. Shlim DR, Cohen MT, Eaton M, et al: An alga-like organism associated with an outbreak of prolonged diarrhea among foreigners in Nepal. Am J Trop Med Hyg 45:383, 1991.
133. Ortega YR, Gilman RH, Sterling CR: A new coccidian parasite (Apicomplexa: Eimeriidae) from humans. J Parasitol 80:625, 1994.
134. Soave R: *Cyclospora*: An overview. Clin Infect Dis 23:429, 1996.
135. Taylor AP, Davis LJ, Soave R: *Cyclospora*. Curr Clin Topics Infect Dis (in press).
136. Long EG, White EH, Carmichael WW, et al: Morphologic and staining characteristics of a cyanobacterium-like organism associated with diarrhea. J Infect Dis 164:199, 1991.
137. Albert MJ, Kabir I, Azim T, et al: Diarrhea associated with *Cyclospora* sp. in Bangladesh. Diagn Microbiol Infect Dis 19:47, 1994.
138. Pape JW, Verdier RI, Boncy M, et al: *Cyclospora* infection in adults infected with HIV: Clinical manifestations, treatment, prophylaxis. Ann Intern Med 121:654, 1994.
139. Hoge CW, Echeverria P, Rajah R, et al: Prevalence of *Cyclospora* species and other enteric pathogens among children less than 5 years old in Nepal. J Clin Microbiol 33:3058, 1995.
139a. Ooi WW, Zimmerman SK, Needham CA: *Cyclospora* species as a gastrointestinal pathogen in immunocompetent hosts. J Clin Microbiol 33:1267, 1995.
139b. Clarke SC, McIntyre M: The incidence of *Cyclospora cayetanensis* in stool specimens submitted to a district general hospital. Epidemiol Infect 117:189, 1996.
139c. Centers for Disease Control and Prevention: Outbreaks of *Cyclospora cayetanensis* infection—United States, 1996. MMWR 45:549, 1996.
139d. Centers for Disease Control and Prevention: Update: Outbreaks of *Cyclospora cayetanensis* infection—United States and Canada, 1996. MMWR Morbid Mortal Wkly Rep 45:611, 1996.
140. Rabold JG, Hoge CW, Shlim DR, et al: *Cyclospora* outbreak

associated with chlorinated drinking water. Lancet 344:1360, 1994.
141. Connor BA, Shlim DR, Sholes JV, et al: Pathologic changes in the small bowel in nine patients with diarrhea associated with a coccidia-like body. Ann Intern Med 119:377, 1993.
142. Bendall RP, Lucas S, Moody A, et al: Diarrhoea associated with cyanobacterium-like bodies: A new coccidian enteritis of man. Lancet 341:590, 1993.
142a. Sifuentes-Osornio J, Porras-Cortes G, Bendall RP, et al: *Cyclospora cayetanensis* infection in patients with and without AIDS: Biliary disease as another clinical manifestation. Clin Infect Dis 21:1092, 1995.
143. Madico G, Gilman RH, Miranda E, et al: Treatment of *Cyclospora* infections with co-trimoxazole. Lancet 342:122, 1993.
144. Berlin OG, Novak SM, Porschen RK, et al: Recovery of *Cyclospora* organisms from patients with prolonged diarrhea. Clin Infect Dis 18:606, 1994.
145. Hoge CW, Shlim DR, Ghimire M, et al: Placebo-controlled trial of co-trimoxazole for *Cyclospora* infections among travellers and foreign residents in Nepal. Lancet 345:691, 1995.
146. Wurtz RM, Kocka FE, Peters CS, et al: Clinical characteristics of seven cases of diarrhea associated with a novel acid-fast organism in the stool. Clin Infect Dis 16:136, 1993.
147. Hart AS, Ridinger MT, Soundaralan R, et al: Novel organism associated with chronic diarrhoea in AIDS. Lancet 335:169, 1990.

Microsporidia

148. Canning EU: Microsporidia. *In* Kreier JP, Baker JR (eds): Parasitic Protozoa, Vol 6. San Diego, CA, Academic Press, 1993, pp 299–370.
149. Canning EU, Lom J, Dykova I: The Microsporidia of Vertebrates. New York, Academic Press, 1986.
150. Matsubayashi H, Koike T, Mikata T, et al: A case of *Encephalitozoon*-like body infection in man. Arch Pathol 67:181, 1959.
151. Bryan RT, Cali A, Owen RL, et al: Microsporidia: Opportunistic pathogens in patients with AIDS. Prog Clin Parasitol 2:1, 1991.
152. Shadduck JA: Human microsporidiosis and AIDS. Rev Infect Dis 11:203, 1989.
153. Mannheimer SB, Soave R: Protozoal infections in patients with AIDS. Infect Dis Clin North Am 8:483, 1994.
154. Weber R, Bryan RT, Schwartz DA, et al: Human microsporidial infections. Clin Microbiol Rev 7:426, 1994.
155. Hartskeerl RA, van Gool T, Schuitema ARJ, et al: Genetic and immunological characterization of the microsporidian *Septata intestinalis* Cali, Kotler and Orenstein, 1993: Reclassification to *Encephalitozoon intestinalis*. Parasitology 110(pt 3):277, 1995.
155a. Silveira H, Canning EU: *Vittaforma corneae* n. comb. for the human microsporidium *Nosema corneum* Shadduck, Meccoli, Davis and Font, 1990, based on its ultrastructure in the liver of experimentally infected athymic mice. J Eukkaryot Microbiol 42:158, 1995.
156. Hollister WS, Canning EU, Weidner E, et al: Development and ultrastructure of *Trachipleistophora hominis*, n.g., n.sp. after in vitro isolation from an AIDS patient and inoculation into athymic mice. Parasitology 112:143, 1996.
157. Cali A: General microsporidian features and recent findings on AIDS isolates. J Protozool 38:625, 1991.
158. Bryan RT, Weber R: Microsporidia: Emerging pathogens in immunodeficient persons. Arch Pathol Lab Med 117:1243, 1993.
159. Eeftinck Schattenkerk JKM, van Gool T, van Ketel RJ, et al: Clinical significance of small-intestinal microsporidiosis in HIV-1–infected individuals. Lancet 337:895, 1991.
160. Kotler DP, Francisco A, Clayton F, et al: Small intestinal injury and parasitic diseases in AIDS. Ann Intern Med 113:444, 1990.
161. Lucas SB, Papadaki C, Conlon N, et al: Diagnosis of intestinal microsporidiosis in patients with AIDS. J Clin Pathol 42:885, 1989.
162. Molina JM, Sarfati C, Beauvis B, et al: Intestinal microsporidiosis in human immunodeficiency virus–infected patients with chronic unexplained diarrhea: Prevalence and clinical and biologic features. J Infect Dis 167:217, 1993.
163. Orenstein JM, Chiang J, Steinberg W, et al: Intestinal microsporidiosis as a cause of diarrhea in human immunodeficiency virus–infected patients: A report of 20 cases. Hum Pathol 21:475, 1990.
164. Kotler DP, Orenstein JM: Prevalence of intestinal microsporidiosis in HIV-infected individuals referred for gastroenterological evaluation. Am J Gastroenterol 89:1998, 1994.
165. Weber R, Bryan RT, Owen C, et al: Improved light microscopical detection of microsporidia spores in stool and duodenal aspirates. N Engl J Med 326:161, 1992.
166. Rabeneck L, Gyorkey F, Genta RM, et al: The role of microsporidia in the pathogenesis of HIV-related chronic diarrhea. Ann Intern Med 119:895, 1993.
167. Bouchaud O, Houze M, Saada J, et al: Intestinal microsporidiosis in AIDS patients: High percentage of asymptomatic carriers (Abstr PO-B10-1509). Presented at the Ninth International Conference on AIDS; June 1993; Berlin, Germany; p 387.
168. Rabeneck L, Genta RM, Gyorkey F, et al: Observations on the pathological spectrum and clinical course of microsporidiosis in men infected with the human immunodeficiency virus: Follow-up study. Clin Infect Dis 20:1229, 1995.
169. Asmuth DM, DeGirolami PC, Federman M, et al: Clinical features of microsporidiosis in patients with AIDS. Clin Infect Dis 18:819, 1993.
170. Avery SW, Undeen AH: The isolation of microsporidia and other pathogens from concentrated ditch water. J Am Mosq Control Assoc 3:54, 1987.
171. Canning EU, Hollister WS: *Enterocytozoon bieneusi* (Microspora): Prevalence and pathogenicity in AIDS patients. Trans R Soc Trop Med Hyg 84:181, 1990.
172. Desportes I, LeCharpentier Y, Galian A, et al: Occurrence of a new microsporidian: *Enterocytozoon bieneusi* n.g., n. sp., in the enterocytes of a human patient with AIDS. J Protozool 32:250, 1985.
173. Kotler DP, Reka S, Chow K, et al: Effects of enteric parasitoses and HIV infection upon small intestinal structure and function in patients with AIDS. J Clin Gastroenterol 16:10, 1993.
174. Orenstein JM, Tenner M, Kotler DP: Localization of infection by the microsporidian *Enterocytozoon bieneusi* in the gastrointestinal tract of AIDS patients with diarrhea. AIDS 6:195, 1992.
175. Pol S, Romana C, Richard S, et al: Microsporidia infection in patients with the human immunodeficiency virus and unexplained cholangitis. N Engl J Med 328:95, 1993.
176. Orenstein JM: Microsporidiosis in the acquired immunodeficiency syndrome. J Parasitol 77:843, 1991.
177. McWhinney PHM, Nathwani D, Green ST, et al: Microsporidiosis detected in association with AIDS-related sclerosing cholangitis. AIDS 5:1394, 1991.
178. Weber R, Herbert K, Keller R, et al: Pulmonary and intestinal microsporidiosis in a patient with the acquired immunodeficiency syndrome. Am Rev Respir Dis 146:1603, 1992.
179. Cali A, Kotler DP, Orenstein JM: *Septata intestinalis* N.G., N. Sp., an intestinal microsporidian associated with chronic diarrhea and dissemination in AIDS patients. J Eukaryot Microbiol 40:101, 1993.
180. Orenstein JM, Tenner M, Cali A, et al: A microsporidian previously undescribed in humans, infecting enterocytes and macrophages, and associated with diarrhea in an acquired immunodeficiency patient. Hum Pathol 23:722, 1992.
181. Orenstein JM, Dieterich DT, Kotler DP: Systemic dissemination by a newly recognized intestinal microsporidia species in AIDS. AIDS 6:1143, 1992.
182. Didier ES, Rogers LB, Orenstein JM, et al: Characterization of *Encephalitozoon (Septata) intestinalis* isolates cultured from nasal mucosa and bronchioalveolar lavage fluids of two AIDS patients. J Eukaryot Microbiol 43:34, 1996.
183. Field A, Hing M, Milliken S, et al: Microsporidia in the small intestine of HIV infected patients: A new diagnostic technique and a new species. Med J Aust 158:390, 1993.
184. Wanke CA, Mattia AR: A 36-year-old man with AIDS, increase in chronic diarrhea, and intermittent fever and chills. N Engl J Med 329:1946, 1993.
185. Cali A, Meisler D, Lowder CY, et al: Corneal microsporidioses: Characterization and identification. J Protozool 38:215S, 1991.
186. Didier ES, Didier PJ, Friedberg DN, et al: Isolation and characterization of a new human microsporidian, *Encephalitozoon hellem* (n sp), from three patients with keratoconjunctivitis. J Infect Dis 163:617, 1991.
187. Friedberg DN, Stenson SM, Orenstein JM, et al: Microsporidial keratoconjunctivitis in the acquired immunodeficiency syndrome. Arch Ophthalmol 108:504, 1990.

188. Metcalfe TW, Doran RML, Rowlands PL, et al: Microsporidial keratoconjunctivitis in a patient with AIDS. Br J Ophthalmol 76:177, 1992.
189. Orenstein JM, Seedor J, Friedberg DN, et al: Microsporidian keratoconjunctivitis in patients with AIDS. MMWR Morbid Mortal Wkly Rep 39:188, 1990.
190. Weber R, Kuster H, Visvesvara GS, et al: Disseminated microsporidiosis due to *Encephalitozoon hellem*: Pulmonary colonization, microhematuria and mild conjunctivitis in a patient with AIDS. Clin Infect Dis 17:415, 1993.
191. Lacey CJN, Clark A, Frazer P, et al: Chronic microsporidian infection in the nasal mucosae, sinuses and conjunctivae in HIV disease. Genitourin Med 68:179, 1992.
192. Schwartz DA, Bryan RT, Hewan-Lowe KO, et al: Disseminated microsporidiosis *(Encephalitozoon hellem)* and acquired immunodeficiency syndrome. Arch Pathol Lab Med 116:660, 1992.
193. Terada S, Reddy R, Jeffers LJ, et al: Microsporidian hepatitis in the acquired immunodeficiency syndrome. Ann Intern Med 107:61, 1987.
194. Zender HO, Arrigoni E, Eckert J, et al: A case of *Encephalitozoon cuniculi* peritonitis in a patient with AIDS. Am J Clin Pathol 92:352, 1989.
195. Chupp GL, Alroy J, Adelman LS, et al: Myositis due to *Pleistophora* (microsporidia) in a patient with AIDS. Clin Infect Dis 16:15, 1993.
196. Ledford DK, Overman MD, Gonzalvo A, et al: Microsporidiosis myositis in a patient with acquired immunodeficiency syndrome. Ann Intern Med 102:628, 1985.
197. Weber R, Sauer B, Luthy R, et al: Intestinal coinfection with *Enterocytozoon bieneusi* and *Cryptosporidium* in a human immunodeficiency virus–infected child with chronic diarrhea. Clin Infect Dis 17:480, 1993.
198. Bergquist NR, Stintzing G, Smedman L, et al: Diagnosis of encephalitozoonosis in man by serological tests. Br Med J 288:902, 1984.
199. Ashton N, Wirasinha PA: Encephalitozoonosis (nosematosis) of the cornea. Br J Ophthalmol 57:669, 1973.
200. Pinnolis M, Egbert PR, Font RI, et al: Nosematosis of the cornea. Arch Ophthalmol 99:1044, 1981.
201. Ryan N, Sutherland G, Coughlan K, et al: A new trichrome-blue stain for detection of microsporidial species in urine, stool, and nasopharyngeal specimens. J Clin Microbiol 31:3264, 1993.
202. Van Gool T, Canning EU, Dankert J: An improved practical and sensitive technique for the detection of microsporidian spores in stool samples. Trans R Soc Trop Med Hyg 88:189, 1994.
203. Van Gool T, Sniders F, Eeftinck Schattenkerk J, et al: Diagnosis of intestinal and disseminated microsporidial infections in patients with HIV by a new rapid fluorescent technique. J Clin Pathol 46:694, 1985.
204. Vavra J, Chalupsky J: Fluorescence staining of microsporidian spores with the brightener "calciofluor white M2R." J Protozool 29:503, 1982.
205. Aldras AM, Didier ES, Orenstein JM, et al: Detection of microsporidia by indirect immunofluorescent antibody test using polyclonal and monoclonal antibodies. J Clin Microbiol 32:608, 1994.
206. Schwartz DA, Visvesvara GS, Diesenhouse MC, et al: Pathologic features and immunofluorescent antibody demonstration of ocular microsporidiosis *(Encephalitozoon hellem)* in seven patients with acquired immunodeficiency syndrome. Am J Ophthalmol 115:285, 1993.
207. Weber R, Muller A, Spycher MA, et al: Intestinal *Enterocytozoon bieneusi* microsporidiosis in an HIV-infected patient: Diagnosis by ileo-colonoscopic biopsies and long-term follow-up. Clin Invest 70:1019, 1992.
208. Peacock CS, Blanshard C, Tovey DG, et al: Histological diagnosis of intestinal microsporidiosis in patients with AIDS. J Clin Pathol 44:558, 1991.
209. Giang TT, Kotler DP, Garro ML, et al: Tissue diagnosis of intestinal microsporidiosis using the chromotrope-2R modified trichrome stain. Arch Pathol Lab Med 117:1249, 1993.
210. Rijpstra AC, Canning EU, van Ketel RJ, et al: Use of light microscopy to diagnose small-intestinal microsporidiosis in AIDS. J Infect Dis 157:827, 1988.
211. Schwartz DA, Visvesvara GS, Leitch GJ, et al: Pathology of symptomatic microsporidial (*Encephalitozoon hellem*) bronchiolitis in AIDS: A new respiratory pathogen diagnosed from lung biopsy, bronchoalveolar lavage, sputum, and tissue culture. Hum Pathol 24:937, 1993.
212. Shadduck JA, Meccoli RA, Davis R, et al: First isolation of a microsporidian from a human patient. J Infect Dis 162:773, 1990.
213. De Groote MA, Visvesvara G, Wilson ML, et al: Polymerase chain reaction and culture confirmation of disseminated *Encephalitozoon cuniculi* in a patient with AIDS: Successful therapy with albendazole. J Infect Dis 171:1375, 1995.
214. Weiss LM, Cali A, Levee E, et al: Diagnosis of *Encephalitozoon cuniculi* infection by Western blot and the use of cross-reactive antigens for the possible detection of microsporidiosis in humans. Am J Trop Med Hyg 47:456, 1992.
215. Blanshard C, Ellis DS, Tovey DG, et al: Treatment of intestinal microsporidiosis with albendazole in patients with AIDS. AIDS 6:311, 1992.
216. Dieterich DT, Lew EA, Kotler DP, et al: Treatment with albendazole for intestinal disease due to *Enterocytozoon bieneusi* in patients with AIDS. J Infect Dis 169:178, 1994.
217. Blanshard C, Gazzard BG: Microsporidiosis in HIV-1–infected individuals (Letter). Lancet 337:1488, 1991.
218. Anwar-Bruni DM, Hogan SE, Schwartz DA, et al: Atovaquone is effective treatment for the symptoms of gastrointestinal microsporidiosis in HIV-1–infected patients. AIDS 10:19, 1996.
219. Diesenhouse MD, Wilson LA, Corrent GF, et al: Treatment of microsporidial keratoconjunctivitis with topical fumagillin. Am J Ophthalmol 115:293, 1993.
220. Yee RW, Tio FO, Martinez JA, et al: Resolution of microsporidial epithelial keratopathy in a patient with AIDS. Ophthalmology 98:196, 1991.
221. Sandfort J, Hannemann A, Stark D, et al: *Enterocytozoon bieneusi* infection in an immunocompetent HIV-negative patient with acute diarrhea. Clin Infect Dis 19:514, 1994.
222. Margileth AM, Strano AJ, Chandra R, et al: Disseminated nosematosis in an immunologically compromised infant. Arch Pathol 95:145, 1973.

Dientamoeba fragilis

223. Weynon CM: Observations on the common intestinal protozoa of man: Their diagnosis and pathogenicity. Lancet 2:1173, 1915.
224. Jepps MW, Dobell C: *Dientamoeba fragilis*, n.g. n.w., a new intestinal amoeba from man. Parasitology 10:352, 1918.
225. Kean BH, Malloch CL: The neglected ameba: *Dientamoeba fragilis*. A report of 100 "pure" infections. Am J Dig Dis 11:735, 1966.
226. Yang J, Scholten T: *Dientamoeba fragilis*: A review with notes on its epidemiology, pathogenicity, modes of transmission, and diagnosis. Am J Trop Med 26:16, 1977.
227. Spencer MJ, Garcia LS, Chapin MR: *Dientamoeba fragilis*. An intestinal pathogen in children? Am J Dis Child 133:390, 1979.
228. Shein R, Gelb A: Colitis due to *Dientamoeba fragilis*. Am J Gastroenterol 78:634, 1983.
229. Grendon JH, Digiacomo RF, Frost FJ: *Dientamoeba fragilis* detection methods and prevalence: A survey of state public health laboratories. Public Health Rep 106:322, 1991.
230. Millet V, Spencer MJ, Chapin M, et al: *Dientamoeba fragilis*, a protozoan parasite in adult members of a semicommunal group. Dig Dis Sci 28:335, 1983.
231. Drugs for parasitic infections. Med Lett Drugs Ther 37:99, 1995.

OTHER PARASITES

293

Intestinal Nematodes

Davidson H. Hamer
Dickson D. Despommier

Roundworms are members of the phylum Nematoda and include free-living and parasitic species that are widely distributed in nature. The diseases they cause rank among the most prevalent communicable diseases, with an estimated 1 billion or more individuals affected.[1] The geographic distribution of roundworms in many tropical and subtropical regions closely parallels socioeconomic and sanitary conditions. In locales where several species of intestinal parasites are found, coinfection with *Ascaris lumbricoides, Trichuris trichiura,* and hookworms is common. Although many subjects may have asymptomatic infections, some individuals with a high worm burden, especially children, may suffer significant morbidity including anemia, malnutrition, and retardation of both physical and cognitive development. Constant reinfection is common in most endemic areas; thus, periodic treatment regimens that result in reductions in parasitic burden may be more practical than attempts to completely eliminate infection.

Understanding the life cycles of roundworms responsible for human infection is important because certain species can be readily transmitted directly from person to person, whereas other species must undergo a cycle of maturation outside of the human host before they can again become infective to humans. Furthermore, pathologic consequences of infection with individual nematode species frequently result from interactions between certain stages of the organism and the host's immune responses. Relevant aspects of the life cycles of the major intestinal nematodes are outlined in Table 293–1. Nematodes reproduce sexually; species identification is frequently dependent on the adult worm's morphologic features. With the exceptions of *Strongyloides stercoralis* and *Capillaria philippinensis*, roundworms are not capable of multiplying within their respective host.

Trichuriasis (*Trichuris trichiura*)

This nematode species is commonly known as the whipworm because of the characteristic shape of the adult worm. It is responsible for an estimated 800 million human infections worldwide, with the greatest frequency in regions that have warm, moist environments. In certain parts of Southeast Asia, Africa, and many island communities in the Caribbean, the prevalence of trichuriasis approaches 80%.[2] Polyparasitism with *Ascaris* and hookworms is common. Children tend to have a greater intensity of infection than do adults living in the same environment and are thus more likely to develop symptomatic disease and to have significant morbidity. This is true even compared with adults with similar worm burdens.

Life Cycle

Humans are the only host of *T. trichuris*, and infection is acquired by direct transmission through the oral route. Although other species of *Trichuris* have been found in a number of mammalian species, they appear to maintain host specificity with the possible exception of *Trichuris vulpis*. This canine species has been rarely described as a cause of human infection.[3] Adult worms reside in the cecum and transverse and descending colon; involvement of the sigmoid and rectum occurs in heavy infections. The female worm has an estimated life span of 1 to 2 years, usually measures 35 to 50 mm in length, and produces 3000 to 10,000 eggs per day.[2] Although the worm appears to disrupt the colonic mucosa, minimal epithelial disruption and little inflammation are visible on histopathologic examination.[4]

After excretion into the external environment, the eggs require about 21 days to embryonate and form an infectious first-stage larva. After the embryonated egg is ingested, the larva hatches in the small intestine and undergoes four molts; then the immature adult is passively transported to the large intestine, where the long, narrow, anterior portion of its body embeds in the intestinal mucosa. It takes approximately 90 days from the time of egg ingestion to the production of new ova by mature worms.

Epidemiology

Infection with *T. trichiura* is most common in areas of the world that are impoverished and lack adequate sanitary facilities. Soil pollution by infected human feces is integral to the continued spread of this ubiquitous organism. Infection results from ingestion of embryonated eggs after direct contamination of hands, food, or drink with infested soil or indirect transmission by insects, domestic animals, or dust. Given appropriate conditions, the *Trichuris* eggs can survive for prolonged periods in moist soil. The intensity of infection in many individuals is light. Young children tend to have

TABLE 293–1 ■ Life Cycle Characteristics of the Major Intestinal Nematodes

ORGANISM	MODE OF TRANSMISSION	INFECTIVE STAGE	HOST TISSUE INVOLVED	FINAL HABITAT	TYPICAL LIFE SPAN
Trichuris trichiura	Direct oral	Eggs	Intestine	Cecum, ascending colon	1–2 y
Ascaris lumbricoides	Direct oral	Eggs	Lung, intestine	Jejunum, ileum	1–2 y
Ancylostoma duodenale	Percutaneous, oral	Filariform larvae	Skin, lung, intestine	Jejunum	5 y
Necator americanus	Percutaneous	Filariform larvae	Skin, lung, intestine	Jejunum	4 y
Enterobius vermicularis	Direct oral	Eggs	Intestine	Colon	37–93 d
Strongyloides stercoralis	Percutaneous, autoinfection	Filariform larvae	Skin, lung, intestine	Duodenum, jejunum	Unknown

TABLE 293–2 ■ Diagnosis and Treatment of Major Intestinal Nematode Infections

ORGANISM	TYPE OF SPECIMEN	SPECIMEN PREPARATION	SIZE OF EGGS OR LARVAE (μm)	DRUG OF CHOICE	ALTERNATIVE THERAPIES
Trichuris trichiura	Stool	Direct smear or concentration	50–54 × 23	Mebendazole, 100 mg orally (PO) twice daily (bid) × 3 d	Albendazole,* 400 mg PO once
Ascaris lumbricoides	Stool	Direct smear or concentration	45–70 × 35–50	Mebendazole, 100 mg PO bid × 3 d *or* Albendazole,* 400 mg PO once *or* Pyrantel pamoate, 11 mg/kg PO once (max 1 g)	Piperazine citrate, 75 mg/kg bid (max 1 g) by nasogastric tube × 2–3 d until resolution of obstruction
Ancylostoma duodenale *Necator americanus*	Stool	Direct smear or concentration	55–70 × 35–45	Mebendazole, 100 mg PO bid × 3 d	Albendazole,* 400 mg PO once *or* Pyrantel pamoate, 11 mg/kg PO × 3 d (max 1 g)
Enterobius vermicularis	Adhesive tape preparation	Direct microscopy	50–60 × 20–30	Mebendazole, 100 mg PO once *or* Pyrantel pamoate, 11 mg/kg PO once Repeat in 2 wk	Albendazole,* 400 mg PO once Repeat in 2 wk
Strongyloides stercoralis	Stool, duodenal aspirate	Concentration or Baermann method	400–500 × 15	Thiabendazole, 25 mg/kg PO bid × 2 d (max 3 g/d)	Ivermectin, 150–200 μg/kg PO × 1–2 d

*Drug has received approval from the U.S. Food and Drug Administration only for the treatment of neurocysticercosis and echinococcosis in the United States.

heavier worm burdens and, consequently, are more likely to suffer from symptomatic infections.

The prevalence of trichuriasis ranges from 1% in the United States, Western Europe, and Japan to as high as 20% to 80% in regions of the developing world. Treatment and control measures initiated earlier in this century resulted in significant reductions in the prevalence of this infection in the United States.[5] Nevertheless, moderate rates of infection still persist in rural areas of the Southeast, young Puerto Rican children, and recent immigrants.

Clinical Manifestations

The majority of *T. trichiura* infections are asymptomatic, with the parasite discovered only on routine stool examinations. Patients with heavy, chronic infections tend to be young children mainly in the 4- to 10-year age range.[2] They may develop a chronic dysentery syndrome characterized by protracted bloody diarrhea, abdominal pain, nausea, vomiting, iron deficiency anemia, and protracted tenesmus leading to rectal prolapse.[6] Prolonged infections may result in clubbing, severe malnutrition, pica, stunting of growth, and congestive heart failure secondary to severe anemia. Eosinophilia is relatively uncommon. Specific anthelmintic chemotherapy results in the resolution of these long-term complications, although reinfection is common.

The anemia associated with trichuriasis, although generally less intense than hookworm anemia, may be severe. Hemorrhage appears to result from local mucosal damage at the site of attachment, but the worm is unable to ingest blood directly because of its capillary esophagus. An estimated 0.005 mL of blood is lost daily for each adult worm.[7] Although this rate of blood loss may not be sufficient to cause severe anemia, the presence of malnutrition and polyparasitism may predispose children to its development.

Diagnosis

The diagnosis is established by the demonstration of characteristic lemon-shaped ova by fecal examination (Table 293–2). The ova have a characteristic barrel shape with a thick outer shell and two terminal polar plugs (Fig. 293–1). A simple smear technique is usually adequate because the rates of egg excretion tend to be high. Although the diagnosis can usually be made with a single specimen, the evaluation of multiple stools is warranted given the high frequency of coinfection with pathogenic protozoa. Heavy infection with *T. trichiura* can be detected by anoscopic visualization of worms embedded in the rectal mucosa.[8]

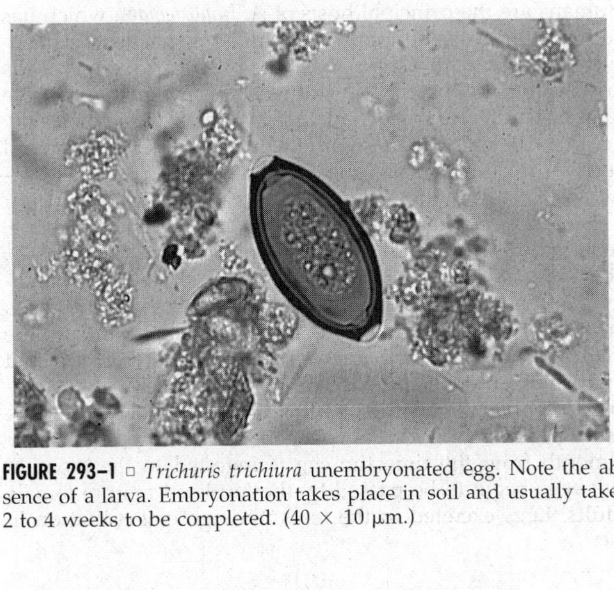

FIGURE 293–1 □ *Trichuris trichiura* unembryonated egg. Note the absence of a larva. Embryonation takes place in soil and usually takes 2 to 4 weeks to be completed. (40 × 10 μm.)

Treatment

Early chemotherapeutic agents for the treatment of this infection including hexylresorcinol enemas, dithiazanine, and thiabendazole were only partially effective. The benzimidazoles mebendazole and albendazole are currently the treatments of choice for trichuriasis (see Table 293–2). These drugs are well tolerated and do not require dosage adjustment for weight because they are poorly absorbed. Their use is not recommended in pregnancy and children younger than 1 year because of possible toxic and teratogenic effects. A 3-day course of mebendazole is highly effective, although rare treatment failures may require an additional round of therapy. Single-dose treatment regimens with albendazole (not an indication approved by the U.S. Food and Drug Administration) are convenient for control programs and may result in significant improvements in physical fitness, appetite, and growth in infected children.[9]

Prevention

Sanitary disposal of human feces is vital to the disruption of this parasite's life cycle. Contamination of produce with human excreta used for fertilization also serves to propagate the organism. Although the eggs are relatively resistant to chemical disinfectants, they can be destroyed by exposure to direct sunlight for 12 hours or temperatures below −80°C and above 40°C for 1 hour.

Ascariasis

The roundworm *A. lumbricoides* has a cosmopolitan distribution and is estimated to infect about one fourth of the world's population.[10] The highest prevalence is in tropical regions; nevertheless, ascariasis remains endemic in the southeastern United States.[5] Although the majority of infections are asymptomatic, *A. lumbricoides* may be responsible for significant morbidity including biliary, pancreatic, or pulmonary disease during larval migration, malabsorption, intestinal obstruction, and growth retardation.

The adult worms, which may attain a length of greater than 30 cm, reside in the small intestine, mainly in the jejunum and ileum. They maintain their position by continuously moving against peristalsis. The worms secrete an antitrypsin protease that allows them to compete for and use proteins ingested by the host.

Life Cycle

Humans are the principal hosts of *A. lumbricoides*, which has no reservoir hosts, although pigs can be infected experimentally. Infection with *Ascaris suum*, the pig ascarid, rarely leads to symptomatic disease.[11] Adult worms have an average life span of 1 to 2 years (see Table 293–1). The female worms lay 2 to 5 $\times$ 10^5 eggs per day, with the number of eggs produced per worm decreasing as the total intestinal worm load increases.[12]

A. lumbricoides larvae, on hatching in the small intestine, penetrate the wall and enter the blood stream (Fig. 293–2). They must then undergo development in the liver parenchyma, where they feed on "liver pâté" before migrating to the lungs. They are now third-stage larvae that return to the small intestine after the infected host coughs them up and complete their development to immature adult worms. Maturation to sexually mature worms takes several weeks. The entire process of worm morphogenesis takes approximately 1 month from the time the egg is ingested to the moment that eggs begin to be passed by the fertilized mature female adults. Eggs excreted in the feces undergo embryonation in soil within 2 to 4 weeks in warm, moist, well-oxygenated soils. In cooler climates, embryonation takes much longer. In any case, the eggs can survive in that state for months to years.

Epidemiology

The majority of the 1 billion people with ascariasis live in Southeast Asia, Africa, and Latin America. An estimated 4 million people are infected in the United States, where the greatest prevalence is in the rural Southeast. Infection with *A. lumbricoides* may occur at any age but is most common in children in the 3- to 14-year age group, which may have prevalence rates of 80% or higher in endemic regions.[10] Transmission is by the fecal-oral route and is sustained by the high egg output of the female worms and the longevity of eggs in the soil. Changes in the soil environment, such as lower temperature or humidity, may be responsible for seasonal breaks in transmission in certain geographic regions.

Clinical Manifestations and Pathogenesis

The intensity of the host response to the migrating *A. lumbricoides* larvae relates directly to the level of infection. Asymptomatic worm migration is common in light infections; heavier infestation may result in pulmonary, intestinal, biliary, and pancreatic manifestations. Infection does not result in meaningful protective immunity.

Previously exposed individuals may experience a hypersensitivity reaction in the lung during the migration of larvae through the lung tissue and tracheobronchial tree. The result is a Löffler-like syndrome characterized by a productive cough, dyspnea, wheezing, and fever that may be accompanied by angioedema or urticaria.[13] Transient pulmonary infiltrates may occur in association with the respiratory symptoms as well as eosinophilia, which may peak as the symptoms and infiltrates resolve. In endemic regions such as Saudi Arabia where the transmission of *A. lumbricoides* peaks from March through May, there may be a seasonal pneumonitis.[14] Histologic examination of the lung tissue reveals a focal alveolar exudate with an eosinophilic reaction and granuloma formation.

Light infections generally do not elicit any clinical or pathologic reactions in the intestine, although vague, crampy abdominal pain may occur. Large worm burdens may result in intestinal obstruction that is clinically manifested by diminished bowel sounds, vomiting, abdominal distention, pain, and radiographic evidence of bowel obstruction.[15] This complication is most common in young children and is usually localized to the ileum. Additional rare intestinal complications in heavily infected individuals include perforation, volvulus, intussusception, and appendicitis.

Aberrant migration of the worms into the biliary tract may lead to symptoms of biliary colic, acalculous cholangitis, ascending cholangitis, and even hepatic abscess formation.[16] Reinvasion of the biliary tree is common on reinfection in treated subjects, especially in those patients who have undergone endoscopic sphincterotomy. Pancreatitis and peritonitis are additional rare complications of errant worm migration.

Intense infections with *A. lumbricoides* in young children may lead to malabsorption and malnutrition secondary to anorexia, increased metabolism, and the consumption of vital nutrients by the worms.[17] Adverse consequences of these events include stunting of growth, vitamin deficiencies, steatorrhea, lactose intolerance, and protein-energy malnutrition. Although it is difficult to distinguish the influence of concomitant parasitic, bacterial, and viral infections on the development of these complications in endemic regions, ascariasis clearly plays a role.

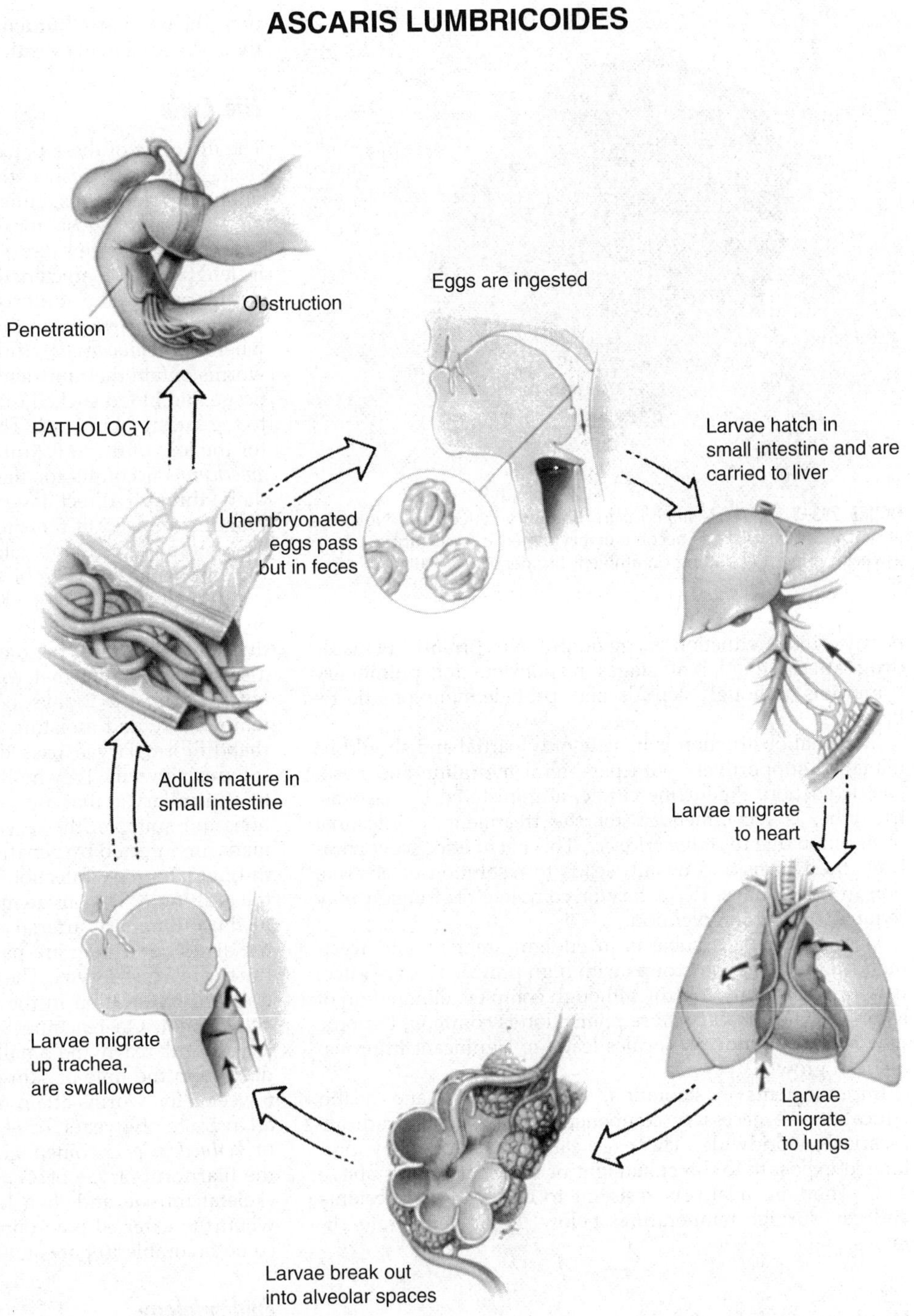
ASCARIS LUMBRICOIDES
Penetration
Obstruction
PATHOLOGY
Eggs are ingested
Larvae hatch in small intestine and are carried to liver
Unembryonated eggs pass but in feces
Adults mature in small intestine
Larvae migrate to heart
Larvae migrate up trachea, are swallowed
Larvae migrate to lungs
Larvae break out into alveolar spaces

FIGURE 293–2 □ *Ascaris lumbricoides* life cycle. (Illustration by John W. Karapelou. From Despommier DD, Gwadz RG, Hotez P: Parasitic Diseases, ed 3. New York, Springer-Verlag, 1995.)

Diagnosis

The high egg output (200,000 per day!) by each fertilized female worm makes a direct smear of stools sufficient for diagnosis in the majority of cases (see Table 293–2). Standard stool concentration techniques may be necessary in light infections. The fertilized, unembryonated eggs are oval with a characteristic thick, irregular cortical layer (Fig. 293–3). Egg counts are useful in clinical studies for estimating worm burden and the response to therapy.

The diagnosis of biliary or pancreatic ascariasis may be difficult because the worm may exit these tracts after producing symptoms. Cholangiography or endoscopic retrograde cholangiopancreatography may demonstrate the parasite. Barium studies of the gastrointestinal tract may reveal a luminal filling defect or ingestion of the barium into the adult worm's intestinal tract. The combination of shifting infiltrates on serial chest radiographs, peripheral eosinophilia, and presence of ascarid larvae in sputum is diagnostic of pulmonary ascariasis. This syndrome may be confused with strongyloidiasis, hookworm disease, tropical pulmonary eosinophilia, and acute schistosomiasis.

Therapy and Prevention

All cases of intestinal ascariasis should be treated because of the potential for multiple complications. Mebendazole and albendazole are the treatments of choice (see Table 293–2), although single-dose therapy with pyrantel pamoate is also highly effective.[18] A 3-day regimen of mebendazole results in

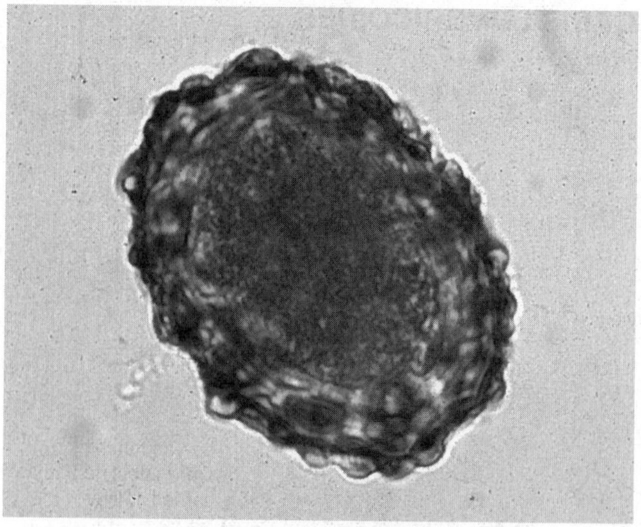

FIGURE 293–3 □ *Ascaris lumbricoides* unembryonated egg. Note the absence of a larva. Eggs become embryonated in soil during a 2- to 4-week period, depending on ambient temperatures. (40 × 10 μm.)

nearly a 100% reduction of egg output. No currently available drug affects the larval stages responsible for pulmonary symptoms, although steroids may provide symptomatic relief.

Intestinal obstruction is usually only partial and should be managed supportively with parenteral hydration and nasogastric suction. Piperazine citrate, administered by nasogastric tube, is recommended for the treatment of intestinal obstruction due to *A. lumbricoides*. This agent effectively paralyzes the worms and usually leads to resolution of obstruction in 2 to 3 days. Refractory or complete obstruction may require surgical intervention.

Mass therapy for subjects in endemic regions and treatments targeted at age groups with high prevalences are effective for community control, although complete elimination of ascariasis is difficult because reinfection is common. Periodic deworming in endemic locales leads to significant improvement in growth.[17]

Improvements in sanitation, water supplies, and health education are necessary components of a plan to eradicate ascariasis worldwide. The eggs can be destroyed by prolonged exposure to direct sunlight or by temperatures above 40°C. They are relatively resistant to chemical disinfectants and can survive temperatures below 0°C in temperate climates.

Hookworm Infection

An estimated 1 billion people worldwide are infected with the hookworms *Ancylostoma duodenale* and *Necator americanus*.[19] *N. americanus* is more commonly found in the Americas, equatorial Africa, Southeast Asia, Polynesia, and Australia; *A. duodenale* is more prevalent in northern Africa and north and southwest Asia.[20] Although the distributions of these two species were formerly thought to be discrete, surveys have shown that there is overlap in parts of Asia, Africa, and South America. *Ancylostoma ceylanicum*, a minor nematode species, is primarily a pathogen of large felines such as panthers and tigers that uncommonly infects humans in parts of Southeast Asia and Suriname. The adult worms of both species reside in the small intestine, mainly in the jejunum, where they feed on intestinal mucosa and blood. Although many individuals have light, asymptomatic infections, heavy worm burdens may result in significant morbidity and occasionally death.

Life Cycle

The life cycle of these parasites is similar to that of *A. lumbricoides* with the nuance that the infective larva penetrates unbroken skin, thus initiating infection (Fig. 293–4). There are no reservoir hosts for either species of hookworm.

The adult worms are small, ranging from 9 to 13 mm in length. The characteristic morphologic appearance of the mouth parts of the adult worms helps to differentiate the two species. *N. americanus* adults have rounded cutting plates, whereas *A. duodenale* adults have cutting teeth. The adult worms obtain their nutrients from the consumption of villous tissue and blood sucked directly from their site of attachment to the intestinal mucosa. The *A. duodenale* adult is responsible for the loss of 0.1 to 0.2 mL of blood per day; the adult of *N. americanus* accounts for the loss of 0.01 to 0.02 mL of blood daily through direct ingestion of blood and focal hemorrhages produced at the site of intestinal attachment.[21] Proteases and anticoagulants released by the worms play a role in the pathogenesis of the blood loss.[22]

Adult females of *A. duodenale* produce approximately 30,000 eggs per day, whereas females of *N. americanus* produce only 9000 eggs per day. Eggs passed in the feces contain a segmented ovum that will undergo larval maturation and hatch within 1 to 2 days in soil if the necessary conditions of temperature and moisture are present.[23] The freshly hatched rhabditiform larvae pass through a free-living cycle in the soil during which they molt twice and then become sheathed, filariform larvae that are infectious to humans. If soil conditions are suitable, the larvae may survive for months. Humans are infected by penetration of the skin, most commonly through the feet. Infection with *A. duodenale* may occur by the oral route. The larvae migrate through the venous system to the pulmonary arterial circulation where they cross into the alveoli and then are passively carried up the bronchi to the trachea and larynx. The migrating larvae of *N. americanus* undergo maturation in the lung, whereas those of *A. duodenale* do not. On reaching the pharynx, the larvae are swallowed and reach the small intestine approximately 3 to 5 days from the time of skin penetration. During the next 4 to 6 weeks, the worms attain full maturity. Intestinal survival is an average of 4 years for *N. americanus* or 5 years in the case of *A. duodenale*. In some regions where reinfection is common, the filariform larvae of *A. duodenale* may remain dormant in skeletal muscle and then later complete their development when the external environmental conditions have again become favorable to parasite development in the soil.[24]

Epidemiology

The prevalence of hookworm infection varies substantially from region to region, with rates as high as 90% described in some locales. The prevalence tends to be higher in rural than in urban areas, and therefore agricultural workers may have high rates of infection. The age-specific prevalence in tropical regions peaks in schoolchildren and then levels off in adulthood. Hookworm infections used to be common in the rural southeast of the United States and Puerto Rico, but the frequency has dropped as socioeconomic conditions have improved. Survival of hookworm larvae is optimal in moist, sandy, or loamy soil with ambient temperatures of 24°C to 32°C. The practices of using the same site for defecation and not wearing footwear facilitate infection. Because *A. duodenale* may also be acquired by the oral route, contamination of fresh produce with nightsoil may result in the transmission of hookworms.

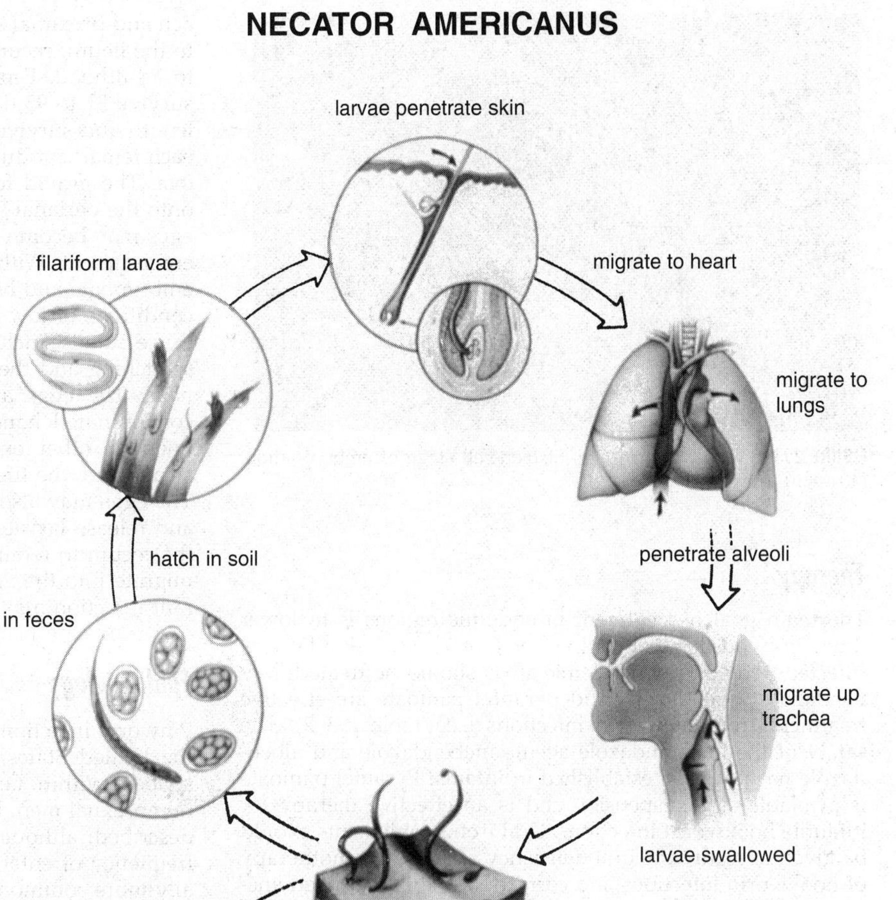

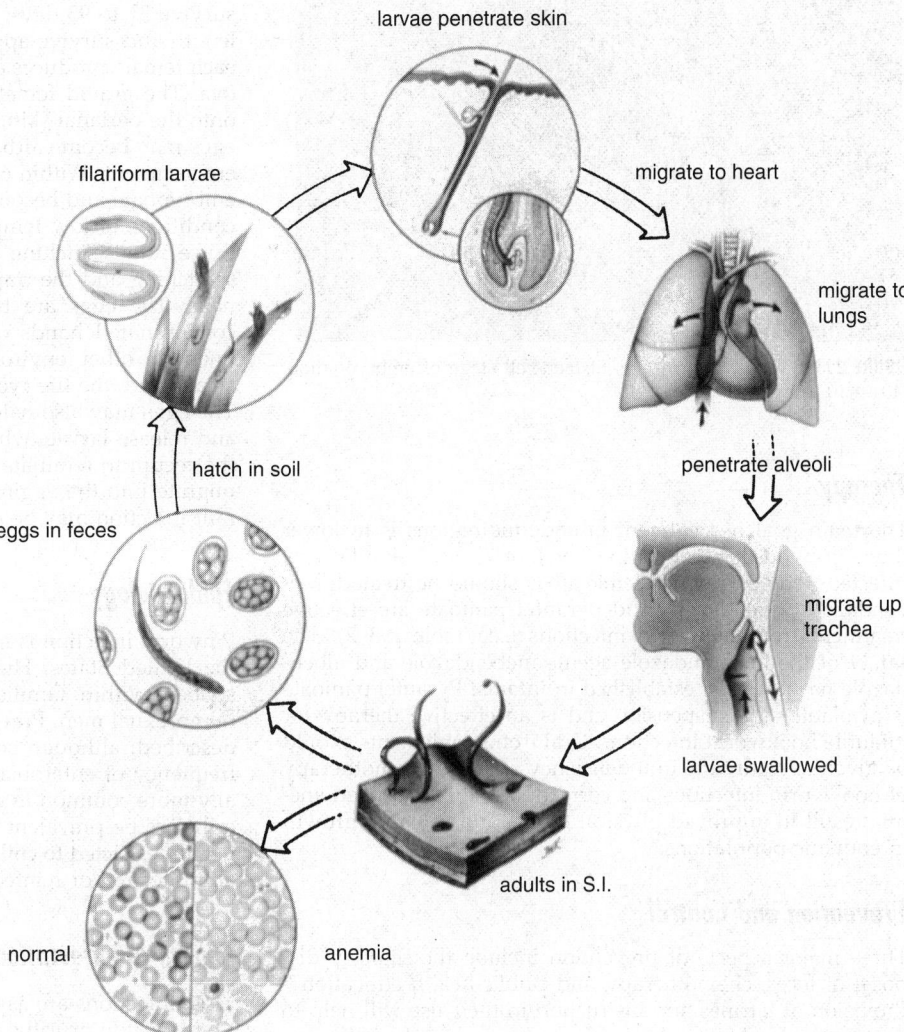

FIGURE 293–4 ▫ *Necator americanus* life cycle. (Illustration by John W. Karapelou. From Despommier DD, Gwadz RG, Hotez P: Parasitic Diseases, ed 3. New York, Springer-Verlag, 1995.)

Clinical Manifestations

A dermatitis characterized by intense pruritus, edema, and erythema followed later by a vesiculopapular eruption may occur at the skin entry site of the filariform larvae. This cutaneous manifestation of infection, known as ground itch or coolie's itch, may last as long as 2 weeks and is more common in individuals in endemic areas who are presensitized to hookworms. Although pulmonary symptoms may occur during the larval migration, they tend to be mild in comparison with *A. lumbricoides* unless the initial infection is heavy, in which case dyspnea and cough may occur.[25] During worm maturation in the small intestine, there may be abdominal pain, steatorrhea, and an intense peripheral eosinophilia with 1000 to 4000 cells per mm^3. Lighter worm burdens tend to result in no or only mild symptoms, whereas heavier infections may be complicated by severe iron deficiency anemia from chronic intestinal blood loss and hypoalbuminemia secondary to a protein-losing enteropathy. These complications may lead to fatigue, peripheral edema, dyspnea, high-output heart failure, loss of normal skin color, and other manifestations of chronic iron deficiency anemia. The hypoproteinemia that results from chronic infection may lead to a kwashiorkor-like state characterized by growth impairment, facial and lower extremity edema, dermatitis, and hair loss. Factors influencing the severity of anemia include the iron content of the individual's diet, the underlying iron stores, and the intensity and duration of infection. Chronic hookworm anemia may result in physical and intellectual growth retardation.[22]

Diagnosis

The diagnosis is established by the identification of characteristic hookworm eggs in direct stool smears (Fig. 293–5). Concentration techniques may be necessary in light infections (see Table 293–2). Fresh or preserved stool specimens should be examined because the eggs may hatch into rhabditiform larvae, which can be misinterpreted as *Strongyloides* larvae. Hookworm ova may be confused with those of *Oesophagostomum* species, which appear identical, or ova of *Trichostrongylus* species, which tend to be much larger. The examination of adult worms or third-stage larvae must be done to differentiate *A. duodenale* from *N. americanus*.

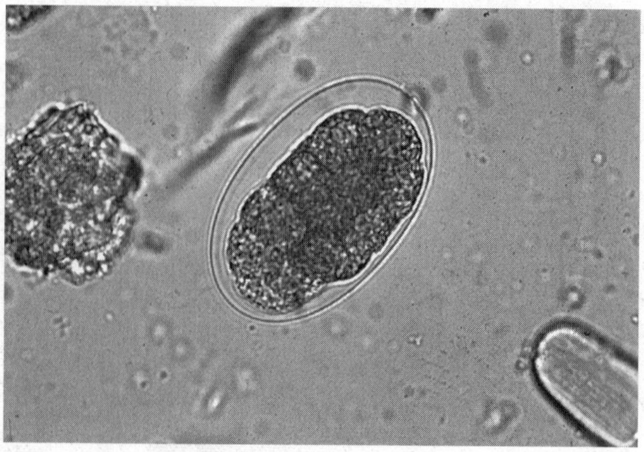

FIGURE 293–5 □ Hookworm egg. Sixteen-cell stage of embryonation. (40 × 10 μm.)

Therapy

The main goal of treatment in endemic regions is to lower the worm burden below the level of clinical significance. Infected people in nonendemic areas should be treated. Mebendazole, albendazole, and pyrantel pamoate are effective treatments for hookworm infections (see Table 293–2). The safety of the benzimidazole agents mebendazole and albendazole has not been established in infants. Pyrantel pamoate is available as a suspension and is an effective therapy for infantile hookworm infections. Oral iron supplements should be given to rectify the iron deficiency anemia. Chemotherapy of hookworm infections and correction of the associated anemia result in improved physical fitness and catch-up growth in endemic populations.[9, 22]

Prevention and Control

Three major aspects of prevention include the sanitary disposal of feces, chemotherapy, and public health education.[23] Provision of latrines and instruction in their use will help to contain the hookworm larvae. In regions where fresh human fecal matter is used as manure, it should be treated to kill the larvae by composting or the addition of chemicals such as sodium nitrate, ammonium sulfate, or calcium superphosphate. Protective footwear and education about the mode of transmission may also be helpful in geographic locales where percutaneous rather than oral transmission is more common.

Enterobiasis

Human infection with *Enterobius vermicularis*, the pinworm, dates back many millennia BC. This organism is found worldwide with a greater prevalence in temperate regions than in the tropics. *E. vermicularis* is the most common intestinal nematode in the United States, where an estimated 20 to 42 million people are infected.[26] This parasite has managed to persist despite modern advances in hygiene, sanitation, and standards of living. Infection with pinworms is generally not associated with significant morbidity, although it may cause social stigmata in certain populations.

Life Cycle

Humans are the only host to *E. vermicularis*; no reservoir host is known. The life cycle is a direct one, beginning with the ingestion of the embryonated eggs. They hatch in the stomach and proximal small intestine, and the larvae then migrate to the ileum, cecum, appendix, and colon where they mature to adulthood. Females measure 8 to 13 mm in length and survive 37 to 93 days; the males are smaller at 2 to 5 mm in length and survive approximately 50 days. After copulation, each female produces about 10,000 fertilized, unembryonated ova. The gravid females migrate at night through the anus onto the perianal skin, lay their eggs, and then die. The light eggs may become airborne and settle on surfaces of the local environment. Within 6 hours of deposition, the eggs rapidly embryonate and become infective. Egg survival is optimal in conditions of low temperature and high humidity. The eggs cause intense itching of the perianal area, which leads to scratching and the trapping of eggs under the host's fingernails. The eggs are transmitted directly to the mouth by contaminated hands or food or by exposure to soiled bed linen or other environmental sources. Once the eggs are swallowed, the life cycle takes 4 to 6 weeks to be completed. The eggs may also hatch on the skin at the site of deposition and release larvae, which migrate in a retrograde fashion to the cecum to reinitiate infection. Freshly hatched larvae may migrate into the vagina of women and girls, where an aberrant infection may be established.

Epidemiology

Pinworm infection is most common in school-age children in the United States. High infection rates have also been described within families, institutionalized populations, and homosexual men. Prevalence rates of 16% to 100% have been described, although some surveys indicate a decline in the frequency of enterobiasis.[27] Although this infection is generally more common in cooler, temperate climates, it may nevertheless be prevalent in some tropical locales where it may not be restricted to children.[28] Persistent infections result from autoinfection or reinfection from family members.

Clinical Manifestations and Pathology

Most infections are asymptomatic. The most common symptoms include pruritus ani and perineal itching. Infected children may rarely be troubled by insomnia, restlessness, irritability, anorexia, weight loss, and emotional lability.[29] Scratching may lead to excoriation and secondary infection. Aberrant migration of the adult pinworms may lead to vulvovaginitis and an increased frequency of urinary tract infections in prepubertal girls. Ectopic migration followed by the death of the worm and the formation of granulomata has been described in the cervix, uterus, fallopian tubes, ovary, peritoneum, prostate, lung, liver, kidney, and spleen.

Although *E. vermicularis* is occasionally found in inflamed appendices, its role in the pathogenesis of appendicitis remains controversial. No significant intestinal disease has been attributed to pinworm infection.

Diagnosis

Identification of adult worms or eggs in specimens taken from the perianal or, less commonly, the vaginal region establishes the diagnosis (Fig. 293–6; see Table 293–2). In suspected cases, transparent adhesive tape preparations should be taken from the perianal skin shortly after the patient awakens on successive days. If five or more consecutive tape test results are negative, the diagnosis is virtually excluded. Stool specimens provide a diagnosis in only 5% to 15% of infected patients and therefore are not reliable. Eosinophilia has not been attributed to enterobiasis.

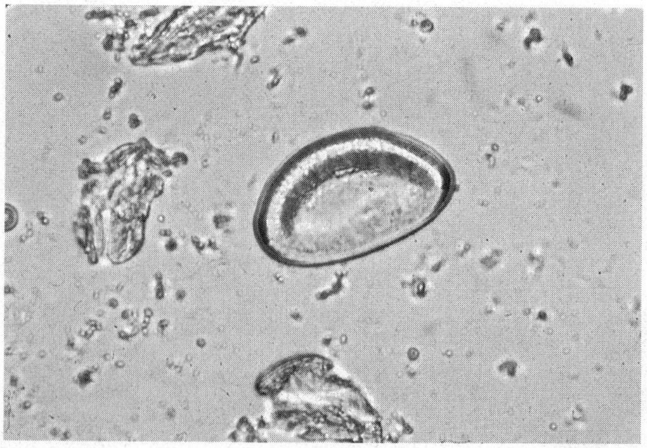

FIGURE 293–6 □ *Enterobius vermicularis* embryonated egg. Note larva inside. (40 × 10 μm.)

Treatment

A single dose of mebendazole or pyrantel pamoate is effective (see Table 293–2) and should be repeated in 2 to 3 weeks to eliminate reinfection. All family members or subjects within an institution should be treated simultaneously to eradicate other reservoirs of infection. Parents of infected children should be reassured that this is not a serious infection and should be educated about the importance of careful hygienic measures.

Strongyloidiasis

S. stercoralis was first described in the 19th century in French army personnel returning from Indochina. It remains a significant cause of disease in many tropical and subtropical regions and, less commonly, in temperate climates such as North America.[30] The unique ability of this nematode to replicate within its host for decades and its potential to cause massive infections with high mortality rates in immunocompromised patients make it a clinically significant pathogen. Although *S. stercoralis* is the usual cause of human strongyloidiasis, *Strongyloides fuelleborni*, an intestinal nematode of primates, may be responsible for occasional human infections in central Africa and New Guinea.

Life Cycle

S. stercoralis has a complex life cycle with a free-living phase and a parasitic phase[3] (Fig. 293–7). The free-living phase is initiated when second-stage rhabditiform larvae are excreted by an infected host into sandy or loamy soil. If the proper conditions of moisture and warmth are present, the larvae molt twice to become free-living adult worms, which then copulate with embryonated eggs deposited by the female into the soil. These then hatch and repeat the cycle, maturing in 3 to 5 days to adults.

Humans acquire the infection when infective third-stage larvae in fecally contaminated soil penetrate the skin of the host. The larvae are transported through the blood stream to the pulmonary circulation where they penetrate the alveoli, migrate up the tracheobronchial tree to the pharynx, and are then swallowed. The larvae undergo a final molt in the duodenum and upper jejunum to become adult females, which live within the intestinal wall. The adult females, measuring 2 mm in length, reproduce by parthenogenesis (i.e., in the absence of male worms). Mature females release small nu… initial skin… mately 25 t… the eggs hatc… colon to beco… may be deposi… additional molt t…

The filariform la… the perianal skin and… just described. This p… *alis* to persist in its ho… hosts may harbor many… which can result in hyp… often fatal complication of…

Epidemiology

As many as 100 to 200 million pe… wide with *S. stercoralis*. Infection… developed, tropical areas of the wo… ture, and poor sanitation are pern… cycle. In addition, some evidence exis… cats, or monkeys may serve as nonhum… tion. In the United States, strongyloidia… recent immigrants from Southeast Asia, t… parts of Appalachia and in institutionaliz… personal hygiene and sanitation are inade… estimates of the prevalence of this pathogen … ing to diagnostic dilemmas posed by the inter… tion of larvae and the low-grade nature of chroni… diasis. The importance of autoinfection has been e… by the detection of symptomatic disease three to fou… after exposure in ex–prisoners of war who had worke… railroad between Myanmar (formerly Burma) and Th… during World War II.[31]

Clinical Manifestations

The clinical manifestations of strongyloidiasis can be re… to stages of the parasite's life cycle, that is, the locatio… type of symptoms depend on whether the larvae ar… ing the skin, migrating through the lung, or penet… intestinal mucosa. Many infections with *S. stercor…* and often asymptomatic. Gastrointestinal symp… clude watery diarrhea alternating with consti… tric pain, nausea, and weight loss. Young chil… infections occasionally develop chronic d… malabsorption, abdominal distention, a… ment. Infants in Papua New Guinea in… *borni* may be afflicted by a swollen bel… ized by persistent diarrhea, ascites, … a protein-losing enteropathy.[1]

Patients with chronic strongyl… tent urticarial eruptions lasting… occur on the buttocks, upper… common but pathognomoni… characterized by a serpigin… a rate of several centimet… phase of larval migrati… like syndrome with… with peripheral e… may be manifeste… nia, and adult re… tions.[32] Gastroi… include indi… chronic dia…

Hyperin… tients who bec… tologic malignant…

XII · PARASITES

STR…

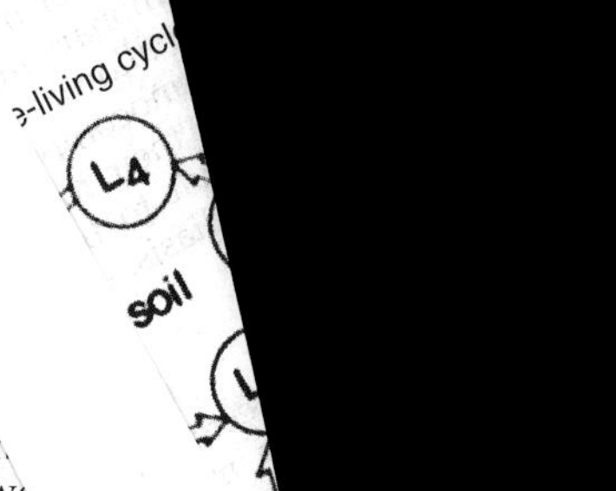

… fr… the… fata…

Diagn…

The dia… motile… mens (se… Baermann… necessary… The use of… test can in… asis. Patient… larvae prese… fluid, urine, a… Patients wit… erate eosinophi… cases of hyperin… *stercoralis*–specifi… linked immunos… assays are both se… available.

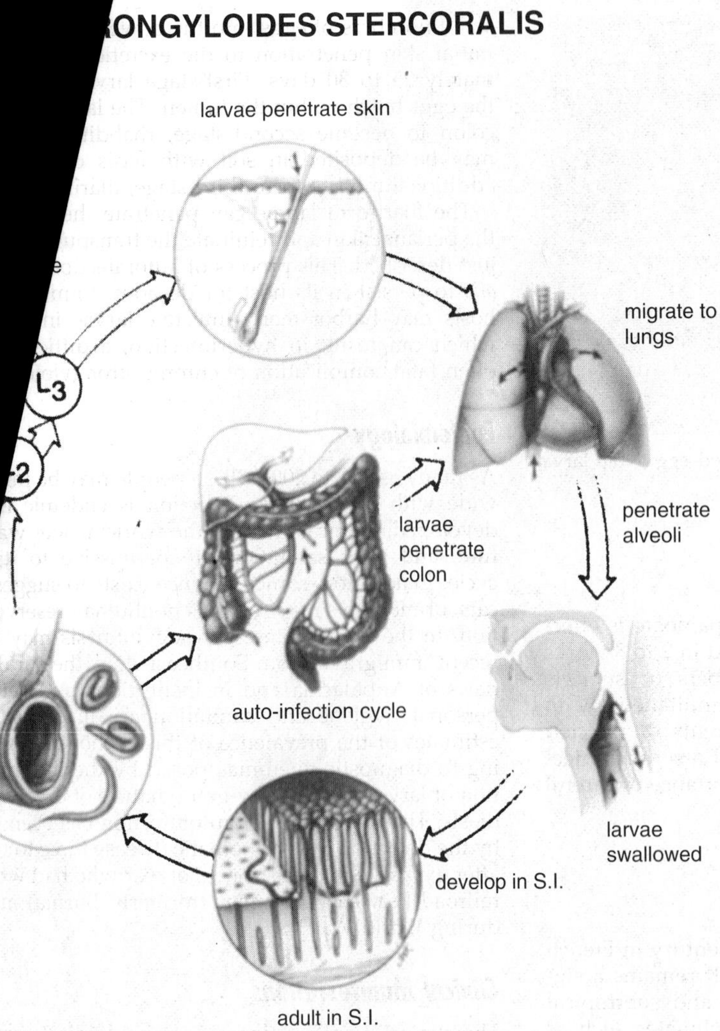

FIGURE 293–7 ▫ *Strongyloides stercoralis* life cycle. (Illustration by John W. Karapelou. From Despommier DD, Gwadz RG, Hotez P: Parasitic Diseases, ed 3. New York, Springer-Verlag, 1995.)

er immunosuppressive agents, and human immunodefi-
ncy virus infection.[33] Individuals with the hyperinfection
drome have heavy worm burdens that can lead to intesti-
obstruction, meningitis, respiratory failure, or gram-nega-
bacteremia. This last complication is believed to result
the carriage of enteric bacteria on the outer surface of
S. stercoralis filariform larvae. Hyperinfection is usually
if it is not promptly diagnosed and treated.

osis

gnosis is established by demonstrating characteristic,
habditiform larvae in stool or duodenal fluid speci-
e Table 293–2). Concentration techniques such as the
method, fecal culture, and serial sampling may be
because larval output is often sporadic and low.[3]
duodenal aspirates, mucosal biopsies, or the string
rease the likelihood of diagnosing strongyloidi-
s with the hyperinfection syndrome may have
t in sputum, bronchial washings, cerebrospinal
nd ascitic fluid.
acute or chronic infections may have a mod-
lia (10% to 25%), but this is usually absent in
fection. Most infected subjects will have *S.*
immunoglobulin G detectable by enzyme-
orbent assays.[34] However, although these
sitive and specific, they are not yet widely

Treatment

Thiabendazole is the drug of choice (see Table 293–2), although its efficacy is variable and its use may be complicated by multiple side effects including nausea, vomiting, dizziness, rash, and hallucinations. Ivermectin is effective therapy for chronic strongyloidiasis and is better tolerated than thiabendazole.[35] Patients with the hyperinfection syndrome tend to be relatively refractory to treatment, which may need to be more prolonged and to be repeated. Intensive supportive therapy, antimicrobial coverage for secondary bacterial infections, and nutritional supplementation are necessary adjuncts to antiparasitic drugs in patients with overwhelming *S. stercoralis* infection.

Zoonotic Intestinal Nematode Infections

Humans are accidental hosts to the intermediate larval stage of several species of zoonotic intestinal nematodes that may cause symptomatic gastrointestinal disease.

Anisakiasis

Anisakiasis is an infection of the stomach or intestine by the larval form of a number of species of marine nematodes that normally infect sea mammals.[36] The intermediate larval stage of four genera (*Anisakis, Pseudoterranova, Contracaecum,* and

Thynnascaris) of the family Anisakidae has been found to cause disease in humans.[37] The adult worm of these marine parasites is found in the stomachs or intestines of whales, dolphins, sea lions, and seals. Eggs released by these final hosts hatch in seawater to form free-living larval stages that infect intermediate hosts, usually crustaceans. These are subsequently ingested by fish such as salmon, herring, cod, haddock, and mackerel or by squid, which serve as transport hosts. Ingestion of the uncooked flesh of the infected fish or squid by the marine mammalian final hosts or humans who are accidental hosts leads to infection.

After ingestion of raw or undercooked saltwater fish by humans, the larva embed themselves in the gastric or intestinal mucosa and then die. The burrowing or dead larva precipitates an intense hypersensitivity reaction characterized by a granulomatous, eosinophilic tissue infiltrate. Infection with *Pseudoterranova* species usually involves only the stomach and tends to be milder than disease due to *Anisakis* species, which may cause symptomatic gastric or intestinal infections. Asymptomatic infections with *Pseudoterranova* species may first come to medical attention when the patient coughs up a live or dead worm. This usually occurs within 48 hours of the ingestion of infected fish and may be preceded by a sensation of feeling a worm crawling in the upper esophagus or pharynx.

Gastric anisakiasis is heralded by the abrupt (generally 1 to 12 hours after ingestion of raw fish) onset of severe epigastric pain, nausea, vomiting, and low-grade fever. There is frequently an accompanying leukocytosis with an intense eosinophilia. Diagnosis and treatment can be accomplished by the gastroscopic or surgical recognition and removal of the larvae. Untreated gastric disease may lead to chronic, ulcer-like symptoms and is more difficult to diagnose because only a granulomatous lesion may be present.

Intestinal anisakiasis is characterized by intermittent or constant abdominal pain that may be severe enough to result in peritoneal signs or evidence of a partial bowel obstruction. The symptoms may not appear until 1 to 3 weeks after ingestion of the anisakid larvae. Leukocytosis without eosinophilia may be present. Diagnosis is made when laparotomy is performed for suspected appendicitis or bowel perforation. Rare cases of intraperitoneal anisakiasis have been described.[36]

The annual occurrence of this seafood-associated parasitic infection is greatest in Japan, where the consumption of raw fish is common. Numerous cases have also been described in northern Europe, especially Holland, which have been attributed to the ingestion of raw herring. Although only about 50 cases have been reported from North America, the frequency may be higher as a result of underreporting or milder forms of disease that go unrecognized. Anisakiasis can be prevented by thorough cooking of fish or freezing at −20°C for 60 hours. Eviscerating fish as soon as possible after catch may decrease the number of larvae in the fish flesh by not allowing them the opportunity to migrate from the intestinal tract into the edible musculature.

Capillariasis

Intestinal disease caused by *C. philippinensis* has been mainly described in coastal regions of the Philippines and Thailand, although scattered cases have been reported from other countries in Southeast Asia and the Middle East.[38] Human infection with this zoonotic nematode may result in severe diarrhea with malabsorption, which can be fatal if it is untreated.

Eggs passed in the feces of infected patients or by migratory fish-eating birds embryonate in fresh or brackish water during a 5- to 10-day period. After ingestion of the embryonated eggs by the intermediate fish host, the eggs hatch and release larvae, which mature in the fish intestine in 3 weeks. After consumption of the parasitized fish by the natural definitive host, fish-eating birds, the larva develops into an adult male or female, which copulate and fertilize. Humans are accidental hosts who acquire infection by eating inadequately cooked or raw fish. The larvae of *C. philippinensis* develop into adult worms in the small intestine 1 to 2 months after ingestion. Adult females appear capable of producing infective larvae in humans, which can lead to an autoinfectious cycle similar to that of *S. stercoralis*.

Clinical disease is manifested by borborygmi, abdominal pain, and intermittent diarrhea, which, if left untreated, may progress to voluminous watery diarrhea. Dehydration, weight loss, steatorrhea, and a protein-losing enteropathy may ensue with the eventual development of muscle wasting, anasarca, and electrolyte disturbances. Death may occur in 4 to 6 months if infected patients are not treated.

The diagnosis should be suspected in patients in endemic regions with the aforementioned symptoms. Direct microscopic examination of stool or duodenal aspirate may reveal the adult worms, larvae, or eggs. The eggs of *C. philippinensis* are thin shelled and peanut shaped. They can be confused with *T. trichiura* eggs by inexperienced technicians. Mebendazole at a dose of 200 mg twice daily administered for 20 days is the current treatment of choice. Preliminary findings with albendazole are promising.

Hepatic capillariasis is a rare zoonotic infection of humans caused by *Capillaria hepatica*, a parasite of rodents.[39] Ingestion of soil or food contaminated with the embryonated eggs of this nematode is followed by hatching of the larvae, which traverse the intestinal wall and migrate to the liver by the portal vein. The larvae mature to adult worms in the liver that deposit thousands of eggs. An intense granulomatous response may ensue and lead to prolonged fever, hepatomegaly, leukocytosis with a relative eosinophilia, and progressive liver failure. The diagnosis is confirmed by the detection of worms or ova in a liver biopsy specimen. Limited experience with thiabendazole and albendazole has demonstrated elimination of adult worms, whereas less favorable results have been observed with the eggs.

Trichostrongyliasis

The genus *Trichostrongylus* is distributed worldwide and includes many species that parasitize the intestinal tracts of herbivorous mammals. Human infection has been described in many less developed countries and has been attributed to at least seven different species of *Trichostrongylus*.[40] People who care for animals such as sheep and goats are more likely to acquire this rare infection.

Ingestion of infectious larvae on fecally contaminated vegetables or hands is the probable mode of transmission. The filariform larvae penetrate the oral mucosa, pass through the lung, and then fully mature in the small intestine. The intensity of infection in humans is usually low, although high worm burdens have been described.[41] Most infections are asymptomatic, although heavy infections may rarely lead to anemia, eosinophilia, and emaciation. Diagnosis is established by the detection of eggs in stool specimens; concentration techniques are needed for lighter infections. The eggs can be confused with those of hookworms, although hookworm eggs tend to be smaller and have more rounded ends. Treatment may be unnecessary in milder infections. Therapy with thiabendazole has been successful in some cases, but resistance has been described. Single-dose therapy with pyrantel pamoate has been effective in cases treated in Japan and Korea, whereas less favorable results have been reported from Iran.

Oesophagostomiasis

Oesophagostomum species, although common parasites of mammals, have rarely been described in humans. Studies in Togo and Ghana have found that as many as 30% of the human populations in some villages are infected with *Oesophagostomum bifurcum*, a nematode of monkeys.[42] The mode of transmission of this parasite remains to be clarified, although close contact with primates may play a role. The larvae and adult worms of this parasite have been found in nodular lesions of the intestinal wall. The eggs of *O. bifurcum* are nearly identical to hookworm eggs, and therefore coproculture with identification of the larvae is needed to establish this diagnosis. The two anthelmintic drugs pyrantel pamoate and albendazole appear capable of eliminating adult worms from infected individuals.

References

1. World Health Organization: Prevention and control of intestinal parasitic infections. World Health Organ Tech Rep Ser 749:1, 1987.
2. Bundy DAP, Cooper ES: *Trichuris* and trichuriasis in humans. Adv Parasitol 28:107, 1989.
3. Despommier DD, Gwadz RW, Hotez PJ: Parasitic Diseases, ed 3. New York, Springer-Verlag, 1995.
4. MacDonald TT, Choy M-Y, Spencer J, et al: Histopathology and immunohistochemistry of the caecum in children with the *Trichuris* dysentery syndrome. J Clin Pathol 44:194, 1991.
5. Warren KS: Helminthic diseases endemic in the United States. Am J Trop Med Hyg 23:723, 1974.
6. Gilman RH, Chong YH, Davis C, et al: The adverse consequences of heavy *Trichuris* infection. Trans R Soc Trop Med Hyg 77:432, 1983.
7. Layrisse M, Aparcedo L, Martinez-Torres C, et al: Blood loss due to infection with *Trichuris trichiura*. Am J Trop Med Hyg 16:613, 1967.
8. Kamath KR: Severe infection with *Trichuris trichiura* in Malaysian children. Am J Trop Med Hyg 22:600, 1973.
9. Stephenson LS, Latham MC, Adams EJ, et al: Physical fitness, growth and appetite of Kenyan school boys with hookworm, *Trichuris trichiura* and *Ascaris lumbricoides* infections are improved four months after a single dose of albendazole. J Nutr 123:1036, 1993.
10. Crompton DWT: Prevalence of ascariasis. *In* Crompton DWT, Nesheim MC, Pawlowski ZS (eds): Ascariasis and Its Prevention and Control. London, Taylor & Francis, 1985, pp 45–69.
11. Davies NJ, Goldsmid JM: Intestinal obstruction due to *Ascaris suum* infection. Trans R Soc Trop Med Hyg 72:107, 1978.
12. Sinniah B: Daily egg production of *Ascaris lumbricoides*: The distribution of eggs in the faeces and the variability of egg counts. Parasitology 84:167, 1982.
13. Spillman RK: Pulmonary ascariasis in tropical communities. Am J Trop Med Hyg 24:791, 1975.
14. Gelpi AP, Mustafa A: *Ascaris* pneumonia. Am J Med 44:377, 1968.
15. Blumenthal DS, Schultz MG: Incidence of intestinal obstruction in children infected with *Ascaris lumbricoides*. Am J Trop Med Hyg 24:801, 1975.
16. Khuroo MS, Zargar SA, Mahajan R: Hepatobiliary and pancreatic ascariasis in India. Lancet 335:1503, 1990.
17. Stephenson LS: The contribution of *Ascaris lumbricoides* to malnutrition in children. Parasitology 81:221, 1980.
18. Drugs for parasitic infections. Med Lett 35:111, 1993.
19. World Health Organization: Intestinal protozoan and helminthic infections. World Health Organ Tech Rep Ser 666:1, 1981.
20. Miller TA: Hookworm infection in man. Adv Parasitol 17:315, 1979.
21. Roche M, Layrisse M: The nature and causes of "hookworm anemia." Am J Trop Med Hyg 15:1031, 1966.
22. Hotez PJ: Hookworm disease in children. Pediatr Infect Dis J 8:516, 1989.
23. Gilles HM: Selective primary health care: Strategies for control of disease in the developing world. XVII. Hookworm infection and anemia. Rev Infect Dis 7:111, 1985.
24. Schad GA, Chowdhury AB, Dean CG, et al: Arrested development in human hookworm infections: An adaptation to a seasonally unfavorable external environment. Science 180:502, 1973.
25. Koshy A, Raina V, Sharma MP, et al: An unusual outbreak of hookworm disease in north India. Am J Trop Med Hyg 27:42, 1978.
26. Russell LJ: The pinworm, *Enterobius vermicularis*. Primary Care 18:13, 1991.
27. Vermund SH, MacLeod S: Is pinworm a vanishing infection? Laboratory surveillance in a New York City medical center from 1971 to 1986. Am J Dis Child 142:566, 1988.
28. Haswell-Elkins MR, Elkins DB, Manjula K, et al: The distribution and abundance of *Enterobius vermicularis* in a south Indian fishing community. Parasitology 95:339, 1987.
29. Cook GC: *Enterobius vermicularis* infection. Gut 35:1159, 1994.
30. Grove DI: Strongyloidiasis: A conundrum for gastroenterologists. Gut 35:437, 1994.
31. Pelletier LL: Chronic strongyloidiasis in World War II Far East ex–prisoners of war. Am J Trop Med Hyg 33:55, 1984.
32. Woodring JH: Pulmonary strongyloidiasis: Clinical and imaging features. AJR 162:537, 1994.
33. Celedon JC: Systemic strongyloidiasis in patients infected with the human immunodeficiency virus. A report of 3 cases and review of the literature. Medicine (Baltimore) 73:256, 1994.
34. Lindo JF: Prospective evaluation of enzyme-linked immunosorbent assay and immunoblot methods for the diagnosis of endemic *Strongyloides stercoralis* infection. Am J Trop Med Hyg 51:175, 1994.
35. Gann PH, Neva FA, Gam AA: A randomized trial of single- and two-dose ivermectin versus thiabendazole for treatment of strongyloidiasis. J Infect Dis 169:1076, 1994.
36. Ishikura H, Kikuchi K, Nagasawa K, et al: Anisakidae and anisakidosis. Prog Clin Parasitol 3:43, 1993.
37. World Health Organization: Parasitic Zoonoses. Report of a WHO expert committee with the participation of FAO. World Health Organ Tech Rep Ser 637:1, 1979.
38. Cross JH, Basaca-Sevilla V: Intestinal capillariasis. Prog Clin Parasitol 1:105, 1989.
39. Choe G, Lee HS, Seo JK, et al: Hepatic capillariasis: First case report in the republic of Korea. Am J Trop Med Hyg 48:610, 1993.
40. Wolfe MS: *Oxyuris*, *Trichostrongylus*, and *Trichuris*. Clin Gastroenterol 7:201, 1978.
41. Ghadirian E, Arfaa F: Present status of trichostrongyliasis in Iran. Am J Trop Med Hyg 24:935, 1975.
42. Polderman AM, Krepel HP, Baeta S, et al: Oesophagostomiasis, a common infection of man in northern Togo and Ghana. Am J Trop Med Hyg 44:336, 1991.

294

Tissue Nematodes

Davidson H. Hamer
Dickson D. Despommier

Filariasis

Filarial parasites infect approximately 200 million humans worldwide. Chronic filariasis, although not responsible for significant mortality, is associated with tremendous suffering and long-term debility in diverse populations, with a resultant adverse socioeconomic impact on afflicted individuals and communities.

All human infections are caused by filariae of the family Onchocercidae. The long, thin adult worms reside in the subcutaneous tissues, lymphatics, or peritoneum. Female adults are usually much larger than males but are rarely observed because of their location within the host. Sexual reproduction yields microfilariae, the diagnostic stage, which migrate in the blood or skin. These first-stage larvae are ingested by an obligate, bloodsucking arthropod that serves as an intermediate host within which the microfilariae develop into third-stage larvae. These infective larvae escape from the insect at the time of feeding and then migrate within the human host to the tissues or lymphatics, where they develop into adult worms. Clinical disease results from the host's immune response to the migrating microfilariae and dying parasites.

Lymphatic Filariasis

Wuchereria bancrofti and *Brugia malayi* are the main causes of lymphatic filariasis in humans, although other minor members of the genus *Brugia*, such as *Brugia timori*, can cause human disease.[1] These threadlike nematodes infect nearly 80 million people worldwide and are responsible for a spectrum of disease ranging from asymptomatic infections with microfilaremia to disfiguring elephantiasis.[2]

LIFE CYCLE

The adult worms live in the lumen of lymphatic vessels. The females measure 4 to 10 cm in length; the *W. bancrofti* females are longer than those of *B. malayi*, whereas the males are about 4 and 1.5 cm long, respectively. The adult parasites are thin; the females measure approximately 250 and 150 μm in diameter, respectively. The adult worms reproduce sexually to yield large numbers of microfilariae or first-stage larvae, which migrate into the blood stream. The microfilariae measure about 270 by 9 μm and are ensheathed. When mosquitoes take a blood meal from infected humans, they ingest the microfilariae, which penetrate the insect's stomach wall and migrate into the thoracic flight muscles where they undergo two molts to become infective third-stage larvae during a 10- to 20-day period. The infective larvae then migrate to the mosquito's biting parts and are deposited onto the skin during its next blood meal. The larvae crawl into the open wound, migrate through the subcutaneous tissues, and finally reach the peripheral lymphatics where they mature into adult worms. Microfilariae are released into the blood stream approximately 6 to 12 months after the infecting bite. Although the adult parasites may survive in their human host for decades, estimates of their life span suggest a shorter existence.[3]

EPIDEMIOLOGY

An estimated 79 million people are infected with *W. bancrofti*, the most widely distributed human filarial parasite. It is endemic in many regions of Africa, Central and South America, the Caribbean, the Indian subcontinent, Southeast Asia, and the western Pacific (Table 294–1). *B. malayi* and *B. timori* are responsible for approximately 6 million human infections. *B. malayi* is endemic in India, Southeast Asia, and the western Pacific; *B. timori* is localized to the Indonesian islands of Timor and Flores. Newer, more sensitive diagnostic techniques suggest that the number of people with lymphatic filariasis is considerably underestimated. Filarial infections are usually first detected in 5- to 10-year-old children in endemic regions.[4] The prevalence of microfilaremia increases progressively with age and then stabilizes in early adulthood.

W. bancrofti usually shows nocturnal periodicity; microfilariae appear in the peripheral circulation late at night. *Culex* and *Anopheles* mosquitos transmit this form of *W. bancrofti*, which is mainly present in Africa, India, Southeast Asia, and Latin America. A diurnal form of infection caused by *W. bancrofti* exists in the South Pacific and is transmitted by day-biting *Aedes* mosquitos. No animal reservoir is known for this parasite. *B. malayi* infections with nocturnal periodicity, transmitted by *Anopheles* and *Mansonia* mosquito species, are found in areas of India, Malaysia, and other parts of Southeast Asia. A less common subperiodic form characterized by less exaggerated fluctuations in microfilarial blood density is found in areas of Southeast Asia where it is associated with numerous animal reservoirs. *B. timori* demonstrates nocturnal periodicity and is transmitted by anopheline mosquitoes.

PATHOGENESIS

Lymphangitis, a common manifestation of infection, may progress to elephantiasis. These pathologic changes appear to be determined by the chronic immune response of the host directed against the dead and dying adult worms rather than the abundant microfilariae. The dead and dying adult worms and released parasite antigens elicit granulomatous and proliferative responses that lead to thickening and distortion of the lymphatic vessels. Plasma cells, macrophages, and eosinophils infiltrate the affected lymphatics, with eventual closure of the lumen and the development of lymphatic obstruction. The blockage of lymphatic channels may be accelerated by intercurrent bacterial infections. As the obstruction evolves, lymphedema and changes of chronic stasis develop in the affected area of the body. Repeated infections for prolonged periods contribute to the gradual process of lymphatic obstruction.

CLINICAL MANIFESTATIONS

The spectrum of clinical presentations of lymphatic filariasis includes asymptomatic microfilaremia, filarial fevers, lymphangitis, lymphatic obstruction, and tropical pulmonary eosinophilia.

Adolescents and young adults may develop a syndrome of filarial fevers characterized by general malaise, low-grade fevers, headaches, and pain associated with lymphangitis or lymphadenitis. Affected lymph nodes may be enlarged and tender; the skin overlying infected lymphatics may be thickened, firm, tender, and edematous. In contrast to bacterial cellulitis, filarial cellulitis does not have a clear demarcation between the affected and healthy skin.

Some individuals have asymptomatic microfilaremia and may spontaneously clear the infection without ever developing symptoms. Others suffer recurrent acute lymphangitis, which will progress to obstructive complications in about one third of cases.

Acute episodes of lymphatic filariasis due to *W. bancrofti* frequently affect the male genitalia and can lead to complications including funiculitis, epididymitis, orchitis, hydrocele, and elephantiasis of the scrotum. Chyluria may develop if the obstructed, swollen lymphatic channels rupture into the urinary tract. The legs are more commonly involved than the upper extremities in bancroftian filariasis. In contrast to the common involvement of male genitalia in bancroftian filariasis, brugian filariasis is more likely to present clinically as lymphadenitis and lymphangitis as a result of a predilection of *Brugia* species to involve the superficial inguinal lymphatics. Elephantiasis of the lower extremities involves the entire leg in bancroftian filariasis, whereas the leg above the knee maintains a relatively normal contour in brugian filariasis. Involvement of the upper extremities, breasts, and other areas of the body is relatively infrequent in both forms of lymphatic filariasis.

Tropical pulmonary eosinophilia is a hypersensitivity syn-

TABLE 294–1 ■ Characteristics of Human Filarial Infections

ORGANISM	GEOGRAPHIC DISTRIBUTION	HABITAT OF ADULT WORMS	VECTOR	LOCATION OF MICROFILARIAE	PERIODICITY OF MICROFILARIAE
Wuchereria bancrofti	Worldwide, tropics and subtropics	Lymphatic system	Mosquitoes: *Aedes, Anopheles, Culex* sp.	Blood	Nocturnal; South Pacific form is subperiodic
Brugia malayi	Southeast Asia, India, western Pacific	Lymphatic system	Mosquitoes: *Anopheles, Mansonia* sp.	Blood	Nocturnal
Brugia timori	Indonesian islands of Timor and Flores	Lymphatic system	Mosquitoes: *Anopheles* sp.	Blood	Nocturnal
Onchocerca volvulus	Africa, Latin America	Subcutaneous tissues	*Simulium* sp. (black flies)	Skin	None
Loa loa	West and Central Africa	Subcutaneous tissues	*Chrysops* sp. (deer flies)	Blood	Diurnal
Mansonella perstans	Africa, Central and South America	Body cavities, mesenteric and retroperitoneal tissues	*Culicoides* sp. (biting midges)	Blood	None
Mansonella streptocerca	West and Central Africa	Subcutaneous tissues	*Culicoides* sp.	Skin	None
Mansonella ozzardi	Caribbean, Central and South America	Subcutaneous tissues	*Culicoides* and *Simulium* sp.	Blood	None

drome found mainly in southern India, where it is most common in young adult men.[5] Symptoms include low-grade fever, nocturnal asthma, cough, fatigue, and weight loss. Associated findings include interstitial infiltrates on chest radiographs, marked eosinophilia, and high levels of serum immunoglobulin E. Subjects with this syndrome mount an intense immune response in vitro to the parasite. If left untreated, tropical pulmonary eosinophilia may result in chronic restrictive lung disease.

DIAGNOSIS

The definitive parasitologic diagnosis is based on the demonstration of microfilariae in blood samples.[6] In patients with lymphatic filariasis from regions where nocturnal periodicity is common, blood specimens should be obtained between 10 PM and 2 AM. Microfilariae in blood may be detected by Giemsa-stained thick smears, although this method is generally less sensitive than are concentration techniques that use centrifugation (Knott test) or filtration. Microfilariae are sometimes demonstrable in hydrocele fluid. Species identification is based on size, staining characteristics of the sheath, and arrangement of nuclei in the tail (Figs. 294–1 and 294–2). Microfilariae may not be detectable in patients with obstructive disease, in which case the diagnosis is made on clinical grounds. The presence of eosinophilia and elevated titers of specific antifilarial antibodies help support the diagnosis. The adult worms in the lymphatics are occasionally observed at autopsy; their identification, therefore, has no diagnostic utility in symptomatic patients. Newer immunologic tests for the direct detection of filarial antigens and polymerase chain reaction for DNA have been developed but are not yet widely available.

TREATMENT

Diethylcarbamazine (DEC) citrate has been used for many years as the main therapy for lymphatic filariasis. Although dosages and administration schedules vary, DEC is usually given as a single oral dose of 6 mg/kg per day for 2 weeks. This treatment effectively eliminates microfilariae from blood within 5 days; however, microfilaremia will recur at lower levels during the next 3 to 6 months.[7] Many treated patients will experience side effects during the first few days of ther-

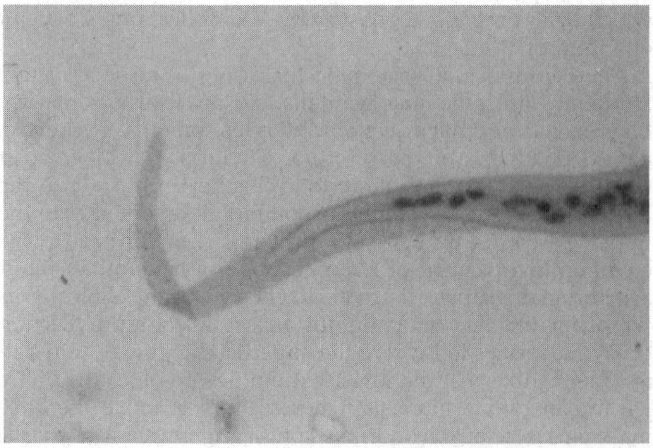

FIGURE 294–1 ▫ *Wuchereria bancrofti* microfilaria. Note that the nuclei are evenly spaced and do not extend to the tip of the tail; the second-stage larva is ensheathed in the first-stage cuticle. (Giemsa stain, 100 × 10.)

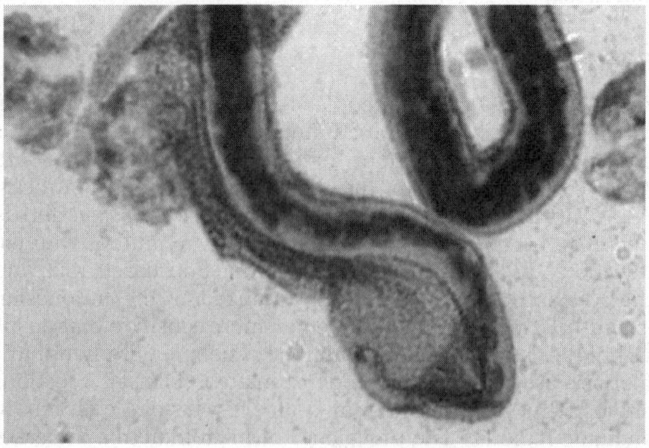

FIGURE 294–2 ▫ *Brugia malayi* microfilaria. Note that the nuclei are unevenly spaced, extending to the tip of the tail, and the second-stage larva is ensheathed in the first-stage cuticle. (Giemsa stain, 100 × 10.)

apy, including fever, chills, nausea, vomiting, headache, dizziness, myalgias, and arthralgias. Local inflammatory reactions of infected lymph nodes may also occur with treatment. These reactions are believed to be due to the rapid microfilaricidal effect of DEC, and therefore a test dose of 25 to 50 mg is frequently administered to patients with high-grade microfilaremia. The effect of DEC on the adult worm appears to be limited; repeated courses of treatment with higher doses at weekly or monthly intervals may reduce or eliminate the adult filaria.[3]

Interest in the use of ivermectin in lymphatic filariasis arose as a consequence of its demonstrated tolerability and efficacy for the treatment of onchocerciasis.[8] Single-dose therapy with ivermectin (20 to 400 μg/kg) rapidly clears microfilaremia and is well tolerated.[7–9] The effectiveness of ivermectin is similar to that of DEC, but it has the advantage of being administered as a single oral dose. Eosinophilia associated with these filarial infections generally resolves with either treatment but may recur if there is a relapse. Combined single-dose therapy with both ivermectin and DEC may prove to be an even more effective treatment for bancroftian filariasis.[10] Like DEC, ivermectin may have a limited effect on the adult worm as evidenced by prolonged suppression of microfilaremia. Side effects experienced by patients are similar with the two drugs; their intensity correlates with the pretreatment level of microfilaremia.[7, 9, 10] Acute inflammatory reactions during therapy should be treated with nonsteroidal antiinflammatory agents.

Treatment of complications due to chronic lymphatic obstruction is difficult. Careful skin care and early antimicrobial therapy can help minimize bacterial superinfections of affected limbs. Hydroceles can be managed successfully with surgery. Surgical bypass shunting plays a limited role in the treatment of elephantiasis. This disfiguring condition is responsible for significant psychosocial trauma, which may require supportive psychologic care.

PREVENTION AND CONTROL

Although it may be difficult for residents of endemic areas to avoid mosquito bites, temporary visitors should use repellants and mosquito nets. Attempts to control the mosquito vectors have failed owing to the development of resistance to insecticides. Recurrent, mass treatment with ivermectin may lead to reductions in the load of microfilariae in treated individuals and thereby to decreased transmission. The long-term use of DEC or ivermectin may also lead to reductions in overt disease.

Onchocerciasis

Chronic infection with the parasite *Onchocerca volvulus* is commonly manifested by dermatologic or ocular disease that may progress to disabling dermatitis and blindness. Onchocerciasis is the fourth leading cause of blindness worldwide. The long-term disability that results from this filarial infection is responsible for a significant socioeconomic burden in endemic areas of equatorial Africa and Latin America.

EPIDEMIOLOGY

An estimated 18 million people worldwide are infected with *O. volvulus*, most of whom live in equatorial Africa in a broad belt stretching from the Atlantic Coast on the west to the Indian Ocean and Red Sea on the east[11] (see Table 294–1). Approximately 100,000 individuals in Latin America suffer from onchocerciasis in scattered foci in Guatemala, Mexico, Venezuela, Brazil, Colombia, and Ecuador. Additional countries with endemic disease include Yemen and southwestern Saudi Arabia.

Humans are the definitive host of this parasite, although similar species are found in other mammals. *O. volvulus* larvae are transmitted to humans by the bite of various species of black fly of the genus *Simulium*.[12] The insect vector breeds along free-flowing waterways that have sufficient forest canopy to protect the black flies from excessively intense sun and heat. The black flies deposit their eggs on rocks, sticks, and vegetation along the rapidly flowing bodies of water from which the larvae and pupae that develop derive their nutrients. Consequently, onchocerciasis, or river blindness, is clustered around rivers and streams that provide the black flies with the necessary conditions for development and survival. The disease has a higher prevalence in men than in women in many communities because of greater exposure during daily activities such as fishing, farming, washing, and water collection.

Approximately 1% to 4% of all infected individuals will become blind; however, as many as half of adults in hyperendemic areas may develop this complication. A much higher prevalence of skin disease and other forms of ocular involvement is found in endemic regions than of blindness. The prevalence of infection rises with age such that almost all members of a village may be infected by early adulthood. The debilitating effects of chronic dermatitis and severe ocular disease tend to affect adults in their third to fifth decades of life at a time when they are the heads of households. The impact of this disease on some rural communities can be devastating in terms of the severe, personal discomfort and negative economic influence.

LIFE CYCLE

Microfilariae in the skin are ingested by female black flies while they are taking a blood meal from an infected individual. Once ingested, the immature worms penetrate the fly's intestinal wall and migrate to the thoracic flight muscles where they molt twice. The infective third-stage larvae migrate into the proboscis after 6 to 12 days of development and are then deposited on human skin when the fly bites. The larvae enter the bite wound and migrate into the subcutaneous tissues, where they molt twice to become mature male and female worms during a period of several months. The adults become encapsulated in fibrous nodules in the subcutaneous tissue and deeper fascial planes during their growth and maturation. The female adult measures 23 to 50 cm in length and about 250 to 450 μm in diameter; the males are 2 to 5 cm long and 125 to 210 μm wide. After a prepatent period of 9 to 18 months, the male and female worms sexually reproduce and release millions of microfilariae during their estimated life span of 8 to 10 years. The microfilariae are motile, are unsheathed, and measure 200 to 360 μm in length. Migration of the microfilariae from the nodules through the subcutaneous and ocular tissues and the host's immune response are responsible for the clinical manifestations of this disease.

PATHOPHYSIOLOGY

The skin, lymph nodes, and ocular tissues are the principal sites of infection. More frequent, intensive exposures lead to greater levels of infection. Histopathologic examination of the skin reveals a low-grade, chronic inflammatory process that may progress to atrophy, loss of elastic fibers, and fibrosis.[13] Live microfilariae do not appear to induce any host response, whereas the dead worms cause inflammation that increases with severity the longer the infection persists. The nodules containing adult worms, known as onchocercomata, have an outer fibrous capsule, a thin layer of chronic inflammation, and an inner inflammatory cell infiltrate around the adult worm.

Neovascularization and scarring of the cornea may lead to blindness. A chronic, nongranulomatous inflammatory process in other parts of the eye can result in anterior uveitis, chorioretinitis, and optic atrophy.

The host reaction to the microfilariae, resulting from cell-mediated immunity to parasite antigens, appears to be the driving force behind the skin and ocular damage. Individuals who manifest the most vigorous immune responses appear more likely to develop severe disease.[13, 14] A multiplicity of factors including host inflammatory mediators and parasite antigens contribute to the complex immunopathogenesis of onchocerciasis.

CLINICAL MANIFESTATIONS

Intense pruritus and intermittent urticarial or papular eruptions localized to one region of the body and conjunctivitis are early manifestations of disease.[11, 12] These may be the only signs and symptoms in nonresidents of endemic areas who usually have lighter infections. Chronic inflammation of the skin may lead to hyperpigmentation and, later, a loss of elasticity, a widespread maculopapular rash, hypopigmentation, scaling, and edema. Depigmentation ("leopard skin"), thickening ("elephant skin"), and eventually a shiny, atrophic epidermis ("lizard skin") may develop in long-standing infections. The increased fragility of the skin may lead to areas of breakdown, which places the patient at risk for bacterial superinfection. A classification and grading system of the cutaneous changes of onchocerciasis has been developed in an attempt to standardize interpretation of skin involvement.[15] The dermal manifestations of the disease in Africa more commonly involve the trunk, buttocks, and lower extremities, whereas they are more prominent around the head and neck in Central America. Lymph node involvement parallels the sites of skin involvement in these two geographic regions.[14] It is usually manifested by enlargement of the lymph nodes; secondary obstructive changes in the groin region or an extremity may occur. A hypergic form of onchocerciasis known as *sowda* (meaning "dark" or "black" in Arabic) characterized by hyperpigmentation, papular eruptions, swelling, and regional lymphadenopathy, usually limited to one extremity, is common in Yemen[16] but has also been observed in Africa and Latin America. In contrast to *sowda*, in which skin snips reveal few microfilariae, the more common, nonreactive form of onchocerciasis tends to be symmetric with many microfilariae present in skin snips.

Onchocercomata are firm, nontender, and freely mobile subcutaneous or dermal nodules that usually measure 1 to 2 cm. If they are attached to periosteum, the nodules may be immobile. They often occur in clusters in areas where lymphatics converge, including the skull, scapula, intercostal areas, iliac crests, and sacrum. The nodules tend to predominate in the lower part of the body in infected Africans, whereas they are more common in the upper regions of the body in Central Americans.

Early ocular involvement is usually manifested by conjunctivitis associated with local irritation, increased tearing, and photophobia. Any part of the eye may be involved from the cornea to the posterior segment, including the retina and optic nerve. Slit-lamp examination may reveal living and dead microfilariae in the cornea, limbus, anterior chamber, retrolental space, vitreous humor, and retina. Associated lesions include punctate keratitis, sclerosing keratitis, iridocyclitis, chorioretinitis (which may cause progressive narrowing of visual fields), and optic neuritis and atrophy. Persistent anterior uveitis may lead to meiosis, pupillary distortion, and glaucoma. Sclerosing keratitis, the primary cause of blindness in onchocerciasis, typically develops after decades of infection.

DIAGNOSIS

A clinical diagnosis of onchocerciasis can be made in infected subjects in endemic regions who have typical skin changes, subcutaneous nodules, or ocular lesions. The diagnosis is confirmed by demonstrating *O. volvulus* microfilariae in skin specimens.[6, 14] Samples of skin are usually taken with a corneoscleral biopsy instrument or razor blade from commonly infected sites, such as the upper portion of the body in Central Americans and the lower part in Africans. The skin is weighed and then placed in saline or tissue culture media. Microfilariae that emerge from the skin specimen are counted after incubation at room temperature for 30 minutes to 3 hours. They must be distinguished microscopically from the smaller microfilariae of *Mansonella perstans*. The skin snipping technique provides a measure of the intensity of infection; less than 10 microfilariae per milligram of skin constitutes a light infection, and more than 100 a heavy one. Multiple biopsy specimens should be taken from different sites to have a reliable sampling.

Serologic tests demonstrating elevated titers of antifilarial antibodies have been developed but, until recently, lacked adequate sensitivity and specificity.[17] In addition, polymerase chain reaction–based diagnosis holds promise for improved detection of onchocerciasis and strain differentiation.[18]

TREATMENT

Although DEC was the standard therapy for nearly half a century, it has largely been supplanted by ivermectin. Suramin has both macrofilaricidal and microfilaricidal activities against *O. volvulus* but is rarely used because of its potential to cause serious toxic effects. DEC is well tolerated in uninfected persons, whereas severe side effects and complications occur in infected persons as a result of the massive killing of microfilariae during the first few days of treatment. The Mazzotti reaction, an exacerbation of pruritus or rash after a test dose of DEC, is common in heavily infected individuals. Complications of treatment with DEC include fever, intense pruritus, prostration, lymph node swelling and pain, hypotension, and arthralgias.[19] Ocular complications include conjunctivitis, keratitis, chorioretinal damage, and optic neuritis. Reactions in the posterior segment of the eye may lead to permanent damage and blindness. Patients treated with DEC should receive escalating doses, and corticosteroids should be considered to help minimize the aforementioned complications. However, as a result of numerous studies in the last decade demonstrating the efficacy of and improved tolerance to ivermectin therapy for onchocerciasis, DEC should be reserved for patients who cannot take ivermectin.

Ivermectin is administered as a single oral dose of 150 to 200 μg/kg on an empty stomach at least 2 hours before the next meal. It has been consistently demonstrated to be well tolerated, acceptable to endemic communities, and highly effective in eliminating microfilariae.[8, 19, 20] Although many treated subjects have little or no reaction to treatment, some may have increased pruritus, fever, headache, edema, and conjunctivitis or blurring of vision. Adverse reactions usually occur in the first 24 to 48 hours of therapy and last for 5 to 10 days. A minority of treated patients will develop a maculopapular rash characteristic of the Mazzotti reaction; more serious reactions such as hypotension or worsening ocular disease are rare. The frequency and severity of adverse reactions to treatment are directly proportional to the intensity of infection. Skin snips should be taken every 6 to 12 months to monitor the response to treatment and to select patients who will need retreatment. Repeated courses of ivermectin at 6-month intervals will lead to a progressive reduction of skin microfilariae counts as well as a decrease in the prevalence of punctate corneal opacities and microfilariae in the anterior chamber of the eye.[20, 21] The intensity and frequency of adverse reactions diminish with later treatments. Although ivermectin is not macrofilaricidal, 3-monthly courses of the drug appear to be effective in reducing the numbers of male *O. volvulus* worms, preventing embryogenesis to the microfilarial stage in females, and progressively reducing the numbers of viable female worms.[22]

Contraindications to ivermectin therapy include pregnancy, breast-feeding during the first 3 months post partum, age younger than 5 years, central nervous system disorders such as meningitis that may increase the permeability of the blood-brain barrier, and a history of allergy to the drug. If a serious Mazzotti-like reaction occurs during treatment, symptomatic therapy with fluids, antipyretics, antihistamines, and corticosteroids should be used.

Surgical removal of nodules containing adult worms should be strongly considered if the nodules are in the head region because of an increased risk for ocular involvement. Nodulectomy has been widely practiced in Latin America but not in Africa, where many nodules are deeper in the subcutaneous tissues or are situated adjacent to bones or joints.

PREVENTION AND CONTROL

No effective prophylactic drugs or vaccines exist. Attempts to avoid the breeding sites of *Simulium* vectors are advisable if they are feasible. Personal protection measures such as protective clothing and insect repellents should be used by visitors to endemic areas. Attempts to eliminate the insect vector with insecticide have met with mixed success in some areas of Africa; evidence of the development of insecticide resistance has begun to appear. Periodic treatment of infected subjects in endemic regions holds promise for the control of onchocerciasis by reduction of the parasite reservoir.

Loiasis

Loa loa is a filarial parasite endemic to the rain forests of equatorial West and Central Africa where an estimated 20 million people are infected[23] (see Table 294–1). It is transmitted to humans by tabanid flies of the genus *Chrysops*. Adult worms migrate and reside in subcutaneous tissues where they cause transient swellings. They occasionally migrate across the eye, hence the name eye worm. The adult females measure about 6 cm in length and 0.5 mm in width; the males are 3.2 cm by 0.4 mm. Sheathed microfilariae deposited by the adult females migrate from the subcutaneous tissues to the blood stream. Peak levels of microfilaremia occur at midday. After ingestion in a blood meal by the vector deerfly, the microfilariae develop into infective third-stage larvae that are released into the bite wound when the fly feeds. The larvae mature to adults in the subcutaneous tissue and reproduce sexually to reinitiate the cycle.

Infected people are frequently asymptomatic despite having heavy microfilaremia and an intense blood eosinophilia. Migration of the adult worms through subcutaneous tissue results in painful, angioedematous eruptions known as Calabar swellings. The forearms, wrists, and periorbital tissues are most commonly affected.[24] These transient skin swellings last 1 to 2 days; are frequently preceded by localized pain and pruritus; and may be associated with fever, arthralgias, and urticaria. Migration of the adult worm across the conjunctiva and sclera may precipitate an intense conjunctivitis. Visitors to endemic regions who develop loiasis often have exaggerated reactions to the migratory worms characterized by more frequent Calabar swellings and cutaneous symptoms as well as higher levels of eosinophilia, parasite-specific immunoglobulin E, and lymphocyte blastogenic responses to parasite antigen.[25] Rare, potentially life-threatening complications include cardiomyopathy, encephalitis, nephropathy, and pulmonary disease.[26] The microfilariae of *L. loa* have been encountered in a variety of aberrant locations including ascites and pleural and joint effusions.

Identification of characteristic microfilariae in thick or thin smears of blood taken during the day and stained with Wright or Giemsa stain establishes the diagnosis of loiasis[6] (Fig. 294–3). Concentration techniques may be necessary in patients with low levels of microfilaremia. Immunodiagnostic tests may be useful in amicrofilaremic patients with eosinophilia in whom the diagnosis is strongly suspected; however, these tests are not widely available and may suffer from low specificity.

DEC effectively eliminates microfilariae; its effect on adult worms remains unclear. Subjects with high levels of microfilaremia may develop intense allergic reactions to the dying parasites characterized by fever, nausea, urticaria, and rarely encephalitis.[27] These patients should be given a test dose of 25 mg of DEC on day 1 followed by 50 mg the following day and then 400 mg/d for 7 to 21 days. Corticosteroids may be given as an adjunct to decrease the initial inflammatory reaction. DEC has also been used successfully as a prophylactic agent in long-term visitors to endemic regions.[28] Single-dose therapy with ivermectin (200 to 400 μg/kg) has been shown to be well tolerated and effective in suppressing microfilaremia.[8, 29] A multidose regimen of albendazole (200 mg twice daily for 21 days) has also been found to effectively reduce microfilaremia without significant adverse effects.[30] Migrating adult worms should be surgically removed, especially if they are found in the conjunctiva.

Mansonella perstans Infection

M. perstans is mainly found in rain forests in tropical Africa, Central and South America, and the Caribbean (see Table 294–1). It is transmitted by midges of the *Culicoides* genus with host reservoirs including humans and chimpanzees.[31] The adult worms live in the peritoneal cavity of their host.[32] Unsheathed microfilariae are released into the blood in a subperiodic fashion. Infected residents of endemic regions are often asymptomatic, although they may have vague joint or cutaneous complaints and eosinophilia. Visitors to en-

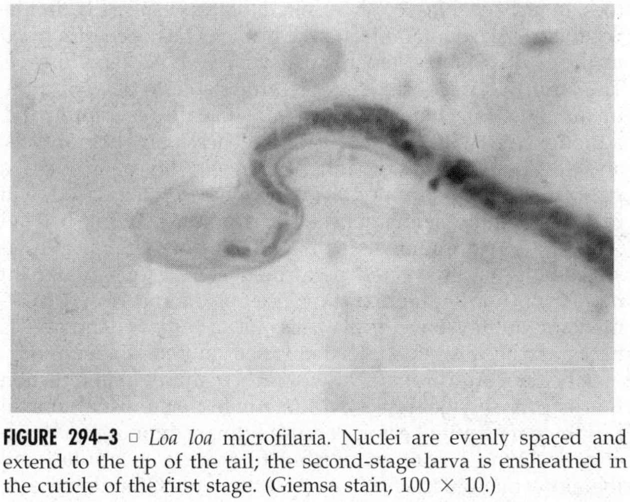

FIGURE 294–3 □ *Loa loa* microfilaria. Nuclei are evenly spaced and extend to the tip of the tail; the second-stage larva is ensheathed in the cuticle of the first stage. (Giemsa stain, 100 × 10.)

demic areas may develop edema, serositis, and fever. Demonstration of characteristic microfilariae in blood smears confirms the diagnosis.[6] High-dose therapy with DEC may eliminate this infection. Therapeutic responses to ivermectin have met with mixed success.[8, 29, 33, 34]

Mansonella streptocerca *Infection*

Streptocerciasis is a common filarial infection in parts of Central and West Africa (see Table 294–1). *M. streptocerca* is transmitted by midges of the genus *Culicoides*. The adult females, which measure approximately 3 cm in length, live in the subcutaneous tissue. The unsheathed microfilariae are about 200 μm long, have a distinctive "shepherd's crook" appearance, and can be found in the skin or blood. Clinical manifestations of infection include pruritus, axillary or inguinal adenopathy, and a chronic dermatitis with hypopigmented macules or papules that resemble those of leprosy but are not anesthetic.[35] Wet mounts of skin snips usually reveal the presence of the microfilariae.[6] Caution must be employed to avoid confusion with the larger microfilariae of *O. volvulus*. Treatment with DEC is effective but may exacerbate the pruritus.

Mansonella ozzardi *Infection*

Mansonelliasis, the filarial infection caused by *M. ozzardi*, is found in parts of Central and South America and in certain Caribbean islands (see Table 294–1). Midges of the genus *Culicoides* or black flies of the *Simulium* group serve as vectors. Adult worms live in the peritoneal cavity, where they produce unsheathed microfilariae with a characteristic sharp tail. The microfilariae are nonperiodic and can be found in the blood.[6] Clinical manifestations of this usually asymptomatic infection are ill-defined but may include chronic arthritis and pruritus. Therapy with DEC is generally ineffective.[36] Single-dose therapy with ivermectin may be effective, but experience with this agent is limited.[8, 37]

Dirofilariasis

Filarial nematodes of the genus *Dirofilaria* are responsible for two syndromes in humans. Transmission of *Dirofilaria immitis* (dog heartworm) larvae from dogs to humans by mosquitoes may lead to the development of a granulomatous pulmonary nodule.[38] Subcutaneous dirofilariasis results from the accidental infection of humans by *Dirofilaria repens*, whose natural hosts are dogs and cats, or by *Dirofilaria tenuis*, a parasite of the subcutaneous tissue of raccoons.[39]

The larvae of *D. immitis* are commonly found in mosquitoes in urban areas of the United States, especially in the Southeast. Accidental infection of humans has been described in the United States, Japan, Australia, and Western Europe. The adult worms of this parasite are unable to develop fully in humans. Infected individuals are usually asymptomatic, although rarely there may be cough, chest pain, hemoptysis, and fever. Chest radiographs commonly reveal a solitary, peripheral pulmonary nodule, which, when it is excised, will reveal a granulomatous reaction surrounding an intact dead worm or worm fragments within an arteriole.[40] Surgical excision of the nodule, often performed to rule out malignant neoplasm, fulfills the dual purposes of diagnosis and treatment of pulmonary dirofilariasis. No additional therapy is necessary because this infection is self-limited.

Subcutaneous dirofilariasis is a rare, cosmopolitan infection that is probably acquired by humans from the usual animal host by a mosquito vector. Because humans represent a dead-end host, the larvae are unable to mature to adults, and therefore microfilariae are never observed. Granulomatous, subcutaneous nodules may be found in the conjunctiva, chest wall, and extremities. The lesion develops slowly during many weeks into a nodule that may be painful and erythematous. Diagnosis is made by identification of the worm in biopsy specimens, a procedure that also serves as treatment.

Other Tissue Nematode Infections

Dracunculiasis

Dracunculiasis, also known as guinea worm disease or dracontiasis, develops after the ingestion of water contaminated with copepods infected with *Dracunculus medinensis*. The disease is manifested by a chronic skin ulcer from which the adult worm protrudes. It is responsible for significant morbidity and decreases in agricultural productivity in endemic populations.

EPIDEMIOLOGY

Dracunculiasis remains endemic in rural populations of India, Pakistan, and sub-Saharan Africa, where an estimated 100 million people are at risk.[41] A worldwide eradication campaign has successfully reduced the incidence of disease to about 221,000 cases in 1993. The prevalence of dracunculiasis exhibits seasonal variation. The frequency of infection increases with age until the second or third decade of life.[42] Greater exposure to infected water through agricultural activities or the collection of water for domestic use places certain groups at higher risk for infection. Sources of drinking water such as step wells or ponds that require people to walk down into the water are necessary for continued transmission of this parasite (Fig. 294–4).

LIFE CYCLE

Human infection is acquired after drinking water containing copepods *(Cyclops)* harboring the third-stage larvae of the parasite. The larvae penetrate the intestinal mucosa to reach the retroperitoneum, where they mature into adult worms during a 12-month period. The adult female migrates to the skin surface to form a blister from which a portion of the worm protrudes. Water exposure leads to the release of many first-stage larvae from the wound, which are in turn ingested by copepods. After a period of about 10 days, the larvae

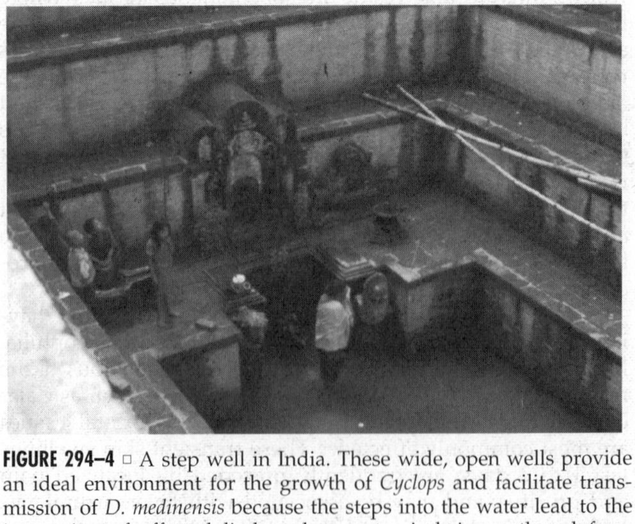

FIGURE 294–4 ▫ A step well in India. These wide, open wells provide an ideal environment for the growth of *Cyclops* and facilitate transmission of *D. medinensis* because the steps into the water lead to the immersion of affected limbs when water is being gathered from the well.

mature to a new infective stage. The adult females of *D. medinensis* range from 70 to 120 cm in length; the males, uncommonly observed in infected humans, measure only 3 to 5 cm.

CLINICAL FEATURES

Prodromal symptoms of urticaria, fever, nausea, vomiting, diarrhea, and dysphoria may precede the formation of a skin blister.[43] The lesion is initially pruritic and erythematous and then progresses to form a vesicle that may measure several centimeters in diameter. After the blister ruptures, the adult female protrudes to a distance of several centimeters. The ulcers are painful and occur most commonly in the lower extremities, although many other locations are possible. Multiple ulcers may be present, with greater numbers directly correlating with the degree of disability suffered. The adult worm intermittently discharges a milky white fluid containing larvae and is gradually resorbed or completely extruded. The healing process may take many weeks or even months, during which the affected person is incapacitated. Secondary bacterial infections including abscess formation are common. Tetanus is a rare complication. If the ulcer formation occurs during a critical agricultural period or the school year for children, the resulting disability can have significant negative social and economic effects.[43, 44] The proximity of an ulcer to a joint may lead to arthritis and long-term disability due to joint contractures.

DIAGNOSIS

The clinical manifestations of the infection are diagnostic. Larvae can be seen on microscopic examination of fluid discharged from the ulcer. Attempts to develop serologic tests for the diagnosis of the infection during the prepatent period have not been successful.

TREATMENT

Treatment consists of manually extracting the worm by winding it around a stick with gentle traction. Accidental rupture of the worm will precipitate severe systemic reactions manifested by fever, anaphylaxis, and urticaria with late complications including abscess formation and chronic ulceration. Surgical extraction of the unerupted worm under local anesthesia effectively shortens the removal time and associated period of disability.[45] Topical or systemic antimicrobial agents help to relieve ulcer-associated pain, improve healing, and facilitate more rapid removal of worms, although no agent has been found to have curative activity against *D. medinensis*.[46] Local care of the wound is necessary to prevent bacterial superinfection. Tetanus precautions are recommended.

PREVENTION

Dracunculiasis can be prevented by teaching people to filter their drinking water through a fine-mesh cloth or to boil the water and to avoid entering drinking water sources when the adult worm is emerging, by providing improved sources of drinking water, and by treating contaminated water supplies with the chemical temefos monthly during the season of transmission. A global campaign to eradicate guinea worm disease, initiated by the World Health Organization in 1986, has resulted in significant reductions in the number of reported cases of the disease.[41]

Gnathostomiasis

Human gnathostomiasis is a sporadic infection principally caused by *Gnathostoma spinigerum*, although at least three other species of *Gnathostoma* have been found in human infections.[47] The disease has been mainly described in Asia, with the highest occurrence in Thailand and Japan. Humans are accidental hosts who acquire infection by the consumption of the raw or undercooked flesh of freshwater fish or other intermediate hosts that contain the encysted, infective larvae. The definitive hosts of *G. spinigerum* include a range of mammals. The adult worms reside in the gastric wall and release eggs that hatch, after passage into the environment, to release first-stage larvae. These larvae are ingested by an intermediate host of the *Cyclops* genus in which they mature to second- or third-stage larvae that may be ingested by a second intermediate host. The larvae migrate to the musculature, complete development, and encyst. The life cycle is completed when a definitive host ingests the flesh of the infected second intermediate host.

Initial clinical manifestations, which occur within 24 to 48 hours after ingestion of the parasite, include malaise, fever, urticaria, nausea, vomiting, diarrhea, and abdominal pain. An intense eosinophilia develops in association with the penetration of the gastric or intestinal wall by the larvae. Cutaneous gnathostomiasis, the most common manifestation of infection, may take 3 to 4 weeks to develop. It is characterized by intermittent episodes of migratory swelling with associated edema, pain, pruritus, and an eosinophilic leukocytosis. These subcutaneous eruptions are caused by the migrating, immature adult worm. The episodes last 1 to 2 weeks and may recur at variable intervals. Ocular complications including anterior uveitis, iritis, intraocular hemorrhage, and even blindness may occur. Less common sites of visceral involvement include the lung, intestine, bladder, and regions of the ear, nose, and throat.

Infection of the central nervous system with *G. spinigerum*, a potentially fatal complication, is manifested by an eosinophilic myeloencephalitis characterized by severe nerve root pain, paralysis, and urinary retention with an associated eosinophilic leukocytosis of the cerebrospinal fluid. Blindness, impairment of visual acuity, paraplegia, and death are serious complications of this infection.

Gnathostomiasis should be suspected in patients from an endemic area who have a positive dietary history, migratory skin lesions, and peripheral eosinophilia. Gnathostomal creeping eruptions are frequently confused with those caused by canine or feline hookworms. Most other diseases characterized by subcutaneous swellings can be differentiated on epidemiologic and clinical grounds. Central nervous system gnathostomiasis can be clinically distinguished from eosinophilic meningitis caused by *Angiostrongylus cantonensis*, which tends to be less severe in terms of nerve root and cranial nerve involvement. The definitive diagnosis of gnathostomiasis is dependent on identification of the worms in surgical specimens or body fluids.

Surgical removal of the worm is the most effective treatment for this infection. Supportive therapy should include antiinflammatory agents and analgesics. A number of anthelmintic drugs have been tried but have not proved effective, although albendazole holds some promise.[48] Adequate cooking of potentially infected intermediate or transport hosts is needed to prevent infection.

Angiostrongylus cantonensis *Infection*

Human eosinophilic meningitis is most commonly caused by *A. cantonensis*, a parasite of rats.[49, 50] The adult worms live in the rat's pulmonary artery, where they lay eggs that hatch in the lung parenchyma. The first-stage larvae penetrate into the alveoli, migrate up the tracheobronchial tree, are swallowed, and are eventually eliminated in the feces. A number of different molluscan species including snails and slugs serve as intermediate hosts. After ingestion by a suitable mollusk, the larvae mature to third-stage larvae that are ingested by rats. The larvae penetrate the intestinal wall and migrate through the venous system to the pulmonary circulation, from which they migrate to the brain and other organs. The larvae undergo additional maturation in the brain before returning to the lungs to complete the cycle. Humans are accidental hosts who acquire infection by ingesting inadequately cooked or raw mollusks or vegetables or other foods contaminated by slugs or planaria.

Human infection with *A. cantonensis* has been principally found in Southeast Asia and some Pacific islands including Guam, American Samoa, and Hawaii. Sporadic cases have been reported from some African countries and Cuba. Infected patients tend to be young people with a history of exposure to snails, raw fish, or prawns.

Invasion of the brain parenchyma and spinal cord by larval stages of the parasite is responsible for clinical symptoms. After an incubation period of about 1 week, infected patients commonly develop the acute onset of severe headache, nausea, vomiting, lethargy, paresthesias, meningismus, and low-grade fever.[49, 51] Physical examination may reveal signs of meningeal irritation, cranial nerve palsies, altered mental status, and a temperature less than 38°C. Characteristic cerebrospinal fluid findings include elevated opening pressure, turbid fluid, eosinophilic pleocytosis (often greater than 20% eosinophils), elevated protein concentration, and normal glucose level. Adult worms are recovered from the cerebrospinal fluid in less than 10% of cases. The parasite is occasionally observed in and may be removed from the eye. The diagnosis can be substantiated by demonstrating elevated titers of antibodies to *A. cantonensis* antigens by enzyme-linked immunosorbent assay.

No anthelmintic therapy has been proved beneficial in treating this form of eosinophilic meningitis. Supportive treatment with fluids and analgesics is indicated. A course of corticosteroids may be justifiable in severe, life-threatening infections of the central nervous system. However, most persons recover after a period of a few weeks and rarely suffer from chronic neurologic sequelae.

Angiostrongylus costaricensis *Infection*

Abdominal angiostrongyliasis has mainly been described in children in Central and South America.[52] The life cycle of *A. costaricensis* is similar to that of *A. cantonensis*. The cotton rat *(Sigmodon hispidus)* and other rodents are the natural host. Human infection is probably acquired by the ingestion of infective larvae contained in tissues of the intermediate host, commonly a slug, or by consumption of vegetables contaminated with extruded mucus of the slug. The larvae develop into adult worms that reside in mesenteric arterioles, especially in the ileocolic area. Eggs released by the female adult result in eosinophilic granulomata, thrombosis, and arteritis of the intestinal wall. The eggs do not appear in the stool. The infection is clinically manifested by acute right lower quadrant abdominal pain, a tumor-like mass, and peritoneal signs that closely resemble acute appendicitis. A visceral larva migrans–like syndrome is a rare complication of the ectopic localization of adult worms in the liver.[53] Marked eosinophilia frequently accompanies the infection. The diagnosis is usually established by histopathologic examination of surgical specimens. Treatment with thiabendazole is recommended but has not been demonstrated to be effective. Surgical resection of infected regions of the ileum, appendix, cecum, and ascending colon is often necessary.

References

1. Despommier DD, Gwadz RW, Hotez PJ: Lymphatic filariae. *In* Parasitic Diseases, ed 3. New York, Springer-Verlag, 1995, pp 40–47.
2. World Health Organization: Lymphatic filariasis: The disease and its control. Fifth report of the WHO Expert Committee on Filariasis. World Health Organ Tech Rep Ser 821:1, 1992.
3. Ottesen EA: Efficacy of diethylcarbamazine in eradicating infection with lymphatic-dwelling filariae in humans. Rev Infect Dis 7:341, 1985.
4. Nanduri J, Kazura JW: Clinical and laboratory aspects of filariasis. Clin Microbiol Rev 2:39, 1989.
5. Ottesen EA, Nutman TB: Tropical pulmonary eosinophilia. Annu Rev Med 43:417, 1992.
6. Eberhard ML, Lammie PJ: Laboratory diagnosis of filariasis. Clin Lab Med 11:977, 1991.
7. Ottesen EA, Vijayasekaran V, Kumaraswami V, et al: A controlled trial of ivermectin and diethylcarbamazine in lymphatic filariasis. N Engl J Med 322:1113, 1990.
8. Campbell WC: Ivermectin as an antiparasitic agent for use in humans. Annu Rev Microbiol 45:445, 1991.
9. Mak JW, Navaratnam V, Grewel JS, et al: Treatment of subperiodic *Brugia malayi* infection with a single dose of ivermectin. Am J Trop Med Hyg 48:591, 1993.
10. Glaziou P, Moulia-Pelat JP, Nguyen LN, et al: Double-blind controlled trial of a single dose of the combination ivermectin 400 μg/kg plus diethylcarbamazine 6 mg/kg for the treatment of bancroftian filariasis: Results at six months. Trans R Soc Trop Med Hyg 88:707, 1994.
11. WHO Expert Committee on Onchocerciasis: Third report. World Health Organ Tech Rep Ser 752:1, 1987.
12. Gibson DW, Duke BOL, Connor DH: Onchocerciasis: A review of clinical, pathologic and chemotherapeutic aspects, and vector control programs. Prog Clin Parasitol 1:57, 1989.
13. Ottesen EA: Immune responsiveness and the pathogenesis of human onchocerciasis. J Infect Dis 171:659, 1995.
14. Greene BM: Modern medicine versus an ancient scourge: Progress toward control of onchocerciasis. J Infect Dis 166:15, 1992.
15. Murdoch ME, Hay RJ, MacKenzie CD, et al: A clinical classification and grading system of cutaneous changes in onchocerciasis. Br J Dermatol 129:260, 1993.
16. Connor DH, Gibson DW, Neafie RC, et al: Sowda-onchocerciasis in North Yemen: A clinicopathologic study of 18 patients. Am J Trop Med Hyg 32:123, 1983.
17. Bradley JE, Trenholme KR, Gillespie AJ, et al: A sensitive serodiagnostic test for onchocerciasis using a cocktail of recombinant antigens. Am J Trop Med Hyg 48:198, 1993.
18. Zimmerman PA, Guderian RH, Araujo E, et al: Polymerase chain reaction–based diagnosis of *Onchocerca volvulus* infection: Improved detection of patients with onchocerciasis. J Infect Dis 169:686, 1994.
19. Greene BM, Taylor HR, Cupp EW, et al: Comparison of ivermectin and diethylcarbamazine in the treatment of onchocerciasis. N Engl J Med 313:133, 1985.
20. Paque M, Munoz B, Greene BM, et al: Community-based treatment of onchocerciasis with ivermectin: Safety, efficacy, and acceptability of yearly treatment. J Infect Dis 163:381, 1991.
21. Greene BM, Dukuly ZD, Munoz B, et al: A comparison of 6-, 12-, and 24-monthly dosing with ivermectin for treatment of onchocerciasis. J Infect Dis 163:376, 1991.
22. Duke BOL, Zea-Flores G, Castro J, et al: Effects of three-month doses of ivermectin on adult *Onchocerca volvulus*. Am J Trop Med Hyg 46:189, 1992.
23. Despommier DD, Gwadz RW, Hotez PJ: *Loa loa*. *In* Parasitic Diseases, ed 3. New York, Springer-Verlag, 1995, pp 53–57.
24. Carme B, Mamboueni JP, Copin N, et al: Clinical and biological study of *Loa loa* filariasis in Congolese. Am J Trop Med Hyg 41:331, 1989.
25. Klion AD, Massougbodji A, Sadeler B-C, et al: Loiasis in endemic and nonendemic populations: Immunologically mediated differences in clinical presentation. J Infect Dis 163:1318, 1991.
26. Klion AD, Eisenstein EM, Smirniotopoulos TT, et al: Pulmonary involvement in loiasis. Am Rev Respir Dis 145:961, 1992.
27. Carme B, Boulesteix J, Boutes H, et al: Five cases of encephalitis during treatment of loiasis with diethylcarbamazine. Am J Trop Med Hyg 44:684, 1991.

28. Nutman TB, Miller KD, Mulligan M, et al: Diethylcarbamazine prophylaxis for human loiasis. Results of a double-blind study. N Engl J Med 319:752, 1988.
29. Martin-Prevel Y, Cosnefroy J-Y, Tshipamba P, et al: Tolerance and efficacy of single high-dose ivermectin for the treatment of loiasis. Am J Trop Med Hyg 48:186, 1993.
30. Klion AD, Massougbodji A, Horton J, et al: Albendazole in human loiasis: Results of a double-blind, placebo-controlled trial. J Infect Dis 168:202, 1993.
31. Nelson GS: *Mansonella perstans* infection. *In* Strickland GT (ed): Hunter's Tropical Medicine, ed 7. Philadelphia, WB Saunders, 1991, pp 745–746.
32. Baird JK, Neafie RC, Lanoie L, et al: Adult *Mansonella perstans* in the abdominal cavity in nine Africans. Am J Trop Med Hyg 37:578, 1987.
33. Van den Enden E, Van Gompel A, Van der Stuyft P, et al: Treatment failure of a single high dose of ivermectin for *Mansonella perstans* filariasis. Trans R Soc Trop Med Hyg 87:90, 1993.
34. Schulz-Key H, Albrecht W, Heuschkel C, et al: Efficacy of ivermectin in the treatment of concomitant *Mansonella perstans* infections in onchocerciasis patients. Trans R Soc Trop Med Hyg 87:227, 1993.
35. Meyers WM, Connor DH, Harman LE, et al: Human streptocerciasis. A clinico-pathologic study of 40 Africans (Zairians) including identification of the adult filaria. Am J Trop Med Hyg 21:528, 1972.
36. Chadee DD, Tilluckdharry CC, Rawlins SC, et al: Mass chemotherapy with diethylcarbamazine for the control of bancroftian filariasis: A twelve-year follow-up in northern Trinidad, including observations on *Mansonella ozzardi*. Am J Trop Med Hyg 52:174, 1995.
37. Nutman TB, Nash TE, Ottesen EA: Ivermectin in the successful treatment of a patient with *Mansonella ozzardi* infection. J Infect Dis 156:662, 1987.
38. Asimacopoulos PJ, Katras A, Christie B: Pulmonary dirofilariasis. The largest single-hospital experience. Chest 102:851, 1992.
39. Neafie RC, Meyers WM: Dirofilariasis. *In* Strickland GT (ed): Hunter's Tropical Medicine, ed 7. Philadelphia, WB Saunders, 1991, pp 748–749.
40. Green LK, Ansari MQ, Schwartz MR, et al: Non-specific fluorescent whitener stains in the rapid recognition of pulmonary dirofilariasis: A report of 20 cases. Thorax 49:590, 1994.
41. Hopkins DR, Ruiz-Tiben E, Ruebush T II, et al: Dracunculiasis eradication: March 1994 update. Am J Trop Med Hyg 52:14, 1995.
42. Abdel-Hameed AA, Ahmed AGM, Elturabi MK, et al: An outbreak of dracunculiasis in central Sudan. Ann Trop Med Parasitol 87:571, 1993.
43. Ilegbodu VA, Ilegbodu AE, Wise RA, et al: Clinical manifestations, disability and use of folk medicine in *Dracunculus* infection in Nigeria. J Trop Med Hyg 94:35, 1991.
44. Ilegbodu VA, Kale OO, Wise RA, et al: Impact of Guinea worm disease on children in Nigeria. Am J Trop Med Hyg 35:962, 1986.
45. Rohde JE, Sharma BL, Patton H, et al: Surgical extraction of Guinea worm: Disability reduction and contribution to disease control. Am J Trop Med Hyg 48:71, 1993.
46. Magnussen P, Yakubu A, Bloch P: The effect of antibiotic- and hydrocortisone-containing ointments in preventing secondary infections in Guinea worm disease. Am J Trop Med Hyg 51:797, 1994.
47. Rusnak JM, Lucey DR: Clinical gnathostomiasis: Case report and review of the English-language literature. Clin Infect Dis 16:33, 1993.
48. Kraivichian P, Kulkumthorn M, Yingyourd P, et al: Albendazole for the treatment of human gnathostomiasis. Trans R Soc Trop Med Hyg 86:418, 1992.
49. Punyagupta S, Juttijudata P, Bunnag T: Eosinophilic meningitis in Thailand. Clinical studies of 484 typical cases probably caused by *Angiostrongylus cantonensis*. Am J Trop Med Hyg 24:921, 1975.
50. Koo J, Pien F, Kliks MM: *Angiostrongylus (Parastrongylus)* eosinophilic meningitis. Rev Infect Dis 10:1155, 1988.
51. Yii CY: Clinical observations on eosinophilic meningitis and meningoencephalitis caused by *Angiostrongylus cantonensis* on Taiwan. Am J Trop Med Hyg 25:233, 1976.
52. Loria-Cortes R, Lobo-Sanahuja JF: Clinical abdominal angiostrongylosis. A study of 116 children with intestinal eosinophilic granuloma caused by *Angiostrongylus costaricensis*. Am J Trop Med Hyg 29:538, 1980.
53. Morera P, Perez F, Mora F, et al: Visceral larva migrans–like syndrome caused by *Angiostrongylus costaricensis*. Am J Trop Med Hyg 31:67, 1982.

295

Schistosoma and Other Trematodes

Charles H. King
Adel A. F. Mahmoud

Several groups of flukes (flatworms) infect humans and are responsible for significant morbidity. Flukes can be classified clinically by the primary sites of involvement in humans (blood, intestines, liver, lungs, brain). Like most other parasitic worms, flukes are characterized by their inability to multiply within the mammalian host and by an association between their tissue migratory phases and significant peripheral as well as tissue eosinophilia.[1]

Blood Flukes: Schistosomiasis

History

Human infection with species of the blood flukes (schistosomes) was first reported in ancient Egypt approximately 3000 to 5000 years ago, and calcified *Schistosoma haematobium* eggs have been found in mummies dating back to 1250 BC. In modern history, the worms were first identified and described by Theodor Bilharz, who found them while performing autopsies in Cairo, Egypt, in 1852. Five species of *Schistosoma* are currently known to infect humans (Table 295–1): *S. haematobium, S. mansoni,* and *S. japonicum* and the less common *S. mekongi* and *S. intercalatum*.[2] Infection is endemic in many parts of Africa, the Middle East, Southeast Asia, South America, and the Caribbean. The total number of infected persons is estimated at 200 to 300 million, and those at risk for acquiring infection range from 600 million to 1 billion.[3]

Characteristics of the Pathogen

The schistosomes are flatworms (platyhelminths) but differ from other flukes that infect humans in that they have separate sexes. Adult worms inhabit the venous system draining the urinary bladder or intestines. Adult male worms measure approximately 1 to 1.5 cm in length; the flattened sides of the body curve anteriorly to form the gynecophoric canal, in which adult females usually live. Adult females are rounded and longer than males (1.5 to 2.0 cm) and produce several hundred eggs daily. Epidemiologic evidence indicates that the mean life span of adult schistosomes is 5 to 10 years, although case reports indicate that viable eggs may be detected in excreta of infected persons as long as 40 years after they depart endemic areas. The life cycle of the schistosome is shown in Figure 295–1.

TABLE 295–1 ■ Clinically Significant Trematode Parasites of Humans

SPECIES	GEOGRAPHIC DISTRIBUTION	INFECTIVE STAGE	DIAGNOSIS	POTENTIAL COMPLICATIONS
Blood Flukes				
Schistosoma haematobium	Africa, Mideast	Cercaria	Urine examination	Hydronephrosis, pyelonephritis, carcinoma
Schistosoma mansoni	Africa, South America, Middle East	Cercaria	Stool examination, biopsy	Portal hypertension, polyposis, splenomegaly
Schistosoma japonicum	Asia, Philippines	Cercaria	Stool examination, biopsy	Seizures, hepatic dysfunction, splenomegaly
Schistosoma mekongi	Southeast Asia	Cercaria	Stool examination, biopsy	As for *S. japonicum*
Schistosoma intercalatum	Africa	Cercaria	Stool and urine examination	Colonic and urinary tract inflammation, prostatitis
Liver Flukes				
Clonorchis sinensis	Asia	Metacercaria	Stool examination	Cholangitis, cirrhosis, cholangiocarcinoma
Opisthorchis felineus	Asia, Eastern Europe	Metacercaria	Stool examination	Cholangitis, cirrhosis, cholangiocarcinoma
Opisthorchis viverrini	Asia	Metacercaria	Stool examination	Cholangitis, cirrhosis, cholangiocarcinoma
Fasciola hepatica	Worldwide	Metacercaria	Stool examination	Fever, hepatomegaly, biliary and pharyngeal obstruction
Fasciola gigantica	Africa, Asia	Metacercaria	Stool examination	Fever, hepatomegaly, biliary obstruction
Tissue Flukes				
Paragonimus westermani	Asia, Africa, Americas	Metacercaria	Sputum and stool examination	Lung abscess, seizures, gastrointestinal ulceration
Other *Paragonimus* spp.	South and Central America	Metacercaria	Sputum and stool examination, biopsy	Lung and cerebral lesions, tissue abscess
Intestinal Flukes				
Fasciolopsis buski	India, Asia	Metacercaria	Stool examination	Intestinal ulceration, diarrhea, ascites
Echinostoma ilocanum	Asia, India, Philippines	Metacercaria	Stool examination	Abdominal pain, diarrhea
Heterophyes heterophyes	Egypt, Asia, India, Philippines	Metacercaria	Stool examination	Diarrhea, central nervous system and cardiac lesions
Metagonimus yokogawai	Asia, Eastern Europe, Spain	Metacercaria	Stool examination	Intestinal ulceration
Nanophyetus salmincola	North America, Siberia	Metacercaria	Stool examination	Nausea, diarrhea, fatigue

Epidemiology

Schistosomiasis is a water-borne infection. The infective larvae, called cercariae, are found in freshwater bodies in areas endemic for the infection. Cercariae infect humans by penetrating intact skin within a few minutes of contact. On maturation in humans, adult worms begin oviposition. A proportion of the ova pass to the environment through human excreta; if they reach freshwater, eggs hatch, releasing free-swimming miracidia that seek the specific snail intermediate host. After a series of multiplications in the snail, cercariae emerge and must find and penetrate the skin of the human definitive host within several hours to complete the life cycle of the parasite.

The geographic distribution of schistosomiasis parallels that of the specific snail intermediate host and is dependent on availability of infected humans who, because of their cultural habits or socioeconomic factors, pass their excreta in or close to freshwater bodies. *S. haematobium* infection is endemic in many parts of Africa and the Middle East; *S. mansoni* in Africa, the Middle East, South America, and some Caribbean islands, including Puerto Rico; *S. japonicum* in the Far East; *S. mekongi* in isolated foci in Southeast Asia; and *S. intercalatum* in Central and West Africa.[4]

The epidemiology of schistosomiasis in human populations has several characteristic features.[5] Infection is gradually acquired as children begin to experience contact with cercariae-contaminated freshwater bodies. Prevalence gradually increases with age until it reaches a peak at approximately 10 to 20 years. The extent of prevalence varies from one endemic community to another and may reach 100% in high-transmission areas. A slight but insignificant decrease in prevalence is usual among persons 30 years and older. Intensity of infection (estimated by egg count in excreta) increases with age, again reaching a maximum at age 15 to 20 years. Thereafter, intensity decreases significantly, so that it is rare to find heavy infection in persons older than 30 years. From this marked reduction of intensity in older persons living in endemic areas, acquisition of protective immunity has been inferred.

Pathogenesis

Disease manifestations due to schistosome infection are a result of stage of parasite in the host and its interaction with specific and nonspecific inflammatory and immune responses.[6] Multiple studies have demonstrated that only a proportion of infected persons exhibit disease. Most of them are heavily infected, but the relationship of disease to intensity of infection is not exact. There is evidence that other factors, such as host genetics,[7] nutrition, and intercurrent infection, participate to varying degrees in determining the susceptibility to and the pathologic outcome of schistosomiasis.

Skin penetration by cercariae and the death of some of these organisms in the subcutaneous tissues result in a popu-

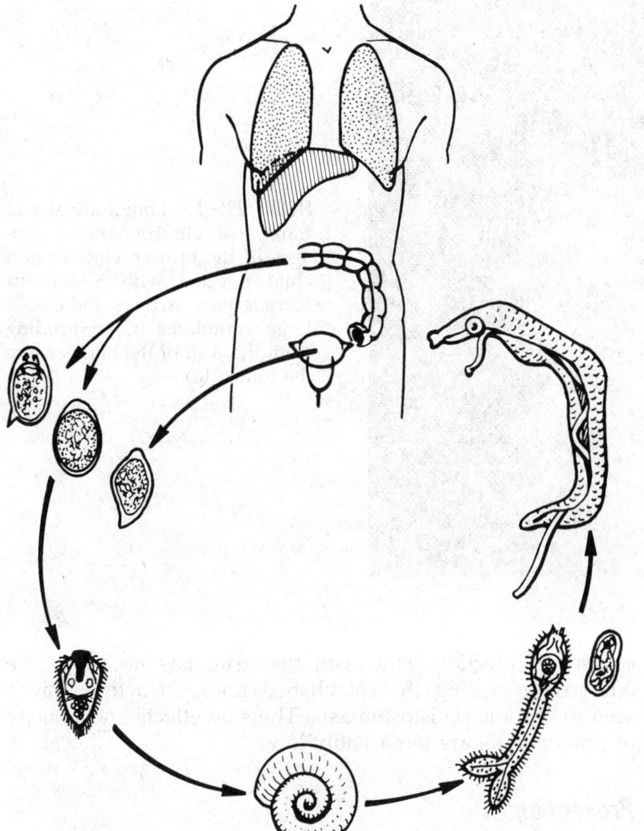

FIGURE 295–1 □ The life cycle of schistosomes (counterclockwise): parasite eggs passed into freshwater in human excreta hatch into miracidia that infect the intermediate host, an aquatic snail. Several weeks later, the snail releases free-swimming cercarial forms that seek and penetrate human skin, transforming into immature male or female larvae. Six to 8 weeks later, mature worms complete the cycle by mating in portal or urinary tract veins and releasing eggs into nearby viscera.

lar eruption called swimmers' itch, which is associated with humoral, cellular, and local infiltrative responses. A serum sickness–like syndrome (acute schistosomiasis or Katayama fever) occurs in some infected individuals at 6 to 8 weeks, particularly those with heavy infection. This syndrome is thought to be due to the formation of antigen-antibody complexes.

The most significant disease manifestations of schistosomiasis follow egg deposition. As mentioned earlier, a proportion of ova escape in excreta; those retained in host tissues elicit a series of immunopathologic reactions. The basic host response to parasite eggs is a delayed-type hypersensitivity granulomatous reaction that far exceeds the size of retained ova. These large granulomata account for some of the early obstructive lesions seen in the lower end of ureters in *S. haematobium*–infected persons and also in the hepatomegaly and interference with portal blood flow seen in *S. mansoni, S. japonicum,* and *S. mekongi* infections. In spite of the multiple immunologic factors that regulate granuloma formation (resulting in smaller granulomatous response in chronically infected persons),[8, 9] another set of more permanent fibrotic responses leads to obstructive and hemodynamic changes that herald significant morbidity.[10]

The multicellular, multistage schistosome infection presents the mammalian host with a variety of antigenic stimuli. The host responds at both systemic and local levels. Serum antibodies and sensitized lymphocytes that react with the different stages of schistosomes are detected after infection. It is remarkable that as long as adult worms live in the venous system, no recognition by the host immune or inflammatory responses can be detected in situ. On the other hand, once ova are deposited, the host recognizes their existence, and the sensitized lymphocytes along with other inflammatory cells and antibodies contribute to granuloma formation. Schistosome egg granulomata are dynamic lesions that are tightly controlled, representing the balance between initiating and down-regulating immune mechanisms. Granuloma formation is further complicated by the subsequent development of fibrosis, which is responsible for the more permanent fibroobstructive and hemodynamic changes seen in schistosomiasis.

Like other worm infections that involve migration through host tissues, schistosome infections are characteristically associated with peripheral as well as tissue eosinophilia. This observation has been related to the role of eosinophils as effector cells in mediating host defense to multicellular organisms.[11] Both oxidative and nonoxidative mechanisms have been linked with eosinophil-induced destruction of schistosome invading stages (schistosomula) and parasite eggs.

Clinical Manifestations

Specific disease manifestations due to schistosomiasis appear in only a proportion of infected individuals.[10] Skin penetration by human schistosomes results in the itchy papular eruption known as swimmers' itch. Acute schistosomiasis manifests as a febrile illness with lymphadenopathy, hepatosplenomegaly, and eosinophilia. The more characteristic clinical manifestations occur after oviposition. In *S. haematobium* infection, the main features are hematuria, dysuria, and frequency as well as laboratory evidence of proteinuria and hematuria. Thickening and irregularity of urinary bladder wall and obstructive uropathy with hydroureter and hydronephrosis may be observed in a significant proportion of infected persons (Fig. 295–2). In *S. mansoni, S. japonicum,* and *S. mekongi* infections, the intestinal phase may be associated with abdominal pain and blood in stools. As egg deposition in the liver increases, hepatomegaly, portal hypertension, splenomegaly, and evidence of portosystemic anastomosis may be seen. These individuals remain asymptomatic for a considerable time, retain good liver function, may bleed several times without progressing to hepatic encephalopathy, but finally succumb to the effects of repeated bleeding or liver failure.

Schistosome eggs can be found in virtually any tissue in the human host. The more common sites are the abdominal organs, the lungs, and more rarely, the spinal cord. Transverse myelitis has been reported with chronic *S. haematobium* or *S. mansoni* infection, and jacksonian epilepsy has been reported with *S. japonicum* infection.

Diagnosis

Parasitologic examination of human excreta or tissue remains the standard procedure for diagnosis of schistosomiasis.[12] Eggs can be detected in urine or stools of infected persons by direct examination—or with greater sensitivity by use of concentration and quantitative methods (Fig. 295–3). The recommended procedures are Nuclepore filtration for urine and the Kato thick smear for fecal examination.

The differential diagnosis of the major clinical features of schistosomiasis is complex because of its protean manifestations. Even the more specific features, such as hematuria, obstructive uropathy, hematemesis, or hepatosplenomegaly, are common manifestations of many diseases. The most help-

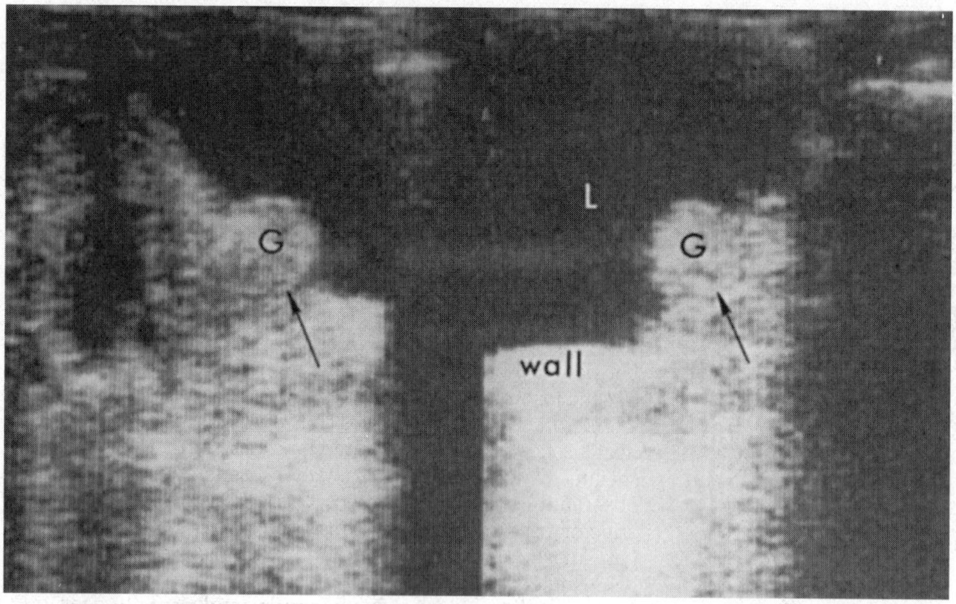

FIGURE 295–2 □ Longitudinal and transverse ultrasonographic images of the urinary bladder of a child infected with *Schistosoma haematobium*. Arrows indicate a large granuloma (G) protruding from the wall of the bladder into the lumen (L).

ful aspect for establishing the correct diagnosis is a thorough geographic history. This provides accurate assessment of the possibility of the infection's having been acquired and suggests the likely species of infecting parasite.

Treatment

The drug of choice for treating all species of schistosomes that infect humans is currently praziquantel.[13] It is administered orally and is extremely effective in either eliminating adult worms or markedly reducing their numbers. The dose and schedule of praziquantel depend on the *Schistosoma* species. For *S. japonicum* and *S. mekongi,* the recommended dosage is 60 mg/kg of body weight orally in two or three divided doses in 1 day. The recommended dose for *S. haematobium, S. mansoni,* and *S. intercalatum* is 40 mg/kg as a single oral dose. Follow-up stool or urine examinations for viable eggs should be performed several weeks after therapy to ensure successful treatment. Praziquantel treatment may also reverse the pathologic process if it is instituted early in the course of infection. However, the drug has no detectable effect on reversing the established fibroobstructive lesions seen in chronic schistosomiasis. The side effects and toxicity of praziquantel are remarkably low.

Prevention

The only reliable method of prevention is to avoid any contact with freshwater bodies in areas known to be endemic for schistosomes. This can easily be achieved for visitors to such areas; the local inhabitants, however, are attracted to these water bodies for many purposes, and in many instances they have no alternative. Another strategy is to stop environmental contamination by excreta of infected persons and so prevent snail infection. In endemic areas, this can be achieved only if cultural and socioeconomic changes are implemented to allow alternative sewage disposal. Several other approaches have been tried, such as the use of widespread chemotherapy and molluscacides. The availability of praziquantel and other safe, effective, and orally administered

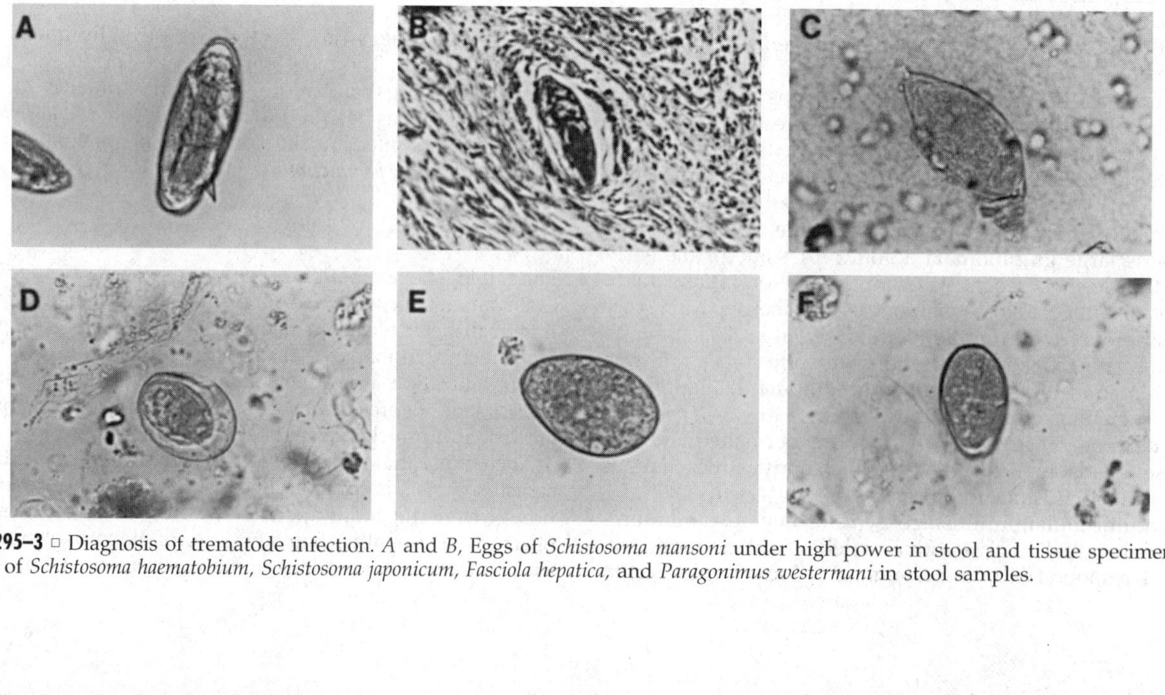

FIGURE 295–3 □ Diagnosis of trematode infection. *A* and *B*, Eggs of *Schistosoma mansoni* under high power in stool and tissue specimens. *C* to *F*, Eggs of *Schistosoma haematobium, Schistosoma japonicum, Fasciola hepatica,* and *Paragonimus westermani* in stool samples.

antischistosomal agents has encouraged the use of chemotherapy as a strategy for parasite control, and such programs have been reasonably successful. Molluscacides, on the other hand, have proved ineffective except under special circumstances.

The hope for the future prevention and control of schistosomiasis is in vaccine production.[14, 15] This is an ambitious goal, but evidence suggests that several characterized, defined parasite antigens are partially protective in experimental animals. Several candidate vaccines are ready for phase I clinical trials in humans.

Other Trematodes

The other human trematode parasites can be grouped according to site of infection (liver, lung, intestine; see Table 295–1).

Characteristics of the Pathogen

Like schistosomes, the liver, lung, and intestinal flukes of humans have complex life cycles that involve one or more intermediate hosts. Infection is established by ingestion of a larval or metacercarial stage found in freshwater plants, insects, fish, or crustaceans. Humans acquire infection through consumption of raw, pickled, smoked, or undercooked foods containing these larval stages. After ingestion, the larvae hatch in the intestine and migrate to their preferred niche in the host's body.

Epidemiology

The epidemiology of tissue and intestinal fluke infections is determined by the distribution of the aquatic intermediate hosts. Transmission occurs in either tropical or temperate regions, but the distribution of individual fluke species is usually limited in range. For the individual patient, a travel history is important for determining exposure risk. The second important feature that determines the prevalence and intensity of infection is the dietary preference of the definitive human host (i.e., could the patient have consumed uncooked or undercooked food known to harbor infective larvae?).

Pathogenesis

Clinical symptoms of tissue fluke infections are the result of inflammatory response to the parasite or its secretions and, less commonly, to eggs.[16] For intestinal flukes, mechanical irritation may also play a role in causing gastrointestinal symptoms such as cramping, diarrhea, and gastrointestinal tract bleeding. In tissue fluke infection, significant symptoms are often noted early, as developing parasites migrate from the intestinal tract into host tissues. Adult flukes range in size from 2 mm *(Heterophyes heterophyes)* to 7.5 cm *(Fasciola)*. Experimental animals have been shown to develop strong humoral and cell-mediated immune responses to parasite antigens, and there is some evidence that these responses can alter the course of a challenge tissue fluke infection.[17] The local inflammatory response to tissue flukes often wanes as parasites encyst in host tissues and become surrounded by fibrosis. In the case of the lung fluke *Paragonimus*, the tissue cyst containing the parasite must rupture into airway spaces so that parasite eggs can be expectorated and reach the environment.[16] In abortive *Paragonimus* infections, tissue fluke encystment may occur in almost any part of the body, including peritoneum, mesenteric lymph nodes, diaphragm, pleura, heart, reproductive organs, and central nervous system. Secondary effects of parasite migration may include effusions, abscess formation, local granuloma formation, fibrosis, calcification, and phlebitis. Biliary tract infection with liver flukes may result in local stenosis and intrahepatic obstruction. Chronic inflammation of biliary structures appears to predispose to formation of cholangiocarcinoma in older patients.

Diagnosis

Infection with any of these trematodes is diagnosed by detection of parasite eggs in stool or sputum. Eggs are characteristically ovoid, spineless, and operculate (lidded). Tissue flukes and their eggs may also be identified in biopsy material. Serologic tests to assist diagnosis are available for some fluke species; however, the specificity of these tests may be limited. In the setting of acute illness, significant travel history, eosinophilia, and characteristic radiographic or sonographic findings may strongly suggest active fluke infection.

Therapy

The drug of choice for liver, lung, and tissue fluke infection is praziquantel, 25 mg/kg of body weight three times a day for 1 or 2 days.[13] Data on praziquantel therapy for *Fasciola hepatica* are limited, and alternative bithionol therapy, 30 to 50 mg/kg every other day for 10 to 15 doses, is recommended.[16]

Prophylaxis

Prevention of tissue and liver fluke infection depends on avoidance of raw or undercooked foods in endemic areas, despite the traditional popularity of many raw food dishes. Advances in food preparation, freezing, and sewage treatment will help break the cycle of transmission of these parasites. Although developed countries such as Japan, Korea, and China have made strides in reducing fluke transmission, technologic progress has been slow in many developing countries, and traditional methods of cultivation and aquaculture continue to foster parasite transmission.

Liver Flukes

The Chinese liver fluke *Clonorchis sinensis* and the various *Opisthorchis* species (found in Southeast Asia and Eastern Europe) produce clinically significant infections.[16] Human infection with *F. hepatica* is less common, having been reported in livestock-raising areas of the Americas, Europe, North Africa, and Asia.

Clonorchiasis

Human infection with *C. sinensis* is endemic in China, Taiwan, Hong Kong, Korea, and the countries of Southeast Asia. The adult worm is approximately 15×3 mm and inhabits the distal branches of the biliary tree or pancreatic duct. Eggs measure 30×14 μm and are passed with the bile into feces. After reaching freshwater, the eggs are ingested by snails. The miracidium hatches and multiplies by asexual division within this intermediate host. After several weeks, cercariae emerge and encyst to form infectious metacercariae under the scales of freshwater fish. Human consumption of raw, pickled, smoked, or incompletely cooked fish allows living metacercariae to reach the intestine, where they hatch and pass through the ampulla of Vater to mature in the biliary tree.

Disease due to clonorchiasis is often minimal, and many infected persons have no symptoms. Acute symptoms include anorexia, epigastric pain, and diarrhea associated with peripheral blood eosinophilia. With chronic infections, cholangitis, cholelithiasis, pancreatitis, and biliary stricture have been reported. Cholangiocarcinoma, often multicentric, may arise as a late sequel to chronic infection, in some cases long after the infection has cleared. Oral treatment with praziquantel, 25 mg/kg three times a day for 1 or 2 days, is highly effective in eliminating infection (87% to 100% cure) but may not prevent or eliminate the late obstructive complications of infection.

Opisthorchiasis

Opisthorchiasis represents human infection with the cat and dog liver flukes *Opisthorchis felineus* and *Opisthorchis viverrini*. *O. felineus* is endemic in Southeast Asia, the Siberian lowlands, and Eastern Europe; *O. viverrini* is endemic in Thailand, western Malaysia, and Laos. The life cycle and clinical features of *Opisthorchis* species are similar to those of *Clonorchis*.[18] The eggs are distinguished from *Clonorchis* eggs by being somewhat narrower (11 × 30 μm). Praziquantel has been found to be effective in treating established infection.

Fascioliasis

Livestock infection with the liver fluke *F. hepatica* is found worldwide, with humans serving only occasionally as accidental hosts. Infections have been reported in all major sheep- and cattle-raising areas of the world. The metacercariae for this parasite encyst on freshwater plants, and human consumption of aquatic plants (such as wild watercress) harvested from contaminated areas leads to infection. After hatching, developing larvae penetrate the gut wall and enter the peritoneal cavity. The young flukes enter the liver by direct penetration of the capsule to the biliary radicles, where they mature and begin to pass eggs. The prolonged tissue migration of the parasite through host tissues is an important aspect of the pathologic process in the host. During this period, the patient may have prolonged fevers, right upper quadrant pain, hepatomegaly, urticaria, and marked eosinophilia. These symptoms abate once the flukes enter the bile ducts, but low-grade biliary symptoms may persist, and local fibrosis may develop around the mature worm. Maturing worms may occasionally fail to reach the liver and may continue to migrate through the peritoneal tissues and retroperitoneum. Rarely, invasion of the subdural space may lead to eosinophilic meningitis and central nervous system tissue inflammation or destruction.

Currently recommended therapy for fascioliasis is bithionol.[19] Therapy may need to be repeated if eggs return in the stool after the first course of treatment.

Lung Fluke and Other *Paragonimus* Infections

Infection with *Paragonimus* species results in fluke encystment in various organs, the most common being the lung fluke infection caused by *Paragonimus westermani*.[16] Different strains of *Paragonimus* are common in different areas of the world; infection with *P. westermani* is common in Asia (China, Japan, Korea, Laos, the Philippines, Taiwan, Thailand) but can also be found in West Africa and in South and Central America, including Mexico, Colombia, Costa Rica, and Peru. Humans are infected by consuming raw or undercooked crustaceans, including freshwater crabs and crayfish. Metacercariae hatch in the intestine, penetrate the gut into the peritoneal cavity, and migrate through the diaphragm and pleural space to invade the lung parenchyma. Acute clinical symptoms of infection include abdominal pain, diarrhea, fever, malaise, and urticaria followed by chest pain or pressure, malaise, dyspnea, and night sweats. Chronic symptoms include hemoptysis and abscess formation due to pulmonary hemorrhage and necrosis in the inflammation surrounding the parasite and pulmonary fibrosis and bronchiolar damage as a consequence of chronic inflammation. Secondary inflammatory response may lead to bronchopneumonia, bronchitis, bronchiectasis, atelectasis, and vasculitis of the lung. Imaging studies may demonstrate the migratory pathway in the lungs. Ectopic worm cysts may also be found in the intestines, peritoneal cavity, lymph nodes, pleura, diaphragm, heart, subcutaneous tissues, and central nervous system. Diagnosis can be made by examination of expectorated sputum for the characteristic 60 × 80 to 120 μm ova. If the patient swallows sputum, eggs may also be noted in the stool. Recommended treatment for paragonimiasis is praziquantel, 25 mg/kg three times daily for 2 or 3 days (reported success rate, 89% to 100%). Resolution of lung fluke infection should be monitored for several months by sputum examination and chest radiographs.

Other *Paragonimus* species may favor encystment in tissues other than the lungs. For example, a syndrome of cerebral hemorrhagic infestation has been described for *Paragonimus mexicanus* in Costa Rica. This syndrome appears to be rare with *P. westermani*. Other significant central nervous system syndromes may include meningitis (acute or chronic); mass lesions; infarction; hemorrhage; and visual disturbances associated with papilledema, nystagmus, or optic atrophy. The most frequent presenting symptoms are seizures, headache, and visual disturbances. Diagnosis of central nervous system involvement may be difficult because of the isolated location of these organisms, far from the gastrointestinal tract and bronchial tree. Travel history, serologic tests, and laboratory evidence of active infection provide only presumptive evidence of central nervous system involvement. Definitive diagnosis depends on tissue biopsy to identify the parasite or its eggs in the affected tissues. Optimal therapy of central nervous system fluke involvement is not established. Surgical removal of the parasite in combination with praziquantel therapy has been recommended. Symptoms of central nervous system infection may also require long-term therapy with anticonvulsants, corticosteroids, or ventricular shunting.

Intestinal Flukes

The metacercariae of intestinal flukes infest various freshwater plants *(Fasciolopsis buski)*, fish *(H. heterophyes, Metagonimus yokogawai, Nanophyetus salmincola)*, and shellfish *(Echinostoma ilocanum)*. These parasites are primarily endemic to Southeast Asia, although *Heterophyes* is also found in the Nile delta of Egypt. To date, transmission to humans of the intestinal fluke *N. salmincola* has been limited to the northwestern United States.[20] Symptoms of light infection with intestinal flukes are generally mild and limited to the intestine; heavy infection may be associated with severe abdominal pain, diarrhea, intestinal ulceration, and even ascites. Diagnosis of individual intestinal flukes is made by identification of parasite eggs on stool examination. Recommended therapy is praziquantel, as listed before for liver flukes.

References

1. Mahmoud AAF: Trematodes (schistosomiasis) and other flukes. *In* Mandell G, Bennett J, Dolin R (eds): Principles and Practice of Infectious Diseases, ed 4. New York, Churchill Livingstone, 1995, pp 2538–2544.
2. Sturrock RF: Biology and ecology of human schistosomes. *In* Mahmoud AAF (ed): Baillière's Clinical Tropical Medicine and

Communicable Diseases, Vol 2. Philadelphia, Baillière Tindall, 1987, pp 249–266.
3. Mahmoud AAF, Abdel Wahab MF: Schistosomiasis. *In* Warren KS, Mahmoud AFF (eds): Tropical and Geographical Medicine, ed 2. New York, McGraw-Hill, 1990, pp 458–473.
4. Atlas of the Global Distribution of Schistosomiasis. Parasitic Diseases Programme. Geneva, World Health Organization, 1987.
5. Anderson RM: Determinants of infection in human schistosomiasis. *In* Mahmoud AFF (ed): Baillière's Clinical Tropical Medicine and Communicable Diseases, Vol 2. Philadelphia, Baillière Tindall, 1987, pp 279–300.
6. Mahmoud AAF: Schistosomiasis. *In* Bennett JC, Plum F (eds): Cecil Textbook of Medicine, ed 20. Philadelphia, WB Saunders, 1996, pp 1927–1931.
7. Abel L, Demenais F, Prata A, et al: Evidence for the segregation of a major gene in human susceptibility/resistance to infection by *Schistosoma mansoni*. Am J Hum Genet 48:959, 1991.
8. Sandor M, Sperling AI, Cook GA, et al: Two waves of γδ T cells expressing different V γδ genes are recruited into schistosome induced liver granuloma. J Immunol 155:275, 1995.
9. Lukacs NW, Boros DL: Lymphokine regulation of granuloma formation in murine schistosomiasis *mansoni*. Clin Immunol Immunopathol 68:57, 1993.
10. Progress in Assessment of Morbidity Due to *Schistosoma mansoni* Infection: A Review of Recent Literature. Geneva, World Health Organization, 1987, pp 3–66.
11. Mahmoud AAF: Eosinophilia. *In* Warren KS, Mahmoud AAF (eds): Tropical and Geographical Medicine, ed 2. New York, McGraw-Hill, 1990, pp 65–70.
12. Peters PAS, Kazura JW: Update on diagnostic methods for schistosomiasis. *In* Mahmoud AAF (ed): Baillière's Clinical Tropical Medicine and Communicable Diseases, Vol 2. Philadelphia, Baillière Tindall, 1987, pp 419–434.
13. King CH, Mahmoud AAF: Drugs five years later: Praziquantel. Ann Intern Med 110:290, 1989.
14. Woolhouse MEJ, Taylor P, Matanhire D, Chandiwana SK: Acquired immunity and the epidemiology of *Schistosoma haematobium*. Nature 351:757, 1991.
15. Butterworth AE: Potential for vaccines against human schistosomes. *In* Mahmoud AAF (ed): Ballière's Clinical Tropical Medicine and Communicable Diseases, Vol 2. Philadelphia, Baillière Tindall, 1987, pp 465–483.
16. Harinasuta T, Bunnag D: Liver, lung, and intestinal trematodiasis. *In* Warren KS, Mahmoud AAF (eds): Tropical and Geographical Medicine, ed 2. New York, McGraw-Hill, 1990.
17. Watanabe N, Kobayashi A: IgE antibody production and cutaneous anaphylactic reactions in rats infected with *Clonorchis sinensis*. Am J Trop Med Hyg 39:74, 1988.
18. Upatham ES, Viyanant V, Kurathong S, et al: Morbidity in relation to intensity of infection in opisthorchiasis *viverrini*: Study of a community in Chon Kaen, Thailand. Am J Trop Med Hyg 31:1156, 1982.
19. Drugs for parasitic infections. Med Lett 37:99, 1995.
20. Eastburn RT, Fritsche TR, Terhune CA Jr: Human intestinal infection with *Nanophyetus salmincola* from salmonid fishes. Am J Trop Med Hyg 36:586, 1987.

296

Cestodes (Tapeworms)

Kaethe Willms

The true tapeworms, class Cestoda, belong to the phylum Platyhelminthes, the most highly specialized of the metazoan parasites (Table 296–1). All adult members of this class are endoparasites of the alimentary tract or associated ducts of vertebrates. Their life cycle includes at least one intermediary host, in which the tapeworm undergoes one phase of development.[1, 2] In this chapter, only tapeworms that cause significant human disease are discussed: *Taenia solium, Taenia saginata*, Asian *Taenia, Echinococcus granulosus* (hydatid cyst), *Hymenolepis nana*, and *Diphyllobothrium latum*.

Within the Cestoda is the order of the Cyclophyllidea, composed of two families that are of medical importance: the Taeniidae and the Hymenolepididae. Within the Taeniidae are three zoonotic tapeworms for which humans are the only natural definitive host, *T. solium*, *T. saginata*, and Asian *Taenia*. Their life cycles require at least one intermediary host, in which the tapeworm undergoes one phase of development, the larval stage or metacestode (also called cysticercus, which has no taxonomic value). A fourth zoonosis caused by the taeniid *E. granulosus* has a similar life cycle; domestic dogs and other carnivores are definitive hosts, and a large number of intermediate hosts (including humans) become infected by the larval stage and develop hydatid disease. All four taeniids still cause widespread disease in developing countries and are zoonoses generally associated with ignorance and poverty. Eggs produced in the *T. solium* tapeworm contain the infective embryos that cause human and porcine cysticercosis in many countries of Latin America, South Africa, and Asia.[3] *T. saginata* tapeworms are the source of bovine cysticercosis and still represent a major public health risk in developing countries and in developed countries, where raw or undercooked beef is consumed and where localized feedlot epidemics have been reported.[4] The adult and larval stages of all cestodes are endoparasites, which lack a digestive system and are therefore able to live only in the intestine.

Taenia Tapeworms

Tapeworms of the genus *Taenia* are flat and exceptionally long parasites measuring 1.5 to 12 m, depending on the species. All species share several morphologic features: a scolex (head with four suckers) and a rostellum, which may be armed with hooks *(T. solium)* or unarmed (*T. saginata* and Asian *Taenia*) (Fig. 296–1). The scolex is attached to the mucosa in the small intestine of the host. Morphologic evidence obtained from adult cestodes has shown that the worm attaches to intestinal epithelium by the scolex suckers, which engulf the host tissue, lysing and destroying the epithelium and submucosal layer. Inspection of the mucosal wall suggests that the worm survives by alternately attaching suckers and obtaining nutrients from the lysis of epithelial cells (Fig. 296–2). From the scolex emerges the neck, from which strobilization (growth of proglottids) occurs. Each proglottid can be considered an independent reproductive unit because it

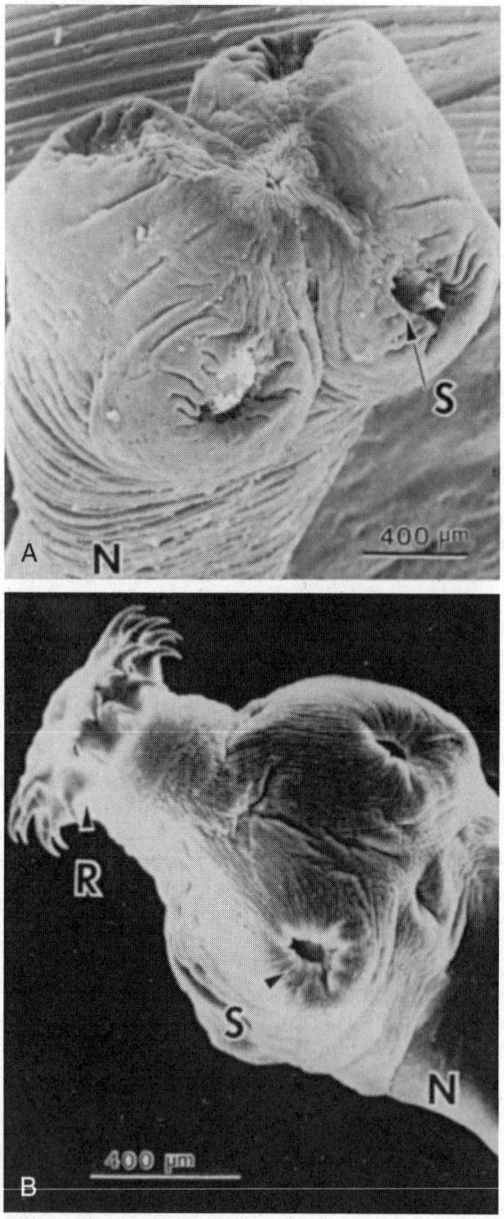

FIGURE 296–1 □ Scanning electron micrographs of *Taenia* scolices. *A, T. saginata.* S, Sucker; N, neck. *B, T. solium.* R, Rostellum with double row of hooks; S, sucker; N, neck. (*A,* Courtesy of Dr. Juan Pedro Laclette, Instituto de Investigaciones Bìomédìcas, UNAM, Mexico. *B,* By permission of Fondo de Cultura Economica, Mexico.)

contains both male and female reproductive organs (Fig. 296–3). The distal proglottids become fertile (gravid proglottids) and contain several thousand eggs, which are at different stages of maturation. Gravid proglottids become detached from the worm and leave the host in feces or by spontaneous migration. When mature eggs are ingested by the intermediate host in contaminated water, food, or fodder, the outer shell of the egg is disrupted by exposure to gastric and intestinal juices and the embryo, called the oncosphere, is released (Fig. 296–4). The oncosphere can traverse the intestinal wall and be transported through the circulation to any organ, where it lodges in the host tissues and develops into a larva or metacestode, a 1- to 2-cm cyst, with an inverted scolex. The larval stage in the intermediate host (cattle or swine) becomes infective for humans in about 8 to 10 weeks. Viable cysticerci ingested by humans from undercooked beef or pork undergo an evagination process in the human intestine, by which the scolex becomes attached to the intestinal wall and matures into a gravid (egg-producing) tapeworm 2 to 6 months after infection. The life cycles of these parasites are entirely dependent on the link between the intermediary host and the definitive host, and any break in this link can end the cycle.

Taenia saginata (Taeniarhynchus saginatus) *(Beef Tapeworm)*

LIFE CYCLE (Fig. 296–5)

The adult tapeworm lives only in the jejunum of humans and so far has never been found naturally in any other host. The worm can measure 4 to 12 m and has been reported to survive up to 30 years in a host. Humans are usually infected with a single *T. saginata* tapeworm. Multiple infections are found only in highly endemic areas.[5] In contrast to *T. solium,* the gravid proglottids of *T. saginata* migrate actively in groups of six to eight segments through the anus, and patients report an unpleasant creeping sensation. Segments (proglottids) can be found in underclothing, in bedding, or on the ground. It has been estimated that approximately 50% of the eggs contained in the gravid proglottids are mature and therefore infective. When they are ingested by cattle, digestive enzymes release the oncospheres (embryos), which then traverse the intestinal wall and enter the blood stream or lymphatics, whence they are carried to various tissues and develop into larvae. The larvae are infective for humans if they are ingested in raw or undercooked beef. In cattle, the cysticerci are most commonly found in the heart and masseters, but they can be found dispersed throughout the musculature and in any organ.[6]

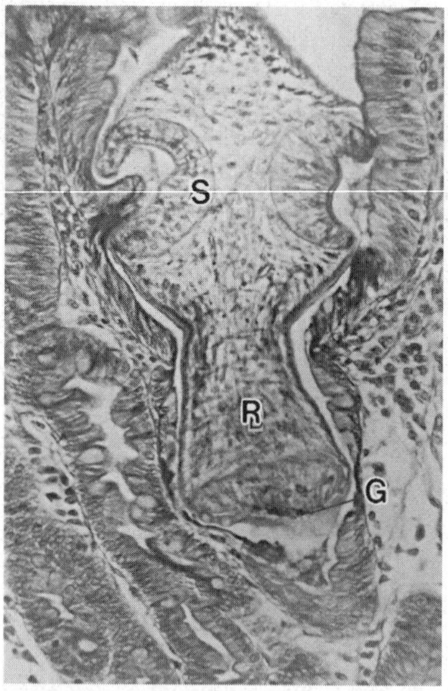

FIGURE 296–2 □ Section of mucosal wall of an experimentally infected dingo *(Canis familiaris dingo)* showing 35-day-old *Echinococcus granulosus* in situ. Rostellum (R) extended into crypt of Lieberkühn and the suckers (S) grasping the epithelium at the base of the villi. G, Rostellar gland. (Magnification, ×40.) (From Thompson RCA: Biology and systematics of *Echinococcus. In* Thompson RCA, Lymbery AJ [eds]: *Echinococcus* and Hydatid Disease. Oxford, CAB International, 1995, pp 1–50.)

TABLE 296–1 ■ Classification of Medically Important Cestodes

Phylum	Platyhelminthes			
Class	Cestoda			
Order	Cyclophyllidea			Pseudophyllidea
Family	Taeniidae		Hymenolepididae	Diphyllobothriidae
Genus	*Taenia*	*Echinococcus*	*Hymenolepis*	*Diphyllobothrium*
Species	*solium* *saginata*	*granulosus*	*nana*	*latum*

Data from Cheng TC: Cestuda. The true tapeworms. *In* Cheng TC (ed): General Parasitology. New York, Academic Press, 1973, pp 474–541; and Schmidt GD: Handbook of Tapeworm Identification. Key to the Genera Taeniidae. Boca Raton, FL, CRC Press, 1986, pp 221–227.

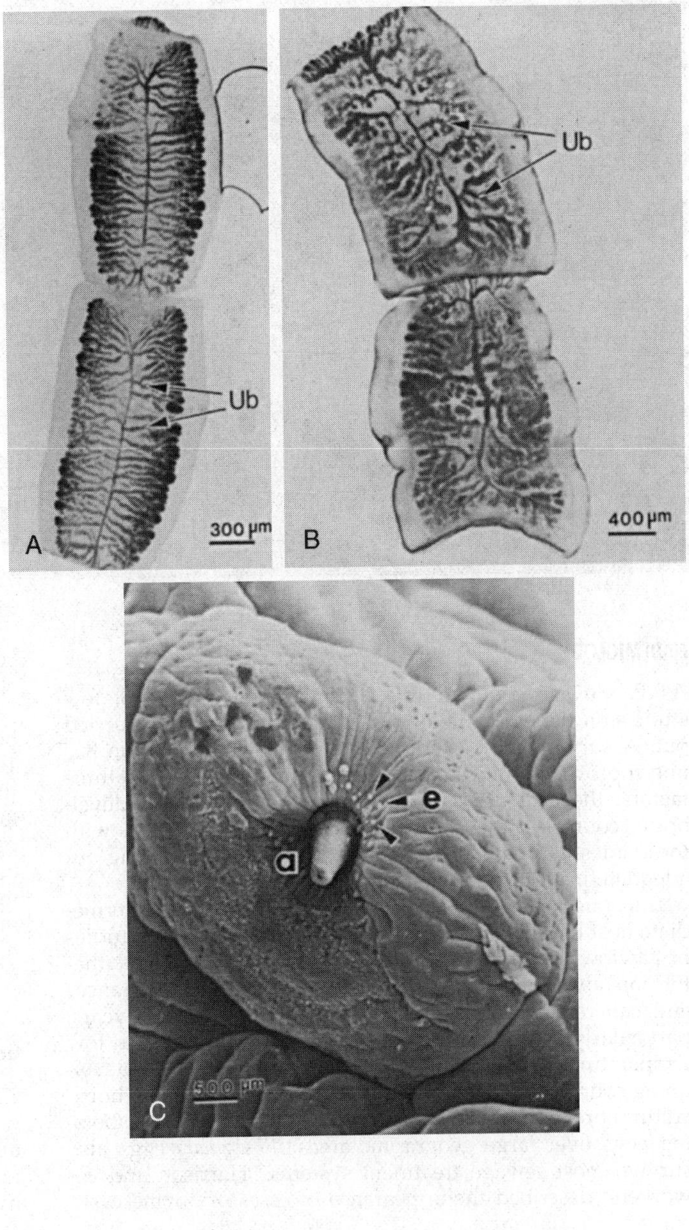

FIGURE 296–3 □ Gravid proglottid segments from *T. saginata (A)* and *T. solium (B)*. Cleared in glycerol and mounted on a slide. Ub, Uterine branches. (*A* and *B* courtesy of Sylvia Paz Diaz Camacho.) C, Scanning electron micrograph of *T. solium* proglottid, showing genital atrium (a) and eggs (e) on surface *(arrows)*. (Courtesy of Dr. Juan Pedro Laclette, Instituto de Investigaciones Bìomédìcas, UNAM, Mexico.)

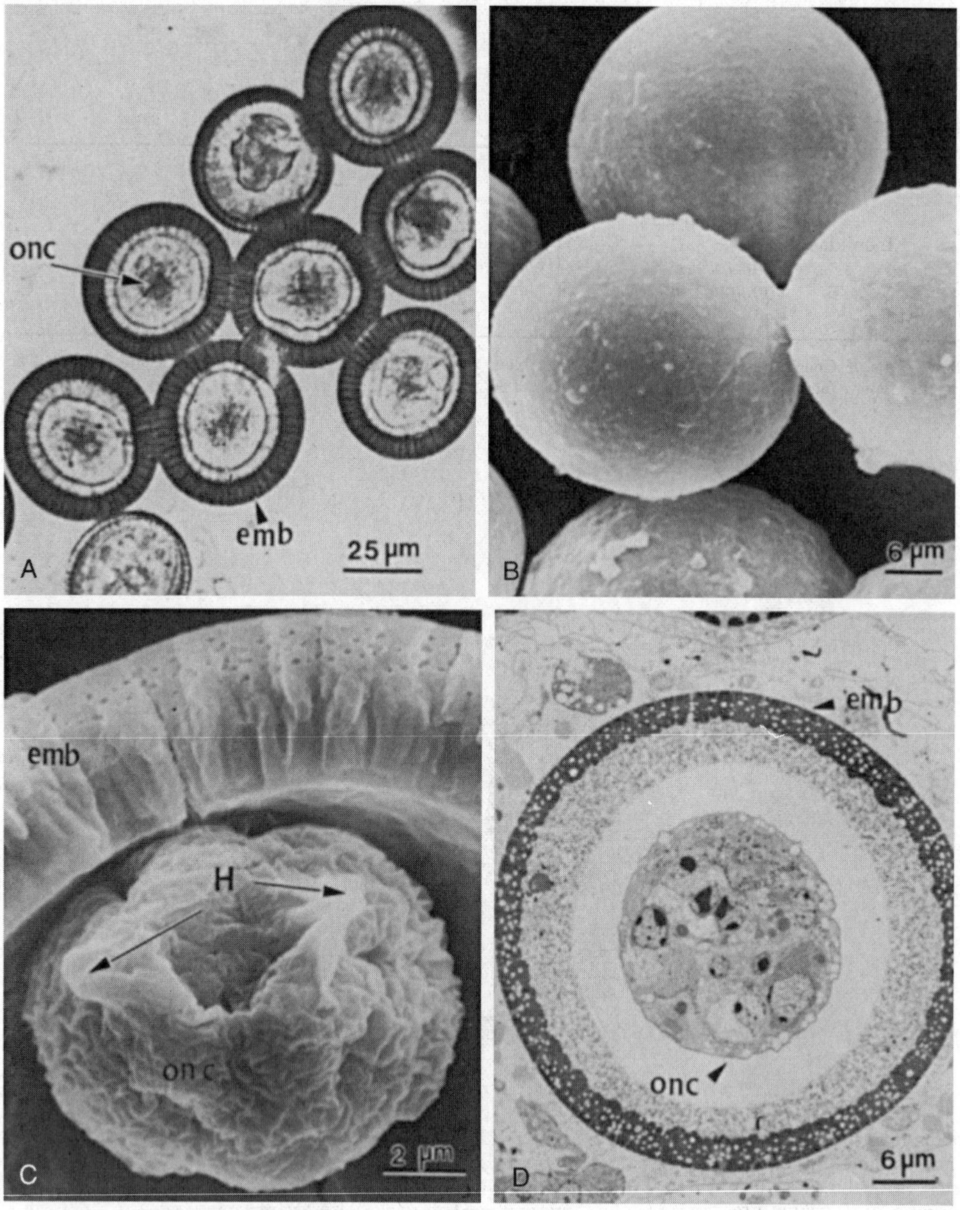

FIGURE 296–4 □ *Taenia* spp. eggs. *A*, Light microscopic appearance of eggs obtained from concentration-flotation method (onc, oncosphere or hexacanth embryo; emb, embryophore shell). *B*, Scanning electron micrograph of *T. solium* eggs. (*B* from Flisser A, Willms K, Laclette JP, et al [eds]: Cysticercosis. New York, Academic Press, 1982.) *C*, Scanning electron micrograph of an open *T. solium* egg, showing outer embryophore shell (emb) and oncosphere (onc) covered by membrane. H, Oncospheral hooks. (*C* courtesy of Dr. Juan Pedro Laclette, Instituto de Investigaciones Bìomédìcas, UNAM, Mexico.) *D*, Transmission electron micrograph of *T. solium* egg. Section stained with lead citrate and uranyl acetate (emb, embryophore shell; onc, oncosphere tissue). (*D* courtesy of Dr. Juan Pedro Laclette, Instituto de Investigaciones Bìomédìcas, UNAM, Mexico.)

EPIDEMIOLOGY

As Pawlowski[7] pointed out a number of years ago, few studies on the epidemiology of *T. saginata* have been carried out. A survey of the literature shows that the situation has not improved significantly. I suggest that this is due to three factors: the difficulties in diagnosing tapeworms in developing countries, the absence of symptoms associated with these intestinal parasites, and the difficulties of carrying out adequate inspection of beef carcasses.

Transmission patterns from humans to the bovine intermediate host have been studied in various locations. The studies of Pawlowski[7] and coworkers in Poland showed clearly that the infective eggs can be disseminated over long distances and can remain infective for many months or even years, particularly under conditions of favorable humidity and low temperatures (4°C to 6°C). The common practice in developing countries of using raw sewage for fertilization of horticultural or agricultural fields is an effective means of dispersing eggs over large geographic areas. *T. saginata* eggs also survive most sewage treatment systems.[8] Harrison and coworkers[9] described the appearance of cases of bovine cysticercosis in Scotland in a group of farms in which sewage sludge had been applied to farm pastures.

It has been estimated that a tapeworm carrier releases between six and nine proglottids daily, each containing about 100,000 eggs, about half of which are probably mature and therefore infective. One infected person may therefore contaminate the environment with more than a half-million eggs per day. The studies of Silverman[10] have shown that under certain climatic conditions, taeniid eggs can survive for many months. The transmission of *T. saginata* from animals to humans depends on the habit of eating raw or undercooked beef. It has been confirmed that the infection rate in humans is closely related to the frequency of ingesting raw beef.[11]

GEOGRAPHIC DISTRIBUTION

T. saginata worms can be found worldwide in countries where cattle are raised for human consumption. The frequency of beef tapeworm has decreased in developed countries owing to stricter meat inspection practices, better hygiene, and significantly better sanitary facilities. In devel-

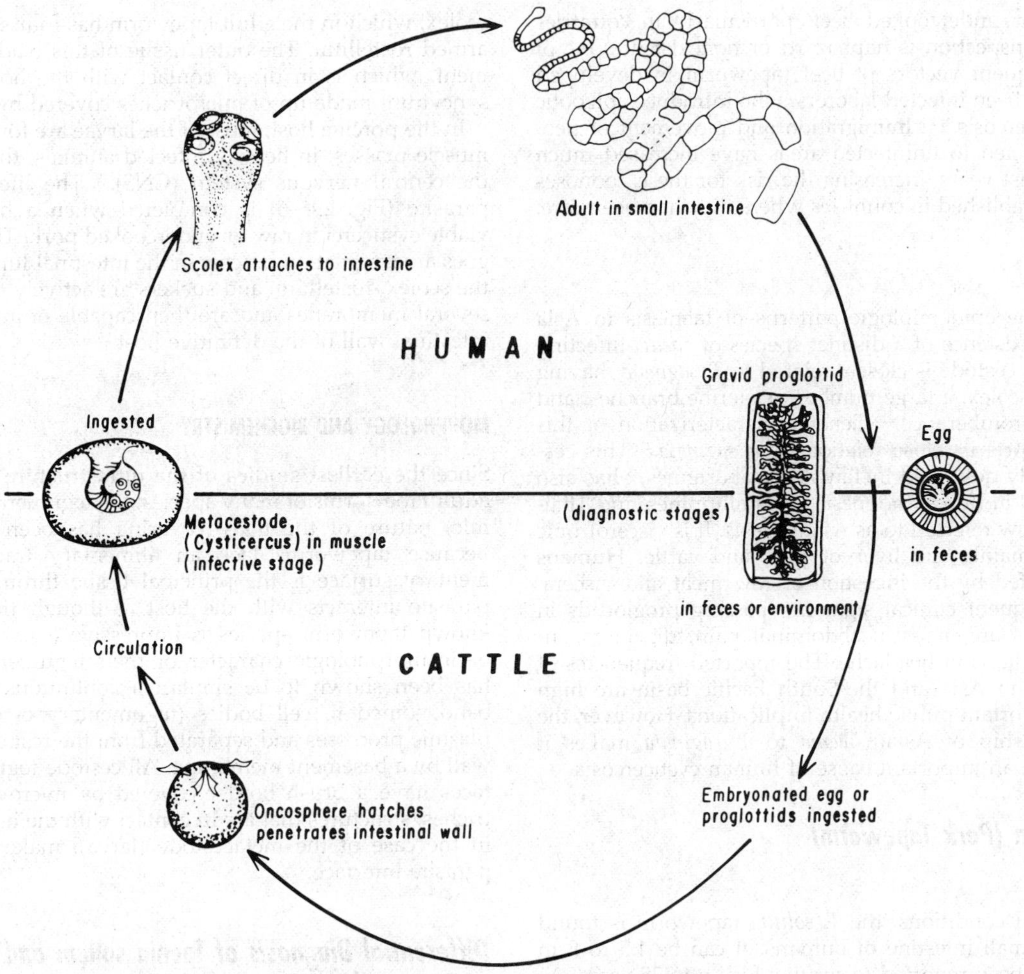

FIGURE 296–5 ▫ Life cycle of *Taenia saginata*.

oping countries, particularly in pastoral societies and rural areas, where sanitary installations are not an element of the culture and where human excrement is disposed of on open ground, used to fertilize, or even used for medicinal purposes,[12] both *T. saginata* and *T. solium* continue to flourish.

CLINICAL MANIFESTATIONS

One of the many paradoxes of taeniasis is the relative absence of symptoms in the definitive host. The symptoms that are usually recorded are vague and include abdominal pain, nausea, weakness, weight loss, increased appetite, headache, constipation, dizziness, pruritus ani, and excitation. The presence of the tapeworm can often be detected by the carrier, who observes proglottids in the stool or senses their active migration through the anus. Many infections may go unnoticed, however.[5] Lenoble and Dumontier[13] described the unusual case of the perforation of the small intestine due to a *T. saginata* infection, the first case reported in the literature in 20 years.

DIAGNOSIS

T. saginata can be suspected by clinical history in a patient who ingests raw beef and who describes elimination of tapeworm segments in stool or active migration of segments through the anus. The diagnosis can be further confirmed by the finding in feces of *Taenia* species eggs or proglottids with more than 12 uterine branches. When the whole worm is retrieved after treatment and an unarmed scolex can be identified, a definite diagnosis can be established. The most effective method reported for diagnosis of *Taenia* species eggs is the perianal swab,[14] or the adhesive tape method, which detects 85% to 95% of eggs from *T. saginata* infections.[15] Other methods reveal between 20% and 80%, depending on the experience of the laboratory. Most parasitologists recommend carrying out three serial stool examinations to increase the probability of detecting taeniid eggs.

The other methods, some of which have been in use for many years,[16–19] are not as reliable as the Graham method for *T. saginata*. However, this method is not dependable for detection of *T. solium* eggs, probably because the proglottids of this tapeworm do not migrate spontaneously. This fact should be kept in mind for patients who live in areas where both pork and beef are consumed and when the specific diagnosis is of consequence, because of the potential risk posed by infections with the *T. solium* tapeworm, the only agent of cysticercosis in humans.

TREATMENT

See the later section on treatment of *Taenia* tapeworms.

PREVENTION AND CONTROL OF *TAENIA SAGINATA* TAENIASIS

Prevention and control of taeniasis are based on health education, diagnosis, and treatment. Health education should be directed to alerting the population to the risk associated with eating raw or undercooked beef, particularly in countries where meat inspection is haphazard or nonexistent. One of the most frequent vectors of beef tapeworm in developed countries has been infected laborers, who introduce epizootic feedlot cysticercosis.[4, 20] Immigration and movement of people from infected to uninfected areas have increased much during the past years, increasing the risk for these zoonoses to become established in countries where they had been rare.

Asian Taenia

Studies on the epidemiologic patterns of taeniasis in Asia indicate the existence of a distinct species of *Taenia* infecting humans. This cestode is closely related to *T. saginata*, having an unarmed scolex, a large number of uterine branches, and a posterior protuberance.[21] Genetic characterization of this cestode supports its close relation to *T. saginata*.[22] This cestode, originally described in Taiwanese aborigines,[23] has also been recorded in Korea, Indonesia, the Philippines, and Thailand and is now referred to as Asian *Taenia*. It is viscerotropic and infects mainly the liver of pigs and cattle. Humans become infected by the ingestion of raw meat and viscera. The most frequent clinical signs are passing proglottids in feces, pruritus ani, nausea, abdominal pain, dizziness, increased appetite, and headache. The reported frequencies of this taeniasis in Asia and the South Pacific basin are high and have important public health implications. However, the close relationship of Asian *Taenia* to *T. saginata* makes it unlikely to be an important cause of human cysticercosis.

Taenia solium *(Pork Tapeworm)*

LIFE CYCLE

Under natural conditions, the *T. solium* tapeworm is found only in the small intestine of humans. It can be 1.5 to 8 m long and has been reported to survive for up to 25 years. As shown in Figure 296–1, it has an armed scolex (head), that is, a rostellum bearing two rows of hooks that vary in number between 22 and 32. The scolex attaches to the intestinal mucosa, from which it derives its nutrients. Growth of the worm (strobilization) proceeds from the distal end of the scolex neck, producing an ever-increasing number of proglottids. As the distal proglottids mature, they become filled with eggs, oncospheres (embryos) surrounded by a keratin-like shell (see Fig. 296–4). The eggs contained in the gravid proglottids have reached different degrees of maturation when the segments are detached from the worm and passively voided in the feces.

Each gravid proglottid contains approximately 50,000 eggs, and because it is estimated that each worm releases four to five proglottids per day, a person with *T. solium* tapeworm is depositing 250,000 eggs a day into the environment. Although not all of the eggs may be infective on release from the host, they may, like other taeniid eggs, mature and survive in humid pastures or sewage for many months. *T. solium* eggs are morphologically indistinguishable from eggs of other *Taenia* species.

When *T. solium* eggs are ingested by their natural intermediate host, the pig, the egg shell or embryophore, made of keratin blocks, becomes progressively disaggregated owing to the effects of pepsin and pancreatin,[24] and the oncosphere is released. The activated oncosphere penetrates the intestinal wall and is then transported through the blood or lymphatics to the tissues.

In the interstitial tissues, the oncosphere develops into a larva (metacestode), a process that takes approximately 8 weeks. The larva is an oval vesicle filled with fluid and measuring 0.2 to 2 cm in diameter, with an invaginated scolex, which in the adult tapeworm has four suckers and an armed rostellum. The outer tissue of this bladder, the tegument, which is in direct contact with the host tissue, is a syncytium made up of microtriches covered by a glycocalyx.

In the porcine host, most of the larvae are found in striated muscle masses; in heavily infected animals, they are also in the central nervous system (CNS).[25] The life cycle of the parasite (Fig. 296–6) is completed when a human ingests viable cysticerci in raw or undercooked pork. The cyst undergoes an evagination process in the intestinal lumen, by which the scolex, rostellum, and suckers are actively extruded from several membranes and are then capable of attaching to the intestinal wall of the definitive host.[26]

MORPHOLOGY AND BIOCHEMISTRY

Since the earliest studies of the ultrastructure of larval and adult tapeworms of many species, the tegumental (protoplasmic) nature of the body covering has been established.[27] Because tapeworms lack an alimentary tract, this tegumentary surface is the principal tissue through which the parasite interacts with the host. Although the number of known tapeworm species is impressive (close to 4000), the basic morphologic character of their tegumentary surfaces has been shown to be similar: a continuous protoplasmic band, joined to cell bodies (tegumentary cytons) by cytoplasmic processes and separated from the rest of the parasite wall by a basement membrane. All cestode tegumentary surfaces have a brush border covered by microvilli or microtriches, structures that are in contact with the host tissue and, in the case of the metacestode (larva), make up the host-parasite interface.

Differential Diagnosis of Taenia solium *and* Taenia saginata *Infestations*

There seems to be general agreement that *T. solium* goes undiagnosed for various reasons: the infected person is not aware of harboring a tapeworm; the infection causes few symptoms and in more primitive or less educated communities is not considered a disease worth treating; few developing countries have the facilities and trained personnel to establish an accurate diagnosis at the primary health care level; the methods presently available for diagnosis of taeniid eggs in stool specimens are not optimal.[14–19] In addition, *T. solium* eggs are identical to *T. saginata* eggs, so that treatment, when given, is seldom followed up by specific identification of the voided tapeworm.

Nevertheless, taeniasis can be diagnosed on the basis of the following findings:

1. A careful clinical history and questioning of patients about ingestion of raw beef or pork (particularly sausages).
2. Discharging of proglottids or worm segments in the stool (loose gravid proglottids in underclothing or bedclothes are indicative of *T. saginata*).
3. Coprologic analysis: three serial stool examinations on three consecutive days by use of perianal swabs[14] or the method of Graham[15] if *T. saginata* is suspected or the method of Faust,[16] Ritchie,[17] or Kato[18] if *T. solium* is suspected. If proglottids become available, an effort should be made to fix them, dehydrate them in glycerol, and count the uterine branches under the microscope. If the number of branches is 12 or fewer, it can be assumed that the patient has *T. solium*. The patient should be advised that he or she is a potential risk to other humans, instructed on hygiene measures, and treated as soon as possible. The patient should also be asked

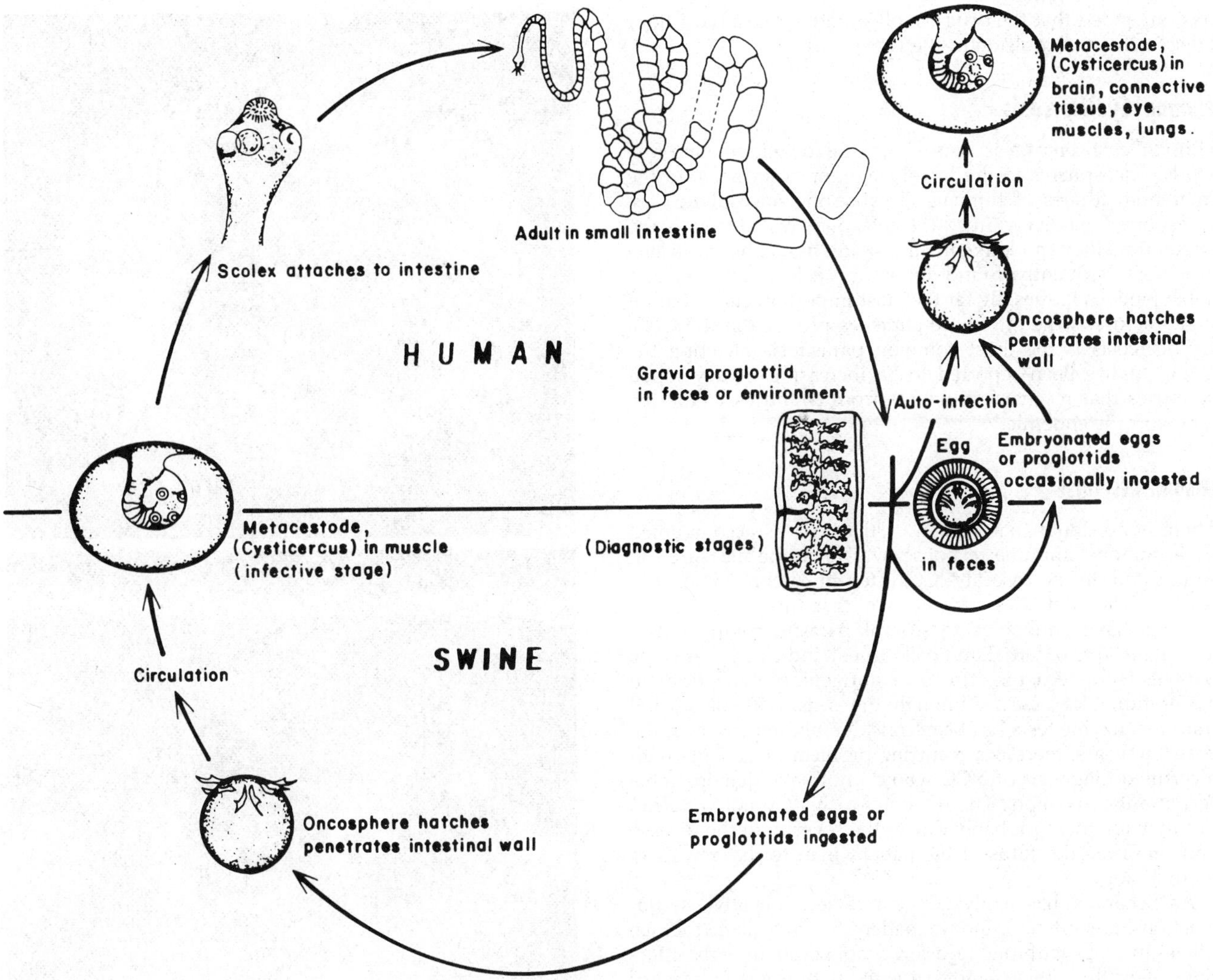

FIGURE 296–6 □ Life cycle of *Taenia solium*.

to recover the tapeworm (taking all safety precautions and using gloves and a disposable or autoclavable container) and bring it into the laboratory for definitive diagnosis.

From the medical point of view, the specific diagnosis and treatment of *Taenia* species infestations are important, because the eggs of *T. solium* and *T. saginata* are indistinguishable, the former being the cause of human cysticercosis (see Fig. 296–6). Although the identification of the scolex and some morphologic features of the proglottids allows precise diagnosis of the tapeworm species, this is frequently not possible. Well-preserved proglottids and trained personnel, which many countries do not have, are required. In addition, when the proglottids are macerated, it is virtually impossible to establish a definitive diagnosis. Two promising new techniques for the detection of taeniid antigens in stool specimens have been worked out by several groups, (1) antigen capture and detection by enzyme-linked immunosorbent assay (ELISA)[28–30] and (2) the preparation of specific DNA probes for the detection of *Taenia* eggs in stool, which promise rapid, highly sensitive and specific assays that could eventually be used for epidemiologic surveys.[31]

Treatment of Taenia Tapeworms

Praziquantel is a broad-spectrum and efficient anthelmintic drug. It has been shown to have a high cure rate[32] in the elimination of intestinal cestodes and in the past 10 years has been used successfully in the treatment of human neurocysticercosis (NCC).[33] It should be used only under medical supervision in patients suspected of having NCC. Its use is also contraindicated for pregnant women, children younger than 2 years, and cirrhosis patients. The recommended dose for treatment of tapeworm in adults is between 2.5 and 10 mg/kg given in a single dose.[34]

Albendazole is a potent anthelmintic drug and is indicated in multiple parasitosis. It should not be used in children younger than 2 years or during pregnancy owing to the embryotoxic and teratogenic effects, which have been observed in experimental animals. The recommended dose for treatment of tapeworms is 6.6 mg/kg (two doses of 200 mg each per day on 3 consecutive days).

Niclosamide is effective in 85% to 95% of cases.[14] It is contraindicated during the first trimester of pregnancy. The dose per adult is 2 g (four tablets) in a single dose, chewed and swallowed with water, preferably after fasting or some hours after a light meal. For children weighing between 11 and 34 kg, the recommended dose is 1 g. Children younger than 2 years of age are given 0.5 g in one dose, the tablets ground to powder and mixed with water. Niclosamide is tolerated well, and less than 10% of patients report nausea, vomiting, abdominal pain, or exanthema, which are transitory. If the species of *Taenia* has not been determined, it is recommended that the drug be followed by a laxative 1 hour later to ensure expulsion of the worm.

Human Cysticercosis

Human cysticercosis is caused by the development of *T. solium* oncospheres to the larval stage, or cysticercus, in the interstitial tissues of humans. Because the oncospheres are transported passively from the intestinal wall through the circulation, they can lodge in almost any tissue, but cysticerci are most frequently found in brain, skeletal muscle, and subcutaneous tissues. By far the most important clinicopathologic picture is the one these parasites produce in the CNS. Cysticercosis is the most common parasitosis affecting the CNS.[35] It has been reported to be increasing in developed countries that receive immigrants from countries where the tapeworm is endemic.[36]

IMMUNE RESPONSE

There is no doubt that human cysticercosis is accompanied by a humoral immune response, which can be measured in serum and, in the case of NCC, often in cerebrospinal fluid (CSF). Various studies have shown that most seropositive patients have antibodies to several parasite components,[37] and the results of Grogl and colleagues[38] indicated that some patients' sera recognize up to 31 antigenic polypeptides in an immunoblot assay. Although the sensitivity of several immunoenzyme tests has been considerably improved in the past few years, there is a recurring problem of patients with a certified diagnosis of NCC who do not have demonstrable serum antibody titers. The reasons for this are not yet clear, but they are more probably due to the severity of the disease and the immune status of the patient than to differences in methodology.

As Schantz[39] has analyzed in a review, negative serum reactions are often found in patients with calcified cysts, others in cases with one or a few viable cysts in early infections. On the other hand, patients with severe cases of NCC—with associated inflammatory processes, involvement of meninges, vasculitis, and increased intracranial pressure, among others—almost always have detectable levels of serum and CSF antibodies.[40, 41]

PATHOLOGY

The pathologic process of NCC is determined by the localization of the parasite in the CNS and by the inflammatory reaction it induces in brain tissue. Macroscopic analysis of brain slices from patients with parenchymatous NCC detects a large variety of localizations (Fig. 296–7) and various degrees of inflammatory infiltrate, which can range from negligible to severe exudative or granulomatous lesions. In early inflammatory lesions, the infiltrates are composed of multifocal groups of lymphocytes, plasma cells, and eosinophils located in a fibrous connective tissue capsule surrounding the parasite.[42] The severity of the reaction appears to be associated with the degree of damage or deterioration of the parasite tissue. As hyalinization and calcification of the parasite progress, the inflammatory infiltrate is found inside the parasite, and mononuclear cells, eosinophils, and polymorphonuclear neutrophils can be observed. The final stages of this process are characterized by the appearance of epithelioid and multinucleated giant cells, which persist until the complete calcification of the parasite.

The composition of the inflammatory exudate clearly suggests the elicitation of a local immune response to this parasite. Other pathologic lesions secondary to the inflammatory response are vasculitis, fibrinoid necrosis, and ischemic necrosis of the neighboring vessels, which may be due to the deposition of immune complexes.

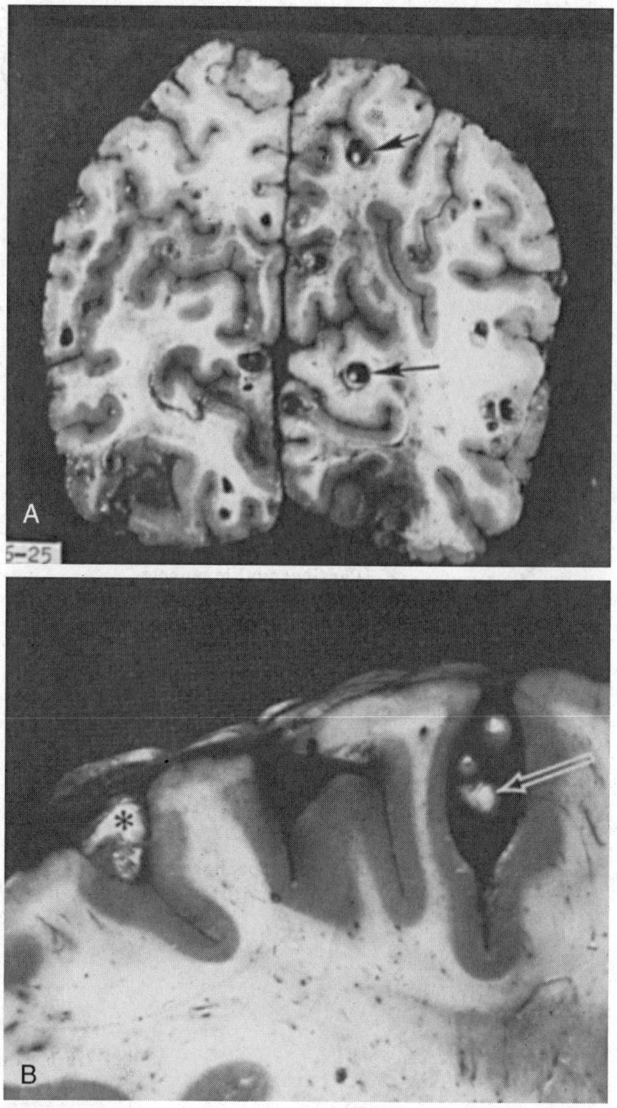

FIGURE 296–7 □ *A,* Coronal section of human brain showing multiple parenchymatous cysticerci *(arrows). B,* Cortical cysticerci: calcified cyst *(asterisk);* viable cyst *(arrow).* (*A* and *B* courtesy of Dr. Alfonso Escobar Izquierdo, Instituto de Investigaciones Biomédicas, UNAM, Mexico.)

CLINICAL MANIFESTATIONS

The clinical manifestations of NCC are secondary to location, number of cysts, and inflammatory response of the host. The clinical signs and symptoms are generally the result of the inflammatory host response to the cysticerci in the brain tissue. The neurologic picture it produces is complex and pleomorphic; often, it can be asymptomatic.[43]

Several studies have pointed out that most viable cysts are accompanied by little or no inflammatory infiltrate and that symptoms appear only after a latent period of several years. The classic description of Dixon and Lipscomb,[44] who studied 450 British soldiers returning from India, found that the average time between their return from the endemic area and the appearance of symptoms was 4.8 years. Various authors have reported the existence of asymptomatic NCC; however, to date, no data have been published on the frequency or distribution of such cases. Escobedo[43] has estimated from his experience in Mexico that approximately one third of NCC patients are asymptomatic.

The principal sites and approximate frequency of brain cysticerci are as follows[43]: parenchyma, approximately 60%; subarachnoid space, meningobasal and cortical, approximately 40%; ventricular system, approximately 10%; mixed areas, more than 50%; spine, approximately 1%. Parenchymal cysts can be single or multiple. The majority of these larvae, when viable, are 1 or 2 cm in diameter, are filled with fluid, and have an invaginated scolex (Fig. 296–8). They are observed in children and young adults and frequently cause no symptoms. It is surmised that a proportion of these infections are resolved spontaneously by the patients' immune response, leaving small granulomata or calcified cysts that are fortuitously detected on radiographs. In other cases, viable, translucent larvae have been seen by computed tomography (CT) in persons without symptoms.

The symptoms of patients with parenchymal cysts are varied, but most induce epilepsy that includes focal or generalized seizures (30% to 92%) and headache. Cysticercosis has been recognized as a major cause of epilepsy in several endemic countries.[43, 45, 46]

When parasites lodge in the ventricular cavities, they may become trapped in lateral ventricles, the fourth ventricle (by far the most frequent ventricular location), or the aqueduct. If the cyst is free, it may cause little inflammatory reaction. The clinical manifestations are the result of obstruction of CSF circulation, which can give rise to hydrocephalus (see Fig. 296–8). Acute hydrocephalus is a syndrome characterized by increased intracranial pressure, headache, vomiting, impaired vision, dizziness, and ataxia. Papilledema and mental disturbances are also common in patients with hydrocephalus. The syndrome progresses if the hydraulic problem is not resolved with a ventricular shunt, causing progressive loss of consciousness, decerebration, and death. Cysticerci that lodge in the fourth ventricle exhibit a syndrome of progressive hydrocephalus, with headache, nausea, vomiting, and papilledema associated with disturbances in the cerebellar functions (dizziness, vertigo, and loss of equilibrium and motor coordination). In other cases, the cyst adheres to the base of the fourth ventricle, inducing an inflammatory response with ependymitis characterized by signs of brain dysfunction.

Cysticerci found in the basal cisternae are frequently in

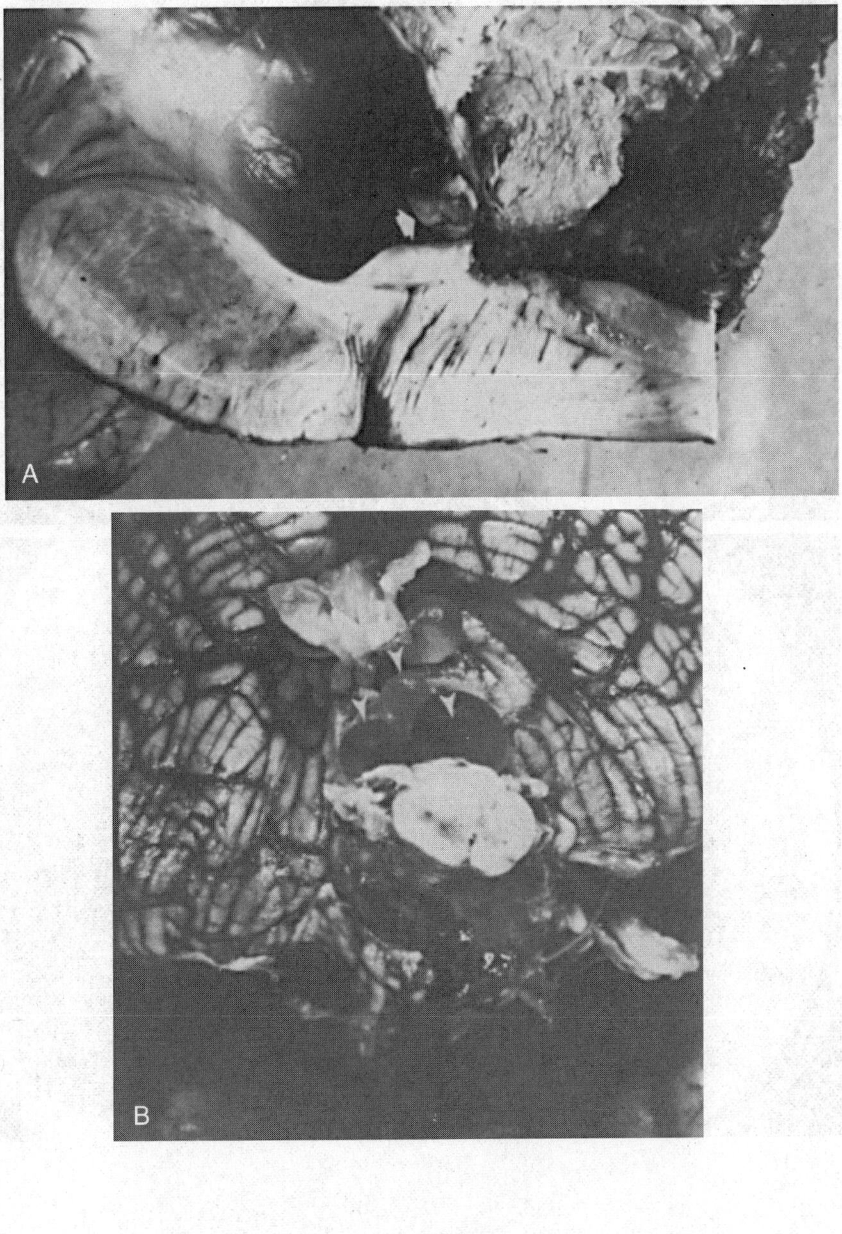

FIGURE 296–8 ▫ *A*, Cysticercus lodged in aqueduct of fourth ventricle *(arrow)*. *B*, *Cysticercus racemosus* in posterior fossa. Arrows point to various lobules of this cyst. (*A* and *B* courtesy of Dr. Alfonso Escobar Izquierdo, Instituto de Investigaciones Bìomédìcas, UNAM, Mexico.)

clumps or of the racemose type. The racemose cysticercus is a large membranous cyst measuring up to 5 cm in diameter. It often does not have a visible scolex, but it is certainly derived from a taeniid because it has the ultrastructural morphologic feature of taeniid tegumentary bladder walls. The work of Rabiela and coworkers[47] has shown by serial sections that these racemose forms do contain vestiges, or sometime whole scolices, unequivocally belonging to the species *T. solium*. For reasons that are at present not understood, the parasite located in the ventricles frequently becomes of the racemose type.

In cases in which the inflammatory process advances or increases, it can induce vasculitis or neuritis with local or distant ischemic phenomena, all of which are responsible for further brain damage and functional deterioration.[48]

Cysticerci located in the subarachnoid space are in close contact with the CSF, and it is assumed that the parasites reach the meninges from the ventricles. This form of NCC is almost always associated with severe inflammatory infiltrates, which eventually give a clinical picture of chronic basal meningitis. This complication gives rise to one of the most frequent signs of NCC: increased intracranial pressure, without focal deficits, which can progress rapidly and cause death if it is not treated. On CT examination, they can be confused with parenchymal cysts.

DIAGNOSIS

NCC should be suspected when the patient is known to live or to have lived in an endemic zone or country or has a clinical history of taeniasis or a family member who does; when there is chronic, persistent, atypical headache that is resistant to ordinary treatment, or seizures in young adults; when there are neurologic symptoms associated with increased intracranial pressure (papilledema); or when a nonsenile person exhibits mental deterioration.[48] CT is the most useful study and in most cases is virtually diagnostic[43, 49] (Fig. 296–9). In some cases, contrast enhancement is necessary.

Subarachnoid or intraventricular cysts are difficult to de-

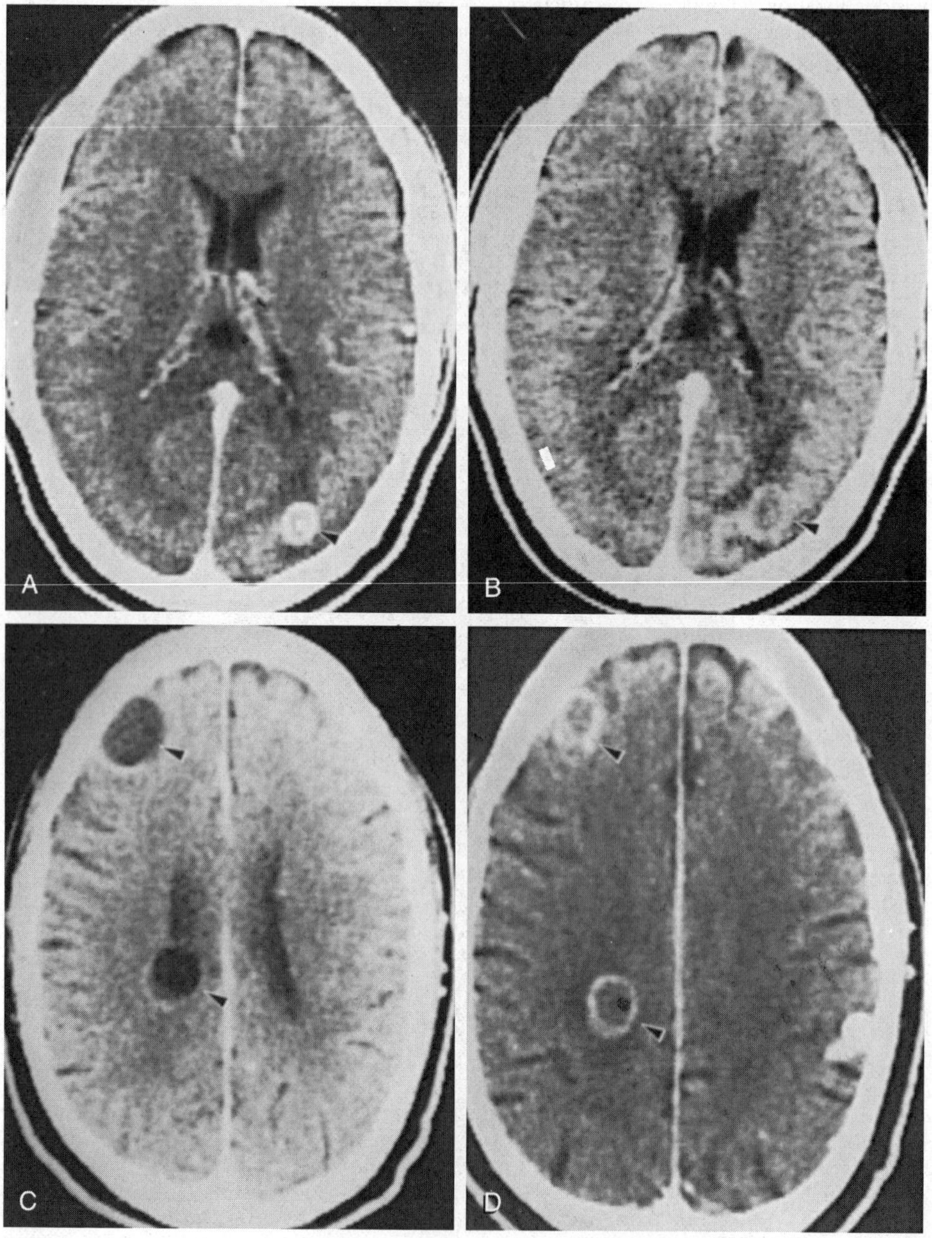

FIGURE 296–9 □ CT scan images. *A,* A patient with an occipital cyst *(arrow).* *B,* Same patient as in *A,* 8 months later, without treatment, showing inflammatory reaction but no reduction in size of lesion. *C,* Patient with two parenchymatous cysts showing as hypodense round areas *(arrows).* *D,* Same patient 4 months after treatment with praziquantel; both lesions are surrounded by an inflammatory infiltrate and are reduced in size. (*A* to *D* courtesy of Dr. Jesus Rodriguez, Instituto Nacional de Neurologia y Neurocirugia, "Manuel Velasco Suarez," Mexico City.)

tect by CT, and other imaging studies must be carried out. Magnetic resonance imaging has turned out to be another powerful technique with a high resolution; parenchymal cysts are clearly outlined in the brain section. The equipment and its cost still limit the study to developed countries—and to a few centers in developing countries where the organism is endemic.

CSF analysis is useful and shows lymphocytic pleocytosis and elevated protein content in most cases, eosinophilia in about 50% of cases, and decreased glucose level in about 25% of cases.[50]

Immunodiagnostic Procedures

Great progress has been made in the development of immunoenzymatic methods for the diagnosis of human cysticercosis. Several ELISAs have been developed. Reproducibility and sensitivity are greatest when larval bladder fluid is used as antigen. The test detects 80% to 90% of seropositive cases in endemic areas and as many as 95% of seropositive cases in nonendemic areas.[51, 52] Indirect hemagglutination is also a sensitive serologic test when bladder fluid is used as antigen and a useful test in countries where enzyme products for the ELISA are more difficult to obtain.[51]

By using a combination of ELISA and immunoblotting (enzyme-linked immunoelectrotransfer blot assay), Gottstein and colleagues[53] have been able to identify specific antibodies against *T. solium* in 92% of serum samples and 100% of CSF samples from patients with cysticercosis. An additional enzyme-linked immunoelectrotransfer blot assay based on affinity of purified glycoprotein antigens and lentil lectin has reported a 98% sensitivity and 100% specificity in detecting antibodies in serum and CSF from patients with confirmed cysticercosis. It is also capable of discriminating cysticercosis from other infections and from no infection.[54] Enzyme-linked immunoelectrotransfer blot assay has been used successfully in numerous field trials.[55, 56] Serodiagnosis with these methods has been extremely useful in epidemiologic studies, and they do aid in the diagnosis of individual cases of suspected NCC. However, definitive diagnosis can be carried out only by CT or magnetic resonance imaging techniques.

TREATMENT

Praziquantel has been shown by various workers in different countries to be an effective drug against parenchymal NCC.[33, 57, 58] Clinical and radiographic improvements have been shown in 70% to 90% of patients with parenchymal cysts.[33] The drug is less effective for patients with chronic arachnoiditis, for whom only 47% remission is reported. The patients are treated with 50 mg/kg daily for 15 days. About 2 or 3 days after the treatment is started, a strong inflammatory reaction occurs, with increased protein levels and cells in CSF, headaches, exacerbation of neurologic symptoms, and edema around cystic lesions, which can be detected by CT. These reactions can be suppressed with steroids and usually last 2 or 3 days. Clinical evidence of improvement is observed about 3 months after treatment.

Albendazole, an imidazole, has been used in several trials and is as effective as praziquantel for parenchymal lesions.[59] It has the additional advantage of being considerably less expensive than praziquantel and should be particularly useful in endemic countries where economy is an important factor in health care. The effective dosage tested by Sotelo and coworkers[59] was 15 mg/kg per day for 1 week. A review of clinical trials indicates that both praziquantel and albendazole are effective drugs in the treatment of parenchymal NCC; albendazole is also effective in the treatment of large subarachnoid cysts.[60]

Extraparenchymal lesions affecting basal or lateral cisternae, lesions caused by *Cysticercus racemosus*, and calcified cysts do not improve with praziquantel or albendazole. These types of NCC require surgery for extirpation of the parasite or insertion of valves to drain CSF and relieve increased intracranial pressure due to hydrocephalus. The specialized surgical techniques are beyond the scope of this chapter.[43]

EPIDEMIOLOGY OF TAENIASIS/CYSTICERCOSIS

The epidemiology of this zoonosis is intimately dependent on the life cycle of the parasite: the adult tapeworm stage, found only in humans; the metacestode or larval stage in the intermediate host, which causes human and porcine cysticercosis; and the egg stage, which is infective and found in the tapeworm proglottids in the intestine of humans or dispersed in the environment, in sewage, or in pastures or other locations, depending on the defecation habits of the local population.

A large number of publications in the last 10 years from a number of endemic countries indicate that human NCC is a significant public health problem in Latin America, Asia, and Africa.[5, 61–69] There is ever-increasing evidence that this disease is now emerging in nonendemic countries, particularly in the United States, because of increased immigration of persons from endemic countries. *T. solium* carriers have been identified among domestic employees from Latin America, and a large number of cases of NCC have been found among immigrants, mostly acquired in their native countries.[70–74]

Clinical data indicate that as many as 10% of CT studies carried out at the National Institute for Neurology and Neurosurgery in Mexico between 1976 and 1981 were diagnosed as cases of intracranial cysticercosis, or NCC.[75] These results are in stark contrast to the prevalence of NCC reported in 1970, when it constituted only 0.08% of all cases seen in a neurologic department in a 12-year period.[76]

Autopsy reports published in the past 20 years indicate that NCC has not diminished[5] in most countries where the tapeworm is endemic. A review of 20,206 autopsies carried out at the General Hospital in Mexico City between 1953 and 1984 revealed 481 cases of NCC (2.38%), of which only 189 (32.29%) were from persons who actually died of NCC, emphasizing again the large number of asymptomatic or relatively benign cases of this disease.[77]

TRANSMISSION PATTERNS

As Mackiewicz[78] has pointed out, the low probability of an egg's developing into an adult has been resolved in the cestodes by three basic strategies: (1) evolution of life cycles interpolated into host biology, (2) presentation of infective stages that increase probability of contact between host and parasite, and (3) increase in reproductive potential. Successful direct cycles are rare and confirm that a key element of cestode survival is the two (or three) host life cycles. Another central element of cestode transmission is the passive incorporation of cestodes into intermediate hosts or through the food chain. In the context of these basic strategies, the life cycles of *T. solium* and *T. saginata* are easily understood, particularly with regard to the transmission of the infection from the adult infective tapeworm eggs to the natural intermediate host.

In the case of *T. solium*, there is no doubt that pigs become infected by ingesting infected human feces. In pastoral or rural communities where sanitary installations do not exist, defecation on open ground is an accepted practice. In small villages or hamlets where pigs are kept as domestic animals, they are usually left to wander and feed freely on garbage and excrement. Aluja[79] has described a widespread practice that consists of having the latrine drain into the pigpen, serving a twofold purpose of feeding the pigs and eliminating the fecal material without a drainage system. Although the development of high-technology farming practices has significantly decreased the number of cysticercotic pigs in large urban slaughterhouses, the life cycle continues to be supported in small rural villages and hamlets, where modern health education is often pitted against century-old cultural patterns.[48] Studies show that porcine cysticercosis can be found in as many as 48% of pigs in villages where no meat inspection is carried out.[80]

Transmission from Human to Human

There are two processes by which infective eggs from a tapeworm carrier can be transmitted to a human intermediary host: ingestion of contaminated food and water and ingestion of eggs from hands contaminated by fecal material. Other mechanisms, such as inhalation of airborne eggs, ingestion of infected insects, and autoinfection by reverse peristalsis, have been suggested but not proved.[5] Little is known about the dynamics of transmission from human to human.

Common features in three epidemiologic studies were poverty, poor personal hygiene and sanitary facilities, the common practice of defecation on open ground, the rearing of domestic pigs that are left free to roam and scavenge through the town and adjacent fields, and the absence of meat inspection at local slaughtering facilities. An important observation derived from these epidemiologic studies carried out in rural villages was a clustered distribution of tapeworm carriers in one house or in neighboring houses. These clusters were associated with significantly higher seropositivity rates to tapeworm antigens in individuals living with a tapeworm carrier. Several studies confirm that seropositive persons are significantly clustered within households in which a member had a history of passing proglottids. The data suggest that transmission from human to human in rural settings is mainly intradomiciliary.[64–66, 81, 82]

Persons who live in daily close contact with a *T. solium* tapeworm carrier, under poor to fair hygiene conditions, may be exposed to frequent minimal doses of tapeworm egg antigens and eventually develop immune resistance to oncosphere infection. This possibility is a reasonable assumption, based on the results of experimental work carried out in other taeniids.[83–85] It has been noted that animals reared from birth in close association with the infected definitive host demonstrate the lightest infection patterns in the intermediate host population.[5]

Molinari and associates[86] have shown that immunization of mice with oncospheral antigens from *T. solium* and *T. saginata* protects these mice from metacestode infection. Although the mouse is not the natural intermediate host, their study does show that *T. solium* oncospheres are highly immunogenic in mammals. The same group[87] has shown that immunization of hogs with cysticercal antigens induces an immune response leading to degeneration and destruction of cysticerci in heavily infected animals.

Such results are encouraging, particularly in relation to the

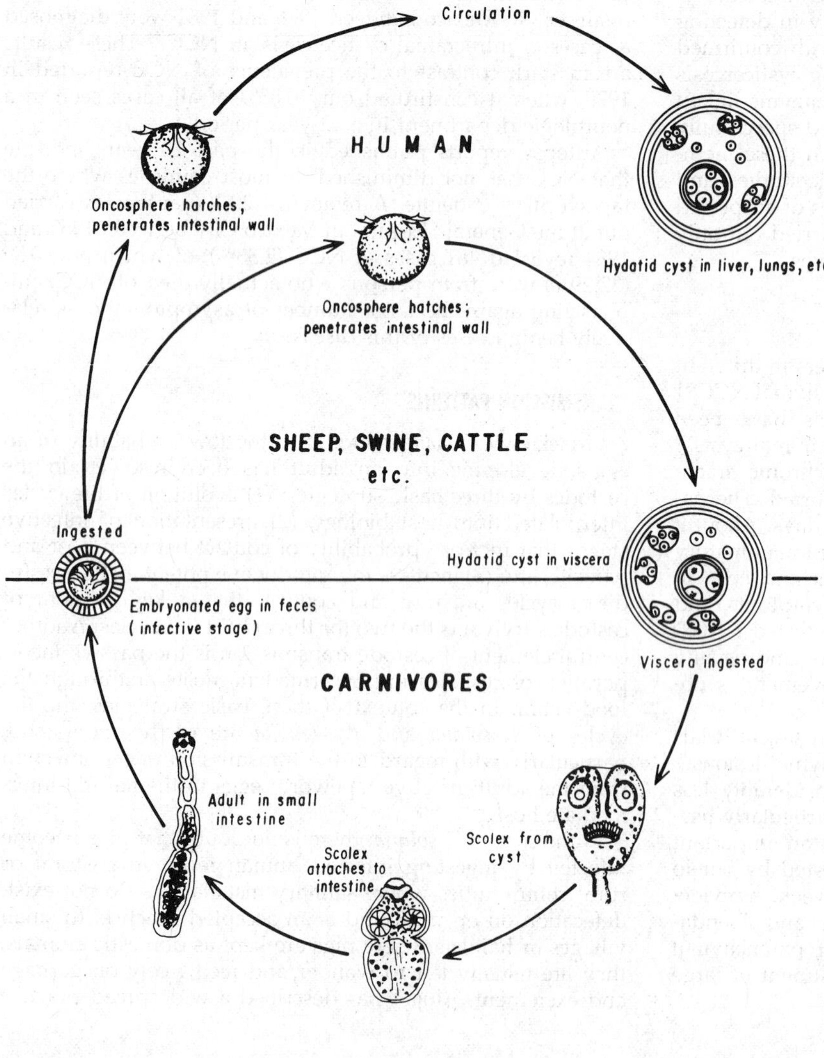

FIGURE 296–10 ▫ Life cycle of *Echinococcus granulosus*.

possibility of developing vaccines, which could be used to protect swine in high-risk areas.

PREVENTION

T. solium has been successfully eradicated in many European and North American countries by strict meat inspection practices, health education, hygiene, and widespread sanitary installations. In some central European countries, taeniasis was eradicated by massive treatment of the population with anthelmintic drugs, a measure that diminished the egg reservoir in the environment.[5] Unfortunately, not all of these measures are immediately applicable in many developing countries. Health education through schools, television, and other programs involving the local population are among the measures suggested by an ad hoc World Health Organization committee. The development of local task forces for the detection, treatment, and proper elimination of tapeworms in small rural communities is a feasible goal and should certainly be considered in areas where porcine cysticercosis is known to exist or where seropositivity of the population to *T. solium* antigens is high (more than 3% or 4%).[66] In addition, Pawlowski[34] and Warren and colleagues[88] have recommended large-scale anthelmintic treatment of the population in endemic areas. Intervention trials carried out in several countries by administration of praziquantel to the population have significantly decreased the prevalence of *T. solium* tapeworms in communities.[66, 89] In spite of the success of these trials, treatment should not be undertaken without strict medical supervision owing to the risk of nonsymptomatic persons with NCC responding to anthelmintic drugs.[90] Reports describing resistance to anthelmintic drugs in livestock and human schistosomiasis[91, 92] should also be given serious consideration, and the detection and treatment of individual cases should be encouraged instead.

Echinococcus granulosus

E. granulosus belongs to the family Taeniidae (see Table 296–1) and is the cause of zoonotic infections by the adult tapeworm found in canids (dogs and other carnivores) and by the larval stage, which produces cystic hydatid disease, found in humans but also in a wide range of mammalian species.[93(pp5–35)]

LIFE CYCLE (Fig. 296–10)

The adult worm is small, measuring between 2 and 7 mm (Fig. 296–11). The scolex bears four suckers and a rostellum with two rows of hooks, one small and one large. Each worm has between two and seven proglottids, the average number being three. The genital pore in all *Echinococcus* species opens laterally. The penultimate segment is mature, containing the eggs, which are ovoid and measure about 30 to 40 μm in diameter. The egg contains the hexacanth embryo (oncosphere) surrounded by the embryophore, a keratin shell, similar to the one found in *T. solium* and *T. saginata*, which also gives it a characteristic dark, striated appearance.

The adult worm parasitizes a wide range of Canidae (carnivores): domestic dogs, wolves, coyotes, jackals, and foxes. When proglottids from infected animals are released into the environment, the infective eggs can survive for long periods under suitable conditions of temperature and humidity.[94, 95]

The intermediate host acquires the infection by ingestion of infective eggs. Under the action of gastric and intestinal enzymes, the oncosphere is released and penetrates the intestinal wall and is transported to the liver or other organs. When the oncosphere reaches its final location, it develops into the larval stage or metacestode, commonly known as the hydatid cyst. The growth time of this cyst is variable but may take several months. Some cysts produce protoscolices and are known as fertile cysts; others do not and are classified as sterile cysts. The life cycle (see Fig. 296–10) is completed when a suitable definitive host ingests raw meat with cysts containing viable protoscolices. These evaginate in the upper duodenum, attach to the intestinal mucosa, and develop into sexually mature tapeworms approximately 6 to 8 weeks after infection.

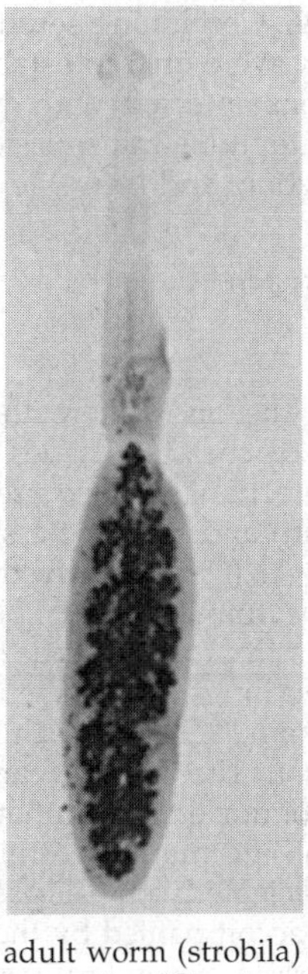

FIGURE 296–11 □ Whole adult worm (strobila) of *E. granulosus* (origin: Argentina), stained with carmine. (Courtesy of Dr. Peter M. Schantz, Centers for Disease Control and Prevention, Atlanta.)

The list of intermediate hosts for *E. granulosus* is long. Suffice it to say that it is maintained primarily in a domestic cycle with the domestic dog as definitive host and sheep the most important intermediate host. Other domestic ungulates, such as cattle, pigs, goats, horses, and camels, are susceptible hosts and may become infected in diverse geographic areas. There exists also a sylvatic cycle involving wolves and moose in North America,[96, 97] foxes and horses in Argentina,[98] and jackals and wild ruminants in Kenya.[99] Among the taeniids that parasitize humans, *E. granulosus* probably has the lowest host specificity of all, both the adult tapeworm and the hydatid cyst.[93(p11)]

EPIDEMIOLOGY AND CONTROL

The spread and maintenance of this zoonosis in rural areas are facilitated by the widespread practice of feeding dogs the viscera of home-slaughtered sheep. Humans acquire hydatid cyst by coming in close contact with infected dogs passing infective eggs in feces. Infective eggs can also be ingested through contaminated water or food. As has been discussed in previous sections, taeniid eggs are resistant to environmental factors and survive particularly well in humid, temperate climates. Desiccation and high temperatures appear to be among the few factors that affect their viability.

The geographic distribution of the disease is cosmopolitan in countries of temperate climates: southern South America, the Mediterranean coast, southern and central Russia, central Asia, Australia, and parts of Africa.[100] In Turkana, Kenya, the highest incidence of clinically recognized hydatid disease has been reported by Nelson,[101] with 198 surgical cases per

100,000 people in 1986. Combining serodiagnosis and mobile ultrasonography, they were able to establish a prevalence of 5% to 10% of persons infected with hydatid cyst. In the United States, autochthonous transmission occurs in Alaska, California, Utah, Arizona, and New Mexico.[100]

Human Hydatid Disease

PATHOLOGY

After penetration of the oncosphere through the intestinal mucosa, the embryo reaches the tissues and develops into a cyst. Most human infections are acquired from the pastoral strain (domestic strain) and produce a single cyst. The most common site is the liver (65%), followed by the lungs (25%), but cysts can also be found in the spleen, bone, kidneys, heart, and CNS. Cysts from the sylvatic strain of this cestode tend to localize in the lungs and cause a less severe disease than the domestic strain.[100] The growth rate of cysts is variable and can range from 1 to 5 cm a year. Transverse sections of the cyst reveal a nonnucleated laminated white membrane about 1 mm thick and an internal germinal membrane 10 to 15 μm thick with nucleated cells (Fig. 296–12). Progressive growth of the cyst is accompanied by the formation of a host connective tissue capsule. Secondary cysts can be generated from the germinal wall of fertile cysts, which contain several hundred to thousands of invaginated, infective protoscolices (see Fig. 296–12). The slowly growing cyst can be tolerated well until its size causes malfunction. Hydatid cysts containing up to 15 L of fluid have been reported and may contain up to 2 million protoscolices, each one of which can develop into a sexually mature worm if it is ingested by an appropriate definitive host. The major risk for patients with hydatid cysts is accidental rupture of the cyst wall. The sudden, massive release of cyst fluid can precipitate allergic reactions that can range from mild to fatal anaphylaxis. Dissemination of protoscolices may generate multiple secondary hydatid cysts.

IMMUNE RESPONSE TO HYDATID CYST

In 1967, Capron and coworkers[102] described a major precipitin band by immunoelectrophoresis found in serum of animals infected with *E. granulosus*. This precipitation band was termed arc 5 and has since been demonstrated to be the immunodominant and most specific antigen of this larval cestode. Its presence in a patient's serum is virtually diagnostic of *Echinococcus* species.[103] Schantz and coworkers[104] later demonstrated that arc 5 could also be found in some patients with NCC; however, this poses differential diagnostic problems only in countries where both infections coexist. Several studies have demonstrated that the more recently developed enzyme-linked immunoelectrotransfer blot tests are capable of discriminating between serologic reactions to hydatidosis and human cysticercosis.[105]

ELISAs developed by Coltorti[106] for the detection of arc 5 have shown a high efficiency. One of the major drawbacks of serologic tests for detection of hydatid cyst is that about a third of the patients with proven disease are seronegative. Studies carried out by Craig and colleagues[107] in Turkana, Kenya, have shown that clinically normal persons living in a highly endemic area had a significantly higher titer of antibodies (by ELISA) to oncospheral antigens than did clinically normal persons living in a nonendemic area. The authors speculated that these differences could be due to the presence, in the endemic areas, of a large number of infected persons who do not develop cystic disease and may, in fact, be exhibiting some degree of protective immunity. Such observations may be important for the eventual development and application of a preventive vaccine in high-risk endemic areas.

CLINICAL MANIFESTATIONS

The clinical manifestations depend on the site and size of the hydatid cyst. They can be variable. The interval between infection and the appearance of symptoms can range from months to years, depending on the growth rate and situation of the cyst. Hepatic cysts may manifest as liver enlargement, with or without a palpable mass, right-sided epigastric pain, nausea, and vomiting. Rupture or leakage may cause allergic reactions and, if massive, may lead to anaphylactic shock.

Unilocular liver cysts can survive for many years in the patient and may be accidentally discovered on radiographs, particularly when the cyst wall is calcified. It is assumed that

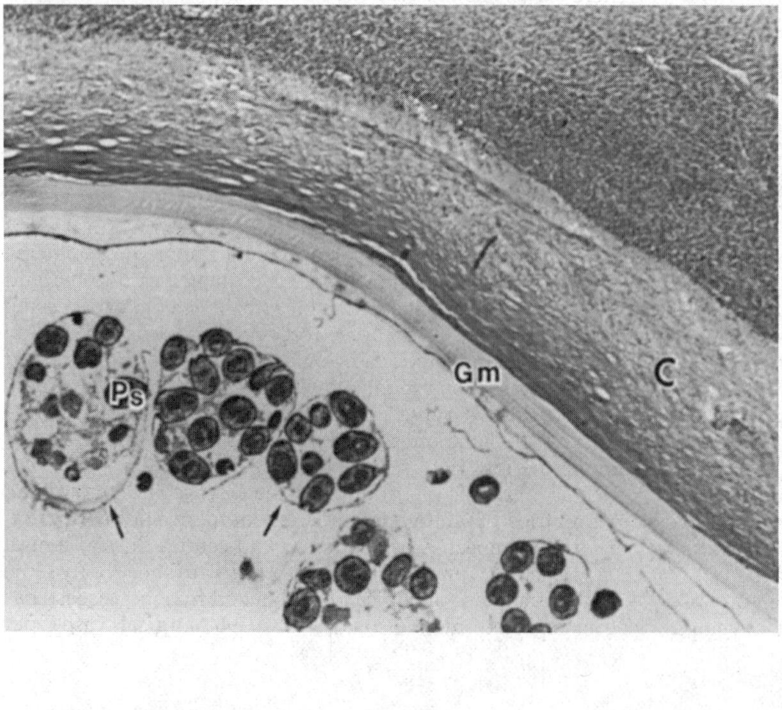

FIGURE 296–12 □ Histologic section of *E. granulosus* hydatid cyst from sheep liver showing protoscolices (Ps) in brood capsules *(arrows)*, germinative membrane (Gm), and host capsule (C). (Courtesy of Dr. Peter M. Schantz, Centers for Disease Control and Prevention, Atlanta.)

most infections are acquired during childhood and are not detected until adult life.[108]

DIAGNOSIS

A history of exposure to sheepdogs in endemic areas and the presence of a cystlike mass in the liver or lung supports the diagnosis of hydatid disease. CT and ultrasonography are the methods of choice for detailed characterization of the cyst. Closed aspiration of cysts should never be attempted because accidental spillage or rupture may cause anaphylaxis or secondary cysts. In lung infections, protoscolices may sometimes be demonstrated in bronchial lavage fluid or sputum. Eosinophilia is present in less than 25% of cases.

Serologic tests are useful and are diagnostic when results are positive, although a significant percentage of patients do not have circulating antibodies. Whenever possible, such sera should be tested for circulating antigen or circulating immune complexes, as described in the previous section.

THERAPY

Surgical removal of the hydatid cyst still remains the most effective treatment.[100] In cases of inoperable hydatid cysts, or when the general condition of the patient precludes surgery, albendazole, 10 to 15 mg/kg per day for 1 month, or mebendazole, 50 to 150 mg/kg per day for 3 months, may be administered, although the results are unpredictable. Okelo[109] in Turkana, Kenya, has reported encouraging results with albendazole in series of patients with large inoperable cysts and extensive secondary involvement. The treatment schedule was 10 mg/kg per day in two divided doses for 8 weeks. Albendazole is also recommended for the prevention of recurrent secondary disease.

PREVENTION AND CONTROL

At present, preventive measures depend mainly on diminishing the infection rate in domestic dogs by avoiding the practice of feeding them sheep offal (viscera) and by periodic mass treatment of dogs with praziquantel (5 mg/kg) in endemic areas. For the prevention of human hydatid disease, measures such as careful personal hygiene and avoidance of infected dogs are essential. Health education and the strict enforcement of meat inspection and proper disposal of infected livestock should be carried out.

In endemic countries, official control programs against *E. granulosus* should be developed and maintained as recommended by the World Health Organization. A control program that has been in operation for more than 30 years has almost extinguished this parasite from New Zealand. The main features of the program were education and systematic deparasitization (dosing) of dogs.[110]

A pilot control program being carried out in Turkana, Kenya, includes case detection of human disease by ultrasonography and serologic tests; treatment of humans with surgery and albendazole; elimination of stray dogs; and registration of remaining dogs for treatment with praziquantel.[111]

Hymenolepis nana

H. nana belongs to the family Hymenolepididae. It was originally described in rats and mice but was later found in humans.

Life Cycle

Among the Cyclophyllidea, it is the only tapeworm that is capable of completing the whole life cycle in one host, but it also sometimes uses the two-host life cycle. The length of the adult worm is inversely proportional to the number of individual worms present in the intestine. Its average length is between 2 and 3 cm. The scolex has four suckers and an armed rostellum with a single row of 8 to 30 hooks. The scolices are attached to the small intestine, and gravid proglottids rupture in the lumen, releasing the embryonated eggs, which have a diameter of 40 to 50 μm. The eggs can hatch in the intestine and lodge between the mucosal microvilli until they develop into cysticercoids. These continue to develop into adult worms, a process that takes 15 to 20 days, when again they begin to release infective eggs.

Epidemiology

Hymenolepiasis is a parasitic disease of populations living under conditions of poor hygiene and is particularly prevalent in children from developing countries with tropical and subtropical climates. The disease is acquired by ingestion of infected mice feces, which contaminate water and food in such areas. Infected children may also contaminate others with infective eggs passed on dirty hands.

H. nana is found mainly in children younger than 8 years. Its prevalence is particularly high in rural communities, where hygiene and sanitation facilities are poor.[112] Experimental work carried out in different laboratories indicates that *H. nana* infections induce humoral immunity[113] and probably have an important cellular immune component,[114] responses that could account for the decreased prevalence of this parasitosis in adults living in endemic areas. Experimental evidence indicates that immunoglobulin E and mast cells participate in the expulsion of *H. nana* adults from the intestine of mice.[115]

Clinical Manifestations

Symptoms are mild (vague abdominal distress) in light infections. Children with multiple infections, however, can have severe disease with abdominal pain, nausea, vomiting, weight loss, diarrhea, and irritability. Erosion of the intestinal mucosa can occur in massive infections.

Diagnosis

The diagnosis can be made on coprologic analysis of serial stool samples by identification of the eggs (which differ from the taeniid egg in that they lack a striated outer embryophore). Adult worms, which can also be found in multiple infections, can be identified by their size and armed scolex.

Treatment

The treatment of choice is niclosamide, 2 g daily for 5 days consecutively. Praziquantel has also been used with good effect, in a single dose of 20 mg/kg.[116]

Prevention

Health education and careful personal hygiene, particularly for children, should diminish the frequency of this parasitosis.

Diphyllobothrium latum (Broad Fish Tapeworm)

Life Cycle (Fig. 296–13)

D. latum belongs to the order of the Pseudophyllidea (see Table 296–1). In contrast to the taeniid tapeworms, Diphyllo-

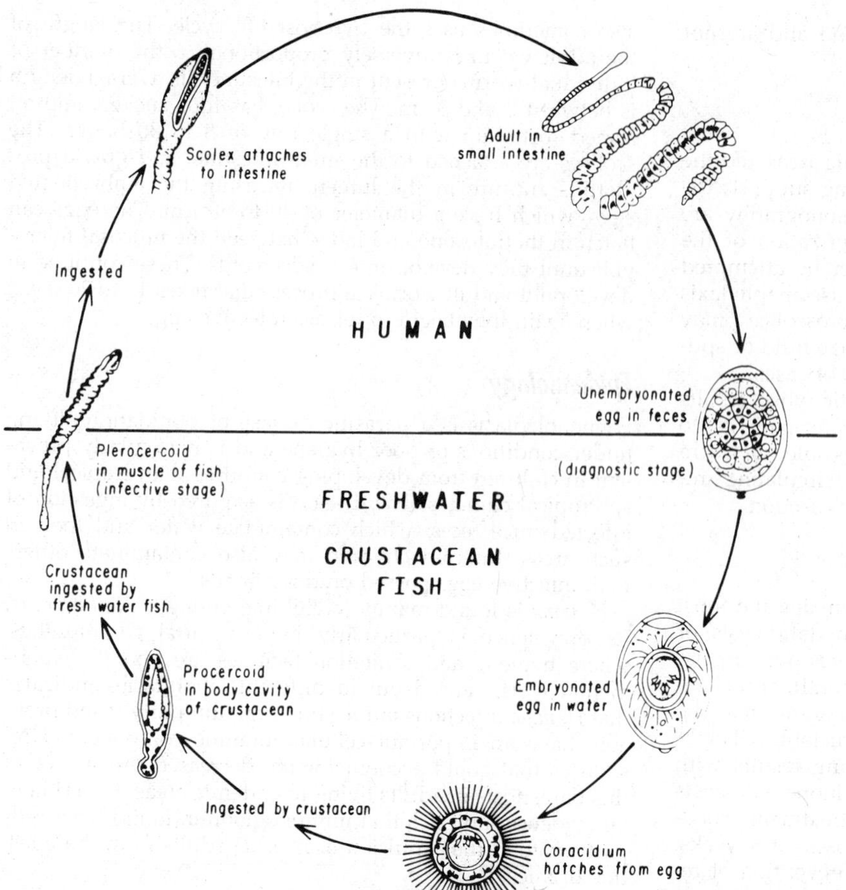

FIGURE 296–13 □ Life cycle of *Diphyllobothrium latum.*

bothriidae organisms require two intermediate hosts to complete their life cycle and in addition have a free-swimming life stage that takes place in freshwater.

The scolex of *D. latum* is variable in shape, with distinct bothria, narrow, deep, and not connected by an apical groove.[2] Adult worms have been reported as long as 6 to 9 m with 3000 to 4000 proglottids, which are wider than long. A single worm can produce about 1 million eggs per day. Von Bonsdorff and Bylund[117] have reported the release of 20 to 40 million eggs per day per worm carrier. Expelled eggs are not completely mature and lie dormant in water after passing from the host. They become fully mature within 8 to 12 days. The egg hatches in water and releases the embryo, known as the coracidium, which is a free-swimming form. The coracidium must then be ingested within 4 or 5 days by its first intermediate host, a copepod (nonspecific microcrustacean). In this host, it becomes an oncosphere and bores through the intestinal wall of the copepod to reach the coelomic cavity, where it metamorphoses into a procercoid larva, measuring about 500 to 600 μm. When the infected microcrustacean is ingested by a fish, the procercoid dislodges and penetrates the intestinal wall of the fish and eventually situates itself in the muscle or one of various viscera. There it develops into a plerocercoid, which may remain viable for the lifetime of the fish. Plerocercoids are visible to the naked eye and measure about 1 to 5 cm. Many freshwater fish species are affected: pike, perch, turbot, ruff, and rainbow trout in Chile, whitefish and salmon in the United States. The life cycle (see Fig. 296–13) is completed when a human or other definitive host ingests raw or undercooked fish. The most suitable definitive host is humans, and the parasite seems to establish itself only in areas where its life cycle includes humans. Other final hosts are dogs, cats, pigs, wolves, foxes, and bears, among others. Worms develop in the small intestine and begin laying eggs about 1 month after infection. They may live for a number of years.

Epidemiology

D. latum is found in various terrestrial and marine fish-eating carnivores. The adult tapeworm also parasitizes humans, and infections have been reported in the subarctic and temperate regions of the Eurasian continent, in the area from the Siberian rivers Yenisei and Ob to the Baltic Sea. There is a high prevalence in the northern European areas of Russia, Volga basin, and Finland. It is also found in the lake districts of northern Italy and western Switzerland and around the Danube River. Immigration has transported the disease to freshwater lakes in North and South America.

Clinical Manifestations

Symptoms include abdominal pain, weight loss, and a unique form of pernicious anemia, which, although not common, is caused by the special capacity of *D. latum* for taking up vitamin B_{12} in the proximal small intestine.

Diagnosis

Diagnosis can be made in persons who report eating raw or undercooked fish by serial stool examinations for proglottids and eggs, which are oval and have a characteristic operculum on one pole.

Treatment

Treatment is a single dose of niclosamide, 2 g, or praziquantel, 5 to 10 mg/kg.

Prevention

Prevention can be achieved by avoiding the ingestion of raw or undercooked fish in endemic areas. The direct drainage of sewage into freshwater lakes or rivers should also be prevented.

Acknowledgment

The author is indebted to Dr. Julio Sotelo for his revision and constructive criticism of the section on human cysticercosis and treatment; to Dr. Jaime Martuscelli for his generous help in revising the manuscript; and to Drs. Jesus Rodriguez Carbajal, Alfonso Escobar Izquierdo, Juan Pedro Laclette, and Peter Schantz for many of the figures included in this chapter. To my long-time collaborator, Marie Therese Merchant, acknowledgment is given for her fine work in the preparation of the photographic material.

References

1. Cheng TC: Cestoda. The true tapeworms. *In* Cheng TC (ed): General Parasitology. New York, Academic Press, 1973, pp 474–541.
2. Schmidt GD: Handbook of Tapeworm Identification. Key to the Genera Taeniidae. Boca Raton, FL, CRC Press, 1986, pp 221–227.
3. Mahajan RC: Geographic distribution of human cysticercosis. *In* Flisser A, Willms K, Laclette JP, et al (eds): Cysticercosis: Present State of Knowledge and Perspectives. New York, Academic Press, 1982, pp 39–46.
4. Schultz MG, Halterman LG, Rich AB, et al: An epizootic of bovine cysticercosis. J Am Vet Med Assoc 155:1708, 1969.
5. Gemmel MM, Matyas Z, Pawlowski Z, et al (eds): Guidelines for the Surveillance, Prevention, and Control of Taeniasis/Cysticercosis. Geneva, World Health Organization, 1983.
6. Slais J: The morphology and pathogenicity of the bladder worms: *Cysticercus cellulosae* and *Cysticercus bovis*. Prague, Academia, 1970.
7. Pawlowski ZS: Epidemiology of *Taenia saginata* infection. *In* Flisser A, Willms K, Laclette JP, et al (eds): Cysticercosis: Present State of Knowledge and Perspectives. New York, Academic Press, 1982, pp 69–85.
8. Bürger HJ, Wilkens S: Infections of cattle with *Cysticercus bovis* and sarcocystic spp. on pastures irrigated with sewage plant effluent. Mol Biochem Parasitol Suppl 274, 1982.
9. Harrison LJ, Holt K, Sewell MM: Serum antibody levels to *Taenia saginata* in cattle grazed on Scottish pastures. Res Vet Sci 40:344, 1986.
10. Silverman PH: The longevity of eggs of *Taenia pisiformis* and *Taenia saginata* under various conditions. Trans R Soc Trop Med Hyg 50:8, 1956.
11. Lisowska M: Epidemiological Analysis of *Taenia saginata* Taeniasis in Poznan [in Polish]. Poznan, Poland, Academy of Medicine, 1979. Thesis. [Cited in reference 6, p 76.]
12. Heinz HJ, Klintworth GK: Cysticercosis in the aetiology of epilepsy. S Afr J Med Sci 30:32, 1965.
13. Lenoble E, Dumontier C: Perforations du grele et parasitoses intestinales. A propos d'un cas de péritonite par perforation du grêle associée à un *Taenia saginata*. J Chir (Paris) 125:350, 1988.
14. Pawlowski ZS, Schultz MG: Taeniasis and cysticercosis (*Taenia saginata*). Adv Parasitol 10:269, 1972.
15. Graham CF: A device for the diagnosis of *Enterobius* infection. Am J Trop Med Hyg 21:159, 1941.
16. Faust EC, D'Antoni JS, Odom V, et al: A critical study of clinical laboratory techniques for the diagnosis of protozoan, cyst and helminth eggs in faeces. Am J Trop Med Hyg 18:169, 1938.
17. Ritchie LS: An ether sedimentation technique for routine stool examinations. Bull US Army Dept 8:326, 1948.
18. Martin LK, Beaner P: Evaluation of Kato thick-smear technique for quantitative diagnosis of helminth infections. Am J Trop Med Hyg 17:382, 1968.
19. David ED, Lindquist WD: Determination of the specific gravity of certain helminth eggs using sucrose density gradient centrifugation. J Parasitol 68:916, 1982.
20. McAninch NH: Case report. An outbreak of cysticercosis in feedlot cattle. Can Vet J 15:120, 1974.
21. Eom KS, Rim HJ: Morphologic descriptions of *Taenia asiatica* sp. Korean J Parasitol 31:1, 1993.
22. Bowles J, McManus DP: Genetic characterization of the Asian *Taenia*, a newly described taeniid cestode of humans. Am J Trop Med Hyg 50:33, 1994.
23. Fan PC, Chung WC, Lin CY, Chan CH: Clinical manifestations of taeniasis in Taiwan aborigenes. J Helminthol 66:118, 1992.
24. Webbe G: The hatching and activation of taeniid ova in relation to the development of cysticercosis in man. Z Trop Parasitol 18:354, 1967.
25. Hernandez-Jauregui PA, Marquez-Monter H, Sastré-Ortiz S: Cysticercosis of the central nervous system in hogs. Am J Vet Res 34:451, 1973.
26. Cañedo L, Laclette JP, Morales E: Evagination of the metacestode of *Taenia solium*. *In* Flisser A, Willms K, Laclette JP, et al (eds): Cysticercosis: Present State of Knowledge and Perspectives. New York, Academic Press, 1982, pp 363–373.
27. Lumsden R, Voge M, Sogandares-Bernal F: The metacestode tegument: Fine structure, development, topochemistry and interactions with the host. *In* Flisser A, Willms K, Laclette JP, et al (eds): Cysticercosis: Present State of Knowledge and Perspectives. New York, Academic Press, 1982, pp 307–361.
28. Allan JC, Craig PS, Garcia Noval J, et al: Coproantigen detection for immunodiagnosis of echinococcosis and taeniasis in dogs and humans. Parasitology 104:347, 1992.
29. Maass M, Delgado E, Knobloch J: Isolation of an immunodiagnostic *Taenia solium* coproantigen. Trop Med Parasitol 43:201, 1992.
30. Allan JC, Mencos F, Garcia Noval J, et al: Dipstick dot ELISA for the detection of *Taenia* coproantigens in humans. Parasitology 107:79, 1993.
31. Chapman A, Vallejo V, Mossie KG, et al: Isolation and characterization of species-specific DNA probes from *Taenia solium* and *Taenia saginata* and their use in an egg detection assay. Clin Microbiol 33:1283, 1995.
32. Groll E: Praziquantel for cestode infections in man. Acta Trop 37:293, 1980.
33. Sotelo J, Torres B, Rubio-Donnadieu F, et al: Praziquantel in the treatment of neurocysticercosis: Long-term follow-up. Neurology 35:732, 1985.
34. Pawlowski ZS: Efficiency of low doses of praziquantel in taeniasis. Acta Trop 48:83, 1989.
35. Grisolia JS, Wiederholt WC: CNS cysticercosis. Arch Neurol 39:540, 1982.
36. Nash TE, Neva FA: Recent advances in the diagnosis and treatment of cerebral cysticercosis. N Engl J Med 311:1492, 1984.
37. Flisser A, Tarrab R, Willms K, et al: Immunoelectroforesis y doble immunodifusion en el diagnostico de la cisticercosis cerebral humana. Arch Invest Med (Mex) 6:1, 1975.
38. Grogl M, Estrada JJ, MacDonald G, et al: Antigen-antibody analysis in neurocysticercosis. J Parasitol 71:433, 1985.
39. Schantz PM: Improvements in the serodiagnosis of helminthic diseases. Vet Parasitol 25:95, 1987.
40. Corona T, Pascoe D, Gonzalez-Barranco D, et al: Anticysticercosis antibodies in serum and cerebrospinal fluid in patients with cerebral cysticercosis. J Neurol Neurosurg Psychiatry 49:1044, 1986.
41. McCormick GF, Zee CS, Heiden J: Cysticercosis cerebri: Review of 127 cases. Arch Neurol 39:534, 1982.
42. Escobar A, Nieto D: Parasitic diseases. *In* Minckler J (ed): Pathology of the Nervous System, Vol 3. New York, McGraw-Hill, 1972, pp 2503–2521.
43. Escobedo F: Neurosurgical aspects of neurocysticercosis. *In* Schmidek HH, Sweet WH (eds): Operative Neurosurgical Techniques. Indications, Methods and Results. Orlando, FL, Grune & Stratton, 1988, pp 93–102.
44. Dixon H, Lipscomb F: Cysticercosis: An Analysis and Follow-up of 450 Cases. Medical Resource Council Special Report 299. London, Her Majesty's Stationery Office, 1961.

45. White AC: Neurocysticercosis: A major cause of neurological disease worldwide. Clin Infect Dis 24:101, 1997.
46. Garcia HH, Gilman R, Martinez M, et al: Cysticercosis as a major cause of epilepsy in Peru. The Cysticercosis Working Group in Peru. Lancet 342:197, 1993.
47. Rabiela MT, Rivas-Hernandez A, Castillo-Medina S, et al: Pruebas morfologicas de que *Cysticercus cellulosae* y *Cysticercus racemosus* son larvas de *Taenia solium*. Arch Invest Med (Mex) 16:83, 1985.
48. Aluja A, Escobar A, Escobedo F, et al: Teniasis y cisticercosis humana: Descripcion de la enfermedad y cuadros clinicos. *In* Cisticercosis, una Recopilacion Actualizada de los Conocimientos Básicos para el Manejo y Control de la Cisticercosis Causada por *Taenia solium*. México, D.F., Biblioteca de la Salud, Fondo de Cultura Económica, 1987, pp 38–43.
49. Rodriguez-Carbajal J, Boleaga-Duran B, Dorfsman J: Cerebral cysticercosis. The role of computed tomography (CT) in the diagnosis of neurocysticercosis. Childs Nerv Syst 3:199, 1987.
50. Del Brutto OH, Sotelo J: Neurocysticercosis: An update. Rev Infect Dis 10:1075, 1988.
51. Larralde C, Laclette JP, Owen CS, et al: Reliable serology of *Taenia solium* cysticercosis with antigens from cyst vesicular fluid: ELISA and hemagglutination tests. Am J Trop Med Hyg 35:965, 1986.
52. Baily GG, Mason PR, Trijssener FE: Serological diagnosis of neurocysticercosis: Evaluation of ELISA tests using cyst fluid and other components of *Taenia solium* cysticerci as antigens. Trans R Soc Trop Med Hyg 82:295, 1988.
53. Gottstein B, Zini D, Schantz PM: Species-specific immunodiagnosis of *Taenia solium* cysticercosis by ELISA and immunoblotting. Trop Med Parasitol 38:299, 1987.
54. Tsang VC, Brand JA, Boyer AE: An enzyme-linked immunoelectrotransfer blot assay and glycoprotein antigens for diagnosing human cysticercosis *(Taenia solium)*. J Infect Dis 159:50, 1989.
55. Montenegro T, Gilman RH, Castillo R, et al: The diagnostic importance of species specific and cross-reactive components of *Taenia solium, Echinococcus granulosus* and *Hymenolepis nana*. Rev Inst Med Trop Sao Paulo 36:327, 1994.
56. Schantz PM, Sarti E, Plancarte A, et al: Community-based epidemiological investigations of cysticercosis due to *Taenia solium*: Comparison of serological screening tests and clinical findings in two populations in Mexico. Clin Infect Dis 18:879, 1994.
57. Botero D, Castaño S: Treatment of cysticercosis with praziquantel in Colombia. Am J Trop Med Hyg 31:810, 1982.
58. Vasconcelos D, Cruz-Segura H, Mateos-Gomez H, et al: Selective indications for the use of praziquantel in the treatment of brain cysticercosis. J Neurol Neurosurg Psychiatry 50:383, 1987.
59. Sotelo J, Escobedo F, Penagos P: Albendazole vs praziquantel for therapy for neurocysticercosis. Arch Neurol 45:532, 1988.
60. Del Brutto OH, Sotelo J, Roman GC: Therapy for neurocysticercosis: A reappraisal. Clin Infect Dis 17:730, 1993.
61. Marty P, Mary C, Pagliardini G, et al: Courte enquête sur la cysticercose et la taeniase à *Taenia solium* dans un village de l'ouest Cameroun. Med Trop (Mars) 46:181, 1986.
62. Fan PC, Chung WC, Chan CH, et al: Studies on taeniasis in Taiwan. V. Field trial on evaluation of therapeutic efficacy of mebendazole and praziquantel against taeniasis. Southeast Asian J Trop Med Public Health 17:82, 1986.
63. Sarti-Gutierrez EJ, Schantz PM, Lara-Aguilera R, et al: *Taenia solium* taeniasis and cysticercosis in a Mexican village. Trop Med Parasitol 29:194, 1988.
64. Keilbach N, Aluja AS, Sarti E: A programme to control taeniasis/cysticercosis *(T. solium)*. Experiences in a Mexican village. Acta Leidensia 57:181, 1989.
65. Diaz Camacho S, Candil Ruiz A, Beltran Uribe M, et al: Serology as an indicator of *Taenia solium* tapeworm infections in a rural community of Mexico. Trans R Soc Trop Med Hyg 84:563, 1990.
66. Diaz Camacho S, Candil Ruiz A, Suate Peraza V, et al: Epidemiological study and control of *Taenia solium* infections with praziquantel in a rural village of Mexico. Am J Trop Med Hyg 45:522, 1991.
67. Kong Y, Ch SY, Cho MS, et al: Seroepidemiological observations of *Taenia solium* cysticercosis in epileptic patients in Korea. J Korean Med Sci 8:145, 1993.
68. Thomson AJ: Neurocysticercosis—Experience at the teaching hospital of the University of Cape Town. S Afr Med J 83:332, 1993.
69. Spina Franca A, Livramento JA, Machado LR: Cysticercosis of the central nervous system and cerebrospinal fluid. Immunodiagnosis of 1573 patients in 63 years (1929–1992). Arq Neuropsiquiatr 51:16, 1993.
70. Schantz PM, Moore AC, Munoz JL, et al: Neurocysticercosis in an Orthodox Jewish community in New York City. N Engl J Med 327:692, 1992.
71. Locally acquired neurocysticercosis—North Carolina, Massachusetts, and South Carolina, 1989–1991. MMWR Morbid Mortal Wkly Rep 41:1, 1992.
72. Ehnert KL, Roberto RR, Barrett L, et al: Cysticercosis: First 12 months of reporting in California. Bull Pan Am Health Organ 26:165, 1992.
73. Sorvillo FJ, Waterman SH, Richards FO, Schantz PM: Cysticercosis surveillance: Locally acquired and travel related infections and detection of intestinal tapeworm carriers in Los Angeles County. Am J Trop Med Hyg 47:365, 1992.
74. Dietrichs E, Tyssvang T, Aanonsen NO, Bakke SJ: Cerebral cysticercosis in Norway. Acta Neurol Scand 88:296, 1993.
75. Rodriguez Carbajal J: La cisticercosis humana en Mexico. Diagnóstico radiológico. Gac Med Mex 124:198, 1988.
76. Macias Sanchez R, Rodriguez Trujillo F, Ordoñez Martinez S: Cisticercosis cerebral: Anatomia patológica y correlación anatomoclinica. Neurol Neurochir Psychiatry 11:271, 1970.
77. Villagran Uribe J, Olvera Rabiela JE: Cisticercosis humana: Estudio clinico y patologico de 481 casos de autopsia. Patologia (Mex) 26:149, 1988.
78. Mackiewicz JS: Cestode transmission patterns. J Parasitol 74:60, 1988.
79. Aluja AS: Frequency of porcine cysticercosis in Mexico. *In* Flisser A, Willms K, Laclette JP, et al (eds): Cysticercosis: Present State of Knowledge and Perspectives. New York, Academic Press, 1982, pp 53–62.
80. The marketing of cysticercotic pigs in the Sierra of Peru. The Cysticercosis Working Group in Peru. Bull World Health Organ 71:223, 1993.
81. Sarti E, Schantz PM, Plancarte A, et al: Epidemiological investigation of *Taenia solium* taeniasis and cysticercosis in a rural village of Michoacan State, Mexico. Trans R Soc Trop Med Hyg 88:49, 1994.
82. Sarti E, Schantz PM, Plancarte A, et al: Prevalence and risk factors for *Taenia solium* taeniasis and cysticercosis in humans and pigs in a village in Morelos, Mexico. Am J Trop Med Hyg 46:677, 1992.
83. Musoke AJ, Williams JF: Immunological response of the rat to infection with *Taenia taeniaeformis*: Protective antibody response to implanted parasites. Int J Parasitol 6:265, 1976.
84. Sewell MMH, Gallie GJ: Immunological studies on experimental infections with the larval stage of *Taenia saginata*. *In* Soulsby EJL (ed): Parasitic Zoonoses. Clinical and Experimental Studies. New York, Academic Press, 1974, pp 187–193.
85. Rickard MD: Immunization against infection with larval taeniid cestodes using oncospheral antigens. *In* Flisser A, Willms K, Laclette JP, et al (eds): Cysticercosis: Present State of Knowledge and Perspectives. New York, Academic Press, 1982, pp 633–646.
86. Molinari JL, Tato P, Aguilar T, et al: Immunity in mice to an oncosphere infection by using oncospheral antigens from *Taenia solium* or *Taeniarhynchus saginatus*. Rev Latinoam Microbiol 30:325, 1988.
87. Molinari JL, Meza R, Tato P: *Taenia solium*: Cell reactions to the larva *(Cysticercus cellulosae)* in naturally parasitized, immunized hogs. Exp Parasitol 56:327, 1983.
88. Warren KS, Bundy DAP, Anderson RM, et al: Helminth Infections, Health Sector Priorities Review. Washington, DC, The World Bank, 1989.
89. Cruz M, Davis A, Dixon H, et al: Operational studies on the control of *Taenia solium* taeniasis/cysticercosis in Ecuador. Bull World Health Organ 67:401, 1989.
90. Flisser A, Madrazo I, Plancarte A, et al: Neurological symptoms in occult neurocysticercosis after single taenicidal dose of praziquantel. Lancet 342:748, 1993.
91. Jackson F: Anthelmintic resistance—The state of play. Br Vet J 149:123, 1993.
92. Brindley PJ: Drug resistance to schistosomiasis and other anthelmintics of medical significance. Acta Trop 56:213, 1994.
93. Eckert J, Gemmel MA, Soulsby EJL (eds): Guidelines for Surveil-

lance, Prevention and Control of Echinococcosis/Hydatidosis. Geneva, World Health Organization, 1981.
94. Sweatman GK, Williams RJ: Survival of *Echinococcus granulosus* and *Taenia hydatigena* eggs in two extreme climatic regions of New Zealand. Res Vet Sci 4:199, 1963.
95. Laws GF: Physical factors influencing survival of taeniid eggs. Exp Parasitol 22:227, 1968.
96. Rausch RL, Nelson GS: A review of the genus *Echinococcus* Rudolphi, 1801. Ann Trop Med Parasitol 57:127, 1963.
97. Rausch RL: Life cycle patterns and geographic distribution of *Echinococcus* species. *In* Thompson RCA, Lymbery AJ (eds): Echinococcus and Hydatid Disease. Oxford, CAB International, 1995, pp 89–134.
98. Schantz PM, Lord RD, de Zavaleta O: *Echinococcus* in the South American red fox *(Dusicyon culpaeus)* and the European hare *(Lepus europaeus)* in the province of Neuquen, Argentina. Ann Trop Med Parasitol 66:479, 1972.
99. Eugster RO: Contribution to the Epidemiology of Echinococcosis/Hydatidosis in Kenya (East Africa) with Special Reference to the Kajiado District. Zürich, University of Zürich, 1978. Doctoral Thesis.
100. Schantz PM: Larval cestodiasis. *In* Hoeprich PD, Jordan MC, (eds): Infectious Diseases. A Modern Treatise of Infectious Processes, ed 4. Philadelphia, JB Lippincott, 1989, pp 829–841.
101. Nelson GS: Hydatid disease: Research and control in Turkana, Kenya. 1. Epidemiological observations. Trans R Soc Trop Med Hyg 80:177, 1986.
102. Capron A, Vernes A, Biguet J: Le diagnostic immunoelectrophoretique de l'hydatidose. *In* Conder J (ed): Le Kyste Hydatique du Foie. Lyon, France, SIMEP, 1967, pp 27–40.
103. Schantz PM: Improvements in the serodiagnosis of helminthic zoonoses. Vet Parasitol 25:95, 1987.
104. Schantz PM, Schanks D, Wilson M: Serologic cross-reactions with sera from patients with echinococcosis and cysticercosis. Am J Trop Med Hyg 21:609, 1980.
105. Moro PL, Guevara A, Verstegui MM, et al: Distribution of hydatosis and cysticercosis in different Peruvian populations as demonstrated by an enzyme-linked immunoelectrotransfer blot (EITB) assay. Am J Trop Med Hyg 51:851, 1994.
106. Coltorti EA: Standardization and evaluation of an enzyme immunoassay as a screening test for the seroepidemiology of human hydatidosis. Am J Trop Med Hyg 35:1000, 1986.
107. Craig PS, Zeyle E, Romig T: Hydatid disease: Research and control in Turkana. II. The role of immunological techniques for the diagnosis of hydatid disease. Trans R Soc Trop Med Hyg 80:183, 1986.
108. Amman R, Eckert J: Clinical diagnosis and treatment of echinococcosis in humans. *In* Thompson RCA, Lymbery AJ (eds): Echinococcus and Hydatid Disease. Oxford, CAB International, 1995, pp 411–463.
109. Okelo GBA: Hydatid disease: Research and control in Turkana, III. Albendazole in the treatment of inoperable hydatid disease in Kenya—A report on 12 cases. Trans R Soc Trop Med Hyg 80:193, 1986.
110. Lawson JR, Roberts MG, Gemmel MA, et al: Population dynamics in echinococcosis and cysticercosis: Economic assessment of control strategies for *Echinococcus granulosus, Taenia ovis* and *Taenia hydatigena*. Parasitology 97:177, 1988.
111. Macpherson CNL, Wachira TM, Zeyle E, et al: Hydatid disease: Research and control in Turkana, IV. The pilot control programme. Trans R Soc Trop Med Hyg 80:196, 1986.
112. Mason PR, Patterson BA: Epidemiology of *Hymenolepis nana* infections in primary school children in urban and rural communities in Zimbabwe. J Parasitol 80:245, 1994.
113. Ito A, Honey RD, Scanlon T, et al: Analysis of antibody responses to *Hymenolepis nana* infection in mice by the enzyme-linked immunosorbent assay and immunoprecipitation. Parasite Immunol 10:265, 1988.
114. Palmas C, Bortolette G, Conchedda M: Immunological memory and lymphoblast migration in mice infected with *Hymenolepis nana*. Z Parasitenkd 72:397, 1986.
115. Watanabe N, Nawa Y, Okamoto K, Kobayashi A: Expulsion of *Hymenolepis nana* from mice with congenital deficiencies of IgE production or of mast cell development. Parasite Immunol 16:137, 1994.
116. Bouree P: Intérêt du praziquantel, un cure unique, comme traitement de *Taenia saginata* et de *Hymenolepis nana*. Pathol Biol (Paris) 36:759, 1988.
117. von Bonsdorff B, Bylund G: The ecology of *Diphyllobothrium latum*. Ecol Dis 1:21, 1982.

297

Arthropods

Andrew Spielman
Mitchell Wachtel

Although many diverse hematophagous arthropods transmit a great variety of pathogenic microorganisms, these jointed-legged creatures themselves may directly compromise human health. Entomologic discussions in public health, however, generally focus on vector-borne infections while only peripherally treating arthropods as agents of disease. Such treatments only infrequently include comprehensive analyses of the direct entomologic causes of human disease. Accordingly, we describe the arthropods that persistently infest people with a focus on the mites, lice, fleas, and myiasis-producing flies and the conditions that they cause. We also describe features of the stings caused by certain Hymenoptera and of the bites of spiders.[1] Our objective is to present a body of information that is useful in the practice of medicine and particularly adapted for temperate parts of the world.

Scabies

The ovoid mite that causes scabies *Sarcoptes scabiei* is colorless and less than 1 mm long.[2] Human scabies infestations perpetuate solely in human skin, forming characteristic sinuous burrows in the stratum corneum. Adult females periodically emerge from these burrows, crawling on their eight legs over the surface of the skin and progressing as rapidly as 25 mm/min.

Epidemiology

Although no population-based estimates of the prevalence of scabies in temperate parts of the world have yet become available, risk may be appreciable. Some 2% to 5% of patients treated by dermatologists suffer from this infestation. In 1983, for example, scabies was the second most common diagnosis in a San Francisco hospital.[3(p36)] The condition is far more frequent, however, in the tropics. Immigrant children from lesser developed nations should therefore be routinely examined for this condition.[4] As many as 300 million cases of scabies are said to occur annually throughout the world.[5]

Because scabies mites die within 2 days when they are isolated from a human host, transmission depends mainly on direct contact between hosts rather than on fomite transfer through contaminated clothing or bedding. Crowding promotes outbreaks. A secondary attack rate of 38% prevails among household contacts, providing a rationale for presumptive community treatment. Scabies affects people of any age but decreases in people older than 40 years. Although scabies infestations frequently burden African villagers, black people are less susceptible to infection than are others.[6]

Nosocomial infections commonly occur in nursing homes and mental hospitals, where health care providers suffer certain occupational risk. Norwegian scabies, discussed later, may pose a particular threat in such settings because of the absence of the characteristic pruritus and the highly infectious nature of the infestation.

Zoonotic scabies frequently afflicts people who experience intimate contact with dogs and where sanitation is poor. Although human disease most commonly results from such canine infection, cats, horses, pigs, and pigeons have also been implicated as sources of infestation.[7, 8] The incubation period of zoonotic scabies is shorter than that of the anthroponosis and is self-limited owing to the failure of these mites to propagate in human skin. Repeated infestations are common, however.

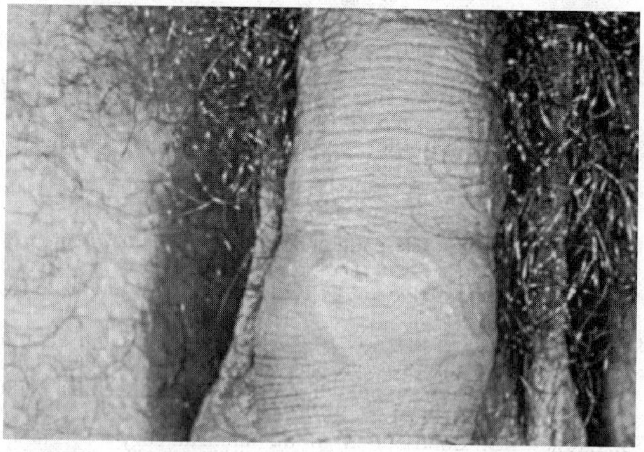

FIGURE 297–1 □ Sinuous burrow of scabies mite in a characteristic site.

Pathogenesis and Histopathology

The inflammatory skin lesions of scabies derive from cell-mediated and humoral immune hypersensitivity responses to the mite's saliva and feces. The immunoglobulin E level tends to be elevated. Although infection is generally silent for some 4 to 6 weeks in people infected for the first time, symptoms may appear almost immediately after subsequent reinfestation.[9(p53), 10] The papular pruritic eruption of scabies derives from immune sensitivity and often bears no relation to the location of the mites. Pruritic nodules may be present for several months after the infestation is eliminated.

For the most part, the burrows of these mites are mainly confined to the stratum corneum of the skin. The blind ends of burrows that contain adult females, however, generally extend into the stratum malpighii. Spongiosis, developing near the mite, may result in vesicle formation. A variable eosinophilic infiltrate characterizes the lesion. Even if no mite is discovered, the mere presence of eggs in the horny layer is pathognomonic for scabies. Papules are characterized by a nonspecific inflammatory reaction that includes no eosinophils and is free of mites.

Chronic nodules, which similarly contain no mites, are characterized by a dense mononuclear infiltrate that may or may not include eosinophils. Typical mononuclear cells may be present, as in lymphoma. The walls of adjacent blood vessels may be thickened.

Norwegian or crusted scabies may develop when the immune response of a patient is impaired. This may occur in leukemia and human immunodeficiency virus infection, after administration of steroids, or when the itch response is flawed as with mental retardation and mental deterioration. Residents of the tropics, however, seem to suffer this syndrome spontaneously. Numerous mites lying in multiple subcorneal burrows characterize biopsy specimens of the crusts of Norwegian scabies. Such lesions are generally characterized by hyperkeratosis, acanthosis, and a marked dermal cellular infiltrate.

Disease Relationships

Scabies is characterized by intense pruritus, often worse at night or after a hot shower.[11] In the usual form of the disease, the symmetric, papulovesicular lesions, 2 to 3 mm in diameter, may be accompanied by macules, pustules, and scaly plaques. Burrows measure 3 to 15 mm and appear as irregular, fine black threads that are often difficult to find (Fig. 297–1).

Scabies lesions are confined to the flexor surfaces of the interdigital spaces in two thirds of patients; nearly nine tenths suffer at least one lesion in these sites. Other affected sites include the breasts, periumbilicus, belt line, buttocks, thighs, penis, scrotum, elbows, feet, ankles, and anterior axillary folds. In children and infants, lesions may appear on any skin surface. In addition, the disease may be present in children as a bullous lesion.

Norwegian scabies is characterized by widespread erythema, hyperkeratosis, and crusting but little or no itching.[12–14] No discrete burrows are evident. Nail involvement is common. Alopecia, generalized hyperpigmentation, pyoderma, and eosinophilia may also occur.

Other atypical forms of the disease may occur.[9(p53)] Patients with a high level of hygiene may develop "scabies of the cultivated." Although burrows are evident in only 7% of such patients and findings may be scant, the patient continues to be infectious. Corticosteroids may suppress symptoms, thereby resulting in a misdiagnosis of fungal infection or impetigo. In nodular scabies, indurated nodules that may be pigmented develop on the groin or axilla but generally contain mites after the first month. Even when treated, infestations may continue for more than a year despite therapy.

Patients infected by human immunodeficiency virus tend to develop papulosquamous lesions in skin cleavage lines, findings similar to pityriasis rosea; other findings tend to be nonexistent. Norwegian scabies has been described in such a human immunodeficiency virus–positive patient.[15, 16]

Zoonotic scabies produces papulovesicular erythematous, pruritic lesions, usually around the waist or on the arms.[9(p53)] No burrows are present. Excoriation from the intense pruritus may produce secondary bacterial infection that confuses the clinical picture. The bleeding that derives from the excoriation constitutes a useful clinical clue to the presence of scabies. Epidemics of poststreptococcal glomerulonephritis have been associated with scabies and secondary bacterial infection.[5]

Diagnosis

Scabies is a highly polymorphic disease, well deserving its reputation as a great imitator, a descriptor once reserved for syphilis.[10] An index of suspicion must be maintained with any patient presenting with pruritus, particularly if more than one household contact suffers from the condition. Primary care physicians more frequently overdiagnose than underdiagnose scabies.[17]

Definitive diagnosis requires discovery of the mites, scybala, or eggs.[3(p4)] Burrows are present in virtually all North American patients and should be sought in the web spaces between the fingers; on the wrists and elbows; and on the sides of the hands, feet, and ankles. Topical application of liquid tetracycline, followed after several minutes by alcohol, causes the burrows to fluoresce yellow-gray with a Wood lamp. Other methods of detecting the burrows include the use of mineral oil to alter the refractive index of the stratum corneum and the ink test, in which ink wiped over an affected area is permitted to penetrate the burrows and the excess wiped away.

The mites, their scybala, or their eggs can be demonstrated by any of various methods. An epidermal shave biopsy or superficial scraping involves placing a drop of sterile mineral oil at the anterior end of a suspected burrow, scraping the epidermal surface with a No. 15 blade, and examining the scrapings microscopically (Fig. 297–2). A magnifying glass may be used to detect the mite within its burrow. It appears as an oval, white object that is darkly pigmented caudally. The mite can be extracted with a needle point and examined under a microscope. An incident light microscope can be used to identify the mites in vivo.[18] In the absence of burrows, a scraping or a shave biopsy of the papulovesicular lesions may yield definitive diagnostic material.

For patients with Norwegian scabies, examination of the crust is diagnostic.[9(p53)] In zoonotic scabies, scrapings of the vesicles into mineral oil often provides diagnostic material. Mites or their products will not always be found, unfortunately, and diagnosis must then rest on clinical features of the lesion.

On the other hand, a diagnosis of scabies does not exclude other conditions. Pediculosis may also be present and should be looked for. Other pruritic and nonpruritic dermatologic diseases may be present as well. Diverse venereal infections must be considered when a diagnosis of scabies or pediculosis is made.

Treatment

Although lindane has been the most frequently used scabicide (the γ-isomer of benzene hexachloride, applied in a vanishing-cream formulation) in the United States,[19] permethrin formulations have largely displaced preparations based on this potentially dangerous neurotoxic insecticide.[20] Permethrin is highly effective and relatively nontoxic.[21, 22] In a double-blind prospective study, for example, 91% of patients treated with 95% permethrin remained free of lesions 1 month after therapy began. The comparable figure for 1% lindane was only 45%, apparently because these mites have developed physiologic resistance against this long-used insecticide.

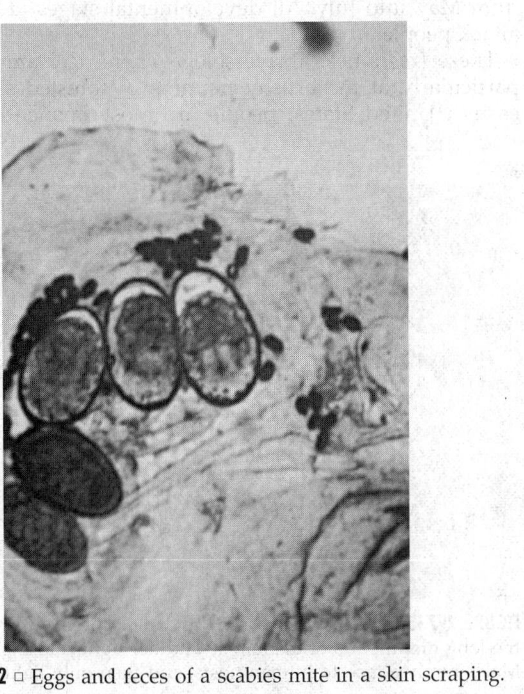

FIGURE 297–2 □ Eggs and feces of a scabies mite in a skin scraping.

A single application of permethrin generally eliminates living scabies mites. The presence of persisting antigens, however, may continue to provoke allergic reactions even months after the mites have been destroyed. Of course, treatment cannot preclude reinfestation, particularly among the homeless, whose close contacts often cannot be identified and treated in a timely fashion.[3(pp44,53)] Treatment with calamine lotion or antihistamines generally reduces the urticaria, but a brief course of steroid therapy may occasionally be required. Patients infected by human immunodeficiency virus may require repeated treatment. Secondary bacterial infections should be treated with topical antibiotics or, when lesions are extensive or adenitis is present, with systemic therapy.

Orally administered ivermectin appears to be effective as a scabicide. At 1 month after administration of a single dose of ivermectin, 70% of 23 originally scabies-infected subjects remained scabies free.[23] Benzyl benzoate, on the other hand, eliminated these mites in only 48% of 21 randomized subjects. Ivermectin appears to be effective in treating Norwegian scabies.[24] This drug has the advantage of simplicity of application and apparent absence of irritation.

Alternative scabicides, including benzyl benzoate, crotamiton cream (Eurax), or sulfur ointment, may be preferred for infants, pregnant women, or nonsupervised mass treatments. For infants, monosulfiram is applied at diagnosis and after a day and a week. Sulfur dermatitis may result. If sulfur ointments are used, alcohol must be avoided because of the possibility of a disulfiram-type reaction. For Norwegian scabies or for nail involvement, a keratolytic agent, such as salicylic acid, may be required before the scabicide is applied. Repeated treatment may be required.

Dust Mites

The Pathogens

House dust mites are minute sarcoptiform organisms that feed mainly on exfoliated human danders.[25] Of the various dust mites, *Dermatophagoides pteronyssinus* and *Dermatophagoides farinae* most commonly cause human disease. All life history stages are similar. The mites are too small to be seen in situ.

Epidemiology

The abundance of dust mites correlates with the quantity of accumulated human dander; their antigens, carried in house dust, directly induce bronchoconstriction in affected asthmatic patients.[26, 27] Dust mites dehydrate when the ambient relative humidity falls below 60%.[28, 29] *D. pteronyssinus* requires exceptionally humid conditions, whereas *D. farinae* is somewhat more tolerant to drying. For this reason, dust mites rarely become abundant at high altitudes or during the winter months. Mite antigens, however, persist in the absence of living mites. Certain housing features permit dust mites to become abundant, particularly inadequate moisture seals in older homes, excessively tight sealing in newer homes, and the presence of fitted carpets.[30] Mites and their secretory products tend to accumulate in carpeting, bedding, mattresses, and upholstered furniture.

Disease Relationships

Three major kinds of antigens derive from dust mites. Those designated Der p I, Der p II, and Der p III are associated with *D. pteronyssinus;* Der f I is associated with *D. farinae.* Der I and II are the best characterized,[31–33] and Der p III has been cloned and sequenced.[34] Der I antigens are associated with mite feces, whereas the Der II moieties are associated with the bodies of these mites; both become airborne in house dust.[35] In sensitized people, these proteins induce an allergic immunoglobulin E–mediated response. In addition, vascular permeability is increased by exposure to the serine proteases that are contained in mite feces.[36, 37] Such exposure, at least in rats, provokes non–immunoglobulin E–mediated mast cell degranulation.[36] Intradermal injection of mite antigen induces expression of the endothelial leukocyte adhesion molecule-1 in susceptible patients, leading to the development of inflammatory cell infiltrates.[38] Ratios of helper to suppressor T cells are altered, and the expression of CD23 on B cells and the serum levels of interleukin-2 are increased in asthmatic children subjected to bronchial allergen provocation.[39]

Exposure to dust mite allergens is associated with asthma,[40] atopic dermatitis,[41] or perennial rhinitis and conjunctivitis.[42–45] Such a dust mite etiology is particularly well supported in the case of asthma.[46] Although asthma was initially associated with childhood disease, adults appear to suffer a similar spectrum of disease.[47] Early childhood exposure seems crucial in the development of these conditions.[48]

Patients with atopic dermatitis experience elevated serum immunoglobulin E levels.[49] Immunoglobulin E receptors in epidermal Langerhans cells[50] present mite antigen to helper T lymphocytes.[51] The risk for atopic dermatitis is greatest in patients who have previously experienced chronically itchy skin and at least three other important signs, including involvement of skin creases or cheeks (in children younger than 10 years), history of asthma or hay fever (or atopy in children younger than 4 years), history of general dry skin in the previous year, visible flexural eczema (or eczema of the cheeks or forehead and outer limbs in children younger than 4 years), and onset in children younger than 2 years unless the child is younger than 4 years.[52, 53] Laboratory tests are available but not required for presumptive diagnosis.

Mite-associated rhinitis and conjunctivitis can be separated from the more common pollen-related allergies by their nonseasonal nature and by the presence of a reactive skin test or antibody against mite antigen.[42–44] The characteristic symptoms are useful in diagnosis, particularly when they are aggravated by the patient's house-cleaning activities. Perennial rhinitis is not associated with nasal polyps. Nasal provocation tests can be used to support the diagnosis.[28] Dust mite–specific immunoglobulin G levels are elevated, for example, in patients suffering from chronic rhinosinusitis.[54]

Treatment

Although specific therapy for atopic disease lies beyond the scope of this discussion, certain general comments are appropriate. Immunotherapy for asthma appears to be a safe and effective treatment of dust mite allergy when it is provided under optimal conditions in certain patients.[55] Exposure to antigen should be minimized by enclosing pillows and mattresses in plastic covers, washing bedding at least once a week, removing carpeting from the bedroom, and reducing upholstered furniture to a minimum. Humidity should be reduced by use of air conditioners and dehumidifiers; outdoor ventilation should be maximized whenever the weather permits.[56] The mites can be destroyed by directly applying chemical acaricides, such as a pyrethroid or tannic acid. Airborne dust can be reduced by the use of portable air filters or, when the patient is absent from the room, by the use of vacuum cleaners. These measures, properly employed, generally reduce the symptoms of house dust allergy.

Ticks

Except in the case of certain residents of Africa who sleep on the ground, people encounter hard (ixodid) ticks far more often than soft (argasid) ticks. Indeed, the few soft ticks that are present in temperate parts of the world are generally closely restricted to the nests of rodents. Hard ticks attach firmly to their hosts and feed continuously for 3 to 10 days; soft ticks attach lightly, mainly on sleeping hosts, and detach within 20 minutes or so. A wide array of viral, rickettsial, bacterial, and protozoal infectious agents are tick-borne, and certain of these are discussed elsewhere in this volume.

Tick saliva contains a complex of chemicals. A thrombin inhibitor, ixin, and an antithromboplastin, ixodin, are present in the salivary glands of *Ixodes ricinus.*[57] An apyrase component of the saliva of a soft tick, *Ornithodoros moubata,* that inhibits platelet aggregation[58] has been dubbed moubatin.[59] An anticoagulant peptide, which affects factor Xa, is also present.[60] This pharmacologically active secretion includes a diverse array of other components that alter humoral and cell-mediated immunity and cytokine function and that suppress various immunoregulatory and immune effector pathways of the host.[61, 62] Antitick salivary components are antigenic in human hosts.[63]

Deer Ticks

The emergence of Lyme disease and human babesiosis in parts of North America and Eurasia[64] has stimulated an intense interest in ticks and an investment of medical attention in these hematophagous organisms. Only certain members of the genus *Ixodes* appear to serve as vectors of zoonotic infection.[65] The deer tick *Ixodes dammini* in the eastern United States (which differs from the more southern *Ixodes scapularis*) and similar *Ixodes pacificus* ticks in the West affect human health in North America. Related ticks (*I. ricinus* and *Ixodes persulcatus*) do so in the Old World. Deer serve as the definitive hosts for these ticks; their larval and nymphal stages feed mainly on mice (Fig. 297–3). *Ixodes* ticks attach firmly, feeding for several days or more and engorging most markedly toward the end of the period of attachment. Adult *I. dammini* ticks quest for hosts from October through April, larvae from August through September, and nymphs mainly from May into July. All developmental stages of these ticks attack people.

These *Ixodes* ticks thrive solely where deer are numerous, particularly at the brushy margins of forested sites. In the eastern United States, people are most frequently attacked

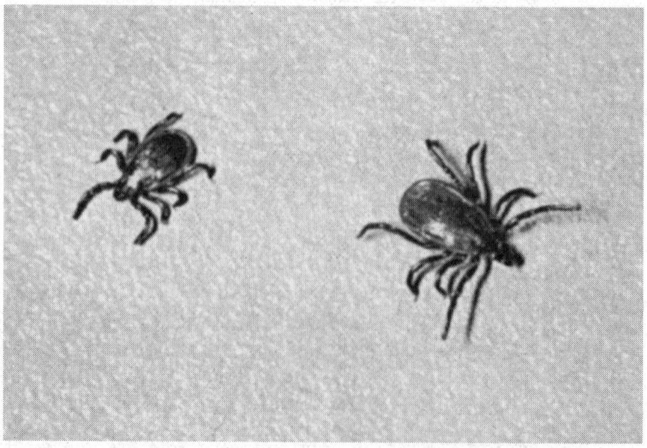

FIGURE 297–3 □ Adult female *(left)* and male *(right)* deer ticks. Note the long mouthparts of the female and her light coloring posteriorly. Males rarely attach to human hosts, and then only lightly.

by the nymphal stage of the deer tick. Although the physical presence of a tick on a person's body is generally distressing, immediate attention is required because of the possibility of consequent microbial infection.

To prevent transmission of the agents of Lyme disease or babesiosis, ticks should be promptly removed from the skin during the first 2 days of attachment, before their rapid phase of engorgement commences. They should be detached by firm traction, with care taken to remove as much of the tick as possible by use of a forceps applied close to the point of attachment to the skin. Although some rotational movement may help dislodge the mouthparts intact, retention of a fragment of the feeding apparatus is inconsequential. The use of heat, burning, or chemical treatment merely delays removal of an attached tick and does not facilitate the process.

The agents of Lyme disease and human babesiosis enter the saliva of the vector tick only after some 2 days of attachment, and saliva is the vehicle of transmission. Spirochetes are delivered to the skin of the host, rather than directly to the blood vasculature, where they remain for 2 days or more.[66] The site of attachment of a tick should therefore be disinfected, as with a substance such as tincture of iodine.[66]

Where the risk of Lyme disease and human babesiosis is great, any poppy seed–sized tick (about 2 mm in diameter) that becomes distended with blood should be considered a potential source of infection.[67] A person bitten by such a tick during May through July should be alert to the possibility of infection if the tick had been feeding for at least 2 days. Presumptive treatment of Lyme disease remains an attractive option. Ticks found attached to a person between October and April would generally be adult deer ticks, and spirochetes generally infect some two thirds of such ticks.[68] Because deer ticks generally attack people less frequently than do other kinds of ticks,[69] because spirochetes infect less than a third of nymphal deer ticks,[70] and because ticks that are discovered tend to be discovered early in their course of attachment, presumptive treatment of any "tick bite" seems inadvisable.[71]

Dog and Wood Ticks

Of the various kinds of ticks that attack residents of the North American continent, dog and wood ticks (of the genus *Dermacentor*) are the most ubiquitous. Wood ticks *(Dermacentor andersoni)* are indigenous to mountainous regions of the West, and dog ticks *(Dermacentor variabilis)* infest more coastal sites. Interestingly, the range of the montane species seems to be diminishing, whereas that of the lowland species is increasing. Where they are abundant, both of these ticks transmit rickettsial infection (Rocky Mountain spotted fever), and either may cause tick paralysis.

The adult stage of the dog tick (Fig. 297–4) feeds mainly on dogs and that of the wood tick on marmots. Larvae and nymphs feed on voles and sometimes mice. All trophic stages feed early in the summer, but only the adult stage attacks people.

Dog ticks infest grassy sites where dogs are numerous. Adults quest most frequently near sources of carbon dioxide, as where automobiles pause on a hill or park on a sandy site; such gaseous emanations suggest the presence of large hosts.

As in the case of deer ticks, attached dog or wood ticks should be promptly removed by gentle traction. In contrast to deer ticks, however, these ticks come away readily and always intact. To avoid contamination by the agent of spotted fever, such ticks should be handled by means of forceps or while wearing rubber gloves. The site of attachment should be disinfected, as with such a substance as tincture of iodine.

Except in southeastern sections of the United States, ticks that are 6 mm or longer and that feed during the summer months should be considered to be dog or wood ticks. Because spotted fever is infrequent, presumptive antibiotic treatment after removal of such a tick seems inadvisable.

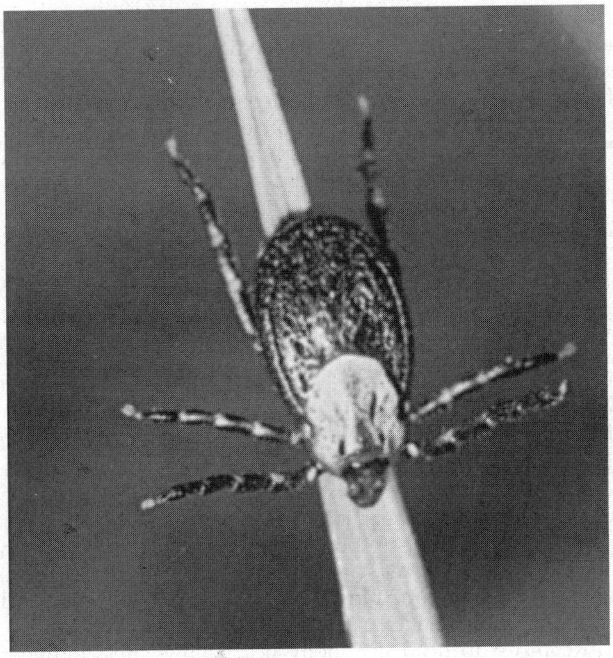

FIGURE 297–4 □ Adult female dog tick. Note the short mouthparts and white sculpturing on the dorsal plate. This plate covers the entire body of a male.

Lone Star Ticks

Lone star ticks *(Amblyomma americanum)* may be abundant locally in forested portions of the southeastern United States and in isolated foci as far north as Prudence Island in Rhode Island. No human infection has conclusively been associated with these ticks. Deer serve as the main host population throughout the entire life cycle of these ticks, and any stage may attack human hosts. They become abundant solely where deer are abundant.

As in the case of *Ixodes* deer ticks, lone star ticks attach so firmly to their hosts that their mouthparts frequently remain in place after the body of the tick is removed. This condition appears to be innocuous, however. Massive infestations by larval lone star ticks occur when people walk near the site where an egg mass has been deposited. Infestations by these "seed ticks" can cause considerable discomfort and may be confused with that of the deer ticks that transmit Lyme disease.

Lice

The Pathogens

The human pediculoses include infestations by head lice *(Pediculus humanus capitis)*, body lice *(Pediculus humanus humanus)*, and pubic lice *(Phthirus pubis)*.[9(p53)] These insects are dorsoventrally flattened and lack wings. The three body regions of the head and body lice are clearly demarcated. The central thorax bears the three pairs of clawed legs. The seven abdominal segments have lateral lobes. All stages of development appear similar, and blood is their only food. Head lice tend to be darker than body lice and somewhat smaller. These insects crawl rapidly, about 23 cm/min.

The mouth of a louse is a toothed tubular structure, the

haustellum, which remains invaginated within the head until feeding begins and contains the feeding apparatus. Blood is aspirated through a pair of stylets. A third such stylet directs the highly antigenic and antihemostatic saliva into the skin of the host. Copious quantities of feces are discharged onto the skin of the host during feeding, thereby providing the vehicle of transmission for louse-borne typhus and relapsing fever.

Pubic lice are crablike and about as broad as they are long. They are shorter than the other anthroponotic lice, and their body appears more fused. Their appendages are unique in that the claws of the forelegs are more slender than the others, enabling this louse to grasp either pubic or facial hairs. They move only about 10 cm/d.

Epidemiology

Head lice most commonly infest the head hair of children. Some 0.3% of North American black children, as opposed to 10% of nonblacks, appear to be infested.[72] Girls are 1.5 times more likely than boys to be infested by head lice. Although direct contact is the most important means of transmission, some infestations are transmitted by shared headgear and grooming implements.

In contrast to head lice, body lice mainly infest indigent people who remain clothed for extended periods. These insects tend to remain in the clothing except when feeding (Fig. 297–5).[3(p45)] Because body lice require frequent feeding, survival in the event of separation from human hosts for more than a day or so is limited. Body lice are transmitted by direct contact between people or by exchange of clothing.

Pubic lice mainly infest the hair of the pubis of sexually active people (Fig. 297–6) but also the eyelids, facial hair, and axillae as well as scalp hair in the case of children. Thus, venereal contact provides the main if not the sole means of transmission.

Histopathology

Early histologic changes after the bites of lice include dermal edema and a mild perivascular lymphocytic, eosinophilic, and neutrophilic infiltrate.[9(p53)] The edema is less prominent than that after other insect bites. Late changes include a lymphocytic histiocytic infiltrate with minimal edema.

Disease Relationships

The saliva of lice produces an intensely pruritic, 2- to 3-mm, erythematous, maculopapular eruption (Fig. 297–7) forming hours to days after feeding.[8] Hives may appear immediately, with flare and wheal formation. Excoriation may produce secondary changes and infection, including crust formation and regional adenopathy. The bites may be inapparent to the patient. A hemorrhagic component is occasionally present, presumably promoted by the salivary product.

The erythematous, maculopapular rash resulting from the bites of head lice is located on the scalp, the nape of the neck, and the shoulders. Secondary changes due to excoriation include crusting, matting of hair, oozing, and bacterial infection. Although the lice may seldom be seen, nits are more readily apparent. These eggs can be differentiated from hair casts, seborrheic material, hair spray, and soap flakes by the impossibility of sliding them along the hair shaft. With a long-wave ultraviolet lamp, infested hair may fluoresce. As with scabies, better hygiene may mask diagnostic findings.

The lesions produced by body lice resemble those of head lice, except that the pruritus tends to be most evident at the neckline, where these lice seem to feed most frequently. Combined malnutrition and intense lousiness can produce a low-grade fever and myalgia. Excoriation and secondary infection frequently occur. Chronic infestation may result in

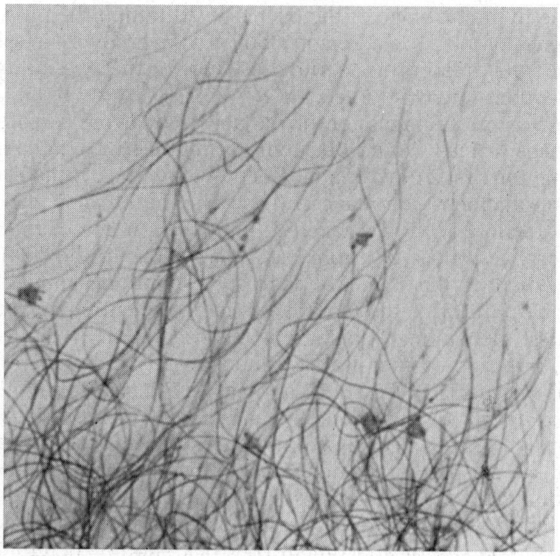

FIGURE 297–6 □ Pubic lice and nits infesting pubic hairs. (From Domonkos AN, Arnold HL Jr: Diseases of the Skin, ed 7. Philadelphia, WB Saunders, 1982, p 556.)

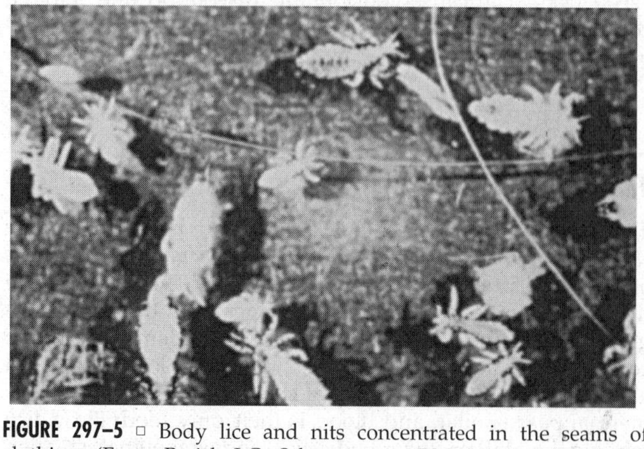

FIGURE 297–5 □ Body lice and nits concentrated in the seams of clothing. (From Parish LC, Schwartzman RM, Nutting WB [eds]: Cutaneous Infestations of Man and Animals. New York, Praeger Publishers, 1983.)

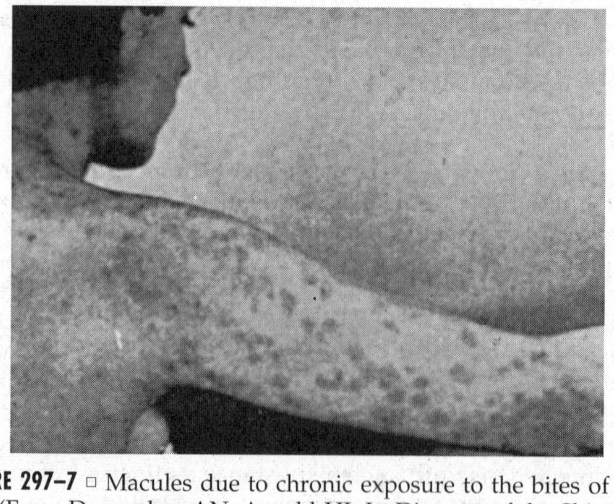

FIGURE 297–7 □ Macules due to chronic exposure to the bites of body lice. (From Domonkos AN, Arnold HL Jr: Diseases of the Skin, ed 7. Philadelphia, WB Saunders, 1982, p 557.)

generalized hyperpigmentation and a characteristic lichenification known as vagabond's disease. In Egypt, a peculiar association of pediculosis and lymphadenopathy has been noted in children, a finding confirmed by serologic studies.[73]

The particularly intense pruritus due to the bites of pubic lice mainly affects pubic, perineal, inguinal, and lower abdominal sites as well as the axillae and eyelids. The rash may present as blue-gray macules, a syndrome known as maculae ceruleae.[74] Excoriation may produce secondary changes, but secondary infection is less likely than with body or head lice. Nits would virtually always be present, and the lice would be visible with the aid of a magnifying glass. Infestations of the eyelids may present with a blepharoconjunctivitis and occasionally with a serosanguineous discharge at the conjunctival margins. Adult lice may be evident at the eyelash roots.

Other sexually transmitted diseases should be considered whenever pubic lice are discovered. An infestation in a juvenile suggests abuse.

Treatment

Head lice may be eliminated by topical applications of insecticide. As in the case of scabies, pyrethroid-based formulations are effective and relatively safe. Although permethrin, the most commonly used pyrethroid, is ovicidal, the continuing presence of dead nits or those that have already hatched frequently misleads patients into repeated applications of the lousicide in the mistaken belief that the prior treatment has failed. Then, too, reports of pyrethroid- and lindane-resistant head lice suggest an increasing pattern of treatment failure.

Synthetic pyrethroid pediculicides are available without prescription. Such permethrin-based shampoos generally constitute highly effective treatments for head lice.[75, 76] In contrast to the lindane-based shampoos, this treatment is ovicidal. Extracts of chrysanthemum flowers (containing pyrethrum) are useful pediculicides but may produce allergic symptoms in people who are sensitized to plant products. One survey of 38,160 patients who received 47,578 permethrin treatments found only 103 adverse side effects.[77] Although formulae based on lindane or malathion require reapplication 2 weeks later, only one pyrethroid treatment is required.[77, 78]

To facilitate detection of head louse infestations and help in the management of individual patients, fine-toothed nit combs should be used to groom all nits from the patient's hair after treatment. Such grooming supports effective surveillance when public health authorities attempt to combat an epidemic in a school. Diagnosis of pediculosis is enhanced by the use of a magnified light source. Because of the wide array of products on the market, comparative studies of efficacy are important.

Infestations by body lice are eliminated by environmental management, supplemented by topical application of pediculicide. Disinfection of all clothing and bedding is crucial; clothing should be placed in a clothes dryer for 30 minutes at a temperature of at least 65°C. Individual patients are then treated from head to foot with a pyrethroid-based pediculicide. Mass treatment of affected populations requires application of dust formulations of any of a variety of insecticides.

Infestations of pubic lice can effectively be eliminated by applications of permethrin-containing shampoo. Although a variety of treatments including petroleum jelly and 1% aqueous malathion shampoo[79] have been suggested for phthiriasis palpebrarum (eyelid infestation), a large study supports the use of 1% yellow oxide of mercury applied four times daily for 2 weeks.[80]

In general, lousiness should be treated environmentally. Grooming equipment should not be shared. Rooms and furniture are best decontaminated by vacuuming. Washable items should be cleaned in hot water and dried for 30 minutes. In the face of an epidemic, close personal contact should be discouraged. The National Pediculosis Association (in Newton, Massachusetts) serves as a clearing-house for information on the treatment and prevention of these infections.

Fleas

The Pathogens

Fleas are wingless, laterally compressed insects, 1 to 4 mm long, that are equipped with powerful jumping legs.[81] In developed regions of the world, the human flea *Pulex irritans* and the cat flea *Ctenocephalides felis* most commonly attack people. The chigoe flea *Tunga penetrans* may do so where conditions are more primitive. The minute, caterpillar-like larvae develop where the host sleeps and feed mainly on the dried pellets of nondigested blood that the adults defecate while feeding. The spatial and seasonal distribution of fleas is limited by the tendency of their larvae to desiccate. Where houses are centrally heated, fleas cannot survive the winter except when the host sleeps on a moist surface, such as a concrete floor. Fleas may live for 1 to 4 months when they are isolated from hosts and for a year or more when suitable hosts are present. Fleas transmit the agents of plague, *Yersinia pestis*, and of murine typhus, *Rickettsia typhi*, as well as the rat tapeworm *Hymenolepis diminuta* and the dwarf tapeworm *Hymenolepis nana*.

Disease Relationships

The bites of fleas induce a pruritic papular urticaria composed of wheals or firm papules with occasional bullae distributed on characteristic parts of the body.[14] In women with exposed legs, the eruption occurs mainly on the lower legs. In children having intimate contact with domestic animals, lesions may occur over the whole body. A generalized allergic response may occur. Extreme pruritus results in secondary changes that may include bacterial infection. Other insects, including bedbugs and mosquitoes, may produce a similar dermatitis. Basophils have been implicated in the production of such lesions.[82] Histologic changes include intercellular and intracellular edema of the stratum malpighii with occasional vesicle formation, a chronic perivascular dermal infiltrate, usually of the superficial and mid-corium. Eosinophils are generally prominent. The microscopic appearance of the lesion may mimic prurigo simplex, except that the presence of eosinophils suggests a papular urticaria. Without sensitization, or with hyposensitization, the clinical and histologic appearances become less pronounced, and the lesion is then mildly edemic with a mild mononuclear perivascular infiltrate.[83]

The chigoe or jigger flea *T. penetrans* may infest travelers who walk barefoot or in sandals in rural sites in the Americas, Africa, and India. The fertilized female penetrates the stratum corneum of the skin, generally in crevices, such as beneath the margins of toenails. The lesion initially appears as a dark furuncular pinpoint that enlarges within 2 weeks as the flea swells to the size of a pea. The lesion is painful but self-limiting. If the flea is permitted to remain in situ, a 0.5-cm section of skin will eventually slough. Developing chigoe fleas should be removed as soon as possible by means of a sterile needle.

Flea infestations may be detected most readily in the host's bedding. Both adults and larvae may be evident.[84] Most often, cat fleas are responsible for infestations that affect residents of North America.

Treatment

Treatment consists of antipruritics and antihistamines. Secondary bacterial infections may be treated with local antibiotics or, if extensive, by systemic therapy.

Flea infestations should be treated mainly by cleaning the nesting site of the host and by ensuring that all bedding is clean and dry. Insecticides may also be applied, but a case report of toxic effects from a commercial-strength pyrethroid flea spray emphasizes the importance of good ventilation in the application of these agents.[85] Recurrence of the flea infestation may result from a new infestation, ineffective treatment, or resistance against the insecticide that was used. Methoprene, a relatively safe synthetic analog of insect juvenile hormone, effectively destroys these fleas.[86]

Myiasis-Producing Flies

The term myiasis designates a group of infections produced by the maggots of certain flies. The myiases include those that produce traumatic, furuncular, intestinal, creeping, and ocular disease.[14, 87]

The Pathogens

The traumatic myiases that affect nonnecrotic tissue are produced by "primary screw-worm" flies, *Cochliomyia hominivorax* in the New World and *Chrysomyia bezziana* in the Old World. Lesions that are generally confined to necrotic tissue are due to the secondary screw-worm flies. The bottle fly *Phaenicia sericata* is the most common cause of such secondary screw-worm fly infection. These conditions are produced by the larvae of brightly metallic flies that do not feed or feed solely on vegetable products in their adult stage and whose larvae develop solely in animal products or in the feces of carnivores. The dull, grayish flies that are anthropophilic as adults are associated with vegetable products as larvae and do not cause traumatic myiasis. The striped, red-marked flesh flies, such as *Wohlfahrtia vigil*, may occasionally produce an adventitious lesion involving nonnecrotic tissue.

Disease Relationships

Traumatic myiasis occurs after the skin has been breached, as by a wound or secondary to a condition such as cancer. An infestation by a primary screw-worm fly would endanger deep tissues and produce a large and suppurating lesion. Although primary screw-worm flies occur mainly in tropical regions, flesh flies are common in North America and Europe. Infections by secondary screw-worm flies may even benefit the host by débriding necrotic tissue and by a bacteriostatic effect. Some systemic illness may result from a screw-worm infection. Prevention involves adequate wound débridement and protection of incompetent or unconscious people.

The secondary screw-worm flies may produce a range of complications in unconscious patients, ranging from a trivial colonization of a tracheotomy tube to a variety of serious complications including oronasal destruction. With restriction by bone or cartilage, pain, edema, and purulent discharge may be seen. Maggot removal may require endoscopy. Aural myiasis may be complicated by deafness, tinnitus, infection, and perforation of the eardrum. Genitourinary or anorectal destruction may occur. Entry into the urinary tract occurs when larvae hatched at the urethral meatus migrate into the bladder; the larvae are then passed in the urine. Clinical manifestations range from urinary distress to bladder and urethral pain, dysuria, and priapism. A diagnosis of urinary myiasis requires certainty that the specimen container had previously been free of flies or their larvae.

In Central and South America, furuncular myiasis is caused by *Dermatobia hominis* (the human botfly).[15, 88, 89] The larvae of these flies penetrate unbroken skin and produce a boil-like lesion on which breathing holes may be evident (Fig. 297–8). Botfly infections occur after the female fly attaches her eggs to the underside of some other insect that she captures while following a large mammal. After a period of embryonation, these eggs hatch in response to the moist heat of the skin of another host. The larva then penetrates the skin to form a flask-shaped boil. Larvae mature in about a month to emerge and pupate in the soil. Extraction of younger maggots may require surgical excision, but pressure generally suffices after the larva begins to mature. Injection of lidocaine into the lesion may facilitate removal.[90]

Another form of furuncular myiasis may afflict people traveling in Africa.[51] Adult female tumbu flies, *Cordylobia anthropophaga*, deposit as many as 100 eggs on urine- or sweat-contaminated clothing. The problem most frequently derives from underclothing that has been laundered traditionally by washing in a stream and drying on vegetation. The eggs become embryonated within 2 days and remain viable for about 2 weeks. Contact with warm, moist skin causes the larvae to emerge and penetrate the victim's skin. Numerous boils may result, from which larvae emerge within 9 days. Tourists should require that their clothes be ironed if they have been traditionally laundered in endemic regions.

Creeping myiasis is due mainly to horse botflies, *Gasterophilus intestinalis*,[14] which deposit their eggs on the flanks of horses and hatch in response to contact with the animal's tongue. The "Lady Godiva" syndrome results when larvae hatch against the bare legs of a rider. The larvae then migrate through the skin, producing pruritic tunnels that are narrow and raised. Differential diagnosis includes subdermal migrating eruptions caused by helminths. Biopsies are most diagnostic if samples are taken from skin just beyond the burrow. The burrows appear to be intraepidermal or subepidermal and may contain debris and desquamated cells in addition to larvae. Although surrounding tissues may appear unaffected, polymorphonuclear leukocytes and eosinophils may be present.

Acute ocular conjunctivitis may result from infestation by

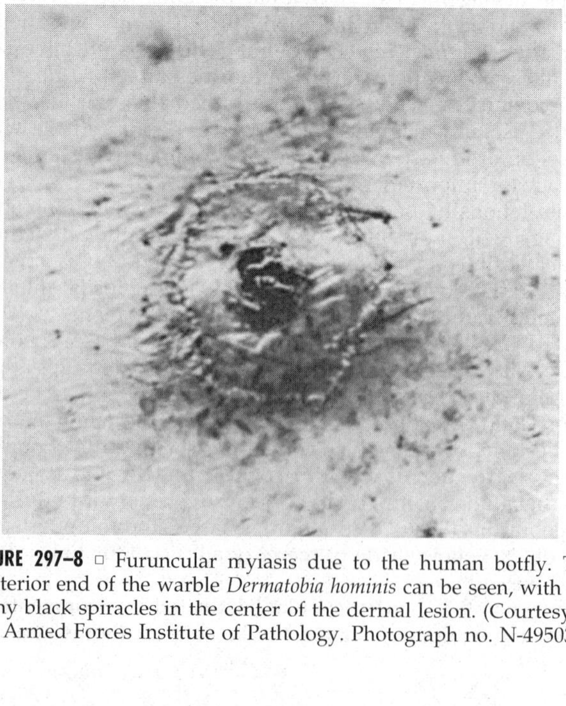

FIGURE 297–8 □ Furuncular myiasis due to the human botfly. The posterior end of the warble *Dermatobia hominis* can be seen, with the shiny black spiracles in the center of the dermal lesion. (Courtesy of the Armed Forces Institute of Pathology. Photograph no. N-49503.)

the sheep botfly *Oestrus ovis*.[87] Ovipositing adult flies "strike" their eggs into the eyes of sheep and, on occasion, people. Motile maggots may be evident in the inflamed area and may invade both the anterior and the posterior chambers. They may be extracted most readily from the anterior chamber. In the posterior chamber, maggots may cause retinal detachment or invade the optic nerve. Acute vitrectomy and photocoagulation have successfully been applied.[91, 92]

Diagnosis and Treatment

Diagnoses of intestinal myiasis tend to be highly controversial.[87] Such a complaint is generally stimulated when maggots are noted in an asymptomatic patient's stool, but this is often due to the rapidly developing maggots of flesh flies that were larviposited on the stool a few hours earlier. Genuine intestinal myiasis is infrequent and generally due to the rat-tail maggots of a drone fly, *Eristalis tenax*. The pathognomonic appearance of the maggot is suggested by its common name. Whereas acute enteritis is the most common complaint, obstruction occasionally results. Before a diagnosis of intestinal myiasis is rendered, however, a fresh stool specimen should be carefully collected in fly-free conditions.

The fly responsible for each myiasis infestation should be identified. Maggots may be placed in 70% ethanol and delivered to a reference laboratory. To facilitate identification, living maggots may be sent to a specialist to be reared to maturity. Except as indicated before, treatment involves removal of maggots from the host.

Spiders

Of the numerous kinds of spiders that have been recognized, including 100 or so that tend to attack people, human disease in general is generated solely by the bites of those in the genera *Latrodectus*, *Loxosceles*, and *Chiracanthium*.[93] Because as many as 80% of attributed spider bites actually appear to have resulted from other causes,[94] diagnosis of spider bite is best limited to episodes in which the offending organism can be examined. Identification may be possible even when the spider has been damaged.

Spiders have two body compartments and eight legs. With few exceptions, they are insectivorous. Venom is delivered through the fangs and is generated by specialized poison glands. Spiders spin webs by means of spinnerets located posteriorly on their ventral surfaces.

Widow Spiders

In the United States, black widow spiders range throughout the East Coast *(Latrodectus mactans)*, through the midwestern and southwestern states *(Latrodectus hesperus)*, and from east Texas to the East Coast *(Latrodectus variolus)*; the red *(Latrodectus bishopi)* and brown *(Latrodectus geometricus)* widow spiders are found in Florida.[93, 95–97] Females (males do not bite people) are black and ornamented ventrally by a red hourglass or circular markings (Fig. 297–9). Males and immature spiders are the more colorful. Adult females can attain more than 1 cm in length, males about 0.5 cm. Widow spiders have eight eyes, with the lateral pairs widely separated. Their webs vary in size and are spun close to the ground.

EPIDEMIOLOGY

Widow spiders live in a variety of sites: behind stones, logs, shutters, windows, and doors and in such littered sites as dumps, barns, and sheds. In the past, widow spiders commonly bit men on the penis while they were seated in an outdoor privy. The vibrations caused by the urine stream's striking its web stimulated the spider as would its insect prey. Today, however, bites most commonly occur when a hand or foot disturbs the web, when a child plays with the spider, or when the spider is trapped against a part of the body.

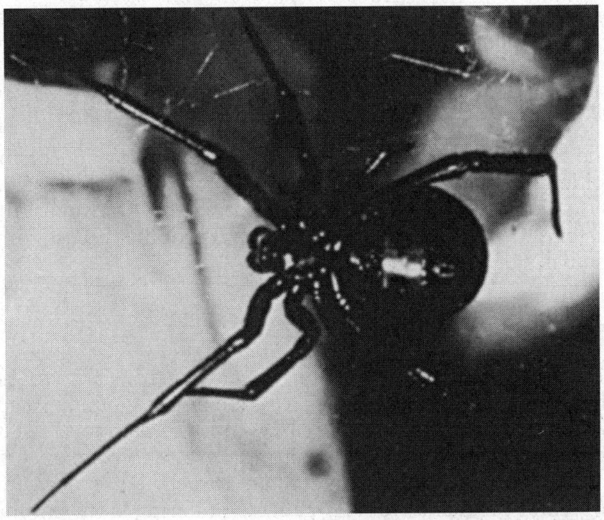

FIGURE 297–9 ▫ Black widow spider. Note the ventral hourglass marking. (From Wong RC, Hughes SE, Voorhees JJ: Spider bites. Arch Dermatol 123:98–104, 1987. Copyright 1987, American Medical Association.)

PATHOPHYSIOLOGY

The venom of widow spiders is an oily yellow fluid containing a mixture of components. Six active components have molecular masses varying from 5 to 130 kDa. Experimental envenomation has resulted in necrosis of a wide variety of organs, but the main effects in vivo relate to the neurotoxic aspects of the venom. The toxin causes acetylcholine, epinephrine, and central nervous system transmitters in presynaptic terminals to release to exhaustion. Antivenin readily blocks the action of the venom.

SYMPTOMS

Local symptoms are minimal; bite pain ranges from a sharp pinprick to none. A pair of small red marks demarcate the fang entrance sites. Slight erythema and edema may also be present.

Nonetheless, within an hour, a dull, cramping, often severe pain and numbness begin to spread from the bite to the entire torso. Generalized muscle cramping and pain result. The abdominal pain is often most prominent; it may be so severe as to be confused with a surgical abdomen, but the history, generalized muscle spasm, and absence of tenderness and distention should point the clinician toward the correct diagnosis. The pain begins to recede after 3 hours but may continue for 2 days. Other symptoms include tachycardia, headache, diaphoresis, salivation, weakness, fever, vomiting, backache, respiratory distress, priapism, impotence, urinary retention, anxiety, increased deep tendon reflexes, proteinuria, paresthesia, hypertension, fetal positioning, and burning (especially of the plantar surfaces). These symptoms generally resolve spontaneously after a few days but may last 1 week to several months. The course may be complicated by renal, cardiac, or respiratory failure; shock; convulsions; and cerebral hemorrhage. Patients who are younger than 16 years or older than 60 years and those with chronic diseases are at greatest risk.

DIAGNOSIS

The most secure diagnosis rests on the identification of the spider. If this is not possible, the patient may be able to select the spider from illustrations. In many cases, however, the history, the physical signs, and the course of the disease form the basis of the diagnosis.

TREATMENT

Tetanus prophylaxis should be administered. The wound should be cleansed. Placing an ice cube on the wound, except when antivenin is administered, will reduce pain at the site.

Hospitalization and antivenin administration are recommended for patients younger than 16 years or older than 60 years, pregnant women, patients suffering from chronic disease, and those with particularly severe symptoms. Vital signs should be closely monitored for the first 12 hours. Hypertension is usually well controlled by analgesics, sedatives, and muscle relaxants but may require antihypertensive drugs. Methocarbamol, diazepam, calcium gluconate, or magnesium sulfate may be useful. Pain control may require morphine sulfate but is usually accomplished with acetaminophen. Vigorous exercise has also been said to be of some help.

Although various insecticides destroy spiders, reinfestation frequently occurs. Gloves and long sleeves should be worn in cleaning infested sites.

Necrotic Arachnidism

Severely necrotic spider bite most frequently results from the bites of recluse spiders of the genus *Loxosceles*.[93, 98, 99] For the various New World species, human disease is most often associated with *Loxosceles reclusa* in the United States and *Loxosceles laeta* in South and Central America. *L. laeta* spiders have established potentially dangerous infestations in the United States.[100] The brownish recluse spiders are distinguished by a fiddle-shaped mark on their dorsal surface and three pairs of eyes arrayed in a curved row (Fig. 297–10). Their legs may span 5 cm, and their bodies more than 1 cm. Females are slightly larger than males, but both bite if

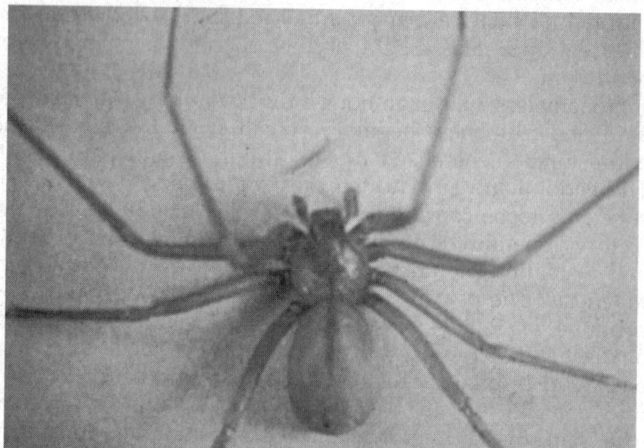

FIGURE 297–10 ▫ Brown recluse spider. Note the fiddle-shaped dorsal marking. (From Wong, Hughes SE, Voorhees JJ: Spider bites. Arch Dermatol 123:98–104, 1987. Copyright 1987, American Medical Association.)

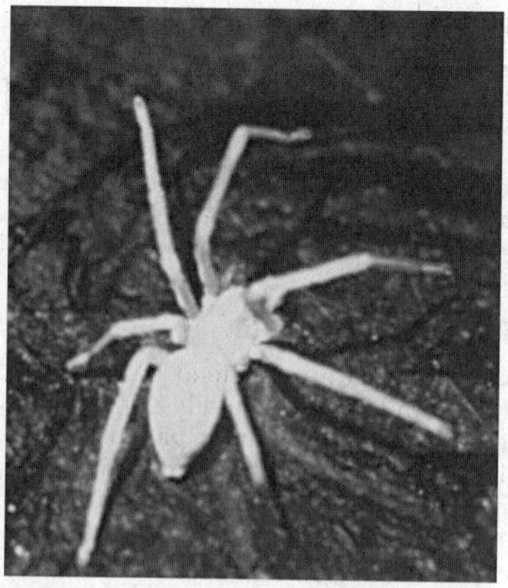

FIGURE 297–11 ▫ The *Chiracanthium* garden spider. (From Wong RC, Hughes SE, Voorhees JJ: Spider bites. Arch Dermatol 123:98–104, 1987. Copyright 1987, American Medical Association.)

disturbed. They spin a funnel-shaped web in dark, secluded locations.

Other necrotic lesions result from the bite of a garden spider, *Chiracanthium mildii* (Fig. 297–11), that was introduced into the United States from Europe during the 1940s. This greenish gray hunting spider has become the most common domestic spider in much of North America. It tends to invade homes in the fall. Garden spiders' tubelike webs may be seen in crevices near windows and porches.

EPIDEMIOLOGY

In out-of-door locations, recluse spiders seek prey beneath rocks and boards and in caves.[93, 98] Indoors, these spiders prefer dark and dry locales, such as closets, garages, storage spaces, areas under furniture, and piled rubbish. Garden spiders seek their prey in more exposed locations. These spiders bite mainly when trapped against a person's body, and bites are generally inflicted when a person is dressing. Necrotic arachnidism, therefore, most commonly affects the face, neck, and hands.

PATHOPHYSIOLOGY

The venom of recluse spiders is a clear, viscous fluid containing hyaluronidase, phospholipase D (sphingomyelinase D), an esterase, alkaline phosphatase, and a protease.[93] The component responsible for dermatonecrosis is unknown but may be sphingomyelinase D, which would interact with erythrocyte and endothelial cell membranes and cause secondary prostaglandin activation.

Various host factors may contribute to the development of the lesion. Age and size of the patient affect severity. Sites having little subcutaneous tissue are most vulnerable.

Microscopic examination reveals a progression to necrosis with subsequent scarring. Neutrophils promote the lesion. Dermatonecrosis may result from platelet aggregation and vascular thrombosis. In severe bites, early changes include dermal edema; arteriolar thrombosis; a polymorphonuclear and eosinophilic infiltrate with possible leukocytoclasis; erythrocyte extravasation; and separation of the dermis and epidermis. Marked necrosis with ulceration follows. A mononuclear infiltrate is seen after several weeks. Granulation tissue underlies the necrotic area. Ultimately, scar formation results.

DISEASE RELATIONSHIPS

Clinical manifestations of necrotic arachnidism are highly variable, ranging from mild pain and erythema to local skin necrosis and systemic viscerocutaneous disease. The bite is frequently painless and the resulting lesion consequently not associated with the spider.

In mild cases, the bite site becomes indurated and erythematous and is mildly painful and pruritic. An ischemic zone of pallor may surround the lesion. These changes occur within hours of envenomation and resolve in several days. Many investigators believe that the mild lesions are the predominant manifestation of recluse spider bites. In general, if necrosis has not developed within 3 days, no scar formation will occur.

More severely affected patients characteristically experience only pain and pruritus for the first 8 to 24 hours. A blue-gray macular halo subsequently develops. A pustule or bulla may also be present at the inoculation site. The generally irregular lesion is often surrounded by erythematous, edematous, and purpuric skin. Progression to necrosis, eschar formation, and ulceration often follows. These changes may be accompanied by edema of the affected limb or portion of the torso. The first changes of severe lesions generally occur within the first day and almost always within the first 3 days.[101] Healing and scar formation may take 6 months. Dermonecrotic lesions are often accompanied by a diffuse eruption of variable appearances. Local complications may include chronic pain, secondary infection, repeated failure of skin grafts, a pyoderma granulosa–like reaction, and upper extremity functional impairment.[102, 103]

The severity and frequency of systemic manifestations are proportional to the size of the lesion. Systemic signs usually appear within 3 days. Mild systemic reactions include leukocytosis, malaise, headache, arthralgia, myalgia, proteinuria, hematuria, vomiting, diarrhea, and generalized urticaria. Severe complications include anuria, delirium, shock, hemolysis, disseminated intravascular coagulation, and coma. All persons with necrosis larger than 1 cm should be screened for hemolysis, renal failure, and disseminated intravascular coagulation. The presence of systemic complications is an indication for hospitalization.

DIAGNOSIS

When the offending spider has not been captured, diagnosis must be presumptive. An increasingly painful plaque with central pallor and surrounding erythema may be suggestive, but the initial signs are sufficiently nonspecific to preclude anything but retrospective diagnosis.

Differential diagnosis involves exclusion of the bites of other arthropods, infections, vasculitides, embolic phenomena, burns, and trauma. Examination of the history and careful exclusion of other diagnostic possibilities may be helpful.

A passive hemagglutination inhibition test detects venom in fluid expressed from the bite as long as 1 day after the bite.[104] A thymidine uptake in vitro test is also available, but it requires acute- and convalescent-phase serum and may take as long as a month to complete.[105]

TREATMENT

Mildly necrotic lesions and those with necrotic areas less than 2 cm across may require only pain medications, antihistamines, sterile dressings, tetanus prophylaxis, ice, and elevation of the affected limb.[106] Although a variety of steroid preparations and protocols have been suggested for more serious lesions, clear-cut evidence of their benefit is lacking. Because it is an inhibitor of neutrophils, dapsone has been suggested.[107, 108] A prospective study demonstrated more rapid healing after administration of dapsone and excision of the necrotic lesion after 6 weeks in place of immediate excision.[109] Administration of antivenin may be helpful. Systemic symptoms warrant hospitalization and treatment of complications.

Bees and Wasps

The Pathogens

The stinging insects belong to the order Hymenoptera, a diverse taxon that includes the ants and numerous entomophagous parasites. People are stung mainly by members of two superfamilies, Apoidea and Vespoidea.[110] The Apoidea includes the honeybees and bumblebees, familiar insects that lose their venom apparatus in the course of stinging. Although they generally attack people only when disturbed, the Africanized bees that have invaded North America are readily provoked. The Vespoidea includes the yellow jackets, whose abdomens are marked with alternating black and yellow bands; the hornets, whose bodies are black but with a white-marked face; and the paper wasps, brownish insects with long legs. Yellow jackets place their nests in burrows that they frequently gnaw into the wooden walls of buildings; hornets construct massive hanging nests; and paper wasps build thin-walled nests, often suspended by a short stalk from the eaves of buildings. Adult Vespoidea generally feed on nectar, and their larvae are fed insects. They are attracted to sugary substances and to meat, leading to their unwelcome appearance at picnics and garbage dumps. Vespoidea retain their stings and can sting repeatedly. About 40 United States residents die each year of anaphylaxis induced by the stings of these insects[2]; between 0.5% and 3.3% of the population are allergic.[111–113]

Pathophysiology

Stinging insects rapidly and efficiently deliver venom into the skin. Honeybees, for example, expel 90% of their venom sac within 20 seconds.[114] Venoms of different insects are biochemically and immunologically distinct,[115, 116] necessitating use of an array of skin tests and individualized venom immunotherapies for allergic people. Venom allergens have been classified into group I (phospholipases), group II (hyaluronidases), group I1 (melitten), and group V (vespid antigen 5).[117–122]

The phospholipase A_1 toxin of these insects is particularly interesting because it induces both hemolysis and edema.[123] Allergic reactions, of course, are mediated by immunoglobulin E antibodies to venom constituents. The pathogenesis of insect sting anaphylaxis is complex, involving plasminogen, the contact system, complement activation, mast cell activation, and basophil degranulation.[124–127] Despite its many components, the pathogenesis of insect sting anaphylaxis seems fundamentally similar to that of other forms of anaphylaxis. The intensity of the allergic reaction to the sting of an insect increases with subsequent exposure only in about 10% of patients, limiting the utility of venom immunotherapy in those whose initial reaction is mild.[128] In other respects, age, the nature of the patient's anaphylactic symptoms, and duration of the interval between stings all contribute to the natural history of the disease.[129]

Disease Relationships and Treatment

Diagnosis of an insect sting is rarely ambiguous. The patient presents with a painful, erythematous, and edematous lesion and relates a history of contact with the offending insect. The condition generally resolves spontaneously within a few hours. Cold compresses and analgesics offer some relief. More extensive local reactions occur, developing in 2 days and lasting as long as a week. Aspirin, antihistamines, and cold compresses may be of use; prednisone may be used if the reaction is particularly disabling.

Anaphylaxis due to insect stings can strike at any age and result from a sting delivered anywhere on the body. The clinical symptoms are variable. Cutaneous signs include generalized urticaria, flushing, and angioedema. Upper airway edema or bronchospasm can result in respiratory failure and shock. Primary vascular collapse occurs in a fourth of all cases of fatal anaphylaxis and may be accompanied by cardiac symptoms.[130] Diarrhea, nausea, vomiting, abdominal pain, tenesmus, and uterine contractions are uncommon. Symptoms usually appear within 20 minutes of a sting but may be delayed for as long as 3 days.[131] Although diagnosis is generally unambiguous, the differential diagnosis may require the exclusion of pulmonary embolism, acute myocardial infarction, cardiac arrhythmia, foreign body aspiration, acute asthma, hereditary angioedema, seizure disorder, and vasovagal reactions. The treatment of this disorder is identical to that for anaphylaxis due to other causes. Epinephrine hydrochloride is immediately administered subcutaneously; intravenous injections, if needed, are diluted 10-fold. Antihistamines may also be administered. Other therapeutic modalities that may be of use include vasopressors, oxygen, and aerosol bronchodilators. Fluid resuscitation may also be required. Airway maintenance is vital and may require intubation.

Skin tests for detecting allergy to hymenopterous antigen can be used to guide specific immunotherapy for patients who have reacted systemically. Although the current criteria for assessing risk generally fail to predict how a patient will react to an insect sting,[132] supplementary laboratory studies improve predictability.[133] Immunotherapy appears to be safe and effective.[129, 134, 135]

A few commonsense preventive measures are in order. People who have experienced an anaphylactic response should carry and learn to use epinephrine kits when exposure seems likely. Neutral-colored clothing should be worn. Patients should not walk barefoot and should wear long pants and gloves when gardening. Cosmetics, perfumes, and hair sprays, which attract wasps, should be avoided. Such a patient, of course, should avoid the site where a previous sting was experienced unless the nest has been identified and destroyed.

Fire Ants

The fire ants illustrate the direct effects of these ubiquitous insects on human health. The fire ants *Solenopsis richteri* and *Solenopsis invicta* that were introduced into Alabama in 1918 have become abundant in 13 southern states in the United States, the Virgin Islands, and Puerto Rico.[136] Although sensitivity to cold limits their range,[137] cold-resistant forms have been identified, and this may permit invasion of more northerly sites.[138] Their expansion has displaced other relatively more docile ants. Thirty percent to 60% of urban residents who live within the range of these ants report being stung each year.[139, 140] In the southwestern United States, fire ants are the most important cause of insect hypersensitivity.[141] Although their effects on human health are important, these insects burden agriculture by stinging animals, eating seeds, and creating mounds that interfere with the operation of farm machinery.[142]

These red-brown, 2- to 5-mm-long ants construct their nests in mounds that may be 50 cm across.[143] Such a colony can include 200,000 members, communicating with the outside world through a system of tunnels extending some 25 m from the center of the mound. Fire ant colonies are constructed in such open sites as fields, yards, or pastures.[144] Stings generally result from direct human contact with their mounds; as many as 10,000 stings have been received in a single such encounter.[143]

Disease Relationships and Treatment

Before stinging, fire ants fasten themselves to their victim by their prominent mandibles. Their bodies then pivot around their heads, successively delivering numerous stings by means of a caudally placed stinging apparatus. This tubular, modified ovipositor serves as an extension of the duct of their venom glands.[145, 146] The wheal and flare reaction that develops 30 minutes to an hour thereafter resolves within another 30 minutes. A sterile pustule generally forms about a day later.[145, 147] Pustule formation is induced by the piperidine component of fire ant venom.[148–150] Two, 6-di–substituted piperidines compose 99% of the alkaloid fraction of this secretion, which in turn composes 95% of the insect's venom. Piperidines possess hemolytic, bactericidal, and cytotoxic properties and have been implicated in the alternative complement pathway. No available treatment for pustules appears to be effective.[147]

Systemic reactions occur in 16% of people who have been stung by fire ants, and anaphylaxis in about 2%.[151] Symptoms and signs of a systemic reaction occur within 30 to 45 minutes after the sting and include urticaria, chest tightness, pruritus, dysphagia, abdominal cramping, nausea, vomiting, diarrhea, and wheezing.[147, 152] Symptoms and signs of anaphylaxis differ little from those described elsewhere. Neurologic reactions, including syncope, convulsions, confusion, mononeuropathy, and seizures, have infrequently been reported.[153] Treatment for these complications is specific to the syndrome.

As with other insects, protein makes up less than 5% of fire ant venom and is responsible for both the systemic and the anaphylactic responses. *S. richteri* has at least three allergen components,[154] and *S. invicta* has at least four.[155]

Although an ideal immunotherapy would be based on the venom itself as antigen, such secretions are difficult to harvest because their volume is so small. Instead, whole-body extracts are used to treat sensitivity to ants. In one such experiment, 65 subjects who received immunotherapy were compared with 11 nontreated subjects.[156] Anaphylaxis followed ant stings in a tenth of these subjects, regardless of treatment. In spite of these inconclusive results, expert opinion tends to support immunotherapy.[146, 157] Definitive studies in the form of double-blinded placebo trials have yet to be produced, however.

Conclusion

The human environment is dynamic, and novel pathogens continue to emerge.[158] The resulting list of "new diseases" includes numerous vector-borne infections of major public health importance. The arthropods that directly affect human health are subject to similar change. Fire ants, Africanized bees, a European wasp, the Asian tiger mosquito, and the garden spider, for example, have invaded North America since midcentury. The future will surely bring other pathogenic arthropods into contact with these and other residents of the temperate zone. New strategies for ameliorating the effects of such contact will be required.

References

1. Natural history of insect sting allergy. Allergy Proc 10:97, 1989.
2. Mellenby K: Scabies. Hampton, England, EW Classey, 1972.
3. Green RW: Infestations: Scabies and lice. *In* Brickner P (ed): Health Care of Homeless People. New York, Springer-Verlag, 1985, pp 33–55.
4. Jenista JA, Chapman D: Medical problems of foreign-born adopted children. Am J Dis Child 141:298, 1987.
5. Reid AF, Poonking T: Epidemic scabies and associated acute glomerulonephritis in Trinidad. Bull Pan Am Health Organ 22:103, 1988.
6. Alexander AM: Role of race in scabies infestation. Arch Dermatol 114:627, 1987.
7. Chakrabari A: Human notoedric scabies from contact with cats infested with *Notoedres cati*. Int J Dermatol 25:646, 1978.
8. Regan AM, Metersky ML, Craven DE: Nosocomial dermatitis and pruritus caused by pigeon mite infestation. Arch Intern Med 147:2185, 1987.
9. Parish LC, Nutting WB, Schwartzman RM: Cutaneous Infestations of Man and Animals. New York, Praeger Publishers, 1983.
10. Arlian LG: Biology, host relations and epidemiology of *Sarcoptes scabiei*. Annu Rev Entomol 34:139, 1989.
11. Orkin M, Maibach HI: This scabies pandemic. N Engl J Med 298:496, 1978.
12. Dick GF, Burgdorf WHC, Gentry WC Jr: Norwegian scabies in Bloom's syndrome. Arch Dermatol 115:212, 1979.
13. Wolf R, Krakowski A: Atypical crusted scabies. J Am Acad Dermatol 17:434, 1987.
14. Binford CH, Connor DH (eds): Pathology of Tropical and Extraordinary Diseases, Vol II. Washington, DC, Armed Forces Institute of Pathology, 1976, pp 626–630.
15. Glover A, Young L, Goltz AW: Norwegian scabies in acquired immunodeficiency syndrome: Report of a case resulting in death from associated sepsis. J Am Acad Dermatol 16:396, 1987.
16. Sadick N, Kaplan MH, Pahwa SG, et al: Unusual features of scabies complicating human T-lymphotropic virus type III infection. J Am Acad Dermatol 15:486, 1986.
17. Pariser RJ, Pariser DM: Primary care physicians' errors in handling cutaneous disorders: A prospective survey. J Am Acad Dermatol 17:239, 1987.
18. Haas N: A simple vital microscopy aid for the detection of scabies mites. Z Hautkr 62:1395, 1987.
19. Mussen JE: Lindane: A prudent approach. Arch Dermatol 123:1008, 1987.
20. Solomon LM, Fahrner L, West DP: Gamma benzene hexachloride toxicity: A review. Arch Dermatol 113:353, 1977.
21. Taplin D, Rivera A, Walker JG, et al: A comparative trial of three treatment schedules for the eradication of scabies. J Am Acad Dermatol 9:550, 1983.
22. Taplin D, Meinking TL, Porcelain SL, et al: Permethrin 5% dermal cream: A new treatment for scabies. J Am Acad Dermatol 9:550, 1983.
23. Glaziou P, Cartel JL, Alzieu P, et al: Comparison of ivermectin and benzyl benzoate for treatment of scabies. Trop Med Parasitol 44:331, 1993.
24. Aubin F, Humber P: Ivermectin for crusted (Norwegian) scabies. N Engl J Med 332:612, 1995.
25. Wharton GW: House dust mites. J Med Entomol 12:577, 1976.
26. Kifuji K, McCullough J, Ownby DR: Relationship between dust mite allergen and human IgA in house dust samples. Ann Allergy 70:219, 1993.
27. M'Raihi L, Charpin D, Thibaudon M, Vervloet D: Bronchial challenge to house dust can induce immediate bronchoconstriction in allergic asthmatic patients. Ann Allergy 65:485, 1990.
28. Platts-Mills TA, Chapman MD: Dust mites: Immunology, allergic disease, and environmental control. J Allergy Clin Immunol 80:755, 1987.
29. Pollart S, Chapman MD, Platts-Mills TA, et al: House dust mite and dust control. Clin Rev Allergy 6:23, 1988.
30. Hyndman SJ, Brown DI, Ewan PW, et al: Humidity regulation in the management of asthma patients sensitized to house dust mites. Q J Med 87:367, 1994.
31. Lind P: Purification and partial characterization of two major allergens from the house dust mite *Dermatophagoides pteronyssinus*. J Allergy Clin Immunol 76:753, 1985.
32. Yasueda H, Mita H, Yiu Y, et al: Isolation and characterization of two allergens for *Dermatophagoides farinae*. Int Arch Allergy Appl Immunol 81:214, 1986.
33. Heymann PW, Chapman MD, Aalberse RC, et al: Antigenic and structural analysis of group II allergens (Der f II and Der p II) from house dust mites (*Dermatophagoides* spp). J Allergy Clin Immunol 83:1055, 1989.
34. Smith WA, Chua KY, Kuo MC, et al: Cloning and sequencing of the *Dermatophagoides pteronyssinus* group III allergen, Der p III. Clin Allergy 24:220, 1994.
35. de Blay F, Heymann PW, Chapman MD, et al: Airborne dust mite allergens: Comparison of group II allergens with group I mite allergen and cat allergen Fel d I. J Allergy Clin Immunol 88:919, 1991.
36. Stewart GA, Boyd SM, Bird CH, et al: Immunobiology of the serine protease allergens from house dust mites. Am J Ind Med 25:105, 1994.
37. Maruo K, Akaike T, Matsumarua Y, et al: Triggering of the vascular permeability reaction by activation of the Hageman factor–prekallikrein system by house dust mite proteinase. Biochim Biophys Acta 1074:62, 1991.
38. Leung DY, Pober JS, Cotran RS: Expression of endothelial-leukocyte adhesion molecule-1 in elicited late phase allergic reactions. J Clin Invest 87:1805, 1991.
39. Schmitt M, Niggemann B, Kleinau I, et al: Lymphocyte subsets, sIL2-r and sICAM-1 in blood during allergen challenge tests in asthmatic children. Pediatr Allergy Immunol 4:208, 1993.
40. Duff AL, Platts-Mills TA: Allergens and asthma. Pediatr Clin North Am 39:1277, 1992.
41. Casimeir GJ, Duchatheau J, Gossart B, et al: Atopic dermatitis: Role of food and house dust mite allergens. Pediatrics 92:252, 1993.
42. Dart JK, Buckley RJ, Monnickendan M, Prasad J: Perennial allergic conjunctivitis: Definition, clinical characteristics and prevalence. Trans Ophthalmol Soc U K 105:513, 1986.
43. Warner JO: Low-dose sublingual therapy in patients with allergic rhinitis due to house dust mite (Editorial). Clin Allergy 16:387, 1986.
44. Scadding GK, Brostoff J: Low-dose sublingual therapy in patients with allergic rhinitis due to house dust mite. Clin Allergy 16:483, 1986.
45. Liu CM, Shun CT, Song HC, et al: Investigation into allergic response patients with chronic sinusitis. J Formos Med Assoc 91:252, 1992.
46. Platts-Mills TA: How environment affects patients with allergic disease: Indoor allergens and asthma. Ann Allergy 72:381, 1994.
47. Gelber LE, Seltzer LH, Bousoukis JK, et al: Sensitization and exposure to indoor allergens as risk factors for asthma among patients presenting to hospital. Am Rev Respir Dis 147:572, 1993.
48. Sporik R, Holgate St, Platts-Mills TA, et al: Exposure to house-dust mite allergen (Der p 1) and the development of asthma in childhood: A prospective study. N Engl J Med 323:502, 1990.
49. Leung DYM: Role of IgE in atopic dermatitis. Curr Opin Immunol 5:956, 1993.
50. Wang B, Rieger A, Kilgus O, et al: Epidermal Langerhans cells from normal human skin bind monomeric IgE via FceRL. J Exp Med 175:1353, 1992.
51. Muddle G, van Reijsen FC, Bolan GF, et al: Allergen presentation by epidermal Langerhans' cells from patients with atopic dermatitis is mediated by IgE. Immunology 69:335, 1990.
52. Collof MJ: Exposure to house dust mites in homes of people with atopic dermatitis. Br J Dermatol 127:322, 1992.
53. Hunter JAA, Herd RM: Recent advances in atopic dermatitis. Q J Med 87:323, 1994.
54. Armenaka MC, Grizzanti JN, Oriel B, Rosentreich DL: Increased immune reactivity to house dust mites in adults with chronic rhinosinusitis. Clin Exp Allergy 23:669, 1993.
55. Bousquet J: Specific immunotherapy in asthma: Is it effective? J Allergy Clin Immunol 94:1, 1994.
56. Corey JP: Environmental control of allergens. Otolaryngol Head Neck Surg 111:340, 1994.
57. Hoffman A, Walmann P, Tiesener G, et al: Isolation and characterization of a thrombin inhibitor from the tick *Ixodes ricinus*. Pharmazie 46:209, 1991.
58. Ribeiro JM, Endris TM, Endris R: Saliva of the soft tick, *Ornitho-*

doros moubata, contains anti-platelet and apyrase activities. Comp Biochem Physiol A Comp Physiol 100:109, 1991.

59. Waxman L, Connolly TM: Isolation of an inhibitor selective for collagen-stimulated platelet aggregation from the soft tick *Ornithodoros moubata*. J Biol Chem 268:5445, 1993.
60. Vlasuk GP: Structural and functional characterization of tick anticoagulant peptide (TAP): A potent and selective inhibitor of blood coagulation factor Xa. Thromb Haemost 70:212, 1993.
61. Wikel SK, Ramachandra RN, Bergman DK: Tick-induced modulation of the host immune response. Int J Parasitol 24:59, 1994.
62. Kubes M, Fuchsberger N, Labuda M, et al: Salivary gland extracts of partially fed *Dermacentor reticulatus* ticks decrease natural killer cell activity in vitro. Immunology 82:113, 1994.
63. Schwartz BS, Nadelman RB, Fish D, et al: Entomologic and demographic correlates of anti-tick saliva antibody in a prospective study of tick bite subjects in Westchester County, New York. Am J Trop Med Hyg 48:50, 1993.
64. Spielman A: The emergence of Lyme disease and human babesiosis in a changing environment. Ann N Y Acad Sci 740:146, 1994.
65. Spielman A: Lyme disease and human babesiosis: Evidence incriminating vector and reservoir hosts. *In* Englund P, Scher A (eds): The Biology of Parasitism. New York, Alan R Liss, 1988, pp 147–165.
66. Shih C-M, Pollack RJ, Telford SR III, Spielman A: Delayed dissemination of Lyme disease spirochetes from the site of deposition in the skin of mice. J Infect Dis 166:827, 1992.
67. Matushchka F-R, Spielman A: The vector of the Lyme disease spirochete. N Engl J Med 327:54, 1992.
68. Treatment of Lyme disease. Med Lett 31:57, 1989.
69. Smith RP, Lacombe EH, Rand PW, et al: Diversity of tick species biting humans in an emerging area for Lyme disease. Am J Public Health 82:66, 1992.
70. Spielman A, Wilson ML, Levine JF, et al: Ecology of *Ixodes dammini*–borne human babesiosis and Lyme disease. Annu Rev Entomol 30:439, 1988.
71. Steere AC, Taylor E, McHugh G, Logigian EL: The overdiagnosis of Lyme disease. JAMA 269:1812, 1993.
72. Lane AT: Scabies and head lice. Pediatr Ann 16:51, 1987.
73. Abdel Fattah SM, el Sedfy HH, el Sayed HL, et al: Seropositivity against pediculosis in children with cervical lymphadenopathy. J Egypt Soc Parasitol 24:59, 1994.
74. Baker RS, Feingold M: *Phthirus pubis* (pubic louse) blepharitis. Am J Dis Child 138:1079, 1985.
75. Palevsky S: Magnified light source assists health staff in nit, lice removal. J School Health 60:396, 1990.
76. Clore ER, Longyear LA: A comparative study of seven pediculicides and their packaged nit removal combs. J Pediatr Health 7:55, 1993.
77. Andrews EB, Joseph MC, Magenheim MJ, et al: Postmarketing surveillance study of permethrin creme rinse. Am J Public Health 82:857, 1992.
78. Burgess IF, Brown CM, Burgess NA: Synergized pyrethrin mousse, a new approach to head lice eradication: Efficacy in field and laboratory studies. Clin Ther 16:57, 1994.
79. Rundle PA, Hughes DS: *Phthirus pubis* infestation of the eyelids. Br J Ophthalmol 77:815, 1993.
80. Ashkenazi I, Desatnik HR, Abraham FA: Yellow mercuric oxide: A treatment of choice for phthiriasis palpebrarum. Br J Ophthalmol 75:356, 1991.
81. Harwood RF, James MT: Entomology in Human and Animal Health, ed 7. New York, Macmillan, 1979.
82. Halliwell REW, Schemmer KR: The role of basophils in the immunopathogenesis of hypersensitivity to fleas (*Ctenocephalides felis*) in dogs. Vet Immunol Immunopathol 15:203, 1987.
83. Lever WF, Schaumberg-Lever G: Histopathology of the Skin. Philadelphia, JB Lippincott, 1983, p 209.
84. Burns DA: The investigation and management of arthropod bite reactions acquired in the home. Clin Exp Dermatol 12:114, 1987.
85. Paton DL, Walker JS: Pyrethrin poisoning from commercial-strength flea and tick spray. Am J Emerg Med 6:232, 1988.
86. Schwinghammer KA, Ballard EM, Knapp FW: Comparative toxicity of 10 insecticides against the cat flea, *Ctenocephalides felis* (Siphonaptera: Pulicidae). J Med Entomol 22:512, 1985.
87. James MT: The Flies That Cause Myiasis in Man. Washington, DC, US Department of Agriculture, 1947. Misccellaneous publication 631.
88. Farrell LD, Wong RK, Manders EK, et al: Cutaneous myiasis. Am Fam Physician 35:127, 1987.
89. Kleeman FJ: *Dermatobia hominis* comes to Boston. N Engl J Med 308:847, 1983.
90. Nunzi E, Rongioletti F, Rebora A: Removal of *Dermatobia hominis* larvae. Arch Dermatol 122:140, 1986.
91. Gjotterberg M, Ingemansson SO: Intraocular infestation by reindeer warble fly larva: An unusual indication for acute vitrectomy. Br J Ophthalmol 106:880, 1988.
92. Laborde RP, Kaufman HE, Beyey WB: Intracorneal ophthalmomyiasis. Case report. Arch Ophthalmol 72:420, 1988.
93. Wong RC, Hughes SE, Voorhees JJ: Spider bites. Arch Dermatol 123:98, 1987.
94. Parrish HM: Analysis of 460 fatalities from venomous animals in the United States. Am J Med Sci 254:129, 1964.
95. Moss HS, Binder LS: A retrospective review of the black widow spider envenomation. Ann Emerg Med 16:188, 1987.
96. Kobernick M: Black widow spider bite. Am Fam Physician 29:241, 1984.
97. Timms PK, Gibbons RB: Latrodectism—Effects of the black widow spider bite. West J Med 144:315, 1986.
98. Young VI, Pin P: The brown recluse spider bite. Ann Plast Surg 20:447, 1988.
99. Bernstein B, Ehrlich F: Brown recluse spider bites. J Emerg Med 4:457, 1986.
100. Levi HE, Spielman A: The biology and control of the South American brown spider, *Loxosceles laeta* (Nicolet), in a North American focus. Am J Trop Med Hyg 13:132, 1964.
101. King LE, Rees RS: Treatment of brown recluse spider bites. J Am Acad Dermatol 14:691, 1986.
102. Delozier JB, Reaves L, King LE, Rees RS: Brown recluse spider bites of the upper extremity. South Med J 81:181, 1988.
103. Pennell TC, Babu SS, Meredith JW: The management of snake and spider bites in the southeastern United States. Am Surg 53:198, 1986.
104. Finke JH, Campbell J, Barrett JT: Serodiagnostic test for *Loxosceles reclusa* bites. Clin Toxicol 7:375, 1974.
105. Berger RS, Millikan LE, Conway F: An in vitro test for *Loxosceles reclusa* spider bites. Toxicon 11:465, 1973.
106. Rees R, Campbell D, Rieger E, et al: The diagnosis and treatment of brown recluse spider bites. Ann Emerg Med 16:654, 1987.
107. Pennell TC, Babu SS, Meredith JW: The management of snake and spider bites in the southeastern United States. Am Surg 51:198, 1987.
108. King LE, Rees RS: Dapsone treatment of a brown recluse bite. JAMA 250:648, 1983.
109. Rees RS, Altenbern P, Lynch JB, et al: Brown recluse spider bites: A comparison of early surgical excision vs dapsone and delayed surgical excision. Ann Surg 202:659, 1985.
110. Barnard JH: Studies of 400 Hymenoptera sting deaths in the United States. J Allergy Clin Immunol 52:259, 1973.
111. Chaffee FH: The prevalence of bee sting allergy in allergic population. Acta Allergol 25:292, 1970.
112. Golden DBK: Epidemiology of allergy to insect venoms and stings. Allergy Proc 16:103, 1989.
113. Charpin D, Birnbaum J, Vervloet D: Prevalence of allergy to Hymenoptera stings in different samples of the general population. J Allergy Clin Immunol 90:331, 1992.
114. Schumacher MJ, Tveten MS, Egen NB: Rate and quantity of delivery of venom from honeybee stings. J Allergy Clin Immunol 93:831, 1994.
115. Mueller U, Elliot W, Reisman RE, et al: Comparison of biochemical and immunologic properties of venoms from the four hornet species. J Allergy Clin Immunol 67:290, 1981.
116. Juarez C, Blanca M, Miranda A, et al: Specific IgE antibodies to vespids in the course of immunotherapy with *Vespula germanica* administered to patients sensitized to *Polistes dominulus*. Allergy 47:299, 1992.
117. Levine MI, Lockey RF (eds): Monograph on Insect Allergy, ed 2. American Academy of Allergy and Immunology, Committee on Insects. Pittsburgh, PA, Dave Lambert Associates, 1986.
118. Hoffman DR: Allergens in Hymenoptera venom XV: The immunologic basis of vespid venom cross-reactivity. J Allergy Clin Immunol 75:611, 1985.
119. Hoffman DR: Allergens in Hymenoptera venom XIII: Isolation and purification of protein components from three species of vespid venoms. J Allergy Clin Immunol 75:599, 1985.

120. King TP: Antigenic cross reactivity of venom proteins from hornets, wasps, and yellow jackets. J Allergy Clin Immunol 75:621, 1985.
121. Hoffman DR: Allergens in Hymenoptera venom XVI: Studies of the structures and cross-reactivities of vespid venom phospholipases. J Allergy Clin Immunol 78:337, 1986.
122. Hoffman DR, Dove DE, Moffit JE, et al: Allergens in Hymenoptera venom XXI: Cross-reactivity and multiple reactivity between fire ant venom and bee and wasp venoms. J Allergy Clin Immunol 82:828, 1988.
123. Ho CL, Hwang LL, Chen CT: Edema-inducing activity of a lethal protein with phospholipase A1 activity isolated from the black-bellied hornet *(Vespa basalis)* venom. Toxicon 31:605, 1993.
124. van der Linden PW, Hack CE, Struyvenberg A, et al: Controlled insect-sting challenge in 55 patients: Correlation between activation of plasminogen and the development of anaphylactic shock. Blood 82:1740, 1993.
125. van der Linden PW, Hack CE, Eerenberg AJ, et al: Activation of the contact system in insect-sting anaphylaxis: Association with the development of angioedema and shock. Blood 82:1732, 1993.
126. van der Linden PW, Hack CE, Poortman J, et al: Insect-sting challenge in 138 patients: Relation between clinical severity of anaphylaxis and mast cell activation. J Allergy Clin Immunol 90:110, 1992.
127. van der Linden PW, Hack CE, Kerckhaert JA, et al: Preliminary report: Complement activation in wasp-sting anaphylaxis. Lancet 336:904, 1990.
128. Reisman RE: Natural history of insect sting allergy: Relationship of severity of symptoms of initial sting anaphylaxis to re-sting reactions. J Allergy Clin Immunol 90:335, 1992.
129. Reisman RE: Stinging insect allergy. Med Clin North Am 76:883, 1992.
130. Delage C, Irey NS: Anaphylactic deaths: A clinicopathologic study of 43 cases. J Forensic Sci 17:525, 1972.
131. Lockey RF, Turkeltaub PC, Baird-Warren A, et al: The Hymenoptera study I, 1979–1982: Demographics and history—Sting data. J Allergy Clin Immunol 82:370, 1988.
132. van der Linden PG, Hack CE, Struyvenberg A, et al: Insect challenge in 324 subjects with a previous anaphylactic reaction: Current criteria for insect-venom hypersensitivity do not predict the occurrence and the severity of anaphylaxis. J Allergy Clin Immunol 94:151, 1994.
133. Li JTC, Yunginger JW: Management of insect sting hypersensitivity. Mayo Clin Proc 67:1988, 1992.
134. Day JH, Buckeridge DL, Welsh AC: Risk assessment in determining systemic reactivity to honeybee stings in sting-threatened individuals. J Allergy Clin Immunol 93:691, 1994.
135. Muller U, Helbling A, Berchold E: Immunotherapy with honeybee venom and yellow jacket venom is different regarding efficacy and safety. J Allergy Clin Immunol 89:529, 1992.
136. Lofgren CS: History of imported fire ants in the United States. *In* Lofgren CS, Vandermeer RD (eds): Fire Ants and Leaf-cutting Ants: Biology and Management. Boulder, CO, Westview Press, 1986, pp 36–47.
137. Stafford CT, Hoffman DR, Rhoades RB: Allergy to imported fire ants. South Med J 82:1520, 1989.
138. Vandermeer RK, Lofgren CS, Alvarez FM: Biochemical evidence for hybridization in fire ants. Fla Entomol 68:501, 1985.
139. de Shazo RD, Griffing C, Kwan TH, et al: Dermal hypersensitivity reactions to imported fire ants. J Allergy Clin Immunol 74:841, 1984.
140. Clemnes DI, Sterling RE: The imported fire ant: Dimensions of the urban problem. South Med J 68:113, 1975.
141. Stablein JJ, Lockey RF: Adverse reactions to ant stings. Clin Rev Allergy 5:161, 1987.
142. Revkin AC: March of the fire ants. Discover 10:70, 1989.
143. Diaz JD, Lockey RF, Stablein JJ, Mines HK: Multiple stings by imported fire ants *(Solenopsis invicta)* without systemic effects. South Med J 82:775, 1989.
144. Hibel JA, Clore ER: Prevention and primary care treatment of stings from imported fire ants. Nurse Pract 17:65, 1992.
145. Rhoades RB, Schafer WL, Schmid WH, et al: Hypersensitivity to the imported fire ant. A report of 49 cases. J Allergy Clin Immunol 56:84, 1975.
146. Rhoades RB, Schafer WL, Newman M, et al: Hypersensitivity to the imported fire ant in Florida. Report of 104 cases. J Fla Med Assoc 64:247, 1977.
147. de Shazo RD, Butcher BT, Banks WA: Reactions to the sting of the imported fire ant. N Engl J Med 323:462, 1990.
148. Blum MS, Walker JR, Callahan PS, Novak AF: Chemical insecticidal and antibiotic properties of fire ant venom. Science 128:306, 1958.
149. Bufkin DC, Russell FE: A study of the venom of the imported fire ant: Physiopharmacology, chemistry and therapeutics. Proc West Pharmacol Soc 17:223, 1974.
150. Rhoades AB: Medical Aspects of the Imported Fire Ant. Gainesville, FL, University Presses of Florida, 1977.
151. Stafford CT, Hutto LS, Rhoades RB, et al: Imported fire ants as a health hazard. South Med J 82:1515, 1989.
152. Adamski DB: Assessment and treatment of allergic response to stinging insects. J Emerg Nurs 16:77, 1990.
153. Candiotti KA, Lamas AM: Adverse neurological reactions to the sting of the imported fire ant. Int Arch Allergy Immunol 102:417, 1993.
154. Jacobsen RS, Hoffman DR: Structural studies of imported fire ant venom allergens. J Allergy Clin Immunol 83:232, 1989.
155. Hoffman DR, Dalton DE, Jacobson RS: Allergies in Hymenoptera venom: Isolation of four allergens from imported fire ants (*Solenopsis invicta*) venom. J Allergy Clin Immunol 82:818, 1988.
156. Freeman TM, Hylander R, Ortiz A, Martin ME: Imported fire ant immunotherapy: Effectiveness of whole body extracts. J Allergy Clin Immunol 90:210, 1992.
157. Triplet RF: Sensitivity to imported fire ants: Successful treatment with immunotherapy. South Med J 66:477, 1973.
158. Spielman A: A commentary on research needs for monitoring and containing emergent vector-borne infections. Ann N Y Acad Sci 740:457, 1994.

INDEX

Note: Page numbers in *italics* refer to illustrations; page numbers followed by t refer to tables.

I

J

K

Q

R

S

U

W

X

Y

ISBN 0-7216-6119-X

90071

9 780721 661193